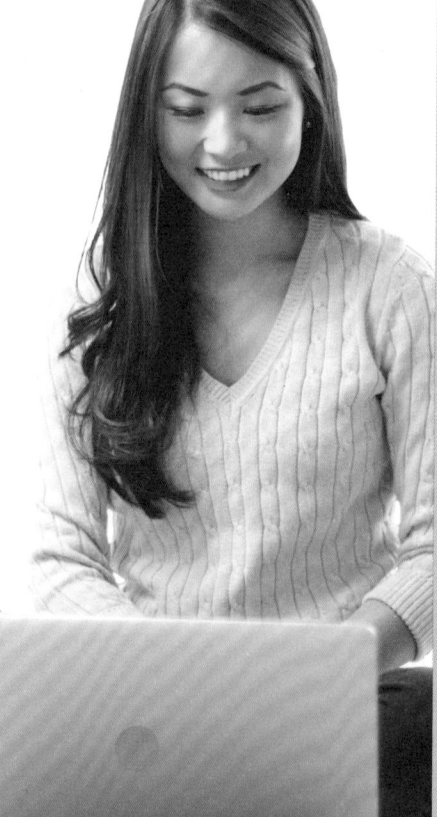
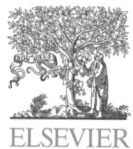

LEWIS'S
Medical-Surgical
Nursing in Canada

Assessment and Management of Clinical Problems

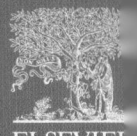

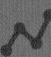

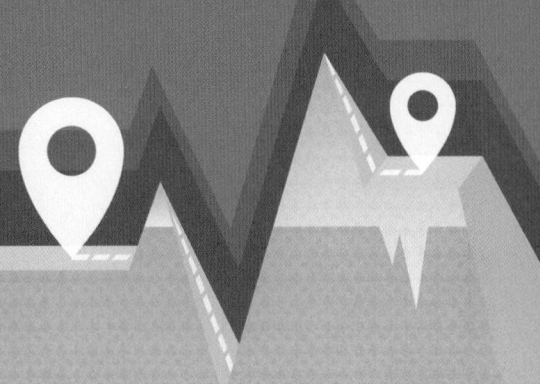

FIFTH EDITION

LEWIS'S
Medical-Surgical
Nursing in Canada

Assessment and Management of Clinical Problems

Jane Tyerman
RN, BA, BScN, MScN, PhD, CCSNE
Assistant Professor
School of Nursing
Faculty of Health Sciences
University of Ottawa
Ottawa, Ontario
Professeure Adjointe
École des sciences infirmières
Faculté des sciences de la santé
Université d'Ottawa
Ottawa, Ontario

Shelley L. Cobbett
RN, BN, GnT, MN, EdD
Assistant Professor, Nursing and BScN Site Administrator
School of Nursing – Yarmouth Campus
Dalhousie University
Yarmouth, Nova Scotia

US Author

Mariann M. Harding, RN, PhD, FAADN, CNE
Professor of Nursing
Kent State University at Tuscarawas
New Philadelphia, Ohio

Section Editors for the US 11th Edition

Jeffrey Kwong, RN, DNP, MPH, ANP-BC, FAAN, FAANP
Professor
Division of Advanced Nursing Practice
School of Nursing
Rutgers University
Newark, New Jersey

Dottie Roberts, RN, EdD, MSN, MACI, OCNS-C, CMSRN, CNE
Executive Director
Orthopaedic Nurses Certification Board
Chicago, Illinois

Debra Hagler, RN, PhD, ACNS-BC, CNE, CHSE, ANEF, FAAN
Clinical Professor
Edson College of Nursing and Health Innovation
Arizona State University
Phoenix, Arizona

Courtney Reinisch, RN, DNP, FNP-BC
Undergraduate Program Director
Associate Professor
School of Nursing
Montclair State University
Montclair, New Jersey

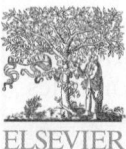

ELSEVIER

LEWIS'S MEDICAL-SURGICAL NURSING IN CANADA:
ASSESSMENT AND MANAGEMENT OF CLINICAL PROBLEMS, FIFTH EDITION

ISBN: 978-0-323-79156-4

Notice

Managing Director, Global Content Partners: Kevonne Holloway
Senior Content Strategist (Acquisitions, Canada): Roberta A. Spinosa-Millman
Content Development Specialists: Tammy Scherer, Suzanne Simpson
Publishing Services Manager: Catherine Jackson
Health Content Management Specialist: Kristine Feeherty
Design Direction: Amy Buxton

Printed in Canada

Last digit is the print number: 9 8 7 6 5 4 3 2 1

CONTENTS

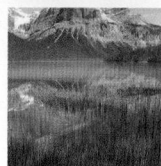

SECTION 1
Concepts in Nursing Practice

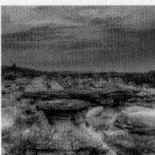

SECTION 2
Pathophysiological Mechanisms of Disease

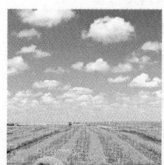

SECTION 3
Perioperative Care

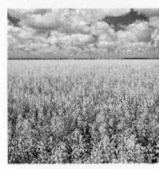

SECTION 4
Conditions Related to Altered Sensory Input

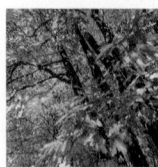

SECTION 5
Conditions of Oxygenation: Ventilation

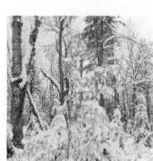

SECTION 6
Conditions of Oxygenation: Transport

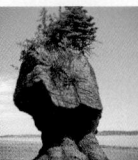

**SECTION 7
Conditions of Oxygenation:
Perfusion**

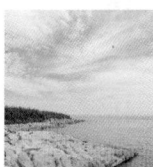

SECTION 8
Conditions of Ingestion, Digestion, Absorption, and Elimination

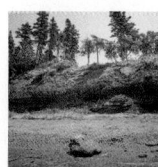

SECTION 9
Conditions of
Urinary Function

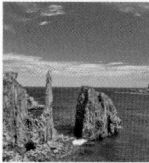

SECTION 10
Conditions Related to
Regulatory and Reproductive
Mechanisms

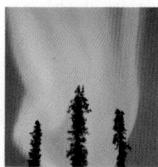

SECTION 11
Conditions Related to Movement and Coordination

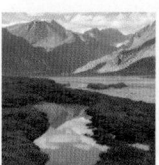

SECTION 12
Nursing Care in
Specialized Settings

Appendix

ABOUT THE AUTHORS

JANE TYERMAN, RN, BA, BScN, MScN, PhD, CCSNE

Jane Tyerman is an Assistant Professor at the University of Ottawa's School of Nursing in Ottawa, Ontario. She holds a diploma in nursing from St. Lawrence College in Ottawa, Ontario; a Bachelor of Arts degree from the University of Ottawa; a Bachelor of Science in nursing from Athabasca University in Alberta; and a Master of Science in nursing and a PhD in nursing from Queen's University in Kingston, Ontario. She has over 25 years of experience in acute care clinical practice and more than 15 years of academic teaching experience at the graduate and undergraduate levels. She is an Advanced Cardiac Life Support (ACLS) and Pediatric Advanced Life Support (PALS) instructor with the Canadian Heart and Stroke Foundation. Dr. Tyerman has contributed to multiple NCLEX textbooks published by Elsevier and has been an HESI Live Review faculty member, delivering in-person and online workshops to graduating students across Canada. She is also an editor for *Edelman and Kudzma's Canadian Health Promotion Throughout the Lifespan*. She has made significant contributions to nursing education by advancing the pedagogy that underpins the effective use of clinical simulation and through her innovative use of technology to expand equity and access to high-quality teaching and learning resources. She is dedicated to developing and researching bilingual virtual simulation games through her role as Co-President of the Canadian Alliance of Nurse Educators Using Simulation (CAN-Sim). Collaborating with nurse educators across Canada and internationally, she has authored multiple publications related to simulation and virtual simulation games.

SHELLEY L. COBBETT, RN, BN, GnT, MN, EdD

Shelley Cobbett began her nursing career at the Yarmouth Regional Hospital School of Nursing diploma program. She received her Post-RN, BN and her MN degrees from Dalhousie University and her EdD from Charles Sturt University. Her clinical practice background is maternal-child nursing, and she has been a nurse educator for over 33 years. Her main research area during the past 15 years has focused on the scholarship of learning and teaching, with over 50 peer-reviewed publications, invited speaker engagements, and oral conference presentations. Dr. Cobbett is President for the Atlantic Region Canadian Association of Schools of Nursing, and she is part of the Education Advisory Committee for the Nova Scotia College of Nursing. She has been recognized for her commitment to the implementation and evaluation of best pedagogical practices within nursing education as recipient of a Dalhousie University Teaching Award and the Canadian Association of Schools of Nursing Excellence in Teaching Award. She is currently an Assistant Professor at Dalhousie University School of Nursing, Site Administrator of the BScN Program at the Yarmouth Campus, and Curriculum Implementation and Evaluation Lead for a new, innovative BScN degree that was initiated in 2016.

11TH US EDITION AUTHOR

Mariann M. Harding, RN, PhD, FAADN, CNE

Mariann Harding is a Professor of Nursing at Kent State University Tuscarawas, New Philadelphia, Ohio, where she has been on the faculty since 2005. She received her diploma in nursing from Mt. Carmel School of Nursing in Columbus, Ohio; her Bachelor of Science in nursing from Ohio University in Athens, Ohio; her Master of Science in nursing as an adult nurse practitioner from the Catholic University of America in Washington, DC; and her doctorate in nursing from West Virginia University in Morgantown, West Virginia. Her 29 years of nursing experience have primarily been in critical care nursing and teaching in licensed practical, associate, and baccalaureate nursing programs. She currently teaches medical-surgical nursing, health care policy, and evidence-based practice. Her research has focused on promoting student success and health promotion among individuals with gout and facing cancer.

SECTION EDITORS FOR THE US 11TH EDITION

Jeffrey Kwong, RN, DNP, MPH, ANP-BC, FAAN, FAANP

Jeffrey Kwong is a Professor at the School of Nursing at Rutgers, the State University of New Jersey. He has worked for over 20 years in the area of adult primary care with a special focus on HIV. He received his undergraduate degree from the University of California–Berkeley, his nurse practitioner degree from the University of California–San Francisco, and his doctoral training at the University of Colorado–Denver. He also has a Master of Science degree in public health with a focus on health education and behavioural sciences from the University of California–Los Angeles, and he was appointed a Hartford Geriatric Interprofessional Scholar while completing his gerontology education at New York University. In addition to teaching, Dr. Kwong maintains a clinical practice at Gotham Medical Group in New York City. He is a Fellow in the American Association of Nurse Practitioners.

Dottie Roberts, RN, EdD, MSN, MACI, OCNS-C, CMSRN, CNE

Dottie Roberts received her Bachelor of Science in nursing from Beth-El College of Nursing, Colorado Springs, Colorado; her Master of Science in adult health nursing from Beth-El College of Nursing and Health Sciences; her Master of Arts in curriculum and instruction from Colorado Christian University, Colorado Springs, Colorado; and her EdD in health care education from Nova Southeastern University, Ft. Lauderdale, Florida. She has over 25 years of experience in medical-surgical and orthopedic nursing and holds certifications in both specialties. She has also taught in two baccalaureate programs in the southeast and is certified as a nurse educator.

She currently serves as contributing faculty for the RN-BSN program at Walden University. For her dissertation, Dottie completed a phenomenological study on facilitation of critical-thinking skills by clinical faculty in a baccalaureate nursing program. She has been Executive Director of the Orthopaedic Nurses Certification Board since 2005 and editor of *MEDSURG Nursing*, official journal of the Academy of Medical-Surgical Nurses, since 2003. Her free time is spent travelling, reading, and cross-stitching.

Debra Hagler, RN, PhD, ACNS-BC, CNE, CHSE, ANEF, FAAN

Debbie Hagler is a Clinical Professor in the Edson College of Nursing and Health Innovation at Arizona State University in Phoenix. She is Deputy Editor of *The Journal of Continuing Education in Nursing*. She received her Practical Certificate in nursing, Associate degree in nursing, and Bachelor of Science in nursing from New Mexico State University. She earned a Master of Science degree from the University of Arizona and a doctorate in learning and instructional technology from Arizona State University. Her clinical background is in adult health and critical care nursing. Her current role focuses on supporting students through the Barrett Honors program and helping faculty members develop their scholarly writing for publication.

Courtney Reinisch, RN, DNP, FNP-BC

Courtney Reinisch is the Undergraduate Program Director and Associate Professor for the School of Nursing at Montclair State University in New Jersey. She earned her Bachelor of Arts in biology and psychology from Immaculata University. She received her Bachelor of Science in nursing and Master of Science in family practice nurse practitioner degree from the University of Delaware. She completed her Doctor of Nursing Practice degree at Columbia University School of Nursing. Courtney's nursing career has focused on providing care for underserved populations in primary care and emergency settings. She has taught in undergraduate and graduate nursing programs in New York and New Jersey. Courtney enjoys playing tennis, snowboarding, reading, and spending time with her family and dogs. She is the biggest fan for her nieces and nephews at their soccer games, cross-country events, and track meets. She is an active volunteer in the Parents Association of her son's school and advocates for the needs of students with learning differences and for the LGBTQ community.

CANADIAN CONTRIBUTORS

Veronique M. Boscart, RN, MScN, MEd, PhD
CIHR/Schlegel Industrial Research Chair for Colleges in Seniors Care
Executive Director, Canadian Institute for Seniors Care
Executive Dean, School of Health & Life Sciences
Conestoga College Institute of Technology and Advanced Learning
Kitchener, Ontario

Wendy Bowles, NP F Vascular Surgery
Royal Columbian Hospital, Fraser Health
New Westminster, British Columbia;
Regional Department Head, Department of Nurse Practitioners
Vice-Chair, Medical Advisory Committee
Adjunct Professor
University of Victoria
Victoria, British Columbia

Myriam Breau, RN, MSN, PhD(C)
Professor
École de science infirmière/Nursing School
Université de Moncton
Moncton, New Brunswick

Danielle Byrne, RN, MN, CCSNE
Adjunct Lecturer, Clinical Instructor, Simulation Specialist
School of Nursing
Dalhousie University
Yarmouth, Nova Scotia

Erica Cambly, RN, MN, CCNE
Associate Professor, Teaching Stream
Lawrence S. Bloomberg Faculty of Nursing
University of Toronto
Toronto, Ontario

Rosemary Cashman, MA, MSc(A), ACNP, NP(A)
Nurse Practitioner
BC Cancer–Vancouver Centre
Vancouver, British Columbia

Ann Mary Celestini, RN, BA, BScN, MHST
Lecturer, Teaching Intensive
Trent/Fleming School of Nursing
Trent University
Peterborough, Ontario

Susan Chernenko, RN(EC), MN
Nurse Practitioner
Toronto Lung Transplant Program
Toronto General Hospital, University Health Network
Toronto, Ontario;
Associate Graduate Lecturer
Lawrence S. Bloomberg Faculty of Nursing
University of Toronto
Toronto, Ontario

Shelley Clarke, RN, MScN, CCSNE
Professor, Nursing Program
Health & Community Studies
Algonquin College
Ottawa, Ontario

Shelley L. Cobbett, RN, BN, GnT, MN, EdD
Assistant Professor, Nursing and BScN Site Administrator
School of Nursing – Yarmouth Campus
Dalhousie University
Yarmouth, Nova Scotia

Sarah Crowe, MN, PMD-NP(F), CNCC(C)
Nurse Practitioner, Critical Care
Surrey Memorial Hospital
Surrey, British Columbia;
Adjunct Professor
School of Nursing
University of British Columbia
Langley, British Columbia

Denise Delorey, BScN, RN, MAdEd
Assistant Professor
Rankin School of Nursing
St. Francis Xavier University
Antigonish, Nova Scotia

Serena Eagland, RN (C), BSN
Clinical Educator
Vancouver Community Primary Care
Vancouver Coastal Health
Vancouver, British Columbia

Laura Fairley, RN, MN, CHPCN(C), CCHN(C)
Assistant Professor, Teaching Stream, Undergraduate Program
Lawrence S. Bloomberg Faculty of Nursing
University of Toronto
Toronto, Ontario

Mary Ann Fegan, RN, MN
Associate Professor, Teaching Stream
Undergraduate Clinical Resource Faculty
Lawrence S. Bloomberg Faculty of Nursing
University of Toronto
Toronto, Ontario

Julie Fraser, RN, MN
Interim Executive Director
Patient Experience Professional Practice
Fraser Health
Surrey, British Columbia

Natasha Fulford, BN, RN, MN
Associate Director, Non-Degree Programs
Centre for Nursing Studies
Memorial University of Newfoundland
St. John's, Newfoundland

Mary Kate Garrity, RN, BScN, EdD
Director of Care
Sienna Senior Living
Toronto, Ontario

Emma Garrod, RN, BScN, MSN
Clinical Nurse Educator–Substance Use
Director
British Columbia Centre on Substance Use
Addiction Nursing Fellowship
Adjunct Professor
University of British Columbia School of Nursing
Vancouver, British Columbia

Renée Gordon, CD, RN, MSc, CMSN(C), CCNE, CCCI, CCSNE
Associate Teaching Professor
Faculty of Nursing
University of New Brunswick
Moncton, New Brunswick

Leslie Graham, RN, MN, PhD(C), CNCC, CHSE, CCSNE
Coordinator, RPN to BScN Nursing Program
Professor, Nursing
Durham College
Oshawa, Ontario;
Adjunct Professor
Ontario Tech University
Oshawa, Ontario

Krista Gushue, BN, RN, MN, CCCI
Nurse Educator
Centre for Nursing Studies
St. John's, Newfoundland

Peggy D. Hancock, RN, MN
Nurse Educator
Western Regional School of Nursing
Corner Brook, Newfoundland

Jackie Hartigan-Rogers, RN, MN
Assistant Professor, Nursing
School of Nursing
Dalhousie University
Yarmouth, Nova Scotia

Kimberly Hellmer, RN, BN, MN
Unit Manager, Medicine
Foothills Medical Centre
Alberta Health Services
Calgary, Alberta

Heather Helpard, RN, BScN, MN, PhD
Assistant Professor
Rankin School of Nursing
Saint Francis Xavier University
Antigonish, Nova Scotia

Sarah Ibrahim, RN, MN, PhD, CHSE
Adjunct Lecturer
Lawrence S. Bloomberg Faculty of Nursing
University of Toronto
Toronto, Ontario

Lynn Jansen, RN, PhD
Assistant Dean and Associate Professor
University of Saskatchewan Prince Albert
    and North Campus College of Nursing
Prince Albert, Saskatchewan

Sarah Johnston, RN, MN
Assistant Professor, Teaching Stream
Lawrence S. Bloomberg Faculty of Nursing
University of Toronto
Toronto, Ontario

Evan Keys, RN, MNSc, ENC(C)
Registered Nurse
Schwartz/Reisman Emergency Centre
Mount Sinai Hospital, Sinai Health
Toronto, Ontario;
Clinical Research Coordinator
Clinical Cardiovascular Physiology Labora-
    tory
Toronto General Hospital Research Institute,
    University Health Network
Toronto, Ontario

Carol A. Kuzio, RN, BScN, CBN
Clinical Practice Lead
Diabetes, Obesity and Nutrition Strategic
    Clinical Network
Alberta Health Services
Edmonton, Alberta

Elizabeth Lee, NP, MN, CGN(C)
Adjunct Lecturer
Lawrence S. Bloomberg Faculty of Nursing
University of Toronto
Toronto, Ontario;
Nurse Practitioner, Hepatology
Toronto General Hospital, University Health
    Network
Toronto, Ontario

Jana Lok, RN, PhD, ENC(C), CHSE
Assistant Professor, Teaching Stream
Lawrence S. Bloomberg Faculty of Nursing
University of Toronto
Toronto, Ontario

Bridgette Lord, RN, MN, NP-Adult
Acute Care Nurse Practitioner
Peter Gilgan Centre for Women's Cancers
Women's College Hospital
Toronto, Ontario

Jean Jacque E. Lovely, BA, BScN, MN, MBA
Director
Core Business Operations–Digital Health
Deloitte Canada
Edmonton, Alberta

Marian Luctkar-Flude, RN, BScN, MScN, PhD, CCSNE
Associate Professor
School of Nursing
Queen's University
Kingston, Ontario

Janet MacIntyre, RN, PhD
Assistant Professor
Faculty of Nursing
University of Prince Edward Island
Charlottetown, Prince Edward Island

Lesley MacMaster, RN, MScN
Nursing Professor
Georgian College
Barrie, Ontario

Lynn McCleary, RN, PhD
Professor
Department of Nursing, Faculty of Applied
    Health Sciences
Brock University
St. Catharines, Ontario

Susannah R. McGeachy, RN(EC), NP-PHC, MN
Nurse Practitioner
University Health Network
Toronto, Ontario

Andrea Miller, MHSc, RD, FDC
Registered Dietitian
Private Practice
Whitby, Ontario

Tess Montada-Atin, RN(EC), MN, CDE, CNeph (C)
Adjunct Lecturer
Lawrence S. Bloomberg Faculty of Nursing
University of Toronto
Toronto, Ontario

Joanne Newell, RN, MN
Adjunct Assistant Professor
School of Nursing
Dalhousie University
Yarmouth, Nova Scotia

Kathryn F. Nichol, RN, MScN, BA, CON(C), CHPCN(C)
Palliative Care Nurse Specialist
Supportive and Palliative Care Team
The Ottawa Hospital
Ottawa, Ontario

Sara Olivier, RN, BScN, MN
Advanced Practice Nurse
Supportive & Palliative Care and Substance
    Use Programs
The Ottawa Hospital
Ottawa, Ontario

Denise K.M. Ouellette, MSN, RN, CNN(C)
Clinical Nurse Specialist, Neurosurgical
    Outreach Activities
St Michael's Hospital, Unity Health Toronto
Toronto, Ontario;
Adjunct Lecturer
Lawrence S. Bloomberg Faculty of Nursing
University of Toronto
Toronto, Ontario

Efrosini Papaconstantinou, RN, PhD
Associate Professor
Faculty of Health Sciences
Ontario Tech University
Oshawa, Ontario

Marie-Noëlle Paulin, RN, BScN, MScN
Clinical Nurse Instructor
School of Nursing
Moncton University
Bathurst, New Brunswick

April Pike, PhD
Associate Professor
Faculty of Nursing
Memorial University of Newfoundland
St. John's, Newfoundland

Dawn Pittman, RN, MScN, PhD(C)
Nurse Educator
Western Regional School of Nursing
Memorial University of Newfoundland and
    Labrador
Corner Brook, Newfoundland

**Debbie Rickeard, RN, DNP, MSN, BScN,
    CCRN, CNE**
Experiential Learning Specialist
Faculty of Nursing
University of Windsor
Windsor, Ontario

**Sheila Rizza, RN(EC), MN NP-Adult,
    CNCC(C), CCN(C)**
Nurse Practitioner
Heart Function Clinic
Trillium Health Partners
Mississauga, Ontario

Anita Robertson, RN
Nursing Instructor
Health and Wellness Programs
Nunavut Arctic College
Iqaluit, Nunavut

**Susan E. Robinson, RN, BScN, MN,
    CON(C)**
Coroner Investigator
Office of the Chief Coroner of Ontario
Toronto, Ontario;
Staff Nurse, Emergency Department
Michael Garron Hospital
Toronto, Ontario

Kathy Rodger, MN, BSN, RN, CMSN(C)
Associate Professor
College of Nursing
University of Saskatchewan
Regina, Saskatchewan

**Kara Sealock, RN, BN, MEd EdD,
    CNCC(C), CCNE**
Senior Instructor
Faculty of Nursing
University of Calgary
Calgary, Alberta

Cydnee Seneviratne, RN, BScN, MN, PhD
Senior Instructor
Faculty of Nursing
University of Calgary
Calgary, Alberta

Catherine Sheffer, RN PhD, PNC(C)
Senior Instructor
School of Nursing
Dalhousie University
Halifax, Nova Scotia

Sarah J. Siebert, RN, MSN, GNC(C)
Director, Primary Care
Fraser Health
Surrey, British Columbia

Catharine R. Simpson, RN, MN
Senior Instructor
Department of Nursing & Health Sciences
University of New Brunswick
Saint John, New Brunswick

Rani H. Srivastava, RN, PhD
Dean, School of Nursing
Thompson Rivers University
Kamloops, British Columbia;
Adjunct Professor
Faculty of Health
York University
Toronto, Ontario;
Adjunct Professor
School of Nursing
Dalhousie University
Halifax, Nova Scotia

**Jane Tyerman, RN, BA, BScN, MScN, PhD,
    CCSNE**
Assistant Professor
School of Nursing
Faculty of Health Sciences
University of Ottawa
Ottawa, Ontario
Professeure Adjointe
École des sciences infirmières
Faculté des sciences de la santé
Université d'Ottawa
Ottawa, Ontario

Christina Vaillancourt, RD, CDE, MHSc
Associate Graduate Faculty, Master of Health
    Sciences, and Adjunct Professor
Faculty of Health Sciences
Ontario Tech University
Oshawa, Ontario

**Brandi Vanderspank-Wright, RN, PhD,
    CNCC(C)**
Associate Professor
School of Nursing, Faculty of Health
    Sciences
University of Ottawa
Ottawa, Ontario

Ellen Vogel, RD, FDC, PhD
Associate Professor
Faculty of Health Sciences
Ontario Tech University
Oshawa, Ontario

Laura Wilding, BScN, RN, MHS, ENC(C)
Advanced Practice Nurse, Regional Program
    Manager
Champlain Regional Medical Assistance in
    Dying (MAiD) Network
The Ottawa Hospital
Ottawa, Ontario

**Barbara Wilson-Keates, RN, PhD,
    CCSNE**
Academic Coordinator
Faculty of Health Disciplines
Athabasca University
Athabasca, Alberta

Kevin Woo, RN, PhD, NSWOC, WOCC(C)
Professor
School of Nursing
Queen's University
Kingston, Ontario

Colina Yim, NP, MN, AF-AASLD
Adjunct Lecturer
Lawrence S. Bloomberg Faculty of Nursing
University of Toronto
Toronto, Ontario;
Nurse Practitioner, Hepatology
Toronto General Hospital, University Health
    Network
Toronto, Ontario

CONTRIBUTORS TO THE US 11TH EDITION

**Vera Barton-Maxwell, PhD, APRN, FNP-
    BC, CHFN**
Assistant Professor, Advanced Nursing
    Practice
Family Nurse Practitioner Program
Georgetown University
Washington, District of Columbia;
Nurse Practitioner
Center for Advanced Heart Failure
West Virginia University Heart and Vascular
    Institute
Morgantown, West Virginia

Cecilia Bidigare, MSN, RN
Professor
Nursing Department
Sinclair Community College
Dayton, Ohio

Megan Ann Brissie, DNP, RN, ACNP-BC, CEN
Acute Care Nurse Practitioner, Neurosurgery
Duke Health
Durham, North Carolina;
Adjunct Instructor
College of Nursing
University of Cincinnati
Cincinnati, Ohio

Diana Taibi Buchanan, PhD, RN
Associate Professor
Biobehavioral Nursing and Health Systems
University of Washington
Seattle, Washington

Michelle Bussard, PhD, RN
RN to BSN Online eCampus Program
    Director
College of Health and Human Services
Bowling Green State University
Bowling Green, Ohio

Kim K. Choma, DNP, APRN, WHNP-BC
Women's Health Nurse Practitioner
Independent Consultant and Clinical Trainer,
    Kim Choma, DNP, LLC
Scotch Plains, New Jersey

Marisa Cortese, PhD, RN, FNP-BC
Research Nurse Practitioner, Hematology/
    Oncology
White Plains Hospital
White Plains, New York

Ann Crawford, RN, PhD, CNS, CEN
Professor
Department of Nursing
University of Mary Hardin-Baylor
Belton, Texas

**Deena Damsky Dell, MSN, RN, APRN,
    AOCN(R), LNC**
Oncology Advanced Practice Registered Nurse
Sarasota Memorial Hospital
Sarasota, Florida

Kimberly Day, DNP, RN
Clinical Assistant Professor
Edson College of Nursing and Health In-
    novation
Arizona State University
Phoenix, Arizona

**Hazel Dennison, DNP, RN, APNc, CPHQ,
    CNE**
Director of Continuing Nursing Education
College of Health Sciences, School of Nursing
Walden University
Minneapolis, Minnesota;
Nurse Practitioner, Urgent Care
Virtua Health System
Medford, New Jersey

Jane K. Dickinson, PhD, RN, CDE
Program Director/Lecturer
Diabetes Education and Management
Teachers College, Columbia University
New York, New York

Cathy Edson, MSN, RN
Nurse Practitioner, Emergency Department
Team Health—Virtua Memorial
Mt. Holly, New Jersey

Jonel L. Gomez, DNP, ARNP, CPCO, COE
Nurse Practitioner
Ophthalmic Facial Plastic Surgery, Special-
    ists, Stephen Laquis, MD
Fort Myers, Florida

**Sherry A. Greenberg, PhD, RN, GNP-BC,
    FGSA**
Courtesy-Appointed Associate Professor,
    Nursing
Rory Meyers College of Nursing
New York University
New York, New York

Diana Rabbani Hagler, MSN-Ed, RN, CCRN
Staff Nurse, Intensive Care Unit
Banner Health
Gilbert, Arizona

Julia A. Hitch, MS, APRN, FNPCDE
Nurse Practitioner, Internal Medicine—
    Endocrinology
Ohio State University Physicians
Columbus, Ohio

Haley Hoy, PhD, APRN
Associate Professor
College of Nursing
University of Alabama in Huntsville
Huntsville, Alabama;
Nurse Practitioner
Vanderbilt Lung Transplantation, Vanderbilt
    Medical Center
Nashville, Tennessee

Melissa Hutchinson, MN, BA, RN
Clinical Nurse Specialist, MICU/CCU
VA Puget Sound Health Care System
Seattle, Washington

**Mark Karasin, DNP, APRN, AGACNP-BC,
    CNOR**
Advanced Practice Nurse, Cardiothoracic
    Surgery
Robert Wood Johnson University Hospital
New Brunswick, New Jersey;
Adjunct Faculty
Center for Professional Development, School
    of Nursing
Rutgers University
Newark, New Jersey

Patricia Keegan, DNP, NP-C, AACC
Director
Strategic and Programmatic Initiatives, Heart
    and Vascular Center
Emory University
Atlanta, Georgia

**Kristen Keller, DNP, ACNP-BC, PMHNP-
    BC**
Nurse Practitioner, Trauma and Acute Care
    Surgery
Banner Thunderbird Medical Center
Glendale, Arizona

Anthony Lutz, MSN, NP-C, CUNP
Nurse Practitioner
Department of Urology
Columbia University Irving Medical Center
New York, New York

Denise M. McEnroe-Petitte, PhD, RN
Associate Professor
Nursing Department
Kent State University Tuscarawas
New Philadelphia, Ohio

**Amy Meredith, MSN, RN, EM Cert/Resi-
    dency**
APN-C Lead and APN
Emergency Department
Southern Ocean Medical Center
Manahawkin, New Jersey

Helen Miley, RN, PhD, AG-ACNP
Specialty Director of Adult Gerontology,
    Acute Care Nurse Practitioner Program
School of Nursing
Rutgers University
Newark, New Jersey

Debra Miller-Saultz, DNP, FNP-BC
Assistant Professor of Nursing
School of Nursing
Columbia University
New York, New York

Eugene Mondor, MN, RN, CNCC(C)
Clinical Nurse Educator, Adult Critical
    Care
Royal Alexandra Hospital
Edmonton, Alberta

Brenda C. Morris, EdD, RN, CNE
Clinical Professor
Edson College of Nursing and Health
    Innovation
Arizona State University
Phoenix, Arizona

Janice A. Neil, PhD, RN, CNE
Associate Professor
College of Nursing, Department of Baccalaureate Education
East Carolina University
Greenville, North Carolina

Yeow Chye Ng, PhD, CRNP, CPC, AAHIVE
Associate Professor
College of Nursing
University of Alabama in Huntsville
Huntsville, Alabama

Mary C. Olson, DNP, APRN
Nurse Practitioner, Medicine
Division of Gastroenterology and Hepatology
New York University Langone Health
New York, New York

Madona D. Plueger, MSN, RN, ACNS-BC, CNRN
Adult Health Clinical Nurse Specialist
Barrow Neurological Institute
Dignity Health, St. Joseph's Hospital and Medical Center
Phoenix, Arizona

Matthew C. Price, MS, CNP, ONP-C, RNFA
Orthopedic Nurse Practitioner
Orthopedic One
Columbus, Ohio;
Director, Orthopedic Nurses Certification Board
Chicago, Illinois

Margaret R. Rateau, PhD, RN, CNE
Assistant Professor
School of Nursing, Education, and Human Studies
Robert Morris University
Moon Township, Pennsylvania

Catherine R. Ratliff, RN, PhD
Clinical Associate Professor and Nurse Practitioner
School of Nursing/Vascular Surgery
University of Virginia Health System
Charlottesville, Virginia

Sandra Irene Rome, MN, RN, AOCN
Clinical Nurse Specialist
Blood and Marrow Transplant Program
Cedars–Sinai Medical Center
Los Angeles, California;
Assistant Clinical Professor
University of California Los Angeles School of Nursing
Los Angeles, California

Diane M. Rudolphi, MSN, RN
Senior Instructor of Nursing
College of Health Sciences
University of Delaware, Newark
Newark, Delaware

Diane Ryzner, MSN, APRN, CNS-BC, OCNS-C
Clinical Nursing Transformation Leader, Orthopedics
Northwest Community Healthcare
Arlington Heights, Illinois

Andrew Scanlon, DNP, RN
Associate Professor
School of Nursing
Montclair State University
Montclair, New Jersey

Rose Shaffer, MSN, RN, ACNP-BC, CCRN
Cardiology Nurse Practitioner
Thomas Jefferson University Hospital
Philadelphia, Pennsylvania

Tara Shaw, MSN, RN
Assistant Professor
Goldfarb School of Nursing
Barnes-Jewish College
St. Louis, Missouri

Cynthia Ann Smith, DNP, APRN, CNN-NP, FNP-BC
Nurse Practitioner
Renal Consultants, PLLC
South Charleston, West Virginia

Janice Smolowitz, PhD, DNP, EdD
Dean and Professor
School of Nursing
Montclair State University
Montclair, New Jersey

Cindy Sullivan, MN, ANP-C, CNRN
Nurse Practitioner
Department of Neurosurgery
Barrow Neurological Institute
Phoenix, Arizona

Teresa Turnbull, DNP, RN
Assistant Professor
School of Nursing
Oregon Health and Science University
Portland, Oregon

Kara Ann Ventura, DNP, PNP, FNP
Director, Liver Transplant Program
Yale University School of Medicine
New Haven, Connecticut

Colleen Walsh, DNP, RN, ONC, ONP-C, CNS, ACNP-BC
Contract Assistant Professor of Nursing
College of Nursing and Health Professions
University of Southern Indiana
Evansville, Indiana

Pamela Wilkerson, MN, RN
Nurse Manager, Primary Care and Urgent Care
Department of Veterans Affairs
Veterans Administration, Puget Sound
Tacoma, Washington

Daniel P. Worrall, MSN, ANP-BC
Nurse Practitioner, Sexual Health Clinic
Nurse Practitioner, General and Gastrointestinal Surgery
Massachusetts General Hospital
Boston, Massachusetts;
Clinical Operations Manager
The Ragon Institute of MGH, MIT, and Harvard
Cambridge, Massachusetts

REVIEWERS

'Lara Alalade, RN, BN, MClSc-WH
Nursing Instructor
Faculty of Health and Community Studies
NorQuest College
Edmonton, Alberta

Jasmina Archambault, RN, BScN, MN
Nursing Instructor
Cégep Héritage
Gatineau, Quebec

Monique Bacher, RN, BScN, MSN/Ed
Semester 3 PN Coordinator and Professor,
    Practical Nursing Program
Sally Horsfall Eaton School of Nursing
George Brown College
Toronto, Ontario

Renee Berquist, RN, BScN, MN, PhD
Professor
School of Baccalaureate Nursing
St. Lawrence College
Brockville, Ontario

Diane Browman, RN, BScN
Nursing Instructor
Faculty of Nursing
John Abbott College
Sainte-Anne-de-Bellevue, Quebec

Lori Carre, RN, MN
Professor
School of Nursing Faculty of Applied Arts &
    Health Sciences
Seneca College
Toronto, Ontario

Sharon R. Cassar, RN, MSN, NP–Primary
    Health Care
Professor
School of Nursing Faculty of Applied Arts &
    Health Sciences
Seneca College
Toronto, Ontario

Annie Chevrier, N, MScA, CMSN(C)
Bachelor of Nursing (Integrated) (BNI)
Program Director, Online Education Initia-
    tives and Continuing Nursing Education
Assistant Professor
Ingram School of Nursing
McGill University
Montreal, Quebec

Sue Coffey, RN, PhD
Associate Professor, Nursing Program
Ontario Tech University
Oshawa, Ontario

Brenda Dafoe-Enns, BA, MN, RN
Nursing Instructor, Baccalaureate Nursing
    Program
School of Health Sciences & Community
    Services
Red River College Polytech
Winnipeg, Manitoba

Laurie Doxtator, RN, BNSc, MSc
Professor, Practical Nursing
Health Sciences
St. Lawrence College
Kingston, Ontario

Donna Dunnet, LPN
Licensed Practical Nurse Instructor Certificate
School of Health Sciences / Practical Nursing
Lethbridge College
Lethbridge, Alberta

Tammy Dwyer, RN, BScN, MEd
Professor, Practical Nursing Program
Faculty of Environmental Studies and Health
    Science
Canadore College
North Bay, Ontario

Arnold Esguerra, RN (NP), BScN, MN
Faculty, Orientation to Nursing in Canada for
    Internationally Educated Nurses
School of Nursing
Saskatchewan Polytechnic – Regina Campus
Regina, Saskatchewan

Natasha Fontaine, RN, BN, PIDP
Professor
Department of Nursing
College of the Rockies
Cranbrook, British Columbia

Caroline Foster-Boucher, RN, MN
Assistant Professor
Department of Nursing Science
MacEwan University
Edmonton, Alberta

Sandra Fritz, RN, BN, MN, CCNE,
    CCSNE(C)
Nursing Instructor
Division of Science and Health
University of Calgary—Medicine Hat
Medicine Hat, Alberta

Monica Gola, RN, MN, CPMHN(C)
Sessional Lecturer
School of Nursing
York University
Toronto, Ontario

Renée Gordon, CD, RN, MSc, CMSN(C),
    CCNE, CCCI, CCSNE
Associate Teaching Professor
Faculty of Nursing
University of New Brunswick
Moncton, New Brunswick

Leslie Graham, RN, MN, PhD(c), CNCC,
    CHSE, CCSNE
Coordinator, RPN to BScN Nursing Program
Professor, Nursing
Durham College
Oshawa, Ontario;
Adjunct Professor
Ontario Tech University
Oshawa, Ontario

Tanya Heuver, BScN, RN, MN
Assistant Professor
Department of Nursing Science, Faculty of
    Nursing
MacEwan University
Edmonton, Alberta

Kerry-Anne Hogan, RN, PhD
Part-Time Professor
Faculty of Health Sciences
University of Ottawa
Ottawa, Ontario;
Registered Nurse, Emergency Department
Queensway Carleton Hospital
Ottawa, Ontario

Tania N. Killian, RN, BScN, BEd, MEd,
    CCN
Professor
School of Nursing Faculty of Applied Arts
    and Health Sciences
Seneca College
King City, Ontario;
Registered Nurse, Emergency Department
Royal Victoria Regional Health Centre
Barrie, Ontario

Natalie McMullin, RN, MN
Nursing Instructor
Faculty of Nursing
Keyano College
Fort McMurray, Alberta

Andrea Miller, RN, BScN, MA
Professor
Faculty of Nursing
McMaster-Mohawk-Conestoga Collaborative
    BScN Program
Conestoga College
Kitchener, Ontario

Kathryn Morrison, RN, BScN, MScN
Nursing Professor and Coordinator, Part-
    Time Practical Nursing and Specialty
    Nursing Programs
Health, Wellness and Sciences
Georgian College
Barrie, Ontario

Melanie Neumeier, RN, BScN, MN
Assistant Professor
Faculty of Nursing
MacEwan University
Edmonton, Alberta

Cindy Pallister, RN, BScN, MScN
Nursing Professor
St. Clair College
Windsor, Ontario

Trina Propp, RN, BSN
Nursing Instructor
Practical Nursing Department
Vancouver Community College
Vancouver, British Columbia

Gabriella Rispoli, RN, BEd, BScN
Nursing Faculty
Heritage College
Gatineau, Quebec

Margot Ellen Rykhoff, RN, BScN, MA(Ed)
Faculty
School of Health Sciences
University of New Brunswick/Humber
    College Collaborative Nursing Degree
    Program
Humber College
Toronto, Ontario

Ali Salman, MD, PhD, DNP, MN, RN
Professor
Faculty of Health Studies
Brandon University
Brandon, Manitoba

Heather Schoenthal, RN, BScN
Year 2 Clinical Instructor
University of Saskatchewan
    College of Nursing
Regina, Saskatchewan

Catherine Schwichtenber, Dip. Nursing, BScN, MSN
GNIE Instructor and Graduate Nurse
Kwantlen Polytechnic University
Surrey, British Columbia

Jennifer Siemens, RN, BSN, MSN
Nurse Educator
Department of Nursing
College of the Rockies
Cranbrook, British Columbia

Richard Snow, RN, BScN, MN
Instructor
School of Nursing
Dalhousie University
Yarmouth, Nova Scotia

Laralea Stalkie, RN, BNSc, MSN
Program Coordinator
Faculty of Nursing
St. Lawrence College/Laurentian University
    Collaborative
St. Lawrence College
Kingston, Ontario

Karen Ursel, RN, BN, MHSA, PhD(C)
Senior Teaching Associate
Faculty of Nursing
University of New Brunswick
Moncton, New Brunswick

Brandi Vanderspank-Wright, RN, PhD, CNCC(C)
Associate Professor
School of Nursing
Faculty of Health Sciences
University of Ottawa
Ottawa, Ontario

Ashley Veilleux, RN, BScN, MN
Professor
Bachelor of Science in Nursing Program
St. Lawrence College
Cornwall, Ontario

Yvonne Mayne Wilkin, RN, BScN, MSc, CEFP, EdD
Year 3 Nursing Faculty Coordinator
Department of Nursing
Champlain College – Lennoxville
Sherbrooke, Quebec

Jim Wohlgemuth, RN, MN, CTN-B
Instructor
Nursing Education & Health Studies
Grande Prairie Regional College
Grande Prairie, Alberta

PHARMD REVIEWER

Tom McFarlane, BScPhm, PharmD, RPh
Clinical Lecturer
School of Pharmacy
University of Waterloo
Kitchener, Ontario;
Clinical Oncology Pharmacist
Odette Cancer Centre, Sunnybrook Health
    Sciences,
and Baruch/Weisz Cancer Centre, North
    York General Hospital
Toronto, Ontario

To the Profession of Nursing and to the Important People in Our Lives

Jane

My husband Glenn, our children Kaitlyn, Kelsey, and Aiden, my grandson Benjamin, and my mother, Jessica Campney. You are my reason for everything.

Shelley

My husband Michael, our children and their partners, our grandsons Jace and Quinn, my mother Bev, and my amazing nursing colleagues at Dalhousie University's Yarmouth Campus.

Mariann

My husband Jeff, our daughters Kate and Sarah, and my parents, Mick and Mary.

Jeff

My parents, Raymond and Virginia, thank you for believing in me and providing me the opportunity to become a nurse.

Dottie

My husband Steve and my children Megan, E. J., Jessica, and Matthew, who have supported me through four college degrees and countless writing projects; and to my son-in-law Al, our grandsons Oscar and Stephen, and my new daughter-in-law, Melissa.

Debbie

My husband James, our children Matthew, Andrew, Amanda, and Diana, and our granddaughter Emma.

Courtney

To future nurses and the advancement of health care globally.

The Fifth Edition of *Lewis's Medical-Surgical Nursing in Canada: Assessment and Management of Clinical Problems* has been thoroughly revised for the Canadian student and incorporates the most current medical-surgical nursing information presented in an easy-to-use format. More than just a textbook, this is a comprehensive resource set in the Canadian context, containing essential information that nursing students need to prepare for lectures, classroom activities, examinations, clinical assignments, and the safe, comprehensive care of patients. In addition to the readable writing style and full-colour illustrations, the text and accompanying resources include many special features to help students learn key medical-surgical nursing content, such as sections that highlight the determinants of health, patient and caregiver teaching, age-related considerations, nursing and interprofessional management, interprofessional care, cultural considerations, nutrition, home care, evidence-informed practice, patient safety, and much more.

The comprehensive content, special features, attractive layout, and student-friendly writing style combine to make this the number one medical-surgical nursing textbook, used in more nursing schools in Canada than any other medical-surgical nursing textbook.

The latest edition of *Lewis's Medical-Surgical Nursing in Canada* retains the strengths of the first four editions, including the use of the nursing process as an organizational theme for nursing management. New features have been added to address some of the rapid changes in practice, and many diagrams and photos are new or improved. The content has been updated using the most recent important research and newest practice guidelines by Canadian contributors selected for their acknowledged excellence in specific content areas, ensuring a continuous thread of evidence-informed practice throughout the text. Specialists in the subject area have reviewed each chapter to ensure accuracy, and the editors have undertaken final rewriting and editing to achieve internal consistency. In other words, all efforts have been made to build on the recognized strengths of the previous Canadian editions.

ORGANIZATION

The content of this book is organized in two major divisions. The first division, Section 1 (Chapters 1 through 13), discusses concepts related to adult patients. The second division, Sections 2 through 12 (Chapters 14 through 72), presents nursing assessment and nursing management of medical-surgical conditions.

The various body systems are grouped in such a way as to reflect their interrelated functions. Each section is organized around two central themes: assessment and management. Each chapter that deals with the assessment of a body system includes a discussion of the following:

1. A brief review of anatomy and physiology, focusing on information that will promote understanding of nursing care
2. Health history and noninvasive physical assessment skills to expand the knowledge base on which decisions are made
3. Common diagnostic studies, expected results, and related nursing responsibilities to provide easily accessible information

Management chapters focus on the pathophysiology, clinical manifestations, laboratory and diagnostic study results in interprofessional care, and nursing management of various diseases and disorders. Nursing management sections are organized into assessment, nursing diagnoses, planning, implementation, and evaluation sections, following the steps of the nursing process. To emphasize the importance of patient care in various clinical settings, nursing implementation of all major health conditions is organized by the following levels of care:

1. Health promotion
2. Acute intervention
3. Ambulatory and home care

CLASSIC FEATURES

- **Canadian context.** Once again, we are pleased to offer the reader a book that reflects the wide range of expertise of nurses from across Canada. In an effort to better reflect the nursing environments across the country, all chapters have been revised with enhanced Canadian research and statistics. SI units and metric measurements are used throughout the text, and the updated APA format, including digital object identifiers (DOIs), is used for the references.
- **Most recent research and clinical guidelines.** Every effort has been made to use the most recent research, statistics, and clinical guidelines available. References older than 5 years at the time of writing are included because they are seminal studies or remain the most recent, authoritative source. Those references are marked "Seminal" in the References list.
- **Nursing management** is presented in a consistent and comprehensive format, with headings for Health Promotion, Acute Intervention, and Ambulatory and Home Care. In addition, over 60 customizable **Nursing Care Plans** on the Evolve website and in the text help students to understand possible nursing diagnoses, goals, and nursing interventions for each condition.
- **Interprofessional care** is highlighted in special Interprofessional Care sections in each of the management chapters and in **Interprofessional Care tables** throughout the text.
- **Patient and caregiver teaching** is an ongoing theme throughout the text. Chapter 4, *Patient and Caregiver Teaching*, and numerous **Patient & Caregiver Teaching Guides** throughout the text emphasize the increasing importance and prevalence of patient management of chronic illnesses and conditions and the role of the caregiver in patient care.
- **Culturally competent care** is covered in Chapter 2, *Cultural Competence and Health Equity in Nursing Care*, which discusses the necessity for culturally competent nursing care; culture as a determinant of health, with particular reference to Indigenous populations; health equity and health equality issues as they relate to marginalized groups in Canada; and practical suggestions for developing cultural competence in nursing care.
- **Coverage of prioritization** includes:
  - Prioritization questions in Case Studies and Review Questions
  - Nursing diagnoses and interventions throughout the text listed in order of priority

- **Focused Assessment boxes** in all assessment chapters provide brief checklists that help students do a more practical "assessment on the run" or bedside approach to assessment.
- **Safety Alerts** highlight important safety issues in relation to patient care as they arise.
- **Pathophysiology Maps** outline complex concepts related to diseases in flowchart format, making them easier to understand.
- **Community-based nursing and home care** are also emphasized in this Fifth Edition. Chapter 6 contains a comprehensive discussion, which is continued throughout the text.
- **Determinants of Health boxes** focus on the determinants of health as outlined by Health Canada and the Public Health Agency of Canada, as they affect a particular disorder. The determinants are introduced and discussed in detail in Chapter 1, and then returned to throughout the text by way of Determinants of Health boxes, which have been extensively updated and revised for the new edition. Each box identifies a health issue specific to the chapter; lists the relevant determinants affecting the issue, supported by the most recent research; and includes references for further investigation.
- **Extensive medication therapy content** includes **Medication Therapy tables** and concise **Medication Alerts** highlighting important safety considerations for key medications.
- **Chronic illness,** which has become Canada's most pressing health care challenge, is discussed in depth in Chapter 5. Nurses are increasingly called on to be active and engaged partners in assisting patients with chronic conditions to live well; this chapter places chronic illness within the larger context of Canadian society.
- **Older persons** are covered in detail in Chapter 7, and issues particularly relevant to this population are discussed throughout the text under the headings "Age-Related Considerations" and also in **Age-Related Differences in Assessment tables**.
- **Nutrition** is highlighted throughout the book, particularly in Chapter 42, *Nutritional Conditions*, and in **Nutritional Therapy tables** throughout that summarize nutritional interventions and promote healthy lifestyles for patients with various health conditions. Chapter 43, *Obesity*, looks in depth at this major factor contributing to so many other pathologies.
- **Complementary and alternative therapies** are discussed in Chapter 12, which addresses timely issues in today's health care settings related to these therapies, and in **Complementary & Alternative Therapies boxes,** where relevant, throughout the rest of the book that summarize what nurses need to know about therapies such as herbal remedies, acupuncture, and biofeedback.
- **Sleep and sleep disorders** are explored in Chapter 9; they are key topics that affect multiple disorders and body systems, as well as nearly every aspect of daily functioning.
- **Genetics in Clinical Practice boxes** build on the foundation of Chapter 15 and highlight genetic screening and testing, as well as the clinical implications of key genetic disorders that affect adults, as rapid advances in the field of genetics continue to change the way nurses practise.
- **Ethical Dilemmas boxes** promote critical thinking with regard to timely and sensitive issues that nursing students contend with in clinical practice, such as informed consent, treatment decision making, advance directives, and confidentiality.
- **Emergency Management tables** outline the emergency treatment of health conditions that are most likely to require rapid intervention.
- **Assessment Abnormalities tables** in the assessment chapters alert the nursing student to abnormalities frequently encountered in practice, as well as their possible etiologies.
- **Nursing Assessment tables** summarize important subjective and objective data related to common diseases, with a sharper focus on issues most relevant to the body system under review. This focus provides for more rapid identification of salient assessment parameters and more effective use of student time.
- **Health History tables** in assessment chapters present relevant questions related to a specific disease or disorder that will be asked in patient interviews.
- **Informatics boxes** throughout the text reflect the current use and importance of technology and touch on everything from the proper handling of social media in the context of patient privacy, to teaching patients to manage self-care using smartphone apps, to using smart infusion pumps.
- **Unfolding assessment case studies** in every assessment chapter are an engaging tool to help students apply nursing concepts in real-life patient care. Appearing in three or four parts throughout the chapter, they introduce a patient, follow that patient through subjective and objective assessment to diagnostic studies and results, and include additional discussion questions to facilitate critical thinking.
- **Student-friendly pedagogy:**
  - **Learning Objectives** at the beginning of each chapter help students identify the key content for a specific body system or disorder.
  - **Key Terms** lists provide a list of the chapter's most important terms and where they are discussed in the chapter. A comprehensive key terms **Glossary** with definitions may be found at the end of the book.
  - **Electronic resources** lists at the start of each chapter draw students' attention to the wealth of supplemental content and exercises provided on the Evolve website, making it easier than ever for them to integrate the textbook content with media supplements such as animations, video and audio clips, interactive case studies, and much more.
  - **Case Studies** bring patients to life. Management chapters have case studies at the end of the chapters that help students learn how to prioritize care and manage patients in the clinical setting. Unfolding case studies are included in each assessment chapter. Discussion questions that focus on prioritization and evidence-informed practice are included in most case studies. Answer guidelines are provided on the Evolve website.
  - **Review Questions** at the end of the chapter correspond to the Learning Objectives at the beginning and thus help reinforce the important points in the chapter. Answers are provided on the same page, making the Review Questions a convenient self-study tool.
  - **Resources** at the end of each chapter contain links to nursing and health care organizations and tools that provide patient teaching and information on diseases and disorders.

EXPANDED AND ENHANCED FEATURES

In addition to the continued classic strengths of this text, we are pleased to include several updated features:

- **Evidence-informed practice content** challenges students to develop critical thinking skills and apply the best available evidence to patient care scenarios in *Evidence-Informed Practice* boxes and questions at the end of many case studies.
- **Medication Alerts** concisely highlight important safety considerations for key medications.
- **Safety Alerts** have been expanded throughout the book to cover surveillance for high-risk situations.
- **New art** enhances the book's visual appeal and lends a more contemporary look throughout.
- Content related to the **COVID-19 pandemic** and the **SARS-CoV-2 virus** is incorporated throughout, focusing on its impacts on nurses and patients alike.
- **Revised Chapter 1:** *Introduction to Medical-Surgical Nursing Practice in Canada* situates nursing practice within the unique societal contexts that continue to shape the profession of nursing in Canada. Patient-centred care, interprofessional practice, and information-communication technologies are forces that have an impact on and are affected by nurses. This chapter includes a section on patient safety and quality improvement and expanded content on teamwork and interprofessional collaboration.

  Nursing education in Canada incorporates clinical decision-making models and guidelines that focus on critical thinking, clinical judgement, and clinical decision-making. These topics are defined along with a comparison between clinical judgement models (including the **NGN Clinical Judgement Measurement Model**) and the nursing process. As the nursing process best fits within Canadian nursing education, this Fifth Edition uses the nursing process as its guiding framework.
- **Revised Chapter 6:** *Community-Based Nursing and Home Care* includes additional content focusing on the impact of the COVID-19 pandemic and changes required in primary care settings, including home health monitoring (HHM) and the integration of virtual care.
- **Revised Chapter 11:** *Substance Use* now includes information about health care provider stigmatizing behaviours that negatively affect patient outcomes. The chapter also includes more detailed information about the impact of substance use experienced by Indigenous peoples of Canada and how health care providers can better meet the needs of this population. Expanded treatment options for opioid use disorder reflect current and innovative approaches to care now available in Canada.
- **Revised Chapter 31:** *Nursing Management: Obstructive Pulmonary Diseases* includes expanded content specific to asthma. Additional content provides a comprehensive overview of environmental and physiological triggers, diagnostic testing, and treatment options. New information includes modifications to infection-control practices and respiratory treatment protocols developed as a result of spread of the SARS-CoV-2 virus.
- **Revised Chapter 72:** *Emergency Management and Disaster Planning* has been expanded to include Canada's Strategic Emergency Management Plan and Emergency Response Plan and updated to include revisions to Canada's Emergency Management Framework and Canada's Incident Command System. Recent Canadian disasters have been included, and new information related to the COVID-19 pandemic has been incorporated. The World Health Organization's Emergency Response Plan has been added in detail, as well as the revised International Council of Nurses Framework of Disaster Nursing Competencies.

A WORD ON TERMINOLOGY

The authors and contributors of the text recognize and acknowledge the diverse histories of the First Peoples of the lands now referred to as Canada. It is recognized that individual communities identify themselves in various ways; within this text, the term *Indigenous* is used to refer to all First Nations, Inuit, and Métis people within Canada unless there are research findings that are presented uniquely to a population.

Knowledge and language concerning sex, gender, and identity are fluid and continually evolving. The language and terminology presented in this text endeavour to be inclusive of all people and reflect what is, to the best of our knowledge, current at the time of publication. Gender pronouns have been removed whenever possible, using the terms *they* and *them* as acceptable singular references to achieve gender neutrality (see https://en/oxforddictionaries.com/usage/he-or-she-versus-they). Patient profiles in Case Studies, Ethical Dilemmas boxes, and Evidence-Informed Practice: Translating Research into Practice boxes include preferred pronouns and employ initials in place of full names.

Throughout the textbook, when information is specific to the role of the RN, "Registered Nurse" or "RN" has been used; in all other instances, the term *nurse* is used to refer to an RN and/or RPN/LPN, depending on jurisdictional regulations.

"Interprofessional collaboration" is used to refer to any collaboration among health care team members and others (for example, spiritual caregivers).

"Health care provider" can include a physician, nurse practitioner, or an RN for whom the prescribing of medications or treatments is within their scope of practice.

A WORD ON LABORATORY VALUES

SI units are used for the laboratory values cited throughout the textbook. The *Laboratory Values* appendix lists SI units first, followed by US conventional units in parentheses in all relevant instances. It is important to note that reference ranges for laboratory values may vary among laboratories, depending on the testing techniques used. If discrepancies should exist between the body of the text and this appendix, the appendix should be considered the final authority.

LEARNING SUPPLEMENTS FOR THE STUDENT

- **Evolve Student Resources** are available online at http://evolve.elsevier.com/Canada/Lewis/medsurg and include the following valuable learning aids that are organized by chapter:
  - **NEW! PN Case Studies for Clinical Judgement**
  - **NEW! NGN-Style Case Studies**
  - Interactive **Student Case Studies** with state-of-the-art animations and a variety of learning activities that provide students with immediate feedback
  - Printable **Key Points** summaries for each chapter
  - **Review Questions**
  - **Answer guidelines** to the case studies in the textbook

- Customizable **Nursing Care Plans**
- **Conceptual Care Map Creator** and **Conceptual Care Maps** for selected case studies in the textbook
- **Managing Multiple Patients case studies for RNs** present scenarios with multiple patients requiring care simultaneously, to develop prioritization and delegation skills. Answer guidelines are also provided.
- Fluids and electrolytes **tutorial**
- **Audio glossary** of key terms, available as a comprehensive alphabetical glossary
- Supporting **animations** and **audio** for selected chapters
- More than just words on a screen, **Elsevier eBooks** come with a wealth of built-in study tools and interactive functionality to help students better connect with the course material and their instructors. Plus, with the ability to fit an entire library of books on one portable device, students can study when, where, and how they want.

TEACHING SUPPLEMENTS FOR INSTRUCTORS

- **Evolve Instructor Resources** (available online at http://evolve. elsevier.com/Canada/Lewis/medsurg) remain the most comprehensive set of instructors' materials available, containing the following:
  - *TEACH for Nurses Lesson Plans* focus on the most important content from each chapter and provide innovative strategies for student engagement and learning. These new lesson plans provide teaching strategies that integrate textbook content with activities for pre-class, in-class, online, group, clinical judgement, and interprofessional collaboration, all correlated with RN-NGN Clinical Judgement Model and PN Clinical Judgement Skills competencies.
  - Two test banks are provided: **Test Bank for RN** and **Test Bank for PN.** Each features examination-format test questions coded for nursing process and cognitive level. The Test Bank for PN is updated to reflect new 2019 PN national competencies, including those for Ontario and British Columbia. The robust ExamView® testing application, provided at no cost to faculty, allows instructors to create new tests; edit, add, and delete test questions; sort questions by category, cognitive level, and nursing process step; and administer and grade tests online, with automated scoring and gradebook functionality.
    - The **Image Collection** contains full-colour images from the text for use in lectures.
    - **PowerPoint® Lecture Slides** consist of customizable text slides for instructors to use in lectures.
- **NEW! Next-Generation NCLEX™ (NGN)**-style case studies for medical-surgical nursing
- **NEW! Concept-Based Curriculum Map**
- **Animations**

Simulation Learning System (SLS)

The Simulation Learning System (SLS) is an online toolkit that helps instructors and facilitators effectively incorporate medium- to high-fidelity simulation into their nursing curriculum. Detailed patient scenarios promote and enhance the clinical decision-making skills of students at all levels. The SLS provides detailed instructions for preparation and implementation of the simulation experience, debriefing questions that encourage critical thinking, and learning resources to reinforce student comprehension. Each scenario in the SLS complements the textbook content and helps bridge the gap between lecture and clinical experience. The SLS provides the perfect environment for students to practise what they are learning in the text for a true-to-life, hands-on learning experience.

Sherpath

Sherpath Book-Organized collections offer digital lessons, mapped chapter-by-chapter to the textbook, so the reader can conveniently find applicable digital assignment content. Sherpath features convenient teaching materials that are aligned with the textbook, and the lessons are organized by chapter for quick and easy access to invaluable class activities and resources.

Elsevier eBooks

This exciting program is available to faculty who adopt a number of Elsevier texts, including *Lewis's Medical-Surgical Nursing in Canada.* Elsevier eBooks is an integrated electronic study centre consisting of a collection of textbooks made available online. It is carefully designed to "extend" the textbook for an easier and more efficient teaching and learning experience. It includes study aids such as highlighting, e-note taking, and cut-and-paste capabilities. Even more importantly, it allows students and instructors to do a comprehensive search within the specific text or across a number of titles. Please check with your Elsevier Canada sales representative for more information.

Next Generation NCLEX™ (NGN)

The National Council for the State Boards of Nursing (NCSBN) is a not-for-profit organization whose members include nursing regulatory bodies. In empowering and supporting nursing regulators in their mandate to protect the public, the NCSBN is involved in the development of nursing licensure examinations, such as the NCLEX-RN®. In Canada, the NCLEX-RN® was introduced in 2015 and is, as of the writing of this text, the recognized licensure exam required for practising RNs in Canada.

As of 2023, the NCLEX-RN® will be changing to ensure that its item types adequately measure clinical judgement, critical thinking, and problem-solving skills on a consistent basis. The NCSBN will also be incorporating into the examination what they call the Clinical Judgement Measurement Model (CJMM), which is a framework the NCSBN has created to measure a novice nurse's ability to apply clinical judgement in practice.

These changes to the examination come as a result of findings indicating that novice nurses have a much higher than desirable error rate with patients (errors causing patient harm) and, upon NCSBN's investigation, that the overwhelming majority of these errors were caused by failures of clinical judgement.

Clinical judgement has been a foundation underlying nursing education for decades, based on the work of a number of nursing theorists. The theory of clinical judgement that most closely aligns with what NCSBN is basing their CJMM on is the work by Christine A. Tanner.

The new version of the NCLEX-RN® is identified loosely as the "Next-Generation NCLEX," or "NGN," and will feature the following:
- Six key skills in the CJMM: recognizing cues, analyzing cues, prioritizing hypotheses, generating solutions, taking actions, and evaluating outcomes.

- Approved item types as of March 2021: multiple response, extended drag and drop, cloze (drop-down), enhanced hotspot (highlighting), matrix/grid, bow tie, and trend. More question types may be added.
- All new item types are accompanied by mini–case studies with comprehensive patient information—some of it relevant to the question, and some of it not.
- Case information may present a single, unchanging moment in time (a "single episode" case study) or multiple moments in time as a patient's condition changes (an "unfolding" case study).
- Single-episode case studies may be accompanied by one to six questions; unfolding case studies are accompanied by six questions.

For more information (and detail) regarding the NCLEX-RN® and changes coming to the exam, visit the NCSBN's website: https://www.ncsbn.org/11447.htm and https://ncsbn.org/Building_a_Method_for_Writing_Clinical_Judgment_It.pdf.

For further NCLEX-RN® examination preparation resources, see *Elsevier's Canadian Comprehensive Review for the NCLEX-RN Examination*, Second Edition, ISBN 9780323709385.

Prior to preparing for any nursing licensure examination, please refer to your provincial or territorial nursing regulatory body to determine which licensure examination is required in order for you to practise in your chosen jurisdiction.

ACKNOWLEDGEMENTS

The editors are grateful to the entire editorial team at Elsevier for their leadership and dedication in the preparation of this very comprehensive, but much needed, Canadian medical-surgical textbook. In particular, we wish to thank Roberta A. Spinosa-Millman, Senior Content Strategist, for her invaluable assistance, and Tammy Scherer and Suzanne Simpson, Content Development Specialists, for their professionalism, sense of humour, patience, and graciousness despite pressing deadlines. We would also like to thank Sarah Ibrahim for her help with the Laboratory Values appendix.

We would like to recognize the commitment and expertise of all the authors, representing diverse areas of practice and regions of Canada. It has been a genuine pleasure to work with both the first-time and returning authors on this project. We are also very grateful to the many reviewers for their valuable feedback on earlier versions of this textbook. It takes a large and coordinated team to create a textbook such as this, and we thank everyone for their individual contributions. We are proud to be able to provide a medical-surgical nursing textbook written from a Canadian perspective that provides current and accurate information to enrich the learning of our nursing students.

SECTION 1

Concepts in Nursing Practice

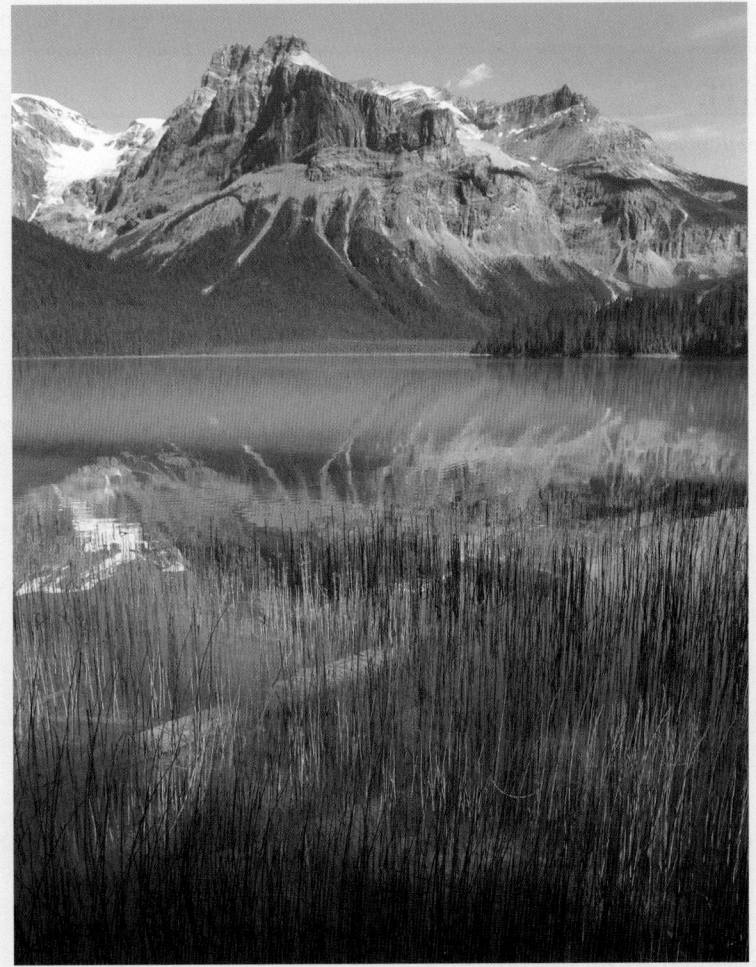

Source: © CanStock Photo / ABBPhoto

CHAPTER

1

Introduction to Medical-Surgical Nursing Practice in Canada

Jane Tyerman

Originating US chapter by Mariann M. Harding

LEARNING OBJECTIVES

1. Describe key challenges facing the current Canadian health care system.
2. Describe the practice of professional nursing in relation to the health care team.
3. Describe the key attributes of the practice of medical-surgical nursing.
4. Explain how teamwork and interprofessional collaboration contribute to high-quality patient outcomes.
5. Discuss the role of integrating patient-centred care and safety and quality improvement processes into nursing practice.
6. Evaluate the role of informatics and technology in nursing practice.
7. Apply concepts of evidence-informed practice to nursing practice.
8. Describe the role of critical thinking and clinical reasoning skills and use of the nursing process to provide patient-centred care.

KEY TERMS

advanced practice nursing (APN)
assessment
clinical (critical) pathway
collaborative problems
continuing competence
critical thinking
determinants of health
electronic health records (EHRs)
evaluation

evidence-informed nursing
expected patient outcomes
implementation
medical-surgical nursing
nursing diagnosis
nursing informatics
nursing intervention
nursing leadership
nursing process

patient-centred approach
patient safety
planning
regulated health care professions
SBAR (situation, background, assessment, and recommendation)
standard of practice
telehomecare
unregulated care providers (UCPs)

THE CANADIAN HEALTH CARE CONTEXT

Health care is a subject of keen interest to the public. In Canada, everyone has access to health care through a government-funded universal program, the costs of which are shared by the federal and the provincial/territorial governments. A multiyear health accord with a long-term funding agreement between the federal and provincial/territorial governments determines the way that health care is delivered in Canada. In addition, the level of health care funding from the federal government to the provinces and territories depends on the economic health of the country.

The *Canada Health Act* health care policy was established to promote, restore, and maintain the physical and mental health of all Canadians through equal access to health services (Government of Canada, 2020). These include most services provided in hospitals and by family health care providers. Because health services have evolved inconsistently across provinces, territories, and regions, however, Canada has a complex health care system. The Canadian health care system continues to struggle with major challenges, including concerns about patient safety, service delivery, fiscal constraints, age-related demographics, the emergence of new infectious diseases such as COVID-19, the prevalence of chronic diseases, and the high cost of new technology and medications. In response, during 2019–2020, Health Canada prioritized the following health initiatives (Health Canada, 2019):

1. Expand resources to address the national opioid crisis and create harm reduction strategies, such as supervised consumption sites and overdose prevention programs
2. Promote smoking cessation (tobacco and vaping) through product regulations that protect youth
3. Improve access to, the affordability of, and appropriate use of prescription medications to all Canadians
4. Increase access to home, community care, and mental health services

TABLE 1.1	PRINCIPLES TO GUIDE HEALTH CARE TRANSFORMATION IN CANADA

- *Patient-centred:* Patients must be at the centre of health care, with seamless access to the continuum of care on the basis of their needs.
- *Quality:* Canadians deserve quality services that are appropriate for patient needs, are respectful of individual choice, and are delivered in a manner that is timely, safe, effective, and according to the most currently available scientific knowledge.
- *Health promotion and illness prevention:* The health system must support Canadians in the prevention of illness and the enhancement of their well-being, with attention paid to broader social determinants of health.
- *Equitable:* The health care system has a duty to Canadians to provide and advocate for equitable access to quality care and commonly adopted policies to address the social determinants of health.
- *Sustainable:* Sustainable health care requires universal access to quality health services that are adequately resourced and delivered across the board in a timely and cost-effective manner.
- *Accountable:* The public, patients, families, providers, and funders all have a responsibility for ensuring that the system is effective and accountable.

Source: Canadian Nurses Association & Canadian Medical Association. (July, 2011). *Principles to guide health care transformation in Canada.* https://www.cna-aiic.ca/~/media/cna/files/en/guiding_principles_hc_e.pdf

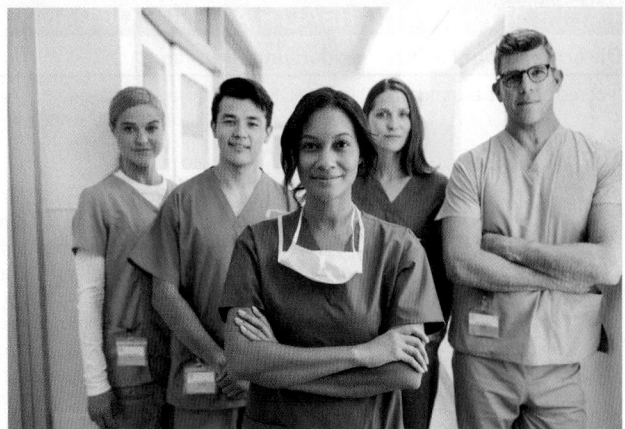

FIG. 1.1 Nurses are frontline professionals of health care. Source: iStock.com/monkeybusinessimages.

ETHICAL DILEMMAS

Social Networking: Confidentiality and Privacy Violation

Situation

A nursing student logs into a closed group on a social networking site and reads a posting from a fellow nursing student. The posting describes in detail the complex care that the fellow student provided to an older patient in a local hospital the previous day. The fellow student comments on how stressful the day was and asks for advice on how to deal with similar patients in the future.

Ethical/Legal Points for Consideration

- Protecting and maintaining patient privacy and confidentiality are basic obligations defined in the *Code of Ethics* (CNA, 2017), which nurses and nursing students should uphold.
- Each province and territory has their own legislation to protect a patient's private health information. Some examples include the *Personal Information Protection Act* (PIPA) in British Columbia and the *Access to Information and Protection of Privacy Act* (ATIPPA) in Newfoundland and Labrador. Private health information is any information about the patient's past, present, or future physical or mental health. This includes not only specific details, such as a patient's name or picture, but also information that gives enough details that someone else may be able to identify that patient.
- A nurse may unintentionally breach privacy or confidentiality by posting patient information (diagnosis, condition, or situation) on a social networking site. Using privacy settings or being in a closed group does not guarantee the secrecy of posted information. Other users can copy and share any post without the poster's knowledge.
- Potential consequences for improperly using social networking vary according to the situation. These may include dismissal from a nursing program, termination of employment, or civil and criminal actions.

Discussion Questions

- How would you address the situation involving a fellow nursing student?
- How would you handle a situation in which you observed a staff member violating the provincial/territorial legislation related to a patient's private health information?

5. Implement a multiyear Healthy Eating Strategy that builds on the revised *Canada's Food Guide* (Government of Canada, 2021)
6. Support the implementation of Indigenous Services Canada (ISC) programs available to Indigenous peoples

Together with the Canadian Medical Association (CMA), the Canadian Nurses Association (CNA) has defined a set of key principles designed to guide health care transformation in Canada. These principles, listed in Table 1.1, are important considerations for all nurses because they will shape the re-engineered health care system of the future.

Complex Health Care Environments

Nurses practice in virtually all health care settings and communities across the country. They are the frontline providers of health care (Figure 1.1). Rapidly changing technology and dramatically expanding knowledge are adding to the complexity of health care environments. Patient acuity is now more complicated because of polypharmacy, chronic health care conditions, and multiple comorbidities, which have paved the way for more research and robust technology to address these needs. Additional health care providers are required to work collaboratively to help restore, maintain, and promote health for all populations with complex health needs. Advanced communication technologies have created a more global environment that affects the delivery of health care worldwide. The number and complexity of advances in patient care technology are transforming how care is delivered. In addition, the Human Genome Project and advances in genetics are affecting the prevention, diagnosis, and treatment of health conditions. With advances in knowledge, ethical dilemmas and controversy arise with regard to the use of new scientific knowledge and the disparities that exist in patients' access to more technologically advanced health care. Throughout this book, expanding knowledge and technology's effects on nursing practice are highlighted in Genetics in Clinical Practice, Informatics in Practice, and Ethical Dilemmas boxes.

Diverse Populations. Patient demographics are more diverse than ever. Canadians are living longer, in part because of advances in medical science, technology, and health care delivery. As the population ages, the number of patients with chronic conditions increases. Unlike those who receive acute, episodic care, patients with chronic conditions have many needs and see a variety of health care providers in various settings over an

TABLE 1.2   PUBLIC HEALTH AGENCY OF CANADA: KEY DETERMINANTS OF HEALTH

Determinant of Health	Underlying Premise
Income and social status	Health status improves at each step up the income and social hierarchy. High income determines living conditions such as safe housing and ability to buy sufficient good food. The healthiest populations are those societies that are prosperous and have an equitable distribution of wealth.
Social support networks	Support from families, friends, and communities is associated with better health. Such social support networks could be very important in helping people solve problems and deal with adversity, as well as in maintaining a sense of mastery and control over life circumstances. The caring and respect that occur in social relationships, and the resulting sense of satisfaction and well-being, seem to act as a buffer against health problems.
Education and literacy	Health status improves with level of education, which is, in turn, tied to socioeconomic status. Education contributes to health and prosperity by equipping people with knowledge and skills for problem solving and helps provide a sense of control and mastery over life circumstances. It increases opportunities for job and income security and job satisfaction. Education also improves people's ability to access and understand information to help keep them healthy.
Employment/working conditions	Unemployment, underemployment, and stressful or unsafe work are associated with poorer health. People who have more control over their work circumstances and fewer stress-related demands of the job are healthier and often live longer than those who have more stressful or riskier types of work and activities.
Social environments	The array of values and norms of a society influences in varying ways the health and well-being of individuals and populations. In addition, social stability, recognition of diversity, safety, good working relationships, and cohesive communities provide a supportive society that reduces or avoids many potential risks to good health. Social or community responses can add resources to an individual's repertoire of strategies to cope with changes and foster health.
Physical environments	The physical environment is an important determinant of health. At certain levels of exposure, contaminants in our air, water, food, and soil can cause a variety of adverse health effects, including cancer, birth defects, respiratory illness, and gastrointestinal ailments. In the built environment, factors related to housing, indoor air quality, and the design of communities and transportation systems can significantly influence physical and psychological well-being.
Personal health practices and coping skills	These refer to those actions by which individuals can prevent diseases and promote self-care, cope with challenges, develop self-reliance, solve problems, and make choices that enhance health. These influence lifestyle choice through at least five domains: personal life skills, stress, culture, social relationships and belonging, and a sense of control.
Healthy child development	Early childhood development is a powerful determinant of health. Early experiences affect brain development and school readiness, which can be affected by the physical environment (housing and neighbourhood), family income, parental education, access to nutritious food, genetics, and access to health care. All of the other determinants of health, in turn, affect the physical, social, mental, emotional, and spiritual development of children and youth.
Biology and genetic endowment	The basic biology and organic makeup of the human body are a fundamental determinant of health. Genetic endowment provides an inherited predisposition to a wide range of individual responses that affect health status. Socioeconomic and environmental factors are important determinants of overall health, but in some circumstances, genetic endowment appears to predispose certain individuals to particular diseases or health problems.
Health services	Health services, particularly those designed to maintain and promote health, to prevent disease, and to restore health and function, contribute to the health of the overall population. The health services continuum of care includes treatment and secondary prevention.
Gender	*Gender* refers to the array of society-determined roles, personality traits, attitudes, behaviours, values, and relative power and influence that society ascribes to the two sexes on a differential basis. Gendered norms influence the health system's practices and priorities. Many health issues are a function of gender-based social status or roles.
Culture	Some persons or groups may face additional health risks due to a socioeconomic environment, which is largely determined by dominant cultural values that contribute to the perpetuation of conditions such as marginalization, stigmatization, loss or devaluation of language and culture, and lack of access to culturally appropriate health care and services.

extended period. Nurses are also caring for a more culturally and ethnically diverse population and must provide culturally safe care (see Chapter 2). Immigrants, particularly undocumented immigrants and refugees, often lack the resources necessary to access health care. Inability to pay for health care is associated with a tendency to delay seeking care; thus, illnesses may become more serious.

Determinants of Health. The determinants of health are the factors that influence the health of individuals and groups. Table 1.2 displays the determinants of health recognized by the Public Health Agency of Canada (PHAC, 2020). The primary factors that shape the health of Canadians are not medical treatments or lifestyle choices but rather the living conditions (the economic, social, and political) that they experience (Alberga et al., 2018; Hancock, 2017). The 12 determinants of health include income and social status, employment and working conditions, education and literacy, childhood experiences, physical environments, social supports and coping skills, healthy behaviours, access to health services, biology and genetic endowment, gender, culture, and race and racism (PHAC, 2020). These determinants of health include biological components and social components. The social components can be further evaluated based on economic, social, and political structures. The determinants of health are used to evaluate components of health for an individual, community, subpopulation, or nation or on a global scale. They help identify many factors that contribute to one's health beyond the biological, innate advantages and disadvantages. These determinants can either improve a person's health status or heighten an individual's risk for disease, injury, and illness. As these factors or determinants intersect with each other, the overall effect can be one of multiple exclusions beyond individual control, leading to compounded adverse effects on health and well-being.

Patient-Centred Care

Nurses have long demonstrated that they deliver patient-centred care based on each patient's unique needs and an understanding of the patient's preferences, values, and beliefs.

TABLE 1.3 QUALITY AND SAFETY EDUCATION FOR NURSES (QSEN) COMPETENCIES

Competency	Knowledge, Skills, and Attitudes
Patient-Centred Care Recognize the patient or designee as the source of control and a full partner in providing compassionate and coordinated care that is based on respect for patient's preferences, values, and needs.	• Provide care with sensitivity and respect, taking into consideration the patient's perspectives, beliefs, and cultural background. • Assess the patient's level of comfort, and treat appropriately. • Engage the patient in an active partnership that promotes health, well-being, and self-care management. • Facilitate patient's informed consent for care.
Teamwork and Collaboration Function effectively within nursing and interprofessional teams, fostering open communication, mutual respect, and shared decision making to achieve quality patient care.	• Value the expertise of each interprofessional member. • Initiate referrals when appropriate. • Follow communication practices that minimize risks associated with handoffs and transitions in care. • Participate in interprofessional rounds.
Safety Minimize risk of harm to patients and providers through both system effectiveness and individual performance.	• Follow recommendations from national safety campaigns. • Appropriately communicate observations or concerns related to hazards and errors. • Contribute to designing systems to improve safety.
Quality Improvement Use data to monitor the outcomes of care and use improvement methods to design and test changes to continuously improve the quality and safety of health care systems.	• Use quality measures to understand performance. • Identify gaps between local and best practices. • Participate in investigating the circumstances surrounding a sentinel event or serious reportable event.
Informatics Use information and technology to communicate, manage knowledge, mitigate error, and support decision making.	• Protect confidentiality of patient's protected health information. • Document appropriately in electronic health records. • Use communication technologies to coordinate patient care. • Respond correctly to clinical decision-making alerts.
Evidence-Based or Evidence-Informed Practice Integrate best current evidence with clinical expertise and the patient/family preferences and values for delivery of optimal health care.	• Read research, clinical practice guidelines, and evidence reports related to area of practice. • Base individual patient care plan on patient's values, clinical expertise, and evidence. • Continuously improve clinical practice on the basis of new knowledge.

Source: Reprinted from *Nursing Outlook, 55*(3), Linda Cronenwett, Gwen Sherwood, Jane Barnsteiner, Joanne Disch, Jean Johnson, Pamela Mitchell, Dori Taylor Sullivan, Judith Warren, "Quality and safety education for nurses," pages 122–131, Copyright 2007, with permission from Elsevier.

Patient-centred care is interrelated with both quality and safety. A **patient-centred approach** focuses on respectful and responsive care to patient preferences, needs, and values, ensuring they are involved in care decisions (Montague et al., 2017). In Canada, numerous provincial initiatives are underway to improve the person's and their family's experience. Many initiatives are partnering with individual users to ensure that the patient (and the patient's family) is the focus of system reform (Registered Nurses' Association of Ontario [RNAO], 2015).

Patient Safety and Quality Improvement. **Patient safety** is defined as the absence of preventable harm to a patient while receiving health care and the unnecessary harm associated with health care (World Health Organization [WHO], 2019). Entry-to-practice nursing competencies recognize the importance of the nurse's ability to assess and manage situations that may compromise patient safety (College of Nurses of Ontario [CNO], 2019). Although patients turn to the health care system for help with their health conditions, there is overwhelming evidence that significant numbers of patients are harmed as a result of the health care they receive, resulting in permanent injury, increased lengths of hospital stay, and even death (WHO, 2019). There are approximately 190 000 patient safety incidences in Canada, resulting in 24 000 preventable deaths yearly, indicating that harmful incidents are a significant issue in Canadian

hospitals (Canadian Patient Safety Institute [CPSI], 2017). The Canadian Patient Safety Institute (CPSI) and other organizations address patient safety by providing safety goals for health care organizations and identifying safety competencies for health care providers. Tools and programs in four priority areas—medication safety, surgical care safety, infection prevention and control, and home care safety—are available from the CPSI (2021).

By implementing various procedures and systems to improve health care delivery to meet safety goals, designers of health care systems are working to attain a culture of safety that minimizes the risk of harm to the patient. Because nurses have the greatest amount of interaction with patients, they are a vital part of promoting this culture of safety by providing care that reduces errors and actively promotes patient safety.

Quality and Safety Education for Nurses. The Quality and Safety Education for Nurses (QSEN) Institute has made a major contribution to nursing by defining specific competencies that nurses need to have to practise safely and effectively in today's complex health care system. Table 1.3 describes each of the QSEN competencies and the knowledge, skills, and attitudes (KSAs) necessary in six key areas: (1) patient-centred care, (2) teamwork and collaboration, (3) quality improvement, (4) safety, (5) informatics and technology, and (6) evidence-informed practice (QSEN, 2014). The rest of this chapter describes how professional nursing practice focuses on acquiring the knowledge, skills, and attitudes for these competencies.

The Profession of Nursing in Canada

Health care in Canada is typically delivered by teams of workers with different responsibilities and scopes of practice. **Regulated health care professions** are governed by a legislative framework and are required to obtain an annual licence to practise in their respective province or territory (Canadian Institute for Health Information [CIHI], 2020). There are four regulated nursing groups: registered nurses (RNs), nurse practitioners, registered psychiatric nurses, and licensed practical nurses/registered practical nurses (LPN/RPNs). In contrast, **unregulated care providers (UCPs)** or unregulated health workers are paid employees who are not licensed or registered by a regulatory body, who have no legally defined scope of practice, for whom education or practice standards may or may not be mandatory, who provide care under the direct or indirect supervision of a nurse, and who are accountable for their own actions and decisions (CNA, 2015, p. 28). Some of the more common titles for UCPs include "health care aides," "personal support workers," "assistive personnel," "care team assistants," and "nursing aides."

Within Canada, nurses are granted the legal authority to use the designation "registered nurse" (RN) in accordance with provincial and territorial legislation and regulation. The provincial regulatory bodies set the standards for practice for RNs to protect the public in their province or territory (CNA, 2015). RN practice is defined by the CNA (2015) in the following way:

> *RNs are self-regulated health-care professionals who work autonomously and in collaboration with others to enable individuals, families, groups, communities and populations to achieve their optimal levels of health. At all stages of life, in situations of health, illness, injury and disability, RNs deliver direct health-care services, coordinate care and support clients in managing their own health. RNs contribute to the health-care system through their leadership . . . in practice, education, administration, research and policy. (p. 5)*

Because RNs work with other regulated providers, as well as with UCPs, they must be aware of both their own and other providers' scopes of practice. This is essential for safely enacting key nursing roles, such as delegation and prioritization and meeting the standards of practice.

Standards of Practice. A **standard of practice** and its guidelines describe nurses' accountabilities to support the safe and ethical provision of care (CNO, 2019). Standards are intended to promote, guide, direct, and regulate professional nursing practice. Standards of practice demonstrate to the public, government, and other stakeholders that a profession is dedicated to maintaining public trust and upholding its professional practice criteria. Standards of practice are based on the values of the profession and articulated in the *Code of Ethics for Registered Nurses* (CNA, 2017). Provincial and territorial regulatory bodies for nursing are legally required to set standards for practice for RNs to protect the public. These standards, together with the *Code of Ethics*, form the foundation for nursing practice in Canada.

Because of the rapid changes in resources, expectations, and technologies that characterize health care in Canada, nursing practice requires a commitment to lifelong learning to promote the highest quality of patient outcomes. **Continuing competence** refers to "the ongoing ability of a nurse to integrate and apply the knowledge, skills, judgement and personal attributes required to

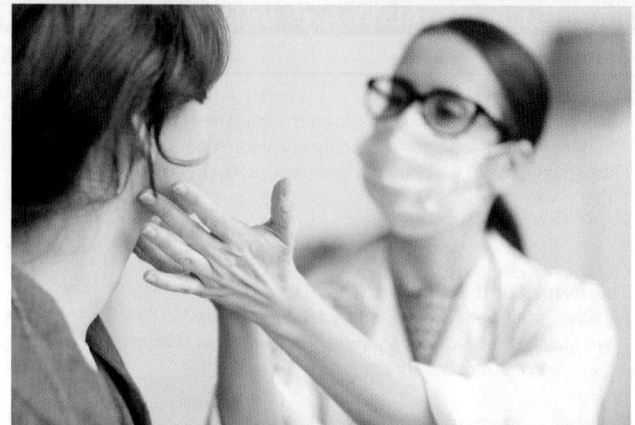

FIG. 1.2 Advanced nursing practice (ANP) plays an important role in primary care delivery. Source: iStock.com/AnnaStills.

practice safely and ethically in a designated role and setting" (CNA/Canadian Association of Schools of Nursing [CASN], 2004).

RNs are initially prepared at the baccalaureate level (except in Quebec) and can pursue further studies at the graduate level. In the province of Quebec, RNs can also be diploma-prepared by receiving nursing education at a college or CEGEP. This diploma is recognized as eligibility to apply for registration with the provincial nursing body if all requirements have been met. Many nurses also seek recognition of their clinical expertise through certification in one of the 20 specialty areas of practice through the CNA (2021). Medical-surgical nursing is one of the newer specialties to be recognized through the certification program.

Advanced Practice Nursing. As Canada's health care system changes, **advanced practice nursing (APN)** roles are also evolving to optimize patient care within the system. According to the Advanced Practice Nursing Pan-Canadian Framework, advanced practice nursing "integrates graduate nursing education preparation with in-depth, specialized clinical nursing knowledge and expertise in complex decision-making to meet the health needs of individuals, families, groups, communities and populations" (CNA, 2019, p. 13). APN roles focus on health assessment, diagnosis, and treatment of conditions previously considered to be the physician's domain (Figure 1.2). It involves analyzing and synthesizing knowledge; critiquing, interpreting and applying nursing theory; participating in and leading research; using advanced clinical competencies; and developing and accelerating nursing knowledge and the profession as a whole (CNA, 2019, p. 13). Examples of roles within APN in Canada include those of the clinical nurse specialist and the nurse practitioner.

In addition to managing and delivering direct patient care, APN nurses have significant roles in health promotion, case management, administration, and research. There is substantial variation among the provinces and territories in the framework for and specific roles of nurses working in APN. Practice settings in which an APN nurse may be employed include primary and tertiary care, such as ambulatory care, long-term care, hospital care, and community care. In the APN role, the nurse's focus may be, for example, the management of primary care and health promotion for a wide variety of health issues in various specialties; activities include physical examination, diagnosis, treatment of health conditions, patient and family education, and counselling. In the management of complex patient care in various clinical specialty areas, the roles of APN may include direct care, consultation, research, education, case management, and administration.

TABLE 1.4	INTERPROFESSIONAL TEAM MEMBERS
Team Member	**Description of Services Provided**
Dietitian	Provides general nutrition services, including dietary consultation about health promotion or specialized diets
Occupational therapist (OT)	May help patient with fine motor coordination, performing activities of daily living, cognitive-perceptual skills, sensory testing, and the construction or use of assistive or adaptive equipment
Pastoral care	Offers interdenominational spiritual support and guidance to patients and caregivers
Pharmacist	Prepares medications and infusion products
Physiotherapist (PT)	Works with patients on improving strength and endurance, gait training, transfer training, and developing a patient education program
Physician (medical doctor [MD])	Practises medicine and treats illness and injury by prescribing medication, performing diagnostic tests and evaluations, performing surgery, and providing other medical services and advice
Nurse practitioner	Diagnoses illness, orders and interprets diagnostic tests, prescribes medications and treatments, and performs specific procedures within their scope of practice
Physician assistant	Conducts physical exams, diagnoses and treats illnesses, and counsels on preventive health care in collaboration with a physician
Respiratory therapist	May provide oxygen therapy in the home, give specialized respiratory treatments, and teach the patient or caregiver about the proper use of respiratory equipment
Social worker	Assists patients with developing coping skills, meeting caregiver concerns, securing adequate financial resources or housing, or making referrals to social service or volunteer agencies
Speech pathologist	Focuses on treatment of speech defects and disorders, especially by using physical exercises to strengthen muscles used in speech, speech drills, and audiovisual aids that develop new speech habits

What Is Medical-Surgical Nursing? Medical-surgical nursing is a challenging and dynamic type of nursing that involves caring for adults experiencing complex variations in health (Canadian Association of Medical and Surgical Nurses [CAMSN], 2020). Because the scope of medical-surgical nursing is very broad, the nurse practising in this area is expected to acquire and maintain a great deal of knowledge and skill. This book provides the beginning nurse with much of the knowledge necessary to become a safe and competent practitioner.

The medical-surgical nurse is considered a leader and a key member of the interdisciplinary team. The medical-surgical nurse's primary responsibilities include prioritization, accountability, advocacy, organization, and coordination of evidence-informed care for multiple patients. Medical-surgical patients and their caregivers come from diverse backgrounds and often possess multiple, complex illnesses; medical-surgical nurses, therefore, must be knowledgeable and well prepared. Because of the rapidly changing and complex health concerns that may affect multiple body systems of medical-surgical patients, safe and effective use of technology is an increasingly important competency required by these nurses. The effective medical-surgical nurse demonstrates adaptability and a strong commitment to ensuring the best possible patient outcomes.

Medical-surgical nurses practise in diverse environments, ranging from outpatient and primary care environments through the continuum of care to tertiary care hospitals (CNA, 2015). As the largest group of nursing professionals in Canada (CAMSN, 2020), they utilize a broad range of evidence-informed knowledge and clinical skills to address acutely ill adults' and their families' needs. The Canadian Association of Medical and Surgical Nurses (CAMSN) is a national organization that promotes excellence through best-practice standards to provide high-quality, safe, and ethical care to patients across the continuum of care. RNs may choose to seek recognition of their expertise in this specialty through post-licensure certification offered by the CNA.

Teamwork and Interprofessional Collaboration

Interprofessional Teams. To deliver high-quality care, nurses need to have effective working relationships with the health care team members. Supporting patients to achieve optimal health, nurses collaborate with a wide range of professionals, including pharmacists, physicians, occupational therapists, physiotherapists, and social workers (Table 1.4).

Successful collaboration with other health care providers has become a cornerstone of nursing practice. To be competent in interprofessional practice, nurses must collaborate in many ways by exchanging knowledge, sharing responsibility for problem-solving, and making patient care decisions. Nurses are often responsible for coordinating care among the team members, taking part in interprofessional team meetings or rounds, and making referrals when expertise is needed in specialized areas to help the patient. To do so, nurses must be aware of other team members' knowledge and skills and be able to communicate effectively with them.

In the position statement *Interprofessional Collaboration,* the CNA (2012) recognized the growing importance of interprofessional collaboration in improving patient-centred access to health care in Canada. The Registered Nurses' Association of Ontario (RNAO, 2013) described a conceptual model for developing and sustaining interprofessional health care whereby outstanding interprofessional care is a result of health care teams demonstrating expertise in six key domains: care expertise; shared power; collaborative leadership; optimizing profession, role, and scope; shared decision making; and effective group functioning (RNAO, 2013).

Nurses function in independent, dependent, and collaborative roles. Each province and territory has a *Nurses' Act* that determines the scope of practice for that region. These acts allow nurses to take on delegated medical responsibilities and have a wider scope of practice when working as nurse practitioners.

Communication Among Health Care Team Members. Effective communication is a key component of fostering teamwork and coordinating care. To provide safe, effective care, everyone involved in a patient's care should understand the patient's condition and needs. Unfortunately, many issues result from a breakdown in communication. Miscommunication often occurs during transitions of care. One structured model used to improve communication is the SBAR (situation, background, assessment, and recommendation) technique (Table 1.5). This technique provides a way for the health care team members to talk about a patient's condition in a predictable, structured manner. Other ways to enhance communication during transitions include

TABLE 1.5	GUIDELINES FOR COMMUNICATION USING SBAR

Purpose: SBAR is a model for effective transfer of information by providing a standard structure for concise factual communications from nurse to nurse, nurse to physician, or nurse to other health professionals.

Steps to Use: Before speaking with a health care provider about a patient issue, assess the patient yourself, read the most recent physician progress and nursing notes, and have the patient's chart available.

Situation	• What is the situation you want to discuss? What is happening right now? • Identify self, unit. State: I am calling about: patient, room number. • Briefly state the challenge: what it is, when it happened or started, and how severe it is. State: I have just assessed the patient and am concerned about: • *Describe why you are concerned.*
Background	• What is the background or what are the circumstances leading up to the situation? State pertinent background information related to the situation that may include: • Admitting diagnosis and date of admission • List of current medications, allergies, intravenous (IV) fluids • Most recent vital signs • Date and time of any laboratory testing and results of previous tests for comparison • Synopsis of treatment to date • Code status
Assessment	• What do you think the issue is? What is your assessment of the situation? State what you think the issue is: • Changes from prior assessments • Patient condition unstable or worsening
Recommendation/**R**equest	• What should we do to correct the problem? What is your recommendation or request? State your request. • Specific treatments • Tests needed • Patient needs to be seen now

Source: Adapted from *SBAR Tool: Situation-Background-Assessment-Recommendation*, developed by Kaiser Permanente, sourced from www.IHI.org with permission of the Institute for Healthcare Improvement, ©2021.

TABLE 1.6	RIGHTS OF DELEGATION

The Five Rights of Delegation
The registered nurse uses critical thinking and professional judgement to be sure that the delegation or assignment is:
1. The right task
2. Under the right circumstances
3. To the right person
4. With the right directions and communication
5. Under the right supervision and evaluation

Rights of Delegation	Description	Questions to Ask
Right Task	One that can be delegated for a specific patient	Is it appropriate to delegate based on legal and facility factors? Has the person been trained and evaluated in performing the task? Is the person able and willing to do this specific task?
Right Circumstances	Appropriate patient setting, available resources, and considering relevant factors, including patient stability	What are the patient's needs right now? Is staffing such that the circumstances support delegation strategies?
Right Person	Right person is delegating the right task to the right person to be performed on the right person	Is the prospective delegatee a willing and able employee? Are the patient needs a "fit" with the delegatee?
Right Directions and Communication	Clear, concise description of task, including its objective, limits, and expectations	Have you given clear communication about the task? With directions, limits, and expected outcomes? Does the delegatee know what and when to report? Does the delegatee understand what needs to be done?
Right Supervision and Evaluation	Appropriate monitoring, evaluation, intervention, and feedback	Do you know how and when you will interact about patient care with the delegatee? How often do you need to directly observe? Will you be able to give feedback to the staff member if needed?

Source: National Council of State Boards of Nursing, Inc. (NCSBN). (2015). *National guidelines for nursing delegation.* https://www.ncsbn.org/1625.htm

performing surgical time-outs, standardizing the change-of-shift process, and conducting interprofessional rounds to identify risks and develop a plan for delivering care.

Delegation and Assignment. Nurses delegate nursing care and supervise other staff members who are qualified to deliver care. *Delegation* is "a formal process through which a regulated health professional (delegator) who has the authority and competence to perform a procedure under one of the controlled acts delegates the performance of that procedure to another individual (delegatee)" (CNO, 2020). The delegation and assignment of nursing activities is a process that, when used appropriately, can result in safe, effective, and efficient patient care.

Delegation typically involves tasks and procedures that UCPs perform. The activities that UCPs perform include feeding and assisting patients at mealtimes, helping stable patients ambulate, and assisting patients with bathing and hygiene. Nursing interventions that require independent nursing knowledge, skill, or judgement (e.g., initial assessment, determining nursing diagnoses, patient teaching, evaluating care) are the nurse's responsibility and cannot be delegated. Nurses need to use professional judgement and follow the Five Rights of Delegation (Table 1.6) to determine appropriate activities to delegate based on the patient's needs. The most common delegated nursing actions occur during the implementation phase of the nursing process and are for patients who are stable with predictable outcomes. For example, the nurse might delegate measuring oral intake and urine output to a UCP, but the nurse uses nursing judgement to decide whether the intake and output are adequate. Delegation is patient-specific, and the UCP can perform the delegated task for only a particular patient.

Assignment is different from delegation. Assignment involves the "allocation of nursing care among providers in order to meet patient care needs" (Nurses Association of New Brunswick/Association of New Brunswick Licensed Practical Nurses, 2015, p. 10). The RN can only assign team members (LPN/UCP) activities that are within the team member's scope of practice. For example, the nurse can assign an LPN/RPN to give a patient medication because it is within their scope of practice. The RN or LPN/RPN cannot assign a UCP to perform a complex dressing change as assessment of the wound, a task when performing dressing changes, is not within their scope of practice.

Whether nurses delegate or are working with staff to whom they assign tasks, they are responsible for the patient's total care during their work period. Nurses are responsible for supervising the UCP who is caring for their patient. It is important to clearly communicate what tasks must be done and to provide necessary guidance. Nurses are accountable for ensuring that delegated tasks are completed competently. This supervision includes evaluation and follow-up as needed by the nurse.

Delegation is a skill that is learned and must be practised to attain proficiency in managing patient care, and it requires the use of critical thinking and professional judgement.

Informatics and Technology

Rapidly changing technologies and dramatically expanding knowledge in the fields of arts and science affect all areas of health care. In telemedicine, telehealth, and telenursing, virtual technologies are used to provide professional education, consultation, and delivery of patient services. **Telehomecare** (digital health) is the delivery of health care and information through digital technologies, including high-speed Internet, wireless, satellite, and video communications. Among the many uses of telehealth are triaging patients, monitoring patients with chronic or critical conditions, helping patients manage symptoms, providing patient and caregiver education and emotional support, and providing follow-up care (CMA, 2019). Telehomecare can increase access to care. The nurse engaged in telehealth can assess the patient's health status, deliver interventions, and evaluate the outcomes of nursing care while separated geographically from the patient.

Nursing Informatics. Nursing informatics is a rapidly growing specialty in nursing. **Nursing informatics** refers to the integration of nursing science, computer science, and information technology to manage and communicate data, information, and knowledge in nursing practice (RNAO, 2012). Nursing is an information-intense profession. Advances in informatics and technology have changed the way that nurses plan, deliver, document, and evaluate care. All nurses, regardless of their setting or role, use informatics and technology every day in practice. Informatics has changed how nurses obtain and review diagnostic information, make clinical decisions, communicate with patients and health care team members, and document and provide care.

Technology advances have increased the efficiency of nursing care, improving the work environment and the care that nurses provide. Computers and mobile devices enable nurses to document at the time they deliver care and give them quick and easy access to information, including clinical decision-making tools, patient education materials, and references. Texting, video chat, and email enhance communication among health care team members and help them deliver the right message to the right person at the right time.

Technology plays a key role in providing safe, quality patient care. Medication administration applications improve patient safety by flagging potential errors, such as look-alike and sound-alike medications and adverse drug interactions, before they can occur. Computerized provider order entry (CPOE) systems can eliminate errors caused by misreading or misinterpreting handwritten orders. Sensor technology can decrease the number of falls by patients at high risk for falls. Care reminder systems provide cues that decrease the amount of missed nursing care.

The ability to use technology skills to communicate and access information is now an essential component of professional nursing practice. Nurses must be able to use word processing software, communicate by email and messaging, access appropriate information, and follow security and confidentiality rules. They need to demonstrate the skills to safely use patient care technologies and navigate electronic documentation systems. The CASN (2012) has outlined three entry-to-practice competencies related to nursing informatics: (1) use of relevant information and knowledge to support the delivery of evidence-informed patient care; (2) use of ICTs in accordance with professional and regulatory standards and workplace policies; and (3) use of ICTs in the delivery of patient care (pp. 6–10). These nursing informatics competencies are considered the minimum knowledge and skills that new graduate nurses require to practise nursing. Throughout this book, Informatics in Practice boxes such as the one below offer suggestions for nurses on how to make information technology part of good nursing practice.

INFORMATICS IN PRACTICE

Responsible Use of Social Media

A nurse wants to post pictures (or videos) of himself and his nursing colleagues from the hospital.
- Before sharing anything on social media, the nurse should ensure that the posts do not negatively reflect the nursing profession, workplace, self, or colleagues as health care providers.
- The nurse should ensure that posts do not cause a breach of confidentiality and privacy for patients, colleagues, or the workplace.
- The nurse should know and follow employer policies on using social media in the workplace.

Nurses have an obligation to ensure the privacy of their patients' health information. To do so, it is necessary to understand their hospital's policies regarding the use of technology. Nurses need to know the rules regarding accessing patient records and releasing personal health information, what to do if the information is accidentally or intentionally released, and how to protect any passwords they use. If nurses are using social media, they must be careful not to place online any personal health information that is individually identifiable and must adhere to certain principles in order to reduce risks to members

TABLE 1.7   **6 *PS* OF SOCIAL MEDIA USE**

Professional: Act professionally at all times
Positive: Keep posts positive
Patient/Person-free: Keep posts patient- or person-free
Protect yourself: Protect your professionalism, your reputation, and yourself
Privacy: Keep your personal and professional life separate; respect privacy of others
Pause before you post: Consider implications; avoid posting in haste or anger

Source: International Nurse Regulator Collaborative. (2016). *Social media use: Common expectations for nurses.* http://www.cno.org/globalassets/docs/prac/incr-social-media-use-common-expectations-for-nurses.pdf

TABLE 1.8   **COMPARISON OF THE NURSING PROCESS WITH TANNER'S CLINICAL JUDGEMENT MODEL AND THE NCSBN MODEL OF CLINICAL JUDGEMENT**

Nursing Process (AAPIE)	Tanner's Clinical Judgement Model	NCSBN Model of Clinical Judgement
Assessment	Noticing	Recognize cues
Analysis	Interpreting	Analyze cues
Analysis	Interpreting	Prioritize hypothesis
Planning	Responding	Generate solutions
Implementation	Responding	Take action
Evaluation	Reflecting	Evaluate outcomes

Source: Ignatavicius, D. (2020). *Getting ready for the Next-Generation NCLEX® (NGN): Transitioning from the nursing process to clinical judgment.* https://evolve.elsevier.com/education/expertise/next-generation-nclex/ngn-transitioning-from-the-nursing-process-to-clinical-judgment/

of the public (Table 1.7). They must also be guided by their professional code of conduct and standards of practice.

Electronic Health Records. Informatics is most widely used in **electronic health records (EHRs)**, also called *electronic medical records.* An EHR is a computerized record of patient information. It is shared among all health care team members involved in a patient's care and moves with the patient—to other providers and across care settings. The ideal EHR is a single file in which team members review and update a patient's health record, document care given, and enter patient care orders, including medications, procedures, diets, and results of diagnostic and laboratory tests. The EHR should contain a patient's medical history, diagnoses, medications, treatment plans, immunization dates, allergies, and test results.

Many agencies have adopted electronic documentation. EHRs and the Canadian Health Outcomes for Better Information and Care (C-HOBIC) project are examples of electronic collection of health care data, and they are being implemented across many parts of Canada (C-HOBIC, 2015). The EHR integrates the output of several information systems. Canada has developed systems that form the essential building blocks of an EHR, such as digital imaging, summaries of drug prescriptions, and laboratory test results. Provinces and territories across Canada are working together with Canada Health Infoway to accelerate the development of these systems through programs such as PrescribeIT, an e-prescribing service, and ACCESS Digital Health, which links patients and their health care providers with access to personal health information and digital health services (Canadian Health Infoway, 2020).

EHRs can reduce medical errors associated with traditional paper records and improve clinical decision making, patient safety, and quality of care. Unfortunately, several obstacles remain in the way of fully implementing EHRs. Systems are expensive and technologically complex, and a number of resources are needed to implement and maintain them. Communication is still lacking among computer systems and software applications in use. Finally, patients must be assured of their privacy and that information is accessed only by members of their care team with a right to know.

Critical Thinking in Nursing

To provide high-quality care in clinical environments of increasing complexity and greater accountability, nurses need to develop higher-level thinking and reasoning skills. **Critical thinking**, the ability to focus one's thinking to get the results needed in various situations, has been described as knowing how to learn, be creative, generate ideas, make decisions, and solve problems (Alfaro-LeFevre, 2017). Critical thinking is not memorizing a list of facts or the steps of a procedure. Instead, it is the ability to make

judgements and solve problems by making sense of information. Learning and using critical thinking is a continual process that occurs inside and outside of the clinical setting.

Clinical reasoning involves critical thinking to examine and analyze patient care issues at the point of care (Alfaro-LeFevre, 2017). It involves understanding the medical and nursing implications of a patient's situation when decisions regarding patient care are made. Nurses use clinical reasoning when they identify a change in a patient's status, take into account the context and concerns of the patient and caregiver, and decide what to do about it.

Clinical judgement is a problem-solving activity in which nurses use critical thinking to apply knowledge, attitudes, and values using both inductive and deductive reasoning (Chin-Yee & Upshur, 2018; Van Graan et al., 2016). It closely aligns to the nursing process and is a core competency of safe nursing care. The Tanner's Clinical Judgement Model and the NCSBN Model of Clinical Judgement are two established paradigms fundamental to nursing. See Table 1.8.

Given the complexity of patient care today, nurses are required to learn and implement critical thinking and clinical reasoning skills long before they obtain those skills through the experience of professional practice. Various experiences in nursing school offer opportunities for students to learn and make decisions about patient care. Various education activities, including interactive case studies and simulation exercises, promote critical thinking and clinical reasoning. Throughout this book, select boxes, case studies, and review questions promote critical thinking and clinical reasoning skills.

Evidence-Informed Practice

Evidence-informed nursing is a problem-solving approach to clinical decision making. The CNA defines evidence-informed decision making as "an ongoing process that incorporates evidence from research findings, clinical expertise, client preferences and other available resources to inform decisions that nurses make about clients" (CNA, 2018, p. 1). Using the best available evidence (e.g., research findings, QI data), combined with nursing expertise and the patient's unique circumstances and preferences, leads to better clinical decisions and improved patient outcomes. Evidence-informed practice (EIP) closes the gap between research and practice, providing more reliable and predictable care than that based on tradition, opinion, and trial and error. Basing health care decisions on evidence is essential for quality care in all domains of nursing practice.

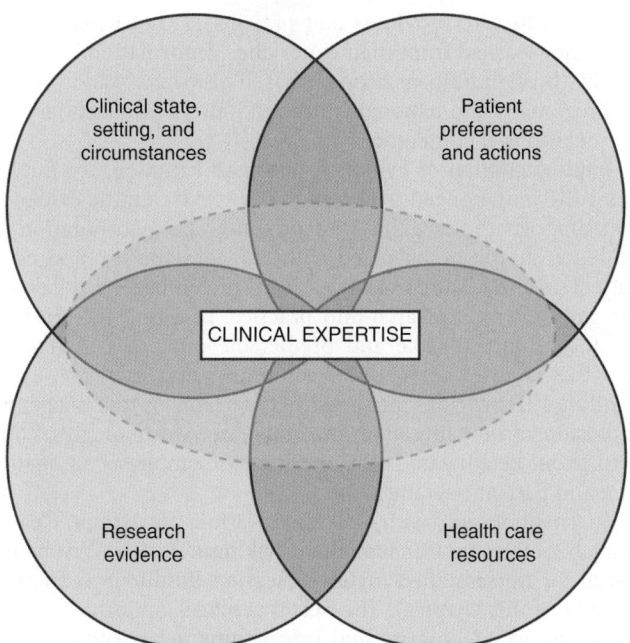

FIG. 1.3 A model for evidence-informed clinical decisions. Source: Adapted by DiCenso, A., Guyatt, G., & Ciliska, D. (2005). In Haynes, R. B., Devereaux, P. J., & Guyatt, G. (2002). Clinical expertise in the area of evidence-based medicine and patient choice. *BMJ Evidence-Based Medicine, 7*(2), 36–38. Copyright © 2002, *British Medical Journal.*

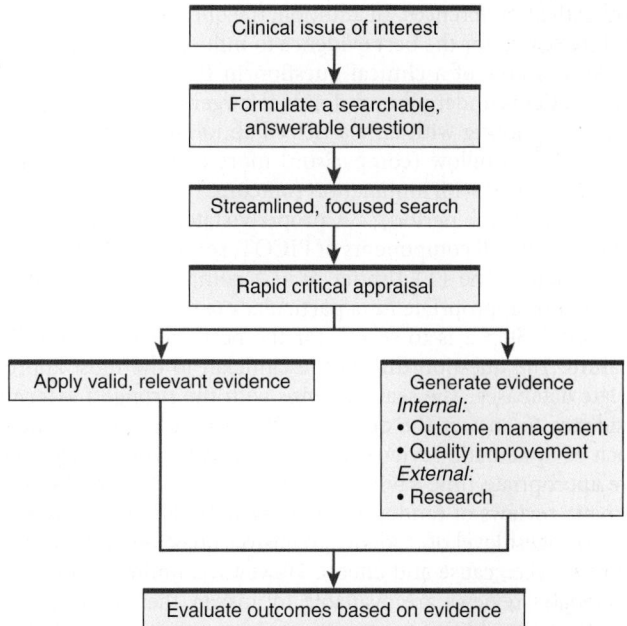

FIG. 1.4 Process of evidence-informed practice.

TABLE 1.9	STEPS OF THE EVIDENCE-INFORMED PRACTICE PROCESS
1. Ask clinical questions by using the **PICOT** format: **P**atients/population of interest **I**ntervention **C**omparison or comparison group **O**utcome(s) **T**ime period (as applicable) 2. Collect the most relevant and best evidence. 3. Critically appraise and synthesize the evidence. 4. Integrate all evidence with your clinical expertise and the patient's preferences and values in making a practice decision or change. 5. Evaluate the practice decision or change. 6. Share the outcomes of the decision or change.	

Four primary elements contribute to the practice of evidence-informed nursing: (1) clinical state, setting, and circumstances; (2) patient preferences and actions; (3) best research evidence; and (4) health care resources (Figure 1.3). *Clinical expertise,* in which these four components are integrated, is the nurse's "ability to integrate their accumulated knowledge from patient care experiences, formal education, and current evidence to make clinical decisions" (Abraham-Settles & Williams, 2019, p. 100). It refers to the nurse's cumulated experience, education, and clinical skills.

EIP produces better outcomes in the most effective and efficient way. Application of EIP results in more accurate diagnoses, the most effective and efficient interventions, and the most favourable patient outcomes. EIP's most distinguishing feature is that the new scientific base for practice is built through a summary of studies on a topic. These summaries are called *evidence syntheses, systematic reviews,* or *integrative reviews,* depending on the organization that produces them. The evidence synthesis summarizes all research results into a single conclusion about the state of the science. From this point, the clinician translates the knowledge into a clinical practice guideline, implements it through individual and organizational practice changes, and evaluates it in terms of the effectiveness and efficiency of producing intended health care outcomes (Figure 1.4). Clinical practice guidelines can take the form of policies, clinical pathways, practice guidelines, policy statements, computer-based policies, or algorithms.

Best-practice guidelines are increasingly used to guide clinical practice in health care. Such guidelines are "systematically developed statements based on best available evidence to assist practitioners' and patients' decisions about appropriate health care" (RNAO, n.d.). Examples of the current best-practice guidelines include *Adult Asthma Care Guidelines for Nurses: Promoting Control of Asthma* (RNAO, 2017); *A Palliative Approach to*

Care in the Last 12 Months of Life (RNAO, 2020); *Person- and Family-Centred Care* (RNAO, 2015); and *Preventing Violence, Harassment and Bullying Against Health Workers* (RNAO, 2019).

Throughout this book, two different types of Evidence-Informed Practice boxes are available for selected topics. Research Highlight boxes provide answers to specific clinical questions. These boxes contain the PICOT (**p**atients/population of interest, **i**ntervention, **c**omparison or comparative group, **o**utcome[s], and **t**ime period as applicable) question (Table 1.9); critical appraisal of the syntheses of evidence or primary studies; implications for nursing practice; and the source of the evidence. Translating Research Into Practice boxes provide an opportunity to practise critical thinking skills in applying evidence to patient scenarios. Evidence can support current practice and increase confidence that nursing care will continue to produce the desired outcome, or evidence may necessitate a change in practice.

Steps in the Evidence-Informed Practice Process. The six steps of the EIP process are provided in Table 1.9 and Figure 1.4.

Step 1. Step 1 is to ask a clinical question in the PICOT format. Developing the clinical question is the most important step in the EIP process (Melynk et al., 2016). A good clinical question sets the context for integrating evidence, clinical judgement, and patient preferences. In addition, the question guides the literature search for the best evidence to influence practice.

An example of a clinical question in PICOT format is "In adult patients undergoing abdominal surgery (**p**atients/population), is splinting with an elasticized abdominal binder (**i**ntervention) or a pillow (**c**omparison) more effective in reducing pain associated with ambulation (**o**utcome) on the first postoperative day (**t**ime period)?" A properly stated clinical question may not have all components of PICOT; some include only four components. The (T) timing or (C) comparison component may not be appropriate for a particular question.

Step 2. Step 2 is to search for the best evidence in the literature. The question directs the clinician to the most appropriate databases. The search begins with the strongest external evidence to answer the question. Preappraised evidence tools, such as systematic reviews and evidence-informed guidelines, are appropriate time-saving resources in the EIP process. Systematic reviews of randomized controlled trials are considered the strongest level of evidence to answer questions about interventions (i.e., cause and effect). However, a limited number of systematic reviews are available to answer the many clinical questions. In addition, systematic reviews or meta-analyses may not always provide the most appropriate answers to all clinically meaningful questions.

If the clinical question is about how a patient experiences or copes with a health issue or lifestyle change, searching for a meta-synthesis of qualitative evidence may be the most appropriate approach. When research is insufficient to guide practice, evidence from opinion leaders or authorities or reports from expert committees may be all that exists. This type of evidence should not be the sole substantiation for interventions. Care based on expert opinions requires diligent, ongoing, rigorous outcome evaluation to generate more robust evidence.

Step 3. Step 3 is to critically appraise and synthesize the data from studies found in the search. A successful critical appraisal process focuses on three essential questions: (1) Are the results of the study valid? (2) What are the results? (3) Are the findings clinically relevant to the clinician's patients? The purpose of critical appraisal is to determine the flaws of a study and the value of the research to practice. To determine best practice, clinicians must determine the strength of the evidence and synthesize the findings in relation to the clinical question.

Step 4. Step 4 involves implementing the evidence in practice. Recommendations that are based on sufficient, strong evidence (e.g., interventions with systematic reviews of well-designed randomized controlled trials) can be implemented in practice in combination with clinicians' expertise and patient preferences. Clinical judgement will influence how patient preferences and values are assessed, integrated, and entered into the decision-making process. For example, although evidence may support the effectiveness of morphine as an analgesic, its use in a patient with renal failure may not be appropriate.

Step 5. Step 5 is to evaluate identified outcomes in the clinical setting. Outcomes must match the clinical project that has been implemented. For example, when the effectiveness of morphine for pain control is compared with that of fentanyl, evaluating the cost of each medication will not provide the required data about clinical effectiveness. Outcomes must reflect all aspects of implementation and capture the interdisciplinary contributions elicited by the EIP process.

Step 6. Step 6 is to share the outcomes of the EIP change. If nurses performing research do not share EIP outcomes, then other health care providers and patients cannot benefit from what they learned from their experience. Information is shared locally through unit- or hospital-based newsletters and posters and regionally and nationally through journal publications and presentations at conferences.

Implementation of Evidence-Informed Practice. To implement EIP, nurses need to continuously seek scientific evidence that supports the care that they provide. The incorporation of evidence should be balanced with clinical expertise and each patient's unique circumstances and preferences. EIP closes the gap between research and practice, resulting in care that produces more reliable and predictable outcomes than does care that is based on tradition, opinion, and a trial-and-error method. EIP provides nurses with a mechanism to manage the explosion of new literature, introduce new technologies, concern about health care costs, and increase emphasis on quality care and patient outcomes.

In collaboration with the First Nations and Inuit Health Branch of Health Canada, the CNA launched a Web-based portal for nurses called myCNA (see the Resources section at the end of this chapter). The portal provides opportunities for nurses to access libraries and information related to EIP and clinical practice issues through a dedicated Web-based portal.

THE NURSING PROCESS

Nurses provide patient-centred care using an organizing framework called the *nursing process*. The nursing process is an assertive, problem-solving approach to the identification and treatment of patient health issues. It provides a nursing process framework to organize the knowledge, judgements, and actions that nurses supply during patient care. Using the nursing process, the nurse can focus on patients' unique responses to actual or potential health issues.

Phases of the Nursing Process

The nursing process consists of five phases: assessment, diagnosis, planning, implementation, and evaluation (Figure 1.5). There is a basic order to the nursing process, beginning with the assessment. Assessment involves collecting subjective and objective information about the patient. *Diagnosis* involves analyzing the assessment data, drawing conclusions from the information, and labelling the human response. Planning consists of setting goals and expected outcomes with the patient and, when feasible, the patient's family and determining strategies

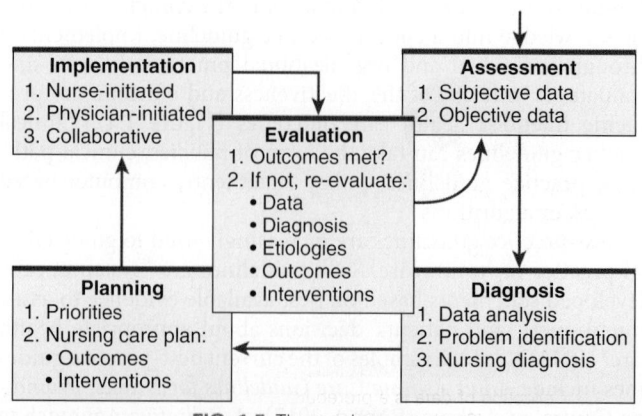

FIG. 1.5 The nursing process.

for accomplishing the goals. Implementation involves the use of nursing interventions to activate the plan. The nurse also promotes self-care and family involvement when appropriate. Evaluation is an extremely important part of the nursing process that is too often not addressed sufficiently. In the evaluation phase, the nurse first determines whether the identified outcomes have been met. Then the overall accuracy of the assessment, diagnosis, and implementation phases is evaluated. If the outcomes have not been met, new approaches are considered and implemented as the process is repeated.

Interrelatedness of Phases

The five phases of the nursing process do not occur in isolation from one another. For example, nurses may gather data about the wound condition (assessment) as they change the soiled dressing (implementation). There is, however, a basic order to the nursing process, which begins with assessment. Assessment provides the data on which planning is based. An evaluation of the nature of the assessment data usually follows immediately, resulting in the formulation of a diagnosis. A plan based on the nursing diagnosis then directs the implementation of nursing interventions. Evaluation continues throughout the cycle and provides feedback on the effectiveness of the plan or the need for revision. Revision may be needed in the data collection method, the diagnosis, the expected outcomes or goals, the plan, or the intervention method. Once initiated, the nursing process is not only continuous but also cyclical in nature.

Assessment Phase

Data Collection. Sound data form the foundation for the entire nursing process. Collection of data is a prerequisite for diagnosis, planning, and intervention (Figure 1.6). Humans have needs and problems in biophysical, psychological, sociocultural, spiritual, and environmental domains. A nursing diagnosis made without supporting data pertaining to all of these dimensions can lead to incorrect conclusions and depersonalized care. For example, if a hospitalized patient does not sleep all night, a disturbed sleep pattern may be mistakenly diagnosed, whereas the patient may have worked nights her entire adult life, and it is normal for her to be awake at night. Information concerning her sleeping habits is necessary to provide individualized care to her by ensuring that sleep medication is not routinely administered to her at 2200 hours. The importance of person-centred assessment in the process of clinical decision making cannot be overemphasized.

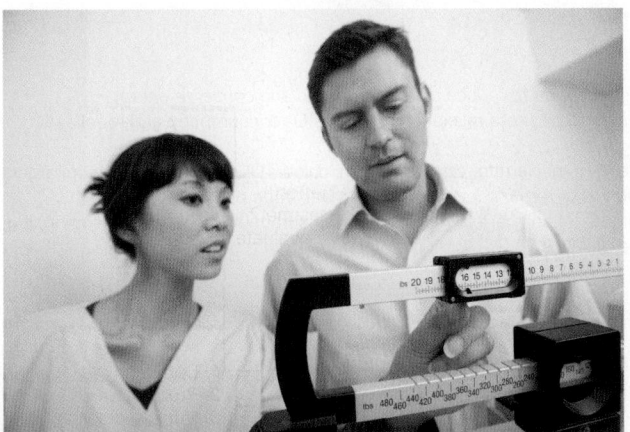

FIG. 1.6 Collection of data is a prerequisite for diagnosis, planning, and intervention. Source: iStock.com/IPGGutenbergUKLtd.

Because nursing interventions are only as sound as the data on which they are based, the database must be accurate and complete. When possible, collateral information obtained from sources such as the patient's record, other health care workers, the patient's family, and the nurse's observations should be validated with the patient. If the patient's statements seem questionable, they should be validated by a knowledgeable person.

Diagnosis Phase

Data Analysis and Problem Identification. The diagnosis phase begins with clustering of information and, after analysis of the assessment data, ends with an evaluative judgement about a patient's health status. Analysis involves sorting through and organizing the information and determining unmet needs, as well as the strengths, of the patient. The findings are then compared with documented norms to determine whether anything is interfering or could interfere with the patient's needs or ability to maintain their usual health pattern.

After a thorough analysis of all available information, one of two possible conclusions is reached: (1) the patient has no health conditions that necessitate nursing intervention or (2) the patient needs nursing assistance to solve a potential or actual health problem.

Nursing Diagnosis. The term *nursing diagnosis* has many different meanings. To some, it merely connotes the identification of a health issue. More commonly, a nursing diagnosis is viewed as the conclusion about an identified cluster of signs and symptoms. The diagnosis is generally expressed as concisely as possible according to specific policies.

Nursing diagnosis is the act of identifying and labelling human responses to actual or potential health issues. Throughout this book, the term *nursing diagnosis* means (1) the process of identifying actual and potential health problems and (2) the label or concise statement that describes a clinical judgement concerning a human response to health conditions/life processes, or susceptibility for that response, by an individual, family, group or community. A nursing diagnosis supports the identification and prioritization of nursing interventions to achieve optimal patient outcomes. Many human responses identified result from a disease process. For example, a patient may have a medical diagnosis of pancreatitis. In this case, the nursing diagnosis would focus on how the illness affects the patient's current health status. Examples of patient responses to pancreatitis might be ineffective breathing pattern, deficit fluid volume, nausea, imbalanced nutrition, and ineffective health maintenance.

Diagnostic Process. The diagnostic process involves analysis and synthesis of the data collected during assessment of the patient. Data that indicate dysfunctional or risk patterns are clustered, and a judgement about the data is made. It is important to remember that not all conclusions resulting from data analysis lead to nursing diagnoses. Nursing diagnoses refer to health states that nurses can legally diagnose and treat. Data may also point to health conditions that nurses treat collaboratively with other health care providers. During this phase of the nursing process, the nurse identifies both nursing diagnoses and treatments that necessitate collaborative nursing intervention.

Nursing diagnostic statements are considered acceptable when written as two- or three-part statements. When written in three parts, the statement is in the PES (**p**roblem, **e**tiology, and **s**igns and symptoms) format. A two-part statement is deemed acceptable if the signs and symptoms data are easily available to other nurses caring for the patient through the nursing history or progress notes. "Risk" nursing diagnoses are also two-part statements because signs and symptoms are not relevant. Use of a three-part statement is recommended during the learning process:

Problem (P): A brief statement of the patient's potential or actual health issue (e.g., pain)

Etiology (E): A brief description of the probable cause of the issue; contributing or related factors (e.g., resulting from surgical incision, localized pressure, edema)

Signs and symptoms (S): A list of the objective and subjective data cluster that leads the nurse to pinpoint the health issue; critical, major, or minor defining characteristics (e.g., as evidenced by verbalization of pain, isolation, withdrawal)

It is important to remember that gathering the "S" comes first in the diagnostic process, even though it is last in the PES statement format.

Identifying the Problem. The NANDA International (NANDA-I; formerly known as the North American Nursing Diagnosis Association) classification system is one framework that is useful for formulating actual nursing diagnoses and at-risk diagnoses. Clinically relevant cues are clustered into functional health patterns based on Gordon's (2014) 11 functional health patterns: health perception–health management pattern; nutritional–metabolic pattern; elimination pattern; activity–exercise pattern; sleep–rest pattern; cognitive–perceptual pattern; self-perception–self-concept pattern; role–relationship pattern; sexuality–reproductive pattern; coping–stress tolerance pattern; and value–belief pattern.

The process of making a nursing diagnosis from clustered cues begins with the recognition of dysfunctional patterns. Checking the definition of nursing diagnoses classified according to the functional pattern helps identify the problem's appropriate label. The nursing diagnosis deemed most accurate is based on the individual patient's data.

Etiology. The etiology underlying a nursing diagnosis is identified in the diagnostic statement. Taking time to properly link the health issue with its etiology directs the nurse to the correct interventions. Interventions to manage the issue are planned by directing nursing efforts toward the etiology. The etiology can be a pathophysiological, maturational, situational, or treatment-related factor (Ladwig, Ackley, & Makic, 2019). The etiology is written after the diagnostic label. These two components are separated by the phrase "related to." For example, in Nursing Care Plan 1.1, the nursing diagnosis is "*Activity intolerance* caused by an *imbalance between oxygen supply/demand*." The etiology directs the nurse to select the appropriate interventions to modify the factor of fatigue. When the etiology is not included in the diagnosis, the nurse cannot plan the correct intervention to treat the specific cause of the condition. When possible, the etiology should be validated with the patient. When the etiology is unknown, the statement reads "related to unknown etiology." When identifying "risk for" nursing diagnoses, the specific risk factors present in the patient's situation are identified as the etiology, and the phrase "as evidenced by" is used rather than "related to."

Signs and Symptoms. Signs and symptoms are the clinical cues that, in a cluster, point to the nursing diagnosis. The signs and symptoms are often included in the diagnostic statement after the phrase "as evidenced by." The complete nursing diagnostic statement in Nursing Care Plan 1.1 is "*Activity intolerance* caused by an *imbalance between oxygen supply/demand* resulting in an *abnormal heart rate response to activity, exertional dyspnea, and fatigue*." Throughout this book, nursing diagnoses are listed for many diseases and patient situations. These diagnoses sometimes include additional explanatory material in parentheses.

Collaborative Problems. Collaborative problems are potential or actual complications of disease or treatment that nurses manage together with other health care providers. A look at the primary nursing goals helps differentiate between nursing and medical diagnoses (see Table 1.4). A medical diagnosis identifies current symptoms associated with a disease to predict the disease course and modify outcomes. A nursing diagnosis involves a clinical judgement about an individual, family, or community response to an actual or potential health issue (Chiffi & Zanotti, 2015). During the nursing process diagnosis phase, the nurse identifies the risks for these physiological

◎ NURSING CARE PLAN 1.1

*Heart Failure**

NURSING DIAGNOSIS	*Activity intolerance* caused by an imbalance between oxygen supply/demand resulting in an abnormal heart rate response to activity, exertional dyspnea, and fatigue

Expected Patient Outcomes	Nursing Interventions and *Rationales*
• Achieves a realistic program of activity that balances physical activity with energy-conserving activities • Vital signs, O$_2$ saturation, and colour are within normal limits in response to activity	*Energy Management* • Encourage alternate rest and activity periods *to reduce cardiac workload and conserve energy.* • Provide calming diversionary activities to promote relaxation to reduce O$_2$ consumption and to relieve dyspnea and fatigue. • Monitor patient's oxygen response (e.g., pulse rate, cardiac rhythm, colour, O$_2$ saturation, and respiratory rate) to self-care or nursing activities *to determine level of activity that can be performed.* • Teach patient and caregiver techniques of self-care to minimize O$_2$ consumption (e.g., self-monitoring and pacing techniques for performance of ADLs). *Activity Therapy* • Collaborate with occupational therapist, physiotherapist, or both *to plan and monitor activity and exercise program.* • Determine patient's commitment to increasing frequency or range of activities, or both, *to provide patient with obtainable goals.*

ADLs, activities of daily living.
*The complete nursing care plan for heart failure is provided in Nursing Care Plan 37.1 in Chapter 37.

complications in addition to nursing diagnoses. Identification of collaborative problems requires knowledge of pathophysiology and possible complications of medical treatment. For example, collaborative problems with heart failure described in Nursing Care Plan 1.1 could include pulmonary edema, hypoxemia, dysrhythmias, cardiogenic shock, or a combination of these. In the interdependent role, nurses use both physician-prescribed and nursing-prescribed interventions to prevent, detect, and manage collaborative problems.

Collaborative problem statements are usually written as "potential complication: _____" (e.g., "potential complication: pulmonary edema") without a "related to" statement. When potential complications are used in this textbook, "related to" statements have been added to increase understanding and link the potential complication to possible causes.

Planning Phase

Priority Setting. After the nursing diagnoses and collaborative problems are identified, the nurse must determine the urgency of the identified problems, with actual problems being prioritized over potential problems. Diagnoses of the highest priority necessitate immediate intervention. Those of lower priority can be addressed later. When setting priorities, the nurse should first intervene for life-threatening conditions involving airway, breathing, or circulation issues.

Maslow's (1954) hierarchy of needs also acts as a useful guide in determining priorities. These needs include the physical needs; safety, love, and belonging; esteem; and self-actualization. Lower-level needs must be satisfied before a higher level can be addressed.

Another guideline in setting priorities is to determine the patient's perception of what is important. When the patient's priorities are not congruent with the actual situation, the nurse may have to give explanations or do some teaching to help the patient understand the need to do one thing before another. Often it is more efficient to meet the need that the patient deems a priority before moving on to other priorities.

Identifying Outcomes. After priorities are established, expected outcomes or goals for the patient are identified. *Outcomes* are simply the results of care. **Expected patient outcomes** are *goals* that articulate what is desired or expected as a result of care. The terms *goals* and *expected outcomes* are often used interchangeably: Both terms describe the degree to which the patient's response, as identified in the nursing diagnosis, should be prevented or changed as a result of nursing care. Expected outcomes should be agreed on with the patient, if feasible, just as priorities of interventions are considered with the patient when possible. Goals are often developed using the **SMART** algorithm: **S**–smart; **M**–measurable; **A**–achievable; **R**–realistic; and **T**–timely. Although the ultimate goal for the patient is to maintain or attain a state of dynamic equilibrium at the highest possible level of wellness, the setting of more specific expected outcomes, both short- and long-term, is necessary for systematic evaluation of the patient's progress. Expected patient outcomes identified in the planning stage indicate which criteria are to be used in the evaluation phase of the nursing process.

The nurse identifies both long-term and short-term goals by writing specific expected patient outcomes in terms of desired, realistic, measurable patient behaviours to be accomplished by a specific date. For example, a short-term expected outcome for the patient in Nursing Care Plan 1.1 might be "The patient will maintain normal vital signs in response to activity in 2 days," whereas a long-term expected outcome might be "The patient will identify a realistic activity level to achieve or maintain by the time of discharge." These outcomes would be evaluated in 2 days and at discharge, and the care plan would be revised as necessary if the outcomes were not met. However, these statements are less than optimal because they provide no criteria by which to evaluate the patient's degree of progress from admission to discharge.

Determining Interventions. After patient outcomes are identified, nursing interventions to accomplish the desired status of the patient should be planned (Saba, 2017). A **nursing intervention** is a single nursing action, treatment, procedure, activity, or service designed to achieve an outcome of a nursing or medical diagnosis for which the nurse is accountable (Ladwig, Ackley & Makic., 2019). Interventions can be independent or dependent nursing actions. Independent interventions can be carried out by the nurse without consultation (e.g., elevating the head of the bed for a patient short of breath). Dependent nursing interventions require an order from a physician or nurse practitioner (e.g., application of oxygen).

Sound knowledge, good judgement, and decision-making ability are necessary to effectively choose the interventions that the nurse will use (Figure 1.7). The nurse should foster the use of a research-based approach to interventions. In the absence of a nursing research base, scientific principles from the behavioural and biological sciences should guide the selection of interventions.

Implementation Phase. Carrying out the specific, individualized plan constitutes the implementation phase of the nursing process. The nurse performs the interventions or may designate and supervise other health care workers who are qualified to intervene. Throughout the implementation phase, the nurse must evaluate the effectiveness of the methods chosen to implement the plan.

Evaluation Phase. All phases of the nursing process must be evaluated (see Figure 1.5). Evaluation occurs after implementation of the plan but also continuously throughout the process. The nurse evaluates whether sufficient assessment data have been obtained to allow a nursing diagnosis to be made. The diagnosis is, in turn, evaluated for accuracy. For example, pain might have actually been related to a wound itself or to pressure from a constricting dressing.

Next, the nurse evaluates, with the patient when possible, whether the expected patient outcomes and interventions are realistic and achievable. If not, a new plan should be formulated.

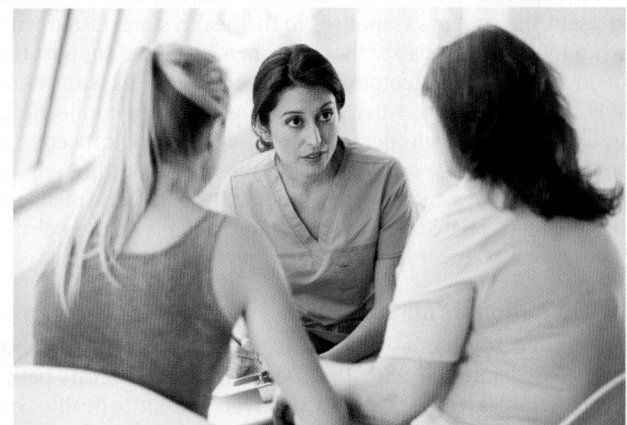

FIG. 1.7 Collaboration among the patient, the family, and the nurse is necessary in setting goals and coordinating high-quality care. Source: iStock. com/monkeybusinessimages.

This may involve revision of expected patient outcomes and interventions. Consideration must be given to whether the plan should be maintained, modified, totally revised, or discontinued in view of the patient's status.

NURSING CARE PLANS

When the nurse has determined the nursing diagnoses, the outcomes, and the interventions for a patient, the plan is recorded to ensure continuity of care by other nurses and health care providers. The plan should contain specific directions for carrying out the planned interventions, including how, when, for how long, how often, where, by whom, and with what resources the activities should be performed.

Various methods and formats are used to record the nursing care plan. One of the important factors influencing a choice of care plan format has to do with the frameworks used in a particular hospital. Care plans are often written on a specific form adopted by an institution, but they may also be entered electronically to organize nursing data. Every nurse who cares for the patient must have access to the plan, whether handwritten or computer generated, to provide the planned care. The care plan is part of the patient's medical record and may be used in legal proceedings. The nurse must document the patient's nursing care requirements, changes that are made as the plan is implemented, and the outcomes of the nursing interventions. Not every activity that the nurse implements with the patient will be recorded on the care plan.

Standardized care plans are sometimes used as guides for routine nursing care and as a basis for developing individualized care plans. When standardized care plans are used, they should be personalized and specific to the unique needs and problems of each patient.

Concept Maps

A concept map is another method of recording a nursing care plan. In a concept map care plan, the nursing process is recorded in a visual diagram of patient issues and interventions that illustrates the relationships among clinical data. Nurse educators use concept mapping to teach nursing process and care planning. There are various formats for concept maps. *Conceptual care maps* blend a concept map and a nursing care plan. On a conceptual care map, assessment data used to identify the patient's primary health concern are centrally positioned. Diagnostic testing data, treatments, and medications surround the assessment data. Positioned below are nursing diagnoses that represent the patient's responses to the health state. Listed with each nursing diagnosis are the assessment data that support the nursing diagnosis, outcomes, nursing interventions with rationales, and evaluation. After completing the map, connections can be drawn between identified relationships and concepts. A conceptual care map creator is available online on the website for this book. For selected case studies at the end of the management chapters, related concept maps are available on the website at http://evolve.elsevier.com/Canada/Lewis/medsurg.

Clinical (Critical) Pathways

Care related to common health issues experienced by many patients is delineated with the use of clinical (critical) pathways. A **clinical (critical) pathway** directs the entire health care team in the daily care goals for select health care conditions. It includes a nursing care plan, specific interventions for each day of hospitalization, and a documentation tool.

The clinical pathway organizes and sequences the caregiving process at the patient level to better achieve desired quality and cost outcomes. It is a cyclical process organized for specific case types by all related health care departments. The case types selected for clinical pathways are usually those that occur in high volume and are highly predictable, such as myocardial infarction, stroke, and angina.

The clinical pathway describes the patient care required at specific times in the treatment. An interprofessional approach helps the patient progress toward desired outcomes within an estimated length of stay. The exact content and format of clinical pathways vary among institutions.

DOCUMENTATION

It is critical that the patient's progress be documented in a systematic way. Proper documentation enables safe and effective patient care. Patient records are also frequently used as evidence when there are legal issues related to negligence and competency. Nurses in Canada should be aware of the Canadian Nurses Protective Society. This is the agency that provides liability coverage and is a source of information and education on issues such as documentation and charting.

Many documentation methods and formats are used, depending on personal preference, hospital policy, and regulatory standards. Many provinces are now moving to implement EHRs (see "Electronic Health Records" earlier in this chapter). Funding and support are available through organizations such as the Canada Health Infoway. Patient progress may be documented by nurses with the use of flow sheets; narrative notes; SOAP (**s**ubjective, **o**bjective, **a**ssessment, **p**lan) charting (described in the next section); clinical pathways; and computer-based charting. Every method or combination of methods is designed to document the assessment of patient status, the implementation of interventions, and the outcome of interventions.

There are several methods of documentation that address the nursing process. The SOAP method is a common way of evaluating and recording patient progress. Some institutions use SOAPIER notes (**s**ubjective, **o**bjective, **a**ssessment, **p**lan, **i**ntervention, **e**valuation, and **r**evision of plan). A SOAP or SOAPIER progress note is issue-specific and incorporates the elements in Table 1.10. The following is the process of SOAP documentation:

1. Additional subjective and objective data related to the area of concern are gathered.
2. On the basis of old and new data, the patient's progress toward the expected patient outcome and the effectiveness of each intervention are assessed.

TABLE 1.10	COMPONENTS OF A SOAP PROGRESS NOTE
SOAP Component	**Explanation**
Subjective	Information supplied by patient or knowledgeable other person
Objective	Information obtained by nurse directly by observation or measurement, from patient records, or through diagnostic studies
Assessment	Nursing diagnosis of issue according to subjective and objective data
Plan	Specific interventions related to a diagnostic or issue with consideration of diagnostic, therapeutic, and patient education needs

3. On the basis of the reassessment of the situation, the initial plan is maintained, revised, or discontinued.

The following is an example of SOAP charting for the nursing diagnosis "*Risk for infection* as evidenced by *alteration in skin integrity and invasive procedure* (surgery)":

S: Wound is more painful today.

O: Temperature of 39.4°C, facial grimacing in response to movement, dressing saturated with purulent drainage

A: Risk for wound infection

P: Notify surgeon, take temperature q2h, reinforce dressing.

A second method of documentation is the PIE (**p**roblem, **i**ntervention, and **e**valuation) method, which is similar to SOAP charting and is also problem-oriented. It does not include assessment data because those are recorded on flow sheets.

A third documentation format is DARP (**d**ata, both subjective and objective; **a**ction or nursing intervention; **r**esponse of the patient; and **p**lan) progress notes. It is also called *focus charting,* and it addresses patient concerns, not just issues.

Charting by exception is another method of documentation that focuses on documenting deviations from predefined normal findings. Assessments are standardized on flow sheets, and nurses make a narrative note only when there are exceptions to the standardized statements.

FUTURE CHALLENGES OF NURSING

Nursing roles continually evolve as society changes and health care providers learn to integrate new knowledge and technology into current practices. Although nursing is defined in different ways, past and current definitions of nursing include commonalities of health, illness, and caring. It is important that these concepts be addressed in nursing education as greater demands are placed on the profession. Future nursing practice will continue to call for the use of reasoning, analytical thinking skills, and synthesis of rapidly expanding knowledge to assist patients in maintaining or attaining optimal health.

An increasing emphasis on leadership, accountability, courage and persistence, innovation and risk taking, and decision making is essential if nursing is to move forward. This has never been more relevant than during the 2020 SARS-CoV-2 global pandemic. Nurses were stressed to maintain standards of nursing practice when resources were scarce. Many of Canada's emergency departments and hospitals that experienced pre-existing capacity issues were further challenged. Nursing roles changed depending on the needs of the community. Nurses were brought out of retirement and deployed to assessment centres that supported the increased need for testing of community members, while others were transitioned into critical care areas based on capacity needs. The unprecedented role that nurses and nursing leaders played in all areas of health care helped to mitigate the impact SARS-CoV-2 had on the country.

Nurses must take a leadership role in creating health care systems that provide safe, high-quality, patient-centred care. Nursing leadership refers not only to people holding certain positions but also to an attitude and approach in which lifelong learning and a commitment to excellence in practice are valued. In its attempt to keep pace, nursing would do well to remember what the Red Queen in *Through the Looking Glass* said to Alice: "Now here, you see, it takes all the running you can do to keep in the same place. If you want to get somewhere else, you must run at least twice as fast as that" (Carroll, 1865/1973). This appears to be the future of nursing. Nursing leaders must ask some fundamental questions about what the contribution of nurses must be for the twenty-first century. Nurses must increasingly challenge the status quo by relying on research and the wisdom that results from asking difficult questions. Nurse leaders must have an attitude of open-mindedness while remaining grounded in values that overcome the tendency to promote self-interest.

Medical-surgical nursing can positively influence the complex health care system in Canada by increasing interprofessional collaboration, improving patient care and safety, utilizing advanced informatics and technology, applying EIP, and continuing to develop nurses' critical thinking and clinical reasoning skills.

REVIEW QUESTIONS

The number of the question corresponds to the same-numbered learning outcome at the beginning of the chapter.

1. Which of the following is a current challenge facing the Canadian health care system?
   a. Lack of long-term funding model between provinces/territories and federal government
   b. Lack of innovation in health care
   c. Expanding knowledge and technology
   d. Health care ranking as a low-priority public health policy issue by Canadians

2. Which of the following is an example of a nursing activity that reflects the Canadian Nurses Association's definition of nursing?
   a. Establishing that the client with jaundice has hepatitis
   b. Determining the cause of hemorrhage in a postoperative client on the basis of vital signs
   c. Identifying and treating dysrhythmias that occur in a client in the coronary care unit
   d. Determining that a client with pneumonia cannot effectively cough up pulmonary secretions

3. Which of the following actions best describes the work of medical-surgical nurses?
   a. Providing care only in acute care hospital settings
   b. Requiring certification by the Canadian Nurses Association in this specialty
   c. Addressing the needs of acutely ill adults and their families
   d. Caring primarily for perioperative clients

4. Which of the following characteristics of health care teams are important for outstanding interprofessional care? (*Select all that apply.*)
   a. Care expertise
   b. Diverse mix of health care providers
   c. Interprofessional leadership
   d. Effective group functioning
   e. Clear differentiation between roles

5. The nurse is caring for a client with diabetes who has just undergone debridement of an infected toe. Which of the following statements best demonstrates client-centred care?
   a. "Administer analgesics every 4 hr prn."
   b. "Keep foot elevated to promote venous return."
   c. "Elicit expectations of client and family for relief of pain, discomfort, or suffering."
   d. "Initiate process of teaching the client and family about self-care management."

6. What are advantages of using informatics in health care delivery? (Select all that apply.)
   a. Reduced need for nurses in acute care
   b. Increased client anonymity and confidentiality
   c. The ability to achieve and maintain high standards of care
   d. Access to standard plans of care for many health issues
   e. Improved communication of the client's health status to the health care team

7. "In adults older than 60 with chronic obstructive pulmonary disease, is structured pulmonary rehabilitation more effective than classroom instruction in reducing the incidence of exacerbation?" In this question, what is the outcome of interest?
   a. Adults older than age 60
   b. Adults with chronic obstructive pulmonary disease
   c. Structured pulmonary rehabilitation
   d. Reduced incidence of exacerbation

8. The nurse identifies the nursing diagnosis of constipation resulting from laxative abuse for a client. What is the most appropriate expected client outcome related to this nursing diagnosis?
   a. The client will stop the use of laxatives.
   b. The client ingests adequate fluid and fibre.
   c. The client passes normal stools without aids.
   d. The client's stool is free of blood and mucus.

1. a; 2. d; 3. c; 4. a, c, d; 5. c; 6. c, d, e; 7. d; 8. c.

evolve

For even more review questions, visit http://evolve.elsevier.com/Canada/Lewis/medsurg.

REFERENCES

Abraham-Settles, B., & Williams, D. N. (2019). Apply Clinical Expertise in the Healthcare Environment. (99). Certified Academic Clinical Nurse Educator (CNE®cl) Review Manual.

Alberga, A. S., McLaren, L., Russell-Mayhew, S., et al. (2018). Canadian Senate report on obesity: Focusing on individual behaviours versus social determinants of health may promote weight stigma. *Journal of Obesity*, 1–7. https://doi.org/10.1155/2018/8645694

Alfaro-LeFevre, R. (2017). *Critical thinking, clinical reasoning and clinical judgment* (6th ed.). Saunders.

Canadian Association of Medical and Surgical Nurses (CAMSN). (2020). *About us*. https://medsurgnurse.ca/about-us/

Canadian Association of Schools of Nursing. (2012). *Nursing informatics competencies: Entry-to-practice competencies for registered nurses*. http://www.casn.ca/wp-content/uploads/2014/12/Nursing-Informatics-Entry-to-Practice-Competencies-for-RNs_updated-June-4-2015.pdf. (Seminal).

Canadian Health Infoway. (2020). *Driving access to care*. https://infoway-inforoute.ca/en/what-we-do/driving-access-to-care

Canadian Health Outcomes for Better Information and Care (C-HOBIC). (2015). *C-HOBIC. Phase 2 final report*. www.cna-aiic.ca/-/media/cna/page-content/pdf-en/2015jan_chobic-phase2-final-report.pdf?la=en&hash=F857EFEFDB59BDE71130CAE-5BA713DEAE45DC724. (Seminal).

Canadian Institute for Health Information. (2020). *Canada's health care providers, 2015 to 2019—Methodology notes*. https://www.cihi.ca/sites/default/files/document/canada-health-care-providers-2015-2019-meth-notes-en.pdf

Canadian Medical Association (CMA). (2019). *CMA health summit: Virtual care in Canada: Discussion paper*. https://www.cma.ca/sites/default/files/pdf/News/Virtual_Care_discussionpaper_v2EN.pdf

Canadian Nurses Association (CNA). (2012). *Interprofessional collaborative teams*. www.cna-aiic.ca/-/media/cna/page-content/pdf-en/interprofteams-virani-en-web.pdf?la=en&hash=8D073AA488 3C9D0AFBD4433D8E02190233BEAC3B. (Seminal).

Canadian Nurses Association (CNA). (2015). *Framework for the practice of registered nurses in Canada, 2015*. https://www.cna-aiic.ca/~/media/cna/page-content/pdf-en/framework-for-the-pracice-of-registered-nurses-in-canada.pdf?la=en. (Seminal).

Canadian Nurses Association(CNA). (2017). *Code of ethics for registered nurses*. https://www.cna-aiic.ca/html/en/Code-of-Ethics-2017-Edition/files/assets/basic-html/page-1.html#

Canadian Nurses Association (CNA). (2018). *Position statement: Evidence-informed decision-making and nursing practice*. https://www.cna-aiic.ca/-/media/cna/page-content/pdf-en/evidence-informed-decision-making-and-nursing-practice-position-statement_dec-2018.pdf

Canadian Nurses Association (CNA). (2019). *Advanced practice nursing—a pan-canadian framework*. https://www.cna-aiic.ca/-/media/cna/page-content/pdf-en/apn-a-pan-canadian-framework.pdf

Canadian Nurses Association (CNA). (2021). *Specialties*. https://mycna.ca/en/my-certification/what-is-certification/competencies-per-specialty-area

Canadian Nurses Association (CNA) & Canadian Association of Schools of Nursing (CASN). (2004). *Joint position statement: Promoting continuing competence for registered nurses*. https://www.cna-aiic.ca/~/media/cna/page-content/pdf-en/promoting-continuing-competence-for-registered-nurses_position-statement.pdf?la=en. (Seminal).

Canadian Nurses Association & Canadian Medical Association. (2011). *Principles to guide health care transformation in Canada*. https://www.cna-aiic.ca/~/media/cna/files/en/guiding_principles_hc_e.pdf. (Seminal).

Canadian Patient Safety Institute (CPSI). (2017). *The case for investing in patient safety in Canada*. https://www.patientsafetyinstitute.ca/en/About/Documents/The%20Case%20for%20Investing%20in%20Patient%20Safety.pdf

Canadian Patient Safety Institute (CPSI). (2021). *About CPSI*. http://www.patientsafetyinstitute.ca/en/About/Pages/default.aspx

Carroll, L. (1973). *Alice's adventures in Wonderland and through the looking glass*. Collier (Original work published 1865).

Chiffi, D., & Zanotti, R. (2015). Medical and nursing diagnoses: a critical comparison. *Journal of Evaluation in Clinical Practice, 21*, 1–6. https://doi.org/10.1111/jep.12146

Chin–Yee, B., & Upshur, R. (2018). Clinical judgement in the era of big data and predictive analytics. *Journal of Evaluation in Clinical Practice, 24*(3), 638–645. https://doi.org/10.1111/jep.12852

College of Nurses of Ontario (CNO). (2019). *Practice standard—Code of conduct*. https://www.cno.org/globalassets/docs/prac/49040_code-of-conduct.pdf

College of Nurses of Ontario (CNO). (2020). *Practice guideline—Authorizing mechanisms*. https://www.cno.org/globalassets/docs/prac/41075_authorizingmech.pdf

Gordon, M. (2014). *Manual of nursing diagnosis* (13th ed.). Jones & Bartlett (Seminal).

Government of Canada. (2020). *Canada Health Act*. https://www.canada.ca/en/health-canada/services/health-care-system/canada-health-care-system-medicare/canada-health-act.html.

Government of Canada. (2021). *Canada's food guide*. https://food-guide.canada.ca/en/

Hancock, T. (2017). Beyond health care: The other determinants of health. *CMAJ: Canadian Medical Association Journal, 189*(50), E1571. https://doi.org/10.1503/cmaj.171419

Health Canada. (2019). *2019-20 Departmental Plan: Health Canada*. https://www.canada.ca/en/health-canada/corporate/transparency/corporate-management-reporting/report-plans-priorities/2019-2020-report-plans-priorities.html#a3

Institute of Medicine. (2011). *The future of nursing: Leading change, advancing health*. National Academies Press. http://books.nap.edu/openbook.php?record_id=12956&page=R1. (Seminal).

Ladwig, G. B., Ackley, B. J., & Makic, M. B. (2019). *Mosby's guide to nursing diagnosis e-book*. Elsevier Health Sciences.

Maslow, A. (1954). *Motivation and personality*. Harper & Row (Seminal).

Melnyk, B. M., Gallagher-Ford, L., & Fineout-Overholt, E. (2016). *Implementing the evidence-based practice (EBP) competencies in healthcare: a practical guide for improving quality, safety, and outcomes*. Sigma Theta Tau.

Montague, T., Gogovor, A., Aylen, J., et al. (2017). Patient-centred care in Canada: Key components and the path forward. *Healthcare Quarterly, 20*(1), 50–56. https://doi.org/10.12927/hcq.2017.25136

Public Health Agency of Canada (PHAC). (2020). *Social determinants of health and health inequalities*. https://www.canada.ca/en/public-health/services/health-promotion/population-health/what-determines-health.html

Quality and Safety Education for Nurses. (2014). *QSEN Institute: Competencies*. http://qsen.org/competencies/pre-licensure-ksas. (Seminal).

Registered Nurses' Association of Ontario (RNAO). (n.d.). *Nursing best practice guidelines: Definition of terms*. https://bpgmobile.rnao.ca/node/1328

Registered Nurses' Association of Ontario (RNAO). (2012). *Nurse educator eHealth resource*. http://rnao.ca/ehealth/educator_resource

Registered Nurses' Association of Ontario (RNAO). (2013). *Developing and sustaining interprofessional health care: Optimizing patients/clients, organizational, and system outcomes*. Registered Nurses' Association of Ontario.

Registered Nurses' Association of Ontario (RNAO). (2015). *Person- and family-centred care*. http://rnao.ca/bpg/guidelines/person-and-family-centred-care. (Seminal).

Registered Nurses' Association of Ontario (RNAO). (2017). *Adult asthma care: Promoting control of asthma*. https://rnao.ca/bpg/guidelines/adult-asthma-care

Registered Nurses' Association of Ontario (RNAO). (2019). *Preventing violence, harassment and bullying against health workers*. https://rnao.ca/bpg/guidelines/preventing-violence-harassment-and-bullying-against-health-workers

Registered Nurses' Association of Ontario (RNAO). (2020). *A palliative approach to care in the last 12 months of life*. https://rnao.ca/bpg/guidelines/palliative-approach-care-last-12-months-life

Saba, V. K. (2017). *Clinical care classification system—Nursing interventions*. https://www.sabacare.com/framework/nursing-interventions/

Van Graan, A. C., Williams, M. J., & Koen, M. P. (2016). Professional nurses' understanding of clinical judgement: A contextual inquiry. *Health SA Gesondheid, 21*(1), 280–293. https://doi.org/10.1016/j.hsag.2016.04.001

World Health Organization (WHO). (2019). *Patient safety*. https://www.who.int/news-room/fact-sheets/detail/patient-safety

RESOURCES

Canadian Association of Medical and Surgical Nurses (CAMSN)
https://medsurgnurse.ca/

Canadian Association of Schools of Nursing (CASN)
https://www.casn.ca

Canada Health Infoway
https://www.infoway-inforoute.ca/

Canadian Health Outcomes for Better Information and Care (C-HOBIC) Project
https://www.cna-aiic.ca/-/media/cna/page-content/pdf-en/2015jan_chobic-phase2-final-report.pdf?la=en&hash=F85-7EFEFDB59BDE71130CAE5BA713DEAE45DC724

Canadian Interprofessional Health Collaborative
http://www.cihc-cpis.com

Canadian Nurses Association (CNA)
https://www.cna-aiic.ca/en

Canadian Nurses Protective Society
https://www.cnps.ca/

Canadian Nursing Students' Association (CNSA)
https://www.cnsa.ca/en/home

Canadian Nursing Informatics Association
https://cnia.ca/

Canadian Patient Safety Institute (CPSI)
https://www.patientsafetyinstitute.ca/en/Pages/default.aspx

myCNA
https://www.myCNA.ca

Registered Nurses' Association of Ontario (RNAO)
https://www.rnao.org/bestpractices

NANDA International (NANDA-I)
https://www.nanda.org/

Quality and Safety Education for Nurses (QSEN)
https://qsen.org/

Sigma Theta Tau International (STT)
https://www.sigmanursing.org

ⓔvolve

For additional Internet resources, see the website for this book at http://evolve.elsevier.com/Canada/Lewis/medsurg.

2

Cultural Competence and Health Equity in Nursing Care

Rani H. Srivastava

ⓔvolve WEBSITE

http://evolve.elsevier.com/Canada/Lewis/medsurg

- Review Questions (Online Only)
- Key Points
- Answer Guidelines for Case Study

- Conceptual Care Map Creator
- Audio Glossary
- Content Updates

LEARNING OBJECTIVES

1. Define the terms *culture, cultural competence, cultural safety, ethnocentrism, cultural imposition, worldview, intersectionality,* and *health equity.*
2. Describe how culture has evolved as a determinant of health.
3. Discuss the factors that lead to health inequities in Indigenous and culturally diverse populations.
4. Examine how culture and social location may influence the approach and delivery of nursing care.
5. Describe strategies for effective cross-cultural communication.
6. Develop strategies for demonstrating cultural competence and promoting health equity in care encounters.
7. Identify the benefits and challenges associated with a diverse workforce.

KEY TERMS

acculturation	diversity	intersectionality
cultural competence	ethnicity	race
cultural imposition	ethnocentrism	racialization
cultural safety	explanatory model	stereotyping
culture	health equity	worldview

Globalization and changes in demographic and cultural compositions of Canada necessitate that health care providers understand the influence of culture on health. Culture influences individual beliefs about health, illness, care, cure, and even expectations of health care providers. As well, just being different from the norm creates challenges that affect health. Understanding these differences is crucial for providing care that is safe, meaningful, and effective for patients and families.

CULTURAL LANDSCAPE OF CANADA

Canada is known as a settler nation and a land of immigrants. Except for the Indigenous people, all other Canadians came to Canada, at some point in time, as newcomers to this land. Canadian society is often described as an ethnocultural mosaic characterized by ethnoracial, linguistic, and religious diversity, as well as diversity in sexual orientation and gender identity. The ethnocultural dimension of diversity is defined by a variety of criteria, including geographic origin, identification with predefined ethnic groups, languages spoken, birthplace, visible minority status, and religion (Morency et al., 2017). Canada's immigration rates have increased from approximately 14% in 1867 to 21.9% in 2016 (Morency et al., 2017). This means that one in five Canadians identifies as immigrant, and this number is expected to increase to nearly 30% by 2036. If second-generation individuals (Canadian-born people whose parents were born outside Canada) are added, the projected number increases to almost 49%. In other words, by 2036, nearly one in two persons will identify as a first- or second-generation immigrant (Morency et al., 2017).

Over the past three decades, Canadian immigration patterns have undergone a significant shift in terms of the countries that people come from and where they settle. Before the 1970s, the majority of immigrants to Canada came from European countries such as the United Kingdom, Italy, Germany, and the Netherlands; however, the proportion of European-born immigrants has continued to decline steadily. By the turn of the twenty-first century most immigrants were coming from Asia, with China, India, and the Philippines being the main source countries. Census data from 2016 show over 250 ethnic origins with nearly

62% of newcomers coming from Asia and 13.4% from Africa. The change in and diversity of newcomers to Canada have had a significant impact on Canada's cultural landscape and have implications for health care. There are also changes to settlement patterns. Large centres such as Toronto, Vancouver, and Montreal continue to be destination cities for most immigrants. While Ontario and Quebec continue to receive large proportions of immigrants, newcomers are settling across Canada in increasing numbers (Statistics Canada, 2017b).

The shift in source countries for immigrants has led to increased linguistic and religious diversity and the proportion of newcomers who identify as visible minorities. The term *visible minority* is a uniquely Canadian term used by Statistics Canada and refers to "persons, other than Aboriginal persons, who are non-Caucasian in race or non-white in colour" (Morency et al., 2017, p. 139). In 2016, visible minorities accounted for over 22% of Canada's population. Of this number, approximately two-thirds were born outside the country and one-third were born in Canada (Statistics Canada, 2017b).

The Black population in Canada, while relatively small in size, is also growing in number and diversity. Between 1996 and 2016, Canada's Black population doubled in size to 3.5% of the total population. Whereas previously much of the Black population came from Haiti and Jamaica, since the 2000s over 60% of Black immigrants have come from Africa. Like other groups, the Black population is also multigenerational, with approximately 35% of the population being born in Canada. This pattern varies across the country. For example, Nova Scotia has the fifth largest Black population in Canada, with nearly 72% being third-generation or more (Statistics Canada, 2019).

Indigenous people have been in Canada long before the European settlers arrived. Until the late eighteenth century, the relationship between First Nations and the British was based on mutual interests. However, in the early 1800s a new perspective, reflecting the presumed cultural superiority of the British, led to intensive efforts to "civilize" the Indian and assimilate First Nations people into Christianity and British society through changes in legislation and the constitution via the1867 *Indian Act* and subsequent establishment of residential schools. The "Sixties Scoop" saw Indigenous children forcibly removed from their families and placed with adoptive or foster families. These initiatives led to restrictions and controls on the lives of First Nations people, resulting in forced abandonment of traditional culture, religion, and ways of life. The long-term negative consequences for children, parents, and the community include loss of land, culture, and cultural identity, as well as trauma (Bombay et al., 2020; Statistics Canada, 2017a/2019; Truth and Reconciliation Commission of Canada [TRC], 2015). In 1996, the findings in the report of the Royal Commission on Aboriginal Peoples began to shed light on the realities and injustices for First Nations communities. The subsequent work, report, and recommendations of the Truth and Reconciliation Commission are charting a new path forward toward understanding, reconciliation, and decolonization (Richmond & Cook, 2016).

It is important to note that Indigenous people's relationship to dominant Canadian society is vastly different from that of newly arrived immigrants and refugees. Understanding the experiences of Indigenous, immigrant, and the many visible minority communities is important toward understanding the larger structural and social processes that lead to exclusion and marginalization and that threaten patient safety and quality care.

Some of these experiences extend to other communities, such as people with nondominant sexual orientation or gender identity, nondominant language, low socioeconomic status, and mental or physical disabilities. While each community and group has a unique history and their own complexities, the impact of discrimination (conscious, unconscious, or structural) can lead to inequities in health.

Culture as a Determinant of Health

The extent to which people are healthy or not depends on many factors, including characteristics, behaviours, and the social, economic, and physical environment. Culture is recognized as one of the 12 determinants of health identified by the Public Health Agency of Canada (PHAC, 2018); however, it also influences all other determinants of health, by mediating the impact of other social factors (Kirmayer & Jarvis, 2019). For example, culture influences how an individual may be perceived with respect to social status; ability to secure stable employment or housing; social supports and obligations; and historical legacies of discrimination, disadvantage, and trauma (Kirmayer & Jarvis, 2019).

Indigenous perspectives on health involve interconnections between physical, social, environmental, and spiritual dimensions and entail three levels of social determinants. *Proximal determinants* are conditions that have a direct impact on health (e.g., health behaviours); *intermediate determinants* constitute factors that are the basis or origins of the proximal determinants (e.g., community infrastructure, kinship networks, ceremonies, and knowledge sharing); and *distal or structural determinants* represent the political, economic, and social contexts, including colonialism, racism, Indigenous worldviews, and self-determination (PHAC, 2018).

Health and illness are inextricably linked to cultural issues. The effect of culture on health is significant and pervasive and can be both positive and negative (Srivastava & Srivastava, 2019). Culture influences an individual's or community's approach to health protection and promotion, perception and experience of illness, what symptoms are reported, what remedies are sought, and who is consulted in the process. For instance, in a 20-year evidence review of Indigenous culture on health and well-being, Bourke et al. (2018) note that "culture is significantly and positively associated with physical health, social and emotional wellbeing, and reduces risk-taking behaviours" (p. 11).

Language barriers can pose a major threat to patient safety and quality of care (Alimezelli et al., 2015; Gil et al., 2016; Minnican & O'Toole, 2020). The resettlement process for immigrants and refugees presents inherent challenges as these individuals experience difficulties in employment, housing, and access to social support. Individuals may also face health risks as a result of marginalization and lack of access to culturally appropriate diet, activity, and health care services. Disruptions in traditional lifestyles along with discrimination can lead to greater social exclusion and increased risk for substance use. Delays in seeking help and lack of culturally competent health care providers and services can result in health concerns and symptoms being minimized or ignored, as well as inadequate follow-up for prescribed treatments (McKenzie et al., 2016). It must be emphasized that although culture is regarded as a determinant of health, it should not be confused with being the *cause* of illness or health inequities; rather, the inequities are rooted in social and structural factors that can and must be addressed.

EXPLORING THE CONCEPTS: DEFINITIONS AND MEANINGS

Terminology related to cultural diversity is subject to multiple interpretations and continues to evolve over time. Culture is an elusive concept. Although many people equate culture with ethnicity, race, country of origin, or religion, this is an erroneous oversimplification. Culture can include many additional dimensions, such as socioeconomic class, professional status, age, sexual orientation, group history, and life experiences (Srivastava & Srivastava, 2019). Culture serves as a guide for people's values, beliefs, and practices, including those related to health and illness, and at the level of the individual, group, and larger society. In the quest for health equity, it is important to recognize that the culture of health care providers and the context of the health care system matter as much as the culture of the patient (Begun, 2015; Berg et al., 2019). Culture exists at the level of the individual, the group or team, or professional discipline, as well as the level of the health care organization or broader society (Srivastava, 2007a).

Cultural values are often unconsciously developed and are responsible for perceptions of acceptable and unacceptable behaviour. Cultural beliefs and ways of being are often referred to as a **worldview**. A *worldview* is a paradigm or a set of assumptions, values, concepts, and practices that influences how people perceive, interpret, and relate to the world around them.

Culture has many distinguishing features, as highlighted in Table 2.1. A key thing to note is that *everyone* has a culture. In fact, as discussed later, we are all part of many cultures. **Culture** is about shared patterns that individuals share with others in a group and can be described as commonly understood learned traditions and unconscious rules of engagement (Srivastava, 2007a). Although individuals within a cultural group have many similarities through their shared values, beliefs, and practices, there is also much diversity within groups. Sometimes the differences within a group can be greater than differences across groups. These variations in group patterns and individual differences mean that each person is both a cultural being and a unique individual. As noted by Murray and Kluckhohn (1953), each person is like no other person, some other persons, and all other persons.

Cultural practices change over time through processes such as acculturation. **Acculturation** is a multidimensional process in which individuals undergo stages of adjustment, as well as

TABLE 2.1   KEY CHARACTERISTICS OF CULTURE

Culture is . . .
Learned through the processes of language acquisition and socialization
Shared by members of the cultural group to varying degrees
Adapted to specific conditions such as context and environmental factors
Dynamic and ever-changing in relation to historical, political, social conditions and experiences
Invisible and often sensed but not seen
Selective and differentiating by creating in-group and out-of-group members, reflecting patterns and experiences of social power or lack of it
Ubiquitous in that it influences all aspects of life including how one is perceived by others

Source: Canadian Nurses Association & Canadian Medical Association. (July, 2011). *Principles to guide health care transformation in Canada.* https://www.cna-aiic.ca/. Adapted from Srivastava, R. (2007). Culture care framework I: Overview and cultural sensitivity. In R. Srivastava (Ed.), *The healthcare professional's guide to clinical cultural competence* (pp. 53–74). Elsevier Canada.

changes in domains such as language, socioeconomic status, values, and attitudes (Delara, 2016). This gradual process results in increased similarity between two cultures.

Ethnocentrism is a tendency of people to believe that their way of viewing and responding to the world is the most correct one (Minnican & O'Toole, 2020). To some extent, this is a universal tendency; each person has the greatest familiarity with, and a preference for, their own way of doing things. However, the conscious or unconscious belief that a particular way is the only way or the best way for everyone may lead to a categorization of other beliefs as unusual, inappropriate, bizarre, and somehow inferior. Ethnocentrism can prevent people from considering alternative perspectives, recognizing the strengths they have, and from respecting others' worldviews. **Cultural imposition**, a closely related concept, is when a person's own cultural beliefs and practices are, intentionally or unintentionally, imposed on another person or group of people. In health care, it can result in disregarding or trivializing a patient's health beliefs or practices.

Ethnicity refers to characteristics of a group whose members share a common social, cultural, linguistic, or religious heritage and often implies a geographic or national affiliation. **Race** is both a biological and social construct and is sometimes used to highlight biological differences and physical characteristics such as skin colour, bone structure, or blood group (Reich, 2018). The biological basis of race is frequently challenged. Children of mixed-race couples can have varying degrees of skin pigmentation and physical characteristics and yet share similar genetic makeup and social culture. So, while there may be some genetic basis for biological differences based on gender and race, any attributions to race must be made with extreme caution (Reich, 2018). In recent years, language has shifted to ancestry. Rather than attributing increasing prevalence of illnesses such as sickle-cell anemia or cystic fibrosis to Black or White race, reference is made to ancestry or descent, such as "sub-Saharan African" or "European" (Chou, 2017). As a social construct, race has been used to categorize people on the basis of physical characteristics and to denote superiority and inferiority. **Racialization** is the process of such categorization, which leads to discrimination. Racialized groups are people who are non-White, visible minorities, or persons of colour (McKenzie et al., 2016). The term *racialized* is often preferred because a racialized community in a particular area may not be a numerical "minority"; as well, it recognizes that barriers faced by people are reflective of historical social prejudice and not individual or group inadequacies.

In a large and growing body of research, racism has been linked to poor health (Paradies et al., 2015). The effect of racism is multifaceted—it may be internalized, reflected in interpersonal relations with respect to how people are treated by others, or be systemic where social structures, processes, and policies lead to exclusion. Individuals experiencing racism may resort to high-risk behaviours such as substance use or self-harm or simply delay seeking health care. Physical health may be challenged by violence and injury or chronic, negative anxiety, depression, and diminished self-esteem or identity, which, in turn, can have direct effects on biological processes such as the cardiovascular and compromised immune systems. Racism also influences health indirectly through differential exposures and opportunities related to other determinants of health such as education and employment (Paradies et al., 2015).

Intersectionality is described as a framework for understanding how multiple social identities such as race, gender,

EQUALITY VERSUS EQUITY

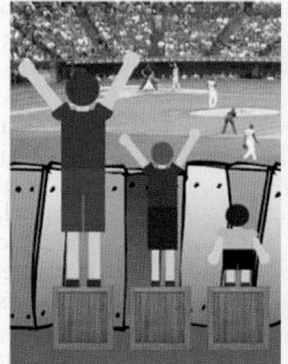 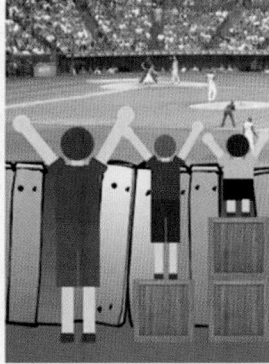 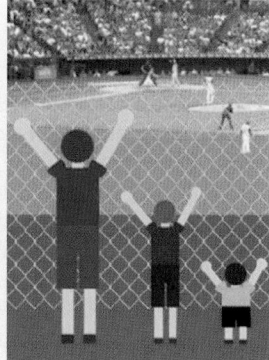

In the first image, it is assumed that everyone will benefit from the same supports. **They are being treated equally.**

In the second image, individuals are given different supports to make it possible for them to have equal access to the game. **They are being treated equitably.**

In the third image, all three can see the game without any supports or accommodations because the cause of the inequity was addressed. **The systemic barrier has been removed.**

FIG. 2.1 The difference between equity and equality. Source: City for All Women Initiative (CAWI). (2015). *Advancing equality and inclusion: A guide for municipalities,* p. 17. https://www.cawi-ivtf.org/sites/default/files/publications/advancing-equity-inclusion-web_0.pdf

sexual orientation, and economic status interact with each other to reflect interlocking systems of privilege and oppression. The multiple disadvantage locations cannot be simply added to one another, rather they interact with each other in ways that something new and specific is created with respect to exclusion and disadvantage (Henry et al., 2016). Think about the social inequality between White males and Black males; now also consider a Black man who may also be gay. While there are only two variables—skin colour and sexual orientation—the combination can drastically change one's experience in different circumstances.

In **stereotyping**, members of a specific culture, race, or ethnic group are automatically assumed to have associated characteristics that are imposed on individuals without further exploration of what the person is like. This oversimplified approach disregards individual differences, imposes a belief, and leads to false assumptions that can lead to poor care.

Diversity is another term that is related to culture. For some people, the term simply refers to differences or variations across individuals and social groups; whereas for others, it represents a sum of differences, usually regarding unequal access to power, privilege, and resources. In the context of health care, diversity usually implies difference from the majority or dominant group that is assumed to be the norm. Diverse groups and communities, in this context, have marginalized status in society, and diversity initiatives often become synonymous with asserting human rights, freedom from discrimination, social justice, and, more recently, health equity (Began, 2015). When thinking about diversity or difference, it is important to recognize *how* differences matter and *which* differences matter more than others.

Equity is the quality of being fair, just, or impartial. It is important to distinguish between equity and equality. The concept of equality refers to sameness in *process* (e.g., everyone gets the same treatment). Equity, on the other hand, focuses on sameness in *outcomes*. To achieve equality in outcomes, people need to be treated differently and in accordance of their needs.

Imagine three people of different heights trying to see over a 122-cm (4-ft) fence to watch a ball game. Kyle is an adult, 183 cm (6 ft) in height; Larry is a preteen, 122 cm (4 ft) in height; and Michael is a child who is 76 cm (2.5 ft) in height. As a way of providing support for onlookers, the park provides 12-inch crates on which people can stand to see over the fence.

In a system in which equality is the driving principle, each person gets one crate to stand on. As a result, Kyle, who is able to see over the fence with no difficulty, is even taller; Larry, who is able to see if he stands on tiptoe, can now stand on the crate and see the game more comfortably. But Michael, even with the crate, still reaches 15 cm (6 inches) below the top of the fence and therefore is still not able to see the game. The outcome is not much different than before the crates were provided, except for some benefit to Larry. The return on investment of crates is minimal, and the crate for both Kyle and Michael is a wasted resource.

In a system in which equity is the driving force, the crates are distributed according to need. Kyle does not receive a crate to stand on, Larry gets one crate, and Michael gets two crates. The outcome is that all three individuals can see over the fence comfortably (Figure 2.1) and the desired goal is achieved. In the first scenario of resource distribution according to the principle of equality, everyone is assumed to be in the same situation and to have the same needs. This is simply not true. Differences in race, gender, income, and other factors means individuals vary in the strengths and needs they bring to every interaction. When these are recognized, interventions can be targeted on the basis of need. The result is optimal outcome with minimal waste. Another option would be to try to remove the barrier. If the wooden fence was removed or replaced by plexiglass or wire mesh that allowed people of all heights to see through the barrier, the supports would not be required. In this example the difference in height is attributed to age; however, if one were to consider the difference based on social or cultural identity, it is important to recognize that the reason people do not have equal access is not their limitation or shortcoming but rather because the ground they are standing on is not level. The tall person begins with considerable advantage and the person who appears "short" or needing support is actually starting from a place of considerable disadvantage created by society.

Health Equity

There are many reasons why population groups may experience differences in health outcomes. These differences are referred to as *health inequalities* if the differences are based on genetics or developmental processes such as aging; however, when these differences are due to social factors such as income, race, or gender, they are identified as *health inequities*, as these factors are modifiable and therefore unfair or unjust. For example, Canadians who live in remote or northern regions do not have the same access to nutritious foods, such as fruits and vegetables, as do other Canadians, and this lack of access to healthy foods results in poor nutrition and poor health—this is an example of heath inequity. Health equity is an important concept in the pursuit of quality care for all individuals, regardless of their background and socioeconomic status. Health equity involves creating equal opportunities for good health for everyone in two ways: (1) by decreasing the negative effect of the social determinants of health, and (2) by improving services to enhance access and reduce exclusion. In Canada, health inequities are evident among Indigenous people, racial and sexual minorities, immigrants, and people living with disabilities (PHAC, 2018).

Indigenous populations in Canada experience many health inequities, as evident from the significantly higher rates of illnesses such as tuberculosis, diabetes, and cardiovascular disease and by higher rates of suicide and self-injury among these groups (PHAC, 2018). Living in remote or northern regions is one contributing factor; however the health of Indigenous Canadians is also affected by the loss of culture, including language and connection to land; racism and stigmatization; social exclusion; and loss of connection with Indigenous identity and spirituality (Fournier et al., 2019; Kim, 2019; Richmond & Cook, 2016).

There is considerable evidence that sexual minority populations (lesbian, gay, bisexual, transgender, queer, intersex, asexual, and two spirited [LGBTQIA2]) experience significant inequities in health (Colpitts & Gahagan, 2016). In 2019, a study focusing on LGBTQIA2 health was undertaken by the Canadian House of Commons Standing Committee on Health. The study noted that while inequities are experienced differently by each of the LGBTQIA2 communities, the individuals overall are more likely to experience poorer mental health, have suicidal thoughts, and attempt suicide (House of Commons Standing Committee on Health, 2019). In particular, the transgender population has considerable vulnerability and unmet needs with respect to health (Giblon & Bauer, 2017).

Racial minorities, immigrant, and refugee populations experience health inequities that can be attributed to lack of provider knowledge, stigmatization, and discrimination, including refusal to provide care or to seek care (McKenzie et al., 2016). Cain et al. (2018) note that palliative care, considered a "gold standard of end-of-life care" continues to be used mainly by Whites and people of northern European descent. Even when the differences are attributed to choice, the researchers point out that it is important to take a nuanced look at factors behind the choice. People of color, of diverse sexual orientations, and who are disabled are less likely to receive care that aligns with their wishes than Whites, and these groups report lower levels of life satisfaction (Cain et al., 2019).

Research from many countries, including Canada, indicates that immigrants report better physical and mental health when they first arrive in the country than their Canadian-born counterparts. This is known as the "healthy immigrant effect." This health advantage is attributed to immigration criteria that favor healthy people; however, this advantage is usually lost as both physical and mental health deteriorates over time to "non-immigrant Canadian levels or worse" (Fung & Guzder, 2018, p. 5). Key factors that lead to this deterioration include social inequities such as poverty, underemployment, or unemployment; racism and discrimination; and inequitable access to services due to difficulties in navigation of the health system, communication challenges, or lack of culturally responsive services (Fung & Guzder, 2018; McKenzie et al., 2016).

Social Justice and Equity in Nursing Care

The growing evidence of health inequities across a variety of groups is challenging previous assumptions about how to provide quality health care for everyone in the context of a culturally diverse society. Without cultural competence, patients, families, and communities are at risk for no care or care that is ineffective or unsafe. A social justice approach requires awareness of and attention to inequities—where culture is understood as patterns but also as power; and racism and discrimination are recognized and challenged at the individual as well as organizational level (Small, 2019; Srivastava & Srivastava, 2019).

The importance of health equity and the role that nurses can and must play is recognized by national and international nursing associations (Canadian Nurses Association, 2018; International Council of Nurses (ICN), 2018). The Truth and Reconciliation Commission of Canada (TRC) has also called for cultural competence education for health care providers to promote cultural safety for Indigenous people (TRC, 2015). Many national and local initiatives are underway to support health equity through research, policy, and in practice. The health equity impact assessment (HEIA) tool is an excellent example of how health care leaders can embed health equity considerations into decision making. When unintended potential effects are recognized, mitigating strategies can be put in place to reduce the negative and maximize the positive effects (Ontario Ministry of Health and Long Term Care, 2021). Nurses, by virtue of their role in the health care system, can promote health equity by recognizing cultural needs and expressions, removing unnecessary complexity in care, supporting informed choices, being sensitive to vulnerability, and drawing on cultural strengths to support and promote health.

Cultural Safety and Cultural Competence

In Canada, both cultural safety and cultural competence are concepts used to guide the provision of safe, effective, equitable patient-centred care. Frameworks for both concepts have different origins but have many similarities regarding key attributes and skills needed by health care providers. The concept of cultural safety is based on the notion of biculturalism and was initially developed in New Zealand to draw attention to the effects of colonization on the health of the Indigenous Maori people. Cultural safety focuses on the impact of colonialism and ongoing power imbalances that lead to a disregard for health and illness beliefs of the Indigenous people and to a privileging of the dominant cultural values. Some authors view cultural safety as an outcome from the process of cultural competence (Sharifi et al., 2019); others view it as a distinct approach that focuses on social and political power and redefines the provider–patient relationship with emphasis on self-determination (Berg et al., 2019). In Canada, the notion of cultural safety continues to be applied largely to health care for Indigenous people.

Cultural competence is a process whereby practitioners recognize the need for the knowledge and skills to modify assessment and intervention strategies in order to achieve equity in health quality and outcomes. Cultural competence in nursing can be traced back to the 1960s, when Madeleine Leininger advocated for the use of culturally based health knowledge and care to ensure appropriate and effective care for individuals and groups with differences in values, beliefs, explanatory models of illness (discussed later in this chapter), and systems of healing (Sharifi et al., 2019). One of the earliest and most widely cited definitions of cultural competence is a "set of congruent behaviors, attitudes, and policies that come together in a system, agency or among professionals and enable that system, agency or those professions to work effectively in cross-cultural situations" (Cross et al., 1989). The International Council of Nurses describes it as care that "respects diversity in race, ethnicity, age, gender, sexual orientation, disability, social status, religious or spiritual beliefs, and nationality; recognizes populations at risk of discrimination; and supports differences in healthcare needs that may result in disparities in healthcare services" (ICN, 2018, p. 1). Both of these definitions denote action based on awareness and knowledge. Cultural competence is recognized as a critical attribute for the provision of safe, effective, quality care and has therefore been declared an entry-to-practice level competency for registered nurses in Canada (Canadian Nurses Association, 2018).

A key difference between cultural competence and cultural safety is the role of cultural knowledge or information associated with specific groups. Because culture is a dynamic concept, the requisite knowledge is not about specific cultural groups but rather the patterns associated with groups and how these patterns may surface in health and illness. In this way, use of cultural knowledge is like the nurse's use of clinical knowledge—to assess, understand, inquire, interpret, and ultimately validate the specific situation with patient, family, or community. Some argue that without knowledge health care providers are at risk for misunderstanding, missing critical information, and placing an undue burden on the patient to educate providers (Jongen et al., 2018). Both frameworks articulate the need for humility and inclusivity; respect for unique history, traditions, and beliefs of individuals and groups; communicating in culturally appropriate ways; and recognizing the effects of the broader social determinants of health on individuals, families, and communities. In this chapter, the term *cultural competence* is used, largely because the notion of competence implies acquisition and use of specific knowledge and skills, in an intentional way, to ensure the provision of quality care. The fundamental tenets underlying culturally competent care include awareness, knowledge, skills, commitment, and application of knowledge in decision making and actions (Table 2.2).

Contrary to some interpretations in the literature, as stated earlier, cultural competence does not mean being an expert in or knowing everything about a particular culture; this is unrealistic and risks stereotyping. Rather, cultural competence is an evolving process that recognizes the dynamic nature of culture created through context and intersectionality and that is grounded in knowledge of a number of concepts, reflection, and action (Sharifi et al., 2019). Outcomes of culturally competent care can be described as culturally congruent care, culturally responsive care, or simply achieving health equity.

TABLE 2.2	FUNDAMENTAL TENETS OF CULTURAL COMPETENCE
Awareness	Develop self-awareness of one's cultural identity, assumptions, biases, and beliefs and how these can impact others
Knowledge	Purposefully seek out and examine similarities and differences between individuals and groups to understand and respect differences, what they mean, and how they impact individuals and communities
Application in practice	Translate awareness and knowledge into actions and skills that include: • Building trust and partnerships • Assessment • Communication • Negotiation and advocacy
Commitment to equity	Identify barriers, facilitators, and strengths in individuals and communities Challenge barriers within one's sphere of influence; promote inclusion and self-determination of goals for individuals and communities

ABCDE of Cultural Competence

There are many frameworks and models of cultural competence, each highlighting a different aspect of culture, attributes of cultural competence, or approach to developing cultural competence (Berg et al., 2019). However, three key domains are evident across these frameworks: (a) an *affective* domain, which reflects an awareness of and sensitivity to cultural values, needs, and biases; (b) a *behavioural* domain, which reflects skills necessary to be effective in cross-cultural encounters; and (c) a *cognitive* domain, which involves cultural knowledge, as well as theory, research, and cross-cultural approaches to care (Brown et al., 2016; Sharifi et al., 2019). Together, these domains can be considered the *ABC's* of cultural competence (Srivastava, 2008). However, to fully understand the complexities of cultural competence and its relationship to health equity, two other domains must also be present. The *dynamics of difference (D)* highlights the fact that difference is not just about differing worldviews; it is also about discrimination and racism associated with minority group status and social power imbalances. The *(E)* domain involves the goal of *equity* in health care and also highlights the importance of the context of care, or the practice *environment*, which may or may not have necessary supports for individual clinicians (Srivastava, 2008).

Understanding and actively addressing the dynamics of difference is consistent with nursing role expectations of social justice and advocacy. Challenging structural and systemic barriers within the care environments and leveraging supports and strengths are essential for effective care. Figure 2.2 shows the ABCDE framework for cultural competence. The framework can serve as road map or guide to developing competencies in each domain. Nurses need to develop and apply awareness and knowledge in ways that effectively navigate the downside of difference and utilize the strengths that come with difference to achieve the goal of equity and quality care. Table 2.3 presents examples of attributes that describe the ABC domains of cultural competence. The influence of the dynamics of difference and the environment is evident throughout the affective, behavioural, and cognitive domains and is thus not highlighted separately in the table.

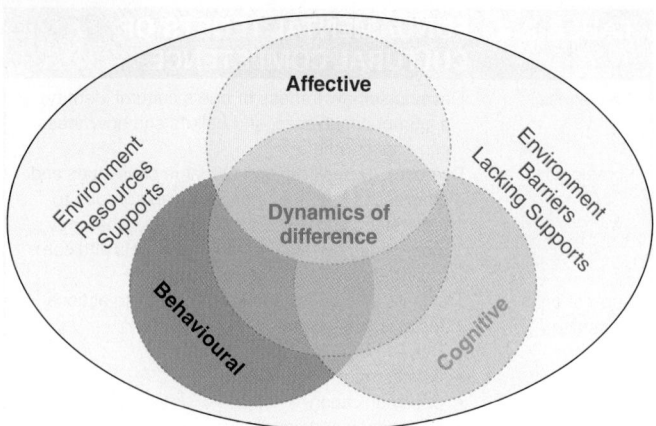

FIG. 2.2 The ABCDE's of cultural competence. Source: Adapted from Srivastava, R. (2008). The ABC (and DE) of cultural competence in clinical care. Ethnicity and Inequalities in Health and Social Care, *8*(11), 25–31 (p. 31).

Affective Domain: Developing Cultural Awareness and Mindset. The affective domain of cultural competence is concerned with both attitude and awareness. This is the first step toward developing cultural competence. Openness, a desire to learn, valuing differences, respect for others, and developing humility are characteristics of this domain (Brown et al., 2016; Sharifi et al., 2019). Developing competencies in this domain means understanding the notion of multiple worldviews and norms, recognizing that no one way is universally superior and yet that we all have a bias toward things that are familiar. Every person is a cultural being; therefore any nurse–patient interaction is affected by the cultures of both the nurse and the patient. Each nurse is influenced by their own cultural identity, the culture of the nursing profession, the culture of the health care team, and the culture of the health care setting in which the interaction occurs. It is important to recognize that within the nursing profession there are different categories (registered nurse, registered/licensed practical nurse, registered psychiatric nurse, and nurse practitioner) and that there are variations in how each category may approach care. The same applies to different disciplines within the interprofessional team. Understanding these differences is critical for effective intra- and interprofessional collaboration.

Awareness can be subcategorized into three components: self-awareness, awareness of others, and awareness of the dynamics of difference (see the "Dynamics of Difference" section later in this chapter). Self-awareness is a critical first step in developing cultural competence. This includes an examination of one's conscious and unconscious biases toward others and exploring one's own cultural identity—both with respect to how one views oneself and how one may be viewed by others (Srivastava, 2007a). Identifying how these views may influence the care encounter is a critical step in recognizing ethnocentrism, avoiding cultural imposition, and building trust. Development of self-awareness requires nurses to engage in ongoing critical self-reflection and being amenable to feedback from other people (see the "Nurse's Self-Assessment" section later in this chapter). Awareness of other people as cultural beings means understanding that people have different worldviews and norms. Cultural differences are not issues of right or wrong; they are simply about being different. Awareness also includes understanding that people have different historical legacies that have an impact on their health and well-being,

including how they interact with the health care system. Understanding the dynamics of differences means going beyond acknowledging the inherent power dynamics that exist in any clinical encounter by recognizing that past experiences of discrimination and exclusion, communication difficulties, and differences in worldviews are also factors that need to be addressed to ensure that patient voice, perspectives, and rights are recognized.

Behavioural Domain: Adding a Cultural Lens to Clinical Skills. The behavioural domain concerns the actual application of knowledge and awareness through interpersonal skills, assessment skills, and communication skills to specific clinical encounters and decisions. Demonstrating humility, intentionality, flexibility, and openness are critical attributes in this domain. Through the intentional use of interpersonal skills to build trust, nurses can partner with patients in performing a comprehensive assessment of not only patients' concerns and symptoms but also their values, beliefs, and practices to develop mutual goals and interventions.

Different cultural groups have different beliefs about the causes of illness and the appropriateness of various treatments. It is important for the nurse to try to determine the patient's **explanatory model** (set of beliefs regarding what causes the disease or illness and the methods that would potentially treat the condition best). It is also important to determine how experiences and beliefs affect health-seeking behaviours. Table 2.4 lists key questions that can be used to learn about the patient's explanatory model of illness and care. These questions do not have to be asked in the order they are listed, and they can be adapted to the situation or incorporated into existing assessment approaches. Through these questions nurses can identify key values, beliefs, and issues that that are important to the patient in each situation (Brown et al., 2016; Jongen et al., 2018)

Cross-Cultural Communication. Communication is foundational for every aspect of the clinical encounter; therefore cross-cultural communication is a key area for cultural skill development (see Table 2.3). Cultural differences are often cited as a barrier to effective communication, leading to poor adherence to treatment regimens, dissatisfaction with care, and adverse health outcomes (Habadi et al., 2019; Ladha et al., 2018). Culturally safe communication that includes communication of cultural understanding and respect is an essential tool in forming a therapeutic relationship with the patient. It is critical for establishing trust, for informed consent, for decision making, for ability to partner in care, and for self-management of chronic illnesses (Brown et al., 2016; Minnican & O'Toole 2020).

Verbal and Nonverbal Communication. Cultural influences on communication are evident in both verbal and nonverbal communication. Verbal communication includes not only the language or dialect but also the voice tone and volume, timing, and a person's willingness to share thoughts and feelings. Nonverbal communication includes silence, eye contact, use of touch, body language, style of greeting, and the spatial arrangement taken up by the participants. Culture influences the ways that feelings are expressed, as well as which verbal and nonverbal expressions are appropriate in given situations, with norms varying across cultures.

For example, many Indigenous people are comfortable with silence and interpret silence as essential for thinking and carefully considering a response. In these interactions,

TABLE 2.3   THE ABC'S OF CULTURAL COMPETENCE

Component	Description
Affective (Awareness) Domain	
Attitude	• Humility and a recognition of the need for ongoing learning and *un*learning • Genuine curiosity and desire to learn; valuing differences • Nonjudgemental stance in encountering situations and perspectives that are different from those of self or the norm • Commitment to the goal of social justice, inclusivity, and equity
Awareness of self, others, and dynamics of difference	• Self-awareness of values, beliefs, and biases, including unconscious bias • Critical reflexivity to examine and critique own beliefs • Awareness of own social location and privilege • Awareness of challenges with cross-cultural communication • Awareness of cultural influences on information seeking, conflict, and decision making • Recognition of the historical effects of racism and discrimination in society and health care
Behavioural (Skills) Domain	
Assessment	• Ask the correct questions in the correct way (knowing what and knowing how) • Establish trust and health care provider's credibility • Elicit patient's explanatory model of illness • Assess for the effect of social determinants on current situation
Cross-cultural communication	• Determine patient's values, strengths, and goals • Adapt own communication style to address cultural nuances and differences in information processing and decision making • Provide information in simple language and in ways that are consistent with patient's language and culture • Become familiar with different communication styles and patterns • Recognize the need for and make use of interpreters for language support
Collaborative decision making Empowering and promoting patient choice Advocacy across differences	• Elicit patient's values, preferences, and explanatory models of health and illness • Engage family and build trust • Accommodate values and preferences and negotiate approaches to obtain mutually agreed-upon goals • Review cultural conflicts as opportunities to learn from differences • Reframe situations to mitigate biases that are held by the health care provider or patient • Acknowledge and support religious and spiritual beliefs • Facilitate participatory decision making and informed patient choices
Development of resources (personal and organizational) to support practice	• Identify own privilege and use it appropriately to further goals of equity • Recognize and address the dynamics of difference at patient–clinician level and at patient–health care system level • Connect patients with resources within their community to promote greater autonomy and self-management • Explore opportunities to partner with and learn from colleagues, patients, and communities that are culturally different from self or own • Seek information on different cultural groups through the Internet, media, movies, and visits to cultural and community centres • Seek out the insider cultural perspectives and meanings of events and traditions • Develop relationship with service agencies that support health for specific cultural groups and communities
Cognitive (Knowledge) Domain	
Generic cultural knowledge	• Understand the effect of culture on health and health-seeking behaviours • Understand the difference between individualistic and collectivist cultures • Recognize dimensions of care that are likely to be influenced by culture in a particular setting (e.g., end-of-life care) • Identify biophysiological determinants of health and illness in minority groups • Identify social determinants of health: effects of race, culture, health status, employment, and so forth • Understand health disparities and health equity issues • Identify the effects of health policy on culturally diverse groups, particularly those whose members are economically disadvantaged • Understand the effect of diversity on team functioning
Specific cultural knowledge	• Develop contextual knowledge of communities served, including cultural strengths and resources; health inequities particular to the group or groups; and incidence and prevalence of major illnesses • Learn about commonly held worldviews and healing traditions • Identify the effect of life events such as migration, settlement, and racism • Review the care process for own clinical specialty and identify processes and treatments that are particularly susceptible to cultural differences • Do not make assumptions on the basis of cultural background; instead, use knowledge as a beginning point for further assessment and inquiry

Sources: Adapted from Srivastava, R. (2008). The ABC (and DE) of cultural competence in clinical care. *Ethnicity and Inequalities in Health and Social Care, 8*(1), 25–31; and from Brown, O., Ham-Baloyi, W., Van Rooyen, D., Aldous, C., & Marais, L. (2016). Culturally competent patient-provider communication in the management of cancer: An integrative literature review. *Global Health Action, 9*(1), 33208.

TABLE 2.4	QUESTIONS FOR DETERMINING THE PATIENT'S EXPLANATORY MODEL OF ILLNESS AND CARE

1. What do you think has caused the problem?
2. Why do you think it started when it did?
3. What do you think the sickness or illness does to you?
4. How severe is the sickness? Will it have a long or short course?
5. What are the major problems or difficulties this sickness has caused in your life?
6. What have you done for this problem up to now?
7. What kind of treatment do you think you should receive?
8. What do you fear most about the sickness?
9. What do you fear most about the treatment?
10. Who else should be consulted or involved in your care?

Source: From Srivastava, R. (2007). Culture care framework I: Overview and cultural sensitivity. In R. Srivastava (Ed.), *The healthcare professional's guide to clinical cultural competence* (p. 89). Elsevier Canada. Adapted from Kleinman, A., Eisenberg, L., & Goode, B. (1978). Culture, illness, and care: Clinical lessons from anthropologic and cross cultural research. *Annals of Internal Medicine, 88,* 251–258.

silence shows respect for the other person and demonstrates the importance of the remarks. In traditional Japanese and Chinese cultures, the speaker may stop talking and leave a period of silence for the listener to think about what has been said before continuing. In other cultures (e.g., French, Spanish, and Russian), silence may be interpreted as meaning agreement.

Differences in communication styles can lead to misinterpretations; what is considered normal and respectful in one culture may be interpreted as rudeness in another (Barker, 2016). Although nurses are often taught to maintain direct eye contact, patients of Asian or Arab descent or who are Indigenous may avoid direct eye contact and consider direct eye contact disrespectful or aggressive. Other factors to consider include the role of sex, age, status, or social position on what is considered as appropriate eye contact. For example, Muslim-Arab women avoid eye contact with men other than their husbands in public situations to exhibit modesty. The degree of physical contact and touch, across gender and age, varies across cultures. In certain cultures (e.g., Muslim), health care providers may be prohibited from touching patients of the opposite sex (Marcus, 2016). Many Asians believe that touching a person's head is a sign of disrespect, especially because the head is believed to be the source of a person's strength.

It is not sufficient for nurses to simply learn about cross-cultural communication issues; they must also develop and adapt their communication skills to connect with different individuals and cultural groups (see Table 2.3). Some groups may respond effectively to direct questions, whereas others respond more comfortably in interactions that are less direct. For example, instead of telling a person what to do, a nurse may phrase the teaching in a less directive way: "Many people who experience this illness find it helpful to do . . . ." Nurses must understand that when a patient says "yes," it can have multiple interpretations, including "Go on," "I hear you," "I understand," or "I agree." Understanding and agreement must be validated through other means. Negotiation skills are also important in cultural competence because nurses are often required to negotiate interventions between mainstream and traditional ways of healing.

Providing Effective Language Support. Effective communication is critical for patient safety. Providing effective

TABLE 2.5	WORKING EFFECTIVELY WITH INTERPRETERS

General Considerations
- Allow extra time for the session.
- Use professionally trained bilingual–bicultural interpreters instead of the patient's family or children.
- Consider personal attributes of the interpreter such as age, gender, ethnicity, and dialect that may influence communication; use the services of an agency interpreter if possible.
- Be aware of common issues such as words that cannot be translated, feeling rushed, interpreter answering for the patient, or conflicts between patient and interpreter.
- Verify translations to avoid misunderstandings, mistakes, and distortions.

Before the Interpretation Session
- Provide an overview of the situation (patient, goals, and procedures) to the interpreter.
- Ask for concerns or issues from the interpreter's perspective.
- Remind the interpreter to interpret *everything*.
- Ask the interpreter to share their cultural insights with you but to differentiate these from the interpretation itself.

During the Interpretation Session
- Introduce everyone who is present.
- Determine the most appropriate person to direct questions to (if relevant).
- Face who you are speaking to and speak to them directly.
- Describe the role of the interpreter, the interpreter service's mandate, and the purpose of the session.
- Use simple language and avoid jargon and technical terminology.
- Speak in one- to two-sentence bursts to allow for easier translation.
- Allow the interpreter to ask open-ended questions, if necessary, to clarify what the patient says.
- Observe the patient for off-target reactions (signalling challenges in interpretation).

After the Interpretation Session and Follow-Up Strategies
- Consider providing written instructions as appropriate.
- Ask the patient whether they have anything to ask or convey.
- Debrief with the interpreter.

language support through language aids, including interpreters, is essential for patient safety. Nurses and other health care providers often feel they can get by without interpreters by using a few words in the patient's language and actions to demonstrate meaning. However, this is a fallacy and compromises quality care (Minnican & O'Toole, 2020). Health care providers must identify encounters where linguistic support is required through trained interpreters (Ladha et al., 2018). Table 2.5 lists strategies for working effectively with interpreters, and Table 2.6 lists strategies for communicating with patients with limited proficiency in English. It is important to recognize that, even though Canada is officially a bilingual country, the francophone community is a language minority in most of the country and requires additional support.

Although in-person interpretation by trained health care interpreters is considered optimal, organizations and individuals can often use technology-aided solutions such as telephone or remote interpretation. Caution is needed for using smartphones and applications such as Google Translate. While these aids are useful in providing basic information, they can pose risks to accuracy and thus patient safety, and such translation must be carefully validated (Ladha et al., 2018).

TABLE 2.6	COMMUNICATING WITH PATIENTS WITH LIMITED ENGLISH PROFICIENCY

1. Introduce yourself and, if possible, greet patient in the patient's preferred language. This indicates that you are aware of and respect the patient's culture.
2. Proceed in an unhurried manner. Pay attention to any effort by the patient or family to communicate.
3. Speak in a low, moderate voice. Avoid talking loudly. Remember that there is a tendency to raise the volume and pitch of your voice when the listener appears not to understand. The listener may perceive that you are shouting or angry, or both.
4. Use simple words, such as *pain* instead of *discomfort.* Avoid medical jargon, idioms, and slang. Avoid using contractions (e.g., "don't," "can't," "won't") and pronouns—refer to people by name or title.
5. Provide information in the proper sequence, outlining steps such as first, second … etc.
6. Focus on one question at a time.
7. Validate understanding by having the patient repeat instructions, demonstrate the procedure, or act out the meaning.

Source: Srivastava, R. (2007). Culture care framework I: Overview and cultural sensitivity. In R. Srivastava (Ed.), *The healthcare professional's guide to clinical cultural competence* (pp. 53–74). Elsevier Canada.

Cognitive Domain: Developing Cultural Knowledge. *Cultural knowledge* is a crucial element of cultural competence. To provide culturally competent care, nurses must identify and seek out the cultural knowledge they need (see Table 2.3). Cultural knowledge can be divided into two categories: generic cultural knowledge and specific cultural knowledge (Brown et al., 2016; Srivastava, 2007b). Generic cultural knowledge is foundational knowledge that applies across a variety of cultural groups. The most fundamental aspect of generic cultural knowledge is understanding the effect of culture on health- and illness-related behaviours. Generic knowledge can be broken down into several broad areas that nurses should be aware of, such as variations in worldviews and explanatory models of illness; beliefs about care, cure, caregivers, and healing systems; family roles and relationships; migration and settlement; norms about time and personal space; and spirituality and religion (Jongen et al., 2018; Sharifi et al., 2019). These areas are discussed in greater detail in the next section.

Specific cultural knowledge focuses on learning about specific population(s) that the nurse is working with. Because of the number of cultural groups in Canada and the dynamic nature of culture, a detailed discussion of specific cultural knowledge is beyond the scope of this chapter. Nurses need to continually educate themselves (see Table 2.3) about specific cultures they encounter frequently in their practice and always be amenable to learning from patients and families. For example, if the nurse is working in a community with large numbers of South Asian and Chinese people, it is important to learn more about the beliefs and issues relevant to these communities. While all nurses need to acquire basic understanding of the legacy of residential schools, Sixties Scoop, and the associated trauma, nurses working with specific Indigenous communities need to acquire knowledge of the specific nation(s) or bands, including their history, current issues, strengths, and challenges, as there are many differences across different Indigenous groups. Other examples of specific cultural knowledge include focusing on specific health issues faced by particular populations, such as immigrant women or the transgender community, or people with a mental illness (Bhugra, 2016; Ferdous et al., 2019;

Suphanchaimat et al., 2015). Table 2.3 lists other attributes of this component of cultural competence.

In addition to determining the kind of generic and specific knowledge that is needed, nurses must critically appraise how knowledge is developed and used. Culture is concerned with shared patterns, not universal truths. Therefore cultural knowledge should not be used to obscure individual differences. Individualized assessments are important to determine the extent to which the patient shares the beliefs and practices ascribed to the culture. Familiarity with cultural norms is helpful but should be used carefully so it does not lead to cultural stereotyping. It is important for nurses to reflect on how they acquired the knowledge and the extent to which the knowledge is unique to the individual, reflective of the broader cultural group, or reflective of cultural processes in general. Cultural knowledge must always be regarded as tentative hypotheses that need to be verified and expanded on by patients and their families.

Generic Cultural Knowledge

Care, Cure, Caregivers, and Healing Systems. Cultural norms have a significant influence on how illness is understood, what remedies are deemed appropriate and desirable, and who provides the care. Whereas in some cultures patients seek professional help, others rely more on family, friends, or spiritual and religious leaders. It is important to ascertain a patient's beliefs about the cause of illness, as well as perceptions of severity, expected treatment, prognosis, and effects (see Table 2.4).

Canadian health care systems and health professions have a cultural basis in the dominant white, Eurocentric culture. The biomedical approach to health care, although regarded as the conventional treatment in North America, is one of several philosophical and scientifically based systems of healing. Other such systems include homeopathy, traditional Chinese medicine, Indigenous medicine, and Ayurvedic medicine (a form of traditional Hindu medicine). Although it is not possible for a health care provider to have expertise in all healing systems, familiarity with basic principles of major systems and traditions can be helpful. Individuals often use multiple healing systems, and a critical part of patient assessment is knowledge of what conventional treatments, as well as other traditional or herbal treatments, are being used. In addition, the use of complementary and alternative therapies continues to increase across Canada (Canizares et al., 2017). Nurses need to understand their role in supporting and providing such therapy (College & Association of Registered Nurses of Alberta, 2018). Complementary and alternative therapies are further discussed in Chapter 12.

Time Orientation. Patient values regarding time orientation and personal space can affect the care delivery process. Health care providers in hospitals and clinics are often frustrated because many patients show up late for appointments and seem to have no regard for appointments and schedules. In reality, this may be a result of several factors, including issues of transportation, ability to navigate the health care system, and time orientation. The value of clock time and punctuality is different across cultures. In Western culture time is viewed as linear with a past–present–future orientation; however, for many people, including Indigenous people, time is structured with respect to cyclical events and associated with seasons or key events. In such an orientation, "when" things happen is not as important as "that" they happen (Janca & Bullen, 2003), thus "lateness" becomes a more relative concept. In collectivist cultures—that is, cultures in which the relationships and interconnectedness between people are valued over the needs of the individual—it is often more important to attend to a social role than to arrive on time for an appointment with a health care provider. Hence, the lack of adherence to the appointment time can be attributed to competing demands or a different time orientation and should not be interpreted as blatant disregard or disrespect for the health care providers or the system. Missed appointment times can also be reflective of a lack of resources, such as access to transportation or dependence on others to get to the appointment.

Biology, Physiology, and Pharmacology. As discussed earlier, racial and ethnic influences on biological and physiological processes are often viewed as controversial because these influences are considered more to be social categories than scientific categories. However, clinical realities should not be ignored. Gender differences exist in the prevalence of illness, expression of illness, and response to pharmaceutical agents. The occurrence of certain diseases in different racial and ethnic populations also varies. Genetic predisposition varies across racial and ethnic lines. For example, sickle cell disease is a common genetic disorder among people of African descent. By being aware of such illness incidences, health care providers can perform a focused and thorough assessment and can avoid stereotypical assumptions. Having knowledge of increased vulnerability can enhance clinical decision making and prevent misdiagnosis or unnecessary delays that lead to poor care.

There is some evidence that ethnicity influences responses to certain medications. These variations are a result of physiological and pathophysiological differences; pharmacogenetics and genetics; environmental factors such as diet, nutritional status, smoking, and alcohol use; and simultaneous use of herbal remedies (Ramamoorthy et al., 2015). Some European and African patients metabolize medications at a slower rate, which leads to high drug levels, whereas some Japanese and Indigenous patients metabolize medications more quickly. Differences in rates of metabolism mean that individuals from Japan, China, Thailand, and Malaysia require lower doses of medications such as codeine than does a European person. Differential response has also been documented for drug classifications such as antihypertensive, antipsychotic, and antianxiety agents. Studies note that Asians often require lower dosages of antipsychotic medications and Blacks have a less favorable response to many antihypertensive medications than that of Whites (Abuatiq, 2018). Although some medications may have population-specific recommendations, it is important for nurses to be vigilant to variations in dosage response and adverse effects. For nurses working in specialty areas, it is important to learn about the ethnocultural variations in response to the classification of medications commonly taken by their clinical population.

Family Roles and Relationships. Family structures and roles differ from one culture to another (Figure 2.3). For this reason, it is important for nurses to determine who should be involved in the communication and decision making related to health care. For example, individualistic cultures emphasize individual rights, goals, and needs, whereas collectivist cultures assign greater priority to the needs of the group (family or community) and there is an emphasis on interdependence rather than independence (Yi, 2018). The Eurocentric health care system is very individualistic focused and places a high value on autonomy; each adult individual is expected to make decisions and sign consent forms when receiving health care. In contrast, in Asian cultures, the head of the household or the eldest son is expected

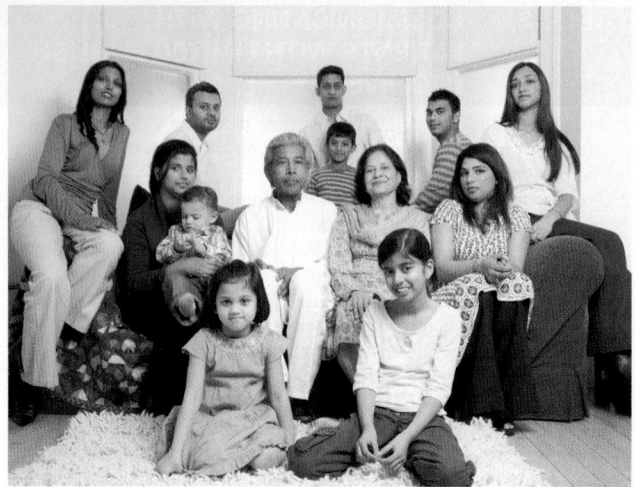

FIG. 2.3 Family roles and relationships differ from one culture to another. Source: iStock.com/Image Source.

to make health care decisions. In collectivist cultures, including Indigenous communities, affiliation is valued over confrontation, and cooperation is preferred to competition. When the nurse encounters a family that values collectivity over individualism, conflicts may arise in how decisions are made. There may be a delay in treatment while the patient waits for significant family members to arrive before giving consent for a procedure or treatment. In other instances, the patient may make a decision that is best for the family but may have negative or adverse consequences for the patient. By being aware of such values, the nurse is better prepared to engage, advocate for, and support the patient.

Spirituality and Religion. Spirituality and religion are aspects of culture that may affect a person's beliefs and decisions about health and illness. Spirituality is related to a person's efforts to find purpose, particularly in challenging situations, and to facilitate healing and wellness (Jiminez & Thal, 2020). Religion is a more formal and organized system of beliefs, including belief in or worship of God, and involves prayer and one or more rituals. Religious and spiritual beliefs have been shown to positively influence health, particularly in the care of patients with mental health and addiction issues (Jimenez & Thal, 2020; Vanderweele et al., 2017). Faith communities have been positively associated with health promotion (Kiger et al, 2017). Thus it is important for health care providers to understand the role of religion, spirituality, and culture in health and illness.

For some ethnocultural groups, culture, spirituality, and religion are inseparable. For example, the Indigenous culture and way of life are intertwined with religious and spiritual beliefs, and these extend to health and wellness. Similarly, Hinduism is as much a way of life as it is a religion and is also associated with a healing system. Spiritual energy in various forms such as *Qi, Kami, Prana*, and "spirit helpers" is associated with many cultures and, in some instances, may be supported by objects that are protective or promote healing (Young & Pompana, 2017). Often these objects, such as sweetgrass, eagle feathers, beads, thread, pictures, or religious figurines and symbols, are placed on or near a person. Nurses can show respect for these beliefs by inquiring about, recognizing, and respecting sacred objects and by seeking permission before touching or removing them from where they are placed. Nurses can also support interventions such as healing ceremonies, prayer, scriptures, listening, and referral to meet a patient's spiritual and religious needs (Drost, 2019; Giske & Cone, 2015).

For many cultures hair is closely connected to spirituality and ancestry (Jahangir, 2015; Stensgar, 2019); it has also been used as an instrument of oppression. Students attending residential schools had their hair cut short. In other situations, athletes have been forced to cut their hair or people have been denied employment because of their long hair (Canadian Broadcasting Corporation, 2017; Johnston, 2018). In some instances, these were deliberate acts of oppression and in others, a lack of knowledge; however, the impact of such actions can be quite traumatic for the individuals concerned and their community.

Migration and Settlement Process. As noted earlier, recent immigrants are at risk for health issues, for many reasons. The settlement process is associated with many losses and can cause physical and mental stress. New immigrants often experience challenges in areas of the social determinants such as employment, housing, social support, and access to services. They are also at risk for social exclusion through underemployment, workplace stress, and unemployment. Older immigrants and women are especially affected by changes in role, social position, and potentially social isolation in a new country. Factors such as fatigue, stress, and racism—and, for refugees, premigratory circumstances—can result in serious physical and psychological trauma. Children and adolescents may experience challenges in negotiating their identity in a new culture. Many newcomers face difficulties in accessing the health care system because of a lack of familiarity with the system, limited English-language proficiency, transportation difficulties, or inability to take time away from other responsibilities related to work and family (Delara, 2016; Kalich et al., 2015). Lack of permanent resident status may also influence if and how health care is accessed. It is important to recognize that while immigrant families face many challenges, they, like other groups, also have strengths such as resilience, optimism, and experience with dealing with challenges, which need to recognized and tapped into for health and wellness (Bonmati-Tomas et al., 2016).

Dynamics of Difference

In the ABCDE framework, *dynamics of difference* is not a distinctly separate domain; rather, these are distinct processes evident across each of the ABC domains. The dynamics of difference must be understood at three levels: (1) the nurse–patient level, (2) the patient–health care organization/system level, and the (3) patient–society level. At the individual level, it is important to note that although power differences exist in all nurse–patient relationships, they are magnified, often through unconscious bias, when clinicians and patients belong to different cultural groups. To ensure that patients' rights and autonomy are respected, it is important for health care providers to be aware of their own biases, to recognize that patients may have biases based on their past experiences, and to intentionally work to build trust while being vigilant in detecting processes that can be marginalizing or exclusionary. At the level of the health care system, factors to consider include the extent to which patients and families feel understood and supported. Are families included in care? Can patients access spiritual care and ceremonies based on their needs, or are there policies prohibiting or discouraging such practices? Are there safe, welcoming spaces for marginalized communities? Are services available at times when and in places where they can be readily accessed?

Is there diversity in the staff and clinicians? Is patient or family voice present in decisions? These are just some of the questions to consider in assessing the dynamics of difference at the level of the organization or system. At the social level, understanding the dynamics of difference means understanding the effect of systemic oppression and institutional racism. Specific actions to address the dynamics of difference are outlined throughout Table 2.3.

Culturally Competent Practice Environment

It is well documented that the culture or context of the health care environment matters as much as the culture of the patient. Effective and equitable care requires that both the clinicians and the health care setting support cultural competence. *Environment* highlights the importance of understanding, developing, and utilizing resources at the individual and organizational levels for ongoing learning, consultation, and referral (Drost, 2019; Jongen et al., 2018). Health care organizations that have policies and resources to support traditional healing practices such as smudging, have flexible hours of service provision, and use welcoming family presence guidelines can greatly facilitate the provision of culturally competent care.

Patients and families are a critical resource for all clinicians to learn cultural needs as well as cultural strengths and resources that may exist within a family and community. Nurses need to be open to and inviting of this knowledge, while recognizing the strengths and limitations of their own expertise. Examples of other resources include colleagues who can share experience and expertise in cross-cultural care, language support aids such as interpreters or telephonic services, hours of service that accommodate different work schedules, and access to spiritual and faith leaders and practices. There are many community and health care agencies that serve minority communities who can serve as a resource for referrals or partnership to better serve patients.

THE NURSE'S SELF-ASSESSMENT

As stated earlier, developing an understanding of one's own culture through reflection and self-assessment is a crucial first step toward practising cultural competence in clinical care. Evidence indicates that health care providers' attitudes, whether they are conscious of them or not, have a significant influence on their interactions with other people. Recognizing and taking conscious steps to address such biases or blind spots is an essential aspect of cultural competence (Srivastava, 2007b; White et al., 2018). This requires critical self-reflection on one's own privilege, identity, values, and beliefs, as well as on one's motivation and the value that one places on cultural competence and social justice. It is also important to reflect on the history and culture of the professions and the health care systems to which nursing students are being socialized. For examples of specific activities that can be undertaken to support one's cultural competence see Anderson-Lain (2017), Rosen et al. (2017), and White et al. (2018). Another helpful tool is Harvard University's Implicit Association Test (IAT), which measures attitudes and beliefs that people may not even know exist within themselves. This tool can be accessed online.

CULTURALLY COMPETENT PATIENT ASSESSMENT

A cultural assessment should be a fundamental part of *all* patient assessments. Conducting a cultural assessment means bringing

TABLE 2.7	CULTURALLY COMPETENT HEALTH ASSESSMENT

- Become aware of your own values, beliefs, and biases.
- Develop humility and a critical awareness that your own expertise is probably ethnocentric.
- Know that racism, heterosexism, classism, sexism, genderism, ageism, ableism, and so forth, are taught, not innate, and that the unlearning process is ongoing.
- Perceive patients and clients as experts of their own realities.
- Work to build trust.
- Communicate in ways that are nonjudgemental and show respect for differences.
- Use open-ended questions to understand patients' priorities and perceptions.
- Pay attention to the economic and social contexts of patients' and families' lives.
- Inquire about health beliefs, practices, and help-seeking behaviours.
- Inquire about the role of religion and spirituality in health and illness.
- Identify sources of cultural support (friends, family, community).
- Advocate with and for patients and learn how to be an ally across diversity and oppression.
- Challenge discrimination, marginalization, and oppression.
- Assist patients in becoming informed, knowledgeable, and empowered.
- Embrace learning as an ongoing process.

TABLE 2.8	LEARN MODEL FOR CROSS-CULTURAL CARE

Listen with sympathy and understanding to the patient's perception of the problem.
Explain your perception of the problem.
Acknowledge and discuss the differences and similarities.
Recommend treatment.
Negotiate agreement.

Source: Ladha, T., Zubairi, M., Hunter, A., Audcent, T., & Johnstone, J. (2018). Cross-cultural communication: Tools for working with families and children. *Pediatrics & Child Health, 23*(1), 66–69. https://doi.org/10.1093/pch/pxxl26

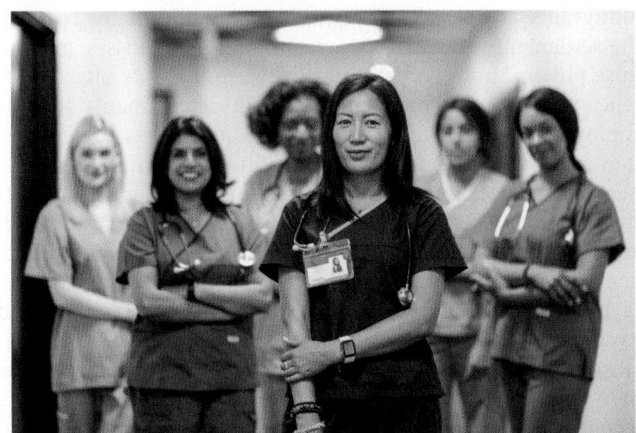

FIG. 2.4 Nurses working together in a multicultural health environment. Source: iStock.com/FatCamera.

a lens of culture and equity to all processes and interactions and asking key questions with regard to language, diet, and religion and eliciting the patient's explanatory model of health and illness (see Table 2.4). Assessments become culturally appropriate through the use of cultural knowledge and skill to determine when, how, and with whom to explore particular issues. It is critical to build trust by adopting an approach that conveys respect, a nonjudgemental attitude, and a genuine desire to understand the patient's perspective. Issues concerning personal space and gender often surface during activities involving physical assessment and personal care. Health care providers can use their position to raise cultural issues, as patients may be hesitant to bring them up. Providers must also be vigilant and sensitive to patient responses and create an environment that facilitates patients being comfortable enough to express their needs and preferences.

Table 2.7 summarizes nursing actions that are part of a culturally competent health assessment.

BRIDGING CULTURAL DISTANCES

Key characteristics of cultural competence are the ability to effectively apply the ABCDEs of cultural competence—cultural awareness, knowledge, and skills in clinical situations; keep in mind the dynamics of difference; access supports available through the practice environment; and continually assess for the goal of equity. Throughout this chapter, strategies that can be used to bridge gaps and differences across cultures have been discussed. One model useful for summarizing this discussion is the LEARN (listen, explain, acknowledge, recommend, and negotiate) model (Table 2.8), which offers simple but comprehensive guidelines for cross-cultural health care (Ladha et al., 2018). The LEARN model enables the nurse to reveal and acknowledge patients' values and perspectives and practise in a professional manner by sharing the nurse's expertise. By listening first, the nurse is

less likely to give the impression of being hurried or too busy and will be able to tailor explanations in ways that are relevant for the patient.

Another approach discussed in the Culture Care Framework (Srivastava 2007b) highlights the importance of acknowledging and validating patient values and beliefs; accommodating and negotiating treatments and approaches to care; and challenging perceptions through reframing interpretations associated with certain practices based on evidence. For example, many collectivist cultures focus on caring for others, thus care that is self-focused may initially be viewed as a self-centred; however, reframing self-care as the ability to have capacity to care for others makes it more acceptable. Throughout this text, special "Culturally Competent Care" sections highlight knowledge and skills relevant to providing culturally competent health care.

WORKING IN DIVERSE TEAMS

Interactions between patients and health care providers are not the only situations in which cross-cultural issues and challenges can arise. The increasing diversity in society also affects the makeup of the health care team (Figure 2.4).

In general, workforce diversity is viewed as a positive attribute and a valuable resource to support the development of cultural competence and the provision of culturally relevant care. A diverse working team creates opportunities for cultural encounters and interactions that can result in greater cultural understanding and better delivery of care. However, diversity in the workforce has its challenges. Although culturally diverse groups have more potential to generate a greater variety of ideas and other resources than do culturally homogeneous groups, racially and ethnically mixed groups can experience more conflict and miscommunication than homogeneous groups. When health care providers from different cultures and countries work together as members of the health care team, opportunities for miscommunication and conflict naturally arise (Adeniranet al., 2015). These challenges can be minimized through the same principles of respect, empathy, and learning from difference that apply to nurse–patient interactions.

CONCLUSION

The need for cultural competence is a fundamental issue of health care quality and patient safety, and achieving it requires a commitment to principles of inclusiveness and equity. Cultural awareness and knowledge must be translated into action. Developing cultural competence is a journey in which nurses begin with strengthening their self-awareness. They develop a generic knowledge base and, with time and experience, acquire additional knowledge specific to populations and aspects of care. They become aware of and sensitively address the dynamics of differences and tap into resources within the practice environment. It is important for nurses to combine the use of this information and knowledge with critical reflection and critical thinking. A commitment to health equity requires that nurses understand vulnerabilities as well as the strengths that exist within individuals and communities. This approach adds both depth and breadth to the nurse's clinical competence and ability to provide care that is truly patient-centred.

CASE STUDY

Communication

Patient Profile

M. J., 45 years old (pronouns she/her), is admitted to the hospital for investigation of a tumour. M. J.'s husband is also present. The healthcare provider explains to the couple that the prognosis is excellent and the treatment involves radiation. She plans to schedule the first treatment the following week.

M. J. and her husband have been in Canada for approximately 3 years, and both speak English, albeit with an accent. There have been no difficulties in communicating in English with either M. J. or M. J.'s husband, although her husband tends to do most of the talking. While the healthcare provider is explaining the diagnosis, they listen intently, nod periodically, and do not raise any questions or objections to the plan. The healthcare provider assumes that the patient is in agreement with her plan.

Discussion Questions

1. Should the nurse who is present for this discussion agree with the healthcare provider's assessment?
2. What factors may be influencing the couple's silence?
3. What actions could be taken by the nurse who is present for this discussion or the doctor that would reflect cultural competence?

ⓔvolve

Answers available at http://evolve.elsevier.com/Canada/Lewis/medsurg.

REVIEW QUESTIONS

The number of the question corresponds to the same-numbered objective at the beginning of the chapter.

1. Which of the following is an example of forcing one's own cultural beliefs and practices on another person?
   a. Stereotyping
   b. Ethnocentrism
   c. Cultural relativity
   d. Cultural imposition

2. Which of the following most accurately describes cultural factors that may affect health?
   a. Diabetes and cancer rates differ by cultural and ethnic groups.
   b. Most clients find that religious rituals help them during times of illness.
   c. There is limited ethnic variation in physiological responses to medications.
   d. Silence during a nurse–client interaction usually means that the client understands the instructions.

3. Which of the following is true about inequities between Indigenous health and the health of the general population? (Select all that apply.)
   a. They result from lifestyle choices.
   b. They result from differences in living conditions, such as housing and education.
   c. They result from conflict between systems of Indigenous medicine and Western health care concepts.
   d. They result from bias and discrimination from the mainstream system.

4. Why is it important for the nurse to develop cultural self-awareness? (Select all that apply.)
   a. This enables the nurse to clearly articulate the nurse's own values to the client.
   b. This enables the nurse to prevent ethnocentrism.
   c. This enables the nurse to prevent cultural imposition.
   d. This enables the nurse to challenge their own assumptions and stereotypes.

5. In communications with a client who speaks a language different from the nurse's, which of the following interventions is important?
   a. Have a family member translate.
   b. Use a trained medical interpreter.
   c. Use specific medical terminology so that there will be no mistakes in the information communicated.
   d. Focus on the translation rather than the nonverbal communication.

6. Which of the following strategies are appropriate for demonstrating cultural competence in clinical care? (Select all that apply.)
   a. Explaining to the client and family how the Canadian health care system works
   b. Exploring economic and social factors affecting the client and family
   c. Pairing the client with a provider from the client's own cultural community
   d. Exploring the client's explanatory model of illness

7. How does a diverse workforce influence a nurse's ability to provide care?
   a. It facilitates matching clients with health care providers of the same ethnicity.
   b. It exposes the nurse to different values, beliefs, and worldviews.
   c. It leads to greater creativity and innovation and to the development of appropriate interventions for diverse clients.

d. It meets mandated objectives of the federal and provincial governments.

1. d; 2. a; 3. c; 4. c; 5. d; 6. b; 7. b.

⊖volve

For even more review questions, visit http://evolve.elsevier.com/Canada/Lewis/medsurg.

REFERENCES

Abuatiq, A. (2018). Cultural competency in ethnopharmacology. *Chronicles of Pharmaceutical Science, 2*(4), 617–621. http://works.bepress.com/DrAbuatiq/11

Adeniran, R. K., Bhattacharya, A., & Srivastava, R. (2015). Facilitators and barriers to advancing in the nursing profession: Voices of U.S.- and internationally educated nurses. *Clinical Scholars Review, 8*(2), 241–248.

Alimezelli, H. T., Leis, A., Denis, W., et al. (2015). Lost in policy translation: Canadian minority francophones and health disparities. *Canadian Public Policy, 41*, 44–52. https://doi.org/10.3138/cpp.2014-073

Anderson-Lain, K. (2017). Cultural identity forum: Enacting the self-awareness imperative in intercultural communication. *Communication Teacher, 31*(3), 131–136.

Barker, G. (2016). Cross-cultural perspectives on intercultural communication competence. *Journal of Intercultural Communication Research, 45*(1), 13–30. https://doi.org/10.1080/17475759.2015.1104376

Beagan, B. (2015). Approaches to culture and diversity: A critical synthesis of occupational therapy literature. *Canadian Journal of Occupational Therapy, 82*(5), 272–282. https://doi.org/10.1177/0008417414567530

Berg, K., McLane, P., Eshkakogan, N., et al. (2019). Perspectives on Indigenous cultural competency and safety in Canadian hospital emergency departments: A scoping review. *International Emergency Nursing, 43*, 133–140. https://doi.org/10.1016/j.ienj.2019.01.004

Bhugra, D. (2016). Social discrimination and social justice. *International Review of Psychiatry, 28*(4), 336–341. https://doi.org/10.1080/09540261.2016.1210359

Bombay, A., McQuaid, R. J., Young, J., et al. (2020). Familial Attendance at Indian Residential School and Subsequent Involvement in the Child Welfare System Among Indigenous Adults Born During the Sixties Scoop Era. *First Peoples Child & Family Review, 15*(1), 62–79. https://doi.org/10.7202/1068363ar

Bonmati-Tomas, A., Malagan-Aguilera, M., Bosch-Farre, C., et al. (2016). Reducing health inequities affecting immigrant women: a qualitative study of their valuable assets. *Globalization and Health, 12*, 37. https://doi.org/10.1186/s12992-016-0174-8

Brown, O., Ham-Baloyi, W., Van Rooyen, D., et al. (2016). Culturally competent patient-provider communication in the management of cancer: An integrative literature review. *Global Health Action, 9*(1), 33208. https://doi.org/10.3402/gha.v9.3208

Bourke, S., Wright, A., Guthrie, J., et al. (2018). Evidence review of Indigenous culture for health and wellbeing. *The International Journal of Health, Wellness, and Society, 8*(4), 11–27. https://doi.org/10.18848/2156-8960/CGP/v08i04/11-27

Cain, C. L., Surbone, A., Elk, R., et al. (2018). Culture and palliative care: preferences, communication, meaning, and mutual decision making. *Journal of Pain and Symptom Management, 55*(5), 1408–1419. https://doi.org/10.1016/j.jpainsymman.2018.01.007

Canadian Broadcasting Corporation. (2017). *The turban that rocked the RCMP*. https://www.cbc.ca/2017/canadathestoryofus/the-turban-that-rocked-the-rcmp-how-baltej-singh-dhillon-challenged-the-rcmp-and-won-1.4110271

Canadian Nurses Association. (2018). *Promoting cultural competence in nursing: Joint position statement*. https://www.cna-aiic.ca/-/media/cna/page-content/pdf-en/position_statement_promoting_cultural_competence_in_nursing.pdf?la=en&hash=4B394DAE5C2138E7F6134D59E505DCB059754BA9

Canizares, M., Hogg-Johnson, S., Gignac, M., et al. (2017). Changes in the use of practitioner-based complementary and alternative medicine over time in Canada: Cohort and period effects. *PLoS ONE, 12*(5), e0177307. https://doi.org/10.1371/journal.pone.0177307

Chou, V. (2017). *April 17). How science and genetics are reshaping the race debate of the 21st century*. Harvard University Science in the News. http://sitn.hms.harvard.edu/flash/2017/science-genetics-reshaping-race-debate-21st-century/

Colpitts, E., & Gahagan, J. (2016). "I feel like I am surviving the health care system": Understanding LGBTQ health in Nova Scotia, Canada. *BCM Public Health, 16*(1), 1–12. https://doi.org/10.1186/s12889-016-3675-8

College & Association of Registered Nurses of Alberta. (2018). *Complementary and Alternative Health Care and Natural Health Products Standards*. https://nurses.ab.ca/docs/default-source/document-library/standards/complementary-and-alternative-health-care-and-natural-health-products.pdf?sfvrsn=2480176b_34

Delara, M. ((2016). *Social determinants of immigrant women's mental health*. Advances in Public Health. https://doi.org/10.1155/2016/9730162. 2016, article ID 9730162.

Drost, J. L. (2019). Developing the alliances to expand traditional Indigenous healing practices within Alberta Health Services. *The Journal of Alternative and Complementary Medicine, 25*(S1), S69–S77. https://doi.org/10.1089/acm.2018.0387

Ferdous, M., Goopy, S., Yang, H., et al. (2019). Barriers to breast cancer screening among immigrant populations in Canada. *Journal of Immigrant and Minority Health, 22*, 410–420. https://doi.org/10.1007/s10903-019-00916-3

Fournier, B., Eastlick Kushner, K., & Raine, K. (2019). "To me, policy is government": Creating a locally driven healthy food environment in the Canadian Artic. *Health and Place, 58*, 1–8. https://doi.org/10.1016/j.healthplace.2019.05.016

Fung, K., & Guzder, J. (2018). Canadian immigrant mental health. In D. Moussaoui, D. Bhugra, & A. Ventriglio (Eds.), *Mental health and illness in migration* (pp. 1–21). Springer. https://doi.org/10.1007/978-981-10-0750-7_11-1

Giblon, R., & Bauer, G. R. (2017). Health care availability, quality, and unmet need: a comparison of transgender and cisgender residents of Ontario, Canada. *BMC Health Services Research, 17*(1), 283. https://doi.org/10.1186/s12913-017-2226-z

Gil, S., Hooke, M., & Niess, D. (2016). The limited English proficiency patient family advocate role: Fostering respectful and effective care across language and culture in pediatric oncology setting. *Journal of Pediatric Oncology Nursing, 33*(3), 190–198. https://doi.org/10.1177/1043454215611082

Giske, T., & Cone, P. H. (2015). Discerning the healing path – how nurses assist patient spirituality in diverse health care settings. *Journal of Clinical Nursing, 24*, 2926–2935. https://doi.org 10.11 1 1/jocn.12907

Henry, F., Dua, E., Kobayashi, A., et al. (2016). Race, racialization and indigeneity in Canadian universities. *Race Ethnicity and Education, 1*(3), 300–314. https://doi.org/10.1080/13613324.2016.1260226

Habadi, A., Mahnashi, F., Alkhundidi, A., et al. (2019). Patient-physician communication: Challenges and skills. *EC Microbiology, 15*(12), 1–10.

House of Commons. Standing Committee on Health. (2019). *The Health of LGBTQIA2 Communities in Canada*. 28th Report. 42nd Parliament, 1st Session. https://www.ourcommons.ca/Content/Committee/421/HESA/Reports/RP10574595/hesarp28/hesarp28-e.pdf

International Council of Nurses (ICN). (2018). *Position statement: Health of migrants, refugees, and displaced persons*. https://www.icn.ch/sites/default/files/inline-files/PS_A_Health_migrants_refugees_displaced%20persons_0.pdf

Jahangir, R. (2015). *How does black hair reflect black history? BBC News*. May 31 https://www.bbc.com/news/uk-england-merseyside-31438273

Janca, A., & Bullen, C. (2003). The Aboriginal concept of time and its mental health implications. *Australian Psychiatry, 11*, s40–s44.

Jimenez, R., & Thal, W. (2020). Culturally competent mental health care. *Nursing Made Incredibly Easy*, May/June, 46–49. https://doi.org/10.1097/01.NME.00000658224.50056.fb

Johnson, M. (2018). *The policing of black hair in sports*. https://theundefeated.com/features/the-policing-of-black-hair-in-sports/

Jongen, C., McCalman, J., & Bainbridge, R. (2018). Health workforce cultural competency interventions: a systematic scoping review. *BMC Health Services Research, 18*, 232. https://doi.org/10.1186/s12913-018-3001-5

Kalich, A., Heinemann, L., & Ghahari, S. (2015). A scoping review of immigrant experience of health care access barriers in Canada. *Journal of Immigrant and Minority Health, 18*(3), 1–13. https://doi.org/10.1007/s10903-015-0237-6

Kiger, A. M., Fagan, D. M., & van Teijlingen, E. R. (2017). *Faith communities and the potential for health promotion*. Oxford Research Encyclopedias. https://doi.org/10.1093/acrefore/9780190228613.013.518

Kim, P. (2019). Social determinants of health inequities in Indigenous Canadians through a life course approach to colonialism and the residential school system. *Health Equity, 3*(1), 378–381 https://doi.org 101089/heq.2019.0041

Kirmayer, L. J., & Jarvis, G. E. (2019). Culturally responsive services as a path to equity in mental health care. *Healthcare Papers, 18*(2), 11–23. https://www.longwoods.com/publications/healthcarepapers

Ladha, T., Zubairi, M., Hunter, A., Audcent, T., et al. (2018). Cross-cultural communication: Tools for working with families and children. *Pediatrics & Child Health, 23*(1), 66–69. https://doi.org/10.1093/pch/pxxl26

Marcus, E. (2016). Muslim women's preferences in the medical setting: How might they contribute to disparities in health outcomes? *Journal of Women's Health, 25*(6), 561–562. https://doi.org/10.1089/jwh.2016.5875

McKenzie, K., Agic, B., Tuck, A., et al. (2016). *The case for diversity: Building the case to improve mental health services for immigrant, refugee, ethno-cultural and racialized populations*. Mental Health Commission of Canada.

Minnican, C., & O'Toole, G. (2020). Exploring the incidence of culturally responsive communication in Australian healthcare: the first rapid review on this concept. *BMC Health Services Research, 20*, 20. https://doi.org/10.1186/s12913-019-4859-6

Morency, J.-D., Malenfant, E. C., & MacIsaac, S. (2017). *Immigration and diversity: Population projections for Canada and its regions, 2011 to 2036*. Statistics Canada Catalogue no. 91-551-X. https://www150.statcan.gc.ca/n1/pub/91-551-x/91-551-x2017001-eng.htm

Murray, H., & Kulckhohn, C. (1953). *Personality in Nature, Society, and Culture*. www.panarchy.org/kluckhohn/personality.1953.html. (Seminal).

Ontario Ministry of Health and Long-Term Care. (2021). *Health equity impact assessment*. http://www.health.gov.on.ca/en/pro/programs/heia/

Paradies, Y., Ben, J., Denson, N., et al. (2015). Racism as a determinant of health: A systematic review and meta-analysis. *PLoS ONE, 10*(9), 1–48. https://doi.org/10.1371/journal.pone.0138511

Public Health Agency of Canada. (2018). Key health inequities in Canada: A national portrait. Pan-Canadian Health Inequities Reporting Initiative. https://www.canada.ca/content/dam/phac-aspc/documents/services/publications/science-research/key-health-inequalities-canada-national-portrait-executive-summary/hir-full-report-eng.pdf

Ramamoorthy, A., Pacanowski, M. A., Bull, J., et al. (2015). Racial/ethnic differences in drug disposition and response: Review of recently approved drugs. *Clinical Pharmacology & Therapeutics, 97*(3), 263–273. https://doi.org/10.1002/cpt.61

Reich, D. (2018, March 23). How genetics is changing our understanding of 'race'. *The New York Times*. https://www.nytimes.com/2018/03/23/opinion/sunday/genetics-race.html

Richmond, C. A. M., & Cook, C. (2016). Creating conditions for Canadian Aboriginal health equity: The promise of healthy public policy. *Public Health Reviews, 37*(2), 1–16. https://doi.org/10.1186/s40985-016-0016-5. (Seminal).

Rosen, D., McCall, J., & Goodkind, S. (2017). Teaching critical self reflection through the lens of cultural humility: an assignment in a social work diversity course. *Social Work Education, 36*(3), 289–298. https://doi.org/10.1080/02615479.2017.1287260

Sharifi, N., Adib-Haijbaghery, M., & Najafi, M. (2019). Cultural competence in nursing: A concept analysis. *International Journal of Nursing Studies, 99*, 1–8. https://doi.org/10.1016/j.ijnurstu.2019.103386

Small, P. M. (2019). Structural justice and nursing: Inpatient nurses' obligation to address social justice needs of patients. *Nursing Ethics, 26*(7-8), 1928–1935. https://doi.org/10.1177/0969733018810764

Srivastava, R. (2007a). Culture care framework I: Overview and cultural sensitivity. In R. Srivastava (Ed.), *The healthcare professional's guide to clinical cultural competence* (pp. 53–74). Elsevier Canada (Seminal).

Srivastava, R. (2007b). Culture care framework II: Culture knowledge, resources, and bridging the gap. In R. Srivastava (Ed.), *The healthcare professional's guide to clinical cultural competence* (pp. 75–100). Elsevier Canada (Seminal).

Srivastava, R. (2008). The ABC (and DE) of cultural competence in clinical care. *Ethnicity and Inequalities in Health and Social Care, 8*(1), 25–31 (Seminal).

Srivastava, R., & Srivastava, R. (2019). Impact of cultural identity on mental health in post-secondary students. *International Journal of Mental Health and Addiction, 17*, 520–530. https://doi.org/10.1007/s11469-018-0025-3

Smith, M. A. (2019). The promotion of social justice. *Nursing Made Incredibly Easy, 17*(2), 26-32. https://doi.org/10.1097/01.NME.0000553091.78584.a9

Statistics Canada. (2017a). *Aboriginal peoples in Canada: Key results from the 2016 Census* (Updated 2019). https://www150.statcan.gc.ca/n1/daily-quotidien/171025/dq171025a-eng.htm

Statistics Canada. (2017b). *Immigration and ethnocultural diversity: Key results from the 2016 Census.* https://www150.statcan.gc.ca/n1/daily-quotidien/171025/dq171025b-eng.htm

Statistics Canada. (2019). *Diversity of the Black population in Canada: An overview. Statistics Canada Catalogue no. 89-657-X. Statistics Canada, Ethnicity, Language and Immigration Thematic Series.* https://www150.statcan.gc.ca/n1/en/pub/89-657-x/89-657-x2019002-eng.pdf?st=p4nh4jOc

Stensgar, B. (2019). *The significance of hair in Native American culture.* https://sistersky.com/blogs/sister-sky/the-significance-of-hair-in-native-american-culture

Suphanchaimat, R., Kantamaturapoj, K., Putthasri, W., et al. (2015). Challenges in the provision of healthcare services for migrants: A systematic review through providers' lens. *BMC Health Services Research, 15*(1), 1–14. https://doi.org/10.1186/s12913-015-1065-z

Truth and Reconciliation Commission of Canada (TRC). (2015). *Truth and Reconciliation Commission of Canada: Calls to action.* Truth and Reconciliation Commission of Canada.

VanderWeele, T., Balboni, T., & Koh, H. (2017). Health and Spirituality. *JAMA, 318*(6), 519–520. https://doi.org/10.1001/jama.2017.8136

White, A. A., Logghe, H. J., Goodenough, D. A., et al. (2018). *Journal of Racial and Ethnic Disparities, 5,* 34–49. https://doi.org/10.1007/s40615-017-0340-6

Yi, J. S. (2018). Revisiting individualism-collectivism: A cross cultural comparison among college students in four countries. *Journal of Intercultural Communication, 47,* 1404–1634.

Young, D., Pompana, C., & Willier, R. (2017). The concept of spiritual power in East Asian and Canadian Aboriginal thought. *Social Compass, 64*(3), 376–387. https://doi.org/10.1177/0037768617713657

RESOURCES

Canadian Institute of Health Research: *Pathways to Health Equity for Aboriginal Peoples: Overview*
https://www.cihr-irsc.gc.ca/e/43630.html

Canadian Psychological Association: *Culturally Competent Care for Diverse Groups*
https://cpa.ca/practice/cultural/

Caring for Kids New to Canada: *Cultural Competence for Child and Youth Health Professionals*
https://www.kidsnewtocanada.ca/culture/competence

Cultural Competence: *A Guide to Organizational Change*
https://albertahumanrights.ab.ca/Documents/CulturalCompetencyGuide.pdf

First Nations Health Authority: *Cultural Safety and Humility*
https://www.fnha.ca/wellness/cultural-humility

Multicultural Mental Health Resource Centre: *Cultural Competence: Tools & Resources*
https://multiculturalmentalhealth.ca/cultural-competence-tools-and-resources/

National Aboriginal Health Organization
https://www.naho.ca/

SickKids Cultural Competence E-Learning Modules Series
https://www.sickkids.ca/tclhinculturalcompetence/index.html

Dimensions of Culture: *Cross Cultural Communications for Health Professionals*
http://www.dimensionsofculture.com/

Ethnicity Online
http://www.ethnicityonline.net/

National Center for Cultural Competence at Georgetown University
https://nccc.georgetown.edu/

Project Implicit: Harvard University Implicit Association Test
https://implicit.harvard.edu/implicit/

The Disparities Solutions Center https://mghdisparitiessolutions.org/

Think Cultural Health
https://www.thinkculturalhealth.hhs.gov/

US Department of Health & Human Services, Office of Minority Health: *Cultural and Linguistic Competence*
http://minorityhealth.hhs.gov/omh/browse.aspx?lvl=1&lvlid=6

⊝volve

For additional Internet resources, see the website for this book at http://evolve.elsevier.com/Canada/Lewis/medsurg.

Health History and Physical Examination

Mary Ann Fegan

Originating US chapter by Courtney Reinisch

ⓔvolve WEBSITE

http://evolve.elsevier.com/Canada/Lewis/medsurg

- Review Questions (Online Only)
- Key Points
- Conceptual Care Map Creator

- Audio Glossary
- Content Updates

LEARNING OBJECTIVES

1. Describe the purpose, components, and techniques of gathering a patient's health history and performing a physical examination.
2. Discuss the functional health pattern framework used for obtaining a nursing history.

3. Explain how the techniques of inspection, palpation, percussion, and auscultation are used during the physical examination of a patient.
4. Differentiate among comprehensive, focused, and emergency types of assessment in terms of indications, purposes, and components.

KEY TERMS

auscultation
database
general survey statement
inspection

nursing history
objective data
palpation
percussion

physical examination
subjective data

During the assessment phase of the nursing process, the nurse documents a patient's health history and performs a physical examination. The findings of this assessment (a) contribute to a database that identifies the patient's current and past health status and (b) provide a baseline against which future changes can be evaluated. The purpose of the nursing assessment is to enable the nurse to make clinical judgements or nursing diagnoses about the patient's health status (Jarvis et al., 2019). While assessment is the first step of the nursing process, it is performed continuously throughout the nursing process to validate nursing diagnoses, evaluate nursing interventions, and determine whether patient outcomes and goals have been met.

Note: This chapter provides a basic overview and review of health assessment and physical examination. A detailed health assessment textbook will provide more information and direction regarding how to perform a physical examination and how to identify and document abnormal findings.

DATA COLLECTION

In the broadest sense, the database is all the health information about a patient. This includes the data from the nursing history and physical examination, the data from the medical history and physical examination, results of laboratory and diagnostic tests, and information contributed by other health care providers.

The focus of nursing care is the diagnosis and treatment of human responses to actual or potential health concerns or life processes. The information obtained from the nursing history and physical examination is used to determine the patient's strengths and responses to a health condition. For example, for a patient with a diagnosis of diabetes, the patient's responses may include anxiety or a lack of knowledge about self-management of the condition. The patient may also experience the physical response of fluid volume deficit because of the abnormal fluid loss caused by hyperglycemia. These human responses to the condition of diabetes are diagnosed and treated by nurses. During the nursing history interview and physical examination, the nurse obtains and records the data to support the identification of nursing diagnoses (Figure 3.1).

The purpose of the health history is to collect both subjective and objective data. Subjective data, also known as *symptoms*, are collected in an interview with the patient (primary source) or caregiver (secondary source), or both, during the nursing history. This type of data includes information that can be described or verified only by the patient or caregiver. It is what the person tells the nurse either spontaneously or in response to a direct question.

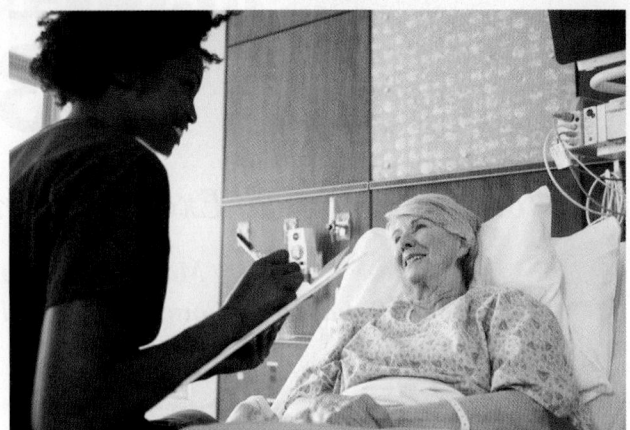

FIG. 3.1 Obtaining a nursing history is an important role of the nurse. Source: iStock.com/monkeybusinessimages.

Objective data, also known as *signs,* are data that can be observed and measured. The nurse obtains this type of data by using inspection, palpation, percussion, and auscultation during the physical examination. Objective data are also acquired by diagnostic testing. Patients often provide subjective data while the nurse is performing the physical examination. The nurse also observes objective signs while interviewing the patient. All findings related to a specific health issue, whether subjective or objective, are known as *clinical manifestations* of that issue.

Interviewing Considerations

The purpose of the patient interview is to obtain a complete health history (e.g., subjective data) about the patient's past and present health status. Effective communication is a key factor in the interview process. Creating a climate of trust and respect is crucial for establishing a therapeutic relationship, as is the nurse's ability to engage in reflective practice. This ability includes the required capacities of self-awareness, self-knowledge, empathy, and awareness of boundaries and limits of the professional role (Registered Nurses' Association of Ontario, 2006). The nurse needs to communicate acceptance of the patient as an individual by using an open, responsive, nonjudgemental approach. Nurses and patients communicate not only through language but also in their manner of dress, gestures, and body language. An awareness of culturally accepted nonverbal communication is important. For example, simple eyebrow-raising indicates a positive response or "yes" answer for the Inuit population. Modes of communication are learned through one's culture and influence—not only the words, gestures, and posture one uses but also the nature of the information that is shared with others (see Chapter 2 for discussion on culture).

The amount of time needed to complete a nursing history may vary with the format used and the experience of the nurse. The nursing history may be completed in one or several sessions, depending on the setting and the patient. For example, several short sessions might be needed for an older patient with a low energy level to allow time for the patient to provide the needed information. The nurse must also make a judgement about the amount of information collected on initial contact with the patient. In interviews with patients with chronic disease, patients in pain, and patients in emergency situations, the nurse should ask only questions that are pertinent to a specific problem. The nurse can complete the health history interview at a more appropriate time.

Before beginning the nursing history, the nurse should explain to the patient that the purpose of a detailed history is to collect information that will provide a health profile for comprehensive health care, including health promotion. This detailed information is collected during the patient's entry into the health care system, and subsequently, only updates are needed. The nurse should explain that personal and social data are needed to individualize the plan of care. This explanation is necessary because the patient may not be accustomed to sharing personal information and may need to know the purpose of such questioning. The nurse should assure the patient that all information will be kept confidential. The Canadian Nurses Association (CNA) requires that nurses protect the confidentiality of all information obtained in the context of the professional relationship and practise within the bounds of relevant laws governing privacy and confidentiality of personal health information. The CNA *Code of Ethics for Registered Nurses* provides helpful guidelines for ensuring confidentiality in nursing practice (CNA, 2017).

To obtain factual, easily categorized information, a direct interview technique can be used. Closed-ended questions such as "Have you had surgery before?" that require brief, specific responses are used. When asking sensitive personal and social questions, the nurse can communicate the acceptance or normality of behaviours by prefacing questions with phrases such as "most people" or "frequently." For example, stating, "Many people taking antihypertensive drugs have concerns about sexual functioning; do you have any you would like to discuss?" shows the patient that a particular situation may not be unique to that patient.

The nurse must judge the reliability of the patient as a historian. An older person may give a false impression about their mental status because of prolonged response time or visual and hearing impairment. The complexity and long duration of health issues may make it difficult for an older person or a chronically ill younger patient to be an accurate historian.

It is important for the nurse to determine the patient's priority concerns and expectations because the nurse's priorities may be different from the patient's. For example, the nurse's priority may be to complete the health history, whereas the patient is interested only in relief from symptoms. Until the patient's priority need is met, the nurse will probably be unsuccessful in obtaining complete and accurate data.

Teamwork and Collaboration

Ongoing data collection is expected of all members of the health care team. In acute-care settings, the initial (admission) nursing assessment must be completed by a registered nurse (RN) and within the time frame determined by the employer. A registered/licensed practical nurse (PN) will often be responsible for collecting and documenting specific patient data as delegated by the RN, after the RN has developed the plan of care on the basis of the admission assessment findings.

Data Organization

Assessment data must be systematically obtained and organized so that the nurse can readily analyze and make judgements about the patient's health status and any health concerns. Information about the patient in various health care settings can be gathered in numerous approaches and formats. The format used in this chapter for obtaining a nursing history includes the following sequence of categories, similar to those outlined by Jarvis et al.

TABLE 3.1   INVESTIGATION OF PATIENT-REPORTED SYMPTOM

Factor	Questions for Patient and Caregiver	Record
Precipitating and **p**alliative	Were there any events that came before the symptom? What makes it better? Worse? What have you done for the symptom? Did this help?	Influence of physical and emotional activities Patient's attempts to alleviate (or treat) the symptom
Quality	Tell me what the symptom feels like (e.g., aching, dull, pressure, burning, stabbing).	Patient's own words (e.g., "Like a pinch or stabbing feeling")
Radiation	Where do you feel the symptom? Does it move to other areas?	Region of the body Local or radiating, superficial or deep
Severity	On a scale of 0–10, with 0 meaning no pain and 10 being the worst pain you could imagine, what number would you give your symptom?	Pain rating number (e.g., 5/10)
Timing	When did the symptom start? Was it sudden or gradual? Any particular time of day, week, month, or year? Has the symptom changed over time? Where are you, and what are you doing when the symptom occurs?	Time of onset, duration, periodicity, and frequency Course of symptoms Where the patient is and what the patient is doing when the symptom occurs
Understanding	Understand the patient's perception of the symptom: What do you think it means?	Patient's own words about what the problem means to them

(2019). These assessment data provide a generic database for all health care providers:

1. Biographical data
2. Reason for seeking care
3. Current health status or history of current illness
4. Past health history
5. Family health history
6. Review of systems
7. Functional assessment

CULTURALLY COMPETENT CARE

ASSESSMENT

The process of obtaining a health history and performing a physical examination is an intimate experience for the nurse and the patient. As noted earlier in the chapter, a person's culture influences patterns of communication and what information is shared with others. During the interview and physical examination, the nurse must be sensitive to issues of eye contact, space, modesty, and touching, as discussed in Chapter 2. Knowing the cultural norms related to male–female relationships is especially important during the physical examination. To avoid violating any culturally based practices, the nurse can ask the patient about cultural values. The nurse should determine whether the patient would like to have someone else present during the history taking or physical examination or would prefer someone of the same gender to perform the history taking and physical examination (Jarvis et al., 2019).

Note: Additional screening or focused assessments may be required during epidemics or pandemics. For example, during the COVID-19 pandemic, advance screenings and assessments were required prior to entering health care facilities.

NURSING HISTORY: SUBJECTIVE DATA

Biographical Data

The nurse records the patient's name, address, contact information, age, birth date, marital status, partner or significant other, ethnocultural background, primary language, and current occupation. Advance care directives can be documented among these data (see Chapter 13). Also important to include here is the source of history: who is providing the information, how reliable the informant seems, and any special circumstances, such as the use of an interpreter (Jarvis et al., 2019).

Reason for Seeking Care

The reason for seeking care is a brief statement in the patient's own words describing the reason for the visit. This statement is documented in quotation marks to indicate the patient's exact words (e.g., "My head has been aching for 3 days"; "My child has a fever and has been vomiting since last evening").

Current Health or History of Current Illness

This section is a chronological record of the reason for seeking care, beginning with the first time the symptom appeared until now. Symptoms experienced by the patient are not observed, so the symptoms must be explored. Table 3.1 shows a mnemonic (PQRSTU) to help remember the areas to explore if a symptom is reported. The information that is obtained may help determine the cause of the symptom. A common symptom assessed is pain (see Chapter 10). For example, if a patient states that he has "pain in his leg at times," the nurse would assess and record the data with the use of PQRSTU:

> Has right midcalf pain that usually occurs at work when climbing stairs after lunch (P). Pain is alleviated by stopping and resting for 2 to 3 minutes. Patient thinks this pain is a "muscle cramp" and states he has been "eating a banana every day for extra potassium" but "it hasn't helped" (U, P). Pain is described as "stabbing" and is nonradiating (Q, R). Pain is so severe (rating 9 on 0–10 scale) that patient cannot continue activity (S). Onset is abrupt, occurring once or twice daily. It last occurred yesterday while he was cutting the lawn (T).

Past Health History

The past health history provides information about the patient's prior state of health. The patient is asked specifically about major childhood and adult illnesses, injuries, hospitalizations, surgeries, obstetrical history (if relevant), immunizations, and allergies. This documentation should include questions about any infectious diseases such as human immunodeficiency virus (HIV) infection, hepatitis, methicillin-resistant *Staphylococcus aureus* (MRSA) infection, and vancomycin-resistant enterococcal (VRE) infection. Specific questions are more effective than simple questions of whether the patient has had any illness or health issues in the past. For example, the question "Do you have a history of diabetes?" elicits better information than does "Do you have any chronic health problems?"

Medications. The nurse should obtain specific details related to past and current medications, including prescription, medical recreational (e.g., cannabis), and over-the-counter drugs; vitamins; herbs; traditional medicines; nutritional supplements; and illegal substance use. The brown-bag technique encourages patients to bring all of their medications, herbs, and supplements with them and is effective in determining what medications the patient is taking and how they are taking them. Indigenous patients should feel safe and respected when asked to share any traditional medicines they are using. It's important for the nurse to ask about all types of medicines because they can interact adversely with existing or newly prescribed medications (see Chapter 12, Table 12.5). Older patients and chronically ill patients should be questioned about medication routines; for these patients, polypharmacy, changes in absorption, distribution, metabolism, and elimination of and reaction to medications can pose serious potential problems (Touhy et al., 2018).

Family Health History

The nurse should ask about the health of family members, as well as the ages at and cause of death of blood relatives, such as parents, siblings, and grandparents. Common questions include those about any family history of heart disease, high blood pressure, stroke, diabetes, blood disorders, cancer, sickle cell disease, arthritis, allergies, obesity, alcoholism, mental health issues or illness, seizure disorder, kidney disease, and tuberculosis (Jarvis et al., 2019). A genogram or family tree will help the nurse accurately document this information. Family health histories may be difficult to obtain from some Indigenous people for a variety of reasons, such as being separated from their families during the Sixties Scoop and relocation to residential schools, not understanding medical terminology, not being aware of relatives' illnesses and hospitalizations, experiencing fragmented care in remote communities, and lacking trust in the health care system.

Review of Systems

The nurse should use a head-to-toe approach to inquire about past and current health states of each body system. This part of the nursing history records subjective data only and provides an opportunity to collect data that may have been omitted in previous categories as well as health promotion practices. System-specific assessment questions are included in the assessment chapters of this text (see, for example, Chapter 34, Table 34.2 for health history of the cardiovascular system). Detailed health assessment textbooks will provide additional information, formats, and examples of completed review of systems documentation.

Functional Health Assessment

The nurse assesses the patient's overall self-care ability, including activities of daily living (ADLs) such as bathing, dressing, toileting, eating, and walking, as well as instrumental activities of daily living (IADLs), or activities needed for independent living such as housekeeping, shopping, cooking, doing laundry, using the telephone, and managing finances; getting adequate nutrition; having social relationships and resources; promoting self-concept; and coping and maintaining a home environment (Jarvis et al., 2019). Assessing functional health enables the nurse to identify positive, dysfunctional, and potentially dysfunctional patterns. Dysfunctional health patterns result in

nursing diagnoses, and potential dysfunctional patterns identify risk conditions for health concerns. Gordon's (2014) functional health pattern framework for assessment can assist the nurse in differentiating between areas for independent nursing intervention and areas necessitating collaboration or referral. The nurse may identify patients with effective health functions who express a desire for a higher level of wellness.

It is also important to consider the social determinants of health to ensure a complete and relevant health history assessment. The nurse should explore the patient's living conditions by asking about employment, working conditions, well-being, health and social services received, and the ability to obtain a quality education, food, and housing, among other factors (Mikkonen & Raphael, 2010).

Health Perception–Health Management. Assessment of the patient's health perception and health management focuses on the patient's perceived level of health and well-being and on personal practices for maintaining health. The nurse should ask the patient to describe their personal health and any concerns they might have. The patient's opinions about the effectiveness of health maintenance practices can be explored with questions about what helps and what hinders their well-being. The nurse should ask the patient to rate their health as excellent, good, fair, or poor. When possible, this information is best recorded in the patient's own words. Asking about the type of health care providers that the patient uses is also important. For example, if the patient is an Indigenous Canadian, a traditional healer may be considered the primary health care provider. If the patient is of Chinese origin, a Chinese healer who practices traditional Chinese medicine may be the primary health care provider.

Other questions are used to identify risk factors, by obtaining a thorough family history (e.g., cardiac disease, cancer, genetic disorders), history of personal health habits (e.g., tobacco, alcohol, drug use), and history of exposure to environmental hazards (e.g., asbestos). If the patient is hospitalized, the nurse should ask about their expectations for this experience. The patient can be asked to describe their understanding of the current health issue, including its onset, course, and treatment. These questions elicit information about a patient's knowledge of their health issue and their ability to use appropriate resources to manage it.

Nutrition–Metabolic. The nurse must assess the patient's processes of ingestion, digestion, absorption, and metabolism. A 24-hour dietary recall should be obtained from the patient to evaluate the quantity and quality of foods and fluids consumed. If a problem is identified, the nurse may ask the patient to keep a 3-day food diary for a more careful analysis of dietary intake. The effect of psychological factors such as depression, anxiety, stress, and self-concept on nutrition should be assessed. In addition, socioeconomic and cultural factors such as food budget, who prepares the meals, and food preferences are also recorded. To determine whether the patient's present condition has interfered with eating and appetite, the nurse can explore any symptoms of nausea, intestinal gas, or pain. Food allergies should be differentiated from food intolerances, such as lactose or gluten intolerance.

Elimination. To assess bowel, bladder, and skin function, the nurse should ask the patient about the frequency of bowel and bladder activity, including laxative and diuretic use. The skin is assessed again in the elimination pattern in terms of its excretory function.

Activity–Exercise. The nurse assesses the patient's usual pattern of exercise, work activity, leisure, and recreation. The patient should be questioned about their ability to perform ADLs and any specific problems identified.

Sleep–Rest. It is important for the nurse to describe the patient's perception of their pattern of sleep, rest, and relaxation in a 24-hour period. This information can be elicited by asking, "Do you feel rested when you wake up?"

Cognitive–Perceptual. Assessment of this area involves a description of all of the senses and cognitive functions. Pain is assessed as a sensory perception in this pattern. (See Chapter 10 for details on pain assessment.) The patient should be asked about any sensory deficits that affect their ability to perform ADLs. Ways in which the patient compensates for any sensory-perceptual problems should be recorded. To plan for patient teaching, the nurse can ask the patient how they learn and communicate best and what they understand about the illness and treatment plan. (See Chapter 4 for details on patient teaching.)

Self-Perception–Self-Concept. The nurse should explore the patient's self-concept, which is crucial for determining the way the person interacts with others. Included are attitudes about self, perception of personal abilities, body image, and a general sense of worth. The nurse should ask the patient for a self-description and about how their health condition affects self-concept. A patient's expressions of helplessness or loss of control frequently reflect an inability to care for themselves.

Role–Relationship. The nurse should explore the patient's roles and relationships, including major responsibilities. The patient should be asked to describe family, social, and work roles and relationships and to rate their performance of the expected behaviours related to these. The nurse should determine whether patterns in these roles and relationships are satisfactory or whether strain is evident. The nurse should note the patient's feelings about how the current condition affects their roles and relationships.

Sexuality–Reproductive. The nurse needs to evaluate the patient's satisfaction or dissatisfaction with personal sexuality, sexual identity, and potential reproductive issues. Assessing these aspects is important because many illnesses, surgical procedures, and medications affect sexual function. A patient's sexual and reproductive concerns may be expressed, and teaching needs may be identified through information obtained in this assessment. The interview should be appropriate for the patient's developmental stage as well as their self-identified gender, sexuality, and expression. The nurse should screen for sexual function and dysfunction in a nonjudgemental way and provide information as appropriate or refer the patient to a more experienced health care provider. It is important to acknowledge that discussing sexual health may be difficult for some patients, especially those who have experienced trauma. Some Indigenous people feel humiliated by a discussion about sexuality, as a result of residential school impacts on sexual health through imposed religious beliefs and Western values, sexual abuse, and shaming about sexuality (O'Brien et al., 2009; Wiebe et al., 2015).

Coping–Stress Tolerance. The nurse should describe the patient's general coping pattern and the effectiveness of the coping mechanisms. Assessment of this pattern involves analyzing the specific stressors or problems that confront the patient, the patient's perception of the stressors, and the patient's response to the stressors. The nurse should document any major losses or stressors experienced by the patient in the previous year.

Strategies used by the patient to deal with stressors and relieve tension should be noted. The nurse should ask about individuals and groups that make up the patient's social support networks.

Value–Belief. The nurse should describe the values, goals, and beliefs (including spiritual) that guide health-related choices. The patient's ethnic background and the effects of culture and beliefs on health practices should be documented. The patient's wishes about the continuation of religious or spiritual practices and the use of religious articles should be noted and respected.

PHYSICAL EXAMINATION: OBJECTIVE DATA

General Survey

After the nursing history, the nurse makes a general survey statement. This reflects a general impression of a patient, including behavioural observations. This initial survey begins with the nurse's first encounter with the patient and continues during the health history interview.

The major areas included in the general survey statement are (a) body features, (b) mental state, (c) speech, (d) body movements, (e) obvious physical signs, (f) nutritional status, and (g) behaviour. Vital signs, height, and weight or body mass index (BMI) (calculated from height and weight [kg/m^2]) may be included. The following is a sample of a general survey statement:

A.H. is a 34-year-old Italian woman, BP 130/84, P 88, R 18. No distinguishing body features. Alert but anxious. Speech is rapid, with trailing thoughts. Wringing hands and shuffling feet during the interview. Skin flushed, hands clammy. Overweight relative to height (BMI = 28.3 kg/m2). Sits with eyes downcast, shoulders slumped, and avoids eye contact.

Physical Examination

The physical examination is the systematic assessment of a patient's physical status. Throughout the physical examination, the nurse explores any positive findings, using the same criteria as those used during the investigation of a symptom in the nursing history (see Table 3.1). A *positive finding* indicates that the patient has or had a particular health issue or sign under discussion (e.g., if the patient with jaundice has an enlarged liver, it is a positive finding). Relevant information about this health issue should then be gathered.

Negative findings may also be significant. A *negative finding* is the absence of a sign or symptom usually associated with a health issue. For example, peripheral edema is common with advanced liver disease. If edema is not present in a patient with advanced liver disease, this should be specifically documented as "no peripheral edema."

Techniques. Four major techniques are used in performing the physical examination: inspection, palpation, percussion, and auscultation. The techniques are usually performed in this sequence, except for the abdominal examination (inspection, auscultation, percussion, and palpation). Performing palpation and percussion of the abdomen before auscultation can alter bowel sounds and produce false findings. Not every assessment area requires the use of all four assessment techniques (e.g., for the musculoskeletal system, only inspection and palpation are required).

Inspection. Inspection is the visual examination of a part or region of the body to assess normal and abnormal conditions. Inspection is more than just looking. This technique is

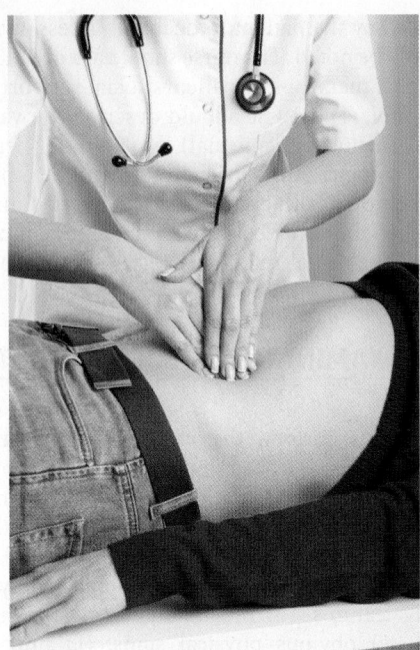

FIG. 3.2 Palpation is the examination of the body using touch. Source: © CanStock Photo Inc. / Bialasiewicz.

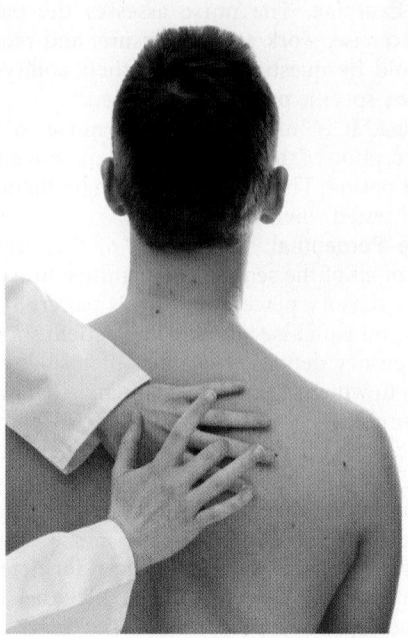

FIG. 3.3 Percussion technique: tapping the interphalangeal joint. Only the middle finger of the nondominant hand should be in contact with the skin surface. Normal percussion sounds for lung tissue are *resonant;* for air-filled viscus (e.g., intestines), *tympany;* for dense organs (e.g., liver), *dull;* and for areas with no air present (e.g., bone, muscle), *flat.* Source: © CanStock Photo Inc. / obencem.

deliberate, systematic, and focused. The nurse must compare what is seen with the known, generally visible characteristics of the body part being inspected. For example, most 30-year-old men have hair on their legs. Absence of hair may indicate a vascular issue and signals the need for further investigation, or it may be normal for a patient of a particular ethnicity (e.g., First Nations men have little body hair).

Palpation. Palpation is the examination of the body through the use of touch. Using light and deep palpation can yield information about masses, pulsations, organ enlargement, tenderness or pain, swelling, muscular spasm or rigidity, elasticity, vibration of voice sounds, crepitus, moisture, and texture. Different parts of the hand are more sensitive for specific assessments. For example, the palmar surface (base of fingers) should be used to feel vibrations; the dorsa (back) of the hands and fingers, to assess skin temperature; and tips of the fingers, to palpate the abdomen (Jarvis et al., 2019) (Figure 3.2).

Percussion. Percussion is a technique of tapping the body directly or indirectly with the fingertips to produce a sound and vibration to obtain information about the underlying area (Figure 3.3). The sounds and the vibrations are specific to the underlying structures. A change from an expected sound may indicate a problem. For example, dullness in the right lower quadrant instead of the normal tympany should be explored. (Specific percussion sounds of various body parts and regions are discussed in the appropriate assessment chapters.)

Auscultation. Auscultation involves using a stethoscope to listen to sounds produced by the body to assess normal and abnormal conditions. This technique is particularly useful in evaluating sounds from the heart, lungs, abdomen, and vascular system. The bell of the stethoscope is more sensitive to low-pitched sounds (e.g., heart murmurs). The diaphragm of the stethoscope is more sensitive to high-pitched sounds (e.g., bowel sounds). Some stethoscopes have only a diaphragm, designed to transmit low- and high-pitched sounds. To listen

for low-pitched sounds, the examiner holds the diaphragm lightly on the patient's skin. For high-pitched sounds, the examiner presses the diaphragm firmly on the skin (Jarvis et al., 2018; Figure 3.4). (Specific auscultatory sounds and techniques are discussed in the appropriate assessment chapters.)

Equipment. The nurse should collect the equipment needed for the physical examination before beginning (Table 3.2). This saves time and energy for the nurse and the patient. (The uses of specific equipment are discussed in the appropriate assessment chapters.)

Organization of the Examination. The physical examination should be performed systematically and efficiently. Explanations should be given to the patient as the examination proceeds, and the patient's comfort, safety, and privacy should be considered. By being confident and self-assured, considerate, and unhurried, the nurse will help reduce any anxiety the patient may be feeling about the examination (Jarvis et al., 2019). Following the same sequence every time helps ensure that the nurse does not forget a procedure, a step in the sequence, or a part of the body. Table 3.3 presents a comprehensive and organized physical examination outline. Adaptations of the physical examination often are useful for older patients, who may have age-related issues such as decreased mobility, limited energy, and perceptual changes.

Recording Physical Examination. At the conclusion of the examination, the nurse records the normal and abnormal findings in the patient's record. Table 3.4 provides an example of how to record the findings of a physical examination of a healthy adult. See Chapter 7, Table 7.2, and the age-related assessment findings in each assessment chapter for helpful references in recording age-related assessment differences.

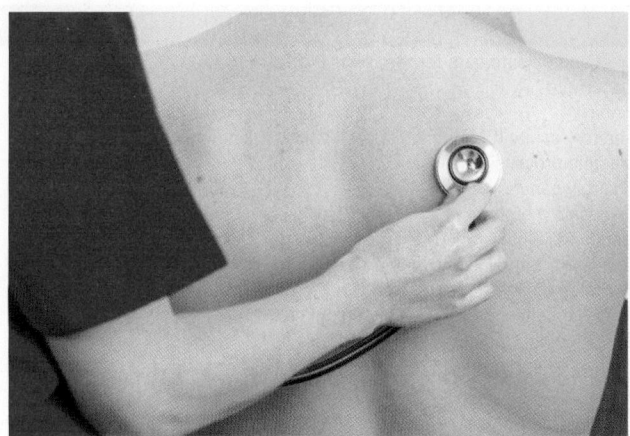

FIG. 3.4 Auscultation is listening to sounds produced by the body to assess normal conditions and deviations from normal. Source: © CanStock Photo Inc. / obencem.

TABLE 3.2	COMMON PHYSICAL EXAMINATION EQUIPMENT

- Alcohol swabs
- Blood pressure cuff
- Cotton balls
- Examining table or bed
- Eye chart (e.g., Snellen eye chart)
- Paper cup with water
- Patient gown
- Pocket flashlight
- Reflex hammer
- Stethoscope (with bell and diaphragm or a dual-purpose diaphragm; 38- to 46-cm tubing)
- Tongue blades
- Watch (with second hand or digital)

TYPES OF ASSESSMENT

Various types of assessment are used to obtain information about a patient. These approaches can be divided into three types: comprehensive, focused, and emergency (Table 3.5). The nurse must decide what type of assessment to perform according to the clinical situation. Sometimes the health care employer provides guidelines, and other times it is a nursing judgement.

Comprehensive Assessment

A *comprehensive assessment* includes detailed documentation of the health history and a physical examination of all body systems. This is typically performed on the patient's admission to the hospital or onset of care in a primary care setting.

Focused Assessment

A *focused assessment* is an abbreviated health history and examination. It is used to evaluate the status of previously identified issues and monitor for signs and symptoms of new issues. It can be performed when a specific condition (e.g., pneumonia) is identified. The patient's clinical manifestations guide a focused assessment. For example, abdominal pain indicates the need for a focused assessment of the abdomen. Some conditions need a focused assessment of more than one body system. A patient with a headache may need

musculoskeletal, neurological, and head and neck examinations. See examples of focused assessments in the appropriate assessment chapters.

Emergency Assessment

In an emergency or a critical care situation, an *emergency assessment* may be performed. This involves a rapid history and examination of a patient while supporting vital functions.

Using Assessment Approaches

Assessment in an inpatient, acute-care hospital setting can be markedly different from assessments in other settings. Focused assessment of the hospitalized patient is frequent and performed by many different people. An interprofessional team approach demands a high degree of consistency among health care providers.

While providing ongoing care for a patient, the nurse constantly refines their mental image of the patient. With experience, the nurse will derive a mental image of a patient's status from a few very basic details, such as "85-year-old Black woman admitted for COPD [chronic obstructive pulmonary disease] exacerbation." Details from a complete verbal report, including the length of stay, laboratory results, physical findings, and vital signs, will help the nurse make a clearer picture. Next, the nurse will perform their own assessment, using a focused approach. During this assessment, the nurse confirms or revises the findings that were read in the medical record and received from other health care providers.

The process does not end once the nurse has completed their first assessment of a patient; rather, the nurse will have to continue to gather information about their patients throughout the shift. Everything that the nurse learned previously about each patient is considered in light of new information. For example, while the nurse is performing a respiratory assessment on a patient with COPD, crackles are heard in the lungs. This finding should lead the nurse to perform a cardiovascular assessment because cardiac issues (e.g., heart failure) can also cause crackles. As the nurse gains experience, the importance of new findings will be more obvious. (See assessment case studies in the appropriate assessment chapters.)

Table 3.6 shows how the nurse can perform different types of assessments on the basis of a patient's progress through a given hospitalization. When a patient arrives at the emergency department with a life-threatening condition, the nurse performs an emergency assessment on the basis of the elements of a primary survey (e.g., airway, breathing, circulation, disability; see Chapter 71, Table 71.5). Once the patient is stabilized, the nurse can begin a focused assessment of the respiratory and related body systems. After the patient is admitted, a comprehensive assessment of all body systems is completed.

PROBLEM IDENTIFICATION AND NURSING DIAGNOSES

After completing the history and physical examination, the nurse analyzes the data and develops a list of nursing diagnoses and collaborative problems. See Chapter 1 for a description of the nursing process, including the identification of nursing diagnoses and collaborative problems.

TABLE 3.3 OUTLINE FOR PHYSICAL EXAMINATION

1. General Survey
Observe general state of health (patient is seated):
- Body features
- Mental state and level of orientation
- Speech
- Body movements
- Physical appearance
- Nutritional status
- Behaviour

2. Vital Signs
Record vital signs:
- Blood pressure—both arms for comparison
- Apical/radial pulse
- Respiration
- Temperature
- Oxygen saturation
- Pain score

Record height and weight; calculate body mass index (BMI)

3. Integument
Inspect and palpate skin for the following:
- Colour
- Integrity (e.g., lesions, breakdown, lacerations)
- Scars, tattoos, piercings
- Bruises, rash
- Edema
- Moisture
- Texture
- Temperature
- Turgor
- Vascularity

Inspect and palpate nails for the following:
- Colour
- Lesions
- Size
- Shape
- Angle
- Capillary refill time

4. Head and Neck
Inspect and palpate head for the following:
- Shape and symmetry of skull
- Masses
- Tenderness
- Condition of hair and scalp
- Temporal arteries
- Temporomandibular joint
- Sensory (CN V; light touch, pain)
- Motor (CN VII; shows teeth, purses lips, raises eyebrows)
- Facial expression (CN VII; looks up, wrinkles forehead)
- Strength (CN XI; raises shoulders against resistance)

Inspect and palpate (occasionally auscultate) neck for the following:
- Skin (vascularity and visible pulsations)
- Symmetry
- Range of motion
- Pulses and bruits (carotid)
- Midline structure (trachea, thyroid gland, cartilage)
- Lymph nodes (preauricular, postauricular, occipital, mandibular, tonsillar, submental, anterior and posterior cervical, infraclavicular, supraclavicular)

Test visual acuity. Inspect and palpate eyes/eyebrows for the following:
- Position and movement of eyelids (CN VII)
- Visual fields (CN II)
- Extraocular movements (CN III, IV, VI)
- Cornea, sclera, conjunctiva
- Pupillary response (CN III)
- Retinal (red) reflex

Inspect and palpate nose and sinuses for the following:
- External nose: shape, blockage
- Internal nose: patency of nasal passages, shape, turbinates or polyps, discharge
- Frontal and maxillary sinuses

Inspect and palpate ears for the following:
- Placement
- Pinna
- Auditory acuity (CN VIII; whispered voice, ticking watch)
- Mastoid process
- Auditory canal
- Tympanic membrane

Inspect and palpate mouth for the following:
- Lips (symmetry, lesions, colour)
- Buccal mucosa (Stensen's and Wharton's ducts)
- Teeth (absence, state of repair, colour)
- Gums (colour, receding from teeth)
- Tongue for strength (CN XII; asymmetry, ability to stick out tongue, move side to side, fasciculations)
- Palates
- Tonsils and pillars
- Uvular elevation (CN IX)
- Posterior pharynx
- Gag reflex (CN IX and X)
- Jaw strength (CN V)
- Moisture
- Colour
- Floor of mouth

5. Extremities
Observe size and shape, symmetry and deformity, involuntary movements. Inspect and palpate arms, fingers, wrists, elbows, shoulders for the following:
- Strength
- Range of motion
- Joint pain
- Swelling
- Pulses (radial, brachial)
- Sensation (light tough, pain, temperature)
- Test reflexes: triceps, biceps, brachioradialis

Inspect and palpate legs for the following:
- Strength
- Range of motion
- Joint pain
- Swelling, edema
- Hair distribution
- Sensation (light touch, pain, temperature)
- Pulses (dorsalis pedis, posterior tibialis)
- Test reflexes: patellar, Achilles, plantar

6. Posterior Thorax
- *Inspect* for muscular development, scoliosis, respiratory movement, an approximation of AP diameter.
- *Palpate* for symmetry of respiratory movement, tenderness of CVA, spinous processes, tumours or swelling, tactile fremitus
- *Percuss* for pulmonary resonance
- *Auscultate* for breath sounds
- *Auscultate* for egophony, bronchophony, whispered pectoriloquy

7. Anterior Thorax
- *Assess* breasts for configuration, symmetry, dimpling of skin
- *Assess* nipples for rash, direction, inversion, retraction
- *Inspect* for apical impulse, other precordial pulsations
- *Palpate* the apical impulse and the precordium for thrills, lifts, heaves, tenderness
- *Inspect* neck for venous distension, pulsations, waves
- *Palpate* lymph nodes in the subclavian, axillary, and brachial areas
- *Palpate* breasts
- *Auscultate* for rate and rhythm, character of S_1 and S_2 in the aortic, pulmonic, Erb's point, tricuspid, and mitral areas; bruits at carotid, epigastrium

8. Abdomen
- *Inspect* for scars, shape, symmetry, bulging, muscular position and condition of umbilicus, movements (respiratory, pulsations, presence of peristaltic waves)
- *Auscultate* for peristalsis (e.g., bowel sounds), bruits
- *Percuss then palpate* to confirm positive findings: check liver (size, tenderness), spleen, kidney (size, tenderness), urinary bladder (distension)
- *Palpate* femoral pulses, inguinofemoral nodes, and abdominal aorta

TABLE 3.3 OUTLINE FOR PHYSICAL EXAMINATION—cont'd

9. Neurological
Observe motor status.
- Gait
- Toe walk
- Heel walk
- Drift

Observe coordination.
- Finger to nose
- Romberg sign
- Heel to opposite shin

Observe the following:
- Proprioception (position sense of great toe)

10. Genitalia
Male External Genitalia
- *Inspect* penis, noting hair distribution, prepuce, glans, urethral meatus, scars, ulcers, eruptions, structural alterations, discharge
- *Inspect* epidermis of perineum, rectum
- *Inspect* skin of scrotum; *palpate* for descended testes, masses, pain

Female External Genitalia
- *Inspect* hair distribution; mons pubis, labia (minora and majora); urethral meatus; Bartholin's, urethral, Skene's glands (may be palpated, if indicated); introitus; any discharge
- *Assess* for presence of cystocele, prolapse
- *Inspect* perineum, rectum

AP, anteroposterior; *CN,* cranial nerve; *CVA,* costovertebral angle; *S₁ and S₂,* first and second heart sounds.

TABLE 3.4 FINDINGS FROM A PHYSICAL EXAMINATION OF A HEALTHY ADULT

Example
Patient's Name: _____
Age:

General Status
Well-nourished, well-hydrated, well-developed White [woman or man] in NAD, appears stated age, speech clear and evenly paced; is alert and oriented × 3; cooperative, calm; BMI 23.8

Skin
Clear s̄ lesions, warm and dry, trunk warmer than extremities, normal skin turgor, no ↑ vascularity, no varicose veins

Nails
Well-groomed, round 160-degree angle s̄ lesions, nail beds pink, capillary refill <2 sec

Hair
Thick, brown, shiny, normal [male, female] distribution

Head
Normocephalic, nontender

Eyes
Visual fields intact on gross confrontation
Visual acuity:
Right eye 20/20
Left eye 20/20
Both eyes 20/20 s̄ glasses
EOM: Intact on all gazes s̄ ptosis, nystagmus
Pupils: PERRLA, negative cover and uncover tests

Ears
Pinnae intact, in proper alignment; external canal patent; small amount of cerumen present bilaterally; TMs intact; pearly-grey LM, LR visible, not bulging; whisper heard at 90 cm (3 ft) bilaterally

Nose
Patent bilaterally; turbinates pink, no swelling
Sinuses nontender

Mouth
Moist and pink, soft and hard palates intact, uvula rises midline on "ahh," 24 teeth present and in good repair

Throat
Tonsils surgically removed, no redness

Tongue
Moist, pink, size appropriate for mouth, no lesions

Neck
Supple, s̄ masses, s̄ bruits, lymph nodes nonpalpable and nontender
Thyroid: Palpable, smooth, not enlarged
ROM: Full, intact, strong
Trachea: Midline, nontender

Breasts
Soft, nonpendulous, s̄ venous pattern, s̄ dimpling, puckering
Nipples: s̄ inversion, point in same direction, areola dark and symmetric, no discharge, no masses, nontender

Axilla
Hair present, no lesions, no palpable lymph nodes

Thorax and Lungs
Respiratory rate 18, regular rhythm, oxygen saturation 98% on room air; AP < transverse diameter, no ↑ in tactile fremitus, no tenderness, lungs resonant throughout, diaphragmatic excursion 4 cm bilaterally, chest expansion symmetric, lung fields clear throughout

Heart
Rate 82, regular rate and rhythm; blood pressure: RA: 122/76, LA: 120/78; no lifts, heaves
Apical impulse: 5th ICS at MCL; no palpable thrills; S₁, S₂ louder, softer in appropriate locations; no S₃, S₄; no murmurs, rubs, clicks
Carotid, femoral, pedal, and radial pulses present; equal, 2+ bilaterally

Abdomen
No pulsations visible, rounded, positive bowel sounds in four quadrants; no bruits or CVA tenderness, no palpable masses

Liver
Lower border percussed at costal margin, smooth, nontender; approx 9-cm span

Spleen
Nonpalpable, nontender

Neurological System
Cranial nerves I–XII intact
Motor (drift, toe stand) intact
Coordination (FN, Romberg) intact
Reflexes: See diagram

Grading Scale
0 No response
1+ Diminished
2+ Normal
3+ Increased
4+ Hyperactive
Sensation (touch, vibration, proprioception) normal bilaterally, upper and lower extremities

Continued

TABLE 3.4 FINDINGS FROM A PHYSICAL EXAMINATION OF A HEALTHY ADULT—cont'd

Musculoskeletal System

Well-developed, no muscle wasting; $\overline{S}$ crepitus, nodules, swelling; no scoliosis

ROM: Full and equal bilaterally, upper and lower extremities

Strength: Equal, strong 5/5 bilaterally, upper and lower extremities

Gait: Walks erect 60-cm (2 ft) steps, arms swinging at side $\overline{S}$ staggering

Female Genitalia*

External genitalia: No swelling, redness, tenderness in BUS; normal hair distribution, no cysts

Vagina: No lesions, discharge, bulging; pink

Cervix: Os closed; pink, no lesions, erosions, nontender

Uterus: Small, firm, nontender

Adnexa: No enlargement; nontender

Rectovaginal: Sphincter intact; confirms above findings

Male Genitalia*

Normal male hair distribution, negative inguinal hernia

Penis: Urethral opening patent; no redness, swelling, discharge; no lesions, structural changes

Scrotum: Testes descended; no redness, masses, tenderness

Rectal: No lesions, redness; sphincter intact; prostate small, nontender

*Some data would be obtained only if the nurse has the appropriate training.

AP, anteroposterior; *BMI*, body mass index; *BUS*, Bartholin's gland, urethral meatus, Skene's duct; *CVA*, costovertebral angle; *EOM*, extraocular movements; *FN*, finger to nose; *ICS*, intercostal space; *LA*, left arm; *LM*, landmark; *LR*, light reflex; *MCL*, midclavicular line; *NAD*, no acute distress; *PERRLA*, pupils equal, round, reactive to light and accommodation; *RA*, right arm; *ROM*, range of motion; $\overline{S}$, without; S_1, S_2, S_3, and S_4, heart sounds; *TM*, tympanic membrane.

TABLE 3.5 TYPES OF ASSESSMENT

The following describes types of assessment that the nurse may use in various situations.

Description	When and Where Performed	Where to Find in Book
Comprehensive • Detailed assessment of all body systems (head-to-toe assessment)	• Onset of care in primary or ambulatory care setting • On admission to hospital, rehabilitation, or long-term care setting • On initial home care visit	• Assessment chapters for each body system • Outline for physical examination (see Table 3.3) • Findings from physical examination of a healthy adult (see Table 3.4)
Focused • Abbreviated assessment that focuses on one or more body systems that are the focus of care • Includes an assessment related to a specific problem (e.g., pneumonia, specific abnormal laboratory findings) • Monitors for signs and symptoms of new problems	• Throughout hospital admission: at beginning of a shift and as needed throughout shift • Revisit in ambulatory care setting or home care setting	• Focused assessment boxes in each assessment chapter • Tables on nursing assessment of specific diseases throughout book
Emergency • Limited to assessing life-threatening conditions (e.g., inhalation injuries, anaphylaxis, myocardial infarction, shock, stroke) • Conducted to ensure survival. Focuses on elements in the primary survey (e.g., airway, breathing, circulation disability) • After life-saving interventions are started, brief systematic assessments are performed to identify any and all other injuries or problems	• Performed in any setting when signs or symptoms of a life-threatening condition appear (e.g., emergency department, critical care unit, surgical setting)	• Chapter 71, Tables 71.3 and 71.5 • Emergency management tables throughout the book and listed in Table 71.1

TABLE 3.6 CLINICAL APPLICATIONS FOR TYPES OF ASSESSMENT

The following is an example of how various types of assessment would be used for a patient progressing from the emergency department to a clinical unit of a hospital.

Timeline	Type of Assessment
Emergency Department	
Patient arrives in acute respiratory distress.	Emergency assessment (see Table 71.3) is performed.
Problem is identified, critical interventions are performed.	Focused assessments of the respiratory and related body systems (e.g., cardiovascular) are performed.
Patient stabilizes.	Comprehensive assessment of all body systems may begin.
Clinical Unit	
Patient is admitted to a monitored clinical unit.	Complete comprehensive assessment of all body systems is performed within proper time frame.
At beginning of each shift, patient is reassessed per orders and more frequently as determined by the nurse.	Focused assessments of respiratory system and other related body systems are performed per hospital policy. Focused assessment of appropriate body system(s) is performed if new symptoms are reported.

REVIEW QUESTIONS

The number of each question corresponds to the same-numbered outcome at the beginning of the chapter.

1. The patient's health history and physical examination findings enable the nurse with information to primarily take which action?
   a. Diagnose a medical condition.
   b. Investigate the client's signs and symptoms.
   c. Classify subjective and objective client data.
   d. Identify nursing diagnoses and collaborative problems.

2. The nurse would place information about the patient's concern that his illness is threatening his job security in which functional health pattern?
   a. Role–relationship
   b. Cognitive–perceptual
   c. Coping–stress tolerance
   d. Health perception–health management

3. The nurse is preparing to examine a patient's abdomen. Place in order the proper steps for an abdominal assessment, using the numbers 1–4, with 1 = the first technique and 4 = the last technique.
   ___ Inspection
   ___ Palpation
   ___ Percussion
   ___ Auscultation

4. Which situation would require the nurse to perform a focused assessment? *(Select all that apply.)*
   a. A patient denies a current health issue.
   b. A patient reports a new symptom during rounds.
   c. A previously identified health issue needs reassessment.
   d. A baseline health maintenance examination is required.
   e. An emergency condition is identified during physical examination.

1. d; 2. a; 3. 1, 4, 3, 2; 4. b, c.

Ⓔvolve

For even more review questions, visit http://evolve.elsevier.com/Canada/Lewis/medsurg.

REFERENCES

Canadian Nurses Association (CNA). (2017). *Code of ethics for registered nurses.* https://www.cna-aiic.ca/~/media/cna/page-content/pdf-en/code-of-ethics-2017-edition-secure-interactive.pdf?la=en

Gordon, M. (2014). *Manual of nursing diagnosis* (13th ed.). Jones & Bartlett. (Seminal).

Jarvis, C., Browne, A., MacDonald-Jenkins, J., et al. (Eds.). (2019). *Physical examination and health assessment* (3rd Canadian ed.) Saunders.

Mikkonen, J., & Raphael, D. (2010). *Social determinants of health: The Canadian facts.* Toronto: York University School of Health Policy and Management. www.thecanadianfacts.org. (Seminal).

O'Brien, B. A., Mill, J., & Wilson, T. (2009). Cervical screening in Canadian First Nation Cree Women. *Journal of Transcultural Nursing, 20*(1), 83–92.

Registered Nurses' Association of Ontario (RNAO). (2006). *Establishing therapeutic relationships. Supplement.* https://rnao.ca/sites/rnao-ca/files/storage/related/943_BPG_TR_Supplement.pdf. (Seminal).

Touhy, T., Jett, K., Boscart, V., et al. (2018). *Ebersole and Hess' gerontological nursing and healthy aging in Canada* (2nd ed.). Mosby.

Wiebe, A. D., Barton, S., Auger, L., et al. (2015). Restoring the blessings of the Morning Star: Childbirth and maternal-infant health for First Nations near Edmonton, Alberta. *Aboriginal Policy Studies, 5*(1), 47–68.

Ⓔvolve

For additional Internet resources, see the website for this book at http://evolve.elsevier.com/Canada/Lewis/medsurg.

4

Patient and Caregiver Teaching

Mary Kate Garrity
Originating US chapter by Brenda C. Morris

evolve WEBSITE

http://evolve.elsevier.com/Canada/Lewis/medsurg

- Review Questions (Online Only)
- Key Points
- Answer Guidelines for Case Study

- Conceptual Care Map Creator
- Audio Glossary
- Content Updates

LEARNING OBJECTIVES

1. Prioritize four specific goals of patient and caregiver teaching.
2. Identify adult learning principles and explore their teaching implications.
3. Analyze specific competencies that enhance the nurse's effectiveness as a teacher.
4. Formulate strategies to manage the challenges to the nurse's teaching effectiveness.
5. Examine the intended role of the family in patient teaching.
6. Explain the basic steps in the teaching–learning process.

7. Relate physical, psychological, and sociocultural characteristics of the patient to the teaching–learning process.
8. Describe the components of a correctly written learning outcome.
9. Appraise advantages, disadvantages, and uses of various teaching strategies.
10. Examine common methods of short- and long-term evaluation.

KEY TERMS

andragogy	learning	stages of behavioural change
demonstration–return demonstration	learning needs	teach-back strategy
empathy	learning outcomes	teaching
geragogy	learning style	teaching plan
facilitator	peer teaching	teaching process
family care conferences	self-efficacy	

ROLE OF PATIENT AND CAREGIVER TEACHING

Teaching patients and caregivers (family members or significant others) is a dynamic and interactive process. It is one of the most important and challenging roles that nurses face in the current health care system. Patient education can occur in any setting—the community, schools, industry, ambulatory care centres, hospitals, long-term care facilities, retirement residences, and homes. Constraints on staff time and resources, coupled with the shortened average length of inpatient hospitalizations, can affect the nurse's ability to engage in patient education.

Inadequate patient teaching frequently results in devastating consequences for the patient and caregiver. For this reason, it is important that the nurse recognize moments when teaching tasks can be delegated. For example, the nurse completes the assessment of the patient, including readiness and motivation

to learn and the most appropriate teaching method, and then delegates a specific task to a registered practical nurse, such as providing written pamphlets to the patient. Teaching patients about promoting, maintaining, and restoring their health is a required nursing skill that often results in improving the overall health care system, better health outcomes, and a reduction in health complications.

Nurses engage in patient education to help patients and their caregivers optimize their health and to assist them in managing acute and chronic health conditions. Specifically, teaching goals include (a) maintenance of health, (b) health promotion and prevention of disease, (c) management of illness, and (d) appropriate selection and use of treatment and resources. Furthermore, these goals facilitate a high level of wellness that is meaningful to and relevant for the patient throughout the lifespan. Effective teaching can assist people in making informed decisions about their lifestyle, health practices, and treatment choices. For patients who have acute health conditions, quality teaching can prevent complications and promote recovery. For patients with chronic illnesses, increased knowledge can promote self-care and independence.

Many patients require assistance from family members or other caregivers in managing their health conditions. **Family care conferences** are held mainly in hospitals, long-term care facilities, and retirement settings. These conferences provide opportunities for patients and their caregivers, along with members of the interdisciplinary health care team, to identify care needs, evaluate care goals, and assist with health care matters (Puurveen et al., 2019). In fact, the involvement of the caregiver is considered one of the key variables influencing patient outcomes (Bastable, 2017). In family conferences, the interdisciplinary team uses knowledge and skills to teach the patient and caregiver about strategies to promote health and prevent complications, assess additional care needs, and share information about community supports.

Every interaction with a patient and a caregiver is a potential *teachable moment*. The teaching episodes expected from nurses are not complex. For example, teaching a patient to cough effectively and to breathe deeply after surgery can help the patient prevent atelectasis. However, when a patient has specific learning needs, such as management of a health issue, a teaching plan should be developed and implemented with the patient. A **teaching plan** includes (1) assessment of the patient's ability and readiness to learn, (2) identification of teaching needs, (3) development of learning goals with the patient, (4) implementation of the teaching, and (5) evaluation of the patient's learning. The nurse, in collaboration with the patient, chooses activities and experiences to facilitate learning to improve the health of the patient. It then becomes necessary to evaluate the achievement of those outcomes (Billings & Halstead, 2016). This chapter describes the steps involved in providing patient and caregiver education and discusses factors that contribute to successful educational experiences.

TEACHING–LEARNING PROCESS

Teaching is a process of deliberately planning experiences and sharing knowledge to meet learner outcomes in the cognitive, affective, and psychomotor domains. Teaching always endeavours to incorporate incidental experiences. Effective teaching can be conducted using a combination of traditional methods, such as printed materials and clinical teaching, and nontraditional methods, such as simulation, mobile applications, and gaming (Farley, 2020).

Learning is the act of a person acquiring knowledge, skills, or attitudes that may result in a permanent change. A vital aspect of the nursing role is to assess a patient's motivation and desire for wellness and understand which factors promote learning (Marshall et al., 2016).

The teaching–learning process involves the patient, the nurse, and the caregiver or social support system. The interdisciplinary team may also participate and can demonstrate accountability and responsibility for patient education based on solid principles of teaching and learning.

Adult Learners

Adult Learning Principles. Through educational research and theoretical development pertaining specifically to adults,

TABLE 4.1	PRINCIPLES OF ADULT EDUCATION APPLIED TO PATIENT TEACHING
Principle	**Teaching Implications for the Nurse**
Adults are independent learners.	• The teacher is a facilitator who directs the patient to resources but is not the source of all information. • Patients expect to make decisions about their own lives and learning experiences and to take responsibility for those decisions. • Respect for the patient's independence can be reflected in statements such as "What do you think you need to learn about this topic?"
Readiness to learn arises from life's changes.	• Patients see life processes as problems to be solved. • Readiness and motivation to learn are high when new tasks are faced. • Crises in health are "teachable moments."
Past experiences are resources for learning.	• Patients have had many life experiences and have engaged in informal learning for years. • Motivation is increased when patients believe that they already know something about the subject from past experiences. • Identifying past knowledge and experiences can familiarize patients with a new situation and increase their confidence.
Adults learn best when the topic is of immediate value.	• Patients need to apply learning immediately. • Long-term goals may have little appeal. • Short-term, realistic goals should be encouraged. • Education should be focused on information that the patient views as being needed right now.
Adults approach learning as problem solving.	• Patients seek out various resources for specific learning to help them deal with an issue • Information that is not relevant to the issue is not readily learned. • When the patient does not recognize relevancy, explanations for the need to learn something should be offered. • Teaching should target the specific issue or circumstance.
Adults see themselves as doers.	• Patients learn better by doing. • Demonstrations, computer activities, and practice of skills should be offered when appropriate.
Adults resist learning when conditions are incongruent with their self-concepts.	• Patients do not learn when they are treated as children and told what they must do. • Patients need control and self-direction to maintain their sense of self-worth.

investigators have identified specific principles and characteristics that differentiate adult's and children's learning styles. These concepts provide a foundation for the effective teaching of adults. Many adult learning theories have arisen from the work of Knowles (1990), who identified seven principles of **andragogy** (methods of teaching adult learners) that are deemed essential for the nurse to consider when teaching adults. These principles and their implications for patient teaching are presented in Table 4.1.

Determinants of Learning. Because of the combined effects of health care trends and population demographics, the nurse must carefully assess all the patient's determinants of learning prior to teaching. The three determinants of learning that require learning assessments are identified in Table 4.2.

TABLE 4.2	DETERMINANTS OF LEARNING

- The needs of the learner—Assist learner to identify, clarify, and prioritize their needs and interests.
- The state of readiness to learn—Seize the moment when the learner demonstrates an interest in learning the material necessary to maintain optimal health. This is the *teachable moment.*
- The preferred learning style for processing knowledge and information—Assess the various teaching techniques and the teaching–learning conditions under which these learners are most likely to perceive, process, store, and recall health-related material.

Source: Bastable, S. B. (2017). *Nurse as educator: Principles of teaching and learning for nursing practice* (5th ed.). Jones & Bartlett.

Motivation of Adult Learners. One important factor that is strongly associated with motivation is *emotional readiness* (Bastable, 2017). When a nurse is teaching an adult, it is important to identify what that adult values so that motivation can be enhanced. If the adult perceives a need for information to enhance health or avoid illness or if the adult believes that a behaviour change has health value, motivation to learn is increased. Humans seek out experiences that stimulate their desire and effort to learn. Therefore learning activities must be stimulating to maintain a desire to reach a goal. *Motivational interviewing* has been shown to promote behaviour change in patients in various health care settings. It is a counselling approach that serves many goals, such as increasing rapport, helping patients feel understood, reducing the likelihood of resistance to change, and allowing patients to explore their inner thoughts and motivation. For example, a common therapeutic intervention for using motivational interviewing is smoking cessation. Helping patients discover their intrinsic motivation(s) demonstrates further readiness for change and, ultimately, more successful outcomes of permanent smoking cessation. This approach supports self-efficacy in patients, meaning that patients' confidence in their ability to change is acknowledged as critical to successful change efforts (Lundahl et al., 2010). (See Chapter 11 for more information regarding motivational interviewing.)

When a change in health-related behaviours is recommended, patients and their families may progress through a series of steps before they are willing or able to accept the need for and make the change. Six stages of change have been identified in the transtheoretical model of health behaviour change developed by Prochaska and Velicer (1997). The **stages of behavioural change** and their implications for patient teaching are described in Table 4.3. It is important to note that individuals progress through these stages at their own pace and that progression through the stages is often cyclic. Therefore it is reasonable to expect a patient to experience periods of relapse, whereby the process must be restarted. Accurate assessment of the patient's stage of change can help the nurse guide the patient through one stage and on to the next.

While much of health teaching focuses on a patient's lifestyle and behaviour, it is important for the nurse to understand that a patient's readiness to learn also involves a reflection of personal beliefs and values that may have a negative effect on health.

Nurse as Teacher

Required Competencies

Knowledge of Subject Matter. Although it is impossible to be an expert in all areas, the nurse can develop confidence as a teacher by acquiring knowledge of the matter that is to be taught. For example, if a nurse is teaching a patient about the management of hypertension, the nurse must be able to explain what hypertension is, why it is important to treat the disease, and what the patient needs to know about exercise, diet, and the effects of medication, both expected and adverse. The nurse should be able to teach the patient how to use blood pressure equipment to monitor their blood pressure and identify situations that should be reported to a health care provider. In addition, the nurse should provide the patient with sources of additional information such as brochures, appropriate websites, and support organizations (e.g., Canadian Heart and Stroke Foundation).

Unique situations can occur when information or policies about health conditions change with time. A prime example of this is COVID-19. Infection with SARS-CoV-2 is a global health concern, with information about the virus and its effects on the population constantly changing. Nurses can offer reassurance to their patients by sharing current information but also adding that information may change as more research is conducted. Nurses can explain to their patients why precautions are being taken. This may provide reassurance to the patient.

It is not unusual for a patient to ask questions that the nurse may not be able to answer. If unsure of the response, the nurse should inform the patient of this, seek additional information to answer the question, and then return to the patient to provide the response.

Communication Skills. Patient education is an interactive and dynamic process. Through effective communication skills, the nurse can establish a valuable partnership with the patient and caregiver. In such a partnership, the nurse can provide a highly supportive environment conducive to the empowerment and self-efficacy of the patient and caregiver (Lind & Mahler, 2019).

Empowerment has become increasingly important in the education of patients and caregivers. *Patient empowerment* may be defined as "a process that enables patients to exert more influence over their individual health by increasing their capacities to gain more control over issues they themselves define as important" (Castro et al., 2016, p. 5). Specifically, nurses can help patients identify their own internal strengths and self-care abilities, both of which can be called on to address health care issues. Nurses can address the need for caregivers to support the rights of patients and ensure that patients have access to the resources necessary to achieve optimal health.

During the teaching process, the nurse should use basic therapeutic communication skills and strategies to support, educate, and empower patients to cope effectively with health-related issues (Arnold & Boggs, 2016). These basic communication skills encompass both verbal and nonverbal components and are described in Chapter 3 in the section "Interviewing Considerations." The value of effective communication skills is to promote safe and empathic ways for patients to explore their illness experience. Terms that convey respect for the culture, spiritual beliefs, and educational level of the patient and of the caregiver are essential. The use of medical jargon is unnecessary and can be omitted (Arnold & Boggs, 2016). To provide positive nonverbal messages, the nurse should sit at eye level with the patient, facing the patient in an open and relaxed position (Figure 4.1).

It is important for the nurse to develop the art of active listening. This means paying attention to what is said as well as observing the patient's nonverbal cues. The nurse needs to concentrate on the patient as a communicator of vital information and not interrupt the patient. Nodding in response to the

TABLE 4.3	STAGES OF CHANGE IN THE TRANSTHEORETICAL MODEL	
Stage	Patient Behaviour	Nursing Implications
1. Precontemplation	Is not considering a change; is not ready to learn	Provide support and increase awareness of condition; describe benefits of change and risks of not changing
2. Contemplation	Thinks about a change; may verbalize recognition of need to change; says, "I know I should" but identifies barriers	Introduce what is involved in changing the behaviour; reinforce the stated need to change
3. Preparation	Starts planning the change, gathers information, sets a date to initiate change, shares decision to change with others	Reinforce the positive outcomes of change, provide information and encouragement, develop a plan, help set priorities, and identify sources of support
4. Action	Begins to change behaviour through practice; is tentative and may experience relapses	Reinforce behaviour with reward, encourage self-reward, discuss choices to help minimize relapses and regain focus, and help patient plan how to deal with potential relapses
5. Maintenance	Practises the behaviour regularly; can sustain the change	Continue to reinforce behaviour; provide additional education on the need to maintain change
6. Termination	Change has become part of lifestyle; behaviour is no longer considered a change	Evaluate effectiveness of the new behaviour; no further intervention is needed

Source: Adapted from Prochaska, J., & Velicer, W. (1997). The transtheoretical model of health behaviour change. *American Journal of Health Promotion, 12*(1), 38–48. https://doi.org/10.4278/0890-1171-12.1.38

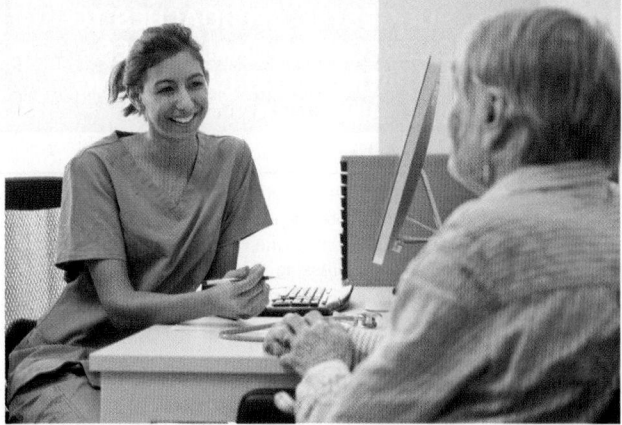

FIG. 4.1 Open, relaxed positioning of the patient and nurse at the same eye level promotes communication in teaching and learning. Source: iStock.com/monkeybusinessimages.

patient's statements and rephrasing and verbally reflecting what the patient is saying can help clarify communication. Allowing time for listening without appearing hurried requires thoughtful organization and planning on the part of the nurse. Listening attentively and red-flagging issues enable the nurse to obtain important information needed for the assessment phase of the teaching process.

Empathy. Empathy can be defined as the quality to enter the world of another so as not to judge, sympathize, or correct but to establish mutual understanding. Empathy means putting aside one's own concerns for a moment and adopting the patient's viewpoint. With respect to patient teaching, empathy means assessing the patient's needs before implementing a teaching plan. For example, a nurse working in a sexual health clinic needs to provide health teaching to an 18-year-old male recently diagnosed with genital herpes. Upon entry to the examination room, the nurse sees the patient crying. An empathic approach to this situation would be for the nurse to sit down beside the patient and say, "I see that you are crying. Would you like to talk about how you are feeling right now?" This approach puts the patient first and may open the path for more effective health teaching.

Challenges to Patient and Caregiver Teaching. The perceived lack of time is a major challenge that detracts from the effectiveness of the teaching effort. When time is limited, the nurse should inform the patient at the beginning of the interaction how much time can be devoted to the session. To make the most of limited time, the nurse and patient must set priorities for the patient's learning so that important teaching can be accomplished during any contact with the patient or caregiver.

Another challenge involves teaching expectations. The patient and nurse may have different expectations about learning outcomes. Patients or caregivers may not be ready to discuss the health issue or its implications or they may hold ideas and values that conflict with those of conventional health care. Although the nurse may face hostility or resentment, the nurse must respect the patient's response to the health issue and explore potential barriers to learning.

Group teaching can become a challenge in an acute, unforeseen event, such as a pandemic. In this situation, the nurse needs to follow directives from Public Health Canada. The nurse also needs to pay attention to the literacy level of the group and adapt to a level that can be understood by everyone in the group.

Another challenge for the patient and for the nurse who is attempting to provide patient education is the current health care system. Decreased length of hospitalization has resulted in discharge of patients into the community with only the basic elements of educational plans established. At the same time, increasingly complex treatment options are being offered. This situation results in greater educational needs of the patient and caregiver. Furthermore, patients and caregivers face greater difficulty using resources as the complexity of the health care system increases. Strategies that can be used to address these challenges are presented in Table 4.4.

Caregiver and Holistic Support

In 2018, over 7 million Canadians aged 15 years and over provided care to a family member or friend with a long-term health condition, a physical or mental disability, or problems related to aging (Statistics Canada, 2020). In this context in particular, the nurse needs to explore how the caregiver feels about providing

TABLE 4.4	SUGGESTED APPROACHES TO OVERCOMING CHALLENGES TO PATIENT AND CAREGIVING TEACHING
Challenge	**Approaches**
Lack of time	Preplan. Set realistic goals. Use time with patient efficiently and use all possible opportunities for teaching, such as when bathing the patient or changing a dressing. Break teaching and practice sessions into small blocks of time. Advocate for time for patient teaching. Carefully document what was taught and the time spent teaching in order to emphasize that it is a primary role of nursing and that it takes time.
Lack of knowledge	Broaden knowledge base. Read, study, and ask questions. Screen teaching materials, participate in other teaching sessions, observe more experienced nurse–teachers, and attend classes.
Incongruent goals	Establish mutually agreed-upon, written goals. Develop a plan in partnership with the patient and incorporate patient's feedback. Revise expectations based on patient's needs.
Diverse patient needs	Ensure teaching methods address the learner's needs (i.e., challenges with communication, education level of patient, geragogy).
Powerlessness, frustration	Recognize personal reaction to stress. Develop a support system. Rely on friends and family for positive encouragement. Network with other nurses, health care providers, and community leaders to change the situation. Become proactive in legislative processes affecting health care delivery. Share knowledge of community resources with patients.

such support, as well as their learning style, cognitive abilities, fears, and current knowledge (Bastable, 2017). Support provided by the caregiver is important to a patient's sense of physical, psychological, and spiritual well-being. Caregivers often bring a wealth of information and personal experience to the teaching encounter. The nurse can initiate conversations about the care and support of the patient and may discover that caregivers provide diagnoses, advice, remedies, and support to their family members in both sickness and health.

To develop a successful teaching plan, the nurse must view the patient's needs within the context of the caregiver's needs. For example, the nurse may teach a patient with right-sided paresis (weakness) self-feeding techniques with the use of special aids, but at a home visit, the nurse finds the patient being fed by the spouse. On questioning, the spouse reveals that it is too difficult to watch the patient struggle with feeding and that it is easier to feed the patient themselves. This is a prime opportunity for the nurse to explore how the family is coping with stress and develop new learning goals that focus on decreasing stress and increasing comfort. Such situations represent opportunities for home care and community health nurses to partner with acute care nurses by evaluating the teaching that is performed in the hospital and providing ongoing patient teaching in the community.

PROCESS OF PATIENT TEACHING

Patient teaching is a distinct and definable activity that includes strategies that help patients and caregivers make informed decisions about the patient's health (Epstein, 2013). These decisions can facilitate proper care for illnesses and the implementation of health-promotion interventions to aid in recovery. In fact, participation in patient education helps patients and caregivers obtain the information and education they want and need (Canadian Partnership Against Cancer, 2019).

Many different approaches are used in patient education. However, the approach used most frequently by nurses parallels the nursing process. Both the teaching process and the nursing process involve development of a plan that includes assessment, diagnosis, patient outcomes or objectives, interventions, and evaluation. The teaching process, like the nursing process, may not always flow in sequential order, but the steps serve as checkpoints that the teaching–learning process has been considered.

The Situated Clinical Decision-Making framework by Gillespie and Paterson (2009) has been adapted specifically for educative nursing practice. This tool encourages the nurse to become an expert educator in working with patients and caregivers in nursing practice (Gillespie, 2010). This framework focuses on the important concepts of respect, reflection, and collaboration. Central to the framework are knowing the patient, understanding the individual's past experiences in relation to health and illness, and understanding their preferences, supports, and resources when making important clinical decisions (Gillespie & Paterson, 2009). Another central component is caring, which provides the interpersonal context in which educative nursing practice occurs with the patient and caregivers (Gillespie, 2010).

Assessment

During the general nursing assessment, the nurse gathers data that determine whether the patient has learning needs that teaching can meet. For example, what does the patient know about the health issue, and how do they perceive the current challenge? If a learning need is identified, a more refined assessment of need is made, and that issue is addressed with an appropriate teaching process (Billings & Hallstead, 2016). The general nursing assessment also identifies many variables that affect the teaching–learning process, such as the patient's physical and mental state of health and sociocultural characteristics. Caregivers may be included in the assessment, and their information can be used to determine their abilities to care for the patient at home. According to Levine (2011), *caregiver assessment* refers to a systematic process of gathering information that not only describes a caregiver situation but identifies particular issues, needs, resources, and strengths of the family caregiver.

The assessment performed for the purpose of developing a teaching plan includes the physical, psychological, educational, and sociocultural characteristics that affect learning, as well as the patient's characteristics that influence the teaching–learning process. Key questions addressing each of these areas are listed in Table 4.5.

Physical Characteristics. The age of the patient is an important factor to consider in the teaching plan. The patient's experiences, rate of learning, and ability to retain information are affected by age. Challenges to effective learning, such as sensory impairments (e.g., hearing or vision loss), decrease sensory input and can alter learning. For the patient with impaired vision, magnifying glasses and bright lighting may help with reading educational materials. Hearing impairment can be compensated for with use of hearing aids or teaching techniques that involve more visual stimuli.

Central nervous system (CNS) function may be affected by disorders of the nervous system, such as stroke and head trauma, but also by other diseases, such as renal disease, hepatic

---

TABLE 4.5	ASSESSMENT OF CHARACTERISTICS THAT AFFECT PATIENT TEACHING: CHARACTERISTICS AND KEY QUESTIONS

Physical
- What is the patient's age and sex?
- Is the patient acutely ill?
- Is the patient fatigued? In pain?
- What is the primary diagnosis?
- Are there other medical problems?
- What is the patient's hearing ability? Visual ability? Motor ability?
- What medications does the patient take? Do they affect learning?
- What is the physical environment in which the teaching will take place: The hospital classroom? The patient's room?

Psychological
- What is the patient's current mental status?
- Does the patient appear anxious, afraid, depressed, or defensive?
- Is the patient in a state of denial?
- What is the patient's level of self-efficacy?
- Is the "timing to teach" appropriate?

Sociocultural
- Is the patient employed?
- What is the patient's current or past occupation?
- How does the patient describe their financial status?
- What is the patient's living arrangement?
- Does the patient have family or close friends?
- What are the patient's beliefs regarding their illness or treatment?
- What is the patient's cultural–ethnic identity?
- Is proposed teaching consistent with the patient's cultural values?
- Has the patient's primary language been assessed for teaching purposes?

Educational
- What is the literacy level of the patient?
- What does the patient already know?
- What does the patient think is most important to learn first?
- What prior learning experiences establish a frame of reference for current learning needs?
- What is the patient's level of motivation?
- What has the patient's health care provider told the patient about the health concern?
- Is the patient ready to change behaviour or learn?
- Can the patient identify behaviours and habits that would make the problem better or worse?
- How does the patient learn best: Through reading? Listening? Physical activities?
- In what kind of environment does the patient learn best: In a formal classroom? In an informal setting, such as home or office? Alone or among peers?
- In what way can the family be involved in patient education?

---

impairment, and cardiovascular failure. Patients with alterations in CNS function have difficulty learning and may require information to be presented in small amounts and with frequent repetitions. Manual dexterity is needed to perform procedures such as self-administered injections or blood pressure monitoring. Problems performing manual procedures might be resolved with the use of adaptive equipment.

Pain, fatigue, and certain medications can also influence the patient's ability to learn. No one can learn effectively when in severe pain. When the patient is experiencing pain, the nurse should provide only brief explanations and follow up with more detailed instruction when the pain has been managed. A fatigued or weakened patient cannot learn effectively because of the inability to concentrate. Such inability can be caused by sleep disruption, which is common during hospitalization, frequently resulting in patients who are exhausted at the time of discharge. Also, many chemotherapeutic medications cause nausea, vomiting, and headaches that affect the patient's ability to assimilate new information. The nurse must adjust the teaching plan and methods to accommodate these factors by setting high-priority goals that are based on needs and are realistic.

Psychological Characteristics. Psychological factors have a major influence on the patient's ability to learn. Anxiety and depression are common reactions to illness. Although mild anxiety increases the learner's perceptual and learning abilities, moderate and severe anxiety limit learning. For example, the patient with newly diagnosed diabetes who is depressed about the diagnosis may not listen or respond to instructions about blood glucose testing. Engaging with the patient in a discussion about these concerns or referring the patient to an appropriate support group may enable the patient to learn that management of diabetes is possible.

Patients also respond to the stress of illness with a variety of defence mechanisms, such as denial, rationalization, and even humour. A patient who denies having cancer is not receptive to information related to treatment options. A patient using rationalization may imagine any number of reasons for avoiding change or for rejecting instruction; for example, a patient with cardiovascular disease who does not want to change dietary habits may relate stories of persons who have eaten bacon and eggs every morning for years and lived to be 100 years of age. Humour is used by some patients as a coping strategy to decrease anxiety. For example, it is not uncommon for patients to assign a name or a characteristic to an intestinal stoma. It is important for nurses to explore whether the patient finds humour as a coping strategy helpful or maladaptive. Humour can be important and useful in the teaching process as well but should focus only on a situation or an idea, not on personal characteristics. It is also important to remember that while some patients respond well to humour, others do not.

One important psychological determinant of successful adoption of new behaviours is the patient's sense of self-efficacy. Self-efficacy refers to an individual's sense of confidence in their ability to perform a set of actions. In fact, the greater a person's confidence, the more likely they are to initiate and persist in that activity. Self-efficacy is the mediator between knowledge and action (Williams et al., 2015). Appropriate teachings by the nurse will provide the patient with the knowledge and skill to cope with upcoming problems, which in turn will decrease the patient's anxiety. Self-efficacy is strongly related to empowerment and better outcomes of illness management.

The nurse should proceed from simple to more complex content to establish a positive experience of success. Both role play, to rehearse new behaviours, and peer learning are teaching strategies that can increase feelings of self-efficacy in patients, caregivers, and family members.

Sociocultural Characteristics. Sociocultural characteristics influence a patient's perception of health, illness, health care, life, and death. Social elements include the patient's lifestyle, status within a family, occupation, income, education, housing arrangement, and living location. Cultural elements include dietary and sleep patterns, exercise, sexuality, language, values, and beliefs. Patients and families whose primary language is not that of the health care provider may value the presence of an interpreter who can decrease the embarrassment of miscommunication.

Socioeconomic Factors. Knowing the patient's current or past occupation may assist the nurse in determining what vocabulary to use during teaching. For example, an auto mechanic might understand the volume overload associated with heart failure through the metaphor of an engine flooding. An engineer may bring the principles of physics associated with gravity and pressures to bear when discussing vascular problems. This technique of teaching requires creativity but can promote a patient's understanding of pathophysiological processes. Knowing socioeconomic status also allows the nurse to identify potential barriers to successful treatment and recovery.

Literacy and Health Literacy. *Health literacy* is the individual's capacity to read, comprehend, and act on health information. A health-literate patient, therefore, has the capacity to acquire, process, and use health information (Spreos, 2011). Health literacy is critical to Canadians' capacity to manage their health (Mitic & Rootman, 2012). As the health care environment has become more complex, individuals with limited literacy lack the basic skills required to function within the twenty-first century health care system (Toronto & Weatherford, 2015). Even patients with high general health literacy can exhibit low health literacy in the presence of complicated health information (Rootman & Gordon-El-Bihbety, 2008). Thus it is imperative that all health education patient resources use plain language. The Canadian Public Health Association (CPHA, n.d) states that use of plain language ensures that health information provided to the public is easy to read, understand, and use.

Knowledge of a person's health literacy level allows the nurse to tailor the teaching plan accordingly. Depending on the patient's health literacy, nonprint teaching materials, such as videos, audio recordings, demonstrations, pictograms, and other visual aids, may provide patients with information concerning their health condition in terms that are understandable. The use of health informatics strategies, such as telehealth, can improve access to health teaching for patients and caregivers in rural or underserviced areas. Virtual education forums are being used extensively as they allow individuals across Canada online access to professionally led educational presentations about how to live well with a particular illness, such as osteoporosis (Osteoporosis Canada, 2019).

Results from an international literacy survey taken by 27 000 adult Canadians in 2012 indicated the following: 17% were at level 1 (poor readers); 32% were at level 2 (material must be simple and clearly laid out); 38% were at level 3 (ability to integrate several sources of information and solve more complex problems); and 14% were at levels 4 and 5 (highest skills in information processing) (CPHA, n.d). Literacy levels also vary between non-Indigenous people and off-reserve First Nations and Metis populations: from the same survey, 65% of off-reserve First Nations and 50% of Metis were below level 3 literacy level as compared to 43% of non-Indigenous people (Arriagada & Hango, 2016). These results underscore the need for the nurse to accurately assess literacy levels of all patients.

The two most widely used health literacy tools in health care settings are the Rapid Estimate of Adult Literacy in Medicine (REALM) and the Test of Functional Health Literacy in Adults (TOFHLA; Altin et al., 2014). The REALM is a test of an individual's ability to recognize and pronounce words, whereas the TOFHLA is a measure of the ability to read, comprehend text, and perform computations involving health-related tasks. However, publications suggest that neither can measure the full breadth of health literacy (Kirk et al., 2012; Pleasant et al., 2011). Newer instruments have been developed for health care providers, including the Newest Vital Sign (NVS) (Stagliano & Wallace, 2013). As a screening tool, NVS identifies patients

at risk for low health literacy. The test result provides information about the patient that allows health care providers to adapt their communication practices to achieve better health outcomes. Another tool is the Brief Health Literacy Screen (BHLS), which is a brief self-report health literacy assessment tool that addresses written and verbal health literacy, as well as the ability of patients to remember health information and instructions provided by a health care provider (Sand-Jecklin & Coyle, 2014).

Housing Arrangements and Living Location. Living arrangements can affect the teaching–learning process. Whether the patient lives alone, with friends, or with caregivers is a determinant of who else is included in the teaching process. If the patient lives in another city, a rural area, or remotely from the site of teaching, the nurse might be expected to plan for continued teaching in the patient's area. For example, if a nurse in an urban hospital was doing discharge teaching to a resident of the Wasagamack First Nation, a remote northern Manitoba community, then she would need to collaborate with an Indigenous Wellness Centre near this community to ensure continuity of care. Similarly, the nurse may have to modify instructions if the patient does not have access to electricity, a phone, or a computer.

Culturally Competent Care. *Cultural competence* is a dynamic learning process that requires nurses to apply knowledge, skills, attitudes, or personal attributes to maximize respectful relationships with diverse populations of patients, their caregivers, and co-workers (Canadian Nurses Association, 2018). A conflict between the patient's cultural beliefs and values and the behaviours promoted by teaching can affect the teaching–learning process. For example, a patient who emigrated to Canada from a country where famine was rampant may view being overweight as a sign of financial success. This patient may have difficulty accepting the need for healthy eating and exercise unless the importance of healthy blood pressure is understood.

As part of the assessment process, patients are encouraged to describe their beliefs regarding health and illness. The use of safe, cultural remedies and traditional healers should be respected and, for teaching to be effective, incorporated into the teaching plan. In addition, it is important to know who has authority in the patient's culture. Whether this is a community leader, a spiritual leader, or a traditional healer, the patient may defer to the authority's decision making. In this case, the nurse could, if feasible, attempt to work with the decision makers in the patient's cultural group.

Learner Characteristics. Finally, the nurse should assess patient characteristics that are directly related to the development of the teaching plan. These factors include the patient's learning needs, readiness to learn, and learning style.

Learning Needs. Learning needs are the new knowledge and skills that an individual must have to meet an objective or a goal. The learning needs of patients with chronic illnesses are different from those of patients with newly diagnosed health problems. A learning needs assessment begins with talking to the patient to determine their existing knowledge of the health condition, what they want to or need to learn, what they are capable of learning, and how they learn best. The patient's thoughts and feelings about making changes in their life also need to be explored to assess readiness to learn. The nurse uses this information to build the teaching plan.

Occasionally, the patient and the nurse may not view the need for health information in the same way. For example, a young adult with a new colostomy may be more concerned with intimacy while the nurse may be focused on colostomy management. In this case, it is necessary for the nurse to explore the patient's thoughts and feelings around body image and intimacy before further teaching can be effective.

To individualize learning needs for a patient, the nurse must include the patient's identified needs. To assist the patient with identifying further learning needs, the nurse may give the patient a list of illness-related topics and ask the patient to number the topics in order of importance. By allowing a patient to prioritize their own learning needs, the nurse can address the patient's most important needs first. When life-threatening complications are a factor, the nurse can encourage the patient to prioritize learning this information by explaining why the item is a "need-to-know" topic.

Readiness to Learn. Before implementing the teaching plan, the nurse needs to determine which stage of change the patient is in (see Table 4.3). If the patient is in the precontemplation stage, the nurse may just provide support and increase the patient's awareness of the issue until the patient is ready to consider a change in behaviour. When the patient leaves the hospital, continuity of care is important; that is, hospital and community nurses should be aware of a transition phase for a patient as adjustment to the community continues. They can share information about the patient's learning stage by means of nurse-to-nurse discharge summaries, continue to evaluate the patient's readiness to learn, and implement the teaching plan as the patient progresses through the stages of change.

Learning Style. Each person has a distinct learning style, which is the way an individual understands and responds to a learning situation (Billings & Hallstead, 2016). The three major learning styles are (1) visual, (2) auditory, and (3) physical or kinesthetic. People often use more than one learning style. To assess a patient's learning style, the nurse might ask how the patient learns best, whether reading or listening is the preferred learning method, and how the patient has learned in the past. Adult learners require a variety of approaches to learning, and nurses must be creative in their delivery of health information. However, if a patient identifies a specific learning style, the nurse should use that method whenever possible. In addition to learning styles, it is valuable to know the patient's worldviews and how the individual perceives their health and illness. Further information on worldviews is found in the discussions on culture in Chapter 2 and on chronic illness in Chapter 5.

Diagnosis

From the assessment, the nurse obtains information about the patient's knowledge, beliefs, and abilities and then compares this information with what the patient wants to know, needs to know, and needs to be able to do. Identifying the gap between the known and unknown helps determine the nursing diagnosis. With teaching, a strength can be validated or a deficiency can be corrected. An example of a desirable outcome that could facilitate validation of a patient's strength is *developing healthy eating patterns*. A common nursing diagnosis for learning needs is *inadequate knowledge*.

Planning

After assessment and identification of the nursing diagnosis, the next steps in the education process include setting goals, determining learning outcomes, and planning the learning experience. Together, the patient and nurse should prioritize the patient's learning needs and agree on the goals and learning outcomes. If the physical or psychological condition of the patient begins to interfere with their participation, the patient's caregiver can assist the nurse in the planning phase.

It is important to write attainable goals and clear learning outcomes. Goals are broad, directional statements of what the patient *wants to accomplish.* Learning outcomes are the *achieved* results of what was learned (Billings & Halstead, 2016)—the competencies and the knowledge that the patient has achieved and can demonstrate successfully after the teaching has occurred. For example, the patient who is diabetic will be able to demonstrate how to give an insulin injection to themselves safely and with precision.

Table 4.6 shows a sample teaching plan that could be adapted to address any patient's learning needs.

Selecting Teaching Strategies. Selecting a teaching strategy is determined by at least three factors: (1) patient characteristics (e.g., age, educational background, degree of illness, culture, learning style); (2) subject matter; and (3) available resources. Some teaching strategies that can be employed to achieve learning objectives follow. Each has advantages and disadvantages that render it suitable to a particular patient and learning situation (Figure 4.2).

Patient Workshop. In the patient workshop, the lecture format is an efficient, versatile, and economical teaching strategy that can be used when time is limited or when a group of patients and family members can benefit from acquiring core information. The nurse presents a series of related ideas or facts to one person or to a group. It is important to remember that the average adult learner can remember five to seven points at a time. Disadvantages of the lecture format are that it often has negative "school learning" connotations, and the extent of individual learning is difficult to evaluate. The lecture–discussion can overcome some of the disadvantages of the lecture alone. With this strategy, the nurse presents specific information by using the lecture technique and follows up with a discussion, during which patients and their caregivers ask questions and exchange points of view with the nurse. This strategy assists the patient in becoming an active learner in the process and creates a more informal reciprocal learning environment. However, some patients may be reluctant to engage in discussions.

Discussion. Discussion provides an opportunity to exchange points of view concerning a topic or to arrive at a decision or conclusion. The nurse discusses content with an individual or with a group, keeping the specific learning objectives in mind and clarifying information as needed. Participants' questions help the nurse identify and correct inaccurate information. This strategy is a good choice when the patient or patients have previous experience with a subject and have information to share, such as smoking cessation or convalescence after coronary artery bypass surgery. The discussion allows the patient or caregivers to participate actively and to apply their own experiences and observations to the learning process.

Group Teaching. There are two main types of group teaching. In the first, the nurse acts as a facilitator, helping the group to share insights about a common issue. As facilitator, the nurse participates by keeping information moving among all group members. The nurse may introduce the patient to an existing group or may recruit a group of patients with similar problems, such as women with multiple sclerosis.

A second kind of group teaching involves peer teaching, which is teaching conducted within the setting of peer groups, such as a self-help or support group. In a peer-teaching setting,

TABLE 4.6	SAMPLE TEACHING PLAN				

Purpose
To provide patient with information necessary to correctly change a colostomy appliance
Goal
The patient will be able to affix accurately and independently a colostomy appliance to a stoma.

Learning Outcomes	Content Outline	Method of Instruction	Time Allotted	Resources	Method of Evaluation
After a 25-min. teaching session, the patient will be able to do the following:					
1. Demonstrate, in order, the steps required to prepare and affix correctly the colostomy appliance (cognitive)	List of the steps Description of the various items required	1:1 instruction	4 min.	Description of equipment	Post-testing • Verbal • Written • Other
2. In the presence of the nurse, accurately measure and affix the colostomy appliance to the stoma (psychomotor)	Technique as per hospital policy and procedure Procedure for measuring stoma and affixing the appliance	Demonstration and return demonstration	13 min.	All equipment required, e.g., colostomy appliance, measuring grid, adhesive paste (Stomahesive), stoma model	Observation of return demonstration
3. Express to the nurse any feelings of discomfort regarding the ostomy and its care (affective)	Discuss common concerns Explore patient's feelings	Discussion	8 min.	Video of patient vignettes Handouts	Question and answer

Source: Modified from Bastable, S. B. (2017). *Nurse as educator: Principles of teaching and learning for nursing practice* (5th ed). Jones & Bartlett. Reprinted with permission.

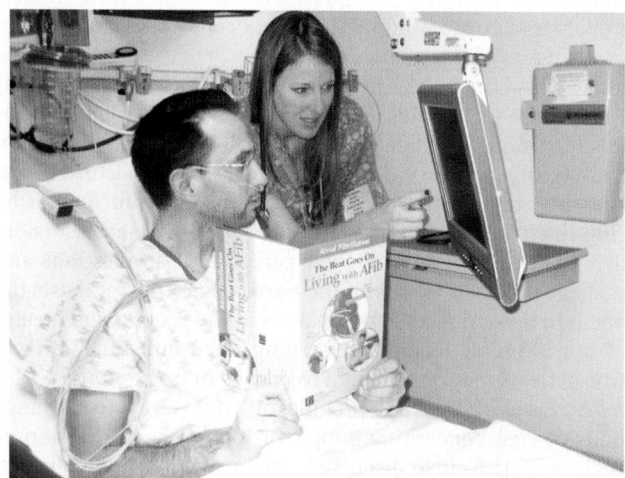

FIG. 4.2 Effective teaching with a variety of materials. Source: Courtesy Linda Bucher, RN, PhD, CEN, CNE, Staff Nurse, Virtua Memorial Hospital, Mount Holly, NJ.

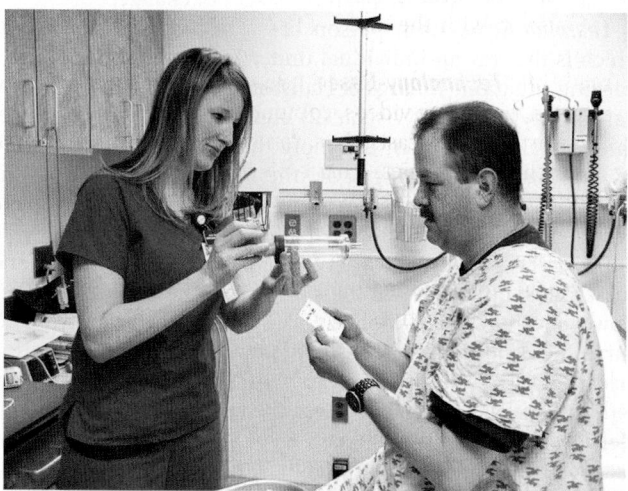

FIG. 4.3 Careful teaching using demonstration–return demonstration has been shown to increase the probability of successful learning by the patient. Source: Courtesy Linda Bucher, RN, PhD, CEN, CNE, Staff Nurse, Virtua Memorial Hospital, Mount Holly, NJ.

the participants learn from one another without the additional input of an instructor.

Nurses need to be mindful of group composition. For example, a nurse may need to look for an Indigenous group for and Indigenous patient, as some Indigenous people may feel uncomfortable in a group if they are the only Indigenous person in the group. Many urban centres have Indigenous Wellness Clinics, such as the Aboriginal Healing Centre in Toronto, Ontario, or the Indigenous Primary Health and Wellness Home in Surrey, British Columbia.

A *support group* is a self-help organization that can provide continuing information, shared experiences, acceptance, understanding, and useful suggestions about a condition or concern. Patients with health issues such as cancer, Parkinson's disease, or compulsive overeating frequently find benefit from

peer-teaching situations. The nurse should actively look for opportunities to refer a patient or caregiver to a support group. This action should be taken in addition to the nurse's planned teaching sessions.

One-to-One Teaching. The **demonstration–return demonstration** is a strategy commonly used by nurses. The purpose is to show the patient how to perform a motor skill–based task, such as a dressing change or injection (Figure 4.3). The focus is on the correct procedure and its application. The nurse demonstrates the procedure in an informal manner, explains unfamiliar terms, and watches the patient for signs of confusion or uncertainty. The nurse clarifies and repeats the teaching as necessary. Then the patient returns the demonstration with the nurse as observer. The entire process should require no more than 15 to 20 minutes. Achieving motor skills requires practice, so the patient must practise the procedure between teaching sessions.

The teach-back strategy is similar to the demonstration–return demonstration, except the focus is on the patient's understanding of the health information being taught. By having the patient repeat the information back to the nurse in their own words, the nurse can assess the patient's level of understanding and determine if further teaching needs to take place (Bastable, 2017). If the patient understands the health information, the nurse has successfully conveyed the information.

Role Play. Role play is another strategy that the nurse might employ, depending on teaching objectives. This format is most often used when patients need to examine their attitudes and behaviours; understand the viewpoints and attitudes of others; or practise carrying out thoughts, ideas, or decisions. The nurse provides information and clear instructions to role players and observers and provides time for feedback and evaluation. Role-playing requires maturity, confidence, and flexibility on the part of the participants. It is important to remember that some patients may feel uncomfortable and inhibited with this method; however, initial discomfort can usually be overcome with patience and support. Role-playing takes time, which must be factored into the teaching plan. An example of role-playing is that of a wife who needs to rehearse how to talk with her husband about his need to quit smoking. In this case, practising the discussion with the nurse ahead of time is often a helpful strategy.

Use of Technology-Based Teaching. Technology-based instruction, including videos, computer-based programs, video chats, charts, or podcasts, is commonly used to supplement other teaching strategies. This type of teaching can enhance the presentation of information because it promotes learning through both visual and auditory stimulation. To use this strategy effectively, the nurse must preview and evaluate the teaching materials for accuracy, completeness, and appropriateness to the learning objectives before showing them. Many older persons are proficient in technology-based instruction and express positive attitudes about its use (Wolfson et al., 2014). Technology-based teaching can be extremely beneficial, particularly when teaching content that is largely visual, such as the steps and processes of procedures (dressing changes, injections, hemodialysis), or if the patient lives a long distance from a health care system. Computer-based programs designed for interactive learning of specific health information are widely available.

Use of the Internet. The Internet is widely used by patients for self-education. Many patients use computers to access health information on the Internet. The Internet also offers established educational programs designed for specific learners. However, the use of the Internet as a source of information can be problematic. While the Internet offers many high-quality health resources and poses seemingly unlimited opportunities to inform, teach, and connect health care providers with patients, it also has much information that is incomplete, misleading, or inaccurate. Therefore it is important that nurses teach patients how to assess websites for credibility. Credible websites usually have the following criteria: an author; current date; are evidence-informed and factual; state a clear purpose; are transparent; and are easy to use (CADTH, 2016).

The nurse is challenged by several factors when using the Internet as a teaching tool. The nurse must have adequate computer competency to review and evaluate information and programs available on the Internet. Personal computer competency is especially necessary to teach patients and caregivers who are unfamiliar with computers how to access information. The nurse should encourage patients to use sites established by the government, universities, or reputable medical or health-related associations (e.g., Canadian Diabetes Association and Public Health Agency of Canada). The list of resources at the end of this chapter includes select reliable patient-education websites for the nurse to review and refer for patient use.

Use of Printed Materials. Printed materials are most often used in combination with other teaching strategies presented in this section. For instance, after a lecture on the physiological effects of smoking, the nurse might distribute a pamphlet from the Canadian Cancer Society that reviews and reinforces the topic. Written materials are always recommended for patients whose preferred learning style is reading.

Written resources must be appropriate for the reading level of the patient. Before written materials are used with patients, the nurse should evaluate the use of plain language. If patients are to understand and benefit from all offered education materials, the information must be selected, revised, or redesigned so that even those patients at the lowest literacy level can comprehend it. Printed materials should also be provided in the patient's preferred language of choice. Asking patients which language they prefer will support their learning and understanding of the materials.

Major resources for acquiring relevant printed materials include the care facility library, the pharmacy, the public library, government agencies, universities, volunteer organizations, websites, and research centres. Written materials, including computer-based programs, should be reviewed by the nurse before being used. In addition to reading level, the following criteria for review are suggested: (a) accuracy, (b) completeness, (c) suitability to meet specific learning goals, (d) inclusion of pictures and diagrams to stimulate interest, (e) focus on one main idea or concept per pamphlet or program, (f) inclusion of information the patient would like to know, and (g) gender and cultural sensitivity of the material (Bastable, 2017).

Games and Simulation. A game provides a framework for inserting content to create learning activities. Frameworks are easily adaptable to a wide variety of content and learning outcomes for patients. Typically, a game requires rules for player moves and termination criteria so that winners can be determined. Simulation games have been shown to enhance educational experience by providing more than a mere review of content. Debriefing, an important aspect of the learning process, occurs after the game in the form of a discussion focused on concepts, generalizations, and the applications of topics covered in the game.

Age-Related Considerations

Of special consideration is teaching of older persons—geragogy. Geragogy is the "method and practice of educating older adults" (Harvey, 2016, para. 2). For nurses to be effective educators, they need to understand how physiological and psychological aging affect learning abilities of older persons (Bastable, 2017). Sensory changes, such as decreased vision, affects a person's ability to read small, printed material. Hearing impairment makes it difficult for the person to hear what the nurse is saying

TABLE 4.7   TECHNIQUES TO ENHANCE PATIENT LEARNING

- Keep the physical environment relaxed and nonthreatening.
- Maintain a respectful, warm, and enthusiastic attitude.
- Let the patient's expressed needs direct what information is provided.
- Focus on "must-know" information; "nice-to-know" information can be added if time allows.
- Involve the patient and family in the process; emphasize active participation.
- Be aware of and take into consideration the patient's previous experiences.
- Emphasize the relevance of the information to the patient's lifestyle and suggest how it may provide an immediate solution to a problem.
- Individualize the teaching plan, even if standardized plans are used.
- Emphasize helping the patient to learn, rather than simply transmitting subject matter.
- Review written materials with the patient.
- Ask frequently for feedback.
- Affirm progress with rewards valued by the patient to reinforce desired behaviours.

and may result in important information being missed. Cognitive changes may result in slower processing and reaction times, and short-term memory loss may make retention of information difficult for some older persons. Chapter 7 also addresses this topic (see Table 7.10).

Implementation

During the implementation phase, the nurse uses the planned strategies to present information and demonstrations. Verbal and nonverbal communication skills, active listening, and empathy are incorporated into the process.

In implementing the teaching plan, the nurse should remember the principles of adult learning and the determinants of learning. Use of reinforcement and reward is important. Techniques to enhance the teaching process with adults are presented in Table 4.7.

Evaluation

Evaluation is the final step in the learning process. Through evaluation the degree to which the patient has mastered the learning objectives is measured. The nurse monitors the performance level of the patient so that changes can be made as needed. The nurse might find that the patient has already achieved their goals. However, if certain goals are not reached, the nurse should reassess the patient and alter the teaching plan. If the patient has developed new needs, the nurse needs to plan new goals, content, and strategies accordingly.

For example, an older man with diabetes mellitus enters the hospital with a blood glucose level of 30.5 mmol/L. Upon observing the patient preparing his insulin injection, the nurse notices that he incorrectly fills the syringe with 20 units of insulin and 20 units of air, instead of 40 units of insulin. After correcting the dosage and questioning the patient, the nurse concludes that the patient could not accurately see the markings on the syringe and may have been administering insufficient insulin to himself for a long time. The patient may require special equipment and new teaching on how to use it so he can administer the insulin safely and accurately.

Evaluation techniques may be short-term or long-term. Short-term evaluation techniques are used to evaluate quickly

the patient's mastery of a concept, skill, or behaviour change; short-term evaluation can be accomplished in the following ways:

1. *Observe the patient directly.* For the example above, the nurse can say, "Let me see how you administer your injection." Through observation, the nurse determines whether the patient has mastered the task, whether further instruction is needed, or whether the patient is ready for new or additional content.
2. *Observe verbal and nonverbal cues.* If the patient asks the nurse to repeat instructions, asks questions, shakes their head, loses eye contact, or otherwise expresses doubt about understanding, the patient may be indicating that further instruction is needed or that an alternative approach should be taken.
3. *Ask direct questions.* For example: "What are the major food groups?" "How often must you change your dressing?" "What should you do if you develop chest pain after returning home?" Open-ended questions almost always provide more information about the patient's understanding than do questions that call for only a "yes" or "no" answer.
4. *Use a written measurement tool, graded for accuracy.* Paper-and-pencil tests can increase anxiety in patients. Many adults "freeze" or "go blank" when given a test or asked to write something that will be graded. Assess the patient's comfort and learning style before using a written method of evaluation.
5. *Talk with a member of the patient's family or support system.* For example, the nurse can ask, "Is he eating regularly?" "How is he handling the walker?" "When is she taking her medications?" Because the nurse cannot observe the patient 24 hours a day, the nurse should receive information from other people who have contact with the patient.
6. *Seek the patient's self-evaluation of progress.* By seeking out a patient's opinion, the nurse is allowing the patient to provide input into the evaluation process. Long-term evaluation necessitates follow-up by the nurse, outpatient clinic, or outside health care organization. The nurse should set up a schedule of visits for the patient before the patient leaves the hospital or clinic or refer the patient to the proper agencies. The nurse keeps written documentation of follow-up telephone calls or emails to urge the patient to maintain the follow-up schedule. The patient's caregivers should be familiar with the follow-up plan so that everyone is involved in the patient's long-term progress.
7. *Use the teach-back method.* The teach-back method is also a way for the nurse to evaluate whether a patient understands health information. For more information about this method, refer to the previous section, "One-to-One Teaching."

Continuity of Educational Care

The nurse is responsible for communicating with the health care providers involved in the patient's long-term follow-up. To ensure continuity, the nurse should telephone, visit, or email these providers and supply them with the patient's education plan. This information needs to be charted and routinely updated in the patient's medical record.

Documentation of the Educational Process

Documentation is an essential component of the entire teaching–learning transaction. The nurse records everything, from the assessment through short- and long-term plans for evaluation. As mentioned, copies of the documentation should be forwarded to the organization or health care provider providing long-term follow-up. The teaching objectives, the content, the strategies, and the evaluation results should be written clearly and completely because many members of the health care team will use these records in different places and for various reasons.

The Standardized Teaching Plan

Standardized teaching plans are often included in care maps and clinical pathways, and they have become an accepted method of developing a teaching plan. Standardized teaching plans contain the widely accepted knowledge and skills that a patient and caregivers need about a specific health problem or procedure. However, the nurse should always individualize these plans to meet the patient's specific needs.

CASE STUDY

Example of the Teaching Process

Patient Profile
E. C., 44 years old (pronouns she/her), is admitted to the hospital for preliminary testing and preparation for a hysterectomy. The nurse is aware that a patient undergoing a hysterectomy is often deeply concerned about her self-concept. The nurse also knows that patients need to express their feelings in an atmosphere of support and understanding. Therefore the nurse has sought to listen attentively and ask questions carefully in order to assess the patient's feelings about and knowledge of the surgical procedure she is about to undergo. The nurse asked open-ended questions, such as "How do you feel about having the surgery?" and "What concerns do you have about undergoing a hysterectomy?" By establishing both a climate of trust and a counselling relationship, the nurse is able to complete the assessment that follows.

Biophysical Dimension
Age 44, high school English teacher and coach of girls' high school basketball team; good general health. Height and weight proportional and average for age. E. C. reports jogging five evenings a week. No sensory impairment; vision, hearing, and reaction time seem normal.

Psychological Dimension
Patient appears mildly anxious about surgery and seems worried about her husband's acceptance of her sexuality. E. C. identifies worry about missing work and leaving classes to a substitute teacher. E. C. states, "I do not let physical problems get me down" and "I don't like pills and hospitals." E. C. is used to "teaching" and not "being taught" and tries to dominate any conversation with or input from the nurse.

Sociocultural Dimension
Married with one child (son), age 23. Mother had a mastectomy at age 51, father healthy. Two younger sisters; both experienced difficult pregnancies but are otherwise healthy. Describes caregiver communication as very good. Describes lifestyle as work-oriented and identifies friends as primarily teaching colleagues. A high priority is placed on work and family.

Learning Style
Responds well to formal lectures. Enjoys reading and group discussions.

Determining Learning Outcomes
After a brief period of rest and adjustment to the unfamiliar hospital environment, E. C. states a desire to learn more about the details of the upcoming planned surgical procedure. Together, E. C. and the nurse identify the following objectives:

After the teaching session, I (E. C.) will be able to do the following:
1. Describe the surgical procedure (hysterectomy) to the nurse.
2. Express to the nurse and my husband my feelings about maintaining an active and fulfilling sex life.
3. Complete arrangements with my family and school principal for convalescence and return to normal activities.
4. List the general recovery experiences that are expected and prioritize circumstances under which to seek medical advice.
5. Discuss "old wives' tales" regarding hysterectomy and verbalize concerns about undergoing the hysterectomy.
6. Identify ways to avoid constipation, weight gain, and potential periods of depression during the recovery period.
7. Propose ways to return comfortably to baseline sexual activities.

Discussion Questions
1. What factors might impede E. C. from learning?
2. What teaching strategies might be most effective for E. C.?
3. What observations will inform the nurse that the teaching session was effective for E. C.? (Consider verbal and nonverbal behaviours.)
4. How can the learning be reinforced?

℮volve
Answers available at http://evolve.elsevier.com/Canada/Lewis/medsurg.

REVIEW QUESTIONS

The number of the question corresponds to the same-numbered objective at the beginning of the chapter.
1. A nurse in a clinic is teaching the client, a middle-aged Italian woman, about methods to relieve her symptoms of menopause. Which of the following is the best goal of this teaching episode?
   a. To prevent early onset of disease
   b. To maintain health promotion
   c. To alter the client's cultural belief regarding the use of herbs
   d. To provide information for selection and use of treatment options

2. What should the nurse do when planning experiences with consideration of adult learning principles?
   a. Present material in an efficient lecture format
   b. Recognize that adults enjoy learning regardless of the relevance to their personal lives
   c. Provide opportunities for the client to learn from other adults with similar experiences
   d. Postpone practice of new skills until the client can independently practise the skill at home

3. Which of the following skills is necessary for the nurse in the role of teacher?
   a. Determining when clients are too distressed physically or psychologically to learn
   b. Assuring the client that the nurse understands what is necessary for the client to learn
   c. Developing standardized teaching plans for use with all clients
   d. Presenting information in medical language to increase the client's vocabulary and understanding of pathophysiology

4. When the nurse is feeling stressed about the limited time available for client teaching, which of the following strategies would be most beneficial? *(Select all that apply.)*
   a. Setting realistic goals that have high priority for the client
   b. Referring the client to a nurse–educator in private practice for teaching
   c. Observing more experienced nurse–teachers to learn how to teach faster and more efficiently
   d. Providing reading materials for the client instead of discussing information the client needs to learn
   e. Rescheduling the client for a later date

5. Which of the following is the best reason the nurse would choose to include family members in client teaching?
   a. They provide most of the care for clients.
   b. Clients have been shown to have better outcomes when caregivers are involved.
   c. The client may be too ill or too stressed by the situation to understand teaching.
   d. Family members might feel rejected and unimportant if they are not included in the teaching.

6. Which step of the teaching process is involved when the nurse, the client, and the client's family decide together what strategies would be best to meet the learning objectives?
   a. Planning
   b. Evaluation
   c. Assessment
   d. Implementation

7. A nurse is spending time with a client who is undergoing a diagnostic procedure. Which of the following comments by the client best indicates a teachable moment?
   a. "I have to email a friend in a few moments."
   b. "How long will this procedure take?"
   c. "I have had this procedure before."
   d. "I'm trying not to think about it."

8. Which of the following is an example of a correctly worded learning outcome?
   a. The client will lose 11.5 kg in 6 weeks.
   b. The client should understand the implications of the condition.
   c. The client will read two pamphlets about breast self-examination.
   d. The client's spouse demonstrates to the nurse how to correctly change a colostomy bag before discharge.

9. What are the benefits of role play as a teaching strategy? *(Select all that apply.)*
   a. Encourages self-reflection
   b. Increased self-efficacy of the client
   c. Rehearses new behaviours
   d. Increases self-efficacy of caregivers

10. Which of these approaches would best provide short-term evaluation of teaching effectiveness?
    a. Observing the client and asking direct questions
    b. Monitoring the client for 3 to 6 months after the teaching
    c. Monitoring for the behaviour change for up to 6 weeks after discharge
    d. Asking the client what they found helpful about the teaching experience

1. d; 2. c; 3. a; 4. a, e; 5. b; 6. a; 7. b; 8. d; 9. b, c, d; 10. a.

ⓔvolve

For even more review questions, visit http://evolve.elsevier.com/Canada/Lewis/medsurg.

REFERENCES

Altin, S., Finke, I., Kautz-Freimuth, S., et al. (2014). The evolution of health literacy assessment tools: A systematic review. *BMC Public Health, 14*, 1–13. https://doi.org/10.1186/1471-2458-14-1207. (Seminal).

Arnold, E., & Boggs, K. (2016). *Interpersonal relationships: Professional communication skills for nurses* (7th ed.). Elsevier.

Arriagado, P., & Hango, D. (2016). *Literacy and numeracy among off-reserve First Nations people and Métis: Do higher skill levels improve labour market outcomes? Insights on Canadian Society*. Minister of Industry, Canada.

Bastable, S. B. (2017). *Nurse as educator: Principles of teaching and learning for nursing practice* (5th ed.). Jones & Bartlett.

Billings, D., & Hallstead, J. (2016). *Teaching in nursing: A guide for faculty* (5th ed.). Saunders.

Canadian Agency for Drugs and Technology in Health (CADTH). (2016). *Evaluating the credibility of health websites: Can you trust Dr. Google?* https://www.cadth.ca/sites/default/files/pdf/CADTH_credible_websites_onepager.pdf

Canadian Nurses Association. (2018). *Promoting cultural competence in nursing*. www.cna-aiic.ca/-/media/cna/page-content/pdf-en/position_statement_promoting_cultural_competence_in_nursing.pdf?la=en&hash=4B394DAE5C2138E7F6134D59E505DCB059754BA9

Canadian Partnership Against Cancer. (2019). *2019-2029 Canadian strategy for cancer control*. https://www.partnershipagainstcancer.ca/cancer-strategy/. (Seminal).

Canadian Public Health Association (CPHA). (n. d). *A plain language service*. https://www.cpha.ca/plain-language-service

Castro, E. M., Van Regenmortel, T., Vanhaecht, K., et al. (2016). Patient empowerment, patient participation and patient-centeredness in hospital care: A concept analysis based on a literature review. *Patient Education & Counseling, 99*(12), 1923–1939. https://doi.org/10.1016/j.pec.2016.07.026

Cullen, M., & Wagner, S. (2015). The nursing process in the 21st century. In D. Gregory, C. Raymond-Seniuk, L. Patrick, et al. (Eds.), *Fundamentals: Perspectives on the art and science of Canadian nursing* (pp. 187–188). Wolters Kluwer Health.

Epstein, R. M. (2013). Whole mind and shared mind in clinical decision-making. *Patient Education and Counseling, 90*(2), 200–206. https://doi.org/10.1016/j.pec.2012.06.035

Farley, H. (2020). Promoting self–efficacy in patients with chronic disease beyond traditional education: A literature review. *Nursing Open, 7*(1), 30–41. https://doi-org.p/10.1002/nop2.382. (Seminal).

Gillespie, M. (2010). Using the Situated Clinical Decision-Making framework to guide analysis of nurses' clinical decision-making. *Nurse Education in Practice, 10*(6), 333–340. https://doi.org/10.1016/j.nepr.2010.02.003

Gillespie, M., & Paterson, B. (2009). Helping novice nurses make effective clinical decisions: The situated clinical decision-making framework. *Nursing Education Perspectives, 30*(3), 164–170 (Seminal).

Harvey, K. (2016). *Critical geragogy in long-term care settings*. International Network for Critical Gerontology. https://criticalgerontology.com/critical-geragogy/

Kirk, J. K., Grzywacz, J. G., Arcury, T. A., et al. (2012). Performance of health literacy tests among older adults with diabetes. *Journal of General Internal Medicine, 27*(5), 534–540.

Knowles, M. (1990). *The adult learner: A neglected species* (4th ed.). Gulf Publishing (Seminal).

Kozier, B., Erb, G., Berman, A., et al. (2014). *Fundamentals of Canadian nursing: Concepts, process, and practice* (3rd Canadian ed.). Pearson Canada (Seminal).

Levine, C. (2011). Supporting family caregivers: The hospital nurse's assessment of family caregiver needs. *The American Journal of Nursing, 111*(10), 47–51. https://doi.org/10.1097/01.NAJ.0000406420.35084.a1. (Seminal).

Lind, J., & Mahler, M. (2019). A systematic mixed methods review: Recovering from a hip fracture in a health promoting perspective. *Nursing Open, 6*(2), 313–329. https://doi.org/10.1002/nop2.214

Lundahl, B., Kunz, C., Brownell, C., et al. (2010). A meta-analysis of motivational interviewing: Twenty-five years of empirical studies. *Research on Social Work Practice, 20*(2), 137–160. https://doi.org/10.1177/1049731509347850. (Seminal).

Marshall, L., Dall'Oglio, L., Davis, D., et al. (2016). *Nurses as educators within health systems. Mastering patient & family education: A healthcare handbook for success.* Sigma Theta Tau.

McAllister, M., Dunn, G., Payne, K., et al. (2012). Patient empowerment: The need to consider it as a measurable patient-reported outcome for chronic conditions. *BMC Health Services Research, 12*(57), 1–8. https://doi.org/10.1186/1472-6963-12-157. (Seminal).

Mitic, W., & Rootman, I. (2012). *An inter-sectoral approach for improving health literacy for Canadians.* https://phabc.org/wp-content/uploads/2015/09/IntersectoralApproachforHealthLiteracy-FINAL.pdf

Organisation for Economic Co-operation and Development. (2008). Adult literacy. www.oecd.org/document/2/0,3343,en_2649_39263294_2670850_1_1_1_1,00.html. (Seminal).

Osteoporosis Canada. (2019). *Bone matters webinars.* https://osteoporosis.ca/what-about-your-bones-and-why-do-they-matter-bone-health-resources-in-small-communities-2/

Pleasant, A., McKinney, J., & Rikard, R. (2011). Health literacy measurement: A proposed research agenda. *Journal of Health Communication, 16*(Suppl. 3), 11–21. 10.1080/10810730.2011.604392. (Seminal).

Prochaska, J. O., & Velicer, W. F. (1997). The transtheoretical model of health behaviour change. *American Journal of Health Promotion, 12*(1), 38. https://doi.org/10.4278/0890-1171-12.1.38. (Seminal).

Puurveen, G., Cooke, H., Gill, R., et al. (2019). A seat at the table: The positioning of families during care conferences in nursing homes. *Gerontologist, 59*(5), 835–844. https://doi.org/10.1093/geront/gny098

Rootman, I., & Gordon-El-Bihbety, D. (2008). *A vision for a health literate Canada: Report of the expert panel on health literacy.* https://www.cpha.ca/sites/default/files/uploads/resources/healthlit/report_e.pdf. (Seminal).

Sand-Jecklin, K., & Coyle, S. (2014). Efficiently assessing patient health literacy: The BHLS instrument. *Clinical Nursing Research, 23*(6), 581–600. https://doi.org/10.1177/1054773813488417. (Seminal).

Stagliano, V., & Wallace, L. (2013). Brief health literacy items predict newest vital sign scores. *Journal of the American Board of Family Medicine, 26*, 558–565. https://doi.org/10.3122/jabfm.2013.05.130096. (Seminal).

Statistics Canada. (2020). *Caregivers in Canada, 2018.* https://www150.statcan.gc.ca/n1/daily-quotidien/200108/dq200108a-eng.htm

Statistics Canada & Organisation for Economic Co-operation and Development. (2005). *Learning a living: First results of the Adult Literacy and Life Skills survey.* https://www.oecd.org/education/innovation-education/34867438.pdf. (Seminal).

Toronto, C., & Weatherford, B. (2015). Health literacy education in health professions schools: An integrative review. *The Journal of Nursing Education, 54*(12), 669–676. https://doi.org/10.3928/01484834-20151110-02

Williams, B. W., Kessler, H. A., & Williams, M. V. (2015). Relationship among knowledge acquisition, motivation to change, and self-efficacy in CME participants. *The Journal of Continuing Education in the Health Professions, 35*(S1), S13–S21. https://doi.org/10.1002/chp.21291

Wolfson, N., Cavanagh, T., & Kraiger, K. (2014). *Older adults and technology-based instruction: Optimizing learning outcomes and transfer* (173). Collected Faculty and Staff Scholarship. https://doi.org/10.5465/amle.2012.0056

RESOURCES

Canadian Association for the Study of Adult Education (CASAE)
https://www.casae-aceea.ca/
Canadian Public Health Agency
https://www.cpha.ca/health-literacy-and-public-health
Health Canada
https://www.hc-sc.gc.ca/index-eng.php
Learning Disabilities Association of Canada
https://www.ldac-acta.ca/

LD Online (Learning Disabilities and Attention-Deficit/Hyperactivity Disorder [ADHD])
https://www.ldonline.org/indepth/adhd
MedicineNet.com
https://www.medicinenet.com
MedlinePlus Health Information
https://www.nlm.nih.gov/medlineplus
MyHealthfinder (Office of Disease Prevention and Health Promotion, US Department of Health and Human Resources)
https://health.gov/myhealthfinder

evolve

For additional Internet resources, see the website for this book at http://evolve.elsevier.com/Canada/Lewis/medsurg.

5

Chronic Illness

Jane Tyerman
With contributions from Susan Robinson

⊘volve WEBSITE

http://evolve.elsevier.com/Canada/Lewis/medsurg

- Review Questions (Online Only)
- Key Points
- Conceptual Care Map Creator

- Audio Glossary
- Content Updates

LEARNING OBJECTIVES

1. Describe the impact of chronic illness in Canada.
2. Define and describe acute and chronic illness and the relationships between these concepts.
3. Identify key factors contributing to the development of chronic illness.
4. Differentiate between chronic illness and disability.
5. Discuss the psychosocial implications of living with a chronic illness.
6. Describe the ways in which chronic illness may affect family members or significant others.
7. Discuss key conceptual models of chronic illness.
8. Describe the role of self-management in chronic illness.
9. Identify emerging models of providing care to individuals with chronic illness.

KEY TERMS

acute illness	health-related hardiness (HRH)	mortality
best buys	health-related quality of life (HRQL)	multimorbidity
caregiver burden	illness	nonmodifiable risk factors
chronic illness	illness behaviour	quality of life
comorbidity	illness trajectory	self-management
disability	informal caregiver	shared decision making
disease	lifestyle	signs
fatigue	modifiable risk factors	stigmatization
health	morbidity	symptoms

Chronic disease is a leading cause of preventable death and disability as it accounts for approximately 41 million deaths globally (Magnussen et al., 2019). **Chronic illness** refers to health conditions that persist over extended periods and that are often (but not always) associated with participation and activity limitations (disability), tobacco use, unhealthy diet, and harmful use of alcohol. The predisposing factors include but are not limited to physiological, environmental, and behavioural factors (Magnussen et al., 2019). The World Health Organization (WHO) considers noncommunicable diseases (NCD) such as cardiac and respiratory disorders, cancer, stroke, and diabetes to be responsible for over 70%

of deaths worldwide. Care for people with chronic illness is ideally embedded within a health care system that promotes patient empowerment.

Unfortunately, the Canadian health care system is still largely built around an acute, episodic model of care that is unable to address the needs of persons with chronic health conditions. The current mismatch between the episodic care orientation of the existing health care system and the needs of people living in the community with chronic illnesses has led to a host of well-documented failures in provision of care. These failures include high rates of hospital readmissions, medical errors, underdiagnosis of conditions, inconsistent monitoring of chronic conditions, lack of patient-centredness, insufficient health education, duplication of resources, inappropriate omission of resources, and preventable injuries (Goodell et al., 2009). Innovative models for providing care for people with chronic illness, such as telemonitoring, are currently being evaluated in Canada and hold promise for improving care in the future (Gordon et al., 2020).

It is critical to recognize that medical diagnosis alone does not predict service needs, length of hospitalization, level of care, or functional outcomes and tells us nothing about the person experiencing the condition or how this person will respond to nursing care. In providing truly holistic and comprehensive care, nurses need to assume a perspective that includes behavioural, psychosocial, and environmental factors. Understanding the illness experience allows for the implementation of effective interventions specific to the needs of the individual, family, or group. This chapter seeks to situate the information contained in the remainder of this textbook within such a framework.

THE EPIDEMIOLOGY OF CHRONIC DISEASES

Almost three-quarters of all NCDs such as heart disease, stroke, cancer, diabetes, and chronic lung diseases occur in low- and middle-income countries, and in 2018, 82% of the 16 million people who died prematurely, before the age of 70 years of age, had NCDs (Magnussen et al., 2019). Worldwide, chronic heart disease, lung diseases, cancer, and diabetes ranked highest among the NCDs, with cardiovascular diseases (17.9 million) being responsible for the highest proportion of global deaths in 2018, followed by cancers (9 million), chronic respiratory disease (3.9 million), and diabetes (1.6 million) (Magnussen et al., 2019).

In Canada, chronic illnesses contribute substantially to morbidity and mortality. **Morbidity** refers to the rates of disease in a population, whereas **mortality** refers to the rates of deaths. One in four Canadian adults lives with obesity, and approximately 1 in 10 children in Canada lives with obesity, a condition that could lead to the development of chronic disease in adulthood (Public Health Agency of Canada [PHAC], 2015). Canada's aging population, along with the rising rates of some risk factors for chronic diseases, is driving the chronic-disease challenge. About two-thirds of deaths in Canada each year result from chronic diseases. Table 5.1 illustrates how chronic illnesses affect Canadians.

Of concern is the fact that chronic diseases and related risk factors are significantly higher among Canada's Indigenous people when compared to the national average. For example, the prevalence of diabetes among First Nations adults living on reserves is 19.7%, compared to 5.2% among the general Canadian population; and the rates of kidney failure compared to non-Indigenous persons are two to four times higher (Ferguson et al., 2017). According to Health Canada 2016 data, common chronic conditions in First Nations adults who live on reserves include diabetes, hepatitis C, and human immunodeficiency virus (HIV), with prevalence rates three times higher than for non-Indigenous Canadians (Health Canada, 2019).

Musculoskeletal conditions such as arthritis and osteoporosis are the most prevalent and costly chronic conditions in Canada. Cancer is the leading cause of death in Canada, although mortality rates have decreased by 14.6% in the past two decades (Statistics Canada, 2019). Despite this decline, in 2015 an estimated 225 800 new cases of cancer and 83 000 cancer-related deaths occurred in Canada, with cancer surpassing cardiovascular disease (heart and cerebrovascular) as the leading cause of death in

Canada (Canadian Cancer Society, 2019). Lung, breast, colorectal, and prostate cancers are the four most common cancer types (excluding non-melanoma skin cancer) in Canada, accounting for over 48% of all new cancer cases (Canadian Cancer Society, 2019). Lung cancer has the highest mortality rate, causing more cancer deaths than the other three cancer types combined. From 2015 to 2019, there was a decline in deaths due to stroke and heart disease (Statistics Canada, 2021).

HEALTH: ACUTE ILLNESS, CHRONIC ILLNESS, AND THE HEALTH–ILLNESS CONTINUUM

Health and illness may be viewed along a continuum on which individuals journey throughout life. **Health**, according to the WHO (2021), is "a state of complete physical, mental, and social well-being and not merely the absence of disease or infirmity." A new conceptualization of health has evolved, in which a person's full state of life needs are met, along with a dynamic quality of living encompassing mind, body, and spirit (Bradley et al., 2018). The state of health is dependent on complex interactions between multiple social and economic factors, the physical environment, and individual behaviour. These factors are referred to as *determinants of health*, and the state of health is a dynamic set of phenomena along the *health–illness continuum*.

Disease is a condition that a health care provider views from a pathophysiological model (Larsen, 2019). **Illness**, conversely, is the human experience of symptoms and suffering. This term refers to how the disease is perceived, lived with, and responded to by individuals and their families (Larsen, 2019). Nursing practice must be informed by both knowledge of disease and understanding of the illness experience.

TABLE 5.1 CHRONIC ILLNESS IN CANADA

Cancer
- About 2 in 5 Canadians will develop cancer in their lifetime; mortality rate is 1 in 4.
- 196 900 people are diagnosed with cancer each year.
- 78 000 Canadians die each year from cancer.

Diabetes
- About 1 in 16 Canadians (6.2%) is living with diabetes, and it is estimated that an additional 0.9% of the population (nearly 300 000) remain undiagnosed.
- The prevalence of diabetes increased by 21% from 2002 to 2007.
- Among adults age 20 years and older, mortality rates for those with diabetes (deaths usually due to a complication of diabetes, such as cardiovascular disease) were twice as high as for those without diabetes.

Cardiovascular Diseases
- 1.6 million Canadians have heart disease or are living with the effects of a stroke.
- In 2007, cardiovascular diseases were responsible for about 70 000 deaths.
- Death rates have decreased since the late 1960s, probably due to lower smoking rates and improved treatment.

Chronic Respiratory Diseases
- Over 3 million Canadians live with a chronic respiratory disease.
- Tobacco remains the most important preventable risk factor for chronic respiratory diseases.

Source: Canadian Cancer Society's Advisory Committee on Cancer Statistics. (2015). *Canadian cancer statistics 2015.* Canadian Cancer Society. http://www.cancer.ca/~/media/cancer.ca/CW/cancer%20information/cancer%20101/Canadian%20cancer%20statistics/Canadian-Cancer-Statistics-2015-EN.pdf?la=en; and Public Health Agency of Canada. (2011). *Chronic diseases in Canada.* Reproduced with permission from the Minister of Health, 2012. https://www.canada.ca/en/public-health/services/chronic-diseases.html

TABLE 5.2	CHARACTERISTICS OF ACUTE AND CHRONIC ILLNESSES	
Description	**Characteristics**	
Acute Illness		
Disease that has a rapid onset and short duration *Examples:* colds, influenza, acute gastroenteritis	• Usually self-limiting • Responds readily to treatment • Complications infrequent • After illness, patient returns to previous level of functioning	
Chronic Illness		
Disease that is prolonged, does not resolve spontaneously, and is rarely cured completely	• Permanent impairments or deviations from normal • Irreversible pathological changes • Residual disability • Special rehabilitation required • Need for long-term medical or nursing management or both	

Table 5.2 compares the characteristics of acute and chronic illness. Acute illness is typically characterized by a sudden onset, with signs and symptoms related to the disease process itself and is described in stages. Signs are typically objective manifestations of a condition, whereas symptoms refer to the subjective reports of the patient. Wagner et al. (2010) describe these stages of acuity, initially cited by Suchman in 1965, as events that persons go through, ranging from shock and disbelief to restitution and resolution. Conversely, chronic illnesses are characterized by exacerbations and remissions and in some cases are persistent. Long-term deleterious effects of a childhood-onset chronic illness such as arthritis, asthma, diabetes, cystic fibrosis, cancer, or epilepsy constitute a significant proportion of adult depression, anxiety disorders, and mental illness (Secinti et al., 2017).

Chronic (or noncommunicable) illnesses are typically characterized as having an uncertain etiology, multiple risk factors, a long latency, prolonged duration, and noninfectious origin and can be associated with impairments or functional disability. The Centers for Disease Control and Prevention (CDC, 2021a) recognizes conditions such as cardiovascular disease, diabetes, arthritis, and other chronic disorders (including depression) as chronic illnesses.

Acute and chronic illnesses can occur in an individual simultaneously. The acute illness may have a profound impact on a person with a pre-existing chronic illness. For example, a person with long-standing, well-controlled diabetes may experience an acute infection that drastically changes blood glucose and insulin requirements. The complexity of caring for patients with multiple illnesses, whether acute or chronic, demands a high standard of nursing knowledge and skill. Nurses frequently have to care for patients with comorbidity, when any two or more disorders occur in the same person either simultaneously or concurrently. One condition or disorder may worsen the other (National Institutes of Health, 2018). Multimorbidity is associated with decreasing quality of life, polypharmacy, and multiple and complex medical treatment regimens in the presence of two to five or more chronic medical conditions (Wallace et al., 2015). Achieving optimal health for a person with multimorbidity is challenging because a treatment targeting one condition may make a coexisting condition worse.

Having multiple chronic medical conditions is associated with many negative outcomes: patients have decreased quality of life, more psychological distress, longer hospital stays, more postoperative complications, functional decline, polypharmacy,

and higher mortality (Wallace et al., 2015). In addition, multimorbidity affects the care process and may result in complex self-care needs; challenging organizational problems (accessibility, coordination, consultation time); polypharmacy; increased use of emergency facilities; difficulty in applying guidelines; and fragmented, costly, and ineffective care (Wallace et al., 2015).

FACTORS CONTRIBUTING TO CHRONIC ILLNESS

The key determinants of health (Government of Canada, 2020; see Chapter 1, Table 1.2) are also critical considerations in the development of chronic illness. Although some chronic conditions have a specific and unique etiology, there are common factors identified by large, longitudinal studies that play an important role in the development of many types of chronic illness.

Lifestyle factors can be harmful to a person's long-term health. There is a clear associations between chronic illness and tobacco use, alcohol misuse, high blood pressure, physical inactivity, obesity, and unhealthy diet (National Institutes of Health [NIH], (n.d.); Nyberg et al., 2020). The term *lifestyle* includes not only the choices made by individuals but also the influence of social, economic, and environmental factors on the decisions people make about their health. A healthy lifestyle is determined by an individual's behaviours within their social environment. As a key determinant of health, the social environment starts with eating well, staying active, not smoking, being immunized, and having access to educational opportunities (Health Canada, 2019). Poverty and socioeconomic disadvantage are recognized as having a major impact on the development of chronic illness (Larsen, 2019). Income and education significantly affect an individual's life expectancy, ability to obtain and provide nutritious food and good housing, and access to health care (Bushnik et al., 2020).

Risk Factors for Chronic Illness

Both individuals and communities may possess risk factors for the development of chronic illness, and as stated earlier, there is a disproportionate rate of chronic illness among socioeconomically disadvantaged populations (Ministry of Health and Long-Term Care [MOHLTC], 2018). The recognition of these common risk factors and conditions is the conceptual basis for an integrated approach to chronic disease.

Individual risk factors can be classified as background, behavioural, or intermediate. Sex, age, level of education, and genetic characteristics are examples of background risk factors. Smoking, unhealthy diet, and physical inactivity would fall into the category of behavioural risk factors. Intermediate risk factors include comorbid conditions such as diabetes, hypertension, and obesity or being overweight. Besides risks that occur at the individual level, community-level factors can also contribute significantly to the development of chronic illnesses. Examples of community-level risk factors include social and economic conditions, such as poverty, employment, and family composition; environmental conditions, such as climate and air pollution; cultural conditions, such as practices, norms, and values; and urbanization, which influences housing and access to products and services (MOHLTC, 2018). In Canada the Indigenous populations face significant challenges in relation to these risk factors, in part due to overcrowding, reserve housing and nutrition insecurity, and lack of access to clean water and sanitation, among other factors. It is important to acknowledge

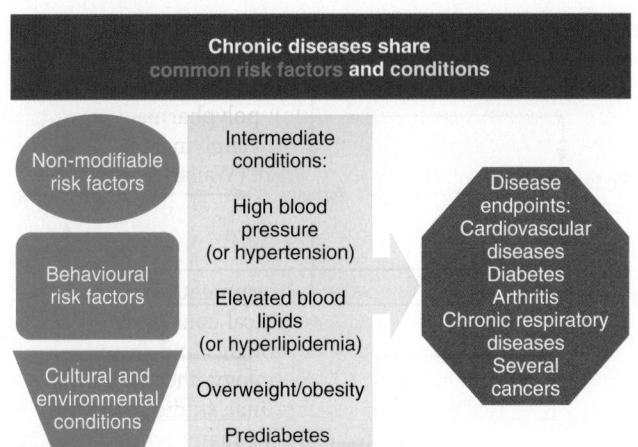

FIG. 5.1 Chronic diseases share common risk factors and conditions. (Source: © All rights reserved. Public Health Agency of Canada. (2015). *Chronic disease risk factors*. Adapted and reproduced with permission from the Minister of Health, 2017.)

that barriers contributing to risk factors are institutional in nature and have been described as systemic bias and racist. The resource The National Collaborating Centre for Aboriginal Health (2013) provides an overview of these concepts.

Figure 5.1 illustrates the conceptual model used by the Centre for Chronic Disease Prevention at the Public Health Agency of Canada (PHAC) to examine risk factors for chronic illness. Although some risk factors, such as age, sex, and genetic makeup, cannot be changed (nonmodifiable risk factors), many behavioural risk factors are considered modifiable. Cultural and environmental risk factors, such as air pollution, may play a significant role in the development of chronic illness and may be modifiable.

PREVENTION OF CHRONIC ILLNESS

Prevention of chronic illness is the best way to deal with the chronic-disease epidemic. Although not all chronic illnesses are preventable, the elimination of four behavioural or modifiable risk factors, such as tobacco use, unhealthy diet, insufficient physical activity, and the harmful use of alcohol, have been cited as effective disease prevention interventions (MOHLTC, 2018). Decades of research have determined the most effective means, or "best buys," of preventing chronic illness. Best buys are actions that should be undertaken immediately to produce accelerated results in terms of lives saved, diseases prevented, and heavy costs avoided. Table 5.3 identifies these best buys.

The Role of Genetics

Genetics has long been recognized to play an important role in the development of certain chronic illnesses. Cystic fibrosis and Huntington's disease are two chronic illnesses for which genetic testing is available. Genetic testing can also show an inherited predisposition to several different types of cancer, including breast and ovarian cancer, melanoma, and colon cancer.

With the completion of human genome sequencing, however, the role of genetic factors will assume increasing importance in prevention, detection, and treatment of many chronic illnesses. Chapter 15 provides an in-depth discussion of genetics in nursing practice.

The Role of Aging

Chronic illnesses are on the increase as populations age and individuals live with one or more chronic conditions for decades. Infectious diseases commonly posed the greatest threat to health in the past, but improved sanitation, vaccination, and public health surveillance and the advent of antibiotics have been key factors in prolonging life expectancy rates. In 2018, life expectancy in Canada was 79.9 years for males and 84.1 years for females. However, the life expectancy for males did not incrementally increase as would normally be expected, owing to premature deaths resulting from the opioid crisis (PHAC, 2019). Prediction is difficult because of this new threat to Canadians. It is anticipated, however, that the number of super-aged individuals, greater than 80 years old, will rapidly increase between 2026 and 2045, and will increase from 1.8 million in 2018 to between 4.7 and 6.8 million by 2068 (Statistics Canada, 2019).

Healthy aging is defined by the WHO as being free of limitations on one's well-being despite the presence of chronic illness (WHO, 2019). However, aging is associated with the development of many chronic illnesses. As people age, they are more likely to have at least one chronic condition; 57% of the world's 80-year-plus population have three or more chronic illnesses (WHO, 2014). The most frequently reported chronic conditions among persons aged 70 years and over are hypertension, heart disease, stroke, cancer, diabetes, and lung diseases (WHO, 2019).

DISABILITY IN CHRONIC ILLNESS

Chronic illness is often associated with disability, although many people are not disabled by their chronic illness. Disability is a term whose definition continues to be refined after significant global debate. It is a complex interaction among health conditions, personal factors, and the environment. As interpreted by the Supreme Court of Canada, disability "includes a wide and evolving range of permanent, temporary or intermittent impairments, both physical and mental, which can result in functional limitations as the person interacts with others and potentially with socially constructed barriers" (Government of Canada, 2014, p. 9).

Worldwide, disabilities affect over 1 billion people. It is reported that a person with a disability is four times more likely to be treated poorly in the health care system, three times more likely to be denied health care, and two times more likely to receive inadequate care (WHO, 2019). Two different conceptual models of disability have shaped the manner in which we think about disability (WHO, 2002): the medical model and the social model. The *medical model* views disability as directly caused by disease, trauma, or another health condition to be medically corrected. This perspective requires the creation of an inclusive community free of physical and systemic barriers (McCain, 2017). The *social model* of disability, conversely, sees disability as a socially created problem and not an inherent attribute of individuals (Barnes, 2012).

The WHO has taken the position that neither the medical nor the social model is fully adequate to define disability, although both models make a significant contribution to the discussion. Disability, according to the WHO (2019), is a phenomenon where there is a complex interaction between the individual with physical or developmental limitations and the physical environment that surrounds them. If that environment is adjusted to meet the individual needs, then no limitations to function or to quality of life are experienced. In other words, both medical and social responses are appropriate and necessary to the problems associated with disability, but a model of disability that synthesizes both approaches is required. The integration of the medical and social approaches is contained in the biopsychosocial model, on which the International Classification of Functioning, Disability and Health, known as the ICF (WHO, 2002), is based. Parallel to the determinants of health (see Chapter 1, Table 1.2), disability and functioning are viewed in the ICF as the outcomes of interactions between health conditions (diseases, disorders, and injuries) and contextual factors. Contextual factors are composed of external environmental factors (i.e., social attitudes, architectural characteristics, and legal and social structures, as well as climate, terrain, and so forth) as well as internal personal factors (i.e., gender, age, coping styles, social background, education, profession, past and current experience, overall behaviour pattern, character, and other factors that influence how disability is experienced by the individual).

Figure 5.2 shows the three levels of human functioning classified by ICF: functioning at the level of the body or body part, at the level of the whole person, and at the level of the whole person in a social context. Disability involves dysfunction at one or more of these same levels: impairments, activity limitations, and participation restrictions.

The ICF acknowledges that every human being can experience a decrement in health and thereby experience some degree of disability. Disability is a universal experience at some point in life and is not something that happens only to a minority of individuals.

PSYCHOSOCIAL DIMENSIONS OF CHRONIC ILLNESS

The interaction between mind and body has received increasing and well-deserved attention in recent years. Because chronic illness affects the whole person, not just a particular body system, the psychosocial dimensions of chronic illness assume great significance. The relational core of nursing practice, which emphasizes nurse–patient dialogue, partnership, and participation, is integral to the care of persons with chronic illness (Robinson, 2016).

The following section will address a number of key concepts related to the psychosocial dimensions of chronic illness and the holistic perspective that shapes the overall experience of chronic illness.

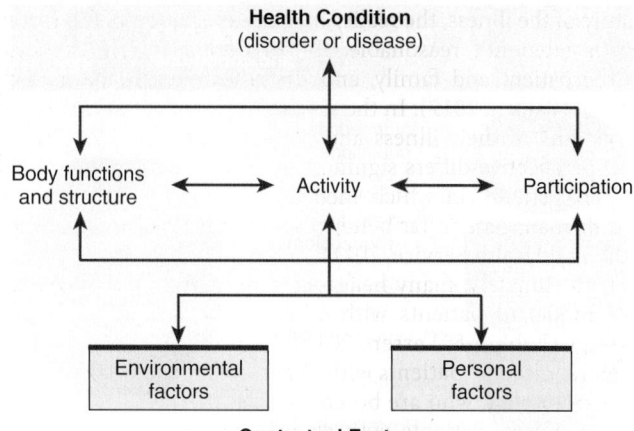

FIG. 5.2 The International Classification of Functioning, Disability and Health (ICF) Bio–Psycho–Social Model. Source: Reprinted from *Towards a common language for functioning, disability and health,* WHO, page no. 9, Copyright 2002.

TABLE 5.4	CHARACTERISTICS OF THE SICK ROLE
Component of the Role	**Associated Behaviours and Expectations**
Sick person is exempt from normal social roles.	Dependent on the nature and severity of illness. More severe illness allows patient to be exempt from more roles. Requires legitimization (validation) by a physician.
Sick person is not responsible for their condition.	Not responsible for becoming sick, the individual therefore has a right to be cared for. Physical dependency and the right to emotional support are therefore acceptable. Patient will need a curative process apart from personal willpower or motivation to get well.
Obligation to want to become well	Being ill is seen as undesirable. Because privileges and exemptions of the sick role can become secondary gains, the motivation to recover assumes primary importance.
Obligation to seek and cooperate with technically competent help	The patient needs technical expertise that the physician and other health care providers have. Cooperation with these providers for the common goal of getting well is mandatory.

Source: Copyright 2001. From *Medical Sociology* by Cockerham, William C. Reproduced by permission of Taylor and Francis Group, LLC, a division of Informa plc., via Copyright Clearance Center.

Illness Behaviour and the Sick Role

Illness behaviour refers to the varying ways that individuals respond to physical symptoms: how they monitor internal states, define and interpret symptoms, make attributions, take remedial actions, and use various sources of informal and formal care (Mechanic, 1995). The "sick role" was first described in 1951 by Talcott Parsons. Sickness was seen by Parsons as a form of deviant behaviour that permitted the avoidance of social responsibilities (Larsen, 2019). A form of learned behaviour, the sick role was achieved through failure to keep well. Table 5.4 describes the characteristics of the sick role.

Parsons's sick-role model, though useful for acute illnesses, has been criticized on many fronts because it does not address important issues related to the experience of chronic illness. It fails to consider characteristics of chronic illness, the long-term nature of the illness, the reality that an expectation of full recovery is often not reasonable, the management role expected of the patient and family, and the adjustment to permanent change (Larsen, 2017). In the sick-role model, patients are seen as victims of their illness and are subordinate to physicians. This perspective differs significantly from the paradigm of the "expert patient," in which the patient knows their condition and its management far better than their health care providers (National Health Service, 2011).

Unfortunately, many health care providers apply the sick-role model to patients with chronic illnesses in acute care settings (Lubkin & Larsen, 2017). The frequent readmissions often required by patients with chronic illness may create frustration for staff, who are bored by what they see as repetitive, tiresome care. Patients with chronic illness who have experience with the health care system may use their knowledge to gain what they want or need from the system, demanding certain treatments, a specific schedule, or particular routines. These patients may be perceived as "disruptive" to the normal routine of a hospital unit. Lack of empathy on the part of health care providers may lay the foundation for frustration and power struggles with the patient (Sternke et al., 2016). Relationships between patients and health care providers tend to be most productive when providers are able to recognize limitations in their own expertise and to respect the expertise of patients and their families. Patients with chronic illness have been found to move from "naive trust" to "disenchantment" and on to a stage of "guarded alliance" in their relationship with health care providers. Nurses must recognize the need to establish credibility and trust with patients who have chronic illness.

Communication between patients with chronic illness and health care providers is critically important in the delivery of patient-centred care. Effective communication must be timely, appropriate, and compassionate (Vennedey et al., 2020). Table 5.5 provides a comparison of effective and problematic communication.

Ensuring clarity, a straightforward approach, receptiveness, and responsiveness to questions and providing written information to complement what was said are helpful characteristics of good communication. Unhelpful communications include those in which there is a mismatch between what patients feel their information needs are at a particular time and the manner in which health care providers supply this information. It is useful for nurses to reflect on the question "Am I treating this patient the way I would want to be treated?"

Given their own expertise and experience with health care, many individuals with chronic illness are demanding a new model of care in which they are truly equal partners. Shared decision making is a decision-making process engaged in jointly by patients and their health care providers (Légaré et al., 2013). It is a central tenet of the patient-centred approach described in Chapter 1. Shared decision making exemplifies the partnership between health care provider and patient and is essential for ethical care, as it respects autonomy (the right to make informed choices), beneficence (the balance between benefits and risk of actions), and nonmaleficence (the avoidance of harm).

Self-Efficacy

The development and maintenance of self-efficacy is critical to effective self-management of chronic illness. Self-management programs based on self-efficacy principles have been demonstrated to be highly effective in reducing symptoms and facilitating behaviour change (Larsen, 2017). Effective self-management relies on a patient-centred care approach in which the individual works in partnership with health care providers to develop solutions to issues related to the patient's chronic condition (Registered Nurses' Association of Ontario [RNAO], 2010). Self-efficacy may be considered a type of self-confidence; it is the belief of an individual that they can successfully execute the behaviour required to produce the desired outcomes (Bandura, 1977). People's beliefs about their personal efficacy constitute a major aspect of their self-knowledge, according to Bandura's social cognitive theory. Judgements about personal self-efficacy can determine which behaviours will be attempted, how much effort will be devoted to the behaviour, and how long a person will persist in continuing that behaviour.

Both outcome expectancies and efficacy expectancies have to be considered in light of self-efficacy. An *outcome expectancy* is the individual's belief that a specific behaviour will lead to certain outcomes. For example, the patient who tells the nurse that exercising helps people to lose weight is voicing an outcome expectancy. An *efficacy expectancy* is the individual's belief that they are able to achieve the outcome. The patient who tells the nurse that they are not able to exercise is voicing an efficacy expectancy. It is helpful if both outcome and efficacy expectancies are positive. A patient who believes that exercise helps other people lose weight but that it will not help them lose weight might benefit from some of the following influences.

Four primary influences shape an individual's self-efficacy beliefs: mastery, vicarious experience, verbal persuasion and other social influences, and physiological and affective states that help us judge our capability and our vulnerability to dysfunction (Larsen, 2017). *Mastery* reflects a belief about whether or not "we have what it takes to succeed" and is considered the most influential source of self-efficacy. Many chronic illnesses necessitate the mastery of certain skills—for example, monitoring heart rate and exertion level during exercise—to achieve a sense of self-efficacy. *Vicarious experience* is the observation of others' performances, from which we

TABLE 5.5	**EFFECTIVE STRATEGIES AND BARRIERS TO COMMUNICATION DURING DIFFICULT CONVERSATIONS**
Effective Strategies	**Barriers to Communication**
• Open and honest communication • Ongoing and early conversations • Communicating about treatment goals • Balancing hope and reality in communicating bad news • Taking cues from the patient about how much information they are able to process at one time	• Provider discomfort with issues (e.g., death and dying) • Lack of experience, training, or knowledge of policies and guidelines • Lack of good mentorship • Patient factors (e.g., reluctance to talk or to face an issue, language barrier, unrealistic prognosis, not ready to hear news) • Age of the patient (e.g., a younger patient can make the discussion more difficult)

Source: Adapted from Kissane, D. W., Bylund, C. L., Banerjee, S. C., et al. (2012). Communication skills training for oncology professionals. *Journal of Clinical Oncology, 30*(11), 1242–1247.

learn through modelling and against which we measure our own performance. These experiences inform our self-efficacy beliefs. In the weight loss example, the patient may be encouraged by the example of fellow participants in a walking program who have achieved weight loss through exercise. When people are *verbally persuaded* that they are capable of performing a certain task, their self-efficacy beliefs may be enhanced. Nurses are in a key position to provide the verbal support that the patient may need to undertake the exercise program. Finally, *physiological and affective states* such as stress have an impact on self-efficacy beliefs. A patient who has just lost their job and is experiencing significant financial stress may not have the energy to begin a walking program.

Health-Related Hardiness

Health-related hardiness (HRH), a concept first described by Kobasa (1979) and expanded by Pollock, Christian, and Sands (1990) to apply to people with chronic illness, is a personality resource that buffers stress and allows people to experience a high degree of stress without falling ill. Hardy people are considered to possess three general characteristics: control, commitment, and challenge. *Control* refers to the belief that the individual can influence the events in their experience. *Commitment* refers to an ability to feel deeply committed to the activities of life. *Challenge* is the anticipation of change. The person with HRH, when confronted with a health stressor, possesses sufficient self-mastery and confidence to appraise and modify responses appropriately (control) and cognitively reappraises the health stressor so it is viewed as stimulating and beneficial or as an opportunity for growth (challenge). This is exemplified by the perception of individuals with diabetes that they have some control over their disease. *Hardiness* has recently been replaced by the term *resilience*, which shifts the emphasis from its being an inherent trait to its being an ability one can develop (Trivedi et al., 2011). Motivation and competence thus develop to enhance the patient's health status and to facilitate coping with the health stressor (Pollock & Duffy, 1990). Higher levels of hardiness or resilience show better psychosocial adaptation to chronic illness; thus nurses can make use of interventions that foster a sense of control, commitment, or challenge.

Mood Disorders

Along with assessments of self-efficacy and health-related hardiness, assessment for the presence of a mood disorder such as depression or anxiety is a key element in the nursing assessment of patients with chronic illness (Barnett et al., 2012). Illness-related anxiety and stress can trigger symptoms of depression. It is estimated that approximately one-third of individuals with at least one chronic disease experience depression (National Institute of Mental Health, 2021). Major depression in particular may adversely affect the course of chronic illness and amplify disability. The presence of a mood disorder in a person with a chronic physical illness has been found to be associated with short-term disability, the need for help with instrumental activities of daily living, and suicidal ideation.

The likelihood of depression increases with the number of chronic conditions affecting a patient. This is due in part to the fact that inflammation has been proved to be an important etiological factor in mood disorders. Individuals with inflammatory illnesses such as inflammatory bowel disease (IBD), cardiovascular disease, rheumatoid arthritis (RA), chronic obstructive pulmonary disease (COPD), and multiple sclerosis (MS) often struggle with depression (Enns et al., 2018; Galecki & Talarowska, 2018; Halaris, 2016). This new understanding of the mechanism by which inflammation influences mood disorders will lead to the development of preventive and therapeutic treatments.

In spite of the evidence that mood disorders are common in persons with chronic physical illness, conditions such as depression remain both under-recognized and undertreated in this population. The nurse must be alert for the presence or development of depressive symptoms when caring for patients with chronic illness.

Fatigue

Fatigue is often associated with chronic illness and has been described as one of the most distressing symptoms people with chronic illness experience. Fatigue may be both a symptom of an underlying condition and an outcome of that condition. It interferes with normal, customary, and desired activities and pervades every aspect of life. The invisibility of fatigue is one of the most frustrating aspects of the experience and can lead to lack of understanding and to misunderstanding by others. The impact of fatigue on functioning is substantial and under-recognized.

Although there is no universally accepted definition of fatigue, it is generally recognized to be a complex, multidimensional experience. Fatigue is "a subjective, unpleasant symptom which incorporates total body feelings ranging from tiredness to exhaustion, creating an unrelenting overall condition which interferes with individuals' ability to function to their normal capacity" (Ream & Richardson, 1996, p. 527). Pain, mood disorders, sleep issues, physical deconditioning, metabolic abnormalities, infection, dietary issues, hypoxia, and medications can lead to profound fatigue. It is important for the patient to incorporate interventions to reduce fatigue such as yoga, acupuncture, and nutritional supplements.

Stigma

People with chronic illness often experience stigmatization, in which they are regarded by others as unworthy or disgraceful. Canadian culture contributes to this stigmatization, as it places value on youth, physical fitness, and productivity. Such stigma can have a significant impact on the quality of life of those who are challenged to meet these standards because of the constraints of illness (PHAC, 2019). They may be set apart and labelled by others according to the disease they have and the treatments they use. Larsen (2017) notes that older persons and chronically ill people are often negatively viewed in health care settings, where caring for these groups is seen as less rewarding in terms of recovery, treatment, and economics than caring for other types of patients. Stigma in health care, overall, is detrimental to the delivery of quality care, undermines diagnosis and treatment, and hinders the patient's ability to achieve optimal health (Nyblade et al., 2019). Stigma is an important concept in nursing because it may influence the manner in which care is provided, cause an unequal power dynamic between nurses and patients, and create an unwillingness of patients to disclose information (PHAC, 2019). Individuals who do not fear being stigmatized if they disclose certain facts are likely to share relevant information.

There are several types of stigma. The stigma of physical deformity relates to situations in which there is a difference between the expected and valued norm of perfect physical condition and the actual physical condition of the person (Larsen, 2017). The changes or deformities in physical appearance that may occur as a result of chronic illness set the individual apart. The person with MS, for example, may have difficulty walking or require the use of a mobility aid, which can create stigmatization. Character blemishes, often associated with undesirable traits such as dishonesty, addiction, lack of control, or mental illness, are another type of stigma (Knaak et al., 2017). Moral judgements are made about the "unworthy" character of the individual. For example, a woman with obesity may experience the stigma of character blemish when others pass judgement about her being responsible for her illness because she is unable to control her appetite and because of her perceived laziness. This leads to the scenario of "blaming the victim" and is not uncommon among health care providers.

Quality of Life

Given the many physical and psychosocial challenges inherent in the experience of living with a chronic illness, quality of life is a primary outcome measure in evaluating treatment for many health conditions. Quality of life, in its broadest definition, refers to subjective evaluations of both the positive and the negative aspects of life (CDC, 2021b). Quality of life is influenced by a host of factors, including financial status, employment, housing, spirituality, social support network, and health. The term health-related quality of life (HRQL) has often been used as a means of focusing on the ways in which health influences and is influenced by overall quality of life. At an individual level, HRQL usually includes perceptions of physical and mental health status and the key variables that are associated with health status, such as health conditions, functional ability, social support, and socioeconomic status (CDC, 2021a). At a community level, HRQL includes resources, conditions, policies, and practices that influence a population's health perceptions and functional status (CDC, 2021a). The concept of HRQL enables health agencies to examine broader areas of healthy public policy around a common theme.

LIVING WITH CHRONIC ILLNESS

Reduced quality of life, depression, fatigue, and stigma, together with physical symptoms, may make living with a chronic illness a daily challenge for many individuals and their families. Over time, the losses a person sustains as a result of living with a chronic illness can cause a decrease in self-esteem. Loss of self is a primary source of suffering for people with chronic illness. Experiencing social isolation, living a restricted life, and being a burden to others all contribute to this loss of self.

People with chronic conditions use various strategies to try to maintain a "normal life." Normalization is a key strategy in living with chronic illness. When individuals fail to exhibit an expected norm, they become viewed as abnormal. Individuals with chronic illness may attempt to conceal their disease from others to pass themselves off as "normal," which is an idealized notion of being the same as the rest of the presumably normal population. Although the objective of this behaviour is to fit in, this strategy may serve as a constant source of stress because of the danger of being discovered.

"Covering" a visible chronic illness is a strategy employed by some individuals. Covering involves acknowledging the condition while attempting to decrease any anxiety and stress experienced by those who do not have the same condition. An example of covering may be making jokes about the condition in an effort to downplay the illness. The nurse must be sensitive to the strategies used by patients with chronic illness and explore with the person whether these strategies are adaptive and helpful or whether they are maladaptive. It is also important for the nurse to recognize that cultural expectations may limit a person's coping strategies. When a culture devalues chronic disease, such as mental illness, people often remain undiagnosed and fail to receive adequate treatment.

CHRONIC ILLNESS AND CAREGIVING

Living with a chronic illness affects not only the individual who has the condition but also those in the patient's immediate social network. Nursing assessment of a person with a chronic illness is incomplete without considering the way in which significant others are affected. Families—and sometimes friends and neighbours—are frequently called on to provide the often complex and long-term care required by some individuals with chronic illnesses. In fact, more than 9 million Canadians (25% of the population) provide care to people with long-term health conditions (Hango, 2020). The term informal caregiver entails anyone who provides care without pay to support an individual with diminishing physical ability, a debilitating cognitive condition, or a chronic life-limiting illness (Carers Canada, 2018).

The vast majority of people with chronic conditions live in the community. The shift away from institutionalization has meant that most of the responsibility for caregiving is left to families and friends, decreasing the costs of health care and social systems but often at the overall health and expense of the care provider. One in five caregivers considers caregiving to have negatively affected their own physical, financial, and emotional health (Ysseldyk et al., 2020). Thus, caregiver burden is defined as the level of multifaceted strain perceived by the caregiver from providing care to a family member or loved one over time (Liu et al., 2020). Issues that can arise include increasing difficulty meeting the physical demands of the caregiving role; lack of time to engage in adequate self-care and health-promotion activities; and the effects of caregiver burden, including fatigue, anxiety, depression, and physical effects such as heart conditions and hypertension (Johansen et al., 2018; Liu et al., 2020; Ringer et al., 2017).

Nurses play a critical role in assessing the level of caregiver distress present, if any, and taking appropriate action to attempt to reduce or eliminate the factors that contribute to the distress.

CONCEPTUAL MODELS OF CHRONIC ILLNESS

Conceptual models are useful in understanding the chronic-illness experience, particularly because caring for a patient with a chronic illness requires a different framework for practice than may be useful in caring for a patient with an acute illness. The following section highlights several of the key models of chronic illness.

Illness Trajectory

The concept of an illness trajectory was first advanced in 1967 by Glaser and Strauss as a way of understanding the complex, dynamic path of chronic illness. An illness trajectory can be defined as an experiential pathway along which the person with an illness progresses. Some illnesses have more predictable

TABLE 5.6	ILLNESS TRAJECTORY PHASES AND GOALS OF MANAGEMENT	
Phase	**Definition**	**Goal of Management**
Pre-trajectory	Genetic factors or lifestyle behaviours that place an individual or community at risk for the development of a chronic condition	Prevent onset of chronic illness
Trajectory onset	Appearance of noticeable symptoms; includes period of diagnostic workup as person begins to discover and cope with implications of diagnosis	Form appropriate trajectory projection and scheme
Stable	Illness course and symptoms are under control. Biography and everyday life activities are being managed within limitations of illness. Illness management centres in the home.	Maintain stability of illness, biography, and everyday activities
Unstable	Period of instability to keep symptoms under control or reactivation of illness. Biographical disruption and difficulty in carrying out everyday life activities. Adjustment is made in regimen; care usually takes place at home.	Return to stable
Acute	Severe and unrelieved symptoms or the development of illness complications necessitating hospitalization or bed rest to bring illness course under control. Biographical and everyday life activities are temporarily placed on hold or drastically cut back.	Bring illness under control and resume normal biographical and everyday life activities
Crisis	Critical or life-threatening situation necessitating emergency treatment or care. Biography and everyday life activities are suspended until crisis passes.	Remove life threat
Comeback	A gradual return to an acceptable way of life within limits imposed by disability or illness	Set in motion and continue the trajectory projection and scheme
Downward	Illness course characterized by rapid or gradual physical decline accompanied by increasing disability or difficulty in controlling symptoms	Adapt to increasing disability with each major downward turn
Dying	Final days or weeks before death. Characterized by gradual or rapid shutting down of body processes, biographical disengagement, and closure and relinquishment of everyday interest and activities	Bring closure, let go, and die peacefully

Source: Corbin, J. (2002). Introduction and overview: Chronic illness and nursing. In R. Hyman & J. Corbin (Eds.), *Chronic illness: Research and theory for nursing practice* (pp. 4–5). Springer.

trajectories than others, but all trajectories are subject to individual variation. There have been a number of conceptualizations of illness trajectories. Rolland (1987) identified three critical time phases within the illness trajectory:

Crisis phase: The period before and immediately after diagnosis, when learning to live with symptoms and illness-related demands takes place

Chronic phase: The time span between initial diagnosis and the final time phase, when the key task is continuing to live as normal a life as possible in the face of the abnormality of having a chronic illness whose outcomes are uncertain

Terminal phase: This phase is marked by issues surrounding grief and death. Depending on the illness, some patients will enter this phase only after many years.

Further important work in the area of illness trajectories was conducted by Corbin (1998). These authors defined a trajectory of the course of an illness over time, identifying nine phases: (a) pre-trajectory; (b) trajectory onset; (c) stable; (d) unstable; (e) acute; (f) crisis; (g) comeback; (h) downward; and (i) dying. Table 5.6 describes the phases and the associated goals of management. Illness trajectory can be altered or shaped by actions that stabilize the disease course, minimize exacerbations, and better control symptoms (Corbin & Strauss, 1992). This model recognizes that each person's illness trajectory is unique.

Shifting Perspectives Model of Chronic Illness

Models that describe living with a chronic illness as a phased process have also been criticized because they imply that an end goal exists and that this goal can be reached only if the person has lived long enough to progress through previous stages. The Shifting Perspectives Model of Chronic Illness (Figure 5.3) described by Paterson (2001) shows living with a chronic illness as an ongoing, continually shifting process. This perspective of chronic illness contains elements of both illness and wellness.

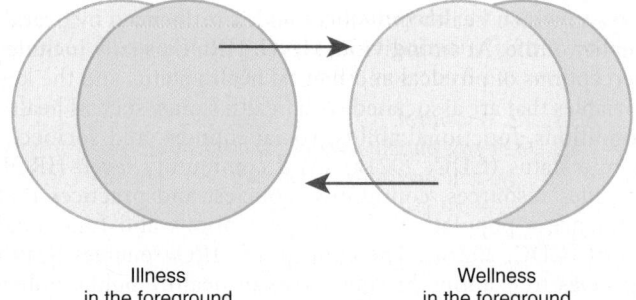

Illness in the foreground — Wellness in the foreground

FIG. 5.3 The Shifting Perspectives Model of Chronic Illness. Source: Paterson, B. (2001). The shifting perspectives model of chronic illness. *Journal of Nursing Scholarship,* 33(1), 21–26. Copyright © 2001, John Wiley and Sons.

As the reality of the illness experience and its context change, the person's perspective shifts in the degree to which illness or wellness is in the foreground or background of their world. Perspectives of chronic illness are not seen as right or wrong but as reflections of people's needs and situations.

When illness is in the foreground, individuals focus on the sickness, suffering, loss, and burden associated with living with a chronic illness. This perspective is marked by self-absorption and difficulty attending to the needs of others. This perspective often occurs in people who are newly diagnosed or overwhelmed by their illness. When wellness is in the foreground, the person attempts to create consonance between self-identity and the identity shaped by the disease and between the construction of the illness by others and by life events. The body is objectified and placed at a distance; it is not allowed to control the person. This perspective can be gained by learning as much as possible about the disease, creating supportive environments, developing skills such as negotiating, identifying the body's unique patterns of response, and sharing with others knowledge about living with the illness. This distance provides for a focus on social, emotional, and spiritual aspects of life, rather than a focus on the diseased body.

The perspective that is in the foreground shifts depending on the circumstances. Emotional distress increases during periods of acute hospitalization and can lead to a loss of control and to humiliation, loneliness, pain, and loss of personal dignity if treated as a "nonperson" (Roger & Hatala, 2018). Returning to having wellness in the foreground may result from changes or interventions that resolve or accommodate the situation that has resulted in the illness focus.

SELF-MANAGEMENT

Self-management is the foundation for optimizing health outcomes for people living with chronic illness. A large body of empirical literature demonstrates that successful self-management is related to better overall physical and psychological health outcomes (Clark, Gong, & Kaciroti, 2014). Self-management is the "intrinsically controlled ability of an active, responsible, informed and autonomous individual to live with the medical, role and emotional consequences of the chronic condition(s) in partnership with their social network and health care provider(s)" (Van de Velde et al., 2019, p. 10). This approach emphasizes the primary role that patients have in managing their illness to achieve the best possible quality of life. Every day, patients decide what they are going to eat, whether they will exercise, and to what extent they will take their prescribed medications. These activities, though usually undertaken in cooperation with a health care provider, go beyond merely adhering to a prescribed behavioural regimen. As Glasgow and Anderson (1999, p. 2090) note:

> Patients are in control. No matter what we as health professionals do or say, patients are in control of these important self-management decisions. When patients leave the clinic or office, they can and do veto recommendations a health professional makes.
>
> The actions people take to manage their conditions are often based on the advice given by health care providers. Sometimes, however, patients choose not to accept this advice, resulting in less than optimal outcomes.

Compliance, adherence, and self-care make up the three levels of patient response to health care recommendations on a continuum of self-care. *Compliance* reflects coercion of the patient to engage in particular recommendations, whereas *adherence* implies conformity of the patient to the recommendations. *Self-care* connotes a therapeutic alliance between the patient and the provider. *Adherence* is now the term most widely accepted because it incorporates the notion of the patient agreeing with the treatment plan presented by the health care provider.

Partnership between the nurse and the patient, which focuses on an open, caring, mutually responsive, and nondirective dialogue, is a key aspect of relational nursing practice and is essential in the promotion of self-management. The process of self-management involves empowering the patient, thereby ensuring some autonomy with respect to adjusting the regimen as necessary. Four tasks related to coping with chronic illness are as follows: (a) processing emotions, including grieving, in response to health or functioning; (b) adjusting to the changes to self and life as a result of the illness; (c) integrating illness into daily life; and (d) determining the meaning of the illness so as to help identify tasks and skills that will promote personal growth and satisfaction.

The nurse must be alert to potential barriers to successful self-management. People of low socioeconomic status and those who are marginalized are more difficult to attract and retain in self-management programs. Similarly, patients who have limited health literacy may be seriously compromised in their ability to self-manage their conditions successfully. In addition to health literacy, other barriers to self-management that the nurse must be sensitive to include poorer health, distress, poor communication, and financial constraints (Adu et al., 2019). The principles of self-management have been the foundation of numerous chronic illness management programs. Evidence-informed self-management (see, for example, the Evidence-Informed Practice box) starts with the premise that there is a partnership

⚡ EVIDENCE-INFORMED PRACTICE

Research Highlight

How Effective Is the Teach-Back Method on Adherence and Self-Management in Health Education for People With Chronic Disease?

Clinical Question

PICO

P—Adults aged 18 years and over with one or more chronic disease(s)
I—Teach-back method used in a chronic disease education program
C—Chronic disease education program that did not use the teach-back method
O—Health outcomes and use of health care services
Research Question: What is the impact of a teach-back chronic disease educational program on health outcomes and use of health care services for adults who have one or more chronic disease(s)?

Best Available Evidence

A systematic review of randomized control trials (RTC), nonrandomized control trials, cohort studies, before–after studies, and case-control studies

Critical Appraisal and Synthesis of Evidence

The reviewers assessed a broad range of studies that used the teach-back method. Four studies found improved disease-specific knowledge; one study showed a statistically significant improvement in medication and diet adherence among type 2 diabetics in the intervention group compared to the control group ($p < 0.001$). Two studies found a statistically significant improvement in self-efficacy ($p = 0.0026$ and $p < 0.001$) in the intervention group. One study examining quality of life in patients with heart failure did not improve with the intervention ($p = 0.59$). Although not statistically significant, five studies found lower hospitalization and readmission rates. Two studies showed improvement in daily weighing among patients with heart failure, and in adherence to diet, exercise, and foot care among those with type 2 diabetes.

Conclusions

The health education teach-back method improves disease-specific knowledge, adherence, and self-efficacy. There was a positive association with self-care, reduction in hospital readmission, hospitalization, or deaths. Teach-back did not improve health-related quality of life or knowledge retention.

Implications for Nursing

Using the teach-back method for educating patients with chronic disease maximizes understanding of the disease and improves self-efficacy and self-care skills.

Reference for Evidence

Dinh, T. T., Bonner, A., Clark, R., et al. (2016). The effectiveness of the teach-back method on adherence and self-management in health educzation for people with chronic disease: a systematic review. JBI Libr Syst Rev, 14(1), 210–247. https://doi.org/10.11124/jbisrir-2016-2296.

P, patient population of interest; *I,* intervention or area of interest; *C,* comparison of interest or comparison group; *O,* outcomes of interest (see Chapter 1).

between patients and health care providers. New paradigms of self-management examine the beliefs and the issues of people with chronic illness, connecting this information with health care providers' views of what knowledge patients must have and what behaviours they must change to manage their condition.

THE EMERGING PARADIGM OF CHRONIC CARE

As stated earlier, our present health care system is organized around an acute, episodic model of care that fails to meet the needs of many patients, including those with chronic illnesses. Patients, families, caregivers, health care providers, and decision makers must recognize that a new model of care must

TABLE 5.7	WHAT PATIENTS WITH CHRONIC ILLNESS WANT FROM THE HEALTH CARE SYSTEM

Access to information concerning:
- Diagnosis and its implications
- Available treatments and their consequences
- Potential impact on the patient's future
- Continuity of care and ready access to it
- Coordination of care, particularly with specialists
- Infrastructure improvements (scheduling, wait times, prompt care)
- Ways to cope with symptoms such as pain, fatigue, disability, and loss of independence
- Ways to adjust to disease consequences such as uncertainty, fear and depression, anger, loneliness, sleep disorders, memory loss, exercise needs, nocturia, sexual dysfunction, and stress

Source: Holman, H., & Lorig, K. (2004). Patient self-management: A key to effectiveness and efficiency in care of chronic disease. *Public Health Reports, 119*, 239–243.

be enacted that better addresses the needs of persons with chronic illness. The shortcomings of the current health care system are well known to the dissatisfied patients, the frustrated families, and the weary staff who have struggled to manage the complexities of chronic illness. In response, the Canadian government has established priorities that will support health care system innovations such as telehealth and that will enhance the integration and coordination of home care services, especially for Indigenous and northern communities (Health Canada, 2015) (see Chapter 6 for further information). Table 5.7 describes what patients with chronic illness want from the health care system and what they believe has been missing. These reasonable expectations are embedded within the chronic care model.

Building on the notion of self-management and the need for an integrated, patient-centred system of care, the chronic care model was first advanced by Bodenheimer, Wagner, and Grumbach (2002). This model predicted that improvements in the following six interrelated components would improve care for persons with chronic illness: (a) self-management support, (b) clinical information systems, (c) delivery system redesign, (d) decision support, (e) health care organization, and (f) community resources. The original model was expanded to include a greater focus on prevention and health promotion by Barr and colleagues (2003). The Expanded Chronic Care Model (ECCM) appears in Figure 5.4.

The ECCM supports the important role that the social determinants of health play in influencing individual, community, and population health. Support of self-management and the development of personal skills for health and wellness in the ECCM may be accomplished by providing information and enhancing life skills.

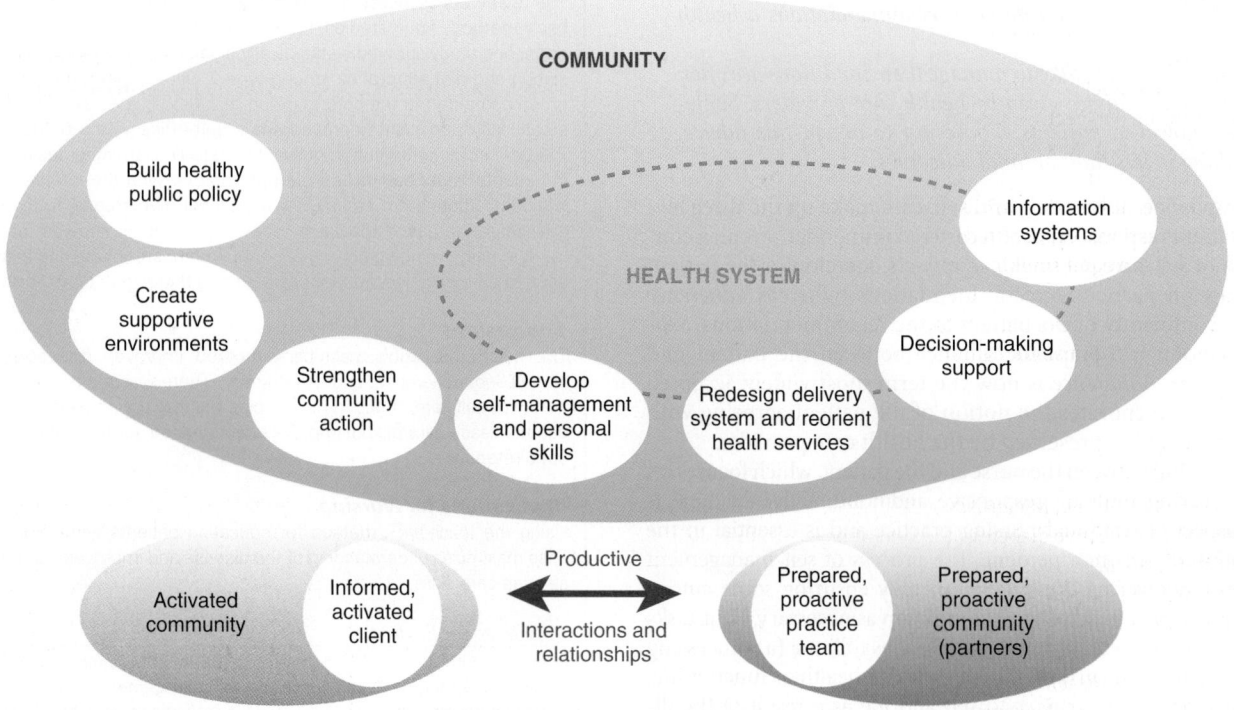

FIG. 5.4 The Expanded Chronic Care Model. Source: Barr, V., Robinson, S., Marin-Link, B., et al. (2003). The Expanded Chronic Care Model: An integration of concepts and strategies from population health promotion and the chronic care model. *Healthcare Quarterly, 7*(1), 73–82.

Delivery system redesign and reorientation of health services encourage health care providers to move beyond the provision of cure-focused services to an expanded mandate that promotes a holistic perspective. Decision support encompasses the gathering of evidence not only on disease and treatment but also on staying healthy. Information systems can be used to evaluate established systems and support new ways of providing care. Healthy public policy involves working toward organizational and governmental legislation and policy that foster greater equity in society and lead to safer and healthier goods, services, and environments. The creation of safe, affordable housing is one example in this area. Finally, strengthening community action involves working together with community groups to set priorities and achieve goals that enhance the health of the community.

Nurses have a vital role to play within the vision of the ECCM and can serve as leaders in the challenge to improve the care of Canadians living with chronic illness.

REVIEW QUESTIONS

The number of the question corresponds to the same-numbered objective at the beginning of the chapter.

1. What is the most common cause of death in Canada?
   a. Cancer
   b. Cardiovascular disease
   c. Respiratory disease
   d. Community-acquired pneumonia
2. Which of the following are characteristics of a chronic illness? (Select all that apply.)
   a. It has reversible pathological changes.
   b. It has a consistent, predictable clinical course.
   c. It results in permanent deviation from normal.
   d. It is associated with many stable and unstable phases.
   e. It always starts with an acute illness and then progresses slowly.
3. Select the modifiable risk factor for developing chronic illness.
   a. Activity level and sex
   b. Age and genetic background
   c. Air pollution and occupation
   d. Smoking and weight
4. According to the World Health Organization, which model best accounts for disability?
   a. The biopsychosocial model
   b. The medical model
   c. The social model
   d. The shifting perspectives model
5. Which statement from a 47-year-old client with COPD reflects her efficacy expectancy?
   a. "I have this disease only because I worked in an auto body shop for years and was exposed to toxic fumes."
   b. "I know I can't quit smoking. I've tried too many times in the past 5 years."
   c. "My mother quit smoking, and she still died from lung disease."
   d. "It's too late to quit smoking now, so what's the point of trying?"

6. Identify the situation in which caregiver burden is most likely to occur.
   a. A husband must administer medications to his cognitively impaired wife.
   b. A daughter must empty her mother's drains following a mastectomy.
   c. A wife with heart failure must assist her husband to the toilet following a cerebrovascular accident.
   d. A neighbour prepares meals for a client recently discharged from hospital following cataract surgery.
7. A client has had multiple sclerosis for the past 2 years and is admitted to hospital to manage symptoms of an exacerbation. According to the illness trajectory model, which phase of chronic illness would she be in?
   a. Trajectory onset
   b. Unstable
   c. Acute
   d. Crisis
8. A 53-year-old with fibromyalgia has followed her prescribed exercise program for the past month. What would this behaviour be an example of?
   a. Compliance
   b. Adherence
   c. Self-management
   d. Chronic care
9. A nurse is part of a citizen group initiative to start a food bank for disadvantaged people. Within the ECCM, in which domain does this work of the nurse fall?
   a. Delivery system redesign
   b. Healthy public policy
   c. Social support
   d. Strengthening community

1. a; 2. c, d; 3. d; 4. a; 5. b; 6. c; 7. c; 8. b; 9. d.

⟳volve

For even more review questions, visit http://evolve.elsevier.com/Canada/Lewis/medsurg.

REFERENCES

Adu, M. D., Malabu, U. H., Malau-Aduli, A. E., et al. (2019). Enablers and barriers to effective diabetes self-management: A multinational investigation. *PloS One, 14*(6), e0217771. https://doi.org/10.1371/journal.pone.0217771

Bandura, A. (1977). *Social learning theory.* Prentice-Hall (Seminal).

Barnes, C. (2012). *Understanding the social model of disability. Routledge handbook of disability studies.* Routledge.

Barnett, K., Mercer, S. W., Norbury, M., et al. (2012). Epidemiology of multimorbidity and implications for health care, research, and medical education: A cross-sectional study. *The Lancet, 380*(9836), 37–43. https://doi.org/10.1016/S0140-6736(12)60240-2

Barr, V. J., Robinson, S., Marin-Link, B., et al. (2003). The Expanded Chronic Care Model: An integration of concepts and strategies from population health promotion and the chronic care model. *Hospital Quarterly, 7*(1), 73–82 (Seminal).

Bodenheimer, T., Wagner, E. H., & Grumbach, K. (2002). Improving primary care for patients with chronic illness. *Journal of the American Medical Association, 288*, 1775–1779. https://doi.org/10.1001/jama.288.14.1775. (Seminal).

Bushnik, T., Tjepkema, M., & Martel, L. (2020). *Socioeconomic disparities in life and health expectancy among the household population in Canada.* Statistics Canada. https://www150.statcan.gc.ca/n1/en/pub/82-003-x/2020001/article/00001-eng.pdf?st=yufIP5s9

Canadian Cancer Society. (2019). *Canadian cancer statistics 2019.* https://www.cancer.ca/~/media/cancer.ca/CW/cancer%20information/cancer%20101/Canadian%20cancer%20statistics/Canadian-Cancer-Statistics-2019-EN.pdf?la=en

Carers Canada. (2018). *Caregiver facts.* https://www.carerscanada.ca/caregiver-facts/

Centers for Disease Control and Prevention (CDC). (2021a). *Health-related quality of life.* https://www.cdc.gov/hrqol/index.htm

Centers for Disease Control and Prevention (CDC). (2021b). *How you can prevent chronic diseases.* National Center for Chronic Disease Prevention and Health Promotion. https://www.cdc.gov/chronicdisease/about/prevent/index.htm

Corbin, J. (1998). The Corbin and Strauss chronic illness trajectory model: An update. *Scholarly Inquiry for Nursing Practice, 12*(1), 33–41 (Seminal).

Corbin, J., & Strauss, A. (1992). A nursing model for chronic illness management based upon the trajectory framework. In P. Woong (Ed.), *The chronic illness trajectory framework.* Springer (Seminal).

Enns, M. W., Bernstein, C. N., Kroeker, K., et al. (2018). The association of fatigue, pain, depression and anxiety with work and activity impairment in immune mediated inflammatory diseases. *PLoS One, 13*(6), e0198975. https://doi.org/10.1371/journal.pone.0198975

Ferguson, T. W., Tangri, N., Tan, Z., et al. (2017). Screening for Chronic Kidney disease in Canadian Indigenous peoples is cost effective. *Kidney International, 92*(1), 192–200. https://doi.org/10.1016/j.kint.2017.02.022

Gałecki, P., & Talarowska, M. (2018). Inflammatory theory of depression. *Psychiatria Polska, 52*(3), 437–447. https://doi.org/10.12740/PP/76863

Glaser, B., & Strauss, A. (1967). *The discovery of grounded theory: Strategies for qualitative research.* Aldine Transaction (Seminal).

Glasgow, R. E., & Anderson, R. M. (1999). In diabetes care, moving from compliance to adherence is not enough. *Diabetes Care, 22*(12), 2090–2092 (Seminal).

Goodell, S., Bodenheimer, T., & Berry-Millett, R. (2009). *Care management of patients with complex health care needs. Research Synthesis Report No. 19.* The Robert Wood Johnson Foundation. https://www.rwjf.org/en/library/research/2009/12/care-management-of-patients-with-complex-health-care-needs.html. (Seminal).

Gordon, K., Gray, C. S., Dainty, K. N., et al. (2020). Exploring an innovative care model and telemonitoring for the management of patients with complex chronic needs: qualitative description study. *JMIR Nursing, 3*(1), e15691. https://doi.org/10.2196/15691

Government of Canada. (2020). *Social determinants of health.* https://www.canada.ca/en/public-health/services/health-promotion/population-health/what-determines-health.html

Halaris, A. (2016). Inflammation-associated co-morbidity between depression and cardiovascular disease. In R. Danzter, L. Capuron (Eds.), *Inflammation-Associated Depression: Evidence, Mechanisms and Implications* (pp. 45–70). Springer.

Hango, D. (2020). *Insights on Canadian society: Support received by caregivers in Canada.* Statistics Canada. https://www150.statcan.gc.ca/n1/pub/75-006-x/2020001/article/00001-eng.htm

Health Canada. (2015). *Health Canada 2015-16 report on plans and priorities.* https://www.hc-sc.gc.ca/ahc-asc/performance/estim-previs/plans-prior/2015-2016/report-rapport-eng.php#a2.1

Johansen, S., Cvancarova, M., & Ruland, C. (2018). The effect of cancer patients' and their family caregivers' physical and emotional symptoms on caregiver burden. *Cancer Nursing, 41*(2), 91–99. https://doi.org/10.1097/NCC.0000000000000493

Knaak, S., Mantler, E., & Szeto, A. (2017). Mental illness-related stigma in healthcare: Barriers to access and care and evidence-based solutions. *Healthcare Management Forum, 30*(2), 111–116. https://doi.org/10.1177/0840470416679413

Kobasa, S. C. (1979). Stressful events, personality and health: An inquiry into hardiness. *Journal of Personality and Social Psychology, 37*(1), 1–11 (Seminal).

Larsen, P. D. (2017). *Lubkin's chronic illness: Impact and interventions* (10th ed.). Jones & Bartlett.

Légaré, F., & Witteman, H. O. (2013). Shared decision making: examining key elements and barriers to adoption into routine clinical practice. *Health Affairs, 32*(2), 276–284. https://doi.org/10.1377/hlthaff.2012.1078

Liu, Z., Heffernan, C., & Tan, J. (2020). Caregiver burden: A concept analysis. *International Journal of Nursing Sciences, 7*(4), 438–445. https://doi.org/10.1016/j.ijnss.2020.07.012

Magnussen, R. S., McGrady, B., Gostin, L., et al. (2019). Legal capacities required for the prevention and control of noncommunicable diseases. *Bulletin of World Health Organization, 97*(2), 108–117. https://doi.org/10.2471/BLT.18.213777

McCain, H. (2017). *Medical Model of Disability versus Social Model of Disability.* https://canbc.org/blog/medical-model-of-disability-versus-social-model-of-disability

Mechanic, D. (1995). The concept of illness behaviour. *Journal of Chronic Diseases, 15*(2), 189–194 (Seminal).

Ministry of Health and Long-Term Care (MOHLTC). (2018). *Chronic Disease Prevention Guideline, 2018.* https://www.health.gov.on.ca/en/pro/programs/publichealth/oph_standards/docs/protocols_guidelines/Chronic_Disease_Prevention_Guideline_2018.pdf

National Collaborating Centre for Aboriginal Health. (2013). *An overview of Aboriginal health in Canada.* https://www.ccnsa.ca/docs/context/FS-OverviewAboriginalHealth-EN.pdf

National Health Service. (2011). *The Expert Patients Programme—What is an expert patient?* https://www.nhs.uk/Conditions/Expert-patients-programme-/Pages/Whatisanexpertpatient.aspx

National Institute of Mental Health. (2021). *Chronic illness and mental health: Recognizing and treating depression.* https://www.nimh.nih.gov/health/publications/chronic-illness-mental-health/index.shtml

National Institutes of Health (NIH), National Heart, Lung and Blood Institute. (n.d.). *What are the key findings of the Farmington Heart Survey?* https://www.nhlbi.nih.gov/science/framingham-heart-study-fhs

Nyblade, L., Stockton, M. A., Giger, K., et al. (2019). Stigma in health facilities: why it matters and how we can change it. *BMC Medicine, 17*(1), 1–15. https://doi.org/10.1186/s12916-019-1256-2

Paterson, B. (2001). The shifting perspectives model of chronic illness. *Journal of Nursing Scholarship, 33*(1), 21–26. https://doi.org/10.1111/j.1547-5069.2001.00021.x. (Seminal).

Pollock, S. E., Christian, B. J., & Sands, D. (1990). Responses to chronic illness: Analysis of psychological and physiological adaptation. *Nursing Research, 39*(5), 300–304. https://doi.org/10.1097/00006199-199009000-00014. (Seminal).

Pollock, S. E., & Duffy, M. E. (1990). The Health-Related Hardiness Scale: Development and psychometric analysis. *Nursing Research, 39*(4), 218–222. https://doi.org/10.1097/00006199-199007000-00008. (Seminal).

Public Health Agency of Canada (PHAC). (2015). *Improving health outcomes—A paradigm shift: Centre for Chronic Disease Prevention strategic plan 2016–2019.* https://www.phac-aspc.gc.ca/cd-mc/ccdp-strategic-plan-2016-2019-plan-strategique-cpmc-eng.php

Public Health Agency of Canada (PHAC). (2019). *Prevalence of chronic diseases among Canadian adults.* https://www.canada.ca/en/public-health/services/chronic-diseases/prevalence-canadian-adults-infographic-2019.html

Ream, E., & Richardson, A. (1996). Fatigue: A concept analysis. *International Journal of Nursing Studies, 33*(5), 519–529. https://doi.org/10.1016/0020-7489(96)00004-1. (Seminal).

Registered Nurses' Association of Ontario (RNAO). (2010). *Nursing best practice guideline: Strategies to support self-management in chronic conditions: Collaboration with clients.* https://rnao.ca/bpg/guidelines/strategies-support-selfmanagement-chronic-conditions-collaboration-clients. (Seminal).

Ringer, T., Hazzan, A. A., Agarwal, A., et al. (2017). Relationship between family caregiver burden and physical frailty in older adults without dementia: a systematic review. *Systematic Reviews, 6*(1), 55. https://doi.org/10.1186/s13643-017-0447-1

Robinson, C. A. (2016). Trust, health care relationships, and chronic illness: a theoretical coalescence. *Global Qualitative Nursing Research, 3,* 1–11. https://doi.org/10.1177/2333393616664823

Roger, K. S., & Hatala, A. (2018). Religion, spirituality & chronic illness: A scoping review and implications for health care practitioners. *Journal of Religion & Spirituality in Social Work: Social Thought, 37*(1), 24–44. https://doi.org/10.1080/15426432.2017.1386151

Rolland, J. S. (1987). Chronic illness and the life cycle: A conceptual framework. *Family Process, 26*(2), 203–211 (Seminal).

Secinti, E., Thompson, E., Richards, M., et al. (2017). Research Review: Childhood chronic physical illness and adult emotional health- a systematic review and meta-analysis. *Journal of Child Psychology and Psychiatry, 58*(7), 753–769. https://doi.org/10.1111/jcpp.12727

Statistics Canada. (2019). *Population projections for Canada (2018–2068), provinces and territories (2018–2043).* https://www150.statcan.gc.ca/n1/en/pub/91-520-x/91-520-x2019001-eng.pdf?st=3cyRYyH3

Statistics Canada. (2021). *Leading causes of death, total population. by age group.* https://www150.statcan.gc.ca/t1/tbl1/en/tv.action?pid=1310039401

Sternke, E. A., Abrahamson, K., & Bair, M. J. (2016). Comorbid chronic pain and depression: patient perspectives on empathy. *Pain Management Nursing, 17*(6), 363–371. https://doi.org/10.1016/j.pmn.2016.07.003

Suchman, E. A. (1965). Stages of illness and medical care. *Journal of Health and Human Behavior,* 114–128 (Seminal).

Trivedi, R. B., Bosworth, H. B., & Jackson, G. L. (2011). Resilience in chronic illness. In B. Resnick, L. Gwyther, & K. Roberto (Eds.), *Resilience in aging* (pp. 181–197). Springer (Seminal).

Van de Velde, D., De Zutter, F., Satink, T., et al. (2019). Delineating the concept of self-management in chronic conditions: a concept analysis. *BMJ Open, 9*(7), 1–15. https://doi.org/10.1136/bmjopen-2018-027775

Vennedey, V., Hower, K. I., Hillen, H., et al. (2020). Patients' perspectives of facilitators and barriers to patient-centred care: insights from qualitative patient interviews. *BMJ Open, 10*(5), e033449. https://doi.org/10.1136/bmjopen-2019-033449

Wallace, E., Salisbury, C., Guthrie, B., et al. (2015). Managing patients with multimorbidity in primary care. *BMJ, 350,* h176. https://doiorg/10.1136/bmj.h176

World Health Organization (WHO). (2002). *Towards a common language for functioning, disability and healthICF: The International Classification of Functioning, Disability and Health.* https://www.who.int/classifications/icf/icfbeginnersguide.pdf. (Seminal).

World Health Organization (WHO). (2014). *Global status report on noncommunicable diseases 2014.* https://apps.who.int/iris/bitstream/10665/148114/1/9789241564854_eng.pdf

World Health Organization (WHO). (2019). *World Health Statistics 2019: Monitoring Health for the SDGs, sustainable development goals.* https://www.who.int.gho/publications/world_health_statistics/2019/EN_WHS2019_TOC_pdf?ua=1

World Health Organization (WHO). (2021). *Constitution.* https://www.who.int/about/governance/constitution

Ysseldyk, R., Kuran, N., Powell, S., et al. (2020). *Original quantitative research—Self-reported health impacts of caregiving by age and income among participants of the Canadian 2012 General Social Survey.* https://www.canada.ca/en/public-health/services/reports-publications/health-promotion-chronic-disease-prevention-canada-research-policy-practice/vol-39-no-5-2019/self-reported-health-impacts-of-caregiving-age-and-income-among-participants.html

RESOURCES

Canada's World Health Organization (WHO) Collaborating Centre on Chronic Noncommunicable Disease
https://www.phac-aspc.gc.ca/about_apropos/whocc-ccoms/index-eng.php

Canadian Lung Association
https://www.lung.ca

Carers Canada
https://www.carerscanada.ca

Heart and Stroke Foundation of Canada
https://www.heartandstroke.ca/

Public Health Agency of Canada: *Chronic Diseases*
https://www.canada.ca/en/public-health/services/chronic-diseases.html

Registered Nurses' Association of Ontario Clinical Best Practice Guidelines: *Strategies to Support Self-Management in Chronic Conditions: Collaboration With Clients*
https://rnao.ca/sites/rnao-ca/files/Strategies_to_Support_Self-Management_in_Chronic_Conditions_-_Collaboration_with_Clients.pdf

Improving Chronic Illness Care (Robert Wood Johnson Foundation)
https://www.rwjf.org/en/library/research/2011/12/improving-chronic-illness-care.html

National ME (Myalgic Encephalomyelitis)/FA (Fibromyalgia Action) Network
http://www.mefmaction.com/

Siteman Cancer Center: *Your Disease Risk interactive questionnaire*
https://siteman.wustl.edu/prevention/ydr/

⊖volve

For additional Internet resources, see the website for this book at http://evolve.elsevier.com/Canada/Lewis/medsurg.

6

Community-Based Nursing and Home Care

Julie H. Fraser and Sarah J. Siebert

ⓔvolve WEBSITE

http://evolve.elsevier.com/Canada/Lewis/medsurg

- Review Questions (Online Only)
- Key Points
- Answer Guidelines for Case Study
- Rationales for Textbook Review Questions
- Conceptual Care Map Creator
- Audio Glossary
- Content Updates

LEARNING OBJECTIVES

1. Distinguish the relevance of community nursing in the patient's health journey.
2. Compare the various community health settings and the related nursing roles.
3. Describe the role that primary and community care plays in promoting the sustainability of Canada's health care system.
4. Differentiate how home care in Canada is organized and funded.
5. Describe the practice of the home health nurse.
6. Examine the key clinical competencies and home health trends.

KEY TERMS

chronic disease management
family-centred care
frailty

home health nursing
primary care
primary health care

public health nursing
virtual care

The community setting offers a diversity of exciting and professionally fulfilling roles in which community health nurses (CHNs) make a meaningful difference to the health of individuals, families, communities, and populations. Home and community care have increasingly been recognized as essential components of the health care system (Canadian Home Care Association [CHCA], 2016). In its report of the 2019 nursing workforce, the Canadian Institute for Health Information (CIHI) indicated that 6.5% of regulated nurses worked in the community health sector, which includes community health centres, home care nursing organizations, nursing stations (outpost or clinic), and public health departments or units (CIHI, 2020). This chapter discusses community-based nursing, including roles and practice, with an emphasis on home health care.

COMMUNITY HEALTH AND THE PATIENT'S HEALTH CARE JOURNEY

The necessity for community health services continues to be relevant in the twenty-first century. The average age of Canadians is increasing. In 2019, Statistics Canada reported that in Canada there were more persons aged 65 years and older (17.5%) than children aged 0 to 14 years (16%) and that the number of older persons will continue to increase to 21%–30% of the population by 2068 (Statistics Canada, 2020). Noncommunicable diseases account for 88% of deaths worldwide (World Health Organization [WHO], 2018b). Management of communicable diseases requires global collaboration as outbreaks continue. Economic factors contributing to the need for more community health services include the fact that over the past 40 years the number of dual-income families has increased from 36% to 69% of the population (Statistics Canada, 2018c), with 15% of individuals reporting a low income (Statistics Canada, 2018b). The societal shift of more individuals working affects the time available for informal caregiving and community development activities. In turn, there is a demand for funded day care for children and for older persons, and the number of private home care companies has grown (IBIS World, 2020). Across the country, governments are working to shift funding and resources to health care services in the community (Health Canada, 2018). The aim of strengthening community health services is to increase proactive approaches to improving health and therefore reduce spending for hospital and facility care (CHCA, 2019; CHCA et al., 2016).

Currently, the average hospital stay, although only 7 days, costs $6 350 or more, depending on the hospital specialty (CIHI, 2021a). Further, 1 in 11 individuals hospitalized found that on discharge community supports were not ready (CIHI, 2021c). The majority of Canadians are in favor of raising taxes to increase the health services received in their home (CHCA, 2016). Providing individuals health care services in the community setting is a strategy to mitigate costs associated with hospital and facility care. **Chronic disease management**, which incorporates strategies to reduce risk factors, could save 600 lives by 2025 (WHO, 2018a). Advanced care planning, which entails proactive conversations about individuals' health care goals, has also been shown to reduce costs associated with hospital and long-term care (Huggins et al., 2019). The outcomes of harm reduction strategies are growing; such strategies are important in supporting marginalized and homeless populations (Wilson et al., 2015). Another priority strategy in the community setting is to close the significant health gaps that have been identified for Indigenous populations (Naqshbandi Hayward et al., 2016; Tompkins et al., 2018). An understanding of community health services is essential for all health care providers to ensure quality handovers in care, judicious use of health resources, and the promotion of self-management.

COMMUNITY HEALTH SETTINGS

According to Community Health Nurses of Canada (CHNC), CHNs "support the health and well-being of individuals, families, groups, communities, populations and systems. . . . Using a capacity-building and strengths-based approach, they provide, facilitate, and coordinate direct care and link people to community resources. . . . Health includes self-determination and a sense of connection to community" (CHNC, 2019, p. 7). A number of roles exist for nurses who work in a variety community-based settings (Table 6.1).

Public Health Care

Public health is built on the foundation of social justice, health equity, and social and ecological determinants of health (Canadian Public Health Association [CPHA], 2017). Public health care focuses on activities and services that increase the health of the population. This includes health protection, health surveillance, disease and injury prevention, population health assessment, health promotion, and emergency preparedness and response (CPHA, 2019). **Public health nursing** recognizes that "a community's health is closely linked to the health of its members and is often reflected first in individual and family health experiences." In turn, "healthy communities and systems that support health contribute to opportunities for health for individuals, families, groups, and populations" (CPHA, 2010, p. 10).

Primary Health Care

As defined by the WHO, "primary health care is essential health care based on practical, scientifically sound, and socially acceptable methods and technology made universally accessible to individuals and families in the community through their full participation and at a cost that the community and country can afford" (WHO, 1978, p.1). Primary health care is the first level of contact that individuals have with a health care system and the first part of the health care process (WHO, 1978, 2018). Community health nursing practice is informed and guided by the philosophy and principles of primary health care and home

TABLE 6.1 EXAMPLES OF COMMUNITY NURSING ROLES

Setting	Nursing Role
Public health	Public health nurse
	Street nurse
	Sexual health nurse
School	Nursing support service
	School health nurse
Place of worship	Faith community nurse
	Parish nurse
Rural	Outpost nurse
	Rural-remote nurse
Corrections	Forensic nurse
	Mental health nurse
Private sector	Occupational health nurse
	Nurse entrepreneur
Primary care	Nurse practitioner
	Chronic disease nurse
	Primary care nurse
	Family practice nurse
	Outreach nurse
Specialized services	Community dialysis nurse
	Sexual assault nurse examiner
Home care	Home care nurse
	Community nurse/Community health nurse

health with nursing theory, social sciences, and public health science (CHNC, 2019) (Table 6.2).

Although the terms *primary care* and *primary health care* are often used interchangeably, there is an important difference between them. **Primary care** has historically been used to describe the clinicians responsible for providing the majority of an individuals' health needs over a continued period of time in the context of their family and community (Molla et al., 1996). **Primary health care** is both a philosophy and a strategy to deliver health care. Its focus is system-wide, and key participants are intersectoral partners in the fields of health, social services, housing, and the environment (Government of Canada, 2012). Primary health care continues to be embraced as a strategy to shift the health system's emphasis from diagnosis and treatment of illness and injury to health promotion and disease prevention (WHO, 2018a). This shift is also known as *transforming the system* (Canadian Foundation for Healthcare Improvement [CFHI], 2012; Canadian Nurses Association [CNA], 2015).

In Canada, there is growing evidence of the deepening adoption of principles of primary health care in policies and service delivery models as well as targeted federal and provincial funding (College of Family Physicians of Canada, 2019 [CFPC]; Misfeldt et al., 2017). Innovative primary care models promote integration between primary care, home care, mental health, and public health services (CFHI, 2012; Kates, 2017). Although there is a plurality of primary care models at the regional and local level, interprofessional team–based care is seen as a critical attribute of models of the future (CFHI, 2012; CFPC, 2019; CNA, 2015). Nurse leaders in primary care (also called *family practice nursing*) have mobilized resources and research to identify for the first time key competencies for nurses working in this setting. This type of practice support and development further strengthen the opportunity to optimize the nursing scope of practice in this setting (Canadian Family Practice Nurses Association, 2019; CNA, 2014, 2015).

TABLE 6.2	KEY PRINCIPLES OF PRIMARY HEALTH CARE

There are six key principles of primary health care:
1. Universal access to health care services on the basis of need
2. Focus on the determinants of health as part of a commitment to health equity and social justice
3. Active participation on the parts of individuals and communities in decisions that affect their health and lives
4. Partnership with other disciplines, communities, and sectors for health (intersectoral approach)
5. Appropriate use of knowledge, skills, strategies, technology, and resources
6. Focus on health promotion–illness prevention throughout the life experience from birth to death

TABLE 6.3	FUNDING MECHANISMS FOR HOME CARE

1. Publicly funded, provincial–territorial health care plan
2. Private insurance (e.g., employment benefit plans)
3. Veterans Affairs Canada
4. First Nations and Inuit Health Branch (FNIHB)
5. Indigenous and Northern Affairs Canada
6. Workers' compensation boards
7. Private payment
8. Associations and foundations (e.g., Canadian Red Cross)

HOME CARE

Definition and Importance of Home Care

In Canada, *home care* is defined as an array of health and support services provided in the home, retirement communities, group homes, and other community settings to people with acute, chronic, palliative, or rehabilitative health care needs. Services offered through publicly funded home care programs include assessments, education, therapeutic interventions (nursing and rehabilitation), personal assistance with activities of daily living (ADLs), help with instrumental activities of daily living (IADLs), and caregiver respite and support (CHCA, 2016, p. 1).

In 2015–2016, 6.4% of Canadians households received home care services (Statistics Canada, 2018a). Home care, however, is *not* one of the insured services covered by the *Canada Health Act*, the legislation that created and protects Canada's universal, publicly funded health care system. Therefore, provinces and territories have no legal obligation to ensure that their citizens have access to home care services. A Nanos poll found that 90% of Canadians consider home care essential to aging at home (CNA, 2015). Although every province and territory now has a home care program, they offer varied access and types of programming (CHCA, 2013). The CHCA (2017) has established national harmonized principles of care: it is (a) patient- and family-centred, (b) accessible, (c) accountable, (d) evidence-informed, (e) integrated, and (f) sustainable. The CNA (2015) and Canadian Medical Association (CMA) (2015) have called on the federal government to adopt national home care standards.

Home Care Services

Home care programs are designed to promote independence; prevent, delay, or substitute for acute or long-term care; assist with the use of community services; and supplement the care and support provided by friends and family (CHCA, 2016). Across the country, these services could be provided by for-profit companies and by organizations that are part of the provincial funded health care system. These services are categorized as acute, chronic, palliative, or rehabilitative. In addition, coordination and management of admission to a facility may be provided when it is no longer possible for the individual to remain at home (CHCA, 2016). Services can be provided in the home, care facility, adult day care centre, workplace, school, shelter, or clinic. Some patients require only intermittent services; others need assistance 24 hours a day. Family members may also receive home care services, such as respite care to support them in their caregiving effort.

Funding and Utilization of Home Care Services

Health care costs range between 6.6% (Yukon) and 30% (Nova Scotia) of provincial and territorial budgets in Canada (CIHI, 2021b). Costs of over $265 billion per year (CIHI, 2021b) have raised an alarm regarding the ability to sustain Canada's health care system and have prompted calls for health care system reform. In particular, elements identified as being in need of change include policies and programs that address the determinants of health, access to a consistent health care provider, and a national strategy on chronic disease prevention and management (Morgan et al., 2007).

The majority of home care is funded by provincial and territorial governments through health budgets that are administered by regional health authorities. The federal government also funds home care services through departments such as the First Nations and Inuit Health Branch and Veterans Affairs Canada (Table 6.3). Persons aged 65 and older accounted for 51.8% of health care expenditures by provincial and territorial governments in 2017 (CIHI, 2021b).

Sometimes the frequency or duration of the government-funded home care services (e.g., the number of nursing visits, the number of hours of supportive care services such as home-making, and length of time on a program) is not deemed sufficient by the patient or family. In those instances, they may purchase additional services either through insurance or with their own financial resources. The Canadian Healthcare Association (2009) reported that between 2% and 5% of Canadians purchase home care services not funded by the government. In addition, it is estimated that 80% of the care of older persons in the community is provided by family and friends, which, if paid, would amount to approximately $31 billion annually (Hollander et al., 2011).

Many Indigenous individuals living on reserves face a number of challenges, such as lack of housing and lack of access to health care services and providers (House of Commons, 2018). There is also a disproportionately high poverty rate among Indigenous communities, as well as infrastructure needs. Indigenous people suffer from chronic conditions earlier in their lives than does the non-Indigenous population; they are also are more likely to suffer from multiple chronic conditions (House of Commons, 2018). Providing home care services on reserves is very different from working with urban populations, as there are staffing shortages, situations where families include many extended family members, political impacts, and cultural considerations (e.g., if there is a death in the community, everything shuts down for the wake and the funeral). There may also be difficulty accessing supplies and equipment as well as a lack of continuity of care from health care providers. The coordination of services on reserves requires the nurse to have a high degree of cultural humility, knowledge of resources and community members, and ability to access services.

Home Health Care Team

Nursing Roles. The home health care team is composed of the *home health nurse* and a variety of team members who work in close collaboration with the patient, family, and medical practitioners (Table 6.4). Nurses on the home health care team may include *registered nurses, licensed practical nurses (RPN/LPNs), nurse practitioners,* and *clinical nurse specialists.* Home health nurses provide a variety of nursing assessments, planning and implementing of interventions, and teaching to assist individuals in optimizing their health. Given the increase in RPN/LPN scope and in order to optimize staff mix, RPNs/LPNs have recently taken on some case management functions in addition to direct care (Fraser et al., 2019).

Nurse practitioners use their in-depth nursing knowledge and advanced scope of practice to diagnose and treat acute and chronic diseases; they provide care for remote and homebound patients who do not have access to a primary care physician (CNA, 2019).

Clinical nurse specialists promote the use of evidence-informed practice and system changes by providing expert consultation and leadership in guideline and policy development in the community setting (CNA, 2019).

Community health workers (CHWs) and *rehabilitative assistants* are unregulated care providers who make an essential contribution to quality of life for the patient by supporting the patient's ADLs, including bathing, preparing meals, and performing household chores and personal errands. They provide an important social connection with patients and often spend the most amount of time with the patient. These individuals can provide delegated or assigned nursing care for patients with frequent and predictable health needs (e.g., daily routine medication).

The role of the *case manager* is to coordinate the comprehensive care plan and services for the patient, including arranging for and funding services. The home health team may also include a physiotherapist, occupational therapist, speech–language pathologist, as well as social worker, pharmacist, dietitian, respiratory therapist, and health care provider. All members of the home health care team work collaboratively to evaluate the patient's progress, make appropriate changes to the care plan, and develop the discharge plan. The home health care team members actively include the patient's family members in all aspects of care. Team-based care is an essential feature for individuals with complex health care needs to ensure a holistic approach.

Populations Served by Home Health Care Providers

Although home health nurses may care for newborns, children, teenagers, and adults of all ages, in the period 2017–2018, 87.4% of individuals who received home care services were 65 years of age or older (CIHI, 2021b). The majority of these individuals live with frailty (CHCA, 2016). **Frailty** is defined as "a medical condition of reduced function and health in older individuals" (Canadian Frailty Network, 2020). Individuals receiving home care may face the physical and cognitive decline associated with many chronic conditions and frailty and may also live alone. Nearly 65% of home care patients (CIHI, 2021a) receive home

Member	Description
TABLE 6.4	**MEMBERS OF THE HOME HEALTH CARE TEAM**
Community health nurse (CHN)	A registered nurse (RN) whose practice specialty is promoting the health and social justice of individuals, families, communities, populations, and systems and an environment that supports health. A CHN practices in diverse community settings, such as homes, schools, shelters, churches, community health centres, and on the street (CHNC, 2019).
Home care or home health nurse	A CHN RN or registered practical nurse/licensed practical nurse (RPN/LPN) who uses knowledge from primary health care (including the determinants of health), nursing science, and social sciences to focus on disease prevention, health restoration and maintenance, or palliation for patients, their caregivers, and families (CHNC, 2019) and who may travel to the patient to provide care.
Case manager	The health care team member who collaborates with individuals, groups, and health care providers to support the client's achievement of safe, purposeful, realistic, and reasonable goals with a complex health, social, culturally diverse, and fiscal environment (National Case Management Network of Canada, 2009)
Community health worker or home support worker	An unlicensed care provider who supports patients with ADLs such as bathing, personal care, dressing, and meal preparation, as well as IADLs such as housekeeping, shopping, and social recreational activities (Canadian Research Network for Care in the Community, 2010)
Nurse practitioner	An advanced-practice nurse who provides autonomous essential health services guided by professional, ethical, and legal standards. "[Nurse practitioners] are registered nurses with advanced education who integrate their in-depth knowledge of advanced nursing practice and theory, health management, health promotion, disease/injury prevention, and other relevant biomedical and psychosocial theories to provide comprehensive health services. Nurse practitioners work in collaboration with their clients and other health care providers in the provision of high-quality patient-centred care. They work with diverse client populations in a variety of contexts and practice settings" (CNA, 2010, p. 5).
Clinical nurse specialist	An advanced-practice nurse who provides expertise for specialized populations. Clinical nurse specialists play a leading role in the development of clinical guidelines and the use of evidence, provide expert consultation, and facilitate system change (CNA, 2008).

ADLs, activities of daily living; *CHCA,* Canadian Home Care Association; *CHN,* community health nurse; *CHNC,* Community Health Nurses of Canada; *CNA,* Canadian Nurses Association; *IADLs,* instrumental activities of daily living.

support services to assist with both their ADLs and IADLs, and close to one-quarter receive nursing services (CIHI, 2021a). The home health nurse must possess knowledge and skill to support individuals living with frailty so that they can age safely at home with dignity (CNA, 2018a, 2018b).

The most common diagnosed health conditions in home care patients in 2019 were cardiovascular, musculoskeletal, and neurological diseases (including dementias); diabetes; chronic obstructive pulmonary disease; and cancer (CIHI, 2021a). The majority of older persons with dementia (61%) in Canada live at home (CIHI, 2021a). Older persons with dementia often have more challenging behaviours, both verbal and physical, and may be resistant to care. However, most of these patients with dementia (75%) do not have any challenging behaviours (CIHI, 2021a).

Home health nurses and all CHNs play an important part in the prevention and management of chronic illness by (a) promoting regular health screening, (b) incorporating health promotion and disease prevention strategies into their practice, and (c) assisting individuals and families in managing chronic illness in the home.

HOME HEALTH NURSING PRACTICE

Overview

Home health nursing is a unique and diverse practice that requires specific clinical competencies. Home health nurses may need to navigate complex traffic and weather conditions and cope with unexpected situations, from power failures to uncooperative pets. In the case of an ice storm or power outage, where the patient, unable to leave their home, is still in need of nursing care, the nurse will need to be creative (CNA, 2018a; Gallo, 2015). Home health nurses have a high level of autonomy and independence (CNA, 2018a) as they work in isolation in a patient's home or a remote community. Such care may include determining the care plan for a complex leg wound, calculating breakthrough hydromorphone doses for a palliative patient, or consulting with a health care provider in another community about an unstable patient. They require knowledge of community resources and proficiency in case management, communication, and physical, psychosocial, and environmental assessment. Many of these competencies differ from those of nurses in other care settings and sectors. Accordingly, standards of practice for CHNs have been developed (CHNC, 2019). The eight interrelated standards of practice presented in Table 6.5 form the core expectations for community health nursing. On the basis of these standards, detailed practice competencies were developed by CHNC in 2010 and are described later in this chapter.

Home Health Nursing and Family-Centred Care

Nursing in the home occurs in a context that is very different from the hospital. In the controlled environment of the hospital, the health care team has the dominant role. Conversely, in the home, the patient, caregiver, or family plays the dominant role; the nurse is a guest in the house and must adapt to the home environment. This includes incorporating infection control practices and use of appropriate personal protective equipment. It is important that the home health nurse demonstrate a holistic, nonjudgemental, and family-centred philosophy.

Family-centred care is "an approach to the planning, delivery, and evaluation of health care that is grounded in mutually beneficial partnerships among patients, families, and health care professionals" (Institute for Patient- and Family-Centered Care [IPFCC], 2017, p. 2) (see Chapter 4). The core concepts of family-centred care include dignity and respect, information sharing, participation, and collaboration (IPFCC, 2017). For the home health nurse, there is an opportunity, while invited into the patient's home, to engage the patient and family in discussion of their goals of care and together co-develop a plan of care. A key factor is the relationship that the nurse has with the patient and family, coupled with strong interpersonal communication skills

TABLE 6.5   COMMUNITY HEALTH NURSING STANDARD

1. Health promotion
2. Prevention and health protection
3. Health maintenance, restoration, and palliation
4. Professional relationships
5. Capacity building
6. Health equity
7. Evidence-informed practice
8. Professional responsibility and accountability

TABLE 6.6   ASSESSMENT OF CAREGIVER BURNOUT

Warning Signs of Stress

Caregiver Stress	Verbalizing
Denial	"My husband is fine. It is the kids who think there is a problem."
Anger	"If my dad calls me again today, I swear I'm going to let him have it."
Withdrawing socially	"I just don't feel like going out or talking to anyone anymore."
Anxiety	"I jump every time my phone rings, fearing the worst."
Depression	"I really don't want to get out of bed or leave the house anymore."
Exhaustion	"I don't have the energy to care for my spouse any longer."
Sleeplessness	"I can only sleep for 2 hours at a time—I constantly feel tired."
Emotional reaction	"I feel like crying all the time. A constant lump is in my throat."
Lack of concentration	"When others are talking, I just can't focus on what they are saying."
Health issues	"Ever since Mom was moved in with me, I feel like I am always fighting a cold or the flu."

Source: Adapted from Alzheimer Society of Canada. (2017). *10 warning signs of stress.* https://alzheimer.ca/en/Home/Living-with-dementia/Caring-for-someone/Self-care-for-the-caregiver/10-warning-signs-of-stress

(Purbhoo & Wojtak, 2018). It is the patient who must direct if and how much they want their family engaged in care (CFPC, 2019).

Home health nursing visits may be several times a day or as infrequent as once a month. Visits may be lengthy to complete an extensive admission assessment or be a short visit to assess health status, including wound healing, pain control, or symptom management. Nursing care during a visit may be administered according to a predetermined routine, such as one specified in a care pathway, or it may be directed toward newly arising symptoms or health concerns.

Assessment of caregiver burnout is a critical role of the home care nurse (Table 6.6). The focus is on empowering the patient and family to meet the identified health care needs while also feeling in control of their lives. One way a nurse can help family members cope with their increased responsibilities is to provide referrals to various support groups in the community, such as the Alzheimer Society, community services, or community seniors programs. Another way to support caregivers is to provide additional home care services to reduce the burden of care, for example, through services of a community health worker, more frequent nursing visits, short-term respite, or support from a social worker.

Culturally Competent Care: Home Health Nursing Practice.
The home health nurse has the opportunity to care for patients and families in Canada's rich ethnocultural mosaic, as noted in Chapter 2. In the home environment, the CHN may need to use an interpreter either in person or through virtual care to optimize language and cultural understanding of health care goals and plans.

In Indigenous remote communities, it is often the CHN who is the on-site health care provider (Tompkins et al., 2018). Engagement and connection are especially important within the Indigenous population as the home health nurse focuses on building a relationship of trust (Prodan-Bhalla et al., 2017). All CHNs can demonstrate and role model respect and care for all patients and identify those who may face health inequities, such as individuals who identify as LGBTQIA2 (Stamler et al., 2016).

The home health nurse is more likely than other nurses to encounter the patient's use of healing practices arising from cultural beliefs and the use of home remedies and complementary and alternative therapies (discussed in Chapter 12). The ability to apply culturally relevant care is embedded in the competencies expected of a CHN (CHNC, 2019). The home health nurse demonstrates culturally sensitive care by having an understanding of how cultural beliefs and values affect care (College of Nurses of Ontario, 2018).

Home Health Nursing Practice Knowledge and Skills

Specific competencies for home care nurses have been established in Canada (CHNC, 2010) and the United States (American Nurses Association, 2008). These competencies reflect the knowledge, skills, judgement, and attitudes associated with home care nursing practice and are outlined in Table 6.7.

Health Assessments and Screening Tools. Health promotion, along with illness prevention, is the foundation to the nurse's approach in home care (CHNC, 2010). The nurse needs to consider the impact of the social determinants of health and support the patient to make informed choices about protective and preventive activities that affect their health (CHNC, 2010). Multiple assessment and screening tools are often used in home care for assessing the physiological, psychological, and functional status of the patient, such as the Resident Assessment Instrument-Home Care (RAI-HC). A thorough head-to-toe assessment is required, as are focused assessments based on the patient's medical and health history. Examples of other assessment tools include the Geriatric Depression Scale, which is completed by the patient and consists of 15 questions (American Psychological Association, 2020). The Clinical Frailty Scale (Table 6.8) can be useful given the high level of frailty in home care patients.

Equipment Skills, Patient and Family Teaching, and Documentation. In addition to assessments, home health nurses need to be proficient in a number of specific skills and require knowledge of the equipment and assistive devices used. Examples include chest and wound drainage tubes; equipment for intravenous therapy, negative pressure wound therapy, or advanced wound-care treatments; enteral feeding equipment; central vascular access devices; and infusion pumps.

Further interventions include teaching self-management strategies to assist individuals in managing chronic disease. Individuals of Indigenous background have experienced a dramatic rise in chronic disease, and the nurse can play a key role in its management (Naqshbandi Hayward et al., 2016). Assigning and delegating care to members of the health care team as part of the overall plan of care is another important competency.

TABLE 6.7	SPECIFIC COMPETENCIES FOR CANADIAN HOME CARE NURSES

Elements of Home Health Nursing
- Assessment, monitoring, and clinical decision making
- Care planning and care coordination
- Health maintenance, restoration, and palliation
- Teaching and education
- Communication
- Relationships
- Access and equity
- Building capacity

Foundations of Home Health Nursing
- Health promotion
- Illness prevention and health protection

Quality and Professional Responsibility
- Quality care
- Professional responsibility

Source: Community Health Nurses of Canada. (2010). *Home health nursing competencies* (version 1.0) Author. http://login.greatbignews.com/UserFiles/289/documents/HomeHealthNursingCompetenciesVersion1March2010.pdf

Documentation is another area of competency for the home health nurse. Documentation may take place in numerous locations, such as the patient's home, the clinic, or the care facility. Increasingly it is done electronically using mobile connectivity. As the nurse is often working independently, having a good knowledge of electronic documentation platforms is necessary.

Establishing and maintaining a therapeutic nurse–patient relationship is fundamental to effective home care nursing practice. Because family members are encouraged to learn how to provide treatments, such as administering end-of-life subcutaneous medications and managing equipment, the nurse must be able to teach both the patient and their family. The home health nurse needs to assess the readiness of the caregiver, teach in a way that is most helpful for the learner, and evaluate the outcomes of care, including the coping of the caregiver.

Palliative Approach. Building on the therapeutic relationship, the palliative approach is another important component of home health nursing practice. The WHO (2021b) defines *palliative care* as an approach used to improve the quality of life of patients and their families facing the issues associated with life-threatening illness, through the prevention and relief of suffering by means of early identification and impeccable assessment and treatment of pain and other issues—physical, psychosocial, and spiritual. In the palliative approach, the principles of palliative care are used not only at the end of life but also throughout the journey for persons with chronic disease conditions (CNA & CHPC, 2015). The home health nurse has the opportunity to initiate discussions with the patient about their advance care planning goals while still at home and before a crisis event occurs. The benefit of this planning is that it decreases unwanted interventions in the hospital at the end of life (Huggins et al., 2019). In addition, the home health nurse often has a central role in achieving the highest possible quality of life for the patient and family throughout the palliative and bereavement experience.

Trends in Home Health Nursing

Virtual Care. Telehealth, or telemedicine, has been used over the last decade as clinicians have provided health care support to patients in a different location, such as through video chat or smartphones. With the expansion of technology has come the broader term *virtual care,* which encompasses any variety of digital health services. In essence, virtual care is any interaction between a patient and their care team that occurs remotely (CMA, 2019).

The COVID-19 pandemic and subsequent need to minimize transmission have driven virtual care at an expedited rate not previously seen. This expansion has occurred not only with the traditional telephone and video chat but also in the use of app-based and remote home monitoring. This growth has not been without challenges, including barriers such as privacy concerns, data integration, lack of infrastructure, and challenges with patient experience (Sherwin et al., 2020).

Home health monitoring (HHM) is a great example of community nursing care that has rapidly expanded during the pandemic. HHM involves the use of remote technology such as a smartphone to record the patient's health information that is then reviewed by the community health nurse. In British Columbia, patients with COVID-19 and those with chronic conditions such as heart failure and chronic obstructive pulmonary disease have been using the provincial HHM system.

The patient benefits associated with virtual care include fewer barriers to accessing care, shortened wait times, less travel time for patients, and increased ability to access one's own health records, therefore increasing the patient's ability to self-manage (Canada Health Infoway, 2021).

Virtual wound-care consultation, a function of community nurses, has increased over the past few years and exponentially during the COVID-19 pandemic. Nurses are able to triage, evaluate, and direct care for patients virtually (Ratliff et al., 2020). The improvements in technology have enabled nurses to remotely visualize the wound to provide direction and co-develop a care plan with the patient.

In addition, CHNs have needed to rely on telehealth systems to communicate with other health care providers in different locations (Bussières et al., 2017). This model has proved to be successful, such as with CHNs who assess patients for tuberculosis and then virtually connect with the health care provider, who is often hundreds of kilometers away (Long et al., 2015). The challenge in remote communities, however, can be the lack of infrastructure to support virtual care (Smith et al., 2016).

During the COVID-19 pandemic, community nurses were able to provide virtual connections with patients who are socially isolated. CHNs also needed to do active screening and triage to establish a safe environment prior to in-person home visits (Yi et al., 2020). As virtual health continues to expand, it is vital that all Canadian nurses be prepared for the technological challenges to manage this changing landscape (Beausejour, 2020).

SUMMARY

Nursing in the community represents a dynamic and fulfilling practice area for nurses. Community-based nursing is an essential component of the health care system and offers the opportunity to positively influence the health and outcomes of individuals, communities, and populations.

TABLE 6.8   THE CSHA CLINICAL FRAILTY SCALE

1	*Very fit*— robust, active, energetic, well motivated and fit; these people commonly exercise regularly and are in the most fit group for their age
2	*Well*—without active disease, but less fit than people in category 1
3	*Well, with treated comorbid disease*— disease symptoms are well controlled compared with those in category 4
4	*Apparently vulnerable* — although not frankly dependent, these people commonly complain of being "slowed up" or have disease symptoms
5	*Mildly frail* — with limited dependence on others for instrumental activities of daily living
6	*Moderately frail*— help is needed with both instrumental and non-instrumental activities of daily living
7	*Severely frail* — completely dependent on others for the activities of daily living, or terminally ill

CSHA, Canadian Study of Health and Aging.

CASE STUDY

Home Health Care for an Older Patient With an Infected Leg Ulcer

Patient Profile

M. T. (pronouns she/her) is 82 years old and has been referred to home care because of an infected leg wound and assessment for other supports. M. T. lives with her disabled son in an apartment in an area of town identified as having a high number of calls to the police. M. T. served in World War II and worked in a department store. She has been the sole caregiver for her son since her husband died 10 years ago. She has a niece an hour's drive away who tries to visit once a month but is busy caring for her own parents. Having access to food, feeling overwhelmed with looking after her son, and now worrying about the wound on her leg has resulted in her visiting her family doctor frequently.

Subjective Data

- Has a history of alcohol use
- Has varicose veins in both legs; worries that, because of these, the home care nurses will want her to wear support stockings, which M. T. finds "ugly"
- Denies pain in the leg but flinches when the nurse takes off the dressing

Objective Data

Physical Examination

- Smells of urine, clothes are dirty
- Dressing to right lower leg: 10 × 10 cm foam dressing with adhesive edges
- Right lower leg ulcer: 10% pink base, 90% yellow base, irregular flat edges. Wound size is 0.5 cm deep, 7 cm long, 4.4 cm wide. Periwound skin is deep pink, and diameter of right lower leg calf is greater than that of the left.

Interprofessional Care

- Referral from patient's family physician, who patient has been seeing for 30 years
- Was previously taking metformin but says she hasn't taken it in a long time
- Acetaminophen with codeine "whenever she thinks of it" and can afford it
- Tea and toast diet

Discussion Questions

1. *Priority decision:* What are the initial priorities for the home health nurse?
2. What other members of the health care team should be involved in the care of M. T.? What are their roles and responsibilities?
3. *Priority decision:* What type of patient education program should be implemented? What are the priority teaching goals to promote self-management?
4. What should the nurse consider in the nutrition assessment? How will the nurse address economic considerations related to M. T.'s diet?
5. How can the nurse address M. T.'s coping skills and use community resources to support M. T. in her feelings of being overwhelmed?
6. What types of supplies will M. T. need? What diagnostics, teaching, and community resources should accompany the use of these supplies?
7. What are the long-term outcomes that M. T. can expect?

evolve
Answers are available at http://evolve.elsevier.com/Canada/Lewis/medsurg.

REVIEW QUESTIONS

The number of the question corresponds to the same-numbered objective at the beginning of the chapter.

1. Primary and community care are relevant in the twenty-first century for which of the following reasons?
   a. The number of older persons is decreasing in Canada.
   b. Strengthening community health services is a proactive approach to improving health and therefore reducing spending for hospital and facility care.
   c. There is less of a societal demand for day care for older persons and children.
   d. The number of noncommunicable diseases are decreasing.
2. Which of the following statements best describes the nurse's role when working in community health settings?
   a. They function autonomously in meeting patient needs.
   b. They focus only on patient needs specific to the setting.
   c. They use the same skills as in acute care settings.
   d. They use case-management skills along the continuum of care.
3. How do primary and community care best contribute to the sustainability of the health care system?
   a. Individuals pay for all of the primary and community care services through private funding.
   b. There is limited use of self-management and limited patient and family involvement.
   c. Life-saving and cost reduction impacts of chronic disease management strategies result.
   d. There is increased use of hospital services by individuals using primary and community care.
4. Which of the following statements best reflects the reality of home care services in Canada?
   a. The use of home health services is increasing.
   b. The use of home health services is decreasing.
   c. Home health services are not yet available in all provinces and territories.
   d. Home health services are used more by families than by single clients.
5. Which of the following is not a common practice of a home health nurse?
   1. End-of-life palliative care in a hospice
   2. Self-management support for chronic diseases in a remote community
   3. Assessment and treatment of chronic wounds for a young adult at a wound clinic
   4. Palliative approach for a client with chronic obstructive pulmonary disease via virtual care platform
6. Which of the following is a home care nurse competency? *(Select all that apply.)*
   a. Appreciate and understand the roles and responsibilities and the contributions of other regulated and unregulated health care workers involved in the client's care plan
   b. Assist the client and their family to recognize their capacity for managing their own health needs according to available resources.
   c. Limit participation in collaborative, interdisciplinary, and intersectoral partnerships to enhance the health of clients and families.
   d. Keep knowledge current to ensure optimal case management.

1. b; 2. d; 3. c; 4. c; 5. a; 6. a, b

Ⓔvolve

For even more review questions, visit http://evolve.elsevier.com/Canada/Lewis/medsurg.

REFERENCES

Alzheimer Society of Canada. (2017). *10 warning signs of stress.* https://alzheimer.ca/en/Home/Living-with-dementia/Caring-for-someone/Self-care-for-the-caregiver/10-warning-signs-of-stress

American Nurses Association. (2008). *Home Health Nursing: Scope and Standards of Practice.* Author (Seminal).

American Psychological Association. (2020). *Geriatric depression scale (GDS).* https://www.apa.org/pi/about/publications/caregivers/practice-settings/assessment/tools/geriatric-depression

Beausejour, W. (2020). *Promising Increase in the Use of Virtual Care Technologies by Canadian Nurses.* Canada Health Infoway. https://www.infoway-inforoute.ca/en/what-we-do/blog/access-to-care/8738-promising-increase-in-the-use-of-virtual-care-technologies-by-canadian-nurses

Bussières, S., Tanguay, A., Hébert, D., et al. (2017). Unité de coordination clinique des services préhospitaliers d'urgence: a clinical telemedicine platform that improves prehospital and community health care for rural citizens. *Journal Telemedicine Telecare, 23*(1), 188–194. https://doi.org/10.1177/1357633X15627234

Canadian Family Practice Nurses Association. (2019). *National Competencies for Registered Nurses in Primary Care.* https://www.cfpna.ca/copy-of-resources-1

Canadian Frailty Network. (2020). What is frailty? https://www.cfn-nce.ca/frailty-matters/what-is-frailty/

Canadian Healthcare Association. (2009). *Home care in Canada: From the margins to the mainstream.* http://www.healthcarecan.ca/wp-content/uploads/2012/11/Home_Care_in_Canada_From_the_Margins_to_the_Mainstream_web.pdf. (Seminal).

Canada Health Infoway. (2021). *Benefits of digital health.* https://www.infoway-inforoute.ca/en/what-we-do/benefits-of-digital-health

Canadian Home Care Association (CHCA). (2013). *Portraits of home care in Canada* (Seminal).

Canadian Home Care Association (CHCA). (2017). *Harmonized home care principles.* https://cdnhomecare.ca/wp-content/uploads/2019/10/CHCA_Harmonized-Principles-2017-web.pdf

Canadian Home Care Association (CHCA). (2019). *Integrated home and community-based care. A vision of health, independence and dignity.* https://cdnhomecare.ca/wp-content/uploads/2020/03/CHCA-Vision-of-Integrated-Home-Care.pdf

Canadian Home Care Association, Canadian Nurses Association, & College of Family Physicians of Canada. (2016). *Better home care in Canada. A national action plan.* http://chca2422.wpengine.com/wp-content/uploads/2020/03/Better-Home-Care-Report-web-EN.pdf

Canadian Institute for Health Information (CIHI). (2020). *Nursing in Canada 2019. Data table.* https://www.cihi.ca/en/nursing-in-canada-2019

Canadian Institute for Health Information (CIHI). (2021a). *Profile of clients in home care, 2019–2020.* https://www.cihi.ca/en/access-data-reports/results?f%5B0%5D=field_primary_theme%3A2054

Canadian Institute for Health Information (CIHI). (2021b). *Quick stats.* https://www.cihi.ca/en/quick-stats

Canadian Institute for Health Information (CIHI). (2021c). *Your health system.* https://yourhealthsystem.cihi.ca/hsp

/inbrief?lang=en&_ga=2.91005850.1422425808.1628726337
-588651406.1628726337#!/indicators/079/hospital-stay-extended--
until-home-care-services-or-supports-ready/;mapC1;mapLevel2;/

Canadian Medical Association (CMA). (2015). *Palliative care—Canadian Medical Association's national call to action.* https://www.cma.ca/sites/default/files/2018-11/palliative-care-report-online-e.pdf. (Seminal).

Canadian Medical Association (CMA). (2019). *Virtual care in Canada: A discussion paper.* https://www.cma.ca/sites/default/files/pdf/News/Virtual_Care_discussionpaper_v2EN.pdf

Canadian Nurses Association (CNA). (2010). *Canadian nurse practitioners: Core competency framework.* https://www.cno.org/globalassets/for/rnec/pdf/competencyframework_en.pdf

Canadian Nurses Association (CNA). (2014). *Optimizing the role of nurses in primary care in Canada.* https://cna-aiic.ca/~/media/cna/page-content/pdf-en/optimizing-the-role-of-nurses-in-primary-care-in-canada.pdf

Canadian Nurses Association (CNA). (2015). *Position statement: Primary health care.* https://www.cna-aiic.ca/~/media/cna/page-content/pdf-en/primary-health-care-position-statement.pdf

Canadian Nurses Association (CNA). (2018a). *Establish standards for home care.* https://www.cna-aiic.ca/-/media/cna/page-content/pdf-en/establish-standards-for-home-care_e.pdf

Canadian Nurses Association (CNA). (2018b). *Fact sheet: nurses and home care.* https://www.cna-aiic.ca/-/media/cna/page-content/pdf-en/fact-sheet-nurses-and-home-care.pdf

Canadian Nurses Association (CNA). (2019). *Advanced practice nursing: A pan-Canadian framework.* https://cna-aiic.ca/-/media/cna/page-content/pdf-en/advanced-practice-nursing-framework-en.pdf?la=en&hash=76A98ADEE62E655E158026DEB45326C8C9528B1B

Canadian Nurses Association & Canadian Hospice Palliative Care Association. (2015). *A joint position statement: Palliative care and the role of the nurse.* https://www.cna-aiic.ca/-/media/cna/page-content/pdf-en/the-palliative-approach-to-care-and-the-role-of-the-nurse_e.pdf

Canadian Public Health Association (CPHA). (2010). *Public health—Community Health Nursing Practice in Canada: Roles and Activities* (4th ed.). Author. https://www.cpha.ca/sites/default/files/assets/pubs/3-1bk04214.pdf. (Seminal).

Canadian Public Health Association (CPHA). (2017). In *Public Health: A conceptual framework* (2nd ed.). https://www.cpha.ca/sites/default/files/uploads/policy/ph-framework/phcf_e.pdf

Canadian Public Health Association (CPHA). (2019). *Public Health in the Context of Health Care Renewal.* https://www.cpha.ca/sites/default/files/uploads/policy/positionstatements/phhsr-positionstatement-e.pdf

Canadian Research Network for Care in the Community. (2010). *Home support workers in the continuum of care for older people.* https://www.ryerson.ca/content/dam/crncc/knowledge/infocus/factsheets/InFocus%20Home%20Support%20Workers.pdf

College of Family Physicians of Canada. (2019). *A new vision for Canada: Family practice—patient medical home 2019.* https://patientsmedicalhome.ca/files/uploads/PMH_VISION2019_ENG_WEB_2.pdf

College of Nurses of Ontario (CNO). (2018). *Standard-guidelines: Culturally sensitive care.* https://www.cno.org/en/learn-about-standards-guidelines/educational-tools/ask-practice/culturally-sensitive-care/

Community Health Nurses of Canada (CHNC). (2010). *Home health nursing competencies (version 1.0).* https://www.chnc.ca/en/competencies

Community Health Nurses of Canada (CHNC). (2019). *Canadian community health nursing: Professional practice model and standards of practice.* https://www.chnc.ca/en/standards-of-practice

Fraser, K., Punjani, N. S., Wilkey, B., et al. (2019). Optimizing Licensed Practical Nurses in home care: Their role, scope and opportunities. *Nursing Leadership (1910-622X), 32*(1), 42–59. https://doi.org/10.12927/cjnl.2019.25849

Gallo, M. (2015). A day in the life of a Canadian nurse in an ice storm. *Home Healthcare Now, 33*(1), 54–55.

Government of Canada. (2012). *About primary health care.* https://www.canada.ca/en/health-canada/services/primary-health-care/about-primary-health-care.html

Health Canada. (2018). *A common statement of principles on shared health priorities.* https://www.canada.ca/en/health-canada/corporate/transparency/health-agreements/principles-shared-health-priorities.html

Hollander, M. J., Lui, G., & Chappell, N. L. (2011). Who cares and how much? The imputed economic contribution to the Canadian health care system of middle-aged and older unpaid caregivers providing care to the elderly. *Healthcare Quarterly, 12*(2), 42–49. http://www.longwoods.com/product.php?productid=20660. (Seminal).

House of Commons. (2018). *The challenges of delivering continuing care in First Nation communitiesReport of the Standing Committee on Indigenous and Northern Affairs.* https://www.ourcommons.ca/Content/Committee/421/INAN/Reports/RP10260656/inanrp17/inanrp17-e.pdf

Huggins, M., McGregor, M. J., Cox, M. B., et al. (2019). Advance care planning and decision-making in a home-based primary care service in a Canadian urban centre. *Canadian Geriatrics Journal, 22*(4), 182–189. https://doi.org/10.5770/cgj.22.377

IBIS World. (2020). *Home Care Providers in Canada—Market research report.* https://www.ibisworld.com/canada/market-research-reports/home-care-providers-industry/

Institute for Patient and Family-Centred Care. (2017). *Advancing the practice of patient-and-family-centred care in hospitals: How to get started.* https://www.ipfcc.org/resources/getting_started.pdf

Kates, N. (2017). Mental health and primary care: contributing to mental health system transformation in Canada. *Canadian Journal Community Mental Health, 36*(4), 33–67.

Long, R., Heffernan, C., Gao, Z., et al. (2015). Do "virtual" and "outpatient" public health tuberculosis clinics perform equally well? A program-wide evaluation in Alberta, Canada. *Plos One, 10*(12), e0144784. https://doi.org/10.1371/journal.pone.0144784

Misfeldt, R., Suter, E., Mallinson, S., et al. (2017). Exploring context and the factors shaping team-based primary healthcare policies in three Canadian provinces: a comparative analysis. *Healthcare Policy, 13*(1), 74–93. https://doi.org/10.12927/hcpol.2017.25190

Molla, S., Donaldson, J., Yordy, D., et al. (1996). *Primary Care: America's Health in a New Era.* Report of a Study by a Committee of the Institute of Medicine, Division of Healthcare Services (Seminal).

Naqshbandi Hayward, M., Paquette-Warren, J., & Harris, S. B. (2016). Developing community-driven quality improvement initiatives to enhance chronic disease care in Indigenous communities in Canada: the FORGE AHEAD program protocol. *Health Research Policy and Systems, 14*(1), 55. https://doi.org/10.1186/s12961-016-0127-y

National Case Management Network of Canada. (2009). Connect, collaborate, communication the power of case management. http://www.ncmn.ca/resources/documents/english%20standards%20for%20web.pdf

Prodan-Bhalla, N., Middagh, D., Jinkerson-Brass, S., et al. (2017). Embracing our "otherness". *Journal Holistic Nursing, 35*(1), 44–52. https://doi.org/10.1177/0898010116642085

Purbhoo, D., & Wojtak, A. (2018). Patient and family-centred home and community care: Realizing the opportunity. *Nursing Leadership 1910-622X, 31*(2), 40–50. https://doi.org/10.12927/cjnl.2018.25604

Ratliff, C., Shifflett, R., Howell, A., et al. (2020). Telehealth for Wound Management During the COVID-19 Pandemic. *Journal Wound Ostomy Continence Nursing, 47*(5), 445–449. https://doi.org/10.1097/WON.0000000000000692

Sherwin, J., Lawrence, K., Gragnano, V., et al. (2020). Scaling virtual health at the epicentre of coronavirus disease 2019: A case study from NYU Langone Health. *Journal of Telemedicine and Telecare, 0*(0), 1–6. https://doi.org/10.1177/1357633X20941395

Smith, S., Hunt, G., & Smith, S. A. (2016). Extending the line: The First Nations Telehealth Expansion Project. *Canadian Journal Rural Medicine, 21*(3), 85.

Stamler, L., Yiu, L., & Dosani, A. (2016). In *Community health nursing: A Canadian perspective* (4th ed.). Pearson.

Statistics Canada. (2018a). *Formal home care use in Canada.* https://www150.statcan.gc.ca/n1/pub/82-003-x/2018009/article/00001-eng.htm

Statistics Canada. (2018b). *The income of Canadians.* https://www150.statcan.gc.ca/n1/pub/11-627-m/11-627-m2018006-eng.htm

Statistics Canada. (2018c). *The rise of the dual-earner family.* https://www150.statcan.gc.ca/n1/pub/11-630-x/11-630-x2016005-eng.htm

Statistics Canada. (2021). *Population and demography statistics.* https://www.statcan.gc.ca/eng/subjects-start/population_and_demography

Tompkins, J. W., Mequanint, S., Barre, D. E., et al. (2018). National survey of indigenous primary healthcare capacity and delivery models in Canada: the Transformation of Indigenous Primary Healthcare Delivery (FORGE AHEAD) community profile survey. *BMC Health Services Research, 18*(1). https://doi.org/10.1186/s12913-018-3578-8

Wilson, D. P., Donald, B., Shallock, A. J., et al. (2015). The cost effectiveness of harm reduction. *International Journal of Drug Policy, 26*, S5–S11. https://doi.org/10.1016/j.drugpo.2014.11.00

World Health Organization (WHO). (1978). *Primary health care: Report of the international conference on primary health care.* USSR: Alma-Ata. https://www.who.int/publications/i/item/9241800011 (Seminal).

World Health Organization (WHO). (2018a). *Declaration on Primary Health Care.* https://www.who.int/primary-health/conference-phc/declaration

World Health Organization (WHO). (2018b). *Noncommunicable diseases country profiles 2018.* https://www.who.int/publications/i/item/ncd-country-profiles-2018

World Health Organization (WHO). (2021a). *Noncommunicable diseases.* https://www.who.int/health-topics/noncommunicable-diseases#tab=tab_1

World Health Organization (WHO). (2021b). *Palliative care.* https://www.who.int/health-topics/palliative-care

Yi, X., Jamil, N., Gaik, I., et al. (2020). Community Nursing Service during the COVID-19 pandemic; the Singapore experience. *British Journal Community Nursing, 25*(8), 390–395.

RESOURCES

Accreditation Canada: Health Care Standards
https://accreditation.ca/standards/
Canadian Gerontological Nursing Association
https://cgna.net
Canadian Home Care Association
https://www.cdnhomecare.ca/
Canadian Hospice Palliative Care Association
https://www.chpca.net/
Canadian Institute for Health Information (CIHI)
https://www.cihi.ca
Canadian Nurses Association
https://www.cna-aiic.ca/
Canadian Patient Safety Institute
https://www.patientsafetyinstitute.ca/
Canadian Research Network for Care in the Community (CRNCC)
https://www.ryerson.ca/crncc/
Community Health Nurses of Canada (CHNC)
https://www.chnc.ca

Institute for Healthcare Improvement
https://www.ihi.org/ihi
National Association for Home Care & Hospice
https://www.nahc.org
National Gerontological Nursing Association (NGNA)
https://www.ngna.org

⊖volve
For additional Internet resources, see the website for this book at http://evolve.elsevier.com/Canada/Lewis/medsurg.

Older Persons

Veronique M. Boscart

Originating US chapter by Sherry A. Greenberg

⊖volve WEBSITE

http://evolve.elsevier.com/Canada/Lewis/medsurg

- Review Questions (Online Only)
- Key Points
- Answer Guidelines for Case Study
- Conceptual Care Map Creator
- Audio Glossary
- Content Updates

LEARNING OBJECTIVES

1. Describe the effects of ageism on the care of older persons.
2. Describe the groups of vulnerable older persons and their needs.
3. Describe nursing interventions to assist acute and chronically ill older persons.
4. Describe challenges and concerns related to the caregiving role.

5. Identify care alternatives to meet specific needs of older persons.
6. Identify the legal and ethical issues related to the care of older persons.
7. Identify the role of the nurse in health screening and promotion and in disease prevention for older persons.

KEY TERMS

ageism
assisted-living facilities (ALFs)
elder abuse

elder mistreatment
ethnogeriatrics
frailty

gerontological nursing
long-term care (LTC) facilities
polypharmacy

Gerontological nursing is a nursing specialty that revolves around the care of older persons. This chapter presents specific information about older persons to assist nurses in providing care in a variety of settings. Gerontological nursing care presents many opportunities and challenges that call for highly skilled assessment and creative adaptations of interventions.

DEMOGRAPHICS OF AGING

Older persons are the fastest-growing population in Canada. There is no absolute chronological age at which a person becomes "old." Most Canadian statistical summaries define older persons as those aged 65 years and older. Psychologists have further divided the "old" into three groups: the young-old, aged 65 to 74 years; the middle-old, aged 75 to 84 years; and the old-old, older than 85 years. As of July 1, 2019, older persons accounted for 17.5% of the Canadian population (Statistics Canada, 2019c). The population aged 65 years and older is projected to reach 22.7% of the Canadian population by 2031 (Statistics Canada, 2019c).

In general, Canada's population is younger than those of most Western industrialized countries, and yet a large proportion of

older persons are immigrants. Currently, one in five Canadians are immigrants, and one in five belong to a visible minority (Statistics Canada, 2018). Approximately 7.3% of the Indigenous population in Canada were aged 65 years or older in 2016 (Statistics Canada, 2019a). Furthermore, there are significant age-related differences between Canada's provinces and territories; the largest share of the older population is in New Brunswick (20.8%), Newfoundland and Labrador (20.5%), and Nova Scotia (20.4%) and the smallest is in Nunavut (3.9%) (Statistics Canada, 2019b).

The most rapidly increasing age group is that of people 85 years and older. Since 1960, this group has increased 250%. In addition, there are approximately 10 795 centenarians in Canada, the vast majority of them women (Statistics Canada, 2019c). Female Canadians born today have a life expectancy of 84 years, and male Canadians have a life expectancy of 79.9 years (Statistics Canada, 2019d).

Because the needs and expectations of the population are changing rapidly, nurses need to acquire and demonstrate the required knowledge, clinical expertise, leadership skills, and a strong understanding of health organizations and policy to deliver the best care possible to older persons and their families.

ATTITUDES TOWARD AGING

Today's health care system promotes the concept of aging from a comprehensive perspective, in which health and wellness are defined as a balance between a person's internal and external environments and the person's emotional, spiritual, social, cultural, and physical processes. According to this perspective, aging is influenced by many factors, including emotional and physical health, developmental stage, socioeconomic status, culture, and ethnicity.

As people age, they are exposed to more and different life experiences. The accumulation of these differences creates a great diversity among older persons. Nurses should acknowledge and incorporate this diversity and older persons' perceptions of aging. Research has indicated that older persons who report a high sense of subjective well-being live longer and healthier lives than those with a low sense of subjective well-being (Ivankina et al., 2016). Age is important, but it may not be the most relevant factor for determining the appropriate care of an individual. In approaching aging from a viewpoint of health and well-being, a person's strengths, resilience, resources, and capabilities are emphasized, rather than existing pathological conditions.

Unfortunately, myths and stereotypes about aging are found throughout society and are often supported by the media (Wilinska & Mosberg Iversen, 2017). These stereotypes provide the basis of commonly held misconceptions that lead to errors in assessments and limitations to interventions. For example, if nurses perceive older persons to be confused or disoriented, necessary assessments for delirium will be neglected, which can result in morbidity and mortality (Cao et al., 2017).

This negative attitude based on age is defined as **ageism**. Ageism leads to discrimination and disparities in the care of older persons. Research has indicated that nurses who demonstrate an ageist attitude provide lower-quality care to older persons (Van Wicklin, 2020). In today's aging society, it is essential for nurses to demonstrate expertise, knowledge, and practice to care for older persons. Nurses can receive a Specialty Certification in Gerontological Nursing with the Canadian Nurses Association (CNA) to demonstrate their capabilities in providing care and services to older persons and their families.

BIOLOGICAL THEORIES OF AGING

Several theories help to explain the aging process. From a biological view, *aging* is defined as the progressive loss of function. The exact cause of biological aging remains to be determined, but aging is clearly a multifactorial process involving genetics, diet, and environment (Yochim, 2017). Nurses' knowledge of biological changes is important because it allows for differentiation between the normal aging process and health conditions that necessitate specific interventions.

Several theories exist regarding biological aging and are presented in Table 7.1. The free radical theory, first proposed in 1956 by Harman, suggests that metabolic byproducts and noxious factors (such as smog, tobacco smoke, and radiation) damage cellular processes through chemical reactions causing *oxidative stress*, which, over time, is responsible for pathological physiological changes such as atherosclerosis and cancer (Yochim, 2017). Two decades of research has focused on the roles of various antioxidants, including vitamins C and E, in slowing down the oxidative process and, ultimately, the aging

TABLE 7.1	SUMMARY OF SOME BIOLOGICAL THEORIES OF AGING
Theory	**Dynamics**
Free radical	Oxidation of fats, proteins, and carbohydrates creates free electrons that attach to other molecules, altering cellular function.
Cross-link	Lipids, proteins, carbohydrates, and nucleic acid react with chemicals or radiation to form bonds that cause an increase in cell rigidity and instability.
Immunological-autoimmunological	Alteration of B and T cells leads to loss of capacity for self-regulation; normal cells or cells with age-related changes are recognized as foreign matter; system reacts by forming antibodies to destroy these cells.

process. A second biological theory is the cross-link theory (Pathath, 2017), which stipulates that repeated exposure to chemicals and radiation in the environment disrupts the natural molecular structure of cells, resulting in tissue damage and rigidity (Pathath, 2017). These changes in cell structure explain the observable changes associated with aging, such as wrinkles and a decreased distensibility of arteries.

SOCIAL THEORIES OF AGING

Several social theories of aging exist. The disengagement theory (Lumen Learning, 2020) suggests that withdrawing from society and social relationships is a natural part of growing old. The activity theory, however, suggests that for individuals to enjoy older age and feel satisfied, they must maintain activities and find a replacement for the statuses and associated roles they have left behind (Lumen Learning, 2020). Continuity theory, then, states that older persons make specific choices to maintain consistency in internal (personality structure, beliefs) and external structures (relationships) and remain active and involved throughout their older years (Lumen Learning, 2020). Lastly, *gerotranscendence* refers to the idea that as people age, they transcend limited views of life they held in earlier times (Lumen Learning, 2020). Gerotranscendence is a natural progression toward maturation and wisdom, in which new meaning or purpose in life is pursued as the individual grows older (Lalani, 2017).

UNIVERSAL HEALTH CARE

The older population requires specific consideration within Canada's health care system. Canada's health care system is based on the *Canada Health Act* (1984) and is publicly funded. Health care is administered and delivered by the provinces and territories. The system is referred to by Canadians as "Medicare" and provides for universal comprehensive coverage for "medically necessary" services, including primary health care, care in hospitals, and surgical–dental services. Each province and territory determines which services are publicly funded, and so there is significant variation in "not urgent" services such as the provision of home care, long-term care (LTC), medications outside of hospital, physiotherapy, optometry services, and other services. As a result of the focus on Canada's health care reform, there has been increased advocacy for more realistic provision of health care for older persons, including an emphasis on health promotion and expanded community care (Hancock et al., 2017; Health Canada, 2016).

AGE-RELATED PHYSIOLOGICAL CHANGES

Age-related changes affect every body system and are part of healthy aging. However, the age at which specific changes become evident differs from person to person. For instance, a person may have greying hair at age 45 but relatively unwrinkled skin at age 80. Recognizing and assessing age-related changes form the basis to differentiation from non–age-related changes. Table 7.2 presents an overview of nursing assessments based on age-related physiological changes and clinical manifestations.

TABLE 7.2   AGE-RELATED DIFFERENCES IN ASSESSMENT
Age-Related Changes and Associated Clinical Manifestations

Function	Normal Age Changes	Clinical Manifestations
Cardiovascular System		
Cardiac output	• Force of contraction decreases • Fat and collagen increase • Heart muscle weakens • Ventricular wall thickens	• Myocardial oxygen demand increases • Stroke volume and cardiac output decrease • Fatigue, shortness of breath, and tachycardia occur • Blood flow to vital organs and periphery decreases
Cardiac rate and rhythm	• Dependence of atrial contraction increases • Fibres from bundle of His are lost • Mitral valve stretching occurs • Ventricles are slower to relax • Sinus node pacemaker cells decrease in number	• HR slows to increase with stress • Maximum HR decreases (e.g., in 80-year-old, HR = 120 bpm; in 20-year-old, HR = 200 bpm) • Possible AV block • Recovery time from tachycardia is prolonged • Frequency of premature beats increases
Structural changes	• Aortic valves become sclerotic and calcify • Baroreceptor sensitivity decreases • Mild fibrosis and calcification of valves occur	• Diastolic murmur is present in 50% of older persons • Heart-position landmarks change
Arterial circulation	• Elastin and smooth muscle are reduced • Vessel rigidity increases • Vascular resistance increases • Aorta becomes dilated	• Systolic BP modestly increases • Rigidity of arteries contributes to coronary artery disease and peripheral vascular disease
Venous circulation	• Vessel tortuosity increases	• Inflamed, painful, or cordlike varicosities appear
Peripheral pulses	• Arteries become more rigid	• Pulses are weaker but equal • Circulation to periphery slows • Feet and hands are cold
Respiratory System		
Structures	• Cartilage degeneration occurs • Vertebral rigidity occurs • Strength of muscles decreases • Respiratory muscles atrophy • Rigidity of thoracic wall increases • Ciliary action decreases	• Kyphosis occurs • Anterior–posterior diameter increases • Use of accessory muscles decreases • Chest becomes rigid and barrel-shaped • Respiratory excursion decreases • Ability to cough and deep breathing ability diminish
Change in ventilation and perfusion	• Pulmonary vascular bed shrinks • Alveoli decrease in number • Alveolar walls thicken • Elastic recoil decreases	• Lung compliance decreases • Total lung volume is unchanged • Vital capacity decreases • Residual lung volume increases • Mucus thickens • PaO_2 and O_2 saturation decreases • Hyperresonance
Ventilation control	• Response to hypoxia and hypercarbia diminishes	• Ability to maintain acid–base balance decreases • Respiratory rate 12–24/min
Integumentary System		
Skin	• Amounts of collagen and subcutaneous fat decrease • Sweat glands decrease in number • Epidermal cell turnover slows • Skin tissue fluid decreases • Capillary fragility increases • Pigment cells decrease in number • Sebaceous gland activity decreases • Sensory receptors diminish • Thresholds for touch, vibration, heat, and pain increase	• Skin elasticity decreases • Wrinkles and folds increase • Extremity fat is lost; fat on trunk increases • Skin heals more slowly • Skin is more dry • Skin tears and bruises easily • Skin colour uneven • Skin lesions increase in number • Ability to respond to heat and cold decreases • Ability to feel light touch decreases • Cutaneous pain sensitivity declines
Hair	• Melanin decreases • Germ centres and hair follicles decrease in size and number	• Hair turns grey or white • Hair quantity decreases and thins • Amounts of scalp, pubic, and axillary hair decrease • Amount of facial hair on men decreases • Amount of facial hair on women increases

TABLE 7.2   AGE-RELATED DIFFERENCES IN ASSESSMENT—cont'd

Function	Normal Age Changes	Clinical Manifestations
Nails	• Blood supply to nail bed decreases • Longitudinal striations increase	• Growth slows • Nails are brittle and thicken • Nails are easily split • Potential for fungal infection increases
Urinary System		
Kidney	• Renal mass decreases • Number of functioning nephrons decreases • Glomerular filtration rate decreases • Renal plasma flow decreases	• Protein in urine increases • Potential for dehydration increases • Creatinine clearance decreases • Serum levels of creatinine and BUN increase • Excretion of toxins and medications decreases • Nocturia increases
Bladder	• Amounts of bladder smooth muscle and elastic tissue decrease	• Capacity decreases • Control decreases; potential for stress incontinence increases
Micturition	• Sphincter control decreases	• Frequency, urgency, and nocturia increase
Reproductive System		
Male structures	• Prostate enlarges • Testicular volume decreases • Sperm count decreases • Seminal vesicles atrophy • Serum testosterone levels remain constant • Estrogen level increases	• Sexual response becomes less intense • Achieving an erection takes longer • Erection is maintained without ejaculation • Force of ejaculation decreases
Female structures	• Estradiol, prolactin, and progesterone levels diminish • Sizes of ovaries, uterus, cervix, fallopian tubes, and labia decrease • Associated glands and epithelium atrophy • Elasticity in the pelvic area decreases • Breast tissue decreases • Vaginal pH becomes alkaline	• Responses to changing hormone levels are altered • Cervical and vaginal secretions decrease • Intensity of sexual response decreases • Potential for vaginal infections increases • Potential for vaginal and uterine prolapse increases
Gastrointestinal System		
Oral cavity	• Dentine decreases • Gingival retraction occurs • Bone density is lost • Papillae of tongue decrease in number • Taste thresholds for salt and sugar increase • Salivary secretions decrease	• Taste perception changes • Potential for loss of teeth is increased • Gingivitis is more likely to occur • Gums may bleed, and dry mouth occurs • Oral mucosa is dry
Esophagus	• Pressure of lower esophageal sphincter decreases • Motility decreases	• Epigastric distress occurs • Dysphagia occurs • Potential for hiatal hernia and aspiration is increased
Stomach	• Gastric mucosa atrophies • Blood flow decreases	• Gastric emptying decreases
Small intestine	• Intestinal villi decrease in number • Enzyme secretions decrease • Motility decreases	• Intestinal transit slows • Absorption of fat-soluble vitamins is delayed
Large intestine	• Blood flow decreases • Motility decreases • Sensation of defecation urge decreases	• Potential for constipation and fecal impaction increases
Pancreas	• Pancreatic ducts become distended • Lipase production decreases • Pancreatic reserve is impaired	• Fat absorption is impaired • Glucose tolerance decreases
Liver	• Number and size of cells decrease • Hepatic protein synthesis is impaired • Ability to regenerate liver cells decreases	• Lower border extends past costal margin • Medication metabolism decreases
Musculoskeletal System		
Skeleton	• Intervertebral disc space narrows • Cartilage of nose and ears increases	• Height diminishes 2.5–10 cm (1–4 inches) • Nose and ears lengthen • Kyphosis occurs • Pelvis widens
Bone	• Amounts of cortical and trabecular bone decrease	• Bone resorption exceeds bone formation • Potential for osteoporotic fractures increases
Muscles	• Number of muscle fibres decreases • Muscle fibres atrophy • Muscle regeneration slows • Contraction time and latency period are prolonged • Flexion of joints increases • Ligaments stiffen • Tendons become sclerotic • Tendon flexor reflexes decrease	• Strength decreases • Agility decreases • Rigidity in neck, shoulders, hips, and knees increases • Potential for restless legs syndrome increases

Continued

TABLE 7.2   AGE-RELATED DIFFERENCES IN ASSESSMENT—cont'd

Function	Normal Age Changes	Clinical Manifestations
Joints	• Cartilage erosion occurs • Calcium deposits increase • Water in cartilage decreases	• Mobility decreases • ROM becomes limited • Osteoarthritis can occur
Nervous System		
Structure	• Neurons in brain and spinal cord are lost • Brain size decreases • Dendrites atrophy • Amount of major neurotransmitters decreases • Size of ventricles increases	• Conduction of nerve impulses slows • Peripheral nerve function is lost • Reaction time decreases • Response time slows • Potential for altered balance, vertigo, and syncope increases • Postural hypotension becomes more common • Proprioception diminishes • Sensory input decreases • EEG alpha waves slow down
Sleep	• Amount of deep sleep decreases • Amount of REM sleep decreases	• Falling asleep becomes more difficult • Period of wakefulness increases
Visual System		
Eye structure	• Orbital fat is lost • Eyebrows and eyelashes turn grey or white • Elasticity of eyelid muscles decreases • Tear production decreases	• Eyes become sunken • Eyes become dry • Potential for ectropion and entropion increases • Potential for conjunctivitis increases
Cornea	• Corneal sensitivity decreases • Corneal reflex decreases • Arcus senilis becomes more common	• Potential for corneal abrasion is increased
Ciliary	• Aqueous humor secretion decreases • Ciliary muscle atrophies	• Ability of lens to accommodate declines • Presbyopia occurs • Peripheral vision decreases
Lens	• Lens becomes less elastic, more dense	• Lens becomes yellow and opaque • Ability to adapt to light and dark lessens • Tolerance of glare decreases • Incidence of cataracts increases • Night vision is impaired
Iris and pupil	• Pigment is lost • Pupil size decreases • Amount of vitreous gel debris increases	• Visual acuity decreases • Pupils appear constricted • Floaters are common
Auditory System		
Structure	• Hairs in external auditory canals of men increase • Ceruminal glands decrease in number	• Potential for conductive hearing loss increases • Cerumen is drier • Sound conduction decreases
Middle ear	• Middle-ear bone joints degenerate • Eardrum thickens	
Inner ear	• Vestibular structures decline • Hair cells are lost • Cochlea atrophies • Organ of Corti atrophies	• Sensitivity to high tones and perception of "s," "t," "f," and hard "g" sounds decrease • Understanding of speech decreases • Discrimination of background voice decreases • Equilibrium–balance deficits occur • Potential for tinnitus increases
Immune system	• Amount of secretory IgA declines • Thymus gland becomes involuted • Amount of lymphoid tissue decreases • Antibody production is impaired • Proliferative response of T and B cells decreases • Number of autoantibodies increases	• Potential for infection on mucosal surfaces increases • Cell-mediated immune response is impaired • Malignancy incidence increases • Response to acute infection is weakened • Recurrence of latent herpes zoster and tuberculosis is more likely • Susceptibility to autoimmune disease increases

AV, atrioventricular; *BP,* blood pressure; *bpm,* beats per minute; *BUN,* blood urea nitrogen; *EEG,* electroencephalographic; *HR,* heart rate; *IgA,* immunoglobulin A; *PaO₂,* arterial partial pressure of oxygen; *REM,* rapid eye movement; *ROM,* range of motion.

OLDER POPULATIONS AT RISK

Some subgroups within the older population are at a higher risk for developing certain conditions or for conditions to be misdiagnosed. Some people belong to several of these subgroups, and their care requires skilled expertise in nursing assessment, interventions, and evaluations.

Older Women

Gender is an important factor that influences the natural history of diseases and determines management and treatment in situations in which gender roles and preferences could influence care-seeking behaviour and treatment. Home care clients and residents in LTC facilities are predominantly female. The progression of dementia is faster in women (Golive et al., 2018), and women are at a higher risk for being prescribed inappropriate medications (Morgan et al., 2016).

In addition to having a high number of chronic health conditions, older persons face challenges such as reduced financial resources, lack of informal caregiving responsibilities, or both; these challenges have a significant effect on the health of older

TABLE 7.3 AGE-RELATED DIFFERENCES IN ASSESSMENT

Effects of Aging on Cognitive Functioning

Function	Manifestations of Healthy Aging
Fluid intelligence (the ability to solve new problems or use logic in new situations)	Declines
Crystallized intelligence (the ability to use learned knowledge and experience)	Improves
Vocabulary and verbal reasoning	Improves
Spatial perception	Remains constant or improves
Synthesis of new information	Declines
Mental performance speed	Declines
Short-term recall memory	Declines
Long-term recall memory	Remains constant

women. As a result, older women often experience disparities in treatment in comparison with men, including unequal access to quality health care. Last but of importance, older women are more likely to be victims of family violence than are older men, in part because they usually live longer (Yon et al., 2017). Several resources, organizations, and programs are in place to raise awareness of, prevent, diagnose, and address the abuse of older persons in Canada. The Registered Nurses' Association of Ontario (RNAO) has created a Best Practice Guideline, "Preventing and Addressing Abuse and Neglect of Older Adults," which is listed at the end of this chapter.

Older Persons With Cognitive Impairment or Dementia

The majority of older persons do not have any noticeable decline in mental abilities. There are some normal age changes, such as a memory lapse or benign forgetfulness, which are significantly different from cognitive impairment. These normal age changes are often referred to as *age-associated memory impairment* (Table 7.3).

An older person who is forgetful can benefit from using memory aids, attempting recall in a calm and quiet environment, and actively engaging in memory improvement techniques. Memory aids include clocks, calendars, notes, marked pillboxes, safety alarms on stoves, and identity necklaces or bracelets. Memory improvement techniques include word association, mental imaging, and mnemonics.

Declining physical health is an important factor in cognitive impairment. Older persons who experience sensory losses or cerebrovascular disease may show a decline in cognitive functioning. An appropriate cognitive assessment includes hearing and vision, functional ability, memory recall, orientation, use of judgement, and appropriateness of emotional state. Standard mental status examinations and behavioural descriptions provide data for determining cognitive status. Cognitive impairment is further discussed in Chapter 62.

Some older persons experience *dementia*, an umbrella term to describe disorders of the brain (Alzheimer Society of Canada, 2021c). There are many types of dementia, but Alzheimer's disease is the most common form of dementia. Dementia is progressive and affects brain cells. As dementia worsens, more cells in the brain become damaged (Alzheimer Society of Canada, 2021c). The Alzheimer Society of Canada (2021b) discusses 10 warning signs of dementia, including struggling to retain new information and difficulty performing familiar tasks.

In Canada, there are 564 000 people currently living with dementia, with the majority of those diagnosed being female (65%) (Alzheimer Society of Canada, 2021c). The prevalence of dementia increases with age. One in four older person age 85 and older are diagnosed with dementia (Canadian Institutes of Health Information [CIHI], 2020b).

As dementia progresses, older persons may need more support with activities of daily living and other health and social needs. This may require moving to an LTC facility to access these services (CIHI, 2020a).

Diagnosing dementia requires collaboration with the interprofessional care team. Dementia is diagnosed by asking questions about symptoms, past illnesses, and family medical information and obtaining any psychiatric information (Alzheimer Society of Canada, 2021a). It is also important to conduct a medication reconciliation to ensure that issues such as medication errors are not the cause of memory changes.

Older Newcomers to Canada

Newcomers to Canada represent almost one-third of Canada's aging population, many of whom are from Arab, South Asian, and African Muslim communities (Salma & Salami, 2020). Unfortunately, newcomers often experience a decline in mental health, comorbidities, and social isolation (Salma & Salami, 2020; Wang et al., 2019). Some newcomers may not access health care services because of barriers such as unawareness of services, lack of health literacy, lack of transportation, language difficulties, cultural differences, health beliefs, cost of services, lack of health insurance, location, socioeconomic status, or a fear of stigma (RNAO, 2007; Wang et al., 2019).

Nurses can develop a welcoming environment that embraces diversity by seeking educational opportunities to become more culturally competent, adhering to policies and guidelines that are respectful of cultural diversity, and learning more about peoples' experiences and values (RNAO, 2007). Nurses can also advocate for government policy changes to increase the access of publicly funded health care services for newcomers in their communities.

Older Persons Living in Rural Settings

Although no recent data are available, studies suggest that many older persons living in rural areas face challenges such as a lack of or limited availability of support to remain independent, as well as limited housing and transportation options (Menec et al., 2015). In addition, older persons in rural and remote areas are frequently required to travel out of their communities for health services, which creates many challenges (Lord et al., 2017). Some research has indicated that older persons living in rural areas present with more symptoms of ill health than do older persons living in urban areas (Vogelsang, 2016).

Nurses working with older persons in rural communities must recognize the lifestyle values and practices of rural life (Figure 7.1) and acknowledge that limited transportation is a possible barrier to providing care. Alternative service approaches such as Internet sources and chat rooms, videos, radio, community centres, and church social events can be used to conduct health screening. Use of telehealth devices for monitoring people in their home environments has enhanced the ability to provide care.

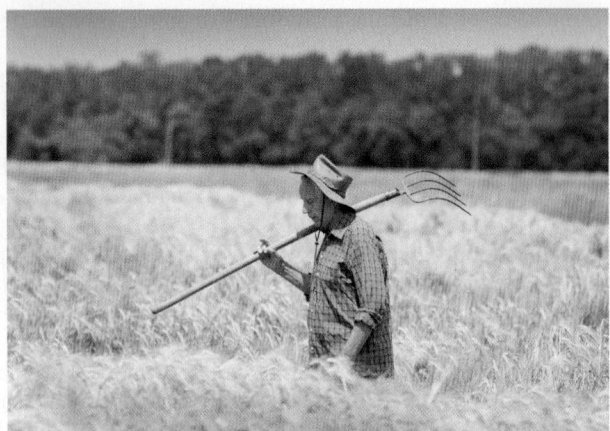

FIG. 7.1 Transportation is a possible barrier to providing service to older persons in rural areas. Source: iStock.com/Jevtic.

Older Persons Who Are Homeless

According to careful estimates, Canada may have as many as 6000 homeless older persons; however, adults over 50 years of age account for only 24% of shelter users, with high rates of mobility impairment, falls, frailty, cognitive impairment, and urinary incontinence (Humphries & Canham, 2019). Key factors associated with homelessness include a low income, reduced cognitive capacity, and living alone. According to Statistics Canada, 3.5% of people 65 years of age and older are living below the low-income cut-off, the point at which a family is spending 70% or more of their income on necessities (i.e., food, clothing, and shelter) (Statistics Canada, 2021). Among older Canadians, single or widowed women are at higher risk for living in poverty. Such low-income older persons may become homeless because of a lack of affordable housing.

When homeless, older individuals may have additional new health issues or experience an exacerbation of existing health conditions because most services provided are not designed for older persons. LTC placement is often an alternative to homelessness, especially when the individual is cognitively impaired and alone. A distinct fear of such institutionalization may explain why older homeless people do not use shelter- and meal-site services.

Frail Older Persons

Frailty is a term used to identify those who, because of declining physical health and resources, are most vulnerable to poor outcomes. Frailty has been defined as the presence of three or more of the following: unplanned weight loss (≥4.5 kg [10 lb] in the past year), weakness, poor endurance and energy, slowness, and low activity (Wilson et al., 2017). Risk factors include disability, multiple chronic illnesses, and the presence of geriatric syndromes. Frailty is not related directly to age per se, although age is a risk factor. Hardiness or psychological strength may be a significant factor in preventing frailty among older persons.

The level of frailty can be determined though assessment with the Clinical Frailty Scale (CFS) (Rockwood & Theou, 2020). The CFS is a nine-point scale, with higher scores indicating greater risk of frailty. The CFS focuses on mobility, balance, use of walking aides, and the ability to perform activities of daily living on one's own.

Most frail older persons have difficulty coping with declining functional abilities and decreasing daily energy. When stressful life events (e.g., the death of a loved one) occur and daily strain

TABLE 7.4	NUTRITIONAL ASSESSMENT OF OLDER PERSONS

The acronym **SCALES** can remind the nurse to assess important nutritional indicators:
Sadness, or mood change
Cholesterol level: high
Albumin level: low
Loss or gain of weight
Eating difficulties
Shopping and food preparation challenges

(e.g., caring for an ill partner) is present, the frail person may have difficulties coping and may become ill. Common health challenges include mobility and strength limitations, sensory impairment, cognitive decline, and falls.

The frail older person is at particular risk for malnutrition and difficulties with hydration (Verlaan et al., 2017). Malnutrition and dehydration are related to sociopsychological factors such as living alone, depression, and low income. Physical factors such as impairment of vision or hearing, declining cognitive status, inadequate dental care, physical fatigue, and limited mobility also add to the risks of malnutrition and dehydration. Because many frail older persons have therapeutic diets and multiple medication regimens, their nutritional state may be altered. It is important for the nurse to monitor for adequate calorie, protein, iron, calcium, vitamin D, and fluid intake. Several assessment tools (Table 7.4) have been developed to monitor older persons for poor nutritional status. Once nutritional needs are identified, interventions can include home-delivered meals, dietary supplements, food stamps, dental referrals, congregate dining sites, home visits by registered dietitians, and vitamin supplements.

Older Persons With Chronic Illness

Daily living with chronic or persistent illness is a reality for many older persons. Although people of all ages have chronic health conditions, illness is most common in older persons. It is estimated that 80% to 92% of older persons have one or more chronic illnesses (Chiaranai et al., 2018).

Chronic illness is composed of multiple health conditions that have a protracted, unpredictable course. Diagnosis and the management of the acute phase of a chronic persistent illness is often managed in a hospital, and all other phases are usually managed at home. Managing chronic illness can profoundly affect the lives and the self-concepts of the older person and their family. Although health status encompasses acute and chronic illness, it also includes an individual's level of daily functioning. Functional health includes activities of daily living (ADLs), such as bathing, dressing, eating, toileting, and transferring. Instrumental activities of daily living (IADLs), such as using a telephone, shopping, preparing food, housekeeping, doing laundry, arranging transportation, taking medications, and handling finances, are also included in a functional health assessment.

Treatment for chronic conditions can often cause new problems. As one disease is treated, another may be affected. For example, the use of a medication with anticholinergic properties, such as a tricyclic antidepressant (e.g., amitriptyline [Elavil]), may cause urinary retention. In older persons, disease symptoms are atypical, and sometimes manifestations of disease are asymptomatic. For example, the only symptom of cardiac

TABLE 7.5	SUPPORTIVE INTERVENTIONS FOR OLDER PERSONS WITH CHRONIC ILLNESS

- Prevent social isolation.
- Control symptoms of the chronic illness.
- Adjust to changes in the course of the disease.
- Prevent and manage episodes of acute illness.
- Carry out prescribed therapies for the chronic illness.
- Use technology to enhance function, independence, and safety.

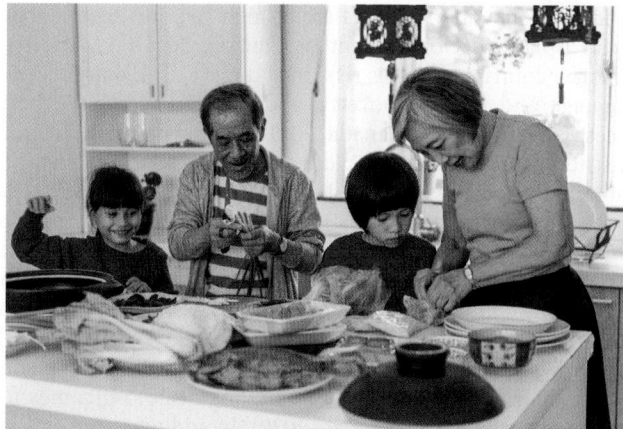

FIG. 7.2 Culture and heritage can be important facets of many older persons' lives. Source: iStock.com/georgeclerk.

disease may be fatigue. Pathological entities with similar symptoms are often confused. Negative consequences of chronic illness include physical suffering, loss, worry, grief, depression, functional impairment, and increased dependence (Han et al., 2018). Daily living with chronic illness can be very difficult for older persons. The nurse must involve the older person in any decision making related to interventions, goals planning, and quality of life and well-being (Table 7.5).

Socially Isolated Older Persons

As people age and social networks contract, they may become increasingly isolated and lonely. Although social isolation and loneliness are related factors, they are distinctly different concepts. *Social isolation* is defined as being separated from one's environment to the point of having few satisfying and rewarding relationships. *Loneliness*, conversely, is one's feeling of dissatisfaction with social contacts in terms of quantity or quality, or both (Bandari et al., 2019). Thus the feeling of loneliness can be present even if an older person is living with another person, with family, or in an LTC facility. It is the quality of the social contacts that is critical for the maintenance of well-being and hardiness.

Both social isolation and loneliness have consistently been found to be associated with poorer physical and psychological health (Bandari et al., 2019). Although many social, personal, and health factors are involved in social isolation and loneliness, it is difficult to predict which older persons are most at risk for poor health. Those who are isolated and lonely should be closely monitored. Keeping these vulnerable older persons engaged in meaningful social relationships and activities is a significant health-promoting intervention, and nurses have an important role to play in this area.

COVID-19 AND THE IMPACT ON OLDER PERSONS

The novel coronavirus disease 2019, or COVID-19, is caused by a coronavirus called SARS-CoV-2. COVID-19 presents similarly to influenza but has a longer incubation period and reproductive number than influenza (World Health Organization [WHO], 2020). Symptoms include fever, cough, and respiratory issues. Approximately 80% of COVID-19 cases have been mild or asymptomatic. However, 15% of individuals with COVID-19 present with more severe infections, requiring oxygen (WHO, 2020). About 5% of infections result in the need to seek critical interventions and admittance into the critical care unit (CCU) for ventilation (WHO, 2020).

In 2019, COVID-19 originated in Wuhan, China, and caused a pandemic, affecting populations over the world (Centers for Disease Control and Prevention [CDC], 2021). Most people who are infected with COVID-19 fully recover. However, this virus has affected older persons disproportionately.

Older persons are more likely to experience comorbidities and thus have weaker immune systems. COVID-19 is more likely to cause serious complications in those with compromised immune systems, such as in residents who live in LTC facilities who experience comorbidities. As of May 2020, LTC residents accounted for 81% of all COVID-19 deaths in Canada (CIHI, 2020c).

Culturally Competent Care. The term ethnogeriatrics is used to describe the specialty area of providing culturally competent care to older persons who are identified with a particular ethnic group (Touhy et al., 2018) (Figure 7.2). Canada is officially a multicultural society, and culturally diverse care is essential in order to provide for the needs of a diverse group of older persons. Vast differences or heterogeneity are found among and within various ethnic groups in relation to health beliefs and practices, access to and utilization of health care, health risks, family dynamics and caregiving, decision-making processes and priorities, and responses to interventions and changes in health care policies (RNAO, 2007). As emphasized throughout this text, nurses are challenged to provide culturally competent care in all types of settings and communities. Although it is unrealistic to expect a health care provider to be proficient in working with every category and subgroup of minority older persons, it is possible to develop levels of awareness, skill, and sensitivity that can be applied to interactions with older persons of ethnic minorities and their families. The nurse must assess each older person's ethnic orientation. Several tools or instruments can assist nurses in eliciting health care beliefs and help identify a patient's perceptions of alternative beliefs (see Resources at the end of this chapter; Kleinman et al., 1978; Touhy et al., 2018). Culturally competent care is further discussed in Chapter 2.

Indigenous Older Persons

Indigenous people are a fast-growing population in Canada (Government of Canada, 2021a) with a growing number of older persons. In 2016, 7% of the Canadian Indigenous population was 65 years old or older, rising from 4.8% in 2006 (Statistics Canada, 2019a). Up to 8.7% of the Métis peoples are 65 years of age and older (Statistics Canada, 2019a). According to population projections, the proportion of the First Nations, Métis, and Inuit populations 65 years of age and older could more than double by 2036 (Statistics Canada, 2020a).

Indigenous older persons are at high risk for experiencing social isolation (Government of Canada, 2021b). Many factors may contribute to this risk, including racism, marginalized language and culture, poverty, and historic negative experiences (Government of Canada, 2021b). Some protective factors exist to ensure Indigenous older persons feel socially engaged and remain socially included (Government of Canada, 2021b). Such factors include participating in ceremonies; having a social support that provides help, positive interaction, and emotional support; feeling part of a community that promotes respect for Indigenous cultural values; having access to social events that respect Elders; and having access to culturally sensitive health care services within the community. Indigenous-led health service collaborations assist in improving health outcomes for Indigenous people (Allen et al., 2020). In addition, nurses providing care for older Indigenous patients must practise cultural competence and remain sensitive to their needs, ensuring that care delivered is person-centred and of the highest quality.

SOCIAL SUPPORT AND THE OLDER PERSON

Social support is essential for all older persons to maintain their level of well-being. Social support occurs at three levels. Family and kinship relations are most often the first level of providers of social support. Second, a semiformal level of support is found in clubs, places of worship, neighbourhoods, and senior citizen centres. Third, older persons may be linked to a formal system of social welfare agencies, health facilities, and government support. In general, the nurse is part of the formal support system.

Caregivers

A *caregiver* is someone who provides supervision and direct care and coordinates services. Caregiving includes many tasks, but focuses mostly on assisting older patients with ADLs and IADLs, providing emotional and social support, and managing health care. In Canada, 7.8 million caregivers provide care to a family member or friend with a long-term health condition, physical or mental disability, or age-related disorder (Statistics Canada, 2020b). In 2018, 70% of caregivers received support from home care or other services (Statistics Canada, 2020b). While the wait time for services varies across Canada, the median wait time for home care services for patients at home is 6 days (Health Quality Ontario [HQO], 2021).

Caregivers often experience their caregiving as rewarding, but it can also be a very physically and emotionally demanding task, even leading to increased medical illnesses and a greater risk of mortality for the caregiver (Hategan et al., 2018) (Table 7.6). Some caregivers may develop a sense of being overwhelmed and have feelings of inadequacy, powerlessness, and depression (Hategan et al., 2018). The burden of caregiving can be isolating, inasmuch as it limits social, emotional, and interactional opportunities. Time commitments, fatigue, and, at times, socially inappropriate behaviours of the dependent older person contribute to the caregiver's social isolation. The socially isolated caregiver must be identified, and plans should be designed to meet their needs for social support and interaction.

Many family members involved in direct caregiving activities also identify rewards associated with this role. Positive aspects of caregiving include knowing that a loved one is receiving good care (often in a home environment), learning and mastering new tasks, and finding opportunities for intimacy. At the same time, the tasks involved in caregiving often provide

TABLE 7.6   CAREGIVER CHALLENGES

- Lack of respite or relief from caregiving
- Conflict in the family unit related to decisions about caregiving
- Lack of understanding of the time and energy needed for caregiving
- Inability to meet personal self-care needs, such as socialization and rest
- Inadequate information about specific tasks of caregiving
- Financial depletion of resources as a result of a caregiver's inability to work and the increased cost of care

opportunities for family members to learn more about one another and strengthen their relationships.

The nurse should always consider the caregiver as a partner in care and plan interventions to reduce caregiver strain if necessary. The caregiver can be taught about age-related changes and diseases and specific caregiving techniques. The nurse can also assist the caregiver in seeking help from the formal social support system regarding matters such as respite care, housing, health coverage, and finances. Finally, the nurse should monitor the caregiver for indications of declining health, emotional distress, and caregiver role strain (Chapter 6).

Elder Mistreatment and Abuse

Elder abuse can be defined as "any action by someone in a relationship of trust that results in harm or distress to an older person. Neglect is a lack of action by that person in a relationship of trust with the same result" (Friedman et al., 2017). The term elder mistreatment is used to describe acts of commission (*elder abuse*) or omission (*elder neglect*) that harm or threaten to harm an older person's health or welfare. Elder abuse may occur in private homes or in any type of care facilities. *Institutional abuse* refers to abuse of people living in LTC facilities. An older person may experience more than one form of abuse (Table 7.7).

Overall, elder abuse is an underreported problem and has been difficult to quantify. According to police reports, in 2015 up to 10% of people older than 65 were victims of family violence, and grown children were most often the perpetrators of violence against older persons (Conroy, 2017). Victims often do not report it because of isolation; impaired cognitive or physical function; feelings of shame, embarrassment, guilt, or self-blame; fear of reprisal; pressure from family members; fear of losing their home and independence; and cultural norms. Health care providers may fail to report it because of lack of confidence in identifying or reporting victims, perceived inability to successfully intervene, and a desire to avoid responsibility for further action.

The nursing approach to a suspected victim of elder abuse should begin with a carefully documented history and a thorough examination for mistreatment. Nurses should assess the individual for the presence of dehydration, malnutrition, pressure injuries, poor personal hygiene, and lack of adherence to the medical regimen. Of importance is that failure to follow the care plan, unauthorized use of restraints, and use of medication or isolation as punishment are also considered forms of abuse.

Key assessment findings include (a) explanations for findings (e.g., injuries) that are not consistent with objective data and (b) contradictory explanations from the patient and the caregiver. The nurse should follow the facility or employer intervention protocol for elder abuse. A screening tool for abuse by a caregiver is available as a pocket tool from the National Initiative for the Care of the Elderly (see the Resources at the end of this chapter).

TABLE 7.7 TYPES OF ELDER MISTREATMENT

Types	Characteristics	Manifestations
Physical abuse	Slapping; restraining; incorrect positioning; oversedation	Bruises, bilateral injuries, repeated injuries in various stages of healing; use of several emergency departments
Physical neglect	Withholding of food, water, medications, clothing, hygiene; failure to provide physical aids such as dentures, eyeglasses, hearing aid; failure to ensure safety	Pressure injuries; loss of body weight; laboratory values showing dehydration (e.g., HCT; serum sodium) and malnutrition (serum protein); poor personal hygiene
Psychological or emotional abuse	Berating; harassment; intimidation, threats of punishment or deprivation; treating older person like a child; isolation	Depression, withdrawn behaviour; agitation; ambivalent attitude toward caregiver
Psychological or emotional neglect	Failure to provide social stimulation; leaving alone for long periods; failure to provide companionship	Depression, withdrawn behaviour; agitation; ambivalent attitude toward caregiver
Sexual abuse	Touching inappropriately; forcing sexual contact	Unexplained vaginal or anal bleeding; bruises; unexplained STIs or genital infections
Financial abuse	Denying access to personal resources; stealing money or possessions; coercing to sign contracts or durable power of attorney; making changes in will or trust	Living situation is below level of personal resources; sudden change in personal finances or transfer of assets
Violation of personal rights	Denying right to privacy or right to make decisions regarding health care or living environment; forcible eviction	Sudden inexplicable changes in living situation; confusion

HCT, hematocrit; *STIs,* sexually transmitted infections.

TABLE 7.8 NURSING MANAGEMENT OF ELDER MISTREATMENT

- It is mandatory to make reports to the appropriate provincial or territorial body about the suspicion of abuse or neglect.
- The nurse should screen for possible elder abuse, including domestic violence.
- A thorough history should be documented and a head-to-toe assessment conducted. It is important to document the findings, including any statements made by the patient or an accompanying adult.
- If an older person appears to be in immediate danger, a safety plan should be developed and implemented in collaboration with the interprofessional team involved in the person's care.
- The nurse should identify, collect, and preserve physical evidence (e.g., dirty or bloody clothing, dressings, or sheets).
- After obtaining consent, photographs should be taken to document physical findings of suspected abuse or neglect. If possible and appropriate, this should be done before the alleged victim is treated or bathed.
- If abuse is suspected, the findings should be reported to the appropriate provincial agency or law enforcement, or both, as mandated by local laws.
- Social work, forensic nursing, and other consultations should be initiated as appropriate.

In LTC facilities, nurses should be alert to patterns of recurrent infections, poor hygiene, lack of interest in activities or eating, behavioural changes, new incontinence, sleep difficulties, and complaints about staff. Specific nursing interventions to reduce the risk of elder abuse include close management of the resident's plan of care and regular review of the use of restraints and psychotropic medications, in addition to the interventions listed in Table 7.8.

When managing elder abuse, the nurse must be familiar with both federal and provincial laws governing reporting procedures and patient privacy. Information on mandatory reporting can be found on the Canadian Network for Prevention of Elder Abuse website.

CARE ALTERNATIVES FOR OLDER PERSONS

Most older persons prefer to continue living at home, but they may have to move to a more restrictive environment at a time of crisis. Several living arrangements and care options for older persons are described here.

Independent Living Options

Many older persons stay in their place of residence and do not move to a different home or geographic location as they age. The community becomes important to older persons as an environment that is safe and that supports social contacts. Older persons need privacy and companionship, as well as a sense of belonging. They may need housing assistance in the form of property tax relief and assistance with home repairs and the cost of utilities (Figure 7.3). A variety of subsidized, low-income housing arrangements are available for older persons in many areas.

For an older person who chooses to remain in their home as functional abilities decline, some home adaptations and modifications can be made, including walker and wheelchair accessibility, increased lighting, and safety devices in bathrooms and kitchens. The *Safe Living Guide—A Guide to Home Safety for Seniors* (see the Resources at the end of this chapter) includes strategies for home adaptations that improve safety and accessibility.

Adult lifestyle communities or *retirement communities* may be an option for some older persons. These communities are age-segregated, self-contained developments and provide social activities, security, and recreational facilities. Some retirement communities offer expanded health care and social support services. An entrance fee and monthly fees for continuing care are charged. Chapter 6 discusses community-based care settings.

Assisted-living facilities (ALFs) are residential care facilities that provide housing and personal care. Because over half of community-based older persons require assistance with ADLs or IADLs, this is a rapidly developing area of care. According to a Canadian Mortgage and Housing Corporation (2016) survey, up to 9.1% of Canadians aged 75 years and older lived in ALFs in 2016. Services vary widely per facility. Nurses working in this area are challenged by questions related to regulations, use of the services of unregulated care providers, assessment to ensure safe "fit of resident to facility," and shared resident decision making. The Canadian Accreditation Council is developing standards for use in accreditation of ALFs (see the Resources at the end of this chapter).

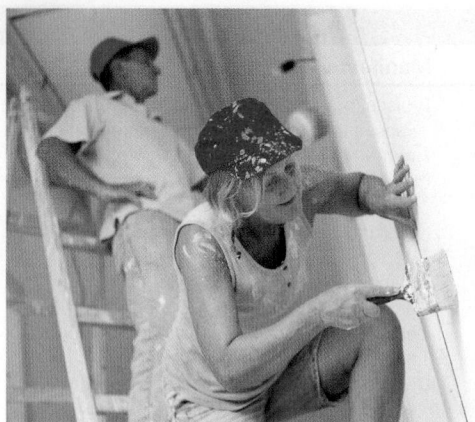

FIG. 7.3 Home maintenance is part of an older person's independent lifestyle. Source: iStock.com/Halfpoint.

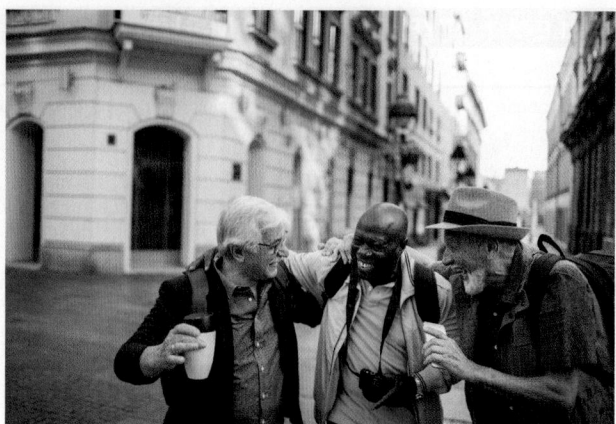

FIG. 7.4 Social interaction and acceptance are important for older persons. Source: iStock.com/Geber86.

Community-Based Care for Older Persons

Many older persons with special care needs can be aided by services in the community, such as adult day care programs or home health care.

Adult Day Care Programs. *Adult day care programs* provide daily supervision, social activities, management of chronic disease, and ADL assistance for older persons who are cognitively impaired. Examples include Alzheimer Society programs and community centre services. The services offered are based on the individual's needs. Restorative programs offer health monitoring, therapeutic activities, one-on-one ADL training, individualized care planning, and personal care services. Programs designed for people with cognitive impairments offer therapeutic recreation, support for family, family counseling, and social involvement. Adult day care programs provide relief to the caregiver, allow continued employment for the caregiver, and delay institutionalization for the older person. Centres are regulated and standards are set by the province. Costs are not covered by health insurance but are tax deductible as dependent care. The nurse's role consists of knowing the available adult day care services and assessing the needs of the older individual.

Home Health Care. Home health care can be a cost-effective care alternative for an older person who is homebound but has health needs that are intermittent or acute. In 2015, 6.4% of households received paid home care services (Gilmore, 2018). Home health care services offer skilled nursing care and care by other regulated health care providers, nonregulated workers, volunteers, friends, and family members, all to help an older person remain in the community. Emphasis of the care and services is often on the management of chronic disease, supporting ADLs, and promoting well-being. Home health care is discussed in more detail in Chapter 6.

Long-Term Care Facilities

Long-term care (LTC) facilities are a placement alternative for people who can no longer live alone, who need continuous supervision, who have three or more disabilities involving ADLs, or who are frail. Three main factors precipitate placement in an LTC facility: (1) rapid deterioration of the person's condition, (2) the caregiver's inability to continue care, and (3) an alteration in or loss of family support system. Changes in orientation (e.g., increased confusion), incontinence, or a major health event (e.g., stroke, fall) can accelerate the need for moving into an LTC facility.

LTC facilities provide care for residents with increasingly complex health care needs (Armstrong et al., 2017). Not only has the prevalence of chronic diseases such as diabetes, heart failure, and arthritis increased, but also conditions such as frailty and dementia necessitate high-quality care by a competent and interprofessional workforce. Nurses are instrumental in the care planning and chronic disease management to address a resident's health care needs while balancing the person's quality of life and wishes. Many LTC facilities provide an environment that truly represents the best of caring and quality of life and an extraordinary commitment and dedication of staff. Several initiatives are underway to shift from an institutional model to LTC facilities as places that nurture quality of life and well-being for older persons (Figure 7.4).

Acute Care Settings

When an emergency arises and a person cannot be cared for at home or in an LTC facility environment, admittance to a hospital might be necessary. Some conditions that might necessitate hospitalization include exacerbations of chronic conditions, stroke, fluid and electrolyte imbalances, pneumonia, and trauma caused by falls. Unfortunately, the complexity of the acute situation often results in the loss of the whole-person perspective with a shift of focus on the diseased part only. Nurses' integrated approach and emphasis on individualized care are essential to restoring an older person's health and well-being within this setting.

In addition, an acute care stay often results in negative consequences for older patients, including functional decline and iatrogenic events, such as falls, pressure injuries, and delirium (Gray et al., 2018). To prevent any of these complications, care of older patients requires an interprofessional approach, including very succinct nursing components. Involvement of the patient and the family is essential in supporting the individualized perspective and creating a support network for when the patient is discharged.

Geriatric Rehabilitation. Geriatric rehabilitation interventions are focused on adapting to a new situation or recovering from trauma. Collaborative and interprofessional teams focus on building up functional reserve and emotional wellness, with the use of appropriate assistive equipment and personal care, and creating a supportive network in which an older person can live as independently as possible. The person can receive rehabilitative assistance through inpatient rehabilitation (limited days are covered), day programs, or home care programs (Figure 7.5).

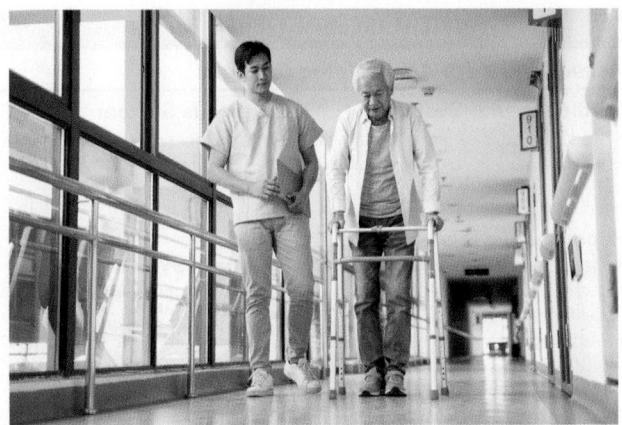

FIG. 7.5 The nurse assists an older person in a geriatric rehabilitation facility. Source: iStock.com/imtmphoto.

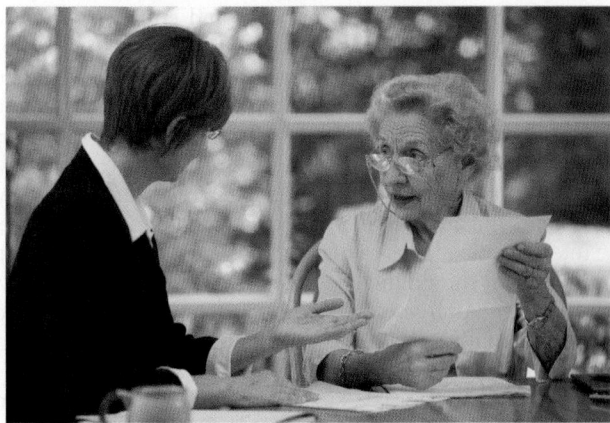

FIG. 7.6 Some residential facilities for older persons post notices announcing when free legal help is available. Source: iStock.com/ebstock.

Rehabilitation of older persons is influenced by several factors. Older persons show greater initial variability in functional capacity than do people at any other age. Pre-existing factors associated with reaction time, visual acuity, fine motor ability, physical strength, cognitive function, and motivation affect the rehabilitation potential of older persons.

Within the interprofessional team, nurses assess and develop interventions for existing chronic illnesses, fears and anxieties specific to falling, fatigue, sensory–perceptual deficits, malnutrition, and social and financial challenges. Many older persons lose functional ability in the hospital because of inactivity and immobility. Older persons can improve flexibility, strength, and aerobic capacity even into very old age. The interprofessional team develops passive and active range-of-motion exercises to prevent deconditioning and subsequent functional decline.

LEGAL AND ETHICAL ISSUES

Legal assistance is an issue for many older persons concerned about advance directives, estate planning, taxation issues, and appeals for denied services. In Canada, legal aid is available for all citizens (Figure 7.6). There is some variation between provinces and territories about legal matters affecting capacity, advance directives, and consent.

Mental capacity is a person's ability to make decisions. It is a legal construct, not a clinical condition (Touhy et al., 2018). To be deemed capable of making a decision, the person must *understand* information that is relevant to making a decision, *evaluate* data, and *appreciate* the consequences of the decision or of not making a decision (Kelly et al., 2020). People are presumed to have capacity unless there is clear evidence to the contrary and the person has been legally deemed incapable. Capacity can improve, decrease, or fluctuate (Kelly et al., 2020).

A *power of attorney* is a legal document and legal device in which one person designates another person (e.g., family member, friend) to act on their behalf.

There are primarily two types of advance directives: instruction directives and those in which a substitute decision maker or proxy is named (RNAO, 2011). An instruction directive (or *living will*) specifies what kinds of interventions are desirable for different health situations. In a proxy directive, the person specifies who is to make health care decisions if they become unable to make their wishes known. Often, these two terms are used interchangeably; however, they serve different purposes (RNAO, 2011). (Advance directives are discussed in Chapter 13.)

The nurse who works with older persons will encounter areas of ethical concern that influence practice and care. Issues may include the need to evaluate the person's ability to make decisions, resuscitation, treatment of infections, issues of nutrition and hydration, and transfer to more intensive treatment units. These situations are often complex and emotionally charged. The nurse can assist the older person, the family, and other health care providers by acknowledging when an ethical dilemma is present, by keeping current on the ethical implications of biotechnology, and by advocating for an institutional ethics committee to help in the decision-making process. For more information, see the Resources section at the end of the chapter.

NURSING MANAGEMENT
OLDER PERSONS

NURSING ASSESSMENT

The assessment of an older person provides the database and baseline information for the rest of the nursing process; however, it is a complex undertaking. First, older persons may face any health issue with fear or anxiety, and the issue may present in an atypical manner. In addition, health care providers may be perceived as helpful, but health care settings may be perceived as negative, potentially harmful places. The nurse beginning an assessment needs to establish a trusting relationship by communicating a sense of concern and care by use of direct and honest statements, appropriate eye contact, and direct touch when appropriate. When beginning the assessment process, the nurse should attend to primary needs first—for example, ensure that the person is free of pain, is adequately hydrated, is wearing appropriate clothing, and does not need to go to the bathroom. All assistive devices such as glasses and hearing aids should be in place. The interview should be short so that the person does not become fatigued. The nurse should allow adequate time to give information, as well as to respond to any questions. The medical history may be lengthy, and the nurse must determine what normal age changes are and which information is relevant. If possible, medical records and any current medications should be reviewed.

To truly assess an older person, a comprehensive geriatric assessment is required (Heckman & Jónsson, 2017). The focus of a comprehensive geriatric assessment is to determine appropriate interventions to maintain and enhance the functional and cognitive abilities of the older person. An example is the interRAI Acute Care instrument for the rapid assessment of functional and psychosocial information of adult patients in hospitals (Gray et al., 2018). This assessment is interprofessional and, at a minimum, includes the medical history, the physical examination, a functional abilities assessment, a cognitive assessment, and an assessment of social and financial resources. The interprofessional team may represent many disciplines, but at minimum it should include the nurse, the physician, and the social worker. After the assessment is complete, the interprofessional team meets with the patient and family to present the team's findings and recommendations.

Nursing assessment is a key component of the comprehensive geriatric assessment, including a history, a functional health pattern format (see Chapter 3), a physical assessment, cognitive assessment, assessment of ADLs and IADLs, and a social–environmental assessment. Evaluation of cognitive status is particularly important for older persons because results of this evaluation often determine the potential for independent living. Evaluation of the results of a comprehensive assessment help determine the services needed.

The comprehensive nursing assessment should be based on instruments that are reliable, valid, and specific to older persons. Several standardized assessment tools for gerontology are available and can be used in accordance with the purpose of the assessment and the status of the person. However, difficulties often arise in the interpretation of the results of findings because of age-related changes and parameters that are not well defined for older persons. The nurse is in an important position to recognize and correct inaccurate interpretation of laboratory test results.

NURSING DIAGNOSES

With few exceptions, the same nursing diagnoses apply to an older person as to a younger individual. However, the causes and defining characteristics are related to age and are unique to older persons. Table 7.9 lists nursing diagnoses that are seen in older persons as a result of age-related changes. The identification and management of nursing diagnoses result in higher-quality care and improved patient–client function.

PLANNING

When setting goals with an older person, the nurse must identify the person's strengths and abilities. Caregivers, if appropriate, should be included in goal development. Personal characteristics such as hardiness, persistence, and the ability to learn contribute to the setting of individualized goals. Priority goals for the older person may be focused on well-being, such as gaining a sense of control, feeling safe, and reducing stress.

NURSING IMPLEMENTATION

When carrying out a plan of action, the nurse may have to modify the approach and techniques used according to the physical and cognitive status of a particular older person. Sensory changes, such as auditory and visual deficits, may interfere with communication. Small body size, common among frail older persons, may necessitate the use of pediatric equipment (e.g., blood pressure cuff). Bone and joint changes often necessitate assistance with transfers, altered positioning, and use of gait belts and lift devices. An older person with declining energy reserves may require additional time to complete tasks. A

TABLE 7.9 NURSING DIAGNOSES
Associated With Age-Related Changes

Cardiovascular System
- Reduced physical activity stamina
- Hypertension or hypotension
- Tiredness

Reproductive System
- Decreased sexual function
- Increased risk of erectile dysfunction (men)
- Perimenopause and menopause (women)

Respiratory System
- Decreased gas exchange
- Potential for dyspnea
- Potential for hypoxemia
- Potential for aspiration
- Potential for pulmonary infection

Gastrointestinal System
- Constipation
- Impaired or delayed absorption of nutrients
- Obesity

Integumentary System
- Reduced tissue integrity
- Delayed or inadequate wound healing

Nervous System
- Cognitive decline (long-term or acute)
- Hyperthermia
- Hypothermia

Urinary System
- Risk of urinary incontinence

Senses
- Reduced self-concept (self-worth, confidence, self-identity)
- Social isolation

Musculoskeletal System
- Chronic pain
- Risk for injury (fractures)
- Decreased mobility
- Sedentary lifestyle

Immune System
- Risk for inflammation or sepsis

slower pace of interaction, more limited scheduling of interventions and activities, and the availability of a bedside commode or other adaptive equipment may be necessary.

Cognitive impairment, if present, mandates careful explanations and a calm approach to avoid producing anxiety in the older person. Depression can result in apathy, malnutrition, and a decline in mobility. Several guidelines and interventions are available to enhance nursing care for people living with cognitive impairment (Touhy et al., 2018).

HEALTH PROMOTION. Health promotion and the prevention of health conditions and challenges in older persons comprise one of the most important areas for nurses. The focus is mainly on three areas: reduction in diseases, increased participation in health promotion activities, and targeted services that reduce health hazards. The Division of Aging and Seniors of the Public Health Agency of Canada (PHAC) provides federal leadership on health issues affecting older persons, including fall prevention, emergency preparedness, and age-friendly communities (PHAC, 2016a).

Within gerontology, nurses need to place a high value on health promotion and positive health behaviours. Several programs have been successfully developed for chronic health condition screening, smoking cessation, geriatric foot care, vision and hearing screening, stress reduction, exercise programs, medication usage, crime prevention, elder mistreatment, delirium prevention and treatment, and home hazards assessment (RNAO, 2017). The nurse can carry out and teach older persons about the need for specific preventive services. The nurse interested in health promotion for older persons can reference Health Canada's "Healthy Living" webpage (see the Resources at the end of this chapter).

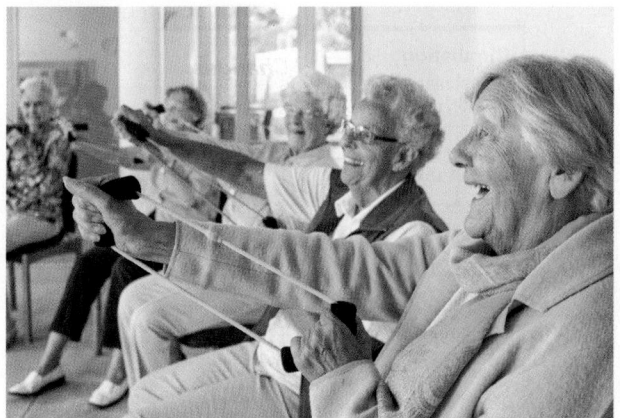

FIG. 7.7 Strength training is an example of a health promotion activity for older persons. Source: iStock.com/Horsche.

TABLE 7.10 PATIENT & CAREGIVER TEACHING GUIDE

Older Persons

Challenges for Older Persons	Specific Strategies
• Time needed to learn is increased. • New learning must relate to the patient's actual experience. • Anxiety and distractions decrease learning. • Lack of willingness to take risks and cautiousness decrease motivation to learn. • Sensory–perceptual deficits and cognitive decline necessitate modifications in teaching techniques.	• Present material at a slower rate. • Use visual aids when possible. • Use peer educators when appropriate. • Encourage participation of a spouse or family member. • Use simple phrases or sentences, and provide for repetition. • Support the belief that change in behaviour is worth the effort. • Emphasize that a person is never too old to learn new things.

Source: Adapted from Rankin, S. H., Stallings, K. D., & London, F. (2004). *Patient education: Principles and practice* (5th ed.). Lippincott.

Health promotion and prevention can be included in nursing interventions at any location where nurses and older persons interact and at any level of care delivery. The nurse can use health promotion activities to strengthen the person's self-care, increase personal responsibility for their own health, and increase independent functioning that will enhance well-being (Figure 7.7).

Teaching Older Persons. Throughout the continuum of care, nurses are involved in instructing and teaching older persons specific self-care practices to enhance health and well-being and modify disease processes (Table 7.10). Individual teaching is discussed in Chapter 4.

Assistive Devices. Using appropriate assistive devices such as dentures, glasses, hearing aids, walkers, wheelchairs, adaptive utensils, elevated toilet seats, and skin protective devices can greatly improve independency for older persons. The need for and use of these devices are assessed by the interprofessional team, and findings are included in the care plan. Electronic monitoring equipment can be used to monitor heart rhythms, blood pressure, and potential falls, as well as to locate the wandering person in the home or LTC facility. Computerized assistive devices can be used to help people with speech difficulties following stroke, and pocket-sized devices can serve as memory aids.

Falls and Safety. Environmental safety is crucial in the maintenance of health and independence by older persons. With normal sensory age changes, slowed reaction time, decreased thermal and pain sensitivity, changes in gait and balance, and medication effects, older persons are prone to accidents. Most accidents, such as trips and falls, occur in or around the home. Older persons' impaired thermoregulating system can cause hypothermia and heat prostration (hyperthermia).

Falls are the leading cause of injury among older persons in Canada (PHAC, 2015). Between 20% to 30% of older persons experience one or more falls each year, and falls cause 85% of injury-related hospitalizations of older persons (PHAC, 2016b). Falls can cause chronic pain and reduced mobility, as well as a loss of independence. Half of all falls happen in the home, and one-third of falls lead to admittance into an LTC facility (PHAC, 2015).

The nurse and the care team can provide valuable counsel regarding environmental safety and changes. Measures such as enhanced lighting, coloured step strips, tub and toilet grab bars, and stairway handrails can be effective in "safety-proofing" the living quarters of an older person. The nurse can also advocate for home fire and security alarms. Uncluttered floor space, railings, increased lighting and night lights, and clearly marked stair edges are some of the easiest and most practical adaptations (PHAC, 2016b).

In addition, an older person who moves to a different location needs a thorough orientation to the environment. The nurse should repeatedly reassure the person that they are safe and attempt to answer all questions. The environment should foster orientation to time and place by displaying large-print clocks, avoiding complex or visually confusing wall designs, clearly designating doors, and using simple bed and nurse-call systems. Beds should be close to the floor to prevent serious injury from falls. Lighting should be adequate while avoiding glare. Environments that provide consistent caregivers and an established daily routine assist older persons.

Medication Use. Medication use in older persons necessitates thorough and regular assessment and care planning. Two-thirds of Canadians 65 years and over are prescribed at least five medications (Sirois et al., 2017). The frequency of adverse medication reactions increases as the number of prescribed medications increases.

Age-related changes alter the pharmacodynamics and pharmacokinetics of pharmacological agents. Medication–medication, medication–food, and medication–disease interactions all influence the absorption, distribution, metabolism, and excretion of medications. Figure 7.8 illustrates the effects of aging on medication metabolism. The most dramatic changes with aging are related to medication metabolism and clearance. Overall, by age 80, there is a 50% decline in the renal clearance of medications. Hepatic blood flow decreases markedly with aging, and the enzymes largely responsible for medication metabolism are decreased as well. Thus, the medication half-life increases for older persons (Jett, 2016).

In addition to changes in the metabolism of medications, older persons may have medication-related difficulties resulting from malnutrition and dehydration, cognitive decline, altered sensory perceptions, limited hand mobility, and the high cost of many prescriptions. Common reasons for medication errors made by older persons are listed in Table 7.11. **Polypharmacy** (the use of multiple medications by a person who has more than one health condition), overdosage, or forgetting to take medications are recognized as major risk factors for adverse effects in older persons (Sirois et al., 2017).

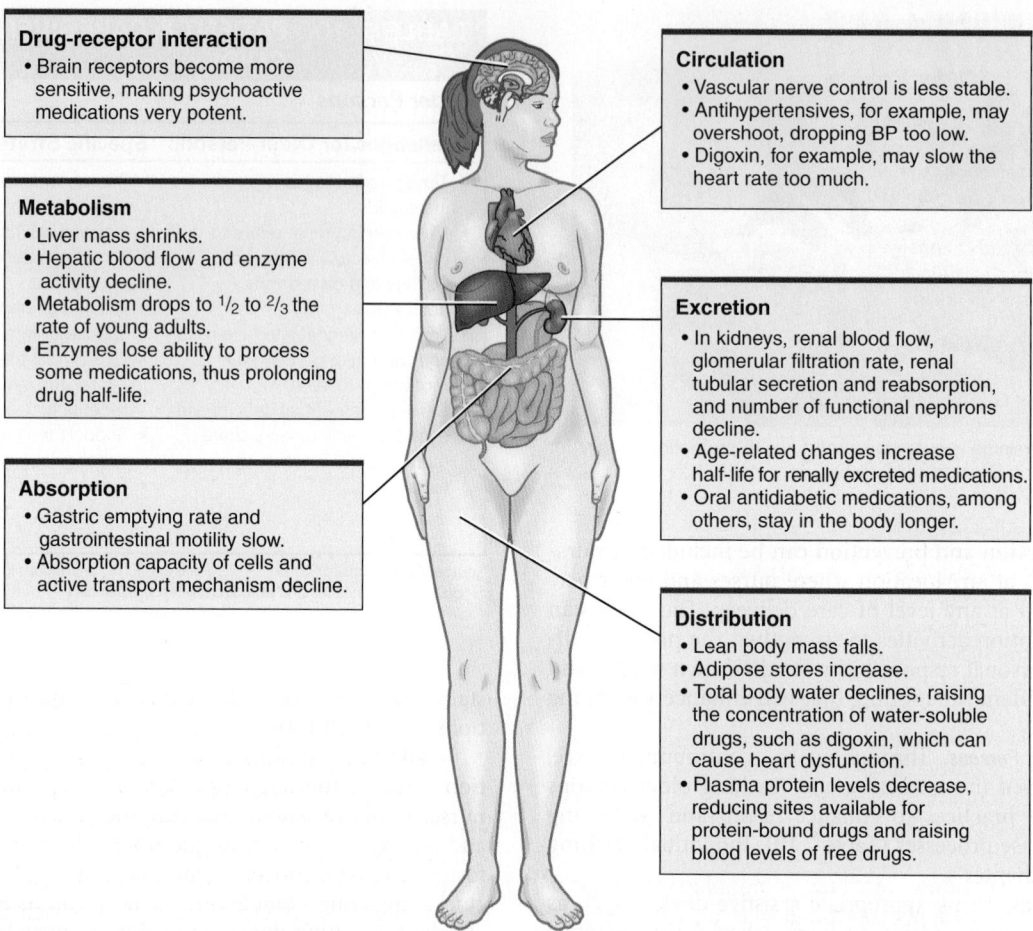

Drug-receptor interaction
• Brain receptors become more sensitive, making psychoactive medications very potent.

Metabolism
• Liver mass shrinks.
• Hepatic blood flow and enzyme activity decline.
• Metabolism drops to $1/2$ to $2/3$ the rate of young adults.
• Enzymes lose ability to process some medications, thus prolonging drug half-life.

Absorption
• Gastric emptying rate and gastrointestinal motility slow.
• Absorption capacity of cells and active transport mechanism decline.

Circulation
• Vascular nerve control is less stable.
• Antihypertensives, for example, may overshoot, dropping BP too low.
• Digoxin, for example, may slow the heart rate too much.

Excretion
• In kidneys, renal blood flow, glomerular filtration rate, renal tubular secretion and reabsorption, and number of functional nephrons decline.
• Age-related changes increase half-life for renally excreted medications.
• Oral antidiabetic medications, among others, stay in the body longer.

Distribution
• Lean body mass falls.
• Adipose stores increase.
• Total body water declines, raising the concentration of water-soluble drugs, such as digoxin, which can cause heart dysfunction.
• Plasma protein levels decrease, reducing sites available for protein-bound drugs and raising blood levels of free drugs.

FIG. 7.8 The effects of aging on medication metabolism. *BP,* blood pressure. Source: Redrawn from Benzon, J. (1991). Approaching drug regimens with a therapeutic dose of suspicion. *Geriatric Nursing, 12*(4), p. 1813.

TABLE 7.11	COMMON CAUSES OF MEDICA-TION ERRORS BY OLDER PERSONS

• Poor eyesight
• Forgetting to take medications
• Use of nonprescription (over-the-counter) medications
• Use of medications prescribed for someone else
• Failure to understand instructions or the importance of medication treatment
• Refusal to take medication because of undesirable adverse effects

To accurately assess medication use and knowledge, many nurses ask patients to bring all medications to the health care appointment (including over-the-counter medications, prescriptions, herbal remedies, and nutritional preparations). The nurse and pharmacist can then accurately assess all medications that the person is taking, including medications that may be overlooked or thought unimportant. Some medications can be tapered or discontinued, especially those medications that may be causing harm or are no longer providing benefit. Specific guidelines for de-prescribing of proton pump inhibitors, benzodiazepines, and antipsychotics in older persons have been developed and can be found at the website of the Ontario Pharmacy Evidence Network (see the Resources at the end of this chapter).

In addition, many older persons have adopted complementary and alternative medicine (CAM) as a means for additional treatment for a condition (Canizares et al., 2017) (see Chapter 12).

One study by Groden and colleagues (2017) indicated that 23% of older persons used CAM. Therapies include acupuncture, herbal supplements, massage, chiropractic care, homeopathy, energy healing, and biofeedback (Esmail, 2017). Additional nursing interventions to assist older persons in following a safe medication routine are listed in Table 7.12.

Several medications are considered inappropriate or dangerous for older persons and are identified on the Beers list (American Geriatrics Society, 2019). This list has been recommended as a "best practice" by several Canadian regulating and professional organizations (see Resources at the end of this chapter for the Web link.)

Depression. Many older persons have experienced multiple, simultaneous stressors, such as loss of loved ones, coping with chronic illness, financial stress, and social isolation. For some older persons, the accumulation of these stressors can result in a mental health issue. The prevalence of mental illness is the same among older as younger people (3%–10%), except for dementia and delirium, which is more prevalent among older persons (RNAO, 2016). Unfortunately, depression is an underrecognized condition for many older persons.

Depression can exacerbate medical conditions by affecting nutritional intake, mobility, or medication regimens. An older person who is at high risk for or exhibits depressive symptoms should be encouraged to seek treatment. Nursing assessment consists of observation of appearance and behaviour and examination of cognitive function, functional abilities, anxiety,

TABLE 7.12 MEDICATION THERAPY

Medication Use by Older Persons

1. Conduct a medication reconciliation review with the physician and the pharmacist.
2. Emphasize medications that are essential.
3. Discuss use of medication that is not essential or counterproductive.
4. Screen use of medications—including over-the-counter medications, herbaceuticals, eyedrops and eardrops, antihistamines, and cough syrups—by using a standard assessment tool.
5. Assess medication interactions.
6. Assess patient's alcohol use.
7. Encourage the use of written or other medication-reminder systems.
8. Monitor medication dosage; normally, the dosage should be less than that for a younger person.
9. Encourage the patient to use one pharmacy.
10. Work with health care providers and pharmacists to establish routine medication profiles on all older patients.
11. Advocate (with pharmaceutical companies) for low-income prescription support services and generic substitutions.
12. Assess financial status and discuss which medications are essential to buy for older patients.

TABLE 7.13 EVALUATING NURSING CARE FOR OLDER PERSONS

Evaluation questions may include the following:
1. Has there been an identifiable change in ADLs, IADLs, cognitive status, or disease signs and symptoms?
2. Does the patient consider their health and well-being state to be improved?
3. Does the patient think the treatment is helpful?
4. Do the patient and the caregiver think the care is worth the time and cost?
5. Can the nurse document positive changes that support interventions?

ADLs, activities of daily living; *IADLs*, instrumental activities of daily living.

adjustment reactions, depression, substance abuse, and suicidal risk. A comprehensive guide to assessment and treatment of depression in older persons is available at the website of the Hartford Institute for Geriatric Nursing (see the Resources at the end of the chapter).

Specific interventions include nonpharmacological approaches and, if needed, pharmacological treatment. Depression is often reversible with prompt and appropriate treatment. Older persons experience improvement with appropriate medication, psychotherapy, or psychosocial interventions (RNAO, 2016), or a combination of these.

Sleep. Adequacy of sleep is often a concern for older persons because of altered sleep patterns. Older persons experience a marked decrease in deep sleep and are easily aroused. In individuals older than 75, the percentage of sleep time spent in the rapid eye movement (REM) stage decreases. In addition, older persons have difficulty maintaining prolonged sleep. Although the demand for sleep decreases with age, older persons may be disturbed by insomnia and complain that they spend more time in bed but still feel tired. Many older persons prefer to spread sleep periods throughout 24 hours with short naps that, combined, provide adequate rest. Other factors that contribute to sleep difficulties include medical conditions, such as sleep apnea and restless legs syndrome, as well as effects of medications (e.g., furosemide [Lasix]). In many cases, a later bedtime promotes a better night's sleep and a feeling of being refreshed on awakening.

Managing Personal Expressions. People living with dementia or a cognitive impairment are often confused and anxious during specific care situations (e.g., while showering) or when left alone. These individuals might respond with certain expressions or behaviours, such as wandering, crying, or pushing away the care provider. In addressing these personal expressions and behaviours, it is important for the nurse to understand that the person with cognitive impairment is responding to a "perceived threat." Ignoring this person's response to the threat and continuing the care task will only cause the person to become more anxious or frightened and result in an exacerbation of the expression or behaviour. In caring for people, nurses need to understand *why* they respond in such a way, and the nurse should intervene with competent and compassionate person-centred care.

The nurse should check for changes in vital signs and urinary and bowel patterns that could account for certain behavioural issues. It is important to use a relational approach with a focus on empathy and nurturing and to keep care assignments consistent. When a person is scared or agitated by the environment, either the person or the stimulus should be changed and responded to. Most personal expressions can be redirected with activities such as holding a towel during the bath or exercising or walking with staff when starting to wander. Reality orientation, if appropriate, can be used to recall the person to time, place, and person. A family member can be asked to stay with the person until they feel more secure and become calmer. The person should be assessed frequently, and all interventions should be documented. An interprofessional approach is important to identify the best redirective strategies.

Use of Restraints. Restraints are physical, environmental, or chemical measures used to limit the activity or control the behaviour of a person or a portion of their body (RNAO, 2012). Devices such as seat belts, "geri-chairs," or side rails that cannot be removed by the person are considered physical restraints, and it has been proved that these actually increase a person's risks for falls and injury (RNAO, 2012). Chemical restraints are any form of psychoactive medication used, not to treat illness, but to intentionally inhibit a person's particular behaviour or movement. Several researchers have indicated that antipsychotic medications have limited effectiveness and pose significant risks for older persons with cognitive impairment (RNAO, 2012). Despite abundant research findings, chemical and physical restraints continue to be used in the care of people with personal expressions or responsive behaviours. The use of evidence-informed nursing interventions significantly reduces the use of any physical and chemical (pharmacological therapy) restraints (RNAO, 2011, 2012).

EVALUATION

The evaluation phase of the nursing process is similar for all care situations and populations. Evaluation is ongoing throughout the nursing process. The results of the evaluation direct the nurse to continue the care plan or revise it as indicated.

When evaluating nursing care for an older person, the nurse should focus on improving or maintaining the person's functional and cognitive status and their quality of life and well-being, rather than on a cure. Useful questions to consider when evaluating the care plan for an older person are included in Table 7.13.

CASE STUDY

Older Persons

Patient Profile

L. X., 79 years old (pronouns she/her), was admitted through the emergency department with shortness of breath. L. X. was diagnosed with community-acquired pneumonia. Her history also indicates chronic obstructive pulmonary disease (COPD), hypertension, diabetes, mild cognitive impairment, depression, macular degeneration, and significant hearing impairment.

Subjective Data

- Had a stroke 5 years ago and has right-sided weakness
- Has a two-pack/week history of tobacco use but quit smoking after the stroke
- Has not seen primary care physician in 1 year
- In past year, has had an unplanned weight loss of 9 kg
- Spends time either in bed or in a recliner watching television

Psychosocial Data

- Came to the Canada 15 years ago from China
- Speaks Mandarin with limited English proficiency
- Lives with unemployed adult son, who provides assistance with ADLs and IADLs
- Has three daughters who live within a 2-hour drive
- Has limited financial resources
- Her son has not visited his mother in the hospital, but her daughters raise concerns about their mother's care and safety at home, given their brother's history of gambling addiction.
- When L. X.'s daughters ask their brother about how he is caring for his mother, he says, "I'm doing the best I can. She refuses help. She refuses to go to the doctor. What do you want me to do? She's old. She does what she wants."

Objective Data

- Matted hair, poor oral hygiene, overgrown toenails
- Two stage III sacral pressure injury
- Unstageable right heel pressure injury
- Multiple small bruises on her forearms and shins
- 5-cm × 10-cm bruise in the middle of her back

Discussion Questions

1. Compare L. X.'s experience as an older woman to known gender differences for older persons.
2. Define *ageism*, and explain how it may be manifested in this situation.
3. What risk factors does L. X. have for development of frailty? Which of these factors are modifiable?
4. **Priority Decision:** On the basis of an assessment of L. X., what are the priority nursing diagnoses?
5. **Priority Decision:** What are the priority nursing interventions for L. X.?
6. Explain ethnogeriatric considerations that affect L. X. and how they will influence nursing care.
7. Based on knowledge of caregiver support and care alternatives for older persons, what nursing care support is required for the son and daughters, and what setting or settings might be appropriate for L. X. on hospital discharge?
8. What risk factors does L. X. have for becoming a victim of elder mistreatment?

ℯvolve

Answers are available at http://evolve.elsevier.com/Canada/Lewis/medsurg.

REVIEW QUESTIONS

The number of the question corresponds to the same-numbered objective at the beginning of the chapter.

1. What is one characteristic of ageism?
   a. Denial of negative stereotypes regarding aging
   b. Positive attitudes toward older persons that are based on age
   c. Negative attitudes toward older persons that are based on age
   d. Negative attitudes toward older persons that are based on physical disability

2. When older persons become ill, which of the following are they more likely to do than younger people?
   a. Complain about the symptoms of their health conditions.
   b. Refuse to carry out lifestyle changes to promote recovery.
   c. Seek medical attention because of limitations on their lifestyle.
   d. Alter their daily living activities to accommodate new symptoms.

3. Which of the following nursing actions would be helpful to a chronically ill older person? *(Select all that apply.)*
   a. Discussing future lifestyle changes
   b. Informing the person that the condition is stable
   c. Engaging with the person as a competent manager of the disease
   d. Encouraging the person to "fight" the disease as long as possible

4. What should the nurse know about an older person's caregivers?
   a. They may need the nurse to assist them in reducing caregiver strain.
   b. They are usually trained health care workers who do not live with the older person.

   c. They are generally strong and healthy, but need teaching to carry out care activities.
   d. They are often reluctant to share the burden of caregiving with other family members.

5. For an older person requiring constant assistance and living with an employed daughter, what is an appropriate care choice?
   a. Adult day care
   b. Nursing home care
   c. A retirement centre
   d. An assisted-living home

6. What is a characteristic of a living will?
   a. Legally binding
   b. Encourages the use of artificial means to prolong life
   c. Allows a person to direct their health care in the event of terminal illness
   d. Designates who can act for the person when the person is unable to do so for themselves

7. In promotion of health for older persons, what is the primary focus of nursing interventions?
   a. Disease management
   b. Controlling symptoms of illness
   c. Teaching positive health behaviours
   d. Teaching the role of nutrition in enhancing longevity

1. c; 2. d; 3. a, c; 4. a; 5. a; 6. c; 7. c

ℯvolve

For even more review questions, visit http://evolve.elsevier.com/Canada/Lewis/medsurg.

REFERENCES

Allen, L., Hatala, A., Ijaz, S., et al. (2020). Indigenous-led health care partnerships in Canada. *CMAJ, 192*(9), E208–E216. https://doi.org/10.1503/cmaj.190728

Alzheimer Society of Canada. (2021a). *How to get tested for dementia.* https://alzheimer.ca/en/about-dementia/do-i-have-dementia/how-get-tested-dementia

Alzheimer Society of Canada. (2021b). *The 10 warning signs of dementia.* https://alzheimer.ca/en/about-dementia/do-i-have-dementia/10-warning-signs-dementia

Alzheimer Society of Canada. (2021c). *What is dementia?* https://alzheimer.ca/en/about-dementia/what-dementia

American Geriatrics Society (AGS). (2019). *For older people, medications are common; Updated AGS Beers Criteria aims to make sure they're appropriate too.* https://www.americangeriatrics.org/media-center/news/older-people-medications-are-common-updated-ags-beers-criterion-aims-make-sure

Armstrong, H., Daly, T. J., & Choiniere, J. A. (2017). Policies and practices: The case of RAI-MDS in Canadian long-term care homes. *Journal of Canadian Studies, 50*(2), 348–367. https://doi.org/10.3138/jcs.50.2.348

Bandari, R., Khankeh, H., Shahboulaghi, F., et al. (2019). Defining loneliness in older adults: protocol for a systematic review. *Systematic Reviews, 8*(26), 1–6. https://doi.org/10.1186/s13643-018-0935-y

Canadian Institute for Health Information (CIHI). (2020a). *Dementia impacts Canadians.* https://www.cihi.ca/en/dementia-in-canada/how-dementia-impacts-canadians

Canadian Institute for Health Information (CIHI). (2020b). *Dementia in long-term Care.* https://www.cihi.ca/en/dementia-in-canada/dementia-care-across-the-health-system/dementia-in-long-term-care

Canadian Institute for Health Information (CIHI). (2020c). *New analysis paints international picture of COVID-19's long-term care impacts.* https://www.cihi.ca/en/new-analysis-paints-international-picture-of-covid-19s-long-term-care-impacts

Canadian Mortgage and Housing Corporation. (2016). *Seniors' housing report—Canada highlights.* https://publications.gc.ca/site/eng/353488/publication.html

Canizares, M., Hogg-Johnson, S., Gignac, M. A. M., et al. (2017). Changes in the use practitioner-based complementary and alternative medicine over time in Canada: Cohort and period effects. *PLoS One, 12*(5). https://doi.org/10.1371/journal.pone.0177307

Cao, F., Salem, H., Nagpal, C., et al. (2017). Prolonged delirium misdiagnosed as a mood disorder. *Dementia & Neuropsychologia, 11*(2), 206–208. https://doi.org/10.1590/1980-57642016dn11-020014

Centers for Disease Control and Prevention (CDC). (2021). *Basics of COVID-19.* https://www.cdc.gov/coronavirus/2019-ncov/your-health/about-covid-19/basics-covid-19.html?CDC_AA_refVal=https%3A%2F%2Fwww.cdc.gov%2Fcoronavirus%2F2019-ncov%2Fcdcresponse%2Fabout-COVID-19.html

Chiaranai, C., Chularee, S., & Srithongluang, S. (2018). Older adults living with chronic illness. *Geriatric Nursing, 39*, 513–520. https://doi.org/10.1016/j.gerinurse.2018.02.004

Conroy, S. (2017). *Section 5: Police-reported family violence against seniors. Statistics Canada.* https://www150.statcan.gc.ca/n1/pub/85-002-x/2017001/article/14698/05-eng.htm

Esmail, N. (2017). *Complementary and Alternative Medicine: Use and Public Attitudes 1997, 2006, and 2016.* Fraser Institute. https://www.fraserinstitute.org/sites/default/files/complementary-and-alternative-medicine-2017.pdf

Friedman, L., Avila, S., Liu, E., et al. (2017). Using clinical signs of neglect to identify elder neglect cases. *Journal of Elder Abuse & Neglect, 29*(4), 270–287. https://doi.org/10.1080/08946566.2017.1352551

Gilmour, H. (2018). *Formal home care use in Canada. Statistics Canada.* https://www150.statcan.gc.ca/n1/pub/82-003-x/2018009/article/00001-eng.htm

Golive, A., May, H., Bair, T., et al. (2018). The impact of gender on atrial fibrillation incidence and progression to dementia. *The American Journal of Cardiology, 122*(9), 1489–1495. https://doi.org/10.1016/j.amjcard.2018.07.031

Government of Canada. (2021a). *Indigenous peoples and communities.* https://www.rcaanc-cirnac.gc.ca/eng/1100100013785/1529102490303

Government of Canada. (2021b). *Social isolation of seniors: A focus on Indigenous seniors in Canada.* https://www.canada.ca/en/employment-social-development/corporate/seniors/forum/social-isolation-indigenous.html

Gray, L., Beattie, E., Boscart, V., et al. (2018). Development and testing of the interRAI Acute Care: A standardized assessment administered by nurses for patients admitted to acute care. *Health Services Insight, 11*, 1–7. https://doi.org/10.1177/1178632918818836

Groden, S. R., Woodward, A. T., Chatters, L. M., et al. (2017). Use of complementary and alternative medicine among older adults: Differences between baby boomers and pre-boomers. *The American Journal of Geriatric Psychiatry, 25*(12), 1393–1401. https://doi.org/10.1016/j.jagp.2017.08.001

Han, K. M., Ko, Y. H., Yoon, H. K., et al. (2018). Relationship of depression, chronic disease, self-rated health, and gender with health care utilization among community-living elderly. *Journal of Affective Disorders, 241*, 402–410. https://doi.org/10.1016/j.jad.2018.08.044

Hancock, T., Kirk, M., MacDonald, M., et al. (2017). The weakening of public health: a threat to population health and health care system sustainability. *Canadian Journal of Public Health, 108*(1), e1–e6. https://doi.org/10.17269/CJPH.108.6143

Harman, D. (1956). Aging: A theory based on free radical and radiation chemistry. *Journal of Gerontology, 11*(3), 298–300. https://doi.org/10.1093/geronj/11.3.298. (Seminal).

Hategan, A., Bourgeois, J. A., Cheng, T., et al. (2018). *Caregiver Burnout. Geriatric Psychiatry Study Guide: Mastering the Competencies.* Cham: Springer.

Health Canada. (2016). *Canada's health care system (Medicare).* https://www.canada.ca/en/health-canada/services/canada-health-care-system.html

Health Quality Ontario (HQO). (2021). *Home care performance in Ontario.* https://www.hqontario.ca/System-Performance/Home-Care-Performance

Heckman, G., & Jónsson, P. V. (2017). *Comprehensive geriatric assessment: the specific assessment technology of InterRAI.* (127). Oxford Textbook of Geriatric Medicine.

Humphries, J., & Canham, S. L. (2019). Conceptualizing the shelter and housing needs and solutions of homeless older adults. *Housing Studies*, 1–23. https://doi.org/10.1080/02673037.2019.1687854

Ivankina, L., Kemasheva, E., & Zeremskaya, Y. (2016). The model of measuring the subjective well-being of a senior age group. *SHS Web of Conferences* (Vol. 28). EDP Sciences:01045.

Jett, K. (2016). Geropharmacology. In P. Ebersole, P. Hess, & A. Luggen (Eds.), *Toward healthy aging: Human needs and nursing response* (9th ed.) (pp. 101–114). Mosby.

Kelly, K., Booth, L., & Miller, P. (2020). *Eliciting consent from patients with dementia in general X-ray departments: Law, ethics and interpretation of context. United Kingdom Imaging and Oncology*

Congress 2020: Pathways and Communication, 1-3 June 2020, ACC, Liverpool. (Unpublished).

Kleinman, A., Eisenberg, L., & Good, B. (1978). Culture, illness, and care: Clinical lessons from anthropologic and cross-cultural research. *Annals of Internal Medicine, 88*(2), 251–258 (Seminal).

Lalani, N. (2017). Positive Aging, Work Retirement, and End of Life: Role of Gerotranscendence Theory and Nursing Implications. *i-Manager's Journal on Nursing, 7*(3), 1. https://doi.org/10.26634/jnur.7.3.13790

Lord, S., Negron-Poblete, P., & Després, M. (2017). Vieillir chez soi dans la diversité des formes urbaines et rurales du Québec, Canada. *Retraite et société* (1), 43–66.

Lumen Learning (2020). *Introduction to sociology: Theoretical perspectives on aging.* https://courses.lumenlearning.com/sociology/chapter/theoretical-perspectives-on-aging/

Menec, V. H., Hutton, L., Newall, N., et al. (2015). How 'age-friendly' are rural communities and what community characteristics are related to age-friendliness? The case of rural Manitoba, Canada. *Ageing & Society, 35*(1), 203–223. https://doi.org/10.1017/S0144686X13000627

Morgan, S., Hunt, J., Rioux, J., et al. (2016). Frequency and cost of potentially inappropriate prescribing for older adults: a cross-sectional study. *CMAJ Open, 4*(2), E346–E351. https://doi.org/10.9778/cmajo.20150131

Pathath, A. W. (2017). Theories of aging. *The International Journal of Indian Psychology, 4*(3), 15–22. https://doi.org/10.25215/0403.142

Public Health Agency of Canada (PHAC). (2015). *Seniors' falls in Canada—Infographic.* https://www.canada.ca/en/public-health/services/health-promotion/aging-seniors/publications/publications-general-public/seniors-falls-canada-second-report/seniors-falls-canada-infographic.html

Public Health Agency of Canada (PHAC). (2016a). *Aging and seniors.* https://www.canada.ca/en/public-health/services/health-promotion/aging-seniors.html

Public Health Agency of Canada (PHAC). (2016b). *You CAN prevent falls!* https://www.canada.ca/en/public-health/services/health-promotion/aging-seniors/publications/publications-general-public/you-prevent-falls.html

Registered Nurses' Association of Ontario (RNAO). (2007). *Embracing Cultural Diversity in Health Care: Developing Cultural Competence.* https://rnao.ca/sites/rnao-ca/files/Embracing_Cultural_Diversity_in_Health_Care_-_Developing_Cultural_Competence.pdf. (Seminal).

Registered Nurses' Association of Ontario (RNAO). (2011). *End-of-life Care During the Last Days and Hours.* https://rnao.ca/bpg/guidelines/endoflife-care-during-last-days-and-hours. (Seminal).

Registered Nurses' Association of Ontario (RNAO). (2012). *Nursing Best Practice Guidelines. Promoting safety: Alternative approaches to the use of restraints.* http://rnao.ca/bpg/guidelines/promoting-safety-alternative-approaches-use-restraints. (Seminal).

Registered Nurses' Association of Ontario. (2016). *Delirium, dementia, and depression in older adults: assessment and care* (2nd ed.). https://rnao.ca/bpg/guidelines/assessment-and-care-older-adults-delirium-dementia-and-depression.

Registered Nurses' Association of Ontario (RNAO). (2017). *Preventing falls and reducing injury from falls* (4th ed.). http://rnao.ca/bpg/guidelines/ prevention-falls-and-fall-injuries.

Rockwood, K., & Theou, O. (2020). Using the clinical frailty scale in allocating scarce health care resources. *Canadian Geriatrics Journal, 23*(3), 254–259. https://doi.org/10.5770/cgi.23.463

Salma, J., & Salami, B. (2020). "We are like any other people, but we don't cry much because nobody listens": The need to strengthen aging policies and service provision for minorities in Canada. *The Gerontologist, 60*(2), 279–290. https://doi.org/10.1093/geront/gnz184

Sirois, C., Ouellet, N., & Reeve, E. (2017). Community-dwelling older adults' attitudes towards deprescribing in Canada. *Research in Social and Administrative Pharmacy, 13*(4), 864–870. https://doi.org/10.1016/j.sapharm.2016.08.006

Statistics Canada. (2018). *Immigration and ethnocultural diversity in Canada.* https://www12.statcan.gc.ca/nhs-enm/2011/as-sa/99-010-x/99-010-x2011001-eng.cfm

Statistics Canada. (2019a). *Aboriginal peoples in Canada: Key results from the 2016 Census.* https://www150.statcan.gc.ca/n1/daily-quotidien/171025/dq171025a-eng.htm

Statistics Canada. (2019b). *Analysis: Population by age and sex.* https://www150.statcan.gc.ca/n1/pub/91-215-x/2018002/sec2-eng.htm

Statistics Canada. (2019c). *Canada's population estimates: Age and sex. July 1, 2019.* https://www150.statcan.gc.ca/n1/daily-quotidien/190930/dq190930a-eng.htm

Statistics Canada. (2019d). *Changes in life expectancy by selected causes of death. 2017.* https://www150.statcan.gc.ca/n1/daily-quotidien/190530/dq190530d-eng.htm

Statistics Canada. (2020a). *2016 Census aboriginal community portrait—Canada.* https://www12.statcan.gc.ca/census-recensement/2016/dp-pd/abpopprof/infogrph/infgrph.cfm?LANG=E&DGUID=2016A000011124&PR=01

Statistics Canada. (2020b). *Caregivers in Canada. 2018.* https://www150.statcan.gc.ca/n1/daily-quotidien/200108/dq200108a-eng.htm

Statistics Canada. (2021). *Low income statistics by age, sex and economic family type.* https://www150.statcan.gc.ca/t1/tbl1/en/tv.action?pid=1110013501

Touhy, T., Jett, K., Boscart, V., et al. (2018). *Ebersole and Hess' gerontological nursing and healthy aging in canada* (2nd ed.). Mosby Elsevier.

Van Wicklin, S. (2020). Ageism in nursing. *Plastic Surgical Nursing, 40*(1), 20–24. https://doi.org/10.1097/PSN.0000000000000290

Verlaan, S., Ligthart-Melis, G., Wijers, S., et al. (2017). High prevalence of physical frailty among community-dwelling malnourished older adults – a systematic review and meta-analysis. *Journal of the American Medical Directors Association, 18*(5), 374–382. https://doi.org/10.1016/j.jamda.2016.12.074

Vogelsang, E. (2016). Older adult social participation and its relationship with health: Rural-urban differences. *Health & place, 42*, 111–119. https://doi.org/10.1016/j.healthplace.2016.09.010

Wang, L., Guruge, S., & Montana, G. (2019). Older immigrants' access to primary health care in Canada: A scoping review. *Canadian Journal on Aging/La Revue canadienne du vieillissement, 38*(2), 193–209. https://doi.org/10.1017/S0714980818000648

Wilinska, M., & Mosberg Iversen, S. (2017). Media and ageism. *Innovation in Aging, 1*(Suppl. 1), 71. https://doi.org/10.1093/geroni/igx004.293

Wilson, D., Jackson, T., Sapey, E., et al. (2017). Frailty and sarcopenia: The potential tole of an aged immune system. *Ageing Research Reviews, 36*, 1–10. https://doi.org/10.1016/j.arr.2017.01.006

World Health Organization (WHO). (2020). *Coronavirus disease (COVID-19): Similarities and differences with influenza.* https://www.who.int/emergencies/diseases/novel-coronavirus-2019/question-and-answers-hub/q-a-detail/q-a-similarities-and-differences-covid-19-and-influenza

Yochim, B. (2017). Biological theories of aging. In B. Yochim, & E. Woodhead (Eds.), *Psychology of aging: A biophysical perspective* (pp. 31–47). Springer.

Yon, Y., Mikton, C., Gassoumis, Z., et al. (2017). The prevalence of self-reported elder abuse among older women in community settings: A systematic review and meta-analysis. *Trauma, Violence, & Abuse, 20*(2). https://doi.org/10.1177/1524838017697308

RESOURCES

Canadian Accreditation Council
https://www.canadianaccreditation.ca/

Canadian Association on Gerontology (CAG)
https://www.cagacg.ca

Canadian Centre for Elder Law
http://www.bcli.org/ccel

Canadian Coalition for Seniors' Mental Health
https://www.ccsmh.ca

Canadian Gerontological Nursing Association
https://www.cgna.net

Canadian Network for the Prevention of Elder Abuse
https://cnpea.ca/en/

Canadian Patient Safety Institute
https://www.patientsafetyinstitute.ca/en/Pages/default.aspx

Canadian Women's Health Network
https://www.cwhn.ca/

Government of Canada: *Seniors' Guide to Staying Cyber Safe During COVID-19*
https://www.getcybersafe.gc.ca/en/resources/seniors-guide-staying-cyber-safe-during-covid-19

Health Canada: Healthy Living: *Seniors*
https://www.hc-sc.gc.ca/hl-vs/seniors-aines/index_e.html

Health Canada: *Just for You—Seniors*
https://www.hc-sc.gc.ca/hl-vs/jfy-spv/seniors-aines_e.html

Health Canada: *Medication Matters: How You Can Help Seniors Use Medication Safely*
http://publications.gc.ca/site/eng/9.695567/publication.html

Health Canada: *Reaching Out: A Guide to Communicating With Aboriginal Seniors*
https://publications.gc.ca/site/eng/9.646842/publication.html

National Initiative for the Care of the Elderly
https://www.nicenet.ca

Oaknet Canadian Law for Older Adults—Legal Resources by Province and Territory
https://www.oaknet.ca/node/112

Ontario Pharmacy Evidence Network
https://www.open-pharmacy-research.ca

Public Health Agency of Canada: *Aging & Seniors*
http://www.phac-aspc.gc.ca/seniors-aines/index_pages/aboutis_e.htm

Public Health Agency of Canada: *The Safe Living Guide—A Guide to Home Safety for Seniors*
http://www.phac-aspc.gc.ca/seniors-aines/publications/public/injury-blessure/safelive-securite/index-eng.php

Registered Nurses' Association of Ontario: *Preventing and Addressing Abuse and Neglect of Older Adults: Person-Centred, Collaborative, System-Wide Approaches*
https://rnao.ca/bpg/guidelines/abuse-and-neglect-older-adults

University of Victoria: *Cultural Safety Learning Modules*
https://web2.uvcs.uvic.ca/courses/csafety/mod1/index.htm
https://web2.uvcs.uvic.ca/courses/csafety/mod2/index.htm
https://web2.uvcs.uvic.ca/courses/csafety/mod3/index.htm

Winnipeg Regional Health Authority: Guide to Health and Social Services for Aboriginal People in Manitoba
https://wrha.mb.ca/wp-content/site-documents/indigenous-health/services/files/AHSGuide.pdf

Hartford Institute for Geriatric Nursing
https://hign.org

evolve

For additional Internet resources, see the website for this book at http://evolve.elsevier.com/Canada/Lewis/medsurg.

8

Stress and Stress Management

Ann Mary Celestini
Originating US chapter by Margaret R. Rateau

evolve WEBSITE

http://evolve.elsevier.com/Canada/Lewis/medsurg

- Review Questions (Online Only)
- Key Points
- Answer Guidelines for Case Study
- Conceptual Care Map Creator
- Audio Glossary
- Content Updates

LEARNING OBJECTIVES

1. Define the terms *stressor, stress, demands, coping, adaptation*, and *allostasis*.
2. Describe the three stages of Hans Selye's general adaptation syndrome.
3. Explain the role of coping in managing stress.
4. Distinguish between the role of the nervous and endocrine systems in the stress process.
5. Discuss the effects of stress on the immune system.
6. Consider the effects of stress on health and illness.
7. Examine coping strategies that can be used by persons experiencing stress.
8. Review variables that may influence an individual's response to stress.
9. Identify the nursing assessment and management of a patient experiencing stress.

KEY TERMS

alarm reaction
allostasis
coping
coping resources
distress
emotion-focused coping

eustress
guided imagery
problem-focused coping
psychoneuroimmunology
resilience
sense of coherence

stage of exhaustion
stage of resistance
stress
stressor

Stress is a reality of daily life that can have a helpful or harmful effect on the mind, body, and spirit of an individual. Stress, particularly if acute or chronic, is linked to numerous psychological and physiological disorders. Anticipating potentially stressful situations, recognizing stress, and implementing appropriate preventative measures to minimize its effect are essential aspects in health promotion and disease prevention. Given the high levels of stress among patients and their caregivers, nurses play a pivotal role in helping them manage stressful events. The aim of this chapter is to focus on the relationship of stress to an individual's physical, emotional, and spiritual health, further considering positive practical coping strategies that can be used during these stressful periods.

DEFINITION OF STRESS

Stress has been defined as a stimulus, process, and response. However, researchers typically define stress as an individualized reaction or response to a stimulus, when real or perceived demands exceed their available coping resources (Arnold, 2020). In the late 1930s, Hans Selye, a researcher at McGill University in Montreal,

described stress as a nonspecific response of the body to any demand, regardless whether it is caused by a pleasant or unpleasant source. An inability to cope with these pressures may further threaten an individuals' mental, emotional, or spiritual well-being.

Sources of Stress

Stress can arise from multiple internal and external sources (Table 8.1). A stressor is defined as any demand, situation, internal stimulus, or circumstance which endangers a person's personal well-being or integrity. Stressors may originate from numerous potential sources, including daily hassles or conditions of daily living that are frustrating or irritating (e.g., traffic, misplacing items), major life events (e.g., death, life-threatening disease, job loss), social isolation, work-related stress, financial concerns, and relationship conflicts (Takahashi et al., 2019). The frequency and intensity of daily hassles have a stronger relationship with somatic illness than do major life events.

Levels of Stress

Regardless of the nature of these stressors, an individual may adapt either negatively or positively to a situation (Lazarus &

Folkman, 1984). While stress is viewed primarily as a negative response to a stressor, it can also serve as a positive protective and adaptative reaction that motivates people to overcome challenges. **Eustress**, a term coined by Selye, is used to describe this mild but motivating and protective form of stress. **Distress** is a negative response to stress that occurs when the demands made exceed a person's normal coping ability.

Behavioural responses to stressors can change over time, as previous stressful experiences and individual contextual factors can produce *adaptation* in stress response systems. Adaptive responses to a stressor are based on the duration (acute or chronic) and intensity (mild, moderate, or severe) of that stimulus. For example, an individual dealing with the chronic stress of caring for a loved one may also be exposed to a multitude of acute episodic stressors (e.g. car accident, influenza).

Theoretical Conceptualizations of Stress

Early ground-breaking theorists such as Walter Cannon (1932) described stress as involving a typical physiological response to a stressor. When people feel well, they are in a state of *homeostasis*. Stress disturbs this delicate physiological balance by

setting the sympathetic nervous system into action to mobilize coping resources within the body. Cannon postulated that people attempt to adapt to a stress through either a fight or flight response. A *fight response* involves a person taking action against the perceived threat. *Flight* becomes an option if an individual believes that they cannot overcome the threat.

Hans Selye (1974) elaborated on this preliminary work, through his classic formulation of the *general adaption syndrome* (GAS), which included three successive stages of physiological responses: alarm or reaction, resistance or adaptation, and exhaustion. This predictable, uniform pattern in the physiological response to various stressors occurs regardless of the type of stressor encountered. Once a stressor stimulates the central nervous system, multiple responses occur because of activation of the hypothalamic–pituitary–adrenal axis and the autonomic nervous system (Figure 8.1). The **alarm reaction** stimulates the central nervous system and mobilizes bodily defences in a fight-or-flight response to the acute stress. When the stressor is of sufficient intensity to threaten the homeostasis of the individual, it leads to a series of physiological changes that promote adaptation. This temporarily decreases the individual's resistance and may even result in disease or death if the stress is prolonged and severe. If the stressor is not resolved during this initial phase, a second adaptive phase, or **stage of resistance** occurs as the body attempts to adapt to the stressor. Overt signs diminish as the immune system attempts to help the body adapt to the stressor demands. Physiological reserves are mobilized to increase the resistance to stress and so that adaptation may occur. Although few overt physical signs and symptoms occur in the resistance stage in comparison to the alarm stage, the person is expending energy to adapt. **Allostasis** is the process of achieving homeostasis in the presence of a challenge (Sterling, 1988). The amount of resistance to the stressor varies among individuals, depending on the level of physical functioning, coping abilities, and total number and intensity of stressors experienced. If homeostasis is not achieved, and if these allostatic responses do not terminate, adaptation does not occur, and the person may move to the final phase, of exhaustion. The **stage of exhaustion** occurs when all the energy for adaptation has been expended. The individual in

TABLE 8.1	**TYPES OF STRESSORS**	
Physiological	**Psychological**	**Spiritual**
• Acute and chronic illness • Trauma or injury • Pain • Insomnia	• Loss of job or job security • Loss of a significant person or pet • Significant change in residence, relationship, work • Personal finances • Work relationships • High-stress work environment • Caregiving (frail older person, children)	• Loss of purpose • Loss of hope • Questioning of values and meaning

Source: Arnold, E. C. (2020). Communication in stressful situations. In E. C. Arnold & K. Underman Boggs (Eds.), *Interpersonal relationships: Professional communication skills for nurses* (8th ed., pp. 310–332). Elsevier Canada.

PATHOPHYSIOLOGY MAP

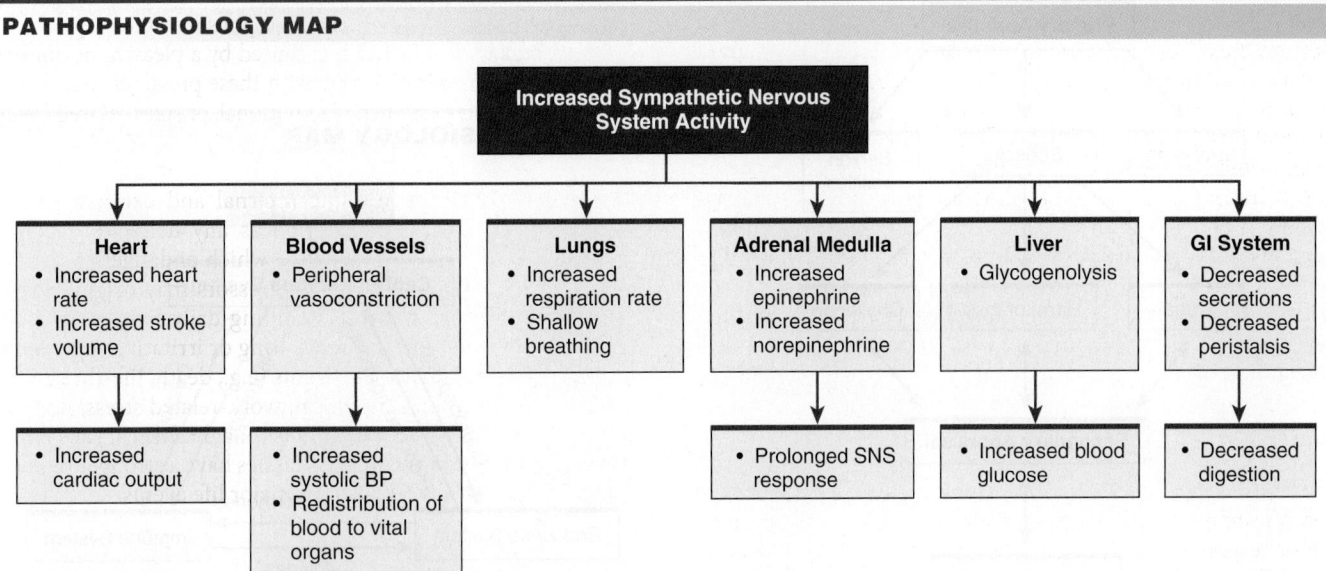

FIG. 8.1 "Fight-or-flight" reaction. Alarm reaction responses resulting from increased sympathetic nervous system activity. *BP,* blood pressure; *GI,* gastrointestinal; *SNS,* sympathetic nervous system.

the stage of exhaustion usually becomes ill and may die if assistance from outside sources is not available. This stage can often be reversed by external sources of adaptive energy.

The *transaction* or *interaction* theory of stress and coping, by Lazarus and Folkman (1984), is another influential stress theory that is widely used in health care. The primary focus is on person–environment interactions. The role of cognitive appraisal (Figure 8.2) in assessing stressful situations and selecting coping options is essential to this theoretical framework. Cognitive appraisal is conceptualized as a judgement or evaluative process whereby the individual recognizes the degree of stress and its effect on well-being. As a result of this appraisal, the individual uses coping resources that respond to the demand placed on them. Cognitive appraisal is divided into two stages: primary and secondary. *Primary appraisal* involves determining whether the stress poses a threat (e.g., you have an exam the next day—identify this is a threat). *Secondary appraisal* involves the individual's evaluation of coping strategies or resources to manage any perceived threat (e.g., access readings and lecture notes, review content—ability to cope with stressor).

Responses to Stress

The perception of and response to the stressor vary greatly among individuals. A multitude of factors may potentially influence this response, including physiological, socioenvironmental, and individual circumstances (Table 8.2).

PHYSIOLOGICAL INFLUENCE

The complex process by which an event is perceived as a stressor and the body responds is not fully understood. A person's response to a stressor ultimately determines the effect it will have on the body. The body responds physiologically to both actual (physiological, or objective) and perceived (emotional–psychological, or subjective) stressors. The nervous, endocrine, and immune systems are three key interrelated physiological responses to stress which may further affect the cardiovascular, respiratory, gastrointestinal, renal, and reproductive systems (Figure 8.3).

Nervous System

Cerebral Cortex. In the cerebral cortex, the emotional–psychological event (stressor) is evaluated with reference to past experiences and future consequences, and a course of action is planned. These functions are involved in the perception of a stressor (Takahashi et al., 2019).

Limbic System. The limbic system lies in the inner midportion of the brain near the base of the skull. The limbic system is an important mediator of emotions and behaviour. When the limbic system is stimulated, emotions, feelings, and behaviours that ensure survival and self-preservation may occur.

Reticular Formation. The reticular formation is located between the lower end of the brainstem and the thalamus. It contains the reticular activating system, which is crucial for the state of wakefulness. When stimulated, the reticular activating system sends impulses to the limbic system and the cerebral

TABLE 8.2   INFLUENCE ON STRESS RESPONSE

Factors influencing the response to stressors:
- Aspects of a structure that influence stress response
- Intensity
- Scope
- Duration
- Number and nature of other stressors
- Past exposure to serious stressors
- Predictability

Characteristics of the individual that influence stress response:
- Age
- Gender
- Perception of personal control or an escape ability
- Availability of social supports
- Feeling of competence
- Cognitive appraisal

Source: Park, T. (2019). Stress and adaptation. In P. A. Potter, A. G. Perry, J. C. Ross-Kerr, M. J. Wood, B. Astle, & W. Duggleby (Eds.), *Canadian fundamentals of nursing* (6th Canadian ed., pp. 508–525). Elsevier Canada.

PATHOPHYSIOLOGY MAP

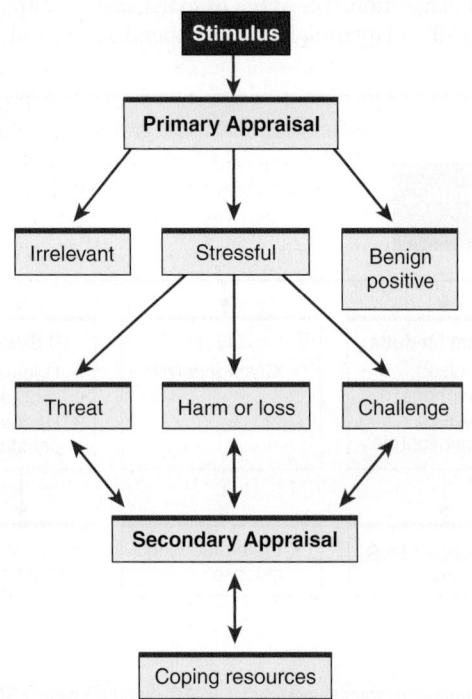

FIG. 8.2 Cognitive appraisal process.

PATHOPHYSIOLOGY MAP

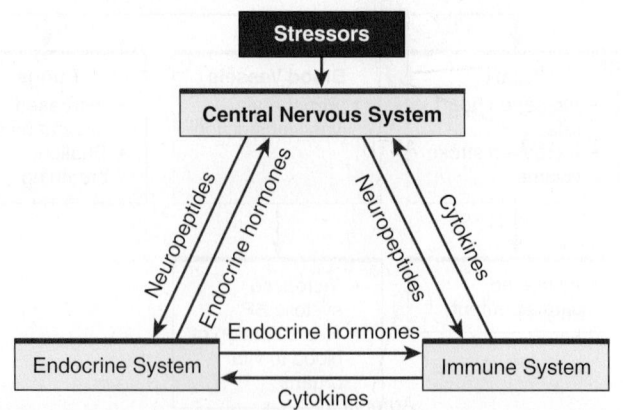

FIG. 8.3 Neurochemical links among the nervous, endocrine, and immune systems. The communication among these three systems is bidirectional.

cortex, which produce arousal and emotional responses to the stressor. Stress usually increases the degree of wakefulness and can lead to sleep disturbances.

Hypothalamus. The hypothalamus, which lies at the base of the brain just above the pituitary gland, has many functions that assist in adaptation to stress. It is the central connection between the nervous and endocrine systems in the stress response. Emotional–psychological (perceived) stressors activate the limbic system, which in turn stimulates the hypothalamus. The hypothalamus sends signals via nerve fibres to stimulate the sympathetic nervous system and releases hormones that regulate the secretion of adrenocorticotrophic hormone (ACTH) by the anterior pituitary gland (Figure 8.4). Physiological (actual) stressors may originate in the limbic system or in portions of the brain that receive sensory information, which in turn then stimulate the hypothalamus (see Chapter 50).

Endocrine System

Once the hypothalamus is activated in response to stress, the endocrine system becomes involved (Takahashi et al., 2019). The sympathetic nervous system stimulates the adrenal medulla to release epinephrine and norepinephrine (catecholamines), which initiates a protective reflex called the *fight-or-flight response* (see Figure 8.1). This, along with the actual response of the body to the catecholamines, is referred to as the *sympathoadrenal response*. Stress activates the hypothalamic–pituitary–adrenal axis (see Figure 8.4). In response to stress, the hypothalamus releases corticotropin-releasing hormone, which stimulates the anterior pituitary to release pro-opiomelanocortin (POMC). Both ACTH (a hormone) and β-endorphin (a neuropeptide) are derived from POMC. Endorphins have analgesic-like effects and blunt pain perception during stress situations involving

pain stimuli. ACTH, in turn, stimulates the adrenal cortex to synthesize and secrete corticosteroids (e.g., cortisol) and, to a lesser degree, aldosterone. The posterior pituitary increases production of antidiuretic hormone, which leads to water retention and a decrease in urine output (Figure 8.5).

Corticosteroids are essential for the stress response. Cortisol, a primary corticosteroid, produces a number of physiological effects that potentiate or blunt aspects of the stress response, such as increasing blood glucose levels, potentiating the action of catecholamines (epinephrine, norepinephrine) on blood vessels, and inhibiting the inflammatory response. The resulting increases in cardiac output, blood glucose levels, oxygen consumption, and metabolic rate enable the fight-or-flight response (see Figure 8.1). Dilation of blood vessels supplying skeletal muscle increases blood supply to the large muscles, which provides for quick movement, and increased cerebral blood flow heightens mental alertness. The increase in blood volume (which results from increases in extracellular fluid and shunting of blood away from the gastrointestinal system) helps maintain adequate circulation to vital organs in case of traumatic blood loss.

By mediating the inflammatory response, cortisol plays an important role in "turning off" aspects of the stress response, which, if uncontrolled, can become self-destructive. The persistent release of such mediators is believed to initiate organ dysfunction in conditions such as sepsis. Thus, corticosteroids act not only to support the adaptive response of the body to a stressor but also to suppress an overzealous and potentially self-destructive response.

Immune System

Psychoneuroimmunology is an interdisciplinary science in which investigators study the interactions among psychological, neurological, and immune responses that affect human health and behaviour (Slavich, 2019). It is now known that the brain is connected to the immune system by neuroanatomical and neuroendocrine pathways; thus, stressors have the potential to cause alterations in immune function (Figure 8.6). The network that links the brain and immune system is bidirectional, allowing for reciprocal communication among these systems. Therefore, emotions modify not only the immune response but also the products of immune cells which send signals back to the brain, altering its activity (see Figure 8.3). Much of the communication from the immune system to the brain is mediated by cytokines, which are crucial in the coordination of the immune response. For example, interleukin-1 (a cytokine made by monocytes) acts on the temperature-regulatory centre of the hypothalamus and initiates the febrile response to infectious pathogens. Nerve fibres extend from the nervous system and reach synapses on cells and tissues (e.g. spleen, lymph nodes) of the immune system. In turn, the cells of the immune system have receptors for many neuropeptides and hormones, which enable them to respond to nervous and neuroendocrine signals. As a result, the mediation of stress by the central nervous system leads to corresponding changes in immune cell activity.

SOCIOENVIRONMENTAL INFLUENCE

Stressful-event responses are not random but influenced by individual differences in socioenvironmental circumstances (Cohen et al., 2019). Low income and poor employment conditions are two primary sources of stress. Low socioeconomic status is evidenced by the likelihood of more frequent and severe

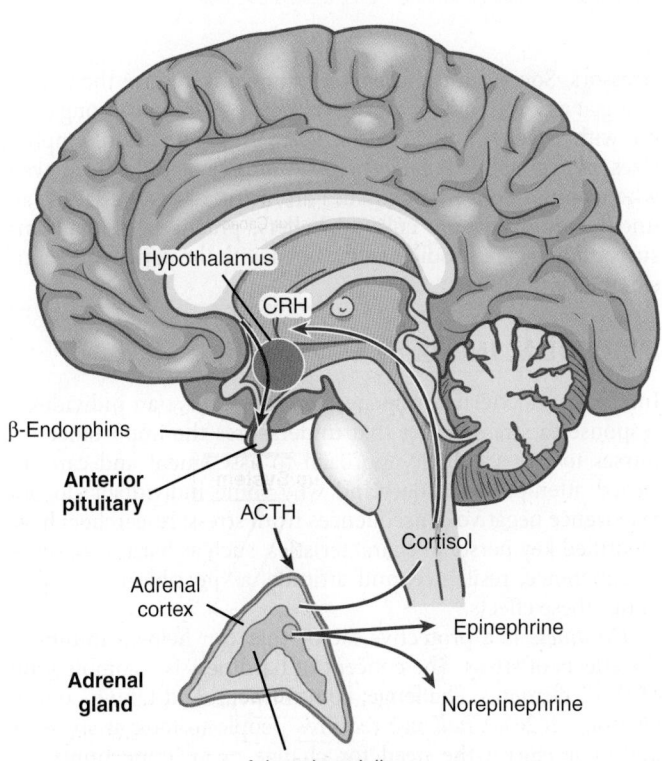

FIG. 8.4 Hypothalamic–pituitary–adrenal axis. *ACTH,* adrenocorticotrophic hormone; *CRH,* corticotropin-releasing hormone.

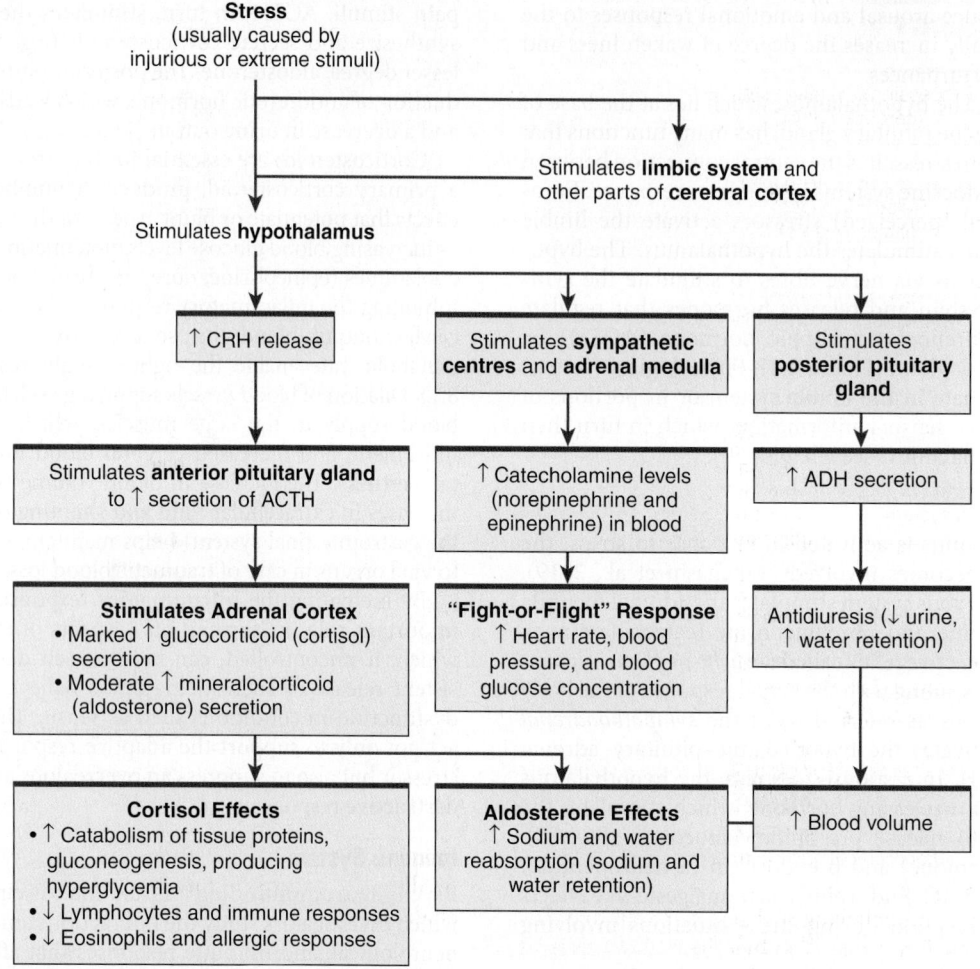

FIG. 8.5 Current concepts of the stress syndrome. *ACTH,* adrenocorticotrophic hormone; *ADH,* antidiuretic hormone; *CRH,* corticotropin-releasing hormone.

stressor exposure, such as overcrowding, violence, and a lack of essential resources. Unemployment is a huge stressor for many people. Canada and other industrialized nations have found an acute rise in mental health challenges as a result of the imposed social isolation practices required to minimize the spread of COVID-19 (Canadian Mental Health Association, 2020). However, problems can also exist among those who are employed and have poor working conditions. Shift work, bullying, and highly pressured work environments caring for patients are a few of many specific occupational problems that may result in stress for nurses and other health care providers. Insufficient staffing trends evident in health care settings further expose health care providers to additional negative health implications.

Individual health practices and coping skills such as sleep, exercise, and social support options can also affect an individual's response to stress. Chronically stressed people are often fatigued, thus ensuring adequate amounts of sleep is important. Regular physical exercise can also supplement well-being by protecting individuals from the harmful effects of stress on physical, mental, and spiritual health. Further to the beneficial effects on depression and anxiety, exercise can also generally reduce stress as long as it remains enjoyable. Although the benefits are clear, nurses must consider patient barriers to accessing resources and motivation.

Being surrounded by a strong social support system and receiving positive encouragement from friends and family has a significant positive effect on an individual's ability to cope with

stressors. Social support has been shown to reduce the risk of dying at any age and affects the chances of survival among people with serious illness (Micozzi, 2019). Each culture emphasizes, interprets, and manages health problems differently, even when similar concerns or issues are being discussed. Thus, an understanding of any cultural beliefs, practices, or concerns surrounding care should be discussed with the patient and considered by the nurse.

INDIVIDUAL INFLUENCE

Internal and external influences can also affect an individual's response to stress, a fact that underscores the importance for nurses to use a holistic approach to assessment and care. In varied attempts to understand why some individuals do not experience negative consequences from stress, researchers have identified key personal characteristics, such as hardiness, sense of coherence, resilience, and attitude, as possible factors that buffer these effects.

Hardiness is a protective factor that can help to minimize the effects of stress. The concept of hardiness is a combination of three elements: challenge, commitment, and taking control (Arnold, 2020). *Challenge* requires people to look at stressors and characterize the need for change as an opportunity for individual growth. *Commitment* is also necessary to develop a sense of purpose and strong involvement in directing one's life.

PATHOPHYSIOLOGY MAP

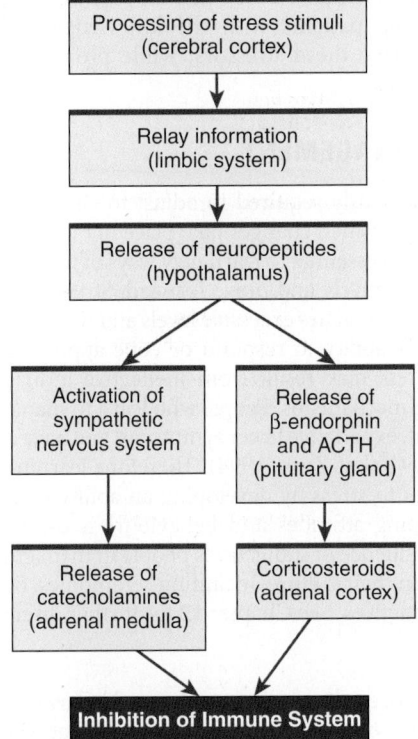

```
Processing of stress stimuli
(cerebral cortex)
          │
          ▼
Relay information
(limbic system)
          │
          ▼
Release of neuropeptides
(hypothalamus)
        ╱   ╲
       ▼     ▼
Activation of        Release of
sympathetic          β-endorphin
nervous system       and ACTH
                     (pituitary gland)
       │                   │
       ▼                   ▼
Release of           Corticosteroids
catecholamines       (adrenal cortex)
(adrenal medulla)
        ╲           ╱
         ▼         ▼
   Inhibition of Immune System
```

FIG. 8.6 The psychological and neuroendocrine response to stress alters immune function. *ACTH,* adrenocorticotrophic hormone.

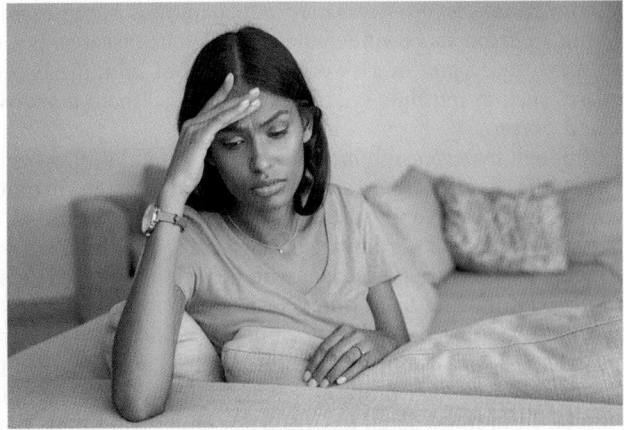

FIG. 8.7 Chronic stress can take a toll on the body, resulting in poor concentration and memory problems. Source: iStock.com/Ridofranz.

TABLE 8.3	**EXAMPLES OF CONDITIONS ASSOCIATED WITH MALADAPTATION TO STRESS**
• Angina	• Insomnia
• Asthma	• Irritable bowel syndrome
• Depression	• Low back pain
• Dyspepsia	• Menstrual irregularities
• Eating disorders	• Peptic ulcer disease
• Headaches	• Sexual dysfunction

Finally, *taking control* and believing that one can help to influence personal life outcomes may also help to reduce stressful challenges. Hardiness is discussed in more detail in Chapter 5.

Sense of coherence, first described by Antonovsky (1987), is a concept closely related to hardiness and represents an individual's ability or capacity to cope with everyday life stressors. Comprehensibility, manageability, and meaningfulness are three indicators of an individual's sense of coherence. An individual with a strong sense of coherence has an enduring tendency to see life as ordered, adaptable, and consequential.

Resilience, a concept linked to well-being and burnout, is another factor that is believed to moderate or buffer the negative effects of stress. Resilience is defined as the ability of an individual to be resourceful, flexible, and recover from exposure to stressful situations, returning to prior levels of functioning. Resilient individuals tend to employ more effective coping and problem-solving strategies, possess higher self-esteem, and be less likely to perceive an event as stressful or taxing. Resilience can be developed through practice, social support, and learning self-efficacy strategies.

Attitude can also influence the effect of stress on a person. People with positive attitudes view situations differently than those with negative attitudes. Individuals with a negative attributional style, such as maladaptive coping, have been found to generate more interpersonal conflicts leading to an increased likelihood of experiencing stressful events. A person's attitude also influences their management of stress. To some extent, positive emotional attitudes can prevent disease and extend life. Optimistic people tend to recover more quickly, whereas pessimistic people are likely to deny the problem, distance themselves from the stressful event, focus on stressful feelings, or allow the stressor to interfere with achieving a goal (Cohen et al., 2019).

EFFECTS OF STRESS ON HEALTH

Stress has the potential to influence the onset of a new illness and holds the possibility to hasten the progression or exacerbation of an existing health condition. Acute stress leads to physiological changes that are important to human adaptation and survival. However, if stress is excessive or prolonged, these physiological responses can be maladaptive and lead to harm and disease. When stress is chronic and unrelieved, the body's defences can no longer keep up with the demands. Over time, stress takes a toll (Figure 8.7) and plays a role in the development or progression of conditions related to maladaptation (Table 8.3).

Chronic and intense stress may have profound effects on brain structure and function, especially the hippocampus. The hippocampus plays an important role in long-term memory and other cognitive functions such as spatial learning (Yaribeygi et al., 2017). The adverse effects of stress on cognition are diverse. While mild stress is believed to facilitate an improvement in cognition, when the intensity surpasses an individual's coping threshold, cognitive disorders specific to memory and judgement may develop. Stress can affect cognitive function, causing deterioration in concentration, memory problems, sleep disturbances, and impairment in decision making.

A relationship between stress and impaired immune function has also been established in the literature. Modulation processes in the central nervous system and neuroendocrine system affect these functions. Severe stress may induce immunosuppression, making a person more vulnerable to infectious diseases, but it also may exacerbate the risk of progression of immune-based diseases such as multiple sclerosis, asthma, rheumatoid arthritis, and cancer.

Although hypertension in acute stress is thought to be transient, studies demonstrate a strong association between chronic, maladaptive stress, and sustained hypertension, which is a major risk factor for cardiovascular disease. In addition, stress can cause a wide variety of changes in behaviour. Such changes include withdrawing from others or becoming unusually talkative, eating disorders, substance misuse, or becoming angry and irritable. Stress can further induce fatigue, and the resulting exhaustion further limits a person's ability to cope. Fatigue is discussed in more detail in Chapter 5. Other conditions that may be either precipitated or aggravated by stress include obesity, migraine headaches, irritable bowel syndrome, and peptic ulcers.

Stress-Related Disorders

Overall, most people who experience stress do not get sick. However, if stress evolves into distress, it can result in stress-related illnesses such as acute stress disorder and post-traumatic stress disorder.

Acute stress disorder (ASD) is a short-term reaction caused by exposure to one or more highly traumatic events. Reactions of intense fear or helplessness typically occur within 1 month of the event and resolve within 4 weeks (Halter et al., 2019). Patients may display symptoms of avoidance or detachment, hyperarousal, or absence of emotional responses. Resulting sleep disturbances further contribute to these problems.

Post-traumatic stress disorder (PTSD) is an acute emotional response to a traumatic situation involving severe environmental stress. Symptoms are more persistent, enduring for at least a month. Problems often begin within 3 months of the trauma but a delay of several months or years is not uncommon. Symptoms are elicited from the persistent re-experiencing of the trauma through recurrent recollections of the event, or flashbacks. Persistent avoidance of stimuli associated with the trauma, numbing of general responsiveness, and persistent symptoms of increased arousal are seen through irritability or difficulty sleeping. Difficulty with relationships and trust are also common issues of concern.

Stressors can have a multilevel impact (Table 8.4), each interacting and potentially magnifying the other in a cumulative effect on an individual's well-being. Harmful stress is essentially the interaction between a negative physiological response, unhealthy lifestyle, negative environment, and self-defeating attitudes or behaviour. Nurses can support healthier practices by empowering patients with the knowledge and resources to better manage these stressors, while promoting improved health outcomes.

STRESS MANAGEMENT

We are continuously required to adjust to changing conditions throughout life. When changes take place in our environment or lives, it becomes essential to learn new ways of thinking or behaving to cope affectively and move forward. Stress only becomes a problem when it reaches excessive levels and the demands exceed an individual's ability to respond or cope appropriately. Symptoms of distress may result from ineffective individual coping and adapting mechanisms. People who learn to manage stress are more resilient, experience fewer symptoms, and have an improved quality of life (Kabat-Zinn, 1994). Therefore, learning to manage our responses to stress by developing an ability to exert control over our coping attitudes and behaviours is essential to well-being. The resilience of Indigenous people in managing stress has been rooted in their culture, including ceremonies, belief system, and health practices. See Chapter 12 for further discussion.

Coping

Coping comprises a person's cognitive and behavioural efforts to manage specific external or internal stressors that seem to exceed available resources (Lazarus & Folkman, 1984). Coping can be either positive or negative. *Positive* coping practices include healthy behaviours such as exercise, eating a proper diet, and the use of social support during times of need. *Negative* coping mechanisms may include substance misuse, overeating, isolation, and denial. The availability of coping resources affects an individual's ability to cope with these stressful situations. Coping resources include internal or external assets, characteristics, or actions that a person draws on to manage stress (Table 8.5).

Types of Coping

Numerous coping strategies exist to help individuals manage stressors. Coping strategies operate generally in two primary ways: as emotion-focused or problem-focused efforts (Table 8.6).

TABLE 8.4	FACTORS THAT INFLUENCE THE IMPACT OF STRESS

- Magnitude and demands of the stressor on self and others
- Multiple stressors occurring at the same time
- Suddenness or unpredictability of a stressful situation
- Accumulation of stressors and duration of the stress demand
- Level of social support available to the patient and family
- Previous trauma, which can activate unresolved fears
- Presence of an associated mental disorder
- Developmental level of the patient
- Normal attitude and outlook
- Knowledge, expectations, and realistic picture

Source: Arnold, E. C. (2020). Communication in stressful situations. In E. C. Arnold & K. Underman Boggs (Eds.), *Interpersonal relationships: Professional communication skills for nurses* (8th ed., pp. 310–332). Elsevier Canada.

TABLE 8.5	EXAMPLES OF COPING RESOURCES	
Internal Coping Resources		
Health, Energy, Morale	**Problem-Solving Skills**	
• Robust health	• Collection of information	
• High energy level	• Identification of problem	
• High morale	• Generation of alternatives	
• Positive beliefs	• Social skills	
• Self-efficacy	• Communication skills	
• Spirituality	• Compatibility	
External Coping Resources		
Social Networks	**Utilitarian Resources**	
• Family members	• Finances	
• Co-workers	• Self-help books	
• Social contacts	• Social agencies	
• Cultural network	• Sweat lodge, smudging, traditional medicine	

TABLE 8.6	EXAMPLES OF EMOTION- AND PROBLEM-FOCUSED COPING	
Stressor	**Emotion-Focused Coping**	**Problem-Focused Coping**
Receiving a diagnosis of terminal cancer	Seeking spiritual guidance from one's place of worship	Preparing advance health care directives
Exacerbation of chronic obstructive pulmonary disease (COPD)	Joining a support group	Quitting smoking
Renal failure that necessitates frequent travel for dialysis	Enjoying relaxing music and reading during travel time	Arranging for a volunteer driver
Extended hospital stay for stem cell transplantation	Communicating on Skype with family and friends regularly while in hospital	Arranging for child or family care before hospital admission

TABLE 8.7	BENSON'S RELAXATION TECHNIQUE

- Choose any word or brief phrase that reflects your belief system, such as *love, unity in faith and love, joy, Shalom, one God, peace.*
- Sit quietly in a comfortable position.
- Close your eyes.
- Deeply relax all your muscles, looking at your feet and progressing up to your face. Keep them relaxed.
- Breathe through your nose. Become aware of your breathing. As you exhale, say your word or phrase silently to yourself, for example, breathe IN . . . OUT (phrase), breathe IN . . . OUT (phrase), and so forth. Breathe easily and naturally.
- Continue for 10 to 20 minutes. You may open your eyes to check the time, but do not use an alarm. When you finish, sit quietly for several minutes, at first with your eyes closed and later with your eyes open. Do not stand for a few minutes.
- Do not worry about whether you are successful and achieving a deep level of relaxation. Maintain a passive attitude and permit relaxation to occur at its own pace. When distracting thoughts occur, try to ignore them by not dwelling on them, and return to repeating your word or phrase. With practice, the response should come with little effort. Practise a technique once or twice daily, but not within 2 hours after any meal, because the digestive process seems to interfere with the elicitation of the relaxation response.

Source: Halter, M., Pollard, C., & Jakubec, S. (Eds.), (2019). *Varcarolis' Canadian psychiatric mental health nursing: A clinical approach* (2nd Canadian ed.). Elsevier. From Benson, H. (1975). *The relaxation response.* William Morrow & Company, Inc.

Problem-focused coping strategies are purposeful, active, task-oriented approaches that are used to reduce stress. Examples include directly confronting a problem, setting priorities, collecting information, seeking advice or support, negotiating for a different solution, and taking action. Emotion-focused coping strategies involve managing the emotions that an individual feels when a stressful event occurs. These strategies are useful when a person needs respite from overthinking about a stressful situation. Two primary purposes of emotion-focused coping are to alleviate negative emotions and to create a sense of well-being. Examples of emotion-focused coping include meditation, yoga, and prayer.

Emotion- and problem-focused strategies can be employed alone or in combination to cope with the same stressor. Although it may not appear to be working toward a solution, emotion-focused coping is a valid and appropriate way to deal with various stressful situations. When a situation is unchangeable or uncontrollable, emotion-focused coping may dominate. If a problem can be changed or controlled, problem-focused coping may be more effective. Problem-focused coping strategies enable an individual to look at a challenge objectively, take action to address the problem, and thereby reduce the stress.

Several coping strategies have been shown to mitigate the effects of stress. Stressful situations are best handled when an individual practises adaptable coping, as certain strategies work more effectively than others, depending on the context of the concern. Thus, an overreliance on one type of coping strategy can be incapacitating. An awareness of personal and external resources provides patients with options to better cope with stressors when they arise.

Coping Strategies

Relaxation Response. In 1975, a book entitled *The Relaxation Response* by Dr. Herbert Benson drew attention to the physical and psychological benefits of relaxation. The *relaxation response* (Table 8.7) was described as a state of deep physiological and psychological rest (Micozzi, 2019). It is characterized by decreased central nervous system and sympathetic nervous system activity, which leads to decreases in heart and respiratory rates, blood pressure, muscle tension, and brain activity and an increase in skin temperature. The relaxation response can be elicited through a variety of relaxation strategies, including relaxation breathing, meditation, mindfulness, guided imagery, hypnosis, biofeedback, muscle relaxation, yoga, prayer, and music and laughter therapies (Table 8.8). Components of relaxation include a quiet space, comfortable position, receptive attitude, and focused attention. It is an effective intervention for stress-related disorders, including chronic pain, insomnia, and hypertension. Individuals who regularly engage in relaxation strategies are able to cope better with their stressors, increase their sense of control over these stressors, and reduce their tension.

Relaxation Breathing. *Relaxation breathing* forms the basis for most relaxation strategies, and an individual can perform it while sitting, standing, or lying down. It is especially useful in reducing stress during a stressful or anxiety-provoking experience. A technique for deep relaxation breathing is presented in Table 8.9. Respiratory retraining, typically through learned diaphragmatic or abdominal breathing practices, is required. Before a person practises relaxation breathing, it is important to assess their normal breathing pattern. To do this, the person begins by placing one hand gently on the abdomen below the waistline and the other hand on the centre of the chest. Without changing the normal breathing pattern, the person takes several breaths. During inhalation, the person takes notice of which hand rises the most. When relaxation breathing is performed properly, the hand on the abdomen should rise more than the hand on the chest. Chest breathing, which involves the upper chest and shoulders, is associated with inefficient breathing, and often occurs during anxiety and distress. Relaxation breathing, which involves the diaphragm, is natural for newborns and sleeping adults and is associated with efficient breathing.

TABLE 8.8 EXAMPLES OF STRESS MANAGEMENT TECHNIQUES

Technique	Description
Thought stopping	A self-directed behavioural approach is used to gain control of self-defeating thoughts. When negative thoughts occur, the individual stops the thought process and focuses on conscious relaxation.
Cognitive reframing	A technique used to modify perceptions of negative, inaccurate, or self-defeating thoughts with the goal of changing behaviours and increasing well-being. Individuals change their perceptions of stress by reassessing stressors and replacing irrational beliefs with more positive self-statements. This practice is associated with greater positive affect and higher self-esteem (Halter, 2019).
Journaling	Maintaining an informal diary or journal of daily events and activities can reveal surprising information about sources of daily stress. Activities that trigger negative feelings are noted and the impact of these events is described. This may enable the individual to increase self-awareness and coping.
Colouring	Colouring is a nostalgic therapeutic activity that can used as a relaxation technique to reduce stress and anxiety at any age. The colouring of mandalas, a circular design with concentric shapes, embraces creativity and has been shown to decrease negative thoughts (Felt et al., 2017).

TABLE 8.9 DEEP BREATHING EXERCISE

1. Find a comfortable position.
2. Relax your shoulders and chest; let your body relax.
3. Shift to relaxed, abdominal breathing. Take a deep breath through your mouth, expanding the abdomen. Hold it for 3 seconds and then exhale slowly through the nose; exhale completely, telling yourself to relax.
4. With every breath, turn attention to the muscular sensations that accompany expansion of the abdomen.
5. As you concentrate on your breathing, you will start to feel focused.
6. Repeat this exercise for 2 to 5 minutes.

Source: Halter, M. (2019). Understanding responses to stress. In M. Halter, C. Pollard, & S. Jakubec (Eds.), *Varcarolis' Canadian psychiatric mental health nursing: A clinical approach* (2nd Canadian ed., pp. 65–78). Elsevier.

TABLE 8.10 BASIC GUIDE TO MEDITATION

- Choose a quiet, calm environment with as few distractions as possible.
- Get in a comfortable position, preferably a sitting position.
- To shift the mind from externally oriented thought, use a constant stimulus, such as a sound, word, phrase, or object. The eyes are closed and a repetitive sound or word is used.
- Pay attention to the rhythm of your breathing.
- When distracting thoughts occur, discard the thoughts and redirect your attention to the repetition of the word or continue gazing at the object. Distracting thoughts will occur and do not mean you are performing the techniques incorrectly. Do not worry about how you are doing. Redirect your focus to the constant stimulus and assume the passive attitude.
- Cease meditation and open your eyes should unbearable feelings arise.

Source: Arnold, E. C. (2020). Communication in stressful situations. In E. C. Arnold & K. Underman Boggs (Eds.), *Interpersonal relationships: Professional communication skills for nurses* (8th ed., pp. 310–332). Elsevier Canada.

depression (Hilton et al., 2017). Meditation also supports calming mental activity, decreasing endless thoughts, and lessening anxiety. Similar to learning other skills, successfully developing meditative abilities requires practice and a determination to attain an effective relaxation response. While the concepts are simple, many people are not initially successful. Therefore, individuals typically start learning the technique with only 5 to 10 minutes of meditation at a time and increase the time as the practice becomes more comfortable.

Mindfulness. *Mindfulness*, an ancient Buddhist practice, involves individuals living consciously and in harmony within the world, while fostering an appreciation for the richness of each moment in life (Kabat-Zinn, 1994). Our current waking state of consciousness is plagued with thoughts virtually all the time, limiting awareness of the present moment. Over time, this can create a buildup of complications that may cause subsequent future health problems for individuals. Mindfulness is a simple but powerful practice that nurtures a greater awareness, clarity, and acceptance of each moment by specifically redirecting attention nonjudgementally toward what is currently occurring in our lives. Being in touch with each moment does not involve changing it in any way, only a conscious attempt to refocus attention on what is occurring at that time. An integral part of practice involves accepting and welcoming stress, pain, anger, frustration, and other negative feelings when present. Acknowledgement of these unpleasant thoughts moves the person toward transforming that reality. While these fundamental principles seem basic to understand, they are often not easy for novices to practise. In the 1970s, Jon Kabat-Zinn founded the Stress Reduction Clinic at the University of Massachusetts Medical Center. At this clinic, an 8-week program offering training in mindfulness and stress reduction continues to be successfully used to treat patients with chronic pain and stress-related disorders.

Guided Imagery. Guided imagery involves the use of directed thoughts or suggestions that guide mental images to positively influence an individual's health and well-being (Table 8.11 and Figure 8.8). It involves the use of mental focus and incorporates all the senses to create physiological and emotional changes (Micozzi, 2019). This simple relaxation technique requires no equipment other than an active imagination. However, a therapist, instructor, or audio or video recordings can be used to guide people into a state of deep relaxation and journey of imagination. Guided imagery can be used to promote relaxation, which in turn may reduce blood pressure, anxiety,

Meditation. *Meditation* is a universal term for self-directed practices that involve calming the mind and relaxing the body. The ultimate goal requires training the mind through the practised regulation of attention and/or emotion to affect bodily functions. Historically, the primary purpose of meditation has been rooted in spiritual or religious practices. It has only been since the 1970s that meditation has been explored as a means to reduce stress (Kabat-Zinn, 1994). Meditation is a discipline that involves training the mind to develop a greater calm that further brings insight into a person's experience. Meditative practice is a simple method that is easy to use in any setting. Many methods of meditation include focusing on a single thought or word for a specific time period; some forms require focus on a physical experience such as breathing, a visual object, or a specific sound or mantra (Table 8.10). However, all forms of meditation have a common objective of stilling the restlessness of the mind so that the focus can be directed inwardly.

There are many techniques that can be used to meditate, some with a mindfulness or awareness focus and others with more spiritual underpinnings. Evidence supports the effectiveness of meditation as an adjunct therapy for PTSD and

TABLE 8.11	SCRIPT FOR GUIDED IMAGERY

- Imagine releasing all the tension in your body and letting it go.
- Now, with every breath you take, feel your body drifting down deeper and deeper into relaxation, floating down, deeper and deeper.
- Imagine a peaceful scene. You are sitting beside a clear, blue mountain stream. You are barefoot and you feel the sun-warmed rock under your feet. You hear the sound of the stream tumbling over the rocks. The sound is hypnotic, and you relax more and more. You see the tall pine trees on the opposite shore bending in the gentle breeze. Breathe the clean, scented air, each breath moving you deeper and deeper into relaxation. The sun warms your face.
- You are very comfortable. There is nothing to disturb you. Experience a feeling of well-being.
- You can return to this peaceful scene by taking time to relax. The positive feelings can grow stronger and stronger each time you choose to relax. You can return to your activities now, feeling relaxed and refreshed.

Source: Halter, M. (2019). Understanding responses to stress. In M. Halter, C. Pollard, & S. Jakubec (Eds.), *Varcarolis' Canadian psychiatric mental health nursing: A clinical approach* (2nd Canadian ed., pp. 65–78). Elsevier.

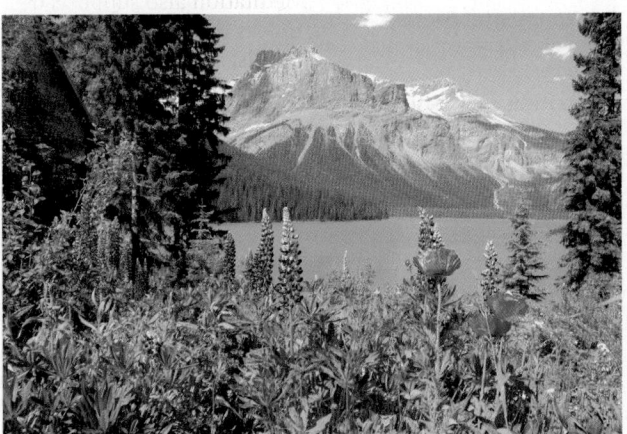

FIG. 8.8 Guided imagery. Creating a "special place" should involve the physical senses, such as a place where rustling leaves can be heard, flowers are smelled, wind is felt, and a colourful landscape is seen. Source: iStock.com/jeu.

depression, and other stress-related problems, such as preparing for a presentation. Sounds, smells, and feelings can be generated from one's creation of safe, relaxing, and peaceful images or places.

Guided imagery can be used in many clinical settings for stress reduction and pain relief. Benefits of imagery may include a reduction in anxiety, decrease in muscle tension, improvement in comfort during medical procedures, enhancement of immune function, decrease in recovery time after surgery, and improvement in sleep. Health care providers may use imagery in their own lives or may use guided imagery with their patients. Imagery is used to create a safe and special place for mental retreat, or it can be used to specifically target a disease, problem, or stressor. For example, mental images can be created to alleviate symptoms (such as pain) or to treat disorders (such as depression). For example, the person may imagine troubles attached to helium balloons and visualize releasing them into the sky.

Hypnosis. *Hypnosis* is widely used by mental health care providers for the treatment of addictions, anxiety disorders, and phobias and for pain control (Micozzi, 2019). The patient enters a state of attentive and focused concentration while becoming relatively dissociated and unaware of their immediate surroundings. During this state of deep concentration, the individual is highly responsive to suggestion.

Hypnosis has three major components: absorption in the words or images presented by the hypnotherapist, dissociation from one's ordinary critical faculties, and responsiveness. A hypnotherapist either leads patients through relaxation, mental imagery, and suggestions or teaches patients to perform the techniques on themselves. Guided audio recordings can help patients practise this therapy at home. Images presented are specifically tailored to the patient's needs and may engage all or one of the senses. Physiologically, hypnosis resembles other forms of deep relaxation, with its effectiveness rooted in the complex connections between the mind and body.

Hypnosis has been successfully used for treatment of skin disorders and can be enhanced with the use of biofeedback. Regular practice of self-hypnosis is also helpful to people with chronic diseases, by reducing bleeding among hemophiliac patients, stabilizing blood glucose levels in diabetic patients, and reducing the severity of asthma attacks. Training in self-hypnosis further enhances the patient's sense of control over stress.

Biofeedback. *Biofeedback* is a mind–body therapy involving the use of special instruments and methods to expand the body's natural internal feedback system to promote well-being (Micozzi, 2019). With initial guidance from a trained professional, patients can monitor, measure, and subsequently learn how to control bodily functions that are not normally within conscious awareness, such as muscle tension, skin temperature, sweat activity, heart rate, and breathing. Patients learn empirically through trial and error by adjusting their thinking and other involuntary bodily processes using feedback received through an attached monitoring device.

There are five common forms of biofeedback therapy: electromyographic or neurofeedback, thermal, electrodermal, finger pulse, and breathing biofeedback therapies. During a typical 30- to 60-minute session, a trained therapist, for example, a nurse, educates the patient on the use of the machine and different relaxation strategies, such as progressive muscle relaxation. Through the provision of feedback, patients learn to use these strategies to monitor and master the techniques, which subsequently change their responses. The number of sessions required to accomplish this is individually dependent.

When practised under the care of certified therapists, biofeedback is a safe technique. However, some patients may experience dizziness or anxiety during a session. Biofeedback is useful in treating Raynaud's disease, certain types of incontinence, headaches, anxiety, teeth clenching, asthma, and blood pressure and muscle disorders (Kennedy & Henrickson Parker, 2019). Additionally, conditions such as epilepsy, attention-deficit disorder, and attention-deficit/hyperactivity disorder have also responded positively to biofeedback therapy.

Muscle Relaxation. Muscle tension is a universal physiological reaction to stress. As the stress response sets in, muscles of the entire body tend to tighten. Muscle relaxation is therefore a common method of eliciting the relaxation response. *Progressive muscle relaxation* (PMR) involves the tensing and relaxing of muscles. This method is intended to help patients differentiate between when a muscle is tensed and when it is relaxed. This recognition enables an individual to reduce overall muscle tension when it occurs during times of stress. PMR is based on the principle that when the muscles are relaxed, the mind relaxes.

In a session of PMR, relaxation typically begins at the extremities and gradually moves across the whole body in a systematic fashion. A typical session lasts approximately 15 minutes and should be practised twice daily for the first few weeks until the individual masters the process. In addition to reducing overall tension, PMR can minimize physical conditions such as stomach aches and headaches and improve sleep (Anxiety Canada, 2019).

Yoga. Evidence supports the effective use of yoga in prevention and management of musculoskeletal and psychological issues, leading to improved quality of life, such as attaining better quality of sleep. A synergistic positive effect can be achieved when yoga is combined with other stress-reducing methods (Cocchiara et al., 2019).

Prayer. *Prayer* is increasingly being recognized as an effective, practical, and readily available coping strategy for managing a variety of stress-related issues, including personal, social, financial, and workplace problems or crises (Achour, 2019). Faith in a divine being or prayers to God can elicit physiological, psychological, and spiritual well-being among believers from a diversity of cultures. See Chapter 12 for additional information.

Music Therapy. Music has been used therapeutically across many cultures throughout history to successfully reduce the effects of stress (Fallon et al., 2020). *Music therapy* is a discipline in which a credentialed music therapist uses evidenced-informed music practices within therapeutic relationships to support the development, health, and well-being of a patient's cognitive, communicative, emotional, musical, physical, social, and spiritual needs (Canadian Association of Music Therapists, 2020). Individuals from various ages, abilities, and musical backgrounds can benefit from the use of this approach. Acquired brain injury, developmental or physical disabilities, emotional trauma, mental health disorders, pain control, cancer, and speech and language impairments are a few of the numerous health conditions that my lead people to seek music therapy. It has also been used in palliative care.

Active and receptive intervention techniques are used by the therapist when working in either private or group sessions. Singing, instrument playing, rhythmic or beat-based sounds, and listening to music are a few of many therapeutic applications available to patients. Music with low-pitch tones, without words, and that has approximately 60 to 80 beats per minute is considered to be soothing. Mozart's compositions are the most popular form of music used for relaxation. In contrast, fast-tempo music can stimulate and uplift a person. Music can be incorporated into clinical practice to help patients achieve relaxation and bring about healthy changes in their emotional, physical, or spiritual states. Listening to relaxing music may act as a diversion from a stressful situation. In addition, healing vibrations from music can return the mind and body to a better balance.

Laughter. The application of laughter-inducing therapies and their effectiveness have risen over the last decade. *Laughter* can be induced through a simulated means of forced self-induced or fake laughter, or in a spontaneous or genuine manner that is triggered by a stimulus such as a joke (van der Wal & Kok, 2019). Laughter produces overall beneficial effects at emotional, biological, psychological, and behavioural levels. While somewhat limited in number, studies support the effective use of laughter-inducing therapies as a valuable, low-cost, simple, complementary therapy that is useful in a variety of settings, with a wide range of patient groups and presenting conditions.

NURSING MANAGEMENT STRESS

NURSING ASSESSMENT

Patients face an array of potential stressors that can have health consequences. Any disruption to an individual's healthy functioning has the potential to create a sense of vulnerability and

---

TABLE 8.12	ASSESSMENT AND INTERVENTION TOOL

Assessment
- Perception of stressors
- Major stress area or health concern
- Present circumstances related to usual pattern
- Experience similar problem? How is it handled?
- Anticipation of future consequences
- Expectations of self
- Expectations of caregivers

Intrapersonal Factors
- Physical (mobility, body function)
- Psychosocial cultural attitudes, values, coping patterns
- Developmental age, factors related to present situation
- Spiritual belief system (hope and sustaining factors)

Interpersonal Factors
- Resources and relationships of family or significant other(s) as they relate to or influence personal factors

Environmental Factors
- Resource is relationships of community as they relate to or influence interpersonal factors

Prevention as Intervention

Primary
- Classify stressor
- Provide information to maintain or reinforce strengths
- Support positive coping mechanisms
- Educate patient and family

Secondary
- Mobilize resources
- Motivate, educate, and involve patient and provide healthcare goals
- Facilitate appropriate interventions, refer to external resources as needed
- Provide information on primary prevention or intervention as needed

Tertiary
- Attain and maintain wellness
- Educate or re-educate as needed
- Coordinate resources
- Provide information about primary and secondary interventions

Source: Arnold, E. C. (2020). Communication in stressful situations. In E. C. Arnold & K. Underman Boggs (Eds.), *Interpersonal relationships: Professional communication skills for nurses* (8th ed., pp. 310–332). Elsevier Canada.

---

result in stress-related issues. When assessing a patient's level of stress and coping resources, the nurse can use a variety of formats (Table 8.12) and tools to obtain needed information.

The Perceived Stress Scale (Roberti et al., 2006) is a popular tool frequently used to measure how stressful a person perceives their life to be at that time. Three major areas are important in assessment of stress: demands, human responses to stress, and coping.

DEMANDS. Stressors, or demands, on the patient may include major life changes, events or situations such as disfiguring or debilitating surgery, or daily hassles. Demands may be categorized as external (e.g., job-related situations, extended hospitalization) or internal (e.g., perception of goals or commitments, physical effects of disease or injury). It is important to keep in mind the many potential stressors that predispose people to stress and take a proactive approach to address them before patients present with stress-related symptoms. The number of simultaneous demands, the duration of these demands, primary appraisal or perception of the demands (see Figure 8.2), previous experience with similar demands, and the patient's family and loved ones' responses to the demands should be considered in the health assessment. Demands may also be categorized as representing harm or loss, threat, or challenge. Eliciting the demand's personal meaning to the patient provides useful insight for planning interventions and self-management strategies with patients.

Distinct groups such as immigrants and Indigenous people may have specific stressors such as language barriers, a limited understanding of Western medical practices, and a lack of available resources that may predispose them to stress. Indigenous people experience stress from intergenerational trauma, poor living conditions, racism, lack of funding and education, and historical factors stemming from residential schools, Indian hospitals, and the Sixties Scoop (Currie et al., 2019). These factors have and continue to negatively impact the health of this population. Therefore, these stressors should be considered when a nursing assessment is performed.

HUMAN RESPONSES TO STRESS. Physiological effects of demands that are appraised as stressful are mediated primarily by the sympathetic nervous system and the hypothalamic–pituitary–adrenal system. Examples of such effects are responses such as increased heart rate, increased blood pressure, loss of appetite, hyperventilation, sweating, and dilated pupils. Symptomatic experiences may include headache, musculoskeletal pain, gastrointestinal upset, skin disorders, insomnia, and chronic fatigue. In addition, the patient may exhibit some of the stress-related illnesses or diseases of adaptation (Table 8.3).

Behavioural manifestations may include accident proneness, anxiety, crying, frustration, and shouting. Behaviour in other aspects of life may include absenteeism or tardiness at work, avoidance of conversations, or procrastination. Observable cognitive responses include self-reports of excessive demand, inability to make decisions, impaired speech, and forgetfulness or inability to concentrate. Some of these responses may also be apparent in stressed caregivers.

COPING. Secondary appraisal, or the patient's evaluation of coping resources and options, is important to assess (see Figure 8.2). Resources such as supportive family members, adequate finances, and the ability to solve problems are examples of positive resources. Knowledge of the patient's resources can assist the nurse in supporting existing resources and developing strategies to expand the patient's sources of support to include family, friends, and community resources.

Coping strategies include cognitive and behavioural efforts to meet demands. The use and effectiveness of problem-focused and emotion-focused coping efforts should be addressed (see Table 8.6). These efforts may be categorized as direct action, avoidance of action, seeking information, defence mechanisms, and seeking the assistance of other people. The probability that a certain coping strategy will bring about the desired result is another important aspect to be assessed. Effective coping skills can be taught, and nurses are in a prime position to teach these skills.

NURSING IMPLEMENTATION

The first step in managing stress is to become aware of its presence. Health-related stressors for patients may include a fear of death or illness, uncertainty or anxiety about a diagnosis, changes in roles or family life, and financial burdens that may arise as a result. Stress can further be exacerbated in hospital settings through the physical discomforts of an illness, strange surrounding noises, unfamiliar people, and use of unfamiliar processes. The role of the nurse is to facilitate and enhance the processes of coping and adaptation, which include identifying and expressing stressful feelings. Nursing interventions depend on the severity of the stress experience or demand. The person with multiple

traumas expends energy in an attempt to physically survive. The nurse's efforts are directed toward life-supporting interventions and the inclusion of approaches aimed at reducing additional stressors to the patient. The individual who has endured significant trauma is much less likely to adapt or recover if faced with additional stressors, such as sleep deprivation or an infection.

The importance of cognitive appraisal in the stress experience should prompt the nurse to assess whether changes in the way a person perceives and labels particular events or situations (cognitive reappraisal) are possible. Some experts also propose that the nurse consider the positive effects that result from successfully meeting stressful demands. Greater emphasis should also be placed on the part that cultural values and beliefs can play to enhance or constrain various coping options.

Because coping with physical, social, and psychological demands is an integral part of daily experiences, the coping behaviours that are used should be adaptive and should not be a source of additional stress to the individual. Generalizing about which coping strategies are most adaptive is not possible. However, in evaluating coping behaviours, the nurse should examine the short-term outcomes (e.g., the effect of the strategy on the reduction or mastery of the demands and the regulation of the emotional response) and the long-term outcomes that relate to health, morale, and social and psychological functioning.

Caregiver stress is a well-identified phenomenon that may occur in a variety of situations, such as caring for a partner or loved one, and thus should also be considered in a stress assessment. To improve the quality of life among caregivers, nurses can provide adequate education regarding patient care and caregiver support. Referrals to appropriate support groups and respite services must also be considered (Piersol et al., 2017). Nurses are well positioned to assess patients and their significant others, to assist them in identifying periods when they are at high risk for stress, and to implement stress management strategies.

Teaching problem-solving skills can equip individuals to better handle present and future encounters with stressful circumstances. Stress-reducing activities can be incorporated into nursing practice (Table 8.13). These activities provide mechanisms through which an individual can develop a sense of control over the situation. As stress-reducing practices are incorporated into daily activities, the individual can increase their confidence and self-reliance, while limiting their emotional response to the stressful circumstance. Possessing a sense of control over one's life, believing that one can overcome adversity, and being

TABLE 8.13 IMPLEMENTING STRESS MANAGEMENT IN CLINICAL PRACTICE

- Learn relaxation–coping techniques by practising them on your own; then practise teaching them to peers before teaching them to patients. Attend seminars and workshops on stress management to learn more.
- Be aware of potential stressors that patients face.
- Assess patients for the demands placed on them, their response to these demands, and coping resources being used or available to them.
- Choose the language you use carefully and be aware of your nonverbal communication. Words or gestures that express overt alarm or ambiguity may increase the stress experience for the patient.
- Choose coping strategies and stress management strategies that are appropriate for your clinical area.
- Take advantage of opportunities to teach coping and relaxation strategies to patients.
- Anticipate setbacks. They provide feedback about what you are doing wrong. Do *not* quit practising!

committed to that end are important characteristics that can avert the harmful effects inherent in the stress response.

The nurse can assume a primary role in planning stress-reducing interventions. Nurses are in an ideal situation to take the lead in integrating stress management into their practice.

Nurses are also well equipped to develop and test the effectiveness of new approaches to manage stress and promote positive health outcomes. However, it is important for the nurse to recognize when the patient, family, or caregivers need to be referred to a professional with advanced training in counselling.

CASE STUDY

Stress Associated With Cancer Diagnosis and Treatment

Patient Profile

M. Z., a Polish immigrant (pronouns she/her), received a diagnosis of stage 2 breast cancer at age 44. Her treatment plan included lumpectomy followed by a regimen of chemotherapy and then radiation therapy. She attributed her breast cancer to her depression, which developed while caring for her mother, who suffered from Alzheimer's disease. M. Z's mother passed away 6 months before her breast cancer diagnosis.

After completion of her lengthy breast cancer therapy, M. Z.'s depression worsened. She no longer had her frequent visits to the breast cancer centre, and she missed the interaction with the nurses and other patients. In addition, M. Z. feared that the cancer would recur and worried it could be "passed on" to her two teenage daughters. She would not discuss her fears with her husband or daughters because she did not want to burden them. M. Z. began to lose weight and constantly felt fatigued. She felt "alone" with her cancer and lost interest in other aspects of her life. She thought about joining a cancer support group but was embarrassed by her Polish accent.

Discussion Questions

1. Consider M. Z.'s situation and describe the physiological and psychological stressors that she is dealing with. Describe the possible effects of these stressors on her health status.
2. What are some other potential stressors that M. Z. may be experiencing that the nurse should anticipate and assess further for?
3. What specific nursing interventions can be included in M. Z.'s management that will enhance her adaptability?
4. On the basis of M. Z.'s profile, what resources are available to her to help her cope with her cancer diagnosis and treatment?
5. Should M. Z. join a cancer support group? If so, how might this be of benefit?
6. **Priority decision:** On the basis of the assessment data provided, what are the priority nursing diagnoses? Are there any interprofessional issues?

evolve

Answers are available at http://evolve.elsevier.com/Canada/Lewis/medsurg.

REVIEW QUESTIONS

The number of the question corresponds to the same-numbered objective at the beginning of the chapter.

1. How does Selye define stress?
   a. Any stimulus that causes a response in an individual
   b. A response of an individual to environmental demands
   c. A physical or psychological adaptation to internal or external demands
   d. The result of a relationship between an individual and the environment that exceeds the individual's resources

2. A client who has undergone extensive surgery for multiple injuries endures a period of increasing blood pressure, heart rate, and alertness. Which stage of general adaptation syndrome are these symptoms most characteristic of?
   a. The resistance state of general adaptation syndrome
   b. The alarm reaction of the general adaptation syndrome
   c. The stage of exhaustion of general adaptation syndrome
   d. An individual response stereotype

3. Which actions best demonstrate that a client is using an emotion-focused coping process? *(Select all that apply.)*
   a. Joining a support group for women with breast cancer
   b. Considering the advantages and disadvantages of the various treatment options
   c. Delaying treatment until her family can take a weekend trip together
   d. Telling the nurse that she has a good prognosis because the tumour is small
   e. Engaging in meditation

4. The nurse would expect which of the following findings in a client as a result of the physiological effect of stress on the limbic system?
   a. An episode of diarrhea while awaiting painful dressing changes
   b. Refusing to communicate with nurses while awaiting a cardiac catheterization

   c. Inability to sleep the night before beginning to self-administer insulin injections
   d. Increased blood pressure, decreased urine output, and hyperglycemia after a car accident

5. Which of the following best demonstrates that the nurse is applying knowledge of the effects of stress on the immune system?
   a. Encouraging clients to sleep for 10 to 12 hours per day
   b. Encouraging clients to receive regular immunizations when they are stressed
   c. Encouraging clients to use emotion-focused rather than problem-focused coping strategies
   d. Encouraging clients to avoid exposure to upper respiratory infections when physically stressed

6. Chronic stress or daily hassles may place a person at higher risk of developing which of the following conditions? *(Select all that apply.)*
   a. Osteoporosis
   b. Colds and flu
   c. Low blood pressure
   d. Irritable bowel syndrome
   e. Depression

7. During a stressful circumstance that is uncontrollable, which type of coping strategy is the most effective?
   a. Avoidance
   b. Coping flexibility
   c. Emotion-focused coping
   d. Problem-focused coping

8. Which of the following clients is least likely to respond to stress effectively?
   a. One who feels that the situation is directing their life
   b. One who sees the situation as a challenge to be addressed
   c. One who has a clear understanding of their values and goals
   d. One who uses more problem-focused than emotion-focused coping strategies

9. Which of the following is an appropriate nursing intervention for a client who has a nursing diagnosis of *reduced coping* resulting from *inadequate resources*?
   a. Controlling the environment to prevent sensory overload and promote sleep
   b. Encouraging the client's family to offer emotional support by frequent visiting
   c. Arranging for the client to phone family and friends to maintain emotional bonds
   d. Asking the client to describe previous stressful situations and how they managed to resolve them

1. d; 2. b; 3. a; 4. c; 5. d; 6. b, d, e; 7. c; 8. a; 9. d.

*e*volve

For even more review questions, visit http://evolve.elsevier.com/Canada/Lewis/medsurg.

REFERENCES

Achour, M., Ghani Azmi, I. B. A., Isahak, M. B., et al. (2019). Job stress and nurses well-being: Prayer and age as moderators. *Community Mental Health Journal*, 55(7), 1226–1235. https://doi.org/10.1007/s10597-019-00410-y.

Antonovsky, A. (1987). *Unraveling the mystery of health. How people manage stress and stay well.* Jossey-Bass (Seminal).

Anxiety Canada. (2019). *How to do progressive muscle relaxation.* https://www.anxietycanada.com/articles/how-to-do-progressive-muscle-relaxation/.

Arnold, E. C. (2020). Communication in stressful situations. In E. C. Arnold, & K. Underman Boggs (Eds.), *Interpersonal relationships: Professional communication skills for nurses* (8th ed) (pp. 310–332). Elsevier Canada.

Benson, H., & Klipper, M. Z. (1975). *The relaxation response.* Morrow. (Seminal).

Canadian Association of Music Therapists. (2020). *About music therapy.* https://www.musictherapy.ca/about-camt-music-therapy/about-music-therapy/.

Canadian Mental Health Association of Canada (CMHAC). (2020). *Mental health in Canada: COVID-19 and beyond: CAMH policy advice.* https://www.camh.ca/-/media/files/pdfs---public-policy-submissions/covid-and-mh-policy-paper-pdf.

Cannon, W. B. (1932). *The wisdom of the body.* Norton (Seminal).

Cocchiara, R. A., Peruzzo, M., Mannocci, A., et al. (2019). The use of yoga to manage stress and burnout in healthcare workers: A systematic review. *Journal of Clinical Medicine*, 8(3), 284–295. https://doi.org/10.3390/jcm8030284.

Cohen, S., Murphy, M. L., & Prather, A. A. (2019). Ten surprising facts about stressful life events and disease risk. *Annual Review of Psychology*, 70, 577–597. https://doi.org/10.1146/annurev-psych-010418-102857.

Currie, C. L., Copeland, J. L., & Metz, A. (2019). Childhood racial discrimination and adult allostatic load: The role of Indigenous cultural continuity in allostatic resiliency. *Social Science and Medicine*, 241, 1–9. https://doi.org/10.1016/j.socscimed.2019.112564.

Fallon, V. T., Warfield, R., Hearn, B., et al. (2020). Stress reduction from a musical intervention. *Psychomusicology: Music, Mind, and Brain*, 30(1), 20–27. https://doi.org/10.1037/pmu0000246.

Halter, M. (2019). Understanding responses to stress. In M. Halter, C. Pollard, & S. Jakubec (Eds.), *Varcarolis' Canadian psychiatric mental health nursing: A clinical approach* (2nd Canadian ed.) (pp. 65–78). Elsevier.

Hilton, L., Ruelaz Maher, A., Colaiaco, B., et al. (2017). Meditation for posttraumatic stress: Systematic review and meta-analysis. *Psychological Trauma: Theory, Research, Practice, and Policy*, 9(4), 453–460. https://doi.org/10.1037/tra0000180.

Kabat-Zinn, J. (1994). *Wherever you go there you are: Mindfulness meditation in everyday life.* Hyperion.

Kennedy, L., & Henrickson Parker, S. (2019). Biofeedback as a stress management tool: A systematic review. *Cognition, Technology & Work*, 21(2), 161–190. https://doi.org/10.1007/s10111-018-0487-x.

Lazarus, R., & Folkman, S. (1984). *Stress, appraisal, and coping.* Springer (Seminal).

Micozzi, M. S. (2019). *Fundamentals of complementary, alternative, and integrative medicine* (6th ed). Elsevier.

Park, T. (2019). Stress and adaptation. In Potter, P. A., Perry, A. G., Ross-Kerr, J. C., et al. (Eds.), (2019). *Canadian fundamentals of nursing* (6th Canadian ed., pp. 508–525). Elsevier Canada.

Piersol, C. V., Canton, K., Connor, S. E., et al. (2017). Effectiveness of interventions for caregivers of people with Alzheimer's disease and related major neurocognitive disorders: A systematic review. *American Journal of Occupational Therapy*, 71(5), 7105180020. https://doi.org/10.5014/ajot.2017.027581.

Roberti, J. W., Harrington, L. N., & Storch, E. A. (2006). Further psychometric support for the 10-item version of the Performance Stress Scale. *Journal of College Counseling*, 9(2), 135–147. http://onlinelibrary.wiley.com/doi/10.1002/j.2161-1882.2006.tb00100.x. (Seminal).

Slavich, G. M. (2019). Psychoneuroimmunology of stress and mental health. In K. Harkness, & E. P. Hayden (Eds.), *The Oxford handbook of stress and mental health.* Oxford University Press. https://doi.org/10.1093/oxfordhb/9780190681777.013.24.

Sterling, P. E. J. (1988). Allostasis: A new paradigm to explain arousal pathology. In S. R. Fisher (Ed.), *Handbook of life stress, cognition and health* (pp. 629–649). Wiley (Seminal).

Takahashi, L. K., McCance, K. L., Margaret, F., et al. (2019). In K. L. McCance, & S. Huether (Eds.), *Pathophysiology: The biologic basis for disease in adults and children* (8th ed.) (pp. 323–344). Elsevier.

van der Wal, N., & Kok, R. N. (2019). Laughter-inducing therapies: Systematic review and meta-analysis. *Social Science & Medicine*, 232(July), 473–488. https://doi.org/10.1016/j.socscimed.2019.02.018.

Yaribeygi, H., Panahi, Y., Sahraei, H., et al. (2017). The impact of stress on body function: A review. *EXCLI Journal*, 16, 1057. https://doi.org/10.171779/excli2017-480.

RESOURCES

Addictions: Centre for Addictions and Mental Health
https://www.camh.ca/en/health-info/mental-illness-and-addiction-index/addiction
Anxiety Canada
https://www.anxietycanada.com/
Canadian Centre for Occupational Health and Safety
https://www.ccohs.ca/
Canadian Institute of Stress
https://www.stresscanada.org
Canadian Nurses Association: myCNA
https://www.mycna.ca/
Centre for Addiction and Mental Health
https://www.camh.net
Centre for the Neurobiology of Stress
https://www.utsc.utoronto.ca/~cnstress
Heart and Stroke Foundation of Canada
https://www.heartandstroke.ca
Psychology Foundation of Canada: Stress Strategies
https://www.stressstrategies.ca/resources
Public Health Agency of Canada
https://www.phac-aspc.gc.ca/chn-rcs/index-eng.php

*e*volve

For additional Internet resources, see the website for this book at http://evolve.elsevier.com/Canada/Lewis/medsurg.

CHAPTER

9

Sleep and Sleep Disorders

Jane Tyerman
Originating US chapter by Diana Taibi Buchanan
With contributions from Efrosini Papaconstantinou

evolve WEBSITE

http://evolve.elsevier.com/Canada/Lewis/medsurg

- Review Questions (Online Only)
- Key Points
- Answer Guidelines for Case Study
- Conceptual Care Map Creator
- Audio Glossary
- Content Updates

LEARNING OBJECTIVES

1. Define *sleep*.
2. Describe physiological sleep mechanisms and stages of sleep.
3. Explain the relationship of various diseases and disorders and sleep disorders.
4. Describe the etiology, clinical manifestations, and interprofessional and nursing management of insomnia.
5. Describe the etiology, clinical manifestations, interprofessional care, and nursing management of obstructive sleep apnea.
6. Describe parasomnias, including sleepwalking, sleep terrors, and nightmares.
7. Select appropriate strategies for managing sleep problems associated with shift work.

KEY TERMS

cataplexy
circadian rhythms
circadian rhythm sleep–wake disorders (CRSWDs)
continuous positive airway pressure (CPAP)
delayed sleep phase disorder (DSPD)

insomnia
narcolepsy
obstructive sleep apnea (OSA)
parasomnias
shift work sleep disorder
sleep

sleep-disordered breathing
sleep disorders
sleep disturbances
sleep hygiene
sleep terrors
wake behaviour

SLEEP

Sleep is a state during which an individual lacks conscious awareness of environmental surroundings and from which the individual can be easily aroused. Sleep is distinct from unconscious states such as coma, from which the individual cannot be aroused. Sleep is a basic, dynamic, highly organized, and complex behaviour that is essential for normal functioning and survival. Over the lifespan of 80 years, a person who sleeps 7 hours per night will spend 24 years sleeping. Both behavioural and physiological functions are influenced by sleep. Some of these include memory, mood, cognitive function, hormone secretion, glucose metabolism, immune function, body temperature, and renal function.

Sleep requirements vary over the lifespan and are affected by health, lifestyle, and gender (Chaput et al., 2017). Most adults require at least 7 to 9 hours of sleep within a 24-hour period (Hirshkowitz et al., 2015; Public Health Agency of Canada [PHAC], 2019). The term sleep disturbances refers broadly to situations of poor-quality sleep. *Insufficient sleep* refers to obtaining less sleep than a person requires to be fully awake and alert during the day (Figure 9.1). *Fragmented sleep* is characterized by frequent arousals or actual awakenings that interrupt sleep continuity. Sleep disturbances can be related to a variety of physical, emotional, environmental, and lifestyle factors.

Sleep disorders are conditions that specifically affect the quality of sleep and wake behaviour. The classification of sleep disorders is complex; 81 different types have been identified. Table 9.1 lists the seven categories of sleep disorders with some examples based on the *International Classification of Sleep Disorders*, third edition (ICSD-3) (Sateia, 2014).

More than one-third of all Canadians report receiving less than the recommended 7 hours of sleep per night (Chaput et al., 2017). On average, one in two adults have trouble going to sleep or staying asleep, one in five adults do not find their sleep refreshing, and one in three adults have difficulty staying awake during waking hours (PHAC, 2019). People with chronic health conditions or physical disability are at greatest risk for sleep disorders (Mathias et al., 2018).

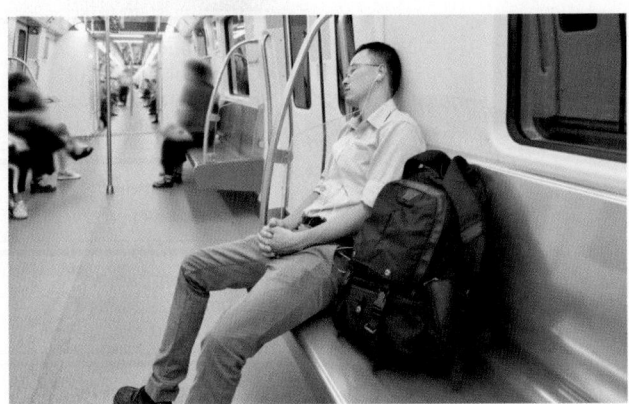

FIG. 9.1 Sleep disorders are common in our society. Source: iStock.com/ baona.

TABLE 9.1	SELECTED SLEEP DISORDERS
Type of Disorder	**Characteristics**
Insomnia	Chronic
	Short-term
Sleep-related breathing disorders	Obstructive sleep apnea
	Central sleep apnea syndromes
Central disorders of hypersomnolence	Types 1 and 2 narcolepsy
	Hypersomnia related to a medical condition
	Hypersomnia related to medication or substance
Sleep-related movement disorders	Periodic limb movement disorder
	Restless legs syndrome
Circadian rhythm sleep–wake disorders	Delayed sleep–wake phase disorder
	Shift work sleep disorder
Parasomnias	Sleepwalking
	Sleep terrors
	Nightmare disorder
Other sleep disorders	

Untreated sleep disorders pose considerable health and economic consequences. Sleepiness during driving has become a national epidemic. An estimated 20% of fatal driving collisions involve driver fatigue (National Highway Traffic Safety Administrations [NHTSA], 2020). Some work-related accidents have been linked to sleep problems (Pilcher & Morris, 2020). Each year, sleep disorders, sleep loss, and excessive daytime sleepiness add billions of dollars to the cost of health care and to the economic effect of work-related accidents and lost productivity (Chattu et al., 2018). Many sleep disorders go untreated because health care providers often do not ask, and patients often do not talk, about sleep problems.

Physiological Sleep Mechanisms

Sleep–Wake Cycle. The nervous system controls the cyclical changes between waking and sleep. Complex networks in the areas of the forebrain (cerebral cortex, hypothalamus, thalamus) and brainstem interact to regulate the sleep–wake cycle.

Wake Behaviour. Wake behaviour is associated with an activated cortical brain wave (electroencephalographic [EEG]) pattern. The reticular activating system in the middle of the brainstem is associated with generalized EEG activation and behavioural arousal. Various neurotransmitters (glutamate, acetylcholine, norepinephrine, dopamine, histamine, serotonin) are involved in wake behaviour. Histamine neurons in the hypothalamus stimulate cortical activation and wake behaviour. The

sedating properties of many over-the-counter (OTC) medications result from inhibiting one of these arousal systems (especially acetylcholine and histamine).

Neuropeptides also influence wake behaviour. *Orexin* (also called *hypocretin*) is found in the lateral hypothalamus. Orexin stimulates wake behaviour through activating the reticular activating system. Decreased levels of orexin or its receptors lead to difficulties staying awake and in the syndrome called *narcolepsy* (Chow & Cao, 2016; Mahoney et al., 2019). (Narcolepsy is discussed later in this chapter.)

Sleep Behaviour. Sleep behaviour is regulated by a variety of neurological structures and neurotransmitters. Ventral lateral and median preoptic areas of the brain interact with other areas of the brain, such as the hypothalamus and the brainstem, to induce sleep by inhibiting the arousal centres. Sleep-promoting neurotransmitters and peptides include melatonin, adenosine, and prostaglandin D2 (Bollu & Kaur, 2019). Proinflammatory cytokines are important in mediating sleepiness and lethargy associated with infectious illness. Certain peptides, such as cholecystokinin, released by the gastrointestinal tract after food ingestion, may mediate the sleepiness that follows eating meals *(postprandial sleepiness).*

Circadian Rhythms. Many biological rhythms of behaviour and physiology fluctuate within a 24-hour period. These circadian rhythms (from the Latin *circa dies,* "approximately a day") persist when people are placed in isolated environments free of external time cues, because the rhythms are controlled by internal (endogenous) clock mechanisms. The suprachiasmatic nucleus in the hypothalamus is the master clock of the body. The 24-hour cycle is synchronized to the environmental light and dark periods through specific light detectors in the retina. Pathways from the suprachiasmatic nucleus innervate sleep-promoting cells in the anterior hypothalamus and wake-promoting cells of the lateral hypothalamus and brainstem.

Light is the strongest time cue for the sleep–wake rhythm. Because of this, light can be used as therapy to shift the timing of the sleep–wake rhythm. For example, bright light used early in the morning causes the sleep–wake rhythm to move to an earlier time; bright light used in the evening causes the sleep–wake rhythm to move to a later time. *Melatonin* is an endogenous hormone produced by the pineal gland in the brain from the amino acid tryptophan. In the central nervous system, melatonin decreases *sleep latency* (time it takes to fall asleep) and increases *sleep efficiency* (time spent asleep in comparison with time spent in bed). The secretion of melatonin is tightly linked to the environmental light–dark cycle. Under normal day–night conditions, more melatonin is released in the evening as it gets dark. Light exposure in the evening hours can suppress the secretion of melatonin (Ostrin, 2019). This can have implications for sleep quality in hospitalized patients, shift workers, and people who are exposed to computer and TV screens in the evening.

Sleep Architecture. On the basis of electrical recordings of brain activity with polysomnography (PSG), sleep can be divided into two major states: *rapid eye movement (REM)* and *non–rapid eye movement (NREM)*. Most adults transition from wake to sleep *(sleep-onset latency)* in approximately 10 to 20 minutes. Once asleep, a person goes through sleep cycles. A typical sleep cycle lasts 90 minutes and is repeated throughout the duration of the person's total sleep time. *Sleep architecture* refers to the pattern of a person's sleep stage cycling.

Non–Rapid Eye Movement Sleep. In healthy adults, the largest percentage of sleep time, approximately 75% to 80%, is spent in NREM sleep. NREM sleep is subdivided into three stages (Berry et al., 2017).

Stage 1 occurs in the beginning of sleep, with slow eye movements, and is a transition phase from wakefulness to sleep. It is short in duration, lasting 1 to 7 minutes, during which the person can be easily awakened.

Stage 2 is a period of sound sleep and accounts for most of the night's sleep. The heart rate slows down and the body temperature drops. This stage lasts 10 to 25 minutes.

Stage 3 is deep sleep, or slow-wave sleep, and is the deepest stage of sleep. During this stage, the sleeper is less responsive to environmental stimuli and unresponsive to sound. This stage lasts 20 to 40 minutes, but this declines as people age. Most adults over 60 years of age have little NREM stage 3 sleep.

Rapid Eye Movement Sleep. REM sleep accounts for 20% to 25% of sleep and occurs more in the later part of a person's total sleep time. REM sleep follows NREM sleep. In a healthy adult, REM sleep occurs four to five times during a period of 7 to 8 hours of sleep. This stage is considered paradoxical because the brain waves resemble wakefulness but movement of the skeletal muscles is inhibited. REM sleep is the period when the most vivid dreaming occurs.

INEFFICIENT SLEEP AND SLEEP DISTURBANCES

Insufficient sleep is associated with changes in body function (Figure 9.2) and health problems (Table 9.2). In patients with chronic illnesses, especially cardiovascular disease and stroke, sleep disorders are directly associated with increased risk for mortality and morbidity (Javaheri & Redline, 2017). Sleep loss is associated with decreases in immune function and body temperature and with endocrine changes, including a decrease in growth hormone levels. Cognitive function and performance on simple behavioural tasks become impaired within 24 hours of sleep loss. The effects of sleep loss are cumulative. Chronic loss of sleep places the individual at risk for a decrease in cognitive function, depression, social isolation, and overall reduction in quality of life (Pavlova & Latreille, 2019).

An insufficient amount of nighttime sleep has a harmful effect on carbohydrate metabolism and endocrine function. Individuals who report less than 6 hours of sleep a night have a higher body mass index (BMI) and are more likely to be obese. Sleep restriction and sleep fragmentation have been linked to decreased insulin sensitivity and increased risk for diabetes (Pavlova & Latreille, 2019). In women with shortened or disturbed sleep, the risk for heart disease was found to be double that of women with adequate sleep (Suh et al., 2018).

Sleep Disturbances in the Hospital

Hospitalization, especially in the critical care unit (CCU), is associated with decreases in total sleep time, sleep efficiency, and REM sleep. Pre-existing sleep disorders may be aggravated or triggered in the hospital. Environmental sleep-disruptive factors, psychoactive medications, and acute and critical illness all contribute to poor sleep. Symptoms such as pain, dyspnea, and nausea can also contribute to sleep loss in acutely ill patients.

Medications commonly used in acutely and critically ill patients can further contribute to sleep loss, by exacerbating sleep-disordered breathing (discussed later in this chapter) or

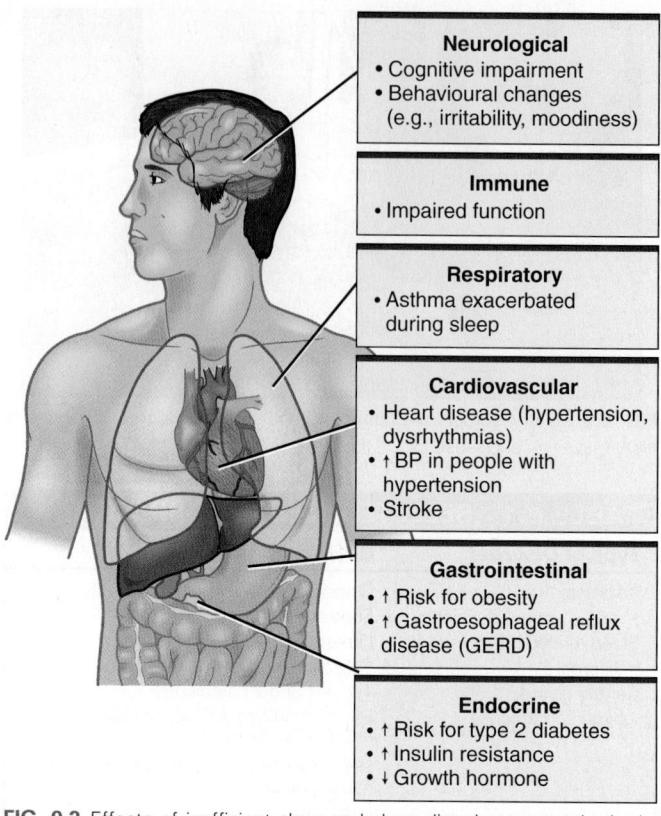

FIG. 9.2 Effects of inefficient sleep and sleep disturbances on the body. *BP,* blood pressure.

by altering sleep architecture. Nightmares can also occur as a result of medication and are commonly reported by patients in the CCU. The longer the stay in the CCU, the more likely the patient is to have nightmares. Drug classes most likely to cause nightmares are sedative–hypnotics, β-adrenergic antagonists, dopamine agonists, and amphetamines.

Hospitalized patients are also at risk for poor sleep partly because of disruptions in circadian rhythm. The hospital or long-term care facility represents a new environment, and thus normal cues linked to sleep may be absent. Bright lights during the night can also disrupt sleep. The hospital and CCU environmental noise (e.g., staff paging system, respirator alarms, bedside monitors, infusion alarms, staff conversations near patients) during both the day and the night can result in sleep difficulties and CCU delirium, previously referred to as *CCU psychosis.* In addition, patient care activities (e.g., dressing changes, blood draws, vital sign monitoring) disrupt sleep. Patients in critical care areas have been found to have poor quantity and quality of sleep (Locihová et al., 2018). Sleep can continue being poor after the patient's hospitalization and can affect their long-term recovery and health. Staff prioritization of sleep over other competing critical care demands and the lack of research into sleep promotion within the CCU can affect use of sleep-promoting strategies (Locihová et al., 2018).

Decreased sleep duration influences pain perception. Psychological factors, such as anxiety and depression, also modify the sleep–pain relationship. Adequate pain management improves the duration and quality of sleep, but medications commonly used to relieve pain, especially opioids, also alter sleep and place the individual at risk for sleep-disordered breathing. Withdrawal of opioids is associated with rebound effects on sleep architecture.

TABLE 9.2 RELATIONSHIP OF SLEEP DISTURBANCES TO SELECTED DISEASES AND DISORDERS

Disease/Disorder	Sleep Disturbance	Disease/Disorder	Sleep Disturbance
Respiratory		Cardiovascular (CV)	With sleep apnea/sleep disorders, increased risk for CV disorders, including hypertension, dysrhythmias, and coronary artery disease
Asthma	Exacerbated during sleep Reports of more insomnia		
Chronic obstructive pulmonary disease (COPD)	Associated with poor sleep quality, nocturnal O_2 desaturation, and coexisting sleep apnea	Heart failure (HF)	Sleep disturbances (insomnia, PLMD, SDB) common Cheyne-Stokes breathing and central apnea are signs of HF exacerbation related to fluid overload Central sleep apnea correlated with poor left ventricle function
Obstructive sleep apnea	Linked to heart disease (hypertension, stroke, coronary artery disease, dysrhythmias) Impairment of glucose control similar to that occurring in type 2 diabetes Associated with cancer	Hypertension	Inadequate sleep in people with hypertension can lead to further elevations in blood pressure
Renal		**Gastrointestinal**	
End-stage renal disease	Disrupted nocturnal sleep with excessive daytime sleepiness In patients on dialysis, high incidence of SDB, PLMD, and RLS, which is a significant predictor of mortality in such patients	Obesity	Short sleep duration may result in metabolic changes that are linked to obesity. Higher BMI in people who sleep <6 hr than in people who sleep >8 hr Risk factor for SDB
Immune Disorders		Gastroesophageal reflux disease (GERD)	Reflux of gastric contents into the esophagus during sleep because of incompetent lower esophageal sphincter Swallowing is depressed during sleep
Human immunodeficiency virus (HIV)	Sleep disturbances and fatigue highly prevalent and associated with lower rates of survival	Chronic liver disease	Associated with excessive sleepiness, nocturnal arousal, and incidence of RLS
Endocrine		Bowel disorders	Associated with increased insomnia
Diabetes	Insufficient sleep linked to increased risk for type 2 diabetes Insulin resistance increased in healthy people with sleep deprivation Sleep duration and quality predictive of HbA1c levels, an important marker of blood glucose control	**Neurological**	
		Parkinson's disease	Associated with difficulty initiating or maintaining sleep, parasomnias, and excessive daytime sleepiness
Musculoskeletal		Alzheimer's disease	SDB (frequently sleep apnea) common Circadian rhythm alterations with nocturnal wandering, daytime sleepiness, and sleep disruption and awakening
Arthritis	Increased rates of RLS and SDB Disease activity linked to sleep complaints		
Fibromyalgia	Comorbid insomnia, especially report of nonrestorative sleep Increased rates of PLMD and RLS Lower levels of sleep-dependent hormones (growth hormone, prolactin)	Pain (acute and chronic)	Decreased quantity and quality of sleep Poor sleep can intensify pain
Chronic fatigue syndrome	Comorbid insomnia Increased rates of SDB	Depression	Can result in insomnia or hypersomnia Amount and quality of REM sleep often affected by antidepressant medication
Cancer	Higher rates of insomnia reported Chemotherapy for cancer treatment associated with fragmented sleep		

BMI, body mass index; *HbA1c*, glycated hemoglobin; *O₂*, oxygen; *PLMD*, periodic limb movement disorder; *REM*, rapid eye movement; *RLS*, restless legs syndrome; *SDB*, sleep-disordered breathing.
Sources: Centers for Disease Control and Prevention. (2011). *Sleep and chronic disease.* https://www.cdc.gov/sleep/about_sleep/chronic_disease.html; and National Sleep Foundation. (2016). *Sleep disorders.* https://sleepfoundation.org/sleep-disorders-problems.

Nurses have a critical role in creating an environment conducive to sleep. This includes the scheduling of medications and procedures during both day and night. Typical sleep architecture should be considered when interventions and care are planned. When any necessary care episodes are scheduled 90 minutes (or a multiple of that) after a patient has fallen asleep, sleep disruption has been decreased. Reducing light and noise levels or use of earplugs can promote opportunities for sleep.

SLEEP DISORDERS

Insomnia

The most common sleep disorder is insomnia. Insomnia is defined as difficulty falling asleep, difficulty staying asleep,

waking up too early, or poor quality of sleep. Insomnia is a common problem, affecting approximately one in three adults.

Acute insomnia refers to difficulties falling asleep or remaining asleep and experiencing daytime fatigue for at least 3 nights per week over a 2-week period. *Chronic insomnia* is defined by the same symptoms and a daytime difficulty (e.g., fatigue, poor concentration, interference with social or family activities) that occur at least three times a week and persist for 3 months or longer. Chronic insomnia occurs in 17% of Canadians and is influenced by age, sex, education, physical health, and mental health status (Garland et al., 2018). Incidence of chronic insomnia increases in people older than 45 years and is higher in divorced, widowed, and separated individuals, as well as in individuals with low socioeconomic status and lower amounts of education (Matheson & Hainer, 2017).

Etiology and Pathophysiology. Behaviours, maladaptive cognitions, lifestyle, diet, and medications contribute to and perpetuate insomnia. *Inadequate sleep hygiene* refers to practices or behaviours that are inconsistent with quality sleep. Consumption of stimulants (e.g., caffeine, nicotine, methamphetamine, other drug misuse), especially before bedtime, results in insomnia. Insomnia is a common adverse effect of many medications (e.g., antidepressants, antihypertensives, corticosteroids, psychostimulants, analgesics). Insomnia can be exacerbated or perpetuated by consumption of alcohol to help induce sleep, smoking close to bedtime, taking long naps in the afternoon, sleeping in until late in the morning, nightmares, exercise near bedtime, and jet lag. *Maladaptive cognitions* concern personal beliefs and interpretations of sleep-related experiences; this is the key area addressed by cognitive–behavioural interventions for sleep (discussed later in this chapter).

Once chronic insomnia is manifested, symptoms are likely to persist over time. Individuals with insomnia may engage in behaviours that perpetuate disturbed sleep by keeping irregular sleep–wake schedules, using OTC medications or alcohol as sleep aids, and spending more time in bed trying to sleep. Increased attention to one's environment, worry or fear about not obtaining sufficient sleep, and poor sleep habits can lead to a conditioned arousal.

Clinical Manifestations. Manifestations of insomnia include (1) difficulty falling asleep *(long sleep latency)*, (2) frequent awakenings *(fragmented sleep)*, (3) prolonged nighttime awakenings or awakening too early and not being able to fall back to sleep, and (4) feeling unrefreshed on awakening (as a result of *nonrestorative sleep*). Daytime consequences of insomnia may manifest as tiredness, trouble concentrating at work or school, altered mood, and falling asleep during the day. Behavioural manifestations of poor sleep include irritability, forgetfulness, confusion, difficulty staying awake during the day, and anxiety.

Diagnostic Studies

Self-Report. The diagnosis of insomnia is based on subjective reports and on an evaluation of a 1- or 2-week sleep diary completed by the patient. A panel of sleep experts created the Consensus Sleep Diary to standardize the type of information that clinicians collect in sleep diaries (Maich et al., 2018). In ambulatory care settings, the evaluation of insomnia requires a comprehensive sleep history to establish the type of insomnia and to screen for possible comorbid psychiatric, medical, or sleep disorder conditions that would necessitate specific treatment. Questionnaires such as the Pittsburgh Sleep Quality Index and the Consensus Sleep Diary are examples of questionnaires commonly used to assess sleep quality (see the Resources at the end of this chapter for additional sleep scales).

Actigraphy. *Actigraphy* is a relatively noninvasive method of monitoring rest and activity cycles. A small actigraph watch, which can be worn on the wrist like a watch, is used to measure gross motor activity (Figure 9.3). The watch continually records the movements. After the data are collected, they are downloaded to a computer, and algorithms are used to analyze the data. Actigraphy is not required to diagnose insomnia but can be used to confirm a patient's sleep self-reports and clarify sleep and activity patterns during treatment.

Polysomnography. A clinical PSG study is not necessary to establish a diagnosis of insomnia. A PSG study is performed only if there are symptoms or signs of a sleep disorder, such as sleep-disordered breathing (discussed later in this chapter). In a PSG study, electrodes simultaneously record physiological

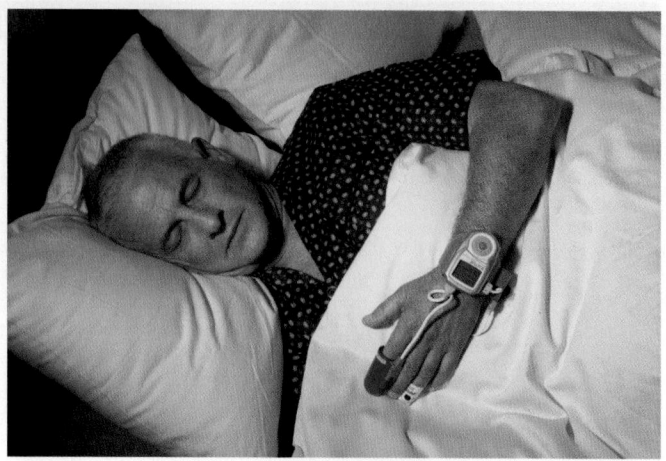

FIG. 9.3 Actigraph watch worn while the patient is sleeping. Source: Courtesy Itamar Medical, Inc.

measures that define the main stages of sleep and wakefulness. These measures include (a) muscle tone, recorded with electromyography; (b) eye movements, recorded with electrooculography; and (c) brain activity, recorded through an EEG study. To determine additional characteristics of specific sleep disorders, other measures are made during PSG. These include airflow at the nose and mouth, respiratory effort around the chest and abdomen, heart rate, noninvasive oxygen saturation, and electromyographic study of the anterior tibialis muscles (used to detect periodic leg movements). In addition, a patient's gross body movements are monitored continuously by audiovisual means.

Interprofessional Care. Treatments are oriented toward symptom management (Table 9.3). A key to management is to change behaviours that perpetuate insomnia. This often encompasses cognitive–behavioural strategies and education about sleep, including sleep hygiene. Sleep hygiene comprises a variety of different practices that are important for normal, quality nighttime sleep and daytime alertness (Table 9.4).

Cognitive–Behavioural Therapies. Cognitive–behavioural therapy for insomnia (CBT-i) is effective in the management of insomnia and should be the first method of therapy (Davidson et al., 2019; Riemann et al., 2017). CBT-i for insomnia includes a structured treatment plan of behavioural routines, relaxation practices, and thought-management strategies related to promoting sleep. Examples of strategies that can be included within CBT-i are relaxation training, guided imagery, and cognitive strategies that address dysfunctional ideas about sleep. CBT-i also includes education about good sleep hygiene practices (see Table 9.4). Often a full lifestyle behaviour plan is devised to include regular exercise (performed several hours before bedtime), regular bedtime routines, and time limits for staying in bed. CBTs require individuals to change behaviour and be able to sustain a change in routine. Supporting a patient's behaviour changes requires evaluation of their motivation and resources for change before treatments are initiated. Full CBT-i treatment requires providers to have training; it is often delivered by nurses working in primary care and mental health settings. Although not all nurses are trained in CBT-i, they can educate people about sleep hygiene and use the principles of CBT-i to help patients set up new routines. For example, individuals with insomnia can be encouraged to avoid watching television, playing video games, or reading in bed. Time in bed should be limited to the actual time that the individual can sleep. Naps and

TABLE 9.3   INTERPROFESSIONAL CARE

Insomnia

Diagnostic Measures	Interprofessional Therapy

• History
• Self-report
  • Sleep assessment (see Table 9.6)
  • Pittsburgh Sleep Quality Index*
  • Epworth Sleepiness Scale*
  • Consensus Sleep Diary
• Physical assessment
• Polysomnography
	Nonpharmacological Therapy
	• Sleep hygiene (see Table 9.4)
	• Cognitive–behavioural therapy for insomnia
	Medication Therapy (see Table 9.6)
	• Benzodiazepines
	• Benzodiazepine receptor–like agents
	• Orexin receptor antagonist
	• Melatonin receptor agonist
	• Antidepressant
	Complementary and Alternative Therapies
	• Melatonin
	• Music therapy
	• Acupuncture
	• Tai chi

*See the Resources for this chapter.

Source: Adapted from American Academy of Sleep Medicine. (2017). *Healthy sleep habits.* https://www.sleepeducation.org/treatment-therapy/healthy-sleep-habits/.

TABLE 9.4   PATIENT & CAREGIVER TEACHING GUIDE

Sleep Hygiene

The nurse should include the following instructions when teaching a patient who has sleep disturbances or disorders:
• Do not go to bed unless you are feeling sleepy.
• If you are not asleep after 20 minutes, get out of bed and do a nonstimulating activity. Return to bed only when you are sleepy.
• Adopt a regular sleep pattern in terms of bedtime and awakening.
• Begin rituals (e.g., warm bath, light snack, reading) that help you relax each night before bed.
• Get a full night's sleep on a regular basis.
• Make your bedroom quiet, dark, and a little bit cool.
• Do not read, write, eat, watch TV, talk on the phone, or use technologies such as smartphones and tablet computers in bed.
• Avoid caffeine, nicotine, and alcohol at least 4–6 hours before bedtime.
• Do not go to bed hungry, but do not eat a big meal near bedtime either.
• Avoid strenuous exercise within 6 hours of your bedtime.
• Avoid sleeping pills, or use them cautiously.
• Practice relaxation techniques (e.g., relaxation breathing) to help you cope with stress.

Source: Arnold, E. C. (2020). Communication in stressful situations. In E. C. Arnold & K. Underman Boggs (Eds.), *Interpersonal relationships: Professional communication skills for nurses* (8th ed., pp. 310–332). Elsevier Canada.

TABLE 9.5   MEDICATION THERAPY

Insomnia

Drug Class	Specific Medication
Benzodiazepines	• Flurazepam • Temazepam (Restoril)
Benzodiazepine receptor–like drugs	• Zopiclone (Imovane) • Zolpidem
Antidepressants	• Amitriptyline • Doxepin
Over-the-counter sleep aids Antihistamines	• Diphenhydramine (Benadryl, Nytol)
Natural health products	• Melatonin • Valerian

Many individuals with insomnia become used to taking OTC or prescription medications to treat insomnia and risk becoming dependent on them, both psychologically and physically (Chapter 11 has more information on substance dependence). *Rebound insomnia* is common with abrupt withdrawal of hypnotic medications. The resulting daytime fatigue can negatively influence the patient's efforts to use nonpharmacological approaches.

Classes of medications used to treat insomnia include benzodiazepines and benzodiazepine receptor–like drugs (Table 9.5). Although antidepressants, antihistamines, and antipsychotics are sometimes used as sleep aids, there is actually insufficient evidence to support their use for insomnia (Murphy et al., 2016).

Benzodiazepines. Benzodiazepines such as diazepam (Valium), serax (oxazepam), and lorazepam (Ativan) work by activating the γ-aminobutyric acid (GABA) receptors to promote sleep. The prolonged half-life of some of these medications (e.g., flurazepam and nitrazepam) can result in daytime sleepiness, amnesia, dizziness, and rebound insomnia so are not recommended. Temazepam and triazolam are benzodiazepines considered to be suitable for short-term treatment of insomnia because of their fast onset and short half-life, which results in less pronounced daytime effects. None of the benzodiazepines are recommended for use in people older than 65 years. Tolerance to these medications develops and increases the risk for dependence (see Chapter 11 for more information on benzodiazepine misuse); therefore, it is recommended that the use of benzodiazepines be limited to less than 7 days or to intermittent use of no more than 3 days a week. In addition, benzodiazepines interact with alcohol and other central nervous system depressants.

Nonbenzodiazepine Hypnotics. Because the safety profile of the so-called Z-drugs (e.g., zolpidem and zopiclone) is better than that of benzodiazepines, Z-drugs are the medication of first choice for insomnia. These medications are effective and safe to use from 3 months to a year (Asnis, 2016). Food has the potential to delay onset of action. These agents have short half-lives, making their duration of action short and reducing the risk for daytime sedation. Newer formulations have improved specific therapeutic uses. A controlled-release formulation of zolpidem (Ambien CR) lengthens the action of the medication, improving its use for sleep maintenance insomnia.

Antidepressants. Trazodone, mirtazapine, and amitriptyline are antidepressants with sedating properties. Trazodone is one of the medications most commonly prescribed in Canada to

consumption of large meals, alcohol, and stimulants need to be avoided. Naps are less likely to affect nighttime sleep if they are limited to 20 to 30 minutes.

Medication Therapy. Despite their perceived usefulness for short-term acute insomnia, medications for sleep are not without risks. Sedatives are associated with increased rates of overall mortality and are linked to adverse events such as falls, motor vehicle accidents, and poisonings. Use of sedatives in Canada has increased sharply in comparison with other prescribed medications (Murphy et al., 2016). The use of sedatives in the management of chronic insomnia, particularly in older persons, is not recommended (Canadian Geriatrics Society, 2019).

treat insomnia. However, there is little evidence supporting their use in nondepressed patients, and the potential for adverse effects such as anticholinergic effects, dizziness, orthostatic hypotension, and cardiac conduction abnormalities is significant (Wilt, 2016).

Antihistamines. Many individuals with insomnia self-medicate with OTC sleep aids. Most OTC agents include diphenhydramine (Benadryl, Nytol, Unisom). These agents are less effective than benzodiazepines, and tolerance develops quickly. In addition, they cause adverse effects, including daytime sedation, impaired cognitive function, blurred vision, urinary retention, and constipation; and they increase the risk for increased intraocular pressure. Agents that contain diphenhydramine are not intended for long-term use and should not be used by older persons.

Complementary and Alternative Therapies. Many types of complementary therapies and herbal products are used as sleep aids. Common herbal medicines used in Canada are chamomile, melatonin, and valerian root. Other therapies include the use of acupuncture, acupressure, tai chi, and music.

Herbal Supplements. Chamomile and valerian are herbs that have been used for many years as a sleep aids and to relieve anxiety. Researchers in only a few small studies have examined chamomile to date, with inconclusive results (Hieu, 2019). Overall, the current available evidence to support the use of chamomile to treat insomnia is lacking and further research is warranted

As noted earlier in the chapter, melatonin is a hormone produced by the pineal gland, which plays an important role in sleep cycle regulation. Melatonin can be somewhat helpful with sleep initiation and quality (Zisapel, 2018). Although effects on insomnia have been found to be less significant than those of other prescription sleep medications, melatonin is considered much safer (Xie et al., 2017). Melatonin has also been used with sleep-phase disorders such as jet lag and shift work disorder, although research evidence for this is weak and further study is required (Iggena et al., 2017).

Other Therapeutic Sleep Aids. Mind–body therapies have been effective interventions to manage insomnia. Examples include mindfulness meditation, tai chi, yoga, relaxation therapy, and musi (Rash et al., 2019). See Chapter 12 for more information and the following Complementary & Alternative Therapies box).

🌿 COMPLEMENTARY & ALTERNATIVE THERAPIES

Effect of Music on Sleep Quality

Scientific Evidence
Several studies, including randomized control trials, have demonstrated the effectiveness of listening to music as a method to improve sleep quality.

Nursing Implications
- Music is a well-tolerated, nonpharmacological intervention.
- Music is accessible to people in both home and hospital environments.

Further research on the use of music for sleep may help specify who can benefit most from the intervention and what factors support its use.

Source: Summarized from Feng, F., Zhang, Y., Hou, J., et al. (2018). Can music improve sleep quality in adults with primary insomnia? A systematic review and network meta-analysis. *International Journal of Nursing Studies, 77,* 189–196. https://doi.org/10.1016/j.ijnurstu.2017.10.011.

TABLE 9.6   NURSING ASSESSMENT
Sleep

The following questions can serve as an initial assessment regarding sleep:
1. What time do you normally go to bed at night? What time do you normally wake up in the morning?
2. Do you often have trouble falling asleep at night?
3. About how many times do you wake up at night?
4. If you do wake up during the night, do you usually have trouble falling back asleep?
5. Does your bed partner say or are you aware that you frequently snore, gasp for air, or stop breathing?
6. Does your bed partner say or are you aware that you kick or thrash about while asleep?
7. Are you aware that you ever walk, eat, punch, kick, or scream during sleep?
8. Are you sleepy or tired during much of the day?
9. Do you usually take one or more naps during the day?
10. Do you usually doze off without planning to during the day?
11. How much sleep do you need to feel alert and function well?
12. Are you currently taking any type of medication or other preparation to help you sleep?

Source: Harrison G. Bloom, Imran Ahmed, Cathy A. Alessi, Sonia Ancoli-Israel, Daniel J. Buysse, Meir H. Kryger, Barbara A. Phillips, Michael J. Thorpy, Michael V. Vitiello, & Phyllis C. Zee. (2009). Evidence-based recommendations for the assessment and management of sleep disorders in older persons, *Journal of the American Geriatrics Society, 57*(5), 761. ©2009, Copyright the Authors. Journal compilation ©2009, The American Geriatrics Society.

NURSING MANAGEMENT INSOMNIA

NURSING ASSESSMENT

Nurses are in a key position to assess sleep problems in patients and their family caregivers. Sleep assessment is important in helping patients to identify environmental factors that may contribute to poor sleep. Family caregivers may experience sleep disruptions because of the necessity of providing care to patients in the home. These sleep disruptions can increase the burden of caregiving.

Both subjective and objective methods are used to assess sleep duration and quality. Report of poor sleep is similar to that of pain in that it is a subjective report. Many patients may not tell their health care provider about their sleep problems. Therefore, the best way to detect sleep problems is for the nurse to ask about sleep on a regular basis. A sleep history should involve characteristics of sleep, such as the duration and pattern of sleep, and of daytime alertness. Before using any questionnaire, the patient's cognitive function, reading level (if a paper form is used), and language abilities need to be assessed.

Examples of questions to assess sleep are presented in Table 9.6. The nurse should also assess lifestyle factors that can influence sleep, such as work schedules, diet, and use of caffeine and other stimulants. In asking about how much alcohol is consumed each week, the nurse should find out whether the patient is using alcohol or other substances as sleep aids.

The nurse should ask the patient about sleep aids, both OTC and prescription medications. It is important to note the medication dose and frequency of use, as well as any adverse effects (e.g., daytime drowsiness, dry mouth). Many individuals also consume herbal or dietary supplements to improve sleep. The exact components and concentrations of herbs and supplements often are unknown, and patients may experience adverse effects. Additional sleep aids include white noise devices or relaxation strategies.

The nurse can encourage individuals to keep a sleep diary for 2 weeks. Other standardized questionnaires such as the Epworth Sleepiness Scale (see the Resources at the end of this chapter) may be used to assess daytime sleepiness.

The patient's medical history can also provide important information about factors that contribute to poor sleep. For example, men with benign prostatic hyperplasia often report frequent awakenings during the night for voiding. Psychiatric conditions such as depression, anxiety, post-traumatic stress disorder, and substance misuse are associated with sleep disturbances. Sleep disturbances often develop as a consequence or complication of a chronic or terminal condition (e.g., heart disease, dementia, cancer, renal failure). Medical conditions that cause pain such as fibromyalgia or arthritis can also disrupt sleep.

The nurse should ask the patient about work schedules, as well as cross-country and international travel. Shift work can contribute to reduced or poor-quality sleep. Work-related effects of poor sleep may include poor performance, decreased productivity, and job absenteeism.

NURSING DIAGNOSES

Specific nursing diagnoses related to sleep include *insomnia, sleep deprivation, disturbed sleep pattern,* and *readiness for enhanced sleep.*

NURSING IMPLEMENTATION

Nursing interventions depend on the severity and duration of the sleep problem, as well as on the characteristics of the individual. Occasional difficulty getting to sleep or awakening during the night is not unusual. However, prolonged sleep disruptions become problematic.

The nurse can assume a primary role in teaching about sleep hygiene (see Table 9.4). An important component of sleep hygiene is reducing dietary intake of substances containing caffeine. To reduce caffeine intake, the patient must be aware of the content of caffeine and related stimulants such as guarana and yerba mate in certain foods and beverages (Health Canada, 2017). Table 9.7 provides examples of the caffeine content of beverages and foods. Health Canada recommends no more than 400 mg of caffeine per day for the general adult population and lower amounts for children and women of childbearing age.

Nurses are also in an ideal position to take the lead in suggesting and implementing change in patients' homes and institutional environments to enhance sleep. Reducing light and noise levels can enhance sleep. Awareness of time passing and watching the clock can add to anxieties about not falling asleep or returning to sleep.

Patients require education about sleeping medications. With the benzodiazepines and zopiclone (Imovane), the patient is taught to take the medication right before bedtime, to be prepared to get a full night's sleep of at least 6 to 8 hours, and not to plan activities the next morning that require highly skilled psychomotor coordination. The patient should also avoid eating high-fat foods that can alter drug absorption. To avoid oversedation, these medications should not be taken with alcohol or other central nervous system depressants. Although sleep hygiene education may be helpful, individuals with chronic insomnia require more in-depth training in cognitive–behavioural strategies so referral to a trained provider may be required.

Patient follow-up with regard to medications is important. The nurse should ask the patient about daytime sleepiness,

TABLE 9.7	CAFFEINE CONTENT OF SELECTED FOODS AND BEVERAGES	
Food/Beverage	**Caffeine (mg)**
Coffee, instant (237 mL)	62
Coffee, decaffeinated	2
Black tea, leaf or bag (237 mL)	47
Green tea	28
Herbal tea, all varieties	0
Citrus (most brand) cola (237 mL)	0
Cola (237 mL)	33
Root beer (most brands) (237 mL)	0
Energy drinks (Red Bull, Monster, Rock Star; 237 mL)	29
Hot chocolate (237 mL)	5

Source: Mayo Clinic. (2017). *Caffeine content for coffee, tea, soda and more.* www.mayoclinic.org/healthy-lifestyle/nutrition-and-healthy-eating/in-depth/caffeine/art-20049372.

nightmares, and any difficulties in activities of daily living. For patients who have been taking sleeping medications for a period of time, withdrawal of the medication should be tapered.

Narcolepsy

Narcolepsy is a chronic degenerative neurological disorder caused by the brain's inability to regulate sleep–wake cycles normally. The onset of narcolepsy typically occurs in adolescence (Mahoney et al., 2019). There are two categories of narcolepsy: type 1 and type 2. With both types of narcolepsy, people experience excessive daytime sleepiness despite adequate sleep. Affected individuals fall asleep for periods lasting from a few seconds to several minutes (Bassetti et al., 2019). In significant contrast to people with other sleep disorders, people with narcolepsy awaken refreshed from sleep but become sleepy in a few hours. This excessive sleepiness interferes with sedentary activities and is accompanied by cognitive impairments in attention and working memory (Mahoney et al., 2019).

Narcolepsy type 1 is characterized by episodes of cataplexy, which is a brief and sudden loss of skeletal muscle tone or muscle weakness. Its manifestations range from a brief episode of muscle weakness to complete postural collapse and falling to the ground. Laughter, anger, or surprise often triggers episodes. Patients with narcolepsy, particularly those with cataplexy, have decreased quality of life because of excessive daytime sleepiness.

Narcolepsy type 2, also known as *secondary narcolepsy*, is characterized by episodes without cataplexy and can result from injury to the hypothalamus. Patients often experience excessive daytime sleepiness without muscle weakness triggered by (National Institute of Neurological Disorders and Stroke [NINDS], 2020). Symptoms are typically less severe than in type 1 and hypocretin hormone levels are normal. Other common symptoms of narcolepsy are listed in Table 9.8.

Etiology and Pathophysiology. Type 1 narcolepsy is caused by a loss of hypothalamic neurons that produce orexin (discussed earlier in the chapter [Mahoney et al., 2019]). The cause of type 2 narcolepsy is thought to be similar but remains unknown.

Diagnostic Studies. Narcolepsy is diagnosed on the basis of a history of sleepiness, PSG findings, and daytime *multiple sleep latency tests* (MSLTs). MSLTs are sleep studies in which the patient is encouraged to fall asleep every 2 hours during the day

TABLE 9.8   COMMON SYMPTOMS OF NARCOLEPSY

Sleep paralysis: a temporary (few seconds to minutes) paralysis of skeletal muscles (except respiratory and extraocular muscles) that occurs in the transition from REM sleep to waking.
Fragmented nighttime sleep
Altered REM sleep regulation (including daytime episodes of REM while awake)
Hypnagogic hallucinations (brief hallucinations that occur at the onset of sleep)
Other sleep disorders such as periodic limb movement disorders, obstructive sleep apnea, REM sleep behaviour disorder
Weight gain
Depression
Anxiety
Chronic pain
Autonomic dysregulation

REM, rapid eye movement.
Sources: Based on Cook, N. (2013). Understanding narcolepsy: the wider perspective. *British Journal of Neuroscience Nursing*, 9(2), 76–82; and Scammell, T. E. (2015). Narcolepsy. *New England Journal of Medicine, 373*(27), 2654–2662. https://doi.org/10.1056/NEJMra1500587.

for approximately 20 minutes. Short sleep latencies and onset of REM sleep in more than two MSLTs are diagnostic signs of narcolepsy.

Interprofessional Care

Medication Therapy. Narcolepsy cannot be cured. But excessive daytime sleepiness and cataplexy, the most disabling symptoms of the disorder, can be controlled with medication treatment in most affected patients. Pharmacological management of narcolepsy includes amphetamine-like stimulants to relieve excessive daytime sleepiness and tricyclic antidepressant medication therapy to control cataplexy (Szabo et al., 2019). Sodium oxybate is sometimes used at night to produce a deep NREM sleep that over time reduces both daytime sleepiness and cataplexy. Because of the significant risk of adverse reactions, this is used only for moderate to severe symptoms of sleepiness and cataplexy.

Behavioural Therapy. None of the current pharmacological therapies cures narcolepsy or allows patients to consistently maintain a full, normal state of alertness. As a result, medication therapy is combined with various behavioural strategies similar to those used for insomnia (discussed earlier in this chapter).

Safety precautions, especially in driving, are crucial for patients with narcolepsy. Excessive daytime sleepiness and cataplexy can result in serious injury or death if not treated. Individuals with untreated narcolepsy symptoms are involved in automobile accidents approximately five times more frequently than is the general population.

Patient support groups are also useful for many patients with narcolepsy and their family members. Social isolation can occur because of symptoms. Patients with narcolepsy can be stigmatized as being lazy and unproductive because of lack of public and professional understanding about this disorder.

Circadian Rhythm Sleep–Wake Disorders

Circadian rhythm sleep–wake disorders (CRSWDs) are characterized by a disruption in the timing of sleep (Gros & Videnovic, 2020). This occurs because of lack of synchrony between the circadian time-keeping system and the environment, which disrupts the sleep–wake cycle. Delayed sleep phase disorder (DSPD) is the most common CRSWD. With

this disorder, people have difficulty falling asleep (staying awake until 0100–0300 hours) and typically sleep later into the morning (waking between 1000 and 1200 hours). Because most people need to get up in the morning for school or work or care responsibilities, chronic sleep restriction and daytime sleepiness result. Typically, DSPD begins in adolescence when there is a normal shift in the sleep–wake drives that then continues into adulthood (Nesbitt, 2018). Attentional and mood-related issues can result from the chronic sleep restriction and be overlooked as inherent traits. The altered sensitivity of the circadian system is thought to be genetic in origin. People with this disorder are at risk for health sequelae of chronic sleep restriction (see the section Effects of Sleep Deprivation earlier in the chapter).

Shift work disorder is another type of CRSWD and is discussed in the section Special Sleep Needs of Nurses later in the chapter.

Sleep-Disordered Breathing

The term sleep-disordered breathing indicates abnormal respiratory patterns associated with sleep. These include snoring, apnea, and hypopnea, characterized by increased respiratory effort that leads to frequent arousals. Sleep-disordered breathing results in frequent sleep disruptions and alterations in sleep architecture. Obstructive sleep apnea is the sleep-disordered breathing problem most commonly diagnosed.

Obstructive Sleep Apnea. Obstructive sleep apnea (OSA), also called *obstructive sleep apnea–hypopnea syndrome,* is characterized by partial or complete obstruction of the upper airway during sleep. *Apnea* is the cessation of spontaneous respirations that lasts longer than 10 seconds. *Hypopnea* is a condition characterized by shallow (30%–90% reduction in airflow) respirations. Airflow obstruction occurs because of narrowing of the air passages with relaxation of muscle tone during sleep, which leads to apnea and hypopnea, or when the tongue and the soft palate fall backward and partially or completely obstruct the pharynx (Figure 9.4).

Each obstruction may last from 10 to 90 seconds. During the apneic period, the patient can experience *hypoxemia* (decreased partial pressure of arterial oxygen or partial oxygen saturation) and *hypercapnia* (increased partial pressure of arterial carbon dioxide). These changes are ventilatory stimulants and cause brief arousals, but the patient may not fully awaken. The patient has a generalized startle response, snorts, and gasps, which cause the tongue and soft palate to move forward and the airway to open. Apnea and arousal cycles occur repeatedly, throughout the night.

Sleep apnea affects 6.4% of Canadians (Statistics Canada, 2018). The risk increases with obesity (BMI >35 kg/m²), age older than 50 years, neck circumference greater than 43 cm (17 inches), craniofacial abnormalities that affect the upper airway, and acromegaly. People who smoke are more likely to have OSA than are those who do not smoke. OSA is twice as common in men as in women until after menopause, when the prevalence is similar.

The STOP-BANG (**s**nore, **t**ired, **o**bstruction, **p**ressure–BMI, **a**ge, **n**eck, **g**ender) questionnaire summarizes the key risk factors and is increasingly used as a quick and reliable screening tool for OSA (Chung et al., 2016) (Table 9.9). In the BANG portion, the more questions that a patient answers "yes," the greater is the patient's risk of having moderate to severe OSA.

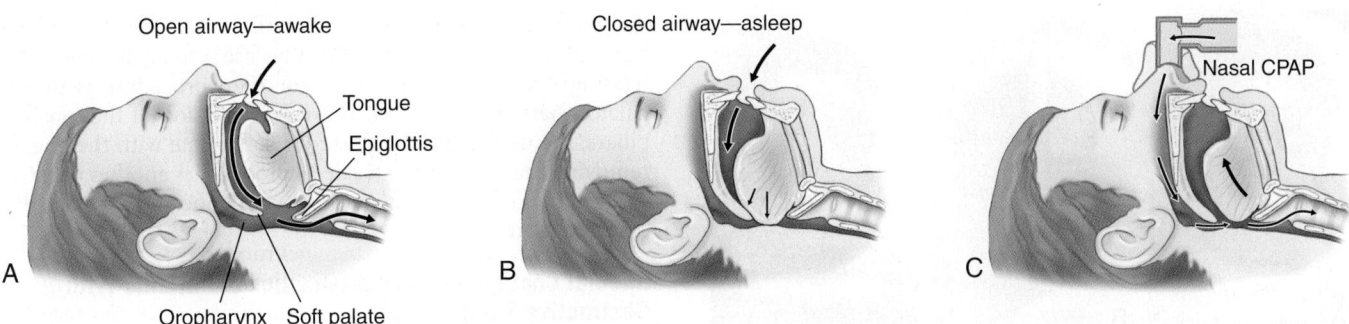

FIG. 9.4 How sleep apnea occurs. **A,** The patient predisposed to obstructive sleep apnea (OSA) has a small pharyngeal airway. **B,** During sleep, the pharyngeal muscles relax, allowing the airway to close. Lack of airflow results in repeated apneic episodes. **C,** With continuous positive airway pressure (CPAP), the airway is splinted open, which prevents airflow obstruction. Source: Modified from LaFleur Brooks, M. (2012). Exploring medical language: A student-directed approach (8th ed.). Mosby.

TABLE 9.9   STOP-BANG

STOP

S (Snore): Have you ever been told that you snore?	Yes	No
T (Tired): Are you often tired during the day?	Yes	No
O (Obstruction): Do you know if you stop breathing, or has anyone witnessed you stop breathing while you are asleep?	Yes	No
P (Pressure): Do you have high blood pressure, or are you on medication to control high blood pressure?	Yes	No

If the person answers "yes" to two or more of the STOP questions, they are at risk for OSA and should contact their primary care provider. The second component of this questionnaire (BANG) provides risk assessment of moderate to severe risk of OSA.

BANG

B (BMI): Is your body mass index (BMI) greater than 28?	Yes	No
A (Age): Are you 50 years or older?	Yes	No
N (Neck): Are you a male with a neck circumference greater than 43 cm or a female with a neck circumference greater than 41 cm?	Yes	No
G (Gender): Are you a male?	Yes	No

OSA, obstructive sleep apnea.
Source: Chung, F., Yegneswaran, B., Liao, P., et al. (2008). STOP questionnaire: A tool to screen patients for obstructive sleep apnea. *Anesthesiology, 108,* 812–821. https://doi.org/10.1097/ALN.0b013e31816d83e4.

Clinical Manifestations and Diagnostic Studies. Clinical manifestations of sleep apnea include frequent arousals during sleep, insomnia, excessive daytime sleepiness, and witnessed apneic episodes. The patient's bed partner may complain about the patient's loud snoring. Other symptoms include morning headaches (from hypercapnia or increased blood pressure that causes vasodilation of cerebral blood vessels), personality changes, and irritability. Women with OSA have higher rates of mortality from the disorder than do men. Hypoxemia associated with OSA is worse in patients with chronic obstructive pulmonary disease (COPD) than in those without COPD.

Complications that can result from untreated sleep apnea include hypertension, right-sided heart failure from pulmonary hypertension caused by chronic nocturnal hypoxemia, and cardiac dysrhythmias, and the risk for stroke is increased. Symptoms of sleep apnea alter many aspects of the patient's life. If problems are identified, appropriate referrals need to be made. Cessation of breathing reported by the bed partner is usually a source of great anxiety because of the fear that breathing may not resume.

Assessment of the patient with OSA includes thorough documentation of sleep and medical histories. The previously mentioned clinical manifestations of OSA should be assessed, as should less obvious symptoms, which may include cardiovascular symptoms, muscle pain, and mood changes.

A diagnosis of sleep apnea is made on the basis of PSG findings. This diagnosis requires documentation of apneic events (no airflow with respiratory effort) or hypopnea (airflow diminished 30% to 50% with respiratory effort) of at least 10 seconds' duration. OSA is defined as more than five apnea/hypopnea events per hour accompanied by a 3% to 4% decrease in oxygen saturation. In severe cases of apnea, apneic events may number more than 30 to 50 per hour of sleep. Typically, PSG studies are performed in a sleep laboratory with technicians monitoring the patient. In some instances, portable sleep studies are conducted in the home setting (see the Informatics in Practice box on sleep apnea diagnosis and monitoring). Overnight pulse oximetry assessment may be an alternative to determine whether nocturnal oxygen supplementation is indicated.

INFORMATICS IN PRACTICE
Sleep Apnea Diagnosis and Monitoring

- Home respiratory monitoring is a cost-effective alternative for diagnosing sleep-related breathing disorders that allows some patients the convenience of sleeping in their own home.
- Home respiratory monitoring is used as part of a comprehensive sleep evaluation and in patients likely to have moderate to severe obstructive sleep apnea but who do not have heart failure, obstructive lung disease, or neuromuscular disease.
- Home respiratory monitoring is used to monitor the effectiveness of non-CPAP therapies for patients with sleep-related breathing disorders.
- Wireless monitors can detect changes in vital signs and pulse oximetry, raising an alarm if values fall outside of set parameters.
- A patient may benefit from telehealth to diagnose and monitor for sleep apnea in the home.

CPAP, continuous positive airway pressure.

NURSING AND INTERPROFESSIONAL MANAGEMENT
SLEEP APNEA

Mild sleep apnea (5 to 10 apneic/hypopneic events per hour) may respond to simple measures. Conservative treatment at home begins with simply sleeping on the side rather than on the back. The patient is instructed to avoid sedatives and consuming

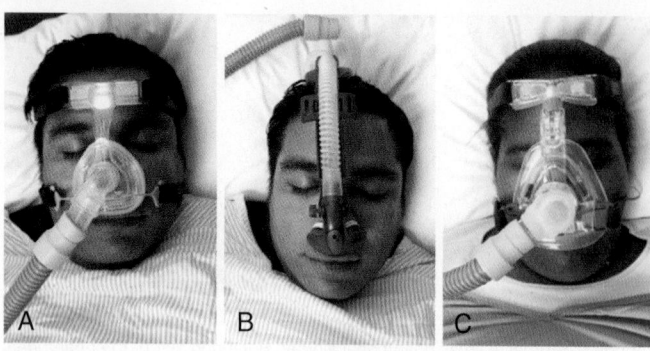

FIG. 9.5 Examples of positive airwave pressure devices for sleep apnea. **A,** Patient wearing a nasal mask and headgear (positive pressure only to nose). **B,** Patient wearing nasal pillows (positive pressure only to nose). **C,** Patient wearing a full face mask (positive pressure to both nose and mouth). Source: Goldman, I., & Schafer, A. I. (2012). *Goldman's Cecil medicine* (24th ed.). Saunders.

alcoholic beverages for 3 to 4 hours before sleep. Sleep medications often make OSA worse. Because excessive weight worsens and weight loss reduces sleep apnea, referral to a weight loss program may be indicated. Bariatric surgery reduces incidence of OSA (Peromaa-Haavisto et al., 2017). It is essential to instruct the patient on the dangers of driving or using heavy equipment as insomnia is commonly experienced by individuals with OSA.

Symptoms may resolve in up to half of patients with OSA who use a special mouth guard, also called an *oral appliance,* during sleep to prevent airflow obstruction. Oral appliances bring the mandible and tongue forward to enlarge the airway space, thereby preventing airway occlusion. Some individuals find beneficial a support group in which concerns and feelings can be expressed and strategies for resolving problems can be discussed.

In patients with more severe symptoms (>15 apneic/hypopneic events per hour), **continuous positive airway pressure (CPAP)** by mask is the treatment of choice. With CPAP, the patient applies a nasal mask that is attached to a high-flow blower (Figure 9.5). The blower is adjusted to maintain sufficient positive pressure (5 to 25 cm H_2O) in the airway during inspiration and expiration to prevent airway collapse. Some patients cannot adjust to wearing a mask over the nose or mouth or to exhaling against the high pressure. With a technologically more sophisticated therapy, bilevel positive airway pressure (BiPAP), a higher inspiration pressure and a lower pressure during expiration can be delivered. With BiPAP, the apnea can be relieved with a lower mean pressure and may be better tolerated.

CPAP is highly effective in reducing apnea, daytime sleepiness, and fatigue. It improves perceived quality of life and returns cognitive functioning to normal. Benefits of CPAP are dose dependent based on how long the device is used at night. It must be used a minimum of 4 hours each night to reduce or reverse the negative cardiovascular effects of OSA (Abuzaid et al., 2017). Approximately two-thirds of patients using CPAP report adverse effects such as nasal stuffiness. Regular cleaning of the mask, tubing, and water chamber should be performed daily with liquid dish soap and hot water or a commercially available CPAP sanitizer.

Surgical Interventions

Tonsillectomy (removal of tonsillar glands) is used if a patient with OSA has large tonsils. If other measures fail, surgical interventions may be attempted to help manage the airway. Patients are carefully selected for these surgeries, inasmuch as there has been no conclusive evidence that they are actually beneficial for treating sleep apnea. The most common procedure is uvulo-palato-pharyngoplasty, which involves excision of the tonsillar pillars, the uvula, and the posterior soft palate with the goal of removing the obstructing tissue. Septoplasty is another effective surgical procedure which straighten the bone and cartilage of a deviated septum.

Special Concerns for Hospitalization of Patients With Obstructive Sleep Apnea

CPAP treatment should be maintained throughout a hospitalization stay. When patients with a history of OSA are hospitalized, health care staff must be aware that the administration of opioid analgesics and sedating medications (benzodiazepines, barbiturates, hypnotics) may worsen OSA symptoms by depressing respiration. This will necessitate that the patient wear the CPAP or BiPAP mask when resting or sleeping (Marshansky et al., 2018).

Perioperative concerns include an increased risk for difficult endotracheal intubation and a need for increased monitoring during the postoperative period. In patients with sleep-disordered breathing, OSA may be exacerbated in the postoperative period in relation to medications they receive during anaesthesia. All patients with OSA should be monitored for pulse oximetry after surgery, and those at increased risk for cardiac events should also receive cardiac monitoring postoperatively.

Sleep Movement Disorders

In sleep movement disorders, involuntary movement during sleep disrupts sleep and leads to daytime sleepiness. *Periodic limb movement disorder (PLMD)* is a type of sleep movement disorder characterized by involuntary, periodic movement of the legs, arms, or both that affects people only during sleep. Sometimes abdominal, oral, and nasal movement accompanies PLMD. Movements typically occur for 0.5 to 10 seconds, in intervals separated by 5 to 90 seconds. PLMD causes poor-quality sleep, which may lead to sleep maintenance insomnia, excessive daytime sleepiness, or both. PLMD and restless legs syndrome often occur simultaneously, but they are distinct disorders. (Restless legs syndrome is discussed in Chapter 61.)

PLMD is diagnosed on the basis of a detailed history from the patient or bed partner, or both, and PSG findings. PLMD is treated by medications aimed at reducing or eliminating the limb movements or the arousals. Dopaminergic medications (pramipexole [Mirapex] and ropinirole [Requip]) are preferred.

Parasomnias. Parasomnias are defined as unusual and often undesirable behaviours that occur during sleep or during arousal from sleep. They can include abnormal movements and dream-related behaviours, emotions, and perceptions. They are divided into three clusters: NREM, REM, and "other."

Rapid Eye Movement Parasomnias. Parasomnias that occur during REM sleep include REM sleep behaviour disorder, nightmare disorder, and recurrent isolated sleep paralysis (Stefani, 2019). Parasomnias may result in fragmented sleep and fatigue. *Nightmare disorder* is a parasomnia characterized by recurrent awakening with recall of the frightful or disturbing dream. *Nightmares* are extended dysphoric dreams that usually involve efforts to avoid threats to survival, security, or physical integrity (Thorpy, 2017). These normally occur during the final third of sleep and in association with REM sleep. In critically ill patients, nightmares are common and likely due to medications.

Drug classes most likely to cause nightmares are sedative–hypnotics, β-adrenergic antagonists, dopamine agonists, and amphetamines.

Treatments for nightmare disorder include psychological interventions such as imagery rehearsal therapy and exposure treatment. Nabilone (a synthetic cannabinoid) has shown promise in people experiencing nightmares related to post-traumatic stress disorder (Babson et al., 2017).

Non–Rapid Eye Movement Parasomnias. NREM parasomnias include sleepwalking, sleep terrors, sleep-related eating disorder, and confusional arousal. *Sleepwalking* behaviours can range from sitting up in bed, moving objects, walking around the room, to driving a car. During a sleepwalking event, the affected individual does not speak and may have limited or no awareness of the event. On awakening, the individual does not remember the event. In the CCU, a parasomnia may be misinterpreted as CCU psychosis. In addition, sedated CCU patients can exhibit manifestations of an NREM parasomnia.

Sleep terrors (night terrors) are characterized by a sudden awakening from sleep along with a loud cry and signs of panic. There is an intense autonomic response, including increased heart rate, increased respiration, and diaphoresis. Factors in the CCU such as sleep disruption and deprivation, fever, stress (physical or emotional), and exposure to noise and light can contribute to sleep terrors.

AGE-RELATED CONSIDERATIONS

Sleep

Sleep, like many physiological functions, changes as people age. Even with healthy aging, there are expected changes in sleep patterns, including a decrease in the amount of deep sleep, overall shorter total sleep time at night, decreased sleep efficiency, more awakenings, and increased napping (Christie et al., 2016). Sleep requirements for older persons are 7 to 8 hours per 24-hour cycle (Centers for Disease Control and Prevention, 2017).

Despite these expected changes, the incidence of sleep disturbances and disorders is also increased in older persons (Figure 9.6). Insomnia, OSA, restless leg syndrome, and PLMD in particular are increased in prevalence among older persons, especially among Indigenous people of Canada (Gulia & Kumar, 2018; Yiallourou et al., 2019).

A key issue is that multiple factors impair the ability of older persons to obtain quality sleep. Chronic conditions that are more common in older persons—including COPD, diabetes, dementia, chronic pain, and cancer—can affect sleep quality and increase the prevalence of insomnia (Gulia & Kumar, 2018). Prescribed and OTC medications used to treat these conditions can contribute to sleep problems. Daily stress and poor social support have also been linked to insomnia in older persons.

Insomnia may have detrimental effects on cognitive function in healthy older persons. Chronic disturbed sleep in an older person can result in disorientation, delirium, impairment of intellect, disturbances in cognition, and increased risk of accidents and injury (see precipitating factors for delirium in Chapter 62).

Getting out of bed during the night to use the bathroom increases the risk for falls. Older persons may use OTC medications or alcohol as a sleep aid (see Chapter 11), which can further increase the risk of falls at night.

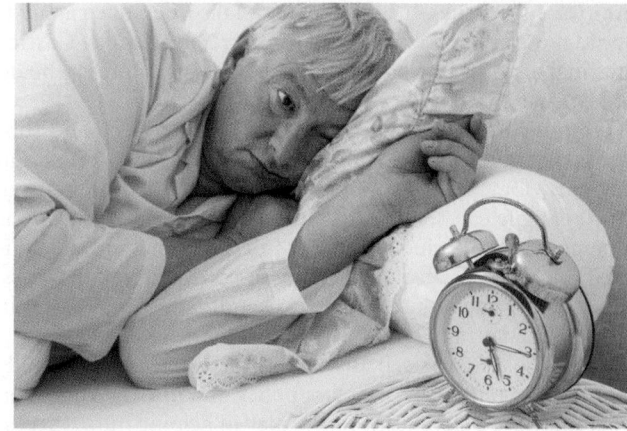

FIG. 9.6 Many older people have sleep difficulties. Source: iStock.com/Studio-Annika.

Because many older persons may not tell their health care providers about their sleep problems, a sleeping assessment (see Table 9.6) can be used to detect sleep disturbances. Napping during the day should not be considered problematic unless the person is reporting insomnia or excessive daytime sleepiness. In the case of insomnia, daytime napping should be restricted. Screening for sleep disorders is important because of their higher prevalence among older persons. Sleep hygiene education and CBT-i are useful interventions for insomnia in older persons. Pharmacological therapies are more challenging for older persons. Whenever possible, long-acting benzodiazepines should be avoided. Older persons receiving benzodiazepines are at increased risk for daytime sedation, falls, and cognitive and psychomotor impairment (see Chapter 62). They also have increased sensitivity to hypnotic and sedative medications. For this reason, medication therapies for sleep disturbances are started at low doses and monitored carefully. Hypnotic drugs should be used for as brief a period as possible, in most cases not exceeding 2 to 3 weeks of treatment.

SPECIAL SLEEP NEEDS OF NURSES

Nursing is one of several professions that necessitate night shift and rotating shift schedules. In many acute-care and long-term care settings, nurses volunteer or are asked to work a variety of day and night shifts, often alternating and rotating them. Unfortunately, many nurses who do shift work report less job satisfaction and more job-related stress (Tahghighi, 2017) than those who do not.

Nurses on permanent night or rapidly rotating shifts are at increased risk of experiencing shift work sleep disorder, characterized by insomnia, sleepiness, and fatigue. Nurses on rotating shifts get the least amount of sleep. With repeated periods of inadequate sleep, the sleep debt grows. Poor sleep is the strongest predictor of chronic fatigue in nurses doing shift work. As a result, rotating and night shift schedules pose specific challenges for the individual nurse's health and for patients' safety.

Shift work alters the synchrony between circadian rhythms and the environment, which leads to sleep disruption. Nurses working the night shift are often too sleepy to be fully alert at work and too alert to sleep soundly the next day. Sustained alterations in circadian rhythms such as that imposed by rotating shift work have been linked to negative health outcomes, including increased risk of morbidity and mortality in association with cardiovascular issues. In addition, mood disorders such as anxiety are more severe in nurses who work rotating shifts. Gastrointestinal disturbances are also more common in nurses who do shift work than in those who do not.

From a patient safety perspective, disturbed sleep and subsequent fatigue can make for a workplace hazard (errors and accidents) for nurses, as well as for their patients (Thompson, 2019). Fatigue can result in diminished memory or distortions in perceptual skills, judgement, and decision-making capabilities. Lack of sleep affects the ability to cope and handle stress. Subsequently, the reduced ability to handle stress may result in physical, mental, and emotional exhaustion.

The problem of sleep disruption is one that is critically important in nursing. Workplace policy and nursing education programs have a significant role to play in helping nurses access strategies to ensure adequate sleep. Several strategies may help reduce the distress associated with rotating shift work. These include brief scheduled periods of on-site napping. Napping during shift has been found to improve recovery time from night shift and to enhance safety on the job of shift workers. Maintaining a consistent sleep–wake schedule even on days off is optimal but perhaps unrealistic. For night shift work, scheduling the sleep period for just before going to work increases alertness and vigilance, improves reaction times, and decreases accidents during night shift work. It is important that nurses self-manage the effect of sleep disruption through the use of sleep hygiene practice. Sleep hygiene skills and self-care practices could be considered as required learning for nursing students because sleep quality has been found to decrease as nurses transition from school to workplace (James et al., 2019).

CASE STUDY

Insomnia

Patient Profile
D. P., 49 years old (pronouns she/her), is seen in the preoperative clinic. D. P. is scheduled for a right shoulder (rotator cuff) repair. She tore her rotator cuff while playing tennis 1 year ago. It is no longer painful, but her range of motion is limited. During the preoperative screening, D. P. reports chronic fatigue. She is postmenopausal, according to her self-report. In the past year, since the end of her periods, D. P. has experienced daily hot flashes and sleep problems. She denies any other health problems. On a usual workday, D. P. drinks two cups of hot tea and one can of diet cola. Currently, she is taking OTC diphenhydramine for sleep. Her partner, who has accompanied her to the clinic, states that D. P.'s snoring has gotten worse and is interfering with his sleep.

Subjective Data
- Reports hot flashes and nighttime sweating
- Reports daytime tiredness and fatigue
- States trouble with getting to sleep and staying asleep

Objective Data
Physical Examination
- Laboratory evaluations within normal limits
- Overweight (20% over ideal body weight for height)
- Blood pressure (BP): 155/92 mm Hg
- Limited lateral and posterior rotation of right shoulder

Diagnostic Studies
- Nighttime polysomnography study reveals episodes of obstructive sleep apnea

Interprofessional Care
- Continuous positive airway pressure (CPAP) nightly
- Referred for weight reduction counselling

Discussion Questions
1. What are D. P.'s risk factors for sleep apnea?
2. What specific sleep hygiene practices could D. P. use to improve the quality of her sleep?
3. How does CPAP work?
4. What are the potential health risks associated with sleep apnea?
5. **Priority decision:** According to the assessment data provided, what are the priority nursing diagnoses? Are there any interprofessional problems?
6. **Priority decision:** For the day of surgery, what are the priority nursing interventions for D. P.?

ℰvolve
Answers are available at http://evolve.elsevier.com/Canada/Lewis/medsurg.

REVIEW QUESTIONS

The number of the question corresponds to the same-numbered outcome at the beginning of the chapter.

1. Sleep is *best* described as a
   a. Loosely organized state similar to coma
   b. State in which pain sensitivity decreases
   c. Quiet state in which there is little brain activity
   d. State in which an individual lacks conscious awareness of the environment

2. Which statement is true regarding rapid eye movement (REM) sleep? *(Select all that apply.)*
   a. The EEG pattern is quiescent.
   b. Muscle tone is greatly reduced.
   c. It only occurs once in the night.
   d. It is separated by distinct physiological stages.
   e. The most vivid dreaming occurs during this phase.

3. Sleep loss is associated with which of the following symptoms? *(Select all that apply.)*
   a. Increased body mass index
   b. Increased insulin resistance
   c. Enhanced cognitive functioning
   d. Increased immune responsiveness

4. Which of the following points should the nurse emphasize when providing education to the client with insomnia?
   a. The importance of daytime naps
   b. The need to exercise before bedtime
   c. The need for long-term use of hypnotics
   d. Avoidance of caffeine-containing beverages before bedtime

5. A client with sleep apnea would like to avoid using a nasal CPAP device if possible. Which of the following suggestions should the nurse make to help him reach his goal?
   a. Lose excess weight.
   b. Take a nap during the day.
   c. Eat a high-protein snack at bedtime.
   d. Use mild sedatives or alcohol at bedtime.
6. A client on the surgical unit has a history of parasomnia (sleepwalking). Which of the following is true with regard to parasomnia?
   a. Hypnotic medications reduce the risk of sleepwalking.
   b. The client is often unaware of the activity on awakening.
   c. The client should be restrained at night to prevent personal harm.
   d. The potential for sleepwalking is reduced by exercise before sleep.

7. Which of the following strategies would reduce sleepiness during nighttime work?
   a. Exercising before work
   b. Sleeping for at least 2 hours before work time
   c. Taking melatonin before working the night shift
   d. Walking for 10 minutes every 4 hours during the night shift

1. d; 2. b, c; 3. a; 4. d; 5. a; 6. b; 7. b.

Ⓔvolve

For even more review questions, visit http://evolve.elsevier.com/Canada/Lewis/medsurg.

REFERENCES

Abuzaid, A. S., Al Ashry, H. S., Elbadawi, A., et al. (2017). Meta-analysis of cardiovascular outcomes with continuous positive airway pressure therapy in patients with obstructive sleep apnea. *American Journal of Cardiology, 120*(4), 693–699. https://doi.org/10.1016/j.amjcard.2017.05.042

Asnis, G. M., Thomas, M., & Henderson, M. A. (2016). Pharmacotherapy treatment options for insomnia: a primer for clinicians. *International journal of molecular sciences, 17*(1), 50. https://doi.org/10.3390/ijms17010050

Babson, K., Sottile, J., & Morabito, D. (2017). Cannabis, cannabinoids, and sleep: A review of the literature. *Current Psychiatry Reports, 19*(4), 23. https://doi.org/10.1007/s11920-017-0775-9

Bassetti, C., Adamantidis, A., Burdakov, D., et al. (2019). Narcolepsy—clinical spectrum, aetiopathophysiology, diagnosis and treatment. *Nature Reviews Neurology, 15*, 519–539. https://doi.org/10.1038/s41582-019-0226-9

Berry, R. B., Albertario, C. L., Harding, S. M., et al. (2017). The American Academy of Sleep Medicine: The AASM scoring manual updates for 2017 (version 2.4). *Journal of Clinical Sleep Medicine, 13*(5), 655–666. https://doi.org/10.5664/jcsm.6576

Bollu, P., & Kaur, H. (2019). Sleep medicine: insomnia and sleep. *Missouri Medicine, 116*(1), 68–75.

Canadian Geriatrics Society. (2019). *Choosing wisely Canada.* https://choosingwiselycanada.org/geriatrics/

Centers for Disease Control and Prevention. (2017). *How much sleep do I need?.* https://www.cdc.gov/sleep/about_sleep/how_much_sleep.html

Chaput, J. P., Wong, S. L., & Michaud, I. (2017). *Duration and quality of sleep among Canadians aged 18 to 79.* https://www150.statcan.gc.ca/n1/pub/82-003-x/2017009/article/54857-eng.htm

Chattu, V., Manzar, M., Kumary, S., et al. (2018). The global problem of insufficient sleep and its serious public health implications. *Healthcare, 7*(1), 1. https://doi.org/10.3390/healthcare7010001

Chow, M., & Cao, M. (2016). The hypocretin/orexin system in sleep disorders: preclinical insights and clinical progress. *Nature and Science of Sleep, 8*, 81–86. https://doi.org/10.2147/NSS.S76711

Christie, A. D., Seery, E., & Kent, J. A. (2016). Physical activity, sleep quality, and self-reported fatigue across the adult lifespan. *Experiential Gerontology, 77*, 7–11. https://doi.org/10.1016/j.exger.2016.02.001

Chung, F., Abdullah, H., & Liao, P. (2016). STOP-BANG Questionnaire: A practical approach to screen for obstructive sleep apnea. *Chest, 149*(3), 631–638. https://doi.org/10.1378/chest.15-0903

Davidson, J. R., Dawson, S., & Krsmanovic, A. (2019). Effectiveness of group cognitive behavioral therapy for insomnia (CBT-I) in a primary care setting. *Behavioral Sleep Medicine, 17*(2), 192–201. https://doi.org/10.1080/15402002.2017.1318753

Feng, F., Zhang, Y., Hou, J., et al. (2018). Can music improve sleep quality in adults with primary insomnia? A systematic review and network meta-analysis. *International Journal of Nursing Studies, 77*, 189–196. https://doi.org/10.1016/j.ijnurstu.2017.10.011

Garland, S. N., Rowe, H., Repa, L. M., et al. (2018). A decade's difference: 10-year change in insomnia symptom prevalence in Canada depends on sociodemographics and health status. *Sleep Health, 4*(2), 160–165. https://doi.org/10.1016/j.sleh.2018.01.003

Gros, P., & Videnovic, A. (2020). Overview of sleep and circadian rhythm disorders in Parkinson disease. *Clinics in Geriatric Medicine, 36*(1), 119–130. https://doi.org/10.1016/j.cger.2019.09.005

Gulia, K., & Kumar, V. (2018). Sleep disorders in the elderly: a growing challenge. *Psychogeriatrics, 18*(3), 155–165. https://doi.org/10.1111/psyg.12319

Health Canada. (2017). *Health Canada is advising Canadians about safe levels of caffeine consumption.* https://healthycanadians.gc.ca/recall-alert-rappel-avis/hc-sc/2017/63362a-eng.php

Hieu, T. H., Dibas, M., Surya Dila, K. A., et al. (2019). Therapeutic efficacy and safety of chamomile for state anxiety, generalized anxiety disorder, insomnia, and sleep quality: A systematic review and meta-analysis of randomized trials and quasi-randomized trial. *Phytotherapy research: PTR, 33*(6), 1604–1615. https://doi.org/10.1002/ptr.6349

Hirshkowitz, M., Whiton, K., Albert, S. M., et al. (2015). National Sleep Foundation's updated sleep duration recommendations. *Sleep Health, 1*(4), 233–243. https://doi.org/10.1016/j.sleh.2015.10.004

Iggena, D., Winter, Y., & Steiner, B. (2017). Melatonin restores hippocampal neural precursor cell proliferation and prevents cognitive deficits induced by jet lag simulation in adult mice. *Journal of Pineal Research, 62*(4), e12397. https://doi-org.proxy.queensu.ca/10.1111/jpi.12397

James, L., Butterfield, P., & Tuell, E. (2019). Nursing students' sleep patterns and perceptions of safe practice during their entrée to shift work. *Workplace Health & Safety, 67*(11), 547–553. https://doi.org/10.1177/2165079919867714

Javaheri, S., & Redline, S. (2017). Insomnia and risk of cardiovascular disease. *Chest, 152*(2), 435–444. https://doi.org/10.1016/j.chest.2017.01.026

Locihová, H., Axmann, K., Padyšáková, H., et al. (2018). Effect of the use of earplugs and eye mask on the quality of sleep in intensive care patients: a systematic review. *Journal of Sleep Research, 27*(3), e12607. https://doi.org/10.1111/jsr.12607

Mahoney, C., Cogswell, A., Koralnik, I., et al. (2019). The neurobiological basis of narcolepsy. *Nature Reviews Neuroscience, 20*, 83–93. https://doi.org/10.1038/s41583-018-0097-x

Maich, K., Lachowski, A., & Carney, C. (2018). Psychometric properties of the consensus sleep diary in those with insomnia disorder. *Behavioral Sleep Medicine, 16*(2), 117–134. https://doi.org/10.1080/15402002.2016.1173556

Marshansky, S., Mayer, P., Rizzo, D., et al. (2018). Sleep, chronic pain, and opioid risk for apnea. *Progress in Neuro-Psychopharmacology and Biological Psychiatry, 87*(20), 234–244. https://doi.org/10.1016/j.pnpbp.2017.07.014

Matheson, E. M., & Hainer, B. L. (2017). Insomnia: pharmacologic therapy. *American Family Physician, 96*(1), 29–35

Mathias, J., Cant, M., & Burke, A. (2018). Sleep disturbances and sleep disorders in adults living with chronic pain: a meta-analysis. *Sleep Medicine Reviews, 52*, 198–210. https://doi.org/10.1016/j.sleep.2018.05.023

Murphy, Y., Wilson, E., Goldner, E., et al. (2016). Benzodiazepine use, misuse, and harm at the population level in Canada: a comprehensive narrative review of data and developments since 1995. *Clinical Drug Investigation, 36*(7), 519–530. https://doi.org/10.1007/s40261-016-0397-8

National Highway Traffic Safety Administration (NHTSA). (2020). *Drowsy Driving.* https://www.nhtsa.gov/risky-driving/drowsy-driving#2271

National Institute of Neurological Disorders and Stroke (NINDS). (2020). *Narcolepsy Fact Sheet.* https://www.ninds.nih.gov/Disorders/Patient-Caregiver-Education/Fact-Sheets/Narcolepsy-Fact-Sheet

Nesbitt, A. (2018). Delayed sleep-wake phase disorder. *Journal of Thoracic Disease, 10*(1), 103–111. https://doi.org/10.21037/jtd.2018.01.11

Ostrin, L. (2019). Ocular and systemic melatonin and the influence of light exposure. *Clinical and Experimental Optometry, 102*(2), 99–108. https://doi.org/10.1111/cxo.12824

Pavlova, M., & Latreille, V. (2019). Sleep disorders. *The American Journal of Medicine, 132*(3), 292–299. https://doi.org/10.1016/j.amjmed.2018.09.021

Peromaa-Haavisto, P., Tuomilehto, H., Kössi, J., et al. (2017). Obstructive sleep apnea: the effect of bariatric surgery after 12 months. A prospective multicenter trial. *Sleep Medicine, 35*, 85–90. https://doi.org/10.1016/j.sleep.2016.12.017

Pilcher, J., & Morris, D. (2020). Sleep and organizational behavior: implications for workplace productivity and safety. *Frontiers in Psychology, 11*(45). https://doi.org/10.3389/fpsyg.2020.00045

Public Health Agency of Canada (PHAC). (2019). *Are Canadian's adults getting enough sleep?.* https://www.canada.ca/en/public-health/services/publications/healthy-living/canadian-adults-getting-enough-sleep-infographic.html

Rash, J. A., Kavanagh, V. A., & Garland, S. N. (2019). A meta-analysis of mindfulness-based therapies for insomnia and sleep disturbance: moving towards processes of change. *Sleep medicine clinics, 14*(2), 209–233. https://doi.org/10.1016/j.jsmc.2019.01.004

Riemann, D., Baglioni, C., Bassetti, C., et al. (2017). European guideline for the diagnosis and treatment of insomnia. *Journal of Sleep Research, 26*(6), 675–700. https://doi.org/10.1111/jsr.12594

Sateia, M. J. (2014). International Classification of Sleep Disorders—Third Edition: Highlights and recommendations. *Chest, 146*(5), 1387–1394. https://doi.org/10.1378/chest.14-0970. (Seminal).

Statistics Canada. (2018). *Health Fact Sheet: Sleep Apnea in Canada, 2016 and 2017.* https://www150.statcan.gc.ca/n1/en/pub/82-625-x/2018001/article/54979-eng.pdf?st=xwDO0mKB

Stefani, A., Holzknecht, E., & Högl, B. (2019). Clinical neurophysiology of REM parasomnias. *Handbook of Clinical Neurology, 161*, 381–396. https://doi.org/10.1016/B978-0-444-64142-7.00062-X

Suh, S., Cho, N., & Zhang, J. (2018). Sex differences in insomnia: from epidemiology and etiology to intervention. *Current Psychiatry Reports, 20*(9), 69. https://doi.org/10.1007/s11920-018-0940-9

Szabo, S., Thorpy, M., Mayer, G., et al. (2019). Neurobiological and immunogenetic aspects of narcolepsy: implications for pharmacotherapy. *Sleep Medicine Reviews, 43*, 23–36. https://doi.org/10.1016/j.smrv.2018.09.006

Tahghighi, M., Rees, C. S., Brown, J. A., et al. (2017). What is the impact of shift work on the psychological functioning and resilience of nurses? An integrative review. *Journal of Advanced Nursing, 73*(9), 2065–2083. https://doi.org/10.1111/jan.13283

Thompson, B. (2019). Does work-induced fatigue accumulate across three compressed 12 hour shifts in hospital nurses and aides? *PloS One, 14*(2), e0211715. https://doi.org/10.1371/journal.pone.0211715

Thorpy, M. (2017). International classification of sleep disorders. In *Sleep Disorders Medicine* (pp. 475–484). Springer.

Wilt, T. J., MacDonald, R., Brasure, M., et al. (2016). Pharmacologic treatment of insomnia disorder: an evidence report for a clinical practice guideline by the American College of Physicians. *Annals of Internal Medicine, 165*(2), 103–112. https://doi.org/10.7326/M15-1781

Xie, Z., Chen, F., Li, W., et al. (2017). A review of sleep disorders and melatonin. *Neurological Research, 39*(6), 559–565. https://doi.org/10.1080/01616412.2017.1315864

Yiallourou, S. R., Maguire, G. P., Eades, S., et al. (2019). Sleep influences on cardio-metabolic health in Indigenous populations. *Sleep Medicine, 59*, 78–87. https://doi.org/10.1016/j.sleep.2018.10.011

Zisapel, N. (2018). New perspectives on the role of melatonin in human sleep, circadian rhythms and their regulation. *British Journal of Pharmacology, 175*(16), 3190–3199. https://doi.org/10.1111/bph.14116

RESOURCES

Canadian Lung Association: *Sleep Disordered Breathing*
https://www.lung.ca/research/sleep-disordered-breathing
Canadian Sleep Society
https://css-scs.ca

American Academy of Sleep Medicine
https://www.aasmnet.org
Better Sleep Council
https://www.bettersleep.org
Centers for Disease Control and Prevention: *Sleep and Sleep Disorders*
https://www.cdc.gov/sleep/index.html
Epworth Sleepiness Scale
https://healthysleep.med.harvard.edu/narcolepsy/diagnosing-narcolepsy/epworth-sleepiness-scale
Narcolepsy Network
https://www.narcolepsynetwork.org
Pittsburgh Sleep Quality Index
http://www.opapc.com/uploads/documents/PSQI.pdf
Sleep Foundation
https://www.sleepfoundation.org

ⓔvolve

For additional Internet resources, see the website for this book at http://evolve.elsevier.com/canada/lewis/medsurg.

Natasha Fulford
Originating US chapter by Debra Miller-Saultz

evolve WEBSITE

http://evolve.elsevier.com/Canada/Lewis/medsurg

- Review Questions (Online Only)
- Key Points
- Answer Guidelines for Case Study

- Conceptual Care Map Creator
- Student Case Study
- Pain

- Audio Glossary
- Content Updates

LEARNING OBJECTIVES

1. Define pain.
2. Describe the neural mechanisms of pain and pain modulation.
3. Differentiate between nociceptive, neuropathic, somatic, and visceral types of pain.
4. Explain the physical and psychological effects of unrelieved pain.
5. Describe the components of a comprehensive pain assessment.
6. Describe effective pain management techniques used across many professional disciplines.

7. Describe pharmacological and nonpharmacological methods of pain relief.
8. Explain the nurse's role and responsibility in pain management.
9. Discuss ethical issues related to pain and pain management.
10. Evaluate the influence of one's own knowledge, beliefs, and attitudes about pain assessment and management.

KEY TERMS

analgesic ceiling
breakthrough pain
ceiling effect
dermatomes
equianalgesic dose
modulation
neuropathic pain

nociception
nociceptive pain
pain
pain perception
patient-controlled analgesia (PCA)
physical dependence
suffering

titration
transduction
transmission
trigger point
windup

PAIN

Pain is a complex experience with sensory-discriminative, motivational–affective, and cognitive–evaluative dimensions. For many people, it is a major problem that causes suffering and reduces quality of life. Pain is one of the major reasons that people seek health care, and effective pain relief is a basic human right (Canadian Pain Task Force, 2019). A thorough understanding of the multiple dimensions of pain is important for effective assessment and management of patients with pain. Nurses have a central role in pain assessment and management. Components of the nursing role include (a) assessing pain and documenting and communicating this information to other health care providers, (b) ensuring delivery of effective pain relief measures, (c) evaluating the effectiveness of these

interventions, (d) monitoring ongoing effectiveness of pain management strategies, and (e) providing education to patients and their families regarding pain management approaches and possible adverse effects. This chapter presents current knowledge about pain and pain management to enable the nurse to assess and manage pain successfully in collaboration with other health care providers.

MAGNITUDE OF THE PAIN PROBLEM

Unrelieved, persistent pain is an epidemic in Canada and the United States. More than 50 million people are affected with musculoskeletal pain, such as back pain and arthritis, that goes unrelieved for 5 years or more (Gaskin & Richard, 2012). In Canada, pain is one of the four most common causes of disability among working-age adults aged 25–64 years. The Canadian Survey on Disability (2017) indicates that pain-related disabilities affect over 4 million Canadians and account for 15% of the total of disabilities in Canada (Clouter et al., 2018). In Canada, 17% of women and 12% of men have a pain-related disability (Clouter et al., 2018). The global prevalence of pain has a major negative economic impact, with estimated annual values of lost productivity ranging from $297.4 billion to $335.5 billion (2010 US dollars). These values include days of work missed (ranging from $11.6 to $12.7 billion), hours of work lost ($95.2 to $96.5 billion), and reduction in wages ($190.6 billion to $226.3 billion) (Institutes of Medicine, 2011). The direct and indirect costs of chronic pain in Canada are estimated to be $60 billion per year (Canadian Pain Task Force, 2019). In Canada, 36% of unemployed Canadians with a pain-related disability have employment potential (Clouter et al., 2018).

Unfortunately, cumulative evidence indicates that, across the lifespan, people in a variety of settings continue to experience considerable acute and persistent pain despite the availability of treatment options (Choinière et al., 2014; McGillion & Watt-Watson, 2015). It has been reported that Indigenous children experience a higher number of pain occurrences than non-Indigenous children (Latimer et al., 2018). Despite management standards and directives from nongovernmental organizations such as the Canadian Pain Society (CPS) and the Registered Nurses' Association of Ontario (RNAO), more than four decades' worth of evidence documents inadequate pain management practices as the norm across health care settings and patient populations. For example, alarming numbers of Canadians are still left in pain after surgery, even in top hospitals. Evidence suggests that up to 50% of patients report pain in the moderate-to-severe range following surgical procedures (Huang et al., 2016).

The prevalence of chronic pain increases with age, with estimates of as many as 65% of community-dwelling older persons and up to 80% of older people in long-term care facilities experiencing chronic pain. Chronic pain in these populations is underrecognized and undertreated. People living with cancer—whether the disease is newly diagnosed, is being actively treated, or is in a more advanced stage—also consistently receive inadequate pain treatment. The prevalence of moderate to severe pain among people with metastatic disease is 66% and 51%, respectively, of all cancer patients, regardless of cancer type and stage (Asthana et al., 2019). It is important to note that Indigenous populations in Canada have the highest prevalence of chronic pain (Canadian Pain Task Force, 2019). Consequences of untreated pain include unnecessary suffering, physical dysfunction, psychosocial distress (which manifests in such forms as anxiety or depression), impairment in recovery from acute illness and surgery, immunosuppression, and sleep disturbances.

In the acutely ill patient, unrelieved pain can result in increased morbidity as a result of respiratory dysfunction, increased heart rate and cardiac workload, increased muscular contraction and spasm, decreased gastrointestinal (GI) motility, and increased catabolism (Table 10.1). Screening for the presence of pain is recommended as an institutional priority. In general, pain should be assessed—in all clinical care settings for all patients—at least once per day (RNAO, 2013).

When left untreated, acute pain can also progress to persistent pain. Common surgical procedures have resulted in

TABLE 10.1	CONSEQUENCES OF UNRELIEVED PAIN	
System	**Responses**
Endocrine	↑ Adrenocorticotrophic hormone (ACTH), ↑ cortisol, ↑ antidiuretic hormone (ADH), ↑ epinephrine, ↑ norepinephrine, ↑ growth hormone, ↑ renin, ↑ aldosterone levels; ↓ insulin, ↓ testosterone levels
Metabolic	Gluconeogenesis, glycogenolysis, hyperglycemia, glucose intolerance, insulin resistance, muscle protein catabolism, ↑ lipolysis
Cardiovascular	↑ Heart rate, ↑ cardiac output, ↑ peripheral vascular resistance, hypertension, ↑ myocardial oxygen consumption, ↑ coagulation
Respiratory	↓ Tidal volume, atelectasis, shunting, hypoxemia, ↓ cough, sputum retention, infection
Genitourinary	↓ Urinary output, urinary retention
Gastrointestinal	↓ Gastric and bowel motility
Musculoskeletal	Muscle spasm, impaired muscle function, fatigue, immobility
Neurological	↓ Cognitive function; mental confusion
Immunological	↓ Immune response

Source: Adapted from McCaffery, M., & Pasero, C. (1999). *Pain: Clinical manual for nursing practice* (2nd ed.). Mosby.

patients experiencing persistent pain after surgery in 5% to 50% of cases; for some (2% to 10%), this pain is moderate to severe (Pergolizzi et al., 2014). Rationales for the undertreatment of pain vary. Among health care providers, frequently cited reasons include a lack of knowledge and skills to adequately assess and treat pain; misconceptions about pain; and inaccurate and inadequate information regarding addiction, tolerance, respiratory depression, and other adverse effects of opioids (Hroch et al., 2019). These reasons are indeed common among nurses, who routinely administer the lowest prescribed analgesic dose when a range of doses is prescribed (McGillion & Watt-Watson, 2015). Such practices do little to provide relief from unremitting pain and are not consistent with current pain management guidelines (RNAO, 2013). The need to improve prelicensure pain education for health care providers in Canada is dire. One national study revealed that the majority of graduate nursing students lack adequate knowledge of pain and how to conduct a thorough pain assessment (Hroch et al., 2019).

DEFINITIONS OF PAIN

McCaffery and Pasero's seminal definition that pain is "whatever and whenever the person says it is" changed practice by focusing health care providers' attention on the subjectivity of pain (McCaffery & Pasero, 1999). Patients' self-reports about their pain are key to effective pain management. This definition at the simplest level may cause problems because patients do not always admit to pain or use the word *pain*. The International Association for the Study of Pain (IASP) has defined **pain** as "an unpleasant sensory and emotional experience associated with actual or potential tissue damage, or described in terms of such damage" (Raja et al., 2020).

Pain is multidimensional and subjective, as the IASP definition emphasizes. The patient's self-report, therefore, is the most valid means of assessment. A person's inability to communicate verbally does not negate the possibility of that individual's

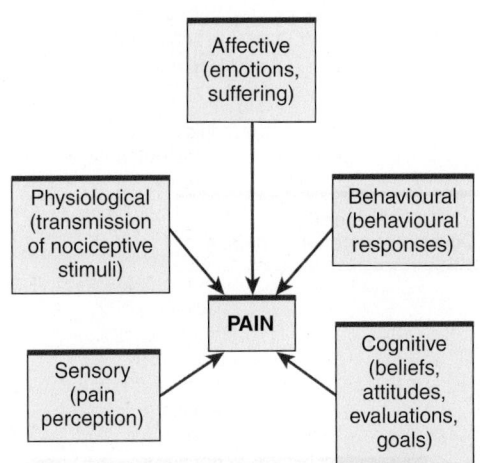

FIG. 10.1 Multidimensional nature of pain. Source: Developed by M. Mc-Caffery, C. Pasero, and J. A. Paice. Modified from McCaffery, M., & Pasero, C. (1999). *Pain: Clinical manual for nursing practice* (2nd ed.). Mosby.

experiencing pain or the need for appropriate pain-relieving treatment. For patients who are nonverbal or cognitively unable to rate pain, gathering nonverbal information is critical for pain assessment.

The IASP definition of pain underscores the fact that pain can be experienced in the absence of identifiable tissue damage. It is important to differentiate pain that involves perception of a noxious (tissue-damaging) stimulus from pain involving nociception, which may not be perceived as painful. Nociception is the activation of the primary afferent nociceptors (PANs) with peripheral terminals (free nerve endings) that respond differently to noxious stimuli. Nociceptors function primarily to sense and transmit pain signals. If nociceptive stimuli are blocked, pain is not perceived.

Pain is not synonymous with *suffering*, although pain can cause substantial suffering. Suffering has been defined as "the state of severe distress associated with events that threaten the intactness (biopsychosocial integrity) of the person" (Cassell, 1982, p. 32). Suffering can occur in the presence or absence of pain, and pain can occur with or without suffering. For example, the woman awaiting breast biopsy may suffer emotionally because of anticipated loss of her breast. She may have acute pain in the breast after the biopsy (due to the procedure itself) without emotional suffering if the biopsy result is negative for malignancy. Conversely, she may have biopsy-related pain with emotional suffering if the biopsy result is positive for malignancy.

DIMENSIONS OF PAIN AND THE PAIN PROCESS

Pain is a complex experience involving several dimensions: *physiological, sensory-discriminative* (i.e., the perception of pain by the individual that addresses the pain location, intensity, pattern, and quality), *motivational–affective, behavioural, cognitive–evaluative,* and *sociocultural* (Figure 10.1). In 1965, Melzack and Wall built on prior understanding of pain mechanisms in order to develop their gate control theory of pain (Melzack & Wall, 1987). Although the gate control theory is limited to providing a basic understanding of acute pain mechanisms, it is seminal work that remains critical to the

understanding of the pain process, including transduction, transmission, perception, and modulation of pain. Pain experience and response result from complex interactions among these dimensions. In the following discussion, each dimension and the ways in which different dimensions influence pain are described.

Physiological Dimension of Pain

Understanding the physiological dimension of pain requires knowledge of neural anatomy and physiology. The neural mechanism by which pain is perceived consists of four major steps: transduction, transmission, perception, and modulation (Fields, 1987). Figure 10.2 outlines these four steps.

Transduction. Transduction is the conversion of a mechanical, thermal, or chemical stimulus to a neuronal action potential. Transduction occurs at the level of the peripheral nerves, particularly the free nerve endings, or PANs. Noxious (tissue-damaging) stimuli can include thermal damage (e.g., sunburn), mechanical damage (e.g., surgical incision, pressure from swelling), or chemical damage (e.g., from toxic substances). These stimuli cause the release of numerous chemicals into the peripheral microenvironment of the PAN. Some of these chemicals—such as histamines, bradykinin, prostaglandins, nerve growth factor, and arachidonic acid—activate or sensitize the PAN to excitation. If the PAN is activated or excited, it fires an action potential to the spinal cord.

An action potential is necessary to convert the noxious stimulus to an impulse and move the impulse from the periphery to the spinal cord. A pain action potential can result from two sources: (a) a release of the sensitizing and activating chemicals *(nociceptive pain)* or (b) abnormal processing of stimuli by the nervous system *(neuropathic pain)*. Both of these sources produce a change in the charge along the neuronal membrane. In other words, when the PAN terminal is transduced, the PAN membrane becomes depolarized. Sodium enters the cell, and potassium exits the cell, thereby generating an action potential. The action potential is then transmitted along the entire length of the neuron to cells in the spinal cord.

Inflammation and the subsequent release of the chemical mediators listed above lower the excitation threshold of PANs and increase the likelihood of transduction. This increased susceptibility is called *sensitization*. Several chemicals, such as leukotrienes, prostaglandins, and substance P, are probably involved in this process of sensitization. It is known that the release of substance P, a chemical stored in the distal terminals of the PAN, sensitizes the PAN and dilates nearby blood vessels, resulting in subsequent development of edema and release of histamine from mast cells (Pelletier et al., 2015).

Therapies directed at altering either the PAN environment or the sensitivity of the PAN are used to prevent the transduction and initiation of an action potential. Decreasing the effects of chemicals released at the periphery is the basis of several pharmacological approaches to pain relief. For example, non-steroidal anti-inflammatory drugs (NSAIDs), such as ibuprofen (Advil, Motrin) and naproxen (Naprosyn, Aleve), and corticosteroids, such as dexamethasone (Decadron), exert their analgesic effects by blocking pain-producing chemicals. NSAIDs block the action of cyclo-oxygenase, and corticosteroids block the action of phospholipase, thereby interfering with the production of prostaglandins.

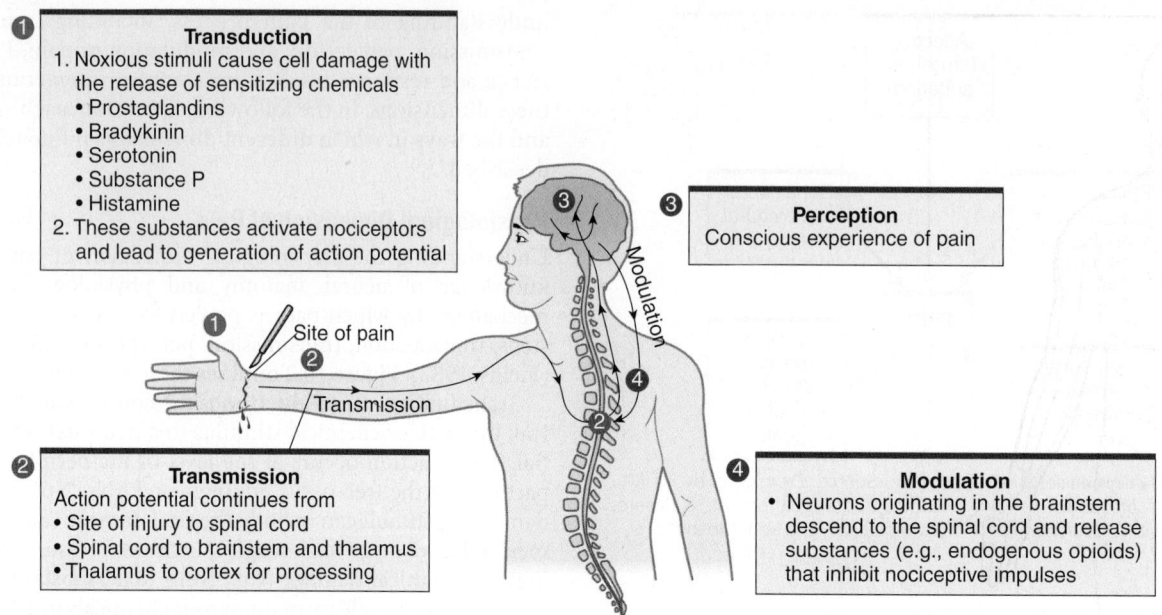

FIG. 10.2 Nociceptive pain originates when the tissue is injured. Transduction *(1)* occurs when chemical mediators are released. Transmission *(2)* involves the conduct of the action potential (short-term change in the electrical potential travelling along a cell) from the periphery (injury site) to the spinal cord and then to the brainstem, thalamus, and cerebral cortex. Perception *(3)* is the conscious awareness of pain. Modulation *(4)* involves signals from the brain going back down the spinal cord to modify incoming impulses. Source: Developed by M. McCaffery, C. Pasero, & J. A. Paice. Modified from McCaffery, M., & Pasero, C. (1999). *Pain: Clinical manual for nursing practice* (2nd ed.). Mosby.

Transmission. Transmission is the movement of pain impulses from the site of transduction to the brain (see Figure 10.2). Three segments are involved in nociceptive signal transmission: (1) transmission along the nociceptor fibres to the level of the spinal cord, (2) processing in the dorsal horn, and (3) transmission to the thalamus and the cortex. Each step in the transmission process is important in pain perception.

Transmission to the Spinal Cord. One nerve cell extends the entire distance from the periphery to the dorsal horn of the spinal cord with no synapses. For example, an afferent fibre from the great toe travels from the toe through the fifth lumbar nerve root into the spinal cord; it is one cell. Once generated, an action potential travels all the way to the spinal cord unless it is blocked by a sodium channel inhibitor or disrupted by a lesion at the central terminal of the fibre (e.g., by a dorsal root entry zone lesion).

Two types of peripheral nerve fibres are responsible for the transmission of pain impulses from the site of transduction to the level of the spinal cord: the A fibres (A-alpha, A-beta, and A-delta) and the C fibres. Neurons that project from the periphery to the spinal cord are also referred to as *first-order neurons*. Each type of fibre has different characteristics that determine its conduction rate (Table 10.2). A-alpha and A-beta fibres are large fibres enclosed within myelin sheaths that allow them to conduct impulses at a rapid rate. A-delta fibres are smaller with thinly myelinated sheaths. Because of their smaller size, however, they conduct at a slower rate than the larger A-alpha and A-beta fibres. C fibres are the smallest fibres and are unmyelinated. They conduct at the slowest rate. The conduction rates have important implications for the modulation of noxious information from A-delta and C fibres.

Stimulation of different fibres results in different sensations. Stimulation of A-delta fibres results in pain described as

TABLE 10.2	CHARACTERISTICS OF PERIPHERAL NERVE FIBRES		
Type of Fibre	**Size**	**Myelinization**	**Conduction Velocity***
A-alpha	Large	Myelinated	Rapid
A-beta	Large	Myelinated	Rapid
A-delta	Small	Myelinated	Medium
C	Smallest	Not myelinated	Slow

*The conduction rates are important because information carried to the spinal cord by the more rapidly conducting nerve fibres reaches dorsal horn cells sooner than does information carried by the fibres that conduct more slowly.

pricking, sharp, well localized, and short in duration. C-fibre activation pain is described as a dull, aching, burning sensation and is characterized by its diffuse nature, slow onset, and relatively long duration. The A-alpha (sensory muscle) and A-beta (sensory skin) fibres typically transmit nonpainful sensations such as light pressure to deep muscles, soft touch to skin, and vibration. All of these fibres extend from the peripheral tissues through the dorsal root ganglia to the dorsal horn of the spinal cord. The manner in which nerve fibres enter the spinal cord is central to the notion of spinal dermatomes. Dermatomes are areas on the skin that are innervated primarily by a single spinal cord segment. Figure 10.3 illustrates different dermatomes and their innervations.

Dorsal Horn Processing. Once the nociceptive signal arrives in the central nervous system (CNS), it is processed within the dorsal horn of the spinal cord. This processing includes the release of neurotransmitters from the afferent fibre into the synaptic cleft. These neurotransmitters bind to receptors on nearby cell bodies and dendrites of cells that may be located elsewhere in the dorsal horn. Some of these neurotransmitters (e.g., aspartate, glutamate, substance P) produce activation of

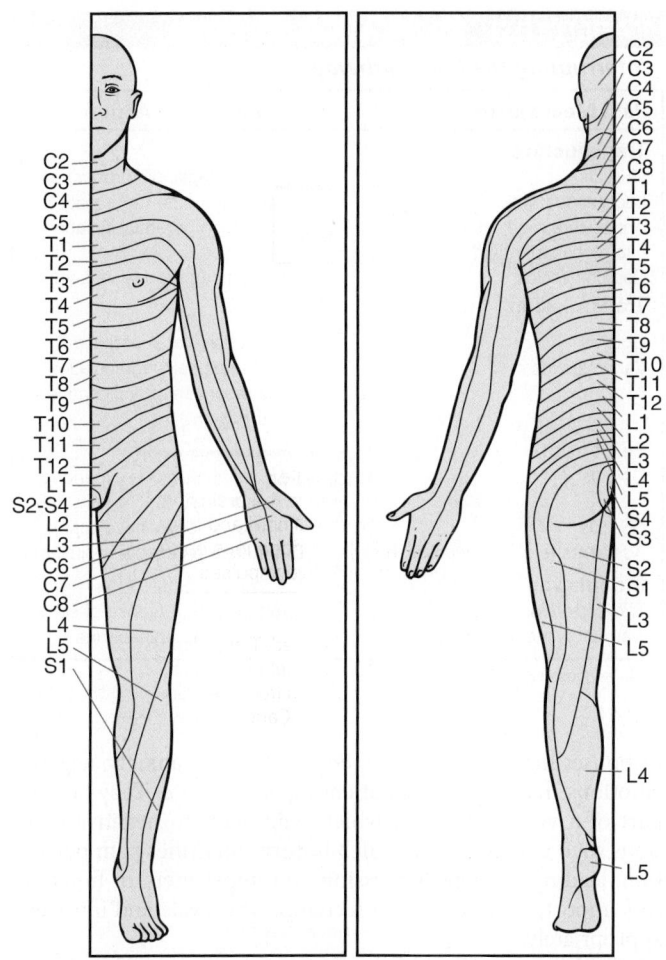

FIG. 10.3 Spinal dermatomes representing organized sensory input carried via specific spinal nerve roots. *C,* cervical; *L,* lumbar; *S,* sacral; *T,* thoracic.

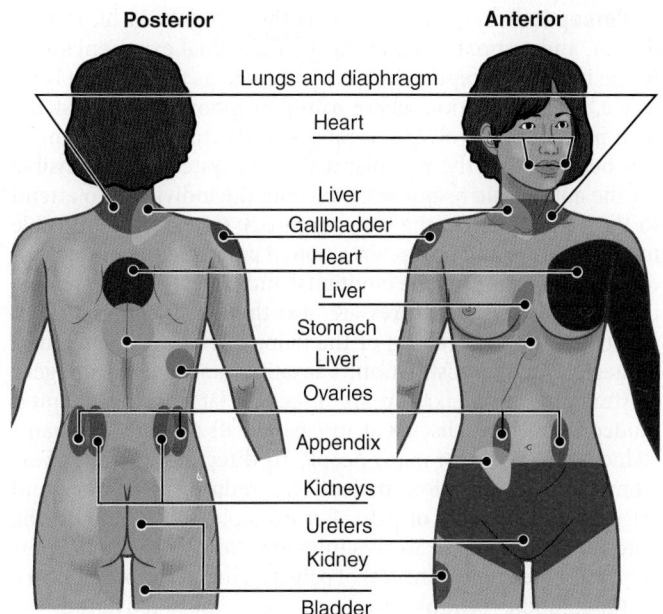

FIG. 10.4 Typical areas of referred pain.

nearby cells, whereas others (e.g., γ-aminobutyric acid, serotonin, norepinephrine) inhibit such activation. In turn, these nearby cells release other neurotransmitters. The effects of the complex neurochemistry can facilitate or modulate (i.e., inhibit) transmission of noxious stimuli. In this area, exogenous and endogenous opioids also play an important role by binding to opioid receptors and blocking the release of neurotransmitters, particularly substance P. Endogenous opioids, which include enkephalins and β-endorphins, are chemicals that are synthesized and secreted by the body. They are capable of producing effects that are similar to those of exogenous opioids such as morphine.

The dorsal horn of the spinal cord contains specialized cells called *wide dynamic range neurons.* These neurons receive input from noxious stimuli primarily carried by A-delta and C-fibre afferent pathways (especially from viscera) and from non-noxious stimuli from A-beta fibres; they also receive indirect input from dendritic projections (Mifflin & Kerr, 2014). These stimuli come from distant areas, providing a neural explanation for referred pain. Inputs from both nociceptive fibres and A-beta fibres converge on the wide dynamic range neuron, and when the message is transmitted to the brain, pain in the originating area of the body becomes poorly localized. The concept of referred pain must be considered when a person with injury to or disease involving visceral organs

reports pain in a certain location. The location of a tumour, for instance, may be distant from the pain location reported by the patient (Figure 10.4). Liver disease is located in the right upper abdominal quadrant, but pain frequently is referred to the anterior and posterior neck region and to a posterior flank area. If referred pain is not considered in the evaluation of a pain location report, diagnostic tests and therapy could be misdirected.

Sensitization, or enhanced excitability, can also occur at the level of the spinal neurons, known as *central sensitization* (Pelletier et al., 2015). Peripheral tissue damage or nerve injury can cause central sensitization, and continued nociceptive input from the periphery is necessary to maintain it. With ongoing stimulation of the slowly conducting, unmyelinated C-fibre nociceptors, firing of specialized dorsal horn neurons gradually increases. This process is known as **windup** and is dependent on the activation of *N*-methyl-D-aspartate (NMDA) receptors. NMDA receptors produce alterations in neural processing of afferent stimuli that can persist for long periods. For this reason, an important goal of therapy is to prevent persistent pain by avoiding central sensitization. Currently, the NMDA antagonist most commonly used is the anaesthetic medication ketamine (Ketalar). Unfortunately, intolerable adverse effects, such as hallucinations, limit its usefulness. Development of newer NMDA-antagonist medications is ongoing and shows promise for potentially blocking central sensitization with fewer adverse effects.

Transmission to the Thalamus and the Cortex. From the dorsal horn, nociceptive stimuli are communicated to the *third-order neurons,* primarily in the thalamus, and several other areas of the brain. Fibres of dorsal horn projection cells enter the brain through several pathways, including the spinothalamic tract and the spinoreticular tract. Distinct thalamic nuclei receive nociceptive input from the spinal cord and have projections to several regions in the cerebral cortex, where the perception of pain is believed to occur.

Perception. Pain perception is the recognition of, definition of, and response to pain by the individual experiencing it. In the brain, nociceptive input is perceived as pain. There is no single, precise location where pain perception occurs. Instead, pain perception involves several brain structures. For example, it is believed that the reticular activating system is responsible for the autonomic response of warning the individual to attend to the pain stimulus; the somatosensory system is responsible for localization and characterization of pain; and the limbic system is responsible for the emotional and behavioural responses to pain. Cortical structures are also thought to be crucial to constructing the meaning of the pain. Therefore, behavioural strategies such as distraction, relaxation, and guided imagery (distraction and relaxation are discussed later in this chapter; guided imagery is discussed in Chapter 8) are effective pain-reducing therapies for many people. By directing attention away from the pain sensation, patients can reduce the sensory and affective components of pain. For example, blood flow to the anterior central gyrus, an area intimately involved with the perception of the unpleasantness of pain, can be altered by hypnosis.

Modulation. Modulation involves the activation of descending pathways that exert inhibitory or facilitatory effects on the transmission of pain. Depending on the type and degree of modulation, the nociceptive stimuli may or may not be perceived as pain. Modulation of pain signals can occur at the level of the periphery, the spinal cord, the brainstem, and the cerebral cortex. Centrally, modulation of nociceptive impulses occurs via descending fibres that influence dorsal horn neuronal activity. Complex neurochemistry involving excitatory and inhibitory neurotransmitters such as enkephalin, γ-aminobutyric acid (GABA), serotonin, and norepinephrine is involved in this nociceptive modulation; as a result, pain transmission is inhibited (Salter, 2014). A number of pain management medications exert their effects through the modulatory systems. For example, tricyclic antidepressants, such as amitriptyline (Elavil), are used in the management of persistent noncancer pain and cancer pain. These medications interfere with the reuptake of serotonin and norepinephrine, thereby increasing their availability to inhibit noxious stimuli and produce analgesia. Baclofen (Lioresal), an analogue of the inhibitory neurotransmitter GABA, can interfere with the transmission of nociceptive impulses and thus produce analgesia for many chronic conditions, particularly those accompanied by muscle spasms. Table 10.3 briefly summarizes how pain-relieving medications can affect pain transduction, transmission, perception, and modulation.

Sensory–Discriminative, Motivational–Affective, Behavioural, Cognitive–Evaluative, and Sociocultural Dimensions of Pain

Pain is subjective; the experience of pain and related responses vary from person to person. Because of the complex neural mechanisms of nociceptive processing, pain is a multidimensional sensory and affective experience that has cognitive, behavioural, and sociocultural aspects.

The *sensory–discriminative* component of pain is the recognition of the sensation as painful. Elements of sensory pain include pattern, area, intensity, and nature (PAIN). Information about these elements and knowledge about the pain process are indispensable to clinical decision making and appropriate pain therapy.

The *motivational–affective* component of pain encompasses the emotional responses to the pain experience. These affective

TABLE 10.3   MEDICATION THERAPY
Interrupting the Pain Pathway

Pain Mechanism	Mechanism of Action
Transduction	
NSAIDs	Block prostaglandin production
Local anaesthetics	Block action potential initiation
Antiseizure medications (e.g., gabapentin [Neurontin])	Block action potential initiation
Corticosteroids	Block action potential initiation
Transmission	
Opioids	Block release of substance P
Cannabinoids	Inhibit mast cell degranulation and response of nociceptive neurons
Perception	
Opioids	Decrease conscious experience of pain
NSAIDs	Inhibit cyclo-oxygenase action
Adjuvants (e.g., antidepressants)	Dependent on specific adjuvant
Modulation	
Tricyclic antidepressants (e.g., amitriptyline [Elavil])	Interfere with reuptake of serotonin and norepinephrine

NSAIDs, nonsteroidal anti-inflammatory drugs.

responses include anger, fear, depression, and anxiety, negative emotions that impair the patient's quality of life. They become part of a vicious cycle in which pain leads to negative emotions such as depression, which in turn intensifies pain perception, leading to more depression and impairment of function. It is important for nurses to recognize this cycle and intervene appropriately.

The *behavioural* component of pain comprises the observable actions used to express or control the pain. For example, facial expressions such as grimacing may reflect pain or discomfort. Posturing may be used to decrease pain associated with specific movements. A person often adjusts their daily physical and social activities in response to the pain. In this way, pain, especially persistent pain, has profound effects on functioning (RNAO, 2013).

The *cognitive–evaluative* component of pain consists of beliefs, attitudes, memories, and the meaning of the pain for the individual. The meaning of the pain stimulus can contribute to the pain experience. For example, a woman in labour may experience severe pain, but for her it is associated with a joyful event; moreover, she may feel control over her pain because of training she received in prenatal classes and the knowledge that the pain is self-limited. In contrast, a woman with persistent, nonspecific musculoskeletal pain may be plagued by thoughts that the pain is "not real." Many people with persistent pain like this experience challenges from health care providers and others who question whether their pain is a legitimate experience (McGillion & Watt-Watson, 2015).

Such anxieties, fears, and stressors have been identified as potential intensifiers of perceived pain and related burden (O'Keefe-McCarthy et al., 2015). The meaning of pain and related responses are critical aspects of nursing pain assessment. The *cognitive* dimension also includes pain-related beliefs and the cognitive coping strategies that people use. For example, some people cope with pain by distracting themselves, whereas others struggle with feelings that the pain is untreatable and overwhelming. People who believe their pain is uncontrolled

TABLE 10.4 COMPARISON OF NOCICEPTIVE AND NEUROPATHIC PAIN

	Nociceptive Pain	Neuropathic Pain*
Definition	Normal processing of stimulus that damages normal tissue or has the potential to do so if prolonged	Abnormal processing of sensory input by the peripheral or central nervous system
Treatment	Usually responsive to nonopioid and/or opioid medications	Usually includes adjuvant analgesics
Types	Superficial Somatic Pain	Central Pain
	Pain arising from skin, mucous membranes, subcutaneous tissue. Tends to be well localized	Caused by primary lesion or dysfunction in the central nervous system
	Examples: Sunburn, skin contusions	*Examples:* Poststroke pain, pain associated with multiple sclerosis
	Deep Somatic Pain	Peripheral Neuropathies
	Pain arising from muscles, fasciae, bones, tendons. Localized or diffuse and radiating	Pain felt along the distribution of one or many peripheral nerves caused by damage to the nerve
	Examples: Arthritis, tendonitis, myofascial pain	*Examples:* Diabetic neuropathy, alcohol-nutritional neuropathy, trigeminal neuralgia, postherpetic neuralgia
	Visceral Pain	Deafferentation Pain
	Pain arising from visceral organs, such as the gastrointestinal tract and bladder. Well or poorly localized. Often referred to cutaneous sites	Pain resulting from a loss of or altered afferent input
		Examples: Phantom limb pain, postmastectomy pain, spinal cord injury pain
		Sympathetically Maintained Pain
	Examples: Appendicitis, pancreatitis, cancer affecting internal organs, irritable bowel and bladder syndromes	Pain that persists secondary to autonomic nervous system dysfunction
		Examples: Phantom limb pain, complex regional pain syndrome

*Some types of neuropathic pain (e.g., postherpetic neuralgia) are caused by more than one neuropathological mechanism.

TABLE 10.5 DIFFERENCES BETWEEN ACUTE AND PERSISTENT PAIN

Characteristic	Acute Pain	Persistent Pain
Onset	Sudden	Gradual or sudden
Duration	Usually within the normal time for healing	May start as acute injury but continues past the normal time for healing to occur
Severity	Mild to severe	Mild to severe
Cause of pain	In general, a precipitating illness or event (e.g., surgery) can be identified	May not be known; original cause of pain may differ from mechanisms that maintain the pain
Course of pain	↓ Over time and goes away as recovery occurs	Typically, pain persists and may be ongoing, episodic, or both
Typical physical and behavioural manifestations	Manifestations reflect sympathetic nervous system activation: • ↑ Heart rate • ↑ Respiratory rate • ↑ Blood pressure • Diaphoresis, pallor • Anxiety, agitation, confusion NOTE: Responses normalize quickly owing to adaptation	Predominantly behavioural manifestations: • Changes in affect • ↓ Physical movement and activity • Fatigue • Withdrawal from other people and social interaction
Usual goals of treatment	Pain control with eventual elimination	Minimizing pain to the extent possible; focusing on enhancing function and quality of life

and overwhelming are more likely to have poor outcomes (Jensen et al., 2017). Cognitions about the pain contribute to patients' goals for and expectations of pain relief and treatment outcomes.

The *sociocultural* dimension of pain encompasses factors such as demographic features (e.g., age, sex, education, socioeconomic status), support systems, social roles, past pain experiences, and cultural aspects that contribute to the pain experience [Yoshikawa et al., 2020]. Female sex, for example, has been found to influence nociceptive processes and the acceptability and usage of and response to analgesics such as NSAIDs and opioids (O'Keefe-McCarthy et al., 2015).

CAUSES AND TYPES OF PAIN

Pain is generally classified as nociceptive, neuropathic, or both, according to the underlying pathological process. Nociceptive pain and neuropathic pain have different characteristics (Table 10.4). Because of its temporal nature, pain may be acute or

persistent; some people may experience both, depending on the situation (Table 10.5).

Nociceptive Pain

Nociceptive pain is caused by damage to somatic or visceral tissue. *Somatic pain,* characterized as aching or throbbing that is well localized, arises from bone, joint, muscle, skin, or connective tissue. *Visceral pain,* which may result from stimuli such as tumour involvement or obstruction, arises from internal organs such as the intestines and the bladder. Examples of nociceptive pain include pain from a surgical incision or a broken bone, arthritis, or cardiac ischemia. Nociceptive pain is usually responsive to both nonopioid and opioid medications.

Neuropathic Pain

Neuropathic pain is caused by damage to nerve cells or changes in the CNS. Typically described as burning, shooting, stabbing, or electrical in nature, neuropathic pain can be sudden, intense, short-lived, or lingering. Neuropathic pain is difficult to treat, and management includes opioids, antiseizure medications, and antidepressants. Neuropathic pain can be either central or peripheral in origin. Although challenging to determine the global burden of neuropathic pain, it is estimated that around 8% of the general population has pain with neuropathic characteristics (Blythe, 2018). Common causes of neuropathic pain include trauma, inflammation, metabolic diseases (e.g., diabetes), alcoholism, nervous system infections (e.g., herpes zoster, human immunodeficiency virus), tumors, toxins, and neurological diseases (e.g., multiple sclerosis). Examples of neuropathic pain conditions include phantom limb sensation, diabetic neuropathy, and trigeminal neuralgia. No single sign or symptom is diagnostic for neuropathic pain.

Neuropathic pain is often not well controlled by opioid analgesics alone. Treatment often requires a multimodal approach combining various adjuvant analgesics from different drug classes. These include tricyclic antidepressants (e.g., amitriptyline), serotonin–norepinephrine reuptake inhibitors (SNRIs) (e.g., bupropion [Wellbutrin, Zyban]), antiseizure medications (e.g., gabapentin [Neurontin]; pregabalin [Lyrica]), transdermal lidocaine, and α_2-adrenergic agonists (e.g., clonidine). NMDA receptor antagonists, such as ketamine, have shown promise in alleviating neuropathic pain refractory to other medications.

Acute and Chronic Pain

Acute pain and persistent pain have different causes, courses, manifestations, and treatment (see Table 10.5). Examples of *acute pain* include postoperative pain, labour pain, pain from trauma (e.g., lacerations, fractures, sprains) and infection (e.g., dysuria), and angina. For acute pain, treatment includes analgesics for symptom control treatment of the underlying cause (e.g., splinting for a fracture, antibiotic therapy for an infection). Normally, acute pain diminishes over time as healing occurs. *Chronic pain* or *persistent pain* continues beyond the normal time expected for healing, often longer than 3 months. The severity and functional impact of chronic pain often are disproportionate to objective findings because of changes in the nervous system not detectable with standard tests. Although acute pain functions as a signal, warning the person of potential or actual tissue damage, chronic pain does not appear to have an

adaptive role. Chronic pain can be disabling and often is accompanied by anxiety and depression.

Cancer pain often is considered separately because its cause can be determined, its course differs from that of nonmalignant pain (cancer pain often worsens with documented disease progression), and the use of opioids in its treatment is more widely accepted than in the treatment of noncancer pain (von Gunten, 2011). Many older persons with advanced cancer experience daily cancer pain, especially at end of life (Booker et al., 2020). An adequate pain assessment for these patients is essential during palliative or end-of-life care (see Chapter 13).

PAIN ASSESSMENT

The goals of a nursing pain assessment are (a) to describe the patient's sensory, affective, behavioural, and sociocultural pain experience for the purpose of implementing pain management techniques and (b) to identify the patient's goal for therapy and resources and strategies for effective self-management. The nurse is responsible for conducting an accurate pain assessment. To conduct an accurate pain assessment, the nurse should consider the principles of pain assessment (Table 10.6). The following sections describe key components in pain assessment.

Initial Pain Assessment

Nurses need to complete an initial pain assessment. The initial pain assessment provides the nurse with a comprehensive overview of the patient's perception of their pain as well as provide a foundation to determine a plan of care and treatment for a patient. The initial pain assessment (Table 10.7) focuses on eight areas, using the acronym OPQRSTUV: **o**nset, **p**rovocative/**p**alliative, **q**uality of the pain, **r**egion of the body/**r**adiation, **s**everity of pain, **t**reatment/**t**iming, **u**nderstanding of pain, and **v**alues (Jarvis, 2019).

Sensory–Discriminative Component

Every pain assessment should include evaluation of the sensory–discriminative component: pattern, area, intensity, and nature (PAIN) of the pain. Information about these elements is essential to identifying appropriate therapy for the type and severity of the pain (RNAO, 2013).

TABLE 10.6 PRINCIPLES OF PAIN ASSESSMENT

Principles	Nursing Implications
1. Patients have the right to appropriate assessment and management of pain.	• Assess pain in *all* patients.
2. Pain is always subjective.	• Patient's self-report of pain is the single most reliable indicator of pain. • Accept and respect this self-report unless there are clear reasons for doubt.
3. Physiological and behavioral signs of pain (e.g., tachycardia, grimacing) are not reliable or specific for pain.	• Do not rely primarily on observations and objective signs of pain unless the patient is unable to self-report pain.
4. Pain is an unpleasant sensory and emotional experience.	• Address physical and psychological aspects of pain when assessing pain.
5. Assessment approaches, including tools, must be appropriate for the patient population.	• Special considerations are needed for assessing pain in patients with difficulty communicating. • Include family members in the assessment process (when appropriate).
6. Pain can exist even when no physical cause can be found.	• Do not attribute pain that does not have an identifiable cause to psychological causes.
7. Different patients have different levels of pain in response to comparable stimuli.	• A uniform pain threshold does not exist.
8. Patients with chronic pain may be more sensitive to pain and other stimuli.	• Pain tolerance varies among and within persons depending on several factors (e.g., genetics, energy level, coping skills, prior experience with pain).
9. Unrelieved pain has adverse consequences. Acute pain that is not adequately controlled can result in physiological changes that increase the chance of developing persistent pain.	• Encourage patients to report pain, especially patients who are reluctant to discuss pain, deny pain when it is probably present, or fail to follow through on prescribed treatments.

TABLE 10.7 INITIAL PAIN ASSESSMENT

Initial Pain Assessment (OPQRSTUV)

O: onset • When did the pain start?	To identify onset of pain (when active, or resting) or whether pain is acute or chronic
P: provocative/palliative • Does your pain increase with movement or activity? • Are the symptoms relieved with rest? • Were any previous treatments effective?	To identify quality of pain and differentiate between nociceptive and neuropathic pain mechanisms To identify alleviating and aggravating factors To evaluate effectiveness of current treatment
Q: quality of the pain • What does your pain feel like? • What words describe your pain?	To identify mechanism of pain (terms such as *throbbing*, *aching*, *shooting*, and *dull* may provide clues)
R: region of the body/radiation • Where is your pain? • Does the pain radiate, or move to other areas?	To identify one or more areas of the body that are affected by pain, inasmuch as there may be several
S: severity of pain • How would you rate your pain on an intensity scale?	To identify intensity (refer to various intensity scales) To identify degree of impairment and effect on quality of life or ability to perform activities of daily living (ADLs)
T: treatment/timing • What treatments have worked for you in the past? • Is it a constant, dull, or intermittent pain?	To identify treatments that have been successful in the past To identify timing of the pain so that treatment can be focused on spikes in pain
U: understanding of pain • To understand patient history of pain. What is your past experience(s) of pain?	To understand patient history of pain To be able to set achievable pain and function goals when reviewing the plan of care
V: values • What is your acceptable level for this pain? • Is there anything else that you would like to say about your pain? • Are there any other symptoms related to the pain?	To understand and discuss other stressors, spiritual pain

Source: Jarvis, C. (2019). *Physical examination and health assessment* (3rd ed. p. 188). Elsevier.

Before beginning any assessment, the nurse must recognize that patients may use words other than *pain* (Table 10.8). For example, older persons may deny that they have pain but respond positively when asked if they have discomfort, soreness, or aching. For these patients, repeatedly using open-ended questions including descriptors to understand pain may elicit more information than closed-ended questions. The words that the patient uses in describing pain must be documented, and when the patient is asked about pain, the patient's words should be used consistently.

Pattern of Pain. Pain onset (when it starts) and duration (how long it lasts) are components of the pain pattern. Acute pain typically increases during wound care, ambulation, coughing, and deep breathing. Acute pain associated with surgery or injury tends to diminish over time, with recovery as tissues heal. In contrast, persistent pain may be ongoing, episodic, or both. For example, a person with persistent osteoarthritis pain may experience increased stiffness and pain on arising in the morning. As the joint is gently mobilized, the pain often decreases.

A patient may have constant, round-the-clock pain or discrete periods of intermittent pain. Breakthrough pain is moderate to severe pain that occurs despite treatment. Many patients with cancer experience breakthrough pain. It is usually rapid in onset and brief in duration, with highly variable intensity and frequency of occurrence. *Episodic, procedural,* or *incident pain* is a transient increase in pain that is caused by a specific activity or event that precipitates the pain (e.g., dressing changes, movement, eating, position changes, and certain procedures such as catheterization).

Area of Pain. The area or location of pain assists in identifying possible causes of the pain and in determining treatment. Some patients may be able to specify one or more precise locations of their pain, whereas others may describe very general areas or comment that they "hurt all over." The location of the pain may also be *referred* from its origin to another site (see Figure 10.4), as described earlier in the chapter. Pain may also *radiate* from its origin to another site. For example, angina pectoris

TABLE 10.8 SOME WORDS USED TO DESCRIBE PAIN

• Pressure • Cramping • Tender • Aching • Burning	• Discomfort • Squeezing • Stabbing • Soreness

is known to radiate from the chest to the jaw, to the shoulders, or down the left arm. Sciatica is pain that originates from compression or damage to the sciatic nerve or its roots within the spinal cord. The pain is projected along the course of the peripheral nerve, causing painful shooting sensations down the back of the thigh and the inside of the leg.

Typically, information about the location of pain is elicited by asking the patient to (a) describe the site or sites of pain, (b) point to painful areas on the body, or (c) mark painful areas on a body diagram (Figure 10.5). Because many patients have more than one site of pain, it is important to make certain that the patient describes every location and identifies which one is most problematic.

Intensity of Pain. An assessment of the severity, or *intensity* of pain provides a reliable measurement for determining the type of treatment as well as for evaluating the effectiveness of therapy. Pain scales are useful in helping the patient communicate the intensity of pain and in guiding treatment. Scales must be adjusted to age and level of cognitive development. Numerical scales (e.g., 0 = "no pain" and 10 = "the worst pain"), verbal descriptor scales (e.g., none, a little [1–3], moderate [4–6], and severe [7–10]), or visual analogue scales (a 10-cm line with one end labelled "no pain" and the other end labelled "worst possible pain") can be used by most adults to rate the intensity of their pain (Figure 10.6). For patients who are unable to respond to other pain intensity scales, a series of faces ranging from "smiling" to "crying" can be used. These scales have been investigated

Initial Pain Assessment Tool

Date _____

Client's Name _____ Age_____ Room _____

Diagnosis_____ Physician _____

Nurse _____

1. LOCATION: Patient or nurse marks drawing.

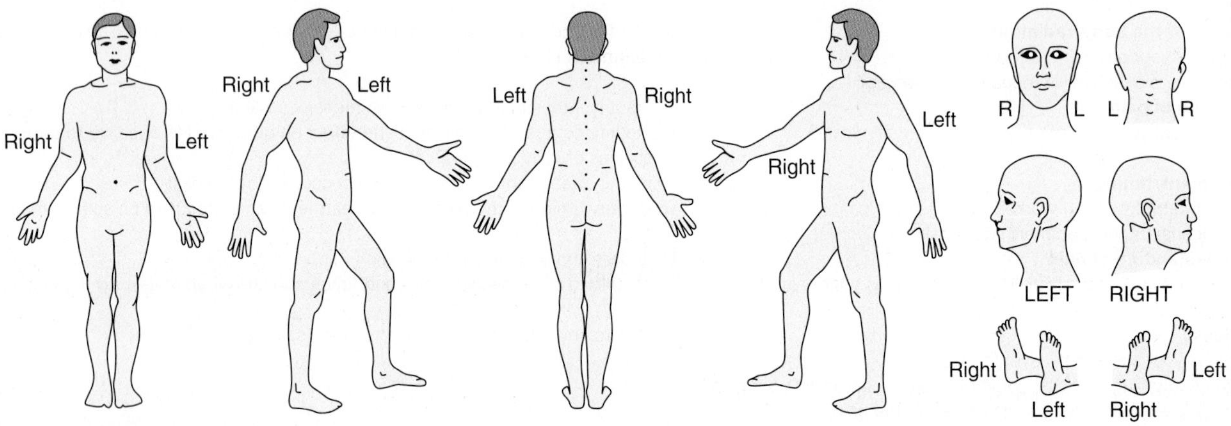

Right   Left

Right   Left   Left   Right

Left

Right

R   L   L   R

LEFT   RIGHT

Right   Left

Left   Right

2. INTENSITY: Client rates the pain. Scale used: _____

  Present: _____

  Worst pain gets: _____

  Best pain gets: _____

  Acceptable level of pain: _____

3. QUALITY: (Use client's own words, e.g., prick, ache, burn, throb, pull, sharp) _____
_____

4. ONSET, DURATION, VARIATIONS, RHYTHMS: _____
_____

5. MANNER OF EXPRESSING PAIN: _____
_____
_____

6. WHAT RELIEVES THE PAIN? _____
_____
_____

7. WHAT CAUSES OR INCREASES THE PAIN? _____
_____
_____

8. EFFECTS OF PAIN: (Note decreased function, decreased quality of life)
  Accompanying symptoms (e.g., nausea)_____
  Sleep _____
  Appetite _____
  Physical activity _____
  Relationship with others (e.g., irritability) _____
  Emotions (e.g., anger, suicidal thoughts and behaviours, crying) _____
  Concentration _____
  Other _____

9. OTHER COMMENTS: _____

10. PLAN: _____
_____

May be duplicated for use in clinical practice. From McCaffery, M., Pasero, C. Pain: Clinical manual, p. 60. Copyright © 1999, Mosby.

FIG. 10.5 Initial pain assessment tool (may be duplicated for use in clinical practice). Source: McCaffery, M., & Pasero, C. (1999). *Pain: Clinical manual for nursing practice* (2nd ed., p. 60). Mosby.

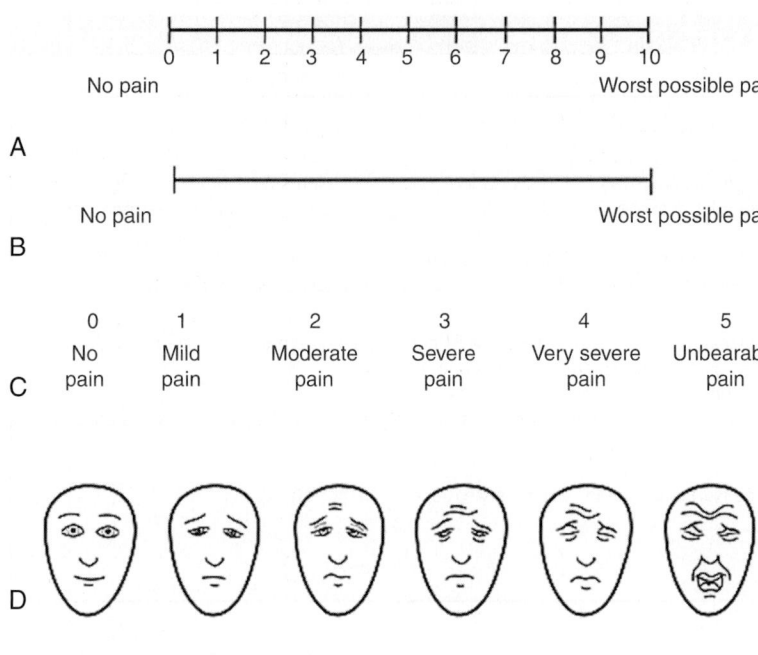

A

B

C

D

FIG. 10.6 Pain intensity scales. **A**, 0 to 10 numeric scale. **B**, Visual analogue scale. **C**, Descriptive scale. **D**, Faces Pain Scale. Modified from Baird, M. (2015). *Manual of critical care nursing: Nursing interventions and collaborative management* (2nd ed.). Elsevier.

for use in a variety of patient populations, including children and older persons.

Although intensity is an important factor in determining analgesic approaches, patients should not be dosed with opioids solely on the basis of reported pain scores (Drew et al., 2018). Opioid "dosing by numbers" without considering a patient's sedation level and respiratory status can lead to unsafe practices and serious adverse events. Safer analgesic administration can be achieved by balancing an amount of pain relief with analgesic adverse effects. Adjustments in therapy can be made to promote better pain control and minimize adverse outcomes.

Nature of Pain

The subjective *nature* of pain refers to the self-reported quality or characteristics of the pain. Many commonly used words to describe the nature of pain are included in the McGill Pain Questionnaire (MPQ; see the Resources at the end of this chapter). The MPQ is a widely used measure of subjective pain experience with well-established reliability, validity, sensitivity, and discriminative capacity in divergent acute and chronic pain populations (Main, 2016). Two major strengths of the MPQ are that (1) it provides a comprehensive assessment of the nature of pain problems in a short time frame (5 to 10 minutes), and (2) it includes subsets of verbal pain descriptors associated with both nociceptive and neuropathic pain.

Motivational–Affective, Behavioural, Cognitive–Evaluative, and Sociocultural Components

Comprehensive pain assessment includes evaluation of all pain dimensions and should be completed upon a patient's admission to a facility and repeated at regular intervals to evaluate response to treatment. In an acute care setting, time limitations may dictate an abbreviated assessment of the affective, behavioural, cognitive, and sociocultural dimensions of pain. At a minimum, patients' expression of pain and the effect of pain on sleep, daily activities, relationships, physical activity, and emotional well-being should be assessed. Strategies that the patient has used or tried to control the pain (effective or not) should also be documented.

When possible and relevant, assessment should also include examination of the psychological and social factors associated with patients' subjective experience of pain and, in particular, the meaning of the pain experience; *pain* meaning may often feature prominently in patients' treatment progress. Data related to meaning may be particularly useful in care planning for patients who exhibit high levels of pain-related behaviour, functional impairment, or pain-related distress. For example, as stated earlier, a woman in labor may have severe pain but can manage it without analgesics because for her it is associated with a joyful event. Moreover, she may feel control over her pain because of the training she received in prenatal classes and the knowledge that the pain is time limited. This may be in contrast to an individual experiencing chronic, undefined musculoskeletal pain who may be stressed by thoughts that the pain is "not real," is uncontrollable, or is caused by their own actions.

Perceptions influence the ways in which an individual responds to pain and must be included in a comprehensive treatment plan. For clinical assessment purposes, key areas of inquiry with patients about the meaning of pain and related beliefs should include effective pain control in relation to current intervention strategies, pain-related disability, value placed on comfort and solace from other people, and the effect of emotions on the experience of pain.

Comprehensive assessment information is necessary to ensure effective treatment, as shown in Table 10.9.

Indigenous Considerations

Indigenous populations in Canada are experiencing high rates of chronic pain. These populations also continue to face many challenges to accessing culturally sensitive health care. It is important for health care providers to acknowledge these challenges, to ensure that Indigenous populations receive appropriate and effective treatment plans for pain. Many of the challenges faced by Indigenous people involve discrimination around the assumption of substance misuse; Indigenous people have expressed being considered a "drug seeker" when they are experiencing legitimate pain issues (Brown et al., 2016). Such discrimination can lead to inadequate treatments for pain experiences (Brown et al., 2016). Health care providers need to acknowledge and

---

TABLE 10.9 NURSING ASSESSMENT:

Pain

Subjective Data
Important Health Information

Health history: Pain history includes onset, location, intensity, quality, patterns, aggravating and alleviating factors, and expression of pain. Coping strategies. Past treatments and their effectiveness. Review health care use related to the pain problem (e.g., emergency department visits, treatment at pain clinics, visits to primary health care providers and specialists).
Medications: Use of any prescription or over-the-counter, illicit, or herbal products for pain relief. Alcohol use
Nonpharmacological measures: Use of therapies, such as massage, heat or ice, Reiki, aromatherapy, acupuncture, hypnosis, yoga, or meditation

Functional Health Patterns

Health perception–health management: Social and work history, mental health history, smoking history. Effects of pain on emotions, relationships, sleep, and activities. Interviews with family members. Records from psychological/psychiatric treatment related to the pain
Elimination: Constipation related to opioid medication use, other medication use, or pain related to elimination
Activity-exercise: Fatigue, limitations in ability to perform activities of daily living (ADLs), instrumental activities of daily living (IADLs), and pain related to use of muscles
Sexuality-reproductive: Decreased libido
Coping–stress tolerance: Psychological evaluation using standardized measures to examine coping style, depression, anxiety

Objective Data

Physical examination, including evaluation of functional limitations
Psychosocial evaluation, including mood

---

understand the historical social issues experienced by Indigenous populations to ensure culturally sensitive care.

PAIN TREATMENT

Basic Principles

All pain treatment is guided by the same underlying principles. Although treatment regimens range from short-term management to multimodal, long-term therapy for many persistent pain problems, all treatment should follow the same basic standards, as stated by the Canadian Pain Society (Watt-Watson et al., 1999) and the RNAO 2013 *Pain Assessment and Management Best Practice Guidelines*:

- Routine assessment is essential for effective pain management. Pain is a subjective experience involving multiple characteristics, including biological and psychosocial factors, all of which must be considered for comprehensive assessment and management.
- Unrelieved acute pain complicates recovery. Unrelieved pain after surgery or injury results in more complications, longer hospital stays, greater disability, and potentially long-term pain.
- Patients' self-report of pain should be used whenever possible. For patients unable to report pain, a nonverbal assessment method must be used.
- Health care providers have a responsibility to assess pain routinely, to accept patients' pain reports and document them, and to intervene in order to manage pain.
- The best approach to pain management involves patients, families, and health care providers. Patients and families must be informed of their right to the best pain care possible and encouraged to communicate the severity of their pain.
- Many patients—in particular, vulnerable populations including infants, children, adolescents, and older adults; individuals from diverse ethnic backgrounds who have limited ability to communicate; and patients with past or current substance use problems—are at high risk for suboptimal or inappropriate pain management. Health care providers must understand that adequate pain relief is a basic human right, must be aware of their own biases and misinformation, and must ensure that all patients

are treated respectfully. Patients with a history of opioid tolerance or addiction may have higher opioid requirements following a new episode of acute pain. Care should be taken that these patients do not experience withdrawal due to undermedication.

- Treatment must be based on the patient's and family's goals for pain treatment, which should be discussed upon initial pain assessment. Sometimes these goals can be described in terms of pain intensity (e.g., the desire for pain intensity to decrease from an "8 out of 10" to a "3 out of 10"). Other patients may express a functional goal (e.g., a person may want the pain to be relieved to an extent that allows them to perform daily activities). Over the course of prolonged therapy, these goals should be reassessed, and progress should be documented. If the patient has unrealistic goals for therapy, such as wanting to be completely rid of all persistent arthritis pain, the nurse should work with the patient to establish a more realistic goal.
- Treatment plans should involve a combination of pharmacological and nonpharmacological therapies. Although medications are often considered the mainstay of therapy, particularly for moderate to severe pain, nonpharmacological strategies should be incorporated to increase the overall effectiveness of the treatment plan and to allow for the reduction of medication dosages to minimize adverse effects. Examples of therapies are discussed later in the chapter.
- A multidimensional and interprofessional approach is necessary for optimal pain management. Multiple perspectives from all members of the interprofessional team, which can include physicians, registered nurses (RNs), registered practical nurses (RPNs), physiotherapy, pharmacy, occupational therapy, and other professional involved in the patient's circle of care, should be incorporated.
- All therapies must be evaluated to ensure that they are meeting the patient's goals. Therapy must be individualized for each patient, and, often, achieving an effective treatment plan requires trial and error. Medications, dosages, and routes are commonly adjusted to achieve maximal benefit while minimizing adverse effects. This trial-and-error process can become frustrating for the patient and family. They need to be

reassured that pain relief is possible and that the health care team will continue to work with them to achieve adequate pain relief.

- Adverse effects of medications must be prevented or managed. Adverse effects are a major reason for treatment failure and nonadherence despite the fact that most patients' pain can be effectively managed (RNAO, 2013). Adverse effects are managed in one of several ways, described in Table 10.10. The nurse plays a key role in monitoring for and treating adverse effects, as well as in teaching the patient and family how to minimize adverse effects.
- Patient and caregiver teaching should be a cornerstone of the treatment plan. Content should include information about the cause or causes of the pain, pain assessment methods, treatment goals and options, expectations for pain management, instruction regarding the proper use of medications, management of adverse effects, and nonpharmacological and self-help measures for pain relief (RNAO, 2013). Teaching should be documented, and the patient's and caregiver's comprehension of this teaching should be evaluated.

Medication Therapy for Pain

Although a physician or nurse practitioner prescribes the medications, it is the nurse's responsibility to evaluate the effectiveness and adverse effects of what is prescribed. It is also a nursing responsibility to document and communicate the outcomes of analgesic therapy and to suggest changes when appropriate, using knowledge and skills related to several pharmacological and pain management concepts. These include calculating equianalgesic doses, scheduling analgesic doses, titrating opioids, and selecting from the prescribed analgesic medications.

Equianalgesic Dose. The term equianalgesic dose refers to a dose of one analgesic that produces pain-relieving effects equivalent to those of another analgesic. The concept of equivalence is important when substituting one analgesic for another in the event that a particular medication is ineffective or causes intolerable adverse effects and when the administration route of opioids is changed (e.g., from parenteral to oral). In general, opioids are administered in equianalgesic doses—which is important to know because no upper dosage limit has been established for many of these medications. Equianalgesic charts and conversion programs are widely available in textbooks, in clinical guidelines, in health care facility pain policies, and on the Internet. Table 10.11 provides an example of common equianalgesic dosages compared with 10 mg of parenteral morphine, which is the standard basis for comparison. Although equianalgesic charts are useful tools, health care providers must understand their limitations: Equianalgesic dosages are approximate, and individual patient response must be routinely assessed. In addition, discrepancies exist among different published equianalgesic charts. All changes in opioid therapy must be carefully monitored and adjusted for the individual patient. When possible, health care providers should use equianalgesic conversions that have been approved for their facility or clinic and should consult a pharmacist before making changes.

Scheduling Analgesics. Appropriate analgesic scheduling should focus on prevention or ongoing control of pain rather than on providing analgesics only after the patient's pain has become moderate to severe. A patient should receive medication before procedures and activities that are expected to produce pain. Similarly, a patient with constant pain should receive analgesics around the clock rather than on an as-needed basis. These strategies control pain before it starts and usually result in lower analgesic requirements. Fast-acting medications should be used for incident or breakthrough pain, whereas long-acting analgesics are more effective for constant pain. Examples of fast-acting and sustained-release analgesics are described later in this section.

Titration. Analgesic titration is dosage adjustment that is based on assessment of the adequacy of analgesic effect versus the adverse effects produced. The amount of analgesic needed to manage pain varies widely, and titration is an important

TABLE 10.10 MEDICATION THERAPY

Examples of Ways to Manage Adverse Effects of Opioids

- Ensuring a schedule for the dosing regimen to maintain blood levels
- Using stool softeners and stimulant laxatives to prevent constipation
- Using an antiemetic to prevent nausea
- Changing to a different medication in the same drug class
- Using an administration route that minimizes drug concentrations at the site of the adverse effect (e.g., intraspinal administration of opioids is sometimes used to minimize high drug levels that produce sedation, nausea, and vomiting)

TABLE 10.11 EXAMPLES OF COMMON EQUIANALGESIC DOSES

Medication	Approximate Equianalgesic Parenteral Dosage	Approximate Equianalgesic Oral Dosage	Alert/Special Considerations
Morphine	10 mg	30 mg	
Hydromorphone (Dilaudid)	1–1.5 mg	4–7.5 mg	
Oxycodone	Not available	20 mg	
Codeine	120 mg	200 mg	
Methadone and tramadol	—	—	Methadone and tramadol conversion morphine dose equivalents have not been reliably established. Methadone conversion requires a licensed expert's assessment based on the patient's history of opioid consumption.
Meperidine (Demerol)	75 mg	300 mg	Prolonged use may increase risk of toxicity (e.g., seizures) from accumulation of the meperidine metabolite, normeperidine.

Source: Adapted from National Opioid Use Guideline Group. (2010). Oral opioid analgesic conversion table. In *Canadian guideline for safe and effective use of opioids for chronic non-cancer pain* (p. 75). https://nationalpaincentre.mcmaster.ca/documents/opioid_guideline_part_b_v5_6.pdf.

strategy in addressing this variability. An analgesic dosage can be titrated upward or downward, depending on the situation. For example, in a postoperative patient, the dosage of analgesic generally decreases over time as the acute pain resolves. On the other hand, opioids for persistent, severe chronic noncancer pain may be titrated upward over the course of therapy to maintain adequate pain control; this titration requires expert specialty care according to the 2017 Canadian Guidelines for Opioids for Chronic Non-Cancer Pain (Busse et al., 2017). The goal of titration is to use the lowest dosage of opioid that provides effective pain control with the fewest adverse effects.

Analgesic Ladder. Several national and international groups have published practice guidelines recommending a systematic plan for using analgesic medications. One widely used system is the analgesic ladder proposed by the World Health Organization (WHO) (Figure 10.7). The WHO treatment plan emphasizes that different medications are administered, depending on the severity of pain, by means of a three-step ladder approach. Step 1 medications are used for mild pain; step 2, for mild to moderate pain; and step 3, for moderate to severe pain. If pain persists or increases, medications from the next higher step are introduced to control the pain. The steps are not meant to be sequential if someone has moderate to severe pain: for this person, the analgesics given would be the stronger analgesics listed in steps 2 and 3.

Medication Therapy for Mild Pain. When pain is mild (1 to 3 on a scale of 0 to 10), nonopioid analgesics (Aspirin and other salicylates, other NSAIDs, and acetaminophen) may be used (Table 10.12). These medications are characterized by the following: (a) their analgesic properties have a ceiling effect, that is, increasing the dose beyond an upper limit provides no greater analgesia; (b) they do not produce tolerance or physical dependence; and (c) many are available without a prescription. It is important to monitor over-the-counter analgesic use to avoid serious problems related to medication interactions, adverse effects, and overdosage.

MEDICATION ALERT—NSAIDs
- NSAIDs (except Aspirin) have been linked to a higher risk for cardiovascular events, such as myocardial infarction, stroke, and heart failure.

- Patients who have just had heart surgery should not take NSAIDs.

A number of nonopioid analgesics such as acetylsalicylic acid (ASA, Aspirin) and NSAIDs inhibit the chemicals that activate the PAN (Figure 10.8). Thus when these medications are used, the PAN is transduced less often, or a larger stimulus is needed to produce transduction.

Aspirin is effective for mild pain, but its use is limited by its common adverse effects, including gastric upset and bleeding. Other salicylates such as choline magnesium trisalicylate cause fewer GI disturbances and bleeding abnormalities. Similarly to Aspirin, acetaminophen (Tylenol) has analgesic and antipyretic effects, but it has no antiplatelet or anti-inflammatory effects. Acetaminophen is well tolerated; however, dosages higher than

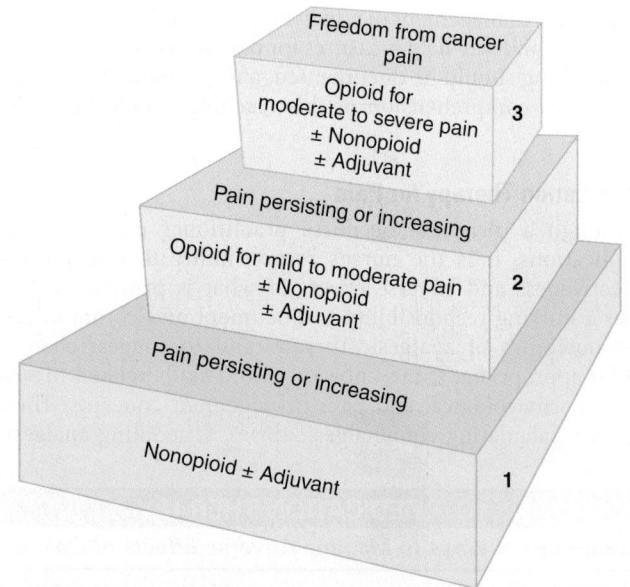

FIG. 10.7 The analgesic ladder proposed by the World Health Organization. Source: Reprinted from *Cancer*, WHO analgesic ladder, WHO, Copyright 2018.

TABLE 10.12 MEDICATION THERAPY

Comparison of Select Nonopioid Analgesics

Medication	Analgesic Efficacy in Comparison to Standards	Nursing Considerations
Acetaminophen (Tylenol)	Comparable to Aspirin	Rectal suppository available; sustained-release preparations available; maximum daily dosage of 4 g
Salicylates		
Acetylsalicylic acid (Aspirin)	Standard for comparison	Rectal suppository available; sustained-release preparations available Possibility of upper GI bleeding
Nonsteroidal Anti-Inflammatory Drugs (NSAIDs)		
Ibuprofen (Motrin, Advil)	Superior at 200–650 mg of Aspirin	Usually well tolerated despite the potential for upper GI bleeding
Indomethacin	25 mg comparable with 650 mg of Aspirin	Not routinely used because of high incidence of adverse effects; rectal, intravenous, and sustained-release oral forms available
Ketorolac (Toradol)	30–60 mg equivalent to 6–12 mg of morphine	Treatment should be limited to maximum of 7 days; may precipitate renal failure in dehydrated patients
Diclofenac (Voltaren)	25–50 mg BID to TID; has a longer duration than 650 mg of Aspirin	Available in oral, ophthalmic, and topical preparations
Cyclo-oxygenase-2 (COX-2) inhibitors (Celecoxib)	Similar to NSAIDs	Fewer GI complaints, including bleeding; more costly than other NSAIDs
Meloxicam (Mobicox)	Similar to other NSAIDs	May cause fewer GI adverse effects, including bleeding, than do other NSAIDs, but risk is still present; is more costly than other NSAIDs

BID, twice per day; *GI,* gastrointestinal; *TID,* three times per day.

4 000 mg per day, acute overdosage, or use by patients with alcoholism or liver disease can result in severe hepatotoxicity.

The NSAIDs represent a broad class of medications with varying efficacy and adverse effects. Some NSAIDs possess analgesic efficacy equal to that of Aspirin, whereas others have somewhat higher efficacy. Patients vary greatly in their responses to a specific NSAID, so when one NSAID does not provide relief, another should be tried. NSAIDs inhibit the cyclo-oxygenase-1 (COX-1) and -2 (COX-2) enzymes, which produce prostaglandins involved in inflammation. Because prostaglandins also play a key role in protecting the lining of the stomach from acids, adverse effects of NSAIDs can be serious and include bleeding tendencies secondary to decreased platelet aggregation, GI issues ranging from dyspepsia to ulceration and hemorrhage, renal insufficiency, and, on occasion, CNS dysfunction. For

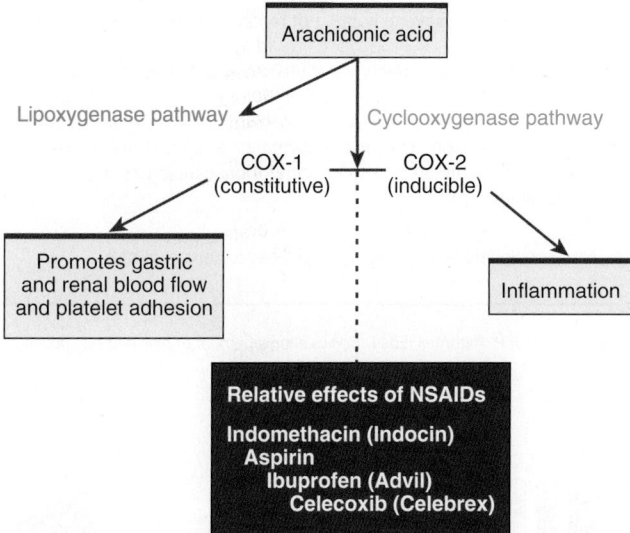

FIG. 10.8 Arachidonic acid is oxidized by two different pathways: lipoxygenase and cyclooxygenase (COX). The cyclooxygenase pathway leads to two forms of the enzyme cyclooxygenase: COX-1 and COX-2. COX-1 is known as constitutive (always present), and COX-2 is known as inducible (its expression varies markedly depending on the stimulus). Nonsteroidal anti-inflammatory drugs (NSAIDs) differ in their actions, with some having more effects on COX-1 and others more on COX-2. Indomethacin acts primarily on COX-1. Ibuprofen is equipotent on COX-1 and COX-2. Celecoxib primarily inhibits COX-2.

certain chronic conditions, such as rheumatoid arthritis and osteoarthritis, NSAIDs that more selectively inhibit COX-2 only are used. The COX-2 enzyme does not play a role in protecting the stomach or intestinal tract; therefore, its selective inhibition is not associated with the same risk for injury to these organs as is the inhibition of COX-1. A common example of a COX-2 inhibitor is meloxicam (Mobicox). Cautious use of anti-inflammatory medications long-term has been recommended because of the increased risk for cardiovascular accidents.

Medication Therapy for Mild to Moderate Pain. When pain is moderate in intensity (4 to 6 on a scale of 0 to 10) or mild but persistent despite nonopioid therapy, step 2 medications are indicated. Medications commonly used for mild to moderate pain are listed in Table 10.13.

One class of step 2 medications is opioids. Opioids include many medications (Table 10.14; also see Table 10.13) that produce their effects by binding to receptors. Opioid receptors are found in the CNS, on the terminals of sensory nerves, and on the surface of immune cells. There are three major opioid receptors, traditionally referred to as *mu, kappa,* and *delta.* The receptors have been reclassified as OP1 (delta), OP2 (kappa), and OP3 (mu). Most clinically useful opioids bind to the mu receptors. Mu agonists include morphine, oxycodone, hydromorphone (Dilaudid), and methadone. Opioid *agonists* (e.g., morphine) bind to the receptors and cause analgesia. *Antagonists* (e.g., naloxone) bind to the receptors but do not produce analgesia; they also block other effects of opioid receptor activation, such as sedation and respiratory depression. *Mixed agonists* naloxone, such as pentazocine (Talwin) and butorphanol, should not be used because they bind as agonists on the kappa receptor and, as weak antagonists or partial agonists, on the mu receptor (Figure 10.9). When a mixed agonist–antagonist is given to someone taking an agonist (e.g., morphine), it will act like an agonist–antagonist, such as naloxone, and reverse any analgesic effect. These opioid agonist–antagonists also cause more dysphoria and agitation. In addition, they have an analgesic ceiling (a dosage at which no additional analgesia is produced regardless of further dosage increases) and can precipitate withdrawal in a patient who is physically dependent on agonist medications.

At step 2, prescriptions for commonly used opioids are often for products combining an opioid with a nonopioid analgesic (e.g., oxycodone [Oxycontin] or codeine plus acetaminophen [Tylenol No. 3]), which may limit the opioid dose that can be given.

TABLE 10.13 MEDICATION THERAPY

Opioid Analgesics Commonly Used for Mild to Moderate Pain

Medication	Comments	Nursing Considerations
Morphine-Like Agonists		
Codeine	Weak opioid: Many preparations are combinations with nonopioid analgesics; codeine is a prodrug and metabolized to morphine; 1%–30% of people metabolize too efficiently and 10%–20% are unable to metabolize it	For mild to moderate pain, preparations of codeine and other opioids are limited by the dosage of nonopioid analgesic (e.g., the maximum dosage of acetaminophen is 4 g in 24 hours)
Tramadol (Ultram)	Maximum dosage: 400 mg in 24 hours	May cause seizures, although rarely
Mixed Agonist–Antagonists		
Butorphanol	Not available orally; not scheduled under *Controlled Drugs and Substances Act*; butorphanol nasal spray is used to treat migraine headaches	May precipitate withdrawal in people taking opioids on a regular basis; may cause psychotomimetic effects; reacts with many other medications; not widely prescribed

Source: Adapted from Inturrisi, C., & Lipman, A. (2010). Opioid analgesics. In S. M. Fishman, J. C. Ballantyne, & J. P. Rathmell (Eds.), *Bonica's management of pain* (4th ed., pp. 1174–1175). Wolters-Kluwer/Lippincott Williams & Wilkins.

TABLE 10.14 MEDICATION THERAPY

Opioids Commonly Used for Severe Pain

Medication	Comments	Nursing Considerations
Morphine	Standard comparison for opioid analgesics; sustained-release preparation (MS Contin) available	For all opioids: Use with caution in people with impaired ventilation, bronchial asthma, increased intracranial pressure, liver failure; in some people, the metabolite M6G may cause excessive vomiting and hallucinations, necessitating a change of opioid.
Morphine-Like Agonists		
Hydromorphone (Dilaudid)	—	Well tolerated; also available in elixir form for patients unable to swallow tablets
Oxycodone (slow-release formulation is OxyNeo)	May be given alone or combined with acetaminophen; immediate- and slow-release preparations are available; formulated to deter potential misuse	For moderate to severe pain; usually well tolerated; physical and psychological dependence can occur with long-term use; withdrawal can occur if medication is abruptly stopped; should be used for short-term pain relief.
Methadone	Good oral potency; 24- to 36-hour half-life, which necessitates careful monitoring	Licence required to prescribe; accumulates with repeated doses; on days 2–5, dosage size and frequency must be reduced
Fentanyl	Available as sublingual tablet, as injection, or, for persistent pain, as transdermal preparation (Duragesic)	Immediate onset after administration by intravenous route; within 7–8 minutes after intramuscular route; onset after transdermal route may take several hours; not recommended for acute pain management
Meperidine (Demerol)	Not recommended as first-line treatment for acute pain and should not be used for persistent pain management	Not well absorbed through oral route and should not be used; normeperidine (toxic metabolite with half-life of 14–21 hours) accumulates with repetitive dosing, causing CNS excitation and seizures; naloxone potentiates excitation and must not be used; avoid in patients taking monoamine oxidase inhibitors (e.g., selegiline)
Mixed Agonist–Antagonists		
Butorphanol	Not available orally; not scheduled under *Controlled Drugs and Substances Act*	May precipitate withdrawal in opioid-dependent patients

CNS, central nervous system.
Source: Adapted from Inturrisi, C., & Lipman, A. (2010). Opioid analgesics. In S. M. Fishman, J. C. Ballantyne, & J. P. Rathmell (Eds.), *Bonica's management of pain* (4th ed., pp. 1174–1175). Wolters-Kluwer/Lippincott Williams & Wilkins.

Oxycodone is now administered for severe pain as well. Although propoxyphene (Darvon) is classified as a step 2 medication, it is not recommended in analgesia guidelines because its effectiveness is limited and its toxic metabolite can cause seizures. Propoxyphene is not approved for use in Canada. A third type of medication available for mild to moderate pain is tramadol (Ultram). Tramadol is a weak mu-receptor agonist and is thought to inhibit the reuptake of norepinephrine and serotonin. It has approximately the same efficacy as acetaminophen plus codeine. The most common adverse effects, which are similar to those of other opioids, include nausea, constipation, dizziness, and sedation.

Medication Therapy for Moderate to Severe Pain. Step 3 medications are recommended for moderate to severe pain (4 to 10 on a scale of 0 to 10) or when step 2 medications do not produce effective pain relief. Most commonly used step 3 analgesics are mu-receptor agonists, although these medications also bind with the other receptors. These medications are effective for moderate to severe pain because they are potent, have no analgesic ceiling, and can be delivered via many routes of administration. Step 3 medications are listed in Table 10.14.

Morphine is one of the opioids most commonly prescribed for moderate to severe pain, although fentanyl (Duragesic), hydromorphone (Dilaudid), methadone (Metadol), and oxycodone also are used extensively. A long-acting morphine formulation (MS Contin) is available to treat moderate to severe persistent pain in patients who require continuous, round-the-clock therapy for an extended period. Meperidine (Demerol), a mu-receptor agonist, is no longer recommended for acute or persistent pain because of the high incidence of neurotoxicity (e.g., seizures) associated with the accumulation of its neurotoxic metabolite, normeperidine.

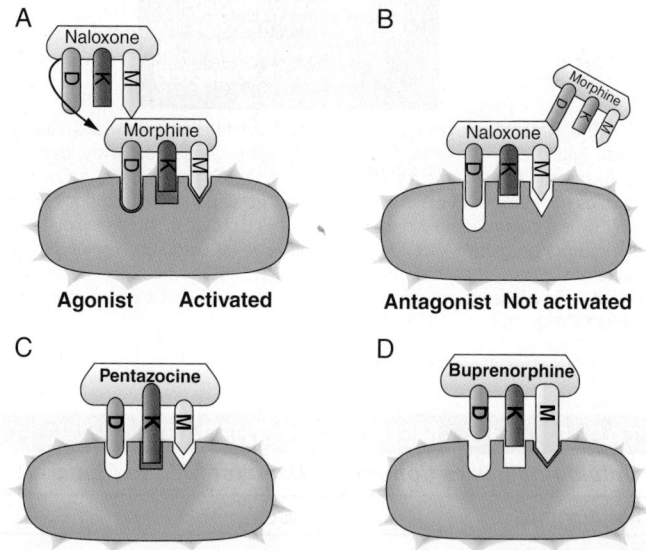

FIG. 10.9 Opioid receptor subtypes. **A,** Agonist action. **B,** Antagonist action. **C,** Agonist–antagonist action. **D,** Partial antagonist action. *D,* delta receptor. *K,* kappa receptor; *M,* mu receptor;

Moreover, any adverse effect cannot be reversed by naloxone, which potentiates the effect of normeperidine. In addition, a hyperpyrexic syndrome with delirium, which can cause death, can occur if meperidine is given to patients taking monoamine oxidase inhibitors. Although step 3 opioids have no analgesic ceiling, people can experience dose-limiting adverse effects. In

TABLE 10.15 MEDICATION THERAPY
Adjuvant Medications Used for Pain Management

Medication	Specific Indication	Nursing Considerations
Corticosteroids	Inflammation	Avoid high dosage for long-term use.
Antidepressants Amitriptyline (Elavil) Bupropion Duloxetine (Cymbalta) Desipramine Doxepin (Sinequan) Imipramine Maprotiline Nortriptyline (Aventyl) Venlafaxine	Neuropathic pain	Monitor for anticholinergic adverse effects.
Antiseizure Medications Carbamazepine (Tegretol) Clonazepam (Rivotril) Gabapentin (Neurontin) Pregabalin (Lyrica) Oxcarbazepine (Trileptal) Topiramate (Topamax) Valproic acid (Epival, Depakene)	Neuropathic pain	Start with low dosages, increase slowly to appropriate level for effect. Clonazepam and carbamazepine: Check liver function, renal function, electrolytes, and blood cell counts at baseline, at 2 weeks and at 6 weeks. Gabapentin: Monitor for idiosyncratic adverse effects (e.g., ankle swelling, ataxia, sedation).
Muscle Relaxant Baclofen (Lioresal)	Neuropathic pain (e.g., trigeminal neuralgia, muscle spasms)	Monitor for weakness, urinary dysfunction; avoid abrupt discontinuation because of CNS irritability.
Anaesthetics: Systemic or Oral Mexiletine	Diabetic neuropathy; neuropathic pain	Monitor for adverse effects, including dizziness, perioral numbness, paresthesias, tremor; can cause seizures, dysrhythmias, and myocardial depression at high dosages; avoid in patients with pre-existing cardiac disease.
Anaesthetics: Local Topical EMLA: lidocaine 2.5% + prilocaine 2.5%	Local skin analgesic before venipuncture, incision; possibly effective for post-herpetic neuralgia	Must be applied under an occlusive dressing (e.g., Tegaderm, DuoDerm) or on an anaesthetic disc; absorption from the genital mucosa is more rapid and onset time is shorter (5–10 min) than after application to intact skin; common adverse effects include mild erythema, edema, skin blanching.
Capsaicin	Pain associated with arthritis, postherpetic neuralgia, diabetic neuropathy	Apply sparingly, rub well into affected area; wash hands with soap and water after application; adverse effects include skin irritation (burning, stinging) at the application site and cough.
Psychostimulants Dextroamphetamine (Dexedrine) Methylphenidate (Ritalin)	Managing opioid-induced sedation	Adverse effect is insomnia; avoid administering late in the day; usually well tolerated at low dosages.
Cannabinoids Nabilone	Neuropathic pain	Recommended as an adjuvant for neuropathic pain in cases where therapeutic effect is not achieved via gabapentin.

EMLA, eutectic mixture of local anaesthetics.

opioid-naive patients, adverse effects include constipation, nausea and vomiting, sedation, respiratory depression, and pruritus. With continued use, most adverse effects diminish; the exception is constipation. Less common adverse effects include urinary retention, myoclonus, dizziness, confusion, and hallucinations.

MEDICATION ALERT—Opioids
- Opioids may cause respiratory depression.
- If respirations are 1 or fewer breaths per minute, withhold medication and contact the ealth care provider.
- Transdermal fentanyl should not be used for management of acute pain.

Methadone has a unique mechanism of action as an NMDA receptor antagonist and mu–opioid receptor agonist. It is used primarily in the treatment of chronic pain but can be used for acute pain. It produces analgesic effects independent of its action as an opioid (Kharasch, 2017).

Constipation is the most common opioid adverse effect. Because tolerance to opioid-induced constipation does not occur, a bowel regimen should be instituted at the beginning of opioid therapy and should continue for as long as the person takes opioids. Although dietary roughage, fluids, and exercise should be encouraged to the extent possible, these measures rarely are sufficient by themselves. Thus, most affected patients should immediately begin taking a gentle stimulant laxative (e.g., senna [Senokot]) plus a stool softener (e.g., docusate sodium [Colace]). Other agents (e.g., milk of magnesia, bisacodyl [Dulcolax], lactulose) can be added if necessary. Left untreated, constipation can lead to fecal impaction and paralytic ileus that can be difficult to differentiate from obstruction.

Nausea often is a problem in opioid-naive patients. The use of antiemetics such as ondansetron (Zofran), metoclopramide, hydroxyzine (Atarax), or a prochlorperazine can prevent or minimize opioid-related nausea and vomiting until tolerance develops, which usually occurs within 1 week. Metoclopramide is particularly effective when a patient reports gastric fullness. Opioids delay gastric emptying, and this effect can be reversed by metoclopramide. If nausea and vomiting are severe and persistent, as with morphine because of the metabolite M6G, changing to a different opioid such as oxycodone or hydromorphone may be necessary.

Two of the most common concerns associated with opioids are sedation and respiratory depression. Sedation may occur initially in opioid-naive patients, although patients handling pain without relief may be sleep deprived. Respiratory depression is rare in opioid-tolerant patients when opioids are titrated to analgesic effect. Individuals at risk for respiratory depression include opioid-naive patients, older patients, and patients with underlying lung disease. If respiratory depression occurs and stimulating the patient (e.g., calling and shaking patient) does not reverse the somnolence or increase the respiratory rate and depth, naloxone (0.4 mg in 10 mL saline), an opioid antagonist, can be administered intravenously or subcutaneously in 0.5-mL increments every 2 minutes. However, if the patient has been taking opioids regularly for more than a few days, naloxone should be used judiciously and titrated carefully because its use can precipitate severe, agonizing pain, profound withdrawal symptoms, and seizures. Because the half-life (60 to 90 minutes) of naloxone is shorter than that of most opioids, nurses should monitor the patient's respiratory rate because it can drop again 1 to 2 hours after naloxone administration.

Itching may occur with opioids, most frequently when they are administered via intraspinal routes. An antihistamine such as diphenhydramine (Benadryl) often is effective. If measures are ineffective, a low-dose opioid antagonist (e.g., naloxone) or a mixed agonist–antagonist can be used, but the patient must be carefully assessed for reversal of analgesia and withdrawal.

SAFETY ALERT
- The most appropriate opioid depends on the patient's clinical profile and the nature of the pain (e.g., mild to moderate, severe).
- Patients should be advised that opioids can cause cognitive effects, impairing their ability to drive.
- It is important to recognize that some women rapidly metabolize codeine to morphine. In the case of postoperative patients who are breastfeeding, the infant may be at risk for fatal opioid toxicity. If codeine is prescribed to breastfeeding mothers, consultation with the physician and other health care team members is crucial to ensure careful monitoring. The patient should be advised to monitor the infant for signs of CNS depression, including poor feeding and limpness, and to contact the health care provider immediately if any such signs are noted.

Adjuvant Analgesic Therapy. Adjuvant analgesic therapies are medications used in conjunction with opioid and nonopioid analgesics. Adjuvants are sometimes referred to as *coanalgesics*. They include medications that enhance pain therapy through one of three mechanisms: (a) enhancing the effects of opioids and nonopioids, (b) possessing analgesic properties of their own, or (c) counteracting the adverse effects of other analgesics. Commonly used analgesic adjuvants are listed in Table 10.15. Figure 10.10 shows the sites of actions of pharmacological and nonpharmacological therapies for pain. Adjuvant medications are used at every step in the WHO ladder.

Antidepressants. Tricyclic antidepressants have analgesic properties at dosages lower than those effective for depression. They enhance the descending inhibitory system by preventing

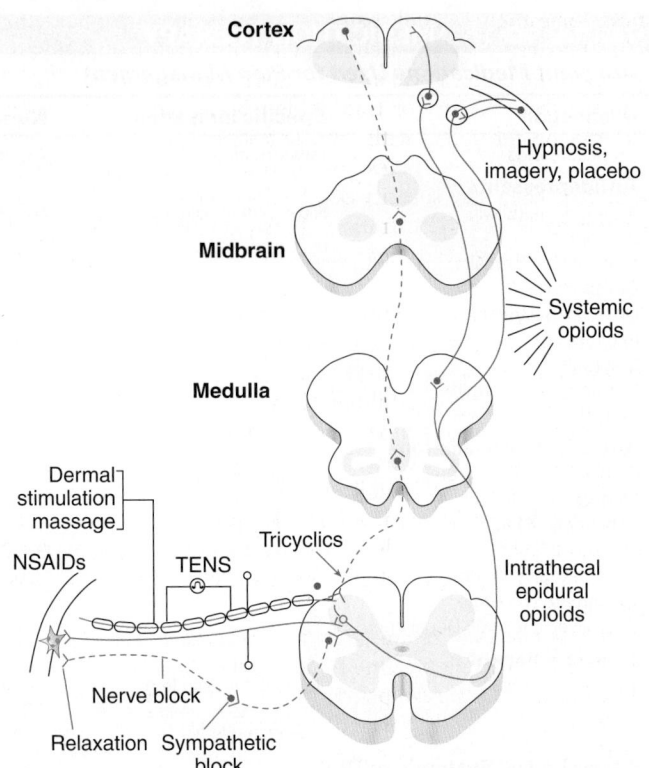

FIG. 10.10 The sites of commonly used pharmacological and nonpharmacological analgesic therapies. *NSAIDs,* nonsteroidal anti-inflammatory drugs; *TENS,* transcutaneous electrical nerve stimulation.

synaptic reuptake of serotonin and norepinephrine. Higher levels of serotonin and norepinephrine in the synaptic cleft inhibit the transmission of nociceptive signals in the CNS. Tricyclic antidepressants have been shown to be effective for a variety of pain syndromes, especially those involving neuropathic pain. Anticholinergic effects such as dry mouth, urinary retention, sedation, and orthostatic hypotension may lessen patients' acceptance of using the medication and adherence to the regimen.

MEDICATION ALERT—Tricyclic Antidepressants
- Tricyclic antidepressants have been implicated in prolonged QT intervals.

Antiseizure Medications. Antiseizure medications such as gabapentin (Neurontin), carbamazepine (Tegretol), and clonazepam (Rivotril) stabilize the membrane of the neuron and prevent transmission. These medications are effective for some neuropathic pain and for prophylactic treatment of headaches.

Corticosteroids. Corticosteroid medications, which include dexamethasone and methylprednisolone (Medrol), are used to treat several types of pain, including acute and persistent cancer pain, pain secondary to spinal cord or brain compression, and some neuropathic pain syndromes. Mechanisms of action are unknown but may involve the ability of corticosteroids to decrease edema and inflammation and, in some cases, to shrink tumours. Corticosteroids have many adverse effects, especially when used chronically in high dosages. Adverse effects include hyperglycemia, fluid retention, dyspepsia and GI bleeding, impairment in healing, muscle wasting, osteoporosis, and susceptibility to infection.

Local Anaesthetics. Oral, parenteral, and topical applications of local anaesthetics are used to interrupt transmission of pain signals to the brain. Local anaesthetics are given for acute pain resulting from surgery or trauma. Persistent neuropathic pain also may be controlled with local anaesthetics. Adverse effects can include dizziness, paresthesias, and seizures (at high dosages). Incidence and severity of adverse effects depend on dosage and route of administration. These medications also affect cardiac conductivity and may cause dysrhythmias and myocardial depression.

Ketamine. Ketamine has traditionally been used as an anaesthetic agent because of its dissociative and amnesic effects. However, ketamine at lower doses displays analgesic effects with opioid-sparing capabilities (Davis et al., 2019). Research has shown that the ketamine is beneficial in the management or both acute and chronic pain.

Ketamine works by inhibiting pain signals to the brain and producing desired analgesic effects (Kremier, 2019). It is water and lipid soluble which allows for crossing of the blood–brain barrier. It can be administered via a variety of routes (Davis et al., 2019).

Adverse effects of ketamine include nausea, vomiting, dizziness, and hallucinations. One benefit noted for the use of ketamine for management of pain is that because of its mechanism of action on receptors it preserves respiratory function, unlike traditional opioids (Davis et al., 2019).

Administration Routes. Opioids and other analgesic medications can be delivered via many routes. This flexibility allows the health care provider to (a) target a particular anatomical source of the pain, (b) achieve therapeutic blood levels rapidly when necessary, (c) avoid certain adverse effects through localized administration, and (d) provide analgesia when patients are unable to swallow. The following discussion highlights the uses of and nursing considerations for analgesics delivered through a variety of routes.

Oral. In general, oral administration is the route of choice for the patient with a functioning GI system. Oral medications are usually less expensive than those delivered by other routes. Many opioids are available in oral preparations, such as liquid and tablet formulations. To obtain analgesia equivalent to that provided by doses administered intramuscularly or intravenously, oral doses must be higher. For example, 10 mg of parenteral morphine is equivalent to approximately 30 mg of orally administered morphine. Generally, oral administration is the route required for opioid-naive patients because of the first-pass effect of hepatic metabolism. This means that oral opioids initially are absorbed from the GI tract into the portal circulation and shunted to the liver. Partial metabolism in the liver occurs before the medication enters systemic circulation and becomes available to peripheral receptors or before it can cross the blood–brain barrier and access CNS opioid receptors, a process necessary to produce analgesia. Many opioids are available in oral preparations, such as liquid and tablet form. Oral opioids are as effective as parenteral opioids if the dose administered is large enough to compensate for first-pass metabolism.

Oral preparations also are available in immediate-release and sustained-release preparations. For example, morphine is available in immediate-release solutions or tablets. These products are effective in providing rapid, short-term pain relief; concentration in the blood typically peaks within 30 to 60 minutes. Sustained-release oral morphine tablets are administered every 8 to 12 hours; the most common preparation is morphine ER

(MS Contin). As with other sustained-release preparations, this product should not be crushed, broken, or chewed. Oxycodone also comes in a sustained-release capsule (OxyNeo). Other opioids with sustained-release formulations include hydromorphone and tramadol. The time to maximum blood plasma dose concentration typically ranges from 30 to 60 minutes and from 2 to 4 hours for immediate-release and sustained-release formulations, respectively.

SAFETY ALERT

Sustained-Release or Extended-Release Preparation
- These medications should not be crushed, broken, dissolved, or chewed. They are to be swallowed whole.
- If all the medicine is released into a person at once, serious adverse effects can occur, including death from overdose.

Sublingual and Buccal. Opioids administered under the tongue or held in the mouth and absorbed into systemic circulation are exempt from the first-pass effect.

Intranasal. Intranasal administration allows delivery of medication to highly vascular mucosa and avoids the first-pass effect. Butorphanol is one of the few intranasal analgesics available. This medication is most commonly indicated for migraine headaches. Several intranasal opioids such as fentanyl drugs are being investigated.

Rectal. The rectal route is often overlooked but is particularly useful when the patient cannot take an analgesic by mouth. Rectal suppositories that are effective for pain relief include hydromorphone (Dilaudid) and morphine.

Transdermal. Fentanyl (Duragesic) is available as a transdermal patch system for application to nonhairy skin. This delivery system is useful for the patient who cannot tolerate oral analgesic medications. Absorption from the patch is slow. Therefore, transdermal fentanyl is not suitable for rapid-dosage titration but can be effective if the patient's pain is stable and the dosage required to control it is known. Patches may have to be changed every 48 hours rather than the recommended 72 hours, depending on individual patient responses.

Currently, creams and lotions containing 10% trolamine salicylate (e.g., Aspercreme, Myoflex) are available. These medications have been recommended by the manufacturers for joint and muscle pain. This Aspirin-like substance is absorbed locally. The topical route of administration precludes gastric irritation, but the other adverse effects of high-dosage salicylate are not necessarily prevented.

Ointments, lotions, gels, liniments, and balms (most of which are over-the-counter products) are sometimes applied topically to achieve pain relief. Common ingredients include methyl salicylate combined with camphor, menthol, or both. On application, these medications usually produce a strong hot or cold sensation and should not be used after massage or a heat treatment, when blood vessels are already dilated. Skin testing is advisable when the patient has not used the particular medication before because the strengths of the medications vary and different intensities of sensation are produced. These products are indicated for arthralgia, bursitis, myalgia, and tendinitis.

Other topical analgesic medications, such as capsaicin (e.g., Flex-ol) and prilocaine plus lidocaine (eutectic mixture of local anaesthetics [EMLA]), and anti-inflammatory medications such as Voltaren (1% diclofenac) also provide analgesia. Derived from red chili pepper, capsaicin depletes and prevents reaccumulation of substance P in the peripheral sensory neurons. It can control pain associated with postherpetic neuralgia, diabetic neuropathy, and arthritis. EMLA is useful for control of pain associated with venipunctures, ulcer debridement, and possibly postherpetic neuralgia. The area to which EMLA is applied should be covered with a plastic wrap for 30 to 60 minutes before a painful procedure begins.

Parenteral Routes. The parenteral route includes subcutaneous and intravenous administration. The only opioid that must be injected intramuscularly is meperidine, and this medication is not recommended because its toxic metabolite, normeperidine, can accumulate with repeated administration, causing CNS excitation. Single-dose administration (subcutaneous or intravenous) is possible via parenteral routes. The intramuscular route, although frequently used, is not recommended because these injections cause significant pain, result in unreliable absorption, and, with chronic use, can result in abscesses and fibrosis. Onset of analgesia after subcutaneous administration is slow, thus the subcutaneous route is rarely used for acute pain management. However, continuous subcutaneous infusions are effective for persistent cancer pain. This route is especially helpful for people with abnormal GI function and limited venous access. Intravenous administration is the best option when immediate analgesia and rapid titration are necessary. Continuous intravenous infusions provide excellent steady-state analgesia through stable blood levels.

Intraspinal Delivery. Intraspinal (epidural or intrathecal) opioid therapy involves inserting a catheter into the subarachnoid space (for intrathecal delivery) or the epidural space (for epidural delivery) and injecting an analgesic, by either intermittent bolus doses or continuous infusion. Percutaneously placed temporary catheters are used for short-term therapy (2 to 4 days), and surgically implanted catheters are used for long-term therapy. Although the lumbar region is the most common site of placement, epidural catheters may be placed at any point along the neuroaxis (cervical, thoracic, lumbar, or caudal). Intraspinally administered analgesics are highly potent because they are delivered close to the receptors in the dorsal horn of the spinal cord. Thus, much lower doses of analgesics are needed for intraspinal delivery in comparison with other routes, including intravenous. Medications delivered intraspinally include morphine, fentanyl, and hydromorphone. Nausea, itching, and urinary retention are common adverse effects of intraspinal opioids.

Complications of intraspinal analgesia include catheter displacement and migration, neurotoxicity (especially of certain medications when infused intraspinally), and infection. Clinical manifestations of catheter displacement or migration depend on catheter location. Movement of a catheter out of the intrathecal or epidural space causes a decrease in pain relief with no improvement even when additional analgesic is administered. Correct placement of an intrathecal catheter can be checked by aspirating cerebrospinal fluid. Migration of a catheter into a blood vessel causes an increase in adverse effects because of systemic medication distribution. A number of medications and chemicals are highly neurotoxic when administered intraspinally, such as preservatives (e.g., alcohol and phenol), antibiotics, potassium, and total parenteral nutrition supplements. To avoid inadvertent injection of intravenous medications into an intraspinal catheter, the catheter should be clearly marked as an intraspinal access device, and only preservative-free medications should be injected.

Infection rarely occurs with intraspinal analgesia. However, it is a serious complication that can be difficult to detect. The skin around the exit site should be carefully assessed for inflammation, drainage, or pain. Signs and symptoms of an intraspinal infection include diffuse back pain, pain or paresthesias during bolus injection, and unexplained sensory or motor deficits. Fever may or may not be present. Acute bacterial infection (meningitis) is manifested by fever, headache, and altered mental status. Infection is avoided with regular, meticulous wound care and with the use of sterile technique in caring for the catheter and injecting medications.

Patient-Controlled Analgesia. A specific type of subcutaneous, intravenous, or intraspinal delivery system is **patient-controlled analgesia (PCA)**, or *demand analgesia*. PCA is an infusion system that allows the patient to self-administer a dose of opioid through a pump when needed: The patient pushes a button to receive a bolus infusion of an analgesic within preprogrammed intervals. PCA is used widely for the management of acute pain, including postoperative pain and cancer pain. Often, the patient also receives an additional continuous basal infusion (known as *PCA plus basal*) at a preset dose and rate. The addition of a continuous basal infusion to a PCA regimen improves nighttime pain relief and promotes better sleep postoperatively. Common opioids used in PCA administration method include morphine, fentanyl, and hydromorphone (Dilaudid).

Use of PCA begins with patient teaching. The patient needs to understand the benefits and principles of PCA therapy, the mechanics of obtaining a medication dose (i.e., the operation of the pump and button), and how to titrate the medication to achieve good pain relief. The patient should be encouraged to use the PCA pump prophylactically by self-administering the analgesic before ambulation, physiotherapy, and dressing changes. The patient also needs to be reminded that apart from the involved health care providers, the patient is the only person who should press the button. The patient should also be assured—for safety reasons and to avoid excessive sedation or respiratory depression—that the pump is programmed to deliver a maximum number of doses per hour; pressing the button after the maximum dose is administered will not result in additional analgesic. If the maximum doses are inadequate to relieve pain, by order of a physician or nurse practitioner, the pump can be reprogrammed to increase the amount or frequency of administration. In addition, bolus doses can be given by the nurse if they are included in the physician's orders. The patient should also be encouraged to report adverse effects such as nausea and vomiting or pruritus so that they can be managed effectively. To make a smooth transition from infusion PCA to oral therapy, the dosage of oral medication should be increased (as ordered) as the PCA analgesic is tapered.

TRADITIONAL MEDICINAL THERAPIES OF INDIGENOUS POPULATIONS IN CANADA

The Indigenous populations in Canada believe in a holistic approach to health and wellness. As the Indigenous populations account for 4% of Canada's population, it is important to understand the traditional medicines used by Indigenous people (Uprety et al., 2016). Many of the traditional medicines come from the Boreal forest in Canada. Health care providers need to be knowledgeable of traditional medicinal practices and seek knowledge of such practices during pain assessments to ensure a comprehensive and holistic approach to planning care. Many medicinal plants are used in Indigenous populations.

Preparation of the plants for medicinal purposes includes paste, poultice, infusion, and eating the plant raw. It is important to note that traditional medicinal practices are usually guided under the direction of an Elder, as some plants are poisonous or can have adverse reactions with other plants or Western medicines (Uprety et al., 2016).

Surgical Therapy for Pain

Nerve Blocks. Nerve blocks are used to reduce pain by temporarily or permanently interrupting transmission of nociceptive input. This is achieved with local anaesthetics or neurolytic drugs (e.g., alcohol, phenol). Neural blockade with local anaesthetics is sometimes used for perioperative pain. For intractable persistent pain, nerve blocks are used when more conservative therapies fail. Nerve blocks have been a successful pain management technique for more localized persistent pain states, such as peripheral vascular disease, trigeminal neuralgia, causalgia, and some cancer pain. A nerve block may be considered advantageous for managing localized pain caused by malignancy and in debilitated patients who could not otherwise withstand a surgical procedure for pain relief.

Interventional Therapy

Therapeutic Nerve Blocks. Nerve blocks generally involve one-time or continuous infusion of local anaesthetics into a particular area to produce pain relief. Such relief is also referred to as *regional anaesthesia*. Nerve blocks interrupt all afferent and efferent transmission to the area and thus are not specific to nociceptive pathways. They include local infiltration of anaesthetics into a surgical area (e.g., for excision of a breast lump, inguinal hernia surgery, intra-articular infiltration after joint surgery, amputation, subcostal incisions) and injection of anaesthetics into a specific nerve (e.g., occipital or pudendal nerve) or nerve plexus (e.g., brachial or celiac plexus). Nerve blocks often are used during and after surgery to manage pain. For longer-term relief of chronic pain, local anaesthetics can be administered via a continuous infusion.

For intractable persistent pain, neuroablative nerve blocks (see next section) with phenol or alcohol may be used. For example, a neurolytic celiac plexus block may be induced for pain caused by pancreatic cancer, or an intercostal neurolytic block may be induced for post-thoracotomy pain. Heat and microwaves, used in many neurolytic procedures, produce nerve tissue destruction.

Neuroablative Techniques. *Neuroablative interventions* are performed for severe pain that is unresponsive to all other therapies. Neuroablative techniques destroy nerves, thereby interrupting pain transmission. Destruction is accomplished by surgical resection or thermocoagulation, including radiofrequency coagulation. Neuroablative interventions that destroy the sensory division of a peripheral or spinal nerve are classified as neurectomies, rhizotomies, and sympathectomies. Neurosurgical procedures that ablate the lateral spinothalamic tract are classified as cordotomies if the tract is interrupted in the spinal cord or as tractotomies if the interruption is in the medulla or the midbrain of the brain stem. Figure 10.11 depicts the sites of neurosurgical procedures for pain relief. Both cordotomy and tractotomy can be performed with the aid of local anaesthesia by a percutaneous technique.

Neuroaugmentation. Neuroaugmentation involves electrical stimulation of the brain and the spinal cord. Spinal cord stimulation is performed much more often than deep brain stimulation. Technological advances have enabled the use of multiple

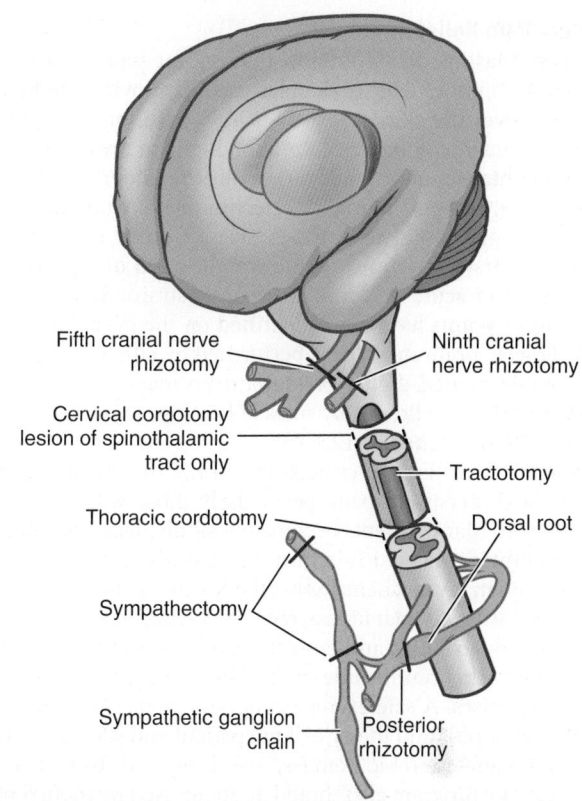

FIG. 10.11 Sites of neurosurgical procedures for pain relief.

TABLE 10.16	NONPHARMACOLOGICAL THERAPIES FOR PAIN	
Physical Therapies		**Cognitive Therapies**
• Acupuncture • Application of heat and cold • Exercise • Massage • Percutaneous electrical nerve stimulation (PENS) • Transcutaneous electrical nerve stimulation (TENS)		• Distraction • Hypnosis • Imagery • Relaxation strategies • Self-management

leads and multiple electrode terminals so as to stimulate large areas. In Canada and the United States, a common use of spinal cord stimulation is for chronic back pain secondary to nerve damage that is unresponsive to other therapies. Other uses include complex regional pain syndrome (CRPS), spinal cord injury pain, and interstitial cystitis. Potential complications include those related to the surgery (bleeding and infection), migration of the generator (which usually is implanted in the subcutaneous tissues of the upper gluteal or pectoralis area), and nerve damage.

Nonpharmacological Therapy for Pain

Use of nonpharmacological pain management strategies can reduce the dose of an analgesic required to control pain and thereby minimize adverse effects of pharmacological therapy. Some strategies are believed to alter ascending nociceptive input or stimulate descending pain modulation mechanisms. Nonpharmacological pain relief methods can be categorized as physical or cognitive strategies (Table 10.16).

Physical Pain Relief Strategies

Massage. Massage is a common therapy for pain, and many massage techniques exist. Examples include moving the hands or fingers over the skin slowly or briskly with long strokes or in circles (*superficial massage*) or applying firm pressure to the skin to maintain contact while massaging the underlying tissues (*deep massage*). Specific massage techniques include acupressure and trigger-point massage. A **trigger point** is a circumscribed hypersensitive area within a tight band of muscle that is the result of acute or persistent muscle strain. Several common trigger points have been identified on the neck, back, and arms. Trigger-point massage is performed by either application of strong, sustained digital pressure, deep massage, or gentler massage with ice followed by muscle heating. (Massage is discussed further in Chapter 12.)

Exercise. Exercise is a critical part of the treatment plan for patients with persistent pain, particularly those with musculoskeletal pain. Many patients become physically deconditioned as a result of their pain, which in turn can exacerbate pain. Exercise acts through many mechanisms to relieve pain: It enhances circulation and cardiovascular fitness, reduces edema, increases muscle strength and flexibility, and enhances physical and psychosocial functioning. This can include both passive and active range-of-motion exercises. A safe exercise program should be tailored to the physical needs and lifestyle of the patient and should include mild to moderate aerobic exercise, stretching, and strengthening exercises. The program also should be supervised by trained personnel (e.g., physiologist, physiatrist, registered nurse with specialty training, exercise physiologist, physiotherapist).

Turning and Positioning. Patients experiencing immobility due to injury or illness can experience pain due to immobility. These patients are unable to turn and position themselves to decrease pressure on pressure points and increase their comfort and reduce the risk of impaired skin integrity (e.g., pressure injuries). Health care providers should turn and position patients frequently, every 2 hours, to promote circulation and comfort (RNAO, 2007).

Transcutaneous Electrical Nerve Stimulation. In *transcutaneous electrical nerve stimulation* (TENS), an electric current is delivered through electrodes applied to the skin surface over the painful region, at trigger points, or over a peripheral nerve. A TENS system consists of two or more electrodes connected by lead wires to a small, battery-operated stimulator (Figure 10.12). Usually, a physiotherapist is responsible for administering TENS therapy, although nurses also can be trained in the technique.

TENS may be used for acute pain, including postoperative pain, visceral pain, and pain associated with physical trauma. Although the effect of TENS on persistent pain is less clear, it may be effective in such cases (Coutaux, 2017).

Heat Therapy. Application of heat for pain management has been used for centuries. The premise is that applying heat to skin will increase blood flow and reduce pain-related neurotransmitter activity. Heat therapy includes application of either moist or dry heat to the skin and can be superficial or deep. Superficial heat can be applied through an electric heating pad (dry or moist), a hot pack, hot moist compresses, or a hot water bottle. For exposure to large areas of the body, patients can immerse themselves in a hot bath, shower, or whirlpool. Physiotherapy departments provide deep-heat therapy through such techniques as shortwave diathermy, microwave diathermy, and ultrasound therapy. Patient teaching regarding heat therapy is described in Table 10.17.

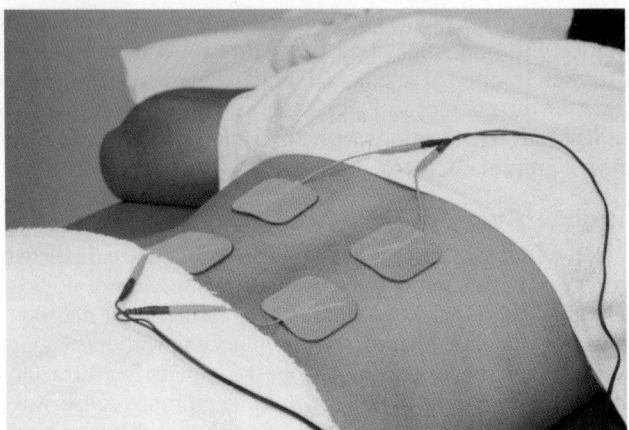

FIG. 10.12 Transcutaneous electrical nerve stimulation (TENS). Source: iStock.com/Praisaeng.

TABLE 10.17	PATIENT & CAREGIVER TEACHING GUIDE

Application of Heat and Cold

When patients use superficial heating techniques, they should be taught the following:
- Do not use heat on an area that is being treated with radiation therapy, is bleeding, has decreased sensation, or has been injured in the past 24 hours.
- Do not use any menthol-containing products (e.g., Vicks VapoRub) with heat applications because this combination may cause burns.
- Cover the heat source with a towel or cloth to prevent burns.
- Do not apply heat directly to transdermal analgesic preparations, such as fentanyl, as heat application may alter drug bioavailability.

When patients use superficial cold techniques, they should be taught the following:
- Cover the cold source with a cloth or towel.
- Do not apply cold to areas that are being treated with radiation therapy, have open wounds, or have poor circulation.
- If it is not possible to apply the cold directly to the painful site, try applying it directly above or below the painful site or on the opposite side of the body on the corresponding site (e.g., left elbow if the right elbow hurts).

Application of Cold. Like heat therapy, application of cold therapy has long been used for pain relief. Cold therapy competes for nerve transmission and reduces sensation, effects that can be especially helpful for pain that resembles a burning sensation (RNAO, 2013). Cold therapy involves the application of either moist or dry cold to the skin. Dry cold can be applied by means of an ice bag, and moist cold by means of towels soaked in ice water, cold hydrocollator packs, or immersion in a cold bath or under running cold water. Icing with ice cubes or blocks of ice made to resemble popsicles is another technique used for pain relief. Cold therapy is believed to be more effective than heat for a variety of painful conditions, including acute pain from trauma or surgery, acute flares of arthritis, muscle spasms, and headache. Patient teaching regarding cold therapy is described in Table 10.17.

Cognitive Techniques. A variety of cognitive strategies and behavioural approaches can alter the affective, cognitive, and behavioural components of pain. Some of these techniques require little training and often are adopted independently by the patient. For others, a trained therapist must administer therapy.

Distraction. The redirection of attention on something other than the pain is a simple but powerful strategy to relieve pain. Distraction-induced analgesia involves introducing competition for attention between a highly salient sensation (pain) and some other information-processing activity. Distraction can be achieved by engaging the patient in any activity that can hold their attention (e.g., watching TV, conversing, listening to music, playing a game).

Relaxation Strategies. Relaxation strategies are used to reduce stress, decrease acute anxiety, distract from pain, alleviate muscle tension, combat fatigue, facilitate sleep, and enhance the effectiveness of other pain relief measures (dos Santos Felix, 2019). Elicitation of the relaxation response requires a quiet environment, a comfortable position, and a mental device as a focus of concentration (e.g., a word, a sound, or the breath). Relaxation strategies include relaxation breathing, music, guided imagery, meditation, and progressive muscle relaxation. (See Chapter 8 for additional information.)

Self-Management. Self-management training is now in widespread use in Canada as an effective, adjunctive strategy for managing the effect of chronic pain on day-to-day functioning and quality of life (Boschen et al., 2016). Through structured rehearsal of various cognitive and behavioural self-management techniques (e.g., energy conservation, pacing, sleep promotion, relaxation, communication skills, safe exercise), patients and family members learn to set realistic weekly goals that are directed at increasing overall functional capacity and emotional well-being. Strong evidence supports the effectiveness of self-management training for (a) improving participants' perceived self-efficacy or ability to achieve selected goals, (b) reducing pain, and (c) improving perceived quality of life.

NURSING AND INTERPROFESSIONAL MANAGEMENT PAIN

The nurse is an important member of the interprofessional pain management team. The nurse acts as planner, educator, patient advocate, interpreter, and supporter of the patient in pain and of the patient's family or caregivers. Because any patient in a wide variety of care settings (e.g., home, hospital, clinic) can be in pain, the nurse must be knowledgeable about current therapies and flexible in trying new approaches to pain management. The extent of the nurse's involvement depends on the unique factors associated with the patient, the setting, and the cause of the pain. Many nursing roles were described earlier in this chapter: conducting pain assessments, administering therapies, monitoring for adverse effects, and teaching patients and caregivers. However, the success of these actions depends on the nurse's ability to establish a trusting relationship with the patient and caregivers and to address the concerns they have regarding pain and its treatment.

Effective Communication

Patients need to feel confident that their reporting of pain will be believed and will not be perceived as "complaining." The patient and family also need to know that the nurse considers the pain significant and is committed to helping the patient obtain pain relief and cope with any unrelieved pain. Pharmacological and nonpharmacological interventions should be incorporated into the treatment plan, and the patient should be supported through the period of trial and error that may be necessary to implement an effective therapeutic plan. It also is important

TABLE 10.18   **NURSING ASSESSMENT**
Pain-Related Nursing Diagnoses

• Anxiety	• Need for health teaching
• Comfort	• Pain
• Constipation	• Reduced functional ability
• Coping	• Reduced stamina
• Discomfort	• Self concept
• Inadequate sleep	• Social isolation

TABLE 10.19   **PATIENT & CAREGIVER TEACHING GUIDE**
Pain Management

Teaching Needs

The goals of teaching related to pain management include the expectation that the patient and the caregivers understand the following:

- The need to maintain a record of pain intensity and effectiveness of treatment
- No need to wait until pain becomes severe to take medications or use nonpharmacological therapies for pain relief
- The possibility that the dosage of medication will have to be adjusted over time to maximize long-term effectiveness
- The potential adverse effects (e.g., nausea and vomiting, constipation, sedation and drowsiness, itching, urinary retention, sweating) and complications associated with opioid therapy or other pain relief therapies
- The need to report when pain is not relieved to tolerable levels

to clarify responsibilities of pain relief. The nurse should help the patient understand the roles of the interprofessional health care team members, as well as the roles and expectations of the patient.

In addition to addressing specific aspects of pain assessment and treatment, the nurse evaluates the total effect that the pain may have on the lives of the patient and family. Thus, other possible nursing diagnoses must also be considered. Table 10.18 lists possible nursing diagnoses that may be appropriate for assessing and managing pain. Table 10.19 addresses teaching needs of patients and caregivers in relation to pain management.

Barriers to Effective Pain Management

Pain is a complex, multidimensional, and subjective experience, and its management is influenced greatly by psychosocial, sociocultural, and legal and ethical factors. These factors include emotions, behaviours, misconceptions, and attitudes of patients and family members about pain and the use of pain therapies. Achieving effective pain management requires careful consideration of these factors.

Concerns regarding tolerance, dependence, and addiction are common barriers to effective pain management, inasmuch as these phenomena are often misunderstood. Patients, family members, and health care providers often share these concerns. It is important for the nurse to understand and be able to explain the differences between these various concepts.

Tolerance. *Tolerance* occurs with chronic exposure to a variety of drugs. In the case of opioids, tolerance to analgesia is characterized by the need for an increased opioid dose to maintain the same degree of analgesia. Although the development of tolerance to adverse effects (except constipation) is more predictable, the incidence of clinically significant analgesic opioid

TABLE 10.20	MANIFESTATIONS OF OPIOID WITHDRAWAL SYNDROME	
	Early Response (6–12 hr)	**Late Response (48–72 hr)**
Psychosocial Secretions	• Anxiety • Lacrimation • Rhinorrhea • Diaphoresis	• Excitation • Diarrhea
Other	• Yawning • Piloerection • Shaking, chills • Dilated pupils • Anorexia • Tremor	• Restlessness • Fever • Nausea and vomiting • Abdominal cramping pain • Hypertension • Tachycardia • Insomnia • Muscle aches

tolerance in patients with chronic pain is unknown, since dosage needs may increase as the disease (e.g., cancer) progresses. It is essential to assess for increased analgesic needs in patients on long-term therapy. The interprofessional team must evaluate and rule out other causes of increased analgesic needs, such as disease progression or infection.

The first sign of tolerance may be that the patient begins to experience regular end-of-dose failure. If manifestations of possible tolerance appear, appropriate evaluations should be made to rule out other causes of increased analgesic needs, such as disease progression or infection. Approaches to managing tolerance are (a) to increase the dosage of the analgesic, (b) to substitute another medication in the same class (e.g., changing from morphine to oxycodone), or (c) to add a medication from a different drug class that will augment pain relief without increasing adverse effects. It is important to note that there is no ceiling effect for opioid-agonist medications and to recognize that drug tolerance is not synonymous with addiction.

Physical Dependence. Like tolerance, physical dependence is an expected physiological response to ongoing exposure to pharmacological agents. It is manifested by a withdrawal syndrome when the drug is abruptly decreased. Manifestations of opioid withdrawal are listed in Table 10.20.

When opioids are no longer needed to provide pain relief, a tapering schedule should be used in conjunction with careful monitoring. A typical tapering schedule involves reducing the dose by 20% to 50% per day. The goal is to reduce the amount of medication and at the same time minimize adverse and withdrawal effects. Despite this slow weaning schedule, the nurse should assess carefully for signs of opioid withdrawal. In addition, it is important to recognize that other commonly prescribed medications for pain also can induce physical dependence and therefore must be slowly tapered. These include benzodiazepines and muscle relaxants.

Substance Misuse. Substance misuse or substance use disorders are complex neurobiological conditions characterized by the use of a substance in high doses or inappropriate situations that can impact one's health or create social problems (McLellan, 2017) (see Chapter 11).

Tolerance and physical dependence are not indicators of addiction or substance misuse. Rather, they are normal physiological responses to chronic exposure to certain drugs, including opioids. For patients without a history of substance use disorder, the risk of addiction or substance misuse is thought to be significantly lower. People with a history of addiction can be managed successfully on opioids for their pain with careful monitoring; however, in this population, the risk for addiction may be higher. Expectations of the health care team and the patient must be discussed openly and documented. Signs and symptoms of possible addiction must be monitored and interventions promptly initiated.

In addition to fears about substance misuse, physical dependence, and tolerance, other barriers hinder effective pain management. These include concern about adverse effects, difficulties with remembering to take medications, desire to handle pain stoically, and not wanting to distract the health care provider from treating the disease. Table 10.21 lists examples of patient-related barriers to effective pain management and includes strategies to address the barriers.

INSTITUTIONALIZING PAIN EDUCATION AND MANAGEMENT

Besides patient and family barriers, other barriers to effective and safe pain management include inadequate health care provider education and lack of institutional support. Traditionally, medical and nursing school curricula have spent little time teaching future physicians and nurses about pain and effective pain management, although this is changing. This lack of emphasis was partially responsible for the insufficiency of health care providers' knowledge of and skills for treating pain adequately.

Over the past few decades, some improvements have been made in overcoming these barriers. Medical and nursing schools now devote more time to addressing pain. Numerous professional organizations have published evidence-informed guidelines for assessing and managing pain in many patient populations and clinical settings. The IASP has published a core curriculum on pain that was developed for the learning needs of a range of health care provider groups. Provincial organizations such as the RNAO (2013) have also developed evidence-informed practice guidelines on pain that are readily accessible (see the Resources section at the end of this chapter for the Web links).

Health care institutions are also directing more, much-needed attention to their support of pain management. Researchers and health care providers have documented the central role of institutional commitment and practices in changing clinical practice; without institutional support, pain outcomes are unlikely to change. The pain management standards from the Canadian Pain Task Force Report (2010) *Chronic Pain in Canada: Laying a Foundation for Action* (see the Resources section at the end of this chapter) emphasize that patients have a right to the best pain relief possible and that measures to prevent or reduce acute pain are a priority. Many large tertiary and quaternary university-affiliated care settings now have specialized teams to manage pain. One such example is the establishment of dedicated acute pain services (APS) that include advanced-practice nurses. These services provide expert management of postsurgical pain and complex pain conditions. Advanced-practice nurses, often nurse practitioners, work collaboratively with anaesthesiologists and allied health care providers to assess and manage pain

TABLE 10.21 PATIENT & CAREGIVER TEACHING GUIDE
Reducing Patient-Related Barriers to Pain Management

Barrier	Nursing Considerations
Fear of addiction	• Provide accurate definition of *addiction*. • Explain that addiction is uncommon in patients taking opioids for pain relief.
Fear of tolerance	• Provide accurate definition of *tolerance*. • Teach that tolerance is a normal physiological response to long-term opioid therapy. If tolerance does develop, the medication may have to be changed (e.g., morphine in place of oxycodone). • Teach that there is no upper limit to pure opioid agonists (e.g., morphine). Dosages can be increased indefinitely, and the patient should not save medication for when the pain is worse. • Teach that tolerance to analgesic effects of opioids develops more slowly than do many adverse effects (e.g., sedation, respiratory depression). Tolerance does not ameliorate constipation; thus a regular bowel program should be started early.
Concern about adverse effects	• Teach methods to prevent and to treat common adverse effects. • Emphasize that adverse effects such as sedation and nausea decrease with time. • Explain that different medications have unique adverse effects and that other pain medications can be tried to reduce the specific adverse effect. • Teach nonpharmacological therapies to minimize the dosage of medication needed to control pain.
Fear of injections	• Explain that oral medicines are preferred. • Emphasize that even if the oral route becomes unusable, transdermal or in-dwelling parenteral routes can be used rather than injections.
Desire to be a good patient	• Explain that patients are partners in their care and that the partnership requires open communication on the parts of both patient and nurse. • Emphasize to patients that they have a responsibility to keep the nurse informed about their pain.
Desire to be stoic	• Explain that although stoicism is a valued behaviour in many cultures, failure to report pain can result in undertreatment and severe, unrelieved pain.
Forgetting to take analgesic	• Provide and teach use of pill containers. • Provide methods of record keeping for medication use. • Recruit family members, as appropriate, to assist with the analgesic regimen.
Fear of distracting the health care provider from treating the disease	• Explain that reporting pain is important for treating both the disease and its symptoms.
Concern that pain signifies disease progression	• Explain that increased pain or analgesic needs may reflect tolerance. • Emphasize that new pain may come from a non–life-threatening source (e.g., muscle spasm, urinary tract infection). • Institute pharmacological and nonpharmacological strategies to reduce anxiety. • Ensure that the patient and family members have current, accurate, comprehensive information about the disease and the prognosis. • Provide psychological support.
Sense of fatalism	• Explain that research has shown that pain can be managed in most patients. • Explain that with most therapies, a period of trial and error is necessary. • Emphasize that adverse effects can be managed.
Ineffectiveness of medication	• Teach that there are multiple options within each category of medication (e.g., opioids, NSAIDs) and that another medication from the same category may provide better relief. • Emphasize that finding the best treatment regimen often requires trial and error. • Incorporate nonpharmacological approaches in the treatment plan.

NSAIDs, nonsteroidal anti-inflammatory drugs.
Source: Adapted from Ersek, M. (1999). Enhancing effective pain management by addressing patient barriers to analgesic use. *Journal of Hospice & Palliative Nursing, 1,* 87–96.

and also to serve in leadership roles to promote best practice guidelines.

ETHICAL ISSUES IN PAIN MANAGEMENT

Fear of Hastening Death by Administering Analgesics

A common concern of health care providers and caregivers is that giving a sufficient amount of medication to relieve pain will hasten or precipitate death of a terminally ill person. However, there is no scientific evidence that opioids can hasten death, even among patients at the very end of life. Moreover, nurses and health care providers have a moral obligation to provide comfort and pain relief at the end of life. The ethical justification for administering analgesics despite the possibility of hastening death follows the bioethical principle of the *rule of double effect*: that if an unwanted consequence (e.g., hastened death)

occurs as a result of an action taken to achieve a moral good (e.g., pain relief), the action is justified according to ethical theory.

Unrelieved pain is one of the reasons that patients make requests for assisted suicide. Aggressive and adequate pain management may decrease the number of such requests. Medical assistance in death, legal in Canada, is a complex issue that extends beyond pain and pain management.

Use of Placebos in Pain Assessment and Treatment

Placebos have been used inappropriately in the past to determine whether patients' pain was "real." Using medication placebos for pain, such as a saline injection instead of an opioid or an oral dosage of an inappropriate medication, is unethical. Many professional organizations condemn the use of placebos to assess or treat pain.

AGE-RELATED CONSIDERATIONS

PAIN

Persistent pain is a common problem in older persons and is often associated with significant physical disability and psychosocial problems. The most common sources of pain among older people are musculoskeletal conditions, such as osteoarthritis and low back pain, and previous fracture sites. Persistent pain often results in depression, sleep disturbance, decreased mobility, increased use of health care services, and physical and social role dysfunction. Despite its high prevalence, pain in older persons often is inadequately assessed and treated. However, there are several barriers to pain assessment in the older patient. In general, the barriers discussed earlier in the chapter are more prevalent among this population. For example, many older patients believe that pain is a normal, inevitable part of aging. They may also believe that nothing can be done to relieve the pain. Older persons may not report pain for fear of being a "burden" or a "bad patient." They may have greater fears of taking opioids than patients in other age groups. Nurses must be vigilant in asking older patients about their pain and its effects.

Additional barriers to pain assessment in older persons include cognitive changes, inconsistency with experience of pain, and acceptance of pain as a normal process in aging (Resnick et al., 2019). Also, hearing and vision deficits may complicate assessment. Therefore, pain assessment tools may have to be adapted for older patients. For example, it may be necessary to use a large-print pain intensity scale. Although there is some concern that older persons have difficulty using pain scales, it has been documented that many older people, even those with mild to moderate cognitive impairment, can use quantitative scales accurately and reliably (see Figure 10.6).

As for other patients with persistent pain, a thorough physical examination should be performed and the history thoroughly documented to identify causes of pain, possible therapies, and potential problems. Because depression and functional impairments are common among older persons with pain, the possibility of these also must be assessed.

Treatment of pain in older people is complicated by several factors. First, older people metabolize medications more slowly than do younger patients and thus are at greater risk for higher blood levels and adverse effects. For this reason, the adage "start low and go slow" is applied to analgesic therapy in this age group. Second, the use of NSAIDs in older persons is associated with a high frequency of serious GI bleeding. For this reason, acetaminophen should be used whenever possible. Third, many older people take multiple medications for one or more chronic conditions. The addition of analgesics can result in dangerous drug interactions and more adverse effects. Fourth, cognitive impairment and ataxia can be exacerbated when analgesics such as opioids, antidepressants, and anticonvulsant medications are used, a possibility that again necessitates health care providers to titrate medications slowly and monitor carefully for adverse effects.

Treatment regimens for older people must incorporate nonpharmacological modalities. Exercise and patient teaching are particularly important nonpharmacological interventions for older persons with persistent pain. The roles of family and paid caregivers should be included in the treatment plan.

SPECIAL POPULATIONS

Cognitively Impaired Individuals

Although patient self-report is a gold standard of pain assessment in most circumstances, severe cognitive impairment often prevents patients from communicating clearly about their pain. For these individuals, behavioural and physiological changes may be the only indicators that they are in pain. Therefore, the nurse must be astute at recognizing behavioural symptoms of pain.

Several scales have been developed to assess pain in cognitively impaired older patients. Typically, these scales help assess pain according to common behavioural indicators, such as the following:

- Vocalization: moaning, grunting, crying, sighing
- Facial expressions: grimacing, wincing, frowning, clenching teeth
- Breathing: noisy, laboured
- Body movements: restlessness, rocking, pacing
- Body tension: clenching fist, resisting movement
- Consolability: inability to be consoled or distracted

Because it is not possible to validate the meaning of the behaviours, nurses should rely on their own knowledge of the patient's usual behaviour. If the nurse does not know the patient's baseline behaviours, the nurse should obtain this information from other caregivers, including family members. When pain behaviours are present, pain therapy should be instituted on an empirical basis, and patients should be carefully reassessed to evaluate treatment effectiveness.

PATIENTS WITH SUBSTANCE USE PROBLEMS

Individuals with a past or current substance use disorder have the right to receive effective pain management. A comprehensive pain assessment is imperative, including a detailed history, physical examination, psychosocial assessment, and diagnostic workup to determine the cause of the pain. The use of screening tools to determine the possible risk for addiction has been described above. The goal of the pain assessment is to facilitate the establishment of a treatment plan that will relieve the individual's pain effectively, as well as prevent or minimize withdrawal symptoms.

Opioids may be used effectively and safely in patients with substance dependence when indicated for pain control. Opioid agonist and antagonist medications (e.g., pentazocine [Talwin], butorphanol) should not be used in this population because they may precipitate withdrawal. The use of "potentiators" and psychoactive medications that do not have analgesic properties should also be avoided. In individuals who are tolerant to CNS depressants, larger doses of opioids or increased frequency of medication administration is necessary to achieve pain relief.

Effective pain management for people with addiction is challenging and requires expert leadership and consultation for assessment and facilitation of a planned, interprofessional team approach. Team members must be aware of their own attitudes and misbeliefs about people with substance use problems, which may contribute to undertreatment of pain.

CASE STUDY

Pain

Patient Profile

S. C., 33 years old (pronouns she/her), is admitted for an incision and drainage of a right renal abscess. S. C.'s renal function is not impaired. She has a history of low back pain and takes oxycodone, 5 to 10 mg, every 6 hours as needed. Her weight is 112 kg and height is 162 cm.

Subjective Data

- Lives alone
- Desires 0 pain during therapy but will accept 1 to 2 on a scale of 0 to 10
- Reports incision-area pain as a 2 or 3 between dressing changes and as a 10 during dressing changes
- States sharp, throbbing pain persists 1 to 2 hours after dressing change
- Reports that pain between dressing changes is controlled by two oxycodone tablets

Objective Data

- Requires twice-a-day dressing changes for 1 week
- Morphine, 2 to 15 mg intravenously, for every dressing change
- Oxycodone, 5 to 10 mg, for breakthrough pain between dressing changes

Discussion Questions

1. Initially, what dosage of intravenous morphine should be given to S. C.?
2. Describe the assessment data that support the dosage selected in Question 1.
3. How long should the nurse wait after the intravenous morphine dose to begin S. C.'s dressing change?
4. If an initial dose of 6 mg intravenous morphine reduces the pain to a 6 during the dressing change, what nursing action is indicated for the next dressing change?
5. What nursing action is indicated if S. C. has pain 5 hours after her dressing change?
6. When S. C. is discharged, needing dressing changes for 3 days at home, how would the home care nurse organize S. C.'s care? (The nurse knows that S. C. has obtained adequate pain relief with 8 mg of intravenous morphine.)

evolve

Answers are available at http://evolve.elsevier.com/Canada/Lewis/medsurg.

REVIEW QUESTIONS

The number of the question corresponds to the same-numbered objective at the beginning of the chapter.

1. Pain is best described as
   a. A creation of a person's imagination
   b. An unpleasant, subjective experience
   c. A maladaptive response to a stimulus
   d. A neurological event resulting from activation of nociceptors

2. Which of the following inhibiting neurotransmitters is known for its involvement in pain modulation?
   a. Dopamine
   b. Acetylcholine
   c. Prostaglandin
   d. Norepinephrine

3. Which of the following words is most likely to be used to describe neuropathic pain? *(Select all that apply.)*
   a. Dull
   b. Mild
   c. Aching
   d. Burning
   e. Sickening
   f. Electric

4. Which of the following is true of unrelieved pain?
   a. It is to be expected after major surgery.
   b. It is to be expected in a person with cancer.
   c. It is dangerous and can lead to many physical and psychological complications.
   d. It is an annoying sensation, but it is not as important as other physical care needs.

5. Which of the following is a critical step in the pain assessment process?
   a. Assessment of critical sensory components
   b. Teaching the client about pain therapies
   c. Conducting a comprehensive pain assessment
   d. Provision of appropriate treatment and evaluation of its effect

6. Which of the following is an example of distraction to provide pain relief?
   a. TENS
   b. Music
   c. Exercise
   d. Biofeedback

7. Which of the following are appropriate nonopioid analgesics for mild pain? *(Select all that apply.)*
   a. Oxycodone
   b. Ibuprofen
   c. Lorazepam
   d. Acetaminophen
   e. Acetaminophen with codeine

8. Which of the following is an important nursing responsibility related to pain?
   a. Encourage the client to stay in bed.
   b. Help the client appear not to be in pain.
   c. Believe what the client says about the pain.
   d. Assume responsibility for eliminating the client's pain.

9. A nurse is administering a prescribed dose of an intravenous opioid titrated for a person with severe pain related to a terminal illness. Which of the following actions is reflective of this practice?
   a. Euthanasia
   b. Assisted suicide
   c. Enabling the client's addiction
   d. Palliative pain management

10. A nurse believes that clients with the same type of tissue injury should have the same amount of pain. Which of the following statements best describes this belief?
    a. It will contribute to appropriate pain management.
    b. It is an accurate statement about pain mechanisms and an expected goal of pain therapy.
    c. The nurse's belief will have no effect on the type of care provided to people in pain.
    d. It is a common misconception about pain and a major contributor to ineffective pain management.

1. b; 2. d; 3. d, f; 4. c; 5. c; 6. b; 7. b, d; 8. c; 9. d; 10. d.

evolve

For even more review questions, visit http://evolve.elsevier.com/Canada/Lewis/medsurg.

REFERENCES

Asthana, R., Goodall, S., Lau, J., et al. (2019). Framing of the opioid problem in cancer pain management in Canada. *Current Oncology, 26*(3), e410. https://doi.org/10.3747/co.26.4517.

Ballantyne, J. C. (2014). Adaptation to continuous opioid use: The role of tolerance, dependence, and memory. In S. N. Raja, & C. L. Sommer (Eds.), *Pain 2014 refresher course: 15th World Congress on Pain* (pp. 375–380). IASP Press.

Blyth, F. M. (2018). Global burden of neuropathic pain. *Pain, 159*(3), 614–617. https://doi.org/10.1016/j.pain.2011.09.014.

Booker, S. Q., Herr, K. A., & Garvan, C. W. (2020). Racial differences in pain management for patients receiving hospice care. *Oncology Nursing Forum, 47*(2), 228–240. https://doi.org/10.1188/20. onf.228-240.

Boschen, K. A., Robinson, E., Campbell, K. A., et al. (2016). Results from 10 years of a CBT pain self-management outpatient program for complex chronic conditions. *Pain Research and Management, 2016*, 1–10. https://doi.org/10.1155/2016/4678083.

Browne, A. J., Varcoe, C., Lavoie, J., et al. (2016). Enhancing health care equity with Indigenous populations: evidence-based strategies from an ethnographic study. *BMC Health Services Research, 16*(544), 1–17. https://doi.org/10.1186/s12913-016-1707-9.

Busse, J. W., Craigle, S., Juurlink, D. N., et al. (2017). Guideline for opioid therapy for chronic noncancer pain. *CMAJ, 189*(18), E652–E658. https://www.cmaj.ca/content/cmaj/189/18/E659.full.pdf.

Canadian Pain Task Force. (2019). *Chronic pain in Canada: Laying a foundation for action.* www.canada.ca/content/dam/hc-sc/documents/corporate/about-health-canada/public-engagement/external-advisory-bodies/canadian-pain-task-force/report-2019/canadian-pain-task-force-June-2019-report-en.pdf.

Cassell, E. J. (1982). The nature of suffering and the goals of medicine. *New England Journal of Medicine, 306*(11), 639–645. https://doi.org/10.1056/NEJM198203183061104. (Seminal).

Choinière, M., Watt-Watson, J., Victor, J. C., et al. (2014). Prevalence of and risk factors for persistent postoperative nonanginal pain after cardiac surgery: A 2-year prospective multicentre study. *Canadian Medical Association Journal, 186*(7), E213–E223. https://doi.org/10.1503/cmaj.131012. (Seminal).

Clouter, E., Grondin, C., & Lévesque, A. (2018). *Canadian survey on disability (2017): Concepts and methods guide.* Statistics Canada. https://www150.statcan.gc.ca/n1/pub/89-654-x/89-654-x2018001-eng.htm.

Coutaux, A. (2017). Non-pharmacological treatments for pain relief: TENS and acupuncture. *Joint Bone Spine, 84*(6), 657–661. https://doi.org/10.1016/j.jbspin.2017.02.005.

Davis, W. D., Davis, K. A., & Hooper, K. (2019). The use of ketamine for the management of acute pain in the emergency department. *Advanced Emergency Nursing Journal, 41*(2), 111–121. https://doi.org/10.1097/TME.0000000000000238.

dos Santos Felix, M. M., Ferreira, M. B. G., da Cruz, L. F., et al. (2019). Relaxation therapy with guided imagery for postoperative pain management: an integrative review. *Pain Management Nursing, 20*(1), 3–9. https://doi.org/10.1016/j.pmn.2017.10.014.

Drew, D. J., Gordon, D. B., Morgan, B., et al. (2018). "As-needed" range orders for opioid analgesics in the management of pain: A consensus statement of the American Society for Pain Management Nursing and the American Pain Society. *Pain Management Nursing, 19*(3), 207–210. https://doi.org/10.1016/j.pmn.2018.03.003.

Fields, H. (1987). *Pain.* Toronto: McGraw-Hill (Seminal).

Gaskin, D. J., & Richard, P. (2012). The economic costs of pain in the United States. *The Journal of Pain, 13*(8), 715–724. https://doi.org/10.1016/j.pain.2012.03.009

Horch, J., VanDerKerkhof, E. G., Sawhney, M., et al. (2019). Knowledge and attitudes about pain management among Canadian nursing students. *Pain Management Nursing, 20*(4), 382–389. https://doi.org/10.1016/j.pmn.2018.12.005.

Huang, A., Azam, A., Segal, S., et al. (2016). Chronic postsurgical pain and persistent opioid use following surgery: the need for a transitional pain service. *Pain management, 6*(5), 435–443. https://doi.org/10.2217/pmt-2016-0004.

Institutes of Medicine of the National Academies. (2011). *Relieving pain in America: A blueprint for transforming prevention, care, education, and research.* National Academies Press, 260. https://books.nap.edu/openbook.php?record_id=13172&page=260.

Jarvis, C. (2019). *Physical Examination and Health Assessment* (3rd ed). Elsevier.

Jensen, M. P., Tomé-Pires, C., de la Vega, R., et al. (2017). What determines whether a pain is rated as mild, moderate, or severe? The importance of pain beliefs and pain interference. *The Clinical Journal of Pain, 33*(5), 414. https://doi.org/10.1097/AJP.0000000000000429.

Kharasch, E. D. (2017). Current concepts in methadone metabolism and transport. *Clinical Pharmacology in Drug Development, 6*(2), 125–134. https://doi.org/10.1002/cpdd.326.

Kremier, N. (2019). Low dose ketamine for chronic pain. *AANLCP Journal of Nurse Life Care Planning, XIX*(3), 10–18.

Latimer, M., Rudderham, S., Lethbridge, L., et al. (2018). Occurrence of and referral to specialists for pain-related diagnoses in First Nations and non-First Nations children and youth. *CMAJ, 190*(49), 1434–1440. https://doi.org/10.1503/cmaj.180198.

Main, C. J. (2016). Pain assessment in context: a state of the science review of the McGill pain questionnaire 40 years on. *Pain, 157*(7), 1387–1399. https://doi.org/10.1097/j.pain.0000000000000457.

McCaffery, M., & Pasero, C. (1999). *Pain: Clinical manual for nursing practice* (2nd ed.). Mosby (Seminal).

McGillion, M. H., & Watt-Watson, J. (2015). Pain Assessment and Management in Canada: We've Come a Long Way but there are Challenges on the Road Ahead. *The Canadian Journal of Nursing Research = Revue Canadienne De Recherche En Sciences Infirmieres, 47*, 9–16. https://doi.org/10.1177/084456211504700102

McLellan, A. T. (2017). Substance misuse and substance use disorders: Why do they matter in healthcare? *Transactions of the American Clinical and Climatological Association, 128*, 112–130.

Melzack, R., & Wall, P. D. (1987). *The challenge of pain.* Penguin Books (Seminal).

Mifflin, K. A., & Kerr, B. J. (2014). The transition from acute to chronic pain: Understanding how different biological systems interact. *Canadian Journal of Anaesthesia, 61*(2), 112–122. https://doi.org/10.1007/s12630-013-0087-4

O'Keefe-McCarthy, S., McGillion, M., Clarke, S., et al. (2015). Pain and anxiety in rural acute coronary syndrome patients awaiting diagnostic cardiac catheterization. *Journal of Cardiovascular Nursing, 30*(6), 546–557. https://doi.org/10.1097/JCN0000000000000203.

Pelletier, R., Higgins, J., & Bourbonnais, D. (2015). Is neuroplasticity in the central nervous system the missing link to our understanding of chronic musculoskeletal disorders? *BMC Musculoskeletal Disorders, 16*(1), 1. https://doi.org/10.1186/s12891-015-0480-y.

Pergolizzi, J. V., Raffa, R. B., & Taylor, R. (2014). Treating acute pain in light of chronification of pain. *Pain Management Nursing, 15*(1), 380–390. https://doi.org/10.1016/j.pmn.2012.07.004.

Raja, S. N., Carr, D. B., Cohen, M., et al. (2020). The revised International Association for the Study of Pain definition of pain: concepts, challenges, and compromises. *Pain, 161*(9), 1976–1982. https://doi.org/10.1097/j.pain.0000000000001939

Registered Nurses' Association of Ontario (RNAO). (2007). *Positioning techniques in long term care: Self-directed learning package for healthcare providers*. https://rnao.ca/sites/rnao-ca/files/Positioning_Techniques_in_Long-Term_Care_-_Self-directed_learning_package_for_health_care_providers.pdf.

Registered Nurses' Association of Ontario (RNAO). (2013). *Assessment and management of pain* (3rd ed.). http://rnao.ca/bpg/guidelines/assessment-and-management-pain.

Resnick, B., Boltz, M., Galik, E., et al. (2019). Pain assessment, management, and impact among older adults in assisted living. *Pain Management Nursing, 20*(3), 192–197. https://doi.org/10.1016/j.pmn.2019.02.008.

Salter, M. W. (2014). Neurobiology of acute and persistent pain: Spinal cord mechanisms. In S. N. Raja, & C. L. Sommer (Eds.), *Pain 2014 refresher course: 15th World Congress on Pain* (pp. 3–12). IASP Press. https://ebooks.iasp-pain.org/pain_2014_refresher_courses. (Seminal).

Sánchez, J. S., Tenias, J. B., Arias, A. A., et al. (2015). Cardiovascular risk associated with the use of non-steroidal anti-inflammatory drugs: cohort study. *Revista espanola de salud publica, 89*(6), 607–613. https://doi.org/10.4321/s1135-57272015000600008.

Uprety, Y., Lacasse, A., & Asselin, H. (2016). Traditional uses of medicinal plants from the Canadian Boreal Forest for the management of chronic pain syndromes. *Pain Practice, 16*(4), 459–466. https://doi.org/10.1111/papr.12284.

Von Gunten, C. F. (2011). Pathophysiology of pain in cancer. *Journal of Pediatric Hematology/Oncology, 33*, S12–S18.

Wang, L., Guyatt, G. H., Kennedy, S. A., et al. (2016). Predictors of persistent pain after breast cancer surgery: A systematic review and meta-analysis of observational studies. *CMAJ, 188*(14), E352–E361. https://doi.org/10.1503/cmaj.151276.

Watt-Watson, J. H., Clark, A. J., Finely, G. A., & Watson, C. P. N. (1999). Canadian pain society position statement on pain relief. *Pain Research and Management, 4*(2), 75–78. https://doi.org/10.1155/1999/643017. (Seminal)

Yoshikawa, K., Brady, B., Perry, M. A., et al. (2020). Sociocultural factors influencing physiotherapy management in culturally and linguistically diverse people with persistent pain: A scoping review. *Physiotherapy, 107*, 292–305. https://doi.org/10.1016/j.physio.2019.08.002.

RESOURCES

Canadian Guideline for Opioids for Chronic Non-Cancer Pain (NOUGG)
https://healthsci.mcmaster.ca/npc/guidelines

Canadian Pain Task Force Report: June 2019
https://www.canada.ca/en/health-canada/corporate/about-health-canada/public-engagement/external-advisory-bodies/canadian-pain-task-force/report-2019.html

Promoting Awareness of RSD and CRPS in Canada: *Charter of Pain Patient's Rights and Responsibilities*
https://www.rsdcanada.org/parc/english/resources/coalition.htm

Winnipeg Regional Health Authority: *Pain Assessment and Management: Clinical Practice Guidelines*
http://www.wrha.mb.ca/extranet/eipt/files/EIPT-017-001.pdf

Agency for Healthcare Research and Quality
https://www.ahcpr.gov

City of Hope Pain & Palliative Care Resource Center
https://prc.coh.org/

Core Curriculum for Professional Education in Pain
https://issuu.com/iasp/docs/core-corecurriculum?mode=embed&layout=http%3A%2F%2Fskin.issuu.com%2Fv%2Fdarkicons%2Flayout.xml&showFlipBtn=true

International Association for the Study of Pain
https://www.iasp-pain.org

McGill Pain Questionnaire
http://www.chcr.brown.edu/pcoc/MCGILLPAINQUEST.PDF

⊜volve

For additional Internet resources, see the website for this book at http://evolve.elsevier.com/Canada/Lewis/medsurg.

Substance Use

Emma Garrod
Originating US chapter by Mariann M. Harding

evolve WEBSITE

http://evolve.elsevier.com/Canada/Lewis/medsurg

- Review Questions (Online Only)
- Key Points
- Answer Guidelines for Case Study
- Conceptual Care Map Creator
- Customizable Nursing Care Plan
  - Alcohol Withdrawal
- Audio Glossary
- Content Updates

LEARNING OBJECTIVES

1. Describe social and biological perspectives on substance use.
2. Describe factors that contribute to substance use.
3. Discuss the nursing role in education, advocacy, offering evidence-informed interventions, and establishing collaborative relationships with people experiencing substance use–related conditions.
4. Describe the harm reduction model.
5. Describe how motivational interviewing can be used to support patients who use substances.
6. Discuss screening, assessment, and treatment planning for people experiencing substance use–related conditions.
7. Identify common substances, their effects, and associated health consequences.
8. Discuss nursing interventions for common substance use disorders and care for patients experiencing substance-induced intoxication or withdrawal.
9. Discuss the nursing management of pain in the patient who has a substance use disorder.
10. Describe nursing management of the surgical patient with a substance use disorder.
11. Discuss substance use considerations specific to the older person.

KEY TERMS

brain reward system
cross-tolerance
Korsakoff syndrome
lapses
motivational interviewing
naloxone
opiates

opioids
opioid agonists
potentiation
relapse
relief craving
reward craving
substance use disorder

tolerance
transtheoretical model of change
Wernicke's encephalopathy
withdrawal
withdrawal management

SUBSTANCE USE IN CANADA

There is a long history of humans consuming psychoactive substances, including alcohol, cannabis, and opioids, for medical use and pleasure. While not all substance use is problematic, there can be harm related to substance use. Thus nurses should routinely assess for substance use with every individual in all practice settings and offer evidence-informed interventions when appropriate. It is important to situate substance use along a continuum of use, capturing a spectrum ranging from non-use or abstinence to substance use disorder. A continuum allows for a broader understanding of the range and severity of substance use behaviours across populations (Figure 11.1). A

substance use disorder is diagnosed by a health care provider and is defined as "a cluster of cognitive, behavioural, and psychological symptoms indicating that the individual continues using despite significant substance-related problems" (American Psychiatric Association [APA], 2013). *Substance use disorder* is the preferred terminology in health care over the word *addiction*. Knowing the severity of substance use allows the health care team to work with the patient, tailoring treatment according to individual needs and preferences. Problematic substance use affects a broad spectrum of Canadians, regardless of age, gender, socioeconomic status, educational level, cultural background, or geographic region.

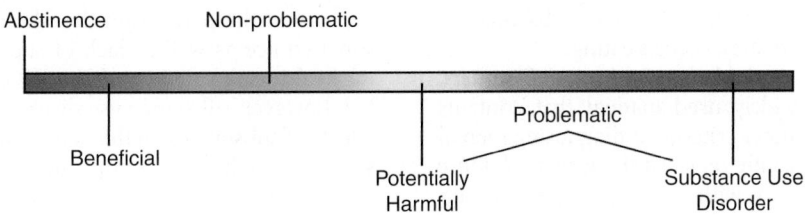

FIG. 11.1 Continuum of substance use. Source: Adapted from First Nations Health Authority, British Columbia Ministry of Health & Health Canada. (2013). *A path forward: A provincial approach to facilitate regional and local planning and action.* http://www.fnha.ca/documents/fnha_mwsu.pdf

In 2017, substance use trends were measured by the Canadian Tobacco, Alcohol and Drugs Survey (Health Canada, 2019). The survey found that 15% of Canadians aged 15 years and older reported current smoking (11% daily smokers); 78% reported past-year consumption of alcohol; 15% reported cannabis use; and 3% reported use of other substances, including cocaine or crack, speed, methamphetamines, ecstasy, heroin, or hallucinogens. Of individuals reporting psychoactive pharmaceutical use (opioids, stimulants, and sedatives), 5% reported nonprescribed use or problematic use.

Substance use trends and related harms shift frequently; most recently, opioid-related deaths have caused significant public health concern. Between 2016 and 2019, 13 900 opioid-related deaths occurred, including overdose; 80% of these involved illicit fentanyl, a very potent opioid (Special Advisory Committee on the Epidemic of Opioid Overdoses, 2019). The opioid overdose crisis has worsened during the coronavirus (COVID-19) pandemic that spread globally in 2020. The United Nations Office on Drugs and Crime (2020) projected that the illicit drug supply would be altered due to COVID-19 restrictions, and this worsening in conjunction with increased isolation has already led to a record spike in overdose deaths in British Columbia (British Columbia Coroner's Report, 2021). Hospital settings are a point-of-care intersection for individuals who are diagnosed with both a substance use disorder and COVID-19.

There are significant personal and social costs of problematic substance use for Canadians and their families, including poor physical and mental health, exacerbated health conditions, and decreased functioning and quality of life. Overall, 4% of Canadians aged 15 years and older report experiencing at least one harm in the past year due to their illegal substance use (Health Canada, 2019). Many of these concerns put individuals in contact with the health care setting, including acute care.

This chapter focuses on the role of the medical-surgical nurse in identifying and working with patients in acute care settings who have a history of substance use or are currently using substances. In this setting, nurses must recognize substance use, understand its effects on the patient's health, provide nonjudgemental care, treat pain, help the patient manage withdrawal, and provide evidence-informed care. The health care setting provides an opportunity for substance use screening and education, as well as the provision of and connection to evidence-informed interventions and services.

FACTORS THAT INFLUENCE SUBSTANCE USE

There are many social and biological factors that contribute to, overlap with, or intersect with substance use. These include but are not limited to genetics, family environment, social environment, trauma (past, current, intergenerational), concurrent mental illness, chronic pain, the social determinants of health, access to health care, and experiences with stigma and discrimination.

For example, about 50% of alcohol use disorder cases are attributable to genetics (Deak et al., 2019). Early adverse childhood experiences such as abuse or neglect also account for a significant portion of risk; one-half to two-thirds of serious substance use issues were found to be correlated with these experiences (Dube et al., 2003). Finally, approximately 50% of individuals with severe mental illness have a concurrent substance use disorder, leading to treatment challenges and poorer outcomes (Khan, 2017). Although any Canadian may be affected, physical and social harms of substance use and substance use disorders are experienced inequitably across social contexts. Indigenous people in Canada are disproportionately affected by harms related to substance use (Firestone et al., 2015), including alcohol-related mortality and opioid overdose death. In one cohort study of Indigenous people aged 14 to 30 years who used substances, the death rate was 12.9 times higher than that of non-Indigenous Canadians of the same age (Jongbloed et al., 2017). Much of this inequity stems from social determinants of health and colonization, which resulted in loss of land, culture, language, and identity. Many Indigenous people were forced to attend residential schools, the devastating impact of which has been linked to higher rates of substance use and mental illness as well as many other health conditions (Wilk et al., 2017). These harms were not only experienced by those who attended residential schools but have affected subsequent generations through intergenerational trauma: psychological, physiological, and social processes which are at the root of substance-related issues facing Indigenous communities (Aguir & Halseth, 2015). Unfortunately, Indigenous people are often portrayed as victims (Nelson et al., 2016), which ignores the resilience and strength of community and culture. In fact, evidence supports the promise of culturally based and community-owned services that reduce health disparities and promote individual and community health (Urbanowski, 2017).

Addressing the harms of substance use is both a health and social issue and requires attention to these many complex factors. Each individual's risk factors for and experience with substance use will be different, as will be their treatment. Understanding these complexities is an important part of nursing care.

Neurophysiology of Substances

Psychoactive substances affect key areas of the brain involved in survival, pleasure, and reinforcement. Many psychoactive substances increase the availability of dopamine in the "pleasure area" of the mesolimbic system of the brain. This mechanism, the **brain reward system**, creates the sensation of pleasure or meaning in reaction to certain behaviours that are required for survival of the human species, such as eating and sex (Burchum & Rosenthal, 2016). Psychoactive substances also increase the activity of the reward pathway by increasing the neurochemical dopamine in the synaptic cleft. Dopamine affects brain processes that control motivation, emotional responses, and the ability to experience pleasure and pain. Substances that act in this area can disrupt normal processes and cause the brain to perceive substances as more important than other activities, such as eating.

The *Diagnostic and Statistical Manual of Mental Disorders*, fifth edition (*DSM-5*) is a widely used manual that contains descriptions, symptoms, and other criteria for diagnosing mental disorders. The *DSM-5* has recently replaced the terms *substance abuse* and *substance dependence* with substance use disorder (APA, 2013), and specific diagnostic criteria determine the level of severity of the disorder as mild, moderate, or severe. Substance use disorders often result from the prolonged effects of psychoactive substances on the brain. Repeated long-term use of substances changes the neural circuitry involving the dopamine neurotransmitter system and reduces the responsiveness of dopamine receptors. This decreased responsiveness leads to tolerance, the need for a larger dose of a substance to obtain the original effects, and also reduces the sense of pleasure from experiences that previously resulted in positive feelings. This also leads to withdrawal; without the substance, the individual may experience physical withdrawal symptoms, or depression, anxiety, and irritability. To feel normal, the individual must take the substance.

A key aspect of substance use is the formation of the memory of the pleasurable experience of the substance that is long-lasting even in periods of nonuse. Relief craving, the intense desire for a substance, usually experienced after decreased use, is the result of the memory aspect related to the brain reward pathway. An important type of craving experienced by people who have experienced problematic substance use or substance use disorder is reward craving, which occurs when in the presence of people, places, or things that they have previously associated with taking the substance. Cue-induced reward craving may occur after long periods of abstinence and is a common cause of relapse, or returning to substance use after a period of abstinence (Koob et al., 2015), as is exposure to stressful circumstances. The goal of medications used to treat substance use disorders is to treat withdrawal symptoms at the level of the synapse, reduce cravings, and prevent relapse, and in time, the brain can recover.

Recovery. Recovery is a process of change through which individuals improve their health and wellness. Recovery is built on access to evidence-informed clinical treatment and recovery support services, available to all populations (Substance Abuse and Mental Health Services Administration [SAMHSA], 2020b).

It is important that a variety of treatment options and approaches are explored, as recovery is an individualized process. Individuals face many barriers when starting the process of recovery, including not believing they have a problem with substances or not believing their use is serious enough to address. They may also not know where to access help. Nurses play an integral role in providing patients hope, support, and access to evidence-informed treatment and services.

Attitudes Toward People Experiencing Substance-Related Problems

People with substance use–related conditions face significant stigma and prejudice, largely perpetuated by characterizations of substance use as a moral issue in the media and society at large. Misunderstanding regarding the biopsychosocial aspects of substance use and associated health complications contributes to the generally accepted perspective that substance use disorders are purely matters of personal choice, which may affect the way health services are delivered. Indeed, studies have indicated that some health care providers have negative attitudes toward people with substance use disorders, in part

because of the perception that the disorder is a matter of personal choice as well as lack of support or adequate education for health care providers (Chu & Galang, 2013). As stated earlier, however, substance use disorder is intimately linked to the effects of substances on the neurophysiology of the brain reward system as well as to environmental and genetic factors; it is a complex biopsychosocial condition that involves the whole person. Substance use disorders are considered chronic, relapsing conditions with relapse rates similar to those of other chronic diseases. For example, relapse rates are similar in people treated for asthma and hypertension when compared to those with substance use disorders—signaling a need for further assessment, support, and potentially a revised treatment plan (McLellan et al., 2000). However, due to associated stigma, relapse to substance use is often viewed more negatively, by both the patient and health care providers. Other chronic conditions add complexity; the co-occurrence of mental illness and substance use disorder (*concurrent disorder*) requires supportive interventions due to the increases in the severity of symptoms and poor outcomes for both disorders (Rush, 2015). Unfortunately, people with substance use disorders frequently report stigmatizing encounters in health care settings (Carusone et al., 2019; van Boekel et al., 2013); this experience may be a contributing factor to patients leaving hospital before completing treatment. Hospitalizations can be a key point of intervention; by offering approaches discussed in this chapter, including harm reduction and evidence-informed medications, health care providers communicate nonjudgement toward substance use and a commitment to meeting patients' needs.

Nurses must explore their own attitudes about people who use substances. It is critical to work with patients in a nonstigmatizing and collaborative way, as upheld by the *CNA Code of Ethics* (Canadian Nurses' Association [CNA], 2017a). Education is an essential place to start; visit the Resources section at the end of this chapter for further resources. An open nurse–patient dialogue about substance use can significantly improve health outcomes and increase the likelihood that the person will attempt to reduce harms associated with substance use. It is important to reduce the stigma related to substance use so that patients access and stay engaged in health care.

KEY CONCEPTS AND APPROACHES

All of the approaches discussed in this section can apply to patients with substance use issues, depending on their current status and goals.

THE HARM REDUCTION PERSPECTIVE

Harm reduction focuses on reducing the harms associated with substance use across the continuum of use, from abstinence to high-risk use (Table 11.1). Harm reduction encompasses policies, programs, and practices that aim to reduce the harms associated with substances in people unable or unwilling to stop; the focus is on prevention of harm as opposed to abstinence (CNA, 2017b). Laws against drinking and driving and nonsmoking bylaws are examples of community harm-reduction strategies to protect people from the harms related to alcohol and smoking. Other examples include evidence-informed interventions such as programs that provide sterile supplies (i.e., syringes) and naloxone (Narcan) kit distribution (Figure 11.2); these measures reduce the harms associated with high-risk substance use without requiring that the person stop such

TABLE 11.1 KEY ELEMENTS OF HARM REDUCTION

Harm Reduction
- Represents a value-neutral view of drug use and of drug user, with no moral, legal, or medical-reductionist limitations
- Targeted at risks and harms
- Evidence-informed and cost-effective
- Incremental success is celebrated
- Accepts that at any given time some people are not ready to choose abstinence
- Promotes multiple services at one site as an alternative to traditional complex multisite service approaches
- Accepts that substance use occurs and works to minimize its harmful effects
- Promotes user participation in planning and creating programs and policies designed to serve them
- Recognizes that users are capable of making choices and taking responsibility in prevention of harm, treatment, and recovery
- Calls for nonjudgemental, noncoercive provision of services and resources for people who use drugs
- Does not attempt to minimize or ignore the many real and tragic harms and dangers associated with drug use
- Does not exclude abstinence as an option

Source: Adapted from Harm Reduction Coalition. (n.d.). *Principles of harm reduction.* http://harmreduction.org/about-us/principles-of-harm-reduction/; Marlatt, G. A. (1996). Harm reduction: Come as you are. *Addictive Behaviours, 21*(6), 779–788. https://doi.org/10.1016/0306-4603(9600042-1;) and UBC Continuing Professional Development. (2020). *Addiction care and treatment online course.* https://elearning.ubccpd.ca/course/view.php?id=164#section-2

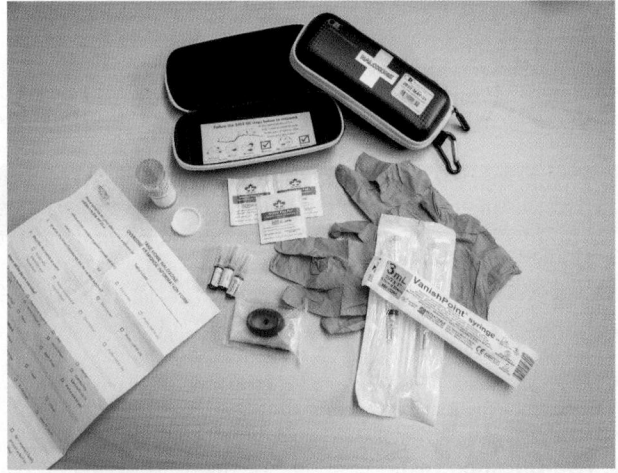

FIG. 11.2 Naloxone kit. Source: The University of British Columbia. (2017, January 23). *Naloxone: The antidote to a public health emergency.* https://students.ubc.ca/ubclife/naloxone-antidote-public-health-emergency

TABLE 11.2 KEY ASPECTS OF SUCCESSFUL MOTIVATIONAL INTERVIEWING

- Express empathy.
- Provide positive reinforcement and encouragement for gains made by the patient.
- Listen rather than tell.
- Understand that change is up to the patient.
- Identify discrepancy between patient's goals or values and current behaviour.
- Help the patient recognize the discrepancies between where they are and where they hope to be.
- Avoid argument and direct confrontation, which can cause defensiveness and a power struggle.
- Adjust to, rather than oppose, patient resistance.
- Focus on the patient's strengths to support the hope and optimism needed to make changes.

Trauma-Informed and Culturally Competent Approaches to Care

As noted above, a history of adverse childhood experiences or intergenerational and historical trauma can lead to greater risk for problematic substance use; such history has also been established as a link to other adverse health outcomes (Felitti et al., 1998). This understanding has led to the creation of trauma-informed approaches to care, which emphasize physical and emotional safety in service delivery, as well as promoting individuals' choice and control in their treatment. This can be as simple as asking permission to perform a blood pressure. It is not necessary to know someone's history in order to provide trauma-informed care and create welcoming services (Nathoo et al., 2018). In Canada, there is also an emphasis on providing culturally competent services that build trust between health care providers and Indigenous people accessing health services, in order to address disparities. See the Resources section for more information on how to engage in trauma-informed and culturally competent practice.

Motivational Interviewing: Engaging in a Supportive Dialogue Around Problematic Substance Use

The nurse is in a unique position to motivate and facilitate behaviour change while caring for patients in primary and acute care settings, as the patient's awareness may be increased. Intervention by nurses at this time can be a crucial factor in promoting behaviour change. Motivational interviewing is "a directive, patient-centred counselling style for eliciting behaviour change by helping patients to explore and resolve ambivalence" (Rollnick & Miller, 1995, p. 326), using nonconfrontational techniques to motivate patients to change behaviour by eliciting talk about substance use. The role of the nurse is to listen and reflect back to the person and to recognize that ambivalence is normal and expected when anyone is confronted with having to make a change. The key aspects of successful motivational interviewing are presented in Table 11.2.

The stages of change identified in the transtheoretical model of change include precontemplation, contemplation, preparation, action, maintenance, and termination (Prochaska & Velicer, 1997), as described in Chapter 4. The stages are not viewed as linear, and during the process of change, relapse and small lapses (very short periods of substance use, followed by quick return to maintaining nonuse) are part of the journey and a normal aspect of behaviour change (Figure 11.3). Patients who do not change behaviours or who return to substance use

use. For example, infections related to injecting substances can be reduced by use of alcohol swabs and sterile syringes. Given the increasing number of opioid-related deaths, naloxone kits are now widely distributed across Canada, including in hospitals. Another approach to reduce overdose risk is supervised consumption, where people use nonprescribed substances they have purchased in the presence of trained staff who can respond if an overdose occurs. Many new supervised consumption facilities are opening across Canada and are often staffed by nurses.

Foundational to harm reduction are respect for patient autonomy and a nonjudgemental approach. Harm reduction is collaborative and honours the patient's inherent dignity and their ability to make informed decisions. There is a broad evidence base to support harm reduction, and it is within nursing scope to engage in these health-promoting activities (CNA, 2017b).

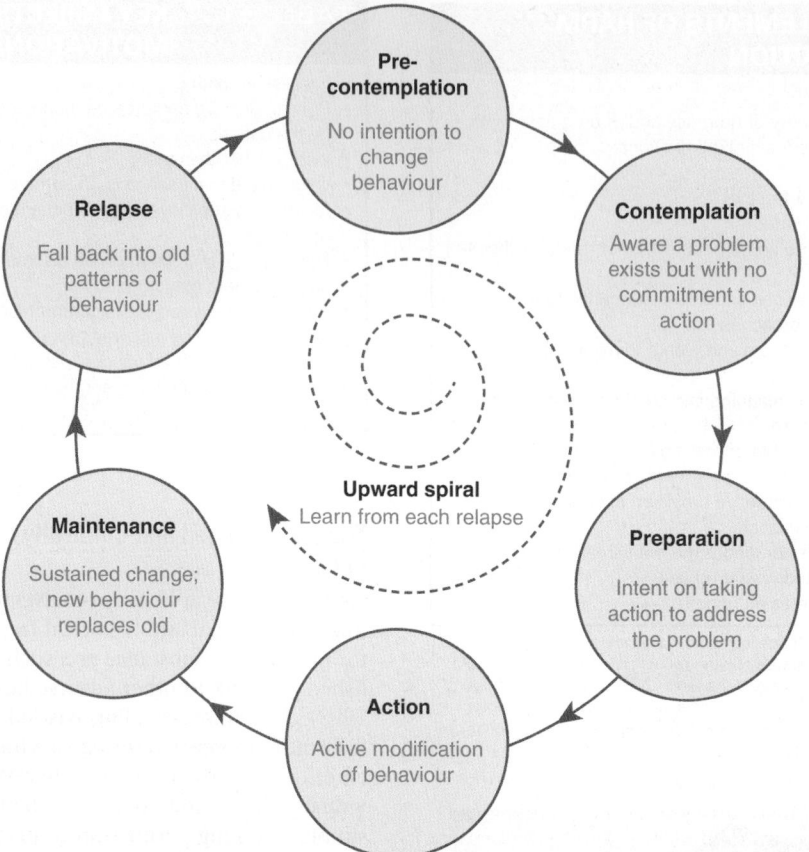

FIG. 11.3 Stages of change model. Source: Adapted from Prochaska, J., & DiClemente, C. (1983). Stages and processes of self-change of smoking: Toward an integrative model of change. *Journal of Consulting and Clinical Psychology, 51*(3), 390–395.

after a period of cessation are often labelled "noncompliant" and "unmotivated." However, this development may reflect a normal relapse or may indicate that the interventions used do not align with the patient's stage of change.

It is important for the nurse to identify the patient's readiness for change and the stage to which the patient is moving. In the precontemplation stage, the nurse can help the patient increase awareness of risks and problems related to current substance use. A patient in the contemplation stage of change often experiences ambivalence and the nurse can help the patient thoughtfully consider the positive and negative aspects of their substance use. As the patient moves from contemplation to preparation, the nurse should support self-efficacy and even the smallest effort to change. The resolution of acute health conditions, or discharge from the hospital may occur before the patient moves to the preparation and action stages of change. In this case, the nurse must support the continuation of the change process by making appropriate referrals to community resources.

NURSING MANAGEMENT SUBSTANCE USE

NURSING ASSESSMENT

The nurse needs to engage with patients to understand if they use substances in ways that place them at risk or may necessitate nursing or medical interventions. Screening, brief intervention, and referral to treatment are recommended in all settings, including acute care (SAMHSA, 2020a). As a baseline, the nurse should ask every patient about the use of all substances, including alcohol, prescribed medications, over-the-counter (OTC) drugs, caffeine,

TABLE 11.3	BRIEF SCREENING TOOL FOR SUBSTANCE USE

1. Single-Question Tests
Use one of the following questions to screen for the presence of alcohol, drug, or tobacco use.
- How often in the past year have you had five (men) or four (women) or more drinks in a day?
- How many times in the past year have you used illegal drugs or prescription medications for nonmedical reasons?
- In the past year, how often have you used tobacco products?

2. Two-Question Tests
Use the following two questions to screen for alcohol or drug use.
- In the past year, have you ever had more alcohol or other drugs than you meant to?
- Have you felt you wanted or needed to cut down on your drinking or drug use in the past year?

Source: Reprinted from *Primary Care: Clinics in Office Practice, 41*(2), Strobbe, S., Prevention and screening, brief intervention, and referral to treatment for substance use in primary care, pages 185–213. Copyright 2014, with permission from Elsevier.

tobacco, and other substances. The nurse may use a simple one- or two-question screening test for substance use (Table 11.3) or a more in-depth tool. Another instrument frequently used is the CAGE-AID questionnaire (Table 11.4). If there are indications of substance use, the nurse determines when the patient last used the substance so that drug interactions or the onset of withdrawal can be anticipated. Screening all patients for substance use with a nonjudgemental manner decreases stigma and results in more patients being offered evidence-informed treatments; a therapeutic relationship with the patient also allows for more accurate

TABLE 11.4	CAGE QUESTIONNAIRE ADAPTED TO INCLUDE DRUGS (CAGE AID)

Have you felt you ought to cut down on your drinking (or drug use)?
_____Yes _____No
Have people annoyed you by criticizing your drinking (or drug use)?
_____Yes _____No
Have you felt bad or guilty about your drinking (or drug use)?
_____Yes _____No
Have you ever had a drink (or used drugs) first thing in the morning to steady your nerves or get rid of a hangover (or to get the day started)?
_____Yes _____No

Note: In the general population, two or more positive answers indicates a need for a more in-depth assessment.
Source: Hinkin, C. H., Castellon, S. A., Dickson-Fuhrman, E., Daum, G., Jaffe, J., & Jarvik, L. (2001). Screening for drug and alcohol abuse among older adults using a modified version of the CAGE. *American Journal of Addiction, 10,* 319–326.

TABLE 11.5	POSSIBLE NURSING DIAGNOSES FOR PATIENTS WITH SUBSTANCE-RELATED CONDITIONS

Acute confusion resulting from substance intoxication (e.g., as evidenced by *alteration in level of consciousness, agitation, disorientation*)
Potential for injury as evidenced by *alteration in cognitive function (impaired judgement)*
Potential for infection as evidenced by *injection drug use*
Imbalanced nutrition as evidenced by *insufficient dietary intake and electrolyte imbalances*
Potential for seizure as evidenced by *signs of alcohol withdrawal: increased heart rate, tremor, confusion*
Potential for opioid overdose as evidenced by *altered level of consciousness, decreased respiratory rate*
Potential for leaving hospital before completing medical treatment as evidenced by *low mood and disengaging from care*

assessments. Biological assessments, including serum and urine drug tests, may indicate substance use. A complete blood count, serum electrolytes, blood urea nitrogen, creatinine, and liver function tests are used to evaluate for electrolyte imbalances and cardiac, kidney, or liver dysfunction, which may be related to acute or chronic effects of substances.

HEALTH COMPLICATIONS OF SUBSTANCE USE. Health complications and harms related to substance use are related to three general factors: the substance, the route, and related high-risk behaviours. First, the inherent properties of the substance itself may have specific physiological harms associated with its use, such as liver damage related to alcohol use and lung damage related to smoking. Second, the route by which the substance is taken will pose specific harms. For example, intravenous (IV) use may expose the individual to bacteria if sterile supplies are not used and cause infections (e.g., endocarditis). Third, high-risk sexual behaviours, exposure to violence and trauma, and placing one's personal safety at risk may occur during substance use. Harm reduction interventions and education can mitigate many of these harms.

PLANNING. Nurses need to effectively assess for, manage, and evaluate patients experiencing intoxication, overdose, and withdrawal symptoms because these clinical situations will arise in all settings, from the emergency department to a surgical environment. A positive, nonjudgemental, supportive, and therapeutic dialogue is fundamental. The nurse and patient should collaborate to establish goals related to achieving the best possible outcome related to their admission diagnosis and nursing diagnoses (Table 11.5) and participation in evidence-informed treatment or harm reduction strategies. Nurses can also coordinate treatment plans that involve the interprofessional team and other important resources, such as family or community support groups.

NURSING IMPLEMENTATION

URGENT CARE SITUATIONS. Urgent care situations precipitated by substance use are acute intoxication, overdose, or withdrawal. The patient may also present with trauma or injuries. Intoxication responses usually last less than 24 hours and are directly related to the ingestion of psychoactive substances. Overdose occurs with the ingestion of an excessive dose of one drug or with a combination of similarly acting drugs. Table 11.6 lists commonly used substances, routes, and effects.

Overdose. An overdose is an emergency situation, and management is based on the type of substance involved. Overdose may include respiratory and circulatory arrest and other

life-threatening complications. If multiple substances have been ingested, a complex and clinical picture can result. The first priority of care in the case of overdose is always the patient's ABC (airway, breathing, and circulation). Emergency management of overdose and toxicity of central nervous system (CNS) stimulants and CNS depressants is presented later in the chapter, in Tables 11.16 and 11.17. As soon as the patient is stable, a thorough history and physical examination must be attempted, which may involve collateral history. A patient who intentionally overdosed should not return home until seen by a psychiatric professional.

Withdrawal. The nurse must be alert to the possibility of withdrawal in any patient who has a history of substance use. Withdrawal is defined as a constellation of physiological and psychological responses that occur upon abrupt cessation or reduced intake of a substance on which an individual is physiologically dependent. Withdrawal from some substances, including alcohol and benzodiazepines, can be life-threatening. Opioid withdrawal is not life-threatening but causes significant discomfort and may cause a patient to leave the hospital before receiving the medical care they need. Specific approaches to withdrawal are discussed in sections on each substance.

HEALTH PROMOTION

Prevention of substance use issues includes primary, secondary, and tertiary prevention. *Primary prevention* targets primarily adolescents and young adults by offering education and harm-reduction strategies. *Secondary prevention* focuses on early detection of substance use and offering evidence-informed interventions to try to prevent severe substance use disorders from developing. *Tertiary prevention* addresses substance use disorders and includes working with patients to match evidence-informed interventions to their goals, including pharmacotherapy and counselling.

COMMON SUBSTANCES, TREATMENT, AND NURSING INTERVENTIONS

NICOTINE

Characteristics

Nurses are very likely to encounter patients with tobacco use disorder, which is diagnosed using *DSM-5* criteria. A

TABLE 11.6   EFFECTS OF SUBSTANCES

Substance and Route of Consumption	Physiological and Psychological Effects	Effects of Overdose	Withdrawal Symptoms
Stimulants			
Nicotine (cigarettes, chewing tobacco, snus, snuff, e-cigarettes, cigars) Smoked, snorted, chewed, vaporized	Increased alertness; increased heart rate and blood pressure; cutaneous vasoconstriction; decreased appetite; increased gastric motility	Nausea, abdominal pain, diarrhea, vomiting, dizziness, weakness, confusion, decreased respirations, seizures, death from respiratory failure or cardiac arrest	Craving, attention difficulties, depression, hyperirritability, headache, insomnia, increased appetite. Onset: 2–4 hours
Cocaine (coke, crack), amphetamine (speed), dextroamphetamine (Dexedrine), methamphetamine (crystal meth, ice, Tina), methylenedioxymethamphetamine (MDMA, Ecstasy), methylphenidate (Ritalin) Oral, snorted, smoked, injected	Euphoria, grandiosity, mood swings, hyperactivity, hyper-alertness, restlessness, anorexia, insomnia, hypertension, tachycardia, marked vasoconstriction, tremor, dysrhythmias, seizures, dilated pupils (cocaine, MDMA), diaphoresis	Agitation; increased temperature, heart rate, respiratory rate, blood pressure; cardiac dysrhythmias; myocardial infarction; hallucinations; seizures; possible death	Craving, severely depressed mood, exhaustion, prolonged sleep, apathy, irritability, disorientation. Onset: ~2 hours for intravenous use
Depressants			
Alcohol Oral, snorted Sedative–hypnotics Oral, snorted, injected • Barbiturates • Benzodiazepines: diazepam (Valium), alprazolam (Xanax) • Gamma-hydroxybutyrate (GHB)	Initial relaxation, decreased inhibitions, drowsiness, lack of coordination, impaired judgement, slurred speech, hypotension, bradycardia, bradypnea	Shallow respirations; cold, clammy skin; weak, rapid pulse; hyporeflexia; coma; possible death	Anxiety, agitation, insomnia, diaphoresis, tremors, delirium, seizures, possible death. Onset: 6–12 hours after last drink for alcohol, 12–16 hours for oral sedatives
Opioids			
Heroin (down), morphine, opium, codeine, fentanyl, meperidine (Demerol), hydromorphone (Dilaudid), oxycodone hydrochloride (Percocet) Methadone Oral, snorted, smoked, injected	Analgesia, euphoria, drowsiness, detachment from environment, relaxation, constricted pupils, nausea, decreased respiratory rate, slurred speech, impaired judgement	Slow, shallow respirations; clammy skin; unresponsive, constricted pupils; coma; possible death	Watery eyes, dilated pupils, runny nose, yawning, tremors, pain, chills, diaphoresis, nausea, vomiting, diarrhea, abdominal cramps, anxiety, restlessness. Onset: 4–6 hours after last use for short-acting, 8–12 hours for longer-acting
Cannabis			
Marijuana: hash, weed, bud, shatter, butter; synthetic: K2, spice Oral, smoked	Relaxation, euphoria, lack of motivation, abrupt mood changes, impaired memory and attention, impaired judgement, reddened eyes, dry mouth, lack of coordination, decreased reflexes, tachycardia, increased appetite	Fatigue, paranoia, panic reactions, psychosis	Insomnia, anxiety, nausea
Hallucinogens			
Lysergic acid diethylamide (LSD) Psilocybin (mushrooms) Dimethyltryptamine (DMT) Mescaline (peyote) Phencyclidine (PCP) Oral, smoked (DMT, PCP), injected (PCP)	Perceptual distortions, hallucinations, depersonalization, heightened sensory perception, euphoria, mood swings, suspiciousness, panic, impaired judgement, increased body temperature, hypertension, flushed face, tremor, dilated pupils; PCP: constricted pupils, nystagmus, delusions, violence	Anxiety, panic, confusion, blurred vision, increases in blood pressure and temperature, paranoia, psychosis PCP only: seizures, coma, death	These substance are not typically used regularly enough to cause dependence, no withdrawal symptoms known
Inhalants			
Solvents, aerosols, and gases found in household products like glue, cleaning products, paint thinner, hairspray, whipping cream (called poppers, whippets) Inhaled through nose or mouth	Euphoria, decreased inhibitions, giddiness, slurred speech, illusions, drowsiness, clouded sensorium, tinnitus, nystagmus, cough, nausea, vomiting, diarrhea; irritation to eyes, nose, mouth	Anxiety, respiratory depression, asphyxiation, cardiac dysrhythmias, loss of consciousness, sudden death, suicide	Nausea, tremors, irritability, difficulties sleeping, mood changes

Sources: Adapted from National Institute on Drug Abuse. (2017). *Commonly abused drugs.* https://www.drugabuse.gov/drugs-abuse/commonly-abused-drugs-charts#alcohol; American Lung Association. (2019). *What it means to be "nic-sick."* https://www.lung.org/about-us/blog/2019/10/nic-sick.html

number of products contain nicotine, including smoked tobacco leaf (cigarettes, cigars, pipes), smokeless tobacco leaf (chew, snuff, dip), and some electronic cigarettes. It is important to differentiate these tobacco products from ceremonial tobacco, which is used by some Canadian Indigenous people

in ceremonies and is rarely inhaled or consumed in a manner that can cause harm (Jetty, 2017). Smoking tobacco is the most popular form of tobacco use in Canada; in 2017, 11% (3.3 million) of Canadians reported smoking daily, and 4% (1.3 million) reported smoking occasionally (Health Canada,

2019). Tobacco smoking is the leading cause of premature death in Canada, with estimated national health care costs due to tobacco exceeding $20 billion per year (Krueger et al., 2014). Most tobacco smokers state that they want to quit, yet relapse occurs frequently. It is estimated that approximately half of current users will die of a tobacco-related disease. Considering the magnitude and severity of the risks associated with tobacco use, it is crucial that nurses screen for tobacco use and offer interventions in all settings, including acute care.

Physiological Effects of Use

Nicotine has a rapid onset of action, especially in smoked form. When nicotine is absorbed, it produces a wide range of effects in the peripheral nervous system and CNS. Responses include increased blood pressure, heart rate, cardiac output, coronary blood flow, and cutaneous vasoconstriction. During inhalation, nicotine is absorbed quickly into the bloodstream and travels to the brain in a matter of seconds. In the brain, the action of nicotine on nicotinic receptors causes general CNS stimulation with increased alertness and arousal. The effects last about 1 to 2 hours before withdrawal symptoms occur, which can leave the person feeling tired, irritable, and anxious. The activity of nicotine on the dopamine reward system can result in ongoing use and cravings and eventual physiological dependence. During withdrawal from nicotine, cue-induced relief craving may cause smoking relapse. Nicotine itself is highly psychoactive and can lead to physiological dependence, but it is the many chemicals contained in tobacco products, especially the smoked form, that cause most of the harm and health complications. These include carbon monoxide, tar, arsenic, and lead, which are poisonous and toxic to the human body.

Electronic Cigarettes

Electronic cigarettes (e-cigarettes) are battery-operated devices that turn nicotine and other chemicals, including propylene glycol, glycerin, and flavourings, into an aerosol or vapour. These devices do not contain tobacco leaf, although some resemble traditional cigarettes. Emerging information indicates that e-cigarettes are not harmless. E-cigarettes containing nicotine have the potential to increase the risk for cardiovascular and respiratory issues (Hajek et al., 2014), and the liquid solutions used in refillable e-cigarettes may cause poisoning or skin irritation and are not subject to quality control. Studies indicate that e-cigarettes are increasing in use, particularly among current smokers, pose less harm to smokers than traditional cigarettes, are being used to reduce or quit smoking, and are widely available (Glasser et al., 2017). However, the long-term health effects of vaping have not been examined and are unknown at this time. Acute effects have included lung injury and a number of associated deaths (Centers for Disease Control and Prevention [CDC], 2020).

Health Complications

The complications of tobacco use are related to dose and method of ingestion. Cigarette smoking is the single most preventable cause of death and also causes significant morbidity, including chronic lung disease, cardiovascular disease, stroke, and cataracts. Smoking during pregnancy can cause stillbirth, low birth weight, sudden infant death syndrome (SIDS), and other serious pregnancy complications (Center for Chronic Disease Prevention and Health Promotion, 2020). Together with the increased

myocardial oxygen consumption that nicotine causes, carbon monoxide significantly decreases the oxygen available to the myocardium. The result is an even greater increase in heart rate and myocardial oxygen consumption that may lead to myocardial ischemia. Users of smokeless tobacco also experience the systemic effects of nicotine on the cardiovascular system.

The chronic respiratory irritation caused by cigarette smoke is the most important risk factor in the development of lung cancer and chronic obstructive pulmonary disease (COPD). Chronic irritation from smoking also is a factor in the increased incidence of cancer of the mouth, larynx, and esophagus in persons who smoke tobacco in any form.

Women are at particular risk for smoking-related diseases. Women who smoke have a 25% higher risk of coronary heart disease than men and have greater risks of reproductive health issues, many forms of gynecological cancer and other types of cancer, chronic obstructive lung disease, and osteoporosis (American College of Obstetricians and Gynecologists, 2011). Lastly, attention should be paid to the inequities in tobacco use patterns, especially among young women, women with a history of trauma, women with mental health issues, and Indigenous women (Greaves et al., 2016), which may affect their ability to have successful quit attempts.

Interprofessional Care: Nursing Interventions for Tobacco Use Disorder

A combination of medications, behavioural approaches, and support has been shown to be most effective in addressing nicotine dependence and long-term tobacco cessation, with immediate benefit to the patient (Figure 11.4).

Tobacco Use Cessation. With each patient encounter, the nurse should ask about tobacco use, assess the person's level of motivation to change, and advise the person about the importance of quitting. The "5 A's" brief intervention (**a**sk, **a**dvise, **a**ssess, **a**ssist, **a**rrange) is an effective approach for working collaboratively with people with nicotine dependence (Tobacco Use and Dependence Guideline Panel, 2008). This approach identifies clinical interventions that can be used at each patient encounter, depending on the time available (Table 11.7). These interventions are designed to identify tobacco users, encourage them to quit, determine their willingness to quit, assist them in quitting, and arrange for follow-up to prevent relapse. Simply screening for and assessing for smoking has a significant impact as an intervention to help people quit smoking. Smoking cessation is the single most effective intervention to increase quality of life and decrease the morbidity and mortality directly caused by smoking. See the Resources section at the end of this chapter for more information on nursing interventions.

Nicotine Replacement Therapy and Pharmacotherapeutic Interventions for Nicotine Dependence. A variety of smoking cessation products are available to help support users in quitting or cutting down, including prescription medicines as well as OTC products such as nicotine patches, inhalers, and gum (Table 11.8). Nicotine replacement therapy (NRT) products reduce the craving and withdrawal symptoms associated with cessation by supplying the body with a safer delivery of nicotine. Because most health care facilities are tobacco-free environments, admitted patients who are dependent on nicotine may experience withdrawal symptoms since they are unable to smoke. Offering NRT to those who desire it will assist in controlling withdrawal symptoms during hospitalization, support patients to stay and get their medical treatment and promote continued cessation after discharge. Many patients with concurrent disorders have tobacco use disorders and often can't smoke due to admission on a secured unit; NRT can be a successful approach to calming patients who wish to leave to smoke. People continuing to smoke while on NRT should not discontinue treatment; in these cases the potential need for increased doses or the addition of a second type of NRT agent should be considered (UBC Continuing Professional Development [CPD], 2020).

Non-nicotine products also support smoking cessation, such as Varenicline (Champix). Varenicline is unique in that it has both agonist and antagonist actions. Its agonist activity at one subtype of nicotinic receptor provides some nicotine effects to ease withdrawal symptoms. If the person does resume smoking, its antagonist action blocks the effects of nicotine at another subtype of nicotinic receptor, which mutes the effects. Bupropion

(Zyban), an antidepressant, reduces the urge to smoke, some symptoms of withdrawal, and helps prevent weight gain associated with smoking cessation. These products can also be used in conjunction with NRT. Varenicline has the strongest evidence for smoking abstinence, but NRT and bupropion are also very effective (Anthenelli et al., 2016).

Along with using a smoking cessation product, individuals who wish to quit are more likely to succeed if they participate in a tobacco cessation program. Nurses should be aware of community resources that assist patients in navigating these services. Many programs teach people skills to decrease triggers and relapse risk and help them develop coping skills, such as cigarette refusal skills, assertiveness, alternative activities, and peer support systems. The advice and motivation provided by health care providers can be a powerful force in smoking cessation. Best Practice Guideline on smoking cessation, available on

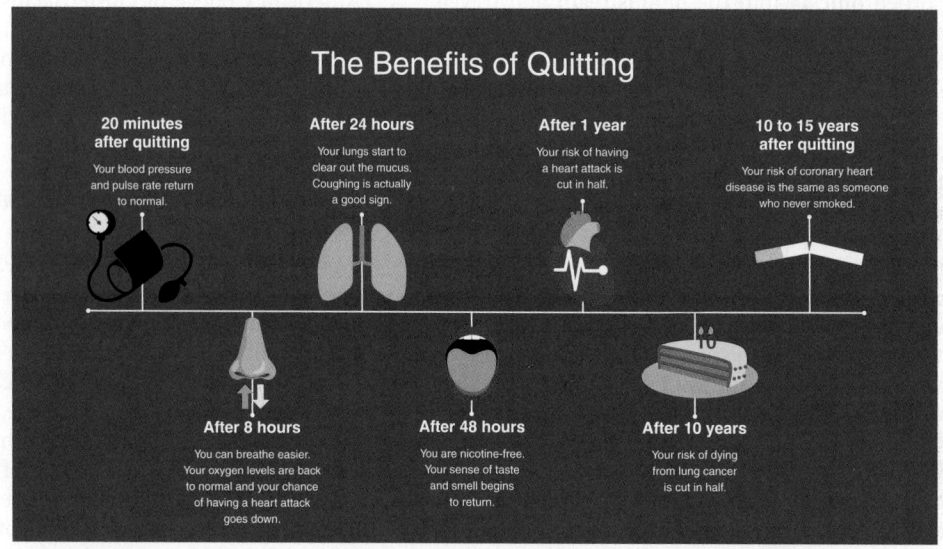

FIG. 11.4 Benefits of quitting smoking. Source: Canadian Cancer Society. [n.d.]. *The benefits of quitting.* https://smokershelpline.ca/quit-plan-public/volume4/static/thinking-about-quitting

TABLE 11.7	CARING FOR THE PATIENT WITH TOBACCO USE DISORDER

The Five A's for Patients Who Desire to Quit
1. **Ask:** Identify all tobacco users at every contact.
   a. "Have you used any form of tobacco in the past 6 months?"
   b. "Do you smoke (even a puff now and again) or use tobacco products of any kind?"
   c. "Have you ever considered stopping?"
2. **Advise:** Strongly urge all tobacco users to quit.
   a. "As your nurse, the most important advice I can give you is to quit smoking."
3. **Assess:** Determine willingness to make a quit attempt.
4. **Assist:** Develop a plan with the patient to help the patient quit (e.g., counselling, medication).
5. **Arrange:** Schedule follow-up or refer patient to smoking cessation program.

Source: Agency for Healthcare Research and Quality. (2008). *AHCPR supported clinical practice guideline: Treating tobacco use and dependence: 2008 update.* U.S. Public Health Service; and Registered Nurses Association of Ontario. (2007). *Best practice guideline: Integrating smoking cessation into nursing practice.* Author. http://rnao.ca/bpg/guidelines/integrating-smoking-cessation-daily-nursing-practice

TABLE 11.8	COMMONLY USED MEDICATIONS TO TREAT NICOTINE USE DISORDER

Medication	Key Features
Nicotine patch	Provides long-acting source of nicotine to help mitigate cravings and other symptoms of nicotine withdrawal
Nicotine gum, inhaler, spray, or lozenge	For prn use; provides short-acting source of nicotine to help mitigate cravings and other symptoms of nicotine withdrawal
Varenicline (Champix®)	Prescription medication that blocks effects of nicotine; most effective approach to helping smokers quit; can be used in conjunction with nicotine patch or prn delivery; monitor for adverse effects including gastrointestinal symptoms and mood changes.
Bupropion (Zyban®)	Prescription medication that makes smoking less pleasurable and reduces cravings; can be used in conjunction with nicotine patch or prn delivery; monitor for adverse effects including mood changes.

Source: Data from QuitNow. *Methods and medications.* https://www.quitnow.ca/quitting/methods-and-medications

RNAO's website, is an excellent resource for the nurse helping patients to quit smoking. A link to this document appears in the Resources section at the end of this chapter. Table 11.8 lists tobacco cessation interventions.

ALCOHOL

Characteristics

Alcohol is the most widely consumed substance in Canada, where 78% of the population aged 15 years and older drinks alcohol (Health Canada, 2019). Canada has low-risk drinking guidelines (Table 11.9), which recommend that women limit consumption to 10 standard drinks per week, with no more than two drinks per day most days and that men limit consumption to no more than 15 standard drinks per week, with no more than three drinks per day most days. In 2017, 21% of Canadians who consume alcohol reported exceeding the guidelines for chronic use and 15% exceeded guidelines for acute use. It is estimated that up to 18% if Canadians aged 18 years and older have met criteria for alcohol use disorder in their lifetime (British Columbia Centre on Substance Use [BCCSU], 2019). Alcohol use contributes to substantial health burden: Nearly 200 disease or injury conditions are wholly or in part attributable to alcohol use, with resulting economic, health care, and social costs.

Numerous factors appear to be interrelated in the development of alcohol use disorder and include genetic, psychosocial, and cultural–environmental factors. Alcohol use disorder is viewed as a chronic, relapsing, and potentially fatal condition if left untreated. Unfortunately, many individuals are not offered evidence-informed treatment. Hospital admissions provide an opportunity for pharmacological and nonpharmacological interventions. In a systematic review, patients who received a brief intervention in hospital had a greater reduction in alcohol consumption compared to usual-care groups at 6 months (McQueen et al., 2011). Nurses play a role in offering these supports. Health teaching about the risks associated with consuming more than the low-risk drinking guidelines (see Table 11.9) is recommended. It is also important to assess patient goals and readiness to change alcohol-related behaviours.

Parts of the Canadian population have been disproportionately affected by alcohol use. Given historical, social, political, and economic factors, Indigenous people have experienced elevated harm related to alcohol use. In one survey 25.1% of Indigenous people reported heavy drinking in the past month, compared to 19.6% of non-Indigenous Canadians, and alcohol-related mortality was estimated to be 5.43 times higher in Indigenous men and 10.11 times higher in Indigenous women than in their non-Indigenous counterparts (Statistics Canada, 2019). As noted in previous sections, there are several contributing factors to these statistics: colonization, the trauma of residential schools, the reserve system, loss, grief, and intergenerational trauma. It is important to understand that many individuals may be using alcohol to cope with trauma and distressing experiences (Brave Heart, 2003; Parappilly et al., 2020).

Adding to these harms, Indigenous people have reported negative experiences and stigma when accessing health care, especially in the context of substance use disorders (Goodman et. al, 2017). Harmful stereotypes around Indigenous people and alcohol use persist and greatly affect their health care experiences. Despite these misconceptions, it is important to note that a higher proportion of Indigenous people over 12 years old reported past-year abstinence from alcohol when compared to the rest of the Canadian population (27.4% vs. 24.6%). In order to address these disparities and not perpetuate stigma or institutionalized racism, health care providers working with individuals with alcohol use disorder should be familiar with and incorporate harm-reduction, trauma-informed, and culturally competent approaches and principles.

TABLE 11.9 CANADA'S LOW-RISK DRINKING GUIDELINES

Drinking is a personal choice. If you choose to drink, these guidelines can help you decide when, where, why, and how much.

Your Limits
Reduce your long-term health risks by drinking no more than:
- 10 drinks per week for women, with no more than two drinks per day most days
- 15 drinks per week for men, with no more than three drinks per day most days.

Plan nondrinking days every week to avoid developing a habit.

Special Occasions
Reduce your risk for injury and harm by drinking no more than three drinks (for women) and four drinks (for men) on any single occasion. Plan to drink in a safe environment. Stay within the weekly limits.

When Zero Is the Limit
Do not drink when you are:
- Driving a vehicle or using machinery and tools
- Taking medicine or other drugs that interact with alcohol
- Doing any kind of dangerous physical activity
- Living with mental or physical health conditions
- Living with alcohol dependence
- Pregnant or planning to be pregnant
- Responsible for the safety of others
- Making important decisions

Pregnant? Zero Is the Safest
If you are pregnant or planning to become pregnant, or if you are about to breastfeed, the safest choice is to drink no alcohol at all.

Delaying Your Drinking
Alcohol can harm the way the body and brain develop. Teens should speak with their parents about drinking. If they choose to drink, they should do so under parental guidance; never more than one to two drinks at a time, and never more than one to two times per week. They should plan ahead, follow local alcohol laws, and consider the safer drinking tips.

Defining "a Drink"
For these guidelines, "a drink" means:
- 341 mL (12 oz.) bottle of 5% alcohol beer, cider, or cooler
- 142 mL (5 oz.) glass of 12% alcohol wine
- 43 mL (1.5 oz.) serving of 40% distilled alcohol (e.g., rye, rum, gin)

Low-risk drinking helps to promote a culture of moderation.
Low-risk drinking supports healthy lifestyles.

Tips
Set limits for yourself and abide by them.
Drink slowly. Have no more than two drinks in any 3 hours.
For every drink of alcohol, have one nonalcoholic drink.
Eat before and while you are drinking.
Always consider your age, body weight, and health issues that might suggest lower limits.
Although drinking may provide health benefits for certain groups of people, do not start to drink, or increase your drinking, for health benefits.

Source: Butt, P., Beirness, D., Gliksman, L., et al. (2011, updated 2018). *Alcohol and health in Canada: A summary of evidence and guidelines for low-risk drinking.* Canadian Centre on Substance Abuse.

Effects of Use

Alcohol is a small, water-soluble molecule that is rapidly absorbed into the bloodstream through the digestive tract; faster absorption occurs when alcohol is mixed with carbonated liquids. Absorption is slower in the presence of water or food, especially proteins and fats. Alcohol has complex CNS effects; it generally acts as a depressant or sedative, but when the blood alcohol level is rising, a period of disinhibition and arousal can occur. With chronic use, the brain becomes tolerant to alcohol and changes activity of excitatory (glutamate) and inhibitory (GABA) neurotransmitters. When alcohol is abruptly stopped, there is an increase in the excitatory activity and the person experiences withdrawal symptoms. The effects of alcohol are related to the blood alcohol concentration (BAC) in the body and individual susceptibility. BAC is affected by the amount consumed, the drinking rate, body size and composition, drink concentration, and hormones. Children and youth or individuals who have lower body mass are more susceptible to the effects of alcohol.

Alcohol Intoxication. Intoxication, as evidenced by increasing BAC, results in behavioural and physical changes. People are at higher risk for self-injurious behaviours while intoxicated, as a result of impaired judgement and impulsivity. People are also at risk for significant mood dysregulation and depression, and risk for suicide is an important consideration. Fatalities caused by drinking and driving, head injuries, physical trauma, and violence are closely linked to alcohol intoxication.

Acute Alcohol Intoxication. It is important to obtain as accurate a history as possible, using collateral information as necessary, and assess for injuries, trauma, diseases, and hypoglycemia. Vital signs and level of consciousness should be monitored. The nurse should remain with the intoxicated patient as much as possible, orienting to reality as necessary. Agitation and anxiety are common, and the patient should be assessed for increasing disorientation and potential for violence. The patient is also at high risk for injury because of lack of coordination and impaired judgement, and protective environmental measures should be used (i.e., supervision). It is critical to continue assessment and interventions until the BAC has decreased to at least 21.7 mmol/L and until any associated disorders or injuries have been ruled out. After acute intoxication, individuals may experience hangovers manifested by malaise, nausea, headache, thirst, and a general feeling of fatigue.

Alcohol Withdrawal. Alcohol withdrawal occurs when an individual with tolerance to alcohol abruptly ceases consumption. Approximately 50% of individuals with long-term, heavy alcohol use will experience some withdrawal symptoms upon cessation of alcohol use (Goodson et al., 2014); for the majority of individuals, symptoms are mild to moderate and resolve quickly. A patient with alcohol dependence who is hospitalized for other health conditions is at risk for alcohol withdrawal. If there is any indication of alcohol or other CNS-depressant use when a patient is hospitalized, the nurse should always assess when the patient last used the substance. This information will help the nurse anticipate drug interactions or the time of possible onset of withdrawal symptoms. The signs and symptoms of alcohol withdrawal generally begin 6 to 12 hours after the patient's last drink and last up to 5 days. Characteristic symptoms include tremors, anxiety, increased heart rate, increased blood pressure, sweating, nausea, vomiting, hyperreflexia, agitation, insomnia, and in some cases hallucinations. Withdrawal hallucinations are not

TABLE 11.10	STAGES OF ALCOHOL WITHDRAWAL
Time of Onset After Last Use	**Symptoms**
6–12 hours	Minor withdrawal symptoms: insomnia, tremors, anxiety, gastrointestinal upset, headache, diaphoresis, palpitations, anorexia, nausea, tachycardia, hypertension
12–14 hours	Visual, auditory, or tactile hallucinations
24–48 hours	Withdrawal seizures: generalized tonic–clonic seizures
48–72 hours	Alcohol withdrawal delirium (delirium tremens): hallucinations (predominantly visual), disorientation, agitation, diaphoresis

Source: Sachdeva, A., Choudhary, M., & Chandra, M. (2015). Alcohol withdrawal syndrome: Benzodiazepines and beyond. *Journal of Clinical and Diagnostic Research, 9*(9), VE01–VE07. https://doi.org/10.7980/JCDR/2015/13407.6538

the same as delirium tremens, developing within 12 to 24 hours and clearing within 24 to 48 hours; during this time the patient is aware they are hallucinating. Severe and life-threatening alcohol withdrawal syndrome include seizures (10%) or delirium tremens (3–5%) (Mirijello et al., 2015). Delirium tremens typically begins 48 to 96 hours after the last drink and presents as severe confusion and autonomic hyperactivity (i.e., hyperthermia) and global clouding of sensorium. Death may be caused by hyperthermia, peripheral vascular collapse, or cardiac failure. Seizures are most likely to occur 24 to 48 hours after the last drink in untreated alcohol withdrawal (Table 11.10). The Predictor of Alcohol Withdrawal Severity Scale is a tool that helps health care providers determine the risk of severe withdrawal and can guide treatment decisions (Maldonado et al., 2015).

Key nursing interventions for and management of alcohol withdrawal are based on early and accurate assessment. Nurses should assess for tachycardia, dehydration, fever, diaphoresis, dysrhythmias, and liver impairment, in addition to cognition and level of consciousness. The Clinical Institute Withdrawal Assessment for Alcohol Scale, Revised (Table 11.11) is a standardized assessment tool that can be used to assess and monitor for withdrawal symptoms caused by alcohol withdrawal. Treatment of intermediate withdrawal usually involves the administration of a benzodiazepine (chlordiazepoxide, diazepam, lorazepam, and oxazepam are most commonly used) to prevent withdrawal-related seizure (Sachdeva et al., 2015). If the person has compromised liver function or is an older person, a short-acting benzodiazepine may be preferred (Hammond et al., 2015). Table 11.12 presents the clinical manifestations of alcohol withdrawal and suggested treatment. A quiet, calm environment is important to preventing exacerbation of symptoms, and frequent reorientation should be provided. The use of restraints and IV lines should be avoided whenever possible. Supportive care is needed to ensure adequate rest and nutrition. Nursing care for the patient in alcohol withdrawal is presented in Nursing Care Plan 11.1.

Complications

The long-term physical effects of alcohol use disorder, outlined in Table 11.13, may be the reason that individuals seek health care. Complications may also arise from the interaction of alcohol with commonly prescribed or OTC drugs. Drugs that interact with alcohol in an additive manner include antihypertensives, antihistamines, antianginals, and salicylates (Aspirin).

TABLE 11.11	CLINICAL INSTITUTE WITHDRAWAL ASSESSMENT FOR ALCOHOL–REVISED (CIWA-AR)

Patient Name:_____ (Last Name, First Name)

Time:_____ Total Score (max score = 67)_____ Temp: _____BP:____/____

Apex rate:_____ Resps:_____

Initials:_____ (print name and credentials) (signature)(dd/mm/yyyy):_____

F0136-20100721 Chart Tab: Assessments/Plans Patient ID Label

Nausea & Vomiting

Ask: "Do you feel sick to your stomach? Have you vomited?"

Observation:

0 No nausea/vomiting
1
2
3
4 Intermittent nausea with dry heaves
5
6
7 Constant nausea, frequent dry heaves and vomiting

Tremor

Arms extended and fingers spread apart

Observation:

0 No tremor
1 Not visible, but can be felt fingertip to fingertip
2
3
4 Moderate, with patient's arms extended
5
6
7 Severe, even with arms not extended

Paroxysmal Sweats

Observation:

0 No sweat visible
1 Barely perceptible sweating, palms moist
2
3
4 Beads of sweat obvious on forehead
5
6
7 Drenching sweats

Anxiety

Ask: "Do you feel nervous?"

Observation:

0 No anxiety, at ease
1 Mildly anxious
2
3
4 Moderately anxious, or guarded, so anxiety is
   inferred
5
6
7 Acute panic as seen in severe delirium or acute
   schizophrenic reactions

Agitation

Observation:

0 Normal activity
1 Somewhat more than normal activity
2
3
4 Moderately fidgety and restless
5
6
7 Paces back and forth during most of interview or
   constantly thrashes about

Tactile Disturbances

Ask: "Have you any itching, pins and needles sensations, any burning, any numbness, or do you feel bugs crawling on or under your skin?"

Observation:

0 None
1 Very mild itching, pins and needles, burning or numbness
2 Mild itching, pins and needles, burning or numbness
3 Moderate itching, pins and needles, burning or numbness
4 Moderately severe hallucinations
5 Severe hallucinations
6 Extremely severe hallucinations
7 Continuous hallucinations

Auditory Disturbances

Ask: "Are you more aware of sounds around you? Are they harsh? Do they frighten you? Are you hearing anything that is disturbing to you? Are you hearing things you know are not there?"

Observation:

0 Not present
1 Very mild harshness or ability to frighten
2 Mild harshness or ability to frighten
3 Moderate harshness or ability to frighten
4 Moderately severe hallucinations
5 Severe hallucinations
6 Extremely severe hallucinations
7 Continuous hallucinations

Visual Disturbances

Ask: "Does the light appear to be too bright? Is its colour different? Does it hurt your eyes? Are you seeing anything that is disturbing to you? Are you seeing things you know are not there?"

Observation:

0 Not present
1 Very mild sensitivity
2 Mild sensitivity
3 Moderate sensitivity
4 Moderately severe hallucinations
5 Severe hallucinations
6 Extremely severe hallucinations
7 Continuous hallucinations

Headache, Fullness in Head

Ask: "Does your head feel different? Does it feel like there is a band around your head?" Do not rate for dizziness or lightheadedness. Otherwise, rate severity.

0 Not present
1 Very mild
2 Mild
3 Moderate
4 Moderately severe
5 Severe
6 Very severe
7 Extremely severe

Orientation & Clouding of Sensorium

Ask: "What day is this? Where are you? Who am I?"

Observation:

0 Oriented and can do serial additions
1 Cannot do serial additions or is uncertain about date
2 Disoriented for date by no more than 2 calendar days
3 Disoriented for date by more than 2 calendar days
4 Disoriented for place and/or person

Source: Brands, B., Kahan, M., Selby, P., et al. (Eds.). (2000). *Management of alcohol, tobacco and other drug problems: A physician's manual* (p. 77). Centre for Addiction and Mental Health.

TABLE 11.12   ALCOHOL WITHDRAWAL TREATMENT

Clinical Manifestations	Pharmacological Treatment

• Minor withdrawal syndrome
  • Tremulousness, anxiety
  • Increased heart rate
  • Increased blood pressure
  • Sweating
  • Nausea
  • Hyperreflexia
  • Insomnia
  • Hallucinations
• Major withdrawal
  • DTs
  • Seizures
• Preventative: Wernicke's encephalopathy
	• Benzodiazepines
	• Gabapentin
	• Haloperidol (Haldol) for hallucinations
	• Naltrexone
	  • Supports individuals to cut down on drinking
	  • Person does not need to be abstinent from alcohol while on this medication
	  • Is an opioid antagonist so can not be concurrently administered with opioids
	• Acamprosate
	  • Preferred if goal is abstinence
	  • Person does not need to be abstinent from alcohol while on this medication
	• Continue to administer benzodiazepines as ordered
	• Additional antiseizure medications for seizures or past history of seizures
	• Thiamine
	• Some individuals may also be administered magnesium sulphate or multivitamins (folic acid, B vitamins)

DTs, delirium tremens.
NOTE: For DTs, provide intravenous fluids (do not overhydrate), cooling blanket, well-lit quiet room, consistent staff, and frequent checks of vital signs; check for hypoglycemia; assess any other health issues.
Source: Data from British Columbia Centre on Substance Use. (2020). *Provincial guideline for the clinical management of high risk drinking and alcohol use disorder.* https://www.bccsu.ca/wp-content/uploads/2020/03/AUD-Guideline.pdf.

⊚ NURSING CARE PLAN 11.1

Alcohol Withdrawal

NURSING DIAGNOSIS	***Potential for injury*** as evidenced by *alteration in psychomotor functioning* (sensorimotor deficits)
Expected Patient Outcomes	**Nursing Interventions and *Rationales***
• Reports no falls or injuries • Experiences decrease in tremors and psychomotor activity • Reports no seizures	• Assess for risk factors such as impaired mobility (e.g., unsteady gait), sensory deficits, tremors, impaired judgement, confusion, seizure activity *to plan appropriate preventive measures.* • Assess for signs of injury such as lacerations, bruises, or burns *to treat appropriately.* • Monitor vital signs frequently, especially heart rate, *because prompt recognition of extreme autonomic nervous system response is necessary for early intervention to prevent progression of symptoms.* • Administer benzodiazepines as ordered *to control hyperactivity,* thiamine *to reduce neurological complications (e.g., Wernicke's encephalopathy),* and antiseizure medications as ordered *to prevent seizures.* • Use seizure precautions *to prevent injury.*
NURSING DIAGNOSIS	***Acute confusion*** resulting from alcohol withdrawal as evidenced by *alteration in cognitive functioning, misperception, agitation, hallucinations* resulting from *sensory overload* as evidenced by *impaired interpretation of environmental stimuli, disorientation, and hallucinations*
Expected Patient Outcomes	**Nursing Interventions and *Rationales***
• Reports no hallucinations • Reports reduced agitation • Remains oriented to person, place, and time	• Assess patient's orientation and cognition *to determine appropriate interventions.* • Provide quiet and nonstimulating environment *to reduce external stimuli and calm overactive CNS.* • Orient to nurse and environment with each contact; use calm, approach; provide consistent staff; explain procedures and what is expected *to assist in orientation and decrease anxiety.* • Administer benzodiazepines as ordered *to reduce CNS stimulation.* • Administer antipsychotic medication (e.g., haloperidol [Haldol]) if ordered *to decrease severity of hallucinations.* (Be aware that Haldol lowers the seizure threshold.)
NURSING DIAGNOSIS	***Ineffective breathing pattern*** resulting from *hyperventilation and respiratory muscle fatigue*
Expected Patient Outcomes	**Nursing Interventions and *Rationales***
• Maintains effective breathing • Reports no indications of hypoxia	• Monitor respiratory rate, depth, and pattern *so appropriate interventions may be taken.* • Position patient on their side and in semi-Fowler's position *to reduce possibility of aspiration and to enhance lung expansion by lowering diaphragm.* • Monitor effects of medications given for withdrawal *to detect respiratory depression.* • Encourage coughing and deep breathing *to prevent complications of hypoventilation.* • Administer supplemental oxygen *to treat hypoxia.*

CNS, central nervous system.

Alcohol taken with Aspirin may cause or exacerbate gastrointestinal (GI) bleeding. Alcohol taken with acetaminophen (Tylenol) may increase the risk for liver damage. Potentiation, a drug interaction causing a response greater than the sum of the individual responses to each drug, occurs when an additional CNS depressant is taken with alcohol, increasing the effect.

People with high alcohol tolerance may also be tolerant (require an increased dose for effect) to other CNS depressants such as benzodiazepines or opioids, even if they have never used these drugs. This is called cross-tolerance.

Complications Associated With Chronic Alcohol Use Disorder. One severe complication of long-term heavy alcohol use

TABLE 11.13 EFFECTS OF LONG-TERM, HEAVY ALCOHOL USE

Body System	System Effects
Central nervous system	Dementia; Wernicke's encephalopathy (confusion, nystagmus, paralysis of ocular muscles, ataxia); Korsakoff syndrome (confabulation, amnesic disorder); impairment of cognitive function, psychomotor skills, abstract thinking, and memory; depression, attention deficit, labile moods, seizures, sleep disturbances
Peripheral nervous system	Peripheral neuropathy including pain, paresthesias, weakness
Immune system	Increased risk for tuberculosis and viral infections, especially pneumonia; increased risk for cancer of oral cavity, pharynx, esophagus, liver, colon, rectum, and possibly breast
Hematological system	Bone marrow depression, anemia, leukopenia, thrombocytopenia, blood clotting abnormalities
Musculoskeletal system	Painful or tender swelling of large muscle groups; painless progressive muscle weakness and wasting; osteoporosis
Cardiovascular system	Elevated pulse and blood pressure; decreased exercise tolerance; cardiomyopathy (irreversible); increased risk for hemorrhagic stroke, coronary artery disease, hypertension, sudden cardiac death
Hepatic system	Steatosis (reversible)—nausea, vomiting, hepatomegaly; hepatitis (reversible)—anorexia, nausea, vomiting, fever, chills, abdominal pain, cirrhosis; cancer
Gastrointestinal system	Gastritis, peptic ulcer, esophagitis, esophageal varices, enteritis, colitis, Mallory–Weiss tear, pancreatitis
Digestive system	Decreased appetite, indigestion, malabsorption, vitamin deficiencies
Urinary system	Diuretic effect from inhibition of antidiuretic hormone
Endocrine and reproductive system	Altered gonadal function, testicular atrophy, decreased beard growth, decreased libido, diminished sperm count, gynecomastia, glucose intolerance, early menopause, fetal alcohol spectrum disorder
Integumentary system	Palmar erythema, spider angiomas, rosacea, rhinophyma

is Wernicke's encephalopathy, an inflammatory, hemorrhagic, degenerative condition of the brain caused by a thiamine deficiency. Because Wernicke's encephalopathy is potentially reversible, IV thiamine is often administered to patients with alcohol use disorder, especially those in withdrawal. Untreated or progressive Wernicke's encephalopathy may lead to Korsakoff syndrome, an irreversible form of amnesia characterized by loss of short-term memory and an inability to learn (Xiong, 2018).

Interprofessional Care

There are many interventions available to individuals with alcohol use disorder, including withdrawal management, pharmacotherapies, and psychosocial interventions. Cessation of drinking is the short-term goal of withdrawal management and consists of interventions and processes aimed at addressing the physiological and psychological symptoms that occur in response to stopping alcohol use. Management of alcohol withdrawal frequently includes the use of medications to decrease symptoms, increase the level of comfort, and decrease the risk of seizures and delirium tremens. Patients should also be offered additional medications that may support goals of alcohol reduction (e.g., naltrexone) and abstinence (e.g., acamprosate) and that treat protracted withdrawal symptoms such as anxiety and insomnia (e.g., gabapentin) (BCCSU, 2019). Lastly, managed alcohol programs are a harm-reduction approach to manage withdrawal symptoms in populations who consume high-risk, non-beverage alcohol such as rubbing alcohol. These are evidence-informed, typically community-based programs that supply regular dosing of safer alcohol sources, such as wine or beer. These treatments are starting to be used in some hospitals (Brookes et al., 2018). Nurses may administer these medications and can provide education on the rationale for these treatments.

Patients should be referred to inpatient or intensive outpatient programs for continued support and treatment if this aligns with their goals. Outpatient options include counselling, Self-Management and Recovery Training (SMART) groups, and Alcoholics Anonymous (AA) meetings.

CANNABIS

Characteristics

According to the Health Canada (2019), about 11% of all Canadians aged 15 years and older had used cannabis at least once in the past year, and about 32% of those who had used cannabis in the past 3 months reported that they used it every day or almost every day. In Canada, 37% of cannabis users report doing so for medical reasons, and there is evidence for the treatment of chronic pain, use as an antiemetic in cancer treatment, and treatment of multiple sclerosis spasticity. However, there are also substantial risks, including prompting the onset of schizophrenia or other psychoses, impairment leading to motor vehicle accidents, newborn low birth weight, respiratory issues, and cannabis use disorder. Adolescents who use cannabis regularly are at higher risk for psychotic symptoms, particularly when there is coexisting or family history of psychosis (George & Vaccarino, 2015).

In 2018, the Canadian government legalized the use of cannabis for recreational use for legal-age adults, while previously it was only legal for specific medical reasons. People may purchase cannabis in several different forms at dispensaries. For medical reasons, pharmaceutical cannabinoids, nabilone (an oral tablet containing a synthetic tetrahydrocannabinol [THC]), or cannabis may still be prescribed. There are illegal synthetic THC derivatives (e.g., K2, Spice), which contain varying amounts of different ingredients, have unpredictable effects, and are more toxic. (See Chapter 12 for further information.)

Effects of Use

Humans have an endocannabinoid system, the receptors of which bind with cannabinoids consumed by taking a natural or synthetic cannabis product orally or by inhalation. Cannabinoids are chemicals found in the cannabis plant, and the chemical most responsible for the psychoactive effects is THC. THC can cause euphoria, relaxation, anxiety, and memory impairment. Cannabidiol (CBD), another chemical in cannabis, mitigates some of these negative effects and has antipsychotic and anti-inflammatory effects. People use cannabis for a variety of desired effects, including euphoria, elation, pain relief, and appetite stimulation, but they may also experience negative effects, such as panic, fear, trouble concentrating, decreased coordination, and lower interest in completing tasks. Signs of intoxication are presented in Table 11.6. In acute intoxication, the nurse should perform a physical examination, a urine or serum drug test, and a thorough history. Cannabis can induce tachycardia and hypertension and, in some users, hypotension, and it can increase cardiovascular risks such as arrythmias (Goyal et al., 2017). Although rare and difficult to diagnose, one presentation that nurses may see in hospital settings is cannabis hyperemesis syndrome, which is characterized by cyclic vomiting and is associated with long-term, heavy cannabis use (Venkatesan et al., 2019).

Withdrawal can occur in a hospitalized patient who is a heavy cannabis user. The patient may experience irritability, anxiety, decreased appetite, disturbed sleep, depressed mood, and one of the following physical symptoms: chills, headache, abdominal pain, fever, or tremors (Livne et al., 2019). No specific pharmacological therapy is effective in treating withdrawal. Supportive care includes measures such as administration of antiemetics, analgesics, and hydration to ensure patient comfort. Benzodiazepines may provide symptom relief.

Interprofessional Care

Nurses should screen for cannabis use as with other substances and determine patient risks, goals, and opportunities for health promotion. Canada has low-risk cannabis use guidelines (see Resources section) which can be shared with patients. The nurse can also support patients with harm reduction strategies, including delaying age of trying cannabis until after 18, limiting use, using edibles instead of smoking, not using high-potency synthetic products, not driving after consumption, and avoiding use for high-risk groups: pregnant women, people with heart disease, and people with a history of psychosis or a family history of psychosis (CNA, 2017c). In the case of cannabis use disorder, there are no currently approved pharmacological treatments, but patients can be supported with inpatient treatment, withdrawal management, counselling, and group therapy. In some hospital settings, cannabis may actually be used therapeutically (e.g., the patient's medical supply may be brought in); the nurse should consult local policies.

OPIOIDS

Characteristics

Opiates are substances that are directly derived from the opium poppy, such as morphine and codeine. Opioids is an umbrella term that includes both opiates and the many semisynthetic and synthetic agents used as analgesics. Commonly used opioids are identified in Table 11.6. Opioids are very effective analgesics, and the majority of people who are prescribed opioid medications for the treatment of acute and chronic pain do not develop problematic use patterns. The risk of nonmedical use is increased by factors discussed earlier in this chapter, including early childhood experiences and mental illness. People may use prescription opioids nonmedically, or purchase illicit opioids such as heroin, oxycodone, or fentanyl. The presence of fentanyl and analogues in the illicit opioid supply has been increasing since 2014, placing users at risk of overdose and death due to its potency. Other risks of opioid use include human immunodeficiency virus (HIV)

infection if injecting equipment is shared, and contact with the criminal justice system if illicit opioids are used.

Effects of Use

Opioids contain opioid agonists, which are chemicals that activate opioid receptors in the brain and exert effects; they include both prescribed medications like morphine or methadone and nonprescribed substances like heroin. Binding to opiate receptors and neurotransmitter systems in the CNS, opioid agonists cause a number of effects, including CNS depression and stimulation of the brain reward system. Opioid antagonists include naloxone (Narcan), which binds to the same receptor but has no activity. Opioids can be consumed orally or intravenously or they can be sniffed or smoked. Initial effects can include euphoria, analgesia, drowsiness, slurred speech, decreased respiratory rate, GI peristalsis, and decreased pupil size. Tolerance to opioids develops quickly; therefore, people who use opioids nonmedically will require increasingly high amounts to achieve the same effect and eventually develop physical dependence as the brain adjusts. Over time, people with opioid use disorder go into withdrawal if they do not use opioids, and they need to use in order to feel normal and alleviate the discomfort of withdrawal. Physiological tolerance to opioids is lost very quickly. After a few days of abstinence, lower tolerance may lead to fatal overdoses should people resume taking the same amount they had been previously accustomed to taking.

Opioid Overdose. Unintentional overdose can occur with illicit opioid use because of the unpredictability in potency. Overdose can also occur with prescribed or nonprescribed opioids if used by someone with lower tolerance. Signs of overdose of opioids include pinpoint pupils, clammy skin, depressed respirations, and decreased level of consciousness that can lead to coma and death if the overdose is not treated (Figure 11.5). Opioid overdose is a medical emergency; treatment can include administering naloxone and maintaining airway. Giving naloxone can put the person into withdrawal temporarily, and when they regain consciousness, they can be reassured that these uncomfortable symptoms will subside soon. Naloxone has a shorter half-life than that of other opioids, meaning it will wear off and repeat doses may be required. Naloxone is a very safe medication, and kits are now available widely across Canada so that individuals can respond to an overdose in the community while waiting for emergency services. In some areas, nurses may train and dispense kits to patients (see Resources section).

Opioid Withdrawal. Withdrawal from opioids occurs with decreased amounts or cessation after a period of moderate to heavy use. Symptoms may include craving, abdominal cramps, diarrhea, tremor, chills, overall body aches, sleep disturbances, anxiety, nausea, and vomiting. Severe withdrawal is extremely uncomfortable (Table 11.14). Opioid withdrawal can begin 4 to 6 hours after last use, depending on the opioid, usually peaks 2 to 3 days after last use, and resolves by days 5 to 7. Interventions to support withdrawal include comfort measures and medications for relief of symptoms (i.e., acetaminophen). Ongoing opioid use despite consequences often results as individuals try to relieve these uncomfortable withdrawal symptoms. In acute care, nurses need to assess for and anticipate opioid withdrawal in patients with regular nonmedical use. This withdrawal should be treated with opioid agonists, discussed below, and in some cases with short-acting opioids. Untreated withdrawal can lead to patients leaving the hospital before completing medical

SIGNS OF AN
OPIOID OVERDOSE

Learn how to spot an overdose and what to do.

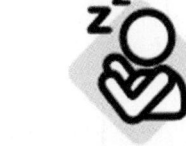

Cannot be woken up
or not moving

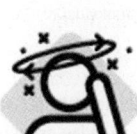

Breathing
slow or absent

Choking
or coughing, gurgling,
or snoring sounds

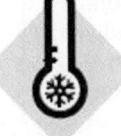

Cold
or clammy skin

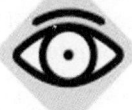

Dizziness
and disorientation

Pupils
extremely small

Discoloration
of lips and nails

CALL 911 IMMEDIATELY!

Your address _____

THEN:

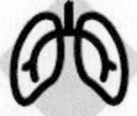

Give breaths
1 breath every
5 seconds

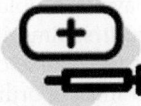

Use naloxone
if you have it

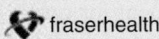 fraserhealth   fraserhealth.ca/overdose   Catalogue#265247 (August 2016) English
To order:Patienteduc.fraserhealth.ca

FIG. 11.5 Opioid overdose signs and symptoms. Source: Reproduced with permission from fraser**health**, Canada (2016). *Recognizing an overdose: Depressants/Opioids. Signs of an Opioid Overdose.* fraser **health**.ca.

TABLE 11.14	SYMPTOMS OF OPIOID WITHDRAWAL
Early Symptoms	**Advanced Symptoms**
• Abdominal cramps • Myalgia (muscle pain) • Lacrimation (teary eyes) • Rhinorrhea (runny nose) • Anxiety • Sweating • Yawning	• Enlarged pupils • Piloerection • Diarrhea • Insomnia • Agitation • Tachycardia • Nausea or vomiting • Tremor • Chills

Note: Each patient's withdrawal looks different. Withdrawal symptoms are measured using the Clinical Opioid Withdrawal Scale (COWS); see Resources section.

TABLE 11.15	COMMONLY USED MEDICATIONS TO TREAT OPIOID USE DISORDER
Medication	**Key features**
Methadone	Long-acting, oral opioid full agonist that reduces withdrawal and cravings with once-daily dosing; usually administered in liquid form; protects against overdose; monitor patients for sedation, especially during titration phase
Buprenorphine-naloxone	Long-acting, opioid partial agonist that reduces withdrawal and cravings with once-daily dosing; most commonly used in sublingual form but injectable forms are also available; protects against overdose; less drug interactions and sedation risk than with methadone
Slow-release oral morphine (Kadian®)	Slow-release oral opioid full agonist that reduces withdrawal and cravings with once-daily dosing; potential safety advantage for patients with cardiac complications (e.g., QTc prolongation) when compared to methadone

Source: Data from Canadian Research Initiative in Substance Misuse (CRISM). (n.d.). *CRISM national guideline for the clinical management of opioid use disorder.* https://crism.ca/wp-content/uploads/2018/03/CRISM_NationalGuideline_OUD-ENG.pdf

treatment (Ti et al., 2015). Treating withdrawal improves care outcomes and nurse–patient interactions.

Other Complications. A key consideration in people with regular, chronic use of opioids is opioid-induced constipation, which can lead to complications such as bowel obstruction. Nurses can support patients to improve bowel health; traditional laxatives such as stool softeners and osmotic, stimulant, and lubricant agents are recommended as initial treatment (Rao et al., 2019). Other health complications are related to route of use, such as contracting hepatitis C or other blood-borne illnesses from sharing injection equipment if there is no access to sterile equipment. Harm reduction interventions are essential to prevent such complications.

Interprofessional Care

Opioid use disorder is considered a chronic and relapsing condition; thus, a long-term treatment approach is taken. Opioid agonist therapy (OAT), such as methadone, has the most evidence for reducing morbidity, mortality, and criminal justice system involvement (Canadian Research Institute in Substance Misuse [CRISM], 2018). Withdrawal management alone (going off all opioids, including OAT) is not recommended because of the risk of relapse and overdose. There are several types of OAT, varying in intensity (Table 11.15). It is recommended that harm reduction be offered across the treatment spectrum, including naloxone kits and access to supervised consumption and sterile supplies if use is ongoing.

In the acute care setting, it is important to review the routine and medication history of patients. A person on OAT should have their daily dose continued while they are in hospital to ensure optimal treatment; on admission it is also essential to confirm when the person last took a dose to avoid double-dosing. If someone starts on methadone for the first time in hospital, doses will be lower and increase during the course of admission. Upon discharge, the health care team must coordinate care to ensure that the patient can continue treatment in the community. A patient can have their care transferred back to their community provider but may need support finding a prescriber if OAT was started in hospital. Not all prescribers provide OAT to patients, so a patient may need a referral to an OAT or methadone clinic to bridge care.

Methadone. Methadone is the most commonly used OAT in Canada. It is a potent long-acting opioid agonist that alleviates withdrawal and cravings for 24 hours at the right dose. Methadone is typically an oral, liquid form that is taken daily. Until a period of stability is achieved, the person undergoes witnessed daily ingestion at a pharmacy. With stability, the patient may be provided take-home doses of methadone, as long as they can be

responsible for ensuring safe storage and handling. Usually a dose of 60 mg or above would be considered therapeutic, but doses can be above 200 mg (CRISM, 2018). Since methadone can be sedating, people on methadone should be advised to avoid using other sedating substances such as alcohol and benzodiazepines.

Buprenorphine. Buprenorphine is a partial opioid agonist that is less sedating than methadone and has less drug interactions. It is available as a sublingual oral tablet and is taken once daily. It is important that the sublingual tablet dissolves completely and is not swallowed. Buprenorphine has a lower risk of overdose than methadone because it is a partial agonist and does not create as much CNS depression (CRISM, 2018). It also binds closely to the receptor and blocks other opioids from binding, so effects are not felt if the individual uses another form of opioids. In Canada, buprenorphine is usually combined with naloxone in the tablet—this does not decrease overdose risk but is included to prevent diversion. If the sublingual tablet is crushed and snorted or injected, the naloxone becomes active and may cause withdrawal. Taken sublingually, the naloxone is inactive.

Specialist Treatments. There are many evolving treatment approaches for opioid use disorder in Canada, including slow-release oral morphine and injectable formulations such as hydromorphone. Slow-release oral morphine, or Kadian®, is an oral alternative that may be prescribed to patients who have not benefitted from methadone or buprenorphine/naloxone; these doses are higher than when used for analgesia (e.g., 1 800 mg) (CRISM, 2018). Injectable treatment for opioid use disorder using diacetylmorphine (the active ingredient in heroin) or hydromorphone has been studied in Canada since 2005 and clinically applied since 2013 for patients who did not benefit from oral medications. Improvements in health outcomes and decrease in illicit opioid use have been observed (Oviedo-Joekes et al., 2016). In community settings, patients self-inject a prescribed dose of the medication; when admitted to an acute care hospital, most often these doses are administered by a nurse. These treatment approaches are becoming more widely available, providing a larger range of treatment options for this chronic disease.

✚ TABLE 11.16 EMERGENCY MANAGEMENT

CNS Stimulant—Cocaine and Amphetamine Toxicity

Assessment Findings	Interventions
Cardiovascular • Palpitations • Tachycardia • Hypertension • Dysrhythmias • Myocardial ischemia or infarction **Central Nervous System** • Euphoria • Agitation • Combativeness • Seizures • Hallucinations • Confusion • Paranoia • Fever	**Initial** • Ensure patent airway • Anticipate need for intubation if respiratory distress evident • Establish IV access and initiate fluid replacement as appropriate • Obtain a 12-lead ECG • Treat ventricular dysrhythmias as appropriate • Administer IV medications for psychosis • Administer IV diazepam (Valium) or lorazepam (Ativan) for seizures • Naloxone IV should be given if CNS depression is present and concurrent opiate use is possible • Anticipate the need for propranolol (Inderal) or labetalol for hypertension and tachycardia **Ongoing** • Monitor vital signs, level of consciousness, cardiac rhythm • Use restraints only if needed to protect the patient and staff

CNS, central nervous system; ECG, electrocardiogram; IV, intravenous.

✚ TABLE 11.17 EMERGENCY MANAGEMENT

CNS Depressant Overdose

Assessment Findings	Interventions

• Agitation
• Confusion
• Lethargy
• Hallucinations
• Slurred speech
• Pinpoint pupils (opioids)
• Nystagmus
• Seizures
• Cold, clammy skin
• Rapid, weak pulse
• Slow or rapid shallow respirations
• Decreased O_2 saturation
• Hypotension
• Dysrhythmia
• ECG changes
• Cardiac or respiratory arrest
	Initial
	• Ensure patent airway
	• Anticipate intubation if respiratory distress evident
	• Establish IV access
	• Obtain temperature
	• Obtain 12-lead ECG
	• Obtain information about substance (name, route, when taken, amount)
	• Obtain specific drug levels or comprehensive toxicology screen
	• Obtain a health history including substance use and allergies
	• Administer antidotes as appropriate:
	  • Opioids: naloxone
	  • Benzodiazepines: flumazenil
	• Perform gastric lavage if no antidote available
	• Administer activated charcoal if within 4–6 hours of consumption
	Ongoing
	• Monitor vital signs, temperature, level of consciousness, O_2 saturation, cardiac rhythm

CNS, central nervous system; ECG, electrocardiogram; IV, intravenous, O_2, oxygen.

STIMULANTS

COCAINE, AMPHETAMINES, AND PRESCRIPTION STIMULANTS

Characteristics

Stimulants may be illicit (i.e. cocaine, crack, amphetamines) or prescribed, such as methylphenidate (treatment of narcolepsy or attention-deficit/hyperactivity disorders). In 2017, 2% of Canadians reported using cocaine within the past year (Health Canada, 2019) and 2% of Canadians aged 15 years and older reported using a prescription stimulant in the past year, with 19% indicating problematic use. In the United States, stimulant-related hospitalizations are increasing (Winkelman et al., 2018).

Acute Effects of Use

All stimulants work in part by increasing the amount of dopamine in the brain, causing euphoria and increasing energy, alertness, and improved performance. This action on the brain reward system enhances pleasure and, over time, can lead to ongoing use despite consequences, by hijacking the reward system. Stimulants also affect the cardiovascular system, causing increased heart rate and blood pressure and increasing cardiovascular risk (Diercks, 2008). There are also acute psychiatric and behavioural effects, including psychosis, agitation and aggression, and skin-picking due to delusions of insects. Stimulants may be used by many routes, including intravenously, snorted, orally, and smoking; smoking and IV methods result in the fastest absorption. Effects of cocaine use are short, which leads to more frequent use, increasing spending and other risks. Amphetamines have a longer half-life than that of cocaine.

During sustained periods of stimulant use, the person may not be sleeping, eating, or performing self-care.

Stimulant Toxicity or Overdose. Currently, there are no recommended pharmacological treatments for stimulant overdose or intoxication. Generally, treatment is supportive and focuses on the system at risk (e.g., cardiovascular). Symptoms of stimulant toxicity and emergency management are presented in Table 11.16.

Withdrawal. Withdrawal from cocaine and amphetamines does not usually cause obvious physical symptoms, but physical and behavioural manifestations do occur. Cravings can be intense during the first hours to days of cessation and may continue for weeks. The nurse may identify withdrawal symptoms in a patient with stimulant use disorder who is hospitalized for management of other health conditions. Abrupt cessation of stimulants can also lead to a "crash," where the patient may be depressed and experience fatigue, prolonged sleep, vivid dreams, irritability, increased appetite, and disorientation. Supportive care includes maintaining a quiet environment and allowing the patient to sleep and eat as desired, clustering care to reduce interruptions, and possibly providing sedating medications to support sleep. If a patient has severe depression, the nurse should initiate suicide precautions and refer the patient for further treatment. With prolonged stimulant cessation, most patients' moods will stabilize.

Complications

Stimulants can lead to a variety of health complications, most significantly those involving the cardiovascular system; psychiatric issues; and subsequent health issues due to route of use or high-risk activity. IV administration may result in collapse and scarring of the veins at the injection site, cellulitis, wound abscess, endocarditis, hepatitis B virus (HBV) and hepatitis C virus (HCV) infection, and HIV infection. With intranasal use, the nasal septum and mucosa may become damaged and pulmonary damage from smoking crack may occur. Over time, stimulant use may lead to paranoia and other forms of persistent psychosis. Persistent psychiatric conditions may be treated with antipsychotics. Elevated mortality also results from overdose, toxicity, and other accidents (Darke et al., 2017).

Interprofessional Care

Treatment will depend on the goals and health status of the patient. Nurses should offer harm reduction to patients with active use, including supervised consumption, sterile supplies, and safer sex supplies. There is an absence of evidence-informed pharmacotherapies at this time (UBC CPD, 2020), so psychosocial interventions are recommended, such as SMART recovery groups, Narcotics Anonymous (NA), or a rewards-based intervention called *contingency management*.

SEDATIVE–HYPNOTICS

Characteristics

Sedative–hypnotic agents include barbiturates, benzodiazepines, and barbiturate-like drugs. Benzodiazepine-class medications are effective in the short-term treatment of panic attacks and severe anxiety and alcohol withdrawal. However, long-term prescription can contribute to the development of tolerance and risk for problematic use. A person who becomes tolerant to the effects may increase the dose and frequency of use without medical advice or indication. People may also purchase illicit sedative–hypnotics. These substances elevate risk for respiratory depression when combined with other CNS depressants.

Effects of Use

Sedative–hypnotic drugs act primarily on the CNS, causing relaxation or sedation at low doses and sleep at high doses. Excessive amounts produce an initial euphoria and an intoxication that includes impaired judgement, slurred speech, and loss of inhibitions and motor coordination. Although benzodiazepines are believed to have a wide margin of safety, they are not without adverse reactions, including rebound anxiety and insomnia with short-acting drugs and confusion and memory loss with long-acting drugs. These drugs are usually taken orally, but barbiturates may be injected intravenously. The effects of sedative–hypnotics are presented in Table 11.6.

Complications

An overdose of a sedative–hypnotic may cause death as a result of respiratory depression. Symptoms of overdose are listed in Table 11.17. Overdoses of benzodiazepines may be treated with flumazenil, a specific benzodiazepine antagonist. There are no known antagonists to counteract the effects of other sedative–hypnotic medications. Emergency life support measures must be taken in cases of overdose.

Withdrawal From Sedative–Hypnotics. Withdrawal from sedative–hypnotics can be highly variable, and the severity and onset of symptoms depend on many factors, including the drug, the pattern of use, the dose and duration of use, and the presence of concurrent alcohol use. Withdrawal from sedative–hypnotics may include anxiety, tremors, weakness, nausea with or without vomiting, muscle cramps, and increased reflexes. Withdrawal from benzodiazepines is potentially life-threatening and necessitates close monitoring in an inpatient setting as it can lead to delirium, seizures, and respiratory and cardiac arrest. Management is symptomatic and includes a gradual reduction in drug dosage; abrupt cessation of the drug is not recommended. Long-acting agents such as diazepam (Valium), chlordiazepoxide (Librax), clonazepam, or phenobarbital may be substituted and tapered after stabilization.

Interprofessional Care

Nurses can work with patients to set goals and monitor symptoms. Medically supervised tapering over an extended period of time is recommended for withdrawal management in people with benzodiazepine use disorder. Inpatient treatment centres or outpatient support groups may support a patient's goals. Underlying mental health diagnoses should be treated.

OTHER SUBSTANCES

INHALANTS

Inhalation (i.e., sniffing, huffing, bagging) is the major route of ingestion for a number of common household and industrial substances. There are four main classes of inhalants: volatile solvents, aerosols, anaesthetic agents, and nitrites. Inhalants are rapidly absorbed and reach the CNS quickly. Most are depressants, and their effects are similar to those of alcohol, including slurred speech, lack of coordination, euphoria, and dizziness. The effects are relatively brief, lasting only 60 to 90 minutes. Long-term use can result in neurological issues, including damage to parts of the brain that control cognition, movement, vision, and hearing. Common agents and their effects are presented in Table 11.6. The patient with inhalant toxicity may experience dizziness, euphoria, disinhibition, nystagmus, slurred speech, and lethargy. The effects usually resolve within minutes to a few hours. Managing inhalant toxicity usually consists of providing supportive care. However, in some cases, users need emergency treatment for dysrhythmias, heart failure, or CNS hyperactivity (e.g., seizures).

HALLUCINOGENS

Hallucinogens are a variety of psychoactive substances that produce a change in level of consciousness, alter mood, and may induce hallucinations; they include psilocybin (magic mushrooms) and lysergic acid diethylamide (LSD). Table 11.6 identifies common hallucinogens and their effects. Hallucinogens do not typically cause physiological dependence, so withdrawal states are not noted. Some hallucinogens (e.g., psilocybin) are being studied for their therapeutic effect in medical settings for the treatment of mental health disorders and substance use disorders.

GAMMA HYDROXYBUTYRATE (GHB)

GHB is a CNS depressant, causing sedation and slowing heart rate and respirations. It is typically in oral solution and difficult to dose, leading to great overdose risk. Chronic use can lead to physical dependence and life-threatening withdrawal, which should be medically managed.

SPECIAL CONSIDERATIONS

Acute Pain Management Considerations

Health care providers may demonstrate reluctance to treat acute pain with opioid medications in people who use substances. However, the effective treatment of acute pain is a key priority for all people, including those who use substances. It is appropriate, therefore, to use opioids to help all people manage acute pain. Untreated pain is more likely to lead to relapse than to exacerbating a substance use disorder (Ries et al., 2015).

If the patient acknowledges opioid use, it is important to determine the type and amount of opioids used. Severe pain may be treated with opioids. The use of one opioid is preferred, and nonopioid and adjuvant analgesics and non-pharmacological pain relief measures may also be used, as appropriate. Withdrawal symptoms can exacerbate pain and need to be addressed in order to provide adequate pain management. Patients need their baseline opioid needs met to treat withdrawal, and acute pain will require additional opioids or other pain management methods. For example, a patient's regular methadone dose will not provide analgesia for acute pain, and they will also have increased tolerance to other opioid medications. To maintain opioid blood levels and prevent withdrawal symptoms, health care providers should give regular doses around the clock or use longer-acting opioids. Supplemental doses should be used to treat breakthrough pain. For adequate pain control in patients with opioid use disorder, the nurse should advocate for much higher doses than those used in opioid-naive patients because of tolerance (Ries et al., 2015). Depending on whether these patients are on OAT to treat their opioid use disorder, these doses can vary widely. Patients on buprenorphine may need specialized care when needing acute pain control, as buprenorphine blocks the effects of other opioids.

Perioperative Care

All patients undergoing emergency surgery must be carefully assessed for signs and symptoms of substance use or overdose that could lead to adverse drug interactions with analgesics or anaesthetics. The prevalence of alcohol use disorders in emergency departments is as high as 40%, and the incidence of symptomatic alcohol withdrawal is two to five times higher in trauma and surgical patients (Ries et al., 2015). Special precautions must be taken for the patient who is intoxicated or alcohol dependent and requires surgery, owing to the risk of withdrawal and postsurgical complications. Vital signs, including body temperature, must be closely monitored to identify signs of withdrawal, possible infections, and respiratory or cardiac problems. Preoperative assessment for elective surgical procedures must include a thorough health history and assessment of substance use, including questions related to alcohol, nicotine, and other substance use. Any type of withdrawal that may be caused by abrupt cessation should be monitored for and treated proactively, including nicotine withdrawal. Other complications may occur as well; respiratory changes in smokers make introduction of endotracheal and suction tubes more difficult and increase the risk for postoperative respiratory problems. Patients on opioid agonist therapy should be continued on their treatment and may need additional doses of opioids to manage acute pain, as discussed above.

ETHICAL DILEMMAS

Situation

> A patient who has been treated for severe alcohol-withdrawal complications discloses to the nurse that he is a long-distance truck driver and has been working for the past 10 years. As part of the substance use assessment, the nurse learns that he seems to have developed high tolerance to alcohol, with daily consumption and only short periods of abstinence since his divorce last year. He has no previous substance use history and had no problematic substance use before last year.
>
> **Important Points for Consideration**
> - Nurses identify ethical issues; consult with the appropriate person or body; and take action to resolve and evaluate the effectiveness of actions.
> - Nurses have an ethical responsibility to promote health and well-being, as well as a responsibility to base their practice on current evidence.
> - Nurses have an ethical obligation to prevent harm to patients and the public.
> - Nurses are responsible for communicating concerns regarding harms to the patient as well as communicating them to the patient's team of health care providers.
> - Nurses must know the legal reporting obligations regarding driver licensing for their province or territory.
>
> **Clinical Decision-Making Considerations**
> More information is needed about this case and a team approach should be taken to determine if this patient's alcohol use needs to be reported and to whom. Involving the patient in care planning is essential, and voluntary acceptance of treatment is ideal. Nurses can contact the Canadian Nurses Protective Society about ethical concerns in the workplace. See Resources section for link.

AGE-RELATED CONSIDERATIONS

Problematic substance use in older persons is under-recognized, for several reasons: patterns of substance use in older persons may be different from that of younger persons; substance use among older persons can be mistaken for other medical or psychiatric conditions, such as insomnia, depression, poor nutrition, heart failure, and frequent falls; and there is a lack of clinician training and comfort in this area (Han, 2018). For example, opioid use disorder in older persons has been under-recognized and undertreated (Canadian Centre on Substance Use and Addiction [CCSA], 2018; Payne et al., 2018), yet there is an increase in older persons seeking treatment for opioid use disorder (both for prescription and illicit opiates) (Huhn et al., 2018). Many specific circumstances place the older person at particular risk for a substance use disorder, including difficulty coping with losses that occur with increasing age, such as retirement, death of family and friends, relocation, social isolation, and poor health. Senior advocacy groups are calling for greater attention to the issue of problematic substance use among older persons.

Aging is associated with cognitive and functional changes that can make the brain more vulnerable to the effects of substances. The effects of alcohol and other psychoactive substances increase with aging. Age-related changes in function, especially in the liver and kidneys, alter circulation, metabolism, and the body's ability to eliminate substances. Older persons tend to have more physical illnesses and be prescribed more medications with exposure to drug combinations; older persons are at increased risk for potentially harmful drug–drug interactions. When taken in combination, alcohol, sedative–hypnotic drugs, and CNS depressants have additive and synergistic effects. Problematic substance use and high rates of prescription medication use in older persons may contribute to confusion, disorientation, delirium, memory loss, and neuromuscular impairment. Older persons have high rates of hospitalization for opiate toxicity in Canada (CCSA, 2018).

As with all patients, it is important for the nurse to discuss all substance use with older patients, including use of OTC medications, and assess the patient's knowledge of the medications they take. Patient education for the older person includes teaching about the desired effects, possible adverse effects, and appropriate use of prescribed and OTC medications. The nurse

should recommend that the patient use only one pharmacy, because many pharmacies maintain a medication profile on each individual that may prevent problems with drug interactions. Patients should be advised about risks of combining CNS depressants. The nurse should monitor people who are experiencing losses and identify those who may need additional supports. Home visits by a nurse provide a good opportunity for assessment of challenges and also provision of valuable support. A nurse who assesses for an alcohol or substance use disorder in an older patient should refer the patient for treatment. Older persons benefit from the treatments discussed in this chapter. Quality of life can be improved significantly by addressing problematic substance use, regardless of a person's age. Older persons can live long, healthy, and productive lives while in recovery.

CASE STUDY

Substance Use

Patient Profile
C. M., 78 years old (pronouns she/her), is admitted to the emergency department after falling and injuring her right shoulder and arm. Her partner died 4 years ago and she lives alone. Recently, her best friend died. Her only family is a daughter who lives out of town. When the nurse contacts C. M.'s daughter by phone, her daughter tells the nurse that C. M. appears to have been more disoriented and confused over the past year when they have talked on the phone.

Subjective Data
- Reports severe pain in her right shoulder and upper arm
- Reports she had some wine in the late afternoon to stimulate her appetite
- Has experienced several falls with minor bruising in the past 2 months
- Reports that she fell after taking her sleeping pill, prescribed by her physician because she does not sleep well
- Speaks with hesitation and slurs
- Says she smokes about half a pack of cigarettes a day

Objective Data
Physical Examination
- Oriented to person and place, but not time
- Blood pressure 162/94, pulse 92, respirations 24

- Bruising and edema of right upper arm
- Tremors of hands

Diagnostic Tests
- Radiographic examination reveals comminuted fracture of the proximal humerus necessitating surgical repair
- Blood alcohol concentration (BAC) 24 mmol/L
- Complete blood count: hemoglobin 106 g/L; hematocrit 0.38 (38%)

Discussion Questions
1. What other information is needed to assess C. M.'s condition?
2. How should questions regarding these areas be addressed?
3. What factors may contribute to C. M.'s use of psychoactive substances?
4. *Priority decision:* What priority nursing interventions are appropriate during C. M.'s preoperative period?
5. What possible complications and other health concerns may become apparent during C. M.'s postoperative recovery?
6. What nursing interventions are appropriate following C. M.'s surgery?
7. *Priority decision:* Based on the assessment data presented, what are the priority nursing diagnoses for C. M.? Are there any interprofessional issues?

evolve
Answers are available at http://evolve.elsevier.com/Canada/Lewis/medsurg.

REVIEW QUESTIONS

The number of the question corresponds to the same-numbered objective at the beginning of the chapter.

1. What term best describes a pattern of continued substance use despite significant harms and withdrawal symptoms?
   a. Abuse
   b. Substance use disorder
   c. Tolerance
   d. Addictive behaviour

2. Which of these statements is true?
   a. Only a small percentage of Canadians are affected by substance use issues.
   b. About 50% of risk for problematic alcohol use is attributable to genetics.
   c. All people are equally susceptible to risk of problematic substance use.
   d. Substance use is more prevalent in urban areas.

3. When engaging a client experiencing substance use or problematic substance use, which of the following is part of the role of the nurse in acute care? *(Select all that apply.)*
   a. Screen all patients for substance use.
   b. Advocate for adequate pain and withdrawal management for patients with opioid use disorder.
   c. Promote a nonjudgemental, collaborative therapeutic relationship that honours client autonomy and choice.
   d. Assess safety concerns and stabilization of acute illness.

4. When using a harm reduction approach with clients experiencing substance use problems, what is the key aim of the nurse?
   a. To provide harm reduction supplies and health teaching
   b. Not to coerce or force the individual to quit their substance use
   c. To ensure that clients have access to health care services
   d. To reduce the harms associated with substance use

5. In which of the following behaviours should the nurse engage during motivational interviewing with a client? *(Select all that apply.)*
   a. Insist that the client maintain abstinence while undergoing therapy.
   b. Relate motivational techniques to the client's stage of behaviour change.
   c. Use any method of communication that will make the client change behaviour.
   d. Identify discrepancies between the client's goals or values and current behaviour.
   e. Ask a prescribed set of questions to increase the client's awareness of negative behaviours.

6. When screening and assessing for substance use, which of the following is the most urgent to cover in acute care in order to determine imminent risks?
   a. Use of substances, pattern of use, route, frequency of use, and date and time of last use
   b. Medical history and psychiatric history
   c. Social supports
   d. Legal history

7. Which of the following is the most appropriate nursing intervention for a client who is seen at the clinic for increasing shortness of breath but who is not interested in quitting smoking?
   a. Accept the client's decision and do not intervene until the client expresses a desire to quit.
   b. Realize that some smokers will never quit and that trying to assist them only increases the client's and the nurse's frustration.
   c. Increase the client's motivation to quit by explaining that continued smoking will only increase the breathing problems.
   d. Ask the client about smoking at every clinic visit, advise of the benefits of quitting smoking, assess reasons for wanting to continue smoking, assist with goal-setting, and arrange a follow-up plan.

8. While caring for a client who is experiencing alcohol withdrawal, what actions should the nurse take? *(Select all that apply.)*
   a. Monitor neurological status on a routine basis.
   b. Administer medications by IV route only.
   c. Pad the side rails and place suction equipment at the bedside.
   d. Orient the client to environment and person with each contact.
   e. Administer antiseizure drugs and sedatives to relieve symptoms during withdrawal.

9. Which of the following is important in pain management of clients with opioid use disorder or other substance use disorders?
   a. The goal is to treat acute pain.
   b. Never administer IV opioids.
   c. Understand that opioid analgesia may worsen a substance use disorder.
   d. These clients should not be prescribed prn opioids.

10. A client who has an opioid use disorder is scheduled for surgery following an automobile accident. What is important for the nurse to recognize in this case?
    a. The client may need less pain medication during the postoperative period.
    b. The client should be continued on any opioid agonist therapy (e.g., methadone) throughout the perioperative period.
    c. The client may have an immediate onset of withdrawal symptoms when given anaesthetic and analgesic agents.
    d. The client has a low risk for physical withdrawal symptoms but is likely to experience craving during the postoperative period.

11. To which factors are substance use issues in older persons most commonly related?
    a. Use of drugs and alcohol as a social activity
    b. Misuse of prescribed and OTC drugs and alcohol
    c. Continued use of illegal drugs initiated during middle age
    d. A pattern of binge drinking for weeks or months with periods of sobriety

1. b; 2. b; 3. a, b, c, d; 4. d; 5. b, d; 6. a; 7. d; 8. a, c, d, e; 9. a; 10. b; 11. b.

evolve

For even more review questions, visit http://evolve.elsevier.com/Canada/Lewis/medsurg.

REFERENCES

Aguiar, W., & Halseth, R. (2015). *Aboriginal Peoples and historic trauma: The process of intergenerational transmission.* https://www.ccnsa-nccah.ca/docs/context/RPT-HistoricTrauma-IntergenTransmission-Aguiar-Halseth-EN.pdf

American College of Obstetricians and Gynecologists. (2011). Committee opinion number 503: tobacco use and women's health. *Obstetrics and Gynecology, 118*(3), 746–750. https://doi.org/10.1097/AOG.0b013e3182310ca9. (Seminal).

American Psychiatric Association (APA). (2013). *Diagnostic and statistical manual of mental disorders* (5th ed.). Author (Seminal).

Anthenelli, R. M., Benowitz, N. L., West, R., et al. (2016). Neuropsychiatric safety and efficacy of varenicline, bupropion, and nicotine patch in smokers with and without psychiatric disorders (EAGLES): a double-blind, randomised, placebo-controlled clinical trial. *The Lancet, 387*(10037), 2507–2520. https://doi.org/10.1016/S0140-6736(16)30272-0

Brave Heart, M. Y. (2003). The historical trauma response among natives and its relationship with substance abuse: a Lakota illustration. *Journal of Psychoactive Drugs, 35*(1), 7–13. https://doi.org/10.1080/02791072.2003.10399988. (Seminal).

British Columbia Centre on Substance Use (BCCSU). (2019). *Provincial Guideline for the Clinical Management of High-Risk Drinking and Alcohol Use Disorder.* https://www.bccsu.ca/wp-content/uploads/2021/01/AUD-Guideline.pdf

British Columbia Coroner's Report. (2021). *Illicit Drug Toxicity Deaths in BC January 1, 2011– May 31, 2021.* https://www2.gov.bc.ca/assets/gov/birth-adoption-death-marriage-and-divorce/deaths/coroners-service/statistical/illicit-drug.pdf

Brooks, H. L., Kassam, S., Salvalaggio, G., et al. (2018). Implementing managed alcohol programs in hospital settings: A review of academic and grey literature: Managed alcohol programs in hospital. *Drug and Alcohol Review, 37*, S145–S155. https://doi.org/10.1111/dar.12659

Burchum, J. R., & Rosenthal, L. D. (2016). *Lehne's pharmacology for nursing care* (9th ed.). Elsevier Saunders.

Canadian Centre on Substance Use and Addiction (CCSA). (2018). *Improving quality of life: substance use and aging.* https://www.ccsa.ca/sites/default/files/2019-04/CCSA-Substance-Use-and-Aging-Report-2018-en.pdf

Canadian Nurses Association (CNA). (2017a). *Code of Ethics for Registered Nurses.* https://www.cna-aiic.ca/~/media/cna/page-content/pdf-en/code-of-ethics-2017-edition-secure-interactive

Canadian Nurses Association (CNA). (2017b). *Harm reduction and illicit substance use: implications for nursing.* https://www.cna-aiic.ca/-/media/cna/page-content/pdf-en/harm-reduction-and-illicit-substance-use-implications-for-nursing.pdf?la=en&hash=5F5BBCDE16C7892D9C7838CF62C362685CC2DDA7

Canadian Nurses Association (CNA). (2017c). *Harm reduction for non-medical cannabis use.* https://www.cna-aiic.ca/~/media/cna/page-content/pdf-en/harm-reduction-for-non-medical-cannabis-use.pdf?la=en

Canadian Research Institute for Substance Misuse (CRISM). (2018). *CRISM National Guideline for the Clinical Management of Opioid Use Disorder.* https://crism.ca/wp-content/uploads/2018/03/CRISM_NationalGuideline_OUD-ENG.pdf

Carusone, S. C., Guta, A., Robinson, S., et al. (2019). "Maybe if I stop the drugs, then maybe they'd care?"—Hospital care experiences of people who use drugs. *Harm Reduction Journal, 16*(1), 16. https://doi.org/10.1186/s12954-019-0285-7

Center for Chronic Disease Prevention and Health Promotion. (2020). *Substance Use During Pregnancy.* https://www.cdc.gov/reproductivehealth/maternalinfanthealth/substance-abuse/substance-abuse-during-pregnancy.htm#tobacco

Centers for Disease Control and Prevention (CDC). (2020). *Outbreak of Lung Injury Associated with the Use of E-Cigarette, or Vaping, Products.* https://www.cdc.gov/tobacco/basic_information/e-cigarettes/severe-lung-disease.html

Chu, C., & Galang, A. (2013). Hospital nurses' attitudes toward patients with a history of illicit drug use. *The Canadian Nurse, 109*(6), 29–33.

Collins, S., Clifasefi, S., Logan, D., et al. (2012). Current status, historical highlights and basic principles. In G. Marlatt, M. Larimer, & K. Witkiewitz (Eds.), *Harm reduction: Pragmatic strategies for management of high-risk behaviours* (2nd ed.). Guilford Press (Seminal).

Darke, S., Kaye, S., & Duflou, J. (2017). Rates, characteristics and circumstances of methamphetamine–related death in Australia: A national 7–year study. *Addiction, 112*(12), 2191–2201. https://doi.org/10.1111/add.13897

Deak, J. D., Miller, A. P., & Gizer, I. R. (2019). Genetics of alcohol use disorder: A review. *Current Opinion in Psychology, 27*, 56–61. https://doi.org/10.1016/j.copsyc.2018.07.012

Diercks, D. B., Fonarow, G. C., Kirk, J. D., et al. (2008). Illicit stimulant use in a United States heart failure population presenting to the emergency department (from the Acute Decompensated Heart Failure National Registry Emergency Module). *American Journal of Cardiology, 102*(9), 1216–1219. https://doi.org/10.1016/j.amjcard.2008.06.045. (Seminal).

Dube, S. R., Felitti, V. J., Dong, M., et al. (2003). Childhood abuse, neglect, and household dysfunction and the risk of illicit drug use: The adverse childhood experiences study. *Pediatrics, 111*(3), 564–572. https://doi.org/10.1542/peds.111.3.564. (Seminal).

Felitti, V. J., Anda, R. F., Nordenberg, D., et al. (1998). Relationship of childhood abuse and household dysfunction to many of the leading causes of death in adults: The adverse childhood experiences (ACE) study. *American Journal of Preventive Medicine, 14*(4), 245–258. https://doi.org/10.1016/S0749-3797(98)00017-8. (Seminal).

Firestone, M., Tyndall, M., & Fischer, B. (2015). Substance use and related harms among Aboriginal people in Canada: A comprehensive review. *Journal of Health Care for the Poor and Underserved, 26*(4), 1110–1131. https://doi.org/10.1353/hpu.2015.0108

Fischer, B., Russell, C., Sabioni, P., et al. (2017). Lower-Risk Cannabis Use Guidelines (LRCUG): An evidence-based update. *American Journal of Public Health, 107*(8). https://doi.org/10.2105/AJPH.2017.303818

George, T., & Vaccarino, F. (2015). *Substance abuse in Canada: The effects of cannabis use during adolescence.* Canadian Centre on Substance Abuse. http://www.ccsa.ca/Resource%20Library/CCSA-Effects-of-Cannabis-Use-during-Adolescence-Report-2015-en.pdf

Glasser, A. M., Collins, L., & Pearson, J. L. (2017). Overview of electronic nicotine delivery systems: A systematic review. *American Journal of Preventive Medicine, 52*(2), e33–e66. https://doi.org/10.1016/j.amepre.2016.10.036

Goodman, A., Fleming, K., Markwick, N., et al. (2017). "They treated me like crap and I know it was because I was Native": The healthcare experiences of Aboriginal peoples living in Vancouver's inner city. *Social Science & Medicine, 178*, 87–94. https://doi.org/10.1016/j.scocscimed.2017.01

Goodson, C. M., Clark, B. J., & Douglas, I. S. (2014). Predictors of severe alcohol withdrawal syndrome: a systematic review and meta-analysis. *Alcoholism: Clinical and Experimental Research, 38*(10), 2664–2677. https://doi.org/10.1111/acer.12529. (Seminal).

Goyal, H., Awad, H. H., & Ghali, J. K. (2017). Role of cannabis in cardiovascular disorders. *Journal of Thoracic Disease, 9*(7), 2079. https://doi.org/10.21037/jtd.2017.06.104

Greaves, L., Hemsing, N., Poole, N., et al. (2016). From fetal health to women's health: expanding the gaze on intervening on smoking during pregnancy. *Critical Public Health, 26*(2), 230–238. https://doi.org/10.1080/09581596.2014.968527

Hajek, P., Etter, J. F., Benowitz, N., et al. (2014). Electronic cigarettes: review of use, content, safety, effects on smokers and potential for harm and benefit. *Addiction, 109*(11), 1801–1810. https://doi.org/10.1111/add.12659 .(Seminal).

Hammond, C., Niciu, M., Drew, S., et al. (2015). Anticonvulsants for the treatment of alcohol withdrawal syndrome and alcohol use disorders. *CNS Drugs, 29*(4), 293–311. https://doi.org/10.1007/s40263-015-0240-4

Han, B. H. (2018). Aging, multimorbidity, and substance use disorders: The growing case for integrating the principles of geriatric care and harm reduction. *The International Journal on Drug Policy, 58*, 135. https://doi.org/10.1016/j.drugpo.2018.06.005

Health Canada. (2019). *Canadian Tobacco, Alcohol and Drugs Survey: Summary of results for 2017.* https://www.canada.ca/en/health-canada/services/canadian-tobacco-alcohol-drugs-survey/2017-summary.html

Hesse, M., & Thylstrup, B. (2013). Time-course of the *DSM-5* cannabis withdrawal symptoms in poly-substance abusers. *BMC Psychiatry, 13*(1), 258. https://doi.org/10.1186/1471-244X-13-258. (Seminal).

Huhn, A. S., Strain, E. C., Tompkins, D. A., et al. (2018). A hidden aspect of the U.S. opioid crisis: rise in first-time treatment admissions for older adults with opioid use disorder. *Drug and Alcohol Dependence, 193*, 142–147. https://doi.org/10.1016/j.drugalcdep.2018.10.002

Jetty, R. (2017). Position statement: Tobacco use and misuse among Indigenous children and youth in Canada. *Paediatrics and Child Health, 22*(7), 395–399. https://doi.org/10.1093/pch/pxx124

Jongbloed, K., Pearce, M. E., Pooyak, S., et al. (2017). The Cedar Project: mortality among young Indigenous people who use drugs in British Columbia. *CMAJ, 189*(44), E1352–E1359. https://doi.org/10.1503/cmaj.160778

Khan, S. (2017). *Concurrent mental and substance use disorders in Canada.* https://www150.statcan.gc.ca/n1/pub/82-003-x/2017008/article/54853-eng.htm

Koob, G., Kandel, D., Baler, R., et al. (2015). Pathophysiology of addiction. In A. Tasman, J. Kay, J. Lieberman, et al. (Eds.), *Psychiatry* (4th ed.). John Wiley & Sons. https://doi.org/10.1002/9781118753378

Krueger, H., Turner, D., Krueger, J., et al. (2014). The economic benefits of risk factor reduction in Canada: tobacco smoking, excess weight and physical inactivity. *Canadian Journal of Public Health, 105*(1), e69–e78 (Seminal).

Livne, O., Shmulewitz, D., Lev-Ran, S., et al. (2019). DSM-5 cannabis withdrawal syndrome: demographic and clinical correlates in US adults. *Drug and alcohol dependence, 195*, 170–177. https://doi.org/10.1016/j.drugalcdep.2018.09.005

Maldonado, J. R., Sher, Y., Das, S., et al. (2015). Prospective validation study of the Prediction of Alcohol Withdrawal Severity Scale (PAWSS) in medically ill inpatients: a new scale for the prediction of complicated alcohol withdrawal syndrome. *Alcohol and Alcoholism, 50*(5), 509–518. https://doi-org.proxy.queensu.ca/10.1093/alcalc/agv043

McLellan, A. T., Lewis, D. C., O'Brien, C. P., & Kleber, H. D. (2000). Drug dependence, a chronic medical illness: implications for treatment, insurance, and outcomes evaluation. *JAMA, 284*(13), 1689–1695. https://doi.org/10.1001/jama.284.13.1689

McQueen, J., Howe, T. E., Allan, L., et al. (2011). Brief interventions for heavy alcohol users admitted to general hospital wards. *Cochrane Database of Systematic Reviews, 10*(8), CD005191 https://doi.org/ 10.1002/14651858.CD005191.pub3. (Seminal).

Mirijello, A., D'Angelo, C., Ferrulli, A., et al. (2015). Identification and management of alcohol withdrawal syndrome. *Drugs, 75*(4), 353–365. https://doi.org/10.1007/s40265-015-0358-1

Mukherjee, S. (2013). Alcoholism and its effects on the central nervous system. *Current Neurovascular Research, 10*(3), 256–262 https://doi.org/10.2174/15672026113109990004. (Seminal).

Nathoo, T., Poole, N., & Schmidt, R. (2018). *Trauma Informed Practice and the Opioid Crisis: A Discussion Guide for Health Care and Social Service Providers.* https://bccewh.bc.ca/2018/05/trauma-informed-practice-and-the-opioid-crisis-a-discussion-guide-for-health-care-and-social-service-providers/

Nelson, S. E., Browne, A. J., & Lavoie, J. G. (2016). Representations of Indigenous peoples and use of pain medication in Canadian news media. *The International Indigenous Policy Journal, 7*(1), 1–26. https://doi.org/10.18584/iipj.206.7.1.5

Oviedo-Joekes, E., Guh, D., Brissette, S., et al. (2016). Hydromorphone compared with diacetylmorphine for long-term opioid dependence: A randomized clinical trial. *JAMA Psychiatry, 73*(5), 447–455. https://doi.org/10.1001/jamapsychiatry.2016.0109

Padwa, H., Larkins, S., Crevecoeur-MacPhail, D. A., et al. (2013). Dual diagnosis capability in mental health and substance use disorder treatment programs. *Journal of Dual Diagnosis, 9*(2), 179–186. https://doi.org/10.1080/15504263.2013.778441. (Seminal).

Parappilly, B. P., Garrod, E., Longoz, R., et al. (2020). Exploring the experience of inpatients with severe alcohol use disorder on a managed alcohol program (MAP) at St. Paul's Hospital. *Harm Reduction Journal, 17*, 28. https://doi.org/10.1186/s12954-020-00371-6

Payne, R. A., Hrisko, S., & Sninivasan, S. (2018). Treatment approaches for opioid use disorders in late life. *Current Treatment Options in Psychiatry, 5*(2), 242–254. https://doi.org/10.1007/s40501-018-0146-0

Prochaska, J. O., & Velicer, W. F. (1997). The transtheoretical model of health behavior change. *American Journal of Health Promotion, 12*, 38–48. https://doi.org/10.4278/0890-1171-12.1.38. (Seminal).

Rao, V., Micic, D., & Davis, A. (2019). Medical management of opioid-induced constipation. *Jama-Journal of the American Medical Association, 322*(22), 2241–2242. https://doi.org/10.1001/jama.2019.15852

Ries, R., Fiellin, D. A., Miller, S. C., et al. (2015). *The ASAM Essentials of Addiction Medicine* (2nd ed.). Wolters Kluwer/Lippincott Williams & Wilkins.

Rollnick, S., & Miller, W. R. (1995). What is motivational interviewing? *Behavioural and Cognitive Psychotherapy, 23*, 325–334. https://doi.org/10.1017/S135246580001643X. (Seminal).

Rush, B. (2015). *Concurrent disorders guidelines: A supplement to the provincial addictions treatments standards.* Newfoundland: Department of Health and Community Services. https://www.health.gov.nl.ca/health/mentalhealth_committee/mentalhealth/pdf/Concurrent_Disorders.pdf

Sachdeva, A., Choudhary, M., & Chandra, M. (2015). Alcohol withdrawal syndrome: Benzodiazepines and beyond. *Journal of Clinical and Diagnostic Research, 9*(9), VE01–VE07. https://doi.org/10.7860/JCDR/2015/13407.6538

Special Advisory Committee on the Epidemic of Opioid Overdoses. (2019). *Joint Statement from the Co-chairs.* https://www.canada.ca/en/public-health/news/2019/12/joint-statement-from-the-co-chairs-of-the-special-advisory-committee-on-the-epidemic-of-opioid-overdoses-on-new-data-related-to-the-opioid-crisis.html

Statistics Canada. (2019). *Table 13-10-0099-01—Health indicator profile, by Aboriginal identity and sex, age-standardized rate, four year estimates (2007–2014).* https://www150.statcan.gc.ca/t1/tbl1/en/tv.action?pid=1310009901

Strobbe, S. (2014). Prevention and screening, brief intervention and referral to treatment for substance use in primary care. *Primary Care Clinic Office Practice, 41*, 185–213. https://doi.org/10.1016/j.pop.2014.02.002. (Seminal).

Substance Abuse and Mental Health Services Administration (SAMHSA). (2020a). *About Screening, Brief Intervention, and Referral to Treatment (SBIRT).* https://www.samhsa.gov/sbirt/about

Substance Abuse and Mental Health Services Administration (SAMHSA). (2020b). *Recovery and Recovery Support.* https://www.samhsa.gov/find-help/recovery

Taber, K., Black, D., Porrino, L., et al. (2012). Neuroanatomy of dopamine: Reward and addiction. *Journal of Neuropsychiatry and Clinical Neuroscience, 24*(1), 1–4. https://doi.org/10.1176/appi.neuropsych.24.1.1. (Seminal).

Ti, L., Milloy, M. J., Buxton, J., et al. (2015). Factors associated with leaving hospital against medical advice among people who use illicit drugs in Vancouver, Canada. *PloS One, 10*(10), e0141594. https://doi.org/10.1371/journal.pone.0141594

Tobacco Use, & Dependence Guideline Panel. (2008). *Treating Tobacco Use and Dependence: 2008 Update.* US Department of Health and Human Services. https://www.ncbi.nlm.nih.gov/books/NBK63952/

UBC Continuing Professional Development (UBC CPD). (2020). *Addiction Care and Treatment Online Course.* https://elearning.ubccpd.ca/course/view.php?id=164#section-2

United Nations Office on Drugs and Crime. (2020). *Research brief: COVID-19 and the drug supply chain: from production and trafficking to use.* https://www.unodc.org/documents/data-and-analysis/covid/Covid-19-and-drug-supply-chain-Mai2020.pdf

Urbanowski, K. (2017). Need for equity in treatment of substance use among Indigenous people in Canada. *CMAJ, 189*(44), E1350–E1351. https://doi.org/10.1503/cmaj.171002

van Boekel, L. C., Brouwers, E. P. M., van Weeghel, J., et al. (2013). Stigma among health professionals towards patients with substance use disorders and its consequences for healthcare delivery: Systematic review. *Drug and Alcohol Dependence, 131*(1), 23–35. https://doi.org/10.1016/j.drugalcdep.2013.02.018. (Seminal).

Venkatesan, T., Levinthal, D. J., Li, B., et al. (2019). Role of chronic cannabis use: Cyclic vomiting syndrome vs cannabinoid hyperemesis syndrome. *Neurogastroenterology and Motility, 31*(Suppl 2), e13606. https://doi.org/10.1111/nmo.13606

Wilk, P., Maltby, A., & Cooke, M. (2017). Residential schools and the effects on Indigenous health and well-being in Canada—a scoping review. *Public Health Reviews*, 38(1), 8. https://doi.org/10.1186/s40985-017-0055-6

Winkelman, T. N., Admon, L. K., Jennings, L., et al. (2018). Evaluation of amphetamine-related hospitalizations and associated clinical outcomes and costs in the United States. *JAMA Network Open*, 1(6) e183758-e183758. https://doi.org.10.1001/jamanetworkopen.2018.3758

Xiong, G. (2018). *Wernicke-Korsakoff syndrome. Medscape.* http://emedicine.medscape.com/article/288379-overview

RESOURCES

10 Ways to Reduce Risks to Your Health When Using Cannabis
https://www.camh.ca/-/media/files/pdfs---reports-and-books---research/canadas-lower-risk-guidelines-cannabis-pdf.pdf

Canadian Cancer Society: Get Help to Quit Smoking
https://www.cancer.ca/en/support-and-services/support-services/quit-smoking/?region=bc

Canadian Centre on Substance Use and Addiction (CCSA)
https://www.ccsa.ca

Canadian Drug Policy Coalition
https://drugpolicy.ca/

Canadian Institute for Health Information
https://www.cihi.ca

Canadian Mental Health Association: Addressing Mental Health and Addictions Needs in Primary Care
http://ontario.cmha.ca/public_policy/addressing-mental-health-and-addictions-needs-in-primary-care/#.WKVQHTvytPY

Canadian Nurses' Association: Harm Reduction & Illicit Substance Use—Implications for Nursing
http://www.cna-aiic.ca/-/media/cna/page-content/pdf-en/harm-reduction-and-illicit-substance-use-implications-for-nursing.pdf?la=en&hash=5F5BBCDE16C7892D9C7838CF62C362685CC2DDA7

Canadian Nurses Protective Society
https://www.cnps.ca/

Canadian Research Institute on Substance Misuse: Guidance Document on the Management of Substance Use in Acute Care
https://crismprairies.ca/wp-content/uploads/2020/02/Guidance-Document-FINAL.pdf

Centre for Addiction and Mental Health
https://www.camh.ca/

Clinical Opioid Withdrawal Scale (COWS)
https://www.bccsu.ca/wp-content/uploads/2017/08/Clinical-Opiate-Withdrawal-Scale.pdf

EQUIP Health Care
https://equiphealthcare.ca/

Harm Reduction Nurses' Association–Canada
https://www.hrna-aiirm.ca/

Indigenous Cultural Safety Training
https://www.sanyas.ca/

Registered Nurses' Association of Ontario (RNAO)
https://rnao.ca

Registered Nurses' Association of Ontario (RNAO) Best Practice Guideline: Engaging Clients Who Use Substances
https://rnao.ca/bpg/guidelines/engaging-clients-who-use-substances

Registered Nurses' Association of Ontario (RNAO) Best Practice Guideline: Integrating Smoking Cessation Into Daily Nursing Practice
https://rnao.ca/sites/rnao-ca/files/Integrating_Smoking_Cessation_into_Daily_Nursing_Practice.pdf

Registered Nurses' Association of Ontario (RNAO): Tobacco
https://rnao.ca/category/topics/tobacco

Respectful Language and Stigma Regarding People Who Use Substances
http://www.bccdc.ca/resource-gallery/Documents/respectful-language-and-stigma-final_244.pdf

Stigma Around Drug Use
https://www.canada.ca/en/health-canada/services/substance-use/problematic-prescription-drug-use/opioids/stigma.html

Trauma-Informed Practice Guide
http://bccewh.bc.ca/wp-content/uploads/2012/05/2013_TIP-Guide.pdf. http://bccewh.bc.ca/wp-content/uploads/2018/06/Opioid-TIP-Guide_May-2018.pdf

UBC Continuing Professional Development: Addiction Care and Treatment Online Course
https://elearning.ubccpd.ca/course/view.php?id=164

Alcoholics Anonymous
https://www.aa.org/

Alcohol Use Disorders Identification Test
https://auditscreen.org/

International Nurses Society on Addictions
https://www.intnsa.org

Take Home Naloxone
https://towardtheheart.com/naloxone

World Health Organization: Mental Health
https://www.who.int/mental_health

evolve

For additional Internet resources, see the website for this book at http://evolve.elsevier.com/Canada/Lewis/medsurg.

Complementary and Alternative Therapies

Ann Mary Celestini

evolve WEBSITE

http://evolve.elsevier.com/Canada/Lewis/medsurg

- Review Questions (Online Only)
- Key Points
- Answer Guidelines for Case Study
- Conceptual Care Map Creator
- Audio Glossary
- Content Updates

LEARNING OBJECTIVES

1. Describe complementary and alternative therapies, including classifications of commonly used therapies such as natural and nonprescription products, mind and body practices, and other related practices.
2. Review natural products such as herbal therapy, including cannabis, while considering the implications for use.
3. Investigate the mind and body practices as part of holistic nursing care.
4. Highlight the health teachings from Indigenous peoples and traditional Chinese medicine practices.
5. Describe the role of the nurse in integrating complementary and alternative therapies into nursing practice.

KEY TERMS

acupuncture
complementary and alternative therapies
herbal therapy

holistic nursing
Indigenous health
massage therapy

prayer
therapeutic touch
traditional Chinese medicine (TCM)

The general health of Canadians is steadily improving, as evidenced by lower mortality rates and increased life expectancy. Biomedical and technological advances have contributed to these improvements. However, conventional therapy has been less helpful in alleviating symptoms of chronic illnesses and associated challenges, which are at an epidemic high. Furthermore, conventional (Western) approaches to health care tend to be depersonalized and often fail to account for all aspects of well-being, including the individual's mind, body, and spirit.

Increasing access to global perspectives has resulted in greater exposure to healing philosophies from many cultures, offering both consumers and health care providers various new ideas about health and healing (Fontaine, 2019). Complementary and alternative therapies is an umbrella term used to describe a broad range of healing philosophies, therapies, and health care approaches that are often considered unconventional in North America. Several terms have been used to describe these methods of care, which are considered outside the conventional biomedical practices dominant in Canada and other Western cultures; such terms include *alternative, complementary, integrative, nontraditional, unconventional, holistic,*

and *natural.* According to the US National Center for Complementary and Integrative Health (NCCIH, 2021), *complementary* care approaches integrate conventional medicine together with unconventional practices. *Alternative* care approaches replace conventional medicine with unconventional practices. *Integrative* care further implies a purposeful action of bringing both conventional and unconventional approaches together in a coordinated manner for care.

Complementary and alternative therapies support many nursing values, including a view of holistic care, an emphasis on healing, a recognition of the importance of therapeutic care partnerships with patients, and a focus on health promotion and illness prevention (Canadian Nurses Association [CNA], 2017; College & Association of Registered Nurses of Alberta, 2018; College of Nurses of Ontario, 2018). Nursing's interest in complementary and alternative perspectives is further reflected in the formation of specialty nursing groups. For example, the Canadian Holistic Nurses Association (CHNA, 2021) was established to recognize holistic nursing as a specialty and to ensure that holistic practices are considered within a health maintenance and promotion framework. Despite this, nurses may face challenges determining their specific role related to the use of complementary and alternative therapies in practice.

In Canada, no national policy or law exists for the regulation of complementary and alternative practitioners, as this power lies within provincial or territorial jurisdictions. To provide direction, the College and Association of Registered Nurses of Alberta (CARNA) (College & Association of Registered Nurses of Alberta, 2018) has published expectations and direction for complementary and alternative health care (CAHC) and use of natural health products (NHPs). The CARNA guideline identifies three standards for registered nurse practice: (a) being responsible and accountable for nursing practice related to CAHC and NHPs; (b) using evidence-informed approaches in the selection of CAHC and NHPs, while considering the benefits and risks to a patient's health and safety; and (c) practising ethically when providing care that includes CAHC and NHPs. Provincial and territorial nurse or practitioner licensure and regulations vary for different therapy practices. Practitioners should refrain from performing any therapy that is not within their scope of professional practice and explain this decision to the patient.

In 2016, a comprehensive longitudinal national study conducted by the Fraser Institute established that there is a steady increase in the number of people using complementary and alternative therapies in Canada. Approximately 80% of Canadians have used one or more complementary or alternative therapy at some point in their lives (Esmail, 2017). This increasing overall use by consumers raises important questions among health care providers about the effectiveness and safety of complementary and alternative approaches. In response to these inquiries, the Canadian Interdisciplinary Network for Complementary and Alternative Medicine Research (INCAM, 2021) was established to foster excellence in complementary and alternative medicine (CAM) research. Its objectives are to build a sustainable network that facilitates and supports research, promotes knowledge transfer among researchers, and thus avoids the duplication of research efforts (see the Resources at the end of this chapter).

Given the vast array of complementary and alternative health practices, categorization becomes difficult. For analytical purposes, the NCCIH (2018) classified these therapies into specific groups: natural products, mind and body practices, and other complementary and alternative practices. Select therapies within each category can be found in Tables 12.1, 12.2, and 12.3. The list of therapies continually changes as practices proven safe and effective become accepted as conventional health care practices.

NATURAL PRODUCTS

An interest in natural and nonprescription therapies has increased in countries whose health care practices are dominated by the biomedical model. Interest in these products is related to several factors, including the high cost of and the potential for severe adverse effects associated with pharmaceutical drugs. Remedies that stem from this category are considered "natural" and therefore may be viewed as safer and more appealing to the public. Since they are directly available to consumers, individuals can assume more autonomy regarding their health care.

In Canada, the Natural and Non-prescription Health Products Directorate is the regulating authority that ensures the safety, efficacy, and quality of NHPs and nonprescription drugs that are available. NHPs are substances that occur naturally from plants, animals, microorganisms, or marine sources and are used to restore or maintain good health. Biologically based, or natural, therapies include herbal therapies (phytotherapy),

TABLE 12.1	**NATURAL PRODUCTS**
Examples	**Description**
Herbal therapy	Use of unrefined plant-based products to treat, prevent, or cure disease. Effects are slow and less dramatic than effects of pharmaceutical drugs.
Nutraceuticals	Vitamin and mineral supplements. The best source of vitamins and minerals is a well-balanced diet.
Nutritional therapy	Special diets for health promotion. Such diets must be studied specifically for their potential benefit.
Aromatherapy	Use of a plants' extracted essential oils for their beneficial effects on stress management, mood regulation, sleep induction, weight reduction, boosting the immune system, promoting speed recovery, and minimizing illness discomfort. They can be used for many antiviral, antibacterial, antifungal, and antiseptic purposes (Fontaine, 2019).
Probiotic therapy	Use of live microorganisms that are similar to those found in the human digestive tract and that aid digestion

nutraceuticals, nutrition therapy, aromatherapy, and probiotic therapy (see Table 12.1) (Fontaine, 2019). For the purposes of classification, cannabis has been grouped with this category, considering the nature of this recently legalized herb in Canada. Natural products come in a wide variety of forms, such as tablets, tinctures, capsules, solutions, creams, ointments, and drops.

Herbal Therapy

Herbal therapy, also known as *botanical medicine* or *phytotherapy*, is the use of individual herbs or combinations of herbs for therapeutic benefit. An *herb* is a plant or plant part (bark, roots, leaves, seeds, flowers, or fruit) that produces and contains chemical substances that act on the body. It is estimated that approximately 25 000 plant species are used medicinally throughout the world, and approximately 30% of modern prescription drugs are derived from plants. Botanical medicine is the oldest known form of medicine; archaeological evidence suggests that Neanderthals used plant-based remedies 60 000 years ago. Today, about 80% of the world's population relies extensively on plant-derived remedies (Fontaine, 2019).

Clinical Applications of Herbal Therapy. Medicinal plants work similarly to medications; both are absorbed and trigger biological effects that can be therapeutic. Many medicinal plants have more than one physiological effect and thus can be used for more than one condition. A number of herbs have been determined to be safe and effective for a variety of conditions. Complementary & Alternative Therapies boxes with descriptions of herbs related to specific diseases are found throughout this book.

COMPLEMENTARY & ALTERNATIVE THERAPIES

Information related to the following complementary and alternative therapies can be found throughout this text.

- Acupuncture
- Bilberry
- Biofeedback
- Echinacea
- Garlic
- Ginger
- Ginkgo biloba
- Ginseng
- Glucosamine
- Goldenseal
- Guided imagery
- Herbs and supplements that affect blood clotting
- Herbs and supplements that affect blood glucose levels
- Herbs and supplements used for menopause
- Herbs for surgical patients
- Herbs that affect healing
- Lipid-lowering agents
- Milk thistle
- Music therapy
- Saw palmetto
- Valerian
- Zinc

TABLE 12.2 MIND AND BODY PRACTICES

Examples	Description
Relaxation breathing	Slow diaphragmatic breathing, and exercises, used to elicit the relaxation response. See Chapter 8 for further information.
Meditation	General term for a wide variety of methods that promote relaxation in the body and preserve tranquility in the mind. State of being with increased concentration and awareness. Focuses on deepening one's attention and increasing self-awareness. Various types of meditation exist, including transcendental, mindfulness, Buddhist, Tibetan, Sufi, and forms of moving meditation, which can be practised individually or in a group.
Biofeedback	Method of learned self-control over physiological responses of the body (Fontaine, 2019). Information about one or more physiological functions is received, interventions are used, and a feedback loop allows for voluntary control of certain functions.
Neurofeedback (formally EEG biofeedback)	A noninvasive drug-free technique whereby electrodes are placed on the scalp to monitor brain activity. Inappropriate brain waveforms are decreased and appropriate waveforms are increased through positive computer-generated visual or auditory reinforcement. It is used for such conditions as epilepsy, stroke, depression, fibromyalgia, PTSD, and ADHD, often improving quality of life during illness (Luctkar-Flude et al., 2019).
Yoga	Part of Ayurveda medical system and widely used for its physical, psychological, and spiritual benefits. Numerous schools of yoga or practices exist but typically combine physical postures, breathing techniques, and relaxation or meditation.
Guided imagery	A state of focused concentration of the mind to generate images that have a calming effect on the body. It involves the use of vision, sound, smell, and taste, as well as movement, position, and the sense of touch.
Hypnotherapy	Application of hypnosis to attain a state of attentive, focused concentration during which individuals become highly responsive to suggestion. It may be applied effectively to a wide variety of medical and psychological disorders.
Music therapy	Clinical and evidenced-informed music interventions developed by a credentialed professional to accomplish individualized goals that promote wellness or improve quality of life.
Animal-facilitated therapy	Use of specifically selected animals for a variety of therapies that have been successfully used as a motivational, educational, and recreational intervention for people with a variety of physical, psychological. and spiritual issues.
Prayer	Communication with a god, or the sacred. Prayer is a frequently used therapy of various forms that is utilized in all cultures.
Chiropractic therapy	Therapy that restores and maintains health by proper alignment of the spine through a variety of adjustment and manipulation techniques. Correct spinal alignment facilitates self-healing and improves health and well-being.
Pressure point therapy	Acupuncture, acupressure, and reflexology are three similar practices of stimulating points on the body, to balance an individual's life energy within the body. It involves application of pressure or stimulation to specific acupuncture points, as defined by energy meridian charts of the body, to improve energy flow, relieve pain, and stimulate the body's innate healing abilities.
Massage therapy	Scientific, purposeful manipulation of soft tissues to improve health, promote healing and help the body heal itself. Outcomes include relaxation, reduced tension, improved immune function, increased flexibility, and pain relief.

ADHD, attention-deficit/hyperactivity disorder; EEG, electroencephalography; PTSD, post-traumatic stress disorder.

TABLE 12.3 OTHER COMPLEMENTARY AND ALTERNATIVE MEDICINE PRACTICES

Examples	Description
Whole Medical Systems	
Indigenous health	Practices based on a domain wherein all things have a "spirit." Community is valued and plays a role in the healing process. Gratitude to and harmony with nature are central themes. Illness occurs when an imbalance occurs. Healers use herbs, natural medicines, spiritual rituals, and ceremonies to support wellness and promote healing.
Ayurvedic medicine	A holistic system developed in India that bases its practice on the balance of mind, body, and spirit. Disease is viewed as an imbalance between a person's life force (prana) and basic metabolic condition (dosha). Interventions include breathing exercises, nutrition, detoxification, herbs, meditation, and yoga.
Traditional Chinese medicine (TCM)	One of the world's oldest, most holistic medical systems. Based on restoring and maintaining the balance of vital energy (qi). Interventions include acupressure, acupuncture, Chinese herbology, cupping, moxibustion, nutrition, meditation, tai chi, and qigong.
Naturopathy	Therapy based on promotion of health rather than on symptom management. Focus is on enhancing the body's natural healing response through a variety of individualized interventions such as nutrition, herbology, homeopathy, physical therapies, and counselling. Naturopathic physicians are graduates of accredited naturopathic medical schools, and licensing varies by province or territory.
Homeopathy	Therapy based on the adage "like cures like." Remedies are specially prepared from the same substance that causes the symptom or health problem. Extremely small amounts of the substance are used for the remedy, which are believed to work through a transfer in energy.
Energy Healing Therapies	
Hand-mediated biofield energies	Designed to balance the body's biofield, or energy field, and increase the flow of energy within an individual by channeling and directing healing energy through the hands of a practitioner. Practices include therapeutic touch, healing touch, and Reiki.
Manipulation of energy fields: bioelectromagnetics	Magnet therapy is based on the principle that every animal, plant, and mineral has an electromagnetic field that allows other objects to interact with it as part of one unified energy system (Fontaine, 2019). Magnets are frequently used to reduce pain, relieve swelling and inflammation, and promote healing of soft tissue and bone.

TABLE 12.4   PATIENT & CAREGIVER TEACHING GUIDE

Herbal Therapies

When teaching patients and caregivers about herbal therapies, the nurse should:
- Ask the patient about use of herbal therapies. Document a complete history of herbal use, including amounts, brand names, and frequency of use. Ask the patient about allergies.
- Investigate whether herbs are used instead of or in addition to traditional medical treatments. Find out whether herbal therapies are used to prevent disease or to treat an existing problem.
- Instruct the patient to inform health care providers of any intention to take herbal treatments before doing so.
- Make the patient aware of the risks and benefits associated with herbal use, including reactions when herbs are taken in combination with other medications.
- Advise the patient using herbal therapies to be aware of any adverse effects while taking herbal treatments and to immediately report them to the health care provider.
- Make the patient aware that moisture, sunlight, and heat may alter the components of herbal products.
- Inform the patient of the need to be aware of the reputation of the manufacturers of herbal products and the safety of the product before buying herbal treatments.
- Encourage the patient to read labels of herbal therapies carefully. Advise the patient not to take more of an herb than is directed.
- Inform the patient that most herbal therapies should be discontinued at least 2 to 3 weeks before surgery.
- Inform the patient that the employees of health food stores may not have any educational background in the actions, interactions, and efficacies of the herbal therapies sold in the store they are working in. It is the responsibility of the patient to ensure that the information received comes from someone who has the appropriate background and education to be providing that information.

Although most herbal therapies can safely be used without professional assistance, nurses should assess for their use to mitigate adverse effects and interactions with prescription drugs. Adverse effects resulting from the use of herbal remedies may be underreported, which can promote the impression that herbal remedies are completely safe to use. Because consumers tend not to discuss their use of herbal therapies with their primary health care provider, herb–drug interactions may also be underreported (Fontaine, 2019). For safety, patients who are scheduled for surgery should be advised to stop taking herbal remedies 2 to 3 weeks before surgery. Patients who are being treated with conventional drug therapy should be advised to discontinue herbal remedies that produce similar pharmacological effects, because the combination may lead to an excessive reaction or to unknown interaction effects. General patient teaching guidelines related to use of herbal therapy are presented in Table 12.4.

Patients who take herbal therapies should be advised to adhere to the suggested dosage. If taken in high doses, herbal preparations can be toxic. The potency of a particular herbal remedy can vary widely because of factors such as where and how it was grown, how it was harvested, and how it was processed. Herbal medicines should be purchased only from reputable manufacturers. Health Canada (2021b) advises Canadians to use only herbal products that have been approved for sale under the Natural Health Products Regulations. If the product has been assessed, it will have a drug identification number (DIN) or natural products number (NPN) on its label. This certifies that the product has passed a review of formulation, labelling, and instructions for use. Because of the potential for adverse effects, pregnant women, nursing mothers, and older persons with liver or cardiovascular disease should use caution in consuming herbal products. Commonly used herbs are listed in Table 12.5, and commonly used dietary supplements are found in Table 12.6.

Cannabis

Cannabis, or *Cannabis sativa*, contains hundreds of chemical substances. Over 100 of these are known as *cannabinoids,* which are produced and stored in trichomes, or tiny clear hairs that protrude from the plant flowers and leaves. Cannabinoids have effects on cell receptors in the brain and body that can change how these cells behave and communicate with each other.

Delta-9-tetrahydrocannabinol (THC), *cannabidiol* (CBD), and *terpenes* are three primary cannabinoids in cannabis. THC, the most researched of the three, is responsible for the physiological response, including the "high" and intoxicating effects of cannabis. THC has both therapeutic and harmful effects that can vary depending on dose, potency, and individual user characteristics. The potency of THC in cannabis, shown in percentage, has increased from 3% in the 1980s to around 15% today, with some strains averaging as high as 30% or greater. Cannabis containing very low amounts of THC (less than 0.3%) is classified as *hemp.* CBD, unlike THC, does not produce a similar "high" or intoxication. Equal or higher amounts of CBD may block or lower some of the THC effects on the mind while offering the possibility of various therapeutic uses. Finally, terpenes are chemicals made and stored in the trichomes of the cannabis plant, with the cannabinoids giving it a distinctive smell and flavour (Health Canada, 2021a).

Cannabis, often known as marijuana, is used for medical, recreational, or religious purposes. Most cannabis products come from or can be made using the flowers and leaves of the cannabis plant. Depending on the plant strain, these products can have a range of potencies of THC and CBD that come in different forms for consumption, such as fresh or dried herbs, oil, concentrated extracts (e.g., hash oil/shatter/budder/wax), physically concentrated extracts (e.g., hash/kief), edibles, tinctures, sprays, and creams (Health Canada, 2021a). Cannabis can be administered by inhalation, oral ingestion, sublingually, topically, and rectally. In Canada, synthetic forms of cannabis such as nabilone and dronabinol are also available through prescriptions (Pratt et al., 2019).

Clinical Applications of Cannabis

Over the last decade there has been increased medical use of cannabis in North America. In Canada, the *Cannabis Act,* which came into effect on October 17, 2018, permitted the legal purchase of cannabis for recreational use. Further, in October 2019, an amendment for cannabis-infused edibles was made to this Act. These recent developments highlight the increasing need for nurses to become familiar with their implications for health and well-being. A Web link to information for health care providers regarding the potential therapeutic uses, dosing, warnings, and adverse effects can be found in the Resources section of this chapter.

TABLE 12.5   COMMONLY USED HERBS*

Name	Uses Informed by Scientific Evidence	Comments
Aloe	Laxative, skin conditions, osteoarthritis, fever	• May lead to abdominal cramping, diarrhea • Can cause electrolyte imbalances • May lower blood glucose level
Black cohosh	Decrease menopausal and menstrual related symptoms	• May cause upset stomach or rash • Can cause liver problems • May increase bleeding
Echinacea	Treat upper respiratory tract infections, wound and skin conditions	• May lead to digestive symptoms • Rash may result from allergic reactions • Only short-term use is recommended
Evening primrose	Treat eczema, skin conditions, rheumatoid arthritis, premenstrual or menopausal symptoms, breast pain	• Contraindicated in individuals on blood thinners and in pregnant and lactating women • May cause mild gastrointestinal upset or headache
Feverfew	Prevent migraine headaches. Used to treat menstruation problems, rheumatoid arthritis, asthma, tinnitus, dizziness, nausea, vomiting, intestinal parasites, and toothaches or as skin cleanser	• May cause gastrointestinal adverse effects • Could increase risk of bleeding • Stopping long-term use may lead to withdrawal symptoms • Avoid use during pregnancy as it can affect uterine contractions
Garlic	Can decrease hypertension cholesterol and low-density lipoproteins Potential anticancer properties	• May increase risk of bleeding • Avoid prior to surgery • Could interfere with effectiveness of some medications
Ginger	Ease nausea and vomiting May help with osteoarthritis, rheumatoid arthritis	• Use cautiously with gallstone disease • May increase risk of bleeding
Ginkgo biloba	Treat symptoms of intermittent claudication, tinnitus, dementia, eye problems	• Can increase risk of bleeding and certain cancers • Could be poisonous if ingesting raw or roasted seeds
Ginseng (Panax species, including Asian and American ginseng)	Improve mental and physical performance, enhance immune system May lower blood glucose level in type 2 diabetes mellitus	• Could increase or decrease blood pressure • May lower blood glucose levels • Can increase risk of bleeding
Hawthorn	Treat mild to moderate heart failure, digestive and kidney problems, anxiety	• May cause dizziness, nausea, and gastrointestinal problems • Could interact harmfully with cardiac medications
Kava	Treat anxiety	• Should be used only under the supervision of a health care provider • Associated with a risk of liver damage • Risk of heart problems and eye irritation with heavy consumption
Milk thistle	Treat liver disorders, high cholesterol, and gallbladder problems	• May lower blood glucose levels
St. John's wort	Treat mild depression, menopausal symptoms	• May lead to serious interactions with herbs, supplements, OTC drugs, or prescription drugs, thus it is important to consult and notify health care provider • Could lead to photosensitivity, anxiety, dry mouth, sexual problems • Not for use with other antidepressants • Not for children
Zinc	Treat upper respiratory tract infections	• Can cause copper deficiency with long-term use • May interact with antibiotics

OTC, over-the-counter.
*Advise patients who are pregnant or lactating to consult a health care provider before they use any herbs. Scientific evidence for the use of most herbs during pregnancy or lactation is limited.
Source: National Center for Complementary and Integrative Health. (2019). *Health topics A–Z.* https://nccih.nih.gov/health/atoz.htm

The flowers and leaves of the cannabis plant are primarily used for their ability to cause short-term positive effects on the mind, including feeling high (euphoria), a sense of well-being, relaxation, and heightened sensory experiences including sight, taste, smell, and sound. Medical cannabis has been used effectively in treating and managing a wide range of health conditions, most notably anxiety, eating disorders, epilepsy, chronic pain management, glaucoma, inflammatory bowel disease, post-traumatic stress disorder, multiple sclerosis, sleep difficulties, and symptom management of several chronic illnesses (NCCIM, 2019; Pratt et al., 2019).

However, despite the diversity of successful applications, certain individuals may experience some of the short-term negative effects on the brain, including confusion; sleepiness (fatigue); impaired ability to remember, concentrate, react quickly, or pay attention; and anxiety, panic, or fear. Short-term effects may also include damaged blood vessels caused by smoking; reduced blood pressure causing people to faint; and increased heart

rate, which can be dangerous for those with heart conditions, increasing their risk for a heart attack. Occasionally, cannabis use can result in psychotic episodes characterized by paranoia, delusions, and hallucinations. Long-term effects of cannabis consumption may develop gradually with daily or near-daily use that continues over months or years. Frequent, excessive use can harm an individual's memory, concentration, intelligence, and ability to think and make decisions. Long-term extreme use may potentially lead to a condition involving recurrent, severe vomiting. If cannabis is smoked, the risks to lung health may be similar to the effects of tobacco smoke.

Similar to cautions with medication administration, pregnant or breastfeeding mothers must be aware of the impact cannabis use can have on the fetus or newborn. Health effects of cannabis use during pregnancy and breastfeeding have been associated with lower infant birth weights (Health Canada, 2021a). With the rising popularity of cannabis-infused edibles, the inherent risks involved should be discussed with users. Responsible use,

TABLE 12.6   COMMONLY USED DIETARY SUPPLEMENTS*

Name	Uses Informed by Scientific Evidence	Comments
Chondroitin sulphate	Treat osteoarthritis	• May interact with anticoagulant • Long-term use could damage kidneys • Should be used with caution in patients who have bleeding disorders or are taking anticoagulants
Coenzyme Q_{10}	Treat hypertension and heart disease and prevent migraines	• May decrease blood glucose levels
Fish oil/omega-3 fatty acids	Treat hypertension or hypertriglyceridemia Prevent cardiovascular disease and relieve symptoms of rheumatoid arthritis	• May increase risk of bleeding • Might increase blood glucose levels in patients with diabetes • Could increase low-density lipoprotein (LDL) level • Can potentiate reaction if allergic to fish or shellfish
Glucosamine	Treat osteoarthritis	• May increase intraocular pressure • Could increase blood glucose and insulin levels and impact effectiveness of diabetes medication • Can increase risk of bleeding • May cause problems in those with shellfish allergies
Melatonin	Treat jet lag Decrease sleep latency	• May increase risk of bleeding • Might alter blood pressure • Should be used with caution in patients with diabetes or hypoglycemia • Should be used with caution by patients with seizure disorder
Probiotics (live bacteria or yeast)	Re-establish gut flora (especially after prolonged antibiotic therapy) Influence immune system	• Should be used with caution in patients with compromised immune system or gastrointestinal disorders

*Advise patients who are pregnant or lactating to consult a health care provider before they use any supplements. Scientific evidence for use during pregnancy or lactation is limited.
Source: National Center for Complementary and Integrative Health. (2019). *Health topics A–Z.* https://nccih.nih.gov/health/atoz.htm

which includes safe storage, should be stressed, to avoid accidental ingestion of cannabis by children or pets (Charlebois et al., 2020). Nurses should be aware of facility policies regarding CBD administration.

MIND–BODY PRACTICES

Mind–body interventions include a variety of techniques designed to facilitate the mind's capacity to affect bodily function. These include behavioural, psychological, social, and spiritual approaches to health. Massage, yoga, meditation, pressure point therapies, relaxation techniques such as breathing exercises, guided imagery, hypnotherapy, biofeedback, neurofeedback, animal-facilitated therapy, chiropractic manipulation, and prayer are examples of mind–body therapies and approaches (see Table 12.2).

Massage Therapy

Massage therapy includes a range of techniques that the practitioner uses to manipulate the soft tissues and joints of the body (Figures 12.1 and 12.2). Involving touch and movement, massage is typically delivered with the hands, although elbows, forearms, or feet may be also used. Massage techniques are used in body work, sports training, physiotherapy, nursing, chiropractic therapy, osteopathy, and naturopathy.

Clinical Applications of Massage Therapy. Until the 1970s, nurses were taught to perform "p.m. care," which consisted of a back rub and other measures to promote relaxation and sleep. After that time, p.m. care and back rubs became the exception rather than the rule. Yet today, with the increased focus on providing holistic care, nurses are again recognizing the benefits of massage. Massage promotes health and wellness and has been shown to improve quality of life (Angelopoulou et al., 2020; Yeun, 2017).

The role of the nurse in massage differs from that of the registered massage therapist. Whereas massage therapists can provide more comprehensive massage therapies, nurses can use specific massage techniques as part of nursing care when indicated by findings in patient assessment. For example, a back massage can be used to help promote sleep. For a bedridden patient, gentle massage can stimulate circulation. When a nurse determines that massage may be indicated in meeting a patient goal, the nurse must first assess the patient's preference regarding touch and massage. The nurse should consider cultural and social beliefs and discuss potential benefits with the patient. The indicated plan of care (e.g., hand massage, back massage) can then be implemented, and reassessment can be performed after the massage.

Prayer

Prayer has been identified as one of the most common and universally used mind–body interventions shared among many cultures, faiths, and religions globally. While prayer may have different implications and meanings within the context of these various perspectives, all have similar intentions of establishing a connection with God, or Creator, to either seek help or give thanks and praise. *Prayer* has been most simply defined as a form of intentional communication with a higher God, or deity. Health challenges or serious illness that arise throughout life may specifically prompt people to look to prayer for guidance, intervention, and healing during these difficult times. Prayer can be initiated on an individual or communal basis, while following a scripted or personalized format in either a public or private forum.

Directed and nondirected prayer are two types that exist. In *directed* prayer, an individual will ask for a specific outcome, in contrast to *nondirected* prayer, which is not focused on the attainment of any specific outcome but on achieving an optimal result considering the circumstances. Further, prayer can be classified according to form, such as meditative, ritualistic, colloquial, and intercessory (or petitionary). Meditative or contemplative prayer, like meditation, requires a process of focusing the mind on an aspect of God over a specified period of time. Ritualistic prayer includes repeated words, phrases, or

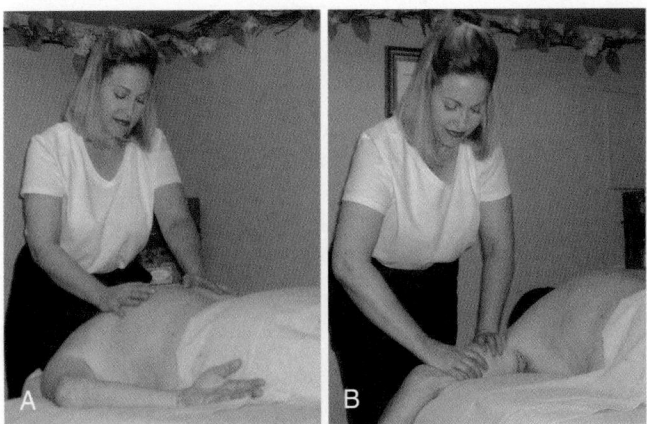

FIG. 12.1 Massage. **A,** Using *effleurage* to relax the back. **B,** Using *pétrissage* to relax arm muscles. Source: Lori Karhu, RMT, RN, San Antonio, Texas.

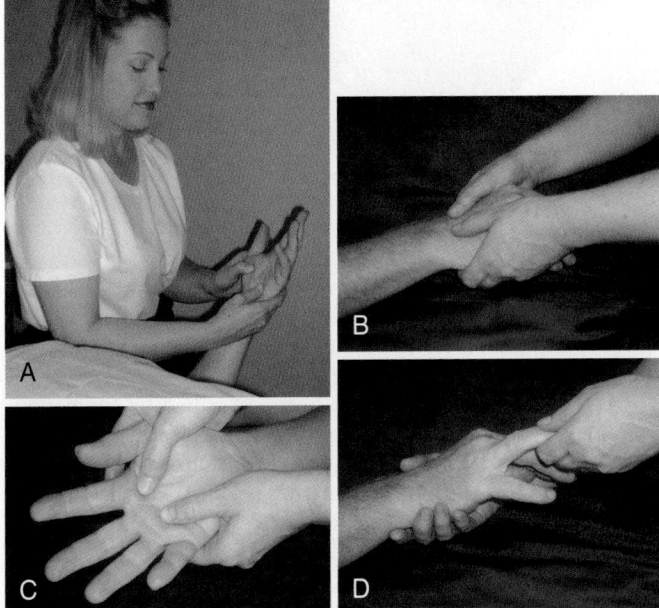

FIG. 12.2 A, Hand massage. **B,** Technique of hand massage: Bend the wrist backward and forward to relax the wrist, then massage the wrist and top of the hand, using circular movements. **C,** Massage the palm of the hand with the cushions of the thumbs, using circular movements. **D,** Massage each finger from the base to the tip. Source: Lori Karhu, RMT, RN, San Antonio, Texas.

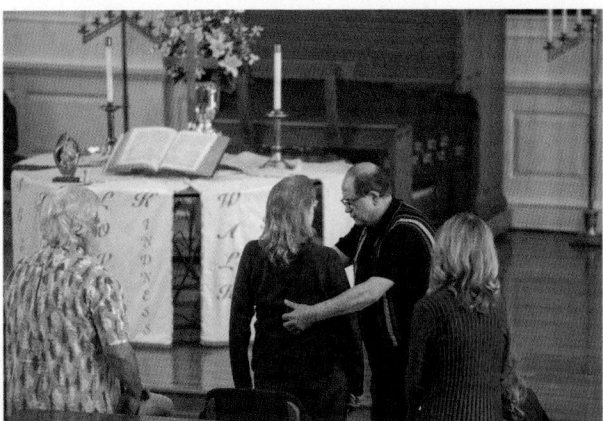

FIG. 12.3 Dr. Issam Nemeh, M.D., a medical physician with an unshakable faith in God's divine intervention and ability to heal through prayer. Source: Path to Faith, Westlake, Ohio.

rituals commonly associated with formal liturgy. Colloquial prayer involves a casual and spontaneous talk with the divine. Petitionary or intercessory prayer involves praying for someone else (Fontaine, 2019).

Clinical Applications of Prayer. Regardless of the method used, prayer supports spiritual health by allowing for the reflective expression of an individual's fears, beliefs, faith, forgiveness, courage, and compassion. Spiritual health problems or crisis may stem from both physical and emotional sources, motivating people to question or search for the meaning or purpose of life. During times of illness, prayer can have positive effects, such as diminishing causes of depression, stress, anxiety, and concern, while in many cases supporting an improvement in the physical functioning and coping patterns among believers (Gonçalves et al., 2015; Mahmodi & Sayehmiri, 2018; Prado Simão et al., 2016). Dr. Issam Nemeh, M.D., a medical physician of unshakable faith,

is globally known for the miraculous recoveries experienced by numerous people after either attending one of his healing services or following treatment in his medical office. With prayer, Dr. Nemeh has and continues to touch many people's lives, from all denominations of faith, with healing, while modestly accrediting these miracles to an intercession from God (Figure 12.3).

Nurses are committed to spiritual care as part of their holistic practice. Nurses need cross-cultural knowledge about prayer practices, awareness of patients' spiritual needs, and engagement in rigorous research that examines the effects of prayer and faith on healing. However, the role of a nurse in supporting the spiritual health of patients is not meant to replace but supplement clergy services. Regardless of personal religious or spiritual beliefs, nurses can promote an atmosphere that accepts and encourages various forms of spiritual expression for patients. Such promotion requires respecting the patient's denominational beliefs and traditions while ensuring that the nurse not force or impose their own views on the patient. Supporting this practice involves fostering self-awareness and education among nurses regarding the clinical relevance of faith and prayer to health, healing, recovery, and even death. Through the development of a caring–healing therapeutic relationship with patients, nurses can honour the inner wisdom of others and promote a deeper level of understanding of their needs. Providing an opportunity and quiet space for holding sacred prayer or rituals can be arranged if needed within a health care organization with the nurse's assistance. If comfortable with prayer, the nurse could offer to pray silently together with the patient (Casterline, 2018). Further, spiritual tools and assessments can guide nurses in identifying patients' needs while establishing the influence and connection of spirituality to their health. Various formal formats or tools for assessment may be useful for nurses to help guide the process, such as the HOPE formatted spiritual assessment questions (Anandaraih & Hight, 2001). The initial letter *H* identified in this spiritual assessment tool requires a nurse to gather information specific to an individual's source of hope, meaning, comfort, strength, peace, love, and connection to others. The letter *O* necessitates the nurse to inquire into any affiliation a patient may have with an organized religion. Next, questions specific to the letter *P* can help the nurse focus on capturing any other personal spirituality and related practices used by the patient to support health and healing. Finally, *E* of the HOPE acronym focuses on obtaining patient input about any effect on medical care and end-of-life issues that need to be considered during care. Following any type of spirituality assessment, the nurse may also offer to contact a chaplain or a personal spiritual leader for the patient if necessary.

OTHER COMPLEMENTARY AND ALTERNATIVE PRACTICES

Alternative Systems of Care

Alternative medical systems are complete methods of health-related theory and practice that were developed outside of the Western biomedical model, often in other cultures. For some countries, these are used as their conventional health care systems. Indigenous health care practices, traditional Chinese medicine (TCM), Ayurvedic, homeopathic, and naturopathic medicine are some of the primary types of whole or alternative systems of care. Within each of these approaches, many individual complementary methods such as healing touch, massage, herbs, and prayers are used in varying combinations to promote or maintain health and treat disease.

Indigenous Health

Indigenous health is viewed as involving a balance of spiritual, emotional, physical, mental, and social aspects of life. To achieve this harmony with all things, maintaining this balance with oneself is a priority. Illness or disease occurs when this crucial equilibrium of life aspects is upset. Most illness is perceived as beginning in the mind; therefore, getting rid of thoughts that contribute to illness is considered key to preventing disease. Disease can also develop as a result of what has been termed *soul loss*, or the loss of one's ability to be generous (Fontaine, 2019). While the term *Indigenous* is used to be inclusive of First Nations, Métis, and Inuit peoples in Canada, each group has a distinctly different healing system. Nonetheless, some commonalities among them can be generalized to gain a better understanding of these main principles.

Medicine Wheel teachings are among the oldest of Indigenous peoples and represent the entirety of Indigenous life, which emphasizes a holistic approach to maintain balance and equilibrium. This circular wheel is specifically balanced in shape, indicating constant movement and change. Generations of various Indigenous communities have utilized divergent versions of the Four Directions in the Medicine Wheel to symbolize their interpretations of the cycles of life and specific dimensions of health. Each of these Four Directions is represented typically by a different colour, such as red, yellow, white, and black (Figure 12.4), which in some Indigenous communities symbolize various races of people in humanity. Each of the Four Directions can also signify (a) stages of life—birth, youth, adult (or elder), and death; (b) seasons of the year—spring, summer, winter, and fall; (c) aspects of life—spiritual, emotional, intellectual, and physical; (d) elements of nature—fire (or sun), air, water, and earth; (e) animals—eagle, bear, wolf, and buffalo; (f) ceremonial plants—tobacco, sweet grass, sage, and cedar; and (g) food groups—fruits and vegetables, meat and fish, wheat and breads, milk and milk products. Movement is circular and typically clockwise within the Medicine Wheel to help align it with the forces of nature, such as gravity and the rising or setting of the sun (Northern College Indigenous Council on Education,

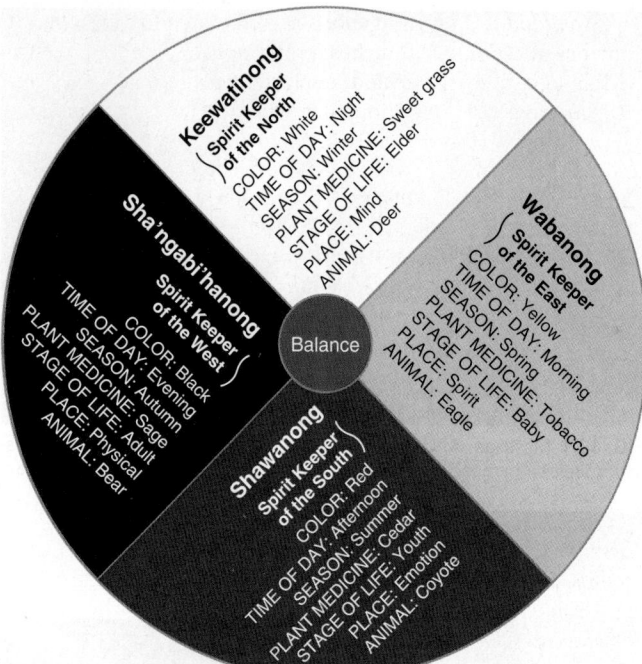

FIG. 12.4 The Medicine Wheel represents teaching that everything is created equal. Source: Anishnaabe Kwewag Gamig: Alderville First Nation Women's Shelter. (2020). *Medicine Wheel.* https://akgshelter.ca/medicine-wheel/

2020). While variants in teachings and representations exist, the underlying themes remain focused on appreciating the continuing interrelatedness of all things.

Four sacred medicines have been described by Indigenous peoples as including tobacco, sweetgrass, sage, and cedar. These four medicines are believed to be sacred because they are provided by the Creator, thus are used in everyday life and ceremonies. All of them can be used to smudge with, although sage, cedar, and sweetgrass also have many other uses. Traditionally, tobacco is burned to communicate with the spirits and thus is offered first to express gratitude toward the land prior to picking medicines or before requesting advice or help of Elders or healers. Tobacco is known to be the main activator of sweetgrass, sage, and cedar. Sweetgrass is usually braided, dried, or burned and is used in prayer, smudging, and purifying ceremonies to attract positive energies. Sage is medicinally stronger than sweetgrass, supporting its use for removing negative energy from homes and sacred items, and in preparing people for ceremonies or teachings. Similarly, cedar has many restorative medicinal uses and can be used in healing baths, to purify the home, or as a form of protection for sweat lodge ceremonies (Northern College Indigenous Council on Education, 2020). The healing properties of plants are acknowledged by Indigenous people. Plants such as those found in the Canadian Boreal Forest have been found to be effective for the management of chronic pain (Uprey et al., 2016).

Clinical Applications of Indigenous Health Practices. Smudging involves a process of cleansing or purifying people and sacred objects using smoke from the burning of sacred herbs, most commonly tobacco, sage, cedar, and sweetgrass in Indigenous health practices. Smoke signifies a prayer to the Creator and is often used in ceremonies or as part of a daily devotion. Negativity can be cleared and the energy field of either people or places can be restored through this form of healing (Fontaine, 2019).

Sweat lodge is an Indigenous sacred ceremony or ritual that purifies the body, mind, heart, and spirit. Typically, a sweat lodge occurs in a heated enclosed, dome-shaped covered structure with a small door flap to seal the inside from outer air and light (Fontaine, 2019). Intense heat or steam, referred to as the *Breath of Spirit*, is generated from pouring water onto heated rocks outside of the lodge to promote the sweating out of toxins and negative energy by individuals seated within it. A variety of herbs can be burned on these heated rocks to treat a range of ailments. Sacred songs and prayer are also used to prevent illness or bring healing. Sweat lodges can be used alone or as part of other ceremonies, each being unique depending on the purpose and context for its use (National Library of Medicine, n.d.).

Traditional Chinese Medicine

Traditional Chinese medicine (TCM) is one of the world's oldest and most comprehensive medical systems. It has evolved over several thousand years of cultural and philosophical developments, as well as extensive clinical observation and testing. Several major concepts constitute Chinese medicine. The principle of *yin and yang* is a core tenet of Chinese art, philosophy, and science, as well as of TCM. Various states are associated with yin energies (feminine energy—cold, heavy, moist, negative) and yang energies (masculine energy—hot, dry, light, positive). Yin and yang are viewed as dynamic, interacting, and interdependent energies, neither of which can exist without the other, each containing some part of the other within it. These energies are a part of everything in nature and must be maintained in a harmonious state of balance to achieve optimal health. Imbalance is associated with illness. TCM modalities are used to restore balance between yin and yang energies (Fontaine, 2019).

Strengths of TCM include its individualized system of diagnosis, treatment, and focus on prevention. Assessment tools include a comprehensive health history, tongue examination, and pulse examination. TCM includes an array of modalities, the most common of which are acupuncture and Chinese herbal medicine. These modalities are used together to replenish and smooth the flow of qi (pronounced "chee") throughout the body. When yin and yang are in balance, qi, or the fundamental life force, flows evenly through the body, leading to good health. Qi is a form of energy found in all life; when it is disrupted, illness and pain can occur. Other TCM interventions include acupressure, moxibustion, cupping, Chinese massage, meditative physical exercise (e.g., tai chi and qigong), and nutrition counselling. Tai chi and qigong are slow-movement exercises that focus on breathing (Fontaine, 2019).

Clinical Applications of Traditional Chinese Medicine. TCM has been used to treat an extensive diversity of medical conditions including respiratory, digestive, blood, urogenital, gynecological, cardiovascular, neurological, and psychiatric disorders (Di et al., 2019). Effectiveness of healing varies individually with health condition and the modality used (NCCIM, 2019).

Acupuncture

Acupuncture is the primary treatment modality used by TCM practitioners. In 1983, the Chinese Medicine and Acupuncture Association of Canada was federally incorporated in order to unite TCM and acupuncture practitioners in Canada. In acupuncture, fine needles are inserted into the circulation of qi underneath the skin's surface. The insertion points depend on the diagnosis and the nature of the health issue. With proper point selection and manipulation, acupuncture corrects disruptions in the flow of qi.

Clinical Applications of Acupuncture. Clinical studies have indicated that acupuncture is effective in reducing pain, fighting inflammation, accelerating wound healing, and promoting nerve regeneration (Liu et al., 2019; Swanson et al., 2015). Acupuncture is considered a safe therapy when the practitioner has been appropriately trained and uses disposable needles. Patients should review the credentials of their practitioners.

ENERGY-BASED THERAPIES

Energy-based therapies are those that involve the manipulation of energy fields. They focus on energy fields originating within the body (biofields, or human energy fields) or those from other sources (electromagnetic fields). Examples of biofield therapies include therapeutic touch, healing touch, Reiki, and bioelectromagnetic, or magnet, therapy. Energy-based therapies (see Table 12.3) are based on the theory that energy systems in the body need to be balanced and repatterned to enhance healing. Some forms of energy therapy manipulate biofields by applying pressure or manipulating the body by placing the hands in, or through, these fields.

Therapeutic Touch

Therapeutic touch is a method of detecting, balancing, and repatterning the human energy field. It is a contemporary interpretation of several ancient healing practices. It involves the conscious use of the hands to direct or modulate human energy fields. Therapeutic touch was developed in the 1970s by a nurse, Dolores Krieger, and a traditional healer, Doris Kunz. According to Krieger (1997), therapeutic touch is based on the assumptions that a human being is an open energy system, a balanced flow of energy underlies good health, and illness is a reflection of an imbalance in an individual's energy field. During the actual treatment, trained nurses or practitioners use their hands to assess the patient's energy field for bilateral similarities or differences in the flow of energy. The practitioner then clears imbalances and smooths the patient's energy field to promote healing and well-being.

Clinical Applications of Therapeutic Touch. Research has been conducted on the effectiveness of therapeutic touch for a wide range of conditions, including wound healing, sleep promotion, enhancement of immune function, and reduction of anxiety, agitation, postoperative pain, tension headache, and stress. The research findings have been inconclusive, which indicates the need for further research. Specialized instruction is needed to perform therapeutic touch. Some individuals can "feel" the energy field more readily than others. However, with patience, determination, and a desire to help others, anyone (including family members) can learn to use therapeutic touch.

AGE-RELATED CONSIDERATIONS

Older persons with non–life-threatening, chronic conditions often use complementary and alternative therapies. For older persons, safety concerns involve herb–drug interactions or toxicity from polypharmacy and age-related changes in pharmacokinetics (Touhy et al., 2019). Decreased renal and liver function may slow metabolism and excretion of herbs and dietary supplements. Because older patients are a more vulnerable population, the nurse must discuss the risks and benefits of using herbal products and also encourage patients to inform their health care provider of any herbal product or dietary supplement that they are taking.

NURSING MANAGEMENT
COMPLEMENTARY AND ALTERNATIVE THERAPIES

The role of the nurse with regard to complementary and alternative therapies is evolving. Roles of the nurse may include (a) assessing patients' use of complementary and alternative therapies, and their risk for complications or adverse interactions with conventional therapies (Table 12.7); (b) serving as a resource about complementary or alternative therapies, including teaching patients about these options, providing information about evidence concerning effectiveness, and making referrals to qualified practitioners; (c) serving as a provider of therapies for which the nurse obtains training and certification, such as therapeutic touch or acupuncture; and (d) conducting research about complementary and alternative approaches. The nurse must be able to perform these roles nonjudgementally. If patients believe they are being judged because of their use of complementary or alternative therapies, they may stop communicating and withhold this vital information from their health care providers.

Collection of data on patients' use of complementary and alternative therapies is part of a thorough nursing assessment. It is especially important because most patients do not voluntarily tell their health care provider about their use of these therapies. However, they usually share this information with a nurse when asked. Nurses must ask general, open-ended questions, while remaining nonjudgemental and respectful of the patient's response. Along with assessing use, the nurse needs to document the effectiveness of interventions that the patient uses.

TABLE 12.7   NURSING ASSESSMENT
Complementary and Alternative Therapies

1. What are you doing to maintain or improve your health and well-being?
2. How involved are you in planning and carrying out your health-related care?
3. What is your view of the ideal relationship between yourself and your primary health care provider?
4. Do you have any conditions that have not responded to conventional medicine? If so, have you tried any other approaches?
5. Are you using any vitamin, mineral, dietary, or herbal supplements or energy-based therapies?
6. Are you interested in obtaining information about alternative or complementary approaches?

Holistic nursing practice is based on the philosophies of holism and humanism, which recognize the entire person while acknowledging the interdependence of differing facets within that whole. A holistic nurse integrates these mind–body–spirit principles into the development of caring and therapeutic relationships with patients that support healing and well-being. With a relationship based on openness, mutuality, and equality, a holistic nurse uses several modalities to deliver care and support focused on restoring power and responsibility to patients, which in turn encourages self-care practices (Jasemi et al., 2017).

Professional nursing has historically considered holistic practice crucial to patient care. However, the influence of a Western, biomedical model rooted in curing has led to a fragmented emphasis on the physical characteristics of an individual's health, missing essential psychological and spiritual aspects of life and well-being. In Canada, a growing trend in the use of complementary and alternative therapies provides an ideal opportunity for nurses to return to their foundations of holistic nursing practice, which honours cultural diversity in the health and well-being of others.

CASE STUDY

Abdominal Distress

Patient Profile

J. C., a 21-year-old university student (pronouns they/them), was seen in the student health centre for increasing episodes of abdominal fullness and discomfort with alternating diarrhea and constipation.

Subjective Data

- Reports that irritable bowel syndrome was diagnosed several years ago
- Was told to eat more fibre, drink at least eight glasses of water per day, and consume foods such as peas, prunes, and oatmeal
- States they have tried to change their diet but due to a limited budget cannot afford fresh fruits and vegetables
- Consumes mainly fast foods because of their busy schedule
- Drinks six to eight colas per day because they do not like water
- Has not been able to effectively reduce abdominal distress
- Is taking a heavy course load this semester
- Has to work 20 hours each week for a work–study contract

Discussion Questions

1. Assess what J. C. is currently doing to help alleviate their symptoms.
2. Explain the psychological stressors that may be contributing to J. C.'s abdominal discomfort.
3. Describe how J. C.'s current diet may be affecting them, both physiologically and psychologically.
4. What complementary or alternative therapy (or therapies) would be appropriate for J. C.?
5. How could the nurse recommend complementary therapies to J. C.'s physician? What arguments could support their use?

⊖volve
Answers are available at http://evolve.elsevier.com/Canada/Lewis/medsurg.

REVIEW QUESTIONS

The number of the question corresponds to the same-numbered objective at the beginning of the chapter.

1. Which of the following statements best describes complementary and alternative therapies?
   a. They are used as a primary form of treatment.
   b. They contradict the values of nursing.
   c. They are based on extensive scientific research.
   d. They were developed outside the Western biomedical model.

2. Which herbs can increase a client's risk of bleeding? *(Select all that apply.)*
   a. Aloe
   b. Kava
   c. Garlic
   d. Ginger
   e. Feverfew

3. Which of the following statements describes holistic nursing? *(Select all that apply.)*
   a. Holistic nursing focuses on physical health.
   b. Holistic nursing is practised only by experienced nurses.
   c. Holistic nursing promotes self-care and self-responsibility.
   d. Holistic nursing is based on the biomedical model of health care.

   e. Holistic nursing incorporates mind–body–spirit principles.

4. Which of the following clients is most likely to benefit from treatment by a traditional Chinese medicine practitioner?
   a. A client with pneumonia
   b. A client with mental illness
   c. A client with chronic back pain
   d. A postoperative client with low blood pressure

5. Which of the following best describes the role of the nurse involved with complementary and alternative therapies?
   a. Caring for clients rather than caring for self
   b. Prescribing the appropriate herbal therapies for a client
   c. Serving as a resource to guide clients in the safe use of therapies
   d. Advocating for use of complementary and alternative therapies instead of conventional health care

1. d; 2. c, d, e; 3. c, e; 4. c; 5. c.

ⓔvolve

For even more review questions, visit http://evolve.elsevier.com/Canada/Lewis/medsurg.

REFERENCES

Anandarajh, G., & Hight, E. (2001). Spirituality and medical practice: Using the HOPE questions as a practical tool for spiritual assessment. *American Family Physician, 63*(1), 81–89. https://www.aafp.org/afp/2001/0101/p81.html

Angelopoulou, E., Anagnostouli, M., Chrousos, P., et al. (2020). Massage therapy as a complementary treatment for Parkinson's disease: A systematic literature review. *Complementary Therapies in Medicine, 49*, 1–8. https://doi.org/10.1016/j.ctim.2020.102340.

Canadian Holistic Nurses Association (CHNA). (2021). *About us.* http://www.chna.ca/about-us/.

Canadian Nurses Association (CNA). (2015). *Framework for the practice of registered nurses in Canada.* https://www.cna-aiic.ca/~/media/cna/page-content/pdf-en/framework-for-the-pracice-of-registered-nurses-in-canada.pdf?la=en. (Seminal).

Canadian Nurses Association (CNA). (2017). *Code of ethics for registered nurses.* https://www.cna-aiic.ca/~/media/cna/page-content/pdf-en/code-of-ethics-2017-edition-secure-interactive.pdf?la=en.

Casterline, G. (2018). Healing, wholeness, & connection through prayer: A guide for nurses. *American Holistic Nurses Association, 1*, 8–9. http://www.ahna.org/Portals/66/Docs/Education/Provider/Beginnings/Articles/Beginnings_CNE_2018_issue_1.pdf?ver=2018-02-19-145220-550.

Charlebois, S., Music, J., Sterling, B., et al. (2020). Edibles and Canadian consumers' willingness to consider recreational cannabis in food or beverage products: A second assessment. *Trends in Food Science and Technology, 98*, 25–29. https://doi.org/10.1016/j.tifs.2019.12.025.

College & Association of Registered Nurses of Alberta. (2018). *Complementary and alternative health care and natural health products standards.* https://www.nurses.ab.ca/docs/default-source/document-library/standards/complementary-and-alternative-health-care-and-natural-health-products.pdf?sfvrsn=2480176b_34.

College of Nurses of Ontario (CNO). (2018). *Complementary therapies.* http://www.cno.org/en/learn-about-standards-guidelines/educational-tools/ask-practice/complementary-therapies/.

Di, Y. M., Yang, L., Shergis, J. L., et al. (2019). Clinical evidence of Chinese medicine therapies for depression in women during perimenopause and menopause. *Complementary Therapies in Medicine, 79*, 1–9. https://doi.org/10.1016/j.ctim.2019.03.019.

Esmail, N. (2017). *Complementary and alternative medicine: Use and public attitudes 1997, 2006, and 2016.* https://www.fraserinstitute.org/sites/default/files/complementary-and-alternative-medicine-2017.pdf.

Fontaine, K. L. (2019). *Complementary and alternative therapies for nursing* (5th ed.). Pearson Education.

Gonçalves, J. P. B., Lucchetti, G., Menezes, P. R., et al. (2015). Religious and spiritual interventions in mental health care: A systematic review and meta-analysis of randomized controlled clinical trials. *Psychological Medicine, 45*, 2937–2949. https://doi.org/10.1017/S0033291715001166 (Seminal).

Health Canada. (2021a). *Health effects of cannabis.* https://www.canada.ca/en/health-canada/services/drugs-medication/cannabis/health-effects/effects.html.

Health Canada. (2021b). *Information on homeopathic products.* https://www.canada.ca/en/health-canada/services/drugs-health-products/natural-non-prescription/regulation/information-homeopathic-products.html. (Seminal).

Interdisciplinary Network for Complementary and Alternative Medicine Research (INCAM). (2021). *About the Interdisciplinary Network for Complementary and Alternative Medicine Research.* www.iscmr.org/content.aspx?page_id=22&club_id=869917&module_id=477001. (Seminal).

Jasemi, M., Valizadeh, L., Zamanzadeh, V., et al. (2017). A concept analysis of holistic care by hybrid model. *Indian Journal of Palliative Care, 23*(1), 71–80. https://doi.org/10.4103/0973-1075.197960.

Krieger, D. (1997). *Therapeutic touch inner workbook: Ventures in transpersonal healing*. Santa Fe, NM: Bear (Seminal).

Liu, F., You, J., Li, Q., et al. (2019). Acupuncture for chronic pain-related insomnia: A systematic review and meta-analysis. *Evidence-Based Complementary and Alternative Medicine*, 1–10. https://doi.org/10.1155/2019/5381028.

Luctkar-Flude, M., Tyerman, J., & Groll, D. (2019). Exploring the use of neurofeedback by cancer survivors: Results of interviews with neurofeedback providers and clients. *Asia-Pacific Journal of Oncology Nursing*, 6(1), 35–42. https://doi.org/10.4103/apjon.apjon_34_18.

Mahmodi, Z., & Sayemiri, K. (2018). The effect of attitude and prayer-related behaviours on depression: A systematic review. *International Journal of Epidemiologic Research*, 5(1), 34–39. https://doi.org/10.15171/ijer.2018.08.

National Center for Complementary and Integrative Health. (2019). *Traditional Chinese medicine: What you need to know*. https://nccih.nih.gov/health/whatiscam/chinesemed.htm.

National Center for Complementary and Integrative Health. (2021). *Complementary, alternative, or integrative health. What's in a name?*. https://nccih.nih.gov/health/integrative-health.

National Library of Medicine. (n.d.). Medicine ways: Traditional healers and healing. https://www.nlm.nih.gov/nativevoices/exhibition/healing-ways/medicine-ways/medicine-wheel.html.

Northern College Indigenous Council on Education. (2020). *Four sacred medicines*. http://www.northernc.on.ca/indigenous/four-sacred-medicines/.

Prado Simão, T., Caldeira, S., & Campos de Carvalho, E. (2016). The effect of prayer on patients' health: Systematic literature review. *Religions*, 7, 1–11 https://doi.org/10.3390/rel7010011 (Seminal).

Pratt, M., Stevens, A., Thuku, M., et al. (2019). Benefits and harms of medical cannabis: A scoping review of systematic reviews. *Systematic Reviews*, 8(320), 1–35. https://doi.org/10.1186/s13643-019-1243-x.

Swanson, B., Keithley, J. K., Johnson, A., et al. (2015). Acupuncture to reduce HIV-associated inflammation. *Evidence-based Complementary and Alternative Medicine*, 5, 1–6 https://doi.org/10.1155/2015/908538 (Seminal work).

Touhy, T. A., Jett, K. F., Boscart, B., et al. (2019). *Ebersole and Hess' gerontological nursing and healthy aging* (2nd Canadian ed.). Toronto: Elsevier.

Uprety, Y., Lacasse, A., & Asselin, H. (2016). Traditional uses of medical plants from the Canadian Boreal Forest for the management of chronic pain syndromes. *Pain Practice*, 16(54), 459–466. https://doi.org/10.11111/paper.12284.

Yeun, Y. (2017). Effectiveness of massage therapy for shoulder pain: A systematic review and meta-analysis. *The Journal of Physical Therapy Science*, 29(2), 365–369 https://doi.org/10.1589/jptd.29.365 (Seminal).

RESOURCES

Acupuncture Canada
https://www.acupuncturecanada.org
Canadian Association for Parish Nursing Ministry
http://www.capnm.ca
Canadian Association of Naturopathic Doctors (CAND)
http://www.naturopathicassoc.ca
Canadian Chiropractic Association
http://www.ccachiro.org
Canadian Holistic Nurses Association
https://www.chna.ca
Canadian Indigenous Nurses Association
http://indigenousnurses.ca/
Canadian Interdisciplinary Network for Complementary and Alternative Medicine Research (INCAM)
https://iscmr.org/content.aspx?page_id=22&club_id=869917&module_id=372144
Chinese Medicine and Acupuncture Association of Canada
http://www.cmaac.ca/public/tcm-regulation-in-canada
College of Traditional Chinese Medicine & Pharmacology Canada
https://www.ctcmpc.ca
Healing Touch Canada
https://www.healingtouchcanada.net
Massage.ca
http://massage.ca/professional_development.html
Natural Health Practitioners of Canada
https://www.nhpcanada.org
Registered Nurses' Association of Ontario (RNAO) Complementary Therapies Nurses' Interest Group (CTNIG)
http://www.rnao-ctnig.org

Healing Beyond Borders
https://www.healingbeyondborders.org
National Center for Complementary and Integrative Health (NCCIH)
https://nccih.nih.gov

For additional Internet resources, see the website for this book at http://evolve.elsevier.com/Canada/Lewis/medsurg.

Palliative and End-of-Life Care

Sara Olivier, Kathryn Nichol, and Laura Wilding
Originating US chapter by Denise M. McEnroe-Petitte

⊖volve WEBSITE

http://evolve.elsevier.com/Canada/Lewis/medsurg

- Review Questions (Online Only)
- Key Points
- Student Case Study

- Chronic Myelogenous Leukemia Including End-of-Life Care
- Conceptual Care Map Creator
- Audio Glossary
- Content Updates

LEARNING OBJECTIVES

1. Describe the philosophy of a palliative approach to care.
2. Describe nursing management of common physical manifestations at the end of life.
3. Describe nursing management of common psychosocial manifestations at the end of life.
4. Explain the process of grief and bereavement.
5. Discuss variables that affect end-of-life care.

6. Discuss key ethical and legal issues related to hospice palliative care.
7. Explore the special needs of family caregivers of a dying patient.
8. Discuss the special needs of nurses who care for dying patients and their families.
9. Understand medical assistance in dying as an end-of-life option.

KEY TERMS

advance care planning
advance directives
bereavement
certification of death
Cheyne-Stokes respiration

death
end-of-life care
grief
hospice palliative care
integrated palliative approach

Medical Assistance in Dying (MAiD)
pronouncement of death
spirituality

HOSPICE PALLIATIVE CARE

The World Health Organization (WHO) describes palliative care as "an approach that improves the quality of life of patients and their families facing the problems associated with a life-threatening illness, through the prevention and relief of suffering by means of early identification and impeccable assessment and treatment of pain and other problems, physical, psychosocial and spiritual" (WHO, 2021). Specific goals of palliative care are listed in Table 13.1.

In Canada, the term hospice palliative care describes the convergence of hospice and palliative care into one movement that has the same principles of practice and that continues to evolve in an effort to reflect changes in people's experience with illness and dying (Canadian Hospice Palliative Care Association [CHPCA], 2013a). A national strategy promotes standardization and consistency through a shared vision for the delivery of care and for the organizational development,

education, and advocacy relating to hospice palliative care across the country (CHPCA, 2013b). Advances in medical treatments have helped people live longer with chronic illnesses. The course of an illness and timing of death are becoming harder to predict as more treatments become available to extend life. Hospice palliative care is available to individuals and families throughout the illness experience. At the beginning of the illness, there is increased focus on treatment and management. Over time, as illness progresses, the role for a palliative approach to care increases to relieve suffering and improve quality of life. Over the course of an illness, the patient's and family's concerns, their goals of care, and treatment priorities should always be taken into consideration (CHPCA, 2013b) (Figure 13.1). Chochinov's model of dignity-conserving care can be used to guide care that specifically targets the maintenance of dignity for those nearing the end of life (Chochinov, 2002).

TABLE 13.1	GOALS OF PALLIATIVE CARE

- Provide relief from symptoms, including pain
- Regard dying as a normal process
- Affirm life and neither hasten nor postpone death
- Support holistic patient care and enhance quality of life
- Offer support to patients to live as actively as possible until death
- Offer support to the family during the patient's illness and in their own bereavement

Source: Reprinted from *Cancer,* WHO, WHO Definition of Palliative Care, Copyright 2018.

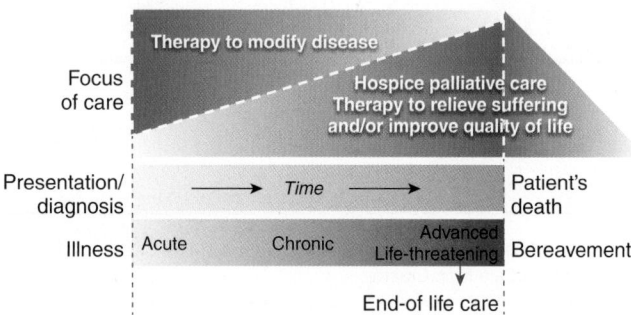

FIG. 13.1 The role of hospice palliative care during illness. Source: Canadian Hospice Palliative Care Association. (2013). *A model to guide hospice palliative care.* Canadian Hospice Palliative Care Association. https://www.chpca.ca/wp-content/uploads/2019/12/norms-of-practice-eng-web.pdf

TABLE 13.2	SUCCESS FACTORS FOR AN INTEGRATED PALLIATIVE APPROACH TO CARE

Vision
- Commitment to person-centred care
- Focus on building capacity in the community
- Focus on changing organizational structure
- Senior management support

People
- Dedicated coordinators
- Interprofessional teams
- Strong role of and more support for family physicians
- Support for health care providers in long-term care facilities
- Key roles for nurses
- Relationships, partnerships, and networks

Delivery of Care
- Integration of primary, secondary, and tertiary care
- Cultural sensitivity
- Single access point and case management
- Around-the-clock community support and care
- Advance care planning

Supportive Tools
- Common frameworks, standards, and assessment tools
- Flexible approaches to education
- Shared records
- Research, evaluation, and quality improvement

Source: Canadian Hospice Palliative Care Association (CHPCA). (2013). *Innovative models of integrated hospice palliative care. The Way Forward Initiative: An integrated palliative approach to care.* http://www.hpcintegration.ca/media/40546/TWF-innovative-models-report-Eng-webfinal-2.pdf

Integrated Hospice Palliative Care Approach

The *Canada Health Act* (1984) is the overarching legislation covering Canada's national medicare program (Madore, 2005). This publicly funded health care system is administered on a provincial or territorial basis; however, developing an integrated palliative approach to care is a priority for Canada (CHPCA, 2013b). In an effort to develop a national standard of palliative care, the CHPCA has produced "The Way Forward" as a national vision (CHPCA, 2013b) (Table 13.2).

Hospice palliative care is best provided as an integral part of health care and should be available in all settings of care, including acute and long-term care facilities, retirement homes, private residences, hospices, palliative care units, and shelters (Quality End-of-Life Care Coalition of Canada [QELCCC], 2010).

An **integrated palliative approach** to care focuses on meeting a patient's and family's full range of needs—physical, psychosocial, and spiritual—at all stages of illness, not just at the end of life. It is a shared-care model—one that shifts hospice palliative care from being a specialized service to a more generalized, integrated service available to people with life-limiting conditions, regardless of where they live and receive care (CHPCA, 2013b). Health care providers—physicians, nurses, home care nurses, personal support workers, long-term care staff, and hospital staff—continue to provide care with support of the expert palliative care team. The expert palliative care team takes the lead only when a patient's and family's needs become increasingly complex and require specialized care (CHPCA, 2015).

The Edmonton Symptom Assessment System (ESAS) (Hui & Bruera, 2017) and Palliative Performance Scale (PPS) (see Resources at the end of this chapter) are standardized tools that support comprehensive assessments and ensure consistent language when providing care and communicating within the health care team.

End-of-Life Care. End-of-life care refers to care provided during the last months, weeks, and days for a person with a life-limiting illness. In June 2000, the Senate of Canada issued a report, "Quality End-of Life Care: The Right of Every Canadian" (Carstairs, 2000), containing recommendations ensuring access to high-quality end-of-life care for all Canadians. The QELCCC (2012) supported these recommendations safeguarding the rights of Canadians "to die with dignity, free of pain, and surrounded by their loved ones, in a setting of their choice." Despite these efforts, well-documented gaps remain between the end-of-life care that Canadians prefer and the care that they receive (Conlon et al., 2019).

Seriously ill individuals in hospitals and their family members have identified the following features of quality end-of-life care: trust in the treating physician, avoidance of unwanted life support, effective communication, continuity of care, and death with dignity (Cook et al., 2013). While most Canadians (75%) state they would prefer to die at home, they also report feeling they would not be able to devote the time required to care for a loved one in a home setting (CHPCA, 2013a). In Canada, caregiver benefits are now available to financially support most individuals who wish to take time away from work to provide care and support a person needing end-of-life care (Government of Canada, 2021). In some cases, the needs of a patient and their family exceed the resources that can be provided in the home, resulting in admission to hospital at the end of life. Residential hospices and palliative care units are alternative settings for patients who are unable to remain at home for the end of their life but do not require an acute-care setting.

PHYSICAL MANIFESTATIONS OF THE END OF LIFE

During the dying process metabolism is altered and body systems gradually slow down until they no longer function.

TABLE 13.3	PHYSICAL MANIFESTATIONS OF APPROACHING DEATH		
System	**Manifestations**	**System**	**Manifestations**
Sensory system • Hearing • Taste and smell • Sight	• Usually last sense to disappear • Decreased with disease progression • Blurring of vision • Sinking and glazing of eyes • Blink reflex absent • Eyelids may remain half open	Gastrointestinal (GI) system	• Loss of appetite and thirst sensations • Slowing or cessation of GI function (opioid medications may contribute to slowed GI transit) • Accumulation of gas and abdominal distension • Nausea • Loss of sphincter control, which may cause incontinence • Bowel movement before imminent death or at time of death
Cardiovascular system	• Increased heart rate; later slowing and weakening of pulse • Irregular rhythm • Decrease in blood pressure • Delayed absorption of drugs administered subcutaneously • Peripheral edema	Musculoskeletal system	• Increasing weakness • Gradual loss of ability to move • Sagging of jaw as a result of loss of facial muscle tone • Difficulty speaking • Difficulty swallowing • Difficulty maintaining body posture and alignment • Loss of gag reflex
Respiratory system	• Increased respiratory rate • Cheyne-Stokes respiration (irregular pattern of respiration characterized by alternating periods of apnea and deep breathing) • Inability to cough or clear upper airway secretions, which results in gurgling, noisy, or congested breathing (terminal secretions) • Irregular breathing, gradually slowing down to terminal gasps (may be described as "guppy breathing")	Integumentary system	• Mottling of hands, feet, arms, and legs • Cold, clammy skin • Cyanosis of nose, nail beds, and knees • "Waxlike" skin when death is very near
Urinary system	• Gradual decrease in urinary output • Incontinent of urine • Inability to urinate		

Respiratory changes are common. Breath sounds may become wet and noisy, both audibly and on auscultation. These *terminal secretions* are caused by mouth breathing and accumulation of mucus in the airways that cannot to be cleared by coughing or repositioning. **Cheyne-Stokes respiration** is an irregular pattern of breathing characterized by alternating periods of apnea and deep breathing.

Dying is a multisystem process that can exhibit a variety of manifestations. Presentation of these changes may vary depending on the comorbidities of the individual. Physical manifestations of approaching death are listed in Table 13.3. Identification and explanation of these changes by the nurse is key in supporting patients and families through the dying process.

Death

Death occurs when all vital organs and body systems cease to function. It is the irreversible cessation of cardiovascular, respiratory, and brain function. When circulation and breathing stop and no attempts are made to restore circulation, after approximately 2 to 5 minutes, cessation of breathing and circulation is permanent and the individual may be determined to be dead.

PSYCHOSOCIAL MANIFESTATIONS OF THE END OF LIFE

A variety of feelings and emotions can affect the patient and family at the end of life. They may experience a wide range of emotions and reactions (Table 13.4). Many people struggle with the news of a terminal diagnosis and the realization that there is no cure or further treatment options. The patient and family may feel overwhelmed, fearful, powerless, and fatigued.

TABLE 13.4	PSYCHOSOCIAL MANIFESTATIONS OF APPROACHING DEATH
• Altered decision making • Anxiety about unfinished business • Decreased socialization • Fear of loneliness • Fear of meaninglessness of one's life • Fear of pain	• Helplessness • Life review • Peacefulness • Restlessness • Saying goodbyes • Unusual communication • Vision-like experiences • Withdrawal

Alternatively, there may be feelings of peace and acceptance if closure has been achieved. A patient-centered approach to understand and support the psychosocial needs of the patient and their family is essential.

GRIEF AND BEREAVEMENT

Bereavement refers to the state of loss, and *grief* refers to the reaction to loss, although the terms are often used interchangeably. **Grief** is a normal reaction to loss and may manifest itself in both psychological and physiological ways. It is a powerful emotional state affecting all aspects of a person's life. Psychological responses may include anger, guilt, anxiety, sadness, depression, despair, or a combination of these. Physiological reactions may include disruption in sleep, changes in appetite, and illness.

Elisabeth Kübler-Ross (1969) was a pioneer in the recognition and description of grief. In her model of grief, she described five stages observed in people who were grieving,

TABLE 13.5	KÜBLER-ROSS'S MODEL OF GRIEF	
Stage	What a Person May Say	Characteristics
Denial	No, not me. It cannot be true.	Denying the loss has taken place and possibly withdrawing. This response may last minutes to months.
Anger	Why me?	Possibly being angry at the person who inflicted the hurt (even after death) or at the world for letting it happen. Possibly being angry with self for letting an event (e.g., car accident) take place, even if nothing could have stopped it.
Bargaining	Yes, me, but...	Making bargains with God, asking, "If I do this, will you take away the loss?"
Depression	Yes, me, and I am sad.	Feeling numb, although anger and sadness may remain subconsciously.
Acceptance	Yes, me, but it is okay.	Tapering off of anger, sadness, and mourning; accepting the reality of the loss.

Source: From *On Death and Dying*, by Dr. Elisabeth Kubler-Ross. Copyright © 1969 by Elisabeth Kubler-Ross; copyright renewed © 1997 by Elisabeth Kubler-Ross. Reprinted with the permission of Scribner, a division of Simon & Schuster, Inc. All rights reserved.

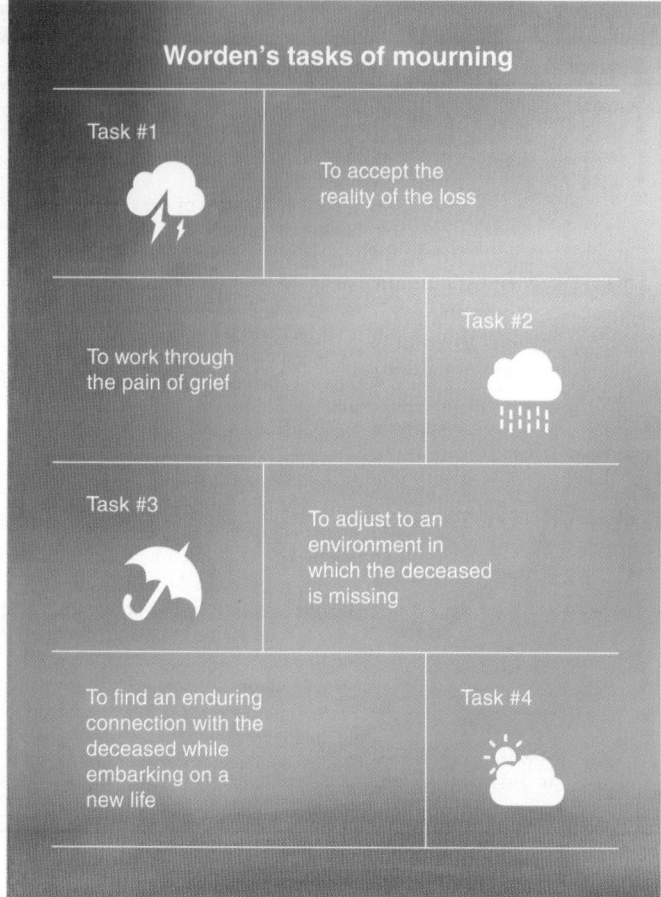

FIG. 13.2 Worden's tasks of mourning. Source: Worden, J. W. (2009). *Grief counselling and grief therapy: A handbook for the mental health practitioner.* http://www.whatsyourgrief.com/wordens-four-tasks-of-mourning/

but also acknowledged hope interwoven in the experience and suggested that some meaning can be taken from the experience (Table 13.5). As other theorists built on this work, they realized that the stages are not linear. Indeed, not every person experiences all the stages of grieving. It is not uncommon to reach a stage and then revert to an earlier stage. William Worden further developed Kübler-Ross's work and began talking about "grief work." He developed a counselling model to assist people in the work of grief. Worden's (2009) model outlines "four tasks of mourning" that must be accomplished in grief work (Figure 13.2).

The way a person grieves depends on factors such as the relationship with the person who has died (e.g., spouse, parent), physical and emotional coping resources, concurrent life stresses, cultural beliefs, and personality. Other factors that affect the grief response include mental and physical health, economic resources, religious influences or spiritual beliefs, family relationships, social support, and time spent preparing for the death.

Anticipatory grief is a form of grieving that takes place before the actual death. Patients nearing the end of life, as well as their family, may experience anticipatory grief. As a patient approaches the end of life, it is common for loved ones to begin to think of what life will be like when the person has died. The extent to which they have explored and experienced anticipatory grief has an influence on their grief after the actual death (National Cancer Institute, 2020).

Working in a positive way through the grief process helps to adapt to the loss. Grief that helps the person accept the reality of death is called *adaptive grief*. It is a healthy response. It may be associated with grieving before death occurs or when the inevitability of the death is known. Indicators of adaptive grief include the ability to see some good resulting from the death and positive memories of the deceased person.

Dysfunctional reactions to loss can occur, and the physical and psychological impact of the loved one's death may persist for years. *Prolonged grief disorder,* formerly called *complicated grief,* is a term used to describe prolonged and intense mourning. Prolonged grief disorder can include symptoms such as recurrent and severe distressing emotions and intrusive thoughts related to the loss of a loved one, self-neglect, and denial of the loss for longer than 6 months. It is estimated that 1 out of 10 bereaved adults is at risk for prolonged grief disorder (Lundorff et al., 2017). Those with prolonged grief disorder have a higher risk for illness and may have work and social impairments.

Bereavement is the period after the death of a loved one during which grief is experienced and mourning occurs. The time spent in bereavement depends on a number of factors, including cultural norms, the nature of the relationship with the deceased person, and the degree to which the surviving person was able to prepare for the loss before death. Bereavement and grief counselling are core components of patient- and family-centered hospice palliative care. Bereavement programs offer support to assist a loved one's transition to a life without the deceased person. An environment in which patients and families can share feelings of anger, sadness, and fear supports individuals as they work through the grieving process.

SPIRITUAL NEEDS

Assessment of spiritual needs in end-of-life care is a key consideration (Table 13.6). Spirituality is defined as the beliefs, values, and practices that relate to the search for existential meaning and purpose (O'Brien, 2018). Spiritual needs do not necessarily equate to religion or belief in a higher power. A person may not be part of a particular religion but may be deeply spiritual. The nurse needs to assess the patient's and family's preferences regarding spiritual guidance or pastoral care services and make appropriate referrals.

Deep-seated spiritual beliefs may surface for some patients when they deal with their progressing illness and related issues. Spiritual distress may arise as they question their beliefs about a higher power, their journey through life, religion, and existence of an afterlife. Characteristics of spiritual distress may include anger toward God or a higher being, change in behaviour and mood, desire for spiritual assistance, or displaced anger toward clergy (Caldeira et al., 2013).

A sense of spirituality has also been associated with decreased despair in patients at the end of life. Some dying patients are secure in their faith about the future. It is common to see patients relinquish material possessions of life and focus on values that they believe will lead them on to another place. Many turn to religion because it gives order to the world even in the presence of physical decline, social losses, suffering, and impending death. Religion may offer an existential meaning that provides a sense of peace and recognition of one's place in the broader cosmic context (O'Brien, 2018).

CULTURALLY COMPETENT CARE

At the End of Life

Although death is universal, the ways in which people understand and experience death vary across cultures. Variations in rituals within cultural groups, religious faiths, and individuals are reminders of the importance of not overgeneralizing culturally attributed qualities.

Some cultural and religious experiences and expressions of death are subdued and intensely private, whereas for others the experience may involve their entire community and be a very public affair with public expressions of grief. Some cultures shield or protect the dying from information about their illness. Effective nurses seek to understand the cultural or religious practices and attitudes toward end-of-life care and death that are specific to each patient (Ganz & Sapir, 2019). This understanding should also include practices or rituals concerning the care of the body upon and immediately after death, including accommodations regarding the patient's language, diet, and cultural beliefs and practices. Families with non–English-speaking members are at risk for receiving less information about their family member's illness and prognosis (Hagerty et al., 2016). When appropriate, the nurse should access interpreter services so that the patient's wishes are known.

In Canada the Indigenous population consists of First Nations, Inuit, and Métis peoples. Leaders within these groups have expressed the importance of culturally appropriate palliative care for their communities (Health Canada, 2019). Ongoing work of Health Canada and national Indigenous organizations is focused on developing a palliative care framework that reflects the specific and unique priorities of Indigenous people.

TABLE 13.6 SPIRITUAL ASSESSMENT

1. Who or what provides you strength and hope?
2. Do you use prayer in your life?
3. How do you express spirituality?
4. How would you describe your philosophy of life?
5. What type of spiritual or religious support do you desire?
6. What is the name of your clergy, minister, chaplain, pastor, rabbi?
7. What does suffering mean to you?
8. What does dying mean to you?
9. What are your spiritual goals?
10. Is there a role of a church, synagogue, mosque, or temple in your life?
11. Has belief in God been important in your life?
12. How does your faith help you cope with illness?
13. How do you keep going day after day?
14. What helps you get through this health care experience?
15. How has illness affected you and your family?

Source: © Joint Commission Resources: Provision of Care, Treatment, and Services (PC) (Critical Access Hospitals/Critical Access Hospitals). Oakbrook Terrace, IL: Joint Commission on Accreditation of Healthcare Organizations, 2018. Reprinted with permission.

In an effort to increase access of Indigenous communities to health care services, Indigenous navigator programs have been developed throughout Canada to support patients and their families navigate the health care system, remove barriers, and increase cultural sensitivity among health care providers. The role of extended family, family gatherings, community leaders, healers, and medicine men and women within Indigenous culture should be explored and integrated into care. Furthermore, it is important to understand the connection to the spirit world, to ceremony, and to sacred ceremonial items such as feathers, tobacco, sweet grass, cloth, and stones and how these elements can be respectfully incorporated into a patient's plan of care (Hampton et al., 2010). (Further considerations around culturally competent care are discussed in Chapter 2.)

LEGAL AND ETHICAL ISSUES AFFECTING END-OF-LIFE CARE

Patients and families struggle with many questions related to a life-limiting illness and the dying experience. Many people decide that the outcomes for their care should be based on their own wishes and values. It is important to provide information to help patients with these decisions. The decisions may involve the choice for (1) organ and tissue donations, (2) advance directives (e.g., medical power of attorney), (3) resuscitation, and (4) medical assistance in dying.

Throughout the COVID-19 pandemic, care settings were required to restrict visitors in order to maintain the safety of patients and staff. This practice brought to light the need for care settings to consider the effects of social isolation on dying patients and to implement safe, compassionate, and inclusive visitation policies allowing those nearing the end of life to say goodbye to their loved ones (CHPCA, 2020).

Advance Care Planning and Advance Directives

Legislation pertaining to advance care planning (ACP) in Canada is specific to each province or territory. However, the principles underlying ACP are common across the country: the intrinsic value and uniqueness of each person, the person's right to self-determination, and autonomous decision making.

ETHICAL DILEMMAS
End-of-Life Care

Case Study
R. S. (pronouns she/her) is a 50-year-old person with metastatic breast cancer. She has developed severe bone pain that is not adequately controlled by her current dosage of intravenous (IV) morphine. She moans at rest and verbalizes severe pain from any movement to reposition her. Even though she appears to sleep at intervals, R. S. requests pain medicine frequently, and her family is demanding additional pain medicine for her. At the interprofessional team conference, the nurses discuss the need for more effective pain control but are concerned that additional medications could hasten her death.

Important Points for Consideration
- Adequate pain relief is an important outcome for all patients, but especially for patients at the end of life. The *principle of beneficence* imposes the obligation to provide the necessary care to benefit the patient.
- One goal of treatment is to provide adequate pain and symptom management to alleviate suffering. This goal is based on the *principle of nonmaleficence:* preventing or reducing harm to the patient. The concern of hastening death should be acknowledged. However, the intent behind adequate management of refractory symptoms is to control the suffering and is a nurse's ethical obligation.
- Adequate pain relief at the end of life continues to be a major concern of health care providers and patients and their families.
- Opportunities for debriefing should be offered to alleviate the potential moral distress of the nurses.

Clinical Decision-Making Questions
1. In R. S.'s situation, what type of discussion needs to occur between the health care team, the patient, and the family as the terminally ill phase of the care approaches?
2. Distinguish between palliative sedation and medical assistance in dying, and the promotion of comfort and relief of pain in dying patients.

TABLE 13.7   DEVELOPING AN ADVANCE CARE PLAN

Steps	Important Considerations
Learn about your condition and medical treatment: Some may improve your quality of life, whereas others may only keep you alive longer. **Think about you:** What are your values, wishes, beliefs, and understanding about your care and specific medical treatments? **Talk about your wishes:** It is important to discuss your wishes with your loved ones, your family physician, and your health care team. **Choose a substitute decision maker:** Choose someone who would honour and follow your wishes if you cannot speak for yourself. **Record your wishes:** It is a good idea to write down or make a recording of your wishes. Give a copy to your health care provider and substitute decision maker.	• What makes each day worthwhile? • What makes you happy? • How do your decisions about your illness, your care, and your treatment affect your loved ones? Does this change the way you feel about treatment? • Do you have fears or worries regarding your treatment? • Do you have a preference regarding location of care (for example, at home, in a health care institution) if your condition gets worse? • Is there anything that feels "undone" about your life? • Whom can you rely on to help you through any challenges? • Do your religious, cultural, or personal beliefs affect your decisions?

Source: Based on Advance Care Planning National Task Group. (2015). *Five steps of advance care planning* (Speak Up campaign video). https://www.youtube.com/watch?v=mPtu-FpY1Kw

Nurses play an important role in educating individuals about their health condition and helping them understand the information they have been given. Patients are encouraged to consider this information in the development of an advance care plan (Table 13.7).

Resuscitation
Do-not-resuscitate (DNR) decisions are unique instructions that have developed in acute care hospitals since the 1970s. Because cardiopulmonary resuscitation (CPR) is the default response to respiratory or cardiac arrest, a DNR decision requires informed consent (Bester & Kodish, 2019). This is a very specific example of an event that can often be anticipated and addressed in an advance care directive.

A physician's DNR order is required and should be specific enough to reflect the patient's expressed wishes, whether through direct discussion with the patient, through the advance directive, or from the patient's SDM. Physicians can reflect this understanding of the patient's wishes with written orders for care that focus on comfort, meaning that treatments associated with pain and symptom management are carried out, but the natural physiological progression to death is not delayed or interrupted. *Allow natural death* (AND) is a term increasingly being used to replace DNR. The use of this type of language means that care is not withheld but rather is supportive while allowing nature to take its course. It is meant to promote comfort and dignity at the end of life. Templates such as the "Goals of Care Designations" from Alberta Health Services are designed to facilitate conversations and documentation of an individual's values and wishes regarding medical care, resuscitative care, and comfort care that is valid across the entire province in all care settings (see Resources section at the end of this chapter).

Health care providers should always speak with patients about their wishes for care and treatment. The intent of an *advance care plan* is that when the patient is no longer able to give direction or consent, the patient's substitute decision maker (SDM) or advance care plan, or both, will ensure that the patient's wishes are known. Each province and territory has legislation outlining who may be designated an SDM.

Advance care planning is the process of thinking about and sharing one's wishes for future health and personal care. It is a means by which an individual can tell others what would be important if they were ill and unable to communicate. An individual may choose an SDM and identify this person through a written document such as a power of attorney (or similar document).

An individual may express their wishes or directions as generally or specifically as they wish through an advance care plan (formerly known as a *living will*). When **advance directives**—legal documents specifying an individual's decisions regarding care—are written, they should be made available to the health care providers and the SDM. The CHPCA has led a national initiative promoting and educating the general public and health care providers on the importance of ACP. The CHPCA website lists a variety of tools, workbooks, and other information regarding ACP (see Resources section at the end of this chapter). In all cases, an SDM must act on a patient's prior expressed wishes, if known, and in a manner that would be consistent with what the patient would have done when capable.

Medical Assistance in Dying. Medical Assistance in Dying (MAiD), legal in Canada since June 2016, involves prescribing or administering medications to intentionally end the life of an adult, at their request. In Canada, federal legislation—Bill C-14—governs who is eligible and the processes under which MAiD can be legally and safely delivered to a patient (Government of Canada, 2016). Specifically, adults who have a serious and incurable illness, disease, or disability; who are in an advanced state of irreversible decline in capability; whose illness, disease, or disability causes them to endure suffering that is intolerable to them and that cannot be relieved under conditions they find acceptable; and whose natural death has become reasonably foreseeable may be eligible to receive MAiD (Government of Canada, 2016). Both nurse practitioners and physicians can assess and provide MAiD in Canada. In order to pursue MAiD, people must be informed of their treatment options, including palliative care, and must make a written request for MAiD that is witnessed by two independent witnesses who meet specific criteria. Mandatory reporting to Health Canada provides oversight of this practice (Government of Canada, 2018). Each province and territory is accountable for the service delivery model of MAiD, which varies considerably across Canada. It is imperative that nurses follow the professional policies and standards for the jurisdiction where they practice.

The choice to pursue MAiD is personal and complex. Psychosocial support for the person, their loved ones, as well as for the health care providers involved in the care of the person is paramount. MAiD-specific grief and bereavement resources may support a positive experience for the patient and family, while mentorship and resiliency resources have been identified as essential components for the wellness of health care providers (Li et al., 2017).

The introduction of Bill C-7, in February 2020, proposed further changes to Canada's law on MAiD (Government of Canada, 2020). However, MAiD remains inaccessible to those under the age of 18 years, to those whose sole underlying medical condition is mental illness, or through an advanced directive.

Palliative Sedation

MAiD should not be confused with palliative sedation. *Palliative sedation* is an infrequent and extraordinary intervention that necessitates interprofessional expertise. Rigorous guidelines are strictly followed to intentionally produce sedation in the last days of a patient's life (Alberta Health Services, 2018) and where the intent is to control refractory symptoms and suffering, not to shorten life or to hasten death (Abarshi et al., 2014).

Promoting the relief of suffering is a nurse's ethical obligation, and it may include appropriate administration of medications that have the potential to cause sedation. The *principle of double effect* justifies the use of medications that cause sedation as an adverse effect—an unintended harm—as its primary role is to relieve suffering and is not intended to hasten death. Careful titration of medication, which is based on the patient's response, can improve the likelihood that the patient will receive appropriate doses of medications to manage symptoms and minimize adverse effects.

The use of opioids for symptom management at the end of life is often misunderstood and feared by patients, families, and some health care providers. For this reason, many patients do not receive adequate medication, which may lead to physical and emotional suffering from uncontrolled pain and symptoms. This presents an opportunity for the nurse to educate the patient and family and address concerns about physical dependence and tolerance of medications. Patients at the end of life should not be concerned with physical dependence when the goal of treatment is comfort until death. (Pain management is discussed in Chapter 10.)

Organ and Tissue Donation

In Canada, oversight and administration of health services, including organ donation, are the responsibility of provincial and territorial governments. Deceased donor services are managed by organ procurement organizations and living donor services are managed by individual hospitals. All people who are 16 years of age or older and are competent may choose organ and tissue donation. Only patients who have sustained a nonrecoverable injury and are on life support may donate organs. However, all patients have the potential to donate tissue (e.g., eyes, bones, heart valves, and skin) after death (Ontario Trillium Gift of Life Network, n.d.). Patients who choose MAiD may also be considered for organ and tissue donation.

Nurses should be aware of ethical and legal issues and the patient's wishes. Advance directives and organ donor information should be in the patient's medical record and identified on that record or in the nursing care plan. All caregivers responsible for the patient need to know the patient's wishes. In addition, nurses are responsible for becoming familiar with provincial or territorial, local, and facility policies regarding documentation of end-of-life care. (Altered immune response and transplantation are discussed in Chapter 16.)

NURSING MANAGEMENT END OF LIFE

Nurses spend more time than any other health care providers with patients nearing the end of life. Nursing care is holistic and encompasses all psychosocial and physical needs. It focuses on what is important for the patient and family, such as respect, dignity, and comfort. Although there is no cure for the person's disease, the treatment plan still consists of assessment, planning, implementation, and evaluation, with the main focus on management of the symptoms of the disease, rather than on the disease itself. In addition, nurses need to recognize their own needs when dealing with grief and dying.

NURSING ASSESSMENT

Assessment of a patient at the end of life varies with the patient's diagnosis, life expectancy, and rate of decline. Depending on the reason for admission, the assessment might be comprehensive or limited to essential data. Nurses must be sensitive and not impose repeated, unnecessary assessments. When possible, health history data that are available in the medical record should be used in the nursing assessment. The nurse documents the specific event or change in condition that caused the patient to enter the health care facility. The patient's medical diagnoses, medication profile, and allergies are recorded.

A comprehensive symptom assessment according to the acronym *OPQRSTUV* (**o**nset, **p**rovoking/**p**alliating, **q**uality, **r**egion/**r**adiation, **s**everity, **t**reatment, **u**nderstanding/impact on person, and **v**alues) and a physical assessment should be completed so that prompt interventions can be initiated. In addition, comorbid conditions or acute episodes of health conditions should be evaluated and managed according to the established goals of care. The nurse should elicit information about the patient's abilities, food and fluid intake, patterns of sleep and rest, and response to the stress of the illness; assess the patient's ability to cope with the diagnosis and prognosis of the illness; and determine the family's capacity to manage care and cope with the illness and its consequences. (Health history and physical assessment are discussed in Chapter 3.)

The physical assessment for patients at the end of life is abbreviated and focuses on changes that accompany the specific disease process (Hui et al., 2015). The frequency of assessment depends on the patient's stability, but a full assessment is completed at least every shift in the institutional setting. For patients cared for in their homes, assessment may occur less frequently. As changes occur, assessment and documentation may be completed more often. If the patient is in the final hours of life, the physical assessment may be limited to gathering essential data.

Key elements of a social assessment include evaluating the goals of the patient and family, assessing what the patient and family know and want to know about the dying process, and determining the relationships and patterns of communication among the family members. If multiple family members are present, the nurse should listen to concerns from different members. Differences in expectations and interpersonal conflict can result in family disruptions during the dying process and after the death of the loved one. As a member of the interprofessional team, the nurse plays a key role in patient and family education, helping them understand what is happening, validating their questions, and advocating for respect of the patient's wishes (Canadian Nurses Association [CNA] et al., 2015).

As the patient nears death, the nurse should monitor multiple systems that often fail at the end of life. This requires vigilance and attention to physical changes that are often subtle. Neurological assessment is especially important and includes evaluation of level of consciousness, presence of reflexes, and pupil responses. Evaluation of vital signs, skin colour, and temperature helps detect changes in circulation. The nurse should monitor and describe respiratory status, character and pattern of respirations, and characteristics of breath sounds. Nutritional and fluid intake, urine output, and bowel function should also be monitored because they provide assessment data for renal and gastrointestinal functioning. Skin condition should be assessed on an ongoing basis because skin becomes fragile and may easily break down.

In the last hours of life, assessments should be limited to only those that are needed to determine the patient's comfort. Assessment of pain and respiratory status may be most important during this time. It may be more peaceful and comforting to the patient and family to refrain from overstimulation that may occur from certain types of assessments, such as measuring blood pressure or checking for pupillary response. As the patient's death approaches, the nurse's efforts may be better spent providing emotional support to the patient and family. (Tools for nursing practice can be found at the Canadian Virtual Hospice and Pallium Canada websites, listed in the Resources section at the end of this chapter.)

NURSING DIAGNOSES

Several nursing diagnoses concern psychosocial manifestations (Table 13.8) and physical manifestations (Table 13.9) associated with end-of-life care.

PLANNING

The patient and family need to be involved in planning and coordinating end-of-life care. In some cases, a family conference may be helpful to develop a coordinated plan of care. The nurse develops a comprehensive plan to support, teach, and evaluate

TABLE 13.8   **NURSING DIAGNOSES**
Psychosocial Manifestations of the End of Life

• Anxiety, death	• Loneliness, potential for
• Confusion, acute	• Sleep pattern, disturbed
• Confusion, chronic	• Social interaction, altered
• Coping, inadequate	• Social isolation
• Denial	• Sorrow, chronic
• Family processes, interrupted	• Spiritual distress
• Fear	• Spiritual well-being, potential to improve
• Grieving, potential for complicated	• Verbal communication, altered
• Grieving, complicated	
• Hopelessness	

TABLE 13.9   **NURSING DIAGNOSES**
Physical Manifestations of the End of Life

• Airway clearance, reduced	• Oral mucous membrane, altered
• Aspiration, potential for	• Pain, acute
• Bed mobility, reduced	• Pain, chronic
• Bowel incontinence	• Mobility, reduced
• Breathing pattern, altered	• Self-care deficits
• Cardiac output, decreased	• Skin integrity, potential for altered
• Constipation	• Skin integrity, altered
• Diarrhea	• Swallowing, altered
• Fatigue	• Thermoregulation, altered
• Gas exchange, inadequate	• Tissue integrity, potential for altered
• Infection, potential for	• Tissue integrity, altered
• Injury, potential for	• Tissue perfusion, reduced
• Nausea	• Incontinence, functional urinary
• Nutrition, altered: less than body requirements	

patients and families. Nursing care goals during the last stages of life involve comfort and safety measures and care of the patient's emotional and physical needs. These goals should also include determining where the patient would prefer to die and whether this is possible. Many factors contribute to the decision of the patient and family; for example, the patient may prefer to die at home, but the family may not be in favour of this because of inadequate support. End-of-life care should always be interprofessional and may include the physician, nurse, social worker, chaplain, and other members of the palliative care team. The nurse should advocate for the patient so that their wishes are met as much as possible (CNA, 2017).

NURSING IMPLEMENTATION

Psychosocial and physical care are interrelated for both the dying patient and the family. Support and education are important components of end-of-life care. Patients and families need ongoing information regarding the disease, the dying process, and any care that will be provided. They need information on how to cope with the many issues during this period of their lives. Anxiety and grief may be barriers to learning and understanding at the end of life for both the patient and their family.

PSYCHOSOCIAL CARE. As the patient's death approaches, the nurse should encourage the family to respond appropriately to the psychosocial manifestations of the end of life. Table 13.10 presents management of psychosocial manifestations near death.

Anxiety and Depression. Patients often exhibit signs of anxiety and depression during the end-of-life period. Anxiety is an uneasy feeling whose cause is not easily identified. Anxiety is frequently a result of fear.

TABLE 13.10   NURSING MANAGEMENT
Psychosocial Care at the End of Life

Characteristic	Nursing Management
Withdrawal A patient near death may seem withdrawn from the physical environment; however, the patient may be able to hear but unable to respond.	• Converse as though the patient were alert, using a soft voice and gentle touch.
Unusual Communication This may indicate that an unresolved issue is preventing the dying person from letting go. The patient may become restless and agitated or perform repetitive tasks (may also indicate terminal delirium).	• Encourage the family to talk with and reassure the dying person.
Vision-Like Experiences The patient may talk to people who are not there or see places and objects not visible. Vision-like experiences assist the dying person in coming to terms with meaning in life and transition from it.	• Affirm the dying person's experience as a part of transition from this life.
Saying Goodbyes It is important for the patient and family to acknowledge their sadness, mutually forgive one another, and say goodbye.	• Encourage the dying person and family to verbalize their feelings of sadness, loss, and forgiveness and to touch, hug, and cry. • Allow the patient and family privacy to express their feelings and comfort one another.
Spiritual Needs The patient or family may request spiritual support, such as the presence of a spiritual care provider.	• Assess spiritual needs. Allow patient to express their spiritual needs. • Encourage visit by appropriate spiritual care service provider such as a chaplain, priest, rabbi, or family member.

Causes of anxiety and depression may include uncontrolled pain and dyspnea, psychosocial factors related to the disease process or impending death, altered physiological states, and medications. Encouragement, support, and teaching decrease some of the anxiety and depression. Management of anxiety and depression may include both medications and nonpharmacological interventions. Relaxation strategies including breathing techniques, muscle relaxation, music, and imagery may be useful. (Complementary and alternative therapies are discussed in Chapter 12.)

Anger. Anger is a common and normal response in the grief process. A grieving person cannot be forced to accept loss. The surviving family members may be angry with the dying loved one who is leaving them. The nurse should encourage the expression of feelings, but at the same time realize how difficult it is to come to terms with loss. The nurse may be the target of the anger; however, it is critical to understand the source of the expressed emotion and not to react on a personal level.

Hopelessness and Powerlessness. Feelings of hopelessness and powerlessness are common during the end-of-life period. The nurse should encourage realistic hope within the limits of the situation. The patient and family should be allowed to deal with what is within their control, and the nurse should help them to recognize what is beyond their control. The nurse should support the patient's involvement in decision making about care, when possible, to foster a sense of control and autonomy.

Fear. Fear is a common emotion associated with dying. Four specific fears associated with dying are fear of pain, fear of shortness of breath, fear of loneliness and abandonment, and fear of meaninglessness.

Fear of Pain. Many people assume that pain always accompanies dying and death. Physiologically, there is no absolute indication that death is always painful. Psychologically, pain may result from the anxieties and separations related to dying. Patients can participate in their own pain control by discussing pain relief measures and their effects. Patients who experience

physical pain should have pain-relieving medications available around the clock (Pereira, 2016). Nurses must assure the patient and family that medications will be given promptly when needed and that adverse effects can and will be managed. Reassessment of pain after medications are given is an important nursing action. Most patients want their pain relieved without the adverse effects of grogginess or sleepiness. Pain relief measures do not have to deprive the patient of the ability to interact with others.

Fear of Shortness of Breath. Respiratory distress and dyspnea occur in some patients near the end of life. The sensation of breathlessness often results in anxiety for both the patient and family. Current therapies may include opioids, bronchodilators, and oxygen, depending on the cause of the dyspnea. Anxiety-reducing medications (anxiolytics) may help produce relaxation.

Fear of Loneliness and Abandonment. Most dying patients fear loneliness and do not want to be alone. Many are afraid that loved ones who are unable to cope with the patient's imminent death will abandon them. The simple presence of someone provides support and comfort. Holding hands, touching, and listening are important nursing interventions. Providing companionship allows the dying person a sense of security.

Fear of Meaninglessness. Fear of meaninglessness leads most people to review their lives. They review their intentions during life, examining actions and expressing regrets about what might have been. *Life review* helps patients recognize the value of their lives. Nurses can assist patients and their families in identifying the positive qualities of the patient's life. Practical ways of helping may include looking at photo albums or collections of important mementos. Sharing thoughts and feelings may enhance spirituality and provide comfort for the patient. A patient may wish to leave a legacy through writing letters to read or making a video to be viewed at future events when they will no longer be present. Nurses must respect and accept the practices and rituals associated with the patient's life review while remaining nonjudgemental.

COMMUNICATION. No two conversations are the same, inasmuch as they are shaped by the unique circumstances, coping styles, and personalities of the individuals involved. Difficult discussions include any information that adversely affects one's expectations for the future. How the person experiences and processes difficult news is dependent on not only the words used but also how the message is delivered (Boles, 2015). Nurses may use several approaches to difficult conversations that share common features. Suggested approaches are "ask–tell–ask," "tell me more," responding to emotions with the NURSE protocol (**n**aming, **u**nderstanding, **r**especting, **s**upporting, and **e**xploring) and the SPIKES six-step protocol (**s**etup, **p**erception, **i**nvitation, **k**nowledge, **e**mpathize, and **s**ummarize and **s**trategize) (Back et al., 2005).

Effective communication techniques used in conversations among the interprofessional team, patient, and family are essential. Empathy and active listening are key communication components in end-of-life care. *Empathy* is the identification with and understanding of another person's situation, feelings, and motives. *Active listening*, an active process required in the development of empathy toward another person's feeling, is paying attention to what is said, observing the patient's nonverbal cues, and not interrupting.

There may also be silence. Silence is frequently related to the overwhelming feelings experienced at the end of life. Silence can also allow time to gather thoughts. Listening to the silence sends a message of acceptance and comfort. The nurse's communication also must show respect for the patient's ethnic, cultural, and religious backgrounds.

Patients and family members may have difficulties expressing themselves emotionally. The nurse must allow time for them to express their feelings and thoughts, making time to listen and interact in a sensitive way. A family conference is one way to create an environment more conducive to large group conversations.

Family members need to be prepared for changes in emotional and cognitive function that occur at end of the patient's life. Unusual communication by the patient may take place at the end of life. The patient's speech may become confused, disoriented, or garbled. Patients may speak to or about family members or others who have predeceased them, give instructions to those who will survive them, or speak of projects yet to be completed. Active, careful listening allows for the identification of specific patterns in the dying person's communication and decreases the risk of inappropriate labelling of behaviours.

PHYSICAL CARE. Nursing management related to physical care at the end of life focuses on symptom management and comfort rather than treatments for cure (Table 13.11). The priority is meeting the patient's physiological and safety needs. Physical care addresses the needs for oxygen, nutrition, pain relief, mobility, elimination, and skin care. People who are dying deserve and require the same physical care as that of patients who are expected to recover. If possible, it is important to discuss with the patient and family the goals of care before treatment begins. Documentation of the discussion regarding wishes and preferences may take the form of an advance directive or simply be recorded in the medical chart to clearly communicate with the interprofessional team.

POSTMORTEM CARE. The pronouncement of death is not a reserved act or a delegated medical function and is within the scope of nursing practice for an expected death related to a terminal illness (Canadian Medical Protective Association, 2019).

Although the death is anticipated, the pronouncement of death should be made with certainty and compassion. Death is considered to have occurred when cardiac and respiratory functions have ceased. The **pronouncement of death** is verification of the absence of an apical pulse and respirations, and the presence of fixed and dilated pupils. A **certification of death**—a legal medical document stating that the patient is dead—is usually required within 24 hours of a death. This function is in the purview of a physician, nurse practitioner, or medical examiner, who is required to both sign the document and indicate the cause of death (Canadian Medical Protective Association, 2019).

After death is pronounced, the nurse prepares or delegates preparation of the body for immediate viewing by the family, with consideration for cultural customs and in accord with employer policies and procedures. In some cultures, it may be important to allow the family to prepare or assist in caring for the body. In general, the nurse should close the eyes, replace dentures, wash the body as needed (placing pads under the perineum to absorb urine and feces), and remove tubes and dressings (if appropriate). The body is straightened, the pillow is positioned to support the head, and a small rolled towel is placed under the chin to hold the mouth closed.

The family should be allowed privacy and as much time as they need with the deceased person. In the case of an unexpected death, preparation of the patient's body for viewing or release to a funeral home depends on provincial law and employer policies and procedures. The deceased person should never be referred to as "the body." Care of and discussion related to the person should continue to be respectful even after death.

SPECIAL NEEDS OF CAREGIVERS IN END-OF-LIFE CARE

Special Needs of Family Caregivers

Family caregivers are important in meeting the patient's physical and psychosocial needs. The role of caregivers includes working and communicating with the patient and family members, supporting the patient's concerns, and helping the patient resolve any unfinished business. Families often face emotional, physical, and economic consequences as a result of caring for a family member who is dying. The caregiver's responsibilities do not end when the person is admitted to an acute care, hospice, or long-term care facility.

Being present during a family member's dying process can be highly stressful. The nurse should recognize signs and behaviours among family members who may be at risk for abnormal grief reactions and be prepared to intervene, if necessary. Warning signs of abnormal grief may include dependency and negative feelings about the dying person, inability to express feelings, sleep disturbances, a history of depression, difficult reactions to previous losses, perceived lack of social or family support, low self-esteem, multiple previous losses, alcoholism, or substance misuse. Caregivers with concurrent life crises (e.g., divorce) may be especially at risk.

Family caregivers and other family members need encouragement to continue their usual activities where possible in order to maintain some control over their lives. The nurse should inform caregivers about appropriate resources for support, including respite care. Resources such as community counselling and local support may assist some people in working through their grief. The nurse should encourage caregivers to accept support from extended family, friends, and community.

TABLE 13.11 NURSING MANAGEMENT
Physical Care at the End of Life

Characteristics	Nursing Management
Pain • May be a major symptom associated with terminal illness and is the one most feared • Can be acute or chronic • Possible causes of bone pain: metastases, fractures, arthritis, and immobility • Aggravated by physical and emotional stressors	• Assess pain thoroughly and regularly to determine the quality, intensity, location, and contributing and alleviating factors. • Minimize possible irritants such as wet skin, heat or cold, and pressure. • Administer medications around the clock in a timely manner and on a regular basis to provide constant relief, rather than waiting until the pain is unbearable and then trying to relieve it. • Provide complementary and alternative therapies such as guided imagery, massage, and relaxation techniques as needed (see Chapter 12). • Evaluate effectiveness of pain relief measures frequently to ensure that the patient is on a correct, adequate drug regimen. • Do not delay or deny pain relief measures to a terminally ill patient.
Delirium • A state characterized by confusion, disorientation, restlessness, clouding of consciousness, incoherence, fear, anxiety, excitement, and often hallucinations • May be misidentified as depression, psychosis, anger, or anxiety • May be caused by use of opioids or corticosteroids, as well as by their withdrawal • May be exacerbated by underlying disease process • Generally considered a reversible process	• Perform a thorough assessment for reversible causes of delirium, including pain, constipation, and urinary retention. • Provide a room that is quiet, well lit, and familiar to reduce the effects of delirium. • Reorient the dying person with delirium to person, place, and time with each encounter. • Administer ordered benzodiazepines and sedatives as needed. • Stay physically close to a frightened patient. Reassure in a calm, soft voice with touch and slow strokes of the skin. • Provide family with emotional support and encouragement in their efforts to cope with the behaviours associated with delirium.
Anxiety/Restlessness • May occur as death approaches and cerebral metabolism slows • May occur with tachypnea, dyspnea, or sweating	• Assess for previous anxiety disorder. • Assess for spiritual distress or concerns related to death as causes of restlessness and agitation. • Assess for urinary retention and stool impaction. • Do not restrain. • Use soothing music; slow, soft touch; and a calm, soft voice. • Limit the number of people at the patient's bedside.
Dysphagia • May occur because of extreme weakness and changes in level of consciousness • Difficulty swallowing • Aspiration of liquids or solids, or both • Drooling/inability to swallow secretions	• Identify the least invasive alternative routes of administration for drugs needed for symptom management. • If necessary, use alternative (rectal, buccal, transdermal) medication routes. • Suction orally as needed. • Modify diet as tolerated or desired (soft, pureed, chopped meats). • Hand-feed small meals. • Elevate the patient's head for meals and for at least 30 minutes after. • Discontinue nonessential medications. • Discuss risk of aspiration with patient and family.
Weakness and Fatigue • Expected at the end of life • Exacerbated by metabolic demands related to disease process	• Assess the patient's tolerance for activities. • Time nursing interventions to conserve the patient's energy. • Help the patient identify and complete valued or desired activities. • Provide support as needed to maintain the patient's positions in bed or a chair. • Provide frequent rest periods for the patient.
Dehydration • May occur during the last days of life • Hunger and thirst are rare in the last days of life • Tendency for dying patients to take in less food and fluid	• Assess mucous membranes frequently for dryness, which can lead to discomfort. • Maintain complete, regular oral care to provide for comfort and hydration of mucous membranes. • Encourage consumption of ice chips and sips of fluids or use moist cloths to provide moisture to the mouth. • Use moist cloths and swabs for an unconscious patient to prevent aspiration. • Apply lubricant to the lips and oral mucous membranes as needed. • Do not force the patient to eat or drink. • Teach the family that hunger and thirst are rare in the last days of life. • Reassure the family that cessation of food and fluid intake is a natural part of the process of dying.

Continued

TABLE 13.11 NURSING MANAGEMENT

Physical Care at the End of Life—cont'd

Characteristics	Nursing Management
Dyspnea • Subjective symptom • Accompanied by fear of suffocation and anxiety • Can be exacerbated by underlying disease process • Progressive difficulty with coughing and expectorating secretions	• Assess respiratory status regularly. • Elevate the patient's head or position the patient on one side to improve chest expansion. • Use a fan or air conditioner to facilitate movement of cool air. • Teach and encourage the use of pursed-lip breathing. • Administer supplemental oxygen as ordered. • Suction as necessary to remove accumulation of mucus from the airways. Suction cautiously when a patient is in the terminal phase. • Administer expectorant as ordered.
Myoclonus • Mild to severe jerking or twitching, sometimes associated with use of high dose of opioids • Possible reports of involuntary twitching of extremities	• Assess for initial onset, duration, and any discomfort or distress experienced by patient. • If myoclonus is distressing or becoming more severe, discuss possible medication therapy modifications with the health care provider. • Changes in opioid medication may alleviate or decrease myoclonus.
Skin Breakdown • Difficulty maintaining skin integrity at the end of life • Risk for development increased by immobility, urinary and bowel incontinence, dry skin, nutritional deficits, anemia, friction, and shearing forces • Skin integrity possibly impaired by disease and other processes • As death approaches, decrease of circulation to the extremities; they become cool, mottled, and cyanotic	• Assess skin for signs of breakdown. • Implement protocols to prevent skin breakdown by controlling drainage and odor and by keeping the skin and any wound areas clean. • Perform wound assessments as needed. • Follow appropriate nursing management policy for dressing wounds. • Follow appropriate nursing management policy for a patient who is immobile but consider realistic outcomes of skin integrity in relation to maintenance of comfort. • Follow appropriate nursing management to prevent skin irritations and breakdown from urinary and bowel incontinence. • Use blankets to cover for warmth. Never apply heat. • Prevent the effects of shearing forces.
Bowel Patterns • Constipation possibly caused by immobility, use of opioid medications, depression, lack of fibre in the diet, and dehydration • Diarrhea possible as muscles relax or as a result of fecal impaction related to the use of opioids and immobility	• Assess bowel function. • Assess for and remove fecal impactions. • Encourage movement and physical activities as tolerated. • Encourage fibre in the diet if appropriate. • Encourage fluid intake if appropriate. • Use suppositories, stool softeners, laxatives, or enemas if ordered. • Assess patient for confusion, agitation, restlessness, and pain, which may be signs of constipation.
Urinary Incontinence • May result from disease progression or changes in level of consciousness • Relaxation of perineal muscles soon before death	• Assess urinary function. • Use absorbent pads for urinary incontinence. • Follow appropriate nursing protocol for the consideration and use of in-dwelling or external catheters. • Follow appropriate nursing management to prevent skin irritations and breakdown from urinary incontinence.
Anorexia, Nausea, and Vomiting • May be caused by complications of disease process • Nausea exacerbated by drugs • All exacerbated by constipation, impaction, and bowel obstruction	• Assess patient for reports of nausea or vomiting. • Assess possible contributing causes of nausea or vomiting. • Have family provide the patient's favorite foods. • Discuss modifications to the drug regimen with the health care provider. • Provide antiemetics before meals if ordered. • Offer and provide frequent meals with small portions of favorite foods. • Offer culturally appropriate foods. • Provide frequent mouth care, especially after the patient vomits. • Ensure uninterrupted mealtimes. • If ordered, administer medications (e.g., megestrol, corticosteroids) to increase appetite. • Teach family that appetite naturally decreases at the end of life.
Candidiasis • White, cottage cheese–like oral plaques • Fungal overgrowth in the mouth as a result of chemotherapy, immunosuppression, or both	• Administer oral antifungal nystatin if ordered. • Clean dentures and other dental appliances to prevent reinfection. • Provide oral hygiene and use a soft toothbrush.

Special Needs of Nurses

Many nurses who care for dying patients do so because they are passionate about providing high-quality end-of-life care. Caring for patients and their families at the end of life is challenging and rewarding but also intense and emotionally charged (Larkin et al., 2019). A bond or connection may develop between the nurse and the patient or family. The nurse should be aware of how grief personally affects them. When the nurse provides care for dying patients, the nurse is not immune to feelings of loss. It is common to feel helpless and powerless when dealing with death. The nurse may need to express feelings of sorrow, guilt, and frustration. It is important to recognize one's own values, attitudes, and feelings about death (Zheng et al., 2018).

Interventions are available that may help ease the nurse's physical and emotional stress. The nurse should be aware of what they can and cannot control. Recognizing personal feelings allows openness in exchanging feelings with the patient and family. Realizing that it is okay to cry with the patient or family may be important for the nurse's well-being.

To meet the nurse's personal needs, they should focus on interventions that will help decrease stress. The nurse can get involved in hobbies or other interests, schedule time for themselves, ensure time for sleep, maintain a peer support system, and develop a support system beyond the workplace. Specialized hospice palliative care teams can help the nurse cope through professionally assisted groups, informal discussion sessions, and flexible time schedules.

REVIEW QUESTIONS

The number of the question corresponds to the same-numbered objective at the beginning of the chapter.

1. What is the purpose of palliative care?
   a. To provide psychological support
   b. To prolong life
   c. To hasten death
   d. To improve quality of life

2. A client with metastatic lung cancer is imminently dying. On assessment, it is noted that she has alternating periods of apnea and deep, rapid breathing. Which of the following is the correct terminology to use in documenting this assessment data?
   a. Tachypnea
   b. Stertorous respirations
   c. Dyspnea
   d. Cheyne-Stokes respirations

3. The client has inoperable pancreatic cancer. Until recently, he has been very active in a book club but no longer wants to attend. Which common end-of-life psychological manifestation is he demonstrating?
   a. Decreased socialization
   b. Decreased disease progression
   c. Decreased sense of helplessness
   d. Decreased perception of pain and touch

4. A client died 2 years ago but his wife refuses to donate his belongings to charity. She often sits in the bedroom, crying and talking to her deceased husband. What type of grief is his wife experiencing?
   a. Adaptive grief
   b. Disruptive grief
   c. Anticipatory grief
   d. Prolonged grief

5. A female client with end-stage renal disease experiences choking when given food or fluids. The family is concerned that she is starving. What is the most helpful response from the nurse? *(Select all that apply.)*
   a. "Allow me to show you how to moisten her mouth."
   b. "If you give her food, she will choke to death."
   c. "I can order you a tray and you can try to feed her if you like."
   d. "People who are dying usually don't experience hunger or thirst."

6. A client did not have an advance directive when he suffered a serious stroke. Who is responsible for identifying end-of-life measures to be instituted when he cannot communicate his specific wishes?
   a. Adult children
   b. Notary and attorney
   c. Physician and substitute decision maker
   d. Physician and nursing staff

7. When a male client was diagnosed with renal failure, his new wife asked his children from a previous marriage to help with their father's care. Each of the children refused to help and his wife cared for him without help until his death. Which factors may predispose the children to an abnormal grief reaction? *(Select all that apply.)*
   a. Negative feelings about the deceased person
   b. Lack of experience with other deaths in the family
   c. Difficulties with substance misuse
   d. Residing geographically far away

8. A nurse has been working full-time with clients with advanced illnesses for 3 years. The nurse has been experiencing irritability and mixed emotions when expressing sadness since four clients died on the same day. What should the nurse change to optimize the quality of her nursing care?
   a. Full-time work schedule
   b. Past feelings toward death
   c. Patterns for dealing with grief
   d. Demands for involvement in care

9. What is an important moral argument supporting medical assistance in dying?
   a. Respect for self-determined choice
   b. Mercy and respect for beneficence
   c. Dignity in dying
   d. All of the above

1. d; 2. d; 3. a; 4. d; 5. a, d; 6. c; 7. a, b, c, d; 8. c; 9. d

Ⓔvolve

For even more review questions, visit http://evolve.elsevier.com/Canada/Lewis/medsurg.

REFERENCES

Abarshi, E. A., Papavasiliou, E. R., Preston, N., et al. (2014). The complexity of nurses' attitudes and practice of sedation at the end of life: A systematic review. *Journal of Pain and Symptom Management, 47*(5), 915–925. https://doi.org/10.1016/j.jpainsymman.2013.06.011. http://www.jpsmjournal.com/article/S0885-3924(13)00396-5/pdf. (Seminal).

Alberta Health Services. (2018). *Provincial clinical knowledge topic; Palliative sedation, adults—All locations. V1.0.* https://extranet.ah

snet.ca/teams/policydocuments/1/klink/et-klink-ckv-palliative-sedation-adult-all-locations.pdf

Back, A. L., Arnold, R. M., Baile, W. F., et al. (2005). Approaching difficult communication tasks in oncology. *A Cancer Journal for Clinicians, 55,* 164–177. https://doi.org/10.3322/canjclin.55.3.164. (Seminal).

Bester, J., & Kodish, E. (2019). Cardiopulmonary resuscitation, informed consent, and rescue: What provides moral justification for the provision of CPR? *The Journal of Clinical Ethics, 30*(1), 67–73.

Boles, J. (2015). Bearing bad news: Supporting patients and families through difficult conversations. *Pediatric Nursing, 41*(6), 306–308.

Caldeira, S., Campos Carvalho, E., & Vieira, M. (2013). Spiritual distress – Proposing a new definition and defining characteristics. *International Journal of Nursing Knowledge, 24*(2), 77–84. https://doi.org/10.1111/j.2047-3095.2013.01234.x. (Seminal).

Canadian Hospice Palliative Care Association (CHPCA). (2013a). *A model to guide hospice palliative care: Based on national principles and norms of practice (revised and condensed ed.).* https://www.chpca.ca/wp-content/uploads/2019/12/norms-of-practice-eng-web.pdf

Canadian Hospice Palliative Care Association (CHPCA). (2013b). *Innovative models of integrated hospice palliative care. The Way Forward Initiative: An integrated approach to care.* http://www.hpcintegration.ca/media/40546/TWF-innovative-models-report-Eng-webfinal-2.pdf. (Seminal).

Canadian Hospice Palliative Care Association (CHPCA). (2015). *The way forward national framework: A roadmap for an integrated palliative approach to care.* http://www.hpcintegration.ca/media/60044/TWF-framework-doc-Eng-2015-final-April1.pdf. (Seminal).

Canadian Hospice Palliative Care Association (CHPCA). (2020). *Saying Goodbye campaign.* https://www.chpca.ca/campaigns/saying-goodbye/

Canadian Medical Protective Association. (2019). *Completing medical certificates of death: Who's responsible?.* https://www.cmpa-acpm.ca/en/advice-publications/browse-articles/2016/completing-medical-certificates-of-death-who-s-responsible

Canadian Nurses Association (CNA). (2017). *Code of ethics for registered nurses.* https://www.cna-aiic.ca/en/nursing-practice/nursing-ethics

Canadian Nurses Association, Canadian Hospice Palliative Care Association, & Canadian Hospice Palliative Care Nurses Group. (2015). *Joint position statement—The palliative approach to care and the role of the nurse.* https://www.cna-aiic.ca/-/media/cna/page-content/pdf-en/the-palliative-approach-to-care-and-the-role-of-the-nurse_e.pdf

Carstairs, S. (2000). *Quality end-of-life care: The right of every Canadian.* Subcommittee to update "Of Life and Death" of the Standing Senate Committee on Social Affairs, Science and Technology. Final report. https://sencanada.ca/content/sen/committee/362/upda/rep/repfinjun00-e.htm. (Seminal).

Chochinov, H. (2002). Dignity-conserving care – A new model for palliative care. *The Journal of the American Medical Association, 287*(17), 2253–2260. https://doi.org/10.1001/jama.287.17.2253. (Seminal).

Conlon, M. S., Caswell, J. M., Santi, S. A., et al. (2019). Access to palliative care for cancer patients living in a northern and rural environment in Ontario, Canada: The effects of geographic region and rurality on end-of-life care in a population-based decedent cancer cohort. *Clinical Medicine Insights: Oncology, 13,* 1–10. https://doi.org/10.1177/1179554919829500

Cook, D., Rocker, G., & Heyland, D. (2013). Enhancing the quality of end-of-life care in Canada. *Canadian Medical Association Journal, 185*(16), 1383–1384. https://doi.org/10.1503/cmaj.130716

Fraser Health Authority. (2009). *Symptom assessment acronym.* https://www.fraserhealth.ca/-/media/Project/FraserHealth/Frase rHealth/Health-Professionals/Professionals-Resources/Hospice-palliative-care/SymptomAssessmentRevised_Sept09.pdf. (Seminal).

Ganz, F. D., & Sapir, B. (2019). Nurses' perceptions of intensive care unit palliative care at end of life. *Nursing in Critical Care, 24*(3), 141–148. https://doi.org/10.1111/nicc.12395

Government of Canada. (2016). *Bill C-14: An act to amend the criminal code and to make related amendments to other acts (Medical Assistance in Dying)* (June 17). Royal Assent. http://www.parl.ca/DocumentViewer/en/42-1/bill/C-14/royal-assent

Government of Canada. (2018). *Regulations for the monitoring of Medical Assistance in Dying.* https://laws-lois.justice.gc.ca/eng/regulations/SOR-2018-166/FullText.html

Government of Canada. (2020). *Bill C-7: An act to amend the criminal code (Medical Assistance in Dying).* https://www.parl.ca/DocumentViewer/en/43-1/bill/C-7/first-reading

Government of Canada. (2021). *EI caregiving benefits and leave: What caregiving benefits offer.* https://www.canada.ca/en/services/benefits/ei/caregiving.html

Hagerty, T., Velázquez, Á., Schmidt, J. M., et al. (2016). Assessment of satisfaction with care and decision-making among English and Spanish-speaking family members of neuroscience ICU patients. *Applied Nursing Research, 29,* 262–267. https://doi.org/10.1016/j.apnr.2015.02.002

Hampton, M., Baydale, A., Bourassa, C., et al. (2010). Completing the circle: Elders speak about end-of-life care with Aboriginal families in Canada. *Journal of Palliative Care, 26*(1), 6–14. https://doi.org/10.1177/082585971002600103. (Limited Publications) (Seminal).

Health Canada. (2019). *Framework on palliative care in Canada. Catalogue no. H22-4/16-2018E-PDF.* https://www.canada.ca/en/health-canada/services/health-care-system/reports-publications/palliative-care/framework-palliative-care-canada.html

Hui, D., & Bruera, E. (2017). The Edmonton Symptom Assessment System 25 years later: Past, present and future developments. *Journal of Pain and Symptom Management, 53*(3), 630–643. https://doi.org/10.1016/j.jpainsymman.2016.10.370

Hui, D., Dos Santos, R., Chisholm, G., et al. (2015). Bedside clinical signs associated with impending death in patients with advanced cancer: Preliminary findings of a prospective, longitudinal cohort study. *Cancer, 121*(6), 960–967. https://doi.org/10.1002/cncr.29048

Kübler-Ross, E. (1969). *On death and dying.* New York: Macmillan (Seminal).

Larkin, P., Errasti-Ibarrondo, M., McCormack, B., et al. (2019). Barriers and facilitators perceived by registered nurses to providing person-centred care at the end of life. A scoping review. *International Practice Development Journal, 9*(2), 1–22. https://doi.org/10.19043/ipdj.92.008

Li, M., Watt, S., Escaf, M., et al. (2017). Medical assistance in dying—implementing a hospital-based program in Canada. *New England Journal of Medicine, 376*(21), 2082–2088.

Lundorff, M., Holmgren, H., Zachariae, R., et al. (2017). Prevalence of prolonged grief disorder in adult bereavement: A systematic review and meta-analysis. *Journal of Affective Disorders, 212,* 138–149. https://doi.org/10.1016/j.jad.2017.01.030

Madore, O. (2005). *The Canada Health Act: Overview and options. Current issue review, 94-4E.* https://publications.gc.ca/collections/Collection-R/LoPBdP/CIR-e/944-e.pdf. (Seminal).

National Cancer Institute. (2020). *Grief, bereavement, and coping with loss (PDQ®)—Health professional version.* http://www.cancer.gov/about-cancer/advanced-cancer/caregivers/planning/bereavement-hp-pdq. (Seminal).

O'Brien, M. E. (2018). *Spirituality in nursing* (6th ed.). Jones & Bartlett Learning.

Ontario Trillium Gift of Life Network. (n.d.). Organ and tissue donation: Frequently asked questions for health professionals. www .giftoflife.on.ca/resources/pdf/FAQ_for_HP_(fact_sheet)_EN.pdf

Pereira, J. L. (2016). *The Pallium palliative pocketbook: A peer reviewed reference resource* (2nd ed.). Pallium Canada.

Quality End-of-Life Care Coalition of Canada (QELCCC). (2010). *Blueprint for action 2010 to 2020.* https://www.chpca.ca/wp-conten t/uploads/2020/01/eng_progress_report_20102012-07-10_2.pdf. (Seminal).

Quality End-of-Life Care Coalition of Canada (QELCCC). (2012). *Executive summary* (Seminal) https://www.chpca.ca/wp-content/uplo ads//2020/01/microsoft_word_-_3_executive_summary_2012.pdf

Worden, J. W. (2009). *Grief counseling and grief therapy: A handbook for the mental health practitioner* (4th ed.). Springer (Seminal).

World Health Organization. (2021). *Palliative care.* http://www.who.in t/cancer/palliative/definition/en/

Zheng, R., Lee, S., & Bloomer, M. (2018). How nurses cope with patient death: A systematic review and qualitative meta-synthesis. *Journal of Clinical Nursing, 27*(1-2), E39–E49. https://doi. org/10.1111/jocn.13975

RESOURCES

Advance Care Planning
https://www.advancecareplanning.ca
Alberta Health Services: Goals of Care Designations
https://myhealth.alberta.ca/health/Pages/HealthVideoPlayer.aspx ?List=fde13c02%2D8aa3%2D41ec%2D920d%2Ded3c17022ba8& ID=762&Web=c310c9f6%2D9976%2D4384%2Db2af%2Dd167d9 8d0966

Canadian Cancer Society
https://www.cancer.ca
Canadian Home Care Association
https://www.cdnhomecare.ca/
Canadian Hospice Palliative Care Association
https://www.chpca.net
Canadian Virtual Hospice
http://www.virtualhospice.ca
Dignity in Care
https://dignityincare.ca
Life and Death Matters
https://www.lifeanddeathmatters.ca/reflecting-on-death-first-nations-people/
Pallium Canada
https://www.pallium.ca
Trillium Gift of Life Network
http://www.giftoflife.on.ca

Casey House Hospice
https://www.caseyhouse.com
Temmy Latner Centre for Palliative Care
http://www.tlcpc.org/
Victoria Hospice
http://www.victoriahospice.org
Victoria Hospice: Palliative Performance Scale
https://victoriahospice.org/how-we-can-help/clinical-tools/
Worldwide Hospice Palliative Care Alliance
http://www.thewhpca.org

evolve
For additional Internet resources, see the website for this book at http://evolve.elsevier.com/Canada/Lewis/medsurg.

Pathophysiological Mechanisms of Disease

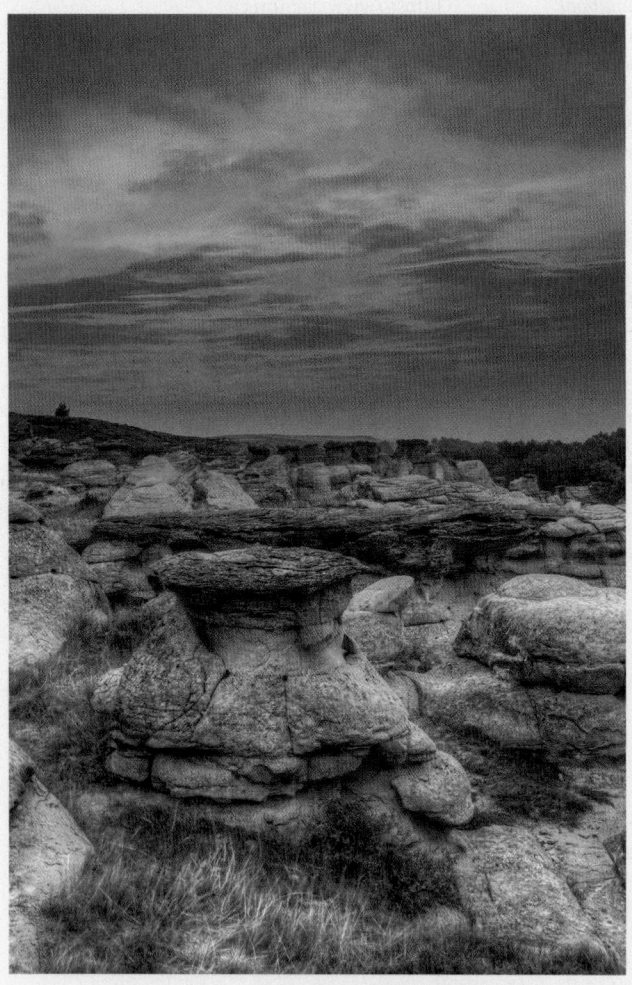

Source: © CanStock Photo/ronniechua

Inflammation and Wound Healing

Kevin Woo
Originating US chapter by Catherine R. Ratliff

ⓔvolve WEBSITE

http://evolve.elsevier.com/Canada/Lewis/medsurg

- Review Questions (Online Only)
- Key Points
- Answer Guidelines for Case Study
- Student Case Study
- Pressure Injuries
- Customizable Nursing Care Plans
- Fever
- Pressure Injury
- Audio Glossary
- Content Updates

LEARNING OBJECTIVES

1. Explain the mechanisms that enable the cell to adapt to sublethal injury.
2. Describe the causes and mechanisms of lethal cell injury.
3. Differentiate among types of cell necrosis.
4. Describe the components and functions of the mononuclear phagocyte system.
5. Describe the inflammatory response, including vascular and cellular responses and exudate formation.
6. Explain local and systemic manifestations of inflammation and their physiological bases.
7. Describe the pharmacological, dietary, and nursing management of inflammation.
8. Differentiate between healing by primary, secondary, and tertiary intention.
9. Describe the factors that delay wound healing and common complications of wound healing.
10. Describe the risk assessment process for pressure injuries.
11. Discuss measures to prevent the development of pressure injuries.
12. Explain the causes and clinical manifestations of pressure injuries.
13. Discuss interprofessional and nursing management of a patient with pressure injuries.

KEY TERMS

adhesions
anaplasia
apoptosis
atrophy
dehiscence
dry gangrene
dysplasia
evisceration
fibroblasts

fistula
hyperplasia
hypertrophic scar
hypertrophy
inflammatory response
integrins
keloid
lethal injury
metaplasia

necrosis
pressure injury
regeneration
repair
selectins
shearing force
sublethal injury
wet gangrene

CELL INJURY

Cell injury can be sublethal or lethal. **Sublethal injury** alters function without causing cell destruction. The changes caused by this type of injury are potentially reversible if the harmful stimulus is removed. **Lethal injury** is an irreversible process that causes cell death.

Cell Adaptation to Sublethal Injury

While cell adaptations to sublethal injuries are common and are part of many normal physiological processes, they may also result from pathological changes. For example, prolonged exposure to sunlight stimulates melanin production, which provides protection of deeper skin layers; increased melanin production causes tanning of the skin. Lack of muscular activity can lead to atrophy and decreased tone of muscles. Adaptive processes of the cell include hypertrophy, hyperplasia, atrophy, and metaplasia. Other responses, which are considered maladaptive, are dysplasia and anaplasia.

Hypertrophy. Hypertrophy is an expansion in the size of cells, which results in increased tissue mass without cell division. *Physiological hypertrophy* results from increased workload on an organ or tissue that is not caused by disease. Examples include an increase in the muscle mass that occurs during weight training, uterine expansion during pregnancy from hormonal stimulation, and enlargement of the sex organs during puberty. *Pathological hypertrophy* occurs as a result of disease—for example, enlargement and thickening of the heart ventricle in a person with severe hypertension in response to increased cardiac workload. *Compensatory hypertrophy* occurs in response to increased workload caused by reduced function. For example, when a kidney is removed, the remaining kidney enlarges as a result of increased work demand.

Hyperplasia. Hyperplasia is a multiplication of cells as a result of increased cellular division. *Physiological hyperplasia* is an adaptive response to normal body changes. For example, cells of the uterus undergo hyperplasia during pregnancy, and the female breast undergoes hyperplasia during puberty and lactation. Examples of *pathological hyperplasia* are endometrial hyperplasia, caused by excessive estrogen secretion, and acromegaly, caused by excessive production of growth hormone. *Compensatory hyperplasia* is a process whereby cells of certain organs regenerate. For example, if portions of the liver are removed, the remaining cells undergo increased mitosis to compensate.

Atrophy. Atrophy is a decrease in the size of a tissue or organ as a result of a reduction in the number or size of individual cells. It is frequently caused by disease (e.g., musculoskeletal disease), lack of blood supply (e.g., thrombus formation), the natural aging process (e.g., atrophy of ovaries after menopause), inactivity (e.g., decreased muscle size), or nutritional deficiency.

Metaplasia. Metaplasia is the transformation of one cell type into another in response to a change in physiological condition or an external irritant. An example of *physiological metaplasia* is the change of circulating monocytes to macrophages as they migrate into inflamed tissues. An example of *pathophysiological metaplasia* is the change of normal pseudostratified columnar epithelium of the bronchi to squamous epithelium in response to chronic cigarette smoking. These squamous cells can later become cancerous.

Dysplasia. Dysplasia is an abnormal differentiation of dividing cells that results in changes in their size, shape, and appearance. Minor dysplasia is found in some areas of inflammation. Dysplasia is potentially reversible if the stimulus for the change is removed. Dysplasia is frequently a precursor of malignancy, as in cervical dysplasia.

Anaplasia. Anaplasia is cell differentiation to a more immature or embryonic form. Malignant tumours are often characterized by anaplastic cell growth.

Causes of Lethal Cell Injury

Many different agents and factors can cause lethal cell injury (Table 14.1). The mechanisms of actual cell death may include deterioration of the nucleus, such as pyknosis (nuclear condensation and shrinking), karyolysis (dissolution of nucleus and contents), disruption of cell metabolism, and rupture of the cell membrane. Microbial invasion often results in cell injury and death. Infection occurs when pathogens invade and multiply in body tissue.

Cell Apoptosis and Necrosis

Apoptosis and necrosis are the two fundamental types of cell death. Programmed cell death, or apoptosis, is a normal, anticipated event that occurs in some regenerating tissues to create homeostasis, such as bone marrow, skin, and gut epithelium. In contrast, necrosis is tissue death that occurs as a result of a traumatic injury, infection, ischemia, or exposure to a toxic chemical that causes a local inflammatory response, which results from the release of intracellular contents after

TABLE 14.1	CAUSES OF LETHAL CELL INJURY
Cause	**Effect on Cell**
Hypoxia or ischemic injury	Compromised cell metabolism, acute or gradual cell death
Physical agents	
• Heat	Denaturation of protein, acceleration of metabolic reactions (see Chapter 27)
• Cold	Decreased blood flow from vasoconstriction, slowed metabolic reactions, thrombosis of blood vessels, freezing of cell contents that forms crystals and can cause cell to burst (see Chapter 71)
• Radiation	Alteration of cell structure and activity, alteration of enzyme systems, mutations (see Chapter 18)
• Electrothermal injury	Interruption of neural conduction, fibrillation of cardiac muscle, coagulative necrosis of skin and skeletal muscle (see Chapter 27)
• Mechanical trauma	Transfer of excess kinetic energy to cells, causing rupture of cells, blood vessels, tissue; examples include the following: *Abrasion:* scraping of skin or mucous membrane *Laceration:* severing of vessels and tissue *Contusion (bruise):* crushing of tissue cells, causing hemorrhage into skin *Puncture:* piercing of body structure or organ *Incision:* surgical cutting
Chemical injury	Alteration of cell metabolism, interference with normal enzymatic action within cells (see Chapter 27)
Microbial injury	
• Viruses	Taking over of cell metabolism and synthesis of new particles that may cause cell rupture; cumulative effect may produce clinical disease
• Bacteria	Destruction of cell membrane or cell nucleus, production of lethal toxins
Immunological*	
• Antigen–antibody response	Release of substances (histamine, complement) that can injure and damage cells
• Autoimmune response	Activation of complement, which destroys normal cells and produces inflammation (see Chapter 16)
Neoplastic growth	Cell destruction from abnormal and uncontrolled cell growth (see Chapter 18)
Normal substances (e.g., digestive enzymes, uric acid)	Release into abdomen, causing peritonitis and crystallization of excess accumulation in joints and renal tissue

*See Chapter 16 for a more detailed discussion.

the rupture of the outer membrane of the dead cells. Various types of tissue necrosis occur in different organs or tissues (Table 14.2; Figure 14.1).

Dry gangrene can result from degenerative changes that occur with certain chronic diseases, such as atherosclerosis or diabetes, when the blood supply to the lower extremities is gradually reduced (see Figure 14.1). Wet gangrene, which can quickly become fatal, occurs as the result of a sudden rapid elimination of blood flow, such as that seen in a severe burn or traumatic crush injury. It is malodorous because of extensive tissue liquefaction, which makes the affected area soft, and the odour is often indicative of a bacterial infection.

DEFENCE AGAINST INJURY

To protect against injury and infection, the body has various defence mechanisms: (a) the skin and mucous membranes (see Chapter 25); (b) the mononuclear phagocyte system; (c) the inflammatory response; and (d) the immune system (see Chapter 16).

Mononuclear Phagocyte System

The *mononuclear phagocyte system* consists of monocytes and macrophages and their precursor cells. In the past, the mononuclear phagocyte system was called the *reticuloendothelial system*. However, it is not a body system with distinctly defined tissues and organs. Rather, it consists of phagocytic cells located in

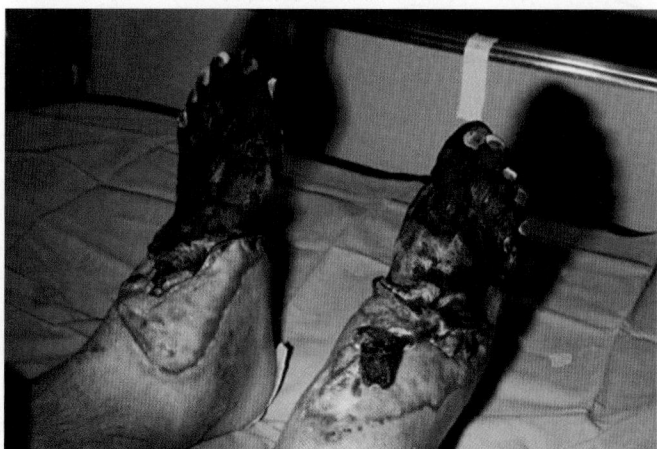

FIG. 14.1 Gangrene of the toes. Gangrenous necrosis 6 weeks after frostbite injury. Source: Courtesy of Cameron Bangs, MD. From Auerbach, P. S. (2007). *Wilderness medicine* (6th ed., p. 201). Elsevier.

various tissues and organs. The phagocytic cells are either fixed or free (mobile). The macrophages of the liver, spleen, bone marrow, lungs, lymph nodes, and nervous system are fixed phagocytes. The monocytes in blood and the macrophages found in connective tissue are mobile, or wandering, phagocytes.

Monocytes and macrophages originate in the bone marrow. Monocytes spend a few days in the blood and then enter tissues and change into macrophages. Tissue macrophages are larger and more phagocytic than monocytes.

The functions of the macrophage system include recognition and phagocytosis of foreign material such as microorganisms, removal of old or damaged cells from circulation, and participation in the immune response (see Chapter 16).

Inflammatory Response

The inflammatory response is a biological response to cell injury caused by pathogens, irritants, or chronic health conditions (e.g., arthritis). Through this response, the inflammatory agent is neutralized and diluted, necrotic materials are removed, and an environment suitable for healing and repair is established. The term *inflammation* should not be confused with *infection*. Infections almost always cause inflammation, but not all inflammations are caused by infections. Furthermore, neutropenic individuals may not mount an inflammatory response to infection. An infection involves invasion of tissues or cells by microorganisms such as bacteria, fungi, and viruses. Inflammation can also be caused by heat, radiation, trauma, chemicals, allergens, or an autoimmune reaction (see Table 14.1). Under these conditions, the presence of an infection represents a superimposed invasion of microorganisms.

The mechanism of inflammation is basically the same regardless of the injuring agent. The intensity of the response depends on the extent and the severity of injury and on the reactive capacity of the injured person. The inflammatory response can be divided into a vascular response, a cellular response, formation of exudate, and healing. Figure 14.2 illustrates the vascular and cellular responses to injury.

Vascular Response. After cell injury, arterioles in the area briefly undergo transient vasoconstriction, which is stimulated by the sympathetic nervous system. Platelets adhere to vessels and aggregate to seal the injured area, forming a fibrin-platelet clot, and they release proinflammatory mediators such as histamine, which cause vasodilation. This results in *hyperemia* (increased blood flow in the area) in which filtration pressure increases, causing endothelial cell retraction and an increase in capillary permeability. These vascular changes will facilitate movement of fluid from capillaries into tissue spaces. Initially

TABLE 14.2	TYPES OF NECROSIS
Type	**Description**
Coagulative necrosis	Caused by ischemia. Ischemia results in decreased levels of adenosine triphosphate (ATP), increased levels of cytosolic Ca^{2+}, and free radical formation, each of which eventually causes membrane damage. A myocardial infarct is an example of a localized area of coagulative necrosis.
Liquefactive necrosis	Usually caused by focal bacterial infections because they can attract polymorphonuclear leukocytes (PMNs). The enzymes in the PMNs are released to fight the bacteria but also dissolve the tissues nearby, which causes pus to accumulate and the tissue to liquefy. An abscess is an example of a liquefactive necrotic process.
Caseous necrosis	A distinct form of coagulative necrosis that occurs in mycobacterial infections (e.g., tuberculosis) or in tumour necrosis, in which the coagulated tissue no longer resembles the cells but is in chunks of unrecognizable debris.
Gangrene	Necrosis of an appendage (usually the limbs). The term may also be used to describe necrosis of an appendix or gallbladder. This form of necrosis applies to ischemic necrosis, usually with superimposed bacterial action (wet gangrene) but sometimes in toes without bacterial effects (dry gangrene or mummification).

Source: Adapted from Krafts, K. (2012). *A quick summary of six types of necrosis*. http://www.pathologystudent.com/?p=5770

PATHOPHYSIOLOGY MAP

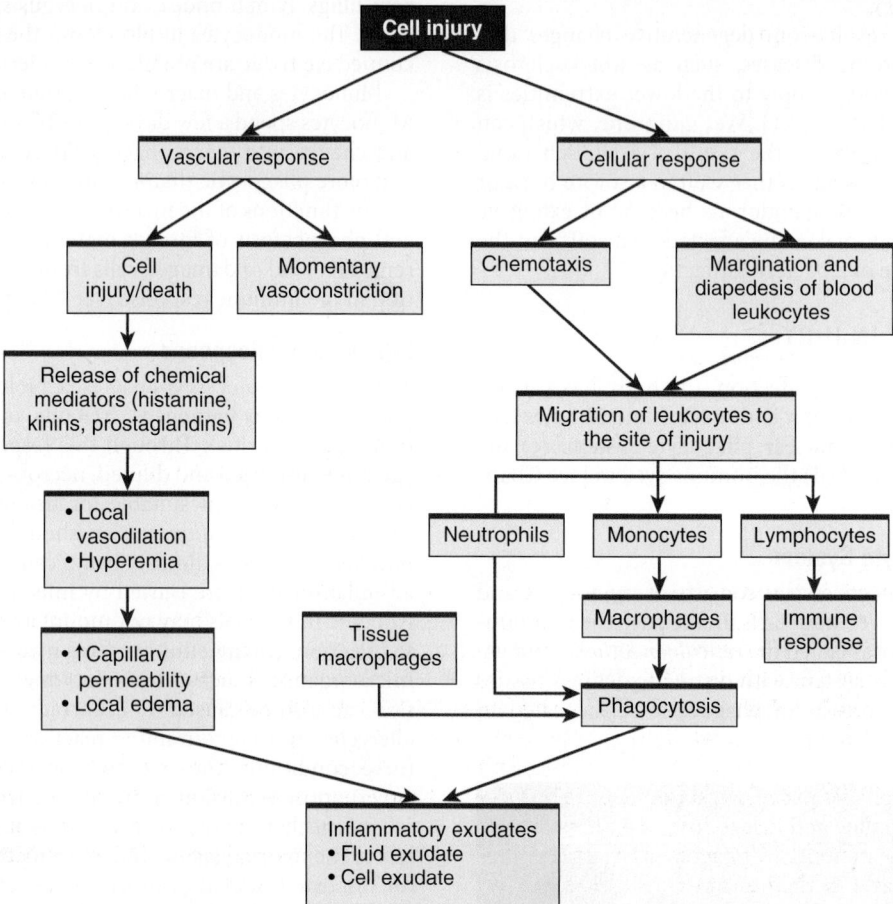

FIG. 14.2 Vascular and cellular responses in inflammation.

composed of serous fluid, this inflammatory exudate later contains plasma proteins, primarily albumin, which exerts oncotic pressure that further draws fluid from blood vessels, and the tissue become edematous.

As the plasma protein fibrinogen leaves the blood, it is activated by the products of the injured cells to become fibrin. Fibrin strengthens the blood clot formed by platelets. In tissue, the clot functions to minimize blood loss, trap bacteria, prevent their spread, and serve as a framework for the healing process. Platelets release growth factors that begin the healing process.

Cellular Response. Phagocytes produce nitric oxide, whose role in the inflammatory response is to inhibit vascular smooth muscle contraction and growth, platelet aggregation, and leukocyte adhesion to endothelium. Cytokines are released by macrophages, which causes endothelial cells to express cellular adhesion molecules: selectins (cell surface carbohydrate-binding proteins that mediate cell adhesion, involved in leukocyte extravasation during the immune response) and integrins (cell receptors that mediate attachment between endothelial cells and surrounding tissues, also involved in leukocyte extravasation during the immune response). The blood flow through capillaries in the area slows as fluid is lost and viscosity increases. Neutrophils and monocytes move to the inner surface of the capillaries (margination) and then, in ameboid manner, through the capillary wall (diapedesis) to the site of injury.

Chemotaxis is the directional migration of white blood cells (WBCs) along a concentration gradient of chemotactic factors, which are substances that attract WBCs to the site of inflammation. Chemotaxis is the mechanism for ensuring accumulation of neutrophils and monocytes at the site of injury.

Neutrophils. Neutrophils are the first leukocytes to arrive at the site of inflammation (within 6 to 12 hours). They phagocytize (engulf) bacteria, other foreign material, and damaged cells. Because of their short lifespan (24 to 48 hours), dead neutrophils soon accumulate. In time, a mixture of dead neutrophils, digested bacteria, and other cell debris collect as a creamy substance (pus).

To keep up with the demand for neutrophils, the bone marrow releases more neutrophils into circulation. This results in an elevated WBC count, especially the neutrophil count. Sometimes the demand for neutrophils increases to the extent that the bone marrow releases immature forms of neutrophils (bands) into circulation. (Mature neutrophils are called *segmented neutrophils.*) The finding of increased numbers of band neutrophils in circulation is called *a shift to the left* and is commonly observed in patients with acute bacterial infections. (See Chapter 32 for a discussion of neutrophils.)

Monocytes. Monocytes are the second type of phagocytic cells that migrate from circulating blood. They are attracted by chemotactic factors and usually arrive at the site within 3 to 7 days after the onset of inflammation. On entering the tissue

TABLE 14.3 MEDIATORS OF INFLAMMATION

Mediator	Source	Mechanisms of Action
Histamine	Stored in granules of basophils, mast cells, platelets	Causes vasodilation and increased vascular permeability by stimulating contraction of endothelial cells and creating widened gaps between cells
Serotonin	Stored in platelets, mast cells, enterochromaffin cells of GI tract	Causes vasodilation and increased vascular permeability by stimulating contraction of endothelial cells and creating widened gaps between cells; stimulates smooth muscle contraction
Kinins (e.g., bradykinin)	Produced from precursor factor kininogen as a result of activation of Hageman factor (XII) of clotting system	Cause contraction of smooth muscle and dilation of blood vessels; result in stimulation of pain
Complement components (C3a, C4a, C5a)	Anaphylatoxic agents generated from complement pathway activation	Stimulate histamine release; stimulate chemotaxis
Fibrinopeptides	Produced from activation of the clotting system	Increase vascular permeability; stimulate chemotaxis for neutrophils and monocytes
Prostaglandins and leukotrienes	Produced from arachidonic acid	Prostaglandins E_1 and E_2 cause vasodilation; leukotriene B_4 stimulates chemotaxis
Cytokines	Secreted by white blood cells and other cells. For more information on cytokines, see Table 16.3.	Act as messengers between cell types; instruct cells to alter their proliferation differentiation, secretion, or activity

GI, gastrointestinal.

spaces, monocytes transform into macrophages. Together with the tissue macrophages, they assist in phagocytosis of the inflammatory debris. The macrophage role is important in cleaning the area before healing can occur. Macrophages have a long lifespan; they may stay in the damaged tissues for weeks and multiply, and they are important in orchestrating the healing process.

In some cases, macrophages perform tasks other than phagocytosis. They may accumulate and fuse to form a *multinucleated giant cell.* The giant cell attempts to phagocytize particles too large for macrophages and is then encapsulated by collagen, which leads to the formation of a granuloma. A classic example of this process occurs in tuberculosis of the lung. Although the *Mycobacterium* bacillus is walled off, a chronic state of inflammation exists. The granuloma formed is a cavity of necrotic tissue.

Lymphocytes. Lymphocytes arrive later at the site of injury. Their primary role is related to humoral and cell-mediated immunity (see Chapter 16).

Eosinophils and Basophils. Eosinophils and basophils have a more selective role in inflammation. Eosinophils are released in large quantities during an allergic reaction. They release chemicals that act to control the effects of histamine and serotonin. They are also involved in phagocytosis of the allergen-antibody complex. Eosinophils contain highly caustic chemicals that are capable of destroying a parasite's cell surfaces. The histamine and heparin that basophils carry in their granules are released during inflammation.

Chemical Mediators. Mediators of the inflammatory response are listed in Table 14.3.

Complement System. The *complement system* is an enzymatic cascade consisting of pathways to mediate inflammation and destroy invading pathogens. Major functions of the complement system are enhanced phagocytosis, increased vascular permeability, chemotaxis, and cellular lysis. All of these activities are important in the inflammatory response.

When the complement system is activated, the components are generated in the sequential order of C1, C4, C2, C3, C5, C6, C7, C8, and C9. The numbering reflects the order of their discovery. Some components have subparts designated by

lowercase letters, such as C3a, C3b, and C5a. The primary pathway for activation of the complement system is through fixation of component C1 to an antigen–antibody complex. Immunoglobulins G and M are responsible for fixing complement. Each activated complex can act on the next component, which creates a cascade effect.

In an alternative pathway, C3 is activated without prior antigen–antibody fixation. Bacterial products, lipopolysaccharides, and neutrophil proteases can stimulate the complement sequence, beginning with C3 and with activation of C5 through C9.

Complement activation increases phagocytosis through opsonization and chemotaxis. *Opsonization* occurs when the antigen, in combination with complement factor C3b and immunoglobulin, sticks to the surface of the foreign particle such as pathogens that are targeted for destruction. This leads to more ready and rapid phagocytosis. In addition, complement component C5a promotes chemotaxis.

The components C3a, C5a, and C4a are termed *anaphylatoxins* and bind to receptors on mast cells and basophils, thus triggering histamine release. Histamine causes smooth muscle contraction, vasodilation, and an increase in vascular permeability.

The entire complement sequence of C1 to C9 must be activated for cell lysis to occur. The final components (C8, C9) act on the cell surface, causing rupture of the cell membrane and lysis. In autoimmune disorders, healthy tissue can be damaged by complement activation and the resulting inflammatory response. Examples of this include rheumatoid arthritis and systemic lupus erythematosus.

Prostaglandins and Leukotrienes. *Prostaglandins* are substances that can be synthesized from the phospholipids of cell membranes of most body tissues, including blood cells. On stimulation by chemotactic factors or phagocytosis or after cell injury, phospholipids can be converted to arachidonic acid, which is then oxidized by two different pathways.

The *cyclo-oxygenase metabolic pathway* leads to the production of prostaglandins of the D, E, F, and I series and of thromboxanes (formed on activation of platelets). Prostaglandins of the E and I series are potent vasodilators and inhibit

TABLE 14.4	TYPES OF INFLAMMATORY EXUDATE	
Type	Description	Examples
Serous	Results from fluid that has low cell and protein content; seen in early stages of inflammation or when injury is mild	Skin blisters, pleural effusion
Serosanguinous	Found during the midpoint in healing after surgery or tissue injury. Composed of RBCs and serous fluid, which is semi-clear pink and may have red streaks.	
Catarrhal	Found in tissues in which cells produce mucus; mucus production is accelerated by inflammatory response	Runny nose in association with upper respiratory tract infection
Fibrinous	Occurs with increasing vascular permeability and fibrinogen leakage into interstitial spaces; excessive amounts of fibrin coating of tissue surfaces may cause tissues to adhere	Adhesions
Purulent (pus)	Consists of WBCs, microorganisms (dead and alive), liquefied dead cells, and other debris	Furuncle (boil), abscess, cellulitis (diffuse inflammation in connective tissue)
Hemorrhagic	Results from rupture or necrosis of blood vessel walls; consists of RBCs that escape into tissue	Hematoma

RBCs, red blood cells; *WBCs,* white blood cells.

platelet and neutrophil aggregation. Prostaglandin E_2 (PGE_2) can sensitize pain receptors in response to stimuli that would normally be painless. PGE_2 is also a potent pyrogen, acting on the temperature-regulating area of the hypothalamus. Thromboxane A_2 is a potent vasoconstrictor and platelet-aggregating agent. Prostaglandins are generally considered proinflammatory, contributing to increased blood flow, edema, and pain. Metabolism of arachidonic acid by the lipoxygenase pathway leads to the production of leukotrienes. Leukotriene B_4 is a potent chemotactic factor. Leukotrienes C_4, D_4, and E_4 form the slow-reacting substance of anaphylaxis, which constricts smooth muscles of bronchi and increases capillary permeability.

Medications that inhibit prostaglandin synthesis are useful clinically. Nonsteroidal anti-inflammatory drugs (NSAIDs) are used to treat many acute and chronic inflammatory conditions. Acetylsalicylic acid blocks platelet aggregation; it also has anti-inflammatory action. Prostacyclin (prostaglandin I_2) has been used to prevent platelet deposition in extracorporeal systems, such as hemodialysis and heart–lung bypass oxygenators.

Another group of medications that inhibit prostaglandins is the corticosteroids. They are valuable in the treatment of asthma because they inhibit leukotriene production and thus prevent bronchoconstriction. (Other mediators of the inflammatory response are described in Table 14.3.)

Exudate Formation. Exudate consists of fluid and leukocytes that move from the circulation to the site of injury. The nature and quantity of exudate depend on the type and the severity of the injury and the tissues involved (Table 14.4).

Clinical Manifestations. The local manifestations of inflammation include redness, heat, swelling, and pain (Table 14.5). Systemic manifestations of inflammation include leukocytosis with a shift to the left, malaise, nausea and anorexia, increased pulse and respiratory rate, and fever. The causes of these systemic changes may be related to complement activation and the release of cytokines from stimulated WBCs. Three of these cytokines—interleukin-1, interleukin-6, and tumour necrosis factor—are important in causing the generalized symptoms of inflammation, such as malaise, as well as inducing fever. A rise in body temperature is accompanied by increased metabolism that is evident by an increase in pulse and respiration. (Cytokines are discussed in Chapter 16.)

Fever. The release of cytokines initiates metabolic changes in the temperature-regulating centre of the hypothalamus, thus causing fever (Figure 14.3). The synthesis of PGE_2 is the most

TABLE 14.5	LOCAL MANIFESTATIONS OF INFLAMMATION
Manifestations	Cause
Redness	Hyperemia from vasodilation
Heat	Increased metabolism at inflammatory site
Pain	Change in pH; nerve stimulation by chemicals (e.g., histamine, prostaglandins); pressure from fluid exudate
Swelling	Fluid shift to interstitial spaces; fluid exudates accumulation

critical metabolic change because it acts directly to increase the thermostatic set point. The hypothalamus then activates the autonomic nervous system to stimulate increased muscle tone and shivering and decreased perspiration and blood flow to the periphery. Epinephrine released from the adrenal medulla increases the metabolic rate. The net result is fever.

With the physiological thermostat fixed at a higher-than-normal temperature, the rate of heat production is increased until the body temperature reaches the new set point. As the set point is raised, the hypothalamus signals an increase in heat production and conservation to raise the body temperature to the new level. At this point, the affected individual feels chilled and shivers. The shivering response is the body's way of raising its temperature until the new set point is reached. The body is hot, and yet the individual paradoxically piles on blankets and may go to bed to get warm. When the circulating body temperature reaches the set point of the core body temperature, the chills and warmth-seeking behaviour cease (Dinarello & Porat, 2015). The febrile response is classified into four stages, described in Table 14.6.

The released cytokines and the fever they trigger activate the body's defence mechanisms. Beneficial aspects of fever include increased killing of microorganisms, increased phagocytosis by neutrophils, and increased proliferation of T cells. Higher body temperatures may also enhance the activity of interferon, the body's natural virus-fighting substance (see Chapter 16).

Types of Inflammation. The basic types of inflammation are acute, subacute, and chronic. In *acute inflammation,* the healing occurs in 2 to 3 weeks and usually leaves no residual damage. Neutrophils are the predominant cell type at the site of inflammation. A *subacute inflammation* has the features of the acute process but lasts longer. For example, infective endocarditis is a

PATHOPHYSIOLOGY MAP

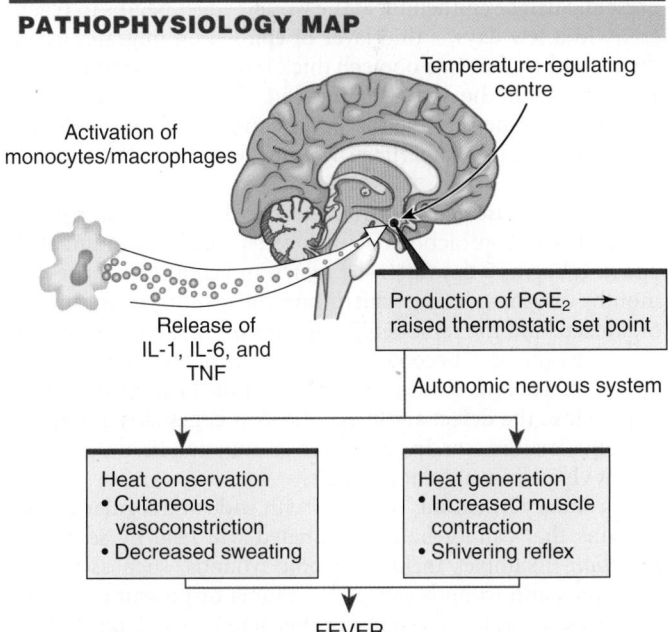

FIG. 14.3 Production of fever. When monocytes or macrophages are activated, they secrete cytokines such as interleukin-1 (IL-1), interleukin-6 (IL-6), and tumour necrosis factor (TNF), which reach the hypothalamic temperature-regulating centre. These cytokines promote the synthesis and secretion of prostaglandin E_2 (PGE$_2$) in the anterior hypothalamus. PGE$_2$ increases the thermostatic set point, and the autonomic nervous system is stimulated, which results in shivering, muscle contraction, and peripheral vasoconstriction.

TABLE 14.7	REGENERATIVE ABILITY OF DIFFERENT TYPES OF TISSUES
Tissue Type	**Regenerative Ability**
Epithelial	
Skin, linings of blood vessels, mucous membranes	Cells readily divide and regenerate.
Connective Tissue	
Bone	Active tissue heals rapidly.
Cartilage	Regeneration is possible but slow.
Tendons and ligaments	Regeneration is possible but slow.
Blood	Cells actively regenerate.
Muscle	
Smooth	Regeneration is usually possible (particularly in GI tract).
Cardiac	Damaged muscle is replaced by connective tissue.
Skeletal	Connective tissue replaces severely damaged muscle; in moderately damaged muscle, some regeneration occurs.
Nerve	
Neurons	Cells of these tissues are generally nonmitotic; they do not replicate or replace themselves if irreversibly damaged.
Glial	Cells regenerate; scar tissue often forms when neurons are damaged.

GI, gastrointestinal.

TABLE 14.6	STAGES OF THE FEBRILE RESPONSE
Stage	**Characteristics**
Prodrome	Nonspecific reports such as mild headache, fatigue, general malaise, muscle aches
Chill	Cutaneous vasoconstriction, "goose pimples," pale skin; feeling of being cold; generalized, shaking chill; shivering that causes body to reach new temperature set by control centre in hypothalamus
Flush	Sensation of warmth throughout body; cutaneous vasodilation; warming and flushing of skin
Defervescence	Sweating; decrease in body temperature

smouldering infection with acute inflammation, but it persists for weeks or months (see Chapter 39).

Chronic inflammation lasts for weeks, months, or even years. The injurious agent persists, causing repeated tissue injuries. The predominant cell types present at the site of inflammation are lymphocytes and macrophages. Examples of chronic inflammation include rheumatoid arthritis, osteomyelitis, and tuberculosis. The prolongation and chronicity of any inflammation may be the result of an alteration in the immune response (e.g., autoimmune disease). C-reactive protein is an acute-phase protein whose plasma concentration increases in response to inflammation, and thus it can be a useful inflammatory marker.

Healing Process. The final phase of the inflammatory response is healing. Healing includes two major components: regeneration and repair. Regeneration is the replacement of lost cells and tissues with cells of the same type. Repair is healing as

a result of lost cells being replaced by connective tissue. Repair is the more common type of healing and usually results in scar formation.

Regeneration. The ability of cells to regenerate depends on the cell type (Table 14.7). Labile cells—such as cells of the skin, lymphoid organs, bone marrow, and mucous membranes of the gastrointestinal, urinary, and reproductive tracts—divide constantly. Injury to these organs is followed by rapid regeneration.

Stable cells retain their ability to regenerate but do so only if the organ is injured. Examples of stable cells are liver, pancreas, kidney, and bone cells.

Permanent cells such as neurons of the central nervous system and cardiac muscle cells do not regenerate. Damage to these cells can lead to permanent loss. Healing occurs by repair with scar tissue.

Repair. Repair is a more complex process than is regeneration. Most injuries heal by connective tissue repair. Repair healing occurs by primary, secondary, or tertiary intention (Figure 14.4).

Primary Intention. *Primary intention* healing takes place when wound margins are neatly approximated, as in a surgical incision or a paper cut. A continuum of processes is associated with primary healing (Table 14.8). These processes include three phases: the initial (inflammatory) phase, the granulation (proliferative/reconstructive) phase, and the maturation phase and scar contraction.

Initial (Inflammatory) Phase. The *initial phase* lasts for 3 to 5 days. The edges of the incision are aligned and sutured (or stapled) in place. The incision area fills with blood from the cut blood vessels, and blood clots form and platelets release growth factors to begin the healing process. This forms a matrix for WBC migration and an acute inflammatory reaction occurs.

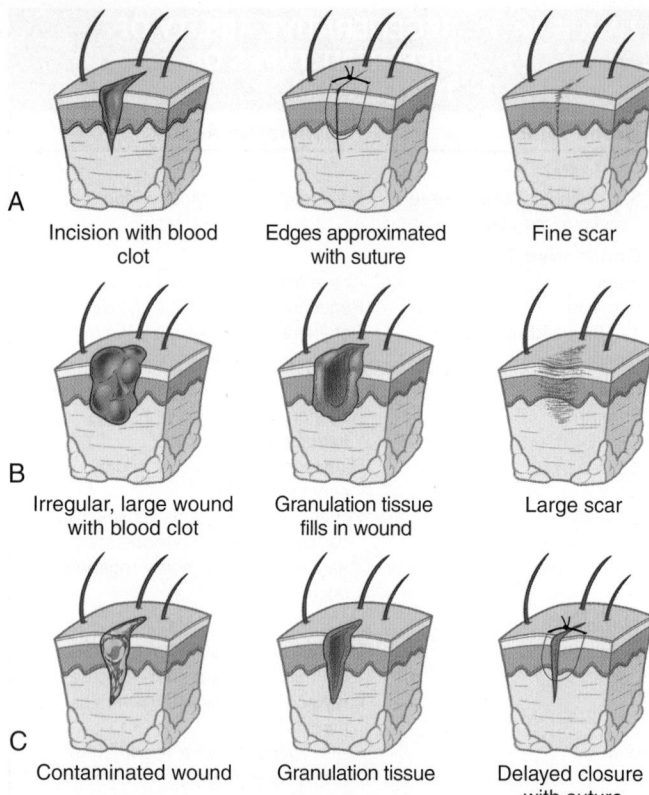

A Incision with blood clot — Edges approximated with suture — Fine scar

B Irregular, large wound with blood clot — Granulation tissue fills in wound — Large scar

C Contaminated wound — Granulation tissue — Delayed closure with suture

FIG. 14.4 Types of wound healing. **A,** Primary intention. **B,** Secondary intention. **C,** Tertiary intention.

TABLE 14.8	PHASES IN PRIMARY INTENTION HEALING
Phase	**Activity**
Initial (3 to 5 days)	Approximation of incision edges; migration of epithelial cells; clot serving as meshwork for starting capillary growth
Granulation (5 days to 4 weeks)	Migration of fibroblasts; secretion of collagen; abundance of capillary buds; fragility of wound
Scar contracture (7 days to several months)	Remodelling of collagen; strengthening of scar

The area of injury is composed of fibrin clots, erythrocytes, neutrophils (dead and dying), and other debris. Macrophages ingest and digest cellular debris, fibrin fragments, and red blood cells. Extracellular enzymes from macrophages and neutrophils help digest fibrin. As the wound debris is removed, the fibrin clot serves as a framework for future capillary growth and migration of epithelial cells.

Granulation (Proliferative/Reconstructive) Phase. The *granulation phase* is the second step and lasts from 5 days to 3 weeks. The components of granulation tissue include proliferating fibroblasts; proliferating capillary sprouts (angioblasts); various types of WBCs; exudate; and loose, semifluid, ground substance.

Fibroblasts are immature connective tissue cells that migrate into the healing site and secrete collagen. In time, the collagen is organized and restructured to strengthen the healing site. At this stage, it is termed *fibrous* or *scar tissue.*

During the granulation phase, the wound is pink and vascular. Numerous red granules (young budding capillaries) are present. Surface epithelium at the wound edges begins to regenerate. In a few days, a thin layer of epithelium migrates across the wound surface in a one-cell thick layer until it contacts cells spreading from the opposite direction. The epithelium thickens and begins to mature, and the wound now closely resembles the adjacent skin. In a superficial wound, re-epithelialization may take 3 to 5 days.

Maturation Phase and Scar Contraction. The *maturation phase,* in which scar contraction occurs, overlaps with the granulation phase. It begins 7 days after the injury and continues for several months or years, during which time collagen fibres are further organized, and the remodelling process occurs. Fibroblasts disappear as the scar becomes stronger. The active movement of the myofibroblasts causes contraction of the healing area, helping to close the defect and bring the skin edges closer together to form a mature scar. In contrast to granulation tissue, a mature scar is virtually avascular and pale.

Secondary Intention. Wounds with wide or irregular wound margins that cannot be approximated will heal by *secondary intention.* Examples include chronic wounds, such as venous leg ulcers, and wounds caused by trauma or pressure. In some instances, a surgical incision may become infected, resulting in dehiscence, and healing by secondary intention must then take place.

The process of healing by secondary intention is essentially the same as that of healing by primary intention. The major differences are the larger defect and the gaping wound edges. The inflammatory reaction that occurs is often greater than in primary healing, which creates more debris, cells, and exudate. The debris may have to be cleaned away (debrided) before healing can take place. Healing and granulation take place from the edges inward and from the bottom of the wound upward until the defect is filled. There is more granulation tissue, and the result is a much larger scar.

Tertiary Intention. *Tertiary intention* (delayed primary intention) healing occurs when a wound is intentionally left open because if the wound is closed immediately, healing could be impaired by contamination (e.g., animal bite or foreign body), infection or high risk of infection, edema, or poor circulation. The wound is later closed surgically after the issue is controlled or resolved. Healing by tertiary intention usually results in a larger and deeper scar than does healing by primary or secondary intention.

Wound Classification. Correctly classifying a wound requires identifying the underlying cause. Wounds can be categorized by cause (surgical or nonsurgical), underlying pathology (vascular, pressure, diabetes related), duration (acute or chronic), level of contamination, or type of tissue affected (superficial, partial thickness, or full thickness). A superficial wound involves only the epidermis. Partial-thickness wounds extend into the dermis. Full-thickness wounds cause destruction to the deepest layer of tissue because they involve the subcutaneous tissue and sometimes even extend into the fascia and underlying structures such as muscle, tendon, or bone (see Figure 27.3). Pressure injuries are the only type of wound that are described and classified using the staging system (European Pressure Ulcer Advisory Panel, National Pressure Injury Advisory Panel, and Pan Pacific Pressure Injury Alliance [EPUAP/NPIAP/PPPIA], 2019); see Table 14.13 later in this chapter).

Another system that is sometimes used clinically to categorize open wounds is based on the colour of the wound bed (red, yellow, black) rather than on the level of tissue destruction

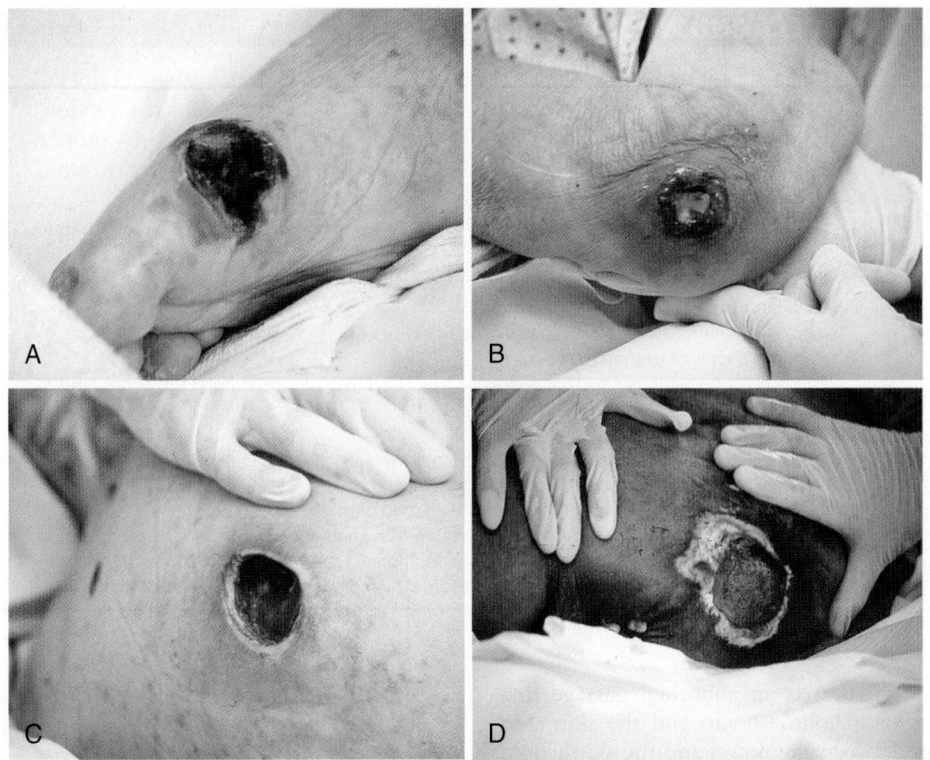

FIG. 14.5 Wounds classified by colour assessment. **A,** Black wound. **B,** Yellow wound. **C,** Red wound. **D,** Mixed-colour wound. Source: Courtesy Molnlyche Health Care, Eddystone, PA. In Potter, P. A., & Perry, A. G. (2009). *Fundamentals of nursing* (8th ed., p. 1285). Elsevier.

(Figure 14.5). It can be used to describe any wound allowed to heal by secondary or tertiary intention. When a wound contains two or three colours at the same time, it should be classified according to the least desirable colour present (e.g., if there is any black in the wound, the wound is deemed "black").

Delay of Healing. In a healthy person, wounds heal at a normal, predictable rate. Little can be done to accelerate this process. However, some factors may delay wound healing. These are summarized in Table 14.9.

Complications of Healing. Complications of wound healing may include adhesions, contractures, dehiscence and evisceration, excess granulation tissue, fistula formation, infection/biofilm, hemorrhage, and formation of hypertrophic scars and keloids.

Adhesions. Adhesions are bands of scar tissue that form between or around organs. They may develop in the abdominal cavity or between the lungs and pleura. Adhesions in the abdomen may cause an intestinal obstruction. Those between the lungs and the pleura necessitate decortication, or stripping of pleura, to enable normal ventilation.

Contractures. Wound contraction is an important part of healing. This process may become abnormal when contraction is excessive, which results in deformity, or *contracture*. Shortening of muscle or scar tissue, especially over joints, results from excessive fibrous tissue formation. Contractures frequently occur in burn injuries, when extensive skin and subcutaneous tissue are lost (see Chapter 27).

Dehiscence and Evisceration. Dehiscence is the separation and disruption of previously joined wound edges. It usually occurs when a primary healing site bursts open (Figure 14.6). Dehiscence has three possible contributing causes. First, an infection may cause an inflammatory process. Second, the

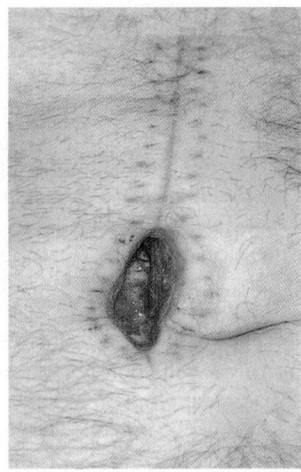

FIG. 14.6 Dehiscence after a cholecystectomy. Source: Bale, S., & Jones, V. (2006). *Wound care nursing: A patient-centered approach* (2nd ed., p. 20). Mosby.

granulation tissue may not be strong enough to withstand the forces imposed on the wound—for example, if a fluid pocket (seroma or hematoma) develops between the tissue layers. Third, individuals with obesity are at a high risk for dehiscence because adipose tissue has less blood supply, which can slow healing. Evisceration occurs when wound edges separate to the extent that intestines protrude through the wound.

Excess Granulation Tissue. *Excess granulation tissue* or hypergranulation tissue ("proud flesh") may protrude above the surface of the healing wound, affecting keratinocyte migration. Hypergranulation tissue may be cauterized or cut off to promote normal healing.

TABLE 14.9	FACTORS DELAYING WOUND HEALING
Factor	**Effect on Wound Healing**
Nutrition	
• Vitamin C deficiency	Delays formation of collagen fibres and capillary development
• Protein deficiency	Decreases supply of amino acids for tissue repair
• Zinc deficiency	Impairs epithelialization
Inadequate blood supply	Decreases supply of nutrients to injured area, decreases removal of exudative debris, inhibits inflammatory response
Smoking	Nicotine is a potent vasoconstrictor and impedes blood flow to healing areas, which results in tissue ischemia and impairs wound healing
Corticosteroid medications	Impair phagocytosis by WBCs, inhibit fibroblast proliferation and function, depress formation of granulation tissue, inhibit wound contraction
Infection	Increases inflammatory response and tissue destruction
Anemia	Reduces supply of oxygen to tissues
Advanced age	Slows collagen synthesis by fibroblasts, impairs circulation, imposes need for longer time for epithelialization of skin, alters phagocytic and immune responses
Obesity	Decreases blood supply in fatty tissue
Diabetes mellitus	Decreases collagen synthesis, retards early capillary growth, impairs phagocytosis (result of hyperglycemia), reduces supply of O_2 and nutrients as a result of vascular disease
Poor general health	Causes generalized absence of factors necessary to promote wound healing
Mechanical friction on wound	Destroys granulation tissue, prevents apposition of wound edges
Cold temperature	Decreases cellular activity and fibroblast proliferation
Excessive moisture	Promotes formation of hypergranulation tissue, which prevents the migration of epithelial cells

WBCs, white blood cells.

Fistula Formation. A fistula is an abnormal passage that forms between organs or a hollow organ and the skin. For example, a connection between the bowel and the skin would be referred to as an *enterocutaneous fistula;* it allows intestinal content or stool to leak through the skin. A connection between the bowel and the bladder would be referred to as an *enterovesical fistula.*

Infection. A wound has an increased risk of *infection* when it contains necrotic tissue, when the blood supply is decreased, when the immune function is depressed, or if a patient is malnourished, has multiple stressors, or is diabetic. Aggregation of microorganisms produce biofilm that can delay wound healing.

Hemorrhage. Bleeding is normal immediately after tissue injury and ceases with clot formation. *Hemorrhage* occurs as abnormal internal or external blood loss caused by suture failure, clotting abnormalities, dislodged clot, infection, or erosion of a blood vessel by a foreign object (tubing, drains) or infection process.

Formation of Hypertrophic Scars and Keloids. Hypertrophic keloid scars form when the body produces excess collagen. A hypertrophic scar is inappropriately large, red, raised, and hard (Figure 14.7). However, it remains confined to the wound edges and regresses in time. In contrast, a keloid is a protrusion of scar tissue that extends beyond the wound edges and may form tumour-like masses of scar tissue (Figure 14.8). Keloids are permanent, without any tendency to subside. A person with keloids often feels tenderness, pain, and hyperesthesia in the area of the scar, particularly in the early stages of development. Keloid formation is thought to be hereditary and occurs more often in dark-skinned people, particularly Black individuals. Neither complication is life-threatening, but both can have serious cosmetic implications.

NURSING MANAGEMENT INFLAMMATION AND HEALING

NURSING IMPLEMENTATION

HEALTH PROMOTION. The best management of inflammation is the prevention of infection, trauma, surgery, and contact with potentially harmful agents. This is not always possible;

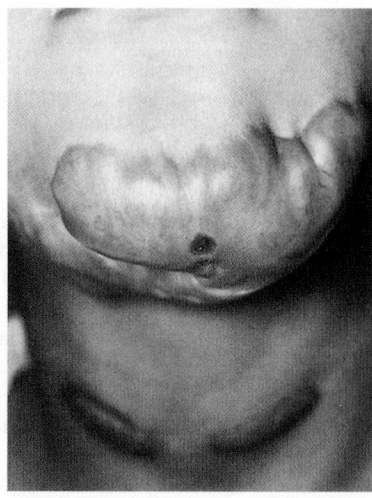

FIG. 14.7 Hypertrophic scarring. Source: Courtesy Dr. C. Lawrence, Wound Healing Research Unit, Cardiff, Wales, UK. In Bale, S., & Jones, V. (2006). *Wound care nursing: A patient-centered approach* (2nd ed., p. 16). Mosby.

for example, a simple mosquito bite causes an inflammatory response. Because occasional injury is inevitable, concerted efforts to minimize inflammation and infection are needed.

Adequate nutrition is essential so that the body has the necessary factors to promote healing when injury occurs. Individuals at risk for wound-healing complications are those with malabsorption problems (e.g., Crohn's disease, gastrointestinal surgery, liver disease), deficient intake or high energy demands (e.g., malignancy, major trauma or surgery, sepsis, fever), or diabetes. An individual should always be considered at risk for delayed wound healing if the following have occurred: (a) loss of 20% or more of total body weight in the preceding 6 months or (b) 10% loss of total body weight in the preceding 2 months.

Special nutritional measures facilitate wound healing. Fluid intake must be high to replace fluid loss from perspiration and exudate formation. An increased metabolic rate intensifies water loss. For every 1°C increase in body temperature above 37.8°C, metabolism increases by 13%. A diet high in protein, carbohydrate,

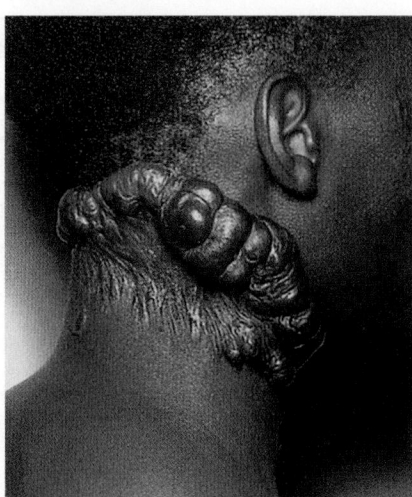

FIG. 14.8 Keloid scarring. Source: Courtesy Dr. C. Lawrence, Wound Healing Research Unit, Cardiff, Wales, UK. In Bale, S., & Jones, V. (2006). *Wound care nursing: A patient-centered approach* (2nd ed., p. 17). Mosby.

and vitamins with moderate fat intake is necessary to promote healing. Protein is needed to correct the negative nitrogen balance that results from the increased metabolic rate. Protein is also necessary for synthesis of immune factors, leukocytes, fibroblasts, and collagen. Carbohydrate is needed for the increased metabolic energy required for inflammation and healing. If carbohydrate intake is deficient, the body breaks down protein for the needed energy. Fats are also a necessary component in the diet to help in the synthesis of fatty acids and triglycerides, which are part of the cellular membrane. Vitamin C is needed for capillary synthesis, capillary formation, and resistance to infection. The B-complex vitamins are necessary as coenzymes for many metabolic reactions. If a vitamin B deficiency develops, metabolism of protein, fat, and carbohydrate is disrupted. Vitamin A is also needed in healing because it aids in the process of epithelialization. It increases collagen synthesis and tensile strength of the healing wound. Patients are sometimes given vitamin A to counteract the effects of steroids on wound healing.

If the patient is unable to eat, enteral feedings and supplements should be the first choice if the gastrointestinal tract is functional. Parenteral nutrition is indicated when enteral feedings are contraindicated or not tolerated. (Enteral nutrition and parenteral nutrition are discussed in Chapter 42.)

The manifestations of inflammation and infection must be recognized early so that appropriate treatment can begin. Treatment may be rest, medication therapy, or specific care of the injured site. Immediate treatment may prevent the extension and complications of prolonged inflammation.

Acute Intervention

Observation and Vital Signs. The ability to recognize the clinical manifestations of inflammation is important. In a patient who is immunosuppressed (e.g., taking corticosteroids or receiving chemotherapy), the classic manifestations of inflammation may be masked. In such a patient, early symptoms of inflammation may be malaise or "just not feeling well."

Observation and recording of wound characteristics are essential. The amount, consistency, colour, and odour of any drainage should be recorded and reported if abnormal. *Staphylococcus* and *Pseudomonas* organisms commonly cause purulent drainage. Exudate from wounds colonized with *Pseudomonas* often has a distinctive bright "highlighter" yellow or green appearance.

Vital signs are important to note with any inflammation, especially when an infectious process is present. When infection is present, temperature may rise, and pulse and respiration rates may increase. If a wound infection develops in a postoperative patient, vital signs change within 3 to 5 days after surgery.

Fever. Although fever is usually regarded as harmful, an increase in body temperature is an important host defence mechanism. Steps are frequently taken to lower body temperature to relieve the anxiety of the patient and medical personnel. Because a mild fever does little harm, imposes no great discomfort, and may benefit host defence mechanisms, antipyretic medications are rarely essential for patient welfare. Moderate fevers (up to 39.5°C) usually produce few problems in most patients. However, if the patient is very young or very old, is extremely uncomfortable, or has a significant medical condition (e.g., severe cardiopulmonary disease, brain injury), the use of antipyretics should be considered. Fever in an immunosuppressed patient should be treated rapidly and antibiotic therapy begun because infections can rapidly progress to septicemia. (Neutropenia is discussed in Chapter 33.)

Fever (especially if the temperature exceeds 40°C) can be damaging to body cells, and delirium and seizures can occur. At temperatures higher than 41°C, regulation by the hypothalamic temperature control centre becomes impaired, and many cells, including those in the brain, can be damaged.

Older persons have a blunted febrile response to infection (El Chakhtoura et al., 2017). The body temperature may not rise to the level expected for a younger adult, or the onset of fever may be delayed. The blunted response can delay diagnosis and treatment. By the time fever (as defined for younger adults) is present, the illness may be severe.

Several medications are commonly used to lower the body temperature set point in the hypothalamus (Table 14.10). Aspirin specifically blocks prostaglandin synthesis in the hypothalamus and elsewhere in the body. Acetaminophen acts on the heat-regulating centre in the hypothalamus. Some NSAIDs (e.g., ibuprofen [Motrin, Advil]) have antipyretic effects. Corticosteroids are antipyretic through the dual mechanisms of inhibiting interleukin-1 production and preventing prostaglandin synthesis. The action of these medications results in dilation of superficial blood vessels, increased skin temperature, and sweating.

Antipyretics should be given around the clock to prevent acute swings in temperature. These agents cause a sharp decrease in temperature. When the antipyretic wears off, the body may initiate a compensatory involuntary muscular contraction (i.e., chill) to raise the body temperature back up to its previous level. To prevent this unpleasant adverse effect, these agents should be administered regularly at 2- to 4-hour intervals. Although sponge baths increase evaporative heat loss, there is no evidence that they decrease the body temperature unless antipyretic medications have been given to lower the set point; otherwise, the body will initiate compensatory mechanisms (e.g., shivering) to restore body heat. The same principle applies to the use of cooling blankets; they are most effective in lowering body temperature when the set point has also been lowered. The nursing care of the patient with a fever is presented in Nursing Care Plan 14.1, available on the Evolve website.

RICE. Rest, ice, compression, and elevation (RICE) constitute a key concept in the treatment of soft tissue injuries and related inflammation.

Rest. Rest helps the body use its nutrients and oxygen for the healing process. The repair process is facilitated when fibrin

TABLE 14.10 MEDICATION THERAPY

Inflammation and Healing

Medication	Mechanisms of Action
Antipyretic Medications	
Salicylates (Aspirin)	Lower temperature by action on heat-regulating centre in hypothalamus, resulting in peripheral dilation and heat loss; interfere with formation and release of prostaglandins; selectively depress CNS
Acetaminophen (Tylenol)	Lowers temperature by action on heat-regulating centre in hypothalamus
NSAIDs (e.g., ibuprofen [Motrin, Advil])	Inhibit synthesis of prostaglandins
Anti-inflammatory Medications	
Salicylates (Aspirin)	Inhibit synthesis of prostaglandins, reduce capillary permeability
Corticosteroids (e.g., prednisone)	Interfere with tissue granulation, induce immunosuppressive effects (decreased synthesis of lymphocytes), prevent liberation of lysosomes
NSAIDs (e.g., ibuprofen [Motrin], naproxen [Naprosyn], celecoxib [Celebrex])	Inhibit synthesis of prostaglandins
Vitamins	
Vitamin A	Accelerates epithelialization
Vitamin B complex	Acts as coenzymes
Vitamin C	Assists in synthesis of collagen and new capillaries
Vitamin D	Facilitates calcium absorption

CNS, central nervous system; *NSAIDs,* nonsteroidal anti-inflammatory drugs.

and collagen are allowed to form across the wound edges with little disruption.

Ice and Heat. At the time of initial trauma, cold application is usually appropriate to promote vasoconstriction and decreases swelling, pain, and congestion from increased metabolism in the area of inflammation. Cold application should be used with caution in areas where vascular flow is compromised. Heat may be used later (e.g., after 24 to 48 hours) and when swelling has subsided to promote healing by increasing the circulation to the inflamed site and subsequent removal of debris. Heat is also used to localize the inflammatory agents. Warm, moist heat may help debride the wound site if necrotic material is present.

Compression and Immobilization. Compression counters vasodilation and development of edema after an injury. Compression by direct pressure over a laceration occludes blood vessels to stop bleeding. Compression bandages provide support to injured joints that have tendons and muscles unable to provide support on their own. Distal pulses and capillary refill should be assessed before and after application of compression to assess whether compression has compromised circulation (e.g., as evidenced by pale colour of skin or loss of sensation).

Immobilization of the inflamed area promotes healing by decreasing the tissues' metabolic need. Immobilization with a cast, splint, or bandage supports fractured bones and prevents further tissue injury from sharp bone fragments that could sever nerves or blood vessels (causing hemorrhage).

Elevation. Elevation of an injured extremity reduces the edema at the inflammatory site by increasing venous and lymphatic return. Elevation helps reduce pain associated with blood engorgement at the injured site. Elevation may be contraindicated in patients with significantly reduced arterial circulation.

Wound Management. The type of wound management and dressings required depend on the type, extent, and characteristics of the wound and the phase of healing (Nurses Specialized in Wound, Ostomy and Continence Canada [NSWOCC], 2021).

The purposes of wound management include (a) cleaning and debriding the wound to remove debris and dead tissue from the wound bed, (b) controlling inflammation and treating infection to prepare the wound for healing, and (c) providing

moisture balance for healable wounds. Tissue debridement and moisture may not always be appropriate for nonhealable and maintenance wounds (Woo, 2017). Treatment of pressure injuries is discussed in more detail later in this chapter.

EVIDENCE-INFORMED PRACTICE
Research Highlight

What Is the Effect of Support Surfaces on Pressure Injury Prevention?
Clinical Question
In patients who are at risk for developing pressure injury (P), what is the effect of therapeutic support surfaces (I) versus standard support surfaces (C) on incidence of pressure injuries (O)?

Best Available Evidence
Randomized controlled trials and quasi-randomized controlled trials

Critical Appraisal and Synthesis of Evidence
- Fifty nine trials (*n* = 12 to 1 171 per trial) involving people who were at risk for pressure injury. Studies included 12 trials that evaluated cushions; 5 evaluating the use of sheepskins; 4 that looked at turning beds/tables; 19 that examined overlays; 28 that looked at mattresses; 3 evaluating use of foam surfaces; 2 examining waffle surfaces; and 1 that examined use of the Heelift suspension boot.
- Foam alternatives to the standard hospital foam mattress reduce the incidence of pressure ulcers in people at risk.
- Pressure-relieving overlays on the operating table and in the postoperative period reduce the incidence of postoperative pressure ulcers.

Conclusion
- Using tap water to cleanse acute wounds does not increase infection rate and, in some cases, it may reduce infection.

Implications for Nursing Practice
- Therapeutic surfaces should be considered for the prevention of pressure injuries.

Reference for Evidence
McInnes, E., Jammali-Blasi, A., Bell-Syer, S. E., et al. (2015). Support surfaces for pressure ulcer prevention. *Cochrane Database of Systematic Reviews 2015* (Issue 9) Art. No. CD001735. doi:10.1002/14651858.CD001735.pub5.
C, comparison of interest or comparison group; *I,* intervention or area of interest; *O,* outcomes of interest; *P,* patient population of interest. (see Chapter 1).

Wound healing management by secondary intention depends on the cause of the wound and the type of tissue in the wound. The red–yellow–black concept of wound care (see Figure 14.5) can be used to describe the wound, and dressing selection depends on the characteristics of the wound. Examples of wound dressing types are presented in Table 14.11.

Red Wound. A *red wound* can be superficial or deep and is clean and red or pink in appearance. Examples include skin tears, pressure injuries, partial-thickness or second-degree burns, and wounds created surgically that are allowed to heal by secondary intention. The goal of treatment is gentle cleansing and protection of the wound (LeBlanc et al., 2019). Wounds should be cleaned with normal saline, water, or noncytotoxic wound cleansers (NSWOCC, 2021). Clean wounds that are granulating and re-epithelializing should be kept slightly moist and protected from further trauma (Jones et al., 2018). A dressing that keeps the wound surface clean and slightly moist is optimal in promoting epithelialization. Unnecessary manipulation during

dressing changes may destroy new granulation tissue and break down fibrin formation.

Yellow Wound. A *yellow wound* has nonviable necrotic tissue, which creates an ideal environment for bacterial growth. The goal of treatment is absorption of excessive drainage and removal of nonviable tissue (described in the next section). Topical antimicrobials and antiseptics (e.g., povidone-iodine, sodium hypochlorite [e.g., Dakin's solution], hydrogen peroxide, acetic acid, and chlorhexidine) may be used to cleanse wounds containing debris that are highly colonized or infected. They are not recommended to clean granulating wounds (NSWOCC, 2021).

Black Wound. A *black wound* is covered with thick, dry, necrotic tissue called *eschar* that is black, brown, or grey. Examples of black wounds include third-degree burns and gangrenous ulcers. The risk of wound infection increases in proportion to the amount of necrotic tissue present. The immediate treatment is removal of the nonviable eschar. The debridement

TABLE 14.11 TYPES OF WOUND DRESSINGS

Type	Description	Examples
Gauze	Provides minimal absorption of exudate. Supports debridement if applied and kept moist. Can be used as filler dressings in sinus tracts.	Nu Gauze (numerous products available)
Nonadherent dressing	Woven or nonwoven dressings may be impregnated with petrolatum or antimicrobial medications. Minimally absorbent. Used on minor wounds or skin tears.	Adaptic, Jelonet, Bactigras, Inadine
Transparent film	Semipermeable membrane that permits gaseous exchange between wound bed and environment. Minimally absorbent so that environment is kept moist in presence of exudate. Bacteria do not penetrate membrane. Used for dry, noninfected wounds, wounds with minimal drainage, or stage 1 pressure injuries to help prevent friction and shear.	Bioclusive, OpSite, Tegaderm, Mefilm
Acrylic clear	Used for superficial and partial-thickness wounds with light drainage. Requires less frequent dressing changes.	Tegaderm Absorbent
Hydrocolloid dressing	Occlusive dressing does not allow O_2 to diffuse from atmosphere to wound bed. Occlusion does not interfere with wound healing and supports debridement. Used for superficial and partial-thickness wounds with light to moderate drainage. Strong adhesive may not be suitable for fragile skin.	Comfeel, DuoDERM, Restore, Tegasorb
Foam	Product comes in many shapes and sizes. Absorbs moderate to heavy amount of exudate. Used for partial- or full-thickness wounds or infected wounds.	Allevyn, Hydrasorb, Lyofoam, Mepilex, Biatain, Tegaderm Foam
Alginate, calcium alginate, and hydrofibre dressings	Large volume of exudate can be absorbed. Dressing forms a gel-like substance that supports autolytic debridement and maintains moistness of wound surface. Fills wound cavities and obliterates dead space. Available in rope or sheet form. For partial- or full-thickness wounds or infected wounds with heavy drainage. Dressing should not be used for lightly draining or dry wounds because it can desiccate the wound bed. A secondary dressing is required. Calcium alginate is a natural hemostatic agent.	Aquacel, Kaltostat, Tegagen, Seasorb, Fibracol, Algisite, Algisite M, Melgisorb
Hypertonic dressing	Sheet, ribbon, or gel impregnated with sodium chloride concentrate. Should not be used on dry wounds (which should be treated with a hydrogel). May be painful on sensitive tissue.	Mesalt, Hypergel
Hydrogel	Facilitates autolytic debridement of necrotic tissue. Maintains moistness of wound surface. Provides limited absorption of exudate. Available as sheet, gel, and impregnated gauze. A secondary dressing is required. Used for partial- or full-thickness wounds with minimal drainage and for necrotic wounds. Has a cooling effect on the wound and thus is effective in managing pain.	IntraSite Gel, DuoDERM Hydroactive Gel, Normlgel, Nu-Gel, Tegagel, Tegaderm Hydrogel wound filler
Charcoal dressing	Dressing that contains odour-absorbent charcoal layered within the product. Some products contain silver to enhance antimicrobial capability.	Actisorb, Carbonet, CarboFlex
Antimicrobial dressing	Broad spectrum against bacteria. Silver, polyhexamethylene biguinide (PHMB), cadexomer iodine, methylene blue/gentian violet, or honey with vehicle for delivery: sheets, foams, alginates, ribbons, gels, or paste. Products are not to be used on patients with known hypersensitivity to any product components.	Acticoat, AMD Antimicrobial Foam, Iodosorb, Allevyn Ag, Mepilex Ag, Aquacel Ag, Contreet, Silvercel, SilvaSorb, Tegaderm Ag Mesh, Hydrofera Blue, Medihoney
Biological dressing	Living human fibroblasts provided in sheets at ambient or frozen temperatures. Extracellular matrix. Collagen-containing preparations. Hyaluronic acid. Not to be used on wounds with infections, sinus tracts, or excessive exudate, or on patients with hypersensitivity to any of the product components.	Apligraf, Dermagraft, Oasis Wound Matrix, Promogran, Tegaderm Matrix

Source: Information on antimicrobials and biological dressings from Wounds Canada. (2017). *Product picker: Wound dressing formulary*. https://www.woundscanada.ca/docman/public/health-care-professional/1113-product-picker-2017-formulary/file method used depends on the amount of debris and the condition of the wound tissue (NSWOCC, 2021). There are several approaches to debridement:

1. *Surgical debridement.* This fast and cost-effective method of debridement is indicated when large amounts of tissue are nonviable and the patient has sepsis. Sharp surgical debridement is selective and can be performed in the operating room or at the patient's bedside, depending on the extent of necrotic material (Woo et al., 2015). Only wounds that have an adequate blood supply and are considered "healable" should be debrided surgically. Conservative sharp wound debridement involves the removal of devitalized tissue with very minimal bleeding (NSWOCC, 2021).

2. *Mechanical debridement.* This method is used when debris is minimal. One example is wet-to-dry dressings, in which open-mesh gauze is moistened with normal saline, placed on the wound surface, and allowed to dry. Wound debris adheres to the dressing. When the dressing is removed, the debris trapped in the gauze is mechanically separated from the wound bed. One disadvantage to this method is that it is nonselective and destroys some healthy tissue. Mechanical debridement can be painful, and the patient should receive appropriate pain management before the removal of a wet-to-dry dressing. Another method of mechanical debridement is pressurized wound irrigation, in which water is delivered at high or low pressure to remove bacteria, foreign matter, and necrotic tissue from the wound. It is important to ensure that an adequate amount of irrigant is used to ensure thorough cleaning of the wound surface and surrounding areas. Whirlpool is another method of mechanical debridement that is no longer recommended because of the risk of tissue maceration and bacterial cross-contamination. Ultrasonic debridement devices are costly but they offer a noncontact debridement method.

3. *Autolytic debridement.* Hydrogels, semi-occlusive dressings, or occlusive dressings (see Table 14.11) may be used to promote softening of dry eschar by autolysis. This is a slow but selective and painless process that enables the body's own endogenous enzymes to selectively rehydrate, soften, and liquefy necrotic tissue. These types of dressings are used in noninfected wounds with necrotic tissue and adequate circulation. The use of a skin protectant around the wound helps prevent maceration.

4. *Enzymatic debridement.* In this method, a topical ointment containing proteolytic enzymes is applied to the necrotic tissue in the wound and then covered with a moist dressing such as saline-moistened gauze and changed daily. Santyl collagenase is the only product in this category currently available in Canada. The wound pH must be between 6 and 8 for optimal enzyme activity; therefore, cleansing products containing detergents or heavy metals such as mercury or silver should not be used.

5. *Biosurgical debridement.* In this debridement method, medical-grade maggots are applied directly to a wound in a controlled and contained environment. The maggots clean the wound by digesting dead tissue with their proteolytic, digestive enzymes. They also kill bacteria by ingesting them and can destroy biofilm.

Negative-Pressure Wound Therapy. This therapy involves the application of negative pressure (suction) to the wound bed. The vacuum creates continuous or intermittent negative pressure at the wound base to remove fluid, exudate, and infectious material and to promote blood flow. The wound is cleansed, and the periwound area is protected with a skin protectant. For deep open wounds, a filler (foam or gauze dressing depending on the manufacturer) may be used to loosely fill to the surface of the wound. A large semi-occlusive dressing is applied over the top to create a sealed environment and then attach to a suction pump (Figure 14.9). Wound types suitable for this therapy include chronic, acute, traumatic, and dehisced wounds; partial-thickness burns; diabetic ulcers; stage 3 and stage 4 pressure injuries; flaps; and grafts. Contraindications include malignancy, untreated osteomyelitis, fistula, eschar, and active bleeding. It is important to count and document the number of pieces of foam or gauze used in the wound. For further information on negative-pressure wound therapy, refer to the Ontario Ministry of Health and Long-Term Care document *Negative Pressure Wound Therapy* (see the Resources at the end of this chapter).

Hyperbaric Oxygen Therapy. Hyperbaric oxygen therapy is the systemic delivery of oxygen at increased atmospheric pressures. The patient is placed in an enclosed chamber in which 100% oxygen is administered at 1.5 to 3.0 times the normal atmospheric pressure. This form of therapy may accelerate granulation tissue formation and wound closure by increasing blood and tissue oxygen content in hypoxic tissues, which stimulates fibroblast proliferation and collagen synthesis.

Electrical Stimulation. With this therapy, a generator connected to electrodes is attached to the periwound skin, and an electrical charge is delivered to the wound tissues to produce a physiological response. Electrical stimulation may be used as an adjunct to regular wound care to promote healing and wound closure with stalled but healable stage 2, 3, and 4 pressure injuries that have not responded to other interventions. It should not be used if a patient has osteomyelitis, cancer, an implanted electronic device, or a blood clot in the leg. It should never be applied over a pregnant uterus, dressings with metallic or ionic components, or excitable tissues.

Psychological Implications. The patient may be distressed at the thought or sight of an incision or wound, because of fear of scarring or disfigurement. Drainage from a wound may also cause alarm. The patient needs to understand the healing process and the normal changes that occur as the wound heals. When a nurse is changing a dressing, their inappropriate facial expressions can alert the patient to problems

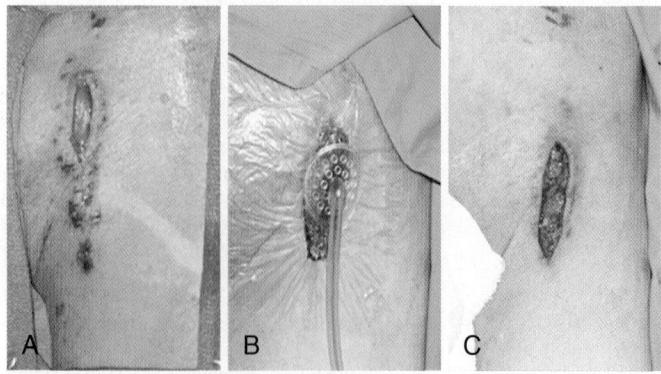

FIG. 14.9 Negative-pressure wound therapy. **A,** Femoral wound that is not healing. **B,** Negative-pressure wound therapy in place. **C,** Granulation tissue formation after therapy. Source: Abai, B., Zickler, R. W., Pappas, P. J, et al. (2007). Lymphorrhea responds to negative pressure wound therapy. *Journal of Vascular Surgery, 45*(3), 610–613. https://doi.org/10.1016/j.jvs.2006.10.043

with the wound or the nurse's ability to care for it. Wrinkling of the nose by the nurse may convey disgust to the patient. The nurse should also be careful not to focus on the wound to the extent that the patient is not treated as a total person.

Ambulatory and Home Care. Because patients are being discharged earlier after surgery and many undergo surgery as outpatients, it is important that the patient, family, or both know how to care for the wound and perform dressing changes. Wound healing may not be complete for 4 to 6 weeks or longer. Adequate rest and good nutrition are essential. Physical and emotional stress should be minimized. The wound should be observed for complications such as infection. The patient should be able to recognize the signs and symptoms of infection and note changes in wound colour and the amount of drainage. The health care provider should be notified of any signs of abnormal wound healing.

Medications are often taken for a period after recovery from an acute infection. Medication-specific adverse effects should be reviewed with the patient, and they should be instructed to contact the health care provider if any of these effects occur. The patient must be taught the necessity to continue the medications for the specified time. For example, a person who is instructed to take an antibiotic for 10 days may stop taking the medication after 5 days because symptoms disappear. However, if a full course of antibiotic is not taken, the infection may not be entirely eliminated and remaining organisms may also become resistant to the antibiotic.

PRESSURE INJURIES

Causes and Pathophysiological Features

A **pressure injury** is a localized injury to the skin or underlying soft tissue, usually over a bony prominence, as a result of excessive or prolonged pressure, shear, and tissue deformation. While most pressure injuries occur from inside out, some of these injuries can be caused by a medical or other device such as catheters. Pressure injuries are generally considered an indicator of the quality of care and most are regarded as avoidable. However, there are instances in which skin breakdown can be considered unavoidable: when patients have limited movement because of hemodynamic instability, when there is inability to provide nutrition and fluids, or at the end of life (Bain et al., 2020).

According to the Canadian Institute for Health Information, pressure injuries are a financial burden to the health care system, in addition to the effect they have on mortality, morbidity, and quality of life. The prevalence of pressure injuries in Canada has been reported to be 0.4% in acute care, 2.4% in home care, 14.1% in complex continuing care, and 6.7% in long-term care (Canadian Institute for Health Information, 2013). The most common sites for development of pressure injury are the sacrum, ischium, trochanter, coccyx, heels, and malleolus.

Factors that influence development of pressure injuries include the amount of pressure (*intensity*), length of time pressure is exerted on the skin (*duration*), and ability of the patient's tissue to tolerate the externally applied stress (Doughty & McNichol, 2016). Besides pressure, shearing force (pressure exerted on the skin when it adheres to the bed and the underlying skin layers slide in the direction of body movement), *friction* (two surfaces rubbing against each other), and *excessive moisture* (incontinence or perspiration) contribute to pressure injury formation (EPUAP/NPIAP/PPPIA, 2019). The tolerance

TABLE 14.12	RISK FACTORS FOR PRESSURE INJURIES

- Advanced age
- Anemia
- Contractures
- Diabetes mellitus
- Elevated body temperature
- Immobility
- Impaired circulation
- Incontinence
- Low diastolic blood pressure (<60 mm Hg)
- Mental deterioration
- Neurological disorders
- Nutritional deficiencies
- Obesity
- Pain
- Prolonged surgery
- Prolonged use of steroids
- Vascular disease

of soft tissue for pressure and shear are affected by microclimate, nutrition, perfusion, comorbidities, and condition of the soft tissue.

Factors that increase a patient's risk for the development of pressure injuries are presented in Table 14.12. Patients at risk include those who are older, incontinent, unable to reposition or unaware of the need to reposition (e.g., spinal cord injury), and bed- or wheelchair-bound. A pressure injury risk assessment and comprehensive skin assessment should be conducted within 8 hours of the patient's admission and with any change in patient condition. A risk-based prevention plan should then be developed (EPUAP/NPIAP/PPPIA, 2019).

Clinical Manifestations

The clinical manifestations of pressure injuries depend on the extent of the tissue that is involved. They are staged according to their deepest level of tissue damage. Table 14.13 illustrates the pressure injury stages according to the EPUAP/NPIAP/PPPIA (2019) guidelines. When slough or necrotic eschar is present, it is not possible to stage the injury until the devitalized tissue is removed by debridement. Clinicians describe such pressure injuries as *unstageable* (EPUAP/NPIAP/PPPIA, 2019).

When full-thickness pressure injuries heal, fat, muscle, and dermis are replaced with granulation tissue, and the original integrity of the tissue is lost. Reverse staging—for example, stating that a stage 3 ulcer has healed into a stage 2 ulcer—is thus not appropriate. Rather, the ulcer would be known as a "healing stage 3 ulcer." It is important to note the location of previously healed pressure injuries in an initial admission assessment because history of a pressure injury is a risk factor for recurrence.

NURSING AND INTERPROFESSIONAL MANAGEMENT PRESSURE INJURIES

Management of a patient with a pressure injury encompasses not only care of the wound itself but also support measures for the whole person, such as adequate nutrition, pain management, control of other medical conditions, and pressure relief. Evidence-informed practice regarding such injuries is to keep a pressure injury slightly moist, rather than dry, to enhance re-epithelialization. In addition to the nurse, other members of the health care team, such as the physician, the dietitian, the physiotherapist, and the occupational therapist, can provide

TABLE 14.13 STAGING OF PRESSURE INJURIES

Deep Tissue Pressure Injury

Intact or nonintact skin with localized area of persistent nonblanchable, deep red, maroon, purple discoloration or epidermal separation revealing a dark wound bed or blood filled blister. Pain and temperature change often precede skin colour changes. Discoloration may appear differently in darkly pigmented skin. This injury results from intense or prolonged pressure and shear forces at the bone–muscle interface. The wound may evolve rapidly to reveal the actual extent of tissue injury, or it may resolve without tissue loss. If necrotic tissue, subcutaneous tissue, granulation tissue, fascia, muscle, or other underlying structures are visible, the injury is a full-thickness pressure injury (unstageable, stage 3, or stage 4). The *term deep tissue pressure injury* does not describe vascular, traumatic, neuropathic, or dermatological conditions.

Diagram   **Clinical Presentation***

Deep Tissue Pressure Injury

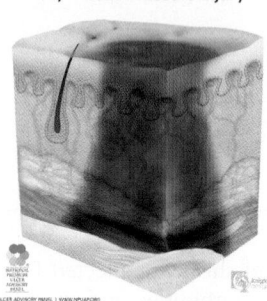
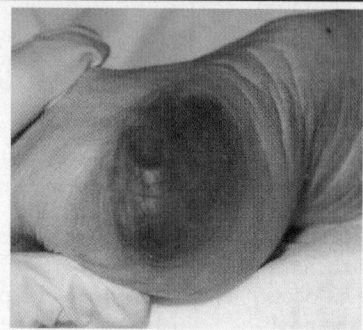
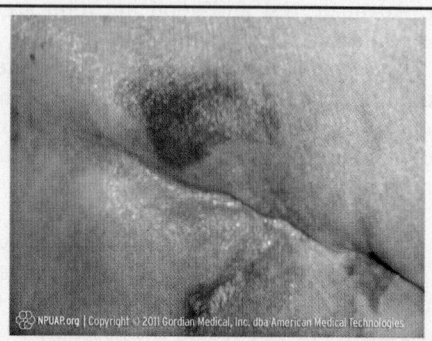

Stage 1

Intact skin with a localized area of nonblanchable erythema, which may appear differently in darkly pigmented skin. Presence of blanchable erythema or changes in sensation, temperature, or firmness may precede visible changes. Colour changes do not include purple or maroon discoloration; these may indicate deep tissue pressure injury.

Diagram   **Clinical Presentation**

Stage 1 Pressure Injury – Darkly Pigmented

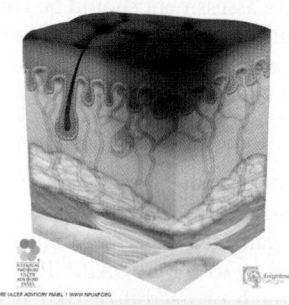
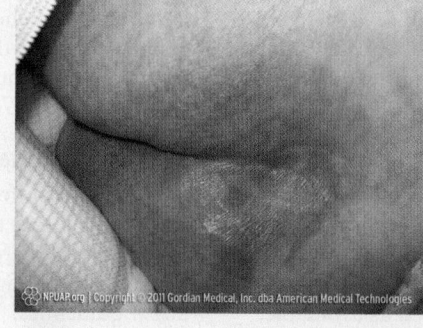

Stage 1 Pressure Injury – Lightly Pigmented

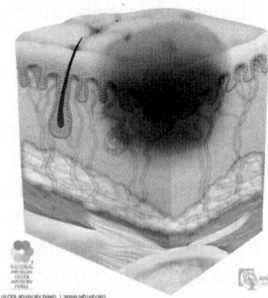
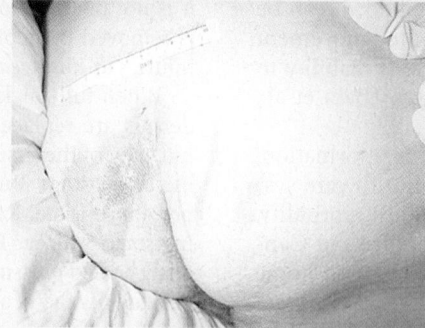

TABLE 14.13 STAGING OF PRESSURE INJURIES—cont'd

Stage 2
Partial-thickness loss of skin with exposed dermis. The wound bed is viable, pink or red, moist, and may also appear as an intact or ruptured serum-filled blister. Neither adipose (fat) nor deeper tissues are visible. Granulation tissue, slough, and eschar are not present. These injuries commonly result from adverse microclimate and shear in the skin over the pelvis and shear in the heel. This stage should not be used to describe moisture-associated skin damage, including incontinence-associated dermatitis, intertriginous dermatitis, medical adhesive–related skin injury, or traumatic wounds (skin tears, burns, abrasions).

Diagram	Clinical Presentation

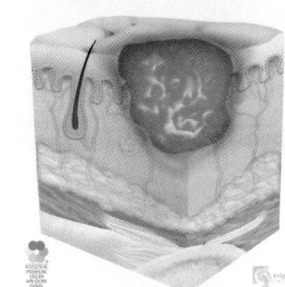
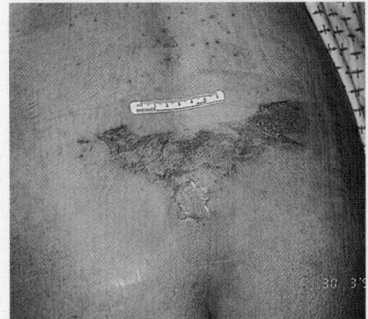
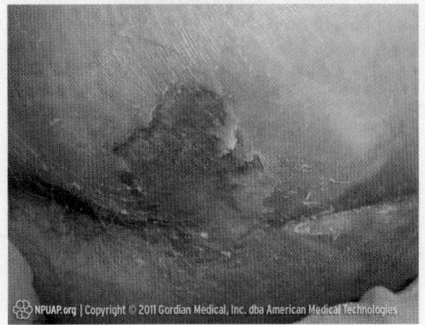

Stage 3
Full-thickness loss of skin, in which adipose (fat) is visible in the ulcer and granulation tissue and epibole (rolled wound edges) are often present. Slough or eschar, or both, may be visible. The depth of tissue damage varies by anatomical location; deep wounds can develop in areas of significant adiposity. Undermining and tunnelling may occur. Fascia, muscle, tendon, ligament, cartilage, and bone are not exposed. If slough or eschar obscures the extent of tissue loss, the injury is considered an unstageable pressure injury.

Diagram	Clinical Presentation

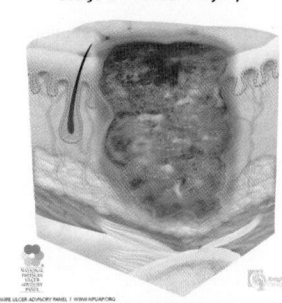
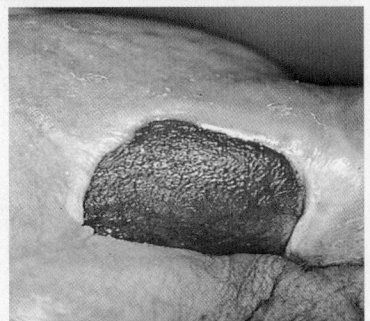
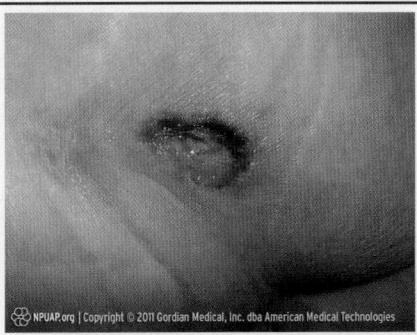

Stage 4
Full-thickness skin and tissue loss with exposed or directly palpable fascia, muscle, tendon, ligament, cartilage, or bone in the ulcer. Slough, eschar, or both may be visible. Epibole (rolled edges), undermining, or tunnelling, or a combination of these, often occurs. Depth varies by anatomical location. If slough or eschar obscures the extent of tissue loss, the injury is considered an unstageable pressure injury.

Diagram	Clinical Presentation

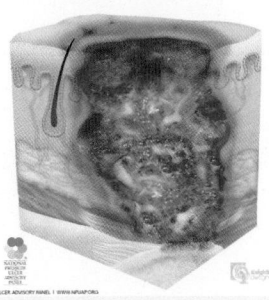
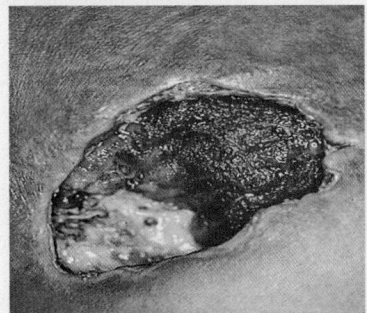
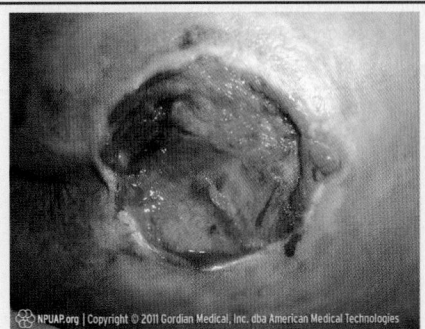

Continued

TABLE 14.13   STAGING OF PRESSURE INJURIES—cont'd

Unstageable

Full-thickness skin and tissue loss in which the extent of tissue damage within the ulcer cannot be confirmed because it is obscured by slough or eschar. If slough or eschar is removed, a stage 3 or stage 4 pressure injury is revealed. Stable eschar (i.e., dry, adherent, intact without erythema or fluctuance) on the heel or ischemic limb should not be softened or removed.

Diagram	Clinical Presentation[†][‡]
Unstageable Pressure Injury – Dark Eschar 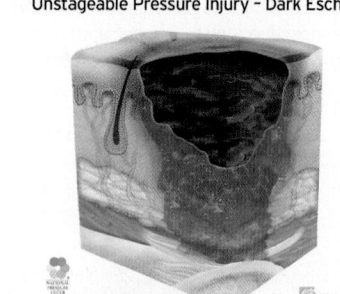 Unstageable Pressure Injury – Slough and Eschar 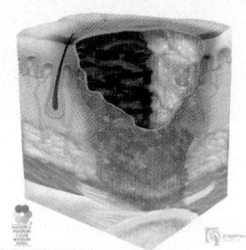	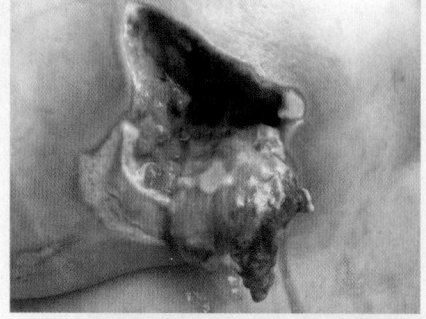 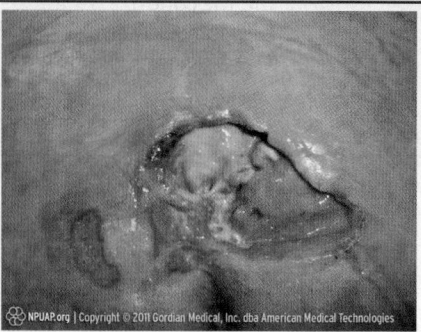 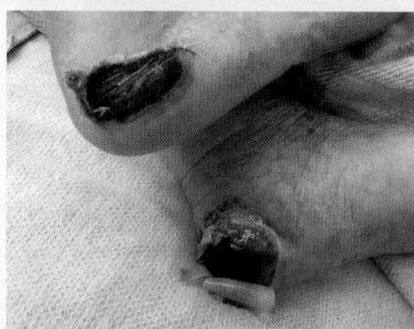

Medical Device–Related Pressure Injury

Medical device–related pressure injuries result from the use of devices designed and applied for diagnostic or therapeutic purposes. The resultant pressure injury generally conforms to the pattern or shape of the device. The injury should be staged according to the staging system just described.

Example

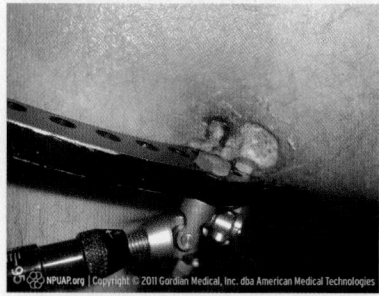

Mucosal Membrane Pressure Injury

Mucosal membrane pressure injury is found on mucous membranes on which a medical device has been in use at the location of the injury. Because of the anatomy of the tissue, these injuries cannot be staged.

Diagram	Clinical Presentation[§]
Mucous Membrane 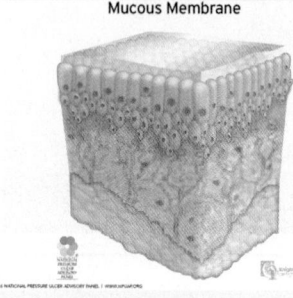	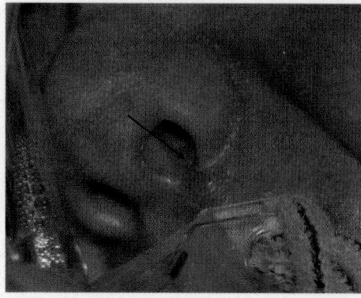

*Photograph of deep tissue injury on heel from Fleck, C. A. (2007). Deep tissue injury: What, why, and when? *Wound Care Canada, 5*(2), 10–53.

[†]Photograph of unstageable pressure injury (first row, middle column) courtesy Kevin Woo, PhD, RN, NSWOC, WOCC(C).

[‡]Photograph of unstageable pressure injury to heel courtesy Kevin Woo, PhD, RN, NSWOC, WOCC(C).

[§]Photograph of mucosal membrane pressure injury used with permission of I. Razmus and L. Lewis.

Note: For additional information regarding the staging of pressure injuries, refer to the European Pressure Ulcer Advisory Panel, National Pressure Injury Advisory Panel, and Pan Pacific Pressure Injury Alliance (EPUAP/NPIAP/PPPIA); Haesler, E. (Ed.). (2019). *Prevention and treatment of pressure ulcers/injuries: Clinical practice guideline. The international guideline*. EPUAP/NPIAP/PPPIA. https://internationalguideline.com

Source: Descriptions, drawings, and photos (with exceptions noted as follows) of pressure injury stages copyrighted by National Pressure Ulcer Advisory Panel (NPUAP) website. (2016). *Educational and clinical resources*. https://www.npuap.org/resources/educational-and-clinical-resources. Used with permission.

valuable input into the complex treatment necessary to prevent and manage pressure injuries. Both conservative and surgical strategies are used in the treatment of pressure injuries, depending on the stage and the condition of the injury. Therapeutic and nursing management are discussed together here because the activities are interrelated.

NURSING ASSESSMENT

Patients should be assessed for pressure injury risk initially on admission to the hospital and at periodic intervals thereafter on the basis of the patient's condition and the care setting. The nurse should conduct a thorough head-to-toe skin assessment on admission to identify and document pressure injuries. The skin and wounds should be reassessed on an ongoing basis and the treatment plan modified accordingly (NSWOCC, 2021).

> **SAFETY ALERT**
> - In acute care, the patient should be reassessed every 24 hours.
> - In long-term care, a resident should be reassessed weekly for the first 4 weeks after admission and at least monthly or every 3 months thereafter.
> - In home care, the patient should be reassessed at each nurse visit.

Risk assessment should be performed with a validated assessment tool such as the Braden scale (Table 14.14). To obtain a patient's pressure injury risk assessment score on the Braden scale, the nurse adds the numerical scores for the factors in each of the six subscales (sensory perception, moisture, activity, mobility, nutrition, and friction and shear). Scores can range from 6 to 23. The lower the numerical score on the Braden scale, the higher is the patient's predicted risk of developing a pressure injury. Incremental changes in the score indicate the level of risk: no risk (19 to 23), at risk (15 to 18), at moderate risk (13 to 14), at high risk (10 to 12), and at very high risk (≤9). Knowing the level of risk can help the health care provider determine how aggressive the preventive measures should be.

Identification of stage 1 pressure injuries may be difficult in patients with dark skin. Table 14.15 presents techniques to help assess darker skin. Subjective and objective data that should be obtained from a person with a pressure injury are presented in Table 14.16.

NURSING DIAGNOSES

Nursing diagnoses for the patient with a pressure injury may include but are not limited to the following:
- *Reduced skin integrity* resulting from *pressure over bony prominence*
- *Reduced tissue integrity* resulting from *inadequate nutrition*

PLANNING. The overall goals are that the patient with a pressure injury will (a) have no deterioration of the ulcer stage, (b) reduce or eliminate the factors that lead to pressure injuries, (c) have improved nutritional status, (d) have increased mobility, (e) not develop an infection in the pressure injury, (f) have healing of pressure injuries, and (g) have no recurrence.

NURSING IMPLEMENTATION

HEALTH PROMOTION. Nurses are responsible for identifying patients at risk for the development of pressure injuries (see Tables 14.12 and 14.14). Once a patient has been identified as being at risk for development of a pressure injury, prevention strategies should be implemented. Prevention remains the best treatment for pressure injuries (Scovil et al., 2019; Suva et al, 2018).

> **SAFETY ALERT**
> - The patient should be repositioned frequently to prevent pressure injuries.
> - Devices to reduce pressure and shearing force (e.g., alternating pressure mattresses, foam dressings, therapeutic mattresses, lift sheets, wheelchair cushions, padded commode seats, heel boots [foam, air]) should be used, as appropriate.
> - These devices are not adequate substitutes for frequent repositioning.

Acute Intervention. Once a pressure injury has developed, the nurse should initiate interventions that are based on the injury characteristics (e.g., stage, size, location, amount of exudate, type of wound tissue, presence of infection or pain) and the patient's general status (e.g., nutritional state, level of mobility).

Measuring the Wound. The size of the pressure injury should be carefully documented. A wound-measuring tape can be used to note the injury's maximum length and width in centimetres (Figure 14.10). To find the depth of the injury, gently place a sterile cotton-tipped applicator into the deepest part of the injury. The length of the portion of the applicator that probed the injury can then be measured.

Documentation. Healing of the wound can be documented with several available pressure injury healing tools such as the NPUAP Pressure Ulcer Scale of Healing (PUSH) tool. Some employers require that pictures of the pressure injury be taken initially and at regular intervals during the course of treatment. See the Informatics in Practice box for suggestions on digital imaging.

Wound Irrigation. Pressure injuries should be cleaned with 100 to 150 mL of a noncytotoxic solution, such as normal saline, that does not damage fibroblasts. It is important to use enough irrigation pressure (4 to 15 psi) to clean the area adequately

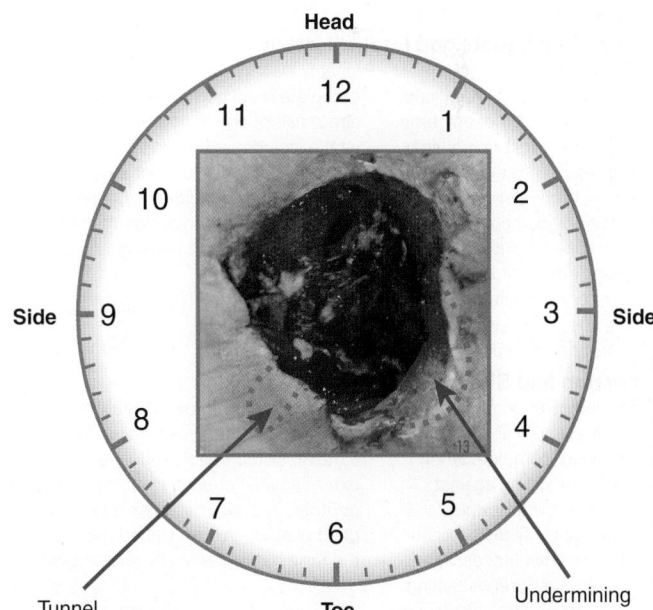

FIG. 14.10 Wound measurements are made in centimetres. The first measurement is oriented from head to toe, the second is from side to side, and the third is the depth (if any). Any tunnelling (when a cotton-tipped applicator is placed in the wound, the applicator moves) or undermining (when a cotton-tipped applicator is placed in wound, there is a "lip" around the wound) is charted like a clock, the 12 o'clock position being toward the patient's head. This wound would be charted as a full-thickness, red wound, 7 cm × 5 cm × 3 cm, with a 3-cm tunnel at the 7 o'clock position and 2-cm undermining from the 3 o'clock to 5 o'clock positions. Source: Courtesy Robert B. Babiak, RN, BSN, CWOCN, San Antonio, TX.

TABLE 14.14   BRADEN SCALE FOR PREDICTING PRESSURE INJURY RISK

Patient's Name _____
Evaluator's Name _____
Date of Assessment _____

Point Value

1	2	3	4	Score
Sensory Perception: Ability to Respond Meaningfully to Pressure-Related Discomfort				
Completely limited: Unresponsive (does not moan, flinch, or grasp) to painful stimuli, due to diminished level of consciousness or sedation or limited ability to feel pain over most of body	Very limited: Responds only to painful stimuli; cannot communicate discomfort except by moaning or restlessness or has a sensory impairment that limits the ability to feel pain or discomfort over half of body	Slightly limited: Responds to verbal commands, but cannot always communicate discomfort or the need to be turned or has some sensory impairment that limits ability to feel pain or discomfort in one or two extremities	No impairment: Responds to verbal commands; has no sensory deficit that would limit ability to feel or to voice pain or discomfort	
Moisture: Degree to Which Skin Is Exposed to Moisture				
Constantly moist: Skin is kept moist almost constantly by perspiration, urine, and so on; dampness is detected every time patient is moved or turned	Very moist: Skin is often, but not always, moist; linen must be changed at least once per shift	Occasionally moist: Skin is occasionally moist, necessitating an extra linen change approximately once per day	Rarely moist: Skin is usually dry; linen requires changing [only] at routine intervals	
Activity: Degree of Physical Activity				
Bedfast: Confined to bed	Chairfast: Ability to walk [is] severely limited or nonexistent; cannot bear own weight or must be assisted into chair or wheelchair	Walks occasionally: Walks occasionally during day, but for very short distances, with or without assistance; spends most of each shift in bed or chair	Walks frequently: Walks outside room at least twice per day and inside room at least once every 2 hours during waking hours	
Mobility: Ability to Change and Control Body Position				
Completely immobile: Does not make even slight changes in body or extremity position without assistance	Very limited: Makes occasional slight changes in body or extremity position but unable to make frequent or significant changes independently	Slightly limited: Makes frequent though slight changes in body or extremity position independently	No limitation: Makes major and frequent changes in position without assistance	
Nutrition: Usual Food Intake Pattern				
Very poor: Never eats a complete meal; rarely eats more than half of any food offered; eats two servings or less of protein (meat or dairy products) per day; takes fluids poorly; does not take a liquid dietary supplement or is NPO and/or maintained on clear liquids or [IV supplements] for more than 5 days	Probably inadequate: Rarely eats a complete meal and generally eats only about half of any food offered; protein intake includes only three servings of meat or dairy products per day; occasionally will take a dietary supplement or receives less than optimum amount of liquid diet or tube feeding	Adequate: Eats over half of most meals; eats four servings of protein (meat or dairy products) per day; occasionally will refuse a meal, but will usually take a supplement when offered or is on a tube feeding or total parenteral nutrition regimen that probably meets most nutritional needs	Excellent: Eats most of every meal; never refuses a meal; eats four or more servings of protein (meat or dairy products); occasionally eats between meals; does not require supplementation	
Friction and Shear				
Problem: Requires moderate to maximum assistance in moving; complete lifting without sliding against sheets is impossible; frequently slides down in bed or chair, necessitating frequent repositioning with maximum assistance; spasticity, contractures, or agitation leads to almost constant friction	Potential problem: Moves feebly or requires minimum assistance; during a move, skin probably slides to some extent against sheets, chair, restraints, or other devices; maintains relatively good position in chair or bed most of the time but occasionally slides down	No apparent problem: Moves in bed and in chair independently and has sufficient muscle strength to lift up completely during move; maintains good position in bed or chair		

IVs, intravenous nutrition; *NPO,* nothing by mouth (status).

EVIDENCE-INFORMED PRACTICE

Translating Research Into Practice

The nurse is caring for S. W. (pronouns she/her), an 86-year-old with obesity and a history of diabetes, hypertension, and chronic kidney disease. S. W. spends most of her time in bed or in a wheelchair and now has a stage 1 pressure injury on her sacral area. The nurse is delivering discharge teaching to the patient's daughter, who is her primary caregiver. The nurse explains the importance of preventing further skin breakdown and that S. W.'s daughter needs to reposition her mother every 2 to 4 hours during the night. S. W.'s daughter tells the nurse that at night, she will reposition her mother only if her mother wakes up to use the commode; otherwise, she must have uninterrupted sleep because she watches her two young grandchildren during the day.

Best Available Evidence	Clinician Expertise	Patient Preferences and Values
Repositioning remains the primary method of reducing risk for pressure injuries. Pressure-reducing devices (e.g., foam dressings and mattress, padded commode seats) can also be used but should not be a substitute for repositioning.	Patients with pressure injuries should be repositioned at least every 2 to 4 hours while in bed and should shift weight every 15 minutes when in a chair. Stage 1 pressure injuries can rapidly deteriorate to stage 2 if proper care is not taken.	S. W.'s caregiver expresses the need to have a certain amount of uninterrupted sleep to maintain multiple family responsibilities. The caregiver states that she will reposition her mother at least every 2–4 hours while she is in bed during the day and every 15 minutes when she is in a wheelchair. S. W.'s caregiver states she will purchase a foam mattress, wheelchair cushion, and padded commode seat to help prevent further skin issues.

Decision and Action

The nurse discusses the importance of repositioning as the primary method to prevent pressure injuries and decrease the progression of existing pressure injuries to more serious ones. S. W.'s daughter reiterates that she will not be able to reposition her mother every 2 to 4 hours during the night. The nurse can understand her decision and documents this discussion in the patient's discharge teaching record.

Reference for Evidence

European Pressure Ulcer Advisory Panel, National Pressure Injury Advisory Panel, & Pan Pacific Pressure Injury Alliance; Haesler, E. (Ed.). (2019). *Prevention and treatment of pressure ulcers/injuries: Clinical practice guideline. The international guideline.* Cambridge Media.

---

without causing trauma or damage to the wound, which can be accomplished with the use of a 100-mL saline squeeze bottle or a 30-mL syringe with a 19-gauge angiocatheter (NSWOCC, 2021).

Local Wound Care. After the pressure injury has been cleansed, it should be covered with an appropriate dressing. Some factors to consider in selecting a dressing are maintenance of a moist environment, prevention of wound desiccation (drying out), ability to absorb the wound drainage, location of the wound, amount of caregiver time, cost of the dressing, presence of infection, pain, and the setting of care delivery. For further information on preparing the wound bed and localized wound care, refer to the Canadian Association of Wound Care website (see the Resources at the end of this chapter). (Dressings are discussed in Table 14.11.)

TABLE 14.15 ASSESSING PATIENTS WITH DARK SKIN

To assess patients with dark skin, the nurse should:
- Look for changes in skin colour, such as skin that is darker (purplish, brownish, bluish) than surrounding skin.
- Use natural light or a halogen light source to accurately assess the skin colour. Fluorescent light casts blue light, which can make skin assessment difficult.
- Assess the skin temperature of the area by using one's hand. The area may feel warm initially and then cooler.
- Touch the skin to feel its consistency. Boggy or edematous observation may indicate a stage 1 pressure injury.
- Ask the patient if they have any pain or itchy sensation.

TABLE 14.16 NURSING ASSESSMENT

Pressure Injuries

Subjective Data
Important Health Information

Past health history: Stroke, spinal cord injury; prolonged bed rest or immobility; circulatory impairment; poor nutrition; altered level of consciousness; history of previous pressure injury; immunological abnormalities; advanced age; diabetes; anemia; trauma
Medications: Use of opioids, hypnotics, systemic corticosteroids, nicotine
Surgery or other treatments: Recent surgery

Symptoms

Incontinence of urine, feces, or both; weakness, debilitation, inability to turn and position body; pain or altered cutaneous sensation in injured area; decreased awareness of pressure on body areas; decreased fluid, calorie, or protein intake; vitamin or mineral deficiencies

Objective Data
General

Obesity; emaciation; clinically significant malnutrition as indicated by low serum albumin level, decreased total lymphocyte count, and decreased body weight (15% less than ideal body weight); contractures

Integumentary

Diaphoresis, edema, and discoloration, especially over bony areas such as sacrum, hips, elbows, heels, knees, ankles, shoulders, and ear rims, progressing to increased tissue damage characteristic of ulcer stages*

Possible Findings

Leukocytosis if infection present, positive cultures for microorganisms from pressure injury

*See TABLE 14.13.

INFORMATICS IN PRACTICE

Digital Images

To monitor wound progress, use digital photography.
For the best images:
- Include a ruler with date, length, width, and depth of the wound in each photo.
- Position the patient the same way for each photo.
- Take the photo from the same angle each time. Pointing perpendicularly at the wound is best.
- Use natural light, without flash, whenever possible.
- Show the wound on a solid background, avoiding shiny underpads.

Stage 2 through stage 4 pressure injuries are considered contaminated or colonized with bacteria. For patients with chronic wounds or who are immunocompromised, the clinical signs of localized infection may be more subtle (UPPER: **U**nhealthy tissue, **P**ain, **P**oor healing, **E**xudate, and **R**eek); typical overt signs of infection including purulent exudate, odour, erythema, induration, warmth, tenderness, edema, pain, fever, and elevated WBC count may not be present even though the wound is infected.

The maintenance of adequate nutrition is an important nursing responsibility for the patient with a pressure injury (NSWOCC, 2021). Many such patients are debilitated and have a poor appetite as a result of inactivity. Clinically significant malnutrition is defined as a body weight decrease of more than 5% over a 6- to 12-month period. Biochemical data including serum albumin level and total lymphocyte count are not sensitive indicators of malnutrition. Oral feedings must be adequate in calories, proteins, fluids, vitamins, and minerals to meet the patient's nutritional requirements. The intake needed to correct and maintain a nutritional balance may be 30 to 35 calories per kilogram per day and 1.25 to 1.50 g of protein per kilogram per day. Nasogastric feedings can be used to supplement the oral feedings. Parenteral nutrition consisting of amino acid and glucose solutions is administered when oral and nasogastric feedings are inadequate. (Parenteral and enteral nutrition are discussed in Chapter 42.) Nursing Care Plan 14.2 (available on the Evolve website) outlines the care for the patient with a pressure injury.

An appropriate support surface for both bed and chair or wheelchair should relieve pressure and keep the patient off of the damaged area. In some circumstances, reconstruction of the pressure injury site by operative repair, including skin grafting, skin flaps, musculocutaneous flaps, or free flaps, may be necessary.

Ambulatory and Home Care. Pressure injuries affect the quality of life of patients and their caregivers. Because recurrence is common, the education of both the patient and the care provider in prevention techniques is extremely important. The care provider needs to know the causes of pressure injuries, prevention techniques, early signs, nutritional support, and best practice for wound management. Because many patients with a pressure injury require extensive care for other health issues, it is important that the nurse support the caregiver in confronting the added responsibility of pressure injury treatment.

Cultural Implications

Issues regarding wound healing among Indigenous people include their high rates of diabetes and other chronic illnesses, as well as social determinants of health inequities such as poor housing, insufficient housing leading to crowding, poverty, and nutritionally poor diets (Jacklin et al., 2017). Issues on reserve, rurally, or in remote areas may include decreased access to wound management services, to sufficient wound healing equipment, or to wound healing dressings, and lack of continuity of care with nurses, health care providers, physiotherapists, and occupation therapists, among others. These inequities, along with cultural considerations, need to be considered when caring for Indigenous patients. Poverty, difficulties accessing pharmacies, transportation difficulties, and housing issues may also affect Indigenous people living in urban areas.

❘ EVALUATION

Expected outcomes for the patient with a pressure injury are presented in Nursing Care Plan 14.2 on the Evolve website.

CASE STUDY

Inflammation and Infection

Patient Profile

F. R. (pronouns he/him), 58 years old, is admitted to the hospital emergency department with partial-thickness burns that involve his face, neck, and upper trunk. He also has a lacerated right lower leg. F. R.'s injuries occurred about 36 hours earlier, when he fell out of a tree onto his gas grill (which was lit) while he was trying to get to his cat.

Subjective Data

- Reports slightly hoarse voice and irritated throat
- States that he tried to treat himself because he does not regularly see the same health care provider
- Has been coughing up sooty sputum
- Reports severe pain in left hip

Objective Data

Physical Examination

- Leg wound is gaping and looks infected; temperature is 38.4°C
- Radiographs reveal a fractured right tibia and a fractured left hip

Laboratory Studies

- WBC count is 26.4×10^9/L with 80% neutrophils (10% bands)

Interprofessional Care

- Surgery is performed to repair the left hip.

Discussion Questions

1. What clinical manifestations of inflammation did F. R. exhibit, and what are their pathophysiological mechanisms?
2. What type of exudate formation developed?
3. What is the basis for F. R.'s elevated temperature?
4. What is the significance of F. R.'s WBC count and differential?
5. Because F. R.'s wound was gaping, primary tissue healing was not possible. How might healing take place? What complications could he develop?
6. What are F. R.'s risk factors for developing a pressure injury?
7. ***Priority Decision:*** On the basis of the assessment data provided, what are the priority nursing diagnoses? Are there any interprofessional issues?

ℯvolve
Answers are available at http://evolve.elsevier.com/Canada/Lewis/medsurg.

REVIEW QUESTIONS

The number of the question corresponds to the same-numbered objective at the beginning of the chapter.

1. In which context is physiological hyperplasia commonly found?
   a. A distended urinary bladder
   b. The female breast during lactation
   c. The bronchi of a chronic cigarette smoker
   d. An enlarged myocardium in heart failure

2. When radiation therapy is used in the treatment of cancer, how does it achieve the desired effect, which is death of cancer cells?
   a. Altering cellular metabolism and activity
   b. Producing mutations that interfere only with cancer cell function
   c. Accelerating metabolic reactions to reduce the normal life-span of cells
   d. Stimulating synthesis of new particles that cause cell rupture and death

3. Which of the following is an example of coagulation necrosis?
   a. Autophagocytosis
   b. Myocardial infarction
   c. Malignant brain tumour
   d. Peripheral vascular disease

4. Which of the following will be experienced by a client with an impaired mononuclear phagocyte system?
   a. Increased circulation of histamine
   b. Decreased susceptibility to infection
   c. Decreased vascular response to cell injury
   d. Decreased surveillance for damaged or mutated cells

5. One day after abdominal surgery a client has incisional pain, 37.5°C temperature, slight erythema at the incision margins, and 30 mL of serosanguineous drainage in the Jackson-Pratt drain. On the basis of this assessment, what conclusion would the nurse make?
   a. The abdominal incision shows signs of an infection.
   b. The client is having a normal inflammatory response.
   c. The abdominal incision shows signs of impending dehiscence.
   d. The client's health care provider must be notified about her condition.

6. The nurse assessing a client with a chronic leg wound finds local signs of erythema and pain at the wound site. What would the nurse anticipate being ordered to assess the client's systemic response?
   a. Serum protein analysis
   b. WBC count and differential
   c. Punch biopsy of centre of wound
   d. Culture and sensitivity testing of the wound

7. A client in the unit has a 39.8°C temperature. Which intervention would be most effective in restoring normal body temperature?
   a. Use a cooling blanket while the client is febrile.
   b. Administer antipyretics on an around-the-clock schedule.
   c. Provide increased fluids and instruct the unregulated care provider to give sponge baths.
   d. Give prescribed antibiotics and provide warm blankets for comfort.

8. A nurse is caring for a client who has a pressure injury that is treated with debridement, irrigations, and moist gauze dressings. How should the nurse anticipate healing to occur?
   a. Tertiary intention
   b. Secondary intention
   c. Regeneration of cells
   d. Remodelling of tissues

9. A nurse is caring for a client with diabetes who is scheduled for amputation of his necrotic left great toe. The client's WBC count is 15.0×10^9/L, and he has coolness of the lower extremities, weighs 34 kg more than his ideal body weight, and smokes two packs of cigarettes per day. Which priority nursing diagnosis addresses the primary factor affecting the client's ability to heal?
   a. Readiness for enhanced nutrition
   b. Impaired tissue integrity resulting from insufficient knowledge about protecting tissue integrity
   c. Ineffective peripheral tissue perfusion related to sedentary lifestyle
   d. Ineffective coping resulting from ineffective tension release strategies

10. An 89-year-old client with end-stage renal disease is assessed to have a score of 16 on the Braden scale. On the basis of this information, how should the nurse plan for this client's care?
    a. Implement a 1-hour turning schedule with skin assessment.
    b. Place a hydrocolloid on the client's sacrum to prevent breakdown.
    c. Elevate the head of bed to 90 degrees when the client is supine.
    d. Continue with weekly skin assessments with no additional special precautions.

11. A 65-year-old client who has had a stroke and has limited mobility has a purple area of suspected deep tissue injury on the left greater trochanter. Which nursing diagnoses are most appropriate? (Select all that apply.)
    a. Acute pain resulting from physical injury agent
    b. Reduced skin integrity resulting from pressure over bony prominence
    c. Reduced tissue integrity resulting from insufficient knowledge about protecting tissue integrity
    d. Potential for infection as evidenced by malnutrition

12. An 82-year-old man is being cared for at home by his family. A pressure injury on his right buttock measures $1 \times 2 \times 0.8$ cm in depth, and pink subcutaneous tissue is completely visible on the wound bed. Which stage would the nurse document on the wound assessment form?
    a. Stage 1
    b. Stage 2
    c. Stage 3
    d. Stage 4

13. Which one of the orders should a nurse question in the plan of care for an older client who is immobile as the result of a stroke and has a stage 3 pressure injury?
    a. Cover the injury with a foam dressing.
    b. Turn and position the client every hour.
    c. Clean the wound every shift with Dakin's solution.
    d. Assess for pain and medicate before dressing change.

1. b; 2, a; 3, b; 4, d; 5, b; 6, b; 7, b; 8, b; 9, b; 10, a; 11, b, c; 12, c; 13, c.

Ⓔvolve

For even more review questions, visit http://evolve.elsevier.com/Canada/Lewis/medsurg.

REFERENCES

Bain, M., Hara, J., & Carter, M. J. (2020). The pathophysiology of skin failure vs. pressure injury: Conditions that cause integument destruction and their associated implications. *Wounds, 32*(11), 319–327.

Braden, B., & Bergstrom, N. (1994). Predictive validity of the Braden scale for pressure sore risk in a nursing home population. *Research in Nursing & Health, 17*, 459. (Seminal).

Canadian Institute for Health Information. (2013). *Compromised wounds in Canada.* https://secure.cihi.ca/free_products/AiB_Compromised_Wounds_EN.pdf. (Seminal).

Dinarello, C. A., & Porat, R. (2015). Fever and hyperthermia. In D. L. Kasper, A. S. Fauci, D. L. Longo, et al. (Eds.), *Harrison's principles of internal medicine* (19th ed.). McGraw-Hill. https://doi.org/10.1001/jama.308.17.1813-b

Doughty, D., & McNichol, L. (2016). *Wound Ostomy Continence Nurses Society core curriculum: Wound management.* Wolters-Kluwer.

El Chakhtoura, N. G., Bonomo, R. A., & Jump, R. L. (2017). Influence of aging and environment on presentation of infection in older adults. *Infectious Disease Clinics, 31*(4), 593–608. https://doi.org/10.1016/j.idc.2017.07.017

European Pressure Ulcer Advisory Panel. (2019). In E. Haesler (Ed.), *National Pressure Injury Advisory Panel, & Pan Pacific Pressure Injury Alliance (EPUAP/NPIAP/PPPIA). Prevention and treatment of pressure ulcers/injuries: Clinical practice guideline. The international guideline:* Cambridge Media. http://www.internationalguideline.com/guideline

Jacklin, K. M., Henderson, R. I., Green, M. E., et al. (2017). Health care experience of Indigenous people living with type 2 diabetes in Canada. *CMAJ, 189*(3), E106–112. https://doi.org/10.1503/cmaj.161098

Jones, R. E., Foster, D. S., & Longaker, M. T. (2018). Management of chronic wounds—2018. *JAMA, 320*(14), 1481–1482. https://doi.org/10.1001/jama.2018.12426

Krafts, K. (2012). *A quick summary of six types of necrosis.* http://www.pathologystudent.com/?p=5770. (Seminal).

LeBlanc, K., Langemo, D., Woo, K., et al. (2019). Skin tears: Prevention and management. *British Journal of Community Nursing, 24*(Suppl 9), S12–S18. https://doi.org/10.12968/bjcn.2019.24.Sup9.S12

McInnes, E., Jammali–Blasi, A., Bell–Syer, S. E., et al. (2015). Support surfaces for pressure ulcer prevention. *Cochrane Database of Systematic Reviews* (9). https://doi.org/10.1002/14651858.CD001735.pub5

Nurses Specialized in Wound, Ostomy and Continence Canada. (2021). *Debridement: Canadian best practice recommendations for nurses.* https://nswoc.ca/wp-content/uploads/2021/05/NSWOCC-Debridement-Best-Practice-Recommendations-April-2021-1.pdf

Scovil, C. Y., Delparte, J. J., Walia, S., et al. (2019). Implementation of pressure injury prevention best practices across 6 Canadian rehabilitation Sites: results from the Spinal Cord Injury Knowledge Mobilization Network. *Archives of Physical Medicine and Rehabilitation, 100*(2), 327–335. https://doi.org/10.1016/j.apmr.2018.07.444

Suva, G., Sharma, T., Campbell, K. E., et al. (2018). Strategies to support pressure injury best practices by the inter–professional team: A systematic review. *International Wound Journal, 15*(4), 580–589. https://doi.org/10.1111/iwj.12901

Woo, K. (2017). HOPES for palliative wounds. *Journal of Palliative Nursing, 23*(6), 264–268. https://doi.org/10.12968/ijpn.2017.23.6.264

Woo, K. Y., Keast, D., Parsons, N., et al. (2015). The cost of wound debridement: A Canadian perspective. *International Wound Journal, 12*(4), 402–407. https://doi.org/10.1111/iwj.12122. (Seminal).

RESOURCES

Infection Prevention and Control Canada
https://ipac-canada.org/

Mount Sinai Hospital Department of Microbiology
https://www.mountsinai.on.ca/care/microbiology

Nurses Specialized in Wound, Ostomy and Continence Canada (NSWOCC)
https://www.nswoc.ca

Ontario Ministry of Health and Long-Term Care
https://www.health.gov.on.ca/en/

Ontario Ministry of Health and Long-Term Care, Medical Advisory Secretariat: Negative Pressure Wound Therapy—An Evidence-Based Analysis
https://www.hqontario.ca/Portals/0/Documents/evidence/reports/rev_npwt_070106.pdf

Ontario Woundcare Interest Group
https://ontwig.ca/

Public Health Agency of Canada
https://www.phac-aspc.gc.ca

Registered Nurses' Association of Ontario (RNAO)—Nursing Best Practice Guidelines
https://rnao.ca/bpg

Regroupement Québécois en Soins de Plaies
www.rqsp.ca

Wounds Canada
https://www.woundscanada.ca

Advances in Skin and Wound Care
https://journals.lww.com/aswcjournal

Agency for Health Care Policy
https://www.ahrq.gov/

Centers for Disease Control and Prevention
https://www.cdc.gov

European Pressure Ulcer Advisory Panel (EPUAP)
https://www.epuap.org

European Wound Management Association
https://www.ewma.org

International Federation of Infection Control
https://www.theific.org/

International Wound Infection Institute
https://www.woundinfection-institute.com/

National Pressure Injury Advisory Panel
https://www.npiap.com

World Council of Enterostomal Therapists
https://www.wcetn.org

World Health Organization
https://www.who.int/en

World Union of Wound Healing Societies (WUWHS)
https://wuwhs2022.org

Wound Management & Prevention
https://www.hmpgloballearningnetwork.com/site/wmp

Wound, Ostomy and Continence Nurses Society
https://www.wocn.org

ℯvolve

For additional Internet resources, see the website for this book at http://evolve.elsevier.com/Canada/Lewis/medsurg.

Genetics

April Pike
Originating US chapter by Janice Smolowitz

WEBSITE

http://evolve.elsevier.com/Canada/Lewis/medsurg

- Review Questions (Online Only)
- Key Points
- Conceptual Care Map Creator
- Audio Glossary
- Content Updates

LEARNING OBJECTIVES

1. Define key terms and principles of genetics and genetic disorders.
2. Distinguish between the two common causes of genetic mutations.
3. Compare and contrast the three most common inheritance patters of genetic disorders.
4. Illustrate how to take a family history or pedigree using the common nomenclature.
5. Describe issues related to genetic screening and testing.
6. Outline the role of the nurse in working with patients and families with genetic and genomic concerns.
7. Explore the complex ethical and social implications of genetic testing.

KEY TERMS

allele	genetics	pharmacogenomics
autosome	genotype	recessive allele
carrier	heterozygous	ribonucleic acid (RNA)
deoxyribonucleic acid (DNA)	homozygous	sex-linked gene
gene therapy	mutation	transcription
genetic counsellor	pharmacogenetics	translation

Genomics, the study of a person's genes (the genome), has the aim of understanding the entire genetic information of an organism, including interactions of these genes with each other and the environment (Genome Canada, 2020b; National Human Genome Research Institute, 2020). There are approximately 30 000 genes in one person's genome. Information about genomes is rapidly becoming available with scientific advancements. Genomics includes the study of complex diseases, such as heart disease, diabetes, and cancer, as these diseases are typically caused by a combination of genetic and environmental factors. At the same time, genomics is creating a paradigm shift in the health care system from one that is disease-focused to one that is more precise, personalized, predictive, preventative, and cost-effective and promotes healthy aging.

Genetics is the study of genes and their role in inheritance. Genetics determines the way that certain traits or conditions are passed down through the genes. *Genes* are the basic units of heredity. They are composed of sequences of deoxyribonucleic acid (DNA) found along a person's chromosomes. Genes are passed down from one generation to the next. The *genome* is the complete set of DNA. It includes all the organism's genes. An organism's genome has all the information it needs to build and maintain itself. A person's genes can have a profound impact on health and disease.

The identification of a genetic basis for many diseases can influence the care of patients at risk for a genetic-linked disease. Nurses are at the interface of translating new human genome research discoveries into clinical practice and will increasingly care for individuals and families who have a genetic condition or a health issue with a genetic component. Nurses must be familiar with the basic principles of genetics and the impact that genetics and genomics can have on the lives of Canadians. They need to be prepared to help the patient and the family navigate genetic concerns.

BASIC PRINCIPLES OF GENETICS: GENES, CHROMOSOMES, AND DNA

Common terms used in genetics and genomics are defined in Table 15.1.

Genes

An individual's genome or genotype is thought to be made up of around 30 000 genes. Genes carry the instructions (encode) for making proteins that direct the activities of cells. Genes control how a cell functions, including how quickly it grows, how often it divides, and how long it lives. To control these functions, genes make proteins that perform specific tasks and act as messengers for the cell. It is essential that each gene have the correct instructions, or "code," for making its protein so that the protein can perform the proper function for the cell. Genes are arranged in a specific linear formation along a chromosome (Figure 15.1). Each gene has a specific location on a chromosome, termed a *locus*. An *allele* is one of two or more alternative forms of a gene that occupy corresponding loci on homologous chromosomes (a pair of chromosomes having corresponding DNA sequences, with one coming from the mother and the other from the father). Each allele codes for a specific inherited characteristic.

When there are two different alleles, the allele that is fully expressed is the *dominant* allele. The other allele that lacks the ability to express itself in the presence of a dominant allele is the *recessive* allele. The actual genetic makeup of the person is called the genotype. The physical and observable characteristics of an individual (e.g., eye colour, weight) are called *phenotypes*.

Chromosomes

Chromosomes occur in pairs and are located within the cell nucleus. Humans have two sets of 23 chromosomes (46 in total). One set is inherited from the mother, and one set is inherited from the father during conception. Twenty-two pairs of chromosomes, called *autosomes,* are the same in both men and women. The twenty-third pair is referred to as the *sex chromosomes*. A male has an X and a Y chromosome, and a female has two X chromosomes. The genetic material on each of the non-sex chromosome pairs is *homologous* to each other, meaning that they have the same position and order (Figure 15.2).

Deoxyribonucleic Acid (DNA)

Genes are made up of deoxyribonucleic acid (DNA), which contains the instructions in cells that drive most cellular processes by synthesizing specific proteins. DNA regulates the rate at which proteins are made. DNA is a double-helix structure in which two strands (polynucleotide chains) run in opposite directions (Figure 15.3). The two strands are held together by hydrogen bonds between pairs of bases: adenine (A), thymine (T), guanine (G), and cytosine (C). DNA is composed of a sugar (deoxyribose), a phosphate group, and one of the four nitrogenous bases. One unit, a sugar group combined with a phosphate group and one of the four bases, is called a *nucleotide*. The bases on each strand of DNA are paired in a specific manner. Adenine

TABLE 15.1	GLOSSARY OF GENETIC TERMS
Term	**Definition**
Allele	One of two or more alternative forms of a gene that can occupy a particular chromosomal locus
Autosome	Any chromosome that is not a sex chromosome
Carrier	An individual who carries a copy of a mutated gene for a recessive disorder
Chromosome	A gene-carrying structure in the nucleus of all human cells that consists of DNA and protein
Codominance	Two dominant versions of a trait that are both expressed in the same individual
Congenital disorder	Condition present at birth
Consanguineous	Reproduction between two people from the same bloodline (e.g., first or second cousins)
Dominant allele	Gene that is expressed in the phenotype of a heterozygous individual
Gene	Unit of hereditary information located on a specific part of a chromosome
Genetic risk	Probability of inheriting a disorder or disease
Genetic counsellor	A health care provider with expertise in genetics and genetic counselling
Genome	An organism's complete set of genetic material present in a cell
Hereditary	A disease or condition being transmitted from parent to offspring
Heterozygous	Having two different alleles for one given gene
Homozygous	Having two identical alleles for one given gene
Locus	Position of a gene on a chromosome
Mutation	A change in the DNA sequence of a gene, affecting expression of the gene (changing the original manner of expression)
Oncogene	Gene that is able to initiate and contribute to the conversion of normal cells to cancer cells
Pedigree	Family tree that contains the genetic characteristics and disorders of that particular family
Pharmacogenomics	The field of genetics that studies how drugs affect and interact with the genome and output expression
Pharmacogenetics	The study of how human genes affect drug metabolism
Phenotype	Clinically expressed traits of an individual
Proto-oncogenes	Normal cellular genes that are important regulators of normal cellular processes; mutations can activate them to become oncogenes
Recessive allele	An allele that has no noticeable effect on the phenotype in a heterozygous individual
Sex-linked gene	A gene located on a sex chromosome
Trait	Physical characteristic that one inherits, such as hair and eye colour

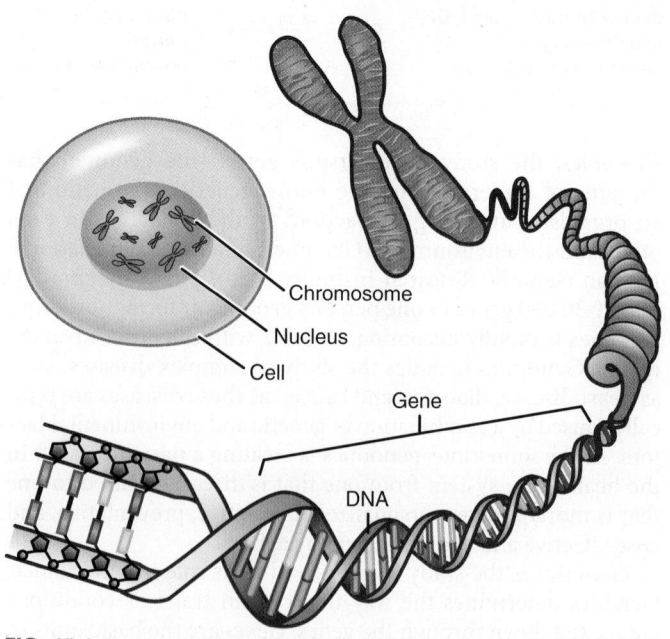

FIG. 15.1 The long, stringy DNA that makes up genes is spooled within chromosomes inside the nucleus of a cell. Note that a gene would actually be a much longer stretch of DNA than what is shown here. Source: National Institute of General Medical Science. National Institutes of Health, US Department of Health and Human Services. (2010). *The new genetics.* https://publications.nigms.nih.gov/thenewgenetics/thenewgenetics.pdf

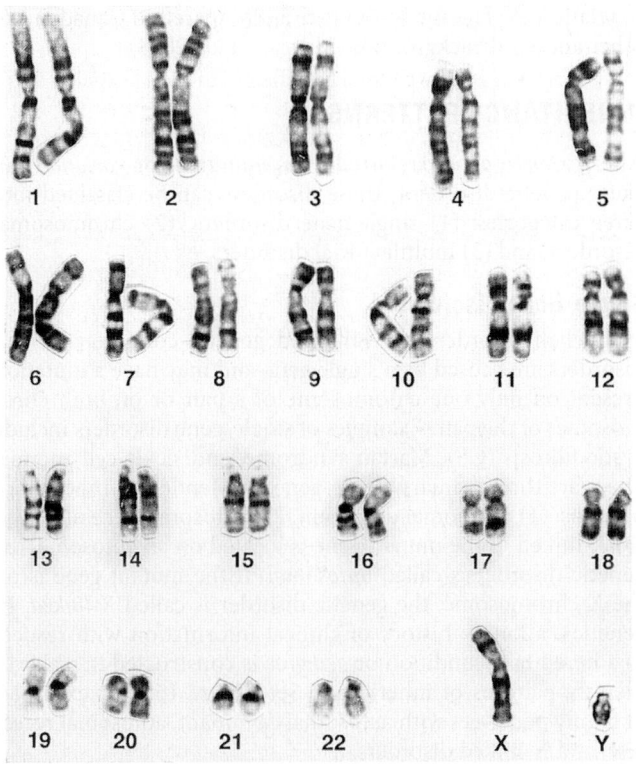

FIG. 15.2 Human chromosomes. Source: Turnpenny, P. D. (2007). *Emery's elements of medical genetics* (13th ed., p. 34). Churchill Livingstone/Elsevier.

always pairs with thymine, and guanine pairs with cytosine. The specific nature of the genetic information encoded in the human genome lies in the nucleotide sequence within the DNA.

DNA can replicate or make copies of itself. Each strand of DNA in the double helix can serve as a pattern for duplicating the sequence of bases. When cells divide, each new cell must have an exact copy of the DNA that was in the parent (original) cell.

Ribonucleic Acid (RNA). RNA is similar to DNA but with some significant differences. Ribonucleic acid (RNA) contains the nitrogenous bases adenine, guanine, and cytosine, but it contains uracil instead of thymine. RNA is single, not double, stranded. It contains ribose instead of deoxyribose sugar. RNA transfers the genetic information obtained from DNA to the proper location for protein synthesis.

Protein Synthesis. Protein synthesis, or the process by which genetic information is converted into proteins, takes place in the cytoplasm and occurs in two steps: transcription and translation (Figure 15.4). Transcription is the creation of a messenger RNA (mRNA) from a single-stranded DNA. The mRNA is complementary to the DNA. The mRNA travels from the cell nucleus into the cytoplasm in preparation for protein synthesis. The ribosome attaches to the mRNA, reads its base sequence, and translates it into its corresponding amino acid. At this point another specialized type of RNA, transfer RNA (tRNA), arranges the amino acids in the correct sequence to assemble the protein. Once the protein is complete, it is released from the ribosome and able to perform its specific function in the cell.

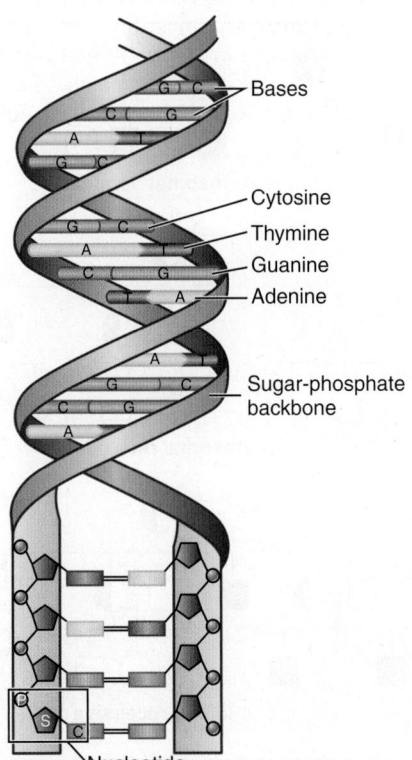

FIG. 15.3 DNA consists of two long, twisted chains made up of nucleotides. Each nucleotide contains one base, one phosphate molecule *(P)*, and the sugar molecule deoxyribose *(S)*. The bases in DNA nucleotides are adenine *(A)*, thymine *(T)*, cytosine *(C)*, and guanine *(G)*. Source: Adapted from National Institute of General Medical Science. National Institutes of Health, US Department of Health and Human Services. (2010). *The new genetics.* https://publications.nigms.nih.gov/thenewgenetics/thenewgenetics.pdf

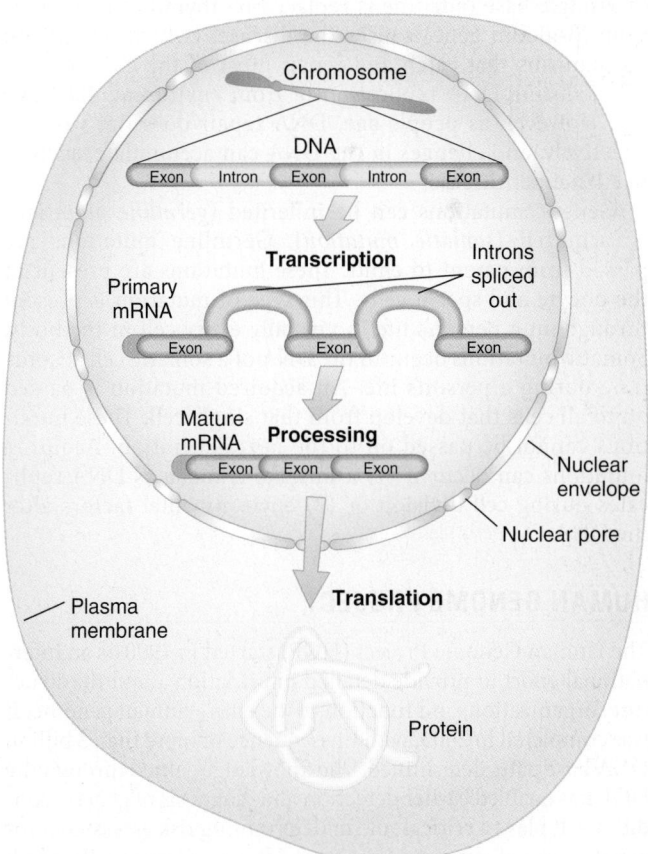

FIG. 15.4 A summary of the steps leading from DNA to protein creation. Replication and transcription occur in the cell nucleus. The mRNA is then transported to the cytoplasm, where translation of the mRNA into amino acid sequences composing a protein occurs. Source: Jorde, L., Cary, J., & Bamshad, M. (2010). *Medical genetics* (4th ed., p. 10). Mosby.

Cell Division

Mitosis. Mitosis results in the formation of genetically identical daughter cells. Before cell division, the chromosomes duplicate, and each new cell (called *daughter cells*) receives an exact replica of the chromosomes from the original cell (called the *parent cell*).

Meiosis. Meiosis occurs only in germline, or sexual reproductive, cells. Two consecutive nuclear divisions, meiosis I and meiosis II, occur without chromosomes replicating in between. This results in the production of four haploid sex cells. Each has a single copy of each chromosome.

Genetic Mutations. A genetic mutation, or variant, permanently changes the usual DNA sequence. Mutations range in size from a single DNA base to a large segment of a chromosome. The change in gene structure may change the type or amount of protein made. The protein may not work at all, or it may work incorrectly. Other mutations can take place during cell division. During replication, the insertion, duplication, deletion, or rearrangement of DNA sequence can take place. Environmental factors such as ultraviolet radiation can damage DNA, leading to skin cancer. Toxins in cigarette smoke can lead to lung cancer. Chemotherapy agents target the DNA of cancer cells and that of healthy cells, thus increasing one's risk of getting secondary cancer.

In some cases, genetic mutations do not have an obvious effect on the people who have them. Some gene variations may result in disease or an increased risk for disease. For example, in people with sickle cell disease, a substitution of a single base (adenine is replaced by thymine) in a single gene (β-globin gene) causes the disease. Cells have built-in mechanisms that catch and repair most of the changes that occur during DNA replication or from environmental damage. However, as people age, DNA repair does not work as effectively, and changes in the DNA can accumulate, such as in Alzheimer disease.

Genetic mutations can be inherited (*germline mutation*) or acquired (*somatic mutation*). Germline mutations are passed from parent to child. These mutations are present in the oocyte and sperm cells. This type of mutation is present throughout a person's life in virtually every cell in the body. Somatic mutations occur in the DNA of a somatic cell at some time during a person's life. An acquired mutation is passed on to all cells that develop from that single cell. These mutations cannot be passed on to the next generation. Acquired mutations can occur if (1) a mistake is made as DNA replicates during cell division or (2) environmental factors alter the DNA.

HUMAN GENOME PROJECT

The Human Genome Project (HGP) started in 1990 as an international effort to provide detailed information about the structure, organization, and function of the entire human genome. It was completed in 2003, with the sequence of more than 3 billion DNA base pairs determined. The knowledge gained through the HGP has enabled earlier detection and diagnosis of genetic conditions. It plays a critical role in determining risk assessment for genetic-related diseases (National Human Genome Research Institute, 2020). However, Canadian First Nations, Métis, and Inuit genomes are virtually absent from the database despite comprising 5.8% of the Canadian population (Statistics Canada, 2020). Consequently, Indigenous Canadians are disadvantaged

in relation to genomic health care as compared to Canadians of other ancestral backgrounds (Morgan et al., 2018).

INHERITANCE PATTERNS

Alterations in genes (referred to as *mutations* or *variants*) can cause genetic disorders. These disorders can be classified into three categories: (1) single-gene disorders, (2) chromosomal disorders, and (3) multifactorial disorders.

Single-Gene Disorders

Mendelian disorders are inherited genetic conditions. These disorders are caused by a single gene and may have a mutation present on only one chromosome of a pair or on both chromosomes of the pair. Examples of single-gene disorders include cystic fibrosis (CF), Marfan syndrome, and sickle cell anemia. There are three primary single-gene, or Mendelian, inheritance patterns: (1) autosomal dominant, (2) autosomal recessive, and (3) X-linked. If the mutant gene is located on an autosome, the genetic disorder is called *autosomal*. If the mutant gene is on the X chromosome, the genetic disorder is called *X-linked*. In genetics, a family history of clinical information with respect to a hereditary condition or *pedigree* is constructed in order to identify patterns of inheritance. See Figure 15.5 for examples of family pedigrees with autosomal dominant, autosomal recessive, and X-linked disorders.

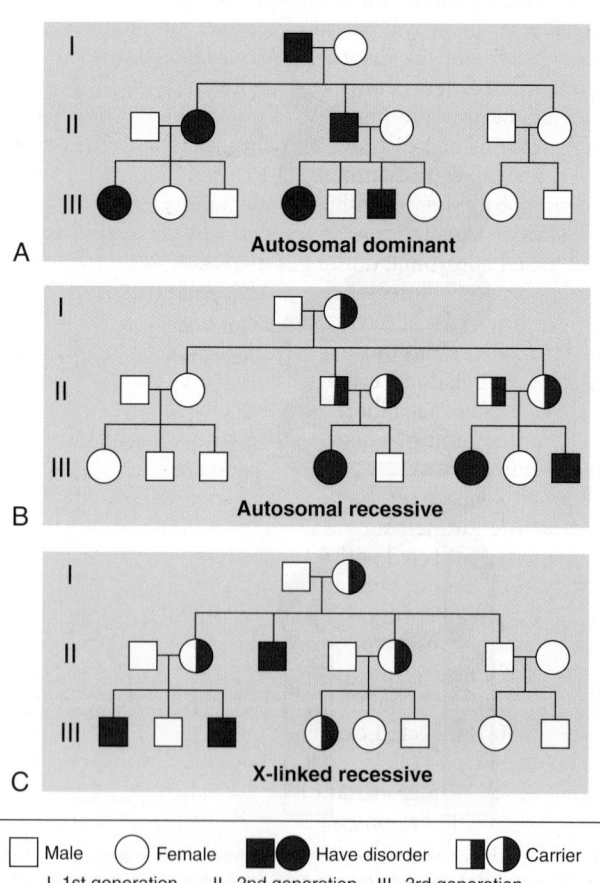

FIG. 15.5 Family pedigrees showing three generations. **A,** Family pedigree suggestive of an autosomal dominant disorder. **B,** Family pedigree suggestive of an autosomal recessive disorder. **C,** Family pedigree suggestive of an X-linked recessive disorder.

🧬 GENETICS IN CLINICAL PRACTICE

Boxes Throughout This Text

Genetic Disorder	Chapter
α_1-Antitrypsin	31
Autoimmune diseases	64
Breast cancer	54
Diabetes mellitus types 1 and 2	52
Familial adenomatous polyposis (FAP)	45
Familial hypercholesterolemia	36
Hemochromatosis	33
Hemophilia A and B	33
Hereditary nonpolyposis colorectal cancer (HNPCC)	45
Huntington's disease	61
Ovarian cancer	56
Polycystic kidney disease	48
Sickle-cell disease	33
Skin malignancies	25

Autosomal Dominant. An autosomal dominant trait is caused by a single gene pair mutation (heterozygous). The affected person has both an abnormal (mutated) and a normal gene. Only one allele of a mutated gene is necessary for the disease. The mutated gene dominates the normal gene. *Penetrance* refers to the chance that a carrier of a dominant mutation will show signs of the disease. *Incomplete penetrance* occurs when a person with a genetic mutation does not have signs of the disorder. It explains why a parent who has a genetic disorder may not have signs of the disorder but the child does. Autosomal dominant disorders show variable expressivity. Expressivity describes the way the phenotype manifests. This accounts for how symptoms of a disorder vary from person to person, even though they have the same mutated gene. Symptoms are also influenced by other, usually unknown, genetic factors, gene–environment interactions, and chance events. An example of an inherited autosomal dominant disorder is Lynch syndrome, or nonpolyposis colorectal cancer (HNPCC). Lynch syndrome increases one's risk of having other types of cancers, including colorectal cancer and those related to the stomach, small intestine, liver, gallbladder, urinary tract, brain, skin, ovaries, and uterus (US National Library of Medicine, 2021a). See Figure 15.5 for an example of a pedigree of a family with another autosomal dominant trait.

Punnett squares can be used to determine inheritance possibilities. The Punnett square in Figure 15.6 illustrates the mating of a parent affected with an autosomal dominant trait (e.g., Huntington's disease) with an unaffected parent. There is a 50% chance that the offspring will have Huntington's disease.

Autosomal Recessive. Autosomal recessive disorders are the result of homozygous (or two gene pair) mutations. In most recessive conditions, an affected offspring results from a mating between two unaffected carriers of the mutated gene. The offspring inherits two alleles of the mutated gene, one from each parent, which results in the offspring exhibiting the disorder. If the person inherits one allele of the recessive gene, they do not develop the disease because the normal allele dominant is a carrier. See Figure 15.5 for an example of a pedigree of a family with an autosomal recessive trait. The Punnett square illustrating the mating of parents who are both carriers of the autosomal recessive gene for CF is shown in Figure 15.6. There is a 25% chance that the offspring will have the disease.

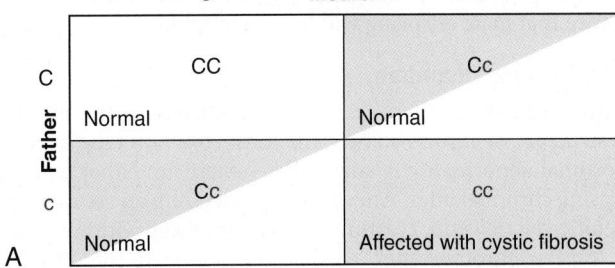

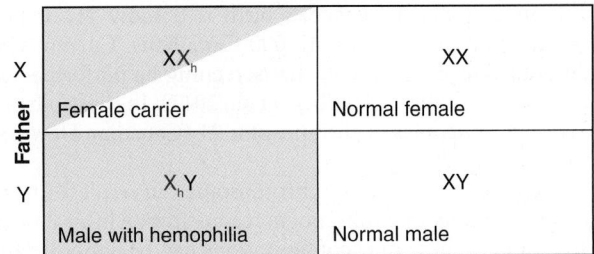

FIG. 15.6 Punnett squares illustrate inheritance possibilities. **A,** If the mother and father are both carriers for cystic fibrosis, there is a 25% chance that offspring will have cystic fibrosis. **B,** If the mother is a carrier for the hemophilia gene and the father has a normal genotype, there is a 50% chance that any male offspring will have hemophilia. There is a 50% chance that any female offspring will be a carrier. **C,** If the mother has a normal genotype and the father has Huntington's disease, there is a 50% chance that offspring will have the disease.

X-Linked. X-linked recessive inheritance is caused by a gene mutation on the X chromosome. Males are primarily affected because they have only one X chromosome. A male with a mutation in a gene on the X chromosome will exhibit the disorder because he has no corresponding normal gene to mask the mutated gene's effects. Women who carry the mutated gene on one X chromosome have another X chromosome to compensate for the mutation, so they are not affected but are a carrier. The female carrier has a 50% chance of passing the gene mutation to male children. Sons will have the disease, whereas daughters, like their mother, will be carriers. Fathers cannot pass X-linked traits to their sons.

Y-linked conditions occur if the mutated gene that causes the disorder is located on the Y chromosome. Given that only males have a Y chromosome, in Y-linked inheritance, an affected father transmits the disorder to all the males; only men are affected. An example of a Y-linked condition is Y chromosome infertility.

See Figure 15.5 for an example of a pedigree of a family with an X-linked recessive trait. The Punnett square in Figure 15.6

illustrates the mating of a female carrier of an X-linked recessive disorder (e.g., hemophilia) and a normal male. There is a 50% chance that male offspring will have hemophilia.

Chromosomal Disorders

Chromosomal disorders result from a change in the number or structure of chromosomes. The most common type of chromosomal abnormality is aneuploidy—there are either extra or missing chromosomes. Aneuploidy results from an error during meiotic cell division, creating a sperm or an egg with too many or too few chromosomes, which is passed on to the offspring during conception. Most aneuploid offspring have either trisomy (three chromosomes) or monosomy (only one chromosome) instead of the normal pair of chromosomes. The most common trisomy that survives birth is trisomy 21, or Down syndrome, affecting nearly 45 000 Canadians. Current Canadian guidelines recommend that screening be performed after 10 weeks of gestation (Audibert et al., 2017). In these offspring, there are three copies of chromosome 21 (Canadian Down Syndrome Society, 2020).

Structural changes in the chromosome can result from chromosome breakage and subsequent reconstitution in an abnormal combination. These new configurations can be either balanced or unbalanced. In balanced rearrangements, the chromosome is complete, with no loss or gain of genetic material. These rearrangements are generally harmless except in rare cases in which one of the break points damages an important functional gene. When a chromosome rearrangement is unbalanced, the chromosomal complement contains an incorrect amount of chromosome material or a different configuration, and the clinical effects are usually serious. Chronic myelocytic leukemia can be caused by a chromosomal translocation, in which portions of two chromosomes (chromosomes 9 and 22) are exchanged. This translocation is called the *Philadelphia chromosome*.

Multifactorial Inheritance

Multifactorial inheritance diseases are the result of the interaction between genes, the environmental, diet, aging, and lifestyle. Multifactorial diseases do not always develop, although the presence of a genetic mutation does increase the person's risk of getting the disease. Multifactorial inheritance is thought to be the basis for most common diseases, including diabetes and heart disease (US National Library of Medicine, 2021b). A primary characteristic of this type of inheritance is familial aggregation of diseases. There is a similar risk for first-degree relatives (offspring, siblings, or parents). While multifactorial conditions tend to run in families, the pattern of inheritance is not as predictable as with single-gene disorders. The chance of recurrence of disease traits within families, though greater than the population risk, is less than that for families with single-gene disorders. The degree of risk for a multifactorial disorder occurring in relatives is related to the number of genes they share in common with the affected individual. The closer the degree of relationship, the more genes they have in common. The greater the number of affected relatives, the higher the recurrence risk. The severity of the disorder and occasionally the sex of the affected individual may modify the risk. The degree of risk also increases with the severity of the disorder. Identical twins may not always have the same condition when inheritance is multifactorial. For instance, the risk for coronary heart disease increases with smoking or obesity, and the risk for emphysema in individuals with α_1-antitrypsin deficiency increases greatly with smoking.

Throughout the book, genetic disorders are highlighted in Genetics in Clinical Practice boxes.

GENETICS IN CLINICAL PRACTICE

Taking a Family History

A detailed three-generation family history, or *pedigree*, offers great insight into possible genetic conditions within a family. A pedigree is a symbolic representation of family members indicating specific details about each individual. Standard nomenclature should be used when constructing a pedigree (see Figure 15.5). When constructing the pedigree, start with the *proband*, or person being interviewed. For each family member, document date of birth, any medical illnesses or health conditions and the age when diagnosed, and if deceased, the age and cause of death. Comment on ancestors' racial and ethnic information, information that is unknown, and presence of consanguinity. After recording the family history or pedigree, review the information to identify key features that may increase a person's risk for genetic-related diseases. This may include the presence of a disease in more than one close relative (e.g., Huntington's disease); a condition that occurs earlier than expected (e.g., sudden cardiac death); diseases that occur in combination with others (e.g., breast and ovarian cancer); and the manifestation of a disease that generally does not affect a gender (e.g., breast cancer in males). This initial pedigree can highlight certain areas, such as those pertinent to a specific condition (e.g., cancer), for further questioning. For example, a pedigree targeting the possibility of a hereditary cancer syndrome will gather even more details about the incidence of cancer, the types of cancer, ages at diagnosis, and outcomes. These persons may benefit from further clinical investigation, screening, and diagnostic testing. As a nurse, you may refer these persons to a specialist for information about the benefits and risks of genetic screening and testing.

Genetic Screening and Testing

Genetic screening and testing refers to the analysis of DNA, chromosomes, proteins, or metabolites, or some combination thereof. Testing can be done on blood, skin, or saliva and involves looking for a genetic mutation that indicates the presence or absence of a genetic condition or predisposition to (i.e., increased risk for) a genetic condition.

Genetic screening is the first level of detection. It is offered to general or targeted populations who are at risk for a disorder but asymptomatic or have a family history of the disorder. An example is screening for α-fetoprotein, which is offered to pregnant women to detect fetal anomalies.

Genetic testing is focused on individuals and families. Genetic testing may also be useful in determining the potential risk for development of a disease in one's lifetime. Test results are used to assess risk or diagnose a disorder, an important step in providing ongoing care for the person and family. It is important to identify people at high risk for conditions that may be preventable. For example, persons who have inherited a gene for familial adenomatous polyposis (FAP) need ongoing monitoring (Kasper et al., 2017).

People get genetic testing to help diagnose the presence of a genetic condition if they are experiencing symptoms. Others seek genetic testing if they have a family history of a genetic condition but have no symptoms of the disease (or presymptomatic). For example, Huntington's disease is an adult-onset

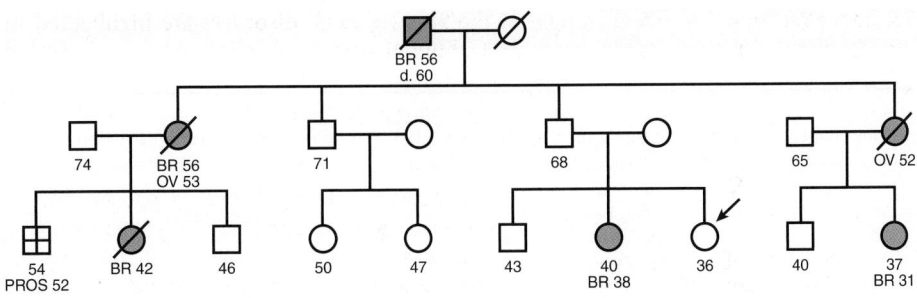

FIG. 15.7 Pedigree for family with the *BRCA1* mutation. Numbers without symbols represent the current ages of family members. Numbers with symbols represent the age at which the diagnosis was made. *BR,* breast cancer; *d.,* age of death; *OV,* ovarian cancer; *PROS,* prostate cancer.

condition characterized by progressive neurological degeneration. The gene responsible for Huntington's disease is 100% penetrant; that is, everyone who inherits this mutation will develop the disease. Other tests are done to determine whether an individual is a carrier of a mutated gene, which may be passed on to offspring. Typically, this testing is done for autosomal recessive and X-linked disorders. Individuals may opt for this type of genetic testing if there is a family history of a genetic disease or if they are in an ethnic group that has a greater risk of carrying a certain genetic mutation. Examples of disorders for which such testing is available are Tay-Sachs disease, CF, and fragile X syndrome. Most tests assess single genes and are used to diagnose genetic disorders, such as CF or Duchenne muscular dystrophy.

Genetic testing is also available to determine an individual's predisposition for developing a genetic condition and is now used in prenatal, pediatric, and adult populations. Many genes, that, when mutated, cause an individual to be predisposed to a disease have been identified. However, not all individuals who have the genetic mutation will get the disease. This is the case with *BRCA1* and *BRCA2*, which are responsible for some types of hereditary breast and ovarian cancers (Kasper et al., 2017). Research has shown that the cumulative breast cancer risk is 72% for *BRCA1* and 69% for *BRCA2* carriers; the cumulative ovarian cancer risk is 44% for *BRCA1* and 17% for *BRCA2* carriers (Kuchenbaecker et al., 2017). Typically, families that carry mutations in these genes have numerous members who have been diagnosed with breast or ovarian cancers (Figure 15.7). Other characteristics that suggest a possible *BRCA1* or *BRCA2* mutation in a family are onset of breast cancer at a young age (less than 50 years), male breast cancer, and bilateral breast cancer. The advantage of testing for mutations in *BRCA1* and *BRCA2* is that women at high risk for developing breast and ovarian cancers can be identified before the development of cancer. These women can then begin vigilant breast and ovarian cancer screening at an earlier age, or they can elect for preventive options (e.g., bilateral mastectomy and bilateral oophorectomy) or chemopreventive medications (e.g., tamoxifen). Each option offers varying cancer risk reduction, and there are both medical and psychological adverse effects that may result.

In summary, examples of uses of genetic testing include the following (Montgomery, 2017):

- Antenatal testing for abnormalities
- Carrier testing to determine which individuals are carriers of a recessive or X-linked disorder
- Diagnostic testing to confirm or rule out a diagnosis
- Predictive testing to determine whether a person is likely to develop a condition
- Pharmacogenetic testing to analyze genetic variants to predict response to specific medications
- Susceptibility testing to determine genetic risk for complex disorders

Genetic testing may raise ethical questions. People considering genetic testing should receive counselling about the various issues. They should be aware that test results in their medical records might not be private. To protect people from discrimination by employers and health insurance companies, the federal government passed the *Genetic Non-Discrimination Act* (GNDA), or Bill S-201, into law in 2017. Amendments in the Canadian Labour Code and the *Canadian Human Rights Act* also prohibit companies or employers from requiring genetic testing or gaining access to genetic test results. The GNDA can be found at www.canlii.org/en/ca/laws/stat /sc-2017-c-3/latest/sc-2017-c-3.html.

Direct-to-Consumer Genetic Tests. Direct-to-consumer genetic tests are marketed directly to people (consumers) via television, print advertisements, or the Internet (such as 23 and Me). The test kit is mailed to the person. The test typically involves collecting a DNA sample at home, often by swabbing the inside of the cheek, and mailing the sample back to the laboratory. In some cases, the person must visit a health clinic to have blood drawn. Participants are notified of their results by mail, over the telephone, or online. In some cases, a genetics counsellor or other health care provider is available to explain the results and answer questions.

Direct-to-consumer genetic tests have significant risks and limitations. People may want their genetic information, but they may not understand what it means. They are vulnerable to being misled by the results of unproven or invalid tests. Without guidance from a health care provider, they may make important decisions about disease treatment or prevention based on inaccurate, incomplete, or misunderstood information about their health. People may experience an invasion of genetic privacy if testing companies use their genetic information in an unauthorized way. When people are considering using these kinds of genetic tests, nurses should provide education and suggest they discuss the issue with their health care provider or a genetics counsellor. Teaching related to genetic testing is outlined in Table 15.2.

Genetic Counselling. *Genetic counselling* is the process of helping people understand and adapt to the medical, psychological, and familial implications of genetic contributions to disease (National Society of Genetic Counselors [NSGC], 2020). Genetic counsellors are health care providers with specialized graduate degrees and experience in the areas of medical genetics and counselling. They provide information and support to families who have members with birth defects or genetic disorders and to families who may be at risk for a variety of inherited conditions. They identify families at risk, investigate the concern that the family has, interpret information about the disorder, analyze inheritance patterns and risks for recurrence, and review available options with the family. Genetic counsellors also provide supportive counselling to families, serve as patient

TABLE 15.2   PATIENT & CAREGIVER TEACHING GUIDE
Genetic Testing

Genetic Counsellors
- People who are considering genetic testing should meet with a genetics counsellor who is specially educated in medical genetics and counselling.
- Counselling is advised to help you understand the purpose of genetic testing, considerations before testing, and the emotional and medical impact of the test results.
- Genetics counselling can help you understand the pros and cons of genetic testing before making a decision to undergo a genetic test.

General Information
The following includes some important general information about genetic testing:
- Genetic testing can be expensive and may not be included in your medical insurance policy.
- Genetic testing may determine whether you are predisposed to developing an inherited disease.
- A particular genetic test will only tell you whether there is a specific genetic variant or mutation. Positive tests do not mean you will develop that disease or disorder. Neither can the results tell you when you will develop the disease.
- If a genetic test shows a genetic predisposition to an inherited disorder, the news may affect your mental health.
- Knowledge of a genetic predisposition to a disease may give you the motivation to take preventive measures (e.g., taking drugs for familial hypercholesterolemia) or make lifestyle changes to lower the risk for a disease (e.g., exercising to decrease the risk for type 2 diabetes).
- If a genetic test reveals you are at risk for a specific genetic disorder, there is the chance that other family members may be at risk.
- If a genetic test reveals you are at risk for developing an inherited disease, whether you decide to share that information with family members is a personal and an ethical decision that you will have to make.
- Genetic testing may provide important information that you can use when making decisions about having children.
- To protect people from discrimination by employers and health insurance companies, refer to the *Genetic Non-Discrimination Act* (GNDA), or Bill S-201. The GNDA can be found at www.canlii.org/en/ca/laws/stat/sc-2017-c-3/latest/sc-2017-c-3.html.

advocates, and provide education about inheritance testing, management, prevention resources, and research. They refer individuals and families to community, provincial, or territorial support services (NSGC, 2020). The Canadian Association of Genetic Counsellors (CAGC) seeks to promote high standards of practice by supporting professional growth and education of genetic counsellors across Canada, including specific Canadian certification. More information about CAGC can be obtained at https://www.cagc-accg.ca/.

Interpreting Genetic Test Results

The results of genetic tests are not always straightforward, which often makes them challenging to interpret and explain. When interpreting test results, health care providers need to consider the reason the test was done, pretest counselling provided, the person's medical history, the family history, and the type of genetic test (Kasper et al., 2017). A positive test result means that the laboratory found a change in a particular gene, chromosome, or protein that was being tested. Depending on the purpose of the test, this result may confirm a diagnosis (e.g., Huntington's disease), show that a person is a carrier of a particular genetic mutation (e.g., CF), identify an increased risk for developing a disease (e.g., breast cancer), or suggest a need for further testing. A positive result of a predictive or presymptomatic genetic test usually cannot establish the absolute risk for developing a disorder. A positive test also cannot predict the course or severity of a condition.

In some situations, it is difficult to interpret a positive result because some people who have the genetic mutation never develop the disease. For example, having the apolipoprotein E-4 (Apo E-4) allele increases the risk for developing Alzheimer's disease. However, many people who test positive for Apo E-4 never develop Alzheimer's disease. A negative test result means that the laboratory did not find an altered form of the gene, chromosome, or protein under consideration. This result generally means a person is not affected by a particular disorder, is not a carrier of a specific genetic mutation, or does not have increased risk for developing a certain disease. It is possible that the test missed a disease-causing genetic alteration. Many tests cannot detect all the genetic changes that cause a particular disorder. Further testing may be needed to confirm a negative result.

Gene Therapy

Gene therapy is a technique used to treat the underlying cause of a disease. Gene therapy may be used to supply a missing gene, avoid the missing gene's role, or enhance treatment of a disease. The goal is to provide a normally functioning gene to a person with a pathogenic gene variant. A carrier molecule called a *vector* must be used to deliver the therapeutic gene to the person's target cells (US National Library of Medicine, 2021c). Currently, the most common vector is a virus that has been genetically altered to carry normal human DNA (Lee et al., 2017). The vector can be injected or given intravenously directly into specific tissue. The vector unloads its genetic material containing the therapeutic human gene into the target cell. If the treatment is successful, the new gene will make a functional protein and restore the target cell to a normal state. A diagram of gene therapy is shown in Figure 15.8. Although gene therapy is a promising treatment for a number of diseases (including inherited disorders, some types of cancer, and certain viral infections), the technique is still under study. In the United States the Food and Drug Administration (FDA) has approved the first two gene therapies. Tisagenlecleucel (Kymriah) is used to treat certain pediatric and young adult patients who have a form of acute lymphoblastic leukemia. The other gene therapy treats vision impairment from a congenital retinal degenerative disorder. Health Canada has approved Kymriah for use in pediatric and young adult patients 3 to 25 years of age with B-cell acute lymphoblastic leukemia (ALL) and for the treatment of adult patients with relapsed or refractory large B-cell lymphoma, the most common type of non-Hodgkin lymphoma, in adults (Health Canada, 2021). In Canada, gene therapy is developing in the fields of stem cell therapeutics and regenerative medicine, transfusion and blood donation, and the treatment of cancer and rare diseases (Sinclair et al., 2018).

Stem Cell Therapy. Stem cells are the subject of much discussion because they may offer treatment for many diseases (Kasper et al., 2017). The use of stem cells may allow for the regeneration of lost tissue and restoration of function in various diseases. *Stem cells* are unspecialized cells in the body that have the ability to (1) remain in their unspecialized state and divide or (2) differentiate and develop into specialized cells. Stem cells

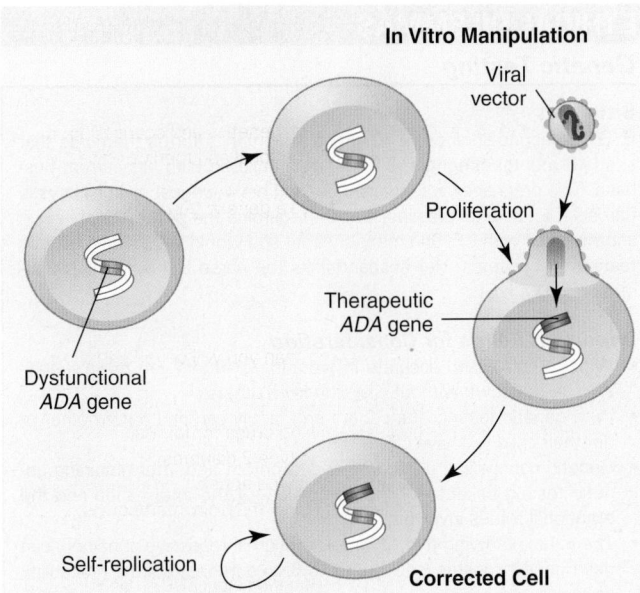

In Vitro Manipulation

Viral vector

Proliferation

Therapeutic *ADA* gene

Dysfunctional *ADA* gene

Self-replication

Corrected Cell

FIG. 15.8 Gene therapy for adenosine deaminase (ADA) deficiency attempts to correct this immunodeficiency state. The viral vector containing the therapeutic *ADA* gene is inserted into the patient's lymphocytes. These cells can then make the ADA enzyme.

can be derived from human embryos or adult somatic tissues. Adult stem cells of an undifferentiated class are found in small numbers in our organs and tissues. Their main function is to maintain and repair the tissues in which they are found. For example, skin stem cells produce new skin cells.

Stems cells are used to treat persons with many different disorders, including severe burns and orthopedic conditions that require bone grafting. For the past 20 years, hematopoietic stem cell transplantation has been a standard for treatment of hematological cancers and bone marrow failure. Medical researchers are investigating the use of stem cells to repair or replace damaged body tissues, similar to whole-organ transplants.

Part of the nurse's role is to safeguard the impact that new and emerging technologies can have on patient privacy and confidentiality (Canadian Nurses Association, 2017).

Pharmacogenomics and Pharmacogenetics. *Pharmacogenomics* is the study of how drugs affect and interact with the genome and output expression. *Pharmacogenetics* is the study of variable drug responses, including adverse events from differences in inheritable genes. Pharmacogenetic and pharmacogenomic studies could lead to the development of drugs that can be tailor-made or adapted to each person's particular genetic makeup. This will make it possible to have personalized medicine by choosing the right drug and the right dose for the right person (Kasper et al., 2017). Health care providers are starting to use pharmacogenomic information to prescribe drugs.

One important area of study has focused on the hepatic cytochrome P450 (CYP450) enzyme system, which is responsible for oxidizing many medications and chemicals (Kasper et al., 2017). The enzymes in this system share certain amino acid sequences, each one coded by a separate gene. People with a less active form of the enzyme (who metabolize the medication slowly) may get too much of the medication. People with a more active form of the enzyme (who metabolize the medication quickly) may get too little of the medication. It may appear that the medication is not effective.

NURSING MANAGEMENT GENETICS

Nurses are often the first point of entry into the health care environment and play an important role in the management and coordination of genetic services. Therefore, nurses must be knowledgeable about the fundamentals of genetics. Although genetics is a part of most nurses' practices, some nurses specialize in genetics. A genetics nurse is a registered nurse who has special education and training in genetics. Genetic nurses help people at risk for or affected by diseases with a genetic component to achieve and maintain good health. They perform risk assessments, analyze the genetic contribution to disease risk, and discuss the impact of risk on health care management for individuals and families. They also provide genetic education, provide nursing care to patients and families, and conduct research in genetics (International Society of Nurses in Genetics [ISONG], 2020). Nurses assist persons and their families seeking information and making decisions related to genetic issues while respecting the patient's right to self-determination and privacy (American Nurses Association Consensus Panel 2009; Montgomery et al., 2017). More information about the ISONG can be found at www.isong.org/page-1325153.

The nurse should be able to give patients and their families accurate information pertaining to genetics, genetic diseases, and probabilities of genetic disorders. Inheritance patterns can be assessed by the nurse and explained to the patient and family through the use of Punnett squares or family pedigrees (see Figures 15.5 and 15.6). Maintaining patient confidentiality and respecting the patient's values and beliefs are critical because the information from the counsellor may have major implications for many people who are involved.

The specialized knowledge and counselling skills of a genetics nurse or genetics counsellor are often important when genetic testing is considered. Genetic testing may raise many psychosocial and ethical issues on a personal and societal level that warrants the expertise of a nurse with a strong foundational knowledge in genetics. Knowledge of carrier status of a genetic disorder may influence a person's career, marriage, and childbearing decisions. It may also affect significant others as they contemplate potentially serious life and health care issues.

On a personal level, genetic test results offer individuals insight into conditions that may already exist or that may develop in the future. This type of information may cause internal ethical dilemmas. Prenatal genetic testing, for example, may raise ethics issues for parents. Parents who learn prenatally that their baby has a genetic condition must consider the future of the pregnancy. A fetus identified as having trisomy 21 (Down syndrome) will be born with physical and developmental abnormalities; however, predicting the severity of these abnormalities is difficult. This complicates the situation for parents who have to decide whether or not to terminate the pregnancy. In addition, for some individuals, cultural and religious beliefs often factor into this decision making.

Another ethical dilemma is who should know the results of a genetic test. Who should protect the privacy of test results and prevent persons from discrimination? People may be reluctant to share or disclose information about family history or genetic test results. They may fear they are vulnerable to stigmatization or discrimination based on their DNA. The nurse needs to understand how different health care policies relate to genetic testing, such as the GNDA, or Bill S-201.

Genetic testing for adult-onset conditions also may raise ethical dilemmas. With testing for adult-onset conditions (e.g., breast cancer), issues related to "duty to warn" may surface. For example, if a woman is told that she has a *BRCA1* mutation, there are significant implications for her blood relatives. Once a *BRCA1* mutation is identified in a family, all blood relatives are eligible to receive genetic testing for the specific mutation. However, if the individual does not share her genetic test results with her family, the family members may be unaware of their chance of having the *BRCA1* mutation and of their significantly increased risk of developing breast and ovarian cancers. The lack of this knowledge may result in a family member's being denied the opportunity to choose a cancer prevention option and may develop cancer as a result.

Many of the ethical concerns described in this chapter can also become a legal issue depending on the jurisdiction of the parties involved. As knowledge of genetic diseases has grown and can better predict what variants mean for the patient (i.e., survival, prognostics), discrimination based on genetic findings in healthy individuals has become a major disadvantage. Nurses need to be well-versed in genetic health care policies. As stated earlier, in Canada, the federal government passed the GNDA, or Bill S-201, into law in 2017, which prevents discrimination by employers and health insurance companies. Changes to the Canadian Labour Code and the *Canadian Human Rights Act* also forbid employers to request genetic testing or access to genetic test results.

Genome Canada has invested in interdisciplinary research looking at genomics and its ethical, environmental, economic, legal, and social features, known as *GE3LS* research. This research provides information for stakeholders and policymakers as they examine policy options that address genomic concerns for Canadians (Genome Canada, 2020a) at an individual, ethical, and societal level. Nurses must be aware of the ethical, environmental, economic, legal, and social implications of genetics when they provide care to individuals.

ETHICAL DILEMMAS
Genetic Testing

Situation

E. G. (pronouns she/her), a 30-year-old woman, informs the nurse that she is 3 months pregnant. She has two children with her current husband. This pregnancy was unplanned, and her youngest child has cystic fibrosis (CF). E. G. expresses concern regarding the possibility of having another child with CF. She mentions that she would like to have genetic testing on her fetus. Her husband asks the nurse if they will have another child with CF.

Important Points for Consideration
- With complete and accurate information, partners can make a decision on their own without coercion from others.
- With genetic testing, the patient and family can find out whether or not their child will have CF.
- Genetic counselling is recommended before and after obtaining genetic testing because of the complexity of the information and the emotional issues involved.
- The nurse, knowing that CF is an autosomal recessive condition, can use Punnett squares (see Figure 15.6) to demonstrate the probability of having another child with CF.
- Genetic testing in the fetus is most informative if the two pathogenic variants are first identified in the affected child. Without the known familial causative variants, prenatal testing cannot rule out the possibility that testing did not find the underlying cause (but may be outside of the tested regions of the gene). Therefore, a negative test result may not mean the fetus will not be born with CF.

Clinical Decision-Making Questions
1. What information should the nurse give the patient regarding genetic testing in order for the patient to make a decision?
2. What options are available for this couple?
3. How should the nurse assist this couple in making a decision about possibly terminating the pregnancy if the results of the genetic testing show that the fetus tested positive for the CF gene?

REVIEW QUESTIONS

The number of the question corresponds to the same-numbered objective at the beginning of the chapter.

1. What is a genetic mutation?
   a. A mutation or variant that permanently changes the usual DNA sequence
   b. A temporary interruption in the DNA sequence
   c. An alteration in the DNA that takes place after cell division occurs
   d. A mutation in the DNA structure that is not transferable to offspring
2. What does it mean if a person is heterozygous for a given gene?
   a. The person is a carrier for a genetic disorder.
   b. The person is affected by the genetic disorder.
   c. The person has two identical alleles for the gene.
   d. The person has two different alleles for the gene.
3. A 53-year-old male client presents with a constellation of symptoms that leads the nurse to believe that his disease is of a genetic etiology. His disease manifested when he was a teenager. The client's 29-year-old son is affected with the same disease. The client's 27-year-old daughter is healthy with an unremarkable clinical history. However, her two sons are similarly affected as their uncle. Which of the following is a mode of inheritance that most likely applies to this family?
   a. Autosomal dominant
   b. Autosomal recessive
   c. Genetic diversity
   d. Genetic drift

4. What is a family pedigree?
   a. The family ancestry traced through the father
   b. The family line of descent through the mother
   c. The depiction of an autosomal recessive gene disorder
   d. A family tree drawn in the form of a diagram
5. Which of the following would be a reason for a client or potential parents to undergo genetic testing?
   a. To determine the sex of an unborn child through amniocentesis
   b. To predict the potential for developing diabetes
   c. To help couples at risk for genetic disorders to make an informed choice before conception
   d. To screen for the possibility of undiagnosed breast cancer
6. A couple who recently had a son with hemophilia A is consulting with a nurse. They want to know if their next child will have hemophilia A. The nurse can tell the parents that if their child is
   a. a boy, he will have hemophilia A.
   b. a boy, he will be a carrier of hemophilia A.
   c. a girl, she will be a carrier of hemophilia A.
   d. a girl, there is a 50% chance that she will be a carrier of hemophilia A.
7. Why might prenatal genetic testing cause ethical, social, or legal dilemmas for parents? *(Select all that apply.)*
   a. The sex of the child would be known.
   b. Decisions about the future of the pregnancy (including termination) would be left to the parents.
   c. Health care providers would know about the genetic conditions of the unborn child.

d. Family members might question the couple's decision to undergo genetic testing.

e. Genetic testing results on the fetus could identify nonpaternity situations and have subsequent legal ramifications.

1 a; 2 d; 3 a; 4 d; 5 c; 6 d; 7 b, e

ⓔvolve

For even more review questions, visit http://evolve.elsevier.com/Canada/Lewis/medsurg.

REFERENCES

American Nurses Association Consensus Panel on Genetic/Genomic Nursing Competencies. (2009). *Essentials of genetic and genomic nursing: Competencies, curricula guidelines, and outcome indicators* (2nd ed.). American Nurses Association. https://www.genome.gov/Pages/Careers/HealthProfessionalEducation/geneticscompetency.pdf. (Seminal).

Audibert, F., De Bie, A., Johnson, J., et al. (2017). No. 348-Joint SOGC-CCMG guideline: Update on prenatal screening for fetal aneuploidy, fetal anomalies, and adverse pregnancy outcomes. *JOGC: Journal of Obstetrics and Gynaecology Canada, 39*(9), 805–817. https://doi.org/10.1016/j.jogc.2017.01.032.

Canadian Down Syndrome Society. (2020). *General information about Down syndrome.* https://cdss.ca/resources/general-information/.

Canadian Nurses Association. (2017). *Code of ethics for registered nurses.* https://www.cna-aiic.ca/~/media/cna/page-content/pdf-en/code-of-ethics-2017-edition-secure-interactive.

Genome Canada. (2020a). *Why Genomics: Societal implications and public policy.* https://www.genomecanada.ca/en/why-genomics/societal-implications-and-public-policy.

Genome Canada. (2020b). *Why genomics? Understanding the code of life.* https://www.genomecanada.ca/en/why-genomics/understanding-code-life.

Health Canada. (2021). *Regulatory decision summary–Kymriah.* https://hpr-rps.hres.ca/reg-content/regulatory-decision-summary-detail.php?lang=en&linkID=RDS00422.

International Society of Nurses in Genetics (ISONG). (2020). *What is a genetics nurse?* https://www.isong.org/page-1325153.

Kasper, C. E., Schneidereith, T. A., & Lashley, F. R. (2017). *Lashley's essentials of clinical genetics in nursing practice* (2nd ed). Springer.

Kuchenbaecker, K. B., Hopper, J. L., Barnes, D. R., et al. (2017). Risks of breast, ovarian, and contralateral breast cancer for BRCA1 and BRCA2 mutation carriers. *JAMA, 317*(23), 2402–2416. https://doi.org/10.1001/jama.2017.7112.

Lee, C. S., Bishop, E. S., Zhang, R., et al. (2017). Adenovirus-mediated gene delivery: Potential applications for gene and cell-based therapies in the new era of personalized medicine. *Genes and Diseases, 4*(2), 43–46. https://doi.org/10.1016/j.gendis.2017.04.001.

Montgomery, S., Brouwer, W. A., Everett, P. C., et al. (2017). Genetics in the clinical setting. *American Nurse Today, 12*(10), 10–18.

Morgan, J., Coe, R. R., Lesueur, R., et al. (2018). Indigenous peoples and genomics: Starting a conversation. *Journal of Genetic Counselling, 10*(2), 407–418. https://doi.org/10.1002/jgc4.1073.

National Human Genome Research Institute. (2020). *The Human Genome Project.* https://www.genome.gov/human-genome-project.

National Society of Genetic Counselors (NSGC). (2020). *About genetic counselors.* https://www.nsgc.org/About/About-Genetic-Counselors.

Sinclair, A., Islam, S., & Jones, S. (2018). *CADTH issues in emerging health technologies. Gene therapy: An overview of approved and pipeline technologies.* CADTH. https://www.ncbi.nlm.nih.gov/books/NBK538378/.

Statistics Canada. (2020). *Population estimates by July 1st, by age and sex.* https://www150.statcan.gc.ca/t1/tbl1/en/tv.action?pid=1710000501.

US National Library of Medicine. (2021a). *Lynch syndrome.* https://ghr.nlm.nih.gov/condition/lynch-syndrome.

US National Library of Medicine. (2021b). *What are complex or multifactorial disorders?.* https://ghr.nlm.nih.gov/primer/mutationsanddisorders/complexdisorders.

US National Library of Medicine. (2021c). *What is gene therapy?* https://ghr.nlm.nih.gov/primer/therapy/genetherapy.

RESOURCES

Canadian Association of Genetic Counsellors
https://www.cagc-accg.ca/

Genome Canada
https://www.genomecanada.ca

Public Health Agency of Canada
https://www.phac-aspc.gc.ca/index-eng.php

American College of Medical Genetics and Genomics
https://www.acmg.net/

Centers for Disease and Control Prevention: Genomics and Precision Health
https://www.cdc.gov/genomics/default.htm

Genetic Alliance
http://www.geneticalliance.org/

Genetic Information Nondiscrimination Act of 2008 (GINA)
https://www.eeoc.gov/statutes/genetic-information-nondiscrimination-act-2008

Genetic Non-Discrimination Act
https://www.canlii.org/en/ca/laws/stat/sc-2017-c-3/latest/sc-2017-c-3.html

Genetic Testing Registry (GTR)
https://www.ncbi.nlm.nih.gov/gtr/

National Human Genome Research Institute
https://www.genome.gov/

National Organization for Rare Disorders
https://rarediseases.org/

Online Mendelian Inheritance in Man (OMIM)
https://www.omim.org/

ⓔvolve

For additional Internet resources, see the website for this book at http://evolve.elsevier.com/Canada/Lewis/medsurg.

Altered Immune Response and Transplantation

Susan Chernenko
Originating US chapter by Haley Hoy and Yeow Chye Ng

evolve WEBSITE

http://evolve.elsevier.com/Canada/Lewis/medsurg

- Review Questions (Online Only)
- Key Points
- Answer Guidelines for Case Study

- Conceptual Care Map Creator
- Audio Glossary

- Supporting Media
  - Function of B Cells
  - Function of T Cytotoxic Cells
- Content Updates

LEARNING OBJECTIVES

1. Describe the components and functions of the immune system.
2. Compare and contrast humoral and cell-mediated immunity regarding lymphocytes involved, types of reactions, and effects on antigens.
3. Characterize the five classes of immunoglobulins.
4. Differentiate among the four types of hypersensitivity reactions in terms of immunological mechanisms and resulting alterations.
5. Identify the clinical manifestations and emergency management of a systemic anaphylactic reaction.
6. Describe the assessment and interprofessional care of a patient with chronic allergies.
7. Explain the relationship between the human leukocyte antigen system and certain diseases.

8. Describe the etiological factors, clinical manifestations, and treatment modalities of autoimmune diseases.
9. Describe the etiological factors and categories of immunodeficiency disorders.
10. Describe the various kinds of organ transplantation and the types of rejection that may be experienced after transplantation.
11. Identify the types of immunosuppressive therapy and their adverse effects.
12. Describe alternative strategies that have been explored to address organ donor shortages.

KEY TERMS

anergy
antigen
apheresis
autoimmunity
cell-mediated immunity

cytokines
human leukocyte antigen (HLA) system
humoral immunity
hypersensitivity reaction
immunity

immunocompetence
immunodeficiency
immunosuppressive therapy
monoclonal antibodies
organ transplantation

This chapter discusses the normal immune response and the altered immune responses of hypersensitivity (including allergies), autoimmunity, and immunodeficiency. Histocompatibility, organ transplantation, and immunosuppressive therapy are also presented.

NORMAL IMMUNE RESPONSE

Immunity is the body's ability to resist disease. Immune responses serve the following three functions (Banasik, 2018):
1. *Defence:* The body protects against invasions by microorganisms and prevents the development of infection by attacking foreign antigens and pathogens.

2. *Homeostasis:* Damaged cellular substances are digested and removed. Through this mechanism, the body's different cell types remain uniform and unchanged.
3. *Surveillance:* Mutations continually arise in the body but are normally recognized as foreign cells and destroyed.

Antigens

An **antigen** is a substance that elicits an immune response. Most antigens are composed of proteins. However, other substances such as large polysaccharides, lipoproteins, and nucleic acids can act as antigens. All of the body's cells have antigens on their surface that are unique to that person and enable the body to recognize itself. The immune system normally becomes

TABLE 16.1 TYPES OF ACQUIRED SPECIFIC IMMUNITY

Active
Natural

Natural contact with antigen through clinical infection (e.g., disease and recovery from chicken pox, measles, and mumps)

Artificial

Immunization with antigen (e.g., immunization with live or killed vaccines)

Passive
Natural

Transplacental and colostrum-mediated transfer from mother to infant (e.g., maternal immunoglobulins in neonate)

Artificial

Injection of serum from immune human (e.g., injection of human γ-globulin)

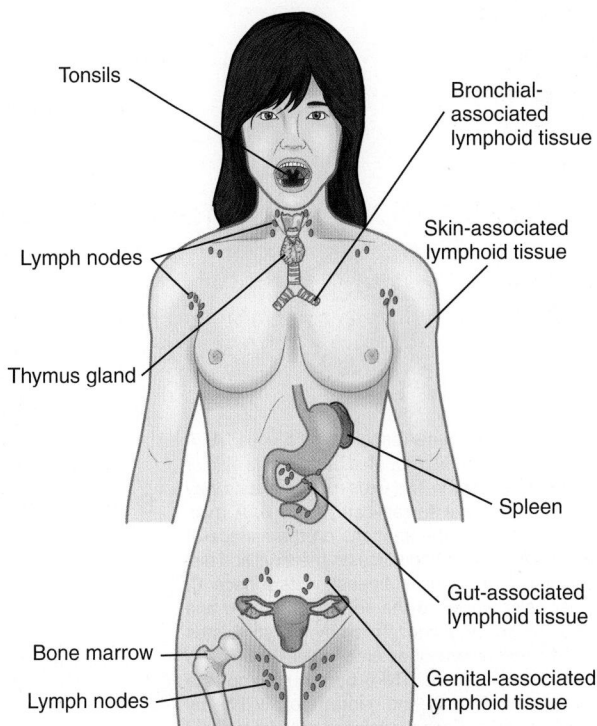

FIG. 16.1 Organs of the immune system.

"tolerant" to the body's own molecules and therefore is nonresponsive to "self" antigens.

Types of Immunity

Immunity is classified as innate or acquired.

Innate Immunity. *Innate immunity* is present at birth, and its primary role is first-line defence against pathogens. This type of immunity produces a nonspecific response, with neutrophils and monocytes being the white blood cells (WBCs) primarily involved. Innate immunity is not antigen-specific, so it can respond within minutes to an invading microorganism without prior exposure to that organism (Banasik, 2018).

Acquired Immunity. *Acquired immunity* is the development of immunity, either actively or passively (Table 16.1).

Active Acquired Immunity. *Active acquired immunity* results from the invasion of the body by foreign substances such as microorganisms, which leads to the development of antibodies and sensitized lymphocytes. With each reinvasion of the microorganisms, the body responds more rapidly and aggressively to fight off the invader. Active acquired immunity may result naturally from a disease or artificially through inoculation of a less virulent antigen (e.g., immunization). Because the body makes antibodies, immunity takes time to develop but is long-lasting.

Passive Acquired Immunity. *In passive acquired immunity,* the host receives antibodies to an antigen rather than making them. This occurs through the transfer of immunoglobulins across the placental membrane from mother to fetus or through injection with γ-globulin (serum antibodies). The benefit of this immunity is its immediate effect; however, its effects are short-lived, as the person does not make the antibodies and therefore does not retain memory cells to the antigen.

Lymphoid Organs

The lymphoid system is composed of central (or primary) and peripheral lymphoid organs. The central lymphoid organs are the thymus gland and bone marrow. The peripheral lymphoid organs are the lymph nodes; tonsils; spleen; and gut-, genital-, bronchial-, and skin-associated lymphoid tissues (Figure 16.1).

Lymphocytes are produced in the bone marrow and eventually migrate to the peripheral organs. The thymus is involved in the differentiation and maturation of T lymphocytes and is therefore essential for a cell-mediated immune response. The thymus is largest during childhood; however, following puberty it shrinks and is replaced with fat. Thus, by the age of 75 years, the thymus is predominantly fatty tissue that produces few T lymphocytes.

When antigens are introduced into the body, they may be carried by the bloodstream or lymph channels to regional lymph nodes. The antigens interact with B and T lymphocytes and macrophages in the lymph nodes. The two major functions of lymph nodes are (1) filtration of foreign material brought to the site and (2) circulation of lymphocytes.

Lymphoid tissue is found in the submucosa of the respiratory (bronchus-associated) (e.g., the tonsils), gastrointestinal (gut-associated), and genitourinary (genital-associated) tracts. This tissue protects the body surface from external microorganisms.

The spleen, a peripheral lymph organ, is the primary site for filtering foreign antigens from the blood.

The skin-associated lymph tissue primarily consists of lymphocytes and Langerhans cells (a type of dendritic cell) found in the epidermis of skin. When Langerhans cells are depleted, the skin cannot initiate an immune response. Therefore, a delayed hypersensitivity reaction (as determined by skin testing with injected antigens) does not occur.

Cells Involved in Immune Response

Mononuclear Phagocytes. The mononuclear phagocyte system includes monocytes in the blood and macrophages throughout the body. Mononuclear phagocytes play a critical role in the immune system by capturing, processing, and presenting the antigen to the lymphocytes. The antigen then stimulates a humoral or cell-mediated immune response. Capturing is accomplished through phagocytosis. The macrophage-bound antigen, which is highly immunogenic, is presented to

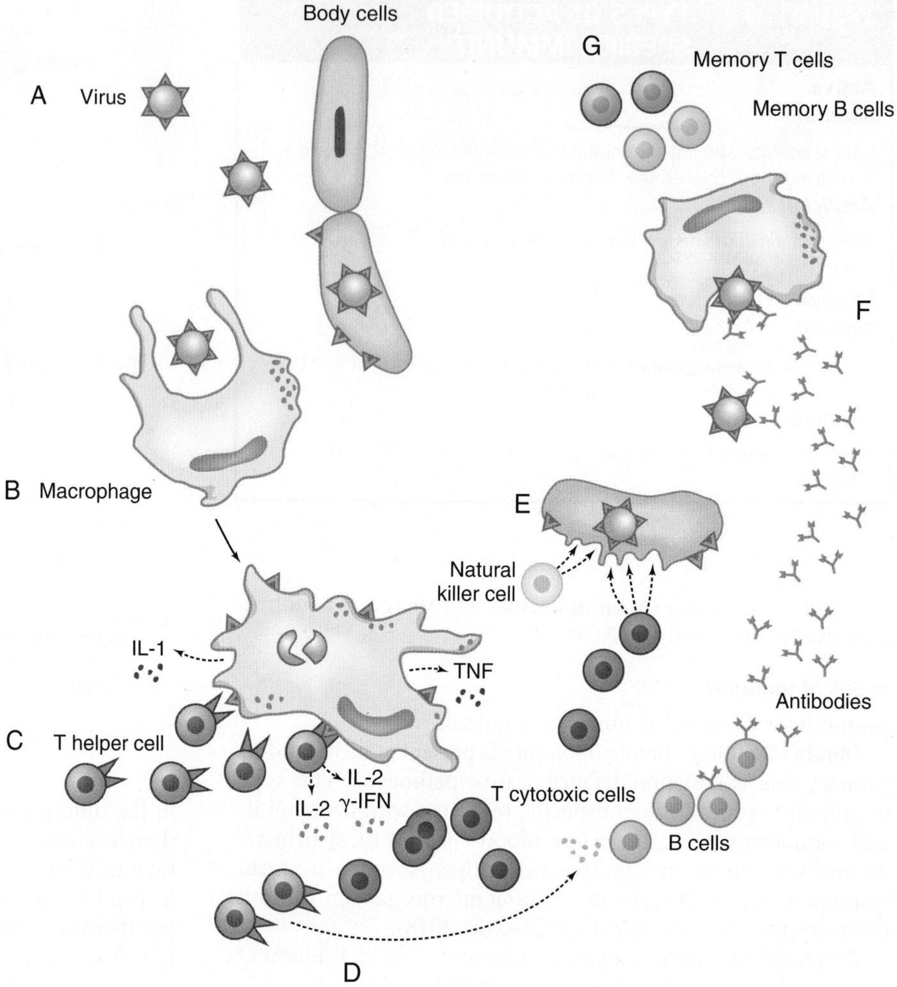

FIG. 16.2 The immune response to a virus. **A,** A virus invades the body through a break in the skin or another portal of entry. The virus must make its way inside a cell in order to replicate itself. **B,** A macrophage recognizes the antigens on the surface of the virus. The macrophage digests the virus and displays pieces of the virus (antigens) on its surface. **C,** T helper cells recognize the antigen displayed and bind to the macrophage. This binding stimulates the production of cytokines (interleukin-1 [IL-1] and tumour necrosis factor [TNF]) by the macrophage and interleukin-2 (IL-2) and γ-interferon (γ-IFN) by the T helper cells. These cytokines are intercellular messengers that provide communication among the cells. **D,** IL-2 instructs other T helper cells and T cytotoxic cells to proliferate (multiply). T helper cells release cytokines, causing B cells to multiply and produce antibodies. **E,** T cytotoxic cells and natural killer cells destroy infected body cells. **F,** Antibodies bind to the virus and mark it for macrophage destruction. **G,** Once the virus is gone, activated T and B cells are turned off by suppressor T cells. Memory B and T cells remain behind to respond quickly if the same virus attacks again.

circulating T or B lymphocytes and thus triggers an immune response (Figure 16.2).

Lymphocytes. Lymphocytes are produced in the bone marrow (Figure 16.3). They then differentiate into B and T lymphocytes.

B Lymphocytes. Early research on B lymphocytes (bursa-equivalent lymphocytes) in birds showed that they mature under the influence of the bursa of Fabricius, hence the name *B cells.* However, this lymphoid organ does not exist in humans. The bursa-equivalent tissue in humans is the bone marrow. B cells differentiate into *plasma cells* when activated and produce antibodies (called *immunoglobulins*) (Table 16.2).

T Lymphocytes. Cells that migrate from the bone marrow to the thymus differentiate into T lymphocytes (thymus-dependent cells). The thymus secretes hormones, including thymosin, that stimulate the maturation and differentiation of T lymphocytes. T cells make up 70% to 80% of the circulating lymphocytes and are primarily responsible for immunity to intracellular viruses, tumour cells, and fungi. T cells live from a few months to an individual's lifespan and account for long-term immunity.

T lymphocytes can be categorized into T cytotoxic and T helper cells. Antigenic characteristics of WBCs have now been classified using monoclonal antibodies. These antigens are classified as *clusters of differentiation,* or *CD, antigens.* Many types of WBCs, especially lymphocytes, are referred

to by their CD designations. All mature T cells have the CD3 antigen (Kellie & Al-Mansour, 2017).

T Cytotoxic Cells. T cytotoxic (CD8) cells are involved in attacking antigens on the cell membrane of foreign pathogens and releasing cytolytic substances that destroy the pathogen. These cells have antigen specificity and are sensitized by exposure to the antigen (Rich & Chaplin, 2019). Much like B lymphocytes, some sensitized T cells do not attack the antigen but remain as memory T cells. As in the humoral immune response, a second exposure to the antigen results in a more intense and rapid cell-mediated immune response.

T Helper Cells. T helper (CD4) cells are involved in the regulation of cell-mediated immunity and the humoral antibody response. T helper cells differentiate into subsets of cells that produce distinct types of cytokines (discussed in a later section). These subsets are called T_H1 cells and T_H2 cells. T_H1 cells stimulate phagocyte-mediated ingestion and killing of microbes, the key component of cell-mediated immunity. T_H2 cells stimulate eosinophil-mediated immunity, which is effective against parasites and is involved in allergic responses.

Natural Killer Cells. Natural killer (NK) cells are also involved in cell-mediated immunity. These cells are not T or B cells but are large lymphocytes with numerous granules in the cytoplasm. Prior sensitization is not required for the generation of NK cells. These cells are involved in the recognition and killing of virus-infected cells, tumour cells, and transplanted grafts;

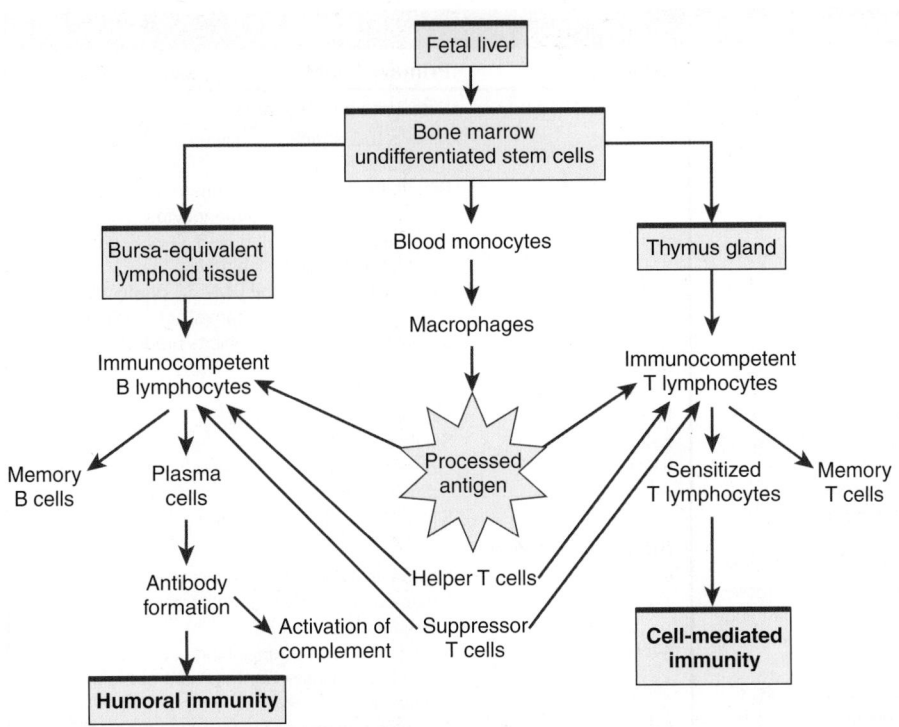

FIG. 16.3 Relationships and functions of macrophages, B lymphocytes, and T lymphocytes in an immune response.

TABLE 16.2   **CHARACTERISTICS OF IMMUNOGLOBULINS**

Class	Relative Serum Concentration (%)	Location	Characteristics
IgG	76	Plasma, interstitial fluid	Is the only immunoglobulin that crosses placenta
			Is responsible for secondary immune response
IgA	15	Body secretions, including tears, saliva, breast milk, colostrum	Lines mucous membranes and protects body surfaces
IgM	8	Plasma	Is responsible for primary immune response
			Forms antibodies to ABO blood antigens
IgD	1	Plasma	Is present on lymphocyte surface
			Assists in differentiation of B lymphocytes
IgE	0.002	Plasma, interstitial fluids	Causes symptoms of allergic reactions
			Fixes to mast cells and basophils
			Assists in defence against parasitic infections

Ig, immunoglobulin.

however, the mechanism of recognition is not fully understood. NK cells have a significant role in immune surveillance for malignant cell changes.

Dendritic Cells. Dendritic cells comprise a system of cells that play a significant role in cell-mediated immune response. They are found in the skin (called *Langerhans cells*), the lining of the nose, the lungs, the stomach, and the intestines; and when in an immature state, they can be found in the blood. Their primary function is to capture antigens at sites of contact with the external environment (e.g., skin, mucous membranes) and then transport this antigen until it encounters a T cell with specificity for the antigen. Dendritic cells have an important function in activating the immune response (Kellie & Al-Mansour, 2017).

Cytokines

The immune response involves complex interactions of T cells, B cells, monocytes, and neutrophils. These interactions depend on **cytokines** (soluble factors secreted by WBCs and a variety of other cells in the body), which act as messengers between

the cell types. Cytokines instruct cells to alter their proliferation, differentiation, secretion, or activity.

Currently more than 100 different cytokines are known and are classified into distinct categories (Rich & Chaplin, 2019). Some of these cytokines are listed in Table 16.3. In general, the interleukins act as immunomodulatory factors, colony-stimulating factors act as growth-regulating factors for hematopoietic cells, and interferons are antiviral and immunomodulatory.

The net effect of an inflammatory response is determined by a balance between proinflammatory and anti-inflammatory mediators. Sometimes cytokines are classified as proinflammatory or anti-inflammatory. However, it is not that straightforward since many other factors (e.g., target cells, environment) influence the inflammatory response to a given injury or insult.

Cytokines serve a beneficial role in hematopoiesis and immune function but can also have detrimental effects such as those observed in chronic inflammation, autoimmune diseases, and sepsis. Cytokines such as erythropoietin (see Chapters 18,

TABLE 16.3   TYPES AND FUNCTIONS OF CYTOKINE

Type	Primary Functions	Type	Primary Functions
Interleukins (ILs)		IL-14	Stimulates proliferation of activated B cells
IL-1	Augments the immune response; mediates the inflammatory response; promotes maturation and clonal expansion of B cells; enhances activity of NK cells; activates T cells; activates macrophages	IL-15	Mimics IL-2 effects; stimulates proliferation of T cells and NK cells
		IL-16	Proinflammatory cytokine; chemoattractant of T cells, eosinophils, and monocytes
IL-2	Induces proliferation and differentiation of T cells; plays role in activation of T cells, NK cells, and macrophages; stimulates release of other cytokines (α-IFN, TNF, IL-1, IL-6)	IL-17	Promotes release of IL-6, IL-8, G-CSF; enhances expression of adhesion molecules
		IL-18	Induces α-IFN, IL-2, and GM-CSF production; plays important role in development of T helper cells; enhances NK activity; inhibits production of IL-10
IL-3 (multi-colony-stimulating factor)	Hematopoietic growth factor for hematopoietic precursor cells	IL-19	Similar to IL-10
IL-4	B-cell growth factor: stimulates proliferation and differentiation of B cells; induces proliferation of T cells; stimulates growth of mast cells	IL-20	Similar to IL-10
		IL-21	Similar to IL-2, IL-4, and IL-5
		IL-22	Similar to IL-10
IL-5	Promotes B-cell growth and differentiation; promotes growth and differentiation of eosinophils	IL-23	Similar to IL-12; also promotes memory T-cell proliferation
		IL-24	Similar to IL-10
IL-6	Enhances the inflammatory response; plays role in B-cell stimulation; promotes differentiation of B cells into plasma cells; stimulates antibody secretion; induces fever; has synergistic effects with IL-1 and TNF	**Interferons (IFNs)**	
		α-IFN	Inhibits viral replication; activates NK cells and macrophages; has antiproliferative effects on tumour cells
IL-7	Promotes growth of T and B cells; increases expression of IL-2 and its receptor	β-IFN	Inhibits viral replication; inhibits certain white blood cells; is used in treatment of multiple sclerosis
IL-8	Involved in chemotaxis of neutrophils and T cells; stimulates superoxide and granule release	γ-IFN	Activates macrophages, neutrophils, and NK cells; promotes B-cell differentiation; inhibits viral replication
IL-9	Acts as mitogen, supporting proliferation in absence of antigen; enhances T-cell survival; plays role in mast cell activation	**Tumour Necrosis Factor (TNF)**	
		TNF	Activates macrophages and granulocytes; promotes the immune and inflammatory responses; kills tumour cells; is responsible for extensive weight loss associated with chronic inflammation and cancer
IL-10	Inhibits cytokine production by T and NK cells; promotes B-cell proliferation and antibody responses; is potent suppressor of macrophage function		
		Colony-Stimulating Factors (CSFs)	
IL-11	Is a multifunctional regulator of hematopoiesis and lymphopoiesis; plays role in osteoclast formation; elevates platelet count; inhibits proinflammatory cytokine production	G-CSF	Stimulates proliferation and differentiation of neutrophils; enhances functional activity of mature PMNs
		GM-CSF	Stimulates proliferation and differentiation of PMNs and monocytes
IL-12	Promotes α-IFN production; plays role in induction of T helper cells; activates NK cells; stimulates proliferation of activated T and NK cells	M-CSF	Promotes the proliferation, differentiation, and activation of monocytes and macrophages
IL-13	Promotes B-cell growth and differentiation; inhibits proinflammatory cytokine production		

G-CSF, granulocyte colony-stimulating factor; *GM-CSF,* granulocyte-macrophage colony-stimulating factor; *M-CSF,* macrophage colony-stimulating factor; *NK,* natural killer; *PMN,* polymorphonuclear neutrophil.

35, and 49), colony-stimulating factors, interferons (see Chapter 18), and interleukin-2 (see Chapter 18) are used clinically.

Interferons help the body's natural defenses attack tumours and viruses (Table 16.4). Three types of interferons have now been identified (see Table 16.3). Interferons are not directly antiviral but produce an antiviral effect in cells by reacting with them and inducing the formation of a second protein termed *antiviral protein* (Figure 16.4). This protein mediates the antiviral action of interferons by altering the cell's protein synthesis and prevents the virus from replicating.

Comparison of Humoral and Cell-Mediated Immunity

Humans need both humoral and cell-mediated immunity to remain healthy. Each type of immunity has unique properties and different modes of action and reactions against particular antigens. Table 16.5 compares humoral and cell-mediated immunity.

Humoral Immunity. Humoral immunity is antibody-mediated immunity. The term *humoral* comes from the Greek word *humor,* which means "body fluid." Since antibodies are produced by plasma cells (differentiated B cells) and found in plasma, the term *humoral immunity* is used. Production of antibodies is an essential component in a humoral immune response. Each of the five classes of immunoglobulins (Igs)—IgG, IgA, IgM, IgD, and IgE—has specific characteristics (see Table 16.2).

When a pathogen (especially bacteria) enters the body, it may encounter a B lymphocyte specific for antigens located on that bacterial cell wall. In addition, a monocyte or macrophage may phagocytize the bacteria and present its antigens to a B lymphocyte. The B lymphocyte recognizes the antigen because it has receptors on its cell surface specific for that antigen. When the antigen meets the cell surface receptor, the B cell becomes activated, and most B cells differentiate into

TABLE 16.4 CLINICAL USES OF CYTOKINES

Cytokine	Clinical Uses
α-Interferon	
(Intron A)	Hepatitis B and C
	Kaposi's sarcoma
	Hairy cell leukemia
	Lymphomas
	Melanoma
	Renal cell carcinoma
	Multiple myeloma
β-Interferon	
β-Interferon-1b (Betaseron)	Multiple sclerosis
β-Interferon-1a (Avonex, Rebif)	
Colony-Stimulating Factors: G-CSF, GM-CSF	
Filgrastim (Neupogen)	Neutropenia
Soluble Tumour Necrosis Factor Receptor	
Etanercept (Enbrel)	Rheumatoid arthritis
Interleukin-2	
Aldesleukin (Proleukin)	Renal cell carcinoma
	Malignant melanoma
	Lymphoma
	Acute myelocytic leukemia
Erythropoietin	
Darbepoetin alfa (Aranesp)	Anemia
Epoetin alfa (Eprex)	
Interleukin-1 Receptor Antagonist	
Anakinra (Kineret)	Rheumatoid arthritis

G-CSF, granulocyte colony-stimulating factor; *GM-CSF,* granulocyte-macrophage colony-stimulating factor.

TABLE 16.5 COMPARISON OF HUMORAL IMMUNITY AND CELL-MEDIATED IMMUNITY

Characteristics	Humoral Immunity	Cell-Mediated Immunity
Cells involved	B lymphocytes	T lymphocytes, macrophages
Products	Antibodies	Sensitized T cells, lymphokines
Memory cells	Present	Present
Protection	Bacteria	Fungi
	Viruses (extracellular)	Viruses (intracellular)
	Respiratory and gastrointestinal pathogens	Chronic infectious agents
		Tumour cells
Examples	Anaphylactic shock	Tuberculosis
	Atopic diseases	Fungal infections
	Transfusion reaction	Contact dermatitis
	Bacterial infections	Graft rejection
		Destruction of cancer cells

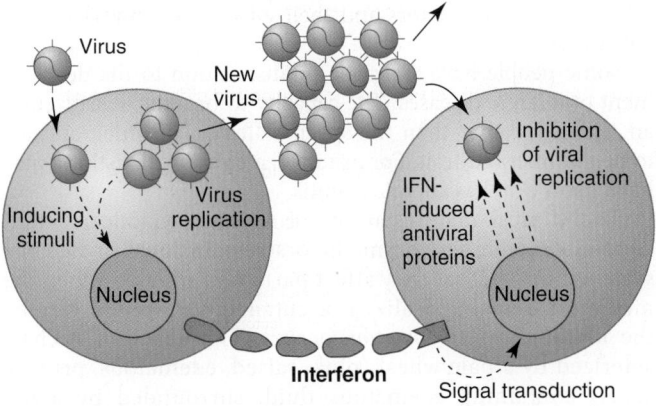

FIG. 16.4 Mechanism of action of interferons. The virus attacks a cell. The cell begins to synthesize viral DNA and interferons. Interferons serve as intercellular messengers. Interferons induce the production of antiviral proteins. The virus is not able to replicate in the cell.

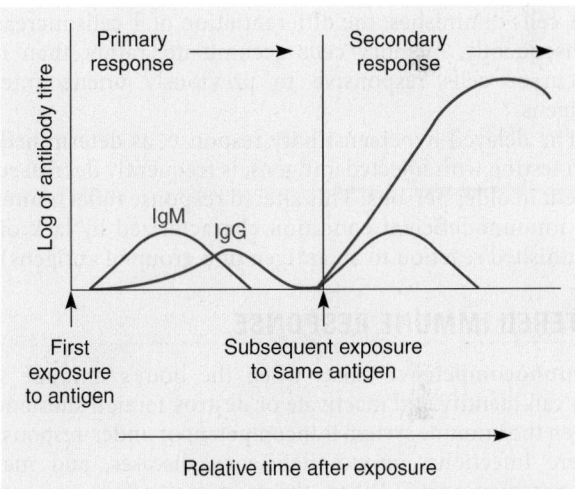

FIG. 16.5 Primary and secondary immune responses. The introduction of antigen induces a response dominated by two classes of immunoglobulins: immunoglobulin M (IgM) and immunoglobulin G (IgG). IgM predominates in the primary response; some amount of IgG appears later. After the host's immune system is primed, another challenge with the same antigen induces the secondary response, in which some IgM and large amounts of IgG are produced.

plasma cells (see Figure 16.3). The mature plasma cell secretes immunoglobulins. Some stimulated B lymphocytes remain as memory cells.

The primary immune response becomes evident 4 to 8 days after the initial exposure to the antigen (Figure 16.5). IgM is the first type of antibody formed. Because of the large size of the IgM molecule, this immunoglobulin is confined to the intravascular space. As the immune response progresses, IgG is produced and can move from intravascular to extravascular spaces.

When a secondary antigenic exposure occurs, the reactive response typically occurs faster (1 to 3 days), is stronger, and lasts for a longer time than the primary response. Memory cells account for the memory of the first exposure to the antigen and

the more rapid production of antibodies. IgG is the primary antibody found in a secondary immune response.

IgG crosses the placental membrane and provides the newborn with passive acquired immunity for at least 3 months. Infants may also get some passive immunity from IgA in breast milk and colostrum.

Cell-Mediated Immunity. Immune responses that are initiated through specific antigen recognition by T cells are termed cell-mediated immunity. Several cell types and factors are involved in cell-mediated immunity, including T lymphocytes, macrophages, and NK cells. Cell-mediated immunity is of primary importance in (a) immunity against pathogens that survive inside of cells, including viruses and some bacteria (e.g., *Mycobacterium* species); (b) immunity against fungal infections; (c) rejection of transplanted tissues; (d) contact hypersensitivity reactions; and (e) tumour immunity.

AGE-RELATED CONSIDERATIONS

Effects of Aging on the Immune System

With advancing age, the effectiveness of the immune system declines (Weyand & Goronzy, 2016) (Table 16.6). The primary clinical evidence for this immunosenescence is the high incidence of malignancies among older persons. Older people become increasingly susceptible to infections (e.g., influenza, pneumonia) from pathogens they were relatively immunocompetent against earlier in life. Bacterial pneumonia is the leading cause of death from infections in older persons. The antibody response to immunizations (e.g., flu vaccine) in older people is lower than in younger adults.

The bone marrow is relatively unaffected by increasing age. Immunoglobulin levels decrease with age, leading to a suppressed humoral immune response in older persons. Thymic involution (shrinking) occurs with aging, along with decreased numbers of T cells. These changes in the thymus gland are a primary cause of immunosenescence. Both T and B cells show deficiencies in activation, transit time through the cell cycle, and subsequent differentiation. However, the most significant changes involve T cells. As thymic output of T cells diminishes, the differentiation of T cells increases. Consequently, memory cells accumulate, rather than new precursor cells responsive to previously unencountered antigens.

The delayed hypersensitivity response, as determined by skin testing with injected antigens, is frequently decreased or absent in older persons. This altered response reflects anergy (an immunodeficient condition characterized by lack of or diminished reaction to an antigen or a group of antigens).

ALTERED IMMUNE RESPONSE

Immunocompetence exists when the body's immune system can identify and inactivate or destroy foreign substances. When the immune system is incompetent or under-responsive, severe infections, immunodeficiency diseases, and malignancies may occur. When the immune system overreacts, hypersensitivity disorders such as allergies and autoimmune diseases may occur.

Hypersensitivity Reactions

Sometimes the immune response is overreactive against foreign antigens or reacts against its own tissue, resulting in tissue damage. This is termed a hypersensitivity reaction. Autoimmune diseases, a type of hypersensitivity response, occur when the body fails to recognize self-proteins and reacts against self-antigens.

Hypersensitivity reactions may be classified according to the source of the antigen, the time sequence (immediate or delayed), or immunological mechanisms causing the injury. Four types of hypersensitivity reactions exist (Table 16.7). Types I, II, and III are immediate and are examples of humoral immunity. Type IV is a delayed hypersensitivity reaction and is related to cell-mediated immunity.

Type I: IgE-Mediated Reactions. Anaphylactic reactions are type I reactions that occur only in susceptible people who are highly sensitized to specific allergens. IgE antibodies, produced in response to the allergen, have a characteristic property of attaching to mast cells and basophils (Figure 16.6; see Figure 31.2 in Chapter 31). Within these cells are granules containing potent chemical mediators (histamine, serotonin, leukotrienes, eosinophil chemotactic factor of anaphylaxis [ECF-A], kinins, and bradykinin). (Chemical mediators of inflammation are discussed in Chapter 14 and Table 14.3. Anaphylaxis is also discussed in Chapter 14.)

On the first exposure to the allergen, IgE antibodies are produced and bind to mast cells and basophils. On any subsequent exposures, the allergen links with the IgE bound to mast cells or basophils and triggers degranulation of the cells and the release of chemical mediators from the granules. These chemical mediators attack target tissues, causing clinical symptoms of allergy (Rich & Chaplin, 2019). These effects include smooth muscle contraction, increased vascular permeability, vasodilation, hypotension, increased secretion of mucus, and itching. Fortunately, the mediators are short-acting and their effects are reversible. The mediators and their effects are summarized in Table 16.8.

Some people have a genetic predisposition to the development of allergic diseases. The capacity to become sensitized to an allergen, rather than the specific allergic disorder, appears to be an inherited trait. For example, a father with asthma may have a son who has allergic rhinitis.

The clinical manifestations of an anaphylactic reaction depend on whether the mediators remain local or become systemic or whether they affect particular organs. When the mediators remain localized, a cutaneous response termed the *wheal-and-flare reaction* occurs. This reaction is characterized by a pale wheal (pink, raised, edematous, pruritic areas) containing edematous fluid, surrounded by a red flare from the hyperemia. The reaction occurs in minutes or hours and is typically not dangerous. A classic example of a wheal-and-flare reaction is the mosquito bite. The wheal-and-flare reaction serves a diagnostic purpose as a means of demonstrating allergic reactions to specific allergens during skin tests.

Common allergic reactions include anaphylaxis and atopic reactions.

Anaphylaxis. Anaphylaxis occurs when mediators are released systemically (e.g., after injection of a medication, after an insect sting). The reaction occurs within minutes and can be life-threatening, resulting in bronchial constriction, airway obstruction, and vascular collapse. The target organs affected are depicted in Figure 16.7. Initial symptoms include edema and itching at the site of the exposure to the allergen. Shock can occur rapidly and is manifested by a rapid, weak pulse; hypotension; dilated pupils; dyspnea; and possibly cyanosis. This is compounded by bronchial edema and angioedema. Death occurs if

TABLE 16.6	AGE-RELATED DIFFERENCES IN ASSESSMENT

Effects of Aging on the Immune System

- ↓ Autoantibodies
- ↓ Cell-mediated immunity
- ↓ Delayed hypersensitivity response
- ↓ Expression of IL-2 receptors
- ↓ IL-1 and IL-2 synthesis
- ↓ Primary and secondary antibody responses
- ↓ Proliferative response of T and B cells
- Thymic involution

IL-1, interleukin-1; *IL-2,* interleukin-2.

TABLE 16.7 TYPES OF HYPERSENSITIVITY REACTIONS

	Type I: Anaphylactic Reactions	Type II: Cytotoxic Reactions	Type III: Immune-Complex Reactions	Type IV: Delayed Hypersensitivity Reactions
Antigen	Exogenous pollen, food, medications, dust	Cell surface of RBCs Basement membrane	Extracellular fungal, viral, bacterial	Intracellular or extracellular
Antibody Involved	IgE	IgG IgM	IgG IgM	None
Complement Involved	No	Yes	Yes	No
Mediators of Injury	Histamine SRS-A	Complement lysis Neutrophils	Neutrophils Complement lysis	Cytokines T cytotoxic cells Monocytes, macrophages Lysosomal enzymes
Examples	Allergic rhinitis Asthma	Transfusion reaction Goodpasture's syndrome	Serum sickness Systemic lupus erythematosus Rheumatoid arthritis	Contact dermatitis Tumour rejection Transplant rejection
Skin Test	Wheal and flare	None	Erythema and edema in 3 to 8 hours	Erythema and edema in 24 to 48 hours (e.g., tuberculin test)

IgE, immunoglobulin E; *IgG,* immunoglobulin G; *IgM,* immunoglobulin M; *RBC,* red blood cell; *SRS-A,* slow-reacting substance of anaphylaxis.

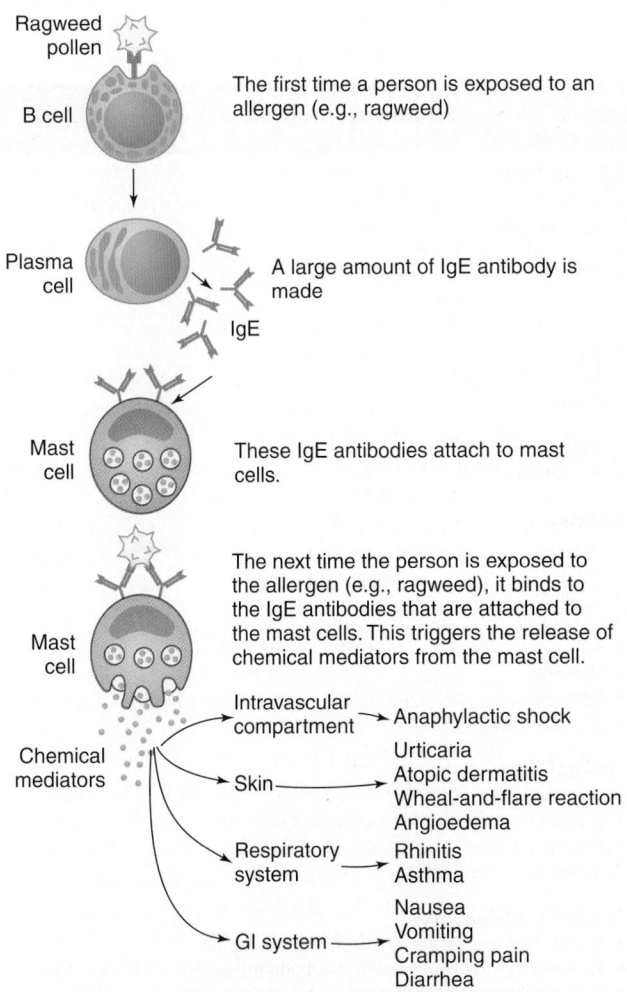

Ragweed pollen

B cell

The first time a person is exposed to an allergen (e.g., ragweed)

Plasma cell

A large amount of IgE antibody is made

IgE

Mast cell

These IgE antibodies attach to mast cells.

Mast cell

The next time the person is exposed to the allergen (e.g., ragweed), it binds to the IgE antibodies that are attached to the mast cells. This triggers the release of chemical mediators from the mast cell.

Chemical mediators

Intravascular compartment → Anaphylactic shock

Skin → Urticaria
Atopic dermatitis
Wheal-and-flare reaction
Angioedema

Respiratory system → Rhinitis
Asthma

GI system → Nausea
Vomiting
Cramping pain
Diarrhea

FIG. 16.6 Steps in a type I allergic reaction. *GI,* gastrointestinal; *IgE,* immunoglobulin E.

emergency treatment is not initiated. Treatment can range from epinephrine administered subcutaneously for mild symptoms to full circulatory support with oxygen and vasopressor therapy (Anagnostou & Turner, 2019). Some of the important allergens leading to anaphylactic shock in hypersensitive people are listed in Table 16.9. Medications are the leading cause of anaphylaxis-related deaths (Turner et al., 2017).

Atopic Reactions. An estimated 20% of the population are atopic, meaning they have an inherited tendency to become sensitive to environmental allergens (Weidinger & Novak, 2016). The atopic diseases that can result are allergic rhinitis, asthma, atopic dermatitis, urticaria, and angioedema.

Allergic rhinitis, or hay fever, is the most common type I hypersensitivity reaction. It can occur year-round (perennial allergic rhinitis) or it may be seasonal (seasonal allergic rhinitis). Airborne substances such as pollens, dust, or moulds are the primary cause of allergic rhinitis. Perennial allergic rhinitis may be caused by dust, moulds, and animal dander. Seasonal allergic rhinitis is commonly caused by pollens from trees, weeds, or grasses. The target areas affected are the conjunctivas of the eyes and the mucosa of the upper respiratory tract. Symptoms include nasal discharge, sneezing, lacrimation, mucosal swelling with airway obstruction, and pruritus around the eyes, nose, throat, and mouth. (Treatment of allergic rhinitis is discussed in Chapter 29.)

Many patients with asthma have an allergic component to their disease. These patients frequently have a history of atopic disorders (e.g., infantile eczema, allergic rhinitis, food intolerances). Inflammatory mediators produce bronchial smooth muscle constriction, excessive secretion of viscous mucus, edema of the mucous membranes of the bronchi, and decreased lung compliance. Because of these physiological alterations, affected patients manifest dyspnea, wheezing, coughing, tightness in the chest, and thick sputum. (Pathophysiology and management of asthma are discussed in Chapter 31.)

TABLE 16.8 MEDIATORS OF ALLERGIC RESPONSE

Type and Source	Biological Activity	Clinical Manifestations
Histamine Mast cell and basophil granules	Increase vascular permeability; constrict smooth muscle; stimulate irritant receptors	Edema of airways and larynx; bronchial constriction; urticaria, angioedema, pruritus; nausea, vomiting, diarrhea; shock
Leukotrienes Metabolites of arachidonic acid by lipoxygenase pathway	Constrict bronchial smooth muscle; increase vascular permeability	Bronchial constriction; enhanced effect of histamine on smooth muscle
Prostaglandins Metabolites of arachidonic acid by cyclo-oxygenase pathway	Stimulate vasodilation; constrict smooth muscle	Wheal-and-flare reaction on skin; hypotension; bronchospasm
Platelet-Activating Factor Mast cell	Aggregates platelets; stimulates vasodilation	Increase in pulmonary artery pressure; systemic hypotension
Kinins Kininogen	Stimulates slow, sustained smooth muscle contraction; increases vascular permeability; stimulates secretion of mucus; stimulates pain receptors	Angioedema with painful swelling; bronchial constriction
Serotonin Platelets	Increase vascular permeability; stimulate smooth muscle contraction	Mucosal edema; bronchial constriction
Anaphylatoxins C3a, C4a, C5a from complement activation	Stimulate histamine release	Edema of airways and larynx; bronchial constriction; urticaria, angioedema, pruritus; nausea, vomiting, diarrhea; shock

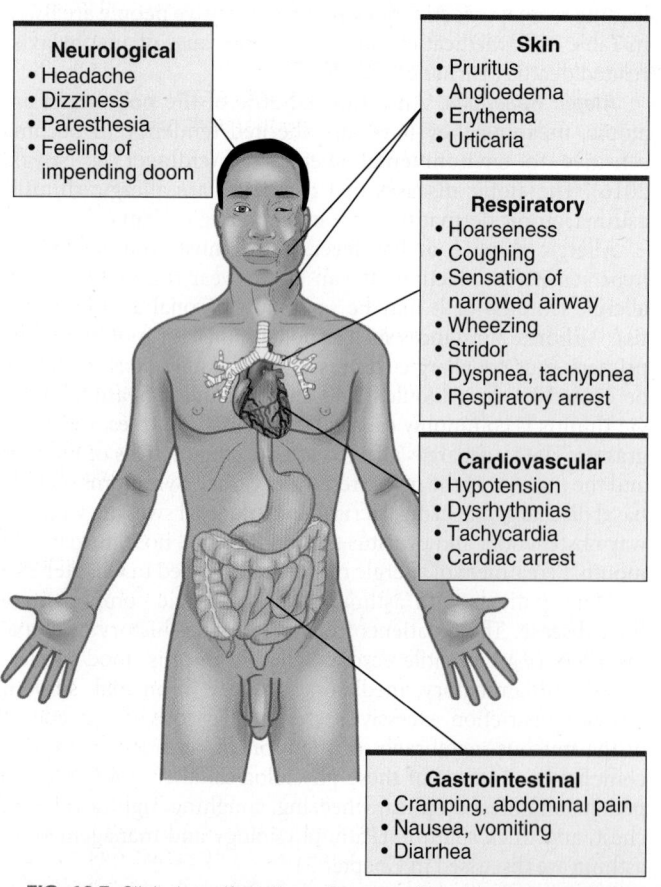

Neurological
- Headache
- Dizziness
- Paresthesia
- Feeling of impending doom

Skin
- Pruritus
- Angioedema
- Erythema
- Urticaria

Respiratory
- Hoarseness
- Coughing
- Sensation of narrowed airway
- Wheezing
- Stridor
- Dyspnea, tachypnea
- Respiratory arrest

Cardiovascular
- Hypotension
- Dysrhythmias
- Tachycardia
- Cardiac arrest

Gastrointestinal
- Cramping, abdominal pain
- Nausea, vomiting
- Diarrhea

FIG. 16.7 Clinical manifestations of a systemic anaphylactic reaction.

TABLE 16.9 ALLERGENS THAT CAUSE ANAPHYLACTIC SHOCK

Medications
- Aspirin
- Cephalosporins
- Chemotherapeutic drugs
- Insulins
- Local anaesthetics
- Nonsteroidal anti-inflammatory drugs
- Penicillins
- Sulfonamides
- Tetracycline

Insect Venoms
- Hymenoptera*

Foods
- Eggs
- Nuts
- Shellfish
- Chocolate
- Milk
- Peanuts
- Fish
- Strawberries

Animal Sera
- Tetanus antitoxin
- Diphtheria antitoxin
- Rabies antitoxin
- Snake venom antitoxin

Treatment Measures
- Blood products (whole blood and components)
- Allergenic extracts in hyposensitization therapy
- Iodine-contrast media for intravenous pyelography or angiography

*Wasps, hornets, yellow jackets, bumblebees, and ants.

Atopic dermatitis is a chronic, inherited skin disorder characterized by exacerbations and remissions. It is caused by several environmental allergens often difficult to identify. Although patients with atopic dermatitis have elevated IgE levels and positive skin tests, the histopathological features do not represent the typical, localized wheal-and-flare type I reactions. The skin lesions are more generalized and involve vasodilation of blood vessels, resulting in interstitial edema with vesicle formation (Figure 16.8). (Dermatitis is discussed in Chapter 26.)

Urticaria (hives) is a cutaneous reaction against systemic allergens that occurs in atopic people. It is characterized by transient wheals that vary in size and shape and may occur throughout the body. Urticaria develops rapidly after exposure to an allergen and may last minutes or hours. Histamine causes localized vasodilation (erythema), transudation of fluid (wheal), and flaring. Flaring is caused by dilation of blood vessels on the edge of the wheal. Histamine is responsible for the pruritus associated with the lesions. (Urticaria is discussed further in Chapter 26.)

Angioedema is a localized cutaneous lesion similar to urticaria but involves deeper layers of the skin and submucosa. The principal areas of involvement include the eyelids, lips, tongue, larynx, hands, feet, gastrointestinal tract, and genitalia. Swelling usually begins in the face and progresses to the airways and other parts of the body. Dilation and engorgement of the capillaries secondary to release of histamine cause the diffuse swelling. Welts are not apparent as in urticaria. The outer skin appears normal or has a reddish hue. The lesions may burn, sting, or itch and, if in the gastrointestinal tract, can cause acute abdominal pain. The swelling may occur suddenly or over several hours and usually lasts for 24 hours.

Type II: Cytotoxic and Cytolytic Reactions (Antibody-Mediated Response). Cytotoxic and cytolytic reactions are type II hypersensitivity reactions involving the direct binding of IgG or IgM antibodies to an antigen on the cell surface. Antigen–antibody complexes activate the complement system, which mediates the reaction. Cellular tissue is destroyed by either (a) activation of the complement cascade resulting in cytolysis or (b) enhanced phagocytosis.

Target cells frequently destroyed in type II reactions are erythrocytes, platelets, and leukocytes. The tissue damage usually occurs rapidly, typically from 2 to 24 hours. Some of the antigens involved are the ABO blood group, rhesus (Rh) factor, and medications. Pathophysiological disorders characteristic of type II reactions include ABO incompatibility transfusion reaction, Rh incompatibility transfusion reaction, autoimmune and medication-related hemolytic anemias, leukopenia, thrombocytopenia, erythroblastosis fetalis (hemolytic disease of the newborn), and Goodpasture's syndrome.

Hemolytic Transfusion Reactions. A classic type II reaction occurs when a recipient receives ABO-incompatible blood from a donor. Naturally acquired antibodies to antigens of the ABO blood group are in the recipient's serum but are not present on the erythrocyte membranes (see Chapter 32, Table 32.9). For example, a person with type A blood has anti-B antibodies, a person with type B blood has anti-A antibodies, a person with type AB blood has no antibodies, and a person with type O blood has both anti-A and anti-B antibodies.

If the recipient receives a transfusion with incompatible blood, antibodies immediately coat the foreign erythrocytes, causing agglutination (clumping). The clumping of cells blocks small blood vessels in the body, using and thus depleting existing clotting factors, which leads to bleeding. Within hours, neutrophils and macrophages phagocytize the agglutinated cells.

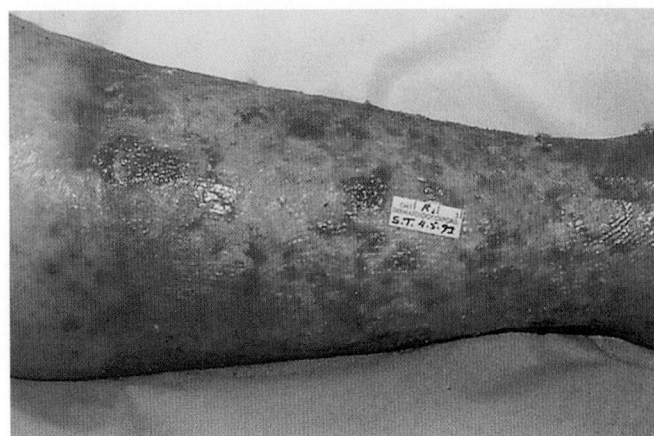

FIG. 16.8 Eczema of the lower leg. Source: Morison, M. J. (2001). *Nursing management of chronic wounds.* Mosby.

As complement is fixed to the antigen, cell lysis occurs, which in turn causes the release of hemoglobin into the urine and plasma. Acute kidney injury can result from hemoglobinuria. (Blood transfusions are discussed in Chapter 33.)

Goodpasture's Syndrome. Goodpasture's syndrome is a rare disorder involving the lungs and the kidneys. An antibody-mediated autoimmune reaction occurs involving the glomerular and alveolar basement membranes. The circulating antibodies combine with tissue antigen to activate the complement system, which causes deposits of IgG to form along the basement membranes of the lungs or the kidneys. This reaction may result in pulmonary hemorrhage and glomerulonephritis. (Goodpasture's syndrome is discussed further in Chapter 48.)

Type III: Immune-Complex Reactions. Tissue damage in immune-complex reactions, which are type III reactions, occurs secondary to antigen–antibody complexes. Soluble antigens combine with immunoglobulins of the IgG and IgM classes to form complexes that are too small to be effectively removed by the mononuclear phagocyte system. Therefore, the complexes deposit in tissue or small blood vessels. They cause activation of the complement system and release of chemotactic factors that lead to inflammation and destruction of the involved tissue.

Type III reactions may be local or systemic and immediate or delayed. The clinical manifestations depend on the number of complexes and their location in the body. Common sites for deposit are the kidneys, skin, joints, blood vessels, and lungs. Severe type III reactions are associated with autoimmune disorders such as systemic lupus erythematosus (SLE), acute glomerulonephritis, and rheumatoid arthritis. (SLE and rheumatoid arthritis are discussed further in Chapter 67, and acute glomerulonephritis is discussed further in Chapter 48.)

Type IV: Delayed Hypersensitivity Reactions. A delayed hypersensitivity reaction—a type IV reaction—is also called a *cell-mediated immune response.* Although cell-mediated immune responses are usually protective mechanisms, tissue damage occurs in delayed hypersensitivity reactions.

The tissue damage in a type IV reaction does not occur in the presence of antibodies or complement. Rather, sensitized T lymphocytes attack antigens or release cytokines, some of which attract macrophages into the area. These macrophages are responsible for most of the tissue destruction. A delayed hypersensitivity reaction takes 24 to 48 hours to occur.

Examples of delayed hypersensitivity reactions include contact dermatitis (Figure 16.9); hypersensitivity reactions to

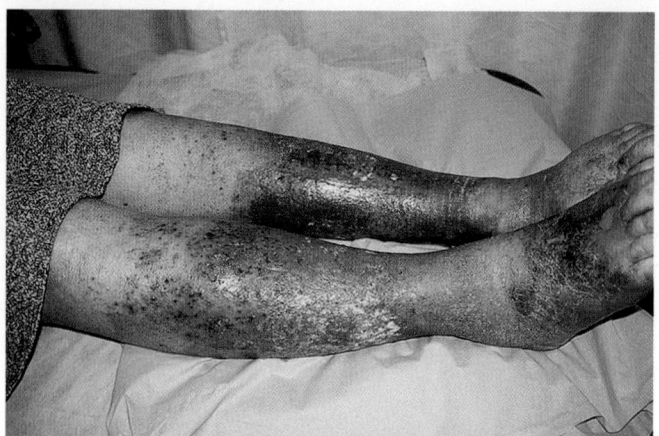

FIG. 16.9 Contact dermatitis in reaction to rubber. Source: Morison, M. J. (2001). *Nursing management of chronic wounds*. Mosby.

bacterial, fungal, and viral infections; and transplant rejection. Some medication sensitivity reactions also fit this category.

Contact Dermatitis. Allergic contact dermatitis is an example of a delayed hypersensitivity reaction involving the skin. The reaction occurs when the skin is exposed to substances that easily penetrate the skin to combine with epidermal proteins. The substance then becomes antigenic, and over a period of 7 to 14 days, memory cells form for the antigen. On subsequent exposure to the substance, a sensitized person develops eczematous skin lesions within 48 hours. The most common antigenic substances encountered are metal compounds (e.g., those containing nickel, mercury); rubber compounds; poison ivy, poison oak, and poison sumac; cosmetics; and some dyes.

In acute contact dermatitis, the skin lesions appear erythematous and edematous and are covered with papules, vesicles, and bullae. The affected area can be pruritic, burn, or sting. When contact dermatitis becomes chronic, the lesions resemble atopic dermatitis because they are thickened, scaly, and lichenified. The main difference between contact dermatitis and atopic dermatitis is that contact dermatitis is localized and restricted to the area exposed to the allergens, whereas atopic dermatitis is usually widespread.

Microbial Hypersensitivity Reactions. The classic example of a microbial cell-mediated immune reaction is the body's defence against the tubercle bacillus. Tuberculosis (TB) results from invasion of lung tissue by the highly resistant tubercle bacillus. The organism itself does not directly damage the lung tissue. However, antigenic material released from the tubercle bacilli reacts with T lymphocytes, initiating a cell-mediated immune response. The resulting response causes extensive caseous necrosis of the lung.

After the initial cell-mediated immune reaction, memory cells persist; therefore, subsequent contact with the tubercle bacillus or an extract of purified protein from the organism causes a delayed hypersensitivity reaction. This is the basis for the purified protein derivative (PPD) TB skin test, which yields results 48 to 72 hours after the intradermal injection. (TB is discussed in Chapter 30.)

ALLERGIC DISORDERS

Although an alteration of the immune system may manifest in many ways, allergies or type I hypersensitivity reactions are seen most frequently.

Assessment

For a thorough assessment of a patient with allergies, a comprehensive health history, physical examination, diagnostic workup, and skin testing for allergens must be performed.

Health History. A comprehensive history must include family allergies, past and current allergies, and social and environmental factors. Identifying the clinical manifestations that may have triggered a reaction and the course of the allergic reaction should be obtained to attempt to control or prevent future allergic reactions. The information may be obtained from the patient or the family about atopic reactions to identify at-risk patients. The patient's use of any over-the-counter (OTC) or prescription medications used to treat the allergies should be documented.

Social factors (patient's lifestyle and stressors), environmental factors, and physical environment should be reviewed in connection with the appearance of allergic symptoms. Questions about pets, trees, plants, air pollutants, floor coverings, and cooling and heating systems in the home or workplace can yield valuable information about potential allergens along with analysis of a daily or weekly food diary. Of particular importance is a screening for any reaction to medications.

Lastly is the need to identify vulnerable populations such as Indigenous people, as differences in their immune systems have shown variability in response to infections (Semple et al., 2019). Indigenous people tend to self-report fewer allergies, which can be a result of multiple factors, such as lack of access to appropriate health care, historical trauma, systemic racism, genetics, or lack of awareness of the allergic response (Currie et al., 2019; Soller et al., 2015).

Physical Examination. A comprehensive head-to-toe physical examination should be undertaken for a patient with allergies with a focus on the site of the allergic manifestations. A comprehensive assessment that includes subjective and objective data should be obtained from the patient (Table 16.10).

Diagnostic Studies

Many specialized immunological techniques can be performed to detect abnormalities of lymphocytes, eosinophils, and immunoglobulins. Studies include a complete blood cell count (CBC) with WBC differential, including an absolute lymphocyte count and eosinophil count. Cellular immunodeficiency is diagnosed if the lymphocyte count is below 1.2×10^9/L. T-cell and B-cell quantification is used to diagnose specific immunodeficiency syndromes. The eosinophil count is elevated with type I hypersensitivity reactions involving IgE. The serum IgE level is also generally elevated in type I hypersensitivity reactions and serves as a diagnostic indicator of atopic diseases.

Sputum and nasal and bronchial secretions may also be tested for the presence of eosinophils. If asthma is suspected, pulmonary function tests (especially forced expiratory volume) are helpful.

Allergy skin testing is the preferred method for determining immediate reactions to allergens, but in some cases blood testing may be ordered. Allergy blood testing is recommended if a person (a) is using a medication that interferes with skin test results (e.g., antihistamines, corticosteroids) and cannot stop taking it for a few days, (b) cannot tolerate the many needle scratches required for skin testing, or (c) has a skin disorder (e.g., severe eczema, dermatitis, psoriasis).

TABLE 16.10   NURSING ASSESSMENT
Allergies

Subjective Data
Important Health Information

Past health history: Recurrent respiratory problems; seasonal exacerbations; unusual reactions to insect bites or stings; past and present allergies; altered home and work environment; presence of pets; family history of allergies
Medications: Unusual reactions to any medications; use of over-the-counter medications; use of medications for allergies

Symptoms

Food intolerances; vomiting; abdominal cramps, diarrhea; fatigue; hoarseness, cough, dyspnea; itching, burning, stinging of eyes, nose, throat, or skin; chest tightness; malaise

Objective Data
Integumentary

Rashes, including urticaria, wheal-and-flare, papules, vesicles, bullae; dryness, scaliness, scratches, irritation

Eyes, Ears, Nose, and Throat

Eyes: Conjunctivitis; lacrimation; rubbing or excessive blinking; dark circles under the eyes ("allergic shiner")
Ears: Diminished hearing; immobile or scarred tympanic membranes; recurrent ear infections
Nose: Nasal polyps; nasal voice; nose twitching; itchy nose; rhinitis; pale, boggy mucous membranes; sniffling; repeated sneezing; swollen nasal passages; recurrent, unexplained nosebleeds; crease across the bridge of nose ("allergic salute")
Throat: Continual throat clearing; swollen lips or tongue; red throat; palpable neck lymph nodes

Respiratory

Wheezing, stridor; thick sputum

Possible Findings

Eosinophilia of serum, sputum, or nasal and bronchial secretions; ↑ serum IgE levels; positive skin tests; abnormal chest and sinus radiographs

IgE, immunoglobulin E.

Skin Tests. Skin testing can be used to identify specific allergens that are causing the allergy symptoms; however, given empiric usage of allergy medications for allergic rhinitis, skin testing is now infrequently performed. Diagnosing an allergy to a specific antigen enables the patient to avoid an allergen and makes the patient a candidate for immunotherapy. Unfortunately, skin testing cannot be done on patients who cannot stop taking medications that suppress the histamine response or on patients with food allergies.

Procedure. Skin testing may be performed by three different methods: (a) a scratch or prick, (b) an intradermal test, or (c) a patch test. Body areas typically used in skin testing are the arms and back. Allergen extracts are applied to the skin in rows with a corresponding control site opposite the test site. Saline or another diluent is applied to the control site. In the *scratch test*, the epidermal skin layer is scratched with a pricking device, and the allergen extract is applied at the site. In the intradermal test, the allergen extract is injected intradermally under the skin, similar to a PPD test for TB. In the patch test, an allergen is applied to a patch that is placed on the skin.

Results. In the scratch and intradermal tests, the reaction typically occurs within 5 to 10 minutes. In the patch test, the patches need to be worn for 48 to 72 hours. If the person is hypersensitive to the allergen, a positive reaction will occur within minutes after insertion in the skin and may last for 8 to 12 hours. A positive reaction is manifested by a local wheal-and-flare response.

The size of the positive reaction does not always correlate with the severity of allergy symptoms. False-positive and false-negative results may occur. Negative results from skin testing do not necessarily mean the person does not have an allergic disorder, and positive results do not necessarily mean that the allergen caused the clinical manifestations. Positive results imply that the person is sensitized to that allergen. Therefore, correlating skin test results with the patient's history is important.

Precautions. A highly sensitive person is always at risk for developing an anaphylactic reaction to skin tests. Therefore, a patient receiving a skin test should never be left alone during the testing period. If a severe reaction does occur with a skin test, the extract is immediately removed and anti-inflammatory topical cream is applied to the site. For intradermal testing, the arm is used so that a tourniquet can be applied during a severe reaction. A subcutaneous injection of epinephrine may also be necessary.

Interprofessional Care

After an allergic disorder is diagnosed, the treatment is aimed at reducing exposure to the offending allergen, treating the symptoms, and, if necessary, desensitizing the person through immunotherapy.

Anaphylaxis. Anaphylactic reactions occur suddenly in hypersensitive patients after exposure to the offending allergen. They may occur after parenteral injection of medications (especially antibiotics), administration of blood products, and after insect stings. The cardinal principle in management is speed in (a) recognizing signs and symptoms of an anaphylactic reaction, (b) establishing and maintaining a patent airway, (c) administering medications, and (d) treating for shock (Turner et al., 2017). Table 16.11 summarizes the emergency treatment of anaphylactic shock.

In severe cases of anaphylaxis, hypovolemic shock may occur because of the loss of intravascular fluid into interstitial spaces secondary to increased capillary permeability (Turner et al., 2017). Peripheral vasoconstriction and stimulation of the sympathetic nervous system occur to compensate for the fluid shift. However, unless shock is treated early, the body will no longer be able to compensate, and irreversible tissue damage will occur, leading to death. (Hypovolemic shock is further discussed in Chapter 69.)

Epinephrine is the medication of choice, given parenterally (intramuscularly, intravenously), to treat an anaphylactic reaction. Patients receiving β-blockers may be resistant to treatment with epinephrine and can develop refractory hypotension and bradycardia. Glucagon should be given to these patients because it has inotropic and chronotropic effects that are not mediated through β-receptors.

All health care workers must be prepared for the rare but life-threatening anaphylactic reaction, which requires immediate medical and nursing interventions. It is extremely important to identify all the patient's allergies and to document them in all appropriate areas in the chart (Turner et al., 2017).

Chronic Allergies. Most allergic reactions are chronic and are characterized by remissions and exacerbations of symptoms. Treatment focuses on identification and control of allergens, relief of symptoms through medication therapy, and hyposensitization of a patient to an offending allergen.

Allergen Recognition and Control. The nurse plays an important role in helping the patient make lifestyle adjustments to minimize exposure to the offending allergens. The nurse can also offer preventive measures that will help control the allergic symptoms. The nurse should reinforce that the patient will never be desensitized or completely symptom-free, even with medication therapy and immunotherapy.

✚ TABLE 16.11   EMERGENCY MANAGEMENT

Anaphylactic Shock

Cause
- Injection of, inhalation of, ingestion of, or topical exposure to substance that produces profound allergic response. See Table 16.9 for a more complete listing.

Assessment Findings
See Figure 16.7.

Interventions

Initial
- Ensure patent airway; prepare for intubation if evidence of impending obstruction.
- Remove insect stinger if it is present.
- IM epinephrine (1 mg/mL preparation): Administer epinephrine 0.3 to 0.5 mg IM, preferably in the mid-outer thigh; repeat every 5 to 15 minutes (or more frequently), as needed.
- IV epinephrine infusion (0.1 mcg/kg/min) titrated to effect if not responsive to IM treatment.
  - IV bolus (0.05 to 1 mg of 0.1 mg/mL) epinephrine over 1 to 10 minutes may be indicated in certain situations, such as (impending) cardiovascular collapse.
- Administer oxygen 8 to 10 L/min or up to 100% oxygen, if needed.
- Administer Albuterol (salbutamol) 2.5 to 5 mg in 3-mL saline via nebulizer for bronchospasm.
- Place patient in recumbent position and elevate legs.
- Keep patient warm.
- Administer diphenhydramine (Benadryl) IM or IV.
- Maintain patient's blood pressure with fluids, volume expanders, vasopressors (e.g., dopamine, norepinephrine bitartrate [Levophed]).

If symptoms are not responding to epinephrine injections, prepare IV epinephrine for infusion.

Ongoing Monitoring
- Monitor vital signs, respiratory effort, oxygen saturation, level of consciousness, and cardiac rhythm.
- Anticipate intubation in cases of severe respiratory distress.
- Anticipate cricothyrotomy or tracheostomy in cases of severe laryngeal edema.

IM, intramuscularly; IV, intravenously.

Of primary importance is the need to identify the offending allergen. With food allergies, an elimination diet can prove helpful. If an allergic reaction occurs, all food previously eaten should be avoided at first and then gradually reintroduced sequentially until the offending food is identified.

Many allergic reactions, especially asthma and urticaria, may be aggravated by fatigue and emotional stress. The nurse can initiate a stress-management program with the patient that includes relaxation techniques when the patient comes for repeated immunotherapy treatments.

Sometimes, control of allergic symptoms necessitates environmental control, including changing an occupation, moving to a different climate, or giving up a pet. In the case of airborne allergens, sleeping in an air-conditioned room, damp-dusting daily, covering mattresses and pillows with hypoallergenic covers, and wearing a mask outdoors may be helpful.

With an identified medication allergy, the patient should be instructed not only to avoid taking the medication but also to notify all health care providers of medication intolerance. The patient should wear a medical alert bracelet listing the medication allergy and have the offending medication listed on all medical and dental records.

For a patient allergic to insect stings, commercial bee-sting kits containing injectable epinephrine and a tourniquet are available. The nurse should instruct the patient and family in the technique of applying the tourniquet and self-injecting the subcutaneous epinephrine. These patients should wear a medical alert bracelet and carry a bee-sting kit whenever they go outdoors.

Medication Therapy. The major categories of medications used for symptomatic relief of chronic allergic disorders include antihistamines, sympathomimetic or decongestant medications, corticosteroids, antipruritic medications, and mast cell–stabilizing medications. Many of these medications may be obtained over the counter.

Antihistamines. Antihistamines are the treatment of choice for allergic rhinitis and urticaria; however, they are less effective for severe allergic reactions (see Chapter 29, Table 29.2). They act by competing with histamine for H_1-receptor sites and thus blocking the effect of histamine. Best results are achieved if they are taken as soon as allergy symptoms appear. Antihistamines can be used effectively to treat edema and pruritus but are relatively ineffective in preventing bronchoconstriction. With seasonal rhinitis, antihistamines should be taken during peak pollen seasons. (Antihistamines are discussed further in Chapter 29.)

Sympathomimetic or Decongestant Medications. The major sympathomimetic medication epinephrine (Adrenalin) is the first-line treatment for an anaphylactic reaction. Epinephrine is a hormone produced by the adrenal medulla that stimulates α- and β-adrenergic receptors. Stimulation of the α-adrenergic receptors causes vasoconstriction of peripheral blood vessels while stimulation of β-adrenergic receptors causes relaxation of the bronchial smooth muscles. Epinephrine also acts directly on mast cells, which stabilizes them against further degranulation. The action of epinephrine lasts only a few minutes. For the treatment of anaphylaxis, the medication must be given parenterally (subcutaneously, intramuscularly, or intravenously).

There are several specific, minor sympathomimetic medications that differ from epinephrine as they can be taken orally or nasally and last for several hours. These medications are used primarily to treat allergic rhinitis and include phenylephrine (Neo-Synephrine) and pseudoephedrine (Sudafed).

Corticosteroids. Nasal corticosteroid sprays are very effective in relieving the symptoms of allergic rhinitis (see Chapter 29, Table 29.2). Occasional patients may experience such severe manifestations of allergies that a brief course of oral corticosteroids is required.

Antipruritic Medications. Topically applied antipruritic medications protect the skin and provide relief from itching. They are most effective when the skin is not broken. Common OTC medications include calamine lotion, coal tar solutions, and camphor. Menthol and phenol may be added to lotions to produce an antipruritic effect.

Mast Cell–Stabilizing Medications. Nedocromil (Alocril) is a mast cell–stabilizing medication that inhibits the release of histamines, leukotrienes, and other agents from the mast cell after antigen–IgE interaction. It is currently available for topical ophthalmic use only.

Leukotriene Receptor Antagonists. Leukotriene receptor antagonists (LTRAs) block leukotriene, one of the major mediators of the allergic inflammatory process. They may be used in the treatment of allergic rhinitis and asthma. These medications can be taken orally. (For more information, refer to Chapters 29 and 31.)

Immunotherapy. Immunotherapy is the recommended treatment for control of allergic symptoms when the allergen cannot be avoided and medication therapy is not effective. Relatively few patients with allergies have symptoms so intolerable that they require allergy immunotherapy. Immunotherapy is indicated only in individuals with anaphylactic reactions to insect venom. It involves administration of small titres of an allergen extract in increasing strengths until hyposensitivity to the specific allergen is achieved. For best results, the patient should continue to avoid the offending allergen whenever possible because complete desensitization is impossible. Unfortunately, not all allergy-related conditions respond to immunotherapy. Food allergies cannot be safely treated with this therapy, and eczema may worsen with immunotherapy.

Mechanism of Action. The IgE level is elevated in atopic individuals. When IgE combines with an allergen in a hypersensitive person, a reaction occurs, releasing histamine in various body tissues. Allergens more readily combine with IgG than with other immunoglobulins. Therefore, immunotherapy involves injecting allergen extracts that will stimulate increases in IgG levels. The goal of long-term immunotherapy is to maintain high levels of "blocking" IgG. By increasing IgG levels, IgE is blocked from binding to the allergen. This prevents mast cell degranulation. In addition, allergen-specific T suppressor cells develop in individuals receiving immunotherapy.

Method of Administration. Allergens included in immunotherapy are chosen on the basis of results of skin testing with a panel of allergens.

Subcutaneous Immunotherapy. Subcutaneous immunotherapy (SCIT) involves the subcutaneous injection of titrated amounts of allergen extracts biweekly or weekly. The initial dose is small and then increased slowly until a maintenance dosage is reached. In general, it takes 1 to 2 years of immunotherapy to reach the maximal therapeutic effect. Therapy may continue for about 5 years; subsequently, discontinuing therapy is considered. In many patients, a sustained decrease in symptoms is seen after the treatment is discontinued. Those with severe allergies or sensitivity to insect stings may continue maintenance therapy indefinitely. Best results are achieved when immunotherapy is administered throughout the year.

Sublingual Immunotherapy. Sublingual immunotherapy (SLIT) involves allergen extracts taken under the tongue. SLIT has been used in Europe for decades and has recently become available in Canada. Products include a five-grass pollen tablet (Oralair), a single-grass pollen tablet (Grastek), and a ragweed pollen tablet (Ragwitek) (Quirt et al., 2018).

SLIT is self-administered (usually daily) by patients at home, although the initial dose is usually given under medical supervision. Some patients experience local application-site reactions (e.g., oral pruritus, throat irritation, tongue swelling), but systemic allergic reactions are markedly fewer than with SCIT. Local reactions subside in many patients within a few days to a week.

SLIT has the advantage of being a convenient, self-administered oral therapy. The main disadvantage of SLIT is that the patient must consistently adhere to the therapy (Quirt et al., 2018).

NURSING MANAGEMENT
IMMUNOTHERAPY

Often the nurse is responsible for administering SCIT. Immunotherapy always carries the risk for a severe anaphylactic reaction; therefore, when injections are given, a health care provider, emergency equipment, and essential medications should be immediately accessible for administration. Adverse reactions should always be anticipated, especially when a new dose strength is applied, after a previous reaction occurred, or after a dose is missed. Early signs and symptoms indicative of a systemic reaction include pruritus, urticaria, sneezing, laryngeal edema, and hypotension. A local reaction should be described according to the degree of redness and swelling at the injection site. If the area is greater than the size of a quarter in an adult, the reaction should be reported to a health care provider so that the allergen dosage may be decreased.

Accurate record keeping is invaluable as it can prevent an adverse reaction to the allergen extract. Before giving the injection, the nurse should check the patient's name against the name on the vial, check the vial strength, the amount of the previous dose, the date of the previous dose, and any reaction information previously identified.

The nurse should always administer the allergen extract in an extremity away from a joint so that a tourniquet can be applied in the event of a severe reaction. The site should be rotated for each injection. Before giving an injection, the nurse must aspirate for blood to ensure the allergen extract is not injected directly into a blood vessel as this can potentiate an anaphylactic reaction. After the injection is given, the patient should be carefully monitored for 20 minutes as systemic reactions typically occur immediately. However, the patient should be warned that a delayed reaction can occur up to 24 hours later.

Latex Allergies

Allergies to latex products have become an increasing problem, affecting both patients and health care providers. The increase in allergic reactions has coincided with the sharp increase in glove use. The more frequent and prolonged the latex exposure, the greater the likelihood is of developing a latex allergy.

In addition to gloves, many other latex-containing products are used in health care, such as blood pressure cuffs, stethoscopes, tourniquets, intravenous (IV) tubing, syringes, electrode pads, oxygen masks, tracheal tubes, colostomy and ileostomy pouches, urinary catheters, anaesthetic masks, and adhesive tape. Latex proteins can become aerosolized through powder on gloves and can result in serious reactions when inhaled by sensitized individuals. It is recommended that all health care facilities use powder-free gloves to avoid respiratory exposure to latex proteins (Canadian Centre for Occupational Health and Safety [CCOHS], 2016).

Types of Latex Allergies. Two types of latex allergies can occur: type IV allergic contact dermatitis and type I allergic reactions. Type IV contact dermatitis is caused by the chemicals used in the manufacturing process of latex gloves. Typically, a person initially develops dryness, pruritus, fissuring, and cracking of the skin, followed by redness, swelling, and crusting at 24 to 48 hours. A delayed reaction can occur within 6 to 48 hours. The dermatitis may extend beyond the area of physical contact with the allergen. Chronic exposure can lead to lichenification, scaling, and hyperpigmentation.

A type I allergic reaction is a response to the natural rubber latex proteins and occurs within minutes of contact with the proteins. These types of allergic reactions can manifest in a variety of ways, from skin redness, urticaria, rhinitis, conjunctivitis, or asthma to complete anaphylactic shock. Systemic reactions to latex may result from exposure to latex protein via various routes, including the skin, mucous membranes, lungs, or blood.

Latex-Food Syndrome. Some proteins in rubber are similar to food proteins; therefore, some foods may cause an allergic reaction in people who are allergic to latex. This is called *latex-food syndrome*. The most common of these foods are banana, avocado, chestnut, kiwi, tomato, water chestnut, guava, hazelnut, potato, peach, grape, and apricot. Most people with a latex allergy have a positive allergy test to at least one related food.

NURSING AND INTERPROFESSIONAL MANAGEMENT: LATEX ALLERGIES

The identification of patients and health care providers who are sensitive to latex is crucial in preventing adverse reactions. A thorough health history including a history of any allergies should be documented, especially for patients with any reports of latex contact symptoms. Risk factors include long-term multiple exposures to latex products (e.g., among health care providers, individuals who have undergone multiple surgical procedures, or rubber-industry workers). Additional risk factors include a patient history of allergic rhinitis, asthma, and allergies to certain foods (listed earlier in the chapter). Despite careful history taking, not all latex-sensitive individuals can be identified. The Canadian Centre for Occupational Health and Safety (CCOHS) has published recommendations for preventing allergic reactions to latex in the workplace (CCOHS, 2016) (Table 16.12).

Latex precaution policies should be used for patients identified as having either a positive reaction to a latex allergy test or a history of signs and symptoms related to latex exposure. Many health care facilities have created latex-free product carts that can be used for patients with latex allergies.

Multiple Chemical Sensitivities

Multiple chemical sensitivities (MCS) comprise a subjective illness marked by recurrent, nonspecific symptoms attributed to low levels of chemical, biological, or physical agents. Common causative substances include smoke, pesticides, plastics, synthetic fabrics, scented products, petroleum products, and paint fumes. Women between the ages of 30 and 50 typically report more symptoms. MCS is a controversial diagnosis and is not formally recognized as an illness by the Canadian Medical Association or other authorities (Rossi & Pitidis, 2018).

The symptoms reported are wide-ranging and nonspecific. They may include headache, fatigue, dizziness, nausea, congestion, itching, sneezing, sore throat, chest pain, breathing problems, muscle pain or stiffness, skin rash, diarrhea, bloating, gas, confusion, difficulty concentrating, memory problems, and mood changes. To date, these subjective symptoms have no evidence of a pathological process or physiological dysfunction. Hence, the diagnosis is solely based on the patient's health history.

Treatment includes minimizing or avoiding the chemicals that may trigger the symptoms and creating a chemical-free and odour-free home and workplace. Psychotherapy is recommended as a primary treatment option. However, if the patient refuses this but is willing to accept medications, antidepressants (such as selective serotonin reuptake inhibitors [SSRIs], e.g., citalopram [Celexa]), anxiolytics, and medications for sleep can been used.

AUTOIMMUNITY

Autoimmunity is an immune reaction to self-proteins: the immune system no longer differentiates self from nonself. For

TABLE 16.12	RECOMMENDATIONS FOR PREVENTING ALLERGIC REACTIONS TO LATEX IN THE WORKPLACE

1. Use alternative nonlatex products.
2. Ensure that workers use good work and housekeeping practices to remove latex-containing dust from the workplace, including avoiding contact with eyes and face, hand hygiene after glove removal, and using HEPA vacuums to clean up dust.
3. Provide workers with education programs about latex allergy.
4. Persons allergic to latex rubber products should consult an allergist to find out if they are allergic to latex (natural) rubber or to chemicals that are in synthetic rubbers. They should also advise their health care providers and dentists so that alternate products can be used.

Sources: Adapted from Canadian Centre for Occupational Health and Safety. (2016). *Latex allergy.* https://www.ccohs.ca/oshanswers/diseases/latex.html; and National Institute for Occupational Safety Health. (n.d.) *NIOSH alert: Preventing allergic reactions to natural rubber latex in the workplace.* http://www.cdc.gov/niosh/docs/97-135/pdfs/97-135.pdf

unknown reasons, immune cells that are normally unresponsive (tolerant of self-antigens) are activated. In autoimmunity, autoantibodies and autosensitized T cells cause pathophysiological tissue damage (Rich & Chaplin, 2019).

The cause of autoimmune diseases remains unknown. Age is thought to play a role since the number of circulating autoantibodies increases in people over age 50 years. However, the principal factors in the development of autoimmunity are (a) the inheritance of susceptibility genes, which may contribute to the failure of self-tolerance, and (b) initiation of autoreactivity by triggers, such as infections, that may activate self-reactive lymphocytes.

Autoimmune diseases tend to occur in clusters, so an individual may have more than one autoimmune disease (e.g., rheumatoid arthritis and Addison's disease), or the same or related autoimmune diseases may be found in other members of the same family. This observation has led to the concept of genetic predisposition to autoimmune disease.

Most of the genetic research in this area correlates certain human leukocyte antigen (HLA) types with an autoimmune condition. (HLAs and disease association are discussed later in this chapter.) Even in a genetically predisposed person, some triggering event is necessary for the initiation of autoreactivity. This event may include infection with an agent such as a virus (Rich & Chaplin, 2019). Viral infections can alter cells or tissues that make them antigenic. Some evidence suggests that viruses may be involved in the development of diseases such as type 1 diabetes mellitus and psychiatric disorders such as obsessive-compulsive disorders (Marazziti et al., 2018). Rheumatic fever and rheumatic heart disease are autoimmune responses triggered by streptococcal infection and mediated by antibodies against group A β-hemolytic streptococci that cross-react with heart muscles, heart valves, and synovial membranes.

Medications can also be precipitating factors in autoimmune diseases. For example, hemolytic anemia can result from methyldopa (Novo-Medopa) administration, and procainamide (Apo-Procainamide) can induce the formation of antinuclear antibodies and cause a lupus-like syndrome.

Gender and hormones also have a role in autoimmune diseases, with more women than men affected. During pregnancy, symptoms of many autoimmune diseases improve; however, after giving birth the disease frequently worsens.

Autoimmune Diseases

In general, autoimmune diseases are grouped according to organ-specific and systemic diseases. (Table 16.13 lists examples of autoimmune diseases.) SLE is a classic example of a systemic autoimmune disease characterized by damage to multiple organs. It occurs most frequently in women, with onset at 20 to 40 years of age. The cause is unknown, but there appears to be a loss of self-tolerance for the body's own deoxyribonucleic acid (DNA) antigens.

In SLE, tissue injury appears to be the result of the formation of antinuclear antibodies. For an unknown reason (possibly a viral infection), the cell membrane is damaged, and DNA is released into the systemic circulation where it is viewed as nonself material. This DNA is normally sequestered inside the nucleus of cells. On release into circulation, the DNA antigen reacts with an antibody. Some antibodies are involved in immune-complex formation, and others may cause damage directly. Once the complexes are deposited, the complement system is activated and further damages the tissue, especially the renal glomerulus. (SLE is discussed further in Chapter 67.)

Apheresis

Apheresis has been effectively used to treat various diseases, including autoimmune diseases. Apheresis is a procedure in which components of the blood are separated and then one or more of those components is removed. Compound words are often used to describe an apheresis procedure, depending on the blood components being collected. For example, *plateletpheresis* is the removal of platelets, usually for collection from healthy individuals to infuse into patients with low platelet counts (e.g., patients taking chemotherapy who develop thrombocytopenia). *Leukocytapheresis* is a term indicating the removal of WBCs, a technique used in chronic myelogenous leukemia to remove high numbers of leukemic cells.

Apheresis is also used in hematopoietic stem cell transplantation to collect stem cells from peripheral blood. These stem cells can then be used to repopulate a person's bone marrow after high-dose chemotherapy (see the section Peripheral Stem Cell Transplantation in Chapter 18).

Plasmapheresis. *Plasmapheresis* is the removal of plasma-containing components that cause or are thought to cause disease. It can also be used to obtain plasma from healthy donors to administer to patients as replacement therapy. When plasma is removed, it is replaced by substitution fluids such as saline, fresh-frozen plasma, or albumin. Therefore, the term *plasma exchange* more accurately describes this procedure.

Plasmapheresis has been used to treat autoimmune diseases such as SLE, glomerulonephritis, Goodpasture's syndrome, myasthenia gravis, thrombocytopenic purpura, rheumatoid arthritis, and Guillain-Barré syndrome. Many disorders for which plasmapheresis is being used are characterized by circulating autoantibodies (usually of the IgG class) and antigen–antibody complexes. The rationale for performing therapeutic plasmapheresis in autoimmune disorders is to remove pathological substances present in plasma. Immunosuppressive therapy has been used to prevent recovery of IgG production, and plasmapheresis has been used to prevent antibody rebound.

In addition to removing antibodies and antigen–antibody complexes, plasmapheresis may remove inflammatory mediators (e.g., complement) that are responsible for tissue damage. In the treatment of SLE, plasmapheresis is usually reserved for patients in an acute attack who are unresponsive to conventional therapy.

TABLE 16.13   EXAMPLES OF AUTOIMMUNE DISEASES*

Systemic Diseases
- Systemic lupus erythematosus (SLE)
- Rheumatoid arthritis
- Progressive systemic sclerosis (scleroderma)
- Mixed connective tissue disease

Organ-Specific Diseases

Blood
- Autoimmune hemolytic anemia
- Immune thrombocytopenic purpura

Central Nervous System
- Multiple sclerosis
- Guillain-Barré syndrome

Muscle
- Myasthenia gravis

Heart
- Rheumatic fever

Endocrine System
- Addison's disease
- Thyroiditis
- Hypothyroidism
- Type 1 diabetes mellitus

Gastrointestinal System
- Pernicious anemia
- Ulcerative colitis

Kidney
- Goodpasture's syndrome
- Glomerulonephritis

Liver
- Primary biliary cirrhosis
- Autoimmune hepatitis

Eye
- Uveitis

*These diseases are discussed in various chapters throughout the book.

Plasmapheresis involves the removal of whole blood through an IV and then the blood circulates through a cell separator. Within the separator, the blood is divided into plasma and its cellular components by centrifugation or membrane filtration. Plasma, platelets, WBCs, or erythrocytes can be separated selectively. The undesirable component is removed and the remainder is returned to the patient. The plasma is generally replaced with normal saline, lactated Ringer's solution, fresh-frozen plasma, plasma protein fractions, or albumin. When blood is manually removed, only 500 mL may be taken at one time. However, with the use of apheresis, more than 4 L of plasma can be removed in 2 to 3 hours.

As with administration of other blood products, nurses must be aware of adverse effects associated with plasmapheresis. The most common complications are hypotension and citrate toxicity. Hypotension is usually the result of a vasovagal reaction or transient volume changes. Citrate is used as an anticoagulant and may cause hypocalcemia, which may manifest as headache, paresthesias, and dizziness.

IMMUNODEFICIENCY DISORDERS

The condition in which the immune system does not adequately protect the body is immunodeficiency. Immunodeficiency disorders involve an impairment of one or more immune mechanisms, which include (a) phagocytosis, (b) humoral response, (c) cell-mediated immune response, (d) complement, and (e) a combined humoral and cell-mediated deficiency. Immunodeficiency disorders are *primary* if the immune cells are improperly developed or absent and *secondary* if the deficiency is caused by illnesses or treatment. Primary immunodeficiency disorders are rare and often serious, whereas secondary disorders are more common and less severe.

Primary Immunodeficiency Disorders

The basic categories of primary immunodeficiency disorders are (a) phagocytic defects, (b) B-cell deficiency, (c) T-cell deficiency, and (d) a combined B-cell and T-cell deficiency (Banasik, 2018) (Table 16.14).

Secondary Immunodeficiency Disorders

Some important factors that may cause secondary immunodeficiency disorders are listed in Table 16.15. Medication-induced immunosuppression is the most common. Immunosuppressive therapy is prescribed for patients to treat autoimmune disorders and to prevent transplant rejection. In addition, immunosuppression is a serious adverse effect of drugs used in cancer chemotherapy. Generalized leukopenia often results from chemotherapeutic drugs, leading to a decreased humoral and cell-mediated immune response. Therefore, secondary infections are common in immunosuppressed patients.

Malnutrition alters cell-mediated immune responses. When protein is deficient over a prolonged period, the thymus gland atrophies, and lymphoid tissue decreases. In addition, an increased susceptibility to infections always exists with malnourishment.

Hodgkin's lymphoma greatly impairs the cell-mediated immune response, and patients may die from severe viral or fungal infections. (Hodgkin's lymphoma is discussed in Chapter 18.) Viruses, especially rubella, may cause immunodeficiency by direct cytotoxic damage to lymphoid cells. Systemic infections can place such a demand on the immune system that resistance to a secondary or subsequent infection becomes impaired.

Radiation can destroy lymphocytes either directly or through depletion of stem cells. As the radiation dose is increased, more bone marrow atrophies, leading to severe pancytopenia and suppression of immune function. Splenectomy in children remains especially dangerous as it may lead to septicemia from a simple respiratory tract infection.

The immune response involves interrelationships among the nervous, endocrine, and immune systems and can be altered by stress (see Chapter 8).

Human Leukocyte Antigen System

The antigens responsible for rejection of genetically dissimilar tissues are called the *major histocompatibility antigens*. These antigens are products of histocompatibility genes. In humans, they are called the human leukocyte antigen (HLA) system. The genes for the HLA antigens are linked and occur together on the sixth chromosome. HLAs are present on all nucleated cells and platelets. The HLA system plays an important part in the body's immune response to foreign substances and, therefore, is used in matching organs and tissues for transplantation.

An important characteristic of HLA genes is that they are highly polymorphic (variable). Each HLA locus can have many different possible alleles and thus many combinations exist. Each person has two alleles for each locus, one inherited from

TABLE 16.14 PRIMARY IMMUNODEFICIENCY DISORDERS

Disorder	Affected Cells	Genetic Basis
Chronic granulomatous disease	PMNs, monocytes	Sex-linked
Job syndrome	PMNs, monocytes	—
Bruton (X-linked) agammaglobulinemia	B	Sex-linked
Common variable hypogammaglobulinemia	B	—
Selective IgA, IgM, or IgG deficiency	B	Some sex-linked
DiGeorge syndrome (thymic hypoplasia)	T	—
Severe combined immunodeficiency disease	Stem, B, T	Sex-linked or autosomal recessive
Ataxia-telangiectasia	B, T	Autosomal recessive
Wiskott–Aldrich syndrome	B, T	Sex-linked
Graft-versus-host disease	B, T	—

IgA, immunoglobulin A; *IgG*, immunoglobulin G; *IgM*, immunoglobulin M; *PMN*, polymorphonuclear neutrophil.

TABLE 16.15 CAUSES OF SECONDARY IMMUNODEFICIENCY

Age
- Infants
- Older persons

Diseases or Disorders
- Acquired immune deficiency syndrome (AIDS)
- Burns
- Malignancies
- Chronic renal disease
- Alcohol-induced cirrhosis
- Diabetes mellitus
- Severe infection
- Systemic lupus erythematosus
- Trauma

Medication-Induced Immunodeficiency
- Chemotherapeutic medications
- Corticosteroids

Malnutrition
- Cachexia
- Dietary deficiency

Stress
- Chronic stress
- Trauma (physical or emotional)

Therapies
- Anaesthesia
- Radiation
- Surgery

each parent. Both alleles of a locus are expressed independently (i.e., they are codominant). The proteins encoded by certain genes are known as *antigens*.

The entire set of A, B, C, and D/DR genes (the HLA genes) is located on one chromosome and is termed a *haplotype*. The complete set is inherited as a unit (haplotype), with one haplotype inherited from each parent (Figure 16.10). This means that a person has HLA genes that are one-half identical from each parent. The HLA genes of one person have a 25% chance of being identical to the HLA genes of a sibling.

In organ transplantation, A, B, and DR are primarily used for compatibility matching. The specific allele at each locus is

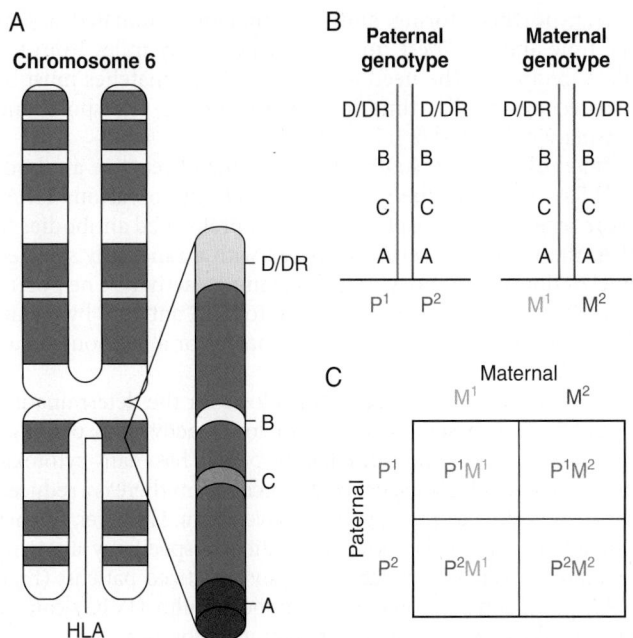

FIG. 16.10 Patterns of human leukocyte antigen (HLA) inheritance. **A,** HLA genes are located on chromosome 6. **B,** The two haplotypes of the father are labelled P¹ and P², and the haplotypes of the mother are labelled M¹ and M². Each child inherits two haplotypes, one from each parent. **C,** Therefore, only four combinations—P¹M¹, P¹M², P²M¹, P²M²—are possible, and the offspring have a 25% chance of having identical HLA haplotypes.

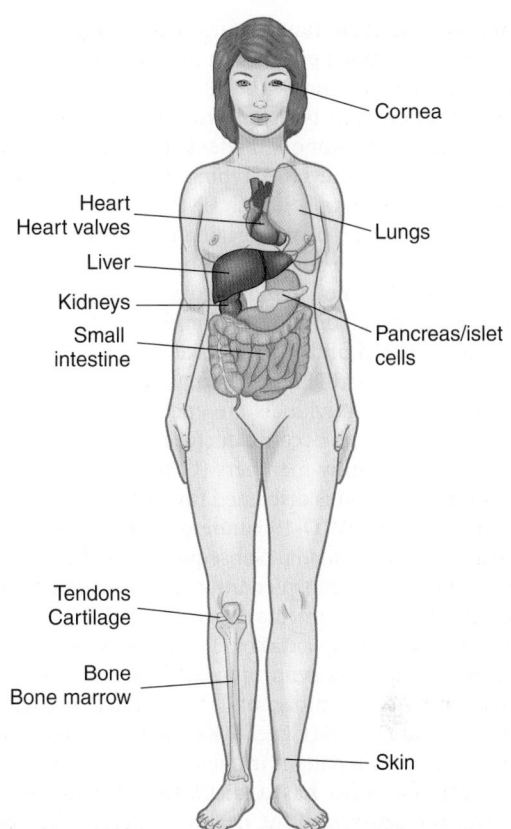

FIG. 16.11 Tissues and organs that can be transplanted.

identified by a number. For example, a person could have an HLA of A2, A6, B7, B27, DR4, and DR7. Currently more than 8 000 HLA alleles have been identified for the various HLA genes.

Human Leukocyte Antigen and Disease Associations. Early interest in HLA occurred because of its potential role in matching donors with organ transplant recipients.

Several diseases show significant associations with specific HLA alleles. People with specific alleles are much more likely to develop the associated disease than those who do not have the allele. However, the possession of a particular HLA allele does not mean that the person will necessarily develop the associated disease—only that the relative risk is greater than in the general population.

Most of the HLA-associated diseases are classified as autoimmune disorders. Examples of associations between HLA types and diseases include (a) the presence of HLA-B27 with ankylosing spondylitis, (b) the presence of HLA-DR2 and HLA-DR3 with SLE, (c) the presence of HLA-DR3 and HLA-DR4 with diabetes mellitus, and (d) the presence of HLA-DR2 with narcolepsy.

The discovery of HLA associations with certain diseases was a breakthrough in understanding the genetic basis of these diseases. It is now known that at least part of the genetic basis of HLA-associated diseases lies in the HLA region, but the actual mechanisms involved in these associations are still unknown. However, most individuals who inherit a specific HLA type associated with a disease never actually develop the disease.

Currently, HLA association with certain diseases is of little practical clinical importance; however, there is promise for the development of clinical applications in the future. For example, in families with certain autoimmune diseases, it may be possible to identify members who are at greater risk for developing the same or a related autoimmune disease. These people would

need close medical supervision, implementation of preventive measures (if possible), and early diagnosis and treatment to prevent chronic complications.

ORGAN TRANSPLANTATION

During the 1960s, organ and tissue transplantation was considered an experimental procedure reserved for patients with critical end-stage medical disease. However, advances in medical technology, including histocompatibility testing, surgical procedures, improved immunosuppressive regimens, and organ transplantation, has resulted in improved survival rates and quality of life. Organ transplantation is the transfer of a whole or partial organ from one individual to another for the purpose of replacing the recipient's damaged or failing organ with a functioning one. Commonly transplanted organs and tissues include the heart, lungs, liver, kidneys, pancreas, corneas, skin, bone marrow, heart valves, bone, and connective tissues (Figure 16.11). Corneas are transplanted to prevent or correct blindness, and skin grafts are used to assist in managing burns. Bone marrow or stem cells are transplanted to help patients with leukemias and other hematological malignancies.

Organs can be successfully transplanted together; for example, a patient with diabetes may receive a pancreas and a kidney transplant due to the diabetes causing pancreatic insufficiency as well as end-stage kidney disease.

Some organs may be transplanted in segments rather than in their entirety. Liver and lung lobes may be transplanted, or an intestine may be used in segments, thus allowing one person's organ donation to benefit multiple recipients. This technique not only enables living donors to donate part of an organ while maintaining their functioning organ but also addresses the mortality rate among patients on the waiting list due to suboptimal organ donation rates.

Organ donations can be taken from two sources: deceased (cadaveric) and living donors. Patients are matched to donors through ABO blood and HLA typing, medical urgency, body size, and, for some organs, length of time on the waiting list. Currently, most donated organs originate from deceased donors. Most living donors are relatives of the recipient, although a number are also unrelated living donors.

To become an organ or tissue donor in Canada, an individual either signs an organ and tissue donor card or registers their consent through the provincial registry. However, despite registering as a donor, individuals are encouraged to discuss the decision with loved ones because doctors will not proceed without the consent of family members (Canadian Blood Services, 2020). (Organ donation is discussed further in Chapter 71.)

With the recent COVID-19 pandemic, organ donation came to a virtual stop in Canada. Subsequent reopening of organ donation centres and transplantation procedures occurred in a graduated approach with mandatory COVID-19 testing for each donor. Lung transplantation for patients with end-stage adult respiratory distress syndrome (ARDS) due to COVID-19 are few in numbers. The impact of COVID-19 currently remains incompletely understood (Cypel & Keshavjee, 2020).

Nurses caring for a patient in the critical care unit or emergency department who has a diagnosis of brain death are encouraged to discuss with the health care team the option of organ donation for the patient's family. The local organ procurement organization should then be contacted to speak with the family.

Tissue Typing

The recipient usually receives a transplant from an ABO blood group–compatible donor (see Chapter 32, Table 32.9). The donor and recipient do not need to share the same Rh factor.

HLA Typing. HLA typing is done on potential donors and recipients. Currently only the A, B, and DR antigens are thought to be clinically significant for transplantation. Because each locus has two alleles that encode for antigens, a total of six antigens are identified. In transplantation, an attempt is made to match as many antigens as possible between the HLA-A, HLA-B, and HLA-DR loci. Antigen matches of five and six antigens and certain four-antigen matches have been found to have better clinical outcomes (i.e., the patient is less likely to reject the transplanted organ), especially in kidney and bone marrow transplants.

The degree of HLA matching deemed suitable for successful solid organ transplantation depends on the type of organ being transplanted. Certain organ and tissue transplants require a closer histocompatibility match than other organs. For example, a cornea transplant can be accepted by nearly any individual because corneas are avascular, therefore no antibodies reach the cornea to cause rejection. In kidney and bone marrow transplantation, HLA matching is very important, since these transplants are at high risk for rejection. On the other hand, for liver transplants, HLA mismatches have little impact on graft survival. Heart and lung transplants fall somewhere in between, although minimizing HLA mismatches significantly improves survival. In addition, for liver, lung, and heart transplants, fewer donors are available; therefore, it can be more difficult to obtain good HLA matches.

Transporting, storing, and then implanting donated organs take time and the "best" match may live many miles from the "ideal" recipient. The need to have the "best" matches must be balanced against the time it takes to retrieve, transport, and transplant a donated organ.

Panel of Reactive Antibodies. A panel of reactive antibodies (PRA) indicates the recipient's sensitivity to various HLAs before receiving a transplant. To detect preformed antibodies to HLA, the recipient's serum is mixed with a randomly selected panel of donor lymphocytes to determine reactivity. The potential recipient may have been exposed to HLA antigens by means of previous blood transfusions, pregnancy, or a previous organ transplant.

PRA, calculated in percentages, allows for the determination of whether a recipient is of high or low reactivity to potential donors. A high PRA indicates that the person has many cytotoxic antibodies and is highly sensitized, which means there is a reduced chance of finding a crossmatch-negative donor. However, further refinement in analysis allows for antibody specificity allowing for a more acceptable match. In highly sensitized patients (high PRA), plasmapheresis and IV immunoglobulin (IVIG) can be used to reduce the number of circulating antibodies.

Crossmatch. A crossmatch is done to determine the existence of antibodies against the potential donor. In a crossmatch, serum from the recipient is mixed with donor lymphocytes to test for any preformed anti-HLA antibodies to the potential donor organ. The crossmatch can be used as a screening test when possible living donors are being considered or once a cadaver donor is selected.

A negative crossmatch indicates absent preformed antibodies and it is safe to proceed with transplantation. A positive crossmatch indicates that the recipient has cytotoxic antibodies to the donor and is an absolute contraindication in living kidney donor transplantation. Live donor transplants may be carried out in patients with a positive crossmatch if no other live donors (with a negative crossmatch) exist. In this situation, plasmapheresis or IVIG can be performed to remove antibodies.

It is not always possible to complete a crossmatch prior to transplantation. If a retrospective crossmatch must be done, the results will have implications for immunosuppression policies after the transplant. A positive crossmatch is particularly important for kidney, heart, and lung transplants but less so for liver transplants.

Transplant Rejection

Rejection is one of the major contributing factors to organ loss after solid organ transplantation. Organ rejection can occur if the HLA profile of the donor organ does not identically match that of the recipient. Rejection can be prevented through close matching of ABO and HLA profiles of the donor and recipient. Unfortunately, because many differing HLA profiles have been found in humans, a perfect match is impossible, except for tissue matching of identical twins. Three forms of rejection can develop: hyperacute, acute, or chronic. Prevention, early diagnosis, and treatment of rejection are essential for long-term graft function.

Hyperacute Rejection. Hyperacute rejection (also called *antibody-mediated* or *humoral rejection*) occurs minutes to hours after transplantation. Hyperacute rejection may result from antibody development through several mechanisms, some of which are not clearly understood. Recipients who have received prior blood transfusions may have antibodies to major histocompatibility complex antigens from the transfused blood

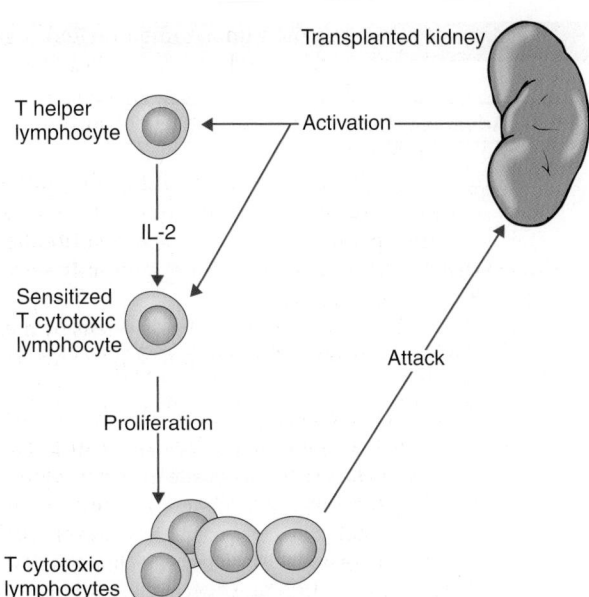

FIG. 16.12 Mechanism of action of T cytotoxic lymphocyte activation and attack of transplanted tissue. The transplanted organ (e.g., kidney) is recognized as foreign, and the immune system is activated. T helper cells are activated to produce interleukin-2 (IL-2), and T cytotoxic lymphocytes are sensitized. After the T cytotoxic cells proliferate, they attack the transplanted organ.

that may match those in the graft (donated organ), which results in hyperacute rejection. Furthermore, multiple prior pregnancies may have exposed a woman to paternal antigens of the fetus, resulting in the development of antibodies. In the absence of these factors, antibody-mediated rejection may occur nonetheless, and the cause often remains unknown.

Acute Rejection. Acute rejection most commonly occurs days to months after transplantation. This type of rejection is mediated by the recipient's T cytotoxic lymphocytes, which attack the foreign organ (Figure 16.12). In addition to cell-mediated rejection, another type of acute rejection occurs when the recipient develops antibodies to the transplanted organ (humoral rejection). Many transplant recipients experience at least one rejection episode after transplantation. These episodes are usually reversible with alteration in or additional immunosuppressive therapy that may include increased corticosteroid doses or polyclonal or monoclonal antibody treatment. Unfortunately, increased doses of immunosuppressants increase the risk for infection. To combat acute rejection, all patients with transplants require lifelong use of immunosuppressants, putting them at a high risk for infection, especially in the first few months after transplantation, when the immunosuppressant doses are highest.

Chronic Rejection. Chronic rejection is a process that occurs over months to years and is considered irreversible. The transplanted organ is infiltrated with large numbers of T and B cells, which is characteristic of an ongoing, low-grade, immune-mediated injury. Chronic rejection results in fibrosis and scarring. In heart transplants, it manifests as accelerated coronary artery disease. In lung transplants, it manifests as bronchiolitis obliterans, which is inflammation and fibrosis of the small airways. In liver transplants, it is characterized by loss of bile ducts. In kidney transplants, it manifests as fibrosis and glomerulopathy.

No definitive therapy is yet available for chronic rejection. Switching immunosuppressive therapy has yielded some improvement for patients; however, treatment has largely been supportive. Ultimately, the prognosis for patients with chronic rejection remains poor, and if possible, such patients should be offered the option of retransplantation.

IMMUNOSUPPRESSIVE THERAPY

The goal of immunosuppressive therapy is to adequately suppress the immune response to prevent rejection of the transplanted organ and yet maintain sufficient immunity to prevent overwhelming infection.

Many of the medications used to achieve immunosuppression have adverse effects. The most common medications, routes of administration, mechanisms of action, and adverse effects are listed in Table 16.16. In a combination of medications that work in different phases of the immune response, lower doses of each medication produce effective immunosuppression and minimize adverse effects. The major immunosuppressive agents are (a) calcineurin inhibitors, which include cyclosporin (Sandimmune, Neoral) and tacrolimus (Prograf); (b) corticosteroids (prednisone, methylprednisolone [Solu-Medrol] by IV route); (c) mycophenolate mofetil (CellCept); and (d) sirolimus (Rapamune). Azathioprine (Imuran) and cyclophosphamide (Procytox) are also used but less frequently, because of the effectiveness of the newer generation of immunosuppressants. Antithymocyte globulin, antilymphocyte globulin, and muromonab-CD3 (OKT3) are medications administered intravenously for short periods to prevent early rejection (induction therapy) or to reverse acute rejection.

Immunosuppressive policies are highly variable among transplant centres, with different combinations of medications being used. Most patients are initially on triple therapy, which includes a calcineurin inhibitor, a corticosteroid, and either mycophenolate mofetil (CellCept) or azathioprine (Imuran). The doses of immunosuppressant medications are reduced over time after the transplant, with some organ groups able to wean off corticosteroids entirely.

Calcineurin Inhibitors

This group of medications, including tacrolimus (Prograf) and cyclosporin (Sandimmune, Neoral), is the foundation of most immunosuppression regimens. These medications prevent a cell-mediated attack against the transplanted organ (Figure 16.13). They are generally used in some combination with corticosteroids, mycophenolate mofetil (CellCept), and sirolimus (Rapamune). Tacrolimus (Prograf) is the most widely used calcineurin inhibitor, with cyclosporin used less frequently. They do not cause bone marrow suppression or alterations of the normal inflammatory response.

Adverse effects of calcineurin inhibitors are dose-related and include nephrotoxicity; therefore, drug levels are closely monitored.

> **MEDICATION ALERT—Tacrolimus (Prograf) and Cyclosporin (Sandimmune, Neoral)**
> • A substance in grapefruit and grapefruit juice prevents metabolism of these medications. Consuming grapefruit or grapefruit juice while using these medications could increase their toxicity.

Mycophenolate Mofetil (CellCept)

Mycophenolate mofetil (CellCept) inhibits purine synthesis with suppressive effects on both T and B lymphocytes. The major limitation of this medication is its gastrointestinal toxicities, including nausea, vomiting, and diarrhea. In many cases,

TABLE 16.16 MEDICATION THERAPY

Immunosuppressive Therapy

Agent	Route	Mechanism of Action	Adverse Effects
Corticosteroids			
Prednisone, methyl-prednisolone (Solu-Medrol)	PO, IV	Suppress inflammatory response; inhibit cytokine production and T-cell activation	Peptic ulcers, hypertension, GI bleeding, osteoporosis, aseptic necrosis, Na+ and H₂O retention, acne, muscle weakness, easy bruising, delayed healing, hyperglycemia, ↑ appetite, mood alterations, leukopenia, cataracts, dyslipidemia, ↓ resistance to infection
Calcineurin Inhibitors			
Cyclosporine (Sandimmune, Neoral*)	PO, IV	Inhibits calcineurin; prevents production and release of IL-2, IL-4, and α-interferon; inhibits production of T cytotoxic lymphocytes	Nephrotoxicity, neurotoxicity, headaches, seizures, tremors, hyperglycemia, hypertension, nausea and vomiting, dyslipidemia, gingival hyperplasia, hirsutism, hepatotoxicity, lymphoma, ↓ resistance to infection
Tacrolimus (Prograf)	PO, IV	Inhibits calcineurin; prevents production and release of IL-2, IL-4, and α-interferon; inhibits production of T cytotoxic lymphocytes	Nephrotoxicity, neurotoxicity, seizures, tremors, nausea and vomiting, hyperglycemia, hypertension, alopecia, lymphoma, ↓ resistance to infection
Cytotoxic (Antiproliferative) Medications			
Azathioprine (Imuran)	PO, IV	Inhibits purine synthesis; suppresses proliferation of T and B cells	Bone marrow suppression (neutropenia, anemia, thrombocytopenia)
Mycophenolate mofetil (CellCept)	PO, IV	Antimetabolite that inhibits purine synthesis; suppresses proliferation of T and B cells	Diarrhea, nausea and vomiting, leukopenia, thrombocytopenia, ↓ resistance to infection, ↑ incidence of malignancies
Sirolimus (Rapamune)	PO	Suppresses lymphocyte proliferation; inhibits B cells from synthesizing antibodies	Diarrhea, dyslipidemia, hypercholesterolemia, arthralgias, delayed wound healing, thrombocytopenia, ↓ resistance to infection, ↑ incidence of malignancies
Monoclonal Antibodies			
Alemtuzumab (Campath)	IV	Monoclonal antibody that targets the CD52 antigen on T and B cells, monocytes, and macrophages; causes prolonged T-cell depletion	Fever, chills, dyspnea, chest pain, nausea, vomiting Neutropenia, anemia, thrombocytopenia Increased risk for opportunistic infections
Basiliximab (Simulect)	IV	Monoclonal antibody that acts as IL-2 receptor antagonist by inhibiting the binding of IL-2; inhibits T-cell activation and proliferation	Generally no adverse effects
Daclizumab (Zenapax)	IV	Same as Basiliximab	Same as Basiliximab
Muromonab-CD3 (OKT3)	IV push	Monoclonal antibody that binds to CD3 receptors on lymphocytes, causing cell lysis; inhibits function of cytotoxic T cells	Fever, chills, tachycardia, pulmonary edema, muscle and joint pain, diarrhea, hypertension or hypotension, aseptic meningitis, ↓ resistance to infection, ↑ incidence of malignancies
Polyclonal Antibodies			
Polyclonal antibody serums: ATG, ALG (Thymoglobulin, ATGAM)	IV	Polyclonal antibodies directed against lymphocytes; particularly deplete T cells	Serum sickness (fever, chills, muscle and joint pain), tachycardia, back pain, shortness of breath, hypotension, anaphylaxis, leukopenia, thrombocytopenia, rash, ↓ resistance to infection, ↑ incidence of malignancies

ALG, antilymphocyte globulin; *ATG,* antithymocyte globulin; *GI,* gastrointestinal; *IL-2,* interleukin-2; *IL-4,* interleukin-4; *IV,* intravenous (route); *PO,* by mouth.
*Neoral is a microemulsion with better absorption than Sandimmune.

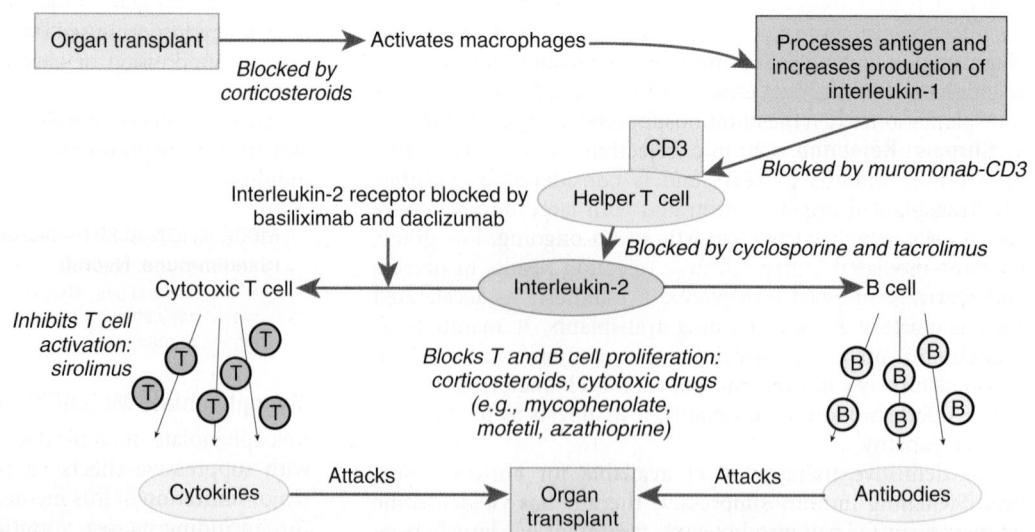

FIG. 16.13 Sites of action for immunosuppressive agents. Source: Adapted from McKenry, L., Tessier, E., & Hogan, M. (2006). *Mosby's pharmacology in nursing* (22nd ed., p. 1161). Mosby.

the adverse effects can be diminished by reduction in the dose or administration of smaller doses more frequently. Myfortic is an enteric-coated form of mycophenolate mofetil that has a similar adverse effect profile.

> **MEDICATION ALERT—Mycophenolate Mofetil (CellCept)**
> - When given intravenously, it must be reconstituted in D_5W and no other solution.
> - Do not give as IV bolus. Give over 2 or more hours.

Sirolimus (Rapamune)

Sirolimus (Rapamune) is an immunosuppressive medication that suppresses T-cell activation and proliferation. At relatively low doses, it has a synergistic effect with cyclosporin (Sandimmune, Neoral), tacrolimus (Prograf), and corticosteroids.

Monoclonal Antibodies

Monoclonal antibodies are used for preventing and treating acute rejection episodes. Muromonab-CD3 (OKT3) was the first monoclonal antibody to be used in clinical transplantation. It is a mouse monoclonal antibody that binds with the CD3 antigen found on the surface of human thymocytes and mature T cells. It interferes with the function of the T lymphocyte, the pivotal cells involved with graft rejection. All T cells are affected, rather than just the subset active in graft rejection. It is administered via IV bolus. Within minutes of the initial infusion of muromonab-CD3 (OKT3), the number of circulating T cells decreases significantly.

A flulike syndrome occurs during the first few days of treatment, as a result of cytokine release. Adverse effects include fever, rigors, headache, myalgias, and various gastrointestinal disturbances. To reduce the expected adverse effects of muromonab-CD3 (OKT3), patients should receive acetaminophen (Tylenol), diphenhydramine (Benadryl), and IV corticosteroids before the dose is administered.

Newer-generation monoclonal antibodies basiliximab (Simulect) (Yeung et al., 2017) and daclizumab (Zenapax) are a hybrid of mouse and human antibodies. They have fewer adverse effects than muromonab-CD3 (OKT3) because large parts of the molecule have been replaced with human IgG. They target the interleukin-2 receptor and impair lymphocyte proliferation. Another monoclonal antibody is alemtuzumab (MabCampath), which targets the CD52 antigen found on T and B cells and the monocytes and macrophages. It can cause prolonged T-cell depletion.

Polyclonal Antibodies

Antilymphocyte globulin and antithymocyte globulin are used as induction therapy or to treat acute rejection. The purpose of induction therapy is to provide significant immunosuppression to an individual immediately after transplantation to prevent early rejection. These agents are prepared by immunizing horses or rabbits with human lymphoid material (thymocytes, lymph nodes, or spleen cells) and then harvesting and purifying the resultant antibody.

Allergic reactions to the foreign proteins from the host animal, manifested by fever, arthralgias, and tachycardia, are common but usually not severe enough to preclude use. These adverse effects can be attenuated by administering the preparation slowly, over 4 to 6 hours, and administering premedication such as acetaminophen (Tylenol), diphenhydramine (Benadryl), and methylprednisolone (Solu-Medrol). The main toxic effects of polyclonal antibodies are lymphopenia and thrombocytopenia, caused by antibody contaminants that are not completely removed during preparation of the antibodies.

Graft-Versus-Host Disease

Graft-versus-host (GVH) disease occurs when an immunoincompetent (immunodeficient) patient receives a transfusion or transplant with immunocompetent cells. A GVH response is most commonly seen in hematopoietic stem cell transplant patients. In most transplant situations, the biggest concern is the patient's (host's) rejection of the organ or transplant. However, in GVH disease, the graft (donated tissue) rejects the host (recipient) tissue (Nassereddine et al., 2017).

The GVH response may begin 7 to 30 days after transplantation. Once the reaction is started, little can be done to modify its course. The exact mechanism involved in this reaction is not completely understood. However, it involves donor T cells attacking and destroying vulnerable host (recipient) cells.

The target organs for the GVH phenomenon are the skin, the gastrointestinal tract, and the liver. The skin disease may be a maculopapular rash, which may be pruritic or painful. It initially involves the palms and the soles of the feet but can progress to a generalized erythema with bullous formation and desquamation (shedding of the outer layer of skin). The liver disease may manifest as mild jaundice with elevated levels of liver enzymes and progress to hepatic coma. The gastrointestinal manifestations may include mild to severe diarrhea, severe abdominal pain, gastrointestinal bleeding, and malabsorption.

The biggest problem with GVH disease is differing types of infection at different time periods. Bacterial and fungal infections predominate immediately after transplantation, when granulocytopenia is occurring. Later, the development of interstitial pneumonitis is the predominant problem.

Once GVH disease is established, there is no satisfactory treatment. Although corticosteroids are often used, the susceptibility to infection then increases. The use of immunosuppressive agents (e.g., methotrexate, cyclosporin [Sandimmune, Neoral]) has been most effective as a preventive rather than as a treatment measure. Use of irradiated blood products before administration is another measure to prevent T-cell replication.

ALTERNATIVE STRATEGIES

In the past decade, there has been a rapid rise in solid organ transplantation worldwide because of the increased incidence of organ failure and improvements in post-transplant outcomes. However, cadaveric organ donation rates have not met demand; thus increasing numbers of patients die waiting for a suitable organ (Black et al., 2018). The number of patients waiting for an organ transplant in Canada in 2018 was 4 351, but only 2 782 organs were transplanted. Approximately 223 people die annually waiting for an organ transplant in Canada (Canadian Institute for Health Information [CIHI], 2020). Various strategies worldwide have been implemented to offset the critical organ shortage, some with modest success, others remaining under scientific investigation and ethical debate (see the Ethical Dilemmas box).

There is an increasing awareness of the need for organ transplantation for Canadian Indigenous people. Social determinants of health have an impact on Indigenous patients' health outcomes, along with differences in their immune response from that of non-Indigenous patients as well as rising rates of diabetes, which then drive the need for organ transplantation. While Canadian Indigenous peoples' knowledge and attitudes toward organ donation and transplantation are positive, donation rates remain low, in keeping with overall Canadian donation rates (Davison & Jhangri, 2014).

ETHICAL DILEMMAS
Transplantation

Situation

A 24-year-old female patient is admitted to hospital with evidence of acute organ rejection. The patient informs the nurse in confidence that she does not take her antirejection medications regularly because she is very busy with work and school. She also states she usually feels so well that she does not feel the need to take them daily. She asks the nurse not to inform the health care team that she has missed taking some of her antirejection medications.

Important Points for Consideration

- Building a trusting relationship with patients is key in the health care environment; however, the larger implications for the patient's health supersede the issue of confidentiality. There are some limits to confidentiality, including potential or real harm to self or others.
- The nurse is a member of the treatment team.
- Organ rejection can cause reduced organ function and potential loss of the graft and subsequent death for the patient. With complete information, the patient can understand the importance of adherence to the medication regimen.

Critical Thinking Questions

1. How should the nurse respond to this patient's request for confidentiality? Should the nurse inform the clinical team treating the patient? If so, should the nurse tell the patient?
2. What information should the nurse give the patient regarding the importance of taking her antirejection medications?
3. How could the nurse work with the patient who has a busy schedule and forgets to take her medications?

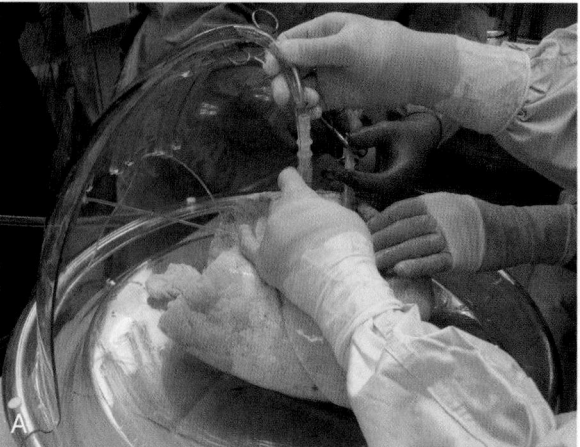

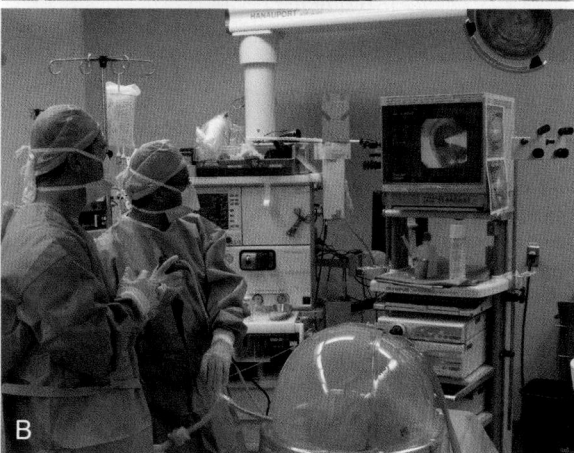

FIG. 16.14 The Toronto Ex Vivo Lung Perfusion (EVLP) System. **A,** Surgeons working on the ex vivo lung. **B,** Thoracic surgeons at Toronto General Hospital, Dr. Marcelo Cypel and Dr. Shaf Keshavjee Director of the Toronto Lung Transplant Program, perform a bronchoscopy on the ex vivo lung for clinical evaluation. Published with permission of Dr. Shaf Keshavjee, Director, Toronto Lung Transplant Program, University Health Network.

Transplantation of Organs from Deceased Donor

One of the most rapid increases in organ recovery rates has been from deceased people who are declared dead on the basis of cardiopulmonary criteria (irreversible cessation of circulatory and respiratory function) rather than neurological criteria of "brain death" (irreversible loss of all functions of the entire brain, including the brainstem) (Ortega et al., 2015). Typically, these patients are on a ventilator because of devastating and irreversible brain injury (not complete brain death) from trauma or intracranial bleeding. In some of these patients, irreversible brain injury occurs due to anoxia (lack of oxygen) from cardiac arrest and subsequent cardiac resuscitation. Further treatment has been deemed futile, and end-of-life care management is implemented. Often, family members express interest in organ donation. The potential donor must meet cardiac death criteria at onset of asystole or absence of a heartbeat. To avoid conflict of interest, those involved in end-of-life care or declaration of death of the potential donor are not involved in the care of the transplant recipient. Organs most commonly recovered for donation include the kidneys, the liver, the pancreas, and the lungs (Ortega et al., 2015). In 2019, a total of 3 014 transplant procedures (all organs) were performed in Canada, an increase of 42% since 2010 (CIHI, 2020).

Ex Vivo Transplantation

A novel strategy to help overcome donor lung shortages has been through the development of normothermic ex vivo lung perfusion (EVLP) (Figure 16.14). The injured donor lungs are reassessed and conditioned through the EVLP system by mimicking the lung's natural physiological environment and by providing oxygen and other substrates necessary for active metabolism. Using EVLP, therapeutic interventions can be performed on the donor lungs that reduce the degree or negative influence of pulmonary edema, pulmonary emboli, gastric aspiration, pneumonia, and lung inflammation (Ali et al., 2017).

Hepatitis C–Infected Organ Transplants

The number of hepatitis C–infected organs in the United States, many attributed to IV drug use and the national opioid crisis, has increased by 250% (Webster, 2018). With a newer generation of medications shown to cure hepatitis C, using these organs for transplantation has opened up new opportunities for patients waiting for this life-saving procedure. Recent studies in Canada have shown the safety of transplanting hepatitis C–positive organs into hepatitis C–negative recipients, following perfusion through the Toronto EVLP System. During the ex vivo process, the donated lungs are treated for 6 hours with medications that reduce the hepatitis C viral load up to 90%. Ongoing research continues to explore preventing viral transmission (Webster, 2018).

Xenotransplantation

Xenotransplantation is transplanting an organ from another species into humans. The pig is believed to be the most appropriate candidate because of its comparable organ size, large litters, and rapid gestation. However, the significant degree of antigen disparity means that there is more for the human immune system to recognize and reject. In addition, the possibility of diseases "jumping" the species barrier and infecting humans, such as porcine endogenous retroviruses or as recently experienced with COVID-19, remains a reason for ongoing skepticism regarding xenotransplantation as an alternative to allogeneic organ transplantation (Cypel & Keshavjee, 2020; Yeung et al., 2017).

Stem Cell Transplantation

Stem cells are cells in the body that can differentiate into other cells. They are divided into two types: embryonic and adult.

Embryonic stem cells are pluripotent and can become any one of the hundreds of types of cells in the human body. Because of their versatility, embryonic stem cells are preferred for use in medical research. Donor eggs, like stem cells, can be used with existing adult tissue to produce new tissue. In a process known as *nuclear transfer* or *therapeutic cloning,* the nucleus is removed from the egg and replaced with the nucleus of the desired tissue. Then, as the egg divides, a 200-cell blastocyst of the desired tissue is created.

Adult stem cells are undifferentiated multipotent cells found in small numbers in most adult tissues. They have been discovered in the skin, the gastrointestinal tract, the bone marrow, and in newborns and can be extracted from umbilical cord blood. Their primary role is to maintain and repair tissues in which they are found. For example, hematopoietic stem cells form all the various cells in blood, whereas skin stem cells produce new skin cells. Scientists hope that adult stem cells can be developed into providing tissue for unrelated organs.

Stem cells found within the bone marrow are the body's site of hematopoiesis. The cells are prolific by design and are used in the treatment of certain diseases, such as leukemia. Studies are ongoing to develop cells that would be capable of becoming other tissues in the body (Elahimehr et al., 2016). With more people needing organ transplants, embryonic stem cell research may be the key to solving the problem of organ shortages through organ regeneration. However, conflicts exist regarding creating embryonic stem cells for therapeutic purposes such as organ development, with much debate over the definition of human life at the earliest stages versus use of stem cells for a potentially life-saving therapy.

NEW TECHNOLOGIES IN IMMUNOLOGY

Hybridoma Technology: Monoclonal Antibodies

Monoclonal antibodies are homogeneous populations of identical antibody molecules produced by specialized tissue cell culture lines. They are manufactured through cell fusion techniques and standard in vitro tissue culture systems (Figure 16.15). The two essential biological components are immunized mice or rats and myeloma tumour cell lines, which are of lymphoid origin. Single antibody-forming cells (lymphocytes) from rodents previously immunized with antigen are fused with myeloma cells to create hybrid cells with properties of both parent cell types. Like the myeloma parent cell, the hybrids have an unlimited capacity to reproduce. The hybrids produce the single type of antibody molecule that they inherited from the normal, antibody-forming parent cell. Hybrid cells derived in this way can produce unlimited quantities of specific antibodies. With appropriate selection techniques, producing monoclonal antibodies to virtually any antigen is possible. Because the monoclonal antibodies are a completely homogeneous population,

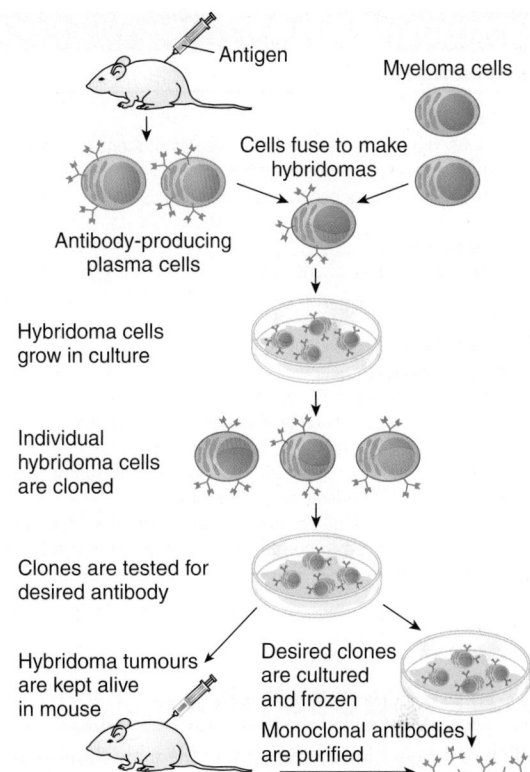

FIG. 16.15 Monoclonal antibodies are identical antibodies made by clones of a single antibody-producing cell. The target antigen is injected into a mouse. Plasma cells are harvested from the spleen of the mouse and fused with myeloma cells. The fused cells, or hybridomas, are then cloned. A clone can secrete monoclonal antibodies over a long period.

their use incurs fewer problems than does that of conventional polyclonal antisera.

Monoclonal antibodies are used widely in many areas of medicine and biological science. Thousands of monoclonal antibodies have been made against many different types of antigens. Monoclonal antibodies have begun to replace conventional antibodies in blood banking and are used in the identification of organisms in bacteriology laboratories. Monoclonal antibodies have also been extensively used in radioimmunoassays to measure serum levels of various substances (e.g., parathyroid hormone). They have been useful in quantifying types of WBCs and subtypes of lymphocytes and in the diagnosis of leukemia. More recently, monoclonal antibodies have been used in the treatment of malignancies (see Chapter 18). They have been used to treat transplant rejection episodes, to purge bone marrow of tumour cells in bone marrow transplants, and to remove mature T cells that cause GVH disease in bone marrow transplant recipients.

A major limitation of monoclonal antibody use for humans is that they are mouse antibodies and therefore can elicit an antibody response by the host against the foreign agent. Human hybridomas have been produced using human myelomas. These hybrids synthesize human monoclonal antibodies and are therefore advantageous for in vivo use in diagnosis and therapy.

CASE STUDY

Anaphylactic Reaction

Patient Profile

K. R. (pronouns she/her), a 21-year-old university student, is brought to the emergency department by ambulance from the school's lunch room after a sudden change in level of consciousness and difficulty with speech.

Subjective Data

Conscious on admission but confused, disoriented, very restless, and anxious

Objective Data

Physical Assessment

- Vital signs on admission: BP 82/58, pulse 124/minute, respirations 8/minute, temp 39.3°C, O2 saturation 84% on 100% oxygen
- Skin: mild facial edema, urticaria, itchy eyes
- Respiratory: tightness of throat, shortness of breath, runny nose
- Gastrointestinal tract: nausea, mild abdominal pain

    K. R.'s friends arrive to the emergency department and report that she had eaten cookies believed to contain peanuts right before the event oc-

curred. Family could not be contacted to determine if K. R. had a previous documented allergy to nuts/peanuts. K.R.'s friends are unaware of a history of such an allergy but do not remember seeing her eating nuts of any kind in the past.

Discussion Questions

1. What kind of reaction is the patient experiencing?
2. **Priority decision:** Based on the assessment data provided, what are the priority nursing diagnoses?
3. **Priority decision:** What are the priority nursing interventions for K. R.?
4. What first-line medication would likely be administered, and how is it going to work to assist the patient?
5. Based on the assessment data provided and the diagnoses, what future nursing care should be provided for this patient?

ⓔvolve

Answers are available at http://evolve.elsevier.com/Canada/Lewis/medsurg.

REVIEW QUESTIONS

The number of the question corresponds to the same-numbered objective at the beginning of the chapter.

1. What is the function of monocytes in immunity?
   a. They stimulate the production of T and B lymphocytes.
   b. They produce antibodies on exposure to foreign substances.
   c. They bind antigens and stimulate natural killer cell activation.
   d. They capture antigens by phagocytosis and present them to lymphocytes.

2. Which of the following is a function of cell-mediated immunity?
   a. Formation of antibodies
   b. Activation of the complement system
   c. Surveillance for malignant cell changes
   d. Opsonization of antigens to allow phagocytosis by neutrophils

3. Which immunoglobulin from maternal transmission protects newborns in the first 3 to 6 months of life from bacterial infections?
   a. IgG
   b. IgA
   c. IgM
   d. IgE

4. Which primary immunological disorder typically occurs in a type I hypersensitivity reaction?
   a. Binding of IgG to an antigen on a cell surface
   b. Deposit of antigen–antibody complexes in small vessels
   c. Release of lymphokines to interact with specific antigens
   d. Release of chemical mediators from IgE-bound mast cells and basophils

5. Which response alerts the nurse that a possible anaphylactic shock reaction may be occurring immediately after a client has received an intramuscular penicillin injection?
   a. Edema and itching at the injection site
   b. Sneezing and itching of the nose and eyes
   c. A wheal-and-flare reaction at the injection site
   d. Chest tightness and production of thick sputum

6. Which is the most appropriate response when a person requests a friend who is a nurse to administer his allergy shot?
   a. It is illegal for nurses to administer injections outside of a medical setting.
   b. The nurse is qualified to do it if the friend has epinephrine in an injectable syringe provided with his extract.
   c. Avoiding the allergens is a more effective way of controlling allergies, and allergy shots are not usually effective.
   d. Immunotherapy should be administered only in a setting where emergency equipment and medications are available.

7. Association between HLA antigens and diseases is most commonly found in what disease conditions?
   a. Malignancies
   b. Infectious diseases
   c. Neurological diseases
   d. Autoimmune disorders

8. A client is undergoing plasmapheresis for treatment of SLE. What effect does plasmapheresis have?
   a. Removes T lymphocytes in the client's blood that are producing antinuclear antibodies
   b. Removes normal particles in the client's blood that are being damaged by autoantibodies
   c. Exchanges the client's plasma that contains antinuclear antibodies with a substitute fluid
   d. Replaces viral-damaged cellular components of the client's blood with replacement whole blood

9. What is the most common cause of secondary immunodeficiencies?
   a. Medications
   b. Stress
   c. Malnutrition
   d. Human immunodeficiency virus

10. Which of the following accurately describes rejection after transplantation?
    a. Hyperacute rejection can be treated with mycophenolate mofetil.
    b. Acute rejection can be treated with sirolimus or tacrolimus.
    c. Chronic rejection can be treated with tacrolimus or cyclosporin.
    d. Hyperacute rejection can usually be avoided if crossmatching is done before transplantation.

11. Which of the following does the nurse understand regarding acute rejection of a transplanted lung? (*Select all that apply.*)
    a. A new transplant should be considered immediately.
    b. Acute rejection can be treated with high-dose corticosteroids.
    c. Acute rejection always leads to chronic rejection.
    d. Acute rejection is treated with muromonab-CD3.
    e. Acute rejection is common after a transplant and is treated with augmentation of immunosuppression.

12. Which of the following statements best describes cardiac death in a deceased donor?
    a. Severe brain damage; coma has progressed to a state of wakefulness without detectable awareness
    b. Irreversible loss of all functions of the entire brain, including the brainstem
    c. Devastating and irreversible brain injuries (not complete brain death) from trauma or intracranial bleeding; complete cessation of the heartbeat may have occurred, and after subsequent cardiac resuscitation, irreversible brain injury results from a long period of lack of oxygen
    d. Inability to be awakened; fails to respond normally to pain or light, does not have sleep–wake cycles, and does not take voluntary actions

1. d; 2. c; 3. a; 4. d; 5. a; 6. d; 7. d; 8. c; 9. a; 10. d; 11. b, e; 12. c.

⊖volve

For even more review questions, visit http://evolve.elsevier.com/Canada/Lewis/medsurg.

REFERENCES

Ali, A., Summers, C., Keshavjee, S., et al. (2017). Normothermic Ex Vivo Lung Perfusion: A Review of the Toronto Protocol. University of. *Toronto Medical Journal, 94*(2), 26–31.

Anagnostou, K., & Turner, P. (2019). Myths, facts and controversies in the diagnosis and management of anaphylaxis. *Archives of Disease in Childhood, 104*(1), 83–90. https://doi.org/10.1136/archdischild-2018-314867.

Banasik, J. L. (2018). *Pathophysiology* (6th ed.). Elsevier.

Black, C. K., Termanini, K. M., Aguirre, O., et al. (2018). Solid organ transplantation in the 21st century. *Annals of Translational Medicine, 6*(20), 409. https://doi.org/10.21037/atm.2018.09.68.

Canadian Centre for Occupational Health and Safety (CCOHS). (2016). *Latex allergy.* https://www.ccohs.ca/oshanswers/diseases/latex.html.

Canadian Institute for Health Information (CIHI). (2020). *Canadian organ replacement in Canada: CORR annual statistics, 2020.* https://www.cihi.ca/en/organ-replacement-in-canada-corr-annual-statistics-2020.

Currie, C. L., Copeland, J. L., & Metz, G. A. (2019). Childhood racial discrimination and adult allostatic load: The role of Indigenous cultural continuity in allostatic resiliency. *Social Science and Medicine, 241*, 112564. https://doi.org/10.1016/j.socscimed.2019.112564.

Cypel, M., & Keshavjee, S. (2020). When to consider lung transplantation for COVID-19. *The Lancet Respiratory Medicine, 8*(10), 944–946. https://doi.org/10.1016/S2213-2600(20)30393-3.

Elahimehr, R., Scheinok, A. T., & McKay, D. B. (2016). Hematopoietic stem cells and solid organ transplantation. *Transplantation Reviews, 30*(4), 227–234. https://doi.org/10.1016/j.trre.2016.07.005.

Kellie, S., & Al-Mansour, Z. (2017). *Overview of the Immune System. Micro and Nanotechnology in Vaccine Development* (pp. 63-81). William Andrew Publishing.

Marazziti, D., Mucci, F., & Fontenelle, L. F. (2018). Immune system and obsessive-compulsive disorder. *Psychoneuroendocrinology, 93*, 39–44. https://doi.org/10.1016/j.psyneuen.2018.04.013.

McKenry, L., Tessier, E., & Hogan, M. (2006). *Mosby's pharmacology in nursing* (22nd ed.). Mosby (Seminal).

Morison, M. J. (2001). *Nursing management of chronic wounds.* Mosby (Seminal).

Nassereddine, S., Rafei, H., Elbahesh, E., et al. (2017). Acute graft vs host disease: A comprehensive review. *Anticancer Research, 37*(4), 1547–1555. https://doi.org/10.21873/anticanres.11483.

Quirt, J., Gagnon, R., Ellis, A. K., et al. (2018). CSACI position statement: Prescribing sublingual immunotherapy tablets for aeroallergens. *Allergy, Asthma, and Clinical Immunology, 14*(1), 1–4. https://doi.org/10.1186/s13223-017-0225-6.

Rich, R. R., & Chaplin, D. D. (2019). *The human immune response. Clinical immunology, principles and practice* (5th ed. pp. 3-17). Elsevier. https://doi.org/10.1016/B978-0-7020-6896-6.00001-6.

Rossi, S., & Pitidis, A. (2018). Multiple chemical sensitivity: Review of the state of the art in epidemiology, diagnosis, and future perspectives. *Journal of Occupational and Environmental Medicine, 60*(2), 138–146. https://doi.org/10.1097/JOM.0000000000001215.

Semple, C., Choi, K. Y. G., Kroeker, A., et al. (2019). Polymorphisms in the P2X7 receptor, and differential expression of Toll-like receptor-mediated cytokines and defensins, in a Canadian Indigenous group. *Scientific Reports, 9*(1), 1–13. https://doi.org/10.1038/s41598-019-50596-0.

Turner, P. J., Jerschow, E., Umasunthar, T., et al. (2017). Fatal anaphylaxis: Mortality rate and risk factors. *The Journal of Allergy and Clinical Immunology. Asthma & Immunology, 5*(5), 1169–1178. https://doi.org/10.1016/j.jaip.2017.06.031.

Webster, P. (2018). Hepatitis C-infected organ transplants offer hope. *The Lancet, 391*(10139), 2485. https://doi.org/10.1016/S0140-6736(18)31424-7.

Weidinger, S., & Novak, N. (2016). Atopic dermatitis. *The Lancet, 387*(10023), 1109–1122. https://doi.org.uhn.idm.oclc.org/10.1016/S0140-6736(15)00149-X.

Weyand, C. M., & Goronzy, J. J. (2016). Aging of the immune system. Mechanisms and therapeutic targets. *Annals of the American Thoracic Society, 13*(Suppl 5), S422–S428. https://doi.org/10.1513/AnnalsATS.201602-095AW.

Yeung, M. Y., Gabardi, S., & Sayegh, M. H. (2017). Use of polyclonal/monoclonal antibody therapies in transplantation. *Expert Opinion on Biological Therapy, 17*(3), 339–352. https://doi.org/10.1080/14712598.2017.1283400.

RESOURCES

Alberta Organ and Tissue Donation Registry
https://myhealth.alberta.ca/Pages/OTDRHome.aspx?utm_source=
redirector
Asthma Society of Canada
https://www.asthma.ca
BC Transplant
http://www.transplant.bc.ca
Canadian Association for Clinical Microbiology and Infectious Diseases
https://www.cacmid.ca
Canadian Blood Services (CBS): Organ and Tissue Donation Transplantation—Privacy Notices
https://www.blood.ca/en/about-us/organ-and-tissue-donation-and-transplantation
Canadian Centre for Occupational Health and Safety (CCOHS)
https://www.ccohs.ca
Canadian Donation and Transplantation Research Program
https://www.cntrp.ca/
Canadian Society of Allergy and Clinical Immunology (CSACI)
https://www.csaci.ca

Transplant Manitoba
https://www.transplantmanitoba.ca/decide/gift-of-life
Transplant Québec
https://www.transplantquebec.ca/en
Trillium Gift of Life Network
https://www.giftoflife.on.ca

Access Excellence: Understanding Gene Testing
http://www.accessexcellence.org/AE/AEPC/NIH
Centers for Disease Control and Prevention: Genomics & Precision Health
https://www.cdc.gov/genomics
National Institute of Nursing Research (NINR), Division of Intramural Research
https://www.ninr.nih.gov/researchandfunding/dir

ⓔvolve
For additional Internet resources, see the website for this book at http://evolve.elsevier.com/Canada/Lewis/medsurg.

Infection and Human Immunodeficiency Virus Infection

Serena Eagland
Originating US chapter by Jeffrey Kwong

⊘volve WEBSITE

http://evolve.elsevier.com/Canada/Lewis/medsurg

- Review Questions (Online Only)
- Key Points
- Answer Guidelines for Case Study
- Student Case Study
- Human Immunodeficiency Virus (HIV) Infection and Acquired Immunodeficiency Syndrome (AIDS)
- Conceptual Care Map Creator
- Audio Glossary
- Content Updates

LEARNING OBJECTIVES

1. Discuss the effect of emerging and re-emerging infections on health care.
2. Review infection prevention and control strategies.
3. List the modes and variables involved in the transmission of the human immunodeficiency virus (HIV).
4. Describe the pathophysiological processes of HIV infection.
5. Outline HIV disease progression against the spectrum of untreated HIV infection.
6. List the diagnostic criteria for acquired immune deficiency syndrome (AIDS).
7. Explain the methods of testing for HIV infection.
8. Discuss the interprofessional management of HIV infection.
9. Discuss the long-term consequences of HIV infection and treatment of HIV infection.
10. Explain the characteristics of opportunistic diseases associated with AIDS.
11. Describe the nursing management of HIV-infected patients and those at risk for HIV infection.
12. Compare and contrast the methods of HIV prevention that eliminate risk and those that decrease risk.

KEY TERMS

acquired immunodeficiency syndrome (AIDS)
acute retroviral syndrome (seroconversion illness)
bacteria
emerging infectious disease
fungi

human immunodeficiency virus (HIV)
opportunistic diseases
oral hairy leukoplakia
protozoa
retroviruses
reverse transcriptase

viral load
viremia
viruses
window period

INFECTIONS

An infection is an invasion of the body by a *pathogen* (any microorganism that causes disease) and the resulting signs and symptoms that develop in response to the invasion. Infections can be divided into two categories: localized and systemic. A *localized* infection is limited to a small area. *Systemic* infections are widespread throughout the body and are often spread via the blood.

Causes of Infections

A number of microorganisms can cause infections. The most common are bacteria, viruses, fungi, and protozoa. Bacteria are one-celled microorganisms that are found virtually everywhere on earth and are involved in fermentation, putrefaction, infectious diseases, and nitrogen fixation. They were first observed by Anton Van Leeuwenhoek, who named them "animalcules." A number of bacteria are considered to be normal flora. Under normal circumstances, they live harmoniously in or on the human body without causing disease. These normal flora act protectively and prevent the overgrowth of other microorganisms. *Escherichia coli* organisms, for example, are bacteria that are normal flora in the large intestine

Bacteria cause disease in two ways. They can enter the body and grow inside human cells (e.g., tuberculosis [TB]), or they can secrete toxins that damage cells. Bacteria are divided into

TABLE 17.1	COMMON DISEASE-CAUSING BACTERIA
Type	**Diseases Caused**
Clostridium organisms	
• *C. botulinum*	Food poisoning with progressive muscle paralysis
• *C. difficile*	Diarrhea, colitis
• *C. perfringens*	Food poisoning, gangrene
• *C. tetani*	Tetanus (lockjaw)
Corynebacterium diphtheriae	Diphtheria
Escherichia coli	Urinary tract infections, cystitis, peritonitis, inflammatory gastrointestinal infections
Haemophilus organisms	
• *H. aegyptius*	Pink eye
• *H. influenzae*	Nasopharyngitis, meningitis, pneumonia, otitis media, upper respiratory tract infections
• *H. pertussis*	Pertussis (whooping cough)
Helicobacter pylori	Peptic ulcers, gastritis
Klebsiella and *Enterobacter* organisms	Urinary tract infections, peritonitis, pneumonia
Legionella pneumophila	Pneumonia (Legionnaires' disease)
Mycobacterium organisms	
• *M. leprae*	Hansen's disease (leprosy)
• *M. tuberculosis*	Tuberculosis
Neisseria organisms	
• *N. gonorrhoeae*	Gonorrhea, pelvic inflammatory disease
• *N. meningitidis*	Meningococcemia, meningitis
Proteus organisms	Urinary tract infections, peritonitis
Pseudomonas aeruginosa	Urinary tract infections, meningitis
Salmonella organisms	
• *S. typhi*	Typhoid fever
• Other *Salmonella* organisms	Food poisoning, gastroenteritis
Shigella organisms	Shigellosis, diarrhea with abdominal pain and fever (dysentery)
Staphylococcus aureus	Skin infections, pneumonia, urinary tract infections, acute osteomyelitis, toxic shock syndrome
Streptococcus organisms	
• *S. epidermidis*	Nosocomial sepsis
• *S. faecalis*	Genito-urinary infection, infection of surgical wounds
• *S. pneumoniae*	Pneumococcal pneumonia, otitis media
• *S. pyogenes* (group A β-hemolytic streptococci)	Pharyngitis, scarlet fever, rheumatic fever, acute glomerulonephritis, erysipelas, pneumonia, upper respiratory tract infections
• *S. pyogenes* (group B β-hemolytic streptococci)	Urinary tract infections
• *S. viridans*	Bacterial endocarditis
Treponema pallidum	Syphilis
Vibrio cholerae	Cholera

TABLE 17.2	COMMON DISEASE-CAUSING VIRUSES
Type	**Diseases Caused**
Adenoviruses	Upper respiratory tract infection, pneumonia
Arbovirus	Syndrome of fever, malaise, headache, myalgia; aseptic meningitis; encephalitis
Coronavirus	Upper respiratory tract infection
Coxsackieviruses A and B	Upper respiratory tract infection, gastroenteritis, acute myocarditis, aseptic meningitis
Ebola virus	Viral hemorrhagic fever
Echoviruses	Upper respiratory tract infection, gastroenteritis, aseptic meningitis
Flaviviruses	Yellow fever, Dengue, West Nile
Hepatitis A, B, C, D, E	Viral hepatitis
Human herpesviruses	
• Cytomegalovirus (CMV)	Gastroenteritis; pneumonia and retinal damage in immunosuppressed individuals; infectious mononucleosis–like syndrome
• Epstein-Barr virus	Mononucleosis, Burkitt's lymphoma (possibly)
• Herpes simplex, type 1	Herpes labialis ("fever blisters"), genital herpes infection
• Herpes simplex, type 2	Genital herpes infection
• Varicella-zoster	Chickenpox; shingles
HIV	HIV infection, AIDS
Influenza A and B	Upper respiratory tract infection
Mumps	Parotitis, orchitis in postpubertal males
Papovavirus	Warts
Parainfluenza types 1–4	Upper respiratory tract infection
Parvovirus	Gastroenteritis
Poliovirus	Poliomyelitis
Poxviruses	Smallpox
Reoviruses 1, 2, 3	Upper respiratory tract infection
Respiratory syncytial virus	Gastroenteritis, respiratory tract infection
Rhabdovirus	Rabies
Rhinovirus	Upper respiratory tract infection, pneumonia
Rotaviruses	Gastroenteritis
Rubella	German measles
Rubeola	Measles
West Nile virus	Flulike symptoms, meningitis, encephalitis

AIDS, acquired immune deficiency syndrome; *HIV,* human immunodeficiency virus.

categories on the basis of the shape of their cells. *Cocci,* including streptococci and staphylococci, are round cells. *Bacilli* are rod-shaped and include tetanus and TB. Bacilli that are curved rods include *Vibrio* bacteria, one of which causes cholera. Table 17.1 lists common pathogenic bacteria and the diseases that they cause (Huether & McCance, 2019).

Viruses can also cause infections. The word *virus* comes from the Latin word *virus,* meaning "poison." Unlike bacteria, viruses are not cells. They consist of either RNA or DNA and a protein envelope. Viruses can reproduce only in the cells of a living organism and are therefore obligate parasites. Examples of diseases caused by viruses are presented in Table 17.2 (Huether & McCance, 2019).

Fungi are organisms similar to plants, but they lack chlorophyll. Mycosis is any disease caused by a fungus. Pathogenic fungi cause infections that are usually localized to a small area, but in an immunocompromised person, they can become disseminated. Athlete's foot and ringworm are two common mycotic infections. Some fungi are normal flora in various places in the body, but when overgrowth occurs, disease can result. Overgrowth of *Candida albicans,* for example, causes oral candidiasis (thrush), esophageal candidiasis, intestinal symptoms, and vaginitis, depending on the affected site. Other fungi and their respective mycotic infections are listed in Table 17.3. Fungal infections of the lungs are presented in Chapter 30 (see Table 30.9) and fungal infections of the skin in Chapter 26 (see Table 26.7).

Protozoa are single-cell, animal-like microorganisms. Protozoa can be divided into four categories: amoebas, ciliates, flagellates, and sporozoa. Protozoa normally live in soil and bodies of water. When they are introduced into the human body, infection can result. Amoebic dysentery and giardiasis are caused by protozoan parasites. Malaria is caused by a sporozoa called *Plasmodium falciparum* (Huether & McCance, 2019).

TABLE 17.3 COMMON DISEASE-CAUSING FUNGI		
Organism	**Diseases Caused**	**Organs Affected**
Aspergillus fumigatus	Aspergillosis	Lungs*
	Otomycosis	Ears
Blastomyces dermatitidis	Blastomycosis	Lungs, various organs
Candida albicans	Candidiasis	Intestines
	Vaginitis	Vagina
	Thrush	Skin,† mouth
Coccidioides immitis	Coccidioidomycosis	Lungs*
Pneumocystis jiroveci	Pneumocystis pneumonia	Lungs*
Sporothrix schenckii	Sporotrichosis	Skin, lymph vessels
Trichophyton species	Tinea pedis	Skin†
Microsporum species	Tinea capitis	Skin
Epidermophyton species	Tinea corporis	Skin†

*See Table 30.9 (Fungal Infections of the Lung).
†See Table 26.7 (Common Fungal Infections of the Skin and the Mucous Membranes).

Emerging Infections

An **emerging infectious disease** is an infectious disease whose incidence has recently increased or threatens to increase in the immediate future. Examples of emerging infections are described in Table 17.4. Emerging infectious diseases can originate from unknown sources, contact with animals, changes in known diseases, natural disasters, or even biological warfare. For example, the coronavirus that causes severe acute respiratory syndrome (SARS), SARS-CoV-2, and the West Nile virus comes from animal sources, whereas other pathogens, such as *Staphylococcus aureus,* have emerged because a previously treatable organism developed resistance to antibiotics. Climate change has resulted in an increase of disease-carrying mosquitoes, as well as increases in rodent numbers and in hantavirus. Earthquakes, such as the large one in Haiti in 2010, are associated with the spread of waterborne diseases such as cholera. The battle against infectious disease is an age-old problem. However, modern technologies have changed how disease spreads. Global travel, population density, encroachment into new environments, and the misuse of antibiotics have all increased the risk for widespread new or untreatable infectious diseases (Public Health Agency of Canada [PHAC], 2015a).

It is interesting that not too long ago, many people believed that science had conquered infectious disease. Unfortunately, infections remain the leading cause of death worldwide. More than 30 newly recognized infectious diseases have emerged since the 1980s, including human immunodeficiency virus (HIV) infection, Lyme disease, hepatitis C, SARS, SARS-CoV-2, avian flu, and Ebola virus disease. In addition, some diseases once thought to be under control, including TB and medication-resistant strains of other bacteria, have re-emerged (PHAC, 2015a).

Results of studies in zoonosis (the science of transmission of diseases from animals to humans) indicate that many known infectious diseases come from animals and insects (vectors). The SARS outbreak in China in 2003, for instance, was linked to the civet cat, a small carnivorous mammal found throughout much of Asia and Africa. (SARS is discussed in Chapters 70 and 72.) Animal-borne infections are difficult to predict and prevent.

West Nile virus is transmitted by a virus carried by mosquitoes. Mosquitoes acquire the virus as they draw blood from infected birds (Government of Canada, 2021a). The virus does not cause illness in the mosquito but can be transferred to

TABLE 17.4 EXAMPLES OF EMERGING INFECTIONS	
Microorganism	**Related Disease**
Bacteria	
Borrelia burgdorferi	Lyme disease
Campylobacter jejuni	Diarrhea
Escherichia coli O157:H7	Hemorrhagic colitis, hemolytic uremic syndrome
Helicobacter pylori	Peptic ulcer disease
Legionella pneumophila	Legionnaires' disease
Vibrio cholerae 0139	New strain associated with epidemic cholera
Viruses	
Coronavirus	COVID-19
Ebola virus	Ebola hemorrhagic fever
Hantavirus	Hantavirus pulmonary syndrome (found in North and South America)
	Hemorrhagic fever with renal syndrome (found mainly in Europe and Asia)
H1N1 virus	H1N1 (swine) flu
Hepatitis A virus	Enterically transmitted hepatitis
Hepatitis C virus	Parenterally transmitted hepatitis
Hepatitis E virus	Enterically transmitted hepatitis
HIV	HIV infection and AIDS
HHV-6	Roseola
HHV-8	Associated with Kaposi's sarcoma and Castleman's disease in immunosuppressed patients, patients with AIDS
West Nile virus	West Nile fever
Avian influenza A (H5N1) virus	Avian flu
Zika virus	Zika fever, microcephaly
Parasites	
Cryptosporidium parvum	Acute and chronic diarrhea

AIDS, acquired immunodeficiency syndrome; *HHV,* human herpesvirus; *HIV,* human immunodeficiency virus.

animals and humans as the mosquito continues to feed. Bird deaths are an indicator of the spread of the West Nile virus and can serve as an early warning sign of an outbreak that can spread quickly if action is not taken in a timely manner (Government of Canada, 2021a). (West Nile virus is discussed in Chapter 59.)

Another serious disease transmitted by animals is Lyme disease, which is caused by the bite of a black-legged tick. In Canada, Lyme disease is most common in British Columbia, Manitoba, Nova Scotia, and certain areas in New Brunswick, Ontario, and Quebec. From 2015 to 2017, the number of Lyme disease cases increased dramatically, with the majority of these cases being in Ontario, Quebec, and Nova Scotia (Government of Canada, 2019a). (See Chapter 67 for further discussion on Lyme disease.)

Sometimes, an organism alters its normal path of transmission. In the past, influenza A viruses were typically spread from birds to pigs to humans. More recently, in cases such as the avian flu outbreak, the virus has been spread directly from chickens to humans. This was first demonstrated in Hong Kong in 1997 and also in the Netherlands in 2003. Infected people generally suffer from conjunctivitis or mild influenza-like symptoms. However, 200 deaths related to avian flu have occurred worldwide (PHAC, 2016a). Upon discovery of an outbreak, all chickens in the area are typically slaughtered to remove the source of the infection.

The disease caused by Ebola virus is an emerging entity that has presented an ongoing challenge to public health since it was first observed in 1976. In 2014 the first cases of Ebola occurred in the United States. These initial cases were primarily from travelers or medical aid workers who were working in Africa. In 2018, the Democratic Republic of Congo reported the second-largest Ebola epidemic recorded, after the outbreak in West Africa between 2014 and 2016 (WHO, 2020b). Ebola virus causes a severe hemorrhagic fever and is usually lethal (World Health Organization [WHO], 2021a). Therapeutic and preventive measures are extremely limited. The natural reservoir and path of transmission of the virus are unknown, which makes it impossible to effectively combat the disease (Government of Canada, 2021b). However, as of 2020, two vaccines were undergoing clinical trials with preliminary positive results (WHO, 2020c). The number of cases has continued to slowly decline, but the virus remains a serious concern at the time of this publication.

A relatively new and emerging entity is the outbreak caused by Zika virus. Originally identified in Africa and Asia in the 1950s and historically occurring in low numbers, it has occurred in a large outbreak in South and Central America, with some cases reported in the United States and Canada. Zika virus generally causes a relatively mild infection, manifested by muscle and joint pain, headache, rash, and conjunctivitis. It is spread primarily by mosquitoes, but there is some evidence of sexual transmission. Zika does not pose a risk to most people; however, women who are infected with the virus during pregnancy are more likely to have a baby with microcephaly and should discuss travel with their health care provider before embarking on a trip to a country where Zika is common. Women should also avoid trying for pregnancy for 2 months after visiting a Zika-infected country, and men for 3 months. (Government of Canada, 2019b).

Re-Emerging Infections. Vaccines and proper medications have led to the near eradication of some infections. However, infective agents can always re-emerge if conditions are right. Table 17.5 illustrates some diseases that have re-emerged in recent decades.

For example, the incidence of TB began to decrease steadily in the mid-1950s (see Chapter 30). However, by 2013, the declining trend stabilized and incidence levelled out to 4.7 cases per 100 000 people in Canada (PHAC, 2015a). One factor that has influenced the continued incidence of TB in Canada is the increase in people with HIV, whose depressed immune systems can allow pathogens such as TB bacilli to cause disease. There has been an increase in medication-resistant TB, although in Canada the rates remain relatively low (PHAC, 2015a). International travel creates a new dilemma for the local eradication of diseases. Measles, for instance, was essentially eradicated in Canada in 1998. However, given historically low immunization rates and global travel, measles re-emerged in Canada in 2018. This re-emergence reiterates the importance of immunization and herd immunity (Government of Canada, 2020). The National Collaborating Centre for Infectious Disease provides up-to-date monitoring information on emerging and re-emerging diseases nationally; its link can be found in the Resources section of this chapter.

Resistant Organisms. Antibiotic-resistant organisms, also called *multidrug-resistant organisms* or *superbugs,* are bacteria whose growth and reproduction are unaffected by particular antibiotics. Microorganisms can become resistant to classic antibiotics (e.g., penicillin) as well as to newer antibiotic and antiviral agents.

Methicillin-resistant *S. aureus* (MRSA), vancomycin-resistant enterococci, health care–associated *Clostridium difficile,* and carbapenem-resistant enterobacteriaceae are four of the most troublesome resistant bacteria in North America (PHAC, 2016a). Table 17.6 lists the most common antibiotic-resistant bacteria.

Bacteria are highly adaptable organisms that have evolved genetic and biochemical means of resisting antimicrobial actions. Genetic mechanisms include mutation and acquisition of new DNA. Biochemically, bacteria resist antibiotics by producing enzymes that destroy or inactivate the drugs. Drug target sites are then altered so that the antibiotic cannot bind to or enter the bacteria. If the medication cannot enter the cell, it cannot kill the bacteria (WHO, 2020a). MRSA can be acquired in a hospital setting and in the community. In health care workers exposed to MRSA, their bodies can become colonized, and they can spread the infection to other health care workers and to patients. The organism can remain viable for days on environmental surfaces

TABLE 17.5	EXAMPLES OF RE-EMERGING INFECTIONS	
Microorganism	**Infection**	**Description**
Bacteria		
Corynebacterium diphtheriae	Diphtheria	Localized infection of mucous membranes or skin
Bordetella pertussis	Pertussis	Acute, highly contagious respiratory disease that is characterized by loud whooping inspiration; also known as *whooping cough*
Mycobacterium tuberculosis	Tuberculosis	Chronic infection transmitted by inhalation of infected droplets (see Chapter 30)
Viruses		
Dengue viruses (flaviviruses)	Dengue fever	Acute infection transmitted by mosquitoes and occurring mainly in tropical and subtropical regions
Parasite		
Giardia	Giardiasis	Diarrheal illness that usually originates in fecal-contaminated water; also known as *travellers' diarrhea*

TABLE 17.6	COMMON ANTIBIOTIC-RESISTANT ORGANISMS AND TREATMENT	
Bacteria	**Resistant To**	**Preferred Treatment**
Clostridium difficile	Associated with the overuse of certain antibiotics, including fluoroquinolones, cephalosporins, and clindamycin	Metronidazole (Flagyl) Vancomycin (Vancocin) Fidaxomicin (Dificid) Stool transplantation
Staphylococcus aureus	Methicillin*	Vancomycin (Vancocin)
Enterococcus faecalis	Vancomycin (Vancocin), streptomycin, gentamicin	Penicillin G or ampicillin
Enterococcus faecium	Vancomycin, streptomycin, gentamicin	Penicillin G or ampicillin
Carbapenem-resistant enterobacteriaceae	Carbapenem class of antibiotics	Fosfomycin (Monurol) Tigecycline (Tygacil)

*No longer used clinically.

and clothing. It is important to understand that many people are colonized with antibiotic-resistant organisms, but they are not infected. However, certain patients are at particular risk of becoming infected, including those who are immunosuppressed (e.g., receiving chemotherapy), have invasive devices (e.g., indwelling catheters), or have breaks in the skin barrier (e.g., surgical or nonsurgical wounds). Vancomycin-resistant enterococci are hardier than MRSA and can remain viable on environmental surfaces for weeks. Alcohol preparations are the most effective antimicrobial agents, followed by chlorhexidine gluconate (PHAC, 2012a). The PHAC (2012b) recommends that infection control for antibiotic-resistant organisms consist of routine practices or standard precautions (see Tables 17.8 and 17.9 later in this chapter), which should be used for all patient care.

Drug resistance is a particularly difficult problem in dealing with infectious diseases. Health care providers contribute to the development of drug-resistant organisms by (a) administering antibiotics for viral infections, (b) succumbing to pressures from patients to prescribe unnecessary antibiotic therapy, (c) using inadequate medication regimens to treat infections, or (d) using broad-spectrum or combination agents for infections that should be treated with first-line medications. Patients who miss doses or do not take antibiotics for the full duration of the prescribed therapy also contribute to the development of resistance. In addition, limited resources or access to medications makes it difficult for some patients to get adequate treatment for infections. Patients and their supports should be taught that the proper use of antibiotics (Table 17.7) is crucial to treatment success and prevention of drug-resistant pathogens.

Health Care–Associated Infections

Health care–associated infections (HAIs; formerly called *nosocomial infections*) are infections that are acquired as a result of exposure to a microorganism in any setting in which health care is delivered (e.g., acute or long-term care facility, ambulatory clinic, home) and are related to receiving health care. While the incidence of HAIs continues to decrease nationally, around 8% of Canadians who are hospitalized still acquire an infection during hospitalization (Mitchell et al., 2019). Approximately 1 in 217 patients acquired an infection while in hospital in 2017 (PHAC, 2019b). Surgical patients are at greater risk. In addition, some bacteria that are not normally pathological can cause infections in patients who are immunocompromised as a result of illness or treatment of illness. HAIs can be caused by any organism, but certain bacteria—including *E. coli, S. aureus, Enterobacter aerogenes, C. difficile,* and various types of streptococci—are the more common culprits. At least 30% of HAIs can be prevented by following infection prevention strategies (PHAC, 2012b). HAIs are often transmitted from patient to patient through direct contact by health care providers. Hand hygiene (handwashing or use of alcohol-based hand rub) between patient visits and procedures and the appropriate use of personal protective equipment (PPE) such as gloves remain the first lines of defence in preventing the spread of HAIs. It is important to remember that *C. difficile* is not killed by alcohol-based hand rub. Handwashing with soap and water must be followed in this instance. Isolated infections can be caused when bacteria that are normally present in one area of the body are introduced into another area. Therefore, nurses must take care to change gloves and use hand hygiene when changing tasks, even when working with one patient.

AGE-RELATED CONSIDERATIONS

Infection in Older Persons

The rate of HAIs is significantly higher among older persons than among younger patients. Individuals in long-term care facilities are at special risk for HAI. Age-related changes (e.g., impaired immune function) and comorbidities such as diabetes and physical disabilities can contribute to higher infection rates (Katz & Roghmann, 2016). HAIs common in older people include pneumonia, urinary tract infections, skin infections, and TB. Urinary tract infections are more common in older people who reside in long-term care facilities than in those who live at home. They are often found in patients who have in-dwelling catheters. Infections in older persons often have atypical manifestations, such as cognitive and behavioural changes, before the emergence of fever, pain, or alterations in laboratory values. Disease should typically be suspected if a patient demonstrates changes in the ability to perform daily activities or in cognitive function. In addition, underlying diseases, increased frequency of medication reactions, and institutionalization can all complicate the management of the older person with infection.

> **SAFETY ALERT**
> Nurses should not rely on the presence of fever to indicate infection in older persons because many have lower core body temperatures and decreased immune responses.

Infection Prevention and Control

Infection Precautions. If a patient develops an infection that is considered a risk to others, infection precautions may be needed. The purpose of these precautions is to prevent the transmission of organisms from patients to health care providers, from health care providers to patients, and from one patient to another. The Centers for Disease Control and Prevention (CDC) have issued isolation precaution guidelines that are

---

TABLE 17.7	**PATIENT & CAREGIVER TEACHING GUIDE**

Decreasing Risk for Antibiotic-Resistant Infection

1. **Do not take antibiotics to prevent illness.** Doing this increases the risk for developing resistant infection.
   - Exceptions include taking antibiotics before certain surgical procedures and taking antibiotics before dental work if the patient has a heart valve disorder.
2. **Wash hands frequently.** Handwashing is the most important way to prevent an infection.
3. **Follow directions.** Not taking antibiotic as prescribed or skipping doses can encourage the development of antibiotic-resistant bacteria.
4. **Finish the antibiotic.** Patients must not stop taking antibiotic when they feel better. If they stop taking the antibiotic early, the hardiest bacteria survive and multiply. Eventually a patient could develop an infection resistant to many antibiotics. Patients should never have leftover antibiotics.
5. **Do not request an antibiotic for flu or colds.** If the health care provider says that an antibiotic is not needed, chances are that this is true. Antibiotics are effective against bacterial infections but not viruses, which cause colds and flus.
6. **Do not take leftover antibiotics.** People often save unfinished antibiotics for later use or borrow leftover medications from family or friends. This is dangerous because (a) the leftover antibiotic may not be appropriate for the patient, (b) the illness may not be a bacterial infection, (c) old antibiotics can lose their effectiveness, and in some cases, ingesting them can even be fatal, and (d) there will not be enough doses in a leftover bottle to allow for a full treatment.

used in many health care institutions in Canada and around the world (CDC, 2016). Health Canada has issued similar recommendations (PHAC, 2019a).

Both sets of guidelines contain two levels of precautions (Table 17.8): *routine practices*, or *standard precautions*, which are designed for the care of all patients in hospitals and health care facilities regardless of their diagnosis or presumed infection status, and *additional precautions*, or *transmission-based precautions*, which are used for patients known to be or suspected of being infected with epidemiologically important pathogens that can be transmitted by airborne or droplet transmission or by contact with dry skin or contaminated surfaces.

The system of routine practices or standard precautions applies to (a) blood; (b) all body fluids, secretions, and excretions regardless of whether they contain visible blood; (c) nonintact skin; and (d) mucous membranes. Routine practices or standard precautions are designed to reduce the risk of transmission of microorganisms from both recognized and

TABLE 17.8	**SUMMARY OF ROUTINE PRACTICES AND ADDITIONAL PRECAUTIONS FOR PREVENTING TRANSMISSION OF INFECTION IN HEALTH CARE**		
Routine Practices or Standard Precautions	**Additional or Transmission-Based Precautions**		
	Airborne*	**Droplet***	**Contact**
When to Use			
All patients	Used in addition to routine practices or standard precautions for patients known to be or suspected of being infected with microorganisms transmitted by airborne droplet (e.g., measles, varicella, tuberculosis). Requires negative-pressure room.	Used in addition to routine practices or standard precautions for patients known to be or suspected of being infected with microorganisms transmitted by droplets (e.g., *Haemophilus influenzae, Neisseria meningitidis, Streptococcus pneumoniae, Mycoplasma pneumoniae*, febrile respiratory illness)	Used in addition to routine practices or standard precautions for specified patients known to be or suspected of being infected with epidemiologically important microorganisms that can be transmitted by direct contact with patient or environmental surfaces (e.g., enteric pathogens, multidrug-resistant bacteria, *Clostridium difficile*, herpes simplex)
Hand Hygiene			
Hand hygiene (the removal or killing of microorganisms on the hands) is done either by handwashing or by use of alcohol-based hand rubs. Using alcohol-based hand rubs is more effective than washing hands (even with antibacterial soap) when hands are not visibly soiled. Hand hygiene should be performed (a) before initial patient contact or contact with the patient's environment, (b) before aseptic procedures, (c) after body fluid exposure risk, and (d) after contact with a patient or the patient's environment.	Same as routine practices or standard precautions	Same as routine practices or standard precautions	Same as routine practices or standard precautions
Gloves			
Nurses wear nonsterile gloves when touching blood, body fluids, secretions, excretions, and contaminated items; they put on clean gloves just before touching mucous membranes and nonintact skin. They remove gloves promptly after use, before touching noncontaminated items or environmental surfaces, or going to another patient.	Same as routine practices or standard precautions	Same as routine practices or standard precautions	In addition to glove use as described in routine practices or standard precautions, nurses wear gloves when entering the patient's room and whenever providing direct patient care or having hand contact with potentially contaminated surfaces or items in the patient's environment.
Mask, Eye Protection, Face Shield			
Nurses wear a mask and eye protection or face shield to protect mucous membranes of eyes, nose, and mouth during procedures and patient care activities likely to generate splashes or sprays of blood, body fluids, secretions, and excretions. These should be worn within 1 m of coughing patient.	In addition to routine practices or standard precautions, nurses wear respiratory protection when entering the room of a patient known to have or suspected of having tuberculosis. *Note:* Nurses should check the facility's policy for use of respirator.	In addition to routine practices or standard precautions, a mask should be worn.	Same as routine practices or standard precautions

TABLE 17.8 SUMMARY OF ROUTINE PRACTICES AND ADDITIONAL PRECAUTIONS FOR PREVENTING TRANSMISSION OF INFECTION IN HEALTH CARE—cont'd

Routine Practices or Standard Precautions	Additional or Transmission-Based Precautions		
	Airborne*	Droplet*	Contact
Gown Nurses wear a clean, nonsterile gown to protect skin and prevent soiling of clothing during procedures and patient care activities likely to generate splashes or sprays of blood, body fluids, secretions, or excretions or likely to cause soiling of clothing. The gown is removed promptly when tasks are completed; hands are washed.	Same as routine practices or standard precautions	Same as routine practices or standard precautions	A clean, nonsterile gown is worn if substantial contact is anticipated with the patient, surfaces, or items in the environment and if the patient is incontinent or has diarrhea, an ileostomy, a colostomy, or uncontained wound drainage. The gown is removed carefully when tasks are completed; hands are washed.
Linen Handle, transport, and process used linen in a manner that prevents skin and mucous membrane exposure, contamination of clothing, and environmental soiling.	Same as routine practices or standard precautions	Same as routine practices or standard precautions	Same as routine practices or standard precautions
Patient Transport	Movement and transport of a patient from their room should be limited to instances of essential purposes only; if transport or movement is necessary, patient dispersal of droplet nuclei is minimized by placement of a surgical mask on the patient, if possible.	Movement and transport of a patient from their room should be limited to instances of essential purposes only; if transport or movement is necessary, patient dispersal of droplet nuclei is minimized by placement of a surgical mask on the patient, if possible.	Movement and transport of a patient from their room should be limited to instances of essential purposes only; if transport is necessary, precautions are maintained to minimize contamination of environmental surfaces or equipment.

*In the case of certain infections (e.g., chicken pox and disseminated zoster), a combination of airborne and contact transmission precautions may be required. For certain other infections (e.g., influenza and invasive group A streptococci), a combination of droplet and contact precautions is required.
Source: © All rights reserved. Routine practices and additional precautions for preventing the transmission of infection in health care settings. Public Health Agency of Canada, 2013. Adapted and reproduced with permission from the Minister of Health, 2017.

unrecognized sources of infection in hospitals. Routine practices or standard precautions should be applied to all patients regardless of diagnosis or infection status.

Additional or transmission-based precautions are designed for patients suspected of or documented as being infected with highly transmissible or epidemiologically important pathogens for which additional precautions beyond routine practices or standard precautions are needed to interrupt transmission in hospitals. The three types of additional or transmission-based precautions are *airborne precautions, droplet precautions,* and *contact precautions.* They may be used in combination for diseases that have multiple routes of transmission. When used either by themselves or in combination, these precautions are used in addition to routine practices or standard precautions.

Preventing Occupational Infections in Health Care Workers. In 2002, Health Canada issued updated standards for preventing and controlling occupational infections in health care workers. These standards mandated that any employer whose employees are potentially exposed to blood from needles and other sharps must implement sharps safety devices wherever feasible. Many provinces have implemented mandatory use of safety-engineered needles and needle-free infusion devices. In addition, employees at risk need to be provided with appropriate PPE. Health care workers must minimize or eliminate exposure to infectious material. When that is not possible, appropriate PPE must be selected. These include gloves, clothing, and facial protection (Table 17.9). Appropriate PPE will vary, depending on the situation.

In the event that a health care worker is exposed to blood or body fluids, as a result of either a needle stick or a mucous membrane splash, the worker should seek immediate medical attention to assess the level of risk for acquiring a bloodborne virus from the incident and complete the appropriate facility critical incident report. Immediate management of an exposure includes allowing the wound to bleed freely, milking the wound if possible, then washing liberally with soap and water. For exposure to skin or mucous membranes, the area should be rinsed using water or saline solution. If the risk is deemed serious enough to put the worker at risk for acquiring HIV, postexposure prophylaxis is initiated. There is no postexposure prophylaxis for hepatitis C virus. Statistics have been compiled since the early 1990s about the rates of HIV seroconversion in health care workers as a result of an accidental exposure, and in fact, the rates are extremely low. However, cases have been documented, so it is important for nurses to use routine practices or standard precautions with every patient with whom they come into contact.

HUMAN IMMUNODEFICIENCY VIRUS INFECTION

The HIV epidemic in Canada and the United States began in the early 1980s. HIV had been circulating in sub-Saharan Africa since the early 1920s (Pepin, 2011), but it was not until 1981 that public health officials documented the presence of a new disease that would become known as the acquired immunodeficiency syndrome (AIDS). Interestingly, people had been dying

TABLE 17.9	HEALTH CANADA RECOMMENDATIONS FOR USE OF PERSONAL PROTECTIVE EQUIPMENT FOR HEALTH CARE WORKERS
Equipment	**Indications for Use**
Medical gloves	Should be worn for all procedures that might involve direct skin or mucous membrane contact with blood or fluids capable of transmitting bloodborne pathogens. May also be indicated for other activities (e.g., procedures involving other infectious agents, toxins, or contaminated equipment).
Masks and protective eyewear (e.g., goggles, safety glasses) or face shields	Should be worn to protect mucous membranes, nonintact skin, and conjunctiva during procedures that are likely to generate splashes of blood or fluids capable of transmitting bloodborne pathogens.
Gowns or aprons	Should be worn during procedures that are likely to generate splashes of blood or fluids capable of transmitting bloodborne pathogens. Assessment of the specific risk will determine the type of gown required (e.g., fluid-resistant).

of AIDS in North America for several decades before it was identified. This first documented case in Canada was in 1959. By 1985, the causative agent, HIV, had been identified, and AIDS was determined to be the end stage of chronic HIV infection. In addition, an antibody test was developed and routes of transmission were determined. Medication therapy to treat the infection became available in 1987 with the release of zidovudine (ZDV, azidothymidine [AZT], Retrovir) and has since expanded. Since 1994, several important advances have been made, including the development of laboratory tests to assess the number of HIV particles in the blood (viral load), the production of new medications, combination medication therapy, the ability to test for antiretroviral medication resistance, treatment to decrease the risk of transmission from mother to baby (Clinical Info.HIV.gov, 2021), the introduction of pre-exposure prophylaxis to prevent HIV acquisition in high-risk individuals, and the use of treatment as prevention (Amico, 2018). In developed countries around the world, these advances have led to significant decreases in the number of HIV-related deaths, improved quality of life, and decreases in the number of cases of congenital HIV infection. Unfortunately, these advances are not effective or available for all people who need them. Although great progress has been made, the HIV epidemic is not over. There are signs that it is levelling off, with fewer new infections each year, but it continues to take its toll, inasmuch as approximately 1.5 million people became newly infected with HIV in 2020 (United Nations AIDS [UNAIDS], 2021). Nursing care for patients with HIV infection continues to be a critical need that will change as new findings and treatment advances emerge.

Significance of the Epidemic

Approximately 37.7 million people were living with HIV globally in 2020. Although there was an estimated 1.5 million new HIV infections diagnosed in 2020, this is a 52% reduction since 1997. Similarly, AIDS-related deaths in 2020 were approximately 680 000; this is a 47% reduction since 1997 (UNAIDS, 2021). In 2015, Saskatchewan faced an HIV epidemic with a 43% annual increase in new HIV diagnoses, 79% of which occurred in Indigenous communities (Government of Saskatchewan, 2017). It is important to consider how inequities in social determinants of health, history of colonial violence, and intergenerational trauma have resulted in the disproportionate numbers of HIV cases in the Canadian Indigenous population and to develop resources to address this health crisis.

Globally, the scale of HIV infection has been devastating. Since the beginning of the pandemic, more than 70 million people have been infected, and more than 30 million of those people have died (UNAIDS, 2021). The burden of HIV is not evenly distributed. Since the beginning of the epidemic, sub-Saharan Africa has been the most devastated, but Asia, Russia, India, Central America, and South America also have rampant epidemics. In developing countries, the major mode of transmission is through heterosexual sex, and women and children bear a large part of the burden of illness. Industrialized countries have fared better but have not been able to eliminate the infection or provide appropriate care to all HIV-infected individuals. For the most part, HIV infection remains a disease of marginalized individuals: those who are disenfranchised by virtue of sex, race, sexual orientation, poverty, drug use, or lack of access to health care.

Transmission of Human Immunodeficiency Virus

HIV is a fragile virus. It can be transmitted only under specific conditions that allow contact with infected body fluids, including blood, semen, vaginal secretions, and breast milk. HIV is transmitted through sexual intercourse with an infected partner, exposure to HIV-infected blood or blood products, as a result of either contaminated transfusion or needle sharing, and perinatally at the time of delivery or through breastfeeding (CDC, 2020).

HIV-infected individuals can transmit HIV to others within a few days after becoming infected. After that, the ability to transmit HIV is lifelong. Transmission of HIV is subject to the same requirements as other microorganisms: A large enough amount of the virus must enter the body of a susceptible host. Duration and frequency of contact, volume of fluid, virulence and concentration of the organism, and host immune status all affect whether infection actually occurs after an exposure. The viral load in the blood, semen, vaginal secretions, or breast milk of the "donor" is an important variable. In HIV infection, large amounts of virus can be found in the blood during the first 2 to 6 months after infection and again during the late stages of the disease (Figure 17.1). Unprotected sexual or blood exposure to an infected individual is more risky during these periods, although HIV can be transmitted during all phases of the disease (CDC, 2020). Throughout 2010–2018, the groundbreaking PARTNER 1 and 2 studies demonstrated definitively that when a person has sustained viral suppression, they cannot transmit HIV to a sexual partner (Harries & Takarinda, 2019). In 2020, the World Health Organization (WHO) endorsed this campaign "U = U," which stands for "undetectable = untransmittable." However, there is still a vast amount of misinformation about HIV transmission, which often leads to social discrimination against people living with HIV.

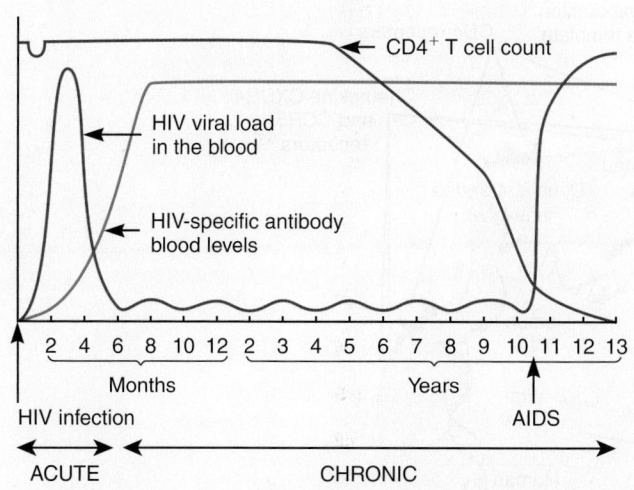

FIG. 17.1 Viral load in the blood and CD4+ T cell counts across the spectrum of untreated human immunodeficiency virus (HIV) infection. *AIDS,* acquired immune deficiency syndrome.

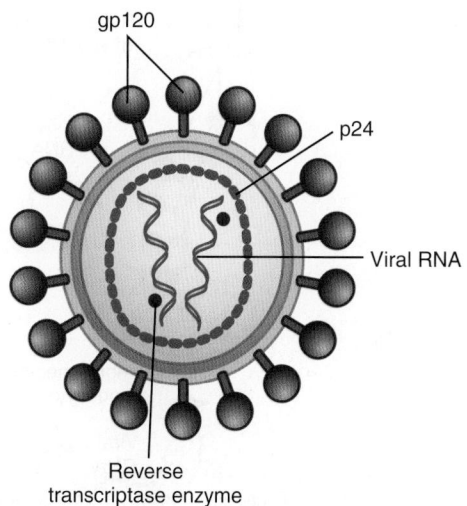

FIG. 17.2 The human immunodeficiency virus (HIV) is surrounded by an envelope made up of proteins (including glycoprotein 120 [gp120]) and contains a core of viral RNA and proteins (including p24).

HIV is not spread casually. The virus cannot be transmitted through hugging, dry kissing, shaking hands, sharing eating utensils, using toilet seats, or attending school or working with an HIV-infected person. It is not transmitted through tears, saliva, urine, emesis, sputum, feces, or sweat. Repeated studies have failed to demonstrate transmission of the virus by respiratory droplets, enteric routes, or casual encounters in any setting. Health care workers have a very low risk of acquiring HIV at work, even after a needle-stick injury (Kuhar et al., 2013). Should a health care worker become exposed, they should follow hospital policy for reporting needle-stick incidents.

Sexual Transmission. The most common mode of HIV transmission is unprotected sexual contact with an HIV-infected partner. Sexual activity involves contact with semen, vaginal secretions, blood, or a combination of these, all of which have lymphocytes that may contain HIV. During any form of sexual intercourse (anal, vaginal, or oral), the risk of infection is greater for the partner who receives the semen, although infection can also be transmitted to the inserting partner. This occurs because the receiver has prolonged contact with infected fluids, and it helps explain why it is easier to infect women than men during heterosexual intercourse. Sexual activities that cause trauma to local tissues can increase the risk of transmission. In addition, genital lesions from other sexually transmitted infections (STIs, e.g., herpes, syphilis) significantly increase the likelihood of HIV transmission.

Contact With Blood and Blood Products. HIV is transmitted by exposure to contaminated blood through the accidental or intended sharing of injection equipment. Sharing equipment to inject illegal drugs is a major means of transmission in many large metropolitan areas and is becoming more common in smaller cities and rural areas. Once used, equipment used to inject any drug, whether prescribed or not, is contaminated, potentially with HIV, other bloodborne organisms, or both, and sharing that equipment can result in disease transmission.

In Canada, an estimated 1 150 individuals were infected with HIV through blood transfusions between 1978 and 1985. In 1985, the practices of routine screening of blood donors to identify at-risk individuals and testing donated blood for the presence of HIV were implemented, which improved the safety of the blood supply. HIV infection as a result of blood transfusions is now rare. In 2001, a new, highly sensitive nucleic acid amplification test (NAAT) was implemented by the Canadian Blood Services to detect HIV genetic material in blood of potential donors. The NAAT has a much shorter window period—the time between exposure to HIV infection and when the test yields an accurate result—than does antibody testing and is now the standard test for donated blood in Canada.

Puncture wounds are the most common means of work-related transmission. The risk of infection after a needle-stick exposure to HIV-infected blood is 0.3% to 0.4% (or 3–4 in 1 000). The risk is higher if the exposure involves blood from a patient with a high viral load, from a deep puncture wound, from a needle with a hollow bore and visible blood, from a device used for venous or arterial access, or from a patient who dies within 60 days. Splash exposure of blood on skin with an open lesion presents some risk, but it is much lower than from a puncture wound (HIV.gov, 2021; PHAC, 2016b).

Perinatal Transmission. Perinatal transmission from an HIV-infected mother to her infant can occur during pregnancy, giving birth, or breastfeeding (CDC, 2021; PHAC, 2011). On average, 25% of infants born to women with untreated HIV infection are born with HIV. Fortunately, the risk of transmission can be reduced to less than 1% in settings where pregnant women are routinely tested for HIV infection. There is a 1 in 1 000 chance of transmitting HIV to a fetus during pregnancy and delivery, when the mother is on antiretroviral treatment (ART) and has a viral load below 50 copies/mL (undetectable) (Beste et al., 2018; Siemieniuk et al., 2017).

Pathophysiology

Human immunodeficiency virus (HIV) is a retrovirus, meaning it carries a single-stranded RNA as its genetic material as opposed to double-stranded DNA cells. It also has the enzyme reverse transcriptase, which allows it to copy RNA into DNA and use that DNA to "copy" to infect human, or host, cells (International Partnership for Microbicides, 2020). HIV cannot replicate unless it is inside a living cell. HIV can enter a cell when the glycoprotein 120 (gp120) "knobs" (Figure 17.2) on

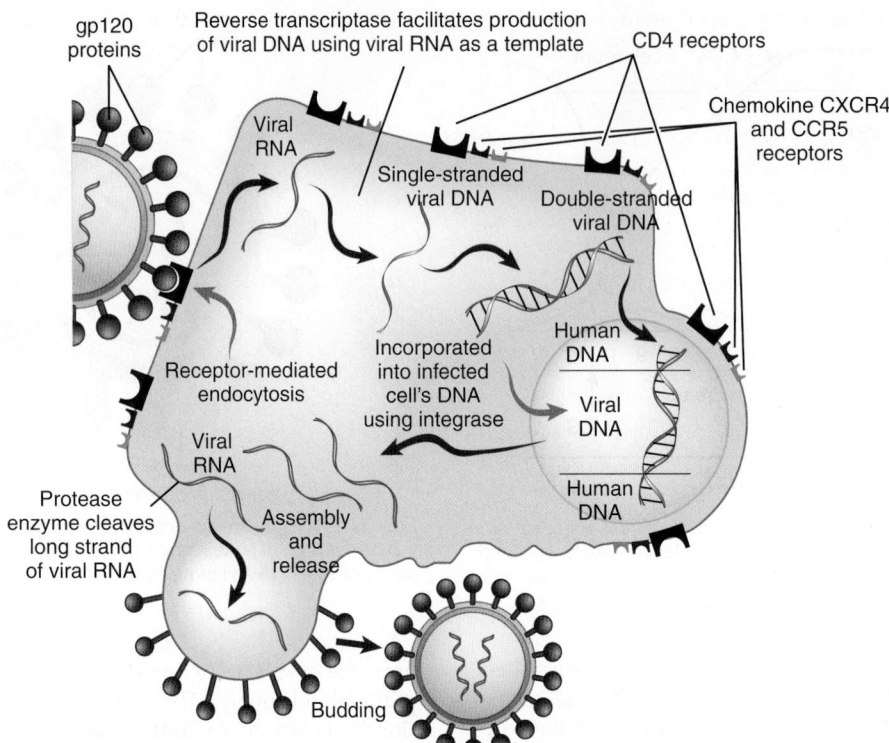

FIG. 17.3 The human immunodeficiency virus (HIV) has glycoprotein 120 (gp120) that attaches to CD4 and chemokine CXCR4 and CCR5 receptors on the surface of CD4⁺ T cells. Viral RNA then enters the cell, produces viral DNA in the presence of reverse transcriptase, and incorporates itself into the cellular genome in the presence of integrase, causing permanent cellular infection and the production of new virions. New viral RNA develops initially in long strands that are cut in the presence of protease and leave the cell through a budding process that ultimately contributes to cellular destruction.

the viral envelope and binds to specific CD4 receptor sites and CCR5 and CXCR4 co-receptor sites on the cell's surface (Figure 17.3). Once bound, viral genetic material enters the cell. In the cell, viral RNA is transcribed into a double strand of viral DNA with the assistance of **reverse transcriptase**, an enzyme made by HIV and other retroviruses. At this point, viral DNA can enter the cell's nucleus and, using an enzyme called *integrase*, splice itself into the genome, becoming a permanent part of the cell's genetic structure. There are two consequences of this action: (a) because all genetic material is replicated during cellular division, all daughter cells from the infected cell will also be infected, and (b) because the genome now contains viral DNA, the cell's genetic codes can direct the cell to make HIV. Production of HIV within the cell is a complicated process that results in long strands of HIV RNA. These are cut into appropriate lengths with the assistance of the enzyme protease during the budding sequence (HIVinfo.NIH.gov, 2019).

Initial infection with HIV results in **viremia** (large amounts of virus in the blood). This is followed within a few weeks by a prolonged period during which HIV levels in the blood remain low even without treatment (see Figure 17.1). During this time, which may last for 10 to 12 years, there are few clinical symptoms. It was initially thought that this phase represented a latency period during which very little viral activity occurred. It is now known that HIV replication occurs at rapid and constant rates in the blood and lymph tissues from early in the infection. A steady-state viral load can be maintained in the body of infected individuals for many years. To do this, 108 to 109 new viruses are produced each day. A major consequence of rapid replication is that errors can occur in the copying process,

causing mutations that can contribute to resistance to ART and limit treatment options.

In a normal immune response, foreign antigens interact with B cells and T cells. In the initial stages of HIV infection, these cells respond and function normally. B cells make HIV-specific antibodies that are effective in reducing viral loads in the blood, and activated T cells mount a cellular immune response to viruses trapped in the lymph nodes (HIVinfo.NIH.gov, 2019).

HIV infects human cells whose surfaces have CD4 receptors. These cells include lymphocytes, monocytes and macrophages, astrocytes, and oligodendrocytes. Immune dysfunction in HIV disease is caused predominantly by damage to and destruction of CD4⁺ T cells (also known as T helper cells or CD4⁺ T lymphocytes). These cells are targeted because they have more CD4 receptors on their surfaces than do other CD4 receptor–bearing cells. This is unfortunate because CD4⁺ T cells play a key role in the ability of the immune system to recognize and defend against pathogens.

Adults without immune dysfunction normally have 800 to 1 200 CD4⁺ T cells per microlitre of blood. The normal lifespan of a CD4⁺ T cell is about 100 days, but HIV-infected CD4⁺ T cells die after an average of only 2 days. The compromise of the immune system is also caused by the chronic state of immune activation that is a result of HIV infection. This activation leads to elevated levels of inflammatory markers and destruction of T helper cells.

Viral activity destroys about 1 billion CD4⁺ T cells every day. Fortunately, the bone marrow and the thymus are able to produce enough CD4⁺ T cells to replace the destroyed cells for many years. Eventually, however, the ability of HIV to destroy CD4⁺ T cells exceeds the body's ability to replace the cells. The result is a decline in the CD4⁺ T-cell count and a decrease in immune capability. In general, the immune system remains healthy with more than 500 CD4+ T cells per microlitre. Difficulties with immunity start to occur when the count drops below this number. Severe health problems develop with fewer than 200 CD4+ T cells per microlitre and a CD4 fraction of less than 15%. Eventually in HIV infection, so many CD4+ T cells are destroyed that not enough remain to regulate immune responses (see Figure 17.1). The major concern related to immune suppression is the development of opportunistic diseases (infections and cancers that occur in immunosuppressed patients that can lead to disability, disease, and death).

Clinical Manifestations and Complications

The typical course of untreated HIV infection follows the pattern shown in Figure 17.4. However, it is important to remember that HIV is highly individualized. The information depicted in Figure 17.4 represents data from large groups of people and should not be used to predict an individual's lifespan after HIV infection.

Acute Infection. Development of HIV-specific antibodies *(seroconversion)* is frequently accompanied by a flulike syndrome of fever, swollen lymph glands, sore throat, headache, malaise, nausea, muscle and joint pain, diarrhea, a diffuse rash, or a combination of these. These symptoms, called acute retroviral syndrome (seroconversion illness), generally occur 1 to 3 weeks after the initial infection and last for 1 to 2 weeks, although some of the symptoms may continue for several months. During this time, a high level of HIV in the blood occurs, and CD4+ T-cell counts fall temporarily but quickly return to baseline (see Figure 17.1). In most infected people, acute retroviral symptoms are moderate and may be mistaken for a cold or flu. In rare cases, neurological complications, such as aseptic meningitis, peripheral neuropathy, facial palsy, or Guillain-Barré syndrome, have developed (Hoenigl et al., 2016).

Chronic Infection

Early Chronic Infection. The median interval between untreated HIV infection and a diagnosis of AIDS is about 10 years. During this time, CD4+ T-lymphocyte counts remain above 500 cells per microlitre (normal) or slightly decreased, and the viral load in the blood remains low. This phase has been referred to as *asymptomatic disease,* but fatigue, headache, low-grade fever, night sweats, persistent generalized lymphadenopathy, and other symptoms often occur.

Because most of the symptoms during early infection are vague and nonspecific for HIV, people with HIV infection may not be aware that they are infected. According to the PHAC (2021), approximately 13% of individuals infected with HIV are estimated to be unaware of their status. During this time, infected people continue activities that may include high-risk sexual and drug-using behaviours, which creates a public health problem because infected people can transmit HIV to others even if they have no symptoms. Personal health is also affected because people who do not know they are infected are unaware of the need to seek treatment and may have a poorer prognosis.

Intermediate Chronic Infection. When the CD4+ T-cell count drops below 500 cells per microlitre (as low as 200 cells per microlitre), the viral load rises, and HIV infection advances to a more active stage. Symptoms and signs that occurred in earlier phases tend to become worse, manifesting as persistent fever, frequent drenching night sweats, chronic diarrhea, recurrent headaches, and fatigue severe enough to interrupt normal routines. Other health issues that may occur at this time include localized infections, lymphadenopathy, and nervous system manifestations.

The most common infection associated with this phase of HIV disease is oropharyngeal candidiasis, or thrush (Figure 17.5). *Candida* organisms rarely cause problems in healthy adults, but such problems do occur in most HIV-infected people at some time. Other infections that can occur at this time include shingles (caused by the varicella-zoster virus), persistent vaginal candidal infections, outbreaks of oral or genital herpes, bacterial infections, and Kaposi's sarcoma (Figure 17.6). Oral hairy leukoplakia, an Epstein-Barr virus infection that causes painless, white, raised lesions on the lateral aspect of the tongue, can also occur (Figure 17.7). Oral lesions may provide the earliest indication of HIV infection.

Late Chronic Infection or Acquired Immune Deficiency Syndrome. A diagnosis of AIDS cannot be made until the HIV-infected patient meets the criteria established by the WHO (2007). These criteria (Table 17.10) are more likely to occur when the immune system becomes severely compromised. As the viral load increases, the absolute number and percentage of

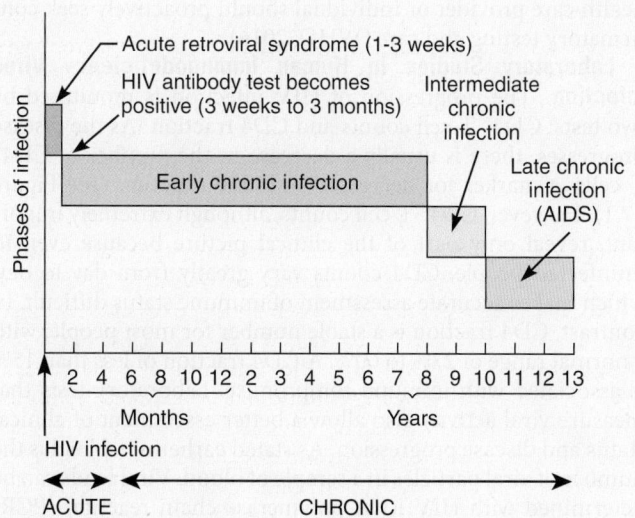

FIG. 17.4 Timeline for the spectrum of untreated human immunodeficiency virus (HIV) infection. The timeline represents the course of the illness from the time of infection to the clinical manifestations of disease. *AIDS,* acquired immune deficiency syndrome.

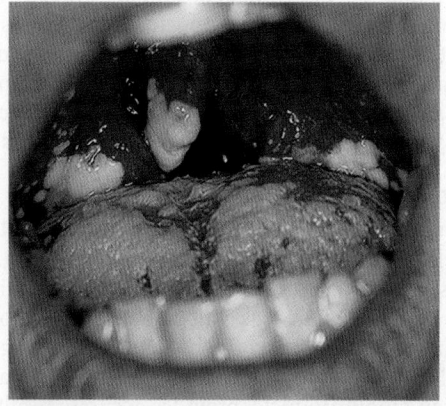

FIG. 17.5 Oral thrush involving the hard and soft palate surfaces. Source: Emond, R., Welsby, P., & Rowland, H. (2003). *Colour atlas of infectious diseases* (4th ed.). Mosby.

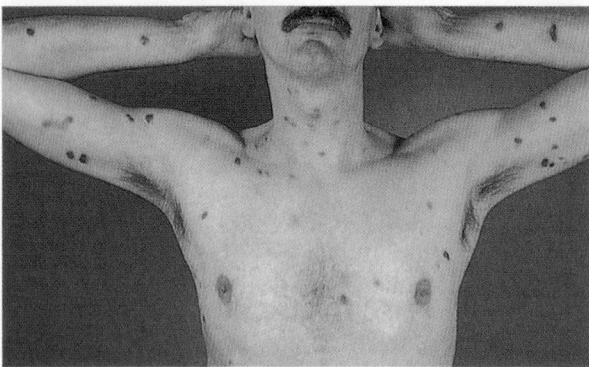

FIG. 17.6 Kaposi's sarcoma: malignant vascular lesion on the torso. The lesions can appear anywhere on the skin surface and on internal organs. Lesions vary in size from pinpoint to very large (several centimetres) and may appear in a variety of shades. Source: Courtesy of Jeffrey Kwong.

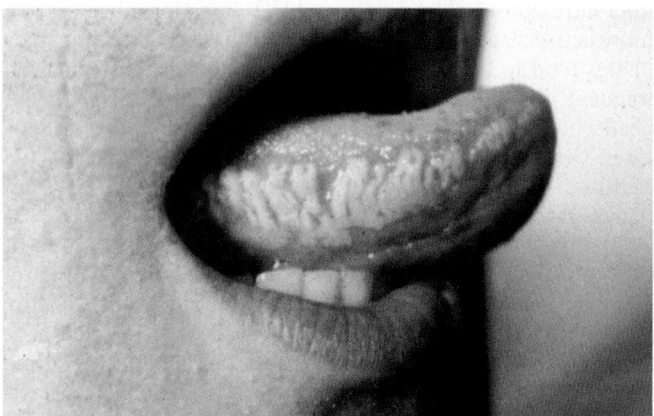

FIG. 17.7 Oral hairy leukoplakia on the lateral aspect of the tongue. Source: Set of slides published in 1992 by Jon Fuller, MD, and Howard Libman, MD, at Boston University School of Medicine, Boston.

TABLE 17.10	**DIAGNOSTIC CRITERIA FOR AIDS**

AIDS is diagnosed when an individual with HIV infection has a CD4 count of under 200 and develops at least one of these conditions:
- Atypical disseminated leishmaniasis
- Central nervous system toxoplasmosis
- Chronic cryptosporidiosis
- Chronic herpes simplex virus infection
- Chronic isosporiasis
- Cytomegalovirus disease (other than liver, spleen, or lymph nodes)
- Disseminated mycosis (coccidiomycosis or histoplasmosis)
- Disseminated nontuberculous mycobacterial infection
- Esophageal candidiasis
- Extrapulmonary cryptococcosis (including meningitis)
- Extrapulmonary tuberculosis
- HIV encephalopathy
- HIV wasting syndrome (*wasting* is defined as a loss of 10% or more of ideal body mass)
- Invasive cervical carcinoma
- Kaposi's sarcoma
- Lymphoma (cerebral or B-cell non-Hodgkin's)
- *Pneumocystis* pneumonia
- Progressive multifocal leukoencephalopathy
- Recurrent bacterial pneumonia
- Recurrent nontyphoid *Salmonella* bacteremia
- Symptomatic HIV-associated cardiomyopathy
- Symptomatic HIV-associated nephropathy

AIDS, acquired immune deficiency syndrome; *HIV*, human immunodeficiency virus. Source: World Health Organization. (2007). WHO case definitions of HIV for surveillance and revised clinical staging and immunological classification of HIV-related disease in adults and children. http://www.who.int/hiv/pub/guidelines/HIVstaging150307.pdf

T cells decrease and the risk of developing opportunistic diseases increases.

Opportunistic diseases, often reactivations of a prior infection, generally do not occur in the presence of a functioning immune system. Numerous infections, a variety of malignancies, wasting, and dementia can result from HIV-related immune impairment (Table 17.11). Organisms that do not usually cause disease in people with functioning immune systems can cause severe, debilitating, disseminated, and life-threatening infections during this stage. Several opportunistic diseases are likely to occur at the same time, further compounding the difficulties of diagnosis and treatment. Advances in HIV treatment have led to significant decreases in opportunistic diseases because successful treatment helps maintain the immune system's function.

Drug Therapy

Diagnosis of Human Immunodeficiency Virus Infection.

HIV testing technologies have come a long way in recent years. Previous tests used to diagnose HIV detected HIV antibodies in the blood. However, there was a median delay of 2 months after infection before antibodies could be detected (see Figure 17.1). The early NAAT/RNA test, described earlier as the standard for all Canadian blood products, provides accurate results as early as 7 days after exposure and may be available in some areas of Canada when acute infection is suspected. However, this test is

rarely used, as it is not cost-effective and the fourth-generation enzyme immunoassay (EIA) is highly accurate. It is important to understand window periods because in an infected individual, an HIV antibody test will not yield positive results during this time even though the individual is infected. Rapid tests are third-generation screening tools discussed in Table 17.12. There are two types of rapid HIV tests approved for use in Canada: the point-of-care (POC) test and the self-test. These rapid tests involve collection of saliva, blood, or urine samples. The sample is applied to the HIV testing device and results are obtained within minutes. Upon confirmation of positive test results, the health care provider or individual should proactively seek confirmatory testing and care (WHO, 2016).

Laboratory Studies in Human Immunodeficiency Virus Infection.

The progression of HIV infection is monitored by two tests: CD4+ T-cell counts and CD4 fraction. As the disease progresses, there is usually a decrease in the number of CD4+ T cells, a marker for decreased immune function (see Figure 17.1). However, CD4+ T-cell counts, although extremely important, reveal only part of the clinical picture because even in uninfected people, CD4 counts vary greatly from day to day, which makes accurate assessment of immune status difficult. In contrast, CD4 fraction is a stable number for most people, with a normal range of 27% to 60%. A CD4 fraction of less than 15% is associated with immune compromise. Laboratory tests that measure viral activity also allow a better assessment of clinical status and disease progression. As stated earlier, viral load is the number of viral particles in a sample of blood. Viral loads can be determined with HIV RNA polymerase chain reaction (PCR) or branched-chain DNA (bDNA) tests. Viral load is reported either as less than 40 copies per millilitre, as a definitive number between 40 and 10 million, or as more than 10 million. These tests provide information that helps determine the efficacy of

TABLE 17.11 MEDICATION THERAPY

Manifestations and Treatment of Common Opportunistic Diseases Associated With HIV Infection

Organism and Disease	Clinical Manifestations	Prophylaxis* and Treatment†
Candida albicans	Thrush, esophagitis, vaginitis; whitish yellow patches in mouth, esophagus, GI tract, vagina	*Treatment:* fluconazole (Diflucan), clotrimazole, nystatin, itraconazole (Sporanox); if infection is resistant to fluconazole: amphotericin B (Fungizone) *Secondary prophylaxis* (only if subsequent episodes are frequent or severe recurrences): fluconazole (Diflucan), itraconazole (Sporanox)
Castleman's disease (caused by HHV-8)	Generalized malaise, night sweats, rigors, fever, anorexia, weight loss Eventually lymphadenopathy, hepatosplenomegaly, ascites, edema, pulmonary and pericardial effusions	*Treatment:* antivirals such as IV ganciclovir (Cytovene) or oral valganciclovir (Valcyte) Chemotherapy, either single drug or combined: the CHOP protocol is most recommended
Cervical cancer	Cancerous lesions in the cervix Vaginal bleeding, pain during intercourse	Surgical excision of the cancerous lesion Chemotherapy Radiotherapy
Coccidioides immitis	Pneumonia: fever, weight loss, cough	*Treatment:* amphotericin B (Fungizone), fluconazole (Diflucan), itraconazole (Sporanox) *Secondary prophylaxis* (to prevent recurrence of documented disease): fluconazole (Diflucan), amphotericin B (Fungizone), itraconazole (Sporanox)
CNS lymphoma	Cognitive dysfunction, motor impairment, aphasia, seizures, personality changes, headache	*Treatment:* radiation, chemotherapy
Cryptococcus neoformans	Meningitis, cognitive impairment, motor dysfunction, fever, seizures, headache	*Treatment:* amphotericin B (Fungizone), fluconazole (Diflucan), itraconazole (Sporanox) *Secondary prophylaxis* (to prevent recurrence of documented disease): fluconazole (Diflucan), amphotericin B (Fungizone), itraconazole (Sporanox) Therapeutic lumbar punctures to reduce intracranial pressure
Cryptosporidium muris	Gastroenteritis, watery diarrhea, abdominal pain, weight loss	*Treatment:* antidiarrheals, nitazoxanide (Alinia), paromomycin (Humatin)
CMV	Retinitis: retinal lesions, blurred vision, loss of vision Esophagitis, stomatitis: difficulty swallowing; colitis, gastritis: bloody diarrhea, pain, weight loss Pneumonitis: respiratory symptoms Neurological disease: CNS manifestations	*Treatment:* ganciclovir (Cytovene), foscarnet (Foscavir), cidofovir (Vistide), valganciclovir (Valcyte) *Secondary prophylaxis* (to prevent recurrence of documented disease): ganciclovir (Cytovene), foscarnet (Foscavir), cidofovir (Vistide), valganciclovir (Valcyte)
Hepatitis B virus (HBV)	Jaundice, fatigue, abdominal pain, loss of appetite, nausea, vomiting, joint pain; 30% of affected patients may have no signs or symptoms	*Primary prevention:* HBV vaccine series; screening and vaccination of people with no evidence of previous HBV infection; encouragement of patients to disclose injection drug use, whether they are sexually active men who have sex with men, sexual partners or household contacts of HBV-infected individuals, and those with HCV; HAV vaccine series should be given to prevent additive effects and advanced liver damage; screening and vaccination of people without evidence of previous HAV infection *Treatment:* adefovir dipivoxil (Hepsera), α-interferon, lamivudine (3TC), entecavir (Baraclude)
Hepatitis C virus (HCV)	Jaundice, fatigue, abdominal pain, loss of appetite, nausea, vomiting, dark urine; 80% may have no signs or symptoms	*Prophylaxis:* none for HCV; HAV and HBV vaccines series should be given to prevent additive effects and advanced liver damage; screening and vaccination of people without evidence of previous HAV or HBV infection *Treatment:* α-interferon, ribavirin (Virazole), boceprevir (Victrelis)
Herpes simplex virus (HSV)	Type 1 (HSV1): orolabial and mucocutaneous vesicular and ulcerative lesions; keratitis: visual disturbances; encephalitis: CNS manifestations Type 2 (HSV2): genital and perianal vesicular and ulcerative lesions	*Treatment:* acyclovir (Zovirax), famciclovir (Famvir), valacyclovir (Valtrex), foscarnet (Foscavir), cidofovir (Vistide) *Secondary prophylaxis* (only if subsequent episodes are frequent or severe): acyclovir (Zovirax), famciclovir (Famvir), valacyclovir (Valtrex)
Histoplasma capsulatum	Pneumonia: fever, cough, weight loss Meningitis: CNS manifestations; disseminated disease	*Treatment:* amphotericin B (Fungizone), itraconazole (Sporanox), fluconazole (Diflucan) *Secondary prophylaxis* (to prevent recurrence of documented disease): itraconazole (Sporanox), amphotericin B (Fungizone)
Influenza virus	Fever (usually high, 38°C–40°C), headache, extreme tiredness, dry cough, sore throat, runny or stuffy nose, muscle aches; nausea, vomiting, and diarrhea can occur	*Primary prevention:* inactivated trivalent influenza virus vaccine; provided annually, before influenza virus season; revaccination if initial vaccine was given when CD4+ T cell count was <200/mcL *Treatment:* supportive therapy
JC papovavirus	Progressive multifocal leukoencephalopathy, CNS manifestations, mental and motor declines	*Treatment:* supportive therapy

Continued

TABLE 17.11 MEDICATION THERAPY

Manifestations and Treatment of Common Opportunistic Diseases Associated With HIV Infection—cont'd

Organism and Disease	Clinical Manifestations	Prophylaxis* and Treatment†
Kaposi's sarcoma (caused by HHV-8)	Vascular lesions on the skin, mucous membranes, and viscera, with wide range of presentation: firm, flat, raised, or nodular; pinpoint to several centimetres in size; hyperpigmented, multicentric; can cause lymphedema and disfigurement, particularly when confluent; not usually serious unless it occurs in the respiratory or GI systems	*Treatment* (dependent on severity of lesions): cancer chemotherapy, α-interferon, local irradiation; cryotherapy for skin lesions
Mycobacterium avium complex	Gastroenteritis, watery diarrhea, weight loss	*Primary prophylaxis* (initiate when CD4+ T cell count is <50/mcL): clarithromycin (Biaxin) or azithromycin (Zithromax), rifabutin (Mycobutin). Prophylaxis may be stopped when CD4+ T cell count of >100/mcL is documented for 6–12 mo; restarted if CD4+ T cell count falls to <50/mcL. Disseminated disease or TB must be ruled out. *Treatment:* clarithromycin (Biaxin), ethambutol (Etibi), rifabutin (Mycobutin), azithromycin (Zithromax), ciprofloxacin (Cipro), levofloxacin (Levaquin), amikacin
Multicentric Castleman's disease (caused by HHV-8)	Fever, anemia, elevated C-reactive protein levels, widespread lymphadenopathy, weight loss, respiratory symptoms, edema, pulmonary and pericardial effusions and splenomegaly	*Treatment:* ganciclovir (Cytovene), systemic chemotherapy (CHOP) and rituximab (Rituxan)
Mycobacterium tuberculosis	Respiratory and disseminated disease; productive cough, fever, night sweats, weight loss	See Chapter 30 (first-line medication therapy for TB; [see Table 30.6], medication regimen options for treatment of TB [see Table 30.7])
Pneumocystis jiroveci pneumonia	Pneumonia, nonproductive cough, hypoxemia, progressive shortness of breath, fever, night sweats, fatigue	*Primary prophylaxis:* initiate when CD4+ T cell count is <200/mcL: TMP/SMX (Septra), dapsone, dapsone with pyrimethamine, folinic acid, aerosolized pentamidine, atovaquone (Mepron). Adverse effects of TMP/SMX and dapsone (especially rash, fever, and anemia) are common and may limit use. *Treatment:* TMP/SMX, pentamidine, dapsone, trimethoprim, clindamycin, primaquine, atovaquone (Mepron); with hypoxia, use corticosteroids
Toxoplasma gondii	Encephalitis, cognitive dysfunction, motor impairment, fever, altered mental status, headache, seizures, sensory abnormalities	*Primary prophylaxis:* (1) TMP/SMX *or* (2) dapsone + pyrimethamine + leukovorin *or* (3) atovaquone ± pyrimethamine + leucovorin *Treatment:* (1) sulphadiazine *or* (2) clindamycin + pyrimethamine + leukovorin *or* (3) atovaquone + pyrimethamine + leukovorin *or* (4) azithromycin + pyrimethamine + leukovorin
Varicella-zoster virus (VZV)	Shingles: erythematous maculopapular rash along dermatomal planes, pain, pruritus Ocular: progressive outer retinal necrosis	*Primary prophylaxis:* varicella-zoster immune globulin administered only after significant exposure to chicken pox or shingles for patients with no history of disease or negative result of VZV antibody test *Treatment:* acyclovir (Zovirax), famciclovir (Famvir), valacyclovir (Valtrex)

*If available. In most cases, effective antiretroviral therapy is the best prevention for all opportunistic diseases.

†In most cases, adequate antiretroviral therapy is the best treatment for all opportunistic diseases.

CHOP, cyclophosphamide, hydroxydaunomycin, Oncovin, prednisone; *CMV,* cytomegalovirus; *CNS,* central nervous system; *GI,* gastrointestinal; *HAV,* hepatitis A virus; *HHV-8,* human herpesvirus 8; *HIV,* human immunodeficiency virus; *IgG,* immunoglobulin G; *IV,* intravenous; *JC,* "John Cunningham" virus; *TB,* tuberculosis; *TMP/SMX,* trimethoprim-sulphamethoxazole.

Source: Data from British Columbia Centre for Excellence in HIV/AIDS. (2009). *Therapeutic guidelines for opportunistic infections.* www.cfenet.ubc.ca/sites/default/files/uploads/docs/Opportunistic_Infection_Therapeutic_Guidelines2009.pdf

therapy, treatment adherence, and whether clinical goals are being met.

Various abnormal results of laboratory tests of the blood are common in untreated HIV infection and may be caused by HIV, opportunistic diseases, or complications of medication or radiation therapy. The white blood cell count is often decreased, especially neutrophil counts (neutropenia); low platelet counts (thrombocytopenia) may be caused by antiplatelet antibodies or medication therapy; and anemia is associated with the chronic disease process, as well as with common adverse effects of some of the antiretroviral agents. Altered results of liver function tests are common. These may be caused by disease processes or medication therapy and may be more common with newer medication therapy. Co-infection with hepatitis B virus (HBV)

or hepatitis C virus must be identified early because these infections may have a more serious course in a patient with HIV infection and may limit options for ART.

It is now possible to test for resistance to antiretroviral medications in people being treated for HIV infection. Two types of assays are used: genotype and phenotype. The *genotype assay* detects drug-resistant viral mutations that are present in the reverse transcriptase and protease genes. The *phenotype assay* is a measure of the growth of the virus in various concentrations of antiretroviral medications (much like bacteria–antibiotic sensitivity tests). These assays are especially useful in making decisions about new medication combinations in patients who are not responding to their current therapies. Genotyping is usually done before the patient starts their first treatment regimen

TABLE 17.12 HIV RAPID TESTING TYPES

Rapid HIV Testing Currently Approved for Use in Canada	

Point-of-Care (POC) Testing
• INSTI HIV-1/HIV-2 antibody test
• Performed in clinic setting
Self-Testing
• INSTI HIV Self Test
• Allows individuals to self-test themselves for HIV
	Results
	• Capillary blood sample
	• Results available within minutes
	• A reactive test result which indicates that a person has HIV
	  • Negative test indicates no further testing required
	  • Positive test requires further testing for diagnostic purposes (public health testing)

Source: CATIE (2020). *HIV testing technologies.* https://www.catie.ca/en/fact-sheets/testing/hiv-testing-technologies

because it is possible to acquire resistant virus. The PHAC (2015b) has estimated that approximately 9.8% of infected individuals have resistant virus at the time of infection.

Another test that is frequently done before patients begin ART is a human leukocyte antigen (HLA) B5701 antigen test. If this test result is positive, the patient will probably have a hypersensitivity to abacavir (Ziagen), one of the nucleoside reverse transcriptase inhibitors.

A test that may be performed is therapeutic medication monitoring. This test is indicated for patients who continue to have replicating virus in the presence of ART without evidence of nonadherence. It indicates whether the patient is effectively metabolizing their ART regimen and has a therapeutic level of medication in their system.

Interprofessional Care

Interprofessional management of the HIV-infected patient focuses on monitoring HIV disease progression and immune function, initiating and monitoring ART, preventing the development of opportunistic diseases, detecting and treating opportunistic diseases, managing symptoms, preventing or decreasing the complications of treatment, and providing comprehensive psychosocial and spiritual care. Ongoing assessment and supportive health care provider–patient interactions are required to accomplish these objectives.

The initial visit provides an opportunity to gather baseline data and to establish rapport. A complete history and physical examination, including an immunization history and psychosocial and dietary evaluations, should be conducted. Findings from the history, assessment, and laboratory tests help determine the patient's needs. This is a good time to initiate patient education regarding the spectrum of HIV disease, treatment, preventing transmission to others, improving health, and family planning. Patient input must be used to develop a plan of care, and necessary referrals can be made. A patient with newly diagnosed infection may be in a state of shock or denial and be unable to understand or retain information. The nurse should be prepared to repeat and clarify information over the course of several months. If case reports are required by the public health department, they should be completed at this time.

Medication Therapy for Human Immunodeficiency Virus Infection. The goals of medication therapy in HIV infection are to (a) decrease the viral load, (b) maintain or raise CD4+ T-cell counts, (c) delay the development of HIV-related symptoms and opportunistic diseases, and (d) prevent transmission. Guidelines on the use of antiretroviral agents are updated

TABLE 17.13 MEDICATION THERAPY

Mechanisms of Action of Medications Used to Treat HIV Infection

Medication Classification	Mechanism of Action
Non-nucleoside reverse transcriptase inhibitors	Combine with reverse transcriptase enzyme to block the process needed to convert HIV RNA into HIV DNA
Nucleoside reverse transcriptase inhibitors	Insert a bit of protein (a nucleoside) into the developing HIV DNA chain, blocking further development of the chain and leaving the production of the new strand of HIV DNA incomplete
Nucleotide reverse transcriptase inhibitors	Inhibit the action of reverse transcriptase
Protease inhibitors	Prevent the protease enzyme from cutting HIV proteins into the proper lengths needed to allow viable virions to assemble and bud out from the cell membrane
Integrase inhibitors	Prevent viral DNA integration into the CD4+ cell chromosome
Fusion inhibitors (entry inhibitors)	Prevent binding of HIV to cells, thus preventing entry of HIV into healthy cells

HIV, human immunodeficiency virus; *RNA,* ribonucleic acid.

regularly (Panel on Antiretroviral Guidelines for Adults and Adolescents, 2019). HIV treatment guidelines incorporate use of the following principles:

1. Treatment should be started immediately upon diagnosis, regardless of CD4+ T-cell counts (BC Centre for Excellence, 2020). A patient's desires for therapy should also guide this decision.
2. Combination ART suppresses HIV replication and limits the potential for antiretroviral resistance, which is the major factor that limits treatment effect. The most effective means to suppress HIV replication is simultaneous initiation of at least three effective antiretroviral medications from at least two different medication classes in optimum schedules and full dosages. In general, therapy begins with two nucleoside (or nucleotide) reverse transcriptase inhibitors and a non-nucleoside reverse transcriptase inhibitor or a protease inhibitor that is boosted with ritonavir. The nucleosides and nucleotides are considered the foundation of ART.
3. Infected women should receive optimal ART even if pregnant.
4. HIV-infected persons with viral loads above detectable limits should be considered infectious and should avoid behaviours associated with transmission of HIV and other infectious pathogens. Recommendations for starting therapy in infected patients have become much more simple in recent years. Treatment is now recommended for everyone, regardless of CD4 count, viral load, or pregnancy status.

Currently approved medications include four groups that inhibit the ability of HIV to make a DNA copy early in replication, one group that inhibits the ability of the virus to reproduce in the late stages of replication, and one group that prevents entry of HIV into the cell (Table 17.13). *Nucleoside reverse transcriptase inhibitors, non-nucleoside reverse transcriptase inhibitors* (NNRTIs), and *nucleotide reverse transcriptase inhibitors*

TABLE 17.14   MEDICATION THERAPY

Antiretroviral Agents Used to Treat HIV Infection* †

Medication	Adverse Effects	Medication	Adverse Effects
Nucleoside Reverse Transcriptase Inhibitors	Common adverse effects: Lactic acidosis with hepatic steatosis, a rare but potentially life-threatening condition; lipodystrophy, especially fat atrophy and mitochondrial toxicity	Entry Inhibitors	
		• Enfuvirtide (Fuzeon)	ISRs, fatigue, nausea, diarrhea, insomnia, peripheral neuropathy, hypersensitivity reaction, pneumonia
• Abacavir (Ziagen)	Nausea; hypersensitivity reaction, including fever, nausea, vomiting, diarrhea, lethargy, malaise, sore throat, shortness of breath, cough, rash; may produce life-threatening event if hypersensitivity is rechallenged	• Maraviroc (Celsentri)	Persistent cough, URT infections, and GI upset
		Combination Therapy	
		• Atripla (tenofovir + emtricitabine + efavirenz)	Nausea and vomiting, cough, increased pigmentation on soles of feet and palms of hands, diarrhea, drowsiness, indigestion, headache, strange dreams, fatigue
• Didanosine (Videx-EC)	Headache, nausea, vomiting, diarrhea, rash		
• Emtricitabine (FTC, Emtriva)	Headache, diarrhea, nausea, rash, skin discoloration	• Biktarvy (bictegravir + tenofovir alafenamide + emtricitabine)	Diarrhea, nausea, headache
• Lamivudine (3TC)	Minimal toxic effects, nausea, nasal congestion	• Combivir (lamivudine + zidovudine)	Headache, nausea, vomiting, unexpected tiredness, diarrhea, loss of appetite, insomnia, muscle pain
• Zidovudine (AZT, Retrovir)	Nausea, vomiting, anemia, leukopenia, fatigue, headache, insomnia, pancreatitis		
Nucleotide Reverse Transcriptase Inhibitor		• Complera (rilpivirine + emtricitabine + tenofovir disoproxil fumarate)	Dizziness, feeling sleepy during the daytime, headache, rash, nausea, stomach pain
• Tenofovir disoproxil fumarate (Viread)	Nausea, vomiting, diarrhea		
Nonnucleoside Reverse Transcriptase Inhibitors	Common adverse effects: rash, erythema multiforme, increased liver enzymes, hepatotoxicity	• Delstrigo (doravirine + lamivudine + tenofovir disoproxil fumarate)	Dizziness, nausea, diarrhea, insomnia, rash, drowsiness
• Doravirine (Pifeltro)	Headache, nausea, fatigue	• Descovy (tenofovir alafenamide +emtricitabine)	Nausea, dizziness
• Efavirenz (Sustiva)	Dizziness, trouble concentrating, unusual dreams, confusion, anxiety, depression, diarrhea, encephalopathy; false-positive cannabinoid test	• Genvoya (elvitegravir + cobicistat + tenofovir alafenamide + emtricitabine)	Headache, fatigue, nausea, diarrhea
• Etravirine (Intelence)	Rash, diarrhea, nausea, flatulence, abdominal pain	• Juluca (dolutegravir + rilpivirine)	Fatigue, diarrhea, headache
• Nevirapine (Viramune)	GI upset, headache, generalized rash	• Kivexa (abacavir + lamivudine)	Unexpected tiredness, diarrhea, nausea, headache
• Rilpivirine (Edurant)	Depression, insomnia, headache		
Protease Inhibitors	Common adverse effects: dysglycemia, hyperlipidemia, lipodystrophy	• Odefsy (rilpivirine + tenofovir alafenamide + emtricitabine)	Headache, dizziness, rash, nausea, diarrhea
• Atazanavir (Reyataz)	Nausea, diarrhea, hyperbilirubinemia		
• Darunavir (Prezista)	Diarrhea, nausea, headache	• Prezcobix (darunavir + cobicistat)	Diarrhea, rash, headache, nausea, vomiting
• Indinavir (Crixivan)	Nausea, diarrhea, asymptomatic hyperbilirubinemia, interstitial nephritis, kidney stones (patient should drink 2–4 L of fluid a day)	• Stribild (elvitegravir + cobicistat + Truvada emtricitabine + tenofovir)	Headache, diarrhea, nausea, vomiting, vivid dreams, anxiety, rash, dizziness, insomnia, loss of appetite
• Ritonavir (Norvir)—most often used in low doses with other protease inhibitors to boost effect	Nausea, diarrhea, vomiting, taste perversion, circumoral and perioral paresthesia, hepatitis	• Symtuza (darunavir + cobicistat + tenofovir alafenamide + emtricitabine)	Diarrhea, rash, nausea, fatigue, headache, gas
• Tipranavir (Aptivus)	Nausea, diarrhea, headache, clinical hepatitis, increased serum transaminases, hepatic decompensation, symptoms of sulpha allergy, rash, or photosensitivity	• Triumeq (dolutegravir + abacavir + lamivudine)	Nausea, vomiting, diarrhea, headache, abdominal discomfort/pain
• Kaletra (lopinavir + ritonavir combination)	Nausea, diarrhea, taste perversion, perioral and circumoral paresthesia, hepatitis	• Trizivir (lamivudine + zidovudine + abacavir)	Diarrhea, nausea, vomiting, loss of appetite, headache, insomnia, unexpected tiredness, muscle pain
Integrase Inhibitors			
• Dolutegravir (Tivicay)	Rash, increased liver enzymes, tiredness, fever, insomnia, headache	• Truvada (tenofovir and emtricitabine)	Dizziness, headache, nausea, vomiting, flatulence
• Raltegravir (Isentress)	Diarrhea, nausea, headache, fever		

*Current recommendations for therapy mandate combinations of three or more of these medications. Treatment with only one medication is rarely acceptable.
†Many of these medications cause serious and potentially fatal interactions when used in combination with other commonly used medications, some of which are available over the counter.
GI, gastrointestinal; ISRs, injection site reactions; URT, upper respiratory tract.
Sources: British Columbia Centre for Excellence in HIV/AIDS. (2019). *Therapeutic guidelines for antiretroviral treatment of adult HIV infection.* http://www.cfenet.ubc.ca/our-work/initiatives/therapeutic-guidelines/adult-therapeutic-guidelines; and Canadian AIDS Treatment Information Exchange (CATIE). http://librarypdf.catie.ca/PDF/ATI-40000s/40247.pdf

work by inhibiting the activity of reverse transcriptase; *protease inhibitors* work by interfering with the activity of the enzyme protease; and *integrase inhibitors* work by interfering with the enzyme integrase. *Fusion inhibitors* (entry inhibitors) work by

inhibiting the binding of HIV to cells. A major problem with most medications used in ART is that resistance develops rapidly when they are used alone or taken in inadequate doses. For this reason, combinations of three or more antiretroviral medications, prescribed at full strength, should be used. Protease inhibitors and NNRTIs also have a number of dangerous and potentially lethal interactions with other commonly used medications, including over-the-counter medications and herbal therapies. For example, St. John's wort can interfere with ART by lowering the blood levels of protease inhibitors and NNRTIs (AIDS InfoNet, 2014). Some herbs (e.g., echinacea, astragalus) should be used only with prescriber permission as they can decrease the efficacy of ART.

Treatment policies can reduce viral loads by 90% to 99% in most cases, but adverse effects and other complications are not uncommon (Panel on Antiretroviral Guidelines for Adults and Adolescents, 2019). Antiretroviral agents used in HIV infection and their adverse effects are detailed in Table 17.14. Some patients are not able to use combination therapies because of the expense, adverse effects, or inability to adhere to required schedules.

MEDICATION ALERT—Efavirenz (Sustiva)

- In pregnant patients, efavirenz can be used after the first 8 weeks of pregnancy.
- Once-a-day doses should be taken at bedtime (at least initially) to help patients cope with adverse effects, including dizziness and confusion.
- Patients should be informed that many people who use the medication have reported vivid and sometimes bizarre dreams.

Preventing Transmission of Human Immunodeficiency Virus. A new and emerging use of ART is pre-exposure prophylaxis (PrEP), which is a comprehensive HIV-prevention strategy to reduce the risk of sexually acquired HIV infection in adults at high risk by around 90% (Underhill et al., 2015; Tan et al., 2017). PrEP should be used in conjunction with other proven prevention interventions such as condoms, risk reduction counselling, and regular HIV testing.

The combination of tenofovir with emtricitabine, known as *Truvada*, is used to reduce the risk of HIV infection in uninfected individuals who are at significant risk of acquiring HIV. PrEP can be taken either daily or on an "on-demand" schedule, where higher doses are taken in the days surrounding a sexual event, rather than every day. Truvada is also currently used in combination with other antiretroviral agents for the treatment of HIV-infected people.

Medication Therapy for Opportunistic Diseases. Management of HIV is complicated by the many opportunistic diseases that can develop as the immune system deteriorates. A preferred approach to treating opportunistic diseases is to prevent their occurrence. A number of opportunistic diseases associated with HIV can be delayed or prevented through the use of adequate ART, vaccines (including hepatitis B, influenza, and pneumococcal), and disease-specific prevention measures. Prophylaxis, used according to established criteria, contributes significantly to preventing morbidity and mortality. Although it is not always possible to eradicate opportunistic diseases once they occur, treatments are available that can control them. Advances in the prevention, diagnosis, and treatment of opportunistic diseases have contributed significantly to increased life expectancy. Table 17.11 lists prophylaxis and treatments for some common HIV-related opportunistic diseases.

Vaccine. Despite considerable research, a vaccine for HIV still eludes scientists. The problems that impede HIV vaccine development are numerous. HIV lives inside cells, where it can "hide" from circulating immune factors. HIV also mutates rapidly, so that infected individuals develop HIV variants that may not all respond to a simple vaccine. In addition, two strains of HIV (HIV-1 and HIV-2) cause AIDS, and at least nine clades (subtypes) of HIV-1 exist around the world. A vaccine developed for one clade may not be effective against the others.

There are also social, ethical, and economic issues related to vaccination. Vaccine efficacy will eventually have to be established in human testing: How will volunteers be recruited? How will true protection be determined? Will volunteers be exposed to HIV after immunization to test immunity? Because HIV is a global problem, with developing countries bearing the brunt of the epidemic, there is also concern about developing a vaccine that can be widely distributed in a short amount of time at an acceptable cost. Will vaccines, once developed, be accepted? Despite the overwhelming nature of these issues, considerable research is in progress. Vaccines in various stages of development are being tested. The development of a successful vaccine would be extremely helpful in controlling the epidemic but would not replace current prevention methods because no vaccine is likely to be 100% effective.

EVIDENCE-INFORMED PRACTICE
Translating Research Into Practice

A nurse in an HIV clinic is counselling M. S. (pronouns he/him), a 25-year-old gay man, and his partner. Mr. S. is receiving antiretroviral therapy. His viral load is very low, and his CD4+ T-cell count is normal. He tells the nurse that since the medications are working, he and his partner (who is not infected with HIV) have decided to forgo the use of condoms. They tell the nurse that they are in a committed relationship and occasionally have other sexual partners, during which they sometimes use condoms. The nurse acknowledges M. S.'s health promotion behaviours and spends time explaining the risks of unprotected sex: They may acquire other STIs, or M. S.'s partner could be at risk for acquiring HIV from an outside partner whose status he does not know. M. S. cannot transmit HIV to his partner with an undetectable viral load, as long as he continues to take his medications. The nurse encourages condom use with outside partners for both parties, and educates M. S.'s partner on the benefits of PrEP as a prevention strategy.

Best Available Evidence	Clinician Expertise	Patient Preferences and Values
The most effective ways to prevent HIV transmission from an infected person to an uninfected person are by using condoms and taking PrEP.	The nurse knows that risk-reducing sexual activities in this situation include the continued use of condoms and PrEP. The nurse also knows that a very low viral load decreases the risk of HIV transmission.	After listening, the patients tell the nurse they do not like using condoms and understand the increased risk of STIs. However, M. S.'s partner is interested in learning more about PrEP on demand.

Decision and Action

The nurse must respect the decision to not use condoms. The nurse reminds M. S. of the importance of maintaining his medication regimen and attending his appointments at the clinic in order to maintain viral suppression and prevent the transmission of HIV to his partner. She rebooks an appointment for M. S.'s partner with herself and the doctor to discuss a PrEP prescription.

Reference for Evidence

Buchbinder, S. P. (2018). Maximizing the benefits of HIV pre-exposure prophylaxis. *Topics in Antiviral Medicine, 25*(4), 138–142.

TABLE 17.15   NURSING ASSESSMENT
HIV-Infected Patient

Subjective Data		Integumentary	Decreased skin turgor, dry skin, or diaphoresis; pallor, cyanosis; lesions, eruptions, discolorations, or bruises of skin and mucous membranes; vaginal or perianal excoriation; alopecia, delayed wound healing
Important health information	*Past health history:* Route of infection; hepatitis; other STIs; tuberculosis; foreign travel; frequent viral, fungal, or bacterial infections; alcohol and drug use		
	Medications: Use of immunosuppressive medications	Eyes	Presence of exudate; retinal lesions or hemorrhage; papilledema
Symptoms	Malaise, chronic fatigue, weight loss, anorexia, nausea, vomiting; lesions, bleeding, or ulcerations of lips, mouth, gums, tongue, or throat; sensitivity to acidic, salty, or spicy foods; difficulty swallowing; abdominal cramping	Respiratory	Tachypnea, dyspnea, intercostal retractions; crackles, wheezing, productive or nonproductive cough
		Cardiovascular	Pericardial friction rub, murmur, bradycardia, tachycardia
	Skin rashes, lesions, or colour changes; pruritus; nonhealing wounds	Gastrointestinal	Mouth lesions, including blisters (HSV), white-grey patches (*Candida*), painless white lesions on lateral aspect of the tongue (hairy leukoplakia), discolorations (Kaposi's sarcoma); gingivitis, tooth decay or loosening; redness or white patchy lesions of throat; vomiting, diarrhea, incontinence; rectal lesions; hyperactive bowel sounds, abdominal masses, hepatosplenomegaly
	Persistent diarrhea, change in character of stools; painful urination		
	Cough, shortness of breath		
	Insomnia; night sweats		
	Headaches, stiff neck, chest pain, rectal pain, retrosternal pain		
	Blurred vision, photophobia, diplopia, loss of vision; hearing impairment; confusion, forgetfulness, attention deficit, changes in mental status, memory loss, personality changes, muscle weakness, difficulty walking; paresthesias, hypersensitivity in feet	Musculoskeletal	Muscle wasting
		Neurological	Ataxia, tremors, lack of coordination; sensory loss; slurred speech, aphasia; memory loss, apathy, agitation, depression, inappropriate behaviour; decreasing levels of consciousness, seizures, paralysis, coma
	Lesions on genitalia (internal or external), pruritus or burning sensation in vagina, painful sexual intercourse, changes in menstruation, vaginal or penile discharge	Reproductive	Genital lesions or discharge, abdominal tenderness secondary to pelvic inflammatory disease
Objective Data		Possible findings	Positive result of HIV antibody assay (EIA or ELISA, confirmed by WB or IFA); viral load levels detectable by bDNA or PCR, ↓ CD4+ lymphocytes, reversal of CD4:CD8 ratio; ↓ WBC count, lymphopenia, anemia, thrombocytopenia; electrolyte imbalances; abnormal results of liver function tests; ↑ cholesterol, triglyceride, and blood glucose levels
General	Lethargy, persistent fever, lymphadenopathy, peripheral wasting, fat deposits in truncal areas and upper back; social withdrawal		

bDNA, branched-chain deoxyribonucleic acid; *EIA*, enzyme immunoassay; *ELISA*, enzyme-linked immunosorbent assay; *HIV*, human immunodeficiency virus; *HSV*, herpes simplex virus; *IFA*, immunofluorescence assay; *PCR*, polymerase chain reaction; *STIs*, sexually transmitted infections; *WB*, Western blot; *WBC*, white blood cell count.

NURSING MANAGEMENT
HUMAN IMMUNODEFICIENCY VIRUS INFECTION

NURSING ASSESSMENT

Nursing assessment for an individual not known to be infected with HIV should focus on behaviours that could put the person at risk for HIV infection and other sexually transmitted and bloodborne diseases. Nurses can help individuals assess risks by asking four basic questions: (1) "Have you ever had a blood transfusion or used clotting factors? If so, was it before 1985?" (2) "Have you ever shared needles, syringes, or other injecting equipment with another person?" (3) "Have you ever been sexually active?" and (4) "Have you ever had an STI?" These questions elicit the minimum data needed to initiate a risk assessment. A positive response to any of these questions necessitates an in-depth exploration of the issues specific to the identified risk.

Further assessment is needed when an HIV infection is diagnosed. Subjective and objective data that should be obtained are presented in Table 17.15. Nursing assessments should be ongoing because early recognition and treatment of problems can decrease the progression of HIV infection. A complete history and a thorough systems review can help the nurse identify issues in a timely manner.

NURSING DIAGNOSES

Nursing diagnoses related to HIV infection are dictated by several variables: the stage (e.g., Is prevention of HIV infection the

TABLE 17.16   NURSING DIAGNOSES: HIV INFECTION

• Anxiety	• Health management, inadequate
• Breathing pattern, inadequate	• Hyperthermia
• Caregiver role strain	• Nutrition, imbalanced: less than body requirements
• Confusion, acute or chronic	• Oral mucous membrane integrity, reduced
• Coping, inadequate	• Pain, acute or chronic
• Decisional conflict	• Powerlessness
• Denial, inadequate	• Relocation stress syndrome
• Diarrhea	• Self-care deficits
• Disuse syndrome, potential for	• Self-concept, reduced
• Family processes, interrupted	• Self-esteem, chronic low
• Fatigue	• Self-esteem, situational low
• Fear	• Sleep pattern, disturbed
• Grieving	• Social isolation
• Headache	• Spiritual distress

issue? Are there concerns related to ongoing infection? Is the patient in a terminal phase of the disease?); presence of specific etiological problems (e.g., respiratory distress, depression, wasting); and social factors (e.g., issues related to self-esteem, sexuality, family interactions, finances). Because HIV infection is a complex disease experienced differently according to the individual, a broad spectrum of nursing diagnoses may include but not be limited to those presented in Table 17.16.

PLANNING

Prevention of HIV infection presents a number of challenges for the patient, many of which are related to challenges with behavioural change and the social and sexual stigma that can come with having HIV. Nurses can be instrumental in this process. Nursing interventions to prevent disease transmission depend on assessment of the patient's individual risk behaviours, knowledge, and skill deficits. Nursing orders based on these assessments will encourage the patient to learn safer, healthier, and less risky behaviours. Infection with HIV affects the entire range of a person's life—not only physical health but also social, emotional, economic, and spiritual well-being. Once a person is infected, current treatment cannot eliminate HIV from the body. The overriding goals of therapy are to keep the viral load as low as possible for as long as possible; to maintain or restore a functioning immune system; to improve the patient's quality of life; to reduce the potential for transmission of the virus; to reduce HIV-related disease, disability, and death; and to prevent reinfection. Nursing interventions can assist the patient to (a) adhere to medication regimens; (b) promote a healthy lifestyle; (c) prevent opportunistic disease; (d) protect others from HIV; (e) maintain or develop healthy, supportive relationships; (f) maintain activities and productivity; (g) come to terms with issues related to disease, death, and spirituality; and (h) cope with the symptoms caused by HIV and its treatments (Canadian Association of Nurses in AIDS Care [CANAC], 2013). Goals are individualized and change as new treatment policies develop or as HIV disease and life circumstances progress.

NURSING IMPLEMENTATION

The complexity of HIV disease is related to its chronic nature. As with most chronic and infectious diseases, primary prevention and health promotion are the most effective health care strategies. When prevention fails, however, disease results. HIV infection has no cure and continues for life. If a patient does not receive ART, it causes increasing physical disability, contributes to impaired health, and ultimately causes death.

Nursing interventions at every stage of HIV disease can be instrumental in improving the quality and quantity of the patient's life. Nurses who emphasize a holistic and individualized approach to care are well suited to and capable of providing optimal care to these patients. Table 17.17 presents a synopsis of nursing goals, assessments, and interventions at each stage of HIV infection.

HEALTH PROMOTION. A major goal of health promotion is to prevent disease. Even with recent successes in the treatment of HIV, prevention is crucial for control of the epidemic. Another goal of health promotion is to detect disease early so that if primary prevention has failed, early intervention can be implemented.

Prevention of Human Immunodeficiency Virus Infection. HIV infection is preventable. At this time, education, harm reduction, and decreases in risk behaviours are the most effective prevention tools. Educational messages should be specific to the patient's need and be trauma-informed, culturally sensitive, language-appropriate, and age-specific. Nurses are excellent resources for this type of education, but nurses must be comfortable with and know how to talk about sensitive topics such as sexuality and substance use (CANAC, 2013).

Prevention behaviours have been known and recommended since the mid-1980s. The nurse must remember that a range of activities can reduce the risk of HIV infection and that individuals will choose different techniques. The goal is for the person to develop safer, healthier, and less risky behaviours than are currently being used. These techniques can be divided into *safe activities* (those that eliminate risk) and *risk-reducing activities* (those that decrease risk but do not eliminate it). The more consistently and correctly prevention methods are used, the more effective they are in preventing HIV infection.

Research shows that the majority of new HIV infections were transmitted by individuals who were not aware that they were infected. As stated earlier, an estimated 21% of HIV-infected people in Canada do not know that they are infected (PHAC, 2015b). In response, British Columbia develop the Seek and Treat for Optimal Prevention of HIV/AIDS (STOP) program. As a result of this program, HIV testing has been expanded to populations not historically considered to be at risk, and the program also ensures that all individuals in whom HIV is diagnosed get rapid access to treatment, which is known to prevent transmission.

Decreasing Risks Related to Sexual Intercourse. Safer sexual activities significantly decrease the risk of exposure to HIV in semen, blood, and vaginal secretions. Abstaining from all sexual activity is the most effective way to accomplish this goal, but there are safe options for those who cannot or do not wish to abstain. *Outercourse* (limiting sexual behaviour to activities in which the mouth, penis, vagina, or rectum does not come into contact with a partner's mouth, penis, vagina, or rectum) is safe because there is no contact with blood, semen, or vaginal secretions. Outercourse includes massage, masturbation, mutual masturbation, telephone sex, and other activities that meet the "no contact" requirements. *Insertive sex* between partners who are not infected with HIV or not at risk of becoming infected with HIV is considered to be safe, although it is important for a person to know their partner's status.

The risk of acquiring HIV from insertive *oral sex* with an HIV positive partner is relatively nonexistent. The risk of acquiring HIV from receptive *oral sex* is also extremely low, but not nonexistent and people may choose to use condoms for this activity.

Reducing the risk of sexual activities through the use of barriers decreases the risk of contact with HIV. Barriers should be used during insertive sexual activity (vaginal or anal) with a partner who is known to be HIV infected or with a partner whose HIV status is not known. The most commonly used barrier is the male condom. Male condoms have been shown to be almost 100% effective in preventing the transmission of HIV when used correctly and consistently. Major points for the correct use of male condoms are discussed in Table 17.18. Female condoms are also available. Use can be complicated, and so careful instruction and practice are necessary (Table 17.19).

Decreasing Risks Related to Substance Use. Use of substances, including alcohol and tobacco, can be harmful. It can cause immune suppression and malnutrition, as well as psychosocial problems. However, substance use in and of itself does not cause HIV infection. The major risk for HIV infection is related to sharing injecting equipment or having unsafe sexual experiences while under the influence of substances. The basic rules are as follows: (a) do not inject illicit drugs; (b) if you do inject illicit drugs, do not share equipment; and (c) do not have sexual intercourse when under the influence of any drug (including alcohol) that impairs decision-making ability.

TABLE 17.17 NURSING INTERVENTIONS IN HIV DISEASE

Levels of Care: Goals	Assess	Interventions
Health Promotion 1. Prevent HIV infection 2. Detect HIV infection early	*Risk factors:* What behaviours or social, physical, emotional, pathological, and immune factors place the patient at risk? Does the patient need to be tested for HIV?	Education, including knowledge, attitudes, and behaviours, with an emphasis on risk reduction, to accomplish the following: • General population: covering general information • Pregnant women: covering general information and information specific to HIV infection and pregnancy; offering prenatal HIV testing in the first trimester Individual patient: specific to assessed need (consider substance use and sexual activities) Empowering patients to take control of prevention measures Providing HIV-antibody testing with pretest and post-test counselling
Acute Intervention 1. Promote health and limit disability 2. Manage problems caused by HIV infection	*Physical health:* Is the patient experiencing problems? *Mental health status:* How is the patient coping? *Resources:* Does the patient have family and social support? Is the patient accessing community services? Is money or housing a problem? Does the patient have access to spiritual support?	Case management Education regarding HIV, the spectrum of infection, options for care, signs and symptoms to watch for, treatment options, immune enhancement, harm reduction, and ways to adhere to treatment regimens Referral to needed resources Establishing long-term, trusting relationship with patient, family, and significant others Providing emotional and spiritual support Providing care during acute exacerbations: recognition of life-threatening developments, life support, rapid intervention with treatments and medications, patient and family emotional support during crisis, comfort, and hygiene needs Developing resources for legal needs: discrimination prevention, wills and powers of attorney, child care wishes Empowering patient to identify needs, direct care, and seek services
Ambulatory and Home Care 1. Maximize quality of life 2. Resolve life-and-death issues	*Physical health:* Are new symptoms developing? Is the patient experiencing medication adverse effects or interactions? *Mental health:* How is the patient coping? What adjustments have been made? *Finances:* Can the patient maintain health care and basic standards of living? *Family, social, and community supports:* Are these available? Is the patient using supports in an effective manner? Do family or significant others need education, encouragement, or stress relief? *Spirituality issues:* Does the patient desire support from a religious organization? Are spirituality issues private and personal? Is the patient seeking cultural connection? What assistance does the patient need?	Continuing case management Educating about changing treatment options and continued adherence Empowering patient to continue to direct care and to make desires known to family members and significant others Continuing physical care for chronic disease process: treatments, medications, comfort, and hygiene needs Supporting patient and family and significant others in a trusting relationship Referral to resources that will assist in meeting identified needs Promoting health maintenance measures Assistance with end-of-life issues: resuscitation orders, comfort measures, funeral plans, and the like Referral to palliative care

HIV, human immunodeficiency virus.

INFORMATICS IN PRACTICE

Use of Internet and Mobile Devices to Manage Human Immunodeficiency Virus Infection

• Reputable websites such as government agencies (e.g., Health Canada) and well-known academic and medical institutions offer resources and support for patients that can assist them in coping with their illness and educate them about signs and symptoms of serious illness. (See also the Resources at the end of this chapter.)
• By monitoring their health and quickly spotting warning signs of serious illnesses, patients are able to alert their health care providers and receive earlier treatment.
• These systems can help the patient manage antiretroviral therapy by sending medication reminders by text or email.

Risk for HIV among people who use drugs can also be eliminated if people do not share injecting equipment. Injecting equipment includes needles, syringes, cookers (spoons or bottle caps used to mix the drug), cotton, and rinse water. None of this equipment should be shared. Another safe tactic is for the person to have access to sterile equipment. This can be accomplished through community needle and syringe exchange programs and supervised injection sites that provide sterile equipment to people who use substances. Opposition to these programs is based in the fear that ready access to injecting supplies will increase drug use. However, studies have shown that in communities where exchange programs and supervised consumption sites have been established, drug use does not

TABLE 17.18	PATIENT & CAREGIVER TEACHING GUIDE

Proper Use of the Male Condom

- Use only condoms ("rubbers") that are made out of latex or polyurethane. "Natural skin" condoms have pores that are large enough for HIV to penetrate.
- Store condoms in a cool, dry place and protect them from trauma. The friction caused by carrying them in a back pocket, for instance, can wear down the latex.
- Do not use a condom if the expiration date has passed or if the package looks worn or punctured.
- Lubricants used in conjunction with condoms must be water soluble. Oil-based lubricants can weaken latex and increase the risk of tearing or breaking.
- Nonlubricated, flavoured, or unflavoured condoms can provide protection during oral intercourse.
- The condom must be placed on the erect penis before any contact is made with the partner's mouth, vagina, or rectum to prevent exposure to pre-ejaculatory secretions that may contain HIV.
- Remove the penis and condom from the partner's vagina or rectum immediately after ejaculation and before the erection is lost. Hold the condom at the base of the penis and remove both penis and condom at the same time. This keeps semen from leaking around the condom as the penis becomes flaccid.
- Remove the condom after use, wrap in tissue, and discard. Do not flush down the toilet because this can cause plumbing problems.
- Condoms are not reusable! A new condom must be used for every act of intercourse.

HIV, human immunodeficiency virus.

TABLE 17.19	PATIENT & CAREGIVER TEACHING GUIDE

Proper Use of the Female Condom

Female condoms consist of a polyurethane sheath with two spring-form rings.
- The smaller ring is inserted into the vagina and holds the condom in place internally. This ring can be removed if the condom is to be used for anal intercourse. It should not be removed if the condom is to be used for vaginal intercourse.
- The larger ring surrounds the opening to the condom. It functions to keep the condom in place while protecting the external genitalia.

Use only water-soluble lubricants with female condoms.
- Female condoms come prelubricated and with a tube of additional lubricant.
- Lubrication is needed to protect the condom from tearing during sexual intercourse and can also decrease the noise that results from friction of the penis against the condom.

Some men have reported that the female condom feels better than the male condom. Other men like male condoms better. The only way to find out which type of condom works best is to try both.

Practise inserting the female condom. Lubrication makes the condom slippery, but do not get discouraged; just keep trying.

During sexual intercourse, ensure that the penis is inserted into the female condom through the outer ring. It is possible for the penis to miss the opening, thus making contact with the vagina and defeating the purpose of the condom.

Do not use a male condom at the same time as a female condom.

After intercourse, remove the condom before standing up.
- Twist the outer ring to keep the semen inside, gently pull the condom out of the vagina, and discard.

Do not flush down the toilet because this can cause plumbing problems.

Do not reuse a female condom.

increase, rates of HIV infection are controlled, and there are overall economic benefits (Health Canada, 2021).

Cleaning equipment before use is also a risk-reducing activity. It decreases the risk for those who share equipment (Table 17.20). This process takes time and may be difficult for a person who begins to suffer drug withdrawal during the process.

Decreasing Risks of Perinatal Transmission. The best way to prevent HIV infection in infants is to prevent HIV infection in women. Women who are already infected with HIV should be asked about their reproductive plans. Women who choose not to have children need to have birth control methods offered.

If HIV-infected pregnant women are appropriately treated during pregnancy, the rate of perinatal transmission can be decreased from 25% to less than 1%. The current standard of care is that all women who are pregnant or contemplating pregnancy should be counselled about HIV infection, informed of their choices, routinely offered access to voluntary HIV-antibody testing, and, if infected, offered optimal ART (Bailey et al., 2018; Burdge et al., 2003).

Decreasing Risks at Work. The risk of infection from occupational exposure to HIV is low but real. The Canadian Centre for Occupational Health and Safety requires employers to protect workers from exposure to blood and other potentially infectious materials. Precautions and safety devices decrease the risk of direct contact with blood and body fluids. Precautions for the prevention of occupational exposure to bloodborne diseases were discussed earlier in this chapter. Should significant exposure to HIV-infected fluids occur, postexposure prophylaxis with combination ART that is based on the type of exposure, the volume of the exposure, and the status of the source patient has been shown to significantly decrease the risk of infection. The possibility of treatment makes reporting of all blood exposures even more critical.

Human Immunodeficiency Virus Testing and Counselling. Testing is the only sure way to determine whether a person has HIV infection. Any individual who is at risk for HIV infection should be encouraged to be tested. When findings are negative, testing

TABLE 17.20	PATIENT & CAREGIVER TEACHING GUIDE

Proper Use of Injection Equipment

- When drugs are injected, it is always preferable to use new, sterile syringes, needles, cookers, and cotton.
- Find out if there is a needle and syringe exchange program in your community. If there is, patients may access unused equipment there.
- If your community has a supervised consumption site, patients should be educated on location and accessibility of these services.
- Swab skin with an alcohol preparation before injecting.
- Use a tourniquet to assist in locating veins.
- Always inject with the bevel facing up on the needle.
- If you must share your equipment, it is very important to clean the equipment thoroughly with bleach before use.
- First, rinse the used needle and syringe twice with tap water.
- Then, fill the syringe with full-strength household bleach, shake for 30 seconds, and squirt the bleach out.
- Repeat the bleaching process a second time, being sure to shake the bleach-filled syringe for 30 seconds.
- Finally, rinse equipment twice with tap water.
- Do not share your bleach or rinse water.
- Do not share your cooker. If you must share your cooker, clean it with bleach and water before using it again.

| TABLE 17.21 | PRETEST AND POST-TEST COUNSELLING ASSOCIATED WITH HIV-ANTIBODY TESTING |

General Guidelines

1. Many people who are being tested for HIV are fearful about the test results:
   - The nurse should establish rapport with the patient.
   - The nurse should assess the patient's ability to understand HIV counselling.
   - The nurse must determine the patient's ability to access support systems.
2. The benefits of testing should be explained:
   - Testing provides an opportunity for education that can decrease the risk of new infections.
   - Infected individuals can be referred for early intervention and support programs.
3. Adverse aspects of testing should be discussed:
   - Confidentiality issues: Breaches of confidentiality have led to discrimination.
   - A positive test result affects all aspects of the patient's life (e.g., personal, social, economic) and can raise difficult emotions (anger, anxiety, guilt, and thoughts of suicide).

Pretest Counselling

1. Determining the patient's risk factors and when the last risk factor occurred. Counselling should be individualized according to these parameters.
2. Providing education to help the patient reduce future risk of exposure
3. Providing education that will help the patient protect sexual and substance-using partners
4. Discussing problems related to the delay between infection and an accurate test, depending on the type of test being used. Discuss the need to use measures to decrease the risks to the patient and the patient's partners during that interval.
5. Discussing the possibility of false-negative tests, which are most likely to occur during the window period
6. Assessing support systems. Provide telephone numbers and resources as needed.
7. Discussing the responses the patient anticipates having to the test results (positive and negative)
8. Outlining assistance that will be offered if the test result is positive

Post-Test Counselling

1. If the test result is negative, pretest counselling and prevention education should be reinforced. The patient should be reminded that the test must be repeated at 3- or 12-month intervals, depending on the individual's ongoing risk factors.
2. If the test result is positive, the nurse needs to understand that the patient may be in emotional shock and not hear much of what the nurse says.
3. The nurse should provide resources for medical and emotional support and help the patient get immediate assistance:
   - Evaluating suicide risk and follow-up as needed
   - Determining need to test others who have had high-risk contact with the patient
   - Encouraging optimism
4. The nurse should remind the patient that effective treatments are available; HIV infection is not a death sentence.
5. Health habits that can improve the immune system and general wellness should be reviewed.
6. The nurse should arrange for the patient to speak to HIV-infected people who are willing to share with and assist patients with new diagnoses during the time between when the test results are available and treatment begins.
7. The nurse should emphasize that a positive HIV test result means that the patient is infected but does not necessarily mean that the patient has AIDS.
8. The patient should be educated to prevent new infections. HIV-infected people should be instructed to avoid donating blood, organs, or semen; to avoid sharing razors, toothbrushes, or other household items that may contain blood or other body fluids; and to protect sexual and needle-sharing partners from blood, semen, and vaginal secretions.

AIDS, acquired immune deficiency syndrome; *HIV,* human immunodeficiency virus.

can relieve anxieties about past behaviours and provide opportunities for prevention education. When findings are positive, testing provides the needed impetus to seek treatment and to protect sexual and substance use partners. All testing for HIV should be accompanied by pretest and post-test counselling (Table 17.21) as mandated by the WHO (2021b).

Acute Intervention

Early Intervention. Early intervention after detection of HIV infection can promote health and limit or delay disability. Because the course of HIV is variable, assessment is very important. Nursing interventions are based on and tailored to patient needs noted during assessment. The nursing assessment in HIV disease should focus on early detection of symptoms, opportunistic diseases, and psychosocial issues (see Table 17.17).

Initial Response to a Diagnosis of Human Immunodeficiency Virus Infection. Reactions to a positive result of an HIV antibody test can vary from immediate acceptance to grief, denial, and suicidal thoughts for both the patient and their loved ones. Immediately upon diagnosis, patients should be given silence and space to absorb the information and to express any immediate emotions or concern. The patient should also be reassured that HIV is no longer life-ending with current treatment options. Despite the improvements in treatment, people with HIV may still experience feelings of loss, anger, powerlessness, depression, and social isolation or stigmatization. The nurse can

help the patient gain control over treatment and life decisions. Empowerment is particularly important because many individuals with HIV infection experience multiple losses, including loss of a sense of control, which can feel overwhelming. Patient empowerment is facilitated by education and honest discussions about the patient's health status and treatment options.

Antiretroviral Therapy. Multidrug therapy policies have been shown to significantly reduce viral loads and reverse clinical progression of HIV. However, nurses must be aware that the policies are complex and the medications may have adverse effects and interactions. These factors, along with a multitude of individual patient factors, can contribute to problems with adherence to treatment regimens, a dangerous situation because of the high risk of developing drug resistance. Nurses are often the health care providers who work most closely with patients who are trying to cope with these issues. Interventions include teaching about (a) advantages and disadvantages of new treatments, (b) dangers of poor adherence to therapeutic regimens, (c) how and when to take each medication, (d) medication interactions to avoid, and (e) adverse effects that must be reported to the health care provider. Table 17.22 provides guidance for patient teaching in these areas.

When to Start Antiretroviral Therapy. ART has been in a state of continuous change since the first antiretroviral drug became available in 1987. When new medications were developed, health care providers had the ability to combine and

TABLE 17.22 PATIENT & CAREGIVER TEACHING GUIDE

Use of Antiretroviral Medications

Resistance to antiretroviral medications is a major problem in treating HIV infection. To decrease the risk of developing resistance:

1. Take at least three different antiretroviral medications at a time; discuss other options with your health care provider.
2. Know what medications you are taking and how to take them (some have to be taken with food, some must be taken on an empty stomach, some cannot be taken together). If you do not understand, ask. Get your nurse to write the instructions clearly for you.
3. Take the full dose prescribed, and take it on schedule. If you cannot take the medication because of adverse effects or other problems, report it to your health care provider.
4. Take all of the medications prescribed. It is important that you take them more than 95% of the time. Do not quit taking one medication while continuing the others. If you cannot tolerate one of your medications, your health care provider will recommend a completely new set of medications.
5. Many of the antiretroviral medications interact with other drugs, including a number of common drugs you can buy without a prescription. Be sure your health care provider and pharmacist know all of the medications that you are taking, and do not take any new medications without checking for possible interactions.
6. The goal of antiretroviral therapy is to decrease the amount of virus in your blood. This is called your viral load. Viral load can be determined by tests such as the PCR or bDNA. The results are reported in absolute numbers. The goal is to get your viral load to an undetectable level. Most health care providers will check this number on a regular basis regardless of whether you are taking antiretroviral agents.
7. In 2 to 4 weeks after you start on medication therapy (or change your therapy), your health care provider will test your viral load to find out whether the medications are working. These results are reported in absolute numbers or in "logs" (logarithms: a mathematical concept). All you have to know is that you want to see the viral load drop. If reports are in logs, you want to see a drop of at least 1 log, which means that 90% of your viral load has been eliminated. If your viral load drops by 2 logs, your viral load will have been 95% eliminated. If your viral load drops by 3 logs, your viral load will have been 99% eliminated.
8. An undetectable viral load means that the amount of virus is extremely low and viruses cannot be found in the blood through the use of the current technology. It does not mean that the virus is gone, for much of the virus will be in lymph nodes and organs where the tests cannot detect it. It means that you are unable to transmit the virus to sexual partners.

AIDS, acquired immune deficiency syndrome; *bDNA,* branched-chain DNA; *HIV,* human immunodeficiency virus; *PCR,* polymerase chain reaction.

TABLE 17.23 PATIENT & CAREGIVER TEACHING GUIDE

Signs and Symptoms That Patients With HIV Infection Need to Report

Report the Following Signs and Symptoms Immediately to a Health Care Provider

- Any change in level of consciousness: lethargy, difficulty arousing, inability to arouse, unresponsiveness, unconsciousness
- Headache accompanied by nausea and vomiting, changes in vision, or changes in ability to perform coordinated activities, or after any head trauma
- Vision changes: blurry or black areas in vision field, new floaters
- Persistent shortness of breath related to activity and not relieved by a short rest period
- Nausea and vomiting accompanied by abdominal pain
- Dehydration: inability to eat or drink because of nausea, diarrhea, or mouth lesions; severe diarrhea or vomiting; dizziness with standing
- Yellow discoloration of the skin
- Any bleeding from the rectum that is not related to hemorrhoids
- Pain in the flank with fever and inability to urinate for more than 6 hours
- New onset of weakness in any part of the body, new onset of numbness that is not obviously related to pressure, new onset of difficulty speaking
- Chest pain not obviously related to cough
- Seizures
- New rash accompanied by fever
- New oral lesions accompanied by fever
- Severe depression, anxiety, hallucinations, delusions, or being a possible danger to self or others

Report the Following Signs and Symptoms Within 24 Hours

- New or different headache; constant headache not relieved by aspirin or acetaminophen
- Headache accompanied by fever, nasal congestion, or cough
- Burning, itching, or discharge from the eyes
- New or productive cough
- Vomiting two or three times a day
- Vomiting accompanied by fever
- New, significant, or watery diarrhea (>6 times a day)
- Painful urination, bloody urine, urethral discharge
- New, significant rash (widespread, painful, itchy, or following a path down the leg or arm, around the chest, or on the face)
- Difficulty eating because of mouth lesions
- Vaginal discharge, pain, or itching

---

substitute medications. However, as new treatments have improved the quality and quantity of patients' lives, problems have emerged. For a while, the preferred treatment strategy was known as "hit it early, hit it hard." This was thought to be appropriate because decreasing the viral load provides for better health outcomes. However, adverse effects and lack of treatment regimen adherence caused many patients to question their ability to sustain ART for long periods of time. Because of this, for several years, treatment was delayed until the CD4+ T-cell count dropped below 500. However, it has become clear that when viral load is suppressed, the possibility of transmission of the virus is reduced. For this reason, current recommendations are that all people infected with HIV should receive treatment, regardless of their CD4+ T-cell count (Gunthard et al., 2014).

Given patient readiness, without which lack of adherence may be a problem, treatment should be initiated at the time of diagnosis to help reduce transmission rates and because a CD4+ T-cell count of less than 500 is associated with non–AIDS-related conditions such as cardiovascular disease, renal disease, and some cancers (Gunthard et al., 2014). Nurses can provide in-depth education and counselling for patients as they struggle to make this decision (CANAC, 2013).

Adherence. Adherence to medication regimens is a critical component of medication therapy for people with HIV infection and an area in which nurses are particularly well prepared to provide assistance. Taking medications as prescribed (right dose and time) is important for all medication therapy, but with HIV infection, missing even a few doses can lead to drug resistance. The difficulty of adhering consistently is clear to anyone who has tried to take a 10-day course of antibiotics. Patients with HIV infection have to take anywhere from one to six pills a day, at precise times during the day. This process must be repeated every day for the rest of their lives. Patients can be helped to adhere to difficult treatment regimens with electronic reminders, beepers, timers on pillboxes, and calendars. Group support and individual counselling can also help, but the best approach is to learn about the patient's lifestyle and assist with problem solving related to taking medications within the daily patterns of their life (CANAC, 2013).

Health Promotion. HIV disease progression may also be delayed by promoting a healthy immune system, regardless of whether the patient chooses to use ART. Useful interventions for HIV-infected patients include (a) nutritional support to maintain lean body mass and ensure appropriate levels of vitamins and micronutrients; (b) moderation or elimination of alcohol intake, smoking, and drug use; (c) adequate rest and exercise; (d) stress reduction; (e) avoidance of exposure to new infectious agents; (f) mental health counselling; and (g) involvement in support groups and community activities. In the absence of ART, however, disease progression can be delayed only for a finite amount of time.

Patients should be taught to recognize symptoms that may indicate disease progression or medication adverse effects so that prompt medical care can be initiated. Table 17.23 provides an overview of symptoms that patients should report. In general, patients should have as much information as needed to make informed decisions about their health care. These decisions then dictate the appropriate interventions.

Acute Exacerbations. Chronic diseases are characterized by acute exacerbations of recurring problems. This is especially true in HIV disease, in which infections, cancers, debility, and psychosocial and economic issues may interact to overwhelm the patient's ability to cope. Nursing care becomes more complex if the patient's immune system deteriorates and new health conditions arise to compound existing difficulties. When opportunistic diseases or difficult adverse effects of treatment develop, symptom management, education, and emotional support are necessary (CANAC, 2013).

Nursing care assumes primary importance in helping patients prevent the many opportunistic diseases associated with HIV infection. The best prevention of opportunistic disease is adequate treatment of the underlying HIV infection.

Ongoing Care. HIV-infected patients share challenges experienced by all individuals with chronic diseases, but these problems are exacerbated by social constructs surrounding HIV. Chronic diseases are often characterized by negative social attitudes that label the patient as weak-willed or immoral for being sick. In HIV, this stigma is compounded by several factors. HIV-infected people may be seen as lacking control over urges to have sex or use drugs. It is then easy to jump to the conclusion that they brought the disease on themselves and, therefore, somehow deserve to be sick. Behaviours associated with HIV infection may be viewed as immoral (e.g., having many sexual partners) and are sometimes illegal (e.g., injecting drugs). The fact that infected individuals can transmit the virus to others furthers the negative, stigmatizing social concept of HIV. Social stigmatization can lead to discrimination in all facets of life. According to the Canadian Human Rights Commission policy on HIV/AIDS, all Canadians have the right to equality and dignity without discrimination, regardless of HIV/AIDS status (Elliot & Gold, 2005).

The chronic nature of HIV infection can cause family stress, social isolation, dependence, frustration, lowered self-image, loss of control over aspects of one's life, and economic pressures. All of these variables may have contributed to the patient's situation surrounding infection in the first place. Low self-esteem, searching for social contact, frustration, and economic difficulties can all contribute to drug use and risky sexual behaviours.

Disease and Medication Adverse Effects. Physical conditions related to untreated HIV disease can interrupt the patient's ability to maintain a desired lifestyle. For instance, a new set of metabolic disorders has emerged among HIV-infected patients, especially

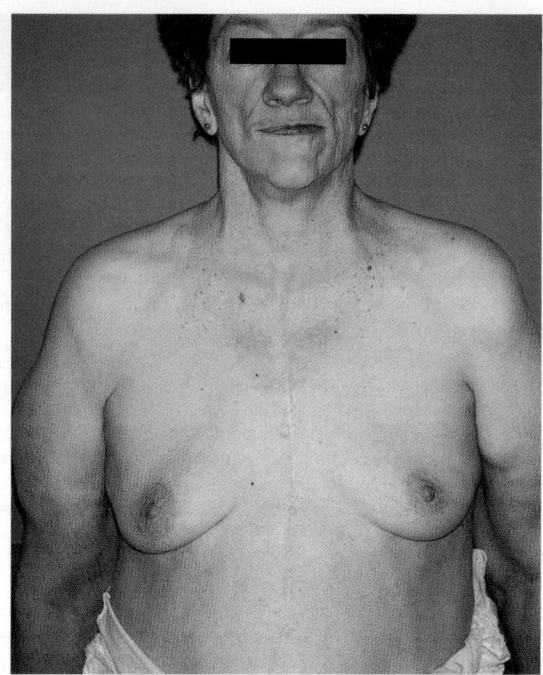

FIG. 17.8 Manifestations of lipodystrophy. Source: James, W. D., Berger, T., & Elston, D. (2006). *Andrews' diseases of the skin: Clinical dermatology* (10th ed.). Saunders.

those who have been infected for a long time and who have been receiving ART. These disorders include changes in body shape (fat deposits in the abdomen, upper back, and breasts, along with fat loss in the arms, legs, and face) caused by lipodystrophy (Figure 17.8); dyslipidemia (elevated triglycerides and decreases in high-density lipoproteins); insulin resistance and hyperglycemia; bone disease (osteoporosis, osteopenia, avascular necrosis); lactic acidosis; and cardiovascular disease. It is still not clear why these disorders develop, but the reason is probably a combination of factors such as long-term infection with HIV, adverse effects of ART, genetic predisposition, and chronic stress.

Management of metabolic disorders currently focuses on detecting problems early, dealing with the symptoms, and helping the patient cope with new health issues and additional medications. It is important to recognize and treat these conditions early, especially because cardiovascular disease and lactic acidosis are potentially fatal complications. A frequent first intervention is to change ART because some medications are more often associated with these conditions than are others (see Table 17.14). Lipid abnormalities are generally treated with lipid-lowering medications, dietary changes, and exercise. Insulin resistance is treated with hypoglycemic medications and weight loss. Bone disease may be improved with exercise, dietary changes, and calcium and vitamin D supplements.

Body changes that combine fat accumulation and wasting are major concerns for patients with this syndrome. Human growth hormone, testosterone, and anabolic steroids have been used to help resolve these changes, but the results are inconclusive. Some patients may undergo plastic surgery procedures such as liposuction or facial implants to deal with the body changes associated with fat redistribution. There is little evidence that exercise or dietary changes make any difference. Nursing interventions must focus on helping the patient make treatment decisions and on coping with negative changes in body image (CANAC, 2013).

End-of-Life Care. Despite new developments in the treatment of HIV infection, some patients eventually experience disease progression, disability, and death. This progression is often due to the inability to access and adhere to treatment because of housing, social, or financial challenges. Mental illness and substance use can also present barriers to accessing care. In addition, ART is now enabling people living with HIV to live longer and to develop diseases of aging, such as cardiovascular and endocrine conditions that lead to death. Nursing care during the terminal phase of any disease must focus on keeping the patient comfortable, facilitating emotional and spiritual acceptance of the finite nature of life, and helping the patient's loved ones with their grief and loss. Nurses become pivotal care providers during the terminal phase of illness, especially in HIV disease, for which patients and families often choose terminal care at home. (End-of-life care is discussed in Chapter 13.)

EVALUATION

The expected outcomes are that the patient at risk for HIV infection will do the following:

- Analyze personal risk factors
- Develop and implement a personal plan to decrease risks
- Get tested for HIV infection

The expected outcomes are that the patient with HIV infection will do the following:

- Describe basic aspects of the effects of HIV on the immune system
- Compare and contrast various treatment options for HIV disease
- Work with a team of health care providers to achieve optimal health
- Prevent transmission of HIV to others

ETHICAL DILEMMAS

Duty to Treat

Situation

A nurse in a community clinic has just discovered that J. M. (pronouns she/her), a patient with respiratory problems, has human immunodeficiency virus (HIV) infection. The nurse is concerned about physical contact with J. M. and her body fluids. The nurse requests that she not be assigned to J. M.'s care. The nurse believes that she has the right to refuse to care for J. M. because she has her own family to support and protect.

Important Points for Consideration

- According to the Canadian Nurses Association's *Code of Ethics*, the nurse must not discriminate in the provision of nursing care on the basis of cultural or socioeconomic background or health status.
- Health care providers have contact with patients every day who may have infectious blood or other body fluids.
- Infection precautions are instituted to protect health care workers from potentially infectious blood or other body fluids.

- There are two situations in which nurses can refuse to care for patients if employers are notified in advance: (a) when caring for a patient would conflict with a nurse's deeply held religious belief, or (b) when there might be greater potential harm to the nurse than benefit to the patient (e.g., if the nurse were immunocompromised).
- The Canadian Human Rights Commission Policy (1996) on HIV/AIDS prohibits discrimination based on HIV/AIDS status.
- If a nurse's primary concern is personal safety, the nurse needs to re-examine their commitment to the nursing profession.

Clinical Decision-Making Questions

1. How should a nurse address this issue if a colleague refused to provide care for a patient with HIV infection?
2. If nurses could select which patients they would care for, how would that affect their ability to care for patients in general?

CASE STUDY

At Risk for Human Immunodeficiency Virus Disease

Patient Profile
E. C. (pronouns they/them), a 20-year-old university student, comes to the student health centre with pain on urination.

Subjective Data
- Describes pain as "Just like it felt when I had the clap last year"
- Provides a history of sexual activity since age 15; reports lifetime sexual partners as six women and two men
- Denies injected-drug use, tobacco use, or corticosteroid therapy
- Uses alcohol (mainly beer) at weekend parties and has smoked cannabis, but not recently
- Recent sexual activity has been on weekends during or after parties

Objective Data
Physical Examination
- 180 cm tall, 76 kg, temperature 38°C, purulent urethral discharge noted

Laboratory Studies
- Urine test for *Neisseria gonorrhoeae* yields positive result

Interprofessional Care
- Intramuscular injection with ceftriaxone, 250 mg
- Doxycycline, 100 mg orally, twice daily for 7 days

Discussion Questions
1. Why should E. C. be encouraged to be tested for human immunodeficiency virus (HIV)?
2. How will the nurse counsel E. C. about the testing process? How can the nurse help them prepare for the test and the test results?
3. What further questions will the nurse need to ask E. C. before the nurse can determine their educational needs?
4. Ask a classmate to be "E. C." and role-play HIV risk assessment, risk-reduction counselling, pretest and post-test counselling.
5. *Priority Decision:* What are the main considerations to cover when teaching about barrier methods of protection? Are there cultural components that may affect the nurse's approach to teaching about condoms?
6. How will the nurse discuss the issue of partner notification with E. C.?
7. *Priority Decision:* E. C.'s HIV test result comes back positive. What are the priority nursing decisions? What psychosocial issues would the nurse consider? What are the most important things for E. C. to know at the first meeting after getting their diagnosis? How might E. C. react, and how should the nurse respond?

℮volve

REVIEW QUESTIONS

The number of the question corresponds to the same-numbered objective at the beginning of the chapter.

1. What are nursing responsibilities regarding emerging and re-emerging infections? *(Select all that apply.)*
   a. Educating clients about risks of developing emerging and re-emerging infections
   b. Maintaining awareness of unusual disease patterns
   c. Participating in immunization programs
   d. Using infection control procedures
   e. Examining prescribing practices to ensure appropriate antibiotic use
2. Which of the following antibiotic-resistant organisms are resistant to normal hand soap?
   a. Vancomycin-resistant enterococci
   b. Methicillin-resistant *Staphylococcus aureus*
   c. Penicillin-resistant *Streptococcus pneumoniae*
   d. β-Lactamase–producing *Klebsiella pneumoniae*
3. How is human immunodeficiency virus (HIV) transmitted?
   a. Most commonly as a result of sexual contact
   b. In all infants born to women with HIV infection
   c. Only when there is a large viral load in the blood
   d. Frequently in health care workers with needle-stick exposures
4. Which is the common physiological change after HIV infection?
   a. The virus replicates mainly in B lymphocytes before spreading to CD4+ T cells in lymph nodes.
   b. The immune system is impaired predominantly by infection and destruction of CD4+ T cells.
   c. Infection of monocytes may occur, but these cells are destroyed by antibodies produced by oligodendrocytes.
   d. A long period develops during which the virus is not found in the blood and there is little viral replication.
5. Which of the following statements is false?
   a. "Infection with HIV results in a chronic disease with acute exacerbations and progression if left untreated."
   b. "Untreated HIV infection can remain in the early chronic stage for a decade or more."
   c. "Late-stage infection is often called *acquired immune deficiency syndrome (AIDS)*."
   d. "Opportunistic diseases occur more often when the CD4+ T-cell count is high and the viral load is low."
6. When is AIDS diagnosed in an HIV-infected person?
   a. When an AIDS-defining illness develops
   b. When the amount of HIV in the blood increases
   c. When the CD4:CD8 ratio is reversed to less than 2:1
   d. When the person has oral hairy leukoplakia, an infection caused by Epstein-Barr virus
7. What does screening for HIV infection generally involve?
   a. Laboratory analysis of blood to detect HIV antigen and antibody
   b. Electrophoretic analysis of HIV antigen in plasma
   c. Laboratory analysis of blood to detect increased T cells
   d. Analysis of lymph tissues for the presence of HIV RNA

8. What is the indication for use of antiretroviral medications?
   a. Cure acute HIV infection
   b. Treat opportunistic diseases
   c. Decrease viral RNA levels
   d. Supplement radiation therapy and surgery
9. Which statement about metabolic adverse effects of ART is true? *(Select all that apply.)*
   a. "These are annoying symptoms that are ultimately harmless."
   b. "ART-related body changes include central fat accumulation and peripheral wasting."
   c. "Lipid abnormalities include increases in triglycerides and decreases in high-density cholesterol."
   d. "Insulin resistance and hyperlipidemia can be treated with medications to control glucose and cholesterol."
   e. "Insulin resistance and hyperlipidemia are more difficult to treat in HIV-infected clients than in uninfected people."
10. Which of the following descriptions of opportunistic diseases in HIV infection is correct?
   a. Usually occur one at a time
   b. Generally slow to develop and progress
   c. Occur in the presence of immunosuppression
   d. Curable with appropriate pharmacological intervention
11. Of the following, which is the most appropriate nursing intervention to help an HIV-infected client adhere to the treatment regimen?
   a. Give the client a DVD and a brochure to view and read at home.
   b. Volunteer to "set up" a medication pillbox for a week at a time.
   c. Inform the client that the adverse effects of the medications are bad but that they go away after a while.
   d. Assess the client's lifestyle and find adherence cues that fit into the client's lifestyle.
12. Which strategy can the nurse teach the client to eliminate the risk of transmission of HIV?
   a. Using sterile equipment to inject drugs
   b. Cleaning equipment used to inject drugs
   c. Taking zidovudine (azidothymidine [AZT], ZDV, Retrovir) during pregnancy
   d. Using latex barriers to cover genitals during sexual contact

1. a, b, c, d, e; 2. a; 3. a; 4. b; 5. d; 6. a; 7. a; 8. c; 9. b, c, d; 10. c; 11. d; 12. a.

For even more review questions, visit http://evolve.elsevier.com/Canada/Lewis/medsurg.

REFERENCES

AIDS InfoNet. (2014). *Fact sheet 729: St. Johns wort (hypericin)* http://www.aidsinfonet.org/fact_sheets/view/729. (Seminal).

Amico, K. R., & Mayer, K. H. (2018). HIV preexposure prophylaxis: A review. *JAMA, 319*(12), 1261–1268. https://doi.org/10.1001/jama.2018.1917

Bailey, H., Zash, R., Rasi, V., et al. (2018). HIV treatment in pregnancy. *The Lancet HIV, 5*(8), e457–e467. https://doi.org/10.1016/S2352-3018(18)30059-6

BC Centre for Excellence in HIV/, A. I. D. S. (2020). *Therapeutic guidelines for antiretroviral (ARV) treatment of adult HIV infection.* http://bccfe.ca/sites/default/files/uploads/Guidelines/2020_06_30-BC-CfE_Adult_ARV_Therapeutic_Guidelines.pdf

Beste, S., Essajee, S., Siberry, G., et al. (2018). Optimal antiretroviral prophylaxis in infants at high risk of acquiring HIV. *The Pediatric Infectious Disease Journal, 37*(2), 169–175. https://doi.org/10.1097/INF.0000000000001700

Burdge, D. R., Money, D. M., Forbes, J. C., & Canadian HIV Trials Network Working Group on Vertical HIV Transmission., et al. (2003). Canadian consensus guidelines for the management of pregnancy, labour and delivery and for postpartum care in HIV-positive pregnant women and their offspring (summary of 2002 guidelines). *Canadian Medical Association Journal, 168*(13), 1671–1674 (Seminal).

Canadian Association of Nurses in AIDS Care. (2013). *Best practice guidelines: Caring for clients who are at risk for or living with HIV/AIDS.* http://www.canac.org/wp-content/uploads/2015/11/CANAC_BPG_v2013.pdf

Centers for Disease Control and Prevention (CDC). (2016). *Infection control basics.* https://www.cdc.gov/infectioncontrol/basics/index.html

Centers for Disease Control and Prevention (CDC). (2020). *HIV transmission.* http://www.cdc.gov/hiv/basics/transmission.html

Centers for Disease Control and Prevention (CDC). (2021). *HIV among pregnant women, infants and children.* https://www.cdc.gov/hiv/group/gender/pregnantwomen/

Clinical Info.HIV.gov. (2021). *Preventing mother-to-child transmission of HIV.* www.hiv.gov/hiv-basics/hiv-prevention/reducing-mother-to-child-risk/preventing-mother-to-child-transmission-of-hiv

Elliot, R., & Gold, J. (2005). Protection against discrimination based on HIV/AIDS status in Canada: the legal framework. *HIV/AIDS Policy and Law Review, 10*(1). http://www.aidslaw.ca/site/wp-content/uploads/2013/04/DiscrProtect-Review10-1-E.pdf. (Seminal).

Government of Canada. (2019a). *Lyme disease.* https://www.canada.ca/en/public-health/services/diseases/lyme-disease.html

Government of Canada. (2019b). *Zika virus: Symptoms and treatment.* https://www.canada.ca/en/public-health/services/diseases/zika-virus.html

Government of Canada. (2020). *Measles: Symptoms and treatment.* https://www.canada.ca/en/public-health/services/diseases/measles.html

Government of Canada. (2021a). *Surveillance of West Nile virus.* www.canada.ca/en/public-health/services/diseases/west-nile-virus/surveillance-west-nile-virus.html

Government of Canada. (2021b). *Update on Ebola outbreaks.* https://www.canada.ca/en/public-health/services/diseases/ebola.html

Government of Saskatchewan: Ministry of Health Population Health Branch. (2017). *HIV prevention and control report,* 1–5. https://pubsaskdev.blob.core.windows.net/pubsask-prod/108029/108029-2017-Saskatchewan-HIV-Prevention-and-Control-Report.pdf

Gunthard, H. F., Aberg, J. A., Eron, J. J., et al. (2014). Antiretroviral treatment of adult HIV infection: 2104 Recommendations of the International Antiviral Society—USA panel. *Journal of the American Medical Association, 312*(4), 410–425. https://doi.org/10.1001/jama.2014.8722

Harries, A., & Takarinda, K. C. (2019). *Prime recommendation of Risk of HIV transmission through condomless sex in serodifferent gay couples with the HIV-positive partner taking suppressive antiretroviral therapy (PARTNER): Final results of a multicentre, prospective, observational study.* Post-Publication Peer Review of the Biomedical Literature. https://doi.org/10.3410/f.735676518.793562292

Health Canada. (2021). *Supervised consumption sites explained.* https://www.canada.ca/en/health-canada/services/substance-use/supervised-consumption-sites/explained.html

HIV.gov. (2021). *Post-exposure prophylaxis (PEP).* https://www.hiv.gov/hiv-basics/hiv-prevention/using-hiv-medication-to-reduce-risk/post-exposure-prophylaxis

HIVinfo.NIH.gov. (2019). *The HIV life cycle.* https://hivinfo.nih.gov/understanding-hiv/fact-sheets/hiv-life-cycle

Huether, S. E., & MacCance, K. L. (2019). *Understanding pathophysiology.* Mosby.

Hoenigl, M., Green, N., Camacho, M., et al. (2016). Signs or symptoms of acute HIV infection in a cohort undergoing community-based screening. *Emerging Infectious Diseases, 22*(3), 532. https://doi.org/10.3201/eid2203.151607

International Partnership for Microbicides. (2020). *How HIV infects a cell.* www.ipmglobal.org/how-hiv-infects-cell#:~:text=HIV%20is%20a%20retrovirus%2C%20which,human%2C%20or%20host%2C%20cells

Katz, M. J., & Roghmann, M. C. (2016). Healthcare-associated infections in the elderly: What's new. *Current Opinion in Infectious Diseases, 29*(4), 388. https://doi.org/10.1097/QCO.0000000000000283

Kuhar, D. T., Henderson, D. K., Struble, K. A., et al. (2013). Updated US Public Health Service guidelines for the management of occupational exposures to human immunodeficiency virus and recommendations for post-exposure prophylaxis. *Infection Control and Hospital Epidemiology, 34*(9), 875–892. https://doi.org/10.1086/672271. (Seminal).

Mitchell, R., Taylor, G., Rudnick, W., et al. (2019). Trends in health care–associated infections in acute care hospitals in Canada: an analysis of repeated point-prevalence surveys. *CMAJ, 191*(36), E981–E988. https://doi.org/10.1503/cmaj.190361

Panel on Antiretroviral Guidelines for Adults and Adolescents. (2019). *Guidelines for the use of antiretroviral agents in adults and adolescents with HIV.* Department of Health and Human Services. https://clinicalinfo.hiv.gov/sites/default/files/guidelines/documents/AdultandAdolescentGL.pdf

Pepin, J. (2011). *The origin of AIDS.* Cambridge University Press (Seminal).

Public Health Agency of Canada (PHAC). (2011). *Chapter 7: HIV/AIDS Epi updates, July 2010—Perinatal HIV transmission in Canada.* http://www.phac-aspc.gc.ca/aids-sida/publication/epi/2010/7-eng.php. (Seminal).

Public Health Agency of Canada (PHAC). (2012a). *Hand hygiene practices in health care settings.* https://publications.gc.ca/collections/collection_2012/aspc-phac/HP40-74-2012-eng.pdf. (Seminal).

Public Health Agency of Canada (PHAC). (2012b). *Routine practices and additional precautions for preventing the transmission of infection in health care settings.* https://publications.gc.ca/collections/collection_2013/aspc-phac/HP40-83-2013-eng.pdf. (Seminal)

Public Health Agency of Canada (PHAC). (2015a). *Canadian Communicable Disease Report* (Vol. 41). http://www.phac-aspc.gc.ca/publicat/ccdr-rmtc/15vol41/index-eng.php

Public Health Agency of Canada (PHAC). (2015b). *AIDS status report: People living with HIV/AIDS—Epidemiological profile of HIV & AIDS in Canada.* Chapter 2: Population-specific HIV/AIDS http://www.phac-aspc.gc.ca/aids-sida/publication/ps-pd/people-personnes/chapter-chapitre-2-eng.php

Public Health Agency of Canada (PHAC). (2016a). *Canadian Antimicrobial Resistance Surveillance System Report 2016.* www.canada.ca/en/public-health/services/publications/drugs-health-products/canadian-antimicrobial-resistance-surveillance-system-report-2016.html#a8-2-8

Public Health Agency of Canada (PHAC). (2016b). *Canadian guidelines on sexually transmitted infections—Management and treatment of specific infections—human immunodeficiency virus infections.* https://www.canada.ca/en/public-health/services/infectious-diseases/sexual-health-sexually-transmitted-infections/canadian-guidelines/sexually-transmitted-infections/canadian-guidelines-sexually-transmitted-infections-36.html

Public Health Agency of Canada (PHAC). (2019a). *Disease present and control guidelines.* https://www.canada.ca/en/public-health/services/reports-publications/disease-prevention-control-guidelines.html

Public Health Agency of Canada (PHAC). (2019b). *Healthcare-associated infection rates in Canadian hospitals.* https://www.canada.ca/content/dam/canada/public-health/services/publications/science-research-data/healthcare-associated-infection-rates-canadian-hospitals-infographic/CNISP-2013-2017-infographic-eng.pdf

Public Health Agency of Canada (PHAC). (2021). *Summary: Estimates of HIV incidence, prevalence and Canada's progress on meeting the 90-90-90 HIV targets, 2016.* https://www.canada.ca/en/public-health/services/publications/diseases-conditions/summary-estimates-hiv-incidence-prevalence-canadas-progress-90-90-90.htm

Siemieniuk, R. A., Foroutan, F., Mirza, R., et al. (2017). Antiretroviral therapy for pregnant women living with HIV or hepatitis B: a systematic review and meta-analysis. *BMJ Open, 7*(9), e019022. https://doi.org/10.1136/bmjopen-2017-019022Open

Tan, D. H., Hull, M. W., Yoong, D., et al. (2017). Canadian guideline on HIV pre-exposure prophylaxis and nonoccupational postexposure prophylaxis. *Canadian Medical Association Journal, 189*(47), E1448–E1458. https://doi.org/10.1503/cmaj.170494

Underhill, K., Morrow, K. M., Colleran, C., et al. (2015). Explaining the efficacy of pre-exposure prophylaxis (PrEP) for HIV prevention: A qualitative study of message framing and messaging preferences among US men who have sex with men. *AIDS and Behavior, 20*(7), 1514–1526. https://doi.org/10.1007/s10461-015-1088-9

United Nations AIDS (UNAIDS). (2021). *Global HIV & AIDS statistics: Fact sheet.* https://www.unaids.org/en/resources/fact-sheet

World Health Organization (WHO). (2007). *WHO case definitions of HIV for surveillance and revised clinical staging and immunological classification of HIV-related disease in adults and children* http://www.who.int/hiv/pub/guidelines/HIVstaging150307.pdf. (Seminal).

World Health Organization (WHO). (2016). *Guidelines on HIV self-testing and partner notification: Supplement to consolidated guidelines on HIV testing services.* https://www.ncbi.nlm.nih.gov/books/NBK401684/

World Health Organization. (2020a). *Antimicrobial resistance.* http://www.who.int/mediacentre/factsheets/fs194/en/

World Health Organization. (2020b). *Ebola outbreak—Democratic Republic of the Congo.* https://www.who.int/emergencies/situations/Ebola-2019-drc-

World Health Organization. (2020c). *Ebola virus: Vaccines.* https://www.who.int/news-room/q-a-detail/ebola-vaccines

World Health Organization. (2021a). *Ebola virus disease.* https://www.who.int/news-room/fact-sheets/detail/ebola-virus-disease

World Health Organization. (2021b). *HIV/AIDS.* https://www.who.int/health-topics/hiv-aids#tab=tab_1

RESOURCES

BC Centre for Excellence in HIV/AIDS
http://bccfe.ca/
Canadian Aboriginal AIDS Network
https://www.caan.ca
Canadian AIDS Society
https://www.cdnaids.ca
Canadian AIDS Treatment Information Exchange (CATIE)
https://www.catie.ca
Canadian Association of Nurses in HIV/AIDS Care
https://www.canac.org
Canadian Blood Services
https://www.blood.ca
Canadian Centre for Occupational Health and Safety
https://www.ccohs.ca
Canadian Lyme Disease Foundation
https://canlyme.com
Canadian Nurses Association: *Code of Ethics for Registered Nurses*
https://www.cna-aiic.ca/~/media/cna/page-content/pdf-en/code-of-ethics-2017-edition-secure-interactive.pdf?la=en
Canadian Public Health Association
https://www.cpha.ca
Health Canada: *HIV and AIDS—Diseases and Conditions*
https://www.canada.ca/en/health-canada/services/health-concerns/diseases-conditions/hiv-aids-diseases-conditions.html
HIV and AIDS: for Health Professionals
https://www.canada.ca/en/public-health/services/diseases/hiv-aids/health-professionals.html
HIV Legal Network
https://www.hivlegalnetwork.ca/site/?lang=en
Infection Prevention and Control Canada (IPAC)
https://ipac-canada.org
National Collaborating Centre for Infection Diseases
https://nccid.ca/
Public Health Agency of Canada
http://www.phac-aspc.gc.ca
Public Health Agency of Canada: *HIV/AIDS Epi Updates*
http://www.phac-aspc.gc.ca/aids-sida/publication/epi/2010/1-eng.php
Public Health Agency of Canada: *Public Health Surveillance*
http://www.phac-aspc.gc.ca/surveillance-eng.php
Realize Canada
https://www.realizecanada.org/en/

Joint United Nations Programme on HIV/AIDS (UNAIDS)
https://www.unaids.org

evolve

For additional Internet resources, see the website for this book at http://evolve.elsevier.com/Canada/Lewis/medsurg.

Cancer

Rosemary Cashman
Originating US chapter by Marisa Cortese

evolve WEBSITE

http://evolve.elsevier.com/Canada/Lewis/medsurg

- Review Questions (Online Only)
- Key Points
- Customizable Nursing Care Plans
  - Radiation
  - Chemotherapy
- Conceptual Care Map Creator
- Audio Glossary
- Content Updates

LEARNING OBJECTIVES

1. List the prevalence, incidence, and death rates of cancer in Canada.
2. Describe the biological processes involved in cancer.
3. Differentiate the three phases of cancer development.
4. Describe the role of the immune system in relation to cancer.
5. Describe the use of the classification systems for cancer.
6. Explain the role of the nurse in the prevention and detection of cancer.
7. Explain the use of surgery, radiation therapy, chemotherapy, and biological therapy in the treatment of cancer.
8. Differentiate between external beam radiation and brachytherapy.
9. Identify the classifications of chemotherapeutic agents and methods of administration.
10. Describe the effects of radiation therapy and chemotherapy on normal tissues.
11. Identify the types and effects of biological therapy agents.
12. Describe the nursing management of patients receiving radiation therapy, chemotherapy, and biological therapy.
13. Describe the nutritional therapy for patients with cancer.
14. Describe the complications that can occur in advanced cancer.
15. Describe the appropriate psychosocial support of a patient with cancer and the patient's family.

KEY TERMS

benign neoplasms
biological therapy
bone marrow transplantation
brachytherapy
cancer
carcinogens
carcinoma
carcinoma in situ

extravasation
histological grading
immunological surveillance
malignant neoplasms
metastasis
nadir
oncogenes
proto-oncogenes

radiation
sarcoma
staging
tumour angiogenesis
tumour-associated antigens
tumour suppressor genes
vesicants

DEFINITION AND INCIDENCE

Cancer is a group of more than 200 diseases characterized by the uncontrolled and unregulated growth of cells. It can occur in persons of all ages and all ethnicities and is a major health problem. In 2019, the Canadian Cancer Statistics Advisory Committee estimated that 220 400 new cancer cases would be diagnosed and that 82 100 people would die from cancer in Canada. As the population ages, the incidence of cancer has risen. It is expected that 90% of new cancer cases will be diagnosed in Canadians 50 years of age and older. Cancer is more common among women between the age of 20 and 59 years, primarily because of breast and thyroid cancer. Nearly 40% of breast cancer cases

are expected to be diagnosed in women aged 30 to 59. In all other age groups, cancer is more common in men. Cancer incidence and death rates also increase from west to east across the country. Although overall mortality has declined in Canada, the number of cancer cases has continued to increase, with significant repercussions on Canadian families, health policy, and the economy (Canadian Cancer Statistics Advisory Committee, 2019). Cancer incidence and mortality are tracked by province and territory through cancer registries. Estimated cancer incidences and mortality rates by site (type) and sex are presented in Tables 18.1 and 18.2. A Canadian cancer statistics report is released every 2 years; the most notable new statistics indicating changing patterns are outlined in Table 18.3.

TABLE 18.1 NEW CASES FOR CANCER BY SITE (TYPE) AND SEX, CANADA, 2019

Type	New Case Estimate	
	Male	Female
Prostate	22 900	N/A
Breast	230	26 900
Lung	14 900	14 500
Colorectal	14 600	11 700
Non-Hodgkin's lymphoma	5 600	4 400
Bladder	9 100	2 700
Kidney	4 700	2 500
Thyroid	2 100	6 100
Uterus	N/A	7 200

Source: Adapted from Canadian Cancer Statistics Advisory Committee. (2019). *Canadian cancer statistics 2019*. Author. cancer.ca/Canadian-Cancer-Statistics-2019-EN

TABLE 18.2 ESTIMATED DEATHS FOR CANCER BY SITE AND SEX, CANADA, 2016

Male		Female	
Type	Deaths	Type	Deaths
Lung	10 900	Lung	10 100
Prostate	4 100	Breast	5 000
Colorectal	5 200	Colorectal	4 400
Pancreas	2 700	Pancreas	2 500
Bladder	1 800	Ovary	1 900

Source: Adapted from Canadian Cancer Statistics Advisory Committee. (2019). *Canadian cancer statistics 2019*. Author. cancer.ca/Canadian-Cancer-Statistics-2019-EN

TABLE 18.3 NOTABLE NEW CANADIAN CANCER STATISTICS FOR 2019

Canadian Cancer Statistical Data Identifying New Patterns
1. Pancreatic cancer is expected to be the third leading cause of cancer death in Canada, surpassing breast cancer.
2. Lung cancer incidence and death mortality rates for females are decreasing.
3. Female breast cancer death rates have decreased approximately 48% since they peaked in 1986.
4. Some of the biggest increase in survival rates since the early 1990s were for blood-related cancers.

Source: Adapted from Canadian Cancer Statistics Advisory Committee. (2019). *Canadian cancer statistics 2019*. Author. cancer.ca/Canadian-Cancer-Statistics-2019-EN

Prevalence is a term used to describe the total number of people who are living with a diagnosis of cancer. Advances in research in the areas of early detection, treatment, and supportive therapies have resulted in more people surviving cancer, especially in the pediatric population. In the context of cancer, therefore, prevalence is more often and more usefully defined as patients still alive 10 years after the initial diagnosis with cancer. Over a lifetime, it is estimated that nearly one in two Canadians (45% of male Canadians and 43% of female Canadians) will develop cancer and one in four (26% of male Canadians and 23% of female Canadians) will die from it (Canadian Cancer Statistics Advisory Committee, 2019). In 2017, cancer was the leading cause of death in Canada, accounting for 30% of all deaths, with cardiovascular diseases (heart and cerebrovascular diseases) in second place (Statistics Canada, 2017). Of the 220 400 new cases of cancer predicted in 2019, the five leading causes of cancer death (lung, colorectal, pancreas, breast, and prostate cancers) accounted for over 50% of all cancer deaths in Canada. Lung cancer remains the leading cause of premature death from cancer (Canadian Cancer Statistics Advisory Committee, 2019).

Tobacco use has long been recognized as a significant risk for the development of lung and other types of cancer. Smoking prevalence and amount have declined in the Canadian population overall; however, smoking rates among Indigenous peoples 15 to 19 years of age are at least three times higher than rates for their non-Indigenous peer group (11% in non-Indigenous vs. 33% in First Nations vs. 65% in Nunavut) (Jetty et al., 2017). Indigenous people in Canada have disproportionately high rates of many cancers and worse cancer outcomes when compared to the non-Indigenous population. Health care policies and systems must address these disparities in cancer incidence and access to treatment and respond appropriately to the social determinants of health affecting Indigenous populations (Horrill et al., 2019; Mazereeuw et al., 2018; National Collaborating Centre for Aboriginal Health, 2013).

While statistics document the incidence and prevalence of cancer, they cannot reveal the physiological and psychosocial effect of cancer on individuals, families, and society. Nurses play a critical role in shaping attitudes and promoting behaviours that prevent the development of cancer and facilitate adjustment to living with cancer.

Progress Made in Cancer Prevention: Modifiable Risk Factors

Many well-known and common cancer risk factors are preventable. For example, in addition to tobacco use, known risk factors include excessive body weight, lack of physical activity, unhealthy eating habits, alcohol consumption, and excessive exposure to the sun. Several of these factors are related to other chronic diseases, such as diabetes, kidney failure, chronic obstructive lung disease, and cardiovascular disease. The Canadian Cancer Society reported a worrisome rising trend in obesity: The percentage of overweight or obese Canadians increased from 61.9% in 2015 to 63.1% in 2018 (Statistics Canada, 2019). In addition, as recently as 2017, only 16.4% of Canadian adults met the recommended physical activity target (Statistics Canada, 2019). All of these risk factors are within the control of each individual. If these lifestyle factors were modified, the rates of cancers and other chronic diseases would be reduced. Concerted efforts in health promotion and disease prevention strategies are required in every province to alert and educate the public about what they can do to achieve improvements in health and longevity.

BIOLOGICAL PROCESSES OF CANCER

The term *cancer* encompasses many diseases of multiple causes that can arise in any cell of the body capable of evading regulatory controls over proliferation and differentiation. Two major dysfunctions present in the process of cancer are defective cellular *proliferation* (growth) and defective cellular *differentiation*.

Defects in Cellular Proliferation

Normally, most tissues of the human adult contain a population of predetermined, undifferentiated cells known as *stem cells*. *Predetermined* means that the stem cells of a particular tissue will ultimately differentiate and become mature, functioning cells of that tissue and only that tissue.

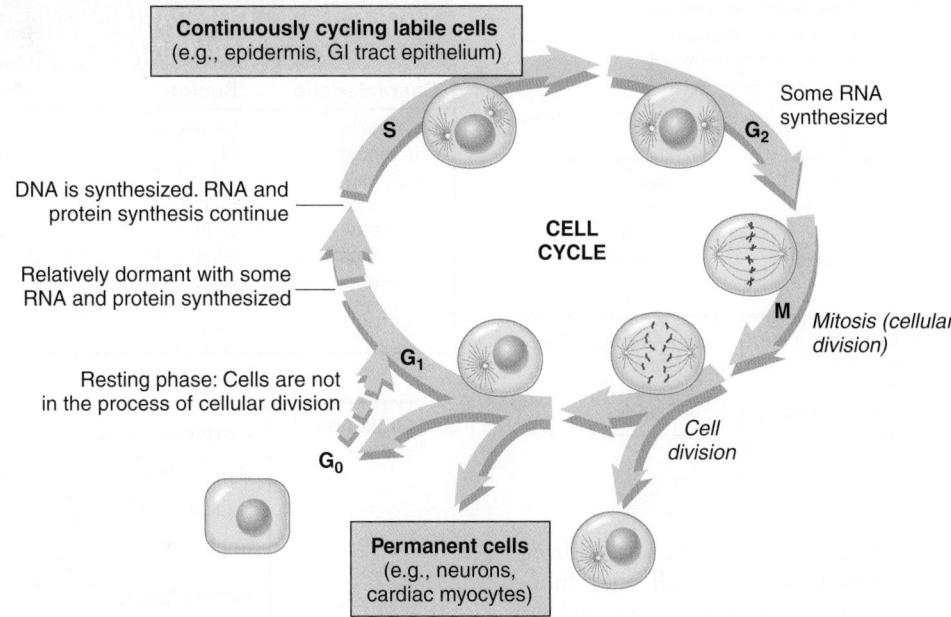

FIG. 18.1 Cell life cycle and metabolic activity. Generation time is the period from one M (mitosis) phase to the next. Cells not in the cycle but capable of division are in the resting phase (G_0). *DNA*, deoxyribonucleic acid; *GI*, gastrointestinal; *RNA*, ribonucleic acid. Source: Adapted from Kumar, V., Abbas, A. K., Fausto, N., et al. (2010). *Robbins and Cotran pathologic basis of disease* (8th ed., p. 86). W. B. Saunders.

Cell proliferation originates in the stem cell and begins when the stem cell enters the cell cycle (Figure 18.1). The time from when a cell enters the cell cycle to when the cell divides into two identical cells is called the *generation time of the cell*. A mature cell continues to function until it degenerates and dies.

All cells of a tissue are controlled by an intracellular mechanism that determines when cellular proliferation is necessary. Under normal conditions, a state of dynamic equilibrium is constantly maintained (i.e., rate of cellular proliferation equals rate of cellular degeneration). Normally, the process of cellular division and proliferation is activated only in the event of cellular degeneration or death. Cellular proliferation also occurs if the body has a physiological need for more cells. For example, the white blood cell (WBC) count normally increases in the presence of infection.

Another mechanism for proliferation control in normal cells is *contact inhibition*. Normal cells "respect" the boundaries and territory of the cells surrounding them; they do not invade a territory that is not their own. The neighbouring cells are thought to inhibit cellular growth through the physical contact of the surrounding cell membranes. Cancer cells grown in tissue culture are characterized by loss of contact inhibition. These cells breach cellular boundaries and will grow on top of one another and also on top of or between normal cells.

The rate of normal cellular proliferation differs in each body tissue. In some tissues, such as bone marrow, hair follicles, and epithelial lining of the gastrointestinal (GI) tract, the rate of cellular proliferation is rapid. In other tissues, such as myocardium, neurons, and cartilage, cellular proliferation is slow or does not occur at all.

Cancer cells usually proliferate in the manner and at the same rate as the normal cells of the tissue from which they arise. However, cancer cells respond differently than normal cells to the intracellular signals that regulate the state of dynamic equilibrium. Whereas normal cell proliferation is regulated according to the body's needs, cell division in cancer is dysregulated and haphazard, and proliferation of cancer cells is indiscriminate and continuous. In this way, with each cell division creating two or more offspring cells, the tumour mass continuously doubles in size: 1 cell → 2 cells → 4 cells → 8 cells → 16 cells, and so on. This is termed the *pyramid effect*. The time required for a tumour mass to double in size is known as its *doubling time*.

According to the stem cell theory, the loss of intracellular control of proliferation results from a mutation of the stem cells. The stem cells are viewed as the target or the origin of cancer development. The DNA of the stem cell is substituted or permanently rearranged. When this happens, the stem cell has mutated. Once the cell has mutated, one of three things can occur: (1) the cell can die, either from the damage resulting from the mutation or from initiation of a programmed cellular suicide called *apoptosis*; (2) the cell can recognize the damage and repair itself; or (3) the mutated cell can survive and pass along the damage to its daughter cells. Mutated cells that survive have the potential to become malignant (i.e., cells with invasive and metastatic potential), especially if the progeny cells acquire additional mutations.

Proliferating cells rely on a genetic blueprint for tissues and organs, which is found on chromosomes within the nucleus of the cell. Structures called *telomeres*, consisting of a repeated DNA code, are found at the end of chromosomes and serve to protect the genetic data within the chromosomes and facilitate normal cell division. Each time a cell divides, the telomere becomes shorter, and a small sequence of genetic material is not copied. Ultimately, the cell is unable to undergo further division, becomes inactive (senescent), and dies. Cancer cells produce an enzyme called *telomerase* that prevents telomere shortening and allows the cells to escape senescence and death. Telomerase thus promotes the immortalization of cells and has a role in the development of cancer, as well as in the process of aging.

Defects in Cellular Differentiation

Cellular differentiation is normally an orderly process in which the cell progresses from a state of immaturity to a state

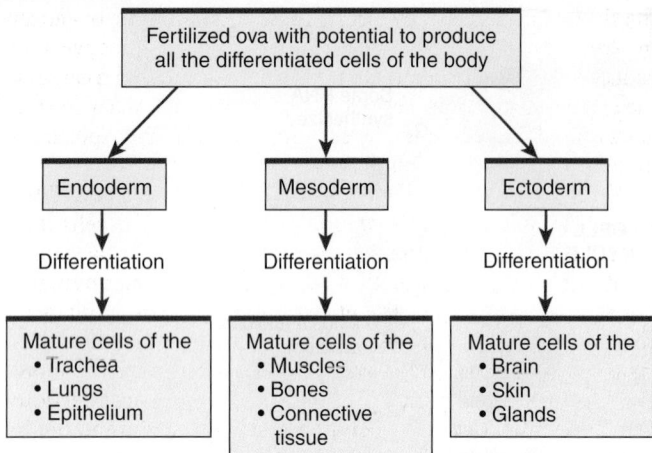

FIG. 18.2 Normal cellular differentiation.

of maturity. Because all body cells are derived from fertilized ova, all cells have the potential to perform all body functions. As cells differentiate, this potential is narrowed, and the mature cell is capable of performing only specific functions (Figure 18.2).

In cellular differentiation, the phasing out of cellular potential is stable and orderly. Under normal conditions, the differentiated cell is stable and does not *dedifferentiate* (i.e., revert to a previous undifferentiated state).

The exact mechanism that controls cellular differentiation and proliferation is not completely understood. Two types of normal genes are important regulators of normal cellular processes: **Proto-oncogenes** promote growth, whereas **tumour suppressor genes**, such as tumour protein 53, suppress growth. Both can be affected by mutations. Those that alter the expression of proto-oncogenes can activate them to function as **oncogenes** (tumour-inducing genes). Mutations that alter tumour suppressor genes render them inactive, which results in a loss of their tumour suppressor ability.

The proto-oncogene has been described as the genetic lock that keeps the cell in its mature functioning state. When this lock is "unlocked," as may occur through exposure to **carcinogens** (cancer-causing agents capable of producing cellular alterations) or oncogenic viruses, genetic alterations and mutations occur. The abilities and properties that the cell had during fetal development are again expressed. Oncogenes interfere with normal cell expression under some conditions, causing the cell to become malignant. This cell regains fetal properties and function. For example, some cancer cells produce new proteins, such as those characteristic of the embryonic and fetal periods of life. These proteins, located on the cell membrane, include carcinoembryonic antigen (CEA) and alpha-fetoprotein. They can be detected in human blood by laboratory studies (see Role of the Immune System section). Other cancer cells, such as small cell carcinoma of the lung, produce hormones (see Complications Resulting From Cancer section) that are ordinarily produced by cells arising from the same embryonic cells as the tumour cells.

Tumours can be classified as benign or malignant. In general, **benign neoplasms** are well-differentiated, and **malignant neoplasms** are undifferentiated. Malignant tumour cells have the ability to invade and metastasize, unlike benign neoplasms. Other differences between benign and malignant neoplasms are listed in Table 18.4.

TABLE 18.4	COMPARISON OF BENIGN AND MALIGNANT NEOPLASMS	
Characteristic	**Benign**	**Malignant**
Encapsulated	Usually	Rarely
Differentiated	Normally	Undifferentiated
Metastasis	Absent	Frequently present
Recurrence	Rare	Possible
Vascularity	Slight	Moderate to marked
Mode of growth	Expansive	Infiltrative and expansive
Cell characteristics	Fairly normal; similar to those of parent cells	Abnormal; bear little resemblance to those of parent cells

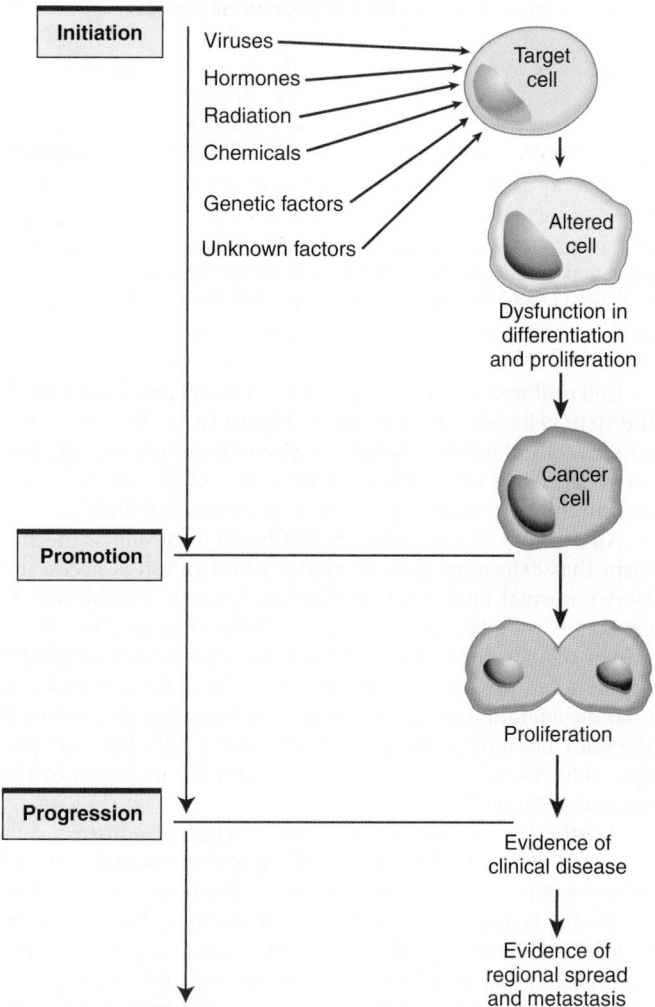

FIG. 18.3 Process of cancer development.

Development of Cancer

In this section, a theoretical model of the development of cancer is described. The cause and development of each type of cancer are likely to be multifactorial. It is not known how many tumours have a chemical, environmental, genetic, immunological, or viral origin. Cancers may arise spontaneously from causes that are thus far unclear.

It is a common misunderstanding that the development of cancer is a rapid, haphazard event. The natural history of cancer is an orderly process comprising several stages and occurring over a period of time. These stages are *initiation, promotion,* and *progression* (Figure 18.3).

Initiation. The first stage, *initiation,* is a mutation in the cell's genetic structure resulting from an inherited mutation, an error that occurs during DNA replication or after exposure to a carcinogen. This altered cell has the potential for developing into a *clone* (progeny of a single cell) of neoplastic cells.

Many carcinogens are detoxified by protective enzymes and harmlessly excreted. If this protective mechanism fails, carcinogens can enter a cell's nucleus and alter its DNA. The cell may die or repair itself. However, if cell death or repair does not occur before cell division, the cell replicates into daughter cells, each with the same genetic alteration. Carcinogens may be chemical, radioactive, or viral in nature. In addition, some genetic anomalies increase the susceptibility of individuals to certain cancers. Common characteristics of carcinogens are that their effects in the stage of initiation are usually irreversible and additive.

Chemical Carcinogens. Chemicals were identified as cancer-causing agents in the latter part of the eighteenth century, when Percival Pott noted that chimney sweeps had a higher incidence of cancer of the scrotum in association with exposure to soot residues in chimneys. Over time, more chemical agents were identified as actual and potential carcinogens. Evidence indicated that individuals undergoing sustained exposure to certain chemicals had a greater incidence of certain cancers than others. Because of the long latency period from the time of exposure to the development of cancer, identifying cancer-causing chemicals is difficult. Chemicals that cause cancer in animals may or may not cause the same specific cancer in humans. Some chemicals are cancer causative in their environmental form, but others must first undergo specific changes to become carcinogenic.

Certain medications have also been identified as carcinogens. Medications that are capable of interacting with DNA (e.g., alkylating agents) and immunosuppressive agents have the potential to cause neoplasms in humans. The use of alkylating agents (e.g., cyclophosphamide and nitrogen mustards), either alone or in combination with radiation therapy, has been associated with an increased incidence of acute myelogenous leukemia in persons treated for Hodgkin's disease, non-Hodgkin's lymphomas, and multiple myeloma. These secondary leukemias are relatively refractory to treatment. Secondary leukemia has also been observed in persons who have undergone transplantation surgery and taken immunosuppressive medications.

Radiation. Early in the twentieth century, ionizing radiation (described later) was found to cause cancer in almost any human body tissue. The safe threshold for exposure to radiation is not known, and there is considerable debate surrounding the effect of exposure to low-dose radiation over time. Radiation damages cellular DNA. Certain malignancies have been linked to radiation:

1. Leukemia, lymphoma, thyroid cancer, and other cancers increased in incidence in the general population of Hiroshima and Nagasaki after the atomic bomb explosions.
2. A higher incidence of bone cancer occurs in persons exposed to radiation in certain occupations, such as radiologists, radiation chemists, and uranium miners.
3. Thyroid cancer has a higher incidence among persons who have received radiation to the head and neck area for treatment of a variety of disorders, such as acne, tonsillitis, sore throat, or enlarged thyroid gland.
4. The incidence of childhood cancer is higher among children exposed to radiation during fetal life.

Ultraviolet radiation has long been associated with melanoma, squamous cell carcinoma, and basal cell carcinoma of the skin. Skin cancer is by far the most common type of cancer in North America. Melanoma is a particularly aggressive skin cancer that responds poorly to treatment. Although the cause of melanoma is probably multifactorial, mounting evidence suggests that ultraviolet radiation secondary to sunlight exposure is linked to the development of melanoma.

Viral and Bacterial Carcinogens. Certain DNA and RNA viruses, termed *oncogenic viruses,* can transform the cells they infect and induce malignant transformation. Viruses have been identified as causative agents of cancer in animals and humans. For example, cells from patients with Burkitt's lymphoma have consistently shown evidence of the presence of the Epstein-Barr virus (EBV) in vitro. This virus also causes infectious mononucleosis; it is unclear which precise process results in infectious disease versus lymphoma. Persons with acquired immunodeficiency syndrome (AIDS), which is caused by a retrovirus, have a higher incidence of Kaposi's sarcoma (see Chapter 17). Other viruses that have been linked to the development of cancer include hepatitis B and C viruses, associated with hepatocellular carcinoma, and human papillomavirus, associated with squamous cell carcinomas such as cervical, anal, and head and neck cancers. *Helicobacter pylori* is a bacterium found in the stomach of two thirds of the world's population and is implicated in the development of gastric and duodenal ulcers, as well as of some gastric cancers.

Genetic Susceptibility. Cancer-related genes have been identified that increase an individual's susceptibility to the development of certain cancers. For example, a woman with mutations in the gene *BRCA1* or *BRCA2* has a 40% to 85% risk of developing breast cancer in her lifetime. However, 95% of women who develop breast cancer do not possess these genetic mutations. It is estimated that only 5% to 10% of cancers are inherited (Canadian Cancer Society, 2021a).

Promotion. A single alteration of the genetic structure of the cell is not sufficient to result in cancer. However, the odds of cancer development are increased with the presence of promoting agents. *Promotion,* the second stage in the development of cancer, is characterized by the reversible proliferation of the altered cells. Consequently, with an increase in the altered cell population, the likelihood of sustained mutagenesis is increased.

An important distinction between initiation and promotion is that the activity of promoters is reversible. This is a key concept in cancer prevention. Promoting factors include dietary fat, obesity, cigarette smoking, and alcohol consumption. The withdrawal or reduction of these factors can reduce the risk of cancer development.

Several promoting factors exert activity against specific types of body tissues or organs, and these agents tend to promote the development of specific kinds of cancer. For example, cigarette smoke is a promoting agent in bronchogenic carcinoma and, in conjunction with alcohol intake, promotes the development of esophageal and bladder cancers. Some carcinogens (*complete carcinogens*) are capable of both initiating and promoting the development of cancer. Tobacco is an example of a complete carcinogen, capable of initiating and promoting the development of cancer.

A period of time, ranging from 1 to 40 years, elapses between the initial genetic alteration and the actual clinical evidence of cancer. This period, called the *latency period,* is now theorized to comprise both the initiation and the promotion stages in the natural history of cancer (DeVita et al., 2018). The variation in the length of time that elapses before the cancer becomes

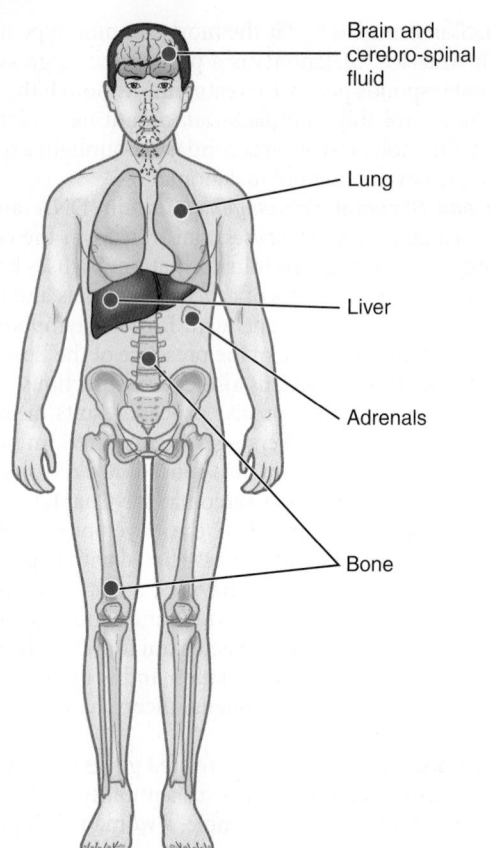

Brain and
cerebro-spinal
fluid

Lung

Liver

Adrenals

Bone

FIG. 18.4 Main sites of bloodborne metastasis. Source: Stevens, A., & Lowe, J. (2000). *Pathology: Illustrated review in color* (2nd ed.). Mosby.

clinically evident is associated with the mitotic rate of the tissue of origin and environmental factors. For most cancers, the process of developing takes years or even decades.

For the disease process to become clinically evident, the cells must reach a "critical mass." A 1-cm tumour (the size usually detectable on palpation) contains 1 billion cancer cells. A 0.5-cm tumour is the smallest that can be detected by current diagnostic measures, such as magnetic resonance imaging (MRI).

Progression. *Progression* is the final stage in the natural history of a cancer. This stage is characterized by increased growth rate of the tumour, as well as by increased invasiveness and spread of the cancer to a distant site (**metastasis**). Certain biochemical and morphological alterations take place during this stage, enabling the tumour to survive and thrive in its primary environment and throughout the process of metastasis.

Some cancers metastasize early in the process of development (e.g., premenopausal breast cancer), whereas others spread regionally and rarely metastasize (e.g., glioblastoma, basal cell carcinoma of the skin). Certain cancers seem to have an affinity for a particular tissue or organ as a site of metastasis (e.g., colon cancer spreads to the liver); other cancers are unpredictable in their pattern of metastasis (e.g., melanoma). Frequent sites of metastasis are the lungs, the brain, the bone, the liver, and the adrenal glands (Figure 18.4). Metastasis is a multistep process beginning with the rapid growth of the primary tumour (Figure 18.5). As the tumour increases in size, development of its own blood supply is crucial for its survival and growth. The process of the formation of blood vessels within the tumour itself is termed **tumour angiogenesis** and is facilitated by tumour angiogenesis factors produced by the cancer cells. As the tumour grows, it

can begin to mechanically invade surrounding tissues, growing into areas of the least resistance.

Certain subpopulations of tumour cells are able to detach from the primary tumour, invade the tissue surrounding the tumour, and penetrate the walls of lymphatic or vascular vessels for metastasis to a distant site. Unique capabilities of some tumour cells facilitate this process. First, rapid proliferation of malignant cells causes mechanical pressure that leads to penetration of surrounding tissues. Second, certain cells have decreased cell-to-cell adhesion in comparison with normal cells. This property allows these cancer cells to physically detach from their site of origin and invade vascular and organ structures. In addition, motility factors are produced by both tumour and normal cells, and changes in the tumour's cytoskeleton further facilitate movement of tumour cells. Some cancer cells produce matrix metalloproteases, a family of lytic enzymes that can erode the basement membrane (a tough barrier surrounding tissues and blood vessels) of the tumour itself, as well as lymph and blood vessels, muscles, nerves, and most epithelial boundaries, which allows for the spread of the tumour. Once free from the primary tumour, metastatic tumour cells frequently travel to distant organ sites via lymphatic and hematogenous routes. Because these two routes are interconnected, it is theorized that tumour cells metastasize via both routes.

Hematogenous metastasis involves several steps, beginning with the penetration of blood vessels by primary tumour cells through the release of metalloproteases, as described previously. The tumour cells then enter the circulation, adhere to small blood vessels of distant organs, and penetrate these vessels, again with the assistance of metalloproteases. Most tumour cells do not survive this process and are destroyed by mechanical mechanisms (e.g., turbulence of blood flow) and cells of the immune system. However, the formation of a combination of tumour cells, platelets, and fibrin deposits may protect some tumour cells from destruction in blood vessels.

In the lymphatic system, tumour cells may be "trapped" in the first lymph node confronted, or they may bypass regional lymph nodes and travel to more distant lymph nodes. This phenomenon, termed *skip metastasis*, is exhibited in certain malignancies, such as esophageal cancers, and is the basis for questions about the effectiveness of dissection of regional lymph nodes for the prevention of some distant metastases. Tumour cells that do survive the process of metastasis must create and maintain an environment in the distant organ site that is favourable to their growth and development. This is facilitated by the ability of tumour cells to evade cells of the immune system and to produce a vascular supply within the metastatic site similar to that developed in the primary tumour site. Vascularization is critical for the supply of nutrients to the metastatic tumour and for the removal of waste products. Metalloproteases contribute to vascularization through release of angiogenesis promoters such as vascular endothelial growth factor (VEGF).

Cells of the primary tumour and metastatic site may develop from a single cell or may be *clones* (cells derived from a single cell of origin). However, as the primary and metastatic sites develop, the cells quickly become more heterogeneous as they repeatedly undergo spontaneous genetic mutations. The heterogeneous nature of the cells in primary and metastatic tumours makes them difficult to treat, inasmuch as they are more likely to become resistant to chemotherapy and radiation therapy. Surgical removal may be effective for some small, circumscribed tumours.

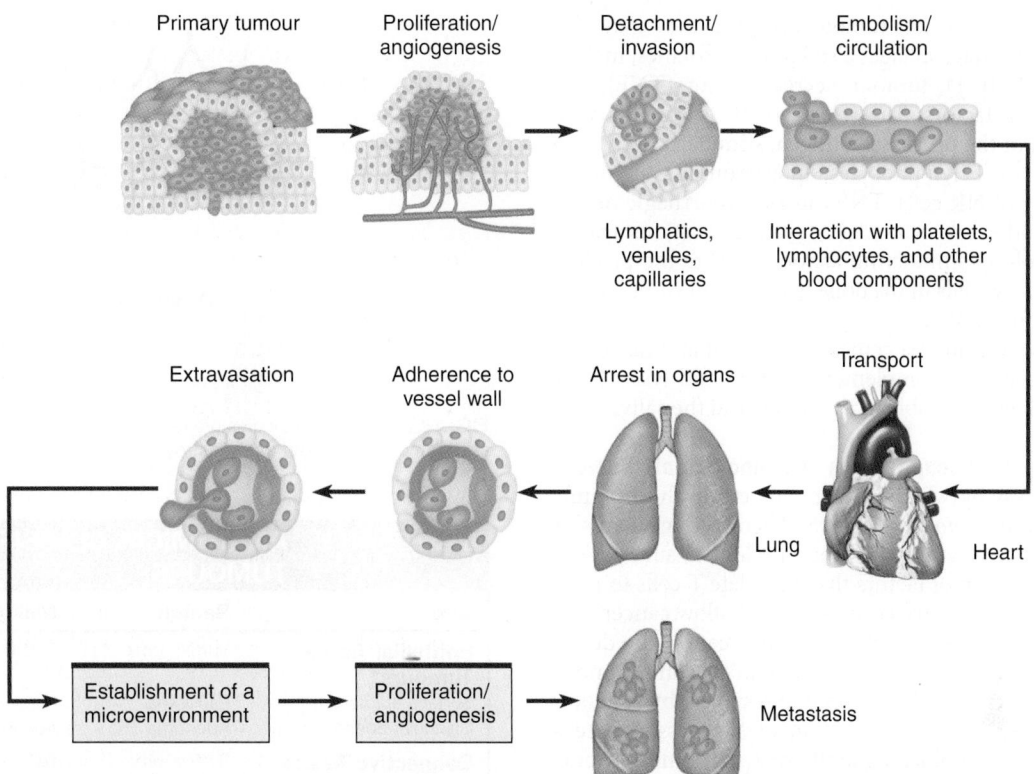

FIG. 18.5 The pathogenesis of cancer metastasis. To produce metastases, tumour cells must detach from the primary tumour and enter the circulation, survive in circulation, adhere to the capillary basement membrane, obtain entrance into the organ parenchyma, respond to growth factors, proliferate and induce angiogenesis, and evade host defences. Source: Reprinted by permission from Macmillan Publishers Ltd: NATURE REVIEWS CANCER, Fidler, I. T. (2003). The pathogenesis of cancer metastasis: the 'seed and soil' hypothesis revisited, *3*, 453-458, copyright © 2003.

Role of the Immune System

This section is limited to a discussion of the role of the immune system in the recognition and destruction of tumour cells. (For a detailed discussion of immune system function, see Chapter 16.)

The immune system has the potential to distinguish normal (self) from abnormal (nonself) cells. For example, cells of transplanted organs can be "perceived" by the immune system as nonself entities and thus elicit an immune response. This response can ultimately result in rejection of the organ. Similarly, cancer cells can be perceived as nonself entities and elicit an immune response that results in their rejection and destruction. However, unlike transplanted cells, cancer cells arise from normal "self" cells, and although mutated and thus different, the immune response that is mounted against cancer cells may be inadequate to reject and destroy the cancer cells.

Some cancer cells have changes on their cell surface antigens as a result of malignant transformation. These altered antigens are termed **tumour-associated antigens** (Figure 18.6). It is believed that one of the functions of the immune system is to respond to tumour-associated antigens. The response of the immune system to antigens of the malignant cells is termed **immunological surveillance**. Lymphocytes continually check cell surface antigens and detect and destroy cells with abnormal or altered antigenic determinants. It has been proposed that malignant transformation occurs continuously and that the malignant cells are destroyed by the immune response. Under most circumstances, immunological surveillance prevents these transformed cells from developing into clinically detectable tumours.

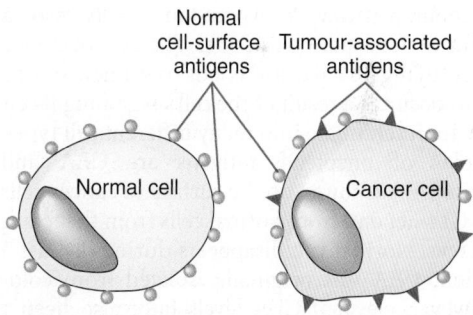

FIG. 18.6 Tumour-associated antigens appear on the cell surface of malignant cells.

Virtually every cell type involved in normal immune responses and every function used to inactivate or remove antigens have been demonstrated in immune responses to tumours. These immune responses involve cytotoxic T cells, natural killer (NK) cells, macrophages, and B lymphocytes.

Cytotoxic T cells are thought to play a dominant role in resisting tumour growth. These cells are capable of killing tumour cells. T cells are also important in the production of cytokines (e.g., interleukin-2 [IL-2] and interferon-γ [IFN-γ], which stimulate T cells), NK cells, B cells, and macrophages.

NK cells are able to directly lyse tumour cells spontaneously without any prior sensitization. These cells are stimulated by IFN-γ and IL-2 (released from T cells), which results in increased cytotoxic activity.

Monocytes and macrophages have several important roles in tumour immunity. Macrophages can be activated by IFN-γ (produced by T cells) to kill tumour cells, but they may also injure normal cells. Macrophages also secrete cytokines, including interleukin-1 (IL-1), tumour necrosis factor (TNF), and colony-stimulating factors. The release of IL-1, coupled with the presentation of the processed antigen, stimulates activation and production of T lymphocytes. Interferon-alfa augments the killing ability of NK cells. TNF causes hemorrhagic necrosis of tumours and exerts cytocidal or cytostatic actions against tumour cells. Colony-stimulating factors regulate the production of various blood cells in the bone marrow and stimulate the function of various WBCs.

B lymphocytes produce specific antibodies that bind to and destroy tumour cells by complement fixation and lysis. These antibodies are often detectable in the serum and the saliva of an affected patient.

Mechanisms of Escape From Immunological Surveillance. The process by which cancer cells evade the immune system is termed *immunological escape*. Theorized mechanisms by which cancer cells can escape immunological surveillance include (a) suppression of factors that stimulate T cells to react to cancer cells, (b) weak surface antigens that allow cancer cells to "sneak through" immunological surveillance, (c) the development of tolerance of the immune system to some tumour antigens, (d) suppression of the immune response by products secreted by cancer cells, (e) induction of suppressor T cells by the tumour, and (f) blocking antibodies that bind tumour-associated antigens, thus preventing their recognition by T cells (Figure 18.7).

Oncofetal Antigens. *Oncofetal antigens* are a type of tumour antigen. They are found on both the surface and the inside of cancer cells, as well as on and inside fetal cells. These antigens are an expression of the shift of cancerous cells to a more immature metabolic pathway, an expression usually associated with embryonic or fetal periods of life. The reappearance of fetal antigens in malignant disease is not well understood, but it is believed to occur as a result of the cell's regaining its embryonic capability to differentiate into many different cell types.

Examples of oncofetal antigens are CEA and alpha-fetoprotein. CEA is found on the surface of cancer cells derived from the GI tract and from normal cells from the fetal gut, liver, and pancreas. Normally, it disappears during the last 3 months of gestation. CEA was originally isolated from colon cancer cells. However, elevated CEA levels have also been found in nonmalignant conditions (e.g., cirrhosis of the liver, ulcerative colitis, and heavy smoking). At present, the major value of CEA is its use as an indicator of the success of cancer treatment. For example, the persistence of elevated preoperative CEA titres after surgery indicates that the tumour was not completely removed. A rise in CEA levels after chemotherapy or radiation therapy may indicate recurrence or spread of the cancer.

Alpha-fetoprotein is produced by malignant liver cells, as well as fetal liver cells. Alpha-fetoprotein levels have also been found to be elevated in some cases of testicular carcinoma, viral hepatitis, and nonmalignant liver disorders. Alpha-fetoprotein has diagnostic value in primary cancer of the liver (hepatoma), but it is also produced in metastases to the liver. The detection of alpha-fetoprotein is of value in tumour detection and determination of tumour progression.

Other examples of oncofetal antigens currently being studied are CA-125, found in ovarian carcinoma; CA-19-9, found in pancreatic, colon, and breast cancer; and prostate-specific antigen (PSA), found in prostate cancer.

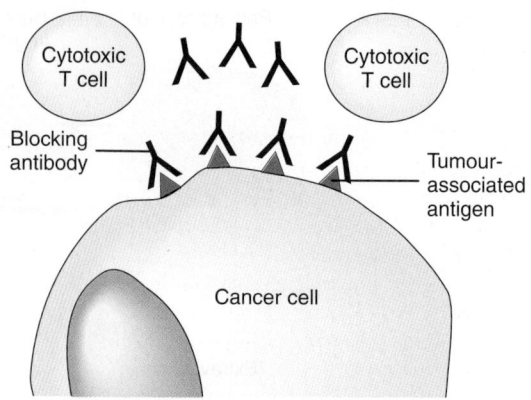

FIG. 18.7 Blocking antibodies prevent T cells from interacting with tumour-associated antigens and from destroying the malignant cell.

TABLE 18.5	ANATOMICAL CLASSIFICATION OF TUMOURS	
Site	**Benign**	**Malignant**
Epithelial Tissue Tumours*	Suffix: *-oma*	Suffix: *-carcinoma*
Surface epithelium	Papilloma	Carcinoma
Glandular epithelium	Adenoma	Adenocarcinoma
Connective Tissue Tumours†	Suffix: *-oma*	Suffix: *-sarcoma*
Fibrous tissue	Fibroma	Fibrosarcoma
Cartilage	Chondroma	Chondrosarcoma
Striated muscle	Rhabdomyoma	Rhabdomyosarcoma
Bone	Osteoma	Osteosarcoma
Nervous Tissue Tumours	Suffix: *-oma*	Suffix: *-oma*
Pineal region	Pineocytoma	Pineoblastoma
Nerve cells	Ganglioneuroma	Neuroblastoma
Hematopoietic Tissue Tumours		
Lymphoid tissue	—	Hodgkin's disease, non-Hodgkin's lymphoma
Plasma cells	—	Multiple myeloma
Bone marrow	—	Lymphocytic and myelogenous leukemia

*Body surfaces, lining of body cavities, and glandular structures.
†Supporting tissue, fibrotic tissue, and blood vessels.

CLASSIFICATION OF CANCER

Tumours can be classified according to anatomical site, histological analysis (grading), and extent of disease (staging). Tumour classification systems are intended to provide a standardized way to (a) communicate the cancer status of a patient to the members of the health care team, (b) assist in determining the most effective treatment plan, (c) evaluate the treatment plan, (d) help determine the prognosis, and (e) compare patients with similar conditions for statistical purposes.

Anatomical Site Classification

In the *anatomical classification* of tumours, the tumour is identified by the tissue of origin, the anatomical site, and the behaviour of the tumour (i.e., benign or malignant; Table 18.5). A **carcinoma** originates from embryonal *ectoderm* (skin and glands) and *endoderm* (mucous membrane linings of the respiratory, GI, and genitourinary tracts). A **sarcoma** originates in the connective tissue of the body (fat, muscles, blood vessels, nerves, bones, or cartilage). Lymphomas and leukemias originate from the hematopoietic system.

Histological Analysis Classification

In histological grading of tumours, the appearance of cells and the degree of differentiation are evaluated. For many tumour cells, four grades are used:

- *Grade I:* Cells differ slightly from normal cells (mild dysplasia) and are well differentiated.
- *Grade II:* Cells are more abnormal (moderate dysplasia) and moderately differentiated.
- *Grade III:* Cells are very abnormal (severe dysplasia) and poorly differentiated.
- *Grade IV:* Cells are immature and primitive (anaplasia) and undifferentiated; the cell of origin is difficult to determine.

Classifying Extent of Disease

Classifying the extent and spread of disease is termed staging. This classification system is based on a description of the extent of the disease rather than on cell appearance. The extent to which the disease has spread has important ramifications for prognosis. Although there are similarities in the staging of cancers, there are many differences between them; thus they are based on a thorough knowledge of the natural history of each specific type of cancer.

Clinical Staging. The clinical staging classification system is used to determine the extent of the disease process of cancer within the body by stages:

- *Stage 0:* cancer in situ
- *Stage I:* tumour limited to the tissue of origin; localized tumour growth
- *Stage II:* limited local spread
- *Stage III:* extensive local and regional spread
- *Stage IV:* metastasis

This classification system has been used as a basis for staging in cancer of the cervix (see Chapter 56, Table 56.11) and Hodgkin's disease (see Chapter 33, Figure 33.14).

TNM Classification System. The *TNM classification system* represents the standardization of the clinical staging of cancer by the Geneva-based International Union Against Cancer. This classification system (Table 18.6) is used to determine the extent of the disease process of cancer according to three parameters: tumour size (T), degree of regional spread to the lymph nodes (N), and metastasis (M).

Staging of the disease may be performed initially and at repeated intervals. Clinical diagnostic staging is performed at the time of diagnosis to determine the most effective treatment plan. Examples of diagnostic studies that may be performed to assess for spread of disease include bone and liver scanning, ultrasonography, computed tomography (CT), positron emission tomography, and MRI.

Surgical staging is used to describe the extent of the disease process after biopsy or surgical exploration. For example, a laparotomy and a splenectomy may be performed in the staging of Hodgkin's disease. During staging laparotomy, lymph node biopsy samples are obtained and margins of any masses are marked with metal clips. These clips are used as markers when radiotherapy is used as a treatment modality.

After the extent of the disease is determined, the stage classification is not changed. The original description of the extent of the tumour remains part of the original record. If additional treatment is needed, or if treatment fails, restaging is performed to determine the extent of the disease process at the time of retreatment.

Carcinoma in situ is a commonly used term in classification of cancer. It is defined as a lesion with all the histological features of cancer except invasion. If left untreated, carcinoma in situ eventually becomes invasive.

In addition to tumour classification systems, there are also classification systems that can be used to describe the functional status of patients with cancer. The Karnofsky Performance Status scale is an example of a functional assessment scale (see the Resources at the end of this chapter).

PREVENTION AND DETECTION OF CANCER

The nurse has a prominent role in the prevention and detection of cancer. Early detection and prompt treatment are directly responsible for increased survival rates among patients with cancer. Public education should include the following recommendations:

1. Reduce or eliminate exposure to carcinogens and cancer promoters, such as cigarette smoke and sun exposure.
2. Eat a balanced diet that includes fresh fruits, vegetables, omega-3 fatty acids, and fibre. Following *Canada's Dietary Guidelines* helps to ensure a healthy diet (Health Canada, 2021; see Chapter 42, Figure 42.1).
3. Participate regularly (e.g., a minimum of 30 minutes, five times per week) in mild to moderate physical activity such as biking, walking, or running.
4. Maintain a healthy weight for your body type.
5. Limit alcohol use to one or two drinks per day.
6. Get to know your body. Learn and practise self-examination (e.g., breast self-examination, testicular self-examination). Report any changes to your health care provider or dentist.
7. Follow cancer screening guidelines (see the Resources at the end of this chapter). Early detection of cancer has a positive effect on prognosis.
8. Know the seven warning signs of cancer (Table 18.7).

When the public is educated about cancer, care should be taken to minimize the fear that surrounds the diagnosis. Teaching strategies that address the specific needs of the target audience (e.g., the needs of older persons in comparison with those of high school students or new immigrants to Canada) are most effective. Although the general public requires information that supports healthy behaviours, those at an increased risk of cancer are the target population for effective cancer control.

TABLE 18.6   TNM CLASSIFICATION SYSTEM

Primary Tumour Size (T)

T_0	No evidence of primary tumour
T_{is}	Carcinoma in situ
T_1–T_4	Ascending degrees of increase in tumour size and involvement
T_X	Primary tumour cannot be assessed

Involvement of Regional Lymph Nodes (N)

N_0	No evidence of disease in lymph nodes
N_1–N_3	Ascending degrees of nodal involvement
N_X	Regional lymph nodes cannot be assessed

Distant Metastases (M)

M_0	No distant metastases
M_1	Distant metastases
M_X	Distant metastases cannot be assessed

TABLE 18.7   SEVEN WARNING SIGNS OF CANCER

C	**C**hange in bowel or bladder habits
A	**A** sore that does not heal
U	**U**nusual bleeding or discharge from any body orifice
T	**T**hickening or a lump in the breast or elsewhere
I	**I**ndigestion or difficulty in swallowing
O	**O**bvious change in a wart or mole
N	**N**agging cough or hoarseness

These individuals must be motivated to learn to change negative health behaviours in order to achieve and maintain an optimal state of health. Nurses can influence people to change lifestyle patterns for a positive effect on their health. To be successful, nurses must identify potential challenges and barriers and develop appropriate strategies to facilitate understanding of information about effective cancer control.

DIAGNOSIS OF CANCER

The threat of a cancer diagnosis creates tremendous anxiety for an individual and their family. Patients typically undergo several days to weeks of diagnostic studies. During this time, fear of the unknown may be more stressful than the actual diagnosis of cancer.

While the patient is waiting for the results of the diagnostic studies, the nurse should be available to actively listen to the patient's concerns. Communication plays a pivotal role in optimal patient care. Essential elements of the establishment of a therapeutic relationship with the patient are the ability to listen, ask questions sensitively, and avoid false reassurances. During this time of high anxiety, the patient needs repetition and reinforcement of information, the opportunity to ask questions, and clarification of the diagnostic workup. Explanations should be clear and tailored to meet the specific needs of patients and families. Content that is particularly threatening or detailed may overwhelm patients, and the nurse should be sensitive to the individual's ability to absorb the information. Written information at the level of the patient's literacy can help with reinforcement of verbal information.

A diagnostic plan for the person in whom cancer is suspected includes health history, potential or actual risk factors, physical examination, and specific diagnostic studies. (The specifics of the health history and the screening physical examination are presented in Chapter 3.)

The health history includes particular emphasis on risk factors, such as family history of cancer, exposure to or ingestion of known carcinogens (e.g., cigarette smoking, exposure to occupational pollutants or chemicals), diseases characterized by chronic inflammation (e.g., ulcerative colitis), and medication ingestion (e.g., hormone therapy). Other important information is related to dietary habits, ingestion of alcohol, lifestyle, and patterns and degree of coping with perceived stressors.

The physical examination should be thorough, with particular attention to the respiratory system, the GI system (including the colon, rectum, and liver), the lymphatic system (including the spleen), the breasts, the skin, the reproductive system (testes and prostate gland in men; cervix, uterus, and ovaries in women), and the musculoskeletal and neurological systems.

The choice of diagnostic studies depends on the suspected primary or metastatic site or sites of the cancer. (Specific procedures related to each body system are discussed in the respective assessment chapters.) Studies that may be conducted in the process of diagnosing cancer include the following:

1. Cytology studies (e.g., Papanicolaou [Pap] test)
2. Hematology and chemistry studies (e.g., complete blood cell count [CBC], liver and renal function tests)
3. Sigmoidoscopic, colonoscopic examination and/or fecal immunochemical test (FIT)
4. Radiological studies (e.g., chest radiography, mammography, CT, MRI)
5. Radioisotope scanning (e.g., bone, lung, liver, brain)
6. Assays for the presence of oncofetal antigens (such as CEA and alpha-fetoprotein) or of genetic markers (such as *BRCA1* and *BRCA2*)
7. Bone marrow examination (if a hematolymphoid malignancy is suspected)
8. Biopsy

Biopsy

The *biopsy* procedure is the definitive means of diagnosing cancer, and the results guide treatment decisions. In a biopsy, a piece of tissue is surgically removed from the suspect area for histological and molecular examination by a pathologist. This examination helps determine whether the tissue is benign or malignant, the anatomical tissue from which the tumour arises, and the degree of cellular differentiation (i.e., how closely the specimen cells resemble the normal cells of the tissue). It may also provide information about response to treatment and prognosis.

The procedure may be a needle biopsy, an incisional biopsy, or an excisional biopsy. In a *needle biopsy*, cells and tissue fragments are obtained through a large-bore needle guided into the tissue of investigation (e.g., bone marrow, prostate gland, breast, liver, or kidney tissues).

Incisional biopsy performed with a scalpel or dermal punch is a common technique for obtaining a tissue sample from, for example, a skin lesion. The premise that incisional biopsy may contribute to the spread of cancer has not been proved.

Excisional biopsy involves removal of the entire tumour. It is usually used for small tumours (<2 cm in diameter), skin lesions, intestinal polyps, and breast masses. This procedure can be therapeutic in addition to diagnostic. When a tumour is not easily accessible, a major surgical procedure (laparotomy, thoracotomy, craniotomy) is necessary to obtain the tumour tissue. Biopsy specimens from the GI tract, respiratory tract, and genitourinary system can usually be obtained by endoscopic procedures, such as flexible sigmoidoscopy.

INTERPROFESSIONAL CARE

Goals and Modalities

The goal of cancer treatment is cure, control, or palliation (Figure 18.8). Factors determining the therapeutic approach include the cell type of the cancer, the location and size of the tumour, and the extent of the disease. The patient's physiological and psychological status and personal desires are also important elements in determining the treatment plan. All factors influence the goals of care, the modalities chosen for treatment, and the length of time the treatment is administered. Evidence-informed treatment guidelines have been developed in a number of provinces and territories to guide treatment decisions (see the Resources at the end of this chapter).

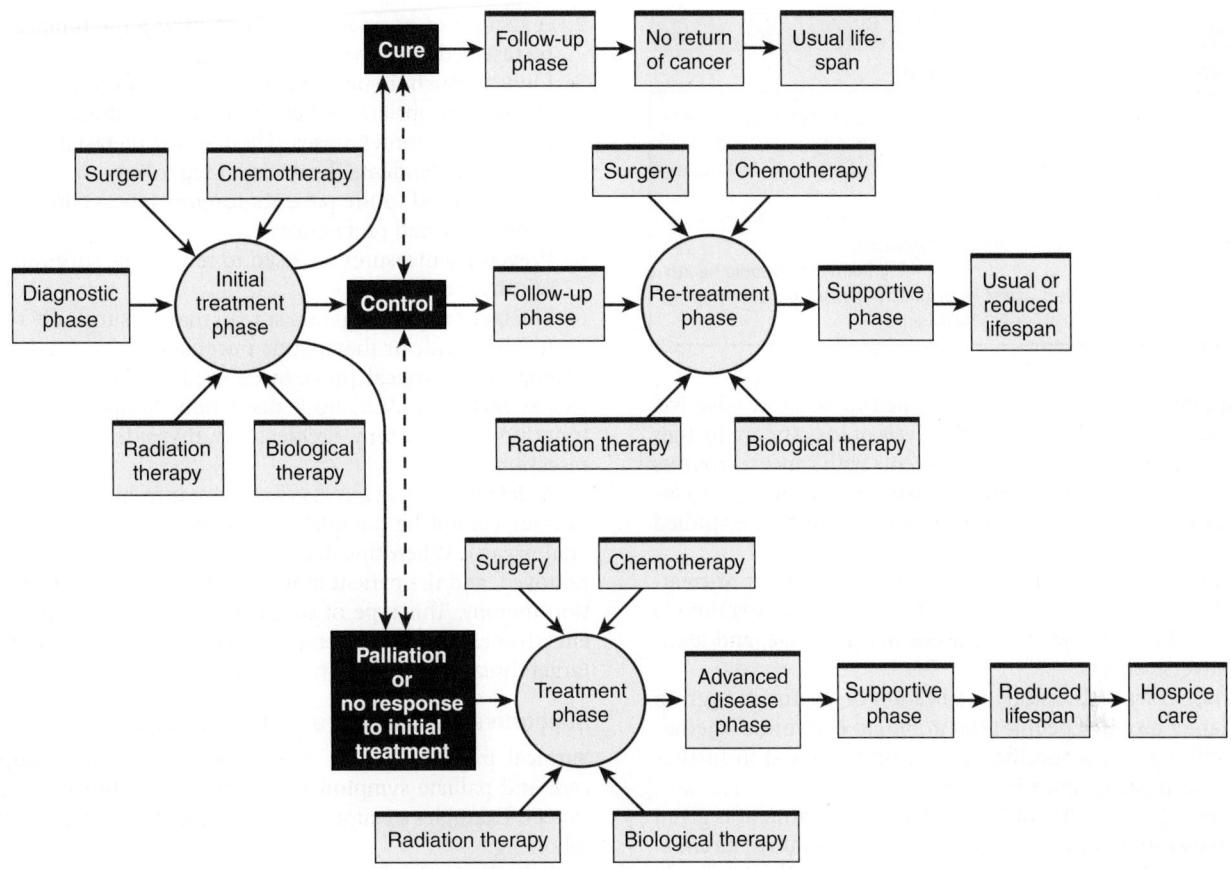

FIG. 18.8 Goals of cancer treatment.

When caring for patients with cancer, the nurse should know the goals of the treatment plan to communicate with and support patients. When cure is the goal, treatment that has the greatest likelihood of eradicating the disease is offered. With many kinds of cancer, therapy has the potential for inducing permanent remission; therapy may be an initial course of treatment or treatment that extends for several weeks, months, or years. Basal cell carcinoma of the skin is usually cured by surgical removal of the lesion or by several weeks of radiation therapy. Acute lymphocytic leukemia in children has the potential for cure. The treatment plan for this type of cancer includes the administration of several chemotherapeutic medications on a scheduled basis over a span of 6 months to several years. Head and neck cancers may be cured with combination therapy that includes surgery and radiation, with or without chemotherapy. The risk of disease recurrence differs according to the tumour type. In general, the risk for recurrent disease is greatest after completion of treatment and gradually decreases with the passage of time. Tumours with a rapid mitotic rate (e.g., testicular cancer) are considered to be in remission if cancer is not detected in a 2-year time span after treatment. For tumours that have a slower mitotic rate (e.g., postmenopausal breast cancer), the patient must be free of disease 20 years or longer before they can be considered cured of cancer.

Control is the goal of the treatment plan for many cancers that cannot be completely eradicated but are responsive to cancer therapies. Such cancers usually are not cured but are controlled by therapy for variably extended periods in a manner similar to other chronic illnesses, such as diabetes mellitus, chronic lung disease, and heart failure. An example of this type of cancer is chronic lymphocytic leukemia (see Chapter 33). The affected patient undergoes the initial course of therapy and continues maintenance therapy for a time or is monitored closely so that early signs and symptoms of disease recurrence or progression can be detected.

Palliation may also be a goal of the treatment plan. With palliation, relief or control of symptoms and the optimization of quality of life are the primary objectives, rather than cure or control of the disease process. Radiation therapy to relieve the pain of bone metastasis is an example of a palliative cancer treatment. Palliative care may be undertaken for days, weeks, months, or years.

The goals of cure, control, and palliation are achieved through the use of four treatment modalities: surgery, radiation therapy, chemotherapy, and biological therapy. These modalities can be used alone or in any combination in the initial treatment phase, as well as in the repeated treatment phases of cancer. For many cancers, two or more of the treatment modalities (referred to as *concurrent, combined-modality,* or *multimodality therapy*) are used to achieve the goal of cure or control for a long period.

Clinical Trials

A *clinical trial* is a research study conducted on humans and designed with the intent of evaluating new treatments or supportive care interventions. The evaluation of treatments in cancer research begins in the laboratory with animal studies. From these studies, the treatments determined to be most effective, with mild or medically manageable levels of toxicity, are further evaluated in a series of studies on patients with cancer. Progress in cancer care depends on research. New medications or treatments, evaluated for the first time in human beings, are studied in three phases:

- In *phase I trials,* researchers test a new medication or treatment in a small group of people (20 to 80) for the first time to evaluate its safety, determine a safe dosage range, and identify adverse effects.
- In *phase II trials,* the study medication or treatment is given to a larger group of people (100 to 300) to determine whether it is effective for a specific medical problem and to further evaluate its safety and adverse effects.
- In *phase III trials,* the study medication or treatment is given to large groups of people (1 000 to 3 000) to confirm its effectiveness, monitor adverse effects, compare it with commonly used treatments, and collect information that will allow the medication or treatment to be used safely.

Institutional review boards in each agency that conducts research closely guard the rights of the patients participating in clinical trials. These boards not only review clinical trials at their inception but also continue to review and monitor each study until its completion. Informed consent is a process in which the clinical trial physician and nurse give the patient full information regarding the nature of the treatment being evaluated and the potential risks and benefits of entering the clinical trial. The patient must understand that they may decide to leave a clinical trial at any time or refuse to participate in the trial without threat of compromised care or treatment.

The guidelines for the administration of a research protocol are included in the study's protocol and are monitored closely by the study investigators and clinical trial nurses to ensure safe and uniform treatment of patients.

SURGICAL THERAPY

Surgery is the oldest form of cancer treatment and was for many years the only method of cancer diagnosis and treatment. Removal of the tumour and a margin of the surrounding normal tissue may cure localized cancers, but it is ineffective if the cancer has metastasized to other locations.

Cure and Control

Several principles are applicable when surgery is used to cure or control the disease process of cancer (Figure 18.9):

1. Cancer that arises from a tissue with a slow rate of cellular proliferation or replication is the most amenable to surgical treatment.

2. A margin of normal tissue surrounding the tumour should be resected along with the tumour.
3. Only as much tissue as necessary is removed.
4. When appropriate, adjuvant therapy is used to eliminate residual micrometastases. The risk for metastatic disease is tumour dependent. The decision regarding adjuvant therapy is customized to the patient's tumour type, stage, comorbid conditions, and preferences.
5. Preventive measures are used to reduce the surgical seeding of cancer cells.
6. The usual sites of regional spread may be surgically removed for diagnostic or therapeutic purposes.

Examples of surgical procedures used for cure or control of cancer include radical neck dissection, lumpectomy, mastectomy, pneumonectomy, orchiectomy, thyroidectomy, and bowel resection.

A *debulking* or *cytoreductive* procedure may be used if the tumour cannot be completely removed (e.g., is attached to a vital organ). When this occurs, as much tumour as possible is removed, and the patient may be given chemotherapy or radiation therapy. This type of surgical procedure may increase the effectiveness of chemotherapy or radiation therapy because the target disease is reduced in volume.

Supportive and Palliative Surgical Procedures

Surgical procedures can also be used to provide supportive care and palliate symptoms throughout the disease process of cancer. Examples of supportive surgical procedures include the following:

1. Insertion of feeding tubes in the stomach for patients with head and neck cancers or cancer of the esophagus
2. Creation of a colostomy to allow healing of rectal abscess
3. Suprapubic cystostomy in cases of advanced prostatic cancer

When cure or control of cancer is no longer possible, relief from distressing symptoms may be achieved through surgical procedures, including the following:

1. Debulking of tumour to relieve pain or pressure
2. Colostomy for the relief of a bowel obstruction (see Chapter 45)
3. Laminectomy for the relief of spinal cord compression

Rehabilitative Management

Cancer surgery may cause a change in a person's body image or function. It may be challenging for patients to cope with these changes on top of the distress of a diagnosis of cancer. As the treatment for certain cancers becomes more effective, the length of time that a patient must live with an alteration created by treatment will be increased. If quality of life is to be maintained, the body image must be one that a patient is able to adapt to and cope with on a daily basis. The rehabilitative role of surgery in cancer care has grown in prominence to improve patients' quality of life. Breast reconstruction after a mastectomy is an example of a rehabilitative surgical procedure. The use of prostheses, such as artificial eyes or limbs, and the care of ostomies are other major contributions to rehabilitative management.

CHEMOTHERAPY

The use of chemicals as a systemic therapy for cancer has been evolving. In the 1940s, chemotherapy was in its infancy. Nitrogen mustard, a chemical warfare agent used in World Wars I and II, was used in the treatment of lymphoma and acute leukemia, and a folic acid antimetabolite (5-fluorouracil) was found to have

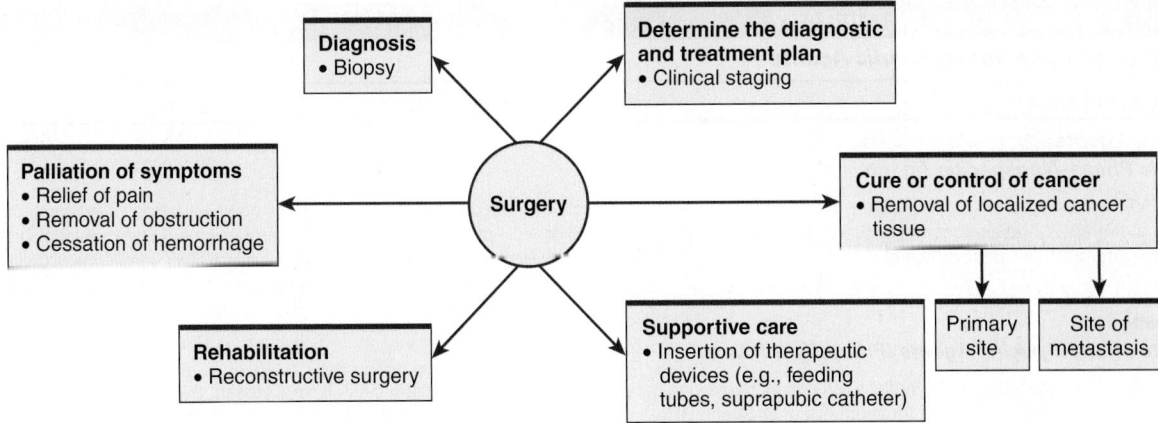

FIG. 18.9 Role of surgery in the treatment of cancer.

antitumour activity. In the 1970s, chemotherapy was established as an effective treatment modality for cancer. Chemotherapy is now used in the treatment of many solid tumours and is the primary therapy for hematological malignancies, including leukemia and lymphoma. Chemotherapy has evolved significantly to become a therapeutic option that can cure some cancers, control others, or palliate symptoms when cure or control is no longer achievable (Figure 18.10). Although practice standards in different provinces and territories vary, nurses administering chemotherapy must be specifically educated in the safe handling, administration, and possible adverse effects of chemotherapy (Canadian Association of Nurses in Oncology, 2017).

Effect on Cells

The effect of chemotherapy is at the cellular level. All cells, whether malignant or normal, enter the cell cycle for replication and proliferation (see Figure 18.1). The effects of the chemotherapeutic agents may be described in relationship to the cell cycle. The two major categories of chemotherapeutic medications are cell cycle phase–nonspecific and cell cycle phase–specific medications.

Cell cycle phase–nonspecific chemotherapeutic medications have their effect on the cells that are in the process of cellular replication and proliferation, as well as those in the resting phase (G_0).

Cell cycle phase–specific chemotherapeutic medications have their effect on cells that are in the process of cellular replication or proliferation (G_1, S_1, G_2, or M). These medications exert their most significant effect during specific phases of the cell cycle. Cell cycle phase–specific and cell cycle phase–nonspecific agents are often administered in combination with one another. The aim of this approach is to promote a better response through the use of agents that function by differing mechanisms and at different points in the cell cycle.

The goal of chemotherapy is to reduce the number of cancer cells present in the primary and metastatic tumour site or sites. Several factors determine the response of cancer cells to chemotherapy:

1. *Mitotic rate of the tissue from which the tumour arises.* The more rapid the mitotic rate, the greater the response to chemotherapy. Chemotherapy is the treatment of choice for acute leukemia, Wilms tumour (in conjunction with surgery), and neuroblastoma. These cancer cells have a rapid rate of cellular proliferation.

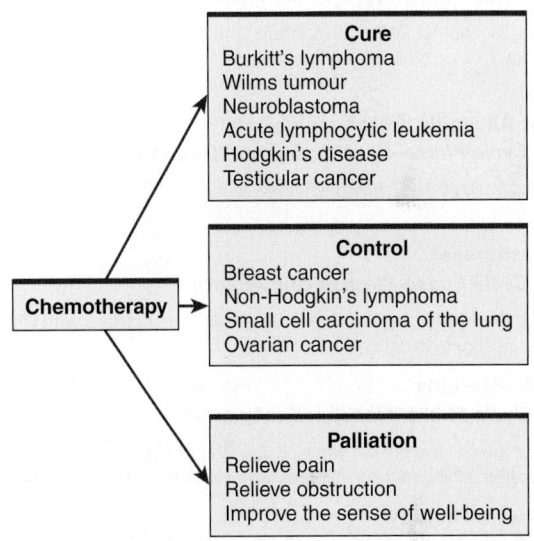

FIG. 18.10 Goals of chemotherapy.

2. *Size of the tumour.* The lower the tumour burden (i.e., the fewer cancer cells), the greater the response to chemotherapy.
3. *Age of the tumour.* The "younger" the tumour, the greater the response to chemotherapy. Developing tumours have a higher percentage of proliferating cells.
4. *Location of the tumour.* Certain anatomical sites provide a protected environment, or "sanctuary," from the effects of chemotherapy. For example, only a few medications (such as nitrosoureas and temozolomide) cross the blood–brain barrier.
5. *Presence of resistant tumour cells.* Mutation of cancer cells within the tumour mass can result in variant cells that are resistant to chemotherapy. Resistance can also occur because of the biochemical inability of some cancer cells to convert the medication to its active form. This resistance is passed on to new daughter cells.

As a tumour first begins to grow, most of its cells are actively dividing. As the tumour increases in size, more cells become inactive and convert to a resting state (G_0). Because many chemotherapeutic agents are most effective against dividing cells, cells can escape death by staying in the G_0 phase. The major challenge of chemotherapy for cancer is overcoming the medication resistance of resting and noncycling cells.

TABLE 18.8 MEDICATION THERAPY
Classification of Chemotherapeutic Agents

Mechanisms of Action	Examples
Alkylating Agents *Cell Cycle Phase–Nonspecific Agents*	
Damage DNA by causing breaks in the double-strand helix (similar to the effect of radiation therapy); if repair does not occur, cells die immediately (cytocidal) or when they attempt to divide (cytostatic)	Mechlorethamine (formerly known as *nitrogen mustard*), cyclophosphamide (Procytox), chlorambucil (Leukeran), melphalan (Alkeran), busulfan (Myleran), dacarbazine (DTIC), lomustine (CCNU, CeeNU), oxaliplatin (Eloxatin), streptozocin (Zanosar), cisplatin, carboplatin
Antimetabolites *Cell Cycle Phase–Specific Agents (Primarily S Phase)*	
Interfere with enzyme function and synthesis of DNA by mimicking naturally occurring metabolites required by the cell for synthesis of DNA and RNA (cytocidal)	Methotrexate, cytarabine (Cytosar), fluorouracil (5-FU), mercaptopurine (6-MP), thioguanine (6-TG), fludarabine (Fludara), hydroxyurea (Hydrea), gemcitabine (Gemzar), cladribine (Leustatin)
Antitumour Antibiotics *Cell Cycle Phase–Nonspecific Agents*	
Modify function of DNA and interfere with transcription of RNA (cytocidal or cytostatic)	Doxorubicin (Adriamycin), bleomycin (Blenoxane), mitomycin, daunorubicin (Daunomycin), dactinomycin (Cosmegen), idarubicin (Idamycin), epirubicin (Ellence), mitoxantrone
Plant Alkaloids (Mitotic Inhibitors) *Cell Cycle Phase–Specific Agents (G$_2$ and M Phases)*	
Interrupt cellular replication in mitosis at metaphase (cytocidal)	Vinblastine, vincristine, etoposide (VePesid), paclitaxel (Taxol), docetaxel (Taxotere), teniposide (Vumon)
Nitrosoureas *Cell Cycle Phase–Nonspecific Agents*	
Similar to alkylating agents; break DNA helix and interfere with DNA replication (cytocidal or cytostatic)	Carmustine (BCNU), lomustine (CCNU, CeeNU)
Corticosteroids *Cell Cycle Phase–Nonspecific Agents*	
Disrupt the cell membrane and inhibit synthesis of protein; decrease circulating lymphocytes; inhibit mitosis; depress immune system; increase feeling of well-being	Cortisone, hydrocortisone (Cortef), methylprednisolone (Medrol), prednisone, dexamethasone
Hormone Therapy *Cell Cycle Phase–Nonspecific Agents*	
Interfere with hormone receptors and proteins, inhibiting tumour growth ***Aromatase Inhibitors***	Androgens (testosterone), estrogens, progestins
Inhibit the enzyme aromatase, a cytochrome P450 enzyme involved in estrogen synthesis ***Selective Estrogen Receptor Modulator (SERM)***	Anastrozole (Arimidex), letrozole (Femara), exemestane (Aromasin)
Selectively modulates estrogen receptors, thus acting as an estrogen antagonist ***Miscellaneous***	Raloxifene (Evista)
Destroys exogenous supply of L-asparagine, which is needed for cellular proliferation; L-asparagine can be synthesized by normal cells but not by cancer cells	L-Asparaginase (Elspar)
Antiestrogens used in breast cancer	Tamoxifen (Nolvadex), fulvestrant (Faslodex)
Suppress mitosis at interphase; appear to alter preformed DNA, RNA, and protein	Procarbazine (Matulane)

Note: Each cancer agency in Canada has a formulary of protocols and practice guidelines; strict adherence to these guidelines is critical in the clinical setting. With new clinical trial research, medication protocols change; thus, the list in this table may not remain current.
DNA, deoxyribonucleic acid; *RNA*, ribonucleic acid.

Classification of Chemotherapeutic Medications

Chemotherapeutic medications are categorized or classified according to their structure and mechanisms of action (Table 18.8). Each medication in a particular classification has many similarities, but major differences among the medications are also evident.

Preparation and Administration of Chemotherapeutic Agents

It is very important to know the specific guidelines for administration of chemotherapeutic medications. These medications may also pose occupational hazards for health care providers. A health care provider preparing or administering chemotherapeutic agents may absorb the medication through inhalation of particles and through skin contact when reconstituting a powder in an open ampule. There may also be some risk in handling the body fluids and excreta of patients receiving chemotherapy. Guidelines for the safe handling of chemotherapeutic agents have been developed by the National Institute for Occupational Safety and Health (NIOSH) and the Oncology Nursing Society (see the Resources at the end of this chapter).

TABLE 18.9 MEDICATION THERAPY
Methods of Administration of Chemotherapeutic Agents

Method	Examples
Oral	Cyclophosphamide
Intramuscular	Bleomycin
Intravenous	Doxorubicin, vincristine
Intracavitary (pleural, peritoneal)	Radioisotopes, alkylating agents, methotrexate
Intrathecal	Methotrexate, cytarabine
Intra-arterial	Dacarbazine (DTIC), 5-fluorouracil (5-FU), methotrexate, floxuridine
Perfusion	Alkylating agents
Continuous infusion	5-FU, methotrexate, cytarabine
Subcutaneous	Cytarabine

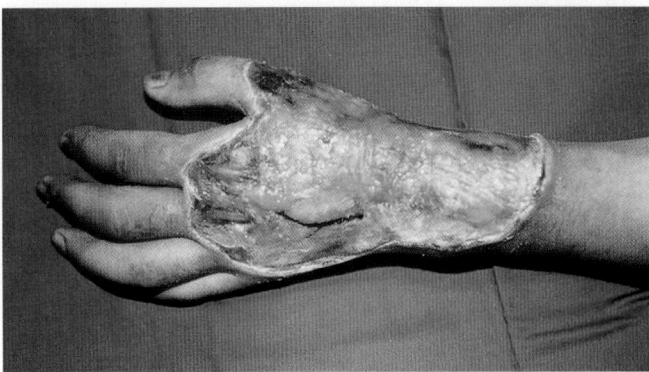

FIG. 18.11 Extravasation injury from infiltration of chemotherapeutic medication. Source: Weinzweig, N., & Weinzweig, J. (2005). *The mutilated hand.* Mosby.

Methods of Administration

Several routes are used to administer chemotherapeutic agents (Table 18.9). The oral and intravenous routes are the most commonly used. The major concerns associated with the intravenous administration of antineoplastic medications are the potential for irritation or damage to the vessels; problems with the venous access device or catheter, including infection; and extravasation (infiltration of medications into tissues surrounding the infusion site), which causes local tissue damage. Many chemotherapeutic medications are irritants or vesicants, agents that cause severe local tissue breakdown and necrosis when accidentally infiltrated into the skin (Figure 18.11).

Pain is the cardinal symptom of extravasation, although extravasation has been known to occur without causing pain. Swelling, redness, and the presence of vesicles on the skin are other signs of extravasation. After a few days, the tissue may begin to ulcerate and necrose, and closure with skin grafts is often required.

To minimize these risks and to avoid physical discomfort, chemotherapeutic medications may be administered by means of a central venous access device. Cancer care increasingly involves combination therapies that entail venous access; therefore, the use of these devices has increased. Central venous access devices are placed in large blood vessels and enable frequent, continuous, or intermittent administration of chemotherapeutic agents, biological therapeutic agents, and other products. They are indicated in instances of limited venous access, intensive chemotherapy, continuous infusion of vesicant agents, and projected long-term need for venous access. (Central venous access devices are discussed further in Chapter 19.)

The advantages of venous access devices are that they provide for rapid dilution of chemotherapeutic agents, decreased incidence of extravasation, and reduced need for venipuncture. In addition to their usefulness in administration of chemotherapeutic agents, venous access devices can be used to administer additional fluids such as blood products, parenteral nutrition, or other medications, as well as for venous blood sampling. The disadvantages are that the presence of central catheters can lead to increased incidence of blood clots, and they can be a source of systemic infection, particularly if a patient becomes immunosuppressed during therapy. Three major types of venous access devices used in oncology care are tunnelled catheters, peripherally inserted central catheters, and implanted infusion ports. (See Chapter 19 for a detailed discussion of these venous access devices.)

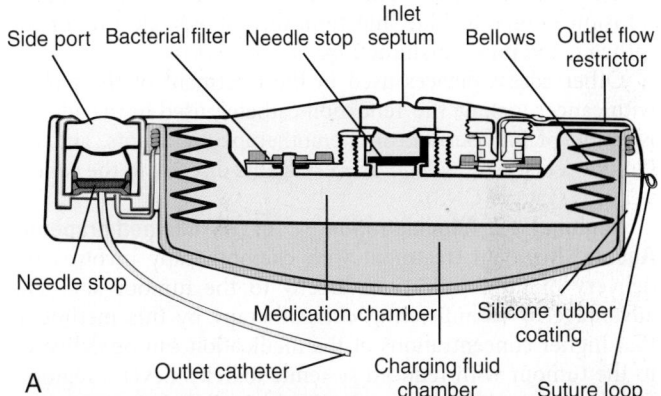

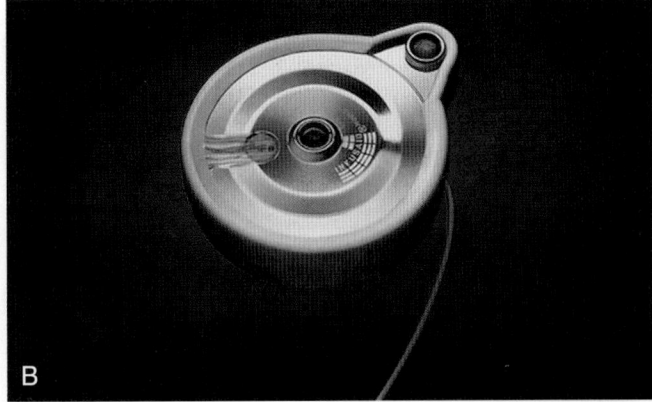

FIG. 18.12 **A,** Cross-section of the implantable pump displaying its two chambers: the medication chamber (inner) and the charging fluid chamber (outer). As the medication chamber is filled, the bellows expand, compressing the charging fluid in the outer chamber. The resulting increased pressure in the outer chamber forces the medication through a membrane filter and preset flow restrictor, thus ensuring a nearly constant flow. **B,** Infusaid pump. Source: Courtesy Strato/Infusaid, Inc., Norwood, MA.

Infusion Pumps. Infusion pumps are used primarily for the continuous infusion of chemotherapeutic agents by intravenous, subcutaneous, intra-arterial, and epidural routes. Infusion pumps can be worn externally or implanted surgically.

Implanted infusion pumps are used primarily for intra-arterial administration of chemotherapeutic agents (Figure 18.12). This approach enables continuous infusion of the chemotherapeutic agent directly to the area of the tumour while sparing patients the systemic effects of the medication. Some implanted pumps have two silicone septa. The second septum can be used for bolus medication administration. The most common use of this method of chemotherapeutic administration has been hepatic artery infusion in the treatment of liver metastasis, usually from primary colon cancer.

Implanted pumps also consist of a catheter that is threaded into the designated artery. The catheter is attached to a pump apparatus that consists of two chambers: an inner chamber that serves as the medication reservoir and an outer chamber that contains vapour pressure, which provides a source of power for the pump. The pump is implanted surgically in a subcutaneous pocket. Access to the pump is via a silicone septum with a Huber point needle. Flow rate of the pump can be affected by medication concentration, the length and diameter of the silicone rubber (Silastic) catheter, and the patient's body temperature. Thus dose alterations may be required if the patient experiences a change in temperature or travels to higher altitudes. Complications that have been associated with implanted infusion pumps include infection, thrombosis, clotting of the catheter, and pump malfunction.

Other access devices used in the treatment of the person with cancer include the Tenckhoff catheter, used in the administration of intraperitoneal chemotherapeutic agents, and the Ommaya reservoir, which delivers agents directly to the central nervous system (CNS).

Regional Administration of Chemotherapeutic Agents. Regional treatment with chemotherapy involves the delivery of the medication directly to the tumour site. The advantage of administering chemotherapy by this method is that higher concentrations of the medication can be delivered to the tumour with reduced systemic toxicity. Several regional delivery methods have been developed, including intra-arterial, intraperitoneal, intrathecal or intraventricular, and intravesical bladder chemotherapy.

Intra-Arterial Chemotherapy. In intra-arterial chemotherapy, the medication is delivered to the tumour via the arterial vessel supplying the tumour. This method has been used for the treatment of osteogenic sarcoma; cancers of the head and neck, the bladder, the brain, and the cervix; melanoma; primary liver cancer; and metastatic liver disease. One method of intra-arterial medication delivery involves the surgical placement of a catheter that is subsequently connected to an external infusion pump or an implanted infusion pump for infusion of the chemotherapeutic agent. In general, intra-arterial chemotherapy results in reduced systemic toxicity. The type of toxic effects experienced by patients depends on the toxicity profile of the chemotherapy agent and the site of the tumour being treated.

Intraperitoneal Chemotherapy. Intraperitoneal chemotherapy involves the delivery of chemotherapeutic agents to the peritoneal cavity for treatment of peritoneal metastases from primary colorectal and ovarian cancers and malignant ascites. Temporary Silastic catheters (e.g., Tenckhoff, Hickman, Groshong) are percutaneously or surgically placed into the peritoneal cavity for short-term administration of chemotherapeutic agents. Alternatively, an implanted port can be used to administer chemotherapeutic agents intraperitoneally. Complications of intraperitoneal chemotherapy delivery include abdominal pain; catheter occlusion, dislodgement, and migration; and infection.

Intrathecal or Intraventricular Chemotherapy. Cancers that metastasize to the CNS—most commonly breast, lung, and GI cancers; leukemia; and lymphoma—are difficult to treat because the blood–brain barrier often prevents distribution of chemotherapeutic agents to this area. One method used to treat metastasis to the CNS is intrathecal chemotherapy. This method involves a lumbar puncture and injection of chemotherapeutic medications into the subarachnoid space. However, this method has resulted in incomplete distribution of the medication in the CNS, particularly to the cisternal and ventricular areas.

To ensure more uniform distribution of chemotherapeutic medications to the cisternal and ventricular areas, an Ommaya reservoir is often inserted. An Ommaya reservoir is a Silastic, dome-shaped disc with an extension catheter that is surgically implanted through the cranium into a lateral ventricle. In addition to providing more consistent medication distribution, the Ommaya reservoir averts the need for repeated painful lumbar punctures.

Complications of intrathecal or intraventricular chemotherapy include meningitis and leukoencephalopathy (Slavc et al., 2018).

Intravesical Bladder Chemotherapy. Many patients with superficial transitional cell cancer of the bladder have recurrent disease after traditional surgical therapy. Instillation of chemotherapeutic agents into the bladder promotes destruction of cancer cells and reduces the incidence of recurrent disease. Additional benefits of this therapy include reduced urinary and sexual dysfunction. The chemotherapeutic agent is instilled into the bladder via a urinary catheter and retained for 1 to 3 hours. Complications of this therapy include dysuria, urinary frequency, hematuria, and bladder spasms.

Effects of Chemotherapy on Normal Tissues

Chemotherapeutic agents cannot selectively distinguish between normal cells and cancer cells. Adverse and toxic effects results from the destruction of normal cells, especially those that proliferate rapidly, such as the cells of the bone marrow, the GI lining, and the integumentary system (Table 18.10). The body's response to the products of cellular destruction in the circulation may cause fatigue, anorexia, and taste alterations.

The adverse effects of these medications can be classified as acute, delayed, or chronic. Acute toxic effects include vomiting, allergic reactions, and dysrhythmias. Delayed effects include mucositis, alopecia, and bone marrow suppression. Mucositis can result in mouth sores, gastritis, and diarrhea. Chronic toxicity involves damage to organs such as the heart, the liver, the kidneys, the peripheral nerves and the lungs.

Treatment Plan

When chemotherapy is used in the treatment of cancer, several medications may be given in combination. Multimedication regimens have proved to be particularly effective in the treatment of many types of cancer. The medications and medication doses are carefully selected to kill the cancer cells most effectively and yet allow the normal cells to repair themselves and proliferate, so that maximal benefit with minimal toxicity is achieved. The dose of each medication is carefully calculated

TABLE 18.10	CELLS WITH RAPID RATE OF PROLIFERATION
Cells and Generation Time	**Effect of Cell Destruction**
Bone marrow stem cell: 6–24 hr	Myelosuppression; infection, bleeding, anemia
Neutrophils: 12 hr	Leukopenia, infection
Epithelial cells lining the gastrointestinal tract: 12–24 hr	Anorexia, stomatitis, esophagitis, nausea and vomiting, diarrhea
Ova or testes: 24–36 hr	Reproductive dysfunction
Cells of the hair follicle: 24 hr	Alopecia

according to the body weight or the body surface area (i.e., body weight and height) of the patient being treated. The principles of combination chemotherapy include the following:

1. The medications used in the treatment plan are effective against the cancer being treated.
2. When medications are given in combination, a synergistic effect occurs.
3. The combination includes cell cycle phase–specific medications, cell cycle phase–nonspecific medications, and medications that have different mechanisms of action.
4. The combination includes medications that have different toxic adverse effects.
5. The combination includes medications that cause nadirs at different time intervals. The nadir is the lowest level of the peripheral blood cell counts (particularly WBC) that occurs secondary to bone marrow depression. The nadir after administration of most chemotherapeutic medications occurs in 7 to 28 days.

An example of a treatment regimen is the FOLFOX (**fol**inic acid, **f**luorouracil, and **ox**aliplatin) regimen (Table 18.11). The agents in this medication protocol differ in mechanisms of action, toxic adverse effects, and nadir, but the combination is synergistic in nature, and the dosage schedule includes a time of medication administration and a time of rest from medication administration. The rest period is necessary to allow the normal cells to proliferate and repair the damaged tissue. The patient is evaluated before the administration of each course of chemotherapy to determine how well they are tolerating the treatment and whether the normal cells have recovered sufficiently for the next dose to be given.

RADIATION THERAPY

Radiation therapy is a local treatment modality for cancer. It is one of the oldest methods of cancer treatment. Historically, workers exposed to radiation had a higher incidence of skin desquamation and developed carcinomas of the fingers. Both Marie Curie and her daughter Irène Joliot-Curie developed leukemia as a result of radiation exposure.

The observation that radiation exposure caused tissue damage led scientists to explore the use of radiation to treat tumours. The hypothesis was that if radiation resulted in the destruction of the highly mitotic skin cells of workers, it could be used in a controlled way to prevent the continued growth of highly mitotic cancer cells. It was not until the 1960s that sophisticated equipment and treatment planning facilitated the delivery of adequate radiation doses to tumours and tolerable doses to normal tissues. Today, radiotherapy has a central role in the treatment of cancer.

Effects of Radiation

Radiation is the emission and distribution of energy through space or a material medium. The energy produced by radiation, when absorbed into tissue, produces ionization and excitation. This local energy and the resultant generation of free radicals break chemical bonds in DNA, which may lead to lethal or sublethal damage. Lethal damage causes sufficient chromosomal disruption that the cell is unable to replicate. Sublethal DNA damage may be repaired between radiation doses or, alternatively, may accumulate with repetitive doses, leading to cell death. Cancer cells are especially vulnerable to the effects of cumulative radiation doses because they are less capable of repairing sublethal damage than are normal cells. When repetitive, *fractionated* (or divided) doses of radiation are delivered to a tumour, damage to malignant cells is maximized, and normal cells are more likely to recover. The principles of radiotherapy dosing and fractionation are guided by cellular response to radiation, known as the *four Rs* of radiobiology: **r**epair of cellular damage, **r**edistribution of cells in the cell cycle, **r**epopulation with normal cells, and **r**eoxygenation of hypoxic tumour areas.

Cellular Death and Tissue Reactions. *Cellular death* related to radiation is defined as an irreversible loss of proliferative capacity. Cells may undergo several mitoses and then die. A cell that retains its proliferative capacity is a clonogenic cell because it is able to produce new clones or colonies of similar cells. After radiation, cancer is considered controlled if the cells that remain are nonclonogenic.

Cellular sensitivity to radiation varies throughout the cell cycle; cells are most sensitive in the M and G_2 phases and least sensitive during the S, or synthesis, phase (see Figure 18.1). Cells treated during the M and G_2 phases of the cell cycle are more likely to suffer lethal damage. The damage to DNA in cells that are not in the M phase is expressed when the cells divide.

The amount of time that is required for the manifestations of radiation damage is determined by the mitotic rate of the tissue. Sufficient numbers of cells within the tissue must be killed to establish a noticeable effect. This is true for both normal and cancer cells. Rapidly dividing cells in the GI tract, oral mucosa, and bone marrow die fast or exhibit other early acute responses to irradiation. Tissues with slowly proliferating cells—such as those of cartilage, bone, and kidneys—manifest late responses to irradiation.

TABLE 18.11 MEDICATION THERAPY

FOLFOX Chemotherapeutic Agent Schedule

Schedule: FOLFOX + bevacizumab (Avastin) is given to treat advanced colon cancer. FOLFOX* includes 5-fluorouracil ("FOL") administered as a continuous intravenous infusion over 46 hours on days 1 and 2; leucovorin (folinic acid; "F") administered intravenously over 2 hours on days 1 and 2; and oxaliplatin (Eloxatin [OX]) administered intravenously over 2 hours on day 1. Bevacizumab is administered intravenously over 2 hours on day 1. This schedule is repeated every 2 weeks. The number of cycles depends on a patient's situation.

Agent	Week 1		Week 3		Week 5		Week 7	
	Day 1	Day 2	Day 1	Day 2	Day 1	Day 2	Day 1	Day 2
5-Fluorouracil	X	X	X	X	X	X	X	X
Leucovorin (folinic acid)	X	X	X	X	X	X	X	X
Oxaliplatin (Eloxatin)	X		X		X		X	
Bevacizumab (Avastin)	X		X		X		X	

*There are slightly different versions of the FOLFOX regimen.

TABLE 18.12	TUMOUR RADIOSENSITIVITY		
High Radiosensitivity	**Moderate Radiosensitivity**	**Mild Radiosensitivity**	**Poor Radiosensitivity**
• Hodgkin's disease • Neuroblastoma • Non-Hodgkin's lymphoma • Ovarian dysgerminoma • Testicular seminoma • Wilms tumour	• Bladder carcinoma • Breast adenocarcinoma • Esophageal carcinoma • Oropharyngeal carcinoma • Prostate carcinoma • Skin carcinoma • Uterine and cervical carcinoma	• Colon adenocarcinoma • Gastric adenocarcinoma • Renal adenocarcinoma • Soft tissue sarcomas (e.g., chondrosarcoma)	• Malignant gliomas • Malignant melanoma • Osteosarcoma • Testicular nonseminoma

This differential rate of cellular death explains the timing of clinical manifestations related to radiation therapy. Normal cells within the radiation field are also affected by treatment. For each normal cell type, there is a maximally tolerated radiation dose. Administration of radiation above the maximally tolerated doses results in limited ability of normal cells to recover from damage and in potentially irreversible adverse effects. Treatment planning, delivery, and computerized dosimetry ensure that normal tissue tolerance is not exceeded (Citrin, 2017).

Table 18.12 lists the relative radiosensitivities of a variety of tumours. In responsive tumours, even a large tumour burden is affected by therapy. In less responsive tumours, a large tumour burden may result in a slower and perhaps incomplete response.

Simulation and Treatment

Simulation is a part of radiation treatment planning used to determine the optimal treatment method. The patient lies on a table in the treatment position. The critical normal structures to be included in the treatment field or portal are identified under fluoroscopy. An image is taken to verify the field, and marks are placed on the skin so that the field can be reproduced on a daily basis. Immobilization devices (e.g., casts, bite blocks, thermoplastic face masks) are typically used to help the patient maintain a stable position (Figure 18.13). Computerized dosimetry, accomplished with CT scanning, is used to produce a treatment plan for delivering the maximum amount of radiation to the tumour within the acceptable dosage limits for normal tissue.

External Radiation. Teletherapy (*external beam irradiation*) is the most common form of radiation treatment delivery. With this technique, the patient is exposed to radiation from a megavoltage treatment machine. The radiation source may include cobalt-60, which emits gamma rays from a radioactive source. Therapy may be delivered by a cyclotron, which produces neutrons or protons, or by a linear accelerator, which generates ionizing radiation from electricity and with which multiple levels of energy can be utilized (Figure 18.14).

Internal Radiation. Another radiation delivery system is brachytherapy ("close" treatment). In this method, radioactive materials are implanted or inserted directly into the tumour or close to the tumour. An implant may be temporary; the source is placed into a catheter or tube that is inserted into the tumour area and left in place for several days. This method is commonly used for tumours of the head and neck and for prostate and gynecological malignancies. Implants may also be permanent, whereby radioactive seeds are inserted into tumours—for example, in the prostate. Brachytherapy is clinically appropriate when the radiation dose necessary to eradicate the tumour exceeds the dose tolerance of nearby normal tissues. The sources used in brachytherapy are not as energetic or penetrating as those used in the external beam machines and thus deliver most of

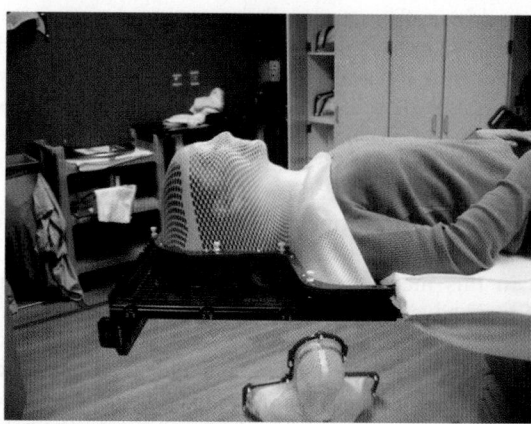

FIG. 18.13 Immobilization device. Use of a head holder and immobilization mask may be used to ensure accurate positioning for daily treatment of head and neck cancer. Source: Courtesy Jormain Cady, Virginia Mason Medical Center, Seattle, WA.

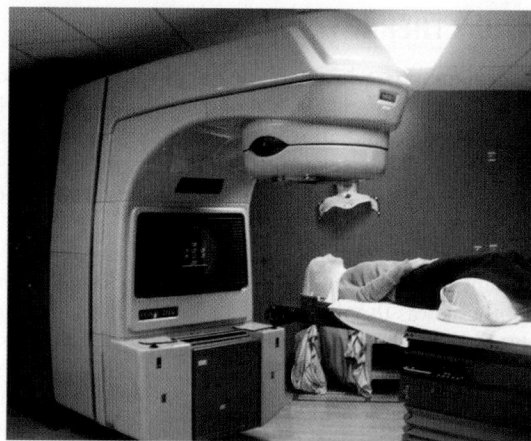

FIG. 18.14 Linear accelerator. Varian Clinac EX linear accelerator with multiple photon and electron energy levels available for use according to the treatment plan. Patient is positioned on radiation treatment table for treatment of head and neck cancer. Source: Courtesy Jormain Cady, Virginia Mason Medical Center, Seattle, WA.

the dose locally. External beam radiation therapy and brachytherapy may be used in combination.

To care for a patient with a radiation implant, the nurse must be aware that the patient is radioactive. Patients with temporary implants are radioactive during the time the source is in place. If the patient has a permanent implant, the radioactive exposure to the outside and to other people is low, and the patient may be discharged with precautions. The principles of time, distance, and shielding are used in caring for the patient with an implant. Nursing care should be organized so that time spent in direct contact with the patient is kept to a minimum. The patient should be informed of these restrictions before the implantation procedure. The radiation safety officer determines how much time at a specific distance can be spent with the patient, according to the dose delivered by the implant. Because the source is nonpenetrating, small differences in distance are critical. Only care that must be delivered near the source, such as checking placement of the implant, is performed in close proximity. Shielding, if available, should be used, and the health care provider should not deliver care without wearing a film badge. This badge indicates any radiation exposure. The film badge should not be shared, should not be worn anywhere other than at work, and should be returned according to the employer's policy.

Measurement of Radiation

Several different units are used to measure radiation (Table 18.13). Grays (Gy) and centigrays (cGy) are the units currently used in clinical practice.

Goals of Radiation Therapy

The goals of radiation therapy are cure, control, and palliation. To accomplish these treatment goals, radiation therapy can be used alone or as an adjuvant treatment modality with surgery, chemotherapy, biological therapy, or some combination of these.

Cure is the goal when radiation therapy is used alone for treating patients with basal cell carcinoma of the skin, tumours confined to the vocal cords, and stage I or IIA Hodgkin's disease. Radiation therapy can be combined with surgery and chemotherapy to cure certain cancers—for example, (a) stages IIB, IIIA, and IIIB Hodgkin's disease (in combination with chemotherapy); (b) Ewing's sarcoma (in combination with chemotherapy); (c) head and neck cancer (in combination with surgery and chemotherapy); and (d) stages I and II breast cancer (in combination with surgery).

Control of the disease process for a time may be a reasonable goal in some situations. Initial treatment is offered at the time of diagnosis, and additional treatment may be instituted if symptoms of disease recur. Most patients enjoy a satisfactory quality of life during the symptom-free period. Radiation therapy can be combined with surgery to further enhance the local control of cancer. It can be given preoperatively to reduce the size of the tumour so that it can be more easily resected, or it can be given postoperatively to destroy any remaining tumour cells. Intraoperative radiation therapy is now available at some research centres. In this procedure, radiation is administered directly to the site of the tumour during surgery.

Inoperable tumours can be treated with radiation therapy. These tumours are large and have extended regionally. An example of an inoperable cancer treated for control with radiation therapy is small cell carcinoma of the lung.

Palliation is often the goal of radiation therapy, with the aim of controlling symptoms resulting from the disease process. Tumours can be reduced in size to relieve symptoms such as pain and obstruction. Examples of the use of radiation therapy for palliation include relief from the following:

1. Pain associated with bone metastasis
2. Pain and neurological symptoms associated with brain metastasis
3. Spinal cord compression
4. Intestinal obstruction

TABLE 18.13	MEASUREMENT OF RADIATION
Unit	**Definition**
Curie (Ci)	A measure of the number of atoms of a particular radioisotope that disintegrate in 1 second
Roentgen (R)	A measure of the radiation required to produce a standard number of ions in air; a unit of exposure to radiation
Rad	Measurement of radiation dosage absorbed by the tissues
Rem	Measurement of the biological effectiveness of various forms of radiation on the human cell (1 rem = 1 rad)
Gray (Gy)	100 rads = 1 Gy
Centigray (cGy)	1 Gy = 100 cGy

5. Superior vena cava obstruction
6. Bronchial or tracheal obstruction
7. Bleeding (e.g., bladder and intrabronchial)

NURSING MANAGEMENT
RADIATION THERAPY AND CHEMOTHERAPY

The nurse has an important role in educating patients about their treatment regimens and the management of adverse effects and disease symptoms. Teaching should be tailored to the needs and abilities of patients and their families. Nurses can also assist patients in coping with the psychosocial issues associated with a cancer diagnosis. Anxiety and fear may pervade a patient's day-to-day experience and become a barrier to their ability to navigate through treatment. The nurse can mobilize an interprofessional team of health care providers, community resources, and the patient's family to provide and reinforce information, facilitate transportation to the cancer centre, and ensure adequate physical, emotional, and spiritual support. One of the most important responsibilities of the nurse is that of differentiating between toxic effects of treatments and progression of the malignant process. The nurse must also distinguish tolerable adverse effects from acute toxic effects of chemotherapeutic agents. For example, nausea and vomiting are expected and controllable adverse effects of many medications. However, if paresthesia occurs with the use of vincristine or if signs of heart failure appear with the use of doxorubicin, these serious reactions must be reported to the health care provider so that medication dosages can be modified or the medication discontinued. Some toxic effects associated with chemotherapy may not be reversible. For example, ototoxicity may be an irreversible effect of cisplatin therapy, especially at high doses. Periodic testing of hearing may be necessary to monitor for this toxic effect. The nurse can also advise patients about the availability of supportive therapies (e.g., antiemetics, antidiarrheals) to optimize quality of life during treatment.

Common adverse effects and specific nursing considerations related to conditions caused by cancer therapy are presented in Table 18.14. Fatigue, anorexia, bone marrow suppression, skin reactions, mucosal reactions, and pulmonary, GI, and reproductive effects are discussed in the following sections. (See Nursing Care Plan 18.1 and Nursing Care Plan 18.2 for care of the patient undergoing radiation or chemotherapy, available on the Evolve website.)

TABLE 18.14	NURSING MANAGEMENT OF CONDITIONS CAUSED BY RADIATION THERAPY AND CHEMOTHERAPY	
Condition	**Cause**	**Nursing Management**
Gastrointestinal System		
Stomatitis, mucositis, esophagitis	Destruction of cells in radiation treatment field Destruction of epithelial cells by chemotherapy Inflammation and ulceration, which result from rapid cell destruction	• Be aware that eating, swallowing, and talking may be difficult and necessitate changes in diet and fluid intake. • Encourage the patient to use artificial saliva. • Assess oral mucosa daily. Teach the patient to do this, and encourage the patient to practise good oral hygiene. • Use evidence-informed policies to minimize the occurrence or reduce the severity of oral mucositis. • Discourage use of irritants such as tobacco and alcohol, spicy foods, and drinks. • Apply topical anaesthetics, such as lidocaine (Xylocaine Viscous) or oxethazaine.
Nausea and vomiting	Cellular breakdown, which stimulates vomiting centre in brain Medications, which also stimulate vomiting centre Destruction of GI lining by radiation and chemotherapy	• Counsel the patient to eat and drink when not nauseated. • Administer antiemetics, and teach the patient and family caregiver when to use antiemetic therapy to maximize symptom control.
Anorexia	Release of TNF and IL-1 from macrophages, which has appetite-suppressant effect General reaction to therapy	• Use diversional activities (if appropriate). • Monitor the patient's weight. • Encourage the patient to eat small, frequent meals of high-protein, high-calorie foods (e.g., Ensure or other supplements). • Reassure family caregivers, and teach them to provide gentle encouragement to the patient.
Diarrhea	Denuding of epithelial lining of intestines	• Suggest low-fibre, low-residue diet. • Increase fluids. • Provide antidiarrheal agents as needed.
Constipation	Autonomic nervous system dysfunction Neurotoxic effects of plant alkaloids (vincristine, vinblastine) Use of opioids	• Encourage the patient to use a diary to monitor bowel movements and report to the health care team as needed. • Provide stool softeners and laxatives as needed. • Encourage intake of high-fibre foods.
Hepatotoxicity	Toxic effects from chemotherapeutic medications	• Monitor liver function values.
Hematological System		
Anemia	Bone marrow depressed as a result of therapy Malignant infiltration of bone marrow by cancer	• Monitor hemoglobin and hematocrit levels. • Encourage intake of foods that promote RBC production (see Chapter 33, Table 33.5).

Leukopenia	Depression of bone marrow as a result of chemotherapy or radiation therapy
	Febrile neutropenia
	Infection resulting from immunosuppression (most frequent cause of morbidity and death in patients with cancer)
	Infection in respiratory and genitourinary systems (usual sites of infection)
		• Monitor WBC count, especially neutrophils.
		• Educate and counsel patients and family caregivers to do the following:
		  • Monitor changes in temperature, and report any elevation immediately to the health care team.
		  • Advise the patient to maintain good personal hygiene, including frequent handwashing.
		  • Recommend that the patient report any signs of infection (swelling, unusual cough, vomiting, severe headache, redness) immediately at the nearest hospital.
		  • Advise the patient to avoid large crowds and people with infections.

Thrombocytopenia	Bone marrow depression secondary to chemotherapy Malignant infiltration of bone marrow Spontaneous bleeding, which can occur with platelet counts at or below 20×10^9/L	• Observe for signs of bleeding (e.g., petechiae, ecchymosis). • Monitor hemoglobin, hematocrit, and platelet counts. • Recommend use of a soft-bristle toothbrush and electric razor.
Integumentary System		
Alopecia (usually temporary with chemotherapy and usually permanent in response to radiation)	Destruction of hair follicles by chemotherapy or radiation to scalp	• Suggest ways to cope with hair loss (e.g., hairpieces, scarves, wigs). • Discuss effect of hair loss on self-image. • Recommend cutting long hair before therapy. • Advise the patient to avoid excessive shampooing, brushing, and combing of hair. • Recommend avoiding use of electric hair dryers, curlers, and curling irons.

TABLE 18.14	NURSING MANAGEMENT OF CONDITIONS CAUSED BY RADIATION THERAPY AND CHEMOTHERAPY—cont'd	
Condition	**Cause**	**Nursing Management**
Skin reactions	Extravasation of vesicant chemotherapeutic medications Radiation therapy damage to skin	• Protect the patient from extravasation through careful attention to delivery of chemotherapeutic medications and assessment of venous access. • Recommend lubricating dry skin with nonirritating creams. • Recommend avoiding the use of harsh soaps. • Advise the patient to wear loose clothing and cotton underwear and to avoid wearing tight garments. • Inform the patient that photosensitivity may occur.
Genitourinary System		
Cystitis	Destruction of cells lining the bladder by chemotherapy Adverse effect of radiation when located in treatment field	• Monitor manifestations such as urgency, frequency, and hematuria. • Discuss these changes with the patient.
Reproductive dysfunction	Damage of cells of testes or ova by therapy	• Provide information about effects on fertility and referral to fertility resources (e.g., sperm banking) before delivery of radiation to the pelvis, high-dose chemotherapy, or bone marrow transplantation.
Nephrotoxicity	Accumulation of medications in the kidney and tumour lysis, which cause necrosis of proximal renal tubules	• Monitor BUN and serum creatinine levels.
Nervous System		
Increased intracranial pressure	Radiation-related edema in central nervous system	• Administer steroids and pain medication. • Monitor neurological status.
Peripheral neuropathy	Paresthesias, areflexia, skeletal muscle weakness, and smooth muscle dysfunction, which can occur as adverse effects of plant alkaloids and cisplatin	• Monitor for such manifestations in patients receiving these medications.
Respiratory System		
Pneumonitis (develops 2–3 mo after start of treatment)	Radiation Adverse effects of some chemotherapeutic medications	• Monitor for dry, hacking cough; fever; and exertional dyspnea.
Fibrosis (develops after 6–12 mo and is evident on radiographs)		
Cardiovascular System		
Pericarditis and myocarditis (complication when chest wall is irradiated; may occur up to 1 yr after treatment)	Inflammation secondary to radiation injury Adverse effect of some chemotherapeutic medications	• Monitor for clinical manifestations of these disorders. • Monitor heart function with ECG studies and cardiac ejection fractions.
Cardiotoxicity	Some chemotherapeutic medications (e.g., doxorubicin, daunorubicin) can cause ECG changes and rapidly progressive heart failure	• Medication therapy may have to be modified.
Biochemical		
Hyperuricemia, secondary gout, and obstructive uropathy	Cell destruction by chemotherapy	• Monitor uric acid levels. • Allopurinol (Zyloprim) may be given as a prophylactic measure. • Encourage high fluid intake.
Multidimensional Effects		
Fatigue	Increased metabolic rate Anabolic processes that result in accumulation of metabolites from cell breakdown	• Counsel the patient that fatigue is an expected adverse effect of therapy but that there are ways to manage fatigue, such as sleep hygiene, moderate exercise, and pacing activities. • Encourage the patient to rest when fatigued, to maintain usual lifestyle patterns as closely as possible, and to pace activities in accordance with energy level.
Pain	Compression or infiltration of tumour involving nerves Inflammation, ulceration, or necrosis of tissues	• Use an analgesic ladder to provide basis for pain medication administration. • Teach use of imagery, relaxation therapy, and other alternative measures (see Chapters 8 and 12).

BUN, blood urea nitrogen (serum urea [nitrogen]); *ECG,* electrocardiographic; *GI,* gastrointestinal; *IL-1,* interleukin 1; *RBC,* red blood cell; *TNF,* tumour necrosis factor; *WBC,* white blood cell.

NURSING IMPLEMENTATION

FATIGUE. Fatigue is a commonly reported adverse effect of cancer therapy, affecting at least 80% of patients with cancer (Charalambous et al., 2019). The pathophysiological mechanisms that result in cancer treatment–induced fatigue are unclear. Accumulation of metabolites from the destruction of cells during treatment is one probable cause. The metabolites include lactate, hydrogen ions, and other end products of cellular destruction and result in decreased muscle strength. Energy production in patients with cancer may also be altered by cachexia, anorexia, fever, and infection. Fatigue associated with radiotherapy generally begins during the third to fourth weeks of treatment, persists after treatment ends, and then gradually subsides. Chemotherapy-related fatigue may become chronic after therapy. Factors such as weight loss, anemia, depression, nausea, and other symptoms exacerbate the sensation of fatigue.

Maintaining good nutrition and adequate hydration, alternating periods of rest and activity, relying on family members for assistance with responsibilities, and managing pain and anxiety may help reduce fatigue. The nurse can prepare patients for the expected adverse effect of fatigue so that they do not assume it is a sign of treatment failure. A patient may report more energy on some days than on others. Encouraging a patient to identify days or times during the day when they feel better may assist in understanding their body's responses and maximizing energy reserves. Ignoring the fatigue or overstressing the body when fatigue is tolerable may lead to an increase in symptoms. Mild physical activity programs are usually within the abilities of patients and have been found to ameliorate symptoms of fatigue, lessen anxiety, and facilitate sleep in persons with cancer (Ebede et al., 2017). Family caregivers of patients with cancer are also prone to fatigue and poor energy levels. Remaining as active as the individual is able has been shown to improve mood and avoid the debilitating cycle of fatigue–depression–fatigue that can occur.

ANOREXIA. Anorexia may develop as a general reaction to treatment. The mechanisms underlying the development of anorexia are unclear, but several theories exist. Macrophages release TNF and IL-1 in an attempt to fight the cancer. Both TNF and IL-1 have an appetite-suppressing (anorexic) effect. It is hypothesized that as tumours are destroyed by therapy, increased levels of these factors are released into the system and cross the blood–brain barrier, affecting the satiety centre. Large tumours produce more of these factors, resulting in the cachexia observed in patients with advanced cancer. In addition, radiation treatments to the head and neck and the GI system exacerbate eating difficulties. Anorexia peaks at about 4 weeks of treatment and seems to resolve more quickly than fatigue when treatment ends.

Patients with anorexia need to be monitored carefully during treatment to ensure that weight loss does not become excessive. Body weight should be measured at least twice weekly. Small, frequent meals of high-protein, high-calorie foods are better tolerated than large meals (see the Resources at the end of this chapter). Nutritional supplements may be required.

BONE MARROW SUPPRESSION. Myelosuppression is a common and significant effect of many chemotherapeutic modalities and may also occur with radiotherapy. Chemotherapy is a systemic treatment with the ability to affect every vulnerable cell in the body, whereas radiotherapy is delivered locally, so that only the cells within the treatment field are affected. Concurrent chemotherapy and irradiation generally increase the risk of toxic effects on the bone marrow. The onset of bone marrow suppression is related to the lifespan of the blood cell type. WBCs are affected within 1 week, platelets in 2 to 3 weeks, and red blood cells (RBCs) in 2 to 3 months. The severity of myelosuppression is related to the type and the dose of chemotherapeutic medication or the specific radiation field and to the extent of bone marrow reserves. In an adult, about 40% of active marrow is in the pelvis, and 25% is in the thoracic and lumbar vertebrae.

Blood cell counts (including WBCs, neutrophils, RBCs, and platelets) must be closely monitored. Neutropenia is most common in patients receiving chemotherapy and puts them at risk for serious infections or sepsis. WBC growth factors may be used to stimulate regeneration of adequate numbers of leukocytes and prevent treatment delays. Thrombocytopenia may cause spontaneous bleeding or hemorrhage and may necessitate a platelet transfusion if counts fall below 20×10^9/L. If anemia occurs and the hemoglobin level drops below 100 g/L, the patient may require blood transfusions.

The novel coronavirus (SARS-CoV-2) pandemic created an international public health crisis in 2020 with particular repercussions for cancer patients. Immunocompromised status due to underlying malignancy and cancer treatments poses a significantly greater risk for the development of SARS-CoV-2 infection and worse outcomes for those infected. Access to diagnostics, treatment, and supportive care was significantly reduced in efforts to control the spread of SARS-CoV-2, leading to greater anxiety and distress for patients with cancer and their families and to exacerbation of social isolation. Recommendations for cancer care during pandemics are being generated and may include guidelines for optimal triage of patients for cancer treatment and supportive services (Al-Shamsi et al., 2020).

SKIN REACTIONS. Like the bone marrow, the skin cells are rapidly proliferating and are therefore vulnerable to the effects of radiation and chemotherapy. Both acute and chronic changes can occur in the skin within the radiation field. The skin-sparing property of modern radiation equipment limits the severity of these reactions. Although the skin reaction begins as early as the first treatment, it is initially transitory. Erythema may develop 1 to 24 hours after a single treatment. Erythema is an acute response followed by dry desquamation (Figure 18.15). If the rate of cellular sloughing is faster than the ability of the new epidermal cells to replace dead cells, a wet desquamation occurs, with exposure of the dermis and oozing of serum (Figure 18.16). Skin reactions are particularly evident in areas subjected to pressure, such as behind the ear and in gluteal folds, the perineum, the breast, the collar line, and bony prominences.

Although skin care policies vary among institutions, they are founded on basic skin care principles. Dry reactions are uncomfortable and result in pruritus. Wet reactions result in discomfort and drainage. Dry skin should be lubricated with a lotion or solution that contains no metal, alcohol, perfume, or additives that would irritate the skin. Wet reactions must be kept clean and protected from further damage. Prevention of infection and facilitation of wound healing are the therapeutic goals.

Irradiated skin should be protected from extremes of temperature to prevent trauma. Heating pads, ice packs, and hot water bottles cannot be used in the treatment field. Constricting garments, rubbing, harsh chemicals, and deodorants may also traumatize the skin and should be avoided. The use of corticosteroids and hydrogen peroxide is controversial because of their interference with wound healing. The guidelines presented in

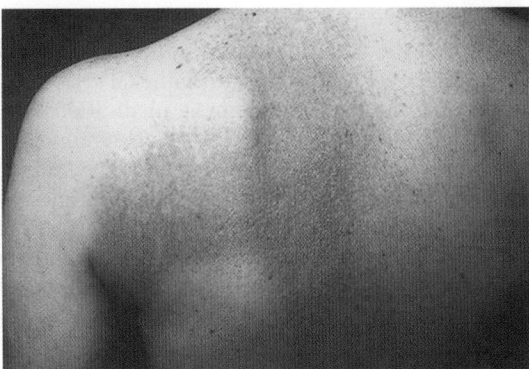

FIG. 18.15 Dry desquamation.

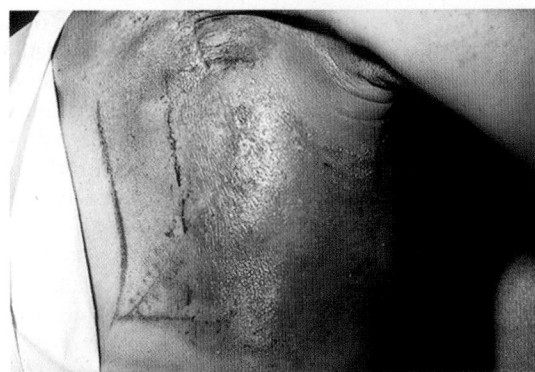

FIG. 18.16 Wet desquamation.

TABLE 18.15	PATIENT & CAREGIVER TEACHING GUIDE

Radiation Skin Reactions

Patient and caregiver teaching for radiation skin reactions should include the following:

1. Gently cleanse the skin in the treatment field with a mild soap (Ivory, Dove), tepid water, and a soft cloth. Rinse thoroughly and gently pat dry.
2. Apply nonmedicated, nonperfumed, moisturizing lotion or creams, such as baby lotion, oil, aloe gel or cream to alleviate dry skin. This substance must be gently cleansed from the treatment field before each treatment and reapplied after. (Note: Care differs from institution to institution.)
3. Rinse the area with saline solution. Expose the area to air as often as possible. If copious drainage is present, nonadhesive absorbent dressings are warranted, and they must be changed as soon as they become wet. Observe the area daily for signs of infection.
4. Avoid wearing tight-fitting clothing such as brassieres, girdles, and belts over the treatment field.
5. Avoid wearing harsh fabrics, such as wool and corduroy. A lightweight cotton garment is best. If possible, expose the treatment field to air.
6. Use gentle detergents such as Ivory Snow to wash clothing that will come in contact with the treatment field.
7. Avoid direct exposure to the sun. If the treatment field is in an area that is exposed to the sun, wear protective clothing such as a wide-brimmed hat during exposure to the sun. (Note: In general, people should avoid sun exposure regardless of whether they are in treatment or not; use of protective clothing and sunscreen on exposed areas should be recommended.)
8. Prevent application of heat from all sources (hot water bottles, heating pads, and sun lamps) on the treatment field.
9. Avoid exposing the treatment area to cold temperatures (ice bags or cold weather).
10. Avoid swimming in salt water or in chlorinated pools during the time of treatment.
11. Avoid the use of all medication, deodorants, perfumes, powders, or cosmetics on the skin in the treatment field. Tape, dressings, and adhesive bandages should also be avoided unless permitted by the radiation therapist. Avoid shaving the hair in the treatment field.
12. Continue to protect sensitive skin after the treatment is completed by doing the following:
    a. Continue to avoid direct exposure to the sun. A sunscreen agent and protective clothing must be worn if there is potential for exposure to the sun.
    b. If shaving is necessary in the treatment field, use an electric razor.

Table 18.15 can be used for managing skin radiation reactions, though they are not intended to replace policies developed by the cancer agency or hospital program.

Alopecia (hair loss) is restricted to the radiation field when caused by radiotherapy but affects all body hair (including eyelashes and eyebrows) when caused by chemotherapeutic agents. For some patients, hair loss causes profound distress. Chemotherapy-induced alopecia is temporary; hair regrowth begins 3 to 4 weeks after therapy is terminated. Radiotherapy-induced hair loss may be temporary or permanent, depending on the dose administered. Patients may be directed to the Canadian Cancer Society's "Look Good, Feel Better" program for support and advice about wigs and head coverings (see the Resources at the end of this chapter).

ORAL, OROPHARYNGEAL, AND ESOPHAGEAL REACTIONS. The mucosal lining of the GI tract is sensitive to the effects of radiation therapy and to certain antineoplastic medications, especially 5-fluorouracil. As a result, nutritional status may be compromised by treatment. Salivary flow often decreases, with resultant xerostomia (dry mouth), during radiotherapy to the head and neck. Food must be dissolved in saliva to be tasted. Taste loss is progressive during therapy, and by the end of treatment, many patients report that all food has lost its flavour. Thick saliva is less able to perform the functions of cleansing teeth and moistening food. Difficulty swallowing, which characterizes esophageal reactions, further impedes eating. Patients report feeling that they have a "lump" as they swallow and that "foods get stuck."

Meticulous oral assessment and prompt intervention are essential to prevent infection and facilitate nutritional intake. Oral care includes pretreatment evaluation by a dentist to perform all necessary dental work before the initiation of treatment. The patient must be taught to examine the mouth and gums daily. Mucous membranes, characteristics of saliva, and ability to swallow must be assessed regularly. The patient should also be taught how to perform oral care at least before and after each meal and at bedtime. A saline solution of 1 teaspoon of salt in 1 L of water is an effective cleansing agent. One teaspoon of sodium bicarbonate may be added to the oral care solution to decrease odour, alleviate pain, and dissolve mucin. Tooth brushing and flossing are critical unless contraindicated by decreased platelet counts. Adherence to this protocol significantly reduces the risk of radiation caries, which develop as a result of loss of saliva. Saliva substitutes are available and may be offered to patients, although many patients find that drinking small amounts of water frequently has an equivalent effect.

Mouthwashes containing corticosteroids, diphenhydramine (Benadryl), and lidocaine (Xylocaine Viscous) are used as a component of oral care. The solutions may be swallowed to alleviate esophagitis. Coating solutions must not be allowed to build up on the mucosa, where they could serve as a medium for infection. Infection, particularly with *Candida albicans,* can occur in individuals receiving head and neck radiation, and its incidence increases dramatically in protocols involving concomitant chemotherapy. Antifungal agents may be prescribed to treat the infection. Alleviation of mucositis may be achieved through the use of coating and analgesic compounds. The use of chlorhexidine and colony-stimulating factor mouthwash is not recommended (Chaveli-Lopez, 2016). Feedings of soft, nonirritating high-protein and high-calorie foods should be offered frequently throughout the day. Extremes of temperature, as well as use of tobacco and alcohol, should be avoided. Nutritional supplements (e.g., Ensure) as an adjunct to meals and fluid intake may be encouraged. Weight should be monitored closely.

Families are an integral part of the health care team. As taste loss increases, the family's role in assisting the patient to eat becomes increasingly critical. If family members are not available, alternative support, such as visits by volunteers and home aides, is indicated.

PULMONARY EFFECTS. Pulmonary effects of cancer therapies may be irreversible and progressive. The effects of radiation on the lung include both acute and late reactions. Radiation doses in the lung are magnified because the dose cannot be reduced through tissue. Pneumonitis can be an acute inflammatory reaction related to radiation. This reaction is often asymptomatic, although cough, fever, and night sweats may increase. Treatment with bronchodilators, expectorants, bed rest, and oxygen is preferable to treatment with corticosteroids.

The most common pulmonary toxic effects associated with chemotherapy include pulmonary edema, interstitial fibrosis, and pneumonitis. The chemotherapeutic agents most strongly associated with these complications include bleomycin, busulfan, carmustine (Bicnu), cyclophosphamide (Procytox), and some targeted agents (e.g., gefitinib [Iressa]). The pulmonary effects of treatments may be difficult to distinguish from those related to the disease and can be frightening to patients because they may involve an exacerbation of the symptoms that precipitated the cancer diagnosis. Cough and dyspnea may increase. The cough becomes more productive because alveoli that had been blocked are opened as the tumour responds to treatment. As treatment continues, the cough can become dry as the mucosa begins to be altered by the radiation. Cough suppressants may be indicated for use at night.

Oxygen, if prescribed for symptomatic pneumonitis, must be used judiciously if a patient has chronic obstructive pulmonary disease (see Chapter 31). Oxygen therapy in such patients can cause carbon dioxide retention and respiratory acidosis and may be lethal. If a patient experiences dyspnea, anxiety may be pronounced. Lying flat on the radiation treatment table and being alone in the room may potentiate anxiety.

GASTROINTESTINAL EFFECTS. The mucosa of the GI tract is highly proliferative: Surface cells are replaced every 2 to 6 days, thus they are highly vulnerable to cancer therapies. The intestinal mucosa is one of the most radiosensitive tissues. Radiation alters gastric secretion by direct injury to cells. The secretion of mucus, hydrochloric acid, and pepsin decreases with further treatment. Nausea, vomiting, and diarrhea are early responses to irradiation of the GI tissue and may occur immediately after the first treatment. The occurrence of these symptoms in response to cancer therapies may be related to the release of serotonin

from the GI tract, which then stimulates the chemoreceptor trigger zone and the vomiting centre in the brain. Further GI irritation is related to direct injury to epithelial cells.

An increasing number of antiemetic medications are available (see Chapter 44 and Table 44.1). Metoclopramide, ondansetron (Zofran), granisetron (Kytril), aprepitant (Emend), and dexamethasone have been used to decrease nausea and vomiting caused by chemotherapy. The introduction of antiemetic clinical practice guidelines facilitates the implementation of methods to manage this undesirable effect of treatment. Administration of antiemetics before treatment prevents or alleviates nausea and vomiting. Patients may find that eating a light meal of nonirritating food before treatment is also helpful. *Anticipatory nausea and vomiting* may develop in patients receiving radiation or chemotherapy when these symptoms are poorly controlled. This conditioned response results in the experience of nausea and vomiting when a patient encounters cues associated with the treatment—for example, walking through the doors of the cancer centre or merely seeing the oncologist, even outside of the treatment centre. In some individuals, this response persists after treatment ends. Aggressive emesis control, including the use of prophylactic antiemetics and antianxiety agents, is recommended.

Patients experiencing nausea and vomiting must be assessed for signs and symptoms of dehydration and alkalosis. Fluid intake is recorded to ensure that the volume consumed and retained is adequate. Diarrhea may be a reaction of the bowel mucosa to radiation. The small bowel is extremely sensitive and does not tolerate significant radiation doses. Administering treatments when a patient has a full bladder may serve to move the small bowel out of the treatment field. Nonirritating diets and low-residue diets, as well as antidiarrheal and antispasmodic medications, are recommended. Lukewarm sitz baths may alleviate discomfort and cleanse the rectal area. The rectal area must be kept scrupulously clean and dry to maintain mucosal integrity. The nurse should inspect the perianal area. Number, volume, consistency, and character of stools per day should be recorded by patients, as should any potentially aggravating or alleviating factors related to bowel movements. Adequate food and fluid intake promote healing and mucosal integrity. Systemic analgesia is warranted for the painful skin irritations that may develop.

REPRODUCTIVE EFFECTS. The effects of radiation and chemotherapy on the ovary and testes are determined by the dose delivered and the type of chemotherapy used. The testes are highly sensitive to radiation, and the testicles are protected whenever possible. Doses of 15 to 30 cGy temporarily decrease the sperm count; aspermia results at 35 to 230 cGy. In some cases, 200 cGy may result in permanent aspermia. In patients receiving 300 to 600 cGy, the sperm count either recovers in 2 to 5 years or does not recover at all. Pretreatment status may be a significant factor because a low sperm count and loss of motility are seen in individuals with testicular cancer and Hodgkin's disease before any therapy. Combined modality treatment or prior chemotherapy with alkylating agents enhances and prolongs the effects of radiation on the testes. When radiation is used alone with conventional doses and appropriate shielding, testicular recovery often occurs. Compromised reproductive function in men may also result from erectile dysfunction after pelvic irradiation and its related vascular and neurological effects.

The radiation dose necessary to induce ovarian failure changes with age. Permanent cessation of menses occurs at 500 to 1 000 cGy in 95% of women younger than 40 years, and at 375 cGy, the percentage is higher in women older than 40 years. Unlike the testes, the ovaries have no avenue for repair; therefore, the ovaries are shielded whenever possible. Other factors that influence reproductive or sexual functioning in women include reactions in the cervix and endometrium. These tissues withstand a high radiation dose with minimal sequelae, which accounts for the ability to treat endometrial and cervical cancer with high external and brachytherapeutic doses. Acute reactions such as tenderness, irritation, and loss of lubrication compromise sexual activity. Late effects of combined internal and external therapy include loss of elasticity, loss of lubrication, and vaginal shortening related to fibrosis. Supportive nursing care during brachytherapy for gynecological cancer is critical to the well-being and psychological functioning of women experiencing this treatment; the patient and the patient's partner require information about the expected effects of treatment on reproductive and sexual issues. Potential infertility can be a significant consequence for the individual, and counselling is indicated. Pretreatment harvesting of sperm or ova may be considered. Specific suggestions to manage adverse effects that have an effect on sexual functioning include use of a water-soluble vaginal lubricant and a vaginal dilator after pelvic irradiation. The nurse needs to be competent in discussing issues related to sexuality, offering specific suggestions and making referrals for ongoing counselling when indicated.

LATE EFFECTS OF RADIATION TREATMENT AND CHEMOTHERAPY

Cancer survivors are achieving higher rates of long-term remission and survival because of advancements in treatment modalities. However, these forms of therapy (especially radiation treatment and chemotherapy) may produce long-term sequelae termed *physiological late effects* that occur months to years after cessation of therapy. Every body system can be affected to some extent by chemotherapy and radiation therapy. The effects of radiation on the body's tissues are caused by cellular hypoplasia of stem cells and alterations in the fine vasculature and fibroconnective tissues. In addition to the acute toxic effects, chemotherapy can have long-term effects related to the loss of cells' proliferative reserve capacity. The additive effects of multiagent chemotherapy before, during, or after a course of radiotherapy can significantly increase the risks of physiological late effects.

Cancer survivors may also be at risk for leukemias and other secondary malignancies resulting from therapy for the primary cancer. However, the potential risk for developing a second malignancy does not contraindicate the use of cancer treatment. The overall risk of developing neoplastic complications is low and the latency period may be long.

The cancer treatments most frequently implicated in causing secondary malignancy are the alkylating chemotherapeutic agents and high-dose radiation, which can induce cancers at the exposure site. The exact mechanism of oncogenesis secondary to irradiation and chemotherapy remains unclear. It could be related to interactions between immunosuppressive factors, direct cellular damage, and carcinogenic effects, along with other environmental carcinogens.

Acute leukemias occurring as secondary malignancies have been most widely reported after treatment for Hodgkin's disease, but they also occur in survivors of ovarian, lung, and breast cancers. Secondary malignancies other than leukemias include multiple myeloma after radiation therapy for breast cancer; non-Hodgkin's lymphoma after treatment for Hodgkin's disease; and cancers of the bladder, the kidney, and the ureters after the use of cyclophosphamide. Radiation therapy for breast, lung, ovarian, uterine, and thyroid cancers, for non-Hodgkin's lymphoma, and for Hodgkin's disease has been linked to secondary osteosarcoma of the rib, scapula, clavicle, humerus, sternum, ilium, and pelvis. Fibrosarcomas have been reported several years after radiation therapy for malignant glioma and pituitary adenoma. Unfortunately, secondary malignancies are usually resistant to therapy, but supportive care and palliative care are options for the patient.

BIOLOGICAL AND TARGETED THERAPY

Biological therapy is treatment involving the use of biological agents such as interferons, interleukins, monoclonal antibodies, and growth factors to modify the relationship between the host and the tumour. Biological agents are assuming a larger role in cancer treatment, either alone or in combination with surgery, radiation therapy, and chemotherapy. An understanding of the principles of cellular interaction underlies the development of agents that modify the relationship between the host and the tumour by altering the biological response of the host to the tumour cells. Biological agents may affect host–tumour response in three ways: (1) They have direct antitumour effects; (2) they restore, augment, or modulate host immune system mechanisms; and (3) they have other biological effects, such as interfering with the cancer cells' ability to metastasize or differentiate (Table 18.16; Figure 18.17).

Tumour cells express tumour antigens on their surfaces that can be recognized and destroyed by the body's immune cells. Cytokines are glycoprotein products of immune cells, such as lymphocytes and macrophages, and are capable of defence functions. Cytokines include interferons, interleukins, colony-stimulating factors, and TNF. Interferons were the first type of cytokine to be studied as a cancer therapy. Interferons protect cells infected by viruses from attack by other viruses and inhibit replication of viral DNA. The antiproliferative effects of interferons are not completely understood. However, they have been shown to inhibit DNA and protein synthesis in some tumour cells and to stimulate the expression of tumour antigens on tumour cell surfaces. Because the interferons have antiviral and antitumour effects, they are used to treat a number of medical conditions, including hepatitis C and Kaposi's sarcoma. The severity of adverse effects of interferons depends on the dose and the route of administration. One of the most common adverse effects is flulike syndrome, which includes fever, chills, myalgia, and headache. Targeted therapy interferes with cancer growth by targeting specific cellular receptors and pathways that are important for tumour growth. The targeted therapies are more selective for specific molecular targets than are cancer medications and are thus able to kill cancer cells without damaging normal cells. Targeted therapies include tyrosine kinase inhibitors, monoclonal antibodies, antiangiogenic agents such as VEGF receptor inhibitors, and interleukins.

Tyrosine kinases are important enzymes that activate the signalling pathways regulating cell proliferation and survival. For example, epidermal growth factor receptor (EGFR) is expressed in cells of epithelial origin, which rely on these receptors for repair and maintenance. EGFR is overexpressed in a wide variety of tumours, including non–small cell lung cancer, head and

TABLE 18.16   MEDICATION THERAPY

Biological and Targeted Therapy

Medication	Mechanism of Action	Indications	Adverse Effects
Cytokines and Immunomodulators			
Interferon alfa-2b (Intron A)	Inhibits DNA and protein synthesis Suppresses cell proliferation Increases cytotoxic effects of NK cells	Hairy cell leukemia, chronic myelogenous leukemia, malignant melanoma, renal cell carcinoma, non-Hodgkin's lymphoma, ovarian cancer, multiple myeloma, Kaposi's sarcoma, pancreatic carcinoma	Flulike syndrome (fever, chills, myalgia, headache), cognitive changes, fatigue, nausea, vomiting, anorexia, weight loss
Interleukin-2 (aldesleukin [Proleukin])	Stimulates proliferation of T and B cells Activates NK cells	Metastatic renal cell cancer, metastatic melanoma	Same as those of interferon alfa-2b; capillary leak syndrome, resulting in hypotension; bone marrow suppression
Levamisole	Potentiates monocytes and macrophage function	Stage III colon cancer (given in combination with 5-fluorouracil)	Diarrhea, metallic taste, nausea, fever, chills, mouth sores, headache
Bacille Calmette-Guérin vaccine	Induces an immune response that prevents angiogenesis of tumour	In situ bladder cancer	Flulike syndrome, nausea, vomiting, rash, cough
Tyrosine Kinase Inhibitors			
Cetuximab (Erbitux)	Inhibits epidermal growth factor receptor, which is coupled with tyrosine kinase	Colorectal cancer, in combination with radiotherapy for head and neck carcinoma	Rash, dry skin, infusion reactions, interstitial lung disease, fatigue, fever
Erlotinib (Tarceva) and gefitinib (Iressa)	Same as for cetuximab	Non–small cell lung cancer	Rash, diarrhea, interstitial lung disease
Imatinib (Gleevec)	Inhibits Bcr-Abl tyrosine kinase	Chronic myeloid leukemia	Nausea, diarrhea, myalgia, fluid retention
Sorafenib (Nexavar)	Inhibits several tyrosine kinases, some of which are involved in angiogenesis	Advanced renal cell carcinoma	Rash, diarrhea, hypertension; redness, pain, swelling, or blisters on hands and feet
Monoclonal Antibody to CD20			
Rituximab (Rituxan)	Binds CD20 antigen, causing cytotoxicity	Non-Hodgkin's lymphoma (B cell)	Fever, chills, nausea, headache, angioedema
Ibritumomab tiuxetan–yttrium-90 (Zevalin)	Binds CD20 antigen, causing cytotoxicity and radiation injury	Non-Hodgkin's lymphoma (B cell)	Bone marrow suppression, fatigue, nausea, chills
Angiogenesis Inhibitor			
Bevacizumab (Avastin)	Binds vascular endothelial growth factor, thereby inhibiting angiogenesis	Colorectal cancer	Hypertension, colon bleeding and perforation, impaired wound healing, thromboembolism, diarrhea
Proteosome Inhibitor			
Bortezomib (Velcade)	Inhibits proteasome activity, which functions to regulate cell growth	Multiple myeloma	Bone marrow suppression, nausea, vomiting, diarrhea, peripheral neuropathy, fatigue
Monoclonal Antibodies			
Gemtuzumab ozogamicin (Mylotarg)	Binds CD33 antigen (expressed on leukemic cells) to deliver cytotoxic medication into the DNA	Acute myeloid leukemia	Bone marrow suppression, fever, chills, nausea
Alemtuzumab (Campath)	Binds CD52 antigen (found on T and B cells, monocytes, NK cells, neutrophils)	Chronic lymphocytic leukemia (B cell)	Bone marrow suppression, chills, fever, vomiting, diarrhea, fatigue
Trastuzumab (Herceptin)	Binds HER2	Breast cancer (HER2 positive)	Cardiotoxicity

HER2, human epidermal growth factor receptor 2; *NK,* natural killer.

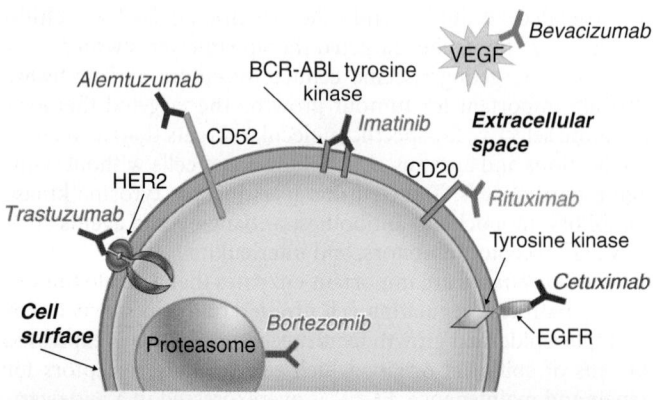

FIG. 18.17 Sites of action of targeted therapy. *EGFR,* epidermal growth factor receptor; *HER2,* human epidermal growth factor receptor 2; *VEGF,* vascular endothelial growth factor.

neck cancers, and pancreatic tumours and gliomas. Overexpression of EGFR is correlated with poor prognosis, increased recurrence rates, and resistance to chemotherapy. As such, it is an appealing target for cancer therapy. Erlotinib (Tarceva) and gefitinib (Iressa) are examples of EGFR tyrosine kinase inhibitors used in the treatment of non–small cell lung cancer.

Produced by B lymphocytes, *monoclonal antibodies* are proteins made by the immune system that bind to a specific target on the surface of tumour cells. Monoclonal antibodies can be unconjugated or conjugated. Unconjugated monoclonal antibodies are used alone to attack tumour cells directly. Conjugated monoclonal antibodies are attached to agents such as radioisotopes, toxins, chemotherapeutic agents, and other biological agents. The goal of this approach is to deliver the monoclonal antibody complex directly to the targeted cancer cells for their ultimate destruction. The antibodies also may stimulate an immune response in patients. Hybridoma technology for the production of monoclonal antibodies is described in Chapter 16.

The first monoclonal antibody approved for use in oncological treatment was rituximab (Rituxan), an unconjugated monoclonal antibody directed against the CD20 antigen found on the surface of B lymphocytes. Human epidermal growth factor receptor 2 (HER2) is overexpressed in certain cancers (especially breast cancer) and is associated with more aggressive disease and decreased rates of survival. Trastuzumab (Herceptin) is an unconjugated monoclonal antibody that binds to HER2 and inhibits the growth of breast cancer cells that express the HER2 protein.

The most common type of conjugated monoclonal antibody is an *immunotoxin*, a molecule formed when a monoclonal antibody is conjugated to a plant or bacterial cell toxin. The most frequently used bacterial toxins to date have been *Pseudomonas* exotoxin and diphtheria toxin. Unfortunately, immunotoxins have shown poor clinical efficacy thus far and are associated with significant toxic effects.

Monoclonal antibodies are administered by infusion. Patients may experience infusion-related symptoms, which can include fever, chills, urticaria, mucosal congestion, nausea, diarrhea, and myalgias. There is also a risk, although rare, of anaphylaxis associated with the administration of monoclonal antibodies. This potential exists because most monoclonal antibodies are produced by mouse lymphocytes and thus represent a foreign protein to the human body. Onset of anaphylaxis can occur within 5 minutes of administration and can be a life-threatening event. (See Chapter 16 for a discussion of nursing management of anaphylaxis.) Other toxic effects of monoclonal antibodies may include hepatotoxicity, bone marrow depression, and CNS effects. Patients who receive trastuzumab may also experience cardiac dysfunction, especially when it is administered in higher doses or in combination with anthracycline antibiotics such as doxorubicin (Adriamycin).

Checkpoint inhibitors are a class of antibodies that target the normal inhibitory immune mechanisms that allow physiological homeostasis. These normal mechanisms may be exploited by tumour cells to elude destruction. PD-1 is a protein on T cells and PD-L1 is a receptor in tumour cells. The interaction between PD-1 and PD-L1 stops the T cell from killing the cancer cell. Blocking either one with antibodies will disrupt the "off" signal and allow the T cell to kill the cancer cell. Nivolumab and pembrolizumab, which target PD-1, and atezolizumab and avelumab, which target PD-L1, are used to treat a number of cancers including lung cancer, melanoma and renal cell carcinoma. Adverse effects are due to a heightened immune response that can attack any tissue and cause symptoms, most commonly diarrhea, pneumonitis, skin rashes, endocrine abnormalities and neuropathy.

Angiogenesis inhibitors work by preventing the mechanisms and pathways necessary for the vascularization of tumours. Bevacizumab (Avastin), a recombinant human monoclonal antibody, is active against the VEGF molecule, a crucial regulator of normal and pathological angiogenesis. Adverse effects of bevacizumab include hypertension, hemorrhage, and thromboembolic events. Its use is indicated in the treatment of colorectal cancer, and trials are being conducted to treat a number of other cancers.

Interleukins are a family of cytokines that act primarily between lymphocytes to induce activation of the immune system or alteration in the functional capacity of tumour cells. To date, 29 interleukins have been discovered, and each is designated by number, but only IL-2 has been approved as an anticancer agent. Aldesleukin (Proleukin) is a recombinant form of IL-2 used in the treatment of metastatic renal cell carcinoma, acute myelogenous leukemia, and lymphoma.

A major toxic effect of IL-2 therapy is capillary leak syndrome, which occurs as a result of changes in capillary permeability and vascular tone. As a consequence of the increase in capillary permeability, fluids shift from intravascular to extravascular compartments. This causes intravascular fluid depletion. Manifestations of capillary leak syndrome include hypotension, peripheral edema, ascites, interstitial pulmonary infiltrates, weight gain, and decreased systemic vascular resistance. Additional toxic effects of IL-2 therapy include renal, cardiovascular, pulmonary, GI, and integumentary toxic effects; bone marrow suppression; and changes in cognitive function. (Note: Provincial and territorial care programs and medication benefits programs may vary; the nurse should consult facility-specific information.)

Hematopoietic Growth Factors

Colony-Stimulating Factors. Colony-stimulating factors are a family of glycoproteins produced by various cells. These glycoproteins stimulate production, maturation, regulation, and activation of cells of the hematological system. After release, colony-stimulating factors attach to receptors on the cell surface of peripheral blood cells and hematopoietic precursors (precursors of mature blood cells). They then stimulate production, maturation, release from the bone marrow, and functional ability of blood cells. The name of the colony-stimulating factor is based on the specific cell line it affects: granulocyte colony–stimulating factor (G-CSF), granulocyte-macrophage colony–stimulating factor (GM-CSF), macrophage colony–stimulating factor (M-CSF), and multicolony-stimulating factor, also known as *interleukin-3* (IL-3).

Colony-stimulating factors have a number of potential clinical uses. They may hasten recovery from bone marrow depression after standard and high-dose chemotherapy and bone marrow transplantation or decrease bone marrow suppression associated with administration of chemotherapeutic agents. Colony-stimulating factors may also re-establish bone marrow function in aplastic anemia, myelodysplastic syndrome, and leukemia and may be effective in the management of sepsis.

G-CSF is available as filgrastim (Neupogen) for the treatment of neutropenia. Pegfilgrastim (Neulasta) is a longer-acting form of filgrastim. G-CSF stimulates the production and function of neutrophils. It can be administered subcutaneously or by intravenous infusion. The most commonly reported adverse effect of G-CSF therapy is medullary bone pain, which occurs most often in the lower back, the pelvis, and the sternum. This pain generally develops at the time the neutrophil count begins to recover and lasts for about 24 hours. The pain associated with G-CSF therapy is usually relieved with nonopioid analgesics.

GM-CSF is available as sargramostim (Leukine, Prokine) for the treatment of (a) neutropenia associated with bone marrow transplantation, (b) bone marrow transplant failure or delay in bone marrow engraftment, and (c) acute myelogenous leukemia after chemotherapy. GM-CSF stimulates the production and function of neutrophils, eosinophils, and monocytes. In addition, GM-CSF stimulates these cells to produce cytokines. GM-CSF can be administered either subcutaneously or by intravenous infusion. The most common adverse effects associated with GM-CSF administration include medullary bone pain (similar to the bone pain associated with G-CSF administration), leukocytosis, and eosinophilia.

IL-3 is a multipotential stimulator of hematopoietic stem cells. IL-3 has been shown to stimulate the growth of neutrophils, monocytes, eosinophils, basophils, and platelet cell lines. IL-3 is being investigated for the treatment of bone marrow failure and for its ability to enhance myeloid recovery after chemotherapy, radiotherapy, and bone marrow transplantation. M-CSF is also undergoing investigation for its potential role in cancer treatment.

Erythropoietin. Erythropoietin is a colony-stimulating factor responsible for stimulating growth of the erythroid precursor cells that ultimately mature into RBCs. Erythropoietin is produced naturally by the kidneys. Erythropoietin was initially approved for the management of chronic anemia associated with end-stage renal disease. Subsequently, approval was expanded to include the use of erythropoietin (Eprex) for the management of chemotherapy-related anemia. Darbepoetin alfa (Aranesp), a long-acting form of erythropoietin, is now available.

Toxic and Adverse Effects of Biological Agents

The administration of one biological agent usually induces the endogenous release of others. The release and action of these biological agents result in systemic immune and inflammatory responses. The toxic effects and adverse effects of biological agents are related to dose and schedule. Common adverse effects, especially with interferons, include constitutional flulike symptoms such as headache, fever, chills, myalgias, fatigue, malaise, weakness, photosensitivity, anorexia, and nausea. The severity of the flulike symptoms associated with interferon therapy generally decreases over time. Acetaminophen administered every 4 hours, as prescribed, often reduces the severity of the flulike syndrome. Many patients undergoing treatment with biological agents receive premedication with acetaminophen in an attempt to prevent or decrease the intensity of these symptoms. In addition, large amounts of fluids help decrease the intensity of symptoms.

Tachycardia and orthostatic hypotension are also commonly reported. IL-2 and monoclonal antibodies can cause capillary leak syndrome, with resulting pulmonary edema. Other toxic and adverse effects may involve the CNS and the renal, hepatic, and cardiovascular systems. These effects are found particularly with interferons and IL-2.

NURSING MANAGEMENT
BIOLOGICAL THERAPY

Adverse effects experienced by patients receiving biological therapy may differ in type or severity from those observed with more traditional forms of cancer therapy. For example, capillary leak syndrome and pulmonary edema are conditions that necessitate expertise in critical care nursing. Bone marrow depression occurring with administration of biological agents is generally more transient and milder than that observed with chemotherapy, but fatigue associated with biological therapy can be so severe that it may constitute a dose-limiting toxic effect.

Nursing interventions for flulike syndrome include the administration of acetaminophen before treatment and every 4 hours after treatment. Intravenous meperidine (Demerol)

has been used to control the severe chills associated with some biological agents. Other nursing measures include monitoring of vital signs and temperature, planning for periods of rest for patients, and assisting with activities of daily living.

With interferon and IL-2 therapy, numerous neurological deficits have been observed. The nature and extent of these conditions have not been completely elucidated. However, these deficits can be frightening to patients and the family, who must be taught to observe for neurological issues (e.g., confusion, memory loss, difficulty making decisions, insomnia), report their occurrence, and institute appropriate safety and support measures. (Note: Provincial care programs and medication benefits programs may vary; the nurse should consult the employer's policies and formulary.)

BONE MARROW AND STEM CELL TRANSPLANTATION

Bone marrow transplantation (BMT) is an effective, life-saving procedure for patients with a number of malignant and nonmalignant diseases (Table 18.17). BMT allows for the safe use of very high doses of chemotherapeutic agents or radiation to patients whose tumours are resistant or unresponsive to standard doses of chemotherapeutic agents and radiation. BMT offers hope to many patients whose disease is responsive to increased doses of systemic therapy. The numbers of BMT and transplantation programs in Canada have increased dramatically since 2005.

Whether the diagnosis is a malignant or nonmalignant disease, the goal of BMT is cure. Cure rates are still low but are steadily increasing. Even if there is no cure, most transplantation procedures result in a period of remission. BMT is an intensive procedure with many risks, and some patients die from complications of BMT or from relapse of the original disease. Because it is a highly toxic therapy, patients must weigh the significant risks of treatment-related death or treatment failure (relapse) against the hope of cure.

Types of Bone Marrow Transplants

Bone marrow transplants can be allogeneic, autologous, or syngeneic. In *allogeneic marrow transplantation,* the infused bone marrow is acquired from a donor who has been matched to the recipient in terms of human leukocyte antigen (HLA) tissue typing. HLA typing involves testing WBCs to identify genetically inherited antigens common to both donor and recipient that are important in compatibility of transplanted tissue. (HLA tissue typing is discussed in Chapter 16.) The donor is often a

TABLE 18.17	USES FOR BONE MARROW TRANSPLANTATION	
Malignant Diseases	**Nonmalignant Diseases**
• Acute and chronic myelogenous leukemia	• Aplastic anemia
• Acute lymphocytic leukemia	• Immunodeficiency diseases
• Hodgkin's lymphoma	• Severe autoimmune diseases
• Multiple myeloma	• Sickle cell disease
• Myelodysplastic syndrome	• Thalassemia
• Neuroblastoma	
• Non-Hodgkin's lymphoma	
• Ovarian cancer	
• Sarcoma	
• Testicular cancer	

family member, but an unrelated donor may be found through a bone marrow registry. The goal is to administer large doses of systemic therapy and then "rescue" the bone marrow through the engraftment and subsequent normal proliferation and differentiation of the donated marrow in the recipient. The most common indication for allogeneic transplantation is leukemia.

In *autologous marrow transplantation,* patients receive their own bone marrow. The aim of this approach is to enable patients to receive intensive chemotherapy or radiation while supporting them with their own bone marrow. In this type of BMT, the patient's own marrow is removed, treated, stored, and reinfused.

A third type of BMT, *syngeneic marrow transplantation,* involves obtaining stem cells from one identical twin and infusing them into the other. Identical twins have identical HLA types and are a perfect match.

Procedures

Harvest Procedures. Bone marrow can be "harvested" through a procedure conducted in the operating room with the patient under general or spinal anaesthesia in which multiple bone marrow aspirations are carried out, usually from the iliac crest but also from the sternum. The entire harvesting procedure usually takes 1 to 2 hours, and the patient can be discharged after recovery. After the procedure, the donor may experience pain at the collection site, which can be treated with mild analgesics. The donor's body replaces the bone marrow in a few weeks.

After harvesting, autologous bone marrow may be treated *(purged)* to remove cancer cells. Many different pharmacological, immunological, physical, and chemical agents have been used for this purpose. The bone marrow is then frozen *(cryopreserved)* and stored until it is used for transplantation. In allogeneic transplantation, the marrow can be harvested, processed, and infused into the recipient within a few hours of donation.

Preparative Regimens. In malignant diseases, the goal of BMT is to rescue the marrow after the patient has received high doses of chemotherapeutic agents, with or without radiation, aimed at treating the underlying disease. After harvesting of the marrow, the patient is given high-dose chemotherapy with or without radiation therapy. Total body irradiation can be used for immunosuppression or to treat the disease.

After the therapy, the marrow that was removed is thawed and administered to the patient intravenously to replace the destroyed marrow. The stem cells reconstitute, or "rescue," the recipient's hematopoietic system. Usually 2 to 4 weeks are required for the transplanted marrow to start producing hematopoietic blood cells. During this pancytopenic period, it is critical for the patient to be in a protective isolation environment and receive supportive care. RBC and platelet transfusions are usually necessary to maintain the necessary quantity of circulating RBCs and platelets.

Complications. Bacterial, viral, and fungal infections are common after BMT. Prophylactic antibiotic therapy may reduce their incidence. A potentially serious complication of allogeneic transplant is graft-versus-host disease. This occurs when the T lymphocytes from the donated marrow (graft) respond to the recipient (host) cells as if they were foreign and begin to attack certain organs such as the skin, the liver, and the intestines. Graft-versus-host disease is discussed in Chapter 16. Another major adverse event is inadequate oral intake, which results in dehydration and malnutrition and thereby necessitates intensive nutritional support through a variety of interventions, such as oral supplementation and enteral feeding.

Peripheral Stem Cell Transplantation

An alternative to the harvest procedure is *peripheral stem cell transplantation* (PSCT). Peripheral (circulating) stem cells are capable of repopulating the bone marrow. PSCT is a type of transplantation that differs from BMT primarily in the method of stem cell collection. Because the blood contains fewer stem cells than does the bone marrow, stem cells from the bone marrow can be mobilized into the peripheral blood through chemotherapy or hematopoietic growth factors. Common growth factors that are used are GM-CSF and G-CSF. The donor's blood is collected, the peripheral stem cells are separated by means of a cell separator machine, and then the blood is returned through a venous line to the patient. This procedure is called *leukapheresis* and usually takes 2 to 4 hours to complete. In autologous transplantation, the stem cells are purged to kill any cancer cells and then frozen and stored until used for transplantation. Although many of the same steps (harvesting, intensive chemotherapy, reinfusion) of BMT are used in PSCT, the hematological recovery period in PSCT is shorter and produces fewer, less severe complications.

Cord Blood Stem Cells

Umbilical cord blood is rich in hematopoietic stem cells, and successful allogeneic transplantation has been performed with the use of this source. Cord blood can be HLA typed and cryopreserved. A disadvantage of cord blood is the possibly insufficient numbers of stem cells for transplantation into adults.

GENE THERAPY

Gene therapy involves the transfer of exogenous genes (transgenes) into the cells of patients in an effort to correct the defective gene. The effect of gene therapy for cancer can be a temporary gene transfer with the additional goal of instigating an immune response to the transgene. The use of this new therapeutic approach for cancer is currently investigational. Several clinical trials are under way to evaluate the safety, tolerability, and efficacy of gene therapy for malignancies such as melanoma, brain tumours, and mesothelioma. (Gene therapy is discussed in Chapter 15.)

COMPLICATIONS RESULTING FROM CANCER

Patients may develop complications related to the continual growth of the malignancy or the adverse effects of treatment.

Nutritional Problems

Malnutrition. Many patients with cancer experience protein and calorie malnutrition, characterized by depletion of fat and muscle. (Assessment of the degree of malnutrition is discussed in Chapter 42.) See the Resources at the end of this chapter for lists of foods suggested for increasing the protein intake to facilitate repair and regeneration of cells, high-caloric foods that provide energy and minimize weight loss, and a sample high-calorie, high-protein diet.

The nurse should suggest a referral to a dietitian as soon as a 5% weight loss is noted or if the patient has the potential for protein and caloric malnutrition. Albumin and prealbumin levels should be monitored. Once a 4.5-kg weight loss occurs, it is difficult to maintain optimal nutritional status. The patient can be taught to use nutritional supplements in place of milk when cooking or baking. Foods to which nutritional supplements can be easily added include scrambled eggs, pudding, custard, mashed potatoes, cereal, and cream sauces. Packages of instant breakfast can be used as indicated or sprinkled on cereals, desserts, and casseroles.

Malnutrition may occur as a result of the effects of cancer and cancer treatments. Patients may also radically alter their diets because of beliefs that certain foods support the growth or treatment of cancer. A discussion about the patient's dietary practices can facilitate mutual understanding and education.

If the malnutrition cannot be treated with dietary intake, it may be necessary to use enteral or parenteral supplementation as an adjunct nutritional measure. (Enteral and parenteral nutrition are discussed in Chapter 42.)

Altered Taste Sensation. It is theorized that cancer cells release substances that resemble amino acids and stimulate the bitter taste buds. Patients may also experience an alteration in the sweet, sour, and salty taste sensations. Meat may taste bitter to patients. The physiological basis of these taste alterations is unclear. It is important to help patients (a) understand the changes that will be experienced and (b) find foods that are appealing. Because many Canadians are from different cultural and ethnic groups, the nurse needs to be aware of possible differences in meal preparation and selection that are acceptable to patients. Patients can be encouraged to experiment with spices and other seasoning agents to taste in an attempt to mask the taste alterations.

Infection

Infection can cause death in a patient whose immune system is suppressed as a result of cancer treatment. The usual sites of infection include the lungs, genitourinary system, mouth, rectum, peritoneal cavity, and blood (septicemia). Infection occurs as a result of the ulceration and necrosis caused by the tumour, compression of vital organs by the tumour, and neutropenia caused by the disease process or the treatment of cancer. A critical aspect of nursing care is teaching about infection risk associated with neutropenia. A patient with a body temperature of 38°C (100.5°F) or higher should be seen at the hospital or cancer centre as soon as possible. Assessment most often includes signs and symptoms of fever, determination of possible cause, and complete blood cell count.

Many patients are neutropenic when an infection develops. In such individuals, infection causes significant morbidity and may be rapidly fatal if not treated promptly. The classical manifestations of infection are often not present in a patient with neutropenia and a depressed immune system. (Neutropenia is discussed in Chapter 33.)

Oncological Emergencies

Oncological emergencies are life-threatening events that can occur as a result of cancer or cancer treatment. These emergencies can be obstructive, metabolic, or infiltrative.

Obstructive Emergencies. Obstructive emergencies are caused primarily by tumour obstruction of an organ or a blood vessel. Obstructive emergencies include superior vena cava syndrome, spinal cord compression syndrome, third space syndrome, and intestinal obstruction.

Superior Vena Cava Syndrome. *Superior vena cava syndrome* results from obstruction of the superior vena cava by a tumour. The clinical manifestations include facial edema, periorbital edema, distension of veins of the neck and chest, headache, and seizures. A mediastinal mass is often visible on chest radiographs. The most common causes are Hodgkin's disease, non-Hodgkin's lymphoma, and lung cancer. Superior vena cava syndrome is considered a serious medical problem, and management usually involves radiation therapy to the site of obstruction and treatment of the primary tumour. Chemotherapeutic agents may be administered concurrently with the radiation therapy.

Spinal Cord Compression. *Spinal cord compression* is a neurological emergency caused by the presence of a malignant tumour in the epidural space of the spinal cord. The most common primary tumours that produce this condition are melanoma and cancers of the breast, lung, prostate, GI system, and kidneys. Lymphomas also pose a risk if diseased lymph tissue invades the epidural space. The manifestations are back pain that is intense, localized, and persistent, accompanied by vertebral tenderness and aggravated by the Valsalva manoeuvre; motor weakness and dysfunction; sensory paresthesia and loss; and autonomic dysfunction. One of the clinical symptoms that reflect autonomic dysfunction is a change in bowel or bladder function. The nurse should carefully assess for potential signs or symptoms related to cord compression. Radiation therapy is used for patients with slowly progressive neurological deficits and radiosensitive tumours. Surgery is usually recommended for patients with rapidly progressive neurological signs, especially if the tumours are relatively radiologically resistant.

Third Space Syndrome. *Third space syndrome* involves a shifting of fluid from the vascular space to the interstitial space that results primarily from extensive surgical procedures, biological therapy, or septic shock. Initially, affected patients exhibit signs of hypovolemia, including hypotension, tachycardia, low central venous pressure, and decreased urine output. Treatment includes fluid, electrolyte, and plasma protein replacement. During recovery, hypervolemia can occur, resulting in hypertension, elevated central venous pressure, weight gain, and shortness of breath. Treatment generally involves reduction in fluid administration and fluid balance monitoring.

Intestinal Obstruction. Intestinal obstruction occurs when partial or complete obstruction of the intestine prevents the passage of the intestinal contents through the GI tract. This can cause nausea, vomiting, abdominal pain, or even more serious conditions, such as bowel necrosis. It necessitates prompt treatment. Chapter 45 contains a complete discussion of intestinal obstruction.

Metabolic Emergencies. Metabolic emergencies are caused by the production of ectopic hormones directly from the tumour or are secondary to cancer treatment. Ectopic hormones can arise in tumours because their cells are less differentiated than normal cells, enabling re-expression of genes that are suppressed in normal development. Metabolic emergencies include syndrome of inappropriate antidiuretic hormone (SIADH), hypercalcemia, tumour lysis syndrome (TLS), septic shock, and disseminated intravascular coagulation.

Syndrome of Inappropriate Antidiuretic Hormone. SIADH results from abnormal or sustained production of antidiuretic hormone (see Chapter 51). SIADH occurs most frequently with carcinoma of the lung but can also occur with cancers of the pancreas, duodenum, brain, esophagus, colon, ovary, prostate, bronchus, and nasopharynx and with leukemia, mesothelioma, reticulum cell sarcoma, Hodgkin's disease, thymoma, and lymphosarcoma. Cancer cells in these tumours are actually able to manufacture, store, and release antidiuretic hormone. The chemotherapeutic agents vincristine and cyclophosphamide

(Procytox) also stimulate the release of antidiuretic hormone from the pituitary or tumour cells. Symptoms of SIADH include weight gain, weakness, anorexia, nausea, vomiting, personality changes, seizures, and coma. Treatment of SIADH includes fluid restriction and, in severe cases, intravenous administration of 3% sodium chloride solution.

Hypercalcemia. Hypercalcemia can occur in the presence of cancer that involves the bone, as in osteolytic metastases or multiple myeloma, or when a parathyroid hormone–like substance is secreted by cancer cells in the absence of bone metastasis (Mirrakhimov, 2015).

Hypercalcemia resulting from malignancies that have metastasized occurs most frequently in patients with lung, breast, kidney, colon, ovarian, or thyroid cancer. Hypercalcemia resulting from secretion of parathyroid hormone–like substance occurs most frequently in patients with hypernephromas; squamous cell carcinoma of the lung; head and neck, cervical, and esophageal cancers; lymphomas; and leukemia. Immobility and dehydration can contribute to or exacerbate hypercalcemia.

The primary manifestations of hypercalcemia include apathy, depression, fatigue, muscle weakness, electrocardiographic changes, polyuria and nocturia, anorexia, nausea, and vomiting. Serum levels of calcium in excess of 3 mmol/L can be life-threatening. Chronic hypercalcemia can result in nephrocalcinosis and irreversible renal failure. The long-term treatment of hypercalcemia is aimed at the primary disease. Acute hypercalcemia is treated by hydration (3 L/day), diuretic administration (particularly loop diuretics), and a bisphosphonate, a medication that inhibits the action of osteoclasts. Infusion of a bisphosphonate is the treatment of choice.

Tumour Lysis Syndrome. Acute TLS is a metabolic complication that occurs in some patients with cancer and is frequently triggered by chemotherapy. It results from the rapid destruction of a large number of tumour cells, which can cause fatal biochemical changes. TLS is often associated with tumours that have high growth rates and are sensitive to the effects of chemotherapy. If not identified and treated quickly, TLS can result in acute renal failure.

The four hallmark signs of TLS are hyperuricemia, hyperphosphatemia, hyperkalemia, and hypocalcemia. TLS usually occurs within the first 24 to 48 hours after the initiation of chemotherapy and may persist for approximately 5 to 7 days. The primary goal of TLS management is preventing renal failure and severe electrolyte imbalances. The primary treatment includes increasing urine production through hydration therapy, and medications to decrease uric acid levels (e.g., allopurinol) and break down uric acid for excretion (e.g., rasburicase) (Canadian Cancer Society, 2021b).

Septic Shock and Disseminated Intravascular Coagulation. Septic shock is discussed in Chapter 69, and disseminated intravascular coagulation is discussed in Chapter 33.

Infiltrative Emergencies. Infiltrative emergencies occur when malignant tumours infiltrate major organs secondary to cancer therapy. The most common infiltrative emergencies are cardiac tamponade and carotid artery rupture.

Cardiac Tamponade. Cardiac tamponade results from fluid accumulation in the pericardial sac, constriction of the pericardium by tumour, or pericarditis secondary to radiation therapy for the chest. Manifestations include a heavy feeling over the chest, shortness of breath, tachycardia, cough, dysphagia, hiccups, hoarseness, nausea, vomiting, excessive perspiration, decreased level of consciousness, pulsus paradoxus, distant or muted heart sounds, and extreme anxiety. Emergency management is aimed at reduction of fluid around the heart and includes surgical establishment of a pericardial window or an indwelling pericardial catheter. Supportive therapy includes administration of oxygen therapy, intravenous hydration, and vasopressor therapy.

Carotid Artery Rupture. Rupture of the carotid artery occurs most frequently in patients with cancer of the head and neck as a result of invasion of the arterial wall by tumour or erosion after surgery or radiation therapy. Bleeding can manifest as minor oozing or, in the case of a bursting of the artery, spurting of blood. In the presence of bursting, pressure should be applied to the site with a finger. Intravenous fluid and blood products are administered in an attempt to stabilize the patient for surgery. Surgical management involves ligation of the carotid artery above and below the rupture site and reduction of local tumour.

MANAGEMENT OF CANCER PAIN

Moderate to severe pain occurs in approximately 50% of patients receiving active treatment for cancer and in 80% of those with advanced cancer. Despite progress made in cancer therapies, the incidence of cancer-related pain has not changed in decades. Cancer pain is commonly undertreated for a number of reasons, and this has a profound effect on the patient's mood, functional status, and quality of life (Scarborough & Smith, 2018).

Inadequate pain assessment is a significant barrier to effective pain management. Data such as vital signs and patient behaviours are not reliable indicators of pain, especially long-standing, chronic pain. Therefore, it is essential that every patient with cancer be assessed for pain by the question "Do you have pain?" If the patient's self-report is affirmative, further data are obtained and documented initially and at regular intervals regarding the onset, location, and intensity of the pain, what it feels like, and how it is relieved. Patterns of change also should be assessed. The patient's pain report must be accepted as the primary source of assessment data. Medication therapy includes nonsteroidal anti-inflammatory medications, opioids, and adjuvant pain medications. Analgesic medications should be administered on a regular schedule, around the clock, with additional doses as needed for breakthrough pain. Oral administration of the medication is preferred. It is important to remember that with opioid medications, such as morphine, the appropriate dose is whatever is necessary to control the pain with the least intrusive adverse effects. Principles of patient-controlled analgesia should also be followed. Fear of addiction is not warranted but must be addressed as part of patient teaching relevant to pain control because, for both the patient and the nurse, it can represent a significant barrier to appropriate pain management.

Nonpharmacological interventions, including relaxation therapy and imagery, can be effectively used to manage pain (see Chapter 12). (Additional strategies to relieve pain are discussed in Chapter 10.) More information on cancer pain management is available from cancer agency clinical practice guidelines, such as those on the BC Cancer website (see the Resources at the end of this chapter).

PSYCHOSOCIAL CARE

Psychosocial care is an important aspect of cancer care. Supportive care includes services and strategies to help cancer patients and their families cope with the cancer experience.

Because of the effectiveness of cancer treatment, cancer is cured in many patients, or the disease is controlled for long periods. In view of this trend in survival, an optimal quality of life must be maintained after the diagnosis of cancer. By understanding the effect of cancer on the patient and the family and by promoting services that can facilitate financial, social, functional, and psychological well-being, the nurse can be more effective in assisting patients and families throughout their cancer experience. Nurses work collaboratively as part of an interprofessional team (e.g., social work and counselling, psychiatry, nutrition, occupational therapy, speech language pathology, community nursing, physiatry, palliative care and primary care) to provide supportive cancer care.

A diagnosis of cancer may precipitate a crisis in the lives of the patient and their family, and repercussions may affect all aspects of their lives. Common fears experienced by the patient with cancer include disfigurement, dependency, unrelieved pain, financial depletion, abandonment, and death.

To cope with these fears, patients with cancer may use and experience different behavioural patterns: shock, anger, denial, bargaining, depression, helplessness, hopelessness, rationalization, acceptance, and intellectualization. These behavioural patterns may occur at any time during the process of cancer. However, some patterns appear to occur more frequently or at a greater intensity at certain stages of the disease process. The following factors may determine how a patient will cope with the diagnosis of cancer:

1. *Ability to cope with stressful events in the past* (e.g., loss of job, major disappointment). By simply asking how the patient has coped with stressful events, the nurse can obtain an understanding of the patient's coping patterns, the effectiveness of the usual coping patterns, and the usual coping time framework.
2. *Availability of significant others.* Patients who have effective support systems tend to cope more effectively than do patients who do not have a meaningful, available support system.
3. *Ability to express feelings and concerns.* Patients who are able to express feelings and needs and who seek and ask for help appear to cope more effectively than do patients who internalize feelings and needs.
4. *Age at the time of diagnosis.* Age determines the coping strategies to a great degree. For example, a young mother with cancer may have concerns that differ from those of a 70-year-old woman with cancer.
5. *Extent of disease.* Cure or control of the disease process is usually easier to cope with than the reality of terminal illness.
6. *Disruption of body image.* Such disruption (e.g., by radical neck dissection, alopecia, mastectomy) may intensify the psychological effect of cancer.
7. *Presence of symptoms.* Symptoms such as fatigue, nausea, diarrhea, and pain may intensify the psychological effect of cancer.
8. *Past experience with cancer.* If past experiences with cancer have been negative, the patient will probably view their current status as negative.
9. *Attitude associated with the cancer.* A patient who feels in control and has a positive attitude about cancer and cancer treatment is better able to cope with the diagnosis and treatment of cancer than a patient who feels hopeless, helpless, and out of control.

To facilitate the development of a hopeful, realistic attitude about cancer and to support the patient and the family throughout the cancer trajectory, the nurse should act on the following suggestions:

1. Be authentically available for discussion with the patient and family, especially during difficult times.
2. Actively assess the patient's needs for counselling and refer them to appropriate services when necessary.
3. Listen actively to fears and concerns.
4. Offer strategies to enhance coping behaviours.
5. Provide essential information as the patient asks for it, and be sensitive to information overload.
6. Establish a therapeutic relationship based on trust and confidence; be open, honest, and caring in the approach.
7. Be "present" with the patient to offer comfort and assurance that the nurse cares about them.
8. Understand and collaborate with the patient to set realistic, reachable short- and long-term goals.
9. Encourage the patient to maintain healthy lifestyle patterns.
10. Maintain hope. Hope varies, depending on the status of the patient—hope that the symptoms are not serious, hope that the treatment is curative, hope for independence, hope for relief of pain, hope for a longer life, or hope for a peaceful death. Hope provides control over what is occurring and is the basis of a positive attitude toward cancer and cancer care. The development of an advanced care plan may help to clarify patients' attitudes and provide reassurance

ETHICAL DILEMMAS
Medical Futility

Situation
K. A. (pronouns she/her), 65 years old, has breast cancer with metastasis to the liver and bone. The family asks the nurse why their mother is not receiving chemotherapy. In addition, family members want to make certain that she will be resuscitated should her heart stop. They are aware of K. A.'s diagnosis and that she may have less than 1 month to live. The nurse was told in morning rounds that K. A. does not want any treatment that would prolong life.

Important Points for Consideration
- If the patient is competent, the patient is legally and ethically the decision maker with regard to their own care in consultation with the patient's family and the health care team as desired.
- Members of the health care team have no obligation to provide care that is medically futile. Care that is futile may be inappropriate, prolong dying, or provide little or no benefit to the patient. Nurses can help patients and families to reconcile their hopes for the future in personally relevant and realistic ways, rather than focusing on futile efforts and unrealistic outcomes.
- Palliative care is health care that provides comfort, controls pain, reduces symptoms, and improves quality of life as defined by the patient.
- The nurse should work in collaboration with the interprofessional team to have discussions with the patient and the family that ease the acceptance of the patient's prognosis, incorporate her goals into the plan of care, and prepares for her eventual death. This may include a discussion about hospice, no CPR (cardiopulmonary resuscitation) orders, and/or medical assistance in dying (MAiD) (Health Canada, 2018).

Clinical Decision-Making Questions
1. How can the nurse help K. A. communicate her wishes to her family?
2. How can the nurse and the health care team help the family plan end-of-life care that incorporates the wishes of their mother?

that their wishes for future care will be respected. Consider the spiritual aspects of care; support patients in exploring their belief systems and in finding meaning that transcends cultural and religious boundaries. Nurses can assist patients in identifying their strengths and developing skills to cope with the emotional aspects of having cancer.

11. Encourage and facilitate patients' participation in their care. This may include considering their interest in the use of integrative therapies such as support groups, mind–body modalities, nutritional supplements, and herbal therapies. The "unofficial" use of complementary and alternative medicines in oncology is widespread and has the potential to help (e.g., by relieving symptoms) or to harm (e.g., through associated toxic effects or by preventing or diminishing the effects of proven therapies). Patients may need support in understanding the difference between complementary and alternative therapies and the risks and benefits associated with these therapies.

Organizations and journals available as resources for the nurse are listed in the Resources section at the end of this chapter. The Ethical Dilemmas box is a description of considerations of nurse–family interactions when treatment is considered medically futile.

AGE-RELATED CONSIDERATIONS

CANCER

Cancer is usually a disease of aging. Most cancers occur in people older than 65 years of age. Cancer is the leading cause of death in people 65 to 74 years of age. Clinical manifestations of cancer in an older person may be mistakenly attributed to age-related changes and ignored by the person.

Older people are particularly vulnerable to the complications of both cancer and cancer therapy because of their decline in physiological functioning, social and emotional resources, and cognitive function. The functional status and comorbid conditions of an older person should be taken into consideration when a treatment plan is selected. Age alone is not a sufficient predictor of tolerance or response to treatment (Koll, 2016).

Because of advances in the treatment of cancer, cancer therapies benefit an increasing number of older persons, including patients with suboptimal health. Some important questions to consider when cancer is diagnosed in an older person include the following: Will the treatment provide more benefit than harm? Will the patient be able to tolerate the treatment safely? What is the patient's choice of therapy?

REVIEW QUESTIONS

The number of the question corresponds to the same-numbered objective at the beginning of the chapter.

1. Which of the following is consistent with trends in the incidence and death rates of cancer?
   a. Lung cancer is the most common type of cancer in men.
   b. Breast cancer is the leading cause of cancer deaths in women.
   c. A higher percentage of women than men have lung cancer.
   d. The incidence of cancer increases as the population ages.

2. What features of cancer cells distinguish them from normal cells? *(Select all that apply.)*
   a. Cells lack contact inhibition.
   b. Cells return to a previous undifferentiated state.
   c. Oncogenes maintain normal cell expression.
   d. Proliferation occurs when there is a need for more cells.
   e. New proteins characteristic of embryonic stage emerge on the cell membrane.

3. Which is a characteristic feature of the stage of progression in the development of cancer?
   a. Oncogenic viral transformation of target cells
   b. A reversible steady growth facilitated by carcinogens
   c. A period of latency before clinical detection of cancer
   d. The proliferation of cancer cells in spite of host control mechanisms

4. What is the primary protective role of the immune system in relation to malignant cells?
   a. Surveillance for cells with tumour-associated antigens
   b. The binding with free antigen released by malignant cells
   c. The production of blocking factors that immobilize cancer cells
   d. The response to a new set of antigenic determinants on cancer cells

5. What is the primary difference between benign and malignant neoplasms?
   a. The rate of cell proliferation
   b. The site of malignant tumour
   c. The requirements for cellular nutrients
   d. The characteristic of tissue invasiveness

6. Which nursing roles are important for the prevention and detection of cancer?
   a. Health promotion in relation to eating low-fibre, refined-carbohydrate diets
   b. Teaching about cancer risk factors
   c. Encouraging the public to participate in regular screening tests for all detectable cancer sites
   d. Using people's natural fear of cancer to motivate changes in unhealthy lifestyles

7. Which principle underpins a therapeutic approach to cancer?
   a. Surgery is the single most effective treatment for cancer.
   b. Initial treatment is always directed toward cure of the cancer.
   c. A combination of treatment modalities is effective for controlling many cancers.
   d. None of the above.

8. Which points would be part of nursing teaching for a client undergoing brachytherapy of the cervix?
   a. The client will learn that she must undergo simulation to locate the treatment area.
   b. The client will be taught about the treatment and need for staff time limitations in relation to her care.
   c. The client will be taught that she may experience desquamation of the skin on the abdomen and upper legs.
   d. The client will require shielding of the ovaries during treatment to prevent ovarian damage.

9. Which is the most effective method of administering a chemotherapeutic agent that is a vesicant?
   a. Giving it orally
   b. Giving it intra-arterially
   c. Using an Ommaya reservoir
   d. Using a central venous access device

10. Why does stomatitis, a common adverse effect of chemotherapeutic agents, occur?
    a. The site of the malignancy is near the oral cavity.
    b. The general health of the client with cancer is poor.

c. Chemotherapeutic medications have a local and irritating effect on epithelial cells.

d. Rapidly dividing cells of the mucous membranes of the mouth are being destroyed.

11. In teaching the client about IL-2, which information will the nurse include?

a. It stimulates the immune system.

b. It inhibits DNA and protein synthesis in tumour cells.

c. It decreases the antigenic expression of antigens on tumour cell surfaces.

d. It prevents bone marrow suppression associated with chemotherapy.

12. Which information will the nurse provide to a client receiving radiation therapy or chemotherapy?

a. Effective birth control methods should be used for the rest of the client's life.

b. Notify the health care team if nausea and vomiting are experienced during treatment so that these can be managed.

c. After successful treatment, the client will return to their previous functional level.

d. The cycle of fatigue-depression-fatigue that may occur during treatment can be reduced by restricting activity.

13. Which is an inappropriate nursing intervention to promote nutrition in the client with cancer?

a. Providing bland, pureed food because the person's taste sensation is altered

b. Providing increased protein for normal cell recovery and immune system function

c. Encouraging the client to eat a high-calorie, high-protein snack every few hours to prevent weight loss

d. Alerting the physician that nutritional supplements may be needed when the client has a 4-kg weight loss

14. What is the primary cause of SIADH in cancer?

a. Autoimmune reaction

b. Gram-negative septicemia

c. Invasiveness of cancer cells

d. Ectopic hormonal production

15. A client has recently received a diagnosis of early-stage breast cancer. Which of the following is most appropriate for the nurse to focus on?

a. Maintaining the client's hope

b. Preparing a will and advance directives

c. Discussing replacement child care for client's children

d. Discussing the client's past experiences with her grandmother's cancer

1. d; 2. a, b, e; 3. d; 4. a; 5. d; 6. b; 7. c; 8. c; 9. d; 10. d; 11. a; 12. b; 13. a; 14. d; 15. a

(e)volve

For even more review questions, visit http://evolve.elsevier.com/Canada/Lewis/medsurg.

REFERENCES

Al-Shamsi, H. O., Alhazzani, W., Alhuraiji, A., et al. (2020). A practical approach to the management of cancer patients during the novel coronavirus disease 2019 (COVID-19) pandemic: An international collaborative group. *Oncologist, 25*(6), e936–e945. https://doi.org/10.1634/theoncologist.2020-0213

Canadian Association of Nurses in Oncology. (2017). *Standards of care, roles, and competencies. Author.*

Canadian Cancer Society. (2021a). *Cancer risk in families.* https://www.cancer.ca/en/cancer-information/cancer-101/what-is-cancer/genes-and-cancer/cancer-risk-in-families/?region=on

Canadian Cancer Society. (2021b). *Tumour lysis syndrome.* https://www.cancer.ca/en/cancer-information/diagnosis-and-treatment/managing-side-effects/tumour-lysis-syndrome/?region=on

Canadian Cancer Statistic Advisory Committee. (2019). *Canadian cancer statistics 2019. Canadian Cancer Society.* https://www.cancer.ca/~/media/cancer.ca/CW/cancer%20information/cancer%20101/Canadian%20cancer%20statistics/Canadian-Cancer-Statistics-2019-EN.pdf?la=en

Charalambous, A., Berger, A. M., Matthews, E., et al. (2019). Cancer-related fatigue and sleep deficiency in cancer care continuum: Concepts, assessment, cluster and management. *Supportive Care Cancer, 27*(7), 2747–2753. https://doi.org/10.1007/s00520-019-04746-9

Chaveli-Lopez, B., & Bagan-Sebastien, J. V. (2016). Treatment of oral mucositis due to chemotherapy. *Journal of Clinical and Experimental Dentistry, 8*(20), 201–209. https://doi.org/10.4317/jced.52917

Citrin, D. (2017). Recent developments in radiotherapy. *New England Journal of Medicine, 377*, 1065–1075. https://doi.org/10.1056/NEJMra1608986

DeVita, V. T., Lawrence, T. S., & Rosenberg, S. A. (2018). *Devita, Hellman, and Rosenberg's cancer: Principles and practice of oncology.* (10th ed.). Lippincott, Williams & Wilkins.

Ebede, C., Jang, Y., & Escalante, C. P. (2017). Cancer-related fatigue in cancer survivorship. *Medical Clinics of North America, 101*(6), 1085–1097. https://doi.org/10.1016/j.mcna.2017.06.007

Health Canada. (2018). *Medical Assistance in Dying.* https://www.canada.ca/en/health-canada/services/medical-assistance-dying.html

Health Canada. (2021). *Canada's food guide resources.* https://www.hc-sc.gc.ca/fn-an/food-guide-aliment/order-commander/index-eng.php#a1

Horrill, T. C., Linton, J., Lavoie, J., et al. (2019). Access to cancer care among Indigenous peoples in Canada: A scoping review. *Social Science Medicine, 238*, 112495. https://doi.org/10.1016/j.socscimed.2019.112495

Jetty, R., & Canadian Paediatric Society, First Nations, Inuit and Metis Health Committee. (2017). Tobacco use and misuse among Indigenous children and youth in Canada. *Paediatrics & Child Health, 22*(7), 395–399. https://doi.org/10.1093/pch/pxx124

Koll, T., Pergolotti, M., Homes, H., et al. (2016). Supportive care in older adults with cancer: Across the continuum. *Current Oncology Reports, 18*(8), 51. https://doi.org/10.1007/s11912-016-0535-8

Mazereeuw, M. V., Withrow, D. R., Nishri, E. D., et al. (2018). Cancer incidence among First Nations adults in Canada: Follow-up of the 1991 Census Mortality Cohort (1992–2009). *Canadian Journal of Public Health, 109*(5-6), 700–709. https://doi.org/10.17269/s41997-018-0091-0

Mirrakhimov, A. (2015). Hypercalcemia of malignancy: An update on pathogenesis and management. *North American Journal of Medical Sciences, 7*(11), 483–493. https://doi.org/10.4103/1947-2714.170600

National Collaborating Centre for Aboriginal Health. (2013). *An overview of Aboriginal health in Canada.* https://www.nccih.ca/495/An_Overview_of_Aboriginal_Health_in_Canada.nccih?id=101

Scarborough, B. M., & Smith, C. B. (2018). Optimal pain management for patients with cancer in the modern era. *A Cancer Journal for Clinicians, 68*(3), 182–196. https://doi.org/10.3322/caac.21453

Slavc, I., Chen-Pfeffer, J. L., Gururangan, S., et al. (2018). Best practices for the use of intracerebroventricular drug delivery devices. *Molecular Genetics and Metabolism, 124*(3), 184–188. https://doi.org/10.1016/j.ymgme.2018.05.003

Statistics Canada. (2017). *Health fact sheets: The 10 leading causes of death, 2013.* https://www150.statcan.gc.ca/n1/pub/82-625-x/2017001/article/14776-eng.htm

Statistics Canada. (2019). *Overweight and obese adults, 2018.* https://www150.statcan.gc.ca/n1/pub/82-625-x/2019001/article/00005-eng.htm

RESOURCES

Advance Care Planning Canada
https://www.advancecareplanning.ca/

BC Cancer: *Cancer Management Guidelines*
http://www.bccancer.bc.ca/HPI/CancerManagementGuidelines/default.htm

BC Cancer: *Pain & Symptom Management*
http://www.bccancer.bc.ca/our-services/services/supportive-care/pain-symptom-management

Canadian Association of Nurses in Oncology (CANO)
https://www.cano-acio.ca

Canadian Association of Provincial Cancer Agencies (CAPCA)
https://www.capca.ca

Canadian Association of Psychosocial Oncology (CAPO)
https://www.capo.ca

Canadian Breast Cancer Research Alliance (CBCRA)
http://www.breast.cancer.ca

Canadian Cancer Society
https://www.cancer.ca

Canadian Cancer Society: *Look Good, Feel Better*
http://www.cancer.ca/en/support-and-services/support-services/look-good-feel-better-qc/?region=qc

Canadian Cancer Society: *Talk to an Information Service*
http://www.cancer.ca/canada-wide/support%20services/cancer%20information%20service.aspx

Canadian Hospice Palliative Care Association
https://www.chpca.net

Canadian Institute of Health Information (CIHI)
https://www.cihi.ca/en

Canadian Oncology Nursing Journal (CONJ)
https://cano.malachite-mgmt.com/?page=CONJOnline

Canadian Partnership Against Cancer
https://www.partnershipagainstcancer.ca

Canadian Virtual Hospice
http://www.virtualhospice.ca

Cancer Care Ontario: *Guidelines & Advice*
https://www.cancercareontario.ca/en/guidelines-advice

Cancernews.com
http://www.cancernews.com

Cancer Research Society
https://www.societederecherchesurlecancer.ca/en

Colorectal Cancer Canada
https://www.colorectalcancercanada.com/

Institute for Clinical Evaluative Studies (ICES)
https://www.ices.on.ca

Psychosocial Oncology Research Training (PORT)
https://www.mcgill.ca/oncology/divisions-programs/psychosocial-oncology

Screening Guidelines for Early Detection of Cancer in Asymptomatic People
http://www.cancer.ca/en/prevention-and-screening/early-detection-and-screening/screening/

American Association for Cancer Education (AACE)
http://www.aaceonline.com

International Society of Nurses in Cancer Care
https://www.isncc.org

Karnofsky Performance Status Scale
https://oncologypro.esmo.org/Guidelines-Practice/Practice-Tools/Performance-Scales

Mayo Clinic: *No Appetite? How to Get Nutrition During Cancer Treatment*
https://www.mayoclinic.org/diseases-conditions/cancer/in-depth/cancer/art-20045046?pg=2

National Coalition for Cancer Survivorship (NCS)
https://www.canceradvocacy.org

National Institute for Occupational Safety and Health (NIOSH): *Preventing Occupational Exposures to Antineoplastic and Other Hazardous Drugs in Health Care Settings*
https://www.cdc.gov/niosh/docs/2004-165/default.html

Nutritional Therapy Protein Foods With High Biological Value
https://www.oncolink.org/support/nutrition-and-cancer/during-and-after-treatment/protein-needs-during-cancer-treatment

OncoLink (cancer information site)
http://www.oncolink.upenn.edu

Oncology Nursing Society
https://www.ons.org

Union for International Cancer Control
http://www.uicc.ch

For additional Internet resources, see the website for this book at http://evolve.elsevier.com/Canada/Lewis/medsurg.

Fluid, Electrolyte, and Acid–Base Imbalances

Joanne Newell
Originating US chapter by Margaret R. Rateau

⊖volve WEBSITE

http://evolve.elsevier.com/Canada/Lewis/medsurg

- Review Questions (Online Only)
- Key Points
- Answer Guideline for Case Study
- Student Case Study
  - Hyponatremia/Fluid Volume Imbalance
- Conceptual Care Map Creator
- Fluids and Electrolytes Tutorial
- Audio Glossary
- Content Updates

LEARNING OBJECTIVES

1. Describe the composition of the major body fluid compartments.
2. Define processes involved in the regulation of the movement of water and electrolytes between the body fluid compartments.
3. Describe the etiology, laboratory diagnostic findings, clinical manifestations, and nursing and interprofessional management of the following disorders:
   a. Water excess and deficit
   b. Sodium and volume imbalances: hypernatremia and hyponatremia
   c. Potassium imbalance: hyperkalemia and hypokalemia
   d. Magnesium imbalance: hypermagnesemia and hypomagnesemia
   e. Calcium imbalance: hypercalcemia and hypocalcemia
   f. Phosphate imbalance: hyperphosphatemia and hypophosphatemia
4. Identify the processes of acid–base regulation.
5. Discuss the etiology, laboratory diagnostic findings, clinical manifestations, and nursing and interprofessional management of the following acid–base imbalances: metabolic acidosis, metabolic alkalosis, respiratory acidosis, and respiratory alkalosis.
6. Describe the composition and indications for use of common intravenous fluid solutions.
7. Discuss types and nursing management of commonly used central venous access devices.

KEY TERMS

acidosis	facilitated diffusion	oncotic pressure
active transport	fluid spacing	osmolality
alkalosis	homeostasis	osmolarity
anions	hydrostatic pressure	osmosis
buffers	hypertonic	osmotic pressure
cations	hypotonic	pH
diffusion	ions	tetany
electrolytes	isotonic	valence

HOMEOSTASIS

Body fluids and electrolytes play an important role in homeostasis. Homeostasis is the state of equilibrium in the internal environment of the body, naturally maintained by adaptive responses that promote healthy survival (Mosby, 2016). Maintenance of the composition and volume of body fluids, electrolytes, and acid–base concentrations within narrow normal limits is necessary to maintain homeostasis (McCance & Huether, 2019). During normal metabolism, the body produces many acids. These acids alter the internal environment of the body, including fluid and electrolyte balances, and must also be regulated to maintain homeostasis. Many diseases and their

treatments have the ability to affect fluid and electrolyte balance. For example, a patient with metastatic breast cancer may develop hypercalcemia. Chemotherapy prescribed to treat the cancer may result in nausea and vomiting and, subsequently, dehydration and acid–base imbalances. Correction of dehydration with intravenous (IV) fluids must be monitored closely to prevent fluid overload.

It is important for the nurse to anticipate the potential for alterations in fluid and electrolyte balance associated with certain disorders and medical therapies, to recognize the signs and symptoms of imbalances, and to intervene with the appropriate actions. This chapter describes the normal control of fluids, electrolytes, and acid–base balance; etiologies that disrupt homeostasis and resultant manifestations; and actions that the health care provider can take to prevent imbalance or restore fluid, electrolyte, and acid–base balance.

WATER CONTENT OF THE BODY

Water is the primary component of the body, accounting for approximately 60% of adult body weight. Water content varies with sex, body mass, and age (Figure 19.1). Lean body mass (muscle) has a higher percentage of water than does adipose tissue (fat); therefore, the more fat present in the body, the less the total water content. Women generally have a lower percentage of body water because they tend to have less lean body mass (more fat) than do men. In older people, the body water content is lower in part because of decreased muscle mass and increased fat. Thus, older people are at an increased risk for fluid-related problems.

Body Fluid Compartments

The two major fluid compartments in the body are intracellular spaces (inside the cells) and the extracellular spaces (outside the cells) (Figure 19.2). Approximately two thirds of body water is

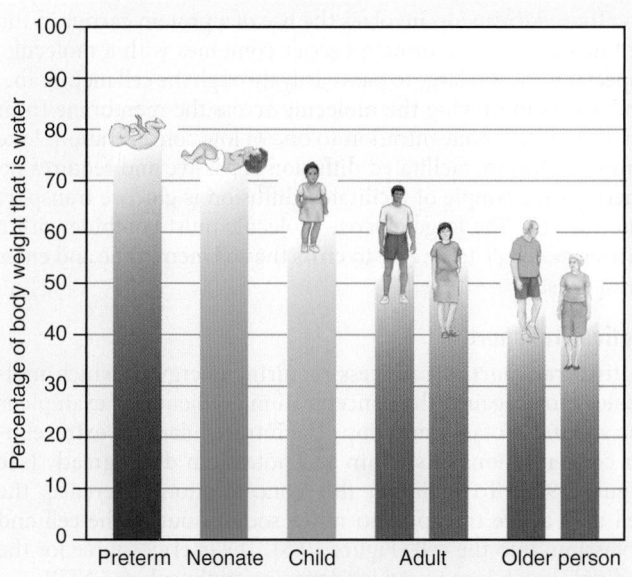

FIG. 19.1 Levels of body water over the lifespan.

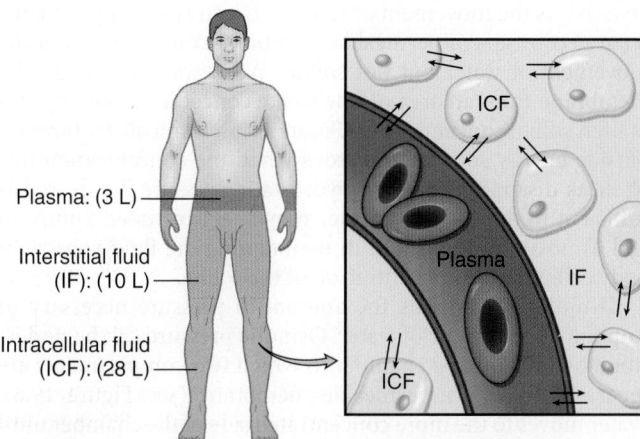

FIG. 19.2 Relative volumes of three body fluids. Values represent fluid distribution in a young male adult. *ICF*, intercellular fluid; *IF*, interstitial fluid.

located within cells and is called *intracellular fluid* (ICF); the ICF constitutes approximately 42% of body weight. The body of a 70-kg man would contain approximately 42 L of water, of which 30 L would be intracellular. *Extracellular fluid* (ECF) consists primarily of interstitial fluid and intravascular fluid (plasma). The ECF constitutes one third of the body water, or approximately 17% of the total weight; this would amount to approximately 11 L in a 70-kg man. Approximately one third of the ECF is in the plasma space (3 L in a 70-kg man), and two thirds is in the interstitial space (8 L in a 70-kg man). Other ECF components include lymph and transcellular fluids. Transcellular fluids account for approximately 1 L and include cerebrospinal fluid; fluid in the gastrointestinal (GI) tract and joint spaces; and pleural, peritoneal, intraocular, and pericardial fluid.

Calculation of Fluid Gain or Loss

One litre of water weighs 1 kg. Body weight change, especially sudden change, is an excellent indicator of overall fluid volume loss or gain. For example, if a patient drinks 240 mL of fluid, weight gain will be 0.24 kg. A patient receiving diuretic therapy who loses 2 kg in 24 hours has experienced a fluid loss of approximately 2 L. Overnight fasting for surgery in a young healthy adult can produce a fluid loss of 820 mL (0.82 kg) (Danielsson et al., 2019).

ELECTROLYTES

Electrolytes are substances whose molecules dissociate or split into ions when placed in solution. Ions are electrically charged molecules. Cations are positively charged ions. Examples include sodium (Na^+), potassium (K^+), calcium (Ca^{2+}), and magnesium (Mg^{2+}) ions. Anions are negatively charged ions. Examples include bicarbonate (HCO_3^-), chloride (Cl^-), and phosphate (PO_4^{3-}) ions. Most proteins bear a negative charge and are thus anions. The electrical charge of an ion is termed its valence. Cations and anions combine according to their valences.

Measurement of Electrolytes

The measurement of electrolytes is important to the nurse in evaluating electrolyte balance, as well as in determining the composition of electrolyte preparations. The concentration of electrolytes can be expressed in milligrams per decilitre (mg/dL), millimoles per litre (mmol/L), or milliequivalents per litre (mEq/L). The international standard symbol for measuring electrolytes is mmol/L. One mole (mol) of a substance is the molecular (or atomic) weight of that substance expressed in grams; hence, a millimole (mmol) of a substance is the atomic weight in milligrams. Sodium's atomic weight is 23 mg; therefore, 23 mg of sodium is 1 mmol of sodium. Sodium and chloride are monovalent elements that carry one electron and will match 1 to 1: 1 mmol of sodium combines with 1 mmol of chloride.

An element with two electrons, such as calcium, requires two monovalent partners. To avoid keeping track of how to match millimoles, the milliequivalent is the favoured unit of measure for electrolytes. The following formula is used to convert millimoles to milliequivalents:

$$mEq = (mmol/L) \times valence$$

Electrolytes in body fluids are active chemicals that unite in varying combinations. Thus, it is more practical to express their

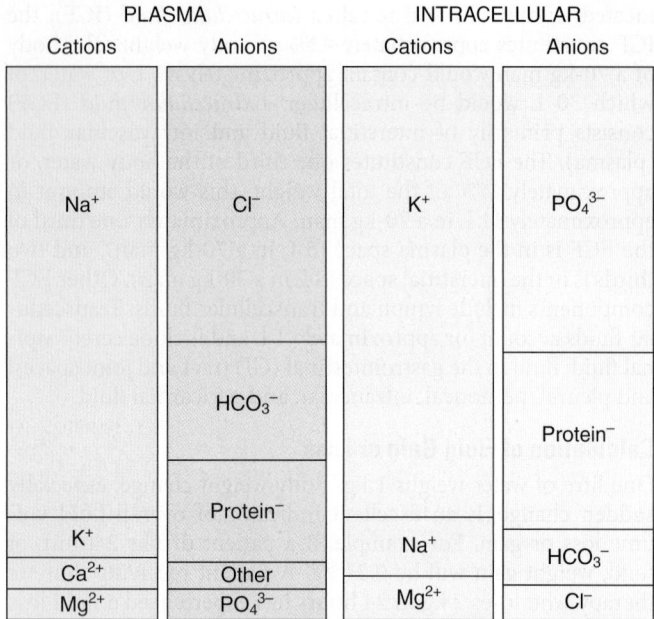

PLASMA / INTRACELLULAR

Cations | Anions — Cations | Anions

FIG. 19.3 The relative concentrations of the major cations and anions in the intracellular space and the plasma.

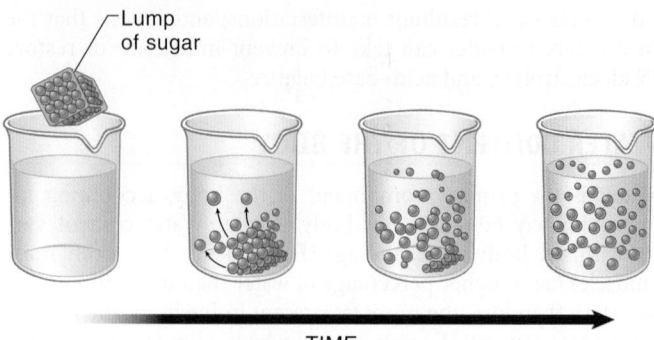

Lump of sugar

TIME

FIG. 19.4 Diffusion is the movement of molecules from an area of high concentration to an area of low concentration. In this example, the sugar molecules eventually are evenly distributed. Source: Patton, K. T., & Thibodeau, G. A. (2019). *Anatomy and physiology* (10th ed., p. 99). Elsevier.

concentration as a measure of chemical activity (or milliequivalents) rather than as a measure of weight. Ions combine milliequivalent for milliequivalent: they match 1 to 1. For example, 1 mEq (1 mmol) of sodium combines with 1 mEq (1 mmol) of chloride, and 1 mEq (0.5 mmol) of calcium combines with 1 mEq (1 mmol) of chloride. This combining power of electrolytes is important for maintaining the balance of positively charged ions (cations) and negatively charged ions (anions) within body fluids.

Electrolyte Composition of Fluid Compartments

Electrolyte composition varies between the ECF and the ICF. The overall concentration of the electrolytes is approximately the same in the two compartments. However, concentrations of specific ions differ greatly (Figure 19.3). In the ECF, the main cation is sodium, with small amounts of potassium, calcium, and magnesium. The primary ECF anion is chloride, with small amounts of bicarbonate, sulphate, and phosphate anions. In the ICF, the most prevalent cation is potassium, with small amounts of magnesium and sodium. The predominant ICF anion is phosphate, with some protein and a small amount of bicarbonate.

MECHANISMS CONTROLLING FLUID AND ELECTROLYTE MOVEMENT

Different processes—such as simple diffusion, facilitated diffusion, and active transport—are involved in the movement of electrolytes and water between the ICF and the ECF. Water movement is driven by two forces: hydrostatic pressure and osmotic pressure.

Diffusion

Diffusion is the movement of molecules from an area of high concentration to one of low concentration (Figure 19.4). The membrane separating the two areas must be permeable by the diffusing substance for the process to occur. Net movement of molecules stops when the concentrations are equal in both

areas. Simple diffusion requires no external energy. Gases (e.g., oxygen, nitrogen, carbon dioxide) and substances (e.g., urea) can permeate cell membranes and are distributed throughout the body.

Facilitated Diffusion

Facilitated diffusion involves the use of a protein carrier in the cell membrane. The protein carrier combines with a molecule, especially one too large to pass easily through the cell membrane, and assists in moving the molecule across the membrane from an area of high concentration to one of low concentration. Like simple diffusion, facilitated diffusion is passive and requires no energy. An example of facilitated diffusion is glucose transport into the cell. The large glucose molecule must combine with a carrier molecule to be able to cross the cell membrane and enter most cells.

Active Transport

Active transport is a process requiring energy in which molecules move against the concentration gradient. An example is the sodium–potassium pump. The intracellular and extracellular concentrations of sodium and potassium differ greatly (see Figure 19.3). To maintain this concentration difference, the cell uses active transport to move sodium out of the cell and potassium into the cell (Figure 19.5). The energy source for the sodium–potassium pump is adenosine triphosphate (ATP).

Osmosis

Osmosis is the movement of water between two compartments separated by a semipermeable membrane, one that allows the movement of water but not solute. Water moves through the membrane from an area of low solute concentration to an area of high solute concentration (Figure 19.6). Osmosis requires no outside energy sources and stops when the concentration differences disappear or when hydrostatic pressure builds and is sufficient to oppose any further movement of water. Diffusion and osmosis are important in maintaining the fluid volume of body cells and the concentration of the solute.

Osmotic pressure is the amount of pressure necessary to stop the osmotic flow of water. Osmotic pressure can be understood by imagining a chamber in which two compartments are separated by a semipermeable membrane (see Figure 19.6). Water moves to the more concentrated side of the chamber until the pressure generated by the height of the higher column of water opposes further movement.

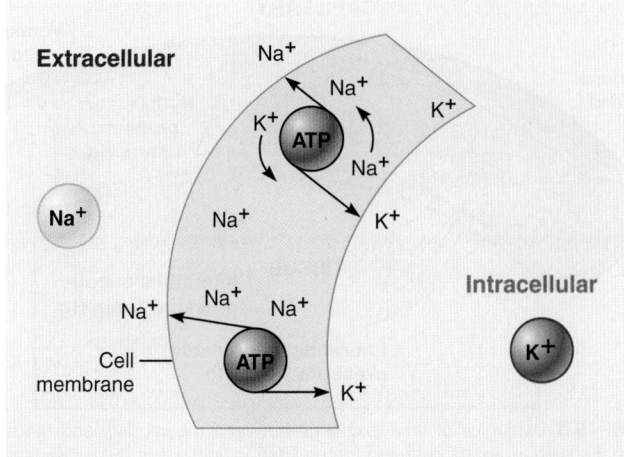

FIG. 19.5 Sodium–potassium pump. As sodium (Na⁺) diffuses into the cell and potassium (K⁺) diffuses out of the cell, an active transport system supplied with energy from adenosine triphosphate (ATP) delivers Na⁺ back to the extracellular compartment and K⁺ to the intracellular compartment.

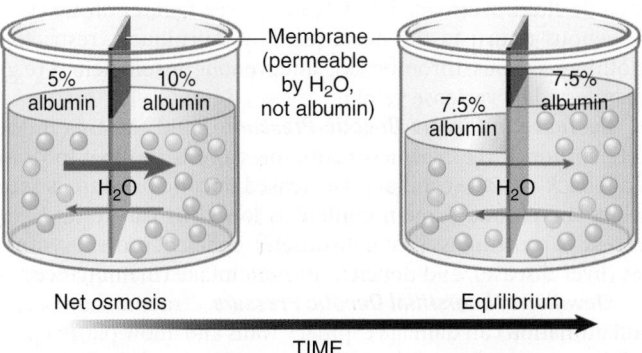

FIG. 19.6 Osmosis is the process of water movement through a semipermeable membrane from an area of low solute concentration to an area of high solute concentration. Source: Patton, K. T., & Thibodeau, G. A. (2019). *Anatomy and physiology* (10th ed., p. 102). Elsevier.

Osmotic pressure is determined by the concentration of solutes in solution. It is measured in milliosmoles (mOsm) and may be expressed as either fluid osmolarity or fluid osmolality. Although the terms *osmolarity* and *osmolality* are often used interchangeably, they are different measurements. Osmolarity is a measure of the total milliosmoles of solute per unit of total volume of solution—that is, the total milliosmoles per litre of solution (mOsm/L), or the concentration of molecules per volume of solution. Osmolality is a measure of the osmotic force of solute per unit of weight of solvent: that is, the number of milliosmoles per kilogram of water (mOsm/kg, or mmol/kg), or the concentration of molecules per weight of water. Osmolality is the preferred measure for evaluating the concentration of plasma, urine, and body fluids (McCance & Huether, 2019).

Measurement of Osmolality. Osmolality is approximately the same in the various body fluid spaces. Determining osmolality is important because it indicates the water balance of the body. To assess the state of the body water balance, the clinician can measure or estimate plasma osmolality. Normal plasma osmolality is between 280 and 295 mmol/kg. A value greater than 295 mmol/kg indicates that the concentration of particles is too great or that the water content is too little. This condition is termed *water deficit*. A value less than 280 mmol/kg indicates

too little solute for the amount of water or too much water for the amount of solute. This condition is termed *water excess*. Both conditions are clinically significant.

Plasma and urine osmolality can be measured in most clinical laboratories. Because the major determinants of the plasma osmolality are sodium, glucose, and urea, the plasma osmolality can be calculated from the concentrations of those compounds with the following equation:

$$\text{Plasma osmolality} = 2 \times (\text{Na}^+) + \text{glucose} + \text{blood urea nitrogen (BUN) (all measurements in mmol/L)}$$

When Na+ is expressed in milliequivalents per litre (mEq/L) and glucose and BUN are measured in mg/dL, conversion to mmol/L is obtained with the following equation (Reddi, 2018):

$$\text{Plasma osmolality} = 2 \times (\text{Na}^+) + (\text{glucose})/18 + \text{BUN}/2.8$$

In both equations the sodium concentration is multiplied by 2 to account for the presence of an equivalent number of anions.

Urea moves freely between body fluid compartments; it has no lasting effect on water movement across cell boundaries and is sometimes dubbed an "ineffective osmole." The concentration of only effective osmoles measures effective osmolality. The measure of the effective plasma osmolality without consideration of the BUN term is the more physiologically meaningful estimate. However, the actual osmolality of plasma is calculated more accurately if BUN is used. Osmolality of urine can range from 100 to 1 300 mmol/kg, depending on fluid intake, the amount of antidiuretic hormone (ADH) released, and the renal response to it.

Osmotic Movement of Fluids. Cells are affected by the osmolality of the fluid that surrounds them. Fluids with the same osmolality as the cell interior are isotonic. Solutions in which the solutes are less concentrated than they are in cells are hypotonic (hypo-osmolar). Those with solutes more concentrated than they are in cells are hypertonic (hyperosmolar).

Normally, the ECF and the ICF are isotonic to one another, so no net movement of water occurs. In the metabolically active cell, there is a constant exchange of substances between the compartments, but no net gain or loss of water occurs.

If a cell is surrounded by hypotonic fluid, water moves into the cell, causing it to swell and possibly to burst. If a cell is surrounded by hypertonic fluid, water leaves the cell to dilute the ECF; the cell shrinks and may eventually die (Figure 19.7).

Hydrostatic Pressure

Hydrostatic pressure is the force within a fluid compartment. In the blood vessels, hydrostatic pressure is the blood pressure generated by the contraction of the heart. Hydrostatic pressure in the vascular system gradually decreases as the blood moves through the arteries until it is approximately 40 mm Hg at the arterial end of a capillary. Because of the size of the capillary bed and fluid movement into the interstitium, the pressure decreases to approximately 10 mm Hg at the venous end of the capillary. Hydrostatic pressure is the major force that pushes water out of the vascular system at the capillary level.

Oncotic Pressure

Oncotic pressure (colloidal osmotic pressure) is osmotic pressure exerted by colloids in solution. The major colloid in the vascular system contributing to the total osmotic pressure is

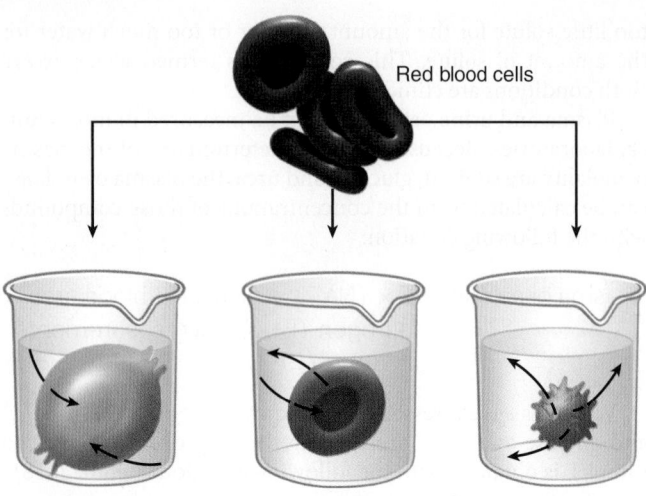

Red blood cells

A Hypotonic solution   **B** Isotonic solution   **C** Hypertonic solution

FIG. 19.7 Effects of water status on red blood cells. **A,** Hypotonic solution (H_2O excess) results in cellular swelling. **B,** Isotonic solution (normal H_2O balance) results in no change. **C,** Hypertonic solution (H_2O deficit) results in cellular shrinking. Source: Patton, K. T., & Thibodeau, G. A. (2019). *Anatomy and physiology* (10th ed., p. 103). Mosby.

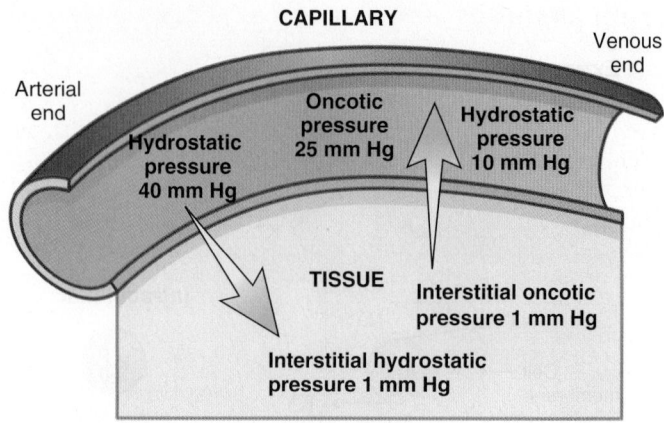

FIG. 19.8 Dynamics of fluid exchange between the capillary and the tissue. Equilibrium exists between forces filtering fluid out of the capillary and forces absorbing fluid back into the capillary. Note that the hydrostatic pressure is greater at the arterial end of the capillary than at the venous end. The net effect of pressures at the arterial end of the capillary causes a movement of fluid into the tissue. At the venous end of the capillary, there is net movement of fluid back into the capillary.

protein. Protein molecules attract water, pulling fluid from the tissue space to the vascular space (Porth, 2018). Unlike electrolytes, proteins have large molecular sizes, which prevents them from leaving the vascular space through pores in capillary walls. Plasma oncotic pressure is approximately 25 mm Hg. Some proteins are found in the interstitial space; they exert an oncotic pressure of approximately 1 mm Hg.

FLUID MOVEMENT IN CAPILLARIES

There is normal movement of fluid between the capillary and the interstitium. The amount and direction of movement are determined by the interaction of (1) capillary hydrostatic pressure, (2) plasma oncotic pressure, (3) interstitial hydrostatic pressure, and (4) interstitial oncotic pressure.

Capillary hydrostatic pressure and interstitial oncotic pressure cause the movement of water out of the capillaries. Plasma oncotic pressure and interstitial hydrostatic pressure cause the movement of fluid into the capillary. At the arterial end of the capillary (Figure 19.8), capillary hydrostatic pressure exceeds plasma oncotic pressure, and fluid is moved into the interstitium. At the venous end of the capillary, the capillary hydrostatic pressure is lower than plasma oncotic pressure, and fluid is drawn back into the capillary by the oncotic pressure created by plasma proteins.

Fluid Shifts

If capillary or interstitial pressures are altered, fluid may abnormally shift from one compartment to another, which results in edema or dehydration.

Shifts of Plasma to Interstitial Fluid. Accumulation of fluid in the interstitium *(edema)* occurs if venous hydrostatic pressure rises, plasma oncotic pressure decreases, or interstitial oncotic pressure rises. Edema may also develop if the lymphatic outflow is obstructed, which causes decreased removal of interstitial fluid.

Elevation of Venous Hydrostatic Pressure. Increasing the pressure at the venous end of the capillary inhibits fluid movement back into the capillary. Causes of increased venous pressure

include fluid overload, heart failure, liver failure, obstruction of venous return to the heart (e.g., by tourniquets, restrictive clothing, venous thrombosis), and venous insufficiency (e.g., manifested by varicose veins).

Decrease in Plasma Oncotic Pressure. Fluid remains in the interstitium if the plasma oncotic pressure is too low to draw fluid back into the capillary. Decreased oncotic pressure is seen when the plasma protein content is low. This can result from excessive protein loss (renal disorders), deficient protein synthesis (liver disease), and deficient protein intake (malnutrition).

Elevation of Interstitial Oncotic Pressure. Trauma, burns, and inflammation can damage capillary walls and allow plasma proteins to accumulate in the interstitium. The resultant increased interstitial oncotic pressure draws fluid into the interstitium and holds it there.

Shifts of Interstitial Fluid to Plasma. Fluid is drawn into the plasma space from the interstitium whenever there is an increase in the plasma osmotic or oncotic pressure. This could happen with administration of colloids, dextran, mannitol, or hypertonic solutions. In turn, water is drawn from cells via osmosis, which causes equilibration of the osmolality between the ICF and the ECF.

Increasing the tissue hydrostatic pressure is another way of causing a shift of fluid into plasma. The wearing of elastic compression gradient stockings or hose to decrease peripheral edema is a therapeutic application of this effect.

FLUID MOVEMENT BETWEEN EXTRACELLULAR FLUID AND INTRACELLULAR FLUID

Changes in the osmolality of the ECF alter the volume of cells. Increased ECF osmolality (water deficit) pulls water out of cells until the two compartments have a similar osmolality. Water deficit is associated with symptoms that result from cell shrinkage as water is pulled into the vascular system. Neurological symptoms are caused by altered central nervous system (CNS) function when brain cells shrink. Decreased ECF osmolality (water excess) develops as the result of gain or retention of excess water. In this case, cells swell when water is pulled into the cell. Again, the primary symptoms are neurological as a result of brain cell swelling.

FLUID SPACING

Fluid spacing is a term sometimes used to describe the distribution of body water. *First spacing* describes the normal distribution of fluid in the ICF and ECF compartments. *Second spacing* refers to an abnormal accumulation of interstitial fluid (edema). *Third spacing* occurs when fluid accumulates in a portion of the body from which it is not easily exchanged with the rest of the ECF. Third-spaced fluid is trapped and essentially unavailable for functional use. Examples of third spacing are ascites, sequestration of fluid in the abdominal cavity with peritonitis, and edema associated with burns, trauma, or sepsis.

REGULATION OF WATER BALANCE

Hypothalamic and Pituitary Regulation

Water balance is maintained by a balance of intake and excretion. A body fluid deficit or an increase in plasma osmolality is sensed by hypothalamic osmoreceptors, which in turn stimulate thirst and ADH release. Thirst causes the patient to drink. Under hypothalamic control, the posterior pituitary gland releases ADH, which induces water reabsorption in the renal distal and collecting tubules. Water is reabsorbed from the tubular filtrate into the blood and not excreted in urine. Together, thirst and hypothalamic ADH result in increased free water in the body and decreased plasma osmolality. Once plasma osmolality is normalized, secretion of ADH is suppressed, and thus urinary excretion is restored.

An intact thirst mechanism is critical because it is the primary protection against the development of hyperosmolality. The patient who cannot recognize or act on the sensation of thirst is at risk for fluid deficit and hyperosmolality. The sensitivity of the thirst mechanism decreases in older persons.

The desire to consume fluids is also affected by social and psychological factors not related to fluid balance. A dry mouth will cause the patient to drink, even when there is no measurable body water deficit. This is normally compensated by equivalent water excretion. A patient with psychiatric issues may display psychogenic polydipsia that may lead to water intoxication.

Under hypothalamic control, the posterior pituitary gland releases ADH, which causes the distal tubules and collecting ducts in the kidneys to regulate water retention by becoming more permeable by water. Factors that stimulate ADH release include increased plasma osmolality, stress, nausea, nicotine, and morphine. For instance, it is common for patients to have a lower serum osmolality after surgery, possibly because of the stress of surgery and opioid analgesia.

A pathological condition seen occasionally is *syndrome of inappropriate antidiuretic hormone* (SIADH; see Chapter 51). Causes of SIADH include abnormal ADH production in CNS disorders (e.g., brain tumours, brain injury) and certain malignancies (e.g., small cell lung cancer). The inappropriate secretion of ADH causes water retention, which causes plasma osmolality to decrease below the normal value and causes a relative increase in urine osmolality with a decrease in urine volume.

Reduction in the release or action of ADH produces diabetes insipidus (see Chapter 51). A copious amount of dilute urine is excreted because the renal tubules and collecting ducts do not appropriately reabsorb water. A patient with diabetes insipidus exhibits extreme polyuria and, if alert, polydipsia (excessive thirst). Symptoms of dehydration and hypernatremia develop if the water losses are not adequately replaced.

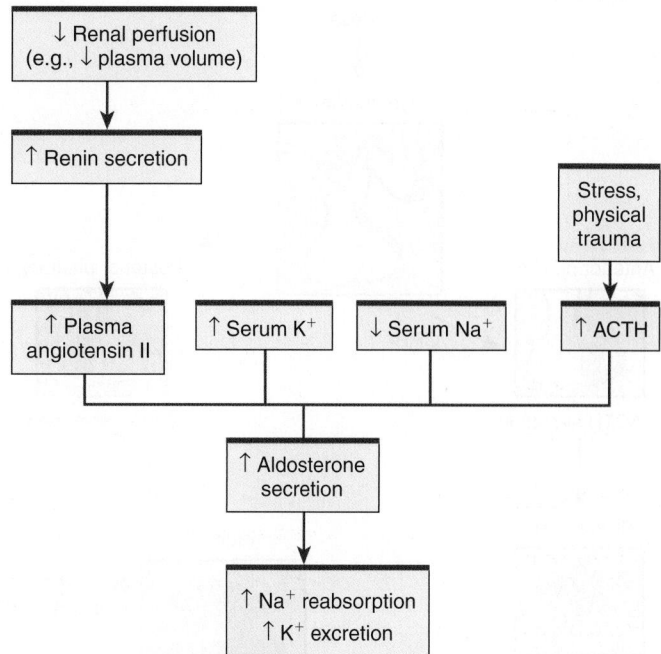

FIG. 19.9 Factors affecting aldosterone secretion. *ACTH,* adrenocorticotrophic hormone.

Adrenal Cortical Regulation

ECF volume is maintained by a combination of hormonal influences. ADH affects only water reabsorption. Hormones released by the adrenal cortex help regulate both water and electrolytes. Two groups of hormones secreted by the adrenal cortex are glucocorticoids and mineralocorticoids. The glucocorticoids (e.g., cortisol) have primarily an anti-inflammatory effect and increase serum glucose levels, whereas the mineralocorticoids (e.g., aldosterone) enhance sodium retention and potassium excretion (Figure 19.9). When sodium is reabsorbed, water follows as a result of osmotic changes.

Cortisol is the most common example of a naturally occurring glucocorticoid. In large doses, cortisol has both glucocorticoid (glucose level–elevating and anti-inflammatory) and mineralocorticoid (sodium-retaining) properties. The adrenocortical hormone cortisol is secreted normally and whenever stress levels are increased. Many body systems, including fluid and electrolyte balance, are affected by stress (Figure 19.10).

Aldosterone is a naturally occurring mineralocorticoid with potent sodium-retaining and potassium-excreting capability. Decreased renal perfusion or decreased sodium in the distal portion of the renal tubule activates the renin–angiotensin–aldosterone system, which results in aldosterone secretion. In addition to this system, increased serum potassium, decreased serum sodium, and adrenocorticotrophic hormone (ACTH) stimulate aldosterone secretion. Aldosterone increases sodium and water reabsorption in the renal distal tubules, which causes plasma osmolality to decrease and fluid volume to be restored (see Figure 19.9).

Renal Regulation

The primary organs for regulating fluid and electrolyte balance are the kidneys (see Chapter 47). The kidneys regulate water balance through adjustments in urine volume. Similarly, urinary excretion of most electrolytes is adjusted so that a balance

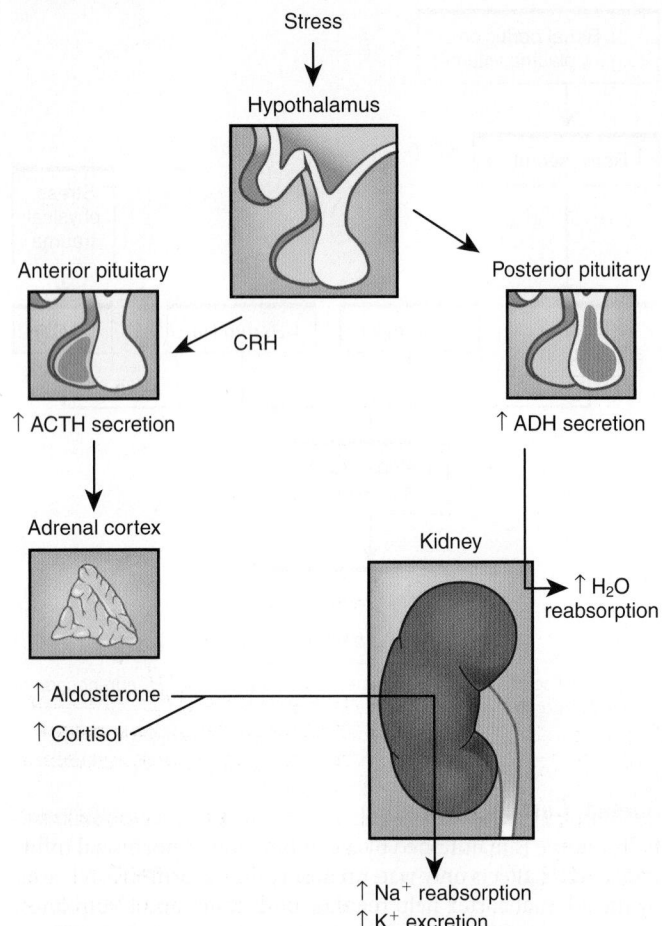

FIG. 19.10 Effects of stress on fluid and electrolyte balance. *ACTH*, adrenocorticotrophic hormone; *ADH*, antidiuretic hormone; *CRH*, corticotropin-releasing hormone.

| Stress |
| Hypothalamus |

Anterior pituitary

Posterior pituitary

CRH

↑ ACTH secretion

↑ ADH secretion

Adrenal cortex

Kidney

↑ H₂O reabsorption

↑ Aldosterone

↑ Cortisol

↑ Na⁺ reabsorption
↑ K⁺ excretion

TABLE 19.1	NORMAL FLUID BALANCE IN THE ADULT	
Substance		**Amount**
Intake		
Fluids		1 200 mL
Solid food		1 000 mL
Water from oxidation		300 mL
Total		2 500 mL
Output		
Insensible loss (skin and lungs)		900 mL
Urine		1 500 mL
In feces		100 mL
Total		2 500 mL

is maintained between overall intake and output. The total plasma volume is filtered by the kidneys many times each day. In the average adult, the kidneys reabsorb 99% of this filtrate, producing approximately 1.5 L of urine per day. As the filtrate moves through the renal tubules, selective reabsorption of water and electrolytes and secretion of electrolytes result in the production of urine, whose composition and concentration are greatly different from those of the plasma. This process helps maintain normal plasma osmolality, electrolyte balance, blood volume, and acid–base balance. The renal tubules are the site for the actions of ADH and aldosterone.

When renal function is severely impaired, the kidneys cannot maintain fluid and electrolyte balance. This condition results in edema, potassium and phosphorus retention, acidosis, and other electrolyte imbalances (see Chapter 49).

Cardiac Regulation

Atrial natriuretic factor (ANF) is a hormone released by the cardiac atria in response to increased atrial pressure (increased volume, such as what occurs in heart failure) and high serum sodium levels. The primary actions of ANF are vasodilation and increased urinary excretion of sodium and water, which decreases blood volume (McCance & Huether, 2019).

Gastrointestinal Regulation

Daily water intake and output are between 2000 and 3000 mL (Table 19.1). The GI tract accounts for most of the water intake.

Water intake includes fluids, water from food metabolism, and water present in solid foods. Lean meat is approximately 70% water, whereas the water content of many fruits and vegetables approaches 100%.

Most of the body's water is excreted by the kidneys, and a small amount of water is eliminated in feces. The GI tract normally secretes approximately 8000 mL of digestive fluids each day, most of which is reabsorbed. Diarrhea and vomiting prevent GI reabsorption of secreted fluid, which can lead to significant fluid and electrolyte loss.

Insensible Water Loss

Insensible water loss, which is invisible vaporization from the lungs and the skin, cannot be measured and the individual is unaware that the loss of water occurred. Normally, approximately 900 mL per day is insensible loss. The amount of water loss is increased by accelerated body metabolism, which occurs with increased body temperature and exercise. Sensible water loss is water loss that the individual is aware of and that can be measured.

Insensible water loss through the skin should not be confused with the water excreted by sweat glands. Excessive sweating *(sensible perspiration)* caused by fever or high environmental temperatures may lead to large losses of both water and electrolytes.

AGE-RELATED CONSIDERATIONS

FLUID AND ELECTROLYTES

Older persons experience normal physiological changes that increase susceptibility to fluid and electrolyte imbalances. Structural changes in the kidneys and a decrease in the renal blood flow lead to a decrease in the glomerular filtration rate, decreased creatinine clearance, the loss of the ability to concentrate urine and conserve water, and narrowed limits for the excretion of water, sodium, potassium, and hydrogen ions. Hormonal changes include decreases in renin and aldosterone and increases in ADH and atrial natriuretic peptide (ANP) (Koch & Fulop, 2017). Loss of subcutaneous tissue and thinning of the dermis lead to increased loss of moisture through the skin and an inability to respond to heat or cold quickly. Older persons experience a decrease in the thirst mechanism, which results in decreased fluid intake despite increases in osmolality and serum sodium level. Frail older people, especially if ill, are at increased risk for free-water loss and subsequent development of hypernatremia secondary to impairment of the thirst mechanism, and increased risk for adverse social and environmental conditions (Koch & Fulop, 2017).

Healthy older people usually consume adequate fluids to remain well hydrated. However, functional changes may occur that affect the individual's ability to independently obtain fluids. Musculoskeletal changes, such as stiffness of the hands and fingers, can lead to a decreased ability to hold a glass or cup. Mental status changes, such as confusion or disorientation, or changes in ambulation status may lead to a decreased ability to obtain fluids. As a result of incontinent episodes, an older person may intentionally restrict fluid intake (Koch & Fulop, 2017).

To help older patients, the health care provider must understand the homeostatic changes that occur in this population. It is important to avoid the pitfalls of ageism, wherein fluid and electrolyte problems may be inappropriately attributed to the natural processes of aging. The nurse needs to adapt assessment and nursing implementation strategies to account for these physiological and functional changes. Suggestions for alterations in nursing care for older persons are presented throughout this chapter and in Chapter 7.

FLUID AND ELECTROLYTE IMBALANCES

Fluid and electrolyte imbalances occur to some degree in most patients with a major illness or injury because illness disrupts the normal homeostatic mechanism. Some fluid and electrolyte imbalances are directly caused by injury or disease (e.g., burns, heart failure). At other times, therapeutic measures (e.g., IV fluid replacement, diuretics) cause or contribute to fluid and electrolyte imbalances.

The imbalances are commonly classified as *deficits* or *excesses*. Each imbalance is discussed here separately. Normal values are listed in Table 19.2. In actual clinical situations, more than one imbalance occurring in the same patient is common. For example, a patient undergoing prolonged nasogastric suction will lose Na^+, K^+, H^+, and Cl^-. These imbalances may result in deficiencies of both Na^+ and K^+, as well as metabolic alkalosis and fluid volume deficit.

Sodium and Extracellular Fluid Volume Imbalances

Sodium plays a major role in maintaining the concentration and volume of the ECF. Sodium is the main cation of the ECF and the primary determinant of ECF osmolality. Sodium imbalances are typically associated with parallel changes in osmolality. Because sodium affects the water distribution between the ECF and the ICF, it affects osmolality. Sodium is also important in the generation and transmission of nerve impulses and the regulation of acid–base balance. Serum sodium is measured in milliequivalents per litre or millimoles per litre.

The GI tract absorbs sodium from foods. Typically, daily intake of sodium far exceeds the body's daily requirements. Sodium leaves the body through urine, sweat, and feces. The kidneys are the primary regulator of sodium balance. The kidneys regulate the ECF concentration of sodium by excreting or retaining water under the influence of ADH. Aldosterone also plays a part in sodium regulation by promoting sodium reabsorption from the renal tubules. The serum sodium level reflects the ratio of sodium to water, not necessarily the loss or gain of sodium. Thus, changes in the serum sodium level may reflect either a primary water imbalance, a primary sodium imbalance, or a combination of the two. Sodium imbalances are typically associated with imbalances in ECF volume (Figures 19.11 and 19.12).

TABLE 19.2	NORMAL SERUM ELECTROLYTE VALUES
Electrolyte	**Normal Value**
Anions	
Bicarbonate (HCO_3^-)	23–29 mmol/L
Chloride (Cl^-)	98–106 mmol/L
Phosphate (PO_4^{3-})	1.0–1.5 mmol/L
Protein	60–80 g/L
Cations	
Potassium (K^+)	3.5–5.1 mmol/L
Magnesium (Mg^{2+})	0.65–1.05 mmol/L
Sodium (Na^+)	136–145 mmol/L
Calcium (Ca^{2+}) (total)	2.10–2.50 mmol/L
Calcium (ionized)	1.15–1.35 mmol/L

Source: Pagana, K. D., Pagana, T. J., & Pike-MacDonald, F. A. (2019). *Mosby's Canadian manual of diagnostic and laboratory tests* (2nd ed.). Elsevier.

Hypernatremia. The serum sodium level may become elevated as a result of water loss or sodium gain. Because sodium is the major determinant of the ECF osmolality, hypernatremia causes hyperosmolality. In turn, hyperosmolality causes a shift of water out of the cells, which leads to cellular dehydration.

As discussed earlier, the primary protection against the development of hyperosmolality is thirst. As the plasma osmolality increases, the thirst centre in the hypothalamus is stimulated, and the individual seeks fluids.

Hypernatremia is not a problem in an alert person who has access to water, can sense thirst, and is able to swallow. Hypernatremia secondary to water deficiency is often the result of an impaired level of consciousness or an inability to obtain fluids. Unconscious patients and certain cognitively impaired patients are at risk because of an inability to express thirst and act on it.

Several clinical states can produce water loss and hypernatremia (Table 19.3). A deficiency in the synthesis of ADH or in its release from the posterior pituitary gland (central diabetes insipidus) or a decrease in kidney responsiveness to ADH (nephrogenic diabetes insipidus) can result in profound diuresis, causing a water deficit and hypernatremia. Hyperosmolality can result from administration of concentrated hyperosmolar tube feedings and osmotic diuretics (mannitol), as well as from hyperglycemia associated with uncontrolled diabetes mellitus. These situations result in osmotic diuresis. Dilute urine is lost, leaving behind a high solute load. Other causes of hypernatremia include excessive sweating and increased sensible losses from high fever.

Sodium intake in excess of water intake can also lead to hypernatremia. Causes of sodium gain include IV administration of hypertonic saline or sodium bicarbonate, use of sodium-containing drugs, excessive oral intake of sodium (ingestion of seawater), and primary aldosteronism (hypersecretion of aldosterone), which in turn is caused by a tumour of the adrenal glands.

Symptoms are primarily the result of changes in the plasma osmolality that lead to changes in the volume of cellular water (see Table 19.3). Dehydration of neurons leads to neurological manifestations such as intense thirst, lethargy, agitation, seizures, and even coma. Sodium excess also has a direct effect on the irritability and conduction of neurons, causing them to be more easily excited. Patients with hypernatremia will also exhibit the symptoms of any accompanying volume imbalance.

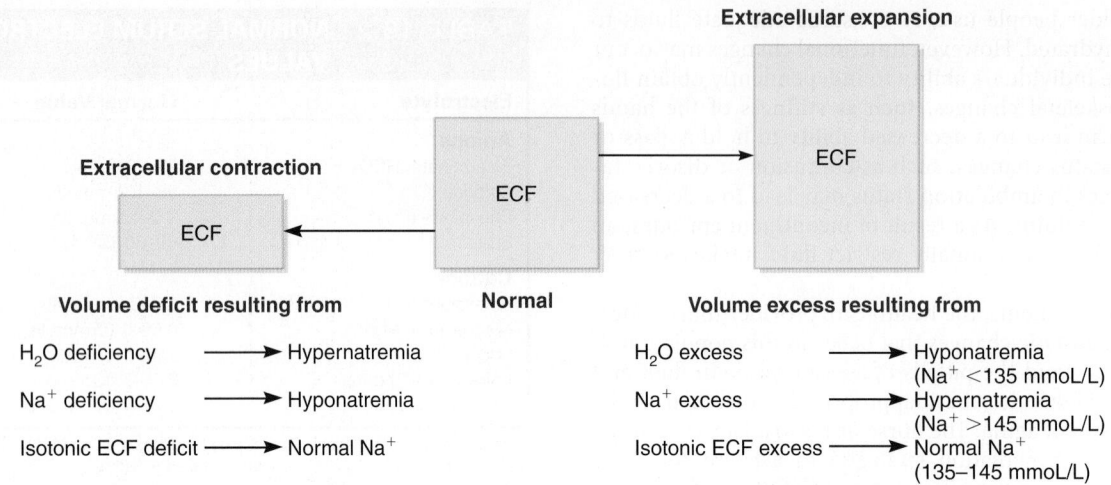

FIG. 19.11 Differential assessment of extracellular fluid (ECF) volume.

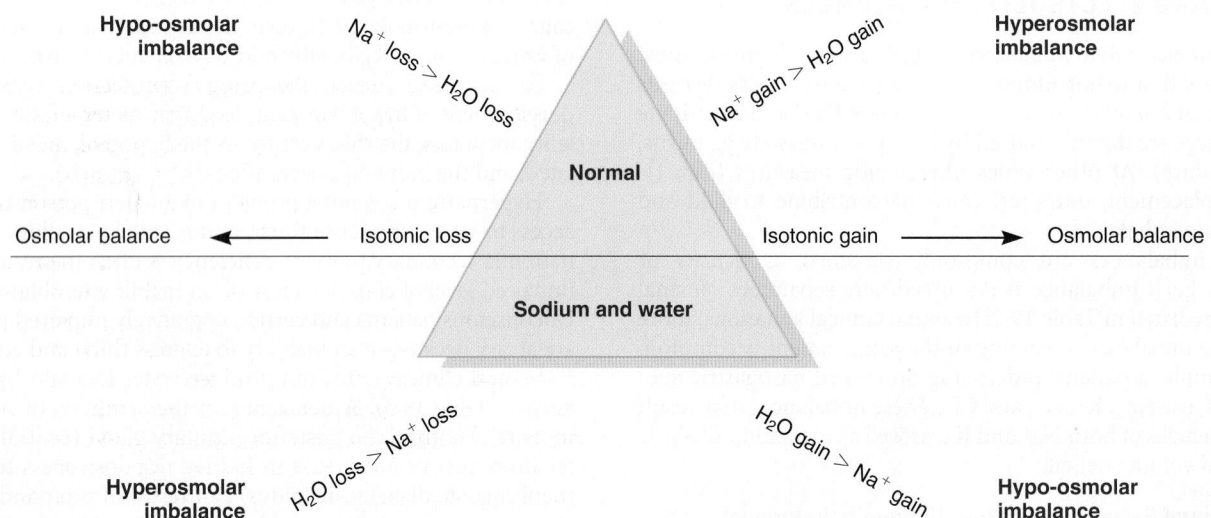

FIG. 19.12 Isotonic gains and losses affect mainly the extracellular fluid (ECF) compartment, with little or no water movement into the cells. Hypertonic imbalances cause water to move from inside the cell into the ECF to dilute the concentrated sodium, which results in cell shrinkage. Hypotonic imbalances cause water to move into the cell, which results in cell swelling.

Interprofessional Care. The goal of treatment in hypernatremia that is caused by either water loss or sodium gain is to treat the underlying cause. In the treatment of primary water deficit, fluid is replaced either orally or by IV infusion with isotonic fluids, such as 0.9% sodium chloride (Reddi, 2018). Serum sodium levels must be reduced gradually to prevent too rapid a shift of water back into the cells. Overly rapid correction of hypernatremia can result in cerebral edema. The risk is greatest in patients who have developed hypernatremia over several days or longer.

The goal of treatment for sodium excess is to dilute the sodium concentration with salt-free IV fluids, such as 5% dextrose in water, and to promote excretion of the excess sodium by administering diuretics. Dietary sodium intake is often restricted. (See Chapter 51 for specific treatment of diabetes insipidus.) To prevent hypernatremia in older persons or cognitively impaired patients, it is important to pay close attention to fluid intake and losses. Regular administration of oral fluids must be incorporated into these patients' plan of care (Kear, 2017).

Hyponatremia. Hyponatremia (low serum sodium) may result from a loss of sodium-containing fluids, water excess in relation to the amount of sodium (dilutional hyponatremia), or a combination of both (see Table 19.3). Hyponatremia is usually associated with ECF hypo-osmolality that results from the excess water. To restore balance, fluid shifts out of the ECF and into the cells, leading to cellular edema. Common causes of hyponatremia caused by water excess are inappropriate use of sodium-free or hypotonic IV fluids. This may occur in patients after surgery or major trauma, during administration of fluids in patients with renal failure, or in patients with psychiatric disorders associated with excessive water intake. In SIADH, dilutional hyponatremia results from abnormal retention of water. (See Chapter 51 for a discussion of the causes of SIADH.)

Losses of sodium-rich body fluids from the GI tract, the kidneys, or the skin indirectly result in hyponatremia. Because these fluids are either isotonic or hypotonic, sodium is lost with an equal or greater proportion of water. However, hyponatremia

TABLE 19.3 WATER AND SODIUM IMBALANCES
Causes and Clinical Manifestations

Water Excess: Hyponatremia (Na⁺ Level <136 mmol/L)	Water Deficit: Hypernatremia (Na⁺ Level >145 mmol/L)
Causes	
Sodium loss	Water loss (sodium concentration)
• GI losses: diarrhea, vomiting, fistulas, NG suction	• ↑ Insensible water loss or perspiration (high fever, heatstroke)
• Renal losses: diuretics, adrenal insufficiency, Na⁺ wasting renal disease	• Diabetes insipidus
• Skin losses: burns, wound drainage	• Osmotic diuresis
Water gain (sodium dilution)	Sodium gain
• SIADH	• IV hypertonic NaCl
• Heart failure	• IV sodium bicarbonate
• Excessive hypotonic IV fluids	• IV excessive isotonic NaCl
• Primary polydipsia	• Primary hyperaldosteronism
	• Saltwater near-drowning
Clinical Manifestations	
Decreased ECF volume (sodium loss)	Decreased ECF volume (water loss)
• Irritability, apprehension, confusion	• Intense thirst; dry, swollen tongue
• Postural hypotension	• Restlessness, agitation, twitching
• Tachycardia	• Seizures, coma
• Rapid, thready pulse	• Weakness
• ↓ CVP	• Postural hypotension, ↓ CVP
• ↓ Jugular venous filling	• Weight loss
• Nausea, vomiting	
• Dry mucous membranes	
• Weight loss	
• Tremors, seizures, coma	
Normal or increased ECF volume (water gain)	Normal or increased ECF volume (sodium gain)
• Headache, lassitude, apathy	• Intense thirst
• Weakness, confusion	• Restlessness, agitation, twitching
• Nausea, vomiting	• Seizures, coma
• Weight gain	• Flushed skin
• ↑ BP, ↑ CVP	• Weight gain
• Muscle spasms, seizures, coma	• Peripheral and pulmonary edema
	• ↑ BP, ↑ CVP

BP, blood pressure; CVP, central venous pressure; ECF, extracellular fluid; GI, gastrointestinal; IV, intravenous; NaCl, sodium chloride; NG, nasogastric; SIADH, syndrome of inappropriate antidiuretic hormone.

TABLE 19.4 CAUSES OF ECF VOLUME IMBALANCES

ECF Volume Deficit	ECF Volume Excess
Increased loss	Increased retention
• Vomiting	• Heart failure
• Diarrhea	• Cushing's syndrome
• Fistula drainage	• Chronic liver disease with portal hypertension
• GI tract suction	• Long-term use of corticosteroids
• Excessive sweating	• Renal failure
• Third-space fluid shifts (e.g., burns, intestinal obstruction)	
• Overuse of diuretics	
• Hemorrhage	
Decreased intake	Increased intake
• Nausea	• Rare when renal function is adequate
• Anorexia	• Excessive IV administration of fluids
• Inability to drink	
• Inability to obtain water	

ECF, extracellular fluid; GI, gastrointestinal; IV, intravenous.

includes fluid replacement with sodium-containing solutions. The nurse must monitor serum sodium levels and the patient's response to therapy to avoid rapid correction or overcorrection. Rapidly increasing levels of sodium can cause osmotic demyelination syndrome with permanent damage to nerve cells in the brain. An accurate record of fluid input and output is essential. Commercially available oral rehydration fluids containing electrolytes may help prevent the development of hyponatremia in the home setting.

Extracellular Fluid Volume Imbalances. ECF volume deficit (hypovolemia) and ECF volume excess (hypervolemia) are commonly occurring clinical conditions (Table 19.4). ECF volume imbalances are typically accompanied by one or more electrolyte imbalances. As previously discussed, volume imbalances are often associated with changes in the serum sodium level. Fluid volume deficit can occur with abnormal loss of body fluids (e.g., through diarrhea, fistula drainage, hemorrhage, polyuria), decreased intake, or a plasma–to–interstitial fluid shift. Although the terms are often used interchangeably, fluid volume deficit and dehydration are not the same; *dehydration* refers to loss of pure water alone without a corresponding loss of sodium. Fluid volume excess may result from excessive intake of fluids, abnormal retention of fluids (e.g., heart failure, renal failure), or interstitial–to–plasma fluid shift. Although shifts in fluid between the plasma and the interstitium do not alter the overall volume of the ECF, these shifts do result in changes in the clinically important intravascular volume.

Interprofessional Care. The goal of treatment for fluid volume deficit is to correct the underlying cause and to replace both water and electrolytes. Balanced IV solutions, such as lactated Ringer's solution, are usually given. Isotonic NaCl is used when rapid volume replacement is indicated. Blood is administered when volume loss is caused by blood loss.

The goal of treatment for fluid volume excess is removal of sodium and water without producing abnormal changes in the electrolyte composition or osmolality of ECF. The primary cause must be identified and treated. IV therapy is usually not indicated for this type of fluid imbalance. Diuretics and fluid restriction are the primary forms of therapy. Restriction of sodium intake may also be indicated. If the fluid excess leads to ascites or pleural effusion, an abdominal paracentesis or thoracentesis may be necessary.

develops as the body responds to the fluid volume deficit with activation of the thirst mechanism and by releasing ADH. The resultant retention of water lowers the sodium concentration.

The manifestations of hyponatremia are due to cellular swelling and first appear in the CNS (see Table 19.3). Mild hyponatremia has minor, nonspecific neurological symptoms, including headache, irritability, and difficulty concentrating. More severe hyponatremia can cause confusion, vomiting, seizures, and even coma. If hyponatremia is severe and develops rapidly, irreversible neurological damage or death from brain herniation can occur (Reddi, 2018).

Interprofessional Care. In hyponatremia that is caused by water excess, fluid restriction is often all that is needed to treat the problem. If severe symptoms (seizures) develop, small amounts of IV hypertonic saline solution (3% sodium chloride [NaCl]) are administered to restore the serum sodium level while the body is returning to a normal water balance. Treatment of hyponatremia associated with abnormal fluid loss

NURSING MANAGEMENT
SODIUM AND VOLUME IMBALANCES

NURSING DIAGNOSES

Nursing diagnoses and interprofessional issues for patients with various fluid and sodium imbalances include but are not limited to the following:

ECF volume excess:
- *Fluid overload* resulting from *excessive sodium intake*
- *Inadequate airway clearance* resulting from *retained secretions*
- *Potential for reduced skin integrity* resulting from *alteration in fluid volume (edema)*
- *Reduced self-concept* resulting from *alteration in self-perception*
- Potential complications: pulmonary edema, ascites

ECF volume deficit:
- *Reduced fluid volume* resulting from *insufficient fluid intake*
- *Inadequate cardiac output* resulting from *excessive ECF losses or decreased fluid intake*
- Potential complication: hypovolemic shock

Hypernatremia:
- *Potential for injury* as a result of *alteration in cognitive functioning (seizures)*

Hyponatremia:
- *Potential for injury* as a result of *alteration in cognitive functioning* (decreased level of consciousness)

NURSING IMPLEMENTATION

INTAKE AND OUTPUT. The 24-hour records of intake and output contain valuable information regarding fluid and electrolyte issues. Sources of excessive intake or fluid losses can be identified on a properly recorded intake-and-output flow sheet. Intake should include oral, IV, and tube feedings and retained irrigants. Fluid output includes urine, excess perspiration, wound or tube drainage, vomitus, and diarrhea. Fluid loss from wounds and perspiration should be estimated. Urine specific gravity can be measured. Readings higher than 1.030 indicate that the urine is concentrated, whereas those lower than 1.005 indicate that the urine is diluted.

CARDIOVASCULAR CHANGES. Monitoring patients for cardiovascular changes is necessary to prevent or detect complications from sodium and volume imbalances. Signs and symptoms of ECF volume excess and deficit are reflected in changes in blood pressure, pulse force, and jugular venous visibility. In fluid volume excess, the pulse is full and bounding. Because of the expanded intravascular volume, the pulse is not easily obliterated by the pressure cuff. Increased volume causes distension of neck veins (jugular venous distension) and increased blood pressure.

In mild to moderate fluid volume deficit, compensatory mechanisms include sympathetic nervous system stimulation of the heart and peripheral vasoconstriction. Stimulation of the heart increases heart rate and, in combination with vasoconstriction, maintains blood pressure within normal limits. A change in position from lying to sitting or standing may elicit a further increase in heart rate or a decrease in blood pressure (orthostatic hypotension). If vasoconstriction and tachycardia provide inadequate compensation, hypotension occurs when the patient is recumbent. Severe fluid volume deficit can cause a weak, thready pulse that is easily obliterated and flattened neck veins. Severe, untreated fluid deficit results in shock.

RESPIRATORY CHANGES. Both fluid excess and fluid deficit affect respiratory status. Fluid excess results in pulmonary congestion and pulmonary edema as increased hydrostatic pressure in the pulmonary vessels forces fluid into the alveoli. Affected patients exhibit shortness of breath, irritative cough, and moist crackles on auscultation. Patients with fluid deficit demonstrate an increased respiratory rate because of decreased tissue perfusion and resultant hypoxia.

NEUROLOGICAL CHANGES. Changes in neurological function may occur with sodium and water imbalances. With increased water volume and hyponatremia, water moves by osmosis into the brain cells. Alternatively, decreased water volume and hypernatremia cause water to shift out of the brain cells, with resultant shrinkage. In addition, profound volume depletion may cause an alteration in sensorium secondary to reduced cerebral tissue perfusion.

Assessment of neurological function includes evaluation of (1) the level of consciousness, which includes responses to verbal and painful stimuli and the determination of a person's orientation to time, place, and person; (2) pupillary response to light and equality of pupil size; and (3) voluntary movement of the extremities, degree of muscle strength, and reflexes. Nursing care focuses on maintaining patient safety.

DAILY WEIGHT MEASUREMENTS. Accurate daily weight measurements are the easiest way to estimate volume status. An increase of 1 kg is equal to 1 000 mL (1 L) of fluid retention (provided that the person has maintained usual dietary intake or has not been on nothing-by-mouth [NPO] status). However, weight changes can be relied on only if obtained under standardized conditions. Obtaining an accurate weight depends on the patient being weighed at the same time every day, with the same garments on, and on the same carefully calibrated scale. Excess bedding should be removed, and all drainage bags should be emptied before the weighing. If bulky dressings or tubes are present, which may not necessarily be used every day, a notation regarding these variables should be recorded on the flow sheet or nursing notes.

SKIN ASSESSMENT AND CARE. Clues to fluid volume deficit and excess can be detected by inspection of the skin. Skin should be examined for turgor and mobility. Normally, a fold of skin, when pinched, moves readily and, on release, rapidly returns to its former position. Skin areas over the sternum, the abdomen, and the anterior forearm are the usual sites for evaluation of tissue turgor (Figure 19.13). In older people, decreased skin turgor is less predictive of fluid deficit because of the loss of tissue elasticity (Sterns, 2020).

In ECF volume deficit, skin turgor is diminished; there is a lag in the pinched skinfold's return to its original state (referred to as *tenting*). In mild fluid deficits, the skin may appear warm, dry, and wrinkled. These signs may be difficult to evaluate in an older person because the patient's skin may be normally dry, wrinkled, and nonelastic. In more severe deficits, the skin may be cool and moist if there is vasoconstriction to compensate for the decreased fluid volume. Oral mucous membranes are dry, the tongue may be furrowed, and many affected individuals report thirst. Routine oral care is critical for the comfort of a patient who is dehydrated or has a fluid restriction order.

Edematous skin may feel cool because of fluid accumulation and a decrease in blood flow secondary to the pressure of the fluid. The fluid can stretch the skin, causing it to feel taut and hard. The nurse assesses edema by pressing with a thumb or forefinger over the edematous area. A grading scale (ranging from 1+ [slight edema; 2-mm indentation] to 4+ [pitting edema; 8-mm indentation]) is used to standardize the description if an

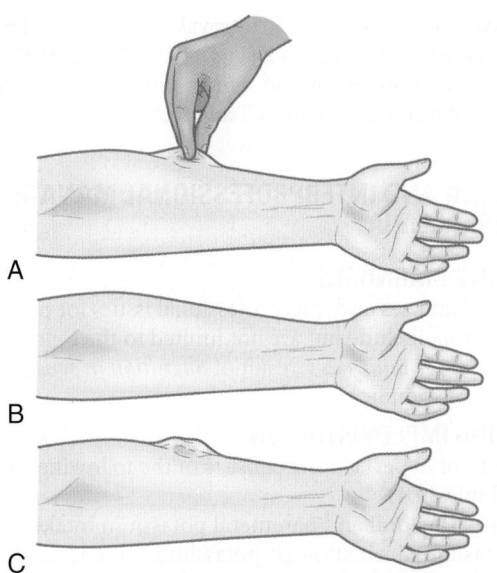

FIG. 19.13 Assessment of skin turgor. **A** and **B,** When normal skin is pinched, it resumes shape in seconds. **C,** If the skin stays wrinkled for 20 to 30 seconds, the patient has poor skin turgor.

indentation remains when pressure is released. The nurse must evaluate for edema in areas where soft tissues overlie a bone, particularly the tibia, fibula, and sacrum.

Good skin care for the person with fluid volume excess or deficit is important. Edematous tissues must be protected from extremes of heat and cold, prolonged pressure, and trauma. Frequent skin care and changes in position protect the patient from skin breakdown. Elevation of edematous extremities helps promote venous return and fluid reabsorption. Dehydrated skin needs frequent care without the use of soap. The application of moisturizing creams or oils increases moisture retention and stimulates circulation.

OTHER NURSING MEASURES. The nurse should administer IV fluids as ordered and carefully monitor the rates of infusion of IV fluid solutions, especially when large volumes of fluid are being given. This is especially true in patients with cardiac, renal, or neurological conditions. Patients receiving tube feedings need supplementary water added to their enteral formula. The amount of water depends on the osmolarity of the feeding and the patient's condition.

Patients with nasogastric suction should not be allowed to drink water because it will increase the loss of electrolytes. On occasion, such patients may be given small amounts of ice chips to suck. A nasogastric tube should always be irrigated with isotonic saline solution and not with water. Water causes diffusion of electrolytes into the gastric lumen from mucosal cells; the electrolytes are then suctioned away.

Nurses in hospital and community settings should encourage and often assist older or debilitated patients in maintaining an adequate oral intake. This may be accomplished by giving patients a drink as part of the morning care, encouraging extra sips of fluid with medications, and including a drink of fluids as part of one-on-one conversations.

Potassium Imbalances

Potassium is the major ICF cation; 98% of the body potassium is intracellular. For example, potassium concentration within muscle cells is approximately 140 mmol/L; potassium concentration in the ECF is 3.5 to 5.1 mmol/L. The sodium–potassium pump in cell membranes maintains this concentration difference by pumping potassium into the cell and sodium out, a process fueled by the breakdown of ATP. The ratio of ECF potassium to ICF potassium is the major factor in the resting neuron's membrane potential. Many of the symptoms related to potassium imbalance are caused by changes in the ratio of ECF and ICF potassium (McCance & Huether, 2019).

Potassium is critical for many cellular and metabolic functions. It is necessary for the transmission and conduction of nerve impulses, maintenance of normal cardiac rhythms, and skeletal and smooth muscle contraction. As the major intracellular cation, potassium regulates intracellular osmolality and promotes cellular growth. Potassium is necessary to promote the storage of glucose in liver and skeletal muscle cells (McCance & Huether, 2019). Potassium also plays a role in acid–base balance, which is discussed with acid–base regulation later in this chapter.

Diet is the source of potassium. The typical Western diet contains approximately 50 to 100 mmol of potassium daily, mainly from fruits, dried fruits, and vegetables. Many salt substitutes contain substantial potassium. Patients may receive potassium from parenteral sources, including IV fluids, stored transfused blood, and potassium–penicillin.

The kidneys are the primary route for potassium loss. Approximately 90% of the daily potassium intake is eliminated by the kidneys; the remainder is lost in the stool and sweat. If kidney function is significantly impaired, toxic levels of potassium may be retained. There is an inverse relationship between sodium and potassium reabsorption in the kidneys. Factors that cause sodium retention (e.g., low blood volume, increased aldosterone level) cause potassium loss in the urine. Large urine volumes can be associated with excess loss of potassium in the urine. The ability of the kidneys to conserve potassium is weak even when body stores are depleted (McCance & Huether, 2019).

Disruptions in the dynamic equilibrium between ICF and ECF potassium often cause clinical problems. Among the factors causing potassium to move from the ECF to the ICF are the following:

- Insulin
- Alkalosis
- β-Adrenergic stimulation (catecholamine release in stress, coronary ischemia, delirium tremens, or administration of β-adrenergic agonist drugs)
- Rapid cell building (administration of folic acid or cobalamin [vitamin B_{12}] to patients with megaloblastic anemia, which results in marked production of red blood cells [RBCs])

Factors that cause potassium to move from the ICF to the ECF include acidosis, trauma to cells (as in massive soft tissue damage or in tumour lysis), and exercise. Both digoxin-like drugs and β-adrenergic–blocking drugs (e.g., propranolol [Inderal]) can impair entry of potassium into cells, which results in the higher ECF potassium concentration. Causes of potassium imbalance are summarized in Table 19.5.

Hyperkalemia. Hyperkalemia (high serum levels of potassium) may be caused by a massive intake of potassium, impaired renal excretion, shift of potassium from the ICF to the ECF, or a combination of these factors. The most common cause of hyperkalemia is renal failure. Hyperkalemia is also common in patients with massive cell destruction (e.g., burn or crush injury, tumour lysis), rapid transfusion of aged blood, and catabolic state (e.g., severe infections). Metabolic acidosis, particularly when the chloride level is normal, is associated with a shift of potassium ions from the ICF to the ECF as hydrogen ions move into the cell. Adrenal insufficiency leads to retention of potassium ions in the serum because of aldosterone deficiency. Certain drugs, such as potassium-sparing diuretics (e.g., spironolactone [Aldactone], triamterene) and angiotensin-converting enzyme (ACE) inhibitors (e.g., enalapril [Vasotec], lisinopril [Prinivil]), may contribute to the development of hyperkalemia. Both types of medications reduce the kidneys' ability to excrete excess potassium (see Table 19.5).

Clinical Manifestations. Hyperkalemia causes membrane depolarization, altering cell excitability. Skeletal muscles become weak or paralyzed. The first symptom may be leg cramping. The most clinically significant issues are the disturbances in cardiac conduction. The initial finding is tall, peaked T waves. As potassium increases, cardiac depolarization decreases, leading to loss

of P waves, a prolonged P–R interval, ST segment depression, and a widening QRS complex (Figure 19.14). Heart block, ventricular fibrillation, or cardiac standstill may occur. Other clinical manifestations are listed in Table 19.5.

NURSING AND INTERPROFESSIONAL MANAGEMENT HYPERKALEMIA

NURSING DIAGNOSES
Nursing diagnoses and interprofessional issues for patients with hyperkalemia include but are not limited to the following:
- *Potential for injury* as a result of *alteration in sensation*
- Potential complication: dysrhythmias

NURSING IMPLEMENTATION
Treatment of hyperkalemia consists of the following (see Chapter 49, Table 49.4):
1. Eliminating oral and parenteral potassium intake
2. Increasing elimination of potassium. This is accomplished with diuretics, dialysis, and use of ion-exchange resins such as sodium polystyrene sulphonate (Kayexalate). Increased fluid intake can enhance renal potassium elimination.

TABLE 19.5   POTASSIUM IMBALANCES
Causes and Clinical Manifestations

Hypokalemia (K⁺ Level <3.5 mmol/L)	Hyperkalemia (K⁺ Level >5.1 mmol/L)
Causes	
Potassium loss	Excess potassium intake
• GI losses: diarrhea, vomiting, fistulas, NG suction	• Excessive or rapid parenteral administration
• Renal losses: diuretics, hyperaldosteronism, magnesium depletion	• Potassium-containing medications (e.g., potassium–penicillin)
• Skin losses: diaphoresis	• Potassium-containing salt substitute
• Dialysis	
Shift of potassium into cells	Shift of potassium out of cells
• Increased insulin (e.g., IV dextrose load)	• Acidosis
• Alkalosis	• Tissue catabolism (e.g., fever, sepsis, burns)
• Tissue repair	• Crush injury
• ↑ Epinephrine (e.g., stress)	• Tumour lysis syndrome
Lack of potassium intake	Failure to eliminate potassium
• Starvation	• Renal disease
• Diet with low potassium content	• Potassium-sparing diuretics
• Failure to include potassium in parenteral fluids if NPO status is in effect	• Adrenal insufficiency • ACE inhibitors
Clinical Manifestations	
• Fatigue	• Irritability
• Muscle weakness	• Anxiety
• Leg cramps	• Abdominal cramping, diarrhea
• Nausea, vomiting, ileus	• Weakness of lower extremities
• Soft, flabby muscles	• Paresthesias
• Paresthesias, decreased reflexes	• Irregular pulse
• Weak, irregular pulse	• Cardiac standstill if hyperkalemia is sudden or severe
• Polyuria	
• Hyperglycemia	
Electrocardiographic Changes	
• ST segment depression	• Tall, peaked T wave
• Flattened T wave	• Prolonged P–R interval
• Presence of U wave	• ST depression
• Ventricular dysrhythmias (e.g., PVCs)	• Loss of P wave
• Bradycardia	• Widening QRS complex
• Enhanced digitalis effect	• Ventricular fibrillation • Ventricular standstill

ACE, angiotensin-converting enzyme; *GI*, gastrointestinal; *IV*, intravenous; *NG*, nasogastric; *NPO*, nothing by mouth; *PVC*, premature ventricular contraction.

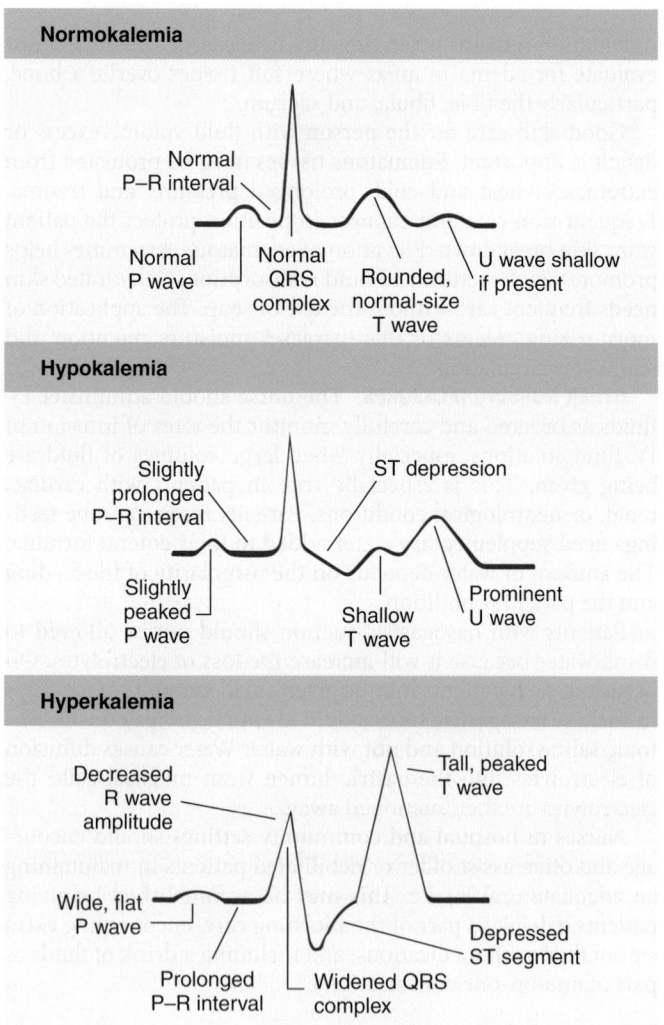

FIG. 19.14 Electrocardiographic changes associated with alterations in potassium status. Source: Redrawn from McCance, K. L., & Huether, S. E. (2019). *Pathophysiology: The biologic basis for disease in adults and children* (8th ed., p. 116). Mosby.

3. Forcing potassium from the ECF to the ICF. This is accomplished by administration of IV insulin (along with glucose so that the patient does not become hypoglycemic) or by administration of IV sodium bicarbonate in the correction of acidosis. In rare cases, a β-adrenergic agonist (e.g., epinephrine) is administered.
4. Reversing the membrane effects of the elevated ECF potassium by administering calcium gluconate intravenously. Calcium ion can immediately reverse the effect of the depolarization on cell excitability.

In cases in which the elevation of potassium level is mild and the kidneys are functioning, it may be sufficient to withhold potassium from the diet and IV sources and increase renal elimination by administering fluids and possibly diuretics. Kayexalate, which is administered via the GI tract, binds potassium in exchange for sodium, and the resin is excreted in feces (see Chapter 49). All patients with clinically significant hyperkalemia should be monitored electrocardiographically to detect dysrhythmias and to monitor the effects of therapy. Patients with moderate hyperkalemia should additionally receive one of the treatments to force potassium into cells, usually IV insulin and glucose. The patient experiencing dangerous cardiac dysrhythmias should receive IV calcium gluconate immediately; this serves to protect the patient while the potassium is being eliminated and forced into cells. Hemodialysis is an effective means of removing potassium from the body in patients with renal failure.

HYPOKALEMIA

Hypokalemia (low serum levels of potassium) can result from abnormal losses of potassium caused by a shift of potassium from ECF to ICF or, in rare cases, by deficient dietary potassium intake. The most common causes of hypokalemia are abnormal losses, via either the kidneys or the GI tract. Abnormal losses occur in patients with diuresis, particularly in patients with an elevated aldosterone level. Aldosterone is released when the circulating blood volume is low; it causes sodium retention in the kidneys but loss of potassium in the urine. Magnesium deficiency may contribute to the development of potassium depletion. Low plasma magnesium stimulates renin release and subsequently increases aldosterone levels, which results in potassium excretion. GI tract losses of potassium secondary to diarrhea, laxative abuse, vomiting, and ileostomy drainage can cause hypokalemia.

Metabolic alkalosis can cause a shift of potassium into cells in exchange for hydrogen, thus lowering the potassium level in the ECF and causing symptomatic hypokalemia. Hypokalemia is sometimes associated with the treatment of diabetic ketoacidosis because of a combination of factors, including an increased urinary potassium loss and a shift of potassium into cells with the administration of insulin and correction of acidosis. A less common cause of hypokalemia is the sudden initiation of cell formation—for example, the formation of RBCs as in treatment of anemia with cobalamin, folic acid, or erythropoietin.

Clinical Manifestations. Hypokalemia alters resting membrane potential. It most commonly is associated with hyperpolarization or an increased negative charge within the cell. This causes excitability problems in many types of tissue. The most serious clinical problems are cardiac. The incidence of potentially lethal ventricular dysrhythmias is increased in hypokalemia. Patients should be monitored with electrocardiography (ECG) for signs of hypokalemia. These changes include impaired repolarization, which results in a flattening of the T wave and eventually in emergence of a U wave. The P-wave amplitude may increase and may become peaked (see Figure 19.14). Patients taking digoxin experience increased digoxin toxicity if their serum potassium level is low. Skeletal muscle weakness and paralysis may occur with hypokalemia. As with hyperkalemia, symptoms are most often observed in the legs. Severe hypokalemia can cause weakness or paralysis of respiratory muscles, leading to shallow respirations and respiratory arrest. Muscle cramping and muscle cell breakdown (known as rhabdomyolysis) can be caused by hypokalemia. This can cause myoglobin to appear in the plasma and the urine, which can, in turn, lead to renal failure.

Smooth muscle function is altered by hypokalemia. Affected patients may experience decreased GI motility (e.g., paralytic ileus), altered airway responsiveness, and impaired regulation of arteriolar blood flow, all of which possibly contribute to muscle cell breakdown. Finally, hypokalemia can impair function in nonmuscle tissue. With prolonged hypokalemia, the kidneys are unable to concentrate urine, and diuresis occurs. Release of insulin is impaired, which often leads to hyperglycemia. Clinical manifestations of hypokalemia are presented in Table 19.5.

NURSING AND INTERPROFESSIONAL MANAGEMENT HYPOKALEMIA

NURSING DIAGNOSES
Nursing diagnoses and interprofessional issues for patients with hypokalemia include but are not limited to the following:
- *Potential for injury as a result of reduced psychomotor functioning* (muscle weakness, hyporeflexia)
- Potential complication: Dysrhythmias

NURSING IMPLEMENTATION
Hypokalemia is treated by administration of potassium chloride (KCl) supplements and increasing dietary intake of potassium. KCl supplements can be given orally or intravenously. Except in severe deficiencies, KCl is never given unless the urine output is at least 0.5 mL/kg of body weight per hour. KCl supplements added to IV solutions should never exceed 60 mmol/L (mEq/L). The preferred level is 40 mmol/L (40 mEq/L). IV KCl infusion rates should not exceed 10 mmol/L per hour unless the patient is in a critical care setting with continuous ECG monitoring and central line access for administration (Mount, 2019). When given intravenously, potassium may cause pain in the area of the vein where it is entering. Because KCl is irritating to the vein, IV sites need to be assessed at least hourly for phlebitis and infiltration. Infiltration can cause necrosis and sloughing of the surrounding tissue. The nurse must teach patients ways to prevent hypokalemia (Table 19.6). Patients at risk for hypokalemia should have serum potassium levels monitored regularly.

SAFETY ALERT
- KCl given intravenously must always be diluted.
- Never give KCl via IV push or in concentrated amounts.
- IV bags containing KCl should be inverted several times to ensure even distribution in the bag.
- Never add KCl to a hanging IV bag, to prevent giving a bolus dose.

Calcium Imbalances
Calcium is obtained from ingested foods. However, only approximately 30% is absorbed in the GI tract. More than 99% of the body's calcium is combined with phosphorus and concentrated in the skeletal system. Bones serve as a readily available store of calcium. Thus, to avoid wide variations in serum calcium levels, the movement of calcium into or out of the bone is regulated.

TABLE 19.6	PATIENT & CAREGIVER TEACHING GUIDE

Prevention of Hypokalemia

1. Teach the patient and caregivers the signs and symptoms of hypokalemia and to report them to the health care provider.
2. For the patient taking potassium-losing diuretics:
   - Explain the importance of increasing dietary potassium intake, especially if the patient is receiving a thiazide or loop diuretic.
   - Teach the patient which foods have high potassium content (see Chapter 49, Table 49.10).
   - Explain that salt substitutes contain approximately 50–60 mmol of potassium per teaspoon and help raise potassium level if the patient is taking a potassium-losing diuretic.
3. For the patient taking potassium-sparing diuretics:
   - Explain that salt substitutes and foods with high potassium content should be avoided.
4. For the patient taking oral potassium supplements:
   - Instruct the patient to take the medication as prescribed to prevent overdosage and to take the supplement with a full glass of water to help it dissolve in the GI tract.
5. For the patient taking digitalis preparations and others at risk for hypokalemia:
   - Explain the importance of having serum potassium levels monitored regularly because a low potassium level enhances the action of digitalis.

GI, gastrointestinal.

Usually, the amounts of calcium and phosphorus found in the serum have an inverse relationship; that is, as one increases, the other decreases (McCance & Huether, 2019). The functions of calcium include transmission of nerve impulses, myocardial contractions, blood clotting, formation of teeth and bone, and muscle contractions.

Calcium is present in the serum in three forms: free or ionized; bound to protein (primarily albumin); and complexed with phosphate, citrate, or carbonate. The ionized form is the biologically active form. Approximately half of the total serum calcium is ionized.

Calcium is typically measured in millimoles per litre (mmol/L). As usually reported, serum calcium levels reflect the total calcium level (all three forms), although ionized calcium levels are sometimes reported separately. The levels listed in Table 19.7 reflect total calcium levels. Changes in serum pH alter the level of ionized calcium without altering the total calcium level. Acidosis decreases calcium binding to albumin, which leads to more ionized calcium, and alkalosis increases calcium binding, which leads to decreased ionized calcium. Alterations in serum albumin levels affect interpretation of total calcium levels. Low albumin levels result in a drop in the total calcium level, although the level of ionized calcium does not change as much.

Calcium balance is controlled by parathyroid hormone (PTH), calcitonin, and vitamin D (McCance & Huether, 2019). PTH is produced by the parathyroid gland. Its production and release are stimulated when serum calcium levels are low. PTH increases bone resorption (movement of calcium out of bones), increases GI absorption of calcium, and increases renal tubule reabsorption of calcium.

Calcitonin is produced by the thyroid gland, and its production and release are stimulated when serum calcium levels are high. It opposes the action of PTH and thus lowers the serum calcium level by decreasing GI absorption, increasing calcium deposition into bone, and promoting renal excretion.

TABLE 19.7	CALCIUM IMBALANCES

Causes and Clinical Manifestations

Hypocalcemia (Ca^{2+} Level <2.10 mmol/L)	Hypercalcemia (Ca^{2+} Level >2.50 mmol/L)
Causes	
Decreased total calcium	Increased total calcium
• Chronic renal failure	• Multiple myeloma
• Elevated phosphorus	• Other malignancy
• Primary hypoparathyroidism	• Prolonged immobilization
• Vitamin D deficiency	• Hyperparathyroidism
• Magnesium deficiency	• Vitamin D overdose
• Acute pancreatitis	• Thiazide diuretics
• Loop diuretics	• Milk–alkali syndrome
• Chronic alcoholism	
• Diarrhea	
• ↓ Serum albumin (patient is usually asymptomatic because of normal ionized calcium level)	
Decreased ionized calcium	Increased ionized calcium
• Alkalosis	• Acidosis
• Excess administration of citrated blood	
Clinical Manifestations	
• Easy fatigability	• Lethargy, weakness
• Depression, anxiety, confusion	• Depressed reflexes
• Numbness and tingling in extremities and region around mouth	• Decreased memory
• Hyperreflexia, muscle cramps	• Confusion, personality changes, psychosis
• Chvostek's sign	• Anorexia, nausea, vomiting
• Trousseau's sign	• Bone pain, fractures
• Laryngeal spasm	• Polyuria, dehydration
• Tetany, seizures	• Nephrolithiasis
	• Stupor, coma
Electrocardiographic Changes	
• Elongation of ST segment	• Shortened ST segment
• Prolonged Q–T interval	• Shortened Q–T interval
• Ventricular tachycardia	• Ventricular dysrhythmias
	• Increased digitalis effect

Vitamin D is formed through the action of ultraviolet rays on a precursor found in the skin or is ingested in the diet. Vitamin D is important for absorption of calcium from the GI tract. Causes of calcium imbalances are listed in Table 19.7.

Hypercalcemia. More than 90% of hypercalcemia cases are caused by hyperparathyroidism and malignancy (Shane, 2021), especially from breast, renal, and squamous cell cancers, multiple myeloma, and lymphomas (Horwitz, 2020). Malignancies lead to hypercalcemia through bone destruction from tumour invasion or through tumour secretion of a parathyroid-related protein, which stimulates calcium release from bones. Hypercalcemia is also associated with vitamin D overdose. Prolonged immobilization results in bone mineral loss and increased calcium concentration. Hypercalcemia rarely occurs as a result of increased calcium intake (e.g., ingestion of antacids containing calcium, excessive administration during cardiac arrest).

Excess calcium blocks the effect of sodium in skeletal muscles, which leads to reduced excitability of both muscles and nerves (McCance & Huether, 2019). Manifestations of hypercalcemia include impaired memory, confusion, disorientation, fatigue, muscle weakness, constipation, cardiac dysrhythmias, and renal calculi (see Table 19.7).

NURSING AND INTERPROFESSIONAL MANAGEMENT
HYPERCALCEMIA

NURSING DIAGNOSES

Nursing diagnoses and interprofessional issues for patients with hypercalcemia include but are not limited to the following:

- *Potential for injury as a result of alteration in sensation*
- Potential complication: dysrhythmias

NURSING IMPLEMENTATION

The basic treatment of hypercalcemia is promotion of excretion of calcium in urine by administration of a loop diuretic (e.g., furosemide [Lasix]), and hydration of the patient with isotonic saline infusions. IV saline therapy necessitates careful monitoring. Fluid overload can occur in patients who cannot excrete the excess sodium because of impaired renal function.

Synthetic calcitonin can also be administered to lower serum calcium levels. A diet with low calcium content may be prescribed. Mobilization with weight-bearing activity is encouraged to enhance bone mineralization. In hypercalcemia associated with malignancy, biophosphates are used to inhibit the activity of osteoclasts. The medication of choice is zoledronic acid (Aclasta) because it does not have cytotoxic adverse effects, it inhibits bone resorption, and it decreases serum calcium and phosphorus levels (Shane & Berenson, 2020).

HYPOCALCEMIA

Any condition that causes a decrease in the production of PTH may result in the development of hypocalcemia. This may occur with surgical removal of a portion of or injury to the parathyroid glands during thyroid or neck surgery. Acute pancreatitis is another potential cause of hypocalcemia. Lipolysis, a consequence of pancreatitis, produces fatty acids that combine with calcium ions, which leads to a decrease in serum calcium levels. A patient who receives multiple blood transfusions can become hypocalcemic because the citrate used to anticoagulate the blood binds with the calcium. Sudden alkalosis may also result in symptomatic hypocalcemia despite a normal total serum calcium level. The high pH increases calcium binding to protein, decreasing the amount of ionized calcium. Hypocalcemia can occur if the diet has low calcium content or if loss of calcium is increased as a result of laxative abuse and malabsorption syndromes. (See Table 19.7 for the clinical manifestations and etiologies of hypocalcemia.)

Low calcium levels allow sodium to move into excitable cells, which increases depolarization. This results in increased nerve excitability and sustained muscle contraction that is referred to as tetany. Clinical signs of tetany include Trousseau's and Chvostek's signs. *Trousseau's sign* refers to carpal spasms induced by inflating a blood pressure cuff on the arm (Figure 19.15). The blood pressure cuff is inflated above the systolic pressure. Carpal spasms become evident within 3 minutes if hypocalcemia is present. *Chvostek's sign* is contraction of facial muscles in response to a tap over the facial nerve in front of the ear (see Figure 19.15). Other manifestations of tetany are laryngeal stridor, dysphagia, and numbness and tingling around the mouth or in the extremities.

Because calcium is necessary for cardiac contractions, hypocalcemia results in decreased cardiac contractility and ECG changes. Clinical manifestations of hypocalcemia are listed in Table 19.7.

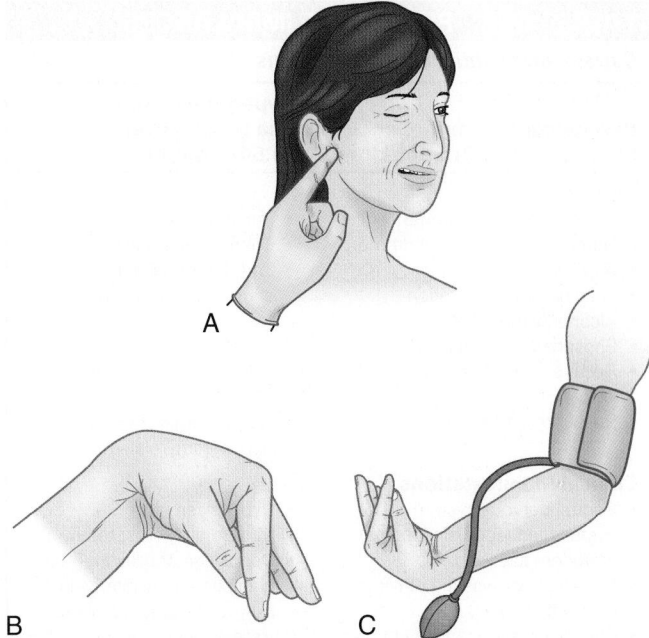

FIG. 19.15 Tests for hypocalcemia. **A,** Chvostek's sign is contraction of facial muscles in response to a light tap over the facial nerve in front of the ear. **B,** Trousseau's sign is a carpal spasm induced by **C,** inflating a blood pressure cuff above the systolic pressure for a few minutes.

NURSING AND INTERPROFESSIONAL MANAGEMENT
HYPOCALCEMIA

NURSING DIAGNOSES

Nursing diagnoses and interprofessional issues for patients with hypocalcemia include but are not limited to the following:

- *Potential for injury* as a result of *alteration in cognitive functioning* (tetany and seizures)
- Potential complications: fracture, respiratory arrest

NURSING IMPLEMENTATION

Treatment of hypocalcemia is aimed primarily at correcting the cause. Treating mild or asymptomatic hypocalcemia involves a diet of calcium-rich foods and calcium and vitamin D supplementation. IV preparations of calcium, such as calcium gluconate, are administered when severe symptoms of hypocalcemia are impending or present. Oral calcium supplements, such as calcium carbonate, may be used when patients are unable to consume enough calcium in the diet, such as those who do not tolerate dairy products. Pain and anxiety must be adequately treated in patients with suspected hypocalcemia because hyperventilation-induced respiratory alkalosis can precipitate hypocalcemic symptoms. Any patient who undergoes thyroid or neck surgery must be observed closely in the immediate postoperative period for manifestations of hypocalcemia because of the proximity of the surgery to the parathyroid glands.

Phosphate Imbalances

Phosphorus is a primary anion in the ICF and is essential to the function of muscle, RBCs, and the nervous system. It is deposited with calcium for bone and tooth structure. It is also involved in the acid–base buffering system, in the mitochondrial energy production of ATP, in cellular uptake and use of glucose, and as an intermediary in the metabolism of carbohydrates, proteins, and fats.

TABLE 19.8   PHOSPHATE IMBALANCES
Causes and Clinical Manifestations

Hypophosphatemia (PO_4^{3-} Level <1.0 mmol/L)	Hyperphosphatemia (PO_4^{3-} Level >1.50 mmol/L)
Causes	
• Malabsorption syndrome	• Renal failure
• Nutritional recovery syndrome	• Chemotherapeutic agents
• Glucose administration	• Enemas containing phosphorus (e.g., Fleet enema)
• Total parenteral nutrition	
• Alcohol withdrawal	• Excessive ingestion (e.g., milk, phosphate-containing laxatives)
• Phosphate-binding antacids	
• Recovery from diabetic ketoacidosis	• Large vitamin D intake
• Respiratory alkalosis	• Hypoparathyroidism
Clinical Manifestations	
• Central nervous system dysfunction (confusion, coma)	• Hypocalcemia
• Rhabdomyolysis	• Muscle problems; tetany
• Renal tubular wasting of Mg^{2+}, Ca^{2+}, HCO_3^-	• Deposition of calcium–phosphate precipitates in skin, soft tissue, corneas, viscera, blood vessels
• Cardiac problems (dysrhythmias, decreased stroke volume)	
• Muscle weakness, including respiratory muscle weakness	
• Osteomalacia	

TABLE 19.9   CAUSES OF MAGNESIUM IMBALANCES

Hypomagnesemia (Mg^{2+} Level <0.65 mmol/L)	Hypermagnesemia (Mg^{2+} Level >1.05 mmol/L)
• Diarrhea	• Renal failure (especially if patient is given magnesium products)
• Vomiting	
• Chronic alcoholism	
• Impaired GI absorption	• Excessive administration of magnesium for treatment of eclampsia
• Malabsorption syndrome	
• Prolonged malnutrition	
• Large urine output	• Adrenal insufficiency
• NG suction	
• Poorly controlled diabetes mellitus	
• Hyperaldosteronism	

GI, gastrointestinal; NG, nasogastric.

For maintenance of normal phosphate balance, renal functioning must be adequate because the kidneys are the major route of phosphate excretion. A small amount is lost in the feces. A reciprocal relationship exists between phosphorus and calcium in that a high serum phosphate level tends to cause a low calcium concentration in the serum.

Hyperphosphatemia. The major condition that can lead to hyperphosphatemia is acute or chronic renal failure that results in an altered ability of the kidneys to excrete phosphate. Other causes include chemotherapy for certain malignancies (lymphomas), excessive ingestion of milk or phosphate-containing laxatives, and large intakes of vitamin D that increase GI absorption of phosphorus (Table 19.8).

Clinical manifestations of hyperphosphatemia (presented in Table 19.8) relate primarily to metastatic calcium–phosphate precipitates. Ordinarily, calcium and phosphate are deposited only in bone. However, an increased serum phosphate concentration along with calcium precipitates readily, and calcified deposits can develop in soft tissue such as those of the joints, arteries, skin, kidneys, and corneas (see Chapter 49). Other manifestations of hyperphosphatemia are neuromuscular irritability and tetany, which are related to the low serum calcium levels often associated with high serum phosphate levels.

Management of hyperphosphatemia is aimed at identifying and treating the underlying cause. Ingestion of foods and fluids with high phosphorus content (e.g., dairy products) should be restricted. Adequate hydration and correction of hypocalcemic conditions can enhance the renal excretion of phosphate. For patients with renal failure, measures to reduce serum phosphate levels include calcium supplements, phosphate-binding agents or gels, and dietary phosphate restrictions (see Chapter 49).

Hypophosphatemia. Hypophosphatemia (low serum phosphate) is seen in patients who are malnourished or have malabsorption syndromes. Other causes include alcohol withdrawal and use of phosphate-binding antacids. Hypophosphatemia may also occur during parenteral nutrition with inadequate phosphorus replacement. Table 19.8 lists causes of phosphorus imbalances.

Most of the clinical manifestations of hypophosphatemia (presented in Table 19.8) are related to a deficiency of ATP or 2,3-diphosphoglycerate (2,3-DPG), an enzyme in RBCs. Both conditions result in impaired cellular energy resources and oxygen delivery to tissues. Hemolytic anemia may occur because of the fragility of the RBCs. Acute manifestations include CNS depression, confusion, and other mental changes. Other manifestations include muscle weakness and pain, dysrhythmias, and cardiomyopathy.

Management of a mild phosphorus deficiency may involve oral supplementation and ingestion of foods with high phosphorus content (e.g., dairy products). Severe hypophosphatemia can be serious and may necessitate IV administration of sodium phosphate or potassium phosphate. Frequent monitoring of serum phosphate levels is necessary to guide IV therapy. Sudden symptomatic hypocalcemia, secondary to increased calcium phosphorus binding, is a potential complication of IV administration of phosphorus.

Magnesium Imbalances

Magnesium, the second most abundant intracellular cation, plays an important role in essential cellular processes. It is a cofactor in many enzyme systems, including those responsible for carbohydrate metabolism, DNA and protein synthesis, blood glucose control, and blood pressure regulation. Magnesium is required for the production and use of ATP, the energy source for the sodium–potassium pump. Muscle contraction and relaxation, normal neurological function, and neurotransmitter release depend on magnesium.

Approximately 50 to 60% of the body's magnesium is contained in bone. Magnesium concentration is regulated by GI absorption and renal excretion. The kidneys conserve magnesium in times of need and excrete excess. Factors that regulate calcium balance (e.g., PTH) appear to influence magnesium balance. Manifestations of magnesium balance are often mistaken for those of calcium imbalances. Because magnesium balance is related to calcium and potassium balance, all three cations should be assessed together. Causes of magnesium imbalances are listed in Table 19.9.

Hypermagnesemia. Hypermagnesemia usually occurs only with an increase in magnesium intake accompanied by renal insufficiency or failure. In patients with chronic renal failure, ingesting products containing magnesium (e.g., Maalox, milk of magnesia) will cause excess magnesium. Magnesium excess could develop in pregnant women who receive magnesium sulphate ($MgSO_4$) for the management of eclampsia.

Excess magnesium inhibits acetylcholine release at the myoneural junction and calcium movement into cells, impairing nerve and muscle function. Initial manifestations include hypotension, facial flushing, lethargy, urinary retention, nausea, and vomiting. As the serum magnesium level increases, deep tendon reflexes are lost, followed by muscle paralysis and coma. Respiratory and cardiac arrest can occur.

Management begins with avoiding magnesium-containing medications and limiting diet intake of magnesium-containing foods (e.g., green vegetables, nuts, bananas, oranges, peanut butter, chocolate). If renal function is adequate, increased fluids and diuretics promote urinary excretion. In patients with impaired renal function, dialysis is required. If hypermagnesemia is symptomatic, calcium gluconate administered by IV infusion opposes the effects of the excess magnesium on cardiac muscle.

Hypomagnesemia. Magnesium deficiency occurs in patients with limited magnesium intake or increased gastrointestinal or renal losses. Causes of hypomagnesemia from insufficient food intake include prolonged fasting or starvation and chronic alcoholism (Table 19.9). Another potential cause is prolonged parenteral nutrition without magnesium supplementation. Fluid loss from the GI tract, inflammatory bowel disease, and proton pump inhibitors interfere with magnesium absorption. Diuretic medications and having uncontrolled diabetes mellitus may cause magnesium loss through increased urinary excretion (Yu, 2020).

Clinically, hypomagnesemia resembles hypocalcemia and may contribute to the development of hypocalcemia as a result of the decreased action of PTH. Neuromuscular manifestations are common, such as muscle cramps, tremors, hyperactive deep tendon reflexes, Chvostek's sign, and Trousseau's sign. Neurological manifestations include confusion, vertigo, and seizures.

Magnesium deficiency can lead to cardiac dysrhythmias, such as ventricular fibrillation. Hypomagnesemia is associated with digitalis toxicity. Hypomagnesemia may also be associated with hypokalemia that does not respond well to potassium replacement. This occurs because intracellular magnesium is crucial for normal function of the sodium–potassium pump.

Mild magnesium deficiencies can be treated with oral supplements and increased dietary intake of foods with high magnesium content (e.g., green vegetables, nuts, bananas, oranges, peanut butter, chocolate). If the condition is severe, parenteral IV or intramuscular magnesium (e.g., $MgSO_4$) should be administered. The nurse should monitor vital signs and use an infusion pump because rapid administration can lead to hypotension and cardiac or respiratory arrest.

Protein Imbalances

Plasma proteins, particularly albumin, are a significant determinant of plasma volume. Because of their large molecular size, they remain in the vascular space and contribute to the colloidal oncotic pressure. Causes of protein imbalances are listed in Table 19.10. Hypoproteinemia can occur over time. Causes related to intake are anorexia, malnutrition, starvation, fad

TABLE 19.10 CAUSES OF PROTEIN IMBALANCES

Hypoproteinemia (Protein Level <60 g/L)	Hyperproteinemia (Protein Level >80 g/L)
• Decreased food intake • Starvation • Diseased liver • Massive burns • Loss of albumin in renal disease • Major infection	• Dehydration • Hemoconcentration

dieting, and imbalanced vegetarian diets. Poor absorption of protein can occur in certain GI malabsorptive diseases, such as pancreatic insufficiency and inflammatory bowel disease. Protein can shift out of the intravascular space with inflammation. Increased breakdown of proteins occurs with elevated basal metabolic rates and catabolic states, such as fever, infection, and certain malignancies. Use of protein increases with cell growth and repair after surgical wounds or burns. Hemorrhage with loss of RBCs can be a cause of protein deficit. Impaired synthesis of albumin occurs in liver failure. The kidneys can lose large amounts of protein, especially albumin, in nephrotic syndrome (see Chapter 48).

Clinical manifestations of protein deficit include edema (caused by decreased oncotic pressure), slow healing, anorexia, fatigue, anemia, and muscle loss that results from the breakdown of body tissue to meet the body's need for protein. Intravascular fluid readily accumulates in the peritoneal cavity, which leads to ascites, when the vascular oncotic pressure is decreased in hypoproteinemia.

Management of protein deficit includes providing a high-carbohydrate, high-protein diet and dietary protein supplements. If the patient cannot meet the needs for protein orally, enteral nutrition or total parenteral nutrition may be used. (Protein-calorie malnutrition is discussed in Chapter 42.)

Hyperproteinemia is rare, but it can occur with dehydration-induced hemoconcentration.

Acid–Base Imbalances

The body normally maintains a steady balance between acids produced during metabolism and bases that neutralize and promote the excretion of the acids. Many health problems may lead to acid–base imbalances in addition to fluid and electrolyte imbalances. Patients with diabetes mellitus, chronic obstructive pulmonary disease, and kidney disease frequently develop acid–base imbalances. Vomiting and diarrhea may cause loss of acids and bases in addition to loss of fluids and electrolytes. The kidneys are an essential buffer system for acids, and in older persons, the kidneys are less able to compensate for an acid load. Older people also have decreased respiratory function, which impairs compensation for acid–base imbalances. In addition, tissue hypoxia from any cause may alter acid–base balance. The nurse must always consider the possibility of acid–base imbalance in patients with serious illnesses.

pH and Hydrogen Ion Concentration. The acidity or alkalinity of a solution depends on its hydrogen ion (H^+) concentration. An increase in H^+ concentration leads to acidity; a decrease leads to alkalinity. (Definitions related to acid–base balance are presented in Table 19.11.)

Although acids are produced by the body daily, the H^+ concentration of body fluids is small (0.0004 mEq/L). This tiny

TABLE 19.11	TERMS IN ACID–BASE PHYSIOLOGY
Acid	Donor of hydrogen ion (H$^+$); separation of an acid into H$^+$ and its accompanying anion in solution
Acidemia	Signifying an arterial blood pH of <7.35
Acidosis	Process that adds acid or eliminates base from body fluids
Alkalemia	Signifying an arterial blood pH of >7.45
Alkalosis	Process that adds base or eliminates acid from body fluids
Anion gap	Calculation approximating normally unmeasured anions in the plasma; helpful in differential diagnosis of acidosis
Base	Acceptor of hydrogen ions; chemical combining of acid and base when hydrogen ions are added to a solution containing a base; bicarbonate (HCO$_3^-$) is most abundant base in body fluids
Buffer	Substance that reacts with an acid or base to prevent a large change in pH
pH	Negative logarithm of the H$^+$ concentration

amount is maintained within a narrow range to ensure optimal cellular function. H$^+$ concentration is usually expressed as a negative logarithm (symbolized as **pH**) rather than in milliequivalents. The use of the negative logarithm reveals an inverse relationship: the higher the pH, the lower the H$^+$ concentration. A high pH of (7 or 8) represents a 10-fold decrease in H$^+$ concentration. In contrast, a low pH indicates a high H$^+$ concentration.

The pH of a chemical solution may range from 1 to 14. A solution with a pH of 7 is considered neutral. Blood is slightly alkaline and thus the normal pH of blood is between 7.35 and 7.45 with 7.4 being neutral. Medically, if a patient's blood pH drops below 7.35, the patient has **acidosis**. If the blood pH is greater than 7.45, the patient has **alkalosis** (Figure 19.16).

Acid–Base Regulation. The body's metabolic processes constantly produce acids. These acids must be neutralized and excreted to maintain acid–base balance. Normally, the body has three mechanisms by which it regulates acid–base balance to maintain the arterial pH between 7.35 and 7.45: the buffer systems, the respiratory system, and the renal system.

The regulatory mechanisms react at different speeds. Buffer systems react immediately; the respiratory system responds in minutes and reaches maximum effectiveness in hours. The renal response takes 2 to 3 days to respond maximally, but the kidneys can maintain balance indefinitely in patients with chronic imbalances.

Buffer System. The buffer system is the fastest-acting system and the primary regulator of acid–base balance. **Buffers** act chemically to change strong acids into weaker acids or to bind acids to neutralize their effect. All body fluids contain buffers. The major buffer system in ECF is carbonic acid–bicarbonate. Other buffers include phosphate, protein, and hemoglobin. The cell itself can act as a buffer by the shifting of H$^+$ in and out of the cell. With an accumulation of H$^+$ in the ECF, the intracellular compartment can accept hydrogen in exchange for another cation (e.g., K$^+$).

When ECF levels of H$^+$ are increased, H$^+$ enters the cell in exchange for potassium. This may result in hyperkalemia. Conversely, with decreased H$^+$ levels, H$^+$ enters plasma in exchange for potassium. This is referred to as an *intracellular buffering response* and the reason why alkalosis can cause hypokalemia and acidosis can cause hyperkalemia.

A buffer consists of a weakly ionized acid or a base and its salt. Buffers function to minimize the effect of acids on blood pH until they can be excreted from the body. The carbonic acid (H_2CO_3)–bicarbonate (HCO_3^-) buffer system neutralizes hydrochloric acid (HCl) in the following manner:

$$\underset{(\text{strong acid})}{HCL} + \underset{(\text{weak base})}{NaHCO_3} \rightarrow \underset{(\text{salt})}{NaCl} + \underset{(\text{weak acid})}{H_2CO_3}$$

In this way, combining a strong acid with a base prevents the acid from causing a large decrease in pH. The carbonic acid is broken down to H_2O and CO_2. The lungs excrete CO_2, either combined with insensible H_2O as carbonic acid or alone as CO_2.

The phosphate, protein, and hemoglobin buffer systems act in the same way as the bicarbonate system. The main components of the phosphate system are monohydrogen phosphate (HPO_4^{2-}) and dihydrogen phosphate ($H_2PO_4^-$). A phosphate, combined with sodium, can neutralize a strong acid such as HCl by forming NaCl and sodium biphosphate (NaH_2PO_4), a weak acid. If a strong base, such as sodium hydroxide (NaOH), is present, sodium biphosphate (NaH_2PO_4) neutralizes it to a weaker base (Na_2HPO_4) and H_2O.

Intracellular and extracellular proteins constitute an effective buffering system throughout the body. The protein buffering system acts like the bicarbonate system. Some of the amino acids of proteins contain free acid radicals such as –COOH, which can dissociate into CO_2 and H$^+$. Other amino acids have basic radicals such as –NH_3OH, which can dissociate into NH^{3+} and OH$^-$; the OH$^-$ can combine with an H$^+$ to form H_2O.

Using the "chloride shift" mechanism, hemoglobin regulates pH by shifting chloride in and out of RBCs in exchange for bicarbonate. This shift is regulated according to the level of oxygen in blood.

The body buffers an acid load better than it neutralizes base excess. Buffers cannot maintain pH without the adequate functioning of the respiratory and renal systems.

Respiratory System. The lungs help maintain a normal pH by excreting CO_2 and water, which are byproducts of cellular metabolism. When released into circulation, CO_2 enters RBCs and combines with H_2O to form H_2CO_3. The carbonic acid dissociates into hydrogen ions and bicarbonate. The free hydrogen is buffered by hemoglobin molecules, and the bicarbonate diffuses into the plasma. In the pulmonary capillaries, this process is reversed, and CO_2 is formed and excreted by the lungs. The overall reversible reaction is expressed as the following:

$$CO_2 + H_2O \rightleftharpoons H_2CO_3 \rightleftharpoons H^+ + HCO_3^-$$

The amount of CO_2 in the blood directly relates to carbonic acid concentration and subsequently to H$^+$ concentration. With increased respirations, less CO_2 remains in the blood. This leads to less carbonic acid and fewer H$^+$ molecules. With decreased respirations, more CO_2 remains in the blood. This leads to increased amounts of carbonic acid and more H$^+$.

The rate of excretion of CO_2 is controlled by the respiratory centre in the medulla in the brainstem. If increased amounts of CO_2 or H$^+$ are present, the respiratory centre stimulates an increased rate and depth of breathing. Respirations are inhibited if the centre senses low H$^+$ or CO_2 levels.

As a compensatory mechanism, the respiratory system acts on the $CO_2 + H_2O$ side of the reaction by altering the rate and depth of breathing to "blow off" (through hyperventilation) or "retain" (through hypoventilation) CO_2. If a respiratory problem

TABLE 19.12   ACID–BASE IMBALANCES

Common Causes	Pathophysiology	Laboratory Findings
Respiratory Acidosis • Chronic obstructive pulmonary disease • Barbiturate or sedative overdose • Chest wall abnormality (e.g., obesity) • Severe pneumonia • Atelectasis • Respiratory muscle weakness (e.g., Guillain-Barré syndrome) • Mechanical hypoventilation	• CO_2 retention by lungs from hypoventilation • Compensatory response to HCO_3^- retention by kidneys	• ↓ Plasma pH • ↑ $PaCO_2$ • HCO_3^- normal (uncompensated) • ↑ HCO_3^- (compensated) • Urine pH <6 (compensated)
Respiratory Alkalosis • Hyperventilation (caused by hypoxia, pulmonary emboli, anxiety, fear, pain, exercise, fever) • Stimulated respiratory centre caused by septicemia, encephalitis, brain injury, salicylate poisoning • Mechanical hyperventilation	• Increased CO_2 excretion by lungs from hyperventilation • Compensatory response of HCO_3^- excretion by kidneys	• ↑ Plasma pH • ↓ $PaCO_2$ • HCO_3^- normal (uncompensated) • ↓ HCO_3^- (compensated) • Urine pH >6 (compensated)
Metabolic Acidosis • Diabetic ketoacidosis • Lactic acidosis • Starvation • Severe diarrhea • Renal tubular acidosis • Renal failure • Gastrointestinal fistulas • Shock	• Gain of fixed acid, inability to excrete acid or loss of base • Compensatory response of CO_2 excretion by lungs	• ↓ Plasma pH • $PaCO_2$ normal (uncompensated) • ↓ PCO_2 (compensated) • ↓ HCO_3^- • Urine pH <6 (compensated)
Metabolic Alkalosis • Severe vomiting • Excess gastric suctioning • Diuretic therapy* • Potassium deficit • Excess $NaHCO_3$ intake • Excessive mineralocorticoids	• Loss of strong acid or gain of base • Compensatory response of CO_2 retention by lungs	• ↑ Plasma pH • $PaCO_2$ normal (uncompensated) • ↑ PCO_2 (compensated) • ↑ HCO_3^- • Urine pH >6 (compensated)

HCO_3^-, bicarbonate; *$NaHCO_3$*, sodium bicarbonate; *$PaCO_2$*, arterial partial pressure of CO_2; *PCO_2*, partial pressure of CO_2.
*Commonly used diuretics such as thiazides and furosemide are known to produce mild alkalosis by affecting tubular excretion of electrolytes and bicarbonate.

is the cause of an acid–base imbalance (e.g., respiratory failure), the respiratory system cannot play its usual role to correct a pH alteration.

Renal System. Under normal conditions, the kidneys reabsorb and conserve the bicarbonate they filter. The kidneys can generate additional bicarbonate and eliminate excess H^+ as compensation for acidosis. The three mechanisms of acid elimination include (1) secretion of small amounts of free hydrogen into the renal tubule, (2) combination of H^+ with ammonia (NH_3) to form ammonium (NH_4^-), and (3) excretion of weak acids.

The body depends on the kidneys to excrete a portion of the acid produced by cellular metabolism. Thus, the kidneys normally excrete an acidic urine (average pH is 6). As a compensatory mechanism, the pH of the urine can decrease to 4 and increase to 8. If the renal system is the cause of an acid–base imbalance (e.g., renal failure), it loses its ability to correct a pH alteration.

Alterations in Acid–Base Balance. An acid–base imbalance is produced when the ratio of 1:20 between acid and base content is altered (Table 19.12; see also Figure 19.16). A primary disease or process may alter one side of the ratio (e.g., CO_2 retention in pulmonary disease). The compensatory process is an attempt to maintain the other side of the ratio (e.g., increased renal bicarbonate reabsorption). When the compensatory mechanism fails, an acid–base imbalance results. The compensatory process may be inadequate because either the pathophysiological process is overwhelming or there is insufficient time for the compensatory process to function.

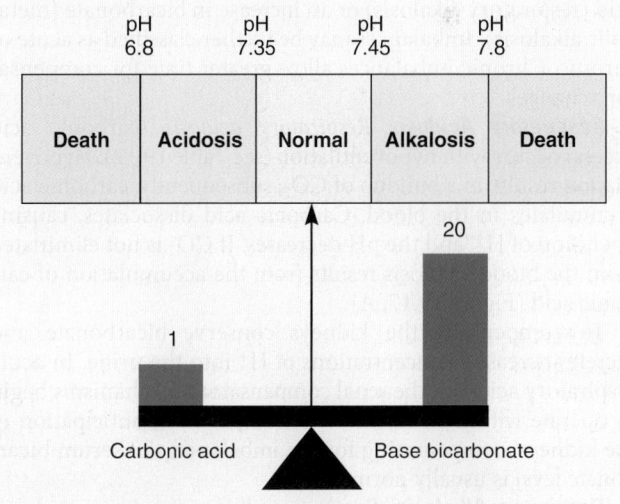

FIG. 19.16 The normal range of plasma pH is 7.35 to 7.45. A normal pH is maintained by a ratio of 1 part carbonic acid to 20 parts bicarbonate.

Acid–base imbalances are classified as respiratory or metabolic. *Respiratory imbalances* affect carbonic acid concentrations; *metabolic imbalances* affect the base bicarbonate. Therefore, acidosis can be caused by an increase in carbonic acid (respiratory acidosis) or a decrease in bicarbonate (metabolic acidosis). Alkalosis can be caused by a decrease in carbonic

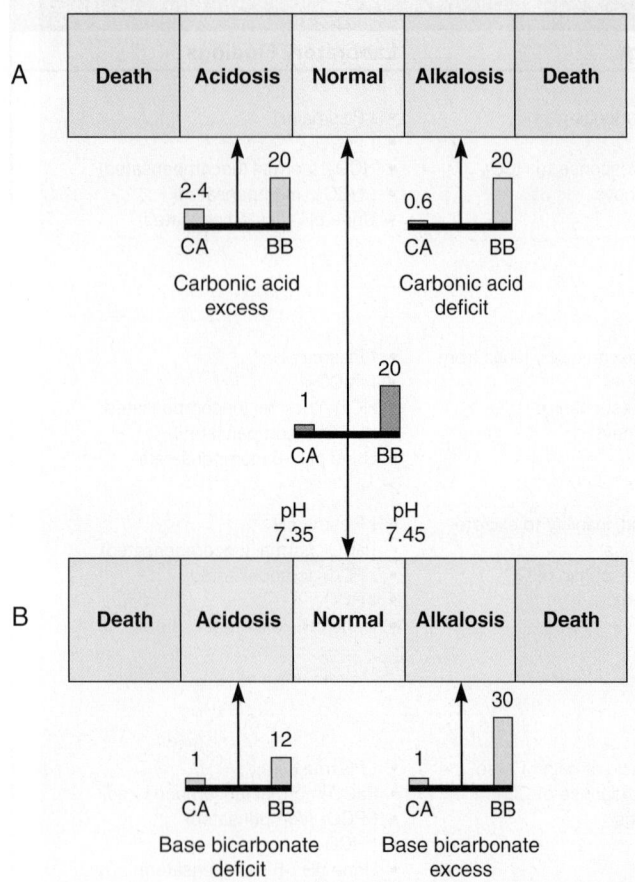

FIG. 19.17 Kinds of acid–base imbalances. **A,** Respiratory imbalances caused by carbonic acid (CA) excess and CA deficit. *BB,* base bicarbonate. **B,** Metabolic imbalances caused by BB deficit and BB excess.

acid (respiratory alkalosis) or an increase in bicarbonate (metabolic alkalosis). Imbalances may be further classified as acute or chronic. Chronic imbalances allow greater time for compensatory changes.

Respiratory Acidosis. *Respiratory acidosis* (carbonic acid excess) occurs with hypoventilation (see Table 19.12). Hypoventilation results in a buildup of CO_2; subsequently, carbonic acid accumulates in the blood. Carbonic acid dissociates, causing liberation of H^+, and the pH decreases. If CO_2 is not eliminated from the blood, acidosis results from the accumulation of carbonic acid (Figure 19.17, *A*).

To compensate, the kidneys conserve bicarbonate and secrete increased concentrations of H^+ into the urine. In acute respiratory acidosis, the renal compensatory mechanisms begin to operate within 24 hours. Therefore, even in anticipation of the kidneys' compensating for the imbalance, the serum bicarbonate level is usually normal.

Respiratory Alkalosis. *Respiratory alkalosis* (carbonic acid deficit) occurs with hyperventilation (see Table 19.12). The primary cause of respiratory alkalosis is hypoxemia from acute pulmonary disorders (e.g., pneumonia, pulmonary embolus). Hyperventilation can occur as a physiological response to metabolic acidosis and increased metabolic demands (e.g., in a state of fever). Pain, anxiety, and some CNS disorders can cause an increase in respirations without a physiological need. The decrease in the arterial CO_2 level leads to a decrease in carbonic acid concentration in the blood and an increase in pH (see Figure 19.17, *A*).

Compensated respiratory alkalosis is uncommon unless the patient has been maintained on a ventilator or has a CNS condition. If the respiratory alkalosis is caused by panic or pain, rebreathing CO_2 from a closed system (e.g., paper bag) can assist in the compensatory process. A decreased bicarbonate level differentiates compensated respiratory alkalosis from acute or uncompensated respiratory alkalosis.

Metabolic Acidosis. *Metabolic acidosis* (base bicarbonate deficit) occurs when an acid other than carbonic acid accumulates in the body or when bicarbonate is lost from body fluids (see Table 19.12 and Figure 19.17, *B*). In both cases, a bicarbonate deficit results. Ketoacid accumulation in diabetic ketoacidosis and lactic acid accumulation with shock are examples of accumulation of acids. Severe diarrhea results in loss of bicarbonate. In renal disease, the kidneys lose their abilities to reabsorb bicarbonate and secrete H^+.

The compensatory response to metabolic acidosis is to increase CO_2 excretion by the lungs. Many affected patients develop Kussmaul's respiration (deep, rapid breathing). In addition, the kidneys attempt to excrete additional acid.

If metabolic acidosis is present, calculating the anion gap helps determine the source of the acidosis. The *anion gap* is the difference between the measured serum cations and anions in ECF. The anion gap is calculated according to the following formula:

$$\text{Anion gap (in mmol/L)} = Na^+ - (HCO_3^- + Cl)$$

A normal anion gap is 8 to 16 mmol/L. The anion gap increases in metabolic acidosis associated with acid gain (e.g., lactic acidosis, diabetic ketoacidosis) but is normal in metabolic acidosis caused by bicarbonate loss (e.g., diarrhea).

Metabolic Alkalosis. *Metabolic alkalosis* (base bicarbonate excess) occurs when acid is lost (as a result of prolonged vomiting or gastric suction) or when bicarbonate increase (from ingestion of baking soda) occurs (see Table 19.12 and Figure 19.17, *B*). The compensatory mechanism is a decreased respiratory rate to increase plasma CO_2. However, once hypoxemia occurs or plasma CO_2 reaches a certain level, stimulation of chemoreceptors increases respirations. Renal excretion of bicarbonate also occurs.

Mixed Acid–Base Disorders. A *mixed acid–base disorder* occurs when two or more acid–base disturbances are present at the same time. The pH will depend on type, severity, and acuity of each of the simple disorders involved. Respiratory acidosis combined with metabolic alkalosis (e.g., chronic obstructive pulmonary disease treated with diuretic therapy) may result in a near-normal pH, whereas respiratory acidosis combined with metabolic acidosis causes a greater decrease in pH than either disorder alone. An example of a mixed acidosis appears in a patient in cardiopulmonary arrest: Hypoventilation elevates the CO_2 level and anaerobic metabolism produces lactic acid. An example of a mixed alkalosis is the case of a patient who is hyperventilating because of postoperative pain and is also losing acid as a result of nasogastric suctioning.

Clinical Manifestations. Clinical manifestations of acidosis and alkalosis are summarized in Tables 19.13 and 19.14. Because a normal pH is vital for all cellular reactions, the clinical manifestations of acid–base imbalances are generalized and nonspecific. The actual compensatory mechanisms also produce some clinical manifestations. For example, the deep, rapid

TABLE 19.13	CLINICAL MANIFESTATIONS OF ACIDOSIS
Respiratory ($\uparrow PCO_2$)	**Metabolic ($\downarrow HCO_3^-$)**
Neurological • Drowsiness • Disorientation • Dizziness • Headache • Coma	**Neurological** • Drowsiness • Confusion • Headache • Coma
Cardiovascular • ↓ Blood pressure • Ventricular fibrillation (related to hyperkalemia from compensation) • Warm, flushed skin (related to peripheral vasodilation)	**Cardiovascular** • ↓ Blood pressure • Dysrhythmias (related to hyperkalemia from compensation) • Warm, flushed skin (related to peripheral vasodilation)
Gastrointestinal • No significant findings	**Gastrointestinal** • Nausea, vomiting, diarrhea, abdominal pain
Neuromuscular • Seizures	**Neuromuscular** • No significant findings
Respiratory • Hypoventilation with hypoxia (lungs are unable to compensate when there is a respiratory problem)	**Respiratory** • Deep, rapid respirations (compensatory action by the lungs)

HCO_3^-, bicarbonate; PCO_2, partial pressure of CO_2.

TABLE 19.14	CLINICAL MANIFESTATIONS OF ALKALOSIS
Respiratory ($\downarrow PCO_2$)	**Metabolic ($\uparrow HCO_3^-$)**
Neurological • Lethargy • Light-headedness • Confusion	**Neurological** • Dizziness • Irritability • Nervousness • Confusion
Cardiovascular • Tachycardia • Dysrhythmias (related to hypokalemia from compensation)	**Cardiovascular** • Tachycardia • Dysrhythmias (related to hypokalemia from compensation)
Gastrointestinal • Nausea • Vomiting • Epigastric pain	**Gastrointestinal** • Anorexia • Nausea • Vomiting
Neuromuscular* • Tetany • Numbness • Tingling of extremities • Hyperreflexia • Seizures	**Neuromuscular*** • Tremors • Hypertonic muscles • Muscle cramps • Tetany • Tingling of fingers and toes
Respiratory • Hyperventilation (lungs are unable to compensate when there is a respiratory problem)	**Respiratory** • Hypoventilation (compensatory action by the lungs)

HCO_3^-, bicarbonate; PCO_2, partial pressure of CO_2.
*Alkalosis decreases calcium binding to protein.

respirations of a patient with metabolic acidosis are an example of respiratory compensation. In alkalosis, hypocalcemia may concurrently be present and accounts for many of the clinical manifestations.

Blood Gas Values

Arterial blood gas (ABG) values provide valuable information about a patient's acid–base status, the origin of the imbalance, an idea of the body's ability to regulate pH, and a reflection of the patient's overall oxygen status. Acid–base disturbances are diagnosed and compensatory processes identified in the following six steps:

1. Determining whether the pH is acidotic or alkalotic. A value of 7.4 is the starting point. Values less than 7.4 characterize the pH as acidotic (7.35–7.4 is normal pH acidic side) and values greater than 7.4 characterize the pH as alkalotic (7.4-7.45 normal pH alkalosis side). If the pH is between 7.35 and 7.45, and the CO^2, HCO_3^-, and arterial partial pressure of oxygen (PaO_2) are within normal limits, the ABG values are normal. If any value is abnormal, then step 2 follows.

2. Analyzing the arterial partial pressure of carbon dioxide ($PaCO_2$) to determine whether the patient has respiratory acidosis or alkalosis. Levels of CO_2 are controlled by the lungs, and CO_2 is thus considered the respiratory component of the ABG. Because carbonic acid forms when CO_2 is dissolved in blood, high CO_2 levels indicate acidosis, and low CO_2 levels indicate alkalosis.

3. Analyzing the HCO_3^- level to determine whether the patient has metabolic acidosis or alkalosis. Levels of HCO_3^-, the metabolic component of the ABG value, are controlled primarily by the kidneys. Because HCO_3^- is a base, high levels of HCO_3^- result in alkalosis, and low levels result in acidosis.

4. Determining whether the CO_2 or the HCO_3^- level matches the acid or base alteration of the pH. For example, if the pH

is acidotic and the CO_2 level is high (respiratory acidosis) but the HCO_3^- level is high (metabolic alkalosis), the CO_2 is the parameter that matches the pH derangement. The patient's acid–base imbalance would be diagnosed as respiratory acidosis.

5. Deciding whether the body is attempting to compensate for the pH change. If the parameter that does not match the pH is opposing the pH imbalance, the body is attempting to compensate. In step 4, the HCO_3^- is alkalotic; this is then opposing or counteracting the respiratory acidosis and is considered compensation. If compensatory mechanisms are functioning, the pH will return toward normal range. When the pH is back to normal, the patient has *full compensation*. The body will not overcompensate for pH changes, meaning a corrected acidosis will result in a pH of 7.35–7.4 and a corrected alkalosis will result in a pH between 7.4 and 7.45. If both parameters match the pH, it is possible that a combined respiratory or metabolic acidosis or alkalosis is present. For example, if the pH is acidotic, the CO_2 level is high (respiratory acidosis) and the HCO_3^- level is low (metabolic acidosis); the patient's underlying acid–base imbalance is combined respiratory-metabolic acidosis.

6. Assessing the PaO_2 and O_2 saturation. If these values are abnormal, hypoxemia is present.

Table 19.15 lists normal ABG values, and Table 19.16 provides a sample ABG value with interpretation. (Refer to Table 19.12 for the laboratory findings of the four major acid–base disturbances.) Table 19.17 explains the ROME (**r**espiratory, **o**pposite, **m**etabolic, **e**quivalent) mnemonic to clarify acid–base imbalances. (Blood gases are discussed further in Chapter 28.)

TABLE 19.15   NORMAL ARTERIAL BLOOD GAS VALUES

Parameter	Arterial
pH	7.35–7.45
PCO₂	35–45 mm Hg
Bicarbonate (HCO₃⁻) level	21–28 mmol/L
PO₂*	80–100 mm Hg
Base excess	0 ± 2.0 mmol/L

PCO_2, partial pressure of carbon dioxide; PO_2, partial pressure of oxygen.
*Decreases above sea level and with increasing age.

TABLE 19.16   ARTERIAL BLOOD GAS (ABG) ANALYSIS

ABG Values
- pH 7.30
- $PaCO_2$ 25 mm Hg
- PaO_2 90 mm Hg
- HCO_3^- 16 mmol/L

Analysis
1. pH of <7.4 indicates acidosis (abnormal range below 7.35).
2. $PaCO_2$ is low, indicating respiratory alkalosis.
3. HCO_3^- level is low, indicating metabolic acidosis.
4. Metabolic acidosis matches the pH.
5. The $PaCO_2$ level does not match the pH but is opposing the acidosis, which indicates the lungs are attempting to compensate for the metabolic acidosis.
6. The PaO_2 indicates adequate oxygenation of the blood.

Interpretation
This ABG value is interpreted as representing metabolic acidosis with partial compensation. If the pH returns to the normal range, the patient is said to have full compensation.

ABG, arterial blood gas; HCO_3^-, bicarbonate; $PaCO_2$, partial pressure of arterial CO_2; PaO_2, partial pressure of oxygen.

TABLE 19.17   ROME: MNEMONIC FOR ACID–BASE IMBALANCES

For acid–base imbalances, the mnemonic ROME can be used.
In **r**espiratory conditions, the pH and the $PaCO_2$ are in **o**pposite directions. (RO)
- In respiratory alkalosis, the pH is ↑ and the $PaCO_2$ is ↓.
- In respiratory acidosis, the pH is ↓ and the $PaCO_2$ is ↑.

In **m**etabolic conditions, the pH and the HCO_3^- go in the same direction (**e**qual or **e**quivalent). (ME)
- In metabolic alkalosis, pH and HCO_3^- are ↑.
- In metabolic acidosis, pH and HCO_3^- are ↓.

Type of Imbalance	RO = Respiratory Opposite		ME = Metabolic Equal	
	pH	$PaCO_2$	pH	HCO_3^-
Acidosis	↓	↑	↓	↓
Alkalosis	↑	↓	↑	↑

HCO_3^-, bicarbonate; $PaCO_2$, arterial partial pressure of carbon dioxide.

ASSESSMENT OF FLUID, ELECTROLYTE, AND ACID–BASE IMBALANCES

Subjective Data

Important Health Information

Past Health History. The patient should be questioned about any health history of past conditions involving the kidneys, the heart, the GI system, or the lungs that could affect the current fluid, electrolyte, and acid–base balance. Medical information about specific diseases such as diabetes mellitus, diabetes insipidus, chronic obstructive pulmonary disease, ulcerative colitis, and Crohn's disease should be obtained from the patient. The patient should also be questioned about the incidence of a prior fluid, electrolyte, or acid–base disorder.

Medications. The patient's current and past use of medications must be assessed. The ingredients in many medications, especially over-the-counter medications, are often overlooked as sources of sodium, potassium, calcium, magnesium, and other electrolytes. Many prescription medications, including diuretics, corticosteroids, and electrolyte supplements, can cause fluid and electrolyte problems.

Surgery or Other Treatments. The patient should be asked about previous or current renal dialysis, kidney surgery, or bowel surgery that resulted in a temporary or permanent external collecting system, such as a colostomy or nephrostomy.

Other Subjective Data. If the patient is currently experiencing a problem related to fluid, electrolyte, and acid–base balance, a careful description of the illness, including onset, course, and treatment, should be obtained.

The nurse should ask the patient about diet and any special dietary practices. Weight reduction diets, fad diets, or any eating disorders, such as anorexia or bulimia, can lead to fluid and electrolyte problems. If the patient is on a special diet, such as one of low sodium content or high potassium content, the nurse should assess the patient's ability to adhere to the dietary prescription.

The patient's usual bowel and bladder habits should be noted. Any deviations from the expected elimination pattern, such as diarrhea, nocturia, or polyuria, should be carefully documented.

The patient's exercise pattern is important to determine because excessive perspiration secondary to exercise could result in a fluid and electrolyte problem. Also, the patient's exposure to extremely high temperatures as a result of leisure or work activity should be determined. The patient should be asked what practices are followed to replace fluid and electrolytes lost through excessive perspiration.

The patient should be queried about any changes in sensations, such as numbness, tingling, fasciculations (uncoordinated twitching of a single muscle group), or muscle weakness, that could indicate a fluid and electrolyte problem. In addition, both the patient and the caregivers should be asked whether any changes in mentation or alertness have been noted, such as confusion, memory impairment, or lethargy.

Objective Data

Physical Examination. There is no specific physical examination to assess fluid, electrolyte, and acid–base balance. Common abnormal assessment findings of major body systems offer clues to possible imbalances (Table 19.18).

Laboratory Values. Assessment of serum electrolyte values is a good starting point for identifying fluid and electrolyte imbalance (see Table 19.2). However, serum electrolyte values often provide only cursory information. Each value reflects the concentration of the electrolyte in the ECF but does not necessarily provide information concerning the concentration of the electrolyte in the ICF. For example, the majority of potassium in the body is located intracellularly. Changes in serum potassium values may be the result of a true deficit or an excess of potassium, or it may reflect the movement of potassium into or out of the cell due to acid–base imbalances.

TABLE 19.18 ASSESSMENT ABNORMALITIES

Fluid and Electrolyte Imbalances

Finding	Possible Cause
Skin	
Poor skin turgor	Fluid volume deficit
Cold, clammy skin	Na$^+$ deficit, shift of plasma to interstitial fluid
Pitting edema	Fluid volume excess
Flushed, dry skin	Na$^+$ excess
Pulse	
Bounding pulse	Fluid volume excess, shift of interstitial fluid to plasma
Rapid, weak, thready pulse	Shift of plasma to interstitial fluid, Na$^+$ deficit, fluid volume deficit
Weak, irregular, rapid pulse	Severe K$^+$ deficit
Weak, irregular, slow pulse	Severe K$^+$ excess
Blood Pressure	
Hypotension	Fluid volume deficit, shift of plasma to interstitial fluid, Na$^+$ deficit
Hypertension	Fluid volume excess, shift of interstitial fluid to plasma
Respirations	
Deep, rapid breathing	Compensation for metabolic acidosis
Shallow, slow, irregular breathing	Compensation for metabolic alkalosis
Shortness of breath	Fluid volume excess
Moist crackles	Fluid volume excess, shift of interstitial fluid to plasma
Skeletal Muscles	
Cramping of exercised muscle	Ca^{2+} deficit, Mg^{2+} deficit, alkalosis
Carpal spasm (Trousseau's sign)	Ca^{2+} deficit, Mg^{2+} deficit, alkalosis
Flabby muscles	K$^+$ deficit
Positive Chvostek's sign	Ca^{2+} deficit, Mg^{2+} deficit, alkalosis
Behaviour or Mental State	
Picking at bedclothes	K$^+$ deficit, Mg^{2+} deficit
Inappropriate indifference	Fluid volume deficit, Na$^+$ deficit
Apprehension	Shift of plasma to interstitial fluid
Extreme restlessness	K$^+$ excess, fluid volume deficit
Confusion and irritability	K$^+$ deficit, fluid volume excess, Ca^{2+} excess, Mg^{2+} excess, H$_2$O excess
Decreased level of consciousness	H$_2$O excess

An abnormal serum sodium level may reflect a sodium problem or, more possibly, a water problem. A reduced hematocrit value could indicate anemia, or it could be caused by fluid volume excess. Other laboratory tests that are helpful in evaluating the presence of or risk for fluid, electrolyte, and acid–base imbalances include serum and urine osmolality, serum glucose level, serum urea nitrogen (BUN) values, serum creatinine level, urine specific gravity, and urine electrolyte concentrations.

In addition to arterial and venous blood gas values, serum electrolyte data can provide important information concerning a patient's acid–base balance. Changes in the serum bicarbonate (often reported as HCO$_3$ content on an electrolyte panel) indicate the presence of metabolic acidosis (low bicarbonate level) or alkalosis (high bicarbonate level). Calculation of the anion gap can help determine the source of metabolic acidosis. The anion gap is increased in metabolic acidosis associated with acid gain (e.g., lactic acidosis, diabetic ketoacidosis) but remains normal in metabolic acidosis caused by bicarbonate loss (e.g., diarrhea).

ORAL FLUID AND ELECTROLYTE REPLACEMENT

In all cases of fluid, electrolyte, and acid–base imbalances, the treatment is directed toward correction of the underlying cause. The specific diseases or disorders that cause these imbalances are discussed in various chapters throughout this text. Mild fluid and electrolyte deficits can be corrected with the use of oral rehydration solutions containing water, electrolytes, and glucose. Glucose not only provides calories but also promotes sodium absorption in the small intestine. Commercial oral rehydration solutions are now available in markets and pharmacies for home use.

INTRAVENOUS FLUID AND ELECTROLYTE REPLACEMENT

IV fluid and electrolyte therapy are commonly used to treat many different fluid and electrolyte imbalances. Many patients need maintenance IV fluid therapy only while they cannot take fluids orally (e.g., during and after surgery). Other patients need corrective or replacement therapy for losses that have already occurred. The amount and the type of solution are determined by the normal daily maintenance requirements and by imbalances identified by laboratory results. Table 19.19 provides a list of commonly prescribed IV solutions. With IV fluid replacement therapy, local complications may occur, including phlebitis, ecchymosis, extravascular fluid infiltration, infection, thrombosis, and venous spasm. Systemic complications may also occur, such as bacteremia and sepsis, air embolism, and pulmonary edema.

Solutions

Hypotonic. A hypotonic solution provides more water than electrolytes, diluting the ECF. Osmosis then produces a movement of water from the ECF to the ICF. After osmotic equilibrium has been achieved, the ICF and the ECF have the same osmolality, and both compartments have been expanded. Examples of hypotonic fluids are listed in Table 19.19. Maintenance fluids are usually hypotonic solutions (e.g., 0.45% NaCl) because normal daily losses are hypotonic. Additional electrolytes (e.g., KCl) may be added to maintain normal levels. Hypotonic solutions have the potential to cause cellular swelling, and patients should be monitored for changes in mentation, which may indicate cerebral edema (Porth, 2018).

Although 5% dextrose in water is considered an isotonic solution, the dextrose is quickly metabolized, and the net result is the administration of free water (hypotonic) with proportionately equal expansion of the ECF and ICF. One litre of a 5% dextrose solution provides 50 g of dextrose, or 170 calories. Although this amount of dextrose is not enough to meet caloric requirements, it helps prevent ketosis associated with starvation. Pure water must not be administered intravenously because it would cause hemolysis of RBCs.

Isotonic. Administration of an isotonic solution expands only the ECF. There is no net loss or gain from the ICF. An

TABLE 19.19	COMPOSITION AND USE OF COMMONLY PRESCRIBED CRYSTALLOID SOLUTIONS			
Solution	Tonicity	Concentration (mmol/kg)	Glucose Content (g/L)	Indications and Considerations
Dextrose in Water				
5%	Isotonic, but physiologically hypotonic	278	50	Provides free water necessary for renal excretion of solutes Used to replace water losses and treat hypernatremia Provides 170 cal/L Does not provide any electrolytes
10%	Hypertonic	556	100	Provides free water only, no electrolytes Provides 340 cal/L
Saline (Sodium Chloride [NaCl])				
0.45%	Hypotonic	154	0	Provides free water in addition to Na^+ and Cl^- Used to replace hypotonic fluid losses Used as maintenance solution, although it does not replace daily losses of other electrolytes Provides no calories
0.9%	Isotonic	308	0	Used to expand intravascular volume and replace extracellular fluid losses Only solution that may be administered with blood products Contains Na^+ and Cl^- in excess of plasma levels Does not provide free water, calories, other electrolytes May cause intravascular overload or hyperchloremic acidosis
3.0%	Hypertonic	1 026	0	Used to treat symptomatic hyponatremia Must be administered slowly and with extreme caution because it may cause dangerous intravascular volume overload and pulmonary edema
Dextrose in Saline				
5% in 0.225%	Isotonic	355	50	Provides Na^+, Cl^-, and free water Used to replace hypotonic losses and treat hypernatremia Provides 170 cal/L
5% in 0.45%	Hypertonic	432	50	Same as 0.45% NaCl except provides 170 cal/L
5% in 0.9%	Hypertonic	586	50	Same as 0.9% NaCl except provides 170 cal/L
Multiple-Electrolyte Solutions				
Ringer's solution	Isotonic	309	0	Similar in composition to plasma except that it has excess Cl^-, no Mg^{2+}, and no HCO_3^- Does not provide free water or calories Used to expand the intravascular volume and replace extracellular fluid losses
Lactated Ringer's (Hartmann's) solution	Isotonic	274	0	Similar in composition to normal plasma except does not contain Mg^{2+} Used to treat losses from burns and lower GI tract May be used to treat mild metabolic acidosis but should not be used to treat lactic acidosis Does not provide free water or calories

GI, gastrointestinal; HCO_3^-, bicarbonate.

Source: Adapted from Heitz, U. E., & Horne, M. M. (2005). *Pocket guide to fluid, electrolyte, and acid–base balance* (5th ed., p. 70). Mosby.

isotonic solution is the ideal fluid replacement for a patient with an ECF volume deficit. Examples of isotonic solutions include lactated Ringer's solution and 0.9% NaCl. Lactated Ringer's solution contains sodium, potassium, chloride, calcium, and lactate (the precursor of bicarbonate) in approximately the same concentrations as those of the ECF. Its use is contraindicated in the presence of lactic acidosis because of the body's decreased ability to convert lactate to bicarbonate.

Isotonic saline (0.9% NaCl) has a sodium concentration (154 mmol/L) somewhat higher than that of plasma (135–145 mmol/L) and a chloride concentration (154 mmol/L) significantly higher than the plasma chloride level (98–106 mmol/L or mEq/L). Therefore, excessive administration of isotonic NaCl can cause elevation of sodium and chloride levels. Isotonic saline may be used when a patient has sustained both fluid and sodium losses or as vascular fluid replacement in hypovolemic shock.

Hypertonic. A hypertonic solution initially raises the osmolality of ECF and expands it. It is useful in treatment of hypovolemia and hyponatremia. Examples are listed in Table 19.19. In addition, the higher osmotic pressure causes water to shift out of the cells and into the ECF. Hypertonic solutions (e.g., 3% NaCl) necessitate frequent monitoring of blood pressure, lung sounds, and serum sodium levels and should be used with caution because of the risk for intravascular fluid volume excess and intracellular dehydration (Porth, 2018).

Although concentrated dextrose and water solutions (≥10% dextrose) are hypertonic solutions, once the dextrose is metabolized, the net result is the administration of water. The free water provided by these solutions ultimately causes both the ECF and the ICF to expand. The primary use of these solutions is in the provision of calories. Concentrated dextrose solutions may be combined with amino acid solutions, electrolytes, vitamins, and trace elements to provide total parenteral nutrition (see Chapter 42). Solutions containing 10% dextrose or less may be administered through a peripheral IV catheter. Solutions with greater concentrations of dextrose must be administered through a central catheter so that dilution is adequate to prevent shrinkage of RBCs.

Intravenous Additives. Additives in basic IV solutions replace specific losses. KCl, calcium chloride (CaCl), $MgSO_4$, and HCO_3^- are common additives. The use of each was described earlier in the discussion of the specific electrolyte deficiencies. Many premixed IV solutions containing specific additives are available. Use of these solutions reduces error inasmuch as they contain the correct amount of the electrolytes in the proper volumes and types of IV solution. Recommendations for administering potassium vary, but in general, no more than 10 mmol/L per hour is considered safe for routine administration. Potassium can be safely diluted as 40 mmol/L of solution, with a maximum of 60 mmol/L. It must never be administered undiluted or by IV push because it can cause fatal cardiac reactions.

Plasma Expanders. Plasma expanders stay in the vascular space and increase the osmotic pressure. Plasma expanders include colloids, dextran, and hetastarch. Colloids are protein solutions such as plasma, albumin, and commercial plasmas. Albumin is available in 5% and 25% solutions. The 5% albumin solution has a concentration similar to that of plasma and expands the intravascular fluid millilitre for millilitre. In contrast, the 25% albumin solution is hypertonic and causes additional fluid to move from the interstitium. Dextran is a complex synthetic sugar. Because dextran is metabolized slowly, it remains in the vascular system for a prolonged period but not as long as a colloid solution. It causes additional fluid to move into the intravascular space. (Indications for plasma volume expanders are discussed in Chapter 69.)

If the patient has lost blood, whole blood or packed RBCs are necessary. Packed RBCs have the advantage of giving the patient primarily RBCs; the blood bank can use the plasma for blood components. Whole blood, with its additional fluid volume, may cause circulatory overload. Although packed cells have a decreased plasma volume, they will increase the oncotic pressure and pull fluid into the intravascular space. Loop diuretics may be administered with blood to prevent symptoms of fluid volume excess in anemic patients who are not volume depleted. (Administration of blood is discussed in Chapter 33.)

CENTRAL VENOUS ACCESS DEVICES

Central venous access devices (CVADs) are catheters that are placed in large blood vessels (e.g., subclavian vein, jugular vein) when access to the vascular system is needed frequently. When the GI tract is nonfunctioning or requires rest, CVADs are used to deliver nutrients and electrolytes. In contrast to CVADs, the basic IV catheter is inserted into a peripheral vein in the hand, inside of the arm, or antecubital fossa and is used for short-term IV access. Central venous access can be achieved by three different methods: centrally inserted catheters, peripherally inserted central catheters (PICCs), or implanted ports. Centrally inserted catheters and implanted ports must be placed by a physician, whereas PICCs can be inserted by a nurse with specialized training.

🔍 EVIDENCE-INFORMED PRACTICE
Research Highlight

Do Heparin Flushes Decrease Occlusions in Central Venous Catheters?
Clinical Question
For patients with intermittently used central venous catheters (P), do heparin solution flushes (I) versus normal saline flushes (C) decrease catheter occlusions (O)?

Best Available Evidence
Cochrane systematic review of six studies with a total of 1 433 participants.

Critical Appraisal and Synthesis of Evidence
- Study participants were adult patients with a central venous catheter (CVC) or a peripherally inserted central catheter (PICC).
- Primary outcomes included occlusion of CVCs and duration (in days) of catheter patency.
- There were wide variations in guideline recommendations and practice surrounding the effectiveness of heparin flushing of CVCs.
- Potential harms were associated with heparin use, especially in critically ill patients.

Conclusions
- No conclusive evidence favours intermittent flushing with heparin over flushing with 0.9% normal saline in relation to safety or efficacy.
- More studies of central venous access maintenance are needed to guide evidence-informed practice.

Implications for Nursing Practice
- Maintenance of catheter patency is critical.
- Flushing devices with saline solution may be a safe and effective alternative to heparin flushes for catheter maintenance.

Reference for Evidence

López-Briz, E., Ruiz Garcia, V., Cabello, J. B., et al. (2018). Heparin versus 0.9% sodium chloride locking for prevention of occlusion in central venous catheters in adults (Review). Health. Cochrane Database of Systematic Reviews (7), CD008462. doi: 10.1002/14651858.CD008462.pub3.
P, patient population of interest; *I*, intervention or area of interest; *C*, comparison of interest or comparison group; *O*, outcome(s) of interest (see Chapter 1 of this textbook).

CVADs enable frequent, continuous, rapid, or intermittent administration of fluids and medications. They allow for the administration of drugs that are potential vesicants, blood and blood products, and parenteral nutrition. They may also be used for hemodynamic monitoring and venous blood sampling. These devices are indicated for patients who have limited peripheral vascular access or who have a projected need for long-term vascular access. Table 19.20 provides examples of medical conditions in which CVADs are used.

Advantages of CVADs include a reduced need for multiple venipunctures, decreased risk of extravasation injury, and immediate access to the central venous system. Although the incidence is decreased, extravasation can nonetheless occur if the device being used is displaced or damaged. The major disadvantages of CVADs are an increased risk of systemic infection and the invasiveness of the insertion procedure.

Centrally Inserted Catheters

The tip of centrally inserted catheters (also called *central venous catheters* [CVCs]) rests in the distal end of the superior vena cava near its junction with the right atrium (Figure 19.18). The other end of the catheter exits through a separate incision on the chest

TABLE 19.20	INDICATIONS FOR USE OF CENTRAL VENOUS ACCESS DEVICES*
Medical Condition	**Indications for Use**
Medication administration	
• Cancer	Chemotherapy, infusion of irritating or vesicant medications
• Infection	Long-term administration of antibiotics
• Pain	Long-term administration of pain medication
• Medications and other substances that increase risk for phlebitis	Epoprostenol (Flolan), calcium chloride, potassium chloride, amiodarone (Cordarone)
Nutritional replacement	Infusion of parenteral nutrition
	Solutions with higher dextrose content can be infused through CVAD (versus peripheral line)
Blood samples	Multiple diagnostic blood tests over a period of time
Blood transfusions	Infusion of blood or blood products in acute situations, as well as over a period of time
Renal failure	Performing hemodialysis (especially on an acute basis) or continuous renal replacement therapy
Shock, burns	Infusion of high volumes of fluid and electrolyte replacement
Hemodynamic monitoring	Measuring CVP to assess fluid balance
Heart failure	Performing ultrafiltration
Autoimmune disorders	Performing plasmapheresis

CVAD, central venous access device; *CVP*, central venous pressure.
*This list is not all-inclusive, and these are examples only.

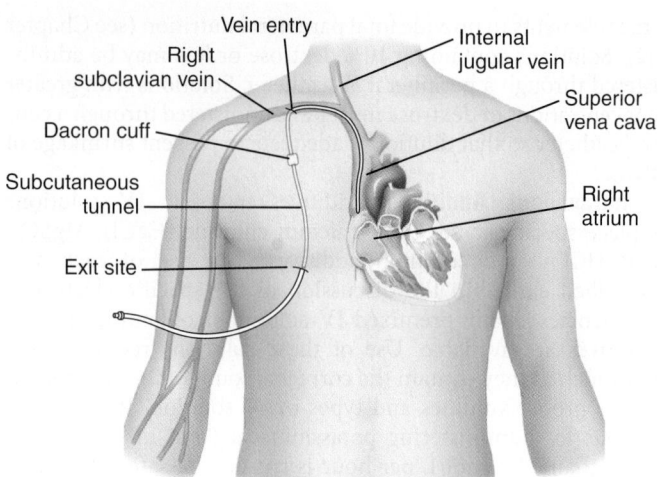

FIG. 19.18 Tunnelled central venous catheter. Note tip of the catheter in the superior vena cava.

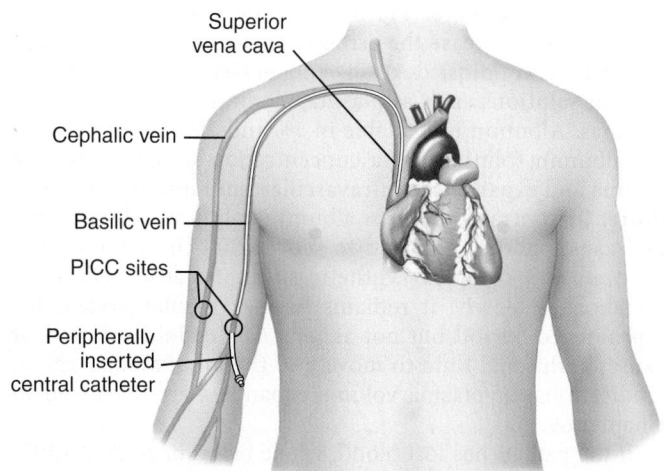

FIG. 19.19 Peripherally inserted central catheter (PICC) can be inserted into the basilic or cephalic vein.

or abdominal wall. Nontunnelled catheters are placed usually in the subclavian or internal jugular vein and more rarely in the femoral vein. They are best for patients with short-term needs in an acute care setting. Surgically placed tunnelled catheters (e.g., Hickman catheters) are suitable for long-term needs. Tunnelling of the catheter through subcutaneous tissue and the synthetic cuff used to anchor the catheter provide stability and decrease infection risk. Accurate placement must be verified by chest radiography before the catheter can be used. After the site heals, the catheter does not require a dressing, which makes it easier for the patient to maintain the site at home. Care requirements include injection cap change, cleansing, flushing, and dressing change.

CVCs are available as single-, double-, triple-, or quadruple-lumen catheters. Multilumen catheters are useful in critically ill patients because each lumen can be simultaneously used to provide a different therapy. For example, incompatible medications can be infused in separate lumens without mixing, and a third lumen can provide access for blood sampling. Specific types of long-term central catheters are Hickman catheters, for which clamps are needed to make sure the valve is closed, and Groshong catheters, which have a valve that opens as fluid is withdrawn or infused and remains closed when not in use.

Peripherally Inserted Central Catheters

PICCs are CVCs inserted into a vein in the arm. The basilic vein is preferred because of its large diameter. PICC lines are inserted at or just above the antecubital fossa and advanced to a position with the tip ending in the distal one third of the superior vena cava (Figure 19.19). Single-, double-, or triple-lumen PICCs are available; those with double lumens are preferred because they allow for simultaneous uses. PICCs are used in patients who need vascular access for 1 week to 6 months, but they can be in place for longer periods.

The technique for placement of a PICC line involves insertion of the catheter through a needle with the use of a guide wire or forceps to advance the line. Advantages of the PICC over a CVC are lower infection rate, fewer insertion-related complications, decreased cost, and ability to be inserted at the patient's bedside or in the outpatient area.

Complications of PICC lines include catheter occlusion and phlebitis (Table 19.21). If phlebitis occurs, it usually happens within 7 to 10 days after insertion. The nurse must not use the arm with the PICC to obtain a blood pressure reading or draw blood. When the blood pressure cuff is inflated, the PICC can touch the vein wall, which increases the risk of vein damage and thrombosis.

Implanted Infusion Ports

An implanted infusion port is a CVC connected to a single or double implanted subcutaneous injection port (Figure 19.20, *A*). The catheter is placed into the desired vein, and the other end is connected to a port that is surgically implanted in a subcutaneous pocket on the chest wall. The port consists of a metal sheath with a self-sealing silicone septum. Medications are injected through the skin into the port. After being filled, the reservoir slowly releases the medicine into the bloodstream.

TABLE 19.21 POTENTIAL COMPLICATIONS OF CENTRAL VENOUS ACCESS DEVICES

Possible Cause	Clinical Manifestations	Nursing and Interprofessional Management
Catheter Occlusion		
Clamped or kinked catheter	Sluggish infusion or aspiration	Instructing patient to change position, raise arm, and cough
Tip against wall of vessel	Inability to infuse or aspirate	Assessing for and alleviating clamping or kinking
Thrombosis		Flushing with normal saline with a 10-mL syringe; do not force flush
Precipitate buildup in lumen		Fluoroscopy to determine cause and site
		Anticoagulant or thrombolytic agents
Embolism		
Catheter breakage	Chest pain	Administering oxygen
Dislodgement of thrombus	Respiratory distress (dyspnea, tachypnea, hypoxia, cyanosis)	Clamping catheter
Entry of air into circulation		Placing patient on left side with head down (air emboli)
	Hypotension	Notifying health care provider
	Tachycardia	
Catheter-Related Infection (Local or Systemic)		
Contamination during insertion or use	Local: redness, tenderness, purulent drainage, warmth, edema	Local
		• Culture of drainage from site
Migration of organisms along catheter	Systemic: fever, chills, malaise	• Warm, moist compresses
		• Catheter removal if indicated
Immunosuppression of patient		Systemic
		• Blood cultures
		• Antibiotic therapy
		• Antipyretic therapy
		• Catheter removal if indicated
Pneumothorax		
Perforation of visceral pleura during insertion	Decrease in or absence of breath sounds	Administering oxygen
	Respiratory distress (cyanosis, dyspnea, tachypnea)	Positioning in semi-Fowler's position
		Preparing for chest tube insertion
	Chest pain	
	Unilateral distension of chest	
Catheter Migration		
Improper suturing	Sluggish infusion or aspiration	Fluoroscopy to verify position
Insertion site trauma	Edema of chest or neck during infusion	Assistance with removal and new CVAD placement
Changes in intrathoracic pressure	Patient report of gurgling sound in ear	
Forceful catheter flushing	Dysrhythmias	
Spontaneous movement	Increased external catheter length	

CVAD, central venous access device.

The port is accessed via the septum by means of a special noncoring needle that has a deflected tip, which prevents damage to the septum that could render the port useless (see Figure 19.20, *B*). Implanted ports are convenient for long-term therapy and can remain in the body for years. Because the port is hidden, it offers cosmetic advantages (Chopra, 2021). Care requirements include regular flushing. Formation of "sludge" (accumulation of clotted blood and drug precipitate) may also occur within the port septum.

Complications

The potential for complications associated with CVADs is always present. Astute monitoring and assessment may assist in early identification of potential complications. Table 19.21 lists potential complications of CVADs.

NURSING MANAGEMENT CENTRAL VENOUS ACCESS DEVICES

Nursing management of CVADs includes assessment, dressing change and cleansing, injection cap changes, and flushing. Although institution policies and procedures may differ for specific types of CVADs, there are some general guidelines to be followed.

Catheter and insertion site assessment includes inspecting the site for redness, edema, warmth, drainage, and tenderness or pain. Observing the catheter for misplacement or slippage is important.

The nurse should perform a comprehensive pain assessment, particularly noting any reports of chest or neck discomfort, arm pain, or pain at the insertion site. Newly placed CVADs should not be used until the tip position is verified with a chest radiograph.

Dressing change and cleansing of the catheter insertion site should be performed according to institution policies and procedures with strict sterile technique. Transparent semipermeable dressings or gauze and tape can be used. If the site is bleeding, a gauze dressing may be preferable; otherwise, transparent dressings are preferred because they allow observation of the site without having to be removed. Transparent dressings may be left in place for up to 1 week. The dressing should be changed immediately if it becomes damp, loose, or soiled.

The skin around the catheter insertion site should be cleansed according to institution policy. A chlorhexidine-based preparation is the cleansing agent of choice. Its effects last longer than either povidone-iodine or isopropyl alcohol, offering improved killing of bacteria (Broadhurst et al., 2017). When chlorhexidine is used, cleansing the skin with friction is critical for preventing infection (Cobbett et al., 2020). When applying a new dressing, the nurse should allow the area to air-dry completely. The lumen ports are secured to the skin above the dressing site. The nurse should document the date and time of the dressing change and initial the dressing.

Injection caps must be changed at regular intervals with the use of strict sterile technique according to institution policy or when

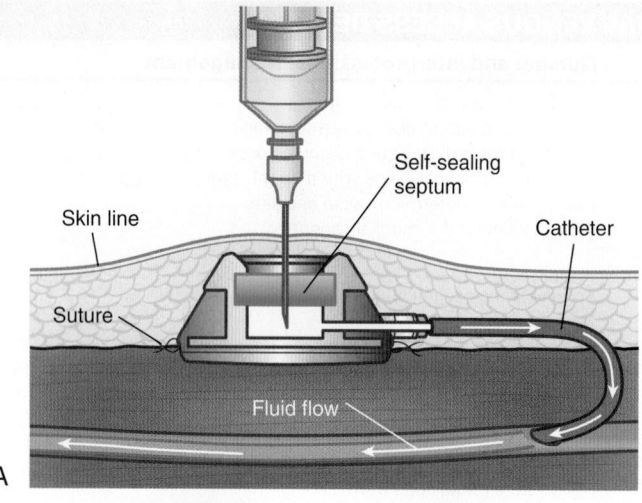

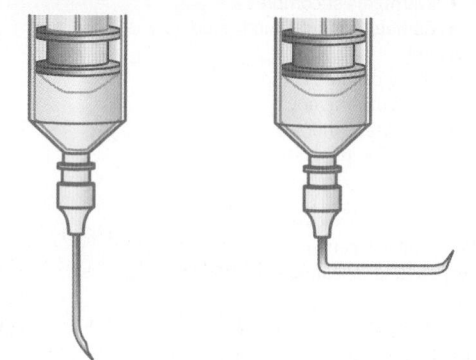

FIG. 19.20 **A,** Cross-section of implantable port displaying access of the port with the Huber-point needle. Note the deflected point of the Huber-point needle, which prevents coring of the port's septum. **B,** Two Huber-point needles used to enter the implanted port. The 90-degree needle is used for top-entry ports for continuous infusion. Source: A, Courtesy Pharmaceia Deltec, Inc., St. Paul, MN.

they are damaged from excessive punctures. The patient should be taught to turn their head to the opposite side of the CVAD insertion site during cap change. If the catheter cannot be clamped and is open to air, the patient should be asked to lie flat in bed and perform the Valsalva manoeuvre to prevent an air embolism.

Flushing is one of the most effective ways to maintain lumen patency and to prevent occlusion of the CVAD. It also keeps incompatible medications or fluids from mixing. The lumen is flushed with a normal saline solution in a syringe that has a barrel capacity of 10 mL or more to avoid excess pressure on the catheter. If resistance is felt, force should not be applied; this could result in rupture of the catheter or in the creation of an embolism if a thrombus is present. Because of the risk of contamination and infection, prefilled syringes or single-dose vials are preferred over multiple-dose vials. During flushing, the push–pause method is preferred over a continual even push of saline into the catheter. The push–pause technique creates turbulence within the catheter lumen, promoting the removal of debris that adheres to the catheter lumen. This technique involves injecting the saline with a rapid alternating push–pause motion, instilling 1 to 2 mL with each push on the syringe plunger.

Removal of Central Venous Access Devices

CVADs should be removed according to institution policy and the nurse's scope of practice. In many agencies, nurses with demonstrated competency can remove PICCs and nontunnelled CVCs. The procedure involves removing any sutures and then gently withdrawing the catheter. The patient is instructed to perform the Valsalva manoeuvre as the last 5 to 10 cm of the catheter is withdrawn. The nurse immediately applies pressure to the site with sterile gauze to prevent air from entering and to control bleeding. The catheter tip is inspected to ensure that it is intact. After bleeding has stopped, an antiseptic ointment and sterile dressing are applied to the site.

CASE STUDY

Fluid and Electrolyte Imbalance

Patient Profile

S. S. (pronouns she/her), a 73-year-old with lung cancer, has been receiving chemotherapy on an outpatient basis. Her third treatment was completed 5 days ago and she has been experiencing nausea and vomiting for 2 days even though taking prochlorperazine as directed. S. S.'s daughter brings her to the hospital, where she is admitted to the medical unit. The admitting nurse performs a thorough assessment.

Subjective Data

• Reports lethargy, weakness, and a dry mouth
• Has been too nauseated to eat or drink anything for 2 days

Objective Data

• Heart rate, 110; pulse, thready
• Blood pressure, 100/65 mm Hg
• Weight loss of 2.2 kg since she received her chemotherapy treatment 5 days ago
• Dry oral mucous membranes

Discussion Questions

1. According to the patient's clinical manifestations, what fluid imbalance does S. S. have?

2. What additional assessment data should the nurse obtain?
3. What are the patient's risk factors for fluid and electrolyte imbalances?
4. The nurse draws blood for a serum chemistry evaluation. What electrolyte imbalances are likely to be found and why?
5. This patient is at risk for which acid–base imbalance? Describe the changes that would occur in the patient's ABG values with this acid–base imbalance. How would S. S.'s body compensate?
6. What is the interprofessional team's priority for S. S.?
7. The health care provider orders dextrose 5% in 0.45% saline to infuse at 100 mL per hour. What type of solution is this, and how will it help the patient's fluid imbalance?
8. ***Priority Decision:*** What are the priority nursing interventions for S. S.?
9. ***Evidence-Informed Practice:*** S. S. has a double-lumen PICC in the left arm. One lumen is connected to the IV infusion; the other is unused. What is the recommended practice for maintaining the patency of the unused lumen?

evolve

Answers are available at http://evolve.elsevier.com/Canada/Lewis/medsurg.

REVIEW QUESTIONS

The number of the question corresponds to the same-numbered objective at the beginning of the chapter.

1. Why are older persons more at risk for fluid related imbalances?
   a. A higher proportion of their fluid is stored intracellularly.
   b. They have an increase in lean body mass as they age.
   c. They have a larger portion of fluid extracellularly which is easily lost.
   d. They have less total body fluid because of a decline in muscle and increase in fat.

2. If a client's extracellular fluid space is hypertonic in comparison to their intracellular fluid compartment, what would occur?
   a. Diffusion of fluid into the cell
   b. Osmotic pull of fluid out of the cell
   c. Active transport of sodium out of the cell
   d. Facilitated diffusion of glucose into the cell

3a. A client was admitted to the medical unit with GI bleeding and fluid volume deficit. What are the clinical manifestations of the latter problem? *(Select all that apply.)*
   a. Weight loss
   b. Dry oral mucosa
   c. Full bounding pulse
   d. Engorged neck veins
   e. Decreased central venous pressure

3b. Which of the following nursing actions is required for clients with hyponatremia?
   a. Fluid restriction
   b. Administration of hypotonic intravenous fluids
   c. Administration of a cation exchange resin
   d. Increased water intake for clients on nasogastric suction

3c. Which of the following should the nurse monitor for when a client is receiving a loop diuretic?
   a. Restlessness and agitation
   b. Paresthesias and irritability
   c. Weak, irregular pulse and poor muscle tone
   d. Increased blood pressure and muscle spasms

3d. Which of the following clients would be at greatest risk for the potential development of hypermagnesemia?
   a. An 83-year-old man with lung cancer and hypertension
   b. A 65-year-old woman with hypertension taking β-adrenergic blockers
   c. A 42-year-old woman with systemic lupus erythematosus and renal failure
   d. A 50-year-old man with benign prostatic hyperplasia and a urinary tract infection

3e. In a client who has just undergone a total thyroidectomy, it is especially important for the nurse to assess which of the following?
   a. Weight gain
   b. Depressed reflexes
   c. Positive Chvostek's sign
   d. Confusion and personality changes

3f. Care of the client experiencing hyperphosphatemia secondary to renal failure includes which of the following?
   a. Calcium supplements
   b. Potassium supplements
   c. Magnesium supplements
   d. Fluid replacement therapy

4. How do the lungs act as an acid–base buffer?
   a. By increasing respiratory rate and depth when CO_2 levels in the blood are high, thereby reducing acid load
   b. By increasing respiratory rate and depth when CO_2 levels in the blood are low, thereby reducing base load
   c. By decreasing respiratory rate and depth when CO_2 levels in the blood are high, thereby reducing acid load
   d. By decreasing respiratory rate and depth when CO_2 levels in the blood are low, thereby increasing acid load

5. A client has the following arterial blood gas results: pH, 7.52; partial pressure of carbon dioxide in the arterial blood ($PaCO_2$), 30 mm Hg; HCO_3^- level, 24 mmol/L. These results indicate the presence of which acid–base disturbance?
   a. Metabolic acidosis
   b. Metabolic alkalosis
   c. Respiratory acidosis
   d. Respiratory alkalosis

6. What is the typical fluid replacement for the client with a fluid volume deficit?
   a. Dextran
   b. 0.45% Saline
   c. Lactated Ringer's solution
   d. 5% Dextrose in 0.45% saline

7. The nurse is unable to flush a central venous access device and suspects occlusion. Which of the following would be the best nursing intervention?
   a. Apply warm moist compresses to the insertion site.
   b. Attempt to force 10 mL of normal saline into the device.
   c. Place the client on the left side with head-down position.
   d. Instruct the client to change positions, raise arm, and cough.

1. d; 2.b; 3a. a, b, e; 3b. a; 3c. c; 3d. c; 3e. c; 3f. d; 4. a; 5. d; 6. c; 7. d.

ⓔvolve

For even more review questions, visit http://evolve.elsevier.com/Canada/Lewis/medsurg.

REFERENCES

Broadhurst, D., Moureau, N., & Ullmna, A. (2017). Management of central venous access device–associated skin impairment. *Journal of Wound Ostomy Continence Nursing*, 44(3), 211–220. https://doi.org/10.1097/WON.0000000000000322

Chopra, V. (2021). *Central venous access devices and approach to device and site selection in adults.* UpToDate. https://www.uptodate.com/contents/central-venous-access-devices-and-approach-to-device-and-site-selection-in-adults

Cobbett, S. L., Perry, A. G., Potter, P. A., et al. (2020). *Canadian clinical nursing skills and techniques* (1st Canadian ed.). Elsevier.

Danielsson, E. J. D., Leibman, I., & Akeson, J. (2019). Fluid volume deficits during prolonged overnight fasting in young health adults. *Acta Anaesthesiologica Scandinavica*, 63, 195–199. https:///doi.org/10.1111/aas.13254

Horwitz, M. J. (2020). *Hypercalcemia of malignancy: Mechanisms.* UpToDate. https://www.uptodate.com/contents/hypercalcemia-of-malignancy-mechanisms

Kear, T. M. (2017). Fluid and electrolyte management across the age continuum. *Nephrology Nursing Journal*, 44(6), 491–496.

Koch, C. A., & Fulop, C. (2017). Clinical aspects of changes in water and sodium homeostasis in the elderly. *Reviews in Endocrine and Metabolic Disorders, 18,* 49–66. https://doi.org/10.1007/s11154-017-9420-5

McCance, K. L., & Huether, S. E. (2019). *Pathophysiology: The biologic basis for disease in adults and children* (8th ed.). Elsevier.

Mosby. (2016). *Mosby's dictionary of medicine, nursing, and health professions* (10th ed.). Mosby.

Mount, D. B. (2019). *Clinical manifestations and treatment of hypokalemia in adults.* UpToDate. https://www.uptodate.com/contents/clinical-manifestations-and-treatment-of-hypokalemia-in-adults

Porth, C. M. (2018). *Pathophysiology: Concepts of altered health states* (10th ed.). Lippincott.

Reddi, A. S. (2018). *Fluid, electrolyte, and acid-based disorders: Clinical evaluation and management* (2nd ed.). Springer.

Shane, E. (2021). *Etiology of hypercalcemia.* UpToDate. https://www.uptodate.com/contents/etiology-of-hypercalcemia

Shane, E., & Berenson, J. R. (2020). *Treatment of hypercalcemia.* UpToDate. https://www.uptodate.com/contents/treatment-of-hypercalcemia

Sterns, R. H. (2020). *Etiology, clinical manifestations, and diagnosis of volume depletion in adults.* UpToDate. https://www.uptodate.com/contents/etiology-clinical-manifestations-and-diagnosis-of-volume-depletion-in-adults

Yu, A. S. L. (2020). *Hypermagnesemia: Causes of hypermagnesemia.* UpToDate. https://www.uptodate.com/contents/hypomagnesemia-causes-of-hypomagnesemia

RESOURCES

Acid–Base Physiology
http://www.anaesthesiamcq.com/AcidBaseBook/ABindex.php
Acid–Base Tutorial
https://www.acid-base.com/
Body Fluid Volumes Calculator
https://www.globalrph.com/body_fluid_volumes.htm

Ⓔvolve

For additional Internet resources, see the website for this book at http://evolve.elsevier.com/Canada/Lewis/medsurg.

Perioperative Care

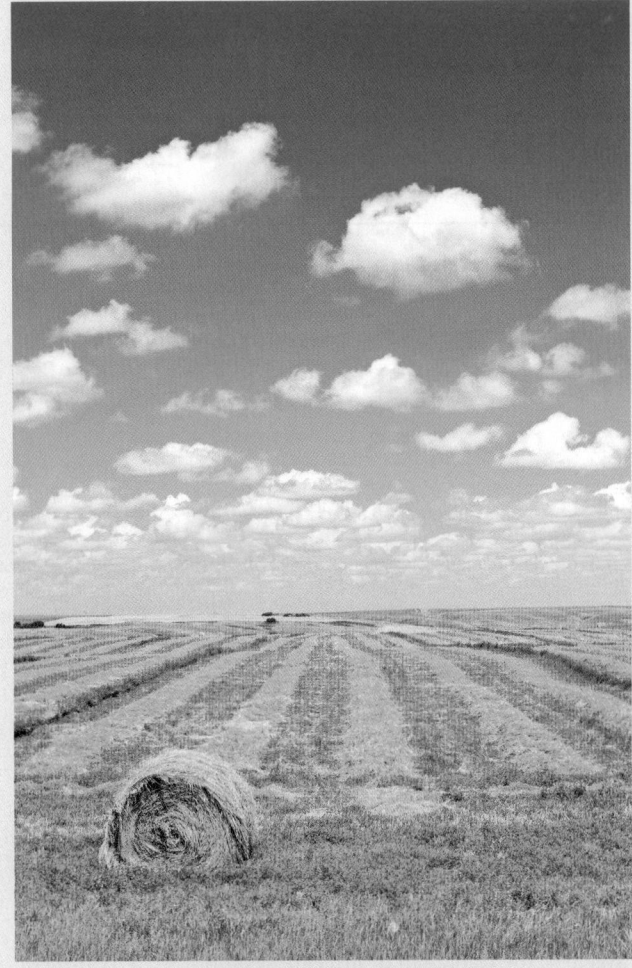

Source: © CanStock Photo/Elenathewise.

Chapter 20: Nursing Management: **Preoperative Care**
Chapter 21: Nursing Management: **Intraoperative Care**
Chapter 22: Nursing Management: **Postoperative Care**

Nursing Management
Preoperative Care

Peggy Hancock
Originating US chapter by Janice A. Neil

evolve WEBSITE

http://evolve.elsevier.com/Canada/Lewis/medsurg

- Review Questions (Online Only)
- Key Points
- Answer Guidelines for Case Study
- Conceptual Care Map Creator
- Audio Glossary
- Content Updates

LEARNING OBJECTIVES

1. Identify the common purposes and settings of surgery.
2. Describe the purpose and components of a preoperative nursing assessment.
3. Interpret the significance of the data related to the preoperative patient's health status and operative risk.
4. Analyze the purpose and components of the patient's informed consent for surgery.
5. Examine the nursing role in the physical, psychological, and educational preparation of the patient undergoing surgery.
6. Prioritize nursing responsibilities related to day-of-surgery preparation for the patient undergoing surgery.
7. Identify the purposes and types of common preoperative medications.
8. Apply knowledge of special considerations in the preoperative preparation for the older surgical patient.

KEY TERMS

ambulatory surgery	emergency surgery	perioperative
elective surgery	informed consent	same-day admission

As stated throughout this text, the Canadian health care system focuses on the health and well-being of all Canadians, through health promotion and illness prevention. Nonetheless, diseases or conditions can occur that require surgical interventions. Surgery may be performed for any of the following purposes:

1. *Diagnosis*—to determine the presence or extent of pathological abnormality (e.g., lymph node biopsy or bronchoscopy)
2. *Cure*—to eliminate or repair a pathological condition (e.g., removal of a ruptured appendix or benign ovarian cyst) or repair anatomy (e.g., fracture fixation)
3. *Palliation*—to alleviate symptoms without cure (e.g., cutting a nerve root [rhizotomy] to remove symptoms of pain or creating a colostomy to bypass an inoperable bowel obstruction)
4. *Prevention*—to reduce the risk of developing a condition (e.g., removal of a mole before it becomes malignant, removal of the colon in a patient with familial polyposis to prevent cancer)

5. *Cosmetic improvement*—to alter physical appearance (e.g., repairing a burn scar, breast reconstruction after a mastectomy)
6. *Exploration*—to determine the nature or extent of a disease (e.g., laparotomy). Exploration is less common because many problems can be identified noninvasively.

The total surgical episode is called the perioperative period. Terminology used in surgical procedures combines anatomical vocabulary with prefixes and suffixes derived primarily from Latin and Greek. The use of this language pattern allows us to determine what operation or procedure is being done. Table 20.1 provides a sampling of suffixes that are commonly combined with an anatomical part or organ in naming surgical procedures.

SURGICAL SETTINGS

Surgery may be a carefully planned event (elective surgery) or may arise with unexpected urgency (emergency surgery).

TABLE 20.1	SUFFIXES DESCRIBING COMMON SURGICAL PROCEDURES			
Suffix	**Meaning**	**General Surgery**	**Orthopedic Surgery**	**Urological Surgery**
-ectomy	Excision/removal	Appendectomy	Discectomy	Nephrectomy
-oscopy	Looking into	Gastroscopy	Knee arthroscopy	Cystoscopy
-ostomy	Creation of opening into	Colostomy		Ureterostomy
-otomy	Cutting into/incision	Tracheotomy	Arthrotomy	Cystotomy
-plasty	Repair/reconstruction	Mammoplasty	Total hip arthroplasty	Ureteroplasty

Regardless of where the surgery is performed or whether it is emergency or elective surgery, nurses are vital in preparing the patient for surgery, caring for the patient during surgery, and facilitating the patient's recovery postoperatively.

Elective Inpatient Surgery

The most common inpatient surgeries in Canada are Caesarean birth, knee replacement, hip replacement, fractures, and coronary artery angioplasty (Canadian Institute for Health Information [CIHI], 2018). Patients requiring hospitalization for surgery are usually admitted the day of their surgery (same-day admission).

Ambulatory Surgery. In Canada, for the majority of surgeries, the patient is discharged on the same day that they undergo surgery. Ambulatory surgery, also called *same-day surgery,* can be conducted in emergency departments, endoscopy clinics, health care provider's offices, and outpatient surgery units in hospitals. These procedures can be performed using general, regional, or local anaesthetic, usually take less than 2 hours, and necessitate less than a 3- to 4-hour stay in the postanaesthesia care unit (PACU); they do not require overnight hospitalization. Sometimes patients are admitted to hospital postoperatively if they experience complications, but many patients go home with a caregiver within hours of surgery.

Health care providers work collaboratively to ensure the safety and well-being of the patient. Several nurses are involved in the surgical patient's continuum of care through the preoperative, intraoperative, and postoperative phases. The following information gathered by the perianaesthesia nurse before surgery assists these nurses in planning care:

- The disorder necessitating surgery
- Awareness of comorbidities
- Identification of the patient's response to the stress of surgery
- Assessment of results of preoperative diagnostic tests
- Consideration of bodily alterations, impact of comorbidities, risks, and potential complications associated with surgery

This preoperative assessment is communicated and documented to ensure continuity of care.

The preoperative nursing measures included in this chapter are applicable to the preparation of any patient undergoing surgery, whether or not the patient is coming from home or previously admitted to hospital. Measures to prepare for specific surgical procedures (e.g., abdominal, thoracic, or orthopedic surgery) are covered in appropriate chapters of this text.

SURGICAL WAIT TIMES

Currently, all provinces in Canada collect and report on surgical wait times for heart, joint replacement, and sight-restoration surgery. Provincial wait times are compared using a pan-Canadian benchmark for the various categories (CIHI, 2020).

Efforts to reduce wait times for elective surgery in Canada had mixed results from 2015 to 2017. For instance, the wait time for cataract and joint replacement surgery increased. Wait times for urgent repair of hip fractures, which is associated with a high mortality risk in older persons, remained stable in those 2 years. The COVID-19 pandemic has had a negative impact on wait time for elective surgeries, with tens of thousands of scheduled surgeries being cancelled across Canada (Wiseman et al., 2020). Despite all the contextual variables, Canada remains committed to reducing surgical and diagnostic wait times and continues to perform well when compared internationally (CIHI, 2021). Interprofessional collaboration and leadership for a strategic management plan of surgical wait lists postpandemic will be imperative (Wiseman et al., 2020).

PREOPERATIVE ADMISSION ASSESSMENT

The patient's initial contact for preoperative evaluation is done at the preoperative admission clinic (PAC), where the patient is interviewed by a perianaesthesia nurse. The interview is done at least 1 day ahead of surgery and can be conducted either in person or by telephone (Campbell, 2019). Patients with complex conditions may require an anaesthesia or interprofessional team consult.

The preoperative assessment typically includes a physical assessment, collection of admission data (including medication and food allergies), reviewing consent forms, a preanaesthesia evaluation, obtaining the patient's weight and airway history, and collecting laboratory and diagnostic tests (Campbell, 2019). This session provides an opportunity to educate the patient and family or caregiver and for them to ask questions regarding the preparation for surgery and anaesthetic policies. The information provided includes the following:

- Policy for taking routine medication on day of surgery
- Which medications (e.g., anticoagulants) or herbal remedies to stop prior to surgery and when to stop them
- Nothing-by-mouth (NPO) instructions
- Pain management options
- Infection prevention and wound care
- Instructions for postoperative exercises
- Postoperative discharge and care (see Chapter 22)

DAY-OF-SURGERY ASSESSMENT

All surgical patients have a physical assessment completed and documented by a physician. The extent of the exam depends on the type of surgery and anaesthesia required.

On the day of surgery, the nurse does a focused preoperative assessment involving review of existing information, reinforcement of teaching, and review of discharge plans (Cartwright & Andrews, 2018). The psychosocial needs of the patient are paramount at this time, as are the needs of the patient's companion or family (O'Brien, 2018). Each hospital or facility has a concise preoperative checklist that can help the nurse meet the following goals:

- Confirm and identify changes to the patient's physical status by reviewing the physical exam, confirming that preoperative consultations are complete (e.g., by a cardiology, internal medicine, physiotherapy, or wound care nurse), and communicate mobility or sensory deficits to the perioperative team.
- Determine the patient's psychological status and reinforce coping strategies.
- Establish baseline data (i.e., vital signs) for comparison in the intraoperative and postoperative periods.
- Review prescription medications, over-the-counter (OTC) medications, and herbal medications that may affect the surgical outcome.
- Ensure that preoperative laboratory and diagnostic test results are documented and communicated to appropriate personnel.
- Support the patient's language, family, culture, and spiritual or religious needs that may affect the surgical experience.
- Determine whether the patient has adequate information from the surgeon to make an informed decision to have the surgery, and ensure that the consent form is signed by the patient and physician.
- Ensure that the patient understands the discharge plan and has postoperative support. This may involve setting up postoperative care with rehabilitative facilities or community nursing agencies.

Subjective Data

Psychosocial Assessment. The meaning of surgery should be explored with the patient, as each person has a different perception and anxiety level regarding the procedure, anaesthesia, and postoperative pain (Schick, 2018). Stress can negatively affect surgical outcomes, such as causing a longer, more painful postoperative recovery (Ashpari & Lakshman, 2018). Many factors can influence the patient's susceptibility to stress, including the use of positive coping strategies, such as taking an active role, relaxation training, using distraction, and practising other pain control techniques. Past experiences, current health, socioeconomic status, and age also affect a patient's level of stress. Calm, confident nursing communication can help allay patients' fears (Schick, 2018). (See Chapter 8 for a discussion of stress.)

Older persons may perceive hospitalization for surgery as a physical decline or loss of mobility and independence. They may fear being placed in a long-term care facility, which some view as a place to die. The nurse is instrumental in alleviating anxieties and restoring the self-esteem of these surgical patients (see Age-Related Considerations at the end of the chapter) by identifying stressors that can negatively affect them (Table 20.2). If the patient and caregivers do not speak English, it is ideal to have an interpreter to disseminate information. Not all hospitals can provide an interpreter, so families may bring an English-speaking representative with them to the preoperative interview, or a language translation software program or phone app may be used. (The use of interpreters is discussed in Chapter 2.)

Anxiety. Patients may be anxious when facing surgery because of lack of knowledge—for example, not knowing what to expect during the surgical experience or having uncertainty about the outcome of surgery and the potential findings of diagnostic procedures. Some may worry about allowing strangers to

TABLE 20.2 PSYCHOSOCIAL ASSESSMENT OF THE PATIENT BEFORE SURGERY

Situational Changes
- Determine support systems, including family, other caregivers, significant others, and religious or spiritual orientation.
- Define degree of personal control, decision making, and independence.
- Consider the impact of surgery and hospitalization on the family and dependents and financial impacts related to recovery time and medical expenses.
- Identify the presence of hope and anticipation of positive results.

Concerns With the Unknown
- Identify specific areas and depth of anxiety and fears.
- Identify expectations of surgery, changes in current health status, and effects on daily living.

Concerns With Body Image
- Identify current roles or relationships and view of self.
- Determine perceived or potential changes in role or relationships and their impact on body image.

Past Experiences
- Review previous surgical experiences, hospitalizations, and treatments.
- Determine responses to those experiences (positive and negative).
- Identify current perceptions of surgical procedure in relation to the above and information from others (e.g., a neighbour's view of a personal surgical experience).

Knowledge Deficit
- Identify what preoperative information this specific patient wants to receive.
- Assess understanding of the surgical procedure, including preparation, care, interventions, preoperative activities, restrictions, and expected outcomes.
- Identify the accuracy of information the patient has received from others, including the health care team, family, friends, and the media.

take control of their life or even have concerns about not waking from anaesthesia. Nurses can minimize anxiety by explaining the anticipated sequence of events, providing time for the patient and their family to discuss concerns, and minimizing exposure to stimuli in the operating room (OR) that may promote anxiety (Devolder, 2019).

Patients may be concerned when surgical or anaesthetic interventions, for example, blood transfusions, are in conflict with religious or cultural beliefs. The requesting physician should discuss the need for blood replacement with the patient and obtain an informed consent, noting patient consent or refusal for transfusion on the patient's chart.

Common Fears. The primary reasons that patients fear surgery are the fear of dying under anaesthesia, permanent disability resulting from the operation, pain, change in body image, or receiving a poor prognosis during a diagnostic procedure (e.g., breast biopsy). Patients can become fearful after independently hearing or reading about the risks of surgery and during the informed-consent process when the surgeon explains all aspects of the operation to the patient.

Fear of death can be extremely stressful for the patient. If the nurse identifies that a patient has a fear of death, this information must be communicated to the surgeon immediately. It is important that the surgeon talk with the patient in order to understand where the fear originates and to assuage anxiety.

Fear of pain and discomfort during and after surgery is common. If the fear appears extreme, the nurse should notify the anaesthesiologist so that appropriate preoperative medication (such as an antianxiety medication) can be ordered. The patient should be reassured that medications are available to minimize or eliminate pain during and after surgery. Medications can be given that provide an amnesic effect so that the patient will not remember what occurs during the surgical episode. These medications can cause temporary cognitive deficits following surgery that the patient must be informed of. The nurse should stress that the patient should ask for pain medications as needed following surgery and that taking these medications will not contribute to an addiction but may assist with postoperative recovery. (Pain is discussed in Chapter 10.)

Fear of mutilation or alteration in body image can occur whether the surgery is minor or radical, such as amputation. Even the presence of just a small scar on the body can be bothersome to some patients. The nurse should assess these concerns with an open, nonjudgemental attitude.

Fear of anaesthesia may arise from fear of the unknown, from reports of others' bad experiences, or from previous personal experience. Some patients are concerned about information provided about hazards or complications (e.g., brain damage, paralysis, family history of malignant hyperthermia). Other patients have a fear of losing control while under the influence of anaesthesia. If these fears or questions are identified, the nurse should inform the anaesthesiologist immediately so that they can reassure the patient and confirm that a nurse and the anaesthesiologist will be present at all times during surgery.

Fear of disruption of life function or patterns can present to varying degrees. A patient may fear permanent disability or loss of life or have concerns about physical limitations after surgery. Also common are concerns about separation from family and worry about how a spouse or children will manage. Financial concerns may surface as a result of an anticipated loss of income because of missed work. If the nurse identifies any of these fears, consultation with a social worker, a spiritual or cultural advisor, a psychologist, or family members may provide valuable assistance to the patient.

Coping With Surgery. The way that patients transition through the perioperative period can affect their postoperative recovery. Many draw on their spirituality, seeking inner peace and sources of hope. As patients, especially outpatients, move through the surgical experience in an accelerated fashion, the perioperative team must be responsive to the patient's health goals, hopes, and fears in order to provide the necessary support. For many people, spirituality and health are interrelated, thus requiring the interprofessional team to implement a holistic preoperative approach to patient care (Adugbire & Aziato, 2020).

Health History. During the preoperative interview, the nurse should ask about the patient's diagnosed medical conditions and current health issues. An organized approach using hospital guidelines and subjective questioning elicits good information regarding the patient's health history. Initially, the nurse should determine whether the patient understands the reason for surgery. For example, the patient scheduled for a total knee replacement may indicate that the reason for surgery is increasing pain and mobility problems. Detailed information on past hospitalizations, previous surgeries, dates of the surgeries, and any adverse reactions or problems with surgery or anaesthetics is documented. As an example, the patient may have experienced a bad wound infection or a reaction to an analgesic following a prior surgery.

Women should be asked about their menstrual and obstetrical history, including the date of their last menstrual period and the number of pregnancies and births they have had. If the patient states that she might be pregnant, this information should be immediately communicated to the surgeon to avoid maternal and subsequent fetal exposure to anaesthetics during the first trimester. Questioning an adolescent regarding her reproductive functioning may be embarrassing for her and should be done in privacy with parents or guardians out of the room.

The nurse may identify inherited conditions by asking about the patient's family health history. A family history of cardiac and endocrine disease should be recorded. If a patient reports a mother or father with hypertension, sudden cardiac death, myocardial infarction, or coronary artery disease, the nurse should be alerted to the possibility that the patient may have a similar predisposition or condition. A family history of diabetes should be investigated because of the familial predisposition to both type 1 and type 2 diabetes mellitus. Tendencies toward these conditions may be exacerbated during surgery and affect physiological function during and after surgery. Family history must be considered, since inherited traits contribute to the choice of anaesthesia and can impact surgical outcomes (Cartwright & Andrews, 2018). Anaesthesia care providers obtain the patient's and family's anaesthetic history, particularly adverse reactions to or problems with anaesthesia, such as malignant hyperthermia. This is a rare metabolic disease triggered by specific anaesthesia that results in hyperthermia, skeletal muscle rigidity, and possible death if uncorrected in a timely manner. The genetic predisposition for malignant hyperthermia susceptibility is well documented, and anaesthetic care plans are preventive (Campbell, 2019). (Malignant hyperthermia is discussed in Chapter 21.)

Medications. As part of the preoperative interview, the nurse documents the patient's current medication use, including the use of OTC medications and herbal products. Patients may be asked to bring their medication bottles when attending the PAC so that the nurse can accurately chart the names and dosages as patients who use a variety of medications may not remember specific details. At this time, it is important also to investigate whether the patient is taking the medication as ordered or has stopped taking it because of cost, adverse effects, or the belief that ongoing therapy is no longer needed.

Medications and herbal products may interact with anaesthetics, often increasing or decreasing potency and effectiveness, or they may be needed during surgery to maintain physiological function. It is important to consider the effects of medications used for heart disease, hypertension, immunosuppression, seizure control, anticoagulation, and endocrine replacement. Insulin or oral hypoglycemic agents may require dosage or agent adjustments during the perioperative period because of increased body metabolism, decreased caloric intake, stress, and anaesthesia. Many patients use OTC acetylsalicylic acid (Aspirin) or are on anticoagulant therapy such as warfarin sodium (Coumadin), heparin, clopidogrel (Plavix), or others that inhibit platelet aggregation and may contribute to postoperative bleeding complications. Surgeons often require that patients stop taking acetylsalicylic acid (Aspirin) for at least 2 weeks before surgery. It is also important to stress that stopping some medications abruptly can cause complications. The preoperative nurse should check with an anaesthesiologist to ensure which medications should be stopped and which should be taken the day of surgery.

The use of herbal therapy and dietary supplements is common, but many patients do not disclose to health care providers that they take these supplements unless specifically asked (Larner, 2019). Therefore, it is essential for the nurse to ask about the use of vitamins, herbal supplements, and other alternative substances (see Chapter 12, Table 12.5). These products may interfere with anaesthesia and potentially cause complications during surgery, such as effects on blood pressure, increased sedation, cardiac effects, electrolyte alterations, and inhibition of platelet aggregation. In patients taking anticoagulants or platelet aggregation inhibitors, the use of specific herbal products can cause excessive postoperative bleeding that may necessitate a return to the OR. It is generally recommended that herbal supplements be discontinued at least 2 weeks before surgery (Larner, 2019). Some effects of specific herbs that can be of concern during the perioperative period are identified in the Complementary & Alternative Therapies box.

In the preoperative interview, the nurse should ask the patient about recreational drug use and any substance use disorder. The most likely used substances include tobacco, alcohol, opioids, marijuana, cocaine, and amphetamines. Questions should be asked matter-of-factly and information given that recreational drug use may affect the type and amount of anaesthesia required. Patients should be asked when and what was last used. When patients are aware of the potential interactions of these drugs with anaesthetics, most will respond honestly about their drug use. Furthermore, if the patient has a history of drug use, medications given during the operative period should be considered in light of the patient's recovery.

The nurse must also gather information about the patient's tobacco use as well as electronic cigarettes, or vaping. Members of the interprofessional team should encourage the patient to stop smoking at least 6 weeks before surgery. Smoking and vaping increase the risk for pulmonary complications during and after surgery.

Chronic alcohol use may place the patient undergoing surgery at risk because of lung, gastrointestinal, or liver damage. When liver function is decreased, metabolism of anaesthetic agents is prolonged, nutritional status is altered, and the potential for postoperative complications is increased. Alcohol withdrawal can also occur during lengthy surgery or in the postoperative period but can be avoided with appropriate planning and management (see Chapter 11).

The nurse should also assess for recent use of cannabis. While the full effect of cannabis use is not fully understood, individuals who use cannabis have been shown to require increased doses of propofol for induction and require higher doses of postoperative analgesia (Alexander & Joshi, 2019).

When assessing medication use, medication intolerance and medication allergies should be considered. Medication intolerance usually results in adverse effects that are uncomfortable or unpleasant for the patient but not life-threatening. These effects can include nausea, constipation, diarrhea, or *idiosyncratic* (opposite from expected) reactions. A true medication allergy produces hives, an anaphylactic reaction, or both, causing cardiopulmonary compromise, including hypotension, tachycardia, bronchospasm, and possibly pulmonary edema. Awareness of medication intolerance and medication allergies, however, makes it possible to maintain patient comfort, safety, and stability. For example, some anaesthetic agents contain sulphur, so the anaesthesiologist should be notified of a history of allergy to sulphur. Any medication intolerance or medication allergy

COMPLEMENTARY & ALTERNATIVE THERAPIES

Effects of Herbs and Supplements During the Perioperative Period

Herb	Perioperative Considerations
Echinacea	May cause immune suppression if taken over long term. Use is to be discontinued as far in advance of surgery as possible.
Ephedra	Stimulant, decongestant, bronchodilator, taken for weight loss. Multiple cardiovascular and GI adverse effects. Use is to be discontinued at least 24 hours preoperatively.
Feverfew	May increase clotting time. Preoperative use is to be avoided.
Garlic	May increase clotting time and potentiate effects of anticoagulants. Use is to be discontinued at least 7 days preoperatively.
Ginger	May increase bleeding. Should be avoided preoperatively.
Ginkgo biloba	May increase bleeding, especially in patients taking anticoagulants. Use is to be discontinued at least 36 hours preoperatively.
Ginseng	May falsely elevate digoxin levels and potentiate MAOIs. Contraindicated for cardiac disorders, hypertension, and hypoglycemia. Use is to be discontinued at least 7 days preoperatively.
Goldenseal	May cause hypotension; may increase edema and potentiate effect of insulin. Preoperative use is to be avoided.
Kava	May prolong the effects of certain anaesthetics and have an adverse effect on motor reflexes. Use is to be discontinued at least 24 hours preoperatively.
Licorice	Certain preparations may cause elevated BP or electrolyte imbalance. Not to be used for more than 7 days.
Saw palmetto	May have additive effects with other hormone therapies.
St. John's wort	May prolong the effects of anaesthetic agents, potentiate opioids, and cause peripheral neuropathy.
Valerian	Potentiates sedative–hypnotics; may prolong anaesthesia recovery time. Dose is to be tapered for 1–2 weeks preoperatively.
Vitamin E	May increase bleeding.

BP, blood pressure; *GI*, gastrointestinal; *MAOI*, monoamine oxidase inhibitor.
Sources: Modified from Braun, L., & Cohen, M. (2015). *Herbs and natural supplements, volume 2: An evidence-based guide* (4th ed.). Elsevier; Wang, C., et al. (2015). Commonly used dietary supplements on coagulation function during surgery. *Medicines (Basel), 2*(3), 157–185; National Center for Complementary and Integrative Health (NCCIH). (2016). *Herbs at a glance.* https://nccih.nih.gov/health/herbsataglance.htm, as found in Larner, R. (2019). Integrative health practices: Complementary and alternative therapies. In J. Rothrock & D. McEwen (Eds.), *Alexander's care of the patient in surgery* (16th ed., pp. 1147–1162). Elsevier Mosby.

identified must be documented and flagged on the patient's chart; on the day of surgery, an allergy wristband is put on the patient. Depending on institutional policy, the nurse may be responsible for entering the identified allergy in the electronic medical record so that all health care providers and the pharmacy have knowledge of any medication or related allergy.

All findings of the medication history are documented and communicated to the intraoperative and postoperative teams. Although the anaesthesiologist will determine the appropriate schedule and dose of the patient's routine medications before and after surgery based on the medication history, the nurse must ensure that all of the patient's medications are identified, administer the medications as ordered, and monitor the patient for potential interactions and complications.

Allergies. The nurse should inquire about nonpharmaceutical allergies to foods, metals, chemicals, tape, and pollen. The patient with a history of any allergic response has a greater potential for demonstrating hypersensitivity reactions to medications administered during anaesthesia. Patients should also be screened for possible latex allergies (Operating Room Nurses Association of Canada [ORNAC], 2019) (see Chapters 16 and 21). The Operating Room Nurses Association of Canada (2019) recommends that patients who report the following be considered at risk for latex allergy:

- History of contact dermatitis and atopic immunological reactions
- Allergies to nuts, bananas, avocados, kiwi, chestnuts, papayas, pitted fruit
- Repeated exposure to latex (multiple operations, spina bifida, or malformations of genitourinary tract)

High-risk groups for latex allergy also include health care providers. Latex allergies produce reactions ranging from mild skin redness to anaphylaxis (ORNAC, 2019).

Review of Systems. A thorough body systems review is performed and documented before surgery by members of the perioperative team. This review of systems is described in detail in Chapter 3. The surgeon does a preoperative physical examination and patient history and orders appropriate preoperative laboratory tests and consultations before the day of surgery. In the immediate preoperative period, there is seldom time for the nurse to do a full physical assessment, so nurses rely on the chart documentation. The following are important points for the nurse to assess immediately before surgery to ensure a seamless, safe experience for the patient.

Nervous System. Preoperative evaluation of neurological functioning includes assessing the patient's ability to respond to questions, follow commands, and maintain orderly thought patterns. Alterations in the patient's hearing (e.g., requiring hearing aids) and vision (e.g., requiring glasses, development of glaucoma) may affect responses and the ability to follow directions. A person's ability to pay attention, concentrate, and respond appropriately is documented to use as the baseline for postoperative comparison.

Impaired cognitive function may affect the patient's ability to prepare for surgery, and the nurse must determine whether all preoperative procedures were carried out—for example, bowel preparations. If confusion is noted and persistent, it is important to determine whether there are appropriate resources and support to assist the patient after surgery.

Cognitive function is of major importance in the assessment of older patients. Although major surgery is a predisposing factor for delirium, other predictive conditions for delirium are dehydration, malnutrition, immobility, urinary catheters, medications, and infection (Allen, 2019). Nonverbal older patients and those with chronic conditions such as Alzheimer's disease must be assessed for their interpretation of pain before surgery so that postoperative pain scales can be used effectively. These preoperative findings are extremely important for postoperative comparison. Older people are at risk for untreated pain because of beliefs that pain must be endured and that they should not disturb nurses with complaints of pain (Allen, 2019).

Cardiovascular System. The purpose of evaluating cardiovascular function is to determine the presence of pre-existing disease or existing concerns so that the patient's condition can be effectively monitored during the surgical and recovery periods. If there is a history of cardiac conditions, including hypertension, angina, dysrhythmias, heart failure, or myocardial infarction, or use of pacemakers or implanted cardiac devices, the patient may need a cardiology and anaesthesia consult before surgery.

If pertinent, clotting and bleeding times and other relevant laboratory results must also be on the chart before surgery, the exact time as determined by facility policy. For example, for the patient who receives digitalis therapy, serum potassium levels must be documented. If the patient has a history of congenital, rheumatic, or valvular heart disease, antibiotic prophylaxis before surgery may be given to decrease the risk for bacterial endocarditis. Further, the nurse should confirm that the patient has not taken anticoagulants, as an international normalized ratio (INR) may need to be drawn before surgery.

Respiratory System. The patient should be asked about any recent or chronic upper respiratory infections. The presence of an upper airway infection may result in the cancellation or postponement of elective surgery because the patient has an increased anaesthetic risk. If the patient has a history of respiratory conditions, they will have an anaesthetic consult before surgery and an appropriate workup.

If a patient has asthma, the nurse should inquire about the patient's recent use of inhaled or oral corticosteroids and bronchodilators. The patient with a severe active airway infection, chronic obstructive pulmonary disease, or asthma is at risk for pulmonary complications, including bronchospasm, laryngospasm, hypoxemia, and atelectasis.

The patient who smokes should be encouraged to stop at least 8 weeks before surgery to decrease the risk for intraoperative and postoperative respiratory complications (Canadian Anesthesiologists' Society, 2021). The greater the patient's pack-years of smoking, the greater the patient's risk is for pulmonary complications.

Obesity; spinal, chest, or airway deformities; and sleep apnea can compromise respiratory function. Depending on the patient's history and physical examination findings, baseline pulmonary function tests and arterial blood gas tests may be ordered before surgery.

Urinary System. Before surgery, the patient's urinary system status should be documented. Results of any renal function tests, such as serum creatinine and blood urea nitrogen (serum urea [nitrogen]), ordered before surgery should be available on the patient's chart.

Male patients who have difficulties voiding may have an enlarged prostate, which would hinder the insertion of a urinary catheter during surgery and also impair voiding in the postoperative period. This information is documented for the perioperative team. The nurse should inform patients if they will have a catheter after surgery.

Integumentary System. Any skin rashes, boils, ulcers, or other dermatological conditions should be noted. A history of pressure injuries may necessitate extra padding during surgery, and skin problems may affect postoperative healing.

Musculoskeletal System. The nurse should note mobility difficulties in any affected joints, as these restrictions influence intraoperative and postoperative positioning and can affect ambulation. Spinal anaesthesia may be difficult if the patient cannot flex their lumbar spine adequately to allow easy needle insertion. If the neck is affected, intubation and airway management may be difficult.

Endocrine System. Diabetes mellitus is a risk factor for both anaesthesia and surgery. The patient with diabetes is at risk for the development of hypoglycemia, hyperglycemia, ketosis, cardiovascular alterations, delayed wound healing, and infection. Preoperative capillary blood glucose tests should be done to determine baseline levels. It is important to clarify with the patient's surgeon or anaesthesiologist whether the patient should take the usual dose of insulin on the day of surgery. Some practitioners prefer that the patient take only half of the usual dose; others ask that the patient take either the usual dose or no insulin at all. Regardless of the preoperative insulin orders, the patient's capillary blood glucose will be determined periodically and managed, if necessary, with regular (short-acting, rapid-onset) insulin.

It should also be determined whether the patient has a history of thyroid dysfunction. Either hyperthyroidism or hypothyroidism can place the patient at surgical risk because of alterations in metabolic rate. If the patient takes a thyroid replacement medication, the nurse should check with the anaesthesiologist about administration of the medication the day of surgery. If the patient has a history of thyroid dysfunction, laboratory tests may be ordered to determine current levels of thyroid function.

Immune System. Patients with active chronic infections, such as hepatitis, acquired immune deficiency syndrome (AIDS), or tuberculosis, may be suitable for surgery; however, if the patient has a history of immunosuppression or takes immunosuppressive medications, this will be noted in the patient chart. Impairment of the immune system can lead to delayed wound healing and postoperative infections. If the patient has an acute infection (e.g., active skin rash, acute sinusitis, flu), elective surgery is frequently cancelled. (Infection control guidelines are discussed in Chapter 17.)

Fluid and Electrolyte Status. The patient should be questioned about vomiting, diarrhea, or difficulty swallowing. Medications that the patient takes that alter fluid and electrolyte status, such as diuretics, should also be identified because serum electrolyte levels may need to be evaluated before surgery. Most patients have restricted fluids because of NPO status before surgery; it is the responsibility of the anaesthesiologist to administer intravenous (IV) fluids and electrolyte therapy to maintain proper hydration.

Nutritional Status. Nutritional extremes in patients require consideration in the perioperative period. For example, if the patient is extremely obese, having notification before surgery allows the perioperative nurse time to prepare the necessary equipment and instrumentation. Obesity stresses the cardiac and pulmonary systems and predisposes the patient to obstructive sleep apnea, which in turn can indicate difficult intubation and postextubation complications. Obesity also increases the risk of deep vein thrombosis (DVT) and surgical site infection (Smith, 2019).

Malnutrition is a result of inadequate intake of protein or calories. Malnutrition has been linked to complications such as delayed wound healing and surgical site infections (Bak, 2019; Odom-Forren, 2019). Many older persons are at risk for malnutrition and fluid volume deficits. If the patient is very thin, the perioperative team should be notified so as to have adequate pressure-reducing positioning devices (pressure points on all patients are protected routinely) on the operating bed. Pressure reduction helps prevent pressure injuries, especially during

TABLE 20.3	HEALTH HISTORY

Patient About to Undergo Surgery

Subjective Data
Past Health History

- Have you had surgeries in the past?* Which ones?* Did you have any complications?*
- Have you or any family members ever experienced any problems with anaesthesia?*
- Do you have any past hospitalizations?*
- Do you have any chronic health conditions?
- Do you have a history of high blood pressure or cardiac disease?*
- Do you have any history of dyspnea, coughing, hemoptysis, COPD, or asthma?*

Current Health History

- What is your usual or present height and weight? Have you had a recent weight gain or loss?*
- Do you at present have an upper respiratory infection?*
- Do you wear glasses, contact lenses, or a hearing aid?*
- Do you smoke?* If yes, how many packs daily? For how many years?
- What is your usual use of alcohol?
- Do you have a history of drug use?
- Do you have any problems healing?*
- Do you have any musculoskeletal issues that might affect positioning during surgery or activity level after surgery?*
- Do you have any limitation in mobility of your neck?* (Might affect intubation for surgery)
- Do you require any special equipment for ambulation?*
- How would you describe your pain tolerance? What methods have you found effective for pain relief?
- Do you have anxiety about the surgery?
- Will you have the support you feel you need following discharge?

Medications

- Are you currently taking any prescribed medications, over-the-counter medications, or herbal or vitamin supplements?*
- Do you have any allergies or sensitivities to any foods or medications?*

*If yes, describe.
COPD, chronic obstructive pulmonary disease.

lengthy procedures. Nutritional deficiencies impair the ability to recover from surgery, so if the nutritional condition is severe, surgery may be postponed until the patient's weight and nutritional deficiencies are corrected.

Impaired nutritional status may affect postoperative recovery and should be identified if the patient will remain in the hospital after surgery. This is particularly true of the undernourished older patient, who is at high risk for poorer surgical outcomes (Allen, 2019).

NURSING ASSESSMENT
PATIENT ABOUT TO UNDERGO SURGERY

The review of the patient's health provides valuable data about the patient's physical and psychological status as well as cultural values and beliefs related to their health care. Questions to ask a patient about to undergo surgery are listed in Table 20.3.

OBJECTIVE DATA

PHYSICAL EXAMINATION. In Canada, the health authority in each province or territory may have its own policies on preoperative health assessments, but it is important to have a physical examination documented on the chart in case surgical

TABLE 20.4   ASA PHYSICAL STATUS CLASSIFICATION SYSTEM

Rating	Examples
ASA I: A normal healthy patient	Healthy, nonsmoking, no or minimal alcohol use
ASA II: A patient with mild systemic disease	Mild diseases only without substantive functional limitations. Current smoker, social alcohol drinker, pregnancy, obesity (30<BMI<40), well-controlled DM/HTN, mild lung disease.
ASA III: A patient with severe systemic disease	Substantial functional limitations; one or more moderate to severe diseases. Poorly controlled DM or HTN, COPD, morbid obesity (BMI ≥40), active hepatitis, alcohol dependence or abuse, implanted pacemaker, moderate reduction of ejection fraction, ESRD undergoing regularly scheduled dialysis, history (>3 months) of MI, CVA, TIA, or CAD/stents.
ASA IV: A patient with severe systemic disease that is a constant threat to life	Recent (<3 months) MI, CVA, TIA or CAD/stents, ongoing cardiac ischemia or severe valve dysfunction, severe reduction of ejection fraction, shock, sepsis, DIC, ARD, or ESRD not undergoing regularly scheduled dialysis
ASA V: A moribund patient who is not expected to survive without the operation	*Examples:* Ruptured abdominal/thoracic aneurysm, massive trauma, intracranial bleed with mass effect, ischemic bowel in the face of significant cardiac pathology or multiple organ/system dysfunction
ASA VI: A declared brain-dead patient	

ARD, acute respiratory disease; *ASA,* American Society of Anesthesiologists; *BMI,* body mass index; *CAD,* coronary artery disease; *COPD,* chronic obstructive pulmonary disease; *CVA,* cerebrovascular accident; *DIC,* disseminated intravascular coagulation; *DM,* diabetes mellitus; *ESRD,* end-stage renal disease; *HTN,* hypertension; *MI,* myocardial infarction; *TIA,* transient ischemic attack.
Source: Based on ASA physical status classification system, 2019, of the American Society of Anesthesiologists. Reprinted with permission of the American Society of Anesthesiologists, 1061 American Lane, Schaumburg, Illinois 60173-4973.

TABLE 20.5   PHYSIOLOGICAL ASSESSMENT OF THE PATIENT BEFORE SURGERY*

Neurological System
- Determine orientation to time, place, and person.
- Identify presence of confusion, disorderly thinking, or inability to follow commands.
- Identify past history of strokes, TIAs, or diseases of the central nervous system such as Parkinson's disease or multiple sclerosis.
- Identify history of headaches or issues with vision or hearing.

Cardiovascular System
- Identify acute or chronic conditions; focus on the presence of angina, hypertension, heart failure, and recent history of myocardial infarction.
- Palpate baseline radial pulse for rate and characteristics.
- Inspect for edema, noting location and severity.
- Take baseline blood pressure.
- Identify any medication or herbal product that may affect coagulation (e.g., acetylsalicylic acid, ginkgo biloba, ginger).
- Review laboratory and diagnostic tests for cardiovascular function when indicated.

Respiratory System
- Identify acute or chronic conditions; note the presence of infection or COPD.
- Assess history of smoking and encourage the patient to stop before surgery by educating them about the increased risk for complications.
- Determine baseline respiratory rate and rhythm, regularity of pattern, and pulse oximetry.
- Observe for cough, dyspnea, use of accessory muscles of respiration, and cyanosis.

Urinary System
- Identify any pre-existing disease and ability of the patient to void. Prostate enlargement may affect catheterization during surgery and ability to void after surgery.
- Review laboratory and diagnostic tests for renal function when indicated.

Hepatic System
- Review any history of substance misuse, especially alcohol and intravenous drug use.
- Review laboratory and diagnostic tests for liver when indicated.

Endocrine and Hematological Systems
- Identify pre-existing conditions with bleeding or hematological and endocrine disorders.

Integumentary System
- Assess mucous membranes for dryness and intactness.
- Determine skin status; note drying, bruising, or breaks in integrity of surface.
- Inspect skin for rashes, boils, or infection, especially around the planned surgical site.
- Assess skin moisture and temperature.
- Inspect mucous membranes and skin turgor for presence of dehydration.
- Identify any history of problems with wound healing.

Musculoskeletal System
- Examine skin–bone pressure points and pressure injuries.
- Assess for limitations in joint pain, range of motion, and muscle weakness.
- Assess mobility, gait, and balance.

Gastrointestinal–Nutritional System
- Identify history of gastrointestinal disorders or problems with elimination.
- Determine food and fluid intake patterns and any recent weight loss.
- Weigh patient.
- Assess for presence of dentures and bridges (loose dentures or teeth may be dislodged during intubation).

*See related body system chapters for more specific assessments and related laboratory studies.
COPD, chronic obstructive pulmonary disease; *TIA,* transient ischemic attack.

complications arise. This examination may be done in advance of surgery or on the day of surgery.

Findings from the patient's history and physical examination will enable the anaesthesiologist to assign the patient a physical status rating for anaesthesia administration reference. The classification system commonly used was developed by the American Society of Anesthesiologists as a way to provide a standardized way to assess the expected anaesthesia outcome for the surgical patient and provide health care providers with a way to measure perioperative risk (Campbell, 2019) (Table 20.4). Many physiological stressors may put the patient at risk

for surgical complications, whether the surgery is an elective or an emergency procedure. A physiological assessment of the patient who is about to undergo surgery is presented in Table 20.5. If the physical examination is done immediately before surgery, it will be a more focused assessment because of the impending procedures that must be completed before surgery. The nurse should review the documentation already present on the patient's chart, including the review of systems and the physician's physical examination report. All findings must be documented, with any relevant findings immediately communicated to members of the perioperative team.

TABLE 20.6   COMMON PREOPERATIVE LABORATORY TESTS

Test	Area Assessed
ABGs, oximetry	Respiratory and metabolic function, oxygenation status
Blood glucose	Metabolic status, diabetes mellitus
Blood urea nitrogen, creatinine	Renal function
CBC: RBCs, Hgb, Hct, WBCs	Anemia, immune status, infection
Electrocardiogram	Heart disease, dysrhythmias
Electrolytes	Metabolic status, renal function, diuretic side effects
hCG	Reproductive status
hCG Liver function tests	Liver status
PT, PTT, INR, platelet count	Coagulation status
Pulmonary function studies	Pulmonary status
Serum albumin	Nutritional status
Type and crossmatch	Blood available for replacement (elective surgery patients may have their own blood available)
Urinalysis	Renal status, hydration, urinary tract infection and disease

ABGs, arterial blood gases; *CBC,* complete blood count, *hCG,* human chorionic gonadotropin; *Hct,* hematocrit; *Hgb,* hemoglobin; *INR,* international normalized ratio; *PT,* prothrombin time, *PTT ,* partial thromboplastin time, *RBC,* red blood cell; *WBCs,* white blood cells.

LABORATORY AND DIAGNOSTIC TESTING. Preoperative laboratory and electrocardiogram testing is obtained on the basis of the patient's history in order to determine their surgical and anaesthetic risk. Diagnostic tests must be ordered judiciously according to hospital policy, to reduce unnecessary testing (Marley & Sheets, 2018). For example, if the patient is taking an antiplatelet medication (e.g., Aspirin), a coagulation profile may be done; a patient on diuretic or digoxin therapy may need to have a potassium level obtained; a patient taking medications for dysrhythmias will have a preoperative electrocardiogram. Blood glucose monitoring should be done for patients with diabetes. Findings may necessitate dosage or medication adjustments during the perioperative period because of increased body metabolism, decreased caloric intake, stress, and anaesthesia. Regulation of the stability of the blood glucose levels during surgery will promote a more positive outcome. Some patients require blood type and crossmatch testing preoperatively. Crossmatch determines the patient's ABO blood group and RhD type (Canadian Blood Services, 2020). As indicated, the preoperative team should ensure adequate reserved crossmatched blood for transfusion during surgery and postoperatively as deemed necessary. Some patients may need to have a complete blood count (CBC) to provide a baseline understanding of blood loss or anemia that may require correction. Additional commonly ordered preoperative laboratory tests can be found in Table 20.6.

Offices and PACs may do the preoperative tests days before surgery. Thus, the nurse must ensure that all laboratory reports are on the chart. Lack of these reports may result in a delay or cancellation of the surgery.

NURSING MANAGEMENT PATIENT ABOUT TO UNDERGO SURGERY

Preoperative nursing interventions are derived from the nursing assessment and must reflect each individual patient's specific needs. Physical preparations are determined by the pending surgery and the routines of the surgery setting. Psychological preparations should be tailored to each patient's needs.

Preoperative teaching may be minimal or extensive. General information for surgery should be given.

PREOPERATIVE EDUCATION

Preoperative education empowers the patient to make informed health decisions and to participate effectively during the surgical experience. Preoperative teaching can increase patient adherence to instructions as well as their satisfaction with the experience. Such teaching may also reduce patients' fear, anxiety, and stress; the duration of hospitalization; and their recovery time following discharge. Given Canada's multicultural society, nurses may encounter challenges in perianaesthesia teaching including language barriers; cultural perceptions of health, hospitals, and surgery; and the individualized time required to allay the patient's concerns and anxiety level.

In most surgical settings, patients attend the PAC within a month of their scheduled surgery. However, even in unplanned surgery, there is time for the nurse to present information to the patient about the surgery and the postoperative period. The only time patients may not receive any information about their surgery is in an emergency situation where there is no time for teaching. In the PAC, information is presented to the patient in verbal, video, and written forms, which patients and caregivers can review at their leisure.

In preparing the patient for surgery, the nurse can identify the patient's educational needs by determining age, language, reading level, emotional status, and motivation to understand the surgery and the perianaesthesia process. Preoperative teaching concerns three types of information: sensory, process, and procedural. Different patients, with varying cultures, backgrounds, and experience, may want different types of information. Patients wanting *sensory information* want to know what they will see, hear, smell, and feel during the surgery. The nurse may tell them that the OR will be cold, but they can ask the perioperative nurse for a warm blanket; the lights in the OR are very bright; or there will be lots of sounds that are unfamiliar and specific smells. Patients wanting *process information* may not want specific details but rather a description of the general flow of what is going to happen. Patients can be advised that a nurse and anaesthesiologist will speak with them in the preoperative unit; then they will go to the OR, and when they wake up, they will be in the PACU. After this, they will be transferred back to their postoperative room or home. With *procedural information,* desired details are more specific: for example, an IV line will be started while the patient is in the holding area, and in the OR, the patient will be asked to move onto the narrow bed and a safety strap will be placed over their thighs.

Preoperative patient teaching is a perianaesthesia nursing team effort; PAC nurses initiate teaching, perioperative nurses continue it, and the postoperative and discharge nurses reinforce and supplement it. Community nurses who visit the patient at home, in the community, or in extended-care facilities after surgery must also be cognizant of the surgical teaching plan. All teaching should be documented in the patient's medical record. A patient and caregiver teaching guide for preoperative preparation is presented in Table 20.7. Additional information related to patient teaching may be found in Chapter 4.

GENERAL SURGERY INFORMATION. The nurse also provides information specific to the operation being performed and the educational needs of the patient (Table 20.8). All patients should receive instruction about deep breathing, incentive spirometry, coughing, and mobilizing after surgery. This education is essential because patients may not want to do these activities after surgery unless they are taught the rationale for them and

TABLE 20.7 PATIENT & CAREGIVER TEACHING GUIDE

Preoperative Preparation

Sensory Information
- Preoperative holding area may be noisy.
- Drugs and cleaning solutions may be odourous.
- Operating room (OR) can be cold. Forced-air warming devices may be used. Warm blankets are available.
- Talking may be heard but may be distorted because of masks. Ask questions if something is not understood.
- OR bed will be narrow. A safety strap will be applied over the thighs.
- Lights in the OR may be very bright.
- Monitoring machines may be heard (e.g., beeping noises) when awake.

Procedural Information
- What to bring and what type of clothing to wear on the day of surgery
- Any changes in time of surgery
- Fluid and food restrictions
- Physical preparation required (e.g., shower, bowel or skin preparation)
- Purpose of frequent vital signs assessment
- Pain control and other comfort measures (including any pain scales that a specific hospital might use to assess pain)
- Why turning, deep breathing, and coughing after surgery are important. Do practice sessions.
- How to use a pillow to assist with splinting after surgery
- Insertion of intravenous lines
- Procedure for anaesthesia administration
- Importance of transferring, mobilizing pain management, and postoperative exercises
- Expected procedure for discharge and postoperative support

Process Information
Information About General Flow of Surgery
- Admission area
- Preoperative holding area, OR, and postanaesthesia care unit (PACU)
- Families can usually stay in holding area until surgery.
- Families may be able to enter recovery area as soon as the patient is awake.
- Identification of any technology that may be present on awakening, such as monitors, central lines, or intermittent pneumatic compression devices

Where Families Can Wait During Surgery and Postoperative Roles
- Patient and family members need to be encouraged to ask questions and express any concerns.
- OR staff will notify the family when surgery is completed.
- Surgeon will usually talk with the family following surgery.
- A competent adult must accompany the patient upon discharge and continue monitoring the patient at home as per the discharge instructions.
- Caregivers need to have requisite information to contact a health care provider with concerns and questions after discharge.

OR, operating room.

practise them before surgery. Patients and caregivers should be told whether there will be tubes, drains, monitoring devices, or special equipment after surgery and that these devices enable the nurse to safely care for the patient.

Examples of individualized teaching may include how to use incentive spirometers or postoperative, patient-controlled analgesia pumps. Examples of surgery-specific information include having an immobilizer (for a patient undergoing a total joint replacement), having an epidural catheter for postoperative pain control, or waking up in the critical care unit (for a patient requiring extensive surgery).

AMBULATORY SURGERY INFORMATION. The ambulatory surgery patient or the patient admitted to hospital the day of surgery will need to receive information before admission. The teaching is generally done in the surgeon's office or PAC and reinforced on the day of surgery. Some ambulatory surgical centres have the staff telephone the patient the evening before surgery to answer last-minute questions and to reinforce teaching.

Information provided includes the need for preoperative shower, bowel prep, or medication; arrival time at the hospital; and the time of surgery. Arrival time is usually a minimum of 2 hours before the scheduled time of surgery to allow for completion of the preoperative assessment and paperwork. Information given can also include the day-of-surgery events such as patient registration, parking, what to wear, what to bring, and the need to have a responsible adult present for transportation home after surgery.

Restriction of fluids and food is necessary preoperatively to minimize the risk for aspiration when administering general anaesthesia and to decrease the risk for postoperative nausea and vomiting. Dobson and colleagues (2019) recommend instituting guidelines that vary according to patient age and pre-existing medical conditions. Guidelines apply to all forms of anaesthesia, including local and monitored anaesthesia care. Patients undergoing emergency surgery must be assessed to determine the risk of delaying surgery versus the risk for gastric content aspiration. The type and amount of food ingested is considered when determining the duration of fasting, and adults and children should be encouraged to drink clear fluids up to 2 hours before surgery (Table 20.9). Educating the patient regarding the rationale for adhering to NPO orders improves patient adherence and leads to a decrease in surgical delays and cancellations.

LEGAL PREPARATION FOR SURGERY

Legal preparation for surgery consists of checking that all required forms have been correctly signed and are present in the chart and that the patient and family clearly understand what is going to happen. The most important of these forms are the signed consent form for the surgical procedure on the correct side (right or left), with no abbreviations, and specific consents for anaesthesia interventions and for blood transfusion. Other forms can include those that have been completed for advance directives and powers of attorney (see Chapter 13).

CONSENT FOR SURGERY. It is critical that nurses, as patient advocates, understand the ethical and legal tenets of informed consent. From an ethical perspective, the patient, at all times, has the right to autonomously make their own health decisions regarding medical, surgical, or diagnostic treatment. Autonomous choice is especially vital for individuals of Indigenous ancestry, who have been historically subjected to inhumane practices such as forced sterilization (Rasmussen, 2019).

Before nonemergency surgery can be legally performed, the patient must voluntarily sign an **informed consent** in the presence of a witness. Informed surgical consent is an active process between the surgeon and the patient that allows the patient to assess information and make an informed decision. Legally, a written, signed, and witnessed surgical consent helps protect the patient, surgeon, hospital, and health care team. Surgical consent forms may vary among facilities; nurses must be familiar with the form and process of obtaining consent in their institution.

According to the Canadian Medical Protective Association (CMPA, 2021), three key elements are required for a consent to be considered valid:
1. It must be voluntary.
2. The patient must have the mental capacity to consent.
3. The patient must be properly informed.

⚙ EVIDENCE-INFORMED PRACTICE

Translating Research Into Practice

G. K. (pronouns she/her) is a 57-year-old scheduled for a knee replacement. G. K. has been NPO since midnight and was scheduled to be the third surgical case of the day. Unfortunately, several emergency surgeries have resulted in delays, and the patient is not expected to leave for surgery for another 4 hours. She tells the nurse that she has a "headache" from missing her "morning coffee." She says she is hungry and thirsty, and, since surgery has been delayed, she would like a cup of coffee.

Best Available Evidence	Clinician Expertise	Patient Preferences and Values
For healthy adults, the minimum fasting period for clear liquids before surgery is 2 hours.	NPO restrictions are meant to prevent aspiration and vomiting during surgery. Patients who are NPO from midnight frequently report hunger and thirst while waiting for surgery. Patients who regularly drink caffeine in the morning often experience a "caffeine withdrawal" headache when fasting. Clear liquids consist of water, fruit juices without pulp, carbonated beverages, clear tea, and black coffee.	Patient is requesting something to drink given the extended period of fast due to the delay in surgery.

NPO, nothing by mouth.

Decision and Action

The nurse knows that the current policy of keeping all patients NPO after midnight for surgery does not reflect the best available evidence and that a multidisciplinary task force is working to review and revise the policy. The nurse decides to call the anaesthesia care provider to discuss G. K.'s situation and request that clear liquids be ordered for her.

References for Evidence

Crenshaw, J. T. (2011). Preoperative fasting: Will the evidence ever be put into practice? *American Journal of Nursing, 111*(10), 38–43. https://doi.org/10.1097/01.NAJ.0000406412.57062.24

Merchant, R., Chartrand, D., Dain, S., et al. (2016). Guidelines to the practice of anaesthesia—Revised edition 2016. *Canadian Journal of Anaesthesia, 63*(1), 86–112. https://doi.org/10.1007/s12630-015-0470

Voluntary Consent. Patients must be free either to consent to or to refuse treatment without duress, fraud, or coercion. It is considered prudent to have the surgical consent signed by the patient before giving any preoperative medications that may interfere with patient comprehension. It is the physician's legal responsibility to obtain consent. Preoperatively, the nurse can be a patient advocate, by verifying that the patient voluntarily signed the consent and understands the consent and its implications. If the patient is unclear about operative plans, the nurse may need to contact the surgeon to offer additional information. The patient must be informed that permission for treatment may be withdrawn at any time, even after the consent has been signed.

Documentation of the consent discussion should be made in the patient chart, and in many Canadian jurisdictions, a signed consent form is a legal requirement before surgery (CMPA, 2021).

Capacity to Consent. Patient understanding is complex. However, the physician must ensure the patient comprehends the consent discussion, taking into consideration such things as emotional state and language difficulties. A patient has the capacity to consent if they understand the nature and effects of the proposed treatment, the consequences of refusing the treatment, and any alternatives to the treatment. Capable patients have a right to refuse to consent.

In all provinces and territories except Quebec, there is no chronological age of consent; capacity to consent is determined by maturity. This means that children and youth are considered capable of consenting to or of refusing treatment if their physical, mental, and emotional development allow them to fully appreciate the consequences of their decisions. Additionally, capable minors must give permission (consent) to the physician to have their parents involved in health care decisions. In Quebec, people 14 years and older can give consent (CMPA, 2021).

The patient who is unconscious or who has diminished capacity may have the consent form signed by a responsible family member or legally appointed representative. Hospital policies should be consulted for clarification.

Life-Threatening Situations. If the patient's life or limb is at risk, the patient is unable to consent, and the substitute decision maker is not available, the physician does what is immediately necessary based on any known wishes of the patient and then obtains consent as soon as possible.

Properly Informing the Patient. The physician relates the diagnosis, also explaining any uncertainty about the diagnosis, the proposed treatment, the risks and consequences, the probability of a successful outcome, and the consequences of leaving the medical condition untreated. The patient must know the availability, benefits, and risks of alternative treatments (see the Ethical Dilemmas box). Depending on the patient's unique condition, the physician may need to discuss uncommon risks, such as permanent disability or death.

ETHICAL DILEMMAS

Informed Consent

Situation

The nurse discusses with a patient of Indigenous ancestry their impending surgery in the preoperative holding area. It becomes obvious that this competent adult patient was not fully informed of the alternatives to this surgery, although she has signed the consent form.

Important Points for Consideration

- Informed consent requires that patients have complete information about the proposed treatment and its possible consequences as well as alternative treatments and possible consequences.
- Risks and benefits of each treatment option must also be explained in order for patients to weigh treatment options.
- It is the surgeon's responsibility to provide this information.
- An important element of informed consent is the opportunity to have questions answered about the various treatment options and their possible outcomes.
- Health care providers must not decide what is best for patients.
- Indigenous people have experienced some horrific situations when seeking health care that have negatively affected many individuals intergenerationally. Past experiences of discrimination by health care providers may create barriers to seeking health care (Kitching et al., 2020) or to making health care decisions. As patient advocate, the nurse must ensure that the patient is not rushed into making an informed decision.

Clinical Decision-Making Questions

1. What should the nurse do?
2. What is the nurse's role as patient advocate in the informed-consent process?

TABLE 20.8   SUMMARY OF PREOPERATIVE TEACHING

Topic	What to Teach the Patient	Rationale
Nutrition	• NPO guidelines • Diet increased slowly • Nausea is common—there are medications to help with this	• NPO guidelines help keep the stomach empty, reducing the potential for aspiration during anaesthesia induction. • Diet is increased slowly to prevent gastric overfilling and prevent nausea.
Ambulation	• Ambulate early • May have immobilizers, have to use assistive devices • Leg exercises • May have to wear antiembolism stockings after surgery	• Early ambulation increases circulation, ventilation, muscle tone, and vital capacity; improves gastrointestinal and urinary function; reduces pain; and supports healing. • Antiembolic stockings reduce the incidence of postoperative formation of deep vein thrombosis.
Breathing	• To perform deep breathing and coughing exercises • Splinting • Use of incentive spirometer	• Postoperative patients are at risk for pulmonary complications (e.g., pneumonia) due to increased respiratory secretions, decreased lung expansion, and depression of the respiratory centre that occurs during general anaesthesia.
Grooming	• Take a bath or shower the morning of surgery—may be required to bathe using chlorhexidine • Remove nail polish, artificial fingernails, hair clips, and jewellery (including from piercings) before surgery • Remove dentures and eyeglasses (stored during surgery) • Remove external prosthetics • Remove contact lenses	• Showers remove soil and reduce the number of transient bacteria on the skin. • Nail polish prevents accurate assessment of nail beds and interferes with pulse oximetry. • Jewellery can interfere with patient positioning, cause pressure points, and get caught on equipment. • Dentures and glasses interfere with administering general anaesthesia. • External prosthetics may impair patient transfer and positioning and interfere with intraoperative equipment. • Contact lenses can cause corneal abrasions if left in during surgery.

Medications	• Take preoperative medication as ordered
	• Consult physician, anaesthesiologist, or surgeon regarding when and what prescribed medications, OTC medications, and herbal remedies should be stopped preoperatively
		• Medication is used preoperatively to:
		  • Assist with reducing anxiety and sedating the patient
		  • Reduce oral secretions
		  • Reduce risk of aspiration of gastric contents
		  • Reduce nausea and vomiting
		• Prescribed and OTC medications and herbal remedies may cause surgical complications (e.g., increased bleeding, hypertension, arrhythmias) and may need to be discontinued prior to surgery.

Pain control	• Ask for pain medication as needed
	• Types of pain control (epidural, PCA)
		• Early and effective analgesia reduces postoperative complications such as:
		  • Decreased lung compliance; risk of atelectasis
		  • Decreased mobility; risk of thromboembolism
		  • Increased risk of myocardial ischemia
		  • Impaired immune system
		  • Delayed return of bowel and gastric function

Drains, dressings, and tubings	• Drains (e.g., Jackson-Pratt, Hemovac) • Dressings (staples, sutures) to be expected • Tubing: IV, NG, or epidural tubing	• Preoperative patient and family teaching prepares them for the presence of postoperative drains and tubes. • Patient instruction and postoperative follow-up regarding routine practices for infection control and wound management can reduce the incidence of SSI.
Safety	• Patient identification and allergy wrist band (if appropriate) in place • Instructed to call for assistance to get out of bed • Use of call bell • Instructed not to climb over the side rails	• Identification and allergy wrist bands are important so that all health care providers can identify the patient and immediately be alerted to any allergies. • Patient injury such as rail entrapment and falls can occur if patients try to climb over bed rails.
Preoperative information	• Parking • Time to be at hospital and time of surgery • Waiting areas for family • Length of expected stay	• Preoperative information provides patients and family with guidelines and can mitigate stress on the day of surgery.

IV, intravenous; *NG,* nasogastric; *NPO,* nothing by mouth; *OTC,* over-the-counter; *PCA,* patient-controlled analgesia; *SSI,* surgical site infection.

TABLE 20.9   PREOPERATIVE FASTING RECOMMENDATIONS OF THE CANADIAN ANESTHESIOLOGISTS' SOCIETY

Liquid and Food Intake	Minimum Fasting Period (hr)
After drinking clear liquids (e.g., water, clear tea, black coffee, carbonated beverages, and fruit juice without pulp)	2
After ingesting breast milk	4
After light meal (e.g., toast and clear liquids) or after drinking infant formula or nonhuman milk	6
After meal including meat, fried or fatty food	8

Source: Dobson et al. (2019). Guidelines to the practice of anesthesia—Revised edition 2019. *Canadian Journal of Anesthesia, 2019*(66), 75–108. https://doi.org/10.1007/s12630-018-1248-2

DAY-OF-SURGERY PREPARATION

NURSING ROLE

Communication is a major consideration in the patient's surgical experience. Nurses can help patients understand the questions posed preoperatively by taking a "teach-back" approach to verify that patients understand the information they are given and that, if necessary, culturally appropriate translators are available (Brega et al., 2015).

Surgery preparation will vary depending on whether the patient is an inpatient or an outpatient. The nurse prepares inpatients for surgery, but for outpatient procedures, the patient or a family member may have the responsibility of preoperative preparation.

Most facilities have preoperative checklists that indicate all pertinent documentation and actions required prior to surgery.

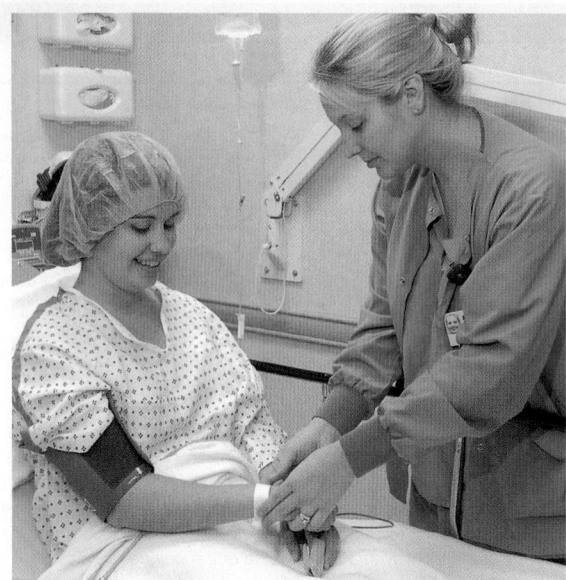

FIG. 20.1 As part of the preoperative preparations, the nurse performs a safety check by verifying that the patient has an identification band (wristband) before going to surgery. Source: Courtesy Susan R. Volk, MSN, RN, CCRN, CPAN, Staff Development Specialist, Christiana Care Health System, Newark, DE.

Nurses, however, must ensure that all required tasks are complete before surgery: final preoperative teaching, readiness assessment, and communication of pertinent findings from diagnostic procedures and consults to appropriate health care providers. This can be challenging for investigations done outside the hospital, as in many provinces there is poor data sharing. The chart should include a patient history, physical examination, lab results, baseline vitals, informed consent, and nurses' notes. All critical documentation must accompany the patient or be accessible electronically in the OR.

Most institutions require that a patient has showered or bathed before surgery and is dressed in a hospital gown; underclothes may or may not be permitted. The patient should not wear cosmetics because observation of skin colour will be important. Nail polish is removed because it may skew the results of the pulse oximeter placed on the patient's fingertip and used to monitor oxygenation. An identification band and, if applicable, an allergy band, is put on the patient. The band(s) must remain on the patient as a means of communicating important information to health care providers (Figure 20.1). If the patient has been typed and screened for possible blood transfusion, a blood band also may be applied to the patient's wrist. All patient valuables are returned to a family member or locked up according to institutional policy. If the patient prefers not to remove a wedding ring, in most circumstances, the ring can be taped securely to the finger to prevent loss. All other jewellery (including body piercings) and prostheses, such as dentures, contact lenses, and glasses, are generally removed to prevent loss or damage. Hearing aids are usually left in place to allow the patient to better follow instructions. Eyeglasses need to be returned to the patient as soon as possible after surgery.

The patient must void shortly before surgery to prevent involuntary elimination under anaesthesia and reduce the possibility of urinary retention during early postoperative recovery. The patient should void before administration of any preoperative medication since many preoperative medications can interfere with balance and possibly lead to a fall when the patient is in the bathroom. Voiding should be documented on the patient record. The nurse should determine that all preoperative preparations have been completed and that the signed consent for surgery is present before giving any preoperative medications.

SAFETY ALERT
Use a preoperative checklist (Figure 20.2) to ensure that all preoperative preparations have been completed before the patient is given any sedating medications. See Chapter 21 for a surgical safety checklist.

PREOPERATIVE MEDICATIONS. Preoperative medications are used for a variety of reasons, and patients may receive a single medication or a combination of medications. The following are examples of preoperative medications:

- *Benzodiazepines* such as midazolam, diazepam (Valium), and lorazepam (Ativan) and *barbiturates* reduce anxiety and are used for their sedative and amnesic properties.
- *Anticholinergics* such as atropine and glycopyrrolate may be given to reduce respiratory and oral secretions.
- *Opioids* such as morphine, meperidine (Demerol), and fentanyl may be given to decrease intraoperative anaesthetic requirements and to decrease pain.
- *Antiemetics* such as metoclopramide may be given to decrease nausea and vomiting after surgery.
- *Antacids* such as sodium citrate increase gastric pH, as do the following histamine H_2-receptor antagonists, in addition to decreasing gastric volume: cimetidine, famotidine (Pepcid), and ranitidine (Zantac).
- *Antibiotics* are routinely given intravenously before surgery or in the OR, with optimal initiation 30 minutes before the incision time. (Some provinces require reporting of prophylactic antibiotic use rates for specific surgical interventions to monitor surgical site infections.)
- *Eye drops* are commonly ordered and administered for the patient undergoing cataract and other eye surgery. The patient may require multiple sets of eye drops to be administered at 5-minute intervals to adequately prepare the eye for surgery.

There is no standard protocol for routine preoperative medications. In order to facilitate patient teaching and eliminate confusion, written preoperative orders clarify which medications should and should not be taken on the day of surgery. If there is any question, the nurse should clarify the orders with the anaesthesiologist. Most patients will be advised to take routine cardiac, antihypertensive, and asthma medications on the day of surgery. In the case of insulin, it is important to clarify the time and amount of the last dose before surgery.

Premedications may be administered by oral, IV, subcutaneous, or intramuscular routes. Oral medications should be given 60 to 90 minutes before the patient goes to the OR. Because patients are fluid restricted before surgery, the patient should swallow these medications with a minimal amount of water. Intramuscular and subcutaneous injections should be given 30 to 60 minutes before arrival at the OR (minimally 20 minutes). IV medications are usually administered to the patient after arrival in the preoperative holding area or the OR. The medication administration must be charted immediately. The patient should be told the effects of the medications, such as relaxation, drowsiness, and dry mouth.

TRANSPORTATION TO THE OPERATING ROOM

If the patient is an inpatient, transport personnel go to the patient's room with a stretcher to transport the patient to surgery. The nurse assists the patient in transferring from the hospital

Preoperative requirements	Initials	Day of surgery	Initials
Height _____ Weight _____		Surgical site marked Y N NA	
Isolation? _____ Type _____		ID band on patient	
Allergies noted on chart		Allergy band on patient Y NA	
Vital signs (Initial) T _____ P _____ R _____ BP _____		Vital signs Time _____ T _____ P _____ R _____ BP _____	
Chart Review		**Procedures**	
H&P on chart		NPO since _____	
H&P within 30 days? Y N		Capillary blood glucose Y N	
Signed and witnessed informed consent form on chart		Preoperative skin prep Y N Shower Scrub Shave	
Signed consent for blood administration Y NA		Makeup, nail polish, false fingernails, and false eyelashes removed Y NA	
Blood type and crossmatch Y NA		Hospital gown applied Y NA	
Name plate on chart		**Valuables** Y N	
Old chart requested and sent Y NA		Dentures _____	
Diagnostic Results		Wig or hairpiece _____	
Hb/Hct _____/_____ NA		Eyeglasses _____	
PT/INR/PTT _____/_____/_____ NA		Contact lenses _____	
CXR _____ NA		Hearing aid _____	
ECG _____ NA		Prosthesis _____	
Other labs		Jewellery _____	
		Clothing _____	
Final chart review: New forms added		Disposition of valuables Family Rings taped Safe	
Signed off		Voided/catheter Time _____	
		Preoperative medications given Time _____ NA	
Time to OR _____ Date _____ Transported to OR by _____ Final check by _____ RN		Preoperative antibiotics given Time _____ NA	

FIG. 20.2 Preoperative checklist. *BP,* blood pressure; *CXR,* chest radiograph (X-ray); *ECG,* electrocardiogram; *H&P,* history and physical examination; *Hb,* hemoglobin; *Hct,* hematocrit; *ID,* identification; *INR,* international normalized ratio; *N,* no; *NA,* not applicable; *NPO,* nothing by mouth; *OR,* operating room; *P,* pulse; *PT,* prothrombin time; *PTT,* partial thromboplastin time; *R,* respiration; *T,* temperature; *Y,* yes.

bed to the OR stretcher, and the side rails of the stretcher are raised and secured. The nurse should ensure that the completed chart goes with the patient.

If the patient is an outpatient, the patient may be transported to the OR by stretcher or wheelchair, or, in the absence of premedication, the patient may walk, accompanied, to the OR. The method of transportation must be safe and documented by the nurse responsible for the transfer.

The family or caregivers are instructed where to wait for the patient during surgery. Many hospitals have a surgical waiting room where OR personnel communicate the status of the patient to the family. It is in this waiting room that the surgeon can locate the family after surgery and where families can be notified when surgery is complete. Some hospitals provide pagers to waiting family members so that they may go eat or run errands during the surgery.

While the patient is in surgery, the patient's room is prepared to accommodate the patient's needs after surgery, the bed is made and raised to stretcher height, and, if necessary, disposable pads are placed for any anticipated drainage. There should be a basin, soap, towels, and clean gown available in the patient's room. Necessary equipment, including those for vital signs, IV administration, oxygen, suction, kidney basin, warm blankets, and additional pillows for positioning, should also be placed in the room and organized to facilitate entry of the stretcher or hospital bed. Having the room ready and equipped ensures a smooth patient transfer from the PACU.

CULTURALLY COMPETENT CARE

PATIENT ABOUT TO UNDERGO SURGERY

In Canada, health care providers must be aware and supportive of cultural perceptions and beliefs of patients when preparing them for surgery. Decisions made because of cultural variations must be respected and valued. For example, Makokis and

Makokis (2018) detail the experience of one of the authors, a 51-year-old Cree woman faced with undergoing a total hysterectomy in the Western medical system. Makokis felt the need to respect and give thanks to her uterus and ovaries, which had given her the gift of two children. She wanted to bring her body parts home from the hospital, wrapped in sage and broadcloth (both have spiritual significance), provide a ceremony for them, and commit them to Mother Earth. Makokis's preparation involved planning ahead with her gynecologist and a First Nations liaison worker. After the surgery, which was uneventful, Makokis was able to carry out her burial ceremony and felt that she had been treated with respect by the interprofessional team.

AGE-RELATED CONSIDERATIONS

OLDER PATIENT ABOUT TO UNDERGO SURGERY

Many surgical procedures are performed on patients older than 65 years of age, and surgery can be safely performed even on those in their 90s. Frequently performed procedures in older persons include cataract extraction, coronary and vascular procedures, prostate surgery, herniorrhaphy, cholecystectomy, total knee and hip replacements, and repair of fractured hips.

The nurse must be particularly alert when assessing and caring for the older patient undergoing surgery. An event that has little effect on a younger patient may be overwhelming to the older patient. As well, the risks associated with anaesthesia and surgery increase in the older patient. The older the patient, the greater the risk for complications after surgery. However, assessment and consideration of the physiological status of older persons, and not simply their chronological age, are essential when planning surgery and assessing risks. A 75-year-old woman may be biologically healthy and more like a 60-year-old in physiological responses. Conversely, a 55-year-old with multiple chronic health problems may biologically resemble a 75-year-old. The risk for surgical complications in the older person relates to physiological

aging (frailty can be predictive of postoperative outcomes) and changes that compromise organ function, reduce reserve capacity, and limit the body's ability to adapt to stress.

When preparing patients for surgery, a detailed history and complete physical examination are obtained. Preoperative laboratory tests and results, an electrocardiogram, and chest radiograph help plan the choice of and technique for anaesthesia. More than one physician may be involved in geriatric care, so the nurse coordinates the care and the physicians' orders for the patient.

Knowledge of family support is important when considering the continuity of care for the older person, especially for same-day surgical patients who may be discharged to a family caregiver.

The nurse must remember that many older people have sensory deficits. Vision and hearing may be diminished, and bright lights may bother those with eye conditions. Physical reactions are often slowed as a result of mobility and balance challenges, so more time should be allowed for the older person to complete preoperative testing. Since thought processes and cognitive abilities also may be slowed or impaired, these patients may need extra time to understand preoperative instructions. However, not every older person has cognitive deficits. Sensory function and cognition must be assessed and documented (Yu & Woo, 2019). If for any reason the patient cannot sign the consent form for themselves, a legal representative of the patient must be present to provide consent for surgery.

Some older people live in long-term care facilities. Transportation from these agencies must be coordinated so that the arrival time allows for surgery preparation. A falls-risk assessment should be completed.

Adding to the stress of the surgical procedure, even a minimally invasive one, the perceived situational change and loss may be overwhelming to the older person. The threat to independence, lifestyle, and self-esteem may result in ineffective coping. The nurse must be particularly supportive and help the older person cope with the surgical experience.

CASE STUDY

Patient About to Undergo Surgery

Patient Profile
M. G. (pronouns she/her), an 82-year-old retired librarian, is admitted to the hospital with compromised circulation of the right lower leg and a necrotic right foot. Her health history includes a diagnosis of diabetes mellitus 40 years ago and insulin administration to maintain appropriate blood glucose levels. She is scheduled for surgery today for a below-knee amputation under spinal anaesthesia. The patient had a light breakfast at 0600 hours and a glass of apple juice at 1000 hours but has not had anything since. It is now 1300 hours on the day of surgery.

Subjective Data
- History of type 2 diabetes mellitus for 40 years
- History of renal conditions
- History of vision conditions
- Surgical history that includes a Caesarean birth at age 30 and a cholecystectomy at age 65; did not heal well following the last surgery
- Blood glucose has not been well controlled
- Pension cheques barely cover the cost of living and medications
- Lives alone but has family who want her to move in with them following surgery
- Uses herbs to control diabetes and frequently refuses to take insulin

Objective Data
Physical Examination
- Alert, cognitively intact, anxious, older person with reports of numbness and lack of feeling in right leg
- Weight, 65 kg; height, 160 cm
- Wears glasses
- Has macular degeneration in right eye

Diagnostic Studies
- Admission laboratory blood glucose level was 29.8 mmol/L
- Morning finger-stick blood glucose level was 5.3 mmol/L
- Doppler pulses for lower right leg very weak; absent in right foot
- Doppler pulses in left leg present, weak in left foot
- Serum creatinine 221 mmol/L

Interprofessional Care
- Scheduled for a below-the-knee amputation of the right leg as the last case of the day

Discussion Questions
1. What factors may influence M. G.'s response to hospitalization and surgery?

Patient About to Undergo Surgery—cont'd

2. **Priority decision:** Given the patient's history, what preoperative nursing assessments should be completed and why?
3. What potential perioperative complications might be expected for this patient?
4. **Priority decision:** What priority topics should be included in M. G.'s preoperative teaching plan?
5. **Priority decision:** Based on the assessment data presented, identify the priority nursing diagnoses and related interventions. Are there any interprofessional problems?

6. **Evidence-informed practice:** M. G. asks why insulin was administered this morning when there has been no food intake since midnight. How should the nurse respond to her?

℮volve

Answers are available at http://evolve.elsevier.com/Canada/Lewis/medsurg.

REVIEW QUESTIONS

The number of the question corresponds to the same-numbered objective at the beginning of the chapter.

1. A client who is overweight is scheduled for laparoscopic cholecystectomy at an outpatient surgical clinic. Which of the following statements is true?
   a. Surgery will involve multiple small incisions.
   b. This setting is not appropriate for this procedure.
   c. Surgery will involve removing part of the liver.
   d. The client will need special preparation because of obesity.
2. The client tells the nurse in the preoperative setting that she has noticed she has a reaction when wearing rubber gloves. What is the *most* appropriate action?
   a. Notify the surgery so that the surgery can be cancelled.
   b. Ask additional questions to assess for a possible latex allergy.
   c. Notify the OR staff at once so they can use latex-free supplies.
   d. No action is needed because the patient's rubber sensitivity has no bearing on surgery.
3. A client is scheduled for a herniorrhaphy in 2 days and reports use of ginkgo daily. What is the priority intervention?
   a. Inform the surgeon, since the procedure may have to be rescheduled.
   b. Notify the anaesthesia care provider, since this herb interferes with anaesthetics.
   c. Ask the client about any side effects from taking this herbal supplement.
   d. Tell the client to continue to take the herbal supplement up to the day before surgery.
4. What is the nurse's role when assisting a client with informed consent before an operative procedure?
   a. Obtains the consent when a surgeon cannot
   b. Asks the client to explain what surgical procedure they are having and ensures that the client understands the operation to be performed
   c. Explains all the risks of the surgical procedure
   d. Ensures that the client signs the consent form before preoperative sedation is given
5. A priority nursing intervention to aid a preoperative client in coping with fear of postoperative pain would include which of the following?
   a. Inform the client that pain medication will be available.
   b. Teach the client to use guided imagery to help manage pain.
   c. Describe the type of pain expected with the client's particular surgery.
   d. Explain the pain management plan, including the use of a pain rating scale.

6. A client is scheduled for surgery requiring general anaesthesia at an ambulatory surgical centre. The nurse asks the client when they ate last. The client replies that a light breakfast was consumed a couple of hours before coming to the surgery centre. What should the nurse do first?
   a. Tell the client to come back tomorrow, since a meal was consumed.
   b. Have the client void before giving any preoperative medications.
   c. Proceed with the preoperative checklist, including site identification.
   d. Notify the anaesthesia care provider of when and what the client last ate.
7. A client who normally takes 40 units of glargine insulin (long-acting) at bedtime asks the nurse what to do about the dose the night before surgery. How should the nurse respond?
   a. Skip her insulin altogether the night before surgery.
   b. Obtain instructions from the health care provider on any insulin adjustments.
   c. Take the usual dose at bedtime and eat a light breakfast in the morning.
   d. Eat a moderate meal before bedtime and then take half of the usual insulin dose.
8. Preoperative considerations for older persons include which of the following? (*Select all that apply.*)
   a. Using only large-print educational materials
   b. Speaking louder for clients with hearing aids
   c. Recognizing that sensory deficits may be present
   d. Providing warm blankets to prevent hypothermia
   e. Teaching important information early in the morning

1. a, 2. b, 3. a, 4. b, 5. d, 6. d, 7. b, 8. c, d

℮volve

For even more review questions, visit http://evolve.elsevier.com/Canada/Lewis/medsurg.

REFERENCES

Adugbire, B. A., & Aziato, L. (2020). Surgical patients' perception of spirituality on the outcome of surgery in Northern Ghana. *Journal of Holistic Nursing, 38*(1). https://doi.org/10.1177/0898010120902916

Alexander, J., & Joshi, G. (2019). A review of the anesthetic implications of marijuana use. *Baylor University Medical Center Proceedings, 32*(3), 364–371. https://doi.org/10.1080/08998280.2019.1603034

Allen, S. (2019). Geriatric surgery. In J. Rothrock & D. McEwen (Eds.), *Alexander's care of the patient in surgery* (16th ed.) (pp. 1069–1090). Elsevier.

Ashpari, A., & Lakshman, K. (2018). Effects of pre-operative psychological status on post-operative recovery: a prospective study. *World Journal of Surgery, 42*(1), 12–18. https://doi.org/10.1007/s00268-017-4169-2

Bak, J. (2019). In J. Rothrock & D. McEwen (Eds.), *Alexander's care of the patient in surgery* (16th ed.) (pp. 244–260). Elsevier.

Brega, A. G., Barnard, J., Mabachi, N. M., et al. (2015). AHRQ health literacy universal precautions toolkit (2nd ed.). AHRQ Publication No. 15-0023-EF. Agency for Healthcare Research and Quality. www.ahrq.gov/sites/default/files/publications/files/healthlit-toolkit2_4.pdf

Campbell, B. (2019). Anesthesia. In J. Rothrock & D. McEwen (Eds.), *Alexander's care of the patient in surgery* (16th ed.) (pp. 108–140). Elsevier.

Canadian Anesthesiologists' Society. (2021). *Stop smoking.* https://www.cas.ca/en/about-cas/advocacy/anesthesia-faq/stop-smoking

Canadian Blood Services. (2020). *Crossmatch.* https://www.blood.ca/en/laboratory-services/crossmatch

Canadian Institute for Health Information (CIHI). (2018). *Inpatient hospitalizations, surgeries, newborns and childbirth indicators, 2016–2017.* https://secure.cihi.ca/free_products/hospch-hosp-2016-2017-snapshot_en.pdf

Canadian Institute for Health Information (CIHI). (2020). *Explore wait times for priority procedures across Canada.* https://www.cihi.ca/en/explore-wait-times-for-priority-procedures-across-canada/

Canadian Institute for Health Information (CIHI). (2021). *Wait times for priority procedures in Canada.* https://www.cihi.ca/en/wait-times-for-priority-procedures-in-canada

Canadian Medical Protective Association (CMPA). (2021). *Consent: A guide for Canadian physicians.* https://www.cmpa-acpm.ca/en/advice-publications/handbooks/consent-a-guide-for-canadian-physicians

Cartwright, S., & Andrews, S. (2018). Perianesthesia nursing as a specialty. In J. Odom-Forren (Ed.), *Drain's perianesthesia nursing: A critical care approach* (7th ed.) (pp. 11–16). Elsevier.

DeVolder, B. (2019). Gastrointestinal surgery. In J. Rothrock & D. McEwen (Eds.), *Alexander's care of the patient in surgery* (16th ed.) (pp. 287–340). Elsevier.

Dobson, G., Chong, M., Chow, L., et al. (2017). Guidelines to the practice of anesthesia. *Canadian Journal of Anesthesia, 64*(1), 65–91. https://doi.org/10.1007/s12630-016-0749-0

Dobson, G., Chow, L., Flexman, A., et al. (2019). Guidelines to the practice of anesthesia—revised edition 2019. *Canadian Journal of Anesthesiology* (66), 75–108. https://doi.org/10.1007/s12630-018-1248-2

Kitching, G., Firestone, M., Schei, B., et al. (2020). Unmet health needs and discrimination by healthcare providers among an Indigenous population in Toronto, Canada. *Canadian Journal of Public Health, 111*, 40–49. https://doi.org/10.17269/s41997-019-00242-z

Larner, R. (2019). Integrative health practices: Complementary and alternative therapies. In J. Rothrock & D. McEwen (Eds.), *Alexander's care of the patient in surgery* (16th ed.) (pp. 1147–1162). Elsevier.

Makokis, P., & Makokis, J. (2018). Practising "the good way of life" from the hospital bed to mother earth. In M. Greenwood, S. de Leeuw, & N. Lindsay (Eds.), *Determinants of Indigenous people's health in Canada: Beyond the social* (2nd ed.) (pp. 257–273). Canadian Scholars' Press.

Marley, R., & Sheets, S. (2018). Preoperative evaluation and preparation of the patient. In J. Nagelhout & S. Elisha (Eds.), *Nurse anesthesia* (6th ed.). Elsevier. 311-345.

O'Brien, D. (2018). Patient education and care of the perianesthesia patient. In J. Odom-Forren (Ed.), *Drain's perianesthesia nursing: A critical care approach* (7th ed.) (pp. 385–397). Elsevier.

Odom-Forren, J. (2019). Postoperative patient care and pain management. In J. Rothrock & D. McEwen (Eds.), *Alexander's care of the patient in surgery* (16th ed.) (pp. 261–285). Elsevier.

Operating Room Nurses Association of Canada (ORNAC). (2019). *Standards, guidelines, and position statements for perioperative registered nursing practice* (14th ed.). Author.

Rasmussen, P. (2019). Colonizing racialized bodies: Examining the forced sterilization of Indigenous women and the shameful history of eugenics in Canada. *University of Victoria Undergraduate Journal of Political Science, 13*(1), 18–29. https://journals.uvic.ca/index.php/onpolitics/article/view/19415

Schick, L. (2018). Assessment and monitoring of the perianesthesia patient. In J. Odom-Forren (Ed.), *Drain's perianesthesia nursing: A critical care approach* (7th ed.) (pp. 385–397). Elsevier.

Smith, J. (2019). Hernia repair. In J. Rothrock & D. McEwen (Eds.), *Alexander's care of the patient in surgery* (16th ed.) (pp. 376–399). Elsevier.

Wiseman, S., Crump, R., & Sutherland, J. (2020). Surgical wait list management in Canada during a pandemic: Many challenges ahead. *Canadian Journal of Surgery, 63*(3), E226–E228. https://doi.org/10.1503/cjs.006620

Yu, R., & Woo, J. (2019). Cognitive assessment of older people. Do sensory function and frailty matter? *International Journal of Environmental Research and Public Health, 16*(4), 662. https://doi.org/10.3390/ijerph16040662

RESOURCES

Additional resources for this chapter are listed in Chapter 22.

evolve

For additional Internet resources, see the website for this book at http://evolve.elsevier.com/Canada/Lewis/medsurg.

21

Nursing Management

Intraoperative Care

Peggy Hancock
Originating US chapter by Mark Karasin

⊖volve WEBSITE

LEARNING OBJECTIVES

1. Describe the roles and responsibilities of the perioperative nurse in the management of patients undergoing surgery.
2. Differentiate the purposes of the three different areas of the surgical suite and the proper attire for each area.
3. Identify characteristics of the operating room environment that contribute to patient safety and infection prevention.
4. Describe the activities and responsibilities of the members of the surgical team.
5. Prioritize the needs of patients undergoing surgery.
6. Describe basic principles of aseptic technique used in the operating room.
7. Discuss the importance of safety in the positioning of patients in regard to surgical procedure, equipment, and anaesthesia.
8. Differentiate between general and regional or local anaesthesia, including advantages, disadvantages, and rationale for choice of the anaesthetic technique.
9. Identify the basic techniques used to induce and maintain general anaesthesia.
10. Discuss techniques for administering local and regional anaesthesia.

KEY TERMS

anaesthesia care team
anaesthesiologist
circulating nurse
epidural block
general anaesthesia
holding area

laryngeal mask airway (LMA)
local anaesthesia
malignant hyperthermia (MH)
moderate sedation
neuraxial blocks
operating room (OR)

regional anaesthesia
scrub nurse
spinal anaesthesia
surgeon
surgical suite

Traditionally, surgery has been performed in hospital operating rooms (ORs). However, the advent of advanced surgical technologies, improvements in the administration of anaesthesia, and changes in the Canadian health care system have altered where and how surgery is provided. Depending on the acuity of the surgical procedure, it can be performed on an outpatient basis in diverse environments like surgi-centres, ambulatory care settings, and clinics. Today, the majority of surgeries are minimally invasive surgery (MIS) and offer the benefits of shorter hospital stays, decreased postoperative pain and incidence of surgical site infection, and, consequently, a faster return to a normal lifestyle (Ball, 2019). The impact of MIS for the surgical team is shorter procedures requiring quicker turnovers and less time available for perioperative teaching of patient and caregivers. Conversely, complex procedures and use of advanced technologies such as robotics may require longer setups and surgical time.

Despite the variety of settings and range of surgical complexity, the principles of intraoperative patient care remain the same and are discussed in detail in this chapter.

PHYSICAL ENVIRONMENT

Department Layout

The surgical suite is a controlled environment designed to maximize infection control and provide a seamless flow of patients, personnel, and operative instruments, equipment, and supplies. The suite is divided into three distinct areas: unrestricted, semi-restricted, and restricted. The *unrestricted* area

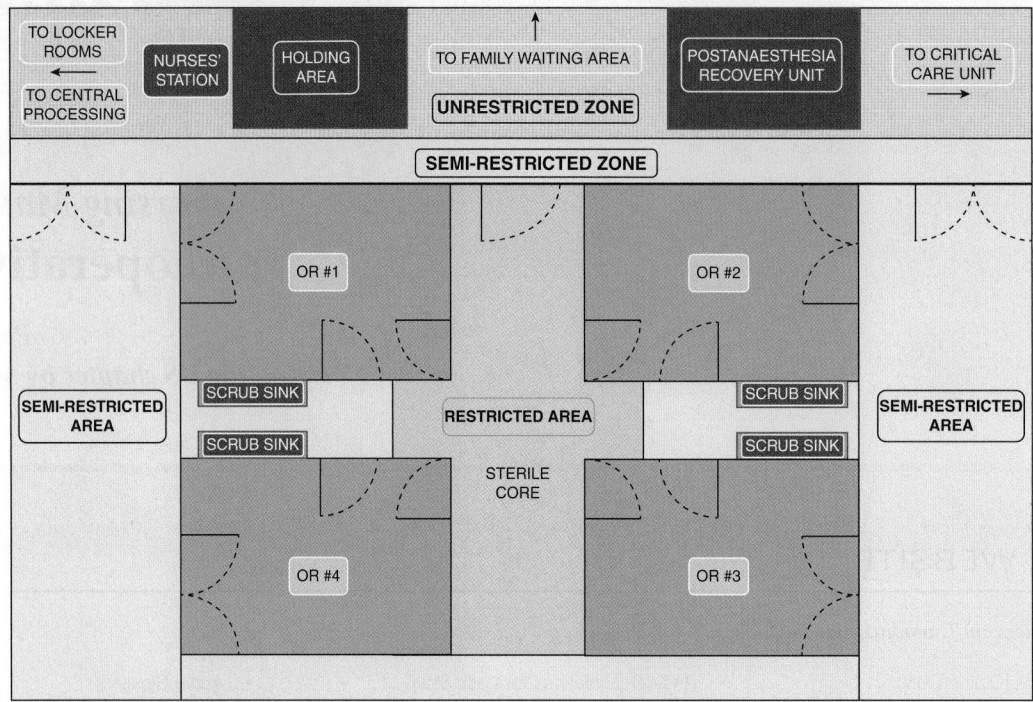

FIG. 21.1 Perioperative department layout.

provides access to all people in street clothes, who can interact with those in scrub uniforms. These areas typically include the patient admissions area, a staff locker room, the communication or control centre, and offices. The *semi-restricted* area includes the peripheral support areas, such as work and storage areas for clean and sterile supplies. Authorized personnel can access semi-restricted areas but must wear surgical attire and cover all head and facial hair. *Restricted* areas include the ORs and all areas where sterile supplies are opened. Personnel wear surgical attire and masks (Operating Room Nurses Association of Canada [ORNAC], 2019). Since the restricted area is designed to reduce cross-contamination, personnel may not bring in personal belongings, food, or beverages (ORNAC, 2019), and clean and sterile items must be separated from contaminated supplies and waste by space, time, and traffic patterns. For example, sterile surgical supplies move from the medical device reprocessing department (MDRD) through the clean core and into the restricted OR. Supplies contaminated after surgery are covered or otherwise contained and transported through the peripheral area to the MDRD decontamination area (ORNAC, 2019).

Preoperative Holding Area

The preoperative holding area is an admission and waiting area inside or adjacent to the surgical suite. This preoperative unit may be a centralized area that accommodates numerous patients or a single-patient area immediately outside the OR designated for the surgical procedure. In the holding area, the perioperative nurse identifies and assesses the patient, gives preoperative medications, and, in some institutions, initiates intravenous (IV) infusions before the patient is transferred into the OR or to an anaesthesia block room. Hospitals that have instituted anaesthesia block rooms have the ability to do neuraxial (spinal and epidural) and peripheral nerve blocks. The presence of these holding rooms reduces anaesthesia prep time in the OR, thus enhancing the provision of efficient, patient-centred care (Brown et al., 2019). Family or caregivers are often permitted to wait in the holding area with the patient until it is time to be transferred to the OR. Their presence helps relieve patient anxiety.

Operating Room

The operating room (OR) is a unique acute care setting specially designed for surgery (Figure 21.1) that, in a hospital, is usually adjacent to the *postanaesthesia care unit* (PACU) and the surgical critical care unit (CCU). This positioning allows for quick patient transport and proximity to anaesthesia and surgical personnel if complications arise.

ORs are designed using infection-control and safety principles. Airborne transmission of microorganisms and dust is controlled by high-efficiency particulate air (HEPA) filters in the ventilating systems, and controlled positive pressure airflow helps remove anaesthetic gas and toxic fumes. Proper air exchange, temperature, and humidity control provide physical comfort and inhibit bacterial proliferation (ORNAC, 2019). OR furniture and equipment are manufactured from materials that resist the corroding effects of disinfectants, are adjustable, and can be moved. Equipment is checked frequently to ensure proper functioning and electrical safety. Lighting provides a low- to high-intensity range for a precise view of the surgical site (Figure 21.2). Effective integrated voice-over Wi-Fi aids communication workflows in the OR: Hands-free communication allows sterile team members to converse without touching anything and provides seamless connectivity between the OR and other support areas.

SURGICAL TEAM

Registered Nurse

The registered nurse (RN) provides individualized nursing to patients throughout the surgical continuum. In order to address the patient's complex physiological, psychological, sociocultural, and spiritual responses to the surgical event, perioperative nurses require basic and expanded knowledge, skills, and

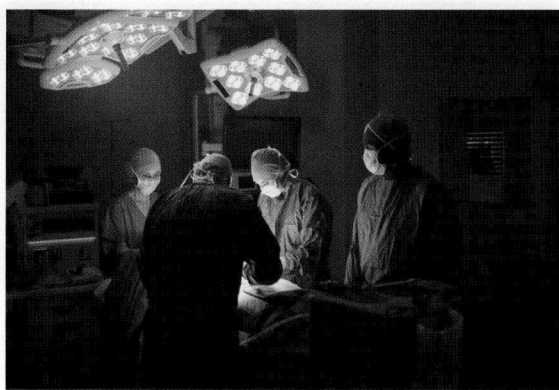

FIG. 21.2 The lighting system in an operating room must provide a range of lighting intensity for a clear view of the surgical site. Source: iStock.com/ shapecharge

abilities. The Operating Room Nurses Association of Canada (ORNAC) Standards for Perioperative Registered Nursing Practice present the evidence-informed rationale for the structure and resources required in the perioperative environment to promote safe, effective patient care through collaboration with the interprofessional team (ORNAC, 2019). Since 1995, perioperative nurses have been able to attain national certification through the Canadian Nurses Association (2021) and the designation Certified Perioperative Nurse (Canada).

The scope of perioperative nursing practice is a continuum of nursing activities that identify and meet the patient's unique needs throughout the perioperative experience (ORNAC, 2019). Competencies include practicing professionally, providing physical and supportive care, promoting a safe environment, responding to urgent situations, and managing resources (ORNAC, 2019). The perioperative nurse orchestrates the preparation of the OR with other members of the surgical team. The nurse is usually the first member of the surgical team to greet the patient on arrival to the surgical suite and advocates for the patient throughout the intraoperative experience by:
- Maintaining privacy, confidentiality, and dignity
- Providing physical care and comfort
- Ensuring safety
- Promoting communication—for example, explaining steps prior to induction and ensuring that patients can hear (e.g., hearing aids left in) (ORNAC, 2019)

Some specific intraoperative activities of the circulating nurse are outlined in Table 21.1.

Perioperative nurses must know that all surgical procedures have a potential for adverse outcomes, so they implement evidence-informed guidelines for surgical care by establishing and maintaining infection-control measures and keeping current on new technologies. The perioperative nurse has a role to play in carrying out the Surgical Safety Checklist—an interprofessional time-out before the surgical incision to verify patient information and status at three points in the operative process (Canadian Patient Safety Institute [CPSI], 2020).

Since the development of this checklist by the World Health Organization (WHO) in 2009, there have been mixed reports on its efficacy. While this tool has been acknowledged to be one of the most useful tools for improving surgical safety, it must be implemented with adequate support in order to provide meaningful patient outcomes (Urbach et al., 2019). (See the Resources at the end of this chapter for the Canadian adaptation of the Surgical Safety Checklist.)

TABLE 21.1	**ACTIVITIES OF THE CIRCULATING NURSE**
Circulating Role	
The perioperative Registered Nurse shall practice in a manner that:	
2.1.1	Assesses the health status of the patient
2.1.2	Develops, modifies, and documents the individualized plan of care, or a clinical pathway to meet the specific needs of the patient
2.1.3	Provides resources for the health care team to function efficiently
2.1.4	Provides physical comfort measures specific to each surgical patient
2.1.5	Provides appropriate care during the admission to the operating room, preinduction, induction, intraoperative, and emergence phases
2.1.6	Performs the surgical count procedure concurrently with the scrub nurse and documents accurately
2.1.7	Uses a surgical conscience to maintain and monitor the integrity of the sterile field
2.1.8	Reduces risk by providing continuous, astute, and vigilant observation of the surgical team throughout the surgical phase, meeting the health care team and patient's needs
2.1.9	Acts as the patient's advocate throughout the perioperative period
2.1.10	Responds to complications and unexpected events during the perioperative period
2.1.11	Demonstrates leadership capabilities and skills to provide a safe and therapeutic environment for the patient
2.1.12	Organizes and coordinates appropriate resources in a timely manner in preparation for the subsequent patient
2.1.13	Provides and assists with procedures and devices required to complete patient care following the surgical procedure
2.1.14	Assists in the patient transfer and postoperative positioning
2.1.15	Accurately and appropriately documents nursing, surgical, and other health care team activities during the perioperative period
2.1.16	Promotes appropriate communication techniques to keep noise levels at a minimum
2.1.17	Assists with patient transport to a receiving unit and communicates pertinent patient information
2.1.18	Organizes and coordinates appropriate resources to ensure an efficient operating room turnover
2.1.19	Has knowledge and awareness of their organization's policies and procedures and implements appropriately

Source: Operating Room Nurses Association of Canada (ORNAC). (2019). *The ORNAC standards, guidelines, and position statements for perioperative registered nurses* (14th ed.). Author.

In the perioperative role, nurses perform either sterile activities (scrub nurse) or unsterile activities (circulating nurse). Canadian ORs comprise a mixture of registered and practical nurses. The scope of practice for practical nurses allows them to assume the scrub role; however, RNs may perform all aspects of perioperative practice.

Circulating Role. Perioperative nurses use critical thinking in assessing patients on an ongoing basis and in responding to changing patient conditions. Examples of nursing activities that characterize each phase of the patient's surgical experience are presented in Table 21.2.

The circulating nurse is not scrubbed, gloved, or gowned and remains in the unsterile field. This nurse documents nursing and medical activities throughout the perioperative period. Intraoperative documentation includes but is not limited to the following (ORNAC, 2019):
- Naming all personnel involved in patient care in the OR
- Recording event times, additional interventions, and the surgical procedure performed

TABLE 21.2	COMMON PERIOPERATIVE NURSING ACTIVITIES THROUGHOUT THE PATIENT'S SURGICAL EXPERIENCE	
Before Surgery	**During Surgery**	**After Surgery**
Home, Clinic, Holding Area • Starts preoperative assessment • Plans teaching appropriate to patient's needs • Involves caregiver **Surgical Unit** • Completes preoperative assessment • Coordinates patient teaching with staff • Develops a plan of care that reflects patient's level of function and ability • Safely gives ordered medications **Surgical Suite** • Conducts preprocedure verification • Assesses patient's level of consciousness, skin integrity, mobility, emotional status, and functional limitations • Reviews chart • Ensures all supplies and equipment needed are available, functioning, and sterile, if appropriate	**Safety Maintenance** • Ensures integrity of sterile field • Ensures that sponge, needle, instrument, and medical device counts are correct • Positions patient to ensure correct alignment, exposure of surgical site, and prevention of injury • Prevents chemical injury from prepping solutions, medications • Ensures safe use of electrical equipment • Safely gives ordered medications **Monitoring Physical Status** • Monitors and reports changes in patient's vital signs • Monitors blood loss and urine output **Monitoring Psychological Status** • Gives emotional support to patient • Ensures patient's right to privacy • Communicates patient's emotional status to health care team	**Postanaesthesia, Discharge Area** • Determines patient's response to surgical intervention • Monitors ABCs, vital signs, level of consciousness • Safely gives ordered medications **Clinical Unit** • Evaluates effectiveness of nursing care in OR using patient outcome criteria • Determines patient's level of satisfaction with care given • Assesses patient's psychological status • Helps with discharge planning **Home, Clinic** • Seeks patient's perception of surgery in terms of effects of anaesthetic agents, impact on body image, immobilization • Determines caregiver's perceptions of surgery

- Documenting the patient's positioning, surgical skin preparation, and placement of dispersive pad
- Documenting patient monitoring devices and type of anaesthesia
- Recording all equipment used on the patient, including settings and serial numbers
- Noting information for prosthetic implants and other devices left in the patient such as catheters and drains
- Logging of specimens and documenting blood loss and the surgical count
- Making note of any untoward events

Practical Nurse

The scrub role is often performed by a practical nurse who has a perioperative certificate. Practical nurses may assume broader responsibilities depending on patient acuity and hospital policy.

Scrub Role. The scrub nurse is often a practical nurse who performs surgical hand asepsis, is gowned and gloved in sterile attire, and remains in the sterile field assisting the surgical team by preparing and handling instruments. The scrub nurse's duties include setting priorities and ensuring an efficient aseptic setup for the surgical procedure. The nurse monitors aseptic technique throughout the procedure, performs the surgical count concurrently with the circulating nurse, and acts as the patient's advocate during the surgical procedure (ORNAC, 2019). Additionally, the scrub nurse implements patient safety protocols through accurate administration of medication, proper handling and counting of surgical instruments and supplies, management and labelling of specimens, and completion of postoperative documentation.

Surgeon and Assistant

The surgeon performs the surgical procedure and is primarily responsible for the following:

- Preoperative medical history and physical assessment, including need for surgical intervention, choice of surgical procedure, and management of preoperative workup
- Informed consent—explaining surgical risks, complications, and alternative treatment options and obtaining written consent

- Patient safety and surgical management in the OR
- Postoperative patient management

The surgeon's assistant holds retractors to expose surgical areas and assists with hemostasis and suturing. The surgeon's assistant is usually a physician but, in educational settings, may be a surgical resident who can perform some portions of the operation under the surgeon's direct supervision. Some institutions employ registered nurse first assistants (RNFAs) to assist in surgery under the direct supervision of the surgeon.

Registered Nurse First Assistant

The RNFA is a registered perioperative nurse with formal surgical education, skills, and knowledge who facilitates and supports the health care needs of the patient through the perioperative continuum. The scope of practice allows the RNFA to collaborate with the surgeon in planning preoperative, intraoperative, and postoperative patient care. Intraoperatively, RNFAs handle instruments, provide exposure, assist with maintaining hemostasis, and suture under direct supervision of the surgeon (ORNAC, 2019).

Anaesthesiologist

An anaesthesiologist is a physician who is responsible for the administration of anaesthetic agents (Dobson et al., 2019). As vital members of the surgical team, anaesthesiologists are experts in administering potent drugs used to deliver general and regional anaesthesia and in ensuring absence of pain during surgery. Anaesthesiologists medically manage the unconscious or insensible patient during interventions requiring anaesthesia. This duty includes protecting vital functions, managing pulmonary and cardiac complications, including cardiopulmonary resuscitation (CPR), and caring for critically ill patients.

In larger ORs and teaching hospitals, respiratory therapists or RNs can take advanced education and training in order to work with the anaesthesia care team as anaesthesia assistants. An anaesthesia care team is an anaesthesiologist-led care model in which anaesthesiologists practise among a team of other professionals such as nurse practitioners in anaesthesia care, anaesthesia assistants, RNs, and respiratory therapists.

Advanced Nursing Practice Roles

Registered Nurse Anaesthesia Assistant. A registered nurse anaesthesia assistant (RNAA) is an RN with advanced education, knowledge, and skills in anaesthesia who works in collaboration with and under the supervision of an anaesthesiologist throughout the perioperative period (ORNAC, 2019).

An additional Canadian category of anaesthesia provider is the nurse practitioner in anaesthesia care (NP-A), which requires master's-level preparation. These nurse practitioners with specialist education in anaesthesia care work as part of the anaesthesia care team, providing a range of services both pre- and postoperatively (University Health Network, 2021).

NURSING MANAGEMENT
PATIENT BEFORE SURGERY

The collection of preoperative assessment data and health information, in partnership with the patient and family, encourages active involvement in the care plan and helps establish baseline data for the perioperative team (Cunning, 2019). Further information on the psychosocial assessment and physical assessment can be found in Chapter 20.

CHART REVIEW

Charting requirements vary with hospital policy, patient condition, and specific surgical procedures; for instance, ambulatory surgery facilities have healthier patients, so fewer preoperative tests may be required. Nursing review of the health record includes validating important findings and verifying that appropriate documentation is present. Of key importance is ensuring that appropriate consent documentation is on the patient chart and has been completed as per agency policy (see Chapter 20 for discussion of consent).

ADMITTING THE PATIENT

The nurse follows hospital protocol for patient admission to the preoperative holding area and OR. The perioperative nurse greets the patient using a respectful, caring communication style and institutes comfort measures to keep the patient warm and relaxed. The identification process includes asking the patient to state his or her name, the surgeon's name, the operative procedure, and the site of surgery. This active communication process reduces the risk for error. The nurse confirms the identity of the patient with the patient using at least two patient-specific identifiers, which can include the patient's name, date of birth, and/or their unique identification number (ORNAC, 2019). The admission procedure verifies items on the preoperative checklist such as NPO status, allergies, presence of dentures or prostheses, and so on. The nurse confirms informed consent, secures personal belongings, and confirms whether preoperative medication was administered (ORNAC, 2019). The patient must have time to get responses to last-minute questions. The nurse completes the chart review, documenting any abnormalities or changes. The patient is seen and assessed by the surgeon and anaesthesiologist before anaesthesia induction.

The patient may be offered complementary or alternative therapies to decrease anxiety and promote relaxation. Therapeutic touch, guided imagery, aromatherapy, music therapy, and controlled breathing are modalities that can be used for surgical patients (Larner, 2019).

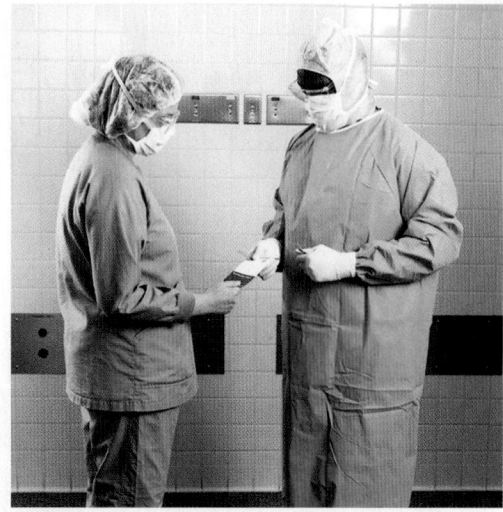

FIG. 21.3 Surgical attire is worn by all persons entering the operating room suite.

NURSING MANAGEMENT
INTRAOPERATIVE CARE

ROOM PREPARATION

Before the patient enters the OR, nurses start implementing the intraoperative care plan by ensuring all case-specific surgical instrumentation and supplies are available, have been properly sterilized, and are aseptically opened onto the sterile field. The scrub nurse sets up the instrument table, placing instruments and supplies in a predesignated spot so they can be handled systematically and accurately during the surgical procedure. The perioperative nurse determines the type of surgical count: full or partial, depending on the probability of leaving an instrument, sponge, or other item in the incision. Counts are conducted and documented in accordance with ORNAC guidelines and hospital policy (ORNAC, 2019).

Nurses verify the proper functioning and safe operation of electrical and mechanical equipment, ensure patient privacy by limiting personnel in the OR, and are infection-control stewards. The circulating nurse ensures that all people entering the OR are wearing surgical attire. Dress protocols include scrub pants and shirt, mask, protective eyewear, a cap or hood that covers all hair, and absence of jewellery or false nails (Figure 21.3).

Once gowned and gloved, nurses create a sterile environment by disinfecting the incision site and placing sterile sheets (drapes) over the patient to expose only the incision area. Sterile team members can touch only items in the sterile field and must keep their hands above waist level.

The circulating nurse remains outside the sterile field (at least 30 cm [1 foot] away from sterile items) and supports the patient by assisting the anaesthesiologist and surgical team, monitoring aseptic practice, providing ongoing supplies and communication, and documenting care.

PATIENT TRANSFER TO THE OR. Once the change-over in the OR is done, the patient is identified for the final time and transported into the room for surgery. If the patient is unable to assist in the transfer to the OR bed, a sufficient number of health care providers must be available to monitor and lift the patient from the stretcher to the OR table. It is essential that the wheels of both be locked to prevent accidents. If the patient was sent to

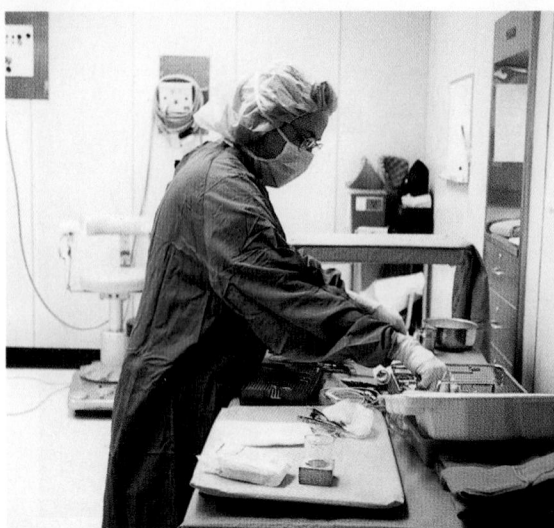

FIG. 21.4 A sterile field is created before surgery. Source: Courtesy the Methodist Hospital, Houston, TX. Photograph by Donna Dahms, RN, CNOR.

the OR with hearing aids or glasses, they should be removed and safely stored at this time. A cultural valuable worn on the body often has spiritually protective significance for Indigenous people undergoing surgery (Vancouver Coastal Health, 2015). Any jewellery that has been taped or secured to the patient's gown should be identified at this time. The nurse should ensure that any requirement to touch personal cultural items or valuables is discussed first with the patient and family. Once the patient is on the operating table, a safety strap is placed across the patient's thighs and the arms secured as appropriate for the procedure. The electrocardiogram monitor leads, oxygen saturation monitor, and blood pressure cuff are applied, and an IV catheter is inserted if it was not started before surgery.

SCRUBBING, GOWNING, AND GLOVING. Although all personnel entering the OR must perform hand hygiene, the surgeon, scrub nurse, and surgical assistant must disinfect their hands and arms using a surgical hand antiseptic or scrub agent. The surgical hand antiseptic or scrub is a broad-spectrum agent that kills microorganisms on contact and supplies persistent protection because it inhibits microbial reproduction. There are different procedures for water-based and waterless hand preparation, and personnel must follow the manufacturer's written instructions and hospital policy (ORNAC, 2019).

After completing the scrub procedure, the team members enter the room and don sterile surgical gowns and gloves, which allow them to manipulate and organize all sterile items for use during the procedure (Figure 21.4).

BASIC ASEPTIC TECHNIQUE

The surgical team adheres to surgical aseptic principles with the intention of eliminating patient exposure to pathogenic microorganisms and thus preventing surgical site infection (King & Spry, 2019). Members of the surgical team share responsibility for monitoring aseptic practice and initiating corrective action if the sterile field is compromised (King & Spry, 2019).

In addition to protecting the surgical patient, the safety of the perioperative interprofessional team must also be considered. Pathogens can spread via airborne, droplet, or contact transmission, so appropriate infection-control precautions addressing specific methods of transmission are implemented to protect the surgical team (ORNAC, 2019). These guidelines emphasize routine

---

TABLE 21.3	**MAINTAINING A STERILE FIELD IN THE OPERATING ROOM**

Practice

2.16.1   Opened sterile supplies and setup shall not be left unattended. They shall be continuously monitored for possible contamination.

2.16.2   Unsterile persons shall not reach over the sterile field. Movement is from unsterile to unsterile areas. They should not pass between sterile fields.

2.16.3   Unsterile health care team members shall remain at a safe distance, at least 30 cm (1 ft.), from the sterile field. When approaching the sterile field, unsterile personnel should face the sterile field. Personnel should not pass between sterile fields.

2.16.4   Sterile persons shall not reach over unsterile areas.

2.16.5   Sterile personnel shall stay within the sterile field. Sterile persons shall not walk around or go outside the operating room.

2.16.6   Sterile personnel shall always face the sterile field. If changes in position are necessary, sterile personnel shall pass face-to-face or back-to-back with each other. When changing positions, the sterile personnel should avoid changing levels; personnel either sit or stand. Hands shall be kept above waist level.

2.16.7   Talking should be kept to a minimum.

2.16.8   The sterile setup shall not be covered.

2.16.9   Unsterile equipment is covered with sterile barriers before placing them over or in the sterile field. For example, C-arms, laparoscopic cameras, certain positioning devices should be draped for use.

2.16.10 Breaks in aseptic technique shall be recognized, monitored, and documented (as per health care facility policy) and corrective action taken as soon as safely possible.

2.16.11 A sterile setup may be covered in circumstances when it is identified that there is an increased risk of a setup becoming contaminated, or in consideration for specific patient care needs (e.g., extended or unanticipated delays between setup and surgery start time). The nurse continues to monitor the sterile field/area when there is a delay; covering a sterile field is not a substitute for continuous monitoring.

2.16.12 The nurse shall know how to properly cover and uncover a sterile field. When covering and uncovering a sterile setup, it shall be done by personnel in a way that prevents drapes that extend below the top of the table from being brought back over the sterile surface.

Source: Operating Room Nurses Association of Canada (ORNAC). (2019). *The ORNAC standards, guidelines, and position statements for perioperative registered nurses* (14th ed.). Author.

and transmission-based precautions (see Table 17.8), engineering and work practice controls, and the use of personal protective equipment such as gloves, gowns, caps, face shields, masks, and protective eyewear (see Table 17.9 and Table 21.3). For example, infection-prevention guidelines have been altered to enhance precautions for aerosolized procedures for individuals with COVID-19. Nurses caring for patients with COVID-19 are expected to adhere to personal protective equipment (PPE) guidelines as provided by provincial/territorial health authorities (ORNAC, 2020).

POSITIONING THE PATIENT

Proper patient positioning is a critical part of every procedure. The perioperative interprofessional team must have in-depth knowledge about the surgical procedure in order to determine the patient's position and optimize surgical exposure. Examples of vulnerable patients who require special consideration when positioning include older persons, patients with respiratory and circulatory disorders, and patients with limited mobility (Fawcett, 2019).

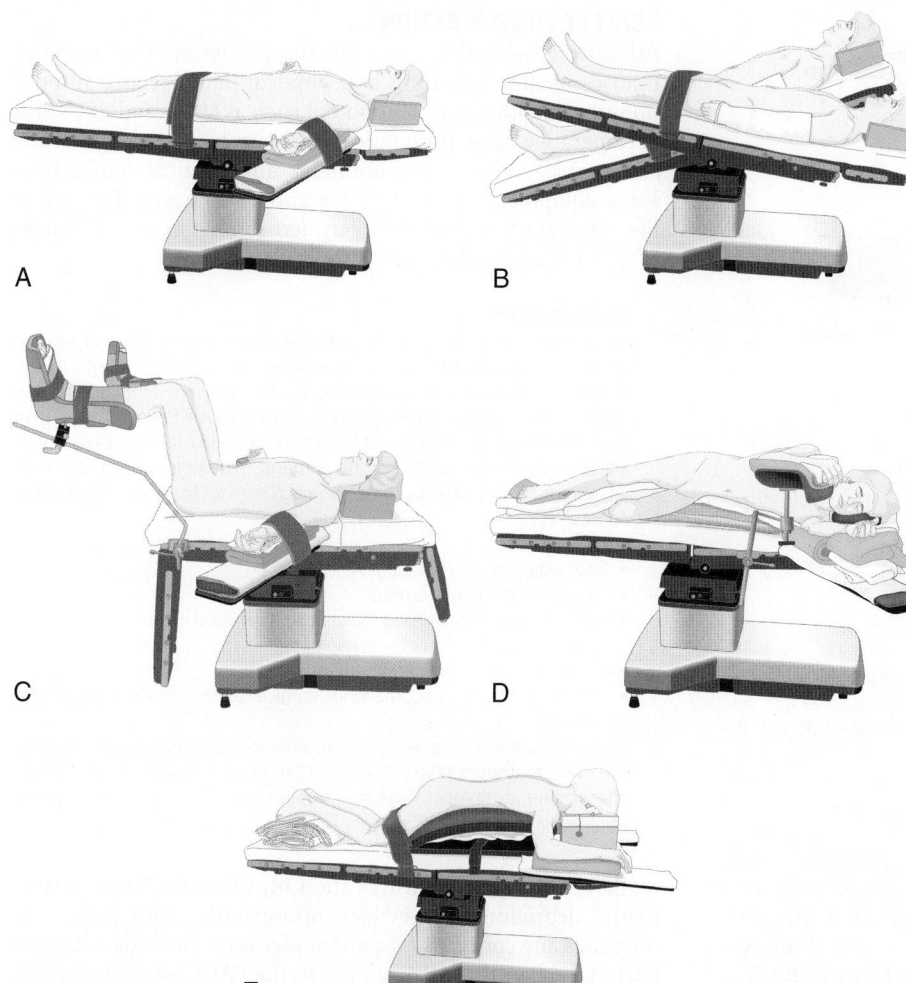

FIG. 21.5 Common intraoperative patient positioning. **A,** Supine position: abdominal surgery. **B,** Trendelenburg position: pelvic surgery. **C,** Lithotomy position: abdominal perineal resection. **D,** Lateral decubitus position: thoracic surgery. **E,** Prone position with a Wilson frame: spinal surgery. Source: Miller, R. D. (Ed.). (2010). *Miller's anesthesia* (7th ed., pp. 1153, 1155, 1157, 1158, & 1160). Churchill-Livingstone.

Anaesthesia blocks sensory nerve impulses, so the patient will not feel pain, discomfort, or stress being placed on nerves, muscles, bones, or skin. Inappropriate positioning, however, may result in muscle strain, joint damage, pressure injuries, and untoward effects like hypotension and oxygen desaturation.

Proper positioning is a team effort that follows administration of the anaesthetic. The patient's position ensures proper anatomical alignment and functioning while allowing access to the operative site, access for anaesthesia medication administration, patient monitoring, and patent airway maintenance. Principles for positioning include (1) ensuring correct skeletal alignment; (2) preventing pressure on nerves, skin over bony prominences, and eyes; (3) providing for adequate thoracic excursion; (4) preventing occlusion of arteries and veins; (5) providing modesty in exposure; and (6) recognizing and respecting individual needs such as previously assessed aches, pains, or deformities. The perioperative nurse must consider the individual needs of the patient, collaborating with the surgical team to plan, implement, and monitor the patient's position throughout the surgical procedure (Fawcett, 2019).

As part of the intraoperative nursing care plan, extremities are secured and appropriate padding and support for at-risk areas (e.g., eyes during prone positioning) are provided. Obtaining sufficient physical or mechanical help in positioning avoids unnecessary strain on either the patient or perioperative interprofessional team (ORNAC, 2019).

Patient positions include supine, prone, Trendelenburg, lateral decubitus, and lithotomy (Figure 21.5). Supine is the most common position and is suited for abdominal, cardiac, and breast surgeries. A variation of the supine is the Trendelenburg position, used in lower abdominal or pelvic surgery, for which it is necessary to see the pelvic organs. The prone position allows easy access for back surgeries (e.g., laminectomies). The lithotomy position is used for genitourinary procedures such as vaginal hysterectomy and transurethral resection of the prostate.

Once the patient is positioned, the circulating nurse applies an adhesive, flexible gel pad called a *dispersive electrode* on a well-muscled, dry, clean area as close to the operative site as possible, avoiding any bony areas, implanted prostheses, or scar tissue (Figure 21.6). The dispersive pad is connected to the electrosurgical unit (ESU) or electrocautery, which is used by the surgeon to cauterize blood vessels and cut tissue. The dispersive electrode is a safety device that acts as a ground. If for any reason the current from the ESU is interrupted in its return through the dispersive electrode, thermal injury can occur (ORNAC, 2019).

PREPARING THE SURGICAL SITE

The purpose of skin preparation, or "prepping," is to reduce the number of transient and resident skin microorganisms at and surrounding the surgical incision site. Skin prep is usually the responsibility of the circulating nurse.

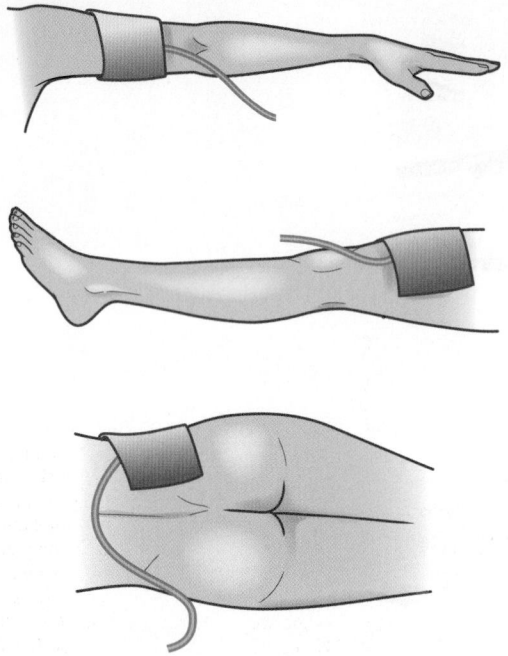

FIG. 21.6 When an electrosurgical unit is used, well-vascularized muscle mass is an optimal site. Safety can be compromised by excessive hair, adipose tissue, bony prominences, fluid (edema), adhesive failure, and scar tissue. Source: Courtesy Covidien, Mansfield, MA.

Before surgical skin preparation, body-piercing jewellery is removed. Hair is not removed unless it interferes with access to the surgical incision site. The rationale is that hair removal can traumatize skin by causing minor abrasions and increase the incidence of surgical site infections (ORNAC, 2019). In light of this evidence-informed information, surgical units must form their own policies and procedures for determining when hair removal is necessary, while considering the following:

- Hair is clipped, not shaved.
- Hair removal is performed close to the time of surgery (within 2 hours of surgical start time) and in an area outside the OR.
- A depilatory agent may be used for hair removal.
- Hair removal should be done with single-use clippers. Clippers with reusable heads must be disinfected between uses (ORNAC, 2019).

Before prepping the skin, the nurse verifies that the surgeon has marked the incision site with an indelible ink marker. Any lesions, irritation, or abrasions on or near the incision site are documented. The incision site is cleansed using a nontoxic agent that has a fast-acting, broad-spectrum, persistent antimicrobial action to which the patient is not allergic (King & Spry, 2019). The area is scrubbed in a circular motion from the clean area (site of the incision) to the dirty area (periphery). If the incision is proximal to the umbilicus, the umbilical area is prepped first to prevent contaminants from splashing onto a previously prepped area (ORNAC, 2019). Prep solution must not be allowed to pool as it may cause chemical skin burns, and it must be allowed to dry thoroughly before draping and using electrocautery or laser because of the risk for fire (alcohol and heat source) (ORNAC, 2019). After preparation of the skin, the sterile members of the surgical team drape the area, leaving the incision exposed.

SAFETY CONSIDERATIONS

All surgical procedures can put the patient at risk for injury. Injuries include infections and physical injury related to positioning, anaesthesia, or equipment such as lasers and ESUs. The perioperative nurse must follow safety protocols to prevent fires and burns. Airborne contaminants and surgical smoke from some equipment produce toxins and carcinogens that irritate the respiratory system and can aerosolize viruses, so smoke evacuators are used during these cases.

SAFETY ALERT

Surgery is one of the services with the highest percentage of adverse events in Canadian hospitals (Canadian Institute for Health Information & Canadian Patient Safety Institute, 2016). Given the serious repercussions of errors made during surgery, the Canadian Patient Safety Institute recommends using the safe-surgery checklist for all cases. Before administration of anaesthesia, the surgeon, anaesthesiologist, and nursing personnel do a briefing to ensure each item on the checklist has been addressed:

- Patient identity
- Site, side, and level of surgery
- Procedure being performed
- Antibiotic prophylaxis: was initial dose given, and is repeat dose necessary?
- Final surgical positioning of patient
- Any questions or concerns from surgical team members before proceeding

Once the patient is anaesthetized, positioned, prepped, and draped, the team members take a "time-out" to reconfirm patient, procedure, site or side, antibiotic dose, and positioning. The operation can then be conducted.

Before the surgeon leaves the OR, the team has a postoperative debriefing that reviews intraoperative patient care and identifies any concerns for patient recovery. These data become part of the hand-off information to the PACU or CCU nursing staff in the transfer of accountability (ORNAC, 2019).

ASSISTING THE ANAESTHESIOLOGIST

It is the perioperative circulating nurse who assists the anaesthesiologist in many ORs. The nurse is familiar with anaesthetic modalities and effects of anaesthetic drugs and can respond to complications and emergency situations with appropriate medication and equipment (ORNAC, 2019).

Before anaesthetic induction, the circulating nurse may help establish the following monitoring:

- Temperature, pulse, and respiration
- Blood pressure
- Electrocardiogram
- Oxygen saturation
- Arterial, central venous pressure, and pulmonary artery lines
- Input and output (urine, blood loss)

During induction of general anaesthesia through an IV, the nurse remains at the patient's side to ensure safety and to assist the anaesthesiologist by ensuring all necessary equipment is available and functional (e.g., suction is on, laryngoscope is fully lighted, monitoring is initiated) (Figure 21.7). After the patient loses consciousness, the anaesthesiologist can insert a **laryngeal mask airway (LMA)**—a supraglottic airway device that is easily placed and used as a method of elective ventilation—or administer a neuromuscular blocking medication intravenously, causing skeletal muscle relaxation and enabling the anaesthesiologist to perform a direct laryngoscopy and tracheal intubation. The circulating nurse will be expected to assist

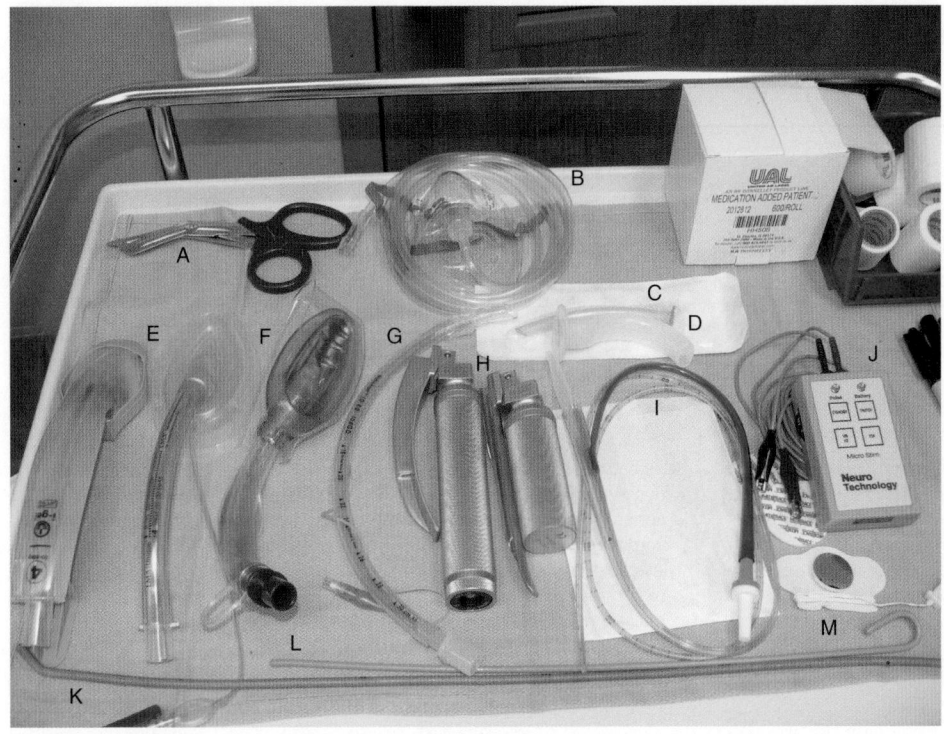

FIG. 21.7 Commonly used anaesthesia equipment: **A,** scissors; **B,** supplemental oxygen mask; **C,** nasal trumpet airway; **D,** Guedel oral airway; **E,** supraglottic airway I-gel laryngeal mask airway (LMA); **F,** Cook intubating LMA; **G,** endotracheal tube (ETT); **H,** long- and short-handled laryngoscopes with curved Macintosh and straight Miller blades; **I,** nasogastric/orogastric tube; **J,** peripheral nerve stimulator; **K,** elastic Bougie ETT introducer; **L,** ETT malleable stylet; **M,** skin temperature probe. Source: Rothrock, J. C. (2019). *Alexander's care of the patient in surgery* (16th ed.), Figure 5.2.

intubation by remaining at the bedside and applying cricoid pressure, supporting head positioning, and administering oxygen (ORNAC, 2019).

When the patient is receiving regional anaesthesia (e.g., spinal, epidural, nerve block), the circulating nurse assists the anaesthesiologist by placing appropriate monitors on the patient and assisting and supporting patient positioning for the insertion (ORNAC, 2019).

CLASSIFICATION OF ANAESTHESIA

The anaesthesiologist selects the anaesthetic technique and drugs in collaboration with the patient and interprofessional team. Considerations for choice of anaesthesia include the patient's physical and mental status, age, and allergy and pain and family history; the length of the surgery; the operative procedure; and discharge plans.

Anaesthesia is classified according to the effect that it has on the patient's central nervous system and pain perception. General anaesthesia is an altered physiological state characterized by reversible loss of consciousness, skeletal muscle relaxation, amnesia, and analgesia. Local anaesthesia is the loss of sensation without loss of consciousness and can be induced topically or via intracutaneous or subcutaneous infiltration. Regional anaesthesia causes a reversible loss of sensation to a region of the body by blocking nerve fibres with the administration of a local anaesthetic. Examples include spinal, epidural, or peripheral nerve blocks. An advantage of this technique is that the patient remains conscious throughout the procedure.

Moderate sedation, or procedural sedation (formerly *conscious sedation*), is a mild depression of consciousness that results from administration of IV sedatives, analgesics, or both so patients can tolerate minor procedures yet still maintain airway control and minimize cardiopulmonary complications

(Dobson et al., 2018). Examples of drugs commonly used for this purpose include ketamine, propofol, and midazolam.

General Anaesthesia

General anaesthesia is the technique of choice for lengthy surgical procedures that require skeletal muscle relaxation and for surgery that requires the patient to be in uncomfortable positions for the duration. General anaesthesia is appropriate for anxious patients and for those who refuse or have contraindications for local or regional anaesthetics.

General anaesthesia can be produced by many different drugs but is primarily administered intravenously or by inhalation. Balanced anaesthetic technique refers to the use of nitrous oxide, neuromuscular blocking medications, and opioids during the maintenance phase of general anaesthesia. Table 21.4 presents common anaesthetic agents along with their advantages and disadvantages and the nursing interventions indicated for patients receiving them.

Intravenous Induction Agents. Routine induction of general anaesthesia in adults usually includes IV drug administration, such as midazolam or propofol (Diprivan). These drugs induce a pleasant sleep, with a rapid onset of action that patients find desirable. A single dose lasts only a few minutes, which is long enough for an endotracheal (ET) tube to be placed and an inhalation drug to be started.

In today's clinical anaesthesia, one or two inhalation drugs, in conjunction with a variety of IV medications, are given to produce an anaesthetic state. Inhalation drugs come as a liquid, are vaporized in an anaesthetic machine, and are then delivered to the brain and body tissues via the lungs (Nagelhout, 2019). These drugs are noted for ease of administration and the ability to monitor their alveolar concentration and thus the level of anaesthesia. When the inhalation gas is discontinued at the end of surgery, the drug leaves the tissues via the bloodstream and is

TABLE 21.4   MEDICATION THERAPY

General Anaesthesia

Medication	Advantage	Disadvantage	Nursing Implications
Preoperative Agents			
Lorazepam (Ativan)	Excellent for patients with anxiety	Must be administered with caution to patients with hepatic or renal disease and to pediatric or older patients	Ensure patients have signed consent before administering any premedication.
			Ensure side rails on stretcher or bed are up.
Midazolam	Short acting; excellent for inducing retrograde amnesia	Has a slower induction than thiopental	Used for premedication and as anaesthetic induction and maintenance agent; no pain on injection; often used in conjunction with regional anaesthetic
Induction Agents			
Propofol (Diprivan)	Ideal for short outpatient procedures because of rapid onset of action and elimination; may be used for induction and maintenance of anaesthesia	May cause bradycardia and other dysrhythmias, hypotension, apnea, phlebitis, nausea and vomiting, hiccups	Short action leads to minimal postoperative effects; monitor injection site for phlebitis; ensure cardiac monitoring if patient condition is unstable.
Ketamine (Ketalar)	Can be administered by IV or IM route; potent analgesic and amnestic	May cause hallucinations and nightmares, increased intracranial and intraocular pressure, increased heart rate, hypertension	—
Inhalation Gases			
Volatile Liquids			
Isoflurane (Forane)	All volatile liquids: muscle relaxation, low incidence of nausea and vomiting	All volatile liquids: myocardial depression, early onset of postoperative pain because of rapid elimination	Assess and treat pain during early anaesthesia recovery; assess for adverse effects such as cardiopulmonary depression with hypotension and prolonged respiratory depression, confusion, and nausea and vomiting.
Desflurane (Suprane)	*Isoflurane:* less cardiac depression, devoid of toxicity to body organs		
Sevoflurane	*Desflurane:* rapid induction and emergence, most widely used volatile agent		
	Sevoflurane: predictable effects on cardiovascular and respiratory systems, smooth, rapid induction, nonirritating to respiratory system		
Gaseous Agents			
Nitrous oxide (N_2O)	Potentiates volatile agents, allowing a reduction in both their dosage and their adverse effects, and accelerates induction	Weak anaesthetic, rarely used alone; must be administered with oxygen to prevent hypoxemia	Produces little or no toxicity; monitor for effects of volatile liquids when N_2O used as an adjunct.
Induction: Depolarizing Muscle Relaxants			
Succinylcholine (Quelicin)	Used with intubation or short cases; rapid onset	Can trigger MH crisis	Requires refrigeration; may cause fasciculation
Induction: Nondepolarizing Muscle Relaxants			
Intermediate Onset and Duration			
Atracurium	Used with intubation; maintains relaxation	May have slight histamine release	Requires refrigeration
Rocuronium (Zemuron)	Rapid onset; maintains relaxation	Can increase heart rate (vagolytic)	Eliminated via the kidneys and the liver
Longer Onset and Duration			
Pancuronium	Onset 1–3 min; maintains relaxation	May increase heart rate and blood pressure	Eliminated via the kidneys
Reversal: Cholinergic Agent			
Neostigmine bromide (Prostigmin)	Reverses nondepolarizing neuro-muscular blocker in 3–15 min	Cardiac arrhythmias	Given with atropine sulphate or glycopyrrolate; prevents breakdown of acetylcholine
Anticholinergics			
Atropine sulphate (Atropine)	Blocks effect of acetylcholine; can decrease vagal tone; increases heart rate, suppresses salivary, gastric, and bronchial secretions	May cause dry mouth, CNS symptoms (dizziness)	Used to treat bradycardia
Glycopyrrolate	Blocks effect of acetylcholine; can decrease vagal tone; increases heart rate; suppresses salivary, gastric, and bronchial secretions	Can have prolonged duration of effects	Does not cross blood–brain barrier; has lower incidence of dysrhythmias than atropine sulphate

CNS, central nervous system; *IM,* intramuscular; *IV,* intravenous; *MH,* malignant hyperthermia.

TABLE 21.5 MEDICATION THERAPY
IV Medications Used in General Anaesthesia

Medications	Uses During Anaesthesia	Adverse Effects	Nursing Interventions
Opioids Fentanyl Morphine sulphate Sufentanil Alfentanil	Induce and maintain anaesthesia, reduce stimuli from sensory nerve endings, provide analgesia during surgery	Respiratory depression, stimulation of vomiting centre, possible bradycardia and peripheral vasodilation (when combined with anaesthetics), high incidence of pruritus with both regional and IV administration	Assess respiratory status, monitor pulse oximetry findings, protect airway in anticipation of vomiting, use standing orders for antipruritics such as diphenhydramine (Benadryl) and low-dose naloxone.
Benzodiazepines Midazolam Diazepam (Valium) Lorazepam (Ativan)	Induce and maintain anaesthesia	Potentiation of the effects of opioids, increasing the potential for respiratory depression; hypotension and tachycardia	Monitor cardiopulmonary status, level of consciousness.
Antiemetics Ondansetron (Zofran) Metoclopramide Dimenhydrinate (Gravol) Promethazine (Histantil) Droperidol	Prevention of vomiting with aspiration during surgery, counteract the emetic effects of inhalation agents and opioids; droperidol often used during surgery; others more often used after surgery	*Droperidol:* dysrhythmias, laryngospasm, bronchospasm, tachycardia, hypotension, CNS alterations, extrapyramidal reactions; contraindicated for use in patients with Parkinson's disease or hypomagnesemia *Other antiemetics:* headache, dizziness, sedation, malaise, fatigue, musculoskeletal pain, shivers, diarrhea, acute dystonic reactions, cardiovascular alterations; contraindicated for use with patients with hypomagnesemia	Monitor cardiopulmonary status, level of consciousness, and ability to move limbs. *Droperidol:* Administer with caution in patients with heart disease.

CNS, central nervous system; *IV,* intravenous.

excreted through the lungs with ventilation, allowing for rapid reversal of anaesthesia. It is routine practice to administer 100% oxygen (O_2) during emergence to assist with recovery (Nagelhout, 2019). Inhalation drugs are most commonly administered through a mask, an LMA, or an ET tube once the patient has been induced with an IV agent. The ET tube permits control of ventilation and airway protection, both to ensure patency and to prevent aspiration. Complications of ET intubation are associated with insertion and removal and include damage to teeth and lips, laryngospasm, laryngeal edema, postoperative sore throat, and hoarseness caused by injury to or irritation of the vocal cords or surrounding tissues.

IV Medications and General Anaesthesia. The administration of general anaesthesia is rarely limited to one agent. For instance, IV opioids, benzodiazepines, and neuromuscular blocking medications (muscle relaxants) result in analgesia, amnesia, and muscle relaxation. Maintenance of general anaesthesia can be achieved with total intravenous anaesthesia (TIVA) (Nimmo et al., 2019). On occasion, reversal agents may be required to speed up the reversal of muscle relaxants and opioids at the end of surgery. See Table 21.4 for nondepolarizing muscle relaxants.

Antiemetic medications may be given preoperatively, intraoperatively, and postoperatively to prevent the nausea and vomiting that can result from anaesthesia. (See Table 21.5 for IV medications used in general anaesthesia.)

Opioids. Opioids are used before surgery for sedation and analgesia, intraoperatively for induction and maintenance of anaesthesia, and after surgery for pain management. Opioids alter the perception and response to painful stimuli. When administered before the end of surgery, the residual analgesia often carries over into the PACU, allowing the patient to awaken relatively pain free.

All opioids produce dose-related respiratory depression. It can be difficult to detect respiratory depression in the OR because of altered level of consciousness; therefore, close observation of

respiratory status and oximetry monitoring are required. Respiratory depression from opioids can be reversed with naloxone.

Benzodiazepines. Benzodiazepines are commonly used before surgery for their sedative and amnestic effects, and less commonly used as induction and maintenance agents. They are used for procedural sedation, as supplemental IV sedation during local and regional anaesthesia, and for postoperative anxiety and agitation. Midazolam is an excellent amnestic medication, has a short duration of action, and causes no pain on injection, so it is frequently used intramuscularly or intravenously for ambulatory surgery and procedural sedation. Flumazenil is a benzodiazepine antagonist that may be used to reverse marked benzodiazepine-induced respiratory depression.

Neuromuscular Blocking Medications. Neuromuscular blocking medications (muscle relaxants) are used during general anaesthesia to facilitate airway control and to optimize surgical working conditions by providing relaxation (paralysis) of skeletal muscles. These medications interrupt the transmission of nerve impulses at the neuromuscular junction. The effects of muscle relaxants are frequently reversed toward the end of the surgery by the administration of anticholinesterase medications (e.g., neostigmine [Prostigmin], pyridostigmine [Mestinon]).

A disadvantage of muscle relaxants of special concern to the anaesthesiologist and postanaesthesia nurse is that their duration of action may outlast the surgical procedure, and reversal agents may not be effective in completely eliminating the residual effects. Patients receiving these medications must be carefully observed for airway patency and adequacy of respiratory muscle movement. Lack of movement or poor return of reflexes and strength may indicate the need for an artificial airway and ventilator. If the patient is intubated, the ET tube should not be removed without careful assessment of return of muscular strength, level of consciousness, and the minute volume (respiratory rate times tidal volume [amount of air inhaled and exhaled during a normal ventilation]).

TABLE 21.6	METHODS FOR ADMINISTERING LOCAL ANAESTHESIA

- Topical application
- Local infiltration
- Regional injection
- Peripheral nerve block
- Intravenous regional block (Bier block)
- Spinal anaesthesia (block)
- Epidural anaesthesia (block)

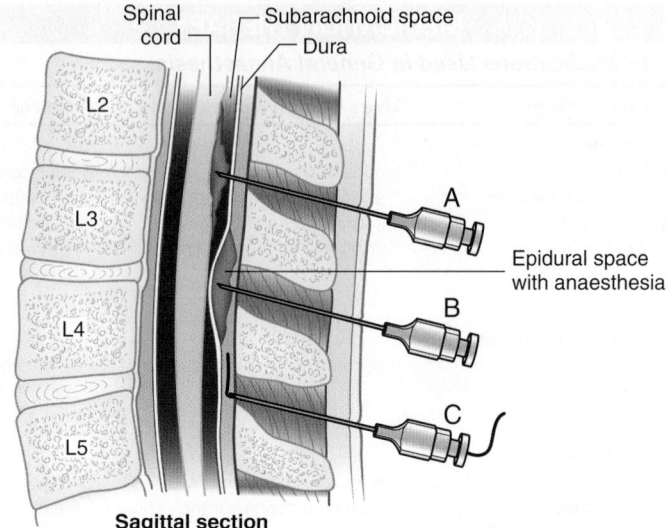

FIG. 21.8 Location of needle point and injected anaesthetic relative to dura. **A,** Epidural catheter. **B,** Single-injection epidural. **C,** Spinal anaesthesia. (Interspaces most commonly used are L4–L5, L3–L4, and L2–L3.)

Antiemetics. Antiemetics, as previously described, are used before, during, and after surgery to prevent and treat nausea and vomiting associated with the administration of anaesthesia. The antiemetics listed in Table 21.5 are most frequently used before and after surgery.

Local Anaesthesia

Local anaesthetics block the initiation and transmission of electrical impulses along nerve fibres. With progressive increases in local anaesthetic concentration, the transmission of autonomic, then somatic sensory, and finally somatic motor impulses is blocked. This produces autonomic nervous system blockade, anaesthesia, and skeletal muscle paralysis in the area of the affected nerve.

Local anaesthesia allows an operative procedure to be performed on a particular part of the body without loss of consciousness or sedation. Because there is little systemic absorption of the drug, recovery is rapid, and the duration of action of the local anaesthetic frequently carries over into the postoperative period, providing continued analgesia. In addition, the use of a local anaesthetic in a regional technique provides an alternative to a general anaesthetic in a physiologically compromised patient.

The disadvantages of local anaesthetics include the technical challenges of performing the block, discomfort that may be associated with injections, inadvertent IV administration producing hypotension and potential seizures, and the inability to precisely match the duration of action of the drugs administered to the duration of the surgical procedure.

Methods of Administration. There are a variety of methods for administering local anaesthetics (Table 21.6). *Topical application* is application of the agent directly to the skin, mucous membranes, or open surface. A mixture of local anaesthetics (lidocaine and prilocaine) in a skin cream form can be applied to the skin to produce localized dermal anaesthesia (see Chapter 10). Anaesthetic cream should be applied to the site 30 to 60 minutes before painful procedures. *Local infiltration* is the injection of the agent into the tissues through which the surgical incision will pass.

Regional (peripheral) nerve block is achieved by the injection of a local anaesthetic into or around a specific nerve or group of nerves. Nerve blocks may be used to provide intraoperative anaesthesia and postoperative analgesia and for the diagnosis and treatment of chronic pain. Examples of common regional nerve blocks include brachial plexus, intercostal, and retrobulbar blocks. *IV regional nerve block* (e.g., Bier block) is the IV injection of a local anaesthetic into an extremity following mechanical exsanguination using a compression bandage and a tourniquet. This type of block provides not only analgesia but also the ability to work in a bloodless field.

Spinal and Epidural Anaesthesia (Neuraxial Blocks). Spinal and epidural anaesthesia are types of regional anaesthesia referred to as neuraxial blocks. Neuraxial anaesthesia blocks pain transmission during surgery and may be used in combination with other techniques (e.g., inhalation or IV anaesthesia) to balance anaesthetic options, thus maximizing benefits and reducing adverse effects of any particular anaesthetic modality (Pellegrini, 2019).

Spinal anaesthesia involves the injection of a local anaesthetic into the cerebrospinal fluid found in the subarachnoid space, usually below the level of L2. The local anaesthetic mixes with cerebrospinal fluid, and depending on the extent of its spread, various levels of anaesthesia are achieved. Because the local anaesthetic is administered directly into the cerebrospinal fluid, a spinal anaesthetic produces an autonomic, sensory, and motor blockade. Patients experience vasodilation and may become hypotensive as a result of the autonomic block, will feel no pain as a result of the sensory block, and will be unable to move as a result of the motor block. The duration of action of the spinal anaesthetic depends on the agent selected and the dose administered. A spinal anaesthetic may be used for intraabdominal surgery; procedures involving the lower extremities, pelvis, or groin (hernia); and back and spinal surgery.

An **epidural block** involves injection of a local anaesthetic into the epidural (extradural) space via either a thoracic or a lumbar approach. The anaesthetic agent does not enter the cerebrospinal fluid but works by binding to nerve roots as they enter and exit the spinal cord. This allows the anaesthesiologist to titrate the dosage of medication and better control the extent of sensory or motor block (Pellegrini, 2019). A low concentration of local anaesthetic ensures that sensory pathways are blocked but allows motor fibres to remain intact. In higher doses, both sensory and motor fibres are blocked (Figure 21.8). Epidural anaesthesia may be the sole anaesthetic for a surgical procedure, or a catheter may be placed to allow for intraoperative use and postoperative analgesia, using lower doses of epidural local anaesthetic, usually combined with an opioid. Epidural anaesthesia is commonly used during labour, as it has minimal impact on maternal and fetal physiology yet offers a comfortable birth while allowing for immediate maternal–infant bonding. Furthermore, it provides flexibility for surgical options if the patient must convert to Caesarean birth (Pellegrini, 2019). Epidurals are also used for lower extremity vascular procedures

TABLE 21.7	DIFFERENCES BETWEEN EPIDURAL AND SPINAL ANAESTHETICS		
Medications	**Injection Space**	**Potential Complications**	**Postoperative Monitoring**
Spinal Anaesthetic (Local)			
Bupivacaine (Marcaine) Lidocaine Tetracaine (Ametop)	Most commonly used interspaces: L4–L5, L3–L4, and L2–L3	Hypotension, total spinal anaesthesia, post–dural puncture headache	Vital signs Motor and sensory block Urinary output and bladder distension Headache assessment
Spinal Anaesthetic (Analgesia)			
Fentanyl Morphine sulphate (preservative-free)	Most commonly used interspaces: L4–L5, L3–L4, and L2–L3	Hypotension; pruritus; urinary retention; nausea, vomiting; infection; epidural hematoma; oversedation *Contraindications:* Septicemia, ↑ ICP, hypovolemia, neurological disease, anticoagulation therapy, spinal fracture	Vital signs Motor and sensory block Urinary output and bladder distension Headache assessment
Epidural Anaesthetic (Local)			
Ropivacaine (Naropin) Lidocaine Bupivacaine	Between the ligamentum flavum and the dura	Bupivacaine can be associated with cardiac toxicity if injected intravascularly	Respiratory assessment Vital signs Sedation score
Epidural Anaesthetic (Analgesia)			
Morphine sulphate (preservative-free) Fentanyl Sufentanil	The dura	Hypotension; pruritus; urinary retention; nausea, vomiting; infection; epidural hematoma; oversedation *Contraindications:* Septicemia, ↑ ICP, hypovolemia, neurological disease, anticoagulation therapy, spinal fracture	Urinary output and bladder distension Assessment for pruritus, nausea, or vomiting Pain assessment Assessment for catheter migration (numbness or tingling) Assessment of dressing and insertion site Headache assessment

ICP, intracranial pressure.

and hip and knee replacements. (Table 21.7 lists some differences between epidural and spinal anaesthetics.)

During the surgical procedure involving use of either spinal or epidural anaesthesia, the patient can remain fully conscious, or sedation can be achieved intravenously. The onset of spinal anaesthesia is faster than that of an epidural, but the results are similar. The patient must be closely observed for signs of autonomic nervous system blockade, including hypotension, bradycardia, nausea, and vomiting. As well, inadvertent high blocks or excessive drug dosages can lead to cardiac and respiratory depression (ORNAC, 2019).

One advantage of epidural (extradural) over spinal (subarachnoid) anaesthesia is a decreased incidence of post–spinal anaesthesia headache due to leakage of spinal fluid at the site of injection. The incidence of headache decreases with the use of smaller-gauge (25- to 27-gauge) and noncutting spinal needles.

Because there are varying perceptions of relative and absolute contraindications for administering neuraxial anaesthesia, it is preferable to formulate an anaesthetic plan specific to the patient's unique health status. The following situations and conditions must be considered when determining whether or not to use spinal or epidural anaesthesia or both (Pellegrini, 2019):

- Patient refusal or inability to cooperate
- Increased intracranial pressure
- Coagulopathies
- Skin infection at injection site
- Musculoskeletal deformities
- Hypovolemia and shock
- Diabetic neuropathies
- Cardiac fixed-volume states

Moderate Sedation

Moderate sedation is achieved through administration of sedatives, with or without analgesics. Historically, moderate sedation was referred to as *conscious sedation*, but that term is no longer in use. The term *moderate sedation* most closely reflects procedural sedation; however, some procedures may require deep sedation (Dobson et al., 2018). The Canadian Anesthesiologists' Society recommends use of the American Society of Anesthesiologists' Continuum of Depth of Sedation tool (Dobson et al., 2018). The levels of sedation include minimal, moderate, deep, and general anaesthesia and are outlined in Table 21.8.

Moderate sedation reduces the patient's anxiety and discomfort when undergoing a noninvasive or minimally invasive procedure (Dobson et al., 2018). Examples of interventions done under procedural sedation include (a) interventional radiology, (b) endoscopy, (c) wound debridement, (d) central line and chest tube placement, (e) dental surgery, and (f) more extensive surgery such as breast biopsy and some cosmetic and reconstructive procedures. Traditionally, this monitored anaesthetic care (MAC) has been provided by and supervised by anaesthesiologists. Practice is changing, however, with many of these surgical and diagnostic procedures being done outside the OR. Patients may be monitored by other health care team members, such as nurses or anaesthesia assistants, with an anaesthesiologist close by in case of a need to convert to a general anaesthetic or in case of complications.

Nurses receive education and training in minimal and moderate sedation, which is an advanced skill (ORNAC, 2019), before implementing the monitoring role. They should not perform circulating duties at the same time because complications can occur quickly.

Patient After Surgery

The anaesthesiologist anticipates the end of the surgical procedure and titrates doses of anaesthetic drugs so there will be minimal effects at the end of the surgical procedure, allowing the patient greater physiological control during the transfer to the PACU or designated recovery area.

TABLE 21.8	AMERICAN SOCIETY OF ANESTHESIOLOGISTS, CONTINUUM OF DEPTH SEDATION			
	Minimal Sedation/ Anxiolysis	**Moderate Sedation/ Analgesia**	**Deep Sedation/ Analgesia**	**General Anaesthesia**
Responsiveness	Normal response to verbal stimuli	Purposeful response to verbal or tactile stimuli	Purposeful response following repeated or painful stimuli	Unarousable even with repeated or painful stimuli
Airway	Unaffected	No intervention required	Intervention may be required	Intervention often required
Spontaneous ventilation	Unaffected	Adequate	May be adequate	Frequently inadequate
Cardiovascular function	Unaffected	Usually maintained	Usually maintained	May be impaired

Source: Dobson et al. (2018). Procedural sedation: A position paper of the Canadian Anesthesiologists' Society. *Canadian Journal of Anesthesiology, 65*, 1372–1384. https://doi.org/10.1007/s12630-018-1230-z

The anaesthesiologist and the perioperative nurse or another member of the surgical team accompany the patient to the PACU. A report of the patient's status and of the procedure is communicated to staff there. The OR nurse evaluates the patient's response to nursing care based on outcome criteria established when the plan of care was developed and transfers nursing care accountability to the health care providers in the PACU using a written and verbal report. The verbal report of nursing care provides continuity of care from one health care provider to another, decreases the risk for error, and provides an opportunity for family-centred care. For instance, the perioperative nurse may have information on where the family is waiting for news of the surgical outcome. Although traditionally, the surgeon, keeping confidentiality issues in mind, is responsible for providing postoperative information to family or significant others, some hospital policies allow a family member or significant other to visit in the PACU once the patient is stable. Hand-off communication with the PACU nurse should include the patient's situation, background, assessment, and recommendations (SBAR). Examples of information included are as follows (Murphy, 2019):

- Name and age of patient
- Preoperative diagnosis and comorbid medical conditions
- Allergies
- Time of next antibiotic dose, surgical medication administration (e.g., local anaesthesia)
- Operative procedure performed
- Intake/output, vital signs
- Drains (e.g., Foley catheter, nasogastric tube, intraoperative drainage), dressing/packing
- Intraoperative complications if any

AGE-RELATED CONSIDERATIONS

PATIENT DURING SURGERY

While anaesthetic drugs are safe and predictable, they must be administered to older persons judiciously. Currently, the majority of patients over 65 have one or more chronic conditions that may be a risk factor during surgery. In conjunction with physiological deficits due to aging, these may cause varying and unique responses to anaesthetics, blood and fluid management, hypothermia, pain, and the tolerance for the surgical procedure and positioning (Allen, 2019).

OR nurses must understand the geriatric assessment data required to formulate an intraoperative plan of care—for example, risk for impaired skin integrity (Allen, 2019):

Risk is related to the patient's current skin condition, such as less elasticity due to decreased collagen, decreased turgor due to dehydration, and decreased peripheral circulation and sensation.

Outcome is that skin integrity remains intact throughout surgery.

Interventions to accomplish this outcome may include assessing the likelihood for pressure injuries, avoiding friction and shearing when moving the patient, ensuring the patient's pressure points are adequately padded when positioned, minimizing tape used to secure devices, and preventing moisture on the linens.

Evaluation takes place immediately postoperatively, when the nurse assesses and documents the patient's skin condition.

EXCEPTIONAL CLINICAL EVENTS IN THE OPERATING ROOM

Unanticipated intraoperative events demand immediate interventions by the interprofessional perioperative team. Such events include anaphylactic reactions, malignant hyperthermia, hemorrhage due to trauma or disseminated intravascular coagulation, cardiac arrest, and intraoperative death (ORNAC, 2019).

Anaphylactic Reactions

Anaphylaxis is a severe form of allergic reaction, manifesting with life-threatening pulmonary and circulatory complications. Initial clinical manifestations of anaphylaxis may be masked by anaesthesia. Anaesthesiologists administer an array of medications to patients, such as anaesthetics, antibiotics, blood products, and plasma expanders, and because they are parenterally administered, they can stimulate an allergic response, so vigilance and rapid intervention are essential. An anaphylactic reaction causes hypotension, tachycardia, bronchospasm, and, possibly, pulmonary edema. Anaesthetics, antibiotics, and latex are responsible for many perioperative allergic reactions. (Anaphylaxis is discussed in Chapter 16.)

Latex allergy remains a concern in the perioperative setting, despite fewer surgical products being manufactured from natural rubber latex. Reactions to natural rubber latex range from urticaria to anaphylaxis, with symptoms appearing immediately or at some time during the surgical procedure.

Policies and procedures must ensure that the health care team can provide a latex-safe environment for patients and staff with potential or actual latex allergy (ORNAC, 2019). (Latex allergies are also discussed in Chapter 16.)

Malignant Hyperthermia

Malignant hyperthermia (MH) is a rare, potentially fatal metabolic disease characterized by hyperthermia with rigidity of skeletal muscles that can affect genetically susceptible patients. It is triggered by commonly administered anaesthetic drugs, particularly succinylcholine (Anectine), which is given during general anaesthesia. MH susceptibility has an inherited autosomal dominant pattern. (Autosomal dominant disorders are discussed in Chapter 15.) The MH defect is hypermetabolism of skeletal muscle resulting from altered control of intracellular calcium, leading to muscle contracture, hyperthermia, hypoxemia, lactic acidosis, and hemodynamic and cardiac alterations that can result in cardiac arrest and death. The first sign of MH is often severe masseter muscle rigidity (MMR) that occurs after the administration of succinylcholine and is noted by the anaesthesiologist when trying to establish an airway. MMR should be considered an indication of MH, and treatment should be initiated immediately. Other signs of MH include a rise in end-tidal carbon dioxide (CO_2), tachycardia, and elevated body temperature (Riazi et al., 2018)

The definitive treatment of MH is prompt administration of dantrolene (Dantrium, Ryanodex), which slows metabolism and provides symptomatic support to correct hemodynamic instability, acidosis, hypoxemia, and elevated temperature.

To prevent an MH episode, the nurse must obtain a careful family history and be alert to MH susceptibility preoperatively. The patient known or suspected to be at risk for MH can be anaesthetized with minimal risk if appropriate precautions are taken. Patients with MH susceptibility should inform family members so they are aware of the health care risks and can wear a medic alert bracelet or choose to be genetically tested by having a muscle biopsy (ORNAC, 2019).

Major Blood Loss

Surgery can pose a risk for blood loss and hemorrhage. While there are a variety of methods for measuring blood loss, it is vital that the surgical team monitor the patient's hemodynamic response to this change in fluid status (Higgins Roche & Schwartz, 2019). Early signs of intraoperative hemorrhage include decreased mixed venous oxygen saturation and increased heart rate (Higgins Roche & Schwartz, 2019). If major blood loss occurs during surgery, the circulating nurse assists the anaesthesiologist with fluid replacement. Initially, nonblood products such as crystalloids and colloid solutions are given to maintain fluid volume, but when hemorrhage is significant, blood or blood components may be administered (Higgins Roche & Schwartz, 2019). Laboratory values, such as hemoglobin and hematocrit, will be assessed to provide feedback on whether or not the patient is responding as expected (Muirhead & Weiss, 2017). Situations involving massive hemorrhage require a coordinated approach by all perioperative team members. Some institutions have massive transfusion protocols in place to ensure adequate communication between the anaesthetist, surgeon, and blood bank during incidences of severe blood loss (Muirhead & Weiss, 2017).

CASE STUDY

Intraoperative Patient

Patient Profile

G. S. (pronouns he/him), a 63-year-old retired accountant, was admitted to the hospital for severe pain from acute cholecystitis. His medical history includes hypertension and type 2 diabetes mellitus. His pain has been managed with hydromorphone (Dilaudid) using patient-controlled analgesia. Intractable nausea and vomiting required the placement of a nasogastric (NG) tube. G. S. is scheduled for a laparoscopic cholecystectomy. The surgery will be done under general anaesthesia.

Subjective Data

- G. S. is awake and able to identify himself, his birth date, procedure, and surgical site
- Rates pain as a 4 on a 0-to-10 scale on arrival to the holding area

Objective Data

- Admitted to the preoperative holding area with an NG tube in place and one peripheral IV catheter
- Capillary blood glucose 1 hour ago was 6.9 mmol/L
- Oxygen saturation 96% on room air

Interprofessional Care

- Vital signs per holding area routine

- 0.9 normal saline solution at 100 mL/hr
- Titrate O_2 therapy to keep O_2 saturation >90%
- NG tube connected to low, intermittent suction

Discussion Questions

1. What are the potential intraoperative problems that the nurse may expect with G. S.?
2. *Priority Decision:* What priority nursing interventions would be appropriate to prevent these complications from occurring?
3. *Collaboration:* What are the interprofessional team's priorities for G. S.?
4. *Evidence-Informed Practice:* G. S. tells the nurse that he is cold despite having a blanket in place. Why is it important that G. S. stay warm?
5. *Safety:* What are two areas of risk for injury to G. S.? What actions can be taken to ensure patient safety?

⊖volve

Answers are available at http://evolve.elsevier.com/Canada/Lewis/medsurg.

REVIEW QUESTIONS

The number of the question corresponds to the same-numbered objective at the beginning of the chapter.

1. What is the perioperative nurse's primary responsibility for the care of the client undergoing surgery?
   a. Developing an individualized plan of nursing care for the client
   b. Carrying out specific tasks related to surgical policies and procedures
   c. Ensuring that the client has been assessed for safe administration of anaesthesia
   d. Performing a preoperative history and physical assessment to identify client needs

2. What is the proper attire for the semi-restricted area of the surgery department?
   a. Street clothing
   b. Surgical attire and head cover
   c. Surgical attire, head cover, and mask
   d. Street clothing with the addition of shoe covers

3. What is one characteristic of the OR environment that facilitates the prevention of infection in the surgical client?
   a. Adjustable lighting
   b. Conductive furniture
   c. Filters in the ventilating system
   d. Explosion-proof electrical plugs

4. Which of the following activities might a nurse perform in the role of a scrub nurse during surgery? (*Select all that apply.*)
   a. Checking electrical equipment
   b. Preparing the instrument table
   c. Passing instruments to the surgeon and assistants
   d. Coordinating activities occurring in the operating room
   e. Maintaining accurate counts of sponges, needles, and instruments

5. What is the priority intervention when a client arrives to the OR with musculoskeletal impairments?
   a. Ensure proper preparation of the skin.
   b. Ensure the anaesthesiologist uses muscle relaxants.
   c. Ensure positioning on the OR bed to prevent injury.
   d. Provide detailed explanations about the surgical activities.

6. The practical nurse in the OR knows that which of the following is not acceptable for ensuring a sterile field?
   a. Unsterile personnel remaining at least 30 cm from the sterile field
   b. Reaching over the sterile field to place sterile items on the sterile back table
   c. Covering unsterile items such as laparoscopic cameras with sterile barriers before placing them on the sterile field
   d. Flipping a sterile item from a paper peel pack onto the sterile field

7. Which of the following is not a consideration when positioning the surgical client?
   a. Providing modesty for the client
   b. Avoiding compression of nerve tissue
   c. Providing correct skeletal alignment
   d. Ensuring that students in the room can see the operative site

8. A client is scheduled for an abdominal hysterectomy. She is extremely anxious and has a tendency to hyperventilate when upset. What is the most appropriate type of anaesthetic for this client?
   a. A spinal block
   b. An epidural block
   c. A general anaesthetic
   d. A local anaesthetic

9. Why is IV induction for general anaesthesia the method of choice for most clients?
   a. The client is not intubated.
   b. The drugs are nonexplosive.
   c. Induction is rapid and pleasant.
   d. The odour of the drug is not offensive.

10. What is the name for the injection of the local anaesthetic into the tissues through the surgical incision?
    a. Nerve block
    b. Local infiltration
    c. Topical application
    d. Regional application

1. a; 2. b; 3. c; 4. b, c, e; 5. c; 6. d; 7. d; 8. c; 9. c; 10. b.

*e*volve

For even more review questions, visit http://evolve.elsevier.com/Canada/Lewis/medsurg.

REFERENCES

Allen, S. (2019). Geriatric surgery. In J. C. Rothrock, & D. R. McEwen (Eds.), *Alexander's care of the patient in surgery* (16th ed., pp. 1069–1090). Elsevier.

Ball, K. (2019). Surgical modalities. In J. C. Rothrock, & D. R. McEwen (Eds.), *Alexander's care of the patient in surgery* (16th ed., pp. 201–242). Elsevier.

Brown, B., Khemani, E., Lin, C., et al. (2019). Improving patient flow in a regional anaesthesia block room. *BMJ Open Quality, 8*, e000346. https://doi.org/10.1136/bmjoq-2018-000346

Canadian Institute for Health Information & Canadian Patient Safety Institute. (2016). *Measuring patient harm in Canadian hospitals.* Author.

Canadian Nurses Association. (2021). *Certification nursing practice specialties.* https://www.cna-aiic.ca/en/certification/get-certified/certification-nursing-practice-specialties

Canadian Patient Safety Institute (CPSI). (2020). *Surgical safety checklist.* https://www.patientsafetyinstitute.ca/en/toolsResources/Pages/SurgicalSafety-Checklist-Resources.aspx

Cunning, R. (2019). Concepts basic to perioperative nursing. In J. C. Rothrock, & D. R. McEwen (Eds.), *Alexander's care of the patient in surgery* (16th ed., pp. 1–13). Elsevier.

Dobson, G., Chong, M., Chow, L., et al. (2018). Procedural sedation: a position paper of the Canadian Anesthesiologists' Society. *Canadian Journal of Anesthesia, 65*, 1372–1384. https://doi.org/10.1007/s12630-018-1230-z

Dobson, G., Chow, L., Flexman, A., et al. (2019). Guidelines to the practice of anesthesia – Revised edition 2019. *Canadian Journal of Anesthesia, 66*(1), 75–108. https://doi.org/10.1007/s12630-018-1248-2

Fawcett, D. (2019). Positioning the patient for surgery. In J. C. Rothrock, & D. R. McEwen (Eds.), *Alexander's care of the patient in surgery* (16th ed., pp. 157–175). Elsevier.

Higgins Roche, B., & Schwartz, P. (2019). Blood and blood component therapy. In J. Nagelhout, & S. Elisha (Eds.), *Nurse Anesthesia* (6th ed., pp. 369–379). Elsevier.

King, C., & Spry, C. (2019). Infection prevention and control. In J. C. Rothrock, & D. R. McEwen (Eds.), *Alexander's care of the patient in surgery* (16th ed., pp. 54–105). Elsevier.

Larner, R. (2019). Integrative health practices. In J. C. Rothrock, & D. R. McEwen (Eds.), *Alexander's care of the patient in surgery* (16th ed., pp. 1147–1162). Elsevier.

Muirhead, B., & Weiss, A. (2017). Massive hemorrhage and transfusion in the operating room. *Canadian Journal of Anesthesiology, 64*, 962–978. https://doi.org/10.1007/s12630-017-0925-x

Murphy, E. (2019). Patient safety and risk management. In J. C. Rothrock, & D. R. McEwen (Eds.), *Alexander's care of the patient in surgery* (16th ed., pp. 15–34). Elsevier.

Nagelhout, J. (2019). Pharmacokinetics of inhalation anesthetics. In J. Nagelhout, & S. Elisha (Eds.), *Nurse anesthesia* (6th ed., pp. 73–79). Elsevier.

Nimmo, A., Absalom, A., Bagshaw, O., et al. (2019). Guidelines for the safe practice of total intravenous anaesthesia (TIVA): Joint guidelines from the Association of Anaesthetists and the Society for Intravenous Anaesthesia. *Anaesthesia, 74*, 211–224. https://doi.org/10.1111/anae.14428

Operating Room Nurses Association of Canada (ORNAC). (2019). *The ORNAC standards, guidelines, and position statements for perioperative registered nurses* (14th ed.). Kingston, ON: Author.

Operating Room Nurses Association of Canada (ORNAC). (2020). *Covid-19, recommendations and links.* https://ornac.ca/en/education/links

Pellegrini, J. (2019). Regional anesthesia. In J. Nagelhout, & S. Elisha (Eds.), *Nurse anesthesia* (6th ed., pp. 1015–1041). Elsevier.

Riazi, S., Kraeva, N., & Hopkins, P. (2018). Updated guide for the management of malignant hyperthermia. *Canadian Journal of Anesthesia, 65*, 709–721. https://doi.org/10.1007/s12630-018-1108-0

University Health Network. (2021). *About nurse practitioners—anesthesia (NP-A).* https://www.uhn.ca/healthcareprofessionals/Meet_Professions/Nurse_Practitioners_Anesthesia

Urbach, D., Dimick, J., Haynes, A., et al. (2019). Is WHO's surgical safety checklist being hyped? *BMJ 2019*, 366. https://doi.org/10.1136/bmj.l4700

Vancouver Coastal Health. (2015). *Aboriginal cultural practices. A guide for physicians and allied health professionals.* http://www.vch.ca/Documents/AH-cultural-practices.pdf

RESOURCES

Association of Nova Scotia PeriAnesthesia Nurses
https://anspan.weebly.com

Canadian Anesthesiologists' Society
https://www.cas.ca

Canadian Nurses Protective Society: *InfoLAW: Operating Room Nursing*
https://cnps.ca/article/operating-room-nursing/

Canadian Patient Safety Institute's Surgical Safety Checklist
http://www.patientsafetyinstitute.ca/en/toolsResources/Pages/SurgicalSafety-Checklist-Resources.aspx

National Association of PeriAnesthesia Nurses of Canada
http://www.napanc.org

Ontario PeriAnesthesia Nurses Association
https://www.opana.org

Operating Room Nurses Association of Canada
http://www.ornac.ca

Ottawa Hospital Malignant Hyperthermia Unit
https://www.ottawahospital.on.ca/wps/portal/Base/TheHospital/ClinicalServices/DeptPgrmCS/Departments/Anesthesiology/MalignantHyperthermiaUnit

PeriAnesthesia Nurses Professional Practice Group of Saskatchewan
http://www.srna.org

PeriAnesthesia Nursing Association of British Columbia
https://panbc.ca

Quebec PeriAnesthesia Nurses Association
https://qpana.org/en-ca/

Malignant Hyperthermia Association of the United States
https://www.mhaus.org

evolve

For additional Internet resources, see the website for this book at http://evolve.elsevier.com/Canada/Lewis/medsurg.

Nursing Management
Postoperative Care

Peggy Hancock
Originating US chapter by Diane M. Rudolphi

evolve WEBSITE

http://evolve.elsevier.com/Canada/Lewis/medsurg

- Review Questions (Online Only)
- Key Points
- Answer Guidelines for Case Study
- Student Case Study
  - Patient Undergoing Surgery

- Customizable Nursing Care Plan
  - Postoperative Patient
- Conceptual Care Map Creator

- Audio Glossary
- Content Updates

LEARNING OBJECTIVES

1. Identify the components of an initial postanaesthesia assessment.
2. Describe the nursing responsibilities in admitting patients to the postanaesthesia care unit (PACU).
3. Explain the etiology and nursing assessment and management of potential complications in patients in the PACU.
4. Describe the initial nursing assessment and management after transfer from the PACU to the general care unit.
5. Explain the etiology and nursing assessment and management of potential complications during the postoperative period.
6. Differentiate discharge criteria from phase I and phase II postanaesthesia care.

KEY TERMS

atelectasis	epidural analgesia	syncope
delayed awakening	hypothermia	
emergence delirium	paralytic ileus	

The postoperative period begins immediately after surgery and continues until the patient is discharged from medical care or until the patient experiences complete recovery. This chapter focuses on the postoperative nursing care required for patients undergoing surgery. After surgery, the primary focus is on protecting the patient, who has been put in physiological risk during surgery, and preventing complications while the body heals. The issues and nursing care related to specific surgical procedures are discussed in the appropriate chapters of this text.

POSTOPERATIVE CARE IN THE POSTANAESTHESIA CARE UNIT

The patient's immediate recovery period occurs in a *postanaesthesia care unit* (PACU), which is sometimes referred to as the *postanaesthetic recovery room* (PARR). It is located adjacent to the operating room (OR) to minimize the transport distance of the patient after surgery and to provide ready access to surgical and anaesthesia personnel.

Admission of the patient to the PACU is a transfer of care from the anaesthesiologist and perioperative nurse to the PACU or perianaesthesia nurse. Interprofessional team members determine what phase of care the patient is assigned. There are three levels of postanaesthesia care, depending on the patient's surgical procedure, anaesthesia, and individualized needs (Table 22.1).

An inpatient or outpatient who is stable and recovering well is admitted to phase I care but may rapidly be discharged to either phase II care or an inpatient unit. An accelerated system of care, *fast-tracking,* involves admitting ambulatory surgery patients who have received general, regional, or local anaesthesia directly to phase II care. The rate at which patients move

TABLE 22.1	PHASES OF POSTANAESTHESIA CARE

Phase I
- Care during the immediate postanaesthesia period
- Focused on the patient's basic life-sustaining needs
- Constant, vigilant monitoring

Goal: Prepare patient for safe transfer to phase II or inpatient unit

Phase II
- Surgery patient is ambulatory

Goal: Prepare patient for transfer to extended-care environment or home with discharge teaching

Extended Observation
- Ongoing care for patients who will be admitted to the unit and those who require observation or interventions

Goal: Prepare patient for self-care

Source: American Society of PeriAnesthesia Nurses. (2016). *Perianesthesia nursing core curriculum* (3rd ed.). Elsevier.

TABLE 22.2	INITIAL PACU ASSESSMENT

Airway
- Patency
- Oral or nasal airway
- Laryngeal mask airway
- Endotracheal tube with ventilator settings

Breathing
- Respiratory rate and quality
- Auscultated breath sounds
- Pulse oximetry
- Capnography or other technology-supported monitoring if indicated
- Supplemental O_2

Circulation
- ECG monitoring: rate and rhythm
- BP: noninvasive or arterial line
- Hemodynamic pressure readings (if applicable)
- Temperature
- Capillary refill
- Color, temperature, moisture of skin
- Apical and peripheral pulses

Neurological
- Level of consciousness
- Orientation
- Sensory and motor status
- Pupil size and reaction

Surgical Site
- Dressings and visible incisions
- Drains: type, patency, and drainage
- IV assessment: location and condition of sites, solutions infusing

Genitourinary
- Urine output

Gastrointestinal
- Nausea, vomiting
- Intake (fluids, irrigations)
- Output (vomitus)
- Bowel sounds

Pain
- Incision or other

Patient Safety Needs
- Patient position
- Fall risk assessment

BP, blood pressure; *ECG,* electrocardiogram; *IV,* intravenous.

TABLE 22.3	CLINICAL MANIFESTATIONS OF INADEQUATE OXYGENATION

Central Nervous System
- Restlessness
- Agitation
- Muscle twitching
- Seizures
- Coma

Cardiovascular System
- Hypertension
- Hypotension
- Tachycardia
- Bradycardia
- Dysrhythmias

Integumentary System
- Cyanosis
- Prolonged capillary refill
- Flushed and moist skin

Respiratory System
- Alterations ranging from increased to absent respiratory effort
- Use of accessory muscles
- Abnormal breath sounds
- Abnormal arterial blood gases

Renal System
- Urine output 30 mL/hour

Initial Assessment

On patient admission to the PACU, the anaesthesiologist and perioperative nurse give a verbal report to the admitting perianaesthesia nurse including general patient information, current vital signs data, intraoperative management, and any unexpected surgical events. While the patient is in the PACU, priority care includes the monitoring and management of respiratory and circulatory functions, pain, temperature, and surgical site and the assessment of the patient's response to the reversal of anaesthetic, such as sedation score and level of spinal block.

Assessment should begin with an evaluation of the patient's airway, breathing, and circulation (ABC) (Table 22.2). The first priority is to establish a patent airway. In order to breathe adequately, the patient may need stimulation, repositioning to the right side, or a chin tilt. If these measures do not work, an oral or nasal airway may be used. Pulse oximetry monitoring is initiated on admission because it provides a noninvasive means of assessing the adequacy of oxygenation and alerts nurses to any respiratory compromise. Residual neuromuscular blockade, opioid use, and patient characteristics such as sleep-disordered breathing (e.g., obstructive sleep apnea [OSA], abnormal airway anatomy) affect oxygenation and ventilation. Nurses must be alert for signs of inadequate oxygenation and ventilation (Table 22.3). Any sign of respiratory distress needs prompt intervention. Oxygen therapy is used if the patient had general anaesthesia or if ordered by the anaesthesiologist. Oxygen therapy, given via nasal cannula or face mask, aids in eliminating anaesthetic gases and meets the increased oxygen demand due to decreased blood volume or increased cellular metabolism. Oxygen saturation should be regularly assessed. If the patient requires postoperative ventilation, a ventilator is provided. During the initial assessment, signs of inadequate oxygenation and ventilation should be identified (see Table 22.3).

Electrocardiographic (ECG) monitoring may be initiated to determine cardiac rate and rhythm. Deviations from preoperative findings must be noted and evaluated. Blood pressure (BP) should be measured and compared with baseline readings. Invasive monitoring (e.g., arterial BP monitoring) initiated in the OR will be monitored in the PACU. Body temperature, skin colour and condition, and capillary refill should also be assessed. Any evidence of inadequate circulatory status requires prompt intervention. Hearing aids and glasses should be returned as soon as appropriate to aid with communication and accurate assessment.

through the phases of care in the PACU depends on their condition. Patients' safety is the primary consideration when determining what level of postoperative care is provided.

The *initial neurological assessment* focuses on level of consciousness; orientation; sensory and motor status; and size, equality, and reactivity of the pupils. Hearing is the first sense to return in the unconscious patient, so the nurse should explain all activities to the patient from the moment of PACU admission, including that the surgery is completed, that the patient is in the recovery room, and that the family or significant other has been notified.

A patient who has had a regional anaesthetic (e.g., spinal or epidural) should be assessed for residual sensory and motor blockade by testing for sensation and movement.

Urinary system assessment focuses on intake, output, and fluid balance. Intraoperative fluid totals are communicated during the anaesthesia report. The PACU nurse should note the presence of all intravenous (IV) lines, irrigation solutions and infusions, and output devices such as catheters. IV infusions are regulated according to postoperative orders. If the patient is nauseated or vomiting, the nurse should administer antiemetic medications as ordered. The colour and amount of emesis should be charted.

The surgical site is assessed by noting the condition of dressings, and the colour and amount of drainage from the incision site or wound drains should be documented. All data obtained in the admission assessment are documented on a specific PACU record.

The goal of PACU care is to identify actual and potential patient complications that may occur as a result of anaesthetic administration and surgical intervention, so the perianaesthesia nurse is continually assessing, adjusting diagnoses, and intervening appropriately. Common postoperative conditions that require nursing interventions are airway compromise (obstruction), respiratory insufficiency (hypoxemia and hypercarbia), cardiac compromise (hypotension, hypertension, and dysrhythmias), neurological compromise (emergence delirium and delayed awakening), hypothermia, pain, and nausea and vomiting (Figure 22.1). Each of these conditions and appropriate nursing interventions are discussed in this chapter.

POTENTIAL ALTERATIONS IN RESPIRATORY FUNCTION

Etiology

Postanaesthesia Care Unit. In the immediate postanaesthetic period, the most common causes of airway compromise include airway obstruction, hypoxemia, and hypoventilation (Table 22.4). Airway obstruction is most commonly caused by the patient's tongue (Figure 22.2). The base of the tongue falls backward against the soft palate and occludes the pharynx. It is most pronounced in the supine position and in the patient who is extremely sleepy after surgery. Often basic airway manoeuvres will relieve the obstruction (e.g., head tilt/chin lift).

Patients at particular risk include those who had general anaesthesia, are older, have a smoking history or lung disease, are obese, or have undergone airway, thoracic, or abdominal surgery. However, respiratory complications may occur in any patient who was anaesthetized.

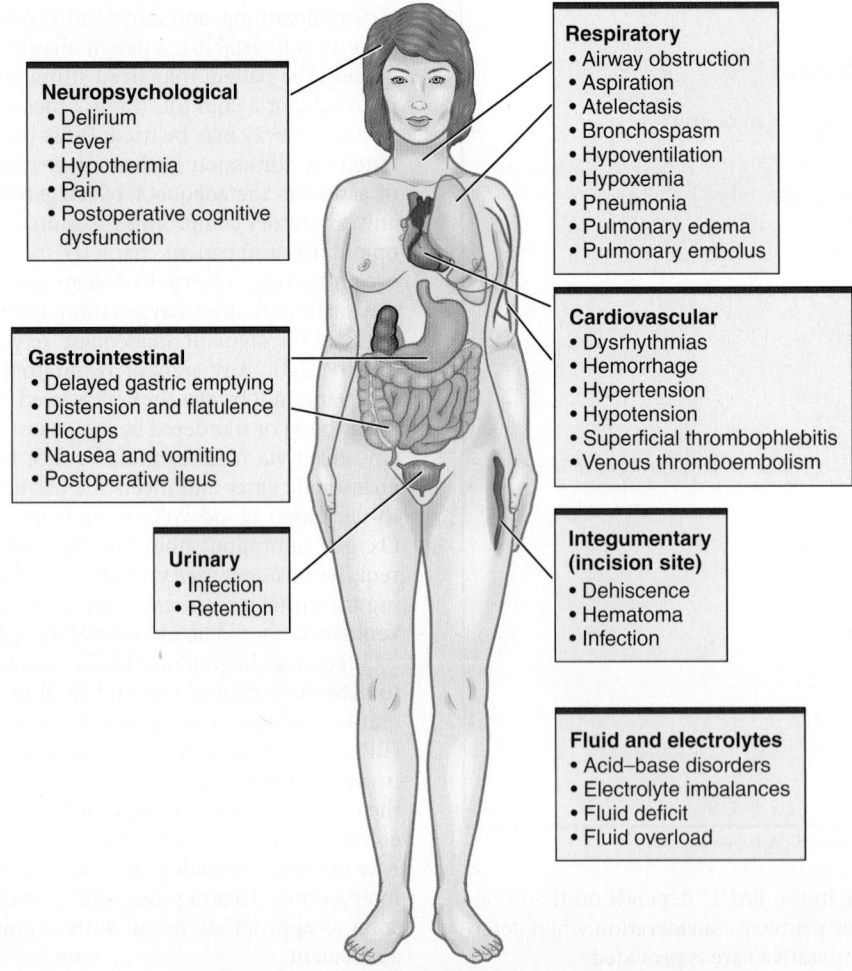

Neuropsychological
- Delirium
- Fever
- Hypothermia
- Pain
- Postoperative cognitive dysfunction

Respiratory
- Airway obstruction
- Aspiration
- Atelectasis
- Bronchospasm
- Hypoventilation
- Hypoxemia
- Pneumonia
- Pulmonary edema
- Pulmonary embolus

Gastrointestinal
- Delayed gastric emptying
- Distension and flatulence
- Hiccups
- Nausea and vomiting
- Postoperative ileus

Cardiovascular
- Dysrhythmias
- Hemorrhage
- Hypertension
- Hypotension
- Superficial thrombophlebitis
- Venous thromboembolism

Urinary
- Infection
- Retention

Integumentary (incision site)
- Dehiscence
- Hematoma
- Infection

Fluid and electrolytes
- Acid–base disorders
- Electrolyte imbalances
- Fluid deficit
- Fluid overload

FIG. 22.1 Potential complications in the postoperative period.

TABLE 22.4 CARING FOR THE POSTOPERATIVE PATIENT

PACU	Clinical Unit
• Assess patient's initial airway, breathing, and circulation status. • Ensure patient is in lateral recovery position unless contraindicated. • Evaluate for the return to consciousness, ability to maintain airway and breathing. • Perform ongoing assessments of vital signs and for postoperative problems (e.g., airway obstruction, hypoventilation, hypotension or hypertension, dysrhythmias, emergence delirium). • Administer and titrate O_2 based on facility policy. • Give analgesics and IV fluids. • Evaluate patient's readiness for transfer to clinical unit or discharge from ambulatory surgery. • Give hand-off report to nurse about patient status when transferring patient to clinical unit. • Provide discharge teaching for patient and caregiver after ambulatory surgery. • Position patient in lateral recovery position unless contraindicated.	• Assess patient on initial admission to the unit. • Assess for complications (e.g., atelectasis, hemodynamic instability, cognitive dysfunction, pain, fluid and electrolyte imbalance, fever or hypothermia, nausea and vomiting, urinary retention, wound infection). • Monitor vital signs. • Reposition and ambulate patient as prescribed. • Assist with deep breathing and coughing exercises. • Develop and implement an individualized plan of care based on identification of patient risk factors and potential complications. • Titrate O_2 administration according to prescribed parameters. • Monitor pain level and administer prescribed analgesics. • Administer medications. • Provide wound care, including dressing changes. • Insert urinary catheter as prescribed for urinary retention. • Develop and implement individualized patient and caregiver education, including discharge teaching.
Collaborate With Interprofessional Team ***Respiratory Therapist***	
• Provide respiratory care modalities that support patient recovery from anaesthesia (e.g., O_2 therapy, nebulizer treatments, pulmonary drainage procedures, mechanical ventilation, and airway support). • Institute extubation protocols. • Monitor pulse oximetry, capnography, or other technology-assisted means of assessing hypoxemia or hypoventilation. • Assist with O_2 and/or ventilation management during patient transport. • Perform arterial blood gas sampling in the absence of an arterial line.	• Institute rapid intubation protocols if required. • Provide respiratory care modalities (e.g., O_2 therapy, nebulizer treatments, pulmonary drainage procedures). • Assist with O_2 and/or ventilation support during patient transport. • Monitor pulse oximetry and capnography and titrate O_2 as needed. • Perform arterial blood gas sampling as needed.
Physiotherapist	
• Perform initial assessment to determine normal functioning level if surgery was emergent. • Support patient motion and joint mobility.	• Support patient motion and joint mobility. • Support patient return to baseline functional mobility following surgery. • Support interprofessional team members on best measures for joint positioning, transferring from bed to chair, and/or ambulation.

Clinical Unit. Common causes of respiratory concerns for postoperative patients in the clinical unit are atelectasis and pneumonia, especially after abdominal or thoracic surgery. Breathing aids in eliminating anaesthetic gasses from the body (Smith, 2019). Postoperatively, bronchial secretions increase when the respiratory passages have been irritated by heavy smoking, acute or chronic pulmonary infection or disease, and the drying of mucous membranes that occurs with intubation, inhalation anaesthesia, and dehydration. Subsequent postoperative development of mucous plugs that block small bronchi and decreased surfactant production are directly related to hypoventilation, constant recumbent position, ineffective coughing, and history of smoking. Without intervention, the affected lung segment can collapse, become infected, and progress to pneumonia within 2 to 3 days postoperatively.

NURSING MANAGEMENT RESPIRATORY COMPLICATIONS

NURSING ASSESSMENT

For an adequate respiratory assessment, nurses in the PACU and clinical unit settings must evaluate airway patency, chest symmetry, and the depth, rate, and character of respirations. The chest wall should be observed for symmetry of movement with a hand placed lightly over the xiphoid process. Slow breathing or diminished chest and abdominal movement during the respiratory cycle may indicate impaired ventilation. The nurse should determine whether abdominal or accessory muscles are being used for breathing, as their use may indicate

respiratory distress. Breath sounds should be auscultated anteriorly, laterally, and posteriorly. Decreased or absent breath sounds are detected when airflow is diminished or obstructed. The presence of crackles or wheezes necessitates notifying the health care provider.

Regular monitoring of vital signs and use of pulse oximetry in conjunction with thorough respiratory assessment enable the nurse to recognize early signs of respiratory complications. Hypoxemia from any cause may be reflected by rapid breathing, gasping, apprehension, restlessness, and a rapid or thready pulse.

The characteristics of sputum or mucus should be noted and recorded. Mucus from the trachea and throat is colourless and thin in consistency. Sputum from the lungs and bronchi can be thick with a slight yellow or pink tinge.

NURSING DIAGNOSES

Nursing diagnoses and interprofessional issues related to potential postoperative respiratory complications for the patient in the PACU or clinical unit include but are not limited to the following:

- *Inadequate airway clearance* resulting from *excessive mucus, retained secretions*
- *Inadequate breathing pattern* resulting from *pain, respiratory muscle fatigue*
- *Reduced gas exchange* as a result of *hypoventilation*
- *Potential for aspiration* resulting from *decrease in level of consciousness, depressed gag reflex*
- Potential complications: pneumonia, atelectasis

NURSING IMPLEMENTATION

POSTANAESTHESIA CARE UNIT. Nursing interventions in the PACU are designed to prevent and treat respiratory conditions. Proper patient positioning facilitates respirations and protects the airway. Unless contraindicated by the surgical procedure, the unconscious patient is positioned in a lateral "recovery" position that keeps the airway open and reduces risk for aspiration if vomiting occurs (Figure 22.3). Once conscious, the patient is usually returned to a supine position with the head of the bed elevated. This position maximizes thoracic expansion by decreasing the pressure of the abdominal contents on the diaphragm.

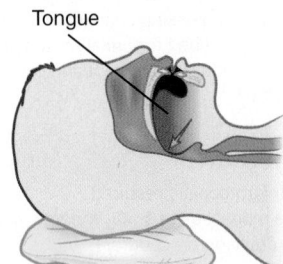

Tongue

Tongue occluding airway

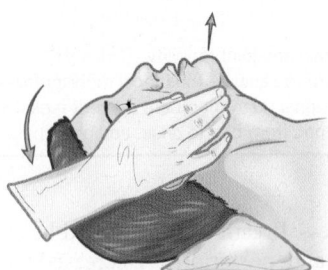

Manually elevate the jaw
while tilting the head back

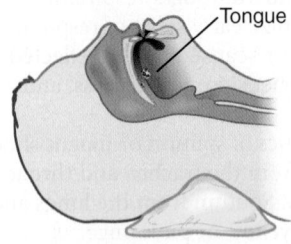

Tongue

Airway cleared

FIG. 22.2 Causes and relief of airway obstruction caused by the patient's tongue.

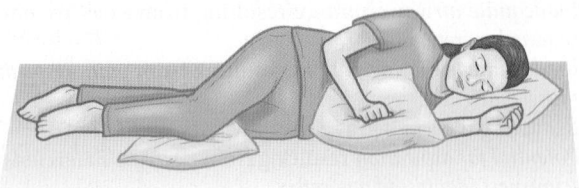

FIG. 22.3 Position of patient during recovery from general anaesthesia.

CLINICAL UNIT. Deep breathing is encouraged to facilitate gas exchange and promote the return to consciousness. The patient should be taught to take in slow, deep breaths, ideally through the nose; to hold the breath; and then to exhale slowly. This type of breathing is also useful as a relaxation strategy when the patient is anxious or in pain. Other nursing interventions appropriate for specific respiratory complications are detailed in Table 22.4.

Deep breathing and coughing techniques in the postoperative phase help the patient prevent alveolar collapse and move respiratory secretions to larger airway passages for expectoration. The patient should be stimulated to take three to four deep breaths every 5 to 10 minutes. As well, the sustained maximal inspiratory (SMI) manoeuvre can be used to increase lung volumes postoperatively. The patient inhales to the limit of their lung capacity and holds air in the lungs for 3 to 5 seconds before exhaling. Using an incentive spirometer is helpful in providing visual feedback of respiratory effort. The patient is taught to use an incentive spirometer preoperatively by inhaling into the mechanism, holding the ball for about 3 seconds, and then exhaling. This is done 10 to 15 times, and then the patient is encouraged to cough. This technique is used to improve oxygenation and prevent or reverse atelectasis (Odom-Forren & Brady, 2018). **Atelectasis** is a complete or partial collapse of a lung or segment of a lung that occurs when the alveoli become deflated (Figure 22.4). Diaphragmatic or abdominal breathing is accomplished by inhaling slowly and deeply through the nose, holding the breath for a few seconds, and then exhaling slowly and completely through the mouth. Placing the patient's hands lightly over the lower ribs and upper abdomen helps the patient to feel the abdomen rise during inspiration and fall during expiration.

Effective coughing is essential in mobilizing secretions (see Chapter 30). If secretions are present in the respiratory passages, deep breathing often will move them up to stimulate the cough reflex, and then they can be expectorated. Splinting an abdominal incision with a pillow or a rolled blanket provides support to the incision and aids in coughing and expectoration of secretions (Figure 22.5).

The patient's position should be changed every 1 to 2 hours to allow full chest expansion and increase perfusion of both lungs. Ambulation, not just sitting in a chair, should be aggressively carried out unless contraindicated by the surgical procedure performed or other concurrent diagnoses. Adequate and regular analgesic medication should be provided because incisional pain often deters patient participation in effective ventilation and ambulation. The patient should be reassured that these activities will not cause the incision to separate. Adequate parenteral or oral hydration is essential to maintain the integrity of mucous membranes and keep secretions thin and loose for easy expectoration.

POTENTIAL ALTERATIONS IN CARDIOVASCULAR FUNCTION

Etiology

Postanaesthesia Care Unit. In the immediate postanaesthetic period, common cardiovascular complications include hypotension, hypertension, and dysrhythmias. Patients at greatest risk for alterations in cardiovascular function include those with altered respiratory function or a cardiac history, older persons, and debilitated or critically ill patients.

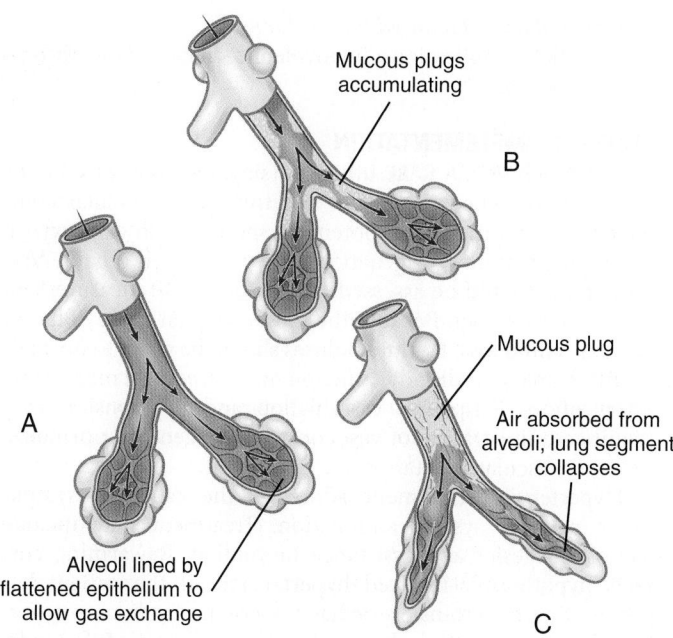

FIG. 22.4 Postoperative atelectasis. **A,** Normal bronchiole and alveoli. **B,** Mucous plugs in bronchioles. **C,** Collapse of alveoli caused by atelectasis following absorption of air.

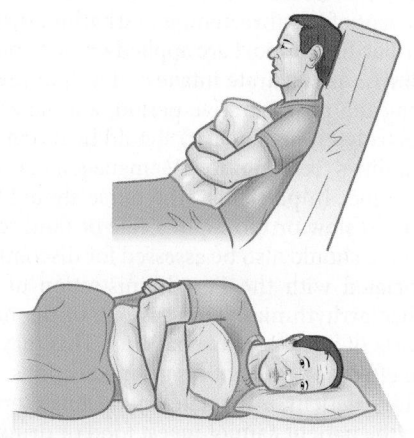

FIG. 22.5 Techniques for splinting wound when coughing.

Hypotension is evidenced by signs of hypoperfusion to the vital organs, especially the brain, heart, and kidneys. Clinical signs of disorientation, loss of consciousness, chest pain, oliguria, and anuria reflect hypoxemia and the loss of physiological compensation. Timely intervention may prevent the devastating complications of cardiac ischemia or infarction, cerebral ischemia, renal ischemia, and bowel infarction.

A common cause of hypotension in the PACU is unreplaced intraoperative fluid and blood loss, or postsurgical internal hemorrhage. If changes in level of consciousness and vital signs are detected, treatment is directed toward restoring circulating volume. If there is no response to fluid administration, cardiac dysfunction should be presumed to be the cause of hypotension. Lab values, such as hemoglobin and hematocrit, can provide additional insight into the patient's hematological status.

Primary cardiac dysfunction, as in myocardial infarction, cardiac tamponade, or pulmonary embolism, results in an acute fall in cardiac output. Secondary myocardial dysfunction occurs

as a result of the negative chronotropic (rate-derived) and negative inotropic (force-derived) effects of medications, such as β-adrenergic blockers, digoxin, or opioids. Other causes of hypotension include decreased or low systemic vascular resistance and dysrhythmias.

Hypertension, a common finding in the PACU, is most frequently the result of sympathetic nervous stimulation resulting from pain, anxiety, bladder distension, or respiratory compromise. Hypertension may result from hypothermia or pre-existing hypertension and be seen after revascularization in vascular and cardiac surgery.

Dysrhythmias are often the result of an identifiable cause other than myocardial injury. The leading causes include hypokalemia, hypoxemia, hypercarbia, alterations in acid–base status, circulatory instability, and pre-existing heart disease. Hypothermia, pain, surgical stress, and many anaesthetic agents are also capable of causing dysrhythmias.

Clinical Unit. Postoperative fluid and electrolyte imbalances contribute to alterations in cardiovascular function. Imbalances develop as a result of a combination of the body's normal response to the stress of surgery, excessive fluid losses, and improper IV fluid replacement, which directly affects cardiac output. Fluid retention during the first 2 to 5 postoperative days can be the result of the stress response (see Chapter 8). This body response maintains both blood volume and BP (see Chapter 8, Figure 8.5). The mechanisms that increase aldosterone lead to significant sodium and fluid retention, which can alter fluid balance and lead to urinary retention and cardiac complications.

Fluid overload may occur during this period of fluid retention when IV fluids are administered too rapidly, when chronic disease (e.g., cardiac or renal) exists, or with older patients. Conversely, fluid deficit may be related to slow or inadequate fluid replacement, which leads to decreases in cardiac output and tissue perfusion. Untreated preoperative dehydration or intraoperative or postoperative losses from vomiting, bleeding, wound drainage, or suctioning may contribute to fluid deficits.

Hypokalemia results when potassium is lost through the urinary and gastrointestinal (GI) tracts and not replaced by IV fluids. Low serum potassium levels directly affect the contractility of the heart, thus contributing to decreased cardiac output and overall body tissue perfusion. Adequate replacement of potassium usually entails administration of 40 mmol/day. However, it should not be given until adequate renal function has been established. A urine output of at least 30 mL/hr is generally considered indicative of adequate renal function. Serum analysis of electrolytes should be obtained for any patients who are at risk for electrolyte imbalances.

Cardiovascular status is affected by the state of tissue perfusion or blood flow. The stress response contributes to an increase in clotting tendencies in the postoperative patient by increasing platelet production. Deep vein thrombosis (DVT) may form in leg veins as a result of inactivity, body position, and pressure, all of which lead to venous stasis and decreased perfusion. DVT, common in older persons and obese or immobilized individuals, is a potentially life-threatening complication because it may lead to pulmonary embolism. Patients with a history of DVT have a greater risk for pulmonary embolism. Pulmonary embolism should be suspected in any patient reporting tachypnea, dyspnea, and tachycardia, particularly when the patient is already receiving oxygen therapy. Manifestations may include chest pain, hypotension, hemoptysis, dysrhythmias, or heart failure. Definitive diagnosis requires pulmonary angiography.

Superficial thrombophlebitis is an uncomfortable but less ominous complication that may develop in a leg vein as a result of venous stasis or in the arm veins as a result of irritation from IV catheters or solutions. If a piece of a clot becomes dislodged and travels to the lung, it can cause a pulmonary infarction of a size proportionate to the vessel in which it lodges.

Syncope (fainting) is another factor that reflects cardiovascular status. It may indicate decreased cardiac output, fluid deficits, defects in cerebral perfusion, or orthostatic hypotension, a fall in BP when the patient sits or stands. This results from peripheral dilation when blood leaves the central body organs, most notably the brain, and moves to the periphery, causing the person to feel faint.

NURSING MANAGEMENT CARDIOVASCULAR CONDITIONS

NURSING ASSESSMENT

Cardiovascular assessment involves frequent monitoring of vital signs, usually every 15 minutes or more often until they stabilize, and then less frequently. Postoperative vital signs are compared with preoperative and intraoperative readings to determine when the signs are stabilized at the patient's normal level. The anaesthesiologist or surgeon should be notified if any of the following occur:

1. Systolic BP is less than 90 mm Hg or greater than 160 mm Hg.
2. Pulse rate is less than 60 beats per minute (bpm) or greater than 120 bpm.
3. Pulse pressure (difference between systolic and diastolic pressures) narrows.
4. BP gradually decreases during several consecutive readings.
5. An irregular cardiac rhythm develops.
6. There is a significant variation from preoperative readings.

Cardiac monitoring is recommended for patients who have a history of cardiac disease and for all older patients who have undergone major surgery, regardless of whether they have cardiac conditions. The apical–radial pulse should be assessed, and irregularities should be reported.

Assessment of skin colour, temperature, and moisture provides valuable information for detecting cardiovascular problems. Hypotension accompanied by a normal pulse and warm, dry, pink skin usually represents the residual vasodilation effects of anaesthesia and suggests a need for continued observation. Hypotension accompanied by a rapid pulse and cold, clammy, pale skin may be caused by impending hypovolemic shock and necessitates immediate treatment.

Assessment of cardiovascular function includes regular monitoring of the patient's BP, heart rate, pulse, and skin temperature and colour. Peripheral circulation, dressing, and drains should also be assessed. Results should be compared with the preoperative status and the immediate postoperative and intraoperative findings.

NURSING DIAGNOSES

Nursing diagnoses and interprofessional problems related to potential cardiovascular complications in the PACU and the clinical unit include but are not limited to:

- *Reduced cardiac output* as a result of *hypovolemia, dysrhythmias*
- *Inadequate peripheral tissue perfusion* resulting from *sedentary lifestyle* (prolonged immobility)
- *Potential for imbalanced fluid volume*
- Potential complications: hypovolemic shock, venous thromboembolism

NURSING IMPLEMENTATION

POSTANAESTHESIA CARE UNIT. Nursing interventions in the PACU are designed to prevent and treat cardiovascular complications. Treatment of hypotension should begin with oxygen therapy to promote oxygenation of hypoperfused organs. Volume status should be assessed, and errors of BP measurement should be ruled out. Because the most common cause of hypotension is fluid loss, IV fluid boluses should be given to normalize BP. Primary cardiac dysfunction may necessitate medication intervention. Peripheral vasodilation and hypotension may require administration of vasoconstrictive agents to normalize systemic vascular resistance.

Hypertension treatment addresses the cause of sympathetic nervous system stimulation. Treatment may include use of analgesics and assistance in voiding. Rewarming corrects hypothermia-induced hypertension. If the patient has pre-existing hypertension or has undergone cardiac or vascular surgery, medication therapy designed to reduce BP may be required.

Most dysrhythmias seen in the PACU have identifiable causes, so treatment is directed toward eliminating the cause. Correcting physiological alterations often corrects the dysrhythmias. In the event of life-threatening dysrhythmias, protocols of advanced cardiac life support are applied (see Chapter 38).

CLINICAL UNIT. An accurate intake and output record should be kept during the postoperative period, and laboratory findings (e.g., electrolytes, hematocrit) should be monitored. Nursing responsibilities relating to IV management are critical during this period. In particular, the nurse should be alert for symptoms of too slow or too rapid a rate of fluid replacement. The infusion site should also be assessed for discomfort and the hazards associated with the IV administration of potassium, such as cardiac arrhythmias. Thirst is one of the most annoying discomforts of postoperative patients. This may be a result of the drying effects of anticholinergic medications, anaesthetic gases, and fluid deficits. Adequate and regular mouth care is helpful while the patient cannot ingest food or drink by mouth.

When confined to bed, patients should alternately flex and extend all joints 10 to 12 times every 1 to 2 hours while awake. The muscular contraction produced by these exercises and by ambulation facilitates venous return from the lower extremities. The ambulating patient should pick up their feet rather than shuffling them so as to maximize muscular contraction. When the patient is sitting in a chair or lying in bed, there should be no pressure to impede venous flow through the popliteal space. Crossed legs, pillows behind the knees, and extreme elevation of the knee gatch must be avoided.

The use of medications such as low-dose unfractionated heparin or low-molecular-weight heparin is a prophylactic measure for prevention of venous thrombosis and pulmonary embolism. Some surgeons routinely prescribe use of elastic stockings or mechanical aids such as sequential compressive devices to stimulate the massaging and milking actions that are transmitted to the veins when leg muscles contract. These devices may actually impair circulation if the legs remain inactive or if the devices are sized or applied improperly. Elastic stockings must be removed and reapplied at least twice daily for skin care and inspection.

Before the patient may ambulate, the nurse should first raise the head of the patient's bed for 1 to 2 minutes and then assist the patient to sit on the side of the bed while monitoring the radial pulse for rate and quality. If no changes or patient discomfort is noted, ambulation can be started. Nurses should use transfer belts or have adequate personnel to assist ambulation if the patient is unsteady or unable to transfer themselves. If the patient reports feeling faint during ambulation, the nurse should provide assistance to ease the patient to a supine position until recovery is evidenced by BP stability. While faintness is often frightening for the patient, it poses no real physiological danger, although injury can result from a fall.

POTENTIAL ALTERATIONS IN NEUROLOGICAL FUNCTION

Etiology

Postanaesthesia Care Unit. Occasionally, patients may wake up from anaesthesia in an agitated state referred to as *emergence delirium* (Figure 22.6). This is a reversible neurological alteration in which patients may be disoriented and exhibit bizarre behaviour (Odom-Forren, 2018,). **Emergence delirium** can include restlessness; agitation; disorientation to place, time, and person; thrashing; and shouting. Primarily pediatric and older patients are affected, and it is usually noted about half an hour after surgery but may manifest in up to 24 hours in older persons. Contributing factors include the following:
- Hypoxia
- Anaesthetic agents
- Bladder distension
- Sensory and cognitive impairments
- Inadequate pain control
- Electrolyte abnormalities
- State of anxiety before surgery

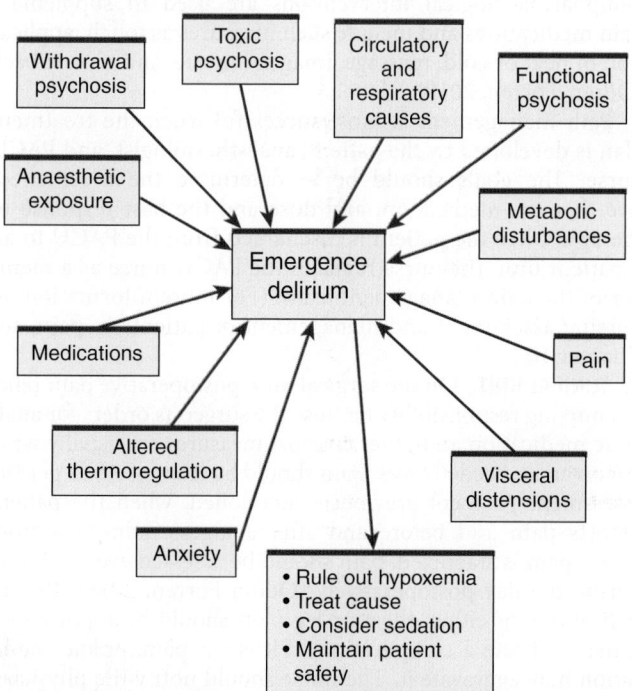

FIG. 22.6 Emergence delirium in the postanaesthesia care unit: contributing factors and treatment. Source: Redrawn from Rothrock, J. C. (2019). Alexander's care of the patient in surgery (16th ed., p. 268). Mosby.

If delirium is suspected, the nurse should first rule out hypoxia. Postoperative electrolyte disorders (e.g., hyponatremia and hypocalcemia) are risk factors for postoperative delirium and should be assessed (Wang et al., 2016). Once the cause is determined, the patient can receive appropriate treatment. Additional treatment involves the consideration of sedation and implementing anxiety-reducing interventions while ensuring patient safety (Odom-Forren, 2018).

Delayed awakening is another possible issue after surgery. Fortunately, the most common cause of delayed awakening is prolonged drug action, particularly of opioids, sedatives, and inhalational anaesthetics, as opposed to neurological injury. Normally, the anaesthesiologist can predict awakening based on the drugs used in surgery.

NURSING MANAGEMENT NEUROLOGICAL COMPLICATIONS

NURSING ASSESSMENT
After surgery, the nursing assessment should include the patient's level of consciousness, orientation, and ability to follow commands; the size, reactivity, and equality of the pupils; and the patient's sensory and motor status. If the patient had a regional anaesthetic, the level of anaesthetic effect should also be determined by assessing the level of numbness and number of dermatomes blocked. If the neurological status is altered, possible causes should be determined.

NURSING DIAGNOSES
Nursing diagnoses related to potential neurological complications for the patient in the PACU and the clinical unit include but are not limited to the following:
- *Potential for acute confusion* resulting from *sensory deprivation, pharmaceutical agent*
- *Potential for injury* resulting from *alteration in cognitive functioning, alteration in sensation*
- *Reduced verbal communication* resulting from *central nervous system impairment, emotional disturbance*

NURSING IMPLEMENTATION
POSTANAESTHESIA CARE UNIT. The most common cause of postoperative agitation is hypoxemia, so the nurse needs to evaluate respiratory function. Once hypoxemia has been ruled out and all potentially known causes have been addressed, sedation may prove beneficial in controlling the agitation and provide patient and staff safety. Emergence delirium and delays in awakening are time-limited and will resolve before the patient is discharged from the PACU. If necessary, benzodiazepines and opioids may be pharmacologically reversed with antagonists.

Until the patient is awake and able to communicate effectively, it is the responsibility of the PACU nurse to act as a patient advocate and to maintain patient safety at all times. Measures to accomplish this include having the side rails up, securing IV lines and artificial airways, verifying the presence of identification and allergy bands, and monitoring physiological status.

Clinical Unit. On the postoperative unit, the nurse can prevent or manage postoperative delirium by maintaining fluid and electrolyte balance, ensuring adequate nutrition and sleep, providing pain management, ensuring proper bowel and bladder function, and aiding early mobilization. Specific aids, such as clocks, calendars, and photographs, can help orient the patient.

Psychological issues in the postoperative period can be limited by providing adequate support for the patient—for example, by listening to and talking with the patient, explaining, reassuring, and encouraging caregiver presence.

Some common alterations in neurological function seen on the clinical unit may be related to medications for pain management, sleep deprivation, or sensory overload. It is important that the nurse complete a central nervous system assessment for all patients who have undergone surgery. For patients who are receiving pain medication, the nurse must ensure that they are responsive and oriented to person, place, and time. For patients who have received a spinal or epidural anaesthetic, the nurse must assess sensation and motor function. An ice pack may be used to check a patient's motor block as the effects of the spinal anaesthetic are resolving.

PAIN AND DISCOMFORT

Etiology

Postanaesthesia Care Unit. Despite the availability of analgesic medications and pain-relieving techniques, pain remains a common problem and a significant fear for the patient in the PACU and during the postoperative period. Pain may be the result of surgical manipulation, positioning, or the presence of internal devices such as an endotracheal tube or a catheter, or it may occur as the patient begins to mobilize after surgery.

Clinical Unit. On the surgical unit, postoperative pain is caused by the interaction of a number of physiological and psychological factors. Skin and underlying tissues have been traumatized during surgery, and there may be reflex muscle spasms around the incision. Anxiety and fear, sometimes related to the anticipation of pain, create tension and further increase muscle tone and spasm. The effort and movement associated with deep breathing, coughing, and changing position may aggravate pain by creating tension or pull on the incisional area.

When the internal viscera are cut, no pain is felt. However, pressure in the internal viscera elicits pain. Therefore, deep visceral pain may signal the presence of a complication such as intestinal distension or bleeding that can occur in the immediate postoperative phase or abscess formation, which can be apparent within 3 to 5 days postoperatively.

NURSING MANAGEMENT
PAIN

NURSING ASSESSMENT

POSTANAESTHESIA CARE UNIT. Pain assessment may be difficult in the PACU and in the early postoperative period on the clinical unit. The patient's self-report is the most important means of measuring pain intensity. Physiological indicators such as vital signs are not good indicators of pain, as research has demonstrated no significant correlation between the patient's self-reported intensity of pain and elevated heart rate and BP (Odom-Forren, 2018). When caring for patients who cannot self-report, the nurse should observe for behavioural clues of pain such as crying, restlessness, a wrinkling face or brow, or moaning.

CLINICAL UNIT. Postoperative pain is usually most severe within the first 48 hours and subsides thereafter. Variation is considerable, however, and is affected by the procedure performed and the patient's individual pain tolerance or perception. A comprehensive pain assessment includes the following:

- Location
- Intensity, assessed using a reliable, valid pain assessment tool (e.g., verbal descriptor, numeric rating, or visual analogue)
- Quality (e.g., neuropathic pain may be described as "burning" or "shooting")
- Factors that relieve and aggravate
- Effect of pain on function
- Comfort–function goal (e.g., for the postoperative patient, link pain control to the ability to deep-breathe, turn, or ambulate)

The nurse assesses the effectiveness of all pain control measures (e.g., epidural catheters, patient-controlled analgesia [PCA]) (Odom-Forren, 2018). (See Chapter 10 for a more detailed discussion of pain assessment.)

NURSING DIAGNOSES

Nursing diagnoses for the patient experiencing pain and discomfort in the PACU and clinical unit include but are not limited to the following:

- *Acute pain* resulting from *physical injury agent* (surgical procedure)
- *Chronic pain* resulting from *injury agent, emotional distress*

NURSING IMPLEMENTATION

POSTANAESTHESIA CARE UNIT. A multimodal, interprofessional team approach to postoperative pain has been shown to lead to better patient outcomes (Odom-Forren, 2019). IV opioids provide the most rapid relief. Medications are administered slowly and titrated to allow for optimal pain management with minimal to no adverse medication effects. Around-the-clock use of nonsteroidal anti-inflammatory drugs (NSAIDs), Cox-2 inhibitors, or acetaminophen can be used to decrease opioid requirements (Odom-Forren, 2019). More sustained relief may be obtained through the use of additional interventions, such as epidural catheters, PCA, or regional anaesthetic blockade. Nonpharmacological interventions are used to supplement pain medications and include such measures as touch, application of heat or cold, massage, imagery, music, and biofeedback (Odom-Forren, 2019).

Pain management is most successful when the treatment plan is developed by the patient, anaesthesiologist, and PACU nurse. The goals should be to determine the most effective therapy, medication, and dose and the best response to therapy. Once the patient is discharged from the PACU to an inpatient unit, the nurse replaces the PACU nurse as a member of the pain management team. (For more information on nursing assessment and management of patients in pain, see Chapter 10.)

CLINICAL UNIT. On the surgical unit, postoperative pain relief is a nursing responsibility because the surgeon's orders for analgesic medication and other comfort measures are usually written on an as-needed basis. Pain should be reassessed, as per the assessment protocol previously mentioned, when the patient reports pain and before and after analgesic administration. When pain is stabilized, pain should be assessed every 2 hours during the day postoperatively (Odom-Forren, 2018). Patient indications of either chest or leg pain should be reported, as it may indicate a complication. If it is gas pain, opioid medication may aggravate it. The nurse should notify the physician and request a change in the order if the analgesic either fails to relieve pain or makes the patient excessively lethargic or somnolent.

During the first 48 hours or longer, opioid analgesics (e.g., morphine) are required to relieve moderate to severe pain. After that, nonopioid analgesics, such as NSAIDs, may be sufficient as pain intensity decreases.

Effective pain management will reduce harmful complications, promote optimal healing, and enable patients to participate in necessary activities such as ambulating (Odom-Forren, 2018). Although opioid analgesics are often essential for the postoperative patient's comfort, adverse effects such as constipation, nausea and vomiting, respiratory depression, and hypotension are common. PCA is one of the most common ways to deliver opioid analgesia. PCA provides immediate analgesia and maintains a constant, steady blood level of the analgesic agent. PCA allows for self-administration of a preset bolus dose of analgesia by the patient (Odom-Forren, 2018). (PCA is discussed in Chapter 10.)

Epidural analgesia is the infusion of pain-relieving medications through a catheter placed into the epidural space surrounding the spinal cord. The goal of epidural analgesia is delivery of medication directly to opiate receptors in the spinal cord. The administration is through a bolus, continuous infusion, or patient-controlled epidural analgesia and is monitored by the nurse (Odom-Forren, 2018).

POTENTIAL ALTERATIONS IN TEMPERATURE

Etiology

Postanaesthesia Care Unit. Hypothermia sets in when a person's core temperature is less than 35°C. The perianaesthesia nurse should monitor the patient's temperature with an electronic oral temperature device (Odom-Forren, 2018). Postoperative hypothermia may be the result of heat loss during long, open surgical procedures due to the low ambient temperature in the OR, the use of cold irrigation fluids, or both.

Patients predisposed to hypothermia include older persons, children under 2 years—especially newborns—burn patients, females, and patients under general or neuraxial anaesthesia (Odom-Forren, 2018). Complications from hypothermia may include prolonged emergence from anaesthesia, increased likelihood of impaired wound healing and surgical site infection, bleeding, and cardiac incidences (Odom-Forren, 2018).

Active rewarming of hypothermic patients is achieved by applying external warming devices to the body and head. Although the application of warm blankets is traditionally done in the PACU, the use of forced-air warmers is an evidence-informed initiative that also effectively rewarms patients (Odom-Forren, 2018). When using any external warming device, the nurse should monitor the patient's body temperature at 15-minute intervals and use care to prevent thermal skin injuries. Oxygen therapy via nasal prongs or mask is used to treat the increased demand for oxygen that accompanies the increase in body temperature. Shivering is usually quickly suppressed by opioids.

Clinical Unit. Temperature variation in the postoperative period provides valuable information about the patient's status. Fever may occur at any time during the postoperative period (Table 22.5). A mild elevation (≤38°C) during the first 48 hours usually reflects the surgical stress response. A moderate elevation (>38°C) is caused more frequently by respiratory congestion or atelectasis and less frequently by dehydration. After the first 48 hours, a moderate to marked elevation (>37.7°C) is usually caused by infection.

TABLE 22.5 SIGNIFICANCE OF POSTOPERATIVE TEMPERATURE CHANGES

Time After Surgery	Temperature	Possible Causes
≤12 hours	Hypothermia to 35°C	Effects of anaesthesia Body heat loss in surgical exposure
First 24–48 hours	Elevation to 38°C	Inflammatory response to surgical stress
	>38°C	Lung congestion, atelectasis
Third day and later	Elevation above 37.7°C	Wound infection Urinary infection Respiratory infection Phlebitis

NURSING MANAGEMENT POTENTIAL TEMPERATURE COMPLICATIONS

NURSING ASSESSMENT

Frequent assessment of the patient's temperature in the days after surgery helps in detecting patterns of hypothermia or fever that may be present postoperatively. The nurse should observe the patient for early signs of inflammation and infection so that any complications that arise may be treated in a timely manner. Infections may include the following:

- Wound infection
- Respiratory tract infection
- Urinary tract infection (secondary to catheterization)
- IV site superficial thrombophlebitis (temperature elevation 7 to 10 days after surgery)
- Hospital-associated diarrhea caused by *Clostridium difficile*
- Septicemia (microorganisms enter bloodstream during surgery, especially in GI or genitourinary procedures)

NURSING DIAGNOSES

Nursing diagnoses related to potential postoperative temperature complications may include but are not limited to the following:

- *Hypothermia* resulting from *decrease in metabolic rate, inactivity*
- *Hyperthermia* resulting from *increase in metabolic activity, dehydration*
- *Potential for hypothermia* as a result of *inefficient non-shivering thermogenesis* (general anaesthesia, surgical procedure)

NURSING IMPLEMENTATION

POSTANAESTHESIA CARE UNIT. Passive rewarming (i.e., shivering) raises basal heat metabolism, so active rewarming using forced-air warmers or other devices, such as radiant warmers or heated water mattresses, is preferable. During rewarming, the nurse should also monitor a patient who has an increase in temperature, specifically for symptoms of malignant hyperthermia, because symptoms may not be evident until the postoperative phase. (See discussion of malignant hyperthermia in Chapter 21). Oxygen therapy via nasal prongs or mask is used to address the increased demand for oxygen that accompanies the increased body temperature. (See Chapter 71 for more on the management of hypothermia.)

Clinical Unit. The nurse's role with respect to postoperative fever may be preventive, diagnostic, therapeutic, or a combination of these. The patient's temperature is usually measured every 4 hours for the first 48 hours after surgery and then less frequently if no problems develop. As well, the nurse must maintain meticulous care of the wound and the IV site and encourage airway clearance. If fever develops, chest X-rays may be taken and antipyretic medications administered. Depending on the suspected cause of the fever, wound, sputum, urine, or blood cultures may be required. If a bacterial infection is the source of the fever, antibiotics are started as soon as cultures are obtained. If temperature rises above 39.4°C, body-cooling measures may be used.

POTENTIAL GASTROINTESTINAL CONDITIONS

Etiology

Postanaesthesia Care Unit. Nausea and vomiting are significant concerns in the immediate postoperative period and are often the reason for unanticipated hospital admission of day-surgery patients, increased patient discomfort, delays in discharge, and patient dissatisfaction with the surgical experience.

Clinical Unit. Slowed GI motility and altered patterns of food intake may lead to the development of several distressing postoperative symptoms that are most pronounced after abdominal surgery. Nausea and vomiting may be caused by the action of anaesthetics or opioids, delayed gastric emptying, slowed peristalsis resulting from the handling of the bowel during surgery, or resumption of oral intake too soon after surgery (Table 22.6).

NURSING MANAGEMENT GASTROINTESTINAL CONDITIONS

NURSING ASSESSMENT

NAUSEA AND VOMITING. Postoperative nausea and vomiting (PONV) is a complex physiological interaction between the following: the vomiting centre in the brainstem, the chemoreceptor trigger zone, the internal ear, the vagus nerve, the limbic system, and the cerebral cortex. PONV occurs in approximately 30% of all surgical patients and 80% of high-risk patients (Peterson, 2018). PONV leads to delayed PACU or hospital discharge and, sometimes, subsequent readmission.

Primary risk factors for PONV include the following (Odom-Forren & Brady, 2018):

Patient-specific
- Age less than 50 years old

TABLE 22.6	**POSTOPERATIVE DIETS**

Clear Fluids
Broth, gelatin, water, tea, black coffee

Fluids
Milk, coffee with cream, cream soups

Soft Diet
Fish, cottage cheese, pasta, eggs, mousse, pudding

Full Diet
Regular diet
Patients can also be placed on special diets, such as diabetic or low sodium.

- Female gender
- History of motion sickness or PONV
- Nonsmoker

Anaesthesia-related
- Use of volatile anaesthetics
- Use of nitrous oxide
- Opioid use postoperatively

Surgery-related
- Duration of surgery greater than 1 hour
- Type of surgery

These risk factors can be determined in the preoperative assessment so that prophylaxis can be planned using either one medication such as ondansetron (Zofran) or a combination of medications that minimize PONV.

Nonpharmacological interventions that may be used in combination for PONV or for postdischarge nausea and vomiting (PDNV) include transcutaneous electrical nerve stimulation, acupuncture, acupressure, acupoint stimulation, and aromatherapy (isopropyl alcohol and peppermint) (Odom-Forren & Brady, 2018). Nurses should document the quantity and characteristics (including colour) of the emesis.

Ileus

Postoperative Ileus. Postoperative ileus (POI) is a delay in the return of the GI system's normal peristalsis, specifically after GI surgery. It is characterized by abdominal distension and tenderness or pain. Stomach motility returns in 1 to 2 days, and bowel motility in 3 to 5 days. Laparoscopic colon surgery is associated with a shorter period of POI than open surgery. Abdominal distension during this time may require insertion of a nasogastric tube for symptomatic relief and the lowering of opioid doses or provision of pain relief with NSAIDs to reduce inflammation (Cagir, 2018).

Paralytic Ileus. Paralytic ileus is impairment of intestinal motility (ileus that persists for more than 2 to 3 days) postoperatively. It can be associated with the large and small intestine and resolves with treatment; it is not a mechanical obstruction. Peristalsis stops and the patient has abdominal pain, distension, nausea, vomiting, and poor appetite. Nursing care on the postoperative unit consists of measuring the patient's abdominal girth for distension and auscultating the abdomen in all four quadrants to determine presence, frequency, and characteristics of bowel sounds. Bowel sounds are frequently absent or diminished, and the abdomen will sound tympanic to percussion. Early bowel sounds may signal return of small intestine motility; however, full return of bowel function is indicated by the passage of flatus or stool (DeVolder, 2019). When paralytic ileus does not resolve spontaneously, the patient may require diagnostic tests to rule out mechanical blockage that would require surgical intervention.

NURSING DIAGNOSES

Nursing diagnoses and interprofessional issues related to potential GI complications in the PACU and clinical unit may include but are not limited to the following:
- *Nausea* resulting from *noxious environmental stimuli*
- *Potential for aspiration* as a result of *delayed gastric emptying, depressed gag reflex, increase in intragastric pressure*
- *Potential for deficient fluid volume* resulting from *active fluid volume loss*
- *Inadequate nutrition* resulting from *inability to ingest food, inability to absorb nutrients*
- Potential complications: fluid and electrolyte imbalance

NURSING IMPLEMENTATION

POSTANAESTHESIA CARE UNIT. Intervention for *nausea and vomiting* is primarily the use of antiemetic or prokinetic medications (see Chapter 44). In the PACU, oral fluids should be given only as indicated and tolerated. IV fluids will provide hydration until the patient is able to tolerate oral fluids. Care should also be taken to prevent aspiration in case the patient vomits while still sleepy from anaesthesia. Having suction equipment readily available at the bedside and positioning the patient in the lateral recovery position will help protect the patient from aspiration (see Figure 22.3). Other interventions that may be effective include placing the patient in the upright position; encouraging slow, deep breathing; doing mouth care; using distraction; and providing emotional support.

CLINICAL UNIT. Depending on the nature of the surgery, the patient may resume oral intake as soon as the gag reflex returns. While the patient is on NPO (nothing-by-mouth) status, IV infusions are given to maintain fluid and electrolyte balance. Once oral intake is allowed, clear liquids are started and the IV infusion is continued, usually at a reduced rate. If oral intake is well tolerated by the patient, the IV is discontinued and the diet is advanced progressively until a regular diet is tolerated.

The nurse should assess the patient regularly to detect the resumption of normal intestinal peristalsis, as evidenced by the return of bowel sounds and the passage of flatus. The patient may need to be encouraged to expel flatus and be reassured that expulsion is necessary and desirable. Gas pains, which tend to become pronounced on the second or third postoperative day, may be relieved by ambulation and frequent repositioning. Positioning the patient on their right side permits gas to rise along the transverse colon and facilitates its release. Resumption of a normal diet after bowel sounds have returned will also enhance the return of normal peristalsis. A patient who does not improve with conservative measures will need to be reassessed and may require additional surgery.

POTENTIAL ALTERATIONS IN URINARY FUNCTION

Etiology

Low Urine Output. In patients with normal renal function, a urinary output of ≈30 mL/hr is expected in the PACU. This lower output is caused by increased aldosterone and antidiuretic hormone secretion resulting from the stress of surgery, fluid restriction before surgery, loss of fluids during surgery, drainage, and diaphoresis. By the second or third day, the patient's urinary output should return to the normal level of 0.5 to 1 mL/kg/hr (≈60 mL/hr). Persistent low urinary output, or *oliguria*, can indicate inadequate renal perfusion and pending renal failure. Restoring renal blood flow and urine production can prevent renal failure.

Acute urinary retention can occur in the postoperative period for a variety of reasons. Surgical genitourinary trauma can cause swelling and bleeding. Anaesthesia depresses the nervous system, allowing the bladder to fill more completely than normal before the urge to void is felt. Neuraxial anaesthesia can cause autonomic blockade of sacral nerves, resulting in a hypotonic bladder. After lower abdominal or pelvic surgery, spasms or guarding of the abdominal and pelvic muscles interferes with their normal function, resulting in urinary retention. Pain may alter perception, interfering with the patient's awareness of the sensation arising as the bladder fills. Voiding may be impaired by lack of skeletal muscle activity (decreased smooth bladder muscle tone). As well, the supine position reduces the ability to relax the perineal muscles and the external sphincter.

Anticholinergic, antispasmodic, and opioid medications are some medications that prevent the complete emptying of the bladder.

NURSING MANAGEMENT
POTENTIAL URINARY CONDITIONS

NURSING ASSESSMENT

The urine of the patient after surgery should be examined for both quantity and quality. The colour, amount, consistency, and odour of the urine should be noted. In-dwelling catheters should be assessed for patency, and urine output should be approximately 60 mL/hr. Most people urinate approximately 200 mL of urine within 6 to 8 hours after surgery. If no voiding occurs, the abdominal contour should be inspected and the bladder palpated and percussed for distension or a bladder scanner used to detect bladder volumes.

NURSING DIAGNOSES

Nursing diagnoses and interprofessional issues related to potential urinary complications for the patient after surgery include but are not limited to the following:
- *Urinary retention* resulting from *anaesthetic drugs, pain*
- Potential complication: acute kidney injury, catheter-associated urinary tract infections (CAUTIs)

NURSING IMPLEMENTATION

There may be a postoperative order to catheterize the patient in 8 to 12 hours if voiding has not occurred; however, there are ways for the nurse to facilitate voiding. Some measures known to help include positioning the patient—sitting for women and standing for men—ambulating, putting a commode in place, providing reassurance, running water, providing water to drink, or pouring warm water over the perineum.

In assessing the need for catheterization, the nurse considers fluid intake during and after surgery and determines bladder fullness (e.g., palpable fullness above the symphysis pubis, discomfort when pressure is applied over the bladder, the presence of the urge to void). Urinary tract infections are the most common complication associated with urinary catheterization and frequently occur in the first postoperative week. Patients should be catheterized only when absolutely necessary, using aseptic protocol, and the catheter should be removed as soon as it is no longer required.

POTENTIAL ALTERATIONS IN THE INTEGUMENT

Etiology

Despite advances in surgical technologies and techniques, environmental conditions, antibiotic regimens, and sterilization methods, surgery remains an invasive procedure that can predispose patients to surgical site infections (SSIs). An SSI is an infection that occurs within 30 days of surgery or up to 1 year after implant surgery. Superficial SSI has at least one of the following signs or symptoms (Bak, 2019):
- Purulent discharge
- Isolation of organisms from wound fluid or tissue
- Pain, tenderness, local edema, warmth
- Health care provider diagnosis

In Canada, SSIs are the most common health care–associated infection experienced by surgical patients, with 77% of patient deaths reported to be related to infection (Canadian Patient Safety Institute, 2020). Having nurses provide leading-edge wound care practice is decreasing the need for patient readmission to hospital and thus saving health care costs (Nurses Specialized in Wound, Ostomy, and Continence Canada, 2020).

Wounds are a significant, costly, and preventable barrier to successful recovery from routine surgical interventions, so reducing the incidence of SSIs is essential, and much evidence is now available to support prevention practices. The Wound Care Instrument provides a set of standards to guide a comprehensive appraisal process for wound management education (Canadian Association of Wound Care and Canadian Association for Enterostomal Therapy, 2011). (Wound healing and complications are discussed in Chapter 14.)

SSIs are believed to be caused by factors that can be considered modifiable or nonmodifiable patient factors, as well as by extrinsic factors (King & Spry, 2019). Examples of modifiable

patient factors include obesity, smoking, glycemic control, and immunosuppression. Nonmodifiable patient factors are history of skin infection, age, and prior radiation to the surgical site. Examples of extrinsic factors include lapses in sterile technique, inadequate ventilation in the OR, and inappropriate antibiotic choice (King & Spry, 2019).

Table 22.7 provides guidelines for the prevention of SSIs.

NURSING MANAGEMENT
SURGICAL WOUNDS

NURSING ASSESSMENT

Wound assessment requires gathering information through questioning, observation, physical examination, and clinical investigation and using this information to formulate a wound care plan. It is recommended that the physical assessment be done in three zones: wound bed, wound edge, and periwound

TABLE 22.7 RECOMMENDATIONS FOR PREVENTION OF SURGICAL SITE INFECTIONS

Intervention	Guidelines for SSI Prevention
Perform holistic preoperative assessment and manage preoperative risk	Document patient's age, weight, general health, medications, coexisting health conditions, glycemic control, recent weight loss or gain, state of being overweight or obese, physical activity levels, present and past smoking history, and previous experiences with anaesthetic. *Example:* Advanced age is associated with decreased healing potential and diminished immune factors. Complete a nutritional assessment or lab analysis for serum albumin and total protein or both. Improve diet preoperatively.
Manage intraoperative risk	Maintain patient homeostasis (e.g., temperature, glucose levels, O$_2$ saturation >95%). Ensure strict adherence to aseptic practice by surgical personnel. Minimize tissue trauma through gentle handling and limited use of electrocautery, and when closing incision, eliminate dead space below the skin. Use antibiotics prophylactically.
Manage postoperative risk	Maintain body temperature. Ensure adequate oxygenation. Use clean, intact wound dressing (e.g., waterproof dressing for 48 hours or aseptic technique for dressing change). Control pain.
Educate patients and families on signs and symptoms of SSIs	Provide information in easy-to-understand verbal and written form, including: • How to recognize an SSI (i.e., a little redness around wound edge is normal and can be expected for the first few days after surgery; redness spreading out more than 2 cm from incision, pain, swelling, or pus are SSI danger signs that must be reported to the health care provider) • Who to contact if infection is suspected • How to care for wound at home • Antibiotic regimen
Identify and treat SSIs	Ensure early diagnosis. Open incision to remove sutures and infected tissue and to drain. Use dressings to promote secondary healing. Follow evidence-informed recommendations for antibiotics.
Debride necrotic tissue	(Necrotic tissue prolongs inflammation and may harbour aerobic and anaerobic bacteria and toxins.) Choose debridement technique based on wound condition, resources, and patient condition.
Choose dressing or device to manage exudate and bacterial burden	Choose a dressing based on: • Depth of wound • Exudate and odour control • Conformability • Antimicrobial efficacy • Ease of removal • Patient safety and comfort
Consider adjunctive therapies	Use topical NPWT (e.g., for sternal and abdominal dehiscence, use growth factors, antibacterial honey, larva therapy [maggots], anti-scarring agents, and antiseptic-impregnated sutures).
Implement a surgical site surveillance program	(Collating infection rates for individual surgeons and surgical procedures reduces infection rates and identifies trends and causative agents. Surveillance programs must be in the community and extend a minimum of 30 days postoperatively and up to 1 year for implants.) Help evaluate effectiveness of preventive strategies. Determine adherence to guidelines (e.g., teamwork, interprofessional collaboration, and effective communication).

NPWT, negative-pressure wound therapy; *SSI,* surgical site infection.
Adapted from Keast, D., & Swanson, T. (2014). Ten top tips: Managing surgical site infections. *Wounds International, 5*(3), 15–16. http://www.woundinfection-institute.com/wp-content/uploads/2014/11/SSI_11422.pdf (Seminal).

skin (Dowsett & von Hallern, 2017). Assessment includes the following:

- *Appearance:* Note the colour of wound, bruising, redness, and approximation of the incision.
- *Size:* Note the length, width, depth and shape of the wound and any signs of the wound opening (i.e., dehiscence or evisceration).
- *Exudate:* Check the wound for exudate type (e.g., watery, purulent), odour, and amount. A small amount of serous drainage is common, and it changes from sanguineous (red) to serosanguineous (pink) to serous (clear yellow). Draining will decrease over time.
- *Edema:* Excessive swelling may indicate wound complications.
- *Pain:* Sudden onset or persistent severe incisional pain may indicate infection, hemorrhage, or hematoma.
- *Drains:* Note the placement and security of drain or tube. Check the collection device; empty as required and document.

Wound dehiscence (separation and disruption of previously joined wound edges) may be preceded by a sudden discharge of brown, pink, or clear drainage. *Wound evisceration* (protrusion of the visceral organs though a wound opening) can occur after surgery and is considered a medical emergency. If evisceration occurs, the nurse needs to place sterile, saline-soaked towels over any extruding tissue, keep the patient on NPO status, observe the patient for signs and symptoms of shock, and call the surgeon immediately.

NURSING DIAGNOSES

Nursing diagnoses related to surgical wounds of the patient after surgery include but are not limited to the following:

- Reduced tissue integrity resulting from chemical injury agent
- Potential for surgical site infection resulting from invasive procedure, type of surgical procedure, comorbidity

NURSING IMPLEMENTATION

When drainage occurs on the dressing, the type, amount, colour, consistency, and odour of drainage should be noted and recorded. Expected drainage from tubes is outlined in Table 22.8. The effect of position changes on drainage should also be assessed. The surgeon should be notified of any excessive or abnormal drainage and significant changes in vital signs.

Immediately after surgery, the incision is usually covered with a dressing. Surgical wound dressings are left dry and untouched for a minimum of 48 hours after surgery. This permits re-establishment of the protective, natural bacteria-proof barrier. The nurse changes the dressing according to employer policy. (Wound healing and care are discussed in Chapter 14.)

POTENTIAL ALTERATIONS IN PSYCHOLOGICAL FUNCTION

Etiology

Anxiety and depression may occur in the postoperative patient. These states may be more pronounced in the patient who has had radical surgery (e.g., colostomy, amputation) or who has received a poor prognosis (e.g., inoperable tumour). A history of a neurotic or psychotic disorder should alert the nurse to the possibility of postoperative anxiety and depression. However, these responses may develop in any patient as part of the grief response to loss of a body organ or disturbance in body image (e.g., mastectomy or hysterectomy) and may be exacerbated by a lowered response to stress.

The patient who lives alone or requires rehabilitation after surgery may also develop anxiety and depression when faced with the need for assistance after surgery until strength and independence can be regained. Discharge planning should be ongoing from the preoperative phase onward (Cuming, 2019).

In caring for the older person, nurses must be cognizant of the increasing incidence of delirium, dementia, and depression in this segment of the population. Nurses must possess the knowledge and skills to screen for and differentiate between these conditions, which can have overlapping clinical features (Registered Nurses' Association of Ontario, 2016).

After surgery, confusion or delirium may arise from physiological sources, including fluid and electrolyte imbalances; hypoxemia; medication effects; sleep deprivation; and sensory alteration, deprivation, or overload.

Delirium tremens may also occur in some patients after surgery as a result of alcohol withdrawal. Delirium tremens is a reaction characterized by restlessness, insomnia, nightmares, tachycardia, apprehension, confusion and disorientation, irritability, and auditory or visual hallucinations. (Management of delirium tremens is discussed in Chapter 11.)

NURSING MANAGEMENT PSYCHOLOGICAL FUNCTION

NURSING DIAGNOSES

Nursing diagnoses related to potential postoperative alterations in psychological function include but are not limited to the following:

- *Anxiety* resulting from *threat to current status*

TABLE 22.8 EXPECTED DRAINAGE FROM TUBES AND CATHETERS				
Substance	**Daily Amount**	**Colour**	**Odour**	**Consistency**
In-dwelling Catheter				
Urine*	500–700 mL, 1–2 days postoperative; 1 500–2 500 mL thereafter (output = 0.5–1 mL/kg/hr)	Clear, yellow	Ammonia	Watery
Nasogastric Tube, Gastrostomy Tube				
Gastric contents	≤1 500 mL/day	Pale, yellow–green, brown Bloody following gastrointestinal surgery	Sour	Watery
Hemovac, Jackson-Pratt				
Wound drainage	Variable with procedure	Variable with procedure Usually serosanguineous	Same as wound dressing	Variable
T Tube				
Bile	500 mL	Bright yellow to dark green	Acid	Thick

*See Chapter 47.

- *Disrupted body image* resulting from *alteration in self-perception*
- *Disrupted sleep pattern* resulting from *environmental barrier (unfamiliar setting, insufficient privacy)*

NURSING IMPLEMENTATION

Nurses must observe and evaluate the patient's behaviour and plan appropriate interventions to ensure proper treatment of symptoms, prevent adverse outcomes, and improve the patient's quality of life on discharge. Supportive measures include taking time to listen to and talk with the patient, offering explanations and reassurance, and working collaboratively with family or significant others for discharge planning.

The nurse should discuss the patient's expectations for activity and the assistance that will be needed following discharge. The older patient may be particularly distressed if an immediate return to home is not feasible. The patient must be included in discharge planning and provided with the information and support to make informed decisions about continuing care.

Recognition of alcohol withdrawal syndrome in a patient not previously known to misuse alcohol presents a particular challenge. Any unusual or disturbed behaviour should be reported immediately so that diagnosis can be made and treatment instituted.

DISCHARGE FROM THE POSTANAESTHESIA CARE UNIT

The patient leaving the PACU may be discharged to a critical care unit, an inpatient unit, an ambulatory care unit, or home. The choice of discharge site is based on patient acuity, access to follow-up care, and the potential for postoperative complications. The decision to discharge the patient from the PACU is based on written discharge criteria, which can take the form of a standardized scoring system used to determine the patient's general condition and readiness for discharge. Examples of discharge criteria are provided in Table 22.9.

CARE OF THE POSTOPERATIVE PATIENT ON THE CLINICAL UNIT

Before discharging the patient from the PACU to the clinical unit, the PACU nurse should provide a verbal report about the patient to the receiving nurse. The report summarizes the operative and postanaesthetic period.

TABLE 22.9	POSTANAESTHESIA AND AMBULATORY SURGERY DISCHARGE CRITERIA

Postanaesthesia Discharge Criteria
- Patient awake (or baseline)
- Vital signs stable
- No excess bleeding or drainage
- No respiratory depression
- Oxygen saturation >90%
- Report given

Ambulatory Surgery Discharge Criteria
- All PACU discharge criteria met
- No IV opioids for last 30 minutes
- Minimal nausea and vomiting
- Voided (if appropriate to surgical procedure or orders)
- Able to ambulate if age appropriate and not contraindicated
- Responsible adult present to accompany patient
- Written discharge instructions given and understood

IV, intravenous; *PACU*, postanaesthesia care unit.

The nurse receiving the patient on the clinical unit assists PACU transport personnel in transferring the patient from the PACU stretcher onto the bed. Care must be taken to protect IV lines, wound drains, dressings, and traction devices. The use of a draw sheet or transfer board and sufficient personnel facilitates transfer of the patient.

On the clinical unit, vital signs should be obtained, and patient status should be compared with the report provided by the PACU. Documentation of the transfer is then completed, followed by a more in-depth assessment (Table 22.10). Postoperative orders and appropriate nursing care are then initiated.

Although many of the health problems that may occur in the PACU are time-limited to the immediate postoperative period, complications may occur during the extended postoperative recovery period on the clinical unit. Nursing assessment and management are based on awareness of the potential complications of surgery in general as well as complications specific to the surgical procedure. (A comprehensive nursing care plan for the postoperative patient is available on the Evolve website.)

PLANNING FOR DISCHARGE AND FOLLOW-UP CARE

Ambulatory and Inpatient Surgery Discharge

Ambulatory Surgery Discharge. Ambulatory surgery is also referred to as *outpatient surgery* or *same-day surgery* (Peng & Anker, 2020). A significant number of surgeries are now performed on an ambulatory basis in Canada. Despite the obvious advantages of ambulatory surgery (e.g., patient convenience, lower health care costs), because these patients are in the health care setting for such a short time, it is difficult to complete all the required teaching. Optimally, the patient and any caregivers should be contacted 1 or more days before surgery to collect assessment data and to provide teaching that will be needed after surgery. The patient's lower anxiety level at this time may enhance learning.

The patient leaving an ambulatory surgery setting must be mobile and alert so as to be able to provide self-care when discharged to home. Postoperative pain must be controlled. Overall, the patient must be stable and near the level of preoperative functioning for discharge from the unit. On discharge, instructions specific to the type of anaesthesia received and the surgery are given to the patient and caregiver verbally and reinforced with written directions. The patient may not drive and must be accompanied by a responsible adult at the time of discharge. A follow-up evaluation of the patient's status is made by telephone, and any specific questions and concerns are addressed.

As more complex surgical procedures are being done on an ambulatory basis, the nurse should carefully determine not only readiness for discharge but also the home care needs of the individual, including availability of assistive personnel (e.g., family, friends), access to a pharmacy for prescriptions, access to a phone in the event of an emergency, and access to follow-up care.

Discharge From the Clinical Unit. Preparation for the patient's discharge should be an ongoing process throughout the surgical experience, beginning during the preoperative period. During the preoperative assessment, the nurse must determine if the patient will need additional health care support upon returning home. Arrangements for home care nurses and community resources are initiated so that they are in place when the patient is discharged. The patient is educated about what they will have to do postoperatively and, as events unfold, gradually assume greater responsibility for self-care. As discharge approaches, the nurse should be certain that the patient and any caregivers have the following information:

- Care requirements for wound site and any dressings, including bathing recommendations

TABLE 22.10 NURSING ASSESSMENT AND CARE OF PATIENT ON ADMISSION TO CLINICAL UNIT

General Anaesthetic Versus Spinal or Epidural Anaesthetic

General Anaesthetic	Spinal or Epidural Anaesthetic

1. Verify patient identification using name band and medical record number.
2. Note any allergies and ensure presence of an allergy bracelet if applicable.
3. Record time of patient's return to unit.
4. Take baseline vital signs.
5. Assess airway and breath sounds.
6. Assess neurological status, including level of consciousness and movement of extremities.
7. Assess wound, wound closure and dressing, and drainage and nasogastric tubes.
  • Note length of tubing where applicable.
  • Ensure all drains and tubings are secured in place (minimizes risk of accidental discontinuation and resulting tissue trauma).
  • Note type and amount of drainage.
  • Note any packing to an open wound.
  • Connect tubing to gravity or suction drainage.
8. Assess colour and appearance of skin.
9. Assess urinary status.
  • Note time of voiding.
  • Note presence of catheter, if any, and total output.
  • Check for bladder distension or urge to void.
  • Note catheter patency; check integrity of insertion site and size of Foley catheter.
10. Assess pain and discomfort.
  • Note last dose and type of pain control.
  • Note current pain intensity.
11. Position for comfort and safety (bed in low position, side rails up).
12. Check IV infusion.
  • Note type of solution.
  • Note amount of fluid remaining.
  • Note flow rate.
13. Attach call light within patient's reach, and orient patient to its use.
14. Ensure that emesis basin and tissues are available.
15. Determine emotional condition and support needed.
16. Check for presence of family member or significant other.
17. Orient patient and family to immediate environment.
18. Check and carry out postoperative orders.
	1. Record time of patient's return to unit.
	2. Take baseline vital signs.
	3. Assess airway and breath sounds.
	4. Assess neurological status, including level of consciousness and movement of extremities.
	  • Assess spinal insertion or epidural insertion site; ensure that there is a continuous epidural infusion in place and that the dressing and catheter are secure.
	  • Assess motor and sensory blockade from spinal anaesthetic.
	5. Assess wound, wound closure, dressing, and drainage tubes.
	  • Note type and amount of drainage.
	  • Note any packing to an open wound.
	  • Connect tubing to gravity or suction drainage.
	6. Assess colour and appearance of skin.
	7. Assess urinary status.
	  • Note time of voiding.
	  • Note presence of catheter, if any, and total output.
	  • Check for bladder distension or urge to void.
	  • Note catheter patency; check integrity of insertion site and size of Foley catheter.
	8. Assess pain and discomfort.
	  • Note last dose and type of pain control.
	  • Note current pain intensity.
	9. Position for comfort and safety (bed in low position, side rails up).
	10. Check IV infusion.
	  • Note type of solution.
	  • Note amount of fluid remaining.
	  • Note flow rate.
	11. Attach call light within patient's reach, and orient patient to its use.
	12. Ensure that emesis basin and tissues are available.
	13. Determine emotional condition and support.
	14. Check for presence of family member or significant other.
	15. Orient patient and family to immediate environment.
	16. Check and carry out postoperative orders.

IV, intravenous.

- Action and possible adverse effects of any medications and when and how to take them
- Activities allowed and prohibited; when various physical activities can be resumed safely (e.g., driving a car, returning to work, sexual intercourse, leisure activities)
- Dietary restrictions or modifications
- Symptoms to be reported (e.g., development of incisional tenderness or increased drainage, discomfort in other parts of the body)
- Where and when to return for follow-up care
- Answers to any individual questions or concerns

The nurse should specifically document in the record the discharge instructions provided to the patient and family. For the patient, the postoperative phase of care continues and extends into the recuperative period. Assessment and evaluation of the patient after discharge may be accomplished by a follow-up call or by a visit from a community-based nurse.

Increasingly, patients with many medical or surgical needs are being discharged from hospital. They may be transferred to transitional care facilities, to long-term care facilities, or directly to their homes (see Chapter 6). When discharged directly to home, it is expected that the patient, with assistance from family, friends, or home health care services, will continue self-care in the home. This may include dressing changes, wound care, catheter or drain care, home antibiotics, or continued physical therapy. Working through the discharge planner for the hospital unit or through the case manager, the nurse can facilitate the transition of care from hospital-based to community-based care without jeopardizing the quality of care.

INFORMATICS IN PRACTICE

Discharge Teaching

If the nurse is discharging a patient who requires a complex dressing change and thinks that written instructions are not adequate, the nurse should consider using a video either on the hospital's television system or from the Internet (e.g., YouTube) or creating a patient-specific video. If using a video from the Internet, the nurse should check it first to ensure that the procedure is properly done. The nurse could also take a series of pictures that demonstrate how to perform the procedure. The patient and caregiver can view the video or pictures at home as a reference when performing the procedure.

AGE-RELATED CONSIDERATIONS

PATIENT AFTER SURGERY

Aging is a chronological, functional, and physiological process, and all these factors must be considered when determining the postoperative needs of the older patient. The nurse should understand that normal aging and chronic disease can affect surgical outcomes (Allen, 2019). The older person has decreased respiratory function and ability to cough, due to reduced thoracic compliance. These alterations in pulmonary status increase the work of ventilation and decrease the ability to eliminate some pharmacological agents. Reactions to anaesthetic agents must be carefully monitored and their postoperative elimination assessed before the patient is left without close supervision. Pneumonia is a common postoperative complication in older persons.

Vascular function in the older person is altered because of atherosclerosis and decreased elasticity in the blood vessels. Cardiac function is often compromised, and compensatory responses to changes in BP and fluid volume are limited. Circulating blood volume is decreased, and hypertension is common. Cardiovascular parameters must be closely monitored throughout surgery and the postoperative period.

Drug toxicity is a potential concern in the older person as renal perfusion decreases, thus reducing elimination of medications excreted by the kidney. Decreased liver function also leads to decreased medication metabolism and thus increased medication activity. Renal and liver function must be carefully assessed in the postoperative phase of the patient's care to prevent medication overdose and toxicity.

Observing for changes in mental status is an important part of postoperative care in older persons. Predisposing factors for postoperative delirium in this population include such things as age greater than 80 years, alcohol misuse, lower education level, polypharmacy, sensory impairments, low mobility, and major surgery. Anaesthetics, notably anticholinergic medications and benzodiazepines, increase the risk for delirium. One way for the nurse to lessen delirium is to ensure adequate postoperative pain control (Allen, 2019). An acute change in mental status can have a potentially reversible cause, such as an infection or an adverse effect of analgesic medication. (Dementia and delirium are discussed in Chapter 62.)

Pain is a multidimensional experience, and assessment should include how pain affects function, mood, activities, and quality of life. Older patients are at great risk for undertreated pain. They may be hesitant to request pain medication, believing that pain is an inevitable consequence of surgery and that acknowledging it is a sign of weakness. Nurses must be alert to nonverbal indications of pain and should also assess pain using a standardized scale that is explained to the patient each time it is used. The presence of postoperative pain should always be assumed in the cognitively impaired patient who cannot reliably respond (Allen, 2019). Surgery will usually result in pain, and, if untreated, pain could have a negative effect on recovery. (Pain is discussed in Chapter 10.)

A comprehensive, interprofessional approach is recommended when caring for older persons, and all health care personnel delivering geriatric care must be educated in it and be competent. When older people undergo surgery, nurses have the opportunity to enhance outcomes and improve the patient's quality of life (Allen, 2019).

CASE STUDY

Patient After Surgery

Patient Profile

E. L. (pronouns he/him), a 74-year-old retired university professor, has just undergone surgery for a fractured hip. He fell off a ladder while painting the family house. E. L.'s medical history includes type 2 diabetes mellitus and chronic obstructive pulmonary disease (COPD). The surgery performed while the patient was under general anaesthesia lasted 3 hours.

Subjective Data

- Walks 30 to 50 km/wk
- Smokes one pack of cigarettes per day × 58 years
- Has always had problems sleeping
- Has difficulty hearing; wears hearing aid
- Is upset with injury and its impact on his life
- Is a widower and has no relatives or friends nearby who are able to assist with care
- Reports pain is 8 on a 0-to-10 scale on arrival to PACU

Objective Data

- Admitted to PACU with abduction pillow between the legs, one peripheral IV catheter, a self-suction drain from the hip dressing, an in-dwelling urinary catheter
- Oxygen (O_2) saturation 91% on 40% O_2 face mask

Interprofessional Care
Postoperative Orders

- Vital signs per PACU routine
- Capillary blood glucose level on arrival and every 4 hours: Call for blood glucose level <3.9 mmol/L to >13.9 mmol/L; follow employer policy for management of hypoglycemia
- 0.45% normal saline at 100 mL/hr
- Morphine via patient-controlled analgesia 1 mg q10min (20 mg max in 4 hr) for pain
- Advance diet as tolerated
- Incentive spirometry q1hr × 10 while awake
- O_2 therapy to keep O_2 saturation >90%
- Respiratory: Ventolin 2.5 mg via nebulizer every 4 hours PRN for wheezing
- Neurovascular checks q1hr × 4 hr
- Empty and measure self-suction drain every shift
- Strict intake and output

Discussion Questions

1. What are the potential postanaesthesia complications for E. L.?
2. **Priority decision:** What priority nursing interventions would be appropriate to prevent these complications from occurring?
3. What factors may predispose E. L. to the following conditions: atelectasis, infection, pulmonary embolism, and nausea and vomiting?
4. What criteria would determine when E. L. is sufficiently recovered from general anaesthesia to be discharged to the clinical unit?
5. What potential postoperative issues on the clinical unit might be expected?
6. **Priority decision:** Based on the assessment data presented, what are two priority nursing diagnoses? Are there any interprofessional issues?

⊝volve
Answers are available at http://evolve.elsevier.com/Canada/Lewis/medsurg/.

REVIEW QUESTIONS

The number of the question corresponds to the same-numbered objective at the beginning of the chapter.

1. When a client is admitted to the PACU, what are the *priority* interventions the nurse performs?
   a. Assess the surgical site, noting presence and character of drainage.
   b. Assess the amount of urine output and the presence of bladder distension.
   c. Assess for airway patency and quality of respirations and obtain vital signs.
   d. Review results of intraoperative laboratory values and medications received.

2. A client is admitted to the PACU after major abdominal surgery. During the initial assessment, the client states, "I am going to throw up." What would be the *priority* nursing intervention?
   a. Increase the rate of the IV fluids.
   b. Obtain vital signs, including O₂ saturation.
   c. Position client in lateral recovery position.
   d. Administer antiemetic medication as ordered.

3. After admission of the postoperative client to the clinical unit, which assessment data require the *most* immediate attention?
   a. O₂ saturation of 85%
   b. Respiratory rate of 13/min
   c. Temperature of 38°C
   d. Blood pressure of 90/60 mm Hg

4. A 70-kg postoperative client has an average urine output of 25 mL/hr during the first 8 hours. Given this assessment, what would the *priority* nursing intervention(s) be?
   a. Perform a straight catheterization to measure the amount of urine in the bladder.
   b. Notify the physician and anticipate obtaining blood work to evaluate renal function.
   c. Continue to monitor the client because this is a normal finding during this time period.
   d. Evaluate the client's fluid volume status since surgery and obtain a bladder ultrasound.

5. The nurse on the postoperative unit is caring for a client who had a laparoscopic partial colectomy. On postoperative day 2, the client reports abdominal distension and discomfort. Which of the following interventions may be appropriate for this client? (*Select all that apply.*)
   a. Increase the dose of opioids for pain relief.
   b. Insert a nasogastric tube.
   c. Reassure the client that this complication should subside in a day or two.
   d. Monitor the client's abdominal girth by measuring for distension and auscultate the abdomen in all four quadrants.

6. Discharge criteria for the phase II client include which of the following? (*Select all that apply.*)
   a. No nausea or vomiting
   b. Ability to drive themselves home
   c. No respiratory depression
   d. Written discharge instructions understood
   e. Opioid pain medication given 45 minutes ago

1. c, 2. c, 3. a, 4. d, 5. b, c, d, 6. c, d, e.

Ⓔvolve

For even more review questions, see the website for this book at http://evolve.elsevier.com/Canada/Lewis/medsurg.

REFERENCES

Allen, S. (2019). Geriatric surgery. In J. Rothrock & D. McEwen (Eds.), *Alexander's care of the patient in surgery* (16th ed., pp. 1069–1090). Elsevier.

Bak, J. (2019). Wound healing, dressings, and drains. In J. Rothrock & D. McEwen (Eds.), *Alexander's care of the patient in surgery* (16th ed., pp. 244–260). Elsevier.

Cagir, B. (2018). *Postoperative ileus*. https://emedicine.medscape.com/article/2242141-treatment

Canadian Association of Wound Care and Canadian Association for Enterostomal Therapy. (2011). *The Wound CARE Instrument: Collaborative Appraisal and Recommendations for Education.* https://www.woundscanada.ca/docman/public/health-care-professional/551-wound-care-instrument-1/file

Canadian Patient Safety Institute. (2020). *Surgical site infection (SSI): Getting started kit.* https://www.patientsafetyinstitute.ca/en/toolsResources/Pages/SSI-resources-Getting-Started-Kit.aspx

Cuming, R. (2019). Concepts basic to perioperative nursing. In J. Rothrock & D. McEwen (Eds.), *Alexander's care of the patient in surgery* (16th ed., pp. 1–13). Elsevier.

DeVolder, B. (2019). Gastrointestinal surgery. In J. Rothrock & D. McEwen (Eds.), *Alexander's care of the patient in surgery* (16th ed., pp. 287–340). Elsevier.

Dowsett, C., & von Hallern, B. (2017). The triangle of wound assessment: A holistic framework from wound assessment to management goals and treatments. *Wounds International 2017, 8*(4), 34–39.

King, C., & Spry, C. (2019). Infection prevention and control. In J. Rothrock & D. McEwen (Eds.), *Alexander's care of the patient in surgery* (16th ed., pp. 54–105). Elsevier.

Nurses Specialized in Wound, Ostomy and Continence Canada. (2020). *The power of 3*. https://nswoc.ca/powerof3/

Odom-Forren, J. (2019). Postoperative pain care and pain management. In J. Rothrock & D. McEwen (Ed.), *Alexander's care of the patient in surgery* (16th ed., pp. 261–285). Elsevier.

Odom-Forren, J., & Brady, J. (2018). Postanesthesia recovery. In J. Nagelhout & S. Elisha (Eds.), *Nurse anesthesia* (6th ed., pp. 1147–1166). Elsevier.

Peng, L., & Anker, A. (2020). *Outpatient surgery instructions, types of anesthesia, risks and complications.* https://www.emedicinehealth.com/outpatient_surgery/article_em.htm#what_is_outpatient_surgery

Peterson, C. (2018). The hepatobiliary and gastrointestinal system. In J. Odom-Forren (Ed.), *Drain's perianesthesia nursing: A critical care approach* (7th ed., pp. 221–226). Elsevier.

Registered Nurses' Association of Ontario. (2016). *Delirium, dementia and depression in older adults: Assessment and care* (2nd ed.). https://rnao.ca/bpg/guidelines/screening-delirium-dementia-and-depression-older-adult

Smith, C. (2019). Workplace issues and staff safety. In J. Rothrock & D. McEwen (Eds.), *Alexander's care of the patient in surgery* (16th ed., pp. 38–53). Elsevier.

Wang, L., Xu, D., Wei, X., et al. (2016). Electrolyte disorders and aging: Risk factors for delirium in patients undergoing orthopedic surgeries. *BMC Psychiatry, 16*, 418. https://doi.org/10.1186/s12888-016-1130-0

RESOURCES

Canadian Allergy, Asthma, and Immunology Foundation
https://www.allergyfoundation.ca
Canadian Anesthesiologists' Society
https://www.cas.ca
Canadian Pain Society
https://www.canadianpainsociety.ca
National Association of PeriAnesthesia Nurses of Canada
http://www.napanc.org

Operating Room Nurses Association of Canada
http://www.ornac.ca
Registered Nurses' Association of Ontario
https://rnao.ca
Wounds Canada
https://www.woundscanada.ca

evolve

For additional Internet resources, see the website for this book at http://evolve.elsevier.com/Canada/Lewis/medsurg.

Conditions Related to Altered Sensory Input

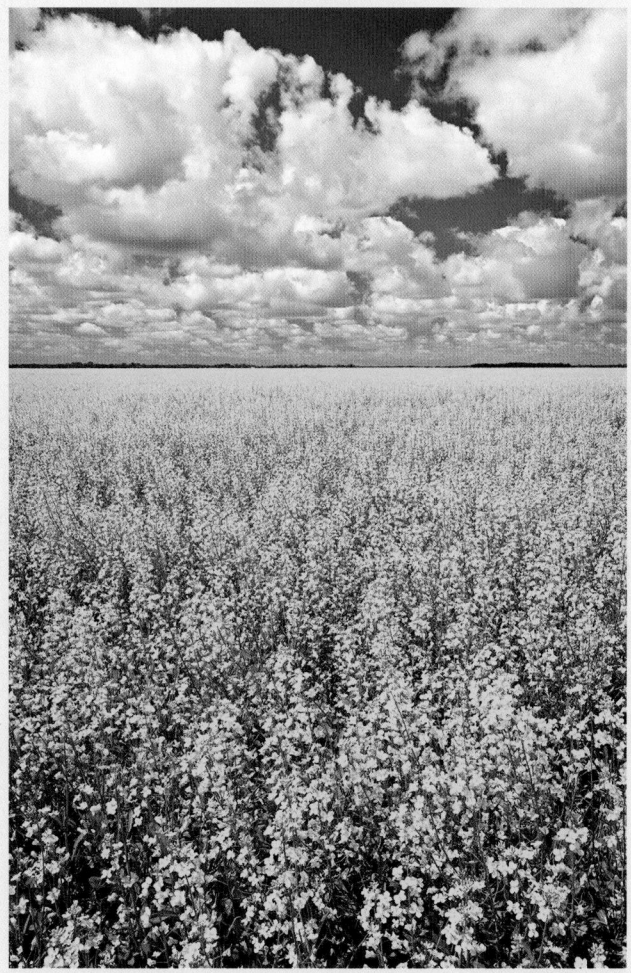

Source: © CanStock Photo/Elenathewise

Nursing Assessment

Visual and Auditory Systems

Marian Luctkar-Flude
Originating US chapter by Jonel L. Gomez and Mariann M. Harding

⊖volve WEBSITE

http://evolve.elsevier.com/Canada/Lewis/medsurg

- Review Questions (Online Only)
- Key Points
- Answer Guidelines for Case Study
- Conceptual Care Map Creator

- Audio Glossary
- Supporting Media—Animation
  - Weber Test
- Content Updates

LEARNING OBJECTIVES

1. Describe the structures and functions of the visual and auditory systems.
2. Describe the physiological processes involved in normal vision and hearing.
3. Identify the significant subjective and objective assessment data related to the visual and auditory systems that should be obtained from the patient.
4. Describe the appropriate techniques used in the physical assessment of the visual and auditory systems.

5. Differentiate normal from common abnormal findings of a physical assessment of the visual and auditory systems.
6. Explain how age-related changes in the visual and auditory systems correspond to differences in assessment findings.
7. Describe the purpose, the significance of results, and the nursing responsibilities related to diagnostic studies of the visual and auditory systems.

KEY TERMS

accommodation	myopia	retina
aqueous humor	nystagmus	sclera
astigmatism	PERRLA	tinnitus
conjunctiva	posterior cavity	vertigo
hyperopia	presbycusis	vitreous humor
lens	presbyopia	

THE VISUAL SYSTEM

STRUCTURES AND FUNCTIONS

The visual system consists of the external tissues and structures surrounding the eye, the external and internal structures of the eye, the refractive media, and the visual pathway. The external structures are the eyebrows, eyelids, eyelashes, lacrimal system, conjunctiva, cornea, sclera, and extraocular muscles. The internal structures are the iris, lens, ciliary body, choroid, and retina. The entire visual system is important for visual function. Light reflected from an object in the field of vision passes through the transparent structures of the eye and, in doing so, is *refracted*

(bent) so that a clear image can fall on the retina. From the retina, the visual stimuli travel through the visual pathway to the occipital cortex, where they are perceived as an image.

Structures and Functions of Vision

Eyeball. The eyeball, or globe, is composed of three layers (Figure 23.1). The tough outer layer is composed of the sclera and the transparent cornea. The middle layer consists of the uveal tract (iris, choroid, and ciliary body). The innermost layer is the retina. The anterior chamber lies between the iris and the posterior surface of the cornea, whereas the posterior chamber lies between the anterior surface of the lens and the posterior

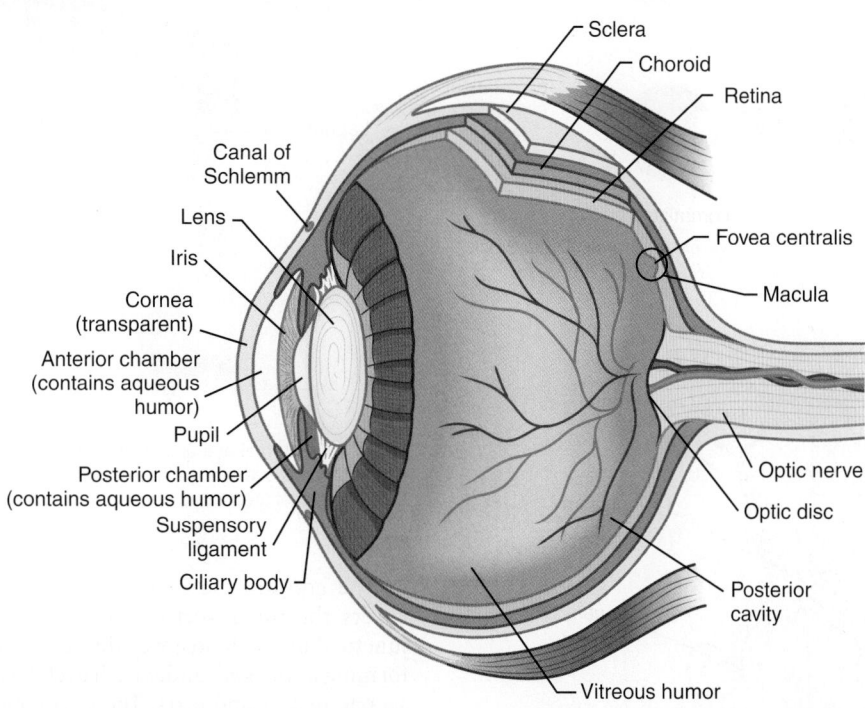

FIG. 23.1 The human eye. Source: Adapted from Patton, K. T., & Thibodeau, G. A. (2013). *Anatomy and physiology* (8th ed., p. 527). Mosby.

surface of the iris. The posterior cavity (vitreous cavity) lies between the posterior lens and the retina.

Refractive Media. For light to reach the retina, it must pass through several structures: the cornea, the aqueous humor, the lens, and the vitreous humor. All these structures must remain clear for light to reach the retina and stimulate the photoreceptor cells. The cornea, which is normally transparent, is the first structure through which light passes. It is responsible for most of the light refraction necessary for clear vision.

Aqueous humor, produced by the ciliary process, is a clear, watery fluid that fills the anterior and posterior chambers of the anterior cavity of the eye. It bathes and nourishes the lens and the endothelium of the cornea. It drains through the trabecular meshwork located in the angle. This circular canal conveys fluid into scleral veins, which enter the circulation of the body. Normal intraocular pressure is between 10 and 21 mm Hg; excess production or decreased outflow of the aqueous humor can cause an elevation in this pressure, a condition termed *glaucoma.*

The lens is a biconvex structure located behind the iris and supported in place by small fibres collectively called the *suspensory ligament* (also called the *zonule*) that connect the lens to the ciliary body. The primary function of the lens is to bend light rays, which enables them to fall onto the retina. Anything altering the clarity of the lens affects light transmission.

The vitreous humor is located in the posterior (vitreous) cavity (see Figure 23.1). Light passing through the vitreous humor may be blocked by any nontransparent substance within, such as the cellular debris (often called *floaters*). The effect on vision varies, depending on the amount, type, and location of the substance blocking the light.

Refractive Errors. *Refraction* is the ability of the eye to bend light rays so that they fall on the retina (Figure 23.2). In the normal eye, parallel light rays are focused through the lens into a sharp image on the retina. The state that enables this process is termed *emmetropia,* which means that light is focused exactly on the retina, not in front of it or behind it. The condition in which the light does not focus properly is called a *refractive error.*

The individual with myopia can see near objects clearly *(nearsightedness),* but objects in the distance appear blurred. The individual with hyperopia can see distant objects clearly *(farsightedness),* but near objects appear blurred. Astigmatism is an imperfection in the curvature of the cornea or in the shape of the eye's lens that causes blurred or distorted vision for both near and far objects. Presbyopia is a normal aging change in which the lens of the eye loses its elasticity and flexibility, resulting in an inability to focus on close objects, usually beginning at approximately age 40.

Visual Pathways. Once the image travels through the refractive media, it is focused on the retina, inverted, and reversed left to right. For example, if the visualized object is in the upper part of the left temporal visual field, it is focused in the lower part of the nasal retina, upside down, and as a mirror image. From the retina, the impulses travel through the optic nerve to the optic chiasm, where the nasal fibres of each eye cross over to the other side. The optic chiasm is the X-shaped space just in front of the pituitary gland where the optic nerve fibres partially cross. Fibres from the left field of both eyes form the left optic tract and travel to the left occipital cortex. The fibres from the right field of both eyes form the right optic

VISION DISORDERS

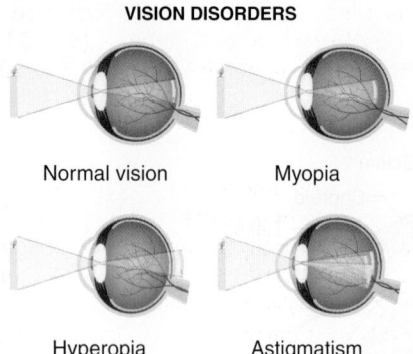

Normal vision   Myopia

Hyperopia   Astigmatism

FIG. 23.2 Vision disorders related to refractive error. Source: © CanStock Photo Inc. / Neokryuger.

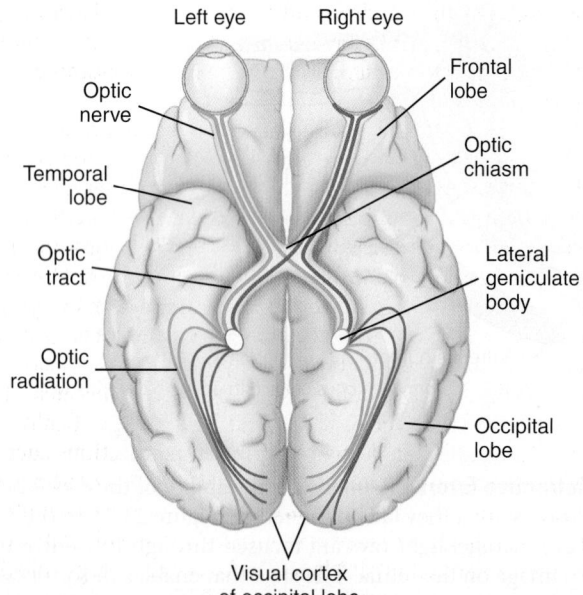

FIG. 23.3 The visual pathway. Fibres from the nasal portion of each retina cross over to the opposite side of the optic chiasm, terminating in the lateral geniculate body of the opposite side. The location of a lesion in the visual pathway determines the resulting visual defect.

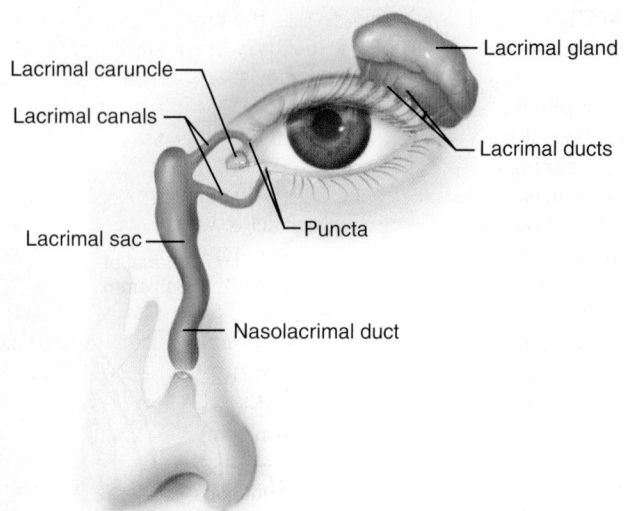

FIG. 23.4 External eye and lacrimal apparatus. Tears produced in the lacrimal gland pass over the surface of the eye and enter the lacrimal canal. From there, the tears are carried through the nasolacrimal duct to the nasal cavity.

tract and travel to the right occipital cortex. Because of this arrangement of the nerve fibres in the visual pathways, it is possible to determine the anatomical location of abnormalities in those nerve fibres from the specific visual field defect (Figure 23.3).

External Structures and Functions

Eyebrows, Eyelids, and Eyelashes. Eyebrows, eyelids, and eyelashes serve an important role in protecting the eye. They provide a physical barrier to dust and foreign particles. The eye is further protected by the surrounding bony orbit and by fat pads located below and behind the globe, or eyeball.

The upper and lower eyelids join at the medial and lateral canthi. The upper eyelid blinks spontaneously approximately 15 times a minute. Blinking distributes tears over the anterior surface of the eyeball and helps control the amount of light entering the visual pathway (Figure 23.4).

The eyelids open and close through the action of muscles innervated by cranial nerve (CN) VII, which is the facial nerve. Muscular action also helps hold the eyelids against the eyeball.

The **conjunctiva** is a transparent mucous membrane that covers the inner surfaces of the eyelids (the palpebral conjunctiva) and extends over the **sclera** (the bulbar conjunctiva), forming a "pocket" under each eyelid. Glands in the conjunctiva secrete mucus and tears. The sclera, an opaque structure commonly referred to as the "white" of the eye, is formed by collagen fibres meshed together. The sclera forms a tough shell that helps protect the intraocular structures.

The transparent and avascular cornea allows light to enter the eye (see Figure 23.1). The curved cornea refracts (bends) incoming light rays to help focus them on the retina. The cornea consists of six layers: the epithelium, Bowman's layer, the stroma, Dua's layer, Descemet's membrane, and the endothelium (Vargas et al., 2019). The epithelium consists of a layer of cells that helps protect the eye. Epithelial cells regenerate when damaged. The stroma consists of collagen fibrils. The cornea is maintained by the lacrimal system, which consists of the lacrimal gland and ducts, the lacrimal canals and puncta, the lacrimal sac, and the nasolacrimal duct (see Figure 23.4). In addition to the lacrimal gland, other glands provide secretions to make up the mucous, aqueous, and lipid layers of the tear film. The tear film moistens the eye and provides oxygen to the cornea.

Each eye is moved by three pairs of extraocular muscles and controlled by three cranial nerves: (a) superior and inferior rectus muscles (CN III), (b) medial (CN III) and lateral rectus muscles (CN VI), and (c) superior (CN IV) and inferior oblique muscles (CN III). Neuromuscular coordination enables simultaneous movement of the eyes in the same direction (conjugate movement).

Internal Structures and Functions

The iris (plural: *irides*) is the colourful part of the eye. This structure has a small, round opening in its centre, the pupil, which allows light to enter the eye. The pupil constricts through action of the iris sphincter muscle (innervated by CN III [oculomotor nerve]) and dilates through action of the iris dilator muscle (innervated by CN V [trigeminal nerve]) to control the amount of light that enters the eye.

The lens is a structure behind the iris whose function is to bend light rays so that they fall onto the retina. The shape of the lens is modified by action of the ciliary body as part of **accommodation**, the convergence of the eyes and the constriction of the pupils that occurs when the eyes refocus from a far object to a near object. This enables a person to focus on near objects, as in reading a book. The choroid is a highly vascular structure that nourishes the ciliary body, the iris, and the outer portion of the retina. It lies inside and parallel to the sclera and extends from the area where the optic nerve enters the eye to the ciliary body (see Figure 23.1). The ciliary body consists of the ciliary muscles, which surround the lens and lie parallel to the sclera; the ciliary zonules, which attach to the lens capsule; and the ciliary processes, which constitute the terminal portion of the ciliary body. The ciliary processes lie behind the peripheral part of the iris and secrete aqueous humor.

The **retina** is the innermost layer of the eye that extends and gives rise to the optic nerve. Neurons make up the major portion of the retina. Therefore, retinal cells cannot regenerate if destroyed. The retina lines the inside the eyeball, extending from the area of the optic nerve to the ciliary body (see Figure 23.1). It is responsible for converting images into a form that the brain can understand and process as vision. The retina is composed of two types of photoreceptor cells: rods and cones. *Rods* are stimulated in dim or darkened environments, and *cones* are receptive to colours in bright environments. The centre of the retina is the *fovea centralis,* a pinpoint depression composed only of densely packed cones (Patton & Thibodeau, 2020). This area of the retina provides the sharpest visual acuity. Surrounding the fovea is the *macula,* an area smaller than 1 square millimetre, which has a high concentration of cones and is relatively free of blood vessels. With the exception of the macula, the retina is nourished by retinal arterioles and veins. This blood supply enters the eye through the optic disc, located nasally from the macula. The *optic disc* is the area where the optic nerve (CN II) exits the eyeball. Within the disc is the *physiological cup*, a depression that can be visualized through the pupil with the ophthalmoscope. The retinal veins and arteries can also be visualized in this way and can provide information about the condition of the vascular system in general.

AGE-RELATED CONSIDERATIONS

THE VISUAL SYSTEM

Every structure of the visual system is subject to changes as the individual ages. Whereas many of these changes are relatively benign, others may compromise visual acuity severely in the older person. The psychosocial effect of poor vision or blindness can be highly significant. Visual impairment increases with age, ranging from 2.7% in those 45 to 54 years old to 15.6% in those 75 to 84 years old (Aljied et al., 2018). Age-related changes in the visual system and differences in assessment findings are presented in Table 23.1. Refractive error is the leading cause of visual impairment among Canadians over the age of 45 years (Aljied et al., 2018).

ASSESSMENT

Assessment of the visual system may be as simple as determining a patient's visual acuity (clarity or sharpness) or as complex as collecting complete subjective and objective data pertinent to the visual system. To perform an appropriate ophthalmic evaluation, the nurse must determine which parts of the data collection are important for each patient. Table 23.2 lists suggested questions to ask to obtain subjective data related to the visual system.

Subjective Data

Past Health History. Information about the patient's health history should include both ocular and nonocular history. The nurse should ask specifically about systemic diseases—such as diabetes mellitus, hypertension, cancer, rheumatoid arthritis, sexually transmitted infections, acquired immune deficiency syndrome (AIDS), muscular dystrophy, myasthenia gravis, multiple sclerosis, inflammatory bowel disease, and hypothyroidism or hyperthyroidism—because many of these diseases have ocular manifestations. It is particularly important to determine whether the patient has any history of cardiac or pulmonary disease because the eye drops often used to treat glaucoma (β-adrenergic blockers) may have serious adverse effects, including bronchospasm, hypotension, and heart failure (Skidmore-Roth & Richardson, 2021).

Medications. If the patient takes any medications, the nurse should obtain a complete list, including over-the-counter medicines, eye drops, herbal therapies, or dietary supplements. Many patients do not think that over-the-counter medications, eye drops, or herbal therapies are "real" medications and may not mention their use unless specifically questioned. However, many of them have ocular effects. For example, many preparations for colds contain a form of epinephrine (e.g., pseudoephedrine) that can dilate the pupil. The nurse should also note the use of any antihistamines or decongestants because they can cause ocular dryness. The nurse should specifically ask whether the patient uses any prescription medications such as corticosteroids, thyroid medications, oral hypoglycemic agents, or insulin. Long-term use of corticosteroids can contribute to development of glaucoma or cataracts. It is especially important to note whether the patient is taking any β-adrenergic blocker eye drops because they may potentiate the effects of corticosteroids. The nurse should ask female patients whether they are taking birth control pills, are pregnant, or are experiencing perimenopause or menopause, because hormonal changes can affect the wearing of contact lenses. Finally, the nurse should determine whether the patient has allergies to medications or other substances, such as dust, pollens, pets, cosmetics, or scents.

Surgery or Other Treatments. Surgical procedures related to the head, eye, or brain should be noted. Brain surgery and subsequent swelling can cause pressure on the optic nerve or tract, which results in alterations in vision. Any laser procedures involving the eye should also be documented, as should the effect of any eye surgery or laser treatment on visual acuity. The nurse should ask the patient about previous trauma to the head. Also, inquiring about headaches is important because migraines may create visual disturbances.

A history of visual acuity tests should be obtained, including the date of the most recent examination and change in glasses or contact lens prescriptions, as well as testing for glaucoma and the results. The nurse should specifically ask about a history of strabismus, amblyopia, cataracts, retinal detachment, refractive surgery, glaucoma, and any trauma to the eye, its treatment, and sequelae.

The patient's dietary intake of vitamins and trace minerals can be important to ocular health. Antioxidants found in

TABLE 23.1   AGE-RELATED DIFFERENCES IN ASSESSMENT

Visual System

Changes	Differences in Assessment Findings
Eyebrows and Eyelashes	
Loss of pigment in the hair	Greying of eyebrows, eyelashes
Eyelids	
Loss of orbital fat, decreased muscle tone	Entropion (eyelid turned inwards), ectropion (eyelid turned outwards), mild ptosis (eyelid drooping)
Tissue atrophy, prolapse of fat into eyelid tissue	Blepharodermachalasis (excessive upper eyelid skin)
Plaques	Xanthelasma
Conjunctiva	
Tissue damage related to chronic exposure to ultraviolet light or to other chronic environmental exposure	Pinguecula (small, yellowish spot seen usually on the medial aspect of the conjunctiva)
Sclera	
Lipid deposition	Yellowish (as opposed to bluish) scleral colour
Cornea	
Cholesterol deposits in peripheral cornea	Arcus senilis (milky or yellow ring encircling periphery of cornea; see Figure 23.1)
Tissue damage related to chronic exposure	Pterygium (thickened, triangular bit of pale tissue that extends from the inner canthus of the eye to the nasal border of the cornea)
Decrease in water content, atrophy of nerve fibres	Decreased corneal sensitivity and corneal reflex
Epithelial changes	Loss of corneal lustre
Accumulation of lipid deposits	Blurring of vision
Lacrimal Apparatus	
Decreased tear secretion	Dryness
Malposition of the eyelid that results in tears overflowing the eyelid margins instead of draining through the puncta	Tearing, irritated eyes
Iris	
Increased rigidity of iris	Decreased pupil size
Dilator muscle atrophy or weakness	Slower recovery of pupil size after light stimulation
Loss of pigment	Change of iris colour
Shrinking and stiffening of ciliary muscle	Decrease in near vision and accommodation
Lens	
Biochemical changes in lens proteins, oxidative damage, chronic exposure to ultraviolet light	Cataracts
Increased rigidity of lens	Presbyopia
Opacities in the lens (may also be related to opacities in the cornea and the vitreous humor)	Reports of glare, impairment of night vision
Accumulation of yellow substances	Yellow colouring of lens
Retina	
Retinal vascular changes related to atherosclerosis and hypertension	Narrowed, pale, straighter arterioles; acute branching
Decrease in cones	Changes in colour perception, especially blue and violet
Loss of photoreceptor cells, retinal pigment, epithelial cells, and melanin	Decreased visual acuity
Age-related macular degeneration as a result of vascular changes	Loss of central vision
Vitreous Humor	
Liquefaction and detachment of the vitreous humor	Increased reports of "floaters" or light flashes

fruits and vegetables including anthocyanins, carotenoids, flavonoids, and vitamins have been shown to reduce the risk of eye-related diseases. Supplementation with vitamins C and E, minerals selenium and zinc, and the phytochemicals lutein and zeaxanthin has been reported in some studies to help delay the progression of eye diseases such as age-related macular degeneration, whereas other studies reported negative findings (Khoo et al., 2019). (See the Determinants of Health box later in this section.)

For a patient who has undergone or will undergo ophthalmological surgical procedures, the nurse should assess the patient's elimination pattern and determine the potential for constipation, as straining to defecate (the Valsalva manoeuvre) can raise intraocular pressure. Although there is some evidence that elevation of the intraocular pressure during normal activities is not detrimental in relation to the surgical incision made during eye surgery, many surgeons do not want such patients to strain.

Social and Occupational Health History. The patient's socioeconomic status can impact their vision health. Lower education and income levels are associated with a higher prevalence of visual impairment (Aljied et al., 2018). The patient's ability to maintain necessary or desired roles and responsibilities in home, work, and social environments can also be negatively affected by vision problems. For example, macular degeneration may decrease the patient's visual acuity to a level inadequate for functioning at work.

Issues related to Indigenous eye health and care for Indigenous people include high rates of diabetes mellitus and other chronic illnesses, as well as inequity in the social

TABLE 23.2 HEALTH HISTORY

Visual System: Questions for Obtaining Subjective Data

Vision Difficulty
- Do you have any visual difficulties or change in your visual acuity?* Describe the change in your vision. Describe how this affects your daily life.
- Did it come on slowly or progress slowly? Does it affect one or both eyes? Is it constant or intermittent? Do you see spots or floaters move in front of your eyes?* Do you see light flashes?*
- Do you have a blind spot?* Do you have any night blindness?*
- For older persons: Are you experiencing any visual difficulties when you climb stairs or drive at night?
- Do you use any visual aids such as glasses or contact lenses?

Eye Pain
- Do you have any eye pain?*

Strabismus or Diplopia
- Have you ever had a history of crossed eyes, or do you have double vision?*

Redness or Swelling
- Do you have redness or swelling in your eyes?*
- Do you have any discharge or watering from your eyes?*

Family History
- Do you have a family or personal history of diseases such as atherosclerosis, diabetes mellitus, thyroid disease, hypertension, arthritis, or cancer that might affect your eyes?*
- Do you have a family or personal history of ocular conditions such as cataracts, tumours, glaucoma, refractive errors (especially myopia and hyperopia), or retinal degenerative conditions (e.g., macular degeneration, retinal detachment, retinitis pigmentosa)?*

Nutrition and Elimination
- Do you take any nutritional supplements?*
- Does your visual problem affect your ability to obtain and prepare food?*
- Do you have to strain to void or defecate?*

Sleep
- Is your vision affected by the amount of sleep you get?*
- Is your sleep affected by your eye condition?*

Reproduction–Sexuality
- Has your eye condition caused a change in your sex life?*
- For women: Are you pregnant? Do you use birth control pills?

Self-Care History
- Do you have regular eye examinations? When was your last test?
- Do you wear glasses or contact lenses? When was the last time your eye prescription was checked? Was it changed?
- Have you ever been tested for colour vision?*
- Do you wear protective eyewear (sunglasses, safety goggles, or hats)?*
- Do you wear contact lenses? If so, how do you take care of them?
- If you use eye drops, how do you instill them?
- Do you spend long periods of time in the sun?* Do you wear sunglasses?
- Do you smoke, or are you regularly exposed to second-hand smoke?
- Have you ever been tested for glaucoma?* Results?

Social and Occupational History
- Do you have any difficulties at work or home because of your eyes?*
- Does your eye condition affect your ability to read?*
- Have you made any changes in your social activities because of your eyes?*
- Are your activities limited in any way by your eye condition?*
- Are there any environmental conditions at home or work that may have an effect on your eyes (e.g., smoke, dust, chemicals, flying sparks)?* If so, do you use goggles for eye protection?
- Do you participate in any leisure activities that have the potential for eye injury?*
- Do you work for long hours at the computer?*

Coping Abilities
- How does your eye condition make you feel about yourself? Has it created stress for you?*
- If you have a vision loss, how do you cope?* Are you able to maintain your same living environment?* Do you use large-print books or Braille?*

Adapted from Jarvis, C., Browne, A. J., MacDonald-Jenkins, J., et al. (2019). *Physical examination & health assessment* (3rd Canadian ed., pp. 308–310). Elsevier.
*If yes, describe.

CASE STUDY

Patient Introduction

F. A. (pronouns she/her), 81 years old, comes to the emergency department noting that her vision "looks like everything is covered with spider webs."

Critical Thinking

Throughout this assessment chapter, think about F. A. with the following questions in mind:
1. What are possible causes of F. A.'s visual disturbances?
2. What type of assessment should be most appropriate: comprehensive, focused, or emergency?
3. What questions should the nurse ask F. A.?
4. What should be included in the physical assessment? What would the nurse be looking for?
5. What diagnostic studies might be ordered?

See Case Study: Subjective Data and Case Study: Objective Data: Physical Examination for more information on F. A.

Answers available at http://evolve.elsevier.com/Canada/Lewis/medsurg.

Self-Care History

The nurse should assess the patient's ocular health care activities, including regular eye examinations and awareness of the importance of eye safety practices, such as wearing protective eyewear during poten-

tially hazardous activities or while playing sports and avoiding noxious fumes and other eye irritants. Information about the use of sunglasses in bright light should be obtained as prolonged exposure to ultraviolet light can affect the retina and may contribute to cataract formation. Nighttime driving habits and any difficulties encountered in nighttime driving should be noted. For a patient who wears contact lenses, the nurse should assess the patient's use and care habits, which may indicate a need for teaching, as true adherence to proper care has been reported in between 1 and 50% of users (Steele, 2018). Similarly, the nurse should assess the patient's use of and technique for eye drop instillation. The nurse should also ask about time spent working on computers or handheld devices because eye strain is a common problem. The 20-20-20 rule can be promoted: Every 20 minutes, patients should look away from their computer screen for 20 seconds and focus their eyes on something at least 6 metres (20 feet) away (Canadian Association of Optometrists, 2020).

Environmental exposures at home or work can cause trauma or irritation to the eyes; eye protection should be discussed. Patients should be asked whether they smoke or are regularly exposed to second-hand smoke. Smokers are at greater risk for developing age-related macular degeneration (see the Determinants of Health box). If patients use eye drops, the nurse should ascertain whether they are aware of correct methods for instilling drops to avoid contamination of the container.

DETERMINANTS OF HEALTH

Macular Degeneration

Gender
- The incidence of macular degeneration is higher among women than among men. Early-onset menopause can also increase the risk for developing macular degeneration.*

Biology and Genetic Endowment
- The risk of developing macular degeneration increases with a family history (first generation).[†]
- White individuals are more likely to develop macular degeneration than any other ethnic group.[†]
- Vision problems are more common among new immigrants and refugees from developing countries than in the general Canadian population.[‡]

Personal Health Practices and Coping Skills
- Smoking increases the risk of developing macular degeneration fourfold. Smokers also develop the disease approximately 10 years earlier than nonsmokers. Twenty percent of vision loss may be avoided by staying smoke-free.[†]
- Adequate exercise and a healthy diet (leafy vegetables, omega-3 fatty acids) reduces the risk of macular degeneration. Antioxidants and zinc can slow the progression of intermediate and advanced macular degeneration and thereby minimize vision loss.[†]
- Ultraviolet radiation damages the retina, which leads to macular degeneration.[†]

References:
*Jarvis, C., Browne, A. J., MacDonald-Jenkins, J., et al. (Eds.). (2019). *Physical examination & health assessment* (3rd Canadian ed.). Elsevier.
[†]Canadian National Institute for the Blind (CNIB). (2019). *Age-related macular degeneration.* https://cnib.ca/en/sight-loss-info/your-eyes/eye-diseases/age-related-macular-degeneration?region=on
[‡]Grenier, D., & Bailon-Poujol, J. (2018). *Caring for kids new to Canada: Vision screening.* https://www.kidsnewtocanada.ca/screening/vision

determinants of health such as poverty, poor housing, and inadequate diet. The high incidence of diabetes mellitus among Indigenous people contributes to an increased risk of diabetic retinopathy. Indigenous Canadians also face a number of barriers to accessing eye care (Canadian Association of Optometrists, 2018), such as living on reserve, rurally, or remotely, where there is decreased access to eye health care, lack of continuity of care, and lack of rehabilitation services for severe vision loss. Poverty, difficulties accessing eyeglasses, and transportation difficulties may also affect urban Indigenous people.

In many occupations, employees work in conditions in which eye injury may occur. For example, factory workers may be at risk from flying debris; health care workers are at risk from splashes of bodily fluids; and cleaners and laboratory technicians are at risk from chemical burns due to splashes of chemicals or inhalation of noxious vapours. Information should be obtained about eye safety practices, such as use of goggles or safety glasses, and knowledge of prevention and treatment protocols such as eyewash stations. Workers can also be exposed to eyestrain in the office from video display terminals, poor lighting, and glare. An ergonomic consultation may be beneficial.

A patient with diabetes mellitus may not be able to see well enough to self-administer insulin. This patient may resent dependence on a family member who takes over this function. The patient with *exophthalmos* (marked protrusion of eyeballs) may be embarrassed by their appearance and avoid usual social

CASE STUDY

Subjective Data

A focused subjective assessment of F. A. revealed the following information.

Vision Difficulty: Had no vision problems until today. Wears eyeglasses for seeing distances and reading. Now having difficulty reading. Reports seeing periodic light flashes and small white spots "floating" in the air. Denies eye pain, itching, or tearing.

Past Health History: Extraocular extraction of cataract on right eye with implantation of intraocular lens 2 months ago. Type 2 diabetes mellitus and hypertension.

Medications: Glyburide (DiaBeta), 5 mg/day; metoprolol (Lopressor), 50 mg PO daily.

Self-Care History: States adherence to postoperative regimen of antibiotic and corticosteroid eye drops and with office follow-up with eye surgeon. Recovery from surgery was uneventful, and eye drops were discontinued 2 weeks ago. Does not have allergies. Walks in the mall at least 1 km three times a week. No resistance or isotonic exercises. Has had difficulty moving bowels with increased straining. Trying prune juice to help.

Coping Abilities: Afraid she is having a stroke.

See Case Study: Patient Introduction and Case Study: Objective Data: Physical Examination for more information on F. A.

activities. The nurse should sensitively inquire whether the patient's preferred roles and responsibilities have been affected by the ocular condition.

The nurse should also inquire about leisure activities during which the patient may incur an ocular injury. For example, during gardening, woodworking, and other craft activities, foreign bodies can scratch or enter the cornea or conjunctiva or even penetrate the globe. Injuries to the globe or the bony orbit can also occur after blows to the head or eye during sports activities such as racquetball, baseball, and tennis. Other leisure activities such as needlepoint, fly tying, watching television, or playing video games may have high-level visual demands and produce eye strain.

Coping Abilities. Patients with temporary or permanent visual difficulties may experience emotional stress. The nurse should assess the patient's coping strategies and availability of support systems and perform a more comprehensive psychosocial assessment if it is indicated.

Objective Data

Physical Examination. Physical examination of the visual system includes inspecting ocular structures and determining their functional status. Assessment of ocular structures should include examining the ocular adnexa, the external eye, and internal structures. Some structures, such as the retina and blood vessels, must be visualized with the aid of equipment, such as the ophthalmoscope. Physiological functional assessment includes determining the patient's visual acuity and ability to judge closeness and distance, assessing extraocular muscle function, evaluating visual fields, observing pupil function, and measuring intraocular pressure.

Assessment of the visual system may include all of the components described in the following text, or it may be as brief as measuring the patient's visual acuity. The nurse assesses what is appropriate and necessary for the specific patient. All of the following assessments are in the nurse's scope of practice, but some require special training. Normal findings of a physical assessment of the visual system are outlined in Table 23.3. Age-related

TABLE 23.3	NORMAL FINDINGS IN PHYSICAL ASSESSMENT OF THE VISUAL SYSTEM

- Visual acuity: 20/20* in both eyes; no diplopia
- External eye structures: symmetrical and without lesions or deformities
- Lacrimal apparatus: nontender and without drainage
- Conjunctiva: clear; sclera: white
- Pupils: equal, round, and reactive to light and accommodation (PERRLA)
- Lens: clear
- Extraocular movements: intact
- Optic disc margins: sharp
- Retinal vessels: normal, with no hemorrhages or spots

*20/20 means that the person sees at 20 feet what the majority of people can see at 20 feet.

visual changes and differences in assessment findings are listed in Table 23.1. Assessment techniques related to vision are summarized in Table 23.4. Common abnormalities found during assessment are listed in Table 23.5.

The initial observation of the patient can provide information that will help the nurse focus the assessment. A patient with impaired colour vision may dress in clothing with unusual colour combinations. A patient with diplopia may hold their head in a skewed position in an attempt to see a single image. A patient with a corneal abrasion or photophobia may cover their eyes with their hands or wear dark glasses to try to block out room light. The nurse can make a rough estimate of depth perception by extending a hand for the patient to shake.

During the initial observation, the nurse should also observe the overall facial and ophthalmic appearance of the patient. The eyes should be symmetrical and normally positioned on the face. The globes should not have a bulging or sunken appearance.

Assessing Functional Status

Visual Acuity. Before the patient receives any care, the nurse should record the patient's visual acuity. To assess distance visual acuity, the patient sits or stands 6 metres (20 feet) from the Snellen chart with the usual correction (glasses or contact lenses) left in place unless they are used solely for reading. The nurse asks the patient to cover the left eye with an eye spoon and to read through the chart to the smallest line of letters that the patient can possibly discern. The nurse notes the smallest line the patient can read with a maximum of one or two errors. The nurse then asks the patient to cover the right eye, and the process is repeated. At the left of most rows of the Snellen chart is a fraction (e.g., "20/30") in which the numerator represents the distance the patient is from the chart and the denominator represents the distance at which a normal eye could see the letters in the row. For example, a patient with a visual acuity of 20/30 sees at 20 feet what the patient with no vision problems would see at 30 feet. The larger the denominator, the worse the visual acuity. If vision is poorer than 20/30, the patient should be referred to an ophthalmologist or optometrist (Jarvis et al., 2019). *Legal blindness* is defined as the best corrected vision in the better eye of 20/200 or worse. If a patient cannot read letters, the nurse can use an eye chart with pictures, numbers, or symbols, such as the STYCAR graded-balls test, the Sheridan-Gardiner letter-matching test, or the Snellen E chart.

To evaluate visual acuity when the patient is unable to see even the largest letters, the nurse holds up a number of fingers in front of the patient at successively closer distances and asks the patient to count them. If the patient cannot count the fingers, the nurse asks the patient to indicate whether they can see hand motion or light from a penlight in front of their face.

If the patient reports near vision problems, and for all patients 40 years of age or older, the nurse tests near visual acuity. The patient is instructed to hold a Jaeger chart 35 cm (14 inches) from their eyes. The nurse covers the patient's left eye with an eye spoon, asks the patient to read successively smaller lines of print from the chart, and records the visual acuity corresponding to the smallest line of print the patient can read comfortably. The procedure is repeated with the right eye covered. A normal result is 14/14. A result of 14/20 means the person can read at 14 inches what someone with normal vision reads at 20 inches. If a screening card is not available, the nurse can assess near vision acuity by asking the patient to read from a newspaper.

Extraocular Muscle Functions. The nurse observes the corneal light reflex to evaluate for weakness or imbalance of the extraocular muscles. In a darkened room, the nurse asks the patient to look straight ahead while a penlight is shone directly on the cornea. The light reflection should be located in the centre of both corneas as the patient faces the light source.

To assess eye movement, the nurse should hold a finger or object 25 to 30 cm from the patient's nose. The patient is asked to follow the movement of the object or finger with only their eyes through the six cardinal positions of gaze (Figure 23.5). This test can indicate weakness or paralysis in the extraocular muscles or dysfunction in a cranial nerve (oculomotor nerve [CN III], trochlear nerve [CN IV], and abducens nerve [CN VI]).

Pupil Function. To determine pupil function, the nurse inspects the pupils and their reactions to light. Pupil size is noted before reaction to light is checked. Normal pupil size is 3 to 5 mm. Pupils should be equal in size and round and should react briskly to light. With age, pupil size decreases (Jarvis et al., 2019). In a small percentage of the population, pupils are unequal in size (*anisocoria*). Pupils should react to light directly (pupil constricts when a light shines into the eye) and consensually (pupil of one eye constricts when a light shines into the opposite eye). Accommodation should also be present: When the patient looks at a distant object 60 to 90 cm away and then is asked to focus on an object 7 to 8 cm from the nose, the nurse should observe convergence, simultaneous inward movement of both eyes toward each other, and constriction of the pupils. Normal pupil function may be documented as PERRLA (**p**upils **e**qual, **r**ound, **r**eactive to **l**ight and **a**ccommodation).

CASE STUDY

Objective Data: Physical Examination

Physical examination findings of F. A. are as follows: PERRLA. No abnormalities noted on visual examination of external eye structures. EOM (extraocular movement) intact and symmetrical.

Diagnostic Studies

Ophthalmoscopic examination identifies a partial retinal detachment, which is confirmed via ultrasonography.

See Case Study: Patient Introduction and Case Study: Subjective Data for more information on F. A.

TABLE 23.4   NURSING ASSESSMENT
Visual System

Technique	Description	Purpose
Basic Techniques		
Visual acuity testing	Patient reads from Snellen chart at a distance of 6 m (distance vision test) and from Jaeger test type at a distance of 35 cm (near vision test); examiner notes smallest print that patient can read on each chart.	To determine patient's distance and near visual acuity
Confrontation visual field test	Patient faces examiner, covers one eye, fixates on examiner's face, and counts number of fingers that the examiner brings into patient's field of vision.	To determine whether patient has a full field of vision, without obvious scotomas
Pupil function testing	Examiner shines light into patient's pupil and observes pupillary response; each pupil is examined independently; examiner also checks for consensual and accommodative response.	To determine whether patient has normal pupillary response
Extraocular muscle functioning	Patient faces examiner, holds head still, and follows (with eyes only) object that examiner moves through six cardinal positions of gaze. Examiner also tests corneal light reflex.	To determine whether muscles and cranial nerves III, IV, and VI are functioning normally
Colour vision testing	Patient identifies numbers or paths formed by pattern of dots in a series of colour plates.	To determine patient's ability to distinguish colours
Advanced Techniques*		
Tono-Pen tonometry	Covered end of probe gently touches the anaesthetized corneal surface several times; examiner records several readings to obtain a mean intraocular pressure (see Figure 23.7).	To measure intraocular pressure (normal pressure is 10–22 mm Hg)
Ophthalmoscopy	Examiner holds ophthalmoscope close to patient's eye, shining light into back of eye and looking through aperture on ophthalmoscope; examiner adjusts dial to select one of the lenses in ophthalmoscope that produces the desired amount of magnification to inspect ocular fundus.	To observe retina and optic nerve head
Keratometry	Examiner aligns the projection and notes the readings of corneal curvature.	To measure the corneal curvature; often performed before fitting of contact lenses, before refractive surgery, or after corneal transplantation

*Performed by qualified health care provider.

TABLE 23.5   ASSESSMENT ABNORMALITIES
Visual System

Finding	Description	Possible Etiology and Significance
Subjective Data		
Pain	Foreign body sensation	Superficial corneal erosion or abrasion; can result from contact lens wear or trauma or from foreign body in the conjunctiva or cornea
	Severe, deep, throbbing	Anterior uveitis, acute glaucoma, infection; acute glaucoma also associated with nausea, vomiting
Photophobia	Persistent abnormal intolerance to light	Inflammation or infection of cornea or anterior uveal tract (iris and ciliary body), conjunctivitis
Blurred vision	Gradual or sudden inability to see clearly	Refractive errors, corneal opacities, cataracts, migraine aura, retinal changes (detachment, macular degeneration)
Appearance of spots, floaters, or light flashes (photopsias)	Seeing spots, "spider webs," "a curtain," or floaters within the field of vision, or flashes or flickers of light	Most common: liquefaction of the vitreous humor (benign phenomenon); other possible causes include hemorrhage into the vitreous humor, retinal holes, or retinal tears
		Light flashes may occur as the retina is being tugged, torn, or detached.
Dryness	Discomfort, sandy or gritty sensation, irritation, or burning	Decreased tear formation or changes in tear composition because of aging or various systemic diseases
Diplopia	Double vision	Abnormalities of extraocular muscle action related to muscle or cranial nerve abnormality
Glare	Headache, ocular discomfort, reduced visual acuity	Related to corneal inflammation or to opacities in cornea, lens, or vitreous humor that scatter the incoming light; can also result from light scatter around edges of an intraocular lens; worse at night, when pupil is dilated
Objective Data		
Eyelids		
Allergic reactions	Redness, excessive tearing, and itching of eyelid margins	Many possible allergens; associated eye trauma can occur from rubbing itchy eyelids
Hordeolum (stye)	Small, superficial white nodule along eyelid margin	Infection of a sebaceous gland of eyelid; causative organism is usually bacterial (most commonly *Staphylococcus aureus*)
Blepharitis	Redness, swelling, and crusting along eyelid margins	Bacterial invasion of eyelid margins; often chronic

TABLE 23.5 ASSESSMENT ABNORMALITIES

Visual System—cont'd

Finding	Description	Possible Etiology and Significance
Ptosis	Drooping of upper eyelid margin; unilateral or bilateral	Mechanical causes as a result of eyelid tumours or excess skin; myogenic causes such as myasthenia gravis or neurogenic causes
Entropion	Inward turning of upper or lower eyelid margin, unilateral or bilateral	Congenital causes resulting in development abnormalities
Ectropion	Outward turning of lower eyelid margin	Mechanical causes as a result of eyelid tumours, herniated orbital fat, or extravasation of fluid
Conjunctiva		
Conjunctivitis	Redness, swelling of conjunctiva; possibly itching	Bacterial or viral infection; may be allergic response or inflammatory response to chemical exposure; may be the first or only symptom of SARS-CoV-2 infection*
Subconjunctival hemorrhage	Appearance of blood spot on sclera; may be small or can affect entire sclera	Conjunctival blood vessels rupture, leaking blood into the subconjunctival space
Cornea and Sclera		
Corneal abrasion	Localized painful disruption of the epithelial layer of cornea; visualized with fluorescein dye	Trauma; overwear or improper fit of contact lenses
Jaundice	Yellow discoloration† of the entire sclera	Related to liver dysfunction or hemolytic disease
Globe		
Exophthalmos	Protrusion of globe beyond its normal position within bony orbit; sclera often visible above iris when eyelids are open	Intraocular or periorbital tumours; hyperthyroidism; Crouzon's syndrome
Pupil		
Anisocoria	Pupils are unequal (constricted)	Central nervous system disorders; in a small percentage of the population, slight difference in pupil size is normal
Abnormal response to light or accommodation	Pupils respond asymmetrically or abnormally to light stimulus or accommodation	Central nervous system disorders, general anaesthesia
Iris		
Heterochromia	Irides are different colours‡	Congenital causes (Horner's syndrome); acquired causes (chronic iritis, metastatic carcinoma, diffuse iris nevus or melanoma)
Extraocular Muscles		
Strabismus	Deviation of eye position in one or more directions	Overaction or underaction of one or more extraocular muscles
Lens		
Cataract	Opacification of lens; pupil can appear cloudy or white when opacity is visible behind pupil opening	Aging, trauma, diabetes mellitus, long-term systemic corticosteroid therapy
Visual Field Defect		
Peripheral	Partial or complete loss of peripheral vision	Glaucoma; interruption of visual pathway (e.g., tumour); migraine headache
Central	Loss of central vision	Macular disease

*Source: Ozturker, Z. (2021). Conjunctivitis as sole symptom of COVID-19: A case report and review of the literature. *European Journal of Ophthalmology, 31*(2), NP161–NP166. https://doi.org/10.1177/1120672120946287
†Yellow colour is normal after a diagnostic study necessitating intravenous fluorescein injection.
‡Most cases of heterochromia occur by chance and are not associated with any other symptoms or conditions.

Assessing Structures. The visual system is unique because the nurse can directly inspect not only the external structures but also many of the internal structures by using special equipment such as the ophthalmoscope and the slit-lamp microscope, which enables examination of conjunctiva, sclera, cornea, anterior chamber, iris, lens, vitreous humor, and retina under magnification. The *ophthalmoscope,* a hand-held instrument with a light source and magnifying lenses, is held close to the patient's eye to visualize the posterior part of the eye. Little pain or discomfort is associated with these examinations.

Eyebrows, Eyelashes, and Eyelids. All structures should be present, symmetrical, and without deformities, redness, or swelling. Eyelashes extend outward from the eyelid margins. In normal closing, the upper and lower eyelid margins just touch. The lacrimal puncta should be open and positioned properly against the globe. If the sac is inflamed, pressure over the lacrimal sac may cause purulent material to ooze from the puncta.

Conjunctiva and Sclera. The nurse can examine the conjunctiva and sclera at the same time, evaluating colour, smoothness, and presence of any lesions or foreign bodies. The conjunctiva covering the sclera is normally clear, with fine blood vessels visible, more commonly in the periphery.

The sclera is normally white, but its colour may become yellowish in older individuals because of lipid deposition in the sclera. A pale blue cast caused by scleral thinning can also be normal in older persons and in infants (who have naturally

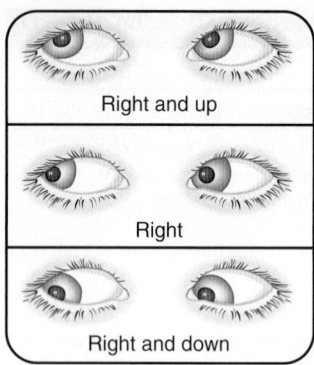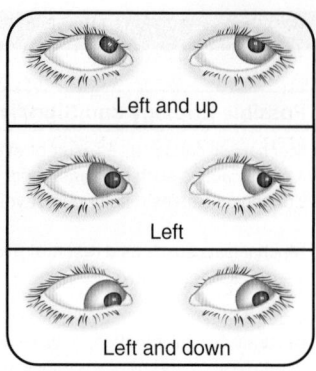

FIG. 23.5 Six cardinal positions of gaze. Source: Adapted from Bowling, B. (2015). *Kanski's clinical ophthalmology: A systematic approach* (8th ed, p. 731). Saunders.

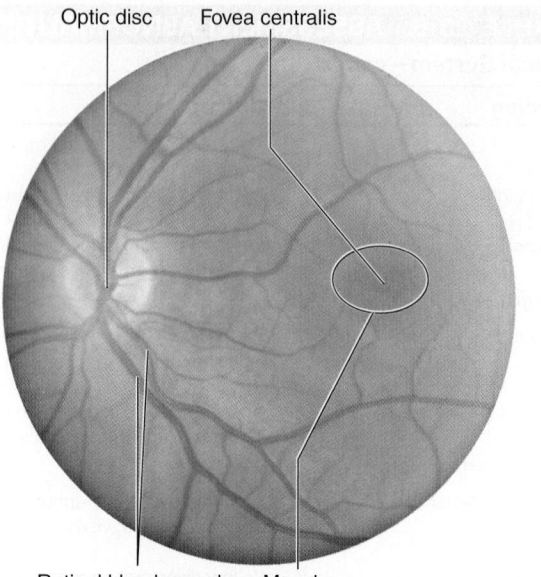

FIG. 23.6 Illustration of magnified view of retina through the ophthalmoscope. Source: Adapted from Patton, K. T., & Thibodeau, G. (2020). *Structure and function of the body* (16th ed., p. 215). Mosby.

thinner sclerae). A slightly yellow cast may also be normal finding in some dark-skinned people.

Cornea. The cornea should be clear, transparent, and shiny. The iris should appear flat and not bulge toward the cornea. The area between the cornea and iris should be clear, with no blood or purulent material visible in the anterior chamber.

Iris. Both irides should be of similar colour and shape. However, a colour difference between the irides is normal in a small proportion of individuals. Round or notched areas of missing iris tissue are often the result of cataract or glaucoma surgery. The nurse should determine the cause of these round, notched, or triangular areas and document the findings.

Retina and Optic Nerve. To assess these structures, the nurse uses an ophthalmoscope to magnify the ocular structures and bring them into crisp focus (Figure 23.6). This enables the examiner to directly view arteries, veins, and the optic nerve. The nurse directs the beam of light from the ophthalmoscope obliquely into the patient's pupils and should note the appearance of a *red reflex*. This reflex is a result of light's reflecting off the retina. Any dense area in the lens or nontransparent material in the vitreous humor decreases the red reflex. The optic nerve or disc is examined for size, colour, and abnormalities. The optic disc is creamy yellow with distinct margins. A slight blurring of the nasal margin is common.

A central depression in the disc, called the *physiological cup*, is the exit site for the optic nerve. The cup should be less than half the diameter of the disc. Normally, no hemorrhages or exudates are present in the fundus (retinal background). Careful inspection of the fundus can reveal the presence of retinal holes, tears, detachments, or lesions. Small hemorrhages can be associated with diabetes mellitus or hypertension and can appear in various shapes, such as dots or flames. Finally, the nurse examines the macula for shape and appearance. This area of high reflectivity is devoid of any blood vessels.

The nurse can obtain important information about the vascular system and the central nervous system through direct visualization with an ophthalmoscope. Skilled use of this instrument requires practice.

Focused Assessment. A focused assessment (see the Focused Assessment box) may be performed by the nurse when a patient is admitted to hospital or an outpatient clinic. Inspection of the eyes may be performed routinely as part of the assessment of a hospitalized patient. In addition, the nurse should assess for and document use of glasses or contact lenses. Assessment for PERRLA may be performed routinely

FOCUSED ASSESSMENT

Visual System

Use this checklist to make sure the key assessment steps have been performed.

Subjective
Ask the patient about any of the following and note responses.

Changes in vision (e.g., acuity, blurred)	Y	N
Eye redness, itching, discomfort	Y	N
Drainage from eyes	Y	N

Objective: Physical Examination
Inspect

Eyes for any discoloration or drainage	✓
Conjunctiva and sclera for colour and vascularity	✓
Lens for clarity	✓
Eyelid for ptosis	✓

Assess

Vision based on patient's looking at nurse or Snellen chart	✓
Extraocular movements	✓
Peripheral vision	✓
Pupil function: PERRLA	✓

PERRLA, pupils equal, round, reactive to light, and accommodation.

as part of neurological assessment of a hospitalized patient (see Chapter 58).

Special Assessment Techniques

Colour Vision. Testing the patient's ability to distinguish colours can be an important part of the overall assessment because some occupations may require accurate colour discrimination. The Ishihara test for colour blindness determines the patient's ability to distinguish a pattern of colour in a series of colour plates. Each plate has a pattern of dots of a specific colour which form a number or shape printed against a background of dots of other colours. A patient with normal colour

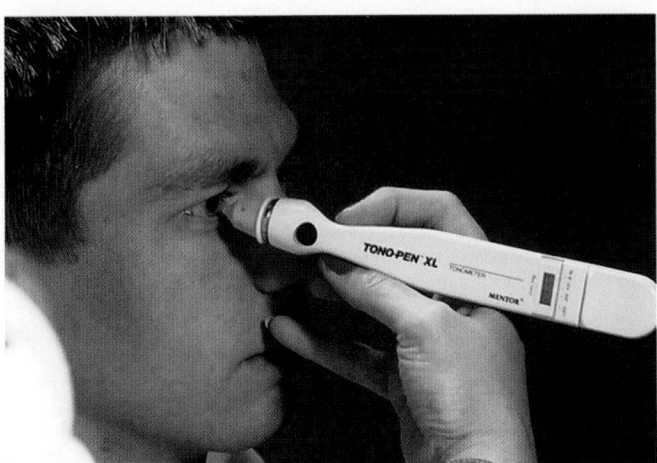

FIG. 23.7 Tono-Pen tonometry. Source: Courtesy the Eye Institute, Department of Ophthalmology and Visual Services, University of Iowa Health Care, Iowa City, Iowa.

vision can see each pattern (Jarvis et al., 2019). Older persons have a loss of colour discrimination at the blue end of the colour spectrum and loss of sensitivity throughout the entire spectrum, especially when cataracts are present.

Stereopsis. *Stereoscopic vision* enables a patient to see objects in three dimensions. Any event causing a patient to have monocular vision (e.g., enucleation, patching) results in loss of stereoscopic vision, which impairs the individual's depth perception. This condition can have serious consequences—for example, if the patient trips over a step when walking or follows too closely behind another vehicle when driving.

Intraocular Pressure. Testing intraocular pressure is important because high intraocular pressure is a major risk factor for glaucoma. Intraocular pressure can be measured by a variety of methods, including the Tono-Pen (Figure 23.7). Use of the Tono-Pen is common because it is simple, and results are very accurate. The surface of the anaesthetized cornea is touched lightly several times with the covered end of the probe. The instrument records several readings and provides a mean measurement on a digital light-emitting diode (LED) screen located on the front surface. Normal intraocular pressure ranges from 10 to 22 mm Hg.

DIAGNOSTIC STUDIES

Diagnostic studies provide important objective data to the nurse monitoring the patient's condition and planning appropriate interventions. Table 23.6 presents the most common basic diagnostic studies of the visual system.

SAFETY ALERT

Nurses should avoid using the abbreviations *OS* for left eye, *OD* for right eye, and *OU* for both eyes when documenting in patients' charts or transcribing medication orders because they can be easily confused with each other and with the abbreviations *AD, AS,* and *AU* for the ear. Use of these abbreviations can contribute to communication errors and potentially serious medication errors (Institute for Safe Medication Practices Canada, 2016).

THE AUDITORY SYSTEM

STRUCTURES AND FUNCTIONS

The auditory system is composed of the peripheral and central auditory systems. The peripheral auditory system includes the structures of the ear itself: external, middle, and inner ear (Figure 23.8). This system is concerned with the reception and perception of sound. The external and middle portions of the ear function to conduct and amplify sound waves from the environment. The inner ear serves functions of hearing and balance. The central auditory system (the brain and its pathways) integrates and assigns meaning to what is heard.

External Ear

The external ear consists of the auricle (pinna) and the external auditory canal. The *auricle* is composed of cartilage and connective tissue covered with epithelium, which also lines the external auditory canal (see Figure 23.8). The *external auditory canal* is a slightly S-shaped tube about 2.5 cm in length in the adult. The skin that lines the canal contains fine hairs (outer half of the canal only) and sebaceous (oil) glands and ceruminous (wax) glands. The cerumen (wax) helps prevent infection and serves as a physical barrier to the external environment (Swain et al., 2018).

The inner half of the external auditory canal is highly sensitive. The function of the external ear and canal is to collect and transmit sound waves to the *tympanic membrane* (eardrum). This shiny, translucent, pearl-grey membrane is composed of epithelial cells, connective tissue, and mucous membrane. It serves as a partition and instrument of sound transmission between the external auditory canal and middle ear.

Middle Ear

The middle ear cavity is an air space located in the temporal bone. Mucosa lines the middle ear and is continuous from the nasal pharynx via the Eustachian (auditory) tube. The *Eustachian tube* functions to equalize atmospheric air pressure between the middle ear and throat and allows the tympanic membrane to move freely. It opens during yawning and swallowing. Blockage of this tube can occur with allergies, nasopharyngeal infections, or enlarged adenoids.

The middle ear contains three tiny bones, or *ossicles: malleus, incus,* and *stapes.* Vibrations of the tympanic membrane cause the ossicles to move and transmit sound waves to the oval window. The resulting vibration in the oval window causes fluid in the inner ear to move and stimulate hearing receptors. The round window sits below the oval window and is covered with a thin membrane called the *fenestra cochlea;* it also opens into the inner ear and acts as a pressure valve that moves outward as fluid pressure builds in the inner ear. The superior part of the middle ear is called the *epitympanum* (attic). It also communicates with air cells within the mastoid bone. The facial nerve (CN VII) passes above the oval window of the middle ear. The thin, bony covering of the facial nerve can become damaged by chronic ear infection, skull fracture, or trauma during ear surgery. Such damage can cause problems with voluntary facial movements, eyelid closure, and taste discrimination. Permanent damage to the facial nerve can also result.

Inner Ear

The inner ear is composed of a bony labyrinth (maze) surrounding a membrane. This complex contains the functional organs for hearing and balance. The receptor organ for hearing is the *cochlea,* a coiled structure. It contains the *organ of Corti,* whose tiny hair cells respond to stimulation of selected portions of the basilar membrane according to pitch. This stimulus is converted into an electrochemical impulse and then transmitted by the cochlear branch of the vestibulocochlear nerve (CN VIII;

TABLE 23.6   DIAGNOSTIC STUDIES

Visual System

Study	Description and Purpose	Patient Education*
Refractometry	Subjective measure of refractive error; multiple lenses are mounted on rotating wheels. While patient sits looking through apertures at Snellen acuity chart, lenses are changed; patient chooses lenses that make acuity sharpest. Cycloplegic medications are used to paralyze accommodation during refraction process.	Procedure is painless; patient may need help holding the head still. Pupil dilation makes it difficult for the patient to focus on near objects; dilation may last 3–4 hr.
Ultrasonography	A-scan probe is placed on patient's anaesthetized cornea; used primarily for axial length measurement for calculating power of intraocular lens implanted after cataract extraction. B-scan probe is applied to patient's closed eyelid; used more often than A-scan for diagnosis of ocular disorders such as intraocular foreign bodies or tumours, opacities in the vitreous humor, and retinal detachments.	Procedure is painless (cornea is anaesthetized).
Fluorescein angiography	Fluorescein (a nonradioactive, non-iodine dye) is intravenously injected into antecubital or other peripheral vein, followed by serial photographs (over 10-min period) of the retina through dilated pupils. Provides diagnostic information about flow of blood through pigment epithelial and retinal vessels; often used in patients with diabetes mellitus to accurately locate areas of diabetic retinopathy before laser destruction of neovascularized area.	Fluorescein is toxic to tissue if extravasation occurs; systemic allergic reactions are rare, but the nurse should be familiar with emergency equipment and procedures. The patient should be informed that dye can sometimes cause transient nausea or vomiting and transient yellow discoloration of urine and skin.
Amsler grid test	Test is self-administered with a hand-held card printed with a grid of lines (similar to graph paper); patient fixates on centre dot and records any perceived abnormalities of the grid lines, such as wavy, missing, or distorted areas. Test is used to monitor macular concerns.	Regular testing is necessary to identify any changes in macular function.

*Patient education regarding the purpose and method of testing is a nursing responsibility for all diagnostic procedures.

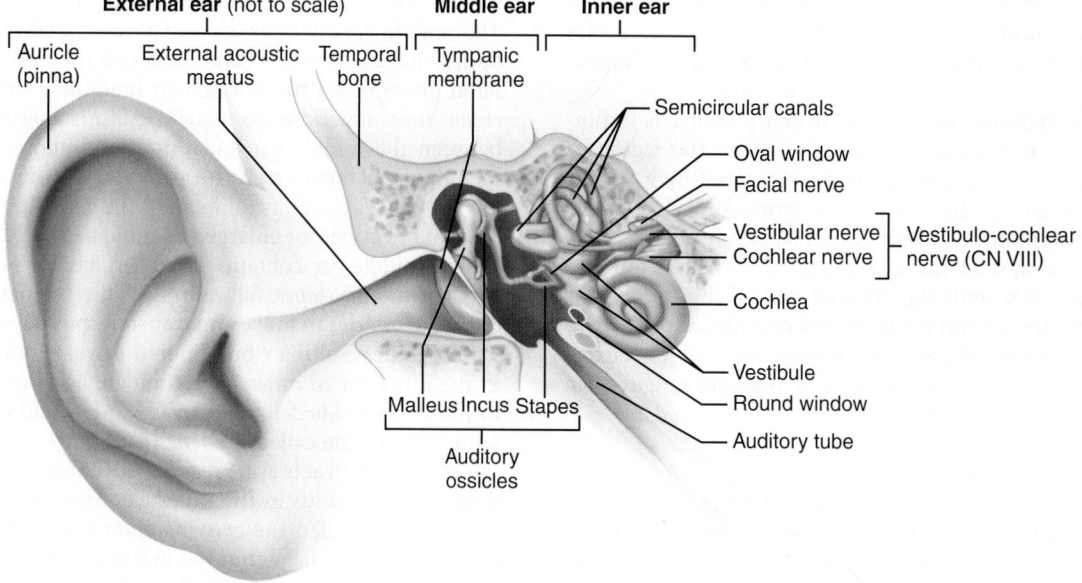

FIG. 23.8 External, middle, and inner ear. *CN,* cranial nerve. Source: Adapted from Patton, K. T., & Thibodeau, G. A. (2020). *Structure and function of the body* (16th ed., p. 217). Mosby.

formerly called the *acoustic nerve*) to the temporal lobe of the brain to process and interpret the sound.

Three semicircular canals and the vestibule make up the membranous labyrinth, which is housed in the bony labyrinth and enables the sense of balance. The membranous labyrinth is filled with endolymphatic fluid, and the bony labyrinth is filled with perilymphatic fluid. This extracellular fluid cushions these two sensitive organs and communicates with the brain and the subarachnoid spaces of the brain. The nervous stimuli are communicated by the vestibular portion of CN VIII. Debris or

excessive pressure within the lymphatic fluid can cause disorders such as vertigo.

Transmission of Sound and Implications for Hearing Loss

Sound waves are conducted by air (air conduction) and picked up by the auricles and the auditory canal. The sound waves strike the tympanic membrane, causing it to vibrate. The central area of the tympanic membrane is connected to the malleus, which also starts to vibrate, transmitting the vibration to the incus and then the stapes. As the stapes moves back and forth, it pushes the membrane of the oval window in and out. Movement of the oval window produces waves in the perilymphatic fluid. Pathological disturbances in the external ear canal or the middle ear may cause a conductive hearing loss, resulting in an alteration in the patient's perception of or sensitivity to sounds.

Once sound has been transmitted to the liquid medium of the inner ear, the vibration is picked up by the tiny sensory hair cells of the cochlea, which initiate nerve impulses. These impulses are carried by nerve fibres to the main branch of the acoustic portion of CN VIII and then to the brain. Disruptions of the inner ear or along the nerve pathway from the inner ear to the brain can result in sensorineural hearing loss. This may result in an alteration of the patient's perception of or sensitivity to specific tones. Impairment within the central auditory system causes *central hearing loss*. This type of hearing loss causes difficulty in understanding the meaning of words that are heard. (Types of hearing loss are discussed further in Chapter 24.)

The bones of the skull can also transmit sound directly to the inner ear (bone conduction). This can be demonstrated by placing the stem of a vibrating tuning fork on the patient's head, against the skull.

AGE-RELATED CONSIDERATIONS

THE AUDITORY SYSTEM

Age-related changes in the auditory system can result in hearing impairment. Presbycusis, or hearing loss caused by aging, can also result from insults from a variety of sources. Noise exposure, vascular or systemic diseases, poor or inadequate nutrition, ototoxic medications, and pollution during the lifespan can damage delicate hair cells of the organ of Corti or cause atrophy of lymph-producing cells. Sound transmission is diminished by calcification of the ossicles. Dry cerumen in the external canal can also interfere with transmission of sound. Tinnitus, or the perception of ringing in the ears, may accompany hearing loss that results from the aging process.

Hearing impairment, especially in an older person, can lead to social and health consequences, including embarrassment, fatigue, anxiety, depression, distress, social isolation, participation restrictions, falls and other injuries, lower quality of life, and mortality (Ramage-Morin et al., 2019). As the average lifespan increases, the number of people with hearing impairment will also increase. As many as 77% of adults aged 40 to 79 years have unperceived hearing impairment (Ramage-Morin et al., 2019). Regular screening and early identification of hearing problems will ensure patients are more active and healthier as they age.

Age-related changes in the auditory system and differences in assessment findings are presented in Table 23.7.

ASSESSMENT

Assessment of the auditory system includes assessment of the *vestibular* (balance) system because the auditory and vestibular systems are so closely related. Initially, the nurse should try to categorize symptoms related to balance and distinguish them from symptoms related to hearing loss or tinnitus. Problems with balance may manifest as nystagmus or vertigo. Nystagmus is abnormal eye movements that may be observed by other people as twitching of the patient's eyeball or may be described by the patient as a blurring of vision with head or eye movement. Vertigo is a sense that the person or objects around the person are moving or spinning and is usually

TABLE 23.7   AGE-RELATED DIFFERENCES IN ASSESSMENT

Auditory System

Changes	Differences in Assessment Findings
External Ear	
Increased production of and drier cerumen	Impacted cerumen; potential hearing loss
Increased hair growth	Visible hair, especially in men
Loss of elasticity in cartilage	Collapsed ear canal
Middle Ear	
Atrophic changes of tympanic membrane	Conductive hearing loss
Inner Ear	
Hair cell degeneration, neuron degeneration in auditory nerve and central pathways, reduced blood supply to cochlea, calcification of ossicles	Presbycusis, diminished sensitivity to high-pitched sounds, impairment in speech reception, tinnitus
Less effective vestibular apparatus in semicircular canals	Alterations in balance and body orientation
Brain	
Decline in ability to filter out unwanted and unnecessary sound	Difficulty hearing in a noisy environment, heightened sensitivity to loud sounds

stimulated by movement of the head. *Dizziness* is a sensation of being off-balance that occurs when the person is standing or walking. It does not occur when the person is lying down. Health history questions to ask a patient with an auditory condition are listed in Table 23.8.

Subjective Data
Important Health History
Current Health of Auditory System. The nurse should inquire about earache or pain in the ear. Such pain may be caused by ear conditions such as middle ear infection or may be referred pain originating in the teeth or temporomandibular joint. If pain is present, the patient should be asked to describe the pain and the treatments used for relief. If the patient has experienced any ear infections or has a history of chronic ear infections, this may contribute to increased hearing loss. Pus or bloody discharge may indicate an ear infection, whereas clear discharge may consist of cerebrospinal fluid, particularly if the patient has experienced any head trauma. Cerebrospinal fluid will feel oily and test positive for glucose (Jarvis et al., 2019). The nurse should note the time of onset of the hearing loss, whether it was sudden or gradual, and the person who noted the onset. Gradual hearing losses are most often noted by people who communicate regularly with the patient. Sudden losses and those exacerbated by some other condition are most often reported by the patient. If a hearing loss is identified in an older patient, the nurse can use the questions from the Hearing Handicap Inventory for Older Persons (Table 23.9). Referral is recommended for individuals scoring 10 or higher on the inventory.

If the patient has experienced any ringing, crackling, or buzzing sensation, the nurse should note time of onset and whether the patient is taking any medications that might cause tinnitus. Symptoms such as dizziness, tinnitus, and hearing loss are recorded in detail in the patient's own words. This careful description could help differentiate the cause.

TABLE 23.8   HEALTH HISTORY

Auditory System: Questions for Obtaining Subjective Data

Earache
- Do you have earache or another kind of pain in your ear?*
- Where is it located? Can you describe the pain?
- Do you have any symptoms of a cold or a sore throat?*
- What measures have you used to relieve the pain?* Were they effective?

Discharge
- Have you experienced discharge from your ears? How much and what colour?
- Have you had ear infections? How frequent? How were they treated?

Hearing Loss
- Was the hearing loss sudden or gradual?*
- Is it all your hearing or just hearing of certain sounds that has decreased?
- Where do you notice the hearing loss (e.g., conversations in a crowd, telephone conversations, watching television)?
- Have you travelled by airplane recently?
- Do you have any allergies that result in ear problems?*
- How does your hearing loss affect your daily life at home and at work?

Environmental Noise
- Do you have loud noise in your home or work environment?*
- Do you work near loud noises such as heavy machinery or drums in a band?

Tinnitus
- Have you ever experienced ringing, crackling, or buzzing in your ears?*
- Does the noise seem louder at certain times?*
- When does it bother you the most?
- What things have you tried that help?

Vertigo
- Have you felt vertigo—a spinning sensation?*
- Have you felt dizzy, as if you were falling or losing your balance?*
- Do you ever experience lightheadedness or giddiness?*
- Have you ever fallen because of the dizziness?*
- How does the dizziness affect your daily life?*

Nutrition and Elimination
- Do you have any food allergies that affect your ears?*
- Do you notice any differences in symptoms with changes in your diet?*
- Does your ear condition cause nausea that interferes with your food intake?*
- Does chewing or swallowing cause you any ear discomfort?
- Does straining during a bowel movement cause you ear pain?*

Activities of Daily Living and Exercise
- Does your ear condition cause you to change your usual activity or exercise?*
- Do you need help with certain activities (e.g., lifting, bending, climbing stairs, driving, speaking) because of symptoms?*
- Do you have any limitations in activities of daily living because of your symptoms?*
- Is your sleep disturbed by symptoms of pain, tinnitus, or dizziness?*

Self-Care History
- When did you last have your ears checked?
- How do you clean your ears?
- Do you use any devices to improve your hearing (e.g., hearing aid, special volume control, headphones for television or audio devices)?*
- How long have you used a hearing aid? Do you have any problems using or maintaining your hearing aid?*
- Do you use any means to protect your ears, such as headphones or earplugs?* When?
- Do you use personal sound systems such as iPhones or MP3 players?*

Coping Abilities
- Is your ability to communicate and understand affected by your symptoms?*
- What effect has your ear condition had on your work, family, or social life?
- How does your ear condition make you feel about yourself?
- Do you consider your ear condition a stressor?*
- How do you cope with your ear condition?

Source: Adapted from Jarvis, C., Browne, A. J., MacDonald-Jenkins, J., et al. (Eds.). (2019). *Physical examination and health assessment* (3rd Canadian ed., pp. 355–358). Elsevier.
*If yes, describe.

Past Health History. Many conditions related to the ear are sequelae of childhood illnesses or result from conditions of adjacent organs. Consequently, a careful assessment of past health conditions is important.

The patient should be questioned about previous conditions regarding the ears, especially those experienced during childhood. The frequency of acute middle ear infections *(otitis media)*, perforations of the eardrum, drainage, and history of mumps, measles, or scarlet fever should be recorded. Congenital hearing loss can result from infectious diseases (e.g., rubella, influenza, or syphilis), teratogenic medications, or hypoxia in the first trimester of pregnancy. Information regarding family members with hearing loss and type of hearing loss is important. Some congenital hearing loss is hereditary. The age at onset of presbycusis also follows a familial pattern. Head injury should be documented because it can result in hearing loss. Information about food and environmental allergies is important because they can cause the Eustachian tube to become edematous and prevent aeration of the middle ear.

Medications. The nurse should obtain information about current or past medications that are ototoxic (cause damage to CN VIII) and can produce hearing loss, tinnitus, and vertigo. The amount and frequency of acetylsalicylic acid (ASA; Aspirin) use is important because tinnitus can result from high ASA (Aspirin) intake. Salicylates and nonsteroidal anti-inflammatory medications, aminoglycoside and macrolide antibiotics, antimalarial agents, platinum-based chemotherapeutics, and loop diuretics are groups of mediations that are potentially ototoxic (Ganesan et al., 2018). Careful monitoring for hearing and balance issues is essential. Many medications produce hearing loss that may be reversible if treatment is stopped. The nurse should also inquire about the use of herbal or alternative therapies, including ear candling. Health Canada does not recommend ear candling because patients have experienced burns and hearing loss as a result (Government of Canada, 2013).

Surgery or Other Treatments. The nurse should obtain information about previous hospitalizations for ear surgery (e.g., myringotomy, tympanoplasty), tonsillectomy, and adenoidectomy. Use of and satisfaction with a hearing aid should

TABLE 23.9	THE HEARING HANDICAP INVENTORY FOR OLDER PERSONS*

Does a hearing problem cause you
1. (E) To feel embarrassed when meeting new people?
2. (E) To feel frustrated when talking to members of your family?
3. (S) To have difficulty understanding when someone speaks in a whisper?
4. (E) To feel handicapped?
5. (S) To have difficulty when visiting friends, relatives, or neighbours?
6. (S) To attend religious services less often than you would like?
7. (E) To have arguments with family members?
8. (S) To have difficulty when listening to television or radio?
9. (E) To feel that your hearing limits or hampers your personal or social life?
10. (S) To have difficulty when in a restaurant with relatives and friends?

Source: Adapted from Ventry, I. M., & Weinstein, B. E. (1982). The Hearing Handicap Inventory for the Elderly: a new tool. *Ear and Hearing, 3,* 128–134.
*Overall scoring: *yes* = 4 points; *sometimes* = 2 points; *no* = 0 points.
(E), question referring to emotional handicap; *(S)*, question referring to social handicap.

be documented. Problems with impacted cerumen should also be noted.

Nutrition and Elimination. Both alcohol and sodium affect the amount of endolymph in the inner ear system. Patients with Ménière's disease generally notice some improvement in their symptoms with alcohol restriction and a low-sodium diet. Improvements and exacerbations associated with food intake should be noted. The patient should also be questioned about any ear pain or discomfort that occurs with chewing or swallowing, which might decrease nutritional intake. This situation is often associated with a problem in the middle ear.

Assessment of clenching or grinding of the teeth helps differentiate conditions of the ear from referred pain of the temporomandibular joint. The nurse should ask about dental issues and dentures.

Elimination patterns and their association with ear conditions are of interest mainly in patients with perilymph fistula or in patients immediately after surgery. Frequent constipation or straining with bowel or bladder elimination may interfere with healing of a perilymph fistula or its repair. A patient who has just undergone stapedectomy especially needs to prevent the increase in intracranial (and consequent inner ear) pressure associated with straining during bowel movements. Stool softeners may be ordered postoperatively for a patient who reports chronic problems with constipation.

Activities of Daily Living and Exercise. Activity and exercise review is most important in assessing a patient with vestibular issues. If vertigo is a problem, the patient should be questioned about the onset, duration, and frequency of this symptom. Patients who have Ménière's disease demonstrate increasing inability to compensate for environmental input as the day progresses. Symptoms are experienced most often in the evening. In contrast, patients with chronic vertigo syndrome (benign paroxysmal positional vertigo) note that the symptoms improve throughout the day as adjustment to the visual and positional input from the environment occurs. The nurse and the patient should identify a list of activities and exercises that aggravate and relieve dizziness and vertigo or cause nausea or vomiting. Frequent repetition of an activity that causes symptoms (*habituation*) may help the body adjust so that the activity is no longer a problem.

A patient with chronic tinnitus should be questioned about sleep problems. Tinnitus can disturb sleep and activities

conducted in a quiet environment. Affected patients should be asked whether they have used or tried any masking devices or techniques to drown out the tinnitus. The nurse should also assess for snoring because it can be caused by swelling or hypertrophy of tissue in the nasopharynx. This excessive tissue can impair the functioning of the Eustachian tube and cause the sensation of ear fullness or pain.

Self-Care History. Patients should be questioned about personal practices such as the most recent ear examination, use of cotton ear swabs, use of earphones for personal listening devices, and measures used to preserve hearing. Patients should be questioned about contact with environments that have excessive noise levels, such as work with jet engines and machinery, firing of firearms, and electronically amplified music. The use of protective ear covers or earplugs is good practice for people in high-noise environments and is important to document.

If the patient is a swimmer, the frequency and duration of swimming and use of ear protection should be documented. It is also important to note the type of water (pool, lake, or ocean) in which the swimming takes place to help identify contact with contaminated water. Placement of any item in the ear, including hearing aids, that can cause trauma to the skin increases risk of infection.

Coping Abilities. Patients should be questioned about the effect the ear condition has had on family life, work responsibilities, and social relationships. Hearing loss can strain family relations and create misunderstandings. Failure to acknowledge hearing loss and failure to seek treatment can further hinder family relationships. Many jobs rely on the ability to hear accurately and respond appropriately. If hearing loss is present, the nurse should gather detailed information of its effect on the patient's job. The patient should be assisted to realistically evaluate the job situation.

The unpredictability of vertigo attacks can have devastating effects on all aspects of a patient's life. Ordinary activities such as driving, childcare, housework, climbing stairs, and cooking all acquire an element of danger. The patient should be asked to describe the effect of the vertigo on the many roles and responsibilities of life. Compensatory practices to avoid the development of dangerous situations should also be noted.

Hearing loss often leaves the patient feeling isolated from valued social relationships. The nurse should historically document social activities such as playing cards, going to movies, and attending religious functions from before and since the hearing loss occurred. Comparison of the frequency and enjoyment of the events can indicate whether a problem is present. The nurse should determine whether hearing loss or deafness has interfered with the patient's establishment of a satisfactory sex life. Although intimacy does not depend on the ability to hear, it could interfere with establishing or maintaining a relationship.

Objective Data

Physical Examination. During the health history interview, the nurse can collect valuable objective data regarding the patient's ability to hear. Clues such as posturing of the head and appropriateness of responses should be noted. Does the patient ask to have certain words repeated? Does the patient intently watch the examiner but miss comments when not looking at the examiner? Such observations are significant and should be recorded. This is also important because many patients are unaware of hearing loss or do not admit to changes in hearing until moderate losses have occurred. A normal assessment of the ear is described in Table 23.10.

TABLE 23.10	NORMAL FINDINGS IN PHYSICAL ASSESSMENT OF THE AUDITORY SYSTEM

- Ears: symmetrical in location and shape
- Auricles and tragus: nontender, without lesions
- Canal: clear; tympanic membrane: intact; landmarks and light reflex: intact
- Ability to hear low whisper at 30 cm; Rinne's test results: air conduction is better than bone conduction; Weber's test results: no lateralization

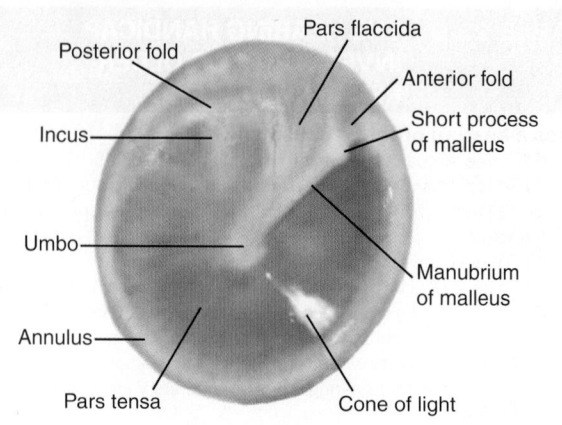

TYMPANIC MEMBRANE

FIG. 23.10 Illustration of normal landmarks of the right tympanic membrane, as seen through an otoscope. Source: Jarvis, C., Browne, A. J., MacDonald-Jenkins, J., et al. (2019). *Physical examination & health assessment* (3rd Canadian ed.). Elsevier.

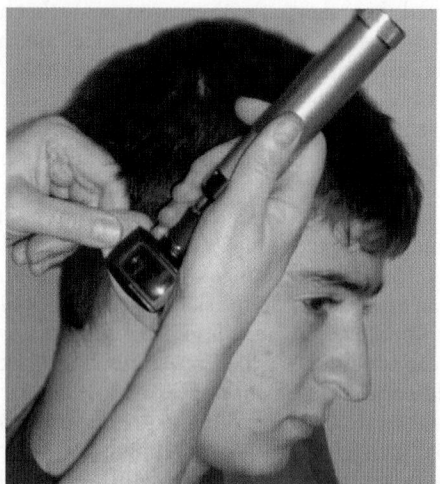

FIG. 23.9 Otoscopic examination of the adult ear. The auricle is pulled up and back. The examiner's hand holding the otoscope is braced against the patient's face for stabilization. Source: Courtesy Maureen Barry.

Age-related changes of the auditory system and differences in assessment findings are listed in Table 23.7.

External Ear. The external ear is inspected and palpated before examination of the external canal and tympanum. The auricle, preauricular area, and mastoid area are observed for symmetry of the ears, colour of skin, temperature, nodules, swelling, redness, and lesions. The auricle and mastoid areas are then palpated for tenderness and nodules. Grasping the auricle may elicit a pain response, especially if inflammation of the external ear or canal is present.

External Auditory Canal and Tympanum. Before inserting an otoscope, the nurse should inspect the canal opening for patency, palpate the tragus, and gently move the auricle to check for discomfort. A speculum only slightly smaller than the size of the ear canal is selected. The patient's head is tipped to the opposite shoulder. The top of the auricle is grasped and gently pulled up and backward in adults and slightly down and backward in children to straighten the canal. The otoscope, held in one of the examiner's hands and stabilized on the patient's head by the fingers of the other hand, is inserted slowly (Figure 23.9). A tight seal of the speculum is essential during this step of the examination. The canal is observed for size and shape and for the colour, amount, and type of cerumen. The tympanic membrane separates the external ear from the middle ear. If a large amount of cerumen is present, the tympanic membrane may not be visible. The tympanic membrane is observed for colour, landmarks, contour, and intactness (Figure 23.10). It is pearl-grey, white, or pink; shiny; and translucent.

The handle *(manubrium)* of the malleus and the end *(umbo)* are formed from the short process of the malleus and should be visible through the membrane. The somewhat anterior position

and concave shape of the tympanic membrane causes the light from the otoscope to reflect back as a cone of light with crisp edges. If the tympanic membrane is bulging or retracted, the edges of the light reflex do not have the cone shape; instead, the reflected light spreads out or moves and has irregular edges (diffuse). The circumference of the tympanum is thickened into a dense, whitish, fibrous ring, or *annulus,* except in the superior area. The tympanum within the annulus *(pars tensa)* is taut. Above the short process of the malleus is the *pars flaccida,* the flaccid part of the tympanum. The malleolar folds are anterior and posterior to the short process of the malleus. The middle and inner ear cannot be examined with the otoscope because of the tympanic membrane. Table 23.11 summarizes common abnormalities of the auditory system that are found in the assessment.

Focused Assessment. A focused assessment (see the Focused Assessment box) may be performed by a nurse when a patient is admitted to a hospital or an outpatient clinic. The ears may be inspected routinely as part of the assessment of a hospitalized patient. In addition, the nurse should assess for the presence of a hearing aid and document whether the patient has been using it.

FOCUSED ASSESSMENT

Auditory System

Use this checklist to make sure the key assessment steps have been performed.

Subjective
Ask the patient about any of the following and note responses.

Changes in hearing	Y	N
Ear pain	Y	N
Ear drainage	Y	N

Objective: Physical Examination

Inspect

Alignment and position of ears on head	✓
Size, shape, symmetry, colour, and skin intactness	✓
External auditory meatus for discharge or lesions	✓

Assess

Hearing, according to ability to respond to conversation, respond to a whisper, or hear a ticking watch	✓

TABLE 23.11   ASSESSMENT ABNORMALITIES

Auditory System

Finding	Description	Possible Cause and Significance
External Ear and Canal		
Sebaceous cyst behind ear	Usually within skin, possible presence of black dot (opening to sebaceous gland)	Removal or incision and drainage if painful
Tophi	Hard nodules in the helix or antihelix, consisting of uric acid crystals	Associated with gout, metabolic disorder; further diagnosis needed
Impacted cerumen	Wax that has not been excreted from the ear normally; no visualization of eardrum	Decreased hearing possible, sensation of fullness in auditory canal; removal necessary before otoscopic examination can be conducted
Discharge in canal	Infection of external ear, usually painful	Swimmer's ear, infection of external ear; possibly caused by ruptured eardrum and otitis media
Swelling of auricle, pain	Infection of glands of skin, hematoma caused by trauma	Aspiration (for hematoma)
Scaling or lesions	Change in usual appearance of skin	Seborrheic dermatitis, squamous cell carcinoma, atrophic dermatitis
Exostosis	Bony growth extending into canal, causing narrowing of canal	Possible interference with visualization of tympanum; usually asymptomatic
Tympanum		
Retracted eardrum	Appearance of shorter, more horizontal malleus; cone of light is absent or bent	Vacuum in middle ear, blockage of Eustachian tube, negative pressure in middle ear
Hairline fluid level, yellow-amber bubbles above fluid level	Caused by transudate of blood and serum; meniscus of fluid produces hairline appearance	Serous otitis media
Bulging red or blue eardrum, lack of landmarks	Middle ear filled with fluid (pus, blood)	Acute otitis media; perforation possible
Perforation of eardrum (central or marginal)	Previous perforations of the eardrum that have failed to heal; thin, transparent layer of epithelium surrounding eardrum	Chronic otitis media, mastoiditis
Recruitment	Disproportionate loudness of sound; difficulty in using hearing aid	Malfunction of inner ear

DIAGNOSTIC STUDIES

Table 23.12 describes diagnostic studies commonly used to assess the auditory system.

Tests for Hearing Acuity

Tests involving the whispered and the spoken voice can provide gross screening information about the patient's ability to hear. Audiometric testing provides more detailed information that can be used for diagnosis and treatment. In the *whispered voice test,* the examiner stands 30 to 60 cm behind the patient and, after exhaling, speaks in a low whisper. A louder whisper is used if the patient does not respond correctly. Spoken voice, increasing in loudness, is similarly used. The patient is asked to repeat numbers or words or answer questions. One ear at a time is tested while hearing in the other ear is masked to prevent sound transmission around the head. During testing, the nontest ear is masked by the patient, who occludes the ear, or by the examiner, who gently occludes the auditory canal with a finger and rubs the tragus in a circular motion.

Tuning-Fork Tests. Tuning-fork tests aid in differentiating between conductive and sensorineural hearing loss. For this examination, 512-Hz tuning forks are generally used. Both skill and experience are necessary to ensure accurate results. If a hearing difficulty is suspected, further evaluation by pure-tone audiometry is essential. The most common tuning-fork tests are the Rinne test and Weber test (see Table 23.12).

Results of tuning-fork tests are subjective. A patient with inconsistent test results or questionable results should be referred for more objective audiometric evaluation.

Audiometry. *Audiometry* is beneficial as a screening test for hearing acuity and as a diagnostic test for determining the degree and type of hearing loss. The audiometer produces pure tones at varying intensities to which the patient can respond. Sound is characterized by the number of vibrations or cycles that occur each second. *Hertz* (Hz) is the unit of measurement used to classify the frequency of a tone; the higher the frequency, the higher the pitch. Hearing loss can affect certain sound frequencies. The specific pattern produced on the audiogram by these losses can assist in the diagnosis of the type of hearing loss. The intensity or strength of a sound wave is expressed in terms of decibels (dB), ranging from 0 to 110 dB. The intensity of a sound required to make any frequency barely audible to the average normal ear is 0 dB. *Threshold* refers to the signal level at which pure tones are detected *(pure tone thresholds)* or the signal level at which the patient correctly hears 50% of the signals *(speech detection thresholds).*

Normal speech is approximately 40 to 65 dB; a soft whisper is 20 dB. Normally, a child and a young adult can hear frequencies from about 16 to 20 000 Hz, but hearing is most sensitive between 500 and 4 000 Hz. This range is similar to the frequencies contained in speech. A 40- to 45-dB loss in these frequencies causes moderate difficulty in hearing normal speech. A hearing aid may be helpful because it makes sound information louder, although not clearer. A hearing aid may not be helpful to a patient who has problems with discrimination of sounds or sound information, because the consonants are still not heard well enough to make speech understandable.

Screening Audiometry. Screening audiometry is the testing of large numbers of people with a fast, simple test to

TABLE 23.12   DIAGNOSTIC STUDIES

Auditory System

Study	Description and Purpose	Nursing Responsibility
Auditory Tests		
Pure tone audiometry	Sounds are presented through earphones in a soundproof room. Patient responds nonverbally when sound is heard. Response is recorded on an audiogram. Purpose is to determine patient's hearing range in terms of decibels (dB) and hertz (Hz) for diagnosing conductive and sensorineural hearing loss. Tinnitus can cause inconsistent results.	Nurse does not usually participate in examination.
Speech audiometry	Includes speech-awareness threshold (SAT) (measure of intensity at which speech is recognized) and speech recognition threshold (SRT) (ability to discriminate among various speech sounds).	Nurse does not usually participate in examination.
Tuning-Fork Tests		
Rinne test	Compares hearing by bone conduction (BC) and air conduction (AC). Stem of vibrating tuning fork is held against mastoid bone and time noted. When the sound is no longer perceived behind the ear (BC of sound), time is noted once again and the still-vibrating fork is moved close to the pinna. Have patient report when sound next to the ear canal (AC) is no longer heard and note time. Normally, sound is heard twice as long in front of the ear as it is on the bone. With conductive hearing loss, the relationship is reversed; BC is longer than AC. With sensorineural hearing loss, both AC and BC are reduced, but AC remains longer.	Nurse may perform test.
Weber test	Stem of vibrating tuning fork is placed on midline of skull or forehead. Patient is asked to indicate where the sound is heard best. In normal auditory function, the patient perceives a midline tone and the sound is heard equally in both ears. If a patient has conductive hearing loss in one ear, the sound will be heard louder (lateralizes) in that ear. If sensorineural loss is present, the sound is louder (lateralizes) in the normal (unaffected) ear.	Nurse may perform test.
Auditory evoked potential (AEP)	Procedure is similar to electroencephalography (see Chapter 58, Table 58.8). Electrodes are attached to patient in a darkened room. Electrodes are placed typically at vertex, mastoid process, or earlobes and forehead. A computer is used to record auditory activity in isolation from other electrical activity of the brain.	Nurse should explain procedure to patient. Nurse should not leave patient alone in the darkened room.
Auditory brainstem response (ABR)	Electrical peaks along auditory pathway of inner ear to brain are measured, and diagnostic information is related to acoustical neuromas, brainstem problems, and stroke.	Nurse does not usually participate in examination.
Electrocochleography	Test is useful for uncooperative patient or for patient who cannot volunteer useful information. Test records electrical activity in the cochlea and auditory nerve.	Nurse does not usually participate in examination.
Tympanometric Tests		
Tympanometry (impedance audiometry)	Useful in diagnosis of middle ear effusions. A probe is placed snugly in the external ear canal, and positive and negative pressures are then applied. Compliance of the middle ear is then noted in response to the pressures.	Nurse does not usually participate in examination.
Vestibular Tests		
Caloric test stimulus	Endolymph of the semicircular canals is stimulated by irrigation of cold (20°C) or warm (36°C) solution into the ear. Patient is seated or in supine position. Observation of type of nystagmus, nausea and vomiting, falling, or vertigo is helpful in diagnosing disease of labyrinth. Decreased response indicates decreased function and thus disease of vestibular system. The other ear is tested similarly, and results from both are compared.	Nurse instructs patient to eat no more than a light meal before test, to prevent nausea. Nurse observes patient for vomiting and assists patient if necessary. Nurse ensures patient safety.
Electronystagmography	Electrodes are placed near patient's eyes, and movement of eyes (nystagmus) is recorded on a graph during specific eye movements and when ear is irrigated. Study aids in diagnosing diseases of vestibular system.	Nurse instructs patient to eat no more than a light meal before test, to prevent nausea. Nurse observes patient for vomiting and assists patient if necessary. Nurse ensures patient safety.
Posturography	A balance test in which one semicircular canal can be isolated from others to determine site of lesion	Nurse informs patient that test is time consuming and uncomfortable but that the test can be discontinued any time at patient's request.
Rotary chair testing	The patient is seated in a chair driven by a motor under computer control. Test is an evaluation of peripheral vestibular system.	Nurse instructs patient to eat no more than a light meal before test, to prevent nausea. Nurse observes patient for vomiting and assists patient if necessary. Nurse ensures patient safety.

detect possible hearing problems. A pass–fail criterion is used to identify people who will need additional diagnostic testing. People who fail the screening should be referred to an audiologist for pure-tone (threshold) audiometry (see Table 23.12).

Specialized Tests

Specialized tests of the auditory system are most often performed in an outpatient setting by an audiologist using audiometers and computers that record electrical activity from the middle ear, the inner ear, and the brain. The test most commonly performed by audiologists is pure-tone audiometry. More sophisticated tests are available to determine the origin of certain hearing losses. These include the auditory evoked potential (AEP), auditory brainstem response (ABR), and electrocochleography (see Table 23.12). Computed tomography (CT) and magnetic resonance imaging (MRI) are used to diagnose the site of a lesion, such as a tumour of the auditory nerve.

Test for Vestibular Function

Table 23.12 describes diagnostic studies commonly used to assess vestibular function. Results of these tests can be altered by use of caffeine, other stimulants, sedatives, and antivertigo agents.

REVIEW QUESTIONS

The number of the question corresponds to the same-numbered objective at the beginning of the chapter.

1. In a client with a hemorrhage in the vitreous cavity of the eye, where is the blood accumulating?
   a. In the aqueous humor
   b. Between the lens and the retina
   c. Between the cornea and the lens
   d. In the space between the iris and the lens
2. Why might intraocular pressure increase?
   a. Edema of the corneal stroma
   b. Dilation of the retinal arterioles
   c. Blockage of the lacrimal canals and ducts
   d. Increased production of aqueous humor by the ciliary process
3. Which of the following should the nurse question clients about if they are using eye drops to treat glaucoma?
   a. Use of corrective lenses
   b. Their usual sleep pattern
   c. A history of heart or lung disease
   d. Sensitivity to opioids or depressants
4. For a client with an ophthalmic condition, the nurse should always assess for which of the following?
   a. Visual acuity
   b. Pupillary reactions
   c. Intraocular pressure
   d. Confrontation visual fields
5. Which of the following normal findings would the nurse expect during assessment of the auditory system?
   a. Absence of the cone of light
   b. Pearl-grey tympanic membrane
   c. Lateralization with Weber's test
   d. Bone conduction greater than air conduction
6. Which of the following are common age-related changes in the auditory system? (Select all that apply.)
   a. Drier cerumen
   b. Tinnitus in both ears
   c. Auditory nerve degeneration
   d. Atrophy of the tympanic membrane
   e. Greater ability to hear high-pitched sounds
7. Before fluorescein is injected for angiography, what should the nurse do? (Select all that apply.)
   a. Obtain an emesis basin.
   b. Ask whether the client is fatigued.
   c. Administer a topical anaesthetic.
   d. Inform the client that skin may turn yellow.
   e. Assess for allergies to iodine-based contrast media.

1. b; 2. d; 3. c; 4. a; 5. b; 6. a, c, d; 7. a, d.

evolve

For even more review questions, visit http://evolve.elsevier.com/Canada/Lewis/medsurg.

REFERENCES

Aljied, R., Aubin, M.-J., Buhrmann, R., et al. (2018). Prevalence and determinants of visual impairment in Canada: Cross-sectional data from the Canadian Longitudinal study on aging. *Canadian Journal of Ophthalmology, 53*(3), 291–297. https://doi.org/10.1016/j.jcjo.2018.01.027

Canadian Association of Optometrists. (2018). *Indigenous access to eye health and vision care in Canada.* https://opto.ca/document/indigenous-access-to-eye-health-and-vision-care-in-canada

Canadian Association of Optometrists. (2020). *The 20-20-20 rule.* https://opto.ca/health-library/the-20-20-20-rule

Ganesan, P., Schmiedge, J., Manchaiah, V., et al. (2018). Ototoxicity: A challenge in diagnosis and treatment. *Journal of Audiology & Otology, 22*(2), 59–68. https://doi.org/10.7874/jao.2017.00360

Government of Canada. (2013). *Ear candling.* https://www.canada.ca/en/health-canada/services/medical-procedures/ear-candling.html

Institute for Safe Medication Practices Canada. (2016). *Do not use: List of dangerous abbreviations, symbols, and dose designations.* https://www.ismp-canada.org/dangerousabbreviations.htm

Jarvis, C., Browne, A. J., MacDonald-Jenkins, J., et al. (2019). *Physical examination & health assessment* (3rd Canadian ed.). Elsevier.

Khoo, H. E., Ng, H. S., Yap, W.-S., et al. (2019). Nutrients for prevention of macular degeneration and eye-related diseases. *Antioxidants, 8*, 85. https://doi.org/10.3390/antiox8040085

Patton, K., & Thibodeau, G. (2020). *Structure and function of the body* (16th ed.). Mosby.

Ramage-Morin, P. L., Banks, R., Pineault, D., et al. (2019). Unperceived hearing loss among Canadians aged 40-79. *Statistics Canada: Health Reports, 30*(8), 11–20. https://doi.org/10.25318/82.003-x201900800002-eng

Skidmore-Roth, L., & Richardson, F. (2021). *Mosby's Canadian nursing drug reference* (1st Canadian ed.). Mosby.

Steele, K. (2018). Contact lens compliance: A review. *Contact lens update. Clinical insights based on current research* (Vol. 44). https://contactlensupdate.com/2018/10/26/contact-lens-compliance-a-review/

Swain, S. K., Sahu, M. C., Debta, P., et al. (2018). Antimicrobial properties of human cerumen. *Apollo Medicine, 15*, 197–200. https://doi.org/10.4103/am.am_69_18

Vargas, V., Arnalich-Montiel, F., & Alió del Barrio, J. L. (2019). Corneal healing. In J. Alió, J. Alió del Barrio, & F. Arnalich-Montiel (Eds.), *Corneal regeneration. Essentials in ophthalmology.* Springer.

RESOURCES

Resources for this chapter are listed after Chapter 24.

For additional Internet resources, see the website for this book at http://evolve.elsevier.com/Canada/Lewis/medsurg.

CHAPTER 24

Nursing Management
Visual and Auditory Conditions

Anita Robertson

Originating US chapter by Jonel L. Gomez and Mariann M. Harding

⊖volve WEBSITE

http://evolve.elsevier.com/Canada/Lewis/medsurg

- Review Questions (Online Only)
- Key Points
- Answer Guidelines for Case Study

- Student Case Study
  - Patient Undergoing Cataract Surgery
- Customizable Nursing Care Plan
  - Patient After Eye Surgery

- Conceptual Care Map Creator
- Audio Glossary
- Content Updates

LEARNING OBJECTIVES

1. Compare and contrast the types of refractive errors and appropriate corrections.
2. Describe the etiology of and interprofessional care for extraocular disorders.
3. Review the pathophysiological features and clinical manifestations of selected intraocular disorders and the nursing management and interprofessional care of affected patients.
4. Discuss the nursing measures that promote health of the eyes and ears.
5. Explain the general preoperative and postoperative care of the patient undergoing ophthalmological or otological surgery.
6. Summarize the action and uses of medication therapy for treating conditions of the eyes and ears.

7. Explain the pathophysiological features and clinical manifestations of common ear conditions and the nursing management and interprofessional care of affected patients.
8. Compare the causes, management, and rehabilitative potential of conductive and sensorineural hearing loss.
9. Explain the use of, care of, and patient teaching regarding assistive devices for eye and ear problems.
10. Describe the common causes and assistive measures for uncorrectable visual impairment and deafness.
11. Describe the measures used to assist the patient in adapting psychologically to decreased vision and hearing.

KEY TERMS

acoustic neuroma
age-related macular degeneration (AMD)
amblyopia
astigmatism
benign paroxysmal positional vertigo (BPPV)
cataract
conjunctivitis
enucleation

external otitis
glaucoma
hordeolum
hyperopia
keratitis
lacrimal puncta
Ménière's disease
myopia

otosclerosis
presbycusis
presbyopia
refractive error
retinal detachment
retinopathy
strabismus

This chapter describes visual and auditory conditions, with an emphasis on their pathophysiological features and clinical manifestations and on the interprofessional care and nursing management of affected patients. Assistive devices for visual and hearing impairment are also discussed.

VISUAL CONDITIONS

The eye contains numerous structures, all of which are critical for proper functioning of the visual system. These components include, most anteriorly, the tear film and cornea; the anterior segment structures, including the iris and lens; and posterior structures, including the vitreous, retina, and optic nerve. The optic nerves of both eyes meet and cross at the optic chiasm. At this point, the information from both eyes is combined and then splits according to the visual field. Information from the visual fields travels via the right or left optic tract, which terminates in the posterior part of the brain in the occipital cortex.

Loss of some or all vision has a significant impact on the lives of those who experience it, as well as their families. Vision loss

449

affect's quality of life, independence, and mobility and has been linked to falls, injury, and worsened status in mental health, cognition, social function, employment, and educational attainment (Welp et al., 2016).

CORRECTABLE REFRACTIVE ERRORS

The most common visual condition is refractive error. In this defect, light rays focus either in front of or behind the retina. The cornea is responsible for two thirds of the refractive power of the eye, and the lens is responsible for one third of refractive power. In addition to their combined refractive power, the length of the eye is an important determinant of potential refractive error. When light rays are out of focus, the patient may experience blurry vision, eye strain (asthenopia), headaches, or generalized eye discomfort. The principal refractive errors of the eye can be corrected by the use of lenses in the form of eyeglasses or contact lenses, by refractive surgery, or by surgical implantation of an artificial lens. Refractive errors in young children should be corrected because such children may develop amblyopia (reduced or no vision in affected eye), also known as "lazy eye," which may result in permanent vision loss if not treated in early childhood (National Eye Institute, 2019a). Undetected and untreated refractive errors and cataracts in persons older than 65 can lead to falls and unintentional injuries. Falls and fractures are of particular concern because of the effect on the individual's independence and long-term health (Welp et al., 2016).

> **SAFETY ALERT**
> Upon admission to hospital, older patients should undergo vision screening and, when it is warranted, be referred to an appropriate eye care specialist.

Myopia (nearsightedness) is an inability to accommodate for objects at a distance. It causes light rays to be focused in front of the retina. Myopia may occur because of excessive light refraction by the cornea or lens or because of an abnormally long eye.

Hyperopia (farsightedness) is an inability to accommodate for near objects. The light rays focus behind the retina, and so the patient must use accommodation to focus the light rays on the retina for near objects. This type of refractive error occurs when the cornea or lens does not have adequate focusing power or when the eyeball is too short.

Presbyopia is the loss of accommodation associated with age. This condition generally appears at approximately age 40. As the eye ages, the lens becomes larger, firmer, and less elastic. These changes, which progress with aging, result in an inability to focus on near objects. The first sign of presbyopia is often the need to hold reading material farther away.

Astigmatism is caused by an irregular corneal curvature. This irregularity causes the incoming light rays to be bent unequally. Consequently, the light rays do not converge in a single point of focus on the retina. Astigmatism can occur in conjunction with any of the other refractive errors.

Aphakia is the absence of the lens, which results in significant refractive error. Without the focusing ability of the lens, images are projected behind the retina. In rare cases, the lens may be absent congenitally, or it may be removed during cataract surgery. A lens that is traumatically injured is removed and replaced with an intraocular lens (IOL) implant. The lens accounts for approximately 30% of ocular refractive power.

Nonsurgical Corrections

Corrective Glasses. Myopia, hyperopia, presbyopia, and astigmatism can be modified by the appropriate corrective lenses. Myopia necessitates a "minus" (concave) corrective lens, whereas hyperopia and presbyopia necessitate a "plus" (convex) corrective lens. Glasses for presbyopia are often called reading glasses because they are usually worn only for close work. The presbyopic correction may also be combined with a correction for another refractive error, such as myopia or astigmatism. In these combined glasses, the presbyopic correction is in the lower portion of the spectacle lens. A traditional bifocal or trifocal has visible lines. A newer type of corrective glasses for presbyopia, the progressive lens, is actually a multifocal lens in which the transition from near to far correction is graduated seamlessly over a range in the middle area of the lens. This eliminates the visible lines between the different corrective lenses. The lower lens in multifocal glasses may predispose older people to falls because viewing the environment through their lower lenses impairs important visual capabilities (contrast sensitivity and depth perception) for detecting environmental hazards, particularly in unfamiliar environments (Gagnon-Roy et al., 2018).

Contact Lenses. Use of contact lenses is another way to correct refractive errors; they are available in rigid and soft types. The rigid types are available in standard and gas-permeable forms. Their care requires separate solutions for cleaning, storing, and wetting. The soft types are available in many forms. The most commonly used soft contact lenses are the standard and disposable forms, which are less durable and more expensive than rigid forms. Contact lenses generally provide better vision than glasses because the patient has more normal peripheral vision without the distortion and obstruction of glasses and their frames. This is especially true with high refractive errors. Contact lenses are made from various plastic and silicone substances, which are very permeable by oxygen, have a high water content, and thus enable longer wearing time with greater comfort. If the oxygen supply to the cornea is decreased, the cornea becomes swollen, visual acuity decreases, and the patient experiences severe discomfort.

Altered or decreased tear formation can make wearing contact lenses difficult. Tear production can be decreased by medications such as antihistamines, decongestants, diuretics, hormone medications such as oral contraceptives, and the hormones produced during pregnancy. Environmental factors such as wind, fans, and dust may also decrease the tear film. Allergic conjunctivitis with itching, tearing, and redness can also affect contact lens wear.

In general, the nurse must know whether the patient wears contact lenses, the pattern of wear (daily versus extended), and care practices. Shining a light obliquely on the eyeball can help the nurse visualize a contact lens. The patient should know the signs and symptoms of contact lens problems that must be managed by the eye care professional. These symptoms are remembered better with the mnemonic device RSVP: redness, sensitivity, vision problems, and pain.

> **SAFETY ALERT**
> The nurse should stress the importance of removing contact lenses immediately when the patient experiences RSVP symptoms.

Surgical Therapy

Surgical procedures are designed to eliminate or reduce the need for eyeglasses or contact lenses and correct refractive errors by changing the focus of the eye. Surgical management for refractive errors includes laser surgery and IOL implantation.

Laser Surgery. *Laser-assisted in situ keratomileusis* (LASIK) may be considered for patients with low to moderately high degrees of myopia, hyperopia, and astigmatism. It has revolutionized refractive surgery, and millions of LASIK procedures have been performed worldwide. The procedure first involves using a laser or surgical blade to create a thin flap in the cornea. Through new "wave-front" technology, the laser is then programmed to use a map of the patient's cornea to sculpt the cornea and correct the refractive error. The flap is then repositioned and adheres on its own without sutures in a few minutes (Artini et al., 2018). Perceptions of glare, halos, double images, and starbursts are negative consequences for some patients despite uncomplicated and successful surgery (Eydelman et al., 2017).

Photorefractive keratectomy is indicated for low to moderate degrees of myopia, hyperopia, and astigmatism and is a good option for a patient with insufficient corneal thickness for a LASIK flap. In this procedure, only the epithelium is removed, and the laser is used to sculpt the cornea to correct the refractive error. *Laser-assisted epithelial keratomileusis* (LASEK) is similar to photorefractive keratectomy except that the epithelium is replaced after surgery.

Implantation. *Intracorneal ring segments* are two semicircular pieces of plastic that are implanted between the layers of the cornea to treat mild forms of myopia. They are designed to change the shape of the cornea by adjusting the focusing power. Intracorneal ring segments can be removed, and the cornea usually returns to its original shape within a few weeks.

Refractive IOL implantation is an option for patients with severe myopia or hyperopia. Like cataract surgery, it involves the removal of the patient's natural lens and implantation of an IOL, which is a small plastic lens to correct a patient's refractive error. Because this requires entering the eye, the risk of complications is higher. New accommodating IOLs correct both myopia and presbyopia.

Phakic IOLs are sometimes referred to as *implantable contact lenses*. They are implanted into the eye without removal of the eye's natural lens. They are used for patients with severe myopia and hyperopia. Unlike the refractive IOL, the phakic IOL is placed in front of the eye's natural lens. Leaving the natural lens in the eye preserves the ability of the eye to focus for reading vision. The Artisan IOL is one type of phakic IOL used for moderate to severe myopia.

UNCORRECTABLE VISUAL IMPAIRMENT

Approximately 5% of Canadians have a *seeing disability,* defined as either difficulty seeing ordinary newsprint with corrective lenses if those are usually worn or difficulty seeing the face of someone 4 m across a room with corrective lenses if those are usually worn (Statistics Canada, 2018). The partially sighted individual may actually have significant vision. It is important in working with a visually impaired patient to understand that a person classified as blind may have useful vision. Appropriate responses and interventions depend on the nurse's understanding of an individual patient's visual abilities.

Levels of Visual Impairment

Total blindness is defined as no light perception and no usable vision. With *functional blindness* the patient has some light perception but no usable vision. A patient with either total or

TABLE 24.1	DEFINITION OF BLINDNESS IN CANADA

Legal blindness is defined as follows:
- Central visual acuity for distance: 20/200 or worse in the better eye (with correction)
- Visual field: no more than 20 degrees in its widest diameter or in the better eye

functional blindness may use vision substitutes such as guide dogs and canes for ambulation. Vision enhancement techniques are not helpful.

Legal blindness is defined as visual acuity 20/200 (6/60) or less in both eyes after correction and/or a visual field of 20 degrees or narrower (Canadian National Institute for the Blind [CNIB], 2019). The more common unit for expressing visual acuity is feet (i.e., 20/20), but some sources use the metric conversion (i.e., 6/6). More than 5.5 million Canadians have a major eye disease that could cause vision loss (Canadian Association of Optometrists [CAO], 2019). Most cases of vision impairment and blindness are caused by conditions such as age-related macular degeneration, glaucoma, diabetic retinopathy, or cataracts. These conditions are preventable, treatable, or both. The prevalence of vision loss in Canada is expected to increase nearly 30% by 2025 (CAO, 2019).

A *legally blind individual* meets the criteria developed by the federal government to determine eligibility for government programs and income tax benefits (Table 24.1). A legally blind individual may have some usable vision. The *partially sighted individual* who is not legally blind has a corrected visual acuity greater than 20/200 in the better eye and more than 20 degrees of visual field, but the visual acuity is 20/50 or worse in the better eye. The patient who is partially sighted but also legally blind can benefit greatly from vision enhancement techniques.

NURSING MANAGEMENT VISUAL IMPAIRMENT

NURSING ASSESSMENT

It is important to determine how long a patient has had a visual impairment because recent loss of vision has particular implications for nursing care. To determine how the patient's visual impairment affects normal functioning, the nurse should question the patient about the level of difficulty encountered when they perform certain tasks. For example, the nurse may ask how much difficulty the patient has when reading a newspaper, writing a cheque, moving from one room to the next, or watching television. Other questions can help the nurse determine the personal meaning that the patient attaches to the visual impairment. The nurse can ask how the vision loss has affected specific aspects of the patient's life, whether the patient has lost a job, or in what activities the patient no longer engages because of the visual impairment. Techniques such as describing where personal items are located, advising the patient when the nurse will be providing direct care, and informing the patient where food items are located on the tray are helpful strategies (Touhy et al., 2019). In older patients in all health care settings, vision should be assessed using a reliable tool.

Patients may attach many negative meanings to the impairment because of societal opinions about blindness. For example, patients may view the impairment as punishment or view themselves as useless and burdensome. It is also important to determine a patient's primary coping strategies, the patient's emotional reactions, and the availability and strength of the patient's support systems.

NURSING DIAGNOSES

Nursing diagnoses depend on the degree of visual impairment and how long it has been present. Nursing diagnoses for a visually impaired patient include but are not limited to the following:

- *Potential for injury* resulting from *alteration in sensation* (visual impairment)
- *Reduced self-care* resulting from *perceptual disorders* (visual impairment)
- *Preparedness for intensified self-care* as demonstrated by *willingness to learn self-care alterations* as a result of visual impairment
- *Potential for grieving* resulting from loss of vision

PLANNING

For a patient with recently impaired vision or a patient with impaired adjustment to long-standing visual impairment, the overall goals are that the patient will (a) make a successful adjustment to the impairment, (b) verbalize feelings related to the loss, (c) identify personal strengths and external support systems, and (d) use appropriate coping strategies. If the patient has been functioning at an appropriate or acceptable level, the goal is to maintain the current level of function.

NURSING IMPLEMENTATION

HEALTH PROMOTION. When a partially sighted patient is at risk for preventable further visual impairment, the nurse should encourage the patient to seek appropriate health care. For example, the patient with vision loss from glaucoma may prevent further visual impairment by adhering to prescribed therapies and suggested ophthalmological evaluations.

ACUTE INTERVENTION. The nurse needs to provide emotional support and direct care to patients with visual impairment of recent onset. Active listening and facilitating are important components of nursing care for these patients. The nurse should allow the patient to express anger and grief and help the patient identify fears and successful coping strategies. The patient's family is intimately involved in the experiences that follow vision loss. With the patient's knowledge and permission, the nurse should include family members in discussions and encourage members to express their concerns.

Many people are uncomfortable around a blind or partially sighted individual because they are not sure what behaviours are appropriate. Sensitivity to the person's feelings without being overly concerned or stifling the person's independence is vital in creating a therapeutic nursing presence.

The nurse should always communicate in a normal conversational tone and manner with the patient and address the patient directly, not the caregiver or friend who may accompany the patient. Common courtesy dictates introducing oneself and any other persons who approach a blind or partially sighted patient and saying goodbye on leaving. Making eye contact with the partially sighted patient accomplishes several objectives. It ensures that the nurse speaks while facing the patient so that the patient has no difficulty hearing the nurse. The nurse's head position confirms that the nurse is attentive to the patient. Also, establishing eye contact ensures that the nurse can observe the patient's facial expressions and reactions.

Orientation to the environment lessens patients' anxiety or discomfort and facilitates independence. In orienting a partially sighted or blind patient to a new area, the nurse should identify one object as the focal point and describe the location of other objects in relation to it. For example, the nurse may say, "The bed is straight ahead, approximately 10 steps. The chair is to the left of the bed, and the nightstand is to the right, near the head of the bed. The bathroom is to the left of the foot of the bed." The nurse should explain any activities or noises occurring in the patient's immediate surroundings.

The nurse should assist the patient in ambulating to each major object in the area, using the *sighted-guide technique*. When using this technique, the nurse stands slightly in front and to one side of the patient and offers an elbow for the patient to hold. The nurse serves as the sighted guide, walking slightly ahead of the patient with the patient holding the back of the nurse's arm. When using this technique, in any situation, the nurse describes the environment to help orient the patient. For example, the nurse may say, "We're going through an open doorway and approaching two steps down. There is an obstacle on the left." To assist the patient to sit, the nurse can place one of the patient's hands on the back of the chair.

The nurse should be familiar with common vision deficits such as cataracts, refractive errors, macular degeneration, glaucoma, and diabetic retinopathy and their associated nursing strategies for care. For example, age-related macular degeneration entails loss of central vision, and the patient is best cared for by being approached from the side. This condition affects a person's ability to see detail required for reading, writing, preparing meals, and recognizing faces. When caring for the patient with glaucoma, which entails loss of peripheral vision, the nurse should directly face the patient. Vision loss from glaucoma primarily affects a person's mobility, especially in a dynamic moving environment (Touhy et al., 2019).

AMBULATORY AND HOME CARE. Rehabilitation after partial or total loss of vision can foster independence, self-esteem, and productivity. The nurse should know what services and devices are available for a partially sighted or blind patient and be prepared to make appropriate referrals for those services and devices. For patients who are legally blind and those with low-degree vision, the primary resource for services is the Canadian National Institute for the Blind (CNIB). A list of agencies that serve the partially sighted or blind patient is available from this institute (see the Resources at the end of this chapter).

Braille or audio books for reading and a cane or guide dog for ambulation are examples of vision substitution techniques. These are usually most appropriate for patients with no functional vision. For most patients who have some remaining vision, vision enhancement techniques can provide enough help for them to learn to ambulate, read printed material, and accomplish activities of daily living.

Optical Devices for Vision Enhancement. A wide range of technological advances have become available to assist people with low-degree vision. These devices include desktop video magnification/closed-circuit units, electronic hand-held magnifiers, text-to-speech scanners, e-readers, and computer tablets (material read aloud, magnification, image zooming, brighter screen, voice recognition). Many of these devices require some training and practice for successful use. The nurse should encourage patients to practise with the device so that they can use it successfully.

Nonoptical Methods for Vision Enhancement. Approach magnification is a simple but sometimes overlooked technique for enhancing the patient's residual vision. The nurse can recommend that the patient sit closer to the television or hold books closer to their eyes, which the patient may be reluctant to do unless encouraged. Contrast enhancement techniques include watching television in black and white, placing dark objects against a light background (e.g., a white plate on a black placemat), using a black felt-tip marker to write, and using contrasting colours (e.g., a red stripe at the edge of steps or curbs). Increased lighting can be provided by halogen lamps, direct sunlight, or gooseneck lamps that can be aimed directly at the reading material or other near objects. Large type is often helpful, especially in conjunction with other optical or nonoptical vision enhancements.

EVALUATION

The overall expected outcomes are that the patient with severe visual impairment will
- Have no further loss of vision
- Be able to use adaptive coping strategies
- Not experience a decrease in self-esteem or social interactions
- Function safely within their own environment

AGE-RELATED CONSIDERATIONS

VISUAL IMPAIRMENT

Older persons are at an increased risk for vision loss caused by eye disease (Touhy et al., 2019). Older people may have other deficits, such as cognitive impairment or limited mobility, that further affect the ability to function in usual ways. Financial resources may meet normal needs but can be inadequate in meeting increased demands of vision services or devices.

Older patients may become confused or disoriented when visually compromised. The combination of decreased vision and confusion increases the risk of falls, which have potentially serious consequences for older persons. Decreased vision may compromise an older person's ability to function, which raises concerns about maintaining independence and damaging the patient's self-image. Because of decreased manual dexterity, some older people may have difficulty instilling prescribed eye drops. It is important to provide proper instruction and demonstration. Having the patient demonstrate the technique is an important aspect of nursing education and reassurance for patients. Eye drop assistive devices are available for purchase at pharmacies in Canada, and their use can be suggested.

EYE TRAUMA

Although the eyes are well protected by the bony orbit and by fat pads, everyday activities can result in ocular trauma. Ocular injuries can involve the ocular adnexa, the superficial structures, or the deeper ocular structures. Eye trauma is one of the leading causes of vision impairment in Canada; an estimated 700 workers experience an eye injury every day (Lian, 2018). Of all Canadian workers, 40% do not get needed visual aids, and approximately 200 per day suffer eye injuries. Furthermore, many of these injuries are serious enough to cause workers to lose work time, and some can lead to permanent eye damage or blindness. A Canadian online eye injury registry has been developed to gather data about the pattern and types of eye injuries that occur. Table 24.2 outlines emergency management of an eye injury. Types of ocular trauma include blunt injuries, penetrating injuries, and chemical exposure injuries. Causes of ocular injuries include automobile accidents, falls, injuries from sports and leisure activity, assaults, and work-related situations. Trauma is often a preventable cause of visual impairment. Almost 90% of all eye injuries could be prevented by the wearing of protective eyewear during potentially hazardous work, hobbies, or sports activities. The nurse's role in individual and community education is extremely important in reducing the incidence of ocular trauma.

EXTRAOCULAR DISORDERS

Inflammation and Infection

One of the most common conditions encountered by ophthalmologists is inflammation or infection of the external eye. Many external irritants or microorganisms can affect the eyelids and conjunctiva and can involve the avascular cornea. The nurse is responsible for teaching the patient appropriate interventions related to the specific disorder.

Hordeolum. An external hordeolum (commonly called a *stye*) is an infection of the sebaceous glands in the eyelid margin (Figure 24.1). The most common bacterial infective pathogen is *Staphylococcus aureus*. The affected area rapidly becomes red, swollen, circumscribed, and acutely tender. The nurse should instruct the patient to apply warm, moist compresses at least four times a day until it improves. This may be the only treatment necessary. If it tends to recur, the patient should be taught to perform eyelid scrubs daily. In addition, use of appropriate antibiotic ointments or drops may be indicated.

Chalazion. A *chalazion* is a chronic inflammatory granuloma of the meibomian (sebaceous) glands in the eyelid. A hordeolum may evolve into a chalazion. A chalazion may also occur as a response to the material released into the eyelid when a blocked gland ruptures. The chalazion usually appears on the upper eyelid as a swollen, tender, reddened area that may be painful. Initial treatment is similar to that for a hordeolum. If warm, moist compresses are ineffective in causing spontaneous drainage, the ophthalmologist may surgically remove the lesion (this is normally an office procedure), or the ophthalmologist may inject the lesion with corticosteroids.

Blepharitis. *Blepharitis* is a chronic inflammatory process of the eyelid margin. It is a common eye disorder throughout the world and can affect any age group. The cause is unknown and probably multifactorial. Bacteria have been implicated in playing a significant role. It may be associated with several systemic diseases such as rosacea or seborrheic dermatitis. It is related to other ocular conditions such as dry eye, chalazion, conjunctivitis, and keratitis. Symptoms include a burning sensation, irritation, tearing, photophobia, blurred vision, and redness of the conjunctiva. These symptoms are usually worse in the morning because the inflamed eyelids are in close contact with the ocular surface and tear production is decreased overnight as a result of less blinking. Basic treatment includes a long-term commitment to eyelid hygiene. Warm compresses and washing the eyelid margins with baby shampoo diluted in water and applied gently with a cotton-tipped swab are recommended. An antibiotic-corticosteroid ointment can be used for short periods only.

Conjunctivitis. Conjunctivitis is an infection or inflammation of the conjunctiva, the mucous membrane that lines the eyelids and covers the conjunctiva. These infections may be

TABLE 24.2 EMERGENCY MANAGEMENT

Eye Injury

Cause	Interventions
Trauma	**Initial**
• *Blunt:* Fist; other blunt objects	• Determine mechanism of injury.
• *Penetrating:* Fragments such as glass, metal, wood; knife, stick, or other large object	• Ensure airway, breathing, and circulation.
	• Assess for other injuries.
Chemical Burn	• Assess for chemical exposure.
• Alkaline	• In case of chemical exposure, begin ocular irrigation *immediately;* do not stop until emergency personnel arrive to continue irrigation. Use sterile saline or water if saline is unavailable.
• Acid	
	• Do not attempt to treat the injury (except as noted above for chemical exposure).
Thermal Burn	• Assess visual acuity.
• Direct burn from curling iron or other hot surface	• Do not put pressure on the eye.
• Indirect burn from ultraviolet light (e.g., welding torch, sun lamp)	• Instruct patient not to blow nose.
	• Stabilize foreign objects.
Foreign Bodies	• Cover injured eye or eyes with dry, sterile patches, and a protective shield.
• Glass	
• Metal	• Do not give the patient food or fluids.
• Wood	• Elevate head of bed to 45 degrees.
• Plastic	• Do not put medication or solutions in the eye unless ordered by physician.
• Ceramic	
Possible Assessment Findings Depending on Cause	• Administer analgesic medications as appropriate.
• Pain	**Ongoing Monitoring**
• Photophobia	• Reassure the patient.
• Redness: diffuse or localized	• Monitor pain.
• Swelling	• Anticipate surgical repair for penetrating injury, globe rupture, or globe avulsion.
• Ecchymosis	
• Tearing	
• Blood in the anterior chamber	
• Absence of eye movements	
• Fluid drainage from eye (e.g., blood, CSF, aqueous humor)	
• Abnormal or decreased vision	
• Visible foreign body	
• Prolapsed globe	
• Abnormal intraocular pressure	
• Visual field defect	

CSF, cerebrospinal fluid.

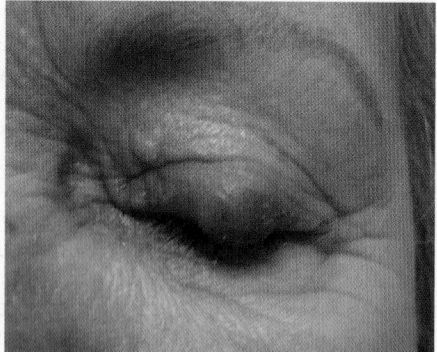

FIG. 24.1 External hordeolum (stye) on the upper eyelid caused by staphylococcal infection. Source: Courtesy Cory J. Bosanko, OD, FAAO, Eye Centers of Tennessee, Crossville, Tennessee.

caused by bacteria or viruses (Varu et al., 2019). Conjunctival inflammation may result from exposure to allergens or chemical irritants. Symptoms include ocular redness, discharge, burning, and sometimes itching and light sensitivity. It can occur in one or both eyes and is contagious, requiring meticulous care not to cross-contaminate the unaffected eye. Careful hand hygiene and the use of individual or disposable towels and preventing close contact with others can help prevent the spread of the condition (Varu et al., 2019).

Bacterial Infections. Acute bacterial conjunctivitis *(pinkeye)* is a common infection. Although it occurs in every age group,

epidemics commonly occur among children because of their limited personal hygiene habits. In adults and children, the most common causative microorganism is *S. aureus. Streptococcus pneumoniae* and *Haemophilus influenzae* are other common causative pathogens, but they are seen more often in children than in adults. A patient with bacterial conjunctivitis may have discomfort, pruritus, tearing, redness, and a mucopurulent drainage. Although this initially occurs in one eye, it generally spreads within 48 hours to the unaffected eye. The infection is usually self-limiting, but treatment with antibiotic drops shortens the course of the disorder.

Viral Infections. Conjunctival infections may be caused by many different viruses. A patient with viral conjunctivitis may experience tearing, foreign-body sensation, redness, and mild photophobia. This condition is usually mild and self-limiting. However, it can be severe, with considerable discomfort and subconjunctival hemorrhaging. Adenovirus conjunctivitis may be contracted in contaminated swimming pools and through direct contact with an infected patient. Treatment is usually palliative. If the patient's symptoms are severe, topical corticosteroids provide temporary relief but do not cure the infection. Antiviral drops are ineffective and therefore not indicated.

Chlamydial Infections. Trachoma is a chronic conjunctivitis caused by *Chlamydia trachomatis* (serotypes A through C). It is a major cause of blindness worldwide. It is responsible for visual impairment in approximately 1.9 million people and is responsible for about 1.4% of all blindness worldwide (World

Health Organization, 2021). This preventable eye disease is transmitted mainly via contact with the hands and by flies. Adult inclusion conjunctivitis (AIC) is caused by *C. trachomatis* (serotypes D through K). Manifestations of both trachoma and AIC are mucopurulent ocular discharge, irritation, redness, and eyelid swelling. For unknown reasons, AIC does not carry the long-term consequences of trachoma. AIC also differs from trachoma in that it is common in economically developed countries, whereas trachoma is most common in underdeveloped countries. Antibiotic therapy is usually effective for trachoma and AIC.

Although antibiotic treatment may be successful in adults with AIC, these patients have a high risk of concurrent chlamydial genital infection, as well as other sexually transmitted infections. The nurse's teaching plan for this patient should include the implications of AIC for sexual activity and reproductive health.

Allergic Conjunctivitis. Conjunctivitis caused by exposure to an allergen can be mild and transitory, or it can be severe enough to cause significant swelling, sometimes causing the conjunctiva to balloon beyond the eyelids. The defining symptom of allergic conjunctivitis is itching. The patient may also experience burning, redness, and tearing. In the acute stage, the patient may have white or clear exudate. If the condition is chronic, the exudate is thicker and becomes mucopurulent. The patient may develop allergic conjunctivitis in response to pollens, in addition to animal dander, ocular solutions and medications, or even contact lenses. The nurse should instruct the patient to avoid the allergen if it is known. Artificial tears can be effective in diluting the allergen and washing it from the eye. Effective topical medications include antihistamines and corticosteroids.

Keratitis. Keratitis is an inflammation or infection of the cornea that can be caused by a variety of microorganisms or by other factors. The condition may involve the conjunctiva, the cornea, or both. When it involves both, the disorder is termed *keratoconjunctivitis*.

Bacterial Infections. When the epithelial layer is disrupted, the cornea can become infected by a variety of bacteria. Topical antibiotics are generally effective but eradicating the infection may require subconjunctival antibiotic injection or, in severe cases, intravenous antibiotics. Risk factors include mechanical or chemical corneal epithelial damage, contact lens wear, debilitation, nutritional deficiencies, immunosuppressed states, and use of contaminated products (e.g., lens care solutions and cases, topical medications, cosmetics).

Viral Infections. Herpes simplex virus (HSV) keratitis is the most frequently occurring infectious cause of corneal blindness in the Western hemisphere. It is a growing problem, especially among immunosuppressed patients. It may be caused by HSV-1 or HSV-2 (genital herpes), although HSV-2 ocular infection is much less common. The resulting corneal ulcer has a characteristic dendritic (tree-branching) appearance (Tognarelli et al., 2019). Pain and photophobia are common. In up to 40% of patients, herpetic keratitis heals spontaneously. The spontaneous healing rate increases to 70% if the cornea is debrided to remove infected cells. Interprofessional management includes corneal debridement, followed by topical therapy with trifluridine for 2 to 3 weeks. Topical corticosteroids are usually contraindicated because they contribute to a longer course and possible deeper ulceration of the cornea. Medication therapy may also include oral acyclovir (Zovirax).

The varicella-zoster virus causes both chicken pox and herpes zoster ophthalmicus (HZO). HZO occurs in approximately 10 to 20% of all cases of herpes zoster (Freund & Chen, 2018). HZO causes a painful vesicular rash and may occur by reactivation of an endogenous infection that has persisted in latent form after an earlier attack of varicella or by contact with a patient with chicken pox or herpes zoster. It occurs most frequently in older persons and in immunosuppressed patients. Interprofessional care of a patient with acute HZO may include analgesics for the pain, topical corticosteroids to reduce inflammation, antiviral medications such as acyclovir (Zovirax) to reduce viral replication, mydriatic medications to dilate the pupil and relieve pain, and topical antibiotics to combat secondary infection. Ideally, antiviral agents should be initiated within 72 hours of onset of the rash to minimize complications. However, given the risk of blindness and other complications with HZO, antiviral agents may be started beyond this time frame (Freund & Chen, 2018). The patient may apply warm compresses and povidone-iodine gel to the affected skin (gel should not be applied too near the eye).

Epidemic keratoconjunctivitis is the most serious ocular adenoviral disease. This condition is spread by direct contact, including sexual activity. In the medical setting, contaminated hands and instruments can be the source of spread. The patient may experience tearing, redness, photophobia, and sensation of a foreign body in the eye. In most patients, the disease involves only one eye. Treatment is primarily palliative and includes ice packs and dark glasses. In severe cases, therapy can include mild topical corticosteroids to temporarily relieve symptoms and topical antibiotic ointment. The nurse's most important role is to teach the patient and caregivers the importance of good hygienic practices to avoid spreading the disease.

Other Causes of Keratitis. Keratitis may also be caused by fungi (most commonly *Aspergillus*, *Candida*, and *Fusarium* species), especially in the case of ocular trauma in an outdoor setting in which fungi are prevalent in the soil and moist organic matter. *Acanthamoeba* keratitis is caused by a parasite that is associated with contact lens wear, probably as a result of using contaminated lens care solutions or cases. Homemade saline solution is particularly susceptible to *Acanthamoeba* contamination. The nurse should instruct all patients who wear contact lenses in good lens care practices. Medical treatment of fungal and *Acanthamoeba* keratitis is difficult. The *Acanthamoeba* organism is resistant to most medications. If antimicrobial therapy fails, the patient may require corneal transplantation.

Exposure keratitis occurs when the patient cannot adequately close the eyelids. The patient with exophthalmos (protruding eyeball) caused by thyroid eye disease or masses posterior to the globe is susceptible to exposure keratitis.

Corneal Ulcer. Tissue loss caused by infection of the cornea produces a *corneal ulcer* (infectious keratitis) (Figure 24.2). The infection can be caused by bacteria, viruses, or fungi. Corneal ulcers are often very painful, and patients may feel as if a foreign body is in the eye. Other symptoms can include tearing, purulent or watery discharge, redness, and photophobia. Treatment is generally aggressive to prevent permanent loss of vision. Antibiotic, antiviral, or antifungal eye drops may be prescribed as frequently as every hour, night and day, for the first 24 hours. An untreated corneal ulcer can result in corneal scarring and perforation (hole in the cornea). Corneal transplantation may be indicated.

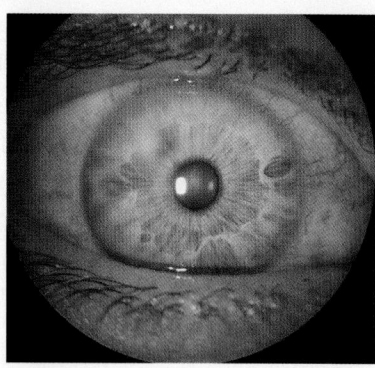

FIG. 24.2 Corneal ulcer. Infection associated with poor contact lens care. Source: Courtesy Cory J. Bosanko, OD, FAAO, Eye Centers of Tennessee, Crossville, Tennessee.

NURSING MANAGEMENT INFLAMMATION AND INFECTION

NURSING ASSESSMENT

The nurse should assess ocular changes—such as edema, redness, decreasing visual acuity, the sensation that a foreign body is present, or discomfort—and document the findings in the patient's record. In the assessment, the nurse should also consider the psychosocial aspects of the patient's condition, especially when the patient's vision is also impaired.

NURSING DIAGNOSES

Nursing diagnoses for the patient with inflammation or infection of the external eye include but are not limited to the following:

- *Acute pain* resulting from *biological injury agent* (infection)
- *Anxiety* resulting from threat to current status (major change in health status)

PLANNING

The overall goals are that the patient with inflammation or infection of the external eye will (a) avoid spread of infection, (b) maintain an acceptable level of comfort and functioning during the course of the specific ocular problem, (c) maintain or improve visual acuity, (d) adhere to the prescribed therapy, and (e) engage in appropriate health-seeking behaviours.

NURSING IMPLEMENTATION

HEALTH PROMOTION. Careful asepsis and frequent, thorough hand hygiene are essential to prevent spread of organisms from one eye to the other, to other patients, to family members, and to the nurse. The patient and family require information about avoiding sources of ocular irritation or infection and responding appropriately if an ocular condition occurs. Patients with infective disorders that may be transmitted sexually or who have an associated sexually transmitted infection need specific information about those disorders. The nurse should inform the patient about the appropriate use and care of lenses and lens care products.

ACUTE INTERVENTION. The nurse can apply warm or cool compresses if indicated for the patient's condition. Darkening the room and providing an appropriate analgesic are other comfort measures. If the patient's visual acuity is decreased, the nurse may need to modify the patient's environment or activities for safety.

The patient may require eye drops as frequently as every hour. If the patient receives two or more different types of drops, the nurse should stagger the eye drop dosing to promote maximum absorption. For example, if two different eye drops are ordered hourly, the nurse should administer one kind of drop on the hour and the other kind of drop on the half-hour unless otherwise prescribed. This staggered schedule promotes maximum absorption. The patient who needs frequent eye drop administration may experience sleep deprivation.

AMBULATORY AND HOME CARE. The patient's primary need in the home environment is for information about required care and how to accomplish that care. The patient and family also need information about proper techniques for medication administration. If the patient's vision is compromised, the nurse should provide suggestions for alternative ways to accomplish necessary daily activities and self-care. A patient who wears contact lenses and develops infections should discard all opened or used lens care products and cosmetics to decrease the risk of reinfection from contaminated products (a common problem and a probable source of infection for many patients).

EVALUATION

The overall expected outcomes are that the patient with inflammation or infection of the external eye will

- Adhere to the treatment plan
- Experience relief from ocular discomfort
- Effectively cope with functional changes if visual acuity is decreased
- Obtain specific information to prevent recurrent disease

DRY EYE DISORDERS

Keratoconjunctivitis sicca (dry eyes) is a common condition, particularly among older persons and individuals with certain systemic diseases such as scleroderma and systemic lupus erythematosus. Patients with dry eyes can experience irritation or the sensation of sand in the eye, and the sensation typically worsens throughout the day. This condition is caused by a decrease in the quality or quantity of the tear film, and treatment is directed at the underlying cause. If it is caused by lacrimal duct dysfunction, the condition may respond to hot compresses and eyelid massage. With decreased tear secretion, the patient may use artificial tears or ointments. They should be used sparingly because preservatives in the drops or overuse can cause further ocular irritation. In severe cases, closure of the lacrimal puncta may be necessary. Patients with dry eyes in association with dry mouth may have Sjögren syndrome (see Chapter 67).

STRABISMUS

Strabismus is a condition in which the patient cannot consistently focus both eyes simultaneously on the same object (Figure 24.3). One eye may deviate inward (esotropia), outward (exotropia), upward (hypertropia), or downward (hypotropia). Strabismus in adults may be caused by thyroid disease, neuromuscular disorders of the eye muscles, retinal detachment repair, or cerebral lesions. The primary symptom with strabismus is double vision.

CORNEAL DISORDERS

Corneal Scars and Opacities

The cornea is a transparent tissue that allows light rays to enter the eye and focus on the retina, thus producing a visual image. Any wound causes the cornea to become abnormally hydrated

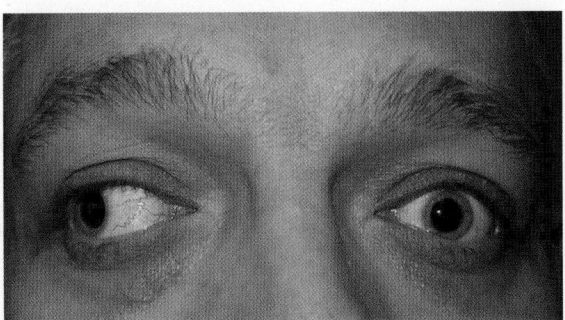

FIG. 24.3 Strabismus with right exotropia and fixation of the left eye. Source: Courtesy Cory J. Bosanko, OD, FAAO, Eye Centers of Tennessee, Crossville, Tennessee.

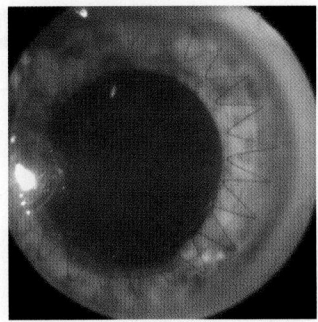

FIG. 24.4 Sutures on a donated cornea after penetrating keratoplasty (corneal transplantation). Source: Courtesy Cory J. Bosanko, OD, FAAO, Eye Centers of Tennessee, Crossville, Tennessee.

and decreases the normal transparency. A rigid contact lens can be effective in correcting the irregular astigmatism that results from corneal scars. In other situations, the treatment for corneal scars or opacities is *penetrating keratoplasty* (corneal transplantation). In this surgical procedure, the ophthalmological surgeon removes the full thickness of the patient's cornea and replaces it with a donor cornea that is sutured into place (Figure 24.4). Vision may not be restored for up to 12 months. Corneal problems leading to blindness are uncommon, but if they occur, corneal transplantation can preserve vision that otherwise would be lost.

Corneal transplantation surgery is one of the fastest and safest of all tissue or organ transplantation procedures (Del Buey et al., 2019). The time between the donor's death and the removal of the tissue should be as short as possible. Most surgeons prefer this interval to be 4 hours or less. The eye banks test donors for human immunodeficiency virus (HIV) and hepatitis B and C viruses. The tissue is preserved in a special nutritive solution, and it can be kept for up to 5 days in the storage medium, if used for transplantation. Improved methods of tissue procurement and preservation, refined surgical techniques, postoperative topical corticosteroids, and careful follow-up have decreased the incidence of graft rejection. Matching the blood type of the donor and the recipient may also improve the success rate (National Eye Institute, 2019b).

Keratoconus

Keratoconus is a noninflammatory, usually bilateral disease that has a familial tendency. It can be associated with Down syndrome, atopic dermatitis, Marfan syndrome, aniridia (congenital absence of the iris), and retinitis pigmentosa (hereditary disease characterized by bilateral primary degeneration of the retina beginning in childhood and progression to blindness by middle age).

The anterior cornea thins and protrudes forward, taking on a cone shape. Keratoconus usually appears during adolescence and slowly progresses between the ages of 20 and 60 years. The only symptom is blurred vision. The astigmatism may be corrected with glasses or rigid contact lenses. Intacs inserts, for example, are two clear plastic lenses surgically inserted on the cornea's perimeter to reduce astigmatism and myopia. Intacs inserts are generally used to delay the need for corneal transplantation when contact lenses or glasses no longer help a patient achieve adequate vision. The cornea can perforate as central corneal thinning progresses. In advanced cases, a penetrating keratoplasty is indicated before perforation.

INTRAOCULAR DISORDERS

Cataract

A cataract is an area of opacity within the lens. The patient may have a cataract in one or both eyes. If cataracts are present in both eyes, one cataract may affect the patient's vision more than the other. Cataracts are one of the leading causes of reversible vision loss worldwide, affecting 95 million people, including nearly 2.5 million Canadians (Jin et al., 2019).

Causes and Pathophysiological Processes. Although most cataracts are age related *(senile cataracts)*, they can be associated with other factors. These include blunt or penetrating trauma, congenital factors such as maternal rubella, exposure to radiation or ultraviolet light, certain medications such as systemic corticosteroids or long-term topical corticosteroids, and ocular inflammation. Patients with diabetes mellitus tend to develop cataracts at a younger age than average.

Cataract development is mediated by a number of factors. In senile cataract formation, it appears that altered metabolic processes within the lens cause an accumulation of water and alterations in the lens fibre structure. These changes affect lens transparency, causing vision changes.

Clinical Manifestations. Patients with cataracts may experience a decrease in vision, abnormal colour perception, and glare. Glare results from light scatter caused by the lens opacities, and it may be significantly worse at night when the pupil dilates. The visual decline is gradual, but the rate of cataract development varies from patient to patient. Secondary glaucoma can also occur if the enlarging lens causes an increase in intraocular pressure (IOP).

Diagnostic Studies. Diagnosis is based on decreased visual acuity or other reports of visual dysfunction. The opacity is directly observable by ophthalmoscopic or slit-lamp microscopic examination. A totally opaque lens creates the appearance of a white pupil. Table 24.3 outlines other diagnostic studies that may be helpful in evaluating the visual effect of a cataract.

Interprofessional Care. The presence of a cataract does not necessarily indicate a need for surgery. For many patients, the diagnosis is made long before they actually decide to have surgery. Nonsurgical therapy may postpone the need for surgery. Interprofessional care for cataracts is described in Table 24.3.

Nonsurgical Therapy. Currently, the only way to "cure" cataracts is through surgical removal. If the cataract is not removed, the patient's vision will continue to deteriorate. However, specific strategies may help the patient. In many cases, changing the patient's eyewear prescription can improve the level of visual acuity, at least temporarily. Other visual aids, such as strong

TABLE 24.3   INTERPROFESSIONAL CARE
Cataract

Diagnostic Studies
- History and physical examination
- Visual acuity measurement
- Ophthalmoscopy (direct and indirect)
- Slit-lamp microscopy
- Glare testing, potential acuity testing in selected patients
- Keratometry and A-scan ultrasonography (if surgery is planned)
- Other tests (e.g., visual field perimetry) may be indicated to determine cause of visual loss

Interprofessional Therapy
Nonsurgical
- Prescription change for glasses
- Strong reading glasses or magnifiers
- Increased lighting
- Lifestyle adjustment

Acute Care: Surgical Therapy
Preoperative
- Mydriatic, cycloplegic medications (see Table 24.4)
- Nonsteroidal anti-inflammatory drugs
- Topical antibiotics
- Antianxiety medications

During Surgery
- Removal of lens:
- Phacoemulsification (see Figure 24.5)
- Extracapsular extraction
- Correction of surgical aphakia
- Intraocular lens implantation (most frequent type of correction)
- Contact lens

Postoperative
- Topical antibiotic
- Topical corticosteroid or other anti-inflammatory medication
- Mild analgesic medication if necessary
- Eye shield and activity as preferred by patient's surgeon

reading glasses or magnifiers of some type, may help the patient with close vision. Increasing the amount of light to read or accomplish other near-vision tasks is another useful measure. The patient may be willing to adjust their lifestyle to accommodate for visual decline. For example, if glare makes it difficult to drive at night, a patient may elect to drive only during daylight hours and to have a family member drive at night. Sometimes, informing and reassuring the patient about the disease process can make the patient comfortable about choosing nonsurgical measures, at least temporarily.

Surgical Therapy. When palliative measures no longer provide an acceptable level of visual function, the patient is an appropriate candidate for surgery. The patient's occupational needs and lifestyle changes are also factors affecting the decision to undergo surgery. In some instances, factors other than the patient's visual needs may influence the need for surgery. Lens-induced conditions such as increased IOP may necessitate lens removal. Opacities may prevent the ophthalmologist from obtaining a clear view of the retina in a patient with diabetic retinopathy or other sight-threatening pathological conditions. In those cases, the cataract may be removed to allow the surgeon to visualize the retina and adequately manage the problem.

Preoperative Phase. The patient's preoperative preparation should include an appropriate documentation of the history and a physical examination. Because almost all patients undergo the procedure under local anaesthesia, many physicians and surgical facilities do not require an extensive preoperative physical assessment. However, most patients with cataracts are older persons and may have several medical conditions that should be evaluated and controlled before surgery. The surgeon may order preoperative antibiotic eye drops. The patient should not have food or fluids for approximately 6 to 8 hours before surgery. Almost all patients with cataracts are admitted to a surgical facility on an outpatient basis. The patient is normally admitted several hours before surgery to allow adequate time for necessary preoperative procedures.

EVIDENCE-INFORMED PRACTICE
Research Highlight

Does the Administration of Perioperative Antibiotic Prophylaxis Prevent Endophthalmitis After Cataract Surgery?

Clinical Question
In adults undergoing cataract surgery (P), does perioperative antibiotic prophylaxis (I) as compared to different antibiotics or no antibiotics perioperatively (C) result in the prevention of endophthalmitis and better visual acuity postoperatively (O)?

Best Available Evidence
Systematic review of randomized controlled trials

Critical Appraisal and Synthesis of Evidence
- Meta-analysis of five randomized controlled trials ($n = 101\,005$)
- The review included a narrative synthesis.
- Primary outcomes were endophthalmitis (presence or absence) and visual acuity within 6 weeks of cataract surgery.
- Intraocular and periocular administration demonstrated that ocular injections had the lowest rates of endophthalmitis.
    Irrigation solution was compared with one group receiving vancomycin and gentamycin in a balanced salt solution (BSS) and the other group receiving the BSS only. The group that had the antibiotics in the BSS reported no incidence of endophthalmitis.
- Comparing topical levofloxacin to no antibiotic perioperatively showed no differences in the incidence of endophthalmitis.
- No studies reported any differences in visual acuity postoperatively.

Conclusions
- Intracameral antibiotics are recommended for reducing endophthalmitis post–cataract surgery.

Implications for Nursing Practice
- Provide information that antibiotics given perioperatively can reduce the incidence of a serious postoperative infection, endophthalmitis.
- Inform the patient that there is no evidence to support a decline in visual acuity postoperatively with the use of antibiotics in the perioperative period.

Reference for Evidence
Fong, E. (2019). Acute endophthalmitis post-cataract surgery: Perioperative antibiotics. JBI Evidence Summary AN: JBI 17117.
P, patient population of interest; *I,* intervention or area of interest; *C,* comparison of interest or comparison group; *O,* outcome or outcomes of interest (see Chapter 1).

The instillation of dilating and nonsteroidal anti-inflammatory eye drops helps maintain pupil dilation and reduce inflammation, respectively. One type of medication used for dilation is a mydriatic, an α-adrenergic agonist that produces pupillary dilation by causing contraction of the iris dilator muscle. Another type of medication is a cycloplegic, an anticholinergic medication that produces paralysis of accommodation (cycloplegia) and thus pupillary dilation (mydriasis) by blocking the effect of acetylcholine on the ciliary body

TABLE 24.4 MEDICATION THERAPY

Topical Medications for Pupil Dilation

Examples	Onset	Duration	Comments
Mydriatic Medications			
Phenylephrine hydrochloric acid (Mydfrin)	45–60 min	4–6 hr	May cause tachycardia and elevation in blood pressure, especially in older patients; can cause a reflexive decrease in heart rate when blood pressure rises Punctal occlusion should be used to limit systemic absorption
Cycloplegic Medications			
Tropicamide (Mydriacyl)	20–40 min	4–6 hr	1% Solution used in cycloplegic refraction; 0.5% solution used in fundus examination
Cyclopentolate HCl acid (Cyclogyl)	30–75 min	6–24 hr	Has been associated with psychotic reactions and behavioural disturbances Used in cycloplegic refraction, fundus examination, and uveitis
Homatropine hydrobromide (Isopto Homatropine)	30–60 min	1–3 days	Used in cycloplegic refraction, uveitis; may be used for pupil dilation to allow patient to see around a central lens opacity
Atropine sulphate (Isopto Atropine)	30–180 min	6–12 days	Used in cycloplegic refraction, uveitis

muscles. Examples of mydriatic and cycloplegic medications are listed in Table 24.4, and nursing considerations are discussed in the Nursing Management: Cataracts section. Many patients receive preoperative antianxiety medication before the injection of local anaesthetic.

> **MEDICATION ALERT—Cycloplegics and Mydriatics**
> - Instruct patient to wear dark glasses to minimize photophobia.
> - Monitor for signs of systemic toxicity (e.g., tachycardia, central nervous system effects).

Intraoperative Phase. Cataract extraction is an intraocular procedure. The anterior capsule is opened and the lens nucleus and cortex are removed, leaving the remaining capsular bag intact. In extracapsular extraction, the surgeon can remove the lens nucleus by "scooping" it out with a lens loop or by *phacoemulsification,* in which the nucleus is fragmented by ultrasonic vibration and aspirated from inside the capsular bag (Mayo Clinic, 2019). In either case, the remaining cortex is aspirated with an irrigation and aspiration instrument. The choice of placement and type of incision varies among surgeons. Corneoscleral incisions necessitate closure with sutures, whereas scleral tunnel incisions are self-sealing and require no closing suture. The incision required for phacoemulsification is considerably smaller than that required with intracapsular or standard extracapsular surgery.

In almost all cases today, an IOL is implanted at the time of cataract extraction surgery (Figure 24.5). Because most patients undergo an extracapsular procedure, the lens of choice is usually a posterior chamber lens that is implanted in the capsular bag behind the iris. However, other patient needs (e.g., financial resources) may dictate an additional type of lens. At the end of the procedure, additional medications such as antibiotics and corticosteroids may be administered. Depending on the type of anaesthetic, the patient's eye is covered with a patch or protective shield. If used, a patch or protective shield is usually worn overnight and removed during the first postoperative visit, which is usually the day after surgery. Patients should be instructed not to drive a vehicle while the eye shield is in place.

Postoperative Phase. Unless complications occur, most patients are ready to go home as soon as the effects of sedative medications have worn off. Postoperative medications usually include antibiotic drops to prevent infection and corticosteroid drops to decrease the postoperative inflammatory response. There is some evidence that postoperative activity restrictions

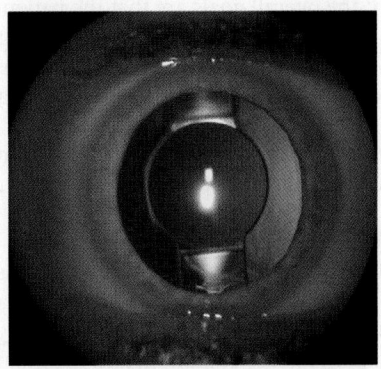

FIG. 24.5 Intraocular lens implant after cataract surgery. Source: Courtesy Cory J. Bosanko, OD, FAAO, Eye Centers of Tennessee, Crossville, Tennessee.

and nighttime eye shielding are unnecessary. However, many ophthalmologists still prefer that the patient avoid activities that increase the IOP, such as bending or stooping, coughing, or lifting.

During each postoperative examination, the ophthalmologist measures the patient's visual acuity, checks anterior chamber depth, assesses corneal clarity, and measures IOP. A flat anterior chamber may cause adhesions of the iris and cornea. The cornea may become hazy or cloudy from intraoperative trauma to the endothelium. Even on the day of surgery, the patient's uncorrected visual acuity in the operative eye may be good. However, it is not unusual or indicative of any problem if the patient's visual acuity is reduced immediately after surgery.

The postoperative eye drops are gradually reduced in frequency and finally discontinued when the eye has healed. When the eye is fully recovered, the patient receives a final prescription for glasses if still required after surgery. The newest innovation is a multifocal IOL that corrects for both near and distance vision. Regardless of the type of IOL used, patients may still need glasses to achieve their best visual acuity.

NURSING MANAGEMENT CATARACTS

NURSING ASSESSMENT

The nurse should assess the patient's distance and near visual acuity. If the patient is to undergo surgery, the nurse should especially note the visual acuity in the patient's nonoperative eye. With this information, the nurse can determine how visually compromised the patient may be while the operative eye is healing. In addition, the nurse should assess the psychosocial effect of the patient's visual disability and the patient's level of knowledge regarding the disease process and therapeutic options. Postoperatively, it is important to assess the patient's level of comfort and ability to follow the postoperative regimen.

NURSING DIAGNOSES

Nursing diagnoses for the patient with a cataract include but are not limited to the following:

- *Reduced self-care* resulting from *perceptual disorders* (visual impairment)
- *Anxiety* resulting from *unmet needs* (knowledge about surgical and postoperative experience)

PLANNING

Preoperatively, the overall goals are that the patient with a cataract will (a) make informed decisions regarding therapeutic options and (b) experience minimal anxiety. Postoperatively, the overall goals are that the patient with a cataract will (a) understand and adhere to postoperative therapy, (b) maintain an acceptable level of physical and emotional comfort, and (c) remain free of infection and other complications.

NURSING IMPLEMENTATION

HEALTH PROMOTION. There are no proven measures to prevent cataract development. However, it is wise (and certainly does no harm) to suggest that the patient wear sunglasses, avoid extraneous or unnecessary radiation, and maintain good nutrition and appropriate intake of antioxidant vitamins (e.g., vitamins C and E). Also, information about vision enhancement techniques should be provided to the patient who chooses not to undergo surgery.

ACUTE INTERVENTION. Preoperatively, patients with cataracts need accurate information about the disease process and the treatment options, especially because cataract surgery is considered an elective procedure. Although cataracts are not a life-threatening condition, patients need to know that without surgery, some degree of visual disability will develop. The nurse should be available to give each patient and the family or caregivers information to help them make an informed decision about appropriate treatment.

For a patient who elects to have surgery, the nurse is able to provide information, support, and reassurance about the surgical and postoperative experience that can reduce or alleviate the patient's anxiety.

When administering topical medications for pupil dilation before surgery (see Table 24.4 for examples), the nurse should note that patients with dark irides may need a larger dose. Photophobia is common; therefore, decreasing the room lighting is helpful. These medications produce transient stinging and burning and are contraindicated for use in patients with narrow-angle glaucoma because angle-closure glaucoma may be produced. Mydriatic medications can produce significant cardiovascular effects.

Table 24.5 outlines patient and caregiver teaching after eye surgery. Patients with a patch should be informed that they will not have depth perception until the patch is removed (usually within 24 hours). This necessitates special considerations to avoid possible falls or other injuries. The patient with significant

| TABLE 24.5 | **PATIENT & CAREGIVER TEACHING GUIDE** |

After Eye Surgery

Include the following information when teaching the patient and the caregiver after eye surgery.
1. Proper hygiene and eye care techniques to ensure that medications, dressings, and surgical wound are not contaminated during eye care
2. Signs and symptoms of infection and when and how to report those to allow early recognition and treatment of possible infection
3. Importance of adhering to postoperative restrictions on head positioning, bending, coughing, and the Valsalva manoeuvre to optimize visual outcomes and prevent increased intraocular pressure
4. How to instill eye medications with the use of aseptic techniques and to adhere to prescribed eye medication regimen to prevent infection
5. How to monitor pain, take pain medication, and report pain not relieved by medication
6. Importance of continued follow-up as recommended to maximize potential visual outcomes

Source: Adapted from Lamb, P., & Simms-Eaton, S. (2008). *Core curriculum for ophthalmic nursing* (3rd ed.). Kendall-Hunt.

visual impairment in the nonoperative eye requires more assistance while the operated eye is patched. Once the patch is removed (usually within 24 hours), most patients with visual impairment in the nonoperative eye have adequate vision for necessary activities because the implanted IOL provides immediate visual rehabilitation in the operated eye. On occasion, a patient may require 1 or 2 weeks for the visual acuity in the operated eye to reach an adequate level for most visual needs. Such a patient also needs some special assistance until the vision improves.

After cataract surgery, most patients experience little or no pain. There may be some scratchy sensation in the operative eye. Mild analgesics are usually sufficient to relieve any pain. If the pain is intense, the patient should notify the surgeon because this may indicate hemorrhage, infection, or increased IOP. The nurse should also instruct the patient to notify the surgeon of increased or purulent drainage, increased redness, or any decrease in visual acuity. (A nursing care plan for the patient after eye surgery is available on the Evolve website.)

AMBULATORY AND HOME CARE. For a patient with cataracts who has not undergone surgery, the nurse can suggest ways in which the patient may modify activities or lifestyle to accommodate the visual deficit caused by the cataract. The nurse should also provide the patient with accurate information about appropriate long-term eye care.

Patients with cataracts who undergo surgery remain in the surgical facility for only a few hours. The patient and the family are responsible for almost all postoperative care. The nurse must give them written and verbal instructions before discharge. These instructions should include information about postoperative eye care, activity restrictions, medications, follow-up visit scheduling, and signs and symptoms of possible complications. The patient's family should be included in the instruction because some patients may have difficulty with self-care activities, especially if the vision in the nonoperative eye is poor. The nurse should provide an opportunity for the patient and family to demonstrate any necessary self-care activities. Most patients experience little visual impairment after surgery.

IOL implants provide immediate visual rehabilitation, and many patients achieve a usable level of visual acuity within a few days after surgery. Also, the patient's eye may remain patched for only 24 hours, and many patients have good vision in the nonoperative eye. A few patients may experience significant visual impairment postoperatively: those who do not have an IOL implanted at the time of surgery, those who require several weeks to achieve a usable level of visual acuity after surgery, or those with poor vision in the nonoperative eye. For these patients, the time between surgery and receiving glasses or contacts can be a period of significant visual disability. The nurse can suggest ways in which the patient and the family can modify activities and the environment to maintain an adequate level of safe functioning. Suggestions may include getting assistance with going up stairs, removing area rugs and other potential obstacles, preparing meals for freezing before surgery, and obtaining audio books for diversion until visual acuity improves.

EVALUATION

The overall expected outcomes are that after cataract surgery, the patient will

- Have improved vision
- Be better able to take care of self
- Have minimal to no pain
- Be optimistic about expected outcomes

AGE-RELATED CONSIDERATIONS

Most patients with cataracts are older persons. When an older patient is visually impaired, even temporarily, they may experience a loss of independence, lack of control over their life, and a significant change in self-perception. Many older patients need emotional support and encouragement, as well as specific suggestions to allow a maximum level of independent function. The nurse should assure older patients that cataract surgery can be accomplished safely and comfortably with minimal sedation. A retrospective case-series study found that very old patients (over 85 years of age) undergoing cataract surgery may be more prone to complications (Sella et al., 2020).

RETINOPATHY

Retinopathy is a process of microvascular damage to the retina. It can develop slowly or rapidly and lead to blurred vision and progressive vision loss. In adults, retinopathy is most often associated with diabetes mellitus or hypertension.

Diabetic retinopathy is a common complication of diabetes mellitus, especially in patients with long-standing uncontrolled diabetes (Chaudhary et al., 2018). It is the leading cause of visual disability and blindness in Canadians with long-standing uncontrolled diabetes (diabetes is discussed in Chapter 52). Because diabetes has been diagnosed in increasing numbers of Canadians, the incidence of diabetic retinopathy will continue to increase. In a Canadian study of diabetic retinopathy in Indigenous and non-Indigenous Canadians, the data indicated that ethnicity plays a significant role in the development and severity of diabetic retinopathy, even though potential risk factors are not significantly different (Altomare et al., 2018).

Nonproliferative retinopathy is the most common form of diabetic retinopathy and is characterized by capillary microaneurysms, retinal swelling, and hard exudates. Macular edema represents a worsening of the retinopathy, inasmuch as plasma leaks from macular blood vessels. As capillary walls weaken they can rupture, which leads to intraretinal "dot and blot"

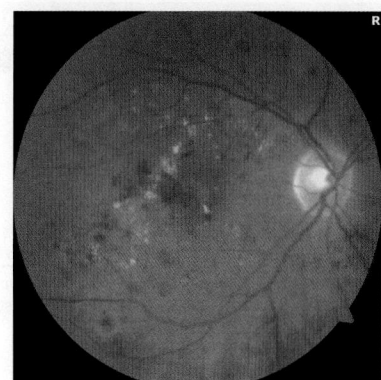

FIG. 24.6 Diabetic retinopathy. Intraretinal "dot and blot" hemorrhages. Source: Courtesy Cory J. Bosanko, OD, FAAO, Eye Centers of Tennessee, Crossville, Tennessee.

hemorrhaging (Figure 24.6). This can lead to a severe loss of central vision. As the disease advances, *proliferative retinopathy* may occur, where new blood vessels grow. However, these blood vessels are abnormal, fragile, and predisposed to leak and thus predispose the patient to severe vision loss. Fluorescein angiography is used to detect diabetic macular edema, which may be treated with laser photocoagulation (National Eye Institute, 2019c).

Hypertensive retinopathy is caused by blockages in retinal blood vessels that result from hypertension. (Hypertension is discussed in Chapter 35.) These changes may not initially affect a person's vision. On a routine eye examination, retinal hemorrhages and macular swelling can be noted. Sustained, severe hypertension can cause swelling of the optic disc and nerve (*papilledema*) and lead to sudden visual loss. Treatment, which may be required on an emergency basis, focuses on lowering the blood pressure. Normal vision is restored in patients with treatment of the underlying cause of the hypertension.

RETINAL DETACHMENT

A **retinal detachment** is a separation of the retina and the underlying pigment epithelium, with fluid accumulation between the two layers. The incidence of nontraumatic retinal detachment is approximately 1 per 15 000 individuals each year. This number is higher when aphakic individuals are included because retinal detachment is more likely to occur in aphakic patients. Almost all patients with an untreated, symptomatic retinal detachment become blind in the involved eye, hence the importance of immediate treatment. On average, 9 out of 10 patients have positive outcomes from retinal detachment treatment and surgery (National Eye Institute, 2020).

Etiology and Pathophysiology

Retinal detachment has many causes, the most common of which is a retinal break. A *retinal break* is an interruption in the full thickness of the retinal tissue, and such breaks can be classified as tears or holes. *Retinal holes* are atrophic retinal breaks that occur spontaneously. *Retinal tears* can occur as the vitreous humor shrinks during aging and pulls on the retina. The retina tears when the traction force exceeds the strength of the retina. Once the retina has a break, liquid vitreous can enter the subretinal space between the sensory layer and the retinal pigment epithelium layer, causing a *rhegmatogenous* retinal detachment. Retinal detachment can also occur when abnormal membranes

TABLE 24.6	RISK FACTORS FOR RETINAL DETACHMENT

- Increasing age
- Severe myopia
- Infection or eye trauma
- Retinopathy (diabetic)
- Eye diseases or tumours
- Cataract or glaucoma surgery
- Family or personal history of retinal detachment

Source: Adapted from National Eye Institute. (2020). *Retinal detachment.* https://www.nei.nih.gov/learn-about-eye-health/eye-conditions-and-diseases/retinal-detachment

TABLE 24.7	INTERPROFESSIONAL CARE

Retinal Detachment

Diagnostic Studies
- History and physical examination
- Visual acuity measurement
- Ophthalmoscopy (direct and indirect)
- Slit-lamp microscopy
- Ultrasonography if cornea, lens, or vitreous humor is hazy or opaque

Interprofessional Therapy
Preoperative
- Mydriatic, cycloplegic eye drops (see Table 24.4)
- Photocoagulation of retinal break that has not progressed to detachment

Surgery
- Laser photocoagulation
- Cryotherapy (cryopexy)
- Scleral buckling procedure
- Draining of subretinal fluid
- Vitrectomy
- Intravitreal bubble

Postoperative
- Topical antibiotic
- Topical corticosteroid
- Analgesia
- Mydriatics
- Positioning and activity as preferred by patient's surgeon

mechanically pull on the retina. Such detachments are called *tractional* detachments and are less common. A third type of retinal detachment is the *secondary* or *exudative* detachment, which occurs in conditions that allow fluid to accumulate in the subretinal space (e.g., choroidal tumours, intraocular inflammation). Risk factors for retinal detachment are listed in Table 24.6.

Clinical Manifestations

Patients with a detaching retina describe symptoms that include *photopsia* (light flashes), floaters, and a "cobweb," "hairnet," or ring in the field of vision. Once the retina has detached, the patient describes a painless loss of peripheral or central vision, "like a curtain" coming across the field of vision. The area of visual loss corresponds to the area of detachment. If the detachment is in the superior nasal retina, the visual field loss is in the inferior temporal area. If the detachment is small or develops slowly in the periphery, the patient may not be aware of a visual problem. The effects of a retinal detachment can be viewed online at VisionSimulations.com (see the Resources at the end of this chapter).

Diagnostic Studies

Visual acuity measurements should be the first diagnostic procedure with any report of vision loss (Table 24.7). The retinal detachment can be directly visualized through direct and indirect ophthalmoscopy or slit-lamp microscopy in conjunction with a special lens to view the far periphery of the retina. Ultrasonography may be useful for identifying a retinal detachment if the retina cannot be directly visualized (e.g., when the cornea, the lens, or the vitreous humor is hazy or opaque).

Interprofessional Care. Some retinal breaks are not likely to progress to detachment. The ophthalmologist monitors the patient, giving precise information about the warning signs and symptoms of impending detachment and instructing the patient to seek immediate evaluation if any of those signs or symptoms occurs. The ophthalmologist usually refers the patient with a detachment to a retinal specialist. Treatment objectives are to seal any retinal breaks and to relieve inward traction on the retina. Several techniques are used to accomplish these objectives (National Eye Institute, 2020).

Surgical Therapy

Laser Photocoagulation and Cryopexy. These techniques seal retinal breaks by creating an inflammatory reaction that causes a chorioretinal adhesion or scar. In *laser photocoagulation,* an intense, precisely focused light beam is used to create an inflammatory reaction. The light is directed at the area of the retinal break. For retinal breaks accompanied by significant detachment, the retinal specialist may use photocoagulation

intraoperatively in conjunction with scleral buckling. Tears or holes without accompanying retinal detachment may be treated prophylactically with laser photocoagulation if there is a high risk of progression to retinal detachment. When used alone, laser therapy is an outpatient procedure for which most patients require only topical anaesthesia. Patients may experience minimal adverse symptoms during or after the procedure.

Another method used to seal retinal breaks is *cryopexy.* This procedure involves the use of extreme cold to create the inflammatory reaction that produces the sealing scar. The ophthalmologist applies the cryoprobe instrument to the external globe in the area over the tear. This is usually done on an outpatient basis and with the use of a local anaesthetic. As with photocoagulation, cryotherapy may be used alone or during scleral buckling surgery. The patient may experience significant discomfort and eye pain after cryopexy. The nurse should encourage the patient to take the prescribed pain medication after the procedure.

Scleral Buckling. *Scleral buckling* is an extraocular surgical procedure that involves compressing the globe so that the pigment epithelium, the choroid, and the sclera move toward the detached retina. The retinal surgeon sutures a silicone implant against the sclera, causing the sclera to buckle inward. The surgeon may place an encircling band over the implant if there are multiple retinal breaks, if suspected breaks cannot be located, or if there is widespread inward traction on the retina (Figure 24.7). To drain any subretinal fluid, a small-gauge needle is inserted to facilitate contact between the retina and the buckled sclera. Scleral buckling is usually done as an outpatient procedure with the patient under local anaesthesia.

Intraocular Procedures. In addition to the extraocular procedures described, retinal surgeons may use one or more intraocular procedures in treating some retinal detachments. *Pneumatic retinopexy* is the intravitreal injection of a gas to form a temporary bubble in the vitreous that closes retinal breaks and provides apposition of the separated retinal layers. Because the intravitreal bubble is temporary, this technique is combined with laser photocoagulation or cryotherapy (cryopexy). A patient with an intravitreal bubble must position their head so that the bubble is in contact with the retinal break. It may be necessary for the patient to maintain this position as much as possible for up to several weeks.

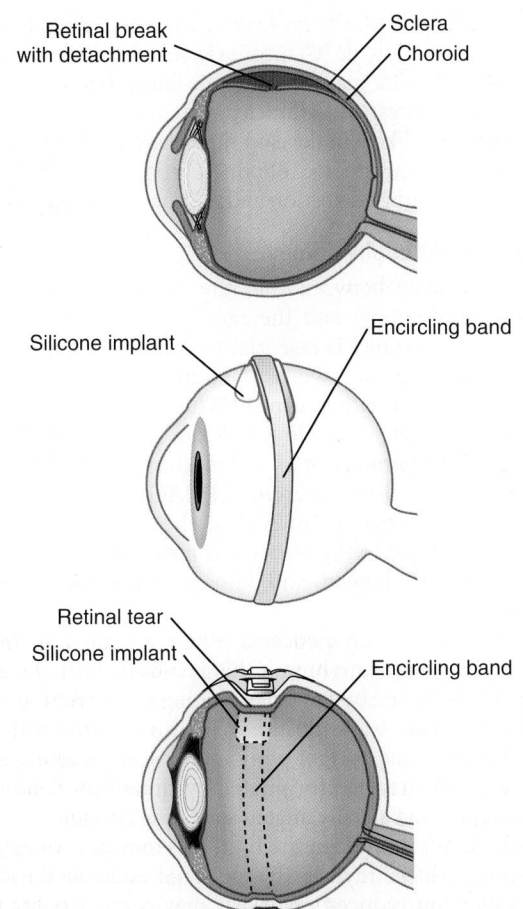

FIG. 24.7 Retinal break with detachment *(top)*; surgical repair by scleral buckling technique *(middle* and *bottom).*

Vitrectomy (surgical removal of the vitreous) may be used to relieve traction on the retina, especially when the traction results from proliferative diabetic retinopathy. Vitrectomy may be combined with scleral buckling to provide a dual effect in relieving traction.

Postoperative Considerations in Scleral Buckling and Intraocular Procedures. Reattachment procedures are successful in 90% of retinal detachments (National Eye Institute, 2020). Visual prognosis varies, depending on the extent, length, and area of detachment. Postoperatively, the patient may be on bed rest and may require special positioning to maintain proper position of an intravitreal bubble. The patient may need multiple topical medications, including antibiotics, anti-inflammatory medications, or dilating medications. The level of activity restriction after retinal detachment surgery varies greatly. The nurse should verify the prescribed level of activity with the patient's surgeon and help the patient plan for any necessary assistance in relation to activity restrictions.

In most cases, retinal detachment is an urgent situation, and the patient is confronted suddenly with the need for surgery. The patient needs emotional support, especially during the immediate preoperative period when preparations for surgery can lead to additional anxiety. When the patient experiences postoperative pain, the nurse should administer prescribed pain medications and teach the patient to take the medication as necessary after discharge. The patient may go home within a few hours of surgery or may remain in the hospital for several days, depending on the surgeon and the type of repair.

Discharge planning and teaching are important, and the nurse should begin these processes as early as possible because the patient does not remain hospitalized long. Patient and caregiver teaching after eye surgery is discussed in Table 24.5. The patient is at risk for retinal detachment in the other eye. Therefore, the nurse should teach the patient the signs and symptoms of retinal detachment. The nurse can also promote use of proper protective eyewear to help avoid retinal detachments related to trauma.

AGE-RELATED MACULAR DEGENERATION

Age-related macular degeneration (AMD) is an eye disease that progressively destroys the macula (the central portion of the retina), causing irreversible central vision loss. It is the leading cause of blindness and vision loss in Canada (Canadian National Institute for the Blind [CNIB], 2021). AMD is a common eye condition, affecting 2 million people in Canada, with the majority aged 50 years or older (Devenyi et al., 2016). Canadians who have AMD outnumber those who have breast cancer, prostate cancer, Parkinson's disease, or Alzheimer's disease combined (CNIB, 2021).

AMD is divided into two forms: dry (nonexudative) and wet (exudative). People with *dry AMD*, which is the more common form (90% of all cases), often notice that close-vision tasks become more difficult. In this form, the macular cells start to atrophy, leading to a slowly progressive and painless vision loss. *Wet AMD* is the more severe form. Wet AMD accounts for 90% of the cases of AMD-related blindness. Wet AMD has a more rapid onset and is characterized by the development of abnormal blood vessels in or near the macula.

Etiology and Pathophysiology

AMD is related to retinal aging. The prevalence increases drastically with age and occurs more often in women than in men. Genetic factors also appear to play a major role, and family history is a major risk factor for AMD (Touhy et al., 2019). People who smoke cigarettes are twice as likely to develop late AMD as are nonsmokers (National Eye Institute, 2021). Other risk factors include long-term exposure to ultraviolet light, hyperopia, and light-coloured irides. Nutritional factors may play a role in the progression of AMD. A dietary supplement of vitamin C, vitamin E, beta-carotene, and zinc decreases the progression of advanced AMD but has no effect on people with minimal AMD or those with no evidence of AMD (Chew, 2017). Mechanisms of protection are also being discovered among non-antioxidant nutrients such as omega-3 fatty acids and the B vitamins. A nutritious diet is thought to be more protective than nutritional supplements. Zinc was found to increase the subretinal fluid and the thickness of the macula, which decrease the risk of acquiring AMD in older patients (Detaram et al., 2019).

The dry form of AMD starts with the abnormal accumulation of yellowish extracellular deposits called *drusen* in the retinal pigment epithelium. The macular cells then undergo atrophy and degeneration. Wet AMD is characterized by the growth of new, fragile blood vessels from their normal location in the choroid to an abnormal location in the retinal epithelium. As the new blood vessels leak, scar tissue gradually forms. Acute vision loss may occur in some cases, with bleeding from subretinal neovascular membranes.

Clinical Manifestations

The patient may experience blurred and darkened vision, the presence of *scotomas* (blind spots in the visual field), and *metamorphopsia* (distortion of vision). Many people may not notice unilateral early changes in their vision if the other eye is not affected.

Diagnostic Studies

In addition to visual acuity measurement, the primary diagnostic procedure is ophthalmoscopy. The examiner looks for drusen and other fundus changes associated with AMD. The Amsler grid test may help define the involved area, and the result provides a baseline for future comparison. Fundus photography and intravenous angiography with fluorescein or indocyanine green dyes, or both, may help to further define the extent and type of AMD.

Interprofessional Care

Vision often does not improve for most people with AMD. Limited treatment options for patients with wet AMD include several medications that are injected directly into the vitreous cavity. Ranibizumab (Lucentis) and bevacizumab (Avastin) are selective inhibitors of endothelial growth factor that help to slow vision loss in wet AMD. Adverse effects can include blurred vision, eye irritation, eye pain, and photosensitivity. The injections are given at 4- to 6-week intervals, depending on which medication is used. Retinal stability is determined by ocular coherence tomography, which enables the physician to identify fluid in the central retina to determine the need for continued intravitreal injections.

Photodynamic therapy entails the use of verteporfin (Visudyne) intravenously and a "cold" laser to excite the dye. This procedure is used for cases of wet AMD and destroys the abnormal blood vessels without permanent damage to the retinal pigment epithelium and photoreceptor cells. Verteporfin is a photosensitizing drug that becomes active when exposed to the low-level laser light wave. Until the drug is completely excreted by the body, it can be activated by exposure to sunlight or other high-intensity light such as halogen; therefore, patients are cautioned to avoid direct exposure to sunlight and other intense forms of light for 5 days after treatment. After receiving therapy, patients must be completely covered because any exposure to skin by sunlight could activate the drug in that area, which would result in a thermal burn.

People at risk for developing advanced AMD should consider supplements of vitamins and minerals (in consultation with their health care provider). The cessation of smoking may also help in halting the progression of dry AMD to a more advanced stage.

Many patients with assistive devices for low-degree vision can continue reading and retain a licence to drive during the daytime and at lowered speeds. The permanent loss of central vision has significant psychosocial implications for nursing care. Nursing management of patients with uncorrectable visual impairment is discussed earlier in the chapter and is appropriate for patients with AMD. The nurse should avoid giving the impression that "nothing can be done" about the condition when caring for a patient with AMD. Although therapy will not recover lost vision, much can be done to augment the remaining vision.

GLAUCOMA

Glaucoma is a group of disorders characterized by elevated IOP and its consequences: optic nerve atrophy and peripheral visual field loss. Glaucoma is the second most common reason for vision loss in Canadians. It affects more than 400 000 Canadians and 80 million people worldwide (Glaucoma Research Society of Canada, 2021). Risk factors for glaucoma include family history, age, near-sightedness, diabetes, and ethnicity (e.g., individuals of African descent are more likely to develop the disease). The incidence of glaucoma increases with age. Blindness from glaucoma is largely preventable with early detection and appropriate treatment.

Etiology and Pathophysiology

A proper balance between the rate of aqueous production (referred to as *inflow*) and the rate of aqueous reabsorption (referred to as *outflow*) is essential to maintain the IOP within normal limits. The place where the outflow occurs is the *angle* where the iris meets the cornea. When the rate of inflow is greater than the rate of outflow, IOP can rise above the normal limits. If IOP remains elevated, vision loss may be permanent.

Primary open-angle glaucoma (POAG) is the most common type of glaucoma. In POAG, the outflow of aqueous humor is decreased in the trabecular meshwork. The drainage channels become clogged, and damage to the optic nerve can then result.

Primary angle-closure glaucoma (PACG) is due to a reduction in the outflow of aqueous humor that results from angle closure. Usually this is caused by the lens's bulging forward as a result of the aging process. Angle closure may also occur as a result of pupil dilation in the patient with anatomically narrow angles. An acute attack may be precipitated by situations in which the pupil remains in a partially dilated state long enough to cause an acute and significant rise in the IOP. This may occur because of medication-induced mydriasis, emotional excitement, or darkness. Medication-induced mydriasis may occur not only from topical ophthalmic preparations but also from many systemic medications (both prescription and over-the-counter medications). The nurse should check medication records and documentation before administering medications to the patient with angle-closure glaucoma and instruct the patient not to take any mydriatic medications.

Clinical Manifestations

POAG develops slowly and without symptoms of pain or pressure. The patient usually does not notice the gradual visual field loss until peripheral vision has been severely compromised. Eventually, patients with untreated glaucoma have "tunnel vision," in which only a small centre field can be seen and all peripheral vision is absent.

Acute angle-closure glaucoma causes definite symptoms, including sudden, excruciating pain in or around the eye. This is often accompanied by nausea and vomiting. Visual symptoms include blurred vision, ocular redness, and seeing coloured halos around lights. The acute rise in IOP may also cause corneal edema, which gives the cornea a frosted appearance.

Manifestations of subacute or chronic angle-closure glaucoma appear more gradually. The patient who has had a previous, unrecognized episode of subacute angle-closure glaucoma may report a history of blurred vision, ocular redness, eye or brow pain, or seeing coloured halos around lights. The effects of glaucoma can be viewed online at VisionSimulations.com (see the Resources at the end of this chapter).

Diagnostic Studies

IOP is usually elevated in glaucoma (normal IOP is 10–21 mm Hg). In cases of elevated pressures, the ophthalmologist usually

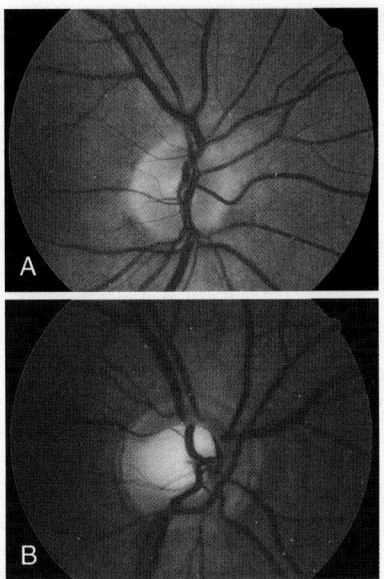

FIG. 24.8 The optic disc. **A,** In the normal eye, the optic disc is pink with little cupping. **B,** In glaucoma, the optic disc is pale, and optic cupping is present. (Note the appearance of the retinal vessels, which travel over the edge of the optic cup and appear to dip into it.)

TABLE 24.8 **INTERPROFESSIONAL CARE**	
Glaucoma	
Diagnostic Studies	**Surgical Therapy**
• History and physical examination	• Argon laser trabeculoplasty (ALT)
• Visual acuity measurement	• Trabeculectomy with or without filtering implant
• Tonometry	
• Ophthalmoscopy (direct and indirect)	**Acute Angle-Closure Glaucoma**
• Slit-lamp microscopy	• Topical cholinergic medication
• Gonioscopy	• Hyperosmotic medication
• Visual field perimetry	• Laser peripheral iridotomy
	• Surgical iridectomy
Interprofessional Therapy **Chronic Open-Angle Glaucoma** **Medication Therapy***	
• β-Adrenergic blockers	
• α-Adrenergic agonists	
• Cholinergic medications (miotics)	
• Carbonic anhydrase inhibitors	

*See Table 24.9.

repeats the measurements over time to verify the elevation. In open-angle glaucoma, IOP is usually between 22 and 32 mm Hg. In acute angle-closure glaucoma, IOP may exceed 50 mm Hg.

In open-angle glaucoma, slit-lamp microscopy reveals a normal angle. In angle-closure glaucoma, the examiner may note a markedly narrow or flat anterior chamber angle, an edematous cornea, a fixed and moderately dilated pupil, and ciliary injection (hyperemia of the ciliary blood vessels produces redness).

Measures of peripheral and central vision provide other diagnostic information. Whereas central acuity may remain 20/20 even in the presence of severe peripheral visual field loss, visual field perimetry may reveal subtle changes in the peripheral area of the retina early in the disease process, long before actual scotomas develop. In acute angle-closure glaucoma, central visual acuity is reduced if corneal edema is present, and the visual fields may be markedly decreased.

As glaucoma progresses, *optic disc cupping* may be one of the first signs of chronic open-angle glaucoma. The optic disc becomes wider, deeper, and paler (light grey or white); these characteristics are visible with direct or indirect ophthalmoscopy (Figure 24.8).

Interprofessional Care

The primary focus of glaucoma therapy is to keep the IOP low enough to prevent optic nerve damage. Therapy varies with the type of glaucoma. The diagnostic studies and interprofessional care of glaucoma are summarized in Table 24.8.

Chronic Open-Angle Glaucoma. Initial treatment in chronic open-angle glaucoma is with medications (Table 24.9). The patient must understand that continued treatment and supervision are necessary because the medications control, but do not cure, glaucoma.

Argon laser trabeculoplasty (ALT) is a noninvasive option to lower IOP when medications are not successful or when the patient either cannot or will not use the medication therapy as recommended. ALT is an outpatient procedure that necessitates

only topical anaesthesia. The laser stimulates scarring and contraction of the trabecular meshwork, which opens the outflow channels. ALT reduces IOP approximately 75% of the time. The patient uses topical corticosteroids for approximately 3 to 5 days after the procedure. The most common postoperative complication is an acute rise in IOP. The ophthalmologist examines the patient 1 week and again 4 to 6 weeks after surgery.

Filtration surgery, also called a *trabeculectomy,* may be indicated if medical management and laser therapy are not successful. The success rate of this surgery is 75 to 85%.

Acute Angle-Closure Glaucoma. Acute angle-closure glaucoma is an ocular emergency that necessitates immediate intervention. Miotics and oral or intravenous hyperosmotic medications are usually successful in immediately lowering the IOP (see Table 24.8). A laser peripheral iridotomy or surgical iridectomy is necessary for long-term treatment and prevention of subsequent episodes. These procedures allow the aqueous humor to flow through a newly created opening in the iris and into normal outflow channels. One of these procedures may also be performed on the other eye as a precaution because many patients often experience an acute attack in the other eye.

SAFETY ALERT
Patients who take miotic medications must be warned that they may experience decreased visual acuity, especially in dim light.

NURSING MANAGEMENT GLAUCOMA

NURSING ASSESSMENT

Because glaucoma is a chronic condition that necessitates long-term management, the nurse must assess the patient's ability to understand and adhere to the rationale and regimen of the prescribed therapy. In addition, the nurse should assess the patient's psychological reaction to the diagnosis of a potentially sight-threatening chronic disorder. The nurse must include the patient's caregiver in the assessment process because the chronic nature of this disorder can affect the family in many ways. Some families

TABLE 24.9   MEDICATION THERAPY

Acute and Chronic Glaucoma

Medication	Action	Adverse Effects	Nursing Considerations
β-Adrenergic Blockers			
Betaxolol (Betoptic)	Cardioselective β₁-adrenergic blocker; probably decreases aqueous humor production	Transient discomfort; systemic reactions (rarely reported) include bradycardia, heart block, pulmonary distress, headache, depression	Topical medications; minimal effect on pulmonary and cardiovascular parameters Contraindicated for use in patients with bradycardia, cardiogenic shock, or overt cardiac failure Systemic absorption can have additive effect with systemic β₁-adrenergic blocking medications.
Levobunolol (Betagan) Timolol maleate (Timoptic)	Noncardioselective β₁- and β₂-blockers; probably decrease aqueous humor production	Transient ocular discomfort, blurred vision, photophobia, blepharoconjunctivitis, bradycardia, decreased blood pressure, bronchospasm, headache, depression	Topical drops; same effects and contraindications as for betaxolol; also contraindicated for use in patients with asthma or severe COPD
α-Adrenergic Agonists			
Apraclonidine (Iopidine) Brimonidine tartrate (Alphagan)	α-Adrenergic agonists; probably decrease aqueous humor production	Ocular redness; irregular heart rate	Topical drops; used to control or prevent acute rise in IOP after laser procedure (used before and immediately after ALT and iridotomy, Nd:YAG laser capsulotomy). For patient at risk for systemic reactions, teaching includes instructions to occlude puncta.
Latanoprost (Xalatan)	Prostaglandin-F analogue	Increased brown iris pigmentation, ocular discomfort and redness, dryness, itching, and sensation of foreign body	Topical drops Teach patient not to take more than 1 drop per evening and to remove contact lens 15 min before instilling.
Cholinergic Medications (Miotics)			
Carbachol (Isopto Carbachol)	Parasympathomimetic; stimulates iris sphincter contraction, causing miosis and opening of trabecular meshwork, facilitating outflow of aqueous humor; also partially inhibits activity of cholinesterase	Transient ocular discomfort, headache, ache in brow area, blurred vision, decreased adaptation to darkness, syncope, excessive salivation, dysrhythmias, vomiting, diarrhea, hypotension, retinal detachment in susceptible individual (rare)	Topical drops Caution patient about decreased visual acuity caused by miosis, particularly in dim light.
Pilocarpine (Isopto Carpine)	Parasympathomimetic; stimulates iris sphincter contraction, causing miosis and opening of trabecular meshwork, facilitating outflow of aqueous humor	Same as those of carbachol	Topical drops Same cautions as for carbachol
Carbonic Anhydrase Inhibitors ***Systemic***			
Acetazolamide Methazolamide	Decreases production of aqueous humor	Paresthesias, especially "tingling" sensation in extremities; hearing dysfunction or tinnitus; loss of appetite; taste alteration; GI disturbances; drowsiness; confusion	Oral nonbacteriostatic sulfonamides Anaphylaxis and other sulpha type of allergic reactions may occur in patient allergic to sulpha drugs. Diuretic effect can lower electrolyte levels. Ask patient about acetylsalicylic acid (ASA; Aspirin) use; medication should not be given to patient receiving high-dose ASA (Aspirin) therapy.
Topical Brinzolamide (Azopt) Dorzolamide (Trusopt)	Decreases production of aqueous humor	Transient stinging, blurred vision, redness	Same as for systemic medications
Combination Therapy			
Timolol maleate and dorzolamide (Cosopt)	Combination of two medications (β-adrenergic blocker and topical carbonic anhydrase inhibitors)	Same as those for timolol maleate and dorzolamide (described previously)	—
Hyperosmolar Medications			
Mannitol solution (Osmitrol)	Increases extracellular osmolarity so that intracellular water moves to the extracellular and vascular spaces, reducing IOP	Nausea, vomiting, diarrhea, thrombophlebitis, hypertension, hypotension, tachycardia	Intravenous solution; used in acute glaucoma attacks or preoperatively when decreased IOP is desired Nurse must assess patient for susceptibility to pulmonary edema and HF before administering hyperosmolar medications.

ALT, argon laser trabeculoplasty; *COPD*, chronic obstructive pulmonary disease; *GI*, gastrointestinal; *HF*, heart failure; *IOP*, intraocular pressure; *Nd:YAG*, neodymium:yttrium–aluminum–garnet (laser).

may become the primary providers of necessary care, such as eye drop administration, if the patient is unwilling or unable to accomplish these self-care activities. The nurse also assesses visual acuity, visual fields, IOP, and fundus changes when appropriate.

NURSING DIAGNOSES

Nursing diagnoses for the patient with glaucoma include but are not limited to the following:
- *Potential for injury* as demonstrated by *sensory integration dysfunction* (visual acuity deficits)
- *Reduced self-care* resulting from *perceptual disorders* (visual impairment)
- *Preparedness for intensified self-care*
- *Acute pain* resulting from *physical injury agent* (surgical process)

PLANNING

The overall goals are that the patient with glaucoma will (a) have no progression of visual impairment, (b) understand the disease process and the rationale for therapy, (c) adhere to all aspects of therapy (including medication administration and follow-up care), and (d) have no postoperative complications.

NURSING IMPLEMENTATION

HEALTH PROMOTION. Loss of vision from glaucoma is preventable. It is important to teach the patient and caregiver about the risk of vision loss from glaucoma and that this risk increases with age. The nurse should stress the importance of early detection and treatment in preventing visual impairment. A comprehensive ophthalmic examination is invaluable in identifying persons with glaucoma or those at risk of developing glaucoma. The Canadian Ophthalmological Society (2007) recommended an eye examination every 3 to 5 years until the age of 40 and then every 2 to 4 years until the age of 65. Patients with risk factors such as family history of glaucoma and those of African descent should have annual eye examinations. Because so many eye diseases tend to occur in older persons, those older than 65 should have an examination every 2 years (annually if they have any risk factors; Canadian Ophthalmological Society, 2007). Even though the Non-Insured Health Benefits for First Nation and Inuit Program provides coverage for biennial eye exams for persons over 18 years of age (Indigenous Services Canada, 2020), Indigenous people may be at higher risk for not receiving screening eye examinations for several reasons—for example, lack of access to health care providers, comorbidities, and economic and cultural barriers (Campbell et al., 2020).

ACUTE INTERVENTION. Acute nursing interventions are directed primarily toward patients with acute angle-closure glaucoma and patients undergoing surgery for glaucoma. A patient with acute angle-closure glaucoma requires immediate IOP-lowering medication, which the nurse must administer in a timely and appropriate manner according to the ophthalmologist's prescription. Most surgical procedures for glaucoma are outpatient procedures. In the acute situation, the patient needs postoperative instructions and may require nursing comfort measures to relieve discomfort related to the procedure. Patient and caregiver teaching after eye surgery is discussed in Table 24.5.

AMBULATORY AND HOME CARE. Because of the chronic nature of glaucoma, the patient needs encouragement to follow the therapeutic regimen and follow-up recommendations prescribed by the ophthalmologist. The patient needs accurate information about the disease process and treatment options, including the rationale underlying each option. In addition, the patient needs information about the purpose, frequency, and technique of administering prescribed antiglaucoma medications. In addition to verbal instructions, all patients should receive written instructions that contain the same information. The nurse can encourage adherence by helping the patient identify the most convenient and appropriate times for medication administration or by advocating a change in therapy if the patient reports unacceptable adverse effects.

EVALUATION

The overall expected outcomes are that the patient with glaucoma will
- Have no further loss of vision
- Adhere to the recommended therapy
- Safely function within their own environment
- Obtain relief from pain associated with the disease and surgery

AGE-RELATED CONSIDERATIONS

Many older patients with glaucoma have systemic illnesses or take systemic medications that may affect their glaucoma therapy. In particular, patients who take a β-adrenergic blocking medication for glaucoma may experience an additive effect if they are also taking a systemic β-adrenergic blocking medication. All β-adrenergic blocking glaucoma medications are contraindicated for use in patients with bradycardia, a greater than first-degree heart block, cardiogenic shock, and overt cardiac failure. The non–cardioselective β-adrenergic blocking glaucoma medications are also contraindicated in patients with severe chronic obstructive pulmonary disease (COPD) or asthma. The hyperosmolar medications may precipitate heart failure or pulmonary edema in susceptible patients. Older patients receiving high-dose acetylsalicylic acid (ASA; Aspirin) therapy for rheumatoid arthritis should not take carbonic anhydrase inhibitors. The α-adrenergic agonists can cause tachycardia or hypertension, which may have serious consequences in older patients. The nurse must teach older patients to occlude the lacrimal puncta to limit the systemic absorption of glaucoma medications.

INTRAOCULAR INFLAMMATION AND INFECTION

The term *uveitis* is used to describe inflammation of the uveal tract, the retina, the vitreous cavity, or the optic nerve. This inflammation may be caused by bacteria, viruses, fungi, or parasites. *Cytomegalovirus retinitis* is an opportunistic infection that occurs in patients with acquired immune deficiency syndrome (AIDS) and in other immunosuppressed patients. The causes of sterile intraocular inflammation include autoimmune disorders, AIDS, malignancies, or disorders associated with systemic diseases such as inflammatory bowel disease. Pain and photophobia are common symptoms.

Endophthalmitis is an extensive intraocular inflammation of the vitreous cavity. Bacteria, viruses, fungi, or parasites can all induce this serious inflammatory response. The mechanism of infection may be endogenous, in which the infecting pathogen arrives at the eye through the bloodstream, or exogenous, in which the infecting pathogen is introduced through a surgical wound or a penetrating injury. Although rare, endophthalmitis is a devastating complication of intraocular surgery (e.g., cataract surgery) or penetrating ocular injury and can lead to irreversible blindness within hours or days. Manifestations include ocular pain, photophobia, decreased visual acuity, headaches, reddened and swollen conjunctiva, and corneal edema. Preoperative administration of prophylactic antibiotics is recommended (see the Evidence-Informed Practice box).

When all the layers of the eye (vitreous humor, retina, choroid, and sclera) are involved in the inflammatory response, the patient has *panophthalmitis*. In the final stages of extensive cases, the scleral coat may undergo bacterial or inflammatory dissolution. Subsequent rupture of the globe spreads the infection into the orbit or eyelids.

Treatment of intraocular inflammation depends on the underlying cause. Intraocular infections must be treated with antimicrobial medications, which may be delivered topically, subconjunctivally, intravitreally, systemically, or in some combination. Sterile inflammatory responses necessitate anti-inflammatory medications such as corticosteroids. The patient with intraocular inflammation is usually uncomfortable and may be noticeably anxious and frightened. The nurse must provide accurate information and emotional support to the patient and the family. In severe cases, enucleation may be necessary. When patients lose visual function or even the entire eye, they grieve over the loss. The nurse's role includes helping patients through the grieving process.

ENUCLEATION

Enucleation is the removal of the eye. The primary indication for enucleation is the combination of blindness and pain in the eye. These may result from glaucoma, infection, or trauma. Enucleation may also be indicated in ocular malignancies, although many malignancies can be managed with cryotherapy, radiation, and chemotherapy. The surgical procedure includes severing the extraocular muscles close to their insertion on the globe, inserting an implant to maintain the intraorbital anatomy, and suturing the ends of the extraocular muscles over the implant. The conjunctiva covers the joined muscles, and a clear conformer is placed over the conjunctiva until the permanent prosthesis is fitted. A pressure dressing helps prevent postoperative bleeding.

Postoperatively, the nurse observes the patient for signs of complications, including excessive bleeding or swelling, increased pain, displacement of the implant, or temperature elevation. Patient teaching should include instructions about the instillation of topical ointments or drops and wound cleansing. The nurse should also instruct the patient how to insert the conformer into the socket in case it falls out. The patient is often devastated by the loss of an eye, even when enucleation occurs after a lengthy period of painful blindness. The nurse should recognize and validate the patient's emotional response and provide support to the patient and the family.

Approximately 6 weeks after surgery, the wound is sufficiently healed for the permanent prosthesis. The prosthesis is fitted by an ocular specialist and designed to match the remaining eye. The prosthesis is gently cleansed with fingertips and warm water using mild soap and then dried lightly with a soft tissue. Solvents or alcohol-based solutions are to be avoided as they can cause damage. The nurse should teach the patient how to remove, cleanse, and insert the prosthesis. Special polishing is required periodically to remove dried protein secretions.

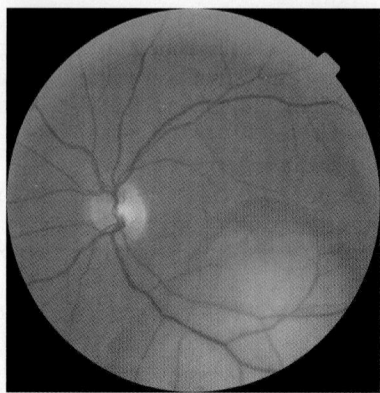

FIG. 24.9 Uveal melanoma. A large tumour in the choroid, the most common location in the eye for melanoma. Source: Courtesy Cory J. Bosanko, OD, FAAO, Eye Centers of Tennessee, Crossville, Tennessee.

OCULAR TUMOURS

Benign and malignant tumours can occur in many areas of the eye, including the conjunctiva, retina, and orbit. Malignancies of the eyelid include basal cell and squamous cell carcinomas (see Chapter 26).

Uveal melanoma is a cancerous neoplasm of the iris, choroid, or ciliary body. It is the most common primary intraocular malignancy in adults, but it is much rarer than skin melanoma. Approximately 200 cases are diagnosed in Canada each year (Melanoma Network of Canada, 2015). It is more frequently found in light-skinned people older than 60 years of age with chronic exposure to ultraviolet light. Genetic factors such as a mutated gene may also increase a person's risk (Nielsen et al., 2015). Uveal melanoma can arise from pre-existing nevi in the eye. Tumours may be asymptomatic or associated with vision loss depending on their size and location and presence of hemorrhage and retinal detachment. As with other cancers, cancer stage and cell type are important variables in the patient's prognosis. Diagnostic testing may include ultrasonography, magnetic resonance imaging (MRI), and fine-needle aspiration biopsy. Uveal melanoma commonly appears as a dome-shaped, well-circumscribed, solid brown to golden pigment in the iris, choroid, or ciliary body (Figure 24.9). Many patients do not lose the affected eye, and some may experience good vision after treatment in that eye.

Depending on the status of the involved eye, treatment options can include enucleation, plaque radiation therapy (brachytherapy), external beam radiation, transpupillary photocoagulation, eye wall resection, and exenteration. Within 15 years, approximately 50% of all patients with uveal melanoma will develop metastases, most commonly in the liver.

OCULAR MANIFESTATIONS OF SYSTEMIC DISEASES

Many systemic diseases are accompanied by significant ocular manifestations. Ocular signs and symptoms may be the first finding in or report by a patient with a systemic disease. One example is the patient with undiagnosed diabetes who seeks ophthalmic care for blurred vision. A thorough history and careful examination of the patient can reveal that the underlying cause of the blurred vision is lens swelling resulting from hyperglycemia. Another example is the patient who seeks care for a conjunctival lesion. The ophthalmologist may be the first health care provider to make the diagnosis of AIDS on the basis of the presence of a conjunctival Kaposi's sarcoma.

AUDITORY CONDITIONS
EXTERNAL EAR AND CANAL

External Otitis
The skin of the external ear and the ear canal is subject to the same problems as skin anywhere on the body. External otitis involves inflammation or infection of the epithelium of the auricle and ear canal. Swimming may alter the flora of the external canal as a result of chemicals and contaminated water. This can result in an infection often referred to as "swimmer's ear." Trauma from picking the ear or using sharp objects (e.g., hairpins) to clean the ear frequently causes the initial break in the skin. Piercing of auricular cartilage carries a greater risk of infection than does soft-tissue piercing (Hoover et al., 2017).

Causes. Infections and skin conditions may cause external otitis. Bacteria or fungi may be the cause. *Pseudomonas aeruginosa* is the most common bacterial cause. Fungi, including *Candida albicans* and *Aspergillus* species, especially thrive in warm, moist climates. The warm, dark environment of the ear canal provides a good medium for the growth of microorganisms.

Malignant external otitis is a serious infection caused by *P. aeruginosa*. It occurs mainly in older patients with diabetes. The infection, which can spread from the external ear to the parotid gland and temporal bone (osteomyelitis), is usually treated with antibiotics.

Clinical Manifestations and Complications. Ear pain *(otalgia)* is one of the first signs of external otitis. Even in mild cases, a patient may experience significant discomfort with chewing, moving the auricle, or pressing on the tragus. Swelling of the ear canal can muffle hearing. Drainage from the ear may be serosanguineous (blood-tinged fluid) or purulent (white to green thick fluid). Fever occurs when the infection spreads to surrounding tissue. Facial nerve paralysis may occur with malignant external otitis.

NURSING AND INTERPROFESSIONAL MANAGEMENT EXTERNAL OTITIS

Diagnosis of external otitis is made by otoscopic examination of the ear canal. The nurse must be careful to avoid pain when pulling on the patient's auricle to straighten out the canal or when inserting the otoscope speculum. The eardrum may be difficult to see because of swelling in the canal. Culture and sensitivity studies of the drainage may be done. Moist heat, mild analgesics, and topical anaesthetic drops usually control the pain. Topical antibiotics include polymyxin B (Polysporin), neomycin (Neosporin), and chloramphenicol (Chlor Palm 250). Nystatin (Nyaderm CRM) is used for fungal infections. Corticosteroids may also be used to decrease inflammation unless the infection is fungal, in which case their use is contraindicated. If the surrounding tissue is involved, systemic antibiotics are prescribed. Improvement should occur in 48 hours, but the patient must adhere to the prescribed therapy for 7 to 14 days for complete resolution.

Hands should be washed before and after otic drops (eardrops) are administered. The drops should be administered at room temperature; cold drops can cause vertigo by stimulating the semicircular canals, and heated drops can burn the

TABLE 24.10 PATIENT & CAREGIVER TEACHING GUIDE
Prevention of External Otitis

Include the following instructions when teaching the patient and caregiver how to prevent external otitis.
1. Do not put anything in your ear canal unless requested by your health care provider.
2. Report itching if it becomes a problem.
3. Cerumen (earwax) is normal.
   - It lubricates and protects the canal.
   - Report chronic excessive cerumen if it impairs your hearing.
4. Keep your ears as dry as possible.
   - Use earplugs if you are prone to swimmer's ear.
   - Turn your head to each side for 30 sec at a time to help water run out of the ears.
   - Do not dry with cotton-tipped applicators.
   - A hair dryer set to low and held at least 6 in from the ear can speed water evaporation.

TABLE 24.11 MANIFESTATIONS OF CERUMEN IMPACTION

- Hearing loss
- Otalgia
- Tinnitus
- Vertigo
- Cough
- Cardiac depression (vagal stimulation)

tympanum. The tip of the dropper should not touch the ear during administration, to prevent contamination of the entire bottle. The ear is positioned so that the drops can run down into the canal. The patient should maintain this position for 2 minutes to allow the drops to spread. Sometimes drops are placed onto a wick of cotton that is placed in the canal. The nurse should instruct the patient not to push the cotton farther into the ear. Careful handling and disposal of material saturated with drainage is important. The nurse should also instruct the patient on methods to reduce the risk of external otitis (Table 24.10).

Cerumen and Foreign Bodies in the External Ear Canal
Impacted cerumen can cause discomfort and decreased hearing. In older persons, the earwax becomes dense and drier. Hair becomes thicker and coarser, entrapping the hard, dry cerumen in the canal. Symptoms of cerumen impaction are outlined in Table 24.11. Management involves irrigation of the canal with body-temperature solutions to soften the cerumen. Special syringes, varying from a simple bulb syringe to special irrigating equipment, can be used. The patient is placed in a sitting position with an emesis basin under the ear. The auricle is pulled up and back, and the flow of solution is directed above or below the impaction. It is important that the ear canal not be completely occluded with the syringe tip. If irrigation does not remove the cerumen, mild lubricant drops may be used to soften it. Severe impaction may need to be removed by the health care provider.

Attempts to remove a foreign object from the ear canal may result in pushing it farther into the canal. Vegetable matter in the ear tends to swell and may create a secondary inflammation, which makes removal more difficult. Mineral oil or lidocaine drops can be used to kill an insect before removal under microscope guidance. Removal of impacted objects should be performed by the health care provider.

Ears should be cleaned with a washcloth and finger. Cotton-tipped applicators should be avoided: Penetration of the middle ear by a cotton-tipped applicator can cause serious injury to the tympanic membrane (TM) and ossicles. The use of cotton-tipped applicators can also cause cerumen to become impacted against the TM and impair hearing.

Trauma

Trauma to the external ear can cause injury to the subcutaneous tissue that may result in a hematoma. If the hematoma is not aspirated, inflammation of the membranes of the ear cartilage (perichondritis) can result. Blows to the ear can also cause a conductive hearing loss if the ossicles in the middle ear are damaged or the TM is perforated. Head trauma that injures the temporal lobe of the cerebral cortex can impair the ability to understand the meaning of sounds.

Malignancy of the External Ear

Skin cancers are the only common malignancies of the ear. Rough sandpaper-like changes to the upper border of the auricle are premalignant lesions (actinic keratoses) associated with chronic sun exposure. They are often removed with liquid nitrogen. Malignancies in the external ear canal include basal cell carcinoma in the auricle and squamous cell carcinoma in the ear canal. If left untreated, they can invade underlying tissue. The nurse should teach the patient about the dangers of sun exposure and the importance of using hats and sunscreen when outdoors.

MIDDLE EAR AND MASTOID

Acute Otitis Media

Acute otitis media (AOM) is an infection of the tympanum, ossicles, and space of the middle ear. Swelling of the auditory tube as a result of colds or allergies can trap bacteria, causing a middle ear infection. Pressure from the inflammation pushes on the TM, causing it to become red, bulging, and painful. AOM is usually a childhood disease; in children the auditory tube that drains fluids and mucus from the middle ear is shorter and narrower and its position is flatter than that in adults (Le Saux & Robinson, 2016). Pain, fever, malaise, and reduced hearing are signs and symptoms of infections. Referred pain from the temporomandibular joint, teeth, gums, sinuses, or throat may also cause ear pain. Clinical practice guidelines include strategies such as observation, antibiotics, and pain control (Deniz et al., 2018).

Interprofessional care involves the use of antibiotics to eradicate the causative organism. Amoxicillin (Amoxil) is the current therapy of choice in North America. Surgical intervention is generally reserved for patients who do not respond to medical treatment. A *myringotomy* involves an incision in the tympanum to release the increased pressure and exudate from the middle ear. A tympanostomy tube may be placed for short- or long-term drainage. Prompt treatment of an episode of AOM generally prevents spontaneous perforation of the TM. In the adult patient for whom allergy may be a causative factor, antihistamines may also be prescribed.

Otitis Media With Effusion

Otitis media with effusion is an inflammation of the middle ear with a collection of fluid in the middle ear space. The fluid may be thin, mucoid, or purulent. If the Eustachian tube does not open and allow equalization of atmospheric pressure, negative

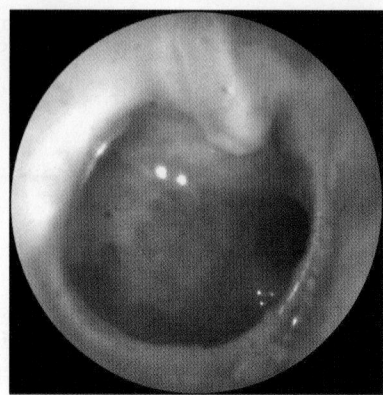

FIG. 24.10 Perforation of the tympanic membrane (TM) Source: Flint, P., Haughey, Lund, V., et al. (Eds.). (2010). *Cummings otolaryngology: Head and neck surgery* (5th ed.). Mosby.

pressure within the middle ear pulls fluid from surrounding tissues. This situation commonly follows upper respiratory tract or chronic sinus infections, barotrauma (caused by pressure change), or otitis media.

Patients can experience a feeling of fullness of the ear, a "plugged" feeling or popping sensation, and decreased hearing. The patient does not experience pain, fever, or discharge from the ear. It is normal to have otitis media with effusion for weeks to months after an episode of AOM. It usually resolves in 75 to 90% of cases without treatment but may recur.

Chronic Otitis Media and Mastoiditis

Etiology and Pathophysiology. Repeated attacks of AOM may lead to chronic otitis media, especially in adults who have a history of recurrent otitis in childhood. Organisms involved in chronic otitis media include *S. aureus, Proteus mirabilis,* and *P. aeruginosa.* Because the mucous membrane is continuous, both the middle ear and the air cells of the mastoid bone can be involved in the chronic infectious process.

Clinical Manifestations. *Chronic otitis media* is characterized by a purulent exudate and inflammation that can involve the ossicles, Eustachian tube, and mastoid bone. It is often painless and may be accompanied by hearing loss, nausea, and episodes of dizziness. Hearing loss is a complication from inflammatory destruction of the ossicles, a TM perforation, or accumulation of fluid in the middle ear space.

Complications. Untreated conditions can result in TM perforation and the formation of a *cholesteatoma* (a mass of epithelial cells and cholesterol in the middle ear). The cholesteatoma enlarges and can destroy the adjacent bones. Unless removed surgically, it can cause extensive damage to the ossicles and impair hearing.

Diagnostic Studies. Otoscopic examination of the TM may reveal colour and mobility changes or a perforation (Figure 24.10). Culture and sensitivity tests of the drainage are necessary to identify the organisms involved so that the appropriate antibiotic therapy can be prescribed. Audiography may demonstrate a hearing loss as great as 50 to 60 decibels (dB) if the ossicles have been damaged or separated. Sinus radiographic studies, MRI, or computed tomography (CT) of the temporal bone may demonstrate bone destruction, absence of ossicles, or the presence of a mass.

Interprofessional Care. The aims of treatment are to clear the middle ear of infection, repair the perforation, and preserve hearing (Table 24.12). Systemic antibiotic therapy is initiated on

TABLE 24.12   INTERPROFESSIONAL CARE
Chronic Otitis Media

Diagnostic Studies	Interprofessional Therapy
• History and physical examination	• Ear irrigations
• Otoscopic examination	• Otic, oral, or parenteral antibiotics
• Culture and sensitivity tests of middle ear drainage	• Analgesics
• Mastoid radiography	• Antiemetics
	• Surgery
	• Tympanoplasty*
	• Mastoidectomy

*See Table 24.13.

TABLE 24.13   PATIENT & CAREGIVER TEACHING GUIDE
After Ear Surgery

Include the following instructions when teaching the patient and caregiver after ear surgery.
1. Avoid sudden head movements.
2. Do not try to get out of bed without assistance.
3. Take medications to reduce dizziness if prescribed.
4. Change positions slowly.
5. Avoid getting the head wet (including showering) until directed by surgeon.
6. Report fever, pain, an increase in hearing loss, or drainage from the ear.
7. Do not cough or blow the nose because this causes increased pressure in the Eustachian tube and middle ear cavity and disrupts healing.
8. If you need to cough or sneeze, leave the mouth open to help reduce the pressure.
9. Avoid crowds because respiratory infections may be contracted.
10. Avoid situations in which pressure or popping in the ears is normally experienced, such as high elevations or airplane travel.

TABLE 24.14   INTERPROFESSIONAL CARE
Otosclerosis

Diagnostic Studies	Interprofessional Therapy
• History and physical examination	• Hearing aid
• Otoscopic examination	• Surgery (stapedectomy or fenestration)
• Rinne test	• Medication therapy
• Weber test	• Sodium fluoride with vitamin D
• Audiometry	• Calcium carbonate
• Tympanometry	

the basis of results of the culture and sensitivity tests. In addition, the patient may need to undergo frequent evacuation of drainage and debris in an outpatient setting. Otic and oral antibiotics are used to reduce infection. In many cases of chronic otitis media, the causative pathogen is resistant to antibiotics.

Surgical Therapy. Chronic TM perforations often do not heal with conservative treatment, and surgery is necessary. *Tympanoplasty (myringoplasty)* involves reconstruction of the TM, the ossicles, or both. A *mastoidectomy* is often performed with a tympanoplasty to remove infected portions of the mastoid bone. Removal of tissue stops at the middle ear structures that appear capable of conducting sound. Sudden pressure changes in the ear and postoperative infections can disrupt the surgical repair during the healing phase or cause facial nerve paralysis.

NURSING MANAGEMENT
CHRONIC OTITIS MEDIA

AFTER TYMPANOPLASTY

Routine preoperative care is provided before tympanoplasty and includes teaching postoperative expectations (Table 24.13).

After surgery, the patient is positioned flat and side-lying with the operated side up. It is normal for hearing to be impaired during the postoperative period if there is packing in the ear. A cotton-ball dressing is used for the incision made through the external auditory canal (endaural incision). The patient should be instructed to change the cotton packing and dressing daily. If a postauricular incision was used and a drain is in place, a mastoid dressing is used. A small gauze pad is cut to fit behind the ear, and fluffs are applied over the ear to prevent the outer circular head dressing from placing pressure on the auricle. The nurse should monitor the amount and type of drainage postoperatively, as well as the tightness of the dressing, to prevent tissue necrosis.

Otosclerosis

Otosclerosis is a hereditary autosomal dominant disease and the most common cause of hearing loss in young adults (Ferri, 2020). Spongy bone develops from the bony labyrinth, causing immobilization of the footplate of the stapes in the oval window. This reduces the transmission of vibrations to the inner ear fluids and results in conductive hearing loss. Although otosclerosis is typically bilateral, hearing loss may progress more rapidly in one ear. The patient is often unaware of the problem until the loss becomes so severe that communication is difficult.

Otoscopic examination may reveal a reddish blush of the tympanum (Schwartz's sign) caused by the vascular and bony changes within the middle ear. Tuning-fork tests help identify the conductive component of the hearing loss. On Rinne test, sound is heard longer when the stem of the tuning fork is touching the mastoid bone (bone conduction) than when placed next to the ear (air conduction). In the Weber test, the sound is heard better through the skull bone in the ear than through air when conductive hearing loss is greater. Audiography demonstrates good hearing by bone conduction but poorer hearing by air conduction (air–bone gap). The difference between air and bone conduction levels of hearing is usually at least 20 to 25 dB in otosclerosis.

Interprofessional Care. The hearing loss associated with otosclerosis may be stabilized by the use of sodium fluoride with vitamin D and calcium carbonate to retard bone resorption and encourage calcification of bony lesions. Amplification of sound by a hearing aid can be effective because the inner ear function is normal. Surgical treatment involves partial removal of the stapes (stapedectomy) or complete removal with prosthesis insertion (fenestration). Interprofessional care of otosclerosis is described in Table 24.14.

These procedures are usually performed with the patient under conscious sedation. The ear with poorer hearing is repaired first, and the other ear may be operated on within a year. An endaural incision is made under visualization through the operating microscope. Gelfoam is used on the incision flap to limit bleeding. A cotton ball is placed in the ear canal, and a small dressing is used to cover the ear.

During surgery, patients often report an immediate improvement in hearing in the operated ear. Because of the accumulation of blood and fluid in the middle ear, the hearing level decreases postoperatively but improves with healing. After stapedectomy, 90% of patients experience an improvement in hearing, in many instances to near normal.

NURSING MANAGEMENT OTOSCLEROSIS

Nursing management of patients undergoing stapedectomy or fenestration is similar to that for patients who have undergone tympanoplasty. Postoperatively, patients may experience dizziness, nausea, and vomiting as a result of intraoperative stimulation of the labyrinth. Some patients demonstrate nystagmus because of disturbance of the perilymph fluid. The patient should take care to avoid sudden movements that may induce or exacerbate dizziness. The patient should avoid actions that increase inner ear pressure, such as coughing, sneezing, lifting, bending, and straining during bowel movements.

INNER EAR CONDITIONS

Three symptoms that indicate disease of the inner ear are vertigo, sensorineural hearing loss, and tinnitus. Symptoms of vertigo arise from the vestibular labyrinth, whereas hearing loss and tinnitus arise from the auditory labyrinth. Manifestations of inner ear conditions overlap with some manifestations of central nervous system disorders.

Ménière's Disease

Ménière's disease (endolymphatic hydrops) is characterized by symptoms caused by inner ear disease, including episodic vertigo, tinnitus, fluctuating sensorineural hearing loss, and a sense of aural fullness. The patient experiences significant disability because of sudden, severe attacks of vertigo with nausea, vomiting, sweating, and pallor. Symptoms usually begin between the ages of 30 and 60 years (Di Berardino et al., 2020).

The cause of the disease is unknown, but it results in an excessive accumulation of endolymph in the membranous labyrinth. The volume of endolymph increases until the membranous labyrinth ruptures. Attacks may be preceded by a sense of fullness in the ear, increasing tinnitus, and muffled hearing. Patients with Ménière's disease may experience the feeling of being pulled to the ground ("drop attacks"). Some patients report that they feel as if they are whirling in space. Attacks may last hours or days and may occur several times a year. The clinical course of the disease is highly variable.

NURSING AND INTERPROFESSIONAL MANAGEMENT MÉNIÈRE'S DISEASE

Interprofessional care of Ménière's disease (Table 24.15) includes diagnostic tests to rule out other causes of symptoms, including central nervous system disease. Audiography demonstrates a mild, low-frequency sensorineural hearing loss. Vestibular tests indicate decreased function.

A glycerol test may aid in the diagnosis. An oral dose of glycerol is given, followed by serial audiography over 3 hours. Improvement in hearing or speech discrimination supports a diagnosis of Ménière's disease. The improvement is attributed to the osmotic effect of glycerol that pulls fluid from the inner ear. Although a positive test result is diagnostic of Ménière's disease, a negative test result does not rule out the condition.

TABLE 24.15   INTERPROFESSIONAL CARE
Ménière's Disease

Diagnostic Studies
- History and physical examination
- Audiometric studies (including speech discrimination, tone decay)
- Vestibular tests (including caloric test, positional test)
- Electronystagmography
- Neurological examination
- Glycerol test

Interprofessional Therapy
Acute Care
Medication Therapy (One or More Agents)
- Sedatives
- Benzodiazepines
- Anticholinergics
- Antiemetics
- Antihistamines

Surgical Therapy
Conservative Surgical Intervention
- Endolymphatic shunt
- Vestibular nerve section

Destructive Surgical Intervention
- Labyrinthotomy
- Labyrinthectomy

Ambulatory or Home Care
- Diuretics
- Antihistamines
- Calcium channel blockers
- Sedatives
- Hydrops diet: restriction of sodium, caffeine, nicotine, alcohol, and foods with monosodium glutamate (MSG)

During the acute attack, antihistamines, anticholinergic medications, and benzodiazepines can be used to decrease the abnormal sensation and lessen symptoms such as nausea and vomiting. Acute vertigo is treated symptomatically with bed rest, sedation, and antiemetics or antivertigo medications for motion sickness. The patient requires reassurance and counselling that the condition is not life-threatening. Management between attacks may include diuretics, antihistamines, calcium channel blockers, and a low-sodium diet. Diazepam (Valium) may be used to reduce the vertigo. Over time, most patients respond to the prescribed medications, but the attacks and hearing loss remain unpredictable.

Frequent and incapacitating attacks are indications for surgical intervention. Decompression of the endolymphatic sac and shunting are performed to reduce the pressure on the cochlear hair cells and to prevent further damage and hearing loss. If relief is not achieved, the vestibular nerve may be resected. When involvement is unilateral, surgical ablation of the labyrinth, resulting in loss of the vestibular and hearing cochlear function, is performed. Careful management can decrease the possibility of progressive sensorineural loss in many patients.

Nursing interventions are planned to minimize vertigo and provide for patient safety. During an acute attack, the patient is kept in a quiet, darkened room in a comfortable position. The patient needs to be taught to avoid sudden head movements or position changes. Fluorescent or flickering lights or television may exacerbate symptoms and should be avoided. An emesis basin should be available because vomiting is common. To minimize the patient's risk of falling, the nurse should keep the side rails up and the bed low in position when the patient is in bed. The patient should be instructed to call for assistance when getting out of bed. Medications and fluids are administered parenterally, and intake and output are monitored. When the attack subsides, the patient should be assisted with ambulation because unsteadiness may remain.

Benign Paroxysmal Positional Vertigo

Benign paroxysmal positional vertigo (BPPV) is a common cause of vertigo. Approximately 50% of cases of vertigo may be due to BPPV. In BPPV, free-floating debris in the semicircular canal causes vertigo with specific head movements, such as those involved with getting out of bed, rolling over in bed, and sitting up from lying down (HealthLink BC, 2019). The debris ("ear rocks") is composed of small crystals of calcium carbonate derived from the utricle in the inner ear. The utricle may be injured by head trauma, infection, or degeneration as a result of the aging process. However, for many patients, a cause cannot be found.

Symptoms include dizziness, vertigo, light-headedness, loss of balance, and nausea. Hearing loss is not characteristic, and symptoms tend to be intermittent. The symptoms of BPPV may be confused with those of Ménière's disease. Diagnosis is based on the results of auditory and vestibular tests.

Although BPPV is bothersome, it is rarely a serious problem unless an affected person falls. The Epley manoeuvre (canalith repositioning procedure) is effective in providing symptom relief for many patients (Balatsouras et al., 2018). In this manoeuvre, the ear debris is moved from areas in the inner ear that cause symptoms and repositioned into areas where they do not cause these problems. The Epley manoeuvre does not address the actual presence of debris; rather, it changes their location. A trained health care provider can instruct the patient in how to perform the Epley manoeuvre.

Acoustic Neuroma

An acoustic neuroma is a unilateral benign tumour that occurs where the vestibulocochlear nerve (cranial nerve VIII) enters the internal auditory canal. Early diagnosis is important because the tumour can compress the trigeminal and facial nerves and arteries within the internal auditory canal. Symptoms usually begin at 40 to 60 years of age.

Early symptoms are associated with compression and destruction of cranial nerve VIII. They include unilateral, progressive, sensorineural hearing loss; reduced touch sensation in the posterior ear canal; unilateral tinnitus; and mild, intermittent vertigo. Diagnostic tests include neurological, audiometric, and vestibular tests; computed tomographic scans; and MRI.

Surgery to remove small tumours generally preserves hearing and vestibular function. Large tumours (>3 cm) and the surgery required to remove them can leave the patient with permanent hearing loss and facial paralysis. The nurse should instruct the patient to report any clear, colourless discharge from the nose. This may be cerebrospinal fluid, and such leaks increase the risk of infection.

Hearing Loss and Deafness

Hearing loss is the fastest growing and one of the most prevalent, chronic conditions facing Canadians today (Hearing Foundation of Canada, 2020). Hearing loss has many causes; age-related presbycusis and noise-induced hearing loss are two of the most common. Nearly half of the persons who need assistance with hearing disorders are 65 years of age or older. With the aging of the population, the prevalence of hearing loss is increasing. At age 50, one of every eight persons is hearing impaired. A disturbing trend is the number of young adults showing signs of hearing loss. The tiny hair cells located inside the ear pick up sound waves and convert them into electrical signals that the brain can interpret. When loud sounds are listened to constantly, the vibrations destroy the tiny hair cells, which contributes to hearing loss. Unlike other cells in the body,

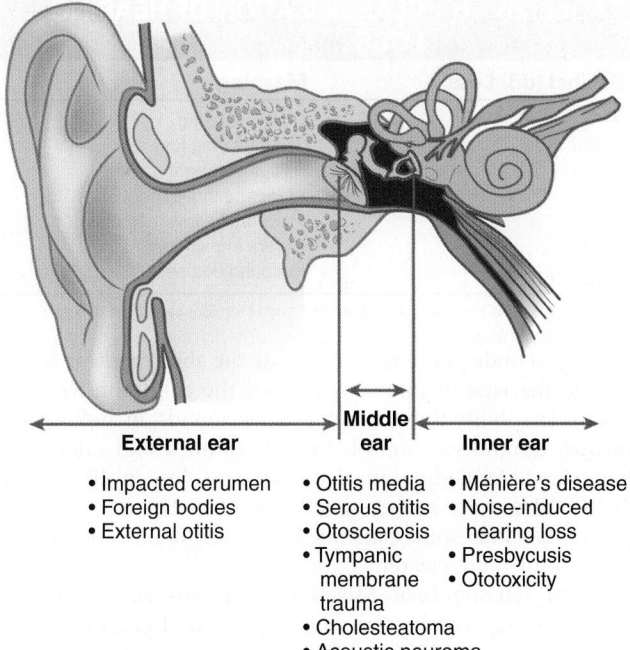

FIG. 24.11 Causes of hearing loss, by location.

- **External ear**
  - Impacted cerumen
  - Foreign bodies
  - External otitis
- **Middle ear**
  - Otitis media
  - Serous otitis
  - Otosclerosis
  - Tympanic membrane trauma
  - Cholesteatoma
  - Acoustic neuroma
- **Inner ear**
  - Ménière's disease
  - Noise-induced hearing loss
  - Presbycusis
  - Ototoxicity

hair cells never grow back once they are damaged (Government of Canada, 2020). Earbuds are of particular concern because volumes must be high in order to block out environmental distractions (Berg et al., 2016). Causes of hearing loss are listed in Figure 24.11.

Types of Hearing Loss

Conductive Hearing Loss. *Conductive hearing loss* occurs when conditions in the outer or middle ear impair the transmission of sound through air to the inner ear. A common cause is otitis media with effusion. Other causes are impacted cerumen, TM perforation, otosclerosis, and narrowing of the external auditory canal (Kandaswamy et al., 2020)).

Audiography demonstrates an air–bone gap of at least 15 dB. The term *air–bone gap* represents the situation in which hearing sensitivity is better by bone conduction than by air conduction. Patients may speak softly because they hear their own voices, which are conducted by bone, as being loud. These patients hear better in a noisy environment. If correction of the cause is not possible, a hearing aid may help if the loss is greater than 40 to 50 dB. Visit the Hearing Loss Sampler online to listen to simulated hearing loss sounds (see the Resources at the end of this chapter).

Sensorineural Hearing Loss. *Sensorineural hearing loss* is caused by impairment of function of the inner ear or the vestibulocochlear nerve (cranial nerve VIII). Congenital and hereditary factors, noise trauma over time, aging (presbycusis), Ménière's disease, and ototoxicity can cause sensorineural hearing loss.

Ototoxic medications include ASA (Aspirin), nonsteroidal anti-inflammatory drugs (NSAIDs), antibiotics (aminoglycosides, erythromycin, vancomycin), loop diuretics, and chemotherapy drugs.

Systemic infections, such as Paget's disease of the bone, immune diseases, diabetes mellitus, bacterial meningitis, and trauma, are associated with this type of hearing loss. The two main problems associated with sensorineural loss are (a) the

TABLE 24.16	**CLASSIFICATION OF HEARING LOSS**
Decibel (dB) Loss	**Meaning**
0–15	Normal hearing
16–25	Slight hearing loss
26–40	Mild impairment
41–55	Moderate impairment
56–70	Moderately severe impairment
71–90	Severe impairment
>90	Profound deafness*

*Most people in this category have been deaf since birth (congenitally deaf).

inability to understand speech despite the ability to hear sound and (b) the lack of understanding of the condition by other people. The ability to hear high-pitched sounds, including consonants, diminishes. Sounds become muffled and difficult to understand. An audiogram demonstrates a loss in dB levels at the 4 000-Hz range and eventually the 2 000-Hz range. A hearing aid may help some patients, but it only makes sounds and speech louder, not clearer.

Mixed Hearing Loss. Mixed hearing loss results from a combination of conductive and sensorineural causes. Careful evaluation is needed if corrective surgery for conductive loss is planned because the sensorineural component of the hearing loss will still remain.

Central and Functional Hearing Loss. Central hearing loss involves the inability to interpret sound, including speech, because of a disorder in the brain (central nervous system). Careful documentation of the history is helpful because there is usually a reference to deafness within the family. The patient should be referred to a qualified hearing and speech service if it is indicated.

Functional hearing loss may be caused by an emotional or a psychological factor. The patient does not seem to hear or respond to pure-tone subjective hearing tests, but no physical cause can be identified. Psychological counselling may help.

Classification of Hearing Loss. Hearing loss can also be classified by the dB level or loss as recorded on the audiogram. Normal hearing is in the 0- to 15-dB range. Table 24.16 describes the levels of hearing loss.

Clinical Manifestations. Common early signs of hearing loss are answering questions inappropriately, not responding when not looking at the speaker, asking others to speak up, and showing irritability with others who do not speak up. Other behaviours that suggest hearing loss include straining to hear, cupping the hand around the ear, reading lips, and an increased sensitivity to slight increases in noise level. Often, the patient is unaware of minimal hearing loss or may compensate by using these mannerisms. Family and friends who get tired of repeating or talking loudly are often first to notice hearing loss.

Deafness is often called the "unseen handicap" because it is not until conversation is initiated with a deaf adult that the difficulty in communication is realized. It is important that the health care provider be aware of the need for thorough validation of the deaf person's understanding of health teaching. Descriptive visual aids can be helpful.

Interference in communication and interaction with others can be the source of many challenges for the patient and caregiver. Often the patient refuses to admit or may be unaware of impaired hearing. Irritability is common because the patient must concentrate very hard to understand speech. The loss of clarity of speech is most frustrating to a patient with sensorineural hearing loss. The patient may hear what is said but not understand it. Withdrawal, suspicion, loss of self-esteem, and insecurity are commonly associated with advancing hearing loss.

NURSING AND INTERPROFESSIONAL MANAGEMENT HEARING LOSS AND DEAFNESS

HEALTH PROMOTION

ENVIRONMENTAL NOISE CONTROL. Noise is the most preventable cause of hearing loss. Figure 24.12 lists the levels of environmental noise generated by common indoor and outdoor sounds. Sudden severe loud noise (acoustic trauma) and chronic exposure to loud noise (noise-induced hearing loss) can damage hearing. Acoustic trauma causes hearing loss by destroying the hair cells of the organ of Corti. Sensorineural hearing loss as a result of increased and prolonged environmental noise, such as amplified sound, is occurring in young adults at an increasing rate. Amplified music (e.g., on iPods or MP3 players) should not exceed 50% of maximum volume. Health teaching must emphasize avoidance of continued exposure to noise levels greater than 70 dB. Young adults should be encouraged to keep amplified music at a reasonable level and limit their exposure time. Hearing loss caused by noise is irreversible.

In work environments known to have high noise levels (>85 dB), ear protection should be worn. Canadian Occupational Health and Safety regulations Part VII, Sections 7.1 to 7.8, address workplace noise (Department of Justice Canada, 2021). A variety of protectors that are worn over the ears or in the ears to prevent hearing loss are available. Periodic audiometric screening should be part of the health maintenance policies of industry. This provides baseline data on hearing to measure subsequent hearing loss.

Employees should participate in hearing conservation programs in work environments. Such programs should include noise exposure analysis, provision for control of noise exposure (hearing protectors), measurements of hearing, and employee–employer notification and education.

IMMUNIZATIONS. Various viruses in utero can cause deafness as a result of damage and malformations affecting the ear. The nurse should promote childhood and adult immunizations, including the measles-mumps-rubella (MMR) vaccine. Rubella infection during the first 8 weeks of gestation is associated with an 85% incidence of congenital rubella syndrome, which causes sensorineural deafness. Women of childbearing age should be tested for antibodies to these viral diseases. Women should avoid pregnancy for at least 3 months after being immunized. Immunization must be delayed if the woman is pregnant. Women who are susceptible to rubella can be vaccinated safely during the postpartum period.

OTOTOXIC SUBSTANCES. Medications commonly associated with ototoxicity include salicylates, NSAIDs, loop diuretics, chemotherapy drugs, and antibiotics. Chemicals used in industry (e.g., toluene, carbon disulphide, mercury) may damage the inner ear. Patients who are receiving ototoxic drugs or are exposed to ototoxic chemicals should be monitored for signs and symptoms associated with ototoxicity, including tinnitus, diminished hearing, and changes in equilibrium. If these symptoms develop, immediate withdrawal of the drug may prevent further damage and may cause the symptoms to disappear.

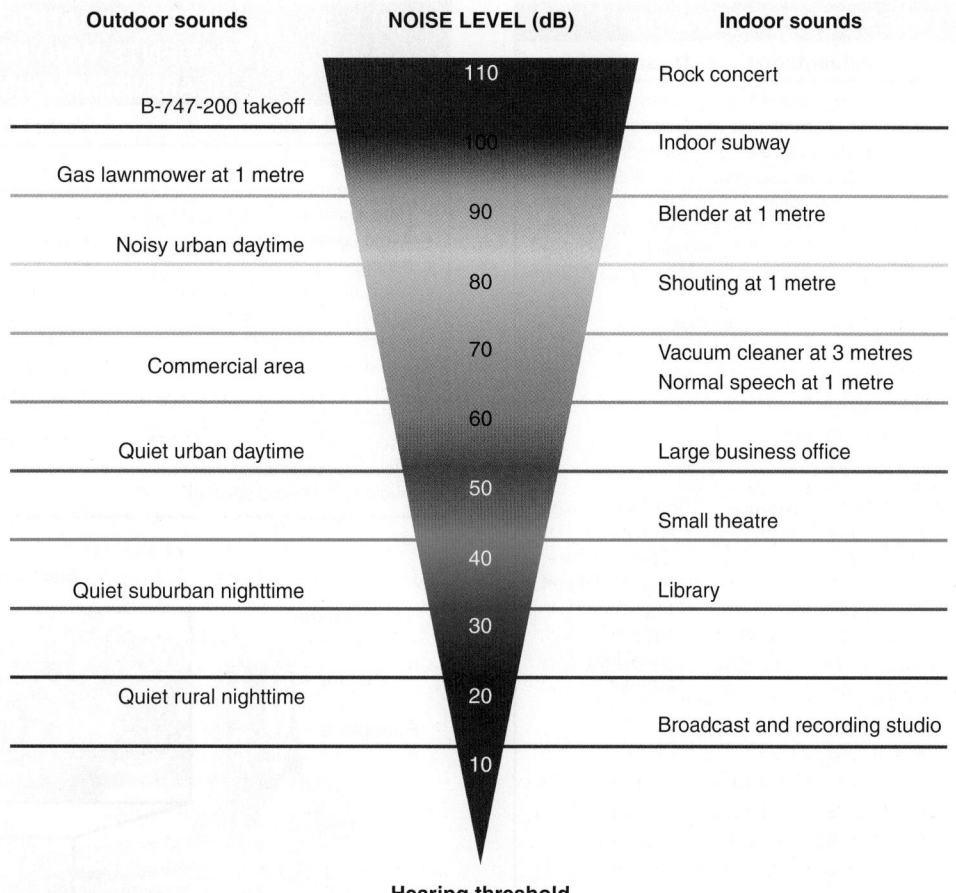

FIG. 24.12 Levels of common environmental sounds.

ASSISTIVE DEVICES AND TECHNIQUES

HEARING AIDS. The patient with a suspected hearing loss should have a hearing assessment by a qualified audiologist. If a hearing aid is indicated, it should be fitted by an audiologist or by a speech and hearing specialist. Many types of hearing aids are available, each with advantages and disadvantages (Table 24.17). The conventional hearing aid serves as a simple amplifier.

For patients with bilateral hearing impairment, binaural hearing aids provide the best sound lateralization and speech discrimination. The nurse must give careful instruction on its use and maintenance and must assist the patient during the period of adjustment. The goal of hearing aid therapy is improved hearing with consistent use. Patients who are motivated and optimistic about using a hearing aid are more successful users. The nurse should determine the patient's readiness for hearing aid therapy, including acknowledgement of a hearing impairment, the patient's feelings about wearing a hearing aid, the degree to which hearing loss affects life, and any difficulties the patient has manipulating small objects, such as putting a battery in a hearing aid.

Initially, use of the hearing aid should be restricted to quiet situations in the home. The patient must first adjust to voices (including the patient's own) and household sounds. The patient should also experiment by increasing and decreasing the volume, as situations require. As the patient adjusts to the increase in sounds and background noise, they can progress to situations in which several people are talking simultaneously. Next, the environment can be expanded to the outdoors and then to such environments as a shopping mall or grocery store. Adjustment to different environments occurs gradually, depending on the individual patient.

When the hearing aid is not being worn, it should be placed in a dry, cool area where it will not be inadvertently damaged or lost. The battery should be disconnected or removed when not in use. Battery life averages 1 week, and patients should be advised to purchase only a month's supply at a time. Ear moulds should be cleaned weekly or as needed. Toothpicks or pipe cleaners may be used to clear a clogged ear tip.

SPEECH READING. *Speech reading,* commonly called *lip reading,* can be helpful in increasing communication. It enables patients to achieve approximately 40% understanding of the spoken word. Individuals are able to use visual cues associated with speech, such as gestures and facial expression, to help clarify the spoken message. In speech reading, many words look alike to the person (e.g., "rabbit" and "woman"). If the person wears glasses, the glasses should be used to facilitate speech reading. The nurse can help the patient by using and teaching verbal and nonverbal communication techniques as described in Table 24.18.

SIGN LANGUAGE. *Sign language* is used as a form of communication for people with profound hearing impairment. It involves gestures and facial features such as eyebrow motion and lip-mouth movements.

There is no one universal sign language. American Sign Language is used in the United States and the English-speaking

TABLE 24.17	TYPES OF HEARING AIDS		
Type	**Advantages**	**Disadvantages**	
Completely in the canal (mild to moderate hearing loss)	Smallest and least visible aid Protected from sounds such as wind noise	Costly No space for add-ons such as directional microphones or volume controls Small, short-lived batteries	
In the canal (mild to severe hearing loss)	More powerful than aids completely in the canal Has adjustable features such as noise reduction	Small size of aid with its additional features may be difficult to operate for patients with visual loss or arthritis	
In the ear (mild to severe hearing loss)	Powerful amplification Inserts and adjusts easily Longer-lasting batteries	Visible May pick up wind noise readily	
Behind the ear (all types of hearing loss)	Most powerful aid Adjusts easily Longest battery life	Largest, most visible aid Newer models may be smaller and less obvious	

TABLE 24.18	COMMUNICATION WITH PATIENTS WHO HAVE HEARING IMPAIRMENTS	
Nonverbal Aids	**Verbal Aids**	
• Draw attention with hand movements. • Have speaker's face in good light. • Avoid covering mouth or face with hands. • Avoid chewing, eating, and smoking while talking. • Maintain eye contact. • Avoid distracting environments. • Avoid careless expression that the patient may misinterpret. • Use touch. • Move close to better ear. • Avoid light behind speaker.	• Speak normally and slowly. • Do not overexaggerate facial expressions. • Do not overenunciate. • Use simple sentences. • Rephrase sentence; use different words. • Write name or difficult words. • Do not shout. • Speak in normal voice directly into better ear.	

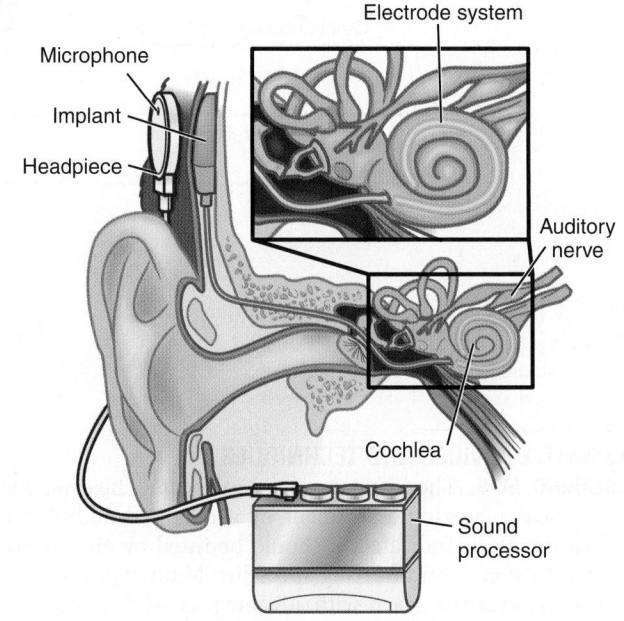

FIG. 24.13 Cochlear implant.

parts of Canada. Quebec Sign Language, known in French as *Langue des signes québécoise* or *Langue des signes du Québec (LSQ)*, is the sign language of deaf communities in francophone Canada, primarily in Quebec. Also, some Indigenous people have created their own sign language (e.g., Oneida sign language) (Albert, 2018).

COCHLEAR IMPLANT. The *cochlear implant* is used as a hearing device for people with severe to profound sensorineural hearing loss in one or both ears. The system consists of an external microphone placed behind the ear, a speech processor and a transmitter implanted under the skin that change sounds into electrical impulses, and a group of electrodes placed within the cochlea that stimulate the auditory nerves in the ear (Figure 24.13). Cochlear implants send information that covers the entire range of sound frequencies. The cochlear implant electrodes are inserted as far as possible into the cochlea to send both high- and low-frequency information. For patients with conductive and mixed hearing loss, the cochlear Baha system may be surgically implanted. The system works through direct bone conduction and becomes integrated with the skull bone over time.

Extensive training and rehabilitation are essential in order to receive maximum benefit from these implants. The positive aspects of a cochlear implant include providing sound to the person who heard none, improving lip-reading ability, monitoring the loudness of the person's own speech, improving the sense of security, and decreasing feelings of isolation. With continued research, the cochlear implant may offer the possibility of aural rehabilitation for a wider range of hearing-impaired individuals.

The U.S. Food and Drug Administration has created an informational website on cochlear implants (see the Resources at the end of this chapter). The site includes an animated movie to help visualize the implants and how they work.

ASSISTED LISTENING DEVICES. Numerous devices are now available to assist hearing-impaired persons. Direct amplification devices, amplified telephone receivers, alerting systems that flash when activated by sound, an infrared system for amplifying the sound of the television, and a combination FM receiver and hearing aid are all devices that the nurse can explore on the basis of the patient's needs. People with profound deafness may be assisted by text-telephone alerting systems that flash when activated by sound, by closed captioning on television, and by specially trained dogs. Such dogs are trained to alert their owners to specific sounds within the environment, which thus increases the person's safety and independence.

AGE-RELATED CONSIDERATIONS

HEARING LOSS

Presbycusis, hearing loss associated with aging, includes the loss of peripheral auditory sensitivity, a decline in word recognition ability, and associated psychological and communication issues. Because consonants (high-frequency sounds) are the letters by which spoken words are recognized, an older person with presbycusis has a diminished ability to understand the spoken word. Vowels are heard, but some consonants fall into the high-frequency range and cannot be differentiated. This may lead to confusion and embarrassment because of the difference in what was said and what was heard (Öberg, 2015).

The cause of presbycusis is related to degenerative changes in the inner ear. Noise exposure is thought to be a common factor. Table 24.19 describes the classification of specific causes and associated hearing changes of presbycusis. Many patients have

TABLE 24.19	CLASSIFICATION OF PRESBYCUSIS	
Type	**Hearing Change**	**Prognosis**
Sensory Atrophy of auditory nerve; loss of sensory hair cells	Loss of high-pitched sounds	Little effect on speech understanding; good response to sound amplification
Neural Degenerative changes in cochlea and spinal ganglion	Loss of speech discrimination	Amplification alone not sufficient
Metabolic Degenerative changes in cochlea and spinal ganglion	Uniform loss for all frequencies accompanied by recruitment*	Good response to hearing aid
Cochlear Stiffening of basilar membrane, which interferes with sound transmission in the cochlea	Range of hearing loss increases from low to high frequencies; speech discrimination affected with higher frequency losses	Ameliorated by appropriate forms of amplification

*Abnormally rapid increase in loudness as sound intensity increases.

more than one type of presbycusis. The prognosis for hearing depends on the cause of the loss. Sound amplification with the appropriate device is often helpful in improving the understanding of speech. In other situations, an audiological rehabilitation program can be valuable.

Many older people are reluctant to use a hearing aid for sound amplification. Reasons cited most often include cost, appearance, insufficient knowledge about hearing aids, amplification of competing noise, and unrealistic expectations. Most hearing aids and batteries are small, and neuromuscular changes such as stiff fingers, enlarged joints, and decreased sensory perception often make the care and handling of a hearing aid a difficult and frustrating experience for an older person. Some older persons may also tend to accept their losses as part of aging and believe there is no need for improvement.

CASE STUDY

Glaucoma and Diabetic Retinopathy

Patient Profile
L. A. (pronouns she/her), 68 years old, has osteoarthritis and type 2 diabetes mellitus, diagnosed 15 years earlier. Her current diagnosis is diabetic retinopathy. L. A. returns to the eye clinic for continued evaluation and care of her primary open-angle glaucoma (POAG) and re-examination for changes in diabetic retinopathy. L. A.'s current medical regimen for POAG includes topical timolol maleate, 0.5% extended (Timoptic XE), once daily in each eye, and latanoprost (Xalatan), 0.005%, in each eye, at bedtime. At L. A.'s last examination, microaneurysms and hard exudates of the retina were noted.

Subjective Data
• Can no longer read the newspaper and reports that medication labels are difficult to read.
• States limited success in getting the eye drops instilled because hands are stiff and painful from osteoarthritis.

Objective Data
• Distant and near visual acuity are stable at 20/60 in the right eye and 20/50 in the left eye. This is a reduction from 20/40 in both eyes since last visit.
• Intraocular pressures (IOPs) are stable at 20 mm Hg in both eyes. Visual field testing in the left eye reveals a new scotoma.
• Fluorescein angiography reveals diabetic macular edema in both eyes.

Interprofessional Care
• Brimonidine (Alphagan), 0.15%, in left eye 15 min before and immediately after argon laser trabeculoplasty (ALT)
• Argon laser treatment in left eye to seal leaking microaneurysm from macular edema
• Checking IOP after ALT
• Continuing previous glaucoma drop regimen
• Follow-up examination for glaucoma in 2 weeks for possible ALT in right eye
• Follow-up examination for diabetic macular edema in 8 weeks

Continued

CASE STUDY

Glaucoma and Diabetic Retinopathy—cont'd

Discussion Questions

1. What is the cause of L. A.'s new nonproliferative retinopathy?
2. Why might laser photocoagulation be an appropriate therapy for macular edema?
3. What is the purpose of the fluorescein angiography?
4. *Priority decision:* What priority topics should be discussed in discharge teaching?
5. In what way could glaucoma cause vision loss if L. A.'s eye pressures are not properly monitored?

6. *Priority decision:* What are the priority nursing interventions for L. A.?
7. *Priority decision:* On the basis of the assessment data, what are the priority nursing diagnoses? Are there any interprofessional problems?
8. *Evidence-informed practice:* L. A. wants to know if glaucoma is related to diabetes. How should the nurse respond to the patient's question?

ⓔvolve

Answers are available at http://evolve.elsevier.com/Canada/Lewis/medsurg.

REVIEW QUESTIONS

The number of the question corresponds to the same-numbered objective at the beginning of the chapter.

1. Why does presbyopia occur in older individuals?
   a. The retina degenerates.
   b. The lens becomes inflexible.
   c. The corneal curvature becomes irregular.
   d. It is associated with cataract development.
2. What is the most important nursing intervention for clients with epidemic keratoconjunctivitis?
   a. Applying patches to the affected eyes
   b. Accurately measuring intraocular pressure
   c. Monitoring near visual acuity every 4 hours
   d. Teaching client and family members good hygiene techniques
3. What should clients with eye inflammation or an eye infection be taught?
   a. Wear dark glasses to prevent irritation from ultraviolet light.
   b. Acute conditions commonly lead to chronic problems.
   c. Apply a cold compress with pressure to the inflamed area frequently.
   d. Regular, careful hand hygiene may prevent the infection from spreading.
4. Which of the following client behaviours would the nurse promote for healthy eyes and ears? *(Select all that apply)*
   a. Wearing protective sunglasses when bicycling.
   b. Supplemental intake of B vitamins and magnesium
   c. Playing amplified music at 75% of maximum volume
   d. Notifying the health care provider if tinnitus occurs during antibiotic therapy
   e. For women, avoiding pregnancy for 4 weeks after receiving measles-mumps-rubella (MMR) immunization
5. What should the nurse do to prepare clients for retinal detachment surgery?
   a. Explain how to care for an ocular prosthesis.
   b. Assure clients that they can expect 20/20 vision after surgery.
   c. Teach the family how to recognize when the client is hallucinating.
   d. Assess the client's level of knowledge about retinal detachment and provide information appropriate to the situation.
6. What should be included in the nursing plan for a client who needs to administer antibiotic eardrops?
   a. Cool the drops so that they decrease swelling in the canal.
   b. Be careful to avoid touching the tip of the dropper bottle to the ear.
   c. Placement of a cotton wick to assist in administering the drops is not recommended.
   d. Keep the head tilted for 5 to 7 minutes after administering the drops to prevent them from running out of the ear canal.

7. The nurse would suspect otosclerosis from assessment findings of hearing loss in which of the following clients?
   a. A 26-year-old woman with three biological children younger than 5 years of age
   b. A 52-year-old man whose hearing loss is accompanied by vertigo and tinnitus
   c. A 42-year-old woman who has a history of serous otitis media
   d. A 63-year-old man who can hear high-pitched sounds more effectively than low-pitched sounds
8. Which of the following statements best describes a client who has a sensorineural hearing loss?
   a. The client has difficulty understanding speech.
   b. The client experiences clearer sounds with the use of a hearing aid.
   c. The client may have a reversal of damage caused by ototoxic drugs.
   d. The client hears low-pitched sounds better than high-pitched sounds.
9. Which of the following would the nurse tell the client who is newly fitted with bilateral hearing aids? *(Select all that apply.)*
   a. Replace the batteries monthly.
   b. Clean the ear moulds weekly or as needed.
   c. Clean ears with cotton-tipped applicators daily.
   d. Disconnect or remove the batteries when not in use.
   e. Initially restrict usage to quiet listening in the home.
10. Which strategies would best assist the nurse in communicating with a client who has a hearing loss? *(Select all that apply.)*
    a. Overenunciate speech.
    b. Exaggerate facial expression.
    c. Raise the voice to a higher pitch.
    d. Write out names or difficult words.
    e. Speak normally and slowly.
11. Which of the following statements best describes clients with permanent visual impairment?
    a. They feel most comfortable with other visually impaired persons.
    b. They may feel threatened when others make eye contact during a conversation.
    c. They usually need others to speak louder so they can communicate appropriately.
    d. They may experience the same grieving process that is associated with other losses.

1. b; 2. d; 3. d; 4. a, d; 5. d; 6. b; 7. a; 8. a; 9. b, d, e; 10. d, e; 11. d.

ⓔvolve

For even more review questions, visit http://evolve.elsevier.com/Canada/Lewis/medsurg.

REFERENCES

Albert, A. (2018). *Oneida sign language created to connect deaf community with their culture*. CBC News. https://www.cbc.ca/news/canada/london/oneida-sign-language-culture-deaf-1.4605295

Altomare, F., Kherani, A., & Lovshin, J. (2018). Diabetes Canada 2018 clinical practice guidelines for the prevention and management of diabetes in Canada: Retinopathy. *Canadian Journal of Diabetes*, 48(Suppl 1). http://www.guidelines.diabetes.ca/cpg/chapter30

Artini, W., Riyanto, S. B., Hutauruk, J. A., et al. (2018). Predictive factors for successful high myopic treatment using high-frequency Laser-in-situ keratomileusis. *The Open Ophthamology*, 12, 214–225. https://doi.org/10.2174/1874364101812010214

Balatsouras, D. G., Koukoutsis, G., Fassolis, A., et al. (2018). Benign paroxysmal positional vertigo in the elderly: current insights. *Clinical Interventions in Aging*, 13, 2251–2266. https://doi.org/10.2147/CIA.S144134

Berg, A. L., Ibrahim, H., Sandler, S., et al. (2016). Music-induced hearing loss: What do college students know? *Contemporary Issues in Communication Science and Disorders*, 43. https://pubs.asha.org/doi/pdf/10.1044/cicsd_43_F_195

Campbell, R., Sutherland, R., Khan, S., et al. (2020). Diabetes-induced eye disease among First Nations people in Ontario: A longitudinal, population-based cohort study. *CMAJ Open*, 8(2), E282–E288. https://doi.org/10.9778/cmajo.20200005

Canadian Association of Optometrists (CAO). (n.d.). *Eye safety at home*. https://opto.ca/health-library/eye-safety-at-home

Canadian Association of Optometrists (CAO). (2019). *CAO Policy and advocacy position statement: Importance of eye health and vision care for healthy aging*. https://opto.ca/sites/default/files/resources/documents/importance_of_eye_health_and_vision_care_to_healthy_aging_jan_14_2019.pdf

Canadian National Institute for the Blind (CNIB). (2021). *Age-related macular degeneration*. http://www.cnib.ca/en/sight-loss-info/your-eyes/eye-diseases/age-related-macular-degeneration?region=ab

Canadian Ophthalmological Society. (2007). Evidence-based clinical practice guidelines for the periodic eye examinations in adults in Canada. *Canadian Journal of Ophthalmology*, 42(1), 39–45. https://doi.org/10.3129/canjophthalmol.06-126e. (Seminal).

Chaudhary, N. A., Hameed, S., Ul Moazzam, M. S., et al. (2018). Diabetic retinopathy: Predictive value of elevated HbA1C levels for the presence of diabetic retinopathy. *The Professional Medical Journal*, 25(8). https://doi.org/10.29309/TPMJ/18.4886

Chew, E. Y. (2017). Nutrition, genes, and age-related macular degeneration: What have we learned from the trials? *Ophthalmologica*, 238, 1–5. https://doi.org/10.1159/000473865

Del Buey, M. A., Casas, P., Caramello, C., et al. (2019). An update on corneal biomechanics and architecture in diabetes. *Journal of Ophthalmology*. Article 7645352. https://doi.org/10.1155/2019/7645352

Deniz, Y., van Uum, R. T., de Hoog, M., et al. (2018). Impact of acute otitis media clinical practice guidelines on antibiotic and analgesic prescriptions: A systematic review. *Archives of Disease in Childhood*, 103(6), 597–602. https://doi.org/10.1136/archdischild-2017-314103

Department of Justice Canada. (2021). *Canada occupational health and safety regulations (SOR/86-304)*. https://laws.justice.gc.ca/PDF/SOR-86-304.pdf

Detaram, H., Franzco, P., Russell, J., et al. (2019). Dietary zinc intake is associated with macular fluid in neovascular age-related macular degeneration. *Clinical and Experimental Ophthalmology*, 48(1), 61–68. https://doi.org/10.1111/ceo.13644

Devenyi, R., Maberley, D., Sheidow, T. G., et al. (2016). Real-world utilization of ranibizumab in wet age-related macular degeneration patients from Canada. *Canadian Journal of Ophthalmology*, 51(2), 55–57. https://doi.org/10.1016/j.jcjo.2015.11.008

Di Berardino, F., Conte, G., Turati, F., et al. (2020). Cochlear implantation in Ménière's disease: a systematic review of literature and pooled analysis. *International Journal of Audiology*, 59(6), 40–415. https://doi.org/10.1080/14992027.2020.1720992

Eydelman, M., Hilmantel, G., Tarver, M. E., et al. (2017). Symptoms and satisfaction of patients in the patient-reported outcomes with laser in situ keratomileusis (PROWL) studies. *JAMA Ophthalmology*, 135(1), 13–22. https://doi.org/10.1001/jamaophthalmol.2016.4587

Ferri, F. (2020). *Ferri's clinical advisor 2020*. Elsevier.

Freund, P., & Chen, S. (2018). Herpes zoster ophthalmicus. *CMAJ*, 190(21), E656. https://doi.org/10.1503/cmaj.180063

Gagnon-Roy, M., Hami, B., Genereaux, M., et al. (2018). Preventing emergency department (ED) visits and hospitalisations of older adults with cognitive impairment compared with the general senior population: What do we know about avoidable incidents? Results from a scoping review (e019908) *BMJ Open*, 8. https://doi.org/10.1136/bmjopen-2017-019908

Glaucoma Research Society of Canada. (2021). *Learning about glaucoma*. https://www.glaucomaresearch.ca/about/about-glaucoma/

Government of Canada. (2020). *Noise and your health*. https://www.canada.ca/en/health-canada/services/noise-your-health.html

HealthLink BC. (2019). *Benign paroxysmal positional vertigo (BPPV)*. https://www.healthlinkbc.ca/health-topics/hw263714

Hearing Foundation of Canada. (2020). *Statistics*. http://www.hearingfoundation.ca/statistics/

Hoover, C., Rademayer, C., & Farleu, C. (2017). Body piercing: Motivations and implications for health. *Journal of Midwifery & Women's Health*, 62(5), 521–530. https://doi.org/10.1111/jmwh.12630

Indigenous Services Canada. (2020). *Guide to vision care benefits*. https://www.sac-isc.gc.ca/eng/1579545788749/1579545817396#s2-2

Jin, S., Chan, S., & Gupta, N. (2019). Distribution gaps in surgery care and impact on seniors across Ontario. *Canadian Journal of Ophthalmology*, 54(4), 451–475. https://doi.org/10.1016/j.jcjo.2018.10.022

Kandaswamy, B., Miane Ng, M. Y., & Nash, R. (2020). Assessing and treating adults with hearing loss in primary care. *Practice Nursing*, 31(3). https://doi.org/10.12968/pnur.2020.31.3.106

Le Saux, N., & Robinson, J. L. (2016). Management of acute otitis media in children six months of age and older. *Paediatrics & Child Health*, 21(1), 39–50. https://www.cps.ca/documents/position/acute-otitis-media

Lian, J. (2018). *Keeping eye injuries at bay. Occupational Health and Safety Canada*. https://www.ohscanada.com/overtime/keeping-eye-injuries-bay/

Mayo Clinic (2019). *Cataract surgery*. https://www.mayoclinic.org/tests-procedures/cataract-surgery/about/pac-20384765

Melanoma Network of Canada. (2015). *A guide to uveal melanoma*. https://www.melanomanetwork.ca/wp-content/uploads/2015/04/140622-MNC_UvealGuideBooklet_FIN2_lr1.pdf

National Eye Institute. (2019a). *Amblyopia (lazy eye)*. https://www.nei.nih.gov/learn-about-eye-health/eye-conditions-and-diseases/amblyopia-lazy-eye

National Eye Institute. (2019b). *Corneal conditions*. https://www.nei.nih.gov/learn-about-eye-health/eye-conditions-and-diseases/corneal-conditions

National Eye Institute. (2019c). *Macular edema.* https://www.nei.nih.gov/learn-about-eye-health/eye-conditions-and-diseases/macular-edema

National Eye Institute. (2020). *Retinal detachment.* https://www.nei.nih.gov/learn-about-eye-health/eye-conditions-and-diseases/retinal-detachment

National Eye Institute. (2021). *Age-related macular degeneration.* https://www.nei.nih.gov/learn-about-eye-health/eye-conditions-and-diseases/age-related-macular-degeneration

Nielsen, M., Dogrusöz, M., Bleeker, J. C., et al. (2015). The genetic basis of uveal melanoma. *Journal Français d'Ophthalmologie, 38*(6), 516–521. https://doi.org/10.1016/j.jfo.2015.04.003

Öberg, M. (2015). Hearing care for older adults: Beyond the audiology clinic. *American Journal of Audiology, 24*(2), 104–107. https://doi.org/10.1044/2015_AJA-14-0077

Sella, R., Chou, L., Schuster, A. K., et al. (2020). Accuracy of IOL power calculations in the very elderly. *Eye.* https://doi.org/10.1038/s41433-019-0752-0

Statistics Canada. (2018). *New data on disability in Canada, 2017.* https://www150.statcan.gc.ca/n1/pub/11-627-m/11-627-m2018035-eng.htm

Tognarelli, E. I., Palomino, T. F., Corrales, N., et al. (2019). Herpes simplex virus evasion of early host antiviral responses. *Frontiers in Cellular and Infection Microbiology, 9*, 27. https://doi.org/10.3389/fcimb.2019.00127

Touhy, T., Jett, K., Boscart, V., et al. (2019). *Ebersole and Hess' gerontological nursing and healthy aging in Canada* (2nd ed.). Elsevier.

Varu, D., Rhee, M., Akpek, E., et al. (2019). Conjunctivitis preferred practice pattern. *Ophthalmology, 126*(1), 94–169. https://doi.org/10.1016/j.ophtha.2018.10.020

Welp, A., Woodbury, R. R., McCoy, M. A., et al. (2016). *Making eye health a population health imperative.* National Academies Press. https://www.ncbi.nlm.nih.gov/books/NBK385157/

World Health Organization. (2021). *Trachoma.* https://www.who.int/news-room/fact-sheets/detail/trachoma

RESOURCES

Alberta Association of the Deaf
http://www.aadnews.ca/

Alliance for Equality of Blind Canadians
http://www.blindcanadians.ca/

BC and Alberta Guide Dog Services.
http://www.bcguidedog.com/

Bob Rumball Canadian Centre of Excellence for the Deaf
https://www2.bobrumball.org/

Canadian Association of the Deaf
http://www.cad.ca/

Canadian Association of Optometrists
http://opto.ca/

Canadian Council of the Blind (CCB)
http://ccbnational.net

Canadian Glaucoma Society
http://www.cgs-scg.org/

Canadian Hard of Hearing Association
http://www.chha.ca/chha/

Canadian Hearing Society
http://www.chs.ca/

Canadian Helen Keller Centre
http://www.chkc.org/

Canadian National Institute for the Blind (CNIB)
http://www.cnib.ca

Canadian Ophthalmological Society
http://www.cos-sco.ca

Foundation Fighting Blindness
http://www.blindness.org/

Hearing Foundation of Canada
http://hearingfoundation.ca

Misericordia Health Centre: Buhler Eye Care Centre
https://misericordia.mb.ca/programs/acute-care/eye-care/

Misericordia Health Centre: Focus on Falls Prevention Vision Screening Program
https://misericordia.mb.ca/programs/clinical-services/focus-on-falls/

Montreal Association for the Blind: MAB-Mackay Rehabilitation Centre
https://www.llmrc.ca/program-and-services/by-impairment/visual-impairment/

The Ottawa Hospital Eye Institute
http://www.ottawahospital.on.ca/wps/portal/Base/TheHospital/ClinicalServices/DeptPgrmCS/Programs/EyeInstitute

Society of Deaf and Hard of Hearing Nova Scotians
http://sdhhns.org/

American Academy of Audiology
http://www.audiology.org

American Academy of Ophthalmology
http://www.aao.org/

American Society of Cataract and Refractive Surgery
http://ascrs.org/

American Society of Ophthalmic Registered Nurses
http://www.asorn.org/

Glaucoma Research Foundation
http://www.glaucoma.org/

Hearing Loss Sampler
http://www.uww.edu/comdis/radio/hlsimulation/

International Hearing Society
http://ihsinfo.org/IhsV2/Home/Index.cfm

The Macula Foundation
http://maculafoundation.org/

National Eye Institute of the National Institutes of Health
http://www.nei.nih.gov/

National Center on Deaf-Blindness
http://www.nationaldb.org/

University of Michigan Kellogg Eye Center
https://www.umkelloggeye.org/

U.S. Food and Drug Administration: Cochlear Implants
http://www.fda.gov/MedicalDevices/ProductsandMedicalProcedures/ImplantsandProsthetics/CochlearImplants/default.htm

VisionSimulations.com
http://visionsimulations.com/

ⓔvolve

For additional Internet resources, see the website for this book at http://evolve.elsevier.com/Canada/Lewis/medsurg.

Nursing Assessment
Integumentary System

Susannah McGeachy
Originating US chapter by Mariann M. Harding

⊖volve WEBSITE

- Review Questions (Online Only)
- Key Points
- Answer Guidelines for Case Study
- Conceptual Care Map Creator
- Audio Glossary
- Content Updates

LEARNING OBJECTIVES

1. Describe the structures and the functions of the integumentary system.
2. Link the age-related changes in the integumentary system to differences in assessment findings.
3. Identify the significant subjective and objective data regarding the integumentary system that should be obtained from a patient.
4. Identify appropriate techniques used in the physical assessment of the integumentary system.
5. Compare the critical components for describing primary and secondary lesions.
6. Differentiate normal from common abnormal findings of a physical assessment of the integumentary system.
7. Summarize the structural and assessment differences in individuals of varying skin tones.
8. Describe the purpose, significance of results, and nursing responsibilities related to diagnostic studies of the integumentary system.

KEY TERMS

alopecia	hirsutism	pallor
clubbing	intertriginous	pruritus
cyanosis	jaundice	sebaceous glands
dermis	keratinocytes	vitiligo
epidermis	melanocytes	
erythema	mole (nevus)	

The integumentary system is the largest body organ and comprises skin, hair, nails, and glands. The skin is further divided into two layers: the epidermis and the dermis. The subcutaneous tissue is immediately under the dermis (Figure 25.1). The skin is as complex as any organ but, unlike the others, it is readily visible. Being able to see and touch the skin assists the nurse in an integumentary assessment, as abnormalities are readily apparent and their detection enables early intervention.

STRUCTURES AND FUNCTIONS OF THE SKIN AND APPENDAGES

Structures

The epidermis is the outermost layer of the skin. The dermis, the second skin layer, contains collagen bundles and supports the nerve and vascular network. Subcutaneous tissue lies below the dermis and is composed primarily of fat and loose connective tissue.

Epidermis. The epidermis, the outer layer of the skin, is relatively thin, ranging from 0.05 mm on the eyelids to 0.1 mm on the soles of the feet (Habif, 2016). There are no lymphatic or vascular structures in the epidermis. It is supported by passive circulation from the dermis.

The epidermis is divided into five distinct but interrelated layers. Two of the layers are the stratum corneum (the surface layer) and the stratum germinativum (deepest, basal layer) (see Figure 25.1). Most epithelial cells are keratinocytes (90%). The remaining cells are melanocytes, Langerhans cells, and Merkel cells.

Keratinocytes form in the basal layer. Initially, they are undifferentiated and shaped like columns. As they mature

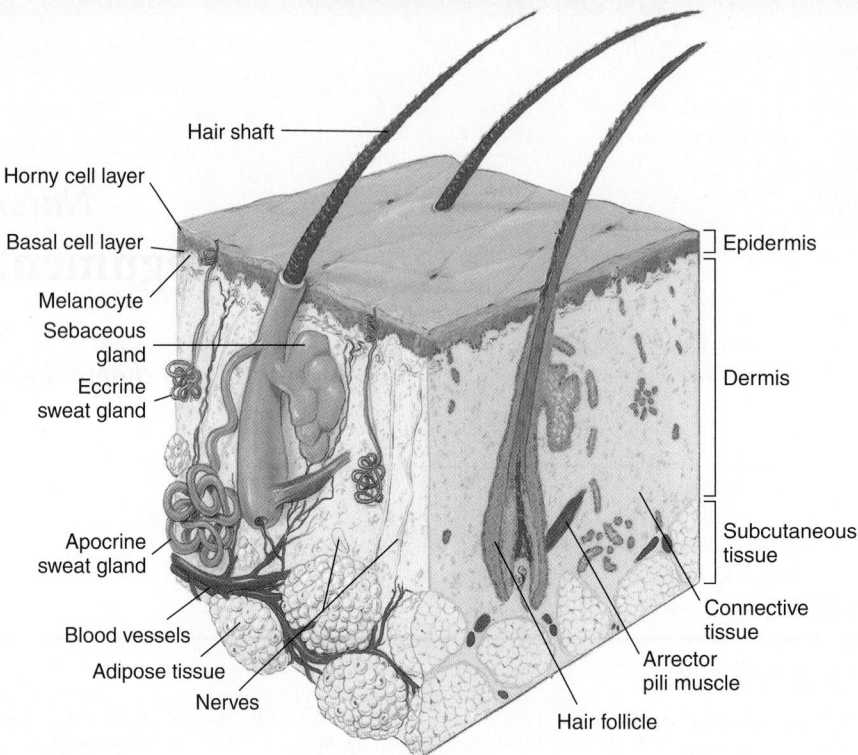

FIG. 25.1 Microscopic view of the skin in longitudinal section. Source: Jarvis, C., Browne, A. J., MacDonald-Jenkins, J. et al. (2019). *Physical examination & health assessment* (3rd Canadian ed., p. 226). Elsevier.

(keratinize), they move to the surface, where they flatten and die to form the outer skin layer (stratum corneum). Keratinocytes make a fibrous protein, *keratin*, which is vital to the skin's protective barrier function. The upward movement of keratinocytes from the basal layer to the outermost levels of the stratum corneum takes about 14 days. The keratinocytes stay there for another 14 days, allowing the epidermis to regenerate every 28 days. Thus, each month, a new layer of skin is created.

Many skin conditions result from changes in this cell cycle. If dead cells slough off too rapidly, the skin appears thin and eroded. If new cells form faster than old cells are shed, the skin becomes scaly and thickened. Failure of the epidermis to function normally occurs with skin cancer and psoriasis (discussed in Chapter 26).

Melanocytes are found in the deep, basal layer. They contain *melanin*, a pigment that gives colour to the skin and hair and protects the body from damaging ultraviolet (UV) sunlight. Sunlight and hormones stimulate the melanosome (within the melanocyte) to increase the production of melanin. People of all skin tones have similar numbers of melanocytes. In darker skin, the melanosomes are larger and more numerous, thus producing more melanin (Gawkrodger & Ardern-Jones, 2016). This increased melanin forms a natural sun shield for dark skin and results in a decreased incidence of skin cancer. *Langerhans cells* are a type of dendritic cell (discussed in Chapter 16). They are immunocompetent cells that recognize antigens. When they are depleted, the skin cannot initiate an immune response. The Langerhans cells in bioengineered skin grafts have been removed to prevent graft rejection. In skin diseases such as psoriasis and sarcoidosis, there are decreased numbers of Langerhans cells. *Merkel cells* are found in the basal layer and are involved in the sensation of light touch. They are used when a person is feeling the texture of an object and figuring out what it is.

The *basement membrane zone* is between the epidermis and dermis. This structure provides for (1) exchange of fluids between the epidermis and dermis and (2) structural support for the epidermis. The basement membrane helps to secure the two layers together. Inflammation and separation of the epidermal and dermal layers result in the blisters seen in conditions such as burns, full-thickness wounds, and mechanical trauma.

Dermis. The **dermis** is the connective tissue below the epidermis. The dermis is highly vascular, with a thickness varying from 0.3 to 3 mm (Habif, 2016). It also contains nerves, lymphatic vessels, hair follicles, sebaceous glands, and specialized cells such as mast cells and macrophages that protect the body from external stimuli.

The dermis has two layers: an upper thin papillary layer and a deeper, thicker reticular layer. The *papillary layer* is arranged haphazardly in ridges, or papillae, which extend into the outer epidermal layer. These elevated surface ridges form fingerprints and footprints. The *reticular layer* forms the bulk of the dermis. It is made up of thick collagen bundles arranged parallel to the skin's surface.

The dermis is made of three types of connective tissue: collagen, elastic fibers, and reticular fibers. Collagen forms the greatest part of the dermis. It gives the skin toughness and strength and is critical in wound healing. The primary cell type in the dermis is the *fibroblast,* which makes collagen and elastin. The dermis also contains nerves, lymphatic vessels, hair follicles, sebaceous glands, and specialized cells such as mast cells and macrophages that protect the body from external stimuli.

Subcutaneous Tissue. While not part of the skin, the subcutaneous tissue is often discussed with the integument because it attaches the skin to underlying tissues such as the muscle and bone. It contains loose connective tissue and fat cells that provide insulation, cushioning, temperature regulation, and energy storage. The distribution of subcutaneous tissue varies with gender, heredity, age, and nutritional status.

Skin Appendages. Skin appendages include the hair, nails, and glands (sebaceous, apocrine, and eccrine). These appendages are epidermal extensions that have their roots in the dermis. These structures receive nutrients, electrolytes, and fluids from the dermis. Hair and nails form from specialized keratin. Systemic diseases can affect the condition and health of both hair and nails. Hair grows on most of the body; the density and pattern of distribution varies depending on age, sex, and race. Hair colour is a result of heredity and determined by the type and amount of melanin in the hair shaft. Hair grows about 1 cm per month. People lose about 100 hairs each day (Alikhan & Hocker, 2016). Alopecia (partial or complete lack of hair) results when lost hair is not replaced, for example, with normal aging or anticancer medications.

Nails are made of heavily keratinized cells. The visible part of the nail is the nail body; the rest is the nail root. A fold of skin, bordered by the cuticle, hides most of the nail root. The portion of the nail root that can be seen is called the *lunula*. This white, crescent-shaped area is the site of mitosis and nail growth (Figure 25.2). Under the nail is a highly vascular area of epidermis called the *nail bed*. Fingernails grow slowly, at a rate of 0.5 to 2 mm per week (Habif, 2016). A lost fingernail usually regenerates in 3 to 6 months, while a lost toenail may require 12 months or longer to regenerate. Nail growth varies on the basis of a person's age and health. Nails grow faster in men and in warm weather. Nail colour ranges from pink to yellow or brown depending on skin colour. Colour and texture variations in the nails may represent normal or abnormal conditions. Pigmented longitudinal bands *(melanonychia striata)* occur in the nail bed of 90% of people with dark skin (Figure 25.3) (Bishop & Tosti, 2017).

There are two major types of glands in the skin: sebaceous and sweat glands. Sebaceous glands secrete *sebum,* which is emptied into the hair follicles. Sebum waterproofs and lubricates the skin and promotes the absorption of fat-soluble substances. Sebum is somewhat bacteriostatic and fungistatic. These glands depend on sex hormones, particularly testosterone, to regulate sebum secretion and production. Actual production varies depending on age, sex, and testosterone and estrogen levels. Sebaceous glands are present on all areas of the skin except the palms and soles and dorsum of the feet. These glands are most abundant on the face, scalp, upper chest, and back.

The *apocrine sweat glands* are mainly found in the axillary, genital, and breast areas. They are always connected to a hair follicle. These glands enlarge and become active at puberty with the increased activity of reproductive hormones. They secrete a thick milky substance that is naturally odorless. Odor occurs when skin surface bacteria alter the secretions.

The *eccrine sweat glands* are found on most of the body, except the lips, ear canals, nail beds, labia minora, glans penis, and prepuce. One square inch of skin has about 3 000 eccrine sweat glands. Their main function is to cool the body by evaporation,

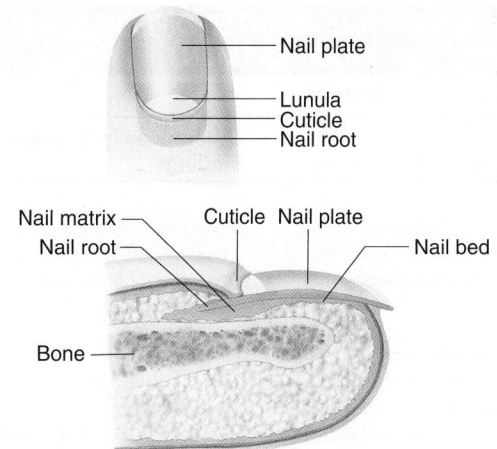

FIG. 25.2 Structure of a nail. Source: Patton, K. T., & Thibodeau, G. A. (2016). *Essentials of anatomy and physiology* (9th ed., p. 196). Mosby.

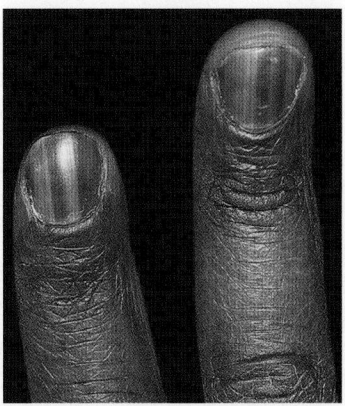

FIG. 25.3 Pigmented nail bed normally seen with dark skin colour. Source: Habif, T. P. (2016). *Clinical dermatology: A color guide to diagnosis and therapy* (6th ed., p. 766). Mosby.

excrete waste products, and moisturize surface cells. Sweat is a transparent watery solution composed of salts, ammonia, urea, and other wastes. In extreme situations, the body can make 2 to 4 L of sweat per hour or up to 12 L in 24 hours. Heat, certain mental stimuli, and ingestion of hot, spicy foods stimulate sweat secretion.

Functions of the Integumentary System

The skin's primary function is to protect the underlying tissues of the body from the external environment. The skin acts as a barrier against invasion by bacteria and viruses and prevents excessive water loss. The fat in the subcutaneous layer insulates the body and provides protection from trauma. Melanin screens and absorbs ultraviolet radiation. Nerve endings and receptors located within the skin provide sensory information on environmental stimuli to the brain related to pain, temperature, touch, pressure, and vibration. In addition, the skin regulates heat loss by responding to changes in internal and external temperature with vasoconstriction, vasodilation, and excretion of sweat. Evaporation of water from the lungs and skin results in the loss of 600 to 900 mL of water daily. Sebum and sweat lubricate the skin surface. Furthermore, endogenous synthesis of vitamin D, which is critical to calcium and phosphorus balance, occurs in the epidermis.

TABLE 25.1   AGE-RELATED DIFFERENCES IN ASSESSMENT

Integumentary System

Changes	Differences in Assessment Findings
Skin	
• Decreased subcutaneous fat, muscle laxity, degeneration of elastic fibres, collagen stiffening	Increased wrinkling, sagging breasts and abdomen, redundant flesh around eyes, slowness of skin to flatten when pinched (tenting)
• Decreased extracellular water, surface lipids, and sebaceous gland activity	Dry, flaking skin with possible signs of excoriation caused by scratching
• Decreased activity of apocrine and sebaceous glands	Dry skin with minimal to no perspiration, uneven skin coloration
• Increased capillary fragility and permeability	Bruising
• Increased focal melanocytes in basal layer with pigment accumulation	Solar lentigines on face and backs of hands
• Diminished blood supply	Decrease in rosy appearance of skin and mucous membranes; skin cool to touch; diminished awareness of pain, touch, temperature, and peripheral vibration
• Decreased proliferative capacity	Diminished rate of wound healing
• Decreased immunocompetence	Increase in neoplasms
Hair	
• Decreased melanin and melanocytes	Grey or white hair
• Decreased oil	Dry, coarse hair; scaly scalp
• Decreased density of hair	Thinning and loss of hair
• Cumulative androgen effect; decreasing estrogen levels	Facial hirsutism, baldness
Nails	
• Decreased peripheral blood supply	Thick, brittle nails with diminished growth
• Increased keratin	Longitudinal ridging
• Decreased circulation	Prolonged return of blood to nails on blanching

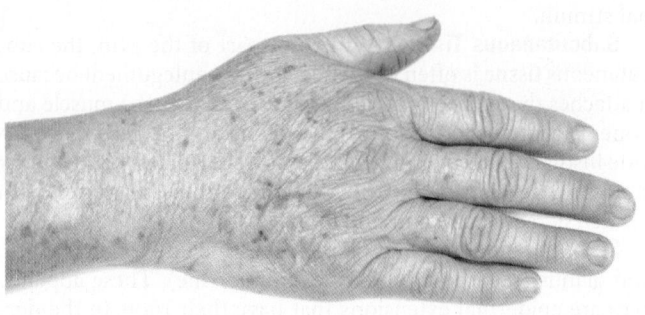

FIG. 25.4 Photoaging. Various pigmented spots, such as freckles, solar lentigines (known as age or liver spots), and uneven skin colour. Source: (c) iStock.com/weerapatkiatdumrong

AGE-RELATED CONSIDERATIONS

EFFECTS OF AGING ON THE INTEGUMENTARY SYSTEM

Skin changes related to aging include decreased turgor, thinning, dryness, wrinkling, vascular lesions, increased skin fragility, and benign neoplasms. Although many changes are only of cosmetic concern, others can be serious and need careful evaluation. Age-related changes of the integumentary system and differences in assessment findings are listed in Table 25.1.

With advancing age, the junction between the dermis and the epidermis becomes flattened, and the epidermis contains fewer melanocytes. In addition, the dermis loses volume and has fewer blood vessels. Scalp, pubic, and axillary hair becomes depigmented and thinner. A loss of melanin results in fading hair colour. The nail plate thins, and nails become brittle, thicker, and more prone to splitting and yellowing.

Chronic UV exposure is the major contributor to photoaging and wrinkling of the skin (Canadian Dermatology Association [CDA], 2021b). Sun damage to the skin is cumulative (Figure 25.4). Inadequate nutrition, with decreased intake of protein, calories, and vitamins, further contributes to aging

of the skin. With aging, collagen fibres stiffen, elastic fibres degenerate, and the amount of subcutaneous tissue decreases. These changes, with the added effects of gravity, lead to wrinkling. The visible effects of aging on the skin and hair may result in an altered self-image and may have a profound psychological effect.

Benign neoplasms related to the aging process can occur. These growths include seborrheic keratoses, vascular lesions such as cherry angiomas, and skin tags. Actinic keratoses appear on areas of chronic sun exposure, especially in people with a light complexion. These premalignant cutaneous lesions place an individual at increased risk for squamous cell and basal cell carcinomas. The photoaged person is more susceptible to skin cancers because of decreased capacity to repair cellular deoxyribonucleic acid (DNA) damage caused by UV exposure (CDA, 2021a). Chronic UV exposure from tanning beds causes the same damage as UV from the sun.

Subcutaneous fat decreases with age, leading to increased risk of traumatic injury, hypothermia, and skin shearing, which may lead to pressure injuries. With aging, the apocrine and eccrine sweat glands atrophy, causing dry skin and decreased body odour. The growth rate of the hair and nails decreases as a result of atrophy of the involved structures. Hormonal and vitamin deficiencies can cause dry, thin hair and alopecia.

ASSESSMENT OF THE INTEGUMENTARY SYSTEM

The general skin assessment begins with the nurse's first contact with the patient and continues throughout the examination. As this is the first meeting with the patient, the overall condition of the patient's skin and hair should be noted. Specific areas of the skin will be assessed when examining other body systems, unless the chief complaint is a skin problem. The nurse needs to record a general statement about the skin's physical condition (Table 25.2). The nurse can investigate further by asking the health history questions presented in Table 25.3 when a skin condition is noted.

Subjective Data

Past Medical History. Past medical history reveals previous trauma, surgery, or disease that involves the skin. Many diseases

TABLE 25.2	**NORMAL PHYSICAL ASSESSMENT OF THE INTEGUMENTARY SYSTEM**

Skin: Evenly pigmented; no petechiae, purpura, lesions, or excoriations; warm; good turgor
Nails: Pink; oval; adhere to nail base with 160° angle
Hair: Shiny and full; amount and distribution appropriate for age and gender; no flaking of scalp, forehead, or pinna

CASE STUDY

Patient Introduction

D. A. (pronouns she/her), 74 years old, comes to the primary care clinic with concerns about various "spots" on her face. She says they have been there for a while and thought they were just "age spots," but she got concerned after a friend was diagnosed with a malignant melanoma.

Critical Thinking
The following questions should be kept in mind while studying this assessment chapter:
1. What are the possible causes of D. A.'s facial lesions?
2. What subjective data should the nurse gather from the patient to help determine possible causes?
3. What should be included in the physical assessment? What specific characteristics of the skin lesions should the nurse look for?
4. What diagnostic studies might be ordered?
    See Case Study: Subjective Data and Case Study: Objective Data for more information on D. A.

⊝volve
Answers available at http://evolve.elsevier.com/Canada/Lewis/medsurg.

have dermatological manifestations. The nurse needs to determine if the patient has noticed any issues such as jaundice (yellowing of the skin and/or sclera associated with increased bilirubin levels), delayed wound healing, cyanosis (bluish colour resulting from hypoxia), erythema (redness), or pallor (paleness). It is important to obtain specific information regarding sensitivities, allergies, and skin reactions to insect bites and stings. Any history of chronic or unprotected exposure to UV light, including tanning bed use or radiation treatments, should be noted.

Medications. A thorough medication history is important. The nurse should ask the patient about skin-related issues that occurred from taking a medication. Many hormones, antibiotics, corticosteroids, and antimetabolites have adverse effects that manifest in the skin. Medications may contain fragrances and preservatives that can cause skin reactions. The nurse should document the use of medications specifically used to treat a primary skin condition, such as acne, or a secondary skin condition, such as itching. The medication's name, length of use, method of application, and effectiveness should be recorded.

Surgery or Other Treatments. The nurse needs to determine if any surgical procedures, including cosmetic surgery, were done on the skin. Biopsy results should be recorded. The nurse needs to note any treatments specific for a skin condition (e.g.,

phototherapy) or for a health condition (e.g., radiation therapy). Any treatments undergone primarily for cosmetic purposes, such as tanning booth use, laser resurfacing, or cosmetic "peels," also need to be documented.

Family History. The nurse should obtain information about any family history of skin diseases or systemic diseases with dermatological manifestations. Any family or personal history of skin cancer, particularly melanoma, must also be noted.

Self-Care History. The patient should be tactfully questioned about health and hygiene practices related to the integumentary system, including the type, quantity, and frequency of use of personal care products (e.g., shampoos, moisturizing agents, cosmetics). Any current skin conditions, including onset, symptoms, course, and treatment, should be recorded, as well as frequency of use and the sun protection factor (SPF) of sunscreen products.

Nutritional History. A diet history reveals the adequacy of nutrients essential to healthy skin, such as vitamins A, D, E, and C; dietary fat; and protein. The nurse should question the patient regarding recent dietary changes, any food allergies that cause a skin reaction, and conditions of the skin such as dryness, edema, erythema, and pruritus (itching), which can indicate alterations in fluid balance. If the patient is experiencing incontinence, the nurse should determine the condition of the skin in the anal and perineal areas.

Social, Environmental, and Occupational Health History. The patient should be questioned about environmental factors that affect the skin, such as occupational exposure to chemicals, irritants, sun, insects, animals, extreme temperatures, and prolonged pressure. For example, during the COVID-19 pandemic, increased facial pressure injuries in health care providers occurred, as a result of prolonged use of personal protective equipment (Desai et al., 2020). Contact dermatitis caused by allergies and irritants is a common condition associated with occupation, as well as with some hobbies. The patient's participation in any recreational activities involving significant sun exposure should be determined and documented.

Indigenous populations in Canada face particular challenges to skin health that result from poor water quality, inadequate housing, lack of access to fresh foods, and limited access to culturally safe health care. Contamination of drinking and bathing water in northern Indigenous communities has been implicated in a higher incidence of eczema, skin cancers (Bradford et al., 2016), and invasive cutaneous infections such as methicillin-resistant *Staphylococcus aureus* (Kirlew et al., 2014).

Cognitive–Perceptual. The patient's perception of the sensations of health, cold, pain, and touch should be determined. The nurse should note any discomfort associated with a skin condition, especially when observed in intact skin. As well, joint pain and the mobility of joints should be assessed and recorded, since a skin condition may cause alterations in mobility.

Coping Abilities. The nurse needs to assess the role that stress may play in creating or worsening the skin condition. The patient should be asked what coping strategies they use to manage the skin condition. For example, pruritus can be distressing and cause major alterations in normal sleep patterns, and acne can be disfiguring and lead to a significant threat to self-image.

TABLE 25.3   HEALTH HISTORY

Integumentary System: Questions for Obtaining Subjective Data

General
- Describe any current skin condition, including when it started, how it has progressed, and how you have treated it.
- Describe any changes in the condition of your skin, hair, and nails.
- Have you noticed any changes in the way sores or lesions heal?*

Past History
- Do you have any history of previous trauma, surgery (including cosmetic surgery), or prior disease that involves the skin?*
- Do you have any body art, piercings, or tattoos?* If yes, were they completed in a regulated business?
- Do you have any chronic diseases that affect your skin health? (For example, liver disease, diabetes mellitus, respiratory disorders, anemia?)
- Do you have a history of significant sun exposure, tanning bed use, or history of radiation treatments?*
- Have you ever had a skin biopsy?* If so, what were the results?
- Have you used prescription or OTC medications to treat a skin condition?*
- Have you had any treatments specifically for a skin condition (e.g., phototherapy, radiation therapy, cosmetic "peels")?

Family History
- Do you have a family history of any skin diseases, including congenital and familial diseases (e.g., alopecia and psoriasis) and systemic diseases with dermatological manifestations (e.g., diabetes, thyroid disease, cardiovascular diseases, immune disorders)?
- Do you have any family or personal history of skin cancer, particularly melanoma?

Self-Care History
- Describe your daily hygiene practices.
- What skin products are you currently using?
- Do you do anything to protect yourself from the sun?* How frequently do you use sun protection, and what is the SPF number of your sunscreen products?

Nutritional History
- Are there any changes in the condition of your skin, hair, or nails that might be related to changes in your diet?*
- Do you have food allergies that cause a skin reaction?

Social, Environment, or Occupational History
- Do you have any pets?
- Do you have any food, pet, or medication allergies, or allergy to insect bites or stings?*
- Do your leisure or work activities involve the use of any chemicals or devices that might irritate your skin?*
- Do you have any close household or sexual contacts with a similar skin condition?*

Cognitive–Perceptual
- Do you have any unusual sensations of heat, cold, or touch?*
- Do you have any pain associated with your skin condition?*
- Do you have any joint pain?*

Coping Abilities
- Are you aware of any situation or stressor that changes your skin condition?
- Does your skin condition keep you awake or awaken you after you have fallen asleep?*
- How does your skin condition make you feel about yourself?
- What strategies have you used to manage your skin condition?

*If yes, describe.
OTC, over-the-counter; *SPF*, sun protection factor; *UV*, ultraviolet.
Source: Based on Jarvis, C., Browne, A., MacDonald-Jenkins, J., et al. (2019). *Physical examination & health assessment* (3rd Canadian ed.). Elsevier.

Objective Data

Physical Examination. A physical examination of the skin begins with a systematic, general inspection and then a more specific assessment of problem areas. The nurse should note changes in the colour, turgor, temperature, dryness, thickness, and vascularity of the skin. The findings may be normal, relative to age, genetic factors, and environmental exposures, or may represent primary or secondary skin lesions. General principles when conducting an assessment of the skin are as follows:

1. Use a private examination room of moderate temperature with good lighting.
2. Ensure that the patient is comfortable and in a gown that allows easy access to all skin areas.
3. Use gloves when palpating nonintact skin and rashes.
4. Perform a general inspection followed by a lesion-specific examination.
5. Use the metric system when taking measurements.
6. Use appropriate terminology when reporting or documenting.

Clinical Photography. Photographs are an adjunct to documentation and promote communication among the interprofessional team. They are used to assess and monitor skin conditions and determine if the condition has improved or declined with treatment. They can be used to track moles and precancerous lesions and detect any changes early. The nurse needs to follow facility policy for obtaining a patient's consent to photograph lesions.

Inspection. The skin is inspected for general colour and pigmentation, vascularity, bruising, and the presence of lesions or discolorations. The critical factor in assessment of skin colour is change. A skin colour that is normal for a particular patient can be a sign of a pathological condition in another patient. The most reliable areas in which to assess erythema, cyanosis, pallor, and jaundice are the areas of least pigmentation, such as sclerae, conjunctivae, nail beds, lips, and buccal mucosa. The true skin colour is best observed in photoprotected areas, such as the buttocks. Activity, sun

CASE STUDY

Subjective Data

A focused subjective assessment of D. A. reveals the following:
- *Past medical history:* Negative except for an appendectomy at age 16.
- *Medications:* None at present. No known allergies.
- *Self-care:* Currently washes face with a skin cleanser in the morning and at nighttime. After cleansing, applies a moisturizer with SPF 15. She has used these facial products for the past 3 years, since small age spots were first noticed. Before that, she used just soap and water.
- *Nutritional:* D. A. reports that skin seems to be drier with age, but otherwise no changes besides the "age spots or whatever they are." Denies any changes in the way cuts or sores heal. No weight loss. Takes 400 IU of vitamin D daily; does not take any other supplemental vitamins or minerals.
- *Elimination:* Although skin is a little dry, does not perceive it to be excessively dry. Denies excessive sweating or any swelling.
- *Social, environmental, and occupational:* Loves to garden and go for walks outdoors. Reports a history of frequent, sometimes severe, sunburns as a child. No use of sunscreen growing up but does remember being made to wear T-shirts over bathing suits to help prevent sunburn. Has used sunscreen for the past 20 years when outdoors. Reapplies as needed.
- *Coping abilities:* Denies any pain or discomfort associated with skin lesions. Fearful of the possibility of skin cancer.

See Case Study: Patient Introduction and Case Study: Objective Data for more information on D. A.

GENETICS IN CLINICAL PRACTICE

Skin Malignancies

- The primary risk factor leading to skin cancers, including melanoma, is environmental exposure to UV radiation. UV radiation damages DNA, causing an error in the genetic code and resulting in abnormal skin cells (Coit et al., 2016).
- Inherited genetic factors can increase the risk for skin cancer. A person has an increased risk for developing melanoma if they have a first-degree relative (e.g., parent, full sibling) who had a melanoma (CDA, 2021a).
- The risk for skin cancer is also increased in people who have a fair complexion (light-coloured skin that easily freckles, red or blond hair, and blue or light-coloured eyes).

(UV) exposure, emotions, smoking, and edema, as well as respiratory, renal, cardiovascular, and hepatic disorders, can all directly affect the skin colour.

In the general inspection, the nurse should note the presence of body art such as piercings and tattoos. The nose, ears, eyebrows, lips, navel, and nipples are common sites of piercing. Tattoos and needle track marks should be identified, and their location and the characteristics of the surrounding skin area noted. Tattoo pigments deposited in the skin may cause itching, pain, and sensitivity for several weeks after the tattoo is placed.

The skin is examined for conditions related to vascularity, including bruising and vascular and purpuric lesions such as *angioma* (benign tumor of blood or lymph vessels), *petechiae* (tiny, flat, purplish red pinpoint lesions on skin), *ecchymosis* (bruise larger than petechiae), or *purpura* (purple-coloured spots and patches characterized by ecchymosis or other small

hemorrhages). The reaction to direct pressure on the lesion should be noted. If a lesion blanches on direct pressure and then refills, the redness is due to dilated blood vessels. If the discoloration stays, it is the result of subcutaneous or intradermal bleeding or a nonvascular lesion. The nurse should note any pattern of bruising, such as discoloration in the shape of the hand or fingers or bruises at different stages of resolution. These may indicate other health concerns or abuse and need further investigation.

The colour, size, height, distribution, location, and shape of any lesions should be noted. Lesions may be primary or secondary lesions. *Primary skin lesions* develop on previously unaltered skin. The common characteristics of primary skin lesions are shown in Table 25.4. *Secondary skin lesions* are lesions that change with time or occur because of scratching or infection. Secondary skin lesions are shown in Table 25.5.

Skin lesions are usually described in terms of their configuration (shape, whether solitary or forming a pattern in relation to other lesions) and distribution (arrangement of lesions over an area of skin) (Table 25.6). For example, herpes zoster (shingles) lesions are characteristically vesicular and have a linear distribution clustered along one or more dermatomes (Figure 25.5). Any unusual odours should also be noted. Skin sites with lesions, such as rashes, may be colonized with yeast or bacteria, which can be associated with distinctive odours in intertriginous areas (Figure 25.6), where skin surfaces overlap and rub on each other (e.g., below the breasts, axillae, and groin).

The nurse needs to inspect all body hair, noting the distribution, texture, and quantity of hair. Changes in the normal distribution of body hair and growth may indicate an endocrine or vascular disorder. Any nail grooves, pitting, ridges, or detachment from nail bed should be noted. Changes in nail smoothness or thickness can occur with anemia, psoriasis, thyroid conditions, decreased vascular circulation, and some infections. Clubbing (a distortion of the nail angle at the cuticle resulting in bulbous-appearing nails and fingertips caused by chronic hypoxemia) may occur with various respiratory and cardiac conditions.

Palpation. Palpating the skin provides information about temperature, turgor and mobility, moisture, and texture. The nurse should use the back of their own hand to gauge skin temperature, since the skin on the back of the examiner's hand is thinner than on the palm and more sensitive to temperature changes. The patient's skin should be warm, not hot. Localized temperature increase occurs with burns and local inflammation. A generalized increase will result from fever. A decreased skin temperature may occur when shock or other circulatory problems, chilling, or infection is present.

Turgor refers to the elasticity of the skin. Turgor is assessed by gently pinching an area of skin under the clavicle or on the back of the hand. Skin with good turgor should move easily when lifted and immediately return to its original position when released. In patients with dehydration and aging, a loss of turgor occurs and can cause tenting of the skin (Table 25.7).

Skin moisture (level of dampness or dryness of the skin) increases in intertriginous areas and with high humidity and varies with environmental temperature, muscular activity, body weight, and body temperature. The skin should be intact with no flaking, scaling, or cracking. Skin generally becomes drier with increasing age.

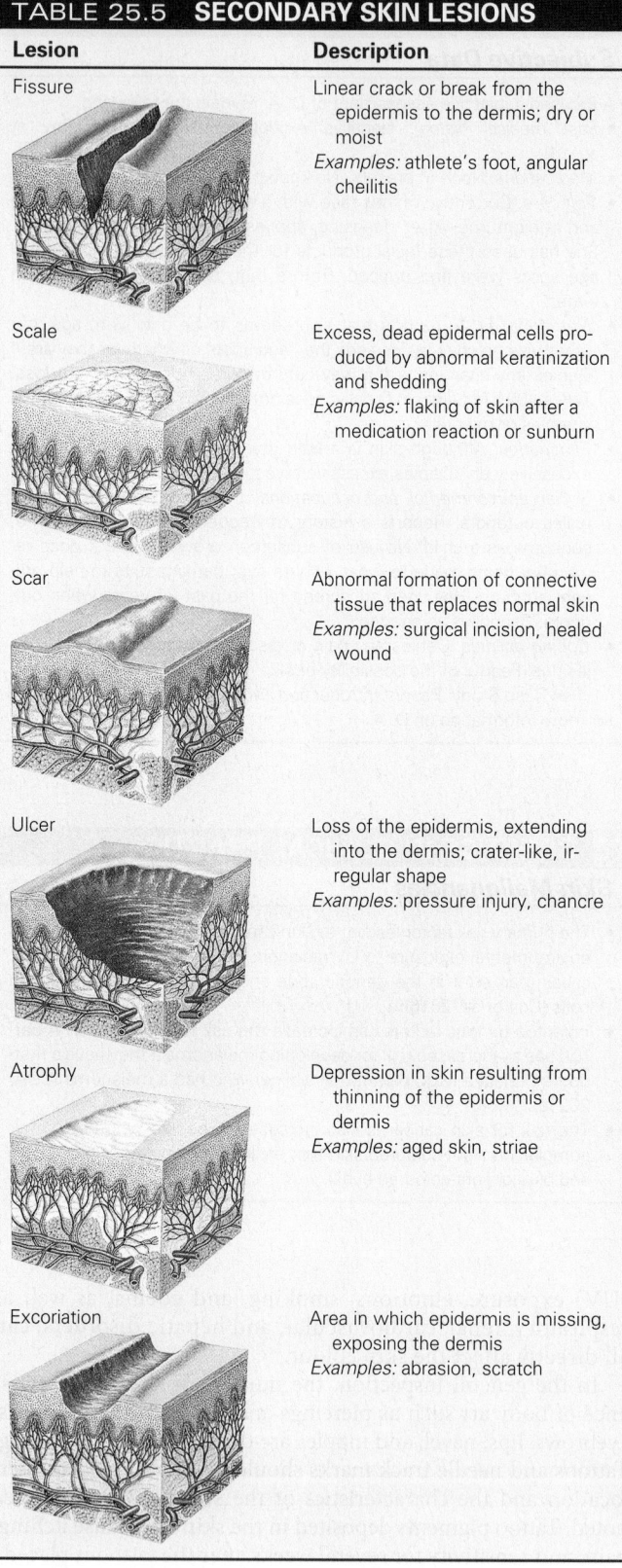

TABLE 25.4	**PRIMARY SKIN LESIONS**
Lesion	**Description**
Macule	Circumscribed, flat area with a change in skin colour; <1.0 cm in diameter *Examples:* freckles, petechiae, measles, flat mole (nevus), café-au-lait spots, vitiligo (complete depigmentation)
Papule	Elevated, solid lesion; <0.5 cm in diameter; if lesion is >0.5 cm in diameter, it is a *nodule* *Examples:* wart (verruca), elevated moles, lipoma, basal cell carcinoma
Vesicle	Circumscribed, superficial collection of serous fluid; <0.5 cm in diameter *Examples:* varicella (chicken pox), herpes zoster (shingles) (see Figure 25.5), second-degree burn
Plaque	Circumscribed, elevated, superficial, solid lesion; >0.5 cm in diameter *Examples:* psoriasis, seborrheic and actinic keratoses
Wheal	Firm, edematous, irregularly shaped area; diameter variable *Examples:* insect bite, urticaria
Pustule	Elevated, superficial lesion filled with purulent fluid *Examples:* acne, impetigo

TABLE 25.5	**SECONDARY SKIN LESIONS**
Lesion	**Description**
Fissure	Linear crack or break from the epidermis to the dermis; dry or moist *Examples:* athlete's foot, angular cheilitis
Scale	Excess, dead epidermal cells produced by abnormal keratinization and shedding *Examples:* flaking of skin after a medication reaction or sunburn
Scar	Abnormal formation of connective tissue that replaces normal skin *Examples:* surgical incision, healed wound
Ulcer	Loss of the epidermis, extending into the dermis; crater-like, irregular shape *Examples:* pressure injury, chancre
Atrophy	Depression in skin resulting from thinning of the epidermis or dermis *Examples:* aged skin, striae
Excoriation	Area in which epidermis is missing, exposing the dermis *Examples:* abrasion, scratch

TABLE 25.6 LESION DISTRIBUTION TERMINOLOGY

Term	Description
Annular	Circular, beginning in centre and spreading to periphery (e.g., tinea corporis [ringworm])
Asymmetrical	Unilateral distribution
Confluent	Merging together (e.g., urticaria [hives])
Diffuse	Wide distribution over large area
Discrete	Distinct individual lesions that are separate (e.g., acne)
Grouped	Cluster of lesions
Gyrate	Twisted, coiled spiral, snakelike
Localized	Limited areas of involvement that are clearly defined
Satellite	Single lesion in proximity to a large grouping
Solitary	A single lesion
Symmetrical	Bilateral distribution
Zosteriform	Bandlike distribution along a dermatome area

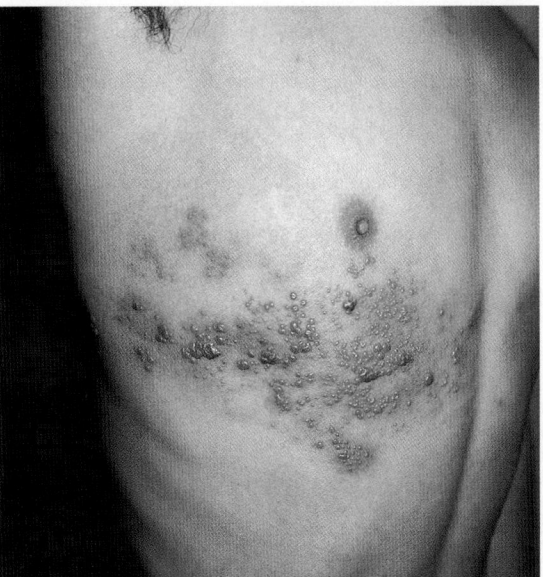

FIG. 25.5 Herpes zoster (shingles) on the anterior chest, classic dermatomal distribution. Source: James, W. D., Berger, T. G., & Elston, D. M. (2011). *Andrews' diseases of the skin* (11th ed.). Philadelphia: Saunders.

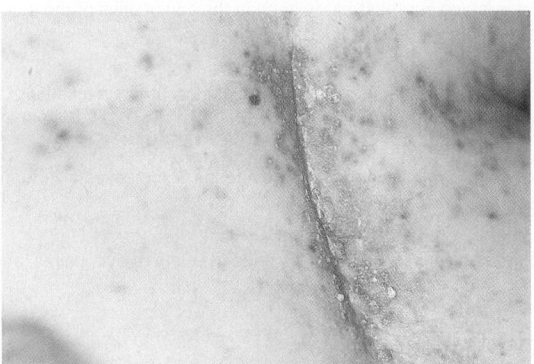

FIG. 25.6 Intertrigo. Candidal rash in body folds. Source: Graham-Brown, R., Bourke, J., & Cunliffe, T. (2008). *Dermatology: Fundamentals of practice*. Mosby.

Texture refers to the fineness or coarseness of the skin. The skin should feel smooth and firm, with the surface evenly thin in most areas. Thickened callous areas are normal on the soles and palms and result from weight bearing. Increased thickness

is often work-related and may be a result of excessive pressure. Excessive calluses on the soles of patients with neuropathy or diabetes predispose them to developing lesions.

Risk assessment to predict a patient's pressure injury risk should be done using a validated assessment tool such as the Braden Scale (see Chapter 14, Table 14.14, for the Braden Scale for Predicting Pressure Sore Risk).

A focused assessment is used to evaluate the status of previously identified integumentary issues and to monitor for signs of new concerns. A focused assessment of the integumentary system is presented in the Focused Assessment box. Common assessment abnormalities of the skin are described in Table 25.7.

FOCUSED ASSESSMENT

Integumentary System

This checklist can be used to make sure the key assessment steps have been done.

Subjective
The patient should be asked about any of the following and responses noted:

Hair loss (unusual or rapid)	Y	N
Changes in the skin (e.g., lesions, bruising)	Y	N
Nail discoloration	Y	N

Objective: Diagnostic
The following should be checked for results and critical values:

Biopsy results	✓
Albumin	✓

Objective: Physical Examination
The following should be inspected:

Skin for colour, integrity, scars, lesions, signs of breakdown	✓
Facial and body hair for distribution, colour, quantity, and hygiene	✓
Nails for shape, contour, colour, thickness, and cleanliness	✓
Dressings if present	✓

Palpation is used to determine the following:

Skin for temperature, texture, moisture, thickness, turgor, and mobility	✓

Assessment of Dark Skin Colour

The structures of dark skin are no different than those of lighter skin, and both normal and abnormal findings may present differently (Table 25.8). Colour variation is easiest to assess in parts of the body where the epidermis is thin and pigmentation is not influenced by sun exposure, such as the lips, mucous membranes, nail beds, palmar and plantar surfaces, and protected areas such as the buttocks.

Rashes are often difficult to observe in darker-skinned individuals and may need to be palpated. Wrinkling also is less apparent in this population.

Individuals with dark skin are predisposed to certain skin and hair conditions. *Keloid* is an overgrowth of collagenous tissue at the site of a skin injury (e.g., ear piercing) (Figure 25.7). Vitiligo is total loss of pigment in the affected area (Figure 25.8). In *dermatosis papulosa nigra*, the person has small, pigmented wartlike papules, commonly on the face. *Traction alopecia* may

TABLE 25.7   ASSESSMENT ABNORMALITIES

Integumentary System

Finding	Description	Possible Etiology and Significance
Alopecia	Loss of hair (localized or general) (see Figure 25.9)	Heredity, friction, rubbing, traction, trauma, stress, infection, inflammation, chemotherapy, tinea capitis, immunological factors
Angioma	Tumour consisting of blood or lymph vessels	Increased incidence is normal with aging; liver disease, pregnancy, varicose veins
Carotenemia (carotenosis)	Yellow discoloration of skin, no yellowing of sclerae, most noticeable on palms and soles	Excessive ingestion of vegetables containing carotene (e.g., carrots, squash), hypothyroidism
Comedone (acne lesion)	Enlarged hair follicle plugged with sebum, bacteria, and skin cells; can be open (blackhead) or closed (whitehead)	Heredity, certain medications, hormonal changes with puberty and pregnancy
Cyanosis	Slightly bluish-grey or purple discoloration of the skin and mucous membranes caused by presence of excessive amounts of reduced hemoglobin in capillaries	Cardiorespiratory conditions; vasoconstriction, asphyxiation, anemia, leukemia, and malignancies
Cyst	Sac containing fluid or semisolid material	Obstruction of a duct or gland, parasitic infection
Ecchymosis	Large, bruise-like lesion caused by collection of extravascular blood in dermis and subcutaneous tissue	Trauma, bleeding disorders
Erythema	Redness occurring in patches of variable size and shape	Heat, certain medications, alcohol, ultraviolet rays, any condition that causes dilation of blood vessels to the skin
Hematoma	Extravasation of blood of sufficient size to cause visible swelling	Trauma, bleeding disorders
Hirsutism	Male-pattern distribution of hair in women	Abnormality of ovaries or adrenal glands, decrease in estrogen level, heredity
Hypopigmentation	Congenital or acquired loss of melanin resulting in lighter depigmented areas	Chemical or pharmacological agents, nutritional factors, burns, inflammation and infection
Intertrigo	Dermatitis of overlying surfaces of the skin (see Figure 25.6)	Moisture, irritation, obesity; may be complicated by *Candida* infection
Jaundice	Yellow or yellowish-brown discoloration of the skin, best observed in the sclera; secondary to increased bilirubin in the blood	Liver disease, red blood cell hemolysis, pancreatic cancer, common bile duct obstruction
Keloid	Hypertrophied scar beyond margin of incision or trauma (see Figure 25.7)	Predisposition more common in dark-skinned individuals
Lichenification	Thickening of the skin with accentuated skin markings	Repeated scratching, rubbing, and irritation usually due to pruritus or neurosis
Mole (nevus)	Benign overgrowth of melanocytes	Defects of development; sometimes hereditary
Petechiae	Pinpoint, discrete deposit of blood <1–2 mm in the extravascular tissues; visible through the skin or mucous membrane	Inflammation, marked dilation, blood vessel trauma, thrombocytopenia
Telangiectasia	Visibly dilated, superficial, cutaneous small blood vessels, commonly found on face and thighs	Aging, acne, sun exposure, alcohol use, liver failure, corticosteroids, radiation, certain systemic diseases, skin tumours
Tenting	Failure of skin to return immediately to normal position after gentle pinching	Aging, dehydration, cachexia
Varicosity	Increased prominence of superficial veins	Interruption of venous return (e.g., from tumour, incompetent valves, inflammation), commonly found on lower extremities with aging
Vitiligo	Complete absence of melanin (pigment) resulting in chalky white patch (see Figure 25.8)	Autoimmune, heredity, thyroid disease

Lighter Skin	Darker Skin
Cyanosis	
Greyish-blue tone, especially in nail beds, earlobes, lips, mucous membranes, and palms and soles of feet	Ashen or greyish colour most easily seen in the conjunctiva of the eye, mucous membranes, and nail beds
Ecchymosis	
Dark red, purple, yellow, or green colour, depending on age of bruise	Purple to brownish-black; difficult to see unless occurring in an area of light pigmentation
Erythema	
Reddish tone, possibly accompanied by increased skin temperature secondary to localized inflammation	Deeper brown or purple skin tone with evidence of increased skin temperature secondary to inflammation
Jaundice	
Yellowish colour of skin, sclera, fingernails, palms of hands, and oral mucosa	Yellowish-green colour most obviously seen in sclera of eye, palms, and soles
Pallor	
Pale skin colour that may appear white or ashen; also evident on lips, nail beds, and mucous membranes	May appear yellowish, ashen, or grey
Petechiae	
Lesions appear as small, reddish purple pinpoints, best observed on abdomen and buttocks	Difficult to see; may be evident in the buccal mucosa of the mouth or the conjunctiva of the eye
Rash	
May be visualized as well as felt with light palpation	Not easily visualized, but may be felt with light palpation
Scar	
Narrow scar line, usually white or pink	Higher incidence of keloid development, resulting in a thickened, raised scar (see Chapter 14, Figure 14.8)

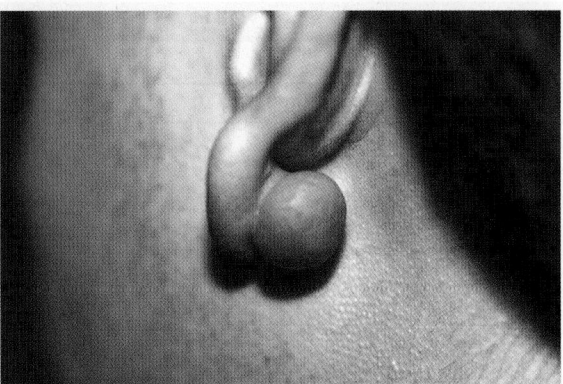

FIG. 25.7 Keloid. Hypertrophic scarring after skin injury. Source: Kliegman, R. M., Stanton, B. F., St. Geme III, J. W., et al. (2011) *Nelson textbook of pediatrics.* Saunders.

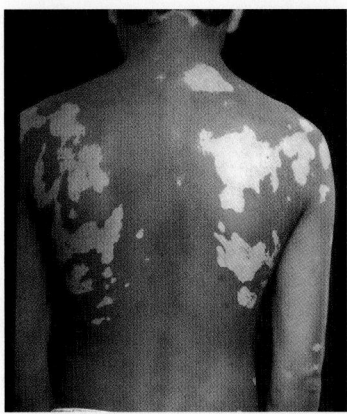

FIG. 25.8 Vitiligo. Total loss of pigment in affected areas. Source: Graham-Brown, R., Bourke, J., & Cunliffe, T. (2008). *Dermatology: Fundamentals of practice.* Mosby.

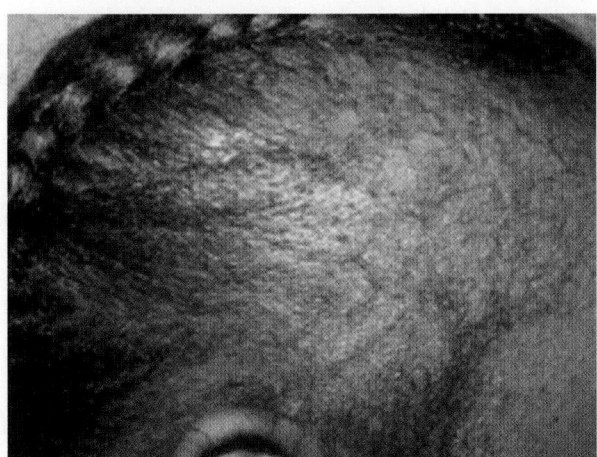

FIG. 25.9 Traction alopecia. Hair loss in scalp because of prolonged tension from hair roller, braiding, or straightening combs. Source: With permission: Sperling, L. C., Sinclair, R. D., & Shabrawi-Caelen, L. E. Alopecias. In J. L. Bolognia, J. L. Jorizzo, & J. V. Schaffer (Eds.). (2012). *Dermatology* (3rd ed.). Saunders.

CASE STUDY

Objective Data

Physical Examination

Physical examination findings of D. A.'s skin are as follows:

- Complexion fair. Wrinkles around eyes, above upper lip, and on sides of cheeks bilaterally. Normal skin temperature and turgor.
- Lesions on upper right forehead measuring 2 × 3 mm; on left forehead near hairline measuring 1 × 2 mm; and on left lower cheek measuring 2 × 2.5 mm.

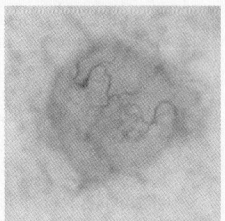

Source: Cheek lesion. From Bolognia, J. L., Schaffer, J. V., Duncan, K. O., et al. (2014). *Dermatology essentials.* Saunders.

- All lesions are slightly erythematous but do not blanch when direct pressure is applied. Borders are distinct. Minimal elevation is noted on palpation.
- No skin lesions are noted on rest of body.

Throughout this chapter, consider which diagnostic studies would likely be performed for D. A., and also identify patient concerns and appropriate nursing interventions while she is a patient at the clinic.

Diagnostic Studies

D. A..'s health care provider examines the lesions via dermatoscopy and also uses a Wood's lamp to rule out a fungal infection. A basal cell carcinoma diagnosis is suspected and is confirmed by a shave biopsy.

See Case Study: Patient Introduction and Case Study: Subjective Data for more information on D. A.

be the result of trauma from tight braiding of the hair or hair extensions (Figure 25.9). The hair loss may be temporary or permanent. *Pseudofolliculitis* is an inflammatory response to ingrown hairs that may occur after shaving, which results in pustules and papules.

In patients with darker skin, colour may not be a reliable indicator of systemic conditions (e.g., flushed skin with fever). Cyanosis may be difficult to determine because a normal bluish hue occurs in dark-skinned people. Dark skin rarely shows a blanch response, making it more difficult to identify pressure injuries.

DIAGNOSTIC STUDIES OF THE INTEGUMENTARY SYSTEM

Table 25.9 presents common diagnostic studies used for the integumentary system. The main diagnostic techniques related to skin conditions are inspection of an individual lesion and a careful history related to the concern. If a definitive diagnosis cannot be made by these techniques, other tests may be needed. With *dermatoscopy*, the health care provider uses a lighted instrument with optical magnification to see skin structures and colours not visible with the naked eye (Russo et al., 2016). These hand-held screening devices can help determine if a lesion should be biopsied.

TABLE 25.9   DIAGNOSTIC STUDIES
Integumentary System

Study	Description and Purpose	Nursing Responsibility
Biopsy		
Punch	Special punch biopsy instrument of appropriate size is used. Instrument is rotated to appropriate level to include dermis and some fat. Suturing may or may not be done. Provides full-thickness skin for diagnostic purposes.	Verify that consent form is signed (if needed). Assist with preparation of site, anaesthesia, procedure, and hemostasis. Apply dressing and give postprocedure instructions to patient. Properly identify specimen.
Excisional	Useful when good cosmetic results or entire removal or both are desired. Skin closed with subcutaneous and skin sutures.	Same as above
Incisional	Wedge-shaped incision made in lesion too large for excisional biopsy. Useful when larger specimen than shave biopsy is needed.	Same as above
Shave	Single-edged razor blade used to shave off superficial lesions or small sample of a large lesion. Provides thin specimen for diagnostic purposes.	Same as above
Microscopic Tests		
Potassium hydroxide (KOH)	Hair, scales, or nails are examined for superficial fungal infection. Put specimen on glass slide and add potassium hydroxide solution of 10%–20%.	Instruct patient regarding purpose of test. Prepare slide.
Culture	Test identifies fungal, bacterial, and viral organisms. For *fungi*, scraping or swab of skin is performed. For *bacteria*, material is obtained from intact pustules, bullae, or abscesses. For *viruses*, vesicle or bulla is scraped and exudate taken from base of lesion.	Instruct patient regarding purpose and procedure. Properly identify specimen. Follow instructions for storage of specimen if not immediately sent to laboratory.
Mineral oil slides	Test checks for infestations. Scrapings are placed on slide with mineral oil and viewed microscopically.	Instruct patient about purpose of test. Prepare slide.
Immunofluorescent studies	Some cutaneous diseases have specific, abnormal antibody proteins that can be identified by fluorescent studies. Both skin and serum can be examined.	Inform patient about purpose of test. Assist in obtaining specimen. For punch biopsy of tissue, place specimen in special fixative (e.g., Michel's), and not formalin.
Miscellaneous		
Wood's lamp (black light)	Examination of skin with long-wave ultraviolet light causes specific substances to fluoresce (e.g., *Pseudomonas* organisms, fungal infections, vitiligo).	Explain purpose of examination and that it is not painful. Darken room for examination.
Patch test	Used to determine whether patient is allergic to specific testing material. Small amount of potentially allergenic material is applied, usually to skin on back.	Explain purpose of test and procedure to patient. Instruct patient to return in 48–72 hr for removal of allergens and evaluation. Inform patient if re-evaluation is needed at 96 hr.

Biopsy is one of the most common diagnostic tests used to evaluate a skin lesion. A biopsy is needed when cancer is suspected or a specific diagnosis is questionable. Techniques include punch, incisional, excisional, and shave biopsies. The method used depends on factors such as the biopsy site, cosmetic result desired, and type of tissue needed.

Other diagnostic procedures include stains and cultures for fungal, bacterial, and viral infections. Direct immunofluorescence is a special diagnostic technique used on biopsy specimens. It may be needed in certain conditions such as bullous diseases and systemic lupus erythematosus. Indirect immunofluorescence is completed on blood samples.

REVIEW QUESTIONS

The number of the question corresponds to the same-numbered objective at the beginning of the chapter.

1. What is the primary function of the skin?
   a. Insulation
   b. Protection
   c. Sensation
   d. Absorption
2. Which of the following are age-related changes in the hair and nails? *(Select all that apply.)*
   a. Oily scalp
   b. Scaly scalp
   c. Thinner nails
   d. Thicker, brittle nails
   e. Longitudinal nail ridging
3. When assessing self-care habits in relation to the skin, what does the nurse question the client about?
   a. Joint pain
   b. Use of sunscreen products
   c. Recent changes in exercise tolerance
   d. Family history of melanoma
4. During the physical examination of a client's skin, which of the following would the nurse do?
   a. Use a flashlight if the room is poorly lit.
   b. Note cool, moist skin as a normal finding.
   c. Pinch up a fold of skin to assess for turgor.
   d. Perform a lesion-specific examination first and then a general inspection.

5. The nurse assessed the client's skin lesions as firm, edematous, and irregularly shaped with variable diameter. What would these lesions be called?
   a. Wheals
   b. Papules
   c. Pustules
   d. Plaques
6. On inspection of the client's skin, the nurse notes the complete absence of melanin pigment in patchy areas on the client's hands. What is this assessment finding called?
   a. Vitiligo
   b. Keloid
   c. Telangiectasia
   d. Lichenification
7. Individuals with dark skin are more likely to develop which of the following?
   a. Keloids
   b. Wrinkles
   c. Rashes
   d. Skin cancer
8. Under what circumstance is diagnostic testing recommended for skin lesions?
   a. When a health history cannot be obtained
   b. When a more definitive diagnosis is needed
   c. When percussion reveals an abnormal finding
   d. When treatment with prescribed medication has failed

1. b, 2. b, d, e; 3. b; 4. c; 5. a; 6. a; 7. a; 8. b

For even more review questions, visit http://evolve.elsevier.com/Canada/Lewis/medsurg.

REFERENCES

Alikhan, A., & Hocker, T. L. (2016). *Review of dermatology*. Elsevier Health Sciences.

Bishop, B., & Tosti, A. (2017). *Melanonychias*. Springer International Publishing.

Bradford, L. E. A., Bharadwaj, L. A., Ukpalauwaekwee, U., et al. (2016). Drinking water quality in Indigenous communities in Canada and health outcomes: A scoping review. *International Journal of Circumpolar Health*, 75, 32336. https://doi.org/10/3402/ijch.v75.32336

Dermatology Association (CDA). (2021a). *Melanoma*. https://dermatology.ca/public-patients/skin/melanoma/

Dermatology Association (CDA). (2021b). *Photoaging*. https://dermatology.ca/public-patients/skin/photoaging/

Coit, D., Thompson, J. A., Algazi, A., et al. (2016). Melanoma. *Journal of the National Comprehensive Cancer Network*, 14(4), 450–473. https://doi.org/10.6004/jnccn.2016.0051

Desai, S. R., Kovarik, C., Brod, B., et al. (2020). COVID-19 and personal protective equipment: Treatment and prevention of skin conditions related to the occupational use of personal protective equipment. *Journal of the American Academy of Dermatology*, 83(2), 675–677. https://doi.org/10.1016/j.jaad.2020.05.032

Gawkrodger, D., & Ardern-Jones, M. (2016). *Dermatology* (6th ed.). Mosby.

Habif, T. P. (2016). *Clinical dermatology* (6th ed.). Mosby.

Kirlew, M., Rea, S., Schroeter, A., et al. (2014). Invasive CA-MRSA in northwestern Ontario: A 2-year prospective study. *Canadian Journal of Rural Medicine*, 19(3), 99–102.

Russo, T., Piccolo, V., Lallas, A., et al. (2016). Recent advances in dermoscopy (F1000 Faculty Review). *F1000 Research*, 5, 184–190. https://doi.org/10.12688/f1000research.7597.1.

For additional Internet resources, see Chapter 26 and the website for this book at http://evolve.elsevier.com/Canada/Lewis/medsurg.

26

Nursing Management

Integumentary Conditions

Susannah McGeachy
Originating US chapter by Mariann M. Harding

---

evolve WEBSITE

http://evolve.elsevier.com/Canada/Lewis/medsurg

- Review Questions (Online Only)
- Key Points
- Answer Guidelines for Case Study

- Customizable Nursing Care Plan
  - Patient with Chronic Skin Lesions
- Conceptual Care Map Creator

- Audio Glossary
- Content Updates

LEARNING OBJECTIVES

1. Specify health promotion practices related to the integumentary system.
2. Explain the etiology, clinical manifestations, and interprofessional management of skin cancers.
3. Explain the etiology, clinical manifestations, and interprofessional management of bacterial, viral, and fungal skin infections.
4. Explain the etiology, clinical manifestations, and interprofessional management of infestations and insect bites.

5. Explain the etiology, clinical manifestations, and interprofessional management of allergic dermatological disorders.
6. Explain the etiology, clinical manifestations, and interprofessional management of benign dermatological disorders.
7. Summarize the psychological and physiological effects of chronic dermatological conditions.
8. Explain the indications for and nursing management of common cosmetic procedures and skin grafts.

KEY TERMS

acne vulgaris
actinic keratosis (AK)
basal cell carcinoma (BCC)
cellulitis
cryosurgery

curettage
dysplastic nevi (DN)
herpes zoster (shingles)
impetigo
lichenification

malignant melanoma
psoriasis
squamous cell carcinoma (SCC)
sun protection factor (SPF)
urticaria

HEALTH PROMOTION

Health promotion practices for the skin often parallel practices appropriate for general good health. The skin reflects both physical and psychological well-being. Specific health promotion practices to maintain good skin health include avoidance of environmental hazards; adequate rest, hygiene, and nutrition; and skin self-examination.

Environmental Hazards

Sun Exposure. Sun exposure comes with serious risk and results in permanent sun damage to skin. Sunlight is made up of visible light and ultraviolet (UV) light. There are two types of UV light that can affect skin: UVA and UVB. Specific wavelengths (Table 26.1) have different effects on the skin. UVA light

is responsible for tanning, UVB for sunburn; exposure to both types increases the risk of skin cancer. The damage caused by UV rays is cumulative. It results in degenerative changes in the dermis and premature aging (e.g., loss of elasticity, thinning, wrinkling, abnormal dryness). Prolonged and repeated sun exposure increases risk for actinic keratosis, basal cell carcinoma (BCC), squamous cell carcinoma (SCC), and melanoma.

Nurses play a crucial role in educating patients on sun-safety strategies. Patient teaching regarding sun protection is important, as people often do not understand the serious risks of sun exposure. Following sun safety guidelines beginning early in life can help people avoid experiencing the damaging effects of the sun and the formation of skin cancer later in life. Fair-skinned persons and those with light-coloured eyes

TABLE 26.1	WAVELENGTHS OF THE SUN AND EFFECTS ON SKIN
Wavelength	**Effect**
Long (UVA)	• Causes elastic tissue damage and actinic skin damage • Responsible for tanning due to increased melanin production • Contributes to formation of skin cancer
Middle (UVB)	• Responsible for sunburn • Major factor in development of skin cancer
Short (UVC)	• Does not reach earth; is blocked by atmosphere

UVA, ultraviolet A light; *UVB,* ultraviolet B light; *UVC,* ultraviolet C light.

should be especially cautious about excess sun exposure. They have less melanin and thus less natural protection against skin damage and disease.

Environment and Climate Change Canada (ECCC) uses the UV index to communicate the risk for harmful UV exposure; it is regularly included in local weather forecasts and is available online. At an index of 3 (moderate) or higher, ECCC (2017) recommends using sun-protective measures, particularly around midday, and if a person will be exposed to sun for 30 minutes or longer. Even on overcast days, serious sunburn can occur, because up to 80% of UV rays can penetrate cloud cover. Other factors that increase sunburn risk include being at high altitudes, where atmospheric protection from UV rays is decreased, and being in or on snow or in or near water, as water and snow reflect a significant portion of the sun's rays back toward the skin.

Sun-protective measures for the skin include carrying an umbrella, wearing a large-brimmed hat and long-sleeved clothing, and applying sunscreen to exposed skin. Two types of sunscreens, chemical and physical, filter both UVA and UVB wavelengths. *Chemical sunscreens* are light creams, lotions, or sprays that absorb or filter UV light, resulting in diminished UV light penetration. In contrast, *physical sunscreens* (e.g., titanium dioxide, zinc oxide) are thick, opaque, heavy creams that reflect UV radiation, blocking all UVA and UVB radiation. Sunscreen products are rated according to their **sun protection factor (SPF)**; SPF measures the effectiveness of a sunscreen in filtering and absorbing UVB radiation. Broad-spectrum products offer protection against UVA radiation as well (Government of Canada, 2017b).

Individuals need to select the right sunscreen for their needs. The Canadian Dermatology Association (CDA) (2021d) and the Government of Canada (2017b) recommend that everyone use daily sunscreen with a minimum SPF of 30 to prevent premature aging of the skin and skin cancer. Patients should be taught to look for the term *broad spectrum* on sunscreen packaging. Those who have a history of skin cancer or have sun sensitivity should use a product with an SPF of at least 30. Sunscreens should be applied 20 to 30 minutes before going outdoors. The SPF value of all sunscreens decreases with time. Sunscreen should be reapplied every 2 hours, or more frequently after swimming or profusely sweating, to maintain good sun protection, even if the product is "waterproof."

Eye protection is also important to consider when spending time in the sun, as UV rays can potentially cause retinal damage and may be a contributing factor in development of cataracts. The nurse should advise patients to use sunglasses with UVA and UVB protection, particularly when the UV index is 3 or above (Government of Canada, 2017a).

EVIDENCE-INFORMED PRACTICE
Translating Research Into Practice

A nurse is working in a skin cancer screening clinic. S. W. (pronouns she/her) is 24 years old and has a fair skin type (blond hair and blue eyes). S. W. is completing the health history before beginning the screening examination and indicates use of an indoor tanning salon every other week because "I feel hot and healthier when I am tanned." The nurse spends time explaining the increased risk for skin cancer associated with the use of tanning booths.

Best Available Evidence	Clinician Expertise	Patient Preferences and Values
The World Health Organization (WHO) and International Agency for Research on Cancer (IARC) report a strong link between exposure to indoor tanning devices and development of skin cancer and melanoma, particularly when use is initiated prior to 35 years of age.	The nurse notes that S. W. has the following skin cancer risk factors: fair skin, blond hair, blue eyes, frequent use of tanning booths.	After listening, the patient tells the nurse that the frequency of tanning visits will decrease—going only when there is an upcoming important event.

Decision and Action
The nurse informs S. W. this is a step in the right direction and encourages consideration of completely stopping tanning bed uses.

References for Evidence
Canadian Dermatology Association. (2021). *Indoor tanning is out.* https://dermatology.ca/public-patients/sun-protection/indoor-tanning-is-out/
Government of Canada. (2019). *Tanning beds and equipment.* https://www.canada.ca/en/health-canada/services/sun-safety/tanning-beds-lamps.html

Tanning booths and sun lamps are still commonly used to artificially tan skin, despite well-known associated risks, including photoaging (see Chapter 25) and skin cancers. Patients should be warned that indoor tanning increases a person's risk of developing melanoma by 59% if used before the age of 35 and increases the risk of developing other skin malignancies such as SCC and BCC (Government of Canada, 2019). Indoor tanning especially increases cancer risk for individuals who are younger than 18 years of age; at present, every province in Canada and two of three territories have banned tanning bed use by minors under 18 or 19 years of age (CDA, 2021b).

Certain medications potentiate the sun's effects, even with brief exposure. The chemicals in these medications absorb light when exposed to natural sunlight and release energy that harms cells and tissues. Common photosensitizing medications are shown in Table 26.2. The manifestations of medication-induced photosensitivity (Figure 26.1) are like those of an exaggerated sunburn. These include swelling, erythema, vesicles, and papular, plaque-like lesions. The photosensitivity of each individual drug should be assessed. Patients taking these medications should be taught about their photosensitizing effect and the need to protect the skin from photosensitivity reactions by using sunscreen products.

The nurse should also teach patients to self-examine their skin monthly. They should have a periodic professional assessment of areas that are hard to see. The cornerstone of skin examination

TABLE 26.2   MEDICATION THERAPY

Medications That May Cause Photosensitivity

Categories	Examples
Anticancer drugs	Methotrexate, vinorelbine tartrate
Antidepressants	Amitriptyline (Elavil), clomipramine (Anafranil), doxepin (Silenor)
Antidysrhythmics	Quinidine, amiodarone
Antifungals	Ketoconazole (Ketoderm, Nizoral)
Antihistamines	Diphenhydramine (Benadryl), chlorpheniramine (Chlor-Tripolon)
Antimicrobials	Tetracycline, sulfamethoxazole-trimethoprim (Septra), azithromycin (Zithromax), ciprofloxacin (Cipro)
Antipsychotics	Chlorpromazine, haloperidol
Diuretics	Furosemide, hydrochlorothiazide
Hypoglycemics	Tolbutamide,
Nonsteroidal anti-inflammatory medications	Diclofenac (Voltaren), piroxicam, sulindac

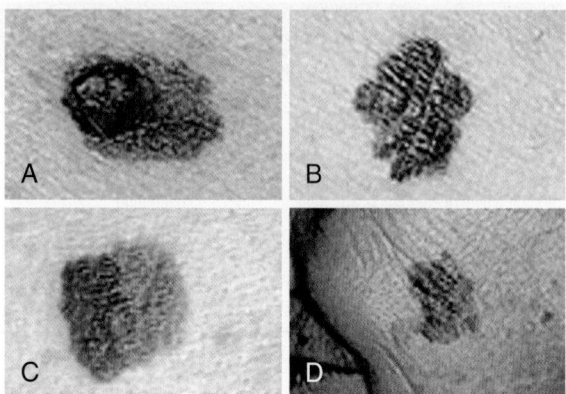

FIG. 26.2 The ABCDEs of melanoma. **A,** Asymmetry: one half is unlike the other half. **B,** Border irregularity: edges are ragged, notched, or blurred. **C,** Colour: varied pigmentation; shades of tan, brown, and black. **D,** Diameter: greater than 6 mm (diameter of a pencil eraser). **E,** Evolving (not pictured); changing appearance (change in shape, size, colour, or other characteristic is noted over a length of time). Source: The Skin Cancer Foundation, New York, NY.

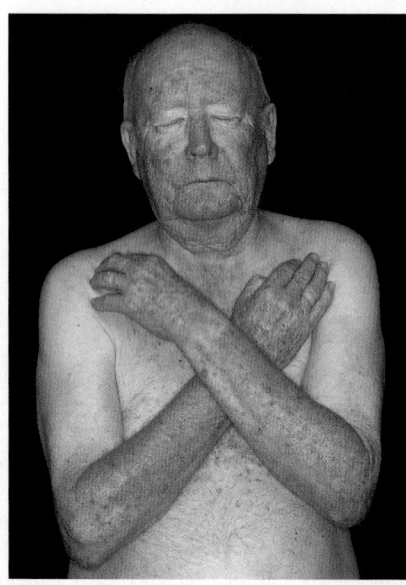

FIG. 26.1 Intense eruption in areas exposed to sunlight after patient started on hydrochlorothiazide. Source: Habif, T. P. (2016). *Clinical dermatology: A color guide to diagnosis and therapy* (6th ed., p. 454). Mosby.

is the ABCDE rule: Skin lesions are examined for **a**symmetry, **b**order irregularity, **c**olour change and variation, **d**iameter of 6 mm or more, and **e**volving in appearance (Figure 26.2). Patients should be taught that a persistent skin lesion that does not heal and lesions once flat and now raised, once small and recently growing, or changing in appearance are warning signs. These should be examined by a health care provider. Skin malignancies generally grow slowly, and early detection and treatment often leads to a highly favourable prognosis.

Cold Exposure. Excessive or prolonged exposure to cold can cause damage to the skin and underlying tissue, or *frostbite*. Assessment and management of frostbite are discussed further in Chapter 71.

Irritants and Allergens. The nurse should counsel patients to avoid known irritants (e.g., ammonia, harsh detergents). Skin patch testing (application of allergens) can sometimes be helpful in determining the most likely sensitizing agent (see Chapter 25). The nurse must also be aware that prescribed and over-the-counter (OTC) topical and systemic medications used to treat a variety of

conditions may contain fragrances and preservatives that cause dermatological reactions. Usually symptoms will resolve with discontinuation of the medication or product.

Rest and Sleep

Sleep is restorative to the skin. Pruritic skin diseases often interfere with sleep. Helping patients obtain high-quality sleep is an important health promotion practice. Adequate rest increases the patient's ability to tolerate itching, thereby decreasing skin damage from scratching.

Exercise

Exercise has numerous psychological and physiological benefits, including dilation of the blood vessels and improved perfusion of the dermis. However, caution must be used to avoid overexposure to heat, cold, and sun during outdoor exercise.

Hygiene

The patient's skin type, lifestyle, culture, age, and gender influence hygienic practices. The normal acidity of the skin and perspiration protect against bacterial overgrowth. Most soaps are alkaline and neutralize the skin surface, leading to a loss of protection. Using mild, moisturizing soaps and lipid-free cleansers and avoiding hot water and vigorous scrubbing can noticeably decrease local skin irritation and inflammation. Skin piercings in which jewellery has been inserted can be cared for with antibacterial soaps that do not contain sulphites.

In general, skin and hair must be washed often enough to remove excess oil and excretions and to prevent odor. Older persons should avoid using harsh soaps and shampoos and frequent bathing because of the dryness of their skin and scalp. Using moisturizers right after a bath or shower (while the skin is still damp) seals in the moisture.

Nutrition

A well-balanced diet adequate in all food groups can produce healthy skin, hair, and nails (see *Canada's Food Guide* in Chapter 42). Important elements of skin nutrition are listed in Table 26.3.

Obesity has an adverse effect on the skin. The increase in subcutaneous fat can lead to stretching and overheating. Overheating secondary to the greater insulation provided by fat causes an

TABLE 26.3 NUTRITIONAL THERAPY

Nutrients Essential for Healthy Skin, Hair, and Nails

Nutrient	Supportive Function	Impact of Nutrient Deficiency
Vitamin A	• Maintenance of normal epithelial cell structure • Wound healing	• Conjunctival dryness • Poor wound healing
Vitamin B complex (niacin, pyridoxine, biotin)	• Complex metabolic functions	• Erythema/rashes • Bullae • Seborrhea-like lesions • Alopecia
Vitamin C (ascorbic acid)	• Connective tissue formation • Wound healing	• Symptoms of scurvy (severe deficiency) • Petechiae • Bleeding gums • Purpura
Vitamin D3 (cholecalciferol)	• Bone health • Produced in skin cells after UVB exposure	• Decreased bone mineral density • Muscle weakness and pain
Vitamin K	• Blood clotting cascade	• Decreased prothrombin synthesis • Easy bruising
Protein	• Cell growth and maintenance • Wound healing	• Poor wound healing • Dry, flaky skin • Brittle nails and hair
Unsaturated fatty acids (e.g., linoleic acid, arachidonic acid)	• Integrity of cellular and subcellular membranes	• Decreased tissue metabolism

increase in sweating, which inflames and dries the skin. Obesity is a risk factor for poor wound healing and type 2 diabetes mellitus. Increased skinfolds contribute to skin conditions. Skin in these intertriginous (skin on skin) areas is predisposed to skin tags *(acrochordons),* candidiasis (yeast), intertrigo (bacteria, fungi, yeast), and erythrasma (bacteria) infections.

MALIGNANT SKIN NEOPLASMS

Skin cancer is the most common cancer diagnosed in Canada, with incidence of both melanoma and nonmelanoma in Canada steadily increasing since the early 1980s (Canadian Cancer Society [CCS], 2021; Canadian Cancer Statistics Advisory Committee, 2019). The fact that skin lesions are so visible increases the likelihood of early detection and diagnosis.

RISK FACTORS

Risk factors for skin malignancies include having fair skin, blond or red hair, light eye colour, history of chronic sun exposure, family or personal history of skin cancer, outdoor occupations, frequent outdoor recreational activities, indoor tanning, and smoking (CCS, 2021). Patients treated with photochemotherapy, which is called *PUVA* and is a combination of oral methoxsalen (psoralen) and UVA radiation, may be at greater risk for melanoma. Individuals with darker skin are less susceptible to skin cancer because of naturally occurring increased melanin. Skin cancers are not common among Indigenous people in Canada despite the high prevalence of prolonged outdoor activities. However, melanoma may still occur in these patients, most often on the palms, the soles, and the mucous membranes. The nurse must be just as vigilant in screening for skin cancers occurring on darker skin as for skin cancers on light skin, as changes may be more subtle and difficult to detect on darker skin.

NONMELANOMA SKIN CANCERS

Nonmelanoma skin cancers (basal cell and squamous cell carcinomas) are the most common forms of skin cancer, accounting for 40% of new cancer diagnoses in Canada (CCS, 2021). Nonmelanoma skin cancers do not develop from melanocytes. They develop in the basement membrane of the skin. Although there are few deaths from nonmelanoma skin cancers, they have the potential for severe local destruction, permanent disfigurement, and disability.

Nonmelanoma skin cancers usually develop in sun-exposed areas, such as the face, head, neck, back of the hands, and arms. The most common causative factor is sun exposure, and the majority of cases are diagnosed between age 80 and 90 (CCS, 2021). There are some differences between basal and squamous cell cancers. SCCs usually occur on the head and neck, where there is the highest degree of UV radiation. BCCs do not follow that pattern and may occur in sun-protected areas.

Actinic Keratosis

Actinic keratosis (AK), also known as *solar keratosis,* is the most common premalignant skin lesion and affects nearly all older individuals with light skin. They appear most often on skin that has been exposed to the sun or to artificial UV light. The clinical appearance of actinic keratoses can be highly varied. The typical lesion is an irregularly shaped, flat, slightly erythematous papule with indistinct borders and an overlying hard keratotic scale or horn (Table 26.4). Because actinic keratosis is impossible to differentiate from SCC, treatment should be aggressive. Nonsurgical procedures are the first-line treatment. Any lesion that persists should be evaluated for a possible biopsy.

Basal Cell Carcinoma

Basal cell carcinoma (BCC) is a locally invasive malignancy arising from epidermal basal cells. It is the most common type of skin cancer but the least deadly. BCC usually occurs in middle-aged to older persons. Most BCCs occur in the head and neck area (e.g., sun-exposed), followed by the trunk and extremities (Verkouteren et al., 2017).

Clinical manifestations are described in Table 26.4. Some BCCs are pigmented, with curled borders and an opaque appearance. They may be hard to distinguish from melanoma. A tissue biopsy is needed to confirm the diagnosis. BCCs rarely

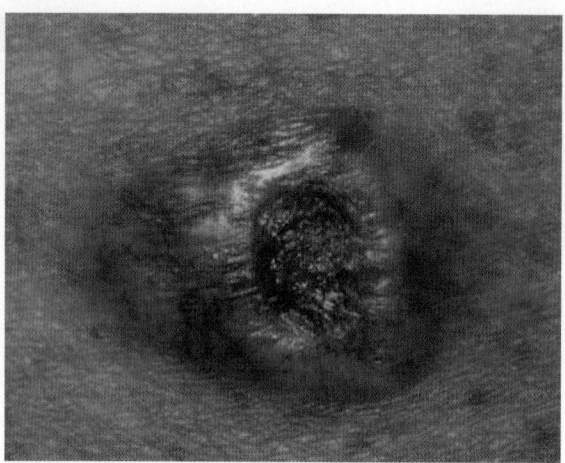

FIG. 26.3 Basal cell carcinoma. Rolled, well-defined border and central erosion Source: Goldman, L., & Schafer, A. (2016). *Goldman-Cecil medicine* (25th ed.). Saunders.

metastasize (Figure 26.3). However, if BCC is left untreated, massive tissue destruction may result. Treatment depends on the tumour location and histological type, history of recurrence, and patient characteristics (see Table 26.4). Location and size are important factors in determining the best treatment.

Squamous Cell Carcinoma

Squamous cell carcinoma (SCC) is a malignant neoplasm of keratinizing epidermal cells. It frequently occurs on sun-exposed skin. While less common than BCC, SCC can be aggressive, has the potential to metastasize, and may lead to death if not treated early and correctly. SCC often occurs at the base of an actinic keratosis or another lesion. The main risk factors are sun exposure and immunosuppression after organ transplantation (Green & Olsen, 2017). Pipe, cigar, or cigarette smoking contributes to the formation of SCC on the mouth and lips. Manifestations and treatment of SCC are described in Table 26.4. A biopsy should always be performed when a lesion is suspected to be SCC.

MELANOMA

Melanoma is a tumour arising in melanocytes, the cells producing melanin. Melanoma causes the majority of skin cancer deaths. Unlike most cancers whose incidence is stable or decreasing, the incidence of melanoma is steadily rising. The Canadian Cancer Statistics Advisory Committee (2019) estimated that nearly 7 800 new cases would be diagnosed in Canada in 2019, and nearly 1 300 Canadians would die from the disease. Melanoma can occur in the eyes, ears, gastrointestinal tract, and oral and genital mucous membranes. When it begins in the skin, it is called *cutaneous melanoma*. Melanoma has the ability to metastasize to any organ, including the brain and heart.

A combination of environmental and genetic factors is likely involved in the development of melanoma. UV radiation from the sun is the main cause of melanoma. Artificial sources of UV radiation, such as sunlamps and tanning booths, also play a role. UV radiation damages the deoxyribonucleic acid (DNA) in skin cells, causing mutations in their genetic code, thus altering the cells. The use of immunosuppressive medications and a history of dysplastic nevi also increase risk.

A person may have a genetic predisposition toward getting melanoma. Of those with melanoma, approximately 9% have

a first-degree relative (e.g., parent, full sibling) who had melanoma (Frank et al., 2017). This risk increases significantly if multiple relatives have had melanoma. Mutated genes have been found in some families who have a high familial incidence of melanoma.

Other factors that affect a person's likelihood for developing melanoma are listed in the Determinants of Health box.

Clinical Manifestations

Melanoma often occurs on the lower legs in women and on the trunk and head in men. About one-fourth of melanomas occur in existing nevi or moles. About 20% occur in dysplastic nevi. Rarely, it occurs in the mouth, intestines, and eyes.

Lesions showing any sudden or progressive change in the ABCDE rule (see Figure 26.2) should be evaluated. Because most melanoma cells continue to produce melanin, melanoma tumours are often deep brown or black (see Table 26.4).

Interprofessional Care

One of the first steps in diagnosing a suspicious lesion is dermoscopic examination. Dermoscopy can help the health care provider decide if a lesion should be biopsied. Biopsy is a critical tool for determining the type of lesion. A biopsy should be done using an excisional biopsy technique. Shave biopsy, shave excision, or electrocauterization should not be done because these techniques do not measure the depth of the lesion.

The most important prognostic factor is tumour thickness at the time of the diagnosis. Two methods to determine thickness are currently being used. The *Breslow measurement* indicates tumour depth in millimetres, and the *Clark level* indicates the number of skin layers involved (one to five); the higher the number, the deeper the melanoma (Figure 26.4).

Treatment depends on the site of the original tumour and the stage of the cancer. Melanoma staging (stages 0 to IV)

TABLE 26.4 PREMALIGNANT AND MALIGNANT CONDITIONS OF THE SKIN

Etiology and Pathophysiology	Clinical Manifestations	Treatment and Prognosis
Actinic Keratosis Actinic (sun) damage. Premalignant skin lesion, precursor of squamous cell carcinoma.	Flat or elevated, dry, hyperkeratotic scaly papule; felt more than seen. Adherent rough scale on red base, which returns when removed. Often multiple. Often on erythematous sun-exposed areas; increase in number with age.	Cryosurgery, chemical caustics, topical application of fluorouracil (Actikerall, Efudex, Tolak) or imiquimod (Aldara), chemical peels, laser resurfacing, photodynamic therapy. Recurrence is possible even with adequate treatment.
Dysplastic Nevi Morphologically between common acquired nevi and melanoma. May be precursor of cutaneous malignant melanoma.	Often >5 mm; irregular border, possibly notched. Variegated colour of tan, brown, black, red, or pink with single mole. Presence of at least one flat portion, often at edge of mole. Frequently multiple. Most common site is the back, but possible in uncommon mole sites such as scalp or buttocks (see Figure 26.5).	Increased risk for melanoma. Careful monitoring of people suspected of familial tendency to melanoma or dysplastic nevi. Excisional biopsy used for suspicious lesions.
Basal Cell Carcinoma (BCC) Change in basal cells. No maturation or normal keratinization. Continuing division of basal cells and formation of enlarging mass. Related to excessive sun exposure, genetic skin type, radiographic radiation, scars, and some types of nevi.	*Nodular and ulcerative:* Small, slowly enlarging papule. Borders are semi-translucent or "pearly," with overlying telangiectasia. Erosion, ulceration, and depression of centre. Normal skin markings are lost (see Figure 26.3). *Superficial:* Erythematous, pearly, sharply defined, barely elevated multinodular plaques; similar to eczema but nonpruritic.	Excisional surgery, chemosurgery, electrosurgery, radiation therapy, laser surgery, Mohs (microscopically controlled) surgery, cryosurgery; 90% cure rate; slow-growing tumour that invades local tissue; metastasis is rare; fluorouracil and imiquimod (Aldara) are used for superficial lesions.
Squamous Cell Carcinoma (SCC) Frequent occurrence on previously damaged skin (e.g., from sun, radiation, scar). Malignant tumour of squamous cell of epidermis. Invasion of dermis, surrounding skin.	Most common on sun-exposed areas such as face and hands. *Superficial:* Thin, scaly, erythematous plaque without invasion into the dermis. *Early:* Firm nodules with indistinct borders, scaling, and ulceration. *Late:* Covering of lesion with scale or horn from keratinization. Most common on sun-exposed areas such as face and hands.	Surgical excision, cryosurgery, radiation therapy, chemotherapy, Mohs surgery, or electrodessication and curettage. Untreated lesion may metastasize to regional lymph nodes. Fluorouracil and imiquimod are used for noninvasive SCC. High cure rate with early detection and treatment.
Cutaneous T-Cell Lymphoma Originates in skin. Localized, chronic, slowly progressing disease. Possibly related to environmental toxins and chemical exposure. Mycosis fungoides is most common form. Prevalence is twice as high in men as in women.	Classic presentation involving three stages—patch (early), plaque, and tumour (advanced). History of persistent macular eruption followed by gradual appearance of indurated erythematous plaques on the trunk. Appears similar to psoriasis. Pruritus, lymphadenopathy.	Treatment usually controls symptoms, not curative. Phototherapy, corticosteroids, topical nitrogen mustard, radiation therapy, imiquimod, retinoids. Systemic chemotherapy, extracorporeal photopheresis. Disease course is unpredictable; 10% will have progressive disease.
Malignant Melanoma Neoplastic growth of melanocytes anywhere on skin, eyes, or mucous membranes. Classification according to major histological mode of spread. Potential invasion and widespread metastases.	Irregular colour, surface, and border. Varying colour including red, white, blue, black, grey, and brown. Flat or elevated. Eroded or ulcerated. Often <1 cm in size. Most common sites are back, chest, and legs.	Wide surgical excision and possible sentinel lymph node evaluation depending on depth. Correlation of survival rate with depth of invasion. Poor prognosis unless diagnosis and treatment are done early. Spreading by local extension, regional lymphatic vessels, and bloodstream. Adjuvant therapy after surgery may be indicated if lesion >1.5 mm in depth.

is based on tumour size (thickness), nodal involvement, and metastasis. In stage 0, melanoma is confined to one place (in situ) in the epidermis. Melanoma is nearly 100% curable by excision if diagnosed at stage 0. Unfortunately, those with deep tumours or disease that has already spread to lymph nodes often develop metastases. The 5-year survival rate for those with advanced disease is less than 10% (Coit et al., 2016).

The initial treatment of malignant melanoma is wide surgical excision. Melanoma that has spread to the lymph nodes or nearby sites usually requires additional (adjuvant) therapy such as chemotherapy, immunotherapy, targeted therapy, radiation therapy, or a combination of therapies.

Atypical/Dysplastic Nevus

Dysplastic nevi (DN), or atypical moles, are nevi that are larger than usual (greater than 5 mm across) with irregular borders and various shades of color (Figure 26.5). DN may have the same ABCDE characteristics as melanoma, but they are less pronounced. Those with DN have an increased risk for developing

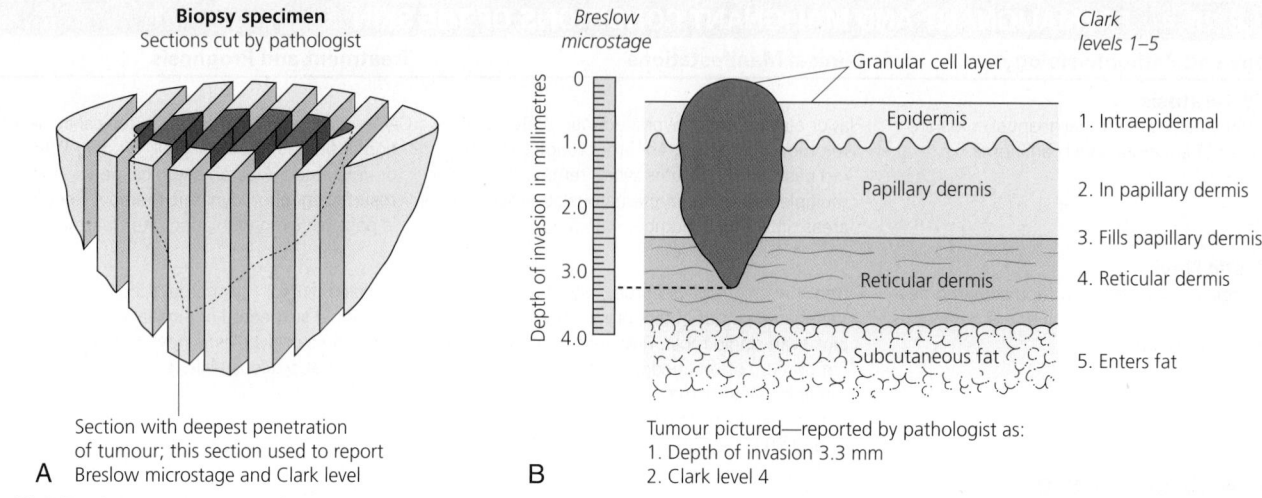

FIG. 26.4 Breslow measurement of tumour thickness. **A,** Thin (0.08-mm) superficial spreading melanoma, good prognosis. **B,** Thick nodular melanoma with lymph node involvement, poor prognosis. Source: Habif, T. P. (2016). *Clinical dermatology: A color guide to diagnosis and therapy* (6th ed.). Mosby.

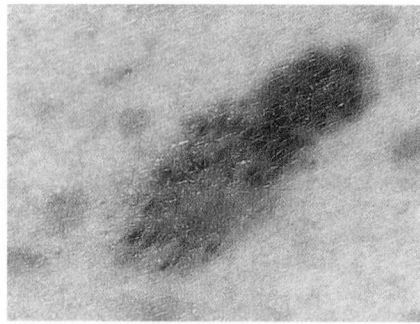

FIG. 26.5 Dysplastic nevus. Irregular border and colour Source: Graham-Brown, R., Bourke, J., & Cunliffe, T. (2008). *Dermatology: Fundamentals of practice.* Mosby.

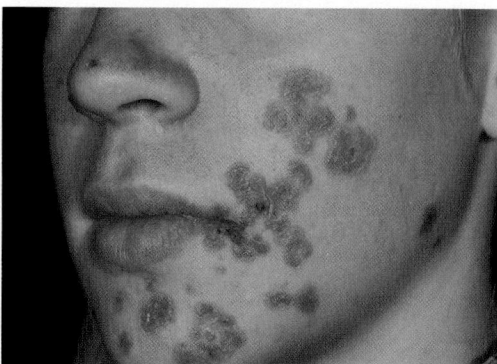

FIG. 26.6 Impetigo. Superficial pustules covered by a thick, honey-coloured crust. Source: Habif, T. P. (2016). *Clinical dermatology: A color guide to diagnosis and therapy* (6th ed., p. 329). Mosby.

melanoma in a mole or elsewhere on the body. The more DN a person has, the higher the risk. Those with 10 or more DN have 12 times the risk for developing melanoma.

SKIN INFECTIONS AND INFESTATIONS

Bacterial Infections

The skin provides an ideal environment for bacterial growth because of its abundant supply of nutrients and water and its warm temperature; it is home to numerous microorganisms, including bacteria. Bacterial infection occurs when the balance between the host and the microorganisms is altered. Infection can be primary, following a break in the skin, or secondary, appearing in already damaged skin or as a sign of a systemic disease. *Staphylococcus aureus* and group A β-hemolytic streptococci are the major types of bacteria responsible for primary and secondary skin infections, including impetigo (Figure 26.6), erysipelas, cellulitis (Figure 26.7), lymphangitis, and furuncles (Table 26.5).

Although infection can develop on healthy skin, factors such as moisture, obesity, atopic dermatitis, systemic corticosteroids and antibiotics, and chronic disease such as diabetes mellitus all increase the likelihood of infection. If an infection is present, the resulting drainage is infectious. Good skin hygiene and infection control practices are necessary to prevent the spread of infection. Lack of clean water for bathing and overcrowded housing conditions in many Indigenous

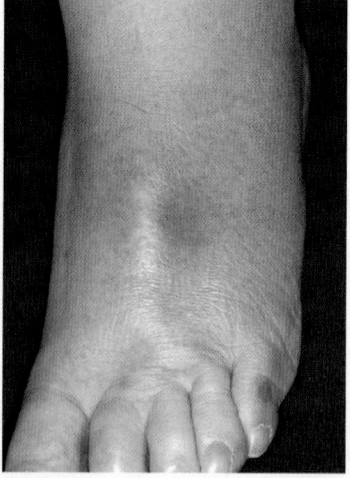

FIG. 26.7 Cellulitis with characteristic erythema, tenderness, and edema Source: Habif, T. P. (2011). *Clinical dermatology: A color guide to diagnosis and therapy* (5th ed.). Mosby.

communities in Canada may be associated with higher rates of bacterial skin infections such as methicillin-resistant *S. aureus* (MRSA) (Porter, 2015), leading to increased antibiotic use and antibiotic resistance in these communities (Kirlew et al., 2014).

TABLE 26.5 COMMON BACTERIAL INFECTIONS OF THE SKIN

Etiology and Pathophysiology	Clinical Manifestations	Treatment and Prognosis
Impetigo Group A β-hemolytic streptococci, staphylococci, or combination of both. Associated with poor hygiene. Primary or secondary infection. Contagious.	Vesiculopustular lesions that develop a thick, honey-coloured crust surrounded by erythema. Pruritic, may be painful. Most common on face as primary infection (see Figure 26.6).	*Local Treatment* Warm saline or aluminum acetate soaks followed by soap-and-water removal of crusts. Topical antibiotic cream or ointment (mupirocin [Bactroban], fusidic acid [Fucidin]). Meticulous hygiene essential. *Systemic Antibiotics* Oral cephalexin, (Keflex), clindamycin, erythromycin (Eryc), cephalosporins, amoxicillin for widespread or systemic manifestations.
Folliculitis Usually staphylococci. Present in areas subjected to friction, moisture, oiliness, or shaving. Increased incidence in patients with diabetes mellitus.	Small pustule at hair follicle opening with minimal erythema. Development of crusting; most common on scalp, beard, extremities and pubic area. Tender to touch.	Warm compresses of water or aluminum acetate solution. Antistaphylococcal soap (e.g., Hibiclens, Lever 2000, Dial) and water cleansing. Topical antibiotics (e.g., mupirocin [Bactroban], fusidic acid [Fucidin]). Heals usually without scarring. If lesions are extensive and deep, with possible scarring and loss of involved hair follicles, treatment is with systemic antibiotics.
Furuncle Deep infection with staphylococci around hair follicle. Often associated with severe acne or seborrheic dermatitis.	Tender, painful erythematous area around hair follicle. Draining pus and core of necrotic debris on rupture. Most common on face, back of neck, axillae, breasts, buttocks, perineum, thighs.	Incision and drainage, possibly with packing. Antibiotics. Meticulous care of involved skin, including frequent application of warm, moist compresses.
Furunculosis Increased incidence in patients with obesity, diabetes, or chronic illness, or in those regularly exposed to moisture or pressure.	Lesions as above. Malaise, regional adenopathy, fever.	Incision and drainage of painful nodules. Warm, moist compresses. Measures to reduce surface staphylococci include antimicrobial cream to nares, armpits, and groin and antiseptic to entire skin. Meticulous personal hygiene. Systemic antibiotic is effective against MRSA after culture and sensitivity study of drainage. Often recurrent with scarring. Prevention or correction of predisposing factors required.
Carbuncle Multiple, interconnecting furuncles.	Many pustules appearing in erythematous area. Most common at nape of neck.	Same as for furuncles. Slow healing with scar formation.
Cellulitis Deep inflammation of subcutaneous tissues due to enzymes produced by bacteria. May be primary infection or secondary complication. Often following break in skin. *Staphylococcus aureus* and streptococci are usual causative agents.	Hot, tender, erythematous, and edematous area with diffuse borders (see Figure 26.7). Chills, malaise, and fever.	Moist heat, immobilization and elevation. Systemic antibiotic therapy. Hospitalization if severe for IV antibiotic therapy based on culture and sensitivity. Progression to gangrene is possible if untreated.
Erysipelas Superficial cellulitis primarily involving the dermis. Group A β-hemolytic streptococci.	Red, hot, sharply demarcated plaque that is indurated and painful. Bacteremia possible. Most common on face and extremities. Toxic signs, such as fever, ↑ WBC count, headache, malaise.	Systemic antibiotics, usually penicillin. Hospitalization is often required.

IM, intramuscular; *MRSA*, methicillin-resistant *Staphylococcus aureus*; *WBC*, white blood cell.

Viral Infections

Like viral infections elsewhere in the body, viral infections of the skin are difficult to treat. When a virus infects a cell, a skin lesion may develop. Lesions can also result from an inflammatory response to the viral infections. Herpes simplex (Figure 26.8), herpes zoster (see Chapter 25, Figure 25.5), and warts (Figure 26.9) are the most common viral infections affecting the skin (Table 26.6).

Fungal Infections

Because of the prevalence of fungi in the environment, it is almost impossible to avoid exposure to some pathological varieties. However, some fungi, including candidiasis and tinea unguium (Figure 26.10), can cause infections of the skin, hair, and nails. Common fungal infections of the skin are presented in Table 26.7. Most infections are relatively harmless in healthy adults, but they can cause embarrassment and distress.

Fungal infections are easy to diagnose. A microscopic examination showing the appearance of hyphae (threadlike structures) in a skin scraping mounted in 10% to 20% potassium hydroxide (KOH) indicates a fungal infection. A Wood's light examination of hair infected with certain fungi will fluoresce blue to green.

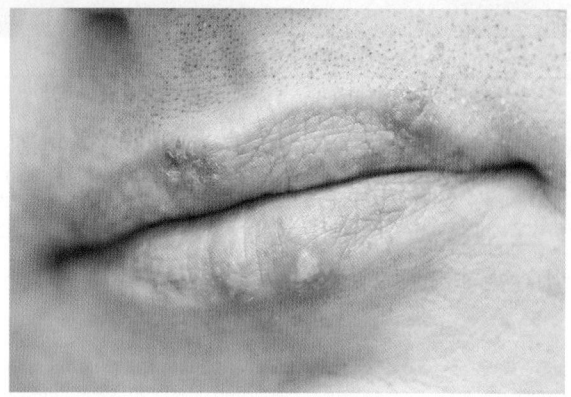

FIG. 26.8 Herpes viral infection on the lips. Source: © CanStock Photo / kadmy.

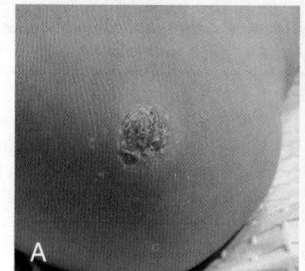 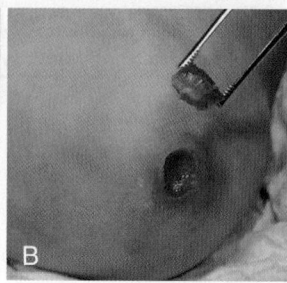

FIG. 26.9 Plantar wart. **A,** Keratotic lesion. **B,** After excision. Source: Swartz, M. H. (2010). *Textbook of physical diagnosis: History and examination* (6th ed.). Saunders.

TABLE 26.6   COMMON VIRAL INFECTIONS OF THE SKIN

Etiology and Pathophysiology	Clinical Manifestations	Treatment and Prognosis
Herpes Simplex Virus (HSV) Types 1 and 2 Oral or genital HSV infections can be serotyped as either HSV-1 or HSV-2. Both are recurrent, lifelong viral infections. Exacerbated by sunlight, trauma, menses, stress, and systemic infection. Contagious to those not previously infected. Transmission by respiratory droplets or virus-containing fluid (e.g., saliva, cervical secretions). Infection in one area is readily transmitted to another area by direct contact.	*First Episode* Symptoms occurring 2–14 days after contact. Painful local reaction. Single or grouped vesicles on erythematous base. Systemic symptoms (e.g., fever, malaise) or asymptomatic presentation possible (see Figure 26.8). *Recurrent Episodes* Typically milder and shorter. Recur in similar location. Characteristic grouped vesicles on erythematous base. Prodrome includes mild burning/tingling 1–2 days before outbreak.	Soothing, moist compresses; petroleum jelly to lesions. Usually no scarring. Antiviral agents (e.g., acyclovir, famciclovir [Famvir], and valacyclovir [Valtrex]) depending on location, frequency of outbreaks.
Herpes Zoster (Shingles) Activation of the varicella-zoster virus. Incidence increases with age and in immunosuppressed patients. Potentially contagious to anyone who has not had varicella.	Linear distribution along dermatome of grouped vesicles on erythematous base. Usually unilateral on trunk, face, and lumbosacral areas. Burning, pain, and neuralgia preceding outbreak. Mild to severe pain during outbreak (see Chapter 25, Figure 25.5).	Symptomatic. Antiviral agents (e.g., acyclovir, famciclovir [Famvir], and valacyclovir [Valtrex]) are effective for prevention of postherpetic neuralgia (PHN) if given within 72 hr of lesion appearance. Wet compresses, silver sulfadiazine (Flamazine) to ruptured vesicles. Analgesia. Gabapentin (Neurontin) or pregabalin (Lyrica) to treat PHN. Usually heals without complications, but scarring and PHN possible. Vaccines (Zostavax, Shingrix) to reduce risk for shingles and PHN are available for adults 50 yr or older who previously had chicken pox.
Verruca Vulgaris Caused by human papilloma virus (HPV). Spontaneous disappearance in 1–2 yr possible. Mildly contagious by autoinoculation. Specific response dependent on body part affected. Prevalence greater in adolescents and immunosuppressed.	Circumscribed, hypertrophic, flesh-coloured papule limited to epidermis. Painful on lateral compression.	Multiple treatments, including surgery using blunt dissection with scissors or curette, liquid nitrogen therapy keratolytic agents (e.g., cantharidin/salicylic acid [Cantharone Plus]), podophyllin (Podofilm), CO_2 laser destruction. Possibility of scarring.
Plantar Warts Caused by human papilloma virus (HPV).	Wart on bottom surface of foot, growing inward because of pressure of walking or standing. Painful when pressure applied. Interrupted skin markings. Cone-shaped with black dots (thrombosed vessels) when wart removed (see Figure 26.9).	Topical immunotherapy (imiquimod [Vyloma]), cryotherapy, salicylic acid, duct tape.

Infestations and Insect Bites

The possibilities for exposure to infestations (harbouring insects or worms) and insect bites are numerous (Table 26.8). In many instances, an allergy to the venom plays a major role in the reaction. In other cases, the clinical manifestations are a reaction to eggs, feces, or body parts of the invading organism. Some individuals react with a severe hypersensitivity (anaphylaxis), which can be life-threatening. (Anaphylaxis is discussed in Chapter 16).

Prevention of insect bites by avoidance or by the use of repellents is somewhat effective. Meticulous hygiene related to personal articles, clothing, bedding, and examination and care of pets, as well as careful selection of sexual partners, can reduce

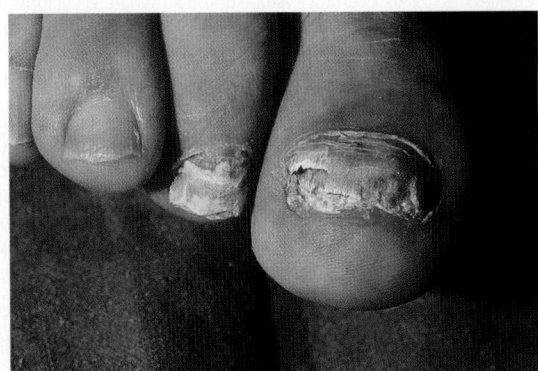

FIG. 26.10 Tinea unguium (onychomycosis). Fungal infection of toenails. Crumbly, discoloured, and thickened nails. Source: Gawkrodger, D., & Ardern-Jones, M. R. (2012). *Dermatology: An illustrated colour text* (5th ed.). Churchill Livingstone.

the incidence of infestations. Routine inspection is necessary in geographic areas where there is a risk of tick bites and Lyme disease (LD) (see Chapter 67).

ALLERGIC DERMATOLOGICAL CONDITIONS

Patients may seek treatment for irritant or allergic dermatitis, which are two types of contact dermatitis. *Irritant contact dermatitis* is produced by direct chemical injury to the skin. *Allergic contact dermatitis* is an antigen-specific, type IV delayed hypersensitivity response. This response requires sensitization and occurs only in individuals who are predisposed to react to a particular antigen. The pathophysiology related to allergic and contact dermatitis is discussed in Chapter 16. Dermatological conditions associated with allergies and hypersensitivity reactions may present a challenge to the clinician (Table 26.9). A careful family history and discussion of exposure to possible offending agents can provide valuable data. Patch testing involves the application of allergens to the patient's skin (usually on the back) for 48 hours and evaluation of the test sites for signs of reaction; this is useful in determining possible causative agents. The best treatment of allergic dermatitis is avoidance of the causative agent. The extreme pruritus (itching) of contact dermatitis and its potential for chronicity make it a frustrating problem for clinicians and patients, especially if the offending agent cannot be identified.

CUTANEOUS MEDICATION REACTIONS

Stevens Johnson syndrome (SJS) and *toxic epidermal necrolysis* (TEN) are rare, life-threatening diseases. They are violent

TABLE 26.7	COMMON FUNGAL INFECTIONS OF THE SKIN AND THE MUCOUS MEMBRANES	
Etiology and Pathophysiology	**Clinical Manifestations**	**Treatment and Prognosis**
Candidiasis Caused by *Candida albicans*; 50% of adults are symptom-free carriers. Appears in warm, moist areas such as groin area, oral mucosa, and submammary folds. Immunosuppression (e.g., from HIV infection, chemotherapy, radiation, and organ transplantation) allows yeast to become pathogenic.	*Mouth:* White, cheesy plaque, resembles milk curds. *Vagina:* Vaginitis, with red, edematous, painful vaginal wall, white patches, vaginal discharge, pruritus, and/or pain on urination and intercourse. *Skin:* Diffuse papular erythematous rash with pinpoint satellite lesions around edges of affected area.	Microscopic examination and culture. Azole antifungals (e.g., fluconazole [Diflucan], ketoconazole [Ketoderm, Nizoral]), nystatin mouthwash or other specific medication, such as vaginal suppository. Abstinence from intercourse or use of condom. Skin hygiene to keep area clean and dry. Powder is effective on nonmucosal skin surfaces to prevent reinfection.
Tinea Corporis Various dermatophytes, commonly referred to as *ringworm*.	Typical annular (ringlike), scaly appearance; well-defined margins. Erythematous.	Cool compresses. Topical antifungals for isolated patches (e.g., miconazole [Monistat], clotrimazole [Canesten], ketoconazole [Ketoderm, Nizoral]).
Tinea Cruris Various dermatophytes, commonly referred to as *jock itch*.	Well-defined, scaly plaques in groin area. Does not affect mucous membranes.	Topical antifungal cream or solution.
Tinea Pedis Various dermatophytes, commonly referred to as *athlete's foot*.	Interdigital scaling and maceration. Scaly plantar surfaces sometimes with erythema and blistering. May be pruritic or painful.	Topical antifungal cream, gel, solution, spray, or powder (e.g., tolnaftate [Tinactin], clotrimazole [Canesten]).
Tinea Unguium (Onychomycosis) Various dermatophytes. Incidence increases with age.	Toenails are more commonly affected than fingernails. Scaliness under distal nail plate. Brittle, thickened, broken, or crumbling nails with yellowish discoloration (see Figure 26.9).	Oral antifungal (terbinafine [Lamisil], itraconazole [Sporanox]). Topical antifungals (e.g., ciclopirox [Penlac], efinaconazole [Jublia]) are minimally effective but are an option if unable to tolerate systemic treatment. Thinning of toenails if needed. Nail avulsion (removal) is an option.

HIV, human immunodeficiency virus.

TABLE 26.8   COMMON INFESTATIONS AND INSECT BITES

Etiology and Pathophysiology	Clinical Manifestations	Treatment and Prognosis
Bees and Wasps Hymenoptera species.	Intense, burning, local pain. Swelling and itching. Severe hypersensitivity, may lead to anaphylaxis.	Cool compresses. Local application of antipruritic lotion. Antihistamines if indicated. Usually uneventful recovery.
Bedbugs *Cimicidae* species. Usually feed at night. Present in furniture, clothing, walls during day.	Wheal surrounded by vivid flare. Firm urticaria transforming into persistent lesion. Severe pruritus. Often grouped in threes appearing on noncovered parts of body.	Bedbug environmental treatments include steam cleaning, vacuuming, heating, freezing, washing, and disposal of items. Lesions usually require no treatment. Severe itching possibly necessitates use of antihistamines or topical corticosteroids.
Pediculosis (Head Lice, Body Lice, Pubic Lice) *Pediculus humanus,* var. *capitis; Pediculus humanus,* var. *corporis; Phthirus pubis.* Obligate parasites that suck blood, leave excrement and eggs on skin, live in seams of clothing (if body lice) and in hair as nits. Transmission of pubic lice is often by sexual contact.	Minute, red, noninflammatory. Points flush with skin. Progression to papular wheal-like lesions. Pruritus with secondary excoriation, especially parallel linear excoriations in intrascapular region. Firmly attached to hair shaft in head and body lice.	Pyrethrins (R&C Shampoo, Pronto), permethrin 1% (Nix Crème Rinse), isopropyl myristate/cyclomethicone (Resultz) to treat various parts of body. Apply as directed. Screen and treat all possible close contacts: bed partners, playmates. Do not share head gear.
Scabies *Sarcoptes scabiei.* Mite penetrates stratum corneum, deposits eggs. Allergic reaction results from presence of eggs, feces, mite parts. Transmission by direct physical contact, only occasionally by shared personal items. Rarely seen in dark-skinned people.	Severe itching, especially at night, usually not on face. Presence of burrows, especially in interdigital webs, flexor surface of wrists, genitalia, and anterior axillary folds. Erythematous papules (may be crusted), possible vesiculation, interdigital web crusting.	5% permethrin topical lotion (Kwellada-P, Nix Dermal Cream), one overnight application with second application 1 week later, may yield 95% eradication. Treat all cohabitants and sexual partners. Treat environment with plastic covering for 5 days, launder all clothes and linen with bleach. Antibiotics if secondary infections are present. Residual pruritus is possible up to 4 weeks after treatment. Recurrence is possible if inadequately treated.
Ticks *Borrelia burgdorferi* (spirochete transmitted by ticks in certain areas) causes Lyme disease. Distribution shifts yearly, but generally endemic in Nova Scotia, southern and eastern Ontario, southeast Manitoba, and southern British Columbia, with isolated occurrences in the southern part of the provinces bordering the United States.	Spreading, ringlike "bull's-eye" rash 3–4 weeks after bite (see Chapter 67, Figure 67.7). Rash commonly in groin, buttocks, axillae, trunk, and upper arms and legs. Rash may be warm, itchy, or painful. Flulike symptoms. Cardiac, arthritic, and neurological manifestations are possible. Serological and molecular assays can detect the three genospecies (*B. burgdorferi, afzelii,* and *garinii*) of Lyme disease (Alberta Health Services, 2020).	Oral antibiotics such as doxycycline. Intravenous antibiotics for arthritic, neurological, and cardiac symptoms. Rest and healthy diet. Most patients recover (see Chapter 67).

immune responses that often occur as a severe adverse reaction to either a medication or, more rarely, an infection. The result is the acute destruction of the epithelium of the skin and mucous membranes. SJS, SJS-TEN overlap, and TEN represent a spectrum of disease severity. SJS involves less than 10% of total body surface area, TEN involves more than 30% of total body surface area, and SJS-TEN overlap involves 10% to 29% of total body surface area.

SJS/TEN typically occurs 4 to 21 days after starting use of the offending medication. Systemic symptoms, including fever, cough, headache, anorexia, myalgia, and nausea, precede skin and mucous membrane findings by 1 to 3 days. Skin involvement starts as an erythematous, macular rash with purpuric centers. Over a period of hours to days, the rash merges to form blisters with sheet-like epidermal detachment. The lesions usually start on the palms, soles, and trunk, then spread to the face and extremities. They are extremely painful. Most people have mucosal lesions in the eye, mouth, and genital areas.

Identifying and stopping the offending medication(s) is the most important action in caring for a patient with SJS/TEN. The most common medications involved include sulfonamides, carbamazepine, nonsteroidal anti-inflammatory drugs (NSAIDs), lamotrigine, allopurinol, phenytoin, and phenobarbital (Habif, 2016). Immunotherapy may play a role in slowing disease progression and promoting skin repair.

The patient receives supportive care, often in a critical care unit. Interventions focus on airway management, preserving renal function, maintaining fluid and electrolyte balance, and pain control. Fluid replacement is given to maintain urine output. Proper wound care helps prevent infection and promote healing. Dressing with petrolatum gauze or other nonadhesive material provides a barrier and offers moisture to help the skin repair. Because of painful oral lesions, most patients need parenteral or enteral nutrition to meet nutrition and caloric demands. Eye drops, lubricating ointment, and antibiotic drops should be applied to those with conjunctivitis.

BENIGN DERMATOLOGICAL CONDITIONS

The list of benign skin conditions is extensive. Some of the most commonly seen and distressing conditions include psoriasis, acne vulgaris (Figure 26.11), and seborrheic keratoses. Benign conditions are summarized in Table 26.10.

TABLE 26.9 COMMON ALLERGIC CONDITIONS OF THE SKIN

Etiology and Pathophysiology	Clinical Manifestations	Treatment and Prognosis
Allergic Contact Dermatitis Type IV delayed hypersensitivity response. Absorbed agent acts as antigen. Sensitization occurs after one or more exposures. Appearance of lesions 2–7 days after contact with allergen.	Red papules and plaques, sharply circumscribed with occasional vesicles. Usually pruritic. Area of dermatitis frequently takes shape of causative agent (e.g., metal allergy and bandlike dermatitis on ring finger).	Elimination of contact allergen. Topical or systemic corticosteroids. Antihistamines. Skin lubrication.
Urticaria Usually allergic phenomenon. Erythema and edema in upper dermis resulting from a local increase in permeability of capillaries (histamine response).	Spontaneously occurring, raised or irregularly shaped wheals. Varying size; usually multiple. May occur anywhere on the body.	Removal of triggering agent, if known. Oral antihistamine. Cool compresses. Systemic corticosteroids if severe.
Medication Reaction May be caused by any medication that acts as antigen and causes hypersensitivity reaction. Certain medications (e.g., penicillin) are more prone to reactions. Not all reactions are allergic; some are intolerance (e.g., gastric upset).	Rash of any morphology. Often red, macular and papular, semiconfluent, generalized rash with abrupt onset. Appearance as late as 14 days after cessation of medication. May be pruritic. Some reactions may be life-threatening, requiring immediate and critical care.	Withdrawal of medication if possible. Antihistamines, topical or systemic corticosteroids may be necessary depending on severity of symptoms.
Atopic Dermatitis Type 1 hypersensitivity response. Genetically influenced, chronic, relapsing disease. Associated with allergic rhinitis and asthma. Usually most severe in childhood.	Multiple presentations include acute, subacute, and chronic stages. All are pruritic. Common in an antecubital and popliteal space in adults. *Acute stage* with bright erythema, oozing vesicles, with extreme pruritus. *Subacute stage* with scaly, light-red to red-brown plaques. *Chronic stage* with thickened skin and accentuation of skin markings (lichenification), possible hypo- or hyperpigmentation. Dry skin.	Lubrication of dry skin; restoration of skin barrier function. Topical immunomodulators (pimecrolimus [Elidel], tacrolimus [Protopic]). Topical corticosteroids. Phototherapy for severe inflammation and pruritus. Reduction of stress reduces flares. Antibiotics for secondary infection as needed.

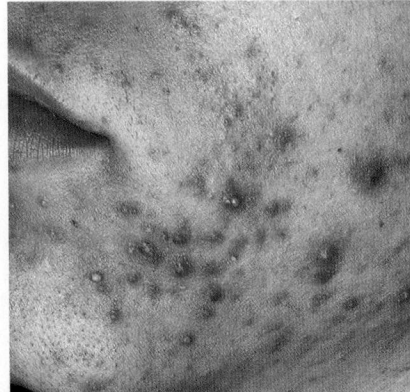

FIG. 26.11 Acne vulgaris. Papules and pustules Source: James, W. D., Berger, T., & Elston, D. (2011). *Andrews' diseases of the skin: Clinical dermatology* (11th ed.). Saunders.

Psoriasis is a common inherited benign disorder that is characterized by the eruption of reddish, silver-scaled maculopapules, predominantly on the elbows, knees, scalp, and trunk. It currently affects 1 million people in Canada (CDA, 2021c) and usually develops in individuals between 15 and 35 years old. One-third of people with psoriasis have at least one relative with the disease. Diagnosis is often based on the skin's appearance (Figure 26.12). Lesions merge to form plaques. The affected area is normally rounded, with adherent silver scales that bleed easily when removed.

While most people with psoriasis have mild disease, many with severe disease often have a weakened immune system,

diabetes mellitus, depression, or cardiovascular disease. Psoriatic arthritis affects up to 40% of all people with psoriasis (Cantrell, 2017) (Psoriatic arthritis is discussed in Chapter 67.) The chronicity of psoriasis can be severe and disabling. People may withdraw from social contacts because of visible lesions, and quality of life can diminish.

MEDICATION ALERT—Isotretinoin (Accutane)

Medication Alert

- Used to treat acne
- Can cause serious damage to fetus
- Contraindicated in women who are pregnant or could become pregnant while on the medication
- Blood donation prohibited for those taking the medication and for 1 month after treatment ends
- Linked to liver function test abnormalities

INTERPROFESSIONAL CARE: DERMATOLOGICAL CONDITIONS

Diagnostic Studies

A careful history is of prime importance in the diagnosis of skin conditions. The health care provider must be skilled at detecting evidence that could reveal the cause of a large number of skin diseases and conditions. Individual lesions must be inspected as part of the physical examination. Thorough history, physical examination, and appropriate diagnostic tests guide therapy.

Treatment

Many different treatment methods are used in dermatology. Advances in this field have brought relief to patients with

TABLE 26.10   COMMON BENIGN CONDITIONS OF THE SKIN

Etiology and Pathophysiology	Clinical Manifestations	Treatment and Prognosis
Acne Vulgaris Inflammatory disorder of sebaceous glands. More common in adolescents but possible development and persistence in adulthood. Flare can occur before menses, with use of corticosteroids, or with use of androgen-dominant oral contraceptives.	Noninflammatory lesions, including open comedones (blackheads) and closed comedones (whiteheads). Inflammatory lesions, including papules, pustules, and cysts. Most common on face, neck, and upper back. Nodular or inflammatory acne produces deeper lesions and can lead to significant scarring (see Figure 26.11).	Mechanical removal of multiple lesions with comedo extractor. Topical benzoyl peroxide, retinoids, or combination. Systemic antibiotics if severe. Aim of treatment is to suppress new lesions and minimize scarring. Spontaneous remission is possible. Use of isotretinoin (Accutane) for severe nodulocystic acne to possibly provide lasting remission (see Medication Alert box for contraindications). Pregnancy testing and monitoring of liver function, lipids, and depression is essential.
Nevi (Moles) Grouping of normal cells derived from melanocyte-like precursor cells.	Hyperpigmented areas that vary in form and colour. Flat, slightly elevated, verrucoid, dome-shaped, sessile, or papillomatous. Preservation of normal skin markings. Hair growth possible.	No treatment necessary except for cosmetic reasons. Skin biopsy for suspicious or changing nevi.
Psoriasis Autoimmune chronic dermatitis. Involves excessively rapid turnover of epidermal cells. Genetic predisposition. Usually develops before age 40.	Sharply demarcated, silvery, scaling plaques on the scalp, elbows, knees, palms, soles, and fingernails. Itching, burning, pain. Localized or general, intermittent or continuous. Symptoms vary from mild to severe (see Figure 26.12).	Goal is to reduce inflammation and suppress rapid turnover of epidermal cells. No cure, but control is possible. Topical treatments including corticosteroids, calcineurin inhibitors (tacrolimus, pimecrolimus). Intralesional injection of corticosteroids for chronic plaques. Sunlight, natural or artificial UVB, PUVA, UVA (alone or with topical or systematic potentiation [psoralen]). Systemic treatments include antimetabolites (e.g., methotrexate), immunosuppressants (e.g., cyclosporin), and biological therapies (e.g., adalimumab [Humira], etanercept [Enbrel], infliximab [Remicade], ustekinumab [Stelara]) for moderate to severe plaque form of disease.
Seborrheic Keratoses Benign, familial growths. Exact etiology is unknown. Increasing number with age; no association with sun exposure.	Irregularly round or oval, often verrucous, flat-topped papules or plaques. Well-defined shape, appearance of being "stuck on." Increase in pigmentation with time. Usually multiple. May be itchy.	Removal by curettage or cryosurgery for cosmetic reasons or to eliminate source of irritation. Biopsy if unable to differentiate from melanoma.
Acrochordons (Skin Tags) Common after midlife. Appearance on neck, axillae, and upper trunk secondary to mechanical friction or redundant skin. Correlated with obesity.	Small, skin-coloured, soft, pedunculated papules, irregularly round or oval. May become irritated.	Surgical removal for cosmetic reasons or to eliminate source of irritation only. Usually just "clipping off" with or without local anaesthesia.
Lipoma Benign tumour of adipose tissue, often encapsulated. Most common in 40- to 60-yr-old age group.	Rubbery, compressible, round mass of adipose tissue. Single or multiple. Variable in size, may be quite large. Most common on trunk, back of neck, and forearms.	Usually no treatment; biopsy to differentiate from liposarcoma; excision only when indicated.
Vitiligo Unknown cause; genetically influenced. Most noticeable in dark-skinned people and those with a tan. Complete absence of melanocytes. Noncontagious.	Focal amelanosis (complete loss of pigment). Macular. Wide variation in size and location. Usually symmetrical and may be permanent.	Topical steroids are often successful in small areas. Attempts at repigmentation of larger areas with exposure to PUVA. Depigmentation of pigmented skin with extensive disease (>50% of body involved). Cosmetics and stains to conceal vitiliginous areas.
Lentigo Increased number of normal melanocytes in basal layer of epidermis. Related to sun exposure and aging. Also called "liver spots" or "age spots."	Hyperpigmented, brown to black, flat macule or patch. Single or multiple. Typically on sun-exposed areas.	Evaluate carefully for progression. Treatment (only for cosmetic purposes) is liquid nitrogen or laser resurfacing. May recur. Biopsy if suspicious of melanoma.

PUVA, psoralen plus ultraviolet A light; *UVA*, ultraviolet A light; *UVB*, ultraviolet B light.

previously chronic, untreatable conditions. Many therapies require specialized equipment and are usually reserved for use by a dermatologist.

Phototherapy. UV light of different wavelengths may be used to treat many dermatological conditions, including psoriasis, cutaneous T-cell lymphoma, atopic dermatitis, vitiligo, and pruritus. One form of phototherapy involves the use of psoralen plus UVA light (PUVA). Psoralen is a photosensitizing medication given to patients for a prescribed amount of time before exposure to UVA.

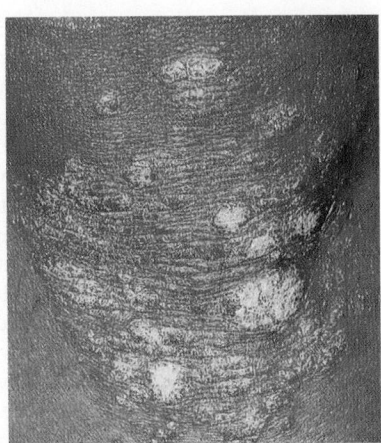

FIG. 26.12 Psoriasis. Characteristic inflammation and scaling. Source: Habif, T. P. (2011). *Clinical dermatology: A color guide to diagnosis and therapy* (5th ed.). Mosby.

TABLE 26.11	SKIN CONDITIONS TREATED BY LASER
• Acne scars	• Port wine stain
• Skin lesions	• Vascular lesions
• Hemangiomas	• Tattoo removal
• Spider veins or telangiectasias	• Rough or scarred skin
• Rosacea	• Psoriasis
• Pigmented nevi	• Wrinkles
• Hair removal	• Pigment discoloration in epidermis

Treatments are generally given two to four times a week. Adverse effects of oral psoralen include nausea and vomiting, sunburn, and persistent pruritus. Nurses should perform frequent skin assessments on all patients receiving phototherapy since erythema is an adverse effect of treatment. Topical corticosteroids may reduce painful erythema. Psoralen is used with extreme caution in patients with liver or renal disease because slower metabolism and excretion can lead to prolonged photosensitivity.

Prior to initiating phototherapy, the patient should understand the risks and benefits associated with UV exposure. Patients should be cautioned about the potential hazards of using photosensitizing chemicals and of further exposure to UV rays from sunlight or artificial UV light during therapy. Because the lens of the eye absorbs psoralen, patients receiving PUVA need prescription protective eyewear that blocks 100% of UV light to prevent cataract formation. Patients should be instructed to use the eyewear for 24 hours after taking the medication when outdoors or even when near a bright window because UVA penetrates glass. Ongoing monitoring is essential because of the immunosuppressive effects of PUVA, including an increased risk of SCC, BCC, and melanoma.

Photodynamic therapy is a special type of phototherapy used to treat actinic keratosis and some malignant skin tumours. This therapy uses a photosensitizing agent in a different way than other phototherapy treatments. The patient receives the photosensitizing agent intravenously or topically, depending on the area being treated. Time is allowed for the drug to be absorbed by the target cells, and light is then applied to the area, causing the medication to react with oxygen. This starts a reaction that kills the cells (Abrahamse & Hamblin, 2016).

Radiation Therapy. The use of radiation therapy to treat BCC and SCC varies. The best candidates are patients with lesions in challenging locations, such as the ear, nose, scalp, neck, and shin; those who may have trouble with wound healing; or those with medical comorbidities who cannot undergo surgery (Stegman, 2017). Use is limited in patients with melanoma to palliative pain control or treating brain metastases.

Radiation therapy usually requires multiple visits to a radiology department. It can produce permanent hair loss *(alopecia)* in the irradiated areas. Other adverse effects, depending on anatomical location and dose of radiation delivered, include telangiectasia, atrophy, hyperpigmentation, depigmentation, ulceration, hearing impairment, ocular damage, atrophy, and mucositis. Careful shielding is necessary to prevent ocular lens damage if the irradiated area is around the eyes. (Radiation therapy is discussed in Chapter 18).

Total-body skin irradiation (in which the body is bombarded with high-energy electrons) is one treatment for cutaneous T-cell lymphoma. Treatment follows a lengthy course. Patients experience varying degrees of hair loss and radiation dermatitis with transient loss of sweat gland function. This treatment causes premature aging of the skin.

Laser Technology. Laser treatment is an efficient surgical tool for many types of dermatological conditions (Table 26.11). Depending on the type of laser and the wavelength, lasers serve a wide variety of functions. Lasers are able to produce measurable, repeatable, consistent zones of tissue damage. They can cut, coagulate, and vaporize tissue to some degree. Laser light does not accumulate in body cells and cannot cause cumulative cellular changes or damage. With less damage to surrounding tissue, there is a decreased risk for scarring.

The surgical use of laser energy requires a focusing device to produce a small, high-density spot of energy. Several types of lasers are available. The CO_2 laser, the most common, has numerous applications as a vaporizing and cutting tool for most tissues. The argon laser emits light that is primarily absorbed by hemoglobin. It helps in the treatment of vascular and other pigmented lesions. Other, less common lasers include copper and gold vapours and neodymium: yttrium–aluminum–garnet (Nd:YAG). Written policies and procedures should cover laser safety and be reviewed by all interprofessional team members working with laser equipment.

Laser technology is increasingly being used for cosmetic treatments such as hair removal. The effectiveness of the treatment depends on a variety of factors, including choice of the correct laser equipment, training and skills of the laser operator, beam wavelength, power settings, duration of the energy pulse, and colour of the skin or hair. The patient must be informed about the risks of laser treatments, which include pain; reddened, bruised, and swollen skin; burns; infection; and temporary scarring and skin discoloration (CDA, 2021a).

Medication Therapy

Antibiotics. Antibiotics are used both topically and systemically to treat dermatological conditions, and they are often used in combination. If used, topical antibiotics should be applied lightly in a thin film to clean skin. The most common OTC topical antibiotics are polymyxin B sulphate–neomycin sulphate and bacitracin zinc (Polysporin). Prescription topical antibiotics include mupirocin (Bactroban; used for superficial *Staphylococcus* such as impetigo) and erythromycin (used for Gram-positive cocci [staphylococci and streptococci] and Gram-negative cocci and bacilli). Topical metronidazole (Metrogel, Flagyl) is used to treat rosacea and bacterial vaginosis. Though used historically, topical antibiotics such as clindamycin (Clindoxyl, Benzaclin) are now rarely recommended for the treatment of acne vulgaris because of ineffectiveness and concerns about antibiotic resistance (Asai et al., 2016).

If there are manifestations of systemic infection, a systemic antibiotic should be used. They have a role in treating bacterial infections, such as erysipelas, cellulitis, abscesses, and certain wound infections. They are also indicated in the treatment of severe or treatment-resistant acne vulgaris (Asai et al., 2016). Culture and sensitivity of the lesion can guide the choice of antibiotic. The most frequently used are cephalexin (Keflex), clindamycin, erythromycin (Eryc), minocycline, and doxycycline (Apprilon, Doxycin). These medications are particularly useful for erysipelas, cellulitis, carbuncles, and severe, infected eczema (see Chapter 16). Patients require medication-specific instructions on the proper technique of taking or applying antibiotics.

Corticosteroids. Corticosteroids are particularly effective in treating a wide variety of dermatological conditions and can be used topically, intralesionally, or systemically. Topical corticosteroids are used for their local anti-inflammatory action as well as for their antipruritic effects. Attempts to diagnose a lesion should be made before a corticosteroid preparation is applied because corticosteroids may alter the clinical manifestations. Once a sufficient amount of medication is dispensed, limits should be set on the duration and frequency of application.

The potency of a particular preparation is related to the concentration of active drug in the preparation. With prolonged use, the more potent corticosteroid formulations can cause adrenal suppression, especially if a large surface area is covered and occlusive dressings are used. High-potency corticosteroids may produce adverse effects when their use is prolonged, including atrophy of the skin resulting from impaired cell mitosis and capillary fragility and susceptibility to bruising. Other adverse effects include rosacea eruptions, severe exacerbations of acne vulgaris, and dermatophyte infections. In general, dermal and epidermal atrophy does not occur until a corticosteroid has been used for 2 to 3 weeks. If medication use is discontinued at the first sign of atrophy, recovery usually occurs in several weeks. Rebound dermatitis is not uncommon when therapy is stopped; this can be reduced by tapering the use of high-potency topical corticosteroids when the patient improves.

Low-potency corticosteroids such as hydrocortisone act more slowly but can be used for a longer period without producing serious adverse effects. Low-potency corticosteroids are safe to use on the face and intertriginous areas, such as the axillae and groin. The most potent delivery system for a topical corticosteroid is an ointment form. Creams and ointments are applied in thin layers and slowly massaged into the site one to three times a day. Accurate and adequate topical therapy is often the key to a successful outcome.

Intralesional corticosteroids are injected directly into or just beneath the lesion. This method provides a reservoir of medication with an effect lasting several weeks to months. Intralesional injection is commonly used in the treatment of psoriasis, alopecia areata (patchy hair loss), hypertrophic scars, and keloids. Triamcinolone acetonide (Kenalog) is the most common medication used for intralesional injection.

Systemic corticosteroids can have remarkable results in the treatment of dermatological conditions. However, they often have undesirable systemic effects (see Chapter 51). Corticosteroids can be administered as short-term therapy for acute conditions such as contact dermatitis caused by poison ivy. Long-term corticosteroid therapy for dermatological conditions is reserved for chronic bullous (blistering) disorders.

Antihistamines. Oral antihistamines are helpful in treating urticaria, angioedema, and pruritus that can occur with conditions such as atopic dermatitis, contact dermatitis, and other allergic cutaneous reactions. Antihistamines compete with histamine for the receptor site, thus preventing its effects. Antihistamines may have anticholinergic or sedative effects or both. Several different antihistamines may have to be tried before the satisfactory therapeutic effect is achieved. Sedating antihistamines such as hydroxyzine hydrochloride and diphenhydramine (Benadryl) are often preferred for pruritus because the tranquilizing and sedative effects offer symptomatic relief. The patient should be warned about sedative effects, a particular problem when driving or operating heavy machinery. Antihistamines such as fexofenadine (Allegra), cetirizine (Reactine), and loratadine (Claritin) bind to peripheral histamine receptors, providing antihistamine action without sedation. These nonsedating antihistamines are generally not effective for controlling pruritus. Antihistamines should be used with caution in older people because of the medications' long half-life and their anticholinergic effects.

Topical Fluorouracil. Fluorouracil (Efudex) is a topical cytotoxic agent with selective toxicity for sun-damaged cells. It is used for the treatment of premalignant (especially actinic keratosis) and some malignant skin diseases. Because systemic absorption of the drug is minimal, systemic adverse effects are virtually nonexistent. Patient adherence can be a challenge because fluorouracil causes erythema and pruritus within 3 to 5 days and painful, eroded areas over the damaged skin within 1 to 3 weeks, depending on skin thickness at the site. Treatment must continue with applications one to two times a day for 2 to 4 weeks. Healing may take up to 4 weeks after medication is stopped (Luger et al., 2017). Low-potency topical steroids are often prescribed and can increase patient adherence to therapy and can be applied 20 minutes after fluorouracil application. Because fluorouracil is a photosensitizing medication, the patient must be educated to avoid sunlight during treatment. Patients should also be informed of the effect of the medication, including a warning that they will look worse before they look better. Adherence depends on thoroughness of the instruction, which should include a written handout. After effective treatment, treated skin is smooth and free of actinic keratosis. Recurrence in treated areas is possible, and multiple courses of therapy may be necessary over the years for individuals with severely sun-damaged skin.

Immunomodulators. Topical immunomodulators, such as pimecrolimus (Elidel) and tacrolimus (Protopic), are used to treat atopic dermatitis, psoriasis, and rosacea (Luger et al., 2017). They work by suppressing an overreactive immune system. The adverse effects are minimal and may include a transient burning or feeling of heat at the application site. An increased risk of skin cancer and precancerous lesions may be associated with long-term use of these medications.

The topical immunomodulator imiquimod (Aldara P) is used to treat external genital warts, AK, and superficial BCC. It stimulates the production of α-interferon and other cytokines to enhance cell-mediated immunity. It boosts the immune response only where applied and is safe for transplant patients.

Most patients using this cream experience skin reactions, including redness, swelling, blistering, peeling, itching, and burning. Dosing varies depending on the type of lesion treated and the strength of medication prescribed (Habif, 2016).

Diagnostic and Surgical Therapy

Skin Scraping. Scraping is done with a scalpel blade to obtain a sample of surface cells (stratum corneum) for microscopic inspection and diagnosis. The most common tests of skin scrapings are KOH for fungus and mineral oil examination for scabies.

Electrodesiccation and Electrocoagulation. Electrical energy can be converted to heat by the tip of an electrode. The heat burns and destroys tissue. The major uses of this type of therapy are point coagulation of bleeding vessels to obtain hemostasis and destruction of small *telangiectasias* (dilation of groups of superficial capillaries and venules). *Electrodesiccation* uses a monopolar electrode and usually involves more superficial destruction. *Electrocoagulation* uses a dipolar electrode and has a deeper effect, with better hemostasis but an increased possibility of scarring. While minor electrosurgery on patients with a pacemaker poses minimal risk, the electrical energy can affect both pacemakers and internal defibrillators.

Curettage. Curettage is the removal and scooping away of tissue using an instrument called a *curette*. A curette looks like a small spoon with very sharp edges. Although a curette is not usually strong enough to cut normal skin, it can remove many types of small, soft skin tumours and superficial lesions, such as warts, AK, seborrheic keratosis, and small BCCs and SCCs. The area to be curetted is anaesthetized before the procedure. The health care provider removes the lesion and then cauterizes the skin. The removed tissue is usually sent for biopsy. A dressing may be applied, and the nurse needs to teach the patient wound care. A small scar and hypopigmentation can result.

Punch Biopsy. Punch biopsy is a common procedure used to obtain a tissue sample for histological study or to remove small lesions (Figure 26.13). The procedure is simple. The health care provider marks the biopsy area and then anaesthetizes it so that the anaesthetic will not obscure the landmarks. The health care provider then rotates the punch into the skin and removes a small cylinder of skin. The core of skin is snipped from the subcutaneous fat and appropriately preserved for examination in a fixative solution. Hemostasis is achieved with pressure or absorbable gelatin (Gelfoam) packing. Sites of 4 mm or larger are usually closed with sutures. Punch biopsies are not done below the knee if other sites are available. Circulatory changes can make evaluating the tissue sample more difficult.

Cryosurgery. Cryosurgery is the use of subfreezing temperatures to destroy epidermal lesions. Cryosurgery is a useful treatment for common benign, precancerous conditions including common and genital warts, cutaneous tags, thin seborrheic keratoses, lentigines, actinic keratoses, BCC, and SCC. Topical liquid nitrogen is the agent most commonly used for cryosurgery (Stegman, 2017). Damage occurs in treated tissue because of intracellular ice formation. It causes the cell to rupture during thaw, leading to cell death and necrosis. The degree of damage depends on the rate of cooling and the minimum temperature achieved.

Liquid nitrogen can be applied topically (directly onto the lesion) with a direct spray or cotton-tipped applicator. Patients usually feel a stinging cold sensation. The lesion will first become swollen and red, and it may blister. A scab forms and

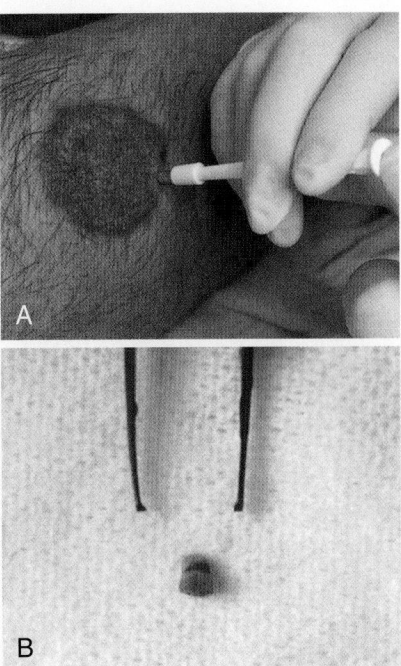

FIG. 26.13 Punch biopsy. **A,** Removal of skin for diagnostic purposes. **B,** Specimen obtained. Source: Graham-Brown, R., Bourke, J., & Cunliffe, T. (2008). *Dermatology: Fundamentals of practice.* Mosby.

falls off in 1 to 3 weeks. The skin lesion is sloughed off along with the scab. Growth of new skin follows. The low temperature of the liquid nitrogen easily destroys melanocytes, leaving an area of hypopigmentation resembling a scar in lighter skinned individuals and hyperpigmentation in darker skinned individuals (Prohaska & Badri, 2020). The size of the area to be treated may limit the use of cryotherapy. Other disadvantages of this treatment are lack of a tissue specimen for histological confirmation of cell type before destruction and potential for destruction of adjacent healthy tissue.

Excision. Excision is an option if the lesion involves the dermis. Complete closure of the excised area usually results in a good cosmetic outcome. One type of excision is *Mohs surgery* (Figure 26.14), which is a microscopically controlled removal of a skin cancer. In this procedure, the health care provider removes tissue sections in thin horizontal layers. All of the specimen's margins are examined to determine whether any malignant cells remain. Any residual tumour not removed by the first surgical excision is removed in serial excisions performed the same day. Benefits of Mohs surgery are preserving normal tissue, producing the smallest possible wound, and completely removing the cancer before surgical closure. Although this can become a lengthy procedure, it is done in an outpatient setting using local anaesthesia.

NURSING MANAGEMENT
DERMATOLOGICAL CONDITIONS

AMBULATORY AND HOME CARE

Dermatological conditions are not usually a primary reason for hospitalization. Nevertheless, many hospitalized patients will exhibit concurrent skin conditions that warrant nursing intervention and patient education. Nursing interventions related to dermatological conditions fall into broad categories. They are

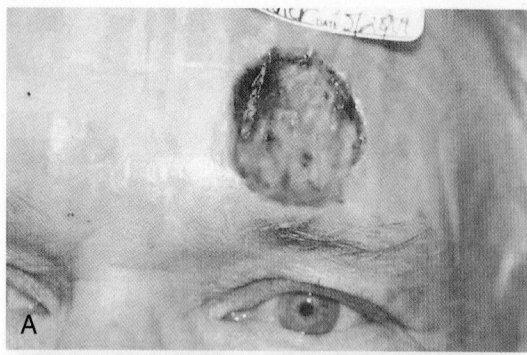
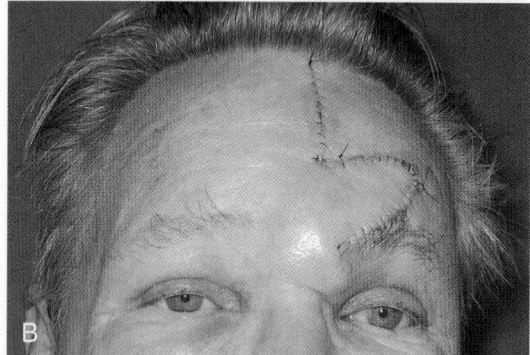

FIG. 26.14 A, Removal of melanoma by Mohs surgery. **B,** Following plastic surgery using a skin flap to repair defect. Source: Courtesy Peter Bonner.

Agent	Therapeutic Considerations
Powder	Promotion of dryness. Lubrication of skinfold areas to prevent irritation. Common base for antifungal preparations. Patient must be protected from inhalation.
Lotion	Oil, alcohol, and water emulsions. Cooling and drying effect, with residual powder film after evaporation of water. Useful in subacute pruritic eruptions.
Cream	Oil and water emulsions. Most common base for topical medications. Affords lubrication and protection.
Ointment	Oil with differing amounts of water added in suspension. Lubrication and prevention of dehydration. Petrolatum most common. Preferred for delivering high-potency medication.
Paste	Mixture of powder and ointment. Useful when drying effect necessary because moisture is absorbed.
Gel	Nongreasy combination of propylene glycol and water. May contain alcohol. Used for acute exudative inflammation (e.g., poison ivy contact dermatitis).

TABLE 26.12   MEDICATION THERAPY
Common Bases for Topical Medications

applicable to many skin conditions in both inpatient and outpatient settings. A nursing care plan for the patient with chronic skin lesions is available on the Evolve website.

Wet Dressings. For superficial skin conditions that involve inflammation, itching, and infection, wet compresses (dressings) are commonly used. They are appropriate for damaged, oozing skin. Wet compresses are an excellent way to remove crusts and scabs that are adhering to the wound surface. Wet compresses provide comfort and treatment of conditions such as poison ivy, insect bites, and skin infections.

It is important to understand how to do a wet dressing correctly. Unless there is a concern about water quality, tap water at room temperature is the best choice. If drinkable water is not available, filtered, bottled, or sterile water may be used. Depending on the skin concern, additives may be used. Common solutions include (1) saline, (2) Burow's solution (Domeboro powder [aluminum acetate; calcium acetate]), (3) acetic acid (vinegar), and (4) silver nitrate (Habif, 2016). Close attention to appropriate concentrations is critical when additives are used. Wet compresses should generally be tepid (lukewarm). However, when an anti-inflammatory effect is desired, the wet dressing should be cool.

The material for wet compresses should be four to eight layers thick and slightly larger than the area being treated. Gauze or any clean material (e.g., thin cotton sheeting, thermal underwear, tube socks) may be used. Ingenuity is sometimes required when covering odd-shaped body parts. Gauze sponges with fillers (abdominal pads) should be avoided for this purpose because they will retain too much solution, and fibres can be left in the wound if the skin is open. Compress material is placed into fresh solution and excess liquid squeezed out. The goal is a *wet* compress—not simply damp and not dripping.

Wet compresses are applied continuously or intermittently. When used continuously, new solution should be used as needed but no additional solution added since doing so can alter the concentration and damage the skin. Depending on the desired effect, intermittent compresses are placed for 10 to 30 minutes two to four times a day, always using clean materials. Careful monitoring of the skin is important. If the skin appears *macerated* (softens and turns white), the dressings should be discontinued for 2 to 3 days. The patient should be protected from discomfort and chilling. A water-resistant pad will help protect the mattress, linens, and furniture.

Baths. Baths are appropriate when large body areas need to be treated. They also have sedative and antipruritic effects. Some medications, such as colloidal oatmeal (Aveeno) and sodium bicarbonate, can be added directly to the bath water. The tub should be filled enough to cover affected areas. Both the bath water and the prescribed solution should be a tepid temperature. The patient can soak for 15 to 20 minutes three or four times a day, depending on the severity of the dermatitis and the patient's discomfort. It is important to stress to the patient that the skin must not be rubbed dry with a towel but gently patted to prevent increasing irritation and inflammation. Adding oils increases the risk for falls and should thus be avoided. To sustain the hydrating effect, cream, ointment emollients (moisturizers), or other prescribed topical agents are applied after the bath. This helps seal the moisture in the hydrated cells and increases the absorption of any topical agents.

Topical Medications. Topical medications are commonly used to treat cutaneous conditions. The effectiveness of topical therapy depends on which base the medication is prepared in. Table 26.12 summarizes the common agents used as bases for topical preparations and their therapeutic considerations. The base selected depends on the properties needed.

Creams are very versatile and most commonly prescribed. Ointments are more lubricating than creams and offer enhanced potency of the active ingredient. They may be too occlusive for conditions with high levels of exudate or in body creases. Gels work well on the scalp, where other compounds may mat the hair, and for acute exudative conditions such as poison ivy. Lotions can be a mix of water, alcohols, and oils. They are also appropriate for the scalp but may cause stinging and drying when used in skinfolds. Pastes are a compound of 50% or more powder in an ointment base. They are good for protecting the skin but are messy. A limited number of foams are available.

Some of these medications are very costly. Proper administration, as directed, will yield best results, maintain consistency, and avoid waste. As a general rule, topical medication should be applied in a thin film to clean skin and spread evenly in a downward motion in the direction of hair growth, using a gloved hand. Thick creams will spread more easily if the skin is still damp. If a secondary dressing is going to be used, the medication may be applied directly onto a dressing. The patient and caregiver will need to be taught proper dosing, application technique, anticipated results, and common reactions. Patients and caregivers should be reminded to wash their hands with soap and water after applying topical medications at home.

Occlusion with a plastic wrap is an effective way of increasing the absorption of topical corticosteroids or simple emollients. The plastic wrap traps perspiration against the outer layer of the epidermis. Applying preparations to moist skin increases absorption 10-fold. Tape or stretch wraps can keep the plastic wrap in place. For conditions on the feet or lower legs, socks can be worn over the plastic wrap. Wraps applied multiple times daily are kept in place for 2 to 8 hours. Some patients choose to use the occlusion technique at bedtime. Occlusion is recommended with discretion because it is not appropriate in areas prone to infection, such as skin creases, or when high-potency corticosteroids or antibiotics are used.

Control of Pruritus. Many conditions cause *pruritus,* including dry skin, almost any physical or chemical stimulus to the skin (such as drugs or insects), and any scaling skin disorder. The itch sensation is carried by the same nonmyelinated nerve fibres as pain and temperature. The patient will have pain rather than an itch if the epidermis is damaged or absent. It is important to assess whether itching preceded a skin lesion. Itching can lead to scratching that results in an excoriated and inflamed lesion.

The itch/scratch cycle must be broken to prevent excoriation and lichenification. Control of pruritus is also important because it is difficult to diagnose a lesion that is excoriated and inflamed. Certain circumstances make itching worse. Anything that causes vasodilation, such as heat or rubbing, should be avoided. Dryness of the skin lowers the itch threshold and increases the itch sensation.

There are several approaches to help break the itch/scratch cycle. A cool environment may cause vasoconstriction and decrease itching. Hydration, wet compresses, and moisturizers (including antipruritic lotions) are normally helpful. Topical and injectable corticosteroids are occasionally ordered. Topically applied menthol, camphor, or phenol can be used to numb the itch receptors. Systemic antihistamines may provide relief while the underlying cause of the pruritus is being diagnosed and treated. The principal adverse effect of most antihistamines is sedation, although this effect may be desirable because pruritus is often worse at night and can interfere with sleep.

Lichenification is a thickening of epidermis with exaggerated markings resembling a washboard. It is caused by chronic scratching or rubbing of the skin. Lichenification is often associated with atopic dermatoses and other pruritic conditions. Although any area of the body may be affected, the hands, forearms, shins, and nape of the neck are common sites. Itching may become habitual. The persistent scratching can cause excoriations. Treating the cause of the itching is the key to preventing lichenification.

Prevention of Spread. Although most skin conditions are not contagious, infection control precautions indicate wearing gloves when working with any open wounds or lesions with drainage. Procedures should be explained to avoid discouraging patients who may be sensitive about skin lesions. Careful hand hygiene and proper disposal of soiled dressings are the best means of preventing the spread of infections or infestations. The most common contagious lesions include impetigo, streptococcal infections, staphylococcal infections (e.g., MRSA), fungal infections, primary chancre, scabies, and pediculosis.

Prevention of Secondary Infections. Open skin lesions are susceptible to invasion by other viral, bacterial, or fungal organisms. Meticulous hygiene, hand hygiene, and dressing changes are important to minimize potential for secondary infections. Patients should be warned against scratching lesions, which can cause excoriations and create a portal of entry for pathogens. The patient's nails should be kept short to minimize trauma from scratching.

Prevention of Pressure Injuries. Prevention and treatment of pressure injuries is an important nursing role, particularly when caring for the hospitalized patient. Pressure injuries tend to develop over boney prominences and where skin and underlying tissue is in prolonged contact with a weight-bearing surface such as a bed or chair. Risk factors include increased moisture, decreased sensation, decreased activity and mobility, poor nutritional status, and friction and shear (see Chapter 14, Table 14.14, for the Braden Scale for Predicting Pressure Sore Risk). Sites where devices (e.g., nasal prongs, masks, intravenous lines, feeding tubes) are in prolonged contact with skin also present risk for pressure injuries. Health care and other essential workers using personal protective equipment such as masks for prolonged periods may experience pressure injuries, often on the face or ears (Desai et al., 2020). Older patients are at particular risk for pressure injury and skin tears due to age-related changes to the skin such as thinning, loss of elasticity, and decreased subcutaneous fat. A variety of devices and care strategies may be used to reduce risk of developing these injuries including offloading, frequent repositioning, and use of skin barriers. If these injuries do occur, the patient is at risk for secondary infection, pain, and loss of function. Wound care and management of these injuries may involve a variety of approaches depending on level of injury and may be complex and prolonged (see Chapter 14).

Specific Skin Care. Nurses are often in a position to advise patients regarding skin care following simple surgical procedures such as skin biopsy, excision, and cryosurgery. Patient follow-up should be individualized. In general, instructions include dressing changes, use of topical medications, and the signs and symptoms of infection. After a dermatological procedure, any oozing wound should be cleansed twice a day with a saline solution or as ordered by the health care provider. Soap and potable (safe for drinking) water can be used to clean a non-oozing wound. An antibiotic ointment or plain petroleum jelly may then be applied with a dressing that is both absorbent and nonadherent.

Wounds that are kept moist and covered heal more rapidly and with less scarring. The initial crust that forms should be left undisturbed as a protective coating for the damaged skin beneath. Healing crusts that have been moisturized and protected will separate naturally from healed epidermis.

A sutured wound may be covered with a variety of dressings. Sutures are generally removed within 4 to 14 days depending on the site. Sometimes alternating sutures are removed after the third day. Incision lines may require daily cleansing, usually with plain tap water. If necessary, a topical antibiotic is applied and the wound either covered with a dry sterile dressing or left open to air. The patient may experience some swelling and discomfort in the first 24 hours during the first phase of wound healing. Intermittent application of cold (ice packs) over the surgical dressing may reduce edema and promote comfort. Mild analgesics such as acetaminophen or a nonsteroidal anti-inflammatory medication should control discomfort. The nurse should instruct the patient on how to differentiate normal inflammation from an infection. A slight red border during the first few days after a procedure is normal inflammation. Redness that persists longer than a week or extends beyond a 1-cm border, a temperature above 38°C, increased pain, pronounced swelling, and purulent drainage are all signs and symptoms of a possible infection. If these occur, they should be promptly reported to the health care provider.

PSYCHOLOGICAL EFFECTS OF CHRONIC DERMATOLOGICAL CONDITIONS

Emotional stress can occur for people who suffer from chronic skin conditions such as psoriasis, atopic dermatitis, or acne. The sequelae of chronic skin conditions can include social and employment problems with subsequent financial implications, a poor self-image, challenges with sexuality, and increasing and progressive frustration. The usual lack of overt systemic illness coupled with the visibility of the skin lesions often presents a real problem to the patient.

Nurses are positioned to help the patient remain optimistic and adhere to the prescribed regimen. The patient must be allowed to verbalize the "Why me?" question, even though there is no ready answer. Dermatology patient support groups are listed on the CDA website (see the Resources at the end of this chapter). These groups are extremely helpful in providing patient support and accurate educational materials.

The location of lesions and scars is the determining factor with respect to cosmetic implications. Facial scars are the most damaging psychologically because they are so visible.

Creative use of cosmetics can do much to mask lesions and scarring. Individual sensitivity to product ingredients must be considered when selecting cosmetics. Oil-free, hypoallergenic cosmetics are available and may be beneficial for the allergic patient. Rehabilitative cosmetics are available to help camouflage and de-emphasize such lesions as *vitiligo* (loss of pigmentation), *melasma* (tan to brown patches on the face), and healed postoperative wound sites. These commercially available products are opaque, smudge resistant, and water resistant.

PHYSIOLOGICAL EFFECTS OF CHRONIC DERMATOLOGICAL CONDITIONS

Scarring and lichenification are the result of chronic dermatological conditions. Scars occur when ulceration takes place and reflect the pattern of healing in the area. Scars are pink and vascular at first. With time, in lighter-skinned people, they become avascular and white, and in individuals with darker skin, they may become hyperpigmented. Different regions of the body scar differently, such as the face and neck, which heal fairly well because they are well vascularized. Scar formation is described in Chapter 14.

COSMETIC PROCEDURES

A vast array of cosmetic procedures is available, including chemical peels, toxin injections, collagen fillers, laser surgery, breast augmentation and reduction (see Chapter 54), laser surgery, facelift, eyelid lift, and liposuction. Common cosmetic topical procedures are presented in Table 26.13. Other types of common cosmetic injection procedures include the injection of botulinum toxins (Botox), collagenase (Xiaflex), deoxycholic acid (Belkyra), and hyaluronic acid fillers (Costa et al., 2016). Transitory adverse effects such as mild redness, pain, swelling, and bruising may occur.

The reasons for undergoing these procedures are as varied as the techniques. The most common reason that people suffer

---

TABLE 26.13   COMMON COSMETIC TOPICAL PROCEDURES

Procedure	Indications	Description	Adverse Effects	Patient Teaching
Tretinoin (Retin-A)	Improves appearance of photodamaged skin, especially fine wrinkling. Reduces actinic keratosis.	Applied initially every other day, nightly as tolerated. Treatment stopped if inflammation is severe. Maximum response in 8–12 mo.	Erythema, swelling, flaking, photosensitivity, pigmentation changes. Teratogenic. Increases phototoxicity if also taking other photosensitive medications (see Table 26.2).	Apply at night as light causes photodegradation. Sunscreen (SPF 30 or higher), sun-avoidance measures. Avoid use of abrasive or drying facial cleanser if severe sensitivity.
Chemical peels	Improves appearance of aged and photodamaged skin, acne scarring, freckles, actinic and seborrheic keratoses.	Solution applied in varying amounts to the skin, causing a controlled burn. Loss of melanin occurs.	Moderate swelling and crusting for 1 wk. Redness persisting 6–8 wk. Pink tone possible for several months. Photosensitivity.	Use sunscreen; avoid sun for 6 mo to prevent hyperpigmentation.
Microdermabrasion	Smooths appearance of photodamaged and wrinkled skin, acne scarring.	Removal of the epidermis and top dermal layer by application of aluminum oxide or baking soda crystals. Re-epithelialization of abraded surface then occurs.	Light pink tone that resolves within 24 hr. Photosensitivity.	Generous application of emollients and sunscreen
Alpha-hydroxy acids (e.g., glycolic acid, lactic acid)	Smooths appearance of photodamaged and wrinkled skin, acne scarring.	Low concentrations (<10%) found in many skin care products that patients can self-administer. Higher concentrations (50%–70%) given only by a health care provider.	Photosensitivity, irritation at lower concentrations. Severe redness, oozing, and flaking skin possible with higher concentrations.	Sunscreen and sun avoidance.

SPF, sun protection factor.

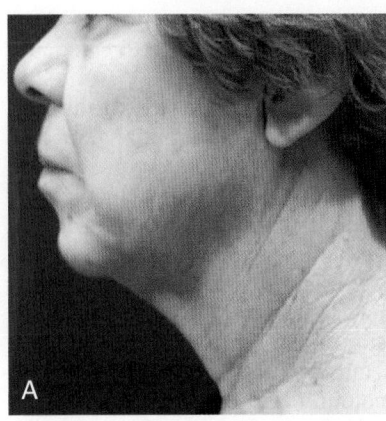 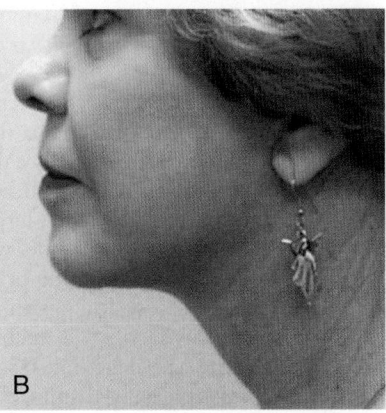

FIG. 26.15 Facelift. **A,** Preoperative. **B,** Postoperative. Source: Cuzalina A., Copty T. V., & Khan, H. (2012). *Current therapy in oral and maxillofacial surgery.* Elsevier.

the discomfort and financial expense (most are not covered by insurance) of a cosmetic procedure is to improve their body image. Many believe that if patients feel better about themselves after having cosmetic procedures, they will often act more confident and self-assured. Often social position and economic considerations are part of the decision. Critics of cosmetic procedures argue that they feed unrealistic societal expectations of maintaining youthful appearance indefinitely. There is no doubt that increased longevity is fueling demand for and popularity of such procedures.

Regardless of the patient's reasons, the nurse should maintain a supportive, nonjudgemental attitude about these cosmetic procedures. If the patient wishes to change or enhance a body feature perceived as unattractive and has realistic expectations about the outcome, it is reasonable to support this decision.

Body Art and Tattoos

Body art through tattoos and skin piercings is a popular means of self-expression. A *tattoo* is a permanent design that is made by injecting dyes into the skin's epidermal layer (Chalmers et al., 2019). Patients should ensure that tattoo and piercing establishments are certified through the local public health unit and that artists use new, sterile equipment and good hand hygiene and gloves. These measures minimize the risk of contracting a bloodborne disease (e.g., human immunodeficiency virus [HIV], hepatitis C) or skin infection. Tattoo dye contains metal, so a magnetic resonance imaging (MRI) scan may be contraindicated over a tattooed site. Patients should be educated on how to care for tattoos and piercings at home in order to minimize infection risk. The nurse should instruct patients to wash their hands thoroughly before applying lotions or ointments to the tattooed or pierced area and before rotating jewellery and teach them to watch for signs of infection (severe pain, swelling, pus, redness, or heat) and allergic reactions. Oral piercings require specific care, including careful mouth hygiene and use of a mouth guard when playing sports.

Tattooing, piercing, and other forms of body art play an important role in some Indigenous cultures. Historically, these were used to communicate family and clan identity, social rank, territorial affiliation, and hunting and fishing rights and were perceived as a kind of "permanent regalia" (Gilpin, 2018). While these practices were often forbidden and silenced as part of colonial suppression of Indigenous identity, traditional tattoos and piercings are seeing a resurgence in Indigenous

communities across Canada (Allford, 2019; Gilpin, 2018). Traditional tattoo practitioners use a variety of techniques, including skin-stitching, hand-poke, and brush and blade tattoos (Gilpin, 2018). Affirming these practices may support patients in fostering an enhanced sense of identity, belonging, and self-worth.

Elective Surgery

Laser Surgery. Laser surgery is used to treat congenital and acquired vascular lesions (cherry angiomas, spider leg veins, hemangiomas, port wine stains, and tattoo removal) and for skin resurfacing and hair removal. Lasers can reduce scarring and fine wrinkles around the lips or eyes and remove facial lesions (see Table 26.11). Swelling, redness, and bruising are common after treatment. The treated areas usually are kept moist with ointment or occlusive dressings for the first few days. The patient must protect treated skin from the sun.

Facelift. A facelift *(rhytidectomy)* is the lifting and repositioning of the lower two-thirds of the face and neck to improve appearance (Figure 26.15). Indications for this procedure include the following:

1. Redundant soft tissue resulting from disease (e.g., acne scarring)
2. Asymmetrical redundancy of soft tissues (e.g., facial palsy)
3. Redundant soft tissue resulting from trauma
4. Preauricular lesions
5. Redundant soft tissues resulting from solar elastosis (sagging of the skin as a result of sun damage), changes in body weight, and the effects of gravity
6. Restoration of body image

The surgical approach and the lines of incisions vary according to the nature of the deformity and the position of the hairline. Eyelid lifts *(blepharoplasty)* with similar indications are performed to remove redundant tissue and possibly improve the field of vision. Preventing hematoma formation is the most important postoperative consideration. Ice packs are usually applied during the first 24 to 48 hours to reduce swelling and decrease the possibility of hematoma formation. Usually pain is minimal. Antibiotics are used at the surgeon's discretion. Infection is not a common concern. Complications can occur if the person smokes or is involved in vigorous exercise.

Liposuction. *Liposuction* is a technique for removing subcutaneous fat to improve facial and body contours. Although not a substitute for diet and exercise, it can be successful in removing areas of fat from virtually any body area that is resistant to other techniques.

Liposuction is relatively free of complications. Possible contraindications include use of anticoagulants, uncontrolled hypertension, diabetes mellitus, and poor cardiovascular status. People younger than 40 years of age with good skin elasticity are the best candidates, but those over 40 can be treated successfully.

The procedure is usually performed on an outpatient basis under local anaesthesia. One or more sessions may be necessary, depending on the size of the area to be treated. A blunt-tipped cannula is inserted through a small incision and pushed into the fat to break it loose from the fibrous stroma. Multiple repeated thrusts disrupt the fat and create tunnels. The loosened fat is removed with a powerful suction. Afterwards, firm pressure is applied to the wounds, until drainage stops (Chia et al., 2017). It may take several months for the results to be evident.

NURSING MANAGEMENT
COSMETIC SURGERY

Many cosmetic surgical procedures are performed in well-equipped day-surgery units or in office surgery suites. Nursing interventions are important, regardless of where the surgery was done.

PREOPERATIVE MANAGEMENT

A major preoperative management consideration involves informed consent and realistic expectations of what cosmetic surgery can accomplish. Although this information is usually provided by the surgeon, the nurse should reinforce this information and answer questions and concerns. For instance, a facelift has little or no effect on deep wrinkling of the forehead and temples, deep nasolabial grooves, or vertical lip wrinkles. Before- and after-treatment photographs of similar cases are often useful in helping the patient to set realistic expectations.

The nurse's teaching plan should include the time frame for healing. The oozing, crusting stage of the abrasive procedure must be explained so the patient can plan time off from work if necessary. Since the third phase of wound healing does not become complete for 1 year, the patient should not anticipate complete results immediately. The final results of the cosmetic procedure are affected by the patient's age, general state of health, extent of procedure, and skin type. Efforts should be made to correct or control any existing health problems before the procedure.

POSTOPERATIVE MANAGEMENT

Most cosmetic procedures are not extremely painful. Usually, mild analgesics are sufficient to keep the patient comfortable. Although infection is not a common concern after cosmetic surgery, the nurse should assess surgical sites for signs of infection. The patient should be educated on signs of infection and know to report any such signs and symptoms immediately so that appropriate intervention can be started.

If the surgery involved a change in the skin's circulation (e.g., face-lift), the nurse needs to carefully monitor for adequate circulation. Warm, pink skin that blanches on pressure shows that adequate circulation is present in the surgical area. Supportive, compressive dressings and ice packs may be necessary early in the postoperative period.

SKIN GRAFTS
Uses

Skin grafts may be necessary to provide protection to underlying structures or to reconstruct areas for functional or cosmetic purposes. They may be used to facilitate rapid closure and minimize complications. Ideally, wounds heal by primary intention. However, large wounds, surgically created wounds, trauma, and chronic wounds can result in extensive tissue destruction, making primary-intention healing impossible. In these cases, skin grafting may be necessary to close the defect. Improved surgical techniques make it possible to graft skin, bone, cartilage, fat, fascia, muscles, and nerves. For cosmetically pleasing results, the colour, thickness, texture, and hair-growing nature of skin used for grafting should match the recipient site. (See Chapter 27 for further discussion of skin grafting.)

Types

The two types of skin grafts are *free grafts* and *skin flaps*. Free grafts are further classified according to the method of providing a blood supply to the grafted skin. One method is to transfer the graft (epidermis and part or all of the dermis) to the recipient site from the donor site. If the graft is an *autograft* (from the patient's own body) or an *isograft* (from an identical twin), it will revascularize and become fixed to the new site. Chapter 27 discusses full- and split-thickness skin grafts in detail. Another method of free skin grafting is by *reconstructive microsurgery*. With the use of an operating microscope, the health care provider establishes circulation immediately in the graft by connecting blood vessels in the skin flap to vessels in the recipient site.

Skin flaps involve moving a section of skin and subcutaneous tissue from one part of the body to another without terminating the vascular attachment (*pedicle*). Skin flaps are used to cover wounds with a poor vascular bed, provide padding when needed, and cover wounds over cartilage and bone. The patient may need intermediate flap placement if the recipient site is far removed from the donor site. For instance, a skin flap from the thigh to the head would require an intermediate graft. The flap is advanced to the recipient site when circulation is well established at the intermediate site. The patient's needs and the type of defect to be repaired determine the type of flap and the route of transfer.

Soft-tissue expansion is a technique for providing skin (1) for resurfacing a defect, such as a burn scar, (2) for removing a disfiguring mark (e.g., a tattoo), or (3) as a preliminary step in breast reconstruction. A subcutaneous tissue expander of an appropriate size and shape is placed under the skin, usually as an outpatient procedure. Weekly expansion with saline solution can be done in a health care setting or by the patient at home. This expansion procedure is repeated until the skin reaches the size needed for the repair. This may take from several weeks to 4 months. Once sufficient skin is available, the old incision is opened, the expander is removed, and the soft tissue is ready to be used as an advancement flap. The tissue expander next to a defect retains the primary tissue characteristics such as colour and texture.

Engineered skin substitutes (e.g., Dermagraft, Alloderm) are gaining popularity. There are a number available, each with its own indications and benefits. Some are two-layered membranes with both dermal and epidermal components. Others are only one layer. The skin is engineered from newborn fore-skins and cadavers. Skin substitutes do not contain structures such as blood vessels, hair follicles, sweat glands, or cells such as melanocytes, Langerhans cells, macrophages, and lymphocytes, therefore reducing the risk of rejection (Bryant & Nix, 2016).

Engineered skin grafts have an extended shelf life. Some are cryopreserved, others are shipped overnight as they are needed. Advantages include ready availability, the avoidance of a donor site, application in outpatient settings, minimal scarring, and less pain.

CASE STUDY

Malignant Melanoma and Dysplastic Nevi

Patient Profile

G. L. (pronouns he/him), 46 years old, is a contract safety officer supervising large industrial construction sites. During his leisure time, G. L. enjoys fishing and kayaking. He has fair skin and has come to the clinic for evaluation of a changing skin lesion on his left arm.

Subjective Data

- History of a basal cell carcinoma (BCC) on left ear in the past 4 years
- Father treated for metastatic malignant melanoma at age 77
- First noted the lesion 5 months ago, when it started changing size
- Anxious the lesion might have spread and might require extensive, disfiguring surgery

Objective Data

Physical Examination

- Has a 4-mm lesion, dark brown/black, scalloped with vaguely defined borders to dorsum of left forearm just distal to the elbow
- Has a large number of small nevi (>50) on back, legs, and arms
- Has four dysplastic nevi on back

Diagnostic Studies

- Excisional biopsy confirmed superficial spreading melanoma.

- Sentinel node biopsy results were negative.
- Diagnostic tests indicate melanoma stage 1.

Discussion Questions

1. What risk factors for malignant melanoma does G. L. have?
2. What are the usual clinical manifestations associated with malignant melanoma?
3. What is the prognosis for a patient with this stage of malignant melanoma?
4. What treatment options are available for him?
5. **Priority decision:** What is the priority of care for G. L.?
6. How would the nurse address his anxiety about the treatment outcomes?
7. Which members of the interprofessional team might the nurse involve to support G. L.'s care?
8. What should the nurse include in the patient teaching plan to address future sun exposure?
9. Evidence-informed practice: G. L. wants to know whether regularly applying sunscreen will reduce the risk of developing a second melanoma. How should the nurse reply?

ⓔvolve

Answers available at http://evolve.elsevier.com/Canada/Lewis/medsurg.

REVIEW QUESTIONS

The number of the question corresponds to the same-numbered objective at the beginning of the chapter.

1. Which sun-safety practices would the nurse include in the teaching plan for a client who has photosensitivity? *(Select all that apply.)*
   a. Wear protective clothing.
   b. Apply sunscreen liberally and often.
   c. Use tanning booths only for short durations.
   d. Avoid exposure to the sun, especially during midday.
   e. Wear any sunscreen as long as it is purchased at a drugstore.

2. What measurement is the prognosis of a client with melanoma most dependent on?
   a. The thickness of the lesion
   b. The degree of asymmetry in the lesion
   c. How much the lesion has spread superficially
   d. The amount of ulceration in the lesion

3. The nurse determines that a client with a diagnosis of which disorder is most at risk for spreading the disease?
   a. Tinea pedis
   b. Impetigo on the face
   c. Candidiasis of the nails
   d. Psoriasis on the palms and soles

4. A mother and her two children have been diagnosed with pediculosis corporis at a health centre. Which of the following is an appropriate measure in treating this condition?
   a. Application of pyrethrins to the body
   b. Topical application of an antifungal ointment

   c. Moist compresses applied frequently
   d. Administration of systemic antibiotics

5. What is a common site for the lesions associated with atopic dermatitis?
   a. Buttocks
   b. Temporal area
   c. Antecubital space
   d. Plantar surface of the feet

6. During assessment of a client, the nurse notes on the client's knee and elbow red, sharply defined plaques covered with silvery scales that the client reports as mildly itchy. What should the nurse recognize this finding to be?
   a. Lentigo
   b. Psoriasis
   c. Actinic keratosis
   d. Seborrheic keratosis

7. A patient with acne vulgaris tells the nurse that she has quit her job as a receptionist because she feels her appearance is disgusting to customers. Which of the following nursing diagnoses best describes this patient's response?
   a. Ineffective coping resulting from insufficient social support
   b. Impaired skin integrity as a result of inadequate nutrition
   c. Anxiety resulting from unmet needs (lack of knowledge about the disease process)
   d. Social isolation due to alteration in physical appearance

8. What important point should client teaching after a chemical peel include?
   a. Avoidance of sun exposure
   b. Application of firm bandages
   c. Limitation of vigorous exercise
   d. Use of moist heat to prevent discomfort

1. a, b; 2. a; 3. b; 4. a; 5. c; 6. b; 7. d; 8. a.

Ⓔvolve

For even more review questions, visit http://evolve.elsevier.com/Canada/Lewis/medsurg.

REFERENCES

Abrahamse, H., & Hamblin, M. R. (2016). New photosensitizers for photodynamic therapy. *Biochemical Journal, 473*(4), 347–364. https://doi.org/10.1042/BJ20150942

Alberta Health Services. (2020). *Laboratory testing for Lyme disease in Alberta–June 2020.* https://www.albertahealthservices.ca/assets/wf/plab/wf-provlab-appendix-laboratory-testing-of-lyme-disease-in-alberta.pdf

Allford, J. (2019). *Reclaiming Inuit culture one tattoo at a time.* CTV News. https://www.ctvnews.ca/lifestyle/reclaiming-inuit-culture-one-tattoo-at-a-time-1.4651750

Asai, Y., Baibergenova, A., Dutil, M., et al. (2016). Management of acne: Canadian clinical practice guidelines. *Canadian Medical Association Journal, 188*(2), 118–126. https://doi.org/10.1503/cmaj.140665

Bryant, R., & Nix, D. (2016). *Acute and chronic wound* (5th ed.). Mosby.

Canadian Cancer Society (CCS). (2021). *Risk factors for non-melanoma skin cancer.* http://www.cancer.ca/en/cancer-information/cancer-type/skin-non-melanoma/risks/?region=on

Canadian Cancer Statistics Advisory Committee. (2019). *Canadian cancer statistics 2019.* https://cdn.cancer.ca/-/media/files/research/cancer-statistics/2019-statistics/canadian-cancer-statistics-2-019-en.pdf

Canadian Dermatology Association (CDA). (2021a). *Hair removal.* https://dermatology.ca/public-patients/hair/hair-removal/#!/skin-hair-nails/hair/hair-removal/lasering

Canadian Dermatology Association (CDA). (2021b). *Indoor tanning is out.* https://dermatology.ca/public-patients/sun-protection/indoor-tanning-is-out/

Canadian Dermatology Association (CDA). (2021c). *Psoriasis.* https://dermatology.ca/public-patients/skin/psoriasis/#!/skin-hair-nails/skin/psoriasis/living-with-psoriasis

Canadian Dermatology Association (CDA). (2021d). *Sun safety for every day.* https://dermatology.ca/public-patients/sun-protection/sun-safety-every-day/

Cantrell, W. (2017). Psoriasis and psoriatic therapies. *The Nurse Practitioner, 42*(7), 35–39.

Chalmers, S., Harwood, A., Morris, N., et al. (2019). Do tattoos impair sweating? *Journal of Science and Medicine in Sport, 22*(11), 1173–1174. https://doi.org/10.1016/j.jsams.2019.08.001

Chia, C. T., Neinstein, R. M., & Theodorou, S. J. (2017). Evidence-based medicine: Liposuction. *Plastic and Reconstructive Surgery, 139*(1), 267–274. https://doi.org/10.1097/PRS.0000000000002859

Coit, D., Thompson, J. A., Algazi, A., et al. (2016). Melanoma. *Journal of the National Comprehensive Cancer Network, 14*(4), 450–473. https://doi.org/10.6004/jnccn.2016.0051

Costa, C. R., Kordestani, R., Small, K. H., et al. (2016). Advances and refinement in hyaluronic acid facial fillers. *Plastic and Reconstructive Surgery, 138*(2), 233–236. https://doi.org/10.1097/PRS.0000000000002008

Desai, S. R., Kovarik, C., Brod, B., et al. (2020). COVID-19 and personal protective equipment: Treatment and prevention of skin conditions related to the occupational use of personal protective equipment. *Journal of the American Academy of Dermatology, 83*(2), 675–677.

Environment and Climate Change Canada. (2017). *The UV index.* https://www.canada.ca/content/dam/eccc/migration/main/meteo-weather/80b0f2af-9697-4bee-ab17-d401ebba5b4b/4281_uv_index_poster_en_print.pdf

Frank, C., Sundquist, J., Hemminki, A., et al. (2017). Risk of other cancers in families with melanoma: Novel familial links. *Scientific Reports, 7*, 42601. https://doi.org/10.1038/srep42601

Gilpin, E. (2018). *Reawakening cultural tattooing of the Northwest. Canada's National Observer.* https://www.nationalobserver.com/2018/08/23/these-five-indigenous-tattoo-artists-are-reawakening-cultural-practices

Government of Canada. (2017a). *Sunglasses.* https://www.canada.ca/en/health-canada/services/sun-safety/sunglasses.html

Government of Canada. (2017b). *Sunscreens.* https://www.canada.ca/en/health-canada/services/sun-safety/sunscreens.html

Government of Canada. (2019). *Tanning beds and equipment.* https://www.canada.ca/en/health-canada/services/sun-safety/tanning-beds-lamps.html

Green, A. C., & Olsen, C. M. (2017). Cutaneous squamous cell carcinoma: An epidemiological review. *British Journal of Dermatology, 177*(2), 373–381. https://doi.org/10.1111/bjd.15324

Habif, T. P. (2016). *Clinical dermatology* (6th ed.). Saunders.

Kirlew, M., Rea, S., Schroeter, A., et al. (2014). Invasive CA-MRSA in northwestern Ontario: A 2-year prospective study. *Canadian Journal of Rural Medicine, 19*(3), 99–102.

Luger, T. A., McDonald, I., & Steinhoff, M. (2017). *Clinical and basic immunodermatology.* Springer.

Porter, J. (2015). Bad water in First Nations leads to high rate of invasive infection, doctor says. *CBC News.* October 26, 2015 https://www.cbc.ca/news/canada/thunder-bay/bad-water-in-first-nations-leads-to-high-rate-of-invasive-infection-doctor-says-1.3286337

Prohaska, J., & Badri, T. (2020). *Cryotherapy. StatPearls.* https://www.ncbi.nlm.nih.gov/books/NBK482319/

Stegman, L. (2017). Electronic brachytherapy for nonmelanoma skin cancer. *Oncology Times, 39*(9), 38–39.

Verkouteren, J. A., Ramdas, K. H., Wakkee, M., et al. (2017). Epidemiology of basal cell carcinoma: Scholarly review. *British Journal of Dermatology, 177*(2), 359–372. https://doi.org/10.1111/bjd.15321

RESOURCES

Canadian Cancer Society
https://www.cancer.ca
Canadian Dermatology Association
https://www.dermatology.ca
Canadian Dermatology Foundation
https://www.cdf.ca
Canadian Society of Aesthetic Specialty Nurses
https://www.csasn.org/
Canadian Society of Plastic Surgeons
https://www.plasticsurgery.ca
Eczema Society of Canada
https://www.eczemahelp.ca
Environment and Climate Change Canada
https://www.canada.ca/en/environment-climate-change.html
International Skin Tear Advisory Panel
https://www.skintears.org

Melanoma Network of Canada
  https://www.melanomanetwork.ca
Nurses Specialized in Wound Ostomy and Continence Canada
  https://nswoc.ca
Psoriasis Society of Canada
  https://www.psoriasissociety.org
Save Your Skin Foundation
  https://www.saveyourskin.ca
Wounds Canada
  https://www.woundscanada.ca

National Pressure Injury Advisory Panel
  https://npiap.com
Wounds International
  https://www.woundsinternational.com

evolve

For additional Internet resources, see the website for this book at
http://evolve.elsevier.com/Canada/Lewis/medsurg.

Nursing Management

Burns

Krista Gushue
Originating US chapter by Cecilia Bidigare

⊖volve WEBSITE

http://evolve.elsevier.com/Canada/Lewis/medsurg

- Review Questions (Online Only)
- Key Points
- Answer Guidelines for Case Study
- Student Case Study
  - Burns
- Customizable Nursing Care Plan
  - Patient with Thermal Burn Injury
- Conceptual Care Map Creator
- Audio Glossary
- Content Updates

LEARNING OBJECTIVES

1. Explain the causes of burn injuries and prevention strategies.
2. Differentiate between partial- and full-thickness burns.
3. Apply the parameters used to determine the severity of burns.
4. Compare the pathophysiological processes, clinical manifestations, complications, and interprofessional management throughout the three burn phases.
5. Compare the fluid and electrolyte shifts during the emergent and the acute burn phases.
6. Differentiate the nutritional needs of the patient with a burn injury throughout the three burn phases.
7. Compare the various burn wound care techniques and surgical options for partial-thickness versus full-thickness burn wounds.
8. Prioritize nursing interventions in the management of the physiological and psychosocial needs of the patient throughout the three burn phases.
9. Examine the various physiological and psychosocial aspects of burn rehabilitation.
10. Design a plan of care to prepare the burn patient and family for discharge.

KEY TERMS

burn	debridement	full-thickness burn
chemical burns	electrical burns	partial-thickness burn
contracture	escharotomy	smoke and inhalation injuries
cultured epithelial autograft (CEA)	excision and grafting	thermal burns

A **burn** is an injury to the tissues of the body caused by heat, chemicals, electric current, or radiation. The resulting effects are influenced by the temperature of the burning agent, the duration of contact time, and the type of tissue that is injured.

A burn injury occurs in more than two to three million people in North America each year (Arno & Knighten, 2020). There is a lack of current, precise data on the number of Canadians burned each year. According to Statistics Canada (Billette & Janz, 2015), 127 000 Canadians over the age of 12 years stated that they had an activity-limiting injury due to a burn, scald, or chemical burn in the previous 12 months. The highest incidence occurred within the 20- to 64-year age group, and treatment occurred predominantly in the emergency department.

An estimated 486 000 Americans seek medical care each year for burns (American Burn Association [ABA], 2016).

Accounting for the 2016 population difference between the United States and Canada (324 million versus 36 million), the burn incidence data appear to be similar. Around the world, nearly 11 million people need medical attention annually for burn injuries, and about 180 000 die as a result of burns (World Health Organization, 2018).

Although burn incidence has decreased over the past 20 years, burn injuries still occur too frequently, mainly to persons living at lower socioeconomic levels and with histories of substance misuse or mental illness. Most burn incidents are preventable (Grant, 2017). The focus of burn prevention has shifted from blaming individuals and changing behaviours to making legislative changes and collecting global burn data to address the unique prevention needs of low- and middle-income countries (Peck & Tophi, 2020).

TABLE 27.1	COMMON LOCATIONS AND SOURCES OF BURN INJURY*

Home Hazards
Kitchen and Bathroom
- Microwaved food
- Steam, hot grease, or liquids from cooking
- Hot water heaters set at 60°C or higher

General Household
- Heat lamps
- Fireplaces (e.g., gas, wood)
- Open space heaters
- Radiators (e.g., home, automobile)
- Outdoor grills (e.g., propane, charcoal)
- Frayed or defective wiring
- Multiple extension cords per outlet

- Flammables (e.g., starter fluid, gasoline, kerosene)
- Carelessness with cigarettes, matches, candles

Occupational Hazards
- Tar
- Cement
- Chemicals
- Hot metals
- Steam pipes
- Combustible fuels
- Fertilizers, pesticides
- Electricity from power lines
- Sparks from live electric sources

*List is not all-inclusive.

Coordinated national programs in developed countries have focused on use of child-resistant lighters, nonflammable children's clothing, tap water anti-scald devices, stricter building codes, hard-wired smoke detectors and alarms, and fire sprinklers. Nurses can advocate for and teach about burn risk–reduction strategies in the home and at work (Tables 27.1 and 27.2).

TYPES OF BURN INJURY

Thermal Burns

Thermal burns are caused by flame, flash fire, scald, or contact with hot objects. They are the most common type of burn injury (Figure 27.1; see Table 27.2). The severity depends on the temperature of the burning agent and duration of contact time. Scald injuries can occur in the bathroom or while cooking. Flash, flame, or contact burns can occur while cooking, smoking, burning leaves in the backyard, or using gasoline or hot oil.

Chemical Burns

Chemical burns are the result of contact with acids and alkalis. Acids can be found in the home and at work—in car batteries, bleach, chemical laboratories, vinegar, and glass polish. The chemical compounds include hydrochloric, sulphuric, acidic, and hydrofluoric acid. Alkali substances are found in cement, drain cleaners, cleaning agents, and fertilizer and include calcium hydroxide (lime), ammonia, or ammonia hydroxide (Ramponi, 2017).

Smoke and Inhalation Injury

Smoke and inhalation injuries from breathing noxious chemicals or hot air can cause damage to the tissues of the respiratory tract. Fortunately, gases are cooled to body temperature before they reach the lung tissue. The vocal cords and glottis close as a protective mechanism, so damage to the respiratory mucosa occurs less often. Smoke inhalation injuries are a major predictor of mortality in burn patients. Rapid initial and

TABLE 27.2	TYPES OF BURN INJURY AND BURN RISK–REDUCTION STRATEGIES

Flame or Contact
- Never smoke in bed.
- Use child-resistant lighters.
- Hold regular fire exit drills in the home.
- Never leave hot oil unattended while cooking.
- Never use gasoline or other flammable liquids to start a fire.
- Never leave candles unattended or near open windows or curtains.
- Consider a flame-retardant smoking apron for older or at-risk people.
- Exercise caution when microwaving food and beverages as they can get very hot.

Scald
- Lower hot water temperature to the "lowest point" or 40°C.
- Use "anti-scald" devices with showerhead or faucet fixtures.
- Supervise bathing of small children, older persons, or anyone with impaired physical movement, physical sensation, or judgement.
- After running bath water, check temperature with back of hand or bath thermometer.

Inhalation
- Install smoke and carbon monoxide detectors and change batteries annually (if appropriate).

Chemical
- Store chemicals safely in approved containers and label clearly.
- Ensure safety of workers and students handling chemicals (e.g., provide education, protective eyewear, gloves, masks, clothing).

Electrical
- Avoid or repair frayed wiring.
- Avoid outdoor activities during electrical (i.e., lightning) storms.
- Ensure electrical power source is shut off before beginning repairs.
- Wear protective eyewear and gloves when making electrical repairs.

TABLE 27.3	MANIFESTATIONS OF RESPIRATORY INJURY ASSOCIATED WITH BURNS

Upper Airway Injury
Edema, hoarseness, difficulty swallowing, copious secretions, stridor, substernal and intercostal retractions, total airway obstruction

Lower Airway Injury
Strongly assumed if patient was trapped in a fire in an enclosed space or clothing caught fire and if patient has facial burns or singed nasal or facial hair; symptoms include dyspnea, carbonaceous sputum, wheezing, hoarseness, altered mental status

ongoing assessment are critical (Table 27.3). Prompt assessment for signs and symptoms of airway compromise is imperative because severe edema, bronchospasm, or a mucous plug can occur within minutes to days after the initial exposure (Dyamenahalli, 2019).

There are three types of smoke and inhalation injuries:
1. *Carbon monoxide poisoning.* Carbon monoxide poisoning and asphyxiation account for the majority of deaths at a fire scene. Carbon monoxide is produced by the incomplete combustion of burning materials. It is subsequently inhaled and displaces oxygen (O_2) on the hemoglobin molecule, causing carboxyhemoglobinemia, hypoxia, and, when the carbon monoxide levels exceed 20%, death. With severe

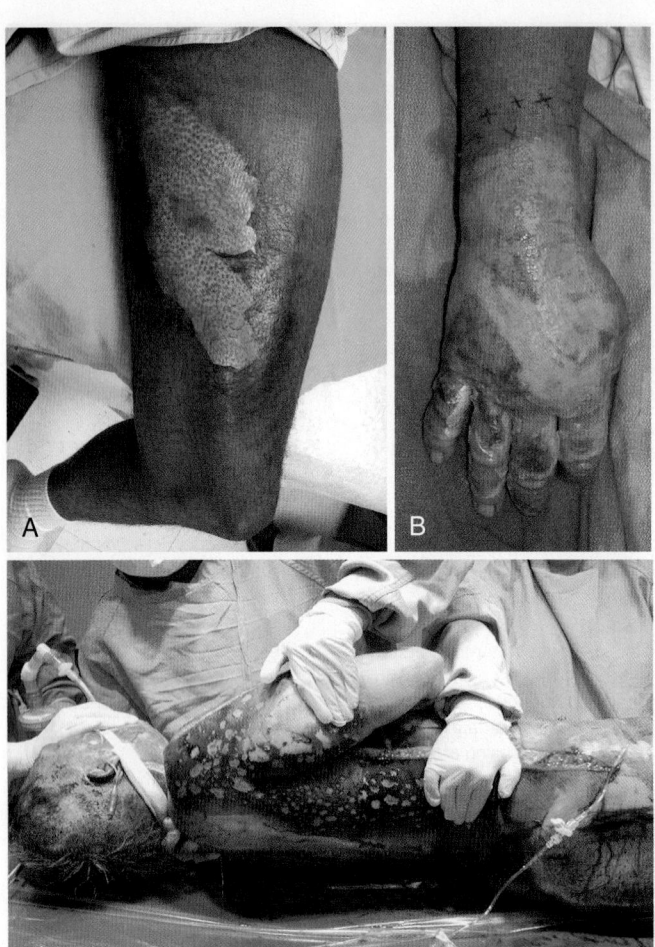

FIG. 27.1 Types of burn injury. **A,** Superficial, partial-thickness scald burn to thigh. **B,** Deep partial-thickness flame burn to hand. **C,** Full-thickness flame burn secondary to posterior chest and arm. Source: Courtesy Judy A. Knighton, RN, MScN, Toronto.

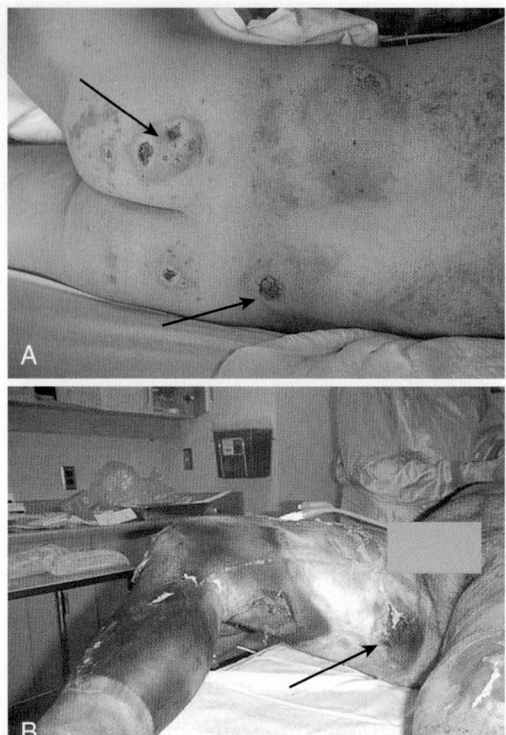

FIG. 27.2 Electrical injury produces heat coagulation of the blood supply and contact area as electric current passes through the skin. **A,** Back and buttock *(arrows)*. **B,** Leg *(arrow)*. Source: Courtesy Judy A. Knighton, RN, MScN, Toronto.

carbon monoxide poisoning, skin colour is often described as "cherry red" in appearance. Carbon monoxide poisoning may occur in the absence of burn injury to the skin (e.g., smoke inhalation during a fire).

2. *Inhalation injury above the glottis.* In general, an inhalation injury above the glottis *(upper airway injury)* is thermally produced and may be caused by the inhalation of hot air, steam, or smoke. Mucosal burns of the oropharynx and larynx are manifested by redness, blistering, and edema. Mechanical obstruction can occur quickly, which represents a true medical emergency. Clues to the occurrence of this injury include the presence of facial burns, singed nasal hair, hoarseness, painful swallowing, darkened oral and nasal membranes, carbonaceous sputum, history of being burned in an enclosed space, and clothing burns around the chest and neck.

3. *Inhalation injury below the glottis.* An inhalation injury below the glottis *(lower airway injury)* is usually chemically produced. Tissue damage is related to the duration of exposure to smoke or toxic fumes. Clinical manifestations such as pulmonary edema may not appear until 12 to 24 hours after the burn, and then they may manifest as acute respiratory distress syndrome (see Chapter 71).

Electrical Burns

Electrical burns result from intense heat generated from an electric current and are considered the most severe type of thermal trauma, generally associated with greater damage of functional structures, such as muscle and bone (Foncerrada et al., 2017). Direct damage to nerves and vessels can cause tissue anoxia and death. The severity of the electrical injury depends on the amount of voltage, tissue resistance, current pathways, surface area in contact with the current, and length of time that the current flow was sustained (Figure 27.2). Tissue density affects the amount of resistance to electric current. For example, fat and bone offer the most resistance, whereas nerves and blood vessels offer the least resistance. Current that passes through vital organs (e.g., brain, heart, kidneys) produces more life-threatening sequelae than that which passes through other tissues. In addition, electric sparks may ignite the patient's clothing, causing a flame injury.

As with inhalation injury, a rapid assessment of the patient with an electrical injury should be performed. Transfer to a burn centre is indicated. The severity of an electrical injury can be difficult to determine since most of the damage is below the skin (known as the *iceberg effect*). Determination of electric current contact points and history of the injury may help reveal the likely path of the current and potential areas of injury. Contact with electric current can cause muscle contractions strong enough to fracture the long bones and vertebrae. Another reason to suspect long bone or spinal fractures is a fall resulting from the electrical injury. For this reason, all patients with electrical burns should be considered at risk for a cervical spine injury. Cervical spine immobilization is used during transport and subsequent diagnostic testing until injury is ruled out.

Electrical injury can range from minor skin burns to life-threatening injuries. Cardiac arrhythmias are the most common complication from electric shock and can be sudden or delayed. Delayed arrythmias can occur without warning during the first 24 hours after injury. Ventricular fibrillation and sudden cardiac death can be caused by both high- and low-voltage currents (Waldmann et al., 2018). Direct nerve damage can result and manifest as a peripheral nerve injury, spinal cord damage, cerebellar ataxia, hypoxic encephalopathy, or intracerebral hemorrhage (Yang et al., 2018). Myoglobin from injured muscle and hemoglobin from damaged red blood cells (RBCs) are released into the circulation whenever massive muscle and blood vessel damage occurs. The released myoglobin travels to the kidneys and can block the renal tubules. This can result in acute tubular necrosis (ATN) and acute kidney injury (see Chapter 49).

Cold Thermal Injury

Cold thermal injury, or *frostbite*, is discussed in Chapter 72.

CLASSIFICATION OF BURN INJURY

Treatment of burns is related to the severity of the injury. Severity is determined by (a) depth of burn, (b) extent of burn calculated in percentage of total body surface area (TBSA), (c) location of burn, and (d) patient risk factors (e.g., age, past medical history). Health Canada uses referral criteria to determine which burn injuries should be treated in burn centres (Table 27.4). Critical Care Services Ontario (CCSO) has adapted the American Burn Association (ABA) "Burn Center Referral Criteria" to develop "Burns Centre Consultation

Guidelines" (see Table 27.4). A list of provincial burn units and centres across Canada is provided in Table 27.5. Goals of care include wound healing, prevention of infection, pain management, prevention of complications, and return to preinjury function.

Depth of Burn

Burn injury involves the destruction of the integumentary system. The skin is divided into three layers: epidermis, dermis, and subcutaneous tissue (Figure 27.3; see Figure 25.1). The *epidermis*, or nonvascular outer layer of the skin, is approximately as thick as a sheet of paper. It is composed of many layers of nonliving epithelial cells that provide a protective barrier to the skin, hold in fluids and electrolytes, help regulate body temperature, and keep harmful agents in the external environment from

---

TABLE 27.4 CRITERIA FOR TRANSFER OF THE PATIENT WITH BURN INJURIES*

Consider transfer to a major burn centre:
- ≥20% TBSA partial- and/or full-thickness at any age
- ≥10% TBSA partial- and/or full-thickness for ages ≤10 and ≥50 years
- Full-thickness burns ≥5% TBSA at any age
- Burns to face, hands, feet, joints, genitalia, perineum
- Electrical burns [including lightning injury]
- Chemical burns
- Inhalation injury
- Burns with comorbidity
- Burns with patients who require special social, emotional, or rehabilitation care

Consider transfer to a minor burn centre:
- Burns >10% but <20% TBSA in adults

Remain at base site:
- Burns <10% TBSA in adults who do not require transfer but seek medical advice or an ambulatory burns clinic referral for assessment

High-risk considerations that may warrant transfer at a lower clinical threshold:
- ≥50 years of age
- Anticoagulation
- Immunosuppression
- Pregnancy
- Diabetes
- Other significant medical problems

TBSA, total body surface area.

Source: Critical Care Services Ontario. (n.d.). *Burns centre consultation guidelines.* https://www.criticalcareontario.ca/EN/Trauma%20and%20Burns%20Consultation%20Guidelines/CCSO_BurnsCentreGuidelines_11x14-EN.pdf

*See also: Health Canada. (2010). *Dermatological emergencies: Burns. Clinical practice guidelines for nurses in primary care: Adult care.* http://www.hc-sc.gc.ca/fniah-spnia/alt_formats/pdf/services/nurs-infirm/clini/adult/skin-peau-eng.pdf; and American Burn Association. (2006). *Guidelines for the operation of burn centers.* http://www.ameriburn.org/Chapter14.pdf

---

TABLE 27.5 CANADIAN BURN UNITS OR CENTRES BY PROVINCE,* 2020

Province	City	Hospital
Alberta	Calgary	Calgary Foothills Medical Centre
	Calgary	Alberta Children's Hospital Burn Treatment Services
	Edmonton	Edmonton Firefighters' Burn Treatment Unit
British Columbia	Vancouver	B.C. Professional Fire Fighters' Burn, Trauma, and High Acuity Unit, Vancouver General Hospital
	Vancouver	B.C. Children's Hospital Burn Unit
	Victoria	Complex Wound and Burn Clinic, Royal Jubilee Hospital
Manitoba	Winnipeg	Manitoba Firefighters' Burn Unit
	Winnipeg	Winnipeg Children's Hospital Burn Unit
New Brunswick	Saint John	Saint John Regional Hospital Plastic and Burns Unit
Newfoundland and Labrador	St. John's	General Hospital Health Sciences Centre
Nova Scotia	Halifax	Queen Elizabeth II Health Sciences Centre
	Halifax	IWK Health Centre
Ontario	Hamilton	Hamilton Health Sciences Centre Burn Unit
	London	London Health Sciences Centre Burn Unit
	Ottawa	Children's Hospital of Eastern Ontario
	Toronto	Hospital for Sick Children (Sick Kids) Burn Unit
	Toronto	Sunnybrook Health Sciences Centre Ross Tilley Burn Centre
Quebec	Montreal	Hôtel-Dieu du CHUM Montreal Burn Unit
	Montreal	CHU Sainte-Justine Burn Clinic
	Montreal	McGill University Health Centre
	Quebec City	Centre d'expertise pour victimes de brulures graves de l'Est du Québec
	Quebec City	Hôpital de L'Enfant-Jésus du CHU de Québec Unité des grands brûlés
Saskatchewan	Regina	South Saskatchewan Firefighters' Burn Unit
	Saskatoon	Royal University Hospital

Source: Developed by Judy Knighton, RN, MScN, clinical nurse specialist—burns. (2015, April). Data collected for Canadian Special Interest Group Meeting, American Burn Association Meeting, Chicago. Adapted by Krista Gushue, BN, RN, MN, 2020.

*There are no known burn centres in Yukon, Northwest Territories, or Nunavut.

injuring or invading the body. The *dermis*, which lies below the epidermis, is approximately 30 to 45 times thicker than the epidermis. The dermis contains connective tissues with blood vessels and highly specialized structures consisting of hair follicles, nerve endings, sweat glands, and sebaceous glands. Under the dermis lies *subcutaneous tissue*, which contains major vascular networks, fat, nerves, and lymphatic vessels. The subcutaneous tissue acts as a heat insulator for underlying structures, which include the muscles, tendons, bones, and internal organs.

Burns continue to be defined by degrees: first-, second-, third-, and fourth-degree. The ABA recommends a more precise definition, classifying them according to depth of skin destruction: **partial-thickness burn** and **full-thickness burn** (see Figure 27.3). Partial-thickness burns have varying degrees of epidermal and dermal skin injury, with some skin elements remaining viable for regeneration. Full-thickness burns involve the destruction of all skin elements and subcutaneous tissues, with the possible involvement of muscles, tendons, and bones. Skin-reproducing (re-epithelializing) cells are located along the shafts of the hair follicles, sweat glands, and sebaceous glands. If there is significant damage to the dermis (e.g., a full-thickness burn), not enough skin cells remain to regenerate new skin. A permanent, alternative source of skin is then needed. In Table 27.6, the various burn classifications are compared according to depth of injury.

Extent of Burn

Two commonly used guides for determining the TBSA affected or the extent of a burn wound are the adult Lund–Browder chart (Figure 27.4, *A*) and the adult rule of nines chart (see Figure 27.4, *B*). (First-degree burns, equivalent to a sunburn, are not included when TBSA burned is calculated.) The Lund–Browder chart is considered more accurate because the patient's age, in proportion to relative body-area size, is taken into account. The rule of nines, which is easy to remember, is considered adequate for initial assessment of an adult patient with burn injury. For irregular or odd-shaped burns, the size of the patient's hand (including the fingers) is approximately 1% TBSA.

An additional tool is the Sage Burn Diagram, a free, Internet-based tool available for estimating TBSA burned (see the Resources at the end of this chapter). There are also mobile applications (e.g., Mersey Burns) available to estimate the percentage of burn and fluid resuscitation needs (https://merseyburns.com/). The extent of a burn is often revised after edema has subsided and demarcation of the zones of injury has occurred.

Location of Burn

The severity of the burn injury is related to the location of the burn wound. Burns to the face and neck and circumferential burns to the trunk or back can result in mechanical obstruction, secondary to edema, and leathery, devitalized tissue formation *(eschar),* both of which may inhibit respiratory function. These injuries may also include possible inhalation injury and respiratory mucosal damage.

Burns to the hands, feet, joints, and eyes are of concern because they make self-care very difficult and may jeopardize future function. Burns to the hands and feet are challenging to manage because of superficial vascular and nerve supply systems that must be protected and because of the need to maintain hand function during healing.

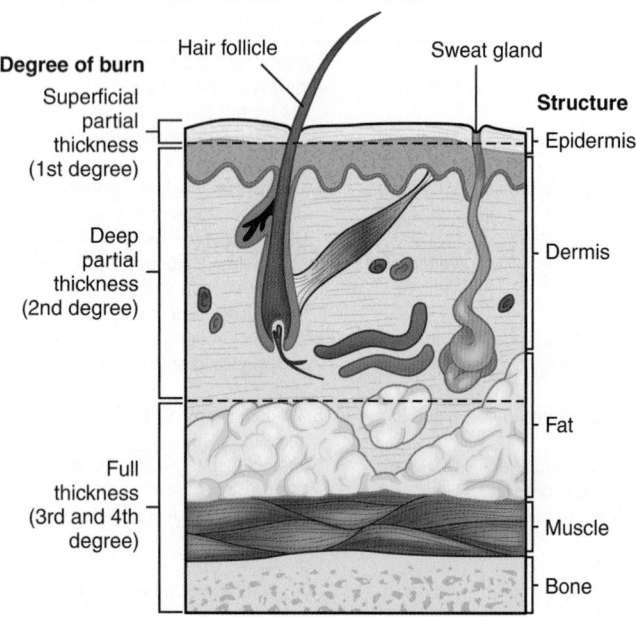

FIG. 27.3 Cross-section of skin indicating the depth of burn and structures involved.

TABLE 27.6	**CLASSIFICATION OF BURN INJURY DEPTH**		
Classification	**Clinical Appearance**	**Possible Cause**	**Structures Involved**
Partial-Thickness Skin Destruction			
Superficial: first-degree burn	Erythema, blanching on pressure, pain and mild swelling, no vesicles or blisters (although after 24 hr, skin may blister and peel)	Superficial sunburn Quick heat flash	Superficial epidermal damage with hyperemia; tactile and pain sensation intact
Deep: second-degree burn	Fluid-filled vesicles that are red, shiny, wet (if vesicles have ruptured); severe pain caused by nerve injury; mild to moderate edema	Flame Flash Scald Contact Chemical Tar Electrical current	Epidermis and dermis involved to varying depth; skin elements from which epithelial regeneration occurs remain viable
Full-Thickness Skin Destruction			
Third- and fourth-degree burns	Dry, waxy-white, leathery, or hard skin; visible thrombosed vessels; insensitivity to pain because of nerve destruction; possible involvement of muscles, tendons, and bones	Flame Scald Chemical Tar Electrical current	All skin elements and local nerve endings destroyed; coagulation necrosis present; surgical intervention advisable for healing

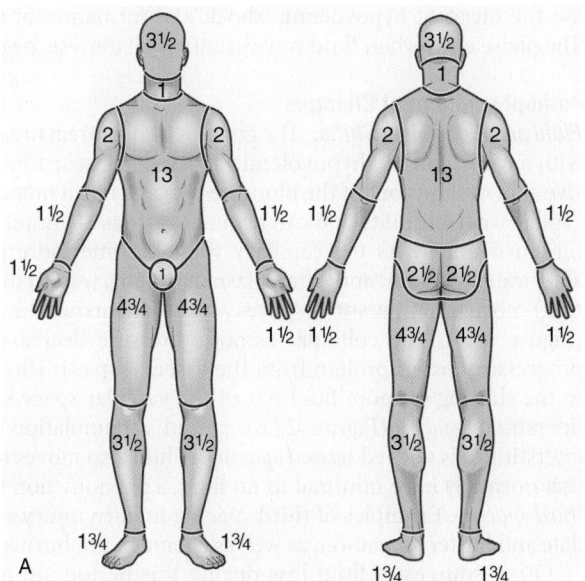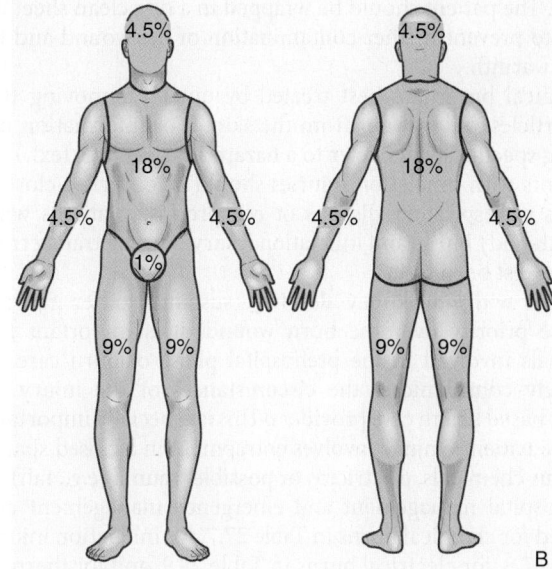

FIG. 27.4 A, Adult Lund–Browder chart. Generally, when the assessor is completing the chart, areas of partial-thickness injury are coloured in blue, and areas of full-thickness in red. Superficial partial-thickness burns are not calculated. **B,** Adult rule of nines chart.

Burns to the ears and nose are susceptible to infection because the skin is very thin and the underlying skeleton frequently exposed. Burns to the buttocks or perineum are at high risk for infection from urine or feces contamination. Circumferential burns to the extremities can cause circulatory compromise distal to the burn and, subsequently, neurological impairment of the affected extremity. Patients may also develop compartment syndrome (see Chapter 65) from direct heat damage to muscles; edema may result, and preburn vascular conditions can be exacerbated.

Patient Risk Factors

The older person heals more slowly and usually experiences more difficulty with rehabilitation than a younger adult. Any patient with pre-existing cardiovascular, respiratory, or renal disease has a poorer prognosis for recovery because of the tremendous demands placed on the body by a burn injury. The patient with diabetes mellitus or peripheral vascular disease is at high risk for poor healing (Okonkwo & DiPietro, 2017), including leg and foot burns. General physical debilitation from any chronic disease—including alcoholism, drug misuse, or malnutrition—renders the patient less physiologically able to recover from a burn injury. In addition, the patient with a burn injury who has concurrently sustained other injuries—fractures, head injuries, or other trauma—has a poorer prognosis for recovery.

PHASES OF BURN MANAGEMENT

Historically, burn management has been organized chronologically into three phases that correspond to the key priority of each particular phase: emergent (resuscitative), acute (wound healing), and rehabilitative (restorative). Care overlaps from one phase to another. For example, although the emergent phase is seen as beginning in the emergency department, care often begins in the prehospital phase, depending on the skill level of paramedics at the scene. Planning for rehabilitation begins on

the day of the burn injury or admission to the burn unit. Formal rehabilitation begins as soon as functional assessment can be performed. Wound care is the primary focus of the acute phase, but it also takes place in both the emergent and rehabilitative phases.

Prehospital Care

At the injury scene, priority is given to removing the person from the source of the burn and stopping the burning process. Rescuers must also protect themselves from being injured. In the case of electrical and chemical injuries, initial management involves removal of the patient from the electrical or chemical source.

Small thermal burns (<10% of TBSA) should be covered with a clean, cool, tap water–dampened towel for the patient's comfort and protection until definitive medical care is instituted. Cooling of the injured area (if small) within 1 minute helps minimize the depth of the injury. If the burn area is large (>10% TBSA) or an electrical or inhalation burn is suspected and the patient is unresponsive, attention needs to be focused first on ABC (**a**irway, **b**reathing, **c**irculation) (NB Trauma Program, 2019):

- *Airway:* Check for patency, soot around nares and on the tongue, singed nasal hair, darkened oral or nasal membranes.
- *Breathing:* Check for adequacy of ventilation.
- *Circulation:* Check for presence of pulses and elevate the burned limb(s) above the heart to decrease pain and swelling.

Airway assessment and management are critical initial steps in caring for burn patients. To prevent hypothermia, large burns should be cooled for no more than 10 minutes. The burned body part should not be immersed in cold water because doing so might lead to extensive heat loss. A burn should never be covered with ice because this can cause hypothermia and vasoconstriction of blood vessels, further reducing blood flow to the injury. As much burned clothing as possible should be gently removed, to prevent further tissue damage. Adherent clothing should be left in place until the patient is transferred to a hospital. The patient should be wrapped in a dry, clean sheet or blanket to prevent further contamination of the wound and to provide warmth.

Chemical burns are best treated by quickly removing the solid particles and powder from the skin. (For information on handling specific agents, refer to a hazardous materials text.)

Patients with inhalation injuries should be observed closely for signs of respiratory distress or compromise. Patients who have both body burns and inhalation injury must be transferred to the nearest burn unit.

Patients with burns may also have sustained other injuries that take priority over the burn wound. It is important for individuals involved in the prehospital phase of burn care to adequately communicate the circumstances of the injury to hospital-based health care providers. This is especially important when the patient's injury involves entrapment in a closed space, hazardous chemicals, electricity, or possible trauma (e.g., fall).

Prehospital management and emergency management are described for chemical burns in Table 27.7, for inhalation injury in Table 27.8, for electrical burns in Table 27.9, and for thermal burns in Table 27.10.

Emergent Phase

The *emergent (resuscitative) phase* is the period of time required to resolve the immediate, life-threatening conditions resulting from the burn injury (Hampson et al., 2012). This phase usually lasts up to 72 hours from the time of the burn. Primary concerns are the onset of hypovolemic shock and formation of edema. The phase ends when fluid mobilization and diuresis begin.

Pathophysiological Changes

Fluid and Electrolyte Shifts. The greatest initial threat to a patient with a major burn is hypovolemic shock. It is caused by a massive shift of fluids out of the blood vessels as a result of increased capillary permeability and can begin as early as 20 minutes after the burn injury. As the capillary walls become more permeable, water, sodium, and, later, plasma proteins (especially albumin) move into interstitial spaces and other surrounding tissue (Figure 27.5). The colloidal osmotic pressure decreases with progressive loss of protein from the vascular space. This results in the shifting of more fluid out of the vascular space into the interstitial spaces (Figure 27.6). (Fluid accumulation in the interstitium is termed *second spacing*.) Fluid also moves to areas that normally have minimal to no fluid, a phenomenon termed *third spacing*. Examples of third spacing in burn injury are exudate and blister formation, as well as edema in nonburned areas.

Other sources of fluid loss during this period are insensible losses by evaporation from large, denuded body surfaces and the respiratory system. The normal insensible loss of 30 to 50 mL per hour is increased in severely burned patients. The net result of the fluid shifts and losses is intravascular volume depletion. Decreased blood pressure (BP), increased heart rate, and other manifestations of hypovolemic shock are clinically detectable signs of intravascular volume depletion

✚ TABLE 27.7   EMERGENCY MANAGEMENT

Chemical Burns

Cause	Assessment Findings	Interventions
• Acids • Alkalis • Organic compounds	• Burning • Redness, swelling of injured tissue • Degeneration of exposed tissue • Discoloration of injured skin • Localized pain • Edema of surrounding tissue • Degeneration of exposed tissue (tissue destruction continuing for up to 72 hr) • Respiratory distress if chemical inhaled • Decreased muscle coordination (if organophosphate is involved) • Paralysis	**Initial** 1. If unresponsive, assess circulation, airway, and breathing before decontamination procedures are done. 2. If responsive, monitor airway, breathing, and circulation before decontamination procedures are done. 3. Stabilize cervical spine. 4. Provide supplemental oxygen as needed. 5. Anticipate intubation with significant inhalation injury, circumferential full-thickness burns to the neck and trunk, or large TBSA burn. 6. Brush dry chemical from skin before irrigation. 7. Remove nonadherent clothing, shoes, watches, jewellery, and, if face was exposed, glasses or contact lenses. 8. Flush chemical from wound and surrounding area with copious amounts of saline solution or water. 9. For chemical burn of the eye, flush from inner to outer corner of eye with water unless lactated Ringer's solution is available. 10. Cover burned areas with dry dressings or clean sheet. 11. Establish IV access with two large-bore catheters if burn >15% TBSA. 12. Begin fluid replacement. 13. Insert urinary catheter if adult burn >15% TBSA. 14. Elevate burned limb above level of heart to decrease edema. 15. Administer IV analgesic drug and assess effectiveness frequently. 16. Contact poison control centre for assistance. **Ongoing Monitoring** • Monitor airway if patient was exposed to chemicals. • Monitor urine output. • Consider possibility of systemic effect of identified chemical, and monitor and treat accordingly. • Monitor pH of eye if eye was exposed to chemicals. • Monitor pain level.

IV, intravenous; *TBSA,* total body surface area.

TABLE 27.8 EMERGENCY MANAGEMENT

Inhalation Injury

Cause	Assessment Findings	Interventions
• Exposure of respiratory tract to intense heat or flames • Inhalation of noxious chemicals, smoke, or carbon monoxide	• History of being trapped in an enclosed space, of being in an explosion, or of clothing catching fire • Rapid, shallow respirations • Increasing hoarseness • Coughing • Singed nasal or facial hair • Darkened oral or nasal membranes • Smoky breath • Carbonaceous sputum • Productive cough with black, grey, or bloody sputum • Irritation of upper airways or burning pain in throat or trunk • Difficulty swallowing • Cherry-red skin colour (carbon monoxide levels >20%) • Restlessness, anxiety • Altered mental status, including confusion, coma • Decreased oxygen saturation • Dysrhythmias	**Initial** 1. If unresponsive, assess circulation, airway, and breathing. 2. If responsive, monitor airway, breathing, and circulation. 3. Stabilize cervical spine. 4. Assess for inhalation injury. 5. Assess for concurrent thermal burn. 6. Provide 100% humidified oxygen. 7. Monitor vital signs, level of consciousness, oxygen saturation, and cardiac rhythm. 8. Remove nonadherent clothing, jewellery, and, if face was exposed, glasses or contact lenses. 9. Establish IV access with two large-bore catheters if burn >15% TBSA. 10. Begin fluid replacement. 11. Insert urinary catheter if burn >15% TBSA. 12. Elevate burned limb(s) above level of heart to decrease edema. 13. Measure arterial blood gas and carboxyhemoglobin levels, and obtain chest radiograph. 14. Administer IV analgesic drug and assess effectiveness frequently. 15. Identify and treat other associated injuries (e.g., fractures, pneumothorax, head injury). 16. Cover burned areas with dry dressings or clean sheet if TBSA is large or patient is hypothermic; can cover with normal saline–moistened gauze and clean sheet if TBSA is small. 17. Anticipate need for fibre-optic bronchoscopy or intubation. **Ongoing Monitoring** • Monitor airway, breathing, and circulation. • Monitor urine output. • Monitor vital signs, level of consciousness, respiratory status, oxygen saturation, and cardiac rhythm. • Monitor pain level.

IV, intravenous; *TBSA*, total body surface area.

(see Chapter 69). If it is not corrected, irreversible shock and death may result. The circulatory status is also impaired because of hemolysis of RBCs. The RBCs are hemolyzed by circulating factors (e.g., oxygen free radicals) released at the time of the burn, as well as by the direct insult of the burn injury. Thrombosis in the capillaries of burned tissue causes an additional loss of circulating RBCs. Elevation of the hematocrit is commonly caused by hemoconcentration, which results from fluid loss. After fluid balance has been restored, hematocrit levels lower as a result of dilution.

Major shifts in sodium and potassium also occur during this phase. Sodium rapidly shifts to the interstitial spaces and remains there until edema formation ceases (Figure 27.7). A potassium shift develops initially because injured cells and hemolyzed RBCs release potassium into the circulation. (Fluid and electrolyte shifts are discussed in Chapter 19.)

Toward the end of the emergent phase, capillary membrane permeability is restored if fluid replacement is adequate. Fluid loss and edema formation cease. Interstitial fluid gradually returns to the vascular space (see Figure 27.7). Clinically, diuresis is noted with low urine specific gravities.

Inflammation and Healing. Burn injury causes coagulation necrosis, in which tissues and vessels are damaged or destroyed. Neutrophils and monocytes accumulate at the site of injury. Fibroblasts and newly formed collagen fibrils appear and begin wound repair within the first 6 to 12 hours after injury. (The inflammatory response is discussed in Chapter 14.)

Immunological Changes. Burn injury causes widespread impairment of the immune system. The skin barrier to invading organisms is destroyed, bone marrow depression occurs, and circulating levels of immunoglobulins decrease. The function of white blood cells (WBCs) becomes defective. The inflammatory cytokine cascade triggered by tissue damage impairs the function of lymphocytes, monocytes, and neutrophils. This impaired function increases the patient's risk for infection.

Clinical Manifestations. Patients with burns are likely to be in shock from hypovolemia. In many cases, areas of full-thickness and deep partial-thickness burns are initially anaesthetic because nerve endings have been destroyed. Superficial to moderate partial-thickness burns are painful. Blisters, filled with fluid and protein, may develop in partial-thickness burns. Fluid is not actually lost from the body as much as it is sequestered in the interstitium and third spaces. Patients with a larger burn area may have signs of adynamic ileus, such as absent or decreased bowel sounds, as a result of the body's response to massive trauma and potassium shifts. Shivering may occur as a result of chilling caused by heat loss, anxiety, or pain. Ongoing nursing assessment of the ABCs, vital signs, cardiac rhythm, oxygenation, and level of consciousness are priorities during the emergent phase of burn care.

TABLE 27.9   EMERGENCY MANAGEMENT

Electrical Burns

Cause	Assessment Findings	Interventions
Alternating Current • Electrical wires • Utility wires **Direct Current** • Lightning • Defibrillator	• Leathery, white, or charred skin • Burn odour • Loss of consciousness • Impaired touch sensation • Minimal or no pain • Dysrhythmias • Cardiac arrest • Location of contact points • Diminished peripheral circulation in injured extremity • Thermal burns if clothing ignited • Fractures or dislocations from force of current • Head or neck injury if fall occurred • Depth and extent of wound difficult to visualize (injury should be presumed more severe than what is seen)	**Initial** 1. Remove patient from electric source while protecting rescuer. 2. If unresponsive, assess circulation, airway, and breathing. 3. If responsive, monitor airway, breathing, and circulation. 4. Stabilize cervical spine. 5. Provide supplemental oxygen as needed. 6. Monitor vital signs, level of consciousness, respiratory status, oxygen saturation, and cardiac rhythm. 7. Check pulses distal to burns. 8. Remove nonadherent clothing, shoes, watches, jewellery, and, if face was exposed, glasses or contact lenses. 9. Cover burned areas with dry dressing or clean sheet if TBSA is large or patient is hypothermic; can cover with normal saline–moistened gauze and dry sheet if TBSA is small. 10. Establish IV access with two large-bore catheters if burn >15% TBSA. 11. Begin fluid replacement. 12. Measure arterial blood gas to assess acid–base balance. 13. Insert urinary catheter if burn >15% TBSA. 14. Elevate burned limb(s) above level of heart to decrease edema. 15. Administer IV analgesic drug and assess effectiveness frequently. 16. Identify and treat other associated injuries (e.g., fractures, pneumothorax, head injury). **Ongoing Monitoring** • Monitor airway, breathing, and circulation. • Monitor vital signs, cardiac rhythm, level of consciousness, respiratory status, oxygen saturation, and neuro-vascular status of injured limbs. • Monitor urine output. • Monitor serum creatine kinase for development of myoglobinuria secondary to muscle breakdown and urine for hemoglobinuria secondary to RBC breakdown. • Anticipate possible administration of $NaHCO_3$ to alkalinize the urine and maintain serum pH >6.0. • Monitor pain level.

IV, intravenous; *$NaHCO_3$*, sodium bicarbonate; *RBC*, red blood cell; *TBSA*, total body surface area.

Most patients with burn injuries are quite alert and can provide answers to questions shortly after the injury or until they are intubated. They are often frightened and benefit from calm reassurance and simple explanations by all health care providers. Unconsciousness or altered mental status in a patient with burn injury is usually not a result of the burn. The most common reason for unconsciousness or altered mental status is hypoxia associated with smoke inhalation. Other possibilities include head trauma, history of substance misuse, or excessive amounts of sedation or pain medication.

Complications. The three major organ systems most susceptible to complications during the emergent phase of burn injury are the cardiovascular, respiratory, and urinary systems.

Cardiovascular System. Cardiovascular system complications include dysrhythmias and hypovolemic shock, which may progress to irreversible shock. Circulation to the extremities can be severely impaired by deep, circumferential burns and subsequent edema formation. These processes occlude the blood supply by acting like a tourniquet. If they are untreated, ischemia, paresthesias, and necrosis can occur. To restore circulation to compromised extremities, an escharotomy (a scalpel or electrocautery incision into necrotic tissue) is frequently performed after the patient's transfer to a burn unit (Figure 27.8).

Initially, blood viscosity increases with burn injuries because of fluid loss occurring in the emergent period. Microcirculation is impaired because of damage to skin structures containing small capillary systems. These two events result in a phenomenon termed *sludging*. Sludging can be corrected by adequate fluid replacement.

Respiratory System. The respiratory system is especially vulnerable to two types of injury: (a) upper airway burns, which cause edema formation and obstruction of the airway, and (b) lower airway injury (see Table 27.3). Upper airway distress may occur with or without smoke inhalation, and airway injury at either level may occur in the absence of burn injury to the skin.

Upper Airway Injury. Upper airway injury results from an inhalation injury to the mouth, oropharynx, or larynx. The injury may be caused by thermal burns or the inhalation of hot air, steam, or smoke. Mucosal burns of the oropharynx and larynx are manifested by redness, blistering, and edema. The swelling can be massive, and the onset rapid. Flame burns to the neck and chest may make breathing more difficult because of burn eschar, which becomes tight and constricting from underlying edema. Swelling from scald burns to the face and neck can also

TABLE 27.10 EMERGENCY MANAGEMENT

Thermal Burns

Cause	Assessment Findings	Interventions
• Hot liquids or solids • Flash flame • Open flame • Steam • Hot surface • UV rays	**Partial-Thickness Burn** ***Superficial; First-Degree Burn*** • Redness • Pain • Moderate to severe tenderness • Minimal edema • Blanching with pressure ***Deep; Second-Degree Burn*** • Moist blebs, blisters • Mottled white, pink to cherry red • Hypersensitive to touch or air • Moderate to severe pain • Blanching with pressure **Full-Thickness; Third- or Fourth-Degree Burn** • Dry, leathery eschar • White, waxy, dark brown, or charred appearance • Strong burn odour • Impaired sensation when touched • Absence of pain with severe pain in surrounding tissues • Lack of blanching with pressure	**Initial** 1. If unresponsive, assess circulation, airway, and breathing. If responsive, monitor airway, breathing, and circulation. 2. Stabilize cervical spine. 3. Assess for inhalation injury. 4. Provide supplemental oxygen as needed. 5. Anticipate endotracheal intubation and mechanical ventilation with circumferential, full-thickness burns to the neck, trunk, or both or with large TBSA. 6. Monitor vital signs, level of consciousness, respiratory status, oxygen saturation, and cardiac rhythm. 7. Remove nonadherent clothing, shoes, watches, jewellery, and, if face was exposed, glasses or contact lenses. 8. Cover burned areas with dry dressings or clean sheet if TBSA is large or patient is hypothermic; cover with normal saline–moistened gauze and dry sheet if TBSA is small. 9. Establish IV access with two large-bore catheters if burn >15% TBSA. 10. Begin fluid replacement. 11. Insert urinary catheter if burn >15% TBSA. 12. Elevate burned limb(s) above level of heart to decrease edema. 13. Administer IV analgesic drug and assess effectiveness frequently. 14. Identify and treat other associated injuries (e.g., fractures, pneumothorax, head injury). **Ongoing Monitoring** • Monitor airway, breathing, and circulation. • Monitor vital signs, cardiac rhythm, level of consciousness, respiratory status, and oxygen saturation. • Monitor urine output. • Monitor pain level.

IV, intravenous; *TBSA*, total body surface area; *UV*, ultraviolet.

be lethal, as can external pressure from edema pressing on the airway. Mechanical obstruction can occur quickly, presenting a true airway emergency.

The patient must be carefully assessed for facial burns, singed nasal hair, hoarseness, painful swallowing, darkened oral and nasal membranes, carbonaceous sputum, history of being burned in an enclosed space, and clothing burns around the neck and trunk.

Lower Airway Injury. An inhalation injury to the trachea, bronchioles, and alveoli is usually caused by breathing in toxic chemicals or smoke. Tissue damage is related to the duration of exposure to toxic fumes or smoke. Clinical manifestations of lower airway lung injury are presented in Table 27.3. Pulmonary edema may not appear until 12 to 48 hours after the burn and may manifest as acute respiratory distress syndrome (ARDS) (see Chapter 71).

Other Cardiopulmonary Complications. Burn-injured patients with pre-existing heart disease (e.g., myocardial infarction) or lung disease (e.g., chronic obstructive pulmonary disease) are at risk for complications. If fluid replacement is too vigorous, these patients can develop heart failure or pulmonary edema. Invasive measures (e.g., hemodynamic monitoring) may be necessary to monitor fluid resuscitation.

Burn-injured patients with pre-existing respiratory conditions are more likely to develop a respiratory infection.

Pneumonia is a common complication of major burns and the leading cause of death in patients with inhalation injury. Debilitation, abundant microbial flora, and relative immobility predispose such patients to development of pneumonia.

Urinary System. The most common complication of the urinary system in the emergent phase is ATN. If the patient becomes hypovolemic, blood flow to the kidneys decreases, causing renal ischemia. If the decreased flow rate continues, acute kidney injury may develop.

With full-thickness and electrical burns, myoglobin (from muscle cell breakdown) and hemoglobin (from RBC breakdown) are released into the bloodstream and occlude renal tubules. Adequate fluid replacement and diuretics can counteract myoglobin and hemoglobin obstruction of the tubules.

NURSING AND INTERPROFESSIONAL MANAGEMENT EMERGENT PHASE

In the emergent phase, patient survival depends on rapid and thorough assessment and intervention (Fahlstrom et al., 2013). The nurse and physician make the initial assessment of depth and extent of the burn and coordinate the actions of the health care team. In a community hospital, decisions must be made as to whether the patient requires inpatient or outpatient care and, in the case of inpatient care, whether the patient remains in that

PATHOPHYSIOLOGY MAP

```
            ┌──────────┐
            │   BURN   │
            └──────────┘
                 │
                 ▼
      ┌────────────────────────┐
      │ ↑ Vascular permeability │
      └────────────────────────┘
          │              │
          ▼              ▼
    ┌──────────┐   ┌──────────────┐
    │  Edema   │   │ ↓ Intravascular │
    │          │   │    volume     │
    └──────────┘   └──────────────┘
         │               │
         ▼               ▼
  ┌────────────────┐  ┌─────────────┐
  │ ↓ Blood volume │  │ ↑ Hematocrit │
  └────────────────┘  └─────────────┘
         │               │
         │               ▼
         │          ┌─────────────┐
         │          │ ↑ Viscosity │
         │          └─────────────┘
         │               │
         ▼               ▼
  ┌──────────────────────────────┐
  │    ↑ Peripheral resistance    │
  └──────────────────────────────┘
                 │
                 ▼
          ┌──────────────┐
          │  Burn shock   │
          └──────────────┘
```

FIG. 27.5 At the time of a major burn injury, there is increased capillary permeability. All fluid components of the blood begin to leak into the interstitium, causing edema and a decrease in blood volume. Hematocrit increases, and the blood becomes more viscous. The combination of decreased blood volume and increased viscosity produces increased peripheral resistance. Burn shock, a type of hypovolemic shock, rapidly ensues, and, if it is not corrected, death can result.

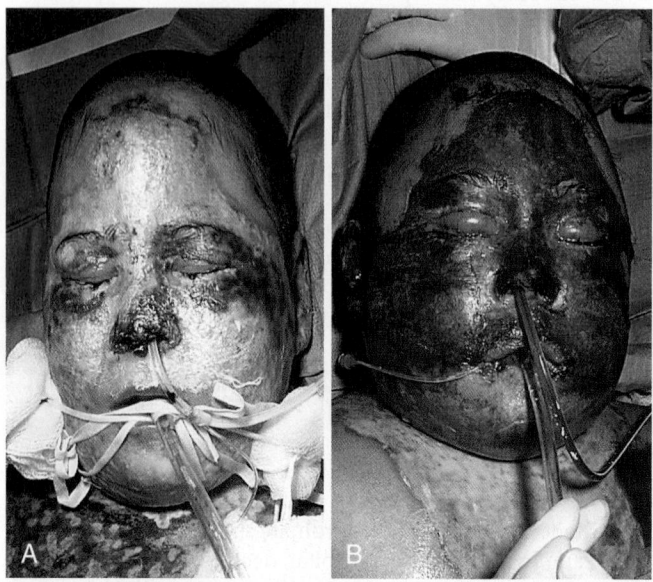

FIG. 27.6 A, Facial edema before fluid resuscitation. **B,** Facial edema after 24 hours. Source: Courtesy Judy Knighton, Toronto, Canada.

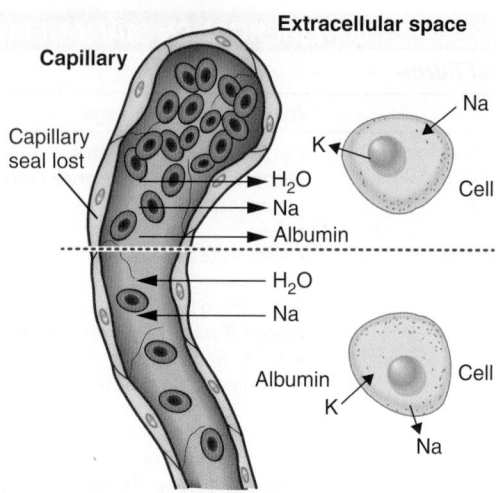

FIG. 27.7 The effects of burn shock are shown above the dotted line. As the capillary seal is lost, interstitial edema develops. The cellular integrity is also altered, with sodium *(Na)* moving into the cell in abnormal amounts and potassium *(K)* leaving the cell. The shifts after the resolution of burn shock are shown below the dotted line. The water and sodium move back into the circulating volume through the capillary. The albumin remains in the interstitium. Potassium is transported into the cell, and sodium is transported out as the cellular integrity returns.

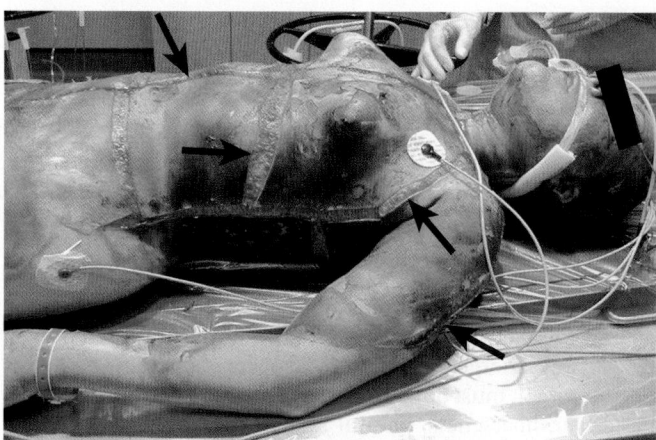

FIG. 27.8 Escharotomies of the anterior chest and arm (indicated by *arrows*). Source: Courtesy Judy A. Knighton, RN, MScN, Toronto.

hospital or is transferred to the closest regional burn unit (see Table 27.5). From the onset of the burn event until the patient is stabilized, nursing and interprofessional management consist predominantly of airway management, fluid therapy, and wound care (Table 27.11).

Although burn management can be chronologically categorized as emergent, acute, and rehabilitative, overall care requirements are not so easily classified. Depending on the severity of the patient's condition, the duration of time spent in each phase varies greatly, and conditions improve and worsen unpredictably on a daily basis. Care changes accordingly. Whereas physiotherapy and occupational therapy are a focus of the acute and rehabilitative phases, proper positioning and splinting begin at the time of admission. Support and teaching of patients and caregivers begin on admission and intensify in the rehabilitative phase. See the accompanying nursing care

TABLE 27.11 INTERPROFESSIONAL CARE
Patient With Burn Injury

Emergent Phase	Acute Phase	Rehabilitation Phase
Fluid Therapy • Assess fluid needs.* • Begin IV fluid replacement. • Insert urinary catheter. • Monitor intake and output. **Wound Care** • Start daily shower/cleansing and wound care. • Debride as necessary. • Assess extent and depth of burns. • Administer tetanus toxoid or tetanus antitoxin. **Pain and Anxiety** • Assess and manage pain and anxiety. **Psychosocial Care** • Provide support to patient and family during initial crisis phase. **Respiratory Therapy** • Assess oxygenation needs. • Provide supplemental oxygen as needed. • Intubate if necessary. • Monitor respiratory status. **Physiotherapy and Occupational Therapy** • Place patient in position that prevents contracture formation and reduces edema. • Assess need for splints or devices such as pressure relief/reduction mattresses to decrease tissue ischemia and potential for skin breakdown. • Turn and reposition patient frequently to allow for appropriate circulation to tissues. **Nutritional Therapy** • Assess nutritional needs and begin feeding patient by most appropriate route as soon as possible.	**Fluid Therapy** • Continue to monitor intake and output. • Continue to replace fluids, depending on patient's clinical response. **Wound Care** • Continue daily shower and wound care. • Assess wound daily and adjust dressing protocols as necessary. • Observe for complications (e.g., infection). • Continue debridement (if necessary). **Pain and Anxiety** • Continue to assess for and treat pain and anxiety. **Psychosocial Care** • Continue to provide ongoing support, counselling, and education to patient and family about physical and emotional aspects of care and recovery. • Begin to anticipate discharge needs. **Respiratory Therapy** • Continue to assess oxygenation needs. • Continue to monitor respiratory status. • Monitor for signs of complications (e.g., pneumonia). **Physiotherapy and Occupational Therapy** • Have patient begin daily therapy program for maintenance of range of motion. • Assess need for splints and anticontracture positioning. • Encourage and assist patient with self-care as possible. **Nutritional Therapy** • Continue to assess diet to support wound healing. **Other Therapy** ***Early Excision and Grafting*** • Provide temporary homografts. • Provide permanent autografts. • Care for donor sites. ***Medication Therapy**** • Assess need for medications. • Continue to monitor effectiveness of and necessity for medications. • Titrate medications and discontinue as appropriate.	• Continue to counsel and teach patient and caregiver about wound care. • Discuss possible need for home care to continue wound care in the community. • Continue to counsel and teach patient and family. • Continue to encourage and assist patient in resuming self-care. • Continue to prevent or minimize contractures (surgery, physiotherapy and occupational therapy, splinting, or pressure garments), and assess likelihood for scarring. • Discuss possible reconstructive surgery. • Prepare for discharge home or transfer to rehabilitation unit or hospital.

IV, intravenous.
*See Tables 27.12, 27.13, and 27.14.

plan NCP 27.1 (Patient With a Thermal Burn Injury) on the Evolve website.

AIRWAY MANAGEMENT
Airway management frequently involves early endotracheal (preferably orotracheal) intubation. Early intubation eliminates the necessity for emergency tracheostomy after respiratory complications have become apparent. In general, patients with major injuries that include burns to the face and neck require intubation within 1 to 2 hours after burn injury. (Intubation is discussed in Chapter 68.) After intubation, such patients are placed on ventilatory assistance, and the delivered oxygen concentration is determined from an assessment of arterial blood gas (ABG) values. Extubation may be indicated when the edema resolves, usually 3 to 6 days after burn injury, unless severe inhalation injury is involved. Escharotomies of the trunk may be needed to relieve respiratory distress secondary to circumferential, full-thickness burns to the neck and trunk (see Figure 27.8).

Within 6 to 12 hours after injury in which smoke inhalation is suspected, a fibre-optic bronchoscopy should be performed to assess the lower airway. Significant findings include the appearance of carbonaceous material, mucosal edema, vesicles, erythema, hemorrhage, and ulceration.

When intubation is not performed, treatment of inhalation injury includes administration of 100% humidified oxygen as needed. Patients should be placed in a high Fowler's position unless it is contraindicated (e.g., because of spinal injury), and coughing and deep breathing every hour should be encouraged. Patients should be repositioned every 1 to 2 hours and chest physiotherapy and suctioning performed as necessary. If respiratory failure develops, intubation and mechanical ventilation are initiated. Positive end-expiratory pressure (PEEP), a method of ventilation in which airway pressure is maintained above atmospheric pressure at the end of exhalation by mechanical means, may be used to prevent collapse of the alveoli and progressive respiratory failure (see Chapter 68). Bronchodilators may be administered to treat severe bronchospasm. Carbon monoxide poisoning is treated by administering 100% oxygen until carboxyhemoglobin levels return to normal. The use of hyperbaric oxygen therapy to treat carbon monoxide poisoning is contraindicated in the presence of a body burn as it delays important burn care.

FLUID THERAPY

Establishing intravenous (IV) access that can accommodate large volumes of fluid is critical for fluid resuscitation and medication administration. At least two large-bore IV access routes must be obtained for patients with burns over more than 15% TBSA. For patients with burns over more than 30% TBSA, a central line for fluid and medication administration, as well as a line for blood sampling, should be considered if frequent ABGs or invasive BP monitoring is needed.

A standardized chart is used to assess the extent of the burn wound (see Figure 27.4), allowing for accurate estimation of fluid resuscitation requirements.

The type of fluid replacement is determined by size and depth of burn, age of the patient, and individual considerations, such as pre-existing chronic illness. Fluid replacement is accomplished with crystalloid solutions (usually lactated Ringer's solution), colloids (albumin), or a combination of the two. Paramedics generally administer IV saline until the patient's arrival at the hospital.

The Parkland (Baxter) formula for fluid replacement is the formula most commonly used to estimate fluid replacement (Table 27.12; see also the Parkland Formula for Burns calculator in the Resources for this chapter). It is important to remember that all formulas yield estimates, which must be titrated on the basis of the patient's physiological response. For example, in patients with an electrical injury or inhalation injury, fluid requirements may be greater than normal and include an osmotic diuretic (mannitol) and sodium bicarbonate to alkalize the urine. Too much fluid and overestimation of TBSA contribute to the development of fluid over-resuscitation or "fluid creep" (Greenhalgh, 2019).

Colloidal solutions (e.g., albumin) may be given. However, administration is recommended in the first 12 to 24 hours after the burn injury, when capillary permeability returns to normal or near normal. After this time, the plasma remains in the vascular space and expands the circulating volume. The replacement volume is calculated on the basis of the patient's body

TABLE 27.12	FLUID RESUSCITATION WITH THE PARKLAND (BAXTER) FORMULA*

Formula
4 mL of lactated Ringer's solution per kilogram of body weight per percentage of TBSA burned = Total fluid requirements for first 24 hr after burn

Application
50% of total in first 8 hr
25% of total in second 8 hr
25% of total in third 8 hr

Example
For a 70-kg patient with a burn on 50% of TBSA:

4 mL × 70 kg × 50% of TBSA burned	=	14 000 mL, or 14 L, in 24 hr
50% of total in first 8 hr	=	7000 mL (875 mL/hr)
25% of total in second 8 hr	=	3500 mL (438 mL/hr)
25% of total in third 8 hr	=	3500 mL (438 mL/hr)

TBSA, total body surface area.
*Formulas are guidelines. Fluid is administered at a rate to produce 0.5–1.0 mL/kg/hr of urine output.

weight and TBSA burned (e.g., 0.3 to 0.5 mL/kg per percentage of TBSA burned).

The adequacy of fluid replacement is best assessed according to clinical parameters. Urine output, the most commonly used parameter, and cardiac parameters are defined as follows:

1. *Urine output:* The goal is generally 0.5 to 1 mL/kg/hour for most patients with burn injuries but increases to 75 to 100 mL/hour for patients with an electrical burn and evidence of hemoglobinuria or myoglobinuria.
2. *Cardiac factors:* Mean arterial pressure is greater than 65 mm Hg, systolic BP is greater than 90 mm Hg, and heart rate is less than 120 beats/minute. Mean arterial pressure and BP are most appropriately measured by means of an arterial line. Peripheral measurement is often invalid because of vasoconstriction and edema.

WOUND CARE

Once a patent airway, adequate circulation, and adequate fluid replacement have been established, the priority is care of the burn wound. Full-thickness burn wounds are dry and waxy white to dark brown or black and have only minor, localized sensation because nerve endings have largely been destroyed. Partial-thickness burn wounds appear pink to cherry red and are wet and shiny with serous exudate. These wounds may or may not have intact blisters and are painful when touched or open to air because of exposed nerve endings.

Cleansing and gentle debridement, with the use of scissors and forceps, can occur on a cart shower (Figure 27.9), a regular shower, or the patient's bed or stretcher. Extensive, surgical debridement (Figure 27.10) is performed in the operating room. During debridement, necrotic skin is removed from the wound to prevent infection and promote healing. Releasing escharotomies and fasciotomies can be carried out in the emergent phase, usually in burn units by burn physicians.

Patients find the initial wound care to be both physically and psychologically demanding. Patients are showered with tap water not exceeding 40°C. A once-daily shower and dressing change in the morning, followed by a dressing change in the patient's room in the evening, are part of a common routine

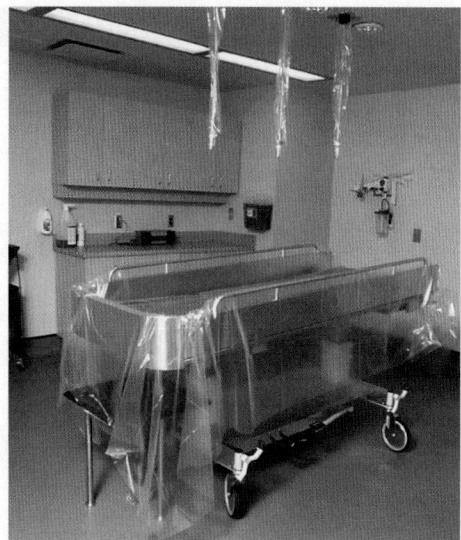

FIG. 27.9 Cart shower. Showering presents an opportunity for wound care and physiotherapy. Source: Courtesy Judy A. Knighton, RN, MScN, Toronto.

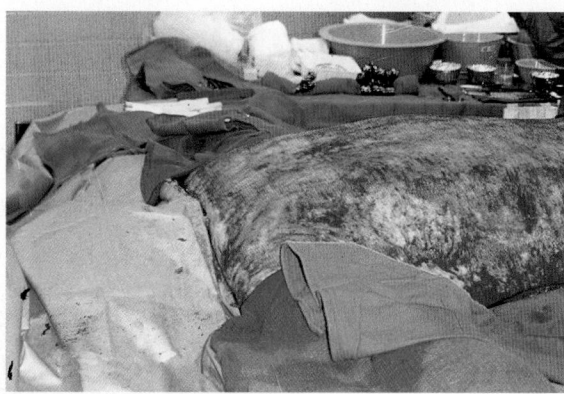

FIG. 27.10 Surgical debridement of full-thickness burns is necessary to prepare the wound for grafting. Source: Courtesy Judy Knighton, Toronto, Canada.

in many burn units. Some of the newer antimicrobial dressings can be left in place from 3 to 14 days, thereby decreasing the frequency of dressing changes.

The source of infection in burn wounds can be the patient's own flora, predominantly from the skin (burned and unburned), respiratory tract, and gastrointestinal tract. Increased opportunity for infection occurs following invasive hospital procedures such as central line placement (Manning, 2018). The prevention of cross-contamination between one patient and another is a priority for all members of the interprofessional health care team.

Two approaches to burn wound treatment are the open method and the closed method, using multiple dressing changes. In the *open method*, the patient's burn is covered with a topical antimicrobial and has no dressing over the wound. In the *multiple–dressing change* or *closed method*, sterile gauze dressings are impregnated with or laid over a topical antimicrobial. These dressings are changed at various intervals, from every 12 to 24 hours to once every 14 days, depending on the product. Most burn units support the concept of moist wound

healing and use dressings to cover the burned areas, except for the burned face.

When the patient's open burn wounds are exposed, staff must wear personal protective equipment (PPE) (e.g., disposable hats, masks, gowns, gloves). Increased levels of PPE are required when caring for burn patients with suspected SARS-CoV-2 infection. When removing contaminated dressings and washing the dirty wound, the nurse may use nonsterile, disposable gloves. Sterile gloves, however, are used when applying ointments and sterile dressings. In addition, the room must be kept warm (approximately 30°C) to prevent the patient from using up valuable calories through shivering. When finished treating one patient, the nurse removes all PPE and dons new PPE before treating another patient to avoid transmitting organisms from one patient to another. Careful hand hygiene and the use of alcohol-based hand rub, both inside and outside each patient room, is also necessary to prevent cross-contamination. After the dressing change is completed, the equipment and immediate environment are thoroughly cleaned and disinfected. The use of plastic liners on equipment is helpful in reducing the potential contamination of the equipment and facilitates cleaning.

Coverage is the primary goal for burn wounds. In the major burn wound (>50% TBSA), there is rarely enough unburned skin for immediate grafting. This necessitates the use of other temporary wound closure methods. *Allograft (homograft) skin* (from a cadaver skin bank) is used, along with newer biosynthetic options, with varying frequency among burn units (Table 27.13).

OTHER CARE MEASURES

For certain parts of the body (e.g., face, eyes, hands, arms, ears, perineum), nursing care must be particularly meticulous. The face is highly vascular and subject to a great amount of edema. It is often covered with ointments and gauze but not wrapped, to limit pressure on delicate facial structures. Eye care for corneal burns or edema includes antibiotic ointments. All patients with facial burns should undergo an ophthalmological examination soon after admission. Periorbital edema can prevent opening of the eyes and be frightening to the patient. The nurse should provide assurance that the swelling is not permanent. Instillation of methyl cellulose drops or artificial tears into the eyes for moisture provides additional comfort for patients.

Burned hands and arms should be extended and elevated on pillows to minimize edema. Splints may need to be applied to maintain them in positions of function. Ears should be kept free of pressure because of their poor vascularization and predisposition to infection. A patient with ear burns should not rest their head on pillows because pressure on the cartilage may cause chondritis and the ear may stick to the pillowcase, causing pain and bleeding. The patient's head can be elevated with a rolled towel placed under the shoulders, with care to avoid pressure necrosis. The same holds true for a patient with neck burns. Pillows are removed and a rolled towel is placed under the shoulders to hyperextend the neck and prevent neck wound contracture.

The perineum must be kept as clean and dry as possible. In addition to providing hourly urine outputs, an in-dwelling catheter prevents urine contamination of the perineal area.

Routine laboratory tests are performed to monitor fluid and electrolyte balance. ABGs are measured to determine adequacy

TABLE 27.13   SOURCES OF GRAFTS

Source	Graft Name	Coverage
Porcine skin	Heterograft or xenograft (different species)	Temporary (3 days to 2 wk)
Cadaveric skin	Homograft or allograft (same species)	Temporary (3 days to 2 wk)
Patient's own skin	Autograft	Permanent
Patient's own skin and cell cultures	Cultured epithelial autograft (CEA)	Permanent
Porcine collagen bonded to silicone membrane	Biobrane	Temporary (10–21 days)
Bovine collagen and glycosaminoglycan bonded to silicone membrane	Integra	Permanent
Acellular dermal matrix derived from donated human skin	AlloDerm	Permanent
Donated neonatal foreskin fibroblasts and keratinocytes in bovine collagen sponge	OrCel	Permanent
Donated neonatal foreskin fibroblasts and keratinocytes in bovine collagen gel	Apligraf	Permanent
Bovine collagen and elastin matrix	MatriDerm	Permanent

TABLE 27.14   MEDICATION THERAPY

Medications Commonly Used in Burn Treatment

Types and Names of Medications	Purpose
Nutritional Support	
Vitamins A, C, E, and multivitamins	Promote wound healing
Minerals: zinc, iron (ferrous sulphate)	Promote cell integrity and hemoglobin formation
Analgesia	
Morphine (Statex)	Promote pain control
Sustained-release morphine (MS Contin)	
Hydromorphone (Dilaudid)	
Sustained-release hydromorphone (Dilaudid)	
Fentanyl	
Acetaminophen (Tylenol)	
Ibuprofen (Advil)	
Adjuvant analgesics (e.g., gabapentin [Neurontin], pregabalin [Lyrica])	
Sedation–Hypnosis	
Quetiapine (Seroquel)	Produce antipsychotic and sedative effects
Haloperidol (Haldol)	
Lorazepam (Ativan)	Diminish anxiety
Midazolam	Provide short-acting
Ketamine (Ketalar)	amnestic effects
Antidepressant Therapy	
Venlafaxine (Effexor XR)	Reduce depression; improve mood
Citalopram (Celexa)	
Anticoagulation Therapy	
Enoxaparin (Lovenox)	Prevent venous thromboembolism
Heparin	
Gastrointestinal Support	
Ranitidine (Zantac)	Decrease stomach acid and risk for Curling's ulcer
Esomeprazole (Nexium)	
Aluminum/magnesium hydroxide (Diovol)	Neutralize stomach acid

of ventilation and perfusion in all patients with suspected or confirmed inhalation or electrical injury.

Physiotherapy is begun immediately, sometimes during showering and dressing changes and before new dressings are applied. Early range-of-motion exercises are necessary to facilitate mobilization of the extravasated fluid back into the vascular bed. Exercise also maintains function, prevents contracture, and reassures the patient that movement is still possible.

MEDICATION THERAPY

ANALGESICS AND SEDATIVES. Analgesics are ordered to promote patient comfort. Early in the postburn period, pain medications should be given intravenously because (a) onset of action is fastest with this route; (b) gastrointestinal function is slowed or impaired as a result of shock or paralytic ileus; and (c) medications injected intramuscularly are not absorbed adequately in burned or edematous areas, and so medications pool in the tissues. When fluid mobilization begins, interstitial accumulation of previous intramuscular medications could cause inadvertent overdose.

Opioids commonly used for pain control are listed in Table 27.14. The need for analgesia must be re-evaluated frequently because patients' needs may change and tolerance to medications may develop over time. Initially, opioids are the drugs of choice for pain control. Sedative–hypnotics and antidepressant drugs can also be given with analgesics to control the anxiety, insomnia, or depression that patients may experience (see Table 27.14). Analgesic requirements can vary tremendously from one patient to another. The extent and depth of burn may not be correlated with pain intensity. Hospital pharmacists, psychiatrists, and multidisciplinary pain services are valuable resources for the more complex patient situations. Effective pain control depends on assessment, prompt analgesia with dosages titrated to achieve effect, and regular evaluation.

TETANUS IMMUNIZATION. Tetanus toxoid is given routinely to all patients with burn injuries because of the likelihood of anaerobic contamination of the burn wound. If the patient has not received an active immunization in the 10 years before the burn injury, tetanus immunoglobulin should be considered.

ANTIMICROBIAL AGENTS. After the wound is cleansed, topical agents are applied and covered with a light dressing. Systemic antibiotics are not routinely used to control burn wound flora because there is little or no blood supply to the burn eschar and, consequently, little delivery of the antibiotic to the wound. In addition, the routine use of systemic antibiotics increases the chance of developing multidrug-resistant organisms. Some topical burn agents penetrate the eschar, thereby inhibiting bacterial invasion of the wound. Silver-impregnated dressings (e.g., Acticoat Flex, Aquacel Ag Burn, Exsalt T7) can be left in place anywhere from 3 to 14 days and are effective against many organisms. Silver sulphadiazine (Flamazine) and mafenide acetate (Sulfamylon) creams are also used (Cartotto, 2017). Sepsis remains a leading cause of death in patients with major burns because it may lead to multiple organ dysfunction syndrome (see Chapter 69). Systemic antibiotic therapy is initiated when invasive burn wound sepsis is clinically diagnosed or when some other source of infection (e.g., pneumonia) is identified.

Fungal infections may develop in the patient's mucous membranes (mouth and genitalia) as a result of systemic antibiotic therapy and low resistance in the host. The offending organism is usually *Candida albicans*. Oral infection is treated with nystatin mouthwash. When a normal diet is resumed, yogourt or *Lactobacillus* may be given by mouth to reintroduce the normal intestinal flora that have been destroyed by antibiotic therapy.

VENOUS THROMBOEMBOLISM PROPHYLAXIS. For burn-injured patients at risk for venous thromboembolism (e.g., those with lower extremity burns, patients with obesity), if there are no contraindications, it is recommended that low-molecular-weight heparin (enoxaparin [Lovenox]) or low-dose unfractionated heparin be started as soon as it is considered safe to do so (see Table 27.14). For any patients who are at high risk for bleeding, it is recommended that mechanical prophylaxis against venous thromboembolism, with sequential compression devices or graduated compression stockings, or both, be used until the bleeding risk decreases and heparin can be started (Weinberger & Cipolle, 2016) (see Table 27.14).

NUTRITIONAL THERAPY

The metabolic rate of burn patients can exceed twice the normal rate, and without early and aggressive nutritional support within several hours of the burn injury, impaired wound healing, organ dysfunction, and susceptibility to infection can occur (Clark et al., 2017). Nonintubated patients with a burn over less than 20% TBSA are generally able to eat enough to meet their nutritional requirements. Intubated patients and those with larger burns require additional support. Enteral feedings (gastric or intestinal) have almost entirely replaced parenteral feeding. Early enteral feeding, usually with smaller-bore tubes, preserves gastrointestinal function, increases intestinal blood flow, promotes optimal conditions for wound healing, and prevents complications (e.g., Curling's ulcer). The patient with a large burn (greater than 20% TBSA) can develop paralytic ileus within a few hours as a result of the body's response to major trauma. If a large nasogastric tube is inserted on admission, gastric residuals should be checked frequently to detect delayed gastric emptying. Bowel sounds should be assessed every 8 hours. In general, feedings can begin slowly at 20 to 40 mL/hour and be increased to the goal rate within 24 to 48 hours.

A *hypermetabolic state* proportional to the size of the wound occurs after a major burn injury. Resting metabolic expenditure may increase by 50 to 100% above normal in patients with major burns. Core temperature is elevated. Catecholamines, which stimulate catabolism and heat production, increase. Massive catabolism can occur and is characterized by protein breakdown and increased gluconeogenesis. Failure to supply adequate calories and protein leads to malnutrition and delayed healing. Calorie-containing nutritional supplements and milkshakes are often administered because of the great need for calories. Protein powder can also be added to food and liquids.

Decreased levels of vitamins A, C, and D and iron, copper, selenium, and zinc have been found to negatively affect wound healing and skeletal and immune function. Supplemental vitamins should ideally be initiated within 24 hours of injury (Clark et al., 2017; see Table 27.14).

ACUTE PHASE

The *acute phase* begins with mobilization of extracellular fluid and subsequent diuresis. This phase concludes when the burned area is completely covered by skin grafts or when the wounds are healed. This may take weeks or many months.

Pathophysiological Changes

Burn injury involves pathophysiological changes in many body systems. Diuresis from fluid mobilization occurs, and the patient becomes less edematous. Areas that are full- or partial-thickness burns are more evident than in the emergent phase. Bowel sounds return. The patient may now become aware of the enormity of the situation and benefit from additional psychosocial support. Some healing begins as WBCs surround the burn wound and phagocytosis occurs. Necrotic tissue begins to slough. Fibroblasts lay down matrices of the collagen precursors that eventually form granulation tissue. A partial-thickness burn wound heals from the edges and the dermal bed below if kept free from infection and *desiccation* (dryness). However, full-thickness burn wounds, unless extremely small, must be covered by skin grafts. In some cases, healing time and length of hospitalization are decreased by early excision and grafting.

Clinical Manifestations

Partial-thickness wounds form eschar, which begins separating fairly soon after injury. Once the eschar is removed, re-epithelialization begins at the wound margins and appears as red or pink scar tissue. Epithelial buds from the dermal bed eventually close in the wound, which then heals spontaneously without surgical intervention, usually within 10 to 21 days.

Margins of full-thickness eschar take longer to separate. As a result, full-thickness wounds necessitate surgical debridement and skin grafting for healing.

Laboratory Values

Because the body is attempting to re-establish fluid and electrolyte homeostasis in the initial acute phase, it is important to monitor serum electrolyte levels closely.

Sodium. *Hyponatremia* can develop from excessive gastrointestinal suction, diarrhea, and excessive water intake. Manifestations of hyponatremia include weakness, dizziness, muscle cramps, fatigue, headache, tachycardia, and confusion. The patient with burn injuries may also develop *water intoxication*, a dilutional form of hyponatremia. To avoid this condition, the patient should drink fluids other than water, such as juice or nutritional supplements.

Hypernatremia may occur after successful fluid replacement if copious amounts of hypertonic solutions were required. Other causes may be related to tube-feeding therapy or inappropriate fluid administration. Manifestations of hypernatremia include thirst; dry, coated tongue; lethargy; confusion; and possibly seizures.

Potassium. *Hyperkalemia* is noted if the patient has renal failure, adrenocortical insufficiency, or massive deep muscle injury (e.g., electrical burn) and if large amounts of potassium are being released from damaged cells. Cardiac dysrhythmias and ventricular failure can occur with elevated potassium levels. Muscle weakness and electrocardiographic changes are observed clinically (see Chapter 19).

Hypokalemia occurs with vomiting, diarrhea, prolonged gastrointestinal suction, and prolonged IV therapy without potassium supplementation. Constant potassium loss occurs through the burn wound. Manifestations of hypokalemia include fatigue, muscle weakness, leg cramps, paresthesias, and decreased reflexes (see Chapter 19).

Complications

Infection. The body's first line of defence, the skin, is destroyed by burn injury. Pathogens often proliferate before phagocytosis has adequately begun. The burn wound becomes colonized with organisms. If the bacterial density at the junction of the eschar with underlying viable tissue rises to greater than 10^5 bacteria/g of tissue, the burn wound is considered infected. In the presence of an infection, localized inflammation, induration, and sometimes suppuration can occur at the burn wound margins. Partial-thickness burns can convert to full-thickness wounds when the infecting organisms invade viable, adjacent, unburned tissue. Invasive wound infections may be treated with systemic antibiotics on the basis of culture results.

Burn wound infection may progress to transient bacteremia and sepsis as a result of burn wound manipulation (e.g., after showering and debridement). Manifestations of sepsis include hypothermia or hyperthermia, increased heart and respiratory rates, decreased BP, and decreased urine output. Patients may exhibit mild confusion, chills, malaise, and loss of appetite. The WBC count is usually between 10 and 20×10^9/L.

There are functional deficits in the WBCs, and the patient remains immunosuppressed for a time after the burn injury. The causative organisms of sepsis are usually Gram-negative bacteria (e.g., *Pseudomonas*, *Proteus* organisms), which increase the risk for septic shock.

When sepsis is suspected, cultures are immediately obtained from all possible sources, including the burn wound, blood, urine, sputum, oropharynx, perineal regions, and any invasive line or tube sites. However, treatment should not be delayed pending results of the culture and sensitivity studies. Therapy begins with antibiotics appropriate for the usual residual flora of the particular burn unit. The topical antibiotic in use may be continued or changed to another medication. At this stage, the patient's condition is critical, and vital signs must be monitored closely. Collaboration with infectious disease specialists is important to ensure appropriate antibiotic coverage.

Cardiovascular and Respiratory Systems. The same cardiovascular and respiratory system complications present in the emergent phase may continue into the acute phase of care. In addition, new complications might arise, necessitating timely intervention.

Neurological System. Neurologically, the patient usually has no physical symptoms, unless severe hypoxia from respiratory injuries or complications from electrical injuries occur. However, some patients may demonstrate certain behaviours that are not completely understood. A patient can become extremely disoriented, become withdrawn or combative, or have hallucinations and nightmare-like episodes. Delirium is more acute at night and occurs more often in older patients. Consultation with psychiatric or geriatric services is helpful in quickly diagnosing and treating delirium or similar behaviours. The nurse can then focus on strategies to orient and reassure a confused or agitated patient. Delirium is a transient state, lasting from a day or two to several weeks. Various causes have been considered, including electrolyte imbalance, stress, cerebral edema, sepsis, sleep disturbances, and the use of analgesics and antianxiety drugs.

Musculoskeletal System. The musculoskeletal system is prone to complications during the acute phase. As the burns begin to heal and scar tissue forms, the skin is less supple and pliant. Range of motion may be limited, and contractures can occur. The muscles in the body tend to shorten in a flexed position. The patient should be encouraged to stretch and move the burned body parts as much as possible. Splinting can be beneficial in preventing or reducing contracture formation. Attention to repositioning and the use of devices such as pressure-redistribution mattresses may also be necessary to decrease the potential for tissue ischemia and skin breakdown.

Gastrointestinal System. The gastrointestinal system may also exhibit complications during this phase. Paralytic ileus results from sepsis. Diarrhea may be caused by the use of enteral feedings or antibiotics. Constipation can occur as an adverse effect of opioid analgesics, decreased mobility, and a low-fibre diet. *Curling's ulcer* is a type of gastroduodenal ulcer characterized by diffuse superficial lesions (including mucosal erosion). It is caused by a generalized stress response to decreased blood flow to the gastrointestinal tract during the emergent phase; this response results in decreased production of mucus and increased secretion of gastric acid. The best measure for preventing Curling's ulcer is feeding the patient soon after the injury. Antacids, H_2-histamine blockers (e.g., ranitidine [Zantac]), and proton pump inhibitors (e.g., esomeprazole [Nexium]) are used prophylactically to neutralize stomach acids and inhibit the secretion of histamine and hydrochloric acid (see Table 27.14).

Endocrine System. A transient increase in blood glucose levels may occur because of stress-mediated cortisol and catecholamine release, which results in increased mobilization of glycogen stores, gluconeogenesis, and subsequent production of glucose. Insulin production and release also increase. However, insulin's effectiveness decreases because of relative insulin insensitivity; consequently, the blood glucose level becomes elevated. Later, hyperglycemia can be caused by the increased caloric intake necessary to meet metabolic requirements. When hyperglycemia occurs, the treatment is supplemental IV insulin, not decreased feeding. Serum glucose levels are checked frequently, and an appropriate amount of insulin is given if hyperglycemia is present. Glucometers may be used to assess blood glucose at the patient's bedside; however, serum glucose samples yield more accurate results. As the patient's metabolic demands are met and less stress is placed on the entire system, this stress-induced condition may be reversed before or at time of discharge.

NURSING AND INTERPROFESSIONAL MANAGEMENT ACUTE PHASE

The predominant therapeutic interventions in the acute phase are (a) wound care, (b) excision and grafting, (c) pain management, (d) physiotherapy and occupational therapy, (e) nutritional therapy, and (f) psychosocial care.

WOUND CARE

The goals of wound care are to (a) prevent infection by cleansing and debriding the area of necrotic tissue that would promote bacterial growth and (b) promote wound re-epithelialization, successful skin grafting, or both.

Wound care consists of daily observation, assessment, cleansing, debridement, and dressing reapplication. Nonsurgical debridement, dressing changes, topical antimicrobial therapy, graft care, and donor site care are performed as necessary, depending on the topical cream or dressing ordered. Wounds are cleansed with soap and water or with normal saline–moistened gauze to gently remove the old antimicrobial agent and any loose necrotic tissue, scabs, or dried blood. During the debridement phase, the wound is covered with topical antimicrobial agents (e.g., silver sulphadiazine, silver-impregnated dressings). When partial-thickness burn wounds have been fully debrided, a protective greasy (paraffin or petroleum) gauze dressing is applied to protect the re-epithelializing cells as they resurface and close the open wound bed. If grafting is necessary, the meshed, split-thickness skin graft may be protected with the same greasy gauze dressings, followed by middle and outer dressings. With facial grafts, the unmeshed sheet graft is left open, so it is possible for *blebs* (serosanguinous exudate) to form between the graft and the recipient bed. Blebs prevent the graft from permanently attaching to the wound itself. The evacuation of blebs is best performed by aspiration with a tuberculin syringe and only by professionals who have received instruction in this specialized skill. (Dressings are discussed in Chapter 14 and Table 14.11.)

EXCISION AND GRAFTING

Current management of full-thickness burn wounds involves early removal of the necrotic tissue, followed by application of split-thickness autograft skin. In the past, patients with major burns had low rates of survival, hypertrophic scars, contractures, and poor functional outcomes and developed sepsis because healing and wound coverage took so long (Douglas et al., 2017). Currently, as a result of earlier intervention, mortality and morbidity rates have been greatly reduced. Many patients, especially those with major burns, are taken to the operating room for wound excision on day 1 or 2 (resuscitation phase). The wounds are covered with a biological dressing or allograft for temporary coverage until permanent grafting can be accomplished (see Table 27.13).

During the procedure of excision and grafting, devitalized tissue (*eschar*) is removed down to the subcutaneous tissue or the fascia, depending on the degree of injury. Surgical excision can result in massive blood loss. Topical application of epinephrine or thrombin, application of extremity tourniquets, or application of a fibrin sealant (ARTISS) all work to decrease surgical blood loss.

Once hemostasis has been achieved, a graft is then placed on clean, viable tissue to achieve good adherence. Whenever possible, the freshly excised wound is covered with *autograft* (the person's own) skin (see Table 27.13). Fibrin sealant has been used to attach skin grafts to the wound bed. Grafts can also be stapled or sutured into place (Figure 27.11, A). Negative-pressure wound therapy dressings are often placed on top of skin grafts to optimize adherence to the excised bed (Mohsin et al., 2017). A temporary *allograft* (from a cadaver skin bank) can be used to test how the recipient site will accept a graft. The allograft is then removed several days later in the operating room and an autograft applied.

With early excision, function is restored and scar tissue formation is minimized. Frequent observation for bleeding and circulation problems and appropriate nursing interventions can help identify and manage complications that would interfere with graft survival. Facial, neck, and hand burns require skillful nursing care to identify and manage clots quickly for the best functional and aesthetic outcomes.

Donor skin from another area of the patient's body is harvested for grafting by means of a dermatome, which removes a thin (14/1000 to 16/1000) split-thickness layer of skin from an unburned site (see Figure 27.11, B). This sample of skin can be meshed (usually a ratio of 1.5:1) to allow for greater wound coverage, or it may be applied as an unmeshed sheet graft for a better cosmetic result when grafting the face, neck, and hands. The site from which this skin was taken now becomes a new open wound.

The goals of donor site care are to promote rapid moist wound healing, decrease pain at the site, and prevent infection. The choices of dressings vary among burn centres and include greasy gauze dressings, silver-impregnated dressings,

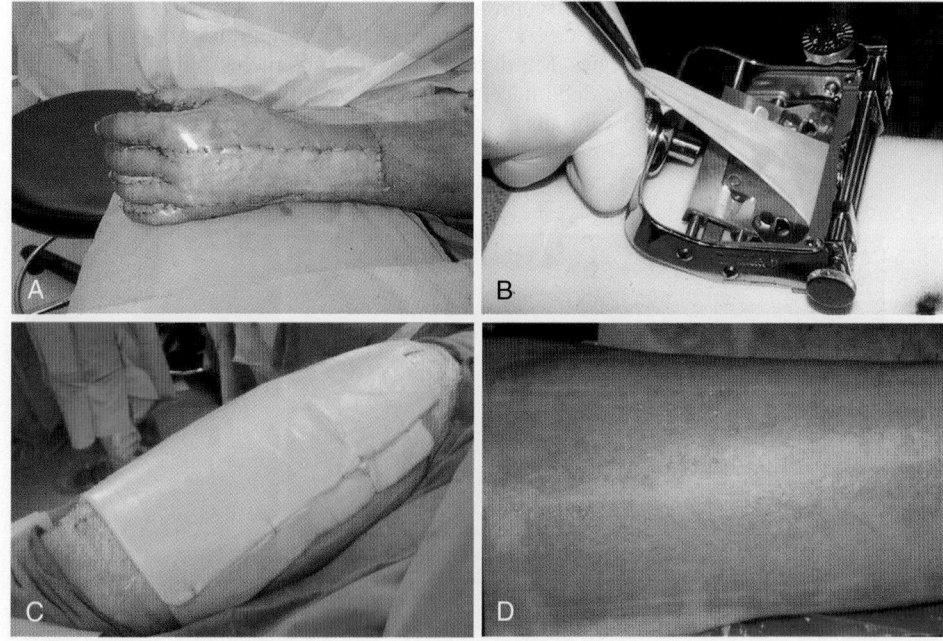

FIG. 27.11 Split-thickness skin grafting. **A,** Freshly applied split-thickness sheet skin graft to the hand. **B,** Split-thickness skin graft is harvested from a patient's thigh using a dermatome. **C,** Donor site is covered with a hydrophilic foam dressing after harvesting. **D,** Healed donor site. Source: Courtesy Judy A. Knighton, RN, MScN, Toronto.

and hydrophilic foam dressings (see Figure 27.11, *C*). Nursing care of the donor site is specific to the dressing selected. Several of the newer dressing materials offer decreased healing time, which facilitates earlier reharvesting of skin at the same site. The average healing time for a donor site is 10 to 14 days (see Figure 27.11, *D*).

CULTURED EPITHELIAL AUTOGRAFTS. In the patient with large body surface area burns, only a limited amount of unburned skin may be available as donor sites for grafting, and some of that available skin may be unsuitable for harvesting. Cultured epithelial autograft (CEA) is a method of obtaining permanent skin from a person with limited available skin for harvesting. CEA is grown from biopsy specimens obtained from the patient's own unburned skin. The specimens are sent to a commercial laboratory, where the keratinocytes from the biopsy sample are grown in a culture medium containing epidermal growth factor. After approximately 18 to 25 days, the keratinocytes have expanded up to 10 000 times and form confluent sheets that can be used as skin grafts. The cultured skin is returned to the burn unit, where it is placed on the patient's excised burn wounds. Because CEA tissue is made only of epidermal cells, meticulous care is required to prevent shearing injury or infection (Figure 27.12). Problems related to CEA include infection, contracture development, and poor graft take as a result of loss of thin epidermal skin during healing.

ARTIFICIAL SKIN. Skin substitutes are an alternative to conventional skin grafting techniques for reconstruction of partial-thickness and full-thickness burn wounds (Sando & Chung, 2017). The Integra dermal regeneration template is an example of a successful skin replacement system available in burn care today. As with CEA, it is indicated for use in the treatment of life-threatening full-thickness or deep partial-thickness burn wounds when conventional autograft is not available or advisable, as in older patients or those at high risk for complications from anaesthesia. It has also been successfully used in surgical burn reconstructive procedures. As with CEA, it needs to be applied within a few days of admission for greatest success.

Integra artificial skin has a bilayer membrane composed of acellular dermis and silicone. The wound is debrided, the bilayer membrane is placed dermal layer down, and the wound is wrapped with dressings in the operating room. The dermal layer functions as a biodegradable template that induces organized regeneration of new dermis by the body. The silicone layer remains intact for 3 weeks as the dermal layer degrades and epidermal autografts become available. At this point, the silicone is removed during a second surgical procedure and replaced by the patient's own epidermal autografts. In some situations, burn units use CEA as the source of epidermis.

Another currently available dermal replacement is Allo-Derm, a cryopreserved allogenic dermis. Human allograft dermis, harvested from cadavers, is decellularized to render it immunogenic, and then it is freeze-dried. Once thawed, Allo-Derm is rehydrated with ultrathin epidermal autografts immediately before placement on a newly excised wound.

PAIN MANAGEMENT

One of the most critical functions a nurse performs on behalf of a patient with burn injuries is individualized and ongoing pain assessment and management. Many aspects of burn care cause pain. However, patients experience moments of relative comfort if they receive adequate analgesia. A coordinated understanding of both physiological and psychological aspects of pain is essential if the nurse is to intervene with actions that are beneficial. (General pain management is discussed in Chapter 10.) Patients with burn injuries experience two kinds of pain: (1) continuous, background pain that might be present throughout the day and night and (2) treatment-induced pain associated with dressing changes, ambulation, and rehabilitation activities. Initial treatment is pharmacological (see Table 27.14). With background pain, a continuous IV infusion of an opioid allows for a steady, therapeutic level of medication. If an IV infusion is not present, slow-release twice-a-day opioid medications (e.g., MS Contin, sustained-release hydromorphone [Dilaudid]) are indicated. Around-the-clock oral analgesics can also be used (ibuprofen, acetaminophen). Breakthrough doses of pain medication need to be available regardless of the regimen selected. Anxiolytics (e.g., lorazepam [Ativan]), which frequently potentiate analgesics, are also indicated.

For treatment-induced pain, premedication with an analgesic and perhaps an anxiolytic via the IV or oral route, is required. For patients with an IV infusion, a potent, short-acting analgesic, such as fentanyl, is useful. During treatment or activity, doses should be low but high enough to keep the patient as comfortable as possible. Elimination of all pain is difficult to achieve, and most patients indicate satisfaction with "tolerable" levels of discomfort.

Pain can also be managed through nonpharmacological strategies. Mind–body interventions such as relaxation, hypnosis, guided imagery, biofeedback, and music therapy are considered adjuncts to traditional pharmacological treatment of pain.

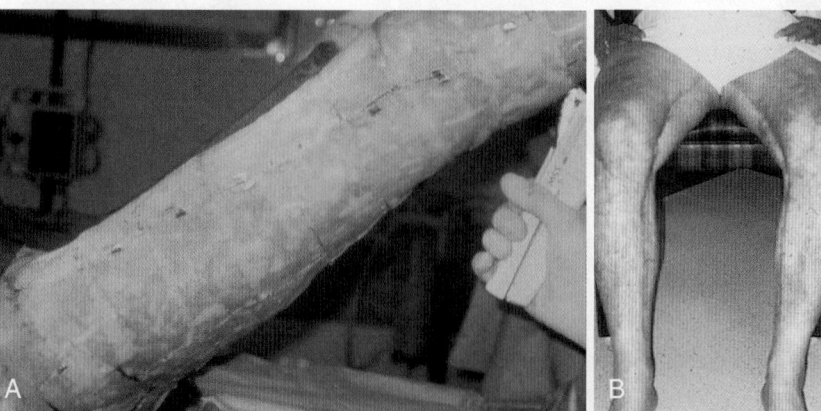

FIG. 27.12 Cultured epithelial autograft (CEA). **A,** Intraoperative application of CEA. **B,** Appearance of healed CEA. Source: Courtesy of Epicel.

They are not meant to be used exclusively to control pain but may help some patients cope with the painful aspects of care, both in the hospital and after discharge (see Chapter 8).

An important point to remember is that the more control the patient has in managing the pain, the more successful the chosen strategies are. Patient-controlled analgesia (PCA) is used in some burn units, with varying degrees of success. (PCA is discussed in Chapters 10 and 22.) Active patient participation has been found to be effective also for some patients in anticipating and coping with treatment-induced pain.

PHYSIOTHERAPY AND OCCUPATIONAL THERAPY

Rigorous physiotherapy throughout burn recovery is imperative to maintain muscle strength and optimal joint function. A good time for exercise is during and after wound cleansing, when the skin is softer and bulky dressings are removed. Passive and active range-of-motion exercises should be performed on all joints. The patient with neck burns must sleep without pillows or with the head hanging slightly over the top of the mattress to encourage hyperextension. Custom-fitted splints are designed to keep joints in a functional position. These must be re-examined frequently to ensure an optimal fit with no undue pressure that might lead to skin breakdown or nerve damage.

NUTRITIONAL THERAPY

The goal of nutritional therapy during the acute burn phase is to provide adequate calories and protein to promote healing. The patient with burn injury is in a hypermetabolic and highly catabolic state. Decreasing catecholamine release by minimizing pain, fear, anxiety, and cold can maximize the patient's comfort and conserve energy. Infection also increases the metabolic rate.

Meeting daily caloric requirements is crucial and should begin within the first 1 to 2 days after the burn injury. The daily estimated caloric needs must be regularly calculated by a dietitian and readjusted as the patient's condition changes (e.g., wound healing, sepsis).

If the patient is on a mechanical ventilator or unable to consume adequate calories by mouth, a small-bore feeding tube is inserted and enteral feedings are initiated. When the patient is extubated, a swallowing assessment should be performed by a speech–language pathologist before oral feeding is commenced. The alert patient should be encouraged to eat high-protein, high-carbohydrate foods to meet increased caloric needs. Family members should be encouraged to bring in favourite foods from home. Ideally, weight loss should not be more than 10% of preburn weight. Daily calorie counts and weekly weights are monitored by the dietitian to evaluate progress.

PSYCHOSOCIAL CARE

The patient and family have many needs for psychosocial support during the often lengthy, unpredictable, and complex course of care. The social worker and nursing staff have important support and counselling roles to play. (Patient and family emotional needs are discussed later in this chapter and in Chapter 6.)

REHABILITATION PHASE

The formal *rehabilitation phase* begins when the patient's burn wounds have healed and the patient is able to resume a level of self-care activity. This can occur as early as 2 weeks or as long as 7 to 8 months after the burn injury. The goal for this period is to assist the patient to regain and maintain function and

---

🔍 EVIDENCE-INFORMED PRACTICE

Research Highlight

Does Cooling Burns With Water as a First Aid Treatment Affect Outcomes in Burn Patients?

Clinical Question

In patients with burns (P), what is the effect of holding a burn under cool, running water (I) versus alternate treatment (C) in reducing skin surface temperature, admission to the critical care unit (CCU), and depth of the wound and pain (O)?

Best Available Evidence

Systematic review of randomized controlled trial (RCT), cohort study, expert opinion, and clinical practice guidelines

Critical Appraisal and Synthesis of Evidence

- One RCT ($n = 96$) with burn patients in the emergency department and a large cohort study ($n = 2\,897$) using burn registry data
- The RCT found that cooling with water as an initial first aid treatment was associated with a significant reduction in skin temperature as compared to hydrogel tea tree burn dressings.
- The cohort study reported an association between 20 to 25 minutes of water cooling as a standard first aid measure and a reduction in surgery and admission to CCU.

Expert opinions reported a decrease in burn depth, faster healing, and less scarring with the use of 20 minutes of running, cool water. Clinical guidelines suggested that cooling significantly reduced pain and wound edema if started within 3 hours of the burn injury.

Conclusion

- It is recommended that a burned wound should be held under running cool tap water for 20 minutes within 3 hours following burn injuries, unless contraindicated (e.g., large burn causing rapid heat loss, hypothermia, multiple trauma).

Implications for Nursing Practice

- Nurses can promote the use of this simple, easy-to-implement first aid measure when educating patients, families, and community groups.
- It is important to stress that the water should be running and cool; ice is contraindicated as it can cause vasoconstriction, hypothermia, and burning if placed directly on the skin.

Reference for Evidence

Gyi, A. A. (2018). Management of burn injuries: Cooling burns with water. JBI Evidence Summary. AN, JBI20528.

P, patient population of interest; *I*, intervention or area of interest; *C*, comparison of interest or comparison group; *O*, outcomes of interest (see Chapter 1).

---

independence (Knighton, 2020). Rehabilitation-focused activities that were taking place during the earlier emergent and acute phases begin in earnest once the patient's wounds have healed.

Pathophysiological Changes and Clinical Manifestations

Burn wounds can heal on their own or through skin grafting. Through epithelialization, the tissue structure destroyed by the burn injury begins to rebuild. Collagen fibres, present in the new scar tissue, assist with healing and add strength to weakened areas. The new skin appears flat and pink. In approximately 4 to 6 weeks, the area may become raised and hyperemic. If adequate range of motion is not instituted, the new tissue shortens, which causes a contracture. Mature healing is reached in about 12 months, by which time suppleness has returned and, in lighter-skinned people, the pink or red colour has faded to a slightly lighter hue than the surrounding unburned tissue. More heavily pigmented skin takes longer to regain its dark colour because many of the melanocytes have been destroyed. In many cases, the skin does not regain its original colour. Paramedical cosmetic camouflage—the topical application of pigment onto the skin—can help even out unequal skin tones and improve the patient's overall appearance and self-image.

Scarring has two components: discoloration and contour. The discoloration of scars fades somewhat with time. However, scar tissue tends to develop altered contours; that is, it is no longer flat or slightly raised but becomes elevated and enlarged above the original burned area. It is believed that pressure can help keep a scar flat. Gentle pressure can be maintained on the healed burn with custom-fitted pressure garments, worn up to 24 hours a day for as long as 12 to 18 months. They should never be worn over unhealed wounds and are removed for bathing.

Patients typically experience discomfort from itching where healing is occurring. Application of water-based moisturizers and use of oral antihistamines (e.g., diphenhydramine [Benadryl]) help reduce the itching. Massage, transcutaneous electrical nerve stimulation (TENS), silicone gel sheeting (e.g., Cica-Care), gabapentin (Neurontin)/pregabalin (Lyrica), beeswax and herbal oil, antipruritic hydrogel, and injectable steroids may also be helpful (Nedelec & LaSalle, 2018). As "old" epithelium is replaced by new cells, flaking occurs. Newly formed skin is extremely sensitive to trauma. Blisters and skin tears are likely to develop from slight pressure or friction. In addition, newly healed areas can be hypersensitive or hyposensitive to cold, heat, and touch. Grafted areas are more likely to be hyposensitive until peripheral nerve regeneration occurs. Healed burn areas must be protected from direct sunlight for 3 to 6 months to prevent hyperpigmentation and sunburn.

Complications

The most common complication during the rehabilitative phase are contractures due to the healing process and scaring and the loss of soft tissue length and extensibility (Godleski & Umraw, 2020). A contracture (an abnormal, usually permanent condition of a joint, characterized by flexion and fixation) develops as a result of the shortening of scar tissue in the flexor tissues of a joint. Areas most susceptible to contracture formation include anterior and lateral neck areas, axillae, antecubital fossae, fingers, groin areas, popliteal fossae, knees, and ankles (Figure 27.13). Not only does the skin over these areas develop contractures, but also the underlying tissues, such as the ligaments and tendons, have a tendency to shorten in the healing process.

Because of pain, patients with burn injuries prefer to assume a flexed position for comfort. This position predisposes wounds to contracture formation. Proper positioning, splinting, and exercise should be instituted to minimize this complication while the skin matures. Burned legs may be wrapped with elastic (e.g., tensor [ACE]) bandages to assist with circulation to leg graft and donor sites before ambulation. This additional pressure prevents blister formation, promotes venous return, and decreases pain and itchiness. Once the skin is completely healed and less fragile, interim tubular gauze (Tubigrip, Coban) and then custom-fitted pressure garments can replace the elastic bandages.

NURSING AND INTERPROFESSIONAL MANAGEMENT REHABILITATION PHASE

During the rehabilitation phase, both the patient and the family are actively encouraged to participate in care. Because the patient may go home with small, unhealed wounds, education and "hands-on" instruction in dressing changes and wound care are needed. If necessary, home care nursing services may be arranged to assist with wound care for the first few weeks after discharge. An emollient, water-based cream (e.g., Vaseline Intensive Care Extra Strength) that penetrates into the dermis should be used routinely on healed areas to keep the skin supple and well moisturized, thereby decreasing itching and flaking. Reconstructive surgery is frequently required after a major burn. It is important for the patient to understand the need for or possibility of further surgery before leaving the hospital.

The continuous role of exercise and physiotherapy or occupational therapy cannot be overemphasized. Computerized gaming devices such as tablets can provide patients with a break from exercise routines and allow access to interactive games, movies, books and puzzles (Burns-Nader et al., 2017). Constant encouragement and reassurance are necessary to maintain morale, particularly once the patient realizes that recovery can be slow and rehabilitation may need to be a primary focus for at least the next 12 months.

Because of the tremendous psychological effect of burn injury, health care providers should be particularly sensitive and attuned to the patient's emotions and concerns. It is essential that patients be encouraged to discuss their fears regarding loss of their lifestyle as they once knew it, loss of function, temporary or permanent deformity and disfigurement, return to work and home life, and financial burdens resulting from a long and potentially costly hospitalization and rehabilitation. Patients may benefit from being assisted toward a realistic and positive

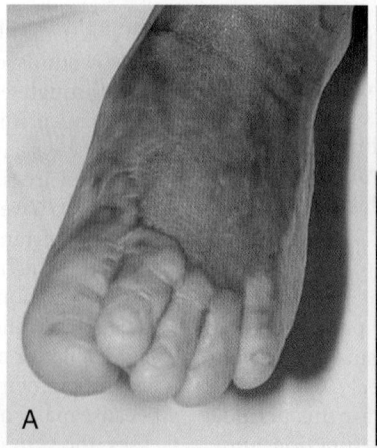
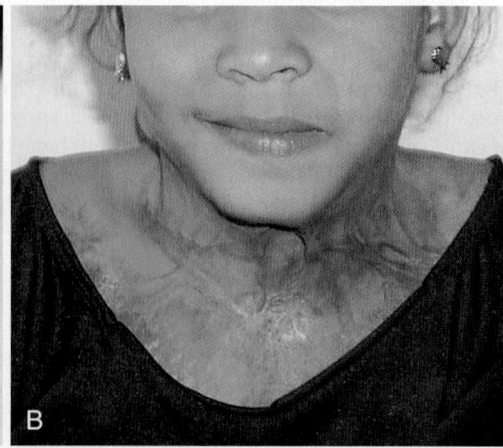

FIG. 27.13 Contractures. **A,** Foot. **B,** Neck. Source: Courtesy Judy A. Knighton, RN, MScN, Toronto, and Linda Bucher, RN, PhD.

appraisal of their particular situation, emphasizing what they can do instead of what they cannot do.

A person's self-esteem may be affected by a burn injury. In some individuals, an overwhelming fear may be the loss of relationships because of perceived or actual physical disfigurement. In a society in which physical beauty is valued, alterations in body image may result in psychological distress. Encouraging appropriate independence, an eventual return to preburn activities, and interactions with other burn survivors will involve the patient in familiar activities that may bring comfort and help restore self-esteem. Counselling, which may have started in the acute phase of care, can be offered after discharge. Patients appreciate reassurance that their emotions during this period of adjustment are normal and that frustration is to be expected as they attempt to resume a normal lifestyle.

AGE-RELATED CONSIDERATIONS

BURNS

Older patients with burns present many challenges for the burn team. The normal aging process puts such patients at risk for injury because of the possibility of an unsteady gait, limited eyesight, and diminished hearing. As people age, skin becomes drier, more wrinkled, and looser. The dermal layer thins, there is a loss of elastic fibres, the amount of subcutaneous adipose tissue lessens, and vascularity decreases. As a result, the thinner dermis, with reduced blood flow, sustains deeper burns with poorer rates of healing.

Once injured, older persons have more complications in the emergent and acute phases of burn resuscitation because of pre-existing medical conditions. For example, among older patients with diabetes, heart failure, or chronic obstructive pulmonary disease, morbidity and mortality rates exceed those of healthy, younger patients. Pneumonia is a frequent complication, burn wounds and donor sites take longer to heal, and surgical procedures are not as well tolerated. Weaning from a ventilator can be a challenge, and delirium from medication and anaesthesia may be a distressing, although usually self-limiting, outcome. It usually takes longer for older patients to become rehabilitated to the point at which they can safely return home. For some, a return home to independent living may not be possible. As the population ages, developing strategies to prevent burn injuries in this age group is a priority.

EMOTIONAL NEEDS OF THE PATIENT AND CAREGIVERS

Treatment of the burn injury often takes priority over psychological assessments and interventions. Close relatives, especially caregivers, may have to cope with many concerns, such as childcare financial issues and changes in family roles and the patient's appearance (Bond et al., 2017). It is important to ensure that correct interventions addressing a patient's coping ability and mental health occur appropriately in each of the stages of the recovery process (Cleary et al., 2018). At any time, emotions of fear, anxiety, anger, guilt, and depression may be experienced (Table 27.15).

A common emotional response is regression. The patient may revert to behaviour that helped with stressful situations in the past. This response can be healthy and is usually short-lived. As more independence is expected from the patient, new fears must be confronted: "Can I do it?" "Am I a desirable partner

TABLE 27.15	EMOTIONAL RESPONSES OF PATIENTS WITH BURN INJURY*
Emotion	**Possible Verbal Expression**
Fear	"Will I die?" "What will happen next?" "Will I be disfigured?" "Will my family and friends still love me?"
Anxiety	"I feel out of control." "What's going to happen to me?" "When will I look normal again?"
Anger	"Why did this happen to me?" "The nurses enjoy hurting me." "I hope the person who did this to me dies."
Guilt	"If only I'd been more careful." "I'm being punished because I did something wrong."
Depression	"It's no use going on like this." "I don't care what happens to me." "I wish people would leave me alone."

*List is not all-inclusive.

or parent?" Open and frequent communication among the patient, family members, close friends, and burn team members is essential.

Burn survivors frequently experience thoughts and feelings that are frightening and disturbing, such as guilt about the burn accident, reliving the experience, fear of death, concern about future therapy and surgery, frustrations with ongoing discomfort and wound breakdown, and, perhaps, hopelessness about the future. Families may share some or all of these feelings. At times, family members may feel helpless to assist their loved one. Continued support from trusted and familiar burn team members is essential. Assisting with aspects of care helps family members reconnect with their loved one and assists with the transition home. Many burn survivors and their families eventually adapt quite well and resume a productive and satisfying life; however, this process of adaptation can continue for several years (Rosenberg et al., 2018). Acknowledgement of a range of possible feelings (e.g., hopelessness, despair, rage, joy, and hope) can provide support for patients and their families.

The stress of the burn injury occasionally precipitates a time-limited psychiatric or psychological crisis. Many patients realize that coping with this experience is beyond their ability. Assessment by a psychiatrist who can prescribe appropriate medication, if needed, and begin short-term counselling is frequently helpful. Early psychiatric intervention is essential if the patient has been previously treated for a psychiatric illness or if the injury resulted from a suicide attempt. The diagnosis of post-traumatic stress disorder is made in a number of patients with burn injuries. However, it has been noted that distress and trauma symptoms can act as a catalyst for positive post-traumatic growth. Social support is a strong predictor of psychological recovery following a burn injury (Bond et al., 2017). Treatment typically begins in the hospital, but links to community resources must be made before discharge to ensure continuity of psychological care. Once the patient is discharged, referral to a psychiatrist, psychologist, mental health counsellor, social worker, or psychiatric clinical nurse specialist may be helpful if concerns are raised at burn clinic follow-up.

Patients with burn injuries benefit from information about sexuality and intimacy (Rosenberg et al., 2018)). Physical appearance is altered in patients who have sustained a major burn, and acceptance of any changes can be difficult at first for both the patient and their significant other. The nature of skin injury causes modifications in processing sexual stimuli. Touch is an important part of sexuality, and immature scar tissue may make the sensation of touch unpleasant or may dull it. This effect is usually transient, but the patient and partner need to know that it is normal, so they will benefit from anticipatory guidance from the health care team to avoid undue emotional strain.

Patient and family support groups may assist patients and families with their emotional needs at any phase of the recovery process. Speaking with other people who have experienced burn trauma can be beneficial, both in terms of reaffirming that their feelings are normal and allowing for sharing of helpful advice (Rosenberg et al., 2018)). The Phoenix Society (see the Resources at the end of this chapter) is an international and highly respected burn survivors' support group that has been offering invaluable support and resources to burn survivors, family members, and burn team personnel for many years.

SPECIAL NEEDS OF THE NURSING STAFF

Warm, trusting, mutually satisfying relationships frequently develop between patients with burn injuries and nursing staff, not only during hospitalization but also during the long-term rehabilitation period. The frequency and intensity of family contact can also be rewarding, as well as draining, for the nurse. Those new to burn nursing often find it difficult at first to cope with not only the deformities caused by burn injury but also the odours, the unpleasant sight of wounds, and the reality of the pain that accompanies the burn and its treatment. With time and positive experiences, those reactions diminish.

Many nurses come to know that the care they provide makes a critical difference in helping patients not only to survive but also to cope with and triumph over a challenging and multifaceted injury. It is this belief that allows and inspires nurses to provide meaningful care to patients with burn injury and their families.

Ongoing support services for the burn nurse or critical incident stress debriefings led by a psychiatrist, psychologist, psychiatric clinical nurse specialist, or social worker may be helpful. Professional burn nursing groups (e.g., American Burn Association, Canadian Association of Burn Nurses, International Society for Burn Injuries) can serve a similar purpose by helping nursing staff cope with difficult feelings they may experience when caring for patients with burn injuries. Burn nursing is physically, psychologically, and intellectually demanding and immensely rewarding. Attention to self-care helps to maintain a positive attitude and healthy work–life balance. Time with family and friends and rest and relaxation at home are essential parts of self-care and living a life with purpose and fulfillment.

CASE STUDY

Burn Injury

Patient Profile
E. C. (pronouns he/him), 65 years old, is brought to the emergency department with burns to his face, neck, torso, right arm and hand, and right foot from a kitchen grease fire. Upon arrival, the nurse notes an 18-gauge IV line with lactated Ringer's solution infusing at 100 mL/hour, and 100% humidified oxygen by mask is being administered.

Subjective Data
- Reports impaired vision and swallowing difficulties
- States burns are painful and is scared
- States has "diabetes and high blood pressure"

Objective Data
Physical Examination
- Patient is awake, alert, and oriented but in some distress
- Eyes are red and irritated
- Voice is hoarse; nasal hair is singed
- Face is reddened, with blisters noted on the nose and forehead
- Right arm, right hand, anterior torso, neck, and right foot have shiny, bright red, wet wounds
- Patient is shivering

Discussion Questions
1. *Priority decision:* What are the priorities of care in the prehospital setting and emergency department? How should E. C.'s airway, breathing, and circulation be managed?
2. *Priority decision:* What signs and symptoms indicate that he likely has an inhalation injury? What priority interventions can be anticipated?
3. What pain medications might be considered to relieve the pain?
4. Which of the criteria for admission to the hospital burn unit does E. C. meet?
5. What metabolic disturbances would be expected soon after his admission? Explain the physiological basis for these changes.
6. How might E. C.'s comorbidities affect burn care and rehabilitation?
7. What measures should be taken to support E. C.'s family?
8. *Priority decision:* What three priority nursing diagnoses and any interprofessional issues can be identified, based on the assessment data presented?
9. *Evidence-informed practice:* What are the most effective wound care strategies to manage E. C.'s burn wounds?

Ⓔvolve
Answers are available at http://evolve.elsevier.com/Canada/Lewis/medsurg.

REVIEW QUESTIONS

The number of the question corresponds to the same-numbered objective at the beginning of the chapter.

1. Knowing the most common causes of household fires, which prevention strategy would the nurse focus on when teaching about fire safety?
   a. Set hot water temperature at 60°C.
   b. Use only hard-wired smoke detectors.
   c. Encourage regular home fire exit drills.
   d. Never permit older persons to cook unattended.

2. Which of the following injuries is least likely to result in a full-thickness burn?
   a. Sunburn
   b. Scald injury
   c. Chemical burn
   d. Electrical injury

3. When assessing a client with a partial-thickness burn, what would the nurse expect to find? *(Select all that apply.)*
   a. Blisters
   b. Exposed fascia
   c. Exposed muscles
   d. Intact nerve endings
   e. Red, shiny, wet appearance
4. A client is admitted to the burn centre with burns on his head and neck, chest, and back after an explosion in his garage. On assessment, the nurse auscultates the lung fields and hears wheezes throughout. On reassessment, the wheezes are gone and the breath sounds are greatly diminished. Which action is the most appropriate for the nurse to take next?
   a. Obtain vital signs and an immediate arterial blood gas.
   b. Encourage the client to cough and auscultate the lungs again.
   c. Document the findings and continue to monitor the client's breathing.
   d. Anticipate the need for endotracheal intubation and notify the physician.
5. Which of the following fluid and electrolyte shifts occurs during the early emergent phase?
   a. Adherence of albumin to vascular walls
   b. Movement of potassium into the vascular space
   c. Sequestering of sodium and water in interstitial fluid
   d. Hemolysis of RBCs from large volumes of rapidly administered fluid
6. Which of the following must the client with a major burn do in order to maintain a positive nitrogen balance?
   a. Eat a high-protein, low-fat, high-carbohydrate diet.
   b. Increase normal adult caloric intake by about three times.
   c. Eat at least 1 500 calories per day in small, frequent meals.
   d. Eat rice and whole wheat for their chemical effect on nitrogen balance.
7. A client has 25% of TBSA burned in a car fire. His wounds have been debrided and covered with a silver-impregnated dressing. What should the nurse's priority intervention for wound care be?
   a. To reapply a new dressing without disturbing the wound bed
   b. To observe the wound for signs of infection during dressing changes
   c. To apply cool compresses for pain relief in between dressing changes
   d. To wash the wound aggressively with soap and water three times a day

8. Which of the following is most effective in terms of pain management for the client with burn injuries? *(Select all that apply.)*
   a. A pain rating tool is used to monitor the client's level of pain.
   b. Painful dressing changes are delayed until the client's pain is completely relieved.
   c. The client is educated about pain management and has some control over its management.
   d. A multimodal approach is used (e.g., sustained-release and short-acting opioids, nonsteroidal anti-inflammatory drugs, adjuvant analgesics).
   e. Nonpharmacological therapies (e.g., music therapy, distraction) replace opioids in the rehabilitation phase of a burn injury.
9. Which of the following therapeutic measures is used to prevent hypertrophic scarring during the rehabilitative phase of burn recovery?
   a. Applying pressure garments
   b. Repositioning the patient every 2 hours
   c. Performing active range of motion at least every 4 hours
   d. Massaging the new tissue with water-based moisturizers
10. A client is recovering from second- and third-degree burns over 30% of his body and is now ready for discharge. What is the first action that the nurse should take when meeting with the client?
    a. Arrange a return-to-clinic appointment and prescription for pain medications.
    b. Teach the client and the caregiver proper wound care to be performed at home.
    c. Review the client's current health care status and readiness for discharge to home.
    d. Give the client written discharge information and websites for additional information for burn survivors.

1. c; 2. a; 3. a, d, e; 4. d; 5. c; 6. a; 7. b; 8. a, c, d; 9. a; 10. c.

evolve

For even more review questions, visit http://evolve.elsevier.com/Canada/Lewis/medsurg.

REFERENCES

American Burn Association (ABA). (2016). *Burn incidence and treatment in the United States: 2016.* https://www.ameriburn.org/resources_factsheet.php

Arno, A., Knighten, J., & F. (2020). Prevention of burn injuries. In F. Sjöberg, et al. (Series Ed.), & M. Jeschke, & L. P. Kamolz (Vol. Eds.) *Handbook of burns: Vol. 1.* (2nd ed.). Springer.

Billette, J.-M., & Janz, T. (2015). *Injuries in Canada: Insights from the Canadian community health Survey. Statistics Canada.* http://www.statcan.gc.ca/pub/82-624-x/2011001/article/11506-eng.htm

Bond, S., Gourlay, C., Desjardins, A., et al. (2017). Anxiety, depression and PTSD-related symptoms in spouses and close relatives of burn survivors: When the supporter needs to be supported. *Burns, 43*(3), 592–601.

Burns-Nader, S., Joe, L., & Pinion, K. (2017). Computer tablet distraction reduces pain and anxiety in pediatric burn patients undergoing hydrotherapy: A randomized trial. *Burns, 43*(6), 1203–1211.

Cartotto, R. (2017). Topical antimicrobial agents for pediatric burns. *Burns Trauma, 5,* 33. https://doi.org/10.1186/s41038-017-0096-6

Clark, A., Imran, J., Madni, T., et al. (2017). Nutrition and metabolism in burn patients. *Burns & Trauma, 5*(1), 1–12.

Cleary, M., Visentin, D. C., West, S., et al. (2018). Bringing research to the bedside: Knowledge translation in the mental health care of burns patients. *International Journal of Mental Health Nursing, 27*(6), 1869–1876.

Douglas, H., Dunne, J., & Rawlins, J. (2017). Management of burns. *Surgery, 35*(9), 511–518.

Dyamenahalli, K., Garg, G., Shupp, J., et al. (2019). Inhalation injury: Unmet clinical needs and future research. *Journal of Burn Care and Research, 40*(5), 570–584.

Fahlstrom, K., Boyle, C., & Makic, M. B. F. (2013). Implementation of a nurse-driven burn resuscitation protocol: A quality improvement project. *Critical Care Nurse, 33*(1), 25–35. https://doi.org/10.4037/ccn2013385

Foncerrada, G., Capek, K., Wurzer, P., et al. (2017). Functional exercise capacity in children with electrical burns. *Journal of Burn Care and Research, 38*(3), E647–E652.

Godleski, M., & Umraw, N. C. (2020). Rehabilitation management during the acute phase. In M. Jeschke, L. P. Kamolz, F. Sjöberg, et al. (Eds.), *Handbook of burns* (2nd ed., Vol. 1). Springer.

Grant, E. (2017). Burn injuries: Prevention, advocacy, and legislation. *Clinics in Plastic Surgery, 44*(3), 451–466.

Greenhalgh, D. G. (2019). Management of burns. *New England Journal of Medicine, 380*(24), 2349–2359. https://doi.org/10.1056/nejmra1807442

Hampson, N. B., Piantadosi, C. A., Thom, S. R., et al. (2012). Practice recommendations in the diagnosis, management, and prevention of carbon monoxide poisoning. *American Journal of Respiratory and Critical Care Medicine, 186*(11), 1095–1101. https://doi.org/10.1164/rccm.201207-1284CI

Knighton, J. (2020). Nursing management of the burn patient. In M. Jeschke, L. P. Kamolz, F. Sjöberg, et al. (Eds.), *Handbook of burns* (2nd ed., Vol. 1). Springer.

Manning, J. (2018). Sepsis in the burn patient. *Critical Care Nursing Clinics of North America, 30*(3), 423–430. https://doi.org/10.1016/j.cnc.2018.05.010

Mohsin, M., Zarger, H., Wani, A., et al. (2017). Role of customized negative-pressure wound therapy in the integration of split-thickness skin grafts: A randomized control trial. *Indian Journal of Plastic Surgery, 50*(1), 43–49. https://doi.org/10.4103/ijps.IJPS_196_16

NB Trauma Program. (2019). *Consensus statement. Clinical practice guidelines for burn injuries.* https://nbtrauma.ca/wp-content/uploads/2020/10/Consensus-Statement-Emergency-Burn-Care-March-2019-Final.pdf

Nedelec, B., & LaSalle, L. (2018). Postburn itch: A review of the literature. *Wounds, 30*(1), 10–16.

Okonkwo, U., & DiPietro, L. (2017). Diabetes and wound angiogenesis. *International Journal of Molecular Science, 18*(7), 1419. https://doi.org/10.3390/ijms18071419

Peck, M. D., & Toppi, J. T. (2020). Epidemiology and prevention of burns throughout the world. In M. Jeschke, L. P. Kamolz, F. Sjöberg, et al. (Eds.), *Handbook of burns* (2nd ed., Vol. 1). Springer.

Ramponi, D. R. (2017). Chemical burns of the eye. *Advanced Emergency Nursing Journal, 39*(3), 193–198.

Rosenberg, L., Rosenberg, M., Rimmer, R., et al. (2018). Psychosocial recovery and reintegration of patients with burn injuries. In D. Herndon (Ed.), *Total burn care* (5th ed., pp. 709–720). Elsevier.

Sando, I., & Chung, K. (2017). The use of dermal skin substitutes for the treatment of the burned hand. *Hand Clinics, 33*(2), 269–276.

Waldmann, V., Narayanan, K., Combes, N., et al. (2018). Electrical cardiac injuries: Current concepts and management. *European Heart Journal, 39*(16), 1459–1465. https://doi.org/10.1093/eurheartj/ehx142

Weinberger, J., & Cipolle, M. (2016). Mechanical prophylaxis for post-traumatic VTE: Stockings and pumps. *Current Trauma Reports, 2*, 35–41. https://doi.org/10.1007/s40719-016-0039-x

World Health Organization. (2018). Burns. https://www.who.int/news-room/fact-sheets/detail/burns

Yang, L., Cui, C., Ding, H., et al. (2018). Delayed cerebellar infarction after a slight electric injury. *The American Journal of Emergency Medicine, 36*(12), 2337.e3–2337.e5. https://doi.org/10.1016/j.ajem.2018.08.064

RESOURCES

Canadian Burn Survivors Community
https://canadianburnsurvivors.ca/
Canadian Skin Patient Alliance
https://canadianskin.ca/burns

American Burn Association
https://www.ameriburn.org
Burn Foundation
https://www.burnfoundation.org
Burn Survivors Throughout the World
http://www.burnsurvivorsttw.org
Changing Faces
https://www.changingfaces.org.uk
International Society for Burn Injuries
http://www.worldburn.org
Parkland Formula for Burns Calculator
https://www.mdcalc.com/parkland-formula-for-burns
Phoenix Society for Burn Injuries
https://www.phoenix-society.org
Sage Burn Diagram
https://www.sagediagram.com

For additional Internet resources, see the website for this book at http://evolve.elsevier.com/Canada/Lewis/medsurg.

Conditions of Oxygenation: Ventilation

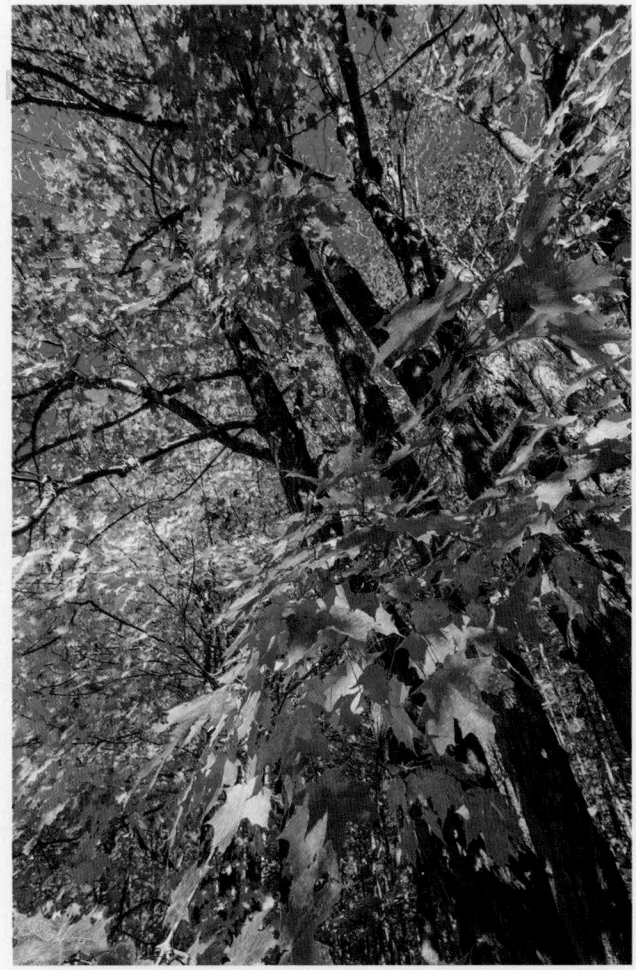

Source: © CanStock Photo/Elenathewise

Nursing Assessment

Respiratory System

Lesley MacMaster
Originating US chapter by Eugene Mondor

evolve WEBSITE

http://evolve.elsevier.com/Canada/Lewis/medsurg

- Review Questions (Online Only)
- Key Points
- Answer Guidelines for Case Study
- Conceptual Care Map Creator
- Audio Glossary
- Supporting Media—Animations
  - Patterns of Respiration

- Percussion Tones Throughout the Chest
- Pulmonary Circulation
- Supporting Media—Audio
- Bronchial Breath Sounds
- Bronchovesicular Breath Sounds
- High-Pitched Crackles
- High-Pitched Wheeze

- Low-Pitched Crackles
- Low-Pitched Wheeze
- Pleural Friction Rub
- Stridor
- Vesicular Breath Sounds
- Content Updates

LEARNING OBJECTIVES

1. Describe the structures and functions of the upper respiratory tract, the lower respiratory tract, and the chest wall.
2. Describe the process that initiates and controls inspiration and expiration.
3. Describe the process of gas diffusion within the lungs.
4. Identify the respiratory defence mechanisms.
5. Describe the significance of arterial blood gas values and the oxygen–hemoglobin dissociation curve in relation to respiratory function.
6. Identify the signs and symptoms of inadequate oxygenation and the implications of these findings.

7. Describe age-related changes in the respiratory system and differences in assessment findings.
8. Identify the significant subjective and objective data related to the respiratory system that should be obtained from a patient.
9. Describe the techniques used in physical assessment of the respiratory system.
10. Differentiate normal from common abnormal findings in a physical assessment of the respiratory system.
11. Describe the purpose, significance of results, and nursing responsibilities related to diagnostic studies of the respiratory system.

KEY TERMS

adventitious sounds	elastic recoil	tidal volume
chemoreceptor	mechanical receptors	ventilation
compliance	pleural friction rub	wheezes
crackles	surfactant	
dyspnea	tactile fremitus	

STRUCTURES AND FUNCTIONS OF THE RESPIRATORY SYSTEM

The primary purpose of the respiratory system is gas exchange, which involves the transfer of oxygen and carbon dioxide from the atmosphere to the blood. The respiratory system is divided into two parts: the upper respiratory tract and the lower respiratory tract (Figure 28.1). The upper respiratory tract includes the nasal cavity, the pharynx, the adenoids, the tonsils, the epiglottis, the larynx, and the trachea. The major structures of the lower respiratory tract are the bronchi, the bronchioles,

the alveolar ducts, and the alveoli. With the exception of the right and left mainstem bronchi, all lower airway structures are contained within the lungs. The right lung is divided into three lobes (upper, middle, and lower) and the left lung into two lobes (upper and lower; Figure 28.2). The structures of the chest wall (ribs, pleura, muscles of respiration) are also essential for respiration.

Upper Respiratory Tract

The nose, made of bone and cartilage, is divided into two nares by the nasal septum. The interior of the nose is shaped into

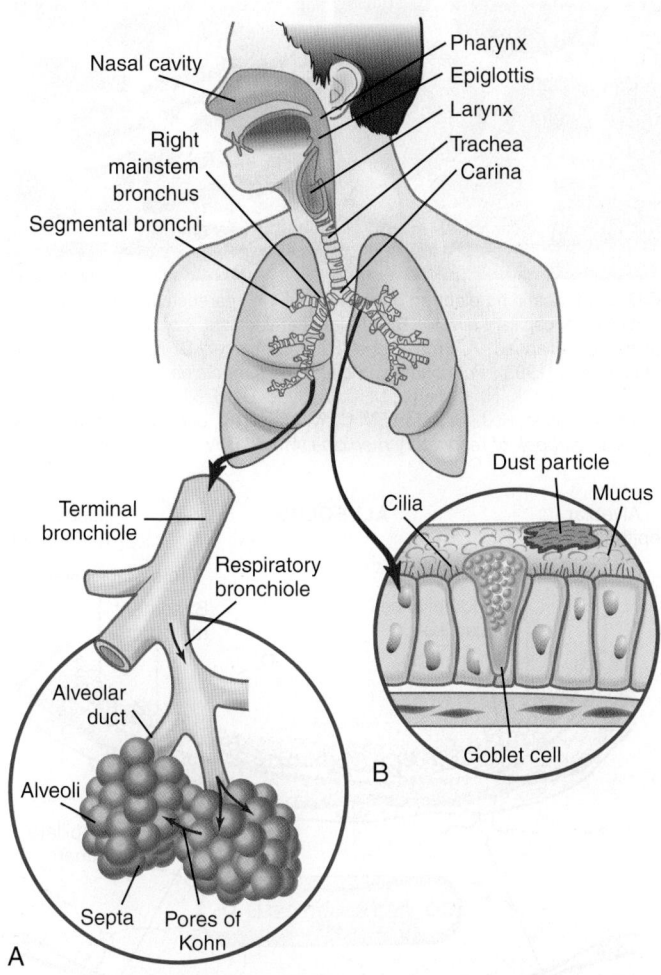

FIG. 28.1 Structures of the respiratory tract. **A,** Pulmonary functional unit. **B,** Ciliated mucous membrane. Source: Redrawn from Price, S. A., & Wilson, L. M. (2003). *Pathophysiology: Clinical concepts of disease processes* (6th ed.). Mosby.

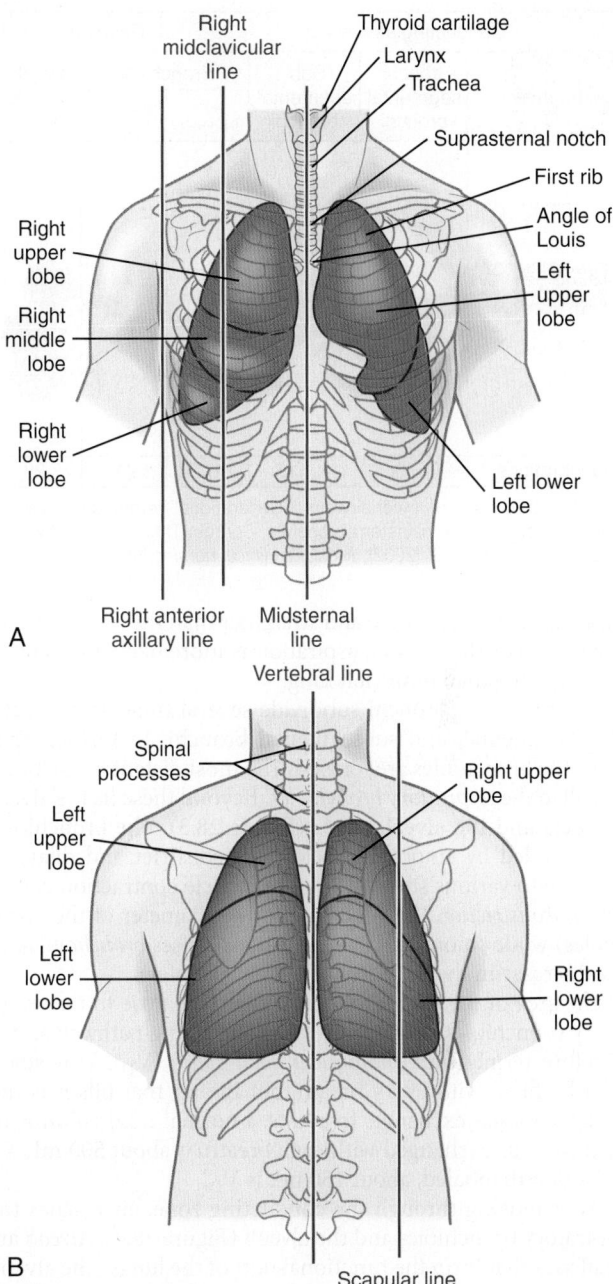

FIG. 28.2 Landmarks and structures of the chest wall. **A,** Anterior view. **B,** Posterior view. Source: Thompson, J. M., McFarland, G., & Tucker, S. (2002). *Mosby's clinical nursing* (5th ed.). Mosby.

rolling projections called *turbinates* that increase the surface area for warming and moistening air. The internal portion of the nose opens directly into the sinuses. The nasal cavity is connected to the *pharynx*, a tubular passageway that is subdivided into three parts: In descending order, they are the *nasopharynx*, the *oropharynx*, and the *laryngopharynx*.

Breathing through the narrow nasal passages (rather than mouth breathing) provides protection for the lower airway. The nose is lined with mucous membrane and small hairs. Air entering the nose is warmed to near body temperature, humidified to nearly 100% water saturation, and filtered to remove particles larger than 10 mcm (e.g., dust, bacteria).

The olfactory nerve endings (receptors for the sense of smell) are located in the roof of the nose. The adenoids and the tonsils, which are small masses of lymphatic tissue, are found in the nasopharynx and the oropharynx, respectively.

The *epiglottis* is a small flap of tissue at the base of the tongue. During swallowing, the epiglottis covers the larynx, preventing solids and liquids from entering the lungs.

After passing through the oropharynx, air moves through the laryngopharynx and the larynx, where the vocal cords are located, and then down into the trachea. The *trachea* is a cylindrical tube about 10 to 12 cm long and 1.5 to 2.5 cm in diameter. The support of U-shaped cartilages keeps the trachea open but allows the adjacent esophagus to expand for swallowing. The trachea bifurcates into the right and left mainstem bronchi at a point called the *carina*, located at the level of the manubriosternal junction, also called the *angle of Louis*. The carina is highly sensitive, and touching it during suctioning causes vigorous coughing (Patton, 2019).

Lower Respiratory Tract

Once air passes the carina, it is in the lower respiratory tract. The mainstem bronchi, the pulmonary vessels, and nerves enter the lungs through a slit called the *hilum*. The right mainstem

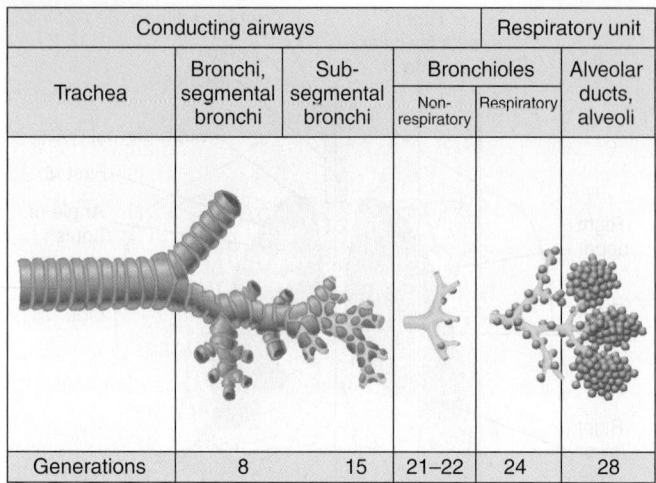

Conducting airways					Respiratory unit
Trachea	Bronchi, segmental bronchi	Sub-segmental bronchi	Bronchioles		Alveolar ducts, alveoli
			Non-respiratory	Respiratory	
Generations	8	15	21–22	24	28

FIG. 28.3 Structures of lower airways. "Generations" refers to the number of subdivisions of the mainstem bronchus. Source: Thompson, J. M., Mc-Farland, G., & Tucker, S. (2002). *Mosby's clinical nursing* (5th ed.). Mosby.

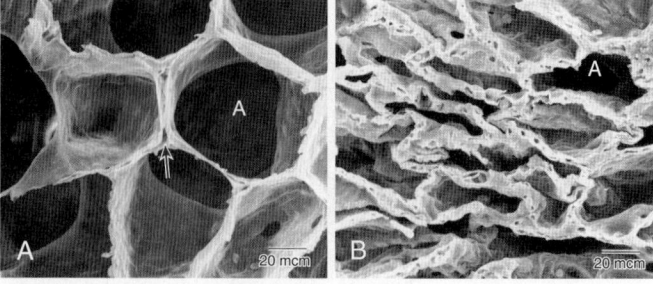

FIG. 28.4 Scanning electron micrograph of lung parenchyma. **A,** Alveoli *(A)* and alveolar capillary *(arrow).* **B,** Effects of atelectasis. Alveoli *(A)* are partially or totally collapsed. A, From Bone, R. C., Dantzker, D. R., George, R. B., et al. (Eds.). (1993). *Pulmonary and critical care medicine* (Vol. 1). Mosby. B, From Albertine, K. H., Williams, M. C., & Hyde, D. M. (2005). Anatomy of the lungs. In Mason, R. J., Broaddus, V. C., Murray, J. F., et al. (Eds.), *Murray and Nadel's textbook of respiratory medicine* (4th ed.). W. B. Saunders.

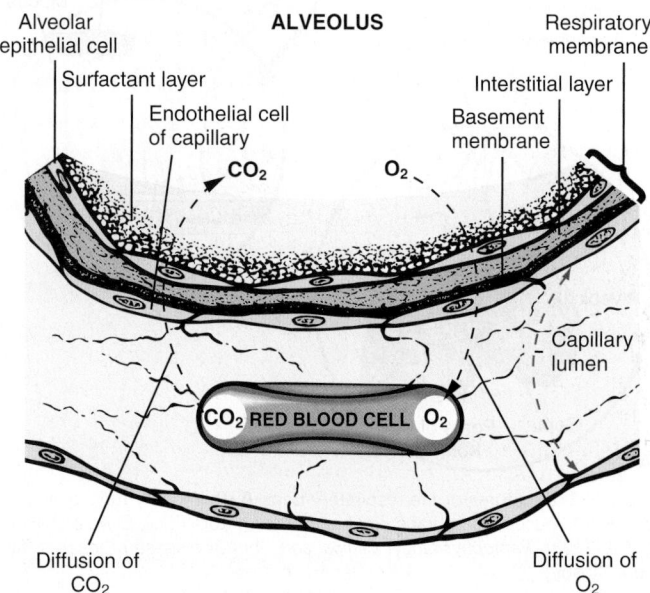

FIG. 28.5 Illustration of a small portion of the respiratory membrane, greatly magnified. An extremely thin interstitial layer of tissue separates the endothelial cell and basement membrane on the capillary side from the epithelial cell and surfactant layer on the alveolar side of the respiratory membrane. The total thickness of the respiratory membrane is less than 5 mcm.

bronchus is shorter, wider, and straighter than the left mainstem bronchus. For this reason, aspiration is more likely to occur in the right lung than in the left lung.

The mainstem bronchi subdivide several times to form the lobar, segmental, and subsegmental bronchi. In further divisions, the bronchioles are formed. The most distant bronchioles are called the *respiratory bronchioles.* Beyond these lie the alveolar ducts and the alveolar sacs (Figure 28.3). The bronchioles are encircled by smooth muscles that constrict and dilate in response to various stimuli. Smooth muscle contraction causes *bronchoconstriction* (i.e., decrease in the diameter of the bronchioles) while smooth muscle relaxation causes *bronchodilation* (i.e., increase in the diameter of the bronchioles).

The area of the respiratory tract from the nose to the respiratory bronchioles serves only as a conducting pathway and is therefore termed the *anatomical dead space* (V_D). This space must be filled with every breath, but the air that fills it is not available for gas exchange. In adults, a normal **tidal volume,** or volume of air exchanged with each breath, is about 500 mL. Of each 500 mL inhaled, about 150 mL is V_D.

After moving through the conducting zone, air reaches the respiratory bronchioles and the alveoli (Figure 28.4). *Alveoli* are small sacs that form the functional unit of the lungs. The alveoli are interconnected by pores of Kohn, which allow movement of air from alveolus to alveolus (see Figure 28.1). Bacteria can also move through these pores; as a result, a respiratory infection can extend to previously noninfected areas. The alveolar–capillary membrane (Figure 28.5) is very thin—less than 5 mcm thick—and is the site of gas exchange. In conditions such as pulmonary edema, excess fluid fills the interstitial space and the alveoli, markedly impairing gas exchange (Patton, 2019).

Surfactant. The alveolar surface is composed of cells that provide structure and cells that secrete surfactant (see Figure 28.5). **Surfactant,** a lipoprotein that lowers the surface tension in the alveoli, reduces the amount of pressure needed to inflate the alveoli and decreases the tendency of the alveoli to collapse. Normally, each person takes a slightly larger breath, termed a *sigh,* after every five to six breaths. This sigh stretches the alveoli and promotes surfactant secretion.

When the amount of surfactant is insufficient, the alveoli collapse. The term *atelectasis* refers to collapsed, airless alveoli

(see Figure 28.4). The patient who has just undergone surgery is at risk for postoperative atelectasis because of the effects of anaesthesia and restricted breathing with pain (see Chapter 22). In acute respiratory distress syndrome, lack of surfactant contributes to widespread atelectasis (McCance & Huether, 2019). Acute respiratory distress syndrome is discussed further in Chapter 70).

Blood Supply. The lungs have two different types of circulation: pulmonary and bronchial. The pulmonary circulation provides the lungs with blood for gas exchange. Deoxygenated blood enters the right atria via the vena cava, flows into the right ventricle and then into the pulmonary artery trunk, which branches into the right and left pulmonary arteries. Further subdivisions form a vast capillary network, where oxygen–carbon dioxide exchange occurs at the alveolar–capillary membrane. The pulmonary veins return the oxygenated blood to the left atrium of the heart, where it enters the systemic circulation via the aorta.

The bronchial circulation perfuses the tracheobronchial tree and other pulmonary tissues. The bronchial arteries branch off the aorta and perfuse structures in the left side of the thorax, while branches from the intercostal, subclavian, or internal mammary artery perfuse structures on the right side. Most deoxygenated venous blood returns to the right side of the heart; however, some venous blood from the bronchial circulation returns into the pulmonary veins and the left atrium.

Chest Wall

The chest wall is shaped, supported, and protected by 24 ribs (12 on each side). The ribs and the sternum protect the lungs and the heart from injury and, collectively, are sometimes called the *thoracic cage.* The structures of the chest wall include the thoracic cage, the pleura, and the respiratory muscles. During exertion or certain diseases, accessory muscles may provide support during inspiration (i.e., sternocleidomastoid, scalene, and trapezius) and expiration (i.e., abdominal and internal intercostals).

The chest cavity is lined with a membrane called the *parietal pleura,* and the lungs are lined with a membrane called the *visceral pleura.* The parietal and visceral pleurae are joined and form a closed, double-walled sac. The visceral pleura does not have any afferent pain fibres or nerve endings. The parietal pleura, however, does have afferent pain fibres. Therefore, irritation of the parietal pleura causes severe pain with each breath.

The space between the pleural layers is termed the *intrapleural space.* In a normal adult, this space is filled with a thin film of 20 to 25 mL of fluid, which serves two purposes: It provides lubrication, allowing the layers of pleura to slide over each other during breathing, and it increases cohesion between the pleural layers, thereby facilitating expansion of the pleura and lung during inspiration.

Fluid is normally drained from the pleural space by the lymphatic circulation. Several pathological conditions may cause the accumulation of greater amounts of fluid; such accumulations are termed *pleural effusions.* Pleural fluid may accumulate because malignant cells block lymphatic drainage or because there is an imbalance between intravascular and oncotic fluid pressures, as occurs in heart failure. The presence of purulent pleural fluid with bacterial infection is called *empyema.* Air in the pleural space (*pneumothorax*) or blood in the pleural space (*hemothorax*) can result in partial or complete collapse of the lung (see Chapter 30 for a full discussion of lower respiratory conditions).

The diaphragm is the major muscle of respiration. During inspiration, the diaphragm contracts, pushing the abdominal contents downward. At the same time, the external intercostal muscles and scalene muscles contract, increasing the lateral and anteroposterior dimension of the chest. This causes the size of the thoracic cavity to increase and intrathoracic pressure to decrease, so that air can enter the lungs.

The diaphragm is made up of two hemidiaphragms, each innervated by the right and left phrenic nerves. The phrenic nerves arise from the spinal cord between the third and fifth cervical vertebrae (C3 and C5). Injury to the phrenic nerve results in hemidiaphragmatic paralysis on the side of the injury. Complete spinal cord injuries above the level of C3 result in total diaphragmatic paralysis, and affected patients are dependent on mechanical ventilation (Herlihy, 2021).

Physiology of Respiration

Ventilation. Ventilation involves *inspiration* (movement of air into the lungs) and *expiration* (movement of air out of the lungs). Air moves in and out of the lungs because intrathoracic pressure changes in relation to pressure at the airway opening. Contraction of the diaphragm and of the intercostal and scalene muscles increases chest dimensions, thereby decreasing intrathoracic pressure. Gas flows from an area of higher pressure (atmospheric) to one of lower pressure (intrathoracic). In forced inspiration, such as during heavy exercise or conditions associated with respiratory distress, accessory muscles (i.e., sternomastoid, scalene, trapezius) assist to heave up the sternum and rib cage (Jarvis et al., 2019). In some conditions such as phrenic nerve paralysis, rib fractures, or neuromuscular disease, diaphragm or chest wall movement may be limited and cause the patient to breathe with smaller tidal volumes. As a result, the lungs do not fully inflate, and gas exchange is impaired. In contrast to inspiration, expiration is passive. The elastic recoil of the chest wall and lungs allows the chest to passively return to its normal position. Intrathoracic pressure rises, causing air to move out of the lungs. Exacerbations of asthma or emphysema cause expiration to become an active, laboured process (see Chapter 31). When there is persistent airflow limitation, such as in chronic obstructive pulmonary disease (COPD), accessory muscles (i.e., the rectus abdominus, internal intercostals) contract to push the abdominal viscera in and up against the diaphragm, causing it to expand and squeeze against the lungs, augmenting the force of expiration (Jarvis et al., 2019).

Elastic Recoil and Compliance. Elastic recoil is the tendency for the lungs to recoil after being stretched or expanded. The elasticity of lung tissue is attributable to the elastin fibres that are found in the alveolar walls and that surround the bronchioles and capillaries.

Compliance (distensibility) is a measure of the elasticity of the lungs and the thorax. When compliance is decreased, inflation of the lungs is more difficult. Examples of conditions in which compliance is decreased include those that increase fluid in the lungs (e.g., pulmonary edema, acute respiratory distress syndrome), diseases that make lung tissue less elastic (e.g., pulmonary fibrosis, sarcoidosis), and conditions that restrict lung movement (e.g., pleural effusion). Compliance is decreased as a result of aging and when there is destruction of alveolar walls and loss of tissue elasticity, as in emphysema.

Diffusion. Oxygen and carbon dioxide move across the alveolar capillary membrane by diffusion. The overall direction of movement is from the area of higher concentration to the area of lower concentration. Thus oxygen moves from alveolar gas (atmospheric air) into the arterial blood, and carbon dioxide from the arterial blood into the alveolar gas. Diffusion continues until equilibrium is reached (see Figure 28.5).

The ability of the lungs to oxygenate arterial blood adequately is determined by examination of the arterial oxygen tension (PaO_2; also referred to as the *partial pressure of oxygen in arterial blood*) and arterial oxygen saturation (SaO_2). Oxygen is carried in the blood in two forms: dissolved oxygen and hemoglobin-bound oxygen. The PaO_2 represents the amount of oxygen dissolved in the plasma and is expressed in millimetres of mercury (mm Hg). The SaO_2 is the amount of oxygen actually bound to hemoglobin, as opposed to the amount of oxygen that the hemoglobin can carry. The SaO_2 is expressed as a percentage. For example, if the SaO_2 is 90%, this means that 90% of the hemoglobin attachments for oxygen have oxygen bound to them.

Oxygen–Hemoglobin Dissociation Curve. The affinity of hemoglobin for oxygen is described by the *oxygen–hemoglobin (oxyhemoglobin) dissociation curve* (Figure 28.6). Oxygen delivery to the tissues depends on the amount of oxygen transported to the tissues and the ease with which hemoglobin gives up oxygen once it reaches the tissues. In the upper flat portion of the curve, fairly large changes in the PaO_2 cause small changes in hemoglobin saturation. For this reason, if the PaO_2 drops from 100 to 60 mm Hg, the saturation of hemoglobin changes only 7% (from the normal 97% to 90%). In other words, the hemoglobin remains 90% saturated despite a 40–mm Hg drop in the PaO_2. This portion of the curve also explains why a patient is considered adequately oxygenated when the PaO_2 is higher than 60 mm Hg. Increasing the PaO_2 above this level does little to improve hemoglobin saturation.

The lower portion of the oxygen–hemoglobin dissociation curve indicates a different type of phenomenon. As hemoglobin is desaturated, larger amounts of oxygen are released for tissue use. This is an important method of maintaining the pressure gradient between the blood and the tissues. It also ensures an adequate oxygen supply to peripheral tissues, even if oxygen delivery is compromised.

Many factors alter the affinity of hemoglobin for oxygen. A shift to the left in the oxygen–hemoglobin dissociation curve indicates that blood picks up oxygen more readily in the lungs but delivers oxygen less readily to the tissues. This occurs in alkalosis, in hypothermia, and with a decrease in arterial carbon dioxide tension ($PaCO_2$; also referred to as the *partial pressure of carbon dioxide in the arterial blood;* see Figure 28.6). A patient with a condition that causes a leftward shift of the curve, such as hypothermia that follows open heart surgery, may be given higher concentrations of oxygen until the body temperature normalizes. This helps compensate for decreased oxygen unloading in the tissues. A shift in the curve to the right indicates the opposite: Blood picks up oxygen less rapidly in the lungs but delivers oxygen more readily to the tissues. This occurs in acidosis, in hyperthermia, and when the $PaCO_2$ is increased.

Two methods are used to assess the efficiency of gas transfer in the lung: analysis of arterial blood gas (ABG) values and oximetry. These measures are usually adequate if the patient is stable and not critically ill. Many critically ill patients have a condition that impairs tissue oxygen delivery. In such patients, cardiac output, tissue oxygen consumption, mixed venous oxygen tension (PvO_2), and venous oxygen saturation (SvO_2) may also be assessed (Urden et al. 2018; see Chapter 68).

Arterial Blood Gases. ABGs are measured to determine oxygenation status and acid–base balance. ABG analysis includes measurement of the PaO_2, the $PaCO_2$, the pH, and the amount of bicarbonate (HCO_3^-) in arterial blood. The SaO_2 is either calculated or measured during this analysis. Blood for ABG analysis can be obtained by arterial puncture or from an arterial catheter in the radial or the femoral artery. Both techniques are invasive and allow only intermittent analysis. Continuous intra-arterial blood gas monitoring is also possible via a fibre-optic sensor or an oxygen electrode inserted into an arterial catheter. An arterial catheter enables ABG sampling without repeated arterial punctures.

Normal ABG values are given in Table 28.1, and ABG analysis and interpretation are further discussed in Chapter 19. The normal PaO_2 decreases with advancing age. The normal PaO_2 also varies in relation to the distance above sea level. At higher altitudes, the barometric pressure is lower, and thus the amount of inspired oxygen pressure and the PaO_2 are lower (see Table 28.1). Most airplanes are pressurized to approximate an altitude of 2 400 m above sea level. A normal person can expect a 16– to

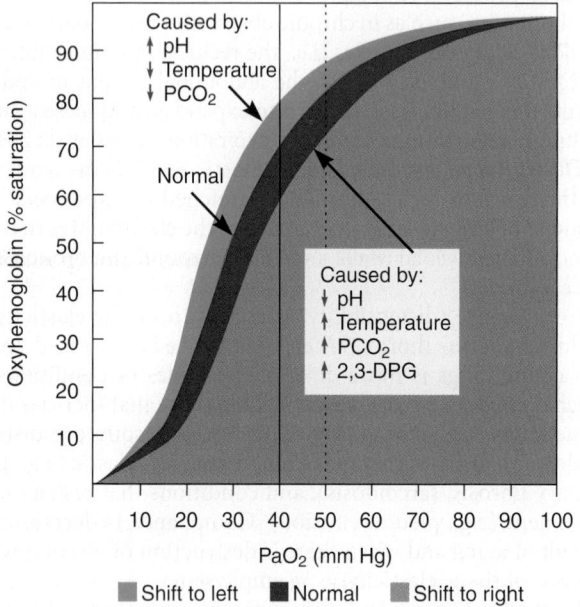

FIG. 28.6 Oxygen–hemoglobin dissociation curve. A shift to the left indicates the hemoglobin's increased affinity for oxygen. A shift to the right indicates the hemoglobin's decreased affinity for oxygen. *2,3-DPG,* 2,3-diphosphoglycerate; *PaO₂,* partial pressure of oxygen in arterial blood; *PCO₂,* partial pressure of carbon dioxide.

TABLE 28.1	NORMAL ARTERIAL AND VENOUS BLOOD GAS VALUES*		
	Arterial Blood Gases		
Laboratory Value	**BP at Sea Level: 760 mm Hg**	**BP at 1609 m Above Sea Level: 629 mm Hg**	**Mixed Venous Blood Gases**
pH	7.35–7.45	7.35–7.45	7.31–7.41
Partial pressure of oxygen	80–100 mm Hg	65–75 mm Hg	40–50 mm Hg
Oxygen saturation	≥95%[†]	≥95%[†]	60%–80%[†]
Partial pressure of carbon dioxide	35–45 mm Hg	35–45 mm Hg	SvO_2 is a better indicator for change in acid–base balance
HCO_3^-	21–28 mmol/L	21–28 mmol/L	21–28 mmol/L

BP, barometric pressure; *HCO_3^-,* bicarbonate; *SvO_2,* venous oxygen saturation.
*Assumes patient is 60 years of age or younger and breathing room air.
[†]The same normal values apply to both the venous oxygen saturation value (obtained through mixed venous blood gas sampling or oximetry via catheter) and the oxygen saturation value (obtained through pulse oximetry).

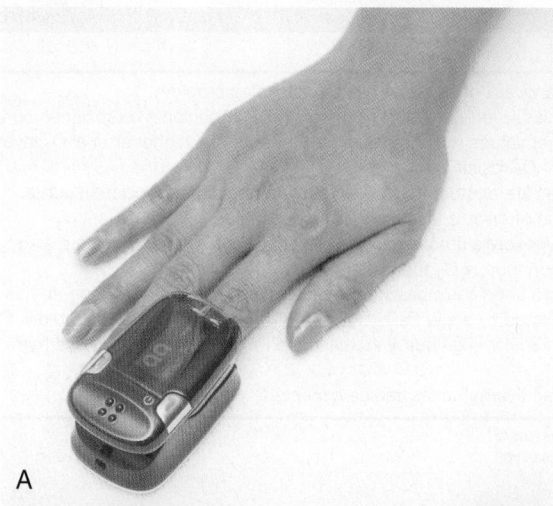

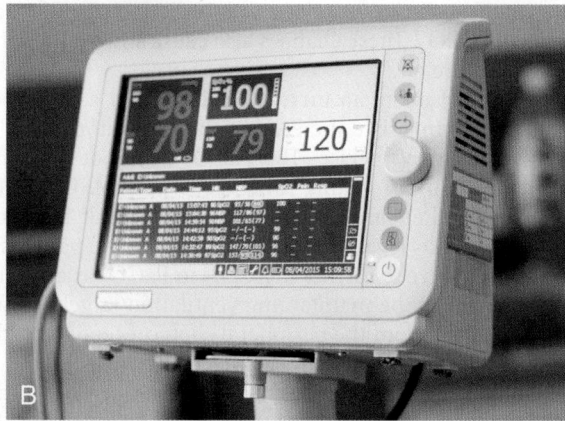

FIG. 28.7 **A,** Portable pulse oximeter displays oxygen saturation (SpO$_2$) and pulse rate. **B,** A pulse oximeter displays the oxygen saturation and pulse rate as a digital reading. Sources: *A,* © Can Stock Photo/praisaeng. *B,* © Can Stock Photo/masuti.

TABLE 28.2	SIGNS AND SYMPTOMS OF INADEQUATE OXYGENATION
Signs and Symptoms	**Onset**
Central Nervous System	
Unexplained apprehension	Early
Unexplained restlessness or irritability	Early
Unexplained confusion or lethargy	Early or late
Combativeness	Late
Coma	Late
Respiratory System	
Tachypnea	Early
Dyspnea on exertion	Early
Dyspnea at rest	Late
Use of accessory muscles	Late
Retraction of interspaces on inspiration	Late
Pause for breath between sentences, words	Late
Cardiovascular System	
Tachycardia	Early
Mild hypertension	Early
Dysrhythmias (e.g., premature ventricular contractions)	Early or late
Hypotension	Late
Cyanosis	Late
Cool, clammy skin	Late
Other Body Systems	
Diaphoresis	Early or late
Decreased urinary output	Early or late
Unexplained fatigue	Early or late

32–mm Hg fall in PaO$_2$ at this altitude (McCance & Huether, 2019). A patient who is already receiving oxygen therapy or whose PaO$_2$ is lower than 72 mm Hg while they are breathing room air needs a careful evaluation before air travel. Supplemental oxygen or a change in litre flow may be required during the flight.

Mixed Venous Blood Gases. For patients with normal or near-normal cardiac status, an assessment of PaO$_2$ or SaO$_2$ is usually sufficient to determine adequate oxygenation. Patients with impaired cardiac output or hemodynamic instability may have inadequate tissue oxygen delivery or abnormal oxygen consumption. The amount of oxygen delivered to the tissues or consumed can be calculated.

A catheter positioned in the pulmonary artery, termed a *pulmonary artery catheter,* is used for mixed venous sampling (see Chapter 68). Blood drawn from a pulmonary artery catheter is termed a *mixed venous blood gas sample* because it consists of venous blood that has returned to the heart from all tissue beds and "mixed" in the right ventricle. Normal mixed venous values are listed in Table 28.1. When tissue oxygen delivery is inadequate or when the amount of oxygen transported to the tissues by the hemoglobin is inadequate, the PvO$_2$ and SvO$_2$ fall.

Oximetry. Arterial oxygen saturation can be monitored continuously by means of a *pulse oximetry* probe on a finger, a toe, an ear, the forehead, or the bridge of the nose (Figure 28.7).

A pulse oximeter emits two wavelengths of light, one red and one infrared, which pass from a light-emitting diode (positioned on one side of the probe) to a photodetector (positioned on the opposite side). Well-oxygenated blood absorbs light differently from deoxygenated blood. The oximeter determines the amount of light absorbed by the vascular bed and calculates the saturation. The oxygen saturation value obtained by pulse oximetry (SpO$_2$) and heart rate are displayed on the monitor as digital readings (see Figure 28.7, *B*). The normal SpO$_2$ is higher than 95%.

Pulse oximetry is particularly valuable in critical care and perioperative areas, in which sedation or decreased consciousness might mask hypoxia (Table 28.2). SpO$_2$ is assessed during each routine check of vital signs in many inpatient areas. Changes in SpO$_2$ can be detected quickly and treated (Table 28.3). Oximetry is also used during exercise testing and when flow rates are adjusted during long-term oxygen therapy.

Values obtained by pulse oximetry are less reliable if the SpO$_2$ is lower than 70%. At this level, the oximeter tends to underestimate saturation and may display an artificially low value. Pulse oximetry is also inaccurate if hemoglobin variants (e.g., carboxyhemoglobin, methemoglobin) are present. Other factors that can alter the accuracy of pulse oximetry include motion, low perfusion, anemia, bright fluorescent lights, intravascular dyes, thick acrylic nails, and dark skin colour. If there is doubt about the accuracy of the SpO$_2$ reading, ABGs should be measured to verify accuracy.

Oximetry can also be used to monitor SvO$_2$ via a pulmonary artery catheter. A decrease in SvO$_2$ suggests that less oxygen is being delivered to the tissues or that more oxygen is being consumed. Changes in SvO$_2$ provide an early warning of a change in cardiac output or tissue oxygen delivery. Normal SvO$_2$ is 60 to 80%.

TABLE 28.3	CRITICAL VALUES FOR PaO₂ AND SpO₂*	
PaO₂	**SpO₂**	**Considerations**
≥70%	≥95%	Adequate unless patient is hemodynamically unstable or has O₂ unloading problem. With a low cardiac output, dysrhythmias, a leftward shift of the oxygen–hemoglobin dissociation curve, or carbon monoxide inhalation, higher values may be desirable. Benefits of a higher arterial O₂ level must be balanced against the risk of O₂ toxicity.
60%	90%	Adequate in almost all patients. Values are at steep part of oxygen–hemoglobin dissociation curve. Oxygenation is adequate, but margin of error is less than for higher values.
55%	88%	Adequate for patients with chronic hypoxemia if no cardiac conditions occur. These values are also used as criteria for prescription of continuous O₂ therapy.
40%	75%	Inadequate but may be acceptable on a short-term basis if the patient also has CO₂ retention. In this situation, respirations may be stimulated by a low PaO₂. Thus, the PaO₂ cannot be raised rapidly. O₂ therapy at a low concentration (24–28%) will gradually increase the PaO₂. Monitoring for dysrhythmias is necessary.
<40%	<75%	Inadequate. Tissue hypoxia and cardiac dysrhythmias can be expected.

PaO₂, partial pressure of oxygen in arterial blood; *SpO₂*, the oxygen saturation value obtained by pulse oximetry.
*The same critical values apply for SpO₂ and arterial oxygen saturation (SaO₂). Values pertain to rest or exertion.

Oxygen Delivery. Information from ABG values or oximetry is used to assess adequacy of oxygenation. Several questions must be asked to determine whether oxygenation is adequate:

1. What is the patient's SpO₂ or PaO₂ in comparison with expected normal values (see Table 28.1)?
2. What is the degree of hypoxemia, and what is the trend? Has SpO₂ or PaO₂ declined rapidly? A sudden drop in blood oxygen level can be life-threatening. A gradual decline is tolerated with fewer symptoms. Critical values for SpO₂ and PaO₂ are given in Table 28.3.
3. Is the patient exhibiting signs or symptoms of inadequate oxygenation? Changes in central nervous system, respiratory, cardiovascular, and renal function occur when tissue oxygen delivery is inadequate (see Table 28.2). Because the brain is highly sensitive to a decrease in tissue oxygen delivery, the first evidence of hypoxemia may be apprehension, restlessness, or irritability. If these signs or symptoms are observed, a change in the management plan is needed.
4. What is the oxygenation status with activity or exercise? To assess for desaturation with activity, pulse oximetry is used to monitor SpO₂ levels during a standardized 6-minute walk distance test or during activities of daily living. An SpO₂ value of 88% or less during exertion indicates the need for supplemental oxygen (McCance & Huether, 2019).

Control of Respiration. In the brainstem, the respiratory centre in the medulla responds to chemical and mechanical signals from the body. Impulses are sent from the medulla to the respiratory muscles through the spinal cord and phrenic nerves.

Chemoreceptors. A chemoreceptor is a receptor that responds to a change in the chemical composition (PaCO₂ and pH) of the fluid around it. Central chemoreceptors are located in the medulla and respond to changes in the hydrogen ion (H+) concentration. An increase in the H+ concentration (acidosis) causes the medulla to increase the respiratory rate and tidal volume. A decrease in H+ concentration *(alkalosis)* has the opposite effect. Changes in PaCO₂ regulate ventilation primarily by their effect on the pH of the cerebrospinal fluid. When the PaCO₂ level is increased, more CO₂ is available to combine with H₂O and form carbonic acid (H₂CO₃). This lowers the pH of the cerebrospinal fluid and stimulates an increase in respiratory rate. The opposite process occurs with a decrease in PaCO₂ level.

Peripheral chemoreceptors are located in the carotid bodies at the bifurcation of the common carotid arteries and in the aortic bodies above and below the aortic arch. The peripheral chemoreceptors respond to decreases in PaO₂ and pH and to increases in PaCO₂. These changes also cause stimulation of the respiratory centre.

In a healthy person, an increase in PaCO₂ or a decrease in pH causes an immediate increase in the respiratory rate. The process is extremely precise. The PaCO₂ does not vary more than about 3 mm Hg if lung function is normal. Conditions such as COPD alter lung function and may result in chronic elevation of PaCO₂ levels. In these circumstances, patients are relatively insensitive to further increases in PaCO₂ as a stimulus to breathe and may be maintaining ventilation largely because of a hypoxic drive from the peripheral chemoreceptors (carbon dioxide narcosis is discussed in Chapter 31).

Mechanical Receptors. Mechanical receptors (juxtacapillary and irritant) are located in lungs, upper airways, the chest wall, and diaphragm. They are stimulated by a variety of physiological factors such as irritants, muscle stretching, and alveolar wall distortion. Signals from the stretch receptors aid in the control of respiration. As the lungs inflate, pulmonary stretch receptors activate the inspiratory centre to inhibit further lung expansion. This is termed the *Hering–Breuer reflex* and prevents overdistension of the lungs. Impulses from the mechanical sensors are sent through the vagus nerve to the brain. Juxtacapillary (J) receptors are believed to cause the rapid respiration (tachypnea) observed in patients with pulmonary edema. These receptors are stimulated by the entry of fluid into the pulmonary interstitial space.

Respiratory Defence Mechanisms

Respiratory defence mechanisms are efficient in protecting the lungs from inhaled particles, microorganisms, and toxic gases. The defence mechanisms include filtration of air, the mucociliary clearance system, the cough reflex, reflex bronchoconstriction, and alveolar macrophages.

Filtration of Air. Nasal hairs filter the inspired air. In addition, the abrupt changes in direction of airflow that occur as air moves through the nasopharynx and larynx increase air turbulence. This causes particles and bacteria to contact the mucosa lining these structures. Most large particles (>5 mcm in diameter) are removed in this manner.

The velocity of airflow slows greatly after it passes the larynx, facilitating the deposition of smaller particles (1–5 mcm in size). They settle like sand in a river, a process termed *sedimentation*. Particles less than 1 mcm in size are too small to settle in this manner and are deposited in the alveoli. One example of small particles that can build up is coal dust, which can lead to pneumoconiosis (see Chapter 30). Particle size is important. Particles larger than 5 mcm are less dangerous because they are removed in the nasopharynx or bronchi and do not reach the alveoli.

Mucociliary Clearance System. Below the larynx, movement of mucus is accomplished by the mucociliary clearance system, commonly referred to as the *mucociliary escalator*. This term is used to indicate the interrelationship between the secretion of mucus and the ciliary activity. Mucus is continually secreted at a rate of about 100 mL per day by goblet cells and submucosal glands. It forms a mucous blanket that contains the impacted particles and debris from distal lung areas (see Figure 28.1). The small amount of mucus normally secreted is swallowed without being noticed. Collectins (glycoproteins that are part of the innate immune system) are secreted and produced by the lungs and contribute to protection against bacteria and viruses (McCance & Huether, 2019).

Cilia cover the airways from the level of the trachea to the respiratory bronchioles (see Figure 28.1). Each ciliated cell contains approximately 200 cilia, which beat rhythmically about 1 000 times per minute in the large airways, moving mucus toward the mouth. The ciliary beat is slower farther down the tracheobronchial tree. As a consequence, particles that penetrate more deeply into the airways are removed less rapidly. Ciliary action is impaired by dehydration, smoking, inhalation of high oxygen concentrations, infection, and ingestion of drugs such as atropine, anaesthetics, alcohol, and cocaine. Cilia are often destroyed by chronic bronchitis and cystic fibrosis, which results in impaired secretion clearance, a chronic productive cough, and frequent upper respiratory infections.

Cough Reflex. The cough is a protective reflex action that clears the airway by a high-pressure, high-velocity flow of air. It is a backup for mucociliary clearance, especially when this clearance mechanism is overwhelmed or ineffective. Coughing is effective in removing secretions only above the subsegmental level (large or main airways). Secretions below this level must be moved upward by the mucociliary mechanism or by interventions such as postural drainage before they can be removed by coughing.

Reflex Bronchoconstriction. Another defence mechanism is reflex bronchoconstriction. In response to the inhalation of large amounts of irritating substances (e.g., dusts, aerosols), the bronchi constrict in an effort to prevent entry of the irritants. In conditions of hyperreactive airways, such as asthma, bronchoconstriction occurs after inhalation of cold air, perfume, or other strong odours.

Alveolar Macrophages. Since ciliated cells are not found below the level of the respiratory bronchioles, the primary defence mechanism at the alveolar level is performed by alveolar macrophages. *Alveolar macrophages* rapidly phagocytize inhaled foreign particles such as bacteria. The debris is moved to the level of the bronchioles for removal by the cilia or is removed from the lungs by the lymphatic system. Particles (e.g., coal dust, silica) that cannot be adequately phagocytized tend to remain in the lungs for indefinite periods and can stimulate inflammatory responses (see Chapter 30). Since alveolar macrophage activity is impaired by cigarette smoke, people who are employed in an occupation with heavy dust exposure (e.g., mining, foundries) and smoke are at an especially high risk for lung disease.

TABLE 28.4	AGE-RELATED DIFFERENCES IN ASSESSMENT

Respiratory System

Changes	Differences in Assessment Findings
Structure	
↓ Elastic recoil	Barrel shape of chest
↓ Chest wall compliance	↓ Chest wall movement
↑ Anteroposterior diameter	↓ Respiratory excursion
↓ Functioning alveoli	↓ Vital capacity*
	↑ Functional residual capacity*
	Diminished breath sounds, particularly at lung bases
	↓ PaO_2 and SaO_2; normal pH and $PaCO_2$
Defence Mechanisms	
↓ Cell-mediated immunity	↓ Cough effectiveness
↓ Specific antibodies	↓ Secretion clearance
↓ Cilia function	↑ Risk of upper respiratory infection, influenza, and pneumonia; respiratory infections may be more severe and last longer
↓ Cough force	
↓ Alveolar macrophage function	
Respiratory Control	
↓ Response to hypoxemia	Greater ↓ in PaO_2 and ↑ in $PaCO_2$ before respiratory rate changes
↓ Response to hypercapnia	Significant hypoxemia or hypercapnia may develop as a result of relatively minor incidents
	Retained secretions, excessive sedation, or positioning that impairs chest expansion may substantially alter PaO_2 or SpO_2 values

$PaCO_2$, arterial carbon dioxide tension; PaO_2, arterial oxygen tension; SaO_2, arterial oxygen saturation; SpO_2, oxygen saturation value obtained by pulse oximetry.
*See Table 28.14 for definitions of terms related to lung volumes and capacities.

AGE-RELATED CONSIDERATIONS

EFFECTS OF AGING ON THE RESPIRATORY SYSTEM

Age-related changes in the respiratory system and related assessment findings can be divided into alterations in structure, defence mechanisms, and respiratory control (Table 28.4).

Within the aging lung, the number of functional alveoli decreases and small airways in the lung bases close earlier in expiration. Consequently, more inspired air is distributed to the lung apices, and ventilation is less matched to perfusion, which causes a lowering of the PaO_2. The PaO_2 associated with a given age can be calculated by means of the following equation:

$$PaO_2 \ (mm \ Hg) = 103.5 - (0.42 \times age \ in \ years)$$

For example, the normal PaO_2 for a patient 80 years of age is 70 mm Hg (103.5 − [0.42 × 80]); in comparison, the normal PaO_2 for a 25-year-old person is 93 mm Hg (103.5 − [0.42 × 25]).

The extent of these changes varies among persons of the same age. Older persons—who have experienced many years of exposure to smoking, air pollutants, and other environmental toxins—are at risk for a host of other conditions (Jarvis et al., 2019).

ASSESSMENT OF THE RESPIRATORY SYSTEM

On admission to acute care, the nurse completes and documents a comprehensive history and physical, including inspection, palpation, percussion and auscultation of the respiratory

TABLE 28.5 HEALTH HISTORY
Respiratory System: Questions for Obtaining Subjective Data

Cough
- Do you have a cough, and if so, when did it start? How often do you cough? Does it wake you up at night? Does activity affect your cough?* What relieves your cough? What makes the cough worse?
- Do you cough up sputum?* How much do you expectorate? What colour is your sputum?
- Are you coughing up blood?*

Shortness of Breath
- Are you ever short of breath?* What brings it on?
- Do you get too short of breath to do the things you want to do?* (Note: To determine the intensity of dyspnea, the Medical Research Council Dyspnea Scale [see Chapter 31, Figure 31.15] or a visual analogue scale may be helpful [Registered Nurses' Association of Ontario, 2005])
- Do breathing problems cause you to awaken during the night?*
- Can you lie flat at night? If not, how many pillows do you use? Do you need to sleep upright in a chair?
- What do you do when you get short of breath?

Chest Pain With Breathing
- Do you experience chest pain with breathing?* Where exactly is the pain located? Can you describe the pain? What brings on the pain? What relieves the pain? Does anything make the pain worse? Can you rate the severity of the pain (NRS 0–10)? When did this pain start? Is the pain continuous or intermittent?

History of Respiratory Infections or Illness
- Do you have any history of breathing trouble or lung disease (e.g., shortness of breath, coughing, blood in your sputum, COPD, bronchitis, emphysema, asthma, pneumonia, sleep apnea)?*
- Have you ever been hospitalized or treated for a respiratory illness?*
- Do you have frequent colds or very severe colds, or both?*
- Do you have any allergies or sensitivities (food, environmental, medications)?*
- Do you have a family history of allergies, tuberculosis, or asthma?*

Self-Care History
- Do you use any equipment or take any medications to manage respiratory symptoms (e.g., home oxygen therapy equipment, metered-dose inhaler with spacer or nebulizer for medication administration, positive airway pressure device for relief of sleep apnea)?*
- Do you smoke?* If yes, how many packs daily? For how many years? Do you smoke cigarettes or cigars? Have you ever tried to quit? Are you living with someone who smokes?
- Are there any environmental conditions at home or work that may have an effect on your respiratory health (e.g., smoke, dust, chemicals)?* If so, do you do anything to protect your lungs or monitor your exposure?
- Have you received immunization for influenza (flu), pneumococcal pneumonia (Pneumovax), tuberculosis skin test, and/or chest radiograph? When?

COPD, chronic obstructive pulmonary disease; *NRS*, numeric rating scale.
Source: Based on Jarvis, C., Browne, A. J., MacDonald-Jenkins, J., et al. (Eds.). (2019). *Physical examination & health assessment* (3rd Canadian ed., pp. 456–458). Elsevier.
*If the answer is "yes," the patient should describe further.

CASE STUDY
Patient Introduction

F. T. (pronouns he/him), 70 years old, comes to the emergency department complaining of increased shortness of breath. F. T. states that he started using a salbutamol (Ventolin) inhaler every 4 hours a few days ago, but it does not seem to be helping. He has been having trouble sleeping or doing any activity because of his shortness of breath.

Critical Thinking
As you read through this assessment chapter, think about F. T.'s symptoms with the following questions in mind:
1. What are the possible causes of F. T.'s shortness of breath?
2. What type of assessment would be most appropriate for F. T.: comprehensive, focused, or emergency?
3. What questions would the nurse ask F. T.?
4. What should be included in the physical assessment? What would the nurse be looking for?
5. What diagnostic studies might be ordered?
   See Case Study: Subjective Data, Case Study: Objective Data: Physical Examination, and Case Study: Diagnostic Studies for more information on F. T.

ⓔvolve
Answers available at http://evolve.elsevier.com/Canada/Lewis/medsurg.

that can provide clues to the presence of respiratory conditions. Nurses collaborate with the interprofessional team, making shared judgements about respiratory health, to achieve the best possible patient outcomes (Registered Nurses' Association of Ontario [RNAO], 2013, 2016).

SAFETY ALERT
Nurses should implement routine and droplet/contact precautions with patients being assessed for acute or novel respiratory illness such as COVID-19 until the epidemiology of the agent has been established (Public Health Agency of Canada [PHAC], 2021c).

Prevention of illness, absenteeism, lost productivity, and even death associated with respiratory illnesses require health care workers to conduct a point-of-care risk assessment and implement additional personal protective equipment, as necessary, prior to conducting any respiratory assessment. During active case finding and surveillance, patients and health care workers should be asked about possible respiratory symptoms on arrival at the health care setting. Screening includes new or worsening cough or shortness of breath, fever, and travel risk assessment (i.e., within the last 14 days or contact with a sick person who has travelled in the past 14 days, and travel destination). Health care personnel asking the initial screening questions should maintain at least a 2-metre distance from the patient or should be protected by a glass or other solid, transparent barrier. On inpatient and residential units in health care facilities, patients and residents should be checked daily for respiratory symptoms and educated to prevent potential transmission of microorganisms. In response to positive screening, appropriate routine practices and droplet/contact precautions are initiated by the nurse and reported to Infection Prevention and Control and Public Health (Public Health Ontario, 2021). The nurse should

system. Correct diagnosis depends on an accurate health history and a thorough physical examination (Table 28.5). Subsequent focused respiratory assessments are performed on the basis of the patient's history, clinical manifestations, or both. If respiratory distress is severe, only pertinent information should be obtained; a thorough assessment should be deferred until the patient's condition stabilizes. Table 28.6 outlines subjective and objective data that may emerge during the assessment and

TABLE 28.6 CLUES TO RESPIRATORY CONDITIONS

Manifestation	Description
Shortness of breath (dyspnea)	Distressing sensation of uncomfortable breathing. Most common report of people with respiratory conditions. Person may become accustomed to the sensation and not recognize its presence. Difficult to evaluate because it is a subjective experience.
Wheezing	May or may not be heard by patient. May be described as "chest tightness."
Pleuritic chest pain	Described on a continuum from discomfort during inspiration to intense, sharp pain at the end of inspiration. Pain is usually aggravated by deep breathing and coughing.
Cough	Characteristics and timing of cough are important diagnostic clues.
Sputum production	Material coughed up from lungs. Contains mucus, cellular debris, or microorganisms and may contain blood or pus. Amount, colour, and constituents of sputum constitute important diagnostic information.
Hemoptysis	Coughing up of blood; sputum may be grossly bloody, frankly bloody, or blood-tinged. Precipitating events should be investigated.
Audible changes	Voice changes such as hoarseness and muffling, stridor (whistling sound during inspiration), or a barking cough may indicate abnormalities of upper airway, vocal cord dysfunction, or gastroesophageal reflux disease.
Fatigue	Sense of overwhelming tiredness, not completely relieved by sleep or rest.

consult best practices for prevention, surveillance, and infection control management of novel respiratory infections in all health care settings, as required (Public Health Ontario, 2021).

Subjective Data

Important Health Information

Past Health History. The nurse should discuss with the patient the types of respiratory illnesses that the patient experienced during childhood (e.g., croup, respiratory syncytial virus, asthma, pneumonia, frequent colds).

The nurse should determine the frequency of upper respiratory conditions (e.g., colds, sore throats, sinus conditions, allergies) and whether weather changes exacerbate these issues. Patients with allergies should be questioned about possible precipitating factors such as medications or exposure to pollen, smoke, or animal dander. Characteristics of the allergic reaction—such as runny nose, wheezing, scratchy throat, or sensation of tightness in the chest—and the severity of the reaction should be documented. The frequency of asthma exacerbations and cause, if known, should also be determined. Prior use of a peak expiratory flowmeter and personal best values can be helpful information in determining the patient's current asthma status.

A history of lower respiratory tract conditions, such as asthma, COPD, pneumonia, and tuberculosis, should also be documented (see the Determinants of Health: Tuberculosis box, Chapter 30). Respiratory symptoms are often manifestations of conditions that involve other body systems; therefore, a full history should be taken. For example, patients with cardiac dysfunction may experience dyspnea (shortness of breath) as a consequence of heart failure. Patients with human immunodeficiency virus (HIV) infection may experience frequent respiratory infections because immune function is compromised.

Medications. Patients should be questioned carefully about prescription and over-the-counter (OTC) medications and herbal remedies used to manage respiratory conditions (e.g., antihistamines, bronchodilators, corticosteroids, cough suppressants, antibiotics, lozenges). The nurse should obtain information about the reason for taking the medication, its name, the dose and frequency, length of time taken, its effect, and any adverse effects.

If a patient is using supplemental oxygen to ease a breathing problem, the amount, the method of administration, and effectiveness of the therapy should be documented. Safety practices related to using supplemental oxygen should also be assessed.

Surgery or Other Treatments. The nurse should assess for and document any reported hospitalizations, surgeries, or interventions for respiratory conditions. The nurse should ask about the use and results of respiratory treatments such as nebulizer, humidifier, airway clearance modalities, high-frequency chest oscillation, postural drainage, and percussion.

Current Health History. The nurse should ask if the patient has a cough and, if present, further evaluate its onset, severity, frequency, timing, pattern, quality, and associated clinical manifestations; the palliating and provoking factors; and the patient's understanding of and concerns related to the cough (Jarvis et al., 2019). Onset/timing and pattern of the cough helps determine a differential diagnosis. For example, a continuous cough lasting 2 to 3 weeks may indicate an acute viral illness, an early morning cough can be a symptom of chronic inflammation and bronchitis related to smoking, and a productive cough during winter months may be an early symptom of COPD. The quality of the cough can reveal underlying associated illness: A hacking cough may indicate mycoplasma pneumonia; barking associated with upper airway obstruction and subglottic edema, croup; congested cough, colds, bronchitis, or pneumonia; and dry cough, early heart failure (Jarvis et al., 2019). The nurse should assess whether the cough is weak or strong and whether it is productive or nonproductive of secretions. If productive, the amount, colour, consistency, and odour of sputum should be evaluated and any recent changes in these findings noted. If sputum contains blood (hemoptysis) the nurse should clarify if there are streaks or frank blood. Sputum production can be characteristic of some conditions: White or clear mucoid production may indicate colds, bronchitis, or viral infections; yellow or green, bacterial infections; rust coloured, tuberculosis (TB) or pneumococcal pneumonia; pink, frothy production, pulmonary edema; grey, a smoker; malodourous, infection; and thick production, dehydration (Jarvis et al., 2019). The nurse needs to explore if further clinical manifestations are brought on by the cough (e.g., chest pain, shortness of breath, ear pain, fatigue), what makes the cough worse (e.g., talking, anxiety, cold air, activity, lying flat) or better (e.g., vaporizer, position change, rest), and what prescriptions or OTC medications or treatments have been tried. The nurse should clarify the patient's perspective related to the cough (e.g., ask, "What concerns you the most about your cough?").

Patients should be questioned about a family history of respiratory conditions that may be genetic or have familial tendencies, such as asthma, emphysema resulting from α_1-antitrypsin deficiency, or cystic fibrosis. A history of family exposure to tubercle bacilli should be noted.

CASE STUDY

Subjective Data

A focused subjective assessment of F. T. revealed the following information:

History of current illness: Has been experiencing increasing difficulty breathing since catching a cold from his granddaughter last week, even with the use of salbutamol (Ventolin). Has had increased shortness of breath on exertion and worsening paroxysmal nocturnal dyspnea. Denies any pain or confusion associated with the shortness of breath.

Past health: COPD, hypertension, and benign prostatic hyperplasia. No history of environmental allergies. Denies history of coronary artery disease or heart failure.

Medications: metoprolol (Lopressor), 50 mg/day orally; finasteride (Propecia, Proscar), 5 mg/day orally; fluticasone and salmeterol (Advair) inhaler, two puffs per day; and salbutamol (Ventolin) inhaler, two puffs every 4 hours as needed. Does not use O_2 at home.

Functional assessment: F. T. usually manages his COPD well with just the fluticasone and salmeterol (Advair) inhaler and occasional use of the salbutamol (Ventolin) inhaler as needed. Has a history of 30 pack-years of smoking, having quit 5 years ago. Had a Pneumovax vaccination 5 years ago and receives the flu vaccine on an annual basis. States he can typically walk at least two blocks and up and down stairs without getting short of breath. However, at this point, he cannot walk 30 metres without feeling short of breath, nor walk up one flight of stairs without stopping for breath. Has been having difficulty sleeping with this most recent episode of shortness of breath. Typically uses just one pillow to sleep with but needed three pillows this week, and slept upright in a recliner last night. Denies any stress or emotional disturbance that could be having an impact on breathing. Feels slightly irritable because of lack of sleep.

See Case Study: Patient Introduction, Case Study: Objective Data: Physical Examination, and Case Study: Diagnostic Studies for more information on F. T.

Indigenous people, health care workers, and residents of long-term care facilities and correctional facilities are at increased risk for TB infection. Further risk factors for TB include prior residence in a developing nation, homelessness, and intravenous drug use. People with certain comorbid conditions such as HIV infection and diabetes and those receiving dialysis have an increased risk of TB reactivation (PHAC, The Lung Association, & Canadian Thoracic Society, 2014).

The nurse should also ask about current and past smoking habits and quantify exposure in pack-years by multiplying the number of packs smoked per day by the number of years smoked. For example, a person who smokes one pack per day for 15 years has a 15 pack-year history. The risk of lung cancer rises in direct proportion to the number of pack-years smoked. Smoking increases the risk of COPD and exacerbates symptoms of asthma and chronic bronchitis. It is also important to investigate history of vaping (PHAC, 2021a) and the use of any other tobacco products, (e.g., cigars, pipes, chewing tobacco). While described as less harmful than smoking burning tobacco, electronic cigarettes, or vapes, have not proven to be harmless, and the short-term and long-term health risks of vaping continue to be studied (Cobb & Solanki, 2020). The *Canadian Tobacco and Vaping Products Act* became law on May 23, 2018, creating a national minimum age of 18 years for access to vaping products and placing significant restrictions on the promotion of vaping products (Health Canada, 2018).

Information about exposure to second-hand smoke is also important. The nurse should ask whether the patient has made efforts, including the use of prescription, OTC, and herbal remedies, to quit use of tobacco products.

The nurse should ask whether the patient has received immunization for influenza (flu) and pneumococcal pneumonia (Pneumovax). Influenza vaccine should be administered yearly in the fall (PHAC, 2019). Pneumococcal vaccine is recommended for persons 65 years of age or older and for individuals with chronic cardiovascular disease, chronic pulmonary disease, or diabetes mellitus. The current recommendation is one dose of Pneumovax vaccine for adults aged 65 or older. Pneumococcal vaccination is also recommended for persons who are immunocompromised or organ transplant recipients, for travellers, and for persons living with underlying chronic disease and asplenia. The immunization status of persons new to Canada should be reviewed by a health care provider and updated as necessary (PHAC, 2021b).

Patients should be asked whether they use equipment to manage respiratory symptoms, such as home oxygen therapy equipment, a metered-dose inhaler (MDI) with spacer or nebulizer for medication administration, and positive airway pressure device for relief of sleep apnea. Patients should be questioned about the type of equipment used, frequency of use, its therapeutic effect, and any adverse effects. Patients who use an MDI should be asked to demonstrate its use, as incorrect technique is common (see Chapter 31).

Objective Data

Physical Examination. Vital signs, including temperature, pulse, respirations, and blood pressure, are important data to collect before examination of the respiratory system. Physical examination includes inspection and assessment of the nose, mouth and pharynx, neck, and thorax and lungs.

Nose. The nose is inspected for patency, inflammation, deformities, symmetry, and discharge. Each naris (nostril) is checked for air patency with respiration while the other naris is briefly occluded. The nurse tilts the patient's head back and pushes the tip of the nose upward gently. With a nasal speculum and a good light, the nurse can inspect the interior of the nose. The mucous membrane should be pink and moist, with no evidence of edema (bogginess), exudate, or bleeding. The nasal septum should be observed for deviation, perforations, and bleeding. Some nasal deviation is normal in an adult. The turbinates should be observed for polyps, which are abnormal, finger-like projections of swollen nasal mucosa. Polyps may result from long-term irritation of the mucosa, as from allergies. Any discharge should be assessed for colour and consistency. The presence of purulent, malodorous, or thick discharge could indicate the presence of a foreign body or infection. Watery discharge could be secondary to allergies or with a recent history of craniofacial trauma could be cerebrospinal fluid. Bloody discharge could be related to a recent trauma, nasal spray or street drug misuse, allergic rhinitis, cancer, or prolonged bleeding times (see Chapter 29 for a more complete discussion of epistaxis).

Mouth and Pharynx. Using a good light source, the nurse can inspect the interior of the mouth for colour, lesions, masses, gum retraction, bleeding, and poor dentition. The tongue is inspected for symmetry and presence of lesions. The pharynx can be observed by pressing a tongue blade against the middle of the back of the tongue. The pharynx should be smooth and moist, with no evidence of exudate, ulcerations, swelling, or postnasal drip. The colour, symmetry, and any enlargement of the tonsils are noted. Eliciting a gag reflex is not usually done in the screening exam, but when there are neurological or swallowing concerns, the gag reflex is assessed on each side of the pharynx. The nurse can stimulate the gag reflex by placing a tongue blade along the side of the pharynx behind the tonsil. A normal response (gagging) indicates that cranial nerves IX (glossopharyngeal nerve) and X (vagus nerve) are intact and that the airway is protected. An absent gag reflex requires the patient to be placed on NPO status until the gag reflex returns or until further investigation is complete.

Neck. The nurse inspects the neck for symmetry and presence of tender or swollen areas. The lymph nodes are palpated while the patient is sitting erect with the neck slightly flexed. Palpation progresses from the nodes around the ears to the nodes at the base of the skull and then to those located under the angles of the mandible to the midline. Normally, the nodes may be small, mobile, and nontender (shotty nodes). Nodes that are tender, hard, or fixed indicate disease. The location and characteristics of any palpable nodes need to be described.

Thorax and Lungs. Chest examination is best performed in a well-lit, warm room, with measures taken to ensure the patient's privacy. Either the anterior or the posterior aspect of the chest may be examined first. Imaginary lines can be pictured on the chest to help in identifying abnormalities (see Figure 28.2). The locations of abnormalities can be described in relation to these lines (e.g., 2 cm from the right midclavicular line).

Inspection. The anterior aspect of the chest should be exposed while the patient is sitting upright or with the head of the bed upright. The patient may need to lean forward on the bedside table for support in order to facilitate breathing. First, the nurse observes the patient's appearance and notes any evidence of respiratory distress, such as tachypnea or use of accessory muscles. Next, the nurse determines the shape and symmetry of the chest. Normally chest movement is equal on both sides, and the anteroposterior diameter is less than the transverse diameter by a ratio of 1:2. An increase in anteroposterior diameter (barrel-shaped chest) may be a normal age-related change or a result of lung hyperinflation, as occurs with emphysema. The nurse needs to observe for abnormalities in the sternum, such as *pectus carinatum* (a prominent protrusion of the sternum) and *pectus excavatum* (an indentation of the lower sternum above the xiphoid process).

Next, the nurse should observe the respiratory rate, depth, and rhythm. The normal rate is 12 to 20 breaths per minute; in older persons, it is 16 to 25 breaths per minute. Inspiration should take half as long as expiration (ratio of inspiration to expiration is 1:2). The nurse should observe for abnormal breathing patterns such as tachypnea, hyperventilation, bradypnea, hypoventilation, Kussmaul's, Cheyne–Stokes, or Biot's respirations (see Table 28.9 later in the chapter) (Jarvis et al., 2019). Skin colour and nail beds provide clues to respiratory status, such as cyanosis caused by hypoxemia and poor cardiac output. In darkly pigmented skin, cyanosis is best observed in the conjunctivae, lips, palms, and soles of the feet. Capillary refill (depressing nail edge to cause blanching and observing color return) taking longer than 1 or 2 seconds and *clubbing* (an increase in the angle between the base of the nail and the fingernail to 180 degrees or more) are associated with cardiovascular and respiratory dysfunction.

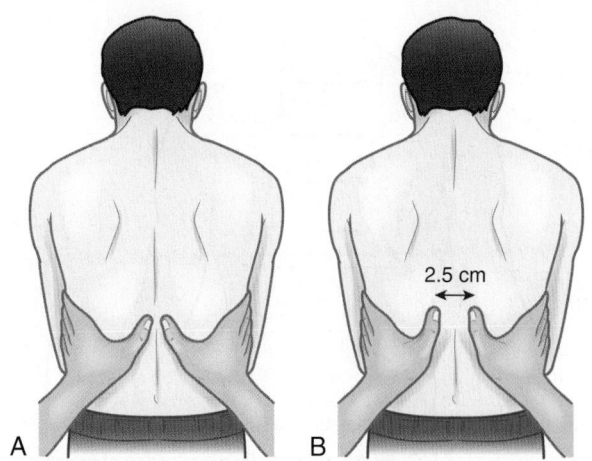

FIG. 28.8 Estimation of thoracic expansion. **A,** Exhalation. **B,** Maximal inhalation.

When the nurse is inspecting the posterior aspect of the chest, the patient should lean forward with arms folded. This position moves the scapula away from the spine so there is more exposure of the area to be examined. The observations made on the anterior part of the chest are made in the same sequence on the posterior part. In addition, any spinal curvature is noted. Spinal curvatures that affect breathing include kyphosis, scoliosis, and kyphoscoliosis.

Palpation. The nurse can determine tracheal position by placing the index fingers on either side of the patient's trachea just above the suprasternal notch and gently pressing back. Normal tracheal position is midline; deviation to the left or right is abnormal. Tracheal deviation occurs away from the side of a tension pneumothorax or a neck mass but toward the side of a pneumonectomy or lobar atelectasis (Urden et al., 2018). Symmetry of chest expansion and extent of movement are determined at the level of the diaphragm. The nurse places both hands over the lower anterior aspect of the patient's chest wall along the costal margin and moves them inward until the thumbs meet at midline. The patient is asked to breathe deeply, and the nurse observes the movement of the thumbs away from each other. Normal expansion is 2.5 cm. On the posterior side of the chest, the nurse places their hands at the level of the patient's tenth rib and moves the thumbs until they meet over the patient's spine (Figure 28.8).

Normal chest movement is symmetrical. Expansion is asymmetrical when air entry is limited by conditions involving the lung (e.g., atelectasis, pneumothorax) or the chest wall (e.g., incisional pain; fractured ribs). Expansion is symmetrical but diminished in conditions that cause the chest to become hyperinflated or barrel-shaped and in neuromuscular conditions (e.g., amyotrophic lateral sclerosis, spinal cord lesions).

Tactile fremitus is a palpable vibration, generated when sounds from the larynx are transmitted through the bronchi and through the lung parenchyma to the chest wall. To assess for tactile fremitus, the nurse asks the patient to repeat "ninety-nine" or "blue moon" while palpating the patient's posterior and anterior chest in a side-to-side pattern, from the lung apices to the bases, using the palmer base (the ball) or ulnar edge of one hand (Figure 28.9). The vibrations normally should be equal on corresponding sides. Palpating over the scapula and female breast tissue is avoided as bone and

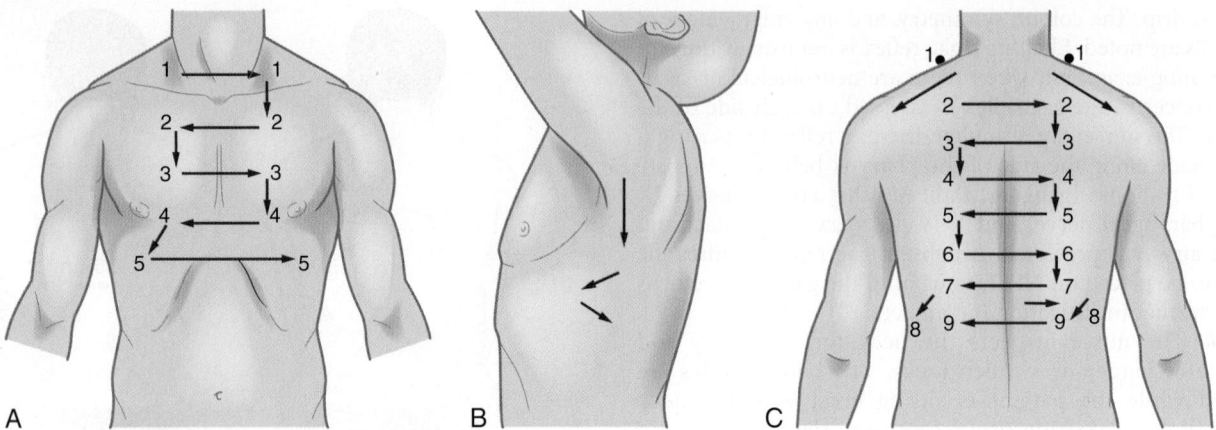

FIG. 28.9 Sequence for examination of the chest. **A,** Anterior sequence. **B,** Lateral sequence. **C,** Posterior sequence. For palpation, the nurse places the palms of the hands in the position designated as *1* on the right and left sides of the chest. The nurse compares the intensity of vibrations. Then the nurse repeats for all positions in each sequence. For percussion, the nurse taps the chest at each designated position, moving downward from side to side, while comparing percussion notes. For auscultation, the nurse places the stethoscope at each position and listens to at least one complete inspiratory and expiratory cycle.

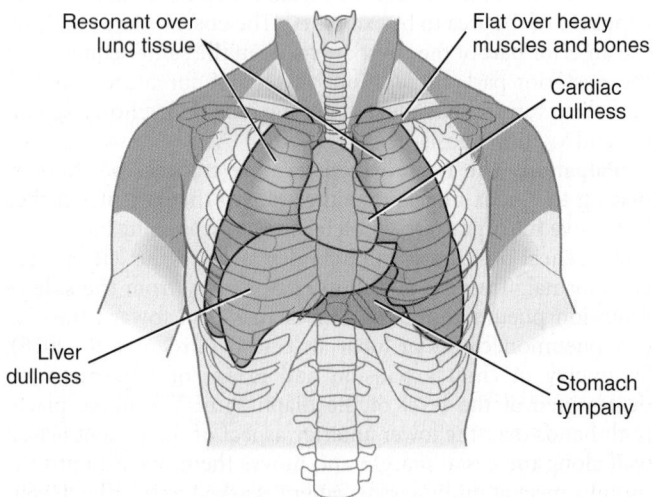

FIG. 28.10 Diagram of percussion areas and sounds in the anterior aspect of the chest. Redrawn from Thompson, J. M., McFarland, G., & Tucker, S. (2002). *Mosby's clinical nursing* (5th ed.). Mosby.

FIG. 28.11 Diagram of percussion areas and sounds in the posterior aspect of the chest. Percussion proceeds from the lung apices to the lung bases, and sounds from opposite areas of the chest are compared. Redrawn from Thompson, J. M., McFarland, G., & Tucker, S. (2002). *Mosby's clinical nursing* (5th ed.). Mosby.

TABLE 28.7	PERCUSSION SOUNDS
Sound	**Description**
Resonance	Low-pitched sound heard over normal lungs
Hyperresonance	Loud, lower-pitched sound than normal resonance heard over hyperinflated lungs, as in chronic obstructive lung disease and acute asthma
Tympany	Drumlike, loud, empty quality heard over gas-filled stomach or intestine or over pneumothorax
Dull	Medium-intensity pitch and duration heard over areas of "mixed" solid and lung tissue, such as over the top area of the liver, partially consolidated lung tissue (pneumonia), or fluid-filled pleural space
Flat	Soft, high-pitched sound of short duration heard over very dense tissue in which air is not present

breast tissue normally dampen the vibration. Tactile fremitus decreases when anything obstructs vibration transmission (e.g., obstructed bronchus, pleural effusion) and increases when there is increased density or consolidation of lung tissue (e.g., lobar pneumonia; tumor) (Jarvis et al., 2019).

Percussion. Percussion is performed to assess density or aeration of the lungs. Percussion sounds are described in Table 28.7. (The technique for percussion is described in Chapter 3).

The anterior aspect of the chest is usually percussed with the patient in a semi-sitting or supine position. Starting above the clavicles, the nurse percusses downward, interspace by interspace (see Figure 28.9). The area over lung tissue should be resonant, with the exception of the area of cardiac dullness (Figure 28.10). For percussion of the posterior chest, the patient should sit leaning forward with arms folded. The posterior chest should be resonant over lung tissue to the level of the diaphragm (Figure 28.11).

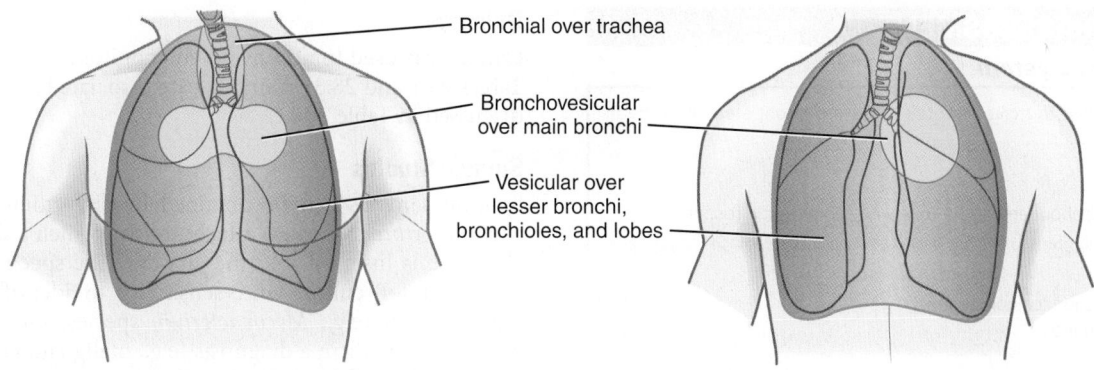

FIG. 28.12 Normal auscultatory sounds. Source: Beare, P. G., & Myers, J. L. (1998). *Adult health nursing* (3rd ed.). Mosby.

TABLE 28.8	**NORMAL PHYSICAL ASSESSMENT OF THE RESPIRATORY SYSTEM**

- Nose is symmetrical with no deformities. Nasal mucosa is pink and moist with no edema, exudate, blood, or polyps. Nasal septum is straight, without perforations.
- Oral mucosa is light pink and moist, with no exudate or ulcerations.
- Tonsils are not inflamed or enlarged.
- Pharynx is smooth, moist, and pink.
- Trachea is midline. No nodes are palpable.
- Chest is elliptical in shape, and chest expansion is symmetrical. Respirations are regular and nonlaboured, at the rate of 14/min. Breath sounds noted throughout both lung fields, without crackles or wheezes. No axillary nodes are palpable.

Auscultation. Using the stethoscope diaphragm, the nurse listens for one full respiration in each location, with side-to-side comparison from the lung apices to the bases, and avoiding placement of the stethoscope over bony prominences (see Figure 28.9). The patient is instructed to breathe slowly and deeply, in through the nose and out through the mouth. The nurse notes the pitch (e.g., high, low), the duration of inspiration versus expiration, and the presence of any abnormal or adventitious sounds. The location of normal auscultatory sounds is more easily understood through visualization of a lung model (Figure 28.12). Normal breath sounds in adults include *bronchial sounds* (harsh, hollow—over the trachea and larynx); *bronchovesicular sounds* (mixed—over major bronchi, posteriorly between the scapula and anteriorly around upper sternum) and *vesicular sounds* (rustling—over peripheral lung fields) (Jarvis et al., 2019). Posteriorly, lungs are auscultated from the apices at C7 to the bases (around T10) and laterally from the axilla down to rib 7 or 8 and during a deep breath to rib 12. Anteriorly, the lungs are auscultated from the supraclavicular areas down to the sixth rib, taking care to displace the female breast to listen directly on the chest wall.

Abnormal breath sounds include decreased or absent sounds caused by conditions that obstruct sound transmission (e.g., secretions, foreign body, hyperinflation in emphysema, pleural effusion or pneumothorax) and increased sounds that are louder than normal because of consolidation or compression of lung tissue (e.g., consolidation in pneumonia). Adventitious sounds are additional breath sounds that are abnormal. Adventitious breath sounds, described more fully in Table 28.9, include crackles (short, low-pitched sounds

CASE STUDY

Objective Data: Physical Examination

Physical examination findings of F. T. are as follows:

BP 170/90, apical pulse 110, respiratory rate 30, temperature 38°C, O_2 saturation 87% on room air. Patient sitting on edge of bed with arms resting on bedside table. Slight use of accessory muscles in neck and shoulders and pursed lips on expiration noted. Barrel-shaped chest with minimal expansion; respirations regular, slightly laboured, with prolonged expiration. Skin colour is pale with no cyanosis. No clubbing noted. Trachea is midline. Lungs: decreased air entry and course crackles right middle lobe and bilateral bases, with low-pitched expiratory wheezing throughout lung fields. Cough: moist, productive with yellow-tinged sputum.

Throughout this chapter, consider diagnostic studies that may be ordered for F. T.

See Case Study: Patient Introduction, Case Study: Subjective Data, and Case Study: Diagnostic Studies for more information on F.T.

caused by the passage of air through an airway intermittently occluded by mucus, unstable bronchial wall, or fold of mucosa), wheezes (continuous high-pitched squeaking sound caused by rapid vibration of bronchial walls), and pleural friction rub (a creaking or grating sound that occurs when roughened, inflamed surfaces of the pleura rub together; it is evident during inspiration, expiration, or both, and does not change with coughing).

A record of normal findings in the physical assessment of the respiratory system is shown in Table 28.8. Assessment abnormalities of the thorax and lungs are listed in Table 28.9. Chest examination findings in common pulmonary conditions are listed in Table 28.10. Age-related changes in the respiratory system and assessment findings are listed in Table 28.4.

A focused assessment is performed to evaluate the status of previously identified respiratory conditions and to monitor for signs of new health problems (see Chapter 3, Table 3.5). A focused assessment of the respiratory system is presented in the Focused Assessment box.

DIAGNOSTIC STUDIES OF THE RESPIRATORY SYSTEM

Blood Studies

Common blood studies used to assess the respiratory system are hemoglobin, hematocrit, and ABGs. Table 28.11 lists nursing responsibilities associated with these tests.

FOCUSED ASSESSMENT
Respiratory System

Use this checklist to make sure the key assessment steps have been done.

Subjective
Ask the patient about any of the following and note the responses:

Shortness of breath	Y	N
Wheezing	Y	N
Sputum production (colour, quantity)	Y	N
Pain with breathing	Y	N
Cough	Y	N

Objective: Diagnostic
Check the following laboratory results for critical values:

Arterial blood gas measurements	✓
Chest radiographic examination	✓
Hematocrit, hemoglobin measurements	✓

Objective: Physical Examination
Observe

Respirations for rate, quality, and pattern	✓
Facial expression, level of consciousness, position patient takes to breathe	

Inspect

Skin and nails for integrity and colour	✓
Accessory muscle use and position of trachea	✓
Shape, symmetry, and movement of chest wall	✓

Palpate

Chest and back for masses	✓
Tactile fremitus	

Auscultate

Lung (breath) sounds	✓

Oximetry

Oximetry is used to noninvasively monitor SpO_2 and SvO_2 (see Tables 28.1 and 28.3). Nursing care associated with oximetry is discussed in Table 28.11.

Sputum Studies

Sputum samples can be obtained by expectoration, tracheal suction, or *bronchoscopy*, a technique in which a flexible bronchoscope is inserted into the airways. The specimens may be examined for culture and sensitivity to identify an infecting organism (e.g., *Mycobacterium* species, *Pneumocystis jiroveci*) or to confirm a diagnosis (e.g., malignant cells). Nursing responsibilities for specimen collection are described in Table 28.11. Regardless of whether specimen tests are ordered, it is important to observe the sputum for colour, blood, volume, and viscosity.

Skin Tests

Skin tests may be performed to test for allergic reactions or exposure to tubercle bacilli or fungi. Usually, 0.1 mL of purified protein derivative is injected intradermally on the ventral surface of the forearm. Skin tests involve the intradermal injection of an antigen. A positive result indicates that the patient has been exposed to the antigen; it does not indicate that disease is currently present. A negative result indicates that the patient has not been exposed or that cell-mediated immunity is depressed, as occurs in HIV infection.

Nursing responsibilities are similar for all skin tests. First, to prevent a false-negative reaction, the nurse should be certain that the injection is intradermal and not subcutaneous. After the injection, the sites should be circled and the patient instructed not to remove the marks. When charting administration of the antigen, the nurse should draw a diagram of the forearm and hand and label the injection sites. The diagram is especially helpful when more than one test is administered.

TABLE 28.9 ASSESSMENT ABNORMALITIES
Respiratory System

Finding	Description	Possible Etiology and Significance*
Inspection		
Pursed-lip breathing	Exhalation through mouth with lips pursed together to slow exhalation	COPD, asthma; suggests ↑ breathlessness; strategy taught to slow expiration, reduce dyspnea
Tripod position; inability to lie flat	Learning forward with arms and elbows supported on overbed table	COPD, asthma in exacerbation, pulmonary edema; indicates moderate to severe respiratory distress
Accessory muscle use; intercostal retractions	Neck and shoulder muscles used to assist breathing; muscles between ribs pull in during inspiration	COPD, asthma in exacerbation, secretion retention; indicates severe respiratory distress, hypoxemia
Splinting	↓ Inspiratory effort (or ↓ in tidal volume) as a result of sharp pain upon inspiration	Thoracic or abdominal incision; chest trauma, pleurisy
↑ Anteroposterior diameter	Anteroposterior chest diameter equal to transverse diameter; slope of ribs more horizontal (90 degrees) to spine	COPD, asthma, cystic fibrosis; lung hyperinflation; advanced age
Bradypnea	A decreased but regular rate <10 breaths/min	Drug-induced depression of the respiratory centre in the medulla, increased intracranial pressure, and diabetic coma
Hypoventilation	Irregular, shallow pattern	Narcotic or anaesthetic overdose; can occur with effort to avoid pain (e.g., rib fracture, chest trauma, thoracic or abdominal surgery)
Tachypnea	Rate >20 breaths/min; >25 breaths/min in older persons	Fever, anxiety, hypoxemia, restrictive lung disease; ↑ above normal respiratory rate reflects increased work of breathing
Hyperventilation	Increase in rate and depth	Extreme exertion, fear or anxiety; diabetic ketoacidosis, hepatic coma, salicylate overdose, midbrain lesions; compensation for metabolic acidosis
Kussmaul's respirations	Regular, rapid, and deep respirations	Metabolic acidosis; ↑ in rate aids body in ↑ CO_2 excretion

TABLE 28.9   ASSESSMENT ABNORMALITIES

Respiratory System—cont'd

Finding	Description	Possible Etiology and Significance*
Cheyne-Stokes respirations	Regular breathing pattern (30–45 sec) with increasing then decreasing rate and depth, followed by periods of apnea (20 sec)	Older persons in sleep; severe heart failure, renal failure, meningitis, drug overdose and increased intracranial pressure
Cyanosis	Bluish coloration of skin, best seen in earlobes, under the eyelids, or in nail beds	↓ Oxygen transfer in lungs, ↓ cardiac output; nonspecific, unreliable indicator
Clubbing of fingers	↑ Depth, bulk, sponginess of distal digit of finger; angle between nail base and nail ≥180°	Chronic hypoxemia; COPD, cystic fibrosis, lung cancer, bronchiectasis
Abdominal paradox	Inward (rather than normal outward) movement of abdomen during inspiration	Inefficient and ineffective breathing pattern; nonspecific indicator of severe respiratory distress
Palpation		
Tracheal deviation	Leftward or rightward movement of trachea from normal midline position	Nonspecific indicator of change in position of mediastinal structures; medical emergency if caused by tension pneumothorax
Altered tactile fremitus	Increase or decrease in vibrations	↑ In pneumonia, pulmonary edema; ↓ in pleural effusion, lung hyperinflation; absent in pneumothorax, atelectasis
Altered chest movement	Diminished movement (can be asymmetrical or symmetrical) of two sides of chest with inspiration	Asymmetrical movement caused by atelectasis, pneumothorax, pleural effusion, splinting; symmetrical but diminished movement caused by barrel shape of chest, restrictive disease, neuromuscular disease
Percussion		
Hyper-resonance	Loud, lower-pitched sound over areas that normally produce a resonant sound	Lung hyperinflation (COPD), lung collapse (pneumothorax), air trapping (asthma)
Dullness	Medium-pitched sound over areas that normally produce a resonant sound	↑ Density (pneumonia, widespread atelectasis), ↑ fluid pleural space (pleural effusion)
Auscultation		
Fine crackles	Series of short, explosive, high-pitched sounds heard just before the end of inspiration; rapid equalization of gas pressure when collapsed alveoli or terminal bronchioles suddenly snap open; sounds similar to rolling hair between fingers just behind ear	Interstitial fibrosis (asbestosis), interstitial edema (early pulmonary edema), alveolar filling (pneumonia), loss of lung volume (atelectasis), early phase of heart failure
Coarse crackles	Series of short, low-pitched sounds on inspiration and sometimes expiration; air passing through airway intermittently occluded by mucus, unstable bronchial wall, or fold of mucosa; sounds similar to blowing through straw under water (increase in bubbling quality with more fluid)	Heart failure, pulmonary edema, pneumonia with severe congestion, COPD
Wheezes	Continuous high-pitched squeaking sound caused by rapid vibration of bronchial walls; first evident on expiration; possibly evident on inspiration as obstruction of airway increases; possibly audible without stethoscope	Bronchospasm (caused by asthma), airway obstruction (caused by foreign body; tumour; viscous, thick increased secretions), COPD, pneumonia, bronchiectasis
Stridor	Continuous musical sound of constant pitch; result of partial obstruction of larynx or trachea	Croup, epiglottitis, vocal cord edema after extubation, foreign body
Absence of breath sounds	No sound evident over entire lung or area of lung	Pleural effusion, mainstem bronchi obstruction, widespread atelectasis, pneumonectomy, lobectomy, severe acute asthma (i.e., silent chest)
Pleural friction rub	Creaking or grating sound occurs when roughened, inflamed surfaces of pleura rub together; evident on inspiration, expiration, or both; no change with coughing; usually painful, especially on deep inspiration	Pleurisy, pneumonia, pulmonary infarct

*Only common causes are listed. (These conditions are discussed further in Chapters 29 through 31.)
COPD, chronic obstructive pulmonary disease.

Tuberculin Skin Testing. When reading tuberculin skin test (TST) results, the nurse should use a good light and the reading should be performed within 48 to 72 hours after the purified protein derivative is administered (PHAC, The Lung Association, & Canadian Thoracic Society, 2014). If an area of induration (i.e., hardness) is present, the widest diameter of the induration is measured in millimetres. Areas of erythema (i.e., redness) without induration are not considered significant. Situations associated with positive reactions are described in Table 28.12. Canadian health care settings use tuberculin purified protein (Tubersol) for skin tests. If any patient has had

a previous bacille Calmette-Guérin vaccination, it will affect results. This is significant especially for people from Quebec, Newfoundland, and Indigenous populations, who regularly received this vaccine from 1940 through the 1970s (PHAC, 2020).

Radiological Studies

Chest Radiography. Chest radiographic examination is the most common method of assessing the respiratory system. It is also used to assess progression of disease and response to treatment. The views most commonly used are posteroanterior and lateral. (See Table 28.11 for nursing responsibilities related to chest radiographic examinations.)

Computed Tomography. Computed tomography (CT) may be used to examine cross-sections of the entire body. CT is used to evaluate areas that are difficult to assess by conventional radiographic study, such as the mediastinum, the hilum, and the pleura. With enhancement by a contrast medium, with a high-resolution technique, or with newer spiral CT, even pulmonary arteries can be inspected for emboli.

Magnetic Resonance Imaging. While in a strong magnetic field, the alignment of spinning nuclei can be changed with a superimposed radiofrequency, and the rate at which they return to alignment with the field can be measured. Magnetic resonance imaging (MRI) is used to produce images of body structures. MRI has limited indications. It is most useful for evaluating images near the lung apex or the spine and for distinguishing vascular from nonvascular structures.

CASE STUDY

Diagnostic Studies

The health care provider orders the following diagnostic studies for F. T.:
- Complete blood cell count, basic metabolic panel (electrolytes, blood urea nitrogen, creatinine)
- ABGs
- Chest radiograph
- Sputum for culture and sensitivity

The ABGs demonstrate a compensated respiratory acidosis (pH, 7.37; $PaCO_2$, 58 mm Hg; HCO_3^-, 29 mEq/L) with hypoxemia (PaO_2, 58 mm Hg; SaO_2, 87%). The white blood cell count is 14.3×10^9/L, and the chest radiograph shows lower lobe pneumonia. F. T. is admitted to the cardiopulmonary medical-surgical nursing unit.

See Case Study: Patient Introduction, Case Study: Subjective Data, and Case Study: Objective Data: Physical Examination for more information on F. T.

Ventilation–Perfusion Scan. A ventilation–perfusion scan is used primarily to check for the presence of a pulmonary embolus. There is no specific preparation or aftercare. A radio-isotope is administered intravenously for the perfusion portion of the test; it outlines the pulmonary vasculature, which is then photographed. For the ventilation portion, the patient inhales a radioactive gas, which outlines the alveoli, and another photograph is taken. Normal scans show homogeneous radioactivity. Diminished appearance or absence of radioactivity is suggestive of lack of perfusion or airflow.

Pulmonary Angiography. Pulmonary angiography is used to confirm the diagnosis of an embolus if findings of the lung scan are inconclusive. A series of radiographs is taken after radiopaque dye is injected into the pulmonary artery. This test can also detect congenital and acquired lesions of the pulmonary vessels.

Positron Emission Tomography. Positron emission tomography (PET) scans involve the use of radionuclides with short half-lives. PET scans are used to distinguish benign from malignant solitary pulmonary nodules. Because uptake of glucose is increased in malignant lung cells, the PET scan, in which an intravenous glucose preparation is used, can demonstrate the presence of malignant lung cells.

Endoscopic Examinations

Bronchoscopy. *Bronchoscopy* is a procedure in which the bronchi are visualized through a fibre-optic tube. Bronchoscopy may be used to obtain biopsy specimens, assess changes resulting from treatment, and remove mucous plugs or foreign bodies. Small amounts (30 mL) of sterile saline may be injected through the bronchoscope, then withdrawn, and examined for cells. This technique, termed *bronchoalveolar lavage*, is used to diagnose *Pneumocystis jiroveci* pneumonia (PCP; see Figure 28.13).

TABLE 28.10	CHEST EXAMINATION FINDINGS IN COMMON PULMONARY CONDITIONS			
Condition	**Inspection**	**Palpation**	**Percussion**	**Auscultation**
Chronic bronchitis	Barrel shape of chest; cyanosis; possible clubbing of fingers	—	Resonant	Crackles over deflated areas; wheeze may be present
Emphysema	Barrel shape of chest; tripod position; use of accessory muscles	↓ Chest expansion	Hyper-resonant or dull if consolidation is present	Crackles diminished if no exacerbation is present
Asthma (during an exacerbation)	Prolonged expiration; tripod position; pursed lips	↓ Chest expansion ↓ Fremitus if hyperinflation is present	Hyper-resonance	Wheezes; ↓ breath sounds are ominous sign if no improvement occurs (represent severely diminished air movement)
Pneumonia	Tachypnea; use of accessory muscles; cyanosis	Unequal movement with lobar involvement; ↑ fremitus over affected area	Dull over affected areas	Early: bronchial sounds Later: crackles; wheezes
Atelectasis	No change unless entire segment or lobe is involved	If area affected is small, no change If area affected is large, ↓ movement on affected side; ↑ fremitus	Dull over affected areas	Crackles (may disappear with deep breaths); absence of sounds if large area is affected
Pulmonary edema	Tachypnea; laboured respirations; cyanosis	↓ Chest expansion or normal movement	Dull or normal, depending on amount of fluid	Fine or coarse crackles
Pleural effusion	Tachypnea; use of accessory muscles	↓ Chest expansion ↑ Fremitus above effusion; absence of fremitus over effusion	Dull	Diminished or absent over effusion; egophony over effusion
Pulmonary fibrosis	Tachypnea	↓ Chest expansion	Normal	Crackles

TABLE 28.11 DIAGNOSTIC STUDIES

Respiratory System

Study	Description and Purpose	Nursing Responsibility
Blood Studies		
Hemoglobin (Hb) measurement	Value reflects amount of hemoglobin available for combination with oxygen. Venous blood is sampled. Normal level for men is 140–180 mmol/L; normal level for women is 120–160 mmol/L.	Explain procedure and its purpose.
Hematocrit (Hct) measurement	Value reflects ratio of red blood cells to plasma cells. Hematocrit is increased (polycythemia) in chronic hypoxemia. Venous blood is sampled. Normal value for men is 0.42–0.52; normal value for women is 0.37–0.47.	Explain procedure and its purpose.
ABG measurements	Values reflect acid–base balance, ventilation status, need for oxygen therapy, change in oxygen therapy, or change in ventilator settings.* Arterial blood is obtained through puncture of radial or femoral artery or through arterial catheter. Continuous ABG monitoring is also possible via a sensor or electrode inserted into the arterial catheter.	Indicate whether patient is using supplemental oxygen (percentage, amount per minute). Avoid change in oxygen therapy or interventions (e.g., suctioning, position change) for 20 min before obtaining sample. Assist with positioning (e.g., palm up, wrist slightly hyperextended if radial artery is used). Collect blood into heparinized syringe. To ensure accurate results, expel all air bubbles, and place sample on ice, unless it will be analyzed in <1 min. Apply pressure to artery for 5 min after specimen is obtained to prevent hematoma at the arterial puncture site.
Oximetry	Test monitors arterial or venous oxygen saturation. Oximetry is used for intermittent or continuous monitoring and exercise testing.†,‡ Device attaches to finger, forehead, earlobe, or nose for SpO_2 monitoring or is contained in a pulmonary artery catheter for SvO_2 monitoring.	Apply probe to finger, forehead, earlobe, or bridge of nose. Before interpreting SpO_2 and SvO_2 values, first assess patient status and presence of factors that can alter accuracy of pulse oximeter reading. For SpO_2, these include motion, low perfusion, bright lights, use of intravascular dyes, acrylic nails, dark skin colour. For SvO_2, these include change in oxygen delivery or consumption. For SpO_2, notify health care provider of ±4% change from baseline or ↓ to <90%. For SvO_2, notify health care provider of ±10% change from baseline or ↓ to <60%.
Sputum Studies		
Culture and sensitivity	Purpose is to diagnose bacterial infection, select antibiotic, and evaluate treatment. Single sputum specimen is collected in a sterile container.	Instruct patient on how to produce a good specimen (see nursing responsibilities for Gram stain). If patient cannot produce specimen, bronchoscopy may be used (see Figure 28.13).
Gram stain	Staining of sputum enables classification of bacteria into Gram-negative and Gram-positive types. Results guide therapy until culture and sensitivity results are obtained.	Instruct patient to expectorate sputum into the container after coughing deeply. Obtain sputum (mucoid-like), not saliva. Obtain specimen in early morning because secretions accumulate during night. If sputum production is unsuccessful, try increasing oral fluid intake unless fluids are restricted. Collect sputum in sterile container (sputum trap) during suctioning or by aspirating secretions from the trachea. Send specimen to laboratory promptly.
Acid-fast smear and culture	Test is performed to collect sputum for acid-fast bacilli (tuberculosis). A series of three early morning specimens is used.	Instruct patient on how to produce a good specimen (see nursing responsibilities for Gram stain). Cover specimen and send to laboratory for analysis.
Cytology study	Purpose is to determine presence of abnormal cells that may indicate malignant condition. Single sputum specimen is collected in special container with fixative solution.	Send specimen to laboratory promptly. Instruct patient on how to produce a satisfactory specimen (see nursing responsibilities for Gram stain). If patient cannot produce specimen, bronchoscopy may be used (see Figure 28.13).
Radiology		
Chest radiograph	Test is used to screen, diagnose, and evaluate change. Most common views are posteroanterior and lateral.	Instruct patient to undress to waist, put on gown, and remove any metal objects (e.g., jewellery, watch) between neck and waist.
Computed tomography (CT)	Test is performed for diagnosis of lesions difficult to assess by conventional radiographic studies, such as those in the hilum, the mediastinum, and the pleura. Images show structures in cross-section.	Same as for chest radiograph.
Magnetic resonance imaging (MRI)	Test is used for diagnosis of lesions difficult to assess by CT (e.g., lung apex near the spine).	Same as for chest radiograph. Instruct patient to remove all metal objects (e.g., jewellery, watch) before test.
Ventilation–perfusion (VQ) scan	Test is used to identify areas of the lung not receiving airflow (ventilation) or blood flow (perfusion). It involves injection of radioisotope and inhalation of small amount of radioactive gas (xenon). A gamma ray–detecting device records radioactivity. Ventilation without perfusion is suggestive of pulmonary embolus.	Same as for chest radiograph. No precautions needed afterward because the gas and isotope transmit radioactivity for only a brief interval.

Continued

TABLE 28.11	**DIAGNOSTIC STUDIES—cont'd**	
Study	**Description and Purpose**	**Nursing Responsibility**
Pulmonary angiography	Study is used to visualize pulmonary vasculature and locate obstruction or pathological conditions such as pulmonary embolus. Contrast medium is injected through a catheter into the pulmonary artery or right side of the heart.	Same as for chest radiograph. Know that contrast injection may cause flushing, warm sensation, and coughing. Check pressure dressing site after procedure. Monitor blood pressure, pulse, and circulation distal to injection site. Report and record significant changes.
Positron emission tomography (PET)	Test is used to distinguish benign and malignant lung nodules. It involves IV injection of a radioisotope with short half-life.	Same as for chest radiograph. No precautions needed afterward because isotope transmits radioactivity for only a brief interval.
Endoscopic Examinations		
Bronchoscopy	Flexible fibre-optic endoscope is used for diagnosis, biopsy, specimen collection, or assessment of changes. It may also be used to suction mucous plugs or to remove foreign objects. Study is typically performed in outpatient procedure room.	Instruct patient to be on NPO status for 6–12 hr. Obtain informed consent. Give sedative if it is ordered. After procedure, keep patient on NPO status until gag reflex returns, and monitor for laryngeal edema; monitor for recovery from sedatives. If biopsy was performed, monitor for hemorrhage and pneumothorax.
Mediastinoscopy	Test is used for inspection and biopsy of lymph nodes in mediastinal area.	Prepare patient for surgical intervention. Obtain informed consent. Afterward, monitor as for bronchoscopy.
Biopsy		
Lung biopsy	Specimens may be obtained by transbronchial or open lung biopsy. This test is used to obtain specimens for laboratory analysis.	Same as for bronchoscopy if procedure is performed with bronchoscope, and same as for thoracotomy (see Chapter 30) if open-lung biopsy is performed. Obtain informed consent.
Other Studies		
Thoracentesis	Test is used to obtain specimen of pleural fluid for diagnosis, to remove pleural fluid, or to instill medication. The physician inserts a large-bore needle through the chest wall into pleural space. A chest radiograph is always obtained after procedure to check for pneumothorax.	Explain procedure to patient, and obtain informed consent before procedure. Position patient sitting upright with elbows on an overbed table and feet supported. Instruct patient not to talk or cough, and assist during procedure. Observe for signs of hypoxia and verify breath sounds in all fields after procedure. Send labelled specimens to laboratory.
Pulmonary function test	Test is used to evaluate lung function. It involves use of a spirometer to diagram air movement as patient performs prescribed respiratory manoeuvres.[†]	Avoid scheduling test immediately after mealtime. Avoid administration of inhaled bronchodilator for 6 hr before procedure. Explain procedure to patient. Allow patient to rest after procedure.

ABG, arterial blood gas; *IV*, intravenous; *NPO*, nothing by mouth; *SpO₂*, the oxygen saturation value obtained by pulse oximetry; *SvO₂*, venous oxygen saturation.
[*]For normal values, see Table 28.1.
[†]For normal values, see Table 28.14.
[‡]For critical values, see Table 28.3.

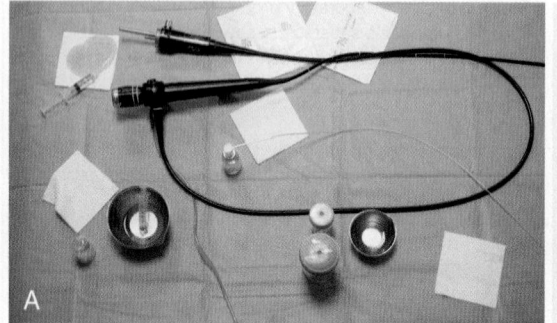
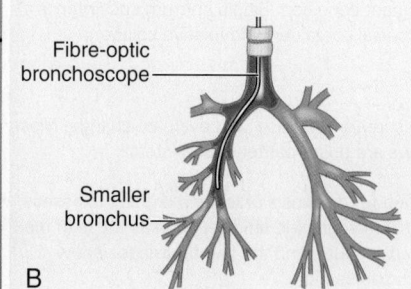
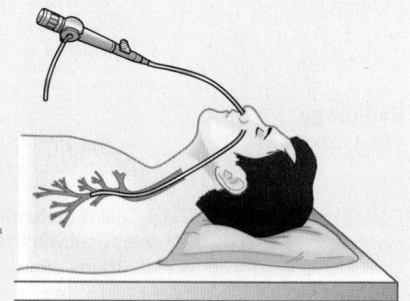

FIG. 28.13 Fibre-optic bronchoscopy. **A,** The transbronchoscopic balloon-tipped catheter and the flexible fibre-optic bronchoscope. **B,** Procedure. The catheter is introduced into a small airway, and the balloon is inflated with 1.5 to 2 mL of air to occlude the airway. To perform bronchoalveolar lavage, 30 mL aliquots of sterile saline solution are injected and withdrawn, with gentle aspiration after each injection. Specimens are sent to the laboratory for analysis. Source: *A,* BSIP SA/Alamy Stock Photo.

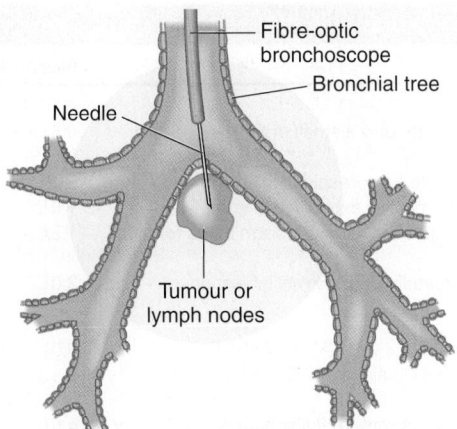

FIG. 28.14 Transbronchial needle biopsy. In this diagram, a transbronchial biopsy needle penetrates the bronchial wall and enters a mass of subcarinal lymph nodes or tumour. Source: Redrawn from Du Bois, R. M., & Clarke, S. W. (1987). *Fiberoptic bronchoscopy in diagnosis and management*. Grune & Stratton.

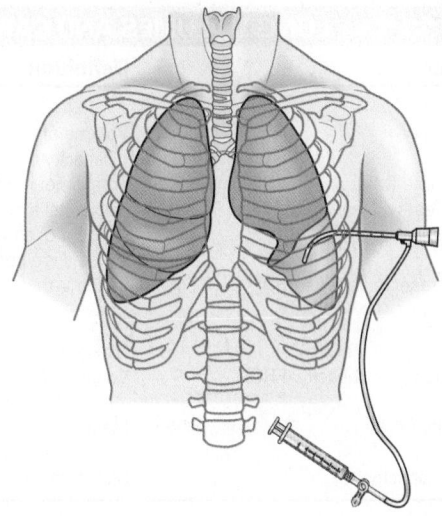

FIG. 28.15 Thoracentesis. A catheter is positioned in the pleural space to remove accumulated fluid.

Bronchoscopy can be performed in an outpatient procedure room, in a surgical suite, or at the patient's bedside in the critical care unit or on a medical-surgical floor, with the patient lying down or seated. After local anaesthetic is applied to the nasal pharynx and oral pharynx, the bronchoscope is coated with lidocaine (Xylocaine) and inserted, usually through the nose, and threaded down into the airways. A bronchoscopy can be performed on mechanically ventilated patients through the endotracheal tube. The nursing care for patients undergoing this procedure is described in Table 28.11.

Mediastinoscopy. For mediastinoscopy, an endoscope is inserted through a small incision in the suprasternal notch and advanced into the mediastinum to inspect lymph nodes and sample them for biopsy. The test is used to diagnose carcinoma, granulomatous infections, and sarcoidosis. The procedure is performed in the operating room and the patient is given a general anaesthetic.

Lung Biopsy

Lung biopsy may be performed transbronchially or as an open lung procedure. The purpose is to obtain tissue, cells, or secretions for evaluation. Transbronchial lung biopsy involves passing a forceps or needle through the bronchoscope for a specimen (Figure 28.14). Specimens can be cultured or examined for malignant cells. A combination of transbronchial lung biopsy and bronchoalveolar lavage is used to differentiate infection and rejection in lung transplant recipients. Nursing care is the same as for fibre-optic bronchoscopy. Open lung biopsy is used when pulmonary disease cannot be diagnosed by other procedures. The patient receives a general anaesthetic, the chest is opened with a thoracotomy incision, and a biopsy specimen is obtained. Nursing care after the procedure is the same as after thoracotomy (see Chapter 30 and NCP 30.2, available on the Evolve website).

Thoracentesis

Thoracentesis is the insertion of a needle through the chest wall into the pleural space to obtain specimens for diagnostic evaluation, remove pleural fluid, or instill medication into the pleural

TABLE 28.12	**SITUATIONS IN WHICH TUBER-CULIN SKIN TEST REACTION IS CONSIDERED POSITIVE**
Test Result	**Situation in Which Reaction Is Considered Positive***
0–4 mm†	In a child younger than 5 years of age and at high risk of TB infection
≥5 mm	HIV infection
	Contact with person with infectious TB case within the past 2 years
	Presence of fibronodular disease on chest radiograph (healed TB, and not previously treated)
	Organ transplantation (related to immunosuppressive therapy)
	Tumour necrosis factor-α inhibitors
	Other immunosuppressive drugs, such as corticosteroids (equivalent of ≥15 mg/day of prednisone for 1 month or more; risk of TB disease increases with higher dosage and longer duration)
	End-stage renal disease
≥10 mm	All others, including the following specific situations: • Test result conversion (within 2 years) • Diabetes, malnutrition, alcohol misuse (3 drinks/day) • Silicosis • Hematological malignancies (leukemia, lymphoma) and certain carcinomas (e.g., head and neck)

HIV, human immunodeficiency virus; *TB*, tuberculosis.
Source: © All rights reserved. Canadian Tuberculosis Standards, 7th Edition. Public Health Agency of Canada, 2013. Adapted and reproduced with permission from the Minister of Health, 2021.
*The goal of testing for latent tuberculosis is to identify individuals who are at increased risk for the development of tuberculosis and therefore would benefit from treatment of latent tuberculosis. Only those who would benefit from treatment should be tested; thus a decision to test presupposes a decision to treat if the test result is positive.
†In general, this level is considered negative, and no treatment is indicated.

space (Figure 28.15). The patient is positioned sitting upright with elbows on an overbed table and feet supported. The skin is cleansed and a local anaesthetic (lidocaine [Xylocaine]) is instilled subcutaneously. A chest tube may be inserted to enable further drainage of fluid. Nursing responsibilities are described in Table 28.11.

TABLE 28.13   LUNG VOLUMES AND CAPACITIES

Parameter	Definition	Normal Value
Volumes		
Tidal volume (V_T)	Volume of air inhaled and exhaled with each breath; only a small proportion of total capacity of lungs	0.5 L
Minute volume (MV)	Total amount of air inhaled and exhaled per minute (V_T × respiratory rate)	5–8 L/min
Expiratory reserve volume (ERV)	Additional air that can be forcefully exhaled after normal exhalation is complete	1.0 L
Residual volume (RV)	Amount of air remaining in lungs after forced expiration; air available in lungs for gas exchange between breaths	1.5 L
Inspiratory reserve volume (IRV)	Maximum volume of air that can be inhaled forcefully after normal inhalation	3.0 L
Capacities		
Total lung capacity (TLC)	Maximum volume of air that lungs can contain (TLC = IRV + V_T + ERV + RV)	6.0 L
Functional residual capacity (FRC)	Volume of air remaining in lungs at end of normal exhalation (FRC = ERV + RV); increase or decrease possible with lung disease	2.5 L
Vital capacity (VC)	Maximum volume of air that can be exhaled after maximum inspiration (VC = IRV + V_T + ERV); generally higher in men	4.5 L
Inspiratory capacity (IC)	Maximum volume of air that can be inhaled after normal expiration (IC = V_T + IRV)	3.5 L

TABLE 28.14   COMMON MEASURES OF PULMONARY FUNCTION

Measure	Description	Normal Value*
Forced vital capacity (FVC)	Amount of air that can be quickly and forcefully exhaled after maximum inspiration	>80% of predicted
Forced expiratory volume in first second of expiration (FEV_1)	Amount of air exhaled in first second of FVC; valuable clue to severity of airway obstruction	>80% of predicted
FEV_1/FVC	Ratio of value for FEV_1 to value for FVC; useful in differentiating obstructive and restrictive pulmonary dysfunction	>80% of predicted
Maximal midexpiratory flow rate (MMEF)	Measurement of airflow rate in middle half of forced expiration; early indicator of disease of small airways	>80% of predicted
Maximal voluntary ventilation (MVV)	Deep breathing as rapidly as possible for specified period; test for airflow, muscle strength, coordination, airway resistance; important factor in exercise tolerance	≈170 L/min
Peak expiratory flow rate (PEFR)	Maximum airflow rate during forced expiration; aids in monitoring bronchoconstriction in asthma	≤600 L/min
Maximum inspiratory pressure (MIP) or negative inspiratory force (NIF)	Amount of negative pressure generated on inspiration; indication of ability to breathe deeply and cough	≤80 cm H_2O

*Normal values vary with height, weight, age, and sex of patient.

Pulmonary Function Tests

Pulmonary function tests (PFTs) are conducted to measure lung volumes and airflow. The results of PFTs are used to diagnose pulmonary disease, monitor disease progression, evaluate disability, and evaluate response to bronchodilators. In PFTs, a spirometer is used. The patient's age, sex, height, and weight are entered into the PFT computer to calculate predicted values. The patient inserts a mouthpiece, takes as deep a breath as possible, and exhales as hard, fast, and long as possible. Verbal coaching is given to ensure that the patient continues blowing out until exhalation is complete. The computer determines the actual value achieved, predicted (normal) value, and percentage of the predicted value for each test. A normal actual value is 80 to 120% of the predicted value. Normal values for PFTs are shown in Tables 28.13 and 28.14, and the relationships between lung volumes and capacities are described in Figure 28.16.

Home spirometry may be used to monitor lung function in persons with asthma or cystic fibrosis, as well as before and after lung transplantation. Changes in spirometry values at home can warn of early lung transplant rejection or infection. Feedback from a peak expiratory flowmeter can increase the sense

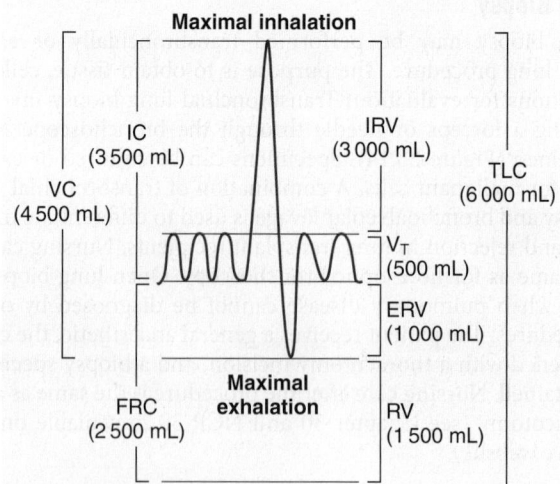

FIG. 28.16 Relationship of lung volumes and capacities. *ERV*, expiratory reserve volume; *FRC*, functional residual capacity; *IC*, inspiratory capacity; *IRV*, inspiratory reserve volume; *RV*, residual volume; *TLC*, total lung capacity; *VC*, vital capacity; *V_T*, tidal volume.

of control achieved when persons with asthma learn to modify activities and medications in response to changes in rates of peak expiratory flow.

Pulmonary function parameters can also be used to determine the need for mechanical ventilation or the readiness to be weaned from ventilatory support. Vital capacity, maximum inspiratory pressure, and minute volume are measured to make this determination (see Tables 28.13 and 28.14).

Exercise Testing

Exercise testing is used in diagnosis, in determining exercise capacity, and for disability evaluation. A complete exercise test involves walking on a treadmill while expired oxygen and carbon dioxide, respiratory rate, heart rate, and rhythm are monitored. A modified test (desaturation test) may also be used. In that case, only SpO_2 is monitored. A desaturation test can also be used to determine the oxygen flow needed to maintain the SpO_2 at a safe level during activity or exercise in patients who use home oxygen therapy.

A timed walk can also be used to measure exercise capacity. The patient is instructed to walk as far as possible during a timed period (6 or 12 minutes), to stop when short of breath, and to continue when able. The distance walked is measured, and the data are used to monitor progression of disease or improvement after rehabilitation.

REVIEW QUESTIONS

The number of the question corresponds to the same-numbered objective at the beginning of the chapter.

1. Which of the following is the mechanism that stimulates the release of surfactant?
   a. Fluid accumulation in the alveoli
   b. Alveolar collapse from atelectasis
   c. Alveolar stretch from deep breathing
   d. Air movement through the alveolar pores of Kohn

2. Which of the following causes air to enter the thoracic cavity during inspiration?
   a. Contraction of the accessory abdominal muscles
   b. Increased carbon dioxide and decreased oxygen in the blood
   c. Stimulation of the respiratory muscles by the chemoreceptors
   d. Decreased intrathoracic pressure relative to pressure at the airway

3. Which of the following measures the lungs' ability to adequately oxygenate the arterial blood?
   a. Arterial oxygen tension
   b. Carboxyhemoglobin level
   c. Arterial carbon dioxide tension
   d. Venous carbon dioxide tension

4. Which of the following is the most important respiratory defence mechanism distal to the respiratory bronchioles?
   a. Alveolar macrophage
   b. Impaction of particles
   c. Reflex bronchoconstriction
   d. Mucociliary clearance mechanism

5. Which of the following is caused by a rightward shift of the oxygen–hemoglobin dissociation curve?
   a. Metabolic alkalosis
   b. Postoperative hypothermia
   c. Release of oxygen at the tissue level
   d. Greater affinity of oxygen for hemoglobin

6. Which of the following are very early signs or symptoms of inadequate oxygenation?
   a. Dyspnea and hypotension
   b. Apprehension and restlessness
   c. Cyanosis and cool, clammy skin
   d. Increased urine output and diaphoresis

7. During the respiratory assessment of an older adult, the nurse would expect to find which of the following? (Select all that apply.)
   a. A vigorous cough
   b. Increased chest expansion
   c. Increased residual volume
   d. Increased breath sounds in the lung apices
   e. Increased anteroposterior (AP) chest diameter

8. Which of the following should the nurse inquire about when assessing activity and exercise related to respiratory health?
   a. Dyspnea during rest or exercise
   b. Recent weight loss or weight gain
   c. Ability to sleep through the entire night
   d. Willingness to wear oxygen equipment in public

9. Which of the following is the best tool to assess for the vibration of tactile fremitus?
   a. Palms
   b. Fingertips
   c. Stethoscope
   d. Index fingers

10. Which of the following is an abnormal finding in the assessment of the respiratory system?
   a. Presence of tactile fremitus
   b. Inspiratory chest expansion of 2.5 cm
   c. Percussion resonance over the lung bases
   d. Symmetrical chest expansion and contraction

11. Which of the following is performed to remove pleural fluid for analysis?
   a. Thoracentesis
   b. Bronchoscopy
   c. Pulmonary angiography
   d. Sputum culture and sensitivity

1. c; 2. d; 3. a; 4. a; 5. c; 6. b; 7. c, e; 8. a; 9. a; 10. a; 11. a.

⊜volve

For even more review questions, visit http://evolve.elsevier.com/Canada/Lewis/medsurg.

REFERENCES

Cobb, N. K., & Solanki, J. N. (2020). E-cigarettes, vaping devices, and acute lung injury. *Respiratory Care, 65*(5), 713–718. https://doi-org.eztest.ocls.ca/10.4187/respcare.07733

Health Canada. (2018). *Health Canada statement on use of vaping products by youth.* https://www.canada.ca/en/health-canada/news/2018/11/health-canada-statement-on-use-of-vaping-products-by-youth.html

Herlihy, B. (2021). *The human body in health and illness* (7th ed.). Elsevier Saunders.

Jarvis, C., Browne, A., MacDonald-Jenkins, J., et al. (2019). *Physical examination & health assessment* (3rd Canadian ed.). Elsevier.

McCance, K. L., & Huether, S. E. (2019). *Pathophysiology: The biologic basis for disease in adults and children* (8th ed.). Mosby.

Patton, K. T. (2019). *Anatomy and physiology* (10th ed.). Mosby.

Public Health Agency of Canada (PHAC). (2019). *An Advisory Committee Statement (ACS) National Advisory Committee on Immunization (NACI): Canadian immunization guide chapter on influenza and statement on seasonal influenza vaccine for 2019–2020,* (pp. 6 12–13). https://www.canada.ca/content/dam/phac-aspc/documents/services/publications/healthy-living/canadian-immunization-guide-statement-seasonal-influenza-vaccine-2019-2020/NACI_Stmt_on_Seasonal_Influenza_Vaccine_2019-2020_v12.3_EN.pdf

Public Health Agency of Canada (PHAC). (2020). *Canadian immunization guide: Bacille Calmette-Guérin (BCG) vaccine.* https://www.canada.ca/en/public-health/services/publications/healthy-living/canadian-immunization-guide-part-4-active-vaccines/page-2-bacille-calmette-guerin-vaccine.html

Public Health Agency of Canada (PHAC). (2021a). *About vaping.* https://www.canada.ca/en/health-canada/services/smoking-tobacco/vaping.html

Public Health Agency of Canada (PHAC). (2021b). *Canadian immunization guide: Part 4—Active vaccines.* https://www.canada.ca/en/public-health/services/publications/healthy-living/canadian-immunization-guide-part-4-active-vaccines.html

Public Health Agency of Canada (PHAC). (2021c). *Coronavirus disease (COVID-19): Symptoms and treatment.* https://www.canada.ca/en/public-health/services/diseases/2019-novel-coronavirus-infection/symptoms.html

Public Health Agency of Canada (PHAC), The Lung Association, & Canadian Thoracic Society. (2014). *Canadian tuberculosis standards* (7th ed.). https://www.canada.ca/en/public-health/services/infectious-diseases/canadian-tuberculosis-standards-7th-edition.html

Public Health Ontario. (2021). *Technical brief: IPAC recommendations of use of personal protective equipment for care of individuals with suspect or confirmed COVID-19.* https://www.publichealthontario.ca/-/media/documents/ncov/updated-ipac-measures-covid-19.pdf?la=en

Registered Nurses Association of Ontario (RNAO) (2005). *Nursing care of dyspnea: the 6th vital sign in individuals with chronic obstructive pulmonary disease (COPD).* https://rnao.ca/sites/rnao-ca/files/Nursing_Care_of_Dyspnea_-The_6th_Vital_Sign_in_Individuals_with_Chronic_Obstructive_Pulmonary_Disease.pdf

Registered Nurses' Association of Ontario (RNAO). (2013). *Best practice guidelines: Developing and sustaining interprofessional health care. Optimizing patient, organizational and system outcomes.* https://rnao.ca/sites/rnao-ca/files/DevelopingAndSustainingBPG.pdf

Registered Nurses' Association of Ontario (RNAO). (2016). *System and healthy work environment best practice guidelines. Intra-professional collaborative practice among nurses* (2nd ed.). https://rnao.ca/sites/rnao-ca/files/bpg/Intra-professional_Collaborative_Practice_042017.pdf

Urden, L. D., Stacy, K. M., & Lough, M. E. (2018). *Critical care nursing: Diagnosis and management* (8th ed.). Elsevier Mosby.

RESOURCES

Resources for this chapter are listed in Chapters 30 and 31.

⊖volve

For additional Internet resources, see the website for this book at http://evolve.elsevier.com/Canada/Lewis/medsurg.

Nursing Management

Upper Respiratory Conditions

Mary Kate Garrity
Originating US chapter by Eugene Mondor

evolve WEBSITE

http://evolve.elsevier.com/Canada/lewis/medsurg

- Review Questions (Online Only)
- Key Points
- Answer Guidelines for Case Study
- Student Case Study
  - Head and Neck Cancer: Laryngectomy With Tracheostomy

- Customizable Nursing Care Plans
  - Tracheostomy
  - Total Laryngectomy and/or Radical Neck Surgery
- Conceptual Care Map Creator
- Audio Glossary

- Supporting Media—Animation
  - Anatomical Location of Sinuses
- Content Updates

LEARNING OBJECTIVES

1. Describe the clinical manifestations and nursing management of conditions of the nose.
2. Describe the clinical manifestations and nursing management of conditions of the paranasal sinuses.
3. Describe the clinical manifestations and nursing management of conditions of the pharynx and the larynx.
4. Discuss the nursing management of the patient who requires a tracheostomy.
5. Identify the steps involved in performing tracheostomy care and suctioning an airway.
6. Describe the risk factors and warning symptoms associated with head and neck cancer.
7. Discuss the nursing management of the patient with a laryngectomy.
8. Describe the methods used in voice restoration for the patient with temporary or permanent loss of speech.

KEY TERMS

allergic rhinitis
deviated septum
epistaxis
esophageal speech

nasal fracture
nasal polyps
rhinoplasty
septoplasty

tracheostomy
tracheotomy

Disorders of the upper respiratory system, including the nose, sinuses, pharynx, and larynx, and the care of patients undergoing surgery for head and neck cancers are the focus of this chapter. The primary concern with these conditions is the impact on ventilation and oxygen (O_2) availability. These disorders can also negatively affect sleep, impair the ability to maintain adequate nutrition, change the senses of both smell and taste, and may lead to depression and changes in body image and sexuality.

STRUCTURAL AND TRAUMATIC DISORDERS OF THE NOSE

DEVIATED SEPTUM

Deviated septum is a misalignment of a normally straight nasal septum. Causes of a deviated septum include trauma to the nose,

normal childhood growth, or a congenital defect. On inspection, the septum is bent to one side, significantly altering air flow and nasal drainage. The patient may experience obstruction to nasal breathing, nasal edema, or dryness of the nasal mucosa with crusting and bleeding (epistaxis). A severely deviated septum may block drainage of mucus from the sinus cavities, resulting in infection (sinusitis) (Patton & Thibodeau, 2016).

For patients with severe symptoms, a nasal septoplasty (surgical realignment of the septum) is performed to reconstruct and properly align the deviated septum. Medical management of deviated septum also includes nasal allergy control, as in allergic rhinitis (discussed later in this chapter).

NASAL FRACTURE

Nasal fracture is most often caused by trauma of substantial force to the middle of the face. Facial fractures occur four to five times more often in Indigenous people in Canada than in the non-Indigenous population (Brennan-Olsen et al., 2017). Some cases of facial trauma can be prevented by using protective sports equipment and protecting against falls. Complications of a nasal fracture include airway obstruction, epistaxis, meningeal tears, and cosmetic deformity.

Nasal fractures are classified as unilateral, bilateral, or complex. A *unilateral fracture* typically produces little or no displacement. *Bilateral fractures,* the most common type, give the nose a flattened look. Powerful frontal blows cause *complex fractures*, which may also shatter the frontal bones. Injury of enough force to fracture nasal bones results in considerable swelling of soft tissues, which can make it difficult to verify the extent of deformity or to repair the fracture until several days later, when the edema subsides. Diagnosis is based on the health history, direct observation, and radiographic findings.

The patient's ability to breathe through each side of the nose needs to be assessed. The nurse should note the presence of edema, bleeding, or hematoma. The nose is inspected internally for evidence of deviated septum, hemorrhage, or clear drainage. Periorbital bruising (*ecchymosis*) involving both eyes is called *raccoon eyes* and often suggests a basilar skull fracture. If the nurse notes periorbital bruising, the patient should be assessed for a cerebrospinal (CSF) leak. Clear, pink-tinged, or persistent drainage from the nose (*rhinorrhea*) or ear (*otorrhea*) suggests a CSF leak. If needed, a specimen should be sent to the laboratory to determine the fluid type.

The goals of nursing management are to reduce edema, prevent complications, and provide emotional support. Ice may be applied to the face and nose to reduce edema and bleeding. When a fracture is confirmed, the goal of management is to realign the fracture using closed or open reduction (septoplasty, rhinoplasty). These procedures are used to re-establish cosmetic appearance and proper function of the nose and to provide an adequate airway. After the patient undergoes nasal surgery, the patient should be assessed for the ability to mouth-breathe. Nasal intubation or use of a nasogastric tube should be avoided in any patient suspected of having a nasal fracture (Rothrock, 2019).

Surgical Procedures

Rhinoplasty refers to surgery performed on the nose to remodel or reconstruct the external nose. Septoplasty refers to rhinoplasty in addition to reconstruction and remodelling of the nasal septum, the internal wall which separates the two sides of the nose. Assessment of the patient's expectations is a critical aspect in preparation for surgery. Expected results of surgery should be explained frankly and truthfully to prepare the patient for any psychosocial or body image changes (Rothrock, 2019).

Interprofessional Care. Rhinoplasty and septoplasty surgeries are performed as an outpatient procedure, using regional anaesthesia. Nasal tissue may be added or removed, and the nose may be lengthened or shortened. Plastic implants are sometimes used to reshape the nose. If the nasal bones are crooked and pushing the septum off to one side, it may be necessary to make cuts in the bones of the nose to reposition them. Small, reinforcing strips of cartilage can be used to help straighten a deviated septum.

After surgery, nasal packing may be inserted to apply pressure and prevent bleeding or septal hematoma formation. Nasal septal splints may be inserted to help prevent formation of scar tissue between the surgical site and the lateral nasal wall. Adhesive-strip skin closures are placed to hold the skin against the septal cartilage. Typically, nasal packing is removed the day after surgery, and the splint is removed in 3 to 5 days. A small dressing under the nostrils is changed as often as every 2 hours during the first 24 hours. The patient is instructed to prevent pressure on the surgical site by sneezing through the mouth (Rothrock, 2019).

NURSING MANAGEMENT
NASAL SURGERY

Before surgery, the patient should be instructed to not take medications containing acetylsalicylic acid (i.e., Aspirin) or nonsteroidal anti-inflammatory drugs (NSAIDs) for 2 weeks to reduce the risk for bleeding. Nursing interventions during the immediate postoperative period include assessment of respiratory status, pain management, and observation of the surgical site for hemorrhage and edema. Discharge teaching is important because the patient must be able to detect complications, such as bright red bleeding lasting more than 10 minutes, heavy bleeding, vision problems, including black eyes, and a fever over 38°C (Rothrock, 2019). There is an interim period while edema and ecchymosis resolve before the final cosmetic effect can be achieved.

EPISTAXIS

Epistaxis (nosebleed) occurs in all age groups, especially in children and older patients. Epistaxis may be caused by trauma, foreign bodies, dry air, nasal spray misuse, alcohol misuse, street drug use, anatomical malformation, allergic rhinitis, or tumours. Any condition that prolongs bleeding time or alters platelet counts will predispose the patient to epistaxis. Bleeding time may also be prolonged if the patient takes NSAIDs or anticoagulants, such as Aspirin. Chronic conditions, such as hypertension, are associated with an increased risk and severity of epistaxis (Byun et al., 2020). Elevated blood pressure, however, makes bleeding more difficult to control.

About 90% of epistaxis cases occur in the anterior portion of the nasal cavity and are easily visualized. Anterior bleeding can be self-treated and usually stops spontaneously. Posterior bleeding occurs more often in older persons, secondary to other health conditions (e.g., hypertension). Since posterior nosebleeds are closer to the throat, it is often hard to determine how much blood loss has occurred. Posterior bleeding may need medical treatment.

NURSING AND INTERPROFESSIONAL MANAGEMENT
EPISTAXIS

Simple first-aid measures should be attempted to control epistaxis. The nurse should (1) keep the patient quiet; (2) place the patient in a sitting position, leaning forward or, if not possible, in a reclining position with head and shoulders elevated; (3) apply direct nasal compression, pinching the soft lower portion of the nose for 10 to 15 minutes; (4) apply ice compresses to the forehead and have the patient suck on ice; (5) apply digital pressure if bleeding continues; and (6) obtain medical assistance if bleeding does not stop.

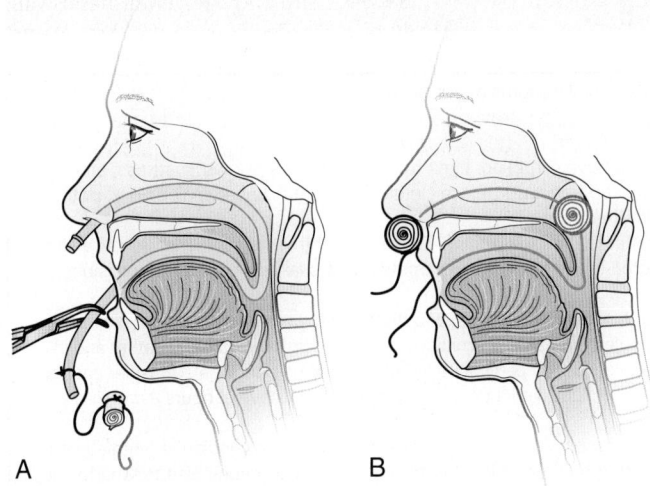

FIG. 29.1 Method for placing posterior nasal pack. **A,** Catheter is passed through the bleeding side of the nose and pulled out through the mouth with a hemostat. Strings are tied to the catheter, and the pack is pulled up behind the soft palate and into the nasopharynx. **B,** Nasal pack in position in the posterior nasopharynx. Dental roll at the nose helps maintain correct position.

Medical management involves localization of the bleeding site and application of a vasoconstrictive agent, cauterization, or anterior packing by a health care provider. Anterior packing may consist of ribbon gauze infused with anaesthetic solution (lidocaine), a vasoconstrictive agent (epinephrine), or both, that is wedged firmly in the desired location and remains in place for 48 to 72 hours. If posterior packing is required, the patient should be hospitalized. Inflatable balloons may be used as a nasal pack, or gauze rolls may be inserted (Figure 29.1). Strings attached to the packing are brought to the outside and taped to the cheek for ease of removal. A nasal sling (a folded 2 × 2–inch gauze pad) should be taped over the nares to absorb drainage. Thermal cauterization is reserved for more severe bleeding and may require the use of local or general anaesthesia (Byun et al., 2020).

Nasal sponges, packing, and balloons can impair respiratory status. The nurse needs to closely monitor level of consciousness, heart rate and rhythm, respiratory rate, and O_2 saturation (SpO_2) using pulse oximetry. The nurse should also observe for any signs of difficulty breathing or swallowing. Because of the increased risk for complications due to location of the injury, all patients with posterior packing should be admitted to a monitored unit for close observation.

Packing is painful because much pressure needs to be applied to stop the bleeding. Nasal packing predisposes to infection from bacteria (e.g., *Staphylococcus aureus*) present in the nasal cavity. The patient should receive a mild opioid analgesic for pain (e.g., acetaminophen with codeine) and an antibiotic effective against staphylococci to protect against infection.

Posterior packs are left in place for no longer than 48 hours because of the incidence of toxic shock syndrome and are usually removed by the surgeon. Before removal, the patient should be medicated for pain because this procedure is extremely uncomfortable. After removal, the nares may be gently cleaned and then lubricated with a petroleum or water-based jelly.

The patient can be discharged after being taught about home care. The patient should be instructed to avoid vigorous nose blowing, strenuous activity, lifting, and straining for 4 to 6 weeks. The patient should be taught to sneeze with the mouth open and to avoid the use of ASA (Aspirin)–containing products or NSAIDs (Rothrock, 2019).

INFLAMMATION AND INFECTION OF THE NOSE AND PARANASAL SINUSES

ALLERGIC RHINITIS

Allergic rhinitis is inflammation of the nasal mucosa due to a specific allergen. Attacks of seasonal rhinitis usually occur in the spring and fall and are caused by an allergy to tree, flower, or grass pollens. A typical attack lasts for several weeks during times when pollen counts are high, then disappears, and recurs at the same time the following year. Perennial rhinitis is present intermittently or constantly. Symptoms are usually caused by specific environmental triggers such as pet dander, dust mites, moulds, or cockroaches. Because symptoms of perennial rhinitis resemble the common cold, the patient may believe the condition is a continuous or repeated cold.

Clinical Manifestations

Manifestations of allergic rhinitis are nasal congestion; sneezing; watery, itchy eyes and nose; altered sense of smell; and thin, watery nasal discharge. The nasal turbinates appear pale, boggy, and swollen. With chronic exposure to allergens, the patient's responses include headache, congestion, pressure, postnasal drip, and nasal polyps. The patient may experience cough, hoarseness, snoring, or the recurrent need to clear the throat.

NURSING AND INTERPROFESSIONAL MANAGEMENT ALLERGIC RHINITIS

Several steps are used in managing allergic rhinitis. The most important step involves identifying and avoiding triggers of allergic reactions (Table 29.1). The patient should be instructed to keep a diary of times when the allergic reaction occurs and the activities that precipitate the reaction. Steps can then be taken to avoid these triggers.

Medication therapy involves using nasal sprays, leukotriene receptor antagonists, antihistamines, and decongestants to manage symptoms (Table 29.2). Intranasal corticosteroid and cromolyn sprays are effective for seasonal and perennial rhinitis. Nasal corticosteroid sprays are used to decrease inflammation locally; there is little absorption in the systemic circulation and, therefore, systemic adverse events are rare. Relief may require combining a nasal corticosteroid spray and an antihistamine. The patient using nasal inhalers needs careful instructions about proper use. Nasal decongestant sprays can be used only for up to 5 days because they can cause a rebound effect from prolonged use.

Immunotherapy ("allergy injections") may be used when a specific, unavoidable allergen is identified and medications are not tolerated or ineffective. Immunotherapy involves controlled exposure to small amounts of a known allergen through frequent (at least weekly) injections, with the goal of decreasing sensitivity. (The mechanisms involved in the allergic response and immunotherapy are discussed in Chapter 16.)

TABLE 29.1   PATIENT & CAREGIVER TEACHING GUIDE

How to Reduce Symptoms of Allergic Rhinitis

Include the following information when teaching the patient and caregiver how to reduce symptoms of allergic rhinitis.

1. Avoidance of allergens is the best treatment.
2. Avoid house dust. Use the approach, "less is best." Focus on the bedroom. Remove carpeting. Limit furniture. Enclose pillows, mattress, and springs in airtight, vinyl encasements. Limit clothing in the bedroom to items used frequently. Place clothing in airtight, zipper-sealed, vinyl clothes bags. Install an air filter. Close the air-conditioning vent into the room. Limit stuffed toys.
3. Avoid house dust mites. Wash bedding in hot water (55°C), weekly. Wear a mask when vacuuming. Double-bag the vacuum cleaner. Install a filter on the outlet port of the vacuum cleaner. Avoid sleeping or lying on upholstered furniture. Remove carpets that are laid on concrete. If possible, have someone else clean the house.
4. Avoid mould spores. The three *D*s that promote growth of mould spores are **d**arkness, **d**ampness, and **d**rafts. Avoid places where humidity is high (e.g., basements, camps on the lake, clothes hampers, greenhouses, stables, barns). Dehumidifiers may be helpful in humid weather and in damp spaces. Ventilate closed rooms, open doors, and install fans. HEPA (high-efficiency particulate air) filters may be beneficial. Consider adding windows to dark rooms. Consider keeping a small light on in closets. A basement light with a timer that provides light several hours a day may decrease mould growth.
5. Avoid pollens. Stay inside, with doors and windows closed, during high-pollen season. Avoid the use of fans. Install an air conditioner with a good air filter. Wash filters weekly during high pollen season. Put the car air conditioner on "recirculate" when driving. Get someone else to tend to your yard.
6. Avoid pet allergens. Remove pets from the interior of the home. Clean the living area thoroughly. Do not expect instant relief. Symptoms usually do not improve significantly for 2 months following pet removal.
7. Avoid exposure to smoke. The presence of a smoker will sabotage the best of all possible symptom-reduction programs.

TABLE 29.2   MEDICATION THERAPY

Allergic Rhinitis and Sinusitis

Preparation	Mechanism of Action	Adverse Effects	Nursing Actions
Corticosteroids **Nasal Spray** Beclomethasone (Apo Beclomethasone) Budesonide (Rhinocort) Flunisolide (Apo-Flunisolide) Fluticasone (Flonase) Triamcinolone (Nasacort) Ciclesonide (Omnaris)	Inhibits inflammatory response. At recommended dosage, systemic adverse effects are unlikely because of low systemic absorption. Systemic effects may occur with greater-than-recommended dosages.	Mild transient nasal burning and stinging; in rare instances, localized fungal infection with *Candida albicans*	• Teach patient correct use. • Instruct patient to use on regular basis and not PRN. • Explain to patient that the spray acts to decrease inflammation over time and does not have an immediate effect. • Discontinue use if nasal infection develops.
Mast Cell Stabilizer **Nasal Spray** Cromolyn spray (Apo-Cromolyn)	Inhibits degranulation of sensitized mast cells that occurs after exposure to specific antigens	Minimal adverse effects; occasional burning or nasal irritation	• Teach patient correct use. • Reinforce that spray prevents symptoms. • Begin 2 wk before pollen season starts and use throughout pollen season. • If isolated allergy, such as to cats, use prophylactically (i.e., 10–15 min before exposure to allergen).
Leukotriene Receptor Antagonists (LTRAs) **Antagonists** Zafirlukast (Accolate) Montelukast (Singulair)	Antagonize or inhibit leukotriene activity, thereby inhibiting airway edema and bronchoconstriction through decreasing inflammatory process	Headaches, dizziness, rash, altered liver function tests, abdominal pain *Zafirlukast:* Monitor PT levels and theophylline levels if patient is taking coumadin or theophylline.	• Monitor liver function tests periodically while on therapy; discontinue if values elevate. • Administer on empty stomach. • Do not discontinue therapy without consulting health care provider. • Not to be used for acute attacks

TABLE 29.2   MEDICATION THERAPY—cont'd

Allergic Rhinitis and Sinusitis

Preparation	Mechanism of Action	Adverse Effects	Nursing Actions
Anticholinergic **Nasal Spray** Ipratropium bromide (Atrovent)	Blocks hypersecretory effects by competing for binding sites on the cell Reduces rhinorrhea in the common cold and allergic and nonallergic rhinitis	Dryness of the mouth and nose may occur Does not cause systemic adverse effects	• Teach patient correct use. • Reinforce that spray prevents symptoms, with onset of action within 1 hr of use. • May reduce need for other rhinitis medications
Antihistamines **First-Generation Agents** Ethanolamines Diphenhydramine (Benadryl) Ethylenediamines Tripelennamine (Vagin-X) Alkylamines Brompheniramine (Dimetane) Chlorpheniramine (Chlor-Tripolon)	Bind with H$_1$ receptors on target cells, blocking histamine binding Relieve acute symptoms of allergic response (itching, sneezing, excessive secretions, mild congestion)	First-generation agents cross blood–brain barrier, bind to H$_1$ receptors in brain, and cause sedation (diminished alertness, slow reaction time, somnolence) and stimulation (restlessness, nervousness, insomnia). Some medications (e.g., ethanolamines) are more likely to cause sedation. Patients vary in their sensitivity to these adverse effects. The next most common adverse effects involve the GI system and include loss of appetite, epigastric distress, constipation, or diarrhea. They may cause palpitations, tachycardia, or urinary retention or frequency.	• Warn patient that operating machinery and driving may be dangerous because of sedative effect. Drowsiness usually passes after 2 wk of treatment. • Teach patient to report palpitations, change in heart rate, change in bowel, bladder habits. • Instruct patient not to use alcohol with antihistamines because of additive depressant effect. • Rapid onset of action, no medication tolerance with prolonged use • Limited use with sinusitis
Second-Generation Agents Loratadine (Claritin) Cetirizine (Reactine) Fexofenadine (Allegra) Desloratadine (Aerius)	—	Second-generation agents have limited affinity for brain H$_1$ receptors; they cause minimal sedation; few effects on psychomotor activities, bladder function.	• Teach patient to expect few, if any, adverse effects. • More expensive than classical antihistamines • Rapid onset of action, no medication tolerance with prolonged use General interactions: • Do not take with alcohol or any form of tranquilizer or sedative. • Do not take with any monoamine oxidase inhibitor.
Decongestants **Oral** Pseudoephedrine (Sudafed)	Stimulate adrenergic receptors on blood vessels, promote vasoconstriction, and reduce nasal edema and rhinorrhea	CNS stimulation, causing insomnia, excitation, headache, irritability, increased blood and ocular pressure, dysuria, palpitations, tachycardia	• Advise patient of adverse reactions. • Advise that use of some preparations is contraindicated for patients with cardiovascular disease, hypertension, diabetes, glaucoma, prostate hyperplasia, and hepatic and renal disease. • Teach patient that these medications should not be used for more than 3 days or more than three or four times a day; longer use increases risk for rebound vasodilation, which can increase congestion.
Topical (Nasal Spray) Oxymetazoline (Dristan) Phenylephrine (Dimetapp)	Same as above Blocks action of histamine	Same as above, plus rhinitis medicamentosa (rebound nasal congestion), headache, bitter taste, somnolence, nasal irritation	—

CNS, central nervous system; *GI*, gastrointestinal; *H$_1$*, histamine 1; *PRN*, as needed; *PT*, prothrombin time.

MEDICATION ALERT—Antihistamines
- First-generation antihistamines (e.g., diphenhydramine) can cause drowsiness and sedation.
- Warn patients that operating machinery and driving may be dangerous because of the sedative effect.

MEDICATION ALERT—Pseudoephedrine
- Large doses may produce tachycardia and palpitations, especially in patients with cardiac disease.
- Overdose in people over 60 years of age may result in central nervous system depression, seizures, and hallucinations.

ACUTE VIRAL RHINITIS

Acute viral rhinitis (common cold or acute coryza) is caused by viruses that invade the upper respiratory tract. It is the most prevalent infectious disease and is spread by airborne droplet sprays emitted by the infected person while breathing, talking, sneezing, or coughing or by direct hand contact. Frequency increases in the winter months, when people stay indoors, and overcrowding is more common. Other factors such as fatigue, physical and emotional stress, and compromised immune status may increase susceptibility. The patient with acute viral rhinitis typically first experiences tickling, irritation, sneezing, or dryness of the nose or nasopharynx, followed by copious nasal secretions, some nasal obstruction, watery eyes, elevated temperature, general malaise, and headache. After the early profuse secretions, the nose becomes more obstructed and the discharge is thicker. Within a few days, the general symptoms improve, nasal passages reopen, and normal breathing is re-established.

NURSING AND INTERPROFESSIONAL MANAGEMENT ACUTE VIRAL RHINITIS

Supportive therapy such as rest, fluids, proper diet, antipyretics, and analgesics is the recommended treatment. Complications of acute viral rhinitis include pharyngitis, sinusitis, otitis media, tonsillitis, and lung infections. Antibiotics do not have a role in the treatment of viral rhinitis during the cold season; the patient with a chronic illness or a compromised immune status should be advised to avoid crowded, close situations and other persons who have obvious cold symptoms. Frequent hand hygiene and avoiding hand-to-face contact may help prevent direct spread.

Interventions are directed toward relieving annoying and uncomfortable symptoms. The patient should be encouraged to drink increased amounts of fluids to liquefy secretions. Antihistamine or decongestant therapy reduces postnasal drip and significantly decreases severity of cough, nasal obstruction, and nasal discharge. The patient should be taught to recognize the symptoms of secondary bacterial infection, such as a temperature higher than 38°C; purulent nasal exudate; tender, swollen glands; and a sore, red throat. In the patient with pulmonary disease, signs of infection include a change in consistency, colour, or volume of the sputum.

INFLUENZA

Approximately 10 to 20% of Canadians become infected with seasonal influenza each year, which runs from October to April. The 2019–2020 influenza season ended in March 2020, which coincided with the start of the COVID-19 pandemic. As of November 10, 2021, a total of 1 740 005 confirmed cases caused by the novel Coronavirus SARS-CoV-2 and 29 249 deaths were reported in Canada (Public Health Agency of Canada, 2021).

🌿 COMPLEMENTARY & ALTERNATIVE THERAPIES
Echinacea

Clinical Uses
Common cold, upper respiratory tract infection, wound healing, urinary tract infections.

Effects
Can reduce cold episodes, pain-killer medicated episodes, recurrent infections and complications of the common cold; anti-inflammatory (Rondanelli et al., 2018)

Nursing Implications
- Echinacea is considered safe when used on a short-term basis in recommended doses.
- Caution patients with autoimmune disorders or a tendency toward allergic reactions about using this herb.
- May be used in conjunction with antibiotics.
- Should not be taken for more than 8 weeks.

🌿 COMPLEMENTARY & ALTERNATIVE THERAPIES
Zinc

Clinical Uses
Common cold, diarrhea, zinc deficiency

Effects
Antiviral effects; if taken within 24 hours of symptom onset may shorten the duration of colds by approximately 33% (Rondanelli et al., 2018)

Nursing Implications
- Intranasal zinc can cause an irreversible loss of the sense of smell.
- Long-term zinc use, especially in high doses, can cause copper deficiency and may increase the risk for urinary tract disorders and reduce immune function.
- Zinc may interact with medications, including antibiotics and penicillamine.

Although the majority recover completely from influenza, an estimated 500 to 1 500 people die from influenza each year (IPAC Canada, 2021). Pneumonia, a common complication of influenza, combined with influenza kills more than 8 000 people a year (IPAC Canada, 2021). Much of the influenza-related morbidity and mortality could be prevented by vaccination of high-risk groups (Table 29.3). Indigenous populations account for less than 5% of Canada's population; however, they are amongst the hardest hit by influenza, including the 2009 H1N1 influenza epidemic, which saw hospitalization rates nearly triple that of non-Indigenous populations (Boggild et al., 2011). Therefore, nurses working with Indigenous populations need to take into account how the social determinants of health affect influenza prevention and management.

There are three groups of influenza viruses—A, B, and C; note that influenza C has little pathogenic potential. Influenza viruses have a remarkable ability to change over time. This ability accounts for widespread disease and the need for annual vaccination against new strains. Fewer cases of influenza result when a minor change in the virus occurs and individuals have partial pre-existing immunity (Public Health Agency of Canada [PHAC], 2018). Birds are natural carriers of influenza A viruses. Avian influenza H5N1 is circulating in some countries, especially in Asia and northeast Africa, and infecting many poultry populations and some humans (Fasanmi et al., 2017). There is no evidence that this virus is transmitted from person to person. Although seasonal influenza immunization will not prevent avian influenza infection, immunization is recommended for those in direct contact with poultry infected with avian influenza during the culling operation. The rationale is that preventing infection with human influenza strains may reduce the theoretical potential for human–avian reassortment of genes should workers become co-infected with both influenza viruses (PHAC, 2015).

The *Canadian Pandemic Influenza Preparedness: Planning Guidance for the Health Sector* document, updated in 2018, provides strategic guidance and a framework for pan-Canadian preparedness and response. It is not a response plan (PHAC, 2018).

Clinical Manifestations

The onset of the flu is typically abrupt, with systemic symptoms of cough, fever, and myalgia often accompanied by a headache and sore throat. Milder symptoms, similar to those of the common cold, may also occur. Physical findings are usually minimal, with normal assessment on chest auscultation. Dyspnea and diffuse crackles are signs of pulmonary complications. In uncomplicated cases, symptoms subside within 7 days. Some patients, particularly older adults, experience weakness or lassitude that persists for weeks. The convalescent phase may be marked by hyperactive airways and a chronic cough. Important diagnostic factors include the patient's health history and clinical findings and the presence of other cases of influenza in the community.

The most common complication of influenza is pneumonia. The patient who develops secondary bacterial pneumonia experiences gradual improvement of influenza symptoms and then worsening cough and purulent sputum. Treatment with antibiotics is usually effective if started early.

NURSING AND INTERPROFESSIONAL MANAGEMENT INFLUENZA

Regular handwashing and annual influenza vaccination are the most effective strategies to reduce the risk for influenza. The nurse should also advocate influenza vaccination for patients at high risk, during routine office visits or, if hospitalized, at the time of discharge (see Table 29.3). The vaccine is 70% to 90% effective in preventing influenza in adults. To be effective, the vaccine must be given in the fall (mid-October), before exposure occurs. Although all healthy people 6 months and older should be encouraged to receive the vaccination, high priority should be given to pregnant women, people who are immunosuppressed, residents of long-term care facilities and retirement settings, and groups that can transmit influenza to high-risk persons, such as health care workers. Vaccination can decrease the risk of transmitting influenza to those who have less ability to cope with the effects of this illness. Despite obvious benefits, many persons are reluctant to be vaccinated. Current vaccines are highly purified, and reactions are extremely uncommon. Soreness at the injection site is usually the only adverse effect. Contraindications to the flu vaccine include children younger than 6 months and people with severe, life-threatening allergies to an ingredient in the flu vaccine. People with a previous history of Guillain-Barré syndrome following a vaccination should avoid future vaccinations.

The primary goals in nursing management are supportive measures directed toward relief of symptoms and prevention of secondary infection. The patient should drink plenty of fluids and get plenty of rest. Older adults and those with a chronic

TABLE 29.3	TARGET GROUPS FOR INFLUENZA IMMUNIZATION

Groups at High Risk

- Indigenous people
- Healthy children between age 6 and 59 months
- Pregnant females, in the third trimester, if their delivery date is in influenza season
- Residents of nursing homes or long-term care facilities
- People with chronic conditions such as diabetes, anemia, cancer, immunodeficiency, immunosuppression, neurological conditions, renal disease, or conditions that compromise management of respiratory secretions
- Health care workers, those who provide essential community services, and other caregivers and household contacts capable of transmitting influenza to the above at-risk groups

Source: Public Health Agency of Canada. (2021). *Canadian immunization guide chapter on influenza and statement on seasonal influenza vaccine for 2020–2021.* https://www.canada.ca/en/public-health/services/publications/vaccines-immunization/canadian-immunization-guide-statement-seasonal-influenza-vaccine-2020-2021.html

illness may require hospitalization. Medication therapy with oral oseltamivir (Tamiflu) and inhaled zanamivir (Relenza) may be given to prevent or decrease symptoms of influenza in high-risk patients. These medications prevent the virus from budding and spreading to other cells. For maximum benefit, they should be initiated as soon as possible and ideally within 2 days of the onset of symptoms. They shorten the duration and severity of influenza and can be used prophylactically for control of outbreaks.

COMPLEMENTARY & ALTERNATIVE THERAPIES
Goldenseal

Clinical Uses
Common cold, respiratory and gastrointestinal infections, wound healing, cirrhosis of the liver, gallbladder inflammation, peptic ulcers

Effects
Has a wide variety of effects, such as anti-inflammatory properties, antimicrobial effects, and immunostimulating actions. Goldenseal can stimulate the flow of bile.

Nursing Implications
Because of the anticoagulant effects, goldenseal should not be used for longer than 2 weeks. Large doses may cause gastrointestinal distress (e.g., diarrhea, vomiting) and possible nervous system effects. Commonly combined with *Echinacea* in preparations. May be used in conjunction with antibiotics. Should not be used concurrently with anticoagulants, antihypertensives, β-adrenergic blockers, or calcium channel blockers. Should not be used if the person has heart or vascular disease, especially hypertension, heart failure, or dysrhythmias.

Source: Rothrock, J. (2019). *Alexander's care of the patient in surgery* (16th ed.). Mosby.

SINUSITIS

Sinusitis affects one in every seven adults. It develops when inflammation or swelling of the mucosa blocks the openings (ostia) in the sinuses, through which mucus drains into the nose (Figure 29.2). The secretions that accumulate behind the obstruction provide a rich medium for growth of bacteria, viruses, and fungi, all of which may cause infection (Tung

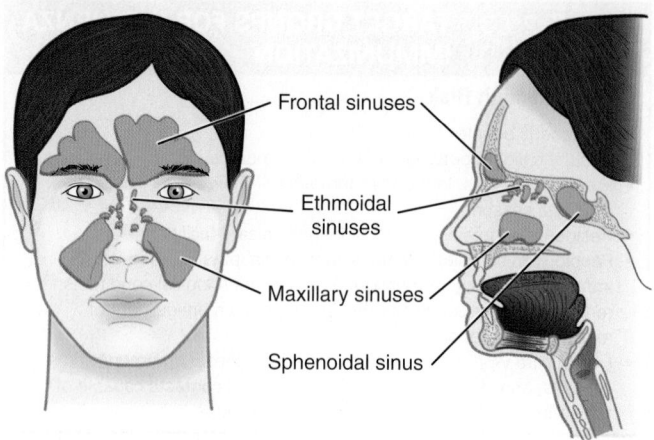

FIG. 29.2 Location of the sinuses.

et al., 2016). Bacterial sinusitis is most caused by *Staphylococcus aureus, Haemophilus influenzae,* or pneumococci (Cash et al., 2020).

Viral sinusitis follows an upper respiratory infection in which the virus penetrates the mucous membrane and decreases ciliary transport. Viral infections usually resolve without treatment in less than 14 days. If symptoms worsen after 3 to 5 days or last for longer than 10 days, a secondary bacterial infection may be present. Only 5 to 10% of patients with viral sinusitis develop a bacterial infection and need antibiotic therapy.

Acute sinusitis usually results from an upper respiratory infection, allergic rhinitis, swimming, or dental manipulation, all of which can cause inflammatory changes and retention of secretions. When acute sinusitis follows viral rhinitis, symptoms worsen after 5 to 7 days and are worse than the original rhinitis. *Chronic sinusitis* is a persistent infection usually associated with allergies and nasal polyps. Chronic sinusitis generally results from repeated episodes of acute sinusitis that result in irreversible loss of the normal ciliated epithelium lining the sinus cavity.

Clinical Manifestations

Acute sinusitis causes significant pain over the affected sinus(es), purulent nasal drainage, nasal obstruction, congestion, fever, and malaise. The patient looks and feels sick. Assessment involves inspection of the nasal mucosa and palpation of the sinus points for pain. Findings that indicate acute sinusitis include a hyperemic and edematous mucosa, enlarged turbinates, and tenderness over the involved sinus(es). The patient may have recurrent headaches that change in intensity with position changes or when secretions drain (Cash et al., 2020).

Chronic sinusitis is difficult to diagnose because symptoms may be nonspecific. The patient is rarely febrile. Although there may be facial pain, nasal congestion, and increased drainage, often severe pain and purulent drainage are absent. Symptoms may mimic those seen with allergies. Radiographic studies of the sinuses or a sinus computed tomographic (CT) scan may be performed to confirm the diagnosis. CT scans may show the sinuses to be filled with fluid or the mucous membrane to be thickened. Nasal endoscopy with a flexible scope may be used to examine the sinuses, obtain drainage for culture, and restore normal drainage.

Many patients with asthma have sinusitis. The link between these conditions is unclear. Postnasal drip associated with sinusitis may trigger asthma by stimulating reflex bronchospasm.

TABLE 29.4	**PATIENT & CAREGIVER TEACHING GUIDE**

Acute or Chronic Sinusitis

The following information should be included when teaching the patient and caregiver about sinusitis.
1. Keep well hydrated by drinking six to eight glasses of water daily to liquefy secretions.
2. Take hot showers twice daily; use a steam inhaler (15-min vaporization of boiled water), bedside humidifier, or nasal saline spray to promote secretion drainage.
3. Report temperature of ≥38°C, which may indicate infection.
4. Follow prescribed medication regimen:
   - Take analgesics to relieve pain.
   - Take decongestants or expectorants, or both, to relieve swelling and to thin mucus.
   - Take antibiotics, as prescribed, for infection. Be sure to take entire prescription and report continued symptoms or a change in symptoms.
   - Administer nasal sprays correctly.
5. Do not smoke, and avoid exposure to smoke—smoke is an irritant and may worsen symptoms.
6. If allergies predispose to sinusitis, follow instructions regarding environmental control, medication therapy, and immunotherapy to reduce the inflammation and prevent sinus infection.
7. Avoid use of nasogastric tube inserted via the nares.

Appropriate treatment of sinusitis often causes a reduction in asthma symptoms (Calhoun et al., 2016).

NURSING AND INTERPROFESSIONAL MANAGEMENT SINUSITIS

If allergies are the precipitating cause of sinusitis, the patient needs to be instructed in ways to reduce sinus inflammation and infection, including environmental control of allergies and appropriate medication therapy (see section on allergic rhinitis earlier in this chapter). Treatment of acute sinusitis includes antibiotics to treat the infection, decongestants to promote drainage, nasal corticosteroids to decrease inflammation, and mucolytics to promote mucus flow (Table 29.4). Classical (first-generation) antihistamines increase the viscosity of mucus and promote continued symptoms, so they should be avoided. Nonsedating (second-generation) antihistamines do not cause this problem. For acute sinusitis, antibiotic therapy is usually continued for 10 to 14 days.

If symptoms do not resolve, the antibiotic should be changed to a broader-spectrum agent. With chronic sinusitis, mixed bacterial florae are often present and infections are difficult to eliminate. Broad-spectrum antibiotics may be used for 4 to 6 weeks.

The patient should be encouraged to increase fluid intake (six to eight glasses daily) and use nasal cleaning techniques. This may include taking a hot shower in the morning and the evening, followed by blowing the nose thoroughly each time. Other interventions to cleanse the nasal passages and promote drainage include irrigating the nose with saltwater (Cooper & Gosnell, 2019).

The patient with persistent or recurrent sinus conditions that are not alleviated by medical therapy may require nasal endoscopic surgery to relieve blockage caused by hypertrophy or deviated septum. This is an outpatient procedure usually performed under local anaesthesia (Cooper & Gosnell, 2019).

OBSTRUCTION OF THE NOSE AND PARANASAL SINUSES

POLYPS

Nasal polyps are benign mucous membrane masses that form slowly in response to repeated inflammation of the sinus or the nasal mucosa. Polyps, which appear as bluish, glossy projections in the naris (nostril), can exceed the size of a grape. The patient may be anxious, fearing the polyps are malignant. Clinical manifestations include nasal obstruction, nasal discharge (usually clear mucus), and speech distortion. Nasal polyps can be removed with endoscopic or laser surgery, but recurrence is common. Topical or systemic corticosteroids may slow polyp growth (Cooper & Gosnell, 2019).

FOREIGN BODIES

A variety of foreign bodies may lodge in the upper respiratory tract. Inorganic foreign bodies such as buttons and beads may cause no symptoms, lie undetected, and be accidentally discovered on routine examination. Organic foreign bodies such as wood, cotton, beans, peas, and paper produce a local inflammatory reaction and nasal discharge, which may become purulent and foul smelling. Foreign bodies should be removed from the nose through the route of entry. Sneezing with the opposite nostril closed may be effective in assisting the removal of foreign bodies. Irrigation of the nose or pushing the object backward should not be done because either could cause aspiration and airway obstruction. If sneezing or blowing the nose does not remove the object, the patient should see a health care provider.

CONDITIONS RELATED TO THE PHARYNX

ACUTE PHARYNGITIS

Acute pharyngitis is an acute inflammation of the pharyngeal walls. It may include the tonsils, palate, and uvula. It can be caused by a viral, bacterial, or fungal infection. Viral pharyngitis accounts for approximately 90% of cases. Acute follicular pharyngitis ("strep throat") results from β-hemolytic streptococcal invasion and accounts for an additional 5 to 15% of episodes (Cooper & Gosnell, 2019). Fungal pharyngitis, especially candidiasis, can develop with prolonged use of antibiotics or inhaled corticosteroids or in immunosuppressed patients, especially those with human immunodeficiency virus (HIV). Other causes of pharyngitis include dry air, smoking, gastroesophageal reflux disease (GERD), allergy and postnasal drip, endotracheal intubation, chemical fumes, and cancer.

Clinical Manifestations

Symptoms of acute pharyngitis range in severity from reports of a "scratchy throat" to pain so severe that swallowing is difficult. Both viral and strep infections appear as a red and edematous pharynx, with or without patchy yellow exudates. Four classic manifestations present in bacterial pharyngitis include (1) fever greater than 38°C (100.4°F), (2) anterior cervical lymph node enlargement, (3) tonsillar or pharyngeal exudate, and (4) absence of cough. However, appearance is not always diagnostic. When two or three of these criteria are present, a rapid antigen detection test, throat culture, or both can help establish the cause and direct treatment. White, irregular patches on the oropharynx suggest fungal infection with *Candida albicans*.

NURSING AND INTERPROFESSIONAL MANAGEMENT ACUTE PHARYNGITIS

The goals of nursing management are infection control, symptomatic relief, and prevention of secondary complications. There is a high incidence of pharyngitis in Indigenous communities, which may lead to rheumatic fever (Gordon et al., 2015). Nurses must consider Indigenous communities' access to necessary medications and treatment.

For viral pharyngitis, antibiotics are not recommended because they do not alter the course of viral infections. For bacterial pharyngitis caused by group A β-hemolytic streptococci, penicillin is the medication of choice. Other antibiotics include azithromycin (Zithromax) or a first-generation cephalosporin. The patient with documented strep throat is treated with antibiotics. Most people with streptococcal infections are contagious until they have been on antibiotics for 24 to 48 hours. Repeat throat cultures after antibiotic therapy are not required.

Candida infections are treated with nystatin, an antifungal antibiotic. The preparation should be swished in the mouth for as long as possible before it is swallowed, and treatment should continue until symptoms are gone. The patient should be encouraged to increase fluid intake. Cool, bland liquids and gelatin will not irritate the pharynx; the patient should avoid drinking citrus juices, which can be irritating to the throat.

PERITONSILLAR ABSCESS

Peritonsillar abscess is a complication of acute pharyngitis or acute tonsillitis, when bacterial infection invades one or both tonsils. The tonsils may enlarge sufficiently to threaten airway patency. The patient experiences a high fever, leukocytosis, and chills. Intravenous antibiotic therapy is given along with needle aspiration or incision and drainage of the abscess. An emergency tonsillectomy may be performed, or an elective tonsillectomy may be scheduled after the infection has subsided.

CONDITIONS RELATED TO THE TRACHEA AND LARYNX

AIRWAY OBSTRUCTION

Airway obstruction may be complete or partial. *Complete airway obstruction* is a medical emergency. *Partial airway obstruction* may occur as a result of aspiration of food or a foreign body. In addition, partial airway obstruction may result from laryngeal edema following extubation, laryngeal or tracheal stenosis, central nervous system (CNS) depression, and allergic reactions. Symptoms include stridor, use of accessory muscles, suprasternal and intercostal retractions, wheezing, restlessness, tachycardia, and cyanosis. Prompt assessment and treatment are essential because partial obstruction may quickly progress to complete obstruction. Interventions to re-establish a patent airway include the obstructed airway (Heimlich) manoeuvre, cricothyroidotomy, endotracheal intubation, and tracheostomy. Unexplained or recurrent symptoms indicate the need for additional tests, such as a chest radiography, pulmonary function tests, and bronchoscopy.

TRACHEOSTOMY

A **tracheotomy** is a surgical incision into the trachea for the purpose of establishing an airway. A **tracheostomy** is the stoma (opening) that results from the tracheotomy. A tracheostomy tube is an artificial airway that is inserted into the trachea during a tracheotomy. Indications for a tracheostomy are to (1) bypass an upper airway obstruction, (2) facilitate removal of secretions, (3) enable long-term mechanical ventilation, and (4) facilitate oral intake and speech in the patient who requires long-term mechanical ventilation. Most patients who require mechanical ventilation are initially managed with an endotracheal tube (ETT), which can be quickly inserted in an emergency (see Chapter 68). A tracheotomy may be performed for patients requiring intubation longer than 7 to 10 days or when an airway is obstructed due to trauma, tumours, or swelling. A tracheostomy may also be required to facilitate airway clearance when spinal cord injury, neuromuscular disease, or severe debilitation is present (Stacy, 2018). A tracheostomy tube is usually inserted by an open procedure in the operating room but can also be inserted emergently in a percutaneous procedure at the bedside (Stacy, 2018).

Several advantages make a tracheostomy a better option than an ETT for long-term nursing management and weaning from the ventilator. Without a tube in the mouth, patient comfort and mobility can be increased, and risk for long-term damage to the vocal cords is decreased. The patient can eat with a tracheostomy and, depending on the type of tracheostomy, can also talk (Stacy, 2018).

NURSING MANAGEMENT
TRACHEOSTOMY

PROVIDING TRACHEOSTOMY CARE

Before the tracheotomy procedure, the nurse should explain to the patient and caregivers the purpose of the procedure and inform them that the patient will not be able to speak while an inflated cuff is used. Several complications can occur with tracheostomies (Table 29.5).

A variety of tubes are available to meet individual patient needs (Table 29.6). All tracheostomy tubes contain a faceplate or flange, which rests on the neck between the clavicle and an outer cannula. In addition, all tubes have an obturator, which is used when inserting the tube (Figure 29.3, *A*). In the event of accidental decannulation, a spare tracheostomy set, obturator, and tracheal dilator should be kept at the bedside, preferably taped at the head of the bed.

Some tracheostomy tubes also have an inner cannula, which can be removed for cleaning (see Figure 29.3, *C*). If an inner cannula is used, whether disposable or nondisposable, tracheostomy care also involves inner cannula care (Stacy, 2018; see Table 29.8). The cleaning procedure involves removal of mucus from the inside of the tube. Acute care settings predominantly use disposable inner cannulas for safety and hygienic purposes. There is also less risk for mucus plugging when using a disposable, inner cannula. If humidification is adequate, mucus may not accumulate and a tube without an inner cannula can be used. Care of the patient with a tracheostomy involves suctioning the airway to remove secretions (Figure 29.4 and Table 29.7) and cleaning around the stoma. In addition, tracheostomy care includes changing tracheostomy ties (Figure 29.5 and Table 29.8). Novice nurses should have another nurse present for safety.

TABLE 29.5	COMPLICATIONS OF TRACHEOSTOMIES	
Complication	**Causes**	**Nursing Management**
Abnormal bleeding	Surgical intervention Erosion or rupture of blood vessel, or both	• Monitor bleeding. • Notify physician if it continues or is excessive.
Tube dislodgement	Excessive manipulation or suctioning	• Ensure ties are secure. • Keep obturator, hemostat, and new tracheostomy tube at bedside.
Obstructed tube	Dried or excessive secretions	• Assess patient's respiratory status. • Suction as necessary. • Maintain humidification. • Perform tracheostomy care. • Ensure adequate hydration.
Subcutaneous emphysema	Air escapes from the incision to the subcutaneous tissue	• Monitor subcutaneous emphysema. • Reassure patient and family.
Tracheoesophageal fistula	Tracheal wall necrosis, leading to fistula formation	• Monitor cuff pressure. • Monitor patient for coughing and choking while eating or drinking.
Tracheal stenosis	Narrowing of tracheal lumen owing to scarring caused by tracheal irritation	• Monitor cuff pressure. • Ensure prompt treatment of infections. • Ensure ties are secure.

Both cuffed and uncuffed tracheostomy tubes are available. A tracheostomy tube with an inflated cuff is used if the patient is at risk for aspiration or needs mechanical ventilation. Because an inflated cuff exerts pressure on tracheal mucosa, it is important to inflate the cuff with the minimum volume of air required to obtain an airway seal. Cuff inflation pressure should not exceed 20 mm Hg or 25 cm H_2O because higher pressures may compress tracheal capillaries, limit blood flow, and predispose to tracheal necrosis. An alternative approach, termed the *minimal leak technique (MLT)*, involves inflating the cuff with the minimum amount of air to obtain a seal and then withdrawing 0.1 mL of air. Disadvantages of MLT are risk for aspiration from secretions leaking around the cuff and difficulty maintaining positive end-expiratory pressure (Stacy, 2018).

In some patients, cuff deflation is performed to remove secretions that accumulate above the cuff. Before deflation, the patient should cough up secretions, if possible, and the tracheostomy tube and mouth should be suctioned (see Figure 29.4 and Table 29.7). This step is important to prevent secretions from being aspirated during deflation. The cuff is deflated during exhalation because the exhaled gas helps propel secretions into the mouth. The patient should also cough or be suctioned after cuff deflation. The cuff should be reinflated during inspiration. The volume of air required to inflate the cuff should be monitored daily because this volume may increase if there is tracheal dilation from cuff pressure. The nurse should assess the patient's ability to protect the airway from aspiration and remain with the patient when the cuff is initially deflated, unless the patient can protect the airway from aspiration and breathe without respiratory distress. Respiratory therapists should also be involved with patients who have a tracheostomy.

Tube	Characteristics	Nursing Management
Tracheostomy tube with cuff and pilot balloon (see Figure 29.3, *A* and *B*)	When properly inflated, low-pressure, high-volume cuff distributes cuff pressure over large area, minimizing pressure on tracheal wall.	**Procedure for Cuff Inflation** • *Spontaneously breathing patient:* Inflate cuff to minimal occlusion pressure by slowly injecting air into the cuff until no sound is heard after deep breath or during inhalation with manual resuscitation bag. If using MLT, remove 0.1 mL of air while maintaining seal. MLT should not be used if there is risk for aspiration. • *Immediately after cuff inflation:* Verify that pressure is within accepted range (≤20 mm Hg or ≤25 cm H_2O) with a manometer. Record cuff pressure and volume of air used for cuff inflation in chart. **Care of Patients With an Inflated Cuff** • Monitor and record cuff pressure q8h. Cuff pressure should be ≤20 mm Hg or ≤25 cm H_2O to allow adequate tracheal capillary perfusion. If necessary, remove or add air to the pilot tubing using a syringe and stopcock. Afterward, verify that cuff pressure is within accepted range with manometer. • Report inability to keep the cuff inflated or need to use progressively larger volumes of air to keep cuff inflated. Potential causes of these problems include tracheal dilation at the cuff site or a crack or slow leak in the housing of the one-way inflation valve. If the leak is caused by tracheal dilation, the physician may intubate the patient with a larger tube. Cracks in the inflation valve may be temporarily managed by clamping the small-bore tubing with a hemostat. The tube should be changed within 24 hr.
Fenestrated tracheostomy tube (Shiley, Portex) with cuff, inner cannula, and decannulation plug (see Figures 29.3, *C* and 29.6, *A*)	When inner cannula is removed, cuff deflated, and decannulation plug inserted, air flows around tube, through fenestration in outer cannula, and up over vocal cords. The patient can then use voice.	• Signs or symptoms of aspiration need further evaluation by a speech pathologist or radiologist. • *Never* insert the decannulation plug in the tracheostomy tube until the cuff is deflated and inner cannula is removed. Prior insertion will prevent the patient from breathing (no air inflow). This may precipitate a respiratory arrest. • Assess for signs of respiratory distress when a fenestrated cannula is first used. If this occurs, the cap should be removed, the inner cannula replaced, and the cuff reinflated. • Cuff management is as described above.
Speaking tracheostomy tube (Portex, National) with cuff, two external tubings (see Figure 29.6, *B*)	Has two tubings, one leading to cuff and one to opening above the cuff. When port is connected to air source, air flows out of opening and up over the vocal cords, allowing voicing with cuff inflated.	• Once tube is inserted, wait 2 days before use so that the stoma can close around the tube and prevent leaks. • When the patient wishes to speak, connect port to compressed air (or oxygen). Be certain to identify correct tubing. If gas enters the cuff, it will overinflate and rupture, necessitating an emergency tube change. Use lowest flow (typically 4–6 L/min) that permits use of the voice. High flows dehydrate mucosa. • Cover port adaptor. This will cause the air to flow upward. Instruct patient to speak in short sentences because voice becomes a whisper with long sentences. • Disconnect flow when patient does not want to speak, to prevent mucosal dehydration. • Cuff management is as described above.
Tracheostomy tube (Bivona Fome-Cuf) foam-filled cuff (see Figure 29.3, *D*)	Cuff is filled with plastic foam. Before insertion, cuff is deflated. After insertion, cuff is allowed to fill passively with air. Pilot tubing is not capped, and no cuff pressure monitoring is required.	• Before insertion, withdraw all air from the cuff, using a 20-mL syringe. Cap pilot balloon tubing to prevent re-entry of air. After tracheostomy is inserted, remove cap from pilot tubing, allowing cuff to passively reinflate. • Do not inject air into tubing or cap pilot balloon tubing while in the patient. Air will flow in and out in response to pressure changes (e.g., with head turning). Place tag on tubing, alerting staff not to cap or inflate cuff. • Deflate cuff daily via pilot balloon to evaluate integrity of cuff. Also assess ability to easily deflate cuff. Difficulty deflating cuff indicates a need for tube change. If aspirate returns with air, the cuff is no longer intact. • Tube can be used for up to 1 mo in patients on home mechanical ventilation. This is a good choice for patients who require an inflated cuff at home because teaching about cuff pressure is simplified.

MLT, minimal leak technique.

When the patient can protect the airway from aspiration and does not require mechanical ventilation, a cuffless tracheostomy tube should be used.

Retention sutures are often placed in the tracheal cartilage when the tracheotomy is performed. The free ends should be taped to the skin in a place and manner that leaves them accessible if the tube becomes dislodged. Care should be taken not to dislodge the tracheostomy tube during the first few days when the stoma is not mature (healed). Because tube replacement can be difficult, several precautions are required: (1) a replacement tube of equal or smaller size is kept at the bedside, readily available for emergency reinsertion; (2) tracheostomy tapes are not changed for at least 24 hours after the insertion procedure; and (3) the first tube change is performed by a physician, usually no sooner than 7 days after the tracheotomy.

If accidental decannulation occurs, the retention sutures (if present) are grasped and the opening is spread with a tracheal dilator or hemostat, and the replacement tube is guided in, using the obturator. To permit airflow, the obturator is immediately removed once the tube is inserted. Another method is to insert a suction catheter to allow passage of air. The new tube is threaded over the catheter, followed by removal of the suction catheter. If the tube cannot be replaced, the level of respiratory distress is assessed. Minor dyspnea may be alleviated by use of semi-Fowler's position until assistance arrives. Severe dyspnea may progress to respiratory arrest; if this situation occurs, the stoma should be covered with a sterile dressing, and the patient should be ventilated with bag–mask ventilation until help arrives.

After the first tube change, the tube should be changed approximately once a month. When a tracheostomy has been

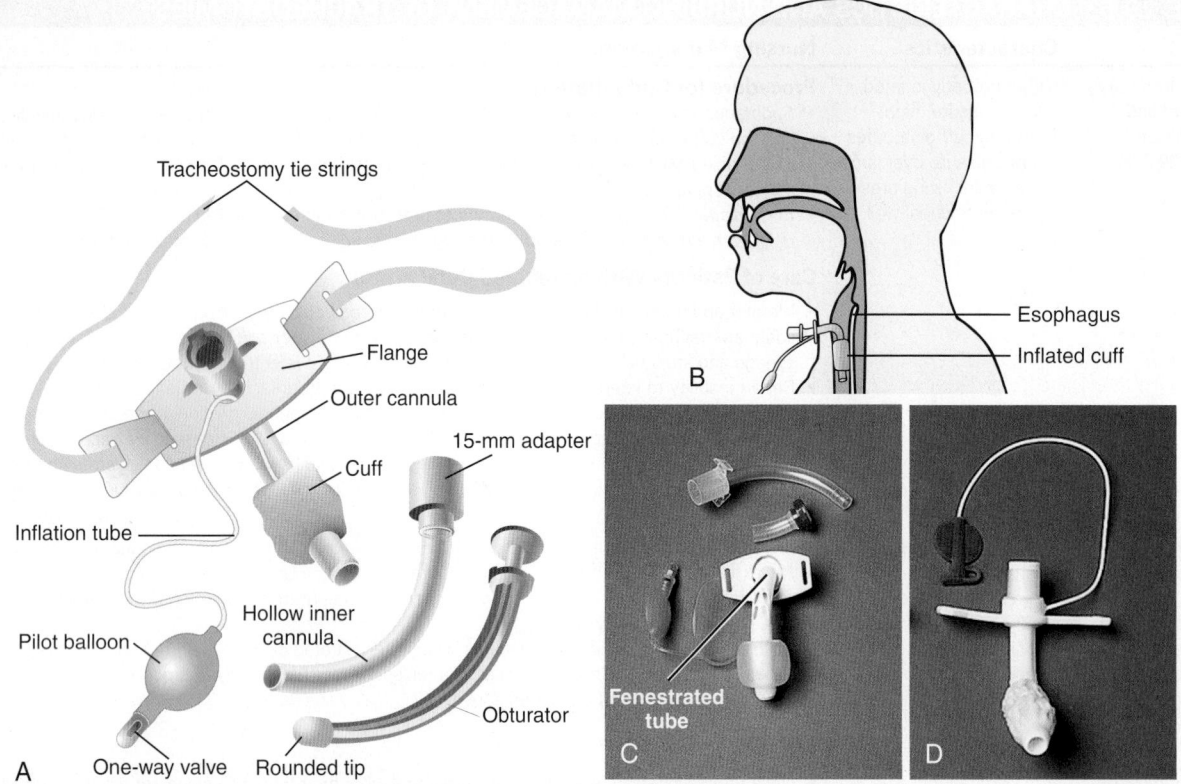

FIG. 29.3 Types of tracheostomy tubes. **A,** Parts of a tracheostomy tube. **B,** Tracheostomy tube inserted in the airway with an inflated cuff. **C,** Fenestrated tracheostomy tube with cuff, inner cannula, decannulation plug, and pilot balloon. **D,** Tracheostomy tube with a foam cuff and obturator (one cuff is deflated on tracheostomy tube). (See Table 29.6 and NCP 29.1 for related nursing management.)

in place for several months, the healed tract will be well formed. The patient can then be taught to change the tube using clean technique at home. Teaching will vary depending on how ill the patient is and what device has been selected.

SWALLOWING DYSFUNCTION

The patient who cannot protect the airway from aspiration requires an inflated cuff. However, an inflated cuff may promote swallowing dysfunction (*dysphagia*) because the cuff interferes with the normal function of the muscles used to swallow. For this reason, it is important to evaluate the risk for aspiration with the cuff deflated. The patient may be able to swallow without aspirating when the cuff is deflated but not when it is inflated. The cuff may then be left deflated or a cuffless tube substituted (Figure 29.6).

VOCALIZATION WITH A TRACHEOSTOMY TUBE

Many techniques promote use of the voice in the patient with a tracheostomy. The patient who can breathe spontaneously may be able to talk by deflating the cuff, which allows exhaled air to flow upward over the vocal cords. This can be enhanced by the patient occluding the tube with a finger or plug. Frequently, a small cuffless tube is inserted so exhaled air can pass freely around the tube. These tracheostomy tubes and valves have been designed to facilitate use of the voice. The nurse can be an advocate in promoting use of these specialized devices. Their use can provide great psychological benefit and facilitate self-care for the patient with a tracheostomy.

A fenestrated tube has openings on the surface of outer cannula that permit air from the lungs to flow over the vocal cords (see Figures 29.3, *C* and 29.6, *A*). A fenestrated tube

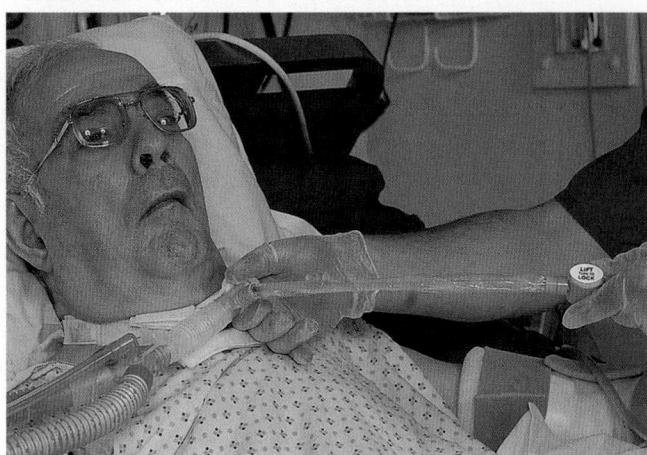

FIG. 29.4 Suctioning tracheostomy with closed system suction catheter. Source: Potter, P. A., Perry, A. G., Stockert, P. A., et al. (2011). *Basic nursing: Essentials for practice* (7th ed., p. 826). Mosby.

allows the patient to breathe spontaneously through the larynx, speak, and cough up secretions with the tracheostomy tube in place. It can be used by the patient who can swallow without risk for aspiration but requires suctioning for secretion removal. It may also be used by the patient who requires mechanical ventilation for less than 24 hours a day (e.g., during sleep).

Before the fenestrated tube is used, the patient's ability to swallow without aspiration is determined (see Table 29.5 and Nursing Care Plan [NCP] 29.1, available on the Evolve website). If there is no aspiration, (1) the inner cannula is removed,

TABLE 29.7   PROCEDURE FOR SUCTIONING A TRACHEOSTOMY TUBE

1. The nurse should assess the need for suctioning q2h. Indications include coarse crackles or wheezes over large airways, moist cough, and restlessness or agitation if accompanied by decrease in SpO_2 or PaO_2. The patient should not be suctioned routinely or if able to clear secretions with cough.
2. If suctioning is indicated, the nurse should explain procedure to the patient.
3. The necessary sterile equipment should be collected: suction catheter (no larger than half the lumen of the tracheostomy tube), gloves, water, cup, and drape. If a closed tracheal suction system is used, the catheter is enclosed in a plastic sleeve and reused. No additional equipment is needed.
4. The next step is to adjust suction pressure until the dial reads between 100 and 150 mm Hg pressure (for adults) with tubing occluded. For infants and children, the pressure should read between 50 and 100 mm Hg, depending on the size of the child. (NOTE: The nurse should check the institution or hospital's policy and procedure manuals for specific guidelines.)
5. The nurse should wash hands and put on goggles, mask, and gloves.
6. Sterile technique should be used to open package, fill cup with water, put on gloves, and connect catheter to suction. One hand should be designated as contaminated for disconnecting, bagging, and operating the suction control, and water should be suctioned through the catheter to test the system.
7. The nurse must assess SpO_2 and heart rate and rhythm to provide baseline for detecting change during suctioning.
8. Preoxygenation should be provided by using a reservoir-equipped MRB connected to 100% oxygen or by asking the patient to take three to four deep breaths while administering oxygen. The method chosen will depend on the patient's underlying disease and acuity of illness. The patient who has had a tracheostomy for an extended period and is not acutely ill may be able to tolerate suctioning without use of an MRB.
9. The nurse should gently insert the catheter *without suction* to minimize the amount of oxygen removed from the lungs and then insert the catheter approximately 13 to 15 cm. Suctioning should be stopped if an obstruction is met.
10. Then the catheter should be withdrawn 1 to 2 cm and suction applied intermittently while withdrawing the catheter in a rotating manner. If secretion volume is large, suctioning should be applied continuously.
11. *Suctioning time should be limited to 10 seconds.* Suctioning should be discontinued if heart rate decreases from baseline by 20 beats per minute, increases from baseline by 40 beats per minute, a dysrhythmia occurs, or SpO_2 decreases to less than 90%.
12. After each suction pass, the nurse should oxygenate with three to four breaths by MRB or deep breaths with oxygen.
13. Single-use catheters should not be reintroduced into the tracheostomy tube. (The nurse should check the institution's policy and procedure manuals.)
14. The procedure should be repeated until airway is clear, and insertions of suction catheter should be limited to as few as needed.
15. Oxygen concentration should be returned to prior setting.
16. The nurse should suction the oropharynx or use mouth suction.
17. The catheter should be disposed of by wrapping it around fingers of gloved hand and pulling glove over catheter. Then equipment should be discarded in a proper waste container.
18. The nurse should auscultate to assess changes in lung sounds and then record time, amount, and character of secretions and response to suctioning.

MRB, manual resuscitation bag.

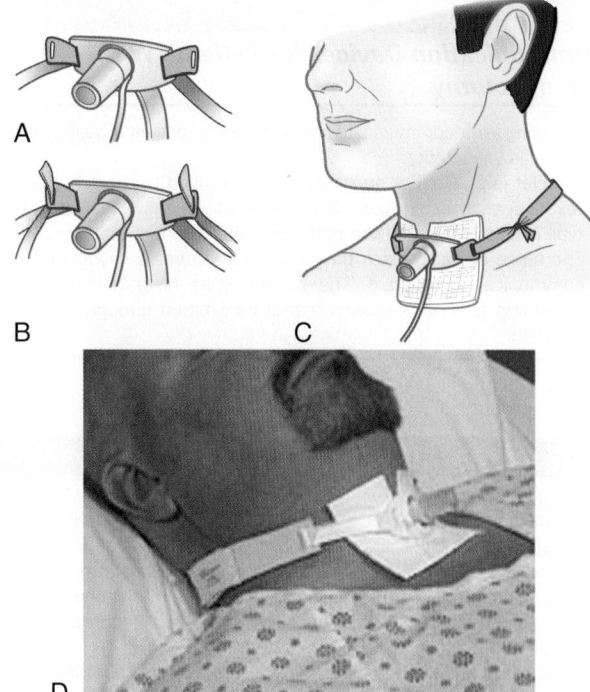

FIG. 29.5 Changing tracheostomy ties. **A,** A slit is cut about 2.5 cm (1 in) from the end. The slit end is put into the opening of the faceplate. **B,** A loop is made with the other end of the tape. **C,** The tapes are tied together with a double knot on the side of the neck, avoiding any blood vessels. **D,** A tracheostomy tube holder can be used in place of twill ties to make tracheostomy tube stabilization more secure. Source: D, Dale Medical Products, Inc.

(2) the cuff is deflated, and (3) the decannulation cap is placed in the tube (see Figure 29.6, *A*). It is important to perform the steps in order because severe respiratory distress may result if the tube is capped before the inner cannula is removed and the cuff deflated. When a fenestrated cannula is first used, the nurse should frequently assess the patient for signs of respiratory distress.

If the patient is not able to tolerate the procedure, the cap should be removed, the inner cannula replaced, and the cuff reinflated. A disadvantage of fenestrated tubes is the potential for development of tracheal polyps from tracheal tissue granulating into the fenestrated openings.

A speaking tracheostomy tube has two pigtail tubes. One tubing connects to the cuff and is used for cuff inflation, and the second connects to an opening just above the cuff (see Figure 29.6, *B*). When the second tubing is connected to a low-flow (4–6 L/min) air source, sufficient air moves up over the vocal cords to produce the voice. The patient can then use the voice, even though the cuff is inflated.

When a speaking tracheostomy valve is used, a cuffless tube must be in place, or the cuff must be deflated, to allow exhalation (Figure 29.7). Ability to tolerate cuff deflation without aspiration or respiratory distress must also be evaluated in patients using this device. If there is no aspiration, the cuff is deflated, and the valve is placed over the tracheostomy tube opening. The speaking valve contains a thin plastic diaphragm that opens on inspiration and closes on expiration. During inspiration, air flows in through the valve. During expiration, the diaphragm prevents exhalation and air flows upward over the vocal cords and into the mouth.

If speaking devices are not used, the patient should be provided with a paper and pencil, a whiteboard with marker, or a computer tablet (e.g., iPad). A word (communication) board can usually be obtained from speech therapy, or one can be devised with pictures of common needs and an alphabet for spelling words. A referral to a speech language pathologist should be considered.

Communication Devices for Patients With Laryngectomy

- Assisting with communication will improve a patient's quality of life after a laryngectomy.
- A tablet (e.g., iPad) or smartphone can be used with a downloaded text-to-speech application. These applications allow the patient to type in text, and then a computer voice says the text aloud.
- The nurse can also teach the patient how to use a keyboard-based communication program. The patient types on a traditional keyboard and generates speech that is transmitted through hand-held speakers.

TABLE 29.8   TRACHEOSTOMY CARE

1. The nurse should explain procedure to patient.
2. A tracheostomy care kit should be used or necessary sterile equipment should be collected (e.g., suction catheter, gloves, water, basin, drape, tracheostomy ties, tube brush or pipe cleaners, 4 × 4–inch gauze pads, normal saline or sterile water, and tracheostomy dressing [optional]). NOTE: Clean rather than sterile technique is used at home.
3. The patient should be positioned in a semi-Fowler's position.
4. The needed materials should be assembled on a bedside table next to the patient.
5. The nurse should wash hands and put on goggles and clean gloves.
6. The next step is to auscultate chest sounds. If wheezes or coarse crackles are present, the patient should be suctioned if unable to cough up secretions (see Table 29.7) and then the nurse should remove soiled dressing and clean gloves.
7. The nurse should open sterile equipment, pour sterile normal saline into basins, and put on sterile gloves.
8. The inner cannula, if present, should be unlocked and removed. Many tracheostomy tubes do not have inner cannulas. Care for these tubes includes all steps except for inner cannula care.
9. If a disposable inner cannula is used, it should be replaced with a new cannula. If a nondisposable cannula is used, the following applies:
   a. Inner cannula should be immersed in sterile normal saline and the inside and outside of the cannula cleaned using a tube brush or pipe cleaners.
   b. Inner cannula should be rinsed in normal saline and shaken to dry.
   c. Inner cannula should be inserted into outer cannula with the curved part downward and then locked in place.
10. Dried secretions should be removed from the stoma, outer cannula, and neck plate, using a 4 × 4–inch gauze pad soaked in normal saline. Then the area around the stoma should be gently patted dry.
11. The nurse should maintain position of tracheal retention sutures, if present, by taping above and below the stoma.
12. Tracheostomy ties should be changed as follows: Secure new ties to flanges before removing the old ones. Tie tracheostomy ties securely with room for one finger between ties and skin (see Figure 29.5). To prevent accidental tube removal, secure the tracheostomy tube by gently applying pressure to the flange of the tube during the tie changes. *Tracheostomy ties should not be changed for first 72 hr after the tracheotomy procedure.*
13. As an alternative, some patients prefer tracheostomy ties made of Velcro, which are easier to adjust.
14. If drainage is excessive, dressings should be placed around tube (see Figure 29.5). A tracheostomy dressing or unlined gauze should be used. The gauze should not be cut because threads may be inhaled or wrap around the tracheostomy tube. Dressing should be changed frequently—wet dressings promote infection and stoma irritation.
15. The nurse should repeat care three times a day and as needed.

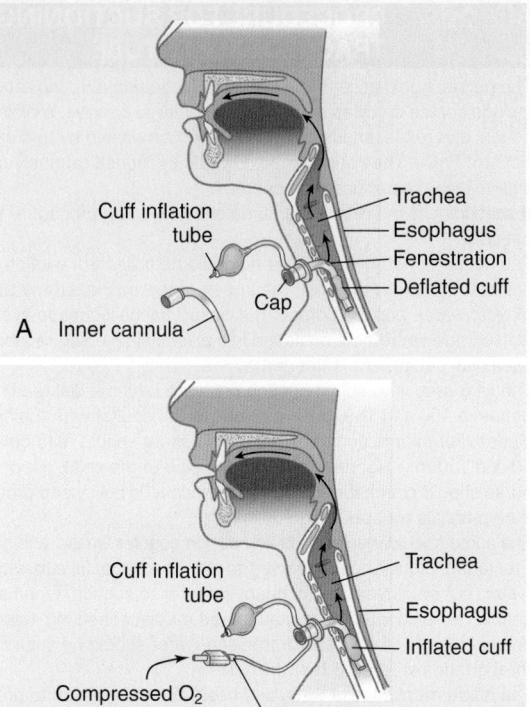

FIG. 29.6 Speaking tracheostomy tubes. **A,** Fenestrated tracheostomy tube with cuff deflated, inner cannula removed, and tracheostomy tube capped to allow air to pass over the vocal cords. **B,** Speaking tracheostomy tube. One tube is used for cuff inflation. The second tube is connected to a source of compressed air or oxygen. When the port on the second tube is occluded, air flows up over the vocal cords, allowing use of the voice with an inflated cuff. (See Table 29.6 and NCP 29.1 for related nursing management.)

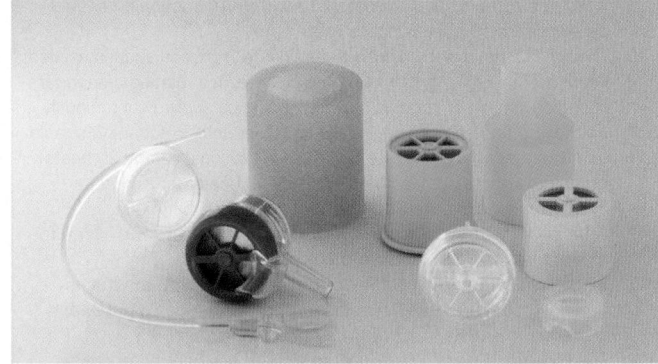

FIG. 29.7 Passy-Muir Tracheostomy & Ventilator Swallowing and Speaking Valve (PMV®). The valve is placed over the hub of the tracheostomy tube after the cuff is deflated. Multiple options are available and can be used for ventilated and nonventilated patients. The PMV is a bias-closed, one-way valve that allows air to enter the lungs during inspiration and redirects air upward over the vocal cords into the mouth during expiration. Source: Image courtesy of Passy Muir, Inc. Irvine, CA.

DECANNULATION

When the patient can adequately exchange air and expectorate secretions, the tracheostomy tube can be removed. The stoma is closed with tape strips and covered with an occlusive dressing. The dressing must be changed if it gets soiled or wet. The patient should be instructed to splint the stoma with the fingers when coughing, swallowing, or speaking. Epithelial tissue begins to form in 24 to 48 hours, and the opening will close in several days. Surgical intervention to close the tracheostomy is not required.

LARYNGEAL POLYPS

Laryngeal polyps may develop on the vocal cords from extensive vocal use (e.g., excessive talking, singing) or irritation (e.g., intubation, cigarette smoking). The most common symptom is hoarseness. Polyps may be treated conservatively with voice rest. Surgical removal may be indicated for large polyps, which may cause dyspnea and stridor. Polyps are usually benign but may be removed because they may later become malignant.

HEAD AND NECK CANCER

Head and neck cancer is a group of cancers that start on mucosal surfaces and is typically squamous cell in origin. This category of tumours includes those of the paranasal sinuses, the oral cavity, and the nasopharynx, oropharynx, and larynx. (Cancer of the oral cavity is discussed in Chapter 44.) Although this type of cancer is uncommon, disability is great because of the potential loss of voice, disfigurement, and social consequences.

Clinical Manifestations

Early signs and symptoms of head and neck cancer vary with the tumour location (Carr, 2016). Cancer of the oral cavity may first be signaled by a painless growth in the mouth, an ulcer that does not heal, or a change in fit of dentures. Pain is a late symptom that may be aggravated by acidic food. Cancers of the oropharynx, hypopharynx, and supraglottic larynx rarely produce early symptoms and are usually diagnosed in late stages. The patient may experience a persistent unilateral sore throat or otalgia (ear pain). Hoarseness may be a symptom of early laryngeal cancer. If a lump in the neck or hoarseness lasts longer than 2 weeks, a medical evaluation is indicated. Some patients experience what feels like a lump in the throat or a change in voice quality.

Late stages of head and neck cancers have easily detectable signs and symptoms, including pain, dysphagia, decreased tongue mobility, airway obstruction, and cranial nerve neuropathies. The nurse should thoroughly examine the oral cavity, including the areas under the tongue and the dentures. The floor of the mouth, the tongue, and the lymph nodes in the neck should be bimanually palpated. There may be thickening of the normally soft and pliable oral mucosa. *Leukoplakia* (white patch) or *erythroplakia* (red patch) may be seen and should be noted for later biopsy. Both leukoplakia and carcinoma in situ (localized to a defined area) may precede invasive carcinoma by many years.

Diagnostic Studies

If lesions are suspected, the upper airways may be examined using indirect laryngoscopy—using a laryngeal mirror to visualize the laryngeal area—or a flexible nasopharyngoscope. The larynx and vocal cords are visually inspected for lesions and tissue mobility. A CT scan, magnetic resonance imaging (MRI), or positron emission tomography (PET) scan may be performed to detect local and regional spread. Neoplastic tissue is identifiable because it contains tissue of greater density or because it distorts, displaces, or destroys normal anatomical structures. Typically, multiple biopsy specimens are obtained to determine the extent of the disease.

Interprofessional Care

The stage of the disease will be determined on the basis of tumour size (T), number and location of involved nodes (N), and extent of metastasis (M). TNM staging classifies disease over the range between stage I through stage IV and guides treatment. Choice of treatment is based on medical history,

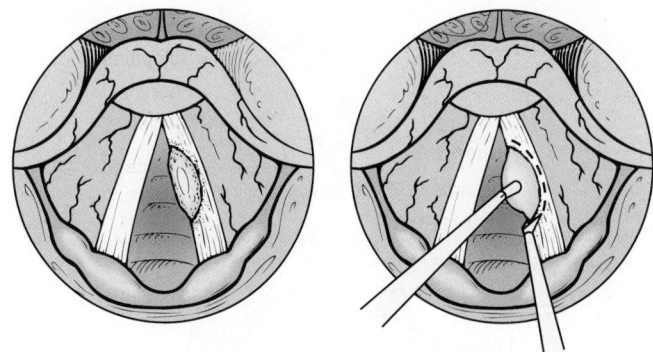

FIG. 29.8 Excision of laryngeal cancer. This cancer of the right vocal cord meets criteria for resection by transoral cordectomy. The cord is fully mobile and the lesion can be fully exposed. It does not approach or cross the anterior commissure.

extent of disease, cosmetic considerations, urgency of treatment, and patient choice. Approximately one third of patients with head and neck cancers have highly confined lesions that are stage I or II at diagnosis. Such patients can undergo radiation therapy or surgery with the goal of cure.

Radiation therapy may be effective in curing early vocal cord lesions. This therapy is usually successful in eliminating the tumour while preserving the quality of the voice. If radiation therapy is not successful or the lesion is too advanced for this therapy, surgery may be performed. A *cordectomy* (partial removal of one vocal cord) is used when there is a superficial tumour involving one cord (Figure 29.8). A *hemilaryngectomy* involves removal of thyroid cartilage, a portion of the larynx, and one vocal cord or part of a cord and necessitates a temporary tracheostomy. A *supraglottic laryngectomy* involves removing structures above the true cords—the false vocal cords and epiglottis. The patient is left at high risk for aspiration following surgery and requires a temporary tracheostomy. Both a hemilaryngectomy and a supraglottic laryngectomy allow the voice to be preserved, but quality is breathy and hoarse.

Advanced lesions are treated by a *total laryngectomy* in which the entire larynx and pre-epiglottic region is removed and a permanent tracheostomy performed. Airflow patterns before and after total laryngectomy are shown in Figure 29.9. *Radical neck dissection* frequently accompanies total laryngectomy to decrease the risk for lymphatic spread. Depending on the extent of involvement, extensive dissection and reconstruction may be performed. This procedure involves wide excision of the lymph nodes and their lymphatic channels (Figure 29.10). The following structures may also be removed or transected: sternocleidomastoid muscle and other closely associated muscles, internal jugular vein, mandible, submaxillary gland, part of the thyroid and parathyroid glands, and the spinal accessory nerve.

A *modified neck dissection* is performed whenever possible as an alternative to a radical neck dissection. The dissection is modified by sparing as many structures as possible to limit disfigurement and functional loss. A modified neck dissection usually involves dissection of the major cervical lymphatic vessels and lateral cervical space, with preservation of nerves and vessels, including the sympathetic and vagus nerves, spinal accessory nerves, and internal jugular vein. Neck dissection with vocal cord cancer usually involves one side of the neck. However, if the lesion is midline, a bilateral neck dissection may be performed. In this case, it is always modified on at least one side to minimize structural and functional deficits (Rothrock, 2019).

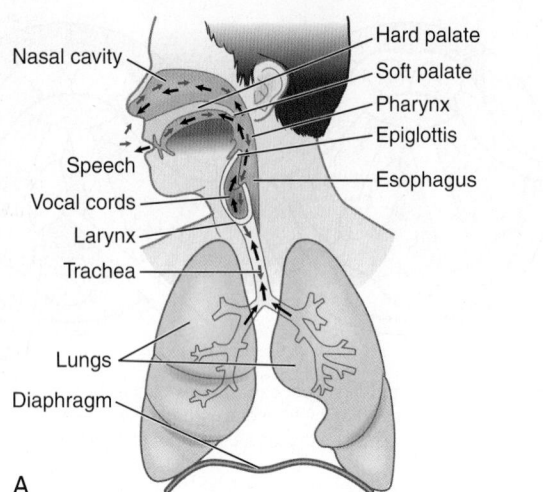
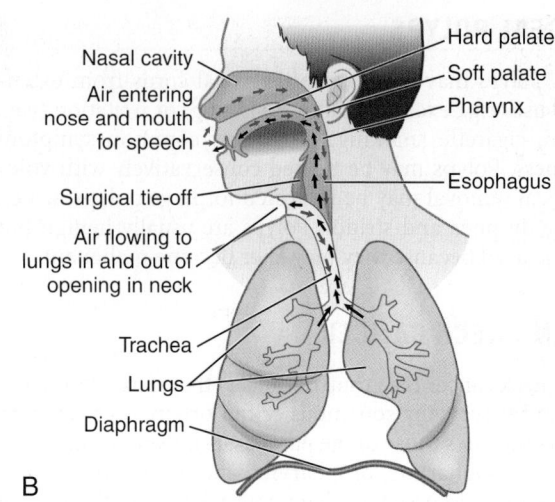

FIG. 29.9 **A**, Normal airflow in and out of the lungs. **B**, Airflow in and out of the lungs after total laryngectomy. Patients use esophageal speech by trapping air in the esophagus and releasing it to create sound. Source: The American Cancer Society.

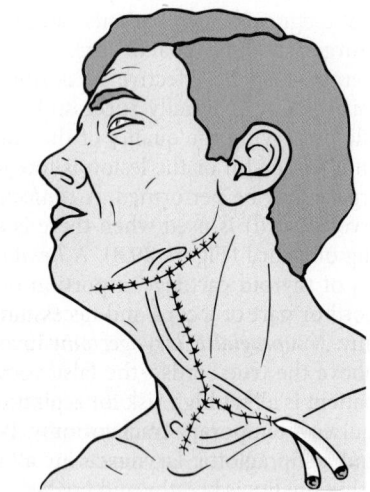

FIG. 29.10 Radical neck incision with drains in place.

The patient may refuse surgical intervention for advanced lesions because of the extent of the procedure, or the patient may be judged to be at too great a medical risk to undergo the procedure. In these situations, external radiation therapy may be used as the sole treatment or in combination with chemotherapy (Rothrock, 2019).

In addition, *brachytherapy*, a concentrated and localized method of delivering radiation that involves placing a radioactive source into or near the tumour, may be used to treat head and neck cancer. The goal of brachytherapy is to deliver high doses of radiation to the target area while limiting exposure of surrounding tissues. Thin, hollow, plastic needles are inserted into the tumour area, and radioactive iridium seeds are placed in the needles. The seeds emit continuous radiation. Brachytherapy can be used alone or combined with external radiation or surgical intervention. (Radiation therapy and brachytherapy are discussed in Chapter 18.)

Nutritional Therapy. The patient's nutritional status should be assessed before surgery as 60% of patients with head and neck cancer initially present with malnutrition (Carr, 2016). After radical neck surgery, the patient may be unable to take in nutrients through the normal route of ingestion because of swelling, the location of sutures, or difficulty swallowing. Parenteral fluids will be given for the first 24 to 48 hours. Tube feedings are usually given via a nasogastric, nasointestinal, or gastrostomy tube that was placed during surgery. (Nasogastric and gastrostomy feedings are described in Chapter 42.) The nurse must observe for tolerance of the feedings and adjust amount, time, and formula if nausea, vomiting, diarrhea, or distension occurs. The patient is instructed about the tube feedings. When the patient can swallow, small amounts of water are given. Close observation for difficulty swallowing is essential. Suctioning may be necessary to prevent aspiration.

Swallowing difficulties should be anticipated when the patient resumes eating. All patients should be referred to a speech pathologist for a dysphagia/swallowing assessment and recommendations during treatment. The type and degree of difficulty vary, depending on the surgical procedure. When a supraglottic laryngectomy is performed, the surgeon excises the upper portion of the larynx, including the epiglottis and the false vocal cords. The patient can speak because the true vocal cords remain intact. However, a new technique, the *supraglottic swallow*, must be learned to compensate for removal of the epiglottis and minimize risk for aspiration (Table 29.9). When the patient is learning this technique, it may be helpful to start with carbonated beverages because the effervescence provides cues about the liquid's position. With this exception, thin, watery fluids should be avoided because they are difficult to swallow and increase the risk for aspiration. A better choice is nonpourable puréed foods, which are thicker and allow more control during swallowing. Swallowing can be enhanced by thickening liquids with a commercially available thickening agent. Consultation with a dietitian can assist in creating an appropriate diet texture while ensuring nutritional and caloric needs are maintained.

Good nutrition is important during radiation therapy because calories and protein are needed for tissue repair. Antiemetics or analgesics may be given before meals to reduce nausea and mouth pain. Bland foods may be better tolerated than more highly flavoured foods. Caloric intake may be increased by adding dry milk to foods during preparation, selecting foods high in calories, and using oral supplements. It is helpful to add sauces and gravies to food, which adds calories and moistens food so that it is more easily swallowed. If an adequate intake cannot be maintained, enteral feedings may be used. When eating, the patient should always be positioned with the head elevated.

TABLE 29.9   PATIENT & CAREGIVER TEACHING GUIDE

Steps for Performing the Supraglottic Swallow

The following information should be included when teaching the patient and caregiver how to perform the supraglottic swallow.

1. Take a deep breath to aerate lungs.
2. Perform the Valsalva manoeuvre to approximate the vocal cords.
3. Place food in the mouth and swallow. Some food will enter the airway and remain on top of the closed vocal cords.
4. Cough to remove food from top of vocal cords.
5. Swallow so food is moved from top of vocal cords.
6. Breathe after cough–swallow sequence to prevent aspiration of food collected on top of vocal cords.

NURSING MANAGEMENT HEAD AND NECK CANCER

NURSING ASSESSMENT

Subjective and objective data that should be obtained from a person with head and neck cancer are presented in Table 29.10.

NURSING DIAGNOSES

Nursing diagnoses for the patient with head and neck cancer include but are not limited to the following:

- *Inadequate airway clearance* resulting from *presence of artificial airway and excessive mucus*
- *Potential for aspiration* resulting from *presence of oral/nasal tube and impaired ability to swallow*
- *Anxiety* resulting from *unmet needs* (lack of knowledge about surgical procedure and pain management)
- *Acute pain* resulting from *physical injury agent* (surgery)
- *Reduced verbal communication* resulting from *physiological condition* (removal of vocal cords)

Additional information on nursing diagnoses for the patient with head and neck cancer is presented in NCP 29.2, available on the Evolve website.

PLANNING

The overall goals are that the patient will have (1) a patent airway, (2) no spread of cancer, (3) no complications related to therapy, (4) adequate nutritional intake, (5) minimal to no pain, (6) the ability to communicate, and (7) an acceptable body image.

NURSING IMPLEMENTATION

HEALTH PROMOTION. Development of head and neck cancer is closely related to personal habits, primarily tobacco use, including the use of cigarettes, vaping, cigars, chewing tobacco, and snuff. Prolonged alcohol use has been implicated as a potentiating factor in head and neck cancer. Excessive sun exposure to the lips also increases the risk for oral cancer.

The nurse should include information about risk factors in health teaching (Carr, 2016). If cancer has been diagnosed, tobacco cessation is still important. The patient with head and neck cancer who continues to smoke during radiation therapy has a lower rate of response and survival than the patient who does not smoke during radiation therapy. In addition, risk for a second primary cancer is significantly increased in patients who continue to smoke.

ACUTE INTERVENTION. The patient and the family must be taught about the type of therapy to be performed and care required. Assessment of concerns is integral to the plan of care.

TABLE 29.10   NURSING ASSESSMENT

Head and Neck Cancer

Subjective Data

Important Health Information

Past health history: Positive family history; prolonged tobacco use (cigarettes, pipes, cigars, chewing tobacco, smokeless tobacco); prolonged, heavy alcohol use

Medications: Prolonged use of over-the-counter medication for sore throat, decongestants

Symptoms

Mouth ulcer that does not heal, change in fit of dentures, change in appetite, weight loss, swallowing difficulty (e.g., sensation of lump in throat, pain with swallowing, aspiration when swallowing)

Fatigue with minimal exertion

Sore throat, hoarseness, change in voice quality, referred ear pain

Objective Data

Respiratory

Hoarseness, chronic laryngitis, nasal voice, palpable neck mass and lymph nodes (tender, hard, fixed), tracheal deviation; dyspnea, stridor (late sign)

Gastrointestinal

White (leukoplakia) or red (erythroplakia) patches inside mouth, ulceration of mucosa, asymmetrical tongue, exudate in mouth or pharynx, mass or thickening of mucosa

Possible Findings

Mass on direct or indirect laryngoscopy; tumour on soft tissue radiographic study, computed tomographic scan, magnetic resonance imaging, or positron emission tomography; positive biopsy

The patient and family must cope with the psychological impact of the diagnosis of cancer, alteration of physical appearance, and possible need for alternative methods of communication (Carr, 2016). The care plan should include assessment of the patient's support system. The patient may not have someone to provide assistance after discharge, may be unemployed, or may be employed in a job that cannot be continued.

Radiation Therapy. The nurse can suggest interventions to reduce adverse effects of radiation therapy. (Radiation is discussed in Chapter 18.) Patients should be encouraged to take frequent rest periods and engage in light, regular exercise, such as walking.

Dry mouth (xerostomia), the most frequent and annoying adverse effect, typically begins within a few weeks of treatment. The patient's saliva decreases in volume and becomes thick. The change may be temporary or permanent. Pilocarpine hydrochloride (Salagen) increases saliva production and should be started before the initiation of radiation therapy and continued for 90 days. Other interventions include fluids, sugarless gum or candy, nonalcoholic mouth rinses (baking soda or glycerin solutions), and artificial saliva.

The patient may also experience stomatitis, especially if the oral cavity is in the field of therapy causing irritation, ulceration, and pain. Normal saline mouth rinses after meals and at bedtime can clean and soothe irritated tissues. Commercial mouthwashes and hot or spicy foods should be avoided because they are irritating. If the problem is severe, a mouthwash mixture of equal parts of antacid, diphenhydramine (Benadryl), and topical lidocaine is suggested.

Skin over the irradiated area often becomes reddened and sensitive to touch. Patients commonly require a break from their scheduled radiation program because of altered skin integrity.

Only prescribed lotions and products should be used during radiation therapy. All exposure to the sun should be avoided to reduce discomfort.

Surgical Therapy. Preoperative care for the patient who is to have a radical neck dissection involves consideration of the patient's physical and psychosocial needs. Physical preparation is the same as for any major surgery, with special emphasis on oral hygiene. Explanations and emotional support are of special significance and should include postoperative measures relating to communication and feeding. The surgical procedure should be explained to the patient and family or caregivers, and the nurse should make sure that the information is understood.

Teaching must be tailored to the planned surgical procedure. For surgeries that involve a laryngectomy, teaching should include information about expected changes in speech. The nurse or speech pathologist should demonstrate means of communicating other than speaking that can be used temporarily or permanently. This may include some type of communication board.

After surgery, maintenance of a patent airway is essential. The inflammation in the surgical area may compress the trachea. A tracheostomy tube will be in place. The patient will be placed in a semi-Fowler's position to decrease edema and limit tension on the suture lines. Vital signs should be monitored frequently because of the risk for hemorrhage and respiratory compromise. Pressure dressings, packing, or drainage tubes (Hemovac, Jackson Pratt) may be used for wound management, depending on the type of surgical procedure. When a radical neck dissection is performed, wound suction using a portable system, such as a Hemovac, is generally used. If skin flaps are employed, dressings are typically not used. This allows better visualization of the incision and helps prevent excessive pressure on tissue (see Figure 29.10). The drainage should be serosanguineous and gradually decrease in volume over 24 hours. Patency of drainage tubes should be monitored every 4 hours to ensure that they are properly removing serous drainage and for the amount and character of drainage. If the tubing becomes obstructed, fluid will accumulate under the skin flap and predispose to impaired wound healing and infection. After drainage tubes are removed, the area should be closely monitored for any swelling. If fluid continues to accumulate, aspiration may be necessary.

Immediately after surgery, the patient with a laryngectomy requires frequent suctioning via the laryngectomy tube. Secretions typically change in amount and consistency over time. The patient may initially have copious blood-tinged secretions that diminish and thicken. Standard administration of saline boluses via the tracheostomy tube to loosen secretions is no longer recommended as it may increase risk for infection (Altobelli, 2017). The patient will benefit from the use of a humidifier while at home.

Following a neck dissection, an exercise program should be instituted to maintain strength and movement in the affected shoulder and the neck. This is especially important when the spinal accessory nerve and the sternocleidomastoid muscles are removed or damaged. Without exercise, the patient will be left with a "frozen" shoulder and limited range of motion in the neck. This exercise program should be continued following discharge to prevent future functional disabilities. The patient may need the neck supported to be able to move the head after surgery.

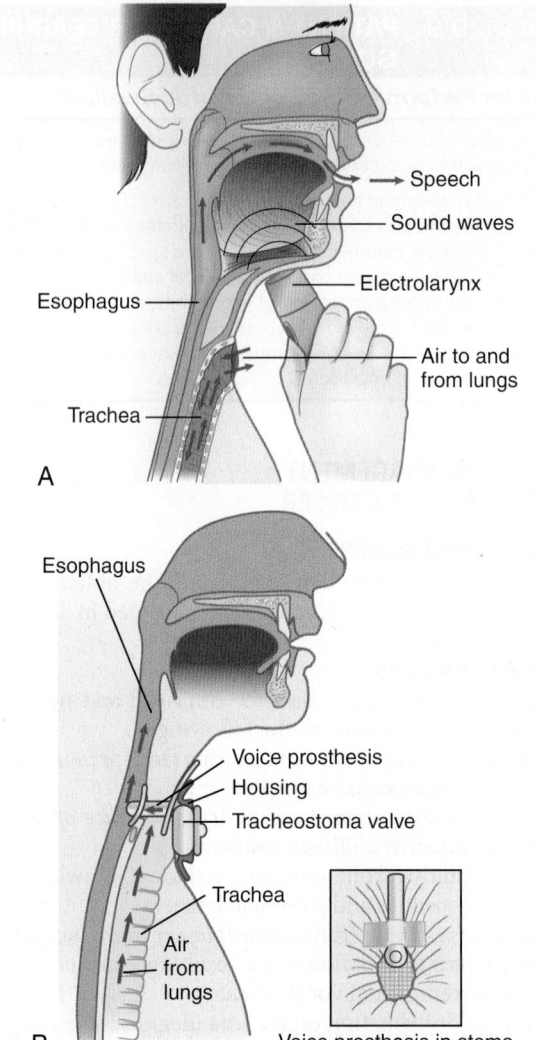

FIG. 29.11 A, The sound waves created by the electrolarynx allow the person to speak. **B,** The Blom–Singer voice prosthesis and valve.

Voice Rehabilitation. A speech pathologist should meet with the patient preoperatively and following a total laryngectomy to discuss voice restoration options. The International Association of Laryngectomees, an association of patients who have had laryngectomies, focuses on assisting patients to re-establish speech. Local groups, called Lost Cord Clubs, often provide member volunteers to visit the patient, preferably before surgery. Several options are available to restore speech. These include use of a voice prosthesis, esophageal speech, and an electrolarynx.

The most used voice prosthesis is the Blom–Singer (Figure 29.11). This soft plastic device is inserted into a fistula made between the esophagus and the trachea. The puncture may be created at the time of surgery or afterward, depending on the preference of the surgeon. A red rubber catheter is placed in the tracheoesophageal puncture and must remain in place until a tract is formed. Once the tract is formed, the voice prosthesis is inserted. This prosthesis allows air from the lungs to enter the esophagus by way of the tracheal stoma. A one-way valve prevents aspiration of food or saliva from the esophagus into the tracheostomy. To produce the voice, the patient manually blocks the stoma with the finger. Air moves from the lungs, through the prosthesis, into the esophagus, and out the mouth. The voice is produced by the air vibrating against the esophagus, and speech

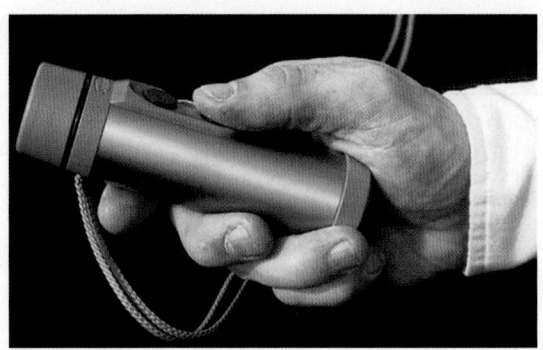

FIG. 29.12 Artificial larynx. Battery-powered electronic artificial larynx for a patient who has had a total laryngectomy. Source: Courtesy CLG Photographics, Inc., St. Louis.

sounds are formed into words by moving the tongue, jaw, and lips. A valve may also be used with this device. When the valve is in place, the stoma does not need to be closed with the finger to speak. The prosthesis must be cleaned regularly and replaced when it becomes blocked with mucus.

An electrolarynx is a handheld, battery-powered device that creates speech with the use of sound waves. There are two main types: the intra-oral type and the neck type. One intra-oral device, the Cooper-Rand, has a plastic tube that is placed in the corner of the roof of the mouth to create vibrations. To create the most normal sound when using this device, the patient should (1) avoid trying to use their tongue to hold the tube in place; (2) compress the tone generator for short intervals and speak in phrases, rather than full sentences; (3) speak using large movements of the lips, tongue, and jaw, rather than keeping the mouth partially closed; (4) talk face-to-face with the listener; and (5) practise because it takes time to develop this skill.

With the neck type of artificial larynx, the device is placed against the neck rather than in the mouth. This device is used after surgical healing is complete and no edema remains (Figure 29.12). With experience, the patient can learn to move the lips in ways that create somewhat normal-sounding speech. With both devices, voice pitch is low, and the sound is mechanical.

Esophageal speech is a method of swallowing air, trapping it in the esophagus, and releasing it to create sound. The air causes vibration of the pharyngoesophageal segment to create sound (which initially is like a belch). With practice, 50% of patients develop some speech skills, but only 10% develop fluent speech.

Stoma Care. Before discharge, the patient should be instructed in the care of the laryngectomy stoma. The area around the stoma should be washed daily with a moist cloth. If a laryngectomy tube is in place, the entire tube must be removed at least daily and cleaned in the same manner as a tracheostomy tube. The inner cannula may have to be removed and cleaned more frequently. A scarf, a loose shirt, or a crocheted shield can be used to shield the stoma.

The patient should cover the stoma when coughing (because mucus may be expectorated) and during any activity (e.g., shaving, applying makeup) that might lead to inhalation of foreign materials. Because water can easily enter the stoma, the patient should wear a plastic collar when taking a shower. Swimming is contraindicated. Initially, humidification will be administered via a tracheostomy mask. After discharge, a bedside humidifier can be used. A high oral fluid intake must be maintained, especially in dry weather.

The patient should be told the importance of wearing a medical alert bracelet or other identification that alerts others in an emergency of the need for neck breathing. Because the patient no longer breathes through the nose, the ability to smell smoke and food may be lost. The patient should be advised to install smoke and carbon monoxide detectors in the home. It is important for food to be colourful, attractively prepared, and nutritious because taste may also be diminished secondary to the loss of smell as well as to radiation therapy.

Depression. Depression is common in the patient who has had a radical neck dissection. The patient may not be able to speak because of the laryngectomy and cannot control saliva. The facial appearance may be significantly altered, with swelling, edema, and deformities. Many physical changes are reversible as the edema subsides and the tracheostomy tube is removed. Depression may also be related to concern about the prognosis. The nurse should encourage verbalization of feelings, conveying acceptance, and help the patient regain an acceptable self-concept. A psychiatric referral for the patient experiencing prolonged or severe depression should be considered.

Sexuality. Surgery and the presence of foreign attachments such as tracheostomy and gastrostomy tubes may affect body image dramatically. The patient may feel less desirable sexually. The nurse can assist the patient by having discussions with the patient regarding sexuality and encouraging them to discuss this problem with the sexual partner. It may be difficult for the patient to discuss sexual issues verbally because of the alteration in communication. The nurse can help the patient plan how to communicate with the sexual partner and offer support and guidance to the sexual partner. Helping the patient see that sexuality involves much more than appearance may relieve some anxiety.

AMBULATORY AND HOME CARE. The patient is often discharged with a tracheostomy and a nasogastric or gastrostomy feeding tube. Home health care may be needed initially as the family's or patient's ability to perform self-care activities is evaluated. The patient and the family must be taught how to manage tubes and whom to call if there are problems.

The patient can resume exercise, recreation, and sexual activity when able. Most patients can return to work 1 to 2 months after surgery. However, many never return to full-time employment. Loss of speech, loss of the ability to taste and smell, inability to produce audible sounds (including laughing and weeping), and the presence of a permanent tracheal stoma that produces undesirable mucus are often overwhelming to the patient. Although changes are discussed before surgery, the patient may not be prepared for the extent of these changes. If the patient has a partner, the reaction of this person to the patient's altered appearance is important.

Reconstructive surgery may be performed at the time of the initial surgery or soon after the tumour is removed. Various types of flaps and grafts are used. It may be necessary to rebuild the nose or the mandible or to close oral cutaneous openings. Prosthetic materials, such as Silastic and Plastigel (which is soft), are often used to reconstruct various deformities.

Metastatic cancer is often painful, leaving the affected person in a severely debilitated state. If pain is significant, a pain control regimen should be instituted to provide comfort, and referral should be made to hospice if indicated.

EVALUATION

Expected outcomes for the patient with head and neck cancer who is treated surgically are addressed in NCP 29.2, available on the Evolve website.

CASE STUDY

Laryngeal Cancer

Patient Profile

T. P., 60 years old (pronoun he/him), was admitted for evaluation of mild pain on swallowing and a persistent sore throat over the past year. He has a history of type 2 diabetes mellitus.

Subjective Data

- States that his symptoms worsened in the past 2 months
- Has used various cold remedies to relieve symptoms, without relief
- Has lost weight because of decrease in appetite and difficulty swallowing
- Has smoked three packs of cigarettes a day for 40 years
- Consumes four to six cans of beer a day

Objective Data

Laryngoscopy

- Subglottic mass

Physical Examination

- Enlarged cervical nodes

Computed Tomographic Scan

- Subglottic lesion with lymph node involvement

Interprofessional Care

- Percutaneous gastrostomy tube inserted preoperatively for enteral tube feeding
- Total laryngectomy with tracheostomy with inflated cuff
- Nasogastric tube postoperatively

Discussion Questions

1. What information in the assessment suggests that T. P. is at risk for cancer of the larynx?
2. What diagnostic tests are typically performed to evaluate the extent of this condition?
3. **Priority decision:** What are the priority teaching strategies for T. P. before and after laryngectomy?
4. Discuss methods used to restore speech after laryngectomy.
5. Is there anything in his history that may affect wound healing after surgery?
6. **Priority decision:** While in the recovery room, T. P. develops shortness of breath. What are the priority nursing interventions?
7. What teaching is required to help this patient assume self-care after his surgery? What precautions should the patient take because of his stoma?
8. While on the medical-surgical unit, T. P. is tearful and is staring at the wall. What should the nurse do?
9. **Priority decision:** Based on the assessment data presented, what are the priority nursing diagnoses? Are there any interprofessional issues?
10. **Evidence-informed practice:** How could the nurse best meet T. P.'s communication needs during the first few postoperative days?

Answers are available at http://evolve.elsevier.com/Canada/Lewis/medsurg.

REVIEW QUESTIONS

The number of the question corresponds to the same-numbered objective at the beginning of the chapter.

1. A client is seen in the clinic for an episode of epistaxis, which is controlled by placement of anterior nasal packing. During discharge teaching, what should the nurse instruct the client to do?
   a. Use ASA (Aspirin) for pain relief.
   b. Remove the packing later that day.
   c. Skip the next dose of antihypertensive medication.
   d. Avoid vigorous nose blowing and strenuous activity.

2. A client with allergic rhinitis reports severe nasal congestion, sneezing, and watery, itchy eyes and nose at various times of the year. What should the nurse advise the client to do?
   a. Avoid all intranasal sprays and oral antihistamines.
   b. Limit the duration of use of nasal decongestant spray to 10 days.
   c. Use oral decongestants at bedtime to prevent symptoms during the night.
   d. Keep a diary of when the allergic reaction occurs and what precipitates it.

3. A client is seen at the clinic with fever, muscle aches, sore throat with yellowish exudate, and headache. Which of the following does the nurse anticipate that the interprofessional management will include? *(Select all that apply.)*
   a. Antiviral agents to treat influenza
   b. Treatment with antibiotics starting ASAP
   c. A throat culture or rapid strep antigen test
   d. Supportive care, including cool, bland liquids
   e. Comprehensive history to determine possible etiology

4. What type of tracheostomy tube prevents the use of the voice?
   a. Cuffless tracheostomy tube
   b. Fenestrated tracheostomy tube
   c. Tube with an inflated foam cuff
   d. Cuffed tube with the cuff deflated

5. Which nursing action related to the tracheostomy tube cuff pressure would prevent excessive pressure on tracheal capillaries?
   a. Monitor pressure every 2 to 3 days.
   b. Ensure pressure is less than 20 mm Hg or 25 cm H_2O.
   c. Ensure pressure is less than 30 mm Hg or 35 cm H_2O.
   d. Ensure pressure is sufficient to fill the pilot balloon until it is tense.

6. Which of the following is not an early symptom of head and neck cancer?
   a. Hoarseness
   b. Change in fit of dentures
   c. Mouth ulcers that do not heal
   d. Decreased mobility of the tongue

7. While in the recovery room, a client with a total laryngectomy is suctioned and has bloody mucus with some clots. Which of the following nursing interventions would apply?
   a. Notify the physician immediately.
   b. Place the client in the prone position to facilitate drainage.
   c. Instill 3 mL of normal saline into the tracheostomy tube to loosen secretions.
   d. Continue the assessment of the client, including oxygen saturation, respiratory rate, and breath sounds.

8. How should the client use a voice prosthesis?
   a. Place a vibrating device in the mouth.
   b. Place a speaking valve over the stoma.
   c. Block the stoma entrance with a finger.
   d. Swallow air using the Valsalva manoeuvre.

1. d; 2. d; 3. c, d, e; 4. c; 5. b; 6. d; 7. d; 8. c.

For even more review questions, visit http://evolve.elsevier.com/Canada/Lewis/medsurg.

REFERENCES

Altobelli, N. (2017). Chapter 36: Airway management. In R. M. Kacmarek, J. K. Stoller, & A. J. Heuer (Eds.), *Egan's fundamentals of respiratory care* (11th ed., pp. 739–789). Mosby Elsevier.

Boggild, A., Yuan, L., Low, D. E., et al. (2011). The impact of influenza on the Canadian First Nations. *Journal of Public Health, 102*(5), 345–348. https://doi.org/10.1007/BF03404174. (Seminal).

Brennan-Olsen, S. L., Vogrin, S., Leslie, W. D., et al. (2017). Fractures in Indigenous compared to non-Indigenous populations: A systematic review of rates and aetiology. *Bone Reports, 6*, 146–158. https://doi.org/10.1016/j.bonr.2017.04.00

Byun, H., Chung, J. H., Lee, S. H., et al. (2020). Association of hypertension with the risk and severity of epistaxis. *JAMA Otolaryngology–Head & Neck Surgery, 147*(1), 1–7. https://doi.org/10.1001/jamaoto.2020.2906

Calhoun, W. J., Omachi, T. A., Reddy, S. R., et al. (2016). Allergic status is associated with increased number of asthma exacerbations. *American Journal of Respiratory and Critical Care Medicine, 193*, A4970. American Thoracic Society. https://doi.org/10.1164/ajrccm-conference.2016.193.1_MeetingAbstracts.A4970

Carr, E. (2016). Head and neck cancers. In J. K. Itano, J. M. Brant, F. A. Conde, et al. (Eds.), *Core curriculum for oncology* (5th ed., pp. 139–157). Elsevier Mosby.

Cash, J. C., Cook, M., & Duke, V. (2020). Acute sinusitis/rhinosinusitis. 7. Nasal guidelines. In J. C. Cash, D. Fraser, L. Corcoran, et al. (Eds.), *Canadian family practice guidelines*. Springer.

Cooper, K., & Gosnell, K. (2019). *Adult health nursing* (8th ed.). Mosby.

Fasanmi, O. G., Odetokun, I. A., Balogun, F. A., et al. (2017). Public health concerns of highly pathogenic avian influenza H5N1 endemicity in Africa. *Veterinary World, 10*(10), 1194–1204. https://doi.org/10.14202/vetworld.2017.1194-1204

Gordon, J., Kirlew, M., Schreiber, Y., et al. (2015). Acute rheumatic fever in First Nations communities in northwestern Ontario: Social determinants of health "bite the heart. *Canadian Family Physician, 61*(10), 881–886. (Seminal).

Infection Prevention and Control (IPAC) Canada. (2021). *Seasonal influenza, avian influenza and pandemic influenza.* https://ipac-canada.org/influenza-resources.php

Patton, K., & Thibodeau, G. (2016). *Anatomy and physiology* (9th ed.). Mosby.

Public Health Agency of Canada (PHAC). (2015). *An Advisory Committee Statement (ACS)-National Advisory Committee on Immunization (NACI): Canadian immunization guide chapter on influenza and statement on seasonal influenza vaccine for 2015-2016.* https://www.phac-aspc.gc.ca/naci-ccni/assets/pdf-flu-2015-grippe-eng.pdf

Public Health Agency of Canada (PHAC). (2018). *Canadian pandemic influenza preparedness: Planning guidance for the health sector.* https://www.canada.ca/en/public-health/services/flu-influenza/canadian-pandemic-influenza-preparedness-planning-guidance-health-sector/table-of-contents.html#pre

Public Health Agency of Canada (PHAC). (2021). *Coronavirus (COVID-19) SARS-CoV-2.* https://ipac-canada.org/coronavirus-resources.php

Rondanelli, M., Miccono, A., Lamburghini, S., et al. (2018). Self-care for common colds: The pivotal role of vitamin D, vitamin C, zinc, and echinacea in three main immune interactive clusters (physical barriers, innate and adaptive immunity) involved during an episode of common colds—Practical advice on dosages and on the time to take these nutrients/botanicals in order to prevent or treat common colds. *Evidence-Based Complementary and Alternative Medicine, 2018*, 36. https://doi.org/10.1155/2018/5813095

Rothrock, J. (2019). *Alexander's care of the patient in surgery* (16th ed.). Mosby.

Stacy, K. M. (2018). Pulmonary therapeutic management. In L. D. Urden, K. M. Stacy, & M. E. Lough (Eds.), *Critical care nursing: Diagnosis and management* (8th ed., pp. 487–519). Elsevier Mosby.

Tung, H. Y., Landers, C., Li, E., et al. (2016). Allergen-encoded signals that control allergic responses. *Current Opinion in Allergy and Clinical Immunology, 16*(1), 51–58. https://doi.org/10.1097/ACI.0000000000000233

RESOURCES

Resources for this chapter are listed in Chapters 30 and 31.

ⓔvolve

For additional Internet resources, see the website for this book at http://evolve.elsevier.com/Canada/Lewis/medsurg.

Nursing Management

Lower Respiratory Conditions

Cydnee Seneviratne
Originating US chapter by Eugene Mondor

ⓔvolve WEBSITE

http://evolve.elsevier.com/Canada/Lewis/medsurg

- Review Questions (Online Only)
- Key Points
- Answer Guidelines to Case Study
- Student Case Studies
  - Lung Cancer
  - Pulmonary Embolism and Respiratory Failure

- Customizable Nursing Care Plans
  - Pneumonia
  - Thoracotomy

- Conceptual Care Map Creator
- Audio Glossary
- Content Updates

LEARNING OBJECTIVES

1. Describe the pathophysiology, types, and clinical manifestations of pneumonia and interprofessional care of patients with pneumonia.
2. Explain the nursing management of the patient with pneumonia.
3. Describe the pathogenesis, classification, clinical manifestations, complications, and diagnostic abnormalities of tuberculosis and the nursing and interprofessional management of the patient with tuberculosis.
4. Identify the causes, clinical manifestations, and nursing and interprofessional management of pulmonary fungal infections.
5. Explain the pathophysiology, clinical manifestations, and nursing and interprofessional management of bronchiectasis and lung abscess.
6. Identify the causative factors, clinical features, and management of environmental lung diseases.
7. Describe the causes, risk factors, pathogenesis, and clinical manifestations of lung cancer and the nursing and interprofessional management of the patient with lung cancer.
8. Identify the mechanisms involved and the clinical manifestations of pneumothorax, fractured ribs, and flail chest.
9. Describe the purpose of chest tubes and the methods of their action, as well as related nursing responsibilities in the care of a patient with a chest tube.
10. Explain the types of chest surgery and appropriate preoperative and postoperative care.
11. Compare and contrast extrapulmonary and intrapulmonary restrictive lung disorders in terms of causes, clinical manifestations, and interprofessional management.
12. Describe the pathophysiology, clinical manifestations, and management of pulmonary hypertension and cor pulmonale.
13. Discuss the use of lung transplantation as a treatment for pulmonary disorders.

KEY TERMS

acute bronchitis
atelectasis
blebs
bronchiectasis
chylothorax
community-acquired pneumonia (CAP)
cor pulmonale
empirical therapy
empyema

flail chest
hemothorax
hospital-acquired pneumonia (HAP)
lung abscess
pleural effusion
pleurisy (pleuritis)
pneumoconiosis
pneumonia
pneumothorax

pulmonary edema
pulmonary embolism (PE)
pulmonary hypertension
tension pneumothorax
thoracentesis
thoracotomy
tuberculosis (TB)

A wide variety of conditions affect the lower respiratory system. Lung diseases that are characterized primarily by an obstructive disorder, such as asthma, emphysema, chronic bronchitis, and cystic fibrosis, are discussed in Chapter 31. All other lower respiratory conditions are discussed in this chapter.

Respiratory tract infections are a common cause of morbidity and mortality worldwide. In Canada, respiratory diseases, including chronic obstructive pulmonary disease (COPD), bronchitis, and pneumonia, account for some of the most common reasons for hospitalization (Canadian Institute for Health

Information, 2021). During the 2019/2020 influenza season, there were up to 52,169 laboratory-confirmed influenza cases by February 2020. The majority of influenza A cases were diagnosed in adults 65 years and older (46%), and influenza B cases diagnosed were in the younger population—children under the age of 19 years (57%) and persons between 20 and 44 years of age (30%) (Government of Canada, 2020). Although information regarding the COVID-19 pandemic is constantly evolving as the world grapples with its impact on individuals and families, it is known that patients with chronic lung disease or recent surgical interventions need to avoid contact with any COVID-19-positive individuals. Finally, tuberculosis (TB), although potentially curable and preventable, is a worldwide public health threat of epidemic proportion.

In many places throughout this chapter, bronchitis, pneumonia, and TB statistics are representative of the Canadian population including the Indigenous people in Canada. However, what the statistics do not show or explain are the challenges that Indigenous populations have faced regarding risk factors, access to health care, and continuity of care for lower respiratory conditions. For example, Indigenous children in Canada between the ages of 5 to 13 years are at higher risk for bronchitis, and Indigenous adults over the age of 18 are at risk for higher rates of pneumonia (Dalcin et al., 2018). Modifiable risk factors such as obesity, exposure to smoke, and mould and dampness in the home are preventable public health factors that have been poorly addressed in Indigenous communities and require further attention. In addition, Indigenous people in Canada have historically experienced a health care system that has been brutal and scarring to Indigenous communities. The most concerning example of stereotyping and improper access to care is TB incidence among Indigenous communities in Canada. First Nations communities are disproportionately affected by TB, with factors such as overcrowding, poor housing, poverty, and inappropriate access to health care contributing to this higher incidence. Canadian history related to the treatment of Indigenous people diagnosed with TB is laden with negative experiences for members of First Nations communities. For example, according to Lux (2018), Indian hospitals such as the Camsell Indian Hospital in Edmonton, Alberta were primary care and research hospitals for TB in Canada. Indigenous people were sent to Indian hospitals, where they were diagnosed with TB and assigned to anti-TB medication trials. After Indian hospitals were shut down, access to proper care did not improve, although unethical experiments decreased. TB remains a rampant and concerning health issue for some Indigenous communities, indicating the need to address determinants of health related to poverty, poor living conditions, and, most importantly, access to appropriate health care.

ACUTE BRONCHITIS

Acute bronchitis is an inflammation of the bronchi in the lower respiratory tract that is usually caused by infection. It is one of the most common conditions seen in primary care. It usually occurs as a sequel to an upper respiratory tract infection. A type of acute bronchitis is acute exacerbation of chronic bronchitis (AECB). AECB represents acute infection superimposed on chronic bronchitis. AECB is a potentially serious condition that may lead to respiratory failure. (Chronic bronchitis is discussed in Chapter 31.)

The cause of most cases of acute bronchitis is viral (rhinovirus, influenza). However, bacterial causes are also common in smokers (e.g., *Streptococcus pneumoniae, Haemophilus influenzae*) and nonsmokers (e.g., *Mycoplasma pneumoniae, Chlamydia pneumoniae*).

In acute bronchitis, persistent cough following an acute upper airway infection (e.g., rhinitis, pharyngitis) is the most common symptom. Cough is often accompanied by production of clear, mucoid sputum, although some patients produce purulent sputum. Associated symptoms include fever, headache, malaise, and shortness of breath on exertion. Physical examination may reveal mildly elevated temperature, pulse, and respiratory rate with either normal breath sounds or expiratory wheezing. Chest radiographic studies can differentiate acute bronchitis from pneumonia because there is no radiographic evidence of consolidation or infiltrates with bronchitis.

Acute bronchitis is usually self-limiting, and the treatment is generally supportive, including fluids, rest, and anti-inflammatory agents. Cough suppressants or bronchodilators may be prescribed for symptomatic treatment of nocturnal cough or wheezing. Antibiotics are generally not prescribed unless the person has a prolonged infection associated with constitutional symptoms (which indicate systemic disease effects), including mild to moderate pain; the person is a smoker; or the person has COPD.

The patient with AECB is usually treated empirically with broad-spectrum antibiotics. Often, the patient with COPD is taught to recognize symptoms of acute bronchitis and to begin a course of antibiotics when symptoms occur. Many health care providers believe that a more severe infection often results if the patient delays taking antibiotics until after a clinical examination. Early initiation of antibiotic treatment in patients with COPD has resulted in a decrease in relapses and a decrease in hospital admissions.

PNEUMONIA

Pneumonia is an acute inflammation of the lung parenchyma caused by a microbial agent. The discovery of sulpha medications and penicillin was pivotal in the treatment of pneumonia. Since that time, there has been remarkable progress in the development of antibiotics to treat pneumonia. However, despite new antimicrobial agents, pneumonia is still common and is associated with significant morbidity and mortality rates.

Etiology

Normally, the airway distal to the larynx is sterile because of protective defence mechanisms. These mechanisms include the following: filtration of air, warming and humidification of inspired air, epiglottis closure over the trachea, cough reflex, mucociliary escalator mechanism, secretion of immunoglobulin A, and alveolar macrophages (see Chapter 28).

Factors Predisposing to Pneumonia. Pneumonia is more likely to result when defence mechanisms become incompetent or are overwhelmed by the virulence or quantity of infectious agents. Decreased consciousness depresses the cough and epiglottal reflexes, which may allow aspiration of oropharyngeal contents into the lungs. Tracheal intubation interferes with the normal cough reflex and the mucociliary escalator mechanism. It also bypasses the upper airways, in which filtration and humidification of air normally take place. The mucociliary escalator mechanism is impaired by air pollution, cigarette smoking, viral upper respiratory infections (URIs), and normal changes of aging. In the presence of malnutrition, the functions

TABLE 30.1	**FACTORS PREDISPOSING TO PNEUMONIA**

- Aging
- Air pollution
- Altered consciousness: alcohol use disorder, head injury, seizures, anaesthesia, drug overdose, stroke
- Altered oropharyngeal flora
- Aspiration
- Bed rest and prolonged immobility
- Chronic diseases: chronic lung disease, diabetes mellitus, heart disease, cancer, end-stage renal disease
- Debilitating illness
- Human immunodeficiency virus (HIV) infection
- Immunosuppressive medications (corticosteroids, cancer chemotherapy, immunosuppressive therapy after organ transplant)
- Inhalation or aspiration of noxious substances
- Intestinal and gastric feedings
- Malnutrition
- Smoking
- Tracheal intubation (endotracheal intubation, tracheostomy)
- Upper respiratory tract infection

of lymphocytes and polymorphonuclear leukocytes are altered. Certain diseases, such as leukemia, alcoholism, and diabetes mellitus, are associated with an increased frequency of Gram-negative bacilli in the oropharynx. (Gram-negative bacilli are not normal flora in the respiratory tract.) Altered oropharyngeal flora can also occur secondary to antibiotic therapy given for an infection elsewhere in the body. A summary of the factors predisposing to pneumonia is provided in Table 30.1.

Acquisition of Organisms. Organisms that cause pneumonia reach the lung by three methods:

1. *Aspiration* from the nasopharynx or oropharynx. Many of the organisms that cause pneumonia are normal inhabitants of the pharynx in healthy adults.
2. *Inhalation* of microbes present in the air (e.g., *M. pneumoniae*, fungal pneumonias)
3. *Hematogenous spread* from a primary infection elsewhere in the body. An example is *Staphylococcus aureus*.

Types of Pneumonia

Pneumonia can be caused by bacteria, viruses, *Mycoplasma*, fungi, parasites, and chemicals. Although pneumonia can be classified according to the causative organism, a clinically effective way to classify pneumonia is as *community-acquired* or *hospital-acquired*. Classifying pneumonia is important because of differences in the likely causative organisms and the selection of appropriate antibiotics.

Community-Acquired Pneumonia. Community-acquired pneumonia (CAP) is defined as a lower respiratory tract infection of the lung parenchyma with onset in the community or during the first 2 days of hospitalization. The incidence of CAP is highest in the winter months. Smoking is an important risk factor. The causative organism in CAP is identified only 50% of the time. Organisms that are commonly implicated in CAP include *S. pneumoniae* and atypical organisms (e.g., *Legionella, Mycoplasma, Chlamydia*, viral). Modifying risk factors include the presence of COPD, recent use of antibiotics, and conditions incurring risk of aspiration.

In 2000, the Canadian Infectious Disease Society and the Canadian Thoracic Society conducted an evidence-informed update of the Canadian guidelines for initial management of CAP (Mandell et al., 2000). Considering that there are over 100

microorganisms that cause pneumonia, in addition to chest radiography and clinical evaluation, assessment and diagnosis need to be based on serology results as well as sputum culture, pleural fluid culture, or both, and blood cultures. Pharmacological intervention should include specific antimicrobial selection based on type of pneumonia, including where acquired, and modifying factors such as pathogens (Table 30.2).

Hospital-Acquired Pneumonia. Hospital-acquired pneumonia (HAP) is pneumonia occurring 48 hours or longer after hospital admission and not incubating at the time of hospitalization. HAP accounts for 25% of all critical care unit infections. It is the second most common hospital-associated infection in Canada and has high mortality and morbidity rates (Wu et al., 2017). The microorganisms responsible for HAP are different from those organisms implicated in CAP. Bacteria are responsible for the majority of HAP infections, including *Pseudomonas, Enterobacter, S. aureus*, methicillin-resistant *Staphylococcus aureus* (MRSA), and *S. pneumoniae*. Many of the organisms causing HAP enter the lungs after aspiration of particles from the patient's own pharynx. Immunosuppressive therapy, general debility, and endotracheal intubation may be predisposing factors. Contaminated respiratory therapy equipment is another source of infection.

Fungal Pneumonia. Fungi may also be a cause of pneumonia (see Pulmonary Fungal Infections section later in this chapter).

Aspiration Pneumonia. *Aspiration pneumonia* refers to the sequelae of abnormal entry of secretions or substances into the lower airway. It usually follows aspiration of material from the mouth or the stomach into the trachea and subsequently the lungs. The person who has aspiration pneumonia usually has a history of loss of consciousness (e.g., as a result of seizure, anaesthesia, head injury, stroke, alcohol intake). With loss of consciousness, the gag and cough reflexes are depressed, and aspiration is more likely to occur. Another risk factor is tube feedings. The dependent portions of the lung are most often affected, primarily the superior segments of the lower lobes and the posterior segments of the upper lobes, which are dependent in the supine position.

The aspirated material—food, water, vomitus, or toxic fluids—is the pathological triggering mechanism for the development of this type of pneumonia. There are three distinct forms of aspiration pneumonia. If the aspirated material is an inert substance (e.g., barium), the initial manifestation is usually caused by mechanical obstruction of airways. When the aspirated materials contain toxic fluids, such as gastric juices, there is chemical injury to the lung with infection as a secondary event, usually 48 to 72 hours later; this is identified as *chemical (noninfectious) pneumonitis*. The most important form of aspiration pneumonia is bacterial infection. The infecting organism is usually one of the normal oropharyngeal flora, and multiple organisms, including both aerobes and anaerobes, are isolated from the sputum of the patient with aspiration pneumonia. Antibiotic therapy is based on an assessment of the severity of illness, where the infection was acquired (community or hospital), and the type of organisms present.

Opportunistic Pneumonia. Patients with altered immune response are highly susceptible to respiratory infections. Specific individuals considered at risk include those with severe protein–calorie malnutrition; those with immune deficiencies; those who have received transplants and been treated with immunosuppressive medications; and patients who are being treated with radiation therapy, chemotherapeutic agents, or

TABLE 30.2 EMPIRICAL ANTIMICROBIAL SELECTION FOR ADULT PATIENTS WITH COMMUNITY-ACQUIRED PNEUMONIA

Type of Pneumonia	Modifying Factors and/or Pathogens	First Choice	Second Choice
Outpatient without modifying factors		Macrolide*	Doxycycline
Outpatient with modifying factors	COPD (no recent antibiotics or oral steroids within past 3 mo)	Newer macrolides†	Doxycycline
	COPD (antibiotics or oral steroids within past 3 mo)—*Haemophilus influenzae* and enteric Gram-negative rods	"Respiratory" fluoroquinolone‡	Amoxicillin–clavulanate + macrolide or second-generation cephalosporin + macrolide
	Suspected macroaspiration—oral anaerobes	Amoxicillin–clavulanate ± macrolide, or fourth-generation fluoroquinolone‡ (e.g., moxifloxacin)	Third-generation fluoroquinolones‡ (e.g., levofloxacin) + clindamycin or metronidazole
Long-term care resident in long-term care facility	*Streptococcus pneumoniae*, enteric Gram-negative rods, *H. influenzae*	"Respiratory" fluoroquinolone‡ alone or amoxicillin–clavulanate + macrolide	Second-generation cephalosporin + macrolide
Long-term care resident in hospital		Identical to treatment for other hospitalized patients (see below)	
Hospitalized patient on medical ward	*S. pneumoniae, Legionella pneumophila, Chlamydia pneumoniae*	"Respiratory" fluoroquinolone‡	Second-, third-, or fourth-generation cephalosporin + macrolide
Hospitalized patient in critical care unit	*Pseudomonas aeruginosa* not suspected (*S. pneumoniae, L. pneumophila, C. pneumoniae*, enteric Gram-negative rods implicated)	IV "respiratory" fluoroquinolone + cefotaxime, ceftriaxone, or β-lactam–β-lactamase inhibitor	IV macrolide + cefotaxime, ceftriaxone, or β-lactam–β-lactamase inhibitor
	P. aeruginosa suspected	Antipseudomonal fluoroquinolone (e.g., ciprofloxacin) + antipseudomonal β-lactam (e.g., ceftazidime, carbapenem, piperacillin–tazobactam) or aminoglycoside (e.g., gentamicin, tobramycin, amikacin)	Triple therapy with antipseudomonal β-lactam + aminoglycoside + macrolide

COPD, chronic obstructive pulmonary disease; *IV*, intravenous.
*Macrolide—erythromycin, azithromycin, clarithromycin.
†Newer macrolide—azithromycin, clarithromycin.
‡Respiratory fluoroquinolone—levofloxacin (third generation), gatifloxacin, and moxifloxacin (fourth generation); trovafloxacin (fourth generation) is restricted because of potential severe hepatoxicity.
Source: Mandell, L. A., & Marrie, T. J. (2000). Canadian guidelines for the initial management of community-acquired pneumonia: An evidence-based update by the Canadian Infectious Diseases Society and the Canadian Thoracic Society. *Clinical Infectious Diseases, 31*(2), 383–421, by permission of Oxford University Press.

corticosteroids (especially for a prolonged period). These individuals have a variety of altered conditions, including altered B- and T-lymphocyte function, depressed bone marrow function, and decreased levels or function of neutrophils and macrophages. In addition to the risk for bacterial and viral pneumonia, immunocompromised patients may develop an infection from microorganisms that do not normally cause disease, such as *Pneumocystis jiroveci* (formerly *P. carinii*) and cytomegalovirus (CMV).

P. jiroveci is an opportunistic pathogen whose natural habitat is the lung. This organism rarely causes pneumonia in healthy individuals. *P. jiroveci* pneumonia (PJP) affects 70% of human immunodeficiency virus (HIV)–infected individuals and is the most common opportunistic infection in patients with acquired immune deficiency syndrome (AIDS). In this type of pneumonia, the chest radiograph usually shows a diffuse bilateral alveolar pattern of infiltration. In widespread disease, the lungs are massively consolidated.

Clinical manifestations are insidious and include fever, tachypnea, tachycardia, dyspnea, nonproductive cough, and hypoxemia. Pulmonary physical findings are minimal in proportion to the serious nature of the disease. Treatment consists of antibiotics. In populations at risk for development of *P. jiroveci* pneumonitis (e.g., patients with hematological malignancies or AIDS), antibiotic prophylaxis may be advocated. (PJP is discussed in Chapter 17.)

CMV is a cause of viral pneumonia in the immunocompromised patient, particularly in transplant recipients. CMV, a type of herpesvirus, gives rise to latent infections and reactivation with shedding of infectious virus. This type of interstitial pneumonia can be a mild disease, or it can be fulminant and produce pulmonary insufficiency and death. Often, CMV coexists with other opportunistic bacterial or fungal agents in causing pneumonia. Ganciclovir (Cytovene) is recommended for treatment of CMV pneumonia.

Pathophysiology

Pneumococcal pneumonia is the most common cause of bacterial pneumonia. However, regardless of causative factors, pneumonia is characterized by four stages of the disease process:

1. *Congestion.* After the pneumococcus organisms reach the alveoli via droplets or saliva, there is an outpouring of fluid into the alveoli. The organisms multiply in the serous fluid, and the infection is spread. The pneumococci damage the host by their overwhelming growth and interference with lung function.
2. *Red hepatization.* There is massive dilation of the capillaries, and alveoli are filled with organisms, neutrophils, red

PATHOPHYSIOLOGY MAP

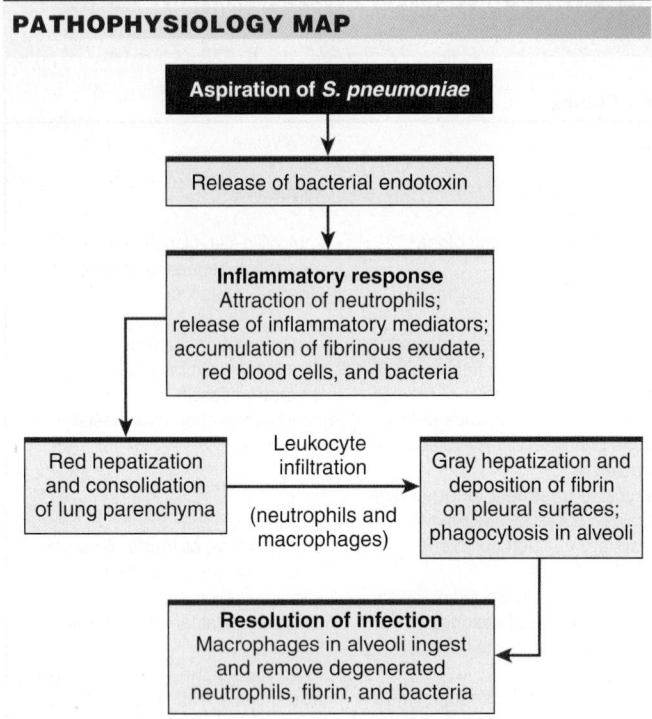

FIG. 30.1 Pathophysiological course of pneumococcal pneumonia.

blood cells, and fibrin (Figure 30.1). The lung appears red and granular, similar to the liver, which is why the process is called *hepatization*.

3. *Grey hepatization.* Blood flow decreases, and leukocytes and fibrin consolidate in the affected part of the lung.

4. *Resolution.* Complete resolution and healing occur if there are no complications.

The exudate becomes lysed and is processed by the macrophages. The normal lung tissue is restored, and the person's gas-exchange ability returns to normal.

Clinical Manifestations

Patients with pneumonia usually have a constellation of symptoms, including sudden onset of fever, chills, a cough producing purulent sputum, and pleuritic chest pain (in some cases). In the older person or debilitated patient, confusion or stupor (possibly related to hypoxia) may be the predominant finding. On physical examination, signs of pulmonary consolidation, such as dullness to percussion, increased fremitus, bronchial breath sounds, and crackles, may be found. The typical pneumonia syndrome is usually caused by the most common pathogen in CAP, which is *S. pneumoniae,* but can also be caused by other bacterial pathogens, such as *H. influenzae.*

Pneumonia may also manifest atypically with a more gradual onset, a dry cough, and extrapulmonary manifestations such as headache, myalgias, fatigue, sore throat, nausea, vomiting, and diarrhea. On physical examination, crackles are often heard. This presentation of symptoms is classically produced by *M. pneumoniae* but can also be caused by *Legionella* and *C. pneumoniae.* Patients with hematogenous *S. aureus* pneumonia may have only dyspnea and fever. This necrotizing infection causes destruction of lung tissue, and these patients are usually very sick.

Manifestations of viral pneumonia are highly variable but may be characterized by chills, fever, dry, nonproductive cough, and extrapulmonary symptoms. Viral pneumonia may be found in association with systemic viral diseases such as measles, varicella-zoster, herpes simplex, or influenza virus infection.

Complications

Most cases of pneumonia run an uncomplicated course. Complications generally develop more frequently in individuals with underlying chronic diseases and may include the following:

1. *Pleurisy* (inflammation of the pleura) is a relatively common accompanying condition of pneumonia.

2. *Pleural effusion* can occur. Usually, the effusion is sterile and is reabsorbed in 1 to 2 weeks. Occasionally, it necessitates aspiration by means of thoracentesis.

3. *Atelectasis* (collapsed, airless alveoli) of one or part of one lobe may occur. These areas usually clear with effective coughing and deep breathing.

4. *Delayed resolution* results from persistent infection and is seen on radiograph as residual consolidation. Usually, the physical findings return to normal within 2 to 4 weeks. Delayed resolution occurs most frequently in patients who are older or malnourished or have alcohol use disorder or COPD.

5. *Lung abscess* is not a common complication of pneumonia. It may be seen with pneumonia caused by *S. aureus* and Gram-negative pneumonias (see Lung Abscess later in this chapter).

6. *Empyema* (accumulation of purulent exudate in the pleural cavity) is relatively infrequent but necessitates antibiotic therapy and drainage of the exudate by a chest tube or by open surgery.

7. *Pericarditis* results from spread of the infecting organism from an infected pleura or via a hematogenous route to the pericardium (the fibroserous sac around the heart).

8. *Bacteremia* can occur with pneumococcal pneumonia, more so in older patients.

9. *Meningitis* can be caused by *S. pneumoniae.* The patient with pneumonia who is disoriented, confused, or somnolent should have a lumbar puncture to evaluate the possibility of meningitis.

10. *Endocarditis* can develop when the organisms attack the endocardium and the valves of the heart. The clinical manifestations are similar to those of acute infective endocarditis (see Chapter 39).

Diagnostic Studies

The common diagnostic measures for pneumonia are presented in Table 30.3. History, physical examination, and chest radiographic study often provide enough information to make management decisions without doing costly laboratory tests.

The chest radiograph often shows a typical pattern characteristic of the infecting organism and is an invaluable adjunct in the diagnosis of pneumonia. Lobar or segmental consolidation suggests a bacterial cause, usually *S. pneumoniae* or *Klebsiella.* Diffuse pulmonary infiltrates are most commonly caused by infection with viruses, *Legionella,* or pathogenic fungi. Cavitary shadows suggest the presence of a necrotizing infection with destruction of lung tissue commonly caused by *S. aureus,* Gram-negative bacteria, or *Mycobacterium tuberculosis.* Pleural effusions, which can occur in up to 30% of patients with CAP, can also be seen on radiographic study.

TABLE 30.3   INTERPROFESSIONAL CARE

Pneumonia

Diagnostic	Interprofessional Therapy
• History and physical examination • Chest radiograph • Gram stain examination of sputum • Sputum culture and sensitivity test (if medication-resistant pathogen or organism not covered by empirical therapy) • Pulse oximetry or ABGs (if indicated) • Complete blood cell count, differential, and routine blood chemistries (if indicated) • Blood cultures (if indicated)	• Appropriate antibiotic therapy • Increased fluid intake (at least 3 L/day) • Limited activity and rest • Antipyretics • Analgesics • Oxygen therapy (if indicated)

ABGs, arterial blood gases.

Sputum cultures are recommended in the case of the suspected presence of a drug-resistant pathogen or an organism that is not covered by the usual empirical therapy (therapy based on observation and experience, implemented when the condition's exact cause is not known). A Gram stain examination of the sputum provides information on the predominant causative organism. A sputum culture should be collected before initiating antibiotic therapy as a means to intervene for patients with community- or hospital-acquired pneumonia. Because of the poor sensitivity and specificity of sputum cultures, any sputum culture results should be correlated with the predominant organisms found on Gram stain examination results. Before treatment, two blood cultures may be done for patients who are seriously ill. Although microbial studies are expected before treatment, initiation of antibiotics should not be delayed.

Arterial blood gases (ABGs), if obtained, usually reveal hypoxemia. Leukocytosis is found in the majority of patients with bacterial pneumonia, usually with a white blood cell (WBC) count greater than 15×10^9/L with the presence of bands (immature neutrophils).

Interprofessional Care

Prompt treatment with the appropriate antibiotic almost always cures bacterial and mycoplasma pneumonia. In uncomplicated cases, the patient responds to medication therapy within 48 to 72 hours. Indications of improvement include decreased temperature, improved breathing, and reduced chest pain. Abnormal physical findings can last for more than 7 days.

In addition to antibiotic therapy, supportive measures may be used, including oxygen therapy to treat hypoxemia, analgesics to relieve the chest pain for patient comfort, and antipyretics such as acetylsalicylic acid (ASA; Aspirin) or acetaminophen (Tylenol) for significantly elevated temperature. During the acute febrile phase, the patient's activity should be restricted, and rest should be encouraged and planned. The Health Quality Ontario and Ministry of Health and Long-Term Care CAP guidelines (2013) recommend airway clearance, supportive therapy, antiviral therapy during flu season, smoking cessation, and vaccinations for CAP in addition to antibiotic therapy.

Most individuals with mild to moderate illness who have no other underlying disease process can be treated on an outpatient basis. If there is a serious underlying disease or if the pneumonia is accompanied by severe dyspnea, hypoxemia, or other complications, the patient should be hospitalized.

Currently, there is no definitive treatment for viral pneumonia. An antiviral medication, amantadine, is approved for oral use in the treatment of influenza A virus. The neuraminidase inhibitors zanamivir (Relenza) and oseltamivir (Tamiflu) are active against both influenza A and B (see Chapter 29). An influenza vaccine is modified annually to reflect the anticipated strains in the upcoming season. The flu vaccine is considered a mainstay of prevention and is recommended annually for individuals considered to be at risk for influenza, including older persons, long-term care residents, patients with COPD or diabetes mellitus, and health care workers (Government of Canada 2016). For older persons with signs and symptoms of influenza, including those who have received the influenza vaccine, treatment with amantadine or a neuraminidase inhibitor is recommended. During epidemics of influenza A, especially in long-term care facilities, chemoprophylaxis with these agents is recommended for unvaccinated patients, immunodeficient patients, or those who have received the vaccine within the past 2 weeks.

Pneumococcal Vaccine. Pneumococcal vaccine is indicated primarily for the individual considered at risk who (1) has a chronic illness such as lung or heart disease or diabetes mellitus, (2) is recovering from a severe illness, (3) is 65 years of age or older, or (4) resides in a long-term care facility. Vaccination is particularly important because the rate of medication-resistant *S. pneumoniae* infections is increasing. Pneumococcal vaccine can be given simultaneously with other vaccines such as the flu vaccine, but each should be administered in a separate site.

The current recommendation is that pneumococcal vaccine is good for a person's lifetime. However, in the immunosuppressed individual at risk for development of fatal pneumococcal infection (e.g., asplenic patient; patient with nephrotic syndrome, renal failure, or AIDS; or transplant recipient), revaccination is recommended every 5 years.

Medication Therapy. The main problems with the use of antibiotics to treat pneumonia are the development of resistant strains of organisms and the patient's hypersensitivity or allergic reaction to certain antibiotics.

Most cases of CAP in otherwise healthy adults do not require hospitalization. The Canadian Infectious Diseases Society and Canadian Thoracic Society have guidelines aimed at classifying patients to determine therapy options (see Table 30.2).

The oral antibiotic therapy administered is frequently empirical treatment with broad-spectrum antibiotics. Once the patient is assigned a treatment classification, therapy can be based on the likely infecting organism.

For HAP, empirical antibiotic therapy should be based on the likely pathogens in the various patient groups. Even with extensive diagnostic testing, an etiological organism is often not identified. It is important to recognize when a patient is not responding to treatment. Therapy may require modification based on the patient's culture results or clinical response. Clinical response is evaluated by factors such as a change in fever, sputum purulence, leukocytosis, oxygenation, or radiographic study patterns. Improvement is often not apparent for the first 48 to 72 hours, and therapy need not be altered during this period unless deterioration is noted or culture results dictate that a different antibiotic should be used. Common antibiotics for HAP include cephalosporins (third-generation antipseudomonal [ceftazidime]), a β-lactam or β-lactamase inhibitor, vancomycin (for MRSA), aminoglycosides (gentamicin), and antipseudomonal quinolones (ciprofloxacin).

Patients with ventilator-associated pneumonia may experience rapid deterioration. Patients who deteriorate or fail to respond to therapy will require aggressive evaluation to assess noninfectious etiologies, complications, other coexisting infectious processes, or pneumonia caused by a resistant pathogen. It may be necessary to broaden antimicrobial coverage while awaiting results of cultures and other studies, such as computed tomographic (CT) scan, ultrasound, or lung scans.

Nutritional Therapy. Fluid intake of at least 3 L/day is important in the supportive treatment of pneumonia. If the patient has heart failure, fluid intake must be individualized. If oral intake cannot be maintained, intravenous (IV) administration of fluids and electrolytes may be necessary for the acutely ill patient. An intake of at least 1 500 calories per day should be maintained to provide energy for the increased metabolic processes in the patient. Small, frequent meals are better tolerated by the patient with dyspnea.

NURSING MANAGEMENT PNEUMONIA

NURSING ASSESSMENT
Subjective and objective data that should be obtained from a patient with pneumonia are presented in Table 30.4.

NURSING DIAGNOSES
Nursing diagnoses for the patient with pneumonia may include but are not limited to the following:
- *Reduced gas exchange* (resulting from fluid and exudate accumulation with the alveoli and surrounding lung tissue)
- *Inadequate breathing pattern* resulting from *pain*
- *Acute pain* resulting from *biological injury agent* (infection)
- *Reduced stamina* resulting from *respiratory condition, physical deconditioning*

Additional information on nursing diagnoses for the patient with pneumonia is presented in Nursing Care Plan (NCP) 30.1, available on the Evolve website.

PLANNING
The overall goals are that the patient with pneumonia will have (a) clear breath sounds, (b) normal breathing patterns, (c) no signs of hypoxia, (d) a normal chest radiograph, and (e) no complications related to pneumonia.

NURSING IMPLEMENTATION
HEALTH PROMOTION. Many nursing interventions are available to help prevent the occurrence of pneumonia as well as the morbidity associated with it. Teaching a patient to practise good health habits, such as proper diet and hygiene, adequate rest, and regular exercise, can help the patient maintain the natural resistance to infecting organisms. If possible, exposure to people with URIs should be avoided. If a URI occurs, it should be treated promptly with supportive measures (e.g., rest, fluids). If symptoms persist for more than 7 days, the person should obtain medical care. Individuals at risk for pneumonia (e.g., people who are chronically ill, older persons) should be encouraged to obtain both influenza and pneumococcal vaccines.

In the hospital, the nursing role involves identifying the patient at risk (see Table 30.1) and taking measures to prevent the development of pneumonia. The patient with altered consciousness should be placed in positions (e.g., side-lying, upright) that will prevent or minimize the risk for aspiration. The patient should be turned and repositioned at least every 2 hours to facilitate adequate lung expansion and to discourage pooling of secretions.

TABLE 30.4   NURSING ASSESSMENT

Pneumonia

Subjective Data

Important Health Information

Past health history: Lung cancer, COPD, diabetes mellitus; cigarette smoking; alcohol use disorder; recent upper respiratory tract infection; chronic debilitating disease; malnutrition; altered consciousness; AIDS; exposure to chemical toxins, dust, or allergens; immobility or prolonged bed rest
Medications: Use of antibiotics, corticosteroids, chemotherapy, or any other immunosuppressants
Surgery or other treatments: Recent abdominal or thoracic surgery, splenectomy, endotracheal intubation, general anaesthesia; tube feedings

Symptoms
- Fatigue, weakness, malaise
- Anorexia, nausea, vomiting
- Fever, chills
- Dyspnea, cough (productive or nonproductive), nasal congestion, pain with breathing
- Chest pain, sore throat, headache, abdominal pain, muscle aches

Objective Data

General

Fever, restlessness, or lethargy; splinting of affected area

Respiratory

Tachypnea; dyspnea, nasal congestion, pharyngitis; asymmetrical chest movements or retraction; decreased excursion; nasal flaring; use of accessory muscles (neck, abdomen); grunting; crackles, friction rub on auscultation; dullness on percussion over consolidated areas, increased tactile fremitus on palpation; pink, rusty, purulent, green, yellow, or white sputum (amount may be scant to copious)

Cardiovascular

Tachycardia

Neurological

Changes in mental status, ranging from confusion to delirium

Possible Findings

Leukocytosis; abnormal ABGs with ↓ or normal PaO_2, ↓ $PaCO_2$, and ↑ pH initially, and later ↓ PaO_2, ↑ $PaCO_2$, and ↓ pH; positive sputum Gram stain examination and culture; patchy or diffuse infiltrates, abscesses, pleural effusion, or pneumothorax on chest radiographic study

ABGs, arterial blood gases; *AIDS,* acquired immune deficiency syndrome; *COPD,* chronic obstructive pulmonary disease; *PaCO₂,* partial pressure of carbon dioxide in arterial blood; *PaO₂,* partial pressure of oxygen in arterial blood.

The patient who has a feeding tube generally requires that measures be taken to prevent aspiration (see Chapter 42). Although feeding tubes are small, an interruption in the integrity of the lower esophageal sphincter still exists and can allow reflux of gastric and intestinal contents. The patient who has difficulty swallowing (e.g., a patient who has had a stroke) needs assistance in eating, drinking, and taking medication to prevent aspiration. The patient who has recently had surgery and others who are immobile need assistance with turning and measures to facilitate deep breathing at frequent intervals (see Chapter 22). The nurse must be careful to avoid overmedication with opioids or sedatives, which can cause a depressed cough reflex and accumulation of fluid in the lungs. Presence of the gag reflex should be ascertained before the administration of fluids or food to the individual who has had local anaesthesia to the throat.

To reduce the incidence of health care–associated infections, the nurse should practice strict medical asepsis and adherence to infection-control guidelines. Poor hand hygiene practices allow spread of pathogens via the hands of the health care worker.

Staff members should wash their hands or, if hands are not visibly soiled, use hand rubs with 60% alcohol before providing care to a patient. Respiratory devices can harbour microorganisms and have been associated with outbreaks of pneumonia. Strict sterile aseptic technique should be used when suctioning the trachea of a patient.

ACUTE INTERVENTION. Although many patients with pneumonia are treated on an outpatient basis, the nursing care plan for a patient with pneumonia (see NCP 30.1, available on the Evolve website) is applicable to outpatients and inpatients. It is important for the nurse to remember that pneumonia is an acute, infectious disease. Although most cases of pneumonia are potentially completely curable, complications can result. The nurse must be aware of these complications and their manifestations. The infection-control nurse can be a valuable resource in assisting with the care of patients with pneumonia.

Therapeutic positioning for patients with pneumonia ensures stable oxygenation status. The "good lung down" position is used for patients with unilateral lung disease, in whom better oxygenation is achieved when the unaffected lung (good lung) is placed in the down (lateral) position to achieve maximum lung expansion. Incentive spirometry, turning, coughing, and deep breathing all increase lung volume, mobilize secretions, and prevent atelectasis. Exercise and early ambulation augment bronchial hygiene and are encouraged as tolerated.

AMBULATORY AND HOME CARE. The patient needs to be reassured that complete recovery from pneumonia is possible. It is extremely important to emphasize the need to take all of any medications prescribed and to return for follow-up medical care and evaluation. The patient needs to be taught about the medication–medication and the food–medication interactions for the prescribed antibiotic. Adequate rest is needed to maintain progress toward recovery and to prevent a relapse. The patient should be told that it may take weeks to feel the usual vigour and sense of well-being. A prolonged period of convalescence may be necessary for the older or chronically ill patient.

The patient considered to be at risk for pneumonia should be told about available vaccines and should discuss them with the health care provider. Deep-breathing exercises should be practised for 6 to 8 weeks after the patient is discharged from the hospital.

EVALUATION. The expected outcomes for the patient with pneumonia are presented in NCP 30.1, available on the Evolve website.

TUBERCULOSIS

Tuberculosis (TB) is an infectious disease caused by *Mycobacterium tuberculosis*. It usually involves the lungs, but it also occurs in the larynx, the kidneys, the bones, the adrenal glands, the lymph nodes, and the meninges and can be disseminated throughout the body. TB is a reportable communicable disease; it kills more people worldwide than any other infectious disease, with an estimated 8.8 million of the world's population having been infected. In Canada, the number of reported cases of active TB has remained relatively stable and low in the global context. In 2020, the Public Health Agency of Canada (PHAC) reported that as of 2017 there was a 2.6% increase from 1 750 to 1 796 of Canadian-born people diagnosed with TB. In addition, foreign-born individuals make up the majority of cases (71.8%), and Canadian-born Indigenous people (21.5 per 100 000 population) continue to have the highest reported number of TB cases

DETERMINANTS OF HEALTH

Tuberculosis

Income and Social Status
Low socioeconomic groups have higher rates of TB.

Physical Environments
Residing in overcrowded institutions (e.g., long-term care facilities, correctional facilities) and urban homelessness increase the risk for acquiring TB.

Personal Health Practices and Coping Skills
Smoking and air pollution increase the risk for TB.

Culture
TB is most prevalent among immigrants and Indigenous people.

References

Public Health Agency of Canada. (2018). *The time is now—Chief Public Health Officer spotlight on eliminating tuberculosis in Canada.* https://www.canada.ca/content/dam/phac-aspc/documents/corporate/publications/chief-public-health-officer-reports-state-public-health-canada/eliminating-tuberculosis/PHAC_18-086_TB_Report_E_forwebcoding.pdf

TB, tuberculosis.

in Canada, with the Inuit population having the highest rate (300 times higher than in the Canadian, non-Indigenous population) (Indigenous Services Canada, 2020; LaFreniere et al., 2019). It is important to note that 80.4% of TB cases reported did result in successful treatment and patient outcomes.

As stated above, the populations most at risk in Canada are the Indigenous and immigrant populations. The rate of TB among Canadian-born Indigenous peoples living on reserve is 40 times higher than the national average. Factors or challenges that Canadian-born Indigenous people face that can influence transmission of TB are food insecurity, overcrowding, poorly ventilated homes, comorbidities (e.g., diabetes, HIV), and smoking (Indigenous Services Canada, 2020).

Etiology and Pathophysiology

M. tuberculosis, a Gram-positive, acid-fast bacillus, is usually spread from person to person via airborne droplets, which are produced when the infected individual with pulmonary or laryngeal TB coughs, sneezes, speaks, or sings. Once released into a room, the organisms are dispersed and can be inhaled. TB is not highly infectious, and transmission usually requires close, frequent, or prolonged exposure. Brief exposure to a few tubercle bacilli rarely causes an infection. The disease cannot be spread by hands, books, glasses, dishes, or other fomites.

The very small droplets, 1 to 5 mcm in size, contain *M. tuberculosis*. Because they are so small, the particles remain airborne indoors for minutes to hours. Once inhaled, these small particles lodge in the bronchiole and alveolus. Factors that influence the likelihood of transmission include the (a) number of organisms expelled into the air, (b) concentration of organisms (small spaces with limited ventilation would mean higher concentration), (c) length of time of exposure, and (d) immune system of the exposed person. *M. tuberculosis* replicates slowly and spreads via the lymphatic system. The organisms find favourable environments for growth primarily in the upper lobes of the lungs, the kidneys, epiphyses of the bone, the cerebral cortex, and adrenal glands.

Healing of the primary lesion usually takes place by resolution, fibrosis, and calcification. The granulation tissue surrounding the lesion may become more fibrous and form a collagenous scar around the tubercle. A *Ghon complex* is formed, consisting of the Ghon tubercle and regional lymph nodes. Calcified Ghon complexes may be seen on chest radiographic studies.

When a TB lesion regresses and heals, the infection enters a latent period in which it may persist without producing clinical symptoms of illness. The infection may develop into clinical disease if the persisting organisms begin to multiply rapidly, or it may remain dormant.

People who are infected with *M. tuberculosis* but do not have TB disease cannot spread the infection to other people. TB infection occurs when the bacteria are inhaled but there is an ineffective immune response and the bacteria become inactive. The majority of people mount effective immune responses to encapsulate these organisms for the rest of their lives, preventing primary infection from progressing to disease. TB infection in a person who does not have the active TB disease is not considered a case of TB and is often referred to as *latent tuberculosis infection* (LTBI). If the initial immune response is not adequate, control of the organisms is not maintained, and clinical disease results. Dormant but viable organisms persist for years. Reactivation of TB can occur if the host's defence mechanisms become impaired. The reasons for reactivation are not well understood, but they are related to decreased resistance found in older persons, individuals with concomitant diseases, and persons who receive immunosuppressive therapy.

Clinical Manifestations

In the early stages of TB, the person is usually free of symptoms. Many cases are found incidentally when routine chest radiographic studies are done, especially in older persons.

Systemic manifestations may initially consist of fatigue, malaise, anorexia, weight loss, low-grade fevers, and night sweats. The weight loss may not be excessive until late in the disease and is often attributed to overwork or other factors.

A characteristic pulmonary manifestation is a cough that becomes frequent and produces mucoid or mucopurulent sputum. Dyspnea is unusual. Chest pain characterized as dull or tight may be present. Hemoptysis is not a common finding and is usually associated with more advanced cases. Sometimes TB has more acute, sudden manifestations: The patient has high fever, chills, generalized flulike symptoms, pleuritic pain, and a productive cough.

The HIV-infected patient with TB often has atypical physical examination and chest radiographic examination findings. Classical signs such as fever, cough, and weight loss may be attributed to PCP or other HIV-associated opportunistic diseases. Clinical manifestations of respiratory conditions in patients with HIV must be carefully investigated to determine the cause.

Complications

Miliary Tuberculosis. If a necrotic Ghon complex erodes through a blood vessel, large numbers of organisms invade the bloodstream and spread to all body organs. This is called *miliary* or *hematogenous* TB. The patient may be either acutely ill with fever, dyspnea, and cyanosis or chronically ill with systemic manifestations of weight loss, fever, and gastrointestinal (GI) disturbance. Hepatomegaly, splenomegaly, and generalized lymphadenopathy may be present.

Pleural Effusion and Empyema. A pleural effusion is caused by the release of caseous material into the pleural space. The bacteria-containing material triggers an inflammatory reaction and a pleural exudate of protein-rich fluid. A form of pleurisy called *dry pleurisy* may result from a superficial tubercular lesion involving the pleura. It appears as localized pleuritic pain on deep inspiration. Empyema is less common than effusion but may occur from large numbers of organisms spilling into the pleural space, usually from rupture of a cavity.

Tuberculosis Pneumonia. Acute pneumonia may result when large amounts of tubercle bacilli are discharged from the liquefied necrotic lesion into the lung or lymph nodes. The clinical manifestations are similar to those of bacterial pneumonia, including chills, fever, productive cough, pleuritic pain, and leukocytosis.

Other Organ Involvement. Although the lungs are the primary site of TB, other body organs may also be involved. The meninges may become infected. Bone and joint tissue may be involved in the infectious disease process. The kidneys, the adrenal glands, the lymph nodes, and the genital tract (in both females and males) may also be infected.

Diagnostic Studies

Tuberculin Skin Testing. The body's immune response can be demonstrated by hypersensitivity to a tuberculin skin test. A positive reaction occurs 2 to 12 weeks after the initial infection, corresponding to the time needed to mount an immune response.

Purified protein derivative (PPD) of tuberculin is used primarily to detect the delayed hypersensitivity response. (The procedure for performing the tuberculin skin test is described in Chapter 28.) Once acquired, sensitivity to tuberculin tends to persist throughout life. A positive reaction indicates the presence of a TB infection, but it does not show whether the infection is latent or active, that is, causing a clinical illness. Because the response to TB skin testing may be decreased in the immunocompromised patient, induration reactions equal to or greater than 5 mm are considered positive. Sometimes, a repeat PPD can cause an accelerated response (the "booster" effect). Thus, two-step testing is recommended for initial screening of health care workers who will be getting regularly retested in the future and for those who have a decreased response to allergens. This procedure helps identify individuals with past disease and prevent a later positive PPD test from being misinterpreted as a new, infection-related PPD conversion. See Chapter 28, Table 28.12, for guidelines in interpreting positive TB skin tests. Recent guidelines for targeted tuberculin testing emphasize targeting only high-risk groups and discourage testing low-risk individuals.

Chest Radiographic Study. Although the findings on chest radiographic examination are important, it is not possible to make a diagnosis of TB solely on the basis of this examination. This is because other diseases can mimic the radiographic appearance of TB. The abnormality most commonly found in TB is multinodular lymph node involvement with cavitation in the upper lobes of the lungs. Calcification of the lung lesions generally occurs within several years of the infection.

Bacteriological Studies. The demonstration of tubercle bacilli bacteriologically is essential for establishing a diagnosis. Microscopic examination of stained sputum smears for acid-fast bacilli (AFB) is usually the first bacteriological evidence of the presence of tubercle bacilli. Three consecutive sputum specimens are collected on different days and sent for smear and culture. In addition to sputum, material for examination can be obtained from gastric washings, cerebrospinal fluid (CSF), or pus from an abscess.

The most accurate means of diagnosis is the culture technique. The major disadvantage of this method is that it may take 6 to 8 weeks for the mycobacteria to grow. The advantage is that it can detect small quantities (as few as 10 bacteria/mL of specimen).

Nucleic acid amplification (NAA) is a rapid diagnostic test for TB. Test results are available in a few hours. They are more sensitive than AFB smears but less sensitive than TB cultures. NAA does not replace routine sputum smears and cultures, but it offers a health care provider increased confidence in the diagnosis.

Since 2007, Canada has been testing using QuantiFERON-TB Gold In-Tube. The patient's blood is mixed with mycobacterial antigens and is then measured using an enzyme-linked immunosorbent assay (ELISA). If the patient is infected with TB organisms, the lymphocytes in the blood will recognize the antigens.

Interprofessional Care

Hospitalization for initial treatment of TB is not necessary in most patients. Most patients are treated on an outpatient basis (Table 30.5), and many can continue to work and maintain their lifestyles with few changes. Hospitalization may be used for diagnostic evaluation, for those who are severely ill or debilitated, and for those who experience adverse medication reactions or treatment failures.

The mainstay of TB treatment is medication therapy. Medication therapy is used to treat an individual with clinical disease and to prevent disease in an infected person.

Medication Therapy

Active Disease. Standard therapy for active TB has been revised because of the global increase in prevalence of multidrug-resistant tuberculosis (MDR TB) (World Health Organization [WHO], 2014). MDR TB occurs when resistance develops to two or more anti-TB medications. In Canada, MDR TB risk factors include previous TB treatment, birth outside of Canada, and exposure to an individual or individuals diagnosed with infectious medication-resistant TB. Prevention over management of MDR TB is recommended to prevent resistance. Treatment is individualized, and an initial phase of treatment for a minimum of 8 months is recommended.

The patient with active TB should be managed aggressively; treatment usually consists of a combination of at least four medications. The reason for combination therapy is to increase the therapeutic effectiveness and decrease the development of resistant strains of *M. tuberculosis*. It has been shown that single-medication therapy can result in rapid development of resistant strains.

Medications are divided into first-line and second-line medications. The four first-line medications used in Canada are isoniazid (INH), rifampin (RMP), pyrazinamide (PZA), and ethambutol (EMB) (Table 30.6). The most commonly used second-line medications include fluoroquinolones (e.g., moxifloxacin, levofloxacin) and injectables (e.g., streptomycin, amikacin). Second-line medications are used in special situations such as medication-resistant tuberculosis.

TABLE 30.5 INTERPROFESSIONAL CARE

Tuberculosis

Diagnostic	Interprofessional Therapy
• History and physical examination • Tuberculin skin test • Chest radiographic study • Bacteriological studies • Sputum smear • Sputum culture	• Long-term treatment with antimicrobial medications (see Tables 30.6 and 30.7) • Follow-up bacteriological studies and chest radiographic examinations

---

TABLE 30.6 MEDICATION THERAPY

First-Line Medication Therapy for Tuberculosis

Medication	Mechanisms of Action	Adverse Effects	Comments
First-Line Medications			
Isoniazid (INH)	Bactericidal; interferes with DNA metabolism of tubercle bacillus	Peripheral neuritis, hepatotoxicity, hypersensitivity (skin rash, arthralgia, fever), optic neuritis	Metabolism primarily by liver and excretion by kidneys; pyridoxine (vitamin B_6) administration during high-dose therapy as prophylactic measure; use as single prophylactic agent for active TB in individuals whose PPD converts to positive; ability to cross blood–brain barrier; safe in pregnancy*
Rifampin (RMP)	Bactericidal; has broad-spectrum effects, inhibits RNA polymerase of tubercle bacillus	Medication interactions, rash, hepatitis, febrile reaction, GI disturbance, peripheral neuropathy, hypersensitivity	Most commonly used with INH; low incidence of adverse effects; suppression of effect of birth control pills; possibility of orange urine and bodily fluids; safe in pregnancy
Pyrazinamide (PZA)	Bactericidal; exact mechanism unknown	Hepatitis, arthralgia, fever, skin rash, hyperuricemia, GI symptoms, jaundice (rare)	High rate of effectiveness when used with streptomycin or capreomycin
Ethambutol (EMB)	Bacteriostatic; inhibits RNA synthesis	Skin rash, GI disturbance, malaise, peripheral neuritis, optic neuritis	Adverse effects uncommon and reversible with discontinuation of medication; most commonly used as substitute medication when adverse effects occur with INH or RMP; safe in pregnancy*

DNA, deoxyribonucleic acid; *GI*, gastrointestinal; *PPD*, purified protein derivative; *RNA*, ribonucleic acid; *TB*, tuberculosis.

*Pyridoxine (vitamin B_6) supplements should be prescribed for patients who may be or are pregnant or who are breastfeeding or are diagnosed with renal failure, diabetes, seizures, malnutrition, or substance use disorder, as these patients are at risk for symptoms of pyridoxine deficiency. Canadian tuberculosis standards suggest pyridoxine dose of 25 mg.

Source: © All rights reserved. *Canadian Tuberculosis Standards*, 7th Edition. Public Health Agency of Canada, 2013. Adapted and reproduced with permission from the Minister of Health, 2021.

TABLE 30.7 MEDICATION THERAPY

Medication Regimen Options for Treatment of Tuberculosis

Standard	Initial Phase (first 2 mo)	Continuation Phase
Regimen 1*	INH + RMP + PZA ± EMB† daily or 5 days/wk	INH + RMP for 4 mo daily or 3 times/wk
Regimen 2	INH + RMP ± EMB daily or 5 days/wk	INH + RMP for 7 mo daily or 3 times/wk

*Regimen 1 is preferred (Nahid et al., 2016; BC Centre for Disease Control, 2019).
†EMB can be stopped as soon as drug susceptibility testing results are available, and the strain is pan-sensitive. PZA is continued for the full 2 months.
EMB, ethambutol; *INH*, isoniazid; *PZA*, pyrazinamide; *RMP*, rifampin.
Source: © All rights reserved. *Canadian Tuberculosis Standards*, 7th Edition. Public Health Agency of Canada, 2013. Adapted and reproduced with permission from the Minister of Health, 2021.

TABLE 30.8 INDICATIONS FOR TREATMENT OF LATENT TUBERCULOSIS INFECTION

Treatment is indicated with positive tuberculin skin tests in people with the following:

- Known or suspected HIV infection
- Recent contact with infectious TB
- Presence of lung scar

Treatment is indicated with significant tuberculin skin test reaction in the following situations:

- Special clinical situations (immunosuppression therapy, use of corticosteroids, diabetes mellitus, silicosis, chronic renal failure, organ transplant, hematological malignancies)
- If the person was born in a high-prevalence country, is a resident of a communal setting, is a health care worker, or is Indigenous

HIV, human immunodeficiency virus; *TB*, tuberculosis.
Source: Adapted from Public Health Agency of Canada & Canadian Lung Association. (2014). *Canadian tuberculosis standards* (7th ed.). https://www.canada.ca/en/public-health/services/infectious-diseases/canadian-tuberculosis-standards-7th-edition.html

Various medication and dosing regimens are available (Table 30.7). Fixed-dose combination anti-TB medications may enhance adherence to treatment recommendations. Patients on antiretroviral treatment for HIV cannot take RMP because it can impair the effectiveness of the antiretroviral medications. Other medications are primarily used for treatment of resistant strains or when the patient develops adverse effects to the primary medications. Many second-line medications carry a greater risk for adverse effects and necessitate closer monitoring.

In follow-up care for patients on long-term therapy, it is important to monitor the effectiveness of medications and the development of adverse effects. Usually, sputum specimens are initially obtained weekly and then monthly to assess the effectiveness of the medication.

Although TB tends to have a rapidly progressive course in the patient co-infected with HIV, it responds well to standard medication. Treatment should occur for at least 6 months beyond the conversion of sputum cultures to negative status.

Follow-up care is important to ensure adherence, as nonadherence is a major factor in the emergence of multidrug resistance and treatment failures. Many individuals do not adhere to the treatment program in spite of understanding the disease process and the value of treatment. Furthermore, completing therapy is crucial because of the danger of reactivation of TB and the development of MDR TB seen in patients who do not complete their full course of therapy. Directly observed therapy (DOT) is recommended for patients known to be at risk for nonadherence to therapy. DOT is an expensive but essential public health issue. DOT involves observing the ingestion of every dose of medication for the TB patient's entire course of treatment. In many regions, the public health nurse administers DOT at a clinic site. The patient needs to have follow-up visits for 12 months after completion of therapy to check for the presence of resistant strains. DOT protocols and options in remote or rural areas and in Indigenous communities remain problematic.

Teaching patients about the adverse effects of these medications and when to seek medical attention is critical. The major adverse effect of INH, RMP, and PZA is hepatitis. Thus liver function tests should be monitored. Baseline liver function tests are done at the start of treatment, and routine monitoring of liver function is done if baseline tests are abnormal.

Latent Tuberculosis Infection. LTBI occurs when an individual becomes infected with *M. tuberculosis* but does not become acutely ill. Medication therapy can be used to prevent a TB infection from developing into a clinical disease. Previously used terms such as *preventive therapy* and *chemoprophylaxis* were confusing. Therefore, *LTBI* is the preferred term. The indications for treatment of LTBI are presented in Table 30.8.

The medication generally used in treatment of LTBI is INH. It is effective and inexpensive and can be administered orally.

Vaccine. Immunization with bacille Calmette–Guérin (BCG) vaccine to prevent TB is currently in use in many parts of the world. Although millions of people have been vaccinated with BCG, the efficacy of the vaccine is not clear. BCG vaccination can result in a positive PPD reaction. The BCG vaccine reaction will wane over time, and the mean PPD reaction size among people who received BCG is less than 10 mm. Because it may be difficult to determine the relevance of increases in individuals who have undergone BCG vaccination, the PHAC and Canadian Lung Association (2014) recommend that a conversion to "positive" be defined as a reaction of 10 mm or greater. People who receive BCG are from high-prevalence areas of the world, and it is important that a positive skin reaction be evaluated for TB.

NURSING MANAGEMENT TUBERCULOSIS

NURSING ASSESSMENT

It is important to determine whether the patient was ever exposed to a person with TB. The patient should be assessed for productive cough, night sweats, afternoon temperature elevation, weight loss, pleuritic chest pain, and crackles over the apices of the lungs. If the patient has a productive cough, an early-morning sputum specimen will be required for an AFB smear to detect the presence of mycobacteria.

NURSING DIAGNOSES

Nursing diagnoses for the patient with TB may include but are not limited to the following:

- *Inadequate airway clearance* resulting from *excessive mucus, retained secretions*
- *Potential for infection* (of others) resulting from *insufficient knowledge to avoid exposure to pathogens*
- *Inadequate health management* resulting from *insufficient knowledge of therapeutic regimen, insufficient social support*

PLANNING

The overall goals are that the patient with TB will (a) adhere to the therapeutic regimen, (b) have no recurrence of disease, (c) have normal pulmonary function, and (d) take appropriate measures to prevent the spread of the disease.

NURSING IMPLEMENTATION

HEALTH PROMOTION. The ultimate goal related to TB in Canada is eradication. Selective screening programs in known risk groups are of value in detecting individuals with TB. The person with a positive tuberculin skin test should have a chest radiographic examination to assess for the presence of TB. Another important measure is to identify the contacts of the individual who has TB. These contacts should be assessed for the possibility of infection and the need for prophylactic medication therapy.

ACUTE INTERVENTION. Acute in-hospital care is seldom required for the patient with TB. If hospitalization is needed, it is usually for a brief period. Patients strongly suspected of having TB should (a) be placed in respiratory isolation, (b) receive four-medication therapy, and (c) receive an immediate medical workup, including chest radiographic examination, sputum smear, and culture. Respiratory isolation is indicated for the patient with pulmonary or laryngeal TB until the patient is considered to be noninfectious (effective medication therapy, clinical improvement, three negative AFB smears). A negative-pressure isolation room that offers six or more exchanges per hour may be used. Ultraviolet radiation of the air in the upper part of the room is another approach for reducing airborne TB organisms. Therefore, ultraviolet lights are commonly seen in clinics and homeless shelters. Masks are needed to filter out droplet nuclei. Use of institution-approved high-efficiency particulate air (HEPA) masks is indicated. The mask must be moulded to fit tightly around the nose and mouth.

The patient should be taught to cover the nose and mouth with paper tissue every time they cough, sneeze, or produce sputum. The tissues should be thrown into a paper bag and disposed of with the trash, burned, or flushed down the toilet. The patient should also be taught careful handwashing techniques to be used after handling sputum and soiled tissues. Special precautions should be taken during high-risk procedures such as sputum induction, aerosolized pentamidine treatments, intubation, bronchoscopy, or endoscopy.

AMBULATORY AND HOME CARE. Patients who have responded clinically are discharged home despite positive smears if their household contacts have already been exposed and the patient is not posing a risk to susceptible people. Determination of absolute noninfection requires negative cultures. Most treatment failures occur because the patient neglects to take the medication, discontinues it prematurely, or takes it irregularly. On discharge, the physician may order a combination of medications to increase the likelihood of adherence, ensure that all medications are taken, and reduce the risk of developing drug resistance.

It is important for the nurse to develop a therapeutic, consistent relationship with each patient. The nurse must understand the patient's lifestyle and be flexible in planning a program that facilitates the patient's participation in and completion of therapy. The nurse should ensure that the patient fully understands the need for dedication to the prescribed regimen. Ongoing reassurance helps the patient understand that adherence can mean cure. If the patient cannot or will not adhere to a self-administered medication regimen, medication may have to be given by a responsible person on a daily or intermittent basis (see the Ethical Dilemmas box). The public health department must be notified if patient adherence to the medication regimen is questionable so that follow-up of close contacts can be accomplished. In some cases, the public health nurse will be responsible for DOT. In other situations, a spouse, grown child, other relative living with the patient, or co-worker may be asked to supervise medication taking.

ETHICAL DILEMMAS
Patient Adherence

Situation
The health clinic for the homeless discovers that a man with tuberculosis has not been adhering to instructions for taking his medication. He tells the nurse that it is hard for him to get to the clinic to obtain the medication, much less to keep on a schedule. The nurse is concerned not only about this patient but also about the risks to the other people at the shelter, in the park, and at the meal sites.

Important Points for Consideration
- Adherence is a complex issue involving a person's culture and values, perceived risk for disease, availability of resources, access to treatment, and perceived consequences of available choices.
- Nurses in the community are concerned not only with providing benefits and supporting decision making for individual patients but also with the health and well-being of the entire community.
- Greater harm may result for the community when more virulent drug-resistant strains of microorganisms develop as a consequence of partial treatment or inability of the patient to complete a course of therapy.
- Advocacy for the patient and the community obliges the nurse to involve other members of the health care team, such as those in social services, to assist in obtaining the necessary resources or support to facilitate the patient's completion of the course of treatment.
- If the patient is unable to adhere to the treatment program, even with necessary supports in place, concern for the public's health would take priority and necessitate placing him in a supervised living situation until his treatment is completed.

Clinical Decision-Making Questions
1. Under what circumstances are health care providers justified in overriding a patient's autonomy or decision making?
2. How would the nurse determine whether there were cultural beliefs interfering with this man's ability to understand the importance of completing the treatment? What would the nurse do about it?

When the treatment regimen has been completed, there is evidence of negative cultures, the patient is improving clinically, and there is radiological evidence of improvement, most individuals can be considered adequately treated. Follow-up care may be indicated during the subsequent 12 months, including bacteriological studies and chest radiographic examinations. Because approximately 5% of individuals experience relapses, the patient should be taught to recognize the symptoms that indicate recurrence of TB. If these symptoms occur, immediate medical attention should be sought.

The patient needs to be instructed about certain factors that could reactivate TB, such as immunosuppressive therapy, malignancy, and prolonged debilitating illness. If the patient experiences any of these events, the health care provider must be told so that reactivation of TB can be closely monitored. In some situations, it may be necessary to put the patient on anti-TB therapy.

EVALUATION
The following are the expected outcomes for the patient with TB:
- Patient will have complete resolution of the disease.
- Patient will have normal pulmonary function.
- Patient will have absence of any complications.
- Patient will have no transmission of TB.

ATYPICAL MYCOBACTERIA

Pulmonary disease that closely resembles TB may be caused by atypical acid-fast mycobacteria. This type of pulmonary disease is indistinguishable from TB clinically and radiologically but can be differentiated by bacteriological culture. These organisms are not believed to be airborne and thus are not transmitted by droplet nuclei.

Atypical mycobacteria may also invade the cervical lymph nodes, causing lymphadenitis. This type of pulmonary disease typically occurs in White men with a history of COPD, cystic fibrosis, or silicosis. *Mycobacterium avium-intracellulare (MAI)* is a common cause of opportunistic infections in the patient with HIV infection (see Chapter 17).

Treatment depends on identification of the causative agent and determination of drug sensitivity. Many of the medications used in treating TB are used in combating infections from atypical mycobacteria.

PULMONARY FUNGAL INFECTIONS

Pulmonary fungal infections are increasing in incidence. They appear most frequently in seriously ill patients being treated with corticosteroids, antineoplastic immunosuppressive medications, or multiple antibiotics. They are also more common in patients with AIDS or cystic fibrosis. Types of fungal infections are presented in Table 30.9. These infections are not transmitted from person to person, and the patient does not have to be placed in isolation. The clinical manifestations are similar to those of bacterial pneumonia. Skin and serology tests are available to assist in identifying the infecting organism. However, identification of the organism in a sputum specimen or in other body fluids is the best diagnostic indicator. In addition, fungal infections in the mouth and throat (thrush) can be prevented if the patient performs an oral rinse after using inhalant therapy, specifically a corticosteroid.

Interprofessional Care

Amphotericin B (Fungizone) is the medication most widely used in treating serious systemic fungal infections. It must be given intravenously to achieve adequate blood and tissue levels because it is poorly absorbed from the GI tract. Amphotericin B is considered a toxic drug with many possible adverse effects, including hypersensitivity reactions, fever, chills, malaise, nausea and vomiting, thrombophlebitis at the injection site, and abnormal renal function. Many of the adverse effects during infusion can be avoided by premedicating with an anti-inflammatory or with diphenhydramine (Benadryl) 1 hour before the infusion. Monitoring renal function and ensuring adequate hydration are essential while a person is receiving this medication. Renal changes are at least partially reversible. Amphotericin infusions are incompatible with most other medications. Amphotericin is frequently administered every other day after daily therapy for an initial period of several weeks. Total treatment with the medication may range from 4 to 12 weeks.

Oral antifungal medications such as ketoconazole (Nizoral), fluconazole (Diflucan), and itraconazole (Sporanox) have also been successful in the treatment of fungal infections. Their effectiveness in treatment allows an alternative to the use of amphotericin B in many cases. Effectiveness of therapy can be monitored with fungal serology titres.

TABLE 30.9	FUNGAL INFECTIONS OF THE LUNG
Organism	**Characteristics**
Histoplasmosis	
Histoplasma capsulatum	Indigenous to soil of the St. Lawrence River valleys; inhalation of mycelia into lungs; infected individual often free of symptoms; generally self-limiting, chronic disease similar to TB
Coccidioidomycosis	
Coccidioides immitis	Indigenous to semi-arid regions of southwestern United States (not normally found in Canada); inhalation of arthrospores into lungs; suppurative (pus-forming) and granulomatous reaction in lungs; symptomatic infection in one third of individuals
Blastomycosis	
Blastomyces dermatitidis	Indigenous to southern Canada; inhalation of fungus into lungs; progression of disease often insidious; possible involvement of skin
Cryptococcosis	
Cryptococcus neoformans	True yeast; indigenous worldwide in soil and pigeon excreta; inhalation of fungus into lungs; possible meningitis
Aspergillosis	
Aspergillus niger or *A. fumigatus*	True mould inhabiting mouth; widely distributed; invasion of lung tissue resulting in possible necrotizing pneumonia; in individual with asthma, allergic bronchopulmonary aspergillosis may necessitate corticosteroid therapy
Candidiasis	
Candida albicans	Leading cause of mycotic infections in hospitalized and immunocompromised hosts; ubiquitous and frequent colonization of upper respiratory and gastrointestinal tracts; infections often follow broad-spectrum antibiotic therapy (systemic or inhaled); possible development of localized pulmonary infiltrate to widespread bilateral consolidation with hypoxemia
Actinomycosis	
Actinomyces israelii	Not a true fungus; anaerobic; Gram-positive bacteria with branching hyphae; presence of necrotizing pneumonia after aspiration; pneumonitis; commonly in lower lobes with abscess or empyema formation
Nocardiosis	
Nocardia asteroides	Not a true fungus; aerobic; soil saprophyte widely distributed in nature; acquisition of infection from nature; rarely present in sputum without accompanying disease
Pneumocystis Pneumonia (PCP)	
Pneumocystis jiroveci	Rarely causes pneumonia in healthy individuals; fungus present in the environment; common opportunistic pneumonia in people with impaired immune systems, HIV infection, or both

HIV, human immunodeficiency virus; *TB,* tuberculosis.

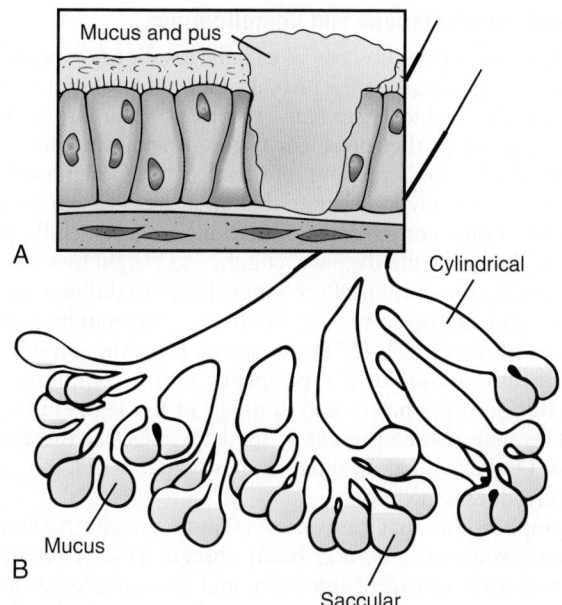

FIG. 30.2 Pathological changes in bronchiectasis. **A,** Longitudinal section of bronchial wall where chronic infection has caused damage. **B,** Collection of purulent material in dilated bronchioles, leading to persistent infection.

BRONCHIECTASIS

Etiology and Pathophysiology

Bronchiectasis is characterized by permanent, abnormal dilation of one or more large bronchi. The pathophysiological change that results in dilation is destruction of the elastic and muscular structures of the bronchial wall. There are two pathological types of bronchiectasis: saccular and cylindrical (Figure 30.2). *Saccular bronchiectasis* occurs mainly in large bronchi and is characterized by cavity-like dilations. The affected bronchi end in large sacs. *Cylindrical bronchiectasis* involves medium-sized bronchi that are mildly to moderately dilated.

Almost all forms of bronchiectasis are associated with bacterial infections. A wide variety of infectious agents can initiate bronchiectasis, including adenovirus, influenza virus, *S. aureus, Klebsiella,* and anaerobes. Infections cause the bronchial walls to weaken, and pockets of infection begin to form. When the walls of the bronchial system are injured, the mucociliary mechanism is damaged, allowing bacteria and mucus to accumulate within the pockets. The infection becomes worse and results in bronchiectasis.

Clinical Manifestations

The hallmark of bronchiectasis is persistent or recurrent cough with production of greater than 20 mL of purulent sputum per day. The cough is paroxysmal and is often stimulated by position changes. Other manifestations include exertional dyspnea, fatigue, weight loss, anorexia, and fetid breath. On auscultation of the lungs, crackle and wheezing may be heard. Sinusitis frequently accompanies diffuse bronchiectasis. The manifestations of advanced, widespread bronchiectasis are generalized wheezing, digital clubbing, and cor pulmonale.

Diagnostic Studies

An individual with a chronic productive cough with copious purulent sputum (which may be blood streaked) should be suspected of having bronchiectasis. Chest radiographic studies are usually done and may show streaky infiltrates or may be normal.

The availability of high-resolution CT scans of the chest, which have excellent sensitivity for detecting bronchiectasis, has made diagnosis easier. Bronchoscopy can also be useful in identifying the source of secretions, in identifying sites of hemoptysis, or for collecting microbiological samples.

Sputum may provide additional information regarding the severity of impairment and the presence of active infection. Pulmonary function studies may be abnormal in advanced bronchiectasis, showing a decrease in vital capacity, expiratory flow, and maximum voluntary ventilation. Complete blood cell count may be normal or show evidence of leukocytosis or anemia from chronic infection.

Interprofessional Care

Bronchiectasis is difficult to treat. Therapy is aimed at treating acute flare-ups and preventing decline in lung function. Antibiotics are the mainstay of treatment and are given on the basis of sputum culture results. Long-term suppressive therapy with antibiotics is occasionally used but is fraught with risks for antibiotic resistance. A form of treatment gaining popularity is the use of nebulized antibiotics. Studies indicate that they are safe and may reduce the number of flare-ups and hospitalizations in bronchiectatic patients (Rubin & Williams, 2014). Antipseudomonal antibiotics, such as tobramycin, are commonly used. Concurrent bronchodilator therapy is given to prevent bronchospasm. Other forms of medication therapy may include mucolytic agents and expectorants. Maintaining good hydration is important to liquefy secretions. Chest physiotherapy and other airway clearance techniques are important to facilitate expectoration of sputum. (These techniques are discussed in Chapter 31.) The individual should reduce exposure to excessive air pollutants and irritants, avoid cigarette smoking, and obtain pneumococcal and influenza vaccinations.

Surgical resection of parts of the lungs, although not used as often as in the past, may be done if more conservative treatment is not effective. Surgical resection of an affected lobe or segment may be indicated for the patient with repeated bouts of pneumonia, hemoptysis, and disabling complications. Surgery is not advisable when there is diffuse or widespread involvement. For select patients who are disabled in spite of maximal therapy, lung transplantation is an option. (Lung transplantation is discussed later in this chapter.)

NURSING MANAGEMENT
BRONCHIECTASIS

The early detection and treatment of lower respiratory tract infections will help prevent complications such as bronchiectasis. Any obstructing lesion or foreign body should be removed promptly. Other measures to decrease the occurrence or progression of bronchiectasis include avoiding cigarette smoking and decreasing exposure to pollution and irritants.

An important nursing goal is to promote drainage and removal of bronchial mucus. Various airway clearance techniques can be effectively used to facilitate secretion removal. The patient should be taught deep-breathing exercises and effective ways to cough (see Chapter 31, Table 31.17). Chest physiotherapy with postural drainage should be done on affected parts of the lung (see Chapter 31, Figure 31.22). Some individuals require elevation of the foot of the bed by 10 to 15 cm to facilitate drainage. Pillows may be used in the hospital and at home to help the patient assume postural drainage positions. A Flutter mucus clearance device is a handheld device that provides airway vibration during the expiratory phase of breathing (see Chapter 31, Figure 31.23). Two to four 15-minute sessions daily by a patient who has been properly trained can provide satisfactory mucus clearance. Positive expiratory pressure therapy is a breathing manoeuvre against an expiratory resistance often used in conjunction with nebulized medications. (Respiratory therapy procedures are explained in Chapter 31.)

Administration of the prescribed antibiotics, bronchodilators, or expectorants is critical. The patient needs to understand the importance of taking the prescribed regimen of medications to obtain maximum effectiveness. The patient should be aware of possible adverse effects and of the adverse effects that must be reported to the health care provider.

Health teaching must include information regarding the importance of getting adequate rest, avoiding overexertion, consuming adequate nutrients, ensuring hydration, and performing oral care. Unless there are contraindications such as concomitant heart failure or renal disease, the patient should be instructed to drink at least 3 L of fluid daily. Generally, the patient should be counselled to use low-sodium fluids to avoid systemic fluid retention.

Direct hydration of the respiratory system may also prove beneficial in the expectoration of secretions. Usually, a bland aerosol with normal saline solution delivered by a jet-type nebulizer is used. The patient with bronchiectasis should avoid using ultrasonic nebulizers because they often induce bronchospasm. At home, a steamy shower can prove effective; expensive equipment that requires frequent cleaning is usually unnecessary. It is important that the patient medicate with an inhaled bronchodilator 10 to 15 minutes before using a bland aerosol, to prevent bronchoconstriction.

The patient and caregivers should be taught to recognize significant clinical manifestations to be reported to the health care provider. These manifestations include increased sputum production, grossly bloody sputum, increasing dyspnea, fever, chills, and chest pain.

LUNG ABSCESS

Etiology and Pathophysiology

A lung abscess is a pus-containing lesion of the lung parenchyma that gives rise to a cavity. The cavity is formed by necrosis of the lung tissue. In many cases, the causes and pathogenesis of lung abscesses are similar to those of pneumonia. Most lung abscesses are caused by aspiration of material from the oral cavity (the gingival crevices) into the lungs. In general, infectious agents including enteric Gram-negative organisms (e.g., *Klebsiella*), *S. aureus,* and anaerobic bacilli (e.g., *Bacteroides*) are responsible for lung abscesses and the associated infection and necrosis of the lung tissue. A lung abscess can also result from a lung infarct secondary to pulmonary embolus, malignant growth, TB, and various parasitic and fungal diseases of the lung.

The areas of the lung most commonly affected are the superior segments of the lower lobes and the posterior segments of the upper lobes. Fibrous tissue usually forms around the abscess in an attempt to wall it off. The abscess may erode into the bronchial system, causing the production of foul-smelling sputum. It may grow toward the pleura and cause pleuritic pain. Multiple small abscesses can occur within the lung.

Clinical Manifestations and Complications

The onset of a lung abscess is usually insidious, especially if anaerobic organisms are the primary cause. A more acute onset occurs with aerobic organisms. The most common manifestation is a cough that produces purulent sputum (often dark brown) that is foul smelling and foul tasting. Hemoptysis is common, especially at the time that an abscess ruptures into a bronchus. Other common manifestations are fever, chills, prostration, pleuritic pain, dyspnea, cough, and weight loss.

Physical examination of the lungs indicates dullness to percussion and decreased breath sounds on auscultation over the segment of lung involved. There may be transmission of bronchial breath sounds to the periphery if the communicating bronchus becomes patent and drainage of the segment begins. Crackles may also be present in the later stages as the abscess drains. Oral examination often reveals dental caries, gingivitis, and periodontal infection.

Complications that can occur include chronic pulmonary abscess, bronchiectasis, and brain abscess as a result of the hematogenous spread of infection, and bronchopleural fistula and empyema as a result of abscess perforation into the pleural cavity.

Diagnostic Studies

A chest radiographic examination will reveal a solitary cavitary lesion with fluid. CT scanning is used if there is suspicion of cavitation not clearly seen. A lung abscess, in contrast to other types of abscesses, does not require assisted drainage, as long as there is drainage via the bronchus. Routine sputum cultures can be collected, but contaminants can confuse the results and it is difficult to isolate anaerobic bacteria. Pleural fluid and blood cultures may be obtained. Bronchoscopy may be used in cases of abscess in which drainage is delayed or in which there are factors that suggest an underlying malignancy.

NURSING AND INTERPROFESSIONAL MANAGEMENT LUNG ABSCESS

Antibiotics given for a prolonged period (up to 2 to 4 months) are usually the primary method of treatment. Penicillin has historically been the medication of choice because of the frequent presence of anaerobic organisms. However, recent studies suggest that the anaerobic bacteria involved in abscesses of the lung produce β-lactamase, which is resistant to penicillin. Clindamycin has been shown to be superior to penicillin and is the standard treatment for an anaerobic lung infection. Patients with putrid lung abscesses usually show clinical improvement with decreased fever within 3 to 4 days of beginning antibiotics.

Because of the need for prolonged antibiotic therapy, the patient must be aware of the importance of continuing the medication for the prescribed period. As well, the patient needs to know about adverse effects to be reported to the health care provider. Sometimes, the patient is asked to return periodically during the course of antibiotic therapy for repeat cultures and sensitivity tests to ensure that the infecting organism is not becoming resistant to the antibiotic. When antibiotic therapy is completed, the patient is re-evaluated.

The nurse should teach the patient how to cough effectively (see Chapter 31, Table 31.17). Chest physiotherapy and postural drainage are sometimes used to drain abscesses located in the lower or posterior portions of the lung. Postural drainage according to the lung area involved will aid in the removal of secretions (see Chapter 31, Figure 31.22). Frequent (every 2 to 3 hours) mouth care is needed to relieve the foul-smelling odour and taste from the sputum. Diluted hydrogen peroxide and mouthwash are often effective.

Rest, good nutrition, and adequate fluid intake are all supportive measures to facilitate recovery. If dentition is poor and dental hygiene is not adequate, the patient should be encouraged to obtain dental care.

Surgery is rarely indicated but occasionally may be necessary when reinfection of a large cavitary lesion occurs or to establish a diagnosis when there is evidence of an underlying neoplasm or chronic associated disease. The usual procedure in such cases is a lobectomy or pneumonectomy. An alternative to surgery is percutaneous drainage, but this has a high risk for contamination of the pleural space.

ENVIRONMENTAL LUNG DISEASES

Environmental or occupational lung diseases result from inhaled dust or chemicals. The duration of exposure and the amount of inhalant have a major influence on whether the exposed individual will have lung damage, as does the susceptibility of the host.

Pneumoconiosis is a general term for lung diseases caused by the inhalation and retention of dust particles. The literal meaning of *pneumoconiosis* is "dust in the lungs." Examples of this condition are silicosis, asbestosis, berylliosis, and hantavirus, a potentially fatal disease transmitted by inhalation of aerosolized rodent excreta particles, which has had outbreaks reported in Canada and the United States. The classical response to the inhaled substance is diffuse parenchymal infiltration with phagocytic cells. This eventually results in diffuse pulmonary fibrosis (excess connective tissue). Fibrosis is the result of tissue repair after inflammation. Pneumoconiosis and other environmental lung diseases are presented in Table 30.10.

Chemical pneumonitis results from exposure to toxic chemical fumes. Acutely, there is diffuse lung injury characterized as pulmonary edema. Chronically, the clinical picture is that of bronchiolitis obliterans, which is usually associated with a normal chest radiograph or one that shows hyperinflation. An example is silo filler's disease. *Hypersensitivity pneumonitis* or extrinsic allergic alveolitis is the response seen when antigens to which an individual is allergic are inhaled. Examples include bird fancier's lung and farmer's lung.

Although the incidence of many occupational respiratory diseases has declined, occupational asthma is the most common occupational lung disease (Canadian Centre for Occupational Health and Safety [CCOHS], 2021a). *Occupational asthma* refers to the development of symptoms of shortness of breath, wheezing, cough, and chest tightness as a result of exposure to dust or fumes that trigger an allergic response. The obstruction may initially be reversible or intermittent, but continued exposure results in permanent obstructive changes. The best-known causative agent in occupational asthma is toluene di-isocyanate (TDI), which is used in the production of rigid polyurethane foam.

Lung cancer, either squamous cell carcinoma or adenocarcinoma, is the most frequent cancer associated with asbestos exposure. People who have experienced more exposure are at a greater risk for disease. There is a minimum lapse of 15 to 19 years between first exposure and development of lung cancer. Mesotheliomas, both pleural and peritoneal, are also associated with asbestos exposure.

Clinical Manifestations

Acute symptoms of pulmonary edema may be seen following early exposure to chemical fumes. However, symptoms of many environmental lung diseases may not occur until at least 10 to 15 years after the initial exposure to the inhaled irritant. Dyspnea and cough are often the earliest manifestations. Chest pain and cough with sputum production usually occur later. Complications that often result are pneumonia, chronic bronchitis, emphysema, and lung cancer. Manifestations of these complications can be the reason the patient seeks health care. Cor pulmonale is a late complication, especially in conditions characterized by diffuse pulmonary fibrosis.

Pulmonary function studies often show reduced vital capacity. A chest radiograph will often reveal lung involvement specific to the primary condition. CT scans have been shown to be useful in detecting early lung involvement.

Interprofessional Care

The best approach to management is to try to prevent or decrease environmental and occupational risks. Well-designed, effective ventilation systems can reduce exposure to irritants. Wearing a mask is appropriate in some occupations. Periodic inspections and monitoring of workplaces by agencies such as the Canadian Centre for Occupational Health and Safety reinforce the obligations of employers to provide a safe work environment (CCOHS, 2021b). In addition, the Canada Labour Code requires that an occupational health and safety committee be established in all workplaces with 20 or more regular employees (Human Resources and Skills Development Canada, 2017).

Cigarette smoking adds increased insult to the lungs, so persons at risk for occupational lung disease should not smoke. In addition, secondhand smoke is an important source of exposure that increases risk for development of lung cancer. This risk has led to regulations requiring a smoke-free workspace for all employees.

Early diagnosis is essential if the disease process is to be halted. Places of employment in which there is a known risk for lung disease may require periodic chest radiographic examinations and pulmonary function studies for exposed employees. This measure can help detect pulmonary changes before symptoms develop.

There is no specific treatment for most environmental lung diseases. The best treatment is to decrease or stop exposure to the harmful agent. Strategies are directed toward providing symptom relief. If there are coexisting conditions, such as pneumonia, chronic bronchitis, emphysema, or asthma, they are treated.

LUNG CANCER

Lung cancer, the most preventable cancer, is the leading cause of cancer-related deaths in men and women in Canada. In 2020, lung cancer accounted for 1.8 million deaths worldwide, making it the deadliest of all cancers (WHO, 2021). In 2020, lung cancer was one of the most commonly diagnosed cancers in Canada and accounted for 2.21 million cases. Lung cancer has a low 5-year survival rate of 19%, based on 2012–2014 data (Canadian Cancer Society, 2021a).

Lung cancer most commonly occurs in people who have a long history of cigarette smoking and who are 40 to 75 years of age, with peak incidence between 55 and 65 years of age.

TABLE 30.10   ENVIRONMENTAL LUNG DISEASES

Agents and Industries	Description	Complications
Asbestosis		
Asbestos fibres present in insulation, construction material (roof tiling, cement products), shipyards, textiles (for fireproofing), automobile clutch and brake linings	Disease appears 15–35 yr after first exposure. Interstitial fibrosis develops. Pleural plaques, which are calcified lesions, develop on pleura. Dyspnea, basal crackles, and decreased vital capacity are early manifestations.	Diffuse interstitial pulmonary fibrosis; lung cancer, especially in cigarette smokers; mesothelioma (rare type of cancer affecting pleura and peritoneal membrane)
Berylliosis		
Beryllium dust present in aircraft manufacturing, metallurgy, rocket fuels	Formation of noncaseating granulomas is seen. Acute pneumonitis occurs after heavy exposure. Interstitial fibrosis can also occur.	Progress of disease possible even after removal of stimulating inhalant
Bird Fancier's, Breeder's, or Handler's Lung		
Bird droppings or feathers	Hypersensitivity pneumonitis is present.	Progressive fibrosis of lung
Byssinosis		
Cotton, flax, and hemp dust (textile industry)	Airway obstruction is caused by contraction of smooth muscles. Chronic disease results from severe airway obstruction and decreased elastic recoil.	Progression of chronic disease after cessation of dust exposure
Coal Worker's Pneumoconiosis (Black Lung)		
Coal dust	Incidence is high (20–30%) in coal workers. Deposits of carbon dust cause lesions to develop along respiratory bronchioles. Bronchioles dilate because of loss of wall structure. Chronic airway obstruction and bronchitis develop. Dyspnea and cough are common early symptoms.	Progressive, massive lung fibrosis; increased risk for chronic bronchitis and emphysema in smokers
Farmer's Lung		
Inhalation of airborne material from mouldy hay or similar matter	Hypersensitivity pneumonitis occurs. Acute form is similar to pneumonia, with manifestations of chills, fever, and malaise. Chronic, insidious form is type of pulmonary fibrosis.	Progressive fibrosis of lung
Hantavirus Pulmonary Syndrome (HPS)		
Rodent droppings inhaled while in rodent-infested areas	Acute hemorrhagic fever associated with severe pulmonary and cardiovascular collapse and death. Incubation period is 1–4 wk with prodrome (3–5 days) of flulike symptoms. No cure or specific treatment exists.	Critical care unit with careful monitoring of fluid and electrolyte balance and blood pressure; supportive therapy and early intervention vital; research on this virus is done in high-level biocontainment facilities
Siderosis		
Iron oxide present in welding materials, foundries, iron ore mining	Dust deposits are found in lung.	—
Silicosis		
Silica dust present in quartz rock in mining of gold, copper, tin, coal, lead; also present in sandblasting, foundries, quarries, pottery making, masonry	In chronic disease, dust is engulfed by macrophages and may be destroyed, resulting in fibrotic nodules. Acute disease results from intense exposure in short period. Within 5 yr, it progresses to severe disability from lung fibrosis.	Increased susceptibility to tuberculosis; progressive, massive fibrosis; high incidence of chronic bronchitis
Silo Filler's Disease		
Nitrogen oxides from fermentation of vegetation in freshly filled silo	Chemical pneumonitis occurs.	Progressive bronchiolitis obliterans

Etiology

Cigarette smoking is the most important risk factor in the development of lung cancer. Smoking is responsible for approximately 85% of all lung cancers in Canada (Canadian Cancer Society, 2021c). Tobacco smoke contains 60 carcinogens in addition to substances (e.g., carbon monoxide, nicotine) that interfere with normal cell development. Cigarette smoking, a lower-airway irritant, causes a change in the bronchial epithelium, which usually returns to normal when smoking is discontinued. The risk for lung cancer is gradually lowered when smoking ceases and it continues to decline with time. After 10 years following cessation of smoking, the risk for lung cancer is cut in half (Canadian Lung Association, 2016). In 2017, 8% of Canadian youth between the ages of 15 and 19 were smokers.

The risk of developing lung cancer is directly related to total exposure to cigarette smoke, measured by total number of cigarettes smoked in a lifetime, age of smoking onset, depth of inhalation, tar and nicotine content, and use of unfiltered cigarettes. Side-stream smoke (smoke from burning cigarettes and cigars) contains the same carcinogens found in mainstream smoke (smoke inhaled by the smoker). According to the Canadian

Cancer Society (2021d) approximately 800 nonsmokers in Canada die from secondhand smoke.

Compared with nonsmokers, those who smoke pipes and cigars have also been shown to have an increased risk of developing lung cancer. Cigar smokers are at higher risk for lung cancer than pipe smokers. In fact, rates of lung cancer caused by heavy smoking of cigars and inhalation of smoke from small cigars have been shown to correlate with the rates of lung cancer caused by cigarette smoking.

Vaping and e-cigarettes, for the short term, have been suggested as an alternative to conventional cigarettes and cigars to help people quit smoking. Although long-term studies have yet to be been conducted, use of vaping and e-cigarette products has been shown to induce exogenous lipoid pneumonia, diffuse alveolar hemorrhage, and vaping-associated bronchiolitis obliterans; long-term use may cause life-threatening lung disease Francesco, 2020). The Canadian Cancer Society (2021e) recommends complete cessation of any type of cigarette or tobacco product use via vape or e-cigarette to decrease risk of lung cancer.

Another major risk factor for lung cancer is inhaled carcinogens. These include asbestos, radon, nickel, iron and iron oxides, uranium, polycyclic aromatic hydrocarbons, chromates, arsenic, and air pollution. Exposure to these substances is common for employees of industries such as mining, smelting, or chemical or petroleum manufacturing. The cigarette smoker who is also exposed to one or more of these chemicals or to high amounts of air pollution is at significantly higher risk for lung cancer.

There are marked variations in a person's propensity to develop lung cancer. To date, no genetic abnormality has conclusively been defined for lung cancer. It is known that the carcinogens in cigarette smoke directly damage deoxyribonucleic acid (DNA). One theory is that people have different genetic carcinogen-metabolizing pathways.

Pathophysiology

The pathogenesis of primary lung cancer is not well understood. More than 90% of cancers originate from the epithelium of the bronchus (bronchogenic). They grow slowly, and it takes 8 to 10 years for a tumour to reach 1 cm in size, which is the smallest detectable lesion on a radiographic study. Lung cancers occur primarily in the segmental bronchi or beyond and have a preference for the upper lobes of the lungs (Figures 30.3 and 30.4). Pathological changes in the bronchial system show nonspecific inflammatory changes with hypersecretion of mucus, desquamation of cells, reactive hyperplasia of the basal cells, and metaplasia of normal respiratory epithelium into stratified squamous cells.

Primary lung cancers are often categorized into two broad subtypes (Table 30.11): non–small cell lung cancer (NSCLC; 85 to 90%) and small cell lung cancer (SCLC; 10 to 15%) (Canadian Cancer Society, 2021b). Lung cancers metastasize primarily by direct extension and via the blood circulation and the lymph system. The common sites for metastatic growth are liver, brain, bones, scalene lymph nodes, and adrenal glands.

Paraneoplastic Syndrome. Certain lung cancers cause *paraneoplastic syndrome*, which is characterized by various systemic manifestations caused by factors (e.g., hormones, enzymes, antigens) produced by the tumour cells. SCLCs are most commonly associated with paraneoplastic syndrome. The systemic manifestations seen are hormonal, dermatological, neuromuscular, vascular, hematological, and connective tissue syndromes.

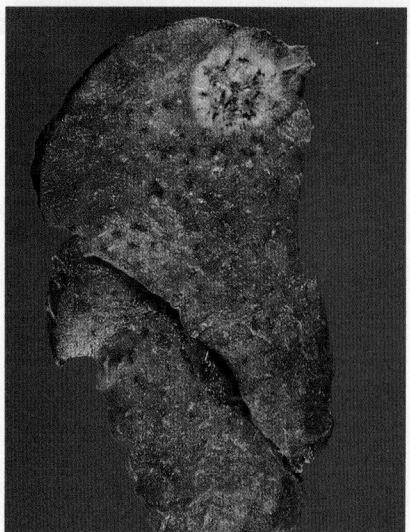

FIG. 30.3 Lung cancer. Peripheral adenocarcinoma. The tumour shows prominent black pigmentation, suggestive of having evolved in an anthracotic scar. Source: Damjanov, I., & Linder, J. (1996). *Anderson's pathology* (10th ed.). Mosby.

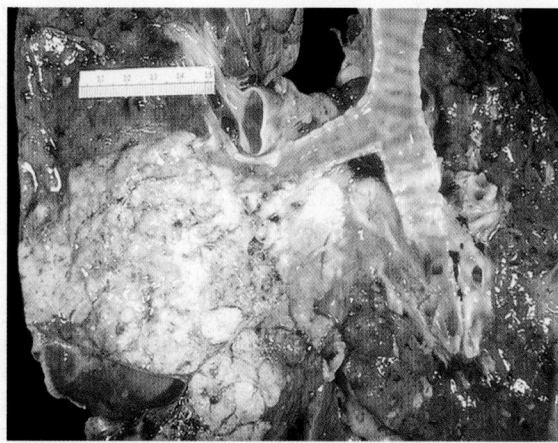

FIG. 30.4 Lung carcinoma. The grey-white tumour tissue is infiltrating the lung. Histologically, this tumour is identified as a squamous cell carcinoma. Source: Kumar, V., Abbas, A. K., Aster, J. C., et al. (2010). *Robbins and Cotran pathologic basis of disease* (8th ed.). Saunders.

Examples of paraneoplastic syndromes include hypercalcemia, syndrome of inappropriate antidiuretic hormone (SIADH) secretion, anemia, leukocytosis, hypercoagulable disorders, and neurological syndromes. These syndromes can respond temporarily to symptomatic treatment, but they are impossible to control without successful treatment of the underlying lung cancer.

Clinical Manifestations

Lung cancer is clinically silent for most individuals for the majority of its course. The clinical manifestations of lung cancer are usually nonspecific and appear late in the disease process. Manifestations depend on the type of primary lung cancer, its location, and metastatic spread. Often, there is extensive metastasis before symptoms become apparent. Persistent pneumonitis that is a result of obstructed bronchi may be one of the earliest manifestations, causing fever, chills, and cough.

One of the most significant symptoms, and often the one reported first, is a persistent cough that may produce sputum. Sputum may be blood-tinged because of bleeding caused by

TABLE 30.11   COMPARISON OF THE TYPES OF PRIMARY LUNG CANCER

Cell Type	Risk Factors	Characteristics	Response to Therapy
Non–Small Cell Lung Cancer (NSCLC)			
Squamous cell (epidermoid) carcinoma	Almost always associated with cigarette smoking; is associated with exposure to environmental carcinogens (e.g., uranium, asbestos)	Accounts for 30% of lung cancers; is more common in men; arises from the bronchial epithelium; produces earlier symptoms because of bronchial obstructive characteristics; does not have a strong tendency to metastasize; metastasizes locally by direct extension; causes cavitating pulmonary lesions	Surgical resection is often attempted; life expectancy is better than for small cell lung cancer.
Adenocarcinoma	Has been associated with lung scarring and chronic interstitial fibrosis; is not related to cigarette smoking	Accounts for approximately 40% of lung cancers; is more common in women; often has no clinical manifestations until widespread metastasis is present; metastasizes via bloodstream; is most commonly located in peripheral portions of lungs*	Surgical resection is often attempted; cancer does not respond well to chemotherapy.
Large cell undifferentiated carcinoma	High correlation with cigarette smoking and exposure to environmental carcinogens	Accounts for 10% of lung cancers; commonly causes cavitation; is highly metastatic via lymphatics and blood; commonly peripheral rather than central	Surgery is not usually attempted because of high rate of metastases; tumour may be radiosensitive but often recurs.
Small Cell Lung Cancer (SCLC)			
Small cell anaplastic undifferentiated (includes oat cell)	Associated with cigarette smoking, exposure to environmental carcinogens	Accounts for 20–25% of lung cancers; is most malignant form; tends to spread early via lymphatics and bloodstream; is frequently associated with endocrine disturbances; predominantly central and can cause bronchial obstruction and pneumonia	This cancer has the poorest prognosis; however, chemotherapy advances have been substantial; radiation is used as adjuvant therapy as well as palliative measure. Average median survival is 12–18 mo.

*See Figure 30.3.

malignancy, but hemoptysis is not a common early symptom. Chest pain may be present and localized or unilateral, ranging from mild to severe. Dyspnea and an auscultatory wheeze may be present if there is bronchial obstruction.

Later manifestations may include nonspecific systemic symptoms such as anorexia, fatigue, weight loss, and nausea and vomiting. Hoarseness may be present as a result of involvement of the recurrent laryngeal nerve. Unilateral paralysis of the diaphragm, dysphagia, and superior vena cava obstruction may occur because of intrathoracic spread of the malignancy. There may be palpable lymph nodes in the neck or the axilla. Mediastinal involvement may lead to pericardial effusion, cardiac tamponade, and dysrhythmias.

Diagnostic Studies

Chest radiographic studies are widely used in the diagnosis of lung cancer. The findings may show the presence of the tumour or abnormalities related to the obstructive features of the tumour such as atelectasis and pneumonitis. The radiograph can also show evidence of metastasis to the ribs or vertebrae and the presence of pleural effusion.

CT scanning is the single most effective noninvasive technique for evaluating lung cancer. CT scans of the brain and bone scans complete the evaluation for metastatic disease. With CT scans, the location and extent of masses in the chest can be identified, as well as any mediastinal involvement or lymph node enlargement. Magnetic resonance imaging (MRI) may be used in combination with or instead of CT scans. Positron emission tomography (PET) can be a useful diagnostic tool in early clinical staging. PET allows measurement of differential metabolic activity in normal and diseased tissues.

A definitive diagnosis of lung cancer is made by identifying malignant cells. Sputum specimens are usually obtained for cytological studies. An early-morning specimen that has been obtained by having the patient cough deeply provides the most accurate results. However, malignant cells may not be obtained even in the presence of a lung cancer.

The use of the fibre-optic bronchoscope is important in the diagnosis of lung cancer, particularly when the lesions are endobronchial or close to an airway. It provides direct visualization and allows biopsy specimens to be obtained. A biopsy is usually the best method for establishing the presence of a malignant tumour.

Mediastinoscopy—the insertion of a scope via a small anterior chest incision into the mediastinum—is done to examine for metastasis in the anterior mediastinum or in the hilum or in the chest extrapleurally. It is also used to determine the stage of the lung cancer, an important step toward preparing a treatment plan. *Video-assisted thoracoscopy* (VAT), which involves the insertion of a scope into a small thoracic incision, may be used to explore areas inaccessible by mediastinoscopy.

Pulmonary angiography and lung scans may be performed to assess overall pulmonary status. Fine-needle aspiration (FNA) may be used to obtain a tissue sample to determine tumour histology. FNA is most useful in cases involving a peripheral lesion near the chest wall, and it is usually attempted to avoid a thoracotomy. If a thoracentesis is performed to relieve a pleural effusion, the fluid should be analyzed for malignant cells. (Table 30.12 summarizes the diagnostic management of lung cancer.)

Staging. Staging of NSCLC is performed according to the tumour–node–metastasis (TNM) staging system in a manner similar to that for other tumours (Table 30.13). Assessment criteria are *T*, which denotes tumour size, location, and degree of invasion; *N*, which indicates regional lymph node involvement; and *M*, which represents the presence or absence of distant metastases. Depending on the TNM designation, the tumour

TABLE 30.12 INTERPROFESSIONAL CARE

Lung Cancer

Diagnostic	Interprofessional Therapy
• History and physical examination	• Surgery
• Chest radiographic examination	• Radiation therapy
• Sputum for cytological study	• Chemotherapy
• Bronchoscopy	• Biological therapy
• CT scan	• Bronchoscopic laser therapy
• MRI	• Phototherapy
• PET	• Airway stenting
• Spirometry (preoperative)	• Cryotherapy
• Mediastinoscopy	• Respiratory therapy
• VAT	• Nutritional therapy
• Pulmonary angiography	
• Lung scan	
• Fine-needle aspiration	

CT, computed tomography; *MRI*, magnetic resonance imaging; *PET*, positron emission tomography; *VAT*, video-assisted thoracoscopy.

TABLE 30.13 LUNG CANCER STAGING

Stage	Grouping		
	Tumour	Node	Metastasis
Occult carcinoma	TX	N0	M0
Stage 0	Tis	N0	M0
Stage IA1	T1a	N0	M0
Stage 1A2	T1b	N0	M0
Stage 1A3	T1c	N0	M0
Stage IB	T2a	N0	M0
Stage IIA	T2b	N1	M0
Stage IIB	T1a–T2b	N1	M0
	T3	N0	M0
Stage IIIA	T1a–T2b	N2	M0
	T3	N1	M0
	T4	N0/N1	M0
Stage IIIB	T1a–T2b	N3	M0
	T3/T4	N2	M0
Stage IIIC	T3/T4	N3	M0
Stage IVA	Any T	Any N	M1a/M1b
Stage IVB	Any T	Any N	M1c

Used with the permission of the American College of Surgeons. The original source for this material is the *AJCC Cancer Staging Manual,* Eighth Edition (2017) published by Springer Science and Business Media LLC, www.springer.com.

is then staged, which assists in estimating prognosis and determining the appropriate therapy.

Staging of SCLC has not been useful because the cancer has usually metastasized by the time a diagnosis is made. Instead, SCLC is determined to be *limited* (confined to one hemothorax and to regional lymph nodes) or *extensive* (any disease exceeding those boundaries).

Screening for Lung Cancer. In 2016, new guidelines were published recommending the screening of asymptomatic adults aged 55 to 74 with at least a 30 pack-year smoking history (who currently smoke or quit smoking less than 15 years ago). Screening is done using a low-dose CT scan every year for 3 consecutive years (Canadian Task Force on Preventive Health Care, 2016).

Interprofessional Care

Cancer Care Ontario has published evidence-informed clinical guidelines for treating lung cancer. The guidelines can be accessed at its website in the Cancer Care Ontario Toolbox, under Guidelines & Advice. (See Resources at the end of the chapter.)

Surgical Therapy. Surgical resection is considered the treatment of choice in NSCLC stages I and II because the disease is potentially curable with resection. For other NSCLC stages, surgery may be indicated in conjunction with radiation therapy, chemotherapy, or both. In limited-stage SCLC, which is rare, surgical resection, chemotherapy, and radiation therapy may be recommended.

When the tumour is considered operable with a potential for cure, the patient's cardiopulmonary status must be evaluated to determine the ability to withstand surgery. This is done by clinical studies of pulmonary function, ABGs, and others, as indicated by the individual's status. Contraindications for thoracotomy include hypercapnia, pulmonary hypertension, cor pulmonale, and markedly reduced lung function. Coexisting conditions such as cardiac, renal, and liver disease may also be contraindications for surgery.

A tumour may be considered inoperable. If operable, the type of surgery performed is usually a lobectomy (removal of one or more lobes of the lung) and, less often, a *pneumonectomy* (removal of one entire lung).

Radiation Therapy. Radiation therapy is used as a curative approach in the individual who has a resectable tumour but who is considered a poor surgical risk. There has been improved survival when radiation therapy is used in combination with surgery and chemotherapy. Adenocarcinomas are the most radioresistant type of cancer cell. Although SCLCs are radiosensitive, radiation (even when used in combination with chemotherapy) does not significantly improve the mortality rate because of the early metastases of this type of cancer.

Radiation therapy is also done as a palliative procedure to reduce distressing symptoms such as cough, hemoptysis, bronchial obstruction, and superior vena cava syndrome. It can be used to treat pain caused by metastatic bone lesions or cerebral metastasis. Radiation used as a preoperative or postoperative adjuvant measure has not been found to significantly increase survival in the patient with lung cancer.

Stereotactic Radiotherapy. Stereotactic radiotherapy (SRT), also called *stereotactic surgery* or *radiosurgery,* is a type of radiation therapy that uses high doses of radiation delivered very accurately to the tumour. SRT provides an option to older patients, patients with severe lung or heart disease, and other patients in poor health who are not good candidates for surgery. SRT is an outpatient procedure that uses special positioning procedures and radiology techniques so that a higher dose of radiation can be delivered to the tumour and a smaller part of the healthy lung is exposed.

Chemotherapy. Chemotherapy may be used in the treatment of nonresectable tumours or as adjuvant therapy to surgery in NSCLC with distant metastases. A variety of chemotherapy agents and multidrug regimens (i.e., policies) including combination chemotherapy have been used. These drugs include etoposide (VePesid), carboplatin, cisplatin, paclitaxel, vinorelbine, cyclophosphamide (Procytox), ifosfamide (Ifex), docetaxel (Taxotere), gemcitabine, topotecan (Hycamtin), and irinotecan (Camptosar). Chemotherapy has improved survival in patients with advanced NSCLC and is now considered standard treatment.

Biological Therapy. Biological (targeted) therapy as adjuvant therapy has been used in individuals with cancer, including malignant lung tumours. (Biological therapy is discussed in Chapter 18.)

Other Therapies

Prophylactic Cranial Radiation. Brain metastasis is a common complication of SCLC. Most chemotherapy agents do not adequately penetrate the blood–brain barrier. Prophylactic cranial radiation may be used as a potential way to improve the prognosis of patients, especially those who have a complete response to chemotherapy. Toxicity of this therapy may include scalp erythema, fatigue, and alopecia.

Bronchoscopic Laser Therapy. Bronchoscopic laser therapy makes it possible to remove obstructing bronchial lesions. The thermal energy of the laser is transmitted to the target tissue. It is a complicated procedure that often requires general anaesthesia to control the patient's cough reflex. Relief of the symptoms from airway obstruction as a result of thermal necrosis and shrinkage of the tumour can be dramatic. However, it is not a curative therapy for cancer.

Phototherapy. Photodynamic therapy is a safe, nonsurgical therapy for lung cancer. Porfimer (Photofrin) is injected intravenously and selectively concentrates in tumour cells. After a set time (usually 48 hours), the tumour is exposed to laser light, producing a toxic form of oxygen that destroys tumour cells. Necrotic tissue is removed through a bronchoscope.

Airway Stenting. Stents can be used alone or in combination with other techniques for palliation of dyspnea, cough, or respiratory insufficiency. The advantage of an airway stent is that it supports the airway wall against collapse or external compression and can impede extension of the tumour into the airway lumen.

Cryotherapy. Cryotherapy is a technique in which tissue is destroyed as a result of freezing. Bronchoscopic cryotherapy is used to ablate (destroy) bronchogenic carcinomas, especially polypoid lesions. A repeat bronchoscopy is performed 8 to 10 days after the first session. The second examination enables assessment of cryodestruction, removal of any slough, and repeat cryotherapy if required for the treatment of large lesions.

NURSING MANAGEMENT LUNG CANCER

NURSING ASSESSMENT

It is important to determine the patient's and family's understanding of the diagnostic tests (those completed as well as those planned), the diagnosis or potential diagnosis, the treatment options, and the prognosis. At the same time, the nurse can assess the level of anxiety experienced by the patient, as well as the support provided and needed by the patient's significant others. Subjective and objective data that should be obtained from a patient with lung cancer are presented in Table 30.14.

NURSING DIAGNOSES

Nursing diagnoses for the patient with lung cancer may include but are not limited to the following:

- *Inadequate airway clearance* resulting from *excessive mucus, retained secretions, foreign body in airway* (tumour)
- *Inadequate breathing pattern* resulting from *body position that inhibits lung expansion* (space-occupying lesion)
- *Reduced gas exchange* resulting from *tumour obstructing airflow*
- *Anxiety* resulting from *unmet needs* (lack of knowledge of the disease process)
- *Grieving* resulting from new cancer diagnosis and therapeutic regimen

TABLE 30.14   **NURSING ASSESSMENT**
Lung Cancer

Subjective Data

Important Health Information

Past health history: Exposure to secondhand smoke; airborne carcinogens (e.g., asbestos, uranium, chromates, hydrocarbons, arsenic) or other pollutants; urban living environment; chronic lung disease, including TB, COPD, bronchiectasis; smoking history; frequent respiratory infections; family history of lung cancer

Medications: Use of cough medicines or other respiratory medications

Symptoms

- Anorexia, nausea, vomiting, dysphagia (late symptom), weight loss
- Persistent cough (productive or nonproductive), dyspnea, hemoptysis (late symptom)
- Fatigue, fever, chills
- Chest pain or tightness, shoulder and arm pain; headache; bone pain (late symptom)

Objective Data

General

Fever, neck and axillary lymphadenopathy, paraneoplastic syndromes (e.g., SIADH secretion)

Integumentary

Jaundice (liver metastasis); edema of neck and face (superior vena cava syndrome), digital clubbing

Respiratory

Wheezing, hoarseness, stridor, unilateral diaphragm paralysis, pleural effusions (late signs)

Cardiovascular

Pericardial effusion, cardiac tamponade, dysrhythmias (late signs)

Neurological

Unsteady gait (brain metastasis)

Musculoskeletal

Pathological fractures, muscle wasting (late sign)

Possible Findings

Observance of lesion on chest radiographic examination, CT scan, lung scan, or PET scan; MRI findings of mediastinal invasion, positive sputum or bronchial washings for cytological studies; positive fibre-optic bronchoscopy and biopsy findings; low serum sodium and hypercalcemia (paraneoplastic syndrome)

COPD, chronic obstructive pulmonary disease; *CT,* computed tomography; *MRI,* magnetic resonance imaging; *PET,* positron emission tomography; *SIADH,* syndrome of inappropriate antidiuretic hormone; *TB,* tuberculosis.

PLANNING

The overall goals are that the patient with lung cancer will have (a) effective breathing patterns, (b) adequate airway clearance, (c) adequate oxygenation of tissues, (d) minimal to no pain, and (e) a realistic attitude toward treatment and prognosis.

NURSING IMPLEMENTATION

HEALTH PROMOTION. The best way to halt the epidemic of lung cancer is for people to stop smoking. Important nursing activities that can work toward this goal include promoting smoking-cessation programs and actively supporting education and policy changes related to smoking. Significant policy changes have taken place as a result of the recognition that side-stream smoke is a health hazard: There are now laws that (a) require designation of nonsmoking areas in most public places, (b) prohibit smoking, and (c) ban smoking on airline flights. Other actions aimed at controlling tobacco use include restrictions on tobacco advertising on television and warning-label requirements for cigarette packaging. These are examples of beginning steps toward the goal of a smokeless society. Despite the small advances being made, tobacco-producer organizations such as marketing boards and tobacco companies still have strong political influences.

The nurse should make an effort to assist patients who smoke to stop smoking. There are many resources available to help in this regard. The Registered Nurses' Association of Ontario's Best Practice Guideline *Integrating Tobacco Interventions into Daily Practice* recommends that nurses advocate for patients and provide or refer them to intensive interventions and counselling as patients contemplate smoking cessation (RNAO, 2017). The six stages of change identified among smokers attempting to quit include precontemplation, contemplation, preparation, action, maintenance, and termination. (The stages of change in relationship to patient teaching [transtheoretical model] are discussed in Chapter 4, Table 4.3.) Each stage requires specific actions to progress to the next stage. Nurses working with patients at their individual stage of change can help them progress to the next stage. For patients unwilling to quit, motivational interviewing is recommended (discussed in Chapter 11). The Canadian Lung Association (2021) provides information on access to counselling, medications, and supports to help Canadians quit smoking. Tobacco use and dependence and strategies to assist patients to stop smoking are discussed in Chapter 11.

Nicotine's addictive properties make quitting a difficult task that requires much support. Nicotine replacement significantly lessens the urge to smoke and increases the percentage of smokers who successfully quit smoking. There is no evidence that one product has better results than another, so the choice of agent is dependent on the health care provider and patient preferences.

The advice and motivation of health care providers can be a powerful force in smoking cessation. Nurses are in a unique position to promote smoking cessation because they see large numbers of smokers who may be reluctant to seek help. Support for the smoker includes education that smoking a few cigarettes during a cessation attempt (a slip) is much different from resuming the full smoking habit (a relapse). Despite the slip, smokers should be encouraged to continue the attempt at cessation without viewing the effort as a failure. Measures to assist an individual in quitting should be directed toward the meaning that smoking has to that individual. The nurse needs to be aware of resources in the community to assist the individual who is interested in quitting.

ACUTE INTERVENTION. Care of the patient with lung cancer will initially involve support and reassurance during the diagnostic evaluation. (Specific nursing measures related to the diagnostic studies are outlined in Chapter 28.)

Another major responsibility of the nurse is to help the patient and the family cope with the diagnosis of lung cancer. The patient may feel guilty about cigarette smoking having caused the cancer and need to discuss this feeling with someone who has a nonjudgemental attitude. Questions regarding the patient's condition should be answered honestly. Additional counselling from a social worker, psychologist, or member of the clergy may be needed. Specific care of the patient will depend on the treatment plan. Postoperative care for the patient having surgery is discussed later in this chapter. Care of the patient undergoing radiation therapy and chemotherapy is discussed in Chapter 18 and in NCP 18.1 and NCP 18.2, on the Evolve website. The nurse has a major role in providing patient comfort, teaching methods to reduce pain, assessing for signs and symptoms of progressive or recurrent disease, and assessing indications for hospitalization.

AMBULATORY AND HOME CARE. Patient teaching needs to include signs and symptoms to report, such as hemoptysis, dysphagia, chest pain, and hoarseness. The patient and caregivers should be encouraged to provide a smoke-free environment, which may include smoking cessation for multiple family members.

If the treatment plan includes the use of home oxygen, teaching must include the safe use of oxygen. The patient who has had a surgical resection with intent to cure should be followed up with carefully, to watch for manifestations of metastasis. The patient and family should be told to contact the physician if symptoms such as hemoptysis, dysphagia, chest pain, and hoarseness develop. For many individuals who have lung cancer, little can be done to significantly prolong their lives. Radiation therapy and chemotherapy can be used to provide palliative relief from distressing symptoms. Constant pain can become a major issue. (Measures used to relieve pain are discussed in Chapter 10. Care of the patient with cancer is discussed in Chapter 18.) The patient and family or caregivers may need information about palliative care options in the community.

EVALUATION

The following are the expected outcomes for the patient with lung cancer:
- Patient will have adequate breathing patterns.
- Patient will have adequate airway clearance.
- Patient will have adequate tissue oxygenation.
- Patient will have minimal to no pain.
- Patient will have a realistic attitude about prognosis.

OTHER TYPES OF LUNG TUMOURS

Other types of primary lung tumours include sarcomas, lymphomas, and bronchial adenomas. Bronchial adenomas are small tumours that arise from the lower trachea or major bronchi and are considered malignant because they are locally invasive and frequently metastasize. Clinical manifestations of bronchial adenomas include hemoptysis, persistent cough, localized obstructive wheezing, and pneumonia. Bronchial adenomas can usually be treated successfully with surgical resection.

The lungs are a common site for secondary metastases and are more often affected by metastatic growth than by primary lung tumours. The pulmonary capillaries, with their extensive network, are ideal sites for tumour emboli. In addition, the lungs have an extensive lymphatic network. The primary malignancies that spread to the lungs often originate in the GI or genitourinary tracts and in the breast. General symptoms of lung metastases are chest pain and nonproductive cough.

Benign tumours of the lung are generally classified as *mesenchymal.* Their occurrence is rare and they have the potential to become malignant. The most common mesenchymal tumours are *chondromas,* which arise in the bronchial cartilage, and *leiomyomas,* which are myomas of smooth, nonstriated muscle fibres. Mesotheliomas may be malignant or benign and originate from the visceral pleura. Benign mesotheliomas are localized lesions.

Hamartomas of the lung are the most common benign tumour. These tumours, composed of fibrous tissue, fat, and

EVIDENCE-INFORMED PRACTICE

Research Highlight

Do Noninvasive Interventions Improve Quality of Life in Patients With Lung Cancer?

Clinical Question

In small cell lung cancer patients (P), what are the effects of preoperative exercise interventions in patients after surgery (I) compared to usual rehabilitation interventions (C) on outcomes related to functional capacity, mental wellness, and medical care (O)?

Best Available Evidence

- Systematic review of randomized controlled trials (RCTs)

Critical Appraisal and Synthesis of Evidence

- Meta-analysis of 10 clinical trials
- Interventions studied included combinations of interventions to manage breathlessness, including aerobic training, inspiratory muscle training, and strength training, inspiratory muscle training, and/or multicomponent training.

Conclusions

- There was a significant beneficial effect of a 6-minute walk distance on dyspnea, postoperative hospitalizations, and postoperative pulmonary complications.
- Physical exercise is an effective treatment to improve exercise tolerance, reduce dyspnea, and improve quality of life in patients with cancer.
- Preoperative exercise is effective in reducing postoperative complications and length of hospital stay in patients undergoing lung cancer surgery.
- Exercise training improves dyspnea in postoperative patients, in particular when aerobic training is part of a postoperative pulmonary rehabilitation program.

Implications for Nursing Practice

- Physical exercise should be considered a standard of preoperative care.
- These interventions may decrease the cost of medical care, which would be beneficial both for patients and for the public.
- Future studies should clearly describe the content of the exercise intervention, as well as the adherence rates to interventions, and they should also report potential adverse events associated with the exercise session.

Reference for Evidence

Rosero, I. D., Ramírez-Vélez, R., Lucía, A., et al. (2019). Systematic review and meta-analysis of randomized, controlled trials on preoperative physical exercise interventions in patients with non-small-cell lung cancer. *Cancers, 11*(7), 944. https://doi.org/10.3390/cancers11070944

P, patient population of interest; *I*, intervention or area of interest; *C*, comparison of interest or comparison group; *O*, outcome(s) of interest (see Chapter 1).

blood vessels, are congenital malformations of the connective tissue of the bronchiolar walls. Hamartomas are slow-growing tumours.

CHEST TRAUMA AND THORACIC INJURIES

Traumatic injuries fall into two major categories: (1) blunt trauma and (2) penetrating trauma. *Blunt trauma* occurs when the body is struck by a blunt object, such as a steering wheel. The external injury may appear minor, but the impact may cause severe, life-threatening internal injuries, such as a ruptured spleen. *Contrecoup trauma*, a type of blunt trauma, is caused by the impact of parts of the body against other objects. This type of injury differs from blunt trauma primarily in the velocity of the impact. Internal organs are rapidly forced back and forth

TABLE 30.15	COMMON TRAUMATIC CHEST INJURIES AND MECHANISMS OF INJURY	
Mechanism of Injury	**Common Related Injury**
Blunt Trauma	
Blunt steering-wheel injury to chest	Rib fractures, flail chest, pneumothorax, hemopneumothorax, cardiac contusion, pulmonary contusion, cardiac tamponade, great vessel tears
Shoulder-harness seat belt injury	Fractured clavicle, dislocated shoulder, rib fractures, pulmonary contusion, pericardial contusion, cardiac tamponade
Crush injury (e.g., heavy equipment, crushing thorax)	Pneumothorax and hemopneumothorax, flail chest, great vessel tears and rupture, decreased blood return to heart with decreased cardiac output
Penetrating Trauma	
Gunshot or stab wound to chest	Open pneumothorax, tension pneumothorax, hemopneumothorax, cardiac tamponade, esophageal damage, tracheal tear, great vessel tears

within the bony structures that surround them so that internal injury is sustained not only on the side of the impact but also on the opposite side, where the organ or organs hit bony structures. If the velocity of impact is great enough, organs and blood vessels can literally be torn from their points of origin. This is the shearing injury that can cause transection of the aorta, hemothorax, and diaphragmatic rupture injuries. Compression injury occurs when the body cannot handle the degree of external pressure during blunt trauma, resulting in contusions, crush injuries, and organ rupture.

Penetrating trauma occurs when a foreign body impales or passes through the body tissues (e.g., gunshot wounds, stabbings). Table 30.15 describes selective traumatic injuries as they relate to the categories of trauma and the mechanism of injury. Emergency care of the patient with a chest injury is presented in Table 30.16.

Thoracic injuries range from simple rib fractures to life-threatening tears of the aorta, vena cava, and other major vessels. The most common thoracic emergencies and their management are described in Table 30.17.

PNEUMOTHORAX

A **pneumothorax** is the presence of air in the pleural space. A complete or partial collapse of a lung results from this accumulation of air. This condition should be suspected after any blunt trauma to the chest wall. Pneumothorax may be closed or open. Pneumothorax associated with trauma may be accompanied by hemothorax, a condition called *hemopneumothorax*.

Types of Pneumothorax

Closed Pneumothorax. *Closed pneumothorax* has no associated external wound. The most common form is a spontaneous pneumothorax, which is accumulation of air in the pleural space without an apparent antecedent event. It is caused by the rupture of small **blebs** (air-filled alveolar dilations less than 1 cm in diameter on the edge of the lung at the apex of the upper lobe or superior segment of the lower lobe) on the visceral pleural space. The cause of the blebs is unknown. This condition

✚ TABLE 30.16 EMERGENCY MANAGEMENT

Chest Trauma

Etiology	Assessment Findings	Interventions
Blunt • Motor vehicle collision • Pedestrian accident • Fall • Assault with blunt object • Crush injury • Explosion **Penetrating** • Knife • Gunshot • Stick • Arrow • Other missiles	**Respiratory** • Dyspnea, respiratory distress • Cough with or without hemoptysis • Cyanosis of mouth, face, nail beds, mucous membranes • Tracheal deviation • Audible air escaping from chest wound • Decreased breath sounds on side of injury • Decreased O_2 saturation • Frothy secretions **Cardiovascular** • Rapid, thready pulse • Decreased blood pressure • Narrowed pulse pressure • Asymmetrical blood pressure values in arms • Distended neck veins • Muffled heart sounds • Chest pain • Crunching sound synchronous with heart sounds • Dysrhythmias **Surface Findings** • Bruising • Abrasions • Open chest wound • Asymmetrical chest movement • Subcutaneous emphysema	**Initial** • Ensure patent airway. • Administer high-flow O_2 with nonrebreather mask. • Establish IV access with two large-bore catheters. Begin fluid resuscitation as appropriate. • Remove clothing to assess injury. • Cover sucking chest wound with nonporous dressing taped on three sides. • Stabilize impaling objects with bulky dressings. Do not remove. • Assess for other significant injuries and treat appropriately. • Stabilize flail rib segment first with hand and then by application of large pieces of tape horizontal across the flail segment. • After cervical spine injury has been ruled out, place patient in semi-Fowler's position or position patient on the injured side if breathing is easier. **Ongoing Monitoring** • Monitor vital signs, level of consciousness, O_2 saturation, cardiac rhythm, respiratory status, and urinary output. • Anticipate intubation for respiratory distress. • Release dressing if tension pneumothorax develops after sucking chest wound is covered.

IV, intravenous; O_2, oxygen.

✚ TABLE 30.17 EMERGENCY MANAGEMENT

Thoracic Injuries

Definition	Clinical Manifestations	Emergency Management
Pneumothorax Air in pleural space (see Figure 30.5)	Dyspnea, decreased movement of involved chest wall, diminished or absent breath sounds on the affected side, hyper-resonance to percussion	Chest tube insertion with chest drainage system; Heimlich (flutter) valve
Hemothorax Blood in the pleural space, usually occurs in conjunction with pneumothorax	Dyspnea, diminished or absent breath sounds, dullness to percussion, shock	Chest tube insertion with chest drainage system; autotransfusion of collected blood, treatment of hypovolemia as necessary
Tension Pneumothorax Air in pleural space that does not escape Continued increase in amount of air shifts intrathoracic organs and increases intrathoracic pressure (see Figure 30.6)	Cyanosis, air hunger, violent agitation, tracheal deviation away from affected side, subcutaneous emphysema, neck vein distension, hyper-resonance to percussion	Medical emergency: needle decompression followed by chest tube insertion with chest drainage system
Flail Chest Fracture of two or more adjacent ribs in two or more places with loss of chest-wall stability (see Figure 30.7)	Paradoxical movement of chest wall, respiratory distress, associated hemothorax, pneumothorax, pulmonary contusion	Stabilization of flail segment with intubation in some patients and taping in others; oxygen therapy; treatment of associated injuries; analgesia
Cardiac Tamponade Blood rapidly collects in pericardial sac, compresses myocardium because the pericardium does not stretch, and prevents heart from pumping effectively	Muffled, distant heart sounds, hypotension, neck vein distension, increased central venous pressure	Medical emergency: pericardiocentesis with surgical repair as appropriate

occurs most commonly in underweight male cigarette smokers between 20 and 40 years of age. There is a tendency for this condition to recur.

Other causes of closed pneumothorax include the following:

- Injury to the lungs from mechanical ventilation
- Injury to the lungs from insertion of a subclavian catheter
- Perforation of the esophagus
- Injury to the lungs from broken ribs
- Ruptured blebs or bullae in a patient with COPD

Open Pneumothorax. *Open pneumothorax* occurs when air enters the pleural space through an opening in the chest wall (Figure 30.5, *B*). Examples include stab or gunshot wounds and surgical thoracotomies. A penetrating chest wound is often referred to as a *sucking chest wound.*

An open pneumothorax should be covered with a vented dressing. (A vented dressing is one secured on three sides with the fourth side left untaped.) This allows air to escape from the vent and decreases the likelihood of tension pneumothorax developing. If the object that caused the open chest wound is still in place, it should not be removed until a health care provider is present. The impaling object should be stabilized with a bulky dressing.

Tension Pneumothorax. Tension pneumothorax is a pneumothorax with rapid accumulation of air in the pleural space, causing severely high intrapleural pressures with resultant tension on the heart and great vessels. It may result from either an open or a closed pneumothorax (Figure 30.6). In an open chest wound, a flap may act as a one-way valve; thus, air can enter on inspiration but cannot escape. The intrathoracic pressure increases, the lung collapses, and the mediastinum shifts toward the unaffected side, which is subsequently compressed. As the pressure increases, cardiac output is altered because of decreased venous return and compression of the vena cava and aorta. Tension pneumothorax can occur with mechanical ventilation and resuscitative efforts. It can also occur if chest tubes are clamped or become blocked in a patient with a pneumothorax. Unclamping the tube or relieving the obstruction will remedy this situation.

Tension pneumothorax is a medical emergency with both the respiratory and the circulatory systems affected. If the tension in the pleural space is not relieved, the patient is likely to die from inadequate cardiac output or marked hypoxemia. Nurses and paramedics are now being trained to insert large-bore needles and chest tubes into the chest wall to release the trapped air.

Hemothorax. Hemothorax is an accumulation of blood in the intrapleural space. It is frequently found in association with open pneumothorax and is then a hemopneumothorax. Causes of hemothorax include chest trauma, lung malignancy, complications of anticoagulant therapy, pulmonary embolus, and tearing of pleural adhesions.

Chylothorax. Chylothorax is the presence of lymphatic fluid in the pleural space because of a leak in the thoracic duct. Causes include trauma, surgical procedures, and malignancy. The thoracic duct is disrupted, and the chylous fluid, milky white with high lipid content, fills the pleural space. Total lymphatic flow through the thoracic duct is 1 500 to 2 400 mL/day. Fifty percent of those affected will heal with conservative treatment (chest drainage, bowel rest, and total parenteral nutrition). Surgery and pleurodesis are options if conservative therapy fails. *Pleurodesis* is the artificial production of adhesions between the parietal and the visceral pleurae, usually done with a chemical sclerosing agent.

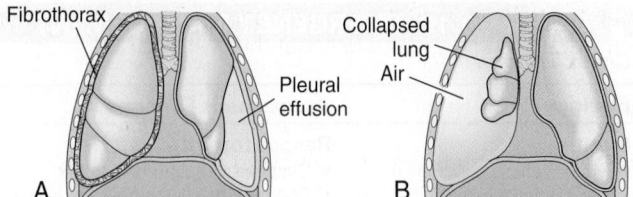

FIG. 30.5 Disorders of the pleura. **A,** Fibrothorax resulting from an organization of inflammatory exudate and pleural effusion. **B,** Open pneumothorax resulting from collapse of the lung caused by disruption of the chest wall and outside air entering.

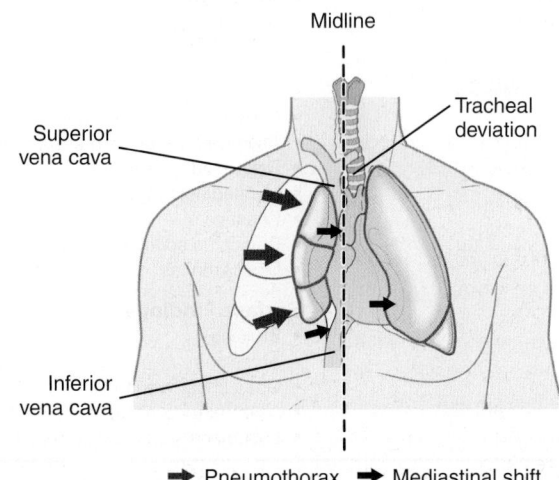

FIG. 30.6 Tension pneumothorax. As pleural pressure on the affected side increases, mediastinal displacement ensues with resultant respiratory and cardiovascular compromise.

Clinical Manifestations

If the pneumothorax is small, mild tachycardia and dyspnea may be the only manifestations. If the pneumothorax is large, respiratory distress may be present, including shallow, rapid respirations; dyspnea; air hunger; and decreased oxygen saturation. Chest pain and a cough with or without hemoptysis may be present. On auscultation, there are no breath sounds over the affected area, and hyper-resonance may be present. A chest radiograph shows the presence of air or fluid in the pleural space. If a tension pneumothorax develops, the patient experiences severe respiratory distress, tachycardia, and hypotension. Mediastinal displacement occurs, and the trachea shifts to the unaffected side. The patient is hemodynamically unstable.

Interprofessional Care

Treatment depends on the severity of the pneumothorax and the nature of the underlying disease. If the patient is stable and the amount of air and fluid accumulated in the intrapleural space is minimal, no treatment may be needed as the pneumothorax resolves spontaneously. If the amount of air or fluid is minimal, the pleural space can be aspirated with a large-bore needle. As a life-saving measure, needle venting (using a large-bore needle) of the pleural space may be used. A Heimlich valve may also be used to evacuate air from the pleural space. The most definitive and common form of treatment of pneumothorax and hemothorax is the insertion of a chest tube that is connected to water-seal drainage. Repeated spontaneous pneumothorax may have to be treated surgically by a partial pleurectomy, stapling, or pleurodesis to promote adherence of the pleurae to one another.

FRACTURED RIBS

Rib fractures are the most common type of chest injury resulting from trauma. Ribs 5 through 10 are most commonly fractured because they are least protected by chest muscles. If the fractured rib is splintered or displaced, it may damage the pleura and the lungs.

Clinical manifestations of fractured ribs include pain (especially on inspiration) at the site of injury. The individual splints the affected area and takes shallow breaths to try to decrease the pain. The person is reluctant to take deep breaths, and the decreased ventilation may cause atelectasis to develop.

The main goal of treatment is to decrease pain so that the patient can breathe adequately to promote good chest expansion. Intercostal nerve blocks with local anaesthesia may be used to provide pain relief. The effect of the anaesthesia lasts for a period of hours to days. It must be repeated as necessary to provide pain relief. Opioid medication therapy must be individualized and used with caution because these medications can depress respirations. Nonsteroidal anti-inflammatory medications are used to reduce pain and aid with deep breathing and coughing. Patient teaching should emphasize deep breathing, coughing, use of incentive spirometry, and use of pain medications. Strapping the chest with tape or using a binder is not common practice. Most health care providers believe that these measures should be avoided because they reduce lung expansion and predispose the individual to atelectasis.

FLAIL CHEST

Flail chest results from multiple rib fractures, causing instability of the chest wall (Figure 30.7). The chest wall cannot provide the bony structure necessary to maintain bellows action and ventilation. The affected (flail) area will move paradoxically to the intact portion of the chest during respiration. During inspiration, the affected portion is sucked in, and during expiration, it bulges out. This paradoxical chest movement prevents adequate ventilation of the lung in the injured area. The underlying lung may or may not have a serious injury. Associated pain and any lung injury giving rise to loss of compliance will contribute to an alteration in breathing patterns and lead to hypoxemia.

A flail chest is usually apparent on visual examination of the unconscious patient. The patient manifests rapid, shallow respirations and tachycardia. A flail chest may not be initially apparent in the conscious patient as a result of splinting of the chest wall. The patient moves air poorly, and movement of the thorax is asymmetrical and uncoordinated. Palpation of abnormal respiratory movements, crepitus of the rib, chest radiography, and ABG assessment assist in the diagnosis.

Initial therapy consists of adequate ventilation, administration of humidified oxygen, careful administration of crystalloid IV solutions, and pain control. The definitive therapy is to re-expand the lung and ensure adequate oxygenation. Although many patients can be managed without the use of mechanical ventilation, a short period of intubation and ventilation may be necessary until the diagnosis of the lung injury is complete. The lung parenchyma and fractured ribs will heal with time. Some patients continue to experience intercostal pain after the flail chest has resolved.

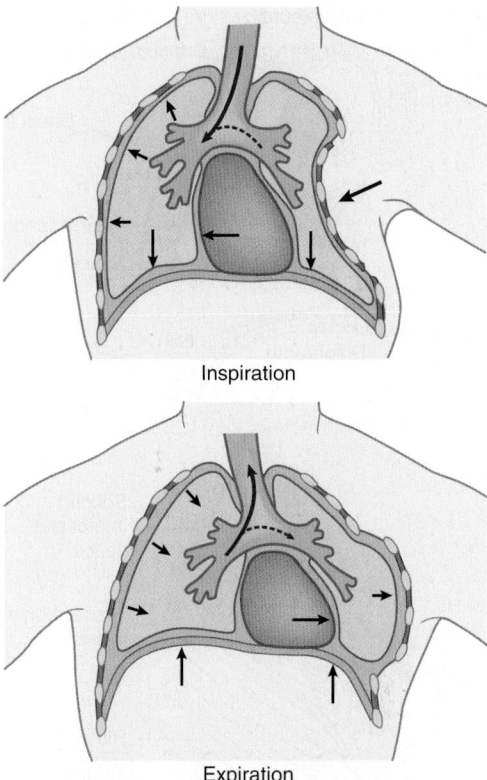

FIG. 30.7 Flail chest produces paradoxical respiration. On inspiration, the flail section sinks in with the mediastinal shift to the uninjured side. On expiration, the flail section bulges outward with the mediastinal shift to the injured side.

CHEST TUBES AND PLEURAL DRAINAGE

The purpose of chest tubes and pleural drainage is to remove the air and fluid from the pleural space and to restore normal intrapleural pressure so that the lungs can re-expand. (Intrapleural pressure, also known as *intrathoracic pressure*, and the intrapleural space are described in Chapter 28.) Small accumulations of air or fluid in the pleural space may not require removal by thoracentesis or chest tube insertion. Instead, the air and fluid may be reabsorbed over time.

Chest Tube Insertion

Chest tubes can be inserted in the emergency department, at the patient's bedside, or in the operating room, depending on the situation. In the operating room, the chest tube is inserted via the thoracotomy incision. In the emergency department or at the bedside, the patient is placed in a sitting position or is lying down with the affected side elevated. Prior to the procedure it is important to have airway, oxygen, suction, and defibrillation equipment available at the bedside in case emergency resuscitation is required. The area is prepared with antiseptic solution, and the site is infiltrated with a local anaesthetic agent. After a small incision is made, one or two chest tubes are inserted into the pleural space. One catheter is placed anteriorly through the second intercostal space to remove air (Figure 30.8). The other is placed posteriorly through the eighth or ninth intercostal space to drain fluid and blood. The tubes are sutured to the chest wall, and the puncture wound is covered with an airtight dressing. During insertion, the tubes are kept clamped. After the tubes are in place in the pleural space, they are connected to drainage tubing and pleural drainage, and the clamp is removed.

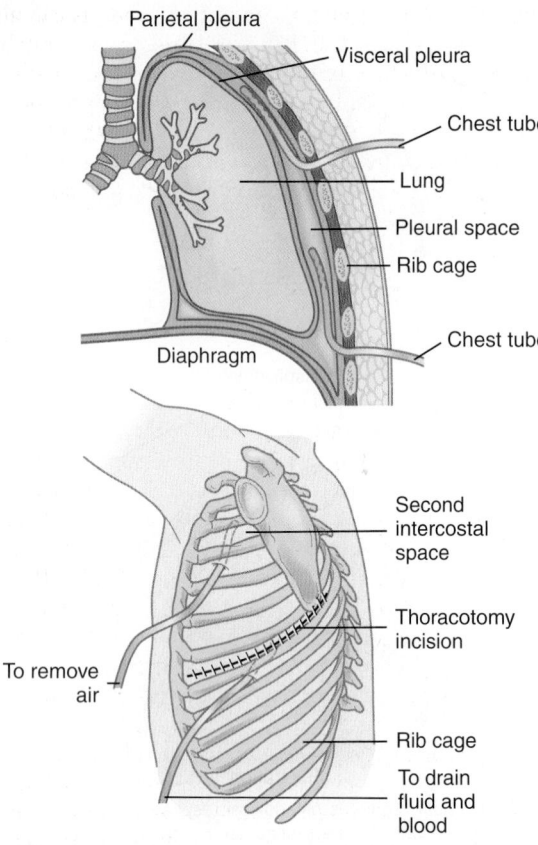

FIG. 30.8 Placement of chest tubes.

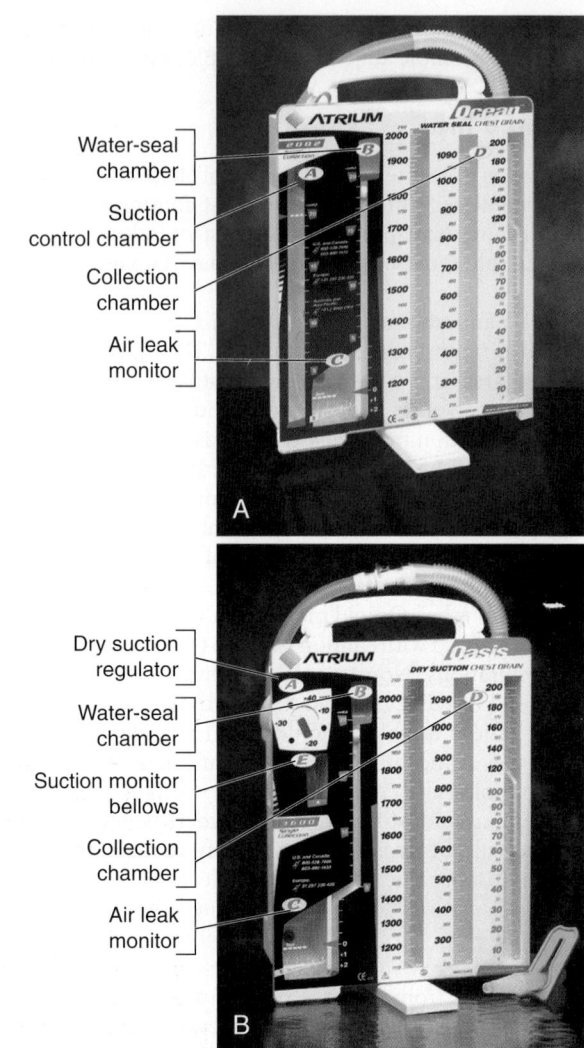

FIG. 30.9 Chest drainage unit. Both units have three chambers: (1) collection chamber; (2) water-seal chamber; and (3) suction control chamber. The suction control chamber requires a connection to a wall suction source that is dialed up higher than prescribed so that the suction will work. **A,** Water suction. This unit uses water in the suction control chamber to control the wall suction pressure. **B,** Dry suction. This unit controls wall suction by using a regulator control dial. Source: Getinge Group, Merrimack, NH.

Each tube may be connected to a separate drainage system and suction. More commonly, a Y-connector is used to attach both chest tubes to the same drainage system.

Pleural Drainage

Most pleural drainage systems have three basic compartments, each with its own separate function.

The first compartment, the *collection chamber*, receives fluid and air from the chest cavity. The fluid stays in this chamber while the air vents to the second compartment (Figure 30.9). The second compartment, called the *water-seal chamber*, contains 2 cm of water, which acts as a one-way valve. The incoming air enters from the collection chamber and bubbles up through the water. (The water acts as a one-way valve to prevent backflow of air into the patient from the system.) Initial bubbling of air is seen in this chamber when a pneumothorax is evacuated. Intermittent bubbling can also be seen during exhalation, coughing, or sneezing because of an increase in the patient's intrathoracic pressure. In this chamber, fluctuations, or "tidalling," will be seen and reflect the pressures in the pleural space. If tidalling is not seen, either the lungs have re-expanded or there is a kink or obstruction in the tubing. The air then exits the water seal and enters the suction chamber.

A third compartment, the *suction control chamber*, applies controlled suction to the chest drainage system. The classic suction control chamber uses tubing with one end submerged in a column of water and the other end vented to the atmosphere. It is typically filled with 20 cm of water. When the negative pressure generated by the suction source exceeds 20 cm, the air from the atmosphere enters the chamber through a vent and begins bubbling up through the water. As a result, excess pressure is

relieved. The amount of suction applied is regulated by the depth of the suction control tube in the water and not by the amount of suction applied to the system. An increase in suction does not result in an increase in negative pressure to the system because any excess suction merely draws in air through the vented tubing. The suction pressure is usually ordered to be -20 cm H_2O.

Two types of suction control chambers are available on the market: wet and dry. The wet suction control chamber system is the classic system outlined previously. Bubbling is one way to tell that suction is functioning. Suction is started by turning up the vacuum source until gentle bubbling appears. Turning the vacuum source higher just makes the bubbling more vigorous and makes the water evaporate faster. Even with gentle bubbling, water evaporates in this chamber, and water must be added periodically. The dry suction control chamber system, by contrast, contains no water. It uses either a restrictive device or a regulator, internal to the chest drainage system, to dial the desired negative pressure. The dry system has a visual alert that

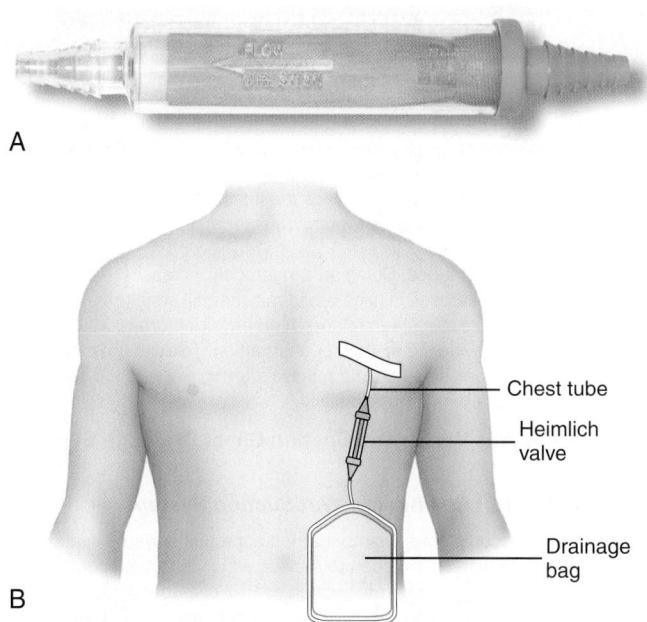

FIG. 30.10 **A,** The Heimlich chest drain valve is a specially designed flutter valve that is used in place of a chest drainage unit for small, uncomplicated pneumothorax with little or no drainage and no need for suction. The valve allows for escape of air but prevents the re-entry of air into the pleural space. **B,** The valve is placed between the chest tube and the drainage bag, which can be worn under a person's clothes.

indicates if the suction is working, so bubbling is not seen in a third chamber. The suction pressures are increased by turning the dial on the drainage system. Increasing the vacuum suction source will not increase the pressure (see Figure 30.9).

A variety of commercial disposable plastic chest drainage systems are available. The manufacturer's suggestions for use are included with the equipment. The plastic units allow the patient mobility and decrease the risk of breaking or spilling the drainage system.

Heimlich Valves. Another device that may be used to evacuate air from the pleural space is the Heimlich valve (Figure 30.10). This device consists of a rubber flutter one-way valve within a rigid plastic tube. It is attached to the external end of the chest tube. The valve opens whenever the pressure is greater than the atmospheric pressure and closes when the reverse occurs. The Heimlich valve functions like a water seal and is usually used for emergency transport or in special home care situations.

Small Chest Tubes. Small chest tubes ("pigtail catheters") are used in selected patients because they are less traumatic. The drains may be straight catheters or "pigtail" catheters (curled at the distal end, resembling a pig's tail). Curled catheters are considered to be less traumatic than straight catheters. These catheters, if occluded, can be irrigated by the health care

provider using sterile water. Chemical pleurodesis can also be performed through this catheter. This system is not suitable for trauma or for drainage of blood. Because of the smaller size, the tube can become kinked, occluded, or dislodged more easily. Small-bore chest tubes and Heimlich valves should be used with caution in patients on mechanical ventilators because there is a potential for rapid accumulation of air and a tension pneumothorax.

NURSING MANAGEMENT
CHEST DRAINAGE

Some general guidelines for nursing care of the patient with chest tubes and water-seal drainage systems are presented in Table 30.18. The traditional practice of routine milking or stripping of chest tubes to maintain patency is no longer recommended because it can cause dangerously high intrapleural pressure and damage to pleural tissue. Drainage and blood are not likely to clot inside chest tubes because the newer chest tubes are made with a coating that makes them nonthrombogenic. The nurse should remember that insertion of the chest tube, as well as its continued presence, can be painful to the patient. Dislodgement of the tube may occur if the tube is not stabilized.

Clamping of chest tubes during transport or when the tube is accidentally disconnected is no longer advocated. The danger of rapid accumulation of air in the pleural space causing tension pneumothorax is far greater than that of a small amount of atmospheric air entering the pleural space. Chest tubes may be momentarily clamped to change the drainage apparatus or to check for air leaks. Clamping for more than a few moments is indicated only for assessing how the patient will tolerate chest tube removal. It is done to simulate chest tube removal and identify if there will be negative clinical repercussions with tube removal. Generally, this is done 4 to 6 hours before the tube is removed, and the patient is monitored closely. If a chest tube becomes disconnected, the most important intervention is immediate re-establishment of the water-seal system and attachment of a new drainage system as soon as possible. In some hospitals, when disconnection occurs, the chest tube is immersed in sterile water (≈2 cm) until the system can be re-established. It is important for the nurse to know the unit policies, individual clinical situation (e.g., whether an air leak exists), and physician preference before resorting to prolonged chest tube clamping.

As with many procedures, the hospital may have policies and procedures referring to the care of chest tubes. The nurse needs to ensure that these are reviewed and followed.

COMPLICATIONS

Chest tube malposition is the most common complication. The nurse does routine monitoring to evaluate whether the chest drainage is successful by observing for tidalling in the water-seal chamber, listening for breath sounds over the lung fields, and measuring the amount of fluid drainage. Re-expansion pulmonary edema can occur after rapid expansion of a collapsed lung in patients with a pneumothorax or with evacuation of large volumes of pleural fluid (>1 to 1.5 L). A vasovagal response with symptomatic hypotension can occur from too-rapid removal of fluid.

Infection at the skin site is also a concern. Meticulous sterile technique during dressing changes can reduce the incidence of infected sites. Other complications include (a) pneumonia from not taking deep breaths, from not using an incentive spirometer,

TABLE 30.18   CLINICAL GUIDELINES FOR CARE OF PATIENT WITH CHEST TUBES AND WATER-SEAL DRAINAGE SYSTEM

1. Keep all tubing loosely coiled below chest level. Tubing should drop straight from bed or chair to drainage unit. Do not let it be compressed.
2. Keep all connections between chest tubes, drainage tubing, and drainage collector tight, and tape at connections.
3. Observe for air fluctuations (tidalling) and bubbling in the water-seal chamber.
   • If no tidalling is observed (rising with inspiration and falling with expiration in the spontaneously breathing patient), the drainage system is blocked, the lungs are re-expanded, or the system is attached to suction.
   • If bubbling increases, there may be an air leak in the drainage system or a leak from the patient (bronchopleural leak).
4. If the chest tube is connected to suction, disconnect from wall suction to check for tidalling.
5. Suspect a system leak when bubbling is continuous.
   • To determine the source of the air leak, momentarily clamp the tubing successively from the chest tube insertion site to the drainage set, observing for the bubbling to cease. When bubbling ceases, the leak is above the clamp.
   • Retape tubing connections.
   • If leak continues, notify physician. It may be necessary to replace the drainage apparatus or to secure the chest tube with an air-occlusive dressing.
6. High fluid levels in the water seal indicate residual negative pressure.
   • The chest system may need to be vented by using the high negativity release valve available on the drainage system to release residual pressure from the system.
   • Do not lower water-seal column when wall suction is not operating or when patient is on gravity drainage.

Patient's Clinical Status

1. Monitor patient's clinical status. Assess vital signs, lung sounds, pain.
2. Assess for manifestations of re-accumulation of air and fluid in the chest (↓ or absent breath sounds), significant bleeding (>100 mL/hr), chest drainage site infection (drainage, erythema, fever, ↑ white blood cell count), or poor wound healing. Notify physician for management plan. Evaluate for subcutaneous emphysema at chest tube site.
3. Encourage patient to breathe deeply periodically to facilitate lung expansion and encourage range-of-motion exercises to the shoulder on the affected side. Incentive spirometry every hour while awake may be necessary to prevent atelectasis or pneumonia.
4. Chest tubes are *not routinely clamped*. A physician order is required. A physician may order clamping for 24 hours to evaluate for re-accumulation of fluid or air before discontinuing the chest tube.

Chest Drainage

1. Never elevate the drainage system to the level of the patient's chest because doing so will cause fluid to drain back into the lungs. Secure the unit to the drainage stand. If the drainage chambers are full, notify the physician and anticipate changing the system. Do not try to empty it.
2. Mark the time of measurement and the fluid level on the drainage unit according to the unit standards. Report any change in the quantity or characteristics of drainage (e.g., clear yellow to bloody) to the physician and record the change. Notify physician if >100 mL/hr drainage.

3. Check position of the chest drainage container. If the drainage system is overturned and the water seal is disrupted, return it to an upright position and encourage patient to take a few deep breaths, followed by forced exhalations and cough manoeuvres.
4. If the drainage system breaks, place the distal end of the chest tubing connection in a sterile water container at a 2-cm level as an emergency water seal.
5. Do not strip chest tubes. Doing so dangerously increases intrapleural pressures. Drainage tubes may be milked (alternately folded or squeezed and then released) on physician order. Milk only if drainage has evidence of clots or obstruction. Take 15-cm strips of the chest tube and squeeze and release starting close to the chest and repeating down the tube distally.

Monitoring Wet Versus Dry Suction Chest Drainage Systems

Suction Control Chamber in Wet Suction System

1. Keep the suction control chamber at the appropriate water level by adding sterile water as needed to replace water lost to evaporation.
2. Keep the muffler covering the suction control chamber in place to prevent more rapid evaporation of water and to decrease noise of the bubbling.
3. After filling the suction control chamber to the ordered suction amount (generally −20 cm water suction), connect the suction tubing to the wall suction.
4. Dial the wall suction regulator until continuous gentle bubbling is seen in the suction control chamber (generally 80–120 mm Hg). Vigorous bubbling is not necessary and will increase the rate of evaporation.
5. If no bubbling is seen in the suction control chamber, (a) there is no suction, (b) the suction is not set high enough, or (c) the pleural air leak is so large that suction is not high enough to evacuate it.

Suction Control Chamber in Dry Suction System (See Manufacturer's Directions)

1. After connecting patient to system, turn the dial on the chest drainage system to amount ordered (generally −20 cm pressure), connect suction tubing to wall suction source, and increase the suction until the correct amount of negative pressure is indicated. There will be a high negative-pressure release valve in the system.

Chest Tube Dressings

1. Dressings are not routinely changed. If there is visible drainage, notify physician for instructions.
2. If ordered to change dressings, remove old dressing carefully to avoid removing unsecured chest tube. Assess the site, and culture site as indicated.
3. Cleanse the site with sterile normal saline. Apply sterile gauze and tape to secure the dressing. Some physicians may prefer use of petroleum gauze dressing around the tube to prevent air leak. Date the dressing and document dressing change.

Obtaining a Sample From the Chest Tube

1. Form a loop in the tubing in an area to get the most recently drained fluid.
2. Swab the sampling site of the tubing with antiseptic and allow to air-dry.
3. Aspirate from the sampling site with a syringe; cap syringe; label with patient name, date, time, and source of specimen.
4. Send to laboratory.

and from splinting on the affected side, and (b) shoulder disuse ("frozen shoulder") from lack of range-of-motion exercises. Poor patient adherence or lack of patient teaching can contribute to these complications. Nurses have a key role in preventing these complications.

CHEST TUBE REMOVAL

The patient with chest tubes may have chest radiographic studies to follow the course of lung expansion. The chest tubes are removed when the lungs are re-expanded and fluid drainage has ceased. Generally, suction is discontinued, and the patient is

TABLE 30.19 CHEST SURGERIES

Type and Description	Indication	Comments
Lobectomy		
Removal of one lobe of lung	Lung cancer, bronchiectasis, TB, emphysematous bullae, benign lung tumours, fungal infections	Most common lung surgery; postoperative insertion of chest tubes; expansion of remaining lung tissue to fill up space
Pneumonectomy		
Removal of entire lung	Lung cancer (most common), extensive TB, bronchiectasis, lung abscess	Done only when lobectomy or segmental resection will not remove all diseased lung; no drainage tubes (generally), fluid gradually fills space where lung was; patient positioned on operative side to facilitate expansion of remaining lung
Segmental Resection		
Removal of one or more lung segments	Lung cancer, bronchiectasis, TB	Technically difficult; done to remove lung segment; insertion of chest tubes; expansion of remaining lung tissue to fill space
Wedge Resection		
Removal of small, localized lesion that occupies only part of a segment	Lung biopsy, excision of small nodules	Need for chest tubes after surgery
Decortication		
Removal of thick, fibrous membrane from visceral pleura	Empyema	Use of chest tubes and drainage after surgery
Exploratory Thoracotomy		
Incision into thorax to look for injured or bleeding tissues	Chest trauma	Use of chest tubes and drainage after surgery
Thoracotomy Not Involving Lungs*		
Incision into thorax for surgery on other organs	Hiatal hernia repair, open-heart surgery, esophageal surgery, tracheal resection, aortic aneurysm repair	
Video-Assisted Thoracoscopic Surgery (VATS)		
VATS under general anaesthesia in OR	Procedures performed using VATS include lung biopsy, lobectomy, resection of nodules, repair of fistulas	Video-assisted technique involving insertion of a rigid scope with a distal lens into the pleura with image shown on a monitor screen, allowing surgeon to manipulate instruments passed into the pleural space through separate small intercostal incisions
Lung Volume Reduction Surgery (LVRS)		
	Advanced bullous emphysema, α_1-antitrypsin emphysema	Involves reducing lung volume by multiple wedge excisions or VATS (see Video-Assisted Thoracoscopic Surgery)

OR, operating room; *TB*, tuberculosis.
*For comments on thoracotomy not involving the lungs, see discussion of individual diseases in text.

placed on gravity drainage for a period of time before the tubes are removed. The tube is removed by cutting the sutures; applying a sterile petroleum jelly gauze dressing; having the patient take a deep breath, exhale, and bear down (Valsalva manoeuvre); and then removing the tube. Pain medication is generally given before chest tube removal. The site is covered with an airtight dressing, the pleura seals itself off, and the wound heals in several days. A chest radiograph is obtained after chest tube removal to evaluate for pneumothorax, re-accumulation of fluid, or both. The wound should be observed for drainage and should be reinforced if necessary. The patient should be observed for respiratory distress, which may signify a recurrent or new pneumothorax.

CHEST SURGERY

Chest surgery is performed for a variety of reasons, some of which are unrelated to primary lung conditions. For example,

a thoracotomy may be performed for heart and esophageal surgery. The types of chest surgery are compared in Table 30.19.

Preoperative Care

Before chest surgery, baseline data are obtained on the respiratory and cardiovascular systems. Diagnostic studies performed are pulmonary function, chest radiography, electrocardiogram (ECG), ABGs, blood urea nitrogen (serum urea [nitrogen]), serum creatinine, blood glucose, serum electrolytes, and complete blood cell count. Additional studies of cardiac function such as cardiac catheterization may be done for the patient who is to undergo a pneumonectomy. A careful physical assessment of the lungs, including percussion and auscultation, should be done. This will allow the nurse to compare preoperative and postoperative findings.

The patient should be encouraged to stop smoking before surgery to decrease secretions and increase oxygen saturation.

In the anxious period before surgery, refraining from smoking is not easy for the habitual smoker to do. Chest physiotherapy may be indicated to help drain the lungs of accumulated secretions. This is especially indicated for the patient with a lung abscess or bronchiectasis.

Preoperative teaching should include exercises for effective deep breathing and incentive spirometry. If the patient practises these techniques before surgery, the techniques will be easier to perform after surgery. The patient should be told that adequate medication will be given to reduce the pain and should be helped to splint the incision with a pillow to facilitate deep breathing.

For most types of chest surgery, chest tubes are inserted and connected to water-sealed drainage systems. The purpose of these tubes should be explained to the patient. In addition, oxygen is frequently given the first 24 hours after surgery. Range-of-motion exercises on the surgical side, similar to those for the mastectomy patient, should be taught (see Chapter 54).

The thought of losing part of a vital organ is frequently frightening. The patient should be reassured that the lungs have a large degree of functional reserve. Even after the removal of one lung, there is enough lung tissue to maintain adequate oxygenation.

The nurse should be available to answer questions asked by the patient and the family, and questions should be answered honestly. The nurse should try to facilitate expression of concerns, feelings, and questions. (General preoperative care and teaching are discussed in Chapter 20.)

Surgical Therapy

Thoracotomy (surgical opening into the thoracic cavity) surgery is considered major surgery because the incision is large and cuts into bone, muscle, and cartilage. The two types of thoracic incisions are median sternotomy, performed by splitting the sternum, and lateral thoracotomy. The median sternotomy is primarily used for surgery involving the heart. The two types of lateral thoracotomy are posterolateral and anterolateral. The posterolateral thoracotomy is used for most surgeries involving the lung. The incision is made from the anterior axillary line below the nipple level posteriorly at the fourth, fifth, or sixth intercostal space. It is rarely necessary to remove the ribs. Strong mechanical retractors are used to gain access to the lung. The anterolateral incision is made in the fourth or fifth intercostal space from the sternal border to the midaxillary line. This procedure is commonly used for surgery or trauma victims, mediastinal operations, and wedge resections of the upper and middle lobes of the lung.

The extensiveness of the thoracotomy incision often results in severe pain for the patient after surgery. Because muscles have been severed, the patient is reluctant to move their shoulder and arm on the surgical side. Chest tubes are placed in the pleural space except in pneumonectomy surgery. In a pneumonectomy, the space from which the lung was removed gradually fills with serosanguinous fluid.

Video-Assisted Thoracoscopic Surgery. Video-assisted thoracoscopic surgery (VATS) is a thoracoscopic surgical procedure that, in many cases, can be done instead of a full thoracotomy. The procedure involves three or four 2.5-cm incisions made on the chest that allow the thoracoscope (a special fibre-optic camera) and instruments to be inserted and manipulated. Video-assisted thoracoscopes improve visualization because the surgeon can view the thoracic cavity from the video monitor. The thoracoscope is equipped with a camera that magnifies the image on the monitor. Thoracoscopy can be used to diagnose and treat a variety of conditions of the lung, the pleura, and the mediastinum.

The candidate for this type of procedure should not have a prior history of conventional thoracic surgery, because of the probability of adhesion formation, which would make access more difficult. The patient whose lesions are in the lung periphery or the mediastinum is a better candidate because of better accessibility. The patient considered for thoracoscopic surgery should have sufficient pulmonary function before surgery to allow the surgeon to perform conventional thoracotomy if complications occur. Complications that may occur are bleeding, diaphragmatic perforation, air emboli, persistent pleural air leaks, and tension pneumothorax.

There are many benefits of thoracoscopic surgery when compared with a conventional thoracotomy procedure. These include less adhesion formation, minimal blood loss, less time under anaesthesia, shorter hospitalization, faster recovery, less pain, and no need for postoperative rehabilitation therapy because of minimal disruption of thoracic structures.

Chest tubes are placed at the end of the procedure through one of the incisions. The incisions are closed with sutures or a wound-approximating adhesive bandage. Nursing assessment and care after surgery include monitoring respiratory status and lung re-expansion with the chest tubes and checking the incisions for drainage or dehiscence. The most common complication is prolonged air leak. A return to prior activities should be encouraged as quickly as possible. The hospital stay averages from 1 to 5 days, depending on the type of surgery.

Postoperative Care

Specific measures related to nursing care after a thoracotomy are presented in NCP 30.2, available on the Evolve website. The specific follow-up care depends on the type of surgical procedure. General postoperative care is discussed in Chapter 22.

RESTRICTIVE RESPIRATORY DISORDERS

Restrictive respiratory disorders are characterized by a restriction in lung volume (caused by decreased compliance of the lungs or chest wall). This is in contrast to obstructive disorders, which are characterized by increased resistance to airflow (see Chapter 31). Pulmonary function tests are the best means of differentiating between restrictive and obstructive respiratory disorders (Table 30.20). Mixed obstructive and restrictive disorders are often manifested. For example, a patient may have both chronic bronchitis (an obstructive condition) and pulmonary fibrosis (a restrictive condition).

Restrictive problems are generally categorized into extrapulmonary and intrapulmonary disorders. Extrapulmonary causes of restrictive lung disease include disorders involving the central nervous system, neuromuscular system, and chest wall (Table 30.21). In these disorders, the lung tissue is normal. Intrapulmonary causes of restrictive lung disease involve the pleura or the lung tissue (Table 30.22).

PLEURAL EFFUSION

Types

The pleural space lies between the lung and the chest wall and normally contains a very thin layer of fluid. **Pleural effusion** is a collection of fluid in the pleural space (see Figure 30.5, *A*). It is not a disease but rather a sign of a serious disease. Pleural effusion is frequently classified as *transudative* or *exudative* according to whether the protein content of the effusion is low or high,

respectively. A transudate occurs primarily in noninflammatory conditions and is an accumulation of protein- and cell-poor fluid. Transudative pleural effusions (also called *hydrothorax*) are caused by (1) increased hydrostatic pressure found in heart failure, which is the most common cause of pleural effusion, or (2) decreased oncotic pressure (from hypoalbuminemia) found in chronic liver or renal disease. In these situations, fluid movement is facilitated out of the capillaries and into the pleural space.

An exudative effusion is an accumulation of fluid and cells in an area of inflammation. An exudative pleural effusion results from the increased capillary permeability characteristic of the inflammatory reaction. This type of effusion occurs secondary to conditions such as pulmonary malignancies, pulmonary infections, pulmonary embolization, and GI disease (e.g., pancreatic disease, esophageal perforation).

The type of pleural effusion can be determined from a sample of pleural fluid obtained via thoracentesis (a procedure to remove fluid from the pleural space). Exudates have a high

TABLE 30.20 RELATIONSHIP OF LUNG VOLUMES TO TYPE OF VENTILATORY DISORDER

Lung Volumes	Restrictive	Obstructive	Restrictive and Obstructive
Vital capacity (VC)	↓	Normal or ↓	↓
Total lung capacity (TLC)	↓	↑	Variable
Residual volume (RV)	Normal or ↓	↑	Variable
Forced expiratory volume in 1 sec (FEV₁)	Normal or ↓	↓	↓
FEV₁/Functional vital capacity (FVC)	Normal or ↑	↓	↓

TABLE 30.21 EXTRAPULMONARY CAUSES OF RESTRICTIVE LUNG DISEASE

Disease or Alteration	Description	Comments
Central Nervous System		
Head injury, CNS lesion (e.g., tumour, stroke)	Injury to or impingement on respiratory centre, causing hypoventilation or hyperventilation; relationship of manifestations to increased intracranial pressure (see Chapters 59 and 60)	Management is directed toward treating the underlying cause, maintaining the airway, using mechanical ventilation for supportive care, and assessing for manifestations of increased intracranial pressure.
Opioid and barbiturate use	Depression of respiratory centre, respiratory rate of <12 breaths/min	Respiratory depression is caused by drug overdose or inadvertent administration of medications to a person with respiratory difficulty. These medications should not be administered to a person with a respiratory rate of <12 breaths/min.
Neuromuscular System		
Spinal cord injury	Complete cervical- and complete upper thoracic–level injuries have restrictive ventilation. The lung volumes are reduced owing to inspiratory muscle weakness.	Patient with a cervical injury may need mechanical ventilator support initially.
Guillain-Barré syndrome	Acute inflammation of peripheral nerves and ganglia; paralysis of intercostal nerves leading to diaphragmatic breathing; paralysis of vagal preganglionic and postganglionic fibres leading to reduced ability of bronchioles to constrict, dilate, and respond to irritants	Patient often has to be put on mechanical ventilation for supportive care (see Chapter 63).
Amyotrophic lateral sclerosis	Progressive degenerative disorder of the motor neurons in the spinal cord, brainstem, and motor cortex; respiratory system involvement as a result of interruption of nerve transmission to respiratory muscles, especially diaphragm	See Chapter 61 for clinical manifestations and management.
Myasthenia gravis	Defect in neuromuscular junction; respiratory system involvement as a result of interruption of nerve transmission to respiratory muscles	See Chapter 61 for clinical manifestations and management.
Muscular dystrophy	Hereditary disease; eventual involvement of all skeletal muscles; paralysis of respiratory muscles, including intercostals, diaphragm, and accessory muscles	Pulmonary difficulties develop late in disease process.
Chest Wall		
Chest-wall trauma (e.g., flail chest, fractured rib)	Rib fracture causing inspiratory pain; voluntary splinting of chest, resulting in shallow, rapid breathing; impaired ventilatory ability caused by paradoxical breathing	Strapping the chest wall to stabilize the fractures is not recommended because this increases the restrictive defect.
Pickwickian syndrome (extreme obesity)	Excess adipose tissue interfering with chest-wall and diaphragmatic excursion, somnolence from hypoxemia and CO₂ retention, polycythemia from chronic hypoxia	Weight loss generally causes reversal of symptoms. Prevention and prompt treatment of respiratory infections is important. Condition is worsened in supine position.
Kyphoscoliosis	Posterior and lateral angulation of the spine; restriction of ventilation as a result of alteration in thoracic excursion; increase in work of breathing; pattern of rapid, shallow breathing; reduction of lung volume; compression of alveoli and blood vessels	Only a small number of people with condition develop severe respiratory conditions. Atelectasis and pneumonia are common complications.

CNS, central nervous system; *CO₂,* carbon dioxide.

TABLE 30.22	INTRAPULMONARY CAUSES OF RESTRICTIVE LUNG DISEASE
Disease or Alteration	**Description**
Pleural disorders	Inflammation, scarring, or fluid in the pleural space causing restriction
Pleural effusion	Accumulation of fluid in pleural space secondary to altered hydrostatic or oncotic pressure; fluid collection >250 mL, showing up on chest radiograph
Pleurisy (pleuritis)	Inflammation of pleura; classification as fibrinous (dry) or serofibrinous (wet); wet pleurisy accompanied by an increase in pleural fluid and possibly resulting in pleural effusion
Pneumothorax	Accumulation of air in pleural space with accompanying lung collapse
Parenchymal disorders	Inflammation, collapse, or scarring of the lung tissue
Atelectasis	Condition of lung characterized by collapsed, airless alveoli; possibly acute (e.g., in postoperative patient) or chronic (e.g., in patient with malignant tumour)
Pneumonia	Acute inflammation of lung tissue caused by bacteria, viruses, fungi, chemicals, dusts, and other factors
Interstitial lung diseases (ILDs)	General term that includes a variety of chronic lung disorders characterized by some type of injury, inflammation, and scarring (or fibrosis); this process occurs in the interstitium (tissue between the alveoli), and the lung becomes stiff (fibrotic); can be caused by occupational and environmental exposures (see Table 30.10), infections (e.g., TB), and connective tissue disorders (e.g., rheumatoid arthritis); when all known causes of ILDs are ruled out, the condition is termed *idiopathic pulmonary fibrosis* (IPF)
Acute respiratory distress syndrome (ARDS)*	Atelectasis, pulmonary edema, congestion, and hyaline membrane lining the alveolar wall; result of variety of conditions, including shock lung, O_2 toxicity, Gram-negative sepsis, cardiopulmonary bypass, and aspiration pneumonia

O_2, oxygen; *TB*, tuberculosis.
*See Chapter 70 for clinical manifestations and management.

protein content, and the fluid is generally dark yellow or amber. Transudates have a low protein content or contain no protein, and the fluid is clear or pale yellow. The fluid can also be analyzed for red and white blood cells, malignant cells, bacteria, and glucose.

An empyema is a pleural effusion that contains pus. It is caused by conditions such as pneumonia, TB, lung abscess, and infection of surgical wounds of the chest. Treatment of empyema is generally chest tube drainage. Appropriate antibiotic therapy is also needed to eradicate the causative organism. A complication of empyema is fibrothorax, in which there is fibrous fusion of the visceral and parietal pleurae (see Figure 30.5, *A*). A condition called *trapped lung* can occur with effusions and empyema. It occurs when the visceral pleura becomes encased with a fibrous peel or rind. The fibrous peel causes severe pulmonary restriction. The pathological process affecting the visceral pleura prevents the lung from expanding and from filling the thoracic cavity. A decortication surgical procedure to remove the pleural peel may be needed.

Clinical Manifestations

Common clinical manifestations of pleural effusion are progressive dyspnea and decreased movement of the chest wall on the affected side. There may be pleuritic pain from the underlying disease. Physical examination of the chest will indicate dullness to percussion and absent or decreased breath sounds over the affected area. The chest radiograph will indicate an abnormality if the effusion is greater than 250 mL. Manifestations of empyema include the manifestations of pleural effusion as well as fever, night sweats, cough, and weight loss. A thoracentesis reveals an exudate containing thick, purulent material.

Thoracentesis

If the cause of the pleural effusion is not known, a diagnostic thoracentesis is needed to obtain pleural fluid for analysis (see Chapter 28, Figure 28.15). If the degree of pleural effusion is severe enough to impair breathing, a therapeutic thoracentesis is done to remove fluid as well as to obtain fluid for analysis.

A thoracentesis is performed by having the patient sit on the edge of a bed and lean forward over a bedside table. The puncture site is determined by chest radiograph, and percussion of the chest is used to assess the maximum degree of dullness. The skin is cleaned with an antiseptic solution and anaesthetized locally. The thoracentesis needle is inserted into the intercostal space. Fluid can be aspirated with a syringe, or tubing can be connected to allow fluid to drain into a sterile collection bag. After the fluid is removed, the needle is withdrawn and a bandage is applied over the insertion site.

Usually, only 1 000 to 1 200 mL of pleural fluid is removed at one time. Because high volumes are removed, rapid removal can result in hypotension, hypoxemia, or pulmonary edema. A follow-up chest radiograph should be obtained to detect a possible pneumothorax that could have been induced by perforation of the visceral pleura. During and after the procedure, the patient should be observed for any manifestations of respiratory distress.

Interprofessional Care

The main goal of management of pleural effusions is to treat the underlying cause. For example, adequate treatment of heart failure with diuretics and sodium restriction will result in decreased pleural effusions. The treatment of pleural effusions secondary to malignant disease represents a more difficult concern. These types of pleural effusions are frequently recurrent and accumulate quickly after thoracentesis. Chemical pleurodesis may be used to sclerose the pleural space and prevent re-accumulation of effusion fluid. Although doxycycline and bleomycin have been used for sclerosing with good results, talc appears to be the most effective agent for pleurodesis. Thoracoscopy can be used to perform talc pleurodesis after inspection of the pleural space. After instillation of the sclerosing agent, patients are usually instructed to rotate their positions to spread the agent uniformly throughout the pleural space. Chest tubes are left in place after pleurodesis until fluid drainage is less than 150 mL/day and no air leaks are noted.

PLEURISY

Pleurisy (pleuritis) is an inflammation of the pleura. The most common causes are pneumonia, TB, chest trauma, pulmonary infarctions, and neoplasms. The inflammation usually subsides with adequate treatment of the primary disease. Pleurisy can be classified as fibrinous (dry), with fibrinous deposits on the pleural surface, or serofibrinous (wet), with increased production of pleural fluid that may result in pleural effusion.

The pain of pleurisy is typically abrupt and sharp in onset and is aggravated by inspiration. The patient's breathing is shallow and rapid to avoid unnecessary movement of the pleura and chest wall. A *pleural friction rub* may occur, which is the sound over areas where inflamed visceral and parietal pleurae rub over one another during inspiration. This sound is usually loudest at peak inspiration but can be heard during exhalation as well.

Treatment of pleurisy is aimed at treating the underlying disease and providing pain relief. Taking analgesics and lying on or splinting the affected side may provide some relief. The patient should be taught to splint the rib cage when coughing. Intercostal nerve blocks may be done if the pain is severe.

ATELECTASIS

Atelectasis is a complete or partial collapse of a lung or segment of a lung that occurs when the alveoli become deflated. The most common cause of atelectasis is airway obstruction that results from retained exudates and secretions, which is frequently observed in the postoperative patient. Normally, the pores of Kohn (see Chapter 28, Figure 28.1) provide for collateral passage of air from one alveolus to another. Deep inspiration is necessary to open the pores effectively. For this reason, deep-breathing exercises are important in preventing atelectasis in the high-risk patient (e.g., postoperative, immobilized patient). (The prevention and treatment of atelectasis are discussed in Chapter 22.)

INTERSTITIAL LUNG DISEASE

Many acute and chronic lung disorders with variable degrees of pulmonary inflammation and fibrosis are collectively referred to as *interstitial lung diseases* (ILDs) or *diffuse parenchymal lung diseases*. ILDs have been difficult to classify because more than 200 known diseases have diffuse lung involvement, either as the primary condition or as a significant part of a multiorgan process, as may occur in connective tissue disorders (e.g., systemic lupus erythematosus, rheumatoid arthritis).

Among the ILDs of known cause, the largest group comprises occupational and environmental exposures, especially the inhalation of dusts and various fumes or gases. The most common ILDs of unknown etiology are idiopathic pulmonary fibrosis and sarcoidosis.

IDIOPATHIC PULMONARY FIBROSIS

Idiopathic pulmonary fibrosis (IPF) is characterized by scar tissue in the connective tissue of the lungs as a sequel to inflammation or irritation. A common risk factor for IPF is environmental or occupational inhalation of organic and inorganic substances (see discussion earlier in this chapter). Other risk factors include cigarette smoking and history of chronic aspiration. There also may be genetic risk factors.

Clinical manifestations of IPF include exertional dyspnea, nonproductive cough, and inspirational crackles with or without clubbing. High-resolution CT scan is the most definitive diagnostic study. Chest radiographic studies show changes characteristic of IPF. Pulmonary function tests show a typical pattern characteristic of restrictive lung disease (see Table 30.20). Open lung biopsy using VATS may help to differentiate the specific pathology.

The clinical course is variable, with a 5-year survival rate of 30 to 50% after diagnosis. Treatment includes corticosteroids, cytotoxic agents (azathioprine [Imuran], cyclophosphamide [Procytox]), and antifibrotic agents (colchicine). However, there is no good evidence that any of these treatments improves survival or quality of life. Lung transplantation is an option that should be considered for those who meet the criteria. (Lung transplantation is discussed later in this chapter.)

SARCOIDOSIS

Sarcoidosis is a chronic, multisystem granulomatous disease of unknown cause that primarily affects the lungs. The disease may also involve skin, eyes, liver, kidney, heart, and lymph nodes. The disease is often acute or subacute and self-limiting, but in many individuals, it is chronic with remissions and exacerbations. Marked pulmonary fibrosis can be present with severe restrictive lung disease. Cor pulmonale and bronchiectasis can develop in the advanced stages.

Corticosteroids are the most commonly used medications for the treatment of pulmonary sarcoidosis. A trial of methotrexate may be considered if the patient does not respond to or cannot tolerate corticosteroid therapy. If methotrexate is ineffective or not tolerated, cyclophosphamide (Procytox) or azathioprine (Imuran) may be initiated. Nonsteroidal anti-inflammatory agents, such as ibuprofen (Motrin), may help decrease acute inflammation or relieve symptoms but are not a treatment of sarcoidosis. Disease progression is monitored by pulmonary function tests, chest radiographic studies, and CT scan.

VASCULAR LUNG DISORDERS

PULMONARY EDEMA

Pulmonary edema is an abnormal, life-threatening accumulation of fluid in the alveoli and the interstitial spaces of the lungs. It is a complication of various heart and lung diseases (Table 30.23) and is considered a medical emergency.

Normally, there is a balance between the hydrostatic and the oncotic pressures in the pulmonary capillaries. If the hydrostatic pressure increases or the colloid oncotic pressure decreases, the net effect will be fluid leaving the pulmonary capillaries and entering the interstitial space, an event referred to as *interstitial edema*. At this stage, the lymphatic system can usually drain away the excess fluid. If fluid continues to leak from the pulmonary capillaries, it will enter the alveoli, an event referred to as *alveolar edema*. Pulmonary edema interferes with gas exchange by causing an alteration in the diffusing pathway between the alveoli and the pulmonary capillaries. The most common cause of pulmonary edema is left-sided heart failure.

TABLE 30.23   CAUSES OF PULMONARY EDEMA

- Heart failure
- Overhydration with intravenous fluids
- Hypoalbuminemia: nephrotic syndrome, hepatic disease, nutritional disorders
- Altered capillary permeability of lungs: inhaled toxins, inflammation (e.g., pneumonia), severe hypoxia, near-drowning
- Malignancies of the lymph system
- Respiratory distress syndrome (e.g., oxygen toxicity)
- Unknown causes: neurogenic condition, opioid overdose, high altitude

(The clinical manifestations and management of pulmonary edema are described in Chapter 37.)

PULMONARY EMBOLISM

Etiology and Pathophysiology

Pulmonary embolism (PE) is the blockage of pulmonary arteries by a thrombus, fat or air embolus, or tumour tissue. The word *embolus* derives from a Greek word meaning "plug" or "stopper." Emboli are mobile clots that generally do not stop moving until they lodge at a narrowed part of the circulatory system. A PE consists of material that gains access to the venous system and then to the pulmonary circulation. The embolus travels with the blood flow through ever-smaller blood vessels until it lodges and obstructs perfusion of the alveoli (Figure 30.11). Because of higher blood flow, the lower lobes of the lung are commonly affected. PE is associated with a mortality rate of up to 30% in patients who are not treated. With diagnosis and anticoagulant therapy, the mortality rate is reduced to 6 to 8% (Hogg et al., 2011). Most PEs arise from deep-vein thromboses (DVT) in the deep veins of the legs. *Venous thromboembolism* (VTE) is the preferred term to describe the spectrum of pathology from DVT to PE (see Chapter 40, Table 40.7). Lethal PEs most commonly originate in the femoral or iliac veins. Generally, the VTEs that are below the knee have not been considered a risk factor for PE because they rarely migrate to the pulmonary circulation without first extending above the knee.

Other sites of origin of PE include the right side of the heart (especially with atrial fibrillation), the upper extremities (rare), and the pelvic veins (especially after surgery or childbirth). Upper-extremity VTE occasionally occurs in the presence of central venous catheters or cardiac pacing wires. These cases may resolve with removal of the catheter. Thrombi in the deep veins can dislodge spontaneously. However, it is more common for mechanical forces (e.g., sudden standing) or changes in the rate of blood flow (e.g., those that occur with Valsalva manoeuvre) to dislodge the thrombus. The majority of patients with PE caused by VTE have no leg symptoms at the time of diagnosis (Thrombosis Canada, 2015). Less common causes of PE include fat emboli (from fractured long bones), air emboli (from improperly administered IV therapy), bacterial vegetations, amniotic fluid, and tumours. Tumour emboli may originate from primary or metastatic malignancies. Risk factors for PE include immobility or reduced mobility, surgery within the past 3 months (especially pelvic and lower-extremity surgery, including hip and knee joint replacement), history of DVT, malignancy, obesity, oral contraceptives, hormone therapy, cigarette smoking, prolonged air travel, heart failure, pregnancy, and clotting disorders.

Clinical Manifestations

The signs and symptoms in PE are varied and nonspecific, making diagnosis difficult. The classic triad—dyspnea, chest pain, and hemoptysis—occurs in only about 20% of patients. Symptoms may begin slowly or suddenly. A mild to moderate hypoxemia with a low partial pressure of carbon dioxide in arterial blood ($PaCO_2$) is a common finding. Other manifestations are cough, pleuritic chest pain, hemoptysis, crackles, fever, accentuation of the pulmonic heart sound, and sudden change in mental status as a result of hypoxemia. Massive emboli may produce abrupt hypotension, pallor, severe dyspnea, and hypoxemia. Chest pain may or may not be present. ECG may indicate tachycardia and right ventricular strain. The mortality rate of people with symptomatic PEs is approximately 10% (Thrombosis Canada, 2015). Medium-sized emboli often cause pleuritic chest pain, dyspnea, slight fever, and a productive cough with blood-streaked sputum. A physical examination may reveal tachycardia and a pleural friction rub. Small emboli frequently are undetected or produce vague, transient symptoms. The exception to this is the patient with underlying cardiopulmonary disease. In these patients, even small or medium-sized emboli may result in severe cardiopulmonary compromise. However, repeated small emboli gradually cause a reduction in the capillary bed and eventual pulmonary hypertension. An ECG and chest radiograph may indicate right ventricular hypertrophy secondary to pulmonary hypertension.

Complications

Pulmonary infarction (death of lung tissue) is most likely when the following factors are present: (a) occlusion of a large or medium-sized pulmonary vessel (>2 mm in diameter), (b) insufficient collateral blood flow from the bronchial circulation, or (c) pre-existing lung disease. Infarction results in alveolar necrosis and hemorrhage. Occasionally, the necrotic tissue becomes infected and an abscess may develop. Concomitant pleural effusion is frequent. *Pulmonary hypertension* results from hypoxemia or from involvement of more than 50% of the area of the normal pulmonary bed. As a single event, an embolus does not cause pulmonary hypertension unless it is massive. Recurrent emboli may result in chronic pulmonary hypertension.

Diagnostic Studies

A spiral (helical) CT scan is the most frequently used test to diagnose PE (Table 30.24). An IV injection of contrast media is required to view the blood vessels. The scanner continuously rotates while obtaining slices and does not start and stop between each slice. This allows visualization of all anatomical regions of the lungs. The computer reconstructs the data to provide a three-dimensional picture and assist in emboli visualization. If a patient cannot have contrast media, a ventilation–perfusion (VQ) scan is done.

The VQ scan has two components and is most accurate when both are performed:
1. Perfusion scanning involves IV injection of a radioisotope. A scanning device images the pulmonary circulation.

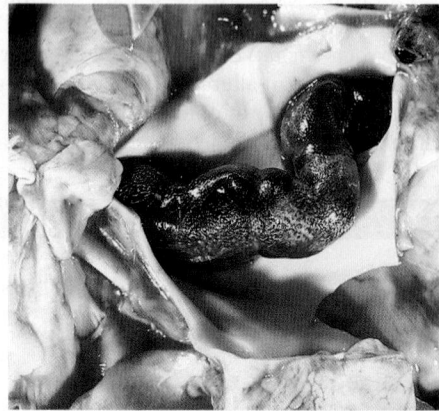

FIG. 30.11 Large embolus from the femoral vein lying in the main left and right pulmonary arteries. Source: From the teaching collection of the Department of Pathology, University of Texas Southwestern Medical School, Dallas.

TABLE 30.24 INTERPROFESSIONAL CARE

Acute Pulmonary Embolism

Diagnostic	Interprofessional Therapy
• History and physical examination • Chest radiographic study • Continuous ECG monitoring • ABGs • Venous ultrasound • CBC count with WBC differential • Spiral (helical) CT scan • Ventilation–perfusion (VQ) scan • Lung scan • D-dimer level • Troponin level, BNP level • Pulmonary angiography	• Supplemental oxygen, intubation may be necessary • Fibrinolytic agent • Unfractionated heparin IV infusion • Low-molecular-weight heparin (e.g., enoxaparin [Lovenox]) • Warfarin (Coumadin) for long-term therapy • Monitoring of aPTT and INR levels • Limited activity • Opioids for pain relief • Inferior vena cava filter • Pulmonary embolectomy in life-threatening situation

ABGs, arterial blood gases; *aPTT*, activated partial thromboplastin time; *BNP*, B-type natriuretic peptide; *CBC*, complete blood cell; *CT*, computed tomography; *ECG*, electrocardiogram; *INR*, international normalized ratio; *IV*, intravenous; *WBC*, white blood cell.

2. Ventilation scanning involves inhalation of a radioactive gas such as xenon. Scanning reflects the distribution of gas through the lung. The ventilation component requires the cooperation of the patient and may be impossible to perform in a critically ill patient, particularly if the patient is intubated.

D-dimer is a laboratory test that measures the amount of cross-linked fibrin fragments. These fragments are found in the circulation after clotting events such as VTE, acute myocardial infarction, unstable angina, and acute stroke. This degradation product is rarely found in healthy individuals. The disadvantage of D-dimer is that it is neither specific (other conditions cause elevation) nor sensitive, because up to 50% of patients with small PEs have normal results. Patients with suspected PE and an elevated D-dimer level but normal venous ultrasound may need a lung scan or spiral CT.

Pulmonary angiography is a sensitive and specific test for PE. However, it is an invasive procedure that involves the insertion of a catheter through the antecubital or femoral vein, advancement to the pulmonary artery, and injection of contrast medium. It allows visualization of the pulmonary vascular system and location of the embolus. However, with spiral CT, pulmonary angiography is now used less frequently.

ABG analysis is important, but not diagnostic. The partial pressure of oxygen in arterial blood (PaO_2) is low because of inadequate oxygenation secondary to an occluded pulmonary vasculature preventing matching of perfusion to ventilation. The pH remains normal unless respiratory alkalosis develops as a result of prolonged hyperventilation or to compensate for lactic acidosis caused by shock. Abnormal findings are usually reported on the chest radiograph (atelectasis, pleural effusion) and on the ECG (ST-segment and T-wave changes), but they are not diagnostic for PE. Serum troponin levels are elevated in 30 to 50% of patients with PE, and, although not diagnostic, they are predictive of an adverse prognosis. Serum B-type natriuretic peptide levels, although not diagnostic, may be helpful in identifying the severity of the clinical course.

Interprofessional Care

Prevention of PE begins with prevention of VTE. VTE prophylaxis includes the use of sequential compression devices, early ambulation, and prophylactic use of anticoagulant medications. To reduce mortality risk, treatment is begun as soon as PE is suspected (see Table 30.24). The objectives are to (a) prevent further growth or multiplication of thrombi in the lower extremities, (b) prevent embolization from the upper or lower extremities to the pulmonary vascular system, and (c) provide cardiopulmonary support if indicated.

Supportive therapy for the patient's cardiopulmonary status varies according to the severity of the PE. The administration of supplemental oxygen by mask or cannula is adequate for some patients. Oxygen is given in a concentration determined by ABG analysis. In some situations, endotracheal intubation and mechanical ventilation are necessary to maintain adequate oxygenation. Respiratory measures such as turning, coughing, deep breathing, and incentive spirometry are important to help prevent or treat atelectasis. If symptoms of shock are present, IV fluids are administered followed by vasopressor agents, as needed, to support perfusion (see Chapter 69). If heart failure is present, diuretics are used. (Heart failure is discussed in Chapter 37.) Pain resulting from pleural irritation or reduced coronary blood flow is treated with opioids, usually morphine.

Medication Therapy. Fibrinolytic medications, such as tissue plasminogen activator (tPA) or alteplase (Activase), dissolve the PE and the source of the thrombus in the pelvis or deep leg veins, thereby decreasing the likelihood of recurrent emboli. Indications for thrombolytic therapy in PE include hemodynamic instability and right ventricular dysfunction. (Thrombolytic therapy is discussed in Chapter 40; see Table 40.10.) Because most deaths are caused by recurrent PEs, treatment should begin immediately. Properly managed anticoagulant therapy is effective in the prevention of further emboli. Heparin works to prevent future clots but does not dissolve existing clots. Although unfractionated heparin IV has traditionally been used, low-molecular-weight heparin (e.g., enoxaparin [Lovenox]) is becoming more common. Warfarin (Coumadin) should be initiated within the first 24 hours and is typically administered for 3 to 6 months. Some health care providers use factor Xa inhibitors and direct thrombin inhibitors in the treatment of PEs. The dosage of heparin is adjusted according to the activated partial thromboplastin time (aPTT), and the dosage of warfarin is determined by the international normalized ratio (INR).

Frequent changes and titrations of heparin doses are needed initially in order to obtain a therapeutic aPTT level. Anticoagulant therapy may be contraindicated if the patient has complicating factors such as blood dyscrasias, hepatic dysfunction causing alteration in the clotting mechanism, injury to the intestine, overt bleeding, a history of hemorrhagic stroke, or neurological conditions.

Surgical Therapy. If the degree of pulmonary arterial obstruction is severe and the patient does not respond to conservative therapy, an immediate embolectomy may be indicated. Pulmonary embolectomy, a rare procedure, has a 50% mortality rate. Preoperative pulmonary angiography is necessary to identify and locate the site of the embolus. When a pulmonary embolectomy is performed, the patient also has placement of a vena cava filter. To prevent further emboli, an inferior vena cava filter may be the treatment of choice in patients who remain at high risk and for patients for whom anticoagulation is contraindicated. This device is placed at the level of the diaphragm in the inferior vena cava via the femoral vein. It prevents migration of large clots into the pulmonary system. Potential complications associated with this device include recurrent VTEs and post-thrombotic syndrome, in addition to misplacement, migration, and perforation.

NURSING MANAGEMENT PULMONARY EMBOLISM

NURSING IMPLEMENTATION

HEALTH PROMOTION. Nursing measures aimed at prevention of PEs are similar to those for prophylaxis of VTEs; see the discussion of venous thrombosis in Chapter 40).

ACUTE INTERVENTION. The prognosis of a patient with PE is good if therapy is promptly instituted. The patient should be kept on bed rest in a semi-Fowler's position to facilitate breathing. An IV line should be maintained for medications and fluid therapy. The nurse should know the adverse effects of medications and observe for them. Oxygen therapy should be administered as ordered. Careful continuous monitoring of vital signs, cardiac dysrhythmia, pulse oximetry (oxygen saturation), ABGs, and lung sounds is critical to assess the patient's status. Laboratory results should be monitored to ensure normal ranges of aPTT and INR. Nursing care includes assessing for the complications of anticoagulant therapy (e.g., bleeding, hematomas, bruising) and for PEs (e.g., hypoxia, hypotension). The nurse should perform appropriate interventions related to immobility and fall precautions. Patients are usually anxious because of pain, a sense of doom, inability to breathe, and fear of death. Explaining the situation and providing emotional support and reassurance can help relieve this anxiety.

AMBULATORY AND HOME CARE. The patient affected by thromboembolic processes may require emotional support. In addition, some patients may have an underlying chronic illness requiring long-term treatment. To provide supportive therapy, the nurse needs to understand and differentiate between the various conditions caused by the underlying disease and those related to thromboembolic disease. Patient teaching regarding long-term anticoagulant therapy is critical.

Anticoagulant therapy continues for at least 3 to 6 months; patients with recurrent emboli are treated indefinitely. INR levels are drawn at intervals and warfarin dosage is adjusted. Some patients are monitored by nurses in an anticoagulation clinic. Long-term management is similar to that for the patient with VTE (see the discussion of VTE in Chapter 40). Discharge planning is aimed at limiting progression of the condition and preventing complications and recurrence. The need for the patient to return to the health care provider for regular follow-up examinations should be reinforced.

EVALUATION

The expected outcomes are that the patient who has a PE will have
- Adequate tissue perfusion and respiratory function
- Adequate cardiac output
- Increased level of comfort
- No recurrence of PE

PULMONARY HYPERTENSION

Pulmonary hypertension comprises a variety of disorders occurring as a primary disease (primary pulmonary hypertension) or as a complication of a large number of respiratory and cardiac disorders (secondary pulmonary hypertension).

Pulmonary hypertension is elevated pulmonary pressure resulting from an increase in pulmonary vascular resistance to blood flow through small arteries and arterioles.

PRIMARY PULMONARY HYPERTENSION

Primary pulmonary hypertension (PPH) is a rare, severe, and progressive disease. PPH is characterized by mean pulmonary arterial pressure greater than 25 mm Hg at rest or greater than 30 mm Hg with exercise, in the absence of a demonstrable cause. PPH is associated with a poor prognosis because there is no definitive therapy.

Etiology and Pathophysiology

The exact etiology of PPH is unknown. PPH has been linked to the use of fenfluramine in the drug Fen-Phen, which was used as an appetite suppressant to treat obesity. The drug was withdrawn from the market in 1996. PPH affects more women than men. It may have a genetic component because the incidence is higher in families. It is a rare and potentially fatal disease; the mean age at diagnosis is 36 years.

Normally, the pulmonary circulation is characterized by low resistance and low pressure. In pulmonary hypertension, the pulmonary pressures are elevated. Until recently, the pathophysiology of PPH was poorly understood. It has been discovered that a key mechanism involved in PPH is a deficient release of vasodilator mediators from the pulmonary epithelium with a resultant cascade of injury (Figure 30.12).

Clinical Manifestations

Classic symptoms of pulmonary hypertension are dyspnea on exertion and fatigue. Exertional chest pain, dizziness, and exertional syncope are other symptoms. These symptoms are related to the inability of cardiac output to increase in response to increased oxygen demand. Eventually, as the disease progresses, dyspnea occurs at rest. Pulmonary hypertension increases the workload of the right ventricle and causes right ventricular hypertrophy (a condition called *cor pulmonale*) and eventually heart failure. A chest radiograph generally shows enlarged central pulmonary arteries and clear lung fields. A heart enlarged on the right may be seen. An echocardiogram usually reveals right ventricular hypertrophy.

Interprofessional Care

Diagnostic evaluation includes an ECG, a chest radiographic study, and an echocardiogram. CT and cardiac catheterization to measure pulmonary artery pressures can be used. Additional tests may be done to exclude secondary factors. Early recognition of pulmonary hypertension is essential to interrupt the self-perpetuation cycle responsible for the progression of this condition (see Figure 30.12). The mean time between onset of symptoms and diagnosis is 2 years. By the time patients become symptomatic, the disease is already in the advanced stages and the size of pulmonary artery pressure is two to three times normal.

Although there is no cure for PPH, treatment can relieve symptoms, improve quality of life, and prolong life. Diuretic therapy relieves dyspnea and peripheral edema and may be useful in reducing right ventricular volume overload. Anticoagulation therapy is recommended for patients with severe pulmonary hypertension to prevent in situ thrombus formation and venous thrombosis.

PATHOPHYSIOLOGY MAP

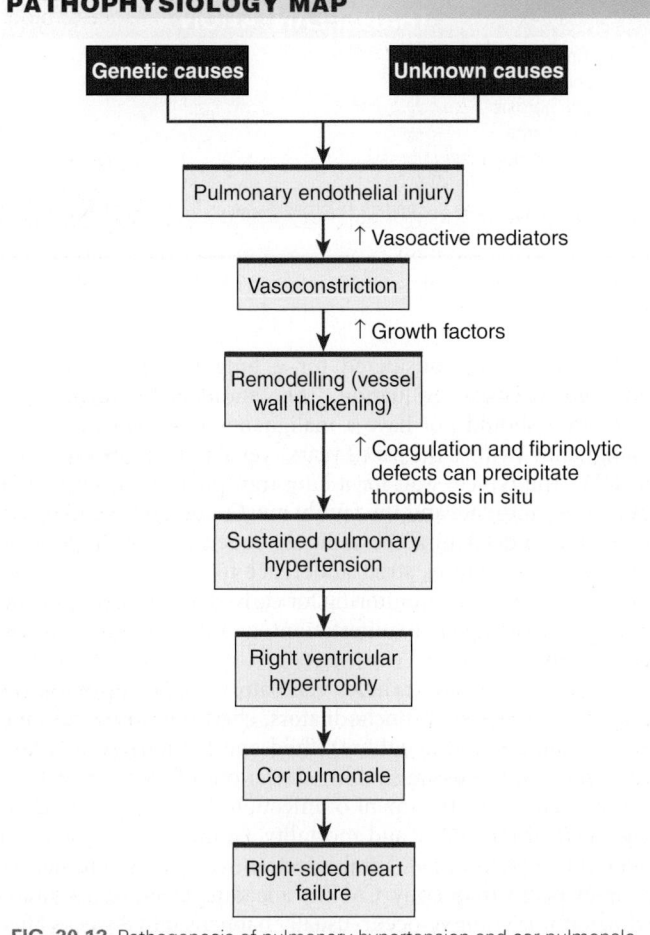

FIG. 30.12 Pathogenesis of pulmonary hypertension and cor pulmonale.

Vasodilator therapy is used to reduce right ventricular overload by dilating pulmonary vessels and reversing remodelling. Many patients with pulmonary hypertension can be effectively managed with calcium channel blocker therapy, such as nifedipine (Adalat) and diltiazem (Cardizem).

Synthetic prostacyclins promote pulmonary vasodilation and reduce pulmonary vascular resistance and have revolutionized the management of PPH. They are now the treatment of choice for select patients unresponsive to calcium channel blockers. They can be administered orally (e.g., bosentan), subcutaneously (e.g., treprostinil), or intravenously (e.g., epoprostenol). Aerosolized forms are not yet available in Canada.

Bosentan (Tracleer) is an oral form of prostacyclin used to treat PPH. It is an active endothelin receptor antagonist. This medication works by blocking the hormone endothelin, which causes blood vessels to constrict. Treprostinil (Remodulin), a prostacyclin, is used as a continuous subcutaneous injection. It causes vasodilation of the pulmonary arterial system and inhibits platelet aggregation.

Surgical interventions include atrial septostomy, pulmonary thromboendarterectomy, and lung transplantation. Lung transplantation is the mainstay of treatment for those patients who do not respond to prostacyclins and progress to severe right-sided heart failure. Recurrence of the disease has not been reported in individuals who have undergone

transplantation. A patient education and support site for pulmonary hypertension is located on the Pulmonary Hypertension Association's website (see the Resources at the end of this chapter).

SECONDARY PULMONARY HYPERTENSION

Secondary pulmonary hypertension (SPH) occurs when a primary disease causes a chronic increase in pulmonary artery pressures. It can develop as a result of parenchymal lung disease, left ventricular dysfunction, intracardiac shunts, chronic pulmonary thromboembolism, or systemic connective tissue disease. The specific primary disease pathology may result in anatomical or vascular changes causing the pulmonary hypertension. Anatomical changes causing increased vascular resistance include (1) loss of capillaries as a result of alveolar wall damage (e.g., COPD), (2) stiffening of the pulmonary vasculature (e.g., pulmonary fibrosis connective tissue disorders), and (3) obstruction of blood flow (chronic emboli).

Vasomotor increases in pulmonary vascular resistance are found in conditions characterized by alveolar hypoxia. Hypoxia causes localized vasoconstriction and shunting of blood away from poorly ventilated alveoli. Alveolar hypoxia can be caused by a wide variety of conditions. It is possible to have a combination of anatomical restriction and vasomotor constriction. This combination is found in the patient with long-standing chronic bronchitis who has chronic hypoxia in addition to loss of lung tissue.

Symptoms can reflect the underlying disease, but some, such as dyspnea, fatigue, lethargy, and chest pain, are directly attributable to the SPH. Physical findings include right ventricular hypertrophy and signs of right ventricular failure (increased pulmonic heart sound, right-sided fourth heart sound, peripheral edema, hepatomegaly). Treatment of pulmonary hypertension caused primarily by pulmonary or cardiac disorders consists mainly of treating the underlying disorder. Treatment of SPH is similar to treatment of PPH.

COR PULMONALE

Cor pulmonale is a hypertrophy of the right side of the heart, with or without heart failure, resulting from pulmonary hypertension. Diseases of the lung or thorax or changes in pulmonary circulation can lead to pulmonary hypertension. Pulmonary hypertension is usually a pre-existing condition in the individual with cor pulmonale. Cor pulmonale may be present with or without overt cardiac failure. The most common cause of cor pulmonale is COPD; however, almost any disorder that affects the respiratory system can cause cor pulmonale. The etiology and pathogenesis of pulmonary hypertension and cor pulmonale are outlined in Figure 30.12.

Clinical Manifestations

Clinical manifestations of cor pulmonale include dyspnea, chronic productive cough, wheezing respirations, retrosternal or substernal pain, and fatigue. Chronic hypoxemia leads to polycythemia and increased total blood volume and viscosity of the blood. (Polycythemia is often present in cor pulmonale secondary to COPD.) Compensatory mechanisms that are secondary to hypoxemia can aggravate the pulmonary hypertension. Episodes of cor pulmonale in a person with underlying

TABLE 30.25	INTERPROFESSIONAL CARE

Cor Pulmonale

Diagnostic	Interprofessional Therapy
• History and physical examination • ABGs • Serum and urine electrolytes • Monitoring with ECG • Chest radiographic study	• O₂ therapy • Bronchodilators • Diuretics • Low-sodium diet • Fluid restriction • Antibiotics (if indicated) • Digitalis (if left-sided heart failure) • Vasodilators (if indicated) • Calcium channel blockers (if indicated)

ABGs, arterial blood gases; *ECG,* electrocardiogram; *O₂,* oxygen.

TABLE 30.26	INDICATIONS FOR LUNG TRANSPLANTATION

- α₁-Antitrypsin deficiency
- Bronchiectasis
- Cystic fibrosis
- Emphysema
- Idiopathic pulmonary fibrosis
- Interstitial lung disease
- Pulmonary fibrosis secondary to other diseases (e.g., sarcoidosis)
- Pulmonary hypertension

chronic respiratory conditions are frequently triggered by an acute respiratory tract infection.

If heart failure accompanies cor pulmonale, additional manifestations such as peripheral edema, weight gain, distended neck veins, full, bounding pulse, and enlarged liver will also be found. (Heart failure is discussed in Chapter 37.) A chest radiograph will show an enlarged right ventricle and pulmonary artery.

Interprofessional Care

The primary management of cor pulmonale is directed at treating the underlying pulmonary condition that precipitated the heart condition (Table 30.25). Long-term low-flow oxygen therapy is used to correct the hypoxemia and reduce vasoconstriction in chronic states of respiratory disorders. If fluid, electrolyte, and acid–base imbalances are present, they must be corrected. Diuretics and a low-sodium diet will help decrease the plasma volume and the load on the heart. Bronchodilator therapy is indicated if the underlying respiratory condition is caused by an obstructive disorder. Digitalis may be used if there is left-sided heart failure. Other treatments include those for pulmonary hypertension and comprise vasodilator therapy, calcium channel blockers, and anticoagulants. Theophylline may help because of its weak inotropic effect on the heart. When medical treatment fails, lung transplantation is an option for some patients.

Management of cor pulmonale resulting from COPD is similar to that described for COPD (see Chapter 31). Continuous low-flow oxygen during sleep, exercise, and small, frequent meals may allow the patient to feel better and be more active.

LUNG TRANSPLANTATION

Lung transplantation has evolved as a viable therapy for patients with end-stage lung disease. A variety of pulmonary disorders are potentially treatable with some type of lung transplantation (Table 30.26). Improved selection criteria, technical advances, and better methods of immunosuppression have resulted in improved survival rates. Various transplant options are available, including single-lung transplant, bilateral-lung transplant, heart–lung transplant, and transplantation of lobes from a living related donor.

Patients being considered for a lung transplant need to undergo extensive evaluation. The candidate for lung transplantation should not have a malignancy or recent history of malignancy (within the past 2 years), renal or liver insufficiency, or HIV. The typical wait for a lung transplant is longer than 1 year. The candidate and the family must undergo psychological screening to determine the ability to cope with a postoperative regimen that requires strict adherence to immunosuppressive therapy, continuous monitoring for early signs of infection, and prompt reporting of manifestations of infection for medical evaluation.

Postoperative care includes ventilatory support, pulmonary clearance measures (bronchodilators, chest physiotherapy, and deep breathing and coughing), fluid and hemodynamic management, immunosuppression, detection of early rejection, and prevention or treatment of infection. Infection is the leading cause of morbidity and mortality. Gram-negative bacterial pneumonia is common. Viral infection with CMV and herpes simplex occur frequently. CMV is a leading cause of mortality, which, if it is going to occur, usually happens 4 to 8 weeks after surgery. Fungal infections are also seen. An empirical antibiotic regimen is routine perioperatively for potential pathogens isolated from the donor or recipient.

Immunosuppressive therapy usually includes a triple-medication regimen of cyclosporine, azathioprine (Imuran), and prednisone. Immunosuppressive medications are discussed in Chapter 16 and Table 16.16.

Acute rejection can be seen as soon as 5 to 7 days after surgery. It is characterized by low-grade fever, fatigue, and oxygen desaturation with exercise. Accurate diagnosis is by transtracheal biopsy. Treatment with bolus corticosteroids results in remission of symptoms.

Bronchiolitis obliterans (an obstructive airway disease causing progressive occlusion) is considered to represent chronic rejection in lung transplant patients. The onset is often subacute, with gradual, progressive obstructive airflow defect, including cough, dyspnea, and recurrent lower respiratory tract infection. Treatment involves optimum maintenance immunosuppression.

Discharge planning begins in the preoperative phase. Patients are placed in an outpatient rehabilitation program to improve physical endurance. The use of home spirometry has been useful in monitoring trends in lung function. Patients are taught to keep logs of medications, laboratory results, and spirometry. Patients need to be able to perform self-care activities, including medication management and ability to identify when to call the health care provider. Over the past decade, lung transplantation has become an increasingly important mode of therapy for patients with a variety of end-stage lung diseases.

CASE STUDY

Pneumonia and Lung Cancer

Patient Profile

J. H. (pronouns he/him), 52 years old, comes to the emergency department reporting shortness of breath. He has not seen a health care provider for many years.

Subjective Data

- Has a 38 pack-year history of cigarette smoking
- States he has always been slender but has had 11-kg weight loss despite a normal appetite in the past few months
- Admits to a "smoker's cough" for the past 2 to 3 years; recently coughing up blood
- Is married and is the parent of three adult children

Objective Data

Physical Examination

- Thin, pale, looking older than stated age
- Height 182 cm; weight 61.2 kg
- Intermittently confused and anxious with rapid shallow respirations
- Vital signs: temperature 39.2°C, heart rate 120, respiratory rate 36
- Chest wall has limited excursion on right side; auscultation of left side reveals coarse crackles but clear with cough; right side has diminished breath sounds

Diagnostic Studies

- Arterial blood gases: pH 7.51, PaO_2 58 mm Hg, $PaCO_2$ 30 mm Hg, HCO_3^- 22 mmol/L, O_2 saturation 84% (room air)
- Chest radiograph: consolidation of the right lung, especially in the base with possible mass in the area of right bronchus; pleural effusion on the right side
- Bronchoscopy with biopsy of mass: small cell lung carcinoma

Interprofessional Care

- Diagnosis: pneumonia with small cell lung cancer
- Follow-up with patient and family to consider treatment options

Discussion Questions

1. How would J. H.'s pneumonia be classified? Why is classification important?
2. What would the nurse's analysis of J. H.'s arterial blood gas results be?
3. *Priority decision:* Based on the assessment data presented, what are the priority nursing diagnoses? Are there any interprofessional issues?
4. *Priority decision:* What are the priority nursing interventions for J. H.?
5. The nurse is planning a meeting with J. H. and his family to discuss their needs. The physician tells the nurse that J. H. is terminally ill. Who should be included in this meeting?
6. *Evidence-informed practice:* J. H.'s children tell the nurse that they are worried they will get lung cancer because their father has it and they grew up around secondhand smoke. They want to know what kind of screening is available for them. How should the nurse respond?
7. What is the goal if radiation therapy is used for J. H.?
8. What issues should be addressed in the nurse's teaching of J. H. and his partner as J. H. is prepared for discharge and care at home?

⊖volve

Answers are available at http://evolve.elsevier.com/Canada/Lewis/medsurg

REVIEW QUESTIONS

The number of the question corresponds to the same-numbered objective at the beginning of the chapter.

1. What clinical manifestations should the nurse expect when assessing a client with pneumococcal pneumonia?
   a. Fever, chills, and a productive cough with purulent sputum
   b. Nonproductive cough and night sweats that are usually self-limiting
   c. Gradual onset of nasal stuffiness, sore throat, and purulent productive cough
   d. Abrupt onset of fever, nonproductive cough, and formation of lung abscesses

2. A client with pneumonia has the nursing diagnosis of *inadequate airway clearance* from an excessive amount of mucus and retained secretions. What would be an appropriate nursing intervention?
   a. Promote fluid hydration, as appropriate, to help liquefy secretions.
   b. Provide analgesics as ordered to promote client comfort.
   c. Administer oxygen as prescribed to maintain optimal oxygen levels.
   d. Teach the client how to cough effectively to bring secretions to the mouth.

3. A client with tuberculosis (TB) has a history of nonadherence to the medication regimen. What is the most common cause of this behaviour in clients with TB?
   a. Fatigue and lack of energy to manage self-care
   b. Lack of knowledge about how the disease is transmitted
   c. Lack of social support systems for the client and family

   d. Feelings of shame and the response to the social stigma associated with TB

4. A client has been receiving high-dose corticosteroids and broad-spectrum antibiotics for treatment of serious trauma and infection. Which of the following infections is the client most susceptible to?
   a. Aspergillosis
   b. Candidiasis
   c. Coccidioidomycosis
   d. Histoplasmosis

5. Which of the following statements best describes the treatment of lung abscess?
   a. It is best treated with surgical excision and drainage.
   b. Antibiotics for a prolonged period is the treatment of choice.
   c. Abscesses are difficult to treat and usually result in pulmonary fibrosis.
   d. Penicillin can effectively eradicate anaerobic organisms.

6. What is a common complication of many types of environmental lung diseases?
   a. Benign tumour growth
   b. Diffuse airway obstruction
   c. Liquefactive necrosis
   d. Pulmonary fibrosis

7. What type of lung cancer is generally associated with the best prognosis because it is potentially surgically resectable?
   a. Adenocarcinoma
   b. Small cell carcinoma

   c. Squamous cell carcinoma

   d. Undifferentiated large cell carcinoma

8. How does the nurse identify in a client a flail chest caused by trauma?

   a. Multiple rib fractures are determined by radiographic study.

   b. Tracheal deviation to the unaffected side is present.

   c. Paradoxical chest movement occurs during respiration.

   d. Decreased movement of the involved chest wall is apparent.

9. The nurse notes tidalling of the water level in the tube submerged in the water-seal chamber in a client with closed chest tube drainage. What should the nurse do?

   a. Continue to monitor this normal finding.

   b. Check all connections for a leak in the system.

   c. Lower the drainage collector further from the chest.

   d. Clamp the tubing at progressively more distal points from the client until the tidalling stops.

10. Which nursing measure should be instituted after a pneumonectomy?

   a. Monitor chest tube drainage and functioning.

   b. Position the client on the operative side or their back.

   c. Perform range-of-motion exercises on the affected upper extremity.

   d. Auscultate frequently for lung sounds on the affected side.

11. What is the cause of respiratory symptoms in clients with Guillain-Barré syndrome?

   a. Central nervous system depression

   b. Deformed chest-wall muscles

   c. Paralysis of the diaphragm secondary to trauma

   d. Interruption of nerve transmission to respiratory muscles

12. A client with chronic obstructive pulmonary disease asks why the heart is affected by the respiratory disease. Which of the following statements regarding cor pulmonale is the basis for the nurse's response to the client?

   a. Pulmonary congestion secondary to left ventricular failure

   b. Excess serous fluid collection in the alveoli caused by retained respiratory secretions

   c. Right ventricular hypertrophy secondary to increased pulmonary vascular resistance

   d. Right ventricular failure secondary to compression of the heart by hyperinflated lungs

13. Which statement(s) describe(s) the management of a client following lung transplantation? *(Select all that apply.)*

   a. High doses of oxygen are administered around the clock.

   b. The use of a home spirometer will help to monitor lung function.

   c. Immunosuppressant therapy usually involves a three-medication regimen.

   d. Most clients experience an acute rejection episode in the first 2 days.

   e. The lung is biopsied using a transtracheal method if rejection is suspected.

1. a; 2. a; 3. d; 4. b; 5. b; 6. d; 7. c; 8. c; 9. a; 10. b; 11. d; 12. c; 13. b, c, e.

For even more review questions, visit http://evolve.elsevier.com/Canada/Lewis/medsurg.

REFERENCES

BC Centre for Disease Control. (2019). *Communicable disease control manual. Chapter 4: tuberculosis.* http://www.bccdc.ca/resource-gallery/Documents/Communicable-Disease-Manual/Chapter%204%20-%20TB/5.0%20Treatment%20and%20Active%20TB%20Disease.pdf.

Canadian Cancer Society. (2021a). *Cancer statistics at a glance.* https://www.cancer.ca/en/cancer-information/cancer-101/cancer-statistics-at-a-glance/?region=ab

Canadian Cancer Society. (2021b). *Lung cancer: Malignant tumours of the lung.* http://www.cancer.ca/en/cancer-information/cancer-type/lung/lung-cancer/cancerous-tumours/?region=on

Canadian Cancer Society. (2021c). *Risk factors for lung cancer.* https://www.cancer.ca/en/cancer-information/cancer-type/lung/risks/?region=ab

Canadian Cancer Society. (2021d). *What is second-hand smoke and how does it affect you?.* https://www.cancer.ca/en/prevention-and-screening/reduce-cancer-risk/make-healthy-choices/live-smoke--free/what-is-second-hand-smoke/?region=on

Canadian Cancer Society. (2021e). *What you need to know about e-cigarettes.* https://www.cancer.ca/en/prevention-and-screening/reduce-cancer-risk/make-healthy-choices/live-smoke--free/what-you-need-to-know-about-e-cigarettes/?region=on

Canadian Centre for Occupational Health and Safety (CCOHS). (2021a). *OSH Answers fact sheets: Asthma, work related.* https://www.ccohs.ca/oshanswers/diseases/asthma.html

Canadian Centre for Occupational Health and Safety (CCOHS). (2021b). *OSH Answers fact sheets: OH&S Legislation in Canada—Basic responsibilities.* https://www.ccohs.ca/oshanswers/legisl/responsi.html

Canadian Institute for Health Information. (2021). *Hospital stays in Canada.* https://www.cihi.ca/en/hospital-stays-in-canada

Canadian Lung Association. (2016). *Smoking and tobacco: Benefits of quitting smoking.* https://www.lung.ca/lung-health/smoking-and-tobacco/benefits-quitting

Canadian Lung Association. (2021). *Smoking and tobacco.* https://www.lung.ca/lung-health/smoking-and-tobacco

Canadian Task Force on Preventive Health Care. (2016). Recommendations on screening for lung cancer. *Canadian Medical Association Journal, 188*(6), 425–432. https://doi.org/10.1503/cmaj.151421

Dalcin, D., Sieswerda, L., Dubois, S., et al. (2018). Epidemiology of invasive pneumococcal disease in Indigenous and non-Indigenous adults in northwestern Ontario, Canada 2006-2015. *BMC Infectious Diseases, 18*(1), 621. https://doi.org/10.1186/s12879-018-3531-9

Francesco, P. (2020). Electronic cigarettes, vaping-related lung injury and lung cancer, where do we stand? *European Journal of Cancer Prevention* (Epub ahead of print). https://doi.org/10.1097/CEJ.0000000000000630

Government of Canada. (2016). *Pneumococcal vaccine: Canadian immunization guide.* https://www.canada.ca/en/public-health/services/publications/healthy-living/canadian-immunization-guide-part-4-active-vaccines/page-16-pneumococcal-vaccine.html

Government of Canada. (2020). *Weekly influenza reports: Flu watch report February 16-22, 2020 Week 8.* https://www.canada.ca/en/public-health/services/publications/diseases-conditions/flu-watch/2019-2020/week-08-february-16-22-2020.html

Health Quality Ontario and Ministry of Health and Long-Term Care. (2013). *Quality-based procedures clinical handbook for community-acquired pneumonia.* http://www.health.gov.on.ca/en/pro/programs/ecfa/docs/qbp_pnemonia.pdf. (Seminal).

Hogg, K., Thomas, D., Mackway-Jones, K., et al. (2011). Diagnosing pulmonary embolism: A comparison of clinical probability scores. *British Journal of Haematology, 153*(2), 253–258. https://doi.org/10.1111/j.1365-2141.2011.08575.x. (Seminal).

Human Resources and Social Development Canada. (2017). *Occupational health and safety and compliance.* https://www.canada.ca/content/dam/esdc-edsc/migration/documents/eng/health_safety/pubs_hs/pdf/compliance.pdf

Indigenous Services Canada. (2020). *Tuberculosis in Indigenous communities*. https://www.sac-isc.gc.ca/eng/1570132922208/1570132959826

LaFreniere, M., Hussain, H., He, N., et al. (2019). Tuberculosis in Canada: 2017. *Canadian Communicable Disease Report, 45*(2/3), 68–74. https://doi.org/10.14745/ccdr.v45i23a04

Lux, M. (2018). Indian hospitals in Canada. *The Canadian Encyclopedia*. https://www.thecanadianencyclopedia.ca/en/article/indian-hospitals-in-canada

Mandell, L. A., Marrie, T. J., Grossman, R. F., et al. (2000). Summary of the Canadian guidelines for the initial management of community-acquired pneumonia: An evidence-based update by the Canadian Infectious Disease Society and the Canadian Thoracic Society. *Canadian Respiratory Journal, 7*(5), 371–382. https://doi.org/10.1086/313959. (Seminal).

Nahid, P., Dorman, S. E., Alipanah, N., et al. American Thoracic Society/Centers for Disease Control and Prevention/Infectious Diseases Society of America Clinical Practice Guidelines: treatment of drug-susceptible tuberculosis. *Clinical Infectious Diseases, 63*(7), e147–e195.

Public Health Agency of Canada (PHAC) & Canadian Lung Association. (2014). *Canadian tuberculosis standards* (7th ed.). https://www.canada.ca/en/public-health/services/infectious-diseases/canadian-tuberculosis-standards-7th-edition.html

Registered Nurses' Association of Ontario. (2017). *Clinical best practice guidelines: Integrating tobacco interventions into daily practice*. https://rnao.ca/sites/rnao-ca/files/bpg/FINAL_TOBACCO_INTERVENTION_WEB.pdf

Rubin, B. K., & Williams, R. W. (2014). Aerosolized antibiotics for non-cystic fibrosis bronchiectasis. *Respiration; International Review of Thoracic Diseases, 88*, 177–184. https://doi.org/10.1159/000366000. (Seminal).

Thrombosis Canada. (2015). *Pulmonary embolism (PE): Diagnosis*. http://thrombosiscanada.ca/wp-content/uploads/2015/11/4A_Pulmonary-Embolism-Diagnosis-2015Oct26-FINAL2.pdf. (Seminal).

World Health Organization (WHO). (2014). *Companion handbook to the WHO guidelines for the programmatic management of drug-resistant tuberculosis*. http://apps.who.int/iris/bitstream/10665/130918/1/9789241548809_eng.pdf?ua=1&ua=1

World Health Organization (WHO). (2021). *Fact sheets: Cancer*. https://www.who.int/news-room/fact-sheets/detail/cancer

Wu, H., Harder, C., & Culley, C. (2017). The 2016 clinical practice guidelines for management of hospital-acquired and ventilator-associated pneumonia. *The Canadian Journal of Hospital Pharmacy, 70*(3). https://doi.org/10.4212/cjhp.v70i3.1667

RESOURCES

BC Cancer
http://www.bccancer.bc.ca

Canadian Cancer Society
https://www.cancer.ca

Canadian Cancer Society: *Get Help to Quit Smoking*
https://www.cancer.ca/en/support-and-services/support-services/quit-smoking/?region=on

Canadian Lung Association
https://www.lung.ca

Cancer Care Ontario
https://www.cancercare.on.ca

Cancer Care Ontario: *Lung Cancer Evidence-Based Guidelines (PEBC)*
https://www.cancercareontario.ca/en/cancer-care-ontario/programs/data-research/evidence-based-care

Cancer Control Alberta
https://www.albertahealthservices.ca/cancer/cancer.aspx

Health Canada
https://www.hc-sc.gc.ca

Public Health Agency of Canada
https://www.phac-aspc.gc.ca

Statistics Canada
https://www.statcan.ca

Centers for Disease Control and Prevention, National Center for Health Statistics
http://www.cdc.gov/nchs/fastats

Centers for Disease Control and Prevention: *Smoking & Tobacco Use*
https://www.cdc.gov/tobacco

National Cancer Institute
https://www.nci.nih.gov

Pulmonary Hypertension Association (PHA)
https://www.phassociation.org

World Health Organization: *International Standards for Tuberculosis Care (ISTC)*
https://www.who.int/tb/publications/ISTC_3rdEd.pdf

evolve
For additional Internet resources, see the website for this book at http://evolve.elsevier.com/Canada/Lewis/medsurg.

Nursing Management
Obstructive Pulmonary Diseases

Kimberly Hellmer
Originating US chapter by Eugene Mondor

℮volve WEBSITE

http://evolve.elsevier.com/Canada/Lewis/medsurg

- Review Questions (Online Only)
- Key Points
- Answer Guidelines for Case Study
- Student Case Studies
  - Asthma
  - Cystic Fibrosis

- Customizable Nursing Care Plans
  - Patient with Asthma
  - Patient with Chronic Obstructive Pulmonary Disease
- Conceptual Care Map Creator

- Conceptual Care Map for Textbook Case Study
- Audio Glossary
- Content Updates

LEARNING OBJECTIVES

1. Explore the etiology, pathophysiology, and clinical manifestations of asthma, and describe the interprofessional care plan of patients with asthma.
2. Explain the nursing management of patients with asthma.
3. Discover the etiology, pathophysiology, and clinical manifestations of chronic obstructive pulmonary disease (COPD), and describe the interprofessional care plan of patients with COPD.
4. Explain the effects of cigarette smoking on the lungs, and formulate a discussion about the benefits of smoking cessation with patients.
5. Outline the nursing management of patients with COPD.
6. Identify the indications for oxygen therapy, the methods of delivery, and the complications of oxygen administration.
7. Determine the etiology, pathophysiology, and clinical manifestations of cystic fibrosis, and describe the interprofessional care plan of patients with cystic fibrosis.

KEY TERMS

absorption atelectasis
α1-antitrypsin (AAT) deficiency
asthma
chest physiotherapy
chronic bronchitis

chronic obstructive pulmonary disease (COPD)
cor pulmonale
cough variant asthma
cystic fibrosis

emphysema
oxygen toxicity
postural drainage
pursed-lip breathing
status asthmaticus

Obstructive pulmonary diseases are the most common chronic lung diseases, which include conditions characterized by increased airflow resistance as a result of airway obstruction or narrowing. Airway obstruction may result from accumulated secretions, edema, inflammation of the airways, bronchospasm of smooth muscle, or destruction of lung tissue, or some combination of these conditions. Asthma, chronic obstructive pulmonary disease (COPD), and cystic fibrosis are obstructive pulmonary diseases.

While breathing is an unconscious effort for most people, individuals living with obstructive pulmonary disease are consciously challenged with breathing. In Canada, there are 3.8 million Canadians over the age of 1 year living with asthma, 2.0 million living with COPD (Government of Canada, 2018),

and more than 4 300 living with cystic fibrosis (Cystic Fibrosis Canada, 2020). Each of the complex disease processes are further explored in this chapter.

ASTHMA

Asthma is a chronic inflammatory disorder of the airways. Inflammation causes varying degrees of obstruction in the airways, which leads to recurrent episodes of wheezing, breathlessness, sensation of chest tightness, and cough, particularly at night and in the early morning. The hyper-responsiveness, or "twitchiness," of the airways is directly related to the degree of airway inflammation. The more airway inflammation present, the more hyper-responsive the airways are to endogenous or exogenous stimuli or triggers. Asthma occurs as a result of environmental (endogenous or exogenous) effects on the airways that trigger a series of events in the immune system of a genetically predisposed individual. These events lead to airway inflammation and bronchoconstriction (airway narrowing). A key characteristic of asthma is the episodic and reversible nature of the airway obstruction and its associated symptoms (cough, wheeze, sensation of chest tightness, dyspnea), so an episode may resolve spontaneously or with treatment.

In 2011, the Public Health Agency of Canada (PHAC) conducted a *Survey on Living with Chronic Disease in Canada* (SLDC), which provided an in-depth analysis of Canadians aged 12 years and over living with asthma. The SLDC identified that more than 2.4 million (8.4%) Canadians older than 12 years were living with asthma, which translates to 9.8% of all female Canadians and 7.0% of all male Canadians (PHAC, 2015). Asthma is 40% more prevalent among Indigenous people when compared to the general Canadian population (Asthma Canada, 2019). The morbidity associated with asthma is dramatic: The SLDC found that 11.1% of Canadians with active asthma reported a minimum of one visit to a hospital emergency room in the previous 12 months because of asthma symptoms (PHAC, 2015). The high rate of morbidity related to asthma may be attributed to practice that is inconsistent with Canadian asthma consensus guidelines, inaccurate assessment of disease severity, a delay in seeking help, inadequate medical treatment, nonadherence to prescribed therapy, an increase in allergens in the environment, limited access to health care, and a lack of knowledge on the part of patients and health care providers.

Pathophysiology

The hallmarks of asthma are airway inflammation and airway hyper-responsiveness. The degree of bronchoconstriction is related to the degrees of airway inflammation, airway hyper-responsiveness, and exposure to endogenous and exogenous triggers (e.g., infections, allergens, histamine, and other cell mediators). Exposure to allergens or irritants initiates an inflammatory cascade involving multiple cell types, mediators, and chemokines. Typically, there are two possible types of asthmatic responses to stimuli: an early-phase response and a late-phase response.

The *early-phase response* in asthma is characterized by bronchospasm (Figure 31.1). This response is triggered when an allergen or irritant attaches to immunoglobulin E (IgE) receptors on mast cells found beneath the basement membrane of the bronchial wall (Figure 31.2). The mast cells become activated and, subsequently, granules are released and the phospholipids' cell membranes are disrupted. Both processes result in the release of inflammatory mediators, including histamine, bradykinin, leukotrienes, prostaglandins, platelet-activating factor, chemotactic factors, and cytokines (e.g., interleukin-4 [IL-4] and interleukin-5 [IL-5]). A similar early-phase response process can occur with exercise. These mediators cause intense inflammation in association with bronchial smooth muscle constriction,

PATHOPHYSIOLOGY MAP

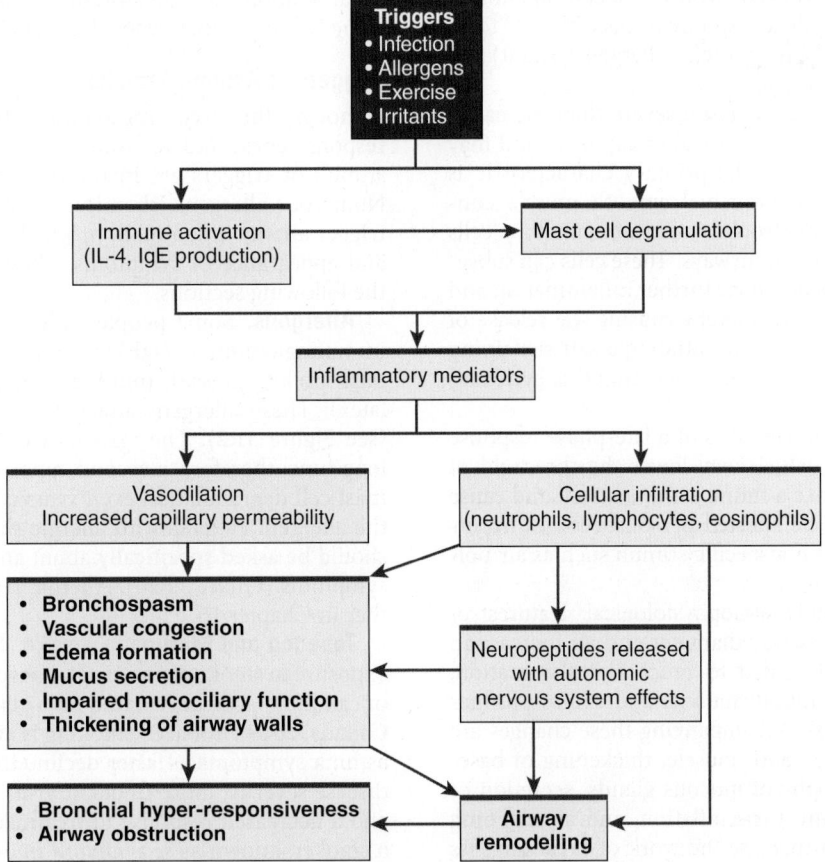

FIG. 31.1 Early- and late-phase responses of asthma. *IgE*, immunoglobulin E; *IL-4*, interleukin-4.

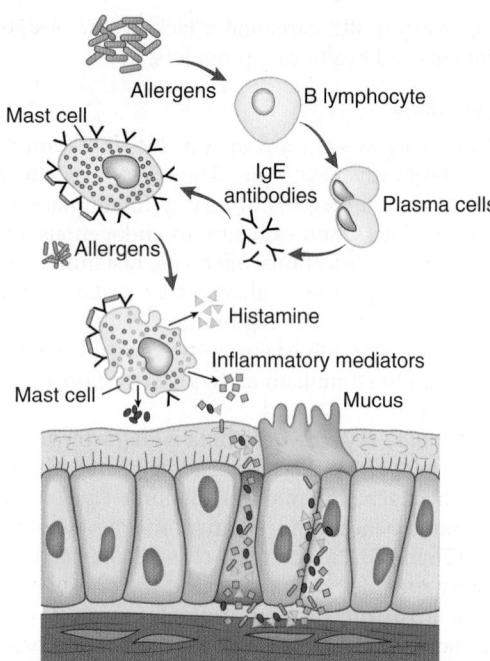

FIG. 31.2 The early-phase response in asthma is triggered when an allergen or irritant attaches to immunoglobulin E (IgE) receptors on mast cells, which are then activated to release histamine and other inflammatory mediators.

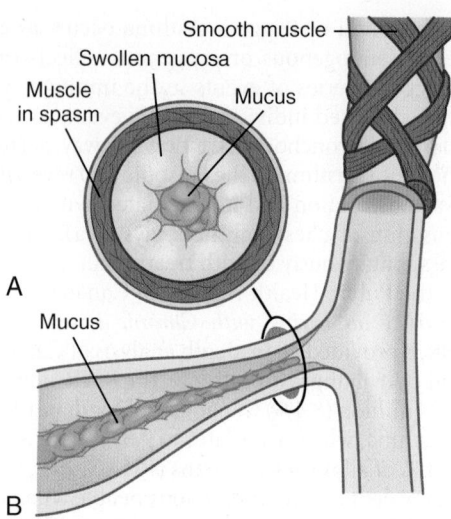

FIG. 31.3 Factors causing obstruction (especially expiratory obstruction) in asthma. **A,** Cross section of a bronchiole occluded by muscle spasm, swollen mucosa, and mucus in the lumen. **B,** Longitudinal section of a bronchiole. Source: Asthma Society of Canada. (2016). *About asthma.* http://www.asthma.ca/adults/about/whatIsAsthma.php

increased vasodilation and permeability, and epithelial damage. Clinically, the effects are bronchospasm, increased mucus secretion, edema formation, and increased amounts of tenacious sputum (see Figure 31.1), which cause wheeze, cough, sensation of chest tightness, shortness of breath, or a combination of these symptoms. This immediate response peaks within 30 to 60 minutes after exposure to the trigger (e.g., allergen, irritant) and subsides in another 30 to 90 minutes.

The *late-phase response* can be more severe than the early-phase response. It peaks 5 to 12 hours after exposure and may last from several hours to days. Its primary characteristic is inflammation as opposed to bronchial smooth muscle contraction. Eosinophils and neutrophils, the inflammatory cells involved in asthma, infiltrate the airways. These cells can subsequently release mediators that induce further inflammation and cause mast cells to degranulate, thereby causing the release of histamine and other mediators and initiating a self-sustaining cycle. Corticosteroids are effective in preventing this cycle and reversing it, if needed.

These inflammatory characteristics of a late-phase response increase airway reactivity, which may lower the threshold of exposure necessary to induce a future asthma attack and cause its symptoms to worsen. The affected person becomes hyperresponsive to allergens and nonspecific stimuli such as air pollution, cold air, and dust.

In summary, prominent pathophysiological features of asthma are a reduction in airway diameter and an increase in airway resistance that are related to mucosal inflammation, constriction of bronchial smooth muscle, and excess production of mucus (Figure 31.3). Accompanying these changes are hypertrophy of bronchial smooth muscle, thickening of basement membrane, hypertrophy of mucous glands, secretion of thick and tenacious sputum, hyperinflation, and air trapping in the alveoli, all of which increase the work of breathing. As a consequence of these events, respiratory muscle function

may be altered, distribution of both ventilation and perfusion may be abnormal, and arterial blood gas (ABG) values may be altered, depending on the severity of the disease. While asthma is considered a disease of the airways, during an asthma attack, eventually all aspects of pulmonary function are compromised. If airway inflammation is not treated or does not resolve, progressive and irreversible lung damage may eventually occur. This irreversible airway obstruction is thought to be the result of inflammation-induced structural changes called *airway remodelling* (Global Initiative for Asthma [GINA], 2020).

Triggers of Asthma Attacks

Although the exact mechanisms that cause airway hyperresponsiveness and inflammation remain unknown, multiple stimuli or triggers are involved (Table 31.1; see Figure 31.1). Numerous allergens, chemicals, and infectious pathogens can trigger airway inflammation, which leads to airway narrowing and appearance of symptoms. These triggers are discussed in the following sections.

Allergens. Some people with asthma have an exaggerated immunoglobulin E (IgE) response to certain allergens (e.g., dust, pollen, grasses, mites, roaches, moulds, animal dander, latex). These allergens attach to IgE receptors on mast cells (see Figure 31.2). The IgE–mast cell complexes remain for a long time; therefore, a second exposure to the allergen triggers mast cell degranulation even years after the initial exposure to the allergen. Patients with allergic rhinitis or atopic dermatitis should be asked specifically about any incidence of respiratory symptoms (GINA, 2020). Allergic reactions are discussed further in Chapter 16.

Tobacco and Marijuana Smoke. Smoke is an air pollutant; exposure to smoke of any kind—tobacco, marijuana, forest fires, or campfire—can be harmful for a person with asthma (Asthma Canada, 2019). Tobacco smoking is associated with the onset of asthma symptoms, a faster decline in lung function, increased disease severity, more frequent visits to a health care provider, and a decreased response to treatment. The smoke exhaled by a smoker, known as *secondhand smoke*, is also a risk factor for an asthma attack. *Tobacco misuse* is a term used to describe the

TABLE 31.1 TRIGGERS OF ASTHMA ATTACKS

Allergens
- Animal dander (e.g., from cats, dogs, horses, mice, guinea pigs)
- Household dust mites
- Cockroaches
- Pollens
- Moulds
- Air pollutants
- Diesel particulates
- Exhaust fumes
- Perfumes
- Ozone
- Sulphur dioxides
- Cigarette smoke
- Aerosol sprays

Viral upper respiratory infection
Sinusitis
Exercise
Cold, dry air
Stress

Hormones or menses
Gastroesophageal reflux disease (GERD)
Medications
- Acetylsalicylic acid (ASA; Aspirin)
- Nonsteroidal anti-inflammatory medications
- β-Adrenergic blockers

Occupational exposure
- Agriculture
- Metal salts
- Wood and vegetable dusts
- Industrial chemicals and plastics (isocyanates)
- Pharmaceutical medications

Food additives
- Sulphites (bisulphites and metabisulphites) found in beer, wine, dried fruit, shrimp
- Monosodium glutamate
- Tartrazine

recreational use of cigarettes, pipes, chewing tobacco, snuff, and electronic cigarettes; use of traditional tobacco by Indigenous people, however, is not considered tobacco misuse. Among Indigenous people, traditional tobacco is used in medicinal and ceremonial contexts and is intended to establish a direct link with the spiritual world; it is not used for inhalation purposes. The rate of smoking is two to five times higher among Indigenous people than among non-Indigenous Canadians (Canadian Partnership Against Cancer, 2019).

Marijuana smoke contains many of the same chemicals that tobacco smoke has and can cause many existing lung conditions to worsen (American Thoracic Society, 2017). Marijuana may be inhaled through a multitude of ways, including joints, electronic cigarettes, water bongs, and vaporizers. None of these delivery devices are considered safe (American Thoracic Society, 2017).

Exercise. Acute airway narrowing that is induced or exacerbated during physical exertion is referred to as *exercise-induced asthma* or *exercise-induced bronchospasm* (EIB). While EIB affects a substantial proportion of patients with an asthma diagnosis, EIB can also be experienced by people who do not have the clinical features or diagnosis of asthma (Cote et al., 2018). Typically, EIB occurs after, not during, vigorous exercise and is characterized by bronchospasm (airway smooth muscle contraction) that causes shortness of breath, cough, wheeze, a sensation of chest tightness, or a combination of these. EIB is pronounced during activities in cold, dry air. Airway hyper-responsiveness may result from changes in the airway mucosa caused by the hyperventilation that occurs during exercise with either the cooling or rewarming of air and capillary leakage in the airway wall.

Several strategies can be incorporated to prevent EIB: an adequate warm-up period before the activity begins, breathing through a scarf or mask during exercise in a cold or dry climate to promote humidification, and using inhaled short-acting β₂-adrenergic agonists either to relieve the symptoms or, 15 minutes before exercising, to prevent symptoms. Too frequent use of β₂-adrenergic agonists indicates poor asthma control, may mask asthma severity, and may cause a reduction in medication effectiveness. In such cases, patients may need escalation of

therapy. (Control criteria and controller therapy are discussed later in this chapter.)

Respiratory Infections. Respiratory infections (particularly viral) are among the most common triggers of worsening asthma. Infections cause increased inflammation in the tracheobronchial system, resulting in increased airway hyper-responsiveness, which can last from 2 to 8 weeks after infection both in individuals with asthma and in those without asthma. Patients with asthma should take steps to reduce the possibility of infections by using proper hand hygiene and receiving an annual influenza vaccination. Influenza vaccines are recommended for patients with asthma aged 6 months and older, especially because of the prevalence of high-risk influenza-related complications in patients with asthma (PHAC, 2019a).

Indigenous communities that have poor housing conditions, overcrowding, and high rates of indoor tobacco use, dampness, and mould are at significant risk for increased respiratory symptoms. Indigenous people (identifying as North American Indian, First Nation, Metis, or Inuit) have 1.5 greater odds of being hospitalized for asthma compared to non-Indigenous people when housing is reported to be in need of major repairs (Carriere et al., 2017). Statistics Canada Census of the Population 2016 reported that one in five Indigenous people in Canada live in a home in need of repairs, and 18.3% live in overcrowded housing (Statistics Canada, 2017).

Nose and Sinus Conditions. Some patients with asthma have chronic sinus and nasal conditions. Nasal conditions include allergic rhinitis, either seasonal or perennial, and nasal polyps. Sinus conditions are usually related to inflammation of the mucous membranes, most commonly from noninfectious causes such as allergies. However, bacterial sinusitis may also occur. It is important to treat these comorbid conditions because they often contribute to poor asthma control. (Sinusitis is discussed further in Chapter 29.)

Medications and Food Additives. Some patients with asthma, especially those with nasal polyps, may have sensitivity to specific medications. Some people with asthma have what is termed the *asthma triad*: nasal polyps, asthma, and sensitivity to acetylsalicylic acid (ASA; Aspirin) and nonsteroidal anti-inflammatory drugs (NSAIDs). Salicylic acid can be found in many over-the-counter medications and some foods, beverages, and artificial flavours. In some asthmatic patients, wheezing develops within 2 hours after they take ASA (Aspirin) or NSAIDs (e.g., ibuprofen [Motrin]). In addition, most affected patients have profound rhinorrhea, congestion, and tearing. Facial flushing, gastrointestinal symptoms, and angioedema can also occur. Although sensitivity to salicylates persists for many years, the nature and severity of the reaction can change over time. These patients should avoid taking ASA (Aspirin) and NSAIDs. However, patients with ASA (Aspirin) sensitivity can, under the care of an allergist, be desensitized by daily administration of the medication (Cortellini et al., 2017). Such patients may be more likely to benefit from antileukotriene medications (further discussed later under Medication Therapy).

β-Adrenergic blockers in oral form (e.g., metoprolol) or topical eye drops (e.g., timolol [Timoptic]) may trigger asthma episodes because they induce bronchospasm. Angiotensin-converting enzyme inhibitors (e.g., lisinopril) may induce cough in susceptible individuals, thus worsening asthma symptoms. Other irritants that may precipitate asthma symptoms in susceptible patients are tartrazine (yellow dye no. 5, found in many foods) and sulphites (e.g., sodium metabisulphite), which are widely used in the food and pharmaceutical industries as preservatives and sanitizing agents. Sulphites are commonly found in fruits, beer, and wine and are used extensively in salad bars to protect vegetables from oxidation.

These medications and food additives are thought to interfere with metabolic pathways, resulting in enhanced production of leukotrienes, some of which are potent bronchoconstrictors. The onset of a typical reaction occurs 15 minutes to 3 hours after ingestion and is marked by profuse rhinorrhea, often accompanied by nausea, vomiting, intestinal cramps, and diarrhea. An acute episode of asthma typically begins after the nasal symptoms appear. Food allergies triggering asthma reactions in adults are rare. Avoidance diets are not recommended until testing has proven an allergy is present.

Gastroesophageal Reflux Disease. The exact mechanism by which gastroesophageal reflux disease (GERD) triggers asthma is unknown. It is postulated that reflux of stomach acid into the esophagus can be aspirated into the lungs, which causes reflex vagal stimulation and bronchoconstriction. Although GERD is involved primarily in nocturnal asthma, it can trigger daytime asthma as well. By monitoring esophageal pH and peak expiratory flow rate (PEFR) simultaneously, the examiner can determine whether GERD is the cause of the asthma symptoms. H_2-histamine blockers or proton pump inhibitors are given to ameliorate symptoms. (GERD is discussed further in Chapter 44.)

Genetics. Asthma has an inherited component, but the genetics are complex. Numerous genes may be involved in the development of asthma. They are likely responsible for varying responses among patients to different types of asthma medications. *Atopy*, the genetic predisposition to develop an allergic (IgE-mediated) response to common allergens, is a major risk factor for asthma.

Air Pollutants. Various air pollutants such as wood smoke, vehicle exhaust, diesel particulate, elevated ozone levels, sulphur dioxide, and nitrogen dioxide can trigger asthma attacks. Ongoing studies are being done to better understand how chronic exposure to urban air pollution and to "hotspots" of air pollution within Canadian cities affects people who work and live in these areas. The Air Quality Health Index (AQHI) was developed by the Government of Canada (2019) as a tool to help alert the public of health risks posed by air pollution (Figure 31.4).

Emotional Stress. Asthma is not a psychosomatic disease. However, physiological stress that elicits emotional responses such as crying, laughing, anger, and fear can lead to hyperventilation and hypocapnia, which can cause airway narrowing (GINA, 2020). An asthma exacerbation can produce panic and anxiety, which are not unexpected emotions during this experience. Panic is a normal response to not being able to breathe. The extent to which psychological factors contribute to the induction and continuation of any given acute exacerbation is unknown, but it probably varies from patient to patient and in the same patient from episode to episode.

Clinical Manifestations

Asthma has an unpredictable, episodic, and variable course. Recurrent episodes of wheezing, breathlessness, sensation of chest tightness, coughing, or a combination of these, particularly at night and in the early morning (typically between 0200 and 0500 hours), are common features. The onset of an attack

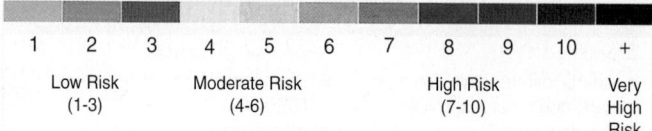

FIG. 31.4 The Air Quality Health Index (AQHI) is measured on a scale ranging from 1 to 10+. The AQHI values are also grouped into health risk categories: 1 to 3 indicates low risk; 4 to 6, moderate risk; 7 to 10, high risk; and 10+, very high risk. These categories help patients easily and quickly identify their level of risk. Source: Courtesy Environment and Climate Change Canada (ECCC).

or episode of asthma may be abrupt (minutes) or more gradual (1 hour to days). Between attacks, the patient may have no symptoms, with normal or near-normal pulmonary function, depending on the severity of disease. However, in some people, prolonged and uncontrolled asthma may result in compromised pulmonary function and chronic debilitation, resulting in irreversible or fixed airway disease.

The characteristic clinical manifestations of asthma are wheezing, cough, dyspnea, and sensation of chest tightness after exposure to a precipitating factor or trigger. Expiration is often prolonged. The inspiratory–expiratory ratio, instead of being the normal 1:2, may be prolonged to 1:3 or 1:4. As a result of bronchospasm, edema, and mucus in the bronchioles, the airways become narrower, taking longer for the air to move out of the bronchioles. This produces the characteristic wheezing, air trapping, and hyperinflation.

Wheezing is an unreliable sign for gauging the severity of an attack. Many patients with minor attacks wheeze loudly, whereas others with severe attacks do not wheeze. A patient with a severe asthma attack may have no audible wheezing because of the marked reduction in airflow. For wheezing to occur, the patient must be able to move enough air to produce the sound. Wheezing usually occurs first on exhalation. As an asthma attack progresses, the patient may wheeze during inspiration and expiration. Severely diminished breath sounds or their absence, often referred to as a "silent chest," is an ominous sign of severe obstruction and impending respiratory failure. During an acute attack, the person with asthma usually sits upright or slightly bent forward and uses the accessory muscles of respiration in an attempt to make breathing easier. The more difficult the breathing becomes, the more anxious the patient feels.

SAFETY ALERT
- If a patient has been wheezing but the wheeze abruptly disappears (i.e., silent chest) and the patient is obviously in distress, the situation has become life-threatening and may necessitate mechanical ventilation.

In some patients with asthma, cough is the only symptom, which is termed cough variant asthma. The bronchospasm may not be severe enough to cause airflow obstruction, but it can increase bronchial tone and cause irritation and stimulation of the cough receptors. The cough may be nonproductive. Mobilizing secretions may be difficult as a result of their thick, tenacious, gelatinous quality.

In patients experiencing an acute attack of moderate or severe asthma, examination usually reveals signs of hypoxemia, which may include restlessness, increased anxiety, inappropriate behaviour, increased pulse and blood pressure, and *pulsus paradoxus* (a drop in systolic pressure during the inspiratory cycle of more than 10 mm Hg). The respiratory rate is significantly increased (usually >30 breaths/minute), and the use of accessory muscles is evident. The patient also has difficulty speaking in complete sentences; typically, they are able to complete only two to five words without requiring another breath. Percussion of the lungs indicates hyper-resonance, and auscultation indicates the presence of inspiratory or expiratory wheezing.

Asthma Control and Severity

A dynamic continuum of treatment is used to manage asthma. With this approach, medication therapy can be adapted to the severity of the underlying illness and the current level of asthma control. The concepts of asthma "control" and "severity" are related to each other but not correlated (GINA, 2020). For example, even severe asthma may be well controlled, whereas mild disease may remain uncontrolled. *Optimal asthma control* is defined by the absence of both asthma symptoms and the need for rescue bronchodilator, as well as by normal pulmonary function; however, this is difficult to achieve in all patients with asthma. According to the Guidelines for Asthma in Adults, treatment needs should be based on achieving acceptable asthma control at the lowest step in the stepwise approach to treatment, which is determined through clinical and physiological criteria (BC Guidelines.ca, Guidelines and Protocols Advisory Committee, 2015; Lougheed et al., 2012) (Table 31.2). Asthma control is obtained through treatment of modifiable risk factor comorbidities (e.g., smoking cessation and increased physical activity), use of written asthma action plans, self-management education and skills training, and pharmacotherapy tailored to the individual (GINA, 2020). Asthma control must be assessed regularly and treatment adjusted accordingly.

The severity of asthma is determined from the frequency and duration of symptoms, the presence of persistent airflow limitation, and the medication required to maintain control (Lougheed et al., 2012). When asthma is well controlled, severity is gauged by level of treatment required to maintain the state of acceptable control (GINA, 2020). Signs of severe or poorly controlled asthma include a history of a previous near-fatal asthma episode (loss of consciousness, need for intubation), recent hospitalization or recent emergency department visit for asthma, nighttime symptoms, limitations in daily activities, and the need for inhaled β_2 agonists several times each day or night.

Asthma severity levels can change for better or worse over the course of a patient's life. This is particularly true for children with asthma, as severity often decreases as the child gets older. When asthma control is good, patients have minimal to no symptoms, are able to sleep through the night, and participate in sports, exercise, and strenuous activity. Once asthma has been kept under control for at least 3 months with a corresponding plateau in lung function, an attempt should be made to reduce medication dosages while maintaining acceptable asthma control (GINA, 2020).

Status Asthmaticus. A life-threatening medical emergency, status asthmaticus is the most extreme form of an acute asthma attack. It is characterized by hypoxia, hypercapnia, and acute respiratory failure. Of the people with asthma admitted to the hospital, approximately 3 to 5% require ventilatory assistance in the critical care unit, as they are unresponsive to bronchodilation and corticosteroid treatment. Common causes of severe acute attacks include viral illnesses, increases in environmental pollutants or other allergen exposure, food allergy, outdoor air pollution, seasonal changes, poor adherence to inhaled

TABLE 31.2 ASTHMA CONTROL CRITERIA

Characteristic	Frequency or Value
Daytime symptoms	<4 days/week
Nighttime symptoms	<1 night/week
Physical activity	Normal
Exacerbations	Mild, infrequent
Absence from work or school because of asthma	None
Need for a fast-acting β_2 agonist	<4 doses/week
FEV_1 or PEF	≥90% personal best
PEF diurnal variation*	<10–15%
Sputum eosinophils†	<2–3%

Diurnal variation is calculated as the highest peak expiratory flow (PEF) minus the lowest peak expiratory flow rate (PEFR), divided by the highest PEFR, multiplied by 100 for morning and night (determined over a 2-week period).
†Considered in adults with uncontrolled moderate to severe asthma who are assessed in specialist centres.
FEV_1, forced expiratory volume in 1 second.
Source: Lougheed, M. D., Lemiere, C., Ducharme, F. M., et al. (2012). Canadian Thoracic Society 2012 guideline update: Diagnosis and management of asthma in preschoolers, children and adults. *Canadian Respiratory Journal, 19*(2), 127–164, Table 16.

corticosteroid (ICS) treatment, and discontinuation of medication therapy (especially corticosteroids) (GINA, 2020). The clinical manifestations of a severe attack are a consequence of increased airway resistance that results from mucosal edema, mucous plugging, epithelial damage, eosinophilic infiltrate, and bronchospasm with subsequent air trapping and hyperinflation. The clinical manifestations are similar to those of nonsevere asthma but are more serious and prolonged. Extreme anxiety, fear of suffocation, severely increased work of breathing, and diaphoresis are common. Absence of diaphoresis may indicate significant dehydration. Sternocleidomastoid, intercostal, and supraclavicular muscle retractions reflect increased work of breathing.

Although wheezing is often audible even without a stethoscope, auscultation may not always be reliable: Airflow obstruction may be so severe and airflow so insufficient that audible wheezing or other abnormal lung sounds may not be produced. As noted earlier, absence of a wheeze (i.e., silent chest) represents a life-threatening situation that may necessitate mechanical ventilation. The chest appears fixed in a hyperinflated position and is often described as "tight," indicating severely decreased movement of air through the constricted bronchial airways.

Forced exhalation with the use of the abdominal musculature can result in increased intrathoracic pressure transmitted to the great vessels and heart. Neck vein distension and pulsus paradoxus with a pressure of 40 mm Hg or higher may result. (Pulsus paradoxus is described in Chapter 39 and Table 39.8.) Hypertension, sinus tachycardia, and ventricular dysrhythmias may occur. These three conditions are related to hypoxemia, to the catecholamines present as a result of an endogenous response to hypoxia, and, in older patients, to underlying coronary artery disease. On the right side of the heart, an electrocardiogram may show sinus tachycardia or signs of strain secondary to pulmonary vasoconstriction, which may appear as cor pulmonale and a right axis deviation.

Hypoxemia with hypocapnia usually occurs initially as the patient attempts to hyperventilate and maintain adequate oxygenation and ventilation. As the severity of the attack increases, the work of breathing increases, which makes it more difficult for the patient to overcome the increased resistance to breathing. The patient becomes fatigued, which causes more carbon

TABLE 31.3   INTERPROFESSIONAL CARE
Asthma

Diagnostic	Interprofessional Therapy
• History and physical examination • Pulmonary function studies (spirometry; methacholine, histamine, exercise challenge test; PEF) • Chest radiograph • Allergy skin testing • Oximetry and measurement of ABGs during acute episodes when patient is in emergency department or hospital	• Establishing partnerships between health care providers and patients and their families • Identification and avoidance or elimination of triggers • Patient and family teaching • Continuous assessment of asthma control and severity • Appropriate pharmacotherapy (see Table 31.5) • Asthma action plan (see Figure 31.11) • Regular follow-up

ABG, arterial blood gases; *PEF,* peak expiratory flow.

TABLE 31.4   DIAGNOSIS OF ASTHMA: PULMONARY FUNCTION CRITERIA

Pulmonary Function Measurement	Children (6 Years of Age and Older)	Adults
Preferred: Spirometry Showing Reversible Airway Obstruction		
Reduced FEV$_1$/FVC	Less than lower limit of normal based on age, sex, height, and ethnicity (<0.8–0.9)*	Less than lower limit of normal based on age, sex, height, and ethnicity (<0.75–0.8)*
	and	*and*
Increase in FEV$_1$ after a bronchodilator or after a course of controller therapy	≥12%	≥12% (and a minimum ≥200 mL)
Alternative: Peak Expiratory Flow Variability		
Increase after a bronchodilator or after course of controller therapy	≥20%	60 L/min (minimum ≥20%)
or	*or*	*or*
Diurnal variation†	Not recommended	>8% based on twice-daily readings; >20% based on multiple daily readings
Alternative: Positive Challenge Test		
Methacholine challenge	PC$_{20}$ <4 mg/mL (4–16 mg/mL is borderline; >16 mg/mL is negative)	
or		*or*
Exercise challenge	≥10–15% decrease in FEV$_1$ postexercise	

*Approximate lower limits of normal ratios for children and adults.
†Difference between minimum morning pre–bronchodilator therapy value in 1 week and maximum nighttime value as percentage of recent maximum.
FEV$_1$, forced expiratory volume in 1 second; *FVC,* forced vital capacity; *PC$_{20}$,* provocative concentration of methacholine producing a 20% fall in FEV$_1$.
Source: Lougheed, M. D., Lemiere, C., Ducharme, F. M., et al. (2012). Canadian Thoracic Society 2012 guideline update: Diagnosis and management of asthma in preschoolers, children and adults. *Canadian Respiratory Journal, 19*(2), 127–164.

dioxide retention. ABG measurements initially reveal hypocapnia due to increased respiratory rate. Ultimately, these measurements deteriorate to manifest hypercapnia and hypoxemia. The patient must move amounts greater than 150 mL of air for air to participate in gas exchange. A moderate elevation in partial pressure of arterial carbon dioxide (PaCO$_2$) may be tolerated without intubation, and mechanical ventilation may be necessary because of respiratory arrest, cardiac arrest, hemodynamic instability, altered level of consciousness, or extreme exhaustion.

Possible complications of a severe asthma attack include pneumothorax, pneumomediastinum, acute cor pulmonale with right ventricular failure, and severe respiratory muscle fatigue that leads to respiratory arrest. Respiratory arrest can be fatal.

Diagnostic Studies for Asthma

Two main features must be considered in the diagnosis of asthma: symptoms and variable airflow obstruction. Several sources of information assist with confirming the diagnosis of asthma along with monitoring severity and control (Table 31.3). A detailed history is important in determining whether a person has had previous attacks of a similar nature, often precipitated by a known cause or trigger, as discussed previously in this chapter. Because asthma and allergies commonly coexist, it is also important to determine whether the patient has a history of nonpulmonary symptoms. Rhinitis, eczema, and conjunctivitis are common but not specific to asthma and indicate a predisposition to allergy.

Of further value is to determine whether the patient has a family history of asthma, allergies, and eczema because such a history increases the likelihood that the patient has asthma. Recurrent symptoms of wheeze, sensation of chest tightness, cough, or breathlessness that improve with treatment are suggestive of asthma. However, wheezing and cough occur with a variety of disorders—COPD, pulmonary embolism, GERD, obesity, vocal cord dysfunction, and heart failure—and their presence can therefore complicate the diagnosis. According to both the Global Initiative for Asthma (GINA) and the Global Initiative for Chronic Obstructive Lung Disease, differentiating between asthma and COPD can be challenging in a small proportion of patients; the term *asthma–COPD overlap syndrome* (ACOS) is used to clinically describe disease features (GINA,

2020). This is discussed further in the section on COPD later in this chapter.

In all patients who are able to perform pulmonary testing, clinically suspected asthma should be confirmed with objective lung measurements that demonstrate post–bronchodilator therapy reversible obstruction, variable airflow limitation over time, or airway hyper-responsiveness (Lougheed et al., 2010). Spirometry is the preferred test for diagnosing asthma; alternative lung testing includes variations in peak expiratory flow and bronchoprovocative challenge testing (Lougheed et al., 2010; Table 31.4).

Spirometry performed before and after bronchodilator treatment can best reveal whether airway obstruction is reversible. The ratio of forced expiratory volume in 1 second to the forced vital capacity (FEV$_1$ to FVC; see Chapter 28, Table 28.14) is a measure of airflow obstruction. For spirometry, the patient is asked to refrain from using bronchodilator medication for 6 to 12 hours before the test. The test is then completed both before and after administration of a bronchodilator to determine the degree of response. Most children 6 years of age and older should be able to perform spirometry, but a standardized clinical score such as the Pediatric Respiratory Assessment Measure (PRAM) can reduce subjectivity of assessment (Ducharme et al., 2015). (The normal values for pulmonary function tests are discussed in Chapter 28.)

An alternative objective pulmonary measurement is peak expiratory flow (PEF), in which variable airflow limitation over time is measured (see Chapter 28, Table 28.14). The PEF is a home measurement, which is not as reliable as spirometry but can be used when spirometry or challenge testing is unavailable. To determine an asthma diagnosis through this method, the patient must measure the PEF four times per day, with the same meter—in the morning and evening both before and after bronchodilator treatment—for several weeks. To determine the PEF variability, the lowest reading is subtracted from the highest reading, the result is divided by the highest reading, and this answer is then multiplied by 100. Variability in PEF of at least 20% is consistent with a diagnosis of asthma (GINA, 2020).

Determining airway hyper-responsiveness with a bronchial provocation test, such as inhaled methacholine, histamine, or exercise challenge, eucapnic voluntary hyperventilation, or inhaled mannitol testing, has moderate sensitivity for asthma diagnosis but limited specificity (GINA, 2020). When a patient is not on ISC therapy, a negative test can help to exclude asthma as a diagnosis, but a positive test does not correlate directly to an asthma diagnosis either; the pattern of symptoms and clinical features need to be taken into account to create a larger diagnostic picture (GINA, 2020). Challenge testing must be performed in a controlled environment by trained staff.

Chest radiographs are not necessary to diagnose asthma; however, they may be used to exclude other diagnoses, such as congenital malformations in children and heart failure in adults (GINA, 2020; Lougheed et al., 2010). A chest radiograph in a patient with asthma with no clinical manifestations is usually normal; however, this radiograph should be used as a baseline on initial diagnosis. A chest radiograph obtained during an acute attack usually shows hyperinflation and may reveal other complications of asthma, such as mucoid impaction, pneumothorax, atelectasis, or pneumomediastinum.

Allergy assessment is warranted in a patient with asthma and must be interpreted in view of the patient's history of exposure and symptom experience. Allergy skin testing can be helpful in determining sensitivity to specific allergens (antigens). (Allergy testing is discussed further in Chapter 16.)

If a patient is in acute distress, it is not feasible to obtain a detailed health history (although a family member may supply some pertinent information). During an acute asthma attack, bedside spirometry (FEV_1 and FVC are preferred, but usually PEF is measured) may be used to monitor obstruction. Serial spirometric parameters, oximetry, and measurement of ABGs help provide information about the severity of the attack and the response to therapy. A complete blood cell count and serum electrolyte measurements are obtained to help monitor the course of therapy because high dosages of inhaled β_2 agonists can cause hypokalemia, resulting from skeletal muscle B-receptor activation due to absorption of short-acting β_2 agonist (SABA) systemically, causing an intracellular potassium shift (Pardue Jones et al., 2020).

In addition to standard measures of asthma control, monitoring of changes in sputum eosinophil counts can be used to measure airway inflammation, which indicates whether treatment for asthma is working (Lougheed et al., 2012). Sputum eosinophils are not normally present in a healthy individual; their levels are increased in individuals with known asthma who are exposed to allergens. These measurements have been used in adults and children and are becoming more easily available and reliable. However, they continue to be used most frequently in major research centres.

Interprofessional Care

In 1990, Canada became the first country to produce asthma practice guidelines. These guidelines provide a medical approach to diagnosing and managing asthma that is informed by the best available evidence. The Registered Nurses' Association of Ontario (RNAO) also developed asthma best practice guidelines for adults (RNAO, 2017) to provide nurses working in diverse settings with an evidence-informed summary of basic asthma care. The RNAO's Best Practice Guidelines build on and complement the Canadian Asthma Consensus Report and remain pertinent with the current Canadian Thoracic Society Asthma Management Guidelines Update (Lougheed et al., 2012). The focus of the nursing guidelines is on promoting asthma control for adults and children affected by asthma. The overall goal of the guidelines is to achieve asthma control with the minimum level of pharmacotherapy while enhancing quality of life of individuals living with asthma and reducing the personal and social burdens inflicted by this condition.

Various health care providers can contribute to development of a care plan for the patient with asthma. A social worker can assist the patient in exploring funding options to pay for medications; a pharmacist can provide counselling about new and previously prescribed medications; a respiratory therapist can teach the patient how to use a metered-dose inhaler (MDI) and spacer (a holding chamber that holds the medication for a few seconds after it has been released from the inhaler) correctly. There are many more examples of how the interdisciplinary team works together to contribute to the patient's care plan.

Some hospitals or outpatient clinics may also provide access to a heath care provider with additional certification specific to respiratory topics. The Canadian Network for Respiratory Care (CNRC) is a certifying organization for health care providers (i.e., nurses, physicians, physiotherapists, occupational therapists, respiratory therapists) who offer health education to patients requiring respiratory care. The CNRC offers certification for providers in becoming a Certified Respiratory Educator (CRE), Certified Asthma Educator (CAE), Certified COPD Educator (CCE), and Certified Tobacco Educator (CTE). This type of certification enables health care providers from a variety of roles to hone their knowledge and skills specific to the topics required in patient education.

Patient education that builds an active partnership between health care providers and patients remains the cornerstone of asthma management (see the Evidence-Informed Practice box). Education should start at the time of asthma diagnosis and be integrated into every aspect of clinical asthma care. Asthma self-management should be tailored to the needs of each patient; patients' cultural beliefs and practices should also be accounted for. Emphasis should be placed on evaluating outcomes in terms of a patient's level of asthma control and their perceptions of improvement, especially quality of life and the ability to engage in their usual activities of living, such as physical activity. A list of centres that provide asthma education to patients can be accessed through the Canadian Network for Respiratory Care (see the Resources at the end of this chapter).

Research Highlight

Adult Asthma Care Guidelines: Promoting Control of Asthma

Clinical Questions

1. What are the appropriate nursing assessment strategies to use with adults living with asthma to achieve optimal asthma control?
2. What are the appropriate nursing management strategies to use with adults living with asthma to achieve optimal asthma control?
3. What education and training do nurses require to assist people living with asthma in achieving optimal asthma control?
4. What organization- or health system–level supports are needed to enable health care providers to assist people living with asthma in achieving optimal asthma control?

Best Available Evidence

- Multiple systematic reviews of asthma management practices
- Synthesis of best available evidence

Recommendations of Clinical Practice Guideline

Assessment

Recommendation 1.0: All individuals identified as having asthma or suspected of having asthma will have their level of asthma control assessed by the nurse.

Recommendation 1.1: At initial encounter, the nurse should identify adults with an asthma diagnosis by reviewing the health record for an established asthma diagnosis, supported by the use of objective lung function measurements, and by asking the following two questions:

1. Have you ever been told by a health care provider that you have asthma?
2. Have you ever used a puffer or inhaler or asthma medication for breathing problems?

Recommendation 1.2a: At every encounter, the nurse should assess the person's current level of asthma control according to the following criteria:

- Need for a fast-acting β_2 agonist <4 doses/week (including for exercise)
- Daytime symptoms <4 days/week
- Nighttime symptoms <1 night/week
- Normal physical activity levels
- Mild, infrequent exacerbations
- No absences from work or school
- Forced expiratory volume in first second (FEV_1) or peak expiratory flow (PEF) ≥90% of personal best*[†]
- Diurnal PEF variation <10–15%*[†]
- Sputum eosinophil [counts] <2–3%*

Recommendation 1.2b: For adults with uncontrolled asthma, the nurse should determine whether the person is currently experiencing an asthma exacerbation and, if so, the severity and need for urgent medical attention.

Recommendation 1.3: At every encounter, the nurse should assess the person's risk of future asthma exacerbations according to the following criteria:

- Current control of asthma
- Severe exacerbations experienced
- Exacerbations necessitating systemic corticosteroids
- Use of emergency care or hospitalizations for asthma

Recommendation 1.4: At every encounter, the nurse should identify factors affecting the complexity of asthma management for the person, including age, sex, smoking habits, social determinants of health, triggers, and comorbid conditions.

Asthma Planning

Recommendation 2.0: The nurse should develop an individualized, person-centred asthma education plan that addresses the following:

- Learning needs
- Culture
- Health literacy
- Empowerment

Implementation

Recommendation 3.1a: The nurse should provide asthma education as an essential component of care.

Recommendation 3.1b: The nurse should educate the person on the es-

sential skills and self-management of asthma based on the person's learning needs, including the following:

- Pathophysiology of asthma
- Medications and device technique
- Self-monitoring
- Action plans
- Trigger identification and management
- Smoking cessation (if applicable)

Recommendation 3.2: The nurse should evaluate nonpharmacological interventions for effectiveness and for potential interactions with pharmacological interventions.

Recommendation 3.3a: At every encounter, the nurse should actively educate the person with asthma on correct inhaler device technique through observation, feedback, physical demonstration, and written instructions.

Recommendation 3.3b: The nurse should engage the person with asthma in shared decision making with regard to the selection of an inhaler device.

Recommendation 3.3c: The nurse should educate the person with asthma on the difference between controller and reliever medications, their indications, and their potential adverse effects.

Recommendation 3.4: When appropriate, the nurse should assist and educate the person with asthma to measure their PEF.

Recommendation 3.5: To support self-management, the nurse should collaborate with the person with asthma to develop and review a documented asthma action plan in one or a combination of the following formats:

- In writing, on paper
- Electronically
- Pictorially

Recommendation 3.6: The nurse should provide integrated asthma self-management support to adults with uncontrolled asthma who are at risk for severe exacerbations through multiple modalities and formats, such as one of the following:

- Home care visits
- Facetime, Skype, WhatsApp, telehealth care

Recommendation 3.7: The nurse should refer and connect persons with asthma to one of the following:

- Health care provider
- Certified asthma educator or certified respiratory educator

Evaluation

Recommendation 4.1: At every encounter, the nurse should evaluate the effectiveness of the overall plan of care in achieving asthma control.

Education

Recommendation 5.1: Develop multifaceted education programs that reinforce standardized, evidence-based asthma care for:

- Health care providers
- Students entering health care professions

Recommendation 5.2: Asthma educators obtain and maintain a certified asthma educator or certified respiratory educator designation

Recommendation 5.3: Provide a quality assurance program and standardized training for health care providers who perform spirometry.

Organization and Policy

Recommendation 6.1: Organizations need to establish a corporate priority focused on the integration and evaluation of best practice asthma care across all care settings.

Recommendation 6.2: Organizations need to provide the resources and professional training necessary to integrate best practices for the assessment and management of adult asthma across all care settings.

Reference for Evidence

Registered Nurses' Association of Ontario (RNAO). (2017). *Adult asthma care: Promoting control of asthma* (2nd ed.). Author. http://rnao.ca/sites/rnao-ca/files/bpg/Adult_Asthma_FINAL_WEB.pdf

*Indicates important objective information for a complete assessment of asthma control, but may not be available.

[†]Performed and interpreted within the health care provider's scope of practice (including appropriate knowledge and skills) and in alignment with organizational policies and procedures.

General Management Approach. Several components enable successful management of asthma: (a) establishment of a confirmed diagnosis through the use of objective measures; (b) development of a partnership between health care providers and the patients and families affected by asthma; (c) limited exposure to triggers; (d) education of patients; (e) appropriate pharmacotherapy; (f) continuous assessment and monitoring of asthma control and severity; (g) implementation of a written action plan; and (h) ensuring regular follow-up.

Asthma treatment and management involve evidence-informed practice based on the Canadian Thoracic Society's Asthma Guidelines, GINA annual reports, and additional up-to-date publications that provide guidance for health care providers. GINA has published the 2020 stepwise approach to initial treatment of asthma (Figure 31.5) and the stepwise approach to personalized management to control and minimize future risks of asthma exacerbation (Figure 31.6). Controlling the disease in order to prevent complications, morbidity, and mortality is the primary goal of asthma management (Lougheed et al., 2010, 2012).

The stepwise approach in personalized management accounts for the fact that the level of control and the severity of asthma change over time. Therefore, a step-up or step-down approach to constant assessment and adjustment of therapy is necessary to achieve and maintain asthma control. Importantly, the stepwise approach to initial asthma treatment (see Figure 31.5) determines on the basis of confirmed diagnosis and symptoms which step is appropriate for initiating therapy. The patient will then have ongoing treatment decisions made on the basis of assessment, treatment adjustments, and review of response, with stepwise adjustment made up or down according to the stepwise approach for personalized management (see Figure 31.6) (GINA, 2020). Overall, the general management approach to asthma includes confirming the diagnosis, monitoring the level of asthma control (see Table 31.3), reducing exposure to environmental triggers, providing appropriate medications, providing asthma education, and providing a written action plan.

All individuals with asthma need to have access to a "rescue medication," sometimes referred to as a *fast-acting β₂ agonist (FABA)* or *reliever;* such medications most commonly consist of an inhaled SABA. In Canada the following inhalers are approved as a FABA/reliever, SABA: salbutamol, terbutaline fenoterol, and one long-acting β₂ agonist (LABA) formoterol (>12 years), but only with an ICS, either in a combination inhaler or separate, when the patient is on an ICS. GINA no longer recommends single SABA therapy for treatment of asthma in adults and adolescents; the recommended practice is prescribing an ICS-containing controller treatment (GINA, 2020).

The GINA asthma management guidelines (see Figures 31.5 and 31.6) emphasize that daily use of ICS in addition to a SABA is necessary for step one controller options; the use of SABA alone places patients at risk for asthma-related death and need for emergency care (GINA, 2020). If symptoms persist and are

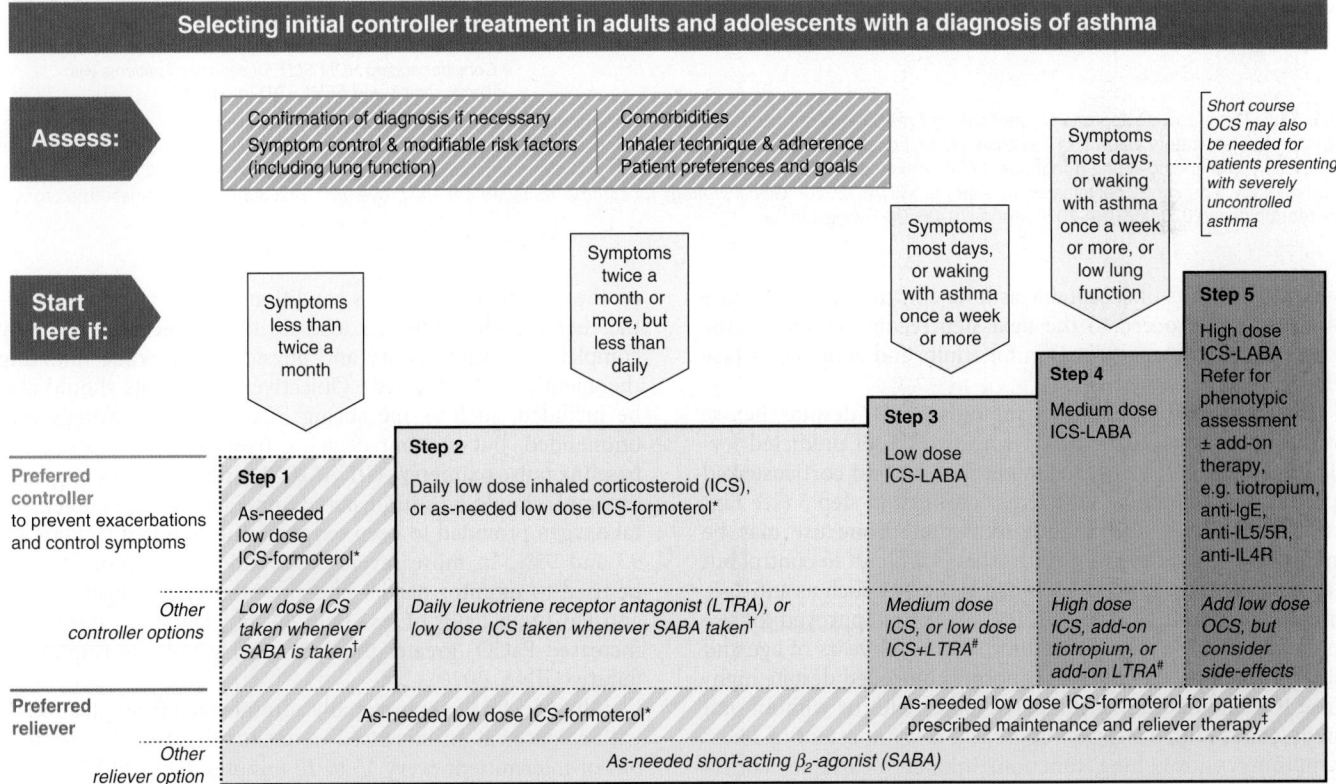

FIG. 31.5 The stepwise approach to initial asthma treatment. *BDP,* beclometasone dipropionate; *FEV₁,* forced expiratory volume in 1 second; *HDM,* house dust mite; *ICS,* inhaled corticosteroid; *IgE,* immunoglobin E, *IL4/IL5,* interleukin 4/5; *IL5R,* interleukin 5 receptor; *LABA,* long-acting β₂ agonist; *LTRA,* leukotriene receptor antagonist; *OCS,* oral corticosteroids; *SABA,* short-acting β₂ agonist; *SLIT,* sublingual immunotherapy. Source: Global Initiative for Asthma (GINA). (2020). *Global strategy for asthma management and prevention* (Box 3-4B). https://ginasthma.org/wp-content/uploads/2020/06/GINA-2020-report_20_06_04-1-wms.pdf

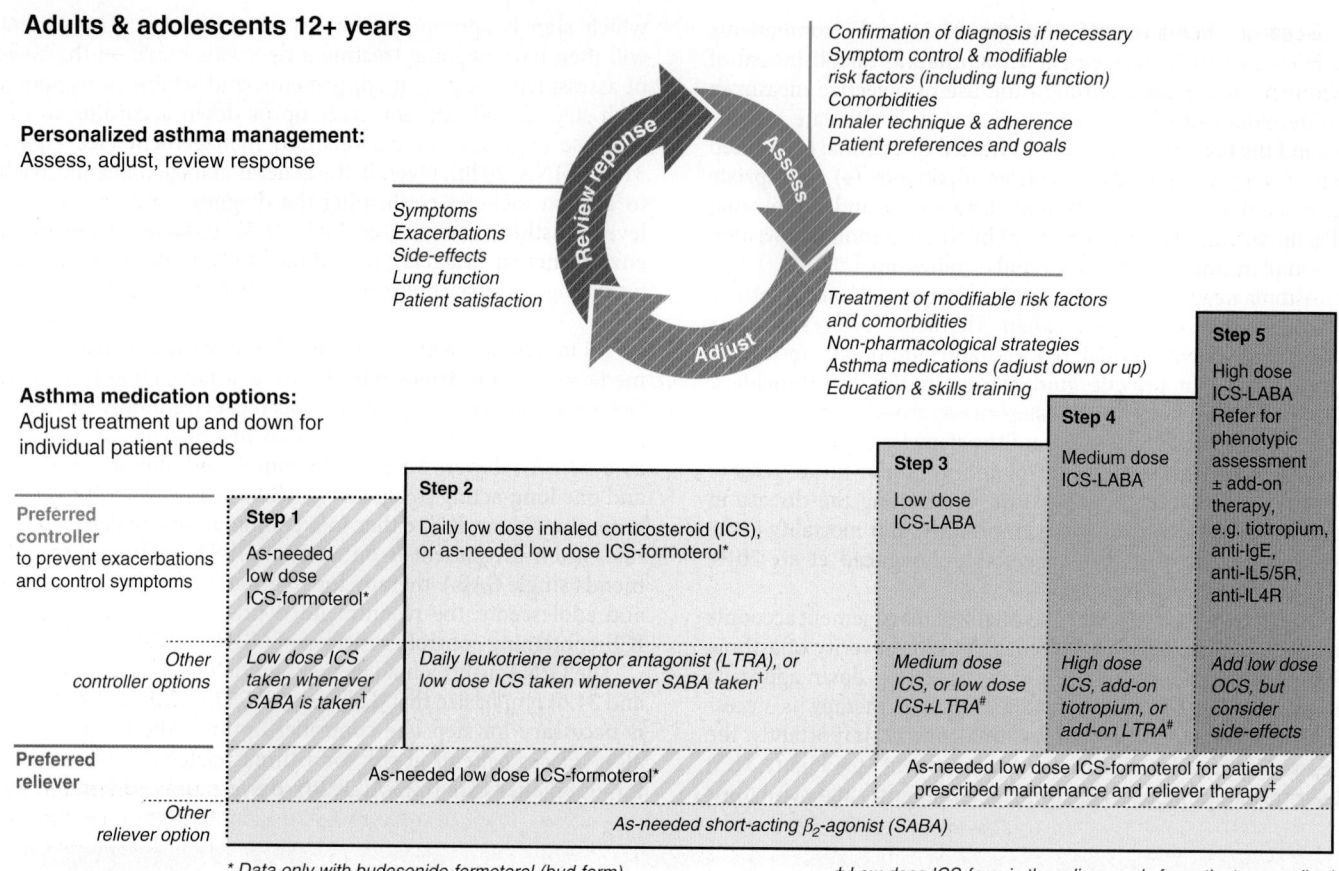

FIG. 31.6 The stepwise approach to personalized management to control and minimize future risk of asthma exacerbation. *BDP,* beclometasone dipropionate; *FEV₁,* forced expiratory volume in 1 second; *HDM,* house dust mite; *ICS,* inhaled corticosteroid; *IgE,* immunoglobin E; *IL4/IL5,* interleukin 4/5; *IL5R,* interleukin 5 receptor; *LABA,* long-acting β₂ agonist; *LTRA,* leukotriene receptor antagonist; *OCS,* oral corticosteroids; *SABA,* short-acting β₂ agonist; *SLIT,* sublingual immunotherapy. Source: Global Initiative for Asthma (GINA). (2020). *Global strategy for asthma management and prevention* (Box 3-5A). https://ginasthma.org/wp-content/uploads/2020/06/GINA-2020-report_20_06_04-1-wms.pdf

outside the limits of acceptable asthma control, the health care provider will proceed to the next step recommended on the personalized management plan for adults and adolescents (see Figure 31.6).

In a minority of patients, symptoms persist despite the use of these therapies. If the FEV_1 is below 60% of predicted levels or of their best value, treatment with an oral corticosteroid (prednisone) should be initiated as outlined in step 5 (see Figure 31.6) (GINA, 2020). Long-term prednisone use may be indicated and effective for asthma that is difficult to control but has many adverse effects. A biological therapy such as anti-IgE, anti-IL5, and anti-IL5R (IL-4R therapy is not approved for use in Canada) may be considered in patients 12 years of age and older with atopic asthma that is poorly controlled despite high-dose ICS and additional therapies, either with or without oral prednisone. With a stepwise approach, it is important to assess symptom control, lung function, inhaler technique, adherence to therapy, avoidance of exposure to asthma triggers, the presence of comorbid conditions, and examination of sputum eosinophils (where available) on a regular basis and before therapy is advanced to the next step (Lougheed et al., 2012).

Acute Asthma Exacerbation. Patients experiencing acute asthma exacerbation should be directed to an emergency department. The choice of treatment of acute asthma depends on the severity of a patient's condition and the response to initial therapy. The examiner assesses the degree of severity by completing a brief history and physical exam while initiating therapeutics (GINA, 2020). Objective assessments should also be included, such as measuring FEV_1 or PEF (strongly recommended, but without delaying treatment) and evaluating baseline pulse oximetry (GINA, 2020). Inhaled SABA (e.g., salbutamol) should be administered immediately and supplemental oxygen provided to keep oxygen saturation (SaO_2) between 93 and 95%. In more severe cases, ABG measurements may be used to monitor partial pressure of arterial oxygen (PaO_2) and $PaCO_2$; a PaO_2 of less than 60 mm Hg and a normal or increased $PaCO_2$ greater than 45 mm Hg indicate respiratory failure (GINA, 2020).

Inhaled SABAs are preferably administered through an MDI with a spacer at an increased frequency that may be continuous or intermittent every 15 to 20 minutes. If the FEV_1 or PEF is below 40% of predicted, one puff every 30 to 60 seconds (up to 20 puffs) may be administered, depending on the patient's response to and tolerance of treatment. Ipratropium bromide (four to eight puffs inhaled every 15 to 20 minutes, repeated three times) may be added to salbutamol during moderate and severe acute asthma episodes. In some emergency departments, bronchodilators are administered via a nebulizer, although a meta-analysis of study results revealed that the MDI with a spacer works faster, is less costly, and is more effective in reducing hospitalization and improving clinical scores (GINA, 2020).

Oral corticosteroids are indicated for treatment of an acute exacerbation that necessitates a visit to the emergency department. Intravenous corticosteroids are generally administered to patients who have difficulty with swallowing. Therapy should be continued until the patient is breathing comfortably, wheezing has disappeared, and pulmonary function measurements are near baseline values.

On occasion, an asthma attack is so severe and unresponsive to treatment that the patient requires mechanical ventilation. Indications for mechanical ventilation are persistent or progressive carbon dioxide retention and respiratory acidosis, clinical deterioration (indicated by fatigue, hypersomnolence), metabolic acidosis, and cardiopulmonary arrest. In life-threatening asthma exacerbation, the goals of initiating mechanical ventilation are to achieve a PaO_2 of 60 mm Hg or higher, an SaO_2 of 90% or higher, and a normal pH.

Audible wheezing may occur in the airways, which indicates a response to therapy as airflow increases. As the patient begins to respond to therapy and symptoms begin to subside, it is important to remember that despite the reversibility of most of the bronchospasm, the edema and cellular infiltration of the airway mucosa and the viscous mucous plugs are still present and improvement may take several days. Intensive therapy includes corticosteroids and must be continued even after clinical improvement has occurred. Patients with moderate or severe acute asthma are typically discharged home with an inhaled SABA, an added LABA or leukotriene receptor antagonist (LTRA), high-dosage ICS, and an oral corticosteroid, and the addition of anti-IgE medications should be considered as well (Lougheed et al., 2010). Discharge instructions should include an action plan detailing use of the medications and the criteria for returning to the emergency department for immediate medical assistance. It is important that patients follow up with their primary asthma care provider after an emergency department visit.

Medication Therapy

Medications used to treat asthma are divided into two categories: (a) relievers and (b) controllers (Table 31.5). They are available in several forms, and various delivery devices are used to administer them. The inhaled route is preferred because the medication is delivered directly to the lungs, which minimizes systemic absorption and also the occurrence of adverse effects. *Relievers* (or rescue medication) are used to ease asthma symptoms and given intermittently as required. *Controllers* are maintenance therapy used on a daily basis, typically twice a day. Because inflammation is considered an early and persistent component of asthma, medication therapy is directed toward long-term suppression of inflammation (see Figure 31.6).

Anti-Inflammatory Medications

Corticosteroids. Chronic inflammation is a primary component of asthma. Corticosteroids are anti-inflammatory medications that reduce bronchial hyper-responsiveness by blocking the late-phase reaction and inhibit migration of inflammatory cells. Corticosteroids are more effective than any other long-term medication in improving asthma control. ICSs are the mainstay therapy for the long-term control of asthma (GINA, 2020) (Figure 31.7). Usually, ICSs must be administered for 1 to

TABLE 31.5 CATEGORIES OF ASTHMA MEDICATIONS

Relievers Versus Controllers

Reliever Medications
Bronchodilators
- Short-acting inhaled β_2-adrenergic agonists (e.g., salbutamol)

Anticholinergics/Short-Acting Muscarinic Antagonists (SAMAs)
- Ipratropium, for example*

Controller Medications
Anti-Inflammatory Medications
- Corticosteroids
  - Inhaled (e.g., fluticasone)
  - Oral (e.g., prednisone)
- Leukotriene modifiers (e.g., montelukast)
- Anti-IgE (e.g., omalizumab)

Bronchodilators
- Long-acting inhaled β_2-adrenergic agonists (e.g., salmeterol inhalation)
- Long-acting oral β_2-adrenergic agonists (e.g., oral salmeterol)
- Methylxanthines (e.g., theophylline)

*Not considered a rescue medication if used alone; commonly used in combination with salbutamol in the emergency department for severe exacerbations.
IgE, immunoglobin E.

2 weeks before maximum therapeutic effects can be observed. However, some ICSs (e.g., fluticasone and budesonide) begin to have a therapeutic effect in 24 hours. Most ICS therapy must be administered on a fixed schedule. The exception is ICS-formoterol combination inhaler, which may be used as a FABA/reliever on an as-needed basis.

ICS therapy is a part of the stepwise treatment throughout the steps 1 through 5. When ICSs are administered, asthma can usually be controlled without significant systemic adverse events because only minimal amounts of drugs are absorbed systemically. However, ICSs administered at the highest dosage levels have been associated with adverse events such as easy bruising and accelerated bone loss (GINA, 2020). Oropharyngeal candidiasis, hoarseness, and dry cough are local adverse effects caused by an ICS (GINA, 2020). Occurrence of these oropharyngeal adverse events can be reduced by mouth rinsing and gargling after every inhalation treatment. If an MDI is used, absorption can be improved, and the intensity of adverse events is reduced with the use of a spacer. However, newer medications (e.g., ciclesonide) that are activated in the lungs (not in the pharynx) appear to minimize the intensity of these adverse events without the need for a spacer or mouth rinsing.

In acute asthma exacerbations, short courses of orally administered corticosteroids are indicated for gaining prompt control (Lougheed et al., 2010). In a minority of cases, maintenance dosages of oral corticosteroids are necessary to control severe chronic asthma. However, long-term use should be avoided in all age groups if possible because of adverse effects. If long-term use is indicated, a single dose in the morning, to coincide with endogenous cortisol production, and alternate-day dosing should be considered; these schedules are associated with fewer adverse effects. Long-term corticosteroid therapy is discussed further in Chapter 51.

Adults using maintenance oral corticosteroids or high dosages of ICS (>500 mcg of fluticasone and beclomethasone; >800 mcg of budesonide), or both, should be monitored for

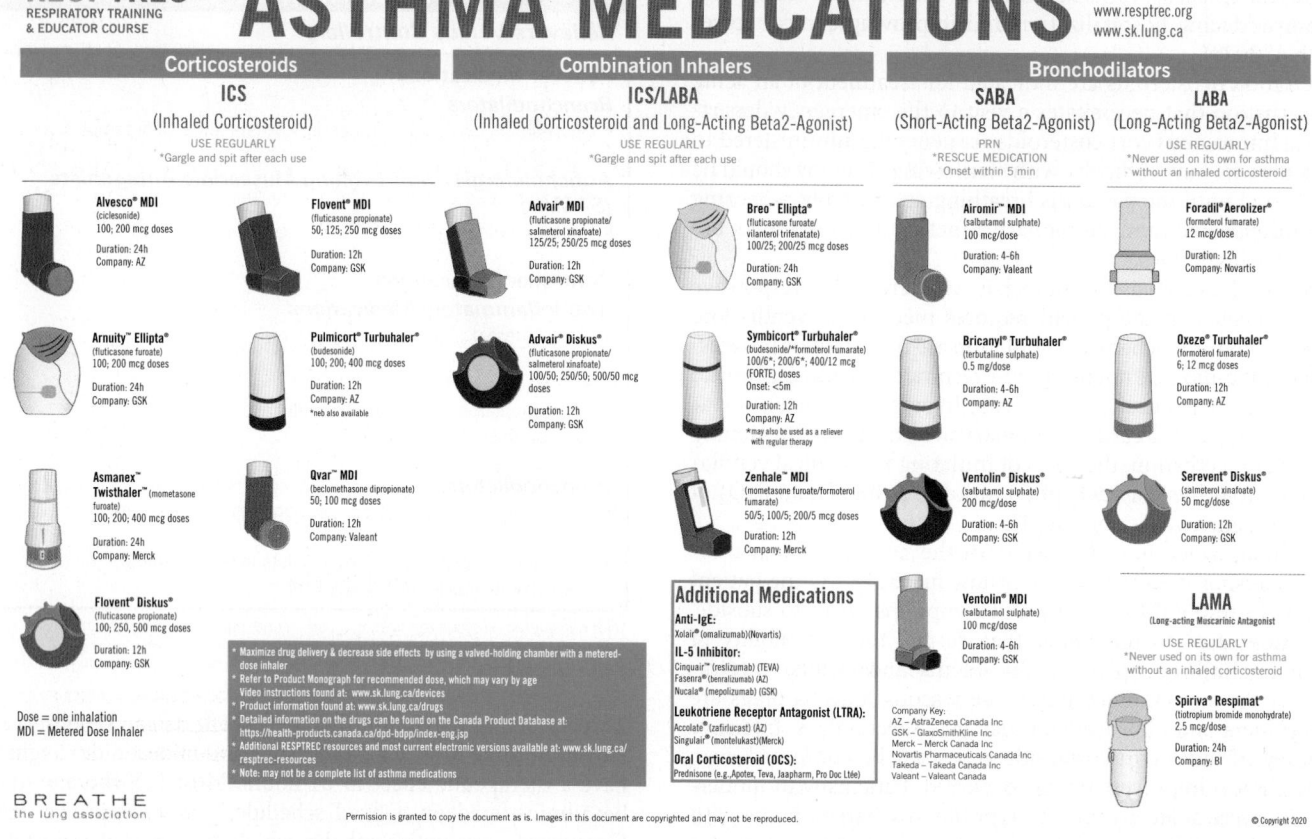

FIG. 31.7 Asthma medications. This is a pictorial guide of the inhaler therapies available for asthma treatment in Canada. Source: Lung Association of Saskatchewan. (2020). *Asthma medications brochure.* https://www.lungsask.ca/healthcare-providers/resptrec-resources

osteoporosis with bone densitometry. Patients should take adequate amounts of calcium and vitamin D and participate in regular weight-bearing exercise. (Osteoporosis is discussed in Chapter 66.)

Antileukotrienes. In Canada, two LTRAs (zafirlukast, montelukast) are available, which block the action of leukotrienes. Leukotrienes are produced as a result of arachidonic acid metabolism (see Chapter 14, Table 14.3). Some leukotrienes are potent bronchoconstrictors, causing airway edema and inflammation, and further contribute to the symptoms of asthma. The anti-inflammatory action of antileukotrienes is not as potent as that of an ICS; therefore, they are not recommended as a single medication in the treatment of persistent asthma. These medications are used as adjuvant or add-on therapy for individuals experiencing symptoms (uncontrolled asthma) or significant adverse events while using higher-dosage ICS. Antileukotrienes may be considered as an alternative to increasing dosages of ICS. They are not used to reverse bronchospasm in acute asthma attacks. An advantage of these medications is that they are administered orally.

Biological Therapy. The only biological anti-IgE therapy available in Canada is omalizumab (Xolair), which is a monoclonal antibody to IgE that decreases circulating free IgE levels (Asthma Canada, 2021a). Omalizumab prevents IgE from attaching to mast cells, which thus prevents the release of chemical mediators. Health Canada has approved this medication for use by patients who have moderate to severe persistent allergic asthma and are 12 years of age and older. This medication is expensive and should be reserved for specific patients: those with asthma that is difficult to control despite adherence to a regimen of high-dosage ICS and at least one additional controller therapy; those who have objectively confirmed asthma; those who have documented allergic perennial asthma; and those whose serum IgE level is 30 to 700 IU/mL. The medication is administered subcutaneously every 2 to 4 weeks and should be part of a well-controlled therapeutic trial supervised by an asthma specialist.

In recent years, Health Canada has approved additional biological therapies, such as the IL-5 inhibitors mepolizumab and benralizumab, and anti-IL-5 receptor alpha monoclonal antibody (IL-5R) benralizumab. IL-5 is a glycoprotein belonging to the cytokine family and is essential for the overall cellular function of eosinophils (Emma et al., 2018). Therefore, the utilization of anti-IL-5 biologicals markedly reduces circulating eosinophils.

IL-5 inhibitors are indicated for add-on maintenance therapy for patients with severe eosinophilic asthma who may or may not have allergies (Emma et al., 2018). Benralizumab also targets the IL-5 pathway but in a different way; ultimately it works to eradicate tissue eosinophilia (Emma et al., 2018). These powerful anti-IL-5 therapies have adverse effects related to a suppressed immune response, such as parasitic, bacterial, and viral infections and sometimes cancer cells (Emma et al., 2018). Regular blood work and physician follow-up are required.

Bronchodilators. Three classes of bronchodilator medications are currently used in asthma therapy: β_2-adrenergic agonists, anticholinergic medications, and methylxanthines.

β₂-Adrenergic Agonists. These medications may be short-acting (SABAs) or long-acting (LABAs). They work by binding to β₂ receptors located on airway smooth muscle, causing relaxation of the bronchial smooth muscle and thus bronchodilation. Fast-acting β₂-adrenergic agonists are the medication of choice for relief of acute symptoms of asthma and are used as rescue or reliever medication for quick relief of symptoms; therefore, they should be carried by the patient at all times. They are also used to prevent bronchospasm precipitated by exercise, with administration 10 to 15 minutes before exercise. In Canada, there are a few SABAs approved for this indication, including salbutamol and terbutaline (Lung Association of Saskatchewan, 2020a). These medications begin to work within a few minutes and cause maximum dilation within 10 to 15 minutes. The duration of effect varies according to the medication, but airflow rates remain significantly elevated for 2 to 6 hours after inhalation. Adverse events from SABAs are few; they include mild tremor and tachycardia, which diminish with repeated use without loss of bronchodilator effect. However, frequent daily use of inhaled SABAs may be associated with decreased control of asthma, which provides the rationale for as-needed dosage. The frequency of use of reliever medications is a good indicator of a patient's level of asthma control.

LABAs provide sustained bronchodilation (approximately 12 hours) and include formoterol and salmeterol. LABAs should be considered as add-on therapy in adults who have persistent symptoms despite low-dosage ICS (GOLD, 2020). Both formoterol and salmeterol can help patients reduce the amount of ICS necessary to control asthma and are useful in controlling nocturnal asthma symptoms. However, LABAs are not to be used as monotherapy but rather in combination with an ICS (Lougheed et al., 2010). Neither salmeterol nor formoterol causes major adverse events when used in conjunction with ICS. Immediate adverse events are similar to those of SABAs. Salmeterol and formoterol cannot be considered interchangeable. Formoterol has a greater bronchopulmonary protective effect and is rapid acting; thus, it can be used as rescue therapy for prompt relief of symptoms when taken in combination with only an ICS. Salmeterol has a narrower therapeutic window and dosage should stay within the recommended range.

Combination therapy inhalers that contain both a LABA and an ICS are available and commonly used (see Figure 31.7). Evidence suggests that combination therapy inhalers can replace the two separate inhalers, thus simplifying therapy and probably increasing adherence to the medication regimen. There is no superior effect over using the two inhalers separately; using the two medications in a combination inhaler is preferred for asthma, if the LABA is always used with the ICS (GINA, 2020).

Anticholinergic Medications. The parasympathetic division of the autonomic nervous system controls airway diameter. The effects of acetylcholine on the airways are increased smooth muscle contraction and mucus secretion, which result in bronchoconstriction. Anticholinergic medications inhibit bronchoconstriction that is related to the parasympathetic nervous system. Anticholinergic bronchodilators are not recommended as first-line therapy in asthma, primarily because their action does not peak until 30 minutes to 1 hour after inhalation; therefore, they are considered a second-line therapy and are not recommended to be used as a reliever outside of the emergency department setting. Anticholinergic medications may be useful in conjunction with FABA treatment when the patient is experiencing adverse effects. The combination of the anticholinergic

ipratropium bromide with salbutamol is commonly used for the emergency management of acute asthma. This combination appears to produce greater bronchodilation than does either medication alone. The most common adverse effect of anticholinergic medications is dry mouth. Systemic adverse events are uncommon because it is poorly absorbed.

A long-acting muscarinic antagonist (LAMA) therapy is an add-on therapy option for asthma patients on ICS-LABA who are still displaying symptoms and the asthma is considered not well controlled (GINA, 2020; Sobieraj et al., 2018). For patients with a diagnosis of asthma–COPD overlap, a LAMA is indicated as an add-on therapy but is never intended as single therapy. It is essential that these patients also receive ICS therapy (GINA, 2020).

Methylxanthines. Sustained-release methylxanthine (theophylline) preparations should be used only as controller medication for asthma that is difficult to control, after ICS, LABA, and LTRAs. Methylxanthines are bronchodilators with mild anti-inflammatory effects. Theophylline should be prescribed only by an asthma specialist because of its narrow toxic/therapeutic ratio and frequent adverse events (Lougheed et al., 2010), which include nausea, headache, insomnia, gastrointestinal distress, tachycardia, dysrhythmias, and seizures. Blood levels must be monitored regularly to determine whether the drug levels are in the therapeutic range.

Patient Education Related to Medication Therapy. Education about asthma medication is an essential component of asthma care (GINA, 2020). Information about medications that the patient should be familiar with should include details such as name, dosage, method of administration, frequency of use, indications, adverse effects, consequences of improper use, and the importance of adherence. Specifically, patients need to be taught about the different roles and indications for using relievers and controllers. In addition to providing information, it is essential that the nurse assess a patient's ability to use inhaler devices accurately and provide coaching in the proper use of the device. All nurses should know the correct use of the various devices and feel confident in their ability to assess and coach patients and their families in their proper use.

Most asthma medications are administered by inhalation. Inhalation of medications is preferred to oral administration because a lower dosage is required and systemic adverse events are fewer and less intense. The onset of action of bronchodilators is faster when they are delivered via inhalation. Inhalation devices include MDIs with or without spacers, dry powder inhalers (DPIs), and jet nebulizers (see Figures 31.8, 31.9, and 31.10).

In response to the outbreak of severe acute respiratory syndrome (SARS) and, recently, COVID-19, the use of jet nebulization (Figure 31.8) has been significantly reduced and avoided when possible, especially in emergency departments, and as much as possible in hospitals. When jet nebulization is used, the patient's sputum can become aerosolized if they contaminate the medication reservoir system with expectorant or saliva, thereby creating airborne particles that are released into the environment, causing infectious risk to persons within proximity to breathe in these aerosol particles (Fink et al., 2020). Specific personal protective equipment (PPE) is required in the presence of an aerosolized generating procedure (AGP)—for example, eye protection (or face shield), an N95 respirator, a gown, and gloves (Fink et. al., 2020). Other preventive measures to reduce infectious aerosolization include ensuring that infectious patients are isolated as per institution policy (most institutions recommend a negative air pressure room when AGPs are

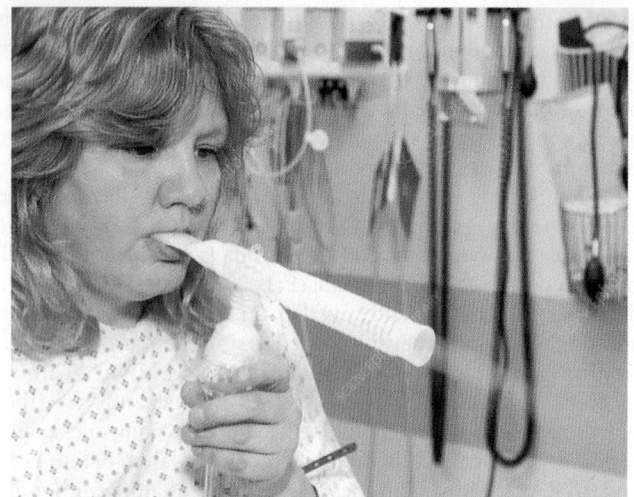

FIG. 31.8 Example of a jet nebulizer. Source: https://www.sciencephoto.com/media/457828/view

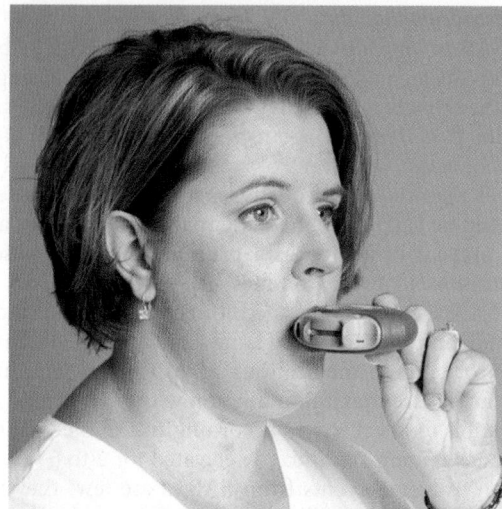

FIG. 31.10 Example of a dry powder inhaler (DPI). Source: Potter, P. A., Perry, A. G., Stockert, P., et al. (2011). *Basic nursing: Essentials for practice* (7th ed.). Mosby.

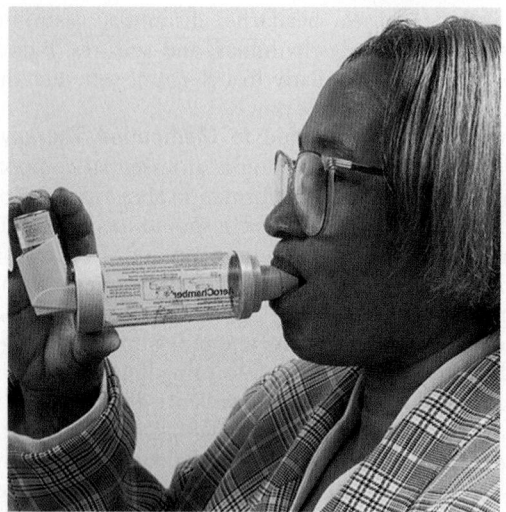

FIG. 31.9 Example of an AeroChamber spacer used with a metered-dose inhaler. Source: Potter, P. A., Perry, A. G., Stockert, P., et al. (2011). *Basic nursing: Essentials for practice* (7th ed.). Mosby.

TABLE 31.6	PROBLEMS ENCOUNTERED WITH USE OF METERED-DOSE INHALER (MDI)

1. Failing to coordinate activation with inspiration
2. Activating MDI in the mouth while breathing through nose
3. Inspiring too rapidly
4. Not holding the breath for 10 sec (or as close to 10 sec as possible)
5. Holding MDI upside down or sideways
6. Inhaling more than one puff with each inspiration
7. Not shaking MDI before use
8. Not waiting a sufficient amount of time between each puff
9. Not opening mouth wide enough, which causes medication to bounce off teeth, tongue, or palate
10. Not having adequate strength to activate MDI
11. Being unable to perform all the necessary steps

in use), cleaning nebulizers or exchanging them after use, using a breath-synchronized device or valved inhalation medication chamber, and placing a filter on the exhalation port of the jet nebulizer (see Figure 31.8). A respiratory therapist or occupational therapist can assess the patient's dexterity and ability to use an alternate handheld device. An alternate strategy is to have a caregiver administer the MDI or DPI.

MDI use must be frequently assessed and teaching provided as needed for patients and family, as inadequate technique in the use of MDIs is a widespread concern, and many patients demonstrate common errors (Table 31.6). If an inhaler technique can be improved and sustained, clinical benefits are likely to result (Table 31.7). Some patients need to add a spacer to the MDI or switch to a DPI to acquire a good technique. Spacers (e.g., AeroChamber, OptiChamber; see Figure 31.9) are used when patients do not have the coordination necessary to use an MDI. Spacers also enhance the delivery of medication to the airways and decrease the intensity of adverse events from ICS because less medication is delivered to the mouth. MDIs with spacers can be considered for all age groups and should be used when ICSs are delivered via an MDI. A spacer with a face mask

is recommended for young children and older persons. When spacers with face masks are used in children, however, a conversion to a spacer with a mouthpiece is recommended as soon as the child is old enough and able to cooperate.

The DPI contains dry, powdered medication and is breath activated (Figure 31.10). No propellant is used; instead, an aerosol is created when the patient inhales quickly and forcefully through a reservoir containing a dose of powder. Patients find DPIs easier to use than MDIs with no spacer. There are several advantages to using DPIs: (a) less manual dexterity is required; (b) the patient does not need to coordinate depressing the canister with inhaling; (c) an easily visible colour or number system indicates the number of doses left in the device; and (d) no spacer is necessary. The biggest issue with DPIs is that the medication may clump if exposed to humidity, so they should be stored in a dry place. The care of DPIs involves wiping off the mouthpiece with a dry tissue. Water or other liquids should never be used to clean the device as they could cause clumping of the medication and cause the device to work improperly.

Various inhalation devices are used to deliver medications to the airways. It is thus important to work with patients individually to identify the inhalation device that best fits their needs.

TABLE 31.7   PATIENT & CAREGIVER TEACHING GUIDE

How to Use a Metered-Dose Inhaler (MDI) and Spacer Correctly

Asthma Canada recommends using a spacer with your puffer if possible, but if you must use it without a spacer then the following steps are recommended for MDI use.
1. Shake the puffer well before use (three or four shakes).
2. Remove the cap.
3. Breathe out, away from your puffer.
4. Bring the puffer to your mouth. Place it in your mouth between your teeth and close your mouth around it.
5. Start to breathe in slowly. Press the top of your puffer once, and keep breathing in slowly until you have taken a full breath.
6. Remove the puffer from your mouth, and hold your breath for about 10 seconds, then breathe out. If you need a second puff, wait 30 sec, shake your puffer again, and repeat steps 3 to 6.

Is the Inhaler Full?

If your puffer doesn't have a built-in dose counter, always write down the number of puffs you have taken so that you can anticipate when you need to refill your prescription. It is a good practice to keep a spare inhaler on hand.

When to Use an MDI With a Spacer

Asthma Canada recommends that anyone, of any age, who is using a puffer should consider using a spacer. A pharmacist, respiratory therapist, asthma educator, or physician can assess how you use your puffer and will recommend the best device for you.
It is recommended that children use a spacer device with their puffer.
Spacers should not be used with dry powder inhalers—only with puffer-style devices.
Puffers with either a rectangular or a round mouthpiece should be able to fit into a spacer—ask your health care provider for a demonstration if you are unsure how to set it up.

Instructions for Using a Spacer With an MDI
1. Shake the puffer well before use (three or four shakes).
2. Remove the cap from your puffer, and from your spacer if it has one.
3. Put the puffer into the spacer.
4. Breathe out, away from the spacer.
5. Bring the spacer to your mouth, put the mouthpiece between your teeth, and close your lips around it.
6. Press the top of your puffer once.
7. Breathe in slowly until you have taken a full breath. (If you hear a whistle sound, you are breathing in too fast.)
8. Hold your breath for about 10 sec; then breathe out.
9. If you need to take more than one puff at a time, wait a minimum of 30 sec between puffs and be sure to shake the puffer (as in step 1) before each puff. Only put one puff of medication into the spacer at a time.

Caring for the Spacer

To clean your spacer, follow the instructions that come with it. In most cases, they will advise you to:
1. Take the spacer apart.
2. Gently move the parts back and forth in warm water using a mild soap. Never use high-pressure or boiling hot water, rubbing alcohol, or disinfectant.
3. Rinse the parts well in clean water.
4. Do **not** dry inside of the spacer with a towel as it will cause static. Instead, let the parts air dry (for example, leave them out overnight).
5. Put the spacer back together.
If you are using your spacer every day, you should replace it about every 12 months (Asthma Canada, 2021b).

Source: Asthma Canada. (2021). *Breathe easy: Medications use as prescribed.* https://asthma.ca/wp-content/uploads/2020/06/BreatheEasy-Medications_optimized_EN.pdf

Poor adherence to asthma therapy regimens is a major challenge in the long-term management of asthma. Patients commonly rely too heavily on their reliever inhalers because they provide immediate relief of symptoms and gratification, whereas no immediate benefit is felt with anti-inflammatory therapy, which must be sustained on a daily basis. It is important to explain to patients the importance and purpose of taking controller therapy regularly, emphasizing that maximum improvement may take more than 1 week. It is also important to emphasize that without regular use, the inflammation in the airways may progress and the asthma is likely to worsen over time.

NURSING MANAGEMENT
ASTHMA

NURSING ASSESSMENT

If a patient can speak and is not in acute distress, a detailed health history, including identification of any precipitating factors and what has helped alleviate attacks in the past, should be documented. If a patient is in acute distress, some of the information may be obtained from the person accompanying the patient. Subjective and objective data to obtain from a patient with asthma are presented in Table 31.8.

NURSING DIAGNOSES

Nursing diagnoses for the patient with asthma may include but are not limited to the following:
- *Inadequate airway clearance* resulting from *excessive mucus, retained secretions*
- *Anxiety* resulting from *threat to current status, threat of death* (difficulty breathing)
- *Inadequate knowledge* as a result of insufficient information, *insufficient knowledge of resources* (asthma education)
Additional information on nursing diagnoses is presented in Nursing Care Plan 31.1.

PLANNING

The overall goals are that patients with asthma will (a) be able to participate in their usual activities (including exercise and other physical activity) with little to no interference; (b) have normal

TABLE 31.8   NURSING ASSESSMENT
Asthma

Subjective Data
Important Health Information
Current health: Assess the level of asthma control (see Table 31.2); frequency and severity of asthma symptoms (wheeze, cough, sensation of chest tightness, dyspnea) in the past week, both during the day and in early morning hours and night; need for reliever medication during the past week; and usual pattern of asthma symptoms. Determine whether the patient experienced a recent worsening of asthma and how it was handled. Identify recent exposure to triggers (e.g., upper respiratory tract infection, pollen, animals, mould, dust, inhaled irritants, weather changes, exercise, smoke).
Past health history: One or more previous asthma attacks and response to treatment; previous visits to the emergency department or hospitalizations for asthma and the need for CCU admission and intubation; recent exposure to pollen, dander, feathers, mould, dust, inhaled irritants, smoke; weather changes; exercise; allergic rhinitis and eczema; sinus infections; gastroesophageal reflux; family history of asthma and allergies
Medications: Last time the reliever medication was used, what level of relief was provided, duration of relief, and frequency of the reliever use in the past week; pattern of use for controller medications; recent use of antibiotics; use of medications that may precipitate asthma, such as ASA (Aspirin), NSAIDs, β-adrenergic blockers; allergies to medications

Symptoms

- Wheezing, cough, sensation of chest tightness, dyspnea
- Decreased level of activity or exercise because of symptoms
- Interrupted sleep, fatigue; fear, anxiety, panic, depression, emotional distress

Objective Data
General

Restlessness or exhaustion, confusion, upright or forward-leaning body position

Integumentary

Eczema, diaphoresis, cyanosis (circumoral, nail beds)

Respiratory

Wheezing, crackles, diminishment or absence of breath sounds on auscultation; hyper-resonance on percussion; sputum character and quantity; increased work of breathing, demonstrated by use of accessory muscle, intercostal, and supraclavicular retractions; tachypnea; prolonged expiration

Cardiovascular

Tachycardia, pulsus paradoxus, jugular venous distension, hypertension or hypotension, premature ventricular contractions

Possible Diagnostic Findings

Abnormal results of pulmonary function tests: decreased flow rates; FVC, FEV_1, PEFR, and FEV_1/FVC ratio that improve with bronchodilators and between exacerbations
↓ O_2 saturation and abnormal ABG values during moderately severe to life-threatening attacks
Serum and sputum eosinophilia
Positive results of skin tests for allergens and allergies to medication

ABG, arterial blood gas; *ASA,* acetylsalicylic acid; *CCU,* critical care unit; *FEV₁,* forced expiratory volume in 1 second; *FVC,* forced vital capacity; *NSAIDs,* nonsteroidal anti-inflammatory drugs; *PEFR,* peak expiratory flow rate.

TABLE 31.9   PATIENT & CAREGIVER TEACHING GUIDE
Basic Asthma Education

Basic asthma education for patients and caregivers should include:

Basic Facts About Asthma
- Basic anatomical and physiological characteristics of the lungs
- Pathophysiological changes of asthma
- Relationship of pathophysiological changes to signs and symptoms
- Asthma control criteria (signs and symptoms)

Trigger Control
- Identification of possible triggers and management strategies
- Avoidance of allergens and other triggers

Medications
- Differences between relievers and controllers
- Indications for using reliever as opposed to controller medication
- Establishing medication schedule
- Adverse effects and strategies to reduce their frequency and intensity

Device Technique
- Good inhaler technique
- Good peak flowmeter and monitoring technique (if applicable)

Self-Monitoring and Action Plan
- Development of an individualized asthma action plan
- Early recognition of worsening asthma
- Actions to take in response to worsening asthma

Follow-Up Care
- Understanding and accepting the need for regular follow-up care

NURSING IMPLEMENTATION

ASTHMA EDUCATION. Nurses play an essential role in preventing and controlling asthma symptoms by developing a partnership with the patient and family, providing information and education, and helping the patient and family develop the necessary skills for controlling asthma. Education is an essential component of asthma care and should occur at every encounter with patients, families, and caregivers. In order to be effective, asthma education must provide information, help develop and refine asthma-related skills, assist with problem solving, and bring about behaviour change. In addition, findings of meta-analyses suggest that self-management asthma education programs can reduce the number of emergency department visits, hospitalizations, urgent care visits, nocturnal awakenings related to asthma, and days of interrupted activity and can improve quality of life (PHAC, 2015). Asthma education programs can also be cost-effective. Table 31.9 details basic asthma education to be provided.

ENVIRONMENTAL CONTROL. Environmental control strategies focus on reducing exposure to asthma triggers specific to the individual. Triggers can be divided into two groups: *allergens* and *irritants.* Patients should be taught to identify known personal triggers for asthma and to reduce exposure to them (see Table 31.1). Sensitization to environmental allergens is clearly linked to asthma in children and adults (PHAC, 2015). However, before patients and families are advised to use environmental control strategies to reduce or manage exposure to allergens, it is important to understand the allergen to which they are sensitized.

House dust mites produce a common allergen that can trigger asthma. House dust mites excrete food and digestive

or near-normal pulmonary function; (c) have the asthma under control; (d) experience as few adverse effects from asthma medication as possible while taking the lowest dosage of medication necessary to keep the asthma under control; and (e) possess the knowledge and skills necessary to participate in management of the asthma.

NURSING CARE PLAN 31.1

Asthma

NURSING DIAGNOSIS	**Inadequate airway clearance** resulting from *excessive mucus, retained secretions* as evidenced by *ineffective cough, adventitious breath sounds*

Expected Patient Outcomes	Nursing Interventions and *Rationales*
• Maintains open airways • Has normal breath sounds and respiratory rate • Has normal or personal best objective lung function measurements (PEFR, FEV₁, FEV₁/FVC) • Participates in normal life activities, including exercise and physical activity (identifying activity that is meaningful to the patient is helpful)	• Position patient to maximize ventilation potential *allowing for adequate chest expansion.* • Monitor respiratory (including spirometry) and oxygenation status *to determine need for intervention or to note improvement.* • Administer medications (e.g., bronchodilators, corticosteroids), as appropriate, *to improve respiratory function.* • Teach patient proper use of prescribed inhalers (see Table 31.7) *to deliver adequate medication to the lungs.* • Auscultate lung sounds after treatments *to note improvement.* • Regulate fluid intake to optimize fluid balance and liquefy secretions *to facilitate removal.* • Provide asthma education *to help patient understand condition and avoid triggers, when possible.* • Establish a written asthma action plan with patient to manage exacerbations, and educate patient about it *to ensure that patient is prepared for emergency situations.*

NURSING DIAGNOSIS	**Anxiety** resulting from *threat to current status* (difficulty breathing, perceived or actual loss of control, fear of suffocation) as evidenced by *restlessness, increase in heart rate, respiratory rate, and blood pressure*

Expected Patient Outcomes	Nursing Interventions and *Rationales*
• Reports reduced anxiety or no anxiety	• Explore patterns of anxiety and feelings, perceptions, and fears to identify precipitating factors and problem areas *so that planning can be concentrated.* • Use a calm, supportive approach *to provide reassurance.* • Stay with patient *to promote safety and reduce fear.* • Provide factual information concerning diagnosis, treatment, and prognosis *to help patient know what to expect.* • Instruct patient on the use of relaxation techniques *to relieve muscle tension and slow respirations.*

NURSING DIAGNOSIS	**Inadequate knowledge** as a result of insufficient information, insufficient knowledge of resources (asthma and treatment) as evidenced by inaccurate follow-through of instruction

Expected Patient Outcomes	Nursing Interventions and *Rationales**
• Demonstrates appropriate use of inhalers, peak flowmeters, spacers, and nebulizers (if used) • Maintains good asthma control • Manages personal triggers • Recognizes worsening asthma and initiates early treatment • Actively participates in management decisions with the asthma care team	• Appraise patient's current level of knowledge and skills related to asthma management *to identify learning needs.* • Teach patient to identify and manage triggers *to prevent asthma attacks.* • Encourage patient to verbalize feelings about diagnosis, treatment, and effect on lifestyle *to offer support and increase adherence to medication regimen to improve asthma control.* • Ensure that patient has an asthma action plan and understands its use to enhance patient's ability to identify worsening asthma and respond appropriately. • Instruct patient in proper administration of each medication and have them complete a return demonstration and teach back* (e.g., inhalers, spacers) *to ensure proper use.* • Evaluate patient's inhaler techniques *to assess correct technique and ensure maximum benefit.* • Instruct patient on purpose, action, dosage, indication, and duration of each medication *to promote understanding of effects and use.* • Teach patient about strategies to decrease the intensity of adverse medication events *to prevent or minimize the intensity of adverse medication events and enhance adherence.* • Assist patient in identifying strategies that incorporate taking medications into daily life, such as taking inhaled steroids before brushing teeth in the morning and at night, *to enhance adherence.* • Include the family and significant others as appropriate *to ensure that a knowledgeable person is available to help when the patient needs it.*

FEV₁, forced expiratory volume; *FVC*, forced vital capacity; *PEFR*, peak expiratory flow rate.
*Refer to Figures 31.7 to 31.11 and to Patient & Caregiver Teaching Guides (see Tables 31.7, 31.8, and 31.9).

enzymes as a fecal particle, which is the major form of mite allergen. They require dead skin and water to survive; thus the bed provides a perfect environment because when humans sleep, they slough off dead skin and provide humidity. As a result, control strategies focus on the bedroom and include keeping the relative humidity below 50%; encasing the mattress, box springs, and pillows in covers that are impermeable to mites and mite allergens; laundering bed linen in hot water and hot (55°C) air to dry it; and removing carpets, when possible (PHAC, 2015).

Pet dander is another common allergen. Strategies to reduce exposure to pet dander have been evaluated. The removal of the pet is the most effective means to reduce exposure. However, this is often not a realistic option for patients and families. As a result, numerous alternative strategies include preventing the pet from entering the bedroom by keeping the door and heating register closed to prevent dander circulation, frequent vacuuming (including furniture) with a high-efficiency particulate air (HEPA)–filtered vacuum, removing carpets, and washing the pet at least twice a week (none of these actions should be performed by the person with the allergies).

Environmental tobacco smoke is the most harmful indoor air irritant and should be avoided. Environmental tobacco smoke is a risk factor for the development of childhood asthma and frequently causes the worsening of asthma in children and adults. Among children with asthma, those whose parents smoke have more severe disease than do those whose parents do not smoke. When parents of a child with asthma stop smoking, the child's asthma improves. Nurses must encourage patients and their family members to stop smoking and assist them in identifying smoking cessation strategies.

Exercise and cold air are very common asthma triggers. Strategies to prevent exposure to cold air include the use of scarves and face masks. Exercise is just as important for individuals with asthma as for those without it because exercise provides multiple health benefits. Asthma is not an excuse for avoiding exercise. If a form of exercise provokes asthma symptoms, the nurse can advise the patient to use a warm-up period and an inhaled SABA 10 to 15 minutes before the activity to prevent bronchospasm.

Work-related asthma (WRA) can account for 15 to 33% of adult asthmatic cases (Lau et al., 2018). WRA includes (1) *occupational asthma,* defined as asthma symptoms induced by exposure to a particular workplace, and (2) *work-exacerbated asthma,* where asthma symptoms are exacerbated but not caused by work exposure. WRA is underreported by workers as they may not connect the work relationship to the exacerbation of asthma symptoms. Therefore, it is of utmost importance for health care providers to include health history questions about a potential work relationship with increased asthma symptoms to hep further determine exacerbation triggers. Objective lung function tests, along with a detailed occupational exposure history, are necessary to confirm the diagnosis of WRA.

SELF-MONITORING AND ACTION PLANS. Every person with asthma should have an asthma action plan (Figure 31.11). An action plan is a written plan developed to provide the patient with a framework for monitoring and determining their level of asthma control and making treatment changes to achieve and maintain control. Often, action plans are designed according to a traffic-light analogy: green, yellow, and red "zones." The green zone represents good asthma control and signals "go" with current therapy. The yellow zone is a time of worsening or uncontrolled asthma and signals "caution" and the need for enhanced anti-inflammatory therapy. The red zone represents a time of danger during which the asthma is severe enough to necessitate urgent medical attention; it signals "stop" current activities in order to address this need.

Nurses must develop a partnership with patients and their families, their primary asthma care provider, and the rest of the asthma care team in order to help patients attain and effectively use an individualized asthma action plan. Systematic reviews have concluded that self-management programs that included self-monitoring, by symptoms or PEF, combined with a written action plan and regular medical review resulted in reduced need for health care services, fewer days lost from work, and fewer episodes of nocturnal asthma (GINA, 2020). Self-monitoring based on symptom experience alone was compared with self-monitoring based on both symptom

experience and PEF monitoring; comparable outcomes were reported (GINA, 2020). PEF provides an objective measurement of lung function (Table 31.10) and, as a result, has been advocated for detecting asthma exacerbations. However, for most people, asthma symptoms are a more sensitive measure and change earlier in the course of an exacerbation than does PEF. The choice of whether an action plan is based on PEF or symptom monitoring may be made according to a patient's ability to perceive symptoms and airflow limitation, the availability of peak flowmeters, and, of most importance, the patient's preferences.

The level of detail in the plan depends on the patient's understanding of asthma and preferences for monitoring (PEF or symptoms). Key components for teaching patients and their families how to use an action plan include the signs and symptoms of worsening asthma, knowing the level of asthma control and how to adjust medications, and when to seek medical attention.

In developing a management plan, it is important to involve the patient's family. Family members and friends should be taught how to help the patient during an asthma exacerbation. They should know where the patient's inhalers and emergency phone numbers are located. Family members can help patients identify deteriorating levels of asthma control, inasmuch as they may notice an increase in symptoms or the need to avoid certain activities before the patient notices.

It is particularly important to provide asthma education, which should occur at every encounter with the patient and family, during emergency department visits, and during hospitalization because this is a time when patients are highly motivated to learn and do not have to schedule an additional visit. The Canadian Lung Association has developed and distributes several excellent resources for individuals affected by asthma. (See the Resources at the end of this chapter.)

EVALUATION. The expected outcomes for the patient with asthma are presented in Nursing Care Plan 31.1.

CHRONIC OBSTRUCTIVE PULMONARY DISEASE

Chronic obstructive pulmonary disease (COPD) is a preventable disease, characterized by persistent airflow limitation that is usually progressive. It is associated with an enhanced chronic inflammatory response in the airways and lungs, caused primarily by cigarette smoking and other noxious particles and gases. COPD exacerbations and other coexisting illnesses or comorbid conditions contribute to the overall severity of the disease (Global Initiative for Chronic Obstructive Lung Disease [GOLD], 2020).

Cardinal symptoms experienced by patients with COPD are dyspnea, difficulty breathing, shortness of breath, and limitations in activity. Symptoms are usually insidious in onset and progressive. Dyspnea is the subjective experience of shortness of breath and is the most disabling symptom in COPD (GOLD, 2020). Initially, COPD is confined to the lungs, but when disease is advanced, skeletal muscle dysfunction, right-sided heart failure, secondary polycythemia, depression, and altered nutrition are commonly observed. Past definitions of COPD included the terms *emphysema* and *chronic bronchitis*. Emphysema describes only one pathological change present in COPD: destruction of the alveoli. Chronic bronchitis, which is the presence of chronic productive cough for 3 months in 2 successive years, remains a useful epidemiological term but it, too, does not convey how

THE ✝ LUNG ASSOCIATION®

My Asthma Action Plan

Name _____   Doctor _____

Date _____   Doctor's Phone Number _____

GREEN LEVEL   My asthma is under control.

SYMPTOMS

- My breathing is normal.
- I have no trouble sleeping.
- I'm not coughing or wheezing.
- I can do all my normal activities.

PEAK FLOW

_____ to _____ (80 to 100% of your personal best)

WHAT SHOULD I DO?

I should continue using my normal medications as directed by my doctor, and re-measure my peak flow every _____ weeks/months.

Medication	Dose	Take it when?

YELLOW LEVEL   My asthma is getting worse.

SYMPTOMS

- I have symptoms, like wheezing or coughing, with activity or at night. They go away when I use my reliever.
- I'm using my reliever more than ___ times a week/day.
- I can't do many of my usual activities.

PEAK FLOW

_____ to _____ (60 to 80% of your personal best)

WHAT SHOULD I DO?

A problem is beginning. I should increase my medication as specified below until I am in the green level for _____ days or more. **If my symptoms do not improve within 4 days, I will call my doctor.**

Medication	Dose	Take it when?

RED LEVEL   I am having an asthma emergency.

SYMPTOMS

- My breathing is difficult.
- I'm wheezing often when resting.
- I'm having difficulty walking and/or talking.
- My lips and/or fingernails are blue or grey.
- My reliever does not help in 10 minutes OR is needed every 4 hours or more.

PEAK FLOW

_____ to _____ (less than 60% of your personal best)

WHAT SHOULD I DO?

I NEED TO GO TO THE HOSPITAL EMERGENCY RIGHT AWAY.

I SHOULD USE MY RELIEVER AS MUCH AS I NEED TO ON THE WAY THERE.

FIG. 31.11 Example of an asthma action plan. Source: Modified from the Canadian Lung Association (n.d.). *Asthma action plan.* https://www.lung.ca/sites/default/files/media/asthma_action_plan.pdf

---

airway limitation so severely affects morbidity and mortality in patients with COPD. People with COPD often display characteristics of both chronic bronchitis and emphysema.

The PHAC (2019b) reported that the prevalence of COPD among the population aged 35 years and older was 9.4% (2 million Canadians). The prevalence among men (9.9%) and that among women (9.1%) are currently comparable, although rates of COPD and of subsequent hospitalization and death are rising more rapidly among women. Compared to the non-Indigenous population, estimated COPD prevalence is 2.3 to 2.4 times greater among First Nations people, 1.86 to 2.10 times higher for Inuit people, and 1.59 to 1.67 times higher among the Métis (Bird et al., 2017). Hospitalization may be required in the treatment of COPD, particularly when symptoms worsen from infection.

Causes

Tobacco Smoke. Exposure to tobacco smoke is the primary cause of COPD cases in Canada (Government of Canada, 2018). Given that smoking prevalence is two to five times

TABLE 31.10 PATIENT & CAREGIVER TEACHING GUIDE

How to Use a Peak Flowmeter

Follow these nine steps to use a peak flowmeter:
1. Attach the mouthpiece to the peak flow monitor.
2. Set the marker (indicator) to the level of zero on the scale.
3. Stand up or, if you cannot stand, sit up straight.
4. Breathe in as deeply as you can.
5. Close your lips around the mouthpiece.
6. Blow out as hard and as fast as you can (i.e., a "fast blast" of air).
7. Note the number next to the marker.
8. Repeat steps 2 through 7 two more times.
9. In a notebook or diary, record the highest of the three numbers. This number is your peak expiratory flow (PEF) for that morning or evening (Asthma Canada, 2021b).

Making Sense of your Results

- Your health care provider or asthma educator will help you determine which of your PEF measurements should be used as a "baseline" – that is, your personal best peak flow. Use your peak flow result with your written asthma action plan to determine the action needed to be taken to manage your asthma.
- Once you know your personal best peak flow, you will be able to know if your asthma is well controlled. If the result of a PEF test is 80% or more of your personal best number, your asthma is likely well controlled.
- If it is less than 80% of your personal best you are not well controlled. Discuss your results with your health care provider.
- Remember that a peak flowmeter can be a useful tool, but monitoring your symptoms is the most important way to assess overall how well your asthma is being managed.

Source: Asthma Canada. (2021). *Peak flow meters.* https://asthma.ca/get-help/living-with-asthma/peak-flow-meters/

higher among Indigenous people, the prevalence of COPD among Indigenous people in Canada is strongly associated with tobacco usage, among other factors (Osipna et al., 2015).

According to the Government of Canada, annually 45 000 Canadians die from tobacco-related diseases (Government of Canada, 2020). For most Canadians who die of lung diseases related to cigarette smoking, death is preceded by a long period of debilitation characterized by frequent hospitalizations and loss of many years of productivity. Cigarette smoking remains the most preventable cause of premature death in Canada. Although the prevalence of cigarette smoking has decreased, it is still a major public health concern. Canada's tobacco strategy has the goal of reaching less than 5% tobacco usage by the year 2035 (Government of Canada, 2020).

When cigarettes are smoked, approximately 4 000 chemicals and gases are inhaled into the lungs. Over 60 carcinogens have been isolated from cigarette smoke, including cyanide, formaldehyde, and ammonia. Nicotine is probably not a carcinogen, but it has deleterious effects. It acts by stimulating the sympathetic nervous system, resulting in increases in heart rate, peripheral vasoconstriction, blood pressure, and cardiac workload. These effects of nicotine compound the health problems in a person with coronary artery disease. (The effects of nicotine are discussed further in Chapter 11.)

Cigarette smoke has several direct effects on the respiratory tract. It simulates an inflammatory response in the lung, which is most evident late in the course of COPD. The irritating effect of the smoke causes hyperplasia of goblet cells, which subsequently results in increased production of mucus and is the basis of chronic cough and sputum accumulation. In airways

smaller than 2 mm in diameter, injury leads to narrowing and obstruction of the airways. Smoking reduces ciliary activity and accelerates loss of ciliated cells. Smoking also produces abnormal dilation of the distal air space with destruction of alveolar walls. Many cells develop large, atypical nuclei, which is considered a precancerous condition. Removal of the inciting stimulus is of greatest benefit early in the process but may be less effective in late disease. However, smoking cessation can prevent or delay the development of airflow limitation or slow its progression.

Carbon monoxide is a component of tobacco smoke. Carbon monoxide has a high affinity for hemoglobin and combines with it more readily than does oxygen, thereby reducing the smoker's oxygen-carrying capacity. Smokers inhale a lower percentage of oxygen than normal; as a result, less oxygen is available at the alveolar level. The heart's need for oxygen is increased because of the stimulatory effect of nicotine on the sympathetic nervous system. Because the blood's oxygen-carrying capacity is reduced, the heart must pump more rapidly to adequately supply tissues with oxygen. Carbon monoxide also seems to impair psychomotor performance and judgement.

Passive smoking (also known as *environmental tobacco smoke* or *secondhand smoke*) is the exposure of nonsmokers to cigarette smoke. In adults, involuntary smoke exposure is associated with decreased pulmonary function, increased risk for lung cancer, and increased rates of mortality from ischemic heart disease.

Smoking, age, low socioeconomic status, and lack of access to health care are strongly associated with a COPD diagnosis among Indigenous people (Bird et al., 2017). Other risk factors for COPD among Indigenous people include exposure to biomass fuel burned for indoor cooking, housing conditions in need of repair, overcrowding, material and social deprivation, lack of education, inadequate nutrition, and childhood and prenatal exposure to secondhand tobacco smoke (Ospina et al., 2015). The nurse needs to take these cultural considerations into effect when completing a nursing care plan that will be successfully implemented.

Occupational Chemicals and Dusts. High levels of urban air pollution are harmful to people with existing lung disease. In a person who has intense or prolonged exposure to various dusts, vapours, irritants, or fumes in the workplace, COPD can develop independently of cigarette smoking (PHAC, 2019b). If the person also smokes, the risk of COPD increases (GOLD, 2020).

Infection. Recurring respiratory tract infection is a major factor contributing to the aggravation and progression of COPD (GOLD, 2020). The pathological destruction of lung tissue and the ensuing progression of COPD results from the recurring infections, which impair normal defence mechanisms, making the bronchioles and alveoli more susceptible to injury, and increase inflammation (GOLD, 2020). The most common causative organisms are *Haemophilus influenzae, Streptococcus pneumoniae,* and *Moraxella catarrhalis,* and in patients with severe to very severe COPD, *Pseudomonas aeruginosa* is probably a causative organism (GOLD, 2020). Retained secretions constitute a good medium for their proliferation.

Severe recurring respiratory tract infections in childhood have been associated with reduced lung function and increased respiratory symptoms in adulthood. It is unclear whether the development of COPD can be related to recurrent infections in adults. People who smoke and also have human immunodeficiency virus (HIV) infection have an accelerated development of COPD. Tuberculosis is also a risk factor for COPD development.

Heredity. α1-Antitrypsin (AAT) deficiency is currently the only known genetic abnormality that leads to COPD; however, research is ongoing to identify other genes that predispose a person to developing this disease (GOLD, 2020). AAT (also termed $α_1$-protease inhibitor) is the major antiprotease in plasma. Its primary function is to inhibit neutrophil elastase. It is produced by the liver and is normally found in the lungs, where it inhibits the action of proteolytic enzymes from neutrophils (neutrophil elastase) and macrophages. Lower levels of AAT result in insufficient inactivation of neutrophil elastase, and the subsequent lysis of lung tissue causes destruction of the alveoli. Severe AAT deficiency leads to early-onset COPD. Smoking greatly exacerbates the disease process in affected patients.

Intravenous or nebulizer-administered AAT (Prolastin) replacement therapy is available for people with AAT deficiency (GOLD, 2020). Infusions are administered weekly. Such therapy should be restricted to AAT-deficient patients who do not smoke and whose postbronchodilator FEV_1 is between 35 and 50% of predicted. Its effectiveness in slowing the progression of the disease continues to be evaluated.

GENETICS IN CLINICAL PRACTICE

α1-Antitrypsin (AAT) Deficiency

Genetic Basis
- Described as an autosomal recessive and codominant genetic disorder; >120 alleles
- A$_1$AT gene, also known as SERPINA 1, is located on chromosome 14.
- Several allelic variants of AAT gene exist.

Incidence and Prevalence
- Severe AAT deficiency occurs in 1 in 5 000 to 1 in 5 500 of the Canadian and North American population.
- Exact prevalence of AAT deficiency in patients with diagnosed COPD is unknown, but estimated prevalence is 1 to 5%.
- Severe AAT deficiency occurs in approximately 1 in 1 600 of the Scandinavian population.
- AAT deficiency is found in equal numbers of male and female patients.

Genetic Testing
- Targeted testing for AAT deficiency is recommended for individuals with COPD diagnosed before the age of 65 years or with a smoking history of less than 20 pack-years.
- DNA testing is available.
- Screening of siblings is useful.
- Serum assay is available to test for AAT deficiency.

Clinical Implications
- Disease predisposes individuals to the development COPD.
- Disease predisposes individuals to early-onset emphysema.
- AAT deficiency is associated with cirrhosis, hepatitis, panniculitis, and anti–proteinase 3 antibody vasculitis.
- AAT deficiency predisposes patients to early-onset COPD (in the third or fourth decade of life).
- Participation in AAT Canadian Registry is encouraged.

Source: Based on Marciniuk, D. D., Hernandez, P., Balter, M., et al. (2012). Alpha-1 antitrypsin deficiency targeted testing and augmentation therapy: A Canadian Thoracic Society clinical practice guideline. *Canadian Respiratory Journal, 19*(2), 109–116. https://doi.org/10.1155/2012/920918

Aging. Aging results in changes in the lung structure and respiratory muscles that cause a gradual loss of the elastic recoil of the lung. As a result, the lungs become smaller and stiffer. The number of functional alveoli decreases as a result of the loss of the alveolar supporting structures. Thoracic cage changes result from osteoporosis and calcification of the costal cartilages. The thoracic cage becomes stiff and rigid, and the ribs are less mobile. These changes result in a decreased compliance of the chest wall and an increase in the work of breathing. These changes are similar to those in patients with emphysema. With fewer capillaries available for gas exchange, arterial oxygen levels decrease. Clinically significant emphysema is usually not caused by aging alone.

Pathophysiology

COPD is characterized by chronic inflammation found in the airways, lung parenchyma (respiratory bronchioles and alveoli), and pulmonary blood vessels (Figure 31.12). The pathogenesis of COPD is complex and involves many mechanisms. The defining features of COPD are (a) airflow limitations during forced exhalation that are caused by loss of elastic recoil and are not fully reversible and (b) airflow obstruction caused by mucus hypersecretion, mucosal edema, and bronchospasm.

In COPD, airflow limitation, air trapping, gas exchange abnormalities, mucus hypersecretion, and, in severe disease, pulmonary hypertension and systemic abnormalities are among the various disease processes that occur (see Figure 31.12). The inflammatory process starts with inhalation of noxious particles and gases (e.g., cigarette smoke) but is magnified in people with COPD. The abnormal inflammatory process causes tissue destruction and disrupts the normal defence mechanisms and repair processes of the lungs.

The predominant inflammatory cells in COPD are neutrophils, macrophages, and lymphocytes. This pattern of inflammatory cells is different from that in asthma. The inflammatory cells in COPD attract other inflammatory mediators (e.g., leukotrienes, interleukins). This cascading inflammatory process results in the activation of proinflammatory cytokines such as tumour necrosis factor. In addition, growth factors are recruited into the area and activated, which results in structural changes in the lungs.

The inflammatory process may also be magnified by oxidative stress. Oxidants are produced by cigarette smoke and other inhaled particles and are released from the inflammatory cells, such as macrophages and neutrophils, during inflammation. The oxidative stress adversely affects the lungs as it inactivates antiproteases (which prevent the natural destruction of the lungs), stimulates mucus secretion, and increases fluid in the lungs (GOLD, 2020).

After the inhalation of oxidants in tobacco or air pollution, the activity of proteases (which break down the connective tissue of the lungs) increases, and the antiproteases (which protect against the breakdown) are inhibited. Therefore, the natural balance of protease/antiprotease is tipped in favour of destruction of the alveoli and loss of the elastic recoil of the lung.

Inability to expire air is a main characteristic of COPD. The airflow limitation occurs primarily in the smaller airways and is caused by remodelling. As the peripheral airways become obstructed, air is progressively trapped during expiration. The residual air becomes significant in severe disease as alveolar attachments to small airways (similar to rubber bands) are destroyed. The residual air, combined with the loss of elastic recoil, makes passive expiration of air difficult and air is trapped in the lungs. The chest hyper-expands and becomes barrel-shaped because the respiratory muscles cannot function effectively. The functional residual capacity is increased, and at this stage, the patient is trying to breathe in when the lungs are in an "overinflated" state; thus, the patient appears dyspneic, and exercise capacity is limited.

As the disease progresses, abnormal gas exchange may occur and results in *hypoxemia* (decreased oxygen in the blood) and *hypercapnia* (increased carbon dioxide). As the air trapping worsens and alveoli are destroyed, *bullae* (large air spaces in the parenchyma) and *blebs* (air spaces adjacent to pleurae) can form (Figure 31.13). Bullae and blebs are not effective in gas exchange because the capillary bed that normally surrounds each alveolus does not exist in the bullae and bleb. Therefore, there is a significant ventilation–perfusion (VQ) mismatch and hypoxemia results. Peripheral airway obstruction also results in

VQ imbalance and, in combination with the respiratory muscle impairment, can lead to carbon dioxide retention, particularly in severe disease (GOLD, 2020).

Excess mucus production, resulting in a chronic productive cough, is a feature of predominant chronic bronchitis and is not necessarily associated with limitation in airflow. However, not all patients with COPD produce sputum. Excess mucus production is a result of an increased number of mucus-secreting goblet cells and enlarged submucosal glands, which respond to the chronic irritation of smoke or other inhalants. In addition,

PATHOPHYSIOLOGY MAP

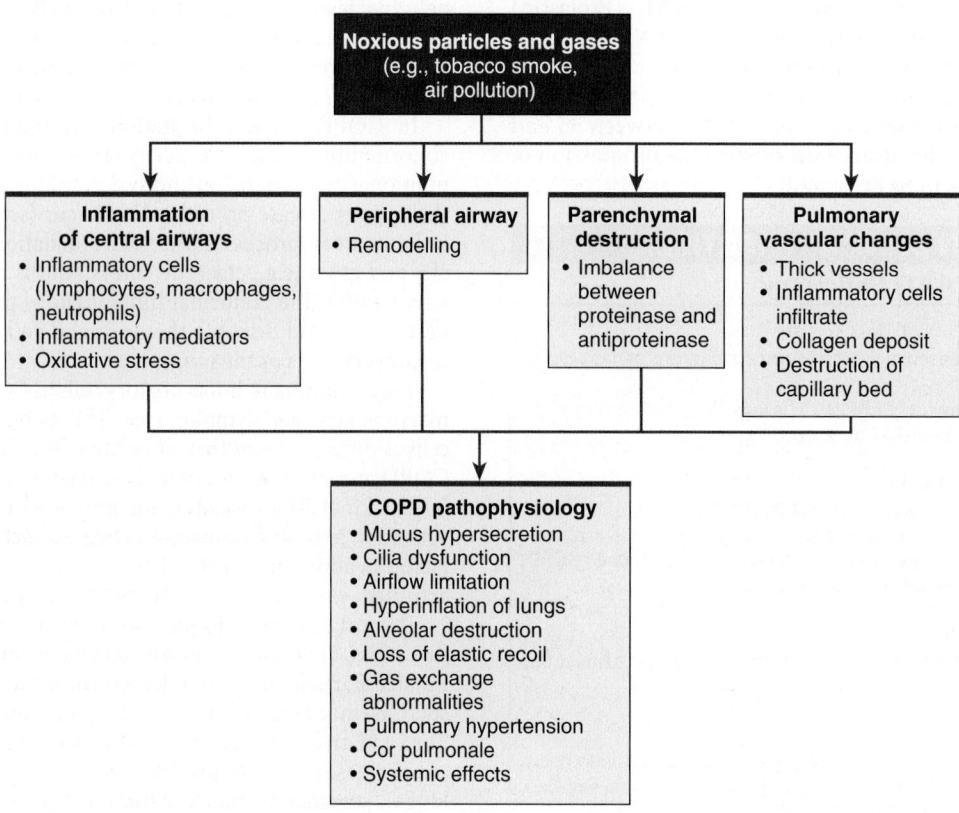

FIG. 31.12 Pathophysiological changes of chronic obstructive pulmonary disease (COPD).

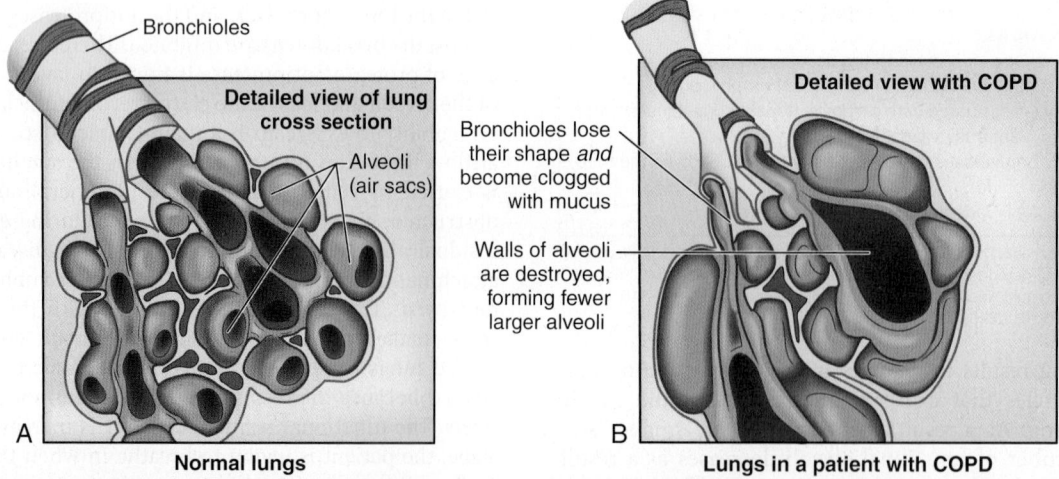

FIG. 31.13 Illustrations of bronchioles and alveoli in the lungs. **A,** Appearance in normal lungs. **B,** Appearance as a result of changes in the lungs of a patient with chronic obstructive pulmonary disease (COPD).

dysfunction of cilia leads to chronic cough and sputum production. Some of the inflammatory mediators also stimulate mucus production.

Pulmonary vasculature changes that result in mild to moderate pulmonary hypertension may occur late in the course of COPD. The small pulmonary arteries undergo vasoconstriction as a consequence of hypoxemia, and their structure changes, which results in thickening of the vascular smooth muscle as the disease advances. Because of the loss of alveolar walls and the capillaries surrounding them, the pressure in the pulmonary circulation increases. Affected patients typically do not have difficulty with hypoxemia at rest until late in the disease. However, hypoxemia may develop during exercise, and such patients may benefit from supplemental oxygen.

Pulmonary hypertension may progress and lead to hypertrophy of the right ventricle of the heart or to cor pulmonale, with or without right-sided heart failure. COPD has been shown to have effects on other body systems, especially in severe disease. These extrapulmonary changes contribute greatly to the clinical findings in affected patients and affect their survival and management. The mechanisms that cause the changes are unclear and are probably multifaceted, but systemic inflammation and inactivity of the patients are probably key factors. Cachexia is common with a loss of skeletal muscle mass (sarcopenia), and weakness probably results from increased *apoptosis* (programmed cell death), muscle disuse, or a combination of both (GOLD, 2020). Patients may have weakness in all muscles of the upper and lower extremities, and the progression of muscle wasting may be gradual or accelerated, depending on the underlying disease state, and it may be accelerated at times of acute exacerbation or during recovery from illness and a time of deconditioning. Consideration must also be given to the presence of exercise intolerance, deconditioning, and osteoporosis. Patients with severe COPD also may develop chronic anemia, anxiety, and depression. The incidence of cardiovascular disease is increased among such patients, probably as a result of an increase in C-reactive protein (another inflammatory marker linked to cardiovascular disease).

Clinical Manifestations

Several common aspects of asthma and COPD cause diagnostic confusion. However, there are clinically important differences between COPD and asthma (Table 31.11). In addition, some patients have a mixture of asthma and COPD (e.g., those with asthma who have a significant smoking history), and it is important to identify such patients because they may benefit from combination therapy of ICS/LABA and anticholinergic medications. In addition, earlier introduction of ICS may be justified if the asthma component is prominent.

A diagnosis of COPD should be considered when a person experiences the symptoms of cough, sputum production, or dyspnea; has a history of smoking or exposure to risk factors for the disease; or demonstrates both. An intermittent cough, often the earliest symptom, usually occurs in the morning with the expectoration of small amounts of mucus. A productive cough (coughing that brings up mucus) during winter months is also a common early symptom that is often exacerbated by respiratory irritants; by cold, damp air; and by respiratory infections. Patients usually seek medical help when they have an acute respiratory infection, dyspnea being the main concern. Dyspnea on exertion may also be one of the earliest symptoms. Dyspnea becomes progressively more severe to the point that it occurs at rest. Patients may dismiss the importance of

TABLE 31.11	**COMPARISON OF CLINICAL FEATURES OF COPD AND ASTHMA**	
Feature	**COPD**	**Asthma**
Age at onset	Usually >40 yr	Usually <40 yr
Smoking history	Usually >10 pack-years	Not causal but can be a trigger
Clinical symptoms	Persistent	Intermittent and variable
Sputum production	Often	Infrequent
Allergies	Infrequent	Often
Spirometry	Findings may improve but never normalize	Findings often normalize
Disease course	Progressive worsening with exacerbations	Stable with exacerbations

COPD, chronic obstructive pulmonary disease.
Source: Adapted from O'Donnell, D. E., Hernandez, P., Kaplan, A., et al. (2008). Canadian Thoracic Society recommendations for the management of chronic obstructive pulmonary disease—2008 Update—Highlights for primary care. *Canadian Respiratory Journal, 15*(Suppl. A), 1–8A.

dyspnea, rationalizing that they are "just getting older." They change behaviours to avoid dyspnea and adapt, such as by using the elevator instead of stairs. The dyspnea gradually interferes with daily activities, such as carrying grocery bags, bathing, and cooking. People with COPD have described acute dyspnea as an experience inextricably related to anxiety and emotional functioning. Patients may describe dyspnea in various terms: "My breath does not go out all the way"; "It's hard work to breathe"; or that breathing feels like "heaviness" or "gasping."

Progressive dyspnea occurs as more alveoli become overdistended, trapping increasing amounts of air. This causes the diaphragm to flatten and the anteroposterior diameter of the chest to increase; as a result, the chest assumes the typical barrel shape. Effective abdominal breathing is decreased because of the flattening of diaphragm, which forces the person to rely on intercostal and accessory muscles. This type of breathing, however, is not very effective because the ribs become fixed in an inspiratory position.

Many people with advanced COPD experience weight loss and anorexia. The exact cause of these developments is not well understood. One possibility is that such patients are in a hypermetabolic state with increased energy requirements, partly because of the increased work of breathing. Even when caloric intake is adequate, weight loss may still occur. (Malnutrition is discussed in Chapter 42.)

During physical examination, a prolonged expiratory phase of respiration, wheezes, or decreased breath sounds, or some combination is noted in some or all lung fields. The patient may sit upright with arms supported on a fixed surface such as a table (tripod position). The patient may naturally purse lips on expiration (pursed-lip breathing) and use accessory muscles, such as those in the neck, to aid with inspiration. Edema in the ankles may be a clue to right-sided heart involvement.

Over time, hypoxemia (PaO_2 <60 mm Hg or SaO_2 <88%) may develop with hypercapnia ($PaCO_2$ >45 mm Hg) later in the disease. The bluish-red colour of the skin results from polycythemia and cyanosis. Polycythemia develops as a result of increased production of red blood cells secondary to the body's attempt to compensate for chronic hypoxemia. Hemoglobin concentrations may reach 200 g/L or more. Cyanosis develops in the presence of at least 50 g/L or more of circulating unoxygenated hemoglobin.

TABLE 31.12   CANADIAN THORACIC SOCIETY CHRONIC OBSTRUCTIVE PULMONARY DISEASE (COPD) CLASSIFICATION OF SEVERITY BY SYMPTOMS, DISABILITY,* AND IMPAIRMENT OF LUNG FUNCTION

COPD Stage	Symptoms	Classification of Function — Spirometry (After Bronchodilator Treatment)
Mild	Shortness of breath from COPD[†] when hurrying on the level or walking up a slight hill (MRC grade 2)	$FEV_1 \geq 80\%$, $FEV_1/FVC < 0.7$
Moderate	Shortness of breath from COPD[†] causing the patient to stop after walking approximately 100 m (or after a few minutes) on the level (MRC grades 3 to 4)	$50\% \leq FEV_1 < 80\%$ predicted, $FEV_1/FVC < 0.7$
Severe	Shortness of breath from COPD[†] resulting in the patient being too breathless to leave the house, being breathless when dressing or undressing (MRC grade 5), or having chronic respiratory failure or clinical signs of right heart failure	$30\% \leq FEV_1 < 50\%$ predicted, $FEV_1/FVC < 0.7$
Very severe		$FEV_1 < 30\%$ predicted, $FEV_1/FVC < 0.7$

*Postbronchodilator FEV_1/FVC ratio of less than 0.7 is required for the diagnosis of COPD to be established.
[†]In the presence of non-COPD conditions that may cause shortness of breath (e.g., cardiac dysfunction, anemia, muscle weakness, metabolic disorders), symptoms may not appropriately reflect COPD disease severity. Classification of COPD severity should be undertaken with care in patients with comorbid disease or other possible contributors to shortness of breath.
FEV_1, forced expiratory volume in one second; *FVC*, forced vital capacity; *MRC*, Medical Research Council Dyspnea Scale.
Source: O'Donnell, D. E., Aaron, S., Bourbeau, J., et al. (2007). Canadian Thoracic Society recommendations for management of chronic obstructive pulmonary disease—2007 Update. *Canadian Respiratory Journal, 14*(Suppl B), 5B–32B, Table 3.

Classification of Chronic Obstructive Pulmonary Disease. The diagnosis of COPD should be considered in any person with exposure to risk factors such as tobacco smoke or environmental or occupational pollutants, chronic cough and dyspnea, or a combination of these. The diagnosis of COPD is confirmed by spirometry, regardless of whether the patient has chronic symptoms. The FEV_1/FVC ratio of less than 70% establishes the diagnosis of COPD. COPD can be classified as mild, moderate, severe, and very severe (Table 31.12); this classification is based on the severity of obstruction (as indicated by FEV_1). The management of COPD is based primarily on a patient's symptoms, but the staging provides a general guideline for the type of interventions.

Complications

Cor Pulmonale. Cor pulmonale is hypertrophy of the right side of the heart, with or without heart failure, that results from pulmonary hypertension. In COPD, pulmonary hypertension is caused primarily by constriction of the pulmonary vessels in response to alveolar hypoxia; acidosis further potentiates the vasoconstriction (Figure 31.14). Chronic alveolar hypoxia causes pulmonary arteriolar muscle hypertrophy. Chronic hypoxia also stimulates erythropoiesis, which causes polycythemia and increases the viscosity of the blood. Cor pulmonale is a late manifestation of COPD with a poor prognosis.

Normally, the right ventricle and the pulmonary circulatory system are low-pressure systems in comparison with the left ventricle and the systemic circulation. When pulmonary hypertension develops, the pressures on the right side of the heart must increase to push blood into the lungs. Eventually, right-sided heart failure develops.

The clinical manifestations of cor pulmonale are related to dilation and failure of the right ventricle with subsequent intravascular volume expansion and systemic venous congestion. Lung sounds are normal, or crackles may be heard in the bases of the lungs. Heart sound changes include accentuation of the pulmonic component of the second heart sound, presence of a right-sided third heart sound (right ventricular gallop), and early systolic ejection click along the left sternal border. Overt manifestations of right-sided heart failure may develop, which include distension of neck veins (jugular venous distension),

hepatomegaly with right upper quadrant tenderness, ascites, epigastric distress, peripheral edema, and weight gain.

Management of cor pulmonale includes continuous administration of low-flow oxygen. Long-term oxygen therapy can slow but not reverse the progression of pulmonary hypertension in patients with COPD. Diuretics are generally used, but serum creatinine level, blood urea nitrogen level, and electrolytes must be monitored because diuretics can cause volume depletion and electrolyte imbalance. (Cor pulmonale is discussed further in Chapter 30.)

Acute Exacerbations of Chronic Obstructive Pulmonary Disease. An acute exacerbation of COPD (AECOPD) is defined as a sustained worsening of COPD symptoms (Canadian Lung Association, 2019). The term *sustained* implies a change from baseline that lasts 48 hours or longer. Exacerbations should be characterized as purulent or nonpurulent to assist in determining the need for antibiotic therapy; purulent exacerbations necessitate antibiotic therapy. The frequency of AECOPD is, in part, related to the underlying severity of airflow obstruction, and patients with a history of frequent exacerbations are more likely to continue experiencing frequent exacerbations. The cause of AECOPD is often difficult to determine. Noninfectious triggers for exacerbations include exposure to allergens, irritants, cold air, and air pollution.

At least half of all exacerbations are thought to be infectious in nature; many of these are viral in origin, whereas the remainder are caused by bacterial infection. The most common organisms causing AECOPD are *H. influenzae, M. catarrhalis,* and *S. pneumoniae.* As COPD becomes more severe, *Pseudomonas* organisms, *Klebsiella pneumoniae,* and *Escherichia coli* are frequent causes of infection (GOLD, 2020). The antibiotics most commonly given are amoxicillin, cefuroxime, cefixime, azithromycin, clarithromycin, trimethoprim-sulphamethoxazole, doxycycline, moxifloxacin, levofloxacin, and amoxicillin with clavulanic acid. Some patients are provided with a written action plan and instructed to self-manage exacerbations by beginning antibiotics at the first signs of change in sputum production and colour. In concept, the COPD action plan is similar to the action plan used for patients with asthma (see Figure 31.11); however, the COPD action plan is specific to COPD and AECOPD. Many action plans are available. An example of an action plan can be

PATHOPHYSIOLOGY MAP

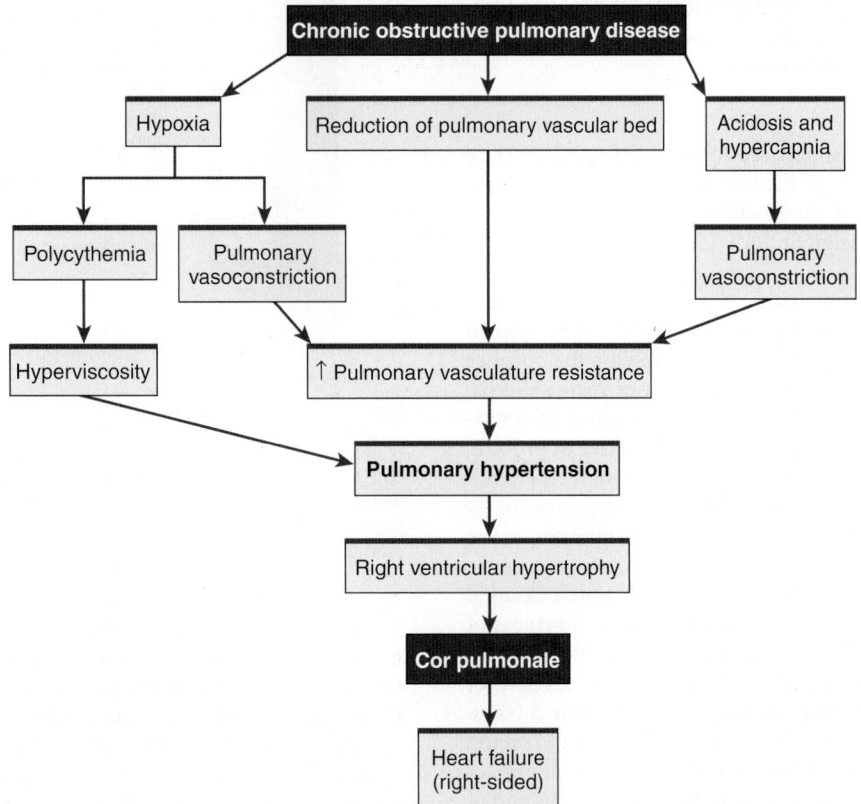

FIG. 31.14 Mechanisms involved in the pathophysiological process of cor pulmonale secondary to chronic obstructive pulmonary disease.

downloaded from the website of the Canadian Lung Association (see the Resources at the end of this chapter).

Pneumonia is a frequent complication of COPD. The most common causative pathogens are *S. pneumoniae, H. influenzae,* and viruses. The most common manifestation is purulent sputum. Systemic manifestations such as fever, chills, and leukocytosis may not be present. (Treatment of pneumonia is discussed in Chapter 30.)

No diagnostic tests currently define AECOPD. A complete history and physical examination are needed to rule out other causes of increased symptoms. In patients who are very dyspneic, SaO$_2$ and ABGs should be measured (if oxygen saturation as measured by oximetry is low). Chest radiography should be performed for patients in the emergency department or who are admitted to the hospital, because they may have pneumonia, heart failure, or pneumothorax. Increased inhaled bronchodilator dosages (β_2 agonists and anticholinergics) are administered to all patients with AECOPD; oral or systemic corticosteroids, to patients with moderate to severe airflow obstruction (FEV$_1$ <50% of predicted); and antibiotics, to those with purulent sputum. Annual influenza vaccination and pneumococcal vaccination should be encouraged unless the patient has a contraindication.

Acute Respiratory Failure. An acute exacerbation leads to increased decline in overall lung function, deterioration in health status, and risk of death (GOLD, 2020). Frequently, patients with COPD wait too long to contact their health care provider when they develop fever, increased cough and dyspnea, or other symptoms suggestive of AECOPD. An exacerbation of cor pulmonale may lead to acute respiratory failure.

Discontinuing bronchodilator or corticosteroid medication may also precipitate respiratory failure. The use of cardioselective β-adrenergic blockers (e.g., atenolol, metoprolol) are underprescribed for patients with a co-diagnosis of COPD and chronic heart failure, although increasing evidence demonstrates that they can be safely prescribed (Mtisi et al., 2020).

Indiscriminate use of sedatives and opioids, especially before or after surgery in a patient who retains carbon dioxide, may suppress ventilatory drive and lead to respiratory failure. The patient with COPD who retains carbon dioxide should be treated with low-flow rates of oxygen, and ABG values should be monitored carefully. Surgery or severe, painful illness involving the chest or abdomen may lead to splinting, ineffective ventilation, and respiratory failure. Careful preoperative screening, which includes pulmonary function tests and ABG monitoring, is important in patients with a history of heavy smoking and COPD, to prevent postoperative pulmonary complications. (Respiratory failure is defined and discussed in Chapter 70.)

Depression and Anxiety. People with COPD experience higher rates of depression and anxiety. Prevalence of depression and COPD ranges from 10 to 42% in patients experiencing stable COPD, and these rates increase from 10 to 86% for persons experiencing an acute exacerbation of COPD (Yohannas, et al., 2018). Patients with COPD are 85% more likely to experience anxiety disorders. Depression may be related to feelings of hopelessness, social isolation, and grief that accompany the progressive course of the disease, and an overall decrease in quality of life is related to reduced physical functioning and sedentary lifestyle. Anxiety can occur when a person is exceptionally dyspneic, particularly if the condition occurs suddenly, and the person becomes anxious and tries to breathe faster, which affects oxygenation status. Proper screening for anxiety and depression and assessment of coping strategies and supports by health care providers are needed to reduce the intensity of these symptoms and improve quality of life.

Clinical Assessment

Goals of the clinical assessment are to determine the severity of the disease and the effect of the disease on the patient's quality of life. Identification of these and other factors enable the health care provider to design an individualized treatment plan (GOLD, 2020).

Clinical assessment begins with a thorough history. Tobacco consumption should be quantified and is typically expressed in pack-years. Pack-years are calculated by multiplying the number of cigarette packs smoked daily by the number of years smoked. Nurses should ask each patient about the experience of symptoms and their effect on the individual's life. A series of probing questions is often necessary to uncover the extent of the patient's breathing difficulty and exercise curtailment. The severity of breathlessness is determined by identifying the magnitude of the task (often an activity of daily living [ADL]) necessary to cause discomfort in breathing. The Modified Medical Research Council (mMRC) Dyspnea Scale is used to assess the level of shortness of breath and disability in COPD (Figure 31.15). The history also should include an assessment of the frequency and severity of exacerbations because the findings may guide treatment choices. Patients should complete a COPD Assessment Test prior to seeing their health care provider in order to measure the overall impact of their current COPD symptoms. (See the Resources at the end of the chapter to access the test.) In addition, nurses should include an assessment of symptoms associated with comorbid conditions or complications of COPD (ankle swelling, weight loss, anxiety, depression) and the current medical treatment.

Physical examination is important for patients with COPD but is not diagnostic. Pulmonary function studies are needed to determine airflow obstruction and, therefore, to determine a diagnosis of COPD and to assess the severity of lung impairment. Spirometry is ordered before and after bronchodilator therapy; when the post-therapy FEV_1/FVC ratio is less than 70% of the predicted value, it confirms the presence of airway obstruction (GOLD, 2020).

Chest radiographic studies are not diagnostic of COPD but are often necessary to confirm or rule out comorbid conditions. This also applies to high-resolution computed tomography, which is not routinely required. Pulse oximetry should be used to assess all patients with an FEV_1 of less than 35% of predicted, and ABGs should be monitored in patients who have a low SaO_2 (<92%) on oximetry, especially in patients in whom respiratory failure is suspected (GOLD, 2020). In the later stages of COPD, typical findings are low PaO_2, elevated $PaCO_2$, decreased pH, and increased bicarbonate levels. The 6-minute walking test is a useful test of functional disability and provides prognostic information. It includes determination of changes in the SaO_2 with exercise.

Interprofessional Care

Primary COPD management goals are to recognize the impact that both symptoms and exacerbations have on the patient's quality of life when determining optimal patient-focused management (Vogelmeier, 2020). This includes the following:
1. Prevent disease progression (smoking cessation)
2. Reduce the frequency and severity of exacerbations

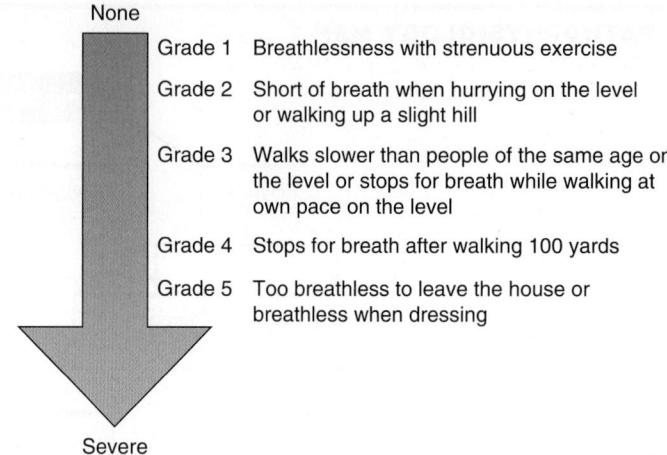

None

Grade 1	Breathlessness with strenuous exercise
Grade 2	Short of breath when hurrying on the level or walking up a slight hill
Grade 3	Walks slower than people of the same age on the level or stops for breath while walking at own pace on the level
Grade 4	Stops for breath after walking 100 yards
Grade 5	Too breathless to leave the house or breathless when dressing

Severe

FIG. 31.15 Medical Research Council (MRC) Dyspnea Scale. This scale can be used to assess shortness of breath and disability in chronic obstructive pulmonary disease. Source: O'Donnell, D. E., Aaron, S., Bourbeau, J., et al. (2004). State of the art compendium: Canadian Thoracic Society recommendations for the management of chronic obstructive pulmonary disease. *Canadian Respiratory Journal, 11*(Suppl. B), 1B–59B, Table 1. Reprinted with permission of D. E. O'Donnell.

3. Alleviate breathlessness and other respiratory symptoms
4. Improve exercise tolerance
5. Treat exacerbations and complications of the disease
6. Improve health status and quality of life
7. Reduce associated mortality and mortality

AECOPD and complications such as respiratory failure, pneumonia, and heart failure necessitate hospitalization; otherwise, patients are treated on an outpatient basis and manage their condition at home. Therapy is expected to escalate in intensity as a patient's disability progresses from the classification of:
• Mild—worsening or new respiratory symptoms without a change in prescribed medications
• Moderate—prescribed antibiotic and/or corticosteroids
• Severe—patient requires hospital admission or emergency department visit
Interprofessional care guidelines are presented in Table 31.13.

Environmental and occupational irritants and triggers should be assessed for a possible negative effect, and ways to control or avoid them should be determined. Patients with COPD should receive an annual influenza vaccination and a pneumococcal vaccine (pneumococcal revaccination is recommended every 5–10 years (O'Donnell et al., 2008). (See the Evidence-Informed Practice: Translating Research Into Practice box.)

Smoking Cessation. Cessation of cigarette smoking is the most significant factor in slowing the progression of COPD. After a patient stops smoking, not only does the accelerated decline in pulmonary function slow but also pulmonary function usually improves. The sooner the patient stops smoking, the less pulmonary function is lost and the sooner the symptoms decrease, particularly cough and sputum production. (See the RNAO's *Best Practice Guideline Integrating Smoking Cessation Into Daily Practice* in the Resources at the end of this chapter.)

Medication Therapy. Medications for COPD can reduce the intensity of symptoms or abolish them altogether, increase the capacity for exercise, improve overall health, and reduce the number and severity of exacerbations. Bronchodilators are the mainstay of pharmacological therapy for COPD (GOLD, 2020).

TABLE 31.13 INTERPROFESSIONAL CARE
Chronic Obstructive Pulmonary Disease

Diagnostic
- History and physical examination
- Pulmonary function tests
- Serum α_1-antitrypsin levels
- Chest radiography (if indicated)
- Sputum specimen for Gram stain and culture (if indicated)
- ABG measurements (if indicated)
- Exercise testing with oximetry (if indicated)
- Electrocardiography (if indicated)
- Echocardiography or cardiac nuclear scans (if indicated)

Interprofessional Therapy
- Smoking cessation
- Bronchodilator therapy (see Tables 31.5 and 31.7)
- β_2-Adrenergic agonists
- Anticholinergic medications
- Long-acting theophylline preparations (rarely used)
- Prompt treatment of exacerbations
- Corticosteroids (oral for exacerbations)

- Nonsteroidal anti-inflammatory drugs (roflumilast)
- Antibiotics for exacerbations with purulent sputum
- Influenza immunization (yearly)
- Pneumovax immunization (every 5–10 yr)
- Pulmonary rehabilitation program
- Progressive plan of exercise, especially walking and upper body strengthening
- Breathing exercises
- Airway clearance techniques
- Hydration of 3 L/day (if not contraindicated)
- Relaxation techniques
- Appropriate pacing and planning of activities
- Patient and family teaching
- Long-term oxygen (if indicated)
- Nutritional supplementation if BMI is low
- Surgery in severe and advanced COPD
- Lung volume reduction
- Lung transplantation

ABG, arterial blood gas; *BMI,* body mass index; *COPD,* chronic obstructive pulmonary disease.

▶ EVIDENCE-INFORMED PRACTICE
Translating Research Into Practice

Physical Activity and Chronic Obstructive Pulmonary Disease

A nurse in the pulmonary clinic is working with a 65-year-old man who has been recently discharged from the hospital after receiving a new diagnosis of COPD. He tells the nurse that he has been mostly inactive for the past few months because his breathing seems to worsen with activity.

Best Available Evidence	Clinician Expertise	Patient Preference and Values
Patients with COPD who participate in regular moderate physical activity (e.g., brisk walking) have fewer severe flare-ups and are less likely to be readmitted to the hospital.	Physical inactivity is common in patients with COPD. Persistent inactivity may place a patient at greater risk for hospital readmissions.	The patient tells the nurse that he misses taking walks every day with his wife and is wondering whether he would be able to resume this activity at a slow pace.

Decisions and Actions
1. What important factors should be discussed with the patient about physical activity and COPD?
2. How would the nurse assess the patient's willingness and motivation to engage in physical activity?
3. How would the nurse involve the interprofessional team members to assist the patient in regular physical activity?

Reference for Evidence

Prieto-Centurion, V., Casaburi, R., Coultas, D. B., & et al (2019). Daily physical activity in patients with COPD after hospital discharge in a minority population. *Chronic Obstructive Pulmonary Diseases, 6*(4), 332. https://doi.org/10.15326/jcopdf.6.4.2019.0136

Bronchodilator medication therapy relaxes smooth muscles in the airway, reduces airway resistance and dynamic hyperinflation of the lungs, and improves the ventilation of the lungs, thus reducing the degree of breathlessness. Although patients with COPD do not respond to bronchodilator therapy as dramatically as those with asthma, a reduction in dyspnea and an increase in FEV_1 are usually achieved.

Bronchodilator medications commonly used are β_2-adrenergic agonists, muscarinic medications, and methylxanthines (Figure 31.16). Short-acting bronchodilators (SABDs), both β_2-adrenergic agonist (SABA) medications and short-acting muscarinic antagonist (SAMA) medications, improve pulmonary function, symptoms, and exercise function (Bourbeau et al., 2019). SABAs and SAMAs can be used separately, but together they produce better bronchodilation than either medication alone. These medications are also available in nebulized combination (i.e., salbutamol and ipratropium [Combivent]). For most patients with mild COPD, SABA and SAMA therapy is best used as maintenance therapy (three or four times per day) with extra puffs on an as-needed basis for breakthrough symptoms. If symptoms are persistent with mild lung function impairment, it is recommended to initiate LAMA or LABA therapy as a step-up therapy.

Long-acting bronchodilators (LABDs) also play a role in COPD treatment and are typically indicated for patients with mild to severe COPD who experience persistent symptoms. Like SABDs, LABDs include both β_2-adrenergic agonist (LABA) and LAMA medications (see Figure 31.16). These two classes of LABDs can be used separately or together in combination therapy. Combination therapy of ICS/LABA is the preferred choice for preventing COPD exacerbation in patients who have higher peripheral eosinophilia counts with previous acute exacerbations (Bourbeau et al., 2019).

The role of ICS in stable COPD has not been found to modify the long-term decline of FEV_1 or overall patient mortality (GOLD, 2020). ICS monotherapy does not have consistent effects on important outcomes (e.g., pulmonary function, symptoms, exacerbations) and is not a recommended therapy. However, ICS in combination with a LABA has been found to reduce the frequency of exacerbations and to improve lung function and health status in patients who are at high risk of AECOPD. The Canadian Thoracic Society guidelines (Bourbeau et al., 2019) suggest either ICS/LABA or LAMA/LABA as minimum maintenance therapy for patients at high risk for AECPOD (see Figure 31.16 and Figure 31.17). For patients who remain symptomatic on dual therapy as previously mentioned, triple therapy of LAMA/LABA/ICS is recommended as the next step up in therapy (Bourbeau et al., 2019).

There are a variety of additional oral therapies that can be added as prevention therapies for patients at high risk for AECOPD. Those who continue to experience exacerbations despite being on optimized LABD therapy may require the addition of a daily macrolide (e.g., azithromycin) as maintenance therapy. The phosphodiesterase 4 inhibitor roflumilast (Daxas) is indicated as add-on therapy for reduction of inflammation with bronchodilators, for the maintenance of COPD in patients with chronic cough and sputum and frequent exacerbations. N-acetylcysteine, a mucolytic, may be added for patients with symptoms of chronic bronchitis to help expectorate tenacious sputum.

Oral or parenteral corticosteroids are used for the treatment of AECOPD. They speed recovery time, reduce relapse

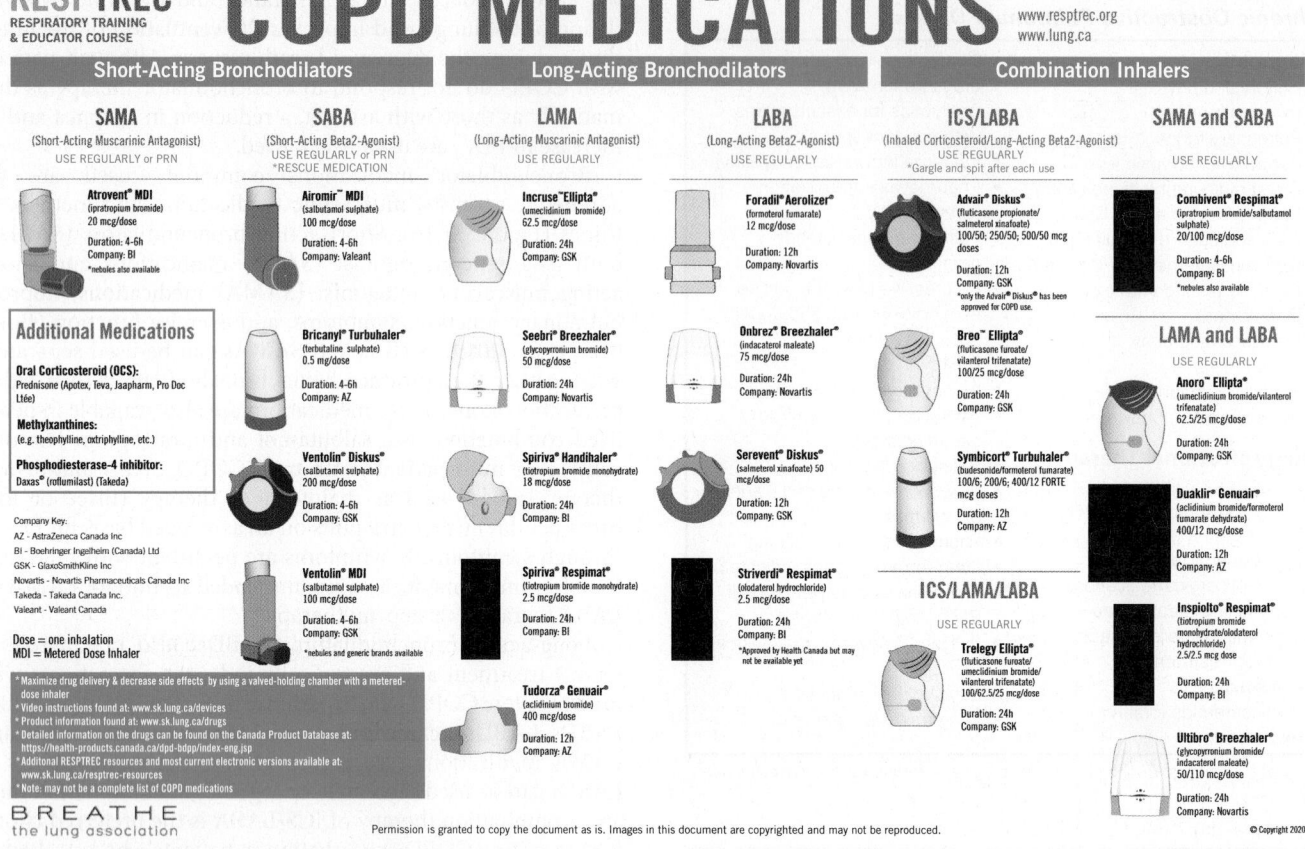

FIG. 31.16 COPD medications. This is a pictorial guide of the inhaler therapies available for COPD treatment in Canada. Source: Lung Association of Saskatchewan. (2020). *COPD medications brochure.* https://www.lungsask.ca/healthcare-providers/resptrec-resources

rates, reduce the need for hospitalization, and improve FEV_1 and partial pressure of oxygen. The dosage and duration should be individualized; treatment periods between 7 and 14 days are recommended for people with moderate to severe COPD (O'Donnell et al., 2008). Continuous use of oral corticosteroids is not recommended for routine use in managing COPD because it can produce deleterious effects (GOLD, 2020).

The use of theophylline in the treatment of COPD is controversial. Although it has some weak bronchodilator effects, its main value may be to improve contractility of the diaphragm and decrease diaphragmatic fatigue. The addition of theophylline to inhaled bronchodilator therapy may provide some benefit in some patients. However, the benefits and the risks need to be weighed because theophylline produces serious cardiovascular and neurological adverse effects.

Oxygen Therapy. Oxygen therapy is frequently used in the treatment of COPD and other conditions associated with hypoxemia. Oxygen is a colourless, odourless, tasteless gas that constitutes 20.95% of the atmosphere. Administering supplemental oxygen raises the PaO_2 in inspired air.

Indications for Use. Oxygen is usually administered to treat hypoxemia caused by respiratory disorders such as COPD, AECOPD, cor pulmonale, pneumonia, atelectasis, and lung cancer. Long-term oxygen therapy (15 hours per day or more to achieve an oxygen saturation of 90% or greater) prolongs life in patients with hypoxemia. Hypoxemia is defined as a PaO_2 lower than 55 mm Hg or lower than 60 mm Hg in the presence of cor pulmonale with a hematocrit higher than 56%. Patients

with COPD are at risk of developing hypoxemia during an exacerbation.

Methods of Administration. The goal of oxygen administration is to supply the patient with adequate oxygen to maximize the oxygen-carrying ability of the blood. There are various methods of oxygen administration (Table 31.14, Figures 31.18 through 31.21). The method selected depends on factors such as the fraction of inspired oxygen, mobility of the patient, humidification requirement, patient cooperation, comfort, cost, and available financial resources.

Oxygen delivery systems are classified as low- or high-flow systems. Because room air is mixed with oxygen, the percentage of oxygen delivered to the patient is not as precise in low-flow systems as in high-flow systems. Most methods of oxygen administration are low-flow devices that deliver oxygen in concentrations that vary in accordance with the patient's respiratory pattern. In contrast, the Venturi mask is a high-flow device that delivers fixed concentrations of oxygen independent of a patient's respiratory pattern. With the Venturi mask, oxygen is delivered to a small jet (Venturi device) in the centre of a wide-based cone (Figure 31.18, C). Air is entrained (pulled) through openings in the cone as oxygen flows through the small jet. The mask has large vents through which exhaled air can escape. The degree of restriction, or narrowness, of the jet determines the amount of entrainment and the dilution of pure oxygen with room air and thus the concentration of oxygen.

Humidification. Oxygen obtained from cylinders or wall systems is dry. A device commonly used for humidification

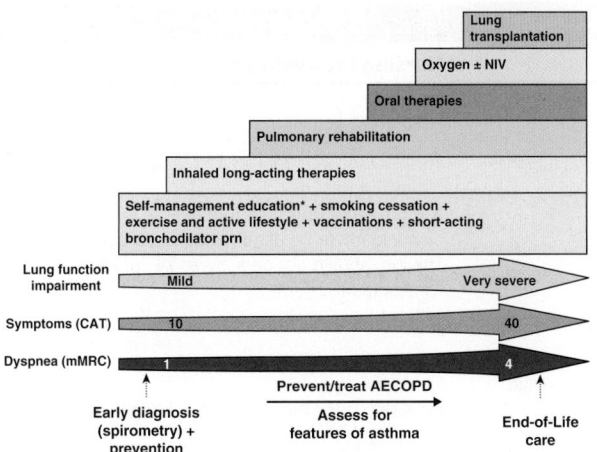

FIG. 31.17 Comprehensive management of chronic obstructive pulmonary disease (COPD). This integrated approach to care includes confirming COPD diagnosis with spirometry; evaluation of symptom burden and risk of exacerbations with ongoing monitoring; assessment for features of asthma; and comprehensive management, both nonpharmacological and pharmacological. *Self-Management Education includes appropriate inhaler device technique and review; breathing techniques and review; early recognition of AECOPD; and written action plan development and implementation (if appropriate). mMRC is a modified (0–4 scale) version of the MRC breathlessness scale that was used in previous Canadian Thoracic Society guidelines. The mMRC aligns with the Global Initiative for Chronic Obstructive Airways Disease (GOLD) 2019 report. *AECOPD,* acute exacerbation of COPD; *CAT,* COPD assessment test; *mMRC,* Modified Medical Research Council; *NIV,* noninvasive ventilation; *prn,* as needed. Inhaled Long-Acting Therapies include long-acting muscarinic antagonist and/or long-acting β2-agonist and/or inhaled corticosteroid. Source: Bourbeau, J., Bhutani, M., Hernandez, P., et al. (2019). Canadian Thoracic Society Clinical Practice Guideline on pharmacotherapy in patients with COPD—2019 Update of evidence. *Canadian Journal of Respiratory, Critical Care, and Sleep Medicine, 3*(4), 210–232. https://doi.org/10.1080/24745332.2019.1668652

when the patient has a catheter, cannula, or low-flow mask is a bubble-through humidifier (Figure 31.19). Cold humidification is delivered through a plastic container filled with sterile distilled water that is attached to the oxygen source by means of a flowmeter. Dry oxygen may have an irritating effect on mucous membranes and can dry secretions; therefore, a bubble through cold humidifier may be added to the oxygen system to counteract this effect. Oxygen passes into the container, bubbles through the water, and then goes through tubing to a patient's catheter, cannula, or mask. The purpose of the bubble-through humidifier is to restore the humidity conditions of room air. However, the need for bubble-through humidifiers at flow rates of less than 5 L/min is debatable when humidity in the environment is adequate.

Caution must be exercised when using humidified high-flow oxygen delivery in a patient with suspected, probable, or confirmed COVID-19. Humified oxygen via an open system such as a high-flow mask system or nasal cannula (>5 L/min) is considered an AGP and requires point-of-care risk assessment and appropriate PPE in this patient setting.

Complications

Combustion. Oxygen supports combustion and increases the rate of burning; thus, it is important that smoking be prohibited in an area where supplemental oxygen is being used. A "No Smoking" sign should be prominently displayed on the patient's door and in their home and car. Patients should also be cautioned against smoking cigarettes when using oxygen.

Carbon Dioxide Narcosis. The drive to breathe is guided by arterial and central chemoreceptors in the respiratory centre that respond to changes in carbon dioxide and oxygen levels. Normally, accumulation of carbon dioxide is the major stimulant of the respiratory centre. In COPD, over time the respiratory

TABLE 31.14 METHODS OF OXYGEN ADMINISTRATION		
Advantages	**Disadvantages**	**Nursing Interventions**
Nasal Cannula		
May be used by a mobile or restless patient Safe and simple method that is relatively comfortable and acceptable Used for patients requiring low O2 concentrations Can be used while patient eats, talks, or coughs (see Figure 31.18, *E*)	Difficult to maintain in position and can be easily dislodged Patient alertness necessary to keep cannula in proper place Dryness of nasal membranes and possible pain in frontal sinuses with high flow rates (>5 L/min) Can cause pressure necrosis or excoriation of nares	Stabilize cannula during care for a restless patient. Flow rate of 2 L/min produces an O2 concentration of approximately 28%. The amount of O2 inhaled depends on room air and patient's breathing pattern. Most patients with COPD can tolerate 2 L/min via cannula.
Simple Face Mask		
Delivers O2 quickly for short periods O2 concentrations of 35–50% achievable with flow rates of 6–12 L/min Provides adequate humidification of inspired air (see Figure 31.18, *A*)	Not as well tolerated as nasal cannula; lack of patient tolerance results in inadequate therapy May be uncomfortable because a tight seal must be maintained between face and mask May produce pressure necrosis of the skin and confines heat radiating from the face to the area around the nose and mouth Must be removed to eat or drink	Wash and dry under mask q2h. Mask must fit snugly. A nasal cannula may be provided while patient is eating. Watch for pressure necrosis at the top of ears from elastic straps. (Gauze or other padding may be used to alleviate this problem.) Method requires at least 5 L/min flow to prevent accumulation of expired air in the mask.
Nasal Catheter		
Allows continuous, uninterrupted O2 therapy Delivers O2 even if patient is a mouth breather Does not interfere with patient care Rarely used except for short-term procedures (e.g., bronchoscopy)	Inserted into nasopharynx through a nostril and can produce excoriation of the nostril Dryness of nasal membranes with high flow rates (>6 L/min) Stomach distension with inadvertent gas flow High degree of humidification not delivered easily; catheter must be taped to patient's face	Catheter should be changed q8h, alternating the nostrils. Distance that catheter is to be inserted is measured from distance between tip of nose and earlobe. A flow rate of 5–6 L/min produces O2 concentration of ≈30%. This method is best for short-term therapy.

Continued

TABLE 31.14	**METHODS OF OXYGEN ADMINISTRATION—cont'd**	
Advantages	**Disadvantages**	**Nursing Interventions**
Partial Rebreathing Mask		
Lightweight and easy to use O_2 conserved by reservoir bag Concentrations of 40–60% achievable with flow rates of 6–10 L/min	Cannot be used when patient requires a high degree of humidity	This method is useful when blood O_2 concentrations must be raised. It is not recommended for patients with COPD and should never be used with a nebulizer. The bag should not be allowed to deflate during inspiration.
Nonrebreathing Mask		
Accurate delivery of high concentrations of O_2 O_2 flow into bag and mask during inhalation Valve in place to prevent expired air from flowing back into bag Concentrations of 60–90% achievable	Cannot be used when patient requires a high degree of humidity	Mask should fit snugly. Flow rate must be sufficient to keep bag from collapsing during inspiration. The bag should not be allowed to deflate during inspiration.
Oxygen-Conserving Cannula		
Has a built-in reservoir that increases O_2 concentration delivered and allows patient to use lower flow rates, usually 30–50%, which increases comfort and lowers cost Reported to be more comfortable than standard nasal cannulas (see Figure 31.20)	Cannot be cleaned: changing cannula weekly recommended More expensive than standard cannulas and requires evaluation with measurement of ABGs and oximetry to determine correct flow Highly visible and heavy on ears	This method is generally indicated when long-term O_2 therapy is used at home rather than during hospitalization. It may be "moustache" or "pendant" type. Cannula may cause necrosis over the tops of the ears; it can be padded.
Transtracheal Catheter		
Less visible than cannula Flow requirement possibly reduced 60–80%, which greatly increases amount of time available from portable source of O_2 Less nasal irritation occurs (see Figure 31.18D)	Necessary for patient and family to learn entire program of care for tracheostoma and how to replace catheter Procedure invasive Equipment more costly	This method may not be appropriate for a patient with excessive mucus production from mucous plugging.
Tracheostomy Collar		
Can deliver high humidity and O_2	Possible for condensed fluid in tubing to drain into tracheostomy Water traps usually inserted Collection of secretions inside collar and around tracheostomy O_2 concentration lost into atmosphere because collar does not fit tightly	The collar attaches to the neck with an elastic strap and should be removed and cleaned at least q4h to prevent aspiration of fluid and infection.
Tracheostomy T Bar		
Better O_2 and humidity delivery than by tracheostomy collar because of tight fit	Possible for condensed fluid in tubing to drain into tracheostomy Water traps usually inserted	T bar must be removed for suctioning. T bar may pull on patient's tracheostomy tube, causing irritation and potential tissue damage. The nurse should monitor this closely.
Tent or Incubator		
Has ability to control temperature and humidity	Limited usefulness Difficult to maintain adequate concentrations of O_2 Isolates patient from environment	The tent should be flushed with O_2 every time it is opened. The nurse should assess for leaks around canopy.
Venturi Mask		
Delivers precise, high flow rates of O_2 Lightweight, cone-shaped plastic device fitted to face Available for delivery of 24%, 28%, 31%, 35%, 40%, and 50% O_2 Possible to apply adaptors to increase humidification (see Figure 31.18, C)	Uncomfortable and must be removed when patient eats Possible to talk while wearing mask, but voice may be muffled Other disadvantages: same as those for the simple face mask	Entrainment device on mask must be changed to deliver higher concentrations of O_2. This method is especially helpful for administering low, constant O_2 concentrations to patients with COPD. Air entrainment ports must not be occluded.

ABGs, arterial blood gases; *COPD,* chronic obstructive pulmonary disease.

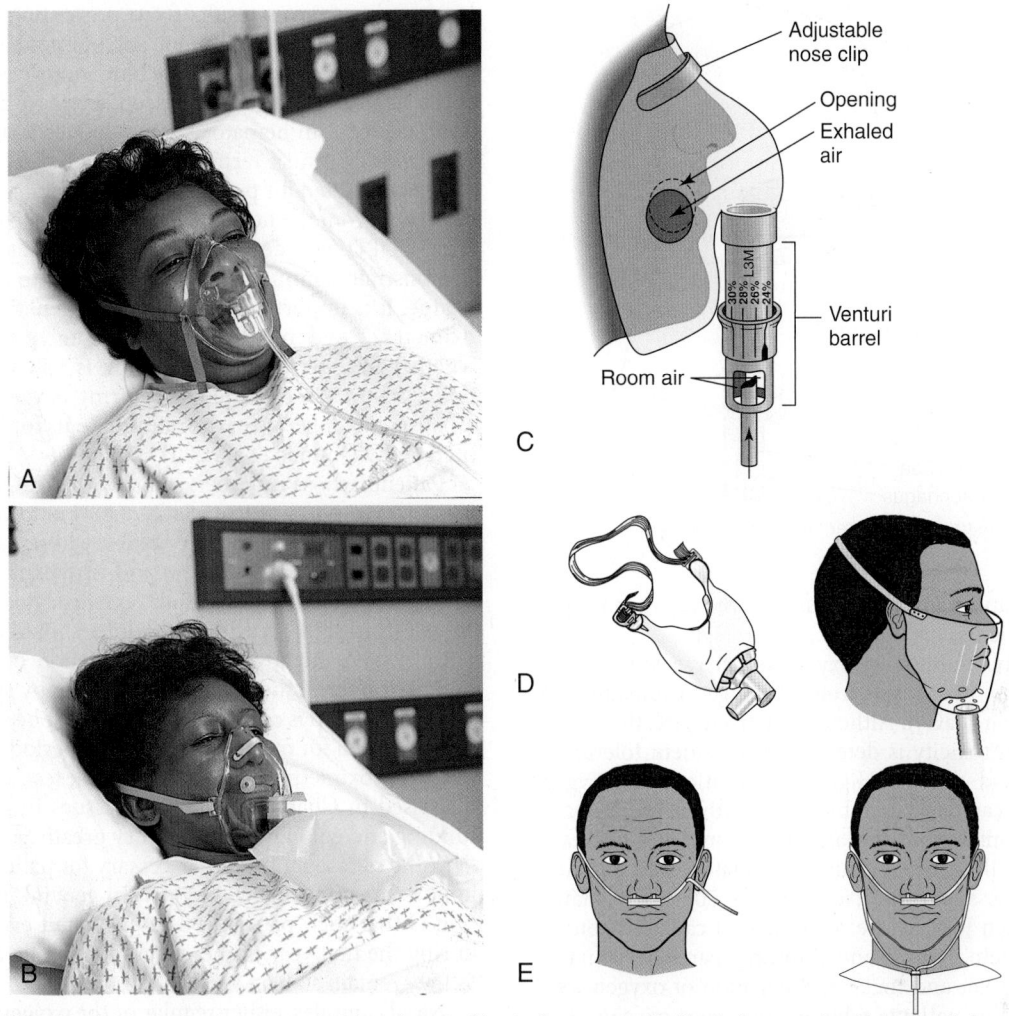

FIG. 31.18 Methods of oxygen administration. **A**, Simple face mask. **B**, Plastic face mask with reservoir bag. **C**, Venturi mask. **D**, Tracheostomy mask. **E**, Standard nasal cannulas. Source: Adapted from Potter, P. A., & Perry, A. G. (2009). *Fundamentals of nursing* (7th ed., pp. 958–959, Figures 40-15, 40-16, and 40-17). Mosby.

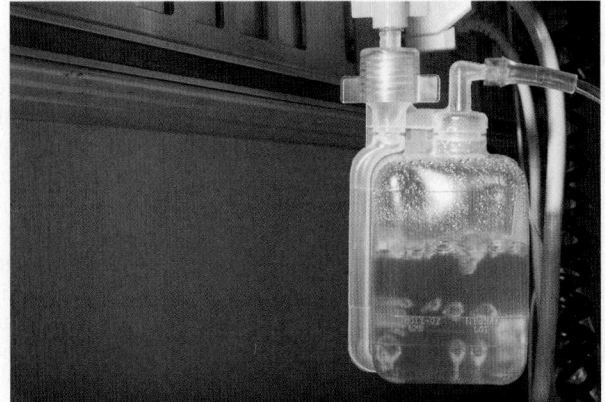

FIG. 31.19 Example of a bubble-through humidifier. Source: CanStock Photo/piedmont_photo.

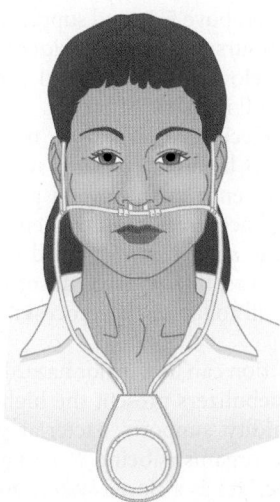

FIG. 31.20 Pendant type of oxygen-conserving cannula.

centre loses its sensitivity to the elevated carbon dioxide levels, and some patients with COPD develop a tolerance for high carbon dioxide levels. In theory, for these individuals the "drive" to breathe is hypoxemia. Therefore, administering oxygen to patients with COPD has been thought to weaken their drive to breathe. This has been a pervasive myth but is not a serious threat. In fact, not providing adequate oxygen to these patients

is much more detrimental. Although oxygen administration should be titrated to the lowest effective dosage, many patients who have end-stage COPD require high flow rates. They may in fact exhibit higher than normal levels of carbon dioxide in their blood, but this is of little concern. What is important is careful,

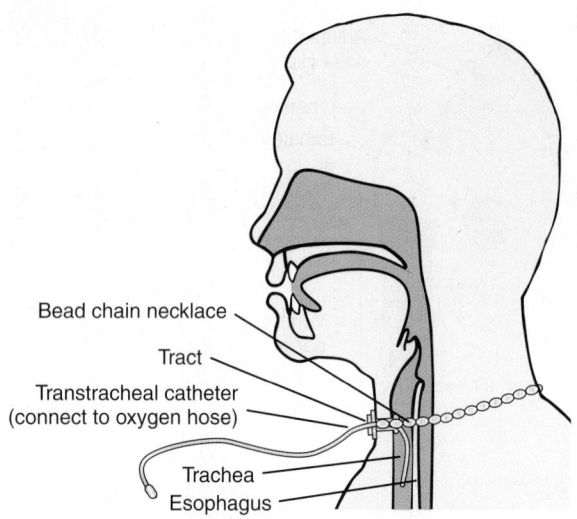

Bead chain necklace

Tract

Transtracheal catheter
(connect to oxygen hose)

Trachea
Esophagus

FIG. 31.21 Transtracheal catheter for oxygen administration.

ongoing physical and cognitive assessment when oxygen is provided to these patients.

Oxygen Toxicity. Pulmonary oxygen toxicity, a condition of oxygen overdosage, may result from prolonged exposure to a high level of oxygen (PaO_2). Although relatively rare, the development of oxygen toxicity is determined by patient tolerance, exposure time, and dosage. High concentrations of oxygen damage alveolar–capillary membranes, inactivate pulmonary surfactant, cause interstitial and alveolar edema, and decrease lung compliance; all of these changes ultimately lead to acute respiratory distress syndrome (see Chapter 70). Early manifestations of oxygen toxicity are reduced vital capacity, cough, substernal chest pain, nausea and vomiting, paresthesia, nasal stuffiness, sore throat, and malaise. Prevention of oxygen toxicity is important in patients who are receiving oxygen. The amount of oxygen administered should be just enough to maintain the PaO_2 within a normal or an acceptable range for each patient. A safe limit of oxygen concentrations has not yet been established. All levels above 50% and supplemental oxygen used for longer than 24 hours should be considered potentially toxic. Levels of 40% and below may be regarded as relatively nontoxic if the exposure period is short.

Absorption Atelectasis. Normally, nitrogen constitutes 79% of the air that is breathed, but it is not absorbed into the bloodstream. Its presence in the alveoli prevents alveolar collapse. When high concentrations of oxygen are given, nitrogen is washed out of the alveoli and replaced with oxygen. If airway obstruction occurs, the oxygen is absorbed into the bloodstream and the alveoli collapse. This process is called absorption atelectasis.

Infection. Infection can be a major hazard of oxygen administration. Heated nebulizers present the highest risk. The constant use of humidity supports bacterial growth, the most common infecting organism being *P. aeruginosa*. Disposable equipment that operates as a closed system should be used. The hospital should have a policy about the required frequency of equipment changes, based on the type of equipment used, and about the use of Gram staining and culturing of both equipment and respiratory secretions.

Long-Term Oxygen Therapy at Home. Improved survival and enhanced quality of life are observed in patients with COPD who receive long-term oxygen therapy to treat hypoxemia. The improved prognosis results from preventing both progression of the disease and subsequent cor pulmonale. The benefits of long-term oxygen therapy include improvements in neuropsychological function and sleep, increase in exercise tolerance, decrease in hematocrit, and reduced rates of pulmonary hypertension. Short-term home oxygen therapy (1 to 30 days) may be indicated for patients in whom hypoxemia persists after discharge from the hospital. For example, a patient with underlying COPD who develops a serious respiratory infection may demonstrate continued hypoxemia for 4 to 6 weeks after discharge. It is important to measure oxygenation status by pulse oximetry 2 to 3 months after an acute episode to determine whether long-term oxygen therapy is still warranted. At that point, up to 50% of patients requiring oxygen during an exacerbation no longer meet the requirements for long-term oxygen therapy (O'Donnell et al., 2007).

Patients whose disease is stable with a PaO_2 of 55 mm Hg or lower (corresponding to an SaO_2 of 88% or lower) should receive long-term oxygen therapy. A patient whose PaO_2 is between 55 and 59 mm Hg (SaO_2 of 89%) and who exhibits signs of tissue hypoxia, such as cor pulmonale, erythrocytosis, and peripheral edema from right-sided heart failure, should also receive long-term oxygen therapy. When desaturation occurs only during exercise or sleep, the use of oxygen therapy specifically during exercise or sleep is controversial and must be assessed individually. The need for oxygen during these periods should be evaluated with oximetry or a 6-minute walk test. (Pulse oximetry is discussed in Chapter 28.) Several issues in Canada related to funding and eligibility criteria vary greatly across jurisdictions. Periodic re-evaluations are necessary for patients who are using long-term supplemental oxygen. In general, the recommendation is that such patients be re-evaluated every 30 to 90 days during the first year of therapy and annually after that, as long as they remain stable.

Nasal cannulas, either regular or the oxygen-conserving type (see Figure 31.18, *E,* Figure 31.20, and Table 31.14) are usually used to deliver oxygen from a central source in the home. The source may be a liquid oxygen storage system, compressed oxygen in tanks, or an oxygen concentrator or extractor, depending on home environment, insurance coverage, activity level, and proximity to an oxygen supply company (Table 31.15). To increase mobility in the home, the patient can use extension tubing (up to 15 m [≈50 ft]) without adversely affecting the oxygen flow delivery if the flowmeter is the back pressure–compensated type. Small portable systems, such as that for liquid oxygen, may be provided for the patient who remains active outside the home.

Reservoir cannulas operate on the principle of storing oxygen in a small reservoir during exhalation. The oxygen is then delivered to the patient during the subsequent inhalation, in a manner similar to a bolus effect. The reservoir cannulas can reduce flow requirements by approximately 50%. A pendant type is available (see Figure 31.20). Other delivery devices for long-term oxygen therapy include transtracheal oxygen delivery and intermittent-demand oxygen delivery systems. Transtracheal oxygen delivery necessitates a surgical procedure to insert the small oxygen catheter into the patient's trachea (Figure 31.21). Nursing care involves teaching the patient and caregivers how to care for the stoma and the transtracheal catheter. The transtracheal catheter is less visible than nasal cannulas and there is no nasal irritation. It also reduces the oxygen flow requirement by 30 to 50%.

TABLE 31.15 HOME OXYGEN DELIVERY SYSTEMS

Advantages	Disadvantages	Comments
Liquid Oxygen		
Portable unit* can be refilled by patient from reservoir. Portable unit holds 6- to 8-hr supply at 2 L/min; reservoir will last approximately 7–10 days when 2 L/min is used continuously.	Liquid system is slightly more expensive, depending on location and is not available everywhere; its use is generally limited to urban areas.	As liquid warms to gas, some is vented from the system. In summer, evaporation is accelerated and may decrease reservoir duration to <1 wk.
Compressed Oxygen Tanks or Cylinders		
Availability is good in most areas. Portability is possible with a cart. Aluminum cylinders available in varying sizes (e.g., D, E, M, H, J) are markedly lighter than steel and easier to manoeuvre.	Duration of large (H or J) tank at 2 L/min flow is approximately 50 hr; storage of four or five large cylinders in the home is necessary to have a 7- to 10-day supply; portable cylinder on the cart is cumbersome and heavy. Duration of E cylinder when 2 L/min is used is approximately 4–5 hr.	Some smaller tanks (D or M) may be used; these can be refilled from large cylinders and weigh approximately 4.5 kg (10 lb). The tank can be carried on a shoulder strap, backpack, or fanny pack or placed on a portable cart.
Concentrator or Extractor		
Because the O_2 supply is made from room air, these devices never need to be "filled." These devices are on wheels, movable from room to room. They provide compact, excellent systems for rural or home-bound patients. They are convenient, safe, and reliable (assuming electricity source is reliable).	—	Concentrator should be kept in a room other than the bedroom if noise disturbs sleep.
Portable Oxygen Concentrator		
These are light-weight devices (3.9–17.7 kg [8.5–17 lb]) that are portable via carts or shoulder straps. Batteries last up to 8 hr with recharging in either AC or DC (e.g., car) outlets. These devices provide the patient with exceptional freedom and are beneficial to an active patient who may use more than the allotted requirement of O_2 cylinders each month.	These devices can be costly. The patient must meet qualifications of O_2 company to use.	—
Pulse or Demand Delivery System (Oxygen-Conserving Device)		
These devices deliver a pulse of O_2 only during inhalation to conserve O_2. They attach to cylinders. Their use increases duration of O_2 supply. There is less drying or irritation to nasal mucosa. These devices save O_2.	These devices may not be able to provide sufficient oxygen during exertion, are costly, are less efficient at higher O_2 flow rates, and are best for low activity levels. Audible pulses may be annoying. Patient must be a nose-breather to trigger the flow of O_2.	Monitor O_2 saturation during rest and exercise to determine whether oxygenation is acceptable. Consult with vendor or a respiratory therapist if O_2 saturation is below the desired level.

*Portable usually refers to units weighing more than 4.5 kg (10 lb); ambulatory units weigh less than 4.5 kg (10 lb).

Intermittent-demand delivery systems or conserver devices are mechanically complex devices that most commonly attach to the oxygen cylinders. They deliver "pulses" of oxygen to the patient, usually during inspiration, and thus eliminate waste of oxygen during exhalation, as is experienced during continuous flow.

Home oxygen systems are usually rented from a company that sends a respiratory therapist or respiratory nurse specialist to the patient's home to teach the patient and caregivers how to use and care for the oxygen system and how to recognize when the supply is running low and must be reordered. A patient and caregiver teaching guide for the use of oxygen at home is presented in Table 31.16.

A patient who uses home oxygen should be encouraged to remain active and to travel. If long-distance travel is by automobile, arrangements can be made for oxygen to be available at the destination point. Oxygen-supply companies can often assist with these arrangements. If a patient wishes to travel by bus, train, or airplane, the patient must notify the transportation company of the need for oxygen during travel when reservations are made. A high-altitude simulation test may be performed or a mathematical formula calculated in a hospital pulmonary function laboratory to determine the oxygen prescription required. Because airplane cabins are pressurized to an elevation of 2 100 or 2 400 m (7 000 or 8 000 ft), a passenger who uses supplemental oxygen should have oxygen provided during flight. The plane's oxygen system must be used. Passengers may not use their own oxygen system during flight because it is not properly pressurized. Airlines allow patients to bring their oxygen system to be carried in the baggage compartment for use at the point of destination, but the reservoirs (liquid or tank) must be empty and the valves left open. Some patients may need to avoid prolonged exposure to high elevations during travel unless they are instructed by their health care provider how to adjust their oxygen flow to attempt to compensate for altitude.

TABLE 31.16   PATIENT & CAREGIVER TEACHING GUIDE

Home Oxygen Use

Mask or Cannula
- Ensure that the straps are not too tight.
- Remove two or three times per day to wash and dry skin where straps are placed.
- Apply pressure-relieving dressings at any pressure points.
- Observe tops of ears, cheeks, and nasal mucosa for skin breakdown from pressure points.

Oral and Nasal Mucous Membranes
- Assess oral and nasal mucous membranes two or three times per day.
- Use water-based gel on the lips and nasal mucosa.
- Practise frequent oral hygiene.
- Avoid dry ambient air; humidity is required whenever oxygen is used.

Decreasing Risk for Infection
- Remove mask or collar, and clean with water two or three times per day.
- Clean skin carefully and observe for cuts, scratches, and bruises.
- Change disposable equipment frequently.
- Remove secretions that are expectorated.

Decreasing Risk of Fire Injuries
- Post "No Smoking" signs in the home where they can be seen.
- Do not use electric razors, portable radios, open flames, wool blankets, or mineral oils in the area where oxygen is in use.
- Do not allow smoking in the home or car.

Note: The Canadian Lung Association has good resources for patients using oxygen at home. See the Resources at the end of this chapter.

Surgical Therapy. Surgical procedures have been used in management of severe COPD. One type of surgery is *lung volume reduction surgery* (GOLD, 2020). The rationale for this surgery is that by reducing the size of the hyperinflated emphysematous lungs, airway obstruction is decreased and room for the remaining normal alveoli to function is increased. The procedure reduces volume by approximately 20 to 35% of the most emphysematous lungs and improves lung and chest wall mechanics. The most common postoperative complication is pneumonia. For a subgroup of patients with severe COPD, however, lung volume reduction surgery may offer improvements in lung function, exercise capacity, quality of life, and possibly length of survival.

Bullectomy is an older surgical procedure, specific to the patient with bullous emphysema (GOLD, 2020). The surgical removal of the bulla is intended to decompress adjacent lung parenchyma.

When all other treatments have failed, the next surgical procedure is *lung transplantation* for selected patients with advanced, severe COPD. In Canada, between 2009 and 2018, 24% of lung transplants were for COPD patients (Canadian Institute for Health Information [CIHI], 2020). Recipients of lung transplants who have COPD tend to have better outcomes than those with other conditions. The major complications affecting long-term morbidity and mortality are (a) chronic graft dysfunction associated with obliterative bronchiolitis and (b) opportunistic infection (GOLD, 2020). Patients with COPD who receive lung transplants can achieve substantial improvements in exercise capacity and improved quality of life, and most recipients no longer need supplemental oxygen. (Lung transplantation is discussed in Chapter 30.)

INFORMATICS IN PRACTICE

Texting for Patients With Chronic Obstructive Pulmonary Disease (COPD)

- Sometimes patients with COPD or those requiring oxygen therapy experience difficulty speaking because of shortness of breath.
- Patients should be encouraged to use typed messages displayed on a handheld electronic device to communicate.
- Texting and instant messaging family and friends are good alternatives to having phone conversations.

Pulmonary Rehabilitation Programs. All patients with COPD should be encouraged to maintain an active lifestyle. Pulmonary rehabilitation programs (PRPs) are used to optimize the functional status of patients with COPD—as well as their quality of life, experience of dyspnea, exercise endurance, psychosocial functioning, and overall autonomy—and to reduce health care costs. The benefits observed with PRPs are often superior to the benefits of pharmacological therapy. These benefits are largely attributable to exercise. In addition, patients who attend a PRP within 1 month of an exacerbation are shown to have improved outcomes (Marciniuk et al., 2011).

Specific components of a PRP can include exercise conditioning (aerobic conditioning and upper and lower body conditioning), breathing exercises, energy conservation, nutrition, smoking cessation, environmental factors, health promotion, patient education and self-management, psychological support, psychological counselling, and vocational rehabilitation. PRPs can be provided as inpatient, outpatient, or in-home programs. The duration of the program is typically 4 to 12 weeks or longer.

Exercise training involves both lower and upper extremity training and improves dyspnea and exercise performance. Lower extremity training focuses on aerobic training and includes walking, treadmill walking, bicycling, and cycling ergometry. Upper extremity training focuses on improving arm strength and endurance. Peripheral muscle wasting and weakness affects approximately 25% of patients with COPD. Exercise training should be performed more than three times per week. Health care providers working in PRPs assess the individual's limitations and conditioning status and develop a customized exercise program that is monitored over the length of the rehabilitation program.

Breathing Exercises. In patients with COPD, the respiratory rate increases and expiration is prolonged, to compensate for airflow obstruction and dyspnea. The accessory muscles of breathing, located in the neck and the upper part of the chest, are used excessively to promote chest wall movement. These muscles are not adapted to long-term use for breathing and, as a result, become fatigued. Breathing exercises can assist the patient during rest and activity (e.g., lifting, walking, stair climbing). The main types of breathing exercises are (a) pursed-lip breathing and (b) diaphragmatic breathing.

Pursed-lip breathing is used to prolong exhalation, prevent bronchiolar collapse and air trapping, and assist with dyspnea. Exhalation should be at least three times longer than inhalation. It is important to demonstrate and teach patients how to use this technique and for them to practise until it works for them and they feel comfortable using it. Patients should be instructed to follow this sequence:
1. Relax neck and shoulder muscles.
2. Inhale slowly through the nose to the count of 2.

TABLE 31.17 PATIENT & CAREGIVER TEACHING GUIDE

Huff Coughing

1. Patient assumes a sitting position with neck slightly flexed, shoulders relaxed, knees flexed, and forearms supported by a pillow and, if possible, with feet on the floor.
2. Patient then drops their head and bends forward while using slow, pursed-lip breathing to exhale.
3. Sitting up again, patient uses diaphragmatic breathing to inhale slowly and deeply.
4. Patient repeats steps 2 and 3 another three or four times to facilitate mobilization of secretions.
5. Before initiating a cough, patient should take a deep abdominal breath, bend slightly forward, and then cough three or four times on exhalation (huff coughing). Patient may need to support or splint the thorax or abdomen to achieve a cough of maximum effectiveness.

3. Pucker lips as if whistling.
4. Exhale slowly and gently through the lips while mentally counting to 6.
5. Always exhale longer than inhaling.

Diaphragmatic (abdominal) breathing focuses on using the diaphragm instead of accessory muscles to achieve maximum inhalation and to slow the respiratory rate. There has been an overall lack of evidence in controlled studies to either support or refute the use of diaphragmatic breathing in PRPs.

Effective Coughing. Many patients with COPD have developed ineffective coughing patterns that do not adequately clear their airways of sputum. In addition, they fear they may develop spastic coughing, which would increase dyspnea. *Huff coughing* is an effective technique that the patient can be taught easily; guidelines are presented in Table 31.17. The main goals of effective coughing are to conserve energy, reduce fatigue, and facilitate removal of secretions.

Nutritional Therapy. Weight loss and malnutrition are common among people with severe COPD and are a result of multiple factors. In these patients, energy expenditure is increased as a result of increased work of breathing (they spend 30–50% more energy on breathing than does the average person); oxygen consumption is increased; gas exchange is inefficient; and dead space ventilation is increased. Other factors further affecting patients' nutritional status may be dyspnea, dysphagia, dyspepsia, depression, anxiety, physical limitations, social isolation, financial considerations, decreased sense of smell and taste, drug and alcohol consumption, medication adverse effects, and a heightened systemic inflammatory response. Eating becomes an effort as a result of dyspnea, especially in the later stages of COPD. In addition, a full stomach presses up on the flattened diaphragm, further increasing dyspnea and causing discomfort. It is difficult for some patients to eat and breathe at the same time; therefore, they eat inadequate amounts of food. The role of a registered dietitian is critical for nutritional screening and intervention.

Patients with COPD should try to keep body mass index (BMI) between 21 and 25 kg/m². Being either overweight or underweight can cause further complications in conjunction with COPD. However, a reduced BMI or weight loss is especially associated with poor outcomes in acute exacerbations and with increased rates of morbidity and mortality among patients with COPD.

To decrease dyspnea and conserve energy, patients may need to rest (30 minutes) before eating, use a bronchodilator before meals, and select foods that can be prepared in advance. Eating five to six small meals per day helps avoid feelings of bloating and early satiety. Patients may want to avoid foods that form intestinal gas, such as cabbage, Brussels sprouts, and beans. Cold foods produce less of a sense of fullness than do hot foods. Foods that require a great deal of chewing can be served in another manner (e.g., grated, pureed). The use of frozen foods and a microwave oven may help conserve a patient's energy in food preparation. Exercises should be avoided for at least 1 hour before and after eating. In patients with late-stage or severe COPD, nutritional requirements for protein and calories may be greater than normal. They may need 1.2 to 1.3 times the normal kilocalorie requirement to even maintain their weight. A high-calorie, high-protein diet is recommended. High-protein, high-calorie nutritional supplements can be offered between meals. (Nutritional supplements are discussed in Chapter 42.)

Fluid intake should be at least 2 to 3 L per day unless contraindicated for other medical conditions, such as heart failure. Fluids should be taken between meals (rather than with them) to prevent excess stomach distension and to decrease pressure on the diaphragm. Sodium restriction may be indicated if a patient also has heart failure. In older patients, corticosteroid use increases the risk of or leads to osteoporosis. As a result, it is important to stress the necessity for adequate calcium and vitamin D intake.

AGE-RELATED CONSIDERATIONS

CHRONIC OBSTRUCTIVE PULMONARY DISEASE

Older people undergo physiological changes, including reduced lean body mass and decreased respiratory muscle strength that may increase the burden of disease from COPD, including more dyspnea and less tolerance of exercise. This causes a poorer ADL status and a higher incidence of acute exacerbations, which necessitate hospitalization. Smoking cessation is a key intervention but can be difficult to achieve.

COPD is frequently complicated by the presence of comorbid conditions such as hypertension, diabetes, obstructive sleep apnea, cardiovascular disease, cerebrovascular disease, psychiatric disorders, gut, renal disorders, musculoskeletal disorders, and cancer (Yin et al., 2017). The presence of comorbid conditions can make it difficult for patients to cope with the stress of an exacerbation. Ongoing assessment of comorbid conditions can assist in ensuring comprehensive and safe management, especially during an exacerbation.

Older patients may have difficulty in handling the increased secretions during an acute COPD exacerbation. The use of additional medications to manage the acute exacerbation can complicate disease management and increase the likelihood of adverse events. The nurse should assess for potential medication–medication interactions, especially in patients being treated for comorbidities.

Some medications used to treat common disorders in older persons, such as hypertension, can worsen COPD symptoms. Nonspecific β-blockers should be avoided because they can also block the α₂ receptors in the airway and cause bronchoconstriction. Angiotensin-converting enzyme inhibitors may cause a dry cough or worsen a current cough.

Older persons may not adhere to medication therapies because of cognitive impairment and complexity of the polypharmacy prescribed. Arthritis in the hands can hinder the patient from using proper technique for MDIs. It is important to review MDI technique during clinic visits and have a DPI or spacers prescribed (if possible) because they are easier to use. For patients with poor memory and visual impairment, an attempt should be made to simplify the medication regimen with written large-font action plans. Long-term use of ICSs has the potential for causing local and systemic adverse effects, lung infection, cataracts, glaucoma, poor diabetes control, oral candidiasis, and osteoporosis (Avdeev et al., 2019). These potential adverse effects should be monitored through ongoing diagnostic assessment to enable early detection and subsequent treatment and intervention.

As the patient with COPD ages, morbidity increases, and comorbidities begin to develop at an earlier age life (GOLD, 2020). With this trajectory in mind, an important role for the nurse is to focus on inventions that will maintain or improve these patients' quality of life. Psychological and emotional support becomes imperative to help them achieve successful outcomes. In the later stages of COPD, the care plan may focus on comfort and end of life, which is best served by consulting a palliative care practitioners or hospice care.

NURSING MANAGEMENT
CHRONIC OBSTRUCTIVE PULMONARY DISEASE

NURSING ASSESSMENT
Subjective and objective data that should be obtained from a patient with COPD are listed in Table 31.18.

NURSING DIAGNOSES
Nursing diagnoses for patients with COPD may include but are not limited to the following:
* *Inadequate breathing pattern* resulting from *hyperventilation, body position that inhibits lung expansion*
* *Inadequate airway clearance* resulting from *excessive mucus, retained secretions* (expiratory airflow obstruction)
* *Reduced gas exchange* (resulting from alveolar hypoventilation)

Additional information on nursing diagnoses is presented in Nursing Care Plan 31.2. See Table 31.12.

TABLE 31.18   NURSING ASSESSMENT
Chronic Obstructive Pulmonary Disease (COPD)

Subjective Data

Important Health Information

Current health: The nurse should assess patient's experience of dyspnea (with activity and at rest) and cough. If cough is productive, the nurse should determine colour, consistency, and quantity of secretions. Current dyspnea should be measured on a quantitative scale such as a visual analogue or a numeric rating scale. (See Chapter 28 with regard to dyspnea.) The usual level of dyspnea that a patient experiences should be measured against the Medical Research Council Dyspnea Scale (see Figure 31.15).

Past health history: The nurse should note whether the patient has had long-term exposure to chemical pollution, respiratory irritants, occupational fumes, and dust; the history and frequency of respiratory infections; previous hospitalizations and emergency department visits related to breathing and cardiac conditions; smoking exposure (pack-years, exposure to secondary smoke, previous attempts at cessation); and personal and family history of respiratory and cardiac conditions.

Medications: The nurse should record the use and duration of supplemental O_2, bronchodilators, anticholinergics, corticosteroids, antibiotics, OTC medications, complementary therapies; effectiveness of bronchodilators; and experience of adverse effects.

Symptoms
* Anorexia, weight loss or gain, early satiety, difficulty eating
* Decreased level of activity and ability to perform ADLs or exercise. Dyspnea, palpitations, recurrent cough, use of sitting-up position for sleeping, paroxysmal nocturnal dyspnea, orthopnea, swelling of feet
* Constipation, gas, bloating
* Headache, loss of memory, inability to concentrate
* Fatigue, insomnia, depression, anxiety, panic

Objective Data

General

Height, weight, BMI

Distress, increased work of breathing, use of compensatory mechanisms for breathing (upright position, pursed-lip breathing), anxiety, depression, restlessness

Integumentary

Cyanosis (bronchitis), pallor or ruddy colour, poor skin turgor, thin skin, easy bruising, peripheral edema (cor pulmonale)

Respiratory

Rapid, shallow breathing; accessory muscle use; inability to speak at all; prolonged expiratory phase; pursed-lip breathing; wheezing, crackles, diminished breath sounds; ↓ chest excursion and diaphragmatic movement; use of accessory muscles; hyper-resonant or dull chest sounds on percussion

Cardiovascular

Tachycardia, dysrhythmias, jugular vein distension, right-sided third heart sound (cor pulmonale), edema (especially in feet)

Gastrointestinal

Ascites, hepatomegaly (cor pulmonale)

Musculoskeletal

Muscle atrophy, ↑ anteroposterior diameter (barrel chest)

Possible Diagnostic Findings

Pulmonary function test results demonstrating airflow obstruction (e.g., ↓ FEV_1, FEV_1/FVC ratio, and PEFR; ↑ RV), ↓ SaO_2 as measured by pulse oximetry, abnormal arterial blood gas values, polycythemia

Chest radiograph showing flattened diaphragm and hyperinflation or infiltrates

ECG showing dysrhythmias

ADLs, activities of daily living; *BMI,* body mass index; *ECG,* electrocardiogram; *FEV_1,* forced expiratory volume in 1 second; *FVC,* forced vital capacity; *OTC,* over-the-counter; *PEFR,* peak expiratory flow rate; *RV,* residual volume; *SaO_2,* arterial oxygen saturation.

⊚ NURSING CARE PLAN 31.2
Chronic Obstructive Pulmonary Disease (COPD)

NURSING DIAGNOSIS	*Inadequate breathing pattern* resulting from body position that inhibits lung expansion, causes fatigue and respiratory muscle fatigue as evidenced by use of three-point position, pursed-lip breathing, use of accessory muscles to breathe

Expected Patient Outcomes

- Returns to baseline respiratory function
- Demonstrates an effective rate, rhythm, and depth of respirations

Nursing Interventions and *Rationales*

Ventilation Assistance
- Monitor respiratory and oxygenation status *to assess need for intervention.*
- Auscultate breath sounds, noting areas of decreased or absent ventilation and presence of adventitious sounds, *to obtain ongoing data on patient's response to therapy.*
- Encourage slow, deep breathing; turning; and coughing *to promote effective breathing techniques and secretion mobilization.*
- Administer medications (e.g., bronchodilators, inhalers) *that promote airway patency and gas exchange.*
- Position to minimize respiratory efforts (i.e., elevate head of the bed and provide overbed table for patient to lean on) *to save energy for breathing and promote chest expansion.*
- Monitor for respiratory muscle fatigue *to detect a need for ventilatory assistance.*
- Initiate a program of respiratory muscle strength and/or endurance training *to establish effective breathing patterns and techniques.*
- Consult dietitian *to ensure adequate caloric intake.*

NURSING DIAGNOSIS	*Inadequate airway clearance* resulting from excessive mucus, retained secretions as evidenced by ineffective cough, absence of cough, diminished breath sounds

Expected Patient Outcomes

- Has normal breath sounds for patient
- Demonstrates effective coughing
- Reports decreased dyspnea
- Maintains clear airway

Nursing Interventions and *Rationales*

- Facilitate deep breathing by sitting patient up *to maximize use of diaphragm and prolong expiratory phase.*
- Ensure adequate hydration (oral intake approximately 2–3 L/day, humidified ambient air) *to liquefy secretions for easier expectoration.*
- Teach effective cough techniques *to minimize the extent of airway collapse and to enhance airway clearance.*
- Assist with inhaled bronchodilator administration *to facilitate clearance of retained secretions.*

NURSING DIAGNOSIS	*Reduced gas exchange* (resulting from alveolar hypoventilation as evidenced by headache on awakening, $PaCO_2$ of ≥45 mm Hg and abnormal for patient's baseline, PaO_2 of <60 mm Hg, or SaO_2 of <90% at rest)

Expected Patient Outcomes

- Has $PaCO_2$ of 35–45 mm Hg or usual compensated baseline value
- Experiences return of PaO_2 to normal range for patient
- Reports improved mental status
- Reports decreased dyspnea
- Performs ADLs

Nursing Interventions and *Rationales*

- Monitor respiratory and oxygenation status *to assess need for intervention.*
- Teach pursed-lip breathing *to prolong expiratory phase and slow respiratory rate.*
- Assist patient to assume position of comfort (e.g., tripod position, elevated back rest, support of upper extremities to fix shoulder girdle) *to maximize respiratory excursion.*
- Administer and teach appropriate use of bronchodilators *to open the airways.*
- Teach signs, symptoms, and consequences of hypercapnia (e.g., confusion, somnolence, headache, irritability, decrease in mental acuity, increase in respiration, facial flush, diaphoresis) *to recognize condition early and initiate treatment.*
- Teach avoidance of central nervous system depressants *because they further depress respirations.*
- Administer O_2 if appropriate *to increase SaO_2 saturation.*
- Select O_2 supply systems and devices (e.g., nasal cannula, mask) that are appropriate for patient's ADLs (rest, sleep, exercise) *to minimize effect on preferred lifestyle.*

NURSING DIAGNOSIS	*Inadequate nutrition: less than body requirements* resulting from insufficient dietary intake, inability to ingest food (decreased energy level, shortness of breath, gastric distention) as evidenced by food intake less than recommended daily allowance

Expected Patient Outcomes

- Maintains body weight within normal range for sex, height, and age
- Has normal serum protein and albumin levels

Nursing Interventions and *Rationales*

- Monitor caloric intake, weight, and serum albumin and protein levels *to determine adequacy of intake.*
- Provide menu suggestions for high-protein, high-calorie foods *to ensure maintenance of weight.*
- Give patient high-protein, high-calorie liquid supplements if necessary, to provide adequate calories and protein *to prevent weight loss and muscle wasting.*
- Plan periods of rest before and after food intake *to assist with controlling fatigue and to compensate for blood flow diversion to the gastrointestinal tract for digestion.*
- Refer to hospital for financial or nutritional assistance as necessary (e.g., Meals-On-Wheels, home care) *to ensure nutritional adequacy after discharge.*
- Discuss benefit of five to six small meals throughout the day *because this reduces bloating.*

Continued

◎ NURSING CARE PLAN 31.2
Chronic Obstructive Pulmonary Disease (COPD)—cont'd

NURSING DIAGNOSIS	**Disturbed sleep pattern** resulting from nonrestorative sleep pattern (dyspnea, orthopnea, paroxysmal nocturnal dyspnea) as evidenced by unintentional awakening, feeling unrested
Expected Patient Outcomes	**Nursing Interventions and Rationales**
• Sleeps at least 5 hr over a 24-hr period • Reports improved sleep pattern • Reports feeling rejuvenated on wakening	• Identify usual sleep habits and elicit reasons for difficulty sleeping *to provide baseline data.* • Monitor patient's sleep pattern, and note physical circumstances (e.g., pain or discomfort and urinary frequency) and psychological circumstances (e.g., fear or anxiety) that interrupt sleep *to initiate appropriate interventions.* • Observe for signs and symptoms of sleep apnea such as frequent awakenings at night or excessive daytime sleepiness, or noting a partner who complains of the patient's snoring or gasping for air *to initiate appropriate diagnostic tests and interventions.* • Identify patient-specific methods of relaxation, and teach patient relaxation methods *to foster sleep.* • Encourage exercise and activity during daylight hours *to ensure improved sleep at night.* • Provide patient with activity that promotes wakefulness *to limit daytime sleep.* • Instruct patient in arranging surroundings (e.g., clothing, temperature, position, noise level) *to produce an environment conducive to sleep.* • Teach patient to avoid alcoholic beverages, caffeine products, or other stimulants before bedtime *to reduce interference with sleep.*
NURSING DIAGNOSIS	**Potential for infection** as evidenced by insufficient knowledge to avoid exposure to pathogens, smoking, malnutrition, stasis of body fluid (increased secretions)
Expected Patient Outcomes	**Nursing Interventions and *Rationales***
• Uses behaviours that minimize risk of infection • Experiences fewer or no respiratory infections	• Monitor for systemic and localized signs and symptoms of infection *to determine whether an infection is present.* • Teach patient to assess indicators of infection: change in sputum colour, quantity, odour, and viscosity; increase in cough and dyspnea; experience of fever, chills, diaphoresis, excessive fatigue; increase in respiratory rate; and abnormal breath sounds (gurgles, wheezing) *to determine whether an infection is present.* • Teach patient to use good handwashing and hygiene techniques and to avoid contact (when possible) with people with respiratory infections *to minimize sources of infection.* • Encourage patient to obtain vaccination for influenza and pneumococcal pneumonia *to decrease occurrence or severity of influenza or pneumonia.* • Teach proper care and cleaning of home respiratory equipment *to eliminate this source of infection.* • Instruct patient to seek medical attention for manifestations of early infection *to initiate treatment promptly.* • Teach patient to follow plan of care for managing exacerbations (e.g., increase fluid intake, initiate antibiotics and oral corticosteroid) *to initiate appropriate self-care promptly.*

ADLs, activities of daily living; *PaCO₂,* partial pressure of arterial carbon dioxide; *PaO₂,* partial pressure of arterial oxygen; *SaO₂,* arterial oxygen saturation.

▌PLANNING

Overall goals for patients with COPD include (a) the prevention of disease progression, (b) the ability to perform ADLs, (c) relief from breathlessness and other respiratory symptoms, (d) improvement in exercise tolerance, (e) the prevention and treatment of exacerbations, (f) improved overall quality of life, and (g) reduction in premature mortality.

▌NURSING IMPLEMENTATION

HEALTH PROMOTION. The best way to prevent COPD is never to smoke, and the next best step is to stop smoking immediately. (See the Nursing Management: Lung Cancer section in Chapter 30.) Avoiding or controlling exposure to occupational and environmental pollutants and irritants is another preventive measure to maintain healthy lungs. (These factors are discussed in the section on environmental lung diseases in Chapter 30.) Early detection of airway disease is important and is the rationale for the use of spirometry or pulmonary function tests. Early identification and treatment of respiratory tract infections is important for improving the long-term prognosis of COPD. Avoiding exposure to large crowds in the peak influenza periods may be necessary, especially for older people and patients with a history of respiratory conditions. Patients should also be taught good handwashing technique, to avoid sharing food and drinks, and to keep their hands away from their nose, mouth, and ears. Influenza and pneumococcal pneumonia vaccinations are recommended.

Families with a history of both COPD and AAT deficiency should be aware of the genetic nature of the disease. Genetic counselling may be appropriate for such patients and their families.

EDUCATION. An important aspect in the long-term care of the patient with COPD is education (Table 31.19). (Patient teaching is discussed in Chapter 4.) One component of education may involve preparation of an advance care plan (see the Ethical Dilemmas: Advance Directives box later in this chapter).

EXERCISE. Walking is by far the best physical exercise for patients with COPD. Coordinated walking with slow, pursed-lip breathing without breath holding is a difficult task that requires conscious effort and frequent reinforcement. During coordinated walking and breathing, the patient is taught to breathe in through the nose while taking one step, then to breathe out through pursed lips while taking two to four steps (the number depends on a patient's tolerance). Walking should occur at a slow pace with rest periods when necessary. If supplemental oxygen has been prescribed, the patient needs to use oxygen while walking or exercising. By walking with the patient, the nurse can help decrease anxiety and help maintain an appropriate pace. Walking also enables the nurse to observe the patient's actions and physiological responses to the activity. Many patients with moderate or severe COPD are anxious and fearful of walking or performing exercise. These patients and their families require much support while they build the confidence they need to walk or to perform daily exercises (GOLD, 2020).

Patients should be encouraged to walk 15 to 20 minutes a day and gradually increase this time. Patients can begin at a slower pace by walking for 2 to 5 minutes three times a day and slowly building up to 20 minutes a day, if possible. Adequate rest periods should be allowed. Some patients benefit from using a SABA (see Figure 31.16) approximately 10 minutes before exercise. Parameters to monitor with exercise include resting pulse and pulse rate after activity. Pulse rate after exercise should not exceed 75 to 80% of the maximum heart rate (maximum heart rate = 220 − age in years). Dyspnea is usually the limiting factor, rather than increased heart rate, for exercise; therefore, the patient's perceived sense of dyspnea should be used as an indication of exercise tolerance. The patient can use the MRC Dyspnea Scale (see Figure 31.15) to determine the intensity of dyspnea.

Patients should be informed that shortness of breath often increases during exercise (as it does for a healthy individual). The activity is not being overdone unless the increased dyspnea does not return to baseline within 5 minutes after the cessation of exercise. Patients should wait approximately 5 minutes after completion of exercise, and if the dyspnea has not returned to baseline levels, then a SABA should be used. During the recovery time, the patient should use pursed-lip breathing. If

---

TABLE 31.19   PATIENT & CAREGIVER TEACHING GUIDE

Chronic Obstructive Pulmonary Disease

Goal: To assist patients and caregivers in improving quality of life through education and to promote lifestyle practices that support successful living with chronic obstructive pulmonary disease (COPD).

Teaching Topic	Strategies and Resources	Teaching Topic	Strategies and Resources
Overall guide to COPD, including topics listed below	Global Initiative for Chronic Obstructive Lung Disease (GOLD): *Patient Guide: What You Can Do About a Lung Disease Called COPD*, available at http://goldcopd.org/wp-content/uploads/2016/04/GOLD_PatientGuide_2012.pdf Canadian Lung Association: *COPD BreathWorks Plan*, available at http://www.lung.ca/lung-health/lung-disease/chronic-obstructive-pulmonary-disease-copd/resources or toll-free helpline at 1-866-717-COPD (2673) Living Well With COPD program: available online (see the Resources at the end of this chapter)	**Medications** Types (include mechanism of action) • β₂-Adrenergic agonists • Anticholinergics • Corticosteroids • Methylxanthines • Phosphodiesterase 4 inhibitor • Antibiotics • Reviewing medication schedule and indications for use in adverse medication events	Written medication list and schedule Having patients explain purpose of the medication and show the medication they are referring to Knowing the various colours of the inhalers, because patients typically refer to them by colour

		Correct Use of Inhalation Devices
		• Metered-dose inhalers with and without spacers
		• Dry powder inhalers
			See Tables 31.6 and 31.7 and Figure 31.9
			Canadian Lung Association
			  • Handouts
			  • Inhalation device videos
			Placebo and demonstration units (provided by pharmaceutical companies) to assist with hands-on training
			Having patients demonstrate inhaler technique, and providing feedback about technique
			Checking periodically to ensure maintenance of proper technique
			Repeating process until accurate technique is demonstrated
			Exploring alternative delivery devices for patients who cannot demonstrate accurate technique

What Is COPD? • Basic anatomy and physiology of lung • Basic pathophysiological changes of COPD • Signs and symptoms of COPD, exacerbations, cold, flu, pneumonia • Tests to assess breathing	Models and posters of the lungs		
Nonpharmacological Therapy • Breathing exercises • Combating breathlessness and shortness of breath with "rescue breathing" techniques • Pursed-lip breathing • Relaxation techniques • Energy conservation techniques • Pacing and planning throughout the day for ADLs (pacing activity and using pursed-lip breathing with activities) • Regular exercise (upper and lower extremity) • Smoking cessation	Demonstration and return demonstration RNAO dyspnea guidelines Developing and using a schedule of daily and weekly activities Pulmonary rehabilitation program See Chapter 11. Smoking cessation guidelines for nurses (e.g., the RNAO's Best Practice Guideline *Integrating Smoking Cessation into Daily Practice*); Quit Smoking helplines	**Home Oxygen** • Explaining need for O₂ • Explaining equipment and rationale for use • Guidance for home O₂ and ambulatory use • Care of oxygen equipment	Canadian Lung Association website (see Resources at the end of this chapter) See Tables 31.15 and 31.16
		Psychosocial/Emotional Issues Concerns about interpersonal relationships • Dependency • Intimacy • Emotional difficulties • Depression • Anxiety and panic • Treatment decisions • Support and rehabilitation groups	Canadian Lung Association website (see the Resources at the end of this chapter) Open discussion (sharing with patient, significant other, and family) Exploring idea of attending social support groups or speaking to another person with COPD

Continued

TABLE 31.19 PATIENT & CAREGIVER TEACHING GUIDE

Chronic Obstructive Pulmonary Disease—cont'd

Teaching Topic	Strategies and Resources	Teaching Topic	Strategies and Resources
COPD Management Plan • Focusing on self-management • A written action plan • Monitoring signs and symptoms • Reporting changes in symptoms • Understanding causes of flares or exacerbations • Recognizing signs and symptoms of respiration infection, heart failure • Reducing the number of risk factors, especially smoking • Pulmonary rehabilitation program • Yearly follow-up	COPD management plan, developed and agreed upon by the nurse and patient, that meets individual needs Assessment of patient's confidence level in managing COPD, and enhancement of skill development and confidence as necessary	**Healthy Nutrition** • Strategies to lose weight (if patient is overweight) • Strategies to gain weight (if patient is underweight) **End-of-Life and Advance Planning** • Identifying concerns and preferences for end-of-life care • Support of problem solving, decision making, and planning	Consultation with dietitian End-of-life planning module in the Living Well With COPD program (see the Resources at the end of this chapter) Open discussion (health care team, patient, and family)

ADLs, activities of daily living; *RNAO,* Registered Nurses' Association of Ontario.

dyspnea takes longer than 5 minutes to return to baseline levels, the patient has probably overdone the exercise and should proceed at a slower pace during the next exercise period. Keeping a diary or log of the exercise program may be beneficial. Diaries provide a realistic evaluation of progress, help motivation, and add to a sense of accomplishment. Stationary bicycles and treadmills can also be used and are particularly valuable when weather prevents walking outside.

Energy-Conserving Strategies. Energy conservation is another important component in COPD rehabilitation. Exercise training of the upper extremities improves function and reduces dyspnea. Many patients have already adapted alternative energy-saving practices for ADLs. Alternative or modified methods of hair care, shaving, showering, and other activities that necessitate over-the-head reaching must be explored. Assuming a tripod posture (elbows supported on a table, chest in fixed position) and placing a mirror on the table while using an electric razor or hair dryer conserves energy in comparison with standing in front of a mirror to perform these activities. If the patient uses home oxygen therapy, it must be used during activities of hygiene because these activities consume energy. Another energy-saving tip is to exhale when pushing, pulling, or exerting effort during an activity and to inhale during rest. Patients should also try to sit as much as possible when performing activities.

Sexual Activity. Modifying but not abstaining from sexual activity can contribute to a feeling of well-being. Using a SABA before sexual activity can help control dyspnea. Patients with COPD also need less energy if these guidelines are followed: (a) have sexual activity during the part of the day when breathing is best, (b) use slow pursed-lip breathing, (c) refrain from sexual activity after eating or other strenuous activity, (d) do not assume a dominant position, and (e) do not prolong foreplay. These aspects of sexual activity require open communication between partners regarding their needs and expectations and the changes that may be necessary as the result of a chronic disease (e.g., changes in body image, role reversal).

Sleep. Adequate sleep is extremely important. Getting adequate amounts of sleep can be difficult for patients with COPD. Medications may cause restlessness and insomnia. If patients experience cough during the night, the use of LABDs may help. Postnasal drip may cause coughing at night and can be treated with nasal saline sprays or rinses, nasal steroids, or both before sleep and in the morning. If a patient snores, stops breathing, or makes gasping breaths while sleeping and has a tendency to fall

asleep during the day, the patient may need to be tested for sleep apnea (see Chapter 9).

Psychosocial Considerations. Healthy coping is often challenging for patients with COPD. Such patients frequently have to deal with many lifestyle changes that may involve a decreased ability to care for themselves and their condition, decreased energy for performing day-to-day activities and social activities, and the loss of a job. These lifestyle changes can put the patient at risk for social isolation.

When a patient first receives a diagnosis of COPD or experiences complications, the nurse should expect a variety of emotional responses. Emotions frequently encountered include guilt, depression, anxiety, social isolation, denial, and dependence. Among patients who still or used to smoke, guilt may result from the knowledge that the disease was caused largely by tobacco smoking. The patient may experience depression as they realize the severity and chronicity of the disease. The nurse should convey a sense of understanding and caring to the patient. Relaxation techniques may provide benefit in terms of relief of dyspnea for some patients, but the evidence for this is unclear. Relaxation techniques include progressive muscular relaxation, positive thinking and visualization, and use of music, yoga, massage, and humour (see Chapters 8 and 12). Progressive relaxation techniques are performed by having the patient listen to music or to their own or another voice, and then gradually begin to slowly tense and relax muscle groups. Support groups at local chapters of the Canadian Lung Association, at hospitals, and at clinics can also be helpful.

End-of-Life Issues. Nurses have a responsibility to discuss with and plan for end-of-life care with patients and their families or caregivers to make sure that the necessary supports are in place to assist them through this critical terminal phase. Patients, their families, and health care providers should be involved in writing advance directives. Nurses must explore and understand the issues facing patients and their families through empathic, honest, and informative conversations. Discussions that highlight the importance of palliative care services and alleviation of terminal dyspnea can lessen anticipatory fear and anxiety. The following Ethical Dilemmas box discusses advance directives.

EVALUATION

The expected outcomes for the patient with COPD are presented in Nursing Care Plan 31.2.

ETHICAL DILEMMAS
Advance Directives

Situation

A 79-year-old man with chronic obstructive pulmonary disease is admitted to the hospital with respiratory failure. He is placed on a mechanical ventilator and responds to stimuli occasionally by opening his eyes. His living will was written 5 years ago, and a copy was given to his wife and health care provider at that time. His wife brings the document to the critical care unit and tells the nurse that the hospital must stop treating her husband and allow him to die as he requested. However, the oldest son is threatening the hospital with a lawsuit if the staff does not provide full care to his father.

Important Points for Consideration

- A living will is one type of advance directive.
- A living will is prepared by the person in advance, indicating the person's treatment wishes should they become terminally ill or in a situation in which there is no hope of recovery.
- Health care providers must determine whether this respiratory crisis is reversible.
- Power of attorney for health care is another form of advance directive in which one person names another person to make health care decisions in the event that the first person is no longer able to do so.
- An advance directive respects the patient's autonomy—that is, the right to self-determination regarding health care at the end of life.
- A legally written living will is legally binding.
- Health care providers are obligated to follow the patient's advance directive when the patient is no longer able to speak for themselves.
- Health care providers are protected from liability when they adhere to advance directives.

Clinical Decision-Making Questions

1. What should the nurse do next with the information provided by the patient's wife?
2. How should the nurse address the needs of each member of this family in the patient's plan of care?
3. What resources can the nurse use to facilitate decision making in this situation?

CYSTIC FIBROSIS

Cystic fibrosis (CF) is an autosomal recessive, multisystem disease characterized by altered function of the exocrine glands involving primarily the lungs, the pancreas, and the sweat glands. (Autosomal recessive disorders are discussed in Chapter 15.) Abnormally thick, abundant secretions from mucous glands lead to a chronic, diffuse, obstructive pulmonary disorder in almost all affected patients. Exocrine pancreatic insufficiency is associated with most cases of CF. Sweat glands excrete increased amounts of sodium and chloride.

CF is a chronic fatal respiratory disease. According to the Canadian Cystic Fibrosis Registry, over 4 370 Canadians had cystic fibrosis in 2018 (representing about 1 in 3 600 live births); 54.7% were male and 45.3% were female, and 93.2% of the total population were White (Cystic Fibrosis Canada, 2019). This autosomal recessive disease has a carrier rate of 1 per 25. If both parents carry the gene, the chance that their offspring will have the disease is 25%. The first signs and symptoms typically occur in early childhood, and in most patients the disease is diagnosed by the age of 5 years. However, some patients tend to have less severe disease, and their cases are not diagnosed until they are adults.

The severity and the progression of the disease vary from person to person. Since the 1990s, the prognosis of this disease has improved dramatically because of early diagnosis and improvements in therapy. The median age of survival for Canadians with CF is currently estimated to be 52.1 years of age, up from 50 years of age in 2012 (Cystic Fibrosis Canada, 2019).

Etiology and Pathophysiology

CF results from mutations in a gene located on chromosome 7. The most common genetic mutation in CF occurs in what is known as the cystic fibrosis transmembrane regulator (CFTR) gene. The CFTR protein localizes to the lining of the exocrine portion of particular organs such as airways, pancreatic duct, sweat gland duct, and reproductive tract. The *CFTR* gene regulates sodium and chloride channels. Mutations in the *CFTR* gene alter this protein in such a way that the channels are blocked. As a result, cells that line the passages of the lungs, the pancreas, and other organs produce abnormally thick, sticky mucus. This mucus obstructs the airways and glands. The glands distal to the duct eventually undergo fibrosis. The high concentrations of sodium and chloride in the sweat of the patient with CF result from decreased chloride resorption in the sweat duct.

In the respiratory system, both upper and lower respiratory tracts can be affected. Upper respiratory tract manifestations include chronic sinusitis and nasal polyposis. The hallmark of respiratory involvement in CF is its effect on the airways. From being a disease of the small airways (chronic bronchiolitis), CF progresses to an entity that eventually involves the larger airways and finally causes destruction of lung tissue. Thick secretions obstruct bronchioles and lead to air trapping and hyperinflation of the lungs. The stasis of mucus provides an excellent growth medium for bacteria, which makes the airways more susceptible to serious lower respiratory tract infections. CF is thus characterized by chronic airway infection. The organisms most commonly cultured from the sputum of a patient with CF are *Staphylococcus aureus* and *P. aeruginosa* (Cystic Fibrosis Canada, 2019). These infections increase the rate of lung destruction through inflammatory mediators such as interleukins, tumour necrosis factor, and leukotrienes.

Lung disorders that can result from this pathological process include pneumonia, bronchiolitis, bronchitis, bronchiectasis, atelectasis, and emphysema. Lung tissue is progressively destroyed by inflammation and scarring, and the resultant chronic hypoxia leads to pulmonary hypertension and cor pulmonale. Blebs and large cysts in the lung are further severe manifestations of lung destruction. Other pulmonary complications include hemoptysis, which can sometimes be fatal, and pneumothorax. The degree of hemoptysis may range from scant streaking to major bleeding.

Initially, CF is an obstructive lung disease caused by the overall obstruction of the airways with mucus. Later, CF progresses to a restrictive lung disease because of the fibrosis, lung destruction, and thoracic wall changes. Death usually results from loss of pulmonary function. Cor pulmonale is a common late complication caused by extensive loss of lung tissue and chronic hypoxia.

Pancreatic insufficiency is caused primarily by mucous plugging of the pancreatic duct and its branches, which results in fibrosis of the acinar glands of the pancreas and leads to the loss of exocrine function. Pancreatic enzymes such as trypsinogen, lipase, and amylase do not reach the intestine to digest ingested nutrients. Fat, protein, and fat-soluble vitamins (vitamins A, D, E, and K) are malabsorbed. Fat malabsorption results in steatorrhea, and protein malabsorption results in malnutrition, failure to grow, and failure to gain weight.

Diabetes mellitus may occur if the islets of Langerhans become fibrotic. CF-related diabetes mellitus affects approximately 15% of all patients with CF. It differs from type 1 diabetes in that some insulin is secreted, the disease is nonketotic, and it is slow in onset. It differs from type 2 diabetes in that affected individuals are underweight (as opposed to being obese), the onset is in a younger age population, and affected individuals are hypoinsulinemic. Routine screening of serum glucose levels is recommended. Insulin may be required for treatment of CF-related diabetes.

The sweat glands of the patient with CF secrete normal volumes of sweat but are unable to absorb sodium and chloride from sweat as it moves through the sweat duct. Therefore, these patients excrete four times the normal amount of sodium and chloride in sweat. This abnormality does not seem to affect the general health of the person, but it is useful as a diagnostic indicator.

Individuals with CF often have gastrointestinal conditions. Intestinal obstruction resulting in meconium ileus is present in 10 to 15% of newborns with CF. GERD, distal intestinal obstructive syndrome (DIOS), and constipation are common. GERD is a major challenge in individuals with CF. The relationship between reflux and exacerbation of respiratory disease is not known, but it is known that these two entities worsen each other.

DIOS is a syndrome that results from intermittent obstruction in the ileocecal area in patients with pancreatic insufficiency. The degree to which the bowel is obstructed may vary with each episode, and a partial obstruction may progress to a complete obstruction. Complete obstruction necessitates gastric decompression and a surgical consultation; partial and uncomplicated episodes of DIOS are treated with ingestion of a balanced polyethylene glycol electrolyte solution. Constipation develops in the sigmoid colon and progresses proximally, whereas DIOS develops in the ileocecal area and progresses distally. Careful monitoring of bowel habits and patterns is essential.

The liver may become involved. Biliary cirrhosis may not be recognized until late in the disease. Hepatobiliary disease is common in adult patients with CF. Chronic cholestasis, inflammation, fibrosis, and portal hypertension can occur.

Clinical Manifestations

The clinical manifestations of CF vary in accordance with the severity of the disease. As mentioned, meconium ileus is present in 10 to 15% of newborns with CF. Early childhood manifestations are failure to grow, digital clubbing, persistent cough with mucus production, tachypnea, and large, frequent bowel movements. The abdomen may become large and protuberant, and the extremities may develop an emaciated appearance.

The first symptom of CF in adults is frequently cough. With time, the cough becomes persistent and produces viscous, purulent, and often greenish sputum. Other respiratory conditions that may be indicative of CF are recurring lung infections such as bronchiolitis, bronchitis, and pneumonia. As the disease progresses, periods of clinical stability are interrupted by exacerbations characterized by increased cough and sputum production, weight loss, and decreases in pulmonary function. Over time, the exacerbations become more frequent and lost lung function is less completely recovered, which ultimately leads to respiratory failure.

DIOS causes pain in the right lower quadrant, loss of appetite, and emesis, and a mass is often palpable. Insufficient pancreatic

enzyme release causes the typical pattern of protein and fat malabsorption with frequent, bulky, foul-smelling stools.

The function of the reproductive system is altered. This finding is important because increasing numbers of people with CF are living to adulthood. Nearly all men with CF have reproductive issues because the vas deferens, which transports the sperm from the storage in the testes to the penile urethra, is congenitally absent. However, men with CF make sperm normally and thus, with assisted reproductive technology, have the capability of fathering children. In women with CF, menarche is usually delayed. During exacerbations, menstrual irregularities and secondary amenorrhea are fairly common. Affected women may be unable to become pregnant because of the increased viscosity of the cervical mucus. Many women with CF do have children, but the fertility rate is lower than among healthy women (Taylor-Cousar, 2020). The baby of such a patient is heterozygous for CF (and hence a carrier of the *CFTR* gene) if the father is not a carrier. If the father is a carrier, the baby has a 50% chance of having CF. Genetic counselling can assist couples in deciding whether they want to have children and whether they want to use assisted reproductive technology to have a baby without the risk of CF. Screening of newborns can identify who will develop CF. Debate about the usefulness of this technology continues. (See Chapter 15 and Figure 15.6 for an explanation of genetic transmission of CF.)

Complications

The most frequent complications experienced are the following (Cystic Fibrosis Canada, 2020):
1. Difficulty digesting fats and proteins with subsequent malnutrition and vitamin deficiencies
2. Progressive lung damage from chronic infections and chronic inflammation
3. Secondary diabetes
4. Chronic sinus infections

Critical life-threatening complication include the following:
1. Pneumothorax is a relatively uncommon but serious complication that is caused by the formation of bullae and blebs.
2. Massive hemoptysis, although rare, is life-threatening. It is often caused by rupture of bronchial arteries in 90% of cases (Monroe et al., 2018).
3. Respiratory failure and cor pulmonale are late complications of CF.

Diagnostic Studies

Diagnostic criteria for CF are evidence of CFTR protein malfunction on the sweat chloride test and characteristic respiratory or gastrointestinal symptoms. The sweat chloride test is performed with the pilocarpine iontophoresis method, which yields abnormal results in more than 90% of adults with CF. Pilocarpine carried by a small electric current is used to stimulate sweat production. The sweat is collected on filter paper or gauze and then analyzed for sodium and chloride concentrations. The test takes approximately 40 to 60 minutes. Values greater than 60 mEq/L for sodium and chloride are suggestive of CF, especially in a person who has other clinical features of the disease (Cystic Fibrosis Canada, 2019). A second sweat chloride test is recommended to confirm the diagnosis unless two CF mutations have been identified by genetic testing. The degree of sodium and chloride elevation is not necessarily correlated with the severity of the disease. Secondary diagnostic studies include chest radiography, pulmonary function tests, fecal analysis for

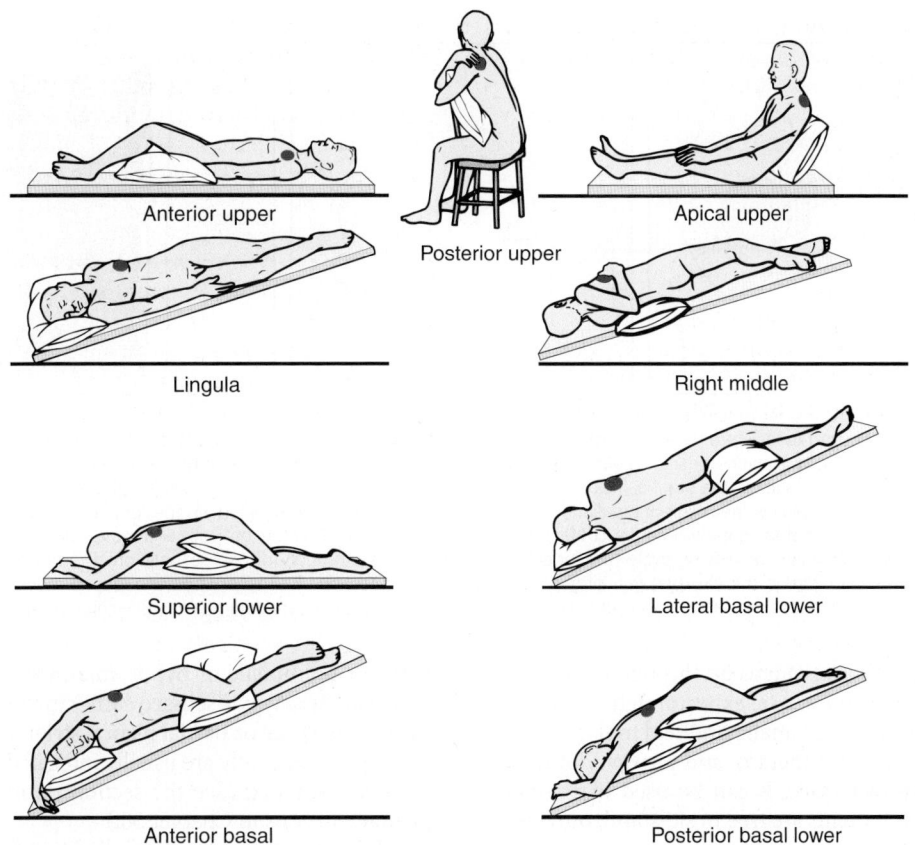

FIG. 31.22 Representative positions for postural drainage. *Shaded areas* in each illustration indicate the segment of the lung in which drainage is promoted.

fat, and duodenoscopy for quantitative determination of pancreatic enzymes.

Because of the large number of CF mutations, DNA analysis is not used for the primary diagnostic test. A positive result of DNA analysis does, however, corroborate the diagnosis. Fetal diagnosis can be performed from specimens obtained by amniocentesis or chorionic villus sampling.

Interprofessional Care

An interprofessional team should be involved in patients' care and should include nurses, physicians, respiratory therapists and physiotherapists, dietitians, pharmacists, and social workers. The major objectives of therapy in CF are to (a) promote clearance of secretions, (b) control infection in the lungs, and (c) provide adequate nutrition. Drainage of thick bronchial mucus is assisted by aerosol and nebulized forms of medications to liquefy mucus and to facilitate coughing. The abnormal viscosity of secretions in CF results primarily from mucus glycoproteins and DNA from degenerated neutrophils. Medications that degrade the high concentrations of DNA in CF sputum (e.g., DNase [Pulmozyme]) decrease sputum viscosity and increase airflow. Bronchodilators (e.g., β_2-adrenergic agonists, theophylline) may be used.

Airway clearance techniques are critical in reducing mucus. These techniques include chest physiotherapy, postural drainage, and positive expiratory pressure (PEP) breathing. **Chest physiotherapy** (CPT) consists of percussion, vibration, and postural drainage. Percussion and vibration are manual or mechanical techniques used to augment postural drainage. In **postural drainage**, the principle of gravity is used to assist in bronchial

clearance (Figure 31.22). Percussion and vibration are used after the patient has assumed a postural drainage position to assist in loosening the mobilized secretions. Percussion, vibration, and postural drainage may assist in bringing secretions into larger, more central airways. Effective coughing is then necessary to help raise these secretions. After each drainage position change, the patient should be given time to cough and breathe deeply. These techniques are individualized on the basis of the patient's pulmonary condition and response to the initial treatment. Sometimes it takes several hours after CPT for secretions to be expectorated. It is important to evaluate the effectiveness of CPT and its relief of symptoms; a physiotherapist who is trained in the proper technique often performs CPT. Complications associated with improperly performed CPT include fractured ribs, bruising, hypoxemia, and discomfort. CPT may not be beneficial and can be stressful for some patients. Some patients may develop hypoxemia and bronchospasm with CPT.

Various *airway clearance devices* are available to mobilize secretions, are easier to tolerate than CPT, and take less time than conventional CPT sessions. These devices include the Flutter device, Acapella device, and TheraPEP Therapy System. These devices involve the use of the principle of PEP and may provide greater benefit to patients with COPD than other airway clearance techniques.

The Flutter mucus clearance device is also effective in promoting mucus removal (Figure 31.23). It is a handheld device that provides PEP. The flutter valve works by (a) causing the airways to vibrate, which loosens mucus from airway walls; (b) intermittently increasing the endobronchial pressure, which helps maintain the patency of the airway; and (c) accelerating

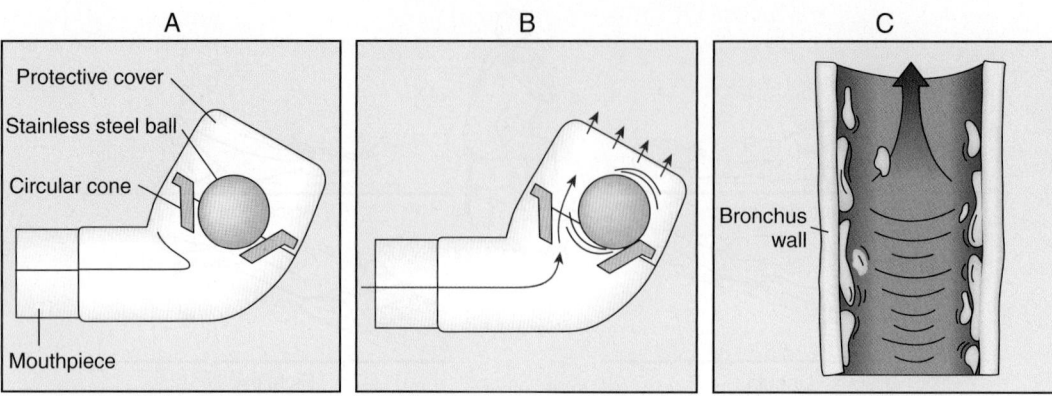

FIG. 31.23 The Flutter mucus clearance device is a small, handheld tool that provides positive expiratory pressure therapy. It is used to facilitate removal of mucus from the lungs. **A,** It consists of a hard plastic mouthpiece, a plastic perforated cover, and a high-density stainless steel ball resting in a circular cone. **B,** The flutter effect occurs during expiration. Before exhalation, the steel ball blocks the conical canal of the Flutter device. During exhalation, the position the steel ball occupies is the result of equilibrium between the pressure of the exhaled air, the force of gravity on the ball, and the angle of the cone where the contact with the ball occurs. As the steel ball rolls and moves up and down, it creates an opening-and-closing cycle that repeats itself many times throughout each exhalation. The net result is that vibrations occur in the airways, resulting in the "fluttering" sensation. **C,** These vibrations loosen mucus from the airway walls and facilitate its movement up the airways. Source: Axcan Scandipharm, Inc., Birmingham, Alabama.

expiratory airflow. It helps move mucus up through the airways to the mouth, where the mucus can be expectorated.

The Acapella device is another small handheld tool that combines the benefits of both PEP therapy and airway vibrations to mobilize pulmonary secretions. It can be used in virtually any setting, inasmuch as patients are free to sit, stand, or recline while using it.

TheraPEP Therapy System can also provide sustained PEP and can simultaneously deliver aerosols so that the patient can inhale and exhale through it. TheraPEP has a mouthpiece attached to tubing connected to a small cylindrical resistor and a pressure indicator. The pressure indicator provides visual feedback about the pressure that the patient needs to hold in an exhalation to receive the PEP. (See the Resources section at the end of this chapter for a description and photo of this system.)

It is important to work collaboratively with families and patients because individuals with CF may have a preference for a certain technique that works well for them. Aerobic exercise seems to be effective in clearing the airways. Important needs to consider in planning an aerobic exercise program for a patient with CF are (a) frequent rest periods interspersed throughout the exercise regimen, (b) meeting increased nutritional demands of exercise, (c) being alert for manifestations of hyperthermia, and (d) drinking large amounts of fluid and replacing salt losses.

Most patients with CF die of complications resulting from lung infection. Rigorous, early treatment of early *P. aeruginosa* infection is of great benefit to these patients to prevent mucoidal biofilm from forming (Smith et al., 2017). Prolonged high-dosage therapy may be necessary because many medications are abnormally metabolized and rapidly excreted by patients with CF. Results of pharmacokinetic and kidney function studies should be monitored closely.

Although combination oral and aerosolized antimicrobial therapy is usually adequate, some patients require a 2- to 4-week course of intravenous antimicrobial therapy. If home care supports are adequate, the patient and family may choose parenteral therapy at home. The usual treatment for an acute infectious exacerbation is either an aminoglycoside combined with penicillin or a third-generation cephalosporin. Aerosolized bronchodilators may be used in selected patients, particularly before CPT. Patients with cor pulmonale or hypoxemia may require oxygen therapy. (Oxygen therapy is discussed earlier in this chapter.) Sclerosing of the pleural space or partial pleural stripping and pleural abrasion performed surgically are usually indicated for recurrent episodes of pneumothorax. (See the section on interprofessional care of pleural effusions in Chapter 30.)

CF has become a leading indication for bilateral lung transplantation, accounting for 24.5% of these operations from 2004 to 2013 (CIHI, 2021). Between 1988 and 2015, 650 people with CF received lung transplants (CIHI, 2020). (Lung transplantation is discussed in Chapter 30.) Lung transplantation for people with CF has resulted in significant improvements in pulmonary function and quality of life, as well as longer life expectancy. The survival rate among lung transplant recipients, including all primary diagnoses, is 86.8% at 1 year and 65.9% at 5 years (CIHI, 2021). The rate of survival after lung transplantation is higher among people with CF than among those with other pulmonary diseases such as COPD.

The management of pancreatic insufficiency includes pancreatic enzyme replacement of lipase, protease, and amylase (e.g., pancrelipase [Cotazym, Creon, Ultrase, Viokase] and zymase, an enzyme complex) administered before each meal and snack. A high-calorie, high-protein diet and multivitamin supplementation are recommended. Fat restriction usually is not necessary. Fat-soluble vitamin supplementation (vitamins A, D, E, and K) is necessary. Use of caloric supplements improves nutritional status. Added dietary salt is indicated whenever sweating is excessive, such as during hot weather, in the presence of fever, or from intense physical activity.

Gene therapy has been used as an experimental therapy for treating CF, but more research is still required (Smith et al., 2017). (Gene therapy is discussed in Chapter 15.)

NURSING MANAGEMENT
CYSTIC FIBROSIS

NURSING ASSESSMENT

Subjective and objective data that should be obtained from a patient with CF are listed in Table 31.20.

TABLE 31.20 NURSING ASSESSMENT

Cystic Fibrosis (CF)

Subjective Data

Important Health Information

Current health: Experience of cough and mucus production (quantity, colour, consistency), dyspnea, and wheeze

Past health history: Past respiratory and sinus infections: typical pattern, how treated, how responded to treatment; past hospitalizations and emergency department visits; when CF was diagnosed; family history of CF

Medications: Use of bronchodilators, antibiotics, enzymes, herbs, and complementary therapies; adverse effects experienced; adherence to treatment regimen

Nonpharmacological therapies: Use of postural drainage, percussion, and vibration

Symptoms

- Runny nose; increased work of breathing; thick, tenacious sputum
- Dietary intolerances, voracious appetite, weight loss, intestinal gas, bulky and foul-smelling stools, abdominal pain
- Fatigue, restlessness, decreased exercise tolerance
- Anxiety, depression
- Delayed menarche, menstrual irregularities, and secondary amenorrhea; fertility issues

Objective Data

General

Restlessness, failure to thrive

Integumentary System

Cyanosis (circumoral, nail beds), digital clubbing, salty skin

Eyes

Scleral icterus

Respiratory System

Runny nose, diminished breath sounds, sputum (amount, colour, tenacious), hemoptysis, increased work of breathing evidenced by use of accessory muscles of respiration, barrel chest

Cardiovascular System

Tachycardia

Gastrointestinal System

Possibility of protuberant abdomen and abdominal distension and of foul, fatty stools

Possible Diagnostic Findings

Abnormal results of the following: pulmonary function tests, sweat chloride test, chest radiography, fecal fat analysis for fatty stools

NURSING DIAGNOSES

Nursing diagnoses for a patient with CF may include but are not limited to the following:

- *Inadequate airway clearance* resulting from *excessive mucus, retained secretions*
- *Inadequate breathing pattern* resulting from *fatigue, respiratory muscle fatigue*
- *Reduced gas exchange* (resulting from recurring lung infection)
- *Inadequate nutrition: less than body requirements* resulting from *insufficient dietary intake, inability to digest food*
- *Inadequate coping* as a result of *high degree of threat* (decreased life expectancy, cost of treatment, limitation of career choices)

PLANNING

Overall goals for patients with CF include (a) adequate airway clearance, (b) reduction in the number of risk factors associated with respiratory infections, (c) ability to perform ADLs, (d) minimizing complications related to CF, (e) adequate nutritional support to maintain appropriate BMI, and (f) active participation in planning and implementing a therapeutic regimen.

NURSING IMPLEMENTATION

Nurses and other health care providers can help young adults with CF obtain independence by helping them assume responsibility for their care. An important issue that should be discussed is sexuality. Delayed or irregular menstruation is not uncommon. There may be delayed development of secondary sex characteristics such as breasts in girls. A patient may use CF as a reason to avoid certain events or relationships. In contrast, healthy individuals may hesitate to make friends with someone who is sick, which can present a challenge for individuals with CF. Normal life transitions can present larger challenges

to young adults with CF, such as building confidence and self-respect on the basis of achievements, persevering with employment goals and opportunities, developing motivation to set and achieve goals, learning to cope with the intensity and chronicity of the treatment program, and adjusting to losing independence when health fails. Disclosing the CF diagnosis to friends, potential spouses, or employers may pose challenges emotionally and financially.

For patients with CF, respiratory intervention targets relief of bronchoconstriction, airway obstruction, and airflow limitation through the use of aggressive CPT, antibiotics, and bronchodilators. Good nutrition, nutritional supplements, and pancreatic enzymes are also important. Advances in long-term vascular access (e.g., implanted ports) have made intravenous access and administration of medication much easier and have eased the transition for intravenous treatment from hospital to home.

CPT is the mainstay of intervention for airway clearance. Home management of CF includes an aggressive plan of postural drainage with percussion and vibration, aerosol nebulization therapy, and breathing retraining. The patient is taught controlled coughing techniques and deep-breathing exercises and is encouraged to perform progressive exercise conditioning, such as a bicycling program.

Individuals and families affected by CF need significant support to cope with the many stresses imposed by the condition. Education and assistance can help them maintain a normal family life while coping with the huge physical demands associated with the condition. It is not uncommon for a person with CF to spend 2 hours a day performing CPT and 1 hour receiving nebulized medication (often antibiotics).

The family and the person with CF have a great financial and emotional burden. The cost of medications, special equipment, and health care is often a financial hardship. Financial support for medications varies considerably across provinces. Some provinces provide complete support, whereas others have much lower levels of subsidy. In addition, some provinces cover only the cost of medications in childhood but stop coverage when the patient becomes an adult. The Canadian Cystic Fibrosis Foundation has established CF centres across the country to provide a comprehensive range of services to patients and families. A major advantage of the centres is the multidisciplinary team of

nurses, physiotherapists, respiratory therapists, nutritionists, and doctors who work very closely with the family to tailor care to meet the family's needs.

As the person continues toward and into adulthood, the nurse and other skilled health professionals should be available to help the patient and family cope with complications resulting from the disease.

CASE STUDY

Chronic Obstructive Pulmonary Disease

Patient Profile

H. M. (pronouns she/her), 68 years old, is a married retired police officer. She has been in the hospital for 3 days with an acute COPD exacerbation and will be discharged tomorrow.

Subjective Data

- Before admission, had 7 days of exceptional shortness of breath and increased volume of sputum, which turned greenish
- Had increased salbutamol use at home to five or six times a day for dyspnea
- Had jitters and racing heart
- Had three or four bouts of exacerbations of COPD in the past year that were treated at home
- Thirty-pack-year history of smoking; smokes half a pack per day now to "clear out lungs" in the morning
- Eats a regular diet but "gets full fast"
- Cannot climb one flight of stairs without stopping; walks down the flat driveway 10 yards without difficulty
- Awakens two or three times per night coughing and short of breath

Objective Data
Physical Examination

- Weight, 58.5 kg (129 lb); height, 1.73 m (5 ft 8 in.); BMI, 20 kg/m²
- Blood pressure, 136/76 mm Hg; pulse, 86; respiratory rate, 28
- Increased anteroposterior diameter of chest (barrel-shaped)
- Slight use of accessory (neck) muscles with breathing
- Diminished breath sounds with occasional wheezes
- No peripheral edema

Diagnostic Studies

- Last spirometry: decreased FEV$_1$ (48%) and FEV$_1$/FVC ratio (62%)
- ABG measurements on admission: pH, 7.34; PaCO$_2$, 49 mm Hg; HCO$_3^-$, 27 mmol/L; PaO$_2$, 70 mm Hg
- WBC count: 14 × 10⁹/L, on admission
- Chest radiograph: hyperinflation, flat diaphragm, no sign of pneumonia
- Sputum: negative for *P. aeruginosa*

Interprofessional Care

- COPD stage: severe COPD with acute exacerbation
- O$_2$, 2 L via nasal catheter while in hospital
- Prednisone, 40 mg daily PO for 5 days
- Levofloxacin, 750 mg PO
- Ipratropium HFA MDI, 2 puffs four times a day
- At discharge: fluticasone, 250 mcg, and salmeterol, 50 mcg (Advair) Diskus 250/50, one inhalation q12hr

Discussion Questions

1. What classic manifestations indicate that the patient had a COPD exacerbation?
2. What are some likely causes of H. M.'s COPD?
3. What symptoms indicate the overuse of inhalers, and which medication would cause the symptoms described?
4. What is the only way H. M. can halt the progression of her lung disease?
5. Why would H. M. "feel full fast" when eating? What could the nurse do to minimize this issue?
6. Interpret the ABG values. What pattern can be seen?
7. *Priority decision:* What are nursing priorities for discharge planning and teaching?
8. *Priority decision:* In view of the assessment data presented, what are the priority nursing diagnoses? Are there any interprofessional issues?
9. *Evidence-informed practice:* H. M.'s son has been trying to persuade his mother to quit smoking for many years without success. He asks the nurse to tell his mother the spirometry results to convince H. M. it is time to quit. Will this approach work?

evolve
Answers are available at http://evolve.elsevier.com/Canada/Lewis/medsurg.

REVIEW QUESTIONS

The number of the question corresponds to the same-numbered objective at the beginning of the chapter.

1. A client is concerned that he may have asthma. Of the following symptoms that he relates to the nurse, which ones suggest asthma or risk factors for asthma? *(Select all that apply.)*
   a. Allergic rhinitis
   b. Prolonged inhalation
   c. History of skin allergies
   d. Cough, especially at night
   e. Gastric reflux or heartburn

2. In evaluating an asthmatic client's knowledge of self-care, the nurse recognizes that additional instruction is needed when the client says which of the following?
   a. "I use my corticosteroid inhaler when I feel short of breath."
   b. "I get a flu shot every year and see my health care provider if I have an upper respiratory tract infection."
   c. "I use my inhaler before I visit my aunt who has a cat, but I visit for only a few minutes because of my allergies."
   d. "I walk 30 minutes every day but sometimes I have to use my bronchodilator inhaler before walking to prevent me from getting short of breath."

3. Which of the following clinical manifestations would the nurse recognize as a key feature of COPD?
   a. Pursed-lip breathing
   b. Smoking history of more than 10 pack-years
   c. History of atopic dermatitis
   d. Increased inspiratory phase

4. When teaching clients about the common adverse effects of cigarette smoke on the respiratory system, the nurse would include which of the following?
   a. Increased proliferation of ciliated cells
   b. Hypertrophy of the alveolar membrane
   c. Destruction of all alveolar macrophages
   d. Hyperplasia of goblet cells and increased production of mucus

5. A plan of care for the client with COPD could include which of the following? *(Select all that apply.)*
   a. Exercise, such as walking
   b. High flow rate of oxygen administration
   c. Low-dose long-term oral corticosteroid therapy
   d. Use of peak flowmeter to monitor the progression of COPD
   e. Breathing exercises such as pursed-lip breathing that focus on exhalation

6. The nurse is preparing a client for transport for a diagnostic test and selects a Venturi mask for oxygen delivery. What is the rationale for choosing a Venturi mask?
   a. It can deliver up to 80% oxygen.
   b. It can provide continuous 100% humidity.
   c. It can deliver a precise concentration of oxygen.
   d. It can be used while a patient eats and sleeps.

7. Which studies would the nurse anticipate that the health care provider would order to diagnose cystic fibrosis?
   a. Pulmonary function test and sweat test
   b. Insulin tolerance and blood glucose
   c. Pancreatic enzymes and hormones
   d. Sweat test and vitamin B tolerance test

1. a, c, d, e; 2. d; 3. b; 4. d; 5. a, e; 6. c; 7. a.

⊖volve

For even more review questions, visit http://evolve.elsevier.com/Canada/Lewis/medsurg.

REFERENCES

American Thoracic Society. (2017). Patient education information series: Smoking marijuana and the lungs. *American Journal of Respiratory and Critical Care Medicine, 195*, 5–6. https://www.thoracic.org/patients/patient-resources/resources/marijuana.pdf

Asthma Canada. (2016). *Breathe easy: Medications: Use as prescribed.* https://asthma.ca/wp-content/uploads/2020/06/BreatheEasy-Medications_optimized_EN.pdf

Asthma Canada. (2019). *Asthma facts and statistics.* https://asthma.ca/wp-content/uploads/2019/02/Asthma-101.pdf

Asthma Canada. (2021a). *Controller medication.* https://asthma.ca/get-help/treatment/controllers/.

Asthma Canada. (2021b). *Delivery devices.* https://asthma.ca/get-help/treatment/how-to-use/

Avdeev, S., Aisanov, Z., Arkhipov, V., et al. (2019). Withdrawal of inhaled corticosteroids in COPD patients: Rationale and algorithms. *International Journal of Chronic Obstructive Pulmonary Disease, 14*, 1267–1280. https://doi.org/10.2147/copd.s207775

BC Guidelines.ca, Guidelines and Protocols Advisory Committee. (2015). *Asthma in adults—Recognition, diagnosis and management.* https://www2.gov.bc.ca/assets/gov/health/practitioner-pro/bc-guidelines/asthma-adults-fullguideline.pdf

Bird, Y., Moraros, J., Mahmood, R., et al. (2017). Prevalence and associated factors of COPD among Aboriginal peoples in Canada: A cross-sectional study. *International Journal of Chronic Obstructive Pulmonary Disease, 12*, 1915–1922. https://doi.org/10.2147/copd.s138304

Bourbeau, J., Bhutani, M., Hernandez, P., et al. (2019). Canadian Thoracic Society clinical practice guideline on pharmacotherapy in patients with COPD—2019 update of evidence. *Canadian Journal of Respiratory, Critical Care, and Sleep Medicine, 3*(4), 210–232. https://doi.org/10.1080/24745332.2019.1668652

Canadian Institute for Health Information (CIHI). (2020). *CIHI snapshot December 2020. Annual statistics on organ replacement in Canada: Dialysis, transplantation and donation, 2010 to 2019.* https://www.cihi.ca/sites/default/files/document/corr-dialysis-transplantation-donation-2010-2019-snapshot-en.pdf

Canadian Institute for Health Information (CIHI). (2021). *Canadian Organ Replacement Register.* https://www.cihi.ca/en/canadian-organ-replacement-register-corr

Canadian Lung Association. (2019). *Chronic obstructive pulmonary disease (COPD).* https://www.lung.ca/lung-health/lung-disease/copd/flare-ups

Canadian Partnership Against Cancer. (2019). *Leading practices in First Nations, Inuit and/or Metis smoking cessation.* https://www.partnershipagainstcancer.ca/topics/leading-practices-first-nations-inuit-metis-smoking-cessation/#:~:text=Rate%20of%20smoking%20among%20First%20Nations%2C%20Inuit%20and,by%20some%20First%20Nations%2C%20Metis%20or%20Inuit%20people

Carriere, G. M., Garner, R., & Sanmartin, C. (2017). Housing conditions and respiratory hospitalizations among First Nations people in Canada. *Health Reports, 28*(4), 9–15. https://www150.statcan.gc.ca/n1/en/pub/82-003-x/2017004/article/14789-eng.pdf?st=OJicJeAk

Cortellini, G., Caruso, C., & Romano, A. (2017). Aspirin challenge and desensitization: How, when and why. *Current Opinion in Allergy and Clinical Immunology, 17*(4), 247–254. https://doi.org/10.1097/ACI.0000000000000374

Cote, A., Turmel, J., & Boulet, L. P. (2018). Exercise and asthma. *Seminars in Respiratory and Critical Care Medicine, 39*(01), 19–28. https://doi.org/10.1055/s-0037-1606215

Cystic Fibrosis Canada. (2019). *The Canadian Cystic Fibrosis Registry: 2018 Annual data report.* https://www.cysticfibrosis.ca/uploads/RegistryReport2018/2018RegistryAnnualDataReport.pdf

Cystic Fibrosis Canada. (2021). *About CF: What is cystic fibrosis.* https://www.cysticfibrosis.ca/about-cf

Emma, R., Morjaria, J. B., Fuochi, V., et al. (2018). Mepolizumab in the management of severe eosinophilic asthma in adults: Current evidence and practical experience. *Therapeutic Advances in Respiratory Disease, 12.* https://doi.org/10.1177/1753466618808490.

Fink, J. B., Ehrmann, S., Li, J., et al. (2020). Reducing aerosol-related risk of transmission in the era of COVID-19: An interim guidance endorsed by the International Society of Aerosols in Medicine. *Journal of Aerosol Medicine and Pulmonary Drug Delivery.* https://doi.org/10.1089/jamp.2020.1615

Global Initiative for Asthma (GINA). (2020). *Global strategy for asthma management and prevention.* https://ginasthma.org/wp-content/uploads/2020/06/GINA-2020-report_20_06_04-1-wms.pdf

Global Initiative for Chronic Obstructive Lung Disease (GOLD). (2019). *GOLD teaching slide set.* https://goldcopd.org/gold-teaching-slide-set/

Global Initiative for Chronic Obstructive Lung Disease (GOLD). (2020). *Global strategy for the diagnosis, management and prevention of chronic obstructive pulmonary disease.* https://goldcopd.org/wp-content/uploads/2019/12/GOLD-2020-FINAL-ver1.2-03Dec19_WMV.pdf

Government of Canada. (2019a). *Air Quality Health Index.* https://www.canada.ca/en/environment-climate-change/services/air-quality-health-index.html

Government of Canada. (2019b). *Asthma and chronic obstructive pulmonary disease (COPD) in Canada, 2018.* https://www.canada.ca/en/public-health/services/publications/diseases-conditions/asthma-chronic-obstructive-pulmonary-disease-canada-2018.html#a1.2.2

Health Canada. (2021). *Canada's tobacco strategy.* https://www.canada.ca/en/health-canada/services/publications/healthy-living/canada-tobacco-strategy.html

Lau, A., & Tarlo, S. M. (2018). Update on the management of occupational asthma and work-exacerbated asthma. *Allergy Asthma Immunology Research, 11*(2), 188–200. https://doi.org/10.4168/aair.2019.11.2.188

Leatherman, J. (2015). Mechanical ventilation for severe asthma. *Chest, 147*(6), 1671–1680. https://doi:10.1378/chest.14-1733

Lougheed, M. D., Lemiere, C., Dell, S., et al. (2010). Canadian Thoracic Society Asthma Committee commentary on long-acting beta-2 agonist use for asthma in Canada. *Canadian Respiratory Journal, 17*(2), 57–60. https://doi.org/10.1155/2010/378289. (Seminal).

Lougheed, M. D., Lemiere, C., Ducharme, F. M., et al. (2012). Canadian Thoracic Society 2012 guideline update: Diagnosis and management of asthma in preschoolers, children and adults. *Canadian Respiratory Journal, 19*(2), 127–164. https://doi.org/10.1155/2012/635624. (Seminal).

Lung Association of Saskatchewan. (2020a). *Asthma medications brochure.* https://www.lungsask.ca/sites/default/files/styles/medium/public/AsthmeBrochure.JPG?itok=6wYOvaAx

Lung Association of Saskatchewan. (2020b). *COPD medications brochure.* https://www.lungsask.ca/sites/default/files/styles/medium/public/copd-brochure-thumb_1.jpg?itok=ZK_-_I7d

Marciniuk, D. D., Goodridge, D., Hernandez, P., et al. (2011). Managing dyspnea in patients with advanced chronic obstructive pulmonary disease: A Canadian Thoracic Society clinical practice guideline. *Canadian Respiratory Journal, 18*(2), 69–78. https://doi.org/10.1155/2011/745047. (Seminal).

Monroe, E. ,J., Pierce, D. B., Ingraham, C. R., et al. (2018). An interventionalist's guide to hemoptysis in cystic fibrosis. *RadioGraphics, 38*(2), 624–641. https://doi.org/10.1148/rg.2018170129

Mtisi, T. F., & Frishman, W. H. (2020). Beta-adrenergic blocker use in patients with chronic obstructive pulmonary disease and concurrent chronic heart failure with a low ejection fraction. *Cardiology in Review, 28*(1), 20–25. https://doi.org/10.1097/CRD.0000000000000284

O'Donnell, D. E., Aaron, S., Bourbeau, J., et al. (2007). Canadian Thoracic Society recommendations for management of chronic obstructive pulmonary disease—2007 update. *Canadian Respiratory Journal, 14*(Suppl B), 5B–32B. (Seminal).

Ospina, M. B., Voaklander, D., Senthilselvan, A., et al. (2015). Incidence and prevalence of chronic obstructive pulmonary disease among Aboriginal peoples in Alberta, Canada. *PLOS ONE, 10*(4), e0123204. https://doi.org/10.1371/journal.pone.0123204

Pardue Jones, B., Fleming, G. M., Otillio, J. K., et al. (2016). Pediatric acute asthma exacerbations: Evaluation and management from emergency department to intensive care unit. *Journal of Asthma, 53*(6), 607–617. https://doi.org/10.3109/02770903.2015.1067323

Public Health Agency of Canada (PHAC). (2015). *Fast facts about asthma: Data compiled from 2011 Survey on Living with Chronic Disease in Canada.* https://www.canada.ca/en/public-health/services/chronic-diseases/chronic-respiratory-diseases/fast-facts-about-asthma-data-compiled-2011-survey-on-living-chronic-diseases-canada.html

Public Health Agency of Canada (PHAC). (2019a). *An Advisory Committee Statement (ACS) National Advisory Committee on Immunization (NACI): Canadian immunization guide chapter on influenza and statement on seasonal influenza for 2019–2020.* https://www.canada.ca/en/public-health/services/publications/vaccines-immunization/canadian-immunization-guide-statement-seasonal-influenza-vaccine-2019-2020.html

Public Health Agency of Canada (PHAC). (2019b). *Fast facts about chronic obstructive pulmonary disease (COPD): Data compiled from 2011 Survey on Living with Chronic Disease in Canada.* https://www.canada.ca/en/public-health/services/chronic-diseases/reports-publications/fast-facts-about-chronic-obstructive-pulmonary-disease-copd-2011.html

Registered Nurses' Association of Ontario (RNAO). (2017). *Adult asthma care: Promoting control of asthma* (2nd ed.). https://rnao.ca/sites/rnao-ca/files/bpg/Adult_Asthma_FINAL_WEB.pdf

Smith, W. D., Bardin, E., Cameron, L., et al. (2017). Current and future therapies for Pseudomonas aeruginosa infection in patients with cystic fibrosis. *FEMS Microbiology Letters, 364*(14). https://doi.org/10.1093/femsle/fnx121

Sobieraj, D. M., Baker, W. L., Nguyen, E., et al. (2018). Association of inhaled corticosteroids and long-acting muscarinic antagonists with asthma control in patients with uncontrolled, persistent asthma: A systematic review and meta-analysis. *JAMA, 319*(14), 1473–1484. https://doi.org/10.1001/jama.2018.2757

Statistics Canada. (2017). *The housing conditions of Aboriginal people in Canada.* https://www12.statcan.gc.ca/census-recensement/2016/as-sa/98-200-x/2016021/98-200-x2016021-eng.pdf

Taylor-Cousar, J. L. (2020). CFTR modulators: Impact on fertility, pregnancy, and lactation in women with cystic fibrosis. *Journal of Clinical Medicine, 9*(9), 2706. https://doi.org/10.3390/jcm9092706

Vogelmeier, C. F., Román-Rodríguez, M., Singh, D., et al. (2020). Goals of COPD treatment: Focus on symptoms and exacerbations. *Respiratory Medicine, 166*, 105938. https://doi.org/10.1016/j.rmed.2020.105938

Yin, H.-L., Yin, S.-Q., Lin, Q.-Y., et al. (2017). Prevalence of comorbidities in chronic obstructive pulmonary disease patients. *Medicine, 96*(19):e6836. https://doi.org/10.1097/md.0000000000006836

Yohannas, A. M., Kaplan, A., & Hanania, N. A. (2018). Anxiety and depression in chronic obstructive pulmonary disease: Recognition and management. *The Journal of Family Practice and Cleveland Clinic Journal of Medicine, 85*(2 Suppl 1), S11–S18. https://doi.org/10.3949/ccjm.85.s1.03

RESOURCES

Alpha 1 Canadian Registry
http://www.alpha1canadianregistry.com

Asthma Canada
https://www.asthma.ca

Canadian Cancer Society
https://www.cancer.ca

Canadian Network for Respiratory Care
http://cnrchome.net/

Canadian Thoracic Society—*Canadian Respiratory Guidelines (CRGC) Library*
https://cts-sct.ca/guideline-library/

Canadian Thoracic Society—*Canadian Respiratory Health Professionals (CRHP)*
https://cts-sct.ca/about-us/assemblies/crhp/

Canadian Thoracic Society Asthma Committee—*Canadian Thoracic Society Asthma Management Continuum—2010 Consensus Summary for Children Six Years of Age and Over, and Adults*
https://www.ncbi.nlm.nih.gov/pmc/articles/PMC2866209/

Cystic Fibrosis Canada
https://www.cysticfibrosis.ca

First Nations Health Authority
https://www.fnha.ca/

Lung Association*
http://www.lung.ca

Lung Association—*Asthma Action Plan*
https://www.lung.ca/lung-health/lung-disease/asthma/asthma-action-plan

---

* Most provinces have their own Lung Association.

Lung Association—*Fact Sheet: Oxygen and COPD*
https://www.lung.ca/sites/default/files/media/Oxygen_COPD_LungAssoc.pdf

Public Health Agency of Canada (includes *Canadian Communicable Disease Reports*)
https://www.phac-aspc.gc.ca/

Registered Nurses' Association of Ontario—*Best Practice Guideline: Integrating Smoking Cessation Into Daily Nursing Practice*
http://rnao.ca/bpg/guidelines/integrating-smoking-cessation-daily-nursing-practice

---

Alpha-1 Foundation
https://www.alpha1.org/

COPD Assessment Test
https://www.catestonline.org/patient-site-test-page-english.html

Cystic Fibrosis Foundation
https://www.cff.org

Global Initiative for Asthma (GINA)
https://ginasthma.org/

Global Initiative for Chronic Obstructive Lung Disease (GOLD)
https://goldcopd.org/

Living Well With COPD Program
http://www.livingwellwithcopd.com/

TheraPEP PEP Therapy System
https://www.smiths-medical.com/catalog/bronchial-hygiene/therapep/therapep-system.html

evolve

For additional Internet resources, see the website for this book at http://evolve.elsevier.com/Canada/Lewis/medsurg.

Conditions of Oxygenation: Transport

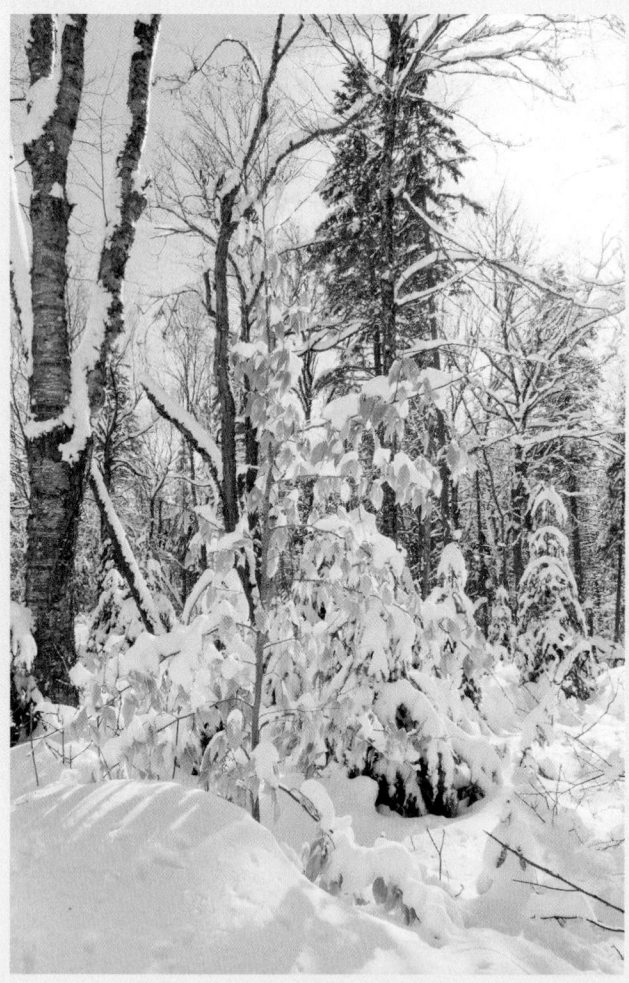

Source: © CanStock Photo / Pierdelune

Chapter 32: Nursing Assessment: **Hematological System**
Chapter 33: Nursing Management: **Hematological Conditions**

Nursing Assessment
Hematological System

Bridgette Lord
Originating US chapter by Sandra Irene Rome

⊝volve WEBSITE

http://evolve.elsevier.com/Canada/Lewis/medsurg

- Review Questions (Online Only)
- Key Points
- Answer Guidelines for Case Study
- Conceptual Care Map Creator
- Audio Glossary
- Content Updates

LEARNING OBJECTIVES

1. Describe the structures and functions of the hematological system.
2. Differentiate among the different types of blood cells and their functions.
3. Explain the process of hemostasis.
4. Link age-related changes in the hematological system to findings of hematological studies.
5. Identify significant subjective and objective assessment data related to the hematological system that should be obtained from a patient.
6. Perform and describe how to conduct physical assessment of the hematological system.
7. Differentiate normal from abnormal physical findings of the hematological system.
8. Describe the purpose and significance of results of diagnostic studies of the hematological system and the nursing responsibilities related to these studies.
9. Differentiate between common normal and abnormal blood laboratory studies.

KEY TERMS

ecchymosis
erythropoiesis
fibrinolysis
hematopoiesis
hemoglobin
hemolysis

leukocytosis
leukopenia
neutropenia
pancytopenia
petechiae
phagocytosis

polycythemia
purpura
stem cell
thrombocytopenia
thrombocytosis

Hematology is the study of blood and blood-forming tissues. This includes the bone marrow, blood, spleen, and lymph system. A basic knowledge of hematology is useful in clinical settings to evaluate a patient's ability to transport oxygen (O_2) and carbon dioxide (CO_2), maintain intravascular volume, coagulate blood, and combat infections. Assessment of the hematological system is based on the patient's health history, physical examination, and results of diagnostic studies.

STRUCTURES AND FUNCTIONS OF THE HEMATOLOGICAL SYSTEM

Bone Marrow

Blood cell production (hematopoiesis) occurs within the bone marrow. *Bone marrow* is the soft material that fills the central core of bones. There are two types of bone marrow: yellow (adipose) and red (hematopoietic). Red marrow actively produces blood cells. In adults, the red marrow is located primarily in the flat and the irregular bones, such as the ends of long bones, pelvic bones, vertebrae, sacrum, sternum, ribs, flat cranial bones, and scapulae. From the early postnatal period onward, red bone marrow is gradually converted to yellow bone marrow. Yellow bone marrow is primarily involved in the storage of fats but can be converted back to red bone marrow to increase blood cell production in times of need. All three types of blood cells— red blood cells (RBCs), white blood cells (WBCs), and platelets—develop from a common hematopoietic stem cell within the bone marrow. This hematopoietic stem cell is best described as an immature blood cell that is able to self-renew and to differentiate

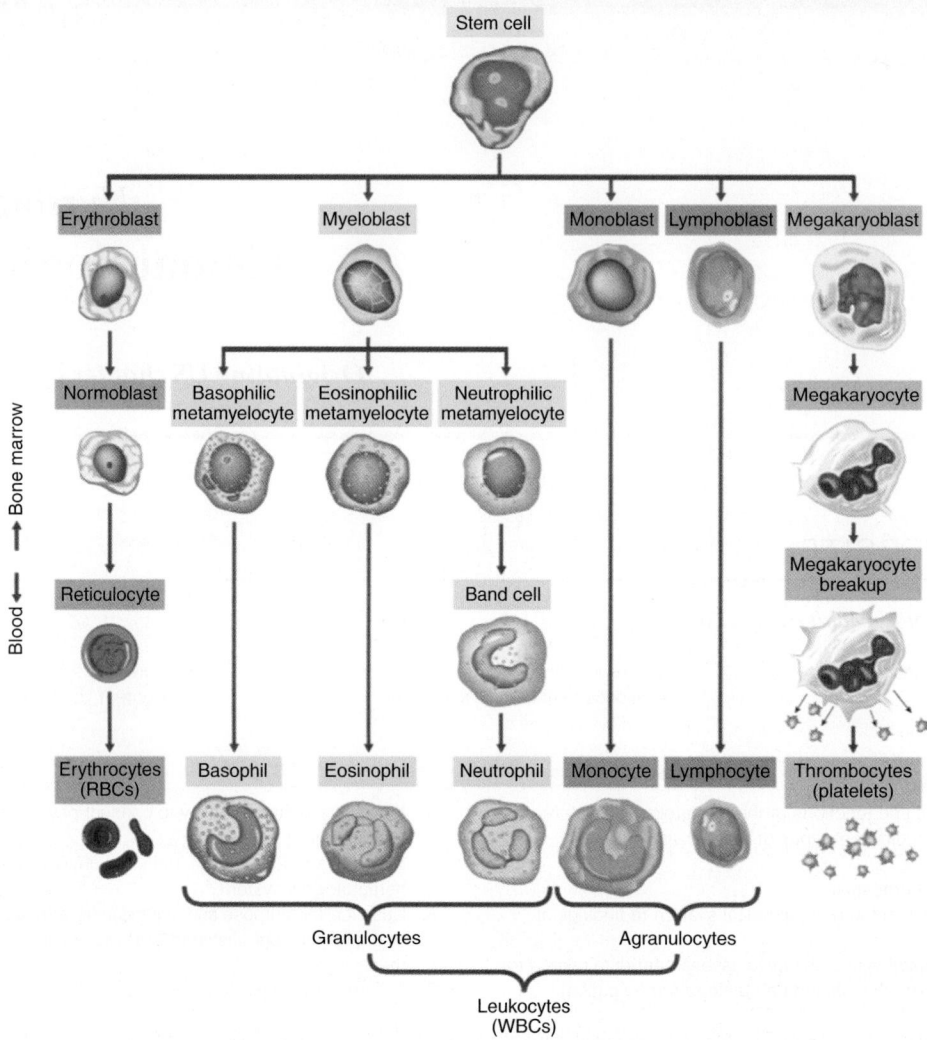

FIG. 32.1 Development of blood cells. *RBCs,* red blood cells; *WBCs,* white blood cells.

into hematopoietic progenitor cells. As blood cells mature and differentiate, several different types of cells are formed (Figure 32.1). The marrow responds to increased demands for various types of blood cells by increasing production by means of a negative feedback system. The bone marrow is stimulated by various factors (e.g., erythropoietin, granulocyte colony–stimulating factor, thrombopoietin) that cause differentiation of the stem cells into one type of the committed hematopoietic cells. For example, when tissue hypoxia occurs, the kidney secretes erythropoietin. It circulates to the bone marrow and causes differentiation of proerythroblasts (earliest RBC precursors) in the bone marrow (Suresh et al., 2020).

Blood

Blood is a type of connective tissue that performs three major functions: protection, regulation, and transportation (Table 32.1). Blood has two major components: plasma and blood cells.

Plasma. Approximately 55% of blood is plasma (Figure 32.2). Plasma is composed primarily of water, but it also contains proteins, electrolytes, gases, nutrients, and waste. The term *serum* refers to plasma without its clotting factors. Plasma proteins include albumin, globulin, and clotting factors (mostly fibrinogen).

TABLE 32.1	**FUNCTIONS OF BLOOD**
Function	**Examples**
Protection	• Maintaining homeostasis of blood coagulation • Combating invasion of pathogens and other foreign substances
Regulation	• Fluid and electrolyte balance • Acid–base balance • Body temperature • Maintaining intravascular oncotic pressure
Transportation	• O_2 from lungs to cells • Nutrients from GI tract to cells • Hormones from endocrine glands to tissues and cells • Metabolic waste products (e.g., CO_2, NH_3, urea) from cells to lungs, liver, and kidneys

CO_2, carbon dioxide; *GI,* gastrointestinal; NH_3, ammonia; O_2, oxygen.

Blood Cells. About 45% of the blood (see Figure 32.2) is composed of formed elements, or blood cells. There are three types of blood cells: *erythrocytes,* or RBCs; *leukocytes,* or WBCs; and *thrombocytes,* or platelets. The primary function of erythrocytes is O_2 transportation, whereas the leukocytes are involved in protection of the body from infection. Thrombocytes mainly function to promote blood coagulation.

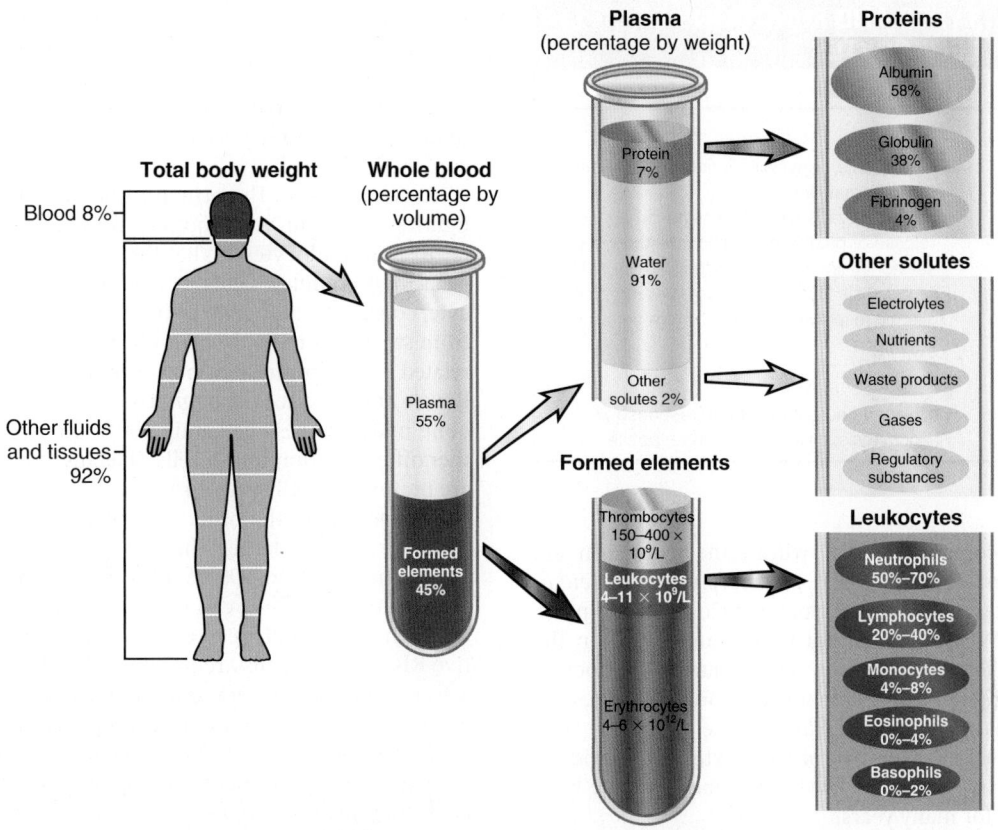

FIG. 32.2 Approximate values for the components of blood in the adult. Normally, 45% of the blood is composed of blood cells, and 55% is composed of plasma.

Erythrocytes. The primary functions of erythrocytes (RBCs) include transport of gases (both O_2 and CO_2) and assistance in maintaining acid–base balance. Erythrocytes are flexible cells with a unique biconcave shape. Flexibility enables the cell to alter its shape so that it can easily pass through tiny capillaries. The cell membrane is also very thin, which facilitates the diffusion of gases. Erythrocytes are composed primarily of a large molecule called hemoglobin, a complex compound composed of heme (an iron compound) and globin (a simple protein) that binds with O_2 and CO_2. As erythrocytes circulate through the capillaries surrounding the alveoli in the lungs, O_2 attaches to the iron on the hemoglobin. The O_2-bound hemoglobin is referred to as *oxyhemoglobin* and is responsible for the bright red appearance of arterial blood. As erythrocytes flow to body tissues, O_2 detaches from the hemoglobin and diffuses from the capillary into tissue cells. CO_2 diffuses from tissue cells into the capillary, attaches to the globin portion of hemoglobin, and is transported to the lungs for removal. Hemoglobin also acts as a buffer and plays a role in maintaining acid–base balance. This buffering function is described further in Chapter 19.

Erythropoiesis (the process of RBC production) is regulated by cellular O_2 requirements and general metabolic activity. Erythropoiesis is stimulated by hypoxia and controlled by *erythropoietin*, a glycoprotein growth factor synthesized and released primarily by the kidneys. Erythropoietin stimulates the bone marrow to increase erythrocyte production. Approximately 2.5 million erythrocytes are produced per second, and the normal lifespan of an erythrocyte is about 120 days. Erythropoiesis is also influenced by the availability of nutrients. Many essential nutrients are necessary for erythropoiesis, including protein, iron, copper, folate (folic acid), cobalamin (vitamin B_{12}), riboflavin (vitamin B_2), pyridoxine (vitamin B_6), pantothenic acid (vitamin B_5), niacin (vitamin B_3), ascorbic acid (vitamin C), and vitamin E. Endocrine hormones, such as thyroxine, corticosteroids, and testosterone, also affect erythrocyte production. For example, hypothyroidism is often associated with anemia (Wopereis et al., 2018).

Several distinct cell types evolve during RBC maturation (see Figure 32.1). The *reticulocyte* is an immature erythrocyte. The reticulocyte count is a measure of the rate at which new RBCs appear in the circulation. Reticulocytes can develop into mature RBCs within 48 hours of their release into circulation. Therefore, assessing the number of reticulocytes is a useful means of evaluating the rate and adequacy of RBC production.

Hemolysis (destruction of RBCs) by monocytes and macrophages removes abnormal, defective, damaged, and old RBCs from circulation. Hemolysis occurs in the bone marrow, liver, and spleen and results in increased levels of bilirubin that must be processed by the body. When hemolysis occurs under normal conditions, the liver is able to conjugate and excrete the bilirubin produced.

Leukocytes. Leukocytes (WBCs) appear white when separated from blood. Like RBCs, WBCs originate from stem cells within the bone marrow (see Figure 32.1). There are several different types of leukocytes, each of which has a different function.

TABLE 32.2	TYPES AND FUNCTIONS OF LEUKOCYTES
Type	**Cell Function**
Granulocytes	
Neutrophil	Phagocytosis, especially during the early phase of inflammation
Basophil	Inflammatory response and allergic response; release of bradykinin, heparin, histamine, serotonin; limited phagocytosis
Eosinophil	Phagocytosis (not as effective as neutrophil); allergic response; protection from parasitic infections
Agranulocytes	
Lymphocyte	Cellular and humoral immune response
Monocyte	Phagocytosis; cellular immune response

Leukocytes that contain granules within the cytoplasm are called *granulocytes* (also known as *polymorphonuclear leukocytes*). Granulocytes include three types: neutrophils, basophils, and eosinophils. WBCs that do not have granules within the cytoplasm are called *agranulocytes* and include lymphocytes and monocytes (Table 32.2). Lymphocytes and monocytes are also referred to as *mononuclear cells* because they have only one discrete nucleus. The lifespan of leukocytes varies widely; granulocytes may live for only a few hours, whereas some lymphocytes may live for many years.

Granulocytes. The primary function of the granulocytes is phagocytosis, a process by which WBCs ingest or engulf an unwanted organism and then digest and kill it. The *neutrophil* is the most common type of granulocyte, accounting for 50 to 70% of all WBCs. Neutrophils are the primary phagocytic cells involved in acute inflammatory responses. Once they engulf the pathogen, they die in 1 to 2 days. Neutrophil production and maturation are stimulated by hematopoietic growth factors (e.g., granulocyte colony–stimulating factor [G-CSF] and granulocyte-macrophage colony–stimulating factor [GM-CSF]) (Rosales, 2018).

A mature neutrophil is called a *segmented neutrophil* ("seg") because the nucleus is segmented into two to five lobes connected by strands. An immature neutrophil is called a *band* (for the band-like or rod-like appearance of the nucleus). Although band cells are sometimes found in the peripheral circulation of healthy people and are capable of phagocytosis, the mature neutrophils are more effective. An increase in neutrophils in the blood is a common diagnostic indicator of infection or tissue injury. The existence of many immature cells is termed a *shift to the left* and may be indicative of active infection or inflammation. (Shift to the left is explained further in the White Blood Cells section later in this chapter.)

Eosinophils account for less than 4% of all WBCs. They have a similar but reduced ability for phagocytosis. One of their primary functions is to engulf antigen–antibody complexes formed during an allergic response. Elevated levels of eosinophils are also seen with some cancers, such as lymphoma, in parasitic infections, and in various skin and connective tissue disorders (Leru, 2019). *Basophils* constitute less than 2% of all WBCs. These cells have cytoplasmic granules that contain chemical mediators such as heparin, serotonin, and histamine. If a basophil is stimulated by an antigen or

by tissue injury, it responds by releasing substances from the granules. This is part of the response in allergic and inflammatory reactions. *Mast cells* are similar to basophils, but they reside in connective tissue and play a central role in inflammation, permeability of blood vessels, and smooth muscle contraction.

Agranulocytes. The primary function of agranulocytes is in fighting infection via acquired immunity. Agranulocytes differ from granulocytes in that their cytoplasm does not contain lysosomal granules. *Lymphocytes*, one type of agranular leukocyte, constitute 20 to 40% of the WBCs. Lymphocytes originate from stem cells in the bone marrow, and their main function is related to the immune response. Two lymphocyte subtypes are B cells and T cells. Although T-cell precursors originate in the bone marrow, these cells migrate to the thymus gland for further differentiation into T cells. (Details of lymphocyte function are presented in Chapter 16.)

Monocytes are the other type of agranular leukocyte. These cells are usually larger than other WBCs and account for approximately 4 to 8% of all WBCs. Monocytes are potent phagocytic cells. They can ingest small or large masses of matter, such as bacteria, dead cells, tissue debris, and old or defective RBCs. These cells are present in the bone marrow for only a short time before they migrate into the tissues and become macrophages. In addition to macrophages that have differentiated from monocytes, resident macrophages can also be found in tissues. These resident macrophages are further differentiated; they include Kupffer cells in the liver, osteoclasts in the bone, and alveolar macrophages in the lungs. These macrophages protect the body from pathogens at these entry points and are more phagocytic than monocytes. Macrophages also interact with lymphocytes to facilitate the humoral and cellular immune responses.

Thrombocytes. The primary function of thrombocytes (platelets) is to initiate the clotting process by producing an initial "platelet plug" in the early phases of the clotting process. Platelets must be available in sufficient numbers and must be structurally and metabolically sound for blood clotting to occur. When capillaries are damaged, platelets adhere to the damaged capillary wall and platelet activation is initiated. Increasing numbers of platelets accumulate to form the platelet plug, which is stabilized with clotting factors. Platelets are also important in the process of clot shrinkage and retraction.

Platelets originate from stem cells within the bone marrow (see Figure 32.1). The stem cell undergoes differentiation by transforming into a *megakaryocyte*, which fragments into platelets. Platelet production is partly regulated by *thrombopoietin*, a growth factor that acts on bone marrow to stimulate platelet production (Songdej & Rao, 2017). Thrombopoietin is produced in the liver, kidneys, smooth muscle, and bone marrow. Typically, platelets have a lifespan of 8 to 10 days.

Iron Metabolism

The body's iron requirement is about 25 mg daily. Iron is obtained from foods and dietary supplements. On average, the body absorbs only 1 mg of every 10 to 20 mg of iron taken in. Absorption primarily takes place in the duodenum and the upper jejunum. Approximately two thirds of the body's iron is found as the heme part of the hemoglobin molecule in RBCs. The other third of iron is stored as ferritin and hemosiderin in

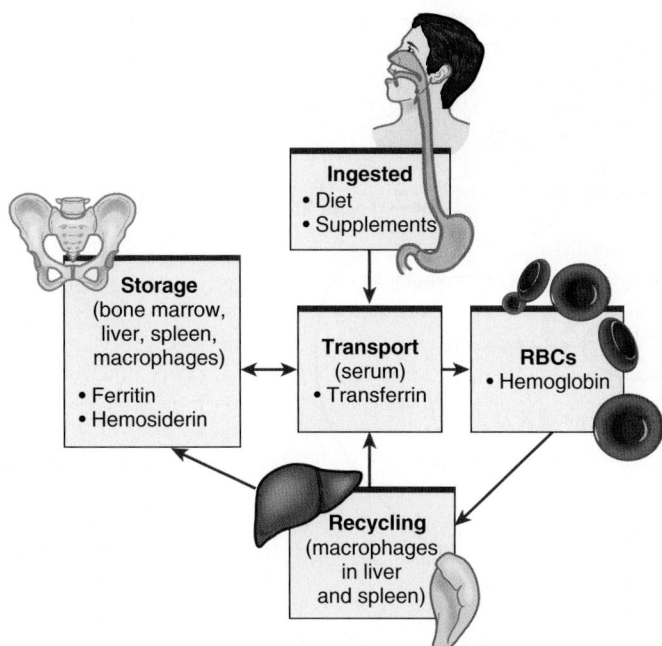

FIG. 32.3 Iron metabolism. Iron is ingested in the diet or from supplements. Macrophages break down ingested red blood cells. Iron is returned to the blood bound to transferrin or stored as ferritin or hemosiderin. *RBC*, red blood cell.

the bone marrow, spleen, liver, and macrophages (Figure 32.3). When stored iron is not replaced, hemoglobin production is reduced.

Transferrin, which is synthesized in the liver, serves as a carrier plasma protein for iron. The degree to which transferrin is saturated with iron is a reliable indicator of the iron supply for developing RBCs.

Iron is recycled in the body after old and damaged RBCs are *phagocytized* (i.e., ingested and destroyed) by macrophages in the liver and spleen. Iron is released into the plasma and transported by transferrin to the bone marrow for RBC production. Alternatively, iron may be stored as ferritin or hemosiderin (see Figure 32.3). Only about 3% of iron is lost daily in urine, sweat, bile, and epithelial cells in the gastrointestinal (GI) tract. Therefore, there is normally very little iron loss except with blood loss.

Clotting Mechanisms

Hemostasis is the stopping of blood flow. This process is important in minimizing blood loss when body structures are injured. The sequence of events is as follows: (1) vascular injury and subendothelial exposure; (2) platelet plug formation involving adhesion, aggregation, and activation; (3) fibrin clot development; and (4) clot retraction and dissolution.

Vascular Injury and Subendothelial Exposure. When a blood vessel is injured, an immediate local vasoconstrictive response occurs. Vasoconstriction reduces the leakage of blood from the vessel not only by restricting the vessel size but also by pressing the endothelial surfaces together. The latter reaction enhances vessel wall stickiness and maintains closure of the vessel even after the vasoconstriction subsides. Vasoconstriction may last for 20 to 30 minutes, allowing time for the platelet response and plasma clotting factors to be activated.

Platelet Plug Formation (Adhesion, Aggregation, Activation). Damage to the endothelial lining of blood vessels exposes glycoproteins, such as collagen and von Willebrand factor (vWF), to which platelets adhere. The stickiness is termed *adhesiveness,* and the formation of clumps is termed *aggregation.* As platelets adhere to the collagen fibres of a wound, platelets become spiked and much stickier. They stick to one another because of fibrin linking their glycoprotein IIb/IIIa receptors. The adhesion process causes platelets to undergo an *activation* process whereby they release their stored granules that contain adenosine diphosphate (ADP), prostaglandin, thromboxane A_2 (TXA_2), serotonin, and other factors that enhance platelet plug formation and limit bleeding (Gomez-Casado et al., 2019).

In addition to their contribution in forming a platelet plug, platelets also facilitate the reactions of the plasma clotting factors within the coagulation cascade. Platelet lipoproteins stimulate necessary conversions in the clotting process (Figure 32.4).

Fibrin Clot Development. The formation of a fibrin clot interlaced with the platelet plug is the conclusion of a complex series of reactions involving different clotting factors. The plasma clotting factors are labelled with both names and Roman numerals (Table 32.3). Plasma proteins circulate in inactive forms until stimulated to initiate clotting through one of two pathways: intrinsic or extrinsic. The *intrinsic pathway* is activated by collagen exposure from endothelial injury when the blood vessel is damaged. The *extrinsic pathway* is initiated when tissue thromboplastin is released extravascularly from injured tissues.

Regardless of whether clotting is initiated by substances inside or outside the blood vessel, coagulation ultimately follows the same final common pathway of the clotting cascade. Thrombin, in the common pathway, is the most powerful enzyme in the coagulation process (Figure 32.5). It converts fibrinogen to fibrin, which is an essential component of a blood clot.

Clot Retraction and Dissolution. Just as some blood elements foster coagulation *(procoagulants),* others interfere with clotting *(anticoagulants).* This counter-mechanism to blood clotting serves to keep blood in its fluid state. Anticoagulation may be achieved by several means: antithrombin activity, fibrinolysis, and vessel and platelet activity. As the name implies, *antithrombins* keep blood fluid by antagonizing thrombin, a powerful coagulant. Endogenous heparin, protein C, and protein S are examples of anticoagulants.

Another method of maintaining blood in its fluid form is fibrinolysis, a continual process resulting in the dissolution of fibrin and thus clots. The fibrinolytic system is initiated when plasminogen is converted to plasmin (see Figure 32.5). Thrombin is one of the substances that can activate the conversion of plasminogen to plasmin, thereby promoting fibrinolysis. The plasmin attacks either fibrin or fibrinogen by splitting the molecules into smaller elements known as *fibrin split products* (FSPs) or *fibrin degradation products* (FDPs). (More information on FSPs can be found in Table 32.8 later in this chapter and in the discussion of disseminated intravascular coagulation in Chapter 33.)

If fibrinolysis is excessive, the patient is predisposed to bleeding. In such a situation, bleeding results from the destruction of fibrin in platelet plugs or from the anticoagulation effects of increased amounts of FSPs. Increased FSPs lead to impairment in platelet aggregation, reduction in prothrombin, and an inability to stabilize fibrin.

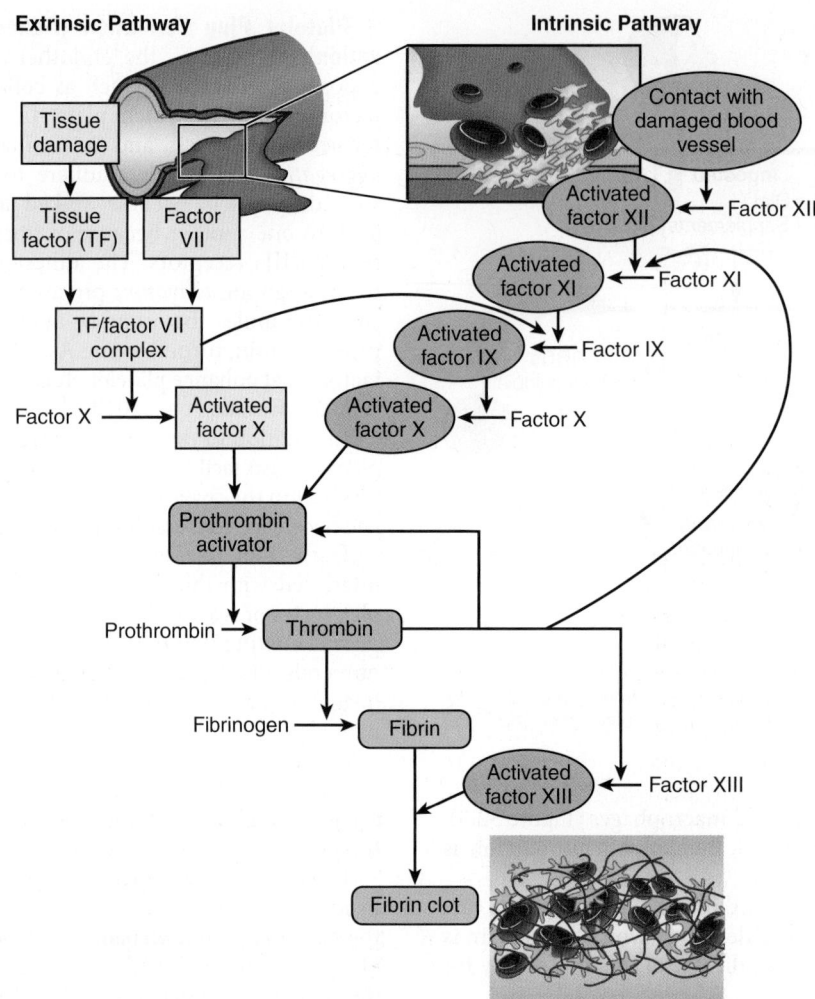

FIG 32.4 Coagulation mechanism showing steps in the intrinsic and the extrinsic pathways as they would occur in the test tube.

TABLE 32.3	COAGULATION FACTORS
Coagulation Factor	**Action**
I Fibrinogen	Source of fibrin to form a clot, made in liver
II Prothrombin	Converted to thrombin, which then activates fibrinogen into fibrin, as well as activating factors V, VII, VIII, XI, XIII; protein C; and platelets
III Tissue factor, tissue thromboplastin	Released from damaged endothelial cells; activates the extrinsic pathway by reacting with factor VII
IV Calcium	Required cofactor at several points in the coagulation cascade
V Labile factor	Binds with factor X to activate prothrombin
VI	Not in use (now obsolete)
VII Stable factor, proconvertin	Forms a complex with factor III and activates factors IX and X
VIII Antihemophilic factor	Works with factor IX and calcium to activate factor X
IX Christmas factor	Together with factor VIII, activates factor X
X Stuart–Prower factor	Activates conversion of factor II (prothrombin) into thrombin
XI Plasma thromboplastin antecedent	Activates factor IX when calcium is present
XII Hageman factor	Activates factor XI, which starts the intrinsic pathway
XIII Fibrin-stabilizing factor	Cross-links fibrin strands and stabilizes fibrin clot

Spleen

Another component of the hematological system is the spleen, which is located in the upper left quadrant of the abdomen. The role of the spleen can be classified into the following four general functions:

1. *Hematopoietic function:* The spleen produces RBCs during fetal development.
2. *Filter function:* The spleen removes old and defective RBCs from circulation by means of the mononuclear phagocyte system. Filtration also involves the reuse of iron—the spleen can catabolize hemoglobin released by hemolysis and return the iron component of the hemoglobin to the bone marrow for reuse. The spleen also plays an important role in filtering circulating bacteria, especially encapsulated organisms such as Gram-positive cocci.
3. *Immune function:* The spleen contains a rich supply of lymphocytes, monocytes, and stored immunoglobulins.
4. *Storage function:* The spleen serves as a storage site for platelets and RBCs. More than 300 mL of blood and one third of platelets can be stored in the spleen.

Lymph System

The lymph system—consisting of lymph fluid, lymphatic capillaries, lymphatic ducts, and lymph nodes—carries fluid from the interstitial spaces to the blood. It is by means of the lymph system that proteins and fat from the GI tract and

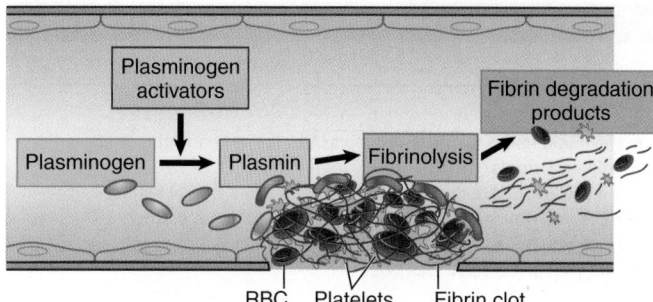

FIG. 32.5 Fibrinolytic system. *RBC*, red blood cell.

certain hormones are able to return to the circulatory system. The lymph system also returns excess interstitial fluid to the blood, which is important in preventing the development of edema.

Lymph fluid is a pale-yellow fluid that circulates through a special vasculature, much as blood moves through blood vessels. Lymph fluid is formed as interstitial fluid diffuses through lymphatic capillary walls. The lymphatic capillaries are thin-walled vessels that have an irregular diameter. They are somewhat larger than blood capillaries. Lymphatic capillaries unite to form lymphatic vessels that carry all lymph fluid to either the right lymphatic duct or to the thoracic duct. The lymphatic vessels are similar to venous blood vessels in that they have valves. These large lymphatic ducts drain into the subclavian veins of the neck. The formation of lymph fluid increases when interstitial fluid increases, thereby forcing fluid into the lymph system. When too much interstitial fluid forms or when something interferes with the reabsorption of lymph, *lymphedema* develops. Lymphedema may occur as a complication following surgery (for example, when axillary lymph nodes are removed as part of a radical mastectomy).

The *lymph nodes* are round, oval, or bean-shaped and vary in size according to their location. Structurally, lymph nodes are small clumps of lymphatic tissue and are found in groups along lymph vessels at various sites in the body. The body contains more than 200 lymph nodes, with the greatest number in the abdomen surrounding the GI tract. Lymph nodes are situated both superficially and deep. The superficial nodes can be palpated, but evaluation of the deep nodes requires radiological examination. A primary function of lymph nodes is the filtration of pathogens and foreign particles that are carried by lymph fluid to the nodes.

Liver

The liver has metabolic, secretory, vascular and storage functions. It makes all the procoagulants that are essential for hemostasis and blood coagulation. The liver secretes bilirubin and bile. In addition, when the amount of iron exceeds tissue needs (which can occur with frequent blood transfusions or with diseases that cause iron overload), the excess is stored in the liver. *Hepcidin*, a protein produced by the liver, is a key regulator of iron balance. The synthesis of hepcidin is regulated by a variety of stimuli, including existent iron stores in the body, inflammation, hypoxia, and RBC requirements (Anderson & Frazer, 2017). Hepcidin reduces the release of stored iron from enterocytes (in the intestines) and macrophages. Thus, when iron is

TABLE 32.4	AGE-RELATED DIFFERENCES IN ASSESSMENT
Effects of Aging on Hematological Studies	
Study	**Changes**
CBC Studies	
Hemoglobin	Normal; possibly slightly decreased
MCV	May be slightly increased
MCHC	May be slightly decreased
WBC count	Diminished response to infection
Platelets	Unchanged
Clotting Studies	
Partial thromboplastin time	Decreased
Fibrinogen	May be elevated
Factors V, VII, VIII, IX	May be elevated
ESR	Increased significantly
D-dimers	Increased
Iron Studies	
Serum iron	Decreased
Total iron-binding capacity	Decreased
Ferritin	Increased
Erythropoietin	May be increased

CBC, complete blood cell count; *ESR*, erythrocyte sedimentation rate; *MCHC*, mean corpuscular hemoglobin concentration; *MCV*, mean corpuscular volume; *WBC*, white blood cell.

deficient, hepatocytes produce less hepcidin, releasing stored iron and increasing dietary absorption. Other functions of the liver are described in Chapter 46.

AGE-RELATED CONSIDERATIONS

HEMATOLOGICAL SYSTEM

Physiological aging is a gradual process that involves cell loss and organ atrophy. Aging leads to a decrease in bone marrow mass and cellularity and an increase in bone marrow fat (Lichtman et al., 2017).). Although older persons can still maintain adequate blood cell levels, the lower reserve capacity leaves them more vulnerable to possible issues with clotting, transporting O_2, and fighting infection. The result is a diminished ability to compensate for an acute or chronic illness. In addition, age-related changes result in an increased risk for clonal myeloid cancers (e.g., acute myeloid leukemia).

Hemoglobin levels begin to decrease in both men and women after middle age. Although iron deficiency is often responsible for the low hemoglobin levels, the cause of anemia in approximately one third of older patients is unknown. Inadequate nutritional intake of iron may be a factor, as may occult inflammation, low testosterone levels, impaired renal function, or incipient myelodysplasia (Stauder et al., 2018). Older persons are also not as able as younger adults to produce reticulocytes in response to hemorrhage or hypoxemia. This is likely due to a blunted response to erythropoietin. Also, the RBC plasma membranes are more fragile in the older person. This fragility may account for a slight increase in mean corpuscular volume (MCV) and a slight decrease in mean corpuscular hemoglobin concentration (MCHC) of RBCs in some older individuals.

The total WBC count and differential are generally not affected by aging (Lichtman et al., 2017). However, humoral

TABLE 32.5   HEALTH HISTORY

Hematological System: Subjective Data

Past History
- Have you had any previous problems with anemia, bleeding disorders, and blood diseases such as leukemia?*
- Have you ever received a blood transfusion?*
- Have you undergone any surgical procedures?

Family History
- Has anyone in your family had anemia, cancer, bleeding, or clotting problems?*

Social and Occupational History
- Does your occupation bring you into contact with hazardous substances?*
- Have you had any past or current occupational or household exposures to radiation or chemicals?*
- Have you had any past exposure to radiation as a medical treatment?
- Do you have a support system to assist you when needed?
- What coping strategies do you use when your symptoms get worse?

Self-Care History
- Do you smoke, or drink alcohol?*
- Do you take any prescribed or over-the-counter medications?*
- Are you undergoing or have you ever had chemotherapy?*
- Do you take any herbal products?* Home remedies?*
- Have you in the past or are you currently consuming illegal drugs? What agents? What route? How frequently? When did you last use them?
- Do you exercise regularly? What type of exercise do you do, and how frequently?*

Activities of Daily Living
- Do you have any difficulty performing daily activities because of a lack of energy?*
- Have you experienced excessive fatigue recently?*
- Do you have any shortness of breath at rest? With activity?*

Nutrition–Metabolic History
- Do you have any difficulties with eating, chewing, or swallowing?*
- Have you had a sore tongue or any mouth sores, swollen or sore gums, or excessive oral bleeding?
- How has your appetite been?
- What kind of diet do you follow? If vegetarian, do you eat eggs, milk products, fish, or chicken? Do you follow a vegan diet?
- Do you take any vitamins, nutritional supplements, or iron?*
- Have you had any changes in your weight in the past year?*
- Are nausea and vomiting a problem for you?*
- Have you ever experienced any unusual bleeding or bruising?*
- Have there been recent changes in the condition of your skin?*
- Have you noticed any swelling in your armpits, neck, or groin?*
- Have you experienced night sweats or cold intolerance?*

Elimination
- Have you had black or tarry stools?* Have you had light- or clay-coloured stools?
- Do you ever have diarrhea or a change in your bowel habits?*
- Have you noticed any blood or a dark tea colour in your urine?*
- Have you been urinating less?*
- Has your urine had a foul odour or cloudiness?

Neurological History
- Do you have any pain, such as bone, joint, or abdominal pain, or abdominal fullness?*
- Do you have pain when moving your joints?*
- Have your muscles been sore or achy recently?*
- Do you have any limitations in joint motion?*
- Do you have an unsteady gait?* Have you fallen recently?*
- Have you experienced any numbness or tingling?*
- Have you had any difficulties with your vision, hearing, or taste?*
- Have you noticed any changes in your mental functions?*

Sleep History
- Do you feel fatigued? Are you more fatigued than usual?*
- Do you feel rested on awakening? If no, explain.

Sexual–Reproductive History
- Has your hematological condition caused any sexual or intimacy problems that concern you?*
- *Women:* When was your last menses? Is your cycle regular? How long does your bleeding usually last? How heavy is the flow? Have you had any increase in cramping or clotting?* Have there been any changes in the amount of flow?
- *Men:* Do you experience erectile dysfunction?*
- Have you had unprotected sex in the past 6 months?* Was your partner someone new, or a person with whom you have had a long-term sexual relationship?

Other
- Has your current illness caused a change in your roles and relationships?*
- Does your health problem make you feel differently about yourself?*
- Do you have any other physical changes that cause you distress?*
- Do you have any personal or religious objection to receiving blood or blood products?*
- Do you have any conflicts between your planned therapy and your value–belief system?*

*If yes, describe.
Adapted from Jarvis, C., Browne, A., MacDonald-Jenkins, J., et al. (Eds.) (2019). *Physical assessment & health assessment* (3rd Canadian ed.). Saunders.

antibody response and T-cell function may decrease. During an infection, an older person may have only a minimal elevation in the total WBC count. This suggests that the bone marrow reserve of granulocytes is diminished in older people and reflects the possible impairment in stimulation of hematopoiesis.

The number of platelets is unaffected by the aging process, but functionally the platelets may have increased adhesiveness. More importantly, the levels of many proteins critical to coagulation increase with age. There is an age-related activation of coagulation and fibrinolytic pathways that favours clot formation. The effects of aging on hematological studies are presented in Table 32.4. Immune changes related to aging are described in Chapter 16.

ASSESSMENT OF THE HEMATOLOGICAL SYSTEM

Much of the evaluation of the hematological system is based on a thorough health history. Key questions to ask a patient with a hematological condition are presented in Table 32.5.

CASE STUDY

Patient Introduction

A. J. (pronouns she/her), 73 years old, is brought to the emergency department by her husband. He found his wife at home, weak and lying in bed after returning from work. A. J. reports slowly getting more "cold and tired" but "that is what happens when you continue to work at this age." A. J.'s husband states that his wife has become more tired over the past couple of weeks and gets short of breath when doing simple errands. A. J. recently developed a "bad cold and sinus infection" that improved only after two courses of antibiotics. She also states, "I've noticed I've had a lot of bruising lately."

Discussion Questions

Throughout this assessment chapter, think about A. J. with the following questions in mind:

1. What are the possible causes of A. J.'s weakness, pallor, and shortness of breath?
2. What would be the nurse's priority assessment?
3. What questions should the nurse ask A. J.?
4. What should be included in the physical assessment? What would the nurse be looking for?
5. What diagnostic studies might be ordered?

A. J. and her condition will be followed throughout this assessment chapter. See Case Study: Subjective Data, Case Study: Objective Data: Physical Examination, and Case Study: Objective Data: Diagnostic Studies for more information on A. J.

ⓔvolve
Answers are available at http://evolve.elsevier.com/Canada/Lewis/medsurg.

Subjective Data

Important Health Information

Past Medical History. It is important to learn whether the patient has had prior hematological conditions or whether the patient's family has any hereditary disorders. Hematological disorders that have a strong genetic link include sickle cell anemia, hemophilia, thalassemia, and hemochromatosis. The nurse should also document other related medical conditions such as mononucleosis, malabsorption, and liver disorders (e.g., hepatitis, cirrhosis), as well as kidney or spleen disorders. A patient may have received a solid organ transplant, may have lost a spleen to traumatic injury, or may have a history of intravenous (IV) drug use that may affect the risk for hematological disorders. A history of recurrent infection or problems with blood clotting should also be noted. In addition, it is important to determine how many, if any, blood transfusions a patient has had, as well as any complications experienced during administration, since the risk for transfusion reactions and iron overload increase with the number of blood transfusions.

Medications. A complete medication history that includes both prescription and over-the-counter medications taken is an important component of a hematological assessment. The use of vitamins, herbal products, or dietary supplements should specifically be addressed because many patients may not consider these to be medications. Many medications and supplements interfere with normal hematological functions. For example, herbal therapies such as *Panax* ginseng can alter clotting times (Xiong et al., 2017). Chemotherapeutic agents used to treat cancer and antiretroviral agents used to treat human immunodeficiency virus (HIV) infection may cause bone marrow depression (see Chapters 17 and 18). A patient previously treated with chemotherapeutic drugs, particularly alkylating

agents, is at a higher risk of developing a secondary malignancy such as leukemia or lymphoma. A patient receiving long-term anticoagulation therapy (e.g., warfarin [Coumadin]) may be at increased risk for bleeding.

Surgery or Other Treatments. The patient should be asked about specific past surgical procedures, specifically splenectomy, tumour removal, prosthetic heart valve placement, surgical excision of the duodenum (where iron absorption occurs), partial or total gastrectomy (in which parietal cells are removed, thus reducing intrinsic factor needed for the absorption of cobalamin [vitamin B_{12}]), gastric bypass (the duodenum may be bypassed and parietal cell surface area decreased), and ileal resection (where cobalamin absorption takes place). The nurse should also ascertain how wound healing progressed postoperatively and if and when any bleeding problems occurred as a result of the surgery. Wound healing and bleeding as responses to past injuries (including minor trauma) and to dental extractions should also be documented.

Approach to Obtaining a Hematological History

Social and Occupational History. The patient should be questioned about any past or current occupational or household exposures to radiation or chemicals. If such exposure has occurred, the type, amount, and duration of exposure should be determined. A person who has been exposed to radiation, as a treatment modality or by accident, is at risk for a higher incidence of certain hematological conditions (see Chapter 18). The same is true for a person who has been exposed to chemicals (e.g., benzene, lead, naphthalene, phenylbutazone). These chemicals are commonly used by potters, dry cleaners, and individuals in occupations involving the use of adhesives. The nurse should assess the effect of the current illness on a patient's usual roles and responsibilities. The patient's support systems and coping skills should also be assessed.

Self-Care History. Risk factors that might disrupt the hematological system, such as alcohol use, illicit drug use, and cigarette smoking, must be assessed. Alcohol is a caustic agent, and damage to the GI tract secondary to alcohol use can cause bleeding. *Hematemesis* (bright-red, brown, or black vomit) can be a symptom of this condition and should be investigated. Alcohol also exerts a damaging effect on platelet function and the liver, in which clotting factors are produced. Consequently, bleeding issues can develop and should be anticipated in patients with a known history of alcohol use disorder. Illicit drug use is important to determine, since many of these drugs may affect hematopoiesis. Cigarette smoking increases low-density lipoprotein cholesterol and levels of CO_2, leading to hypoxia. Chronic hypoxia can lead to elevated RBC levels and increased blood viscosity. Smoking also alters the anticoagulant properties of the endothelium and increases platelet reactivity, plasma fibrinogen, and hematocrit levels, all of which increase the risk of developing blood clots.

Activities of Daily Living. Because fatigue is a prominent symptom in many hematological disorders, the patient should be asked about feeling chronically tired. The nurse should also ask whether the patient experiences weakness and a feeling of heavy extremities. Symptoms of apathy, malaise, dyspnea, or palpitations should be documented. Any change in a patient's ability to perform activities of daily living (ADLs) should also be noted. Whether or not the patient exercises should be determined, as well as any history of falls.

Nutritional–Metabolic History. During the patient interview and assessment, the nurse should measure the patient's weight and determine whether the patient has experienced any anorexia, nausea, vomiting, or oral discomfort. A dietary history may provide clues about the cause of anemia. It is important to assess whether the patient has access to clean water and a secure source of food. Iron, cobalamin, and folic acid are necessary for the development of RBCs. Iron and folic acid deficiencies are associated with inadequate dietary intake. Foods containing these substances include the following:

- Proteins and alternatives—liver, meat (duck, chicken, beef), tofu, eggs, seafood (sardines, oysters), soybeans, lentils
- Fruit and vegetables—leafy green vegetables (kale, spinach, bok choy), dried fruits, potatoes, asparagus, palm hearts
- Grains—whole-grain and enriched breads, fortified cereals

Folic acid deficiencies may be offset by a diet that includes foods that are also high in iron.

Any changes in the skin's texture or colour should be explored. The patient should be asked about any bleeding of gum tissue. Any **petechiae** (small, purplish-red lesions) or **ecchymosis** (bruising) on the skin should be noted; if they are present, the frequency, size, and cause (if known) should be documented. The location of petechiae can indicate an accumulation of blood in the skin or mucous membranes. Small vessels leak under pressure, and if platelet numbers are insufficient to stop the bleeding, petechiae may result. Petechiae may also occur in areas where clothing constricts the circulation.

The patient should also be questioned about any lumps or swelling in the neck, the armpits, or the groin. Specifically, the patient must be asked what the lumps feel like (i.e., hard or soft, tender or nontender) and if they are mobile or fixed. Primary lymph tumours are usually not painful. A nontender swollen lymph node may be a sign of Hodgkin's disease or non-Hodgkin's lymphoma. Lymph nodes that are enlarged and tender are usually associated with an acute infection. Any incidents of fever should be explored thoroughly. It should be determined whether the patient currently has a fever, recurring fevers, chills, or night sweats.

Elimination Pattern. The patient should be asked whether blood has been noted in the urine or stool or whether stools have been black and tarry. The nurse should also ask the patient whether they have had a recent fecal occult blood test, fecal immunochemical test (FIT), or colonoscopy. Also, any decrease in urinary output or diarrhea should be documented.

Neurological History. *Arthralgia* (joint pain) may be caused by a hematological condition and should be assessed. Pain in the joint may be indicative of an autoimmune disorder or may be caused by gout secondary to increased uric acid production, which in turn may be secondary to a hematological malignancy or hemolytic anemia. Aching bones may result from pressure of expanding bone marrow with diseases such as leukemia. *Hemarthrosis* (blood in a joint) can occur in patients with bleeding disorders and can be painful.

Paresthesias, numbness, and tingling may be related to a hematological disorder and should be noted. Any changes in vision, hearing, taste, or mental status should also be assessed carefully.

Sleep History. The patient's feeling of being rested after a night's sleep should be determined. Fatigue secondary to a hematological condition often does not resolve after sleep.

Sexual–Reproductive History. A careful gynecological history should be obtained from women, including the ages at menarche and menopause, duration and amount of bleeding, incidence of clotting and cramping, and any associated health issues. Patients should also be questioned about sexual

behaviour because HIV infection is potentially a concern, particularly among populations at high risk for acquiring this disease.

Values and Beliefs. Some hematological conditions are treated with blood transfusions or bone marrow transplantation. The nurse should determine whether any treatment plans may conflict with a patient's values or beliefs.

Objective Data

Physical Examination. A complete and thorough physical examination is necessary to assess all the body systems that affect or are affected by the hematological system (see Chapter 3). Disorders of the hematological system can manifest in various ways; thus a patient's presenting symptoms may not immediately point to a hematological disorder. For example, paresthesias of the lower extremities may not appear to reflect a hematological condition, but when they are accompanied by other clinical findings or risk factors, cobalamin deficiency and resulting pernicious anemia may be suspected. Although a full examination should be performed on patients suspected of a hematological disorder, certain aspects of the physical examination are specifically relevant in hematological disorders; these include the skin, the lymph nodes, the spleen, and the liver. Examination of the skin is discussed in Chapter 25; spleen and liver examinations are described in Chapter 41.

CASE STUDY

Subjective Data

A focused subjective assessment of A. J. revealed the following information:

Past history: History of mild osteoarthritis. Denies any personal history of anemia, cancer, or bleeding. No surgical history. Prefers to take care of self with "natural therapy" and has not seen a health care provider for 5 years, except for a recent sinus infection.

Medications: Metamucil 1 tbsp. PO daily; vitamins C, E, and D with calcium.

Family history: A. J. denies any family history of anemia, cancer, or bleeding disorders. She believes in coming from a family with great genes for longevity because they "eat organic foods."

Self-care history: A. J. admits to drinking one glass of red wine with the evening meal. She is a nonsmoker and just cannot understand the gradual increase in shortness of breath with exertion. A. J. states not being able to do anything anymore without having to stop for breath. She says, "It's tough getting old."

Activities of daily living: A. J. is having difficulty performing ADLs without having to stop for breath. Denies dyspnea at rest.

Nutritional–metabolic history: A. J. and her husband eat a lot of pasta "because it is cheap." She uses a lot of garlic for flavouring and the "health benefit of it." Although not a vegetarian, she states that she eats little meat.

Elimination: Denies black or tarry stool. Occasional constipation. No difficulties with urination. Urine without odour.

Neurological history: A. J. states that her joints are stiff on arising in the morning and after sitting, but is able to get around okay and work at her secretarial job. States that walking is steady but weak. No history of falling. Denies any numbness or tingling. Admits to being a little hard of hearing but that she can still see "pretty good."

Sleep history: Typically sleeps 8 to 9 hr/night with no difficulty falling asleep. However, she still feels tired and needs to nap during lunch break and on days off.

Other: Prefers natural therapies over traditional medication.

See Case Study: Patient Introduction, Case Study: Objective Data: Physical Examination, and Case Study: Objective Data: Diagnostic Studies for more information on A. J.

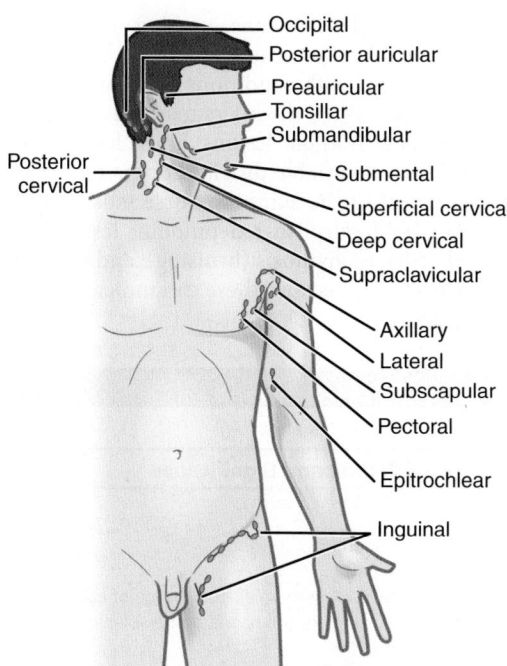

FIG. 32.6 Palpable, superficial lymph nodes.

Labels on figure:
Occipital
Posterior auricular
Preauricular
Tonsillar
Submandibular
Posterior cervical
Submental
Superficial cervical
Deep cervical
Supraclavicular
Axillary
Lateral
Subscapular
Pectoral
Epitrochlear
Inguinal

Lymph Node Assessment. Lymph nodes are distributed throughout the body. Superficial lymph nodes can be evaluated by light palpation (Figure 32.6). Deep lymph nodes cannot be palpated and are best evaluated with radiological examination. Lymph nodes should be assessed with regard to symmetry in location, size, degree of fixation (i.e., movable, fixed), tenderness, and texture. To assess superficial lymph nodes, the nurse lightly palpates the nodes with the pads of the fingers and then gently rolls the skin over the area and concentrates on feeling for possible lymph node enlargement. To be considered normal, a palpable node should be small (0.5 to 1 cm), mobile, firm, and nontender. A node that is tender, hard, fixed, or enlarged (regardless of whether it is tender or not) is abnormal and warrants further investigation. Tender nodes are usually a result of inflammation, whereas hard or fixed nodes are suggestive of malignancy (Ball et al., 2019).

It is important to develop a sequence for examining the lymph nodes. A convenient sequence for examination is to start at the head and neck. First, preauricular, posterior auricular, occipital, tonsillar, submandibular, submental, superficial cervical, posterior cervical chain, deep cervical chain, and supraclavicular nodes are palpated. Next, the axillary lymph nodes and pectoral, subscapular, and lateral groups of nodes are palpated. The epitrochlear nodes, located in the antecubital fossa between the biceps and triceps muscles, are then examined. Last, the inguinal lymph nodes, found in the groin are palpated.

A focused assessment of the hematological system is used to evaluate previously identified hematological conditions and to monitor for signs of new conditions. An example of such an assessment is presented in the Focused Assessment box.

Palpation of the Liver or the Spleen. The liver and the spleen are not usually detectable through palpation of the abdomen.

Hematological System

Use this checklist to make sure the key assessment steps have been performed.

Subjective
Ask the patient about any of the following and note the responses:

Unusual bleeding (e.g., gums) or bruising	Y	N
Black, tarry stool	Y	N
Blood in vomit	Y	N
Swelling in neck, armpits, groin	Y	N
Dark-coloured urine	Y	N
Fatigue	Y	N
Heart palpitations	Y	N
Dyspnea	Y	N

Objective: Diagnostic
Check the following laboratory results for critical values:

CBC	✓
Clotting: PT, INR, aPTT, platelets	✓
Hematocrit and hemoglobin	✓

Objective: Physical Examination

Inspect

Skin for lesions or colour changes	✓

Auscultate

Blood pressure for alteration or orthostasis	✓

Palpate

Pulse for tachycardia	✓
Liver and spleen for enlargement	✓
Lymph nodes for lymphadenopathy	✓

aPTT, activated partial thromboplastin time; *CBC,* complete blood cell count; *INR,* international normalized ratio; *PT,* prothrombin time.

CASE STUDY

Objective Data: Physical Examination

Physical examination findings for A. J. are as follows:
BP 100/70 (lying), 88/60 (standing); apical pulse 110 (lying), 124 (standing), but regular in rhythm. Respiratory rate 26, temperature 36°C (96.8°F), O₂ saturation 90% on room air. No jugular venous distension. Weight: 48 kg. Height: 155 cm. Skin pale with two ecchymoses on her arms and one on the left lower leg. A few scattered petechiae on both ankles. No jaundice noted. Conjunctivas pale. Tongue smooth and shiny. Lungs clear but diminished breath sounds in the bases bilaterally. No visible bleeding. No enlarged lymph nodes, spleen, or liver noted. General weakness with dyspnea on exertion. No numbness or tingling or peripheral edema.

Throughout this chapter, consider diagnostic studies that the nurse may order for A. J.

See Case Study: Patient Introduction, Case Study: Subjective Data, and Case Study: Objective Data: Diagnostic Studies for more information on A. J.

When they are enlarged, however, they may be detectable through percussion or palpation. The degree of enlargement of the liver is measured by the number of centimetres (cm) it extends below the rib border. The spleen may be more difficult to palpate because of its deep location in the abdomen.

Skin Assessment. Assessment of the skin may yield valuable information about the hematological system. The skin should be examined over the entire body in a systematic manner (e.g., starting with the face and oral cavity and moving downward over the body). In patients with RBC disorders, the skin may be pale, as in the case of anemia, or have a cyanotic tinge, in the case of polycythemia. Colour changes in dark-skinned patients are best assessed in the sclera, conjunctiva, buccal mucosa, tongue, lips, nail beds, and palms (Ball et al., 2019). Erythrocytosis often produces small vessel occlusions, causing a purple, mottled appearance of the face, the nose, the fingers, or the toes. Digital clubbing can occur with conditions of chronic anemia, such as sickle cell disease. WBC disorders may cause infectious skin lesions or malignant nodular lesions. These lesions may occur anywhere and have a variable distribution pattern. During the physical assessment of the skin, the nurse must look carefully for petechiae (small purplish-red pinpoint lesions), **purpura** (purplish-red rash), ecchymosis (bruising), and spider nevus (a form of *telangiectasia*) because these can indicate bleeding disorders (Table 32.6).

TABLE 32.6   ASSESSMENT ABNORMALITIES

Hematological System

Finding	Description	Possible Etiology and Significance
Skin		
Pallor of skin or nail beds	Paleness; decrease in or absence of skin coloration (varies with patient's natural skin colour)	Low Hb level (anemia)
Flushing	Transient, episodic redness of skin (usually around face and neck)	Increase in RBC (polycythemia), congestion of capillaries Flushing of the palms of the hands or the soles of the feet may indicate anemia
Jaundice	Yellow appearance of skin and mucous membranes	Accumulation of bile pigment caused by rapid or excessive hemolysis or liver damage
Cyanosis	Bluish discoloration of skin and mucous membranes in lighter-skinned people; greyish/whitish discoloration of skin and mucous membranes in darker-skinned people	Excessive concentration of RBC (polycythemia) in blood (more likely) Reduced Hb (anemia)
Excoriation	Scratch or abrasion of skin	Scratching from intense pruritus
Pruritus	Unpleasant cutaneous sensation that provokes desire to rub or scratch the skin	Hodgkin's lymphoma Cutaneous lymphomas Infiltrative leukemias Increased bilirubin level
Leg ulcers	Prominent on malleoli on the ankles	Sickle cell disease
Angioma	Benign tumour consisting of blood or lymph vessels	Most are congenital; some may disappear spontaneously
Telangiectasia	Small angioma with tendency to bleed; focal red lesions, coarse or fine red lines	Dilation of small vessels
Spider nevus	Form of telangiectasia characterized by a round, red central portion and branching radiations resembling the profile of a spider; usually develop on face, neck, or chest	Elevated estrogen levels as in pregnancy or liver disease
Petechiae	Pinpoint, nonraised, perfectly round area <2 mm; purple, dark red, or brown in colour	Decreased numbers of platelets or clotting factors, resulting in hemorrhage into the skin Vascular abnormalities Break in blood vessel walls as a result of trauma
Purpura	Small hemorrhages in the surface of the skin or mucous membranes resulting in rash of purple, red, or brown spots measuring 2–10 mm in diameter	Same as for petechiae
Ecchymosis (bruise)	Small hemorrhagic spot, larger than purpura; nonelevated; round or irregular	Same as for petechiae
Hematoma	A localized collection of blood, usually clotted	Same as for petechiae
Chloroma	A tumour arising from myeloid tissue and containing pale-green pigment	Acute myelogenous leukemia that has infiltrated the skin
Plasmacytoma	A tumour arising from abnormal plasma cells	Multiple myeloma that has infiltrated tissue
Eyes		
Jaundiced sclera	Yellow appearance of the sclera	Accumulation of bile pigment resulting from rapid or excessive hemolysis or liver disease or infiltration
Conjunctival pallor	Paleness; decreased or absence of coloration in the conjunctiva	Low Hb level (anemia)
Blurred vision, diplopia, visual field cuts	Decreased visual acuity or areas of blindness (field cuts)	Anemia, extreme leukocytosis, and polycythemia may cause visual abnormalities. Thrombocytopenia may cause intraocular hemorrhage with visual abnormalities. Excessive clotting may cause thromboses in the circulation to the brain that cause visual field cuts.
Nose		
Epistaxis	Spontaneous bleeding from the nares	May occur with low platelet counts, especially if patient bends down for a long period, tries to lift a heavy item, or attempts an intense Valsalva manoeuvre

TABLE 32.6	**ASSESSMENT ABNORMALITIES**	
Hematological System—cont'd		
Finding	**Description**	**Possible Etiology and Significance**
Mouth		
Gingival and mucous membrane changes	Pallor	Low Hb level (anemia)
	Gingival or mucosal ulceration, swelling, or bleeding	Neutropenia; inability of impaired leukocytes to combat oral infections; thrombocytopenia
		Gingival hyperplasia may be present with some types of leukemia
Smooth tongue	Tongue surface is smooth and shiny; mucosa is thin and red from decreased papillae	Pernicious anemia, iron-deficiency anemia
Lymph Nodes		
Lymphadenopathy	Lymph nodes are enlarged (>1 cm diameter)	Infection, foreign infiltrations, or systemic disease such as leukemia, lymphoma, Hodgkin's lymphoma, or metastatic cancer
Heart and Chest		
Tachycardia	Heart rate >100 beats/min	Compensatory mechanism in anemia to increase cardiac output
Palpitations	Sensation of feeling the heartbeat, flutter, or pound in the chest	Anemia, fluid volume overload, hypotension with impending syncope, hypertension, or dysrhythmias may cause palpitations
Altered blood pressure	*Orthostasis:* >20/min increase in heart rate or >20 mm Hg decrease in blood pressure from baseline value when moving from a lying position to either sitting or standing	Orthostasis is a common manifestation in anemia, especially if accompanied by low blood volume.
	Hypotension: <90 mm Hg systolic or >40 mm Hg drop in systolic reading from baseline BP	Hypotension may indicate an infectious process, blood loss, or compromised cardiovascular compensatory mechanisms.
	Hypertension: >130/90 mm Hg	Hypertension may occur initially as a compensatory mechanism for anemia.
Sternal tenderness	Abnormal sensitivity to touch or pressure on sternum	Leukemia, as a result of increased bone marrow cellularity, which causes an increase in pressure and bone erosion; multiple myeloma, as a result of stretching of periosteum
Low oxygen saturation	Oxygen-carrying capacity is reflected by the oxygen saturation as measured with pulse oximetry.	Oxygen saturation may be decreased in cases of severe anemia.
Abdomen		
Hepatomegaly	Palpable liver	Leukemia, cirrhosis, or fibrosis secondary to iron overload from sickle cell disease or thalassemia
Splenomegaly	Palpable spleen	Anemia, thrombocytopenia, leukemia, lymphomas, leukopenia, mononucleosis, malaria, cirrhosis, trauma, portal hypertension
Distended abdomen	Distended abdomen is an abdominal profile that is larger than normal; it may be soft or firm, tender or nontender, and accompanied by other symptoms such as nausea, vomiting, or rebound tenderness.	Lymphoma may manifest as abdominal adenopathy, mass(es), or bowel obstruction.
Nervous System		
Paresthesias of feet and hands; ataxia	Numbness sensation and extreme sensitivity experienced in central and peripheral nerves; impaired muscle movement	Cobalamin (vitamin B_{12}) deficiency or folate deficiency
Weakness	Lacking physical strength or energy	Low Hb level (anemia)
Headache, nuchal rigidity	Pain in the cranium, potentially involving one area or extending from the frontal area to the back of the neck	Generalized headache is a common manifestation of mild to moderate anemia.
		Severe headache with or without visual disturbances may signal intracranial hemorrhage caused by thrombocytopenia.
Musculoskeletal System		
Bone pain	Pain in pelvis, ribs, spine, sternum	Multiple myeloma, in relation to enlarged tumours that stretch periosteum
		Bone invasion by leukemia cells
		Bone demineralization that results from various malignancies
		Sickle cell disease
Joint swelling	Fluid-filled spaces surrounding the joints	Occurs with sickle cell anemia as bleeding into the joint (hemarthrosis) causes inflammation
Arthralgia	Joint pain	Sickle cell disease, as a result of hemarthrosis

Hb, hemoglobin.

DIAGNOSTIC STUDIES OF THE HEMATOLOGICAL SYSTEM

The most direct means of evaluating the hematological system is through laboratory analysis and other diagnostic studies. Diagnostic tests of the hematological system are presented in Tables 32.7 through 32.9 and Table 32.11.

Laboratory Studies

Complete Blood Cell Count. The complete blood cell count (CBC) involves several laboratory tests (Table 32.7), each of which serves to assess the three major blood cells formed in the bone marrow. In addition to the CBC, a *peripheral blood smear* may be ordered. The smear is used to look at the morphological

TABLE 32.7   COMPLETE BLOOD CELL COUNT STUDIES

Study	Description and Purpose	Normal Values
Hemoglobin (Hb)	Measurement of gas-carrying capacity of RBCs	Women: 120–160 g/L Men: 140–180 g/L
Hematocrit (Hct)	Measurement of packed cell volume of RBCs, expressed as a percentage of the total blood volume	Women: 0.37–0.47 Men: 0.42–0.54
Total RBC count (erythrocyte count)	Count of number of circulating RBCs	Women: $4.2–5.4 \times 10^{12}$/L Men: $4.7–6.2 \times 10^{12}$/L
RBC indices		
• MCV (Hct/RBC)	Determination of relative size of RBC; low MCV is reflection of microcytosis, high MCV is reflection of macrocytosis	76–100 fL
• MCH (Hb/RBC)	Measurement of average weight of Hb/RBCs; low MCH is indication of microcytosis or hypochromia, high MCH is indication of macrocytosis	27–31 pg
• MCHC	Evaluation of RBC saturation with Hb; low MCHC is indication of hypochromia, high MCHC is evident in spherocytosis	32–36 g/dL
• RBC morphology	Examination of the shape and size of RBCs	No variation in RBC structure
• Reticulocyte count	Number of immature RBCs released from the bone marrow into the blood	0.5–2.0% of RBCs
• WBC count	Measurement of total number of leukocytes	$3.5–12.0 \times 10^9$/L
• WBC differential	Determination of whether each kind of WBC is present in proper proportion; absolute value is determined by multiplying percentage of cell type by total WBC count and dividing by 100	*Neutrophils:* $3.0–5.8 \times 10^9$/L *Eosinophils:* $0.00–0.25 \times 10^9$/L *Basophils:* $0.01–0.05 \times 10^9$/L *Lymphocytes:* $1.5–3.0 \times 10^9$/L *Monocytes:* $0.3–0.5 \times 10^9$/L
• Platelet count	Measurement of number of platelets available to maintain platelet clotting functions (not measurement of quality of platelet function)	$150–400 \times 10^9$/L

Hb, hemoglobin; *Hct,* hematocrit; *MCH,* mean corpuscular hemoglobin; *MCHC,* mean corpuscular hemoglobin concentration; *MCV,* mean corpuscular volume; *RBC,* red blood cell; *WBC,* white blood cell.

features (shape and appearance) of the blood cells and may assist with diagnosis. For example, a large number of immature *blast* WBCs may indicate acute leukemia.

Although the status of each cell type is important, the entire system may be disrupted by diseases, as well as by the treatment of diseases. Suppression of the entire CBC is termed pancytopenia (marked decrease in the number of RBCs, WBCs, and platelets). In such cases, care is directed toward the management of anemia, infection, and hemorrhage (see Chapter 33).

Red Blood Cells. The total RBC count is reported as $RBC \times 10^{12}$/L. However, the total RBC count is not fully reliable in determining the adequacy of RBC function. Instead, other data such as hemoglobin, hematocrit, and RBC indices must be evaluated. It is also important to note that normal values of some RBC tests are reported separately for men and for women because normal values are based on body mass, and men usually have a larger body mass than women.

The *hemoglobin* (Hb) value is reduced in cases of hemorrhage, low RBC production (e.g., aplastic anemia), RBC destruction (e.g., sickle cell anemia), and states of hemodilution, such as those that occur when the fluid volume is excessive. RBCs are increased in polycythemia or in states of hemoconcentration, which can develop from volume depletion (dehydration).

The *hematocrit* value is determined by spinning blood in a centrifuge, which causes RBCs and plasma to separate. The RBCs, being the heavier elements, settle to the bottom. The hematocrit value is the percentage of RBCs compared to the total blood volume. The hematocrit value is reduced and elevated in the same conditions that raise and lower the hemoglobin value.

RBC indices are special indicators that reflect RBC volume, colour, and Hb saturation (see Table 32.7). These parameters may provide insight into the cause of anemia. (The significance of these parameters is discussed further in Chapter 33.)

White Blood Cells. The WBC count provides two different sets of information. The first is a total count of WBCs per litre of peripheral blood. Elevations in WBC count (leukocytosis)

to more than 10×10^9/L are associated with infection, inflammation, tissue injury or death, and malignancies (e.g., leukemia, lymphoma). Although the degree of WBC elevation is not necessarily predictive of the severity of illness, it can provide clues to the cause. Certain types of leukemias are more likely to produce extremely high WBC counts (e.g., $>25 \times 10^9$/L). A total WBC count lower than 4×10^9/L (leukopenia) is associated with bone marrow depression, severe or chronic illness, viral infections, and other types of leukemia.

The second aspect of the WBC count, the *differential count,* is the percentage of each type of leukocyte. The information from the WBC differential provides valuable clues to the cause of illness. When infections are severe, more granulocytes are released from the bone marrow as a compensatory mechanism. To meet the increased demand, many young, immature polymorphonuclear neutrophils (bands) are released into circulation. More mature neutrophils are called *polymorphonuclear segmented neutrophils* ("segs"). The usual laboratory procedure is to report WBCs in order of maturity, with the less mature forms (i.e., band neutrophils) on the left side of the written report; hence, the existence of many immature cells is termed a *shift to the left.* A shift to the left may be indicative of active infection or inflammation (e.g., postsurgically). The WBC differential count is of considerable significance because it is possible for the total WBC count to remain essentially normal despite a marked change in one type of leukocyte. For example, a patient may have a normal WBC count of 8.8×10^9/L, but the differential count may reveal a relative proportion of lymphocytes to be reduced to 10%—an abnormal finding that warrants further investigation.

When the bone marrow does not produce enough neutrophils, neutropenia occurs. Neutropenia is a condition associated with an absolute neutrophil count (ANC) lower than 1×10^9/L to 1.5×10^9/L; severe neutropenia is associated with an ANC lower than 0.5×10^9/L. The ANC is determined as the total WBCs multiplied by the percentage of neutrophils. Neutropenia

TABLE 32.8 CLOTTING STUDIES

Study	Description and Purpose	Normal Values
Activated clotting time (ACT)	Evaluation of intrinsic coagulation status; more accurate than aPTT; used during dialysis, coronary artery bypass procedure, arteriography	70–120 sec
Activated partial thromboplastin time (aPTT)	Assessment of intrinsic coagulation by measuring factors I, II, V, VIII, IX, X, XI, and XII; longer with the use of heparin	25–40 sec
Antithrombin	Naturally occurring protein synthesized by the liver that inhibits coagulation through inactivation of thrombin and other factors; is depleted in DIC	170–300 mg/L or 0.80–1.2 of standard
Capillary fragility test (tourniquet test, Rumpel–Leede test)	Reflection of capillary integrity when positive or negative pressure is applied to various areas of the body; positive result is indication of thrombocytopenia, toxic vascular reactions	No petechiae, or negative
D-dimer	Assay to measure a fragment of fibrin that is formed as a result of fibrin degradation and clot lysis; used in diagnosis of hypercoagulable conditions (e.g., DIC, pulmonary embolism)	<3.0 nmol/L
Fibrin split products (FSP) or fibrin degradation products (FDPs)	Reflection of degree of fibrinolysis and predisposition to bleeding (if present); screening test for DIC; elevated levels associated with DIC, advanced malignancy, severe inflammation	<10 mg/dL
Fibrinogen (factor I)	Reflection of level of fibrinogen; increase in fibrinogen may indicate enhancement of fibrin formation, which renders patient hypercoagulable; decrease in fibrinogen indicates that patient may be predisposed to bleeding	2–5 g/L
International normalized ratio (INR)	Standardized system of reporting PT that is based on a reference calibration model and calculated by comparison of patient's PT with a control value	0.9–1.1
Plasminogen	Assessment of adequacy of plasminogen in patients who have multiple thromboembolic episodes	2.4–4.4 units/mL
Platelet count	Count of number of circulating platelets	150×10^9/L to 400×10^9/L
Prothrombin time (PT)	Assessment of extrinsic coagulation by measurement of factors I, II, V, VII, and X	11–12.5 sec
Thrombin time	Reflection of adequacy of thrombin; prolonged thrombin time indicates that coagulation is inadequate secondary to decreased thrombin activity	10–15 sec

DIC, disseminated intravascular coagulation.

TABLE 32.9 ABO BLOOD GROUP NAMES AND PATIENT/DONOR COMPATIBILITIES*

Recipient's Blood Group	RBC Antigen	Plasma/Serum Antibody	Compatible Donor for RBC Transfusions	Compatible Donor for Plasma Transfusions
A	A	Anti-B	A and O	A and AB
B	B	Anti-A	B and O	B and AB
AB (universal recipient)	Both A and B	Neither anti-A nor anti-B	A, B, AB, and O	AB
O	Neither A nor B	Both anti-A and anti-B	O (universal donor)	A, B, AB, and O

RBC, red blood cell.
*ABO blood groups are named for the antigen found on the RBCs. Donor compatibility is based on the antibodies present in the serum.

results from a number of disease processes, such as leukemia, or from bone marrow depression (see Chapter 33) and is associated with an increased risk for infection and death from sepsis.

Platelet Count. The platelet count is the number of platelets per microlitre of blood. Normal platelet counts are between 150×10^9/L and 400×10^9/L; counts lower than 150×10^9/L signify a condition termed thrombocytopenia. Bleeding may occur with thrombocytopenia. Spontaneous hemorrhage is probable once platelet counts fall below 10×10^9/L. A more extensive description of clotting studies is presented in Table 32.8. Thrombocytosis, in contrast, is an excess of platelets, a disorder that occurs with inflammation and some cancers. The complication related to thrombocytosis that is most likely to occur is excessive clotting.

Blood Typing and Rh Factor. Blood group antigens (A and B) are found only on RBC membranes and form the basis for the ABO blood typing system. The presence or absence of one or both of the two inherited antigens is the basis for the four blood groups: A, B, AB, and O. People with blood group A have A antigens, those with group B have B antigens, those with group AB have both A and B antigens, and those with group O have neither A nor B antigens. People with blood types A, B, or O have antibodies in the serum, termed *anti-A* and *anti-B*, that react with A or B antigens. These antibodies are found when the corresponding antigen is absent from the RBC membrane. For example, anti-B antibodies are found in the plasma of people with blood group A (Table 32.9).

Blood reactions caused by ABO incompatibilities result in intravascular hemolysis of the RBCs. RBCs *agglutinate* (or clump) when a serum antibody that reacts with the antigens on the RBC membrane is present. For example, agglutination would occur in the blood of a person with type A blood if they received blood from a donor with B antigens (i.e., type B or AB). The anti-B antibodies in the serum of the person with type A blood would react with the B antigens on the donor RBCs, thus initiating the process that results in RBC hemolysis.

The Rhesus (Rh) system is based on a third antigen, D, which is also found on the RBC membrane. Rh-positive people have the D antigen, whereas Rh-negative people do not. Rh-positive blood is indicated with a plus sign after the ABO group name (e.g., "AB+"). A Coombs test is used to evaluate the person's Rh status (Table 32.10).

As a result of transfusion therapy or during childbirth, an Rh-negative person may be exposed to Rh-positive blood. If an Rh-negative mother gives birth to an Rh-positive infant, the mother forms an antibody, anti-D, which acts against Rh antigens. (Rh-positive people normally have no anti-D antibody.) In subsequent pregnancies, the mother's anti-D antibodies can cross the placenta and attack the RBCs of a fetus who is Rh-positive, thus causing hemolysis of the RBCs. A pregnant Rh-negative woman should receive Rho(D) immune globulin (WinRho) injections during pregnancy to prevent anti-D antibodies from forming.

TABLE 32.10   MISCELLANEOUS LABORATORY BLOOD STUDIES

Study/Substance Studied	Description and Purpose	Normal Values
Bilirubin	Measurement of degree of RBC hemolysis or liver's inability to excrete normal quantities of bilirubin	Total: 3.0–22 mcmol/L Direct: 1.7–5.1 mcmol/L
	Increase in indirect bilirubin with hemolytic issues; increase in direct bilirubin with obstructive conditions (e.g., gallstones, tumour)	Indirect: 3.4—12 mcmol/L
Blood smear (peripheral blood smear)	Reviews colour, size, shape, and quantity of cells in peripheral blood; can provide significant information regarding disorders affecting RBCs, WBCs, or platelets	Normal quantity of each cell type; normal size, shape, and colour of RBCs; normal WBC differential
Coombs test	Differentiation among types of hemolytic anemias; detection of immune antibodies; detection of Rh factor	Negative finding (no agglutination)
• Direct	Detection of antibodies that are attached to RBCs	Negative finding
• Indirect	Detection of antibodies in serum	Negative finding
Cobalamin (vitamin B_{12})	Level of vitamin B_{12} available for production of new RBCs	148–616 pmol/L
Erythrocyte sedimentation rate (ESR)	Measurement of sedimentation, or settling, of RBCs in 1 hr	Female:
	Inflammatory process causes an alteration in plasma proteins, resulting in aggregation of RBCs and making them heavier; the faster the RBCs settle, the higher the ESR.	• Up to 20 mm/hr Male: • Up to 15 mm/hr
Erythropoietin	Measurement of degree of hormonal stimulation of the bone marrow to release RBCs	5–35 mU/mL
Ferritin	Major iron storage protein; is normally present in blood in concentrations directly related to iron storage	Female: 20–150 mcg/L Male: 20–200 mcg/L
Folic acid (folate)	Amount of folic acid or folate available for RBC production	11–57 nmol/L
Haptoglobin	A serum glycoprotein that binds to Hb released into the bloodstream by hemolysis; decreased with RBC hemolysis; increased with infection, inflammation, cancer	0.5–2.2 g/L
Hemoglobin (Hb) electrophoresis	Proteins involved in development of the hemoglobin molecule have a definitive pattern of separation on electrophoresis; this pattern is altered with abnormal Hb synthesis, as occurs in thalassemia or in sickle cell anemia, in which sickle Hb (HbS) is increased.	Normal HbA_1: 95–98% HbA_2: 2–3% HbF: 0.8–2% HbS: 0% HbC: 0%
Homocysteine	Amino acid formed from methionine	0–30 years: 4.6-8.1 mcmol/L
	Rapidly metabolized through pathways that require cobalamin (vitamin B_{12}) and folic acid; increased in deficiencies of cobalamin and folic acid	30–59 years: • Female 4.5–7.9 mcmol/L • Male 6.3–11.2 mcmol/L >59 years: 5.8–11.9 mcmol/L
Iron		
• Serum iron	Reflection of amount of iron combined with proteins in serum; accurate indication of status of iron storage and use	Female: 5–29 mcmol/L Male: 13–31 mcmol/L
• Total iron-binding capacity (TIBC)	Measurement of all proteins available for binding iron	45–73 mcmol/L
	Transferrin represents the largest quantity of iron-binding proteins; therefore, TIBC is an indirect measure of transferrin.	
Lactic dehydrogenase (LDH)	Intracellular enzyme present in almost all body tissues	45–90 IU/L
	Levels rise in response to cell damage; increased levels confirm diagnosis of injury or disease	
	May be used as a nonspecific marker of hematological malignancy growth and response to treatment	
Methylmalonic acid (MMA)	Indirect test for cobalamin: MMA metabolism requires cobalamin; test helps differentiate cobalamin deficiency from folic acid deficiency	<2.4 mcg/dL
Microglobulin (β_2 microglobulin)	Protein found on the surface of all cells	Urine: <3.6 mcmol/L
	Increased in patients with malignancies such as lymphoma, leukemia, or multiple myeloma; may be used as a tumour marker	
Reticulocyte count	Measurement of immature RBCs; reflection of bone marrow activity in producing RBCs	0.5–2.0% of RBC count (0.005–0.020 of RBC count)
Serum protein electrophoresis (SPEP)	Separates proteins in the blood on basis of electrical charge; helps detect hyperglobulinemic states, as in multiple myeloma or some lymphomas	Normal banding pattern of albumin and globulins; an increase in any protein ("protein spike") is abnormal
Transferrin	The largest of proteins that bind to iron; increased in majority of people with iron-deficiency anemia	Female: 2.5–3.8 g/L Male: 2.15–3.65 g/L
Transferrin saturation (%)	Decreased in iron-deficiency anemia and increased in hemolytic and megaloblastic anemia	Female: 15–50% Male: 20–50%

HbA, hemoglobin alpha; *HbC,* abnormal hemoglobin that shows reduced plasticity of the erythrocyte causing hemoglobinopathy; *HbF,* fetal hemoglobin; *HbS,* sickle hemoglobin; *RBC,* red blood cell.

A blood sample may be obtained from a patient for a "group and screen" and/or "crossmatch" if they may require blood. *Group* refers to determining a patient's blood group (e.g., ABO and RH status). The patient's blood is also "screened" for significant antibodies. *Crossmatch* is a compatibility test that ensures that no antibodies are present in the patient's sample that will react with a specific unit of blood that is being prepared for transfusion.

TABLE 32.11   DIAGNOSTIC STUDIES

Hematological System

Study/Substance Studied	Description and Purpose	Nursing Responsibility
Urine Studies		
Bence Jones protein	An electrophoretic measurement is used to detect the presence of the Bence Jones protein, which is found in most cases of multiple myeloma. Negative finding is considered normal.	Acquire random urine specimen early in the morning. If a 24-hour urine collection is ordered, discard first specimen and collect all urine voided during the 24 hr, keeping on ice or refrigerated.
Radioisotope Studies		
Bone scan	Radioactive isotope is injected by IV. Used for evaluating structure of the bones. Patient is not a source of radioactivity.	IV access is required. Patient needs to lie still during imaging.
SPECT (**s**ingle-**p**hoton **e**mission **c**omputed **t**omography) scan	Radioactive isotope is injected by IV. Images from the radioactive emissions are used to evaluate structure of the spleen, liver, bone, and possible tumours. Patient is not a source of radioactivity.	IV access is required. Patient needs to lie still during imaging. Following the procedure, have patient drink fluids to aid in the excretion of the isotope.
Radiological Studies		
Skeletal radiograph (X-ray)	Radiographic studies performed as a bone survey to detect lytic lesions associated with multiple myeloma. Bone scans do not identify lytic lesions very well in this condition; because of lack of blood supply, there is no uptake of radioactive isotopes.	No specific nursing responsibilities.
Liver, spleen, or abdominal ultrasonography	Noninvasive probe is lubricated and slid across the abdomen to detect the density and borders of the abdominal organs. Irregular borders, masses, vascular structure, and biliary tree can be detected.	Patients must be comfortable lying flat, and the probe must compress the abdomen.
Positron emission tomography (PET) scan	A nuclear tracer substance is injected and is taken up by metabolically active cells. The follow-up scan shows tissues in different colours based on the metabolic rate. "Hot spots" reflect increased glucose consumption that may reflect tumours.	IV access is required for injection of the tracer substance. Patients should ingest nothing by mouth except water and medications for at least 4 hr before the test. IV solutions containing glucose may be held. Patients who are glucose intolerant or diabetic may need adjustments to their medications. Bowel preparation may also be needed, depending on the area being studied.
Computed tomographic (CT) scan	Noninvasive examination in which computer-assisted radiography is used to evaluate the lymph nodes. Contrast medium often is used in abdominal studies of the liver or the spleen. Spiral CT is used to evaluate lymph nodes.	If contrast medium is used, investigate whether patient has iodine sensitivity. IV, oral contrast, or both may be given prior to the procedure, depending on the area being studied. Patient may need to be NPO.
Magnetic resonance imaging (MRI)	Noninvasive procedure that produces sensitive images of soft tissue without the use of contrast medium. No ionizing radiation is required.	Instruct patient to remove all metal objects and ask about any history of surgical insertion of staples, plates, or other metal appliances. Patient may need to lie still in a small chamber for the scan.
Biopsies/Procedures		
Bone marrow biopsy/aspirate	Removal of bone marrow through a locally anaesthetized site to evaluate the status of the blood-forming tissue. Used to diagnose multiple myeloma, leukemia, and some lymphomas and to stage some solid tumours. Also performed to assess efficacy of leukemia therapy.	Explain procedure to patient. Obtain signed consent form. Ensure that a time-out* is done before procedure. Consider preprocedure analgesic administration to enhance patient comfort and cooperation. Apply pressure dressing after procedure. Assess biopsy site for bleeding.
Lumbar puncture (LP)	Purpose is to obtain cerebrospinal fluid for testing for malignancy or infection. It may also be used to administer chemotherapy to central nervous system.	Assist in positioning patient and provide support. Observe site for bleeding and signs of infection.
Lymph node biopsy	Purpose is to obtain lymph tissue for histological examination to determine diagnosis and therapy.	Explain procedure to patient. Obtain signed consent form.
• Open	Excision of lymph node and surrounding tissue through an incision. Performed in the operating room or procedure area; either local or general anaesthesia is administered.	Observe site for bleeding, and monitor vital signs, especially if platelet count is low. The sterile dressing should be changed as ordered, and the wound should be inspected for healing and infection.
• Closed (needle) or fine needle	Performed at patient's bedside or in an outpatient area.	
Molecular, Cytogenic, and Gene Analysis Studies		
Fluorescent in situ hybridization (FISH)	Tests performed on malignant cells, either peripheral blood (e.g., leukemia) or biopsy specimen (bone marrow, lymph node), to assess genetic or chromosomal abnormalities of cancer cells. May be useful in confirming diagnosis and determining treatment modalities and prognosis.	Explain purpose of testing to patient.
Comparative genomic hybridization (CGH)		
Spectral karyotyping (SKY)		

IV, intravenous; *NPO,* nothing by mouth.
*A time-out is done just before a surgical procedure starts in order to verify patient identification, surgical procedure, and surgical site.

Iron Metabolism. The laboratory tests used in evaluating iron metabolism include serum iron, total iron-binding capacity (TIBC), serum ferritin, and transferrin saturation. Additional tests for nutritional deficiencies leading to defective RBC production may also be performed (see Table 32.10).

Serum iron is a measurement of the amount of protein-bound iron circulating in the serum. TIBC provides a measurement of all proteins that bind or transport iron between the tissues and the bone marrow. Although this indirect measurement is a general reflection of the amount of transferrin present in the circulation, it overestimates transferrin levels by 16 to 20% because it also measures other proteins that can bind iron. These alternative proteins bind iron only when transferrin is more than half saturated. Also, TIBC varies inversely with tissue iron stores; it is higher when iron stores are low and lower when iron stores are high.

Transferrin saturation is a better indicator of the availability of iron for erythropoiesis than is serum iron because, unlike serum iron, the iron bound to transferrin is readily available for the body to use. To calculate transferrin saturation, the serum iron value is divided by TIBC, and the result is multiplied by 100. For example, a patient with a serum iron level of 18 mcmol/L and a TIBC of 57 mcmol/L would have a transferrin saturation of about 31.6%. Under normal conditions, the serum ferritin concentration is correlated closely with body iron stores.

Radiological Studies

Radiological studies for the hematological system involve primarily the use of computed tomography (CT) or magnetic resonance imaging (MRI) for evaluating the spleen, the liver, and the lymph nodes. Nursing responsibilities related to these studies are presented in Table 32.11.

Biopsies

Biopsy procedures specific to hematological assessment are bone marrow examination (biopsy and/or aspirate) and lymph node biopsy.

Bone Marrow Examination. Bone marrow examination is important in the evaluation of many hematological disorders. The examination of the marrow may involve aspiration alone or aspiration with biopsy. The benefits of bone marrow examination include the ability to (a) fully evaluate hematopoiesis and (b) obtain specimens for cytopathological chromosomal analysis. The preferred site for both aspiration and biopsy of bone marrow is the posterior superior iliac crest. Bone marrow aspiration and biopsy are performed by a physician nurse practitioner or physician's assistant. Local anaesthesia and sedation may be used to minimize anxiety and pain.

For bone marrow aspiration, the skin over the puncture site is cleansed with a bactericidal agent. The skin, subcutaneous tissue, and periosteum are infiltrated with a local anaesthetic drug (Figure 32.7). Once the area is anaesthetized, a bone marrow needle is inserted through the cortex of the bone. The stylet of the needle is then removed, the hub is attached to a 10-mL syringe, and 0.2 to 0.5 mL of the marrow fluid is aspirated. The patient may experience pain when the periosteum is penetrated and with aspiration. Although it generally lasts for only a few seconds, the pain may be quite uncomfortable. After the marrow aspiration, the needle is removed. Pressure is applied over the aspiration site to ensure hemostasis. If the patient is thrombocytopenic, pressure may be required for 5 to 10 minutes or longer. With severe thrombocytopenia, platelets may be infused before the procedure. If a bone biopsy is required, the preparatory procedure remains the same, but a different needle is used. The needle has a cutting blade that allows a specimen of the bone to be removed. A bone marrow biopsy and aspirate are often done at the same time. They offer different but complementary information about the status of the bone marrow cells.

Although complications of bone marrow aspirations or biopsies are minimal, there is a possibility of penetrating the bone and damaging underlying structures. Other complications include hemorrhage (particularly if the patient is thrombocytopenic) and infection (particularly if the patient is leukopenic). Following a bone marrow biopsy or aspirate, a patient's vital signs should be monitored (if appropriate) and analgesic provided as required. The patient should be assessed for excess drainage or bleeding. Pressure can be applied to the site by having the patient lie on a rolled-up towel for 20 to 30 minutes.

Lymph Node Biopsy. Lymph node biopsy involves obtaining lymph tissue for histological examination to determine the diagnosis and to help plan therapy. This may be done by either an open biopsy or a closed (needle) biopsy. Negative

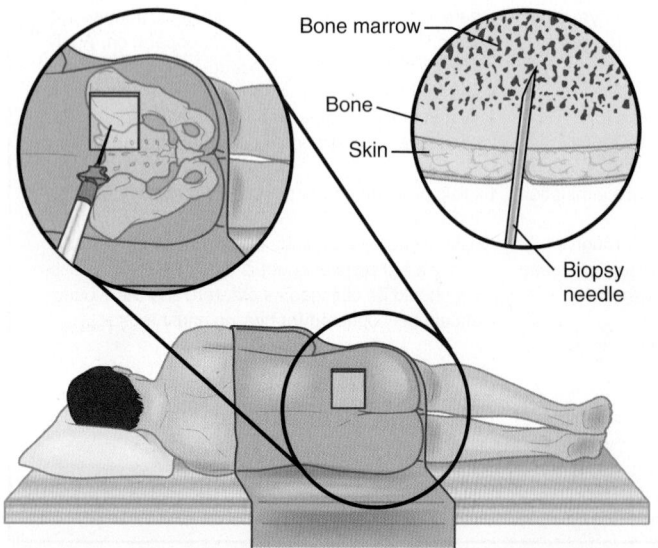

FIG. 32.7 Bone marrow aspiration from the posterior superior iliac crest.

CASE STUDY

Objective Data: Diagnostic Studies

The health care provider orders the following initial diagnostic studies for A. J.:
- CBC, basic metabolic panel (electrolytes, blood urea nitrogen [BUN], creatinine), PT/PTT
- Arterial blood gases
- Chest X-ray

A. J.'s CBC reveals a Hb of 59 g/L, Hct of 0.18, WBC of 2.6×10^9/L, platelet count of 72×10^9/L, PT = 18 sec, aPTT = 37. A. J.'s arterial blood gases are normal, as is the chest X-ray. The health care provider orders more blood work, including a WBC differential and RBC indices, and admits A. J. to the hospital for further evaluation.

See Case Study: Patient Introduction, Case Study: Subjective Data, and Case Study: Objective Data: Physical Examination for more information on A. J.

results from a needle biopsy may indicate only that the cancer cells were not part of the tissue specimen obtained. A repeated needle biopsy or a larger tissue specimen (open biopsy) may be subsequently required. An open (excisional) biopsy is usually done to confirm an initial diagnosis because larger specimens are usually needed for cytopathological tests.

Molecular Cytogenetics and Gene Analysis

Testing for specific genetic or chromosomal variations in hematological conditions is often helpful in diagnosis, in determining the treatment options, and in determining prognosis. If a large number of abnormal cells are circulating in the blood, as in acute leukemia, these tests may be performed with peripheral blood samples. However, testing is usually performed on samples from bone marrow, lymph node biopsies, and sometimes cerebrospinal fluid (CSF). For example, fluorescent in situ hybridization (FISH) can be used to identify specific genes or portions of genes that are abnormal by attaching a probe to a targeted region of deoxyribonucleic acid (DNA). It may be used to reveal an abnormal extra chromosome 8 that is common in certain leukemias. Chromosomal karyotyping allows each set of chromosomes to be painted different colours. This helps to identify normal from abnormal banding patterns. For example, it can be used to identify the 9;22 translocation in the Philadelphia chromosome of chronic myelogenous leukemia. More information on genetics is available in Chapter 15.

REVIEW QUESTIONS

The number of the question corresponds to the same-numbered objective at the beginning of the chapter.

1. Why might a client who lives at a high altitude normally have an increased RBC count?
   a. High altitudes cause vascular fluid loss, leading to hemoconcentration.
   b. Hypoxia caused by decreased atmospheric oxygen stimulates erythropoiesis.
   c. The function of the spleen in removing old erythrocytes is impaired at high altitudes.
   d. Impaired production of leukocytes and platelets leads to proportionally higher RBC counts.
2. What is the primary effect of malignant disorders that arise from granulocytic cells in the bone marrow?
   a. Risk for hemorrhage
   b. Altered oxygenation
   c. Decreased production of antibodies
   d. Decreased phagocytosis of bacteria
3. An anticoagulant such as warfarin that interferes with prothrombin production will alter the clotting mechanism during what process?
   a. Platelet aggregation
   b. Activation of thrombin
   c. Release of tissue thromboplastin
   d. Stimulation of factor activation complex
4. When reviewing laboratory results of an 83-year-old client with an infection, what should the nurse expect to find?
   a. Minimal leukocytosis
   b. Decreased platelet count
   c. Increased hemoglobin and hematocrit levels
   d. Decreased erythrocyte sedimentation rate (ESR)
5. What significant information related to the hematological system should be obtained from a client's health history?
   a. Jaundice
   b. Bladder surgery
   c. Early menopause
   d. Tonsillectomy

6. What technique should the nurse use when assessing the lymph nodes?
   a. Applying gentle, firm pressure to deep lymph nodes
   b. Palpating the deep cervical and supraclavicular nodes last
   c. Lightly palpating superficial lymph nodes with the pads of the fingers
   d. Using the tips of the second, third, and fourth fingers to apply deep palpation
7. When a lymph node is palpated, which of the following is a normal finding?
   a. Hard, fixed nodes
   b. Firm, mobile nodes
   c. Enlarged, tender nodes
   d. Hard, nontender nodes
8. Nursing care for a client immediately after a bone marrow biopsy and aspiration includes which of the following? (*Select all that apply.*)
   a. Administering analgesics as necessary
   b. Preparing to administer a blood transfusion
   c. Instructing on the need to lie still with a sterile pressure dressing intact
   d. Monitoring vital signs and assessing the site for excess drainage or bleeding
   e. Instructing on the need for preprocedure and postprocedure antibiotics
9. A nurse is taking care of a male client who has the following laboratory values from his CBC: WBC 6.5×10^9/L, Hb 134 g/L, Hct 40%, platelets 50×10^9/L. What should the nurse be most concerned about?
   a. The client is neutropenic.
   b. The client has an infection.
   c. The client is at risk for bleeding.
   d. The client is at risk of falling due to his anemia.

1. b; 2. d; 3. b; 4. a; 5. a; 6. c; 7. b; 8. a, c, d; 9. c

ⓔvolve

For even more review questions, visit http://evolve.elsevier.com/Canada/Lewis/medsurg.

REFERENCES

Anderson, G. J., & Frazer, D. M. (2017). Current understanding of iron homeostasis. *American Journal of Clinical Nutrition, 106*(6), 1559S–1566S. https://doi.org/10.3945/ajcn.117.155804

Ball, J. W., Dains, J. E., Flynn, J. A., et al. (2019). *Seidel's guide to physical examination* (9th ed.). Mosby.

Gomez-Casado, C., Villaseñor, A., Rodriguez-Nogales, et al. (2019). Understanding platelets in infectious and allergic lung diseases. *International Journal of Molecular Sciences, 20*(7), 1730. https://doi.org/10.3390/ijms20071730

Leru, P. M. (2019). Eosinophilic disorders: Evaluation of current classification and diagnostic criteria, proposal of a practical diagnostic algorithm. *Clinical and Translation Allergy, 9*(36), 1–9. https://doi.org/10.1186/s13601-019-0277-4

Lichtman, M. A., Kaushansky, K., Prchal, J. T., et al. (2017). *Williams manual of hematology* (9th ed.). McGraw-Hill.

Rosales, C. (2018). Neutrophil: A cell with many roles in inflammation or several cell types? *Frontiers in Physiology, 10*, 1534. https://doi.org/10.3389/fphys.2018.00113

Songdej, N., & Rao, A. (2017). Hematopoietic transcription factor mutations: Important players in inherited defects. *Blood, 129*(21), 2873–2881. https://doi.org/10.1182/blood.2016.11.709881

Stauder, R., Valent, P., & Theuri, I. (2018). Anemia at older age: Etiologies, clinical implications, and management. *Blood, 131*(5), 505–514. https://doi.org/10.1182/blood.2017.07.746446

Suresh, S., Rajvanshi, P. K., & Noguchi, C. T. (2020). The many facets of erythropoietin physiologic and metabolic response. *Frontiers in Physiology, 17*(10), 1534. https://doi.org/10.3389/fphys.2019.01534

Wopereis, D. M., Du Puy, R. S., van Heemst, D., et al. (2018). The relation between thyroid function and anemia: A pooled analysis of individual participant data. *Journal of Clinical Endocrinology & Metabolism, 103*(10), 3658–3667. https://doi.org/10.1210/jc.2018-00481

Xiong, L., Qi, Z., Zheng, B., et al. (2017). Inhibitory effect of triterpenoids from *Panax* ginseng on coagulation factor X. *Molecules, 22*(4), 649. https://doi.org/10.3390/molecules22040649

RESOURCES

Resources for this chapter are listed in Chapter 33.

🔵volve

For additional Internet resources, see the website for this book at http://evolve.elsevier.com/Canada/Lewis/medsurg.

Nursing Management
Hematological Conditions

Bridgette Lord
Originating US chapter by Sandra Irene Rome

⊖volve WEBSITE

LEARNING OBJECTIVES

1. Describe the general clinical manifestations and complications of anemia.
2. Describe the etiologies, clinical manifestations, diagnostic findings, and nursing and interprofessional management of iron-deficiency, megaloblastic, and aplastic anemias and anemia of chronic disease.
3. Explain the nursing and interprofessional management of anemia from blood loss.
4. Describe the pathophysiology, clinical manifestations, and nursing and interprofessional management of anemia caused by increased erythrocyte destruction,
5. Describe the pathophysiology and nursing and interprofessional management of polycythemia.
6. Explain the pathophysiology, clinical manifestations, and nursing and interprofessional management of various types of thrombocytopenia.
7. Describe the types, clinical manifestations, diagnostic findings, and nursing and interprofessional management of hemophilia and von Willebrand disease.
8. Explain the pathophysiology, diagnostic findings, and nursing and interprofessional management of disseminated intravascular coagulation.
9. Describe the etiology, clinical manifestations, and nursing and interprofessional management of neutropenia.
10. Describe the pathophysiology, clinical manifestations, and nursing and interprofessional management of myelodysplastic syndrome.
11. Compare and contrast the major types of leukemia in terms of age of onset, clinical manifestations, and diagnostic findings.
12. Explain the nursing and interprofessional management of acute and chronic leukemias.
13. Compare Hodgkin's lymphoma and non-Hodgkin's lymphoma in terms of clinical manifestations, staging, and nursing and interprofessional management.
14. Describe the pathophysiology, clinical manifestations, and nursing and interprofessional management of multiple myeloma.
15. Describe the spleen disorders and related interprofessional care.
16. Describe the nursing management of transfusing blood and blood products.

KEY TERMS

anemia
aplastic anemia
disseminated intravascular coagulation (DIC)
hemochromatosis
hemolytic anemia
hemophilia
Hodgkin's lymphoma

iron-deficiency anemia
leukemia
lymphomas
megaloblastic anemias
multiple myeloma
myelodysplastic syndrome (MDS)
neutropenia

non-Hodgkin's lymphomas (NHLs)
pernicious anemia
polycythemia
sickle cell disease (SCD)
thalassemia
thrombocytopenia

ANEMIA

DEFINITION AND CLASSIFICATION

Anemia is a deficiency in the number of erythrocytes (red blood cells [RBCs]), the quantity or quality of hemoglobin (Hb), the volume of packed RBCs (hematocrit [Hct]), or a combination of these. It is a common condition and affects approximately a third of the world's population. It has many diverse causes, such as blood loss, impaired production of RBCs, or increased destruction of RBCs. Because RBCs transport oxygen (O_2), erythrocyte disorders can lead to tissue hypoxia; this accounts for many of the signs and symptoms of anemia. Anemia is not a specific disease; it is a manifestation of a pathological process.

Anemia is diagnosed on the basis of a complete blood count (CBC), reticulocyte count, and peripheral blood smear. Once anemia is identified, further investigation is done to determine its specific cause.

Anemia can result from primary hematological disorders or can develop as a secondary consequence of defects in other body systems. The various types of anemia can be grouped according to either a morphological classification (by cellular characteristics) or an etiological one (by underlying cause). Morphological classification is based on descriptive, objective laboratory information such as RBC size and colour (Table 33.1). Etiological classification is related to the clinical conditions causing the anemia (Table 33.2). Although the morphological system is the most accurate means of classifying anemias, it is easier to discuss patient care by focusing on the cause or etiology of the anemia.

CLINICAL MANIFESTATIONS

The clinical manifestations of anemia are caused by the body's response to tissue hypoxia. Specific manifestations vary depending on the rate at which anemia evolved, its severity, and the presence of coexisting disease. Hb levels are often used to determine the severity of anemia. Mild states of anemia (Hb 100–120 g/L) may exist without causing symptoms. If symptoms develop, it is because the patient has an underlying disease or is experiencing a compensatory response to heavy exercise. Symptoms include palpitations, dyspnea, and mild fatigue. In cases of moderate anemia (Hb 60–100 g/L), the cardiopulmonary symptoms are increased and the patient may experience them while resting as well as with activity. The patient with severe anemia (Hb <60 g/L) displays many clinical manifestations involving multiple body systems (Table 33.3).

Integumentary Changes

Integumentary changes may depend on the underlying cause of anemia. They may include pallor, jaundice, and pruritus. *Pallor* results from reduced amounts of Hb and reduced blood flow to the skin. *Jaundice* occurs when hemolysis of RBCs results in an increased concentration of serum bilirubin. In addition to the skin, the sclera of the eyes and the mucous membranes should be evaluated for jaundice because they reflect the integumentary changes more accurately, especially in dark-skinned individuals. The pathogenesis of *pruritus* is poorly understood but has been reported with iron-deficiency anemia.

Cardiopulmonary Manifestations

Cardiopulmonary manifestations of severe anemia result from additional attempts by the heart and lungs to provide adequate

TABLE 33.1	RELATIONSHIP OF MORPHOLOGICAL CLASSIFICATION AND ETIOLOGIES OF ANEMIA	
Morphology	**Etiology**
Normocytic, normochromic (normal size and colour) MCV 80–100 fL, MCH 27–34 pg	Acute blood loss, hemolysis, chronic renal disease, chronic disease, cancers, aplastic anemia, endocrine disorders, sickle cell anemia, pregnancy, starvation
Macrocytic (megaloblastic), normochromic (large size, normal colour) MCV >100 fL, MCH >34 pg	Vitamin B_{12} deficiency, folate deficiency, liver disease (including effects of alcohol use disorder)
Microcytic, hypochromic (small size, pale colour) MCV <80 fL, MCH <27 pg	Iron-deficiency anemia, vitamin B_6 deficiency, copper deficiency, thalassemia, lead poisoning

DNA, deoxyribonucleic acid; *MCH,* mean corpuscular hemoglobin; *MCV,* mean corpuscular volume.

TABLE 33.2	ETIOLOGICAL CLASSIFICATION OF ANEMIA

Decreased Erythrocyte Production
Decreased Hemoglobin Synthesis

- Iron deficiency
- Thalassemias (decreased globin synthesis)
- Sideroblastic anemia (decreased porphyrin)

Defective DNA Synthesis
- Cobalamin (vitamin B_{12}) deficiency
- Folic acid deficiency

Decreased Number of Erythrocyte Precursors
- Aplastic anemia and inherited disorders (e.g., Fanconi syndrome)
- Anemia of myeloproliferative disorders and myelodysplasia
- Chronic diseases or disorders
- Medications (e.g., chemotherapy)
- Radiation

Blood Loss
Acute
- Trauma
- Blood vessel rupture
- Splenic sequestration crisis

Chronic
- Gastritis
- Menstrual flow
- Hemorrhoids

Increased Erythrocyte Destruction
Intrinsic
- Abnormal hemoglobin (e.g., sickle cell disease)
- Enzyme deficiency (G6PD)
- Membrane abnormalities (paroxysmal nocturnal hemoglobinuria, hereditary spherocytosis)

Extrinsic
- Physical trauma (prosthetic heart valves, extracorporeal circulation)
- Acquired antibodies against RBCs
- Infectious agents, medications, and toxins (malaria)
- Disseminated intravascular coagulopathy (DIC)
- HELLP syndrome
- Thrombotic thrombocytopenic purpura (TTP)
- Widespread cancer

DNA, deoxyribonucleic acid; *G6PD,* glucose-6-phosphate dehydrogenase; *HELLP,* **h**emolysis, **e**levated **l**iver enzymes, **l**ow **p**latelet count; *RBCs,* red blood cells.

TABLE 33.3 MANIFESTATIONS OF ANEMIA

Body System	Severity of Anemia		
	Mild (Hb 100–120 g/L*)	Moderate (Hb 60–100 g/L*)	Severe (Hb <60 g/L*)
Integument	None	None	Pallor, jaundice,[†] pruritus[†]
Eyes	None	None	Icteric conjunctiva and sclera, retinal hemorrhage, blurred vision
Mouth	None	None	Glossitis, smooth tongue
Cardiovascular	Palpitations	Increased palpitations, "bounding pulse"	Tachycardia, increased pulse pressure, systolic murmurs, intermittent claudication, angina, HF, MI
Pulmonary	Exertional dyspnea	Dyspnea	Tachypnea, orthopnea, dyspnea at rest
Neurological	None	"Roaring in the ears"	Headache, vertigo, irritability, depression, impaired thought processes
Gastrointestinal	None	None	Anorexia, hepatomegaly, splenomegaly, difficulty swallowing, sore mouth
Musculoskeletal	None	None	Bone pain
General	None or mild	Fatigue	Sensitivity to cold, weight loss, lethargy

Hb, hemoglobin; *HF*, heart failure; *MI*, myocardial infarction.
*Applies to female values; will be slightly higher in males.
[†]Caused by hemolysis.

amounts of O_2 to the tissues. Cardiac output is maintained by increasing the heart rate and the stroke volume. The low viscosity of the blood contributes to the development of systolic murmurs and bruits. In extreme cases or when concomitant heart disease is present, angina pectoris and myocardial infarction (MI) may occur if myocardial O_2 needs cannot be met. Heart failure (HF), cardiomegaly, pulmonary and systemic congestion, ascites, and peripheral edema may develop if the heart is overworked for an extended period.

NURSING MANAGEMENT
ANEMIA

This section discusses general nursing management of anemia. Specific care related to various types of anemia is discussed later in this chapter.

NURSING ASSESSMENT
Subjective and objective data that should be obtained from a patient with anemia are presented in Table 33.4.

NURSING DIAGNOSES
Nursing diagnoses for the patient with anemia include but are not limited to those presented in Nursing Care Plan (NCP) 33.1.

PLANNING
The overall goals are that the patient with anemia will (a) assume normal activities of daily living, (b) maintain adequate nutrition, and (c) develop no complications related to anemia.

NURSING IMPLEMENTATION
The numerous causes of anemia necessitate different nursing interventions specific to the needs of the patient. Nevertheless, there are certain general components of care for all patients with anemia; these are presented in NCP 33.1.

Correcting the cause of anemia is ultimately the goal of therapy. Acute interventions may include blood or blood product transfusions, medication therapy, volume replacement, and O_2 therapy to stabilize the patient. Dietary and lifestyle changes can reverse some types of anemias. The plan of care should include an ongoing assessment of the patient's knowledge regarding adequate

nutritional intake and medication therapies and of the patient's adherence to safety precautions to prevent falls and injury.

AGE-RELATED CONSIDERATIONS
ANEMIA
Modest changes in RBC mass occur in older persons. In healthy older men, a decline in Hb of about 10 g/L between ages 70 and 88 years is common, in part because of the decreased production of androgens. Only a minimal decrease in Hb occurs between these ages in healthy women (≈2 g/L) (Hoffman et al., 2018).

Anemia is not a normal finding in older persons. However, its prevalence increases starting from the seventh decade of life. For many older people, anemia is related to an underlying cause such as iron or folate deficiency, bleeding, cancer, chronic disease or inflammation, renal insufficiency, or a hematological disorder. For persons with no identifiable cause, it may be due to cytokine dysregulation with aging (Lichtman et al., 2017).

Manifestations of anemia in the older person may include pallor, confusion, ataxia, fatigue, and worsening cardiovascular and respiratory conditions. Unfortunately, anemia may go unrecognized in the older person because these manifestations may be mistaken as normal aging changes or be overlooked because of another health condition. By recognizing signs of anemia, the nurse can play a pivotal role in appropriate health assessment and related interventions for older persons.

ANEMIA CAUSED BY DECREASED ERYTHROCYTE PRODUCTION

Normally, RBC production (termed *erythropoiesis*) is in equilibrium with RBC destruction and loss. This balance ensures that an adequate number of erythrocytes are available at all times. The normal lifespan of an RBC is 120 days. Three alterations in erythropoiesis may occur that decrease RBC production: (1) decreased Hb synthesis may lead to iron-deficiency anemia, thalassemia, and sideroblastic anemia; (2) defective deoxyribonucleic acid (DNA) synthesis in RBCs (e.g., cobalamin or folic acid deficiency) may lead to megaloblastic anemias; and (3) diminished availability of erythrocyte precursors may result in aplastic anemia and anemia of chronic disease (see Table 33.2).

TABLE 33.4   NURSING ASSESSMENT

Anemia

Subjective Data

Important Health Information

Past health history: Recent blood loss or trauma; chronic liver, endocrine, or renal disease (including dialysis); GI disease (e.g., malabsorption syndrome, ulcers, gastritis, or hemorrhoids); inflammatory disorders (especially Crohn's disease); smoking, exposure to radiation or chemical toxins (arsenic, lead, benzenes, copper); infectious disease (e.g., HIV) or recent travel suggesting exposure to infection; angina, myocardial infarction; history of falling

Medications: Use of vitamin and iron supplements, acetylsalicylic acid (ASA), anticoagulants, oral contraceptives, phenobarbital, penicillins, nonsteroidal anti-inflammatory medications, phenacetin, omeprazole, phenytoin (Dilantin), sulfonamides, herbal products, cannabis

Surgery or other treatments: Recent surgery, small bowel resection, gastrectomy, prosthetic heart valves, chemotherapy, radiation therapy

Dietary history: General dietary patterns, alcohol consumption

Symptoms

- Nausea, vomiting, anorexia, dysphagia, dyspepsia, heartburn, painful tongue
- Night sweats, cold intolerance, weight loss, pruritus, pain
- Hematuria, decreased urinary output, diarrhea, constipation, flatulence, tarry stools, bloody stools
- Fatigue, muscle weakness, and decreased strength
- Dyspnea, orthopnea, cough, hemoptysis, palpitations, shortness of breath with activity
- Headache; paresthesias of feet and hands; disturbances in vision, taste, or hearing; vertigo
- Menorrhagia, metrorrhagia; recent or current pregnancy in women; male impotence

Objective Data

General

Lethargy, apathy, general lymphadenopathy, fever

Integumentary

Pale skin and mucous membranes; blue, pale white, icteric sclera; cheilitis (inflammation of the lips); poor skin turgor; brittle, spoon-shaped fingernails; jaundice; petechiae; ecchymoses; nose or gingival bleeding; poor healing; dry, brittle, thinning hair

Respiratory

Tachypnea

Cardiovascular

Tachycardia, systolic murmur, dysrhythmias; postural hypotension, widened pulse pressure, bruits (especially carotid); intermittent claudication, ankle edema

Gastrointestinal

Hepatosplenomegaly; glossitis; beefy, red tongue; stomatitis; abdominal distension; anorexia

Neurological

Headache, roaring in the ears, confusion, impaired judgement, irritability, ataxia, unsteady gait, paralysis, loss of vibration sense

Possible Diagnostic Findings

↓ RBCs; ↓ Hb; ↓ Hct; ↓ or ↑ reticulocytes, MCV; ↓ serum iron, ferritin, folate, or cobalamin (vitamin B_{12}); heme-positive stools; ↓ serum erythropoietin level; ↓ or ↑ LDH, bilirubin, transferrin (see Table 33.6)

GI, gastrointestinal; *Hb,* hemoglobin; *Hct,* hematocrit; *HIV,* human immunodeficiency virus; *LDH,* lactate dehydrogenase; *MCV,* mean corpuscular volume; *RBCs,* red blood cells.

IRON-DEFICIENCY ANEMIA

Iron-deficiency anemia is the most common nutritional disorder in the world. It is a subtype of an anemia caused by decreased RBC production. It is a microcytic hypochromic anemia caused by inadequate supplies of the iron needed to synthesize Hb.

People most susceptible to iron-deficiency anemia are the very young, those with nutritionally inadequate diets, and women in their reproductive years (Camaschella, 2019). Among the Indigenous population it is very important to consider social determinants of health when looking at causative factors of iron deficiency anemia (Kenny et al., 2019).

Etiology

Iron deficiency may develop from inadequate dietary intake, malabsorption, blood loss, or hemolysis. Iron is obtained from food and dietary supplements. Dietary iron is usually adequate to meet the needs of men and older women, but it may be inadequate for individuals with higher iron needs (e.g., menstruating or pregnant women). Table 33.5 lists nutrients needed for erythropoiesis. Iron malabsorption may occur after certain types of gastrointestinal (GI) surgery and in malabsorption syndromes. Iron absorption occurs primarily in the duodenum. Consequently, surgical procedures that involve removal or bypass of the duodenum may result in malabsorption. Malabsorption syndromes may also occur if disease of the duodenum alters or destroys the absorption surface.

Blood loss is a major cause of iron deficiency in adults. The major sources of chronic blood loss are from the GI and genitourinary (GU) systems. GI bleeding is often not obvious and, therefore, may be present for a considerable period of time before the disorder is identified. Loss of 50 to 75 mL of blood from the upper GI tract is required for stools to appear black *(melena).* The black colour results from the iron in the RBCs.

Common causes of GI blood loss are peptic ulcer, gastritis, esophagitis, diverticula, hemorrhoids, and neoplasia. GU blood loss occurs primarily from menstrual bleeding. The average monthly menstrual blood loss is about 45 mL and causes the loss of about 22 mg of iron. Pregnancy also contributes to iron deficiency because of the diversion of iron to the fetus for erythropoiesis, blood loss at delivery, and lactation (Tang et al., 2019). Chronic kidney disease can lead to anemia; dialysis treatment may also cause iron-deficiency anemia because of the blood lost in the dialysis equipment and frequent blood sampling.

Clinical Manifestations

In the early course of iron-deficiency anemia, the patient may be symptom free. As the disease becomes chronic, any of the general manifestations of anemia may develop (see Table 33.3). In addition, specific clinical symptoms may occur related to iron-deficiency anemia. Pallor is the most common finding, and *glossitis* (inflammation of the tongue) is the second most common; another finding is *cheilitis* (inflammation of the lips). In addition, the patient may report headache, paresthesias, and a burning sensation of the tongue, all of which are caused by a lack of iron in the tissues.

Diagnostic Studies

Iron-deficiency anemia will lead to a number of characteristic laboratory abnormalities, shown in Table 33.6. Other diagnostic studies are done to determine the cause of the iron deficiency (e.g., stool occult blood test). Endoscopy and colonoscopy may be used to detect GI bleeding. A bone marrow biopsy may be done if other tests are inconclusive.

Interprofessional Care

The main goal of the interprofessional care of iron-deficiency anemia is to treat the underlying disease that is causing iron loss or reduced intake (e.g., malnutrition, alcoholism) or poor absorption of iron. In addition, efforts are directed toward

NURSING CARE PLAN 33.1

Anemia

NURSING DIAGNOSIS	**Fatigue** resulting from *anemia (inadequate oxygenation of the blood)* as evidenced by insufficient energy, *increase in physical symptoms* (pulse rate and blood pressure)

Expected Patient Outcomes

- Participates in activities of daily living (e.g., bathing, dressing, grooming, feeding) without abnormal increases in pulse and blood pressure
- Reports increased endurance of activity

Nursing Interventions and *Rationales*

- Correct physiological status deficits (e.g., chemotherapy-induced anemia) *to help mitigate the underlying cause of anemia.*
- Encourage alternate periods of rest and activity *to provide activity without tiring the patient.*
- Monitor cardiorespiratory response to activity (e.g., tachycardia, dysrhythmias, dyspnea, diaphoresis, pallor, respiratory rate) *to evaluate activity intolerance.*
- Limit environmental stimuli *to reduce demands placed on patient.*
- Assist patient in assigning priority to activities *to accommodate energy levels for important activities.*
- Arrange physical activities (e.g., avoid activity immediately after meals) *to reduce competition for O_2 supply to vital body functions.*
- Assist with regular physical activities (e.g., ambulation, transfers, turning, personal care) *to minimize fatigue and risk for injury from falls.*
- Instruct patient, caregiver(s), and family member(s) to recognize signs and symptoms of fatigue that require reduction in activity *to promote self-care.*
- Instruct patient, caregiver(s), and family member(s) to notify health care provider if signs and symptoms of fatigue persist *to review treatment plan.*

NURSING DIAGNOSIS	**Imbalanced nutrition: less than body requirements** resulting from insufficient dietary intake as evidenced by insufficient interest in food, inability to absorb nutrients

Expected Patient Outcomes

- Maintains dietary intake that provides minimum daily requirements of nutrients
- Experiences normal blood values of nutrients necessary to prevent anemia

Nursing Interventions and *Rationales*

- Determine, in collaboration with dietitian, number of calories and type of nutrients needed to meet nutritional requirements *to plan interventions.*
- Teach patient how to use a food diary *to help evaluate nutritional intake.*
- Monitor recorded intake for nutritional content and calories *to evaluate nutritional status.*
- Instruct patient about nutritional needs (i.e., encourage increased intake of protein, iron, vitamin C) *to help ensure patient gets nutrients needed for maximum iron absorption and hemoglobin production.*
- Adjust diet, as necessary, *to adapt to changes in nutritional requirements.*

NURSING DIAGNOSIS	**Inadequate health management** as a result of insufficient knowledge of therapeutic regimen as evidenced by difficulty with prescribed regimen

Expected Patient Outcomes

- Verbalizes knowledge necessary to maintain adequate nutrition and management of medication regimen

Nursing Interventions and *Rationales*

Nutritional Counselling
- Facilitate identification of eating behaviours to be changed.
- Use accepted nutritional standards *to assist patient in evaluating adequacy of dietary intake.*
- Discuss nutritional requirements and patient's perceptions of prescribed or recommended diet.
- Provide referral or consultation with other members of the health care team *to help patient achieve goals and make adjustments throughout recovery.*
- Review with patient measurements of hemoglobin values *to evaluate response to therapeutic plan.*

Teaching: Prescribed Medication
- Instruct patient on the purpose and action of each medication.
- Instruct patient on dosage, route, and duration of each medication *to improve adherence.*
- Instruct patient on possible adverse effects of each medication *to ensure early detection of adverse responses to medication.*

replacing iron (Table 33.7). The patient should be taught which foods are good sources of iron (see Table 33.5). If nutrition is already adequate, increasing iron intake by dietary means may not be practical. Consequently, oral or parenteral iron supplements may be recommended. If the iron deficiency is from acute blood loss, the patient may require a transfusion of packed RBCs.

Medication Therapy. Oral iron should be used whenever possible because it is inexpensive and convenient. Many iron preparations are available. When giving iron, consider the following factors:

1. Iron is absorbed best from the duodenum and the proximal jejunum. Therefore, enteric-coated or sustained-release capsules, which release iron farther down in the GI tract, are counterproductive.

2. The daily dosage should provide 150 to 200 mg of elemental iron. This can be taken in three or four daily doses, with each tablet or capsule of the iron preparation containing between 50 and 100 mg of iron. Common iron preparations and amounts of elemental iron are provided in Table 33.8.

3. Iron is best absorbed in an acidic environment. For this reason and to avoid binding the iron with food, iron should be taken about an hour before meals, when the duodenal mucosa is most acidic. Taking iron with vitamin C (ascorbic acid) or orange juice, which contains ascorbic acid, also enhances iron absorption. GI adverse effects such as nausea, however, may necessitate ingesting iron with meals.

4. Undiluted liquid iron may stain the patient's teeth; therefore, it should be diluted and ingested through a straw.

TABLE 33.5   NUTRITIONAL THERAPY
Nutrients Needed for Erythropoiesis

Nutrient	Role in Erythropoiesis	Food Sources
Amino acids (protein)	Hemoglobin and plasma membrane synthesis and structure	Eggs, meat, milk and milk products, poultry, fish, legumes, nuts, soy
Cobalamin (vitamin B$_{12}$)	Synthesis of DNA, RBC maturation, facilitates folate metabolism	Red meats (especially liver), eggs, enriched grain products, milk and dairy, fish, fortified rice and soy beverages
Copper	Mobilization of iron from tissues to plasma	Shellfish, whole grains, beans, nuts, potatoes, organ meats, sesame seeds, kale, fermented soy foods, dried fruits
Folic acid	Synthesis of DNA and RNA, RBC maturation	Leafy green vegetables, okra, liver, meat, fish, legumes, whole grains, orange juice, peanuts, avocado, lentils
Iron	Hemoglobin synthesis	Liver and muscle meats, eggs, dried fruits, legumes, leafy dark-green vegetables, whole-grain and enriched bread and cereals, beans, soy
Niacin (vitamin B$_3$)	RBC maturation	Peanut butter, beans, meats, avocado, enriched and fortified grains, yeast extract
Pantothenic acid (vitamin B$_5$)	Hemoglobin synthesis	Meats, leafy green vegetables, cereal grains, legumes, eggs, milk, mushrooms
Pyridoxine (vitamin B$_6$)	Hemoglobin synthesis	Meats, wheat germ, legumes, potatoes, cornmeal, bananas, nuts, fish (salmon, sardines)
Riboflavin (vitamin B$_2$)	Oxidative reactions	Dairy, enriched bread, salmon, chicken, eggs, leafy green vegetables
Vitamin C (ascorbic acid)	Conversion of folic acid to its active forms; aids in iron absorption	Citrus fruits, leafy green vegetables, strawberries, cantaloupe, kiwi, chili peppers
Vitamin E	Hemoglobin synthesis	Vegetable oils, meat, eggs, wheat germ, whole-grain products*, seeds, nuts (pine nuts, almond butter), fish (salmon, eel)

RBC, red blood cell.

*A variety of healthy food choices such as different types of whole-grain products can be found in *Canada's Food Guide,* available at https://food-guide.canada.ca.

5. GI adverse effects of iron administration may occur, including heartburn, constipation, and diarrhea. The patient should stay upright for 30 minutes after taking oral forms. If adverse side effects develop, the dosage and type of iron supplement may be adjusted. For example, many individuals who need supplemental iron cannot tolerate ferrous sulphate because of the effects of the sulphate base. However, ferrous gluconate may be an acceptable substitute. All patients should know that the use of iron preparations will cause their stools to become black because the GI tract excretes excess iron. Constipation is also common, so patients should be started on stool softeners and laxatives, if needed, when taking iron.

MEDICATION ALERT—Iron

- Some preparations of intravenous iron have a risk of allergic reaction; the patient should be monitored accordingly.
- Oral iron should be taken about 1 hour before meals.
- Vitamin C (ascorbic acid) enhances iron absorption.

In some situations, it may be necessary to administer iron parenterally. Parenteral use of iron is indicated for malabsorption, intolerance of oral iron, a need for iron beyond oral-intake limits, or patient nonadherence in taking the oral preparations of iron. Parenteral iron may be given intramuscularly or intravenously. Because intramuscular (IM) iron solutions may stain the skin, separate needles should be used for drawing up the solution and for injecting the medication. A Z-track injection technique should be used.

NURSING MANAGEMENT IRON-DEFICIENCY ANEMIA

Certain groups of individuals are at an increased risk for the development of iron-deficiency anemia. These include premenopausal and pregnant women, persons from low socioeconomic backgrounds, older persons, and individuals experiencing blood loss. Nutritional education, with an emphasis on foods high in iron and on ways to maximize absorption, is important for these groups, as is adherence to both dietary and medication therapy. The patient should be informed of the need for diagnostic studies to identify the underlying cause, and the Hb and RBC counts should be reassessed periodically to evaluate the response to therapy. To replenish the body's iron stores, the patient needs to continue to take iron therapy for 2 to 3 months after the Hb level returns to normal. Patients who require lifelong iron supplementation should be monitored for potential

TABLE 33.6   LABORATORY RESULTS IN ANEMIA

Etiology of Anemia	Hb/Hct	MCV	Reticulocytes	Serum Iron	TIBC	Transferrin	Ferritin	Bilirubin	Serum B$_{12}$	Folate
Acute blood loss	↓	N or ↓	N or ↑	N	N	N	N	N	N	N
Aplastic anemia	↓	N or slight ↑	↓	N or ↑	N or ↑	N	N	N	N	N
Chronic blood loss	↓	↓	N or ↑	↓	↓	N	N	N or ↓	N	N
Chronic disease	↓	N or ↓	N or ↓	N or ↓	↓	N or ↓	N or ↑	N	N	N
Cobalamin deficiency	↓	↑	N or ↓	N or ↑	N	Slight ↑	↑	N or slight ↑	↓	N
Folic acid deficiency	↓	↑	N or ↓	N or ↑	N	Slight ↑	↑	N or slight ↑	N	↓
Hemolytic anemia	↓	N or ↑	↑	N or ↑	N or ↓	N	N or ↑	↑	N	N
Iron deficiency	↓	↓	N or slight ↓ or ↑	↓	↑	N or ↓	↓	N or ↓	N	N
Sickle cell anemia	↓	N	↓	N or ↑	N or ↓	N	N	↑	N	↓
Thalassemia major	↓	N or ↓	↑	↑	↓	↓	N or ↑	↑	N	↓

Hb, hemoglobin; *Hct,* hematocrit; *MCV,* mean corpuscular volume; *N,* normal; *TIBC,* total iron-binding capacity.

TABLE 33.7   INTERPROFESSIONAL CARE
Iron-Deficiency Anemia

Diagnostic	Therapy
• History and physical examination	• Identification and treatment of underlying cause
• Hct and Hb levels	• Medication therapy
• RBC count, including morphology	• Oral: ferrous sulphate or ferrous gluconate
• Reticulocyte count	• IM or IV: iron dextran, iron sucrose, sodium ferric gluconate (Ferrlecit)
• Serum iron	
• Serum ferritin	
• Serum transferrin	• Nutritional therapy (see Table 33.5)
• TIBC	• Transfusion of packed RBCs
• Stool examination for occult blood	

Hb, hemoglobin; *Hct*, hematocrit; *IM*, intramuscular; *IV*, intravenous; *RBC*, red blood cell; *TIBC*, total iron-building capacity.

TABLE 33.8   COMMON IRON PREPARATIONS AND ELEMENTAL IRON PROVIDED

Iron Preparation	Amount of Elemental Iron (mg)
Ferrous sulphate (300-mg tablet)	60
Ferrous gluconate (300-mg tablet)	35
Ferrous fumarate (300-mg tablet)	100
Polysaccharide iron complex	150

Source: Adapted from Alberta Doctors Organization. (2018). *Iron deficiency anemia (IDA): Clinical practice guidelines.* https://actt.albertadoctors.org/download/2256/IDA%20cpg.pdf?_20180409163326

liver conditions related to the iron storage. Appropriate nursing measures are presented in NCP 33.1.

THALASSEMIA

Etiology

Thalassemia is a group of diseases involving inadequate production of normal Hb and, therefore, decreased RBC production. Thalassemia is caused by an absent or reduced globulin protein. Alpha-globulin chains are absent or reduced in alpha thalassemia, and beta-globin chains are absent or reduced in beta thalassemia. Hemolysis also occurs in thalassemia, but insufficient production of normal Hb is the predominant issue. Thalassemia is commonly found in members of ethnic groups whose origins are near the Mediterranean Sea and equatorial or near-equatorial regions of Southeastern Asia, the Middle East, India, Pakistan, China, Southern Russia, and Africa. The prevalence of thalassemia in the Canada is not known but is thought to be increasing, likely due to immigration patterns.

Thalassemia has an autosomal recessive genetic basis. An individual with thalassemia may have a heterozygous or homozygous form of the disease. A person who is heterozygous has one thalassemic gene and one normal gene and is said to have *thalassemia minor* (or *thalassemic trait*), a mild form of the disease. A homozygous person has two thalassemic genes, causing a severe condition known as *thalassemia major* (Angastiniotis & Lobitz, 2019).

Clinical Manifestations

Thalassemia minor is frequently asymptomatic. A person with thalassemia minor may exhibit mild to moderate anemia with microcytosis (small RBCs), hypochromia (pale cells), mild splenomegaly, bronze-coloured skin, and bone marrow hyperplasia.

Thalassemia major is a life-threatening disease in which growth, both physical and mental, is often affected. A person who has thalassemia major may be pale and display other general symptoms of anemia (see Table 33.3). Symptoms often develop by 2 years of age. In addition, pronounced splenomegaly may be noted as the spleen continuously tries to remove the damaged RBCs. Jaundice from RBC hemolysis is prominent. Hepatomegaly and cardiomyopathy may occur from iron deposition. As the bone marrow responds to the reduced O$_2$-carrying capacity of the blood, RBC production is stimulated and the marrow becomes packed with immature erythroid precursors that die. The death of these erythroid precursors stimulates further erythropoiesis, leading to chronic bone marrow hyperplasia and expansion of the marrow space. This expansion may cause thickening of the cranium and the maxillary cavity. Other complications of the disease include endocrinopathies, lung disease, osteoporosis, and thromboses.

Interprofessional Care

The laboratory abnormalities of thalassemia major are summarized in Table 33.6. No specific medication or diet therapies are effective in treating thalassemia. Thalassemia minor requires no treatment because the body adapts to the reduction of normal Hb; however, genetic counselling is advised.

Thalassemia major is managed with blood transfusions in conjunction with chelating agents that bind to iron. Transfusions are administered to keep the Hb level at approximately 100 g/L in order to foster the patient's own erythropoiesis without enlarging the spleen. Chelating agents reduce the iron overloading that occurs with chronic transfusion therapy. Medications used include oral deferasirox (Exjade) or deferiprone (Ferriprox) or intravenous (IV) or subcutaneous deferoxamine (Desferal). During chelation therapy, ascorbic acid supplementation may be used to increase urine excretion of iron; ascorbic acid should not otherwise be taken because it increases the absorption of dietary iron. Zinc supplementation may be needed with transfusion therapy, though supplement amounts are reduced with chelation therapy. Regular folic acid may be given if the patient's diet is poor. Iron supplements should not be given.

Although hematopoietic stem cell transplantation (HSCT) is the only cure for thalassemia, issues such as the risk of the procedure, donor availability, and access make HSCT a reasonable option for only a small number of patients. Regular transfusions and proper iron chelation therapy remain the mainstay of therapy for thalassemia major.

There are also biological and genetic factors (see the Determinants of Health box) that should be considered when caring for a patient with anemia.

MEGALOBLASTIC ANEMIAS

Megaloblastic anemias are a group of disorders caused by impaired DNA synthesis and characterized by the presence of large RBCs. When DNA synthesis is impaired, defective RBC maturation results. The RBCs are abnormal, large (macrocytic), and referred to as *megaloblasts*. Macrocytic RBCs are easily destroyed because they have fragile cell membranes. Although the overwhelming majority of megaloblastic anemias result from cobalamin (vitamin B$_{12}$) and folic acid deficiencies, this type of RBC deformity can also occur from suppression of DNA

TABLE 33.9	CLASSIFICATION OF MEGALOBLASTIC ANEMIA	
Cobalamin (Vitamin B$_{12}$) Deficiency	**Medication-Induced Suppression of DNA Synthesis**
• Chronic alcoholism • Dietary deficiency • Deficiency of gastric intrinsic factor • Celiac disease • Gastrectomy • Gastric bypass • *Helicobacter pylori* • Pernicious anemia • Increased requirement (pregnancy) • Intestinal malabsorption	• Alkylating agents • Folate antagonists • Metabolic inhibitors **Inborn Errors** • Defective folate metabolism • Defective transport of cobalamin **Erythroleukemia**
Folic Acid Deficiency	

• Chronic alcoholism
• Chronic hemodialysis (folic acid lost during dialysis)
• Dietary deficiency (e.g., leafy green vegetables, citrus fruits)
• Medications interfering with absorption or use of folic acid
  • Methotrexate
  • Antiseizure medications (e.g., phenobarbital, phenytoin [Dilantin])
• Increased requirement (pregnancy)
• Malabsorption syndromes
  • Celiac disease
  • Crohn's disease
  • Small bowel resection	

synthesis by medications, inborn errors of cobalamin and folic acid metabolism, and *erythroleukemia* (a malignant blood disorder characterized by a proliferation of erythropoietic cells in bone marrow) (Table 33.9).

Cobalamin Deficiency

The most common cause of cobalamin deficiency is pernicious anemia, which is caused by an absence of intrinsic factor (IF). Pernicious anemia is a disease of insidious onset that begins in middle age or later (usually after age 40), with 60 years being the most common age at diagnosis. Pernicious anemia occurs frequently in people of African or Northern European ancestry (particularly Scandinavians).

Etiology

Normally, a protein termed *intrinsic factor* (IF) is secreted by the parietal cells of the gastric mucosa. IF is required for cobalamin (vitamin B$_{12}$) absorption. Cobalamin is normally absorbed in the distal ileum and if IF is not secreted, cobalamin will not be absorbed. In pernicious anemia, the gastric mucosa does not secrete IF because of either gastric mucosal atrophy or autoimmune destruction of parietal cells and possibly also because of IF itself.

Cobalamin deficiency can also occur in patients who have had GI surgery such as gastrectomy or gastric bypass; patients who have had a small bowel resection involving the ileum; and patients with Crohn's disease, ileitis, celiac disease, diverticulitis of the small intestine, chronic atrophic gastritis, or a combination of these. In these cases, cobalamin deficiency results from the loss of IF-secreting gastric mucosal cells or impaired absorption of cobalamin in the distal ileum. Cobalamin deficiency is also found in long-term users of histamine (H$_2$)-receptor blockers and proton pump inhibitors and in strict vegetarians (Wolffenbuttel et al., 2019).

Clinical Manifestations

General symptoms of anemia related to cobalamin deficiency develop because of tissue hypoxia (see Table 33.3). GI manifestations include a sore, red, shiny tongue; anorexia; nausea; vomiting; and abdominal pain. Neurological manifestations of cobalamin deficiency are not related to hypoxia but are due to progressive demyelination of nerve fibers. Symptoms may include weakness, paresthesias of the feet and hands, reduced vibratory and position senses, ataxia, muscle weakness, and impaired thought processes ranging from confusion to dementia. Because cobalamin deficiency–related anemia has an insidious onset, it may take several months for these manifestations to develop.

Diagnostic Studies

Laboratory data reflective of cobalamin-deficiency anemia are presented in Table 33.6. The RBCs appear large (macrocytic) and have abnormal shapes. This structure contributes to erythrocyte destruction because the cell membrane is fragile. Serum cobalamin levels are reduced. It is important also to know serum folate levels, because if they are normal and cobalamin levels are low, it suggests that megaloblastic anemia is caused by a cobalamin deficiency. A serum test for anti-IF antibodies may be done that is specific for pernicious anemia. Because the potential for gastric cancer is increased in patients with pernicious anemia, a gastroscopy and biopsy of the gastric mucosa may also be done. Testing of serum methylmalonic acid (MMA) (high in cobalamin deficiency) and serum homocysteine (high in both cobalamin and folic acid deficiencies) helps determine the cause of the anemia.

Interprofessional Care

If IF is lacking or if absorption in the ileum is impaired, the patient will not be able to absorb cobalamin regardless of how much is ingested. For this reason, increasing dietary cobalamin does not correct this type of anemia. Parenteral or intranasal administration of cobalamin (cyanocobalamin or hydroxocobalamin) is the treatment of choice. Without cobalamin administration, the patient will die in 1 to 3 years. A typical treatment schedule consists of 1 000 mcg/day of cobalamin IM for 2 weeks and then weekly until the Hb is normal, and then monthly for life. High-dose oral cobalamin and sublingual cobalamin are also available for those whose GI absorption is intact. As long as supplemental cobalamin is used, the anemia can be reversed. However, long-standing neuromuscular complications that a patient has experienced due to cobalamin deficiency may not be reversible.

Folic Acid Deficiency

Folic acid (folate) deficiency also causes megaloblastic anemia. Folic acid is required for DNA synthesis leading to RBC formation and maturation. Common causes of folic acid deficiency are listed in Table 33.9.

The clinical manifestations of folic acid deficiency are similar to those of cobalamin deficiency. The disease develops insidiously, and the patient's symptoms may be attributed to other, coexisting conditions such as cirrhosis or esophageal varices. GI conditions may include stomatitis, cheilosis, dysphagia, flatulence, and diarrhea. The absence of neurological issues is an important diagnostic finding and may help differentiate folic acid deficiency from cobalamin deficiency.

The diagnostic findings for folic acid deficiency are presented in Table 33.6. In addition, the serum folate level is low (normal is 11–57 mmol/L), and the serum cobalamin level is normal. Folic acid deficiency is treated by replacement therapy. The usual dose is 1 mg/day by mouth. The patient with malabsorption or chronic alcoholism may need up to 5 mg/day. The duration of treatment depends on the reason for the deficiency. In addition to supplements, the patient should be encouraged to eat foods containing large amounts of folic acid (see Table 33.5).

NURSING MANAGEMENT MEGALOBLASTIC ANEMIA

Because there is a familial predisposition for pernicious anemia (the most common type of cobalamin deficiency), patients with a positive family history of pernicious anemia should be evaluated for symptoms. Although disease development cannot be prevented, early detection and treatment can help reverse symptoms more easily.

The nursing measures presented in NCP 33.1 for the patient with anemia are appropriate for the patient with cobalamin-deficiency anemia. In addition to these measures, the nurse should ensure protection against injuries such as falls, burns, and trauma because the patient will have diminished sensations to heat and pain resulting from the neurological impairment. If heat therapy is required, the patient's skin must be evaluated at frequent intervals to detect redness.

Ongoing care is focused on ensuring patient adherence to treatment. There must also be careful follow-up to assess for neurological difficulties that were not fully corrected by adequate cobalamin replacement therapy. Because the potential for gastric cancer may be increased in patients with atrophic gastritis–related pernicious anemia, the patient should have frequent and appropriate screening.

ANEMIA OF CHRONIC DISEASE

Anemia of chronic disease (also called *anemia of inflammation*) can be caused by cancer, autoimmune and infectious disorders, HF, or chronic inflammation. Bleeding episodes can contribute to anemia of chronic disease.

Anemia of chronic disease is associated with an underproduction of RBCs and mild shortening of RBC survival. The RBCs are usually normocytic, normochromic, and hypoproliferative. The anemia is usually mild, but it can be more severe if the underlying disorder is not treated.

This type of anemia, which usually develops after 1 to 2 months of disease activity, has an immune basis. Cytokines released with inflammatory, autoimmune, infectious, or malignant disease cause an increased uptake and retention of iron within macrophages. This leads to a diversion of iron from the circulation into storage sites and subsequent limitation of the availability of iron for erythropoiesis.

For any chronic disease, additional factors may contribute to the anemia. For example, with renal disease, the primary factor causing anemia is decreased erythropoietin, a hormone made in the kidneys that is necessary for erythropoiesis. With impaired renal function, erythropoietin production is decreased (see Chapter 49).

Anemia of chronic disease must first be recognized and differentiated from anemias of other etiologies. High serum ferritin and increased iron stores distinguish it from iron-deficiency anemia. Normal folate and cobalamin blood levels distinguish it from megaloblastic anemias secondary to folate and cobalamin deficiencies.

The best treatment of anemia of chronic disease is to correct the underlying disorder. Unless the anemia is severe, blood transfusions are rarely indicated. Erythropoietin therapy may be used for anemia related to renal disease (see Chapter 49) or anemia related to cancer therapies. However, erythropoietin therapy is used conservatively because of the increased risk for thromboembolism and mortality in some patients.

APLASTIC ANEMIA

Aplastic anemia is a disease in which the patient has peripheral blood *pancytopenia* (decrease of all blood cell types—RBCs, white blood cells [WBCs], and thrombocytes [platelets]) and hypocellular bone marrow. The spectrum of the anemia can range from a chronic condition managed with erythropoietin or blood transfusions to a critical condition with hemorrhage and sepsis. The incidence of aplastic anemia is low, with an annual rate of two to five new cases per million per year (Lichtman et al., 2017).

Etiology

About 70% of aplastic anemias are due to autoimmune activity by autoreactive T lymphocytes. The cytotoxic T cells target and destroy the patient's own hematopoietic stem cells. Other aplastic anemias may be *acquired* from toxic injury to bone marrow stem cells or result from a *congenital* stem cell defect (Table 33.10).

Clinical Manifestations

Aplastic anemia can manifest acutely (over days) or insidiously over weeks to months. It can vary from mild to severe. The patient may have symptoms caused by suppression of any

TABLE 33.10	CAUSES OF APLASTIC ANEMIA
Congenital (Chromosomal Alterations)	**Acquired**
• Fanconi's syndrome • Congenital dyskeratosis • Amegakaryocytic thrombocytopenia • Schwachman-Diamond syndrome	• Chemical agents and toxins (e.g., benzene, insecticides, arsenic) • Medications (e.g., gold, antimicrobials) • Idiopathic/autoimmune • Radiation • Viral and bacterial infections

TABLE 33.11	MANIFESTATION OF ACUTE BLOOD LOSS	
Volume Lost*		
%	**mL**	**Manifestations**
10	500	None, or rare vasovagal syncope
20	1000	No detectable signs or symptoms at rest; tachycardia with exercise and slight postural hypotension
30	1500	Normal supine blood pressure and pulse at rest; postural hypotension and tachycardia with exercise
40	2000	Blood pressure, central venous pressure, and cardiac output below normal at rest; air hunger; rapid, thready pulse and cold, clammy skin
50	2500	Shock, lactic acidosis, and potential death

*Based on an adult with a total blood volume of 5L.

or all bone marrow elements. General manifestations of anemia, such as fatigue and dyspnea, as well as cardiovascular and cerebral responses may be seen (see Table 33.3). Patients with neutropenia (low neutrophil counts) are susceptible to infection and are at risk for septic shock. Even a low-grade fever should be considered a medical emergency in neutropenic patients. Thrombocytopenia manifests as a predisposition to bleeding (e.g., petechiae, ecchymosis, epistaxis).

Diagnostic Studies

The diagnosis is confirmed by laboratory studies. Because all marrow elements are affected, Hb, WBC, and platelet values are often decreased in aplastic anemia. Other RBC indices are generally normal (see Table 33.6). The condition is therefore classified as a normocytic, normochromic anemia. The reticulocyte count is low.

Aplastic anemia can be further evaluated by assessing various iron studies. The serum iron and total iron-binding capacity (TIBC) may be elevated as indicating signs of erythropoiesis suppression. Bone marrow biopsy, aspiration, and pathological examination may be done. The marrow in aplastic anemia is hypocellular, with increased yellow marrow (fat content).

NURSING AND INTERPROFESSIONAL MANAGEMENT APLASTIC ANEMIA

Management of aplastic anemia is based on identifying and removing the causative agent (when possible) and providing supportive care until the pancytopenia reverses. Nursing interventions appropriate for the patient with pancytopenia from aplastic anemia are presented in NCP 33.1, earlier in this chapter. (See also NCP 33.2 for thrombocytopenia and NCP 33.3 for neutropenia, both available on the Evolve website.) Nursing actions are directed at preventing complications from infection and hemorrhage.

The prognosis for severe untreated aplastic anemia is poor. However, advances in medical management, including HSCT and immunosuppressive therapy with antithymocyte globulin (ATG), steroids, and cyclosporine (Neoral) or cyclophosphamide have improved outcomes significantly. ATG is a horse or rabbit serum that contains polyclonal antibodies against human T cells. The rationale for this therapy is that aplastic anemia is an immune-mediated disease resulting from the upregulation of T cells actively targeting and destroying the patient's own hematopoietic stem cells. ATG can cause anaphylaxis, but with premedications and careful infusion, most patients can complete the prescribed course of treatment.

The treatment of choice for younger adults who have a human leukocyte antigen (HLA)–matched, half-matched, or unrelated

donor is an HSCT. (HSCT is discussed in Chapter 18.) The best results occur in younger patients who have not had previous blood transfusions (Georges et al., 2018). Prior transfusions increase the risk of graft rejection.

For the older person or the patient without an HLA-matched donor, the treatment of choice is immunosuppression with ATG or cyclosporine. High-dose corticosteroids may also be used. However, this therapy may be only partially beneficial.

ANEMIA CAUSED BY BLOOD LOSS

Anemia resulting from blood loss may be caused by either acute or chronic conditions.

ACUTE BLOOD LOSS

Acute blood loss occurs as a result of sudden hemorrhage. Causes of acute blood loss include trauma, complications of surgery, and conditions or diseases that disrupt vascular integrity. There are two clinical concerns in such situations. First, a sudden reduction in the total blood volume can lead to hypovolemic shock. Second, if the acute loss is more gradual, the body maintains its blood volume by slowly increasing the plasma volume. Although the circulating fluid volume is preserved, the number of RBCs available to carry O_2 is significantly diminished.

Clinical Manifestations

The clinical manifestations of anemia from acute blood loss are caused by the body's attempts to maintain an adequate blood volume and meet O_2 requirements. Table 33.11 summarizes the clinical manifestations of patients with varying degrees of blood volume loss. It is essential to understand that the signs and symptoms that the patient is experiencing are more important than the laboratory values. For example, an adult with a bleeding peptic ulcer who had a 750-mL hematemesis (15% of a normal total blood volume) within the past 30 minutes may have postural hypotension but have normal values for Hb and Hct. Over the ensuing 36 to 48 hours, most of the volume deficit will be repaired by the movement of fluid from the extravascular into the intravascular space. Only then will the Hb and Hct reflect the blood loss.

The nurse should be alert to the patient's expression of pain when assessing for blood loss. Internal hemorrhage may cause pain because of tissue distension, organ displacement, and nerve compression. Pain may be localized or referred. In the case of retroperitoneal bleeding, for example, the patient may not experience abdominal pain. Instead, the patient may have numbness and pain in a lower extremity secondary to compression of the lateral cutaneous nerve, which is located in the region of the first to third lumbar vertebrae. The major complication of acute blood loss is shock. (Shock and its management are discussed in Chapter 69.)

Diagnostic Studies

When blood volume loss is sudden, plasma volume has not yet had a chance to increase, the loss of RBCs is not reflected in laboratory data, and values may seem normal or high for 2 to 3 days. However, once the plasma is replaced, the RBC mass is less concentrated. At this time, RBC, Hb, and Hct levels are low, reflecting the actual blood loss.

NURSING AND INTERPROFESSIONAL MANAGEMENT ACUTE BLOOD LOSS

Interprofessional care is initially concerned with (a) replacing blood volume to prevent shock and (b) identifying the source of the hemorrhage and stopping the blood loss. In order to correct volume loss, IV fluids may be used in emergencies, including isotonic crystalloid solutions such as lactated Ringer's solution or normal saline. The amount of infusion varies with the solution used. (Management of shock is discussed in Chapter 69.) Once volume replacement is established, attention can be directed to correcting the RBC loss. The body needs 2 to 5 days to manufacture more RBCs in response to increased erythropoietin. Consequently, blood transfusions (packed RBCs) may be needed if the blood loss is significant. The nursing care for the patient with anemia resulting from acute blood loss will most likely include administration of blood products (described at the end of this chapter). In addition, if the bleeding is related to a platelet or clotting disorder, replacement of that deficiency must be addressed. If a large volume of blood is lost, platelets, plasma, and possibly cryoprecipitate will also be infused, because large volumes of RBCs would dilute the patient's own coagulation system. As previously mentioned, identifying the source of hemorrhage is also very important. If the patient is postoperative, blood loss from various drainage tubes and dressings should be closely monitored and appropriate actions implemented.

The patient with acute blood loss may need supplemental iron because the availability of iron affects the marrow production of erythrocytes. When anemia exists after acute blood loss, dietary sources of iron will probably not be adequate to maintain iron stores. Therefore, oral or parenteral iron preparations are administered.

CHRONIC BLOOD LOSS

The sources of chronic blood loss are similar to those of iron-deficiency anemia (e.g., bleeding ulcer, hemorrhoids, menstrual and postmenopausal blood loss). The effects of chronic blood loss are usually related to the depletion of iron stores and are usually considered as iron-deficiency anemia. Management of chronic blood loss anemia involves identifying the source and stopping the bleeding. Supplemental iron may be required. The nursing measures presented in NCP 33.1 are relevant to anemia of chronic blood loss.

ANEMIA CAUSED BY INCREASED ERYTHROCYTE DESTRUCTION

The third major cause of anemia is termed hemolytic anemia, a condition caused by the destruction or hemolysis of RBCs at a rate that exceeds production. Hemolysis can occur because of disorders intrinsic or extrinsic to the RBCs. Intrinsic hemolytic anemias, which are usually hereditary, result from defects in the RBCs themselves. More common are the extrinsic acquired hemolytic anemias, which are acquired. In this type of anemia, the patient's RBCs are normal, but external factors are causing damage (see Table 33.2). Macrophages, particularly those in the spleen, liver, and bone marrow, destroy RBCs that are old, defective, or moderately damaged. Figure 33.1 shows the sequence of events involved in extravascular hemolysis.

The patient with hemolytic anemia manifests the general symptoms of anemia and clinical manifestations specific to this type of anemia (see Table 33.3). Jaundice is likely because the increased destruction of RBCs causes an elevation in bilirubin levels. The spleen and the liver may enlarge because of their hyperactivity, which is related to macrophage phagocytosis of the defective erythrocytes.

A major focus of treatment of hemolysis, no matter its cause, is to maintain renal function. When an RBC is hemolyzed, the Hb molecule is released and filtered by the kidneys. The accumulation of Hb molecules can obstruct the renal tubules and lead to acute tubular necrosis (see Chapter 49).

SICKLE CELL DISEASE

Sickle cell disease (SCD) is a group of inherited, autosomal recessive disorders characterized by the presence of an abnormal form of Hb in the RBC. (Autosomal recessive genetic disorders are discussed in Chapter 15.) This abnormal Hb, *hemoglobin S* (HbS), causes the erythrocyte to stiffen and elongate and take on a sickle shape in response to low levels of O_2 in the blood.

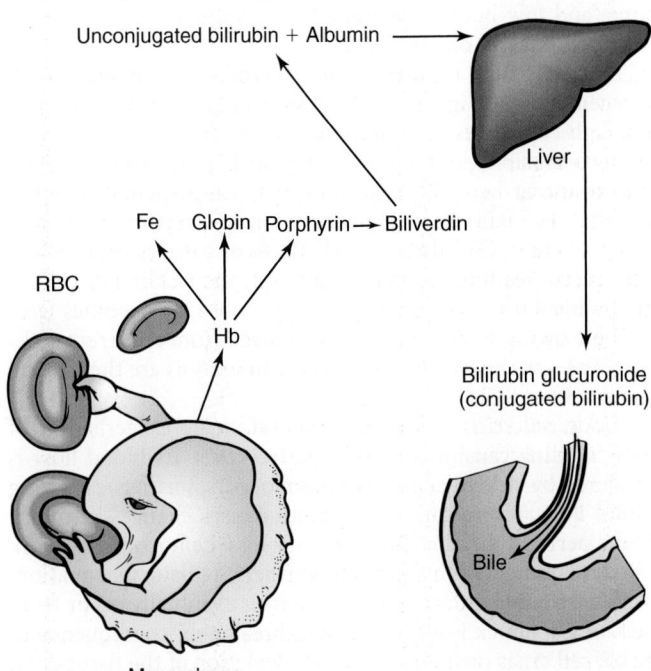

FIG. 33.1 Sequence of events in extravascular hemolysis. *Fe,* iron; *Hb,* hemoglobin; *RBC,* red blood cell.

Because it is a genetic disorder, SCD is usually identified during infancy or early childhood. The disease often results in irreversible damage of the lungs, kidneys, brain, retina, or bones that significantly affects patients' quality of life. It is an incurable disease that is often fatal by the time the affected individual reaches middle age. Death usually results from renal failure, infection, or stroke (Payne et al., 2017).

SCD is common in the African-descended population of Canada. It affects millions of people around the world, mainly those whose ancestors come from sub-Saharan Africa, Spanish-speaking regions (South America, Cuba, Central America), Saudi Arabia, India, and Mediterranean countries.

Etiology and Pathophysiology

Types of Sickle Cell Disease. Types of SCD disorders include sickle cell anemia, sickle cell–thalassemia, sickle cell–HbC disease, and sickle cell trait. *Sickle cell anemia,* the most severe of the SCD syndromes, occurs when a person is homozygous for HbS (HbSS), meaning the person has inherited HbS from both parents. *Sickle cell–thalassemia* and *sickle cell–HbC* occur when a person inherits HbS from one parent and another type of abnormal Hb (such as thalassemia or HbC) from the other parent. Both of these forms of SCD are less common and less severe than sickle cell anemia. *Sickle cell trait* occurs when a person is heterozygous for hemoglobin S (HbAS), meaning the person has inherited HbS from one parent and normal Hb (HbA) from the other parent. Sickle cell trait is typically a very mild or even asymptomatic condition.

Sickling Episodes. The major pathophysiological event of SCD is the sickling of RBCs. Sickling episodes are most commonly triggered by low O_2 tension in the blood. Hypoxia or deoxygenation of the RBCs can be caused by viral or bacterial infection, high altitude, emotional or physical stress, surgery, or blood loss. Infection is the most common precipitating factor. Other events that can trigger or sustain a sickling episode include dehydration, increased hydrogen ion concentration (*acidosis*), increased plasma osmolality, decreased plasma volume, and low body temperature. A sickling episode can also occur without an obvious cause.

Sickled RBCs become rigid and take on an elongated, crescent shape (Figure 33.2). Sickled cells cannot easily pass through capillaries or other small vessels and can cause vascular occlusion, leading to acute or chronic tissue injury. The resulting hemostasis promotes a self-perpetuating cycle of local hypoxia, deoxygenation of more erythrocytes, and more sickling. Circulating sickled cells are also hemolyzed by the spleen, leading to anemia. Initially, the sickling of cells is reversible with reoxygenation, but it eventually becomes irreversible owing to cell membrane damage from recurrent sickling. Vaso-occlusive phenomena and hemolysis are the clinical hallmarks of SCD.

Sickle cell crisis is a severe, painful, acute exacerbation of RBC sickling causing a vaso-occlusive crisis. As blood flow is impaired by sickled cells, vasospasm occurs, further restricting blood flow. Severe capillary hypoxia causes changes in membrane permeability, leading to plasma loss, hemoconcentration, the development of thrombi, and further circulatory stagnation. Tissue ischemia, infarction, and necrosis eventually occur from lack of O_2. Shock is a possible life-threatening consequence of sickle cell crisis owing to severe O_2 depletion of the tissues and a reduction of the circulating fluid volume. Sickle cell crisis can begin suddenly and persist for days to weeks.

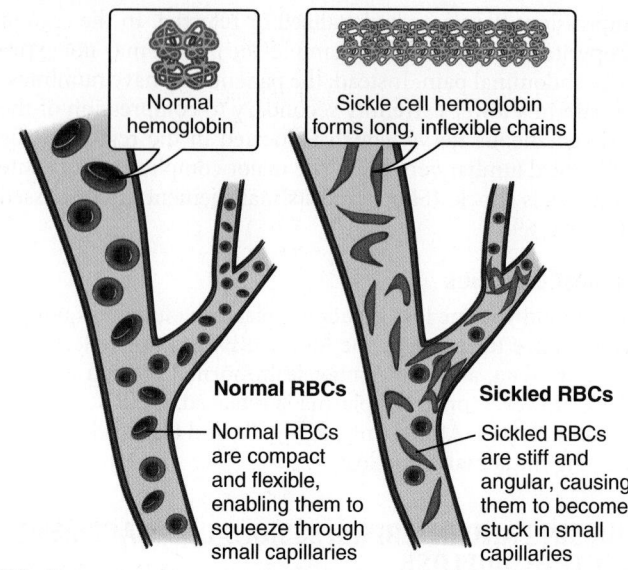

FIG. 33.2 Sickle cell hemoglobin aggregates into long chains and alters the shape of the red blood cell (RBC).

The frequency, extent, and severity of sickling episodes are highly variable and unpredictable but are largely dependent on the percentage of HbS present. Individuals with sickle cell anemia have the most severe form because the RBCs contain a high percentage of HbS.

Clinical Manifestations

The effects of SCD vary greatly from person to person, with their severity believed to result from genetic variants. Many people with sickle cell anemia are in reasonably good health most of the time. However, they may have chronic health conditions and pain because of organ tissue hypoxia and damage (e.g., involving the kidneys or liver). The typical patient is anemic but asymptomatic except during sickling episodes. Because most individuals with sickle cell anemia have dark skin, pallor is more readily detected by examining the mucous membranes. The skin may have a greyish cast. Because of the hemolysis, jaundice is common and patients are prone to gallstones (cholelithiasis).

The primary symptom associated with sickling is pain. The pain can range from mild to excruciating. The episodes can affect any area of the body or several sites simultaneously, with the back, chest, extremities, and abdomen most commonly affected. Pain episodes are often accompanied by objective clinical signs such as fever, swelling, tenderness, tachypnea, hypertension, nausea, and vomiting.

Complications

With repeated episodes of sickling, there is gradual involvement of all body systems, especially the spleen, lungs, kidneys, and brain. Organs that have a high need for O_2 are most often affected, and their involvement forms the basis for many of the complications of SCD (Figure 33.3). Infection is a major cause of morbidity and mortality in patients with SCD. One reason for this is the failure of the spleen to phagocytize foreign substances as it becomes infarcted and dysfunctional (usually by 2 to 4 years of age) from the sickled RBCs. The spleen becomes small because of repeated scarring, a phenomenon termed *autosplenectomy*.

Pneumonia is the most common infection and often is of pneumococcal origin. Infections can be severe enough to cause

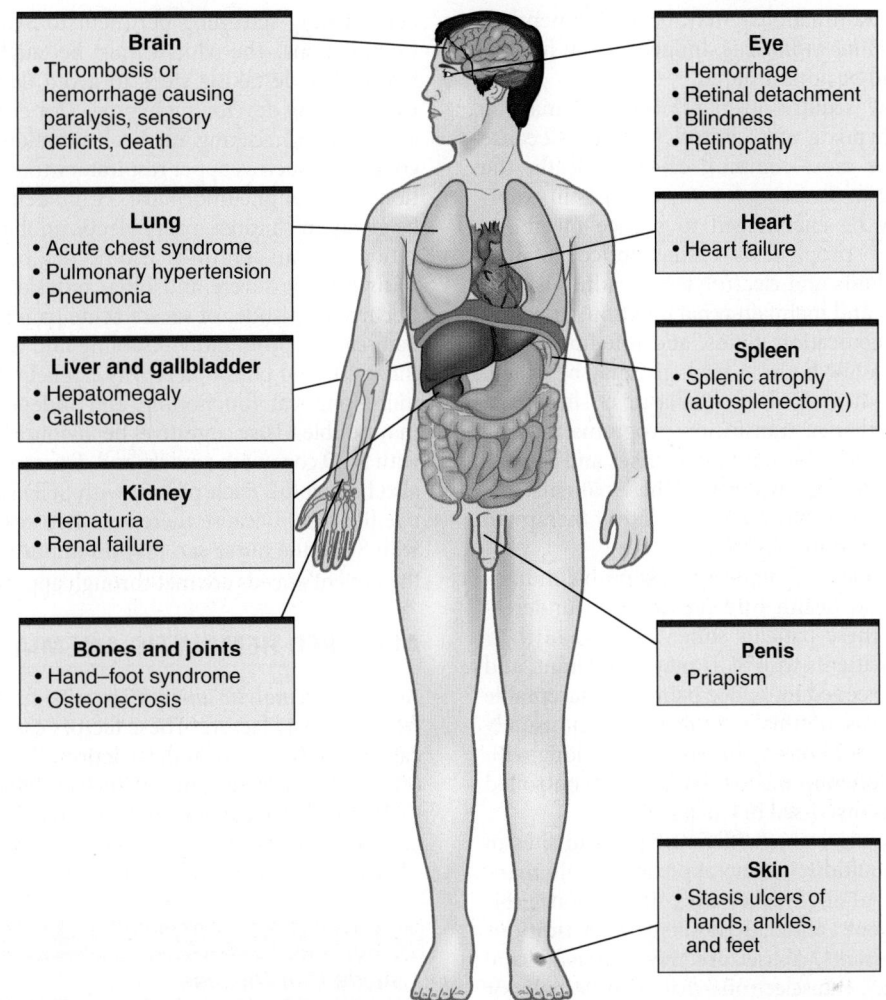

Brain
• Thrombosis or hemorrhage causing paralysis, sensory deficits, death

Lung
• Acute chest syndrome
• Pulmonary hypertension
• Pneumonia

Liver and gallbladder
• Hepatomegaly
• Gallstones

Kidney
• Hematuria
• Renal failure

Bones and joints
• Hand–foot syndrome
• Osteonecrosis

Eye
• Hemorrhage
• Retinal detachment
• Blindness
• Retinopathy

Heart
• Heart failure

Spleen
• Splenic atrophy (autosplenectomy)

Penis
• Priapism

Skin
• Stasis ulcers of hands, ankles, and feet

FIG. 33.3 Clinical manifestations and complications of sickle cell disease. Source: Modified from McCance, K.L., & Huether, S. E. (2014). *Pathophysiology: The biologic basis for disease in adults and children* (7th ed.). Mosby.

an aplastic and hemolytic crisis and gallstones. An *aplastic crisis* can be so severe as to cause a temporary shutdown of RBC production in the bone marrow.

Acute chest syndrome is a term used to describe acute pulmonary complications that include pneumonia, tissue infarction, and fat embolism. It affects 30% of patients with SCD, is characterized by fever, chest pain, cough, pulmonary infiltrates, and dyspnea, and may be life-threatening. Pulmonary infarctions may cause pulmonary hypertension, MI, HF, and ultimately cor pulmonale. The heart may become ischemic and enlarged, leading to HF. Retinal vessel obstruction may result in hemorrhage, scarring, retinal detachment, and blindness. The kidneys may be injured from the increased blood viscosity and the lack of O$_2$, which can lead to renal failure. Pulmonary embolism or stroke can result from thrombosis and infarction of blood vessels. Bone changes may include osteoporosis and osteosclerosis after infarction. Chronic leg ulcers can result from hypoxia and are especially prevalent around the ankles. *Priapism* (persistent penile erection) may occur if penile veins become occluded.

Diagnostic Studies

A peripheral blood smear may reveal sickled cells and abnormal reticulocytes. Hb electrophoresis may be done to determine the amount of HbS and other SCD variants. Because of

the accelerated RBC breakdown, the patient has characteristic findings of hemolysis (jaundice, high serum bilirubin levels) and abnormal laboratory test results. Skeletal X-rays demonstrate bone and joint deformities and flattening. Magnetic resonance imaging (MRI) can be used to diagnose a stroke caused by blocked cerebral vessels from sickled cells. Doppler studies can assess for deep-vein thrombosis (DVT). Other tests may be indicated, such as a chest X-ray, to diagnose infection or organ malfunction.

NURSING AND INTERPROFESSIONAL MANAGEMENT SICKLE CELL DISEASE

Interprofessional care for a patient with SCD is directed toward (a) preventing sequelae from the disease, (b) alleviating manifestations from the complications of the disease, (c) minimizing end–target organ damage, and (d) promptly treating serious sequelae, such as acute chest syndrome that can lead to immediate death. Patients with SCD should be taught to minimize triggers of the disease by avoiding high altitudes, avoiding extreme temperatures, minimizing stress, maintaining adequate fluid intake, and treating infections promptly. Ongoing screening is also pertinent to patients with SCD. Screening for retinopathy should begin at age 10 years. In addition, brain scans (transcranial Doppler examinations) may be recommended. Pneumococcal, *Haemophilus influenzae,* influenza, and hepatitis immunizations should be administered.

Sickle cell crises may require hospitalization. O_2 may be administered to treat hypoxia and control sickling. Because respiratory failure is the most common cause of death, the nurse should be vigilant in assessing for any changes in respiratory status. Rest may be encouraged to reduce metabolic requirements, and DVT prophylaxis (using anticoagulants) should be prescribed. Fluids and electrolytes are administered to reduce blood viscosity and maintain renal function. Priapism is managed with pain medication, fluids, and nifedipine. If it does not resolve within a few hours, a urologist may be called. Transfusion therapy is indicated when an aplastic crisis occurs; aggressive total RBC exchange transfusion programs may be implemented for patients who have frequent crises and serious complications such as acute chest syndrome. These patients, like those with thalassemia major, may require chelation therapy to reduce transfusion-produced iron overload.

Undertreatment of sickle cell pain is a major problem. Lack of understanding can lead health care providers to underestimate how much pain these patients suffer. Because of their prior opioid treatment, patients with SCD may be tolerant, and thus large doses may be needed to reduce pain to an acceptable level. During an acute crisis, optimal pain management usually includes large doses of continuous opioid analgesics along with breakthrough analgesia, often in the form of patient-controlled analgesia (PCA). (PCA is discussed in Chapter 10.)

Because patients may experience different types and sites of pain, a multimodal and multidisciplinary approach to pain management is often needed. Adjunctive measures, such as nonsteroidal anti-inflammatory agents, antineuropathic pain medications (e.g., tricyclic antidepressants, antiseizure medications), local anaesthetics, nerve blocks, transelectrodermal nerve stimulator (transcutaneous electrical nerve stimulation [TENS]), acupuncture, or some combination of these strategies may be used.

Infection is frequent complication of patients with SCD. Any febrile illness in a patient with SCD is an emergency. Infections, such as chronic leg ulcers, may be treated with rest, antibiotics, warm saline soaks, debridement, or grafting if necessary. Patients with acute chest syndrome are treated with broad-spectrum antibiotics, O_2 therapy, fluid therapy, and possibly exchange transfusion. Blood transfusions have little, if any, role in the treatment between crises because patients develop antibodies to RBCs and iron overload. However, because chronic hemolysis results in increased utilization of folic acid stores, routine folic acid supplements should be taken.

Although many antisickling medications have been tried, hydroxyurea (Hydrea) is the only one that has been shown to be clinically beneficial. This medication increases the production of fetal hemoglobin (HbF), which alters the adhesion of sickle erythrocytes to the endothelium. The increase in HbF is accompanied by a reduction in hemolysis, an increase in Hb concentration, and a decrease in sickled cells and painful crises (Meier, 2018). HSCT is the only available treatment that can cure some patients with SCD; however, it is very rarely done in Canada. The selection of appropriate recipients, the scarcity of appropriate donors, the risks involved, and the high cost/benefit ratio limit the use of HSCT for SCD. (Bone marrow transplants are discussed in Chapter 18.)

Patient teaching and support are important in the long-term care of the patient with SCD. The patient and family must understand the basis of the disease and the reasons for supportive care

and ongoing screening pertinent to SCD patients, such as eye examinations. The patient must be taught ways to avoid crises, which include taking steps to avoid dehydration and reducing the chance of developing hypoxia (for example, by avoiding high altitudes and seeking medical attention quickly to counteract conditions such as upper respiratory tract infections). Immunizations such as pneumococcal, *H. influenza,* and hepatitis should be given. In children, prophylactic antibiotics may be used. Education on pain control is also needed because the pain during a crisis may be severe and often requires considerable analgesia. Recurrent episodes of severe acute pain and unrelenting chronic pain can be profoundly disabling and depressing. Occupational therapists and physiotherapists can help the patient achieve optimum physical functioning and independence; a psychologist may be able to use cognitive–behavioural therapy to help patients with SCD cope with anxiety and depression. Support groups may also be helpful. Each person with SCD should have a reproductive life plan. Because there are often many quality-of-life issues with SCD, the nurse can play an important role in ensuring that the patient's needs are met through appropriate referrals.

ACQUIRED HEMOLYTIC ANEMIA

Acquired hemolytic anemia results from hemolysis of RBCs from extrinsic factors. These factors can be separated into three categories: (a) physical destruction, (b) immune reactions, and (c) infectious agents and toxins (see Table 33.2).

Physical destruction of RBCs results from the exertion of extreme force on the cells. Traumatic events causing disruption of the RBC membrane include hemodialysis, extracorporeal

---

🧬 GENETICS IN CLINICAL PRACTICE

Sickle Cell Disease

Genetic Basis
- Autosomal recessive disorder (see Chapter 15, Figure 15.5)
- Mutation in beta-globin gene *(HBB)* found on chromosome 11
- Various versions of beta globin result from different mutations in the *HBB* gene
- HbS variant involves substitution of valine for glutamic acid in the beta-globin gene

Incidence
- Most common inherited blood disorder in Canada
- More commonly affects people of African descent
- Also affects people of Mediterranean, Caribbean, South and Central American, Arabian, and Middle Eastern descent
- Affects 8 of every 100 000 people

Genetic Testing
- DNA testing is available.
- Electrophoresis of hemoglobin and sickling screening test are more commonly used.

Clinical Implications
- SCD requires ongoing continuity of care and extensive patient education.
- Sickle cell trait is the carrier state for SCD and represents a mild type of sickle cell disease.
- If both parents have the trait, there is a one in four chance that their child will have SCD.
- Management of SCD should focus on the prevention of sickle cell crisis.
- Genetic counselling is recommended for people with a family history of SCD so they can understand the risks of transmitting the genetic mutation.

SCD, sickle cell disease.

ETHICAL DILEMMAS
Pain Management

Situation

A 21-year-old (pronouns he/him) is admitted to the emergency department (ED) in sickle cell crisis with reports of excruciating pain. He is known to several of the nurses and health care providers in the department. One of the nurses remarks that it must be time for his "fix" of pain medications.

Important Points for Consideration

- The standard of care for pain management requires that (1) a pain assessment is done on the basis of patient's self-report, (2) the best possible pain relief is provided under the circumstances, and (3) competent and compassionate care is provided to all patients.
- The pain assessment also includes reviewing the patient's medical record to determine if there are health care issues or conditions (e.g., frequent ED visits to request pain medication) that may affect the patient's response to pain and pain management.
- Patient behaviours related to pain management must be documented. Nurses must be objective (factual observation) rather than subjective ("the patient is in withdrawal").
- Somnolence assessment is essential as part of pain assessment.

Clinical Decision-Making Questions

1. How can the nurse educate peers regarding pain assessment and management?
2. What important factors would need to be included in the nurse's assessment and management in consultation with the patient?

circulation used in cardiopulmonary bypass, and prosthetic heart valves. In addition, the force needed to push blood through abnormal vessels, such as those that have been burned, radiated, or affected by vascular disease (e.g., diabetes mellitus), may also physically damage RBCs. RBCs can also be fragmented and destroyed as they try to pass through abnormal arterial or venous microcirculation. The RBCs are sheared as they try to pass by excessive platelet aggregation or fibrin polymer formation, such as seen in thrombotic thrombocytopenic purpura (TTP) and disseminated intravascular coagulation (DIC).

Antibodies may destroy RBCs by the mechanisms involved in antigen–antibody reactions. The reactions may be of an isoimmune or autoimmune type. *Isoimmune reactions* occur when antibodies develop against antigens from another individual of the same species—in the case of humans, that is, from another person. Blood transfusion reactions typify this response, when the recipient's antibodies hemolyze donor cells.

Autoimmune reactions result when individuals develop antibodies against their own RBCs. Autoimmune hemolytic reactions may be idiopathic, developing with no prior hemolytic history, or secondary to other autoimmune diseases (e.g., systemic lupus erythematosus), leukemia, lymphoma, or reactions to medications (e.g. penicillin, ibuprofen, metformin).

Infectious agents and toxins constitute the third category of acquired hemolytic disorders. Infectious agents foster hemolysis in three ways: (1) by invading the RBC and destroying its contents (e.g., parasites such as in malaria), (2) by releasing hemolytic substances (e.g., *Clostridium perfringens*), and (3) by generating an antigen–antibody reaction (e.g., *Mycoplasma pneumonia*). Various agents may be toxic to RBCs and cause hemolysis. These hemolytic toxins involve chemicals such as oxidative medications, arsenic, lead, copper, bee stings, spider bites and snake venom.

Laboratory findings in hemolytic anemia are presented in Table 33.6. Treatment and management of acquired hemolytic anemias involve general supportive care until the causative agent can be eliminated or at least rendered less injurious to the RBCs. Because a hemolytic crisis is a potential consequence, the nurse must be ready to institute appropriate emergent therapy. This includes aggressive hydration and electrolyte replacement to reduce the risk for kidney injury caused by Hb clogging the kidney tubules and, subsequently, shock. Additional supportive care may include administering corticosteroids and blood products or removing the spleen. For chronic hemolytic anemia, folate may have to be replaced. To suppress the RBC destruction, immunosuppressive medications such as rituximab (Rituxan) may be used.

HEMOCHROMATOSIS

Hemochromatosis is an iron overload disorder. Although it is primarily caused by a genetic defect, hemochromatosis occurs secondary to diseases such as sideroblastic anemia. It may also be caused by liver disease and the multiple blood transfusions used to treat thalassemia and SCD.

The genetic disorder *(hereditary hemochromatosis)* is autosomal recessive and characterized by increased intestinal iron absorption and, as a result, increased tissue iron deposition (see the Genetics in Clinical Practice box). In Canada, it is one of the most common genetic disorders (Canadian Hemochromatosis Society, 2020). It affects Canadians of mostly Northern European descent. One in 250 to 300 Canadians is at risk of developing the full-blown disease (homozygous with two recessive genes), and approximately 1 in 9 is a potential carrier with one recessive gene. Approximately 80 000 Canadians have type I hemochromatosis, the most common form of hereditary hemochromatosis (Canadian Hemochromatosis Society, 2020).

GENETICS IN CLINICAL PRACTICE
Hemochromatosis

Genetic Basis

- Autosomal recessive disorder
- Caused by mutations in *HAMP, HFE, HFE2, SLC40A1,* and *TFR2* genes
- These genes play an important role in regulating the absorption, transport, and storage of iron.
- Mutations in these genes impair the control of the iron absorption during digestion and alter the distribution of iron to other parts of the body; as a result, iron accumulates in tissues and organs.

Incidence

- Most common genetic disease in people of European ancestry
- Affects approximately 1 in 300 Canadians of Northern European ancestry
- C282Y mutation of the *HFE* gene is the most common
- Very low prevalence in other ethnic populations

Genetic Testing

- DNA testing is recommended for all first-degree relatives of people with the disease.
- Genetic testing can be performed on either blood or buccal swab samples.

Clinical Implications

- Early treatment can prevent serious complications.
- Clinical expression is variable depending on dietary iron, blood loss, and other modifying factors.
- If untreated, progressive iron deposits can lead to multiple organ failure.

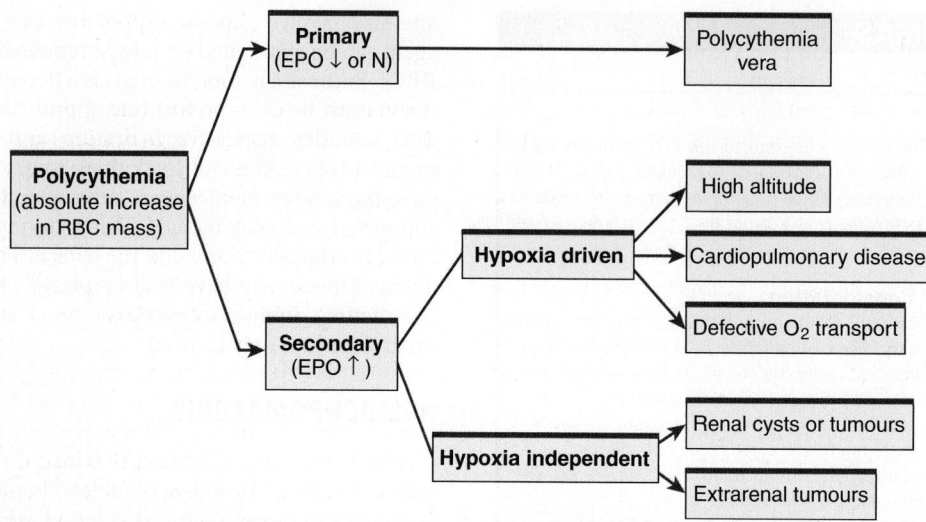

FIG. 33.4 Differentiating between primary and secondary polycythemia. *EPO*, erythropoietin; *N*, normal; *O₂*, oxygen; *RBC*, red blood cell.

The normal range for total body iron is 2 to 6 g. Individuals with hemochromatosis accumulate iron at a rate of 0.5 to 1.0 g each year and may accumulate total iron concentrations exceeding 50 g. Symptoms of hemochromatosis usually develop between 40 and 60 years of age. Early symptoms are nonspecific and include fatigue, arthralgia, erectile dysfunction, abdominal pain, and weight loss. Later, the excess iron accumulates in the liver and causes liver enlargement and eventually cirrhosis. Patients with hemochromatosis are at increased risk for hepatocellular carcinoma. Other organs also become affected, resulting in diabetes mellitus, skin pigment changes (bronzing), cardiac changes (e.g., cardiomyopathy), arthritis, and testicular atrophy. Physical examination reveals an enlarged liver and spleen and pigmentation changes in the skin. Laboratory values demonstrate an elevated serum iron, TIBC, and serum ferritin. Testing for known genetic mutations confirms the diagnosis. A liver biopsy can quantify the amount of iron and is the definitive way to establish the diagnosis.

The goal of treatment is to remove excess iron from the body and minimize any symptoms. Iron removal is achieved by removing 500 mL of blood regularly. The treatment schedule will vary and depend on ferritin levels and underlying cause. Iron chelating agents, which form a complex with iron and promote its excretion from the body, may also be used to remove excess iron.

Management of organ involvement (e.g., diabetes mellitus, HF) is the same as conventional treatment for these conditions. Dietary modifications, such as avoidance of vitamin C and iron supplements, uncooked seafood, and iron-rich foods, may also assist in the reduction of iron accumulation.

The most common causes of death in people with hemochromatosis are cirrhosis, liver failure, liver cancer, and HF. With early diagnosis and treatment, life expectancy is normal. However, many cases go undetected and untreated.

POLYCYTHEMIA

Polycythemia is an abnormal condition characterized by increased RBCs. This increase in RBCs can be so great that blood circulation is impaired as a result of the increased blood viscosity (*hyperviscosity*) and volume (*hypervolemia*).

Etiology and Pathophysiology

There are two types of polycythemia: primary polycythemia (or *polycythemia vera*) and secondary polycythemia (Figure 33.4). Their etiologies and pathogenesis differ, although their complications and clinical manifestations are similar. Polycythemia vera (PV) is a chronic myeloproliferative disorder arising from a chromosomal mutation (e.g., Janus kinase 2 [JAK2]) in a single pluripotent stem cell. The *JAK2* gene provides instructions for making a protein that promotes proliferation of cells, especially blood cells from hematopoietic stem cells. Therefore, not only are RBCs involved but also WBCs and platelets, leading to increased production of each of these blood cells. PV develops insidiously and follows a chronic, vacillating course. The median age at diagnosis is 60 years old, and it has a slight male predominance. With PV, the patient has enhanced blood viscosity and blood volume and congestion of organs and tissues with blood. The increased blood viscosity predisposes these patients to clotting. Splenomegaly and hepatomegaly are also common.

Secondary polycythemia can be either hypoxia driven or hypoxia independent. In the former, hypoxia stimulates erythropoietin (EPO) production in the kidney, which in turn stimulates RBC production. The need for O₂ may be because of high altitude, pulmonary disease, cardiovascular disease, alveolar hypoventilation, defective O₂ transport, or tissue hypoxia. EPO levels may return to normal once the Hb is stabilized at a higher level. In this situation, secondary polycythemia is a physiological response in which the body tries to compensate for a problem rather than a pathological response. (Hypoxia-driven polycythemia is discussed in the section on chronic obstructive pulmonary disease in Chapter 31.) In hypoxia-independent secondary polycythemia, EPO is produced by malignant or benign tumour tissue. Serum EPO levels often remain elevated in these situations. Splenomegaly does not accompany secondary polycythemia.

Clinical Manifestations and Complications

Circulatory manifestations of PV occur because of the hypertension caused by hypervolemia and hyperviscosity. They are often the first symptoms and include subjective complaints of headache, vertigo, dizziness, tinnitus, and visual disturbances.

Generalized pruritus (often exacerbated by a hot bath) may be a striking symptom and is related to histamine release from an increased number of basophils. Paresthesias and *erythromelalgia* (painful burning and redness of the hands and feet) may also be present. In addition, the patient may experience angina, HF, intermittent claudication, and thrombophlebitis, which may be complicated by embolization. These manifestations are caused by blood vessel distension, impaired blood flow, circulatory stasis, thrombosis, and tissue hypoxia caused by the hypervolemia and hyperviscosity. The most common serious complication is stroke secondary to thrombosis.

Hemorrhagic phenomena caused by either vessel rupture from overdistension or inadequate platelet function may result in petechiae, ecchymoses, epistaxis, or GI bleeding. Hemorrhage can be acute and catastrophic. Hepatomegaly and splenomegaly from organ engorgement may contribute to patient complaints of satiety and fullness. The patient may also experience pain from peptic ulcer caused by either increased gastric secretions or liver and spleen engorgement. *Plethora* (ruddy complexion) may also be present. Because uric acid is one of the products of cell destruction, the increase in RBC destruction that accompanies excessive RBC production causes a similar increase in uric acid production, thus leading to hyperuricemia. This condition may cause a form of gout.

Although the incidence is low, myelofibrosis and leukemia may develop in patients with PV. These disorders may be caused by medications used to treat the PV or they may be caused by a disorder in the stem cells that progresses to erythroleukemia.

Diagnostic Studies

The following laboratory manifestations are seen in a patient with PV: (a) high Hb and RBC count with microcytosis; (b) low to normal EPO level (secondary polycythemia will have a high level); (c) high WBC count with basophilia; (d) high platelet count (thrombocytosis) and platelet dysfunction; (e) high leukocyte alkaline phosphatase, uric acid, and cobalamin levels; and (f) high histamine levels. Bone marrow examination in PV shows hypercellularity of RBCs, WBCs, and platelets.

Interprofessional Care

Treatment is directed toward reducing blood volume and viscosity and bone marrow activity. Phlebotomy is the mainstay of treatment. The aim of phlebotomy is to reduce the Hct and keep it less than 45%. Generally, from the time of diagnosis, 300 to 500 mL of blood may be removed every other day until the Hct is reduced to an acceptable level. A person managed with repeated phlebotomies eventually becomes deficient in iron, although this effect is rarely symptomatic. Iron supplementation should be avoided. Hydration therapy is used to reduce the blood's viscosity. Myelosuppressive agents such as busulfan (Myleran) and hydroxyurea (Hydrea) may be given to inhibit bone marrow activity. Interferon alfa may be used in high-risk patients. Targeted therapies such as ruxolitinib (Jakavi), which targets the *JAK2* mutation, may also be used (McMullin et al., 2019). Antiplatelet agents, such as acetylsalicylic acid (ASA; Aspirin), may also be used for erythromelalgia or antithrombotic primary prophylaxis. Allopurinol may reduce the number of acute gout attacks, and antihistamines may be used to alleviate pruritus. Anagrelide (Agrylin) may be used to reduce the platelet count and inhibit platelet aggregation.

NURSING MANAGEMENT POLYCYTHEMIA VERA

Primary polycythemia vera is not preventable. However, because secondary polycythemia is generated by any source of hypoxia, maintaining adequate oxygenation may prevent health problems. Therefore, controlling chronic pulmonary disease, stopping smoking, and avoiding high altitudes may be important.

When acute exacerbations of PV develop, the nurse has several responsibilities. Depending on the institution's policies, the nurse may assist with or perform the phlebotomy. Fluid intake and output must be evaluated during hydration therapy to avoid fluid overload (which further complicates the circulatory congestion) and underhydration (which can cause the blood to become even more viscous). If myelosuppressive agents are used, the nurse must administer the medications as ordered, observe the patient, and teach the patient about medication adverse effects.

Assessment of the patient's nutritional status in collaboration with the dietitian may be necessary to offset the inadequate food intake that can result from GI symptoms of fullness, pain, and dyspepsia. Activities, medications, or both must be instituted to decrease thrombus formation. Active or passive leg exercises and ambulation, when possible, should be initiated.

CONDITIONS OF HEMOSTASIS

Hemostasis involves the vascular endothelium, platelets, and coagulation factors, which normally function together to stop hemorrhage and repair vascular injury. (These mechanisms are described in Chapter 32.) Disruption in any of these components may result in bleeding or thrombotic disorders.

Three major disorders of hemostasis discussed in this section are (1) thrombocytopenia (low platelet count), (2) hemophilia and von Willebrand disease (inherited disorders of specific clotting factors), and (3) disseminated intravascular coagulation (DIC).

THROMBOCYTOPENIA

Etiology and Pathophysiology

Thrombocytopenia is a reduction of platelets to an amount below 150×10^9/L. Acute, severe, or prolonged decreases from this normal range can result in abnormal hemostasis that manifests as prolonged bleeding from minor trauma to spontaneous bleeding without injury.

Platelet disorders occur because of impaired production, increased destruction, or abnormal distribution. While they can be inherited (e.g., Wiskott–Aldrich syndrome), most are acquired (Table 33.12). A common cause of acquired abnormalities is the ingestion of certain medications. Although some medications are directly myelosuppressive (e.g., chemotherapeutic agents, ganciclovir [Cytovene]), the usual mechanism of medication-related thrombocytopenia is accelerated platelet destruction caused by antibodies. Antibodies attack the platelets when the drug binds to the platelet surface.

A careful review of the patient's history can help to identify the causes of thrombocytopenia. For example, quinine may cause thrombocytopenia and is found in tonic water and in many herbal preparations.

TABLE 33.12 CAUSES OF THROMBOCYTOPENIA

Inherited
- Fanconi's syndrome (pancytopenia)
- Hereditary thrombocytopenia

Acquired
Impaired Platelet Production
- Cancers and other disorders
  - Aplastic anemia
  - Leukemia, lymphoma, myeloma, myelodysplastic disorders
  - Marrow metastases by solid tumours
- Medications (chemotherapy, others)
- Immune thrombocytopenic purpura (ITP)
- Infections, bacterial, fungal or viral (hepatitis C, HIV, cytomegalovirus, COVID-19) (Yang et al., 2020)
- Nutritional deficiencies, alcoholism
- Radiation

Increased Platelet Destruction
- Artificial surfaces (e.g. cardiopulmonary bypass, hemodialysis)
- Disseminated intravascular coagulation (DIC)
- Heparin-induced thrombocytopenia (HIT)
- Pregnancy related
- Thrombotic microangiopathy
  - Thrombotic thrombocytopenic purpura (TTP)
  - Atypical hemolytic uremic syndromes (aHUS)

Abnormal Platelet Distribution
- Dilution (massive blood transfusion, fluids)
- Splenic sequestration

HIV, human immunodeficiency virus.

Immune Thrombocytopenic Purpura. The most common acquired thrombocytopenia is a syndrome of abnormal destruction of circulating platelets termed *immune thrombocytopenic purpura* (ITP). ITP is an acquired immune disorder in which the thrombocytopenia results from antiplatelet antibodies, impaired platelet production, and T-cell-mediated destruction of platelets. In ITP, platelets are coated with antibodies. These platelets function normally; however, when they reach the spleen, the antibody-coated platelets are mistaken as foreign and are destroyed by macrophages. Platelets normally survive 8 to 10 days. However, in ITP, survival of platelets is only 1 to 3 days. Generally, the clinical syndrome manifests as an acute condition in children and a chronic condition in adults.

Thrombotic Thrombocytopenic Purpura. *Thrombotic thrombocytopenic purpura* (TTP) is an uncommon syndrome characterized by hemolytic anemia, thrombocytopenia, neurological abnormalities, fever (in the absence of infection), and renal abnormalities. Not all features are present in all patients. Because it is almost always associated with hemolytic–uremic syndrome (HUS), it is often referred to as TTP–HUS. The disease is associated with enhanced agglutination of platelets, which form microthrombi that deposit in arterioles and capillaries. In most cases, the syndrome is caused by a deficiency of a plasma enzyme (ADAMTS-13) that usually breaks down the von Willebrand clotting factor (vWF) into normal size. vWF is the most important protein that mediates platelet adhesion to damaged endothelial cells. Without the enzyme, unusually large amounts of vWF attach to activated platelets, thereby promoting platelet aggregation.

TTP is seen primarily in adults between 20 and 50 years of age and has a slight female predominance. The syndrome may be idiopathic (thought to be due to an autoimmune disorder against ADAMTS-13), or it may due to certain drug toxicities (e.g., chemotherapy), pregnancy, or infection. It may also be the result of a known autoimmune disorder such as systemic lupus erythematosus or scleroderma (Lichtman et al., 2017). TTP is a medical emergency because bleeding and clotting occur simultaneously.

Heparin-Induced Thrombocytopenia. One of the risks associated with the broad and increasing use of heparin is the development of the life-threatening condition called *heparin-induced thrombocytopenia* (HIT), also called *heparin-induced thrombocytopenia and thrombosis syndrome* (HITTS). Typically, patients develop thrombocytopenia 5 to 10 days after the onset of heparin therapy. HIT should be suspected if the platelet count falls by more than 50% or falls below 150×10^9/L. As many as 5% of patients on heparin therapy develop HIT (Arepally, 2017).

Although the major clinical concern of HITTS is venous thrombosis, arterial thrombosis can also develop. DVT and pulmonary emboli most commonly result as a complication of the thromboses. Additional complications may include arterial vascular infarcts resulting in skin necrosis, stroke, and end-organ damage.

In HIT, platelet destruction and vascular endothelial injury are the two major responses to what is believed to be an immune-mediated response to heparin. Platelet factor 4 (PF4) binds to heparin. This PF4–heparin complex then binds to the platelet surface, leading to further platelet activation and release of more PF4, thus creating a positive feedback loop. Antibodies are created against this PF4–heparin complex, and they are removed prematurely from circulation, leading to thrombocytopenia and platelet-fibrin thrombi.

Clinical Manifestations

Many patients with thrombocytopenia are asymptomatic. The most common symptom is bleeding, usually mucosal or cutaneous. Mucosal bleeding may manifest as epistaxis and gingival bleeding, and large bullous hemorrhages may appear on the buccal mucosa owing to the lack of vessel protection afforded by the submucosal tissue. Bleeding into the skin is manifested as petechiae, purpura, or superficial ecchymoses (Figure 33.5).

Petechiae are small, flat, pinpoint, red or reddish-brown microhemorrhages. When the platelet count is low, RBCs may leak out of the blood vessels and into the skin to cause petechiae. When petechiae are numerous, the resulting reddish skin bruise is called *purpura* (see Figure 33.5). Larger purplish lesions caused by hemorrhage are termed *ecchymoses* (Figure 33.6). Pain and tenderness sometimes are present.

The major complication of thrombocytopenia is hemorrhage. The hemorrhage may be insidious or acute and internal or external. It may occur in any area of the body, including the joints, retina, and brain. Cerebral hemorrhage may be fatal. Insidious hemorrhage may first be detected by discovering the anemia that accompanies blood loss. The nurse must be aware of manifestations that reflect this type of blood loss, including weakness, fainting, dizziness, tachycardia, abdominal pain and hypotension.

Diagnostic Studies

The platelet count is decreased in thrombocytopenia. Any reduction below 150×10^9/L may be termed *thrombocytopenia*.

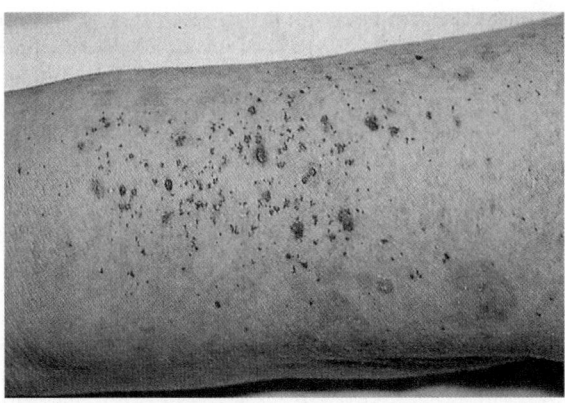

FIG. 33.5 Acute idiopathic thrombocytopenic purpura commonly manifests with purpuric lesions of this kind, although they may often be widespread by the time medical attention is sought. Source: Forbes, C. D., & Jackson, W. F. (2003). *Color atlas and text of clinical medicine* (3rd ed., p. 437). Mosby.

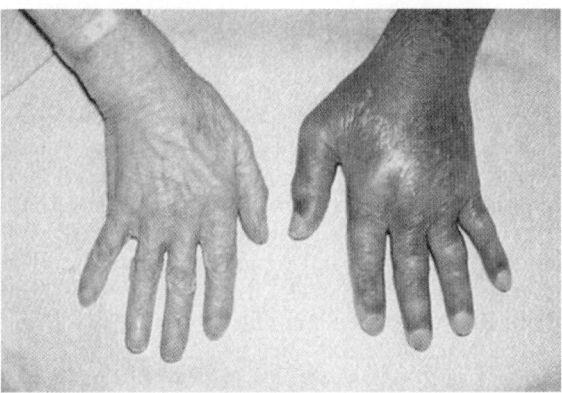

FIG. 33.6 Severe ecchymosis of the left hand.

However, prolonged bleeding from trauma or injury does not usually occur until platelet counts are less than 50×10^9/L. When the count drops below 10×10^9/L, spontaneous, life-threatening hemorrhages (e.g., intracranial bleeding) can occur. Platelet transfusions are generally not recommended until the count is below 10×10^9/L unless the patient is actively bleeding or critically ill with fever or sepsis.

The patient's medical history and clinical examination, along with comparisons of laboratory parameters, help to determine the etiology of the thrombocytopenia. Table 33.13 compares the types of thrombocytopenia.

Laboratory tests that assess secondary hemostasis or coagulation, such as the prothrombin time (PT) and activated partial thromboplastin time (aPTT), can yield normal results even in severe thrombocytopenia. Elevated values may point toward DIC. Specific assays, such as the ITP antigen-specific assay, platelet activation/function assay, or PF4–heparin complex for HIT, can be done to assist with the diagnosis. In TTP, testing for deficiency of ADAMTS-13 is not always diagnostic, so an increase of lactic dehydrogenase (LDH) may help to establish the diagnosis. When thrombocytopenia occurs with anemia characterized by altered RBC morphology, including *sphe-rocytes* (small, globular, completely hemoglobinated RBCs), fragmented cells *(schistocytes)*, and pronounced reticulocytosis, a diagnosis of TTP should be suspected. These findings

are partially a result of intravascular fibrin deposition causing a "slicing" of RBCs. In TTP, thrombocytopenia may be severe, but coagulation studies are normal.

Examination of the peripheral blood smear may help distinguish acquired disorders such as ITP and TTP from congenital disorders, which may be indicated by abnormally sized platelets. Bone marrow examination is done to rule out production problems as the cause of thrombocytopenia (e.g., leukemia, aplastic anemia, other myeloproliferative disorders). It is performed if the other tests are inconclusive, especially in older patients suspected of having an underlying bone marrow disorder. When destruction of circulating platelets is the cause, bone marrow analysis shows *megakaryocytes* (precursors of platelets) to be normal or increased, even though circulating platelets are reduced. The absence or decreased numbers of megakaryocytes on bone marrow biopsy is consistent with thrombocytopenia caused by decreased bone marrow production (e.g., aplastic anemia).

Interprofessional Care

Interprofessional care of thrombocytopenia differs according to the etiology of the thrombocytopenia. Discussion of management strategies for these different etiologies appears in Table 33.14.

Immune Thrombocytopenic Purpura. Multiple therapies are used to manage the patient with ITP. If the patient is asymptomatic, therapy may not be used unless the patient's platelet count is less than 30×10^9/L. Corticosteroids (e.g., prednisone) are used to treat ITP because of their ability to suppress the phagocytic response of splenic macrophages. This suppression alters the spleen's recognition of platelets and increases the lifespan of the platelets. In addition, corticosteroids depress antibody formation and reduce capillary leakage.

Splenectomy is indicated if the patient does not respond to prednisone initially or requires unacceptably high doses to maintain an adequate platelet count. A splenectomy results in a complete or partial remission in approximately 60 to 70% of patients. The effectiveness of splenectomy is based on four factors. First, the spleen contains an abundance of the macrophages that sequester and destroy platelets. Second, structural features of the spleen enhance the interaction between antibody-coated platelets and macrophages. Third, some antibody synthesis occurs in the spleen; thus, antiplatelet antibodies decrease after splenectomy. Fourth, the spleen normally sequesters approximately one third of the platelets, so its removal increases the number of platelets in circulation.

High doses of intravenous immunoglobulin (IVIG) and a component of IVIG, anti-Rho (D) (anti-D, WinRho), may be used to treat the patient who is unresponsive to corticosteroids or splenectomy. These agents work by competing with the antiplatelet antibodies for macrophage receptors in the spleen. They effectively raise the platelet count, but the beneficial effects are temporary. Rituximab (Rituxan) may be used for its ability to lyse activated B cells, thereby reducing the immune recognition of platelets. Romiplostim (Nplate) is used for patients with chronic ITP who have had an insufficient response to the other treatments or who have a contraindication to splenectomy. As a thrombopoietin receptor agonist, this medication increases platelet production. Immunosuppressive therapy (e.g., cyclosporine) may be used in refractory cases (see Table 33.14).

TABLE 33.13	COMPARISON OF DISORDERS CAUSING THROMBOCYTOPENIA			
Laboratory Test	**ITP**	**TTP**	**HIT**	**DIC**
Platelets	↓↓↓ ↓↓	↓↓↓	↓↓	↓↓↓
Hemolysis				
Haptoglobin	N	↓	N	↓
Hb	N	↓↓	N	N or ↓
Indirect bilirubin	N	↑	N	N or ↑
LDH	N	↑↑↑	N	↑
Reticulocytes	N	↑	N	N or ↑
Schistocytes	N	↑↑↑	N or ↑	N or ↑
Coagulopathy				
PT	N	N	N	↑
aPTT	N	N	N	↑
D-dimer	N	N or ↑	↑	↑↑
Other Tests	ITP IgG assay; platelet activation/ function assay, *Helicobacter pylori*, hepatitis C, HIV, bone marrow biopsy	ADAMTS-13, creatinine	Platelet activation/function assay PF4–heparin complex	

aPTT, activated partial thromboplastin time; *DIC*, disseminated intravascular coagulation; *Hb*, hemoglobin; *HIT*, heparin-induced thrombocytopenia; *ITP*, idiopathic thrombocytopenic purpura; *LDH*, lactic dehydrogenase; *N*, normal; *PF4*, platelet factor 4; ↑, increased; ↓, decreased; *PT*, prothrombin time; *TTP*, thrombotic thrombocytopenic purpura.

TABLE 33.14	INTERPROFESSIONAL CARE
Thrombocytopenia	

Diagnostic
- History and physical examination
- Bone marrow aspiration and biopsy
- CBC including platelet count
- Specific laboratory studies

Interprofessional Therapy
Immune Thrombocytopenic Purpura
- Corticosteroids
- Intravenous immunoglobulin (IVIG)
- Anti-Rho(D)
- Romiplostim (Nplate)
- Tranexamic acid
- Splenectomy
- Platelet transfusions (if life-threatening)
- Immunosuppressives (e.g., rituximab [Rituxan], cyclosporine)
- High-dose cyclophosphamide (Procytox) or combination chemotherapy
- Splenectomy

Thrombotic Thrombocytopenic Purpura
- Identification and treatment of cause
- Plasmapheresis (plasma exchange)
- High-dose corticosteroids
- Immunosuppressives (e.g., cyclophosphamide, cyclosporine)
- Rituximab [Rituxan]
- Splenectomy

Heparin-Induced Thrombocytopenia
- Discontinuation of heparin
- Direct thrombin inhibitor (e.g. argatroban)
- Indirect thrombin inhibitor (e.g., fondaparinux [Arixtra])
- Plasmapheresis (plasma exchange)
- Warfarin (Coumadin) (later-stage treatment)

Decreased Platelet Production
- Identification and treatment of cause
- Corticosteroids
- Platelet transfusions

CBC, complete blood count.

Platelet transfusions may be used to increase platelet counts in cases of life-threatening hemorrhage. Platelets should not be given prophylactically because of the possibility of antibody formation. The usual indication for administering platelets is a platelet count less than 10×10^9/L or the presence of bleeding before a procedure. Antifibrinolytic medications such as tranexamic acid may be used to treat severe bleeding.

Thrombotic Thrombocytopenic Purpura. TTP may be treated in a variety of ways. The first step is to treat the underlying disorder (e.g., infection) or to remove the causative agent, if identified. If untreated, TTP usually results in irreversible renal failure and death. Plasma exchange (plasmapheresis) (see Chapter 16) is used to aggressively reverse platelet consumption by supplying the appropriate vWF and enzyme (ADAMTS-13) and removing the large vWF molecules binding with the platelets. Treatment should be continued daily until the patient's counts normalize and hemolysis has ceased. Corticosteroids may be added to this treatment. Monoclonal antibody therapy (e.g., rituximab), immunosuppressants (e.g., cyclosporine or cyclophosphamide), and splenectomy have also been used with success. The administration of platelets is generally contraindicated because it may lead to new vWF–platelet complexes and increased clotting.

Heparin-Induced Thrombocytopenia. Heparin must be discontinued when HITTS is first recognized, including heparin flushes for vascular catheters.

To maintain anticoagulation, the patient should be started on a direct thrombin inhibitor, such as dabigatran (Pradaxa). Warfarin (Coumadin) should be started only when the platelet count has reached 150×10^9/L. If clotting is severe, the most commonly used treatment modalities are plasmapheresis to clear the platelet-aggregating IgG from the blood, protamine sulphate to interrupt the circulating heparin, thrombolytic agents to treat the thromboembolic events, and surgery to remove clots. Platelet transfusions are not effective because they may enhance thromboembolic events. Patients who have had HITTS should never be given heparin or low-molecular-weight heparin. This should be clearly marked in their chart.

Acquired Thrombocytopenia From Decreased Platelet Production. The management of acquired thrombocytopenia is based on identifying the cause and treating the disease or removing the causative agent. If the precipitating factor is unknown, the patient may receive corticosteroids. Platelet transfusions are given if life-threatening hemorrhage develops. Splenectomy is not used because the spleen does not contribute to this type of thrombocytopenia.

Often, acquired thrombocytopenia is caused by another underlying condition (e.g., aplastic anemia, leukemia) or therapy used to treat another condition. For example, in acute leukemia, all blood cell types may be depressed. In addition, the patient may receive chemotherapeutic agents that cause bone marrow suppression. If the patient can be adequately supported throughout the course of chemotherapy-induced thrombocytopenia, the thrombocytopenia will also resolve.

NURSING MANAGEMENT THROMBOCYTOPENIA

NURSING ASSESSMENT

Subjective and objective data that should be obtained from a patient with thrombocytopenia are presented in Table 33.15.

NURSING DIAGNOSES

Nursing diagnoses for the patient with thrombocytopenia may include but are not limited to the following:

- *Potential for bleeding* as evidenced by *inherent coagulopathy*
- *Potential for impaired oral mucous membrane integrity* as evidenced by *decrease in platelets and treatment regimen*
- *Inadequate knowledge* as a result of *insufficient information, insufficient knowledge of resources*

Additional information on nursing diagnoses is presented in NCP 33.2, available on the Evolve website.

PLANNING

The overall goals are that the patient with thrombocytopenia will (a) have no bleeding, (b) maintain vascular integrity, and (c) manage home care to prevent any complications related to an increased risk for bleeding.

NURSING IMPLEMENTATION

HEALTH PROMOTION. It is important for the nurse to discourage excessive use of over-the-counter medications known to be possible causes of acquired thrombocytopenia. Many medications contain ASA (Aspirin) as an ingredient. ASA reduces platelet adhesiveness, thus contributing to bleeding. It is also important for the nurse to encourage the patient to have a complete medical evaluation if manifestations of bleeding tendencies (e.g., prolonged epistaxis, petechiae) develop. In addition, the nurse must observe for early signs of thrombocytopenia in the patient receiving chemotherapeutic agents.

ACUTE INTERVENTION. The goal during acute episodes of thrombocytopenia is to prevent or control hemorrhage (see NCP 33.2 on the Evolve website). In the patient with thrombocytopenia, bleeding is usually from superficial sites; deep bleeding (into muscles, joints, and abdomen) usually occurs only when clotting factors are diminished. It is important to emphasize to the patient that a seemingly minor nosebleed or new petechiae may indicate potential hemorrhage and that the health care provider should be notified. Bleeding from the posterior nasopharynx may be difficult to detect because the blood may be swallowed. If a subcutaneous injection is unavoidable, a small-gauge needle should be used and direct pressure applied for at least 5 to 10 minutes after injection; IM injections should be avoided. The patient needs to understand the importance of adherence to self-care measures that reduce the risk of bleeding (Table 33.16).

TABLE 33.15 NURSING ASSESSMENT

Thrombocytopenia

Subjective Data

Important Health Information

Past health history: Recent hemorrhage, excessive bleeding, or viral illness; HIV infection; cancer (especially leukemia or lymphoma); aplastic anemia; SLE; cirrhosis; exposure to radiation or toxic chemicals; DIC; family history of bleeding disorders

Medications: e.g., chemotherapeutic agents, furosemide, gold, penicillin

Surgeries or other treatments: Recent surgery, splenectomy

Symptoms

- Bleeding gingiva; coffee-ground or bloody vomitus; epistaxis; hemoptysis; easy bruising, hematuria; dark or bloody stools; menorrhagia, metrorrhagia
- Headache; fatigue, weakness, general malaise; fainting
- Dyspnea
- Fever

Objective Data

General

Fever, lethargy

Integumentary

Petechiae, ecchymoses, purpura

Gastrointestinal

Splenomegaly, abdominal distension, heme-positive stools

Possible Findings

Platelet count <150 × 10^9/L (150 000/mcL) or prolonged bleeding time, decreased hemoglobin and hematocrit; normal or increased megakaryocytes in bone marrow examination

DIC, disseminated intravascular coagulation; *HIV,* human immunodeficiency virus; *SLE,* systemic lupus erythematosus.

In a woman with thrombocytopenia, menstrual blood loss may exceed the usual amount and duration. Counting sanitary napkins used during menses is another important intervention to detect excess blood loss; 50 mL of blood will completely soak a sanitary napkin. Suppression of menses with hormonal agents may be indicated during predictable periods of thrombocytopenia to reduce blood loss from menses (e.g., during chemotherapy and bone marrow transplantation).

The platelet count, coagulation studies, Hb, and Hct need to be closely monitored. Together these provide important information regarding potential or actual bleeding.

The proper administration of platelet transfusions is an important nursing responsibility. This is discussed under Blood Component Therapy later in this chapter.

AMBULATORY AND HOME CARE. The patient with ITP who is receiving treatment should be monitored for response to therapy. The person with acquired thrombocytopenia must be taught to avoid causative agents when possible (see Table 33.12). If the causative agents cannot be avoided (e.g., chemotherapy), the patient should learn to avoid injury or trauma during these periods and to detect the clinical signs and symptoms of bleeding caused by thrombocytopenia (see Table 33.16). Patients with either ITP or acquired thrombocytopenia should have periodic medical evaluations so the health care provider can assess the patient's status and intercede in situations in which exacerbations and bleeding are likely to occur. The impact of either an acute or a chronic condition on the patient's quality of life should also be addressed appropriately.

TABLE 33.16   PATIENT & CAREGIVER TEACHING GUIDE

Thrombocytopenia

This instruction sheet explains precautions you should take to protect yourself when your platelet count is low. Please make sure to ask your health care provider about specific precautions you should take that relate to your bleeding risk factors.

- Notify your health care provider of any manifestations of bleeding. These include the following:
  - Black, tarry, or bloody bowel movements
  - Black or bloody vomit, sputum, or urine
  - Bruising or small red or purple spots on the skin
  - Bleeding from the mouth or anywhere in the body
  - Headache or changes in how well you can see
  - Difficulty talking, sudden weakness of an arm or leg, confusion
- Ask your health care provider about restrictions in your normal activities, such as vigorous exercise or lifting weights. Generally, walking can be done safely and should be done while wearing sturdy shoes or slippers. If you are weak and at risk for falling, get help or supervision when getting out of bed.
- Do not blow your nose forcefully; gently pat it with a tissue if needed. For a nosebleed, keep your head up and apply firm pressure to the nostrils and the bridge of your nose. If bleeding continues, place an ice bag over the bridge of your nose and the nape of your neck. If you are unable to stop a nosebleed after 10 minutes, call your health care provider.
- Do not bend down with your head lower than your waist.
- Prevent constipation by drinking plenty of fluids, and do not strain when having a bowel movement. Your health care provider may prescribe a stool softener. Do not use a suppository, an enema, or a rectal thermometer without the permission of your health care provider.
- Shave only with an electric razor; do not use blades.
- Do not pluck your eyebrows or other body hair.
- Do not puncture your skin, such as by getting tattoos or body piercing.
- Avoid using any medication (e.g., ASA [Aspirin]) or herbal product that can prolong clotting time. If you are unsure about a connection between any medication or herbal product and your thrombocytopenia, check with your health care provider or pharmacist.
- Use a soft-bristle toothbrush to prevent injuring the gums. Flossing is also usually safe if it is done gently using the thin tape floss. Do not use alcohol-based mouthwashes because they can dry your gums and increase bleeding.
- Women: If you are menstruating, keep track of the number of pads that you use per day. When you start using more pads per day than usual or bleed more days, notify your health care provider. Do not use tampons; use sanitary pads only.
- Ask your health care provider before you have any invasive procedures done, such as a dental cleaning, manicure, or pedicure.

ASA, acetylsalicylic acid.

EVALUATION. The expected outcomes for the patient with thrombocytopenia are presented in NCP 33.2, available on the Evolve website.

HEMOPHILIA AND VON WILLEBRAND DISEASE

Hemophilia is an X-linked recessive genetic disorder caused by a defective or deficient coagulation factor (see the Genetics in Clinical Practice box, and Figure 15.6; X-linked genetic disorders are discussed in Chapter 15.) The two major forms of hemophilia, which can occur in mild to severe forms, are hemophilia A (classic hemophilia, factor VIII deficiency) and hemophilia B (Christmas disease, factor IX deficiency);

GENETICS IN CLINICAL PRACTICE
Hemophilia A and B

Genetic Basis
- X-linked recessive disorder
- *Hemophilia A:* Caused by mutations in the *F8* gene that provide instructions for making coagulation factor VIII
- *Hemophilia B:* Caused by mutations in the *F9* gene that provides instructions for making coagulation factor IX
- Mutations in the *F8* or *F9* gene lead to the production of an abnormal version of or reduced amounts of these coagulation factors.

Incidence
- *Hemophilia A:* 1 in 5000 to 10000 male births
- *Hemophilia B:* 1 in 25000 to 30000 male births

Genetic Testing
- DNA testing is available.

Clinical Implications
- Female carriers will transmit the genetic defect to 50% of their sons, and 50% of their daughters will be carriers.
- Men with hemophilia will not transmit the genetic defect to their sons, but all of their daughters will be carriers.
- Though rare, female hemophilia can occur if a man with hemophilia mates with a female carrier. Clinical manifestations of hemophilias A and B are very similar.
- Replacement therapy is available for factors VIII and IX (see Table 33.19 later in the chapter).

von Willebrand disease is a related disorder involving a deficiency of the von Willebrand coagulation protein. Factor VIII is synthesized in the liver and circulates as a complex with vWF.

Hemophilia A is the most common form of hemophilia, accounting for approximately 80% of all cases. In Canada, both hemophilia A and hemophilia B are rare disorders. About 2500 Canadians are known to be affected by hemophilia A and about 600 Canadians by hemophilia B. von Willebrand disease is considered the most common congenital bleeding disorder and is estimated to affect as many as 1 in 1000 Canadians (Canadian Hemophilia Society, 2018). This disease can exist in mild to severe forms; however, life-threatening hemorrhage is rare. The deficiency and inheritance patterns of these three forms of inherited coagulopathies are compared in Table 33.17.

Clinical Manifestations and Complications

Clinical manifestations and complications related to hemophilia include (a) slow, persistent, prolonged bleeding from minor trauma and small cuts; (b) delayed bleeding after minor injuries (the delay may be several hours or days); (c) uncontrollable hemorrhage after dental extractions or irritation of the gingiva with a hard-bristle toothbrush; (d) epistaxis, especially after a blow to the face; (e) GI bleeding from ulcers and gastritis; (f) hematuria from GU trauma and splenic rupture resulting from falls or abdominal trauma; (g) ecchymoses and subcutaneous hematomas and possible compartment syndrome (Figure 33.7); (h) neurological signs, such as pain, anaesthesia, and paralysis, that may develop from nerve compression caused by hematoma formation; and (i) hemarthrosis (bleeding into the joints) (Figure 33.8), which may lead to joint deformity severe enough to cause crippling (most commonly in knees, elbows, and ankles).

These symptoms in children may lead to diagnosis during childhood. In adults, these developments may be the first sign

TABLE 33.17 COMPARISON OF TYPES OF HEMOPHILIA

Disorder	Deficiency	Inheritance Pattern
Hemophilia A	Factor VIII	Recessive X-linked (transmitted by female carriers, displayed almost exclusively in men)
Hemophilia B	Factor IX	Recessive X-linked (transmitted by female carriers, displayed almost exclusively in men)
von Willebrand disease	vWF; variable factor VIII deficiencies and platelet dysfunction	Autosomal dominant, seen in both genders Recessive (in severe forms of the disease)

vWF, von Willebrand factor.

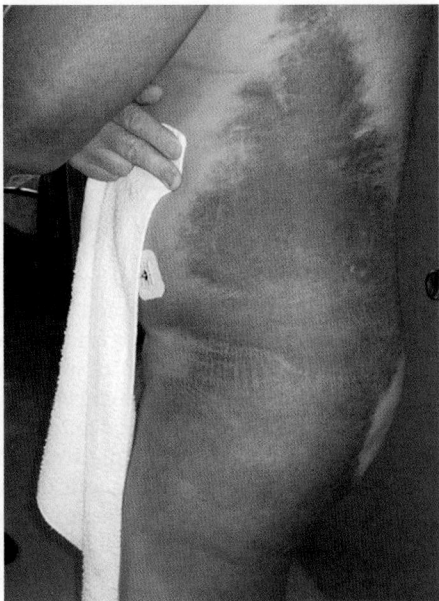

FIG. 33.7 Severe ecchymoses in a person with hemophilia following a fall. Source: Courtesy Peter Bonner.

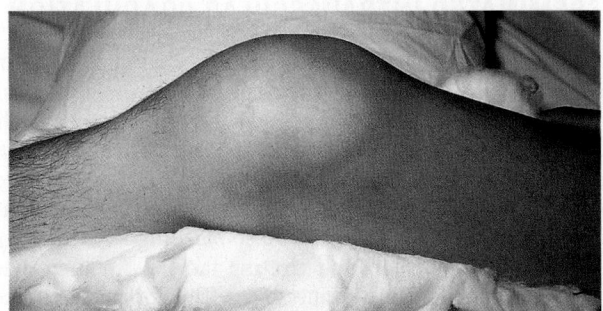

FIG 33.8 Acute hemarthrosis of the knee is a common complication of hemophilia. Source: Forbes, C. D., & Jackson, W. F. (2003). *Color atlas and text of clinical medicine* (3rd ed., p. 441). Mosby.

of a mild form of the disease that escaped detection because of a childhood free of major injuries, dental procedures, or surgeries. All clinical manifestations relate to bleeding, and any bleeding episode in people with hemophilia may lead to a life-threatening hemorrhage.

Diagnostic Studies

Laboratory studies are used to determine the type of hemophilia present. Any factor deficiency within the intrinsic system (factors VIII, IX, XI, or XII or vWF) will yield the laboratory results presented in Table 33.18.

Interprofessional Care

The goals of interprofessional care are to prevent and treat bleeding. Interprofessional care for people with hemophilia or von Willebrand disease requires (a) preventive care, (b) the use of replacement therapy during acute bleeding episodes and as prophylaxis, and (c) the treatment of the complications of the disease and its therapy.

Replacement of deficient clotting factors is the primary means of supporting a patient with hemophilia. In addition to treating acute crises, replacement therapy may be given before surgery and dental care as a prophylactic measure (Srivastava et al., 2020). Examples of replacement therapy are listed in Table 33.19. Fresh-frozen plasma, once commonly used for replacement therapy, is rarely used today.

For mild hemophilia A and certain subtypes of von Willebrand disease, desmopressin acetate (also known as DDAVP), a synthetic analogue of vasopressin, may be used to stimulate an increase in factor VIII and vWF. This medication acts on platelets and endothelial cells to cause the release of vWF, which subsequently binds with factor VIII, thus increasing their concentration. It can be administered intravenously, subcutaneously, or intranasally. Beneficial effects (e.g., decreased bleeding time) of DDAVP, when administered by IV, are seen within 30 minutes and can last for more than 12 hours. Because the effect of DDAVP is relatively short-lived, the patient must be closely monitored, and repeated doses may be necessary. It is an appropriate therapy for minor bleeding episodes and dental procedures. The intranasal form may be indicated for home therapy for some patients with mild to moderate forms of the disease.

Antifibrinolytic therapy (e.g., tranexamic acid [Cyklokapron]) inhibits fibrinolysis by inhibiting plasminogen activation in the fibrin clot, thereby enhancing clot stability. These agents are used to stabilize clots in areas of increased fibrinolysis, such as the oral cavity, and in patients with difficult-to-manage episodes of epistaxis and menorrhagia. Topical thrombin and fibrin sealants may also be used for mucosal bleeding.

Complications of treatment of hemophilia include development of inhibitors to factors VIII or IX, transfusion-transmitted infectious disorders (hepatitis, HIV), allergic reactions, and, with the use of factor IX, thrombotic complications, because it contains activated coagulation factors. Patients with vWF may also develop antibodies against vWF concentrates, the infusion of which could cause life-threatening anaphylaxis; thus, replacement factors for these patients should be devoid of vWF. The most common difficulties with acute management are starting factor replacement therapy too late and stopping it too soon. Generally, minor bleeding episodes should be treated for at least 72 hours. Surgery and traumatic injuries may need longer therapy. Chronically, development of inhibitors to the factor products has occurred and necessitates individualized expert patient management.

Designated treatment centres have been established in Canada as well as in many other countries to provide multidisciplinary care of hemophilia and related disorders. Gene therapy has been used on an experimental basis to treat hemophilia. (Gene therapy is discussed in Chapter 15.)

TABLE 33.18   LABORATORY RESULTS IN HEMOPHILIA

Test	Comments
Bleeding time	Prolonged in von Willebrand disease because of structurally defective platelets; normal in hemophilias A and B because platelets not affected
Factor assays	Reduction of factor VIII in hemophilia A; vWF in von Willebrand disease; factor IX in hemophilia B
Partial thromboplastin time	Prolonged because of deficiency in any intrinsic clotting system factor
Platelet count	Normal. Adequate platelet production
Prothrombin time	Normal. No involvement of extrinsic system
Thrombin time	Normal. No impairment of thrombin–fibrinogen reaction

vWF, von Willebrand factor.

TABLE 33.19   MEDICATION THERAPY

Replacement Factors Used in Treating Hemophilia

Factor VIII	Factor VIII and von Willebrand	Factor IX	von Willebrand	For Patients Who Have Inhibitors
Adynovate	Humate P	Alprolix	Vonvendi	Feiba NF
Eloctate	Wilate	Benefix		NiaStase RT
Kovaltry		Immunine		
Nuwiq		Idelvian		
Xyntha		Rebinyn		
Zonovate		Rixubis		

Source: Adapted from Canadian Hemophilia Society. (2019). *Clotting factor concentrates.* http://www.hemophilia.ca/en/bleeding-disorders/clotting-factor-concentrates

NURSING MANAGEMENT HEMOPHILIA

NURSING IMPLEMENTATION

HEALTH PROMOTION. Genetic counselling referral is especially important now that many people with hemophilia live into adulthood. Reproductive concerns and long-term effects are issues that the nurse should include in the patient's care plan.

ACUTE INTERVENTION. Interventions are related primarily to controlling bleeding and include the following:

1. Stop the topical bleeding as quickly as possible by applying direct pressure or ice, packing the area with fibrin foam or Gelfoam, and applying a topical hemostatic medication such as thrombin.
2. Administer the specific coagulation factor to raise the patient's level of the deficient coagulation factor. Monitor the patient for signs and symptoms, such as hypersensitivity.
3. When joint bleeding occurs, in addition to administering replacement factors, it is important to totally rest the involved joint to prevent crippling deformities from hemarthrosis. Pack the joint in ice. Analgesics (e.g., acetaminophen [Tylenol], codeine) are given to reduce severe pain. However, ASA (Aspirin) and ASA-containing compounds should never be used. As soon as bleeding ceases, it is important to encourage mobilization of the affected area through range-of-motion exercises and physical therapy. Weight bearing is avoided until all swelling has resolved and muscle strength has returned.

4. Manage any life-threatening complication that may develop as a result of hemorrhage or adverse effects from coagulation factors or other medications, such as hyponatremia from use of desmopressin. For example, nursing interventions may include preventing or treating airway obstruction from hemorrhage into the neck and pharynx, recognition of compartment syndrome in an extremity, and early assessment and treatment of intracranial bleeding.

AMBULATORY AND HOME CARE. Home management is a primary consideration for the patient with hemophilia because the disease follows a progressive, chronic course. The quality and the length of life may be significantly affected by the patient's knowledge of the illness and how to live with it. The patient and family can be referred to a local treatment centre or the provincial chapter of the Canadian Hemophilia Society to encourage associations with other individuals who are living with the challenges of hemophilia. The nurse must provide ongoing assessment of the patient's adaptation to the illness. Psychosocial support and assistance should be readily available as needed.

Most of the needed long-term care measures are related to patient teaching. The nurse should teach the patient to recognize disease-related symptoms and to know which symptoms can be resolved at home and which require hospitalization. Immediate medical attention is required for severe pain or swelling of a muscle or joint that restricts movement or inhibits sleep and for a head injury, a swelling in the neck or the mouth, abdominal pain, hematuria, melena, and skin wounds in need of suturing.

Daily oral hygiene must be performed without causing trauma. Understanding how to prevent injuries is another consideration. The patient can learn to participate in noncontact sports (e.g., golf) and wear gloves when doing household chores to prevent cuts or abrasions from knives, hammers, and other tools. The patient should wear medical alert identification to ensure that health care providers know about the hemophilia in case of an accident. Patients or their caregivers can also be taught to self-administer the factor replacement therapies at home.

EVALUATION. The overall expected outcomes are similar to those for the patient with thrombocytopenia and are presented in NCP 33.2 (see the Evolve website).

DISSEMINATED INTRAVASCULAR COAGULATION

Disseminated intravascular coagulation (DIC) is a serious bleeding and thrombotic disorder that results from abnormally initiated and accelerated clotting and anticlotting processes that occur in response to disease or injury. The term *disseminated intravascular coagulation* can be misleading because it suggests that blood is clotting. In fact, the paradox of this condition is that it is characterized by the profuse bleeding resulting from the depletion of platelets and clotting factors. An underlying disease or condition always causes DIC. The underlying disease must be treated for the DIC to resolve.

Etiology and Pathophysiology

DIC is not a disease; it is an abnormal response of the normal clotting cascade stimulated by a disease process or disorder. The diseases and disorders known to predispose a patient to DIC are listed in Table 33.20. DIC can occur as an acute, catastrophic condition, or it may exist at a subacute or chronic level. Each condition may have one or multiple triggering mechanisms to start the clotting cascade. For example, tumours and

TABLE 33.20	PREDISPOSING CONDITIONS TO DEVELOPMENT OF DISSEMINATED INTRAVASCULAR COAGULATION

Acute Disseminated Intravascular Coagulation (DIC)
- Cancers
- Acute leukemia
- Metastatic solid tumours
- Hemolytic processes
- Acute hemolysis from infection or immunologic disorders
- Transfusion of mismatched blood
- Obstetric conditions
- Abruptio placentae
- Amniotic fluid embolism
- HELLP syndrome
- Septic abortion
- Septicemia
- Shock
- Anaphylactic
- Cardiogenic
- Hemorrhagic
- Tissue damage
- Acute anoxia (e.g., after cardiac arrest)

- Extensive burns and trauma
- Fulminant hepatitis
- Heatstroke
- Postoperative damage, especially after extracorporeal membrane oxygenation
- Severe head injury
- Snakebites
- Transplant rejections
- Vascular disorders (e.g., aortic aneurism)

Subacute DIC
- Cancer
- Metastatic cancer
- Myeloproliferative and lymphoproliferative cancers
- Obstetric
- Retained dead fetus

Chronic DIC
- Cancer
- Liver disease
- SLE

HELLP, **h**emolysis, **e**levated **l**iver enzymes, **l**ow **p**latelet count; *SLE,* systemic lupus erythematosus.

traumatized or necrotic tissue release tissue factors into circulation. Endotoxin from Gram-negative bacteria activates several steps in the coagulation cascade.

Tissue factor is released at the site of tissue injury and by some cancers, such as leukemia, and enhances normal coagulation mechanisms. Abundant intravascular thrombin, the most powerful coagulant, is produced (Figure 33.9). It catalyzes the conversion of fibrinogen to fibrin and enhances platelet aggregation. There is widespread fibrin and platelet deposition in capillaries and arterioles, resulting in thrombosis that can lead to multiorgan failure. In addition, clotting inhibitory mechanisms, such as antithrombin III (AT III) and protein C, are depressed. This excessive clotting activates the fibrinolytic system, which in turn breaks down the newly formed clot, creating *fibrin split products* (FSPs); these products have anticoagulant properties and inhibit normal blood clotting. Ultimately, with FSPs accumulating and clotting factors being depleted, the blood loses its ability to clot. Therefore, a stable clot cannot be formed at injury sites, which predisposes the patient to hemorrhage.

Chronic and subacute DIC are most commonly seen in patients with long-standing illnesses such as malignant disorders or autoimmune diseases. Occasionally, these patients have subclinical disease manifested only by laboratory abnormalities. However, the clinical spectrum ranges from easy bruising to hemorrhage and from hypercoagulability to thrombosis.

Clinical Manifestations

There are both bleeding and thrombotic manifestations in DIC. Bleeding manifestations of DIC are multifactorial (see Figure 33.9) and result from consumption and depletion of platelets and coagulation factors as well as from clot lysis and formation of FSPs that have anticoagulant properties. Bleeding manifestations include manifestations in the (a) skin, such as pallor, petechiae, purpura (Figure 33.10), oozing blood, venipuncture site bleeding, hematomas, and occult hemorrhage; (b) respiratory system, such as tachypnea, hemoptysis, and orthopnea; (c) cardiovascular system, such as tachycardia and hypotension; (d) GI tract, such as upper and lower GI bleeding and bloody stools; (e) urinary tract, such as hematuria; (f) neurological system, such as vision changes, dizziness, headache, changes in mental status, and irritability; and (g) musculoskeletal system, such as bone and joint pain.

Thrombotic manifestations are a result of fibrin or platelet deposition in the microvasculature (see Figure 33.9). The manifestations affect the (a) skin, such as cyanosis, ischemic tissue necrosis (e.g., gangrene), and hemorrhagic necrosis; (b) respiratory system, such as tachypnea, dyspnea, pulmonary emboli, and acute respiratory distress syndrome (ARDS); (c) cardiovascular system, such as electrocardiographic (ECG) changes and venous distension; (d) GI tract, such as abdominal pain and paralytic ileus; and (e) urinary system, such as acute kidney injury and oliguria.

Diagnostic Studies

Tests used to diagnose acute DIC and their findings are listed in Table 33.21. As more clots are made in the body, more breakdown products from fibrinogen and fibrin are also formed. These FSPs interfere with blood coagulation by (a) coating the platelets and interfering with platelet function, (b) interfering with thrombin and thus disrupting coagulation, and (c) attaching to fibrinogen, which interferes with the polymerization process necessary to form a stable clot. D-dimer, a polymer resulting from the breakdown of fibrin (and not fibrinogen), is a specific marker for the degree of fibrinolysis. In general, tests that measure raw materials needed for coagulation (e.g., platelets, fibrinogen) are reduced and tests that measure clotting times are prolonged. Fragmented erythrocytes *(schistocytes),* indicative of partial occlusion of small vessels by fibrin thrombi, may be found on blood smears.

Interprofessional Care

It is important to diagnose DIC quickly, stabilize the patient (e.g., oxygenation, volume replacement), treat the underlying causative disease or condition, and provide supportive care for the manifestations resulting from the pathology of DIC itself. Depending on its severity, a variety of different methods are used to manage DIC (Figure 33.11). First, if chronic DIC is diagnosed in a patient who is not bleeding, no therapy for DIC is necessary. Treatment of the underlying disease may be sufficient to reverse the DIC (e.g., chemotherapy when DIC is caused by malignancy). Second, when the patient with DIC is bleeding, therapy is directed toward providing support with necessary blood products while treating the primary disorder.

Blood products are administered cautiously on the basis of specific component deficiencies. Blood product support with platelets, cryoprecipitate, and fresh-frozen plasma is usually reserved for a patient with life-threatening hemorrhage. The concern is that one is adding "fuel to the fire" of already activated coagulation. However, it may be the only method to prevent death in some patients with severe hemorrhage. Therapy will stabilize a patient, prevent exsanguination or massive thrombosis, and permit institution of definitive therapy to treat the underlying cause.

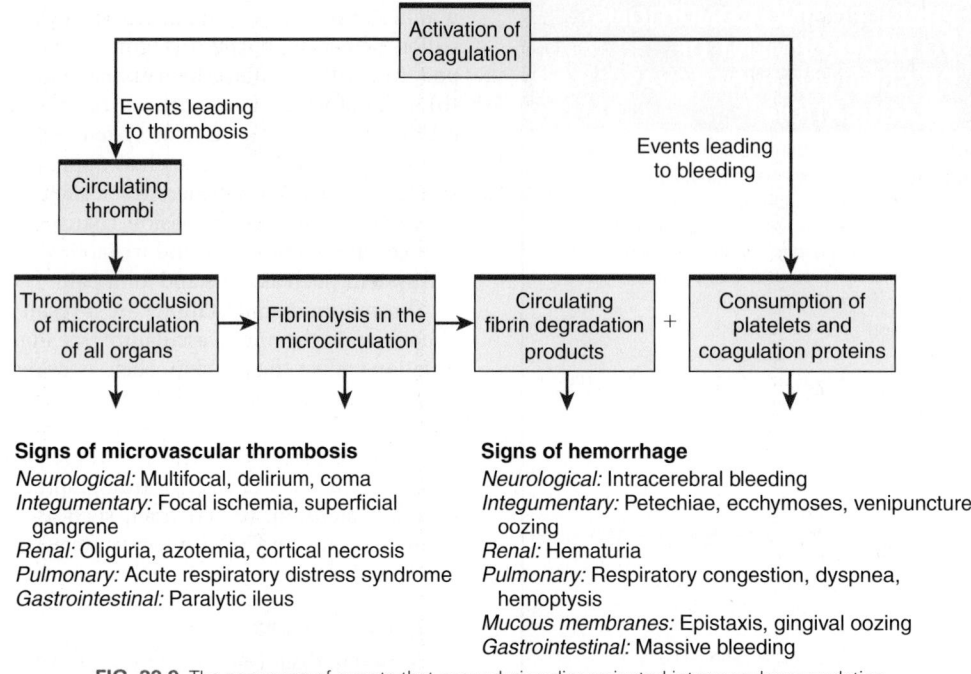

Signs of microvascular thrombosis
Neurological: Multifocal, delirium, coma
Integumentary: Focal ischemia, superficial
  gangrene
Renal: Oliguria, azotemia, cortical necrosis
Pulmonary: Acute respiratory distress syndrome
Gastrointestinal: Paralytic ileus

Signs of hemorrhage
Neurological: Intracerebral bleeding
Integumentary: Petechiae, ecchymoses, venipuncture
  oozing
Renal: Hematuria
Pulmonary: Respiratory congestion, dyspnea,
  hemoptysis
Mucous membranes: Epistaxis, gingival oozing
Gastrointestinal: Massive bleeding

FIG. 33.9 The sequence of events that occur during disseminated intravascular coagulation.

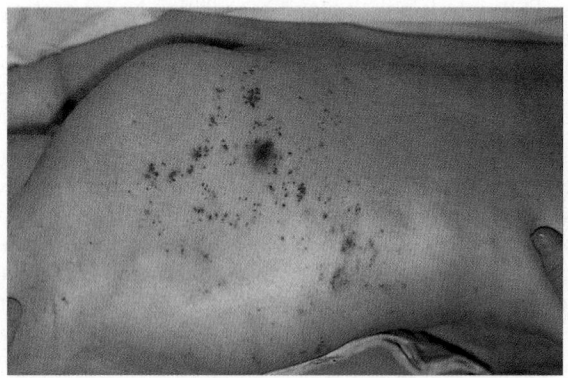

FIG. 33.10 Disseminated intravascular coagulation resulting from staphylococcal septicemia. Note the characteristic skin hemorrhage ranging from small purpuric lesions to larger ecchymoses. Source: Forbes, D. D., & Jackson, W. F. (2003). *Color atlas and text of clinical medicine* (3rd ed., p. 443). Mosby.

TABLE 33.21	**LABORATORY ABNORMALITIES OF ACUTE DISSEMINATED INTRAVASCULAR COAGULATION**
Test	**Finding**
Screening Tests	
Prothrombin time (PT)	Prolonged
Partial thromboplastin time (PTT)	Prolonged
Activated partial thromboplastin time (aPTT)	Prolonged
Fibrinogen	Reduced
Platelets	Reduced
Thrombin time	Prolonged
Special Tests	
Antithrombin III (AT III)	Reduced
D-dimers (cross-linked fibrin fragments)	Elevated
Factor assays (for factors V, VIII, X, XIII)	Reduced but may give misleading results, as V and VIII rise with inflammation
Fibrin split products (FSPs)	Elevated
Peripheral blood smear	Schistocytes present
Plasminogen, tissue activator	Reduced
Protein C and S	Reduced

A patient with manifestations of thrombosis is often treated by anticoagulation with heparin or low-molecular-weight heparin. However, these medications are used in the treatment of DIC only when the benefit (e.g., reduce clotting) outweighs the risk (e.g., further bleeding). AT III is sometimes used in fulminant DIC, although it increases the risk of bleeding. Chronic DIC does not respond to oral anticoagulants, but it can be controlled with long-term use of heparin.

NURSING MANAGEMENT
DISSEMINATED INTRAVASCULAR COAGULATION

NURSING DIAGNOSES
Nursing diagnoses for the patient with DIC may include but are not limited to the following:
- *Potential for bleeding* (ineffective tissue perfusion)
- *Inadequate cardiac output* (resulting from fluid volume deficit)
- *Acute pain* resulting from *physical injury agent* (bleeding)
- *Anxiety* resulting from *unmet needs* (fear of the unknown)

NURSING IMPLEMENTATION
Nurses must be alert to the possible development of DIC and especially to the precipitating factors listed in Table 33.20. The nurse must also remember that, because DIC is secondary to an underlying disease, appropriate care for managing the causative condition must be provided while also providing supportive care related to the manifestations of DIC.

Appropriate nursing interventions are essential to the survival of a patient with acute DIC. Astute, ongoing assessment,

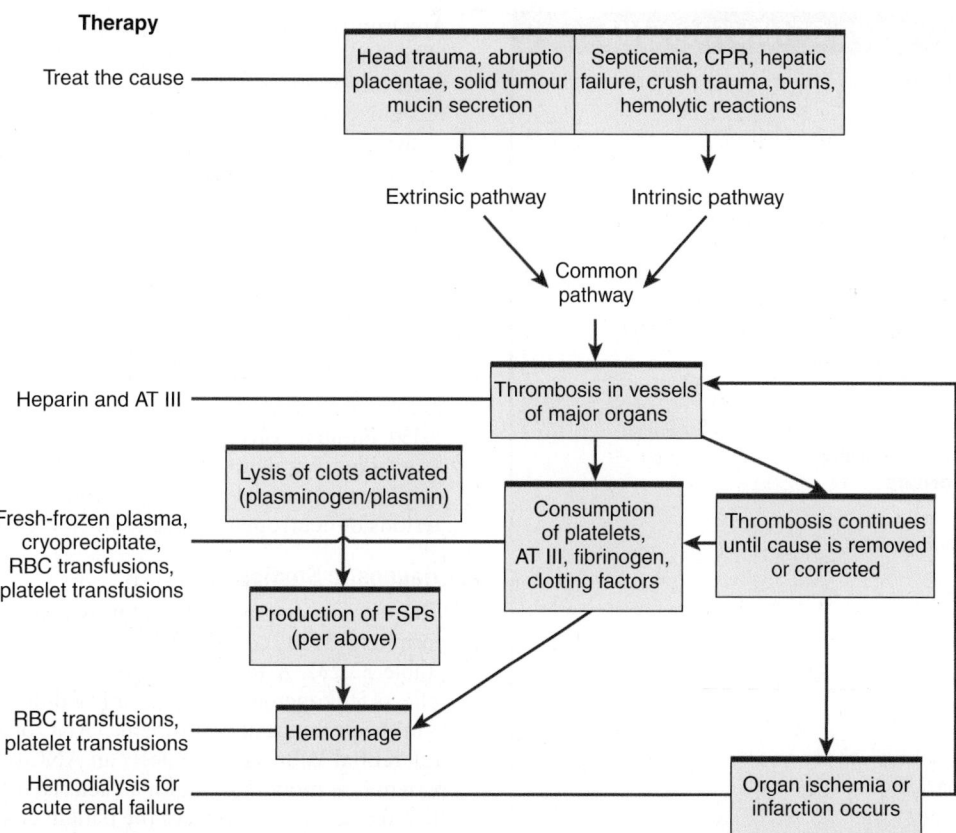

FIG. 33.11 Intended sites of action for therapies in disseminated intravascular coagulation (DIC). *AT III,* antithrombin III; *CPR,* cardiopulmonary resuscitation; *FSPs,* fibrin split products; *RBC,* red blood cell.

active attention to manifestations of DIC, and prompt administration of prescribed therapies are crucial. Table 33.14 and NCP 33.2 (see the Evolve website) provide assessments and interventions appropriate for the patient with DIC. Early detection of bleeding, both occult and overt, must be a primary goal. The nurse must assess for signs of external bleeding (e.g., petechiae, oozing at IV or injection sites) and signs of internal bleeding (e.g., increased heart rate, changes in mental status, increasing abdominal girth, pain) as well as indications that microthrombi may be causing significant organ damage (e.g., decreased urinary output). Tissue damage should be minimized and the patient protected from additional sources of bleeding.

An additional nursing responsibility is to administer blood products and medications correctly. (Blood product transfusion is discussed later in this chapter.)

NEUTROPENIA

Leukopenia refers to a decrease in the total WBC count (granulocytes, monocytes, and lymphocytes). *Granulocytopenia* is a deficiency of granulocytes, which include neutrophils, eosinophils, and basophils. The neutrophilic granulocytes, which play a major role in phagocytizing pathogenic microbes, are closely monitored in clinical practice as an indicator of a patient's risk for infection. A reduction in neutrophils is termed *neutropenia*. (Some clinicians use the terms *granulocytopenia* and *neutropenia* interchangeably because neutrophils constitute the largest proportion of granulocytes.) The *absolute neutrophil count* (ANC) is determined by multiplying the total WBC count by

the percentage of neutrophils. Neutropenia is defined as a neutrophil count of less than 1 to 1.5×10^9/L. Normally, neutrophils range from 2.2 to 7.7×10^9/L. *Severe neutropenia* is defined as an ANC less than 0.5×10^9/L.

In considering the clinical significance of neutropenia, it is important to know whether the decrease in the neutrophil count was gradual or rapid, as well as the degree and the duration of neutropenia. The faster the drop and the longer the duration, the greater the likelihood is of developing life-threatening infection, sepsis, and death. Other factors and comorbid conditions—such as immune disorders, being older than 60 years of age, having an existing infection, being in a hospital, having diabetes, and other factors—can increase the risk of a serious infection.

Neutropenia is not a disease; it is a clinical consequence that occurs with a variety of conditions or diseases (Table 33.22). It can also be a predictable or an unanticipated adverse effect of taking certain medications. The most common cause of neutropenia is iatrogenic, resulting from widespread use of chemotherapeutic and immunosuppressive therapy in the treatment of cancer and autoimmune diseases.

Clinical Manifestations

It is important to note that neutropenia itself produces no symptoms. Instead, the patient with neutropenia is predisposed to infection with nonpathogenic organisms that constitute normal body flora as well as opportunistic pathogens. When the WBC count is low or immature WBCs are present, normal phagocytic mechanisms are impaired. Also, because of the diminished phagocytic response, the classic signs of inflammation—redness,

TABLE 33.22 CAUSES OF NEUTROPENIA

Autoimmune Disorders
- Felty syndrome
- SLE

Medication Therapy
- Alkylating agents (nitrogen mustards, busulfan [Myleran])
- Anti-inflammatory medications (phenylbutazone)
- Antimicrobial agents (ganciclovir, penicillin G, trimethoprim–sulphamethoxazole)
- Antimetabolites (methotrexate, 6-mercaptopurine, cytarabine)
- Antitumour antibiotics (daunorubicin [Cerubidine], doxorubicin [Adriamycin])
- Cardiovascular medications (captopril, procainamide)
- Diuretics (furosemide [Lasix])
- Psychotropics and antidepressants (clozapine, imipramine)
- Miscellaneous (gold, penicillamine)

Hematological Disorders
- Aplastic anemia
- Congenital (cyclic neutropenia)
- Fanconi's anemia
- Idiopathic neutropenia
- Leukemia
- Myelodysplastic syndrome

Infections
- Fulminant bacterial infection (e.g., typhoid fever, miliary tuberculosis)
- Parasitic
- Rickettsial
- Viral (e.g., hepatitis, influenza, HIV, measles)

Miscellaneous
- Bone marrow infiltration (e.g., carcinoma, tuberculosis, lymphoma)
- Hemodialysis
- Hypersplenism (e.g., portal hypertension, storage diseases [e.g., Gaucher's disease])
- Nutritional deficiencies (cobalamin, folic acid)
- Severe sepsis

HIV, human immunodeficiency virus; *SLE,* systemic lupus erythematosus.

heat, and swelling—may not occur. WBCs are the major component of pus. Therefore, in the patient with neutropenia, pus formation (e.g., as a visible skin lesion or as pulmonary infiltrates on a chest radiograph) is also absent.

SAFETY ALERT
- A low-grade fever in a neutropenic patient is of great significance because it may indicate infection and quickly lead to septic shock and death unless treated promptly.
- A fever greater than 38°C and/or new signs or symptoms suggesting an infection and a neutrophil count less than 0.5×10^9/L is a medical emergency.
- Neutropenic patients with signs or symptoms of infection should go to the hospital.
- Blood cultures should be drawn STAT and antibiotics started within 1 hour.

When fever occurs in a neutropenic patient, it is assumed to be caused by infection and calls for immediate attention. The immunocompromised, neutropenic patient has little or no ability to fight infection. Thus, minor infections can lead rapidly to sepsis and death. The mucous membranes of the throat and mouth, skin, perianal area, and pulmonary system are common entry points for pathogenic organisms in susceptible hosts. Manifestations related to infection at these sites include sore throat and dysphagia, ulcerative lesions of the pharyngeal and the buccal mucosa, diarrhea, rectal tenderness, vaginal itching or discharge, shortness of breath, and a nonproductive cough.

Any minor complaint by the patient of pain or any other symptom should be taken seriously. These seemingly minor conditions can progress to fever, chills, sepsis, and septic shock if not recognized and treated in the early stages.

Systemic infections caused by bacterial, fungal, and viral organisms are common in patients with neutropenia. The patient's own flora (normally nonpathogenic) contributes significantly to life-threatening infections such as pneumonia. Organisms that are known to be common sources of infection in neutropenic patients with cancer include Gram-negative organisms such as *Escherichia coli, Klebsiella, Enterobacter,* and *Pseudomonas aeruginosa.* More recently, Gram-positive organisms such as coagulase-negative staphylococci and viridans group streptococci have become more prevalent (Zimmer & Freifeld, 2019). Fungi involved include *Candida* (usually *C. albicans*) and *Aspergillus.* Viral infections caused by reactivation of herpes simplex and herpes zoster are common following prolonged periods of neutropenia, such as in HSCT patients.

Diagnostic Studies

The primary diagnostic tests for assessing neutropenia are the peripheral WBC count and bone marrow aspiration and biopsy (Table 33.23). A total WBC count of 4×10^9/L or 4000/mcL reflects leukopenia. However, only a differential count can confirm the presence of neutropenia (ANC of $1–1.5 \times 10^9$/L). If the differential WBC count reflects an ANC of 0.5 to 1×10^9/L, the patient is at moderate risk for a bacterial infection. An ANC less than 0.5 to 1×10^9/L places the patient at severe risk. Note that patients with acute leukemia who present with a high WBC may in fact have neutropenia, because the majority of the WBCs are ineffective leukemia blast cells.

A peripheral blood smear is used to assess for immature forms of WBCs (e.g., bands). The Hct level, the reticulocyte count, and the platelet count are performed to evaluate bone marrow function. A review of the patient's recent past and current medication history should also be done. If the cause of neutropenia is unknown, bone marrow aspirations and biopsies are performed to examine cellularity and cell morphology. Additional studies may be done as indicated to assess spleen and liver function.

NURSING AND INTERPROFESSIONAL MANAGEMENT NEUTROPENIA

The factors involved in the nursing and interprofessional care of neutropenia include (a) determining the cause of the neutropenia; (b) identifying the offending organisms if an infection has developed; (c) instituting prophylactic, empirical, or therapeutic antibiotic therapy; (d) administering hematopoietic growth factors (e.g., granulocyte colony–stimulating factor [G-CSF] and granulocyte-macrophage colony–stimulating factor [GM-CSF]) after chemotherapy; and (e) instituting protective practices (e.g., strict handwashing, skin and oral hygiene) (see Table 33.23).

Occasionally, the cause of the neutropenia can be easily treated (e.g., nutritional deficiencies). However, neutropenia can also be an adverse effect that must be tolerated as a necessary step in therapy (e.g., chemotherapy, radiation therapy). In some situations, the neutropenia resolves when the primary disease is treated (e.g., tuberculosis).

The nurse must monitor the neutropenic patient for signs and symptoms of infection (any fever ≥38°C) and early sepsis.

TABLE 33.23	INTERPROFESSIONAL CARE

Neutropenia

Diagnostic	Interprofessional Management
• History and physical examination • Risk assessment for severity and duration of neutropenia • WBC count with differential • WBC morphology • Hct and Hb values • Reticulocyte and platelet count • Bone marrow aspiration or biopsy • Cultures of nose, throat, sputum, urine, stool, obvious lesions, blood (as indicated) • Chest X-ray or other diagnostic tests	• Identification and removal of cause of neutropenia (if possible) • Identification of site of infection (if present) and causative organism • Antimicrobial therapy (prophylactic or empiric) • Blood cultures STAT (prior to administration of antimicrobials) • Hematopoietic growth factors (G-CSF, and GM-CSF) • Strict adherence to handwashing and patient hygiene policies • Single-patient room and positive-pressure or HEPA filtration, depending on risk • Community isolation and home precautions if outpatient • Nutritional therapy and dietary instructions on foods to avoid and safe food handling

G-CSF, granulocyte colony–stimulating factor; *GM-CSF,* granulocyte-macrophage colony–stimulating factor; *Hb,* hemoglobin; *Hct,* hematocrit; *HEPA,* high-efficiency particulate air; *WBC,* white blood cell.

Early identification of a potentially infective organism depends on acquiring cultures from various sites. Serial blood cultures (at least two) or one from a peripheral site and one from a venous access device should be done promptly and antibiotics started immediately. In addition, cultures of sputum, throat, lesions, wounds, urine, and feces may be required. It may also be necessary to do a computed tomographic (CT) scan, tracheal aspiration, bronchoscopy with bronchial brushings, or lung biopsy to diagnose the cause of pneumonic infiltrates. Despite these many tests, the causative organism is identified in only approximately half of patients with neutropenia.

When a febrile episode occurs in a patient with neutropenia, antibiotic therapy must be initiated immediately (within 1 hour), even before determination by culture of a specific causative organism. Broad-spectrum antibiotics are usually ordered by the IV route because of the potential lethal effects of infection. However, some oral antibiotics are highly effective and routinely used for prophylaxis against infection in some patients with neutropenia. Antibiotics are often used in combinations because of their synergistic effects and in the event that multiple organisms are responsible for the infectious symptoms. Regardless of the combination, the nurse must initiate therapy promptly and observe for adverse effects of antimicrobial agents.

The longer the neutropenia lasts, the greater the risk of a fungal infection. Antifungal therapy is initiated in patients who produce a positive culture or in patients who do not become afebrile with broad-spectrum antibiotic coverage.

G-CSF (filgrastim [Neupogen]) and GM-CSF can be used to prevent neutropenia or to reduce its severity, its duration, or both. They should be considered for patients receiving chemotherapy based on their risk factors for neutropenia. G-CSF stimulates the production and function of neutrophils. GM-CSF stimulates the production and function of neutrophils and monocytes. These agents can be given by IV or subcutaneously. Keratinocyte growth factor may also be used to reduce the duration

and severity of mucositis, which may contribute to infection. An important consideration in the care of a patient with neutropenia is determination of the best means to protect the patient, whose own defences against infection are compromised. To accomplish this goal, the following principles must be kept in mind: (a) the patient's normal flora is the most common source of microbial colonization and infection; (b) transmission of organisms from humans most commonly occurs by direct contact with the hands; (c) air, food, water, and equipment provide additional opportunities for infection transmission; and (d) health care providers with transmissible illnesses and other patients with infections can also be sources of infection under certain conditions.

Hand hygiene is the single most important preventive measure in minimizing the risk of infection in the patient with neutropenia. Strict adherence to hand hygiene guidelines by all people coming in contact with the compromised patient is the major method to prevent transmission of harmful pathogens.

Immunocompromised patients should be separated from those who are infected or who have conditions that increase the probability of transmitting infections. A patient who is hospitalized, therefore, should be in a private room. Often, patients can be managed on an outpatient basis if the patient and caregivers can astutely monitor for fevers and other signs of infection and then report promptly to a nearby health care facility (Table 33.24). Although it is expensive to install, high-efficiency particulate air (HEPA) filtration, an air-handling method with a high-flow filtering system, can reduce or eliminate the number of aerosolized pathogens in the environment. It is often used for a patient with severe, prolonged neutropenia (e.g., patients who have undergone HSCT). Care routines in a HEPA environment are essentially the same as care in any other private room. Prophylactic antibiotics and antifungals may also be used for severely immunocompromised patients. The patient and caregiver should be instructed regarding a diet that restricts potentially hazardous foods, such as raw and undercooked meats and eggs and soft cheeses with moulds. Fresh flowers should be prohibited.

Quality-of-life issues for the patient with neutropenia should not be overlooked. Potential patient experiences of social isolation, depression, and perceived lack of support require appropriate interventions.

AGE-RELATED CONSIDERATIONS

THROMBOCYTOPENIA AND NEUTROPENIA

About 55 to 60% of cancer diagnoses are currently made in individuals older than 65 years. This proportion is expected to further increase in the next two decades as the baby boomers move into this age group. Age-related changes of bone marrow function are rather subtle and probably not significant for the hematopoietic function of normal older individuals. These changes, however, may become clinically evident under conditions of severe hematopoietic stress, such as the administration of repeated courses of chemotherapy, radiation therapy, or both and the resultant sequelae of myelosuppression. The use of supportive therapies, such as hematopoietic growth factors, increases the likelihood that older individuals will be treated with standard and even aggressive therapies, leading to neutropenia and thrombocytopenia. The nurse also needs to be aware that older individuals may have signs and symptoms different from those of a younger individual. For example, the older person may have delirium as compared with cough as a clinical manifestation of pneumonia.

TABLE 33.24 PATIENT & CAREGIVER TEACHING GUIDE

Neutropenia

This instruction sheet for patients explains protective precautions they should take when their neutrophil count is low. Patients should ask their health care provider about specific precautions to follow related to their particular risk factors for infection.

- *Wash your hands* frequently and make sure those around you wash their hands frequently, particularly if they help with your care. An antibacterial hand gel may also be used.
- Notify your nurse or health care provider if you have any of the following:
  - A fever greater than 38°C
  - Chills or feeling hot
  - Redness, swelling, discharge, or new painful area either on the skin or deeper in your body
  - Changes in urination or bowel movements
  - A cough, sore throat, mouth sores, or blisters
- If you are at home, take your temperature as directed and follow instructions on what to do if you have a fever.
- Avoid crowds and people with colds, flu, or infections. If you are in a public area, wear a mask and use hand-sanitizing gel frequently.
- Avoid eating uncooked meats, seafood, eggs, and unwashed fruits and vegetables. Ask your health care provider about specific dietary guidelines for you.
- Bathe or shower daily. A moisturizer may be used to prevent skin from drying and cracking.
- Maintain some daily activity as instructed by your health care team. This may include walking and moderate exercise while avoiding crowds.
- Brush your teeth with a soft toothbrush four times daily. You may floss once daily if it does not cause excessive pain or bleeding. Avoid using alcohol-based mouthwashes.
- Do not perform gardening or clean up after pets. Feeding and petting your dog or cat is fine as long as you wash your hands well after handling.

MYELODYSPLASTIC SYNDROME

Myelodysplastic syndrome (MDS) is a group of related hematological disorders characterized by a change in the quantity and quality of bone marrow elements. Peripheral blood cytopenias in combination with a hypercellular bone marrow exhibiting dysplastic changes is the hallmark of MDS. In MDS, hematopoiesis is disorderly and ineffective. In Canada, it is estimated that the incidence is about 4 per 100 000 adults (Slack et al., 2018). Although it can occur in all age groups, the highest prevalence is in people over 80 years of age.

Etiology and Pathophysiology

The exact etiology of MDS is unknown. People who have received radiation or chemotherapy or who were exposed to industrial solvents are at higher risk for developing MDS. About 50% of MDS patients have an overt chromosome abnormality. Rarely, genetic disorders are responsible for the disease.

MDS is referred to as a *clonal disorder* because some bone marrow stem cells continue to function normally whereas others (a specific clone) do not. The abnormal clone of the stem cells is usually found in the bone marrow but eventually may be found in circulation. Occasionally, one type of MDS transforms into another. Depending on the subtype, MDS may progress to acute myelogenous leukemia (AML) (Steensma, 2018). In contrast to AML, in which the leukemic cells show little normal maturation, the clonal cells in MDS always display some degree of maturity. Disease progression is slower than in AML and sometimes treatment is not needed.

Clinical Manifestations

MDS commonly manifests as infection and bleeding caused by inadequate numbers of ineffectively functioning circulating granulocytes or platelets. MDS is often discovered in the older person in the course of investigating symptoms of anemia, thrombocytopenia, or neutropenia. It may also be diagnosed incidentally from a routine CBC. During the advanced stage of MDS, life-threatening anemia, thrombocytopenia, and neutropenia occur.

Diagnostic Studies

Bone marrow biopsy with aspirate analysis is essential for both the diagnosis and the classification of the specific types of myelodysplasia. In MDS, the bone marrow is hypocellular or hypercellular and the patient has peripheral cytopenia. Laboratory data and bone marrow studies will help rule out other causes of the dysplasia, such as nonmalignant disorders, cobalamin and folate deficiencies, and infectious causes.

INFORMATICS IN PRACTICE

- Use of the Internet to access information on unfamiliar diseases. From an educational perspective, technology enables nurses to have quick access to a lot of information.
- Nurses assigned the care of a patient with a disease or disorder that they are not familiar with, such as thalassemia, can find evidenced-informed information to help guide clinical care.
- Trusted resources such as the Cochrane Database of Systematic Reviews can be accessed to provide evidence-informed information. Clinical guidelines are also available to help guide practice; however, BEWARE, the process of guideline development is unregulated.
- Guidelines accessed need to be carefully evaluated prior to changing practice to ensure that there is a rigorous, objective process for developing recommendations based on the best available evidence.

NURSING AND INTERPROFESSIONAL MANAGEMENT MYELODYSPLASTIC SYNDROME

Treatment of MDS is based on the premise that the aggressiveness of the treatment should match the aggressiveness of the disease. The recommended treatment depends on the amount and type of dysplasia in the bone marrow, specific genetic mutations, anticipated patient tolerance, and patient preference. Low-intensity treatments consist of hematological monitoring (serial bone marrow and peripheral blood examinations), antibiotic therapy, and transfusions with blood products, including iron chelators to prevent iron overload, if required.

Low-risk patients often can be treated with EPO, myeloid growth factors (e.g., G-CSF), and immunomodulators, such as lenalidomide (Revlimid). Low-intensity chemotherapeutic agents may be used, such as azacitidine (Vidaza) or decitabine. Immunosuppression therapy may be used with medications such as cyclosporine and ATG. High-intensity treatments include the use of intensive chemotherapeutic regimens, HSCT, or both. High-intensity treatments are not recommended for all patients, and only about one third of high-risk patients are treated with intensive chemotherapy, HSCT, or both.

Nursing care of a patient with MDS is similar to that for a patient with manifestations of anemia (see NCP 33.1, earlier in this chapter, for patients with anemia; see NCP 33.2 for thrombocytopenia and NCP 33.3 for neutropenia, both available on the Evolve website).

LEUKEMIA

Leukemia is a broad term given to a group of malignant diseases that affect the blood and blood-forming tissues of the bone marrow, lymph system, and spleen. Leukemia occurs in all age groups. It is characterized by diffuse replacement of bone marrow with proliferating leukocyte precursors. This loss of regulation in cell division results in an accumulation of dysfunctional cells. Leukemia follows a progressive course that is eventually fatal if untreated. It is estimated that, in 2020, there were 6 900 new cases and 3 000 deaths in Canada due to leukemia and that males accounted for almost 60% of new cases (Canadian Cancer Society, 2021b).

Etiology and Pathophysiology

Regardless of the specific type of leukemia, there is generally no single causative agent in the disease's development. Most leukemias result from a combination of factors, including genetic and environmental influences. Chromosomal changes, first recognized in chronic myelogenous leukemia, have led to discoveries of how normal genes, once transformed, can result in abnormal genes (oncogenes) capable of causing many types of cancers, including leukemias (see Chapter 18). Chemical agents (e.g., benzene), chemotherapeutic agents (e.g., alkylating agents), viruses, radiation, and immunological deficiencies have all been associated with the development of leukemia. The incidence of leukemia is increased in radiologists, people who have lived near nuclear bomb test sites or nuclear reactor accidents (e.g., Chernobyl), and people previously treated with radiation therapy or chemotherapy.

Although ribonucleic acid (RNA) retroviruses cause a number of leukemias in animals, a viral cause for a human leukemia has been established only for some patients with adult T-cell leukemia/lymphoma. This form of leukemia is endemic in southwestern Japan and parts of the Caribbean and central Africa and is caused by the human T-cell leukemia virus type 1 (HTLV-1).

Classification

Leukemia can be classified as either acute or chronic. The terms acute and chronic refer to cell maturity and the nature of the disease's onset. Acute leukemia is characterized by the clonal proliferation of immature hematopoietic cells. The leukemia develops following malignant transformation of a single type of immature hematopoietic cell, followed by cellular replication and expansion of that malignant clone. Chronic leukemias involve more mature forms of WBCs, and the disease onset is more gradual.

Leukemia can also be classified by identifying the type of leukocyte involved—that is, whether it is of myelogenous origin or of lymphocytic origin. By combining the acute and chronic categories with the cell type involved, specific types of leukemia can be identified. Four major types of leukemia are acute lymphocytic leukemia (ALL), acute myelogenous leukemia (AML), chronic myelogenous (granulocytic) leukemia (CML), and chronic lymphocytic leukemia (CLL). The defining features of these leukemic subtypes are presented in Table 33.25.

Acute Myelogenous Leukemia. AML represents only one third of all leukemias, but it makes up approximately 80% of the acute leukemias in adults. Its onset is often abrupt and dramatic. A patient may have serious infections and abnormal bleeding from the onset of the disease (Figure 33.12).

AML is characterized by uncontrolled proliferation of myeloblasts, the precursors of granulocytes. There is hyperplasia of the bone marrow and the spleen. The manifestations are usually related to replacement of normal hematopoietic cells in the marrow by leukemic myeloblasts and, to a lesser extent, to infiltration of other organs and tissue (see Table 33.25).

TABLE 33.25 TYPES OF LEUKEMIA

Type	Age of Onset	Clinical Manifestations	Diagnostic Findings
Acute myelogenous leukemia (AML)	Increase in incidence with advancing age; peak incidence between 60 and 70 yr of age	Fatigue and weakness, headache, mouth sores, anemia, bleeding, fever, infection, sternal tenderness, gingival hyperplasia, mild hepatosplenomegaly	Low RBC count, Hb, Hct; low platelet count; low to high WBC count with myeloblasts; high LDH; greatly hypercellular bone marrow with myeloblasts
Acute lymphocytic leukemia (ALL)	Peak prevalence between ages 2 and 5 yr and after age 50 yr	Fever; pallor; bleeding; anorexia; fatigue and weakness; bone, joint, and abdominal pain; generalized lymphadenopathy; infections; weight loss; hepatosplenomegaly; headache; mouth sores; neurological manifestations, CNS involvement, increased intracranial pressure secondary to meningeal infiltration	Low RBC count, Hb, Hct; low platelet count; low, normal, or high WBC count; high LDH; hypercellular bone marrow with lymphoblasts; lymphoblasts also possible in cerebrospinal fluid; presence of Philadelphia chromosome (up to 30% of patients)
Chronic myelogenous leukemia (CML)	Increase in incidence with advancing age, with median age at diagnosis of 67 yr	No symptoms early in disease; then fatigue and weakness, fever, sternal tenderness, weight loss, joint pain, bone pain, massive splenomegaly, increase in sweating	Low RBC count, Hb, Hct; high platelet count early, lower count later; increase in polymorphonuclear neutrophils, normal number of lymphocytes, and normal or low number of monocytes in WBC differential; low leukocyte alkaline phosphatase; presence of Philadelphia chromosome (90% of patients)
Chronic lymphocytic leukemia (CLL)	50–70 yr of age; rare below 30 yr of age; predominance in men	No symptoms frequently; detection of disease often during examination for unrelated condition; chronic fatigue, anorexia, splenomegaly and lymphadenopathy and hepatomegaly; may progress to fever, night sweats, weight loss, fatigue, and frequent infections	Mild anemia and thrombocytopenia with disease progression; total WBC count >100 × 10⁹/L; increase in peripheral lymphocytes; increase in presence of lymphocytes in bone marrow; hypogammaglobulinemia; may have autoimmune hemolytic anemia (4–11%), idiopathic thrombocytopenia purpura (2–4%)

CNS, central nervous system; Hb, hemoglobin; Hct, hematocrit; LDH, lactic dehydrogenase; RBC, red blood cell; WBC, white blood cell.

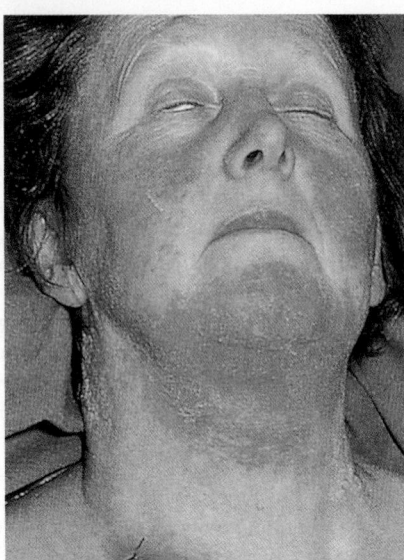

FIG. 33.12 Complications of acute leukemia. Spreading cellulitis of the neck and chin in this woman with acute myelogenous leukemia results from streptococcal and candidal infection. She is at risk because of previous chemotherapy and prolonged neutropenia. Source: Skarin, A. T. (1996). *Atlas of diagnostic oncology* (2nd ed.). Mosby-Wolfe.

Acute Lymphocytic Leukemia. ALL is the most common type of leukemia in children and accounts for about 20% of acute leukemia in adults. In ALL, immature, small lymphocytes proliferate in the bone marrow; most are of B-cell origin. Fever is present in the majority of patients at the time of diagnosis. Signs and symptoms may appear abruptly with bleeding or fever, or they may be insidious with progressive weakness, fatigue, and bleeding tendencies.

Central nervous system (CNS) manifestations are especially common in ALL and represent a serious concern. Leukemic meningitis caused by arachnoid infiltration occurs in many patients with ALL (Lenk et al., 2020). ALL patients with CNS involvement generally have a poorer prognosis. Clinical manifestations of CNS involvement vary but can manifest as headache, nausea, vomiting, lethargy, and visual changes related to increased intracranial pressure.

Chronic Myelogenous Leukemia. CML is caused by excessive development of mature neoplastic granulocytes in the bone marrow. The excess neoplastic granulocytes move into the peripheral blood in massive numbers and ultimately infiltrate the liver and the spleen. These cells contain a distinctive cytogenetic abnormality, the *Philadelphia chromosome*, which serves as a disease marker and results from translocation of genetic material between the *BCR* gene on chromosome 22 and the *ABL* gene on chromosome 9. The protein that is encoded by the newly created *BCR–ABL* gene on the Philadelphia chromosome interferes with normal cell cycle events, such as the regulation of cell proliferation.

The natural history of CML is a chronic stable phase followed by the development of a more acute, aggressive phase referred to as the *blastic phase*. The chronic phase of CML can last for several years and can usually be well controlled with treatment. Even with treatment, the chronic phase of the disease will eventually progress to the accelerated phase, ending in a blastic phase. Once CML transforms to an acute or blastic phase, it must be treated aggressively, similar to an acute leukemia.

Chronic Lymphocytic Leukemia. CLL is the most common leukemia in adults in Western countries. CLL is characterized by the production and accumulation of functionally inactive but long-lived, mature-appearing lymphocytes. The type of lymphocyte involved is usually the B cell. The lymphocytes infiltrate the bone marrow, spleen, and liver. Lymph node enlargement (lymphadenopathy) is present throughout the body, and there is an increased incidence of infection because of T-cell deficiencies or hypogammaglobulinemia. Complications from early-stage CLL are rare but may develop as the disease advances. Pressure on nerves from enlarged lymph nodes causes pain and even paralysis. Mediastinal node enlargement can lead to pulmonary symptoms. Because CLL is usually a disease of older persons, treatment decisions must be made by considering the progression of the disease and the adverse effects of treatment. Many individuals in the early stages of CLL require no treatment. Others may be followed closely and receive treatment only when the disease progresses. About one third need immediate treatment at the time of diagnosis.

Other Leukemias. Occasionally, the subtype of leukemia cannot be identified. The cancerous leukemic cells may have lymphoid, myeloid, or mixed characteristics. Frequently, these patients do not respond to treatment and have a poor prognosis. Other rare types include hairy cell and biphenotypic leukemias.

Clinical Manifestations

The manifestations of leukemia are varied (see Table 33.25). Essentially, they relate to problems caused by bone marrow failure and the formation of leukemic infiltrates. Bone marrow failure results from (a) bone marrow overcrowding by abnormal cells and (b) inadequate production of normal marrow elements. The patient is predisposed to anemia, thrombocytopenia, and decreased number and function of WBCs.

As leukemia progresses, fewer normal blood cells are produced. The abnormal WBCs continue to accumulate because they do not go through the normal cell life cycle to death (*apoptosis*). The leukemic cells may infiltrate the patient's organs, leading to conditions such as splenomegaly, hepatomegaly, lymphadenopathy, bone pain, meningeal irritation, and oral lesions. Solid masses called *chloromas* can result from collections of leukemic cells. A high leukemia WBC count in the peripheral blood can cause the blood to thicken and potentially block circulatory pathways. This is called *leukostasis* and can be life-threatening.

Diagnostic Studies

Peripheral blood evaluation and bone marrow examination are the primary methods of diagnosing and classifying the subtypes of leukemia. Morphological, histochemical, immunological, and cytogenetic methods are all used to identify cell subtypes, stage of development, and significant genetic mutations. This is important because different subtypes have different prognoses and treatment options. Other studies such as lumbar puncture and CT scan can be used to determine the presence of leukemic cells outside of the blood and the bone marrow.

Interprofessional Care

Once a diagnosis of leukemia has been made, interprofessional care is focused on the initial goal of attaining remission. Age and cytogenetic analysis often help form the basis of important treatment decisions. Because chemotherapy is the mainstay of the treatment, the nurse must understand the principles of cancer chemotherapy, including cellular kinetics, the use of multiple medications rather than single medications, and the cell cycle. (See the section on chemotherapy in Chapter 18.)

In some cases, such as asymptomatic patients with CLL, watchful waiting with active supportive care may be appropriate. Although a patient may not be cured, attaining remission or disease control is a realistic option for the majority of patients. In some cases, cure is a realistic goal. In *complete remission,* there is no evidence of overt disease on physical examination, and the bone marrow and peripheral blood appear normal. A lesser state of control is known as *partial remission,* which is characterized by a lack of symptoms and a normal peripheral blood smear, but there is still evidence of disease in the bone marrow. *Minimal residual disease* is defined as tumour cells that cannot be detected by morphological examination but can be detected by molecular testing. *Molecular remission* indicates that all molecular studies are negative for residual leukemia. The patient's prognosis is directly related to the ability to maintain a remission and becomes more unfavourable with each relapse. Each time there is a relapse, the succeeding remission may be more difficult to achieve and shorter in duration.

Sometimes patients have such a high WBC count that initial emergent treatment may include the use of leukapheresis and hydroxyurea administration. The purpose of these treatments is to reduce the WBC count and the risk of leukemia-induced thrombosis.

The chemotherapeutic treatment of acute leukemia is divided into stages. The first stage, *induction therapy,* is the attempt to induce or bring about a remission. Induction is aggressive treatment that seeks to destroy leukemic cells in the tissues, peripheral blood, and bone marrow in order to eventually restore normal hematopoiesis on bone marrow recovery. During induction therapy, a patient may become critically ill because the bone marrow is severely depressed by the chemotherapeutic drugs. Throughout the induction phase, nursing interventions focus on neutropenia, thrombocytopenia, and anemia management as well as on providing psychosocial support to the patient and family. Common chemotherapeutic agents for induction of AML include cytarabine (Cytosar) and antitumour antibiotics (anthracyclines) such as daunorubicin (Cerubidine), idarubicin (Idamycin), or mitoxantrone. After one course of induction therapy, approximately 70% of newly diagnosed patients achieve complete remission. There is one subtype of AML, called *promyelocytic leukemia* (M3), for which tretinoin (Vesanoid) and arsenic trioxide (Trisenox) may also be used to induce a remission. It is generally assumed that leukemia cells persist undetected after induction therapy. As a result, relapse is possible within a few months if no further therapy is administered.

Terms used to describe postinduction or postremission chemotherapy include *intensification, consolidation,* and *maintenance. Intensification therapy,* or high-dose therapy, may be given immediately after induction therapy for several months. This therapy may use the same agents as those used in induction, but at higher dosages. Other drugs that target the cell in a different way than those administered during induction may also be added.

Consolidation therapy is started after a remission is achieved. It may consist of one or two additional courses of the same drugs given during induction or involve high-dose therapy *(intensive consolidation).* The purpose of consolidation therapy is to eliminate remaining leukemic cells that may not be clinically or pathologically evident.

Maintenance therapy is treatment with lower doses of the same agents used in induction or other agents given every 3 to 4 weeks for a prolonged period of time. Like consolidation or intensification, the goal is to keep the body free of leukemic cells. Each leukemia calls for different maintenance therapy. In AML, maintenance therapy is rarely effective and, therefore, rarely administered.

In addition to chemotherapy, corticosteroids and radiation therapy can also have a role in the complex therapeutic plans for the patient with leukemia. Total body radiation may be used to prepare a patient for HSCT, or radiation may be restricted to certain areas (fields) such as the liver and spleen or other organs affected by infiltrates. In ALL, prophylactic intrathecal methotrexate is given to decrease the chance of CNS involvement, which is common in this particular type of leukemia. When CNS leukemia does occur, cranial radiation may be given. Immunotherapy and targeted therapy, such as monoclonal antibodies and chimeric antigen receptor (CAR) T cells, may be indicated for specific leukemias. (Immunotherapy is discussed in Chapter 18.)

Medication Therapy Regimens. Therapeutic medications used to treat leukemia vary. Table 33.26 gives examples of treatment regimens used in various types of leukemia.

TABLE 33.26 MEDICATION THERAPY
Treatments Used in Leukemia*

Medication Therapy	Other Therapy
Acute Myelogenous Leukemia	
Cytarabine (Cytosar), daunorubicin (Cerubidine)[†], idarubicin (Idamycin)[†], mitoxantrone, tretinoin (Vesanoid)[†], etoposide (Vepesid)[†], clofarabine (Clolar), arsenic trioxide (Trisenox), fludarabine (Fludara), azacitidine (Vidaza)	Autologous or allogeneic hematopoietic stem cell transplant (HSCT) (see Chapter 18)
Combination chemotherapy of cytarabine and antitumour antibiotic (most common)	
Acute Lymphocytic Leukemia	
Doxorubicin (Adriamycin), vincristine sulphate, prednisone, dexamethasone, L-asparaginase (Kidrolase) ponatinib (Iclusig), dasatinib (Sprycel), cyclophosphamide (Procytox), methotrexate, 6-mercaptopurine (Purinethol), cytarabine, imatinib (Gleevec), rituximab (Rituxan), clofarabine (Clolar)	Cranial radiation therapy, intrathecal methotrexate or cytarabine, allogeneic HSCT, CAR-T cell therapy (see Chapter 18)
Combination chemotherapy of several agents is common	
Chronic Myelogenous Leukemia	
Imatinib (Gleevec), dasatinib (Sprycel), ponatinib (Iclusig), nilotinib (Tasigna), bosutinib (Bosulif), hydroxyurea (Hydrea)	Radiation, HSCT, interferon alfa, leukapheresis
Combination chemotherapy including any of the following: cytarabine, daunorubicin, methotrexate, prednisone, vincristine, L-asparaginase, 6-mercaptopurine, busulfan (Myleran)	
Chronic Lymphocytic Leukemia	
Chlorambucil (Leukeran), cyclophosphamide (Procytox), prednisone, vincristine, fludarabine (Fludara), rituximab (Rituxan), alemtuzumab (MabCampath), bendamustine (Treanda), oxaliplatin (Eloxatin), methotrexate, ofatumumab (Arzerra), idelalisib (Zydelig), obinutuzumab (Gazyva), ibrutinib (Imbruvica), lenalidomide (Revlimid)	Radiation, splenectomy, colony-stimulating factors, allogeneic hematopoietic stem cell transplant

*The classification and mechanism of action of these medications are presented in Table 18.8 (Medication Therapy: Classification of Chemotherapeutic Agents).
†Used for acute promyelocytic leukemia.

Combination chemotherapy is the mainstay of treatment for leukemia. The three purposes for using multiple drugs are to (a) decrease drug resistance, (b) minimize the drug toxicity to the patient by using multiple drugs with varying toxicities, and (c) interrupt cell growth at multiple points in the cell cycle.

Some therapeutic medications are aimed at affecting small molecules that promote the growth and differentiation of leukemic cells. For example, Imatinib mesylate (Gleevec) and other tyrosine-kinase inhibitors target BCR–ABL protein that is present in nearly all patients with CML. Thus, this drug kills only cancer cells, leaving healthy cells alone.

The use of specific targeted therapy in the form of monoclonal antibodies is an exciting new treatment modality in hematopoietic malignancies, but cures with these therapies alone are rare. Rituximab (Rituxan) binds to the B-cell antigen (CD20) and has been used with CLL. Alemtuzumab (MabCampath) binds to CD52, a panlymphocyte antigen present on both T and B cells, and is used to treat CLL.

Hematopoietic Stem Cell Transplantation. HSCT is another type of therapy used for patients with different forms of leukemia. The goal of HSCT is to totally eliminate leukemic cells from the body using combinations of chemotherapy with or without total body irradiation. This treatment eradicates the patient's hematopoietic stem cells, which are then replaced with those of an HLA-matched sibling, HLA-half-matched relative, volunteer donor (allogeneic), or identical twin (syngeneic), or with the patient's own (autologous) stem cells that were removed (harvested) before the intensive therapy. (HSCT is discussed in Chapter 18.)

The primary complications of patients who undergo allogeneic HSCT are graft-versus-host (GVH) disease, relapse of leukemia (especially ALL), and infection (especially interstitial pneumonia). GVH disease is discussed in Chapter 16. Because HSCT has serious associated risks, the patient must weigh the significant risks of treatment-related death or treatment failure (relapse) with the hope of cure.

NURSING MANAGEMENT LEUKEMIA

NURSING ASSESSMENT

Subjective and objective data that should be obtained from a patient with leukemia are presented in Table 33.27.

NURSING DIAGNOSES

Nursing diagnoses for the patient with leukemia include those appropriate for anemia, thrombocytopenia, and neutropenia (see NCP 33.1 in this chapter and NCPs 33.2 and 33.3 on the Evolve website).

PLANNING

The overall goals are that the patient with leukemia will (a) understand and follow the treatment plan, (b) experience minimal adverse effects and complications associated with both the disease and its treatment, and (c) establish realistic hopes and goals, and feel supported during the periods of treatment, relapse, or remission.

NURSING IMPLEMENTATION

ACUTE INTERVENTION. The nursing role during acute phases of leukemia is extremely challenging because the patient has many physical and psychosocial needs. As with other forms of cancer,

TABLE 33.27 NURSING ASSESSMENT
Leukemia

Subjective Data

Important Health Information

Past health history: Exposure to chemical toxins (e.g., benzene, arsenic), radiation, or viruses (Epstein-Barr, HTLV-1); chromosome abnormalities (Down, Klinefelter's, and Fanconi's syndromes); immunological deficiencies; organ transplantation; frequent infections; bleeding tendencies; family history of leukemia
Medications: Chemotherapy
Surgery or other treatments: Radiation exposure; prior radiation and chemotherapy for cancer

Symptoms

- Weight loss, chills, night sweats
- Fatigue with progressive weakness; bone pain, joint pain; muscle cramps
- Dyspnea, cough
- Nausea, vomiting, anorexia, dysphagia, early satiety; mouth sores, sore throat
- Hematuria, decreased urine output
- Diarrhea, dark or bloody stools
- Headaches, confusion, numbness, tingling, visual disturbances
- Easy bruising; epistaxis; prolonged menses; menorrhagia; erectile dysfunction

Objective Data

General

Fever, generalized lymphadenopathy, lethargy

Integumentary

Pallor or jaundice; petechiae, ecchymoses, purpura, reddish-brown to purple cutaneous infiltrates, macules, and papules

Cardiovascular

Tachycardia, systolic murmurs

Gastrointestinal

Gingival bleeding and hyperplasia; oral ulcerations, herpes and *Candida* infections; perirectal irritation and infection; hepatomegaly, splenomegaly

Neurological

Seizures, disorientation, confusion, decreased coordination, cranial nerve palsies, papilledema

Musculoskeletal

Muscle wasting, bone pain, joint pain

Possible Findings

Low, normal, or high WBC count with shift to the left (↑ blast cells); anemia, ↓ hematocrit and hemoglobin, thrombocytopenia, specific chromosome abnormalities; hypercellular bone marrow aspirate or biopsy with myeloblasts, lymphoblasts, and markedly ↓ normal cells

HTLV-1, human T-cell leukemia virus, type 1; *WBC,* white blood cell.

the diagnosis of leukemia can evoke great fear and be equated with death. It may be viewed as a hopeless, horrible disease with many painful and undesirable consequences. The treatment and prognosis of each patient with leukemia are driven by many factors, such as age and type of leukemia. For each patient, it is important that the nurse has an understanding of the patient's type of leukemia, prognosis, treatment plan, and goals. With this information, the nurse can help the patient realize that, although the future may be uncertain, they can have a meaningful quality of life while in remission or with disease control and that, in some cases, there is reasonable hope for cure. The family also needs help adjusting to the stress of this abrupt onset of serious illness (e.g., with the patient's dependence, withdrawal, changes in role responsibilities, and alterations in body image) and the losses imposed by the sick role. The diagnosis of leukemia often brings with it the need to make difficult decisions at a time of profound stress for the patient and family.

Patients may have comorbid conditions that affect treatment decisions. Important nursing interventions include (a) maximizing the patient's physical functioning, (b) teaching patients that acute adverse effects of treatment are usually temporary, and (c) encouraging patients to discuss their quality-of-life issues. The nurse is an important advocate in helping the patient and family understand the complexities of treatment decisions and manage the adverse effects and toxicities. This may include making sure that fertility concerns are addressed. A patient may require long hospitalization or may need to temporarily relocate to an appropriate treatment centre. These situations can lead a patient to feel deserted and isolated at a time when support is most needed. The nurse has contact with the patient many hours a day and can help minimize feelings of abandonment and loneliness by balancing the demanding technical needs with a humanistic, caring approach. The needs of the patient with leukemia are best met by a multidisciplinary team (e.g., psychiatric and oncology clinical nurse specialists, case managers, dietitians, chaplains, and social workers).

From a physical care perspective, the challenge is to make astute assessments and plan care to help the patient manage the severe adverse effects of chemotherapy. The life-threatening results of bone marrow suppression (neutropenia, thrombocytopenia, and anemia) require aggressive nursing interventions (see NCP 33.1, earlier in this chapter, and NCPs 33.2 and 33.3 on the Evolve website). These patients may be at risk for oncological emergencies such as tumour lysis syndrome, DIC, leukostasis, and cytokine release syndrome. Additional complications of chemotherapy may affect the patient's GI tract, nutritional status, skin and mucosa, cardiopulmonary status, liver, kidneys, and neurological system. (Nursing interventions related to chemotherapy are discussed in Chapter 18 and NCP 18.2 on the Evolve website.)

The nurse must be knowledgeable about all medications being administered. This knowledge must include mechanism of action, purpose of the medication, routes of administration, doses, safe-handling considerations, and potential adverse effects of the medications. In addition, the nurse must know how to assess laboratory data reflecting the effects of the medications. Patient survival and comfort during aggressive chemotherapy are significantly affected by the quality of nursing care.

AMBULATORY AND HOME CARE. Ongoing care for the patient with leukemia is necessary to monitor for signs and symptoms of disease control or relapse. For a patient requiring long-term or maintenance chemotherapy, long-term chronic disease management can become discouraging. Therefore, the patient and the family must be taught to understand the importance of the continued diligence in disease management and the need for follow-up care. Teachings must also include information about the medications and self-care measures and when to seek medical attention.

The goals of rehabilitation for long-term survivors of leukemia are to manage the physical, psychological, social, and spiritual consequences and delayed effects from the disease and its treatment. (Delayed effects from treatment are discussed in Chapter 18.) The patient may need assistance re-establishing some relationships, and friends and family may need help learning how to interact with the patient. The patient and the family

must learn to regain attitudes of health and life while facing the real fear of relapse of disease. Involving the patient in survivor networks and support groups may help the patient adapt to living after a life-threatening illness. Exploring community resources (e.g., Canadian Cancer Society) may reduce the financial burden and the feelings of dependence. Spiritual support may give the patient inner strength and peace.

Vigilant follow-up care helps to ensure that the cancer survivor's unique needs are recognized and treated. Often, these needs require referral or consultation. For example, physiotherapists may be asked to develop an exercise program to prevent post-treatment deficits caused by drug-induced peripheral neuropathy. Some patients' needs may include, for instance, growth and development concerns for childhood survivors, vocational retraining, and reproductive concerns for a patient of childbearing age.

EVALUATION

The expected outcomes are that the patient with leukemia will (a) cope effectively with diagnosis, treatment regimen, and prognosis; (b) experience minimal complications related to the disease or its treatment; and (c) feel comfortable and supported throughout treatment.

LYMPHOMAS

Lymphomas are cancers originating in the bone marrow and lymphatic structures resulting in the proliferation of lymphocytes. Lymphomas make up approximately 5% of all cancers in Canada (Canadian Cancer Society, 2021a, 2021d). Two major types of lymphoma—Hodgkin's disease and non-Hodgkin's lymphoma (NHL)—are discussed in this chapter. A comparison of these two types of lymphoma is presented in Table 33.28.

HODGKIN'S LYMPHOMA

Hodgkin's lymphoma, also called *Hodgkin's disease,* makes up about 10% of all lymphomas. It is characterized by proliferation of abnormal, giant, multinucleated cells, called *Reed–Sternberg cells,* which proliferate in lymph nodes. The disease has a bimodal age-specific incidence, occurring most frequently in people from 20 to 34 years of age and older than 60 years (Zhou et al., 2019). In adults, it is twice as prevalent in men than in women. It is estimated that, in 2020, 1 000 people were diagnosed with Hodgkin's lymphoma in Canada (Canadian Cancer Society, 2021a).

Etiology and Pathophysiology

Although the cause of Hodgkin's lymphoma remains unknown, several key factors are thought to play a role in its development. The main interacting factors include infection with Epstein-Barr virus (EBV), genetic predisposition, and exposure to occupational toxins. The incidence of Hodgkin's lymphoma is also increased in patients with HIV.

The disease likely starts in a single location (it starts in the cervical lymph nodes in 60–70% of patients) and then spreads along adjacent lymphatics. However, in recurrent disease, it may be more diffuse. It eventually infiltrates other organs, especially the lungs, spleen, and liver. When the disease begins above the diaphragm, it remains confined to lymph nodes for a variable time. Disease originating below the diaphragm frequently spreads to extralymphoid sites such as the liver.

TABLE 33.28	COMPARISON OF HODGKIN'S DISEASE AND NON-HODGKIN'S LYMPHOMA	
	Hodgkin's Disease	**Non-Hodgkin's Lymphoma**
Cellular origin	B lymphocytes	B lymphocytes (88%) T or natural killer lymphocytes (12%)
Extent of disease	Localized to region, but may be more widespread	Disseminated
B symptoms*	Common	Uncommon
Extranodal involvement	Rare	Common

*B symptoms include fever, night sweats, and weight loss.

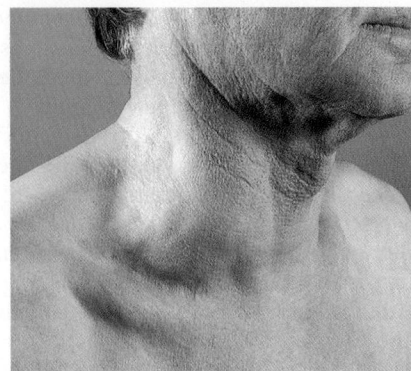

FIG. 33.13 Enlarged cervical lymph node in the neck of a man with Hodgkin's lymphoma. Source: Howard, M. R., & Hamilton, P. J. (2013). *Haematology: An illustrated colour atlas* (4th ed.). Churchill Livingston.

Clinical Manifestations

The onset of symptoms in Hodgkin's lymphoma is usually gradual. The initial development is most often enlargement of cervical, axillary, or inguinal lymph nodes (Figure 33.13); a mediastinal node is the second most common location. This lymphadenopathy affects discrete nodes that remain movable and nontender. The enlarged nodes are not painful unless they exert pressure on adjacent nerves.

The patient may notice weight loss, fatigue, weakness, fever, chills, tachycardia, or night sweats. A group of initial findings including fever, night sweats, and weight loss (termed *B symptoms*) correlates with a worse prognosis. After the ingestion of even small amounts of alcohol, individuals with Hodgkin's disease may experience a rapid onset of pain at the site of disease. The cause for the alcohol-induced pain is unknown. Generalized pruritus without skin lesions may develop. Cough, dyspnea, stridor, and dysphagia may all reflect mediastinal node involvement.

In more advanced disease, there is hepatomegaly and splenomegaly. Anemia results from increased destruction and decreased production of RBCs. Other physical signs vary depending on where the disease is located; for example, (a) intrathoracic involvement may lead to superior vena cava syndrome, (b) enlarged retroperitoneal nodes may cause palpable abdominal masses or interfere with renal function, (c) jaundice may occur from liver involvement, (d) spinal cord compression leading to paraplegia may occur with extradural involvement, and (e) bone pain may occur as a result of bone involvement.

Diagnostic and Staging Studies

Peripheral blood analysis, excisional lymph node biopsy, bone marrow examination, and radiological evaluation are important means of evaluating Hodgkin's lymphoma. Peripheral blood analysis may reveal microcytic hypochromic anemia; however, this is variable and not diagnostic. Leukopenia and thrombocytopenia may develop, but they are usually a consequence of treatment, advanced disease, or superimposed hypersplenism. Other blood studies may show an elevated erythrocyte sedimentation rate, hypoferremia caused by excessive iron uptake by the liver and spleen, high leukocyte alkaline phosphatase from liver and bone involvement, hypercalcemia from bone involvement, and hypoalbuminemia from liver involvement.

Excisional lymph node biopsy offers a definitive means of diagnosis. The removed peripheral lymph node is examined for the presence of the diagnostic Reed–Sternberg cells. Reed–Sternberg cells may also be found in the patient's bone marrow, and a bone marrow biopsy may be performed as an important aspect of staging.

Radiological evaluation can help define all sites and determine the clinical stage of the disease. Positron emission tomographic (PET) and CT scans are used as initial staging tools and then to assess response to therapy and to distinguish residual tumour from fibrotic masses after treatment.

NURSING AND INTERPROFESSIONAL MANAGEMENT HODGKIN'S LYMPHOMA

The information from the various diagnostic studies is used to determine the stage of the disease (Figure 33.14). The nomenclature used in staging includes a Roman numeral (I to IV) that reflects the location and extent of the disease, followed by an *A* or *B* classification (meaning B symptoms are absent or present, respectively). Treatment depends on the nature and the extent of the disease.

Once the stage of Hodgkin's lymphoma is established, management focuses on selecting a treatment plan. The standard for chemotherapy is the ABVD regimen: doxorubicin (**A**driamycin), **b**leomycin, **v**inblastine, and **d**acarbazine. Patients with early-stage disease with favourable characteristics will receive two to four cycles of chemotherapy. Patients with early-stage but unfavourable prognostic features (e.g., the presence of B symptoms) or intermediate-stage disease will be treated with four to six cycles of chemotherapy. Advanced-stage Hodgkin's lymphoma is treated more aggressively using six to eight cycles of chemotherapy. A more aggressive chemotherapy regimen for Hodgkin's lymphoma is BEACOPP (**b**leomycin, **e**toposide, doxorubicin [**A**driamycin], **c**yclophosphamide, vincristine (former trade name **O**ncovin), **p**rocarbazine, and **p**rednisone (Ansell, 2018). The role of radiation as a supplement to chemotherapy varies depending on sites of disease and the presence of resistant disease after chemotherapy.

A variety of chemotherapy regimens and newer medications, such as brentuximab vedotin (Adcetris), are used to treat patients with relapsed or refractory disease. Ideally, once remission is achieved, a curative option may be intensive chemotherapy with the use of autologous or allogeneic HSCT. HSCT has allowed patients to receive higher, potentially curative doses of chemotherapy while reducing life-threatening leukopenia.

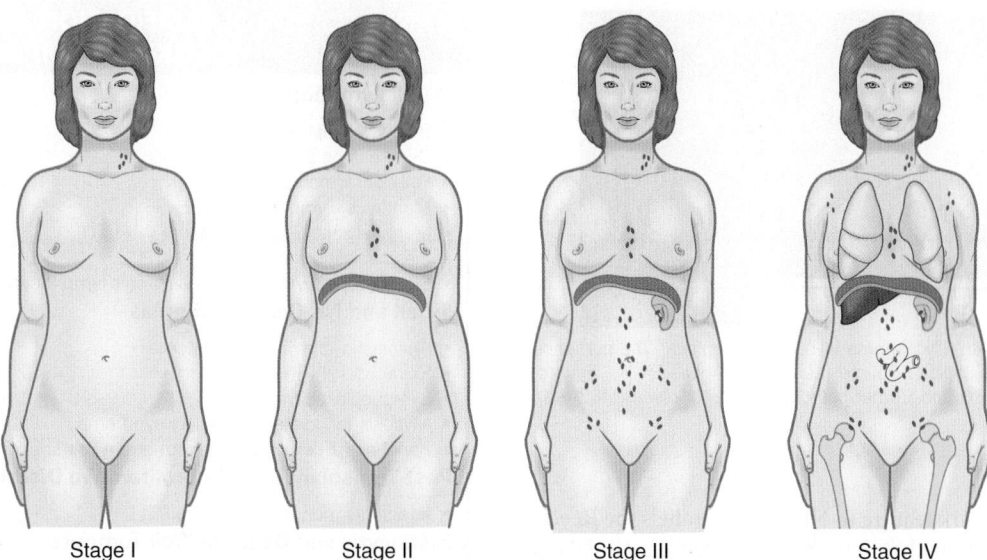

| Stage I | Stage II | Stage III | Stage IV |

FIG. 33.14 Staging system for Hodgkin's lymphoma and non-Hodgkin's lymphoma. **Stage I,** involvement of single lymph node (e.g., cervical node). **Stage II,** involvement of two or more lymph nodes on one side of diaphragm. **Stage III,** lymph node involvement above and below the diaphragm. **Stage IV,** involvement outside the lymph nodes (e.g., liver, bone marrow). The stage is followed by the letter *A* (absence) or *B* (presence) to indicate significant systemic symptoms (e.g., fever, night sweats, weight loss).

Combination chemotherapy works well because, as with leukemia, agents are used that have an additive antitumour effect without increased adverse effects. Therapy must be aggressive, thus potentially life-threatening conditions are risked for the sake of attempting to achieve a remission.

Maintenance chemotherapy does not contribute to increased survival once a complete remission is achieved. Occasionally, single medications may be administered palliatively to patients who cannot tolerate intensive combination therapy. A serious consequence of the treatment for Hodgkin's lymphoma is the later development of secondary malignancies (see Chapter 18) as well as potential long-term toxicities from the treatment, such as endocrine, cardiac, and pulmonary dysfunction. Secondary cancers often occur 10 years after treatment for Hodgkin's lymphoma, the most common of which are breast cancer and lung cancer. Patients should undergo screening for early detection of these diseases.

The nursing care for patients with Hodgkin's lymphoma is largely focused on managing health conditions related to the disease (e.g., pain caused by the tumour), pancytopenia, and other adverse effects of therapy. Because the survival of patients with Hodgkin's lymphoma depends on their response to treatment, supporting the patient through the immunosuppressive state is extremely important.

Psychosocial considerations are just as important as they are with leukemia. However, the prognosis for Hodgkin's lymphoma is better than that for many other forms of cancer. The physical, psychological, social, and spiritual consequences of the patient's disease must be addressed. Fertility issues may be of particular concern because this disease is frequently seen in adolescents and young adults. The nurse must help ensure that these issues are addressed soon after diagnosis. Evaluation of patients for long-term effects of therapy is important because delayed consequences of disease and treatment may not be apparent for many years. (Secondary malignancies and delayed effects of treatment are discussed in Chapter 18.)

NON-HODGKIN'S LYMPHOMA

Non-Hodgkin's lymphomas (NHLs) are a heterogeneous group of cancers of primarily B-, T-, natural killer (NK), histiocytic, and dendritic cell origin. They affect people of all ages. There are more than 30 different types. They are classified by the level of differentiation, (maturity) cell of origin, immunophenotype (cell surface markers), and genetic and clinical features. A variety of clinical presentations and courses are recognized, from indolent (slowly developing) to rapidly progressive disease. NHL is the most commonly occurring hematological cancer. It is estimated that, in 2020, there were 10 400 new cases of NHL diagnosed in Canada and approximately 2 900 deaths due to NHL (Canadian Cancer Society, 2021d). Survival depends on a multitude of factors: age, stage, LDH level in the blood, extranodal spread, and performance status. It is important to note that survival has been reported to be lower in Indigenous people in Canada (Chiefs of Ontario et al., 2017). Further research is warranted.

Etiology and Pathophysiology

As with Hodgkin's lymphoma, the cause of NHL is usually unknown. It may result from chromosomal translocations, infections, environmental factors, or immunodeficiency states. Chromosomal translocations have a key role in the pathogenesis of many NHLs. Some viruses and bacteria are implicated in the pathogenesis of NHL, including HTLV-1, EBV, human herpesvirus 8, hepatitis B and C, *H. pylori*, *Chlamydophila psittaci*, *Campylobacter jejuni*, and *Borrelia burgdorferi*. Environmental factors linked to the development of NHL include chemicals such as pesticides, herbicides, solvents, organic chemicals, and wood preservatives. NHL is also more common in individuals who have inherited immunodeficiency syndromes and who have used immunosuppressive medications or received chemotherapy or radiation.

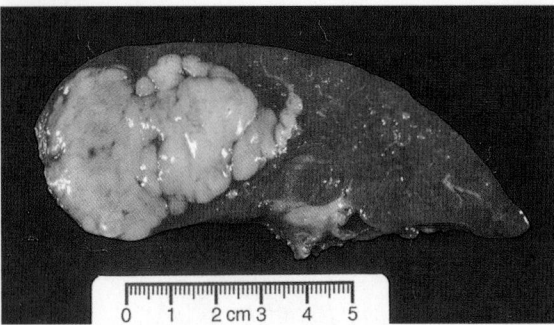

FIG. 33.15 Non-Hodgkin's lymphoma involving the spleen. The presence of an isolated mass is typical. Source: Kumar, V., Abbas, A. K., Fausto, N., et al. (2010). *Robbins and Cotran pathologic basis of disease* (8th ed., p. 607). Saunders.

TABLE 33.29	CLASSIFICATION OF NON-HODGKIN'S LYMPHOMA*

B-Cell Lymphomas

- Burkitt's lymphoma
- Diffuse large B-cell lymphoma (DLBCL)
- Follicular lymphoma
- Mantle cell lymphoma
- Marginal zone B-cell lymphoma (MALT)
- Plasmablastic lymphoma
- Small lymphocytic lymphoma/chronic lymphocytic leukemia

T-Cell and NK-Cell Lymphomas

- Anaplastic large T-cell lymphoma
- Extranodal NK/T-cell lymphoma
- Lymphoblastic lymphoma
- Mycosis fungoides and Sézary syndrome
- Peripheral T-cell lymphoma, not otherwise specified (NOS)

Post-Transplant Lymphoproliferative Disorders (PTLD)

- Infectious mononucleosis-like PTLD

Histiocytic and Dendritic Cell Tumours

- Langerhans cell histiocytosis

MALT, mucosa-associated lymphoid tissue; *NK*, natural killer.
*This is only a partial list.

There is no hallmark feature in NHL that parallels the Reed–Sternberg cell of Hodgkin's lymphoma. However, all NHLs involve lymphocytes arrested in various stages of development and may mimic a leukemia. For example, small lymphocytic lymphoma (SLL) and CLL result from malignant proliferation of small B lymphocytes, with most CLL disease within the bone marrow versus the lymph nodes. Diffuse large B-cell lymphoma, the most common aggressive lymphoma in adults, starts in the lymph nodes, usually in the neck or abdomen. Burkitt's lymphoma is a highly aggressive disease thought to originate from B-cell blast cells in the lymph nodes.

Clinical Manifestations

NHLs can originate outside the lymph nodes, the method of spread can be unpredictable, and the majority of patients have widely disseminated disease at the time of diagnosis (Figure 33.15). The primary manifestation is painless lymph node enlargement. Because the disease is usually disseminated when it is diagnosed, other symptoms will be present depending on where the disease has spread (e.g., hepatomegaly with liver involvement or neurological symptoms with CNS disease). NHL can also manifest in nonspecific ways, such as an airway obstruction, hyperuricemia, renal failure or acute kidney injury from tumour lysis syndrome, pericardial tamponade, or GI symptoms. Patients with high-grade lymphomas may have lymphadenopathy and constitutional symptoms (B symptoms) such as fever, night sweats, and weight loss.

Diagnostic and Staging Studies

Diagnostic studies used for NHL resemble those used for Hodgkin's disease. However, because NHL is more often in extranodal sites, more diagnostic studies may be done, such as an MRI or lumbar puncture to rule out CNS disease, a bone marrow biopsy to determine bone marrow infiltration, or a barium enema or upper endoscopy to visualize suspected GI involvement. Clinical staging, as described for Hodgkin's lymphoma, is used to help guide therapy (see Figure 33.14), but establishment of the precise histological subtype through biopsy is extremely important. NHL is classified on the basis of morphological, genetic, immunophenotypic (i.e., cell surface antigens, CD20, CD52), and clinical features.

The World Health Organization has categorized more than 30 unique types of NHL. A simple modification of the classification system is presented in Table 33.29.

Treatment is guided by cell type, cytogenetic studies, and clinical behaviour: *indolent* (low grade), *aggressive* (high grade), or *highly aggressive* (very high grade). Additional factors, known as the International Prognostic Index (IPI), may be considered for each subtype. These include the clinical stage, number of extranodal sites, age, serum LDH, and patient's performance status.

NURSING AND INTERPROFESSIONAL MANAGEMENT NON-HODGKIN'S LYMPHOMA

Treatment for NHL involves chemotherapy, biotherapy, radiation, and sometimes phototherapy and topical therapy (Table 33.30). Ironically, more aggressive lymphomas are more responsive to treatment and more likely to be cured. In contrast, indolent lymphomas have a naturally long course but are difficult to treat effectively.

Patients with low-grade (indolent) lymphoma may live 10 years or more without treatment. However, some initial therapies are well tolerated and delay the time to progression of the disease. Lymphomas that have an infectious basis, such as *H. pylori* gastric lymphomas, may be treated with antibiotic or antiviral therapy. HSCT may have some benefit in certain subtypes of aggressive or refractory lymphomas. CAR T-cell immunotherapy may also be used.

Rituximab, a monoclonal antibody against the CD20 antigen on the surface of normal and malignant B cells, is used to treat NHL in combination with other agents. Once bound to the cells, rituximab causes lysis and cell death. Numerous chemotherapy combinations have been used to try to overcome the resistant nature of this disease. Recently, targeted therapies have become more prevalent.

MEDICATION ALERT—Rituximab (Rituxin)

- Monitor patients for signs of severe hypersensitivity infusion reactions, especially with the first infusion.
- Manifestations may include hypotension, bronchospasm, dysrhythmias, angioedema, and cardiogenic shock.
- Screen patients for history of hepatitis as the drug may reactivate the disease.

TABLE 33.30   TREATMENT OF NON-HODGKIN'S LYMPHOMA*

Recommended Therapies	Common Chemotherapy Combinations
Indolent (Low Grade) (e.g., follicular lymphoma, marginal zone B-cell lymphoma [MALT])	
• Observation until disease progression for asymptomatic patients with low-volume tumours and normal blood counts • External beam irradiation for local, limited disease • Single-agent rituximab (Rituxan) • Single-agent chemotherapy (chlorambucil, cyclophosphamide, bendamustine, or idelalisib) • Rituximab with another agent (bendamustine, cyclophosphamide, fludarabine, cladribine, lenalidomide, chlorambucil) • Combination chemotherapy (R-CHOP or other) • Radioimmunotherapy • Hematopoietic stem cell transplant (HSCT)	• **R-CHOP: r**ituximab, **c**yclophosphamide, doxorubicin **h**ydrochloride, vincristine (former trade name **O**ncovin), **p**rednisone • **R-CVP: r**ituximab, **c**yclophosphamide, **v**incristine, **p**rednisone • **RFND: r**ituximab, **f**ludarabine, mitoxantrone (former trade name **N**ovantrone), **d**examethasone ± rituximab
Aggressive (Intermediate or High Grade) (e.g., mantle cell, diffuse large B-cell, T-cell, natural killer cell lymphomas)	
• Combination chemotherapy with localized radiation if needed • Aggressive combination chemotherapy for 3–8 cycles with rituximab with local radiation if needed • Intrathecal chemotherapy if needed • Single-agent or other combination treatment, depending on subtype and response (e.g., bendamustine, bortezomib, cladribine, ibrutinib, lenalidomide, gemcitabine, alemtuzumab, oxaliplatin, romidepsin) • HSCT	• **R-CHOP** (see above) • **ICE** (or **RICE** with **r**ituximab): **i**fosfamide, **c**yclophosphamide, **e**toposide • **R-EPOCH: r**ituximab, **e**toposide, **p**rednisone, vincristine (former trade name **O**ncovin), **c**yclophosphamide, doxorubicin **h**ydrochloride • **ESHAP ± R: e**toposide, methylprednisolone (**S**olu-Medrol), **h**igh-dose cytarabine (former trade name **A**ra-C), cisplatin (former trade name **P**latinol), with or without **r**ituximab • **Hyper-CVAD ± R:** hyperfractionated **c**yclophosphamide, **v**incristine, doxorubicin hydrochloride (**A**driamycin), **d**examethasone alternating with high-dose methotrexate and cytarabine with or without rituximab • **DHAP ± R: d**examethasone, **h**igh-dose cytarabine (former trade name **A**ra-C), cisplatin (former trade name **P**latinol), with or without **r**ituximab
Highly Aggressive (e.g., Burkitt's lymphoma)	
• Aggressive combination chemotherapy for 3–8 cycles • HSCT	• **R-EPOCH** (see above) • **Hyper-CVAD ± R** (see above) • **CODOX-M: c**yclophosphamide, vincristine (former trade name **O**ncovin), **dox**orubicin, high-dose **m**ethotrexate, with or without rituximab (includes intrathecal methotrexate)

MALT, mucosa-associated lymphoid tissue.
*Not all-inclusive.

⟳ EVIDENCE-INFORMED PRACTICE

Translating Research Into Practice

A nurse is caring for G. R. (pronouns he/him), a 59-year-old with non-Hodgkin's lymphoma who is receiving chemotherapy. Because of a decrease in red blood cells and platelets, he was advised to rest and avoid the high level of physical exercise he once enjoyed. He misses his active lifestyle and now admits to the nurse that he is "somewhat depressed."

Best Available Evidence	Clinician Expertise	Patient Preferences and Values
Aerobic exercise, especially walking and stretching, to maintain mobility may improve physical functioning, fatigue, and depression in patients with hematological cancers.	The nurse knows that recommendations to decrease intensive physical exercise may result in a diminished quality of life for many patients, especially for individuals who are used to being physically active.	Gerard is considering joining a neighbourhood bicycling club so that he can "feel better."

Decision and Action

1. Why is intensive or extreme exercise contraindicated in someone who is receiving chemotherapy or who is acutely ill?
2. What precautions should the nurse suggest G. R. take before he increases his exercise level?
3. How should the nurse involve G. R. in monitoring his fatigue?
4. As G. R. seeks ways to improve his quality of life, how should the nurse support him?

Reference for Evidence

Knips, L., Bergenthal, N., Streckmann, F., et al. (2019). Aerobic physical exercise for adult patients with haematological malignancies. *Cochrane Database of Systematic Reviews, 1.* https://doi.org/10.1002/14651858.CD009075.pub3

Another therapy for NHL is the monoclonal antibody ibritumomab tiuxetan (Zevalin). It contains a radioactive particle than can kill cancer cells. The therapy targets the CD20 antigen, which is on the surface of mature B cells and B-cell tumours. This targeting allows for the delivery of radiation directly to the cancer cells. Adverse effects of these medications include pancytopenia. Nurses must be aware of the precautions to take in caring for these patients and must educate patients about safety issues to minimize the risk of radiation exposure to staff and others.

In general, T-cell lymphomas are more difficult to treat and are often treated aggressively up front, followed by HSCT. Cutaneous T-cell lymphomas may be treated with topical corticosteroids or topical chemotherapy for limited-stage disease.

For more diffuse disease, treatment may include methotrexate, interferon alfa, or other medications.

The nursing care for NHL is similar to that for Hodgkin's lymphoma. It is largely focused on managing conditions related to the disease (e.g., pain caused by the tumour, spinal cord compression, tumour lysis syndrome), pancytopenia, and other adverse effects of therapy. However, because NHL can be more extensive and involve specific organs (e.g., CNS, spleen, liver, GI tract, bone marrow), it is important that the nurse have an understanding of the subtype and the extent of the disease. For example, a patient with known involvement of the colon may report acute abdominal pain. The patient may have abdominal guarding and an enlarged and tympanic abdomen. This could indicate a bowel perforation and be considered a medical emergency. A patient with Burkitt's NHL starting chemotherapy would be at high risk for tumour lysis syndrome and would require frequent laboratory studies and monitoring, as well as strict documentation of intake and output. (For oncological issues, refer to Chapter 18.) Because most of these patients receive therapy that is potentially myelosuppressive, NCP 33.1, NCP 33.2, and NCP 33.3 would apply to these patients as well.

A patient undergoing radiation therapy has special nursing needs. The skin in the radiation field requires attention. In addition, the nurse must understand the concepts related to administration of and safety issues regarding radiation therapy (see Chapter 18 and NCP 18.1 on the Evolve website).

Psychosocial considerations are very important. Helping the patient and the family understand the disease, the treatment, and expected and potential adverse effects is paramount in enlisting their help in ensuring the patient's well-being and safety. Some aggressive treatments require close follow-up and even inpatient admission. In young patients, fertility concerns may need to be addressed. As with Hodgkin's lymphoma, evaluation of patients with NHL for long-term effects of therapy is important because delayed consequences of disease and treatment may not be apparent for many years. (Secondary malignancies and delayed effects of treatment are discussed in Chapter 18.)

MULTIPLE MYELOMA

Multiple myeloma, or *plasma cell myeloma,* is a condition in which cancerous plasma cells infiltrate the bone marrow and destroy bone. The disease is more common in men than in women with a median age at diagnosis of 65 years (Rajkumar, 2020). Myeloma has a higher incidence in Black ethnic groups than in White people. It is estimated that, in 2020, 3 400 new cases of multiple myeloma were diagnosed in Canada (Canadian Cancer Society, 2021c).

Etiology and Pathophysiology

The cause of multiple myeloma is unknown. Exposure to radiation, organic chemicals (such as benzene), herbicides, and insecticides may play a role. Genetic factors, viral infection, and obesity may also influence the risk of developing multiple myeloma.

The disease process involves excessive production of plasma cells. Normal plasma cells are activated B cells, which make immunoglobulins (antibodies) that protect the body. However, in multiple myeloma, instead of a variety of plasma cells producing antibodies to fight different infections, myeloma tumours produce monoclonal antibodies. *Monoclonal* means they are all of one kind, making them ineffective and even harmful. Not only

do they not fight infections, but they also infiltrate the bone marrow. These monoclonal proteins (called *M proteins*) are made up of two light chains and two heavy chains. *Bence Jones proteins* are the light-chain part of these monoclonal antibodies. They show up in the urine in many patients with multiple myeloma.

In multiple myeloma, plasma cell production of excessive amounts of cytokines (interleukins [ILs]; IL-4, IL-5, and IL-6) plays an important role in the pathological process of bone destruction. As myeloma protein increases, normal plasma cells are reduced, a decrease that further compromises the body's normal immune response. Proliferation of cancer plasma cells and the overproduction of immunoglobulin and proteins result in the end-organ effects of myeloma to the bone marrow, bone, and kidneys and possibly the spleen, lymph nodes, liver, and even heart muscle.

Clinical Manifestations

Multiple myeloma develops slowly and insidiously. The patient often does not manifest symptoms until the disease is advanced, at which time skeletal pain is the major manifestation. Pain in the pelvis, spine, and ribs is particularly common and is triggered by movement. Diffuse osteoporosis develops as the myeloma protein destroys bone. Osteolytic lesions are seen in the skull, vertebrae, long bones, and ribs (Figure 33.16). Vertebral destruction can lead to collapse of vertebrae with ensuing compression of the spinal cord. Loss of bone integrity can lead to the development of pathological fractures.

Bony degeneration causes calcium to be lost from bones, eventually causing hypercalcemia. Hypercalcemia may cause renal, GI, or neurological manifestations such as polyuria, anorexia, confusion, and cardiac conditions. A serum *hyperviscosity syndrome* can occur in some patients, leading to cerebral, pulmonary, renal, and other organ dysfunction. Even without hyperviscosity, high protein levels caused by the presence of the myeloma protein can result in renal tubular obstruction, interstitial nephritis, and renal failure. The patient may have anemia, thrombocytopenia, neutropenia, and immune dysfunction, all of which are related to the replacement of normal bone marrow with plasma cells. Neurological abnormalities may be caused by regional myeloma cell growth that compresses the spinal cord or cranial nerves or by perineuronal or perivascular deposition of the abnormal protein.

Diagnostic Studies

Evaluating multiple myeloma involves laboratory, radiological, and bone marrow examination. M protein is often found in the blood and urine. Pancytopenia, hypercalcemia, the presence of Bence Jones protein in the urine, and a high serum creatinine are possible findings.

Skeletal bone surveys, MRI and/or PET scan, and CT scan show distinct areas of destroyed bone, generalized thinning of the bones, or fractures, especially in vertebrae, ribs, pelvis, and bones of the thigh and the upper arms. Bone marrow analysis shows significantly increased numbers of plasma cells in the bone marrow. The simplest measure of staging and prognosis in multiple myeloma is based on the blood levels of two markers: β_2-microglobulin and albumin. In general, higher levels of β_2-microglobulin and lower levels of albumin are associated with a poorer prognosis. Cytogenetic studies of the bone marrow play an important role in prognostic stratification. For example, deletion of chromosome 17p is considered a high-risk feature (Rajkumar, 2020).

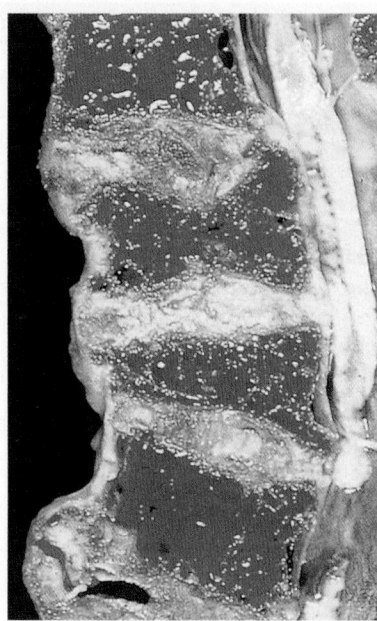

FIG. 33.16 Multiple myeloma. This segment of the lower thoracic spine has been sectioned to show the extensive replacement of the bone and the marrow with red gelatinous tissue. Source: Skarin, A. T. (1996). *Atlas of diagnostic oncology* (2nd ed.). Mosby-Wolfe.

Interprofessional Care

Interprofessional care involves managing both the disease and its symptoms. The current treatment options include corticosteroids, chemotherapy, immunotherapy, targeted therapy, and HSCT (Rajkumar, 2020). Multiple myeloma is seldom cured, but treatment can relieve symptoms, produce remission, and prolong life. Ambulation and adequate hydration are used to treat hypercalcemia, dehydration, and potential renal damage. Weight bearing helps the bones reabsorb some calcium, and fluids dilute calcium and prevent protein precipitates from causing renal tubular obstruction. Control of pain and prevention of pathological fractures are other goals of management. Analgesics, orthopedic supports, and localized radiation help reduce the skeletal pain.

Kyphoplasty is sometimes used to control spinal vertebral disease. *Kyphoplasty* is a minimally invasive procedure in which cement is injected to stabilize the vertebral compression.

Bisphosphonates, such as pamidronate and zoledronic acid (Zometa), inhibit bone breakdown and are used for the treatment of skeletal pain and hypercalcemia. They inhibit bone resorption without inhibiting bone formation and mineralization. They are given monthly by IV infusion and are recommended for all patients with symptomatic multiple myeloma.

MEDICATION ALERT—Zoledronic acid (Zometa)
- Patients must be adequately hydrated prior to administering zoledronic acid (Zometa).
- Renal toxicity may occur if IV zoledronic acid is infused in less than 15 minutes.
- Patients should have a dental exam prior to the first dose and ongoing monitoring for osteonecrosis of the jaw (Willan et al., 2016).

Chemotherapy with corticosteroids is often recommended for multiple myeloma. It is used to reduce the number of plasma cells. Initial treatment depends on whether the patient is a future bone marrow transplant candidate and on anticipated tolerance of therapy. The treatment usually includes a corticosteroid plus one or two chemotherapy agents, such as melphalan (Alkeran), cyclophosphamide, doxorubicin (Adriamycin), and vincristine. High-dose chemotherapy followed by autologous HSCT has evolved as the standard of care in eligible patients.

Immunotherapy and targeted therapy are also used to treat multiple myeloma. Immunomodulator medications include thalidomide (Thalomid), lenalidomide (Revlimid), and pomalidomide (Pomalyst). Proteasome inhibitors include bortezomib (Velcade). Monoclonal antibodies may also be used in the treatment of multiple myeloma.

Other medications may be used to treat complications of multiple myeloma. For example, allopurinol (Zyloprim) may be given to reduce hyperuricemia, and IV furosemide (Lasix) promotes renal excretion of calcium. In some patients, the levels of plasma proteins are so high that a hyperviscosity syndrome results, leading to neurological changes, renal insufficiency, and other disorders related to the lack of blood flow. In this instance, plasmapheresis is used.

NURSING MANAGEMENT MULTIPLE MYELOMA

A major focus of care relates to the bone involvement and the sequelae from bone breakdown. Maintaining adequate hydration is a primary nursing consideration to minimize symptoms from hypercalcemia. Fluids are administered to attain a urinary output of 1.5 to 2 L/day if the patient does not have renal compromise. In addition, weight bearing helps bones reabsorb some of the circulating calcium, and corticosteroids may augment the excretion of calcium. Once chemotherapy is initiated, the uric acid levels may rise because of the increased cell destruction. Hyperuricemia is treated by ensuring adequate hydration and using allopurinol to prevent any renal damage. Because of the myeloma proteins, the patient is at additional risk for renal dysfunction. The nurse must monitor electrolytes and fluid balance.

Because of the potential for pathological fractures, the nurse must be careful when moving and ambulating the patient. A slight twist or strain in the wrong area (e.g., a weak area in the patient's bones) may be sufficient to cause a fracture. In addition, the development of peripheral neuropathy is common with several therapies for multiple myeloma and can contribute to discomfort, the inability to perform basic activities of daily living, and the risk for injury from falling.

Pain management requires innovative and knowledgeable nursing interventions. Analgesics, such as nonsteroidal anti-inflammatory medications, acetaminophen, or an acetaminophen–opioid combination, may be more effective than opioids alone in diminishing bone pain. Braces, especially for the spine, may also help control pain. As in any situation necessitating pain management, the nurse is responsible for assessing the patient and for implementing necessary measures to alleviate the pain. (Pain management is discussed in Chapter 10.) Patients may also be at risk for DVT related to chemotherapy and immobility and should have preventive measures employed.

Assessment and prompt treatment of infection are important in the care of patients with multiple myeloma. Recurrent infections may be caused by a decrease in the production of normal immunoglobulins, the ineffectiveness of the overproduced and abnormal immunoglobulins, corticosteroids, and/or neutropenia that results from the bone marrow infiltration or as an adverse effect of treatment. NCP 33.1 for anemia, NCP 33.2 for thrombocytopenia, and NCP 33.3 for neutropenia apply to the patient with multiple myeloma. (NCPs 33.2 and 33.3 are available on the Evolve website.)

The patient's psychosocial needs require sensitive, skilled management. It is important to help the patient and significant others adapt to changes fostered by chronic sickness and adjust to the losses related to the disease process while helping to maximize functioning and quality of life. The symptoms of multiple myeloma go through remission and exacerbation periods. Consequently, acute care is needed at various times during the course of the illness. The final acute phase is unresponsive to treatment and usually short. The way in which patients and families deal with confronting death may be affected by the manner in which they learned to accept and live with the chronic nature of the disease.

DISORDERS OF THE SPLEEN

The spleen can be affected by many illnesses, most of which cause some degree of *splenomegaly* (enlarged spleen) (Table 33.31). The term *hypersplenism* refers to the occurrence of splenomegaly and peripheral cytopenias (anemia, leukopenia, and thrombocytopenia). The degree of splenic enlargement varies with the disease. For example, massive splenic enlargement may occur with chronic myelogenous leukemia, hairy cell leukemia, and thalassemia major. Mild splenic enlargement occurs with HF and systemic lupus erythematosus.

When the spleen enlarges, its normal filtering and storage capacity increases. Consequently, there is often a reduction in the number of circulating blood cells. In addition, there are unusual findings in the peripheral smear, such as pitted or pocked erythrocytes or Howell–Jolly bodies. These findings aid in diagnosing a malfunctioning spleen. A slight to moderate enlargement of the spleen is usually asymptomatic and found during a routine examination of the abdomen. While massive splenomegaly can be well tolerated, the patient may have abdominal discomfort and early satiety. Other techniques to assess the size of the spleen include radionuclide colloid liver–spleen scan, CT or PET scan, MRI, and ultrasound scan.

Occasionally, a splenectomy is done as part of the evaluation or treatment of splenomegaly. Another major reason for splenectomy is splenic rupture. The spleen may rupture from trauma, inadvertent tearing during other surgical procedures, and diseases such as mononucleosis, malaria, and lymphoid neoplasms. After a splenectomy, there may be a dramatic increase in peripheral RBC, WBC, and platelet counts.

Nursing responsibilities for the patient with spleen disorders vary depending on the disorder. Splenomegaly may be painful and may necessitate analgesic administration; care in moving, turning, and positioning; and evaluation of lung expansion because spleen enlargement may impair diaphragmatic excursion. If anemia, thrombocytopenia, or leukopenia develops from splenic enlargement, nursing measures must be instituted to support the patient and prevent life-threatening complications. If splenectomy is performed, observation for hemorrhage and shock is required.

After splenectomy, immunological deficiencies may develop. Patients who have had splenectomy have a lifelong risk for infection, especially from encapsulated organisms such as pneumococcus (Tahir et al., 2020). This risk is reduced by immunization with pneumococcal vaccine (e.g., Pneumovax).

TABLE 33.31   CAUSES OF SPLENOMEGALY

Congestion
- Acquired hemolytic anemia
- Cirrhosis of the liver
- HF (portal hypertension)
- Portal or splenic vein thrombosis
- Sickle cell disease
- Thalassemia

Infections and Inflammations
- Autoimmune diseases: SLE, RA
- Bacterial infections: endocarditis, splenic abscess, syphilis, salmonella, tuberculosis, Lyme disease, Rocky Mountain spotted fever, typhoid fever
- Fungal infections: histoplasmosis, systemic candidiasis
- Parasitic infections: malaria, trypanosomiasis, schistosomiasis, leishmaniasis, toxoplasmosis
- Viral infections: hepatitis, human immunodeficiency virus, cytomegalovirus, mononucleosis

Infiltrative Diseases and Tumours or Cysts
- Acute and chronic leukemia
- Amyloidosis
- Gaucher disease
- Lymphomas
- Polycythemia vera
- Other primary or secondary neoplasms and cysts
- Sarcoidosis

HF, heart failure; *RA,* rheumatoid arthritis; *SLE,* systemic lupus erythematosus.

BLOOD COMPONENT THERAPY

Blood component therapy is frequently used in managing hematological diseases. Many therapeutic and surgical procedures depend on blood product support. However, blood component therapy supports the patient only temporarily until the underlying condition is resolved. Because transfusions are not free from hazards, they should be used only if necessary.

Nurses must be careful to avoid developing a complacent attitude about this common but potentially dangerous therapy. Nurses also must make sure that the health care provider has discussed the risks, benefits, and alternatives with the patient and that this conversation is documented in the patient's medical record.

Traditionally, the term *blood transfusion* meant the administration of whole blood. Blood transfusion now has a broader meaning because of the ability to administer specific components of blood such as platelets, packed red blood cells (PRBCs), or plasma. Usually, a specific component is ordered, although whole blood may be used rarely with massive hemorrhage or for an exchange transfusion (Table 33.32).

Administration Procedure

Blood components may be administered with a 22-gauge IV needle, cannula, or catheter. However, larger needles (e.g., 18- or 16-gauge) may be preferred if rapid transfusions are given or if the infusion is sluggish. Smaller needles can be used for platelets, albumin, and clotting factor replacement. Whatever type of venous access used, it is important to assess patency prior to requesting the blood component from the blood bank. Most blood product administration tubing is of a "Y type" with a 170- to 260-micron filter. One branch of the Y is for the isotonic saline solution and the other branch for the blood product. Infusion pumps are usually used for blood administration according to institutional policy.

TABLE 33.32 BLOOD PRODUCTS*

Description	Special Considerations	Indications for Use
Albumin		
Albumin is prepared from plasma. It is available in 5% or 25% solution. It can be stored for 5 years.	Albumin 25 g/100 mL is osmotically equal to 500 mL of plasma. Hyperosmolar solution acts by moving water from extravascular to intravascular space. It is heat treated and does not transmit viruses.	Hypovolemic shock, hypoalbuminemia, after large-volume paracentesis, replacement in plasmapheresis
Cryoprecipitates and Commercial Concentrates		
Cryoprecipitate is prepared from fresh-frozen plasma, with 10–20 mL/bag. Once thawed, it must be used.	See Table 33.19.	Replacement for fibrinogen deficiency, usually due to DIC, severe liver disease, or massive transfusion. Replacement of clotting factors, especially factor VIII, and von Willebrand factor
Fresh-Frozen Plasma		
Liquid portion of whole blood is separated from cells and frozen. One unit contains about 250 mL. Plasma is rich in clotting factors but contains no platelets. It may be stored for >1 yr, depending on storage, but must be used within 24 hr after thawing.	Use of plasma in treating hypovolemic shock is being replaced by use of pure preparations such as albumin plasma expanders.	Bleeding caused by deficiency in clotting factors (e.g., DIC, hemorrhage, massive transfusion, liver disease, vitamin K deficiency, excess warfarin)
Frozen Red Blood Cells		
Frozen RBCs are prepared using glycerol for protection. They can be stored for 10 years.	They must be used within 24 hr of thawing. Successive washings with saline solution remove the majority of WBCs and plasma proteins.	Autotransfusion; stockpiling; or rare donors for patients with allobodies. Infrequently used because filters remove most WBCs
Packed RBCs		
Packed RBCs are prepared from whole blood by sedimentation or centrifugation. One unit contains 250–350 mL. They can be stored up to 42 days depending on processing.	Use of RBCs for treatment allows remaining components of blood (e.g., platelets, albumin, plasma) to be used for other purposes. There is less danger of fluid overload.	Severe or symptomatic anemia; acute blood loss. In general, one unit of packed RBCs can be expected to increase a patient's Hb level by 10 g/L or Hct by 3%. One unit of RBCs can replace a blood loss of 500 mL.
Platelets		
Platelets are prepared from fresh whole blood. Platelets may be pooled from multiple donors. A single donation by apheresis is usually 200–400 mL in volume.	Multiple units of platelets can be obtained from one donor by plateletpheresis. They can be kept at room temperature for 1–5 days depending on type of collection and storage. For patients who receive frequent transfusions or who have not responded to previous platelet transfusions, platelets that are leukocyte-reduced or HLA- or type-specific may be given to prevent alloimmunization to HLA antigens.	Bleeding caused by thrombocytopenia or platelet levels <10–20 × 10⁹/L; use may be contraindicated in the presence of thrombocytopenic purpura, thrombotic thrombocytopenic purpura, and heparin-induced thrombocytopenia except for life-threatening hemorrhage. Expected increase is 10 000 mcL per unit. Failure to obtain a rise may be caused by fever, sepsis, splenomegaly, or DIC.

DIC, disseminated intravascular coagulation; *Hb*, hemoglobin; *Hct*, hematocrit; *HLA*, human leukocyte antigen; *RBCs*, red blood cells; *WBCs*, white blood cells.
*Component therapy has replaced the use of whole blood, which accounts for less than 10% of all transfusions. Granulocyte transfusions are not included here because they are rarely used.

SAFETY ALERT
- Dextrose solutions or lactated Ringer's solution must not be used for administering blood because they will cause RBC hemolysis.
- Additives (including medications) must not be given via the same tubing as the blood unless the tubing is first cleared with saline solution.

When the blood or blood components have been obtained from the blood bank, positive identification of the blood donor and the recipient must be made. Improper product-to-patient identification causes 90% of hemolytic transfusion reactions, thus placing a great responsibility on nursing personnel to carry out the identification procedure appropriately. The nurse must follow the policy and procedures of the institution where care is being provided; many institutions have implemented a dual-checking system with two licensed individuals checking patient identification with the labelled blood component. The blood bank is responsible for typing and crossmatching the donor's blood with the recipient's blood; the result of the compatibility testing should be noted on the product bag or tag, if pertinent.

ABO compatibility is not a prerequisite for platelet transfusions. However, after multiple platelet transfusions, a patient may develop anti-HLA antibodies to the transfused platelets. With the use of lymphocyte typing to match HLA types of the donor and the recipient, multiple platelet transfusions can be given with fewer complications to those who develop antibodies to platelets. Patients with a history of reactions to platelet transfusions may be premedicated with an antihistamine and hydrocortisone to decrease the possibility of reaction.

The nurse takes the patient's vital signs before the beginning of the transfusion to obtain a baseline measure; if the patient has abnormal vital signs, such as an elevated temperature, the health care provider is called to clarify when the blood component may be administered. The blood should be administered as soon as it is brought to the patient. Blood products should not be refrigerated on the nursing unit. Products that are not used within 30 minutes of being issued should be returned to the blood bank. During the first 15 minutes or 50 mL of blood infusion, the nurse should remain with the patient. If there are any untoward reactions, they are most likely to occur at this time. The rate of infusion during this period should be no more than 2 mL/min. PRBCs should not be infused quickly unless an emergency exists. Rapid infusion of cold blood may cause the patient to become chilled. If rapid replacement of large amounts of blood is necessary, a blood-warming device may be used. Other blood components, such as fresh-frozen plasma and platelets, may be infused over 15 to 30 minutes. The nurse needs to refer to the institution's policy and procedure for such infusions.

After the first 15 minutes, vital signs are usually retaken, and the rate of infusion is governed by the prescriber's orders, the clinical condition of the patient, and the product being infused. The nurse should observe the patient periodically throughout the transfusion (e.g., every 30 minutes) and up to 1 hour after the transfusion. Most patients not in danger of fluid overload can tolerate the infusion of one unit of PRBCs over 2 hours. The transfusion should not take more than 4 hours to administer because of the increased risk for bacterial growth in the product once it is out of refrigeration.

Blood Transfusion Reactions

A *blood transfusion reaction* is an adverse reaction to blood transfusion therapy that can range in severity from mild symptoms to a life-threatening condition. Because complications of transfusion therapy may be significant, careful evaluation of the patient is required. Blood transfusion reactions can be classified as acute or delayed (Tables 33.33 and 33.34).

If an *acute transfusion reaction* occurs, the following steps should be taken: (a) stop the transfusion; (b) maintain a patent IV line with saline solution; (c) notify the blood bank and the health care provider immediately; (d) recheck identifying tags and numbers; (e) monitor vital signs and urine output; (f) treat symptoms as per health care provider order; (g) save and return the blood bag and tubing to the blood bank for examination; (h) collect blood and urine samples at intervals as stipulated by hospital policy to evaluate for hemolysis; and (i) document the incident on a transfusion reaction form and the patient's chart. The blood bank and laboratory are responsible for identifying the type of reaction.

Acute Transfusion Reactions

Acute Hemolytic Reactions. The most common cause of hemolytic reactions is transfusion of ABO-incompatible blood (see Table 33.33). This is an example of a type II cytotoxic hypersensitivity reaction (see Chapter 16). Severe hemolytic reactions are rare. Mislabelling specimens and administering blood to the wrong individual cause most acute hemolytic reactions. This again points to the importance of using proper patient identifiers when drawing blood samples and when administering medications and blood products.

When an acute hemolytic reaction occurs, antibodies in the recipient's serum react with antigens on the donor's RBCs. This reaction results in agglutination of cells, which can obstruct capillaries and block blood flow. Hemolysis of the RBCs releases free Hb into the plasma. The Hb is filtered by the kidneys and may be found in the urine (hemoglobinuria). Hb may obstruct the renal tubules, leading to acute kidney injury, DIC, and death (see Chapter 49).

The clinical manifestations of an acute hemolytic reaction may be mild or severe and usually develop within 15 minutes of transfusion. Free Hb in blood and urine specimens obtained at the onset of the reaction will provide evidence of an acute hemolytic reaction.

Febrile Reactions. Febrile reactions are most commonly caused by leukocyte incompatibility. Many individuals who receive five or more transfusions develop circulating antibodies to the small amount of WBCs in the blood product. Febrile reactions can often be prevented by using additional filters in the tubing to leukocyte-deplete RBCs and platelets. Donated blood in Canada is processed to reduce the number of circulating WBCs (i.e., leukodepleted), a process that has helped decrease the incidence of the febrile nonhemolytic and minor allergic reactions. Medications such as acetaminophen (Tylenol) and diphenhydramine (Benadryl) may be ordered and given 30 minutes before blood administration to reduce these reactions.

Allergic Reactions. Allergic reactions result from the recipient's sensitivity to plasma proteins of the donor's blood. These reactions are more common in an individual with a history of allergies. Administration of antihistamines may help prevent allergic reactions. Epinephrine or corticosteroids may be used to treat a severe reaction.

Circulatory Overload. An individual with cardiac or renal insufficiency is at risk for developing circulatory overload, especially if a large quantity of blood is infused over a short period, particularly in an older person. PRBCs can be split by the blood bank, allowing for one half of a unit to be given over a time frame of up to 4 hours. A fluid balance assessment, including baseline auscultation of the patient's lungs, is performed. Reports of shortness of breath and the presence of adventitious breath sounds may indicate fluid overload in a patient.

Sepsis. Blood products can become infected from improper handling and storage. Bacterial contamination of blood products can result in bacteremia, sepsis, or septic shock.

Transfusion-Related Acute Lung Injury. Transfusion-related acute lung injury (TRALI) is characterized by the sudden development of noncardiogenic pulmonary edema (acute lung injury). It usually occurs within hours of the transfusion of blood products. With the reduction of clerical errors, leukocyte-reduced products, more effective screening, and the prevention of the transmission of infectious agents, TRALI has surpassed hemolytic reactions as the leading cause of transfusion-related death. It is thought to be caused by an antibody-mediated reaction between the recipient's leukocytes and antileukocyte antibodies from donors who were sensitized during pregnancy or by previous transfusions. TRALI causes pulmonary capillary inflammation and increased permeability, leading to respiratory distress and potentially death.

Massive Blood Transfusion Reaction. An acute complication of transfusing large volumes of blood products is termed *massive blood transfusion reaction*. Massive blood transfusion reactions can occur when replacement of RBCs or blood exceeds the total blood volume within 24 hours. In this situation, an imbalance of normal blood elements results because clotting factors, albumin, and platelets are not found in RBC transfusions. Thus, appropriate monitoring of hemostatic laboratory parameters must be done concurrently.

Additional complications such as hypothermia, citrate toxicity, hypocalcemia, and hyperkalemia may occur when massive blood transfusions are given. Hypothermia and cardiac dysrhythmias can result from rapid infusion of large quantities of cold blood. Blood-warming equipment prevents this problem. Citrate toxicity can occur when large quantities of blood products are used, because citrate is part of the storage solution; calcium binds to the citrate. Citrate toxicity is likely to develop when blood is transfused at a rate of 1 unit in 10 minutes (or 8–10 units of RBCs within a few hours). Manifestations such

TABLE 33.33   ACUTE TRANSFUSION REACTIONS

Cause	Clinical Manifestations	Management	Prevention
Acute Hemolytic Reaction			
Infusion of ABO-incompatible whole blood, RBCs, or components containing 10 mL or more of RBCs. Antibodies in the recipient's plasma attach to antigens on transfused RBCs, causing RBC destruction.	Reaction usually occurs in first 15 minutes. Fever with or without chills; low back, abdominal, chest or flank pain; flushing, tachycardia, dyspnea, tachypnea, hypotension, vascular collapse, hemoglobinuria, acute jaundice, dark urine, bleeding, acute kidney injury, shock, cardiac arrest, DIC, death	Treat shock and DIC if present. Draw blood samples—slowly to avoid hemolysis—for serological testing. Send urine specimen to the laboratory. Maintain BP with IV colloid solutions. Give diuretics as prescribed to maintain urine flow. Insert in-dwelling urinary catheter or measure voided amounts to monitor hourly urine output. Dialysis may be required if renal failure occurs. Do not transfuse additional RBC-containing components until blood bank has provided newly cross-matched units.	Meticulously verify and document patient identification at each step from sample collection to component infusion.
Febrile, Nonhemolytic Reaction (Most Common)			
Sensitization to donor WBCs, platelets, or plasma proteins	Sudden chills and fever (rise in temperature of >1°C), headache, flushing, anxiety, vomiting	Give antipyretics as prescribed—avoid ASA in patients with thrombocytopenia. *Do not restart transfusion* unless health care provider orders it.	Consider leukocyte-poor blood products (filtered, washed, or frozen) for patients with a history of two or more such reactions. Give acetaminophen or diphenhydramine 30 min before transfusion.
Mild Allergic Reaction			
Sensitivity to foreign plasma proteins. More common in people with history of allergies	Flushing, itching, pruritus, urticaria (hives)	Give antihistamine, corticosteroid, epinephrine as directed. If symptoms are mild and transient, transfusion may be restarted slowly with health care provider's order. Do not restart transfusion if fever or pulmonary symptoms develop.	Treat prophylactically with antihistamines and steroids. Consider using washed RBCs and platelets.
Anaphylactic and Severe Allergic Reaction			
Sensitivity to donor plasma proteins. Infusion of IgA proteins to IgA-deficient recipient who has developed IgA antibody	Anxiety; urticaria; dyspnea, wheezing, progressing to cyanosis; bronchospasm; hypotension, shock, and possible cardiac arrest	Initiate CPR if indicated. Administer O$_2$. Have epinephrine ready for injection. Antihistamines, corticosteroids, β$_2$-agonists may also be prescribed. *Do not restart transfusion.*	Transfuse extensively washed RBC products, from which all plasma has been removed. Use blood from IgA-deficient donor. Use autologous components.
Circulatory Overload Reaction			
Fluid administered faster than the circulation can accommodate. People with cardiac or renal disease at risk	Cough, dyspnea, pulmonary congestion, adventitious breath sounds, headache, hypertension, tachycardia, distended neck veins	Place patient upright with feet in dependent position. Obtain chest X-ray STAT if ordered. Administer prescribed diuretics, O$_2$, and/or morphine.	Adjust transfusion volume and flow rate based on patient size and clinical status. Have blood bank divide unit into smaller aliquots for better spacing of fluid input.
Sepsis Reaction			
Transfusion of bacterially infected blood components	Rapid onset of chills, high fever, vomiting, diarrhea, marked hypotension, or shock	Obtain culture of patient's blood and send bag with remaining blood and tubing to blood bank for further study. Treat septicemia as directed—administration of antibiotics, IV fluids, and/or vasopressors.	Collect, process, store, and transfuse blood products according to blood banking standards, and infuse within 4 hr of starting time.
Transfusion-Related Acute Lung Injury (TRALI) Reaction			
Reaction between transfused antileukocyte antibodies and recipient's leukocytes, causing pulmonary inflammation and capillary leak	Fever, chills, hypotension, tachypnea, frothy sputum, dyspnea, hypoxemia, respiratory failure. Noncardiogenic pulmonary edema. Leading cause of transfusion-related deaths. Arises within 1–6 hr of transfusion	Draw blood to analyze ABGs and HLA or antileukocyte antibodies; obtain chest X-ray STAT. Provide O$_2$ and administer corticosteroids (diuretics of no value). Initiate CPR if needed, and provide ventilatory and BP support if needed.	Provide leukocyte-reduced products. Identify donors who are implicated in TRALI reactions, and do not allow them to donate.

Continued

TABLE 33.33   ACUTE TRANSFUSION REACTIONS—cont'd

Cause	Clinical Manifestations	Management	Prevention
Massive Blood Transfusion Reaction			
Can occur with replacement of 10 or more RBC units within 24 hours. RBC transfusions do not contain clotting factors, albumin, and platelets.	Hypothermia and cardiac dysrhythmias (from massive infusion of large quantities of cold blood) Citrate toxicity and hypocalcemia (from the use of citrate as a storage solution) Hyperkalemia (from potassium leaking from stored RBCs)	When patients receive massive transfusions of blood products, monitor clotting status and electrolyte levels.	Use blood-warming equipment. Infusion of 10% calcium gluconate. Because of dilution effect on coagulation due to massive RBC transfusion, platelets and plasma will also be administered.

ABGs, arterial blood gases; *ASA,* acetylsalicylic acid (Aspirin); *BP,* blood pressure; *CPR,* cardiopulmonary resuscitation; *DIC,* disseminated intravascular coagulation; *HLA,* human leukocyte antigen; *IgA,* immunoglobulin A; *IV,* intravenous; *O₂,* oxygen; *RBC,* red blood cell; *WBC,* white blood cell.

TABLE 33.34   DELAYED TRANSFUSION REACTIONS

Manifestations	Prevention and Management
Delayed Hemolytic	
Fever, mild jaundice, decreased hemoglobin. Occurs as early as 3 days or as late as several months post-transfusion as the result of destruction of transfused RBCs by alloantibodies not detected during crossmatch.	Generally, no acute treatment is required. Hemolysis may be severe enough to warrant further transfusions.
Hepatitis B*	
Elevated liver enzymes (AST and ALT), anorexia, malaise, nausea and vomiting, fever, dark urine, jaundice. Usually resolves spontaneously within 4–6 wk. Chronic carrier state can develop and result in permanent damage to the liver.	Hepatitis B virus can be detected in donated blood by the presence of hepatitis B surface antigen (HBsAg). Treat symptomatically (see Chapter 46).
Hepatitis C*	
Similar to hepatitis B, but symptoms are usually less severe. Chronic liver disease and cirrhosis may develop.	Before anti-HCV testing of donated blood began, this accounted for 90–95% of all post-transfusion hepatitis. Treat symptomatically (see Chapter 46).
Iron Overload	
Excess iron is deposited in heart, liver, pancreas, and joints, causing dysfunction. HF, dysrhythmias, impaired thyroid and gonadal function, diabetes, arthritis, cirrhosis. Occurs in patients receiving >20 units for chronic anemia (e.g., sickle cell anemia, beta thalassemia) over time.	Treat symptomatically. Deferoxamine (Desferal), which chelates and removes accumulated iron via the kidneys, administered IV or subcutaneously. Deferasirox (Exjade) and deferiprone (Ferriprox) are oral agents that chelate iron and may be used. Phlebotomy may also be used.
Other	
CMV, HIV, HSV-6, Epstein-Barr virus, HTLV-1, and malaria. Most recent threats have been agents that primarily affect animals but have been transmitted to the blood supply through the food supply, or vectors such as mosquitoes or ticks. These include *Plasmodium* species (malaria), dengue fever virus, West Nile virus, *Trypanosoma cruzi* (Chagas's disease), *Babesia* species (babesiosis), human herpesvirus 8 (KS virus), and variant Creutzfeldt-Jakob disease ("mad cow disease").	Treatment is based on the cause. Ways of detecting some of these agents are now available and required, such as the nucleic acid test for West Nile virus, Zika virus, HIV, and *T. cruzi.* Donor screening has been the only available method to reduce the risk for donor-contaminated blood for others.

ALT, alanine aminotransferase; *AST,* aspartate aminotransferase; *CMV,* cytomegalovirus; *HCV,* hepatitis C virus; *HIV,* human immunodeficiency virus; *HSV-6,* human herpesvirus, type 6; *HTLV-1,* human T-cell leukemia virus, type 1; *KS,* Kaposi sarcoma.
*New cases of transfusion-related hepatitis B and C are not common.

as muscle tremors and ECG changes may be observed with hypocalcemia but can be prevented or reversed by the infusion of 10% calcium gluconate (10 mL with every litre of citrated blood). Hyperkalemia results when potassium leaks from RBCs in stored blood. Mild to severe signs and symptoms can occur, including nausea, muscle weakness, diarrhea, paresthesias, flaccid paralysis of the cardiac or respiratory muscles, and cardiac arrest. Electrolyte monitoring is an important aspect of the care of the patient receiving massive transfusions of blood products.

Delayed Transfusion Reactions. Delayed transfusion reactions include delayed hemolytic reactions (discussed previously), infections, and iron overload (see Table 33.34). These are defined as those occurring 24 hours to 14 days after the administration of blood.

Autotransfusion

Autotransfusion, or autologous transfusion, involves removing whole blood from a person and transfusing that blood back into the same person. Through this method, the issues of incompatibility, allergic reactions, and transmission of disease can be avoided. Methods of autotransfusion include the following:

- *Autologous donation* or *elective phlebotomy* (predeposit transfusion). A person donates blood before a planned surgical procedure. The blood can be frozen and stored for up to 10 years. Usually, the blood is stored without being frozen and is given to the person within a few weeks of donation. This technique is especially beneficial to the patient with a rare blood type or for any patient who might be expected to require limited blood product support during a major surgical procedure (e.g., elective orthopedic surgery).

- *Autotransfusion.* A method for replacing blood volume involves safely and aseptically collecting, filtering, and returning the patient's own blood that is lost during a major surgical procedure or from a traumatic injury. This system was originally developed in response to patients' concerns about the safety of blood from blood products. However, today it provides an important way to safely replace volume and stabilize the condition of bleeding patients. Collection devices are most often used during surgeries. Some systems allow blood to be automatically and continuously reinfused; others require collection for some period (usually no longer than 4 hours), after which the blood is reinfused. Sometimes the collected blood is depleted of its normal coagulation factors, so monitoring coagulation studies in the patient is important. Hospitals in Canada are now required to have a blood conservation program in place.

CASE STUDY

Leukemia

Patient Profile
A. S. (pronouns he/him), 35 years old, went to the emergency department because of severe bruising caused by a fall while hiking.

Subjective Data
- Reports oral pain and white patches covering tongue
- Has had a 2-month history of fatigue, malaise, and flu symptoms
- Reports shortness of breath while doing activities that previously required no exertion
- Has taken numerous prescribed antibiotics and has increased rest and sleep in the past 2 months without relief of symptoms

Objective Data
Physical Examination
- Has bruises and ecchymoses from fall
- Gingiva has petechiae and patchy white spots
- Temperature 39°C, respiratory rate 26/min, pulse 110
- Has splenomegaly

Laboratory Results
- Hematocrit 0.2
- White blood cell (WBC) count 120 × 10⁹/L
- Hemoglobin (Hb) 69 g/L
- Platelet count 25 × 10⁹/L

Bone Marrow Biopsy
- Multiple myeloblasts (>50%)

Discussion Questions
1. What components of the laboratory test results suggest acute leukemia?
2. How is acute myelogenous leukemia treated?
3. What is the prognosis for A. S.?
4. What are the life-threatening conditions that can occur as a result of this disease and treatment? How can the nurse anticipate and assess for these conditions?
5. *Priority decision:* What are the priority nursing interventions?
6. *Priority decision:* What are the priorities for patient teaching of a newly diagnosed young adult with leukemia?
7. *Priority decision:* Based on the assessment data presented, what are the priority nursing diagnoses? Are there any interprofessional issues?
8. *Evidence-informed practice:* A. S. becomes very fatigued after starting chemotherapy. He wants to know if exercise is possible even while so fatigued. What should the nurse tell the patient?

ⓔvolve
Answers are available at http://evolve.elsevier.com/Canada/Lewis/medsurg.

REVIEW QUESTIONS

The number of the question corresponds to the same-numbered objective at the beginning of the chapter.

1. In a severely anemic client, what would the nurse expect to find?
   a. Dyspnea at rest and tachycardia
   b. Cyanosis and pulmonary edema
   c. Cardiomegaly and pulmonary fibrosis
   d. Ventricular dysrhythmias and wheezing
2. When obtaining assessment data from a client with a microcytic, hypochromic anemia, what would the nurse question the client about?
   a. Folic acid intake
   b. Dietary intake of iron
   c. History of gastric surgery
   d. History of sickle cell anemia
3. Nursing interventions for a client with severe anemia related to peptic ulcer disease include which of the following? (*Select all that apply.*)
   a. Giving instructions in high-iron diet
   b. Taking vital signs every 8 hours
   c. Monitoring stools for occult blood
   d. Teaching self-injection of erythropoietin
   e. Administering cobalamin (vitamin B₁₂) injections

4. Which nursing management actions apply for a client in sickle cell crisis? (*Select all that apply.*)
   a. Monitoring CBC
   b. Providing optimal pain management and O₂ therapy
   c. Administering blood transfusions if required and iron chelation
   d. Recommending rest as needed and deep-vein thrombosis (DVT) prophylaxis
   e. Administering IV iron and a diet high in iron content
5. Which is a complication of the hyperviscosity of polycythemia?
   a. Thrombosis
   b. Cardiomyopathy
   c. Pulmonary edema
   d. Disseminated intravascular coagulation (DIC)
6. When caring for a client with thrombocytopenia, the patient teaching should include which instruction?
   a. To wipe their nose gently instead of blowing
   b. To be careful when shaving with a safety razor
   c. To continue with physical activities to stimulate thrombopoiesis
   d. To avoid acetylsalicylic acid because it may mask the fever that occurs with thrombocytopenia

7. The nurse would anticipate that a client with von Willebrand disease who is undergoing surgery would be treated with administration of von Willebrand factor (vWF) and which of the following?
   a. Thrombin
   b. Factor VI
   c. Factor VII
   d. Factor VIII

8. What physiological process occurs in a person with DIC?
   a. The coagulation pathway is genetically altered, leading to thrombus formation in all major blood vessels.
   b. An underlying disease depletes hemolytic factors in the blood, leading to diffuse thrombotic episodes and infarcts.
   c. A disease process stimulates coagulation processes with resultant thrombosis, as well as depletion of clotting factors, leading to diffuse clotting and hemorrhage.
   d. An inherited predisposition causes a deficiency of clotting factors that leads to overstimulation of coagulation processes in the vasculature.

9. Which of the following is (are) a priority nursing action when caring for a hospitalized client with a new-onset temperature of 39°C and severe neutropenia? (Select all that apply.)
   a. Administering the prescribed antibiotic STAT
   b. Drawing peripheral and central line blood cultures
   c. Ensuring ongoing monitoring of the client's vital signs for septic shock
   d. Taking a full set of vital signs and notifying the health care provider immediately
   e. Administering transfusions of WBCs to decrease immunogenicity

10. Because myelodysplastic syndrome arises from the pluripotent hematopoietic stem cell in the bone marrow, which laboratory results would the nurse expect to find?
    a. An excess of T cells
    b. An excess of platelets
    c. A deficiency of granulocytes
    d. A deficiency of all cellular blood components

11. Which is the most common type of leukemia in older persons?
    a. Acute myelocytic leukemia
    b. Acute lymphocytic leukemia
    c. Chronic myelocytic leukemia
    d. Chronic lymphocytic leukemia

12. Why are multiple medications often used in combinations to treat leukemia and lymphoma?
    a. There are fewer toxic and adverse effects.
    b. The chance that one medication will be effective is increased.
    c. The medications are more effective and cause fewer adverse effects.
    d. The medications work by different mechanisms to maximize killing of cancerous cells.

13. What is the major difference between Hodgkin's lymphoma and non-Hodgkin's lymphoma?
    a. Hodgkin's lymphoma occurs only in young adults.
    b. Hodgkin's lymphoma is considered potentially curable.
    c. Non-Hodgkin's lymphoma can manifest in multiple organs.
    d. Non-Hodgkin's lymphoma is treated only with radiation therapy.

14. A patient with multiple myeloma becomes confused and lethargic. What indications would the nurse expect from the diagnostic results?
    a. Hyperkalemia
    b. Hyperuricemia
    c. Hypercalcemia
    d. CNS myeloma

15. What would the nurse expect to find when reviewing a client's hematological laboratory values after a splenectomy?
    a. Deceased WBC count
    b. RBC abnormalities
    c. Decreased hemoglobin
    d. Increased platelet count

16. Which complications of transfusions can be decreased by the use of leukocyte depletion or reduction of red blood cell transfusion?
    a. Chills and hemolysis
    b. Leukostasis and neutrophilia
    c. Fluid overload and pulmonary edema
    d. Transmission of cytomegalovirus and fever

1. a; 2. b; 3. a; 4. a, b, c, d; 5. a; 6. a; 7. d; 8. c; 9. a, b, c, d; 10. d; 11. d; 12. d; 13. c; 14. c; 15. d; 16. d.

For even more review questions, visit http://evolve.elsevier.com/Canada/Lewis/medsurg.

REFERENCES

Angastiniotis, M., & Lobitz, S. (2019). Thalassemias: An overview. *International Journal of Neonatal Screening, 5*(16), 1–11. https://doi.org/10.3390/ijns.5010016

Ansell, S. M. (2018). Hodgkin lymphoma: 2018 update on diagnosis, risk-stratification, and management. *American Journal of Hematology, 93*(5), 704–715. https://doi.org/10.1002/ajh.25071

Arepally, G. M. (2017). Heparin-induced thrombo-cytopenia. *Blood, 129*(21), 2864–2872. https://doi.org/10.1182/blood.2016.11.709873

Camaschella, C. (2019). Iron deficiency. *Blood, 133*(1), 30–39. https://doi.org/10.1182/blood.2018.05.815944

Canadian Cancer Society. (2021a). *Hodgkin lymphoma statistics.* https://cancer.ca/en/cancer-information/cancer-types/hodgkin-lymphoma/statistics

Canadian Cancer Society. (2021b). *Leukemia statistics.* https://www.cancer.ca/en/cancer-information/cancer-type/leukemia/statistics/?region=on

Canadian Cancer Society. (2021c). *Multiple myeloma statistics.* http://www.cancer.ca/en/cancer-information/cancer-type/multiple-myeloma/statistics/?region=on

Canadian Cancer Society. (2021d). *Non-Hodgkin lymphoma statistics.* http://www.cancer.ca/en/cancer-information/cancer-type/non-hodgkin-lymphoma/statistics/?region=on

Canadian Hemochromatosis Society. (2020). *Hemochromatosis—How common is it?* https://www.toomuchiron.ca/hemochromatosis/faqs/

Canadian Hemophilia Society. (2018). *Hemophilia A and B.* https://www.hemophilia.ca/hemophilia-a-and-b/

Chiefs of Ontario. (2017). Cancer Care Ontario, and Institute for Clinical Evaluative Sciences. *Cancer in First Nations People in Ontario: Incidence, mortality, survival and prevalence.* https://www.cancercareontario.ca/sites/ccocancercare/files/assets/CancerFirstNationsReport.pdf

Georges, G., Doney, K., & Storb, R. (2018). Severe aplastic anemia: allogenic bone marrow transplantation as first-line treatment. *Blood Advances, 2*(15), 2020–2028. https://10.1182/bloodadvances.2018021162

Hoffman, R., Benz, E. J., Silberstein, L. E., et al. (2018). *Hematology: Basic principles and practice* (7th ed.). Elsevier.

Kenny, T., Hu, X., Jamieson, J., et al. (2019). Potential impact of restricted caribou (*Rangifer tarandus*) consumption on anemia prevalence among Inuit adults in northern Canada. *BMC Nutrition, 5*(30), 1–11. https://doi.org/10.1186/s40795.019.0292.9

Lenk, L., Alsadeq, A., & Schewe, D. M. (2020). Involvement of the central nervous system in acute lymphoblastic leukemia: opinions on molecular mechanisms and clinical implications based on recent data. *Cancer Metastasis Rev, 39*, 173–187. https://doi.org/10.1007/s10555-020-09848-z

Lichtman, M. A., Prchal, J. T., Kaushansky, K., et al. (2017). *Williams manual of hematology* (9th ed.). McGraw-Hill.

McMullin, M. F., Harrison, C. N., Ali, S., et al. (2019). A guideline for the diagnosis and management of polycythaemia vera. *British Journal of Haematology, 184*(2), 176–191. https://doi.org/10.1111/bjh.15648 file

Meier, E. R. (2018). Treatment options for sickle cell disease. *Pediatric Clinics of North America, 65*(3), 427–443. https://doi.org/10.1016/j.pcl.2018.01.005

Payne, A., Mehal, J., Chapman, C., et al. (2017). Mortality trends and causes of death in persons with sickle cell disease in the United States, 1979-2014. *Blood, 130*(1), 865. https://doi.org/10.1182/blood.V130.Suppl1.865.865

Rajkumar, S. V. (2020). Multiple myeloma: 2020 Update on diagnosis, risk-stratification and management. *American Journal of Hematology, 95*(5), 548–567. https://doi.org/10.1002/ajh.25791

Slack, J., Nguyen, L., Naugler, C., et al. (2018). Incidence of myelodysplastic syndromes in a major Canadian metropolitan area. *Journal of Applied Laboratory Medicine*, 378–383. https://doi.org/10.1373/jalm.2018.026500

Srivastava, A., Santagostino, E., Dougall, A., et al. (2020). WFH guidelines for the management of haemophilia. *Haemophilia, 26*(Suppl 6), 1–158. https://doi.org/10.1111/hae.14046

Steensma, D. (2018). Myelodysplastic syndromes current treatment algorithm 2018. *Blood Cancer Journal, 8*(47), 1–7. https://doi.org/10.1038/s41408.018.0085.4

Tahir, F., Ahmed, J., & Malik, F. (2020). Post-splenectomy sepsis: A review of the literature. *Cureus, 12*(2), e6898. https://doi.org/10.7759/cureus.6898

Tang, G., Lausman, A., Abdulrehman, J., et al. (2019). Prevalence of iron deficiency anemia during pregnancy: A single centre Canadian study. *Blood, 134*(1), 3389. https://doi.org/10.1182/blood-2019-127602

Willan, J., Eyre, T., Sharpley, F., et al. (2016). Multiple myeloma in the very elderly patient: Challenges and solutions. *Clinical Interventions in Aging, 11*, 423–435. https://doi.org/10.2147/CIA.S89465

Wolffenbuttel, B., Wouters, H., Heiner-Fokkema, M., et al. (2019). The many faces of cobalamin (vitamin B12) deficiency. *Mayo Clinic Proceedings: Innovations, Quality and Outcomes, 3*(2), 200–214. https://doi.org/10.1016/j.mayocpiqo.2019.03.002

World Health Organization. (2021). *Anaemia.* https://www.who.int/health-topics/anaemia#tab=tab_1

Yang, M., Deng, H., Yang, L., et al. (2020). Coagulation dysfunction and hematological changes in 633 patients with COVID-19. *Blood, 136*(Suppl 1), 22–23. https://doi.org/10.1182/blood-2020-140274

Zhou, L., Deng, Y., Li, N., et al. (2019). Global, regional, and national burden of Hodgkin lymphoma from 1990 to 2017: estimates from the 2017 Global Burden of Disease study. *Journal of Hematology and Oncology, 12*, 107. https://doi.org/10.1186/s13045.019.0799.1

Zimmer, A., & Freifeld, A. (2019). Optimal management of neutropenic fever in patients with cancer. *Journal of Oncology Practice, 15*(1), 19–24. https://doi.org/10.1016/j.mayocpiqo.2019.03.002

RESOURCES

BC Cancer
http://www.bccancer.bc.ca

Canadian Blood Services
https://www.blood.ca

Canadian Cancer Society
https://www.cancer.ca

Canadian Hemochromatosis Society
https://www.toomuchiron.ca/

Canadian Hemophilia Society
https://www.hemophilia.ca

Cancer Care Ontario
https://www.cancercareontario.ca

Childhood Cancer Foundation Canada
https://www.childhoodcancer.ca

Fanconi Canada
http://www.fanconicanada.org

Health Canada: *Canada's Food Guide*
https://food-guide.canada.ca/

Leukemia & Lymphoma Society of Canada
https://www.llscanada.org

Lymphoma Canada
https://www.lymphoma.ca

Myeloma Canada
https://www.myelomacanada.ca

Sickle Cell Association of Ontario
https://sicklecellontario.ca

Sickle Cell Disease Association of Canada
https://www.sicklecelldisease.ca/

Thalassemia Foundation of Canada
https://www.thalassemia.ca

Global Sickle Cell Disease Network
https://www.globalsicklecelldisease.org/

National Cancer Institute
https://www.cancer.gov

National Heart, Lung, and Blood Institute
https://www.nhlbi.nih.gov

National Hemophilia Foundation
https://www.hemophilia.org

evolve

For additional Internet resources, see the website for this book at http://evolve.elsevier.com/Canada/Lewis/medsurg.

Conditions of Oxygenation: Perfusion

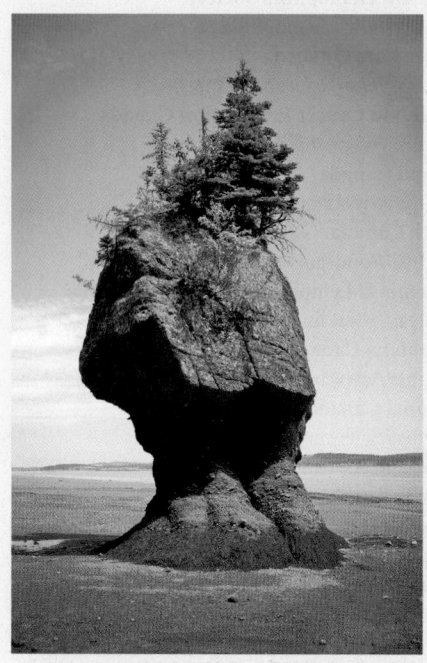

Source: © CanStock Photo / desireephoto

Nursing Assessment
Cardiovascular System

Leslie Graham
Originating US chapter by Debra Hagler and Diana Rabbani Hagler

⊖volve WEBSITE

http://evolve.elsevier.com/Canada/Lewis/medsurg

- Review Questions (Online Only)
- Key Points
- Answer Guidelines for Case Study
- Conceptual Care Map Creator
- Audio Glossary
- Supporting Media—Animations
  - Auscultation of Heart Valves
  - Blood Flow: Circulatory System

- Cardiac Cycle During Systole and Diastole
- Pulse Variations
- Supporting Media—Audio
  - Diastolic Murmur
  - Fourth Heart Sound (S_4)
  - Murmurs: Blowing, Harsh or Rough, and Rumble
  - Murmurs: High, Medium, and Low

- First Heart Sound (S_1) at Various Locations
- Second Heart Sound (S_2) at Various Locations
- Single S_1
- Single S_2
- Systolic Murmur
- Third Heart Sound (S_3)
- Content Updates

LEARNING OBJECTIVES

1. Differentiate the anatomical locations and functions of the following cardiac structures: pericardial layers, atria, ventricles, semilunar valves, and atrioventricular valves.
2. Explain the relation between the coronary circulation and the areas of heart muscle supplied by each blood vessel.
3. Explain the normal sequence of events involved in the conduction pathway of the heart.
4. Differentiate the structures and functions of arteries, capillaries, and veins.
5. Describe the mechanisms involved in blood pressure regulation.
6. Select essential assessment data related to the cardiovascular system that should be obtained from a patient or caregiver.

7. Select the appropriate techniques used in the physical assessment of the cardiovascular system.
8. Discuss the differences between normal and common abnormal findings of a physical assessment of the cardiovascular system.
9. Explain the links between age-related changes of the cardiovascular system and differences in assessment findings.
10. Describe the purpose and significance of and nursing responsibility related to diagnostic studies of the cardiovascular system.
11. Explain the relationship of the various waveforms on an electrocardiogram with the associated cardiac event.

KEY TERMS

action potential
afterload
arterial blood pressure (BP)
atrial kick
cardiac index
cardiac output (CO)
cardiac reserve

coronary angiography
diastole
diastolic blood pressure (DBP)
ejection fraction
heaves
Korotkoff sounds
mean arterial pressure (MAP)

murmurs
point of maximal impulse (PMI)
preload
pulse pressure
systole
systolic blood pressure (SBP)

STRUCTURES AND FUNCTIONS OF THE CARDIOVASCULAR SYSTEM

Heart

Structure. The heart is a four-chambered, hollow, muscular organ normally about the size of a fist. It lies within the thorax in the mediastinal space that separates the right and left pleural cavities. The heart is composed of three layers: a thin inner lining, the *endocardium;* a layer of muscle, the *myocardium;* and an outer layer, the *epicardium.* The heart is covered by a fibroserous sac called the *pericardium.* This sac consists of two layers: the inside *(visceral)* layer of the pericardium (part of the epicardium) and the outer *(parietal)* layer. A small amount of pericardial fluid (approximately 10–15 mL) lubricates the space between the pericardial layers *(pericardial space)* and prevents friction between the surfaces as the heart contracts (Huether et al., 2020).

The heart is divided vertically by the septum. The interatrial septum divides the right and left atria, and the interventricular septum divides the right and left ventricles. The thickness of the wall of each chamber is different. The atrial myocardium is thinner than that of the ventricles, and the left ventricular wall is two or three times thicker than the right ventricular wall (Huether et al., 2020). The left ventricle must be thick in order to produce the force needed to pump the blood into the systemic circulation.

Blood Flow Through the Heart. The blood flow through the heart is illustrated in Figure 34.1.

Cardiac Valves. The four valves of the heart serve to keep blood flowing in a forward direction. The mitral and tricuspid valves' cusps are attached to thin strands of fibrous tissue termed *chordae tendineae* (Figure 34.2). Chordae are anchored in the papillary muscles of the ventricles. This support system prevents the eversion of the leaflets into the atria during ventricular contraction. The pulmonic and aortic valves (also known as *semilunar valves*) prevent blood from regurgitating into the ventricles at the end of each ventricular contraction.

Blood Supply to the Myocardium. The myocardium has its own blood supply, the *coronary circulation* (Figure 34.3). Blood flow into the coronary arteries occurs primarily during diastole. The right coronary artery and its branches usually supply the right atrium, the right ventricle, and a portion of the posterior wall of the left ventricle. The left coronary artery and its branches (left anterior descending artery and left circumflex artery) supply the left atrium and the left ventricle. In 90% of people, the atrioventricular node and the bundle of His (part of the cardiac conduction system) receive blood supply from the right coronary artery. For this reason, obstruction of this artery often causes serious defects in cardiac conduction.

Collateral circulation in the heart involves a network of channels or vessels to reroute blood flow around an obstruction or blockage in the artery. The primary function of collateral circulation is to protect the heart from ischemia by improving perfusion to the region of the heart (Sole et al., 2017).

The divisions of coronary veins parallel the coronary arteries. Most of the blood from the coronary system drains into the coronary sinus, emptying into the right atrium near the entrance to the inferior vena cava (see Figure 34.3).

Conduction System. The conduction system comprises specialized nerve tissue responsible for initiating and conducting the electrical impulse; this impulse is called the **action potential**. This impulse initiates depolarization and, subsequently, cardiac contraction. The electrical impulse is initiated by the sinoatrial node (the dominant pacemaker of the heart; Figure 34.4). The impulse generated at the sinoatrial node travels through the atria via the internodal pathways to the atrioventricular node. Mechanical contraction of the atria follows the depolarization of the cells.

From the atrioventricular node, excitation then moves through the bundle of His and the left and right bundle branches. The left bundle branch has an anterior and a posterior fascicle. The action potential diffuses widely through the walls of both ventricles through *Purkinje fibres*. The efficient ventricular conduction system delivers the impulse within 0.12 seconds. This triggers a uniform ventricular contraction.

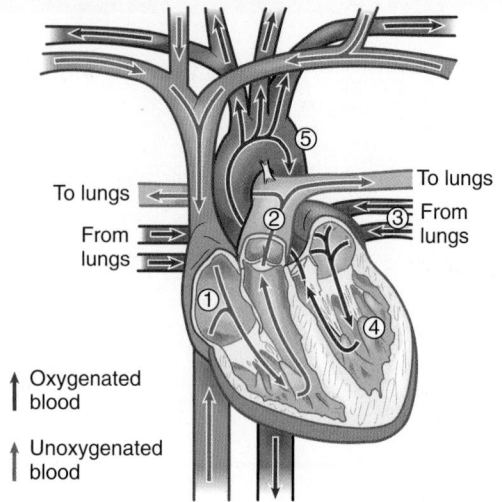

FIG. 34.1 Schematic representation of blood flow through the heart. *Arrows* indicate direction of flow. *1,* The right atrium receives venous blood from the inferior and superior venae cavae and the coronary sinus. The blood then passes through the tricuspid valve into the right ventricle. *2,* With each contraction, the right ventricle pumps blood through the pulmonic valve into the pulmonary artery and to the lungs. *3,* Oxygenated blood flows from the lungs to the left atrium by way of the pulmonary veins. *4,* It then passes through the mitral valve and into the left ventricle. *5,* As the heart contracts, blood is ejected through the aortic valve into the aorta and thus enters the systemic circulation.

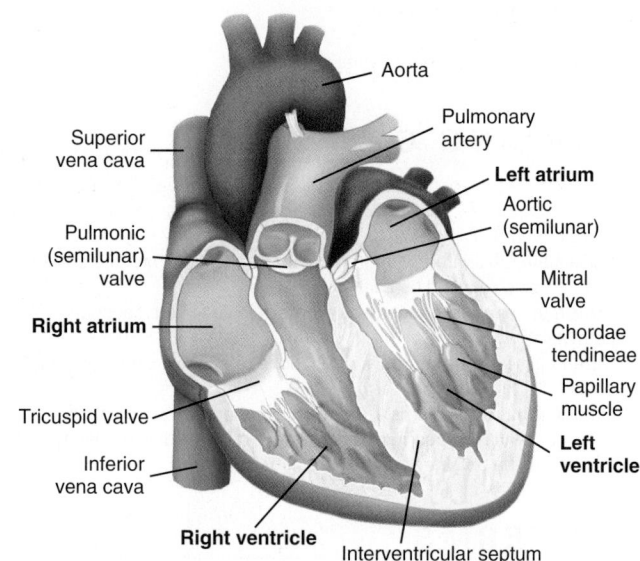

FIG. 34.2 Anatomical structures of the heart.

Lastly, repolarization occurs when the contractile fibre cells and the conduction pathway cells regain their resting polarized condition. Cardiac muscle cells have a compensatory mechanism that makes them unresponsive or refractory to restimulation during the action potential. There is an absolute refractory period during systole when cardiac muscle does not respond to any stimuli. After this period, cardiac muscle gradually recovers its excitability and a relative refractory period occurs by early diastole.

Electrocardiography. The electrical activity of the heart can be detected on the body surface and recorded on an electrocardiogram (ECG). The letters *P, QRS, T,* and *U* are used to identify the separate waveforms (see Figure 34.4, *B*). The first

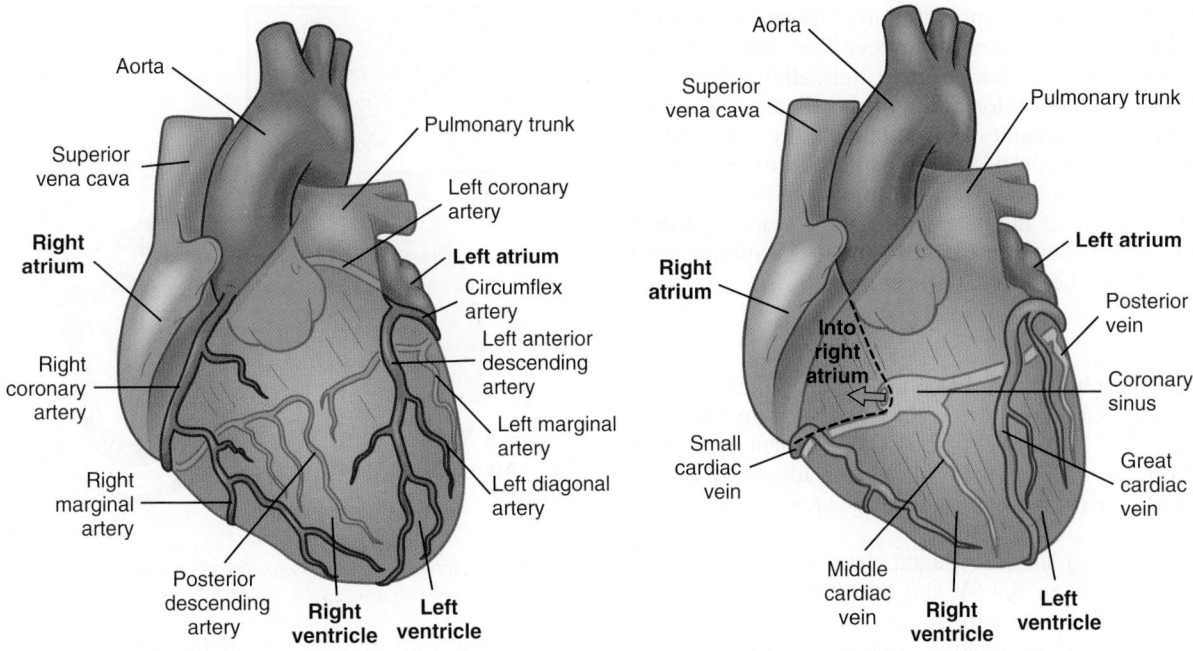

FIG. 34.3 Coronary arteries and veins.

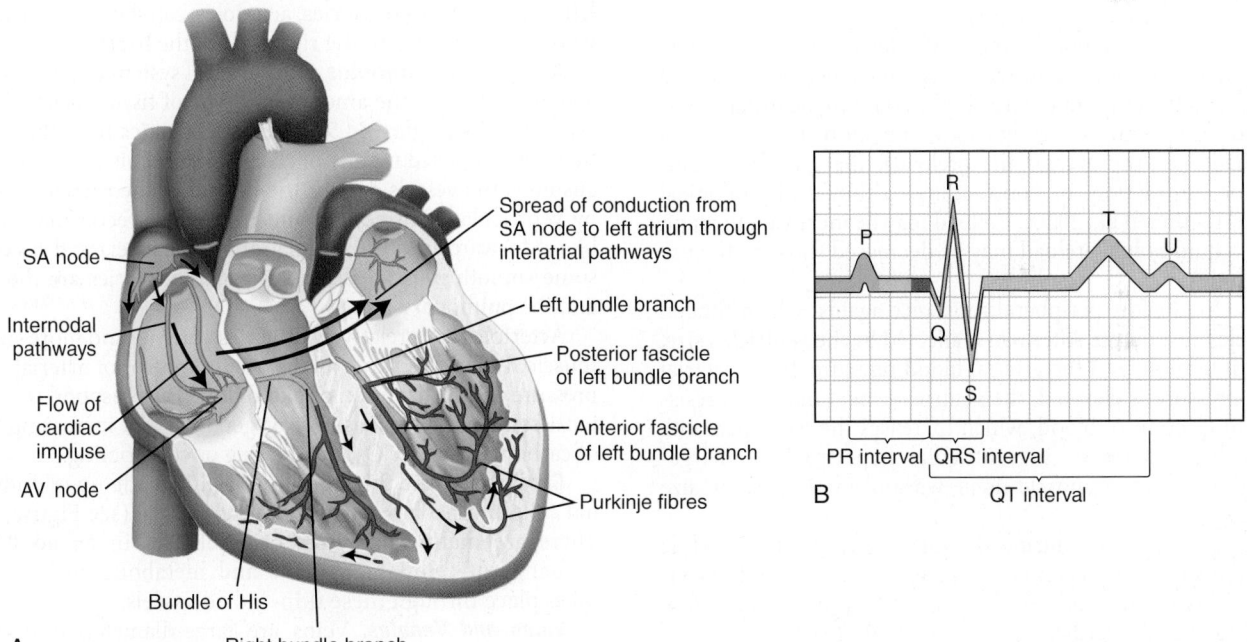

FIG. 34.4 A, Conduction system of the heart. AV, atrioventricular; SA, sinoatrial. B, The normal electrocardiogram pattern. The P wave represents depolarization of the atria. The QRS complex indicates depolarization of the ventricles. The T wave represents repolarization of the ventricles. The U wave, if present, may represent repolarization of the Purkinje fibres or may be associated with hypokalemia. The PR, QRS, and QT intervals reflect the length of time it takes for the impulse to travel from one area of the heart to another.

waveform, the P wave, begins with the firing of the sinoatrial node and represents depolarization of the atria. The QRS complex represents depolarization from the atrioventricular node throughout the ventricles. There is a delay of impulse transmission through the atrioventricular node that accounts for the time sequence between the end of the P wave and the beginning of the QRS complex. The T wave represents repolarization of the ventricles. If present, the U wave represents delayed ventricular repolarization and may be associated with

electrolyte imbalance (i.e., hypokalemia, hypomagnesemia, hypercalcemia) and is most typically observed in different types of bradycardia.

Intervals between these waves (PR, QRS, and QT intervals) reflect the length of time it takes for the impulse to travel from one area of the heart to another. These time intervals have been referenced, and deviations from these time references often indicate pathological conditions (Sole et al., 2017). For a detailed discussion, see Chapter 38.

Mechanical System. Depolarization triggers mechanical activity. Systole, contraction of the myocardium, results in ejection of blood from the cardiac chamber. Relaxation of the myocardium, diastole, allows for filling of the chamber. Cardiac output (CO) is the amount of blood pumped by the ventricle in 1 minute, reflecting the heart's mechanical ability (Sole et al., 2017). The stroke volume (SV) is the amount of blood ejected by the left ventricle of the heart during each systolic cardiac contraction, which may be calculated—the stroke volume (SV) is multiplied by the heart rate (HR) per minute:

$$CO = SV \times HR$$

For a normal adult at rest, CO is maintained in the range of 4 to 8 L/minute. Cardiac index is the CO divided by the body mass index (BMI). A measure of the CO of a patient per square metre of body surface area, the cardiac index adjusts the CO to the body size. The normal cardiac index is 2.8 to 4.2 L/minute/m^2.

Factors Affecting Cardiac Output. Numerous factors can affect either the HR or the SV and thus the CO. The HR is regulated primarily by the autonomic nervous system. The factors affecting the SV are preload, contractility, and afterload (Huether et al., 2020). Increases in preload, contractility, and afterload increase the workload of the myocardium, which results in increased oxygen demand.

The volume of blood in the ventricles at the end of diastole, before the next contraction, is called preload. Preload determines the amount of stretch placed on myocardial fibres. According to Frank-Starling's Law, the more the fibres are stretched (i.e., the greater the preload), the greater is their force of contraction, or contractility, within a physiological range (Huether et al., 2020). Preload may be increased through use of a fluid bolus; preload may be decreased through the use of diuretics.

Afterload is the peripheral resistance against which the left ventricle must pump. Afterload is affected by the ventricle's size, the wall tension, and the arterial blood pressure. If the arterial blood pressure is elevated, the ventricles meet increased resistance to ejection of blood, which increases the work demand. Eventually, this results in ventricular hypertrophy (enlargement of the cardiac muscle tissue without increasing the size of cavities).

Atrial kick occurs during the final phase of atrial systole when the atria contract and eject a bolus of blood into the ventricles. This ejection of blood contributes approximately 30% more blood to the cardiac output (Sole et al., 2017).

Cardiac Reserve. The cardiovascular system must respond to numerous situations in health and illness (e.g., exercise, stress, hypovolemia). The heart's ability to respond to these demands by increasing CO as much as three-fold or four-fold is termed cardiac reserve.

The increase in CO results from an increase in HR or SV. The HR can increase to as high as 180 beats per minute for short periods without deleterious effects. The SV can be increased by an increase in either preload or contractility.

Vascular System

Blood Vessels. The three major types of blood vessels in the vascular system are the arteries, the veins, and the capillaries. *Arteries* carry blood away from the heart and, except for the pulmonary artery, carry oxygenated blood. *Veins* carry blood

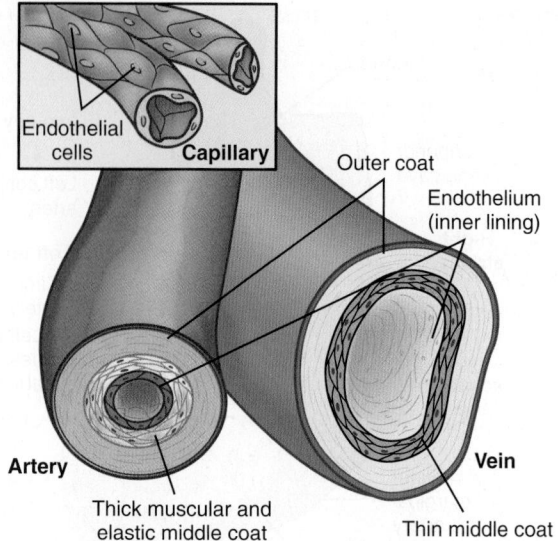

FIG. 34.5 Comparative thicknesses of layers of an artery, a vein, and a capillary.

toward the heart and, except for the pulmonary veins, carry deoxygenated blood. Small branches of arteries and veins are *arterioles* and *venules*, respectively. Blood circulates from the left side of heart into arteries, arterioles, capillaries, venules, and veins and then back to the right side of the heart.

Arteries and Arterioles. The arterial system differs from the venous system by the amount and type of tissue that makes up arterial walls (Figure 34.5). The large arteries have thick walls that are composed mainly of elastic tissue. This elastic property cushions the vessels against the impact of the pressure created by ventricular contraction, and it provides recoil that propels blood forward into the circulation. Large arteries also contain some smooth muscle. Examples of large arteries are the aorta and the pulmonary artery.

Arterioles have relatively little elastic tissue and more smooth muscle. Arterioles serve as the major control of arterial blood pressure and distribution of blood flow. They respond readily to local conditions, such as low oxygen (O_2) and increasing levels of carbon dioxide (CO_2), by dilating or constricting.

Capillaries. The thin capillary wall is made up of endothelial cells and has no elastic or muscle tissue (see Figure 34.5). There are many kilometres of capillaries in an adult. The exchange of cellular nutrients and metabolic end products takes place through these thin-walled vessels.

Veins and Venules. Veins are large-diameter, thin-walled vessels that return blood to the right atrium (see Figure 34.5). The venous system is a low-pressure, high-volume system. The larger veins contain semilunar valves at intervals to maintain the blood flow toward the heart and to prevent backward flow. The amount of blood in the venous system is affected by several factors, including arterial flow, compression of veins by skeletal muscles, alterations in thoracic and abdominal pressures, and right atrial pressure.

The largest veins are the *superior vena cava*, which returns blood to the heart from the head, neck, and arms, and the *inferior vena cava*, which returns blood to the heart from the lower part of the body. These large-diameter vessels are affected by the pressure in the right side of the heart. Elevated right atrial pressure can cause neck veins to become distended or the liver to become engorged from resistance to blood flow.

Venules are relatively small vessels made up of a small amount of muscle and connective tissue. Venules collect blood from various capillary beds and channel it to the larger veins.

Regulation of the Cardiovascular System

Autonomic Nervous System. The autonomic nervous system consists of the sympathetic nervous system and the parasympathetic nervous system.

Effect on the Heart. Stimulation of the sympathetic nervous system increases the HR, the speed of impulse conduction through the atrioventricular node, and the force of atrial and ventricular contractions. This effect is mediated by specific sites in the heart called *β-adrenergic receptors,* which are receptors for norepinephrine and epinephrine.

In contrast, stimulation of the parasympathetic system (mediated by the vagus nerve) causes a decrease in HR by the action on the sinoatrial node and slows conduction through the atrioventricular node.

Effect on the Blood Vessels. The source of neural control of blood vessels is the sympathetic nervous system. The *α-adrenergic receptors* are located in vascular smooth muscles. Stimulation of the α-adrenergic receptors results in vasoconstriction. Decreased stimulation to the α-adrenergic receptors causes vasodilation. (Sympathetic nervous system receptors that influence blood pressure are presented in Chapter 35, Table 35.1.)

The parasympathetic nerves have selective distribution in the blood vessels. Blood vessels in skeletal muscle do not receive parasympathetic input.

Baroreceptors. *Baroreceptors* in the aortic arch and the carotid sinus (at the origin of the internal carotid artery) are sensitive to stretch or pressure within the arterial system. Stimulation of these receptors sends information to the vasomotor centre in the brainstem. This results in temporary inhibition of the sympathetic nervous system and enhancement of the parasympathetic influence, which cause a decrease in HR and peripheral vasodilation. Decreased arterial pressure causes the opposite effect.

Chemoreceptors. *Chemoreceptors* are located in the aortic arch and the carotid bodies. They are capable of initiating changes in HR and arterial pressure in response to decreased arterial O_2 pressure (*hypoxia*), increased arterial CO_2 pressure (*hypercapnia*), and decreased plasma pH (*acidosis*). When the chemoreceptor reflexes in the medulla are triggered, they stimulate the vasomotor centre to increase blood pressure and, in turn, to increase cardiac activity (Huether et al., 2020).

Blood Pressure

The arterial blood pressure (BP) is a measure of the pressure exerted by blood against the walls of the arterial system. The systolic blood pressure (SBP) is the peak pressure exerted against the arteries when the heart contracts. The diastolic blood pressure (DBP) is the residual pressure of the arterial system during ventricular relaxation. BP is usually expressed as the ratio of SBP to DBP.

The two main factors influencing BP are CO and systemic vascular resistance (SVR):

$$BP = CO \times SVR$$

SVR is the force opposing the movement of blood. This force is created primarily in small arteries and arterioles.

Measurement of Arterial Blood Pressure. BP can be measured by invasive and noninvasive techniques. The invasive technique consists of catheter insertion into an artery. The catheter is attached to a recording device, and the pressure is measured directly (see Chapter 68).

Noninvasive, indirect measurement of BP can be done with a sphygmomanometer and a stethoscope. The sphygmomanometer consists of an inflatable cuff and a pressure gauge or an electronic cuff. The examiner measures BP externally by listening for turbulent blood flow sounds through a compressed artery (termed Korotkoff sounds). The brachial artery is the usual site for measuring BP (Jarvis et al., 2019).

After the appropriate-size cuff is placed on the extremity, the cuff is inflated to a pressure in excess of the SBP. This causes blood flow in the artery to cease. As the pressure in the cuff is lowered, the artery is auscultated for Korotkoff sounds. There are five phases of Korotkoff sounds. The first phase is a tapping sound caused by the spurt of blood into the constricted artery as the pressure in the cuff is gradually deflated. The pressure when this sound is heard is considered the SBP. The fifth phase occurs when the sound disappears, and this pressure is known as the DBP (Jarvis et al., 2019). Clinically, the BP is recorded as SBP/DBP (e.g., 120/80 mm Hg). On occasion, an auscultatory gap is heard. An *auscultatory gap* is a loss of sound between the SBP and the DBP. The BP could be measured incorrectly if the cuff is not inflated to exceed the true SBP.

In addition to the manual technique, another noninvasive way to measure BP indirectly is to use automatic BP monitors (see Chapter 35). The monitor consists of a BP cuff and a lightweight microprocessing unit. This system, which records a patient's BP at preset intervals during routine activities over 24 to 48 hours, enables ambulatory BP monitoring and may help clinicians diagnose hypertension more accurately in some patients.

Another method to measure BP is with the use of a Doppler ultrasonic flowmeter, which amplifies the Korotkoff sounds. An appropriate-size cuff is placed on the extremity and the brachial artery palpated. Then gel is applied to the transducer probe. The probe is placed perpendicular to the artery and the cuff inflated until the pulsatile sound is no longer audible. The cuff is inflated 20 to 30 mm Hg beyond the last sound. The cuff is slowly deflated until the sound returns, indicating the SBP (Jarvis et al., 2019).

Pulse Pressure and Mean Arterial Pressure. Pulse pressure is the difference between the SBP and the DBP. Normally it is approximately one third of the SBP. If the BP is 120/80 mm Hg, the normal pulse pressure is 40 mm Hg. The pulse pressure may be elevated during exercise or in individuals with atherosclerosis of the larger arteries because of increased SBP. The pulse pressure may be decreased in cardiac failure or hypovolemia.

Another measurement related to BP is mean arterial pressure (MAP). MAP reflects the pressure during one cardiac cycle that is exerted on vital organs. If the MAP is low for a prolonged period, the organs may exhibit ischemia. MAP is calculated as follows:

$$MAP = (SBP + 2\,DBP) \div 3$$

A person with a BP of 120/60 mm Hg has an MAP of 80 mm Hg.

AGE-RELATED CONSIDERATIONS

EFFECTS OF AGING ON THE CARDIOVASCULAR SYSTEM

One of the greatest risk factors for cardiovascular disease is age. Cardiovascular disease remains the leading cause of death in adults older than 85 years. It is the most common cause of hospitalization and the second leading cause of death in adults younger than age 85. The most common cardiovascular condition is coronary artery disease (CAD) secondary to atherosclerosis. It is difficult to distinguish normal aging changes from the pathophysiological changes of atherosclerosis. Many of the physiological changes in the cardiovascular system of older persons are a result of the combined effects of the aging process, disease, psychosocial stress, environmental factors, and lifetime health behaviours, rather than just age alone (Deley et al., 2019).

Age-related changes in the cardiovascular system and differences in assessment findings are presented in Table 34.1. With increased age, the amount of collagen in the heart increases and elastin decreases. These changes affect the myocardium's ability to stretch and contract. One of the major changes in the cardiovascular system is the response to physical or emotional stress. In times of increased stress, CO and SV decrease because of reduced contractility and HR response. The resting supine HR is not markedly affected by aging. When an older person changes positions (e.g., sits upright), the sympathetic nerve pathway may be affected by fibrous tissue and fatty deposits, manifested as a blunted HR response (Touhy & Jett, 2020).

Cardiac valves become thicker and stiffer from lipid accumulation, degeneration of collagen, and fibrosis. The aortic and mitral valves are most frequently affected, while aortic stenosis is the most common abnormality in adults over 65 years old (Huether et al., 2020). This narrowing of the orifice of the valve (stenosis) causes regurgitation of blood when the valve is closed. When the valve is open, turbulent blood flow across the affected valve results in a murmur.

The number of pacemaker cells in the sinoatrial node decreases with age. By age 75, a person may have only 10% of the normal number of pacemaker cells. Although this is compatible with adequate sinoatrial node function, it may account for the frequency of some sinus dysrhythmias in older persons. Similar decreases also occur in the number of conduction cells in the internodal tracts, bundle of His, and bundle branches. These changes contribute to the development of atrial dysrhythmias and heart blocks. The autonomic nervous system control of the cardiovascular system changes with aging. The number and function of β-adrenergic receptors in the heart decrease with age. Thus, the older person not only has a decreased response to physical and emotional stress but also is less sensitive to β-adrenergic agonist drugs. The lower maximum HR during exercise results in only a two-fold increase in CO, in contrast to the three- or four-fold increase observed in younger adults.

Arterial and venous blood vessels thicken and become less elastic with age. Arteries increase their sensitivity to vasopressin (antidiuretic hormone). With aging, both of these changes contribute to a progressive increase in SBP and a decrease or no change in DBP. Thus, an increase in the pulse pressure is found. Hypertension is not a normal consequence of aging and should be treated. Valves in the large veins in the lower extremities have a reduced ability to return the blood to the heart, which often results in dependent edema.

Orthostatic hypotension, which is estimated to be present in more than 30% of patients older than 70 years with systolic hypertension, may be related to medications, decreased baroreceptor function, or both. *Postprandial hypotension* (decrease in BP of at least 20 mm Hg that occurs within 75 minutes after eating) may also occur in about a third of otherwise healthy older adults. Both orthostatic and postprandial hypotension may be related to falls among older people. Despite the changes associated with aging, the heart is able to function adequately under most circumstances.

TABLE 34.1 AGE-RELATED DIFFERENCES IN ASSESSMENT

Cardiovascular System

Changes	Differences in Assessment Findings
Chest Wall	
Kyphosis	Altered chest landmarks for palpation, percussion, and auscultation; distant heart sounds
Heart	
Myocardial hypertrophy, ↑ collagen and scarring, ↓ elastin	↓ Cardiac reserve, slight ↓ HR
Downward displacement	Difficulty in isolating apical pulse
↓ CO, HR, and SV in response to exercise or stress	Slowed, ↓ response to stress; slowed recovery from activity
Cellular aging changes and fibrosis of conduction system	↓ Amplitude of QRS complex and lengthening of PR, QRS, and QT intervals; left axis deviation; irregular cardiac rhythms
Valvular rigidity from calcification, sclerosis, or fibrosis, impeding complete closure of valves	Systolic murmur (aortic or mitral) possible without being indication of cardiovascular disease
Blood Vessels	
Arterial stiffening caused by loss of elastin in arterial walls, thickening of intima of arteries, and progressive fibrosis of media	Elevation in systolic and possibly diastolic BP (e.g., 160/90 mm Hg); possibly, widened pulse pressures; more pronounced arterial pulses; diminished pedal pulses

BP, blood pressure; *CO,* cardiac output; *HR,* heart rate; *SV,* stroke volume.

CASE STUDY

Patient Introduction

Patient Profile

L. T. (pronouns he/him), 63 years old, is brought to the emergency department by ambulance at 0600 hours after calling 911 with reports of chest pain, shortness of breath, palpitations, and dizziness. The paramedics started an intravenous infusion and administered oxygen at 2 L/min via nasal cannula. They also administered four chewable baby acetylsalicylic acid (ASA) tablets and a nitroglycerin spray, and they obtained a 12-lead ECG. L. T. is pain-free on arrival but still reports palpitations and dizziness.

Critical Thinking

Throughout this assessment chapter, think about L. T.'s symptoms with the following questions in mind:

1. What are the possible causes of L. T.'s chest pain, shortness of breath, palpitations, and dizziness?
2. What would be the nurse's priority assessment of L. T.?
3. What questions would the nurse ask L. T.?
4. What should be included in the physical assessment? What would the nurse be looking for?
5. What diagnostic studies would the nurse expect to be ordered?

See Case Study: Subjective Data, Case Study: Objective Data: Physical Examination, and Case Study: Objective Data: Diagnostic Studies for more information on L. T.

evolve

Answers available at http://evolve.elsevier.com/Canada/Lewis/medsurg.

ASSESSMENT OF THE CARDIOVASCULAR SYSTEM

Subjective Data

A careful health history and physical examination (Table 34.2) should aid the nurse in distinguishing symptoms that reflect a cardiovascular condition from those that reflect conditions of other body systems. For instance, it is important to determine whether weight gain results from overeating or is a manifestation of fluid retention.

Important Health Information

History of Current Illness. The nurse should ask the patient what health concern has brought them to the hospital or provider and should fully explore all symptoms the patient is experiencing.

Past Health History. Many illnesses affect the cardiovascular system directly or indirectly. The nurse should inquire about a history of chest pain, shortness of breath, alcohol use or misuse, anemia, rheumatic fever, streptococcal sore throat, congenital heart disease, stroke, syncope, hypertension, thrombophlebitis, intermittent claudication, varicosities, obesity, and edema.

Medications. An assessment of the patient's current and past use of medications should be made. This includes both over-the-counter drugs and prescription medications. For example, acetylsalicylic acid (ASA; Aspirin), which prolongs the blood clotting time, is contained in many medications used to alleviate cold symptoms.

A medication assessment should include the names of medications the patient is taking and the patient's understanding of their purpose and adverse effects. Medications that may adversely affect the cardiovascular system should also be assessed. Some of these and examples of their effects on the cardiovascular system are listed in Table 34.3.

Surgery or Other Treatments. The patient should also be asked about specific treatments, past surgical procedures, and hospital admissions related to cardiovascular issues. Any hospitalizations for diagnostic workups or cardiovascular symptoms should be explored. It should be noted whether an ECG or a chest radiograph was obtained for baseline data.

TABLE 34.2 HEALTH HISTORY

Cardiovascular System—Questions for Obtaining Subjective Data

Chest Pain

- Do you have any chest pain or discomfort? Please show me where it is.
- Is the pain in one spot, or does it move around?
- How long have you had this pain?
- Does it come and go, or is it constant? Does it get worse before or after meals? When is the pain worst (e.g., with a certain position or activity, with stress)?
- Can you describe how it feels (e.g., burning, stabbing, aching, heaviness, squeezing)?
- What brings the pain on (e.g., activity, stress)?
- Do any other symptoms occur when you get the pain (e.g., shortness of breath, weakness, nausea, vomiting)?*
- What works to relieve the pain (e.g., rest, change of position, medication)?*
- On a scale of 0 to 10, how would you rate your pain?

Dyspnea

- Have you experienced any shortness of breath? If yes, what kind of activity precipitates your shortness of breath?
- Is your shortness of breath dependent on your position (e.g., lying down)?*
- How does the shortness of breath affect your daily activities?*

Orthopnea

- How many pillows do you sleep on at night? Has this number changed recently?*

Cough

- Do you have a cough? If yes, describe the duration, the frequency, and the kind of cough (e.g., dry, hoarse, congested).
- Do you cough up mucus? If yes, describe the colour and the amount.
- Is coughing associated with any activity such as talking, lying down, stress, and so on?*
- Is the coughing relieved by anything (e.g., walking, exercise, rest, medication)?*

Fatigue

- Do you tire easily?* If yes, when did you notice a change in your level of fatigue?
- Is your energy level related to the time of the day?*

Cyanosis or Pallor

- Have you ever noticed a bluish or ashen colour to your face?*

Edema

- Have you ever noticed any swelling in your feet and legs?*
- When did you first experience swelling, and have there been any recent changes?*
- Are both feet swollen to the same degree?*

Nocturia

- How many times a night do you awaken to urinate?*

Cardiac History

- Do you have any past history of hypertension, elevated cholesterol or triglycerides, heart murmur, congenital heart diseases, rheumatic fever or unexplained joint pains in your youth, recurrent tonsillitis, or anemia?
- Do you have any history of heart disease?*
- When was your last ECG, serum cholesterol blood work, or other heart-related tests?*

Family History

- Do you have any family history of heart disease, high blood pressure, obesity, diabetes, or sudden death at a young age?*

Self-Care History

- Describe your usual daily diet, including sodium and fluid intake. What is your current weight? What was your weight 1 year ago?
- Have you ever used tobacco? If yes, in what form, how much, and for how long? Have you ever tried to quit? If yes, what methods have you tried? Does anyone close to you smoke?*
- How often do you drink alcohol, and how much? Have you ever been told that you have a problem with alcohol?*
- What is your usual amount of exercise per week?
- Do you take any cardiac medications (e.g., antihypertensives, diuretics, aspirin, anticoagulants), over-the-counter medications, herbal products, or street drugs?*

ECG, electrocardiogram.
*If yes, describe.
Source: Adapted from Jarvis, C., Browne, A. J., MacDonald-Jenkins, J., & Luctkar-Flude, M. (2020). *Physical examination & health assessment* (3rd Canadian ed., pp. 505–510). Elsevier Inc.

TABLE 34.3   CARDIOVASCULAR EFFECTS OF NONCARDIAC MEDICATIONS*

Medication Classification	Examples	Cardiovascular Effects
Anticancer agents	Doxorubicin (Caelyx)	Dysrhythmias, tachycardia, heart failure, cardiomyopathy
Antipsychotics	Chlorpromazine Haloperidol	Dysrhythmias, orthostatic hypotension, hypertension, cardiac arrest, prolongation of QT
Corticosteroids	Cortisone Prednisone	Hypotension, edema, potassium depletion, hypertension, thrombophlebitis
Hormone therapy, oral contraceptives	Ethinylestradiol/drospirenone	Myocardial infarction, thromboembolism, stroke, hypertension
Nonsteroidal anti-inflammatory drugs (NSAIDs)†	Ibuprofen (Motrin) Celecoxib (Celebrex)	Hypertension, myocardial infarction, stroke, heart failure
Psychostimulants	Cocaine Amphetamines	Tachycardia, angina, myocardial infarction, hypertension, dysrhythmias
Tricyclic antidepressants	Amitriptyline (Elavil) Doxepin (Sinequan, Silenor)	Dysrhythmias, orthostatic hypotension

*List is not all-inclusive.
†Second-generation NSAIDs, known as cyclo-oxygenase 2 (COX-2) inhibitors, have been linked to an increased risk of serious adverse cardiovascular events.

CASE STUDY

Subjective Data

A focused subjective assessment of L. T. revealed the following information:

Past medical history: History of hypertension, mitral valve prolapse with mild regurgitation, heart failure, and type 2 diabetes mellitus

Medications: Lisinopril (Prinivil), 10 mg/day PO; metoprolol (Lopressor), 50 mg PO bid; ASA, 325 mg/day PO; furosemide (Lasix), 40 mg/day PO; and metformin (Glucophage), 500 mg PO qid

Current history: L.T. denies any previous history of chest pain or CAD. He was feeling fine until this morning, when he experienced shortness of breath, chest pain, palpitations, and dizziness while walking to the bathroom after waking up. L. T. became frightened that he was having a heart attack, so called 911. He denies smoking or alcohol intake. Shortness of breath and chest pain are now gone, but L. T. continues to feel palpitations and dizziness when sitting up.

L. T. denies any edema. He takes Lasix in the morning and typically "pees until lunchtime." Denies nocturia.

See Case Study: Patient Introduction, Case Study: Objective Data: Physical Examination, and Case Study: Objective Data: Diagnostic Studies for more information on L. T.

Objective Data

Physical Examination

Vital Signs. After the patient's general appearance has been observed, vital signs—including BP, heart and respiratory rate, and temperature—are measured. The BP should be measured while the patient is sitting, lying, and standing. An appropriate cuff size should be used for accurate readings. Normally, there is a reduction of up to 15 mm Hg in the SBP and 3 to 5 mm Hg in the DBP in the standing position. BP measurements should be taken in both arms. These readings may vary by 5 to 15 mm Hg. BP in the lower extremities is expected to be about 10 mm Hg higher than in the upper extremities.

Peripheral Vascular System

Inspection. The skin colour, hair distribution, and venous blood flow provide information about arterial blood flow and venous return. The extremities should be inspected for conditions such as edema, thrombophlebitis, varicose veins, and lesions such as stasis ulcers. Edema in the extremities can be caused by gravity, interruption of venous return, or elevation of right atrial pressure.

A measure used for assessing arterial flow to the extremities is the *capillary filling time*. The patient's nail bed is depressed to produce blanching and observed for the return of colour. When arterial capillary perfusion is normal, the colour returns within 3 seconds.

The large veins in the neck (internal and external jugular) should be inspected while the patient is gradually elevated to an upright position. Distension and prominent pulsations of these neck veins can be caused by right atrial pressure elevation. To measure jugular venous distention, a ruler is held vertically on the sternal angle. Then a straight edge is placed at the height of the jugular venous pulsation, reading at the level of intersection with the patient elevated to 45 degrees. Normal jugular venous pulsation should be 2 cm or less (Jarvis et al., 2019).

Palpation. Palpation of the pulses in the neck and extremities also provides information on arterial blood flow. The pulses should be palpated to assess the contour, amplitude, and strength of each beat. Characteristics of the arteries on the right and left sides of the body should be compared. It is important to palpate each carotid pulse separately to avoid compromise of arterial blood flow to the brain.

When palpating the arteries identified in Figure 34.6, the nurse should note the pressure of the pulse wave, or how far the vessel wall distends when the pulse occurs. This judgement of the pulsation volume is recorded as normal, bounding, thready, or absent. A scale may be used to document pulse volume or amplitude (Jarvis et al., 2020):

0: Absent
1+: Weak, thready
2+: Normal
3+: Full, bounding

The *rigidity* (hardness) of the vessel should also be noted. The normal pulse feels as if it is tapping, whereas a vessel wall that is narrowed or bulging vibrates. A term for a palpable vibration is known as a *thrill*.

Auscultation. An artery that has a narrowed or bulging wall may cause blood flow to be turbulent. This abnormal flow can sound like a buzzing or humming, termed a *bruit*. It can be heard with the bell of the stethoscope placed over the vessel. Auscultation of major arteries such as the carotid arteries, the abdominal aorta, and the femoral arteries should be part of the initial cardiovascular assessment. Abnormalities of the cardiovascular system are described in Table 34.4.

Thorax

Inspection and Palpation. An overall inspection and palpation of the bony structures of the thorax is the initial step

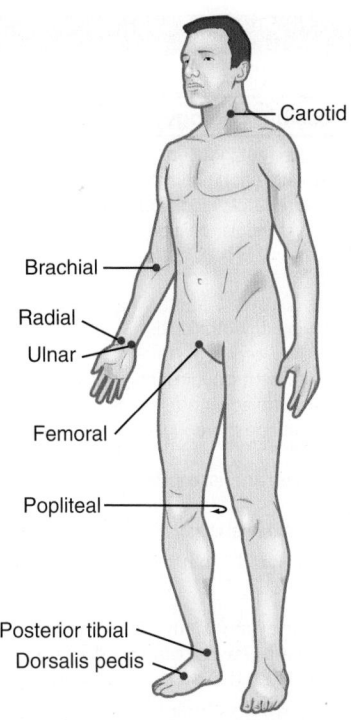

FIG. 34.6 Common sites for palpating arteries.

in the examination. Next, the areas where the cardiac valves project their sounds are inspected and palpated by identifying the intercostal spaces (ICSs). The raised notch, the angle of Louis, where the manubrium and the body of the sternum are joined, is readily palpable in the midline of the sternum. The angle of Louis is at the level of the second rib and can therefore be used to count ICSs and locate specific auscultatory areas.

The following auscultatory areas can be located (Figure 34.7): the aortic area, in the second ICS to the right of the sternum; the pulmonic area, in the second ICS to the left of the sternum; the tricuspid area, in the fifth left ICS close to the sternum; and the mitral area, in the left midclavicular line (MCL) at the level of the fifth ICS. A fifth auscultatory area is Erb point, located at the third left ICS near the sternum. Normally, no pulsations are felt in these areas unless the patient has a thin chest wall.

A valvular disorder may be suspected if abnormal pulsations or thrills are felt. Next, the epigastric area, which lies on either side of the midline just below the xiphoid process, is inspected and palpated. In a thin person, the pulsation of the abdominal aorta may be visible and can normally be palpated here. Next, the precordium, which is located between the apex and the sternum, is inspected for heaves. **Heaves** are sustained lifts of the chest wall in the precordial area that can be seen or palpated,

TABLE 34.4 ASSESSMENT ABNORMALITIES

Cardiovascular System

Finding	Description	Possible Etiology and Significance*
Inspection		
Distended neck veins	Vertical distance between intersection of angle of Louis and level of jugular distension >3 cm with patient sitting at 30- to 45-degree angle	Elevated right atrial pressure; right-sided heart failure
Central cyanosis	Bluish or purplish tinge in central areas such as tongue, conjunctivae, inner surface of lips	Inadequate O_2 saturation of arterial blood as result of pulmonary or cardiac disorders (e.g., congenital defects)
Peripheral cyanosis	Bluish or purplish tinge in extremities or nose and ears	Reduced blood flow because of heart failure, vasoconstriction, cold environment
Splinter hemorrhages	Small red to black streaks under fingernails	Infective endocarditis (infection of endocardium, usually in area of cardiac valves)
Clubbing of nail beds	Obliteration of normal angle between base of nail and skin	Endocarditis, congenital defects, prolonged O_2 deficiency
Colour changes in extremities with postural change	Pallor, cyanosis, mottling of skin after limb elevation; glossy skin	Chronic decreased arterial perfusion
Ulcers	*Venous:* Necrotic crater-like lesions usually found on lower leg at medial malleolus; characterized by slow wound healing *Arterial:* Lesions with pale ischemic base and well-defined edges; usually found on toes, heels, lateral malleoli	Poor venous return, varicose veins, incompetent venous valves; arteriosclerosis, diabetes
Varicose veins	Visible dilated, tortuous vessels in lower extremities	Incompetent valves in vein
Palpation		
Pulse		
Bounding	Sharp, brisk, pounding pulse	Hyperkinetic states (anxiety, fever), anemia, hyperthyroidism
Thready	Weak, slowly rising pulse; easily obliterated by pressure	Blood loss, decreased cardiac output, aortic valve disease, peripheral arterial disease
Irregular	Regularly irregular or irregularly irregular; skipped beats	Cardiac dysrhythmias
Pulsus alternans	Regular rhythm, but strength of pulse varies with each beat	Heart failure
Absent	Lack of pulse	Atherosclerosis, thrombus, trauma, embolus
Thrill	Vibration of vessel or chest wall	Aneurysm, aortic regurgitation, arteriovenous fistula
Rigidity	Stiffness or inflexibility of vessel wall	Atherosclerosis
>100 bpm	Tachycardia	May be exercise induced; may reflect anxiety or shock; may indicate need for increased cardiac output, hyperthyroidism

Continued

TABLE 34.4   ASSESSMENT ABNORMALITIES

Cardiovascular System—cont'd

Finding	Description	Possible Etiology and Significance*
<50 bpm	Bradycardia	May be rest induced; SA or AV node damage, athletic conditioning, adverse effect of drugs (e.g., β-adrenergic blockers), hypothyroidism
Displaced point of maximal impulse (apical pulse)	Point of maximal impulse is palpated (or auscultated) below the fifth ICS and to the left of the MCL	Left ventricular dilation
Extremities		
Unusually warm extremities	Hands and feet warmer than normal	Possible thyrotoxicosis
Cold extremities	Hands or feet, or both, cold to touch; external covering necessary for comfort	Intermittent claudication, peripheral arterial obstruction, low cardiac output, severe anemia
Pitting edema of lower extremities or sacral area	Visible finger indentation after application of firm pressure	Interruption of venous return to heart, fluid in tissues
Abnormal capillary filling time	Blanching of nail bed for >3 sec after release of pressure	Reduced arterial capillary perfusion, anemia
Asymmetry in limb circumference	Measurable swelling of involved limb	Thrombophlebitis, varicose veins, lymphedema
Percussion		
Abnormal cardiac borders	Left border of cardiac dullness extends beyond MCL in fifth ICS; right border of cardiac dullness extends beyond sternal border	Cardiac enlargement due to coronary heart disease, heart failure, cardiomyopathy
Auscultation		
Pulse deficit	Apical heart rate exceeds the peripheral pulse rate	Cardiac dysrhythmias
Arterial bruit	Turbulent flow sound in artery	Arterial obstruction or aneurysm
Third heart sound (S_3)	Extra heart sound, low-pitched, heard in early diastole, similar to sound of a gallop	Left ventricular failure; volume overload; mitral, aortic, or tricuspid regurgitation; hypertension (possible)
Fourth heart sound (S_4)	Extra heart sound, low-pitched, heard in late diastole, similar to sound of a gallop	Forceful atrial contraction from resistance to ventricular filling (e.g., in left ventricular hypertrophy, aortic stenosis, hypertension, coronary artery disease)
Cardiac murmurs	Turbulent sounds occurring between normal heart sounds; characterized by loudness, pitch, shape, quality, duration, timing	Cardiac valve disorder, abnormal blood flow patterns
Pericardial friction rub	High-pitched, scratchy sound heard during S_1 or S_2 or both at the apex; heard best with patient sitting and leaning forward, and at the end of expiration	Pericarditis

AV, atrioventricular; *bpm,* beats per minute; *ICS,* intercostal space; *MCL,* midclavicular line; *SA,* sinoatrial.

*Limited to common etiological factors. (Further discussion of conditions listed may be found in Chapters 35 through 40 and 68.)

Source: Adapted from Jarvis, C., Browne, A. J., MacDonald-Jenkins, J., & Luctkar-Flude, M. (2020). *Physical examination & health assessment* (3rd Canadian ed., pp. 505–510). Elsevier Inc.

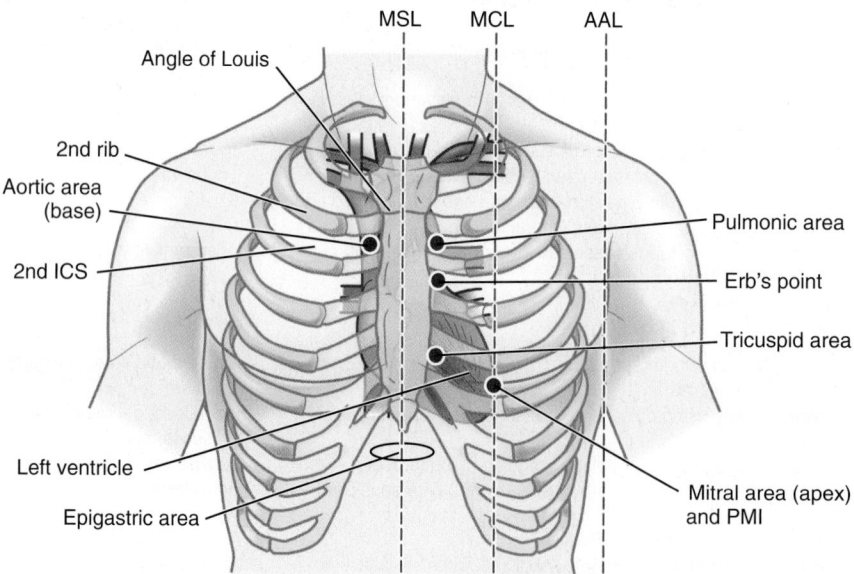

FIG. 34.7 Orientation of the heart within the thorax and cardiac auscultatory areas. Red lines indicate the midsternal line (MSL), midclavicular line (MCL), and anterior axillary line (AAL). *ICS,* intercostal space; *PMI,* point of maximal impulse.

often caused by left ventricular enlargement. Normally, no pulsations are seen or felt in the precordial area.

When the patient is recumbent, the mitral valve area at the apex of the heart is inspected and palpated for the **point of maximal impulse (PMI)**, the site of strongest pulsation. This pulsation or ventricular thrust lies within the MCL in the fifth ICS. If the PMI is palpable, its position is recorded in relation to the MCL and ICSs. When the PMI is to the left of the MCL, the heart may be enlarged.

Percussion. While percussion is a useful skill, percussion to outline cardiac borders has proven to be moderately accurate and has been replaced with chest radiography or echocardiogram. Often breast mass, especially with women, interferes with usefulness of percussion (Jarvis et al., 2019).

Auscultation. The movement of the cardiac valves creates some turbulence in the blood flow; the resulting heart sounds are normal (Figure 34.8). These sounds can be heard through a stethoscope placed on the chest wall. The first heart sound (S_1), which is associated with the closure of the tricuspid and mitral (atrioventricular) valves, sounds like a soft "lubb." The second heart sound (S_2), which is associated with the closure of the aortic and pulmonic (semilunar) valves, sounds like a sharp "dupp." S_1 signals the beginning of systole. S_2 signals the beginning of diastole (see Figure 34.8). The nurse should listen to the auscultatory areas in sequence with both the diaphragm and the bell of the stethoscope.

S_1 and S_2 are heard best with the diaphragm of the stethoscope placed firmly on the surface of the chest, as they are high-pitched sounds. Extra heart sounds (S_3 or S_4), if present, are heard best with the bell of the stethoscope gently placed on the chest, as they are considered low-pitched sounds. If the patient leans forward while sitting, sounds from the second ICSs (aortic and pulmonic areas) are accentuated, whereas in the left lateral decubitus position, sounds produced at the mitral area are accentuated.

The nurse can listen at the apical area with the diaphragm of the stethoscope while simultaneously palpating the radial pulse. When fewer radial than apical pulses are counted, the difference between those numbers is called a *pulse deficit*. A judgement about the rhythm (regular or irregular) is also made when listening at the apex.

Palpating one carotid artery while auscultating allows the examiner to distinguish between S_1 and S_2 and between systole and diastole. Because S_1 ("lubb") occurs almost simultaneously with ventricular ejection, it is heard when the carotid pulse is palpated.

Normally, no sound is heard between S_1 and S_2 during the periods of systole and diastole. Sounds that are heard during these periods may represent abnormalities and should be described in the assessment. An exception to this is a normal splitting of S_2, which is best heard at the pulmonic area during inspiration. Splitting of this heart sound can be abnormal if it is heard during expiration or if it is constant (fixed) during the respiratory cycle.

S_3 is a low-intensity vibration of the ventricular walls usually associated with ventricular filling. S_3 may occur in patients with left ventricular failure or mitral valve regurgitation. It is heard closely after S_2 and is known as a *ventricular gallop*. S_4 is a low-frequency vibration caused by atrial contraction. It precedes S_1 of the next cycle and is known as an *atrial gallop*. S_4 may occur in patients with CAD, left ventricular hypertrophy, or aortic stenosis.

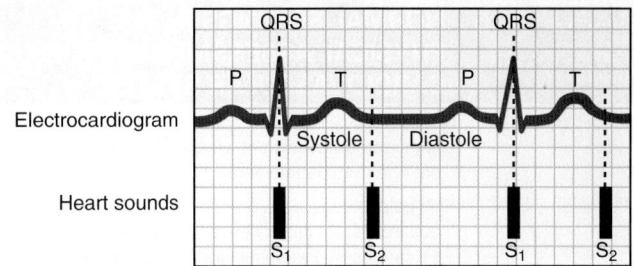

FIG. 34.8 Relationship of electrocardiogram, cardiac cycle, and heart sounds (S_1, S_2).

Murmurs are sounds produced by turbulent blood flow through the heart and are graded on a six-point Roman numeral scale based on loudness and recorded as a ratio. The numerator is the intensity of the murmur, and the denominator is always VI, which indicates that the six-point scale is being used. A grade I/VI murmur is soft and faint; a grade VI/VI murmur can be heard without a stethoscope. Most murmurs are the result of cardiac abnormalities such as valve disease (e.g., aortic stenosis), structural defects (e.g., endocarditis), or flow-related murmurs (e.g., hyperthyroidism).

If an abnormal sound is heard, it should be documented. The description should include the timing (during systole or diastole); the location (the site on the chest where it is heard the loudest); the pitch (heard best with the diaphragm or the bell of the stethoscope); the position (heard best when the patient is recumbent, sitting and leaning forward, or in the left lateral decubitus position); the characteristic (harsh, musical, soft, short, long); and any other abnormal findings (irregular cardiac rhythms or palpable chest wall heaves) associated with the sound.

The most common abnormal sounds and abnormal assessment findings are described in Table 34.4. A method of recording data from the cardiovascular assessment is presented in Table 34.5.

A focused assessment is used to evaluate the status of previously identified cardiovascular conditions and to monitor for signs of new conditions (see Chapter 3, Table 3.5). A focused assessment of the cardiovascular system is presented in the Focused Assessment box.

CASE STUDY

Objective Data: Physical Examination

Physical examination findings of L. T. are as follows:
- BP, 98/70; apical pulse rate, 164; pulse irregular; respiratory rate, 20; temperature, 36.8°C; O_2 saturation, 93% on room air
- Awake, alert, and oriented ×3
- Lungs clear on auscultation; systolic murmur present
- Cardiac monitor shows atrial fibrillation with a rapid ventricular response
- +1 pedal pulses bilaterally
- No peripheral edema, jugular venous distention, or heaves noted

See Case Study: Patient Introduction, Case Study: Subjective Data, and Case Study: Objective Data: Diagnostic Studies for more information on L. T.

TABLE 34.5 NORMAL FINDINGS IN THE PHYSICAL ASSESSMENT OF THE CARDIOVASCULAR SYSTEM

Inspection	Normal skin colour with capillary refill <3 sec; thorax symmetrical with no visible PMI; no JVD with patient at 45-degree angle
Palpation	PMI palpable in fifth ICS at MCL; no forceful pulsations, thrills, or heaves; slight palpable pulsations of abdominal aorta in epigastric area; carotid and extremity pulses 2+ and equal bilaterally; no evidence of impaired arterial flow or venous return in lower extremities, skin is warm and dry
Auscultation	S_1 and S_2 heard; HR, 72 and regular; no murmurs or extra heart sounds

HR, heart rate; *ICS,* intercostal space; *JVD,* jugular venous distension; *MCL,* midclavicular line; *PMI,* point of maximal impulse.

FOCUSED ASSESSMENT

Cardiovascular System

Use this checklist to make sure the key assessment steps have been done.

Subjective
Ask the patient about any of the following and note responses:

Chest pain or discomfort	Y	N
Shortness of breath (especially when lying down)	Y	N
Edema in legs or any part of body	Y	N
Leg pain during exercise	Y	N
Excess urination at night	Y	N
Palpitations	Y	N

Objective: Diagnostic
Check the following laboratory test results for critical values:

Hematocrit and hemoglobin
Cardiac biomarkers (CK-MB, troponin)
Electrocardiogram

Objective: Physical Examination
Inspect and Palpate

Anterior chest wall for contour, lifts, and heaves
Check pulses for symmetry, quality, and rhythm

Auscultate

Blood pressure
Heart for rate, rhythm, and sounds

CK-MB, MB isoenzyme of creatine kinase.

DIAGNOSTIC STUDIES OF THE CARDIOVASCULAR SYSTEM

Numerous diagnostic procedures add to the information obtained from the history and physical examination of the cardiovascular system. These procedures are usually classified as noninvasive or invasive. Procedures in which only a needle is inserted to withdraw blood or inject contrast media are usually considered noninvasive. Catheter insertion for angiography is considered an invasive procedure. The most common studies used to assess the cardiovascular system are presented in Table 34.6.

Noninvasive Studies

Chest Radiography. A radiograph can depict cardiac contours, heart size and configuration, and anatomical changes in individual chambers (Figure 34.9). The radiographic image records any displacement or enlargement of the heart, the presence of extra fluid around the heart (pericardial effusion), and pulmonary congestion.

Electrocardiography. The basic P, QRS, and T waveforms (see Figure 34.4) are used to assess cardiac function. Deviations from normal sinus rhythm can indicate abnormalities in heart function. There are many types of electrocardiographic monitoring, including resting ECG, ambulatory ECG monitoring, and exercise or stress testing.

A resting ECG helps identify at one point in time primary conduction abnormalities, cardiac dysrhythmias, cardiac hypertrophy, pericarditis, myocardial ischemia, site and extent of myocardial infarction (MI), pacemaker performance, and effectiveness of medication therapy. It is also used to monitor recovery from an MI. (See Chapter 38 for a complete discussion of ECG monitoring.)

Ambulatory Electrocardiographic Monitoring. Continuous ambulatory ECG (Holter monitoring) can provide diagnostic information over a longer period than can a standard resting ECG. In Holter monitoring, a recorder is worn by the patient for 24 to 48 hours, and the resulting ECG information is then stored until it is played back for printing and evaluation. Holter monitoring gives the patient freedom to perform usual activities of daily living and those that may be associated with cardiovascular symptoms. The patient maintains a record of activities, symptoms, and sleep, and this record is correlated with the ECG events recorded by the device (see Table 34.6).

Transtelephonic Event Recorders. This type of recorder is helpful for monitoring less frequent ECG events. The monitor is a portable unit with which electrodes are used to transmit a limited ECG over the phone to a receiving device. A disadvantage of this type of monitoring is that if the event is of short duration, the symptoms may end before the patient puts on the device and calls the assigned number. Likewise, if patients are extremely symptomatic (e.g., syncopal), they may not be physically able to transmit the ECG.

Exercise or Stress Testing. Cardiac symptoms frequently occur only with activity because of the demand on the coronary arteries to provide more oxygen. Exercise testing is used to evaluate the heart's response to physical stress. This helps to assess cardiovascular disease and set limits for exercise programs. Exercise testing is used for individuals who do not have restrictions related to walking or using a bicycle. It is also helpful for patients with normal ECGs that limit diagnostic interpretation (e.g., those with pacemakers; see Table 34.6). If the individual is unable to perform exercise testing because of physical limitations such as arthritis, neurological conditions, or pulmonary impairment, the heart is chemically stressed with the use of medications such as dobutamine (Dobutrex) or dipyridamole (Persantine) (Pagana et al., 2019).

Echocardiography. In echocardiography, ultrasound waves are used to record the movement of the structures of the heart. In the normal heart, ultrasonic sound waves directed at the heart are reflected back in typical configurations. The echocardiogram provides information about abnormalities of (a) valvular structure and motion, (b) cardiac chamber size and contents, (c) ventricular muscle and septal motion and thickness, (d) the pericardial sac, and (e) the ascending aorta. The

TABLE 34.6   DIAGNOSTIC STUDIES

Cardiovascular System

Study	Description and Purpose	Nursing Responsibility
Blood Studies*		
MB isoenzyme of creatine kinase (CK-MB)	Cardiospecific isoenzyme that is released in the presence of myocardial tissue injury. Concentrations >4–6% of total CK are highly indicative of MI. Serum levels increase within 4–6 hr after MI.	Explain to patient the purpose of serial sampling (e.g., q6–8h until peaks) in conjunction with serial ECGs.
Troponin (cardiac-specific)	Contractile proteins that are released after an MI. Both troponin T and troponin I are highly specific to cardiac tissue. *Reference intervals:* **Troponin I (cTnI)** Negative: <0.35 mcg/L **Troponin T (cTnT)** Negative: <0.1 mcg/L	Rapid point-of-care (bedside) assays are available. Serial sampling is often done in conjunction with CK-MB measurements and ECGs.
Myoglobin	Low-molecular-weight protein that is 99–100% sensitive for myocardial injury. Serum concentrations rise 30–60 min after MI. *Reference interval:* Normal: 1.0–5.3 nmol/L	Myoglobin is cleared from the circulation rapidly, and the test is most diagnostic if measurements are made within first 12 hr of onset of chest pain.
C-reactive protein (CRP)	Marker of inflammation that can predict risk of cardiac disease and cardiac events, even in patients with normal lipid values. CRP assay is highly sensitive. *Reference intervals:* Lowest risk: <1.1 mg/L Moderate risk: 1.2–1.9 mg/L High risk: 2.0–3.8 mg/L	CRP levels are stable and can be measured nonfasting and any time during the day. In women, CRP levels may be a more predictive risk factor of cardiac disease than LDLs.
Homocysteine	Amino acid produced during protein catabolism that has been identified as a risk factor for cardiovascular disease. Homocysteine may cause damage to the endothelium or have a role in formation of thrombi. *Reference intervals:* 0–30 years: 4.6–8.1 mcmol/L 30–59 years: *Male:* 6.3–11.2 mcmol/L *Female:* 4.5–7.9 mcmol/L >59 years: 5.8–11.9 mcmol/L	Hyperhomocysteinemia resulting from dietary deficiencies is treated with folic acid, vitamin B_6, and vitamin B_{12} supplements.
B-type natriuretic peptide (BNP)	Peptide that causes natriuresis. Elevation indicates presence of heart failure and may help distinguish cardiac from respiratory cause of dyspnea. *Reference interval:* Levels <100 ng/L are diagnostic for heart failure	Continue to monitor for signs and symptoms of heart failure.
N-terminal–pro B-type natriuretic peptide (NT–pro-BNP)	Aids in assessing the severity of heart failure in symptomatic and asymptomatic patients. In patients with renal insufficiency, concentrations may increase and may not correlate with New York Heart Association functional classification of heart failure. *Reference interval:* <100 mcg/L	
Serum Lipids		
Cholesterol	A blood lipid. Elevated levels are considered a risk factor for atherosclerotic heart disease. *Reference interval:* <5 mmol/L (varies with age and gender)	Cholesterol levels can be measured in a nonfasting state.
Triglycerides	Mixtures of fatty acids. Elevations are associated with cardiovascular disease and diabetes. *Reference interval:* <1.7 mmol/L (varies with age and sex)	Triglyceride levels and lipoproteins must be measured in a fasting state (at least 12 hr, except for water); alcohol should be withheld for 24 hr before testing.
Lipoproteins (HDL, LDL)	Soluble proteins that combine with and transport lipids in the plasma. Electrophoresis is performed to distinguish HDL from LDL. Serum lipid levels may fluctuate markedly from day to day. More than one determination is needed for accurate diagnosis and treatment. *Reference intervals* (vary with age): **HDL** • Recommended, adult: >0.91 • Low risk for CAD: >1.55 mmol/L • High risk for CAD: <0.91 mmol/L **LDL** • Optimal: <3.34 mmol/L • Near optimal: 2.6–3.34 mmol/L • Borderline high: 3.37–4.11 mmol/L • High risk for CAD: >4.14 mmol/L	After test is completed, risk for cardiac disease is assessed by dividing the total cholesterol level by the HDL level and obtaining a ratio. *Low risk:* Ratio <3 *Average risk:* Ratio 3–5 *Increased risk:* Ratio >5

Continued

TABLE 34.6   DIAGNOSTIC STUDIES

Cardiovascular System—cont'd

Study	Description and Purpose	Nursing Responsibility
Lipoprotein (a) (Lp[a])	Lipoprotein that contains one molecule of apolipoprotein B. Increased levels are associated with an increased risk of premature CAD and stroke. *Reference intervals:* Male: 0.22–4.94 g/L Female: 0.21–5.73 g/L	Lp(a) levels can be obtained in a nonfasting state. There are gender and genetic variations.
Lipoprotein-associated phospholipase A_2 (Lp-PLA$_2$)	Enzyme that catalyzes release of arachidonic acid. Elevated levels are associated with vascular inflammation and increased risk for CAD. Serum levels of Lp-PLA$_2$ are measured by the PLAC test. *Reference intervals:* Low risk: ≤151 nmol/min/mL Moderate risk: 152–194 nmol/min/mL High risk: ≥195 nmol/min/mL	Lp-PLA$_2$ levels can be obtained during a nonfasting state. Gender variations exist.
Chest radiograph	X-ray imaging. Patient is placed in two upright positions to examine the lung fields and size of the heart. The two common positions are posteroanterior and lateral. Normal heart size and contour for the individual's age, sex, and size are noted.	The nurse should inquire about frequency of recent radiographic studies and possibility of pregnancy. Lead shielding is applied to areas not being viewed. Any jewellery or metal objects that may obstruct the view of the heart and lungs must be removed.
Electrocardiography (ECG)	Electronic graphing of cardiac activity. Electrodes are placed on the chest and extremities, allowing the ECG machine to record cardiac electrical activity from different views. This study can reveal rhythm of the heart, activity of pacemaker, conduction abnormalities, position of the heart, size of atria and ventricles, presence of injury, and history of MI.	The patient's skin is prepared, and electrodes and leads are applied. The nurse should inform patient that no discomfort is involved. Patient should be instructed to avoid moving, to decrease motion artifact.
Signal-averaged electrocardiography (SAECG)	High-resolution ECG that can identify electrical activity called *late potentials* that indicate a patient is at risk for developing ventricular dysrhythmias (e.g., ventricular tachycardia).	Same as for ECG.

Ambulatory ECG Monitoring

Study	Description and Purpose	Nursing Responsibility
Holter monitoring	Recording of ECG rhythm for 24–48 hr; rhythm changes are then correlated with symptoms recorded in patient's diary. Normal patient activity is encouraged to simulate conditions that produce symptoms. Electrodes are placed on the chest, and a recorder is used to store information until it is recalled, printed, and analyzed for any rhythm disturbance. It can be performed on an inpatient or outpatient basis.	The patient's skin is prepared, and electrodes and leads are applied. The nurse should explain the importance of keeping an accurate diary of activities and symptoms. The patient should take no bath or shower during monitoring. Electrodes may cause skin irritation.
Event monitor or loop recorder	Recording of rhythm disturbances that are not frequent enough to be recorded in one 24-hr period. It allows more freedom than does a regular Holter monitor. Some units have electrodes that are attached to the chest and have a loop of memory that captures the onset and end of an event. Other types are placed directly on the patient's wrist, chest, or fingers and have no loop of memory but record the patient's ECG in real time. Recordings may be transmitted over the phone to a receiving unit.	The patient needs instruction in use of equipment for recording and transmitting (if appropriate) of transient events. The nurse should teach patient about skin preparation for lead placement or steady skin contact for units not requiring electrodes. This will ensure reception of optimal ECG tracings for analysis. The nurse should instruct patient to initiate recording as soon as symptoms begin or as soon thereafter as possible.
Exercise or stress testing	Study of the effect of exercise tolerance on cardiovascular function. Various policies are used. A common policy is to use 3-min stages at set speeds and with elevation of the treadmill belt. The patient can exercise to either predicted peak heart rate (calculated as the patient's age subtracted from 220) or to peak exercise tolerance, at which time the test is terminated. The test is also terminated for chest discomfort, significant increase or decrease in vital signs from baseline, or significant ECG changes indicating cardiac ischemia. Vital signs and ECG are monitored. The ECG is monitored after exercise for rhythm disturbances or, if ECG changes occurred with exercise, for return to baseline. Continual monitoring of vital signs and ECG rhythms for ischemic changes is important in the diagnosis of CAD. An exercise bike may be used if the patient is unable to walk on the treadmill.	The nurse should instruct patient (a) to wear comfortable clothes and shoes that can be used for walking and running and (b) about the procedure and importance of reporting any symptoms that may occur. The nurse monitors vital signs and obtains 12-lead ECG before patient's exercise, during each stage of exercise, and after exercise until all vital signs and ECG changes have returned to normal. The nurse monitors patient's response throughout procedure. Contraindications include any reasons patient is unable to reach peak exercise. β-Adrenergic blockers may be withheld 24 hr before the test because they will blunt the heart rate and limit the patient's ability to achieve maximal heart rate. Caffeine-containing food and fluids are also withheld for 24 hr. Patients must refrain from smoking and strenuous exercise for 3 hr before the test.
6-Minute walk test	Measurement of distance patient is able to walk on a flat surface in 6 min. It is used to measure response to treatments and determine functional capacity for activities of daily living. The test is useful for patients who are unable to perform treadmill or exercise bike testing.	The nurse instructs patient to wear comfortable shoes and informs patient to carry or pull oxygen if it is used routinely. Patient should be encouraged to walk as quickly as possible.

TABLE 34.6   DIAGNOSTIC STUDIES
Cardiovascular System—cont'd

Study	Description and Purpose	Nursing Responsibility
Echocardiography • Contrast • M-mode • Two-dimensional • Colour-flow imaging (duplex) • Real-time three-dimensional	Ultrasound imaging of cardiac activity. Transducer that emits and receives ultrasound waves is placed in four positions on the chest above the heart. Transducer records sound waves that are bounced off the heart. Also records direction and flow of blood through the heart and transforms it to audio and graphic data that reflect valvular abnormalities, congenital cardiac defects, wall motion, ejection fraction, and cardiac function. IV contrast medium may be used to enhance images.	The patient is placed in a supine position on their left side, facing equipment. The nurse instructs patient about procedure and expected sensations (pressure and mechanical movement from head of transducer). No contraindications to procedure exist.
Stress echocardiography	Combination of exercise testing and echocardiography. Resting images of the heart are taken with ultrasonography, and then the patient exercises. Postexercise images are taken immediately after exercise (within 1 min of stopping exercise). Differences in left ventricular wall motion and thickening before and after exercise are evaluated.	The nurse instructs and prepares patient for treadmill or exercise bicycle. The nurse also informs patient of importance of timely return to examination table for imaging after exercise. Contraindications include any reasons patient is unable to reach peak exercise.
Pharmacological echo-cardiography	Echocardiography with the use of pharmacological agent. Used as a substitute for the exercise stress test for patients unable to exercise. While echocardiography is performed, dobutamine or dipyridamole is infused intravenously, and dosage is increased in 5-min intervals to detect wall motion abnormalities at each stage.	The nurse starts IV infusion. Medication is administered per policy. The nurse monitors vital signs before, during, and after test until baseline achieved. The nurse also monitors patient for signs and symptoms of distress during procedure. The patient is observed for adverse effects (e.g., shortness of breath, dizziness, nausea). Aminophylline may be given to prevent or reverse adverse effects of dipyridamole. Contraindications include any known allergies to medications.
Transesophageal echo-cardiography (TEE)	Echocardiography with an internal probe. A probe with an ultrasound transducer at the tip is swallowed while the physician controls angle and depth. As the probe passes down the esophagus, it sends back clear images of heart size, wall motion, valvular abnormalities, endocarditis vegetation, and possible source of thrombi without interference from lungs or chest ribs. Contrast medium may be injected intravenously for evaluating direction of blood flow if an atrial or ventricular septal defect is suspected. Doppler ultrasonography and colour-flow imaging can also be used concurrently.	The nurse instructs patient to avoid eating for at least 6 hr before test. Removable dentures are taken out of patient's mouth, and a bite block is placed in the mouth. IV sedative is administered, and local anaesthetic is applied to throat. The nurse monitors vital signs and oxygen saturation levels and performs suctioning as needed during procedure. The nurse also assists patient to relax. Patient may not eat or drink until gag reflex returns. Sore throat is temporary. A designated driver is needed for patient if test is done in outpatient department.
Nuclear cardiology	Radiological study with radioactive isotope (technetium-99m sestamibi). Isotope is injected intravenously. Radioactive uptake is counted over the heart by scintillation camera. Study supplies information about myocardial contractility, myocardial perfusion, and acute cell injury.	The nurse explains procedure to patient. An IV line is established for injection of isotopes. The nurse must explain that radioactive isotope is used in a small, diagnostic amount and will lose most of its radioactivity in a few hours. Patient is informed that they will be lying still on their back with arms extended overhead for 20 min. Repeat scans are performed within a few minutes to hours after the injection.
Multigated acquisition (MUGA) (cardiac blood pool) scan	Imaging with a radioactive isotope. A small amount of the patient's blood is removed, mixed with isotope (e.g., technetium-99m sestamibi with Cardiolite kit), and reinjected intravenously. The ECG is used for timing, and images are acquired during the cardiac cycle. Indicated for patients with MI, heart failure, or valvular heart disease. It also can be used to evaluate the effect of various cardiac or cardiotoxic medications on the heart.	Procedure is explained to patient. The nurse establishes an IV line for removal of blood sample and reinjection of isotope and then establishes ECG monitoring. Patient is informed that procedure involves little risk.
Single-photon emission computed tomography (SPECT)	Computed tomography with radioactive isotope. Used to evaluate myocardium at risk of infarction and to determine infarction size. Small amounts of isotope (e.g., technetium-99m tetrofosmin [Myoview] or thallium-201) are injected intravenously, and recordings are made of the radioactivity emitted over a specific area of the body. Circulation of the isotope can be used to detect coronary artery blood flow, intracardiac shunts, motion of ventricles, ejection fraction, and size of the heart chambers.	The nurse explains procedure to patient, establishes IV line for injection of isotope, and establishes ECG monitoring. Patient must be informed that procedure involves little risk.
Exercise (stress) nuclear imaging	Nuclear imaging performed while patient is at rest and after exercise. The injection is given when patient reaches maximum heart rate on a bicycle or treadmill. Patient is then required to continue exercise for 1 min to circulate the radioactive isotope. Scanning is done 15–60 min after exercise. A resting scan is performed 60–90 min after initial infusion or 24 hr later.	Explain procedure to patient. Instruct patient to eat only a light meal between scans. Certain medications may need to be held for 1–2 days before the scan.

Continued

TABLE 34.6   DIAGNOSTIC STUDIES

Cardiovascular System—cont'd

Study	Description and Purpose	Nursing Responsibility
Pharmacological nuclear imaging	Nuclear imaging performed with vasodilating drugs. Dipyridamole or adenosine is used to produce vasodilation when patients are unable to tolerate exercise. Vasodilation will increase blood flow to well-perfused coronary arteries. Scanning procedure is same as for exercise nuclear imaging. Aminophylline may be given to prevent or reverse adverse effects of dipyridamole (e.g., shortness of breath, dizziness, nausea). Dobutamine is used if vasodilators are contraindicated.	The nurse explains procedure to patient and instructs patient to avoid all caffeine products for 12 hr before procedure. Calcium channel blockers and β-adrenergic blockers should be avoided 24 hr before the test. The nurse observes patient for adverse effects (e.g., shortness of breath, dizziness, nausea).
Positron emission tomography (PET)	Tomographic imaging with two radionuclides. PET is highly sensitive in distinguishing viable and nonviable myocardial tissue. Nitrogen-13 ammonia is injected intravenously first, and scanning is performed to evaluate myocardial perfusion. A second radioactive isotope, fluorine-18 fludeoxyglucose, is then injected, and scanning is performed to show myocardial metabolic function. If the heart is normal, the two scans will match, but if the heart is ischemic or damaged, they will differ. The patient may undergo this test with or without conditions of stress. A baseline resting scan is usually obtained for comparison.	The nurse instructs patient on procedure, explaining that patient will be scanned by a machine and will need to stay still for a period of time. Patient's glucose level must be between 3.3 and 7.8 mcmol/L for accurate glucose metabolic activity. If exercise is included as part of testing, patient will need to fast and refrain from tobacco and caffeine for 24 hr before test.
Cardiovascular magnetic resonance imaging (CMRI)	Noninvasive imaging technique that obtains information about cardiac tissue integrity, aneurysms, ejection fractions, cardiac output, and patency of proximal coronary arteries. It does not involve ionizing radiation and is an extremely safe procedure. It provides images in multiple planes with uniformly good resolution.	The nurse explains procedure to patient, informing patient that the small diameter of the cylinder, along with loud noise of the procedure, may cause panic or anxiety. Antianxiety drugs and distraction strategies (e.g., music) may be recommended. Patient must lie still during MRI. CMRI is contraindicated for patients with implanted metallic devices or other metal fragments. The nurse must discern presence of any implants before scan.
Magnetic resonance angiography (MRA)	Imaging of vascular occlusive disease and abdominal aortic aneurysms. Same as MRI but with use of gadolinium as IV contrast medium.	Contraindications include any known allergies to contrast medium and the presence of implanted metallic devices or other metal fragments.
Cardiac computed tomography (CT)	Heart-specific CT imaging technology with or without IV contrast media. It is used to visualize heart anatomy, coronary circulation, and blood vessels.	The nurse explains procedure to patient.
Computed tomographic angiography (CTA)	Use of CT with injected IV contrast medium to obtain images of blood vessels and diagnose CAD.	The nurse explains procedure to patient. Metal objects should be removed before examination. The patient may be asked not to eat or drink for several hours before the procedure.
Calcium-scoring CT scan • Electron beam computed tomography (EBCT)	Also known as *ultrafast CT*; a scanning electron beam is used to quantify calcification in coronary arteries and heart valves (see Figure 34.12). Used primarily for risk assessment in asymptomatic patients and to assess for heart disease in patients with atypical symptoms potentially resulting from cardiac causes.	The nurse explains procedure to patient and informs patient that procedure is quick and involves little or no risk.
Cardiac catheterization	Insertion of catheter into heart, via artery, to obtain information about O$_2$ levels and pressure readings within heart chambers. Contrast medium is injected to assist in examining structure and motion of the heart.	The nurse checks patient for iodine sensitivity. Food and fluids are withheld for 6–18 hr before procedure. The nurse administers sedative and other drugs, if ordered, and informs patient about use of local anaesthesia, insertion of catheter, feeling of warmth when dye is injected, and possible fluttering sensation of heart as catheter is passed. Patient may be instructed to cough or take a deep breath when dye is injected and then is monitored by ECG throughout procedure. After the procedure, the nurse assesses circulation to extremity used for catheter insertion. The nurse checks peripheral pulses, colour, and sensation of extremity every 15 min for 1 hr and then with decreasing frequency. The puncture site is observed for hematoma and bleeding. A compression device is placed over arterial site to achieve hemostasis, if indicated. The nurse monitors vital signs and ECG and assesses for hypotension or hypertension, abnormal heart rate, dysrhythmias, and signs of pulmonary emboli (e.g., respiratory difficulty).
Coronary angiography	Imaging during a cardiac catheterization in which contrast medium is injected directly into coronary arteries. Used to evaluate patency of coronary arteries and collateral circulation.	Same as for cardiac catheterization.

TABLE 34.6 DIAGNOSTIC STUDIES
Cardiovascular System—cont'd

Study	Description and Purpose	Nursing Responsibility
Noninvasive coronary computed tomographic angiography (CCTA)	A noninvasive imaging modality that can be used to evaluate the anatomy of the coronary arteries. Unlike coronary artery calcium scoring, in which non-contrast CT is used to assess atherosclerotic disease burden, CCTA allows direct visualization of the coronary artery wall and lumen with the administration of IV contrast medium.	Same as for cardiac catheterization.
Intracoronary ultrasonography	Ultrasound imaging in which a small ultrasound probe is introduced into coronary arteries during cardiac catheterization. Data are used to assess size and consistency of plaque, arterial walls, and effectiveness of intracoronary artery treatment.	Same as for cardiac catheterization.
Fractional flow reserve	Measurement of blood pressure and flow. During cardiac catheterization, a special wire is inserted into the coronary arteries to gather these measurements. Information is used to determine need for angioplasty or stent placement on nonsignificant blockages.	Same as for cardiac catheterization.
Electrophysiology study (EPS)	Invasive study used to record intracardiac electrical activity. Catheters (with multiple electrodes) are inserted via the femoral and jugular veins into the right side of the heart. The catheter electrodes record the electrical activity in different cardiac structures. In addition, dysrhythmias can be induced and terminated.	Antidysrhythmic medications may be discontinued several days before study. Patient should be on NPO status 6–8 hr before test. The nurse administers premedication to promote relaxation, if ordered. IV sedative is often used during procedure. Patient must have frequent monitoring of vital signs and continuous ECG monitoring after the procedure.
Peripheral arteriography and venography[†]	Radiographic study involving injection of radiopaque contrast medium into either arteries or veins. Serial radiographs are taken to detect and visualize any atherosclerotic plaques, occlusion, aneurysms, or traumatic injury.	The nurse checks for iodine allergy and administers a mild sedative, if ordered. The nurse checks extremity with puncture site for pulsation, warmth, colour, and motion after procedure. Insertion site is inspected for bleeding or swelling. The nurse observes patient for allergic reactions to dye.
Hemodynamic monitoring	Hemodynamic monitoring of arterial blood pressures, pulmonary artery pressure, pulmonary artery wedge pressure, and cardiac output is used to evaluate cardiovascular status and response to treatment.	Patients requiring hemodynamic monitoring are critically ill and are monitored in critical care units. See Chapter 68 for complete information on hemodynamic monitoring.

CAD, coronary artery disease; *CK*, creatine kinase; *ECG*, electrocardiogram; *HDL*, high-density lipoprotein; *IV*, intravenous; *LDL*, low-density lipoprotein; *MI*, myocardial infarction; *NPO*, nothing by mouth; O_2, oxygen.
*Reference ranges for the laboratory tests vary by institution because of differences in equipment and reagents used.
†Additional peripheral vascular diagnostic studies are found in Table 40.9.

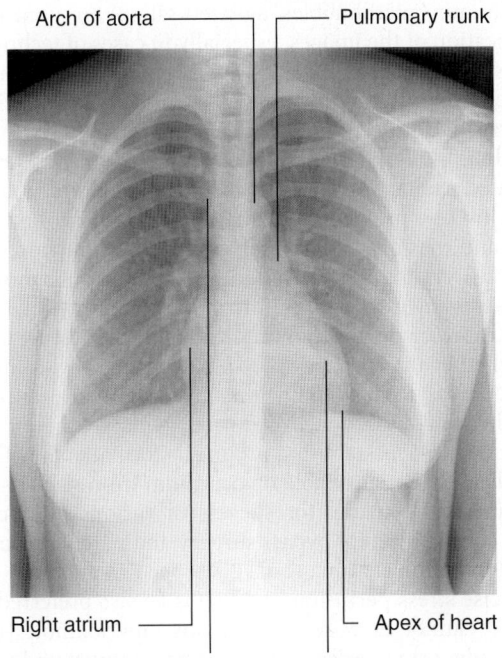

Arch of aorta — — Pulmonary trunk

Right atrium — — Apex of heart

Superior vena cava   Left ventricle

FIG. 34.9 Chest radiograph: standard posteroanterior view. Source: Drake, R. L., Vogl, A. W., & Mitchell, A. W. M. (2010). *Gray's anatomy for students* (2nd ed.). Churchill Livingstone.

ejection fraction, or the percentage of end-diastolic blood volume that is ejected during systole, can also be measured. The ejection fraction provides information about the function of the left ventricle during systole.

Two commonly used types are M-mode (motion mode) and two-dimensional echocardiography. In the M-mode type, a single ultrasound beam is directed toward the heart, and the motion of the intracardiac structures is recorded, as are wall thickness and chamber size. In two-dimensional echocardiography, the ultrasound beam sweeps through an arc, producing a cross-sectional view, and shows correct spatial relationships among the structures.

Doppler technology allows for sound evaluation of the flow or motion of the scanned object (heart valves, ventricular walls, blood flow). Colour-flow (duplex) imaging is the combination of two-dimensional echocardiography and Doppler technology (Figure 34.10). Colour changes demonstrate the velocity and direction of blood flow. Pathological conditions, such as valvular leaks and congenital defects, can be diagnosed more effectively. Stress echocardiography, a combination of treadmill test and ultrasound images, is used to evaluate segmental wall motion abnormalities (Pagana et al., 2019). A digital computer system is used to compare images before and after exercise, and wall motion and segmental function can be clearly seen. This diagnostic test provides the information of an exercise stress test combined with that obtained from an echocardiogram.

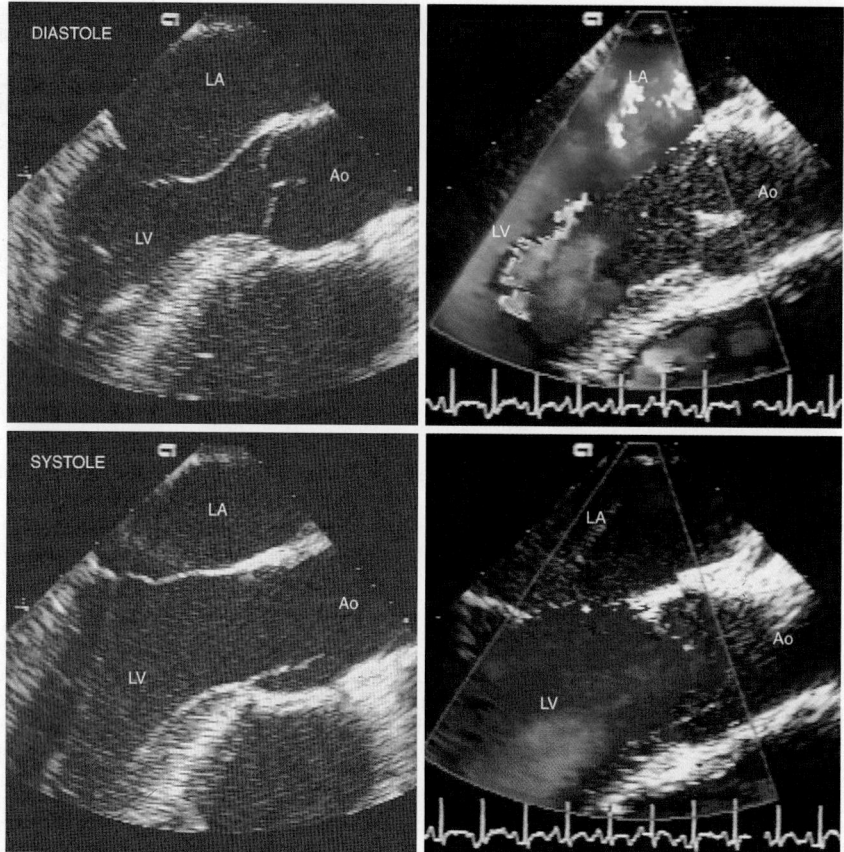

FIG. 34.10 Long-axis images of the aortic *(Ao)* and mitral valve with the depth adjusted to optimize evaluation of valve anatomy and motion. The two-dimensional images *(left)* in diastole *(top)* and systole *(bottom)* show normal aortic and mitral opening and closure. The colour flow images *(right)* show normal left ventricular *(LV)* inflow with no aortic regurgitation in diastole *(top)* and normal antegrade flow in the left ventricular outflow tract and no mitral regurgitation in systole *(bottom)*. *LA,* left atria. Source: Otto, C. (2004). *Textbook of clinical echocardiography* (3rd ed.). Saunders.

For patients unable to exercise, infusion of a pharmacological agent—usually dobutamine (Dobutrex) or dipyridamole (Persantine)—induces stress on the heart while the patient is resting. The same ultrasound technology is used.

In comparison with surface two-dimensional echocardiography, transesophageal echocardiography (TEE) is used to provide more precise images of the heart by eliminating interference from the chest wall and the lungs. TEE involves the use of a modified, flexible endoscope probe with an ultrasound transducer in the tip for imaging of the heart and great vessels. The probe is introduced into the esophagus to the level of the heart, and M-mode, two-dimensional, pulsed Doppler, and colour-flow images can be obtained.

TEE is used frequently in an outpatient setting primarily for evaluation of mitral regurgitation, to detect the presence of thrombus before cardioversion is performed, to identify areas of muscle wall hypokinesia, or to locate the source of cardiac emboli. In addition, TEE has applications in the operating room for assessment of presurgical and postsurgical cardiac function and in the emergency department for detecting potential aortic dissection.

The risks with TEE are minimal. However, complications may include perforation of the esophagus, hemorrhage, dysrhythmias, vasovagal reactions, and transient hypoxemia. TEE is contraindicated if the patient has a history of esophageal disorders, dysphagia, or radiation therapy involving the chest wall. Patients must be sedated during TEE.

In contrast echocardiography, intravenous contrast agents (e.g., albumin microbubbles, agitated saline) are used to assist in delineation of the images, especially in cases of technical difficulties (Pagana et al., 2019). When these agents are injected into the cardiac blood pool, they greatly enhance reflectivity for the ultrasound procedure.

Nuclear Cardiology. A common nuclear imaging test is the multigated acquisition (MUGA), or cardiac blood pool, scanning. This test provides information on wall motion during systole and diastole, cardiac valves, and ejection fraction (see Table 34.6). As it is a three-dimensional picture, it is most accurate in assessing cardiac function and ejection fraction.

Perfusion imaging is also used with exercise testing to determine whether the coronary blood flow changes with increased activity. Stress perfusion imaging may show an abnormality even when a resting image is normal. This procedure is used to diagnose CAD, establish a prognosis for patients with existing CAD, differentiate viable myocardium from scar tissue, and determine the potential for success of various interventions, such as coronary artery bypass surgery and percutaneous coronary intervention (Pagana et al., 2019; see Chapter 36).

Exercise stress perfusion imaging is always preferred, but if a patient cannot exercise, intravenous dipyridamole (Persantine) or adenosine (Adenocard) can be administered to dilate the coronary arteries and simulate the effect of exercise. After the drug takes effect, the isotope is injected and the imaging is performed.

Cardiovascular Magnetic Resonance Imaging. Cardiovascular magnetic resonance imaging (CMRI) can reveal areas of MI in a three-dimensional view. CMRI is considered an important diagnostic procedure as it is sensitive enough to find even small MIs, as well as pericardial disease, intracardiac masses, and many forms of congenital heart disease. CMRI aids in the final diagnosis of an MI, as well as in assessment of cardiac function such as ejection fraction, valvular abnormalities, and ventricular changes due to ischemia (Pagana et al, 2019).

One major advantage of CMRI is that it does not require any irradiation of the patient. In general, the use of CMRI in patients with pacemakers and internal cardioverter-defibrillators (ICDs) is discouraged because the magnets can alter the function of the devices. Some newer models of these devices are approved for use with MRI (Sole et al., 2017).

Cardiac Computed Tomography. Cardiac computed tomography (CT) is a heart imaging test in which CT technology, with or without intravenous contrast medium (dye), is used to visualize the heart anatomy, coronary circulation, and great blood vessels (e.g., aorta, pulmonary veins, artery). This technology is often called *multidetector CT scanning.* Types of CT scans used to diagnose heart disease include coronary CT angiography (CTA) and calcium-scoring CT scan (see Table 34.6).

Coronary CTA is a noninvasive test. It can be performed faster than cardiac catheterization with less risk and discomfort to the patient (Pagana et al., 2019). Although the use of coronary CTA is increasing, cardiac catheterization (discussed in the next section) remains the gold standard for diagnosing coronary artery stenosis. Furthermore, when a cardiac catheterization is done, interventions (e.g., angioplasty, stent placement) can be performed if coronary blockages are found.

The calcium-scoring CT scan is used to find calcium deposits in plaque in the coronary arteries. The most common method used is electron beam CT (Figure 34.11). It can detect early coronary calcification before symptoms develop. The amount of coronary calcium is a predictor of future cardiac events.

Blood Studies. Many blood studies provide information about the cardiovascular system. For example, some reflect the O_2-carrying capacity (red blood cell count and hemoglobin) and coagulation properties (clotting times) of the blood. (See Chapter 32 and Tables 32.7 and 32.8 for hematology studies.) The studies most commonly used to assess the cardiovascular system are listed in Table 34.6.

Cardiac Biomarkers. When cells are injured, they release their contents, including enzymes and other proteins, into the circulation. These *biomarkers* are useful in the diagnosis of myocardial injury and infarction.

Cardiac-specific troponin is a myocardial muscle protein released into circulation after injury or infarction. Two subtypes, cardiac-specific troponin T (cTnT) and cardiac-specific troponin I (cTnI), are specific to myocardial tissue. Normally the level in the blood is very low, and so a rise in level is diagnostic of myocardial injury. Rising levels of cTnT and cTnI are detectable within hours (on average 4 to 6 hours) of myocardial injury; these levels peak at 10 to 24 hours and can be detected for up to 10 to 14 days (see Chapter 36, Figure 36.10). Troponin is the biomarker used in the diagnosis of MI. The development of high-sensitivity troponin (hs-cTnT, hs-cTnI) assays may provide even earlier detection of a cardiac event (Andruchow et al., 2018). Creatine kinase (CK) enzymes are found in a variety of organs and tissues and occur as three isozymes. These isozymes are specific to skeletal muscle (CK-MM), brain and nervous tissue (CK-BB), and

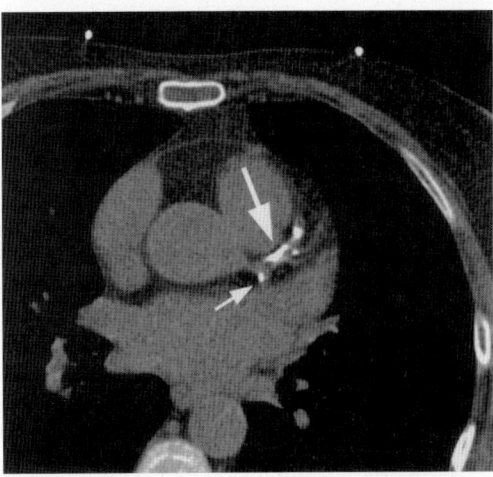

FIG. 34.11 Examples of coronary calcification of the left anterior descending coronary artery *(large arrow)* and left circumflex artery *(small arrow)* as seen on electron beam computed tomography. Source: Libby, P., Bonow, R., Zipes, D., et al. (Eds.). (2008). *Braunwald's heart disease: A textbook of cardiovascular medicine* (8th ed.). Saunders.

the heart (CK-MB). CK-MB elevation is specific for myocardial injury or infarction. CK-MB levels begin to rise 3 to 6 hours after symptom onset, peak in 12 to 24 hours, and return to baseline within 12 to 48 hours after MI (Pagana et al., 2019). The peak level and return to normal can be delayed in cases of large MI. Levels drop more rapidly in patients who are quickly and successfully treated for an MI. (Figure 36.10 in Chapter 36 depicts the changes in cardiac markers related to an MI.)

Myoglobin is a low-molecular-weight heme protein found in cardiac and skeletal muscle. Elevation in myoglobin levels is a sensitive indicator of very early myocardial injury but lacks specificity for MI. Its usefulness in diagnosing MI is limited (Pagana et al., 2019).

To interpret diagnostic test results correctly, the time of onset of symptoms and the time of the expected presence and elevation of the biomarkers must be considered. Additional data (patient symptoms, history, and ECG changes) complete the diagnostic picture for the patient with suspected myocardial injury or MI.

C-Reactive Protein. C-reactive protein (CRP) is a protein produced by the liver during periods of acute inflammation. CRP can be measured with a high-sensitivity test (hs-CRP). An increased level of CRP is an independent risk factor for CAD. The level of CRP may also be predictive of the risk for future cardiac events in patients with unstable angina and MI, but studies have produced conflicting results.

Homocysteine. Homocysteine is an amino acid that is produced during protein catabolism. Elevated homocysteine levels can be either hereditary or acquired from dietary deficiencies of vitamin B_6, vitamin B_{12}, or folate. Elevated levels of homocysteine have been linked to a higher risk of CAD, peripheral vascular disease, and stroke. It is recommended that homocysteine testing be performed in patients with a familial predisposition for early cardiovascular disease or a history of cardiovascular disease in the absence of other common risk factors (Pagana et al., 2019).

Cardiac Natriuretic Peptide Markers. There are three natriuretic peptides: (a) atrial natriuretic peptide (ANP) from the atrium, (b) b-type natriuretic peptide (BNP) from the ventricles, and (c) c-type natriuretic peptide from endothelial and renal epithelial cells. BNP is the marker of choice for distinguishing a cardiac or respiratory cause of dyspnea. When diastolic blood pressure increases (e.g., heart failure), BNP is released and increases natriuresis (excretion of sodium in the urine). ANP and BNP are also discussed in Chapter 37.

Serum Lipids. Serum lipids consist of triglycerides, cholesterol, and phospholipids. They circulate in the blood bound to protein. Thus they are often referred to as *lipoproteins.*

Triglycerides are the main storage form of lipids and make up about 95% of fatty tissue. Cholesterol, a structural component of cell membranes and plasma lipoproteins, is a precursor of corticosteroids, sex hormones, and bile salts. In addition to being absorbed from food in the gastrointestinal tract, cholesterol can also be synthesized in the liver. Phospholipids contain glycerol, fatty acids, phosphates, and a nitrogenous compound. Although formed in most cells, phospholipids usually enter the circulation as lipoproteins synthesized by the liver. Apoproteins are water-soluble proteins that combine with most lipids to form lipoproteins.

Different classes of lipoproteins contain varying amounts of the naturally occurring lipids. These include the following:

1. *Chylomicrons:* primarily exogenous triglycerides from dietary fat
2. *Low-density lipoproteins (LDLs):* mostly cholesterol with moderate amounts of phospholipids
3. *High-density lipoproteins (HDLs):* approximately 50% protein and 50% phospholipids and cholesterol
4. *Very-low-density lipoproteins (VLDLs):* primarily endogenous triglycerides with moderate amounts of phospholipids and cholesterol

A lipid panel usually includes measurements of cholesterol, triglyceride, LDL, and HDL. Elevations in triglyceride and LDL levels are strongly associated with CAD. An increased HDL level is associated with a decreased risk of CAD (Huether et al., 2020). High levels of HDLs serve a protective role by mobilizing cholesterol from tissues.

Although an association exists between elevated serum cholesterol levels and CAD, a measure of total cholesterol alone is not sufficient for an assessment of CAD. To calculate a risk assessment, the ratios of total cholesterol to HDL ratio are compared over time. An increase in the ratio indicates increased risk. This provides more information than either value alone. The patient must fast before blood is drawn for a lipid panel so that food intake does not affect the results.

Plasma levels of apolipoprotein A-I (the major HDL protein) and the ratio of apolipoprotein A-I to apolipoprotein B (the major LDL protein) are stronger predictors of CAD than is the HDL cholesterol level alone. Measurements of these lipoproteins can be useful in identifying patients at risk for CAD (Pagana et al., 2019).

Lipoprotein (a) has been studied for its role as a risk factor for CAD. Increased levels of lipoprotein (a), especially with increased levels of lactate dehydrogenase, have been linked with the progression of atherosclerosis, especially in women (Huether et al., 2020).

Lipoprotein-Associated Phospholipase A_2. Lipoprotein-associated phospholipase A_2 (Lp-PLA$_2$) is an inflammatory enzyme expressed in atherosclerotic plaques. Elevated levels of Lp-PLA$_2$ are related to an increased risk of CAD (Pagana et al., 2019).

Invasive Studies

Invasive studies are performed if definitive information is required. These studies include cardiac catheterization, coronary angiography, electrophysiology (see Table 34.6), intracoronary ultrasonography, and hemodynamic monitoring.

Cardiac Catheterization and Coronary Angiography. Cardiac catheterization is a common outpatient procedure. It provides information about CAD, coronary spasm, congenital and valvular heart disease, and ventricular function. Cardiac catheterization is also used to measure intracardiac pressures and O_2 levels, as well as CO and ejection fraction. With injection of contrast media and fluoroscopy, the coronary arteries are visualized, chambers of the heart can be outlined, and wall motion can be observed.

In cardiac catheterization, a radiopaque catheter is inserted into the right or left side of the heart, or both sides. For the right side of the heart, a catheter is inserted through an arm vein (basilic or cephalic) or a leg vein (femoral). Pressures are recorded as the catheter is moved into the vena cava, the right atrium, the right ventricle, and the pulmonary artery. The catheter is then moved until it is wedged in the pulmonary artery. This blocks the blood flow and pressure from the right side of the heart and looks ahead through the pulmonary capillary bed to the pressure in the left side of the heart *(pulmonary artery wedge pressure).* This pressure is used to assess the function of the left side of the heart.

In left-sided cardiac catheterization, a catheter is inserted into a femoral, brachial, or radial artery. The catheter is passed in a retrograde manner up to the aorta, across the aortic valve, and into the left ventricle.

Coronary angiography is performed with a left-sided heart catheterization. The catheter is positioned at the origin of the coronary arteries (see Figure 34.3) and contrast medium is injected into the arteries. Patients often feel a temporary flushed sensation with dye injection. The images identify the location and severity of any coronary blockages (Figure 34.12; see also Figure 36.9). Complications of cardiac catheterization include bleeding or hematoma at the puncture site; allergic reactions to the contrast media; looping or kinking of the catheter; infection; thrombus formation; aortic dissection; dysrhythmias; MI; stroke; and puncture of the ventricles, cardiac septum, or lung tissue.

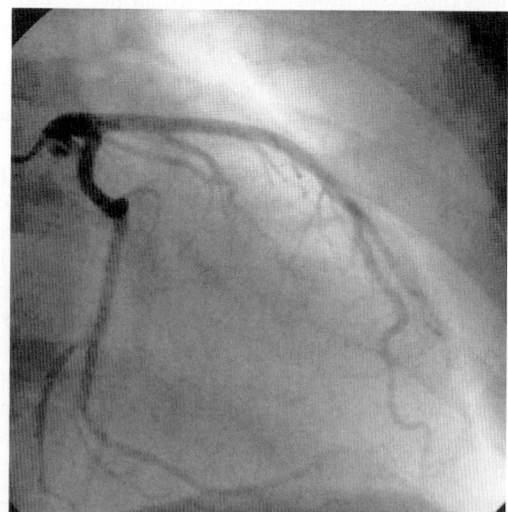

FIG. 34.12 Normal left coronary artery angiogram. Source: Drake, R. L., Vogl, A. W., & Mitchell, A. W. M. (2010). *Gray's anatomy for students* (2nd ed.). Churchill Livingstone.

Intracoronary Ultrasonography. Intracoronary ultrasonography (ICUS), also known as *intravascular ultrasonography* (IVUS), is an invasive procedure performed in the catheterization laboratory with coronary angiography. The two- or three-dimensional ultrasound images provide a cross-sectional view of the arterial walls of the coronary arteries. In this procedure, a miniature transducer or camera attached to a small catheter is moved to the artery to be studied. Once it is in the artery, ultrasound images are obtained. The health of the arterial layers is assessed, including the composition, location, and thickness of any plaque. ICUS can be used to help evaluate vessel response to treatments such as stent placement and atherectomy, as well as any complications that may have occurred during the procedure. Patients most often undergo ICUS in addition to angiography or a coronary intervention. Thus, nursing care is similar to that after cardiac catheterization (see Table 34.6).

Fractional Flow Reserve. Fractional flow reserve is a procedure that is performed during a cardiac catheterization. It involves using a special wire that can measure pressure and flow in the coronary artery. Fractional flow reserve helps to determine the need to perform angioplasty or stent placement on nonsignificant blockages.

Hemodynamic Monitoring. Bedside hemodynamic monitoring of pressures of the cardiovascular system is frequently used to assess cardiovascular status. Invasive hemodynamic monitoring with the use of intra-arterial and pulmonary artery catheters can be performed to monitor arterial blood pressure, intracardiac pressures, and CO (see Chapter 68). The central venous pressure (CVP) is a measurement of preload and can be used to monitor the pressure in the right atrium and right ventricle. The CVP is influenced by the function of the left side of the heart, pressures in the pulmonary vessels, venous return

to the heart, and the position of the patient when the reading is taken. The last factor must be kept in mind to obtain an accurate reading. The CVP can be used as a guide in fluid volume management of fluid overload or hypovolemia.

CVP can be measured with a pulmonary artery catheter (see Chapter 68) or a central venous catheter threaded through the jugular or the subclavian vein into the superior vena cava. The normal CVP is 2 to 9 mm Hg.

CASE STUDY

Objective Data: Diagnostic Studies

The health care provider orders the following initial diagnostic studies for L. T.:
- 12-lead ECG
- Complete blood cell count, basic metabolic panel (glucose, electrolytes, blood urea nitrogen, creatinine)
- Partial thromboplastin time, prothrombin time, international normalized ratio
- BNP measurement
- Troponin, CK-MB measurement
- Thyroid-stimulating hormone, free thyroxine
- Chest radiograph

L. T.'s initial troponin and CK-MB levels are within normal limits. His ECG demonstrates atrial fibrillation with a rapid ventricular response. Results of the chest radiograph, complete blood cell count, basic metabolic panel, BNP measurement, and coagulation studies are all within normal limits. The health care provider orders intravenous diltiazem (Cardizem) and heparin to be started in the emergency department. L. T. will be admitted to the progressive care unit and will have a consult with a cardiologist.

See Case Study: Patient Introduction, Case Study: Subjective Data, and Case Saudy: Objective Data: Physical Examination for more information on L. T.

REVIEW QUESTIONS

The number of the question corresponds to the same-numbered objective at the beginning of the chapter.

1. A client has a tricuspid valve disorder. Between which of the following chambers will the blood flow be impaired?
   a. Vena cava and right atrium
   b. Left atrium and left ventricle
   c. Right atrium and right ventricle
   d. Right ventricle and pulmonary artery

2. A client has a severe blockage in his right coronary artery. Which cardiac structures are most likely to be affected by this blockage? *(Select all that apply.)*
   a. Atrioventricular node
   b. Left ventricle
   c. Coronary sinus
   d. Right ventricle
   e. Pulmonic valve

3. Where is the conduction impairment when the Purkinje system is damaged?
   a. Atria
   b. Atrioventricular node
   c. Ventricles
   d. Bundle of His

4. Describe the differences between an artery and a vein.
   a. Arteries are thin-walled with capacity to hold large quantities of blood.
   b. Arteries are where cellular nutrients are exchanged.
   c. Veins mainly carry oxygenated blood and have rigid walls.
   d. Veins are thin-walled and contain valves for unidirectional flow.

5. When a person's blood pressure rises, which compensatory homeostatic mechanism is stimulated?
   a. Chemoreceptors that inhibit the sympathetic nervous system, causing vasodilation
   b. Baroreceptors that inhibit the parasympathetic nervous system, causing vasodilation
   c. Baroreceptors that inhibit the sympathetic nervous system, causing a decrease in heart rate
   d. Chemoreceptors that stimulate the sympathetic nervous system, causing an increase in heart rate

6. If a client's capillary refill assessment shows that the colour is greater than 3 seconds, what does this indicate?
   a. A normal response
   b. Thrombus formation in the veins
   c. Lymphatic obstruction of venous return
   d. Impaired arterial flow to the extremities

7. Which auscultatory area is found at the left midclavicular line at the level of the fifth intercostal space?
   a. Aortic area
   b. Mitral area
   c. Tricuspid area
   d. Pulmonic area
8. When a palpable precordial thrill is found on assessment, what could this indicate?
   a. Heart murmurs
   b. Gallop rhythms
   c. Pulmonary edema
   d. Right ventricular hypertrophy
9. Which of the following may be found on assessment of a 79-year-old client?
   a. A narrowed pulse pressure
   b. Diminished carotid artery pulses
   c. Difficulty in isolating the apical pulse
   d. An increased heart rate in response to stress
10. Which of the following is an important nursing responsibility for a client undergoing an invasive cardiovascular diagnostic study?
    a. Checking the peripheral pulses and percutaneous insertion site
    b. Instructing the client about radioactive isotope injection
    c. Informing the client that general anaesthesia will be given
    d. Assisting the client to do a surgical scrub of the insertion site
11. Which of the following statements best describe the P-wave impulse?
    a. Arising at the sinoatrial node and repolarizing the atria
    b. Arising at the sinoatrial node and depolarizing the atria
    c. Arising at the atrioventricular node and depolarizing the atria
    d. Arising at the atrioventricular node and spreading to the bundle of His

1. c; 2. a, b, d; 3. c; 4. d; 5. c; 6. d; 7. b; 8. a; 9. c; 10. a; 11. b.

ⓔvolve

For even more review questions, visit http://evolve.elsevier.com/Canada/Lewis/medsurg.

REFERENCES

Andruchow, J., Kavsak, P., & McRae, A. (2018). Contemporary emergency department management of patients with chest pain: A concise review and guide for the high-sensitivity troponin era. *Canadian Journal of Cardiology, 34*(2), 98–108. https://doi.org/10.1016/j.cjca.2017.11.012

Deley, G., Culas, C., Blonde, C., et al. (2019). Physical and psychological effectiveness of cardiac rehabilitation: Age is not a limiting factor. *Canadian Journal of Cardiology, 35*(10), 1353–1358. https://doi.org/10.1016/j.cjca.2019.05.038

Huether, S., McCance, K., & Brashers (2020). *Understanding pathophysiology* (7th ed.). Mosby.

Jarvis, C., Browne, A., MacDonald-Jenkins, J., et al. (2019). *Physical examination & health assessment* (3rd ed.). Elsevier.

Pagana, K., Pagana, T., & Pike-MacDonald, S. (2019). *Mosby's Canadian manual of diagnostic and laboratory tests* (2nd Canadian ed.). Elsevier.

Sole, M., Klein, D., & Moseley, M. (2017). *Introduction to critical care nursing* (7th ed.). Elsevier.

Touhy, T., & Jett, K. (2020). *Ebersole & Ness' toward healthy aging: Human needs and nursing response* (10th ed.). Elsevier.

RESOURCES

Resources for this chapter are listed in Chapter 36.

Nursing Management
Hypertension

Kara Sealock
Originating US chapter by Pamela Wilkerson and Melissa Hutchinson

LEARNING OBJECTIVES

1. Relate the pathophysiological mechanisms associated with primary hypertension to the clinical manifestations and complications.
2. Select appropriate strategies for the prevention of primary hypertension.
3. Describe the interprofessional care for primary hypertension, including medication therapy and lifestyle modifications.
4. Explain the interprofessional care of the older person with primary hypertension.
5. Prioritize the nursing management of the patient with primary hypertension.
6. Describe the interprofessional care of a patient with hypertensive crisis.

KEY TERMS

baroreceptors
blood pressure (BP)
cardiac output (CO)
hypertension

hypertensive crisis
isolated systolic hypertension (ISH)
orthostatic hypotension
primary (essential) hypertension

secondary hypertension
systemic vascular resistance (SVR)

Hypertension, or high blood pressure (BP), is one of the most important modifiable risk factors that can lead to the development of cardiovascular disease. As BP increases, so does the risk for myocardial infarction (MI), heart failure, stroke, and renal disease. This chapter discusses the nursing and interprofessional care of patients who are at risk for or who have hypertension.

NORMAL REGULATION OF BLOOD PRESSURE

Blood pressure (BP) is the force exerted by the blood against the walls of the blood vessel and must be adequate for tissue perfusion to be maintained during activity and rest. The maintenance of normal BP and tissue perfusion requires the integration of both systemic factors and local peripheral vascular effects. Arterial BP is primarily a function of cardiac output (CO) and systemic vascular resistance (SVR) (see Chapter 34). The relationship between the two is summarized by the following equation: arterial blood pressure = cardiac output multiplied by systemic vascular resistance (arterial BP = CO × SVR).

Cardiac output (CO) is the volume of blood ejected from the heart per minute. CO can be described as the stroke volume (SV, or the amount of blood pumped out of the left ventricle per beat [~70 mL]) multiplied by the heart rate (HR) for 1 minute. Systemic vascular resistance (SVR) is the force opposing the movement of blood within the blood vessels. The radius of the small arteries and arterioles is the principal factor determining vascular resistance. A small change in the radius of the arterioles creates a major change in the SVR. If SVR is increased and CO remains constant or increases, arterial BP will increase.

The mechanisms that regulate BP can affect either CO or SVR, or both. Regulation of BP is a complex process involving nervous, cardiovascular, renal, and endocrine functions (Figure 35.1). BP is regulated by both short-term (over seconds to hours) and long-term (over days to weeks) mechanisms. Short-term mechanisms, including the effects exerted by the sympathetic nervous system (SNS) and the vascular endothelium, are active within a few seconds. Long-term mechanisms include renal and hormonal processes that regulate arteriolar resistance and blood volume.

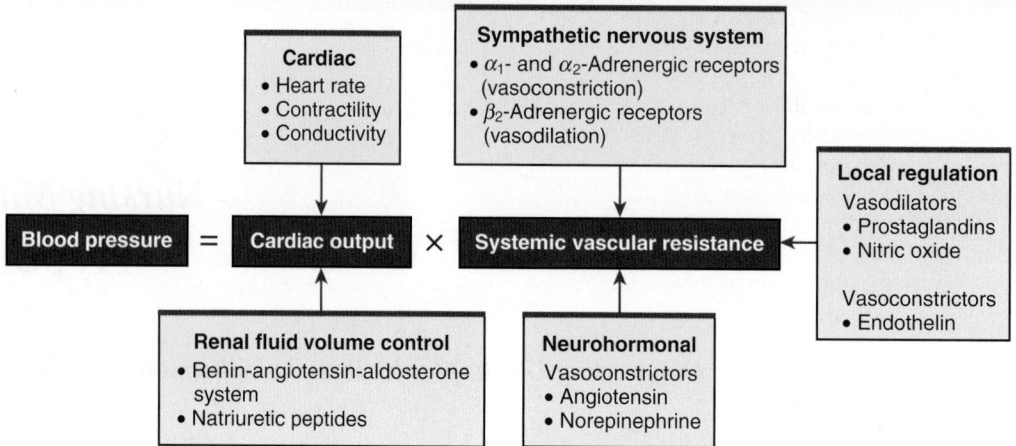

FIG. 35.1 Factors influencing blood pressure (BP). Hypertension develops when one or more of the BP-regulating mechanisms are defective.

Sympathetic Nervous System

The nervous system, which reacts within seconds after a decrease in arterial pressure, increases BP primarily by activation of the SNS. Increased SNS activity increases HR and cardiac contractility, produces widespread vasoconstriction in the peripheral arterioles, and promotes the release of renin from the kidneys. The net effect of SNS activation is to increase arterial pressure by increasing both CO and SVR.

Changes in BP are sensed by specialized nerve cells called *baroreceptors* and transmitted to the vasomotor centres in the brainstem. Information received in the brainstem is relayed throughout the brain by complex networks of interneurons that excite or inhibit efferent nerves, thereby influencing cardiovascular function. Sympathetic efferent nerves innervate cardiac and vascular smooth muscle cells. Under normal conditions, a low level of continuous sympathetic activity maintains tonic vasoconstriction. BP may be reduced by withdrawal of SNS activity or by stimulation of the parasympathetic nervous system, which decreases the HR (via the vagus nerve) and thereby decreases CO.

The neurotransmitter norepinephrine (NE) is released from sympathetic nerve endings. NE activates receptors located in the sinoatrial node, the myocardium, and vascular smooth muscle. The response to NE depends on the type and the density of receptors present. SNS receptors are classified as α_1, α_2, β_1, and β_2 (Table 35.1). α-Adrenergic receptors located in peripheral vasculature cause vasoconstriction when stimulated by NE. β_1-Adrenergic receptors in the heart respond to NE with increased HR (chronotropic effect), increased force of contraction (inotropic effect), and increased speed of conduction (dromotropic effect). Diminished responsiveness of cardiovascular cells to sympathetic stimulation is one of the most significant cardiovascular effects of aging. The smooth muscle of the blood vessels has β_1-adrenergic and β_2-adrenergic receptors. β_2-Adrenergic receptors are activated primarily by epinephrine released from the adrenal medulla and cause vasodilation.

The sympathetic vasomotor centre, located in the medulla, interacts with many areas of the brain to maintain normal BP under various conditions. During exercise, the motor area of the cortex is stimulated, activating the vasomotor centre and the SNS through neuronal connections. This causes an appropriate increase in BP to accommodate the increased oxygen demand

Adrenergic Receptor	Location	Response When Activated
α_1	Vascular smooth muscle	Vasoconstriction
	Heart	Increased contractility
α_2	Presynaptic membrane	Inhibition of norepinephrine release
	Vascular smooth muscle	Vasoconstriction
β_1	Heart	Increased contractility (positive inotropic effect)
		Increased heart rate (positive chronotropic effect)
		Increased conduction (positive dromotropic effect)
	Juxtaglomerular cells	Increased renin secretion
β_2	Smooth muscle of peripheral blood vessels in skeletal muscle, coronary arteries, lungs, kidneys, liver, islet cells, bladder, liver	Vasodilation Relaxation Gluconeogenesis Increase in secretion
Dopaminergic receptors	Primarily kidney and mesenteric blood vessels	Vasodilation

TABLE 35.1 SYMPATHETIC NERVOUS SYSTEM RECEPTORS INFLUENCING BLOOD PRESSURE

of the exercising muscles. During postural change from lying to standing, there is a transient decrease in BP. The vasomotor centre is stimulated and activates the SNS, causing peripheral vasoconstriction and increased venous return to the heart. If this response did not occur, there would be inadequate blood flow to the brain, resulting in dizziness. Cerebral cortical perceptions such as pain and stress activate the vasomotor centres through the neuronal connections.

Baroreceptors. Baroreceptors (pressoreceptors) are specialized nerve cells located in the carotid sinus at the bifurcation of the external and internal carotid arteries and the arch of the aorta. They are sensitive to stretching and, when stimulated by an increase in BP, send inhibitory impulses to the sympathetic vasomotor centre in the brainstem. Inhibition of sympathetic activity results in decreased HR, decreased force of contraction, and vasodilation in peripheral arterioles. Increased parasympathetic activity (vagus nerve) also reduces HR.

A fall in BP, sensed by the baroreceptors, leads to activation of the SNS. The result is constriction of the peripheral arterioles, increased HR, and increased contractility of the heart. The baroreceptors have an important role in the maintenance of BP stability during normal activities. In the presence of long-standing hypertension, the baroreceptors become adjusted to elevated levels of BP and recognize this level as "normal." Consequently, the long-term regulation of arterial pressure requires activation of other mechanisms (primarily hormonal and renal) to maintain normal BP. The baroreceptor reflex is less responsive in some older persons.

Vascular Endothelium

The vascular endothelium is a single cell layer that lines the blood vessels. Previously considered inert, it is now known to have the ability to produce vasoactive substances and growth factors. Nitric oxide, an endothelium-derived relaxing factor (EDRF), helps maintain low arterial tone at rest, inhibits growth of the smooth muscle layer, and inhibits platelet aggregation. Other substances released by the vascular endothelium with local vasodilator effects include prostacyclin and endothelium-derived hyperpolarizing factor.

Endothelin (ET), produced by the endothelial cells, is an extremely potent vasoconstrictor. There are three subclasses of ETs: ET-1, ET-2, and ET-3. ET-1 is the most potent ET in producing vasoconstriction. ET-1 also causes adhesion and aggregation of neutrophils and stimulates smooth muscle growth. Endothelial function and dysfunction is an area of ongoing investigation. There is some evidence that vascular endothelial dysfunction may contribute to atherosclerosis and primary hypertension. The prevention or reversal of endothelial dysfunction may become important for therapeutic interventions in the future.

Renal System

The kidneys contribute to BP regulation by controlling sodium excretion and extracellular fluid (ECF) volume (see Chapter 47). Sodium retention results in water retention, which causes an increased ECF volume. This increases the venous return to the heart, increasing the stroke volume, which elevates the BP through an increase in CO.

The renin–angiotensin–aldosterone system (RAAS) also plays an important role in BP regulation. In response to sympathetic stimulation, decreased blood flow through the kidneys, or decreased serum sodium concentration, renin is secreted from the juxtaglomerular apparatus in the kidney. Renin is an enzyme that converts angiotensinogen to angiotensin I. Angiotensin-converting enzyme (ACE) converts angiotensin I into angiotensin II (A-II), which can increase BP by two different mechanisms (see Chapter 47, Figure 47.6). First, A-II is a potent vasoconstrictor and increases vascular resistance, resulting in an immediate increase in BP. Second, over a period of hours or days, A-II increases BP indirectly by stimulating the adrenal cortex to secrete aldosterone, which causes sodium and water retention by the kidneys, resulting in increased blood volume and increased CO.

A-II also functions at a local level within the heart and the blood vessels. The local vasoactive effects of A-II (vasoconstriction and growth promotion) may contribute to atherosclerosis and primary hypertension.

Prostaglandins (PGs) E_2 (PGE$_2$) and I_2 (PGI$_2$), secreted by the renal medulla, have a vasodilator effect on the systemic circulation. This results in decreased SVR and lowering of BP. (PGs are discussed in Chapter 14.)

Endocrine System

Stimulation of the SNS results in release of epinephrine along with a small fraction of NE by the adrenal medulla. Epinephrine increases CO by increasing HR and myocardial contractility. Epinephrine activates β_2-adrenergic receptors in peripheral arterioles of skeletal muscle, causing vasodilation. In peripheral arterioles with only α_1-adrenergic receptors (skin and kidneys), epinephrine causes vasoconstriction.

The adrenal cortex is stimulated by A-II to release aldosterone. (Release of aldosterone is also regulated by other factors, such as low sodium levels [see Chapters 50 and 51].) Aldosterone stimulates the kidneys to retain sodium and, therefore, water. This increases BP by increasing CO.

An increased blood sodium osmolarity level stimulates the release of antidiuretic hormone (ADH) from the posterior pituitary gland. ADH increases the ECF volume by promoting the reabsorption of water in the distal and the collecting tubules of the kidneys. The resulting increase in blood volume can cause an elevation in BP.

In the healthy person, these regulatory mechanisms function in response to the demands of the body. When hypertension develops, one or more of the BP-regulating mechanisms are defective.

HYPERTENSION

Hypertension is sustained elevation of systemic arterial BP and is the leading cause for visits to primary care physicians (Nerenberg et al., 2018). *Hypertension* is defined as a systolic blood pressure (SBP) equal to or greater than 140 mm Hg or a diastolic blood pressure (DBP) equal to or greater than 90 mm Hg. The American Joint National Committee 7 (JNC-7) defines normal BP as an SBP less than 120 mm Hg and a DBP less than 80 mm Hg. Based on JNC-7, patients with sustained hypertension are further divided into stage 1 hypertension (SBP 140–159 or DBP 90–99 mm Hg) and stage 2 hypertension (SBP =160 or DBP =100 mm Hg). According to Diabetes Canada and Hypertension Canada, for persons diagnosed with hypertension and diabetes mellitus, target BPs for SBP should be less than or equal to 130 mm Hg and DBP should be less than or equal to 80 mm Hg (Tobe et al., 2018). This is the established level at which antihypertensive therapy is effective at decreasing cardiovascular morbidity and mortality. Canadian targets for BP are shown in Table 35.2.

High BP is the most significant modifiable risk factor for cardiovascular disease and mortality in Canada (Oparil et al., 2018). Globally, high BP remains a significant cardiovascular risk factor; in 2015 it affected 24.1% of men and 20.1% of women of the world's population ≥18 years of age (World Health Organization [WHO], 2021a). Even small incremental changes in systolic and diastolic pressures have a direct effect on mortality—for every 20-mm Hg increase in SBP to >115 mm Hg (or a 10-mm Hg increase in DBP to >75 mm Hg), the risk for cardiovascular mortality doubles (Padwal et al., 2015). Women with high BP have a greater risk of developing cardiovascular disease than women with normal BP (Heart and Stroke Foundation, 2018). Given the inequities in social determinants of health, Indigenous people have a significantly higher burden of cardiovascular disease than non-Indigenous people in Canada (Anand et al., 2019). Refer to Table 35.3 for statistics on hypertension in selected ethnic groups.

TABLE 35.2   TARGET VALUES FOR BLOOD PRESSURE*

Setting	Target (mmHg)
Out-of-Office Assessments (Home or Pharmacy)	
Home blood pressure and daytime ambulatory blood pressure measurement (ABPM)*	≤135/85
24-hour ambulatory blood pressure measurement	<130/80
Office	
Diastolic and/or systolic hypertension	<140/90
Isolated systolic hypertension	<140/90 (age <80)
	<150/90 (age >80)
Diabetes (with microalbuminuria, renal disease, cardiovascular disease, or additional cardiovascular risk factors)	<130/80
Nondiabetic chronic kidney disease	<140/90
Automated office oscillometric device	<130/80
Awake	<135/85
24-hr	<130/80

*Automated blood pressure method (preferred).
Source: Adapted from Rabi, D. M., McBrien, K. A., Sapir-Pichhadze, R., et al. (2020). Hypertension Canada's 2020 comprehensive guidelines for the prevention, diagnosis, risk assessment, and treatment of hypertension in adults and children. *Canadian Journal of Cardiology*, 36(5), 596–624.

DETERMINANTS OF HEALTH

Hypertension

Ethnicity: Education and Literacy

- 50% of all Canadians are not aware of the impact of hypertension on kidneys, of the need to adhere to antihypertensive medication, and that hypertension is a chronic condition.
- Chinese Canadians are less aware than other Canadians of the relationship between hypertension and heart attacks; Canadians originating from India are less knowledgeable than other Canadians of the association between hypertension and weight.
- Hypertension education needs to be promoted in populations of people from all ethnic backgrounds and should target individuals of lower socioeconomic status.
- Educational materials need to be available in multiple languages and use multimodal delivery (e.g., television, radio, brochures).

Source: Cunningham, C. T., Sykes, L. L., Metcalfe, A., et al. (2014). Ethnicity and health literacy: A survey on hypertension knowledge among Canadian ethnic populations. *Ethnicity & Disease*, 24(3), 276–282.

According to the Canadian Health Measures Survey (CHMS), approximately 24% of males and 23% of females aged 20 to 79 years have hypertension (DeGuire et al., 2019). Twenty-five percent of adult Canadians are affected by hypertension, which is also a major risk factor for cardiovascular disease, chronic kidney disease, and death (Nerenberg et al., 2018). However, since 2000, there has been a decline in the incidence of hypertension among the Canadian population, largely due to early diagnosis and treatment of at-risk individuals. This decline has contributed to a decrease in the number of people living with ischemic heart disease, heart failure, and all-cause mortality (Public Health Agency of Canada, 2018). Consequently, new recommendations appeared in the 2018 Hypertension Canada guidelines (formerly the Canadian Hypertension Education Program [CHEP] guidelines).

Globally, 40% of the world's population older than 25 years of age is affected by hypertension and it is a leading risk factor for death (Schiffrin et al., 2016). The World Health Organization

(WHO) (2021b) identified hypertension as a silent killer requiring increased global public awareness necessary for early detection. Canada has increased awareness and treatment of hypertension through implementation of community-based programs with a focus on primary prevention (Schiffrin et al., 2016). Large-scale education programs, such as the Hypertension Canada and Heart and Stroke Foundation, have increased people's awareness of hypertension.

Adults with high-normal BP (also called *prehypertension*) require annual BP assessment. Health care providers who have been specifically trained to measure BP accurately should assess BP in all adult patients, at all appropriate visits, to determine cardiovascular risk and monitor antihypertensive treatment. Home measurement of BP has been recommended since the 2008 CHEP guidelines to encourage patient self-efficacy and is consistent with the 2020 Hypertension Canada guidelines (Rabi et al., 2020). Out-of-office BP readings, including ambulatory and home readings, are recommended by Hypertension Canada to identify higher BP readings, prompting patients to seek treatment and earlier diagnosis (Rabi et al., 2020). Patient instructions for purchasing and using home BP measurement devices are available at both the Hypertension Canada and the Heart and Stroke Foundation of Canada websites. A comprehensive instructional video on home measurement of BP was developed in 2009 and can be viewed at the Hypertension Canada website (see the Resources at the end of this chapter).

The recommendations for diagnosis of hypertension and follow-up are shown in Figure 35.2. It should be emphasized that, when using BPs recorded during office visits to diagnose hypertension, the thresholds given refer to readings averaged over a specified range of visits and are not one-time measurements from the last visit.

Subtypes of Hypertension

Isolated systolic hypertension (ISH) is defined as a sustained elevation in SBP equal to or greater than 140 mm Hg with a DBP less than 90 mm Hg. (A one-time isolated reading of increased SBP is not classified as ISH.) Arterial BP increases with advancing age.

An increase of the SBP without an increase of the DBP, as occurs in ISH, increases the pulse pressure. The *pulse pressure* is the difference between the SBP and the DBP. Loss of elasticity of the large arteries contributes to this widening of the pulse pressure. Once considered to be harmless, a high pulse pressure is now considered an independent risk factor for cardiovascular disease and end-organ damage. ISH is associated with a two- to four-fold increased future risk for cardiomegaly, MI, or stroke. There is compelling evidence that treatment of ISH with a reduction in the SBP of 20 to 30 mm Hg results in significant cardiovascular benefits. Figure 35.3 presents the treatment algorithm for ISH.

Etiology

Hypertension can be classified etiologically as either primary or secondary.

Primary Hypertension. **Primary (essential) hypertension** is elevated BP and accounts for the majority of all cases of hypertension. Although the exact cause of primary hypertension has not been identified, it is considered to be a complex interaction between genes and the environment (Manosroi & Williams, 2019). Several contributing factors, including increased SNS activity, overproduction of sodium-retaining hormones and

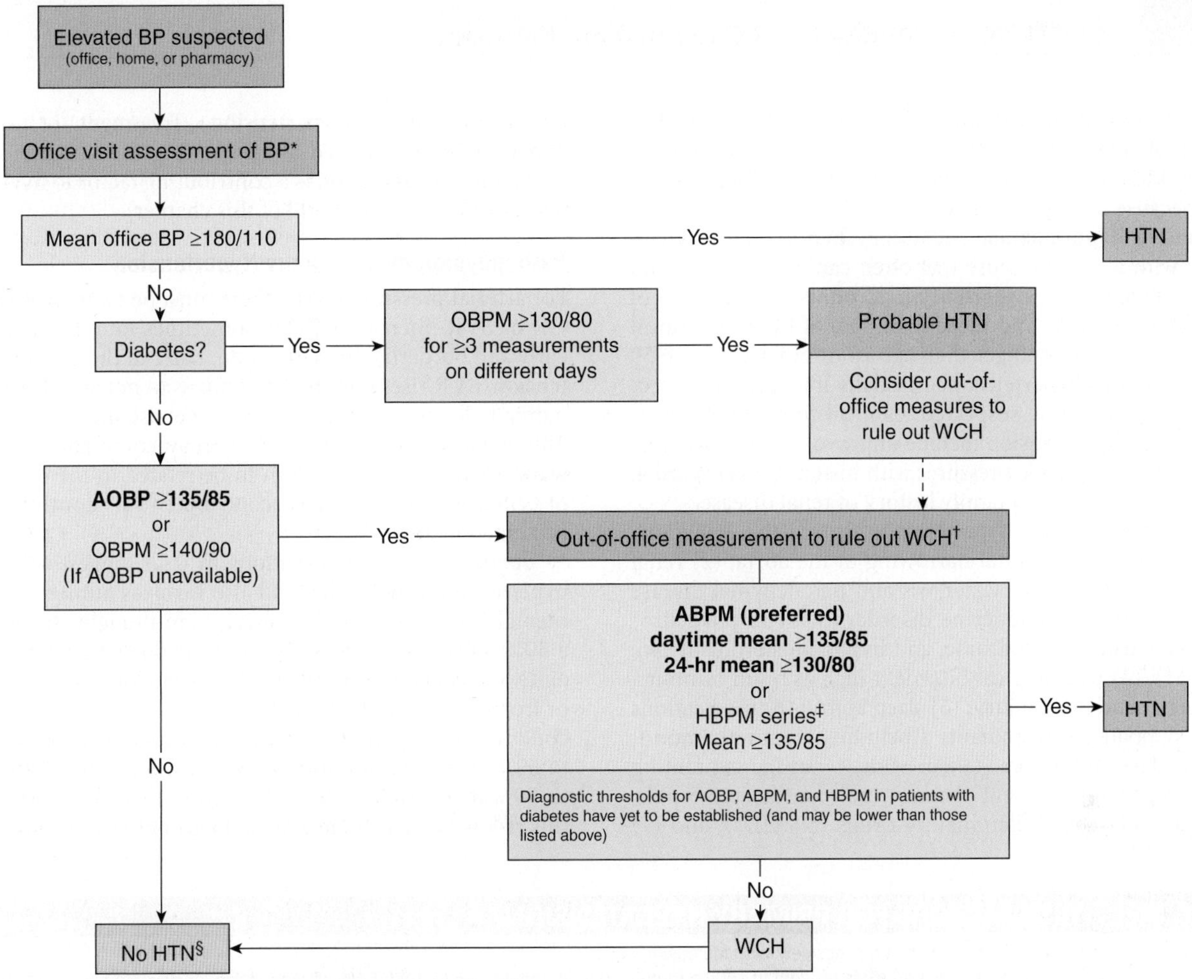

FIG. 35.2 Diagnosis flowchart

Elevated BP suspected (office, home, or pharmacy)

↓

Office visit assessment of BP*

↓

Mean office BP ≥180/110 — Yes → **HTN**

↓ No

Diabetes? — Yes → **OBPM ≥130/80 for ≥3 measurements on different days** — Yes → **Probable HTN** — Consider out-of-office measures to rule out WCH

↓ No

AOBP ≥135/85 or OBPM ≥140/90 (If AOBP unavailable) — Yes → **Out-of-office measurement to rule out WCH†**

ABPM (preferred) daytime mean ≥135/85 24-hr mean ≥130/80 or HBPM series‡ Mean ≥135/85 — Yes → **HTN**

Diagnostic thresholds for AOBP, ABPM, and HBPM in patients with diabetes have yet to be established (and may be lower than those listed above)

↓ No → **WCH**

↓ No (from AOBP box)

No HTN§ ← WCH

FIG. 35.2 Criteria for the diagnosis of hypertension and recommendations for follow-up. The thresholds shown here are blood pressure (BP) values that are averaged across the corresponding number of visits and are not one-time measurements taken at the most recent office visit. All BP measurements are in millimetres of mercury. *ABPM,* ambulatory blood pressure monitoring; *AOBP,* automated office blood pressure; *BPM,* blood pressure monitoring; *HBPM,* home blood pressure monitoring; *HTN,* hypertension; *OBPM,* office blood pressure measurement; *WCH,* white coat hypertension.
*If AOBP is used, use the mean calculated and displayed by the device. If OBPM is used, take at least three readings, discard the first, and calculate the mean of the remaining measurements. A history and physical exam should be performed and diagnostic tests ordered.
†Serial office measurements over three to five visits can be used if ABPM or HBPM are not available.
‡Home BP series: Two readings taken each morning and evening for 7 days (28 total). Discard first-day readings and average the last 6 days.
§In a patient with suspected masked hypertension, ABPM or HBPM could be considered to rule out masked hypertension.
Source: Rabi, D. M., McBrien, K. A., Sapir-Pichhadze, R., et al. (2020). Hypertension Canada's 2020 comprehensive guidelines for the prevention, diagnosis, risk assessment, and treatment of hypertension in adults and children. *Canadian Journal of Cardiology, 36*(5), 596–624. https://doi.org/10.1016/j.cjca.2020.02.086

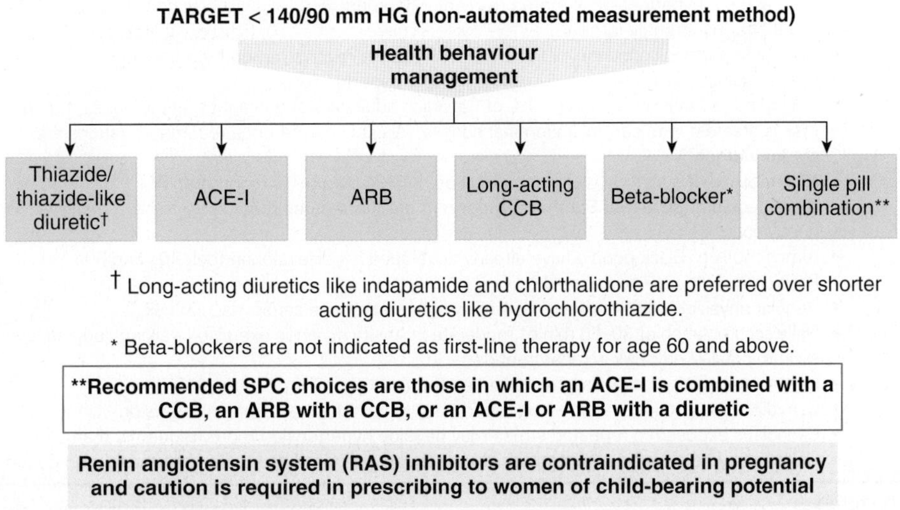

TARGET < 140/90 mm HG (non-automated measurement method)

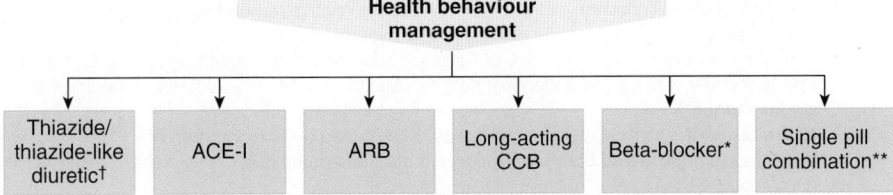

Health behaviour management

| Thiazide/ thiazide-like diuretic† | ACE-I | ARB | Long-acting CCB | Beta-blocker* | Single pill combination** |

† Long-acting diuretics like indapamide and chlorthalidone are preferred over shorter acting diuretics like hydrochlorothiazide.

* Beta-blockers are not indicated as first-line therapy for age 60 and above.

**Recommended SPC choices are those in which an ACE-I is combined with a CCB, an ARB with a CCB, or an ACE-I or ARB with a diuretic

Renin angiotensin system (RAS) inhibitors are contraindicated in pregnancy and caution is required in prescribing to women of child-bearing potential

FIG. 35.3 Treatment of systolic/diastolic hypertension (HTN) without other compelling indications. *ACE-I,* angiotensin-converting enzyme inhibitor; *ARB,* angiotensin II receptor blocker; *CCB,* calcium channel blocker; *SPC,* single pill combination. Source: Hypertension Canada. (2020). *2020 Hypertension highlights.* https://hypertension.ca/wp-content/upl oads/2018/07/Hypertension-Guidelines-English-2018-Web.pdf vasoconstrictors, increased sodium intake, greater-than-ideal body weight, diabetes mellitus, and excessive alcohol intake, have been identified. Primary hypertension is the focus of this chapter because of its prevalence in clinical practice.

Secondary Hypertension. Secondary hypertension is elevated BP with a specific cause that often can be identified and corrected. This type of hypertension accounts for 5 to 10% of hypertension in adults and more than 80% of hypertension in children. If a person younger than age 20 or older than age 50 suddenly develops hypertension, especially if it is severe, a secondary cause should be suspected. Clinical findings that suggest secondary hypertension include unprovoked hypokalemia, abdominal bruit, variable pressures with history of tachycardia, sweating, and tremor, or a family history of renal disease.

Causes of secondary hypertension include the following: (1) coarctation or congenital narrowing of the aorta; (2) renal disease such as renal artery stenosis and parenchymal disease (see Chapter 48); (3) endocrine disorders such as pheochromocytoma, Cushing's syndrome, and hyperaldosteronism (see Chapter 51); (4) neurological disorders such as brain tumours, quadriplegia, and head injury; (5) sleep apnea; (6) medications such as sympathetic stimulants (including cocaine), monoamine oxidase inhibitors taken with tyramine-containing foods, estrogen replacement therapy, oral contraceptive pills, and nonsteroidal anti-inflammatory drugs (NSAIDs); and (7) pregnancy-induced hypertension. Treatment of secondary hypertension is directed at eliminating the underlying cause. Secondary hypertension is a contributing factor to hypertensive urgency (see section at end of this chapter).

Pathophysiology of Primary Hypertension

For arterial pressure to rise, there must be an increase in either CO or SVR. Increased CO is sometimes found in people with early and borderline hypertension. Later in the course of hypertension, SVR rises and the CO returns to normal. The hemodynamic hallmark of hypertension is persistently increased SVR. This persistent elevation in SVR may come about in various ways. Factors that are known to be related to the development of primary hypertension or contribute to its consequences are presented in Table 35.3.

Genes. Genetic observations to date suggest that primary hypertension is polygenic and also involves numerous environmental influences. Genetic factors are thought to account for a 30 to 60% variability in BP in individuals (Patel et al., 2017) and vary depending on the study population, from 15 to 20% or from 65 to 70%. Familial heritability is a significant factor. A child with both parents and a sibling with hypertension has a 40 to 60% chance of developing hypertension. This risk increases to 80% if the child is a monozygotic twin. It is unlikely that this risk is from a single genetic locus but rather from multiple

TABLE 35.3   RISK FACTORS FOR PRIMARY HYPERTENSION

Advancing age	• BP rises progressively with increasing age. • Elevated BP is present in approximately 50% of people >65 yr, with 90% of the remainder developing hypertension during their lifespan.
Heavy alcohol consumption	• Excessive alcohol intake is strongly linked to hypertension. • Canadians with hypertension should limit their daily intake to 30 mL of alcohol.
Cigarette smoking	• The incidence of hypertension is increased among those who smoke ≥15 cigarettes/day. • Canadians with hypertension and who smoke have a greater risk for secondary cardiovascular disease.
Glucose intolerance (diabetes mellitus)	• Hypertension is diagnosed three times more often in individuals diagnosed with diabetes. • When hypertension and diabetes coexist, hypertension augments the already raised risk for cardiovascular diseases and worsens outcomes.
Elevated serum lipids	• Elevated levels of cholesterol and triglycerides are primary risk factors in atherosclerosis. • Hyperlipidemia is more common in Canadians with hypertension.
High dietary sodium intake	• High sodium intake can contribute to hypertension in some patients and can decrease the efficacy of certain antihypertensive medications. • For prevention of hypertension, the daily recommended dietary sodium intake is 1 500 mg for adults ages 14–50 yr of age, 1 300 mg for adults ages 50–70 yr, and 1 200 mg for adults >70 yr.
Gender	• In young adulthood and early middle age, hypertension is more prevalent in men. • After age 55, hypertension is more prevalent in women.
Family history	• Level of BP is strongly familial. • Risk for hypertension increases for those with a close relative having hypertension.
Obesity	• Weight gain is associated with increased risk for hypertension. • According to Statistics Canada, 59% of Canadian adults are at a weight that increases their risk for hypertension. • Risk is greatest with central abdominal obesity. Waist circumference recommendations are <102 cm for men and <88 cm for women.* • Maintenance of a healthy weight and BMI of 18.5–24.9 kg/m² is recommended.*
Ethnicity	• Black people or people of South Asian descent are three times more likely to have hypertension than the general population. • Almost 50% of Black people have already developed hypertension in their 40s and 50s.
Sedentary lifestyle	• Physical activity may decrease BP. • Regular physical activity can help control weight and reduce cardiovascular risk. • Daily accumulation of 30–60 min of moderate-intensity dynamic exercise (walking, jogging, cycling, or noncompetitive swimming) 4–7 days/wk is recommended. • Higher intensities of exercise are no more effective.
Socioeconomic status	• Canadians living in low-income neighbourhoods have higher rates of hypertension.
Psychosocial stress	• Canadians exposed to repeated stress may develop hypertension more frequently than others. • Canadians who develop hypertension may respond differently to stress from those who do not.

BP, blood pressure; *BMI*, body mass index.

*Leung, A. A., Daskalopoulou, S. S., Dasgupta, K., et al. (2017). Hypertension Canada's 2017 guidelines for diagnosis, risk assessment, prevention, and treatment of hypertension in adults. *Canadian Journal of Cardiology, 33*(5), 557–576. https://doi.org/10.1016/j.cjca.2017.03.005

genes. Similarities across populations have not been established; ongoing research is needed in the area of genetic susceptibility to hypertension.

Sodium and Water Retention. Excessive dietary intake of sodium is the most studied environmental factor and is strongly linked to the initiation of hypertension in some people. Studies of populations with a low sodium intake (usually primitive hunter–gatherer societies) show little or no hypertension and no progressive increase in BP with age as is found in industrialized societies. In addition, the prevalence of hypertension increases when people from these societies adopt industrialized lifestyles. In many people with hypertension, when sodium is restricted, their BP falls. A high sodium intake may alter the pressure–natriuresis relationship and cause water retention. Although almost everyone in Western countries consumes a high-sodium diet, only about 20% develop hypertension. This indicates that some degree of sodium sensitivity must be present for high sodium intake to trigger the development of hypertension.

Altered Renin–Angiotensin–Aldosterone Mechanism. The RAAS is a significant mechanism in the regulation of blood volume and pressure. Its role in hypertension is complex. High plasma renin activity (PRA) results in the increased conversion of angiotensinogen to angiotensin I (see Chapter 47, Figure 47.6). A-II causes direct arteriolar constriction, promotes vascular hypertrophy, and induces aldosterone secretion. Thus, altered renin–angiotensin mechanisms may contribute to the development and maintenance of hypertension. However, only about 20% of patients with primary hypertension have high PRA.

Stress and Increased Sympathetic Nervous System Activity. The SNS also plays a critical role in BP control. It has long been recognized that arterial pressure is influenced by factors such as anger, fear, and pain. Physiological responses to stress, which are normally protective, may persist to a pathological degree, resulting in prolonged increase in SNS activity. Increased sympathetic stimulation produces increased vasoconstriction, increased HR, and increased renin release. Increased renin activates the angiotensin mechanism and increases aldosterone secretion, both leading to elevated BP. People exposed to high levels of repeated psychological stress develop hypertension to a greater extent than those who do not experience as much stress.

Insulin Resistance and Hyperinsulinemia. Abnormalities of glucose, insulin, and lipoprotein metabolism are common in primary hypertension. Insulin resistance is present in 50% of patients with primary hypertension; a strong genetic component is associated with hyperinsulinemia-associated hypertension. Insulin resistance is associated with endothelial dysfunction. High insulin concentration in the blood stimulates SNS and RAAS activity and impairs nitric oxide–mediated vasodilation. Additional pressor effects of insulin include vascular hypertrophy and increased renal sodium reabsorption.

Endothelial Cell Dysfunction. Vascular endothelial cells are known to be a source of multiple vasoactive substances such as nitric oxide and ET. Some people with hypertension have a reduced vasodilator response to nitric oxide. ET produces pronounced and prolonged vasoconstriction. The role of endothelial dysfunction in the pathogenesis and treatment of hypertension is an area of ongoing investigation.

Obesity. Obesity is a well-known risk factor for hypertension. Hypertension and central (visceral) obesity are major components of cardiometabolic syndrome. The relationship between hypertension and obesity is multifaceted; the etiology is complex, and it is not well elucidated. Several hormone abnormalities associated with obesity are linked to the development of hypertension. Enlarged adipocytes or fat cells secrete leptin, proinflammatory cytokines, and reactive oxygen species. This dysfunctional adipose tissue may induce activation of the SNS and RAAS.

Clinical Manifestations

Hypertension is a lanthanic, or silent, disease because it is frequently asymptomatic until it becomes severe and target-organ disease has occurred. A patient with severe hypertension may experience a variety of symptoms secondary to effects on blood vessels in the various organs and tissues or to the increased workload of the heart. These secondary symptoms include fatigue, reduced activity tolerance, dizziness, palpitations, angina, and dyspnea. In the past, symptoms of hypertension were thought to include headache, nosebleeds, and dizziness. However, unless BP is extremely high or low, these symptoms are not more frequent in people with hypertension than in the general population.

Complications

The most common complications of hypertension are *target-organ diseases* (Table 35.4) occurring in the heart (hypertensive heart disease), the brain (cerebrovascular disease), the

TABLE 35.4 PATHOLOGICAL EFFECTS OF SUSTAINED, COMPLICATED PRIMARY HYPERTENSION

Site of Injury	Mechanism of Injury	Potential Pathological Effect
Heart		
• Myocardium	Increased workload combined with diminished blood flow through coronary arteries	Left ventricular hypertrophy, myocardial ischemia, left heart failure
• Coronary arteries	Accelerated atherosclerosis (coronary artery disease)	Myocardial ischemia, myocardial infarction, sudden death
Aorta	Weakened vessel wall	Aneurysms, acute aortic syndromes
Kidneys	Renin and aldosterone secretion stimulated by reduced blood flow	Retention of sodium and water, leading to increased blood volume and perpetuation of hypertension
	Inflammation and ischemia	Tissue damage that compromises filtration
	High pressures in renal arterioles	Nephrosclerosis leading to renal failure
Brain	Reduced blood flow and oxygen supply; weakened vessel walls, accelerated atherosclerosis	Transient ischemic attack, cerebral thrombosis, aneurysm, hemorrhage, acute brain infarction
Eyes (retinas)	Reduced blood flow High arteriolar pressure	Retinal vascular sclerosis Exudation, hemorrhage
Arterial vessels of lower extremities	Reduced blood flow and high pressures in arterioles, accelerated atherosclerosis	Intermittent claudication, arterial thrombosis, gangrene

Source: McCance, K. L., & Huether, S. E. (2014). *Pathophysiology: The biologic basis for disease in adults and children.* (7th ed., p. 1138). Mosby.

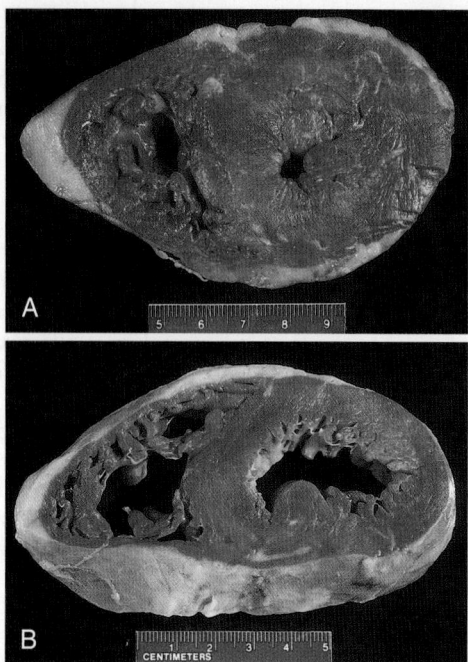

FIG. 35.4 **A,** Massively enlarged heart caused by hypertrophy of the muscle in the left ventricle. **B,** Compare with the thickness of the normal left ventricle. The patient suffered from severe hypertension. Source: Kumar, V., Cotran, R. S., & Robbins, S. L. (2007). *Robbins basic pathology* (8th ed.). Saunders.

peripheral vasculature (peripheral arterial disease), the kidneys (nephrosclerosis), and the eyes (retinal damage).

Hypertensive Heart Disease

Coronary Artery Disease. Hypertension is an established major risk factor for coronary artery disease, almost doubling the risk. The mechanisms by which hypertension contributes to the development of atherosclerosis are multifactorial. The shear stress (response-to-injury hypothesis of atherogenesis) results in endothelial dysfunction, causing impairment in the synthesis and release of the potent vasodilator, nitric oxide. A decreased nitric oxide level promotes the development and acceleration of atherosclerosis and plaque formation.

The intimal layer is exposed to activated white blood cells and platelets. Growth factors released by the vascular endothelium and platelets may induce smooth muscle proliferation within the lesion. These arteriolar changes may account for a high incidence of coronary artery disease and the resulting conditions of angina and MI.

Left Ventricular Hypertrophy. Sustained high BP increases the cardiac workload and produces left ventricular hypertrophy (LVH) (Figure 35.4). The risk for LVH doubles with associated obesity. Initially, LVH is an adaptive or compensatory mechanism that strengthens cardiac contraction and increases CO. However, increased contractility increases myocardial work and oxygen consumption. When the heart can no longer meet the demands for myocardial oxygen, heart failure develops. Progressive LVH, especially in association with coronary artery disease, is associated with the development of heart failure.

Heart Failure. Heart failure is a common complication of a chronically elevated BP and occurs when the heart's compensatory adaptations are overwhelmed and the heart can no longer pump enough blood to meet the metabolic needs of the body (see Chapter 37). Contractility is depressed, and SV and CO are decreased. The patient may complain of shortness of breath on exertion, paroxysmal nocturnal dyspnea, and fatigue. Signs of an enlarged heart may be present on a radiograph, and an electrocardiogram (ECG) may show electrical changes indicative of LVH.

Cerebrovascular Disease. Atherosclerosis is the most common cause of cerebrovascular disease. Hypertension is a major risk factor for cerebral atherosclerosis and stroke. Even in people with mild hypertension, the risk for stroke is four times higher than in people with normal BP. Adequate control of BP effectively diminishes the risk for stroke.

Atherosclerotic plaques are commonly distributed at the bifurcation of the common carotid artery into the internal and external carotid arteries. Portions of the atherosclerotic plaque, or the blood clot that forms on the plaque, may break off and travel to intracerebral vessels, producing a thromboembolism. The patient may experience transient ischemic attacks or a stroke. (These conditions are discussed in Chapter 60.)

Hypertensive encephalopathy may occur after a marked rise in BP if the cerebral blood flow is not decreased by autoregulation. *Autoregulation* is a physiological process that maintains constant cerebral blood flow despite fluctuations in arterial BP. Normally, as pressure in the cerebral blood vessels rises, the vessels constrict to maintain constant flow. When arterial BP exceeds the body's ability to autoregulate, the cerebral vessels suddenly dilate and cerebral edema develops, producing a rise in intracranial pressure. If left untreated, patients die quickly from brain damage. (Cerebral blood flow and autoregulation are discussed in Chapter 59.)

Peripheral Arterial Disease. As it does with other vessels, hypertension speeds up the process of atherosclerosis in the peripheral arterial blood vessels, leading to the development of aortic aneurysm, aortic dissection, and peripheral arterial disease (see Chapter 40). *Intermittent claudication* (ischemic muscle pain precipitated by activity and relieved with rest) is a classic symptom of peripheral arterial disease.

Nephrosclerosis. Hypertension is one of the leading causes of end-stage renal disease (ESRD). Some degree of kidney dysfunction is usually present in the patient with hypertension, even one with a minimally elevated BP. One of the earliest markers of nephropathy is microalbuminuria, the presence of protein in the urine. Kidney dysfunction is the direct result of ischemia caused by the narrowed lumen of the intrarenal blood vessels. Gradual narrowing of the arteries and arterioles leads to atrophy of the tubules, destruction of the glomeruli, and eventual death of nephrons. Initially intact nephrons can compensate, but these changes may eventually lead to renal failure. Common laboratory indications of kidney dysfunction are microalbuminuria, macroalbuminuria, elevated blood urea nitrogen (BUN), serum creatinine levels, and microscopic hematuria.

Retinal Damage. The appearance of the retina provides important information about how severe and long-standing the hypertensive process has been. The retina is the only place in the body where the blood vessels can be directly visualized. Damage seen to have occurred to retinal vessels thus provides an indication of vessel damage in the heart, the brain, and the kidneys. An ophthalmoscope is used to visualize the blood vessels of the eye. Manifestations of severe retinal damage include blurring of vision, retinal hemorrhage, and loss of vision.

Diagnostic Studies

The diagnosis of hypertension is not based on a single elevated reading (if <80/110 mm Hg) but requires several elevated

TABLE 35.5 INTERPROFESSIONAL CARE

Hypertension

Diagnosis
- History and physical examination
- Routine laboratory tests should be performed for the investigation of all patients with hypertension, including the following:
  - Urinalysis
  - Blood chemistry (potassium, sodium, creatinine, blood urea and nitrogen)
  - Fasting blood glucose
  - Fasting total cholesterol and high-density lipoprotein cholesterol, low-density lipoprotein cholesterol, and triglycerides
  - Standard 12-lead electrocardiography
- Assess urinary albumin excretion in patients with diabetes
- All patients with treated hypertension need to be monitored for the appearance of diabetes, according to the Canadian Diabetes Association (CDA) guidelines (Canadian Diabetes Association Clinical Practice Guidelines Expert Committee, 2013).

Interprofessional Therapy
- Periodic monitoring of BP
- Home BP monitoring
- Ambulatory BP monitoring
- Every 3–6 mo once BP is stabilized
- Nutritional therapy (see Table 35.7)
- Restricted sodium intake (reduce to 2 000 mg per day)*
- Restricted intake of cholesterol and saturated fats
- Maintenance of adequate intake of potassium
- Maintenance of adequate intake of calcium and magnesium
- Weight management
- Regular, moderate physical activity
- Tobacco cessation
- Moderation in alcohol consumption
- Antihypertensive medications (see Table 35.8)
- Patient and caregiver teaching

BP, blood pressure.
*Leung, A. A., Daskalopoulou, S. S., Dasgupta, K., et al. (2017). Hypertension Canada's 2017 guidelines for diagnosis, risk assessment, prevention, and treatment of hypertension in adults. *Canadian Journal of Cardiology, 33*(5), 557–576. https://doi.org/10.1016/j.cjca.2017.03.005
NOTE: During the maintenance phase of hypertension management, tests (including those for electrolytes, creatinine, and fasting lipids) should be repeated with a frequency reflecting the clinical situation.

readings over several weeks (see Figure 35.2). (Measurement of BP is discussed in Chapter 34.)

Table 35.5 provides a list of basic laboratory studies that are performed in a person with sustained hypertension. Routine urinalysis and serum creatinine levels are used to screen for kidney involvement and to provide baseline information about kidney function. (Serum creatinine is discussed in Chapters 47 and 49.)

Measurement of serum electrolytes, especially potassium levels, is important to detect hyperaldosteronism, a cause of secondary hypertension. Blood glucose levels should be assessed to assist in the diagnosis of diabetes mellitus. Serum cholesterol and triglyceride levels provide information about additional risk factors that predispose to atherosclerosis. An ECG provides baseline information about the cardiac status. It is helpful in identifying the presence of LVH and myocardial ischemia. If the patient's age, history, physical examination findings, or severity of hypertension points to a secondary cause, further diagnostic tests may be indicated.

Ambulatory Blood Pressure Monitoring. Twenty-four–hour ambulatory BP readings are useful in the diagnosis of uncomplicated mild-to-moderate hypertension and are more accurate in predicting cardiovascular risk than office BP. This method of measuring BP is incorporated into the Hypertension Canada diagnostic algorithm to facilitate more rapid diagnosis of hypertension and reduce the risk of patients being left untreated for long periods of time while a diagnosis is being made over numerous office visits.

A fully automated system that measures BP at preset intervals over a 24-hour period is used. The equipment includes a BP cuff and a small microprocessing unit that fits into a pouch worn on a shoulder strap or belt. Patients are asked to maintain a diary of activities that may affect BP. This procedure may be helpful in patients with suspected white coat hypertension, masked hypertension, apparent medication resistance, hypotensive symptoms with hypertensive medications, episodic hypertension, or autonomic nervous system dysfunction.

Some patients have elevated BP readings in a clinical setting and normal readings when BP is measured elsewhere. This phenomenon is referred to as *white coat hypertension*. Other patients have normal BP in the office and elevated BP at home. This condition is called *masked hypertension*.

As with most physiological phenomena, BP demonstrates diurnal variability, expressed as sleep–wakefulness difference. For day-active people, BP is highest in the early morning, decreases during the day, and is lowest at night. Some patients with hypertension do not show a normal, nocturnal fall in BP—they are called "nondippers." A decrease in nocturnal BP of less than 10% is associated with increased risk for cardiovascular events. The presence or absence of diurnal variability can be determined by continuous ambulatory BP monitoring.

Canadians with hypertension should be encouraged to use an approved BP-measuring device and use proper technique to assess BP at home. BP measured at home is a stronger predictor of cardiovascular events than office-based readings. Home measurement can help to confirm the diagnosis of hypertension, improve BP control, reduce the need for medications, help to identify white coat and masked hypertension, and improve medication adherence in nonadherent patients. An Internet-based toolbox to assist patient self-management for home BP measurement and lifestyle change can be found at the Heart and Stroke Foundation of Canada's website.

Canadian adults with high-normal BP require annual BP assessment. All Canadian adults need to have BP assessed at all appropriate clinical visits. One in five adult Canadians has hypertension, and for those age 55 with normal BP, 90% will develop hypertension if they live to an average age. Thus all adults require ongoing assessment of BP throughout their lives.

Interprofessional Care

Since the establishment of CHEP in 1999, evidence-informed recommendations for the management of hypertension have been updated annually. In 2011, CHEP joined with Hypertension Canada and Blood Pressure Canada with the goal of providing a stronger, united approach to the prevention and control of hypertension. Each year, new evidence is reviewed and integrated into previous evidence-informed guidelines to develop new guidelines (now known as Hypertension Canada guidelines), where appropriate. In order for health care providers to remain informed of updates, the guidelines and other hypertension resources are available at the Hypertension Canada website.

TABLE 35.6 ASSESSMENT OF OVERALL CARDIOVASCULAR RISK

Search for Target-Organ Damage
- Cerebrovascular disease
  - Stroke
    - Ischemic stroke and transient ischemic attack
    - Intracerebral hemorrhage
    - Aneurysmal subarachnoid hemorrhage
  - Dementia
    - Vascular dementia
    - Mixed vascular dementia and dementia of the Alzheimer's type
- Hypertensive retinopathy
- Left ventricular dysfunction
- Left ventricular hypertrophy
- Coronary artery disease
  - Myocardial infarction
  - Angina pectoris
- Heart failure
- Renal disease
  - Chronic kidney disease (GFR <60 mL/min/1.73 m²)
  - Albuminuria
- Peripheral artery disease
  - Intermittent claudication

Search for Key Cardiovascular Risk Factors for Atherosclerosis
Nonmodifiable
- Age ≥55 yr
- Male
- Family history of premature cardiovascular disease (<55 yr in men and <65 yr in women)

Modifiable
- Sedentary lifestyle
- Poor dietary habits
- Abdominal obesity
- Diabetes mellitus
- Smoking
- Dyslipidemia
- Stress
- Nonadherence

Search for Exogenous, Potentially Modifiable Factors That Can Induce or Aggravate Hypertension
- Prescription medications
  - NSAIDs, including "coxibs"
  - Corticosteroids and anabolic steroids
  - Oral contraceptives and sex hormones
  - Vasoconstricting/ sympathomimetic decongestants
  - Calcineurin inhibitors (cyclosporin, tacrolimus)
  - Erythropoietin and analogues
  - Antidepressants: MAOIs, SNRIs, SSRIs
  - Midodrine
- Other
  - Licorice root
  - Stimulants, including cocaine
  - Salt
  - Excessive alcohol use

GFR, glomerular filtration rate; *MAOIs*, monoamine oxidase inhibitors; *NSAIDs*, nonsteroidal anti-inflammatory drugs; *SNRIs*, serotonin–norepinephrine reuptake inhibitors; *SSRIs*, selective serotonin reuptake inhibitors.
Source: Adapted from Leung, A. A., Daskalopoulou, S. S., Dasgupta, K., et al. (2017). Hypertension Canada's 2017 guidelines for diagnosis, risk assessment, prevention, and treatment of hypertension in adults. *Canadian Journal of Cardiology, 33*(5), 557–576 (Supplemental tables). https://doi.org/10.1016/j.cjca.2017.03.005. Reprinted with permission.

Risk Stratification. The risk for cardiovascular disease in people with hypertension is determined by the level of BP; the presence of target-organ damage; risk factors such as diabetes, dyslipidemia, smoking, and obesity; and other exogenous, potentially modifiable factors that can induce or aggravate hypertension (Table 35.6). Over 90% of Canadians with hypertension have other cardiovascular risks. Hypertension Canada guidelines recommend that global cardiovascular risk be assessed in all patients. Simply counting risk factors may lead to underestimating risk.

Follow-up monitoring of BP is important. The frequency of monitoring varies initially with the level of BP. After the BP has stabilized, follow-up visits should be scheduled every 3 to 6 months to ensure continued control of BP, provide support for lifestyle changes, assess for target-organ damage, and detect adverse effects of medications.

Lifestyle Modifications. All patients with hypertension should use lifestyle modifications as either definitive or adjunctive therapy. Lifestyle modifications are directed toward reducing BP and overall cardiovascular risk factors. Modifications include (1) dietary changes, including reduced sodium intake, (2) limitation of alcohol intake, (3) regular physical activity, (4) avoidance of tobacco use (smoking and chewing), (5) stress management, and (6) weight reduction (see Figure 35.3).

Nutritional Therapy. Hypertension Canada and the Heart and Stroke Foundation of Canada recommend consumption of the Dietary Approaches to Stop Hypertension (DASH) diet, which emphasizes consumption of fruits, vegetables, and low-fat dairy products; dietary and soluble fibre; whole grains; and protein from plant sources and that is reduced in saturated fat and cholesterol. The DASH diet is recommended for both patients with hypertension and individuals with normal BP who are at increased risk of developing hypertension. Dietary management of hypertension consists of restriction of sodium; maintenance of dietary potassium, calcium, and magnesium intake; and calorie restriction if the patient is overweight (Table 35.7). (See the Government of Canada's recommended intake for sodium, and the DASH diet to lower high BP, in the Resources at the end of this chapter.)

Hypertension Canada recommendations include a reduction in salt intake for the prevention and treatment of hypertension in accordance with recommendations from Health Canada (Hypertension Canada, 2021). According to the WHO, reducing salt intake is the most cost-effective measure to improve population health outcomes for all individuals, with or without hypertension (WHO, 2020).

High dietary salt causes an estimated 32% of hypertension (Rabi et al., 2020). The daily adequate intake (AI) for sodium is 1 200 mg (52 mmol) to 1 500 mg (65 mmol) for healthy adults, decreasing with age (WHO, 2012). The upper tolerable intake level (UL) for sodium is 2 000 mg/day. There is a large discrepancy between recommended levels of sodium intake and actual sodium intake levels by Canadians. The average sodium consumption in Canada is 3 500 mg/day. Eighty percent of sodium intake comes from processed and restaurant foods, whereas only 10% is added at the table or in cooking. See Sodium 101 and the Government of Canada's Recommended Intake of Sodium in the Resources at the end of this chapter for more educational resources about salt. (See also Chapter 37, Tables 37.6 through 37.9.)

The patient and caregivers, especially those who prepare the meals, should be taught about sodium-restricted diets. Instruction should include reading labels of over-the-counter medications, packaged foods, and health products (e.g., baking soda–containing toothpaste) to identify hidden sources of sodium. It is helpful to review the patient's normal diet and to identify foods high in sodium. Analysis of a 3-day diet history will help in identifying foods high in sodium in the patient's usual diet.

Sodium restriction may be enough to control BP in some patients with stage 1 hypertension. If medication therapy is needed, a lower dose may be effective if the patient also restricts sodium intake. Furthermore, moderate sodium restriction lessens the risk for hypokalemia associated with diuretic therapy. However, people with hypertension respond differently to salt restriction. This heterogeneity of response has led to attempts to define subgroups of people with hypertension as "salt sensitive" or "salt resistant." Patients with low renin activity are more likely to respond to salt restriction with a reduction in BP.

The significance of other dietary elements for the control of hypertension is not certain. There is evidence that greater levels of dietary potassium, calcium, magnesium, and vitamin D are associated with lower BP in the general population and in those with hypertension. Based on available evidence, the

TABLE 35.7   NUTRITIONAL THERAPY

Hypertension

Food Group	Daily Servings	Examples	Significance to DASH Eating Pattern
Whole grains	7–8	Whole wheat breads, cereals; oatmeal; brown rice; pasta; quinoa; barley; low-fat, low-sodium crackers	Major sources of energy and fibre
Vegetables	4–5	Dark green and orange fresh or frozen vegetables, tomatoes, leafy greens, carrots, peas, squash, spinach, peppers, broccoli, sweet potatoes	Rich sources of potassium, magnesium, and fibre
Fruits	4–5	Have fruit more often than juice: apples, apricots, bananas, dates, grapes, oranges, grapefruit, melons, peaches, berries, pineapple	Important sources of potassium, magnesium, and fibre
Low-fat or fat-free dairy foods or alternatives	2–3	Skim milk, 1% milk, fortified soy beverage or yogourt, 6–18% modified-fat cheese	Major sources of calcium and protein
Lean meats, poultry, and fish	≤170 g	Lean meats; choose fish such as char, herring, mackerel, salmon, sardines, and trout; trim fat; broil, roast, or boil; no frying; remove skin from poultry; low-sodium, low-fat deli meats	Rich sources of protein and magnesium
Nuts, seeds, and dry beans	4–5/wk	—	Rich sources of energy, magnesium, potassium, protein, and fibre
Fats and oils*	2–3 tsp	Soft margarine, mayonnaise, vegetable oil (olive, corn, canola, or safflower), salad dressing	Added fat and high-fat sources should be minimal. DASH has 27% of calories as fat, including fat in or added to foods.
Sweets	≤5/wk	Sugar, jelly, jam, hard candy, syrups, sorbet, chocolate	Sweets should be low in fat.

DASH, Dietary Approaches to Stop Hypertension. The DASH eating plan is based on approximately 2 000 calories/day. The number of daily servings in a food group may vary from those listed, depending on specific caloric needs.

*Fat content changes serving counts for fats and oils: For example, 1 tablespoon of regular salad dressing equals 1 serving, 1 tablespoon of low-fat salad dressing equals a half serving, and 1 tablespoon of fat-free salad dressing equals 0 servings.

Source: National Heart, Lung, and Blood Institute. (2006). *The DASH diet*. NIH Publication No. 06-4082. National Institutes of Health. https://www.nhlbi.nih.gov/files/docs/public/heart/hbp_low.pdf

Hypertension Canada 2017 guidelines advise the maintenance of adequate potassium, magnesium, and calcium intake from food sources (Leung et al., 2017). Supplementation of potassium, calcium, and magnesium is not recommended for the prevention or treatment of hypertension. Caffeine may raise BP acutely, but there is no long-term relationship between caffeine intake and elevated BP.

Weight Reduction. Overweight individuals have an increased incidence of hypertension and increased cardiovascular disease risk. Height, weight, and waist circumference should be measured and body mass index (BMI) calculated for all adults. Maintenance of a healthy body weight (BMI 18.5–24.9 kg/m² and waist circumference <102 cm for men and <88 cm for women) is recommended for individuals who are normotensive to prevent hypertension and for Canadians with hypertension to reduce BP. All individuals with hypertension who are overweight should be advised to lose weight. Weight reduction has a significant effect on lowering BP, and the effect is seen with even moderate weight loss. When a person decreases caloric intake, sodium and fat intake may also be reduced. Although reducing the fat content of the diet has not been shown to produce sustained benefits in BP control, it may slow the progress of atherosclerosis and reduce overall cardiovascular disease risk (see Chapter 36). Weight-loss strategies should have a multidisciplinary approach that includes dietary education, increased physical activity, and behavioural intervention.

Modification in Alcohol Consumption. Excessive alcohol consumption is strongly associated with hypertension. To reduce BP, alcohol consumption should be in accordance with Canadian low-risk drinking guidelines for both adults with hypertension and those with normal BP. Healthy adults should limit alcohol consumption to 2 drinks or fewer per day, and consumption should not exceed 14 standard drinks per week for men and 9 standard drinks per week for women. (One standard drink is considered 13.6 g or 17.2 mL of ethanol, or approximately 44 mL of 80-proof [40%] spirits, 148 mL of 12% wine, or 355 mL of 5% beer [Leung et al., 2017].)

Physical Activity. Recommendations for individuals with normal BP (to reduce the possibility of developing hypertension) and for patients with hypertension (to reduce their BP) include the accumulation of 30 to 60 minutes of moderate-intensity dynamic exercise (such as walking, jogging, cycling, or swimming) 4 to 7 days per week, in addition to the routine activities of daily living (Leung et al., 2017). Higher intensities of exercise are no more effective.

Moderately intense activity can lower BP, promote relaxation, and decrease or control body weight. Regular activity of this type can reduce SBP in the patient with hypertension by approximately 10 mm Hg. Sedentary people should be advised to increase activity levels gradually. People with heart disease or other serious health concerns need a thorough examination, possibly including a stress test, before beginning an exercise program.

Avoidance of Tobacco Products. Nicotine contained in tobacco causes vasoconstriction and increases BP in people with hypertension. In addition, smoking tobacco is a major risk factor for cardiovascular disease. The cardiovascular benefits of discontinuing tobacco use can be seen within 1 year in all age groups. Everyone, especially people with hypertension, should be strongly advised to avoid tobacco use. The lower amounts of nicotine contained in smoking cessation aids usually will not raise BP and may be used as indicated. People who continue to use tobacco products should be advised to monitor their BP during use. (See Chapter 11 and the Resources at the end of this chapter for links to smoking cessation materials.)

Stress Management. For patients with hypertension in whom stress may be contributing to BP elevation, stress management should be considered as an intervention. Individualized cognitive–behavioural interventions are more likely to be effective when relaxation techniques are used.

Medication Therapy. The implementation of the CHEP and Hypertension Canada recommendations has resulted in an increased use of antihypertensive medications, increased use of multiple antihypertensive medications, and improved persistence with medication use. The general goal of medication therapy is to achieve a BP of less than 140/90 mm Hg. For patients

with chronic kidney disease or diabetes, target BP is less than 130/80 mm Hg. The medications currently available for treating hypertension have two main actions: (1) to reduce SVR and (2) to decrease the volume of circulating blood (Table 35.8). The medications used in the treatment of hypertension include diuretics, adrenergic (sympathetic) inhibitors, direct vasodilators, angiotensin inhibitors, and calcium channel blockers. The sites where the medications exert their action and the methods of action are shown in Figure 35.5.

TABLE 35.8	**MEDICATION THERAPY**		

Hypertension

Medication	Mechanism of Action	Adverse Effects	Nursing Considerations
Diuretics			
Thiazide and Related Diuretics			
Indapamide (Lozide) Metolazone (Zaroxolyn)	Inhibit NaCl reabsorption in the distal convoluted tubule; increase excretion of Na^+ and Cl^-. Initial decrease in ECF; sustained decrease in SVR. Lower BP moderately in 2–4 wk.	Fluid and electrolyte imbalances (volume depletion, hypokalemia, hyponatremia, hypochloremia, hypomagnesemia, hypercalcemia, hyperuricemia, metabolic alkalosis); CNS effects (vertigo, headache, weakness); GI effects (anorexia, nausea, vomiting, diarrhea, constipation, pancreatitis); sexual issues (impotence and decreased libido); blood dyscrasias; dermatological effects (photosensitivity, skin rash); decreased glucose tolerance	Monitor for orthostatic hypotension, hypokalemia, and alkalosis. Thiazides may potentiate cardiotoxicity of digoxin by producing hypokalemia. Dietary sodium restriction reduces risk for hypokalemia. NSAIDs can decrease diuretic and antihypertensive effect of thiazide diuretics. Advise patient to supplement with potassium-rich foods. Current doses are lower than previously recommended. Indapamide should be administered with caution to patients with renal failure.
Loop Diuretics			
Bumetanide (Burinex) Ethacrynic acid (Edecrin) Furosemide (Lasix)	Inhibit NaCl reabsorption in the thick ascending limb of the loop of Henle. Increase excretion of Na^+ and Cl^-. More potent diuretic effect than thiazides, but shorter duration of action; less effective for hypertension.	Fluid electrolyte imbalance as with thiazides, except no hypercalcemia; ototoxicity (hearing impairment, deafness, vertigo) that is usually reversible; metabolic effects, including hyperuricemia, hyperglycemia, increased LDL cholesterol and triglycerides with decreased HDL cholesterol	Monitor for orthostatic hypotension and electrolyte abnormalities. Loop diuretics remain effective despite renal insufficiency. Diuretic effect of medication increases at higher doses.
Potassium-Sparing Diuretics			
Amiloride hydrochloride (Midamor, Novamilor)	Reduce K^+ and Na^+ exchange in the distal and collecting tubules. Reduce excretion of K^+, H^+, Ca^{2+}, and Mg^{2+}.	Hyperkalemia, nausea, vomiting, diarrhea, headache, leg cramps, and dizziness	Monitor for orthostatic hypotension and hyperkalemia. Potassium-sparing diuretics are contraindicated for use in patients with renal failure and used with caution in patients on ACE inhibitors or angiotensin II blockers. Avoid using potassium supplements.
Spironolactone (Aldactone)	Inhibit the Na^+-retaining and K^+-excreting effects of aldosterone in the distal and collecting tubules.	Same as amiloride; may cause gynecomastia, impotence, decreased libido, and menstrual irregularities	
Adrenergic Inhibitors			
Central-Acting Adrenergic Antagonists			
Clonidine hydrochloride (Catapres)	Reduce sympathetic outflow from CNS. Reduce peripheral sympathetic tone, produce vasodilation; decrease SVR and BP.	Dry mouth, sedation, impotence, nausea, dizziness, sleep disturbance, nightmares, restlessness, and depression; symptomatic bradycardia in patients with conduction disorder	Sudden discontinuation may cause withdrawal syndrome, including rebound hypertension, tachycardia, headache, tremors, apprehension, and sweating. Chewing gum or hard candy may relieve dry mouth. Alcohol and sedatives increase sedation. May be given transdermally with fewer adverse effects and better patient adherence.
Methyldopa	Same as clonidine.	Sedation, fatigue, orthostatic hypotension, decreased libido, impotence, dry mouth, hemolytic anemia, hepatotoxicity, sodium and water retention, psychological depression	Instruct patient about daytime sedation and avoidance of hazardous activities. Administration of a single daily dose at bedtime minimizes sedative effect.

TABLE 35.8 MEDICATION THERAPY

Hypertension—cont'd

Medication	Mechanism of Action	Adverse Effects	Nursing Considerations
α₁-Adrenergic Blockers			
Doxazosin mesylate (Cardura) Prazosin hydrochloride (Minipress) Terazosin hydrochloride (Hytrin)	Block α₁-adrenergic effects, producing peripheral vasodilation (decrease SVR and BP).	Variable amount of orthostatic hypotension, depending on the plasma volume; may see profound orthostatic hypotension with syncope within 90 min after initial dose; retention of salt and water	Reduced resistance to the outflow of urine occurs in benign prostatic hyperplasia. Taking medication at bedtime reduces risks associated with orthostatic hypotension. Medication has beneficial effects on lipid profile.
Phentolamine mesylate (Rogitine)	Block α₁-adrenergic receptors, resulting in peripheral vasodilation (decrease SVR and BP).	Acute, prolonged hypotension, cardiac dysrhythmias, tachycardia, weakness, flushing; abdominal pain, nausea, and exacerbation of peptic ulcer	This is used in short-term management of pheochromocytoma. It is also used locally to prevent necrosis of skin and subcutaneous tissue after extravasation of an α-adrenergic medication. There is no oral formulation.
β-Adrenergic Blockers			
Acebutolol hydrochloride (Sectral) Atenolol (Tenormin) Betaxolol hydrochloride Bisoprolol fumarate Carvedilol Metoprolol tartrate Nadolol Propranolol hydrochloride Timolol maleate	Reduce BP by antagonizing β₁-adrenergic effects. Decrease CO and reduce sympathetic vasoconstrictor tone. Decrease renin secretion by kidney.	Bronchospasm, atrioventricular conduction block, impaired peripheral circulation; nightmares, depression, weakness, reduced exercise capacity; may induce or exacerbate heart failure in susceptible patients; sudden withdrawal of β-adrenergic blockers may cause rebound hypertension and exacerbate symptoms of ischemic heart disease	β-Adrenergic blockers vary in lipid solubility, selectivity, and presence of partial sympathomimetic effect, which explains different therapeutic and adverse effect profiles of specific agents. Monitor pulse regularly. Use with caution in patients with diabetes mellitus because medication may mask signs of hypoglycemia.
Esmolol hydrochloride (Brevibloc)	Reduce BP by antagonizing β₁-adrenergic effects.	—	Use IV administration; medication has a rapid onset and brief duration of action.
Combined α- and β-adrenergic blocker			
Labetalol hydrochloride (Trandate)	α₁-, β₁-, and β₂-Adrenergic blocking properties, producing peripheral vasodilation and decreased heart rate. Reduces CO, SVR, and BP.	Dizziness, fatigue, nausea, vomiting, dyspepsia, paresthesia, nasal stuffiness, impotence, edema; hepatic toxicity	Same as β-adrenergic blockers. IV form is available for hypertensive crisis in hospitalized patients. Patients must be kept supine during IV administration. Assess patient tolerance of upright position (severe orthostatic hypotension) before allowing upright activities (e.g., use of commode).
Direct Vasodilators			
Diazoxide (Proglycem)	Reduce SVR and BP by direct arterial vasodilation.	Reflex sympathetic activation, producing increased HR, CO, and salt and water retention; hyperglycemia, especially in patients with type 2 diabetes	IV use only for hypertensive crisis in hospitalized patients. Administer only into peripheral vein.
Hydralazine hydrochloride (Apresoline)	Reduce SVR and BP by direct arterial vasodilation.	Headache, nausea, flushing, palpitation, tachycardia, dizziness, and angina; hemolytic anemia, vasculitis, and rapidly progressive glomerulonephritis	IV use for hypertensive crisis in hospitalized patients. Twice-daily oral dosage. Not used as monotherapy because of adverse effects. Medication is contraindicated for use in patients with coronary artery disease; used with caution in patients >40 yr of age.
Minoxidil (Loniten)	Reduce SVR and BP by direct arterial vasodilation.	Reflex tachycardia, marked sodium and fluid retention (may require loop diuretics for control), and hirsutism; may cause ECG changes (flattened and inverted T waves) not related to ischemia	Reserved for treatment of severe hypertension associated with renal failure and resistant to other therapy. Use once- or twice-daily dosage.
Nitroglycerin	Relax arterial and venous smooth muscle reducing preload and SVR. At low dose, venous dilation predominates; at higher dose, arterial dilation is present.	Hypotension, headache, vomiting, flushing IV use for hypertensive crisis in hospitalized patients with myocardial ischemia	Nitroglycerin is administered by continuous IV infusion with pump or control device.

Continued

TABLE 35.8   MEDICATION THERAPY

Hypertension—cont'd

Medication	Mechanism of Action	Adverse Effects	Nursing Considerations
Sodium nitroprusside (Nipride)	Direct arterial vasodilation reduces SVR and BP.	Acute hypotension, nausea, vomiting, muscle twitching; signs of thiocyanate toxicity include anorexia, nausea, fatigue, disorientation	IV use for hypertensive crisis in hospitalized patients. Administered by continuous IV infusion with pump or control device. Use intra-arterial monitoring of BP. Light-resistant bags, bottles, and administration sets must be used; stable for 24 hr. Monitor thiocyanate levels with prolonged (>24–48 hr) use.

Angiotensin Inhibitors

Angiotensin-Converting Enzyme (ACE) Inhibitors

Benazepril hydrochloride (Lotensin) Captopril Enalapril sodium (Vasotec) Fosinopril sodium Lisinopril (Prinivil, Zestril) Perindopril erbumine (Coversyl) Quinapril hydrochloride (Accupril) Ramipril (Altace) Trandolapril (Mavik, Tarka) Enalaprilat injection (Vasotec IV)	Inhibit ACE; reduce conversion of angiotensin I to angiotensin II (A-II); prevent A-II–mediated vasoconstriction. Inhibit ACE when oral medications are not appropriate.	Hypotension, loss of taste, cough, hyperkalemia, acute kidney injury, skin rash, angioneurotic edema; same as with oral forms	ASA and NSAIDs may reduce medication effectiveness. Addition of diuretic enhances medication effect. ACE inhibitors should not be used with potassium-sparing diuretics. They can cause fetal morbidity or mortality. Captopril may be given orally for hypertensive crisis. Medication is given by IV route over 5 min; it may be given every 6 hr.

Angiotensin II Receptor Blockers

Candesartan cilexetil (Atacand) Eprosartan mesylate (Teveten) Irbesartan (Avapro) Losartan potassium (Cozaar) Telmisartan (Micardis) Valsartan (Diovan)	Prevent action of A-II and produce vasodilation and increased salt and water excretion.	Hyperkalemia, decreased kidney function	Full effect on BP may not be seen for 3–6 wk.

Calcium Channel Blockers

Amlodipine besylate (Caduet, Norvasc) Diltiazem hydrochloride (Tiazac) Felodipine (Plendil) Nifedipine (Adalat) Verapamil hydrochloride (Isoptin)	Block movement of extracellular calcium into cells, causing vasodilation and decreased SVR.	Nausea, headache, dizziness, peripheral edema; reflex tachycardia (with dihydropyridines); reflex decrease HR (with diltiazem); constipation (with verapamil)	Use with caution in patients with heart failure. Contraindicated for use in patients with second- or third-degree heart block. Sustained-release formulations are available for some medications. Avoid grapefruit consumption when on nifedipine.

ASA, acetylsalicylic acid (Aspirin); *BP*, blood pressure; *CNS*, central nervous system; *CO*, cardiac output; *ECF*, extracellular fluid; *ECG*, electrocardiogram; *GI*, gastrointestinal; *HDL*, high-density lipoprotein; *HR*, heart rate; *IV*, intravenous; *LDL*, low-density lipoprotein; *NSAIDs*, nonsteroidal anti-inflammatory drugs; *SVR*, systemic vascular resistance.

Although the precise action of diuretics in the reduction of BP is unclear, it is known that they promote sodium and water excretion, reduce plasma volume, decrease sodium in the arteriolar walls, and reduce the vascular response to catecholamines. Adrenergic-inhibiting medications act by diminishing the sympathetic effects that increase BP. Adrenergic inhibitors include medications that act centrally on the vasomotor centre and peripherally to inhibit NE release or to block the adrenergic receptors on blood vessels. Direct vasodilators decrease the BP by relaxing vascular smooth muscle and reducing SVR. Calcium channel blockers increase sodium excretion and cause arteriolar vasodilation by preventing the movement of extracellular calcium into cells.

There are two types of angiotensin inhibitors. The first type is angiotensin-converting enzyme (ACE) inhibitors, which prevent the conversion of angiotensin I to A-II and thus reduce A-II–mediated vasoconstriction and sodium and water retention. The second type is A-II receptor blockers (ARBs), which prevent A-II from binding to its receptors in the walls of the blood vessels.

Medication therapy is recommended for all patients at low risk with stage 1 hypertension (140–159/90–99 mm Hg), although lifestyle management may be the sole therapy. As stated earlier, for patients with diabetes or chronic kidney disease, target BP is less than 130/80 mm Hg. Many younger Canadians with hypertension have multiple cardiovascular risks and are not treated with antihypertensive medications. Currently, this is a gap in treatment. See the treatment algorithm of systolic–diastolic hypertension without other compelling indications in Figure 35.3 and Tables 35.9 and 35.10.

The initial medication may be started at a low dosage for several weeks. The full effects of antihypertensive medication may not be apparent for up to 6 weeks. If the BP is not controlled, the dosage of the first-line medication can be increased. A second medication from a different class can be substituted or added if the initial medication is ineffective or if there are adverse effects from the initial medication. For most patients, at least two medications (probably taken in a single tablet) are necessary in addition to lifestyle changes. Before proceeding with the addition or substitution of medication, consideration should be given to possible reasons for the lack of response to medication therapy.

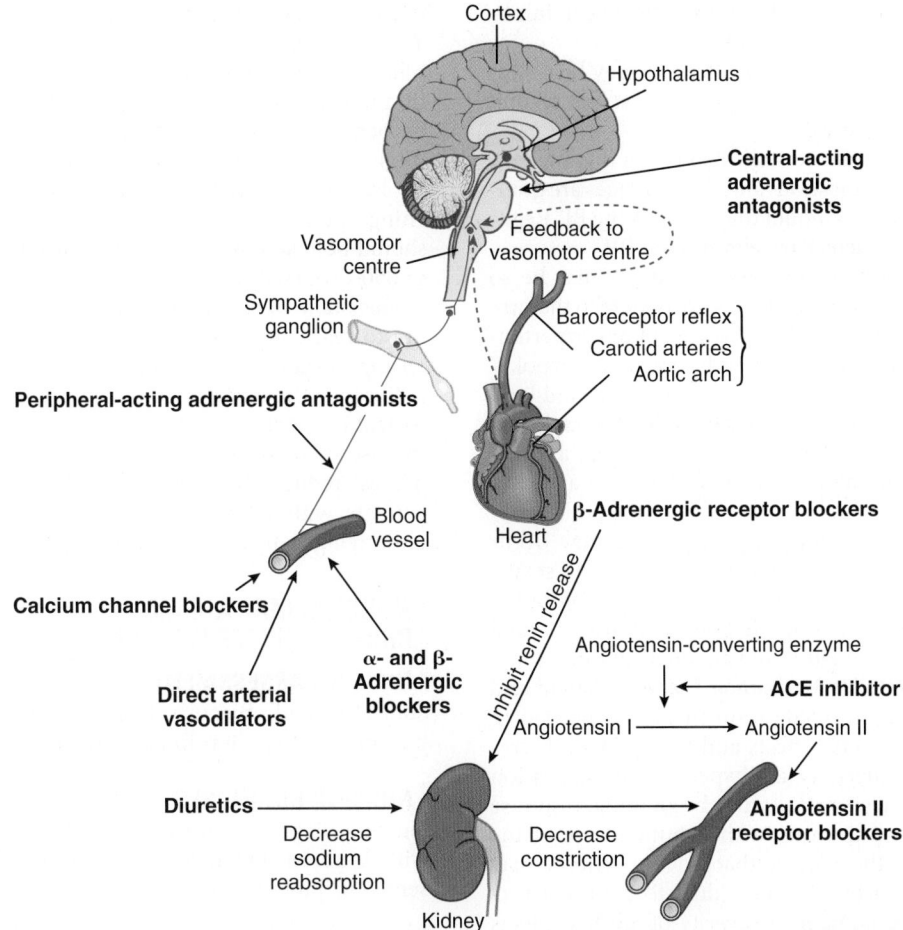

FIG. 35.5 Site and method of action of various antihypertensive medications. *ACE*, angiotensin-converting enzyme. Source: U.S. Department of Health and Human Services. (2003). *The seventh report of the Joint National Committee on Detection, Evaluation, and Treatment of High Blood Pressure (JNC-7)*. National Institutes of Health.

TABLE 35.9	**CONSIDERATIONS REGARDING THE CHOICE OF FIRST-LINE THERAPY**

- Low-dose single pill combinations are preferred as first-line therapy to reduce BP and prevent cardiovascular events and reduce the risk of adverse events.
- Use caution when initiating therapy with two medications in patients in whom adverse events are more likely (e.g., frail older person, patients with orthostatic hypotension or who are dehydrated).
- ACE inhibitors, renin inhibitors, and ARBs are contraindicated in pregnancy, and caution is required in prescribing to women of childbearing potential.
- β-Adrenergic blockers are not recommended for patients ≥60 yr without another compelling comorbid condition (such as diabetes mellitus or heart disease).
- Diuretic-induced hypokalemia should be avoided through the use of potassium-sparing agents, if required.
- ACE inhibitors are not recommended (as monotherapy) for patients who are Black, without another compelling comorbid condition.

ACE, angiotensin-converting enzyme; *ARB*, angiotensin II receptor blocker. Sources: Canadian Hypertension Education Program (CHEP). (2015). *2015 Canadian Hypertension Education Program recommendations. Part 2, Recommendations for hypertension treatment* (Slide 32). https://guidelines.hypertension.ca/chep-resources/; and Leung, A. A., Daskalopoulou, S. S., Dasgupta, K., et al. (2017). Hypertension Canada's 2017 guidelines for diagnosis, risk assessment, prevention, and treatment of hypertension in adults. *Canadian Journal of Cardiology, 33*(5), 557–576. https://doi.org/10.1016/j.cjca.2017.03.005

TABLE 35.10	**MEDICATION COMBINATIONS**

To achieve optimal blood pressure targets:
- Multiple medications are often required to reach target levels, especially in patients with type 2 diabetes.
- Replace multiple antihypertensive agents with single pill combination therapy.
- Low doses of multiple medications may be more effective and better tolerated than higher doses of fewer medications.
- Reassess patients with uncontrolled blood pressure at least every 2 months.
- A combination of two first-line agents may also be considered as initial treatment of hypertension.
- The combination of ACE inhibitors and ARBs should not be used.

ACEIs, angiotensin-converting enzyme inhibitors; *ARBs*, angiotensin II receptor blockers. Source: Hypertension Canada. (2017). *What's new? 2017 Hypertension Canada guidelines for the management of hypertension*. https://www.hypertension.ca/images/CHEP_2017/HTN_Whats_New_2017_EN.pdf

A new medication therapy has been marketed recently in Canada. Although long-term mortality and morbidity studies have yet to be published, it has been authorized for use in Canada. Aliskiren fumarate (Rasilez) is an oral direct renin inhibitor (DRI). Renin inhibition acts on the conversion of angiotensinogen to angiotensin I. This is the rate-limiting step in the production of A-II, which is a key mediator of BP, body fluid volume, and vascular remodelling. DRIs may be more effective in inhibiting RAAS than ACE inhibitors or ARBs.

The addition of a third or fourth medication may be necessary, but only after the maximum doses of the first and second medications have been achieved.

After 1 year of optimum BP control, step-down therapy may be tried. The number of medications and their dosages are gradually decreased to the lowest amount that controls the BP. Regular follow-up is needed to detect any elevation of BP.

Adverse effects of antihypertensive medications may be so severe or undesirable that the patient does not adhere to therapy. Table 35.8 describes the major adverse effects of antihypertensive medications. Hyperuricemia, hyperglycemia, and hypokalemia are common adverse effects with both thiazide and loop diuretics. ACE inhibitors can lead to high levels of bradykinin, which can cause coughing. An individual who develops a cough with the use of ACE inhibitors may be switched to an ARB. Hyperkalemia can be a serious adverse effect of the potassium-sparing diuretics and ACE inhibitors. Impotence may occur with some of the diuretics. Orthostatic hypotension and sexual dysfunction are two undesirable effects of adrenergic-inhibiting agents. Tachycardia and orthostatic hypotension are potential adverse effects of both vasodilators and angiotensin inhibitors.

Patient Teaching Related to Medication Therapy. Patient and caregiver teaching related to medication therapy is needed to identify and minimize adverse effects and to cope with therapeutic effects. Adverse effects of antihypertensive medication therapy are common. Adverse effects may be an initial response to a medication and may decrease with continued use of the medication. Informing the patient that adverse effects may lessen with time may enable the individual to continue taking the medication. The number or severity of adverse effects may be related to the dosage, and it may be necessary to change the medication or decrease the dosage. In this case, the patient should be advised to report the adverse effects to the health care provider who prescribed the medication.

A common adverse effect of several of these medications is orthostatic hypotension. This condition is caused by an alteration in the autonomic nervous system's mechanisms for regulating BP, which are required for position changes. Consequently, the patient may feel dizzy, weak, and faint when assuming an upright position after sitting or lying down. (Specific measures to control or decrease orthostatic hypotension are presented later, in Table 35.15.)

Sexual dysfunction may occur with many of the antihypertensive medications (see Table 35.8) and can be a major reason for nonadherence to the treatment plan. Often, the nurse must approach the patient on this sensitive subject and encourage discussion of any sexual dysfunction the patient may be experiencing. It may be easier for the patient to discuss sexual issues once it has been explained that the medication may be the source of the problem and that the adverse effects can be decreased or eliminated by changing to another antihypertensive medication. The patient should be encouraged to discuss adverse effects with the health care provider who prescribed the medication. If the patient is reluctant to do so, the nurse may offer to alert the health care provider to the sexual adverse effect that the patient is experiencing. There are many options for treating hypertension; a plan that is acceptable to the patient should be achievable.

Some unpleasant effects of medications result from their therapeutic effect, but the impact can be minimized. For example, dry mouth and frequent voiding are unpleasant effects of diuretics. Sugarless gum or candy may relieve the dry mouth. The nurse can assist the patient in developing a medication schedule to minimize unpleasant effects. When frequent urination interrupts sleep, taking the diuretic earlier in the day may be beneficial. Adverse effects of vasodilators and adrenergic inhibitors decrease if the medications are taken in the evening. BP is lowest during the night and highest shortly after awakening; therefore, medications with 24-hour duration of action should be taken as early in the morning as possible (e.g., 0400 or 0500 hours, if the patient awakens to void).

Resistant Hypertension. *Resistant hypertension* is the failure to reach goal BP in patients who are taking full doses of an appropriate three-medication therapy regimen that includes a diuretic. The nurse should carefully explore reasons why the patient is not at goal BP (Table 35.11). Studies have shown that the use of *renal denervation* (destruction of overactive renal nerves) reduces BP and muscle sympathetic nerve activity in patients with resistant hypertension. The exact mechanisms underlying sympathetic neural inhibition are not clear.

NURSING MANAGEMENT PRIMARY HYPERTENSION

NURSING ASSESSMENT
Subjective and objective data that should be obtained from a patient with hypertension are presented in Table 35.12.

NURSING DIAGNOSES
Nursing diagnoses and interprofessional issues for the patient with hypertension include but are not limited to those presented in Table 35.13.

PLANNING
The overall goals for the patient with hypertension are that the patient will (1) achieve and maintain the individually

---

TABLE 35.11	CAUSES OF RESISTANT HYPERTENSION

Improper BP measurement
- Volume overload
- Excess salt intake
- Volume retention from kidney disease
- Inadequate diuretic therapy

Medication induced or other causes
- Nonadherence
- Illegal drugs (e.g., cocaine, amphetamines)
- Inadequate medication dosages
- Inappropriate combinations of medication therapy
- Nonsteroidal anti-inflammatory drugs
- Sympathomimetics (e.g., decongestants, diet pills)
- Oral contraceptives
- Corticosteroids
- Cyclosporin and tacrolimus (Prograf)
- Erythropoietin
- Licorice (including some chewing tobacco)
- Selected over-the-counter dietary or herbal supplements and medicines (e.g., ma huang, bitter orange)

Associated conditions
- Increasing obesity
- Excess alcohol consumptionIdentifiable causes of secondary hypertension

Source: National Heart, Lung, and Blood Institute. (2004). *Seventh report of the Joint National Committee on Prevention, Detection, Evaluation, and Treatment of High Blood Pressure (JNC-7)*. NIH Publication No. 04-5230. Author. https://www.nhlbi.nih.gov/guidelines/hypertension/jnc7full.pdf

TABLE 35.12   NURSING ASSESSMENT

Hypertension Data

Subjective Data
Important Health Information

Current health history: Family history of hypertension or cardiovascular disease; smoking or other tobacco use, alcohol use; sedentary lifestyle; usual salt and fat intake; weight gain or loss
Past health history: Known duration and past workup of high BP; cardiovascular, cerebrovascular, renal, or thyroid disease; diabetes; pituitary disorders; obesity; dyslipidemia; menopause or hormone replacement status
Medications: Use of any prescription or over-the-counter, illicit, or natural health products; previous use of antihypertensive medication therapy

Symptoms
- Dyspnea on exertion, palpitations on exertion, anginal chest pain
- Fatigue
- Intermittent claudication, muscle cramps
- Nocturia
- Dizziness; blurred vision, paresthesias
- Erectile dysfunction, decreased libido

Objective Data
Cardiovascular

BP consistently >140 mm Hg systolic or 90 mm Hg diastolic, orthostatic change in BP and pulse; abnormal heart sounds; laterally displaced, sustained, forceful, apical pulse; diminished or absent peripheral pulses; carotid, kidney, ischial, or femoral bruits; presence of edema

Musculoskeletal

Truncal obesity

Neurological

Mental status changes

Possible Findings

Abnormal serum electrolytes (especially potassium); increased creatinine, glucose, cholesterol, and triglyceride levels; proteinuria, microalbuminuria; evidence of ischemic heart disease and left ventricular hypertrophy on ECG

BP, blood pressure; *ECG,* electrocardiogram.

TABLE 35.13   NURSING ASSESSMENT

Hypertension

Nursing Diagnoses

- *Inadequate health main*tenance as a result of *insufficient resources* (lack of knowledge)
- *Anxiety* resulting from *stressors, threat to current status* (lifestyle changes associated with hypertension)
- *Sexual dysfunction* resulting from *vulnerability* (effects of antihypertensive medications)
- *Inadequate health management* related to:
  - *Insufficient knowledge of therapeutic regimen*
  - *Difficulty managing complex treatment regimen*
  - *Perceived barrier* (cost of medications)
  - *Insufficient social support*
  - *Difficulty navigating complex health care systems*
  - *Powerlessness*
- *Disturbed body image* resulting from *alteration in self-perception*
- *Inadequate peripheral tissue perfusion* resulting from *insufficient knowledge of disease process* (hypertension)

Interprofessional Issues

- Potential complication: adverse effects from antihypertensive therapy
- Potential complication: hypertensive crisis
- Potential complication: stroke

---

determined target BP; (2) understand, accept, and implement the therapeutic plan; (3) experience minimal or no unpleasant adverse effects of therapy; and (4) be confident about the ability to manage and cope with this condition.

NURSING IMPLEMENTATION

HEALTH PROMOTION. Primary prevention of hypertension provides an attractive alternative to the costly cycle of managing hypertension and its complications. Current recommendations for primary prevention are based on lifestyle modifications that have been shown to prevent or delay the expected rise in BP in susceptible people. A diet rich in fruits, vegetables, and low-fat dairy foods, with reduced saturated and total fats, significantly lowers BP (see Table 35.7). This diet has been recommended for primary prevention in the general population. Dietary modifications that do not require active participation of the individual, such as a reduction in the amount of salt added to processed foods, may be even more effective.

Individual Patient Evaluation. The majority of cases of hypertension are identified through routine screening procedures such as insurance and pre-employment or premilitary physical examinations. The nurse in these settings, as well as in most other practice settings, is in an ideal position to assess for the presence of hypertension, identify the risk factors for hypertension and coronary artery disease, and teach the patient about these conditions. In addition to measuring BP, a complete health assessment should include such factors as age, sex, and race; diet history (including sodium and alcohol intake); weight patterns; and family history of heart disease, stroke, renal disease, and diabetes mellitus. Medications taken, both prescribed and over the counter, should be noted. The patient should be asked about a previous history of high BP and the results of treatment (if any) (see Table 35.12).

Initially, the BP is taken two or three times, at least 2 minutes apart, with the average pressure recorded as the value for that visit. Waiting for at least 2 minutes between readings allows the venous blood to drain from the arm and prevents inaccurate readings. Size and placement of the BP cuff are important considerations for accurate measurement. The width of the inflatable bladder should be 40% of the upper arm circumference and the length should be 80%. Use of a cuff that is too small or too large will result in readings that are falsely high or low, respectively. The cuff needs to be placed 2.5 cm above the antecubital fossa.

BP measurements of both arms should be performed initially to detect any differences between arms. Atherosclerotic narrowing of the subclavian artery can cause a falsely low reading on the side where the narrowing occurs. Therefore, the arm with the higher reading should be used for all subsequent BP measurements. The patient's arm is uncovered and placed at the level of the heart. The cuff should be inflated until no pulse is felt in the brachial artery located in the antecubital fossa of the arm being used. The cuff is then inflated an additional 10 to 20 mm Hg to ensure vascular occlusion. The pressure is released at 2 mm Hg per second. Releasing the pressure any more slowly or quickly may create inaccurate readings. Both SBP and DBP should be recorded, with the DBP recorded as the disappearance of sound (Table 35.14).

The BP and the pulse are initially measured with the patient in either the supine or sitting position after at least 5 minutes of

TABLE 35.14 APPROPRIATE TECHNIQUE FOR MEASURING BLOOD PRESSURE

1. The use of electronic (oscillometric) measurement methods is preferred to manual measurement. The patient should be seated with the arm bared, supported, and positioned at heart level. The patient should have neither smoked nor ingested caffeine within 30 min before measurement. The patient should also not have used substances containing adrenergic stimulants, such as phenylephrine or pseudoephedrine, which may be found in decongestants or ophthalmic drops.
2. The patient's bowel and bladder should be comfortable. A quiet environment at a comfortable room temperature should be provided.
3. The patient should stay quiet before and during the procedure.
4. For initial readings, the nurse should take the blood pressure in both arms, and subsequently measure in the arm with the highest reading. Thereafter, two measurements should be taken on the side where the blood pressure is highest. Out-of-office measurement should be performed to confirm the initial diagnosis of hypertension.
5. The appropriate cuff size must be used to ensure an accurate measurement. The rubber bladder should reach nearly around (at least 80% of the circumference) or completely encircle the arm. Cuff width should be at least 40% of the arm circumference. Several sizes of cuffs (e.g., child, adult, and large adult) should be available.
6. Measurements should be taken with a mercury sphygmomanometer, a recently calibrated anaeroid manometer, or a calibrated electronic device. Electronic measurement methods are preferred.
7. Both systolic and diastolic pressures should be recorded. The disappearance of sound should be used for the diastolic reading.
8. Two or more readings (taken at least 2 min apart) should be averaged. If the first two readings differ by >5 mm Hg, additional readings should be obtained.
9. The patient should be informed of the reading and advised of the need for periodic remeasurement.

Source: Adapted from Leung, A. A., Daskalopoulou, S. S., Dasgupta, K., et al. (2017). Hypertension Canada's 2017 guidelines for diagnosis, risk assessment, prevention, and treatment of hypertension in adults. *Canadian Journal of Cardiology, 33*(5), 557–576. https://doi.org/10.1016/j.cjca.2017.03.005

TABLE 35.15 PATIENT & CAREGIVER TEACHING GUIDE

Hypertension

When presenting information to the patient or caregiver, the nurse should do the following:
1. Provide the numerical value of the patient's BP and explain what it means.
2. Inform the patient that hypertension is usually asymptomatic and symptoms do not reliably indicate BP levels.
3. Explain that hypertension means elevated BP and does not relate to a "hyper" personality.
4. Explain that long-term follow-up and therapy are necessary to treat hypertension.
5. Explain that therapy will not cure, but should control, hypertension.
6. Tell the patient that controlled hypertension is usually compatible with an excellent prognosis and a normal lifestyle.
7. Explain the potential dangers of uncontrolled hypertension.
8. Be specific about the names, the actions, the dosages, and the adverse effects of prescribed medications.
9. Tell the patient to plan regular and convenient times for taking medications.
10. Tell the patient not to discontinue medications abruptly because withdrawal may cause a severe hypertensive reaction.
11. Tell the patient not to double up on doses when a dose is missed.
12. Inform the patient that, if BP increases, the patient should not take an increased medication dosage before consulting with the health care provider.
13. Tell the patient not to take a medication belonging to someone else.
14. Inform the patient that adverse effects of medication often diminish with time.
15. Tell the patient to consult with the health care provider about changing medications or dosages if impotence or other sexual issues develop.
16. Tell the patient to supplement the diet with foods high in potassium (e.g., citrus fruits and green leafy vegetables) if taking potassium-losing diuretics.
17. Tell the patient to avoid taking hot baths, consuming excessive amounts of alcohol, and doing strenuous exercise within 3 hr of taking medications that promote vasodilation.
18. Explain that, to decrease orthostatic hypotension, the patient should arise slowly from bed, sit on the side of the bed for a few minutes, stand slowly, not stand still for prolonged periods, do leg exercises to increase venous return, sleep with the head of the bed raised or on pillows, and lie or sit down when dizziness occurs.
19. Caution patient about potentially high-risk over-the-counter medications, such as high-sodium antacids, appetite suppressants, and cold and sinus medications. Advise patient to read warning labels and to consult with a pharmacist.

BP, blood pressure.

rest. BP and pulse should be measured again after 2 minutes, in the standing position. Usually, the SBP decreases on standing, whereas the DBP and the pulse increase. A decrease of more than 10 mm Hg in SBP, or any decrease in DBP when standing, is abnormal and should prompt further investigation. Common causes of abnormal postural BP values include intravascular volume loss (e.g., with diuretic therapy or dehydration) and inadequate vasoconstrictor mechanisms related to disease or medications. Postural changes in BP and pulse should be measured in older persons, people taking antihypertensive medications, and when orthostatic hypotension is suspected. The common definition for orthostatic hypotension is a decrease of 20 mm Hg (or more) in SBP or a decrease of 10 mm Hg (or more) in DBP that occurs when an individual assumes a standing position.

Screening Programs. Screening programs in the community are widely used to assess BP. At the time of the BP measurement, each person should be informed in writing of the numerical value of the reading and, if necessary, why further evaluation is important. Effort and resources should be focused on controlling BP in the person already identified as having hypertension; identifying and controlling BP in high-risk groups such as people who are Black or of Southeast Asian descent, people with obesity, and blood relatives of people with hypertension; and screening persons with limited access to the health care system.

Cardiovascular Risk Factor Modification. Education regarding cardiovascular risk factors is appropriate for individual and targeted screening programs. Modifiable cardiovascular risk factors include hypertension, obesity, diabetes mellitus, elevated serum lipids, tobacco use, and physical inactivity. Risk factors can easily be identified and modification discussed with the patient. (Health-promoting behaviours for cardiovascular risk factors are presented in Chapter 36, Table 36.4 and Figure 36.5.)

AMBULATORY AND HOME CARE. The primary nursing responsibilities for long-term management of hypertension are to assist the patient in reducing BP and adhering to the treatment plan. Nursing actions include patient and family teaching, detection and reporting of adverse treatment effects, adherence assessment and enhancement, and evaluation of therapeutic effectiveness (Table 35.15). Patient and caregiver teaching includes the following: (1) nutritional therapy, (2) medication therapy, (3) physical activity, (4) home monitoring of BP (if appropriate), (5) tobacco cessation (if applicable), and (6) stress management.

EVIDENCE-INFORMED PRACTICE
Translating Research Into Practice

The nurse is caring for T. N. (pronouns he/him), a 46-year-old with a history of poorly controlled hypertension and chronic kidney disease. The nurse notes that he is taking three antihypertensive medications. He tells the nurse that he can no longer live with the adverse effects of these medications (e.g., fatigue, dry mouth, erectile dysfunction). T. N. states that he wants to stop taking the medications. He believes that if he changes his lifestyle by reducing salt from his diet, losing weight, and beginning exercise, he can control his hypertension.

Best Available Evidence	Clinician Expertise	Patient Preferences and Values
Uncontrolled BP places persons with concurrent risk for cardiovascular disease (e.g., diabetes, kidney disease) at highest risk for a cardiovascular event (e.g., stroke). Most patients with hypertension will need two or more medications to achieve their goal BP, in addition to lifestyle changes.	The nurse knows that lifestyle changes can help reduce and control BP in many patients. However, patients with poorly controlled hypertension and target-organ disease require medications to control BP and prevent further complications.	T. N. wishes to eliminate antihypertensive medications because of unpleasant and unacceptable adverse effects that are interfering with his quality of life.

Decision and Actions
The nurse discusses the role of lifestyle changes and medications in the treatment of hypertension and prevention of (further) target-organ disease with T. N. The nurse supports his intention to make lifestyle changes and validates his concerns regarding the adverse effects of the medications. They discuss these adverse effects and the nurse explains that it may be possible to change some of his medications to eliminate or reduce the unpleasant adverse effects. However, given the severity of his hypertension and the chronic kidney disease, T. N. will need to be on medications on a long-term basis. Any of his plans to discontinue medications need to be discussed with his health care provider.

Reference for Evidence
Rabi, D. M., McBrien, K. A., Sapir-Pichhadze, R., et al. (2020). Hypertension Canada's 2020 comprehensive guidelines for the prevention, diagnosis, risk assessment, and treatment of hypertension in adults and children. *Canadian Journal of Cardiology, 36*(5), 596–624. https://doi.org/10.1016/j.cjca.2020.02.086

INFORMATICS IN PRACTICE
Monitoring Blood Pressure

- Patients with hypertension who have a smartphone or computer access should be encouraged to use applications ("apps") aimed at helping them manage their care, including BP self-monitoring and appointment tracking.
- Patients enter their SBP and DBP, heart rate, and other information, including the arm measured. They also indicate whether they were standing, sitting, or lying down, as well as the time the BP was taken.
- At appointment time, the nurse can review the reports generated from the application to assist in determining how well the patient's BP has been controlled.

DBP, diastolic blood pressure; *SBP*, systolic blood pressure.

Physical Activity. *Physical activity* is bodily movement produced by skeletal muscles that requires energy expenditure. Health benefits from physical activity can be achieved with moderate-intensity activities. The goal for all adults is to accumulate 30 minutes of moderate-intensity activity daily. Generally, physical activity is more likely to be sustained if it is safe and enjoyable, fits easily into the daily schedule, and does not generate financial or social costs.

Shopping malls in many communities are open early in the morning (before shopping hours) and provide a warm, safe, flat area for walking. In some communities, health clubs offer special "off-peak" rates to encourage physical activity among older people. Cardiac rehabilitation programs offer supervised exercise with education about reduction of cardiovascular risk factors. Nurses can assist people with hypertension to increase their physical activity by identifying and communicating the need for increased activity, explaining the difference between physical activity and exercise, assisting in initiating activity, and following up appropriately.

Home Blood Pressure Monitoring. Some patients benefit from regularly monitoring their BP at home. Home BP measurement may give a more valid indication of the BP because the patient is more relaxed. It is important to emphasize to the patient that a single reading is not as important as a series of readings over time. The patient should be instructed to take BP readings weekly (unless otherwise instructed), once the BP has stabilized. A log of the BP measurements should be maintained by the patient and brought to office visits.

Home BP readings may help achieve patient adherence by reinforcing the need to continue therapy. A patient may become excessively concerned with the BP readings when using home monitoring. Generally, however, this practice should reassure the patient that the treatment is effective.

Patient Adherence. A major challenge in the long-term management of the patient with hypertension is poor adherence to the prescribed treatment plan. The reasons are many and include inadequate patient teaching, unpleasant adverse effects of medications, return of BP to normal range while on medication, lack of motivation, high cost of medications, and lack of a trusting relationship between the patient and the health care provider. In addition to using BP determinations as an indicator of adherence, the nurse should also assess the patient's diet, activity level, and lifestyle.

Individual assessment to determine the reasons the patient does not adhere to the treatment plan as well as the development of an individualized plan with the patient's assistance are essential. The plan should be compatible with the patient's personality, habits, and lifestyle. Active patient participation increases the likelihood of adherence to the treatment plan. Measures such as involving the patient in scheduling medication convenient to a daily routine, helping the patient link pill-taking with another daily activity, and involving family members (if necessary) can help increase patient adherence. Substituting combination tablets for multiple medications once the BP is stabilized may also facilitate adherence because the patient has to take fewer pills each day and the cost may be less. It is important to help the patient and the family understand that hypertension is a chronic condition that cannot be cured but can be controlled with medication therapy, diet therapy, physical activity, periodic evaluation, and other relevant lifestyle changes (Table 35.16).

TABLE 35.16	RECOMMENDATIONS TO IMPROVE ADHERENCE TO ANTIHYPERTENSIVE PRESCRIPTIONS

Adherence can be improved by using a multipronged approach. The nurse should:
- Assess adherence to pharmacological and nonpharmacological therapy at every health care provider visit.
- Simplify medication regimens to once-daily administration and use electronic medication adherence aids. Use fixed-dose combinations where available and appropriate.
- Tailor pill-taking to fit the patient's daily habits.
- Encourage greater patient responsibility and autonomy in monitoring blood pressure and adjusting prescriptions.
- Coordinate with work-site health care providers to improve monitoring of adherence to pharmacological and lifestyle modification prescriptions.
- Educate patients and families about disease or treatment regimens.

EVALUATION

The overall expected outcomes are that the patient with hypertension will (1) achieve and maintain desired BP as defined for the individual; (2) understand, accept, and implement the therapeutic plan; and (3) experience minimal or no unpleasant adverse effects of therapy.

AGE-RELATED CONSIDERATIONS

HYPERTENSION

Hypertension is common in people 60 years of age and older in industrialized countries. The SBP rises throughout the lifespan and DBP rises until age 55 or 60 years and then levels off. The following age-related physical changes play a role in the pathophysiology of hypertension in the older person: (1) loss of tissue elasticity; (2) increased collagen content and stiffness of the myocardium; (3) increased peripheral vascular resistance; (4) decreased β-adrenergic receptor sensitivity; (5) blunting of baroreceptor reflexes; (6) decreased kidney function; and (7) decreased renin response to sodium and water depletion.

In older persons taking antihypertensive medication, absorption of some medications may be altered as a result of decreased splanchnic blood flow. Metabolism and excretion of medications may also be prolonged.

Careful technique is important in assessing BP in older persons. In some older people, there is a wide gap between the first Korotkoff sound and subsequent beats. This is called the *auscultatory gap*. Failure to inflate the cuff enough may result in seriously underestimating the SBP. This problem can be avoided by palpating the brachial or radial artery while inflating the cuff to a level above the disappearance of the pulse.

Older persons are sensitive to BP changes; therefore, reducing SBP to less than 120 mm Hg in a person with long-standing hypertension could lead to inadequate cerebral blood flow. Medical therapy should be considered for adults when DBP is greater than or equal to 100 mm Hg or SBP is greater than or equal to 160 mm Hg, regardless of age but excluding those with macrovascular tent organ damage or other cardiovascular risks (Rabi et al., 2020).

Because of varying degrees of impaired baroreceptor reflex mechanisms, orthostatic hypotension occurs often in older persons, especially in those with ISH. Orthostatic hypotension in this age group is often associated with volume depletion or chronic disease states, such as decreased renal and hepatic function or electrolyte imbalance. To reduce the likelihood of orthostatic hypotension, antihypertensive medications should be started at low doses and increased cautiously. BP and pulse should be measured in the sitting and standing positions at every visit.

HYPERTENSIVE CRISIS

Hypertensive crisis is a severe and abrupt elevation in BP, arbitrarily defined as a DBP above 120 to 130 mm Hg. The rate of the rise of BP is more important than the absolute value in determining the need for emergency treatment. Prompt recognition and management of hypertensive crisis is essential to decrease the threat to organ function and life.

Hypertensive crisis occurs most commonly in patients with a history of hypertension who have failed to adhere to their prescribed medication regimen or who have been undermedicated. In this setting, rising BP is thought to trigger endothelial damage and the release of vasoconstrictor substances. A vicious cycle of BP elevation ensues, leading to life-threatening damage to target organs. Hypertensive crisis related to cocaine or crack use is becoming a more frequent occurrence. Other drugs, such as amphetamines, phencyclidine (PCP), and lysergic acid diethylamide (LSD), may also precipitate hypertensive crisis that may be complicated by drug-induced seizures, stroke, MI, or encephalopathy. Hypertensive crisis is classified by the degree of organ damage and the rapidity with which the BP must be lowered. *Hypertensive emergency,* which develops over hours to days, is a situation in which a patient's BP is severely elevated, with evidence of acute target-organ damage, especially damage to the central nervous system. Hypertensive emergencies include hypertensive encephalopathy, intracranial or subarachnoid hemorrhage, acute left ventricular failure with pulmonary edema, MI, renal failure, and dissecting aortic aneurysm. *Hypertensive urgency,* which develops over days to weeks, is a situation in which a patient's BP is severely elevated but there is no clinical evidence of target-organ damage.

Clinical Manifestations

A hypertensive emergency may be manifested as *hypertensive encephalopathy,* a syndrome in which a sudden rise in BP is associated with headache, nausea, vomiting, seizures, confusion, stupor, and coma. Other common manifestations are blurred vision and transient blindness. The manifestations of encephalopathy are probably the results of cerebral edema and spasms of cerebral vessels.

Renal insufficiency ranging from minor impairment to complete renal shutdown may occur. Rapid cardiac decompensation, ranging from unstable angina to infarction and pulmonary edema, is also possible with associated chest pain and dyspnea. Aortic dissection causes excruciating chest and back pain, often accompanied by diaphoresis and the loss of pulses in an extremity.

Patient assessment is extremely important, especially monitoring for signs of neurological dysfunction, retinal damage, heart failure, pulmonary edema, and renal failure. The neurological manifestations are often similar to the presentation of a stroke. However, a hypertensive crisis does not show the focal or lateralizing signs often seen with a stroke.

NURSING AND INTERPROFESSIONAL MANAGEMENT HYPERTENSIVE CRISIS

BP level alone is a poor indicator of the seriousness of the patient's condition and is not the major factor in deciding the treatment for a hypertensive crisis. The association between elevated BP and signs of new or progressive end-organ damage (e.g., cerebrovascular, cardiac, retinal, or renal involvement) determines the seriousness of the situation.

Hypertensive emergencies necessitate hospitalization, parenteral administration of antihypertensive medications, and critical care monitoring. Generally, the initial treatment goal is to decrease mean arterial pressure (MAP) 10 to 20% in the first 1 to 2 hours, with further gradual reduction over the next 24 hours. Lowering the BP too far or too fast may decrease cerebral perfusion and could precipitate a stroke. A patient who has aortic dissection, unstable angina, or signs of MI must have the SBP lowered to 100 to 120 mm Hg as quickly as possible.

The intravenous (IV) medications used for hypertensive emergencies include vasodilators (e.g., sodium nitroprusside, nitroglycerin, diazoxide [Proglycem], hydralazine hydrochloride [Apresoline]), adrenergic inhibitors (e.g., phentolamine mesylate [Rogitine], labetalol [Trandate], esmolol hydrochloride [Brevibloc]), and the ACE inhibitor enalapril (Vasotec). Sodium nitroprusside is the most effective parenteral medication for the treatment of hypertensive emergencies. Oral agents may be administered in addition to the parenteral medications to help make an earlier transition to long-term therapy. The mechanisms of action and the adverse effects of these medications are shown in Table 35.8.

Administered intravenously, the medications have a rapid (within seconds to minutes) onset of action. The patient's BP and pulse should be taken every 2 to 3 minutes during the initial administration of these medications. The use of an arterial line (see Chapter 68) or an automated BP monitoring machine (e.g., Dynamap) to monitor the BP is ideal. The rate of medication administration is titrated according to the level of BP. It is important to prevent hypotension and its effects in a person whose body has adjusted to hypertension. An excessive reduction in BP may cause stroke, MI, or visual changes. Frequently, continual ECG monitoring is done to observe for cardiac dysrhythmias. Extreme caution needs to be exercised in treating

the patient with coronary artery disease or cerebrovascular insufficiency. Hourly urinary output should be measured to assess renal perfusion. Careful monitoring of vital signs and urinary output provides information regarding the effectiveness of these medications and the patient's response to therapy. Patients receiving IV antihypertensive medications may be restricted to bed; getting up (e.g., to use the commode) may cause severe cerebral ischemia and fainting.

Regular, ongoing assessment is essential to evaluate the patient with severe hypertension. Frequent neurological checks, including level of consciousness, pupillary size and reaction, movement of extremities, and reactions to stimuli, help in detecting any changes in the patient's condition. Cardiac, pulmonary, and renal systems should be monitored for decompensation caused by the severe elevation in BP (e.g., pulmonary edema, heart failure, angina, renal failure).

Hypertensive urgencies usually do not require IV administration of medications but can be managed with oral agents. The patient with a hypertensive urgency may not need hospitalization but requires frequent follow-up. The oral medications most frequently used for hypertensive urgencies are captopril and clonidine (Catapres) (see Table 35.8). The disadvantage of oral medications is the inability to regulate the dosage from moment to moment, as can be done with IV medications. If a patient with hypertensive urgency is not hospitalized, outpatient follow-up should be arranged within 24 hours.

A patient with severe elevation of BP but without target-organ damage may not require emergent medication therapy or hospitalization. Allowing the patient to sit for 20 or 30 minutes in a quiet environment may significantly reduce BP. Oral medications may then be instituted or adjusted. Additional nursing interventions include encouraging the patient to verbalize fears, answering questions concerning the hypertension, and eliminating excess noise in the patient's environment.

Once the hypertensive crisis is resolved, it is important to determine the cause. The patient will need appropriate management and extensive education to avoid future crises.

CASE STUDY

Primary Hypertension

Patient Profile

F. W. (pronouns he/him), 45 years old, has no previous history of hypertension. At a screening clinic, his BP was found to be 180/120 mm Hg.

Subjective Data

- Father died of stroke at age 60
- Mother is alive but has type 2 diabetes
- States that he feels fine and is not a "hyper" person
- Smokes one pack of cigarettes daily
- Drinks a six-pack of beer on Friday and Saturday nights
- Does not enjoy physical activity
- Has had type 2 diabetes for 5 years and is nonadherent to his diabetic treatment plan
- Has been told that some medications interfere with sexual relationships

Objective Data

Physical Examination

- Moderately obese
- Sustained apical impulse palpable in the fourth intercostal space, just lateral to the midclavicular line

Diagnostic Studies

- ECG: left ventricular hypertrophy

- Urinalysis: protein 0.3 g/L
- Serum creatinine level: 141 mmol/L

Interprofessional Care

- Low-sodium diet
- Hydrochlorothiazide (HCTZ) 12.5 mg daily PO
- Enalapril sodium (Vasotec) 5 mg daily PO

Discussion Questions

1. What risk factors for hypertension does F. W. have?
2. What evidence of target-organ damage is present?
3. What misconceptions about hypertension should be corrected?
4. What are the nursing priorities for F. W.? What resources are available to assist in promoting health for F. W.?
5. **Priority decision:** Based on the assessment data presented, what are the priority nursing diagnoses? Are there any interprofessional issues? How will they affect F. W.'s treatment?
6. **Evidence-informed practice:** F. W. wants to know the most effective nonpharmacological strategies to lower BP. What should the nurse tell him?

ℯvolve

Answers are available at http://evolve.elsevier.com/Canada/Lewis/medsurg.

REVIEW QUESTIONS

The number of the question corresponds to the same-numbered objective at the beginning of the chapter.

1. Which BP-regulating mechanism(s) can result in the development of hypertension if defective? *(Select all that apply.)*
   a. Release of norepinephrine
   b. Secretion of prostaglandins PGE_2 and PGI_2
   c. Stimulation of the sympathetic nervous system
   d. Stimulation of the parasympathetic nervous system
   e. Activation of the renin–angiotensin–aldosterone system

2. While obtaining subjective assessment data from a client with hypertension, the nurse recognizes which of the following as a modifiable risk factor for the development of hypertension?
   a. Hyperlipidemia
   b. Excessive alcohol intake
   c. A family history of hypertension
   d. Consumption of a high-carbohydrate, high-calcium diet

3. The nurse includes which of the following ideas in teaching a client with hypertension about controlling the condition?
   a. All clients with elevated BP require medication.
   b. It is not necessary to limit salt in the diet if taking a diuretic.
   c. People with obesity must achieve a normal weight in order to lower BP.
   d. Lifestyle modifications are indicated for all people with elevated BP.

4. What is a major consideration in the management of an older person with hypertension?
   a. Prevent pseudohypertension from converting to true hypertension.
   b. Recognize that older people are less likely to adhere to the medication therapy than younger adults.
   c. Ensure that the client receives larger initial doses of antihypertensive medications because of impaired absorption.
   d. Use careful technique in assessing the BP of the client because of the possible presence of an auscultatory gap.

5. A client with newly diagnosed hypertension has a blood pressure of 158/98 mm Hg after 12 months of exercise and diet modifications. How does the nurse advise the client?
   a. Medication may be required because the BP is still not within the normal range.
   b. Continued monitoring of the BP every 3 to 6 months is all that will be necessary for treatment.
   c. Because lifestyle modifications were not effective, they do not need to be continued and medications will be used.
   d. The client will have to make more vigorous changes in lifestyle if the client wants to stay off medication for hypertension.

6. A patient is admitted to the hospital in hypertensive emergency (BP 244/142 mm Hg). Sodium nitroprusside is started to treat the elevated BP. Which management strategy or strategies would be appropriate for this patient? *(Select all that apply.)*
   a. Measuring hourly urine output
   b. Decreasing the MAP by 50% within the first hour
   c. Continuous BP monitoring with an intra-arterial line
   d. Maintaining bed rest and providing sedation to lower the BP
   e. Assessing the patient for signs and symptoms of heart failure and changes in mental status

1. a, c, e; 2. b; 3. d; 4. d; 5. a; 6. a, c, e.

ⓔvolve

For even more review questions, visit http://evolve.elsevier.com/Canada/Lewis/medsurg.

REFERENCES

Anand, S. S., Abonyi, S., Arbour, L., et al. (2019). Explaining the variability in cardiovascular risk factors among First Nations communities in Canada: A population-based study. *The Lancet Planetary Health, 3*(12), e511–e520.

Canadian Diabetes Association Clinical Practice Guidelines Expert Committee. (2013). Clinical practice guidelines: Treatment of hypertension. *Canadian Journal of Hypertension, 37*(2013), S117–S118. www.canadianjournalofdiabetes.com/article/S1499-2671%2813%2900034-8/pdf

DeGuire, J., Clarke, J., Rouleau, K., et al. (2019). *Blood pressure and hypertension.* https://www150.statcan.gc.ca/n1/pub/82-003-x/2019002/article/00002-eng.htm

Heart and Stroke Foundation. (2018). *Stroke report.* https://www.heartandstroke.ca/what-we-do/media-centre/stroke-report. (Seminal).

Hypertension Canada. (2021). *What can I do: Limiting salt intake.* https://hypertension.ca/hypertension-and-you/managing-hypertension/what-can-i-do/#limiting-salt-intake

Leung, A. A., Daskalopoulou, S. S., Dasgupta, K., et al. (2017). Hypertension Canada's 2017 guidelines for diagnosis, risk assessment, prevention, and treatment of hypertension in adults. *Canadian Journal of Cardiology, 33*(5), 557–576. https://doi.org/10.1016/j.cjca.2017.03.005

Manosroi, W., & Williams, G. H. (2019). Genetics of human primary hypertension: Focus on hormonal mechanisms. *Endocrine Reviews, 40*(3), 825–856. https://doi.org/10.1210/er.2018-00071

Nerenberg, K., Zamke, K., Leung, A., et al. (2018). Hypertension Canada's 2018 Guidelines for diagnosis, risk, assessment, prevention, and treatment of hypertension in adults and children. *Canadian Journal of Cardiology, 34*, 506–525. https://doi.org/10.1016/j.cjca.2018.02.022

Oparil, S., Acelajado, M. C., Bakris, G. L., et al. (2018). Hypertension. *Nature Reviews Disease Primers, 4*(18014). https://doi.org/10.1038/nrdp.2018.14

Padwal, R. S., Bienek, A., McAlister, F. A., et al. (2015). Epidemiology of hypertension in Canada: An update. *Canadian Journal of Cardiology.* https://doi.org/10.1016/j.cjca.2015.07.734. (Seminal).

Patel, R. S., Masi, S., & Taddei, S. (2017). Understanding the role of genetics in hypertension. *European Heart Journal 28*(29), 2309-2312. https://doi.org/10/1093/euheartj/ehx273

Public Health Agency of Canada (PHAC). (2018). *Report from the Canadian Chronic Disease Surveillance System: Heart disease in Canada.* 2018. https://www.canada.ca/en/public-health/services/publications/diseases-conditions/report-heart-disease-Canada-2018.html

Rabi, D. M., McBrien, K. A., Sapir-Pichhadze, R., et al. (2020). Hypertension Canada's 2020 comprehensive guidelines for the prevention, diagnosis, risk assessment, and treatment of hypertension in adults and children. *Canadian Journal of Cardiology, 36*(5), 596–624. https://doi.org/10.1016/j.cjca.2020.02.086

Schiffrin, E. L., Campbell, N. R. C., Feldman, R. D., et al. (2016). Hypertension in Canada: Past, present, and future. *Annals of Global Health, 82*(2), 288–289. https://doi.org/10.1016/j.aogh.2016.02.006

Tobe, S. W., Gilberg, R. E., Jones, C., et al. (2018). Treatment of hypertension. *Canadian Journal of Diabetes, 42*(1), S186–S189. https://doi.org/10.1016/j.jcjd.2017.10.011

World Health Organization (WHO). (2012). *Sodium intake for adults and children.* https://www.who.int/elena/titles/guidance_summaries/sodium_intake/en/

World Health Organization (WHO). (2020). *Salt reduction.* https://www.who.int/en/news-room/fact-sheets/detail/salt-reduction

World Health Organization (WHO). (2021a). *Cardiovascular diseases (CVDs): Key facts.* https://www.who.int/news-room/fact-sheets/detail/cardiovascular-diseases-(cvds)

World Health Organization (WHO). (2021b). *Hypertension: Key facts.* https://www.who.int/news-room/fact-sheets/detail/hypertension

RESOURCES

Health Canada—*Sodium in Canada*
https://www.canada.ca/en/health-canada/services/food-nutrition/healthy-eating/sodium.html

Healthy Families BC—*Sodium 101*
https://www.healthyfamiliesbc.ca/home/articles/what-is-high-sodium

Heart and Stroke Foundation of Canada
https://www.heartandstroke.ca

Heart and Stroke Foundation of Canada—*Managing Your Blood Pressure*
https://www.heartandstroke.ca/-/media/pdf-files/canada/health-information-catalogue/en-managing-your-blood-pressure.ashx?la=en&hash=96DF8F3C8D87DDFC5E0DB328E6FE2418AEC684AF

Heart and Stroke Foundation of Canada—*The DASH Diet to Lower High Blood Pressure*
https://www.heartandstroke.ca/healthy-living/healthy-eating/dash-diet

Hypertension Canada—Most recent guidelines for diagnosis, assessment, prevention, and treatment of hypertension, along with summary documents, including downloadable slide kits, are available free of charge on the website.
https://www.hypertension.ca

Hypertension Canada—*Video: Home Blood Pressure Measurement*
https://www.youtube.com/watch?v=eqajdX5XU9Y

Registered Nurses' Association of Ontario—*Best Practice Guideline: Integrating Tobacco Interventions Into Daily Practice*
https://rnao.ca/bpg/guidelines/integrating-tobacco-interventions-daily-practice

Registered Nurses' Association of Ontario—*Best Practice Guideline: Nursing Management of Hypertension*
https://rnao.ca/bpg/guidelines/nursing-management-hypertension

SCORE (Systematic COronary Risk Evaluation) Risk Charts (the SCORE risk calculator uses Canadian data)
https://www.escardio.org/Education/Practice-Tools/CVD-prevention-toolbox/SCORE-Risk-Charts

---

Myhealthcheckup—*Do you know your cardiovascular age?*
Programs that compare risk by using terms such as *cardiovascular age, vascular age,* and *heart age* have been shown to improve risk perception by patients and risk factor management by physicians.
https://myhealthcheckup.com/cvd/?lang=en

World Hypertension League
https://www.whleague.org/

(e)volve

For additional Internet resources, see the website for this book at http://evolve.elsevier.com/Canada/Lewis/medsurg.

Nursing Management

Coronary Artery Disease and Acute Coronary Syndrome

Leslie Graham
Originating US chapter by Rose Shaffer

⊖volve WEBSITE

http://evolve.elsevier.com/Canada/Lewis/medsurg

- Review Questions (Online Only)
- Key Points
- Answer Guidelines for Case Study

- Customizable Nursing Care Plan
  - Patient with Acute Coronary Syndrome
- Conceptual Care Map Creator

- Conceptual Care Map for Textbook Case Study
- Audio Glossary
- Content Updates

LEARNING OBJECTIVES

1. Describe the prevalence of heart disease in Canada.
2. Explain the etiology and the pathophysiology of coronary artery disease (CAD), angina, and acute coronary syndrome (ACS).
3. Identify risk factors for CAD and the nursing role in the promotion of therapeutic lifestyle changes for patients at risk.
4. Differentiate the precipitating factors, the clinical manifestations, and the interprofessional care and nursing management of patients with CAD and ACS.
5. Explain the clinical manifestations, complications, diagnostic study results, and interprofessional care of patients with ACS.

6. Describe the pathophysiology of myocardial infarction from the onset of injury through the healing process.
7. Evaluate medication therapy commonly used in treating patients with CAD and ACS.
8. Prioritize key components to include in the rehabilitation of patients recovering from ACS and coronary revascularization procedures.
9. Describe the precipitating factors, the clinical presentation, and the collaborative care of patients who are at risk for or have experienced sudden cardiac death.

KEY TERMS

acute coronary syndrome (ACS)
angina
atherosclerosis
chronic stable angina
collateral circulation

coronary artery disease (CAD)
coronary revascularization
myocardial infarction (MI)
NSTEMI
percutaneous coronary intervention (PCI)

Prinzmetal's angina
silent ischemia
STEMI
sudden cardiac death (SCD)
unstable angina (UA)

Heart disease is the second major cause of death in Canada, accounting for 27.5% (52 541) of all deaths in 2018 (Statistics Canada, 2021). In Canada, approximately 2.4 million adults over the age of 20 are living with heart disease, which will cost billions of health care dollars in treatment and other expenses (Canadian Institute for Health Information [CIHI], 2017). While advances have been made in the treatment of IHD with improvement with patient outcomes, the prevalence of IHD continues to increase (Public Health Agency of Canada, 2019).

Patients with coronary artery disease (CAD) can be asymptomatic or can develop chronic stable angina. Unstable angina (UA) and myocardial infarction (MI), more serious manifestations of CAD, are termed *acute coronary syndrome* (ACS). Cardiovascular disease is one of the more common reasons for

hospitalization in Canada (CIHI, 2021). Cardiovascular disease rates for Indigenous people of Canada are 50% higher than in the general Canadian population (Heart and Stroke Foundation of Canada, 2021d). The Determinants of Health box discusses culture and social status as determinants of CAD in Canada.

CORONARY ARTERY DISEASE

Coronary artery disease (CAD) is a type of blood vessel disorder that is included in the general category of atherosclerosis; it may affect the heart's arteries and produce various pathological effects, especially the reduced flow of oxygen and nutrients to the myocardium. The term *atherosclerosis* is derived from two Greek words: *athere*, meaning "fatty mush," and *skleros*, meaning "hard."

DETERMINANTS OF HEALTH

Coronary Artery Disease in Canada

- Rates of cardiovascular disease are greater in communities with poor access to health care as result of financial, geographic, cultural, social, and educational barriers.*
- Higher income through greater employment opportunities, access to quality education and health care, and social support through meaningful relationships have the potential to improve health outcomes for Indigenous people in Canada.*
- To decrease modifiable cardiovascular risk factors for Indigenous populations, culturally sensitive health care needs to be provided by local service providers to identify and treat individuals while broader community health issues are addressed.*
- The Truth and Reconciliation Commission has recommended that Canada needs "to establish measurable goals to identify and close the gaps in health outcomes between Aboriginal and non-Aboriginal communities" (p. 2).†
- Immigrants from South Asia have a higher risk for cardiovascular disease. Cardiovascular risk increases proportionally with length of stay in Canada.‡
- Members of minority and low-income populations experience a disproportionate burden of death and disability from cardiovascular disease.*

References

*Anand, S., Arbour, L., Balasubramarian, K., et al. (2019). Explaining the variability in cardiovascular risk among First Nations communities in Canada: A population-based study. *Lancet Planet Health, 3*, e511–e20. https://www.thelancet.com/action/showPdf?pii=S2542-5196%2819%2930237-2
†Truth and Reconciliation Commission of Canada, 2012. (2015). *Calls to action.* http://trc.ca/assets/pdf/Calls_to_Action_English2.pdf
‡Tu, J. V., Chu, A., Rezai, M. R., et al. (2015). Incidence of major cardiovascular events in immigrants to Ontario, Canada: The CANHEART Immigrant Study. *Circulation, 132*(16), 1549–1559. https://doi.org/10.1161/CIRCULATIONAHA.115.015345

This word combination indicates that atherosclerosis begins as soft deposits of fat that harden with age. Atherosclerosis is often referred to as "hardening of the arteries." Although this condition can occur in any artery in the body, the atheromas have a preference for the coronary arteries. *Arteriosclerotic heart disease (ASHD), cardiovascular heart disease (CVHD), ischemic heart disease,* and *coronary heart disease* are synonymous terms used to describe CAD.

ETIOLOGY AND PATHOPHYSIOLOGY

Atherosclerosis is the major cause of CAD. It is characterized by deposits of lipids within the intima of the artery. Endothelial injury and inflammation play a central role in the development of atherosclerosis.

The endothelium (the inner lining of the vessel wall) is normally nonreactive to platelets and leukocytes, as well as to coagulation, fibrinolytic, and complement factors. However, the endothelial lining can be injured as a result of tobacco use, hyperlipidemia, hypertension, toxins, diabetes, hyperhomocysteinemia, and infection causing a local inflammatory response (Huether et al., 2020) (Figure 36.1, *A*).

C-reactive protein (CRP), a protein produced by the liver, is a nonspecific marker of inflammation. It is increased in many patients with CAD (Huether et al., 2020) (see Chapter 34, Table 34.6). The level of CRP rises when there is systemic inflammation. Chronic elevations of CRP are associated with unstable plaques and the oxidation of low-density lipoprotein (LDL) cholesterol.

Developmental Stages

CAD is a progressive disease that develops over many years. By the time it becomes symptomatic, the disease process is usually well advanced. The stages of development in

Endothelium   Intima

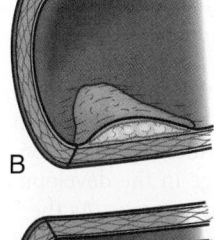

Chronic Endothelial Injury
- Hypertension
- Tobacco use
- Hyperlipidemia
- Hyperhomocysteinemia
- Diabetes
- Infections
- Toxins
- **Damaged endothelium**

A

Fatty Streak
- Lipids accumulate and migrate into smooth muscle cells

B

Fibrous Plaque
- Collagen covers the fatty streak
- Vessel lumen is narrowed
- Blood flow is reduced
- Fissures can develop

C

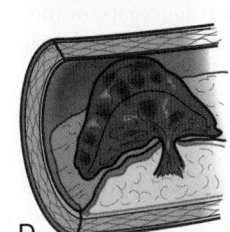

Complicated Lesion
- Plaque rupture
- Thrombus formation
- Further narrowing or total occlusion of vessel

D

FIG. 36.1 Pathogenesis of atherosclerosis. **A,** Damaged endothelium. **B,** Fatty streak and lipid core formation. **C,** Fibrous plaque. Raised plaques are visible: some are yellow; others are white. **D,** Complicated lesion: thrombus is red; collagen is blue. Plaque is complicated by red thrombus deposition.

atherosclerosis are (a) fatty streak, (b) fibrous plaque, and (c) complicated lesion.

Fatty Streak. *Fatty streaks,* the earliest lesions of atherosclerosis, are characterized by lipid-filled smooth muscle cells. As streaks of fat develop within the smooth muscle cells, a yellow tinge appears (Huether et al., 2020) (see Figure 36.1, *B*). Fatty streaks can be seen in the coronary arteries by age 15 and involve an increasing amount of surface area as a person ages. Treatment that lowers LDL cholesterol may reverse this process.

Fibrous Plaque. The *fibrous plaque* stage is the beginning of progressive changes in the endothelium of the arterial wall. These changes can appear in the coronary arteries by age 30 and increase with age.

Normally, the endothelium repairs itself immediately. However, this does not happen in people with CAD. LDLs and growth factors from platelets stimulate smooth muscle proliferation and thickening of the arterial wall. Once endothelial injury has taken place, lipoproteins (carrier proteins within the bloodstream) transport cholesterol and other lipids into the arterial intima. Collagen covers the fatty streak and forms a fibrous plaque that has a greyish or whitish appearance. These plaques can form on one portion of the artery or in a circular fashion involving the

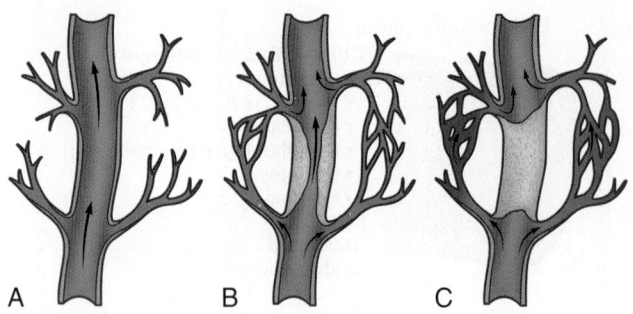

FIG. 36.2 Vessel occlusion with collateral circulation. **A,** Open, functioning coronary artery. **B,** Partial coronary artery closure with collateral circulation being established. **C,** Total coronary artery occlusion with collateral circulation bypassing the occlusion to supply the myocardium.

TABLE 36.1	RISK FACTORS FOR CORONARY ARTERY DISEASE	
Nonmodifiable Risk Factors	**Modifiable Risk Factors**
Increasing age Sex (men > women until 65 yr of age) Ethnicity (Black people > White people) Genetic predisposition and family history of heart disease	**Major** Serum lipid alterations: elevated triglyceride and LDL cholesterol levels, decreased HDL levels Blood pressure ≥140/90 mm Hg Tobacco use Physical inactivity Obesity: waist circumference ≥102 cm (40 inches) in men and ≥88 cm (35 inches) in women **Contributing** Diabetes mellitus Elevated fasting blood glucose level Psychosocial risk factors (e.g., depression, hostility and anger, stress) Elevated homocysteine levels Substance use

HDL, high-density lipoprotein; *LDL,* low-density lipoprotein.

entire lumen. The borders can be smooth or irregular with rough, jagged edges. The result is a narrowing of the vessel lumen and a reduction in blood flow to the distal tissues (see Figure 36.1, *C*).

Complicated Lesion. The final stage in the development of the atherosclerotic lesion is the most dangerous. As the fibrous plaque grows, continued inflammation can result in plaque instability, ulceration, and rupture. Once the integrity of the artery's inner wall is compromised, platelets accumulate in large numbers, leading to a thrombus. The thrombus may adhere to the wall of the artery, leading to further narrowing or total occlusion of the artery. Activation of the exposed platelets causes expression of the glycoprotein IIb/IIIa receptors that bind fibrinogen. This, in turn, leads to further platelet aggregation and adhesion, further enlarging the thrombus. At this stage, the plaque is referred to as a *complicated lesion* (see Figure 36.1, *D*).

Collateral Circulation

Normally, some arterial anastomoses or connections, termed **collateral circulation**, exist within the coronary circulation. Two factors contribute to the growth and extent of collateral circulation: (1) the inherited predisposition to develop new blood vessels *(angiogenesis)* and (2) the presence of chronic ischemia. When an atherosclerotic plaque occludes the normal flow of blood through a coronary artery and the resulting ischemia is chronic, increased collateral circulation develops (Figure 36.2). When occlusion of the coronary arteries occurs slowly over a long period, there is a greater chance that adequate collateral circulation will gradually develop, and the myocardium may continue receiving an adequate amount of blood and oxygen.

However, when CAD has a rapid onset (as in familial hypercholesterolemia) or coronary spasm occurs, there is not enough time for collateral circulation development, and the diminished arterial blood flow results in more severe ischemia or infarction.

CAD usually develops over many years, and clinical manifestations are not apparent in the early stages of the disease. Therefore, it is extremely important to identify people at risk and initiate therapeutic lifestyle changes and treatment strategies early.

RISK FACTORS FOR CORONARY ARTERY DISEASE

Many risk factors—characteristics or conditions that are statistically associated with a high incidence of a disease—have been associated with CAD. Cardiac risk factors are categorized as either *nonmodifiable* or *modifiable* (Table 36.1).

Nonmodifiable Risk Factors

Age, Sex, and Ethnicity. Genetic predisposition is an important factor in the occurrence of CAD, although the exact mechanism of inheritance is not fully understood. Some congenital

🧬 GENETICS IN CLINICAL PRACTICE

Familial Hypercholesterolemia

Genetic Basis
- Autosomal dominant disorder
- Mutation in gene coding for the LDL receptor
- Multiple mutant alleles

Incidence
- Heterozygotes: 1 per 500
- Homozygotes: rare

Genetic Testing
- Disorder characterized by elevated serum LDL level
- Serum lipid profile can be used to measure total cholesterol, triglyceride, LDL, and HDL levels
- DNA testing available

Clinical Implications
- Common genetic disease
- Leading cause of coronary artery disease
- High cholesterol levels are a result of defective function of the LDL receptors.
- Plasma levels of LDL remain elevated throughout life.
- Those affected develop severe atherosclerosis in early to middle years.

DNA, deoxyribonucleic acid; *HDL,* high-density lipoprotein; *LDL,* low-density lipoprotein.

defects in coronary artery walls predispose some people to the formation of plaques. Familial hypercholesterolemia, an autosomal dominant disorder, has been strongly associated with CAD at early ages (see the Genetics in Clinical Practice box). In most cases, patients with angina or MI can identify a parent or sibling who has died of CAD. Indigenous people have a higher incidence of cardiovascular risk factors than non-Indigenous people, which is strongly linked to lack of access to health care as well as socioeconomic factors (Anand et al., 2019)

Women differ from men in nontraditional risk factors, such as age of menarche, contraceptive use, pregnancy, and menopause. Reproductive influences such as early age of menarche or premature menopause are associated with increased risk of cardiovascular disease. Other comorbid conditions such as depression, polycystic ovary disease, breast cancer, and autoimmune disorders also increase the risk of cardiovascular disease in women (Norris et al., 2020). Indigenous women have a

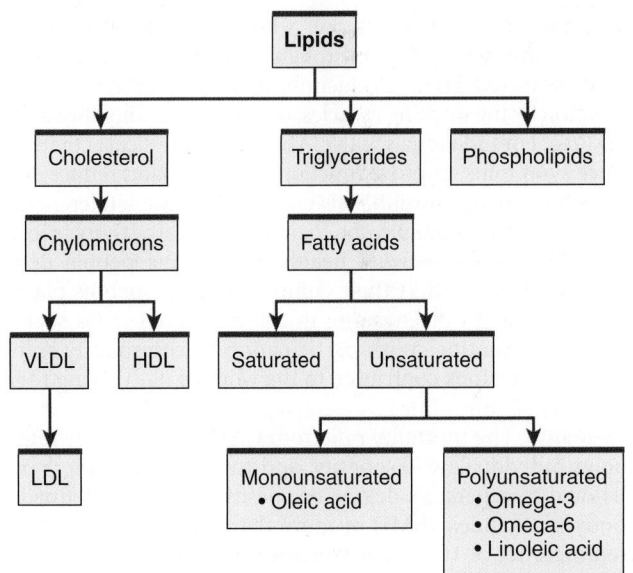

FIG. 36.3 Types of serum lipids. *HDL*, high-density lipoprotein; *LDL*, low-density lipoprotein; *VLDL*, very-low-density lipoprotein.

Who to screen

Men ≥ 40 years of age; women ≥ 50 years of age or postmenopausal (consider screening earlier in ethnic groups at increased risk, such as South Asian or Indigenous individuals);
and
all patients with any of the following conditions, regardless of age:

- Current cigarette smoking
- Diabetes
- Arterial hypertension
- Family history of premature CVD
- Family history of hyperlipidemia
- Erectile dysfunction
- Chronic kidney disease

- Inflammatory disease*
- HIV infection
- Chronic obstructive pulmonary disease
- Clinical evidence of atherosclerosis or abdominal aneurysm
- Clinical manifestation of hyperlipidemia
- Obesity (body mass index > 27)

How to screen

For all: history and examination, LDL, HDL, TG, non-HDL (will be calculated from profile), glucose, eGFR
Optional: apoB (instead of standard lipid panel), urine albumin : creatinine ratio (if eGFR < 60, hypertension, diabetes)

Framingham risk score < 5%
Repeat every 3–5 years

Framingham risk score ≥ 5%
Repeat every year

FIG. 36.4 Patients whose plasma lipid profile should be screened. *Data on inflammatory bowel diseases are lacking. *apoB*, apolipoprotein; *CVD*, cardiovascular disease; *eGFR*, estimated glomerular filtration rate; *HDL*, high-density lipoprotein; *HIV*, human immunodeficiency virus; *LDL*, low-density lipoprotein; *TG*, triglycerides. Source: Reprinted from *Journal of Cardiology, 29*(2), Anderson, T., Grégoire, J., Hegele, R., et al., Society Guidelines 2012 update of the Canadian Cardiovascular Society guidelines for the diagnosis and treatment of dyslipidemia for the prevention of cardiovascular disease in the adult, pp. 151–167, Copyright 2013, with permission from Elsevier.

higher burden of chronic disease than do Indigenous men, and they are more likely to have two chronic health conditions, such as diabetes and cardiac disease (CIHI, 2017; Diffey et al., 2019).

Major Modifiable Risk Factors

Elevated Serum Lipid Levels. As dyslipidemia is an important risk factor for the development of cardiovascular disease, the current guidelines suggest a collaborative and individualized approach to its management (Anderson et al., 2016). It is recommended that persons over 40 years of age undergo lipid screening every 5 years. Screening should be done even earlier in at-risk ethnic groups such as people of South Asian descent or Indigenous people. Earlier screening criteria are also be advised for women with a history of pregnancy-induced hypertension. For ease of access and convenience for the patient, a nonfasting blood sample for lipid and lipoprotein is considered part of a cardiovascular risk assessment. Individuals with a triglyceride level greater than 4.5 mmol/L should have lipid levels tested in a fasting state. The various types of serum lipids are presented in Figure 36.3.

Clinical practice guidelines for the diagnosis, treatment, and prevention of dyslipidemia are available (Anderson et al., 2016). The current Canadian guidelines for treating dyslipidemia include a description of patients whose plasma lipid profile should be screened (Figure 36.4) and target lipid levels associated with the risk level (Anderson et al., 2016). In addition to lipid management, the 2016 guidelines recommend smoking cessation; diet modification focusing on dietary patterns such as those in the Mediterranean, DASH, or Portfolio diets and avoiding intake of trans fats and decreased intake of saturated fats; exercise regimens that include 150 minutes of moderate to vigorous activity; stress management; and (in patients at high risk) pharmacological therapy. Statin therapy is indicated for high-risk conditions such as atherosclerosis, abdominal aortic aneurysm, diabetes mellitus, and LDL levels greater than 5.0 mmol/L to decrease the risk of developing cardiovascular disease (Anderson et al., 2016).

Hypertension. Hypertension is one of the most common chronic health condition affecting individuals across the lifespan (Rabi et al., 2020). Hypertension Canada's 2018 guidelines for diagnosis, risk assessment, prevention, and treatment of hypertension are presented in Figure 35.2 in Chapter 35.

A blood pressure (BP) is considered high when it is greater than 135/85 mmHg, depending on the method of monitoring. If the health care provider is using a manual cuff and stethoscope, hypertension is diagnosed at 140/90 mmHg (Nerenberg et al., 2018). The stress of a constantly elevated BP accelerates the rate of atherosclerotic development. The pressure in the vessel is related to the shearing stress that causes endothelial injury. Atherosclerosis, in turn, causes narrowing and thickening of the arterial walls and decreases the dispensability and elasticity of vessels. More force is required to pump blood through diseased arterial vasculature, and this increased force is reflected in a higher BP. This increased workload is also manifested by left ventricular hypertrophy and decreased stroke volume with each contraction.

Salt intake is positively correlated with elevated BP, adding volume and increasing systemic vascular resistance (SVR) to the cardiac workload. (See Chapter 35 for a complete discussion of hypertension.) Lifestyle modifications are a critical component of hypertension management. Lifestyle factors that increase risk for hypertension include obesity, dietary habits that can increase BP such as high sodium intake, low activity level, high alcohol consumption, and high stress levels (Hypertension Canada, 2018).

Tobacco Use. A third major risk factor in CAD is tobacco use. The risk of developing CAD is two to six times higher in persons who smoke tobacco or use smokeless tobacco than for those who do not. Further, tobacco smoking decreases estrogen levels, placing premenopausal women at greater risk for CAD. Risk is proportional to the number of cigarettes smoked. Changing to lower nicotine or filtered cigarettes does not affect risk.

Nicotine in tobacco smoke causes catecholamine (e.g., epinephrine, norepinephrine) release. These neurohormones cause an increased heart rate (HR), peripheral vasoconstriction, and increased BP, increasing the cardiac workload. Tobacco smoke is also related to an increase in LDL level, a decrease in high-density lipoprotein (HDL) level, and a release of toxic oxygen radicals. All of these factors add to vessel inflammation and thrombosis (Huether et al., 2020).

Carbon monoxide, a byproduct of combustion found in tobacco smoke, affects the oxygen-carrying capacity of hemoglobin by reducing the sites available for oxygen transport. This results in increased cardiac workload, combined with the oxygen-depleting effect of carbon monoxide, significantly decreasing the oxygen available to the myocardium. There is also some indication that carbon monoxide is a chemical irritant and causes injury to the endothelium.

The benefits of smoking cessation are dramatic and almost immediate. CAD mortality rates drop to those of nonsmokers within 12 months. However, nicotine is highly addictive, and often intensive intervention is required to assist people to quit. Individual and group counselling sessions, nicotine replacement therapy, smoking cessation medications (e.g., bupropion [Zyban], varenicline [Champix]), and hypnosis are examples of smoking cessation strategies. (For information on smoking cessation, see Chapter 11, Tables 11.7 and 11.8, and the Resources at the end of the chapter.)

Chronic exposure to environmental tobacco (secondhand smoke) also increases the risk for CAD (Öberg et al., 2010). People who live in the same household as the patient should be encouraged to stop smoking. By doing so, they reinforce the patient's effort and decrease the risk for ongoing exposure to environmental smoke. Pipe and cigar smokers, who often do not inhale, have an increased risk of CAD, similar to those exposed to environmental tobacco smoke. Evidence is emerging on the effects of electronic cigarettes on hemodynamic reactions, inflammatory influences, and thrombogenic effects; more research is needed on this topic (Fischer et al., 2017; MacDonald & Middlekauf, 2019).

For Indigenous people, tobacco use has great cultural significance, as tobacco is a sacred plant that is used in many Indigenous communities in ceremonies. In some communities, tobacco misuse is prevalent and has lead to chronic lung disorders in addition to cardiovascular disease (Jetty, 2017).

Physical Inactivity. Physical inactivity is the fourth major modifiable risk factor for CAD. The Heart and Stroke Foundation of Canada recommends that adults engage in a minimum of 150 minutes of moderate to vigorous physical activity each week, in increments of 10 minutes or more (Heart and Stroke Foundation of Canada, 2021e). Older people should include muscle- and bone-strengthening activities, minimally twice per week. Examples of health-promoting, regular physical activity are brisk walking, jogging, cycling, or swimming, 4 to 7 days per week (Nerenberg et al., 2018).

The mechanism by which physical inactivity predisposes a person to CAD is mostly still unknown. Physically active people have increased HDL levels and exercise improves thrombolytic activity, thus reducing the risk for clot formation. Exercise may also encourage the development of collateral circulation in the heart.

Exercise training for those who are physically inactive decreases the risk for CAD through more efficient lipid metabolism, increased HDL production, and more efficient oxygen extraction by the working muscles, thereby decreasing the cardiac workload. For individuals with CAD, regular physical activity can reduce symptoms, improve functional capacity, and reduce other risk factors, such as insulin resistance and glucose intolerance.

For Indigenous people, the focus of physical activity is intertwined with their view of health. Indigenous people define physical activity within their cultural context, such as playing traditional games or engaging in traditional activities such as fishing and hunting. With participation in community activities, all generations contribute to the work of daily living (Teng & Jardine, 2016).

Obesity. The mortality rate from CAD is statistically higher among individuals with obesity, and the risk for CAD is proportional to a person's degree of obesity. *Obesity* is defined as a body mass index (BMI) of more than 30 kg/m^2 and a waist circumference of 102 cm or larger for men and 88 cm or larger for women (Heart and Stroke Foundation of Canada, 2021c). BMI is a calculation of body fat based on height and weight that can be calculated using online resources (see the Resources section at the end of this chapter). In the past, BMI was the key indicator of health risk related to obesity, but waist circumference is now regarded as the factor that indicates the greatest health risk related to obesity (Heart and Stroke Foundation of Canada, 2021c). Persons with obesity may produce more LDLs and triglycerides, which are strongly related to atherosclerosis. Obesity is also often associated with hypertension. As well, evidence suggests that people who tend to store fat in the abdomen (i.e., have an "apple" figure) rather than in the hips and buttocks (i.e., have a "pear" figure) have a higher incidence of CAD (see Table 43.2). As obesity increases, the heart grows and uses more oxygen. In addition, there is an increase in insulin resistance in persons with obesity (Huether et al., 2020).

Obesity rates are far higher among Indigenous people in Canada than in non-Indigenous populations, owing to inequities in social determinants of health, intergenerational trauma, and food insecurity. Indigenous women are more likely than men to have obesity. Cultural regeneration, such as use of Indigenous language, and eating traditional foods are shown to be factors in decreasing obesity rates among Indigenous populations (Batal & Decelles, 2019).

Modifiable Contributing Risk Factors

Diabetes Mellitus. The incidence of CAD is two to four times greater among persons who have diabetes, even those with well-controlled blood glucose levels, than in the general population. Patients with diabetes manifest CAD not only more frequently but also at a younger age (Huether et al., 2020), with no age difference noted in the onset of symptoms between male and female patients. The presence of diabetes virtually eliminates the lower incidence of CAD in premenopausal women. Diabetes is endemic in the Indigenous population in Canada, which is among the highest-risk population to develop diabetes-related complications (Crowshow et al., 2018).

Undiagnosed diabetes is frequently discovered at the time a person has an MI. People with diabetes have an increased tendency toward endothelial dysfunction, which may account for the development of fatty streaks in these patients. Patients with diabetes also have alterations in lipid metabolism and tend to have high cholesterol and triglyceride levels. Management of diabetes should include lifestyle changes and medication therapy to achieve a glycosylated hemoglobin (A1C or Hb A1C) level of less than 7% (Pagana et al., 2019).

Metabolic Syndrome. *Metabolic syndrome* refers to a cluster of risk factors for CAD whose underlying pathophysiology may be related to insulin resistance. These risk factors include obesity as defined by large waist circumference, hypertension, abnormal serum lipids, and an elevated fasting blood glucose (Huether et al., 2020) (see Table 43.5). These interrelated risk factors of metabolic origin appear to promote the development of CAD. Higher rates of metabolic syndrome are seen in Indigenous people in Canada because of genetic factors, low socioeconomic status contributing to limited access to healthy foods and health care, and lifestyle changes (Kaler et al., 2006) (Chapter 43 discusses metabolic syndrome.)

Psychological States. The Framingham study, a multigenerational research project, provided early evidence that certain behaviours and lifestyles contribute to the development of CAD and correlate with CAD. However, the study of these behaviours remains controversial and complex. One type of behaviour, referred to as *type A,* includes perfectionism and a hardworking, driven personality. Type A people often suppress anger and hostility, feel a sense of time urgency, are impatient, and create stress and tension. These people may be more prone to MIs than people who are *type B,* characterized by being more easygoing, taking upsets in stride, knowing personal limitations, taking time to relax, and not being overachievers. However, findings from studies regarding these relationships are inconsistent (Framingham Heart Study, n.d.). Indigenous people experience large amounts of stress in their lives from a variety of sources, such as intergenerational trauma, impacts of deficient living conditions, poor health, lack of education and funding, racism both personal and systemic, as well as institutional (National Collaborating Centre for Aboriginal Health, 2011).

Studies now are focusing on specific psychological risk factors thought to increase risk for CAD. These include depression, acute and chronic stress (e.g., poverty, serving as a caregiver), anxiety, hostility, anger, and lack of social support (Heart and Stroke Foundation of Canada, 2021f). In particular, depression is a risk factor for both the development and the worsening of CAD. Patients with depression have elevated levels of circulating catecholamines that may contribute to endothelial injury and inflammation and platelet activation. Depression is also a risk factor for adverse outcomes post-ACS (Vaccarino et al., 2019). More research on the treatment of depression and other negative psychological states (e.g., anger) in patients with or at risk for CAD is needed to improve the emotional and physical health of these patients.

Stressful states correlate with the development of CAD (Hagstrom et al., 2017). Sympathetic nervous system (SNS) stimulation—and its effect on the heart—is the physiological mechanism by which stress predisposes a person to the development of CAD. SNS stimulation causes an increased release of catecholamines (e.g., epinephrine, norepinephrine). This stimulation increases HR and intensifies the force of myocardial contraction, resulting in increased myocardial oxygen demand. Also, stress-induced mechanisms can cause elevated lipid and glucose levels and changes in blood coagulation, which can lead to increased atherogenesis.

Homocysteine. High homocysteine levels in the blood have been linked to an increased risk for CAD and other cardiovascular diseases (American Heart Association, 2021; Cardosa, 2018). Homocysteine is produced by the breakdown of the essential amino acid methionine, which is found in dietary protein. High homocysteine levels possibly contribute to atherosclerosis by (a)

damaging the inner lining of blood vessels, (b) promoting plaque buildup, and (c) altering the clotting mechanism to make clots more likely to occur (see Chapter 34, Table 34.6).

Research is ongoing to determine whether a decline in homocysteine can reduce the risk for heart disease. B-complex vitamins (B_6, B_{12}, folic acid) have been shown to lower blood levels of homocysteine. Generally, a screening test for homocysteine is limited to those suspected of having elevated levels, such as older patients with pernicious anemia or people who develop CAD at an early age.

Substance Use. The use of illicit drugs, such as cocaine and methamphetamine, can produce coronary spasm resulting in myocardial ischemia and chest pain. Most people who are seen in the emergency department (ED) with drug-induced chest pain have symptoms that are initially indistinguishable from those of people with CAD. Although MI can occur, these patients more often have sinus tachycardia, high BP, angina, and anxiety (Kim & Park, 2019).

Since the legalization of cannabis for recreational use in Canada, little research has been conducted to study its effects on the cardiovascular system (Fisher et al., 2017). Some reports have linked cannabis to alterations in BP, influences on inflammation, possible arrhythmias, as well as cardiac emergencies such as MI (Heart and Stroke Foundation of Canada, 2021a).

Intergenerational trauma, as well as the historical, community, and personal trauma experienced by Indigenous peoples, has led to much of the substance misuse that is seen in Indigenous communities. There are trends of increasing substance misuse among Indigenous people, which can also be linked to long-standing disparities in the social determinants of health (Firestone et al., 2015).

Health Promotion

The appropriate management of risk factors in CAD may prevent, modify, or slow down the progression of the disease. Emphasis on prevention and early treatment of heart disease must be ongoing.

Identification of People at High Risk for Coronary Artery Disease. Clinical manifestations of CAD are not apparent in the early stages of the disease. Therefore, regardless of the health care setting, it is extremely important to identify people at risk for CAD. Risk screening involves obtaining a thorough health history that includes questioning the patient about (a) family history of heart disease in parents and siblings; (b) the presence of any cardiovascular symptoms; (c) environmental factors, such as eating habits, type of diet, and level of exercise; (d) psychosocial factors, such as tobacco use, alcohol intake, recent stressful events (e.g., loss of a spouse), and any negative psychological states (e.g., anxiety, depression, anger); and (e) the patient's place and type of employment to determine the kind of activities performed, exposure to pollutants or noxious chemicals, and the degree of stress associated with work.

Identifying the patient's attitudes and beliefs about health and illness can give some indication of how disease and lifestyle changes may affect the patient and can also reveal possible misconceptions about heart disease. Knowledge of the patient's educational background can help to determine teaching needs. If the patient is taking medications, it is important to know the names and dosages and whether the patient adheres to the medication regimen.

Management of Patients at High Risk for Coronary Artery Disease. Preventive measures should be recommended for all persons at risk for CAD. Risk factors such as age, sex, ethnicity,

TABLE 36.2	**PATIENT & CAREGIVER TEACHING GUIDE**

Decreasing Risk Factors for Coronary Artery Disease

Risk Factor	Health-Promoting Behaviours
Hypertension	• Monitor BP and report when greater than 140/90 mm Hg or as discussed with health care provider. • Take prescribed medications for BP control. • Take in no more than 2 300 mg of sodium per day. • Never smoke, or stop smoking. • Control or reduce weight to healthy BMI of 18.5 to 24.9. • Exercise regularly to meet targets of 150 min of moderate to vigorous exercise in bouts of 10 min each week.
Elevated serum lipids	• Reduce total fat intake. • Reduce animal (saturated) fat intake. • Adjust total caloric intake to achieve and maintain ideal body weight. • Engage in a regular exercise program. • Increase amount of complex carbohydrates and vegetable proteins in diet. • Consider Mediterranean, DASH, or Portfolio patterns of eating.
Smoking*	• Enroll in a program to stop smoking. • Change daily routines associated with smoking to reduce desire to smoke. • Substitute other activities for smoking. • Ask family members to support efforts to stop smoking.
Physical inactivity	• Develop and maintain routine for physical activity that is done at least three or four times a week. • Increase activities to a level compatible with physical fitness.
Stressful lifestyle	• Increase awareness of behaviours that are detrimental to health. • Alter patterns that are conducive to stress reduction (e.g., get up 30 min earlier so that breakfast is not eaten on the way to work). • Set realistic goals for yourself. • Reassess priorities in view of health needs. • Learn effective coping strategies. • Avoid excessive and prolonged stress. • Plan time for adequate rest and sleep.
Obesity	• Change eating patterns and habits. • Reduce caloric intake for weight reduction. • Exercise regularly to increase caloric expenditure. • Avoid fad and crash diets, which are not effective over the long term. • Avoid large, heavy meals.
Diabetes mellitus†	• Follow the recommended diet. • Reduce weight and control diet. • Monitor blood glucose levels regularly.

BP, blood pressure.

*See Registered Nurses' Association of Ontario. (2017). *Nursing Best Practices Guideline: Integrating smoking cessation into daily nursing practice.* http://rnao.ca/bpg/guidelines/integrating-smoking-cessation-daily-nursing-practice.

†See Chapter 52 for additional health-promoting behaviours.

and genetics cannot be modified. However, people with these risk factors can still reduce their risk for CAD by controlling the additive effects of modifiable risk factors. For example, a young man with a family history of heart disease can decrease his risk by maintaining an ideal body weight, getting adequate physical exercise, reducing intake of saturated fats, and avoiding tobacco use.

Nurses can play a major role in teaching health-promoting behaviours and in encouraging patients who have modifiable risk factors to make lifestyle changes to reduce their risk

for CAD (Table 36.2). First, the nurse should assist patients in clarifying personal values and beliefs for goal-setting purposes. When health care plans are based on patient goals, there is an increased likelihood that the patient will engage in risk-modifying behaviours. Highly motivated people may simply need to know how to reduce their risk in order to get started. For people who are less motivated to take charge of their health, the idea of reducing risk factors may be so remote that they are unable to perceive a threat of CAD. Few people want to make lifestyle changes, especially in the absence of symptoms. First, the nurse should assist these patients in clarifying their personal values. Then, by explaining the risk factors, the nurse may help them recognize their susceptibility to CAD. This information may help patients set realistic goals and enable them to choose which risk factor(s) to change first. Some people are reluctant to make changes until they begin to manifest overt symptoms or actually suffer an MI. Others, having suffered an MI, may find the idea of changing lifelong habits still unacceptable. The nurse can help them identify such choices and then needs to respect their final decision.

Physical Activity. A physical activity program should be designed to improve physical fitness by following the FITT formula: **f**requency (how often), **i**ntensity (how hard), **t**ime (how long), and **t**ype (isotonic). Everyone should aim for at least 150 minutes of moderate to vigorous activity each week (Anderson et al., 2016). This would include 30 to 60 minutes of moderate to vigorous activity, 4 to 7 days per week. In addition, adding weight training to an exercise program 2 days a week can help treat metabolic syndrome and improve muscle strength. Examples of moderate physical activity include brisk walking, hiking, biking, and swimming. Regular physical activity contributes to weight reduction, a reduction in systolic BP, and, in men more than in women, an increase in HDL cholesterol. The American Heart Association (AHA) has developed a program to encourage people, especially women, to increase their daily physical activity. (See the Resources at the end of this chapter.)

In Canada, the interest in attaining and maintaining health has made physical activity a field of major importance. Communities are developing or promoting exercise programs, such as aerobic exercise classes and cardiac walking and jogging groups, for people of all ages and with varying health needs. Local YMCAs often sponsor jogging, bicycling, swimming, and related courses. Many shopping malls open their doors in the early morning to allow people to walk indoors. The Heart and Stroke Foundation of Canada organizes many events that emphasize the need for physical activity in the promotion of health. Many large corporations provide gymnasiums in which their employees can exercise. For many people, running may be inadvisable; however, these people should be encouraged to pursue walking, swimming, or whatever exercise will accommodate their individual physical abilities (Canadian Society of Exercise Physiology, 2021)

Nutritional Therapy. The Heart and Stroke Foundation of Canada recommends eating a healthy, balanced diet to improve one's heart health and lower cardiovascular risk; potential benefits of such a diet include decreasing cholesterol levels, reducing BP, and maintaining a healthy weight (Heart and Stroke Foundation of Canada, 2021b). Heart-healthy choices include decreasing intake of saturated fats and cholesterol and increasing intake of complex carbohydrates (e.g., whole grains, fruit, vegetables) and fibre (Anderson et al., 2018; Heart and Stroke

TABLE 36.3 NUTRITIONAL THERAPY
Therapeutic Lifestyle Changes in Diet

Nutrient	Recommended Daily Intake
Total fat (includes saturated fat calories)	25–35% of total daily calories
Saturated fat	<7% of total daily calories
Cholesterol	<200 mg
Plant stanols or sterols (e.g., margarines, nuts, seeds, legumes, vegetable oils)*	2 g
Dietary fibre*	10–25 g of soluble fibre
Total calories	Only enough calories to reach or maintain a healthy weight
Physical activity	At least 150 min per week of a moderate-intensity physical activity (e.g., brisk walking) in bouts of 10 min

*Diet options for additional lowering of low-density lipoprotein (LDL).
Source: Anderson, T. J., Gregoire, J., Pearson, G. J., et al. (2016). 2016 Canadian Cardiovascular Society guidelines for the management of dyslipidemia for the prevention of cardiovascular disease in the adult. *Canadian Journal of Cardiology, 32*(11), 1263–1282. https://doi.org/10.1016/j.cjca.2016.07.510.

Foundation of Canada, 2021b) (Tables 36.3 and 36.4). Dietary patterns such as the Mediterranean, Portfolio, or DASH diets are examples of ways to lower LDL levels and maintain a healthy body weight (Anderson et al., 2018). Fat intake should account for about 30% of calories, with most coming from mono- and polyunsaturated fats (Figure 36.5). Red meat, egg yolks, and whole-milk products are major sources of saturated fat and cholesterol and should be reduced or eliminated from the diet. If a person's serum triglyceride level is elevated, the guidelines recommend reducing or eliminating alcohol intake and simple sugars.

Omega-3 fatty acids, when eaten regularly, reduce the risks associated with CAD. For individuals without CAD, the AHA recommends eating fatty fish such as salmon and tuna twice a week as it contains two types of omega-3 fatty acids: eicosapentaenoic acid (EPA) and docosahexaenoic acid (DHA). Patients with CAD are encouraged to take EPA and DHA supplements with their diet. The AHA also recommends eating tofu and other forms of soybean, canola, walnut, and flaxseed because these products contain alpha-linolenic acid, which becomes omega-3 fatty acid in the body. (For more information on the AHA's nutritional recommendations, see its website, listed in the Resources at the end of this chapter.)

Lifestyle changes, including eating a low–saturated fat, high-fibre diet, avoiding tobacco, and increasing physical activity, can promote the reversal of CAD and reduce coronary events.

Cholesterol-Lowering Medication Therapy
Statins are a pharmacological intervention indicated for individuals considered to be at high risk of developing cardiovascular disease. Conditions such as atherosclerosis, abdominal aneurysm, diabetes, chronic kidney disease, and elevated serum lipids require statins treatment (Anderson et al., 2016). A complete lipid profile should be obtained every 5 years, beginning at age 40 for men and 50 for women. The lipid profile should be checked more often if the individual has CAD or diabetes. A person with a serum cholesterol level exceeding 5.2 mmol/L is at risk for CAD and should be treated.

The Canadian guidelines for treatment focus on LDL levels (Figure 36.6). Treatment usually begins with smoking cessation, dietary caloric restriction (if overweight), decreased dietary fat

TABLE 36.4 NUTRITIONAL THERAPY
Tips to Implement Diet and Lifestyle Recommendations

General Tips
- Know your caloric needs to achieve and maintain a healthy weight.
- Know the calorie content of the foods and beverages you consume.
- Track your weight, physical activity, and caloric intake.
- Prepare and eat smaller, more frequent meals.
- Track your activities and, whenever possible, decrease sedentary activities (e.g., television watching, computer time).
- Incorporate physical movement into daily activities (e.g., take extra steps when possible).
- If you consume alcohol, do so in moderation (i.e., no more than two drinks for women or three drinks for men a day).

Tips Related to Food Choices and Preparation
- Use the Nutrition Facts panel on food labels and ingredients list when choosing foods to buy.
- Select frozen and canned vegetables and fruits without high-calorie sauces or added salt and sugars.
- Replace high-calorie foods with fresh fruits and vegetables.
- Increase fibre intake by eating beans (legumes), whole-grain products, fruits, and vegetables.
- Use liquid vegetable oils in place of solid fats.
- Limit beverages and foods high in added sugars (e.g., sucrose, glucose, fructose, maltose, dextrose, corn syrups, concentrated fruit juice, honey).
- Choose foods made with whole grains (e.g., whole wheat, oats/oatmeal, rye, barley, corn, popcorn, brown rice, wild rice, buckwheat, cracked wheat, sorghum).
- Eliminate pastries and high-calorie bakery products (e.g., muffins, doughnuts).
- Select milk and dairy products that are either fat free or low fat.
- Reduce salt intake by:
  - Comparing the sodium content of similar products (e.g., different brands of tomato sauce) and choosing products with less sodium
  - Choosing versions of processed foods that are reduced in salt, including cereals and baked goods
  - Limiting condiments (e.g., soy sauce, ketchup)
- Use lean cuts of meat and remove skin from poultry before cooking or eating.
- Avoid processed meats that are high in saturated fat and sodium (e.g., deli meats).
- Grill, bake, or broil fish, meat, and poultry.
- Incorporate vegetable-based meat substitutes into favourite recipes (e.g., soy).
- Consume whole vegetables and fruits in place of juices.

Source: Adapted from Heart and Stroke Foundation of Canada. (2020). *Healthy eating.* https://www.heartandstroke.ca/get-healthy/healthy-eating.

and cholesterol intake, increased physical activity, and stress management (Anderson et al., 2016). Serum cholesterol levels are reassessed after 6 months of diet therapy. If they remain elevated, additional dietary options or medication therapy may be started (Table 36.5).

Medications That Restrict Lipoprotein Production. The *statin* medications (e.g., lovastatin, pravastatin [Pravachol], simvastatin [Zocor], atorvastatin [Lipitor], and rosuvastatin [Crestor]) are the most widely used and studied lipid-lowering medications. These medications inhibit the synthesis of cholesterol in the liver by blocking 3-hydroxy-3-methylglutaryl coenzyme A (HMG-CoA) reductase. An unexplained result of the inhibition of cholesterol synthesis is an increase in hepatic LDL receptors. Consequently, the liver is able to remove more LDLs from the blood. Serious adverse effects of these medications can include liver damage and myopathy that can progress to rhabdomyolysis (breakdown of skeletal muscle), but these are rare.

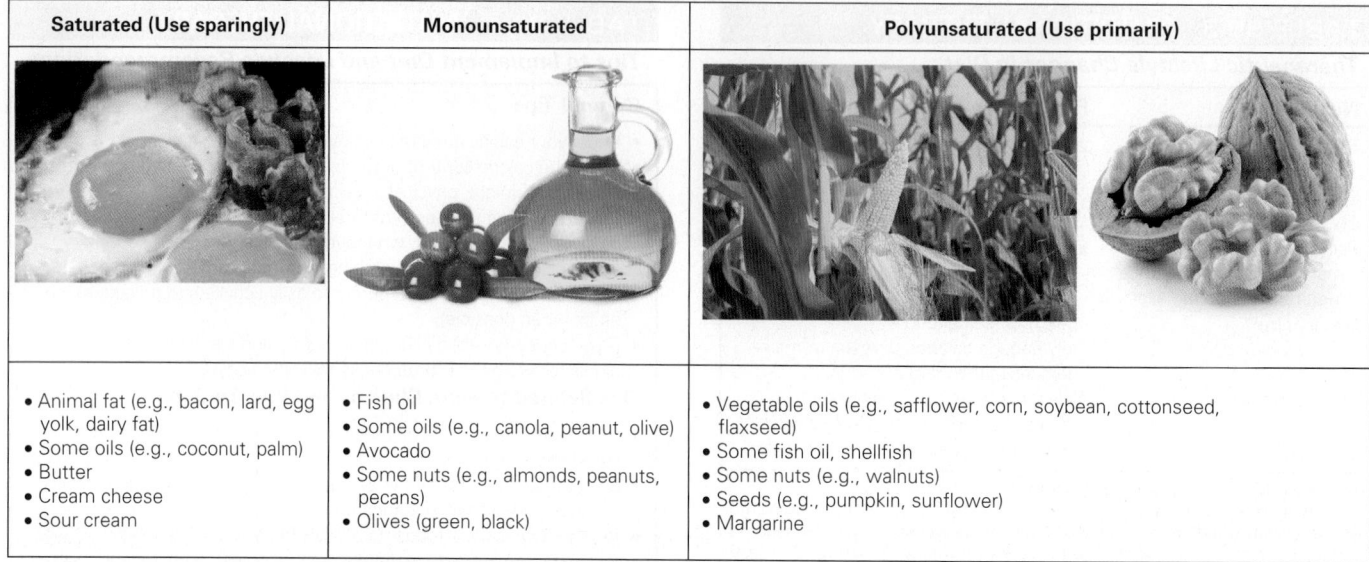

Saturated (Use sparingly)	Monounsaturated	Polyunsaturated (Use primarily)
• Animal fat (e.g., bacon, lard, egg yolk, dairy fat) • Some oils (e.g., coconut, palm) • Butter • Cream cheese • Sour cream	• Fish oil • Some oils (e.g., canola, peanut, olive) • Avocado • Some nuts (e.g., almonds, peanuts, pecans) • Olives (green, black)	• Vegetable oils (e.g., safflower, corn, soybean, cottonseed, flaxseed) • Some fish oil, shellfish • Some nuts (e.g., walnuts) • Seeds (e.g., pumpkin, sunflower) • Margarine

FIG. 36.5 Types of dietary fat. Source: Photos © *(left to right):* iStock.com/onlyyouqj; iStock.com/angelsimon; iStock.com/kowit1982; iStock.com/Tim UR.

Liver enzymes (e.g., aspartate aminotransferase, alanine aminotransferase) must be monitored regularly and checked any time dosage is increased. Creatine kinase (CK) enzymes are assessed if symptoms of myopathy (e.g., muscle aches, weakness) occur (Ward et al., 2019).

Medications That Increase Lipoprotein Removal. The major process of cholesterol elimination begins with its conversion to bile acids in the liver. Bile acid sequestrants such as cholestyramine and colestipol (Colestid) increase conversion of cholesterol to bile acids and decrease hepatic content of total cholesterol and LDLs.

Adverse effects associated with these medications are related to palatability and a variety of upper and lower gastrointestinal (GI) symptoms, including belching, heartburn, nausea, abdominal pain, and constipation. Bile acid sequestrants may interfere with absorption of other medications (e.g., warfarin [Coumadin], thiazides, thyroid hormones, β-adrenergic blockers). Administering these medications at a different time than other medications may decrease this adverse effect (Skidmore, 2020).

Medications That Decrease Cholesterol Absorption. Medication therapy for hyperlipidemia is likely to be prolonged, perhaps continuing for a lifetime. It is essential that diet be modified in order to minimize the need for medication therapy. The patient must fully understand the rationale and goals of treatment, as well as the safety and adverse effects of lipid-lowering medication therapy (Anderson et al., 2016).

Antiplatelet Therapy

Acetylsalicylic acid (ASA; Aspirin) is recommended for most people at risk for cardiovascular disease. Low-dose ASA (81 mg) is recommended for adults 50 to 59 years old who have a calculated 10-year cardiovascular disease risk of 10% or more, are not at increased risk for bleeding (e.g., history of GI bleeding), have a life expectancy of at least 10 years, and are willing to take low-dose ASA for at least 10 years. For adults 60 to 69 years old who have a calculated 10-year cardiovascular disease risk of 10% or more, the decision to take low-dose ASA is an individual one. Adults who have no contraindications (e.g., history of stroke), have a life expectancy of at least 10 years, and are willing to take low-dose ASA daily for at least 10 years are more likely to benefit. Currently, there is insufficient evidence

to recommend low-dose ASA for persons younger than 50 or older than 70 (Wein et al., 2020).

CHRONIC STABLE ANGINA

CAD is a progressive disease, and patients may be asymptomatic for many years, or they may develop chronic but stable chest pain syndromes. When the demand for myocardial oxygen exceeds the ability of the coronary arteries to supply the heart with oxygen, myocardial ischemia occurs. Angina, or chest pain, is the clinical manifestation of reversible myocardial ischemia. Either an increased demand for oxygen or a decreased supply of oxygen can lead to myocardial ischemia (Table 36.6). The primary reason for insufficient blood flow is narrowing of coronary arteries by atherosclerosis (Huether et al., 2020).

On the cellular level, the myocardium becomes hypoxic within the first 10 seconds of coronary occlusion. With total occlusion of the coronary arteries, contractility ceases after several minutes, depriving the myocardial cells of oxygen and glucose for aerobic metabolism. Anaerobic metabolism begins, and lactic acid accumulates. Myocardial nerve fibres are irritated by the increased lactic acid and transmit a pain message to the cardiac nerves and the upper thoracic posterior nerve roots. This is known as *referred pain,* as it is interpreted to be pain in the left shoulder and arm. In ischemic conditions, cardiac cells are viable for approximately 20 minutes. With restoration of blood flow, aerobic metabolism resumes, contractility is restored, and cellular repair begins.

Chronic stable angina refers to chest pain that occurs intermittently over a long period with the same pattern of onset, duration, and intensity of symptoms, therefore having a predictable onset. When questioned (Table 36.7), some patients may deny feeling pain but instead describe a pressure or ache in the chest. It is an unpleasant feeling, often described as a "constrictive," "squeezing," "heavy," "choking," or "suffocating" sensation. Angina is rarely sharp or stabbing, and it usually does not change with position or breathing. Many people with angina experience indigestion or a burning sensation in the epigastric region. Although most of the pain experienced by people with angina is substernal, the sensation may occur in the neck or radiate to various locations, including the jaw, the shoulders,

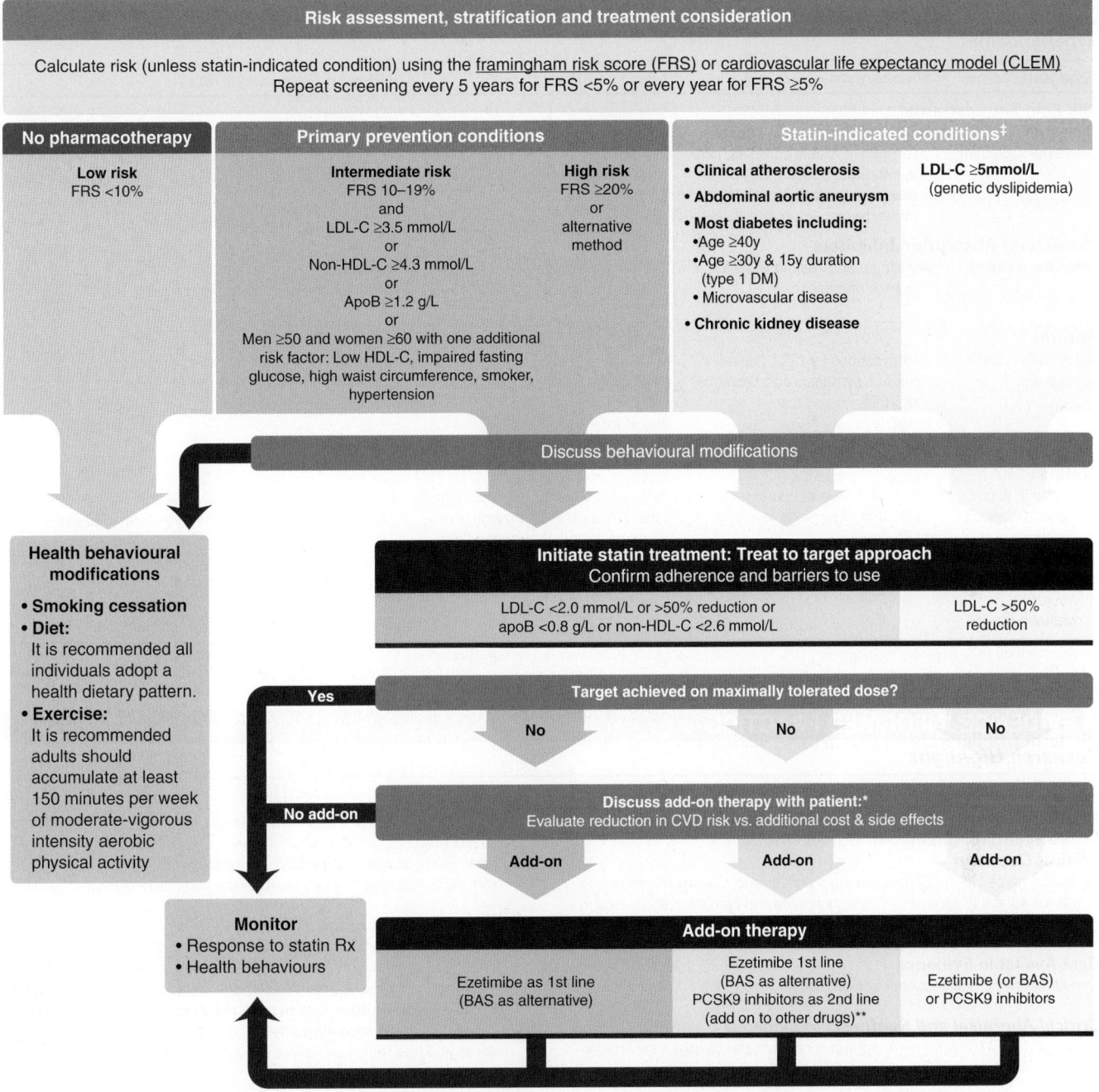

FIG. 36.6 Treatment decisions for high blood cholesterol. ‡Statins are first-line therapy but add-on or alternative therapy might be required as per the algorithm. *Consider more aggressive targets for recent ACS patients. **PCSK9 inhibitors have not been adequately studied as add-on to statins for patients with diabetes and other comorbidities. *ACS*, acute coronary syndrome; *ApoB*, apolipoprotein B; *BAS*, bile acid sequestrants; *CLEM*, Cardiovascular Life Expectancy Model; *CVD*, cardiovascular disease; *DM*, diabetes mellitus; *FRS*, Framingham Risk Score; *HDL-C*, high-density lipoprotein cholesterol; *LDL-C*, low-density lipoprotein cholesterol; *PCSK9*, proprotein convertase subtilisin kexin 9; *Rx*, prescription. Source: Anderson, T. J., Gregoire, J., Pearson, G. J., et al. (2016). 2016 Canadian Cardiovascular Society guidelines for the management of dyslipidemia for the prevention of cardiovascular disease in the adult. *Canadian Journal of Cardiology, 32*(11), 1263–1282. https://doi.org/10.1016/j.cjca.2016.07.510.

and down the arms (Figure 36.7). Sometimes the person may have pain between the shoulder blades and dismiss it as not being related to their heart.

The pain is usually brief (lasting 3 to 5 minutes) and commonly subsides when the precipitating factor is relieved (Table 36.8). Pain at rest is unusual. Electrocardiography (ECG) may reveal transient ST-segment depression, indicative of ischemia (see Chapter 38).

Chronic stable angina can be controlled with medications on an outpatient basis. Because episodes of chronic stable angina are often predictable, medications can be timed to provide peak effects during the time of day when angina is likely to occur. For example, if angina occurs on rising, the patient can take medication upon awakening and wait 30 minutes to 1 hour before engaging in activity. (The different types of angina are compared in Table 36.9.)

TABLE 36.5   MEDICATION THERAPY

Hyperlipidemia

Type and Name	Mechanism of Action	Adverse Effects	Nursing Considerations
Bile Acid Sequestrants			
Cholestyramine Colestipol (Colestid)	Binds with bile acids in intestine, forming insoluble complex, and is excreted in feces. Bile binding results in removal of LDL and cholesterol	Unpleasant gritty quality to taste GI disturbances (e.g., nausea, dyspepsia, constipation)	Effective and safe for long-term use; side effects diminish with time; interferes with absorption of digoxin, thiazides, β-adrenergic blockers, fat-soluble vitamins, folic acid, and some antibiotics (e.g., vancomycin) Monitor liver function tests
Cholesterol Absorption Inhibitors			
Ezetimibe (Ezetrol)	Acts in small intestine to inhibit uptake of cholesterol	Infrequent, but may include mild GI disturbance (e.g., diarrhea) fatigue, headache, cough	When used with a statin, further reduces LDL. Avoid use in patients with moderate to severe liver disease, and pregnant or breast-feeding persons
Fibrates			
Fenofibrate (Lipidil) Gemfibrozil	↓ Triglycerides by ↓ VLDL level ↓ Hepatic synthesis and secretion of VLDL ↑ HDL level	Mild GI disturbances (e.g., nausea, diarrhea) Myopathy Rhabdomyolysis Angioedema	May ↑ effects of anticoagulants and hypoglycemic medications Monitor liver function tests
Statins			
Atorvastatin (Lipitor) Fluvastatin (Lescol) Lovastatin Pravastatin (Pravachol) Rosuvastatin (Crestor) Simvastatin (Zocor)	Block synthesis of cholesterol ↓ LDL and triglyceride levels ↑ HDL level	Rash, mild GI disturbances, insomnia, elevated liver enzyme levels, lens opacities, rhabdomyolysis (specifically with lovastatin)	Well tolerated with few adverse effects Monitoring includes liver function tests and eye examinations Increases bleeding when concurrent use with warfarin Interactions with some antibiotics

GI, gastrointestinal; *HDL,* high-density lipoprotein; *LDL,* low-density lipoprotein; *VLDL,* very-low-density lipoprotein.

🔍 **EVIDENCE-INFORMED PRACTICE**

Research Highlight

Influence of the Workplace on Physical Activity and Cardiometabolic Health: Results of the Multi-Centre Cross-Sectional Champlain Nurses' Study

Clinical Question

To assess nurses in the Champlain region of Ontario, Canada (P), influence of the workplace (I) on overall physical activity and cardiometabolic health (C) to determine cardiovascular risk (O)

Best Available Evidence

A multi-centre, cross-sectional design study.

Critical Appraisal and Synthesis of Evidence

- Nurses (*n* = 410) wore an Actigraph accelerometer to objectively measure levels of moderate to vigorous activity documented in minutes per day.
- On average, nurses reported being overweight, being normotensive, and having a low-risk waist circumference.
- Most nurses were female and reported the following cardiovascular risk factors: poor mental health (depression and anxiety), smoking, hypertension, high cholesterol, and diabetes. Twenty-three percent of nurses met current physical activity guidelines; physical activity was most often accumulated outside of the workplace.

Conclusions

- On average, nurses in the study had lower blood pressure, cholesterol, and glucose.
- Better PWE scores resulted when nurses worked 8-hour shifts and fixed shifts resulting in more flexible hours and schedules.

Implications for Nursing Practice

- As nurses spend considerable amounts of time in the workplace, targeted interventions to reduce sedentary time should be implemented, such as promoting active breaks, reimbursement of recreation/fitness memberships, redesign of hospital flow to encourage taking the stairs, childcare for after work hours to encourage physical activity, changes to nursing schedules, as well as a shift in workplace culture to include more physical activity.

Reference for Evidence

Reed, J., Prince, S., Pipe, A., et al. (2018). Influence of the workplace on physical activity and cardiometabolic health: Results of the multi-centre cross-sectional Champlain Nurses' study. (Clinical report). *International Journal of Nursing Studies, 81,* 49–60. https://doi.org/10.1016/j.ijnurstu.2018.02.001

P, patient population of interest; *I,* intervention or area of interest; *C,* comparison of interest or comparison group; *O,* outcomes of interest (see Chapter 1); *PWE,* perceived workplace environment.

PRINZMETAL'S ANGINA

Prinzmetal's angina (also called *variant angina*) often occurs at rest, usually in response to spasm of a major coronary artery. It is a rare form of angina and occurs in many patients with a history of migraine headaches and Raynaud's phenomenon. The spasm may occur in the absence of CAD, as well as with documented disease. Prinzmetal's angina is not usually precipitated by increased physical demand. *Coronary spasm* can be described as a strong contraction of smooth muscle in the coronary artery caused by an increase in intracellular calcium.

Factors that may precipitate coronary artery spasm include increased myocardial oxygen demand and increased levels of certain substances (e.g., histamine, angiotensin, epinephrine, norepinephrine, prostaglandins, cocaine [Kim et al.,

TABLE 36.6 FACTORS DETERMINING MYOCARDIAL OXYGEN NEEDS

Decreased Oxygen Supply	Increased Oxygen Demand or Consumption
Noncardiac Factors	
Anemia	Anxiety
Hypoxemia	Cocaine use
Pneumonia	Hypertension
Asthma	Hyperthermia
Chronic obstructive pulmonary disease	Hyperthyroidism
Low blood volume	Physical exertion
Cardiac Factors	
Coronary artery spasm	Aortic stenosis
Coronary artery thrombosis	Cardiomyopathy
Dysrhythmias	Dysrhythmias
Heart failure	Tachycardia
Valve disorders	

TABLE 36.7 PQRST ASSESSMENT OF ANGINA

PQRST can be used as a mnemonic to assist in obtaining information from the patient who has chest pain, as follows:

	Factor	Questions to Ask Patient
P	Precipitating events	What events or activities precipitated the pain or discomfort (e.g., argument, exercise, resting)?
Q	Quality of pain	What does the pain or discomfort feel like (e.g., pressure, dull, aching, tight, squeezing)?
R	Radiation of pain	Where is the pain or discomfort located? Does the pain radiate to other areas (e.g., back, arms, jaw, teeth, shoulder, elbow)?
S	Severity of pain	On a scale of 0 to 10, with 10 being the most severe pain you could imagine, how would you rate the pain or discomfort?
T	Timing	When did the pain or discomfort begin? Has the pain or discomfort changed since this time? Have you had pain like this before?

TABLE 36.8 FACTORS PRECIPITATING ANGINA

Physical Exertion
- Increased HR reduces the time the heart spends in diastole (the time of greatest coronary blood flow) and results in an increase in myocardial oxygen demand.
- Isometric exercise of the arms (e.g., raking, lifting heavy objects, or shovelling snow) can cause exertional angina.

Temperature Extremes
- Workload of the heart is increased.
- Blood vessels constrict in response to a cold stimulus.
- Blood vessels dilate and blood pools in the skin in response to a hot stimulus.

Strong Emotions
- The sympathetic nervous system is stimulated.
- The workload of the heart is increased.

Consumption of Heavy Meal
- The workload of the heart may be increased.
- During the digestive process, blood is diverted to the GI system, which reduces blood flow in the coronary arteries.

Tobacco Use
- Nicotine stimulates catecholamine release, causing vasoconstriction and an increase in HR.
- Tobacco diminishes available oxygen by increasing the level of carbon monoxide.

Sexual Activity
- The cardiac workload and sympathetic stimulation are increased.
- In a person with CAD, the extra cardiac workload may precipitate angina.

Stimulants*
- HR and subsequent myocardial oxygen demand are increased.

Circadian Rhythm Patterns
- These patterns are related to the occurrence of chronic stable angina, Prinzmetal's angina, myocardial infarction, and sudden cardiac death.
- Manifestations of CAD tend to occur in the early morning after the patient awakens.

CAD, coronary artery disease; *GI*, gastrointestinal; *HR*, heart rate.
*For example, cocaine and amphetamines.

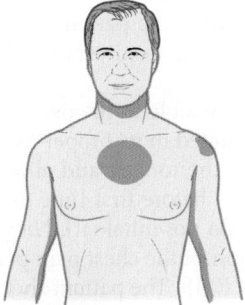

- Midsternal
- Left shoulder and down both arms
- Neck and arms

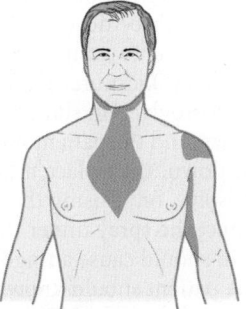

- Substernal radiating to neck and jaw
- Substernal radiating down left arm

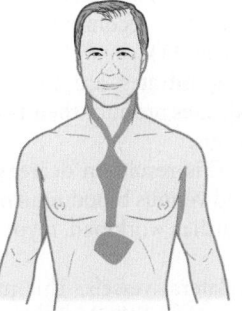

- Epigastric
- Epigastric radiating to neck, jaw, and arms

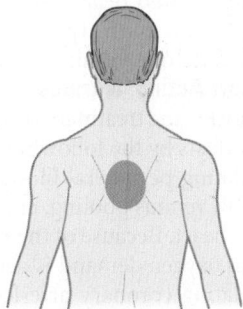

- Intrascapular

FIG. 36.7 Common locations of pain during angina or myocardial infarction.

TABLE 36.9	COMPARISON OF MAJOR TYPES OF ANGINA	
Type	**Etiology**	**Characteristics**
Chronic stable angina	Myocardial ischemia, usually secondary to CAD	• Episodic pain lasting 5–15 min • Provoked by exertion • Relieved by rest or nitroglycerin
Prinzmetal's angina	Coronary vasospasm	• Occurs primarily at rest • Triggered by smoking and increased levels of some substances (e.g., histamine, epinephrine, cocaine) • May occur in presence or absence of CAD
Microvascular angina	Myocardial ischemia secondary to microvascular disease affecting the small, distal branches of the coronary arteries	• More common in women • Triggered by activities of daily living (e.g., shopping, work), not physical exercise (exertion) • Treatment may include nitroglycerin
Unstable angina	Rupture of thickened plaque, exposing thrombogenic surface	• New-onset angina • Chronic stable angina that increases in frequency, duration, or severity • Occurs at rest or with minimal exertion • Pain refractory to nitroglycerin

CAD, coronary artery disease.

2019]). When spasm occurs, the patient experiences angina, and the ECG demonstrates transient ST-segment elevation (see Chapter 38). The pain may occur during rapid eye movement (REM) sleep, when myocardial oxygen consumption increases. The pain may be relieved by moderate exercise, or it may disappear spontaneously. Cyclic, short bursts of pain at a consistent time each day may also occur with this type of angina. It is usually treated with calcium channel blockers, nitrates, or both.

INTERPROFESSIONAL MANAGEMENT

The treatment of chronic stable angina is aimed at decreasing oxygen demand, increasing oxygen supply, or both. Continued emphasis on the reduction of risk factors is a priority and should include those strategies discussed for patients with CAD. In addition to antiplatelet and cholesterol-lowering medication therapy, the most common therapeutic intervention for the management of chronic stable angina is the use of nitrate therapy to enhance coronary blood flow (Table 36.10, Figure 36.8).

Medication Therapy

Medication therapy for chronic stable angina is aimed at preventing MI and death and reducing symptoms. Acetylsalicylic acid (ASA; Aspirin) (previously discussed) is recommended in the absence of contraindications (Table 36.11).

Short-Acting Nitrates. Short-acting nitrates are first-line therapy for the treatment of angina. Nitrates produce their principal effects by the following mechanisms:

1. Dilating peripheral blood vessels. This results in decreased SVR, venous pooling, and decreased venous blood return to the heart. Because of the reduced cardiac workload, myocardial oxygen demand is decreased.
2. Dilating coronary arteries and collateral vessels. This may increase blood flow to the ischemic areas of the heart. However, when the coronary arteries are severely atherosclerotic, coronary dilation is difficult to achieve.

Sublingual   Nitroglycerin. Nitroglycerin   administered sublingually (Nitrostat) or by translingual spray (Nitrolingual) usually relieves pain in approximately 3 minutes, and its action has a duration of approximately 30 to 60 minutes.

TABLE 36.10	MAJOR TREATMENT ELEMENTS OF CHRONIC STABLE ANGINA
	Strategies for the patient with chronic stable angina should address all of the treatment elements in the *ABCDEF* mnemonic:
A	Antiplatelet agent Antianginal therapy ACE inhibitor*
B	β-Adrenergic blocker Blood pressure
C	Cigarette smoking Cholesterol
D	Diet Diabetes
E	Education Exercise
F	Flu vaccination*

ACE, angiotensin-converting enzyme.
*Source: Smith, S., Benjamin, E., Bonow, R., et al. (2011). *AHA/ACCF secondary prevention and risk reduction therapy for patients with coronary and other atherosclerotic vascular disease: 2011 Update.* http://circ.ahajournals.org/content/124/22/2458.

The recommended dosage for symptoms of angina is one tablet taken sublingually (SL) or one metered spray. If symptoms are unchanged or worse, dosage is repeated every 5 minutes to total of three doses in 15 minutes, then the patient should be instructed to contact the emergency medical services (EMS) system (Skidmore, 2020).

Nitroglycerin should be easily accessible to the patient at all times, and the patient must be instructed in its proper use: first, sit down, then place a tablet under the tongue and allow it to dissolve, or, if using the spray, prime before first time use, and direct the spray under the tongue (do not inhale it). Nitroglycerin should cause a tingling sensation. If the chest pain persists, the patient should know to contact EMS. The patient should be warned that the HR may increase and a pounding headache, dizziness, or flushing may occur. The patient should be advised against quickly rising to a standing position because orthostatic hypotension may occur after nitroglycerin use. Patients must be cautioned not to mix erectile dysfunction products (i.e., sildenafil) with nitrates as the reaction may produce intractable hypotension and death (Skidmore, 2020).

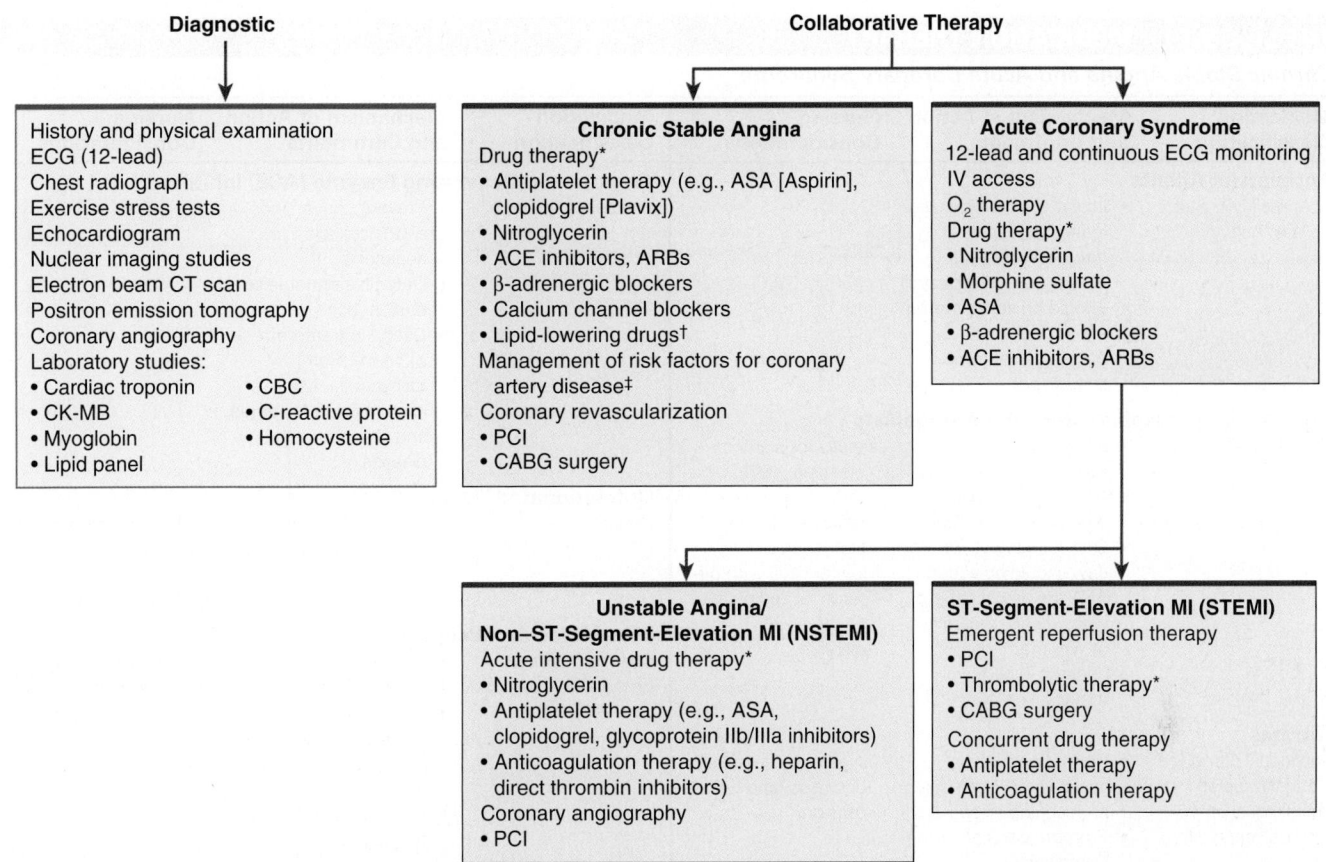

Diagnostic

History and physical examination
ECG (12-lead)
Chest radiograph
Exercise stress tests
Echocardiogram
Nuclear imaging studies
Electron beam CT scan
Positron emission tomography
Coronary angiography
Laboratory studies:
• Cardiac troponin   • CBC
• CK-MB   • C-reactive protein
• Myoglobin   • Homocysteine
• Lipid panel

Collaborative Therapy

Chronic Stable Angina
Drug therapy*
• Antiplatelet therapy (e.g., ASA [Aspirin],
  clopidogrel [Plavix])
• Nitroglycerin
• ACE inhibitors, ARBs
• β-adrenergic blockers
• Calcium channel blockers
• Lipid-lowering drugs†
Management of risk factors for coronary
  artery disease‡
Coronary revascularization
• PCI
• CABG surgery

Acute Coronary Syndrome
12-lead and continuous ECG monitoring
IV access
O_2 therapy
Drug therapy*
• Nitroglycerin
• Morphine sulfate
• ASA
• β-adrenergic blockers
• ACE inhibitors, ARBs

**Unstable Angina/
Non–ST-Segment-Elevation MI (NSTEMI)**
Acute intensive drug therapy*
• Nitroglycerin
• Antiplatelet therapy (e.g., ASA,
  clopidogrel, glycoprotein IIb/IIIa inhibitors)
• Anticoagulation therapy (e.g., heparin,
  direct thrombin inhibitors)
Coronary angiography
• PCI

ST-Segment-Elevation MI (STEMI)
Emergent reperfusion therapy
• PCI
• Thrombolytic therapy*
• CABG surgery
Concurrent drug therapy
• Antiplatelet therapy
• Anticoagulation therapy

FIG. 36.8 Interprofessional care: chronic stable angina and acute coronary syndrome. *See Table 36.11. †See Table 36.5. ‡See Tables 36.2, 36.3, and 36.4. *ACE*, angiotensin-converting enzyme; *ARBs,* angiotensin II receptor blockers; *ASA,* acetylsalicylic acid; *CABG,* coronary artery bypass graft; *CBC,* complete blood cell count; *CK-MB,* creatine kinase, muscle and brain; *CT,* computed tomography; *ECG,* electrocardiogram; *IV,* intravenous; *O2,* oxygen; *PCI,* percutaneous coronary intervention.

Nitroglycerin tablets are marketed in light-resistant bottles with metal caps and, for protection from degradation, should be kept in the tightly closed bottle. Because they tend to lose potency once a bottle has been opened, the patient should be advised to purchase a new supply every 6 months.

Long-Acting Nitrates. Nitrates, such as isosorbide dinitrate and isosorbide mononitrate (Imdur), are longer acting than SL or translingual nitroglycerin and can be used to reduce the incidence of anginal attacks. The predominant adverse effect of all nitrates is headache, caused by the dilation of cerebral blood vessels. Patients can be advised to take acetaminophen (Tylenol) with their nitrate to relieve the headache. Over time, the headaches may decrease, but the principal antianginal effect remains the same.

Orthostatic hypotension is a complication of all nitrates. Nurses should monitor BP after the initial dose because the venous dilation that occurs may cause a drop in BP, especially in volume-depleted patients. In addition, tolerance to nitroglycerin-induced vasodilation can develop. It is recommended that patients schedule an 8-hour nitrate-free period every day, usually during the night, except for patients who experience nocturnal angina (Sole et al., 2017).

Transdermal Controlled-Release Nitrates. Currently, a system provides for a slow delivery of transdermal nitroglycerin through a polymer matrix. These systems allow for slow release of nitroglycerin over 24 hours. These preparations may be removed in the evening to allow for a 10- to 14-hour nitrate-free interval to reduce the risk for nitroglycerin tolerance.

β-Adrenergic Blockers. β-Adrenergic blockers (e.g., propranolol [Inderal], metoprolol [Lopressor], and atenolol [Tenormin]), are the preferred medications for the management of chronic stable angina. These medications cause decreases in myocardial contractility, HR, SVR, and BP, all of which reduce the myocardial oxygen demand. β-Adrenergic blockers also have been shown to decrease morbidity and mortality in patients with CAD, especially following MI (Skidmore, 2020).

β-Adrenergic blockers have many adverse effects and are sometimes poorly tolerated. Adverse effects may include bradycardia, hypotension, wheezing, and GI complaints. Many patients also experience weight gain, depression, and sexual dysfunction. β-Adrenergic blockers should be avoided by patients with asthma and used with caution by patients with diabetes because their effects mask signs of hypoglycemia. Abrupt discontinuation of β-adrenergic blockers may precipitate an increase in the frequency and intensity of angina attacks, so medical supervision during discontinuation is necessary.

Calcium Channel Blockers. If use of β-adrenergic blockers is contraindicated or if they are poorly tolerated or do not control anginal symptoms, calcium channel blockers (e.g., verapamil, diltiazem [Cardizem]) are used. These medications are also used to manage Prinzmetal's angina. Most of these medications are available in sustained-release formulations for longer action, which has the advantages of helping increase patient adherence to therapy and of stabilizing blood levels of the medication. The three primary effects of calcium channel blockers

TABLE 36.11 MEDICATION THERAPY

Chronic Stable Angina and Acute Coronary Syndrome

Medication Classification	Mechanism of Action and Comments	Nursing Considerations
Antiplatelet Agents		
Acetylsalicylic acid (ASA; Aspirin)	• Inhibit cyclo-oxygenase (which produces thromboxane A_2, a potent platelet activator) • Should be administered as soon as acute coronary syndrome is suspected	
Adenosine Diphosphate Receptor Antagonists		
Clopidogrel (Plavix)	• Inhibit platelet aggregation • Alternative for patient who cannot use ASA • Oral clopidogrel, 75 mg/day, should be added to ASA therapy in patients with STEMI, regardless of whether they undergo reperfusion therapy	Assess for signs of bleeding, stroke, thrombocytopenia, renal dysfunction, and fever. Monitor CBC with differential and platelet count, serum bilirubin.
Nitrates		
Sublingual nitroglycerin (Nitrostat) Translingual spray nitroglycerin (Nitrolingual) Transdermal nitroglycerin (Transderm-Nitro, Minitran) Extended-release buccal tablets mononitrate (Imdur) IV nitroglycerin (Nitroject)	• Promote peripheral vasodilation, decreasing preload and afterload • Promote coronary artery vasodilation	Assess for headache, dizziness, and hypotension.
β-Adrenergic Blockers*		
Atenolol (Tenormin) Esmolol (Brevibloc) Metoprolol (Lopressor) Propranolol (Inderal)	• Inhibit sympathetic nervous stimulation of the heart • Reduce both heart rate and contractility • Decrease afterload	Monitor apical heart rate and BP prior to administration. Assess for hypotension, dizziness, and signs of heart failure (dyspnea, crackles, weight gain, peripheral edema).
Calcium Channel Blockers*		
Amlodipine (Norvasc) Diltiazem (Cardizem) Felodipine (Plendil) Verapamil (Isoptin)	• Prevent calcium entry into vascular smooth muscle cells and myocytes (cardiac cells) • Promote coronary and peripheral vasodilation • Reduce both heart rate and contractility	Monitor BP and pulse prior to administration. Monitor ECG. Assess for signs of heart failure (dyspnea, peripheral edema, crackles).

Medication Classification	Mechanism of Action and Comments	Nursing Considerations
Angiotensin-Converting Enzyme (ACE) Inhibitors*		
Enalapril (Vasotec)	• Prevent conversion of angiotensin I to angiotensin II • Decrease endothelial dysfunction • Useful in treatment of heart failure, tachycardia, MI, hypertension, diabetes, and chronic kidney disease	
Unfractionated Heparins†		
Heparin	• Prevent conversion of fibrinogen to fibrin and of prothrombin to thrombin	Monitor for signs of bleeding (bleeding gums, epistaxis, black tarry stools).
Low-Molecular-Weight Heparins†		
Dalteparin (Fragmin) Enoxaparin (Lovenox)	• Bind to antithrombin III, enhancing its effect • Heparin–antithrombin III complex inactivates activated factor X and thrombin • Prevent conversion of fibrinogen to fibrin	Monitor for signs of bleeding.
Glycoprotein IIB and IIIA Inhibitors		
Eptifibatide (Integrilin) Tirofiban (Aggrastat)	• Prevent binding of fibrinogen to platelets, thereby blocking platelet aggregation • Standard antiplatelet therapy in combination with ASA for patients at high risk for unstable angina	Monitor for signs of bleeding.
Opioid Analgesics		
Morphine, morphine sulphate	• Function as analgesic and sedative • Act as vasodilator to reduce preload and myocardial O_2 consumption	Monitor respiratory rate; assess for respiratory depression, CNS depression, and hypotension.
Fibrinolytic Therapy		
Alteplase (Activase) Tenecteplase (TNK, TNKase)	• Break up fibrin meshwork in clots • Used only in STEMI	Monitor for signs of bleeding. Monitor for intracranial bleeding.

BP, blood pressure; *CBC*, complete blood cell count; *CNS*, central nervous system; *ECG*, electrocardiogram; *IV*, intravenous; *MI*, myocardial infarction; *O₂*, oxygen; *STEMI*, ST-segment elevation myocardial infarction.
*See Chapter 35, Table 35.8.
†See Chapter 40, Table 40.10.

are (1) systemic vasodilation with decreased SVR, (2) decreased myocardial contractility, and (3) coronary vasodilation.

Cardiac muscle and vascular smooth muscle cells are more dependent on extracellular calcium than are skeletal muscles and are therefore more sensitive to calcium channel blockers. Calcium channel blockers cause smooth muscle relaxation and relative vasodilation of coronary and systemic arteries, thus increasing blood flow.

Calcium channel blockers potentiate the action of digoxin by increasing serum digoxin levels during the first week of therapy. Therefore, serum digoxin levels should be closely monitored after starting this therapy. The patient should be taught the signs and symptoms of digoxin toxicity, such as disorientation, blurred vision, yellow-green halos, nausea, and vomiting (Skidmore, 2020).

Angiotensin-Converting Enzyme Inhibitors. Certain high-risk patients with chronic stable angina may benefit from the addition of an angiotensin-converting enzyme (ACE) inhibitor (e.g., ramipril) to the medication regimen. Such patients include those with diabetes, significant CAD as determined by coronary angiography (e.g., multivessel disease), or previous history of MI with left ventricular dysfunction (Burchum & Rosenthal, 2016.) (ACE inhibitors are discussed further later in this chapter and in Chapter 35 and Table 35.8.)

Diagnostic Studies

When a patient has a history of CAD or if CAD is suspected, the health care provider orders a variety of studies (see Figure 36.8). After a detailed health history is documented and a physical examination is performed, a chest radiograph is usually taken to look for cardiac enlargement, aortic calcifications, and pulmonary congestion. A 12-lead ECG is obtained and, when possible, compared with an earlier tracing. Certain laboratory tests (e.g., lipid profile) and diagnostic studies (e.g., Holter monitoring, echocardiography) are ordered to confirm CAD and identify specific risk factors for CAD.

For patients with known CAD and chronic stable angina, common diagnostic studies include 12-lead ECG, echocardiography, exercise stress testing, pharmacological nuclear imaging, and coronary angiography (Pagana et al., 2019). (See Chapter 34 and Table 34.6 for a discussion of these studies, including nursing considerations.) Electrocardiography and coronary angiography are discussed in further detail in the section Diagnostic Studies of the Cardiovascular System in Chapter 34.

ACUTE CORONARY SYNDROME

When myocardial ischemia is prolonged and not immediately reversible, acute coronary syndrome (ACS) develops. This syndrome encompasses the spectrum of unstable angina, non–ST-segment elevation myocardial infarction (NSTEMI), and ST-segment elevation myocardial infarction (STEMI). Although each remains a distinct diagnosis, this nomenclature (ACS) reflects the relationships among pathophysiology, diagnosis, prognosis, and interventions for these disorders.

ETIOLOGY AND PATHOPHYSIOLOGY

ACS is associated with deterioration of an atherosclerotic plaque that was once stable. The plaque ruptures, exposing the intima to blood, stimulating platelet aggregation and local vasoconstriction with thrombus formation. This unstable lesion may be partially occluded by a thrombus (manifesting as UA or NSTEMI) or totally occluded by a thrombus (manifesting as STEMI). What causes a coronary plaque to suddenly become unstable is not well understood, but systemic inflammation (described earlier) is thought to play a role. Patients with suspected ACS require immediate hospitalization.

MANIFESTATIONS OF ACUTE CORONARY SYNDROME

Unstable Angina

Chest pain that is new in onset, occurs at rest, or has a worsening pattern is called unstable angina (UA). Patients with chronic stable angina may develop UA, or UA may be the first clinical manifestation of CAD. Unlike chronic stable angina, UA is unpredictable and represents an emergency. Patients with previously diagnosed chronic stable angina describe a significant change in the pattern of angina. It occurs with increasing frequency and is easily provoked by minimal or no exertion, during sleep, or even at rest. Patients without previously diagnosed angina describe anginal pain that has progressed rapidly in the past few hours, days, or weeks, often culminating in pain at rest.

Women with symptoms of UA seek medical attention more often than do men. Studies have shown that women have prodrome symptoms that are early manifestations of CAD, but because they are not recognized as such, what brings these women to first seek care is UA, before CAD is diagnosed. These symptoms include fatigue, shortness of breath, indigestion, and anxiety. Fatigue is the most prominent symptom. Because fatigue can be a symptom of many different diseases and syndromes, a thorough history of CAD risk factors should be obtained to identify these women (Heart and Stroke Foundation of Canada, 2021g).

MYOCARDIAL INFARCTION

A myocardial infarction (MI) occurs as a result of sustained ischemia, causing irreversible myocardial cell death (Figure 36.9). Between 80 and 90% of all acute MIs occur secondary to thrombus formation. When a thrombus develops, perfusion to the myocardium distal to the occlusion is halted, resulting in necrosis. Contractile function of the heart stops in the necrotic areas. The degree of altered function depends on the area of the heart involved and the size of the infarction. Most MIs involve some portion of the left ventricle.

The acute MI process takes time. Cardiac cells can withstand ischemic conditions for approximately 20 minutes before cellular death begins. The tissue to become ischemic earliest is the subendocardium (the innermost layer of tissue in the cardiac muscle). If ischemia persists, the entire thickness of the heart muscle becomes necrotic in approximately 5 to 6 hours.

Descriptions of infarctions are usually based on the location of damage (e.g., anterior, inferior, lateral, or posterior wall infarction). Damage can occur in more than one location (e.g., anterolateral MI, anteroseptal MI). The location of the infarction correlates with the involved coronary circulation. For example, inferior wall infarctions result from occlusions in the right coronary artery. Anterior wall infarctions result from occlusions in the left anterior descending artery. Occlusions in the left circumflex artery usually cause MIs in the lateral or posterior wall or both.

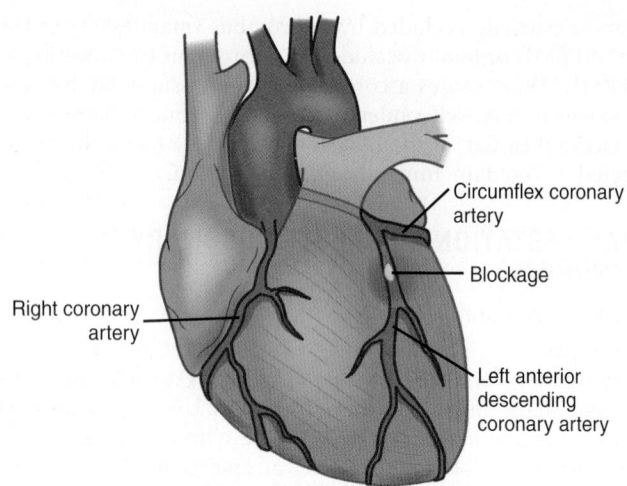

FIG. 36.9 Diagram of occlusion of the left anterior descending coronary artery, resulting in a myocardial infarction.

The degree of pre-established collateral circulation also influences the severity of infarction (see Figure 36.2). In an individual with a history of CAD, collateral circulation may be well established, so the area surrounding the infarction site develops a blood supply. This is one explanation for why a younger person who has an MI often experiences more serious impairment than an older person with the same degree of occlusion.

Clinical Manifestations of Myocardial Infarction

Pain. Severe, immobilizing chest pain not relieved by rest, position change, or nitrate administration is the hallmark of an MI. Persistent and unlike any other pain, it is usually described as a feeling of heaviness, pressure, tightness, burning, or constriction or as a crushing sensation. Common locations are substernal, retrosternal, and epigastric areas. The pain may radiate to the neck, the jaw, and the arms or to the back (see Figure 36.7). It may occur while the patient is active or at rest or when the patient is asleep or awake. However, it commonly occurs in the early morning hours. It usually lasts for 20 minutes or more and is described as more severe than usual anginal pain. When epigastric pain is present, the patient may relate it to indigestion and take antacids without relief.

Not everyone has classic symptoms. Some patients may not experience pain but may have "discomfort," weakness, or shortness of breath. Although symptoms of an acute MI in women and men have more similarities than differences, some women may experience atypical discomfort, shortness of breath, or fatigue. Patients with diabetes are more likely to experience silent (asymptomatic) MIs as a result of neuropathy and seek care with atypical symptoms (e.g., dyspnea). Older patients may experience a change in mental status (e.g., confusion), shortness of breath, pulmonary edema, dizziness, or a dysrhythmia.

Sympathetic Nervous System Stimulation. During the initial phase of MI, catecholamines (norepinephrine and epinephrine) are released from the ischemic myocardial cells that normally contain varying quantities of these substances. The increased SNS stimulation results in release of glycogen, diaphoresis, and vasoconstriction of peripheral blood vessels. On physical examination, the patient's skin may be ashen, clammy, and cool to the touch.

Cardiovascular Manifestations. In response to the release of catecholamines, the BP and HR may initially be elevated. Later,

the BP may drop because of decreased cardiac output (CO). If the patient experiences profound hypotension, renal perfusion and urine output may decrease. Crackles may be noted in the lungs, persisting for several hours to several days and suggesting left ventricular dysfunction. Jugular venous distension, hepatic engorgement, and peripheral edema may indicate right ventricular dysfunction.

Cardiac examination may reveal abnormal heart sounds that may seem distant. Careful auscultation may reveal a third heart sound (S_3) or fourth heart sound (S_4) suggestive of ventricular dysfunction. In addition, a loud holosystolic murmur may develop and may indicate a septal defect or mitral valve dysfunction.

Nausea and Vomiting. Nausea and vomiting can result in some patients due to reflex stimulation of the vomiting centre by the severe pain. These symptoms can also result from vasovagal reflexes initiated in the area of the infarcted myocardium.

Fever. The patient's temperature may increase within the first 24 hours up to 38°C and occasionally as high as 39°C. The temperature elevation may last for as long as 1 week. This increase in temperature is a systemic manifestation of the inflammatory process caused by myocardial cell death.

Healing Process

The body's response to cell death is the inflammatory process (see Chapter 14). Within 24 hours, leukocytes infiltrate the area. Enzymes are released from the dead cardiac cells and are important diagnostic indicators of MI. (See the section Serum Cardiac Markers later in this chapter.) The proteolytic enzymes of the neutrophils and macrophages remove all necrotic tissue by the second or third day, leaving the necrotic muscle wall very thin. The development of collateral circulation improves areas of poor perfusion and may limit the zones of injury and infarction. Once infarction takes place, catecholamine-mediated lipolysis and glycogenolysis occur. These processes allow the increased amounts of plasma glucose and free fatty acids to be used by the oxygen-depleted myocardium for anaerobic metabolism. For this reason, serum glucose levels are frequently elevated after MI.

The necrotic zone is identifiable by ECG changes (e.g., ST-segment elevation, pathological Q wave) and on nuclear scanning after the onset of symptoms. At this point, the neutrophils and monocytes have cleared the necrotic debris from the injured area, and the collagen matrix that will eventually form scar tissue is laid down.

Ten to 14 days after MI, the scar tissue beginning to form is still weak. The myocardium is considered to be especially vulnerable to increased stress because of the unstable state of healing within the heart wall. It is also at this time that the patient's activity level may be increasing, and so special caution and assessment are necessary. By 6 weeks after MI, scar tissue has replaced necrotic tissue. At this time, the injured area is said to be healed. The scarred area is often less malleable than the surrounding fibres. This condition may be manifested by uncoordinated wall motion, ventricular dysfunction, or pump failure.

These changes in the infarcted muscle also cause changes in the unaffected myocardium. In an attempt to compensate for the infarcted muscle, the normal myocardium hypertrophies and dilates. This process is called *ventricular remodelling*. Remodelling of normal myocardium can lead to the development of late heart failure, especially in individuals with atherosclerosis of other coronary arteries, an anterior MI, or both.

Complications of Myocardial Infarction

Dysrhythmias. The most common complication after an MI is a dysrhythmia, which is present in 80% of patients who have had an MI. Dysrhythmias are the most common cause of death in patients in the prehospitalization period. Dysrhythmias are caused by any condition that affects the myocardial cell's sensitivity to nerve impulses, such as ischemia, electrolyte imbalances, and SNS stimulation. The intrinsic rhythm of the heartbeat is disrupted, causing a fast HR *(tachycardia),* a slow HR *(bradycardia),* or an irregular beat, any of which adversely affects the ischemic myocardium.

Life-threatening dysrhythmias occur most often with anterior wall infarction, HF, or shock. A massive infarction can lead to a complete heart block. Ventricular fibrillation, a common cause of sudden cardiac death (SCD), is a lethal dysrhythmia that most often occurs within the first few hours after the onset of pain. As result of ischemia, cardiac cells lack oxygen and become depolarized, causing an alteration in impulse formation or conduction. Premature ventricular contractions (PVCs) may precede ventricular tachycardia and fibrillation. Life-threatening ventricular dysrhythmias must be treated immediately. (See Chapter 38 for a detailed description of dysrhythmias and their management.)

Heart Failure. Heart failure (HF) is a complication of MI in which the pumping action of the heart has diminished. Depending on the severity and extent of the injury, HF occurs initially with subtle signs such as mild dyspnea, restlessness, agitation, or slight tachycardia. Other signs indicating the onset of HF include pulmonary congestion, seen on chest radiograph; S_3 or S_4 heart sounds, heard on auscultation; crackles, heard on auscultation of breath sounds; and jugular vein distension, caused by right-sided HF (Sole et al., 2017). (The treatment of acute decompensated HF is discussed in Chapter 37.)

Cardiogenic Shock. Cardiogenic shock is a condition in which inadequate oxygen and nutrients are supplied to the tissues because of severe left ventricular failure. Cardiogenic shock has occurred less often since the advent of early and rapid treatment of MI with fibrinolytic therapy and percutaneous coronary intervention (PCI), an intervention in which a catheter equipped with an inflatable balloon tip is inserted into a narrowed coronary artery and the balloon is inflated. The rate of mortality from cardiogenic shock is high. Cardiogenic shock necessitates aggressive management, including control of dysrhythmias, intra-aortic balloon pump (IABP) counterpulsation therapy to maintain perfusion, and vasoactive medications to improve contractility. The goal of therapy is to maximize oxygen delivery, reduce oxygen demand, and prevent complications such as acute kidney injury (Urden et al., 2018). (Cardiogenic shock is discussed in Chapter 69.)

Papillary Muscle Dysfunction. Papillary muscle dysfunction may occur if the infarcted area includes or is adjacent to the papillary muscle that attaches to the mitral valve (see Chapter 34, Figure 34.2). Papillary muscle dysfunction causes mitral valve regurgitation, which increases the volume of blood in the left atrium. This condition aggravates an already compromised left ventricle by reducing CO even further. Papillary muscle dysfunction is detected by a systolic murmur at the cardiac apex radiating toward the axilla.

Papillary muscle rupture is a rare but life-threatening complication that causes massive mitral valve regurgitation, which results in dyspnea, pulmonary edema, and decreased CO. The patient's condition deteriorates rapidly. Treatment consists of rapid afterload reduction with a medication such as nitroprusside, IABP counterpulsation therapy, and immediate open-heart surgery with mitral valve replacement, or both (Urden et al., 2018). (See Chapter 39 for discussion of valvular disorders.)

Ventricular Aneurysm. Ventricular aneurysm results when the infarcted myocardial wall becomes thinned and bulges during contraction. The patient with a ventricular aneurysm may experience refractory HF, dysrhythmias, and angina. Besides ventricular rupture, which is fatal, ventricular aneurysms harbour thrombi, which can cause an embolic stroke.

Pericarditis. Acute *pericarditis*—an inflammation of the visceral or parietal pericardium or both—may result in cardiac compression, decreased ventricular filling and emptying, and HF. It may occur 2 to 3 days after an acute MI as a common complication. Pericarditis is characterized by chest pain, which may vary from mild to severe, and is aggravated by inspiration, coughing, and movement of the upper body. The pain may be relieved by sitting in a forward position. The pain is usually different from the pain associated with an MI.

Assessment of a patient with pericarditis may reveal a friction rub over the pericardium. The sound may be best heard with the diaphragm of the stethoscope at the midsternal to lower sternal border. It may be persistent or intermittent. Fever may also be present.

Diagnosis of pericarditis can be made with serial 12-lead ECGs. Characteristic ECG changes are diffuse and reflect the inflammation of the pericardium. Treatment may include pain relief by ASA, corticosteroids, or nonsteroidal anti-inflammatory drugs (NSAIDs). (Pericarditis is discussed further in Chapter 39.)

Dressler's Syndrome. Dressler's syndrome is characterized by pericarditis with effusion and fever that develops 4 to 6 weeks after MI. It may also occur after open-heart surgery. It is thought to be caused by an antigen–antibody reaction to the necrotic myocardium. The patient experiences pericardial pain, fever, a friction rub, pleural effusion, and arthralgia. Laboratory findings include an elevated white blood cell count and an elevated sedimentation rate. Short-term courses of corticosteroids are used to treat this condition. (Dressler's syndrome is discussed further in Chapter 39.)

DIAGNOSTIC STUDIES

Unstable Angina and Myocardial Infarction

In addition to the patient's history of pain, risk factors, and health history, the primary diagnostic studies used to determine whether a person has UA or an MI include an ECG and measurement of serum cardiac markers (see Figure 36.8).

Electrocardiographic Findings. ECG is the primary tool to rule out or confirm UA or an MI. Changes in the QRS complex, the ST segment, and the T wave caused by ischemia and infarction can develop quickly with UA and MI. Whenever possible, it should be compared to a previous ECG recording. Changes in the QRS complex, ST segment, and T wave caused by injury, ischemia, and infarction can develop slowly or quickly with UA and MI. The pattern of the ECG changes among the 12 leads provides information on which of the coronary arteries is involved.

For diagnostic and treatment purposes, it is important to distinguish among STEMI, UA, and NSTEMI. Patients with STEMI tend to have more extensive damage associated with prolonged and complete coronary occlusion and the development of ST

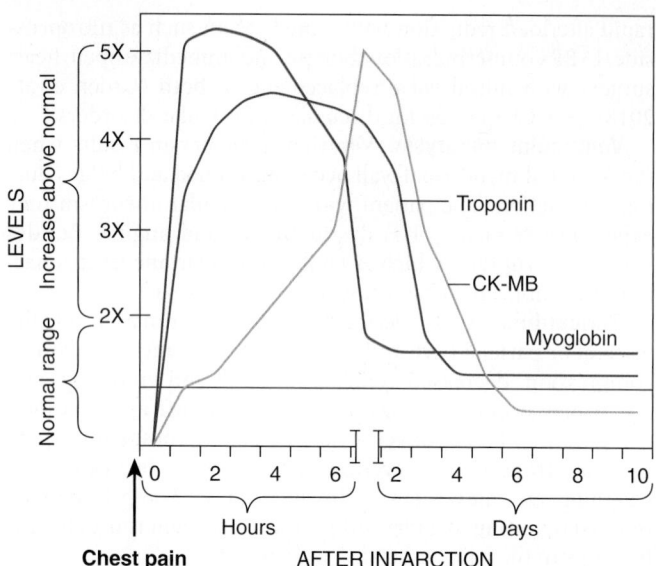

FIG. 36.10 Levels of serum cardiac markers in the blood after myocardial infarction. *CK-MB,* MB isoenzyme of creatine kinase.

elevation in the leads facing the infarction. Within hours to days, the ST segments return to baseline, with T-wave inversion and pathological Q waves in the same leads. A pathological Q wave is defined as a deep Q wave greater than or equal to one third the height of the R wave in the same lead. The Q wave will remain forever on the ECG (Urden et al., 2018). Patients with UA or NSTEMI usually have transient thrombosis or incomplete coronary occlusion and usually do not develop pathological Q waves. Areas of ischemia or infarction may be noted on the ECG.

The ECG may also be normal or nondiagnostic when the patient comes to the ED with chest pain. Within a few hours, the ECG may change to reflect the infarction process. These changes take place when cellular damage has occurred, interrupting the normal electrical depolarization of the ventricles. When the initial ECG is nondiagnostic, serial ECGs are to be obtained. (See Chapter 38 for discussion of ECG changes associated with ischemia and MI.)

Serum Cardiac Markers. After an MI, certain proteins called *serum cardiac markers* are released into the blood in large quantities from necrotic heart muscle. These markers, specifically serum cardiac enzymes and troponin, are important in the diagnosis of MI. When cardiac cells die, their intracellular enzymes are released into circulation. The increase in serum cardiac markers that occurs after cellular death can indicate whether cardiac damage is present and the approximate extent of the damage. CK and troponin are typically measured to diagnose an MI. Figure 36.10 indicates the peak levels and durations of these markers in the presence of MI.

CK levels begin to rise approximately 3 to 12 hours after an MI, peak in 24 hours, and return to normal within 2 to 3 days. The CK enzymes may be fractionated into bands, including the MB band. The MB isoenzyme of creatine kinase (CK-MB) band is specific to myocardial cells and can help in quantifying myocardial damage.

Cardiac-specific troponin is a myocardial muscle protein released into circulation after myocardial injury. In the heart, there are two subtypes: cardiac-specific troponin T (cTnT) and cardiac-specific troponin I (cTnI). These markers are highly

specific indicators of MI, and their tests have greater sensitivity and specificity for myocardial injury than that for CK-MB (Pagana et al., 2019). The troponin level rises as quickly as the CK level. Troponins are usually measured for diagnostic purposes in conjunction with total CK and the MB fraction. Serum levels of cTnI and cTnT increase 3 to 12 hours after the onset of MI, peak at 24 to 48 hours, and return to baseline over 5 to 14 days.

Myoglobin is released into circulation within a few hours after an MI. Although it is one of the first serum cardiac markers to rise after an MI, it lacks cardiac specificity. In addition, it is rapidly excreted in urine so that blood levels return to normal range within 24 hours after an MI, making it of limited diagnostic value (see Chapter 34, Table 34.6).

Coronary Angiography. The patient with UA or NSTEMI may undergo coronary angiography to evaluate the extent of the disease and to determine the most appropriate therapeutic modality. If appropriate, PCI may be performed at this time. Other patients may be treated with conservative medical management (Urden et al., 2018). Coronary angiography is the only way to confirm the diagnosis of Prinzmetal's angina.

Other Measures

When the ECG and serum cardiac marker levels do not confirm MI, other measures for diagnosing UA may be considered (see Chapter 34, Table 34.6). Nuclear testing and echocardiography may be conducted when a patient has an abnormal but nondiagnostic baseline ECG. Dobutamine or persantine stress echocardiography can be performed in patients unable to exercise to increase the HR, which aids in identifying ischemia or cardiac wall dysfunction (Pagana et al., 2019). (See Chapter 34 for additional information on cardiac assessment.)

INTERPROFESSIONAL CARE

It is extremely important that ACS be rapidly diagnosed and treated to preserve cardiac muscle. Initial management of chest pain most often occurs in the ED. Emergency care of patients with chest pain is described in Table 36.12. An intravenous (IV) route is established to provide an accessible means for emergency medication therapy. Sublingual nitroglycerin and chewable ASA (Aspirin) are administered in the ED if the patient has not received them in the prehospital phase by the emergency personnel. Morphine sulphate is given by IV route for pain unrelieved by nitroglycerin, as well as to decrease the workload of the heart (Urden et al., 2018). Oxygen is administered to maintain the oxygen saturation at 90 to 94% (Wong et al., 2019). Patients receive ongoing care in a critical care unit or telemetry unit, in which continuous ECG monitoring is available to detect dysrhythmias and institute appropriate treatment. The interprofessional care of ACS is described in Figure 36.8.

Vital signs, including pulse oximetry, are monitored frequently during the first few hours after admission and are monitored closely thereafter. Bed rest and limitation of activity for 12 to 24 hours are initially ordered, with a gradual increase in activity unless it is contraindicated.

For patients with UA or NSTEMI who have increased levels of cardiac markers and ongoing angina, a combination of ASA (Aspirin), heparin (unfractionated [UH] or low-molecular-weight [LMWH] heparin), and a glycoprotein IIb/IIIa inhibitor (i.e., abciximab [ReoPro], eptifibatide [Integrilin]) is recommended. PCI is a common elective procedure considered once

TABLE 36.12 EMERGENCY MANAGEMENT

Chest Pain

Etiology	Assessment Findings	Interventions
Cardiovascular • Angina • Myocardial infarction • Dysrhythmia • Pericarditis • Aortic aneurysm • Aortic valve disease **Respiratory** • Costochondritis • Pleurisy • Pneumonia • Pneumothorax • Pulmonary edema • Pulmonary embolus **Chest Trauma** • Rib or sternal fracture • Flail chest • Cardiac tamponade • Pneumothorax • Pulmonary contusion • Great vessel injury **Gastrointestinal** • Esophagitis • GERD • Hiatal hernia • Peptic ulcer • Cholecystitis **Others** • Stress • Strenuous exercise • Drugs • Acute anxiety	• Pain in chest, neck, arm, or shoulder • Cold, clammy skin • Diaphoresis • Nausea and vomiting • Epigastric pain • Indigestion or heartburn • Dyspnea • Weakness • Anxiety • Feeling of impending doom • Tachycardia • Irregular HR, murmurs • Palpitations • Dysrhythmias • Decreased BP • Narrowed pulse pressure • Unequal BP readings in upper extremities • Syncope, loss of consciousness • Decreased O_2 saturation • Decreased or absent breath sounds • Crackles, wheezes • Pericardial friction rub	**Initial** • Ensure patent airway. • Assess vital signs. • Administer O_2 by nasal cannula or nonrebreather mask. • Obtain 12-lead ECG. • Insert two IV catheters. • Assess pain, using PQRST mnemonic (see Table 36.7). • Medicate for pain as ordered (e.g., morphine, nitroglycerin). • Initiate continuous ECG monitoring and identify underlying rhythm. • Obtain baseline blood test results (e.g., cardiac markers). • Obtain portable chest radiograph. • Assess for antiplatelet, anticoagulation, or fibrinolytic therapy or for PCI as appropriate. • Administer ASA (Aspirin) and β-adrenergic blockers for cardiac-related chest pain unless contraindicated. • Administer antidysrhythmic medications as indicated. **Ongoing Monitoring** • Monitor vital signs, level of consciousness, cardiac rhythm, and O_2 saturation. • Monitor response to medications (e.g., decrease in chest pain) and readminister or titrate medications (e.g., nitroglycerin) as needed. • Provide reassurance and emotional support to patient and family. • Explain all interventions and procedures to patient in simple terms. • Anticipate need for intubation if respiratory distress is evident. • Prepare for CPR, defibrillation, transcutaneous pacing, or cardioversion.

ASA, acetylsalicylic acid; *BP*, blood pressure; *CPR*, cardiopulmonary resuscitation; *GERD*, gastroesophageal reflux disease; *HR*, heart rate; *IV*, intravenous; *O₂*, oxygen; *PCI*, percutaneous coronary intervention.

the patient is stabilized with angina controlled or if angina returns and increases in severity.

For patients with STEMI or NSTEMI with elevated levels of cardiac markers, reperfusion therapy is initiated (see Figure 36.8). *Reperfusion therapy*, which is an intervention to open the coronary artery that was occluded to restore blood flow to the myocardium, may include emergent PCI or fibrinolytic (thrombolytic) therapy. The goal of treatment is to salvage as much myocardial muscle as possible.

Emergent Percutaneous Coronary Intervention

Emergent PCI is recommended as the first line of treatment for patients with confirmed MI (i.e., definitive ECG changes, presence of cardiac markers, or both). The goal is to open the affected artery within 90 minutes of the patient's arrival at the ED. In this situation, the patient undergoes cardiac catheterization to locate the blockage or blockages (Figure 36.11), to assess the severity of the blockages, to determine the presence of collateral circulation, and to evaluate left ventricular function. With actual visualization of the coronary artery system and left

ventricular function, treatment modalities most beneficial to the patient can be selected. Usually PCI with the placement of one or more stents will be performed (Sole et al., 2017). Stents, either "bare metal" or "drug-eluting" are expandable mesh-like frames to open the vessel for blood flow. Drug-eluting stents are coated with slow-released medication to prevent intimal lining overgrowth and prevent reocclusion of the vessel. Aggressive anticoagulation assists in preventing occlusion of the stents through thrombus formation. Patients with severe left ventricular dysfunction may require the addition of IABP counterpulsation therapy, and a small percentage of patients may require emergency coronary artery bypass graft (CABG) surgery.

The advantages of PCI are that (a) it is an alternative to surgical intervention; (b) it is performed with the use of local anaesthetic; (c) the patient is ambulatory 24 hours after the procedure; (d) the length of hospital stay is approximately 1 to 3 days compared with the 4- to 6-day stay necessary with CABG surgery, thus reducing hospital costs; and (e) the patient can make a rapid return to work (approximately 5 to 7 days after PCI) instead of the 2- to 8-week convalescence period after CABG.

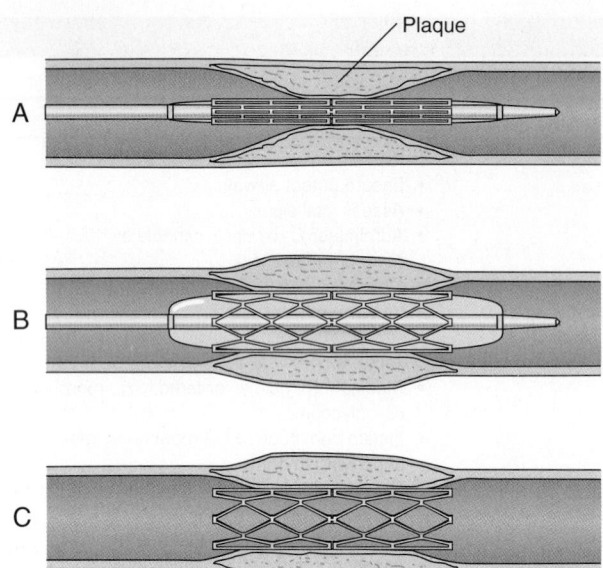

FIG. 36.11 Placement of a coronary artery stent. **A,** The stent is positioned at the site of the lesion. **B,** The balloon is inflated, expanding the stent. The balloon is then deflated and removed. **C,** The implanted stent is left in place. Source: From Lewis, S. L. (2014). *Medical-surgical nursing: Assessment and management of clinical problems* (9th ed). Mosby.

TABLE 36.13	CONTRAINDICATIONS FOR THE USE OF FIBRINOLYTIC THERAPY	
Absolute Contraindications	**Relative Contraindications**
• Active internal bleeding or bleeding diathesis (except for menstruation) • Known history of cerebral aneurysm or arteriovenous malformation • Known intracranial neoplasm (primary or metastatic) • Previous cerebral hemorrhage • Ischemic stroke within past 3 mo • Significant closed-head or facial trauma within past 3 mo • Suspected aortic dissection	• Active peptic ulcer disease • Current use of anticoagulants • Pregnancy • Prior ischemic stroke not within past 3 mo; dementia; or known intracranial disease not covered under absolute contraindications • Surgery (including laser eye surgery) or puncture of noncompressible vessel within past 3 wk • Internal bleeding within past 2–4 wk • Serious systemic disease (e.g., advanced or terminal cancer, severe liver or kidney disease) • Severe uncontrolled hypertension (BP >180/110 mm Hg) on patient's arrival for care or chronic, severe, poorly controlled hypertension • Traumatic or prolonged (>10 min) cardiopulmonary resuscitation

BP, blood pressure.

The most serious complication of PCI is dissection of the newly dilated coronary artery. If the damage is extensive, the coronary artery could rupture, resulting in cardiac tamponade, ischemia and infarction, decreased CO, and possibly death. There is also danger of infarction if the lesion is calcified and a portion of the plaque becomes dislodged, occluding the vessel distal to the catheter. Coronary spasm can occur from the mechanical irritation of the catheter or the balloon or from chemical irritation from the contrast medium used to visualize the artery. Abrupt closure is a complication that can occur in the first 24 hours after PCI. Restenosis after PCI can also occur, and risk is greatest in the first 30 days after the procedure. Nursing care of the patient after PCI is similar to that after cardiac catheterization (Sole et al., 2017) (see Chapter 34, Table 34.6).

Fibrinolytic Therapy

Fibrinolytic therapy offers the advantages of availability and rapid administration for patients who attend facilities without an interventional cardiac catheterization laboratory or for patients who are too unstable for a safe transfer. Treatment of MI with fibrinolytic therapy is aimed at stopping the infarction process by dissolving the thrombus in the coronary artery and reperfusing the myocardium. To be of most benefit, fibrinolytic therapy must be given as soon as possible, no greater than 12 hours and ideally within 2 to 3 hours after the onset of symptoms. The goal is door-to-needle time or the first medical contact, 30 minutes or less (Wong et al., 2019).

Indications and Contraindications. As fibrinolytics are given by IV, it is important to establish a minimum of two access sites (see Table 36.11). The choice of a thrombolytic agent is guided by considerations of cost, efficacy, and ease of administration. Although these medications have different mechanisms of action and different pharmacokinetics, they all open the artery by lysis of the thrombus in the coronary artery. Because all the fibrinolytics produce lysis of the pathological clot, they may also lyse other clots (e.g., a postoperative site, trauma). Therefore, patient selection is important because minor or major bleeding

may be a complication of therapy. Inclusion criteria for fibrinolytic therapy include (a) chest pain typical of acute MI and less than 12 hours in duration, (b) 12-lead ECG findings consistent with acute MI or new onset of a bundle-branch block, and (c) no absolute contraindications (Sole et al., 2017) (Table 36.13).

Procedure. Each hospital has a policy to follow for administration of fibrinolytic therapy. However, all policies have several common factors. Baseline assessments are completed, blood samples for baseline laboratory studies are collected, all other invasive procedures are performed before the fibrinolytic agent is given. This sequence reduces the possibility of bleeding in the patient.

Depending on the medication selected, therapy may be administered in a single IV bolus or over time (30 to 90 minutes). The time at which therapy begins is noted, and the patient is monitored during and after administration. ECG, vital signs measurement, pulse oximetry, and heart and lung assessments are completed frequently to evaluate the patient's response to therapy. When reperfusion occurs, several clinical markers may change. The most reliable marker is the return of the ST segment to baseline on the ECG. Other markers include a resolution of chest pain and a rapid rise of the CK-MB enzyme levels that occurs within 3 hours of therapy and peaks within 12 hours. The CK-MB levels increase as the necrotic myocardial cells release CK-MB enzymes into the circulation after perfusion has been restored to the area. The presence of reperfusion dysrhythmias (e.g., accelerated idioventricular rhythm) is a less reliable marker of reperfusion. These dysrhythmias are generally self-limiting and do not necessitate aggressive treatment (Urden et al., 2018). (See Chapter 38 for management of dysrhythmias.)

A major concern with fibrinolytic therapy is reocclusion of the artery. The site of the thrombus is unstable, and another clot may form, or spasm of the artery may occur. Because of these possibilities, IV heparin therapy is initiated in conjunction with antiplatelet agents (Kosar et al., 2016). If another clot develops, the patient reports similar symptoms of chest pain, and ECG changes return (Urden et al., 2018). The patient is re-evaluated and may receive a second dose of the fibrinolytic or be transferred to a cardiac catheterization laboratory for rescue PCI.

The major complication with fibrinolytic therapy is bleeding. Ongoing nursing assessment is essential. Minor bleeding (e.g., surface bleeding from IV sites or gingival bleeding) is expected and can be controlled by applying a pressure dressing or ice packs. If signs and symptoms of major bleeding occur (e.g., a drop in BP, an increase in HR, a sudden decrease in the patient's level of consciousness, blood in the urine or stool), the physician should be notified, and the therapy should be stopped.

Medication Therapy

IV nitroglycerin, ASA, β-adrenergic blockers, and systemic anticoagulation with either subcutaneous LMWH or IV UH are the initial medication treatments of choice for ACS (Wong et al., 2019). IV antiplatelet medications (e.g., glycoprotein IIb/IIIa inhibitor) may also be used if PCI is anticipated. ACE inhibitors are added for select patients after MI (discussed in the section Angiotensin-Converting Enzyme Inhibitors). Calcium channel blockers or long-acting nitrates can be added if the patient is already receiving adequate doses of β-adrenergic blockers, cannot tolerate β-adrenergic blockers, or has Prinzmetal's angina. Medication therapy for patients with ACS is described in Table 36.11. These medications are discussed in the Medication Therapy section. ACS-specific medications are discussed in the following sections.

Intravenous Nitroglycerin. IV nitroglycerin is used in the initial treatment of patients with ACS. The goal of therapy is to reduce anginal pain and improve coronary blood flow. Nitroglycerin has an immediate onset of action and can be titrated to prevent, treat, and stop UA (Sole et al., 2017).

IV nitroglycerin is used to decrease preload and afterload while increasing the myocardial oxygen supply. The dose is usually titrated to relieve pain. Because hypotension is a common adverse effect, BP is closely monitored during this time. Tolerance is another adverse effect of IV nitroglycerin therapy. An effective strategy to manage this phenomenon is to administer a lower dosage at night and during sleep and a higher dosage during the day.

Morphine Sulphate. Morphine is given for chest pain that is unrelieved by nitroglycerin. As a vasodilator, it decreases cardiac workload by lowering myocardial oxygen consumption, reducing contractility, and decreasing BP and HR. In addition, morphine can help reduce anxiety and fear. In rare situations, morphine can depress respiration. Patients should be monitored for signs of bradypnea or hypoxia, a condition to be prevented when at all possible in myocardial ischemia and infarction.

β-Adrenergic Blockers. IV β-adrenergic blockers should be given to patients with STEMI to decrease myocardial workload and prevent dysrhythmias from occurring (Sole et al., 2017). Oral β-adrenergic blocker therapy should be initiated within 24 hours of STEMI in patients with no contraindications. β-Adrenergic blockers are used to decrease myocardial oxygen demand by reducing HR, BP, and contractility. (See Table 36.11 and Chapter 35, Table 35.8 for a discussion of β-adrenergic blockers.)

Angiotensin-Converting Enzyme Inhibitors. ACE inhibitors (i.e., ramipril) are recommended within the first 24 hours after anterior wall MIs or MIs that result in decreased left ventricular function (ejection fraction <40%) or pulmonary congestion.

The use of ACE inhibitors can help prevent ventricular remodelling and prevent or slow the progression of HF (Sole et al., 2017), ideally continued indefinitely. For patients who cannot tolerate ACE inhibitors, angiotensin receptor blockers (e.g., losartan [Cozaar]) should be considered (see Table 36.11 and Chapter 35, Table 35.8).

Antidysrhythmia Medications. Dysrhythmias are the most common complications after an MI. In general, they are not treated aggressively unless they are life-threatening. (Medications used in the treatment of dysrhythmias are discussed in Chapter 38.)

Cholesterol-Lowering Medications. A fasting lipid panel should be obtained for all patients admitted with ACS. Cholesterol-lowering medications are recommended for all patients with elevated LDL cholesterol levels (see Figure 36.6 and Table 36.5).

Stool Softeners. After an MI, patients may be predisposed to constipation as a result of bed rest and opioid administration. Stool softeners such as docusate sodium (Colace) are given to facilitate and promote the comfort of bowel evacuation. These medications prevent straining and the resultant vagal stimulation from the Valsalva manoeuvre. Vagal stimulation produces bradycardia and can provoke dysrhythmias.

Nutritional Therapy

Initially, patients may be kept NPO (nothing by mouth) except for sips of water until stable (e.g., pain alleviated, nausea resolved). Diet is advanced as tolerated to one of low salt, low saturated fats, and low cholesterol.

Coronary Surgical Revascularization

Coronary revascularization (an intervention to restore blood flow to the affected myocardium) with CABG surgery is recommended for patients who (a) continue to have symptoms despite medical management, (b) have left main coronary artery or three-vessel disease, (c) are not candidates for PCI (e.g., lesions are long or difficult to access), (d) continue to have chest pain despite undergoing PCI, (e) have left ventricular failure, or (f) are expected to have longer-term benefits with CABG than with PCI (Urden et al., 2018).

Coronary Artery Bypass Graft Surgery. CABG surgery consists of the placement of conduits to transport blood between the aorta or other major arteries and the myocardium distal to the blocked coronary artery (or arteries). The procedure may involve one or more grafts using the internal mammary artery (IMA), saphenous vein, or radial artery, to bypass the occlusion (Figure 36.12).

The traditional approach to CABG surgery requires a sternotomy (opening of the chest cavity) and the patient is placed on the *cardiopulmonary bypass* (CPB) machine. During CPB, blood is diverted from the patient's heart to a machine, where it is oxygenated and returned (via a pump) to the patient. This allows the surgeon to operate on a still, nonbeating, bloodless heart while perfusion to vital organs is maintained.

The IMA is the most common artery used for bypass grafting. It is left attached to its origin (the subclavian artery) then dissected from the chest wall where it is *anastomosed* (connected with sutures) to the coronary artery distal to the blockage. As an arterial graft, the IMA tends to have longer-term patency than vein grafts (Sole et al., 2017).

When using the saphenous vein for a bypass graft, the surgeon removes the vein from one or both legs endoscopically

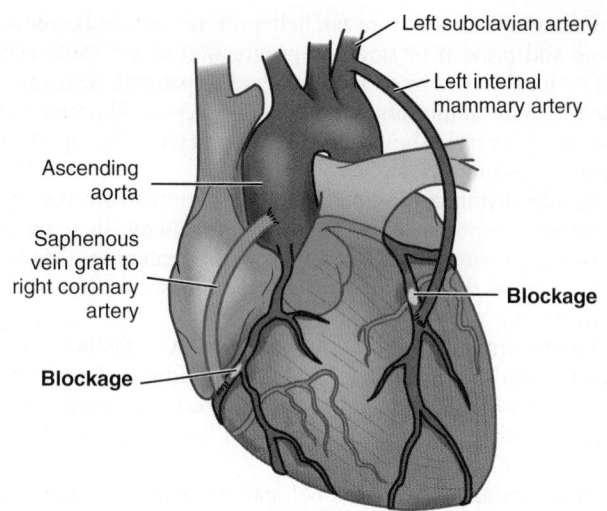

FIG. 36.12 The distal end of the left internal mammary artery is grafted below the area of blockage in the left anterior descending artery. The proximal end of the saphenous vein is grafted to the aorta, and the distal end is grafted below the area of blockage in the right coronary artery.

or by the traditional method (Sole et al., 2017). Sections are attached to the ascending aorta and then to a coronary artery distal to the blockage. Saphenous vein grafts develop diffuse intimal hyperplasia, which contributes to future stenosis and graft occlusions. The use of antiplatelet therapy and statins after surgery improves vein graft patency. (Radial graft patency was shown to be superior to vein grafts after 5 years and has 5-year patency rates as high as 84% [Guandino et al., 2018].)

CABG surgery remains a palliative treatment for CAD and not a cure. Studies have shown improved patient outcomes, quality of life, and survival after CABG surgery. However, postoperative complications and mortality increase with age.

Women have higher operative mortality rates than men. This has been attributed to the late treatment of CAD in women, as women first present with the disease at an older age and are more ill (e.g., decreased left ventricular function) at the time of surgery. Other possible factors include smaller-diameter coronary vessels and the less frequent use of the IMA (Norris et al., 2020)

Minimally Invasive Direct Coronary Artery Bypass. *Minimally invasive direct coronary artery bypass* (MIDCAB) offers patients with limited disease an approach to surgical treatment that does not involve a sternotomy and CPB. In many cases, these patients are too high risk for traditional bypass surgery (Sole et al., 2017). The technique requires several small incisions between the ribs. A thoracoscope is used to dissect the IMA. The heart is slowed using a β-adrenergic blocker (e.g., esmolol [Brevibloc]) or stopped temporarily with adenosine. A mechanical stabilizer immobilizes the operative site. The IMA is then sutured to the left anterior descending or right coronary artery. A radial artery or saphenous vein graft can be used if the IMA is not available.

Off-Pump Coronary Artery Bypass. The *off-pump coronary artery bypass* (OPCAB) procedure involves full or partial sternotomy to access all coronary vessels. OPCAB is performed on a beating heart using mechanical stabilizers and without CPB. It is usually reserved for patients who have limited disease but are at high risk for traditional surgery secondary to multiple comorbidities. Patients who are typically candidates for OPCAB have a very low ejection fraction, severe lung disease, acute or chronic kidney disease, a high risk for stroke, or a calcified aorta (Urden et al., 2018).

Robot-Assisted Cardiothoracic Surgery. This technique incorporates the use of a robot in performing CABG or mitral valve replacement. The benefits of robotic surgery include increased precision, smaller incisions, decreased blood loss, less pain, and shorter recovery time.

Transmyocardial Laser Revascularization. *Transmyocardial laser revascularization* (TMR) is an indirect revascularization procedure. It is used for patients with advanced CAD who are not candidates for traditional CABG surgery and who have persistent angina after maximum medical therapy. The procedure involves the use of a high-energy laser to create channels in the heart to allow blood flow to ischemic areas. The procedure is performed during cardiac catheterization as a percutaneous TMR or during surgery using a left anterior thoracotomy incision as an adjunct to CABG.

NURSING MANAGEMENT
CHRONIC STABLE ANGINA AND ACUTE CORONARY SYNDROME

NURSING ASSESSMENT
Subjective and objective data that should be obtained from a patient with ACS are listed in Table 36.14.

NURSING DIAGNOSES
Nursing diagnoses for the patient with ACS may include but are not limited to those presented in Nursing Care Plan (NCP) 36.1.

PLANNING
The overall goals for a patient with ACS include (a) relief of pain, (b) preservation of the myocardium, (c) immediate and appropriate treatment of ischemia, (d) effective coping with illness-associated anxiety, (e) participation in a rehabilitation plan, and (f) reduction of risk factors.

NURSING IMPLEMENTATION: CHRONIC STABLE ANGINA
HEALTH PROMOTION. Behaviours to reduce the risk for CAD are presented in Table 36.2 and discussed under Health Promotion.

ACUTE INTERVENTION. If a nurse is present during an anginal attack, the following measures should be instituted: (a) administration of supplemental oxygen; (b) measurement of vital signs; (c) 12-lead ECG; (d) prompt pain relief, first with a nitrate and then, if necessary, an opioid analgesic; (e) auscultation of heart sounds; and (f) comfortable positioning of the patient. The patient is likely to appear distressed and to have pale, cool, clammy skin. The BP and HR are probably elevated, and an atrial gallop sound (S_4) may be heard. A ventricular gallop sound (S_3) may indicate left ventricular dysfunction. A murmur heard during an anginal attack may be secondary to ischemia of a papillary muscle of the mitral valve. The murmur is likely to be transient and to disappear with the cessation of symptoms.

The nurse should ask the patient to rate the pain on a scale of 0 to 10 before and after treatment, to evaluate the effectiveness of the interventions. It is important to use the same words that patients use to describe their pain. Some patients may not always verbalize pain. The nurse must be attuned to other manifestations of pain, such as restlessness; elevated HR, respiratory rate, or BP; clutching of the bedclothes; or other nonverbal cues. Supportive and realistic reassurance with a calm, soothing manner can help reduce the patient's anxiety during an anginal attack.

TABLE 36.14 NURSING ASSESSMENT

Acute Coronary Syndrome

Subjective Data

Important Health Information

Current health history: Family history of heart disease; sedentary lifestyle; tobacco use
Past health history: Previous history of CAD, angina, MI, aortic stenosis, HF, or cardiomyopathy; hypertension; diabetes; anemia; lung disease; hyperlipidemia
Medications: Use of ASA (Aspirin), nitrates, β-adrenergic blockers, calcium channel blockers, ACE inhibitors, antihypertensive medications, cholesterol-lowering medications, vitamin or herbal supplements

Symptoms

- Substernal chest pain or pressure (squeezing, constricting, aching, sharp, tingling), possible radiation to jaw, neck, shoulders, back, or arms
- Indigestion, heartburn, nausea, belching, vomiting
- Palpitations, dyspnea, dizziness, weakness
- Fatigue, anxiety, feeling of impending doom

Objective Data

General

Anxiety, fear, restlessness

Integumentary

Cool, clammy, pale skin

Cardiovascular

Tachycardia or bradycardia, pulsus alternans (alternating weak and strong heartbeats), dysrhythmias (especially ventricular), S_3, S_4, higher or lower BP, murmur

Possible Findings

Elevated or nonelevated levels of serum cardiac markers, increased levels of serum lipids; increased WBC count; positive results of exercise stress test and thallium scans; ST-segment and T-wave abnormalities on ECG; cardiac enlargement, calcifications, or pulmonary congestion on chest radiograph; evidence of abnormal wall motion on stress echocardiogram; positive findings on coronary angiogram

ACE, angiotensin-converting enzyme; *ASA,* acetylsalicylic acid; *BP,* blood pressure; *CAD,* coronary artery disease; *ECG,* electrocardiogram; *HF,* heart failure; *MI,* myocardial infarction; S_3, third heart sound; S_4, fourth heart sound; *WBC,* white blood cell.

AMBULATORY AND HOME CARE. Prevention of angina is preferable to its treatment, and this is why teaching is important. Patients and health care providers should be provided information regarding CAD, angina, precipitating factors for angina, risk-factor reduction, and medications.

Patient teaching can be handled in a variety of ways. One-to-one interaction between the nurse and the patient is often the most effective strategy. The time spent providing daily care is often an ideal teaching period. Teaching tools such as pamphlets, video recordings, heart models, online sources, and especially written information are necessary components of patient and family teaching. The nurse should always begin with a needs assessment to determine the plan for health teaching and evaluate the effectiveness of the teaching (i.e., teach-back) (Edelman & Kudzma, 2018) (see Chapter 4).

Patients should be assisted in identifying factors that precipitate angina (see Table 36.8) and given instruction on how to avoid or control precipitating factors. For example, patients should be taught to avoid exposure to extremes of weather and to avoid consumption of large, heavy meals. If a heavy meal is ingested, adequate rest should be planned for 1 to 2 hours after the meal because blood is shunted to the GI tract to aid in digestion and absorption.

Patients should be assisted in identifying personal risk factors for CAD. Once these are known, methods of decreasing any modifiable risk factors should be discussed (see Table 36.2). Teaching the patient and the family or caregivers about diets with low sodium and saturated fat content may be appropriate (see Tables 36.3 and 36.4). Maintaining ideal body weight is an effective strategy in controlling angina, as increased weight increases the myocardial workload.

Adhering to a regular, individualized program of physical activity that conditions the heart rather than overstressing the myocardium is important. As well, the patient and caregivers must be instructed in the proper use of nitroglycerin (see Short-Acting Nitrates and Long-Acting Nitrates). Nitroglycerin may be used prophylactically before an emotionally stressful situation, sexual intercourse, or physical exertion (e.g., climbing a long flight of stairs) to prevent ischemic chest pain.

Counselling should be provided to assess the psychological adjustment of the patient and family to the diagnosis of CAD and the resulting angina. Many patients feel a threat to their identity and self-esteem because they may be unable to fill their usual roles in society. These emotions are normal and real as patients adjust to their health challenge.

NURSING IMPLEMENTATION: ACUTE CORONARY SYNDROME

ACUTE INTERVENTION. Priorities for nursing interventions in the initial phase of ACS include pain assessment and relief, physiological monitoring, promotion of rest and comfort, alleviation of stress and anxiety, and understanding of the patient's emotional and behavioural reactions. Effective management of these priorities decreases the oxygen needs of a compromised myocardium and reduces the risk of complications. In addition, the nurse should institute measures to avoid the hazards of immobility and yet encourage rest.

Pain. Nitroglycerin, morphine sulphate, and supplemental oxygen should be provided as needed to eliminate or reduce chest pain. Ongoing evaluation and documentation of the effectiveness of the interventions are important. Once pain is relieved, the nurse may have to address denial in a patient who interprets the absence of pain as an absence of cardiac disease.

Monitoring. Patients undergo continuous ECG monitoring while in the ED, the critical care unit, and usually after transfer to a step-down or general unit. The nurse should be educated in interpretation of the ECG so that dysrhythmias causing further deterioration of the cardiovascular status can be identified and treated. During the initial period after MI, ventricular fibrillation is the most common lethal dysrhythmia. In many patients, this dysrhythmia is often preceded by PVCs or ventricular tachycardia. The nurse should also monitor the patient for the presence of silent ischemia by monitoring the ST segment for shifts above or below the baseline of the ECG. Silent ischemia occurs without clinical symptoms such as chest pain. It is noted by ST-segment changes only and may place a patient at higher risk for adverse outcomes and even death. Individuals with diabetes are especially at risk due to autonomic neuropathy and may not interpret chest pain (Urden et al., 2018). If episodes of silent ischemia are observed, the physician should be notified. (See Chapter 38 for a complete discussion of ECG monitoring).

In addition to frequent assessment of vital signs, intake and output should be evaluated at least once per shift, and physical

◎ NURSING CARE PLAN 36.1

Acute Coronary Syndrome

NURSING DIAGNOSIS	**Decreased cardiac output** (resulting from altered contractility and altered heart rate and rhythm as evidenced by decrease in BP, elevation in HR, dyspnea, dysrhythmias, diminished pulses, peripheral edema, pulmonary edema, or a combination of these)

Expected Patient Outcomes	Nursing Interventions and *Rationales*
• Maintains stable signs of effective cardiac perfusion	*Cardiac Care* • Monitor vital signs frequently *to determine baseline and ongoing changes.* • Monitor for cardiac dysrhythmias, including disturbances of both rhythm and conduction, *to identify and treat significant dysrhythmias.* • Monitor respiratory status for symptoms of heart failure *to maintain appropriate levels of oxygenation and to detect signs of pulmonary edema.* • Monitor fluid balance (e.g., intake and output, daily weight) *to monitor renal perfusion and observe for fluid retention.* • Arrange exercise and rest periods *to prevent fatigue and decrease the oxygen demand on the myocardium.*

NURSING DIAGNOSIS	**Acute pain** resulting from a biological injury agent (imbalance between myocardial O_2 supply and demand) as evidenced by self-report of pain characteristics using standard pain instrument

Expected Patient Outcomes	Nursing Interventions and *Rationales*
• Reports relief of pain	*Cardiac Care* • Evaluate chest pain (e.g., PQRST [see Table 36.7]) *to accurately evaluate, treat, and prevent further ischemia.* • Monitor vital signs frequently *to determine baseline and detect ongoing changes.* • Obtain 12-lead ECG during pain episode *to help differentiate angina from extension of MI or pericarditis.* *Pain Management* • Provide optimal pain relief with prescribed analgesics *because pain exacerbates tachycardia and increases BP.* • Consider the type and source of pain when selecting pain relief strategy *because angina responds to opioids and measures that increase myocardial perfusion.*

NURSING DIAGNOSIS	**Anxiety** resulting from a threat of death, threat to current status (pain, lifestyle changes) as evidenced by restlessness, distress, helplessness

Expected Patient Outcomes	Nursing Interventions and *Rationales*
• Reports decreased anxiety and increased sense of self-control	*Anxiety Reduction* • Observe for verbal and nonverbal signs of anxiety. • Identify changes in level of anxiety *because anxiety increases the need for oxygen.* • Use a calm, reassuring approach *so as not to increase patient's anxiety.* • Instruct patient in use of relaxation techniques (e.g., relaxation breathing, imagery) *to enhance the patient's self-control.* • Encourage family members to stay with patient *to provide comfort.* • Encourage verbalization of feelings, perceptions, and fears *to decrease anxiety and stress.* • Provide factual information concerning diagnosis, treatment, and prognosis *to decrease fear of the unknown.* *Coping Enhancement* • Provide the patient with realistic choices about certain aspects of care *to support decision making.* • Assist the patient in identifying positive strategies *to cope with limitations and manage needed lifestyle or role changes.* • Help the patient to grieve and work through the losses of chronic illness *to provide support.*

NURSING DIAGNOSIS	**Reduced stamina** resulting from physical deconditioning (decreased cardiac output, poor lung perfusion) as evidenced by fatigue, generalized weakness, abnormal heart rate response to activity

Expected Patient Outcomes	Nursing Interventions and *Rationales*
• Achieves a realistic program of activity that balances physical activity with energy-conserving activities	*Cardiac Care* • Monitor patient's response to antidysrhythmia medications before activity *because these medications affect blood pressure and pulse.* • Arrange exercise and rest periods *to prevent fatigue and to increase activity tolerance without rapidly increasing cardiac workload.* *Energy Management* • Assist patient in understanding energy conservation principles (e.g., the requirement for restricted activity) *to promote healing by conserving energy.* • Teach patient and significant others techniques of self-care that will minimize oxygen consumption (e.g., self-monitoring and pacing techniques for performance of activities of daily living) *to promote independence as well as minimize O_2 consumption.*

NURSING CARE PLAN 36.1

Acute Coronary Syndrome—cont'd

NURSING DIAGNOSIS	**Inadequate health management** as a result of insufficient knowledge of therapeutic regimen (rehabilitation process, home activities, medications) as evidenced by difficulty with prescribed regimen

Expected Patient Outcomes	Nursing Interventions and *Rationales*
• Describes risk factors, the disease process, and rehabilitation activities necessary to manage the therapeutic regimen	**Cardiac Care: Rehabilitative** • Encourage realistic expectations for the patient, caregiver(s), and family member(s) *to promote realistic decision making.* • Instruct the patient, caregiver(s), and family member(s) on appropriate prescribed and over-the-counter medications *to promote adherence to medication regimens.* • Instruct the patient and caregiver on cardiac risk-factor modification (e.g., smoking cessation, diet, exercise) *to increase patient's control of the illness.* • Instruct the patient on self-care of chest pain (e.g., take sublingual nitroglycerin every 5 minutes three times; if chest pain is unrelieved, seek emergency medical care). • Instruct the patient and caregiver on the exercise regimen, including warm-up, endurance, and cool-down, *to reduce cardiac risk factors.* • Instruct the patient and caregiver in wound care and precautions (e.g., sternal incision or catheterization site), if appropriate, *to prevent infection and promote healing after invasive therapies.* • Instruct the patient and caregiver on access to emergency services available in their community *to enable them to obtain immediate care if needed.*

assessment should be carried out to detect deviations from a patient's baseline parameters. Included is an assessment of lung sounds and heart sounds with evaluation of early HF (e.g., dyspnea, tachycardia, pulmonary congestion, distended neck veins).

Assessment of the patient's oxygenation status to maintain an oxygen saturation greater than 90% is important, especially if the patient is receiving oxygen (Urden et al., 2018). Also, the nares should be checked for irritation or dryness, which can cause considerable discomfort if the nasal route is used for oxygen administration.

Rest and Comfort. With a severe insult to the myocardium, as in the case of ACS, it is important for the nurse to promote rest and comfort. Bed rest may be ordered for the first few days after an MI involving a large portion of the ventricle. A patient with an uncomplicated MI (e.g., angina resolved, no signs of complications) may rest in a chair within 8 to 12 hours after the event. The use of a commode or bedpan is based on patient preference.

When sleeping or resting, the body requires less work from the heart than it does when active. It is important to plan nursing and therapeutic actions to ensure adequate rest periods free from interruption. Comfort measures that can promote rest include frequent oral care, adequate warmth, a quiet atmosphere, use of relaxation therapy (e.g., guided imagery), and assurance that personnel are nearby and responsive to the patient's needs.

It is important that patients understand the reasons for limited activity. However, in spite of this limitation, patients are not completely restricted. Gradually, the cardiac workload is increased through more demanding physical tasks so that patients can achieve a discharge activity level adequate for home care. Phases of cardiac rehabilitation are outlined in Table 36.15.

Anxiety. Anxiety is present to various degrees in all patients with ACS. The nurse's role is to identify the source of anxiety and assist the patient in reducing anxiety. If the patient is experiencing anxiety, such as being afraid of being alone, the nurse can provide a supportive environment by enlisting a family

TABLE 36.15	**PHASES OF REHABILITATION AFTER ACUTE CORONARY SYNDROME**

Phase I: Hospital
- Phase occurs while the patient is still hospitalized.
- Activity level depends on severity of angina or MI.
- Patient may initially sit up in bed or a chair, perform range-of-motion exercises and self-care (e.g., washing, shaving), and progress to ambulation in hallway and limited stair climbing.
- Attention focuses on management of pain, anxiety, dysrhythmias, and complications.

Phase II: Early Recovery
- Phase begins after the patient is discharged.
- Phase usually lasts 2–12 wk and is conducted in an outpatient facility.
- Activity level is gradually increased under the supervision of the cardiac rehabilitation team and with electrocardiographic monitoring.
- The team may suggest that physical activity (e.g., walking) be initiated at home.
- Information regarding risk-factor reduction is provided at this time.

Phase III: Late Recovery
- Long-term maintenance program is followed.
- Individual physical activity programs are designed and implemented at home, a local gym, or the rehabilitation centre.
- The patient and family may restructure lifestyles and roles as possible.
- Lifestyle changes should become lifelong habits.
- Medical supervision is still recommended.

MI, myocardial infarction.

member to sit quietly with the patient. If a source of anxiety is fear of the unknown, the nurse should explore these concerns with the patient and identify a plan.

If anxiety is caused by lack of information, the nurse should provide teaching appropriate to the patient's stated need and level of understanding. The nurse should answer the patient's questions with clear, simple explanations sufficient to reduce the patient's anxiety.

It is important to provide health teaching at the patient's level, using nonmedical language to assist in understanding. Many patients are not yet ready to hear about the pathogenesis of CAD and lifestyle changes. The earliest questions usually relate to how the disease affects perceived control and independence. These questions include the following:

- When will I leave the critical care unit?
- When can I be out of bed?
- When will I be discharged?
- When can I return to work?
- How much change will I have to make in my life?
- Will this happen again?

The nurse should advise patients to begin a more complete teaching program once they are feeling stronger. Many patients may not be able to consciously examine the most pervasive and typical concern: "Am I going to die?" Even if a patient denies this concern, it is helpful for the nurse to initiate conversation by remarking that fear of dying is a common concern reported by most patients who have experienced ACS. This information gives the patient "permission" to talk about an uncomfortable and frightening topic (Table 36.16).

Emotional and Behavioural Reactions. The emotional and behavioural reactions of a patient are varied and frequently follow a predictable response pattern (see Table 36.16). The role of the nurse is to provide a supportive environment, listening to the patient's concerns. The nurse may need to advocate for pharmacological and nonpharmacological interventions to treat depression and anxiety (Vaccarino, 2019). It is useful for the nurse to recognize that denial is often a coping mechanism in the early recovery phase of ACS.

The nurse has a duty to maximize and enhance the patient's social support systems. This begins with assessing the support structure of the patient and family, providing guidance to individual roles and function. Often the patient is separated from the most significant support system at the time of hospitalization. The family's greatest need is for information, therefore the nurse's role is to create a trusting relationship with the family. The nurse should encourage conversation with the patient and their family and involve the family in the patient's care, as appropriate (Sole et al., 2017). Open visitation is helpful in decreasing anxiety and increasing support for the patient with ACS. The nurse may also help the patient identify additional support systems (e.g., spiritual care) that can help the patient after discharge.

CORONARY REVASCULARIZATION. Patients with ACS may undergo coronary revascularization with PCI or CABG surgery. The major nursing responsibilities for the care of the patient after PCI involve monitoring for signs of recurrent angina; frequently assessing vital signs, including HR and rhythm; evaluating the groin site for signs of bleeding; and maintaining bed rest per institution policy.

Patients undergoing CABG surgery receive care in the critical care unit for the first 24 hours. Ongoing and intensive monitoring of patients' hemodynamic status is critical during this phase of the postoperative period. Much technology is used to closely monitor patients post-CABG (see Chapter 68). This equipment includes a pulmonary artery catheter for measuring CO and other hemodynamic parameters, an intra-arterial line for continuous BP monitoring, pleural and mediastinal chest tubes for chest drainage, ECG leads for continuous monitoring to detect dysrhythmias, an endotracheal tube connected to mechanical ventilation, epicardial pacing wires for emergency pacing of the heart, and a urinary catheter to monitor urine output. Most patients are extubated within 12 hours after surgery

TABLE 36.16	EMOTIONAL AND BEHAVIOURAL RESPONSES TO ACUTE CORONARY SYNDROME

Denial

- May have history of ignoring symptoms related to heart disease
- Minimizes severity of medical condition
- Ignores activity restrictions
- Avoids discussing illness or its significance

Anger

- Is commonly expressed as "Why did this happen to me?"
- Possibly directed at family, staff, or medical regimen

Anxiety and Fear

- Fears long-term disability and death
- Overtly manifests apprehension, restlessness, insomnia, tachycardia
- Less overtly manifests increased verbalization, projection of feelings to others, hypochondriasis
- Fears activity
- Fears recurrent angina, heart attacks, and sudden death

Dependency

- Is totally reliant on staff
- Is unwilling to perform tasks or activities unless approved by health care provider
- Wants to be monitored by ECG at all times
- Is hesitant to leave the critical care unit or hospital

Depression

- Mourns loss of health, altered body function, and changes in lifestyle
- Realizes seriousness of situation
- Begins to worry about future implications of health problem
- Shows manifestations of withdrawal, apathy
- May be more evident after hospital discharge

Realistic Acceptance

- Focuses on optimum rehabilitation
- Plans changes compatible with altered cardiac function

ECG, electrocardiogram.

and transferred to a step-down unit within 24 hours for continued monitoring of cardiac status.

Many of the postoperative complications that develop after CABG surgery are related to the use of the CPB machine. Major consequences of CPB include bleeding and anemia from damage to red blood cells and platelets, fluid and electrolyte imbalances, and hypothermia because blood is cooled as it passes through the CPB machine. Nursing care focuses on assessing the patient for bleeding (i.e., chest tube drainage, incision sites), monitoring fluid status, replacing electrolytes as needed, assessing neurological function, and restoring temperature (with use of warming blankets).

Postoperative dysrhythmias, specifically atrial dysrhythmias, are common in the first 3 days after CABG surgery. Between 20 and 40% of patients develop postoperative atrial fibrillation. Discharge is often delayed for these patients as a result of the need for anticoagulation. (See Chapter 38 for information on treatment of atrial fibrillation.)

Nursing care for patients with a CABG also involves attention to the surgical sites: the chest, arm, leg, abdomen, or some combination of these. Care of the radial artery harvest site includes careful observation of the incision site, as well as monitoring of sensory and motor function of the distal thumb and fingers. The patient with radial artery harvest should receive therapy with a calcium channel blocker for approximately 3 months to decrease the incidence of arterial spasm at the arm or the anastomosis site.

The care of the leg wound is similar to the postoperative care after the stripping of varicose veins (see Chapter 40). The management of the chest wound, which involves a sternotomy, is similar to that for other chest surgical procedures, with careful attention to prevention of infection, especially from respiratory secretions (see Chapter 30).

Elective CABG is generally well tolerated by older patients. However, the nurse caring for older persons must be aware that although the benefits of treatment may outweigh risks in this population, the incidence of complications (e.g., dysrhythmias, stroke, kidney failure, and infection) is higher than that in younger individuals.

Postoperative nursing care of patients who have undergone a MIDCAB or OPCAB procedure is similar to that for patients who have undergone CABG surgery. Pain management is essential, as patients with thoracotomy incisions report higher levels of pain than those with sternotomy incisions. The recovery time is somewhat shorter with these procedures, and patients often resume routine activities sooner than do patients who have CABG surgery.

AMBULATORY AND HOME CARE. *Rehabilitation* may be defined as the process of helping the patient adjust to a disability by teaching integration of all resources and concentrating more on existing abilities than on permanent disabilities. *Cardiac rehabilitation* is the restoration of a person to an optimal state of function in six areas: physiological, psychological, mental, spiritual, economic, and vocational. Many people recover from ACS physically, but they may never attain psychological well-being because of misconceptions about the illness or a need to practice illness behaviours. Returning to work and resuming all activities have long been outcome measures of cardiac rehabilitation and are important in terms of the cost-effectiveness of cardiac care and rehabilitation. The nurse can provide contact information for the various methods of cardiac rehabilitation.

In considering rehabilitation, the nurse and the patient must recognize that CAD is a chronic disease. It will not be cured, nor will it disappear by itself. Therefore, basic changes in lifestyle must be made to promote recovery and health. In many cases, these changes must be made at a time when the patient is middle-aged or older. The patient must also realize that recovery takes time. Resumption of physical activity after ACS or CABG surgery is slow and gradual. However, with appropriate and adequate supportive care, recovery is possible.

PATIENT TEACHING. Patient- and family-centred care begins with patient teaching by the nurse in the ED, progresses through the care provided by the staff nurse, and continues with the community nurse. The purpose of teaching is to provide the patient and the family with the tools they need to make informed decisions about attainment of health and quality of life. For teaching to be meaningful, the patient must be aware of the need to learn. Careful assessment of the patient's learning needs can help the nurse collaborate with the patient and set goals and objectives that are realistic.

The timing of the teaching is important. When patients or families are in crisis (either physiological or psychological), they may not be able to learn new information. It is important to remember that their early questions should be answered initially in simple, brief terms, without detailed elaboration, and that the answers to these questions often require repetition with

elaboration later. When the shock and disbelief accompanying a crisis subside, the patient and the family are better able to focus on new information.

In addition to teaching the patient and family what they wish to know, the nurse should recognize that several types of information are necessary for achieving optimal health. A teaching guide for the patient with ACS is presented in Table 36.17.

When medical terminology is used, its meaning should be explained in lay terms. For example, it can be explained that the heart, a four-chambered pump, is a muscle that, like all other muscles, needs oxygen to work properly. When blood vessels supplying the heart muscle with oxygen become narrowed by atherosclerosis, less oxygen reaches the heart muscle. It is a good idea for the nurse to have a model of the heart or to use a sketch of what is being explained. Literature written for a nonmedical audience is available through the Heart and Stroke Foundation of Canada. Video recordings are also helpful tools that can be used to teach patients.

Anticipatory guidance involves preparing the patient and the family for what to expect in the course of recovery and rehabilitation. By learning what to expect during treatment and recovery, the patient gains a sense of control over their life. This sense of perceived control allows the patient to consider stressors that may possibly promote recovery.

Physical Activity. Physical activity is an integral part of the rehabilitation program; it is necessary for optimal physiological functioning and psychological well-being. It has a direct, positive effect on maximal oxygen uptake, increasing CO, decreasing blood lipids, decreasing BP, increasing blood flow through the coronary arteries, increasing muscle mass and flexibility, improving the patient's psychological state, and assisting in weight loss and control. A regular schedule of physical activity, even when begun after many years of sedentary living, is beneficial. The Canadian Guidelines for Physical Activity outline recommended activities and their duration for all ages (Canadian Society for Exercise Physiology, 2021).

TABLE 36.17 PATIENT & CAREGIVER TEACHING GUIDE

Acute Coronary Syndrome

The following guidelines should be included when teaching the patient and caregiver about acute coronary syndrome.
- Signs and symptoms of angina and MI and reasons why they occur*
- Anatomy and physiology of the heart and vessels
- Cause and effect of atherosclerosis
- Definitions of terms (e.g., CAD, angina, MI, sudden cardiac death, HF)
- Healing after MI
- Identification of risk factors and ways to decrease risk* (see Table 36.2)
- Rationale for tests and treatments, including ECG, blood tests, and angiography, and for monitoring, rest, diet, and medications*
- Appropriate expectations about recovery and rehabilitation (anticipatory guidance)
- Resumption of work, physical activity, sexual activity
- Measures to take to promote recovery and health
- Importance of the gradual, progressive resumption of activity*
- When and how to seek help (e.g., contact EMS)

CAD, coronary artery disease; *ECG,* electrocardiogram; *EMS,* emergency medical services; *HF,* heart failure; *MI,* myocardial infarction.
*Identified by patients as most important to learn before discharge.

TABLE 36.18	PATIENT & CAREGIVER TEACHING GUIDE

FITT: Physical Activity Guidelines After Acute Coronary Syndrome

Warm-Up and Cool-Down

Mild stretching for 3–5 min before the physical activity and 5 min after the activity is important. Activity should not be started or stopped abruptly.

Frequency

The patient should perform physical activity five or more times per week.

Intensity

Activity intensity should be determined by the patient's HR. If a treadmill test has not been performed, the person recovering from MI should not exceed 20 beats/min over the resting HR.

Type of Physical Activity

Physical activity should be regular, rhythmic, and repetitive; large muscles should be used to build up endurance (as in walking, cycling, swimming, and rowing).

Time

Duration of physical activity can be 30–60 min. It is important to begin slowly according to personal tolerance (perhaps only 5–10 min) and build up to 30 min.

FITT, frequency, intensity, time, and type; *HR,* heart rate; *MI,* myocardial infarction.

In the hospital, the patient's activity level is gradually increased so that by the time of discharge, the patient can tolerate moderate-energy activities of 3 to 6 metabolic equivalents (METs). Many patients with resolved UA or with an uncomplicated MI are in the hospital for approximately 3 to 4 days. By day 2, patients can ambulate in the hallway and begin limited stair climbing (e.g., three to four steps). Because of the short hospital stay, it is critical to give patients specific guidelines for physical activity so as to avoid overexertion. The nurse should stress to patients that they must "listen to what their body is saying" as the most important facet of recovery.

Teaching patients to check their pulse rate is a nursing responsibility. Patients should be taught the parameters within which to exercise. They should be told the maximum rate that the heart should beat at any point. If the HR exceeds this level or does not return to the rate of the resting pulse within a few minutes, patients should stop and rest. Patients should also be instructed to stop exercising if angina or dyspnea occurs. Basic physical activity guidelines for patients after ACS are based on the formula for frequency, intensity, time, and type (FITT) and are presented in Table 36.18.

The basic categories of physical activity are static *(isometric)* and dynamic *(isotonic)*. Most daily activities are a mixture of the two. *Static activities* involve the development of tension during muscular contraction but produce little or no change in muscle length or joint movement. Lifting, carrying, and pushing heavy objects are primarily isometric activities. Because the HR and BP increase rapidly during isometric work, exercise programs involving isometric exercises should be limited.

Isotonic activities involve changes in muscle length and joint movement with rhythmic contractions at relatively low muscular tension. Walking, jogging, swimming, bicycling, and jumping rope are examples of activities that are predominantly isotonic. Isotonic exercise can put a safe, steady load on the heart and lungs and improve the circulation in many organs.

Many patients are referred to an outpatient cardiac rehabilitation program (see Table 36.15). These programs have been found to be beneficial to patients, but not all patients choose or are able to participate in them. Home-based cardiac rehabilitation programs have been developed, as well as gender-specific classes, as alternatives. Maintaining contact with patients appears to be the key to the success of these programs.

Older women (65 years or older) who experience MI frequently have poor adherence to a regular physical activity program. These women often describe a continued post-MI fatigue that is poorly understood. Another factor that has been linked to poor adherence to a physical activity program after MI is depression. Depression is common among patients with CAD, especially women (Norris et al., 2020). All patients with CAD should routinely be screened for depression and treatment should be recommended as appropriate.

Resumption of Sexual Activity. It is important to include sexual counselling for cardiac patients and their partners. This often-neglected area of discussion may be difficult for both the patient and the health care provider to approach. However, the patient's concern about resumption of sexual activity after hospitalization for ACS often produces more stress than the physiological act itself. Most of these patients change their sexual behaviour not because of physical challenges but because they are concerned about sexual inadequacy, death during intercourse, and impotence. A concerned and knowledgeable health care provider can clarify any misconceptions with specific counselling.

Before providing suggestions on resumption of sexual activity, the nurse must know the patient's physiological status, the physiological effects of sexual activity, and the psychological effects of having a heart attack. Sexual activity for most middle-aged men and women with their usual partners is considered a moderate-energy activity equivalent to climbing two flights of stairs.

Nurses may feel uncertain about how and when to begin counselling about resumption of sexual activity. It is helpful to consider sex a physical activity and to discuss or explore feelings about it when discussing other physical activities with the patient. The dialogue may be opened with, for example, "Many people who have had a heart attack wonder when they will be able to resume sexual activity. Has this been of concern to you?" The nurse might also state, "Sexual activity is like other forms of activity and should be gradually resumed after MI. If your ability to perform sexually is concerning you, the energy you use is no more than that when walking briskly." Providing the patient with reading material on resumption of sexual activity can also facilitate discussion, introduced as follows: "If resuming sexual activity has been of concern to you, this information should be helpful." This type of nonthreatening statement brings up the topic, allows the patient to explore personal feelings, and gives the patient an opportunity to raise questions with the nurse or another health care provider (Boothby et al., 2018). Common guidelines are presented in Table 36.19.

TABLE 36.19 SEXUAL ACTIVITY AFTER ACUTE CORONARY SYNDROME

- When planning for resumption of sexual activity, the patient's goal should correspond to sexual activity before hospitalization for acute coronary syndrome.
- Physical training seems to improve the physiological response to coitus; therefore, daily physical activity during recovery should be encouraged.
- Consumption of food and alcohol should be reduced before intercourse is anticipated (e.g., waiting 3 to 4 hr after ingesting a large meal before engaging in sexual activity).
- Familiar surroundings and a familiar partner reduce anxiety.
- Masturbation may be a useful sexual outlet and may reassure the patient that sexual activity is still possible.
- Hot or cold showers should be avoided just before and just after intercourse.
- Foreplay is desirable because it allows a gradual increase in heart rate before orgasm.
- Positions during intercourse are a matter of individual choice.
- Orogenital sex places no undue strain on the heart.
- A relaxed atmosphere free of fatigue and stress is optimal.
- Prophylactic use of nitrates is effective in decreasing angina during sexual activity.
- Use of erectile agents (e.g., sildenafil [Viagra]) is contraindicated if the patient is taking nitrates in any form.
- Anal intercourse may cause undue cardiac stress because of the possibility of inducing a vasovagal response.

EVALUATION

The expected outcomes for the patient with ACS are presented in NCP 36.1.

SUDDEN CARDIAC DEATH

Sudden cardiac death (SCD) is unexpected death resulting from various causes, including cardiac arrest. In many cases, SCD is not actually sudden. Teaching people about the symptoms of impending cardiac arrest and the actions to take can save lives. Rapid cardiopulmonary resuscitation (CPR) and defibrillation with an automated external defibrillator (AED), in combination with early advanced cardiac life support, can enhance the chances for long-term survival after a witnessed arrest.

Etiology and Pathophysiology

In SCD, cardiac function is disrupted abruptly, causing immediate loss of CO and cerebral blood flow. The affected person may or may not have a known history of CAD. SCD is the first sign of illness for 25% of people who die from heart disease (Urden et al., 2018). Death usually occurs within 1 hour of the onset of acute symptoms (e.g., angina, palpitations).

Acute ventricular dysrhythmias (e.g., ventricular tachycardia, ventricular fibrillation) cause the majority of cases of SCD. Less commonly, SCD occurs because of a primary left ventricular outflow obstruction (e.g., aortic stenosis, hypertrophic cardiomyopathy), genetic predisposition such as Brugada syndrome, or long QT syndrome (Urden et al., 2018).

People who experience SCD because of CAD are categorized as (a) those who did not have an acute MI and (b) those who did have an acute MI. The first group accounts for the majority of cases of SCD. In this instance, victims usually have no warning signs or symptoms. Patients who survive are at risk for another episode of SCD because of the continued electrical instability of the myocardium that led to the initial event. The second, smaller group of patients includes those who have had an MI and have suffered SCD. In these cases, patients usually do have prodrome symptoms, such as chest pain, palpitations, and dyspnea.

It is difficult to predict who is at risk for SCD. Risk factors for SCD include (a) male sex, (b) family history of premature atherosclerosis, (c) tobacco use, (d) diabetes mellitus, (e) hypercholesterolemia, (f) hypertension, and (g) cardiomyopathy.

NURSING AND INTERPROFESSIONAL MANAGEMENT SUDDEN CARDIAC DEATH

People who survive an episode of SCD generally require a diagnostic workup to determine whether they have had an MI. Thus, serial analyses of cardiac markers and ECGs are done, and treatment is planned accordingly. (See section on interprofessional care of ACS.) In addition, because most people with SCD have CAD, cardiac catheterization is indicated to determine the possible location and extent of coronary artery occlusion. PCI or CABG surgery may also be indicated.

Most patients with SCD have a lethal ventricular dysrhythmia that has a high incidence of recurrence. Thus it is useful to know when those people are most likely to have a recurrence and what medication therapy is the most effective treatment. Assessment of dysrhythmias in these patients includes 24-hour Holter monitoring or other type of event recorder, exercise stress testing, signal-averaged ECG, and electrophysiological study (EPS) performed with fluoroscopy. Pacing electrodes are placed in select intracardiac areas, and stimuli are selectively used to attempt to produce dysrhythmias. The patient's response to various antidysrhythmic medications is determined and monitored in a controlled environment. (EPS is discussed in Chapters 34 and 38.)

The most common approach to preventing a recurrence is the use of an implantable cardioverter-defibrillator (ICD). Medication therapy with amiodarone may be used in conjunction with an ICD to decrease episodes of ventricular dysrhythmias.

When caring for these patients, the nurse should be alert to the patient's psychosocial adaptation to this sudden "brush with death." Many of these patients develop a "time bomb" mentality. They fear the recurrence of cardiopulmonary arrest and may become anxious, angry, and depressed. Their caregivers are likely to experience the same feelings.

Patients and caregivers may need to cope with additional issues, such as possible driving restrictions and change in occupation. The grief response varies among patients and caregivers. The nurse should be attuned to the specific needs of the patient and caregiver and teach them accordingly while providing appropriate emotional support.

CASE STUDY

Myocardial Infarction

Patient Profile

O. M. (pronouns he/him), a 61-year-old business executive, is rushed to the hospital by ambulance after experiencing crushing substernal chest pain that radiates down his left arm. He also reports having dizziness and nausea.

Subjective Data

- Has a history of chronic stable angina and hypertension
- States is "borderline diabetic"
- Overweight but recently lost 3 kg
- Rarely exercises
- Has three teenage children who are causing "problems"
- Recently experienced loss of best friend and business partner, who died from cancer

Objective Data
Physical Examination

- Diaphoresis, shortness of breath, nausea
- BP 165/100 mm Hg; pulse rate, 120 beats/min; respiratory rate, 26/min

Diagnostic Studies

- ECG shows occasional premature ventricular contractions and ST elevation in leads II, III, aV_F, V_5, and V_6.
- Cardiac-specific troponin I is 5 ng/mL.
- Cholesterol level is 9.1 mmol/L.
- Hb A1C level is 9.0%.
- Inferolateral wall MI is diagnosed.

Interprofessional Care
Emergency Department

- Oxygen, 2 L/min via nasal cannula, titrated to keep O_2 saturation >93%
- Continuous ECG monitoring
- ASA, 160 mg (chewable)
- Eptifibatide (Integrilin), IV
- Weight-based heparin, IV
- Nitroglycerin intravenously, titrated to relieve chest pain; withheld for systolic BP <100 mm Hg
- Morphine, 2 to 4 mg, IV q5min PRN for chest pain unrelieved by nitroglycerin
- Metoprolol (Lopressor), 5 mg IV q5min × 3 doses
- Vital sign measurements and pulse oximetry q15min until stable, then q1h
- Preparation of patient for transfer to cardiac catheterization laboratory for possible PCI

Discussion Questions

1. Which coronary arteries are probably occluded in O. M.'s coronary circulation?
2. What risk factors contribute to its development? What risk factors were present in O. M.'s life?
3. What is angina? How does angina differ from myocardial infarction?
4. What is the pathophysiological basis for the clinical manifestations that O. M. exhibited?
5. What is the significance of the results of the laboratory tests and ECG findings?
6. What is the rationale for each treatment measure ordered for O. M.?
7. *Priority decision:* What are the priority nursing interventions for O. M. immediately after the MI?
8. *Priority decision:* Based on the assessment data presented, what are the priority nursing diagnoses? Identify any interprofessional issues.
9. *Evidence-informed practice:* Two days after an uncomplicated PCI and the placement of two stents, O. M. wants to know what the most effective strategies are to prevent another MI. Based on O. M.'s clinical situation, what should the nurse recommend?

*e*volve

Answers are available at http://evolve.elsevier.com/Canada/Lewis/medsurg.

REVIEW QUESTIONS

The number of the question corresponds to the same-numbered objective at the beginning of the chapter.

1. A nursing student placed on medicine telemetry asks the preceptor how common is heart disease in Canada. What is the best response?
   a. It is more common in people experiencing stress.
   b. It claims the life of 50 000 Canadians each year.
   c. It is the second major cause of all deaths in Canada.
   d. It is not very common at all.
2. A nurse is teaching a client about coronary artery disease. Which changes occur in this disorder? *(Select all that apply.)*
   a. Diffuse involvement of plaque formation in coronary veins
   b. Abnormal levels of cholesterol, especially low-density lipoproteins
   c. Accumulation of lipid plaques or calcification within the coronary arteries
   d. Development of angina due to a decreased blood supply to the heart muscle
   e. Chronic vasoconstriction of coronary arteries leading to permanent vasospasm

3. Which statement indicates that the client requires additional instruction in reducing cardiac risk factors?
   a. "I would like to add weightlifting to my exercise program."
   b. "I can't keep my blood pressure normal without medication."
   c. "I can change my diet to decrease my intake of saturated fats."
   d. "I will change my lifestyle to reduce activities that increase my stress."
4. A hospitalized client with angina tells the nurse that she is having chest pain. What are the nurse's priorities?
   a. Perform vital signs and obtain an ECG.
   b. Administer sublingual nitroglycerin and intravenous morphine.
   c. Call the rapid response team and the physician.
   d. Inform the cardiac catheterization lab and interventional cardiologist.
5. What does the clinical spectrum of ACS include?
   a. Unstable angina and STEMI
   b. Unstable angina and NSTEMI
   c. Stable angina and sudden cardiac death
   d. Unstable angina, STEMI, and NSTEMI

6. In a client recovering from an MI, in which period is the heart most vulnerable to stress?
   a. 3 weeks after the infarction
   b. 4 to 6 days after the infarction
   c. 10 to 14 days after the infarction
   d. When healing is complete, at 6 to 8 weeks
7. A client is admitted to the ED with chest pain of 2 hours' duration, ECG findings consistent with an acute MI, and occasional ventricular dysrhythmias. With what pharmacological therapy would the nurse expect the client to be managed initially?
   a. Diuretics
   b. Nitroglycerin spray
   c. β-Adrenergic blockers
   d. Thrombolytic therapy with tissue plasminogen activator
8. Five days after an MI, a client is restless and apprehensive. How can the nurse assist the client?
   a. By providing all care and doing everything for the client
   b. By structuring the environment and the routine so that the client can rest
   c. By allowing the client to participate in planning and carrying out activities
   d. By encouraging the family to provide for the client's physical care and give emotional support

9. What is the most common pathological finding in individuals experiencing SCD?
   a. Cardiomyopathies
   b. Mitral valve disease
   c. Atherosclerotic heart disease
   d. Left ventricular hypertrophy

1. c; 2. b, c, d; 3. a; 4. a; 5. d; 6. c; 7. b; 8. c; 9. c.

ℯvolve

For even more review questions, visit http://evolve.elsevier.com/Canada/Lewis/medsurg.

REFERENCES

American Heart Association. (2021). *Understand your risk of excessive blood clotting.* https://www.empoweredtoserve.org/en/health-topics/venous-thromboembolism/understand-your-risk-for-excessive-blood-clotting

Anand, S., Arbour, L., Balasubramanian, K., et al. (2019). Explaining the variability in cardiovascular risk factors among First Nations communities in Canada: A population-based study. *The Lancet, 3*(12), E511–E520. https://doi.org/10.1016/S2542-5196(19)30237-2

Anderson, T., Gregoire, J., Pearson, G., et al. (2016). 2016 Canadian Cardiovascular Society guidelines for the management of dyslipidemia for the prevention of cardiovascular disease in the adult. *Canadian Journal of Cardiology, 32,* 1263–1282. https://doi.org/10.1016/j.cjca.2016.07.510

Batal, M., & Decelles, S. (2019). A scoping review of obesity among Indigenous peoples in Canada. *Journal of Obesity, 2019,* 1–20. https://doi.org/10.1155/2019/9741090

Boothby, C. A., Dada, B. R., Rabi, D. M., et al. (2018). The Effect of cardiac rehabilitation attendance on sexual activity outcomes in cardiovascular disease patients: A systematic review. *Canadian Journal of Cardiology, 34*(12), 1590–1599. https://doi.org/10.1016/j.cjca.2018.08.020

Burchum, J., & Rosenthal, L. (2016). *Lehne's pharmacology for nursing care* (9th ed.). Elsevier.

Canadian Institute for Health Information (CIHI). (2017). *Cardiac Care Quality Indicators Report.* https://secure.cihi.ca/free_products/cardiac-care-quality-indicators-report-en-web.pdf

Canadian Institute for Health Information (CIHI). (2021). *Top five reasons for hospital stays.* https://www.cihi.ca/en/hospital-stays-in-canada

Canadian Society for Exercise Physiology. (2021). *Canadian 24-hour movement guidelines: An integration of physical activity, sedentary behaviour, and sleep.* https://csepguidelines.ca/

Cardosa, L. (2018). Hyperhomocysteinemia: How does it affect the development of cardiovascular disease? *International Archives of Cardiovascular Diseases, 2*(1), 1–12.

Crowshoe, L., Dannenbaum, D., Green, M., et al. (2018). Clinical practice guidelines: Type 2 diabetes and Indigenous peoples. *Canadian Journal of Diabetes, 42,* S296–S306. https://doi.org/10.1016/j.jcjd.2017.10.022

Diffey, L., Fontaine, L., & Schultz, A. H. S. (2019). *Understanding First Nations women's heart health.* National Collaborating Centre for Indigenous Health. https://www.nccih.ca/docs/emerging/RPT-Womens-Heart-Health-Diffey-Fontaine-Schultz-EN.pdf

Edelman, C., & Kudzma, E. (2018). *Health promotion across the lifespan* (9th ed). Elsevier.

Firestone, M., Tyndall, M., & Fischer, B. (2015). Substance use and related harms among Aboriginal People in Canada: A comprehensive review. *Journal of Health Care for the Poor and Underserved, 26*(4), 1110–1131. https://doi.org/10.1353/hpu.2015.0108

Fischer, B., Russell, C., Sabioni, P., et al. (2017). Lower-risk cannabis use guidelines (LRCUG): An evidence-based update. *American Journal of Public Health, 107*(8). https://doi.org/10.2105/AJPH.2017.303818

Framingham Heart Study. (n.d.). The Framingham Heart Study. https://framinghamheartstudy.org/

Gaudino, M., Benedetto, U., Fremes, S., et al. (2018). Radial-artery or saphenous-vein grafts in coronary-artery bypass surgery. *New England Journal of Medicine, 378*(22), 2069–2077. https://doi.org/10.1056/NEJMoa1716026

Hagström, E., Norlund, F., Stebbins, A., et al. (2017). Psychosocial stress and major cardiovascular events in patients with stable coronary heart disease. *Journal of Internal Medicine, 283*(1), 83–92. https://doi.org/10.1111/joim.12692

Heart and Stroke Foundation of Canada. (2016). *2016 report on the health of Canadians.* http://www.heartandstroke.ca/-/media/pdf-files/canada/2017-heart-month/heartandstroke-reportonhealth-2016.ashx?la=en

Heart and Stroke Foundation of Canada. (2021a). *Cannabis, heart disease and stroke.* https://www.heartandstroke.ca/heart/risk-and-prevention/lifestyle-risk-factors/heavy-alcohol-use/cannabis-heart-disease-and-stroke

Heart and Stroke Foundation of Canada. (2021b). *Healthy eating.* https://www.heartandstroke.ca/get-healthy/healthy-eating

Heart and Stroke Foundation of Canada. (2021c). *Healthy weight.* https://www.heartandstroke.ca/get-healthy/healthy-weight

Heart and Stroke Foundation of Canada. (2021d). *Helping to close the gap in Indigenous health.* https://www.heartandstroke.ca/what-we-do/our-impact/helping-to-close-the-gap-in-indigenous-health

Heart and Stroke Foundation of Canada. (2021e). *How much physical activity do you need?.* https://www.heartandstroke.ca/get-healthy/stay-active/how-much-physical-activity-do-you-need

Heart and Stroke Foundation of Canada. (2021f). *Stress basics.* https://www.heartandstroke.ca/get-healthy/reduce-stress/stress-basics

Heart and Stroke Foundation of Canada. (2021g). *Women: Risks and signs.* https://www.heartandstroke.ca/women/risk-and-signs

Huether, S., McCance, K., & Brashers (2020). *Understanding pathophysiology* (7th ed.). Mosby.

Hypertension Canada. (2018). *Hypertension Canada guidelines.* https://guidelines.hypertension.ca/about/about-chep/

Jetty, R. (2017). Position statement: Tobacco use and misuse among Indigenous children and youth in Canada. *Paediatrics and Child Health, 22*(7), 395–399. https://doi.org/10.1093/pch/pxx124

Kim, S., & Park, T. (2019). Acute and chronic effects of cocaine on cardiovascular health. *International Journal of Molecular Science, 20*(3), 584–606. https://doi.org/10.3390/ijms20030584

Kosar, L., Koziol, K., Martens, A., et al. (2016). *Duration of dual antiplatelet therapy (DAPT) and triple antiplatelet therapy for cardiovascular and cerebrovascular indications.* https://www.rxfiles.ca/rxfiles/uploads/documents/DAPT%20and%20Triple%20Therapy%20Newsletter%20and%20Chart.pdf

MacDonald, A., & Middlekauff, H. (2019). Electronic cigarettes and cardiovascular health: What do we know so far? *Vascular Health Risk Management, 15*, 159–174. https://doi.org/10.2147/VHRM.S175970

National Collaborating Centre for Aboriginal Health. (2011). *An overview of Aboriginal health in Canada.* https://www.ccnsa-nccah.ca/docs/context/FS-OverviewAbororiginalHealth-EN.pdf (Seminal).

Nerenberg, K., Zamke, K., Leung, A., et al. (2018). Hypertension Canada's 2018 guidelines for diagnosis, risk, assessment, prevention, and treatment of hypertension in adults and children. *Canadian Journal of Cardiology, 34*, 506–525. https://doi.org/10.1016/j.cjca.2018.02.022

Norris, C., Nerenberg, K., Clavel, M., et al. (2020). State of the science in women's cardiovascular disease: A Canadian perspective on the influence of sex and gender. *Journal of American Heart Association, 9*(4), 1–27. https://doi.org/10.1161/JAHA.119.015634

Öberg, M., Woodward, A., Jaakkola, J. A., et al. (2010). *Global estimate of the burden of disease from second-hand smoke.* https://apps.who.int/iris/bitstream/handle/10665/44426/9789241564076_eng.pdf

Pagana, K., Pike-MacDonald, S., & Pagana, T. (2019). *Mosby's Canadian manual of diagnostic and laboratory tests* (2nd ed.). Elsevier.

Prince, S., Comber, L., Turek, M., et al. (2017). Charting the course for women's heart health in Canada: Recommendations from the first Canadian women's heart health summit. *Canadian Journal of Cardiology, 33*(6), 693–700. https://doi.org/10.1016/j.cjca.2017.04.009

Public Health Agency of Canada. (2019). *Report from the Canadian Chronic Disease Surveillance System: Heart disease in Canada, 2018.* https://www.canada.ca/en/public-health/services/publications/diseases-conditions/report-heart-disease-Canada-2018.html

Rabi, D. M., McBrien, K. A., Sapir-Pichhadze, R., et al. (2020). Hypertension Canada's 2020 comprehensive guidelines for the prevention, diagnosis, risk assessment, and treatment of hypertension in adults and children. *Canadian Journal of Cardiology, 36*(5), 596–624. https://doi.org/10.1016/j.cjca.2020.02.086

Skidmore, L. (2020). *Mosby's 2017 Nursing drug reference* (33rd ed.). Elsevier.

Sole, M., Klein, D., & Moseley, M. (2017). *Introduction to critical care nursing* (7th ed.). Elsevier.

Statistics Canada. (2021). *Leading causes of death, total population, by age group.* https://www150.statcan.gc.ca/t1/tbl1/en/tv.action?pid=1310039401

Tang, K., & Jardine, C. (2016). Our way of life: Importance of indigenous culture and tradition to physical activity practices. *International Journal of Indigenous Health, 11*(1). https://doi.org/10.18357/ijih11120161601

Urden, L., Stacey, K., & Lough, M. (2018). *Critical care nursing: Diagnosis and management.* (8th ed.). Elsevier.

Vaccarino, V., Badmimon, L., Bremner, D., et al. (2019). Depression and coronary heart disease: 2018 position paper of the ESC working group on coronary pathophysiology and microcirculation. *European Heart Journal, 41*(17), 1687–1696. https://doi.org/10.1093/eurheartj/ehy913

Ward, N., Watts, G., & Eckel, R. (2019). Statin toxicity. *Circulation Research, 124*, 328–350. https://doi.org/10.1161/CIRCRESAHA.118.312782

Wein, T., Lindsay, P., Gladstone, D., et al. (2020). Canadian stroke best practice recommendations, seventh edition: Acetylsalicylic acid for prevention of vascular events. *Canadian Medical Association Journal, 23*, 302–311. https://doi.org/10.1503/cmaj.191599

Wong, G., Welsford, M., Ainsworth, C., et al. (2019). 2019 Canadian Cardiovascular Society of interventional cardiology guidelines on the acute management of ST-elevation myocardial infarction: Focused update on regionalization and reperfusion. *Canadian Journal of Cardiology, 35*, 107–132. https://doi.org/10.1016/j.cjca2018.11.031

RESOURCES

Canadian Council of Cardiovascular Nurses
https://www.cccn.ca

Canadian Sudden Cardiac Arrest Network (CSCAN)
https://clinicaltrials.gov/ct2/show/NCT03642587

Heart and Stroke Foundation of Canada
https://www.heartandstroke.ca

Hypertension Canada—Guidelines
https://guidelines.hypertension.ca

Public Health Agency of Canada
https://www.phac-aspc.gc.ca/chn-rcs/saa-toxicomanie-eng.php

Registered Nurses' Association of Ontario—Best Practice Guideline: Integrating Smoking Cessation Into Daily Nursing Practice
https://rnao.ca/sites/rnao-ca/files/Integrating_Smoking_Cessation_into_Daily_Nursing_Practice.pdf

---

American College of Cardiovascular Nurses (ACCN)
https://www.accn.net

American Heart Association
https://www.heart.org

Framingham Heart Study
https://www.framingham.com/heart/index.htm

Health Central—Let's Talk About Heart Disease
https://www.healthcentral.com/heart-disease

National Heart, Lung, and Blood Institute—Calculate Your Body Mass Index
https://www.nhlbi.nih.gov/health/educational/lose_wt/BMI/bmicalc.htm

evolve

For additional Internet resources, see the website for this book at http://evolve.elsevier.com/Canada/Lewis/medsurg.

Nursing Management
Heart Failure

Barbara Wilson-Keates
Originating US chapter by Vera Barton-Maxwell

℮volve WEBSITE

http://evolve.elsevier.com/Canada/Lewis/medsurg

- Review Questions (Online Only)
- Key Points
- Answer Guidelines for Case Study
- Customizable Nursing Care Plan

- Heart Failure
- Conceptual Care Map Creator
- Conceptual Care Map for Textbook Case Study

- Audio Glossary
- Content Updates

LEARNING OBJECTIVES

1. Compare the pathophysiology of heart failure with preserved and reduced ejection fraction.
2. Relate the compensatory mechanisms involved in heart failure to the development of acute decompensated heart failure and chronic heart failure.
3. Select the appropriate nursing and interprofessional interventions to manage a patient with acute decompensated heart failure.
4. Select the appropriate nursing and interprofessional interventions to manage a patient with chronic heart failure.
5. Describe the indications for cardiac transplantation and the nursing management of cardiac transplant recipients.

KEY TERMS

cardiac transplantation
heart failure (HF)
heart failure with preserved ejection fraction (HFpEF)

heart failure with mid-range ejection fraction (HFmEF)
heart failure with reduced ejection fraction (HFrEF)

paroxysmal nocturnal dyspnea
pulmonary edema

HEART FAILURE

Heart failure (HF) is an abnormal clinical syndrome involving impaired cardiac pumping or filling, or both. *Heart failure,* formerly called *congestive heart failure,* is the term preferred today because not all patients with HF have pulmonary congestion or volume overload. HF is associated with numerous types of cardiovascular diseases, particularly long-standing hypertension, coronary artery disease (CAD), and myocardial infarction (MI) (Table 37.1). HF is characterized by ventricular dysfunction, reduced exercise tolerance, diminished quality of life, and shortened life expectancy.

Globally, HF has become a major health problem. In contrast to other cardiovascular diseases, HF is projected to increase in incidence. The prevalence of HF increases with age, which is of particular concern to Canada's aging population (Heart and Stroke Foundation of Canada, 2021).

In Canada, it is estimated that one in five people older than 40 years will suffer from HF during their lifetime. Currently, 600 000 Canadians are affected by HF, which is a leading cause of hospitalization. At least $2.8 billion dollars per year is spent on direct health care costs of this disease, creating a significant economic burden on communities (Virani et al., 2017). Canadians hospitalized with HF have a 30-day readmission rate of greater than 20%. Despite improvements in therapy since the late 1980s, the mortality rate 1 year after diagnosis remains high, at 30% (Atzema et al., 2018).

Etiology and Pathophysiology

CAD and hypertension are the primary risk factors for HF. In Canada, CAD and hypertension are responsible for up to 45% and 27.5% of patients, respectively (Di Giuseppe et al., 2019).

Diabetes mellitus predisposes an individual to HF regardless of the presence of concomitant CAD or hypertension. The

TABLE 37.1	COMMON CAUSES OF HEART FAILURE	
Chronic	**Acute**	
Coronary artery disease	Acute myocardial infarction	
Hypertension	Dysrhythmias	
Rheumatic heart disease	Pulmonary embolus	
Congenital heart disease	Thyrotoxicosis	
Ventricular septal defect	Hypertensive crisis	
Pulmonary disease	Rupture of papillary muscle	
Cardiomyopathy	Myocarditis	
Anemia	Bacterial endocarditis	
Bacterial endocarditis		
Valvular disorders		

TABLE 37.2	PRECIPITATING CAUSES OF HEART FAILURE
Cause	**Mechanism**
Anemia	↓ Oxygen-carrying capacity of the blood, stimulating ↑ in CO to meet tissue demands
Infection	↑ Oxygen demand of tissues, stimulating ↑ CO
Thyrotoxicosis	Changes in the tissue metabolic rate; ↑ HR and workload of the heart
Hypothyroidism	Indirectly predisposes to ↑ atherosclerosis; severe hypothyroidism decreases myocardial contractility
Dysrhythmias	May ↓ CO and ↑ workload and oxygen requirements of myocardial tissue
Bacterial endocarditis	Infection: ↑ metabolic demands and oxygen requirements
	Valvular dysfunction: causes stenosis and regurgitation
Myocarditis	↑ HR, ↓ CO, acute right and left ventricular failure
Pulmonary embolism	↑ Pulmonary pressure and exerts pressure on the RV, leading to right ventricular hypertrophy and failure
Pulmonary disease	↑ Pulmonary pressure and exerts a pressure load on the RV, leading to right ventricular hypertrophy and failure
Paget's disease	↑ Workload of the heart by ↑ vascular bed in the skeletal muscle
Nutritional deficiencies	May ↓ cardiac function by ↓ myocardial muscle mass and myocardial contractility
Hypervolemia	↑ Preload, causing volume load on the RV

CO, cardiac output; *HR*, heart rate; *LV*, left ventricle; *RV*, right ventricle.

etiology is thought to be complex and related in part to insulin resistance and its effect on ventricular remodelling (Ezekowitz et al., 2017). Other risk factors for the development of HF include tobacco smoking, obesity, and high serum levels of cholesterol (Heart and Stroke Foundation of Canada, 2021). Diabetes mellitus is particularly endemic in the Indigenous population, mainly because of the impact of social determinants of health, intergenerational trauma, and food insecurity. HF may be caused by any interference with the normal mechanisms regulating cardiac output (CO). CO depends on (a) preload, (b) afterload, (c) myocardial contractility, and (d) heart rate (HR). (Preload, afterload, and other hemodynamic parameters are discussed in Chapter 34.) Any alteration in these factors can lead to decreased ventricular function and the resultant manifestations of HF.

In general, major causes of HF may be divided into two subgroups: primary causes (see Table 37.1) and precipitating causes (Table 37.2). Precipitating causes often increase the workload of the ventricles, which results in a decompensated condition that leads to decreased myocardial function. Certain precipitation causes are reversible if cardiac cells have not hypertrophied or remodelled.

Pathology of Ventricular Failure. HF is described as being accompanied by either reduced ejection fraction (EF; the percentage of total amount of end-diastolic blood volume that is ejected during each systole), mid-range EF, or preserved EF (Ezekowitz et al., 2017).

Heart Failure With Reduced Ejection Fraction. Heart failure with reduced ejection fraction (HFrEF), the most common form of HF, results from an inability of the heart to pump blood effectively. It is caused by impaired contractile function (e.g., myocardial ischemia), increased afterload (e.g., hypertension), cardiomyopathy, and mechanical abnormalities (e.g., valvular heart disease). The left ventricle loses its ability to generate enough pressure to eject blood forward through the aorta. The hallmark of HFrEF is a reduction in the left ventricular EF. Normal EF is higher than 55% of the ventricular volume. Patients with HFrEF requiring specialist intervention generally have an EF of 40% or lower (Ezekowitz et al., 2017).

Heart Failure With Preserved Ejection Fraction. Heart failure with preserved ejection fraction (HFpEF) is the inability of the ventricles to relax and fill during diastole. Decreased filling of the ventricles results in decreased stroke volume and CO. HFpEF is characterized by high filling pressures, which are increased because of poorly compliant ventricles. This results in venous engorgement in both the pulmonary and systemic vascular systems. HFpEF is often the result of left ventricular hypertrophy from hypertension (most common), myocardial ischemia, valve disease (e.g., aortic, mitral), or cardiomyopathy. However, many affected patients do not have identifiable heart disease. The diagnosis of HFpEF is based on the presence of HF symptoms with an EF of 50% or greater (Ezekowitz et al., 2017).

Heart Failure With Mid-Range Ejection Fraction. Heart failure with mid-range ejection fraction (HFmEF) represents many different characteristics of HF with a left ventricular EF of 41 to 49%. (Ezekowitz et al., 2017). This term applies to patients transitioning to and from HFpEF. *Recovered EF* is a new term that refers to individuals who originally had HFrEF but, with treatment and management, now have EF greater or equal to 40%.

Mixed Heart Failure. HF of mixed origin occurs in disease states such as dilated cardiomyopathy. Dilated cardiomyopathy is a condition in which poor systolic function (weakened muscle function) is further compromised by dilated left ventricular walls that are unable to relax and hence fill effectively. Affected patients often have an extremely poor EF (<35%), high pulmonary pressures, and biventricular failure (both ventricles may be dilated and have poor filling and emptying capacity).

Patients with HF of any type have low systemic arterial blood pressure (BP), low CO, and poor renal perfusion. Poor exercise tolerance and ventricular dysrhythmias are also common. Whether a patient arrives at this point acutely as a result of MI or chronically from worsening cardiomyopathy or hypertension, the body's response to this low CO is to mobilize its compensatory mechanisms to maintain CO and BP.

Compensatory Mechanisms. HF can have an abrupt onset, as with acute MI, or it can be a subtle process resulting from slow, progressive changes. The overloaded heart uses compensatory mechanisms to try to maintain adequate CO. The main compensatory mechanisms include (a) sympathetic nervous system (SNS) activation, (b) neurohormonal responses, (c) ventricular dilation, and (d) ventricular hypertrophy.

DETERMINANTS OF HEALTH

Heart Disease Rehabilitation

Barriers to cardiac rehabilitation utilization, particularly for ethnic minorities, include competing priorities (lack of time, work, family responsibilities, and distance to the facility), lack of health care provider endorsement, and lack of knowledge or misinformation.[*]

Gender
- Women are less likely to enroll in a cardiac rehabilitation program.[†]
- Use of cardiac rehabilitation is associated with a more significant reduction in mortality among women than among men.[†]

Culture
- Use of cardiac rehabilitation is lower among members of minority groups because of variations in cultural beliefs, diet, and exercise.[*]

Education and Literacy
- Educated and higher-income individuals are more likely to use cardiac rehabilitation because of availability of resources and their motivation.[*]

Personal Health Practice and Coping Skills
- After diagnosis of a cardiovascular-related illness, fewer than 5% of Canadians who smoked quit.[‡]

Health Services
- Use of cardiac rehabilitation is associated with a 64% reduction in mortality in women and a 49% reduction in mortality in men.[†]
- Only 40% of participants eligible to receive cardiac rehabilitation enroll in such programs.[†]

[*]Data from Mead, H., Ramos, C., & Grantham, S. C. (2016). Drivers of racial and ethnic disparities in cardiac rehabilitation use: Patient and provider perspectives. *Medical Care Research and Review, 73*(3), 251–282. doi:10.1177/1077558715606261
[†]Colbert, J. D., Martin, B. J., Haykowsky, M. J., et al. (2015). Cardiac rehabilitation referral, attendance and mortality in women. *European Journal of Preventive Cardiology, 22*(8), 979–986. https://doi.org/10.1177/2047487314545279
[‡]Heart and Stroke Foundation of Canada. (2021). *Heart failure.* https://www.heartandstroke.ca/heart/conditions/heart-failure

Sympathetic Nervous System Activation. SNS activation is often the first mechanism triggered in low-CO states. However, it is the least effective compensatory mechanism. In response to an inadequate stroke volume and CO, SNS activation increases, resulting in the increased release of catecholamines (epinephrine and norepinephrine). This results in increased HR, increased myocardial contractility, and peripheral vasoconstriction. Initially, this increase in HR and contractility improves CO. Over time, however, these factors are harmful, inasmuch as they increase the already failing heart's workload and need for oxygen. The vasoconstriction causes an immediate increase in preload, which may initially increase CO, but an increase in venous return to the heart, which is already volume overloaded, actually worsens ventricular performance.

Neurohormonal Responses. As the CO falls, blood flow to the kidneys decreases. The juxtaglomerular apparatus in the kidneys sense decreased volume from the reduced blood flow. In response, the kidneys release renin, which converts angiotensinogen to angiotensin I (see Chapter 47 and Figure 47.6). Angiotensin I is subsequently converted to angiotensin II by angiotensin-converting enzyme (ACE) made in the lungs. Angiotensin II causes (a) the adrenal cortex to release aldosterone, which results in sodium and water retention, and (b) increased peripheral vasoconstriction, which increases BP. This response is the *renin–angiotensin–aldosterone system* (RAAS).

Low CO causes a decrease in cerebral perfusion pressure. In response, the posterior pituitary gland secretes antidiuretic hormone (ADH; also called *vasopressin*). ADH increases water reabsorption in the kidneys, which causes water retention. As a result, blood volume is increased when a volume overload state already exists.

Other factors also contribute to the development of HF. The release of ADH, catecholamines, and angiotensin II stimulates the production of endothelin, a potent vasoconstrictor produced by the vascular endothelial cells. Endothelin results in further arterial vasoconstriction and an increase in cardiac contractility and hypertrophy.

Locally, proinflammatory cytokines are released by heart cells in response to various forms of cardiac injury (e.g., MI). Two cytokines, tumour necrosis factor (TNF) and interleukin-1 (IL-1), further depress heart function by causing hypertrophy, contractile dysfunction, and cell death. Over time, a systemic inflammatory response also occurs. This accounts for the cardiac and skeletal muscle myopathy and fatigue that accompany advanced HF.

Activation of the SNS and the neurohormonal response lead to elevated levels of norepinephrine, angiotensin II, aldosterone, ADH, endothelin, and proinflammatory cytokines. Together, these factors result in an increase in cardiac workload, myocardial dysfunction, and ventricular remodelling. Remodelling involves hypertrophy of the ventricular myocytes, which causes contractile cells to become enlarged and abnormally shaped. This altered geometric shape of the ventricles eventually leads to increased ventricular mass, increased wall tension, increased oxygen consumption, and impaired contractility. Although the ventricles become larger, they become less effective pumps. Ventricular remodelling is a risk factor for life-threatening dysrhythmias and sudden cardiac death.

Ventricular Dilation. *Dilation* is an enlargement of the chambers of the heart. It occurs when pressure in the heart chambers (usually the left ventricle) becomes chronically elevated. The muscle fibres of the heart stretch in response to the volume of blood in the heart at the end of diastole. According to Starling's Law, the degree of stretch is directly related to the force of the contraction (systole). Initially, dilation is an adaptive mechanism to cope with increasing blood volume, and this increased contraction leads to increased CO and maintenance of arterial BP and perfusion. Eventually, this mechanism becomes inadequate because the elastic elements of the muscle fibres are overstretched and can no longer contract effectively and CO diminishes (Figure 37.1, *A*).

Ventricular Hypertrophy. *Hypertrophy* is an increase in the muscle mass and cardiac wall thickness in response to overwork and strain (see Figure 37.1, *B*). It develops slowly because it takes time for muscle tissue to thicken. Initially, the increased contractile power of the muscle fibres leads to an increase in CO and maintenance of tissue perfusion. Over time, hypertrophic heart muscle has poor contractility and requires more oxygen to perform work, coronary artery circulation becomes poor (tissue becomes ischemic more easily), and the heart is prone to dysrhythmias due to altered electrical pathways.

Counterregulatory Mechanisms. The body's attempts to maintain balance are demonstrated by several counterregulatory processes. Natriuretic peptides (atrial natriuretic peptide and brain, or B-type, natriuretic peptide [BNP]) are hormones produced by the heart muscle. Atrial natriuretic peptide is

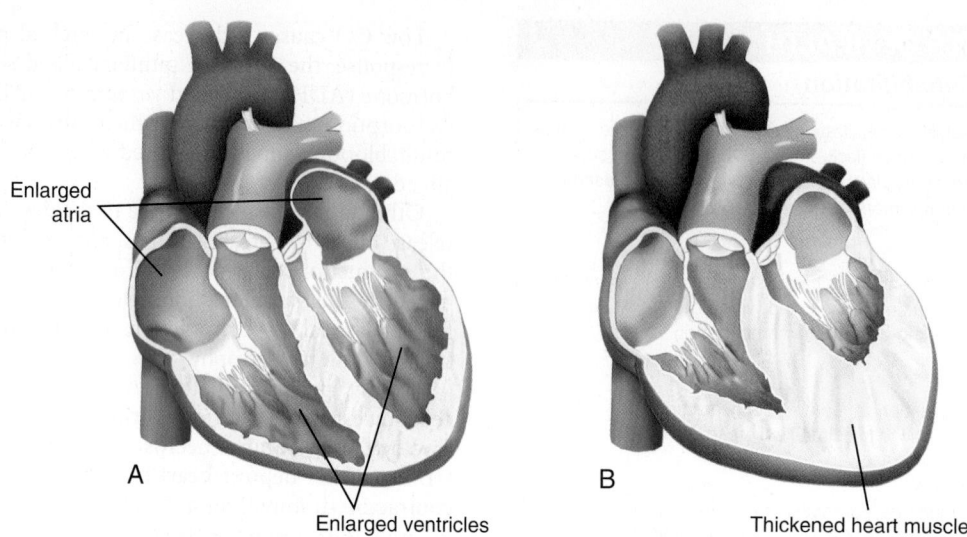

FIG. 37.1 **A,** Dilated heart chambers. **B,** Hypertrophied heart chambers.

released from the atria and BNP is released from the ventricles in response to increased blood volume in the heart (Hannon & Porth, 2017).

The natriuretic peptides have renal, cardiovascular, and hormonal effects. Renal effects include (a) increased glomerular filtration rate and diuresis and (b) excretion of sodium (natriuresis). Cardiovascular effects include vasodilation and decreased BP. Hormonal effects include (a) inhibition of aldosterone and renin secretion and (b) interference with ADH release. The combined effects of atrial natriuretic peptide and BNP help counter the adverse effects of the SNS and RAAS in patients with HF (Hannon & Porth, 2017).

Cardiac compensation occurs when compensatory mechanisms succeed in maintaining a CO that is adequate for essential tissue perfusion. Cardiac decompensation occurs when these mechanisms can no longer maintain adequate CO and tissue perfusion becomes insufficient.

Types of Heart Failure

HF is usually evidenced by biventricular failure, although one ventricle may become dysfunctional before the other. Normally, the pumping actions of the left and right sides of the heart complement each other, producing a continuous flow of blood. However, due to pathological conditions, one side may fail, and the other side continues to function normally for a time. Because of the prolonged strain, both sides of the heart eventually fail, resulting in biventricular failure.

Left-Sided Heart Failure. The most common form of initial HF is left-sided failure (Figure 37.2). Left-sided failure results from left ventricular dysfunction, which causes blood to back up through the left atrium and into the pulmonary veins. The increased pulmonary pressure causes fluid extravasation from the pulmonary capillary bed into the interstitium and then the alveoli, which is manifested as pulmonary congestion and edema with pink, frothy sputum.

Right-Sided Heart Failure. Right-sided HF causes backward blood flow to the right atrium and venous circulation. Venous congestion in the systemic circulation results in peripheral edema, hepatomegaly, splenomegaly, vascular congestion of the gastrointestinal tract, and jugular venous distension. The primary cause of right-sided failure is left-sided failure. In this

situation, left-sided failure results in pulmonary congestion and increased pressure in the blood vessels of the lungs (pulmonary hypertension). Eventually, chronic pulmonary hypertension results in right-sided hypertrophy and failure. Cor pulmonale (right ventricular dilation and hypertrophy caused by pulmonary disease) can also cause right-sided failure. (Cor pulmonale is discussed in Chapter 30.) Right ventricular infarction may also cause right ventricular failure.

Clinical Manifestations of Heart Failure

Regardless of etiology, acute decompensated heart failure (ADHF) typically manifests as pulmonary edema, an abnormal, life-threatening accumulation of fluid in the alveoli and interstitial spaces of the lungs (Figure 37.3). The most common cause of pulmonary edema is acute left ventricular failure secondary to acute myocardial ischemia. (Other etiological factors for pulmonary edema are listed in Chapter 30, Table 30.24.)

In most cases of ADHF, the pulmonary venous pressure increases as a result of decreased efficiency of the left ventricle. This results in engorgement of the pulmonary vascular system. As a result, the lungs become less compliant and there is increased resistance in the small airways. In addition, the lymphatic system increases its flow to help maintain a constant volume of the pulmonary extravascular fluid. This early stage is clinically associated with a mild increase in the respiratory rate and a decrease in partial pressure of arterial oxygen (PaO_2).

If pulmonary venous pressure continues to increase, the increase in intravascular pressure causes more fluid to move into the interstitial space than the lymphatic vessels can drain. Interstitial edema occurs at this point. Tachypnea develops, and the patient becomes symptomatic (short of breath out of proportion to activity level). If the pulmonary venous pressure increases further, the tight alveoli lining cells are disrupted, and a fluid containing red blood cells moves into the alveoli (alveolar edema). As the disruption becomes worse from further increases in the pulmonary venous pressure, the alveoli and the airways are flooded with fluid (see Figure 37.3). This is accompanied by a worsening of the blood gas values (i.e., lower PaO_2 and possible increase in partial pressure of arterial carbon dioxide [$PaCO_2$] and progressive respiratory acidemia).

PATHOPHYSIOLOGY MAP

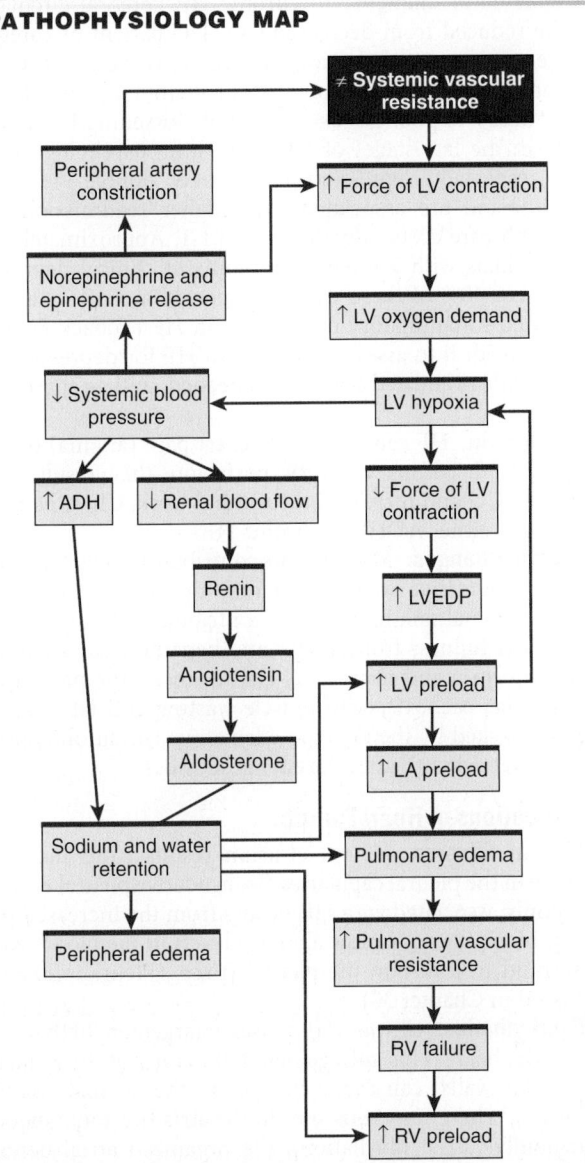

FIG. 37.2 Illustration of how left-sided heart failure results from elevated systemic vascular resistance. Left-sided heart failure leads to right-sided heart failure. Systemic vascular resistance and preload are exacerbated by renal and adrenal mechanisms. *ADH,* antidiuretic hormone; *LA,* left atrial; *LV,* left ventricular; *LVEDP,* left ventricular end-diastolic pressure; *RV,* right ventricular. Source: Adapted from Huether, S. E., & McCance, K. L. (2004). *Understanding pathophysiology* (3rd ed.). Mosby.

Clinical manifestations of pulmonary edema are distinct. Most affected patients are anxious, pale, and possibly cyanotic. The skin is clammy and cold from vasoconstriction caused by stimulation of the SNS. The patient has severe dyspnea, as evidenced by the use of accessory muscles of respiration, a respiratory rate greater than 30 breaths per minute, and orthopnea. There may be wheezing and coughing with the production of frothy, blood-tinged sputum. Auscultation of the lungs may reveal crackles, wheezes, and rhonchi throughout the lungs. The patient's HR is rapid, and BP may be elevated or decreased, depending on the severity of the HF.

Clinical Manifestations of Chronic Heart Failure

Chronic HF is characterized as a progressive worsening of ventricular function and chronic neurohormonal activation that leads to ventricular remodelling. This process involves changes in the size, shape, and mechanical performance of the ventricle. The clinical manifestations of chronic HF depend on the patient's age, the underlying type and extent of heart disease, and which ventricle is failing to pump effectively. Table 37.3 lists the manifestations of right-sided HF and left-sided HF. Patients with chronic HF usually have manifestations of biventricular failure.

Fatigue. Fatigue is one of the earliest symptoms of chronic HF. The patient notices fatigue after activities that normally are not tiring. Decreased CO, impaired perfusion to vital organs, decreased oxygenation of the tissues, and anemia may cause the fatigue. Anemia can result from poor nutrition, renal disease, or medication therapy (e.g., ACE inhibitors).

Dyspnea. *Dyspnea* (shortness of breath) is a common manifestation of chronic HF. It is caused by increased pulmonary pressures secondary to interstitial and alveolar edema. Dyspnea can occur with mild exertion or at rest. *Orthopnea* is shortness of breath that occurs when the patient is in a recumbent position.

Paroxysmal Nocturnal Dyspnea. Paroxysmal nocturnal dyspnea occurs when the patient is asleep. It results from the reabsorption of fluid from dependent body areas when the patient is flat. The patient awakens in a panic, has feelings of suffocation, and has a strong desire to sit or stand up.

A cough is often associated with HF and may be the first clinical symptom. It begins as a dry, nonproductive cough and may be misdiagnosed as asthma or other lung disease. Position change or over-the-counter cough medicines do not relieve the cough.

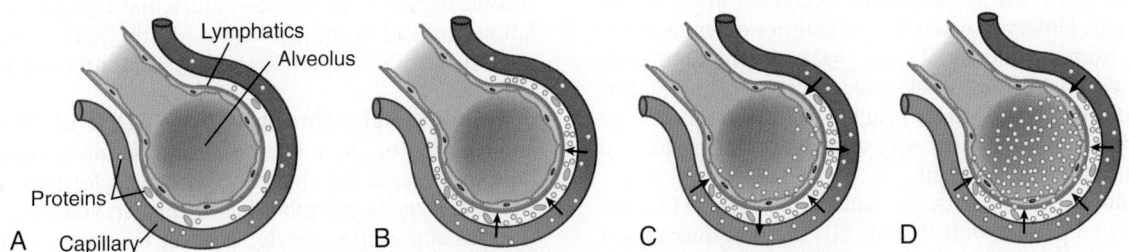

FIG. 37.3 As pulmonary edema progresses, it inhibits oxygen and carbon dioxide exchange at the alveolar capillary interface. **A,** Normal relationship. **B,** Increased pulmonary–capillary hydrostatic pressure causes fluid to move from the vascular space into the pulmonary interstitial space. **C,** Lymphatic flow increases in an attempt to pull fluid back into the vascular or lymphatic space. **D,** Failure of lymphatic flow and worsening of left-sided heart failure result in further movement of fluid into the interstitial space and into the alveoli. Source: Redrawn from Urden, L. D., Stacy, K. M., & Lough, M. E. (2010). *Critical care nursing: Diagnosis and management* (6th ed., p. 462, Figure 19-17). Mosby.

TABLE 37.3   CLINICAL MANIFESTATIONS OF HEART FAILURE

Right-Sided Heart Failure	Left-Sided Heart Failure
Signs	
RV heaves	LV heaves
Murmurs	Cheyne-Stokes respirations
Peripheral edema	Pulsus alternans (alternating
Weight gain	pulses: strong, weak)
↑ HR	↑ HR
Edema of dependent body parts	PMI displaced inferiorly and pos-
(sacrum, anterior tibias, pedal	teriorly (LV hypertrophy)
edema)	↓ PaO₂, slight ↑ PaCO₂ (poor O₂
Ascites	exchange)
Anasarca (massive generalized	Crackles (pulmonary edema)
body edema)	S₃ and S₄ (see Easy Auscultation
Jugular venous distension	website listed in the Resources
Hepatomegaly (liver enlargement)	at the end of this chapter)
Right-sided pleural effusion	
Symptoms	
Fatigue	Fatigue
Dependent edema	Dyspnea (shallow respirations
Right upper quadrant pain	≤32–40/min)
Anorexia and GI bloating	Orthopnea (shortness of breath in
Nausea	recumbent position)
	Dry, hacking cough
	Pulmonary edema
	Nocturia
	Paroxysmal nocturnal dyspnea

GI, gastrointestinal; *HR*, heart rate; *LV*, left ventricular; *PaO₂*, arterial partial pressure of oxygen; *PaCO₂*, arterial partial pressure of carbon dioxide; *PMI*, point of maximal impulse; *RV*, right ventricle/ventricular; *S₃* and *S₄*, third and fourth heart sounds.

Tachycardia. Tachycardia is an early clinical sign of HF. One of the body's first mechanisms to compensate for a failing ventricle is to increase the HR. Because of diminished CO, SNS stimulation increases, which in turn increases HR. However, many patients with chronic HF take β-blocker medications and may not show an increase in response to SNS stimulation.

Edema. Edema is a common sign of HF. It may occur in dependent body areas (peripheral edema), the liver (hepatomegaly), the abdominal cavity (ascites), and the lungs (pulmonary edema and pleural effusion). If the patient is in bed, sacral and scrotal edema may develop. Pressing on the edematous skin may leave a transient indentation (pitting edema). The development of dependent edema or a sudden weight gain of more than 1.5 kg over 1 to 2 days or 2.5 kg in a single week is often indicative of exacerbated HF (Heart and Stroke Foundation of Canada, 2021).

Nocturia. A patient with chronic HF who has decreased CO also has impaired renal perfusion and decreased urine output during the day. However, when the patient lies down at night, fluid moves from the interstitial spaces back into the circulatory system. In addition, cardiac workload is decreased at night during rest. These combined effects result in increased renal blood flow and diuresis. The patient may experience having to void frequently throughout the night.

Skin Changes. Because tissue capillary oxygen extraction is increased in a patient with chronic HF, the skin may appear dusky. Often the lower extremities are shiny and swollen, and hair growth on them is diminished or absent. Chronic swelling may result in pigment changes. This causes the skin to appear brown or brawny in areas covering the ankles and lower legs (hemosiderin staining).

Behavioural Changes. In chronic HF, cerebral circulation may be reduced from decreased CO. The patient or caregiver may report unusual behaviour, including restlessness, confusion, and decreased attention span or memory. This may also be secondary to poor gas exchange and worsening HF. It often occurs in the late stages of HF. Coexisting psychological disorders, especially depression and anxiety, double the risk of mortality and are associated with higher readmission rates and health care costs in patients with HF. Approximately 35% of individuals with HF have symptoms of clinical depression and almost 40% of these patients reported anxiety as a result of elevated inflammatory biomarkers in HF (Toback & Clark, 2017). It is ideal to assess patients with HF for depression and anxiety with a validated scale and, if needed, initiate appropriate consults.

Chest Pain. HF can precipitate chest pain (angina) because of decreased coronary artery perfusion that results from decreased CO and increased myocardial work. Chest pain may accompany either ADHF or chronic HF.

Weight Changes. Many factors contribute to weight changes. First, a progressive weight gain may occur because of fluid retention. Renal failure may also contribute to fluid retention. Abdominal fullness from ascites and hepatomegaly frequently causes anorexia and nausea. As HF advances, the patient may have cardiac cachexia, with muscle wasting and fat loss. This may be masked by the patient's edematous condition and may not be detected until after the edema subsides.

Complications of Heart Failure

Pleural Effusion. Pleural effusion results from increasing pressure in the pleural capillaries. Transudative pleural effusion, commonly associated with HF, occurs from the increased pressure in blood vessels or low albumin levels in the blood, which cause fluid to leak into the pleural space. (Pleural effusion is discussed in Chapter 30.)

Dysrhythmias. Chronic HF causes enlargement of the chambers of the heart. This enlargement (stretching of the atrial and ventricular walls) can cause changes in the normal electrical pathways. When numerous sites in the atria fire spontaneously and rapidly (atrial fibrillation), the organized atrial depolarization (contraction, or "atrial kick") no longer occurs. Atrial fibrillation also promotes thrombus formation within the atria. Thrombi may break loose and form emboli. This increases the risk for stroke in patients with atrial fibrillation. They require treatment with cardioversion, antidysrhythmics, anticoagulants, or a combination of these (see Chapter 38).

Patients with HF are also at risk for ventricular dysrhythmias (e.g., ventricular tachycardia, ventricular fibrillation) and second-degree heart blocks. Ventricular tachycardia and fibrillation can lead to sudden cardiac death. (Sudden cardiac death is discussed in Chapter 36, and dysrhythmias are discussed in Chapter 38.)

Left Ventricular Thrombus. With ADHF or chronic HF, the enlargement of the left ventricle and the decrease in CO combine to increase the chance of thrombus formation in the left ventricle. Once a thrombus has formed, its volume may decrease the area of the left ventricle, reducing left ventricular contractility, and cause a decrease in CO and worsening of the patient's perfusion. The development of emboli from the thrombus also increases the patient's risk for stroke.

Hepatomegaly. HF can lead to severe hepatomegaly, especially with right ventricular failure. Because the venous system

TABLE 37.4	**NEW YORK HEART ASSOCIATION FUNCTIONAL CLASSIFICATION OF PEOPLE WITH CARDIAC DISEASE**
Class I	No limitation of physical activity. Ordinary physical activity does not cause fatigue, dyspnea, palpitations, or anginal pain.
Class II	Slight limitation of physical activity. No symptoms at rest. Ordinary physical activity results in fatigue, dyspnea, palpitations, or anginal pain.
Class III	Marked limitation of physical activity. Usually comfortable at rest. Ordinary physical activity causes fatigue, dyspnea, palpitations, or anginal pain.
Class IV	Inability to carry on any physical activity without discomfort. Symptoms of cardiac insufficiency or of angina may be present even at rest. If any physical activity is undertaken, discomfort is increased.

Source: Criteria Committee of the New York Heart Association. (1994). Functional capacity and objective assessment. In M. Dolgin (Ed.), *Nomenclature and criteria for diagnosis of diseases of the heart and great vessels* (9th ed., pp. 253–255). Little, Brown.

is backed up, the liver lobules become congested with venous blood. The hepatic congestion leads to impaired liver function. Eventually, liver cells die, fibrosis occurs, and cirrhosis can develop (see Chapter 46).

Renal Failure. The decreased CO that accompanies acute and chronic HF results in decreased perfusion to the kidneys and can lead to renal insufficiency or failure (see Chapter 49).

Classification of Heart Failure

The New York Heart Association (NYHA) has developed a system for classifying symptoms experienced by patients with HF. The classification is widely used across Canada and the United States (Table 37.4).

Diagnostic Studies

Diagnosing HF is often difficult because neither the signs nor symptoms are highly specific, and both may mimic many other medical conditions, such as anemia or lung disease. The primary goal in diagnosis is to determine the underlying etiology of HF. Measures to assess the cause and degree of HF are presented in Figure 37.4 (Ezekowitz et al., 2017). Echocardiography and measurement of EF can differentiate between HFrEF and HFpEF, an important distinction to make in the early treatment of HF. Chest X-ray, echocardiogram, and 12 lead electrocardiogram (ECG) do not confirm but can contribute to a diagnosis.

Measurement of either BNP or N-terminal–pro-BNP (NT–pro-BNP) levels is recommended to assist in the diagnosis of HF. In general, levels are positively correlated with the degree of left ventricular dysfunction and can help to differentiate dyspnea caused by HF from other causes of dyspnea (Ezekowitz et al., 2017; Table 37.5).

NURSING AND INTERPROFESSIONAL MANAGEMENT ACUTE DECOMPENSATED HEART FAILURE

The goal of therapy is to improve left ventricular function by decreasing intravascular volume, decreasing venous return (preload), decreasing afterload, improving gas exchange and oxygenation, and increasing CO (Ezekowitz et al., 2017).

DECREASING INTRAVASCULAR VOLUME

Decreasing intravascular volume with the use of diuretics reduces venous return. A loop diuretic (e.g., furosemide [Lasix]) may be used to decrease volume because it may be administered by the direct intravenous (IV) route and its action within the kidney occurs rapidly. By decreasing venous return to the left ventricle and thereby reducing preload, the overfilled left ventricle may contract more efficiently and thus contribute to improving CO. This improves left ventricular function, decreases pulmonary vascular pressures, and improves gas exchange.

Ultrafiltration may be an option for a patient with volume overload. Ultrafiltration has generally been achieved through hemodialysis or with ultrafiltration by way of central venous access. (Ultrafiltration is discussed in Chapter 49.)

DECREASING VENOUS RETURN

Decreasing venous return (preload) reduces the amount of volume returned to the LV during diastole. This can be accomplished by placing the patient in high Fowler's position with the feet horizontal in the bed or dangling at the bedside. This position helps decrease venous return because of the pooling of blood in the extremities. This position also increases the thoracic capacity by decreasing intra-abdominal pressure on the lungs, allowing for improved ventilation. IV nitroglycerine is a vasodilator used in the treatment of ADHF. It reduces circulating volume by decreasing preload and also increases coronary artery circulation by dilating the coronary arteries. In addition to reducing preload, it slightly reduces afterload (in high doses) and increases myocardial oxygen supply. Furosemide (Lasix) may also help decrease venous return through reduction of intravascular volume.

DECREASING AFTERLOAD

Afterload is the resistance against which the LV must pump; that is, it is the amount of work it takes for the left ventricle to eject blood into the systemic circulation. Systemic vascular resistance (SVR) is a determinant of afterload, as is left ventricular filling. If afterload is reduced, the CO improves and pulmonary congestion thereby decreases. Great care should be taken to ensure that the patient's BP is adequate to provide cerebral and renal perfusion. Careful monitoring of vital signs is crucial.

IMPROVING GAS EXCHANGE AND OXYGENATION

Gas exchange may be improved by several measures. IV morphine reduces preload and afterload and may decrease myocardial oxygen demands, which can be raised as a result of anxiety and subsequent increased musculoskeletal and respiratory activity. Administration of oxygen could be considered if the oxygen saturation falls below 90% (Ezekowitz et al., 2017). Care must be taken to avoid using oxygen if it is not required because it can reduce CO and increase SVR. (Oxygen therapy is discussed in Chapter 31.) In severe pulmonary edema, the patient may need noninvasive ventilatory support (e.g., bilevel positive airway pressure) or intubation and mechanical ventilation. (Ventilatory support is discussed in Chapter 68.)

IMPROVING CARDIAC FUNCTION

In a patient who is or becomes hemodynamically unstable—that is, becomes progressively hypotensive, has an HR that is abnormally fast or slow, develops dysrhythmias, or becomes hypoxic with cool and clammy skin—nursing care is more urgent, and treatment policies may call for aggressive, complex therapies. The use of diuretics, morphine sulphate, and vasodilators may not be sufficient to control symptoms. The addition

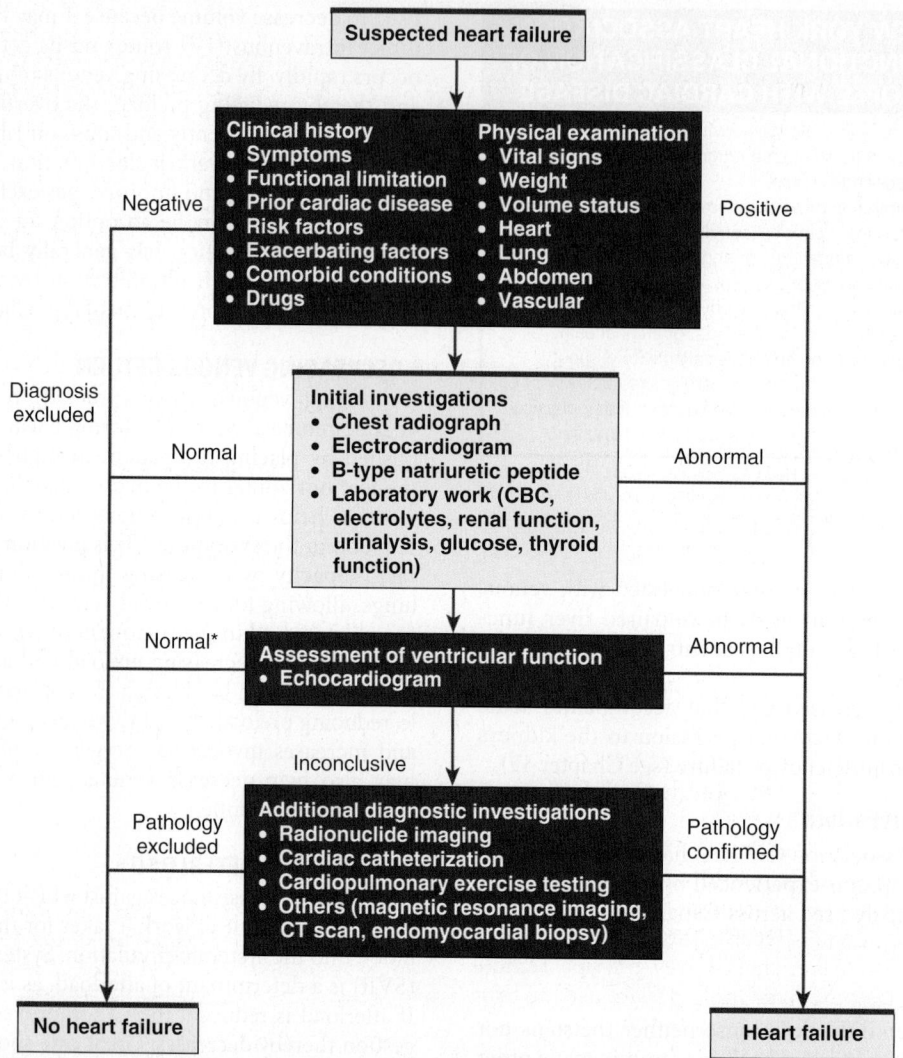

FIG. 37.4 Algorithm for diagnosis of heart failure. *Normal ejection fraction does not rule out heart failure with preserved ejection fraction. *CBC,* complete blood count; *CT,* computed tomography. Source: Reprinted from *Canadian Journal of Cardiology, 29*(2), McKelvie, R. S., Moe, G. W., Ezekowitz, J. A., et al., The 2012 Canadian Cardiovascular Society heart failure management guidelines update: Focus on acute and chronic heart failure, pp. 168–181, Copyright 2013, with permission from Elsevier.

TABLE 37.5	NATRIURETIC PEPTIDES CUT POINTS FOR THE DIAGNOSIS OF HEART FAILURE*			
Peptide	Age in Years	HF Unlikely	HF Possible	HF Probable
BNP	All	<100 pg/mL	100–400 pg/mL	>400 pg/mL
NT–pro-BNP	<50	<300 pg/mL	300–450 pg/mL	>450 pg/mL
	50–75	<300 pg/mL	450–900 pg/mL	>900 pg/mL
	>75	<300 pg/mL	900–1 800 pg/mL	>1 800 pg/mL

BNP, B-type natriuretic peptide; *HF,* heart failure; *NT–pro-BNP,* N-terminal pro-BNP.
*Levels can be increased in the presence of renal dysfunction or sepsis and be decreased in obese patients.
Source: Ezekowitz, J. A., O'Meara, E., McDonald, M. A., et al. (2017). 2017 Comprehensive updates of the Canadian Cardiovascular Society Guidelines for the management of heart failure. *Canadian Journal of Cardiology, 33,* 1342–1433. https://doi.org/10.1016/j.cjca.2017.08.022 Copyright 2015, with permission from Elsevier.

of positive inotropic therapy may be warranted, as well as initiation of hemodynamic monitoring to evaluate the effectiveness of interventions. Once a pulmonary artery catheter is in position, CO, pulmonary artery pressure, and pulmonary artery occlusive pressure should be measured, and therapy should be instituted and titrated to maximize CO. A pulmonary artery occlusive pressure of 14 to 18 mm Hg generally achieves the goal of increasing CO. (Hemodynamic monitoring is discussed in Chapter 68.)

Inotropic medications (e.g., dobutamine, milrinone) that increase myocardial contractility without increasing oxygen consumption may be effective. Dobutamine and milrinone also increase peripheral vasodilation and reduce afterload. There is no evidence that inotropic medications improve mortality rates. Milrinone has been linked to more frequent atrial arrhythmias, increased hypotension, and worsening HF. Therefore, use of inotropic medications should be reserved for hemodynamically unstable patients only (Ezekowitz et al., 2017).

REDUCING ANXIETY

Anxiety is reduced by the sedative action of morphine administered intravenously. When morphine is used, the patient must be watched closely for respiratory depression. In addition, a calm approach in providing care can help reduce anxiety.

Once the patient is more stable, the cause of the pulmonary edema should be determined. Diagnosis of HFrEF or HFpEF then guides further management policies. Aggressive medication therapy may continue with IV forms of diuretics, inotropic medications, vasodilators, and oral ACE inhibitors. Nursing care focuses on continual physical assessment, hemodynamic monitoring, and monitoring the patient's response to treatment.

INTERPROFESSIONAL CARE: CHRONIC HEART FAILURE

The main goal in the management of HF is to treat the underlying cause and contributing factors, maximize CO, and alleviate symptoms. The management of dysrhythmias is discussed in Chapter 38, hypertension in Chapter 35, valvular disorders in Chapter 39, and coronary artery disease in Chapter 36.

Referral to Multidisciplinary Clinics or Specialist Care for Heart Failure

It is recommended that patients with newly diagnosed HF and patients at higher risk for the development of HF be referred to a multidisciplinary heart failure clinic. These clinics, in Canada often referred to as *heart function clinics,* consist of an interprofessional team providing self-management coaching and a mechanism for assessment for more advanced therapies (Kapoor et al., 2018). Because these services are not accessible to some patients, many centres provide remote monitoring, whereby telehealth technologies are used to provide care.

Nonpharmacological Therapies

Oxygen. In a patient with HF, oxygen saturation of the blood may be reduced because the blood is not adequately oxygenated in the lungs. If oxygen saturation is less than 90%, administration of oxygen can improve tissue oxygenation. Thus, appropriate use of oxygen therapy can help relieve dyspnea and fatigue. Pulse oximetry should be used to monitor the effectiveness of oxygen therapy.

Self-Management Teaching. An important part of HF care is helping the patient and family understand that HF is a chronic condition and become proficient in avoiding risks for decompensation and detecting the early signs and symptoms. The Heart and Stroke Foundation of Canada has many useful tools that are available to help support patients in learning to manage their illness (Heart and Stroke Foundation of Canada, 2021; see the Resources at the end of this chapter).

Exercise and Activity. Regular activity and exercise periods should be prescribed for all patients with stable chronic HF. Even patients with NYHA class III symptoms (see Table 37.4) should exercise three to five times per week for 30 to 45 minutes at a time. A cardiac rehabilitation program provides the patient with an individualized exercise regimen (Ezekowitz et al., 2017). To ensure the patient's adherence to regular exercise, the medical team must be realistic about what the patient can achieve and must work around possible barriers, to enable the patient to succeed.

Devices

Cardiac Resynchronization Therapy. For patients with HF who are receiving maximum medical therapy, continue to have NYHA functional class III or IV symptoms (see Table 37.4), and have a widened QRS interval, one therapy is biventricular pacing and cardiac resynchronization therapy (CRT). Traditional pacemakers pace one or two chambers (e.g., atrium or ventricle, or both). CRT coordinates contractility of the right ventricle and left ventricle through biventricular pacing. Normal electrical conduction within the right ventricle and left ventricle improves left ventricular performance and CO. This additional therapy enables patients to increase their exercise capacity and decrease their overall symptoms. CRT has been shown to prolong life and improve quality of life in patients with NYHA functional class III and class IV HF (Ezekowitz et al., 2017). CRT can be combined with an implantable cardioverter–defibrillator (ICD).

Implantable Cardioverter–Defibrillator. If a patient has NYHA functional class II or III HF, is on optimal medical therapy, and has an EF of less than 35%, the implementation and use of an ICD with CRT may be warranted. Life-threatening ventricular dysrhythmias (e.g., ventricular tachycardia) are a complication of the ischemic myocardium and can cause sudden cardiac death. The addition of the ICD in these patients has reduced the overall rate of mortality from sudden cardiac death (Ezekowitz et al., 2017). (Pacemakers and defibrillators are discussed in Chapter 38.)

Mechanical Circulatory Support. Several devices are available to sustain patients with HF in deteriorating conditions, especially those awaiting cardiac transplantation. The intra-aortic balloon pump is used for short-term support for HF patients with acute decompensation. However, the limitations of bed rest, infection, and vascular complications preclude its long-term use (see Chapter 68 for nursing management of circulatory assist devices).

Extracorporeal membrane oxygenation is a support device similar to a bypass machine used in cardiac surgery procedures. This system can be used to support critically ill patients with HF who are being assessed for more advanced therapy, such as a ventricular assist device (VAD) (Figure 37.5). In Canada, VADs are used in carefully selected patients, primarily as a bridge to cardiac transplantation. They provide highly effective long-term support for more than 2 years, allowing patients to live at home and even return to work while waiting for a transplant, and their use has become standard care for candidates for cardiac transplantation with acute decompensation. (Intra-aortic balloon pumps, extracorporeal membrane oxygenation, and VADs are discussed further in Chapter 68.)

Cardiac Transplantation

Cardiac transplantation—the transfer of a heart from one person to another—is the treatment of choice in carefully selected patients with end-stage HF. Because of the lack of donor hearts, however, it is an option for only a small number of patients with HF. (Cardiac transplantation is discussed later in this chapter.)

Advance Care Planning and Goals of Care

HF is a chronic condition suffered primarily by older persons, and the prognosis is worse than that of most cancers. For many patients, therapies such as mechanical support and cardiac transplantation are not indicated.

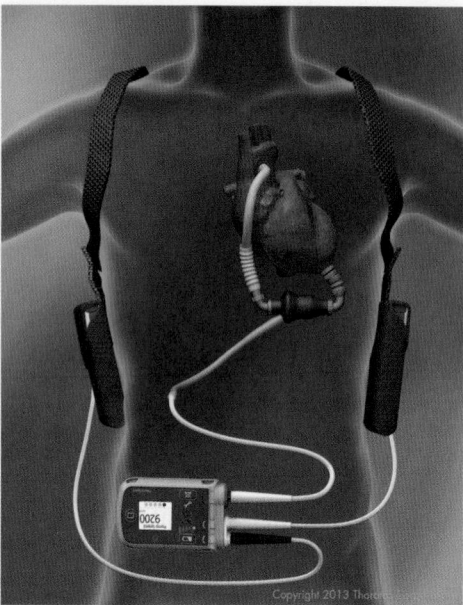

FIG. 37.5 The HeartMate II ventricular assist device (Thoratec Corp., Pleasanton, CA), one of the devices used in transplantation centres across Canada as a bridge to heart transplantation. Source: HeartMate II and St. Jude are trademarks of St. Jude Medical, LLC, or its related companies. Reproduced with permission of St. Jude Medical, © 2018. All rights reserved.

HF is typically characterized by periods of stability interspersed with exacerbations and readmissions to hospital. In the end stages, the patient's quality of life can be limited by the symptoms, and many patients and families are not prepared for death.

The goal of care should be directed toward optimizing guideline-driven therapies outlined in this chapter and, in addition, early discussions with the patient and their loved ones about advance care planning (Figure 37.6). This includes goal setting according to the patient's preferences, as well as planning for end of life. The role of the ICD and other life-prolonging interventions should be discussed regularly between the HF team and the patient.

Early intervention with palliative care support has shown to be effective at improving quality of life and helping patients and their families through these final stages (Heart and Stroke Foundation of Canada, 2021).

MEDICATION THERAPY: CHRONIC HEART FAILURE

General therapeutic objectives for medication management of chronic HF include the following: (a) identification of the type of HF and the underlying causes, (b) correction of sodium and water retention and volume overload, (c) reduction of cardiac workload, (d) improvement of myocardial contractility, and (e) control of precipitating and complicating factors. The aims of treating HF are to improve symptoms, minimize adverse effects of treatment, prevent morbidity, and prolong survival. Current therapeutic approaches stress the importance of diuretics, ACE inhibitors, angiotensin-II receptor blockers (ARBs), neprilysin inhibitors, β-adrenergic blockers, and mineralocorticoid receptor antagonists (MRAs; previously known as *aldosterone antagonists*) (Ezekowitz et al., 2017). Recent guidelines recommend that most people with HFrEF be managed with an ACE inhibitor (or an ARB in people who are intolerant of ACE inhibitors), a β-adrenergic blocker, and an MRA (Ezekowitz et al., 2017) (see Figure 37.6).

Diuretics

Diuretics are used in patients with HF to mobilize edematous fluid, reduce pulmonary venous pressure, and reduce preload (see Chapter 35, Table 35.8). If excess extracellular fluid is excreted, blood volume returning to the heart can be reduced and cardiac function improved.

Diuretics act on the kidneys by promoting excretion of sodium and water. Many varieties of diuretics are available, and some have specific indications for use. Thiazide diuretics may be the first choice for chronic HF because of their convenience, safety, low cost, and effectiveness. They are particularly useful in treating edema secondary to HF and in controlling hypertension. The thiazides inhibit sodium reabsorption in the distal tubule, thus promoting excretion of sodium and water.

Loop diuretics (e.g., furosemide [Lasix]) are potent diuretics. These medications act on the ascending loop of Henle to promote sodium, chloride, and water excretion. Furosemide is more commonly used in cases of acute HF and pulmonary edema because its effects are slightly more predictable. Problems in using loop diuretics include reduction in serum potassium levels, ototoxicity, and possible allergic reaction in patients who are sensitive to sulpha-containing medications (sulphonamides).

Angiotensin-Converting Enzyme Inhibitors

ACE inhibitors are the first-line therapy in the treatment of HF. Examples of ACE inhibitors include ramipril (Altace) and enalapril (Vasotec). Other examples of ACE inhibitors are discussed in Chapter 35 and listed in Table 35.8.

The conversion of angiotensin I to the potent vasoconstrictor angiotensin II requires the presence of ACE (see Chapter 47, Figure 47.6). ACE inhibitors exert their effects by blocking production of this enzyme, which results in decreased levels of angiotensin II. As a result, plasma aldosterone levels are also reduced.

Because CO is dependent on afterload in chronic HF, the reduction in SVR seen with the use of ACE inhibitors produces a significant increase in CO. Furthermore, the improvement of CO and the redistribution of regional blood flow that result from the use of ACE inhibitors help maintain tissue perfusion, even though BP may be decreased. Other hemodynamic changes include reductions in pulmonary artery pressure, right arterial pressure, and left ventricular filling pressure. Adverse effects of ACE inhibitors include symptomatic hypotension, chronic cough, and, when it is used in high doses, renal insufficiency. Aging and baseline renal insufficiency slow the metabolism of ACE inhibitors, and their toxicity may therefore be increased (Ezekowitz et al., 2017). It is recommended that these medications be started at the lowest dose and slowly increased over a 2- to 3-month period and that BP and renal function be monitored at regular intervals. Overall, ACE inhibitors are well tolerated by patients.

In patients who are unable to tolerate the ACE inhibitors because of angioedema or cough, ARBs such as losartan (Cozaar) or valsartan (Diovan) may be prescribed (see Chapter 35, Table 35.8).

Neprilysin Inhibitors

A relatively new combination medication is available in Canada containing an ARB and a neprilysin inhibitor (Sacubitril), which blocks the enzyme that degrades natriuretic peptides. This drug combination has shown that it can significantly reduce rates of

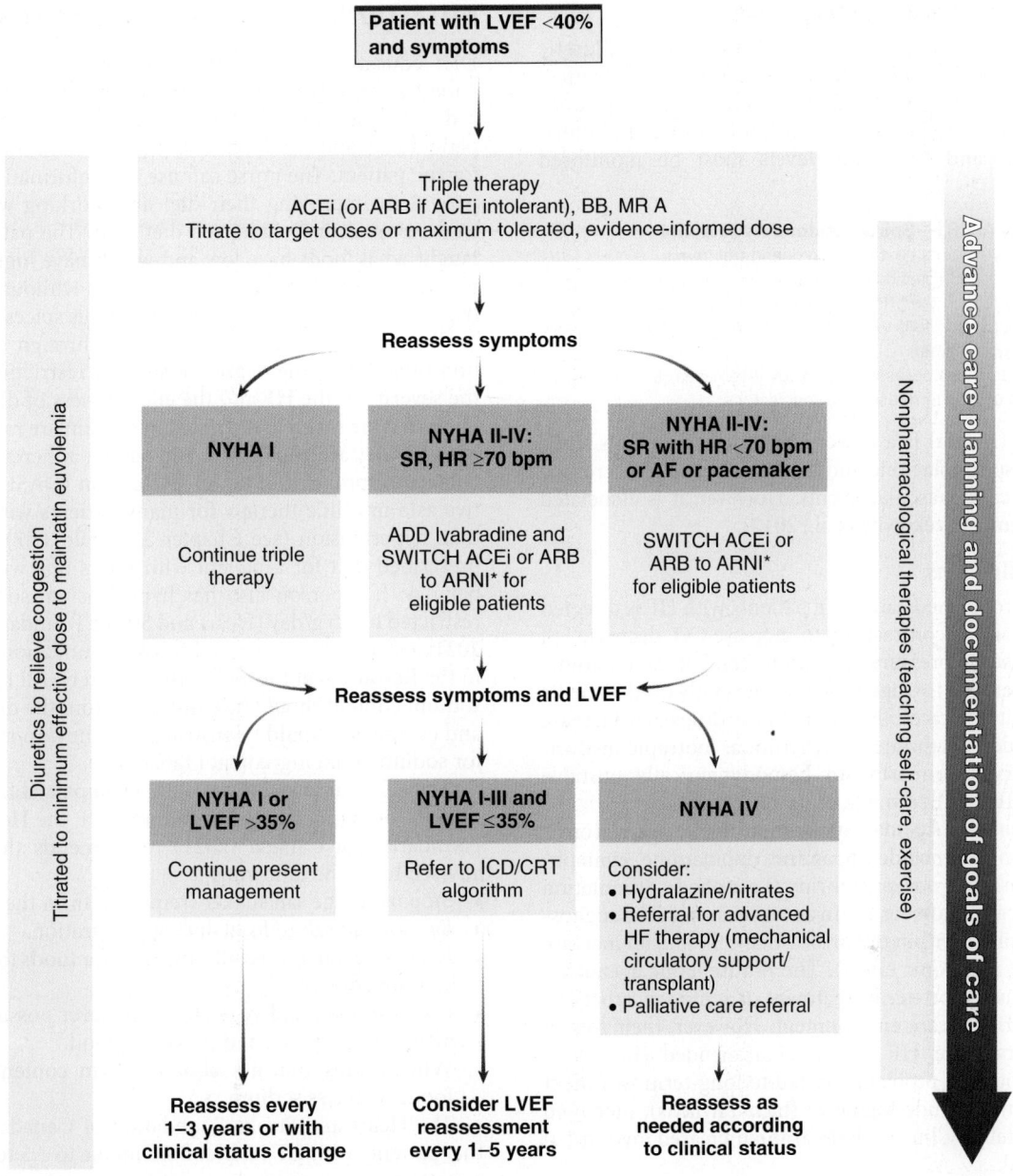

*Sacubitril or valsartan

FIG. 37.6 Therapeutic approach to patients with heart failure (HF) and reduced ejection fraction (EF). *ACEi,* angiotensin-converting enzyme inhibitor; *AF,* atrial fibrillation; *ARB,* angiotensin receptor blocker; *ARNI,* angiotensin receptor neprilysin inhibitor; *BB,* β blocker; *bpm,* beats per minute; *CRT,* cardiac resynchronization therapy; *HF,* heart failure; *HR,* heart rate; *ICD,* implantable cardioverter–defibrillator; *LVEF,* left ventricular ejection fraction; *MRA,* mineralocorticoid receptor antagonist; *NP,* natriuretic peptides; *NYHA,* New York Heart Association class; *SR,* sinus rhythm. Source: Reprinted from *Canadian Journal of Cardiology, 32*(3), Howlett, J. G., Chan, M., Ezekowitz, J. A., et al., The Canadian Cardiovascular Society heart failure companion: Bridging guidelines to your practice, pp. 296–310, Copyright 2016, with permission from Elsevier.

death from and rehospitalizations for HF in selected patients with HF. This medication is beginning to replace the use of ACE inhibitors (Jhund & McMurray, 2016).

β-Adrenergic Blockers

The use of β-adrenergic blockers (or β blockers) in combination with ACE inhibitors in the management of HF has become standard therapy for most patients. Examples include carvedilol and metoprolol (Lopressor). Marked improvement in rates of patient survival has been shown with the use of β-adrenergic blockers. β-Adrenergic blockers directly block the negative effects of the SNS

on the failing heart, such as increased HR. Because β-adrenergic blockade can reduce myocardial contractility, care must be taken to start the medication gradually, the dosage being increased slowly (typically every 2 weeks) as tolerated by the patient, until it reaches the maximum. Major adverse effects include edema, hypotension, fatigue, asthma exacerbations, and bradycardia.

MEDICATION ALERT—β-Adrenergic Blockers
- Overdosage can produce profound bradycardia, hypotension, bronchospasm, and cardiogenic shock.
- Abrupt withdrawal may result in sweating, palpitations, and headaches.

Mineralocorticoid Receptor Antagonists

Spironolactone (Aldactone) is a potassium-sparing diuretic that promotes sodium and water excretion but blocks potassium excretion by blocking the action of aldosterone. Spironolactone appears to be additive to the benefits of ACE inhibitors. Renal function and potassium levels must be monitored carefully.

> **MEDICATION ALERT—Spironolactone (Aldactone)**
> - Potassium levels must be monitored during treatment.
> - It must be used with caution in patients taking digoxin, because hyperkalemia may reduce the effects of digoxin.
> - Patients must avoid foods with high potassium content (e.g., bananas, oranges, dried apricots).
> - Male patients must be assessed for gynecomastia, a common adverse effect of long-term use of spironolactone.

Eplerenone (Inspra) is a newer MRA that has effects similar to those of spironolactone and has been linked to decreased mortality and cardiovascular events. However, it is associated with hyperkalemia (Ezekowitz et al., 2017).

Inotropic Medications

The use of inotropic medications in patients with HF is directed at improving cardiac contractility to increase CO, decrease left ventricular diastolic pressure, and decrease SVR. Dobutamine and milrinone are the two agents most commonly used. Patients should be monitored carefully because these drugs may increase the risk of sudden death due to arrhythmia. Inotropic medications are reserved primarily for hemodynamically unstable patients with HFrEF (Ezekowitz et al., 2017).

Sympathomimetic Agents. Sympathomimetic agents (or β-adrenergic agonists) include dopamine, dobutamine, epinephrine (Adrenalin), and norepinephrine (Levophed). Stimulation of β-adrenergic receptors results in an increase in cyclic adenosine monophosphate within the myocardial cells and an increase in contractility (inotropic effect). The β-adrenergic agents are typically used as a short-term treatment of acute exacerbations of HF in the critical care environment. However, their role in long-term therapy for HF is not recommended (Ezekowitz et al., 2017). Potential problems related to long-term treatment with these agents include tolerance (tachyphylaxis), increased ventricular irritability, limb ischemia, and increased myocardial oxygen demand.

Phosphodiesterase Inhibitors. Inhibition of phosphodiesterase enhances calcium entry into the cell and improves myocardial contractility. Phosphodiesterase inhibitors are also potent vasodilators. They increase CO and reduce arterial pressure (decrease afterload).

Milrinone increases myocardial contraction, increases CO, promotes peripheral vasodilation, and decreases SVR, thus augmenting performance of the left ventricle. Adverse reactions include dysrhythmias, thrombocytopenia, and gastrointestinal effects.

There is little evidence that inotropic medications have a beneficial effect on mortality rates. Therefore, their use should be confined to short-term therapy only in patients in cardiogenic shock with volume overload and who have diuretic resistance (Ezekowitz et al., 2017).

Vasodilator Medications. Vasodilator medications are a class of medications that have been shown to reduce symptoms of dyspnea in HFrEF (Ezekowitz et al., 2017). Their vasodilator effects are found not to improve survival or reduce cardiovascular events.

NUTRITIONAL THERAPY: HEART FAILURE

Diet education and weight management are critical in the patient's control of HF. The nurse or the dietitian should obtain a detailed diet history, determining not only what foods the patient eats and when but also the sociocultural value of food for the patient. The nurse can use this information to assist the patient in improving their diet and working with a dietitian to develop an individualized diet plan. The patient should be taught what foods have low and which have high sodium content and ways to enhance food flavours without the use of salt (e.g., substituting lemon juice and various spices).

The edema of HF is often treated through dietary restriction of sodium. The degree of sodium restriction depends on the severity of the HF and the effectiveness of diuretic therapy. Diets that are severely restricted in sodium are rarely prescribed because they are unpalatable and patient adherence is poor. The Dietary Approach to Stop Hypertension (DASH) diet is effective as a first-line therapy for many patients with isolated systolic hypertension (see Chapter 35, Table 35.7). A commonly prescribed diet for a patient with HF is one with 2 g sodium per day. If a person also has hypertension, sodium intake is restricted to 1.5 g/day (Heart and Stroke Foundation of Canada, 2021; see also the Heart and Stroke Foundation website listed in the Resources at the end of this chapter). All foods with high sodium content should be eliminated from the diet. The patient and caregivers should be instructed on how to read food labels for sodium as an ingredient (Table 37.6).

Typically, a low-sodium diet is unpalatable. In order to increase adherence to a low-sodium diet, the Heart and Stroke Foundation of Canada (2021) recommends that patients be advised to do the following:
- Stop using the salt shaker (remove it from the dinner table).
- Do not add salt to food during preparation.
- Read food labels carefully and look for foods that claim lower sodium content.
- Eat fresh fruit and vegetables whenever possible, and try to avoid pre-prepared and processed food.
- When eating out, ask about sodium content, and choose foods with less sodium.

The Heart and Stroke Foundation of Canada recommends that patients with HF restrict fluid intake to 1.5 to 2 L/day. That equates to six to eight glasses of fluid per day. At least 50% of fluid should be water. Patients should be reminded that fluid is hidden in foods such as fruits and ice cream.

It is vital that patients weigh themselves daily to monitor fluid retention. Patients should be instructed to weigh themselves at the same time each day, preferably before breakfast, while wearing the same type of clothing, and to keep a written record of their weight. This practice helps ensure valid comparisons from day to day and helps reveal early signs of fluid retention. If a patient experiences a weight gain of 2 kg or more over a day or 2.5 kg or more over a week, the patient should contact their health care provider or the heart failure clinic.

General Principles

According to *Canada's Food Guide* (Health Canada, 2021), which contains dietary recommendations endorsed by Health Canada, all Canadians should follow a diet with low sodium content. The guide recommends that the patient read the "Nutrition Facts" label, which is mandatory on all packaged foods, before purchasing foods (see Chapter 42, Figure 42.4).

TABLE 37.6 NUTRITIONAL THERAPY
Sodium Label Language*

Claim	What It Means
Free of sodium or salt	The food contains <5 mg of sodium per serving.
Low in sodium or salt	The food contains ≤140 mg of sodium per serving (or per 100 g, if the food is a prepackaged meal).
Reduced or lower in sodium or salt	The food is processed, formulated, reformulated, or otherwise modified so that it contains at least 25% less sodium than regular foods of its type.
No added sodium or salt	The food contains no added salt, other sodium salts, or ingredients that contain sodium that functionally substitute for added salt.
Lightly salted	The food contains at least 50% less sodium added than the sodium added to the similar reference food.
Words to the effect that the food is "for use in a sodium-restricted diet"	The food meets the criteria for the first three claims in this table.
Words to the effect that the food is "for special dietary use" with respect to the sodium (salt) content	The food meets the criteria for either of the first two items in this table.

*Products advertised as salt replacements should be used with caution; they may contain high quantities of potassium.
Source: Adapted from Canadian Food Inspection Agency. (2019). *Sodium (salt) claims* [summary table]. Retrieved from https://inspection.gc.ca/food-label-requirements/labelling/industry/nutrient-content/specific-claim-requirements/eng/1389907770176/1389907817577?chap=9#s7c9.

Only a small amount of sodium occurs naturally in foods. Most sodium is added during processing. Table 37.7 gives examples of varying amounts of sodium in Western foods before and after processing.

Chinese diets are usually very high in sodium. Patients with HF who adhere to a Chinese diet should be taught to consider the advice in Table 37.8. When teaching the patient with HF who adheres to an East Indian diet, the nurse should take into account the considerations presented in Table 37.9.

NURSING MANAGEMENT HEART FAILURE

NURSING ASSESSMENT
Subjective and objective data that should be obtained from a patient with HF include those listed in Table 37.10.

NURSING DIAGNOSES
Nursing diagnoses for patients with HF include but are not limited to those presented in Nursing Care Plan (NCP) 37.1.

PLANNING
The overall goals are that the patient with HF will (a) have decreased peripheral edema, (b) have decreased shortness of breath, (c) have increased exercise tolerance, (d) adhere to the medication regimen, and (5) have no complications related to HF.

NURSING IMPLEMENTATION
HEALTH PROMOTION. Treatment or control of the underlying heart disease is an important measure to prevent HF. For example, in valvular disease, valve replacement should be planned

TABLE 37.7 NUTRITIONAL THERAPY
Sodium Content in Different Food Groups

Food Groups	Sodium (mg)
Grains and Grain Products	
Cooked cereal, rice, pasta, unsalted, ½ cup	0–5
Ready-to-eat cereal, 1 cup	100–360
Bread, 1 slice	110–175
Vegetables	
Fresh or frozen, cooked without salt, ½ cup	1–70
Canned or frozen with sauce, ½ cup	140–460
Tomato juice, canned, ¾ cup	820
Fruit	
Fresh, frozen, or canned, ½ cup	0–5
Low-Fat or Fat-Free Dairy Foods	
Milk, 1 cup	120
Yogurt, 250 mL	160
Natural cheeses, 45 g	110–450
Processed cheeses, 45 g	600
Nuts, Seeds, and Dry Beans	
Peanuts, salted, ⅓ cup	120
Peanuts, unsalted, ⅓ cup	0–5
Beans, cooked from dried or frozen, without salt, ½ cup	400
Meats, Fish, and Poultry	
Fresh meat, fish, and poultry, 85-g serving	30–90
Tuna, canned, water pack, no salt added, 85-g serving	34–45
Tuna, canned, water pack, 85-g serving	250–350
Ham (lean) roasted, 85-g serving	1020

EVIDENCE-INFORMED PRACTICE
Translating Research Into Practice

T. F. (pronouns she/her) is a 62-year-old patient recovering from an episode of heart failure with reduced EF (HFrEF). Her HF is class III according to the New York Heart Association Functional Classification of Heart Disease (see Table 37.4). Her physician has recommended cardiac resynchronization therapy (CRT) for treatment of her HF symptoms. She tells the nurse that she does not want any artificial implants and that she has researched the use of hawthorn for treatment of her heart disease.

Best Available Evidence	Clinician Expertise	Patient Preferences and Values
Strong evidence supports the use of CRT to improve symptoms, exercise capacity, quality of life, ejection fraction, and survival and to decrease hospitalizations in patients like T. F.	The nurse knows the benefits of and possible complications related to CRT in patients with T. F.'s situation. The nurse also knows that there is evidence supporting the use of hawthorn in patients with mild to moderate HF.	Patient does not want any artificial implants. She wants to consider alternative (herbal) therapy.

Decision and Action
The nurse reviews the risks and benefits of CRT and herbal (hawthorn) therapy for the treatment of HF with T. F. T. F. remains committed to the use of hawthorn—at least for a trial period. The nurse supports her decision and informs the physician of her wishes.

Reference for Evidence
Cicero, A., & Colletti, A. (2017). Nutraceuticals and dietary supplements to improve quality of life and outcomes in heart failure patients. *Current Pharmaceutical Design, 23*(8), 1265–1272.

Heart Failure

NURSING DIAGNOSIS	**Reduced gas exchange** (resulting from increased preload and alveolar–capillary membrane changes as evidenced by abnormal O_2 saturation, hypoxemia, dyspnea, tachypnea, tachycardia, restlessness, and patient's statement about being short of breath)

Expected Patient Outcomes	Nursing Interventions and *Rationales*
• Maintains adequate O_2/CO_2 exchange at the alveolar–capillary membrane to meet O_2 needs of the body	**Respiratory Monitoring** • Monitor pulse oximetry, respiratory rate, rhythm, depth, and effort of respirations *to detect changes in respiratory status.* • Auscultate breath sounds, noting areas of decreased or absent ventilation and presence of adventitious sounds *to detect presence of pulmonary edema.* • Monitor for increased restlessness, anxiety, and work of breathing *to detect increasing hypoxemia.* **Oxygen Therapy** • Administer supplemental O_2 or other noninvasive ventilator support (e.g., bilevel positive airway pressure) as needed *to maintain adequate O_2 levels.* • Monitor the O_2 litre flow rate and placement of O_2 delivery device *to ensure O_2 is adequately delivered.* • Change O_2 delivery device from mask to nasal prongs during meals as tolerated *to sustain O_2 levels while patient is eating.* • Monitor effectiveness of O_2 therapy *to identify hypoxemia and establish range of O_2 saturation.* **Positioning** • Position patient to alleviate dyspnea (e.g., semi-Fowler's position), as appropriate, *to improve ventilation by decreasing venous return to the heart and increasing thoracic capacity.*

NURSING DIAGNOSIS	**Inadequate cardiac output** (resulting from altered contractility, altered preload, altered stroke volume, or a combination of these as evidenced by decreased ejection fraction, increased CVP, decreased peripheral pulses, JVD, orthopnea, chest pain, S_3 and S_4, and oliguria)

Expected Patient Outcomes	Nursing Interventions and *Rationales*
• Maintains adequate blood pumped by the heart to meet metabolic demands of the body	**Cardiac Care** • Perform a comprehensive assessment of peripheral circulation (e.g., check peripheral pulses, edema, capillary refill, colour, and temperature of extremity) *to determine circulatory status.* • Note signs and symptoms of decreased cardiac output (e.g., chest pain, S_3, S_4, jugular venous distension) *to detect changes in status.* • Monitor fluid balance (e.g., input/output and daily weight) *to evaluate patient's fluid status.* • Monitor cardiac rhythm *to detect dysrhythmias.* • Monitor respiratory status for symptoms of heart failure (e.g., dyspnea, fatigue, tachypnea, orthopnea) *to identify involvement of respiratory system.* • Instruct patient and caregivers about activity restriction and progression *to allay fears and anxiety.* • Establish a supportive relationship with patient and caregivers *to promote adherence to the treatment plan.* • Inform patient of the purpose and benefits of the prescribed activity and exercise *to enhance adherence.*

NURSING DIAGNOSIS	**Excess fluid volume** resulting from excessive fluid intake, excessive sodium intake (decreased renal perfusion secondary to heart failure) as evidenced by weight gain over short period of time, edema, adventitious breath sounds, oliguria

Expected Patient Outcomes	Nursing Interventions and *Rationales*
• Experiences reduction or absence of edema and stable baseline weight	**Hypervolemia Management** • Administer prescribed medications to reduce preload (e.g., furosemide, spironolactone, morphine, and nitroglycerine) *to treat hypervolemia.* • Monitor for therapeutic effects of medications (e.g., increased urine output, decreased CVP, decreased adventitious breath sounds) *to assess response to treatment.* • Monitor potassium levels after diuretic medications *to detect hypokalemia.* • Weigh patient daily and monitor trends *to evaluate effect of treatment.* • Monitor intake and output *to assess fluid status.* • Monitor respiratory pattern for symptoms of anxiety, air hunger, orthopnea, dyspnea, tachypnea, cough, frothy sputum production, and shortness of breath *to detect signs and symptoms of pulmonary edema.* • Monitor hemodynamic status, including HR, BP, MAP, PAP, PAWP, CO, and CI, if available, *to evaluate effectiveness of therapy.* • Monitor adventitious breath sounds, adventitious heart sounds, JVD, and peripheral edema *to assess response to treatment.*

NURSING DIAGNOSIS	**Reduced stamina** resulting from imbalance between oxygen supply/demand as evidenced by abnormal heart rate response to activity, exertional dyspnea, and fatigue

Expected Patient Outcomes	Nursing Interventions and *Rationales*
• Achieves a realistic program of activity that balances physical activity with energy-conserving activities • Vital signs, O_2 saturation, and colour are within normal limits in response to activity	**Energy Management** • Encourage alternating rest and activity periods *to reduce cardiac workload and conserve energy.* • Provide calming diversionary activities to promote relaxation *to reduce O_2 consumption and to relieve dyspnea and fatigue.* • Monitor patient's O_2 response (e.g., pulse rate, cardiac rhythm, and respiratory rate) to self-care or nursing activities *to determine level of activity that can be tolerated.* • Teach patient and caregiver techniques of self-care (e.g., self-monitoring and pacing techniques for performance of ADLs) *to minimize O_2 consumption.* • Teach patient to change positions slowly from lying or sitting to standing because patient may experience a postural BP drop that causes dizziness and increases risk of falling. **Activity Therapy** • Collaborate with occupational therapists and physiotherapists *to plan and monitor activity or exercise program.* • Determine patient's commitment to increasing frequency and range of activities or exercise *to provide patient with obtainable goals.*

ADLs, activities of daily living; *BP*, blood pressure; *CI*, cardiac index; *CO*, cardiac output; *CVP*, central venous pressure; *HR*, heart rate; *JVD*, jugular venous distension; *MAP*, mean arterial pressure; *PAP*, pulmonary artery pressure; *PAWP*, pulmonary artery wedge pressure; S_3, and S_4, third and fourth heart sounds.

TABLE 37.8 CONSIDERATIONS FOR SODIUM INTAKE IN A CHINESE DIET

Consideration	High Sodium Content	Recommended Alternatives
Protein	Barbecued meats, Chinese sausages, salted fish, dried shrimp, salted eggs, century eggs, canned fish with black beans	Fresh or frozen unsalted meats, fish, poultry, seafood, eggs, tofu
Condiments and sauces	Monosodium glutamate (MSG), soy sauce, oyster sauce, fish sauce, shrimp paste, Hoisin sauce, Teriyaki sauce, Chinese cooking wine, bean paste, miso, fermented tofu, ketchup	Fresh herbs, spices, and other flavoured substances, such as ginger, onion, garlic, garlic powder, green onion, curry powder, pepper, lemon, vinegar, honey, sesame oil, low-sodium soy sauce
Other foods	Instant noodles, instant rice with seasonings, salty soups, bouillon (cubes or powder)	Unprocessed grain products (e.g., fresh rice, rice noodles, udon noodles, congee, pasta, bread), low-sodium soups
Dining-out tips	Most food served in Chinese restaurants has high sodium content; eat in restaurants only occasionally.	Plain rice rather than rice or noodles mixed with sauces (especially soy sauce or teriyaki sauce)

TABLE 37.9 CONSIDERATION FOR SODIUM INTAKE IN AN EAST INDIAN DIET

Consideration	High Sodium Content	Recommended Alternatives
Protein	Canned beans and lentils	Fresh beans and lentils to make daal
Condiments and sauces	Achaars (pickles); chutneys (made with salt); relish; tomato, curry, or mustard paste; black salt	Fresh herbs and spices: curry powder, turmeric, chili powder, mustard seeds, ginger, garlic, pepper, cumin, fenugreek (methi), garam masala
Dining-out tips	Most food served in East Indian restaurants is high in sodium; eat in restaurants only occasionally.	Ask for foods prepared without salt. Avoid salty chutneys or relishes.

TABLE 37.10 NURSING ASSESSMENT

Heart Failure

Subjective Data
Important Health Information

Family, cultural and psychosocial history: Availability of caregivers, living situation, pets at home, smoking, alcohol, illicit drug use, advance directives if available
Past health history: CAD (including recent MI), hypertension, cardiomyopathy, valvular or congenital heart disease, diabetes mellitus, thyroid or lung disease, rapid or irregular heart rate
Medications: Use of and adherence to any cardiac medications; use of diuretics, estrogens, corticosteroids, nonsteroidal anti-inflammatory medications, over-the-counter medications, herbal supplements

Symptoms
- Fatigue, depression, anxiety
- Nausea, vomiting, anorexia, stomach bloating
- Weight gain, ankle swelling, nocturia, decreased daytime urinary output
- Dyspnea, orthopnea, cough
- Chest pain or heaviness; palpitations, dizziness, fainting
- RUQ pain, abdominal discomfort, constipation
- Behavioural changes, visual changes

Objective Data
Integumentary

Cool, diaphoretic skin; cyanosis or pallor, peripheral edema (right-sided heart failure)

Respiratory
Tachypnea, crackles particularly at the bases, rhonchi, wheezes; frothy, blood-tinged sputum (see Chapter 28 for detailed respiratory assessment)

Cardiovascular
Tachycardia, S_3, S_4, murmurs, PMI displaced inferiorly and posteriorly, jugular vein distension (see Chapter 34 for detailed cardiac assessment)

Gastrointestinal
Abdominal distension, hepatosplenomegaly, ascites

Neurological
Restlessness, confusion, decreased attention or memory

Possible Findings
Altered levels of serum electrolytes (especially Na+ and K+), ↑ BUN, ↑ BNP or NT–pro-BNP, creatinine, or liver function test results; chest radiograph demonstrating cardiomegaly, pulmonary congestion, and interstitial pulmonary edema; echocardiogram showing increased chamber size and decreased wall motion; ECG showing atrial and ventricular enlargement; ↓ O$_2$ saturation

BNP, brain or B-type natriuretic peptide; *BUN,* blood urea nitrogen; *CAD,* coronary artery disease; *ECG,* electrocardiogram; *MI,* myocardial infarction; *NT–pro-BNP,* N-terminal pro-BNP; *PMI,* point of maximal impulse; *RUQ,* right upper quadrant; *S$_3$,* and *S$_4$,* third and fourth heart sounds.

before lung congestion develops. Coronary revascularization procedures should be performed in patients with CAD. Early and continued treatment of hypertension is another important preventive measure. Hyperlipidemic states in people with CAD should be managed with diet, exercise, and medication. The use of antidysrhythmic agents or an ICD–pacemaker is indicated for people with continuing low EF, even if they are receiving optimal medical therapy or are at risk for sudden cardiac death. In addition, patients with HF need to be counselled to quit smoking and obtain yearly influenza vaccinations.

When HF is diagnosed, slowing the disease progression is the focus. The patient must understand the importance of following the medication, diet, and exercise regimens. Exercise training (e.g., cardiac rehabilitation) improves symptoms of chronic HF but is often unavailable or underprescribed.

ACUTE INTERVENTION. Successful HF management depends on several important principles: (a) HF is a progressive disease, and treatment plans are established with quality-of-life goals; (b) symptoms are managed by the patient with self-management tools (daily weights, medication regimens, exercise plans); (c) intake of salt and water must be restricted; (d) a regular, prescribed level of exercise should be maintained; and (e) use of support systems is essential to the success of the entire treatment plan (Ezekowitz et al., 2017).

TABLE 37.11 PATIENT & CAREGIVER TEACHING GUIDE

Heart Failure

What Is Heart Failure?
1. Provide individually tailored information about what heart failure is and how it is treated.
2. Discuss how people make the most of life with a chronic illness.

Health Promotion
1. Instruct patient to obtain annual flu vaccination.
2. Instruct patient to obtain pneumococcal vaccine (e.g., Pneumovax) and revaccination after 5 yr (for people at high risk of infection or serious disease).
3. Provide counselling regarding smoking cessation and weight reduction, if relevant.

Exercise and Rest
1. Once patient is cleared by physician, discuss the benefits of regular exercise and dispel myths.
2. Instruct patient to plan a regular activity program and scheduled rest periods throughout the day.
3. Support communication of concerns and fears and provide encouragement.

Medication Therapy
1. Teach patient to take each medication as prescribed by the health care provider.
2. Help patient develop a system (e.g., daily chart) to ensure medications have been taken.
3. Instruct patient to take pulse and BP each day before taking medications. Know what is normal for the patient.
4. Ensure that patient knows signs and symptoms of orthostatic hypotension and how to prevent them.
5. Ensure that patient knows own INR if taking warfarin (Coumadin) and how often to have blood monitored.
6. If relevant, teach patient signs and symptoms of over-administration of anticoagulation agents.

Dietary Therapy
1. Instruct patient to consult the written diet plan and list of permitted and restricted foods.
2. Teach patient to examine labels to determine sodium content and examine the labels of over-the-counter medications such as laxatives, cough medicines, and antacids.

3. Encourage patient not to use salt in cooking or at the dining table.
4. Instruct patient to measure weight in the early morning every day after emptying bladder. Ensure that patient knows to use the same scale and wear similar clothes.
5. Help patient keep track of daily weight and report weight gain of more than 2 kg (4 lb) over the course of 1 to 2 days.
6. Instruct patient to restrict fluid intake to no more than 6 to 8 cups per day and to remember that fluid can be hidden in many foods. These hidden fluids should be counted in the daily restriction.

Other Topics
1. If adverse effects are bothersome, discuss ways in which timing of medications may help to manage them.
2. Instruct patient to avoid extremes of heat and cold.
3. Encourage patient to keep regular appointments with their health care provider.
4. Discuss end-of-life planning and the importance of advance directives.

Ongoing Monitoring
1. Educate patient about the signs and symptoms of recurring or progressing heart failure.
2. Instruct patient to report immediately to the health care provider the development or worsening of any of the following:
   - Difficulty breathing, especially with exertion or when lying flat
   - Waking up breathless at night
   - Frequent dry, hacking cough, especially when lying down
   - Fatigue, weakness
   - Swelling of ankles, feet, or abdomen
   - Nausea with abdominal swelling, pain, and tenderness
   - Dizziness or fainting
3. Encourage patient to join local support networks such as cardiac rehabilitation or chronic disease management programs.
4. Recognize depression as a major issue, and help patient seek treatment if signs and symptoms of depression occur.
5. Teach caregivers to recognize signs of cognitive impairment.

BP, blood pressure; *INR*, international normalized ratio.

Many patients with HF experience one or more episodes of acute decompensation. When they do, they may be initially managed in a critical care unit and later transferred to a general medical or cardiology unit when their condition has stabilized. NCP 37.1 for patients with HF applies to patients with stabilized HF.

AMBULATORY AND HOME CARE. HF is a chronic illness. Important nursing responsibilities are (a) teaching the patient about the physiological changes that have occurred, (b) assisting the patient to adapt to both the physiological and the psychological changes, and (c) integrating the patient and the patient's family or support system into the overall care plan (Ezekowitz et al., 2017). Patients with HF are at risk for depression, and those who are depressed are more likely to be rehospitalized and die prematurely (Toback & Clark, 2017). Appropriate treatment for depression is needed for patients to adhere to medical therapy and lifestyle changes. The nurse needs to emphasize to the patient and caregivers that it is possible to live productively with this chronic illness. Managing patients with HF out of the hospital setting is a priority of care. A patient and caregiver teaching guide is presented in Table 37.11.

Patients with chronic HF are required to take medication for the rest of their lives. This often becomes difficult because a patient may be asymptomatic when HF is under control. The

nurse should stress to the patient and family that because the disease is chronic, medication administration must be continued even through stable periods to prevent acute decompensation.

The patient and caregivers should learn to evaluate how the patient is feeling, to recognize symptoms of possible decompensation, and to report them early. They need to understand that the medications the patient is taking may cause adverse effects that, especially in the initiation phase, can make the patient feel worse for some weeks after initiation and upward titration. The patient, caregivers, and primary health care providers need to know that simply stopping some HF medications may not be appropriate. For example, a reported pulse rate of 50 beats/minute (especially in a patient who is also taking β-adrenergic blockers) may be acceptable and does not necessarily mean that the patient should stop taking the prescribed medication.

Use of community care services is essential in the care of patients with HF and their caregivers to help the patient maintain as much autonomy as possible and find alternate strategies, if needed, to maintain their independence and activities of daily living. An interprofessional health care team, including family physicians, nurse practitioners, pharmacists, dieticians, nurses, and physiotherapists, can instruct the patient in energy-saving and energy-efficient behaviours for daily activities. Many patients have multiple comorbidities, and a degree of cognitive impairment is common. Frequent physical assessments, including vital signs and weight, are extremely important. The team can coach the patient and the patient's caregivers to implement systems to remember medications and when to take them; identify health concerns, such as an increase in weight as evidence of worsening failure; and institute interventions to prevent hospitalization. The team can also refer the patient to a cardiac rehabilitation or chronic disease program, as well as help identify the need for respite services to reduce caregiver burden.

EVIDENCE-INFORMED PRACTICE
Research Highlight

What Factors Predict Adherence to Self-Care in Rural Patients With Heart Failure?

Clinical Question
For patients with heart failure living in a rural area, what are the predictors of adherence to heart failure (HF) self-care management at baseline and 3 months?

Best Available Evidence
Secondary analysis of data from a randomized controlled trial (RCT) of improving self-care for rural patients with heart failure

Critical Appraisal and Synthesis of Evidence
Analyzed survey data from 349 rural patients with stable chronic heart failure who were randomized to the intervention group of a larger RCT study
- Intervention was an individually tailored education and counselling session with the patient and spouse/caregiver to enhance self-care modelling and to motivate patients to seek prompt care to prevent decompensation.
- At baseline and 3 months, outcome measures were adherence to HF symptom management behaviours, depressive and anxiety symptoms, and perceived control.
- Being male, having less anxiety and depression, and reporting higher perceived control were predictors of improved self-adherence at 3 months.

Conclusion
- Reducing depression and anxiety and improving perceived control result in greater adherence to self-care management of HF behaviours.

Implications for Nursing Practice
- The nurse should consider the patient's gender, anxiety and depression levels, and perception of perceived control to promote adherence to HF self-care behaviours among rural patients.
- The nurse should advise rural patients to seek mental health counselling in order to reduce anxiety and depression to improve adherence to self-care HF management.

Reference for Evidence
Biddle, M. J., Moser, D. K., Pelter, M. M., et al. (2020). Predictors of adherence to self-care in rural patients with heart failure. *The Journal of Rural Health, 36*(1), 120–129. https://doi.org/10.1111/jrh.12405

EVALUATION
The expected outcomes for the patient with HF are presented in NCP 37.1.

CARDIAC TRANSPLANTATION

Heart transplantation was first performed in 1967. Since that time, cardiac transplantation has become the treatment of choice for carefully selected patients with end-stage HF. The

TABLE 37.12	INDICATIONS FOR AND CONTRAINDICATIONS TO CARDIAC TRANSPLANTATION

Indications: Transplantation Centre–Specific
- End-stage heart disease refractory to medical therapy
- Refractory, life-threatening cardiac dysrhythmias
- Functional NYHA class III or IV status with demonstrated poor exercise capacity

Contraindications
- Pulmonary hypertension unrelieved by medication
- Primary systemic disease that would limit survival (e.g., malignancies)
- Renal dysfunction (creatinine level >200 mmol/L): patient could be considered for combined transplantation
- Active infection
- Technical issues
- Smoking, inhaling or vaping use (6-mo abstinence recommended)
- Active alcohol or illicit drug use (6-mo abstinence required)
- Mental illness or other cognitive factors
- Documented life-threatening, repeated nonadherence to medical regimen
- Malignancy (generally must be cancer free for 5 yr)
- Severe osteoporosis
- Significant peripheral vascular disease
- Diabetes mellitus with end-organ damage
- Insufficient social support

NYHA, New York Heart Association.
Source: Chih, S., McDonald, M., Dipchand, A., et al. (2020). Canadian Cardiovascular Society/Canadian Cardiac Transplant Network position statement on heart transplantation: Patient eligibility, selection, and post-transplantation care. *Canadian Journal of Cardiology, 36,* 335–356. https://doi.org/10.1016/j.cjca.2019.12.025

main indications for transplantation are ischemic heart disease and dilated cardiomyopathy. Indications for and contraindications to heart transplantation are listed in Table 37.12.

Among the patients who meet the criteria for cardiac transplantation, the goal of the evaluation process is to identify patients who would most benefit from a new heart. After a complete physical examination and diagnostic workup, the patient and family undergo a comprehensive psychological profile that includes assessment of coping skills, family support systems, and motivation to follow the rigorous regimen that is essential to a successful transplantation. The complexity of the transplantation process may be overwhelming to a patient with inadequate support systems and a poor understanding of the lifestyle changes required after transplantation.

Transplant outcomes are significantly worse for Indigenous patients than for non-Indigenous patients, mainly because of social determinants of health, including lack of access to health care services and post-transplant medications, and existing comorbidities (McGuire et al., 2019).

Once an individual is accepted as a transplantation candidate (this may happen rapidly during an acute illness or over a longer period, depending on the patient's condition), they are placed on a transplant list. Patients may wait at home and receive ongoing medical care if their medical condition is stable. If their condition is not stable, they may require hospitalization for more intensive therapy, including long-term mechanical cardiac support with a VAD. Unfortunately, the overall waiting period for a cardiac transplant is difficult to define but is usually between 6 and 9 months, depending on donor availability.

Donor and recipient matching is based on body and heart size and ABO blood type. Negative lymphocyte crossmatch (explained in Chapter 16) is also important.

Most donor hearts are obtained at sites away from the institution where the transplantation is performed. The maximum acceptable ischemic time for cardiac transplantation is 4 to 6 hours.

The recipient is prepared for surgery, and cardiopulmonary bypass is used. The usual surgical procedure involves removing the recipient's heart, except for the posterior right and left atrial walls and their venous connections. The recipient's heart is then replaced with the donor heart, which has been trimmed to match. Care is taken to preserve the integrity of the donor sinoatrial node so that a sinus rhythm may be achieved postoperatively.

Immunosuppressive therapy begins in the operating room. Some transplantation centres administer medications to rapidly induce immunosuppression in the operating room and critical care area because the regimens most commonly used are nephrotoxic and, hence, cannot be started for a few days after the surgery. This induction therapy (usually with a monoclonal antibody) buys time to allow the kidneys to recover from the insult of surgery. (The mechanisms of action and adverse effects of these and other immunosuppressants are discussed in Chapter 16 and Table 16.16.) Regimens vary, but tacrolimus [Prograf]) with mycophenolate mofetil (Cellcept) and prednisolone are most frequently used for maintenance immunosuppression. In many Canadian programs, cardiac transplant recipients are weaned off prednisolone over a number of months, and after a year, it is uncommon for such patients to be taking prednisolone. The use of today's immunosuppressants has resulted not only in reduced rates of rejection but also in slowing the rejection process so that early treatment can be instituted. Because of the use of immunosuppressants, however, infection is a major complication after transplantation. Patients are advised to stay away from unwell individuals and large crowds and to receive annual influenza vaccinations.

Endomyocardial biopsies via the right internal jugular vein are performed at repeated intervals to detect rejection in the first year. After 3 months, the incidence of acute rejection decreases dramatically; however, a type of CAD known as *cardiac allograft vasculopathy* (also known as *chronic rejection*) develops in a significant proportion of heart transplant recipients over the long term. As a result, regular surveillance of the transplanted heart by means of diagnostic tests such as coronary angiography and echocardiography is performed for the rest of the recipient's life.

Advances in surgical technique and postoperative care have improved survival rates after cardiac transplantation. Approximately 75% of transplant patients will be living after 5 years and 62% will be living after 10 years (Moayedi et al., 2019). This number is an overall average and varies greatly, depending on such factors as age at transplantation, severity of illness, adherence to medication regimens and risk factor modification, and social support systems. In the first year after transplantation, acute rejection, infection, and sudden cardiac death are the major causes of death. Later on, malignancy (especially lymphoma) and allograft vasculopathy are major causes of death.

One factor that may affect morbidity and mortality in heart transplantation is the patient's ability to adhere to medication regimens. In a survey of international transplant centres, 34% of transplant patients were nonadherent to their immunosuppressant regimen. Smoking, lack of family or social support, and financial barriers were factors associated with nonadherence (Denhaerynck et al., 2018).

Nursing management throughout the post-transplantation period focuses on promoting patient adaptation to the transplantation process, monitoring health, managing lifestyle changes, and providing ongoing teaching to the patient and caregivers.

Mechanical Cardiac Support Devices

Temporary support of one or both failed ventricles has been available for many years in the form of intra-aortic balloon pumps or extracorporeal membrane oxygenation. These circulatory support devices are designed for short-term use (days to weeks).

More recently, longer-term devices (for use over months to years) are being used in Canada as a bridge to heart transplantation or recovery of the native heart. These pumps are called *ventricular assist devices* (VADs). A number of VADs are available in Canada. Some examples include the HeartMate II (made by Thoratec Corp., Pleasanton, California; see Figure 37.6) and HeartWare HVAD (made by HeartWare Inc., Framingham, Massachusetts) electronic devices. These pumps are designed to support the left ventricle. In many carefully selected patients, support of the left ventricle alone will alleviate symptoms of right-sided HF by unloading the left side.

Patients carry around a battery pack with a small computer attached to their belt. With adequate social support, patients are able to live at home with these devices and, in some cases, return to work while waiting for a heart transplant. This improved mobility—the ability to live out of the hospital—and the improvement that results in the patient's nutritional state allow the patient to undergo transplantation in much improved physical condition. In the United States and Europe, instead of a transplant, some patients who are ineligible for transplantation use these devices. This practice is commonly referred to as *destination therapy* or *permanent therapy*.

A totally artificial heart is available; however, it is not currently in use in Canada. For more information on mechanical cardiac support, see Chapter 68.

ETHICAL DILEMMAS
Transplant Recipient Requests

Situation
A 60-year-old woman has been awaiting heart transplantation for 6 months. At her recent clinic appointment, she asks if there is any possibility of receiving only a woman's heart. She tells the nurse that she does not want to receive a man's heart as she feels her personality would change.

Important Points for Consideration
- Hearts are not allocated on the basis of gender except as determined by size matching. Specifically, a large man is unlikely to receive a woman's heart because women in general are smaller; however a woman could receive a man's heart if they are the same size.
- There is no evidence that people assume the personalities of their donor.
- Heart transplantation programs do not respond to requests for specific attributes of organ donors such as race, gender, or cultural or religious practices.
- Heart transplantation programs do not give heart transplant recipients information about the characteristics of their donors.
- When heart transplantation candidates make these requests, it is often due to misinformation that has been published in the media. The nurse should explore with the patient her concerns and work with the psychosocial team to help her address them.

Clinical Decision-Making Questions
1. How might the nurse respond to the patient about such a request?
2. What supports should the nurse offer to the patient to assist her in working through her concerns?

CASE STUDY

Heart Failure

Patient Profile
M. E. (pronouns she/her), 70 years old, was admitted to the medical unit with complaints of increasing dyspnea on exertion.

Subjective Data
- Had a myocardial infarction (MI) at 58 years of age
- Has a 25-year history of hypertension
- Has experienced increasing dyspnea on exertion during the last 2 years
- Recently had a respiratory tract infection
- Has moist, productive cough
- Has edema in both legs up to the knees
- Cannot walk two blocks without getting short of breath
- Has to sleep with head elevated on three pillows
- Does not always remember to take medication
- 5-kg weight gain in 3 days

Objective Data
Physical Examination
- In respiratory distress; use of accessory muscles; respiratory rate, 36 breaths/min
- Moist crackles at both lung bases
- Skin cool and diaphoretic
- 2+ Pitting edema in both legs
- HR, 95 bpm and regular
- BP, 160/90 mm Hg
- Oxygen saturation, 88%

Diagnostic Studies
- Chest radiographic examination results: cardiomegaly; fluid in lower lung fields
- Echocardiogram results: ejection fraction (EF), 20%

Interprofessional Care
- Enalapril, 5 mg PO (orally) daily
- Furosemide (Lasix), 40 mg PO bid
- Potassium, 40 mEq PO bid
- 2-g sodium diet
- Oxygen, 6 L/min to maintain O_2 saturation >90%
- Daily weight measurements
- Daily 12-lead electrocardiography (ECG); cardiac enzyme measurements, q8h three times; continuous cardiac monitoring
- Measurements of serum electrolytes, urea, creatinine, and BNP; complete blood cell count (CBC)

Discussion Questions
1. Explain the probable pathophysiological process of M. E.'s heart disease.
2. What clinical manifestations of heart failure did M. E. exhibit?
3. What is the significance of the findings of the diagnostic studies?
4. Explain the rationale for each of the medical orders prescribed for M. E.
5. **Priority decision:** What are the nurse's priority nursing interventions for M. E.?
6. **Priority decision:** What priority patient teaching measures should be instituted to prevent recurrence of an acute episode of heart failure?
7. **Priority decision:** On the basis of the assessment data presented, write one or more appropriate nursing diagnoses. Are there any interprofessional issues?
8. **Evidence-informed practice:** M. E. asks the nurse why it is so important to "watch her salt." M. E. tells the nurse that food tastes better with salt. How might the nurse respond to this patient?

Answers are available at http://evolve.elsevier.com/Canada/Lewis/medsurg.

REVIEW QUESTIONS

The number of the question corresponds to the same-numbered objective at the beginning of the chapter.

1. What are the manifestations of HFrEF that the nurse should recognize?
   a. ↓ Afterload and ↓ left ventricular end-diastolic pressure (LVEDP)
   b. ↓ Ejection fraction (EF) and ↑ pulmonary artery occlusive pressure (PAOP)
   c. ↓ PAOP and ↑ left ventricular EF
   d. ↑ Pulmonary hypertension associated with normal EF

2. Which compensatory mechanism leads to inappropriate sodium and fluid retention?
   a. Ventricular dilation
   b. Ventricular hypertrophy
   c. Neurohormonal response
   d. Sympathetic nervous system activation

3. Which medication used in the management of a client with acute pulmonary edema will decrease both preload and afterload and provide relief of anxiety?
   a. Morphine
   b. Amiodarone
   c. Dobutamine
   d. Aminophylline

4. How can a client with chronic HF best decrease the chances of having an acute decompensation?
   a. Resting and not making any exertions except under medical supervision
   b. Documenting fluid intake and urinary output each day
   c. Monitoring weight daily and reporting changes outside of recommended parameters
   d. Taking extra furosemide when shortness of breath occurs

5. Clients with a heart transplant are at risk for which complications in the first year after transplantation? (Select all that apply.)
   a. Cancer
   b. Infection
   c. Rejection
   d. Vasculopathy
   e. Sudden cardiac death

1. b; 2. c; 3. a; 4. c; 5. b, c, e.

For even more review questions, visit http://evolve.elsevier.com/Canada/Lewis/medsurg.

REFERENCES

Atzema, C. L., Austin, P. C., Yu, B., et al. (2018). Effect of early physician follow-up on mortality and subsequent hospital admissions after emergency care for heart failure: A retrospective cohort study. *Canadian Medical Association Journal, 190*(50), E1468–E1477. https://doi.org/10.1503/cmaj.180786

Denhaerynck, K., Berben, L., Dobbels, F., et al. (2018). Multilevel factors are associated with immunosuppressant nonadherence in heart transplant recipients: The international BRIGHT study. *American Journal of Transplantation, 18*(6), 1446–1460. https://doi: 10.1111/ajt.14611

Di Giuseppe, G., Chu, A., Tu, J. V., et al. (2019). Incidence of heart failure among immigrants to Ontario, Canada: A CANHEART immigrant study. *Journal of Cardiac Failure, 25*(6), 425–435. https://doi.org/10.1016/j.cardfail.2019.03.006

Ezekowitz, J. A., O'Meara, E., McDonald, M. A., et al. (2017). 2017 Comprehensive updates of the Canadian Cardiovascular Society Guidelines for the Management of Heart Failure. *Canadian Journal of Cardiology, 33*, 1342–1433. https://doi.org/10.1016/j.cjca.2017.08.022

Hannon, R. A., & Porth, C. (2017). *Porth pathophysiology: Concepts of altered health states* (2nd ed.). Philadelphia: Wolters Kluwer.

Health Canada. (2021). *Canada's food guide.* https://food-guide.canada.ca/en/

Heart and Stroke Foundation of Canada. (2021). *Heart failure.* https://www.heartandstroke.ca/heart/conditions/heart-failure

Jhund, P., & McMurray, J. J. V. (2016). The neprilysin pathway in heart failure: A review and guide on the use of sacubitril/valsartan. *Heart, 102*, 1342–1347. https://doi.org/10.1136/heartjnl-2014-306775

Kapoor, A., Koul, R., Singh, A., et al. (2018). Economic impact assessment of reducing heart failure related hospitalizations in Alberta, Canada by a community-based outpatient heart failure clinic – A pilot study. *Circulation, 138*(Suppl 1), S137–S138. https://doi/abs/10.1161/circ.138.suppl_1.16048

McGuire, C., Kannathasan, S., Lowe, M., et al. (2019). Patient survival following renal transplantation in Indigenous populations: A systematic review. *Clinical Transplantation, 34*(1), e137760. https://doi.org/10.1111/ctr.13760

Moayedi, Y., Fan, C. P. S., Cherikh, W. S., et al. (2019). Survival outcomes after heart transplantation: Does recipient sex matter? *Circulation: Heart Failure, 12*(10), e006218. https://doi.org/10.1161/CIRCHEARTFAILURE.119.006218

Toback, M., & Clark, N. (2017). Strategies to improve self-management in heart failure patients. *Contemporary Nurse, 53*(1), 105–120. https://doi.org/10.1080/10376178.2017.1290537

Virani, S., Bain, M., Code, J., et al. (2017). The need for heart failure advocacy in Canada. *Canadian Journal of Cardiology, 33*(11), 1450–1454. https://doi.org/10.1016/j.cjca.2017.08.024

RESOURCES

Canadian Association of Cardiovascular Prevention and Rehabilitation (CACPR)
https://www.cacpr.ca

Canadian Cardiovascular Society (CCS)
https://www.ccs.ca

Canadian Council of Cardiovascular Nurses
http://www.cccn.ca

Easy Auscultation: Extra Heart Sounds (S3 and S4)
https://www.easyauscultation.com/course-contents?courseid=25

Heart and Stroke Foundation of Canada—*Healthy Living: Health eTools*
https://www.heartandstroke.ca/get-healthy/health-etools

evolve

For additional Internet resources, see the website for this book at http://evolve.elsevier.com/Canada/Lewis/medsurg.

Nursing Management

Dysrhythmias

Shelley Clarke
Originating US chapter by Kimberly Day

⊖volve WEBSITE

http://evolve.elsevier.com/Canada/Lewis/medsurg

- Review Questions (Online Only)
- Key Points
- Answer Guidelines for Case Study
- Student Case Study
- Atrial Fibrillation
- Conceptual Care Map Creator
- Audio Glossary
- Content Updates

LEARNING OBJECTIVES

1. Identify the clinical characteristics and electrocardiographic (ECG) patterns of normal sinus rhythm, common dysrhythmias, and acute coronary syndrome (ACS).
2. Describe the nursing management of patients requiring continuous ECG monitoring.
3. Describe the nursing and interprofessional management of patients with common dysrhythmias and ECG changes associated with ACS.
4. Differentiate between defibrillation and cardioversion, identifying indications for their use and nursing implications.
5. Describe the management of patients with implantable cardioverter–defibrillators.
6. Describe the management of patients with temporary and permanent pacemakers.
7. Explain the management of patients undergoing electrophysiological testing and radiofrequency ablation therapy.

KEY TERMS

asystole
atrial fibrillation
atrial flutter
automatic external defibrillators (AEDs)
automaticity

cardiac pacemaker
complete heart block
dysrhythmias
electrocardiogram (ECG)
premature atrial contraction (PAC)

premature ventricular contraction (PVC)
ventricular fibrillation
ventricular tachycardia (VT)

RHYTHM IDENTIFICATION AND TREATMENT

The ability to recognize normal and abnormal cardiac rhythms is an essential nursing skill. Nurses have a significant role to play in patient assessment, early identification of arrythmias and acute symptoms, and collaboration with the interprofessional team. Cardiac monitoring is now used in a wide range of hospital, clinic, and home settings. Prompt assessment of abnormal cardiac rhythms, called dysrhythmias, and of the patient's response to them is critical. This chapter describes basic principles of electrocardiographic (ECG) monitoring and recognition of common dysrhythmias, as well as ECG changes that are associated with acute coronary syndrome (ACS). For more detailed information on ECG interpretation, the reader should refer to dedicated texts on this topic.

Conduction System

The properties of cardiac cells enable the conduction system to initiate an electrical impulse, which is transmitted through the cardiac tissue and stimulates muscle contraction (Table 38.1). The conduction system of the heart consists of specialized neuromuscular tissue located throughout the heart (see Chapter 34, Figure 34.4). A normal cardiac impulse begins in the sinoatrial (SA) node in the upper right atrium. It is transmitted throughout the atrial myocardium via the bundle of Bachmann and internodal pathways, which causes atrial contraction. The impulse then travels to the atrioventricular (AV) node through the bundle of His and down the left and right ventricular bundle branches, ending in the Purkinje fibres.

TABLE 38.1	PROPERTIES OF CARDIAC CELLS
Automaticity	Ability to initiate an impulse spontaneously and continuously
Contractility	Ability to respond mechanically to an impulse
Conductivity	Ability to transmit an impulse along a membrane in an orderly manner
Excitability	Ability to be electrically stimulated

Conduction to the point just before the impulse leaves the Purkinje fibres takes place within the time of the PR interval of the ECG. When the impulse emerges from the Purkinje fibres, ventricular depolarization occurs, producing mechanical contraction of the ventricles and the QRS complex on the ECG. The electrical activity of the heart is illustrated in Chapter 34, Figure 34.4.

Nervous Control of the Heart

The autonomic nervous system plays an important role in the rate of impulse formation, the speed of conduction, and the strength of cardiac contraction. The components of the autonomic nervous system that affect the heart are the right and left vagus nerve fibres of the parasympathetic nervous system and the fibres of the sympathetic nervous system.

Stimulation of the vagus nerve causes a decrease in the rate of firing of the SA node, a slowing of impulse conduction of the atrioventricular node, and a decrease in the force of cardiac muscle contraction. Stimulation of the sympathetic nerves that supply the heart has essentially the opposite effect on the heart.

The membrane of a cardiac cell is semipermeable, allowing the intracellular concentration of potassium to remain high and the intracellular concentration of sodium to remain low. A high concentration of sodium and a low concentration of potassium are maintained outside the cell. The inside of the cell, when the cell is at rest or in the polarized state, is negative compared with the outside. When a cell or groups of cells are stimulated, each cell membrane changes its permeability and allows sodium to move rapidly into the cell, making the inside of the cell positive compared with the outside (*depolarization*). A slower movement of ions across the membrane restores the cell to the polarized state; this restoration is called *repolarization*. The phases of the cardiac action potential are as follows: phase 0 is the upstroke of rapid depolarization; phases 1, 2, and 3 represent repolarization; and phase 4 is a polarized state. Antidysrhythmia medications have a direct effect on the various phases of the action potential. When antidysrhythmia medications are used in a clinical setting, it is important to understand the ionic shifts in the cardiac cell and the action potential mechanism (Aehlert, 2018).

Electrocardiographic Monitoring

The electrocardiogram (ECG) is a graphic tracing of the electrical impulses produced in the heart. The waveforms on the ECG are produced by the movement of charged ions across the membranes of myocardial cells, representing depolarization and repolarization.

ECG lead wires are attached to the patient's chest wall by means of an electrode pad fixed with electrical conductive gel. These lead wires enable viewing of the heart's electrical activity. Before placing the electrodes and leads on a patient, the nurse must properly prepare the patient's skin. Excessive hair on the chest wall should be clipped with scissors. The nurse should prepare the skin by rubbing gently with dry gauze until the skin is slightly pink. If the skin is oily, alcohol may be used first. For a diaphoretic patient, a skin protectant should be applied before

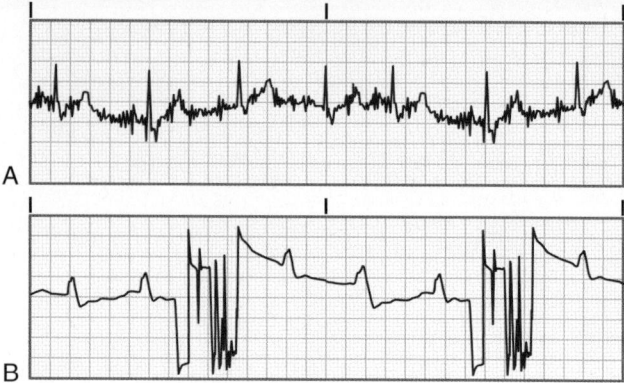

FIG. 38.1 A, Electrocardiogram (ECG) demonstrating muscle tremor. **B,** ECG reflecting loose electrodes.

the electrode secured. If leads and electrodes are not firmly placed or if there is muscle activity or electrical interference from an outside source, an artifact may be seen on the monitor. *Artifact* is a distortion of the baseline and waveforms seen on the ECG (Figure 38.1). If artifact occurs, the nurse should check for loose connections in the equipment. The electrodes on the patient may need to be replaced or moved to areas that are less affected by movement (Aehlert, 2018).

Types of Monitoring

When a patient's ECG is being continuously monitored, between 1 and 12 ECG leads may be used. Most patient monitoring involves using a three- or five-lead system, using the leads I, II, III, or MCL$_1$ (Figures 38.2 and 38.3). The monitoring leads used are determined by the patient's clinical status.

The ECG can be visualized continuously on a monitor oscilloscope. A recording of the ECG (i.e., rhythm strip) is obtained on ECG paper attached to the monitor. The recording provides documentation of the patient's rhythm. It also allows for measurement of complexes and intervals and for assessment of dysrhythmias.

A 12-lead ECG views the surfaces of the left ventricle from 12 different angles (Aehlert, 2018). Six of the 12 ECG leads (leads I, II, III, aV$_R$, aV$_L$, and aV$_F$) measure electrical forces in the frontal plane (see Figure 38.2). The remaining six leads (V$_1$ through V$_6$) measure the electrical forces in the horizontal plane (precordial leads). The 12-lead ECG may show changes indicative of structural changes or damage, such as ischemia, infarction, enlarged cardiac chambers, electrolyte imbalance, or drug toxicity (Aehlert, 2018). An example of a normal 12-lead ECG appears in Figure 38.4; 12-lead ECGs will be discussed later in this chapter.

Telemetry Monitoring. Telemetry monitoring is the observation of a patient's heart rate and rhythm to rapidly diagnose dysrhythmias, ischemia, or infarction. Two types of systems are used for telemetry monitoring. The first type, a centralized monitoring system, requires a nurse or telemetry technician to continuously observe all patients' rhythms at a central location. The second system of telemetry monitoring does not require constant surveillance by the nurse or technician. These systems have the capability of detecting and storing data. Sophisticated alarm systems provide different levels of detection of dysrhythmias, ischemia, or infarction, depending on the severity of each. However, computerized monitoring systems are not fail-proof. Frequent nursing assessment is important in caring for monitored patients.

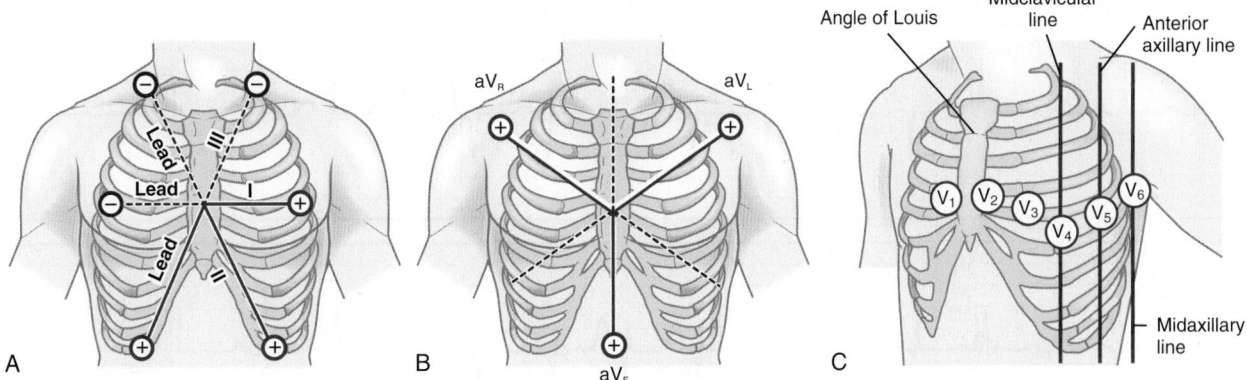

FIG. 38.2 **A,** Limb leads I, II, and III. These bipolar leads are located on the extremities. Illustrated are the angles from which these leads view the heart. **B,** Limb leads aV_R, aV_L, and aV_F. These unipolar leads use the centre of the heart as their negative electrode. **C,** Placement for the unipolar chest leads: V_1, fourth intercostal space at the right sternal border; V_2, fourth intercostal space at the left sternal border; V_3, halfway between V_2 and V_4; V_4, fifth intercostal space at the left midclavicular line; V_5, fifth intercostal space at the left anterior axillary line; V_6, fifth intercostal space at the left midaxillary line.

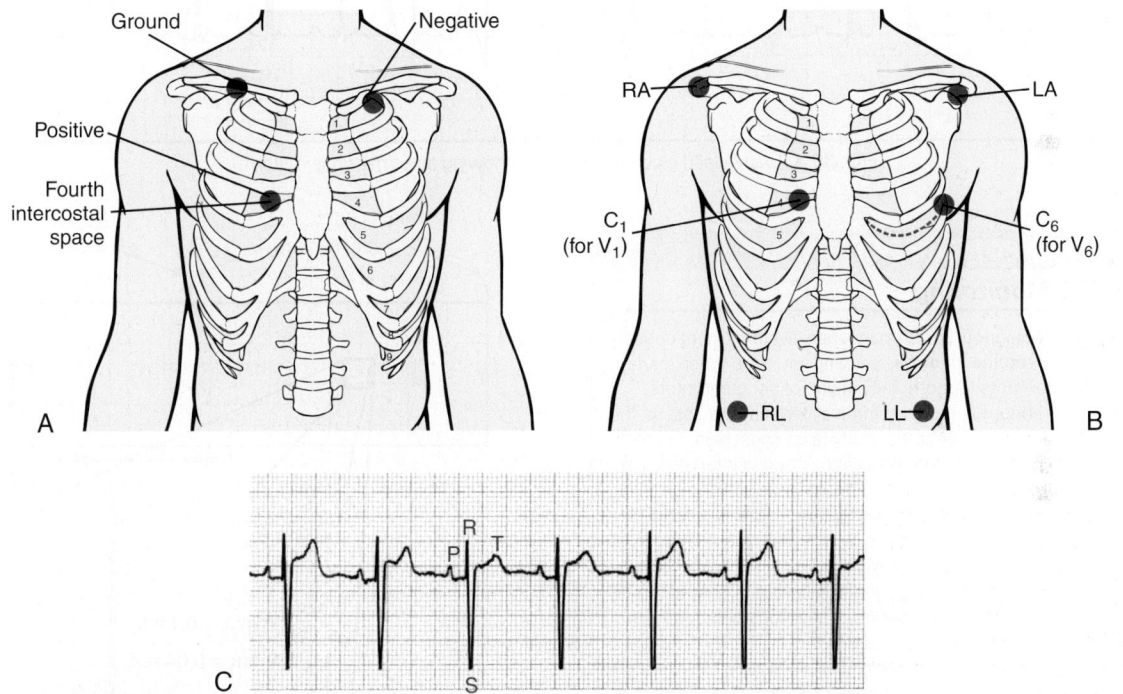

FIG. 38.3 **A,** Lead placement for MCL_1 when a three-lead system is used. **B,** Lead placement for V_1 or V_6 when a five-lead system is used. **C,** Typical electrocardiographic tracing for lead MCL_1. *C,* chest; *LA,* left arm; *LL,* left leg; *RA,* right arm; *RL,* right leg. Source: Adapted from Urden, L. D., Stacy, K. M., & Lough, M. E. (2010). *Critical care nursing: Diagnosis and management* (6th ed., p. 370). Mosby.

The Holter monitor is a device that records the ECG while the patient is ambulatory. The device can record heart rhythm for 24 to 48 hours while the patient performs daily activities. The patient maintains a diary in which activities and any symptoms are recorded. Events in the diary can later be correlated with any dysrhythmias observed on the recording. The monitor is generally a useful device for detecting significant dysrhythmias and evaluating the effects of medications during a patient's normal activities. It can also be used for detecting ischemia by analyzing ST segments. A limitation of the device is that patients who have frequent ventricular dysrhythmias, some of which may be lethal, may not have these dysrhythmias during the monitored time. (Holter monitoring is also discussed in Chapter 34.)

Use of event monitors has greatly improved the evaluation of outpatient dysrhythmias. Event monitors are recorders that

are activated by the patient and can be used only at the time the patient experiences symptoms. The recorder is placed over the patient's chest during symptoms. The patient then transmits the rhythm to a central monitoring company via a phone. This is an easier method of documenting a dysrhythmia than the 24-hour monitor, especially if symptoms are not occurring daily. (Ambulatory ECG monitoring is discussed in Chapter 34.)

Exercise treadmill testing is used for evaluation of cardiac rhythm response to exercise. Exercise-induced dysrhythmias can be reproduced and analyzed, and medication therapy can be evaluated. These tests are performed with routine treadmill testing policies. Diagnostic procedures for assessment of the cardiovascular system are presented in Chapter 34, Table 34.6.

New technology allows for continuous cardiac monitoring in certain patient conditions where early detection of arrhythmias

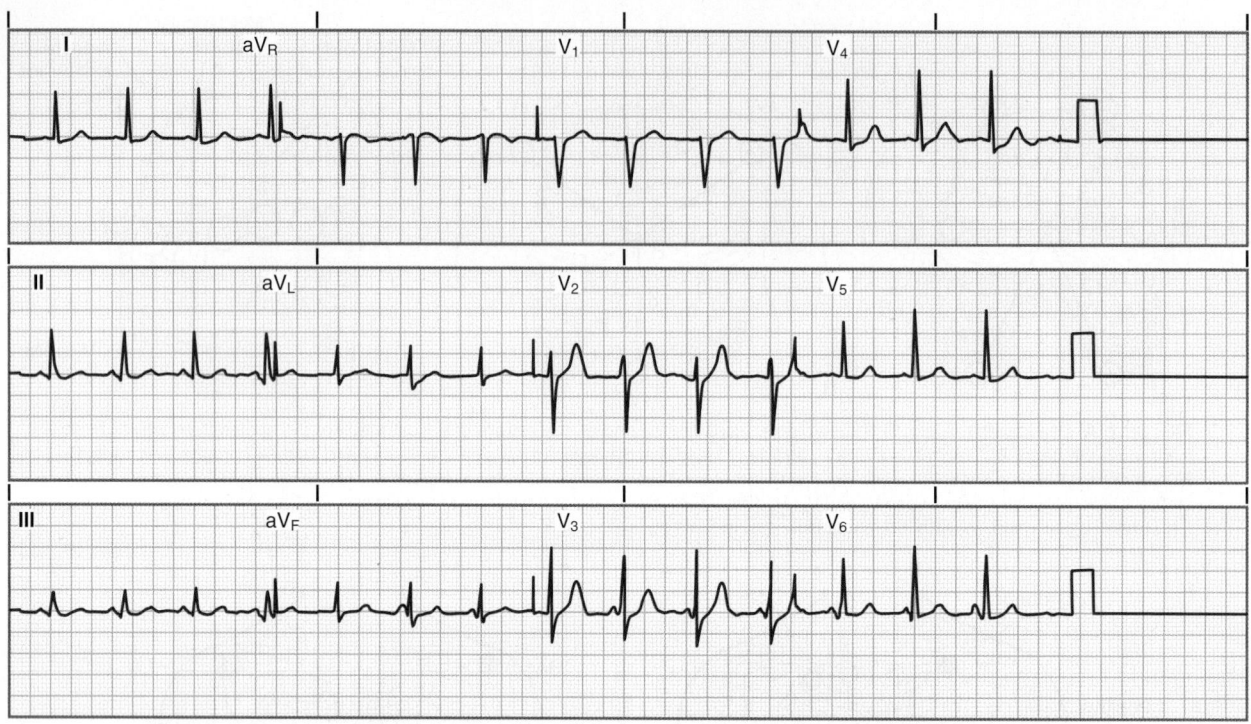

FIG. 38.4 Twelve-lead electrocardiogram showing a normal sinus rhythm.

INFORMATICS IN PRACTICE

Wireless ECG Monitoring

- Wireless electrocardiogram (ECG) monitoring systems continuously monitor and interpret the findings, sending an alert when patient rhythm or measurements (or both) fall outside of set parameters.
- Early detection of abnormal heart rhythms allows time to assess the patient for signs of hemodynamic instability (e.g., chest pain, hypotension, palpitations, dyspnea) and determine the need to intervene (e.g., call the rapid response team).
- These systems can automatically save the pre-event portion of the ECG while continuing to record the post-event portion and send all of the information to the health care provider.
- Computerized monitoring systems are not fail-proof. The nurse must frequently assess all monitored patients for any signs of hemodynamic instability.

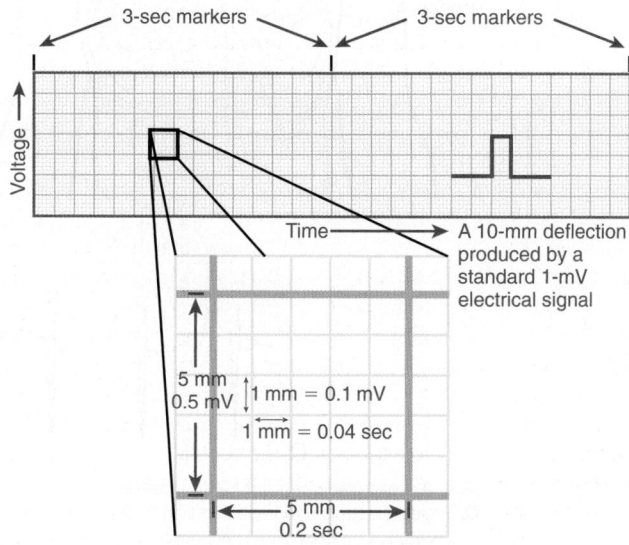

FIG. 38.5 Time and voltage on the electrocardiogram. Source: Adapted from Wesley, K. (2011). *Huszar's basic dysrhythmias and acute coronary syndromes: Interpretation and management* (4th ed., p. 19). Mosby.

contribute to earlier treatment and better outcomes. Insertable cardiac monitors (ICMs) are small, subcutaneously implanted devices offering continuous ambulatory ECG monitoring with a lifespan up to 3 years. ICMs have been studied and proven useful in monitoring patients' ECG in selected cases of unexplained syncope and palpitations, as well as in management of atrial fibrillation (Giancaterino et al., 2018).

Assessment of Cardiac Rhythm

In Figure 38.5 a systematic approach to assessing a cardiac rhythm is presented. To correctly interpret an ECG, the nurse must know how to measure time and voltage on the ECG paper. ECG paper consists of large squares (heavy lines) and small squares (light lines; see Figure 38.5). Each large square incorporates 25 smaller squares (five horizontal and five vertical). Each small square represents 0.04 seconds horizontally and 0.1 millivolt (mV) vertically. This means that the large square represents 0.20 seconds and that 300 large squares represent 1 minute. Vertically, one large square is equal to 0.5 mV. These squares

are used to calculate the heart rate (HR) and intervals between different ECG complexes.

A variety of methods can be used to calculate the HR from an ECG. Probably the most accurate way is to count the number of QRS complexes in 1 minute. However, this method is time consuming. If the rhythm is regular, a simpler process can be used: Every 3 seconds, a marker appears on the ECG paper. An R wave is the first upward (or positive) deflection of the QRS complex. The nurse can count the number of R–R intervals in 6 seconds and multiply that number by 10. This calculation yields the approximate number of beats/minute (Figure 38.6).

Another rapid method for calculating the HR when the rhythm is regular is to count the number of small squares within

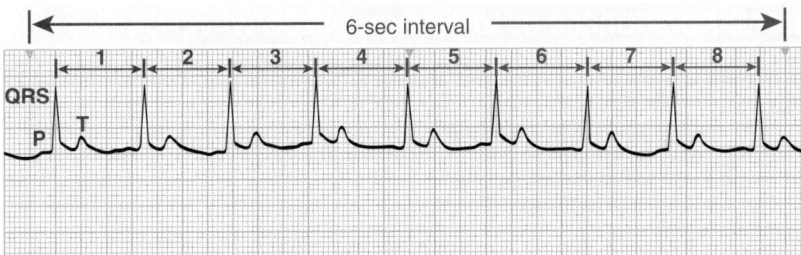

FIG. 38.6 The heart rate is calculated according to the interval between first upward (or positive) deflection (R wave) of one QRS complex to the R wave of the next. When the rhythm is regular, heart rate can be determined at a glance. The estimated heart rate is 80. The actual heart rate is 86. Source: Adapted from Wesley, K. (2011). *Huszar's basic dysrhythmias and acute coronary syndromes: Interpretation and management* (4th ed., p. 56). Mosby.

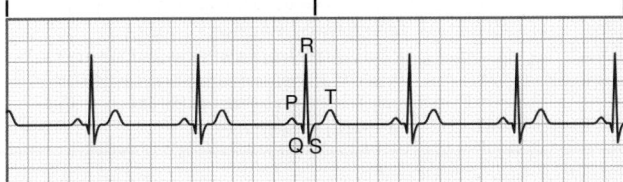

FIG. 38.7 Electrocardiogram depicting normal sinus rhythm in lead II.

one R–R interval. Dividing this number by 1 500 yields the HR. The number of large squares within one R–R interval can also be counted and divided by 300 (see Figure 38.6). These methods are accurate only if the rhythm is regular.

Normal sinus rhythm is a rhythm that originates in the SA node and follows the normal conduction pattern of the cardiac cycle (Figure 38.7). Figure 38.8 shows the normal electrical pattern of the cardiac cycle. Table 38.2 provides a description of ECG waveforms, intervals, normal durations, and possible sources of disturbances in these features. The P wave represents the depolarization of the atria (passage of an electrical impulse through the atria), causing atrial contraction. The PR interval represents the period when the impulse spreads through the atria, the AV node, the bundle of His, and the Purkinje fibres. The QRS complex represents depolarization of the ventricles (ventricular contraction), and the QRS interval represents the time it takes for depolarization. The ST segment represents the time between ventricular depolarization and repolarization. This segment should be flat, or isoelectric, representing the absence of any electrical activity between these two events. The T wave represents repolarization of the ventricles. The QT interval represents the total time for depolarization and repolarization of the ventricles (see Figure 38.8).

Electrophysiological Mechanisms of Dysrhythmias

The heart has specialized cells found in the SA node, parts of the atria, the AV node, and the bundle of His and Purkinje fibres (His–Purkinje system) that are able to discharge spontaneously. This situation is termed automaticity. Normally, the main pacemaker of the heart is the SA node, which spontaneously discharges 60 to 100 times per minute (Table 38.3). A pacemaker from another site may be discharged in two ways. If the SA node discharges more slowly than a secondary pacemaker, the electrical discharges from the secondary pacemaker may passively "escape." The secondary pacemaker then discharges automatically at its intrinsic rate. These secondary pacemakers may originate from the AV node or the His–Purkinje system at rates of 40 to 60 times per minute and 20 to 40 times per minute, respectively.

Another way that secondary pacemakers can originate is when they discharge more rapidly than the normal pacemaker of the SA node. Early or late beats may be triggered at an ectopic

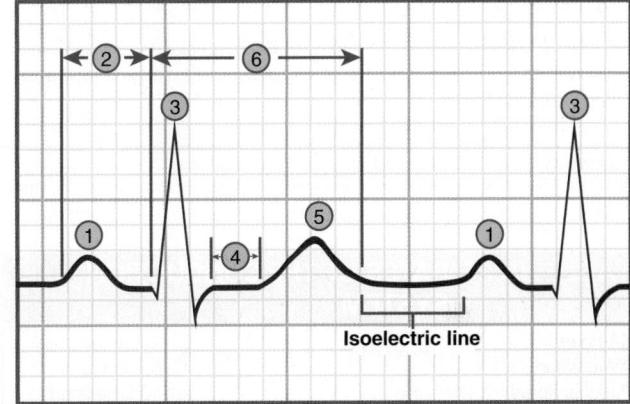

FIG. 38.8 The electrocardiogram tracing as seen in normal sinus rhythm. *1,* P wave; *2,* PR interval; *3,* QRS complex: Q wave, R wave, S wave; *4,* ST segment; *5,* T wave; *6,* QT interval. Isoelectric (flat) line or baseline represents the absence of electrical activity in the heart cells.

focus (area outside the normal conduction pathway) in the atria, the AV node, or the ventricles. This may result in a dysrhythmia, which replaces the normal sinus rhythm.

The impulse started by the SA node or an ectopic focus must be conducted to the entire heart chamber. The property of myocardial tissue that allows it to be depolarized by a stimulus is called *excitability*. This is an important part of the transmission of the impulse from one fibre to another. The level of excitability is determined by the length of time after depolarization that the tissues can be reactivated. The recovery period after stimulation is called the *refractory phase* or *refractory period*. The absolute refractory phase or period occurs when excitability is zero and heart tissue cannot be stimulated. The relative refractory period occurs slightly later in the cycle, and excitability is more likely to occur. In states of full excitability, the heart is completely recovered. Figure 38.9 shows the relationship between the refractory period and the ECG.

If conduction is depressed and if some areas of the heart are blocked (e.g., by necrosis), the unblocked areas are activated earlier than the blocked areas. When the block is unidirectional, this uneven conduction may allow the initial impulse to re-enter areas that were previously not excitable but have recovered. The re-entering impulse may be able to depolarize the atria and ventricles, causing a premature beat. If the re-entrant excitation continues, tachycardia occurs (Aehlert, 2018).

Evaluation of Dysrhythmias

Dysrhythmias occur as the result of various abnormalities and disease states (Aehlert, 2018). The cause of a dysrhythmia influences the treatment of the patient. Common causes of dysrhythmias are listed in Table 38.4.

Description	Normal Duration (sec)	Source of Possible Variation
P wave: Represents time for the electrical impulse that causes atrial depolarization (contraction) to pass through the atrium; should be upright	0.06–0.12	Disturbance in conduction within atria
PR interval: Measured from beginning of P wave to beginning of QRS complex; represents time taken for impulse to spread through the atria, the AV node and bundle of His, the bundle branches, and Purkinje fibres to a point immediately before ventricular contraction	0.12–0.20	Disturbance in conduction usually in AV node, bundle of His, or bundle branches but can be in atria as well
QRS interval: Measured from beginning to end of QRS complex; represents time taken for depolarization (contraction) of both ventricles (systole)	0.06–0.10	Disturbance in conduction in bundle branches or in ventricles
ST segment: Measured from the S wave of the QRS complex to the beginning of the T wave; represents the time between ventricular depolarization and repolarization (diastole); should be isoelectric (flat)	N/A	Disturbances usually caused by ischemia, injury, or infarction
T wave: Represents time for ventricular repolarization; should be upright	N/A	Disturbances usually caused by electrolyte imbalances, ischemia, or infarction
QT interval: Measured from beginning of QRS complex to end of T wave; represents time taken for entire electrical depolarization and repolarization of the ventricles	0.34–0.43	Disturbances usually affecting repolarization more than depolarization and caused by medications, electrolyte imbalances, and changes in heart rate

TABLE 38.2   DEFINITION AND SOURCES OF VARIATION IN ECG WAVEFORMS AND INTERVALS*

AV, atrioventricular; *ECG,* electrocardiogram; *N/A,* not applicable.
*Heart rate influences the duration of these intervals, especially those of the PR and QT intervals (e.g., QT interval decreases in duration as heart rate increases).

TABLE 38.3   RATES OF THE CONDUCTION SYSTEM

SA node	60–100 times/min
AV junction	40–60 times/min
Purkinje fibres	20–40 times/min

AV, atrioventricular; *SA,* sinoatrial.

When assessing the cardiac rhythm, the nurse must make an accurate interpretation and immediately evaluate the consequences of the findings for an individual patient. In Table 38.5, a systematic approach to assessing a cardiac rhythm is presented. Assessment of the patient's hemodynamic response to any change in rhythm is essential because this information guides the selection of therapeutic interventions. Determination of the cause of dysrhythmias should be a priority. For example, tachycardias may be the result of fever and may cause a decrease in cardiac output (CO) and hypotension. Certain dysrhythmias may be a result of electrolyte disturbances and may lead to a life-threatening dysrhythmia. At all times, the patient must be assessed and abnormalities treated.

Types of Dysrhythmias
Examples of the ECG tracings of common dysrhythmias are presented in Figures 38.10 through 38.18. Descriptive characteristics of common dysrhythmias are presented in Table 38.6, and emergency care of the patient with a dysrhythmia is outlined in Table 38.7.

Sinus Bradycardia. In sinus bradycardia, the conduction pathway is the same as that in sinus rhythm, but the SA node fires at a rate less than 60 beats/minute (Figure 38.10, *A*). *Symptomatic bradycardia* refers to an HR that is less than 60 beats/minute and causes the patient to have symptoms of inadequate perfusion (e.g., fatigue, dizziness, chest pain, syncope).

Clinical Associations. Sinus bradycardia may be a normal sinus rhythm in aerobically trained athletes and in other individuals during sleep. It also occurs in response to carotid sinus massage, the Valsalva manoeuvre, increased vagal tone, and certain medications (e.g., beta blockers, calcium channel blockers).

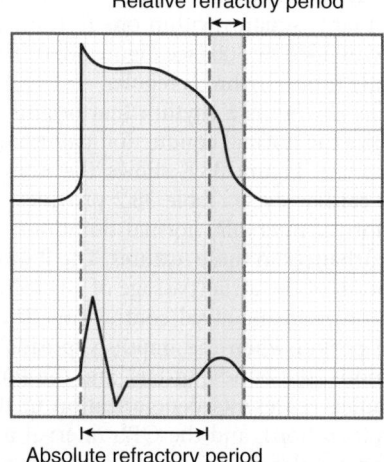

Relative refractory period

Absolute refractory period

FIG. 38.9 Diagram of absolute and relative refractory periods correlated with the cardiac muscle's action potential and with an electrocardiogram tracing. Source: Adapted from Urden, L. D., Stacy, K. M., & Lough, M. E. (2010). *Critical care nursing: Diagnosis and management* (6th ed., p. 368). Mosby.

Disease states associated with sinus bradycardia are hypothyroidism, increased intracranial pressure, and inferior wall myocardial infarction (MI).

Electrocardiographic Characteristics. In sinus bradycardia, the HR is less than 60 beats/minute and the rhythm is regular. The P wave precedes each QRS complex and has a normal shape and duration. The PR interval is normal, and the QRS complex has a normal shape and duration.

Clinical Significance. The clinical significance of sinus bradycardia depends on how the patient tolerates it hemodynamically. Signs of symptomatic bradycardia can include pale, cool skin; hypotension; weakness; angina; dizziness or syncope; confusion or disorientation; and shortness of breath.

Treatment. If bradycardia is due to certain medications, these may have to be reduced or temporarily or permanently stopped. For the patient with symptoms from bradycardia, treatment consists of administration of atropine (an anticholinergic

TABLE 38.4	COMMON CAUSES OF DYSRHYTHMIAS
Cardiac Conditions	**Other Conditions**
• Accessory pathways • Conduction defects • Heart failure • Hypertrophy of cardiac muscle • Myocardial cell degeneration • Myocardial infarction	• Acid–base imbalances • Alcohol • Coffee, tea, tobacco • Connective tissue disorders • Drug effects or toxicity • Electric shock • Electrolyte imbalances • Emotional crisis • Hypoxia, shock • Metabolic conditions (e.g., thyroid dysfunction) • Near-drowning • Poisoning

TABLE 38.5	SYSTEMATIC APPROACH TO ASSESSING CARDIAC RHYTHMS

When assessing a cardiac rhythm, always assess the patient first, and then proceed with a systematic approach to interpreting the rhythm. A recommended approach is as follows:
1. Evaluate the rhythm (ventricular and atrial).
2. Determine the rate (ventricular and atrial).
3. Assess the presence and configuration of P waves.
4. Calculate the duration of the PR interval.
5. Calculate the QRS duration.
6. Calculate the QT interval.
7. Assess for changes in ST segment, T wave, or both.
8. Interpret the rhythm (e.g., atrial fibrillation).
9. Determine the clinical significance of this rhythm. Is the patient stable or unstable?
10. Determine the treatment for the rhythm.

medication). If atropine is ineffective, pacemaker therapy or epinephrine or dopamine infusions may be required (American Heart Association [AHA], 2015).

Sinus Tachycardia. The conduction pathway is the same in sinus tachycardia as that in normal sinus rhythm. The discharge rate from the sinus node is increased as a result of vagal inhibition or sympathetic stimulation. The sinus rate is greater than 100 beats/minute and regular (see Figure 38.10, *B*).

Clinical Associations. Sinus tachycardia is associated with physiological and psychological stressors such as exercise, fever, pain, hypotension, hypovolemia, anemia, hypoxia, hypoglycemia, myocardial ischemia, heart failure (HF), hyperthyroidism, anxiety, and fear. It can also be an effect of medications or drugs such as epinephrine (EpiPen), norepinephrine (Levophed), atropine, caffeine, theophylline, nifedipine, or hydralazine (Apresoline). In addition, many over-the-counter cold remedies have active ingredients (e.g., pseudoephedrine [Sudafed]) that can cause tachycardia.

Electrocardiographic Characteristics. In sinus tachycardia, the HR is greater than 100 beats/minute and the rhythm is regular. The P wave is normal, precedes each QRS complex, and has a normal shape and duration. The PR interval is normal, and the QRS complex has a normal shape and duration.

Clinical Significance. The clinical significance of sinus tachycardia depends on the patient's tolerance of the increased HR. The patient may have symptoms of dizziness, dyspnea, and hypotension. Increased myocardial oxygen consumption is associated with an increased HR. Angina or an increase in

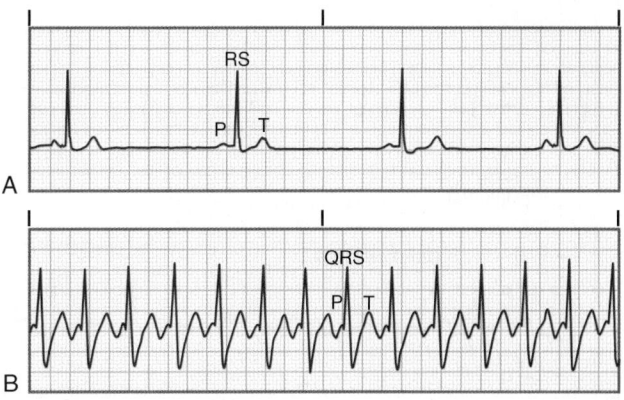

FIG. 38.10 A, Electrocardiogram (ECG) demonstrating sinus bradycardia. **B,** ECG demonstrating sinus tachycardia.

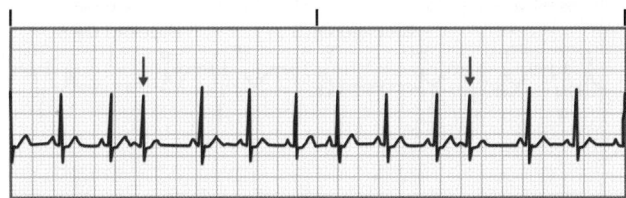

FIG. 38.11 Electrocardiogram demonstrating premature atrial contractions *(arrows)*.

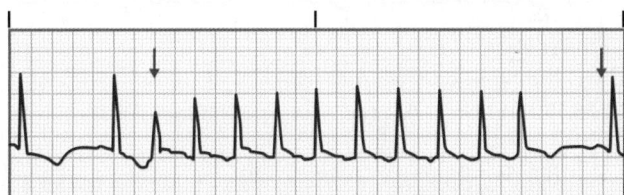

FIG. 38.12 Electrocardiogram demonstrating paroxysmal supraventricular tachycardia (PSVT). *Arrows* indicate beginning and ending of PSVT.

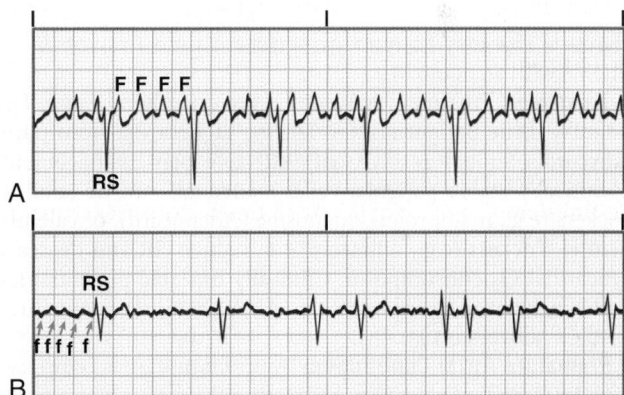

FIG. 38.13 A, Atrial flutter with a 4:1 conduction (four flutter *[F]* waves to each QRS complex). **B,** Atrial fibrillation with a controlled ventricular response. Note the chaotic fibrillatory *(f)* waves *(arrows)* between the RS complexes. NOTE: Recorded from lead V₁.

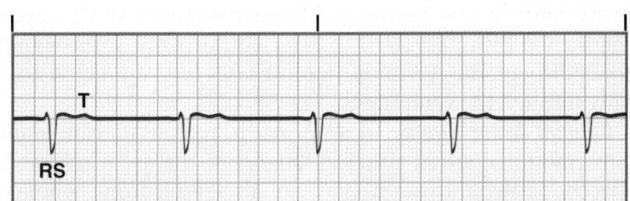

FIG. 38.14 Electrocardiogram demonstrating junctional escape rhythm. The P wave is hidden in the QRS complex. NOTE: Recorded from lead V₁.

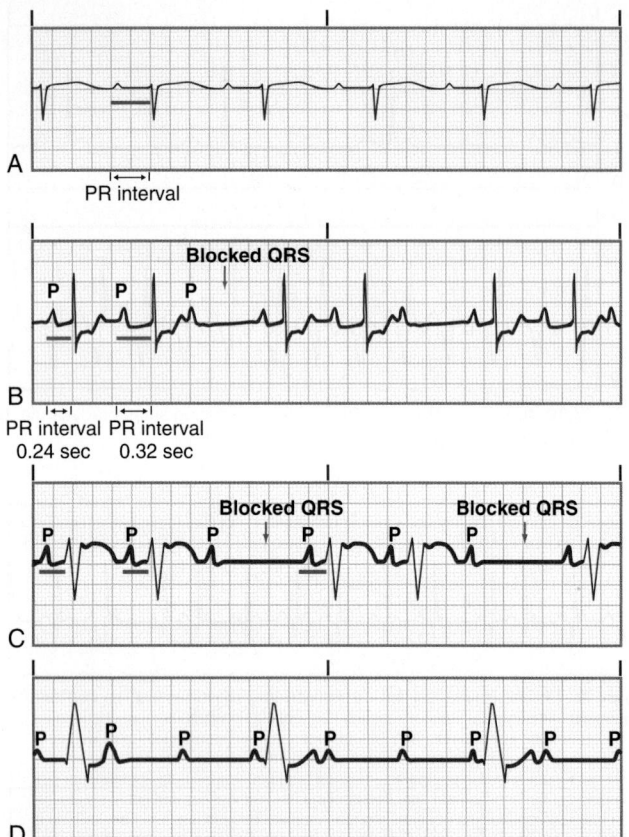

FIG. 38.15 Heart block. **A,** First-degree atrioventricular (AV) block with a PR interval of 0.40 seconds. **B,** Second-degree AV block, type I, with progressive lengthening of the PR interval until a QRS complex is blocked. **C,** Second-degree AV block, type II, with constant PR intervals and variable blocked QRS complexes. **D,** Third-degree AV block. Note that there is no relationship between P waves and QRS complexes.

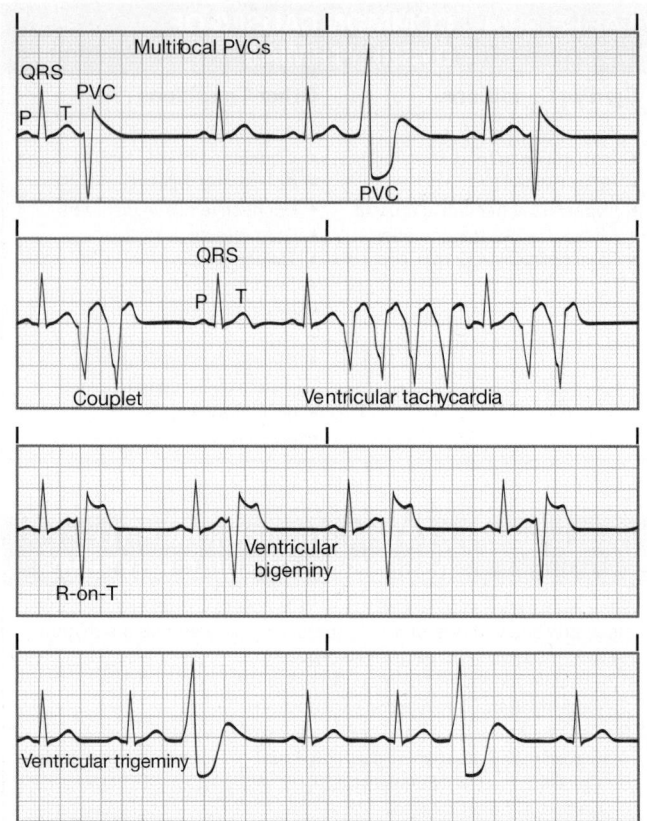

FIG. 38.16 Various forms of premature ventricular contractions (PVCs).

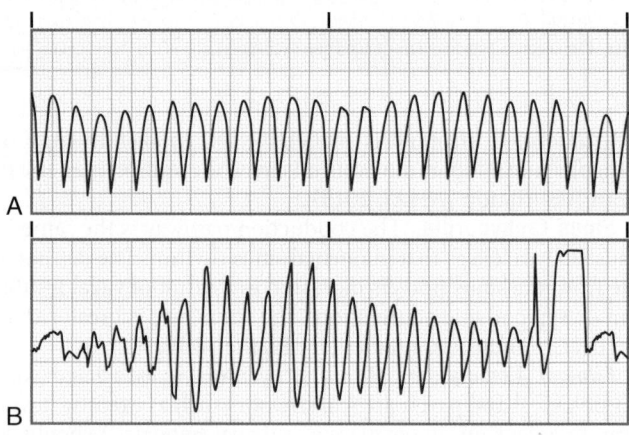

FIG. 38.17 Electrocardiograms demonstrating ventricular tachycardia. **A,** Monomorphic. **B,** Torsades de points (polymorphic).

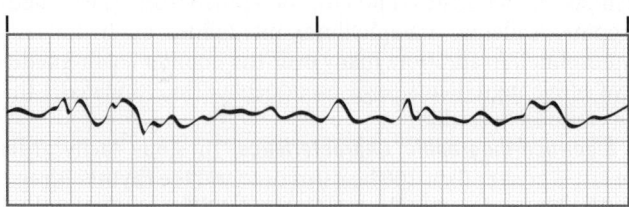

FIG. 38.18 Electrocardiogram demonstrating ventricular fibrillation.

infarction size may accompany persistent sinus tachycardia in patients with an acute MI.

Treatment. Treatment is based on the underlying cause. For instance, if the patient is experiencing tachycardia from pain, tachycardia should resolve with effective pain management. In clinically stable patients, vagal maneuvers can be tried. β Blockers (e.g., metoprolol), adenosine (Adenocard), or calcium channel blockers (e.g., diltiazem) can reduce HR and decrease myocardial O_2 consumption. Clinically unstable patients may need synchronized cardioversion (AHA, 2015). (See Synchronized Cardioversion.)

Premature Atrial Contraction. A **premature atrial contraction (PAC)** is a contraction originating from an ectopic focus in one atrium in an area other than the sinus node before the next expected beat. The ectopic signal originates in the left or the right atrium and travels across both atria by an abnormal pathway, causing the P wave to be distorted (Figure 38.11). At the AV node, it may be stopped (nonconducted PAC), delayed (lengthened PR interval), or conducted normally. If the signal moves through the AV node, in most cases it is conducted normally through the ventricles.

Clinical Associations. In a normal heart, a PAC can result from emotional stress, physical fatigue, or the use of caffeine, tobacco, or alcohol use. A PAC can also result from hypoxia, electrolyte imbalances, and disease states such as hyperthyroidism, chronic obstructive pulmonary disease (COPD), and heart disease, including coronary artery disease (CAD) and valvular disease.

Electrocardiographic Characteristics. HR varies with the underlying rate and frequency of the PAC, and the rhythm is irregular. The P wave may have a different shape from that of

TABLE 38.6 CHARACTERISTICS OF COMMON DYSRHYTHMIAS

Pattern	Rate and Rhythm	P Wave	PR Interval	QRS Complex
Normal sinus rhythm	60–100 beats/min and regular	Normal	Normal	Normal
Sinus bradycardia	<60 beats/min and regular	Normal	Normal	Normal
Sinus tachycardia	>100 beats/min and regular	Normal	Normal	Normal
Premature atrial contraction	Usually 60–100 beats/min and irregular	Abnormal shape	Normal or variable	Normal (usually)
Paroxysmal supraventricular tachycardia	150–250 beats/min and regular	Abnormal shape, may be hidden	Variable	Normal (usually)
Atrial flutter	*Atrial:* 250–350 beats/min and regular *Ventricular:* >100 beats/min and irregular	Sawtooth shape	Variable	Normal (usually)
Atrial fibrillation	*Atrial:* 350–600 beats/min and irregular *Ventricular:* >100 beats/min and irregular or possibly any rate	Chaotic, fibrillatory	Not present	Normal (usually)
Junctional rhythms	40–140 beats/min and regular	Inverted (may be hidden)	Variable	Normal (usually)
First-degree AV heart block	Normal and regular	Normal	>0.20 sec, constant	Normal
Second-degree AV heart block				
Type I (Mobitz I, Wenckebach's)	*Atrial:* Normal and regular *Ventricular:* Slower and irregular	Normal	Progressively lengthened	Normal width, with pattern of one nonconducted QRS complex
Type II (Mobitz II)	*Atrial:* Usually normal and regular or irregular *Ventricular:* Slower and regular or irregular	More P waves than QRS complexes	Normal or prolonged	Widened, preceded by two or more P waves
Third-degree AV heart block	Ventricular rate 20–40 beats/min and regular	Normal, but no connection with QRS complex	None; PR interval not related to QRS complex; more P waves than QRS complexes	Normal or widened; no connection with P waves
Premature ventricular contraction	60–100 beats/min and irregular	None	Not present	Wide and distorted
Ventricular tachycardia	100–250 beats/min and regular or irregular	None	None	Wide and distorted
Ventricular fibrillation	Not measurable and irregular	Absent	Not present	Not measurable

AV, atrioventricular.

✚ TABLE 38.7 EMERGENCY MANAGEMENT

Dysrhythmias

Etiology	Assessment Findings	Interventions
See Table 38.4	• Chest, neck, shoulder, or arm pain • Cold, clammy skin • Decreased blood pressure • Decreased level of consciousness • Decreased O₂ saturation • Diaphoresis • Dizziness, syncope • Dyspnea • Extreme restlessness • Feeling of impending doom • Irregular rate and rhythm, palpitations • Nausea and vomiting • Numbness, tingling of arms • Pallor • Weakness and fatigue	**Initial** • Ensure patent airway • Administer O₂ via nasal cannula • Establish IV access • Apply cardiac monitoring electrodes • Identify underlying rhythm • Identify ectopic beats **Ongoing Monitoring** • Monitor vital signs, level of consciousness, O₂ saturation, and cardiac rhythm • Anticipate need for intubation if respiratory distress is evident • Prepare to initiate CPR or defibrillation, or both

CPR, cardiopulmonary resuscitation; *IV,* intravenous.

the P wave originating from the SA node. It may be notched or have downward (or negative) deflection, or it may be hidden in the preceding T wave. The PR interval may be shorter or longer than the PR interval originating from the SA node, but its length is within normal limits. The QRS complex is usually normal.

Clinical Significance. In people with healthy hearts, isolated PACs are not significant. In people with heart disease, frequent PACs may indicate enhanced automaticity of the atria or a re-entry mechanism. Such PACs may warn of or initiate more serious dysrhythmias (e.g., supraventricular tachycardia).

Treatment. Treatment of PAC depends on the patient's symptoms. Withdrawal of sources of stimulation such as caffeine or sympathomimetic medications may be warranted.

Paroxysmal Supraventricular Tachycardia. *Paroxysmal supraventricular tachycardia* (PSVT) is a dysrhythmia originating in an ectopic focus anywhere above the bifurcation of the bundle of His (Figure 38.12). Identification of the ectopic focus is often difficult even with a 12-lead ECG because the dysrhythmia must be recorded as it is initiated.

PSVT occurs because of a re-entrant phenomenon (re-excitation of the atria when there is a one-way block). Usually, a PAC triggers a run of repeated premature beats. *Paroxysmal* refers to an abrupt onset and termination. The termination is sometimes followed by a brief period of asystole. Some degree of AV block may be present. PSVT can occur in the presence of Wolff–Parkinson–White (WPW) syndrome, or "pre-excitation." In this syndrome, extra conduction pathways or accessory pathways are present.

Clinical Associations. In the normal heart, PSVT is associated with overexertion, emotional stress, deep inspiration, and stimulants such as caffeine and tobacco. PSVT is also associated with rheumatic heart disease, digitalis toxicity, CAD, and cor pulmonale.

Electrocardiographic Characteristics. In PSVT, the HR is 151 to 220 beats/minute, and rhythm is regular or slightly irregular. The P wave is often hidden in the preceding T wave, but if seen, it may have an abnormal shape. The PR interval may be shortened or normal, and the QRS complex is usually normal.

Clinical Significance. The clinical significance of PSVT depends on symptoms and HR. A prolonged episode and rapid HR may precipitate a decrease in CO, resulting in hypotension, dyspnea, and angina.

Treatment. Treatment for PSVT includes vagal stimulation and medication therapy. Common vagal manoeuvres include Valsalva manoeuvres and coughing. Intravenous (IV) adenosine is the medication of first choice to convert PSVT to a normal sinus rhythm. This medication has a short half-life (1.5–10 seconds) and is well tolerated by most patients (DeSimone, 2018). IV β-adrenergic blockers, calcium channel blockers (e.g., diltiazem [Cardizem]), and amiodarone can also be used. For a patient with WPW syndrome, amiodarone should be used. If vagal stimulation and medication therapy are ineffective and the patient becomes hemodynamically unstable, direct-current (DC) cardioversion may be used (Honarbakhsh et al., 2017). (See Synchronized Cardioversion.) If PSVT recurs in patients with WPW syndrome, they may ultimately be treated with radiofrequency ablation of the accessory pathway. (See Radiofrequency Ablation Therapy.)

MEDICATION ALERT—Adenosine (Adenocard)
- The injection site should be as close to the heart as possible (e.g., antecubital area).
- IV dose should be given rapidly (over 1–2 seconds) and followed with a rapid 20-mL normal saline flush.
- The patient's ECG must be monitored continuously. A brief period of asystole can occur.
- The patient should be observed for flushing, dizziness, chest pain, or palpitations.

Atrial Flutter. Atrial flutter is an atrial tachydysrhythmia identified by recurring, regular, sawtooth-shaped flutter (F) waves that originate from a single ectopic focus in the right atrium (Figure 38.13, *A*).

Clinical Associations. Atrial flutter rarely occurs in a normal heart. It is associated with disease states such as CAD, hypertension, mitral valve disorders, pulmonary embolus, chronic lung disease, cor pulmonale, cardiomyopathy, and hyperthyroidism and with the use of medications such as digoxin, quinidine, and epinephrine.

Electrocardiographic Characteristics. In atrial flutter, atrial rate is 250 to 350 beats/minute. The ventricular rate varies according to the conduction ratio. In 2:1 conduction, the ventricular rate is typically found to be approximately 150 beats/minute. Atrial rhythm is regular, and ventricular rhythm is usually regular. The atrial flutter waves represent atrial depolarization followed by repolarization. The PR interval is variable and cannot be measured. The QRS complex is usually normal.

Because of the ability of the AV node to delay signals from the atria, there is usually some AV block in a fixed ratio of flutter waves to QRS complexes (e.g., 2:1, 3:1).

Clinical Significance. The high ventricular rates (>100 beats/minute) and loss of the atrial "kick" (atrial contraction) that are associated with atrial flutter can decrease CO and cause serious consequences such as HF, especially in patients with underlying heart disease. Patients with atrial flutter are at increased risk for stroke because of the risk for thrombus formation in the atria from the stasis of blood. Warfarin (Coumadin) or a non–vitamin K antagonist oral anticoagulant (NOAC) such as rivaroxaban (Xarelto) is used to prevent stroke in patients with atrial flutter of longer than 48 hours' duration (Canadian Cardiovascular Society [CCS], 2018).

Treatment. The primary goal in treatment of atrial flutter is to slow the ventricular response by increasing AV block. Medications used to control ventricular rate include calcium channel blockers and β-adrenergic blockers. Electrical cardioversion may be used to convert the atrial flutter to sinus rhythm in an emergency situation (i.e., the patient is hemodynamically unstable) and electively. Antidysrhythmia medications used to convert atrial flutter to sinus rhythm or to maintain sinus rhythm include procainamide, amiodarone, propafenone (Rythmol), and ibutilide (Corvert) (CCS, 2018).

Radiofrequency ablation is increasingly being used as curative therapy for atrial flutter. With radiofrequency ablation therapy, the tissue with the abnormal atrial automaticity is located and then destroyed. When successful, the abnormal or competitive automaticity is stopped and normal sinus rhythm can be restored (CCS, 2018). (See Radiofrequency Ablation Therapy.)

Atrial Fibrillation. Atrial fibrillation is characterized by a total disorganization of atrial electrical activity caused by multiple ectopic foci, resulting in loss of effective atrial contraction (see Figure 38.13, *B*). Atrial fibrillation is the most common dysrhythmia encountered in the emergency department. The focus of treatment is the rapid assessment of potential hemodynamic instability and identification and treatment of the underlying cause (Parkash, 2018). The dysrhythmia may be chronic or intermittent. The Canadian government estimates that between 350 000 and 700 000 Canadians, or about 1 to 2% of the country's population, are living with atrial fibrillation (Networks of Centres of Excellence in Canada, 2017).

Clinical Associations. Atrial fibrillation usually occurs in patients with underlying heart disease, such as CAD, rheumatic heart disease, cardiomyopathy, hypertension, HF, and pericarditis. It is often acutely caused by factors such as thyrotoxicosis, alcohol intoxication, caffeine use, electrolyte disturbances, stress, and cardiac surgery.

Electrocardiographic Characteristics. During atrial fibrillation, the atrial rate may be as high as 600 beats/minute. The ventricular rate can vary from as low as 50 beats/minute to as high as 180 beats/minute. Atrial fibrillation with ventricular rates greater than 100 are described as atrial fibrillation with a rapid ventricular response. When ventricular rates are less than 100, the condition is described as atrial fibrillation with a slow or controlled ventricular response. P waves are replaced by chaotic, fibrillatory waves in atrial fibrillation. The ventricular rhythm is usually irregular. The PR interval is not measurable, but the QRS complex usually has a normal shape and duration. At times, atrial flutter and atrial fibrillation may coexist.

Clinical Significance. Atrial fibrillation can often result in a decrease in CO because of ineffective atrial contractions or loss of atrial kick, a rapid ventricular response, or both. Thrombi may form in the atria as a result of blood stasis. An embolized clot may develop and travel to the brain, causing a stroke. Overall risk for stroke is increased three to five times with atrial fibrillation (CCS, 2018).

Treatment. The goals of treatment for atrial fibrillation include a decrease in ventricular response (to <100/minute) and prevention of cerebral embolic events (CCS, 2018). Ventricular rate control is a priority for patients with atrial fibrillation. Medications used for rate control include calcium channel blockers (e.g., diltiazem) and β-adrenergic blockers (e.g., metoprolol).

For some patients, conversion of atrial fibrillation to a normal sinus rhythm may be a consideration (e.g., reduced exercise tolerance with rate control medications, contraindications to warfarin). Antidysrhythmia medications used for conversion to and maintenance of sinus rhythm include procainamide, ibutilide (Corvert), amiodarone, and vernakalant (CCS, 2018). In unstable patients with severe left ventricular dysfunction or HF, amiodarone or DC cardioversion should be used (CCS, 2018).

Cardioversion may be used to convert atrial fibrillation to a normal sinus rhythm. If a patient is in atrial fibrillation for longer than 48 hours, anticoagulation therapy with warfarin or an NOAC (Xarelto) for 3 to 4 weeks should be prescribed before the cardioversion (CCS, 2018). Anticoagulation therapy continues for several weeks after the cardioversion because the procedure can cause clots to migrate from the atria, placing the patient at risk for a stroke. A transesophageal echocardiogram (TEE) may be done to rule out clots in the atria.

If medications or cardioversion do not convert atrial fibrillation to normal sinus rhythm, long-term anticoagulation therapy is required. Long-term follow-up with patients experiencing atrial fibrillation or flutter is recommended to assess the need for long-term antithrombotic therapy or antiarrhythmic therapy. (See Chapter 40 for discussion of anticoagulation therapy.)

Other treatment strategies exist for drug-refractory atrial fibrillation and for patients who cannot or choose not to have long-term anticoagulation. These include the use of radiofrequency ablation, which is similar to the procedure for atrial flutter (CCS, 2018; Parkash, 2018).

The role of the nurse in the early identification of atrial fibrillation is key. Nurses are often the first provider to identify the new onset of atrial fibrillation and can report findings and seek early interventions with better outcomes for returning to normal sinus rhythm.

Junctional Dysrhythmias. Junctional dysrhythmias are dysrhythmias that originate in the area of the AV node. The AV node can be seen as a backup pacemaker for the heart when the SA node has failed to fire. The impulse from the AV node usually moves in a retrograde (backward) manner that produces an abnormal P wave occurring just before or after the QRS complex or that is hidden in the QRS complex. The impulse usually moves normally through the ventricles. Junctional premature beats may occur, and they are treated in a manner similar to that for PACs. Other junctional dysrhythmias include junctional escape rhythm (Figure 38.14), accelerated junctional rhythm, and junctional tachycardia. These dysrhythmias are treated according to the patient's tolerance of the rhythm and the patient's clinical condition.

Clinical Associations. Junctional dysrhythmias are often associated with CAD, HF, cardiomyopathy, electrolyte imbalances, inferior MI, and rheumatic heart disease. Certain medications and drugs (e.g., digoxin, amphetamines, caffeine, nicotine) can also cause junctional dysrhythmias (Aehlert, 2018).

Electrocardiographic Characteristics. In junctional escape rhythm, the HR is 40 to 60 beats/minute; in accelerated junctional rhythm, it is 61 to 100 beats/minute; and in junctional tachycardia, it is 101 to 150 beats/minute. Rhythm is regular. The P wave is abnormal in shape and inverted, or it may be hidden in the QRS complex (see Figure 38.14). The PR interval is less than 0.12 seconds when the P wave precedes the QRS complex. The QRS complex is usually normal.

EVIDENCE-INFORMED PRACTICE
Translating Research Into Practice

G. D. (pronouns she/her) is 82 years old and has a new onset of atrial fibrillation and a history of mitral stenosis (high-risk factor). Her physician has ordered the initiation of warfarin (Coumadin). The nurse begins to teach her about the purpose and adverse effects of warfarin. G. D. stops the nurse and states that she will not take the medicine—she has heard too many stories about people bleeding from this medication. Furthermore, she says that she does not want to deal with the blood tests that are needed nor worry about what she eats. She states that she will continue to take her aspirin once a day as usual.

Best Available Evidence	Clinician Expertise	Patient Preferences and Values
Warfarin (Coumadin) is the medication of choice to treat patients with atrial fibrillation who have one or more high-risk factors, in order to prevent stroke. For patients for whom oral anticoagulation with warfarin is considered unsuitable (e.g., patient preference), the addition of clopidogrel (Plavix) to ASA (Aspirin) reduces the risk for major vascular events (especially stroke) but increases the risk for major hemorrhage.	Bleeding is a potential and serious adverse effect of warfarin and of dual antiplatelet therapy (ASA; Aspirin and clopidogrel). When taking warfarin, INR blood levels need to be checked on a regular basis. Patients should avoid drastic changes in diet, especially foods high in vitamin K (they interfere with the action of warfarin).	G. D. does not want to take warfarin or clopidogrel because she is afraid of bleeding. In addition, she does not want to change her lifestyle to accommodate the changes that would be needed to use warfarin.

Decision and Action

The nurse explains the risks of not taking the prescribed medicine (warfarin) or adequate medication (adding clopidogrel to her ASA [Aspirin] therapy). G. D. tells the nurse that she understands completely. The nurse supports her choice and informs the physician of G. D.'s decision.

References for Evidence

Canadian Cardiovascular Society (CCS). (2018). 2018 Focused update of the Canadian Cardiovascular Society guidelines for the management of atrial fibrillation. *Canadian Journal of Cardiology, 34,* 1371–1392. https://doi.org/10.1016/j.cjca.2018.08.026; and Zeballos-Palacios, C. L., Hargraves, I. G., Noseworthy, P. A., et al. (2019). Developing a conversation aid to support shared decision making: Reflections on designing anticoagulation choice. *Mayo Clinic Proceedings, 94*(4). https://doi.org/10.1016/j.mayocp.2018.08.030

ASA, acetylsalicylic acid; *INR,* international normalized ratio.

Clinical Significance. Junctional escape rhythms serve as a safety mechanism for when the SA node has not been effective in firing. Escape rhythms such as this should not be suppressed. Accelerated junctional rhythm and junctional tachycardia, however, indicate a more serious problem with the SA node. These rhythms may result in a reduction of CO, causing the patient to become hemodynamically unstable (e.g., hypotensive).

Treatment. Treatment varies according to the type of junctional dysrhythmia. If a patient has symptoms with an escape junctional rhythm, atropine can be administered. In accelerated junctional rhythm and junctional tachycardia caused by digoxin toxicity, the digoxin is withheld. In the absence of digoxin toxicity, β-adrenergic blockers, calcium channel blockers, and amiodarone can be used for rate control.

First-Degree Atrioventricular Block. *First-degree atrioventricular (AV) block* is a type of AV block in which every impulse is conducted to the ventricles but the duration of AV conduction is prolonged (Figure 38.15, *A*). After the impulse moves through the AV node, it is usually conducted normally through the ventricles.

Clinical Associations. First-degree AV block is associated with MI, CAD, rheumatic fever, hyperthyroidism, vagal stimulation, and medications such as digoxin, β-adrenergic blockers, calcium channel blockers, and flecainide.

Electrocardiographic Characteristics. In first-degree AV block, the HR is normal and the rhythm is regular. The P wave is normal, the PR interval is prolonged to more than 0.20 seconds, and the QRS complex usually has a normal shape and duration.

Clinical Significance. First-degree AV block is usually not serious but can be a precursor of higher degrees of AV block. Patients with first-degree AV block are often asymptomatic (Aelhert, 2018).

Treatment. There is no treatment for first-degree AV block. Modifications to causative medications may be considered. Patients should continue to be monitored for any new changes in heart rhythm.

Second-Degree Atrioventricular Block, Type I. *Type I second-degree AV block (Mobitz I or Wenckebach's heart block)* includes a gradual lengthening of the PR interval. It occurs because of a prolonged AV conduction time until an atrial impulse is not conducted and a QRS complex is blocked (missing) (see Figure 38.15, *B*). Type I AV block most commonly occurs in the AV node, but it can also occur in the His–Purkinje system.

Clinical Associations. Type I AV block may result from the use of medications such as digoxin or β-adrenergic blockers. It may also be associated with CAD and other diseases that can slow AV conduction.

Electrocardiographic Characteristics. The atrial rate is normal, but the ventricular rate may be slower as a result of non-conducted atrial impulses or blocked QRS complexes. Once a ventricular beat is blocked, the cycle repeats itself with progressive lengthening of the PR intervals until another QRS complex is blocked. The rhythm appears on the ECG in a pattern of grouped beats. Ventricular rhythm is irregular. The P wave has a normal shape. The QRS complex has a normal shape and duration.

Clinical Significance. Type I AV block is usually a result of myocardial ischemia or infarction. It is usually transient and well tolerated. However, in some patients (e.g., after an MI), it may be a warning signal of a more serious AV conduction disturbance.

Treatment. If the patient is symptomatic, atropine may be used to increase the HR, or a temporary pacemaker may be needed, especially if the patient has experienced an MI. If the patient has no symptoms, the rhythm should be closely observed with a transcutaneous pacemaker on standby. Bradycardia is more likely to become symptomatic when one or more of the following are present: (a) hypotension, (b) HF, or (c) shock.

Second-Degree Atrioventricular Block, Type II. In *type II second-degree AV block (Mobitz II heart block),* a P wave is not conducted without progressive antecedent PR lengthening. This almost always occurs when a block in one of the bundle branches is present (see Figure 38.15, *C*). On conducted beats, the PR interval is constant. Type II second-degree AV block is a more serious type of block, in which a certain number of impulses from the SA node are not conducted to the ventricles. This occurs in ratios of 2:1, 3:1, and so on (i.e., two P waves to one QRS complex, three P waves to one QRS complex). It may occur with varying ratios. Type II AV block almost always originates in the His–Purkinje system.

Clinical Associations. Type II AV block is associated with rheumatic heart disease, CAD, anterior MI, and digitalis toxicity.

Electrocardiographic Characteristics. The atrial rate is usually normal. The ventricular rate depends on the intrinsic rate and the degree of AV block. The atrial rhythm is regular, but the ventricular rhythm may be irregular. The P wave has a normal shape. The PR interval may be normal or prolonged in duration and remains constant on conducted beats. The QRS complex is usually more than 0.12 seconds because of bundle-branch block.

Clinical Significance. Type II AV block often progresses to third-degree AV block and is associated with a poor prognosis. The reduced HR often results in decreased CO with subsequent hypotension and myocardial ischemia. Type II AV block is an indication for therapy with a permanent pacemaker.

Treatment. Temporary treatment before the insertion of a permanent pacemaker (see Pacemakers) may be necessary if the condition becomes symptomatic (e.g., hypotension, angina). Such treatment involves the use of a temporary transvenous or transcutaneous pacemaker (Aehlert, 2018).

Third-Degree Atrioventricular Block. Third-degree AV block, or complete heart block, constitutes one form of AV dissociation in which no impulses from the atria are conducted to the ventricles (see Figure 38.15, *D*). The atria are stimulated and contract independently of the ventricles. The ventricular rhythm is an escape rhythm, and the ectopic pacemaker may be above or below the bifurcation of the bundle of His.

Clinical Associations. Third-degree AV block is associated with severe heart disease, including CAD, MI, myocarditis, cardiomyopathy, and some systemic diseases such as amyloidosis and progressive systemic sclerosis (scleroderma). Some medications can also cause third-degree AV block, such as digoxin, β-adrenergic blockers, and calcium channel blockers.

Electrocardiographic Characteristics. The atrial rate with third-degree AV block is usually a sinus rate of 60 to 100 beats/minute. The ventricular rate depends on the site of the block. If it is in the AV node, the rate is 40 to 60 beats/minute, and if it is in the His–Purkinje system, it is 20 to 40 beats/minute. Atrial and ventricular rhythms are regular but unrelated to each other. The P wave has a normal shape. The PR interval is variable, and there is no time relationship between the P wave and the QRS complex. The QRS complex is normal if an escape rhythm is initiated at the bundle of His or above. It is widened if an escape rhythm is initiated below the bundle of His.

Clinical Significance. Third-degree AV block almost always results in reduced CO with subsequent ischemia, HF, and shock. Syncope from third-degree AV block may result from severe bradycardia or even periods of asystole.

Treatment. When patients are unstable in the presence of a bradycardia, a transcutaneous pacemaker is typically used as first-line treatment (AHA, 2018). The use of medications such as atropine, epinephrine, isoproterenol, and dopamine is a temporary measure to increase the HR and support blood pressure (BP) until temporary pacing is initiated. Patients need a permanent pacemaker implanted as soon as possible.

Premature Ventricular Contractions. A premature ventricular contraction (PVC) is a contraction originating in an ectopic focus in the ventricles. It is the premature occurrence of a QRS complex, which is wide and whose shape is distorted in comparison with a QRS complex initiated from the normal conduction pathway (Figure 38.16). PVCs that are initiated from different foci appear different in shape from each other and are called *multifocal* PVCs. PVCs that appear to have the same shape are called *unifocal* PVCs. When every other beat is a PVC, it is called *ventricular bigeminy*. When every third beat is a PVC, it is called *ventricular trigeminy*. Two consecutive PVCs are called a *couplet*. When three or more consecutive PVCs occur, it is called *ventricular tachycardia*. A PVC that falls on the T wave of a preceding beat is called the *R-on-T phenomenon*. This phenomenon is considered especially dangerous because the PVC is occurring during the relative refractory phase of ventricular repolarization. Excitability of the cardiac cells is increased during this time, and the risk for the PVC to initiate ventricular tachycardia or ventricular fibrillation is high.

Clinical Associations. PVCs are associated with stimulants such as caffeine, alcohol, nicotine, aminophylline, epinephrine, isoproterenol, and digoxin. They are also associated with electrolyte imbalances, hypoxia, fever, exercise, and emotional stress. Disease states associated with PVCs include MI, mitral valve prolapse, HF, and CAD.

Electrocardiographic Characteristics. HR varies according to intrinsic rate and number of PVCs. The rhythm is irregular because of premature beats. The P wave is absent in a PVC. The QRS complex is wide and distorted in shape, lasting more than 0.12 seconds. The T wave is generally large and opposite in direction to the major direction of the QRS complex.

Clinical Significance. PVCs are usually a benign finding in the patient with a normal heart. In heart disease, depending on frequency, PVCs may reduce the CO and precipitate angina and HF if they are frequently occurring (>10/minute). Because PVCs in CAD or acute MI represent ventricular irritability, the patient's physiological response to PVCs must be monitored. The nurse must take the patient's apical-radial pulse rate and determine the pulse deficit, since PVCs often do not generate a sufficient ventricular contraction to result in a peripheral pulse.

Treatment. Treatment is often based on the cause of the PVCs (e.g., oxygen therapy for hypoxia, electrolyte replacement); however, infrequent PVCs are not typically treated. Assessment of the patient's hemodynamic status is important to guide treatment. Most importantly, the patient must be assessed for signs of decreased CO and whether the PVCs are causing the patient to be symptomatic (e.g., chest pain, dizziness) to determine whether treatment is indicated. If medication therapy is warranted, medications such as β blockers, lidocaine, or amiodarone would be considered.

Ventricular Tachycardia. The diagnosis of ventricular tachycardia (VT) is made when a run of three or more PVCs occurs. It occurs when an ectopic focus or foci fire repetitively and the ventricle takes control as the pacemaker. VT appears in different forms, depending on the QRS configuration. Monomorphic VT (Figure 38.17, *A*) has QRS complexes that are the same in shape, size, and direction. In polymorphic VT, the QRS complexes gradually change back and forth from one shape, size, and direction to another over a series of beats. *Torsades de pointes* (French, "twisting of the points") is polymorphic VT associated with a prolonged QT interval of the underlying rhythm (see Figure 38.17, *B*).

VT may be sustained or nonsustained. Sustained VT lasts for more than 30 seconds. Nonsustained VT lasts for 30 seconds or less. The development of VT is an ominous sign. It is considered a life-threatening dysrhythmia because of decreased CO and the possibility of deterioration to ventricular fibrillation, which is a lethal dysrhythmia.

Clinical Associations. VT is associated with MI, CAD, significant electrolyte imbalances, cardiomyopathy, mitral valve prolapse, long QT syndrome, digitalis toxicity, and central nervous system disorders. This dysrhythmia has also been observed in patients who have no evidence of cardiac disease.

Electrocardiographic Characteristics. The ventricular rate in VT is 150 to 250 beats/minute. The rhythm is regular. The QRS complex is distorted in appearance, with a duration exceeding 0.12 seconds and with the ST–T wave in the opposite direction to that of the QRS complex (see Figure 38.17). The R–R interval may be irregular or regular. The P wave is usually buried in the QRS complex.

Clinical Significance. VT can be stable (patient has a pulse) or unstable (patient is pulseless). Sustained VT causes a severe decrease in CO as a result of decreased ventricular diastolic filling times and loss of atrial contraction. Results include hypotension, pulmonary edema, decreased cerebral blood flow, and cardiopulmonary arrest. The dysrhythmia must be treated quickly, even if it occurs only briefly and stops abruptly, because episodes may recur if prophylactic treatment is not begun. Ventricular fibrillation may also develop.

Treatment. Precipitating causes of VT must be identified and treated (e.g., electrolyte imbalances, ischemia). If the VT is monomorphic and the patient is hemodynamically stable (e.g., pulse is present) and has preserved left ventricular function, IV amiodarone or lidocaine is typically used. If the patient becomes hemodynamically unstable or has poor left ventricular function, IV amiodarone is given, followed by cardioversion if the original medication therapy alone is ineffective.

If the VT is polymorphic with a normal baseline QT interval, any one of the following medications is used: β-adrenergic blockers, amiodarone, or sotalol. Cardioversion is performed if medication therapy is ineffective (AHA, 2020).

If the VT is polymorphic with a prolonged baseline QT interval, therapies include IV magnesium and antitachycardia pacing (discussed later in this chapter). Medications that prolong the QT interval should be discontinued. If the rhythm is not converted, cardioversion may be needed.

VT without a pulse is a life-threatening situation and is treated in the same manner as ventricular fibrillation—cardiopulmonary resuscitation (CPR) and rapid defibrillation are the first lines of treatment, followed by the administration of epinephrine if defibrillation is unsuccessful (AHA, 2020).

An *accelerated idioventricular rhythm* (AIVR) can develop when the intrinsic pacemaker rate (SA node or AV node) becomes lower than that of a ventricular ectopic pacemaker; the rate is between 40 and 100 beats/minute. It is most commonly associated with acute MI and reperfusion of the myocardium after fibrinolytic therapy or angioplasty of coronary arteries. It can also occur with digitalis toxicity. In the setting of acute MI, AIVR is usually self-limiting and well tolerated and requires no treatment. If it becomes symptomatic (e.g., hypotension, angina), atropine can be considered. Temporary pacing may be required. Medications that suppress ventricular rhythms (e.g., lidocaine) should not be used because they can terminate the ventricular rhythm and further reduce the HR.

Ventricular Fibrillation. Ventricular fibrillation is a severe derangement of the heart rhythm, characterized by irregular undulations of varying shapes and amplitude on the ECG (Figure 38.18). This presentation represents the firing of multiple ectopic foci in the ventricle. Mechanically, the ventricle is simply "quivering," and no effective contraction—and consequently no CO—occurs.

Clinical Associations. Ventricular fibrillation occurs in acute MI and myocardial ischemia and in chronic diseases such as CAD and cardiomyopathy. It may occur during cardiac pacing or cardiac catheterization procedures as a result of catheter stimulation of the ventricle. It may also occur with coronary reperfusion after fibrinolytic therapy. Other clinical associations are accidental electric shock, hyperkalemia, hypoxemia, acidosis, and drug toxicity.

Electrocardiographic Characteristics. In ventricular fibrillation, the HR is not measurable. The rhythm is irregular and chaotic. The P wave is not detectable, and the PR and the QRS intervals are not measurable.

Clinical Significance. Ventricular fibrillation results in an unresponsive, pulseless, and apneic state. If it is not rapidly treated, the patient will die.

Treatment. Treatment consists of assessment of circulation, airway, and breathing (CAB), and if no pulse is found, high-quality CPR and advanced cardiac life support (ACLS) measures are initiated immediately with the use of defibrillation and definitive medication therapy such as epinephrine, amiodarone, and lidocaine. If a defibrillator is immediately available, it must be used without delay (AHA, 2020).

Asystole. Asystole represents the total absence of ventricular electrical activity. On occasion, P waves are detected. No ventricular contraction occurs because depolarization does not occur. Patients are unresponsive, pulseless, and apneic. This is a lethal dysrhythmia that necessitates immediate treatment. Ventricular fibrillation may masquerade as asystole; thus the rhythm should be assessed in more than one lead. The prognosis of a patient with asystole is extremely poor.

Clinical Associations. Asystole is usually a result of advanced cardiac disease, a severe cardiac conduction system disturbance, or end-stage HF.

Clinical Significance. In general, patients with asystole have end-stage cardiac disease or have a prolonged cardiac arrest and cannot be resuscitated.

Treatment. Treatment consists of high-quality CPR (see Chapter 71) with initiation of ACLS measures, which include IV/intraosseous (IO) access, early administration of epinephrine 1 mg every 3 to 5 minutes, consideration of advanced airway, and capnography. While CPR is in progress, the health care team should look for reversible causes: hypovolemia, hypoxia, hydrogen ion (acidosis), hypo- or hyperkalemia, hypothermia, tension pneumothorax, tamponades, or pulmonary thrombosis (AHA, 2020).

Pulseless Electrical Activity. Pulseless electrical activity (PEA) is a situation in which electrical activity can be observed on the ECG but there is no mechanical activity of the ventricles and the patient has no pulse. The prognosis is poor unless the underlying cause can be identified and quickly corrected. The most frequent causes of PEA include hypovolemia, hypoxia, metabolic acidosis, hyperkalemia or hypokalemia, hypothermia, drug overdose, cardiac tamponade, MI, tension pneumothorax, and pulmonary embolus. Treatment begins with assessment of CAB and if no pulse is detected, high-quality CPR is initiated and followed by IV/IO access, epinephrine 1 mg every 3 to 5 minutes, consideration of advanced airway, and capnography. Treatment is aimed at potential treatable causes (AHA, 2020).

Sudden Cardiac Death. The term *sudden cardiac death (SCD)* refers to death from a cardiac cause. The majority of SCDs result from ventricular dysrhythmias, specifically VT or ventricular fibrillation. (SCD is discussed further in Chapter 36.)

Antidysrhythmia Medications

An increasing number of antidysrhythmia medications have become available. Table 38.8 categorizes major medication classes by primary effects on the cardiac cells.

Defibrillation

Defibrillation is the most effective method of terminating ventricular fibrillation and pulseless VT. It is most effective when the myocardial cells are not anoxic or acidotic, making rapid defibrillation crucial for a successful patient outcome. Defibrillation is accomplished by the passage of a DC electric shock through the heart that is sufficient to depolarize the cells of the myocardium. The intent is that subsequent repolarization of myocardial cells allows the SA node to resume the role of pacemaker (AHA, 2020).

Research has shown that biphasic defibrillators are preferred over monophasic defibrillators and deliver successful shocks at lower energies and with fewer post-shock ECG abnormalities than monophasic defibrillators (Figure 38.19) (AHA, 2020).

The output of a defibrillator is measured in joules (J), or watts per second. The recommended energy for initial shocks in defibrillation depends on the type of defibrillator. Biphasic defibrillators deliver all shocks of 150 to 200 J. After the initial shock, CPR should be started immediately, beginning with chest compressions.

Rapid defibrillation can be performed with a manual or automatic device (Figure 38.20). Manual defibrillators require health care providers to interpret cardiac rhythms, determine the need for a shock, and deliver a shock. Automatic external defibrillators (AEDs) are defibrillators that have rhythm detection capability and the ability to advise the operator to deliver a shock with hands-free defibrillator pads. Proficiency in use

TABLE 38.8 MEDICATION THERAPY

Antidysrhythmia Medications: Classifications, Actions, and Effects on ECG

Classification	Actions	Effects on ECG
Class I: Sodium channel blockers	Decrease conduction velocity in the atria, ventricles, and His–Purkinje system	—
Class IA • Procainamide (Procan) • Quinidine	Delay repolarization	Widened QRS and prolonged QT interval
Class IB • Lidocaine (Xylocaine) • Mexiletine • Phenytoin (Dilantin)	Accelerate repolarization	Little or none
Class IC • Flecainide (Tambocor) • Propafenone (Rythmol)	Decrease impulse conduction	Pronounced pro-dysrhythmic actions, widened QRS, prolonged QT interval
Class II: β-Adrenergic blockers • Atenolol (Tenormin) • Carvedilol • Esmolol (Brevibloc) • Metoprolol (Lopressor) • Sotalol*	Decrease automaticity of the SA node; decrease conduction velocity in AV node; reduce atrial and ventricular contractility	Bradycardia, prolonged PR interval, AV block
Class III: Potassium channel blockers • Amiodarone • Ibutilide (Corvert) • Sotalol* • Vernakalant†	Delay repolarization, which results in prolonged duration of action potential and prolonged refractory period	Prolonged PR and QT intervals, widened QRS, bradycardia
Class IV: Calcium channel blockers • Diltiazem (Cardizem) • Verapamil	Decrease automaticity of SA node; delay AV node conduction; reduce myocardial contractility	Bradycardia, prolonged PR interval, AV block
Other antidysrhythmia medications • Adenosine (Adenocard) • Digoxin • Magnesium	Decrease conduction through AV node; reduce automaticity of SA node	Prolonged PR interval, AV block

AV, atrioventricular; *ECG,* electrocardiogram; *SA,* sinoatrial.
*Sotalol has both class II and class III properties.
†Vernakalant is used mostly for fast heart rates; therefore, it is best used for converting atrial fibrillation/flutter.

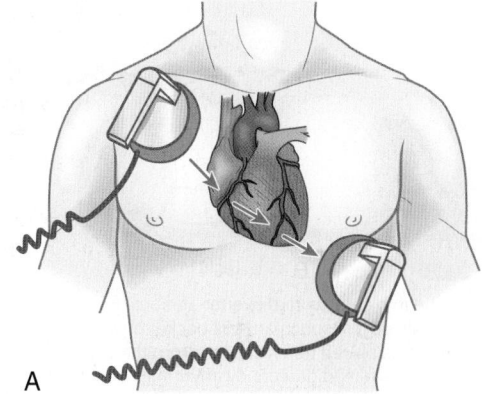

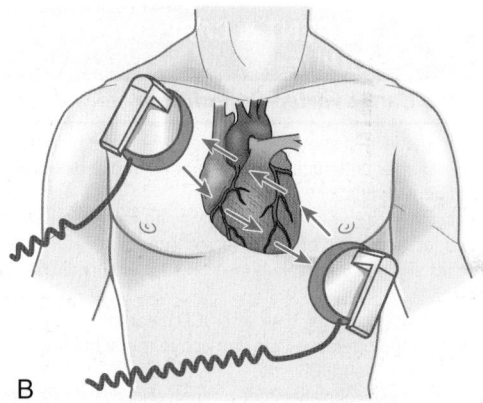

FIG. 38.19 Paddle placement and current flow in monophasic defibrillation **(A)** and biphasic defibrillation **(B).**

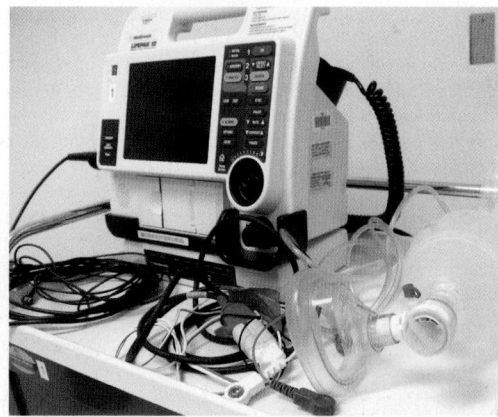

FIG. 38.20 The LifePak device contains a monitor, a defibrillator, and a transcutaneous pacemaker. Source: Science History Images/Alamy Stock Photo.

of the AED is incorporated in many basic life support (CPR) courses for health care workers (AHA, 2000). The nurse should be familiar with the operation of the type of defibrillator that is used in the clinical setting and must be certified to use this equipment. Many communities have implemented a public access defibrillation (PAD) program in locations such as arenas and pools, in order to enhance the provision of early advanced cardiac care to save lives (Heart and Stroke Foundation, 2012).

Synchronized Cardioversion. *Synchronized cardioversion* is the therapy of choice for patients with hemodynamically unstable ventricular or supraventricular tachydysrhythmias. A synchronized circuit in the defibrillator is used to deliver a countershock that is programmed to occur on the R wave of the QRS complex.

The procedure for synchronized cardioversion is the same as for defibrillation, with the following exceptions. If synchronized cardioversion is performed, the operator must ensure

the "synchronize" option is selected. On a nonemergency basis (i.e., the patient is awake and hemodynamically stable), the patient is sedated before the procedure. Strict attention to maintenance of a patent airway is important in this situation. When a patient with supraventricular tachycardia or VT with a pulse is hemodynamically unstable, synchronized cardioversion is performed as quickly as possible. In addition, the energy needed for synchronized cardioversion is generally less than the energy needed for defibrillation. Energy levels are started at 50 J on a defibrillator and increased (e.g., 100 J, 200 J) if needed.

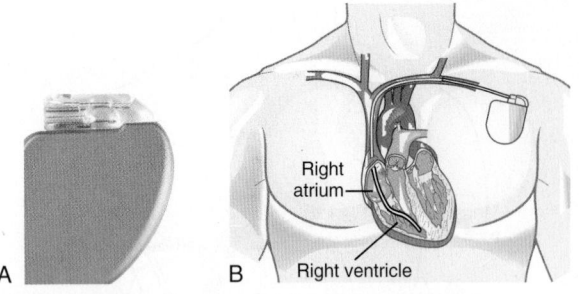

FIG. 38.21 **A,** The implantable cardioverter–defibrillator (ICD) pulse generator. **B,** The ICD is placed in a subcutaneous pocket over the pectoral muscle. A single-lead system is placed transvenously from the pulse generator to the endocardium. The single lead detects dysrhythmias and delivers an electric shock to the heart muscle. Source: A, © Can Stock Photo/CarolinaSmith.

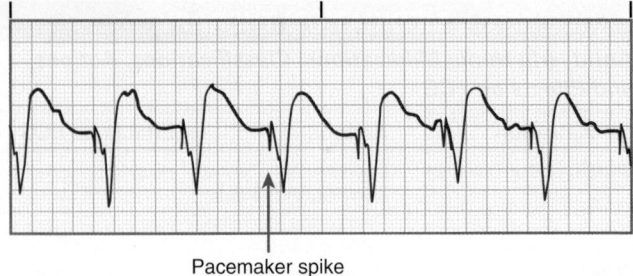

FIG. 38.22 Electrocardiogram demonstrating ventricular capture (depolarization) secondary to signal (pacemaker spike) from pacemaker lead in the right ventricle.

TABLE 38.9	**PATIENT & CAREGIVER TEACHING GUIDE**

Implantable Cardioverter–Defibrillator

The following guidelines should be included when teaching the patient and caregiver after undergoing insertion of an implantable cardioverter–defibrillator (ICD):

1. Maintain close follow-up with the physician for testing of ICD function and for inspection of ICD insertion site.
2. Watch for signs of infection at incision site (e.g., redness, swelling, drainage).
3. Keep the incision dry for 1 wk after ICD insertion.
4. Avoid lifting the operative-side arm above the shoulder for 1 wk.
5. Avoid direct blows to ICD site.
6. When travelling by airplane, inform airport security of the presence of the ICD because it may set off the metal detector. If a handheld screening wand is used, it should not be placed directly over the ICD.
7. When the ICD fires:
   • Lie down.
   • If you lose consciousness or if there is repetitive firing, someone should call 911.
   • If you are feeling well and there is repetitive firing, contact your physician's office for ICD interrogation, including battery checks and safety and diagnostic checks.
8. Ensure routine ICD check with an interrogator–programmer device, which is needed every 2 to 3 months.
9. Wear a medical alert bracelet at all times.
10. Make sure an information card about the ICD is easily accessible in your wallet.
11. Ensure that your family members learn CPR.
12. Speak with your nurse, who can assist you with developing positive coping strategies to reduce stress.
13. Avoid large electromagnetic and vibratory forces because they may turn off the device.
14. In general, do not drive until cleared by your physician. The approval to drive is based on the presence of dysrhythmias, the frequency of ICD firings, your overall health, and provincial or territorial laws regarding drivers with ICDs.

CPR, cardiopulmonary resuscitation.

Implantable Cardioverter–Defibrillator. The implantable cardioverter–defibrillator (ICD) is important technology for patients who (a) have survived SCD, (b) have spontaneous sustained VT, (c) demonstrate syncope with inducible VT or fibrillation during electrophysiology study (EPS), and (d) are at high risk for future life-threatening dysrhythmias (e.g., have cardiomyopathy). Use of the ICD has significantly decreased cardiac mortality rates among such patients and has added a new dimension to the management of life-threatening dysrhythmias and the prevention of SCD (Bun et al., 2019).

The ICD consists of a lead system placed via a subclavian vein to the endocardium. A battery-powered pulse generator is implanted subcutaneously, usually over the pectoral muscle on the patient's nondominant side. The pulse generator is similar in size to a cardiac pacemaker. The newest systems are single-lead systems instead of earlier multi-lead or patch systems (Figure 38.21). The ICD sensing system monitors the heart rate and rhythm and identifies VT or ventricular fibrillation. Approximately 25 seconds after the sensing system detects a lethal dysrhythmia, the defibrillating mechanism delivers a 25-J or milder shock to the patient's heart. If the first shock is unsuccessful, the generator recycles and can continue to deliver shocks.

In addition to defibrillation capabilities, ICDs are equipped with antitachycardia and antibradycardia pacemakers. These sophisticated devices use dysrhythmia algorithms that detect dysrhythmias and determine the appropriate programmed response. These devices can initiate overdrive pacing of supraventricular and ventricular tachycardias, sparing the patient painful defibrillator shocks. They also provide backup pacing for bradydysrhythmias that may occur after defibrillation discharges. Pre-procedure and post-procedure nursing care of patients undergoing ICD placement is similar to the care of patients undergoing permanent pacemaker implantation.

Education of patients who receive an ICD is of extreme importance. Patients experience a variety of emotions, including fear of body image change, fear of recurrent dysrhythmias, expectation of pain with ICD discharge (described as a feeling of a blow to the chest), and anxiety about going home. Table 38.9 describes the teaching guidelines for the patient with an ICD and the patient's caregivers. Participation in an ICD support group should be encouraged. Online resources for patients with an ICD include support groups and the Sudden Cardiac Arrest Network (see the Resources at the end of Chapter 36.)

Pacemakers

The artificial **cardiac pacemaker** is an electronic device used to pace the heart when the normal conduction pathway is damaged or diseased. The basic pacing circuit consists of a power source (battery-powered pulse generator), one or more conducting leads (pacing leads), and the myocardium. The electrical signal (stimulus) travels from the pacemaker, through the leads, to the wall of the myocardium. The myocardium is "captured" and stimulated to contract (Figure 38.22).

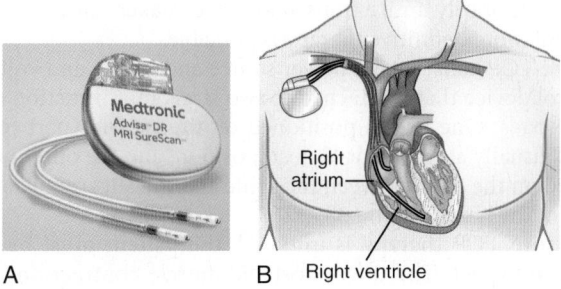

FIG. 38.23 A, A dual-chamber rate-responsive pacemaker from Medtronic, Inc., is designed to treat patients with chronic heart conditions in which the heart beats too slowly to adequately support the body's circulation needs. **B,** Pacing leads in both the atrium and the ventricle enable a dual-chamber pacemaker to sense and pace in both heart chambers. Source: *A,* © 2017 Medtronic. Reproduced with permission of Medtronic.

TABLE 38.10	INDICATIONS FOR PERMANENT PACEMAKER THERAPY

- Chronic atrial fibrillation with slow ventricular response
- Fibrosis or sclerotic changes of cardiac conduction system
- Hypersensitive carotid sinus syndrome
- Sick sinus syndrome
- Sinus node dysfunction
- Tachydysrhythmias
- Third-degree AV block

Current pacemakers are small, sophisticated, and physiologically precise. They pace the atrium and/or one or both ventricles. Most pacemakers are demand pacemakers; this means that they sense the heart's electrical activity and fire only when the HR drops below a preset range. Demand pacemakers have two distinct features: (1) a sensing device that inhibits the pacemaker when the HR is adequate and (2) a pacing device that triggers the pacemaker when no QRS complexes occur within a preset time (Aehlert, 2018). Pacemakers were initially indicated for symptomatic bradydysrhythmias; however, advances now include pacing for antitachycardia and overdrive pacing. Antitachycardia pacing involves the delivery of a stimulus to the ventricle to terminate tachydysrhythmias (e.g., VT). Overdrive pacing involves pacing the atrium at rates of 200 to 500 impulses/minute in an attempt to terminate atrial tachycardias (e.g., atrial flutter, atrial fibrillation).

A *permanent pacemaker* is one that is implanted totally within the body (Figure 38.23). The permanent pacemaker power source is implanted subcutaneously, usually over the pectoral muscle on the patient's nondominant side. It is attached to pacing leads, which are threaded transvenously to the right atrium and one or both ventricles. Indications for insertion of a permanent pacemaker are listed in Table 38.10.

New technology and research are focused on miniaturized, leadless permanent pacemakers and ICDs. Single-component devices have the battery, sensors, electronics, and stimulating electrodes inside a small capsule, about the size of a medication capsule that is placed in the ventricle. A multicomponent device has a small "seed" that is placed in a cardiac chamber. It acts as an energy transducer while an outside piece beams ultrasound (or radio waves) to the seed. The seed converts the energy to a pacing pulse (Bun et al., 2019; Verma & Knight, 2019).

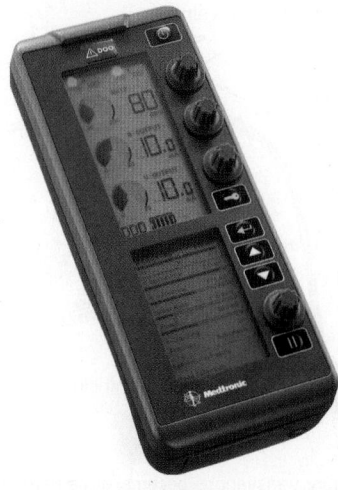

FIG. 38.24 Temporary external, dual-chamber demand pacemaker. Source: © 2017 Medtronic. Reproduced with permission of Medtronic.

TABLE 38.11	INDICATIONS FOR TEMPORARY PACING

- Maintenance of adequate heart rate and rhythm during special circumstances such as surgery and postoperative recovery, cardiac catheterization, or coronary angioplasty; during medication therapy that may cause bradycardia; and before implantation of a permanent pacemaker
- As prophylaxis after open-heart surgery
- Acute anterior MI with second- or third-degree AV block or bundle-branch block
- Acute inferior MI with symptomatic bradycardia and AV block
- Termination of AV nodal re-entry or reciprocating tachycardia associated with WPW syndrome, atrial flutter, or ventricular tachycardia
- Suppression of ectopic atrial or ventricular rhythm
- EPS to evaluate patient with bradydysrhythmias and tachydysrhythmias

AV, atrioventricular; *EPS,* electrophysiology study; *MI,* myocardial infarction; *WPW,* Wolff–Parkinson–White.

Another specialized type of cardiac pacing has been developed for the management of HF. More than 50% of patients with HF have intraventricular conduction delays that cause abnormal ventricular activation and contraction and subsequent asynchrony between the right and left ventricles. This asynchrony can result in reduced systolic function, pump inefficiency, and worsened HF. Cardiac resynchronization therapy (CRT) is a pacing technique that resynchronizes the cardiac cycle by pacing both ventricles, thus promoting improvement in ventricular function. Several devices are available in which CRT is combined with an ICD for maximum therapy. (HF is discussed in Chapter 37.)

There is no research on use of pacemakers in Indigenous people in Canada. However, it should be recognized that many Indigenous people live on reserve, rural or remotely, and may live far from health care services. They may need additional support emotionally and financially and for finding appropriate resources and services.

Temporary Pacemaker. A *temporary pacemaker* is one with a power source outside the body (Figure 38.24). There are three types of temporary pacemakers: transvenous, epicardial, and transcutaneous. Indications for temporary pacing are listed in Table 38.11.

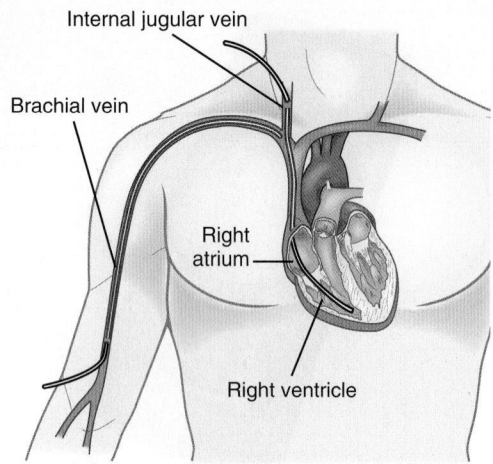

FIG 38.25 Temporary transvenous pacemaker catheter insertion. A single lead is positioned in the right ventricle through the brachial, subclavian, jugular, or femoral vein.

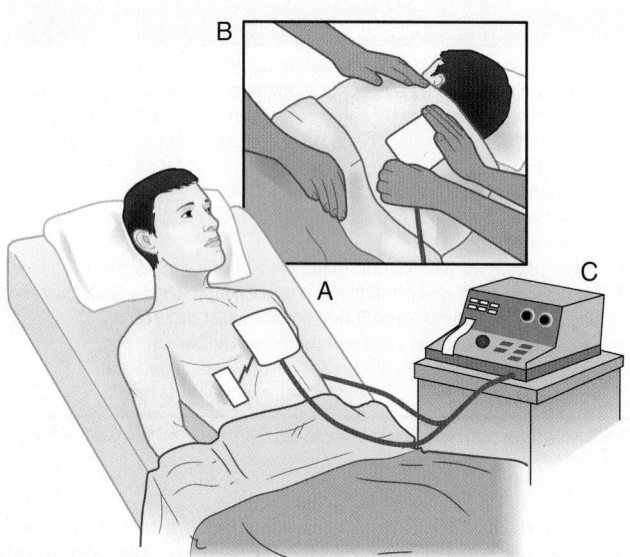

FIG. 38.26 Transcutaneous pacemaker. Pacing electrodes are placed on the patient's anterior **(A)** and posterior **(B)** chest walls and attached to an external pacing unit **(C)**.

A *transvenous pacemaker* consists of a lead or leads that are threaded transvenously to the right atrium, the right ventricle, or both and attached to the external power source (Figure 38.25). Most temporary transvenous pacemakers are inserted in critical care units in emergency situations. They are used until a permanent pacemaker can be inserted or the underlying cause of the dysrhythmia has been resolved.

To achieve *epicardial pacing*, an atrial pacing lead and a ventricular pacing lead are attached to the epicardium during heart surgery. The leads are passed through the chest wall and attached to the external power source. Epicardial pacing leads are placed prophylactically in case any bradydysrhythmias or tachydysrhythmias occur early in the postoperative period.

A *transcutaneous pacemaker* (TCP) is used to maintain adequate heart rate and rhythm in an emergency situation. Placement of the TCP is a noninvasive procedure. This pacemaker is used temporarily until a transvenous pacemaker can be inserted or until more definitive therapy is available.

The TCP consists of a power source and a rate- and voltage-control device that is attached to two large, multifunction electrode pads. One pad is positioned on the anterior part of the chest, usually at the V_2 or V_5 lead position, and the other pad is placed on the back between the spine and the left scapula at the level of the heart (Figure 38.26).

Before TCP therapy is initiated, the patient must be told what to expect. The uncomfortable muscle contractions that the pacemaker creates when the current passes through the chest wall should be explained. The patient should be reassured that the therapy is temporary and that the TCP will be replaced with a transvenous pacemaker as soon as possible. Whenever possible, an analgesic, sedative, or both should be provided.

Patient Monitoring. Patients with temporary or permanent pacemakers are monitored by ECG to evaluate the status of the pacemaker. Pacemaker malfunction is manifested primarily by a failure to sense or a failure to capture. *Failure to sense* is the situation in which the pacemaker fails to recognize spontaneous atrial or ventricular activity and it fires inappropriately. Failure to sense may be caused by pacer lead damage, battery failure, or dislodgement of the electrode. *Failure to capture* is the situation in which the electrical charge to the myocardium is insufficient to produce atrial or ventricular contraction. Failure to capture may also be caused by pacer lead damage, battery failure, or dislodgement of the electrode, as well as by fibrosis at the electrode tip.

Complications of invasive temporary (i.e., transvenous) or permanent pacemaker insertion include infection and hematoma formation at the site of insertion of the pacemaker power source or leads, pneumothorax, failure to sense or capture with possible symptomatic bradycardia, perforation of the atrial or the ventricular septum by the pacing lead, and appearance of "end-of-life" battery parameters when the pacemaker is tested. Several measures are taken to prevent or assess for complications, including prophylactic IV antibiotic therapy before and after insertion, postinsertion chest radiographic study to check lead placement and to rule out the presence of a pneumothorax, careful observation of insertion site, and continuous ECG monitoring of the patient's rhythm.

After pacemaker insertion, the patient is permitted out of bed once the heart rate and rhythm are stable. Arm and shoulder activity is limited to prevent dislodgement of the newly implanted pacing leads. The nurse needs to observe the insertion site for signs of bleeding and to check that the incision is intact. Any temperature elevation should be reported, and pain at the insertion site should be treated. Most patients are discharged the next day if the heart rate and rhythm are stable.

The nurse must provide patient teaching in addition to observing for complications after pacemaker insertion. The patient with a newly implanted pacemaker may have questions about activity restrictions and concerns about body image after the procedure. The goal of pacemaker therapy should be to enhance physiological functioning and the patient's quality of life. Patient and caregiver teaching for the patient with a pacemaker is outlined in Table 38.12.

After discharge, pacemaker function should be checked regularly during outpatient visits to a pacemaker clinic or by home monitoring using telephone transmitter devices. Another

TABLE 38.12 PATIENT & CAREGIVER TEACHING GUIDE

Pacemaker

The following guidelines should be included when teaching the patient and their caregiver after undergoing insertion of a pacemaker:

1. Maintain follow-up care plan with a physician to check the pacemaker site and begin regular pacemaker function checks with interrogator or programmer device.
2. Watch for signs of infection at incision site—for example, redness, swelling, or drainage.
3. Keep the incision dry for 1 week after pacemaker implantation.
4. Avoid lifting operative-side arm above shoulder level for 1 week.
5. Avoid direct blows to generator site.
6. Avoid close proximity to high-output electrical generators or large magnets such as an MRI scanner. These devices can reprogram a pacemaker.
7. Do not be concerned about using microwave ovens, which are safe to use and do not threaten pacemaker function.
8. Be aware that you may travel without restrictions. The small metal case of an implanted pacemaker rarely sets off an airport security alarm.
9. Ensure that you are taught how to take your pulse.
10. Carry a pacemaker information card at all times.
11. Watch for return of preimplantation symptoms (i.e., chest pain, excessive sweating, dizziness).

MRI, magnetic resonance imaging.

TABLE 38.13 ECG EVIDENCE AND ASSOCIATED CORONARY ARTERY IN ACUTE CORONARY SYNDROME

Area of Involvement of Left Ventricle	ECG Evidence		Associated Coronary Artery
	Leads Facing Area	Leads Opposite Area	
Septal wall	V_1, V_2	II, III, aV_F	Left anterior descending
Anterior wall	V_2, V_3, V_4	II, III, aV_F	Left anterior descending
Lateral wall, low	V_5, V_6	II, III, aV_F	Left anterior descending or circumflex
Lateral wall, high	I, aV_L	II, III, aV_F	Circumflex
Inferior wall	II, III, aV_F	I, aV_L, V_5, V_6	Right coronary artery

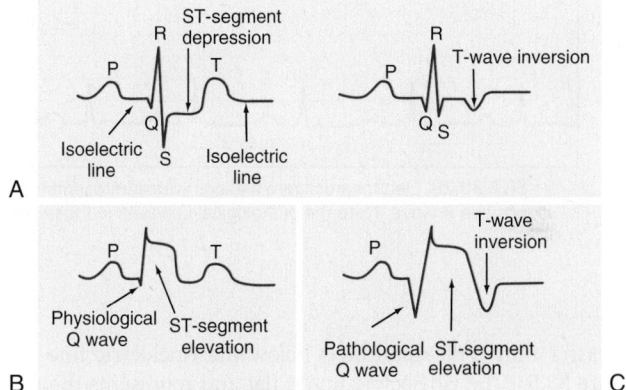

FIG. 38.28 Diagrams of changes in ST segment, T wave, and Q wave in association with myocardial ischemia **(A)**, injury **(B)**, and infarction **(C)**.

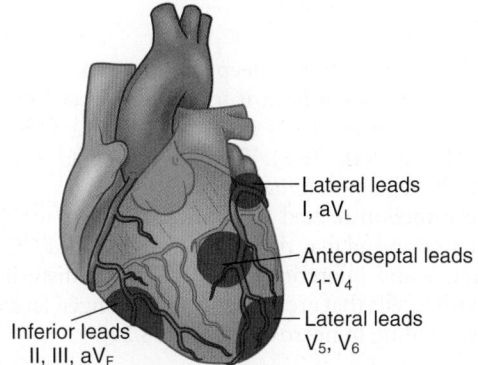

FIG. 38.27 Diagram showing where leads detect electrocardiogram (ECG) changes. Definitive ECG changes occur in leads that face the area of ischemia, injury, or infarction. Reciprocal changes may occur in leads facing opposite the area of ischemia, injury, or infarction.

method to evaluate pacemaker performance is noninvasive program stimulation, which is done on an outpatient basis in the electrophysiology laboratory.

Radiofrequency Ablation Therapy

Radiofrequency ablation (RFA) therapy is a relatively new development in the area of antidysrhythmia therapy. Radiofrequency energy (produced by a low-voltage, high-frequency form of electrical energy) is used to "burn" or ablate areas of the conduction system as definitive treatment of tachydysrhythmias.

Ablation therapy is performed after EPS has identified the source of the dysrhythmia. An electrode-tipped ablation catheter is used to ablate accessory pathways or ectopic sites in the atria, the AV node, and the ventricles. Catheter ablation is considered the nonpharmacological treatment of choice for AV nodal re-entrant tachycardia or for re-entrant tachycardia related to accessory bypass tracts and to control the

ventricular response of certain tachydysrhythmias. In some cases of uncontrolled ventricular response in atrial fibrillation or cases of atrial flutter that is unresponsive to medical therapy, the AV node or bundle of His may be ablated completely. If this is done, the patient must have a permanent pacemaker inserted at the same time. The ablation procedure is a successful therapy with a low complication rate. Care of the patient undergoing ablation therapy is similar to that of a patient undergoing cardiac catheterization (see Chapter 34).

ELECTROCARDIOGRAPHIC CHANGES ASSOCIATED WITH ACUTE CORONARY SYNDROME

The 12-lead ECG is the primary diagnostic tool used to evaluate patients receiving care for ACS. Many treatment decisions are directed by the ECG changes that occur with ACS. These definitive changes are in response to ischemia, injury, or infarction of myocardial cells and are detected in the leads that face the area of involvement (Figure 38.27). Reciprocal (opposite) ECG changes are often detected in the leads facing opposite the area involved in ACS. In addition, the pattern of ECG changes provides information on the coronary artery involved in ACS (Table 38.13).

Ischemia

Typical ECG changes that are seen in myocardial ischemia include ST-segment depression, T-wave inversion, or both (Figure 38.28, *A*). ST-segment depression is significant if it is

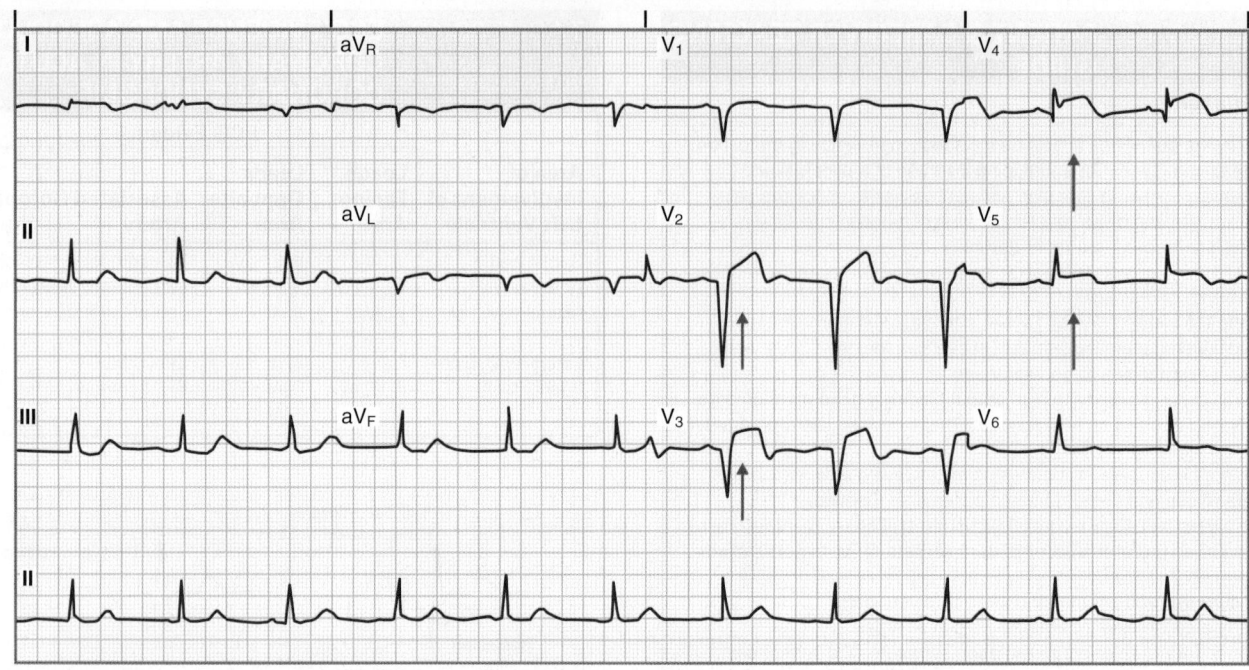

FIG. 38.29 Electrocardiogram findings with anteroseptal lateral wall myocardial infarction. Normally, leads I, aV$_L$, and V$_1$ to V$_3$ have a positive R wave. Note the pathological Q waves in these leads and the ST-segment elevation in leads V$_2$ to V$_5$ *(arrows)*.

at least 1 mm (one small box) below the isoelectric line (see Figure 38.5). The isoelectric line is flat and represents the normal times in the cardiac cycle when the ECG is not recording any electrical activity in the heart. These times are as follows: (a) from the end of the P wave to the start of the QRS complex, (b) the entire ST segment, and (c) from the end of the T wave to the start of the next P wave (see Figure 38.8). ST-segment depression, T-wave inversion, or both occur in response to the electrical disturbance in the myocardial cells that is caused by an inadequate supply of blood and oxygen. Once the cause of the disturbance is treated (adequate blood flow is restored), the ECG changes resolve and the ECG returns to the patient's baseline (Aehlert, 2018). (See Chapter 36 for a complete discussion of ACS.)

Injury and Infarction

Myocardial injury represents a stage of worsening ischemia that is potentially reversible but may evolve to infarction (necrosis) of myocardial cells. The typical ECG change seen during injury is ST-segment elevation. ST-segment elevation is significant if it is at least 1 mm above the isoelectric line (see Figure 38.28, *B*). If treatment is prompt and effective, it is possible to restore oxygen to the myocardium and avoid infarction. Avoidance of infarction is confirmed by the absence of serum cardiac markers. If serum cardiac markers are present, infarction has occurred and is referred to as an *ST-segment–elevation myocardial infarction* (STEMI).

In addition to ST-segment elevation, a pathological Q wave may be seen on the ECG with infarction (see Figure 38.28, C). A physiological Q wave is the first negative deflection (wave) after the P wave (see Figure 38.8). It is normally very small and narrow (<0.04 seconds in duration). A pathological Q wave that

develops during infarction is deep and more than 0.03 seconds in duration. If it does appear, it indicates that at least half the thickness of the heart wall is involved, which is referred to as a *Q-wave MI* (Aehlert, 2018). The pathological Q wave may be present on the ECG indefinitely.

T-wave inversion related to infarction occurs within hours after an infarction and may persist for months. The ECG changes seen in injury and infarction reflect electrical disturbances in the myocardial cells that are caused by a prolonged lack of blood and oxygen leading to necrosis (Figure 38.29).

Patient Monitoring

Monitoring guidelines for patients with suspected ACS include continuous, multi-lead ECG and ST-segment monitoring (AHA, 2017). The leads selected for monitoring should minimally include the leads that reflect the area of ischemia, injury, or infarction.

SYNCOPE

Syncope—a brief lapse in consciousness accompanied by a loss in postural tone (fainting)—is a common diagnosis in the emergency department and the hospital. The causes of syncope can be categorized as cardiovascular or noncardiovascular. The most common cardiovascular causes of syncope include (a) neurocardiogenic syncope or "vasovagal" syncope (e.g., carotid sinus sensitivity) and (b) primary cardiac dysrhythmias (e.g., tachycardias, bradycardias). Other causes can be related to prosthetic valve malfunction, pulmonary emboli, aortic dissection, and hypertrophic cardiomyopathy. Noncardiovascular causes are varied and can include hypoglycemia, hysteria, unwitnessed seizure, and vertebrobasilar transient ischemic attack (Potter et al., 2019).

A diagnostic workup for a patient with syncope from a suspected cardiac cause begins with ruling out structural or ischemic heart disease or both. This is done with echocardiography and stress testing. In older patients, who are more likely to have ischemic and structural heart disease, EPS is used to diagnose atrial and ventricular tachydysrhythmias, as well as conduction system disease causing bradydysrhythmias, all of which can cause syncope. These conditions can be treated with antidysrhythmia medication therapy, pacemakers, ICDs, catheter ablation therapy, or a combination of these treatments.

In patients without structural heart disease or in whom the results of EPS testing are not diagnostic, head-upright tilt-table testing may be performed. Normally, an upright position results in gravity displacing 300 to 800 mL of blood to the lower extremities. Specialized nerve fibres called *mechanoreceptors* are located throughout the vascular system. These receptors respond to the increased blood volume by initiating a reflex increase in sympathetic stimulation and decrease in parasympathetic output. The end results are slight increases in HR and diastolic BP and a slight decrease in systolic BP.

In neurocardiogenic syncope, the increase in venous pooling that occurs in the upright position reduces venous return to the heart. This results in a sudden, compensatory increase in ventricular contraction. This reaction is misinterpreted by the brain as a hypertensive state, and sympathetic stimulation is consequently withdrawn. This produces a paradoxical vasodilation and bradycardia (vasovagal response). The end results are bradycardia, hypotension, cerebral hypoperfusion, and syncope (Al-Busaidi & Jardine, 2019).

In the head-upright tilt-table test, the patient is placed supine on a table and supported by belts across the torso and the feet. Baseline ECG, BP, and HR are obtained in the horizontal position. Next, the table is tilted 60 to 80 degrees, and the patient is maintained in this upright position for 20 to 60 minutes. The ECG and HR are recorded continuously, and BP is measured every 3 minutes throughout the test. In healthy individuals, venous pooling activates the mechanoreceptors, resulting in the normal response just described.

If the patient's BP and HR responses are abnormal and clinical symptoms are reproduced (e.g., faintness), the test result is considered positive. If after 30 minutes there is no response, the table is returned to the horizontal position and an IV infusion of low-dose isoproterenol may be started in an attempt to provoke a response. Neurocardiogenic syncope that recurs frequently and interferes with normal activities can be treated with a variety of medications (e.g., metoprolol) (Albassam et al, 2019).

Other diagnostic tests for syncope include various recording devices. Holter monitors and event monitors are used and are discussed in this chapter and Chapter 34. A subcutaneously implanted loop-recording device can also be used to record the ECG during presyncopal and syncopal events. The device can be interrogated after a syncopal event in order to determine the ECG rhythm at the time of the event (Kim et al., 2019).

CASE STUDY

Dysrhythmia

Patient Profile
J. S. (pronouns he/him), a 78-year-old retired postal worker, is admitted to the cardiac care unit after a STEMI. While in the emergency department, J. S. had two episodes of ventricular tachycardia (VT). The first VT resolved after 20 seconds, and the second episode needed defibrillation to resolve the pulseless state. He is awake and lethargic, responding appropriately.

Subjective Data
- Has had two MIs and a history of HF
- Has shortness of breath, even in a sitting position

Objective Data
Physical Examination
- Appears anxious
- BP 92/60 mm Hg, pulse 98/min, respirations 28/min
- Lungs: bilateral coarse crackles
- Heart: S_3 gallop at apex

Diagnostic Studies
- ECG: frequent PVCs
- Echocardiogram: severe left ventricular dysfunction with ejection fraction of 20%
- Serum potassium level: 2.9 mmol/L

Interprofessional Care
- Amiodarone infusion
- Scheduled for electrophysiology study (EPS)

Discussion Questions
1. Why is J. S. at risk for ventricular fibrillation?
2. Why is amiodarone used after ventricular fibrillation?
3. What methods may be used to assess the effectiveness of an antidysrhythmia medication?
4. Would J. S. be a candidate for an ICD?
5. If ventricular fibrillation recurred while J. S. was receiving amiodarone infusion, what other IV medications would be tried?
6. What is the significance of the serum potassium value?
7. **Priority decision**: On the basis of these nursing diagnoses, what are the priority nursing interventions for J. S.?
8. **Evidence-informed practice**: J. S. is scheduled for the insertion of a CRT/ICD once stable. On the nurse's rounds, J. S. asks why he needs two devices.

ⓔvolve
Answers are available at http://evolve.elsevier.com/Canada/Lewis/medsurg.

REVIEW QUESTIONS

The number of the question corresponds to the same-numbered objective at the beginning of the chapter.

1. The nurse is monitoring the ECG of a client admitted with ACS. Which of the following ECG characteristics would be most suggestive of ischemia?
   a. Sinus rhythm with a pathological Q wave
   b. Sinus rhythm with an elevated ST segment
   c. Sinus rhythm with a depressed ST segment
   d. Sinus rhythm with premature atrial contractions

2. A client with a stable blood pressure and no symptoms has the following ECG characteristics: atrial rate, 74 beats/minute and regular; ventricular rate, 62 beats/minute and irregular; P wave, normal contour; PR interval, lengthens progressively until a P wave is not conducted; QRS complex, normal contour. What would be the appropriate treatment for this rhythm?
   a. Epinephrine, 1 mg IV push
   b. Isoproterenol, IV continuous drip
   c. Immediate insertion of a temporary pacemaker
   d. Careful observation for signs of further heart block

3. The cardiac monitor of a client in the cardiac care unit after an acute myocardial infarction indicates ventricular bigeminy. What would be the most appropriate intervention from the following list?
   a. Performing defibrillation
   b. Treatment with intravenous amiodarone
   c. Insertion of a temporary pacemaker
   d. Continuing to monitor and attempt to determine the underlying cause

4. How does defibrillation differ from cardioversion?
   a. Defibrillation requires a greater dose of electrical current.
   b. Defibrillation is synchronized to countershock during the QRS complex.
   c. Cardioversion is indicated only for treatment of atrial tachydysrhythmias.
   d. Cardioversion may be done on a nonemergency basis with sedation of the client.

5. Which of the following is true when the client has an implantable cardiac defibrillator?
   a. Antidysrhythmia medications can be discontinued.
   b. All members of the client's family should learn CPR.
   c. The client should not drive until the physician approves it after the ICD has been implanted.
   d. The client is usually relieved to have the device implanted to prevent dysrhythmias.

6. Which client teaching points should the nurse include when providing discharge instructions to a client with a new permanent pacemaker and their caregiver? *(Select all that apply.)*
   a. Avoid or limit air travel.
   b. Take and record a daily pulse rate.
   c. Obtain and wear a medical alert bracelet at all times.
   d. Avoid lifting the arm on the side of the pacemaker above shoulder height.
   e. Avoid microwave ovens because they interfere with pacemaker function.

7. Which of the following would be essential to teach a client before they undergo electrophysiological monitoring?
   a. A catheter will be placed in each of the femoral arteries to allow double-catheter use.
   b. The client will be given a general anaesthetic to prevent the awareness of "near-death" experiences.
   c. Ventricular tachycardia and ventricular fibrillation may be induced and treated during the procedure.
   d. The procedure is used to "burn" or ablate areas of the conduction system that are causing tachydysrhythmias.

1. c; 2. d; 3. d; 4. d; 5. c; 6. b, c; 7. d.

e̶volve

For even more review questions, visit http://evolve.elsevier.com/Canada/Lewis/medsurg.

REFERENCES

Aehlert, B. (2018). *ECGs made easy* (6th ed.). Mosby.

Albassam, O., Redelmeier, R., Shadowitz, S., et al. (2019). Did this patient have cardiac syncope? The Rational Clinical Examination Systematic Review. *JAMA, 321*(24), 2448–2457. https://doi.org/10.1001/jama.2019.8001

Al-Busaidi, I., & Jardine, D. (2019). Different types of syncope presenting to clinic: Do we miss cardiac syncope? *Heart, Lung & Circulation, 29*(8), 1129–1138. https://doi.org/10.1016/j.hlc.2019.09.008

American Heart Association (AHA). (2000). Part 4: The automated external defibrillator (key link in the chain of survival). *Circulation, 102*(Suppl), I60–I76. https://doi.org/10.1161/circ.102.suppl_1.I-60

American Heart Association (AHA). (2015). American Heart Association Guidelines for cardiopulmonary resuscitation and emergency cardiovascular care science. *Circulation, 122*(18), S639. https://doi.org/10.1161/CIR.0b013e3181fdf7aa

American Heart Association (AHA). (2017). Update to practice standards for electrocardiographic monitoring in hospital settings: A scientific statement. *Circulation, 136*, e273–e344. https://doi.org/10.1161/CIR.0000000000000527

American Heart Association (AHA). (2018). 2018 American Heart Association focused update on advanced cardiovascular life support use of antiarrhythmic drugs during and immediately after cardiac arrest (an update to the American Heart Association guidelines for cardiopulmonary resuscitation and emergency cardiovascular care). *Circulation, 138*, e740–e749. https://doi.org/10.1161/CIR.0000000000000613

American Heart Association (AHA). (2020). Highlights of the 2020 American Heart Association guidelines for CPR & ECC (Heart and Stroke Foundation of Canada edition). *Circulation, 142*(16), S366–S468. https://doi.org/10.1161/CIR.0000000000000916

Bun, S. S., Squara, F., Scarlatti, D., et al. (2019). Technological advances in cardiac pacing and defibrillation. *Heart, Vessels and Transplantation, 3*(3), 95–101. https://doi.org/10.24969/hvt.2019.129

Canadian Cardiovascular Society (CCS). (2018). 2018 Focused update of the Canadian Cardiovascular Society guidelines for the management of atrial fibrillation. *Canadian Journal of Cardiology, 34*(11), 1371–1392. https://doi.org/10.1016/j.cjca.2018.08.026

DeSimone, C., Naksuk, N., & Asirvatham, S. (2018). Supraventricular arrhythmias: Clinical framework and common scenarios for the internist. *Mayo Clinic Proceedings, 93*(12), 1825–1841. https://doi.org/10.1016/j.mayocp.2018.07.019

Giancaterino, S., Lupercio, F., Nishimura, M., et al. (2018). Current and future use of insertable cardiac monitors. *JACC: Clinical Electrophysiology, 4*(11), 1383–1396.

Heart and Stroke Foundation. (2012). *Position Statement: Public access to automated external defibrillators (AEDs).* https://www.heartandstroke.ca/-/media/pdf-files/canada/other/pad-eng-final.ashx. (Seminal).

Honarbakhsh, S., Baker, V., Kirkby, C., et al. (2017). Safety and efficacy of paramedic treatment of regular supraventricular tachycardia: A randomised controlled trial. *Heart, 103*(18), 1413–1418. https://doi.org/10.1136/heartjnl-2016-309968

Kim, Y. H., Paik, S. H., Jeon, N. J., et al. (2019). Cerebral perfusion monitoring using near-infrared spectroscopy during head-up tilt table test in patients with orthostatic intolerance. *Frontiers in Human Neuroscience, 13*, 55. https://doi.org/10.3389/fnhum.2019.00055

Networks of Centres of Excellence of Canada. (2017). *"Fixing" atrial fibrillation earlier would benefit millions of Canadians.* Government of Canada. https://www.nce-rce.gc.ca/Research-Recherche/Stories-Articles/2017/CANet-CANet_eng.asp

Parkash, R. (2018). Does lifestyle impact risk, burden and symptomatology of atrial fibrillation? *Canadian Journal of General Internal Medicine, 13*(SP1). https://doi.org/10.22374/cjgim.v13iSP1.310

Potter, P., Perry, A., Stockert, P., & Hall, A. (2019). *Canadian fundamentals of nursing* (6th ed.). Elsevier.

Verma, N., & Knight, B. (2019). Update in cardiac pacing. *Arrhythmia Electrophysiology Review, 8*(3), 228. https://doi.org.10.15420/aer.2019.15.3

RESOURCES

Heart and Stroke Foundation of Canada
https://www.heartandstroke.ca

ACLS Training Center
https://www.acls.net/aclsalg.htm

American Heart Association
https://www.heart.org

Practical Clinical Skills—*EKG*
https://www.practicalclinicalskills.com/ekg

Skill Stat—*The 6 Second ECG* (rhythm interpretation)
https://www.skillstat.com/tools/ecg-simulator/

Nursing Management
Inflammatory and Structural Heart Disorders

Sheila Rizza
Originating US chapter by Patricia Keegan

℮volve WEBSITE

http://evolve.elsevier.com/Canada/Lewis/medsurg

- Review Questions (Online Only)
- Key Points
- Answer Guidelines for Case Study
- Student Case Study
  - Rheumatic Fever and Heart Disease
- Conceptual Care Map Creator

- Supporting Media—Audio
  - Pericardial Friction Rub
- Customizable Nursing Care Plans
  - Patient with Infective Endocarditis
  - Patient with Valvular Heart Disease

- Audio Glossary
- Content Updates

LEARNING OBJECTIVES

1. Describe the etiology, pathophysiology, and clinical manifestations of infective endocarditis and pericarditis.
2. Discuss the interprofessional care and nursing management of infective endocarditis and pericarditis.
3. Explain the importance of prophylactic antibiotic therapy in infective endocarditis.
4. Explain the etiology and clinical manifestations of myocarditis, along with the interprofessional care and nursing management of patients with myocarditis.
5. Describe the etiology, pathophysiology, and clinical manifestations of rheumatic fever and rheumatic heart disease.
6. Discuss the interprofessional care and nursing management of patients with rheumatic fever and rheumatic heart disease.
7. Identify the etiologies of congenital and acquired valvular heart diseases.
8. Discuss the pathophysiology and clinical manifestations of the various types of valvular heart conditions and the diagnostic studies used in connection with them.
9. Describe the interprofessional care and nursing management of patients with valvular heart disease.
10. Describe surgical interventions used in management of patients with valvular heart conditions.
11. Describe the pathophysiology and clinical manifestations of the different types of cardiomyopathies.
12. Discuss the nursing care and interprofessional management of patients with different types of cardiomyopathies.

KEY TERMS

acute rheumatic fever (ARF)
aortic stenosis
aortic valve regurgitation (AR)
Aschoff bodies
cardiac tamponade
cardiomyopathy
dilated cardiomyopathy (DCM)

endomyocardial biopsy (EMB)
hypertrophic cardiomyopathy (HCM)
infective endocarditis (IE)
Janeway's lesions
mitral valve prolapse (MVP)
myocarditis
Osler's nodes

pericardial effusion
pericardial friction rub
pericardiocentesis
pericarditis
regurgitation
rheumatic fever
rheumatic heart disease

▎INFLAMMATORY DISORDERS OF THE HEART

INFECTIVE ENDOCARDITIS

Infective endocarditis (IE), previously known as *bacterial endocarditis*, is an infection of the heart valves or the endocardial surface of the heart. The name of this disorder has changed because it is now recognized that organisms other than bacteria may cause the disease (Heart and Stroke Foundation of Canada, 2021a). The *endocardium*, the inner layer of the heart (Figure 39.1), is contiguous with the valves of the heart. Therefore, inflammation from IE affects the cardiac valves.

Before the era of antibiotics, IE was almost always fatal. The advent of penicillin therapy changed the prognosis dramatically and mortality rates decreased appreciably.

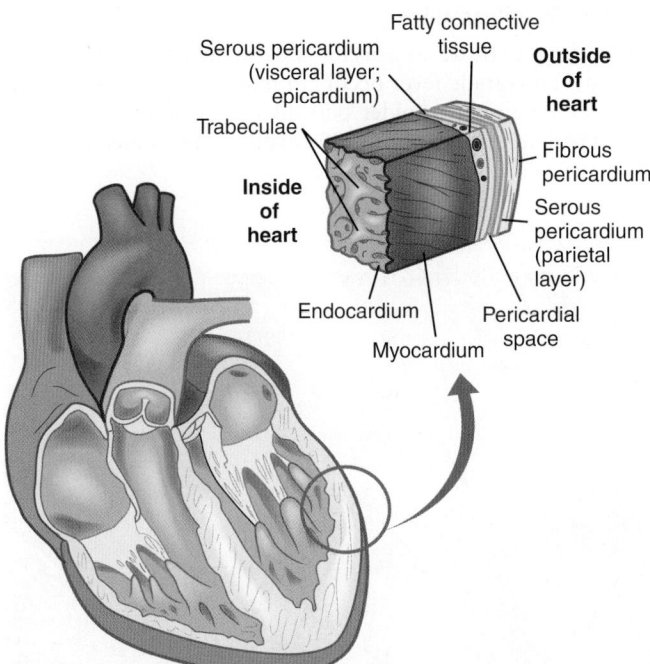

FIG. 39.1 Layers of the heart muscle and pericardium. Source: Adapted from Patton, K. T., & Thibodeau, G. A. (2014). *The human body in health and disease* (6th ed., p. 371). Mosby.

Classification

Four different categories of IE describe the site of infection, the presence of cardiovascular devices, and how the individual acquired the infection: left-sided native valve IE, left-sided prosthetic valve IE, right-sided IE (includes intravenous [IV] drug use), and intracardiac and intravascular devices (e.g., pacemaker/defibrillator wires, hemodialysis). IE is identified as being community-acquired IE or health care–associated IE. With the changing landscape of health care and patient populations, more than 25% of IE cases are now health care associated (Cahill et al., 2017).

Etiology and Pathophysiology

The most common causative organisms of IE, *Staphylococcus aureus*, oral *Streptococcus*, and *Enterococci*, are Gram-positive bacterial organisms, which are responsible for more than 80% of IE cases (Table 39.1). Other possible pathogens include fungi and viruses. Newly identified pathogens, which are difficult to cultivate (e.g., *Bartonella, Tropheryma whippelii*), have been found to cause IE. Resistant organisms (e.g., methicillin-resistant *S. aureus*) also cause IE and are challenging conventional antibiotic therapy.

IE occurs when blood flow turbulence within the heart allows the causative organism to infect previously damaged valves or other endothelial surfaces. It can occur in individuals with a variety of underlying cardiac conditions. The principal risk factors for IE are prior endocarditis, prosthetic valves, acquired valvular disease, and cardiac lesions. Several noncardiac conditions and procedures also can allow large numbers of organisms to enter the bloodstream and initiate the infectious process (Tables 39.2 and 39.3).

Vegetations, the primary lesions of IE, consist of fibrin, leukocytes, platelets, and microbes that adhere to the valve surface or the endocardium (Figure 39.2). The loss of portions of these friable vegetations into the circulation results in emboli. As

TABLE 39.1	CAUSATIVE ORGANISMS ASSOCIATED WITH INFECTIVE ENDOCARDITIS

Bacteria
- *Bartonella quintana*
- Chlamydiae
- Coagulase-negative staphylococci
- Enterococci
- HACEK group (*Haemophilus, Actinobacillus, Cardiobacterium, Eikenella, Kingella* species)
- Methicillin-resistant *Staphylococcus aureus*
- Vancomycin-resistant *S. aureus*
- Rickettsiae
- *S. aureus*
- *Staphylococcus epidermidis*
- *Streptococcus bovis*
- Groups A, B, and C streptococci
- *Streptococcus pneumoniae*
- Viridans streptococci
- *Tropheryma whippelii*

Fungi
- *Candida albicans*
- *Candida parapsilosis*
- *Aspergillus*

Viruses
- Coxsackievirus B

TABLE 39.2	PREDISPOSING CONDITIONS FOR THE DEVELOPMENT OF INFECTIVE ENDOCARDITIS

Cardiac Conditions
- Prior endocarditis
- Prosthetic valves
- Cardiac valvulopathy in cardiac transplant recipients
- Native valve disease, including rheumatic heart disease, mitral valve prolapse, and degenerative heart disease
- Unrepaired cyanotic congenital heart disease, including palliative shunts and conduits
- Repaired congenital heart defect with prosthetic material or device, surgically or through catheterization, during the first 6 months when endothelialization occurs
- Implanted cardiac devices, e.g., pacemaker, cardioverter–defibrillator

Noncardiac Conditions
- Intravenous drug use
- Hospital-acquired bacteremia

Procedure-Associated Risks
- Intravascular devices (e.g., hemodialysis catheters)
- Procedures listed in Table 39.3

many as 22 to 50% of patients with IE will experience systemic embolization. These emboli arise from left-sided heart vegetations and progress to various organs (particularly the brain, the kidneys, and the spleen), causing infarction, and to the extremities, causing limb infarction. Right-sided heart lesions embolize to the lungs. The risk of embolization is greatest within the first few days of commencing antimicrobial therapy.

The infection may spread locally to cause damage to the valves or to their supporting structures. This damage results in dysrhythmias, valvular incompetence, and eventual invasion of the myocardium, leading to heart failure (HF), sepsis, and heart block (Figure 39.3).

At one time, rheumatic heart disease was the most common cause of IE; it now accounts for fewer than 20% of cases. Currently, the main contributing factors include (1) degenerative valve sclerosis; (2) recreational IV drug use; (3) use of prosthetic valves; (4) proliferation of intravascular device placement, resulting in health care–associated infections; and (5) renal dialysis (Cahill et al., 2017). Left-sided endocarditis is more common in patients with bacterial infections and underlying heart disease. The primary cause of right-sided endocarditis is IV use of illicit drugs. However, the incidence of affected left-sided valves has increased, especially with cocaine use. *S. aureus* is the most common causative organism in IE caused by IV drug use.

TABLE 39.3	PROCEDURES NECESSITATING ANTIBIOTIC PROPHYLAXIS TO PREVENT INFECTIVE ENDOCARDITIS*

Oropharyngeal
- All dental procedures likely to produce gingival or mucosal bleeding (not simple adjustment of orthodontic appliances or shedding of deciduous teeth), including professional cleaning
- Tonsillectomy or adenoidectomy

Respiratory
- Surgical procedures or biopsy involving respiratory mucosa

Integumentary
- Procedures on infected skin, skin structures, or musculoskeletal tissues with incision of the tissue

Gastrointestinal/Genitourinary
- Prophylactic administration of antimicrobial agents to prevent infective endocarditis in patients undergoing genitourinary or gastrointestinal procedures is no longer recommended (Otta et al., 2020).

*This table lists select procedures and is not all-inclusive.

Clinical Manifestations

The findings in IE are nonspecific and can involve multiple organ systems. Low-grade fever occurs in more than 90% of patients but may be absent in older persons and in immunocompromised patients. Other nonspecific manifestations include chills,

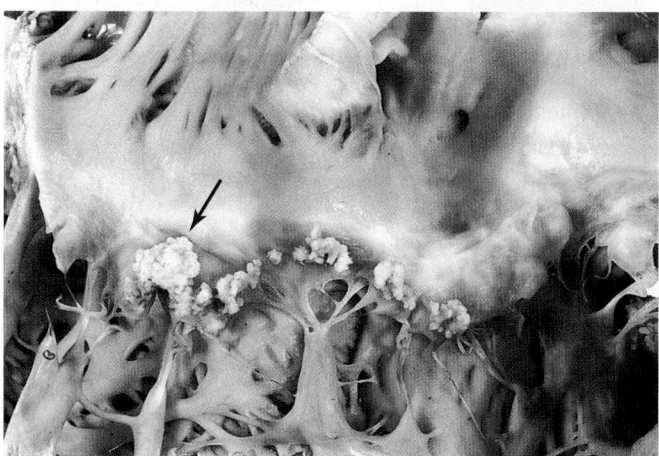

FIG. 39.2 Bacterial endocarditis of the mitral valve. The valve is covered with large, irregular vegetations (*arrow*). Damjanov, I., & Linder, J. (2000). *Pathology: A color atlas.* Mosby.

PATHOPHYSIOLOGY MAP

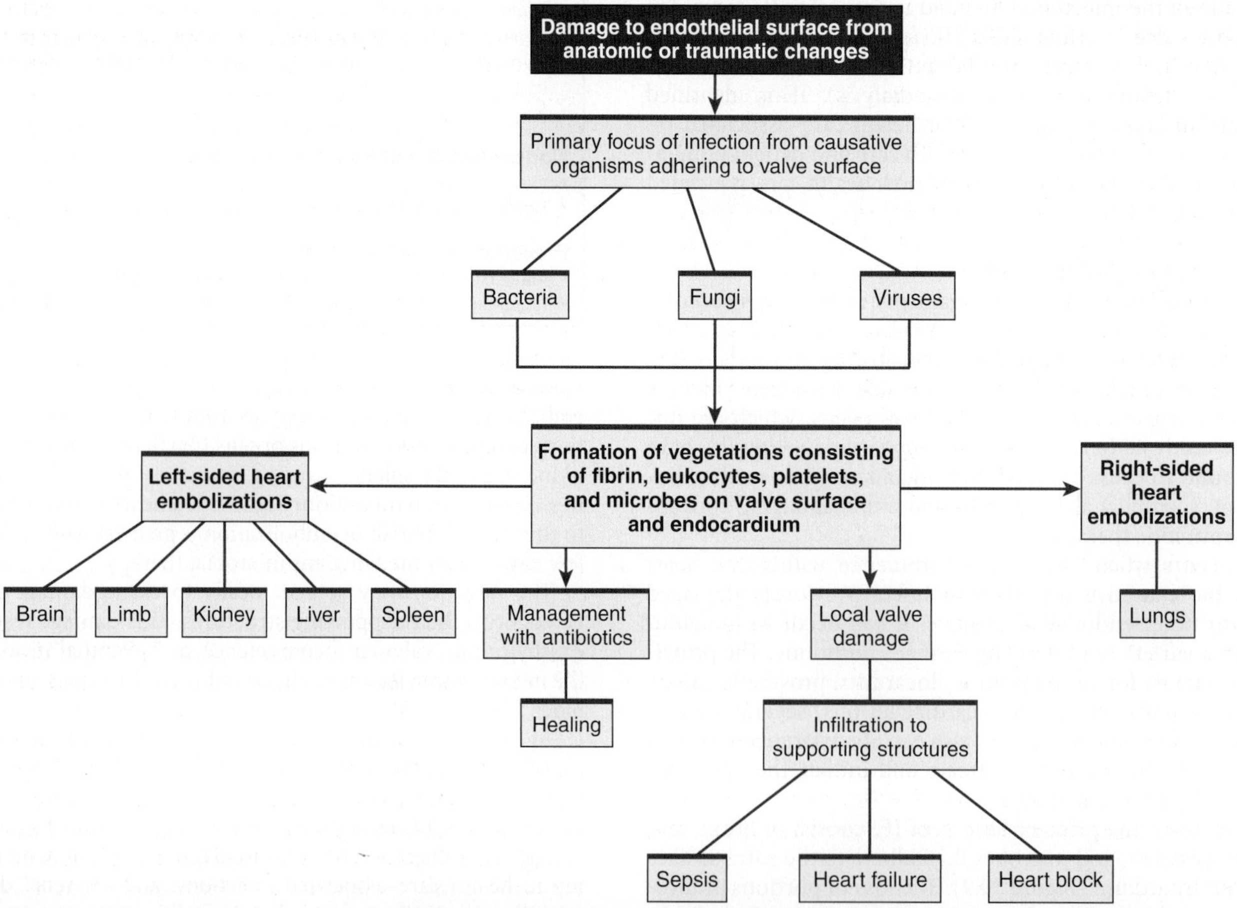

Damage to endothelial surface from anatomic or traumatic changes
→ Primary focus of infection from causative organisms adhering to valve surface
→ Bacteria | Fungi | Viruses
→ Formation of vegetations consisting of fibrin, leukocytes, platelets, and microbes on valve surface and endocardium

Left-sided heart embolizations → Brain | Limb | Kidney | Liver | Spleen

Management with antibiotics → Healing

Local valve damage → Infiltration to supporting structures → Sepsis | Heart failure | Heart block

Right-sided heart embolizations → Lungs

FIG. 39.3 Pathogenesis of infective endocarditis.

weakness, malaise, fatigue, and anorexia. Arthralgias, myalgias, back pain, abdominal discomfort, weight loss, headache, and clubbing of fingers may occur in subacute forms of endocarditis.

Vascular manifestations of IE include *splinter hemorrhages* (longitudinal black streaks) that occur in the nail beds. Petechiae may occur as a result of fragmentation and microembolization of vegetative lesions and are common in the conjunctivae, the lips, the buccal mucosa, and the palate and over the ankles, the feet, and the antecubital and popliteal areas. Osler's nodes (painful, tender, red or purple, pea-size lesions that last 1 to 2 days) may be found on the fingertips or the toes. Janeway's lesions (flat, painless, small, red spots) may be found on the palms and the soles. Funduscopic examination may reveal hemorrhagic retinal lesions called *Roth's spots.*

The onset of a new or changing murmur is noted in most patients with IE, with the aortic and mitral valves most commonly affected. The mitral murmur of endocarditis is generally a mid-tolate systolic regurgitant type. The aortic murmur may be early diastolic. Murmurs are often absent in tricuspid endocarditis because right-sided heart pressures are too low to be heard. HF is observed in 42 to 60% of patients with IE, more often in those with aortic valve endocarditis (29%) than in patients with mitral valve endocarditis (20%) (Habib et al., 2015).

Clinical manifestations secondary to embolization in various body organs may also be present. Embolization to the spleen may result in sharp, left upper quadrant pain and splenomegaly. Local tenderness and abdominal rigidity may be present. Embolization to the kidneys may cause pain in the flank, hematuria, and azotemia. Emboli may lodge in small peripheral blood vessels of the arms and legs and may cause gangrene. Embolization to the brain may cause neurological conditions such as hemiplegia, ataxia, aphasia, visual changes, and change in the level of consciousness. Pulmonary emboli may occur in right-sided endocarditis.

Diagnostic Studies

Obtaining the patient's recent health history is important in assessing IE. Inquiry should be made regarding any recent (within the past 3–6 months) dental, urological, surgical, or gynecological procedures, including normal or abnormal obstetrical delivery. Previous history of use of illicit IV drugs, previous valvular or congenital heart disease, presence of an intracardiac prosthetic device, recent cardiac catheterization, and skin, respiratory, or urinary tract infections should be documented.

Laboratory data, especially blood cultures, should also be assessed. Two blood cultures drawn 60 minutes apart will be positive in more than 90% of patients. Culture-negative endocarditis is often associated with antibiotic usage within the previous 2 weeks or caused by a pathogen not easily detected by standard culture procedures (e.g., *Bartonella* species). Negative cultures should be kept for 3 weeks if the clinical diagnosis remains endocarditis, because of the possibility that a slow-growing causative organism may be detected.

A mild leukocytosis occurs in acute endocarditis (but is uncommon in the subacute form), with average white blood cell (WBC) counts ranging from 10 to 11×10^9/L. The erythrocyte sedimentation rate (ESR) and C-reactive protein (CRP) levels may be elevated.

Echocardiography is valuable in the diagnostic workup for a patient with IE when the blood cultures are negative or for

TABLE 39.4 INTERPROFESSIONAL CARE

Cardiac Conditions* Necessitating Antibiotic Prophylaxis to Prevent Infective Endocarditis

- Prosthetic cardiac valves
- History of endocarditis
- Surgically constructed systemic–pulmonary shunts
- Complex cyanotic congenital heart disease
- Vascular grafts (first 6 mo after implantation)
- Cardiac transplantation requiring valvulopathy

*This table lists common cardiac conditions associated with high risk for infective endocarditis but is not all-inclusive.
Source: Habib, G., Lancellotti, P, Antunes, M., et al. (2015). Guidelines for the management of infective endocarditis. *European Heart Journal, 36*(44), 3075–3128. https://doi.org/10.1093/eurheartj/ehv319

the patient who is a surgical candidate and has an active infection. Transesophageal echocardiograms and digital imaging using two-dimensional transthoracic echocardiograms can detect vegetation, destructive lesions, and abscesses on valves (Habib et al., 2015). A chest radiograph is done to detect the presence of *cardiomegaly* (an enlarged heart). An electrocardiogram (ECG) may show first- or second-degree atrioventricular (AV) block because the cardiac valves lie in proximity to cardiac conductive tissue, especially the AV node. Cardiac catheterization may be used to evaluate coronary artery patency and valvular function when surgical intervention is being considered for patients with IE.

Interprofessional Care

Prophylactic Treatment. Antibiotic prophylaxis is recommended for patients with specific cardiac conditions before they undergo certain dental or surgical procedures (Dayer & Thornhill, 2018). Procedures for which endocarditis prophylaxis is recommended are summarized in Table 39.4. Specific antibiotic regimens are recommended for dental procedures that require manipulation of the gingival or periapical region of the teeth or perforation of the oral mucosa and respiratory tract. Current guidelines suggest that routine activities of oral hygiene contribute to bacteremia that may result in IE (Habib et al., 2015).

Medication Therapy. Accurate identification of the infecting organism is key to successful treatment of IE. Long-term treatment is necessary to kill dormant bacteria clustered within the valvular vegetations. Complete eradication of the organism generally takes weeks to achieve and relapses are common. Initially, patients are hospitalized and IV antibiotic therapy is started. Table 39.5 outlines suggested antibiotic regimens for patients with IE from various causative organisms and with different clinical circumstances.

Subsequent blood cultures may be performed to evaluate the effectiveness of antibiotic therapy. Blood cultures that remain positive indicate inadequate or inappropriate antibiotic administration, aortic root or myocardial abscess, or the wrong diagnosis (e.g., an infection elsewhere). Serum antibiotic drug levels are often monitored to establish therapeutic dosages. Renal function is monitored when antibiotics are used that are nephrotoxic (e.g., vancomycin [Vancocin]) and for patients with poor kidney function.

Fungal infection and prosthetic valve endocarditis (PVE) are most frequently observed in IV drug users and immunocompromised patients and respond poorly to antibiotic therapy alone. Early prolonged (≥6 weeks) medication therapy is recommended in these situations (Habib et al., 2015). Valve

TABLE 39.5   MEDICATION THERAPY

Treatment of Infective Endocarditis With Outpatient Antibiotic Therapy*

Causative Agent	Antibiotic Regimen Options
Streptococcal endocarditis involving native valve	IV penicillin G or IV or IM ceftriaxone; IV penicillin G or IV or IM ceftriaxone plus IV or IM gentamicin; or IV vancomycin (Vancocin)
Enterococcal endocarditis involving native or prosthetic valve	IV ampicillin plus IV or IM gentamicin; or IV penicillin G plus IV or IM gentamicin; or IV vancomycin plus IV or IM gentamicin
Staphylococcal endocarditis in absence of prosthetic materials	IV cloxacillin or IV cefazolin for penicillin allergy
Fungal endocarditis in native or prosthetic valves	IV amphotericin B (Fungizone)
HACEK group	IV ceftriaxone

HACEK, Haemophilus, Actinobacillus, Cardiobacterium, Eikenella, Kingella; IM, intramuscular; IV, intravenous.
*This table lists common medication regimens but is not all-inclusive.

TABLE 39.6   NURSING ASSESSMENT

Infective Endocarditis

Subjective Data
Important Health Information
Past health history: Valvular, congenital, or syphilitic cardiac disease (including valve repair or replacement); previous endocarditis, childbirth, staphylococcal or streptococcal infections, health care–associated bacteremia
Medications: Immunosuppressive therapy, recreational IV drug use
Surgery or other treatments: Recent obstetrical or gynecological procedures; invasive techniques including catheterization, cystoscopy, intravascular procedures; recent dental or surgical procedure; GI procedures (endoscopy)

Symptoms
- Exercise intolerance, generalized weakness, fatigue, malaise
- Cough, dyspnea on exertion, orthopnea, paroxysmal nocturnal dyspnea
- Palpitations, night sweats
- Chest, back, or abdominal pain
- Headache, joint tenderness, muscle tenderness
- Weight gain or loss; anorexia
- Chills, diaphoresis
- Bloody urine

Objective Data
General
Fever

Integumentary
Osler's nodes on extremities; splinter hemorrhages under nail beds; Janeway's lesions on palms and soles; petechiae of skin, mucous membranes, or conjunctivae; purpura; peripheral edema, finger clubbing

Respiratory
Tachypnea, crackles

Cardiovascular
Dysrhythmias, tachycardia, new or enhanced murmurs, S_3, S_4, retinal hemorrhages

Possible Findings
Leukocytosis, anemia, ↑ ESR, ↑ CRP and cardiac enzymes; positive blood cultures; microscopic hematuria; echocardiogram showing chamber enlargement, valvular dysfunction, and vegetations; chest radiograph showing cardiomegaly and pulmonary infiltrates; ECG demonstrating ischemia and conduction defects, signs of systemic embolization or pulmonary embolism

CRP, C-reactive protein; ECG, electrocardiogram; ESR, erythrocyte sedimentation rate; GI, gastrointestinal; IV, intravenous; S_3, third heart sound; S_4, fourth heart sound.

replacement has become an important adjunct procedure in the management of IE. It is used in more than 25% of cases. (Valve replacement is discussed later in this chapter.)

Fever may persist for 5 to 10 days after treatment has been started and can be treated with acetylsalicylic acid (ASA; Aspirin), acetaminophen (Tylenol), ibuprofen (Motrin), fluids, and rest. Complete bed rest is usually not indicated unless the temperature remains elevated or there are signs of HF. Endocarditis coupled with HF responds poorly to both medication therapy and valve replacement and is often life-threatening.

NURSING MANAGEMENT
INFECTIVE ENDOCARDITIS

NURSING ASSESSMENT
Subjective and objective data that should be obtained from a patient with IE are presented in Table 39.6. Heart sounds should be assessed together with vital signs to detect a murmur or a change in the character of a pre-existing murmur and the presence of extradiastolic sounds.

Arthralgia is common, may involve multiple joints, and may be accompanied by myalgias. The patient should be assessed for joint tenderness, decreased range of motion, and muscle tenderness. The oral mucosa, conjunctivae, upper chest, and lower extremities should be examined for petechiae. A general systems assessment should be completed to facilitate recognition of hemodynamic and embolic complications.

NURSING DIAGNOSES
Nursing diagnoses for the patient with IE may include but are not limited to the following:
- *Decreased cardiac output* (resulting from altered heart rhythm, valvular insufficiency, and fluid overload)
- *Reduced stamina* resulting from *physical deconditioning* (generalized weakness, arthralgia, valvular dysfunction)

Additional information on nursing diagnoses for the patient with IE is presented in Nursing Care Plan (NCP) 39.1, available on the Evolve website for this chapter.

PLANNING
The overall goals for the patient with IE include (a) normal or baseline cardiac function, (b) performance of activities of daily living without fatigue, and (c) knowledge of the therapeutic regimen to prevent recurrence of endocarditis.

NURSING IMPLEMENTATION
HEALTH PROMOTION. The incidence and recurrence of IE can be decreased by identifying individuals who are at risk for developing endocarditis (see Tables 39.2 and 39.4) and those who have had IE in the past and by providing relevant teaching to them. Assessment of a patient's history and an understanding of the disease process are crucial for planning and implementing appropriate health-promotion strategies. Teaching is necessary for patients with IE so that they understand and

adhere to the planned treatment regimen. The following measures should be stressed:

- Avoiding people with infection, especially upper respiratory infection, and reporting cold, flu, and cough symptoms
- Avoiding excessive fatigue and planning rest periods before and after activity
- Good oral hygiene, including daily care and regular dental visits
- Informing health care providers performing dental, medical, or surgical procedures of IE history
- The significance of prescribed prophylactic antibiotic therapy before undergoing any invasive procedure
- Drug treatment program if there is history of IV drug use

AMBULATORY AND HOME CARE. Patients with IE will require nursing management (see NCP 39.1 for nursing diagnoses and interventions, available on the Evolve website for this chapter). IE generally requires treatment with antibiotics for 4 to 6 weeks, depending on the results of blood cultures (see Table 39.5). After initial treatment in the hospital, a patient who is hemodynamically stable and adherent to treatment may continue their treatment in the home setting. The adequacy of the home environment in terms of in-home support and hospital access must be determined for successful management. Patients who receive outpatient IV antibiotics will require vigilant home nursing care.

Assessment findings are often nonspecific (see Table 39.6) but can help assist with the treatment plan. Fever, chronic or intermittent, is a common early sign. The patient or the caregiver needs instructions about the importance of monitoring body temperature because persistent, prolonged temperature elevations may mean that the medication therapy is ineffective. Patients with IE are at risk for life-threatening complications, such as cerebral emboli, pulmonary edema, and HF. Patients and caregivers must be taught to recognize signs and symptoms of these complications (e.g., change in mental status, dyspnea, chest pain).

Patients with IE need adequate periods of physical and emotional rest. Bed rest may be necessary when fever is present or when there are complications (e.g., heart damage). Otherwise, the patient may ambulate and perform moderate activity. To prevent complications of immobility, the patient should wear elastic compression stockings, perform range-of-motion exercises, and cough and deep-breathe every 2 hours. Patients may experience anxiety and fear associated with the illness. The nurse must recognize such feelings and implement strategies to help the patient cope with the illness.

Laboratory data should be monitored to determine the effectiveness of the antibiotic therapy. Ongoing monitoring of blood cultures is necessary to ensure eradication of the infecting organism. IV lines should be monitored for patency, and antibiotics should be given according to schedule. Patients should be monitored continuously for adverse medication reactions.

During the course of therapy in either the home or the hospital setting, management will also focus on teaching the patient about the nature of the disease and on reducing the risk for reinfection. The nurse must explain to the patient the relationship of follow-up care, good nutrition, and early treatment of common infections (e.g., colds) to maintaining good health. The patient should be instructed about symptoms that may indicate recurrent infection, such as fever, fatigue, malaise, and chills. If any of these symptoms occur, the patient should be aware of the importance of notifying a health care provider. Finally, the patient must be instructed about the need for and importance of prophylactic antibiotic therapy before undergoing invasive procedures (see Table 39.3).

EVALUATION

Expected outcomes for the patient with IE are presented in NCP 39.1.

ACUTE PERICARDITIS

Pericarditis, which may occur on an acute basis, is a condition caused by inflammation of the pericardial sac (the pericardium). The *pericardium* is composed of the inner serous membrane (visceral pericardium), which closely adheres to the epicardial surface of the heart, and the outer fibrous (parietal) layer (see Figure 39.1). The *pericardial space* is the cavity between these two layers, and in the normal state, it contains 10 to 30 mL of serous fluid. Although the pericardium may be congenitally absent or surgically removed, it serves a useful anchoring function, provides lubrication to decrease friction during systolic and diastolic heart movements, and assists in preventing excessive dilation of the heart during diastole.

Etiology and Pathophysiology

The common causes of acute pericarditis are listed in Table 39.7. Acute pericarditis is most often (>70% of the time) idiopathic in higher-income countries, while infectious etiologies such as tuberculosis are more common in lower-income countries. With a variety of suspected viral causes, the coxsackievirus B group is the most commonly identified virus. In addition to idiopathic or viral pericarditis, causes of this syndrome include bacterial infection, fungal infection, acute myocardial infarction (MI), tuberculosis, neoplasm, autoimmune conditions, medication reactions, metabolic disorders, and trauma (Andreis et al., 2019; McNamara et al., 2019).

Pericarditis in the patient with acute MI may be described as two distinct syndromes: (a) *acute pericarditis*, which may occur within the initial 48 to 72 hours after an MI, and (b) *Dressler's syndrome* (late pericarditis), which appears 4 to 6 weeks after an MI (see Chapter 36).

An inflammatory response—including an influx of neutrophils, increased pericardial vascularity, and eventually fibrin deposition on the visceral pericardium—is the characteristic pathological finding in acute pericarditis (Figure 39.4).

Clinical Manifestations

Characteristic clinical manifestations found in acute pericarditis include progressive, frequently severe chest pain that is sharp and pleuritic in nature. The pain is generally worse with deep inspiration and when lying supine. It is relieved by sitting upright. The pain may radiate to the neck, arms, or left shoulder, making it difficult to differentiate from angina. One distinction is that the pain from pericarditis can be referred to the trapezius muscle (shoulder, upper back) because the phrenic nerve innervates these two regions. Pericarditis is diagnosed in 5% of people presenting to the emergency department with chest pain (McNamara et al., 2019). The dyspnea that accompanies acute pericarditis is related to the patient's need to breathe in rapid, shallow breaths to avoid chest pain and may be aggravated by fever and anxiety.

The hallmark finding in acute pericarditis is the pericardial friction rub. The rub is a scratching, grating, high-pitched

TABLE 39.7   ETIOLOGIES OF PERICARDITIS

Infectious
- Viral: coxsackievirus A and B, echovirus, adenovirus, mumps, rubella, Epstein-Barr, varicella-zoster, hepatitis B, hepatitis C, human immunodeficiency virus (HIV)
- Bacterial: *Mycobacterium tuberculosis* (most common; rarely other bacteria); pneumococci, staphylococci, streptococci, *Neisseria gonorrhoeae, Legionella pneumophila,* septicemia from Gram-negative organisms
- Fungal: *Histoplasma, Candida* species
- Infections: toxoplasmosis, Lyme disease

Noninfectious
- Uremia
- Myxedema
- Acute myocardial infarction
- Neoplasms: lung cancer, breast cancer, leukemia, Hodgkin's lymphoma, non-Hodgkin's lymphoma
- Trauma: thoracic surgery, pacemaker insertion, cardiac diagnostic procedures
- Radiation
- Dissecting aortic aneurysm

Hypersensitive or Autoimmune
- Delayed post–myocardial-pericardial injury
- Post–myocardial infarction (Dressler's) syndrome
- Postpericardiotomy syndrome
- Rheumatic fever
- Medication reactions: procainamide, hydralazine (Apresoline), isoniazid, doxorubicin, and daunorubicin (often associated with cardiomyopathy)
- Rheumatological diseases: rheumatoid arthritis, systemic lupus erythematosus, systemic sclerosis (scleroderma), ankylosing spondylitis

TABLE 39.8   MEASUREMENT OF PULSUS PARADOXUS

1. Make determination during quiet breathing with stable rhythm.
2. Determine systolic blood pressure.
3. Inflate blood pressure cuff until no sounds are heard with stethoscope.
4. Deflate cuff slowly until systolic sounds are heard on expiration and note the pressure.
5. Deflate cuff until systolic sounds are heard throughout the respiratory cycle and note the pressure.
6. Determine the difference between the measurements taken in Steps 4 and 5. This will equal the amount of paradox:

Sounds heard in expiration at	110 mm Hg
Sounds heard throughout cycle at	82 mm Hg
Amount of paradox	28 mm Hg

The difference is usually <10 mm Hg. If the difference is >10 mm Hg, cardiac tamponade may be present.

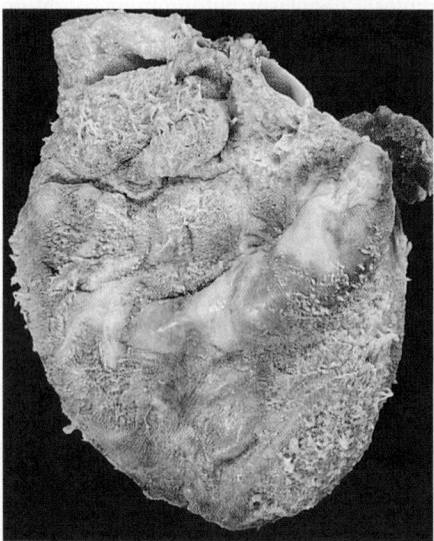

FIG. 39.4 Acute pericarditis. Note the shaggy coat of fibrin covering the surface of the heart. Source: Damjanov, I., & Linder, J. (2000). *Pathology: A color atlas.* Mosby.

sound believed to arise from friction between the roughened pericardial and epicardial surfaces. It is best heard with the stethoscope placed at the lower left sternal border of the chest with the patient leaning forward. Since it is difficult to tell a pericardial friction rub from a pleural friction rub, patients can be asked to hold their breath. If the rub is still heard, then it is cardiac. Pericardial friction rubs may require frequent attempts to identify because they are often intermittent and short-lived.

Complications

Two major complications that may result from acute pericarditis are pericardial effusion and cardiac tamponade. Pericardial effusion is an accumulation of excess fluid in the pericardium. It can occur rapidly (e.g., chest trauma) or slowly (e.g., tuberculous pericarditis). Large effusions may compress adjoining structures. Pulmonary tissue compression can cause cough, dyspnea, and tachypnea. Phrenic nerve compression can induce hiccups, and compression of the recurrent laryngeal nerve may result in hoarseness. Heart sounds are generally distant and muffled, although blood pressure (BP) is usually maintained by compensatory mechanisms.

Cardiac tamponade, also referred to as *pericardial tamponade*, develops as fluid accumulates in the pericardial sac (pericardial effusion), causing an increase in intrapericardial pressure and producing compression of the heart. The speed of fluid accumulation affects the severity of clinical manifestations. Cardiac tamponade can occur acutely (e.g., rupture of heart, trauma) or subacutely (e.g., secondary to uremia, malignancy). The patient with cardiac tamponade may report chest pain and is often confused, anxious, and restless. As the compression of the heart increases, heart sounds become muffled and the pulse pressure is narrowed. The patient will develop tachypnea, tachycardia, and a decreased cardiac output (CO). The neck veins are usually markedly distended because of increased jugular venous pressure, and a significant pulsus paradoxus is present. *Pulsus paradoxus* is a decrease in systolic BP with inspiration that is exaggerated in cardiac tamponade. (See Table 39.8 for the measurement technique.) In a patient with a slow onset of a cardiac tamponade, dyspnea may be the only clinical manifestation.

Diagnostic Studies

The ECG is useful in the diagnosis of acute pericarditis, with changes noted in approximately 90% of cases. The most sensitive ECG changes include diffuse (widespread) ST-segment elevations or PR-segment depression. This reflects the abnormal repolarization that develops secondary to the pericardial inflammation. It is important to differentiate these changes from the ST changes seen in MI. (See Chapter 38 for more

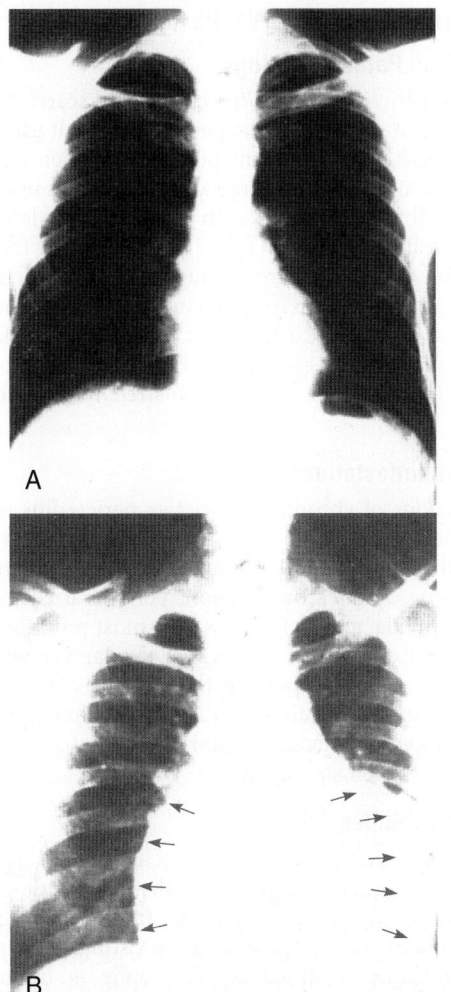

FIG. 39.5 **A,** Radiograph of a normal chest. **B,** Pericardial effusion is present and the cardiac silhouette is enlarged with a globular shape (*arrows*). Source: Guzetta, C. E., & Dossey, B. M. (1992). *Cardiovascular nursing: Holistic practice.* Mosby.

TABLE 39.9 INTERPROFESSIONAL CARE
Acute Pericarditis

Diagnostic	Interprofessional Therapy
• History and physical examination • Auscultation of chest • ECG • Laboratory: CRP, ESR, white blood cell count, BUN*, serum creatinine • TB test • Chest radiographic examination • Echocardiogram • Pericardiocentesis • Pericardial biopsy • CT scan • Cardiac nuclear scan	• Treatment of underlying disease • Bed rest • ASA (Aspirin) • NSAIDs • Colchicine • Corticosteroids • Pericardiocentesis (for large pericardial effusion or tamponade) • Pericardial window (for tamponade or ongoing pericardial effusion)

ASA, acetylsalicylic acid; *BUN,* blood urea nitrogen; *CRP,* C-reactive protein; *CT,* computed tomography; *ECG,* electrocardiogram; *ESR,* erythrocyte sedimentation rate; *NSAIDs,* nonsteroidal anti-inflammatory drugs; *TB,* tuberculosis.
*Serum urea (nitrogen).

information on ECG monitoring.) The chest radiographic findings are generally normal, but cardiomegaly may be seen in a patient who has a large pericardial effusion (Figure 39.5). Echocardiographic findings are more useful in determining the presence of a pericardial effusion or cardiac tamponade. Newer methods such as tissue Doppler imaging and colour M-mode Doppler imaging of early left ventricular flow help to assess diastolic function and diagnose constrictive pericarditis (discussed later in the chapter). Computed tomography (CT) and cardiac magnetic resonance imaging (CMRI) provide for visualization of the pericardium and pericardial space (McNamara et al., 2019).

Common laboratory findings include leukocytosis and elevation of CRP and ESR. Troponin levels may be elevated in patients with ST-segment elevation and acute pericarditis, a reading that would indicate concurrent myocardial damage. The fluid obtained during pericardiocentesis or the tissue from a pericardial biopsy may also be analyzed to determine the cause of the pericarditis.

Interprofessional Care

Management of acute pericarditis is directed toward identification and treatment of the underlying issue (Table 39.9). Antibiotics should be used to treat bacterial pericarditis. Corticosteroids

may be used for patients with pericarditis secondary to systemic inflammatory diseases such as systemic lupus erythematosus, patients already taking corticosteroids, or patients whose symptoms do not respond to nonsteroidal anti-inflammatory drugs (NSAIDS) or for certain populations where NSAIDS are contraindicated (e.g., patients with renal failure, who are pregnant, or on anticoagulation with increased bleeding risk) (Imagzio & Gaita, 2017). When necessary, prednisone is usually given according to a tapering dosage schedule. Corticosteroids are administered with caution because of their numerous adverse effects, such as upper gastrointestinal bleeding, sodium retention, hyperglycemia, hypokalemia, and Cushing's syndrome (see Chapter 51).

The chest pain and inflammation of acute pericarditis are usually treated with ASA or NSAIDs plus Colcrys (Colchicine). Corticosteroids may be added as a second-line option. The use of Colchicine with anti-inflammatories may reduce the recurrence rate of pericarditis by up to half. For patients with recurrences despite usual therapy, alternative therapies such as azathioprine (Imuran), intravenous immunoglobulin (IVIG), and anakinra (Kineret) may be considered (Imazio & Gaita, 2017)

If surgical drainage is necessary, a **pericardiocentesis** may be performed. During this procedure, a 16- to 18-gauge needle is inserted into the pericardial space to remove fluid for analysis and to relieve cardiac pressure. The procedure is rapid and safe and done using a percutaneous approach that is guided by ECG and echocardiography (Figure 39.6). It is usually performed for pericardial effusion with acute cardiac tamponade, purulent pericarditis, and a high index of suspicion of neoplasm. Hemodynamic support for the patient being prepared for the pericardiocentesis may include administration of volume expanders and inotropic medications (e.g., dopamine) and the discontinuation of any anticoagulants (see Figure 39.6). Complications from pericardiocentesis include dysrhythmias, further cardiac tamponade, pneumomediastinum, pneumothorax, myocardial laceration, and coronary artery laceration.

NURSING MANAGEMENT
ACUTE PERICARDITIS

The management of the patient's pain and anxiety during acute pericarditis is a primary nursing consideration.

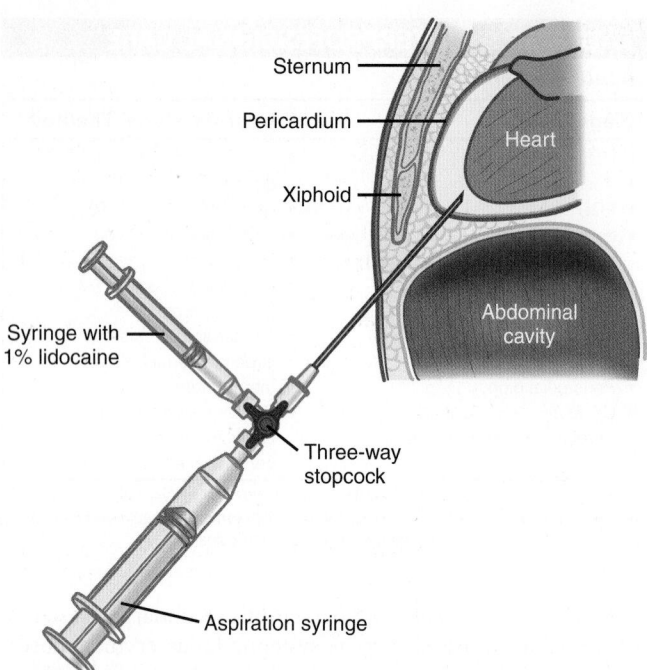

FIG. 39.6 Pericardiocentesis performed under sterile conditions in conjunction with electrocardiogram (ECG) and hemodynamic measurements.

Assessment of the amount, quality, and location of the pain is important, particularly in distinguishing the pain of myocardial ischemia (angina) from the pain of pericarditis. Pericarditic pain is usually located in the precordium or left trapezius ridge and has a sharp, pleuritic quality that increases with inspiration. Pain is often relieved by sitting or leaning forward, and the pain is worsened when lying supine. ECG monitoring can aid in distinguishing these types of pain because ischemia usually involves localized ST-segment changes, as compared with the diffuse ST-segment changes present in acute pericarditis.

Pain relief measures include maintaining the patient on bed rest with the head of the bed elevated to 45 degrees and providing an overbed table for support. Anti-inflammatory medications help alleviate the patient's pain; however, at high doses they can cause upper gastrointestinal bleeding. Nursing interventions, therefore, should be directed toward identification and management of this potential adverse effect. Specific interventions include administering these medications with food or milk and instructing the patient to avoid any alcoholic beverages while taking the medications.

Other medications, such as misoprostol, or a proton pump inhibitor may be ordered to protect the gastric mucosa. Anxiety-reducing measures for patients with acute pericarditis include providing simple, complete explanations of all procedures performed and the possible cause of the pain. These explanations are particularly important for patients whose diagnosis of acute pericarditis is being established and for patients who have already experienced angina or an acute MI.

The potential for decreased CO exists for patients with acute pericarditis because of the possibility of cardiac tamponade. Monitoring for the signs and symptoms of tamponade and preparing for possible pericardiocentesis are important nursing responsibilities.

CHRONIC CONSTRICTIVE PERICARDITIS

Etiology and Pathophysiology

Chronic constrictive pericarditis results from scarring with consequent loss of elasticity of the pericardial sac. It usually begins with an initial episode of acute pericarditis (often secondary to idiopathic causes, cardiac surgery, or radiation) and is characterized by fibrin deposition with a clinically undetected pericardial effusion. Resorption of the effusion slowly follows, with progression toward the chronic stage of fibrous scarring, thickening of the pericardium from calcium deposition, and eventual obliteration of the pericardial space. The fibrotic, thickened, and adherent pericardium encases the heart, thereby impairing the ability of the atria and ventricles to stretch adequately during diastole.

Clinical Manifestations

Manifestations of chronic constrictive pericarditis occur over an extended period and mimic those of HF and cor pulmonale. Many of the clinical manifestations are related to decreased CO. They include dyspnea on exertion, peripheral edema, ascites, fatigue, anorexia, and weight loss. The most prominent finding on physical examination is elevated jugular venous pressure. Unlike with cardiac tamponade, the presence of significant pulsus paradoxus is uncommon. Auscultatory findings include a *pericardial knock,* which is a loud, early diastolic sound often heard along the left sternal border.

Diagnostic Studies

ECG results are often nonspecific in chronic constrictive pericarditis. The cardiac silhouette on the chest radiograph may be normal or enlarged depending on the degree of pericardial thickening and the presence of a coexisting pericardial effusion. Two-dimensional echocardiography is insensitive for determining pericardial thickness but may inform the health care provider about the physiology. Colour M-mode and tissue Doppler imaging are used to confirm constrictive pericarditis. CT and MRI provide measurement of pericardial thickness and assessment of diastolic filling patterns. Cardiac catheterization is indicated when noninvasive investigation such as Doppler echocardiography, CT, or MRI do not provide definitive diagnosis (Welch, 2018).

NURSING AND INTERPROFESSIONAL MANAGEMENT CHRONIC CONSTRICTIVE PERICARDITIS

Unless the patient is free of symptoms or the condition is inoperable, the treatment of choice for chronic constrictive pericarditis is a *pericardiectomy.* This procedure involves complete resection of the pericardium through a median sternotomy with the use of cardiopulmonary bypass. Some patients show immediate improvement after surgery, but others may take weeks. The postoperative prognosis is improved when the surgery is performed before severe clinical disability has developed.

MYOCARDITIS

Etiology and Pathophysiology

Myocarditis is a focal or diffuse inflammation of the myocardium. Possible causes include viruses, bacteria, fungi, parasites, radiation therapy, pharmacological or chemical factors, and immune-mediated disease. Viruses, particularly coxsackievirus types A and B, are the most common causative agents of myocarditis in Canada and the United States. Autoimmune disorders (e.g., polymyositis) also have been associated with the development of myocarditis. In some cases, no causative agent or factor can be identified (i.e., *idiopathic* myocarditis). Myocarditis can be seen with pericardial involvement, *myopericarditis* (mostly pericarditis with myocardial involvement), as well as *perimyocarditis*, which is primarily myocarditis with pericarditis (Fardman et al., 2016). When the myocardium becomes infected, the causative agent invades the myocytes and causes cellular damage and necrosis. The immune response is activated, and cytokines and oxygen free radicals are released. As the infection progresses, an autoimmune response is activated, leading to further destruction of myocytes. Myocarditis results in cardiac dysfunction and has been linked to the development of dilated cardiomyopathy (DCM) (discussed later in this chapter).

Clinical Manifestations

The clinical features of myocarditis are variable, ranging from a benign course without any overt manifestations to severe heart involvement or sudden cardiac death (SCD). Fever, fatigue, malaise, myalgias, pharyngitis, dyspnea, lymphadenopathy, and nausea and vomiting are early systemic manifestations of the viral illness.

Early cardiac manifestations appear 7 to 10 days after viral infection. These include pleuritic chest pain with a pericardial friction rub and effusion, because pericarditis often accompanies myocarditis. Late cardiac signs relate to the development of HF and may include a third heart sound (S_3), crackles, jugular venous distension, syncope, peripheral edema, and angina.

Diagnostic Studies

The ECG changes for a patient with myocarditis are often nonspecific and reflect associated pericardial involvement (e.g., diffuse ST-segment abnormalities). Dysrhythmias and conduction disturbances may be present. Laboratory findings are also often inconclusive. They may include mild to moderate leukocytosis and atypical lymphocytes, increased ESR and CRP levels, elevated levels of myocardial markers such as troponin, and elevated viral titres (virus is generally present in tissue and fluid samples only during the initial 8–10 days of illness). Histological confirmation of myocarditis is done through endomyocardial biopsy (EMB). This technique involves removing several small pieces of myocardial tissue percutaneously from the right ventricle with a special instrument called a *bioptome* and microscopically examining the samples (Ammirati et al., 2018). A biopsy done during the initial 6 weeks of acute illness is most diagnostic because, in this period, lymphocytic infiltration and myocyte damage indicative of myocarditis are present. Other studies to evaluate cardiac function include echocardiography, nuclear scans, and MRI.

Interprofessional Care

The treatment for myocarditis in patients with fulminant HF includes cardiovascular support with inotropic or vasopressor therapy, or both, and mechanical circulatory support (e.g., left ventricular assist device [LVAD]). Care of patients with both myocarditis and HF with reduced ejection fraction (HFrEF) is the same usual care for HFrEF patients: β blockers, angiotensin-converting enzyme (ACE) inhibitor/angiotensin receptor blocker (ARB) or angiotensin-neprolysin inhibitor (ARNI), mineralocorticoid receptor antagonist (MRA), and diuretic

therapy, the last of which may help to reduce fluid volume and decrease preload (Ezikowitz et al., 2017). Immunosuppressive therapy with medications such as prednisone and azathioprine (Imuran) may be used in management of the patient with biopsy-proven giant-cell myocarditis or eosinophilic myocarditis or when viral genome has been excluded (Ammirati et al., 2018). For patients with systemic immune-mediated disease, with proven myocarditis, immunosuppressive and/or immunomodulatory therapies are targeted to the level of disease activity. Oxygen therapy, bed rest, restricted activity, and maintenance of standby emergency equipment are general supportive measures in the management of myocarditis.

NURSING MANAGEMENT
MYOCARDITIS

Decreased CO is an ongoing nursing diagnosis in the care of the patient with myocarditis. Interventions focus on assessment for the signs and symptoms of HF. Important nursing measures to decrease cardiac workload include using semi-Fowler's position, spacing out activity and rest periods, and providing a quiet environment. Prescribed medications that increase the heart's contractility and decrease the preload, afterload, or both require careful monitoring. Ongoing evaluation of the effectiveness of these interventions is necessary.

Patients may be anxious about the diagnosis of myocarditis, recovery from myocarditis, and the therapeutic plan. Nursing measures include assessing the patient's level of anxiety, instituting measures to decrease anxiety, and keeping the patient and caregivers informed about therapeutic measures.

Patients who receive immunosuppressive therapy have additional concerns of alterations in the immune response with the potential for infection and complications related to the therapy. Guidelines for care include monitoring for complications and providing the patient with a clean, safe environment by following proper infection-control procedures. Most patients with myocarditis recover spontaneously, although some may develop DCM. If severe HF occurs, the patient may require heart transplantation.

RHEUMATIC FEVER AND HEART DISEASE

Rheumatic fever is defined by the Heart and Stroke Foundation of Canada (2021b) as "an inflammatory disease that may affect several connective tissues of the body, especially those of the heart, brain, joints, or skin." Rheumatic fever potentially involves all layers of the heart (endocardium, myocardium, and pericardium). Rheumatic heart disease is a chronic condition resulting from rheumatic fever that is characterized by scarring and deformity of the heart valves.

Etiology and Pathophysiology

Acute rheumatic fever (ARF) is a complication that occurs as a delayed result (usually after 2–3 weeks) of group A streptococcal pharyngitis (Watkins et al., 2018). Manifestations of ARF appear to be related to an abnormal immunological response to group A streptococcal cell membrane antigens. The incidence of ARF has declined in higher-income countries as a result of the effective use of antibiotics to treat streptococcal infections. However, it remains an important public health problem in lower-income countries. The sequela of ARF, rheumatic heart disease, is found primarily in young adults.

Cardiac Lesions and Valvular Deformities. About 40% of ARF episodes are marked by carditis, and all layers of the heart (endocardium, myocardium, and pericardium) may be involved (see Figure 39.1). This generalized involvement gives rise to the term *rheumatic pancarditis.*

Rheumatic endocarditis is found primarily in the valves, with swelling and erosion of the valve leaflets. Vegetations form from deposits of fibrin and blood cells in areas of erosion. The lesions initially create fibrous thickening of the valve leaflets, fusion of commissures and chordae tendineae, and fibrosis of the papillary muscle. Valve leaflets may fuse and become thickened or even calcified, resulting in stenosis. Reduction in the mobility of valve leaflets may occur with failure of the leaflets, resulting in regurgitation. The mitral and aortic valves are most commonly affected.

Myocardial involvement is characterized by Aschoff bodies, which are tiny, rounded, or spindle-shaped nodules formed by a reaction to inflammation with accompanying swelling and fragmentation of collagen fibres. As the Aschoff bodies age, they become more fibrous and scar tissue forms in the myocardium. In addition to Aschoff bodies, a diffuse cellular infiltrate is present in interstitial tissues. Rheumatic pericarditis affects both layers of the pericardium, which become thickened and covered with a fibrinous exudate, and a serosanguineous pericardial effusion may develop. When healing occurs, fibrosis and adhesions develop that partially or completely obliterate the pericardial sac, but constrictive pericarditis does not occur.

These pathophysiological changes in the heart may occur as a result of an initial attack of rheumatic fever. However, recurrent infections may cause further structural damage.

Extracardiac Lesions. The lesions of rheumatic fever are systemic, involving the connective tissues especially. The joints (polyarthritis), skin (subcutaneous nodules), and central nervous system may be involved in rheumatic fever.

Clinical Manifestations

Symptoms of ARF can include chest pain, excessive fatigue, heart palpitations (the heart fluttering or missing beats), a thumping sensation in the chest, shortness of breath, and swollen ankles, wrists, or stomach (Heart and Stroke Foundation of Canada, 2021b). The diagnosis of ARF is suggested by a clustering of signs and symptoms as well as by laboratory findings. When not observed in its most severe form, the disease may be difficult to differentiate from many illnesses with similar clinical manifestations. Criteria established by T. D. Jones in 1944 have been revised by the American Heart Association and provide a basis for diagnosis (Gewitz et al., 2015) (Table 39.10). The presence of two major criteria or one major and two minor criteria plus evidence of a preceding group A streptococcal infection indicates a high probability of ARF.

Major Criteria. *Carditis* is the most important manifestation of ARF and results in three signs: (a) an organic heart murmur or murmurs of mitral or aortic regurgitation or mitral stenosis; (b) cardiac enlargement and HF occurring secondary to myocarditis; and (c) pericarditis resulting in muffled heart sounds, chest pain, a pericardial friction rub, or signs of effusion.

Mono- or *polyarthritis* is the most common finding in rheumatic fever. The inflammatory process affects the synovial membranes of the joints, causing swelling, heat, redness, tenderness, and limitation of motion. The larger joints are most frequently affected, particularly knees, ankles, elbows, and wrists.

TABLE 39.10	MODIFIED JONES CRITERIA FOR ACUTE RHEUMATIC FEVER	
Major Criteria	**Minor Criteria**	**Evidence of Group A Streptococcal Infection**
• Carditis • Mono- or polyarthritis • Sydenham chorea • Erythema marginatum • Subcutaneous nodules	• Clinical findings: fever, polyarthralgia • Laboratory findings: ↑ ESR, ↑ WBC count, ↑ CRP • ECG findings: prolonged PR interval	• Laboratory findings: ↑ antistreptolysin • O titre, positive throat culture, positive rapid antigen test for group A streptococci

CRP, C-reactive protein; *ECG*, electrocardiogram; *ESR*, erythrocyte sedimentation rate; *WBC*, white blood cell.

Chorea (Sydenham chorea) is the major central nervous system manifestation of ARF, often a delayed sign occurring several months after the initial infection. It is characterized by involuntary movements, especially of the face and the limbs, muscle weakness, and disturbances of speech and gait.

Erythema marginatum lesions are a less common feature of ARF. The bright pink map-like macular lesions occur mainly on the trunk and the proximal extremities and may be exacerbated by heat (e.g., warm bath). Subcutaneous nodules, usually associated with severe carditis, are firm, small, hard, painless swellings located over extensor surfaces of the joints, particularly knees, wrists, and elbows.

Minor Criteria. Minor clinical manifestations (see Table 39.10) are frequently present and are helpful in diagnosing the disease. The minor criteria are used as supplemental data to confirm the presence of rheumatic fever when only one major criterion is present.

Complications

A complication that can result from ARF is *chronic rheumatic carditis.* It results from changes in valvular structure that may occur months to years after an episode of ARF. Rheumatic endocarditis can result in fibrous tissue growth in valve leaflets and chordae tendineae with scarring and contractures. The mitral valve is most frequently involved; the aortic or tricuspid valve or both may also be affected.

Diagnostic Studies

No single diagnostic test exists for rheumatic fever (see Table 39.10). An echocardiogram may show valvular insufficiency and pericardial fluid or thickening. A chest radiographic study may show an enlarged heart if HF is present. The most consistent ECG change is delayed AV conduction as evidenced by prolongation of the PR interval.

Interprofessional Care

Treatment consists of medication therapy and supportive measures (Table 39.11). Antibiotic therapy does not modify the course of the acute disease or the development of carditis. It does eliminate residual group A streptococci remaining in the tonsils and the pharynx and prevent the spread of organisms to close contacts. Salicylates, NSAIDs, and corticosteroids are the anti-inflammatory medications most widely used in the management of ARF. All are effective in controlling the fever

TABLE 39.11 INTERPROFESSIONAL CARE
Rheumatic Fever

Diagnostic	Interprofessional Therapy
• History and physical examination	• Bed rest (modified)
• Laboratory findings (see Table 39.10)	• Benzathine penicillin (1.2 million units IM) daily for 10 days
• Throat culture	• Acetylsalicylic acid
• Chest radiograph	• Corticosteroids
• Echocardiogram	• Codeine
• ECG	• Carbamazepine, valproic acid, phenobarbital

ECG, electrocardiogram; *IM,* intramuscularly.

TABLE 39.12 NURSING ASSESSMENT
Rheumatic Fever and Rheumatic Heart Disease

Subjective Data
Important Health Information
Past health history: Recent β-hemolytic streptococcal infection, previous rheumatic fever or rheumatic heart disease, family history of rheumatic fever

Symptoms
- Malaise, generalized weakness, fatigue
- Anorexia; weight loss
- Palpitations
- Ataxia; migratory joint pain and tenderness (especially large joints)
- Chest pain

Objective Data
General
Low-grade fever

Integumentary
Subcutaneous nodules and erythema marginatum

Cardiovascular
Tachycardia, pericardial friction rub, distant heart sounds; gallop rhythm, diastolic and systolic murmurs, peripheral edema

Neurological
Chorea (involuntary, purposeless, rapid motions; facial grimaces)

Musculoskeletal
Signs of polyarthritis including swelling, heat, redness, limitation of motion (especially of knees, ankles, elbows, shoulders, and wrists)

Possible Findings
Cardiomegaly on chest radiographic study; delayed AV conduction on ECG; valve abnormalities, chamber dilation, and pericardial effusion on echocardiogram; ↑ ASO titre, ↑ ESR, ↑ CRP, leukocytosis

ASO, antistreptolysin O; *AV,* atrioventricular; *CRP,* C-reactive protein; *ECG,* electrocardiogram; *ESR,* erythrocyte sedimentation rate.

and joint manifestations. Salicylates or NSAIDs are used when arthritis is the main manifestation, and corticosteroids are used if severe carditis is present.

NURSING MANAGEMENT RHEUMATIC FEVER AND HEART DISEASE

NURSING ASSESSMENT
Subjective and objective data that should be obtained from a patient with rheumatic fever and heart disease are presented in Table 39.12. It is important to note that rheumatic fever is more likely to reoccur in a person with a previous history of rheumatic fever than to occur in the general population. The skin of the patient should be assessed for subcutaneous nodules and erythema marginatum. The procedure involves palpation for subcutaneous nodules over all bony surfaces and along extensor tendons of the hands and feet. The nodules range in size from 1 to 4 cm and are hard, painless, and freely movable. Erythema marginatum can occur on the trunk and the inner aspects of the upper arm and the thigh. The erythematous map-like macules do not itch and are not raised. The possible presence of these bright pink macules should be assessed in good light because the rash is difficult to observe, especially if the patient is dark skinned.

NURSING DIAGNOSES
Nursing diagnoses for the patient with rheumatic fever and heart disease may include but are not limited to the following:
- *Decreased cardiac output* (resulting from valve dysfunction or HF)
- *Reduced stamina* resulting from *physical deconditioning* (arthralgia, arthritis, pain from pericarditis)
- *Inadequate health management* as a result of *insufficient knowledge of therapeutic regimen* (need for long-term prophylactic antibiotic therapy)

PLANNING
The overall goals for a patient with rheumatic fever include (a) normal or baseline heart function, (b) resumption of daily activities without joint pain, and (c) verbalization of the ability to manage the disease.

NURSING IMPLEMENTATION
HEALTH PROMOTION. Rheumatic fever is a preventable cardiovascular disease. Prevention involves early detection and immediate treatment of group A β-hemolytic streptococcal pharyngitis. Adequate treatment of streptococcal pharyngitis prevents initial attacks of rheumatic fever. Treatment consists of intramuscular injection of penicillin G benzathine (Bicillin L-A) or oral penicillin V potassium. If the patient is allergic to penicillin, erythromycin or azithromycin (Zithromax) may be substituted. Oral therapy requires faithful adherence to the full course of treatment. The nurse's role is to educate people in the community to seek medical attention for symptoms of streptococcal pharyngitis and to emphasize the need for adequate treatment of this infection.

ACUTE INTERVENTION. The primary goals of managing a patient with ARF are to control and eradicate the infecting organism; prevent cardiac complications; relieve joint pain, fever, and other symptoms; and support the patient psychologically and emotionally. The nurse should administer antibiotics as ordered to treat the streptococcal infection and should teach the patient that oral antibiotic therapy requires faithful adherence to the full course of therapy. Antipyretics, NSAIDs, and corticosteroids should be administered as prescribed and fluid intake monitored. Promotion of optimal rest is essential to reduce the cardiac workload and diminish the metabolic needs of the body. Relief of joint pain is an important nursing goal. Painful joints should be positioned for comfort and proper alignment. Heat may be applied and salicylates or NSAIDs administered to relieve joint pain. After the acute symptoms have subsided, the patient without carditis should ambulate. If the patient has carditis with HF, bed rest restrictions should be maintained. (See Chapter 37 for care of a patient with HF.)

Nonstrenuous activities should be encouraged once recovery has begun.

AMBULATORY AND HOME CARE. The aim of secondary prevention is to prevent the recurrence of rheumatic fever. The patient with a previous history of rheumatic fever should be taught about the disease process, possible sequelae, and the ongoing or permanent need for prophylactic antibiotics. Prior history of rheumatic fever makes the patient more susceptible to a second attack after a streptococcal infection. The best prevention is monthly injections of long-acting penicillin. Alternative treatment is administration of oral penicillin or erythromycin one or two times a day. Rheumatic fever without carditis may require 5 to 10 years of prophylactic antibiotic therapy or up until age 21 years, or longer in high-risk patients. Secondary prophylaxis for those with rheumatic fever with carditis should continue for 10 years or up until age 40. Those with chronic carditis should continue prophylaxis for life (Zuhlke et al., 2017).

The dosage of antibiotics used in maintenance prophylaxis of rheumatic fever is not adequate to prevent IE when invasive procedures are performed. Additional prophylaxis is necessary if a patient with known rheumatic heart disease has a dental procedure or an invasive respiratory tract procedure (e.g., tonsillectomy) that involves perforation of the mucosa (see Table 39.3). The nurse must explain the difference between these two prophylactic programs.

Patient teaching should encourage good nutrition, hygienic practices, and adequate rest. The patient should also be cautioned about the possibility of developing valvular heart disease. The nurse should teach the patient to seek medical attention if symptoms such as excessive fatigue, dizziness, palpitations, or exertional dyspnea develop.

▌EVALUATION

The following are expected outcomes for patients with rheumatic fever and heart disease:

- Ability to perform activities of daily living with minimal fatigue and pain
- Adherence to treatment regimen
- Expression of confidence in managing disease
- Prevention of complications

▌VALVULAR HEART DISEASE

The heart contains two AV valves, the mitral and the tricuspid, and two semilunar valves, the aortic and the pulmonic, that are located in four strategic locations to control unidirectional blood flow (see Figure 34.2). Valvular heart disease is defined according to the valve or valves affected and the types of functional alteration: stenosis or regurgitation.

The pressure on either side of an open valve is normally equal. However, in a stenotic valve, the valve orifice is restricted, impeding the forward flow of blood and creating a pressure gradient across an open valve. The degree of *stenosis* (constriction or narrowing) is reflected in the degree of the pressure gradient (i.e., the higher the gradient, the greater the stenosis). In **regurgitation** (also called *valvular incompetence* or *insufficiency*), incomplete closure of the valve leaflets results in the backward flow of blood.

Valve disorders occur in children and adolescents primarily when congenital conditions such as tricuspid atresia, pulmonary stenosis, and aortic stenosis are present. Valvular heart disease has remained prevalent because of an increase in the number of older persons, many of whom have some form of cardiovascular disease. Aortic stenosis and mitral regurgitation (MR) are common valve disorders in older people. Other causes of valve disease in adults include inflammatory disorders, drug-induced disease, and radiation exposure (Lung & Kappetein, 2018).

MITRAL VALVE STENOSIS

Etiology and Pathophysiology

Most cases of adult mitral valve stenosis result from rheumatic heart disease; rheumatic mitral stenosis is most prevalent in low-income countries. Degenerative calcific mitral stenosis is more common in older patients (Vahanian, 2018). Less common causes include congenital mitral stenosis, rheumatoid arthritis, and systemic lupus erythematosus. Rheumatic endocarditis causes scarring of the valve leaflets and the chordae tendineae. Contractures and adhesions develop between the commissures (the junctional areas) of the two leaflets (Figure 39.7). These structural deformities cause obstruction of blood flow and create a pressure difference between the left atrium and the left ventricle during diastole. Left atrial pressure and volume elevations cause increased pulmonary vasculature pressure and subsequent hypertrophy of the pulmonary vessels. In chronic mitral stenosis, pressure overload occurs in the left atrium, the pulmonary bed, and the right ventricle.

Clinical Manifestations

The primary symptom of mitral stenosis is exertional dyspnea owing to reduced lung compliance (Table 39.13). Fatigue and palpitations from atrial fibrillation may occur. Heart sounds include a loud first heart sound and a low-pitched, rumbling

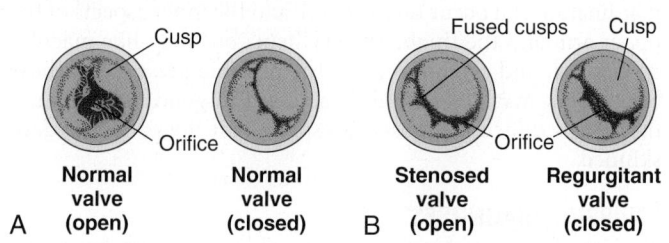

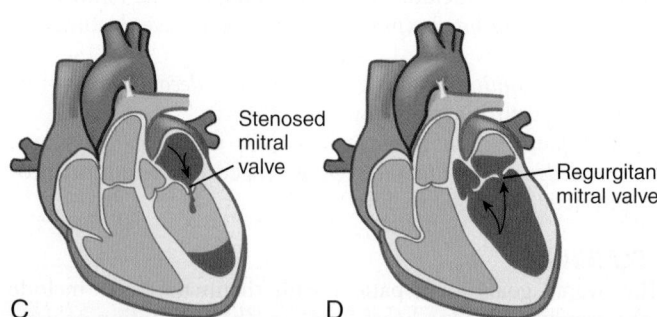

FIG. 39.7 Valvular stenosis and regurgitation. **A,** Normal position of the valve leaflets, or cusps, when the valve is open and closed. **B,** Open position of a stenosed valve *(left)* and closed position of regurgitant valve *(right)*. **C,** Hemodynamic effect of mitral stenosis. The stenosed valve is unable to open sufficiently during left atrial systole, inhibiting left ventricular filling. **D,** Hemodynamic effect of mitral regurgitation. The mitral valve does not close completely during left ventricular systole, permitting blood to re-enter the left atrium. At the same time, blood is moving forward through the aortic valve. Source: Huether, S. E., McCance, K. L., Brashers, V. L., et al. (2014). *Pathophysiology: The biologic basis for disease in adults and children* (7th ed., p. 1167). Mosby.

TABLE 39.13   CLINICAL MANIFESTATIONS AND DIAGNOSTIC FINDINGS OF VALVULAR HEART DISEASES

	Clinical Manifestations	Electrocardiogram	Echocardiogram	Cardiac Catheterization
Mitral valve stenosis	Exertional dyspnea, hemoptysis; fatigue; palpitations; loud, accentuated S₁; opening snap; low-pitched, rumbling diastolic murmur	Right axis deviation, left atrial enlargement, right ventricular hypertrophy, P mitrale (wide, M-shaped P wave), atrial flutter or fibrillation	Restricted movement of mitral valve leaflets; decreased size of orifice; diastolic turbulence	Left atrial pressure increased at end of diastole, reduction in CO
Mitral valve regurgitation	*Acute:* generally poorly tolerated with fulminating pulmonary edema and shock developing rapidly; systolic murmur	Left atrial enlargement, atrial fibrillation	Hyperdynamic left ventricular contraction in association with shock; regurgitant jets and flail* chordae or leaflets	Contrast medium injection in left ventricle showing regurgitation of blood into left atrium
	Chronic: weakness, fatigue, exertional dyspnea, palpitations; an S₃ gallop, holosystolic or pansystolic murmur	P mitrale, left ventricular hypertrophy, atrial flutter or fibrillation	Left atrial enlargement; left ventricular hypertrophy; flail leaflets	Contrast medium injection in left ventricle showing regurgitation of blood into left atrium
Mitral valve prolapse	Palpitations, dyspnea, chest pain, activity intolerance, syncope; mobile midsystolic nonejection click and a late or holosystolic murmur	Usually normal; occasionally T-wave inversion or biplasticity in leads II, III, and aVF are noted; PVCs and tachydysrhythmias possible	On the M-mode echocardiogram, late-systolic posterior motion or holosystolic billowing of the mitral leaflets; on two-dimensional echocardiogram, systolic billowing of the mitral leaflets	Left ventricular angiogram reveals mitral leaflets with prominent scalloping as the leaflets billow into the left atrium during systole
Aortic valve stenosis	Angina pectoris, syncope, heart failure, normal or soft S₁, prominent S₄, crescendo–decrescendo murmur	Left ventricular hypertrophy, left bundle branch block, complete atrioventricular heart block	Restricted movement of aortic valve; diminished orifice; systolic turbulence	Left ventricular systolic pressure increased, reduction in CO
Aortic valve regurgitation	*Acute:* abrupt onset of profound dyspnea, transient chest pain, progression to shock	Left ventricular strain	Normal-sized left ventricle with hyperdynamic systolic contraction; aortic dissection can be seen, if cause of acute process	Significant elevation of left ventricular diastolic pressure
	Chronic: fatigue, exertional dyspnea; water-hammer pulse; heaving precordial impulse; diastolic high-pitched soft decrescendo diastolic murmur, characteristic Austin Flint murmur at diastolic rumble, systolic ejection click	Left ventricular hypertrophy	Enlarged left ventricle and dilated aortic root	Increase in left ventricular diastolic pressure, aortic root contrast medium injection demonstrating regurgitation of blood into left ventricle
Tricuspid stenosis and regurgitation	Peripheral edema, ascites, hepatomegaly; diastolic low-pitched decrescendo murmur with increased intensity during inspiration (stenosis); pansystolic murmur with increased intensity at inspiration (regurgitation)	Tall, peaked P waves; atrial fibrillation	Right ventricular dilation and paradoxical septal motion; usually poor visualization of tricuspid valve itself	Pressure gradient across tricuspid valve and increased right atrial pressure (stenosis); reflux of contrast medium into right atrium (regurgitation)

aVF, augmented vector foot; *CO,* cardiac output; *PVCs,* premature ventricular contractions; *S₁,* first heart sound; *S₃,* third heart sound; *S₄,* fourth heart sound.
*Flail mitral leaflet is a complication of mitral valve prolapse, which can lead to severe mitral regurgitation and left ventricular dysfunction.

diastolic murmur (best heard at the apex with the stethoscope bell). Less frequently, patients may have hoarseness (from atrial enlargement pressing on the laryngeal nerve), hemoptysis (from pulmonary hypertension), chest pain (from decreased CO), and seizures or a stroke (from emboli). Emboli can arise from blood stasis in the left atrium.

MITRAL VALVE REGURGITATION

Etiology and Pathophysiology

Mitral valve function depends on intact mitral leaflets, mitral annulus, chordae tendineae, papillary muscles, left atrium, and left ventricular function. A defect in any of these structures can result in regurgitation. Most cases of MR are caused by MI, chronic rheumatic heart disease, mitral valve prolapse (MVP), ischemic papillary muscle dysfunction, or IE. MI with left ventricular failure increases the risk for rupture of the chordae tendineae and for acute MR.

MR allows blood to flow backward from the left ventricle to the left atrium because of incomplete valve closure during systole. The left ventricle and the left atrium both work harder to preserve an adequate CO. In chronic MR, the additional volume load results in atrial enlargement, ventricular dilation, and eventual ventricular hypertrophy. In acute MR, the left atrium and ventricle do not abruptly dilate. The sudden increase in pressure and volume is transmitted to the pulmonary bed, resulting in pulmonary edema and shock.

Clinical Manifestations

The clinical course of MR is determined by the nature of its onset (see Table 39.13). Patients with acute MR will have thready peripheral pulses and cool, clammy extremities. A low CO may obscure a new systolic murmur. Rapid assessment (e.g., cardiac catheterization) and intervention (e.g., valve repair or replacement) are critical for a positive outcome.

Patients with chronic MR may remain asymptomatic for many years until the development of some degree of left ventricular failure. Initial symptoms of left ventricular failure may include weakness, fatigue, palpitations, and dyspnea that gradually progress to orthopnea, paroxysmal nocturnal dyspnea, and peripheral edema. Accentuated left ventricular filling leads to an audible S_3, even with normal left ventricular function. The murmur is a loud holosystolic or pansystolic murmur at the apex radiating to the left axilla. Patients with asymptomatic MR should be monitored carefully because the natural history for MR can be variable, and surgery (valve repair or replacement) should be considered before significant left ventricular failure or pulmonary hypertension develops (Nishimura et al., 2017). Patients with symptomatic secondary, or functional, MR may be considered a candidate for percutaneous mitral valve repair (PMVR) or MitraClip (Figure 39.8) (O'Meara et al., 2020).

MITRAL VALVE PROLAPSE

Etiology and Pathophysiology

Mitral valve prolapse (MVP) is a structural abnormality of the mitral valve leaflets and the papillary muscles or chordae that allows the leaflets to prolapse, or buckle, back into the left atrium during ventricular systole (Figure 39.9). The etiology of MVP is unknown but is related to diverse pathogenic mechanisms of the mitral valve apparatus. The term *prolapse* is misleading because, in some cases, the valvular anomaly permits normal function. MVP is one of the most common forms of valvular heart disease.

MVP is usually benign, but serious complications can occur, including MR, IE, SCD, and cerebral ischemia. There is an increased familial incidence (autosomal dominant) among some patients.

Clinical Manifestations

MVP covers a broad spectrum of severity. Most patients are asymptomatic and remain so for their entire lives. A characteristic of MVP is a murmur from regurgitation that gets more intense through systole. This could be a late or holosystolic murmur. Another major sign is one or more clicks usually heard in midsystole to late systole. MVP does not alter the first (S_1) or second (S_2) heart sounds. Severe MR is an uncommon complication of MVP.

M-mode echocardiography confirms MVP by demonstrating late-systolic prolapse, and two-dimensional echocardiography reveals leaflet billowing into the left atrium. Dysrhythmias, most commonly ventricular premature contractions, paroxysmal supraventricular tachycardia, and ventricular tachycardia, may cause palpitations, light-headedness, and dizziness. IE may occur in patients with MR associated with MVP.

Patients may or may not have chest pain. The cause of the chest pain is not known, but it may be caused by abnormal

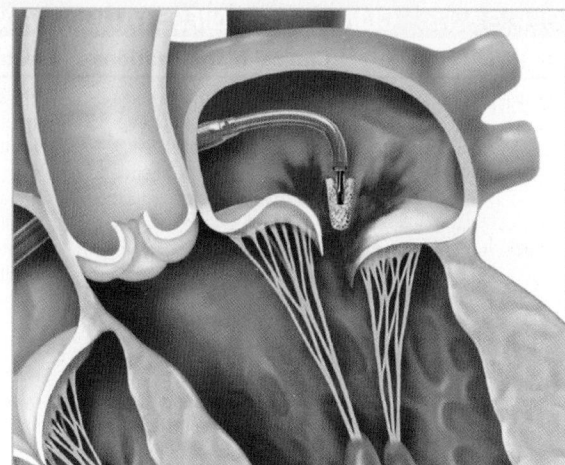

FIG. 39.8 MitraClipTM. ©Abbott.

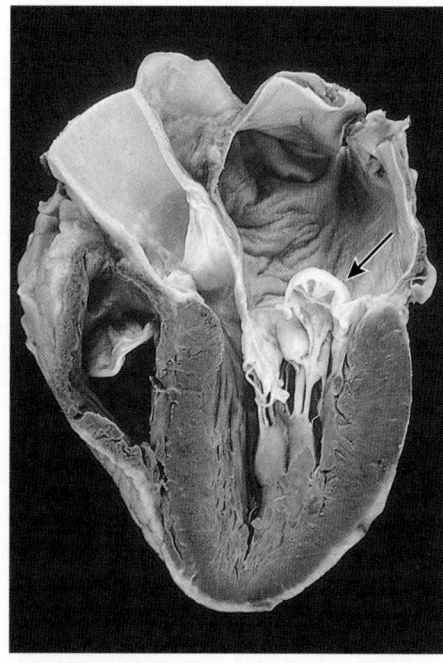

FIG. 39.9 Mitral valve prolapse. In this valvular abnormality, the mitral leaflets have prolapsed back into the left atrium. They also demonstrate hooding (*arrow*). The left ventricle is on the right. Source: Kumar, V., Abbas, A. K., & Aster, J. (2013). *Robbins basic pathology* (9th ed., p. 391). Elsevier Saunders.

tension on the papillary muscles. If chest pain occurs, it tends to occur in clusters, especially during periods of emotional stress. Dyspnea, palpitations, and syncope may occasionally accompany the chest pain and do not respond to antianginal treatment (e.g., nitrates). β-Adrenergic blockers may be prescribed to control palpitations and chest pain. Patients with MVP generally have a benign, manageable course unless conditions associated with MR are present. A teaching plan for patients with MVP appears in Table 39.14.

AORTIC VALVE STENOSIS

Etiology and Pathophysiology

Congenitally abnormal stenotic aortic valves are generally discovered in childhood, adolescence, or young adulthood. In older patients, aortic stenosis is a result of rheumatic fever or degeneration that may have an etiology similar to that of coronary artery disease. In rheumatic valvular disease, fusion of the commissures and secondary calcification cause the valve leaflets to stiffen and retract, resulting in stenosis. If aortic stenosis does occur owing to rheumatic heart disease, mitral valve disease accompanies it. Isolated aortic valve stenosis is almost always nonrheumatic in origin. The incidence of rheumatic aortic valvular disease has been decreasing, but senile or degenerative stenosis is expected to increase as the population ages.

Aortic stenosis causes obstruction of blood flow from the left ventricle to the aorta during systole. The effect is left ventricular hypertrophy and increased myocardial oxygen consumption because of the increased myocardial mass. As the disease course progresses and compensatory mechanisms fail, reduced CO leads to decreased tissue perfusion, pulmonary hypertension, and HF.

Clinical Manifestations

Symptoms of aortic stenosis (see Table 39.13) develop when the valve orifice becomes approximately one third its normal size. Symptoms include the classic triad of angina, syncope, and exertional dyspnea, reflecting left ventricular failure. The prognosis is poor for a patient with symptoms and whose valve obstruction is not relieved. Use of nitroglycerin is contraindicated for patients with significant aortic stenosis because it would reduce preload, and preload is necessary to help open the stiffened aortic valve. Auscultation of aortic stenosis typically reveals a normal or soft S_1; a diminished or absent S_2; a systolic, crescendo–decrescendo murmur that ends before S_2; and a prominent S_4.

> **MEDICATION ALERT—Nitroglycerin**
> - This medication must be used with caution in patients with aortic stenosis because it may cause significant hypotension.
> - Chest pain can worsen because of a decrease in preload and drop in BP.

AORTIC VALVE REGURGITATION

Etiology and Pathophysiology

Aortic valve regurgitation (AR) may be the result of a primary disease of the aortic valve leaflets, of the aortic root, or of both. Acute AR is caused by IE, trauma, or aortic dissection and constitutes a life-threatening emergency. Chronic AR is generally the result of rheumatic heart disease, a congenital bicuspid

aortic valve, syphilis, or chronic rheumatic conditions such as ankylosing spondylitis or Reiter's syndrome.

AR entails retrograde blood flow from the ascending aorta into the left ventricle when the valve should be closed, resulting in volume overload. The left ventricle initially compensates for chronic AR through dilation and hypertrophy. Myocardial contractility eventually declines, and blood volumes increase in the left atrium and the pulmonary bed. This increase results in pulmonary hypertension and right ventricular failure.

Clinical Manifestations

Patients with acute AR have sudden clinical manifestations of cardiovascular collapse (see Table 39.13). The left ventricle is exposed to aortic pressure during diastole. The patient develops severe dyspnea, chest pain, hypotension (indicating left ventricular failure), and shock, all of which constitute a medical emergency.

Patients with chronic, severe AR develop a *water-hammer pulse* (a strong, quick beat that collapses immediately). Heart sounds may include a soft or absent S_1, presence of S_3 or S_4, and a soft, decrescendo, high-pitched diastolic murmur. A systolic ejection click may also be heard as well as a low-frequency diastolic murmur known as an *Austin Flint murmur*.

The patient with chronic AR generally remains asymptomatic for years and is seen with exertional dyspnea, orthopnea, and paroxysmal nocturnal dyspnea only after considerable myocardial dysfunction has occurred (see Table 39.13). Angina occurs less frequently with AR than with aortic stenosis.

TRICUSPID AND PULMONIC VALVE DISEASE

Etiology and Pathophysiology

Diseases of the tricuspid and pulmonic valves are uncommon, with stenosis occurring more frequently than regurgitation. *Tricuspid valve stenosis* occurs almost exclusively in patients who have had rheumatic fever, have used IV drugs, have had multiple myocardial biopsies, have had radiation treatment, have used anorectic medications, or have been treated with a dopamine receptor agonist (e.g., pergolide). *Pulmonic valve stenosis* is almost always congenital.

Tricuspid and pulmonic stenosis both result in an increase in blood volume in the right atrium and the right ventricle, respectively. Tricuspid stenosis results in right atrial enlargement and elevated systemic venous pressures. Pulmonic stenosis results in right ventricular hypertension and hypertrophy (see Table 39.13).

DIAGNOSTIC STUDIES FOR VALVULAR HEART DISEASE

Diagnosis of valvular heart disease is generally based on the results of history, physical examination, echocardiogram, and cardiac catheterization (especially if surgery is considered) (Table 39.15). Chest radiograph results, ECG findings, and the clinical manifestations exhibited by the patient also aid in establishing the correct diagnosis.

An echocardiogram reveals valve structure, function, and chamber size. Transesophageal echocardiography and Doppler colour-flow imaging are valuable in diagnosing and monitoring the progression of valvular heart disease. Real-time three-dimensional echocardiography may be helpful in qualitative assessments of mitral valve and congenital heart disease. Cardiac catheterization is used to detect pressure changes in the cardiac chambers, measure pressure gradients across the

TABLE 39.15   INTERPROFESSIONAL CARE

Valvular Heart Disease

Diagnostic • History and physical examination • Chest radiograph • CBC • ECG • Echocardiogram • Cardiac catheterization **Interprofessional Therapy** **Nonsurgical** • Prophylactic antibiotic therapy • Rheumatic fever • Infective endocarditis (see Table 39.5) • Medications to treat or control HF • Vasodilators* (e.g., nitrates, ACE inhibitors) • Positive inotropes (e.g., digoxin)	• Diuretics (see Chapter 35, Table 35.8) • β-Adrenergic blockers (see Chapter 35, Table 35.8) • Sodium restriction • Anticoagulation therapy (see Chapter 40, Table 40.13) • Antidysrhythmia medications • Percutaneous transluminal balloon valvuloplasty • Percutaneous valve replacement **Surgical** • Valve repair • Commissurotomy (valvulotomy) • Valvuloplasty • Annuloplasty • Valve replacement

Use with caution in patients with aortic stenosis.
ACE, angiotensin-converting enzyme; *CBC,* complete blood cell count; *ECG,* electrocardiogram; *HF,* heart failure.

valves, and quantify the size of valve openings. An ECG shows heart rate and rhythm and provides information about any ischemia or chamber enlargement. Chest radiograph reveals the heart size, alterations in pulmonary circulation, and calcification of valves.

Interprofessional Care of Valvular Heart Disease

Conservative Therapy. An important aspect of conservative management of valvular heart disease is prevention of recurrent rheumatic fever and IE (see Table 39.15). Treatment depends on the valve involved and the severity of the disease. It focuses on preventing exacerbations of HF, acute pulmonary edema, thromboembolism, and recurrent endocarditis. If manifestations of HF develop, vasodilators, positive inotropes, β-adrenergic blockers, diuretics, and a low-sodium diet are recommended (see Chapter 37). Anticoagulant therapy is used to treat systemic or pulmonary embolization. It is also used prophylactically for stroke prevention in patients with atrial fibrillation. Atrial dysrhythmias are common and are treated with digoxin, antidysrhythmia medications, or electrical cardioversion. β-Adrenergic blockers may be used to slow the ventricular response in patients with atrial fibrillation. (Dysrhythmias are discussed in Chapter 38.)

Percutaneous Aortic Valve Replacement. Percutaneous, or transcatheter aortic valve replacement (TAVR) is the standard of care for select patients with severe symptomatic aortic stenosis who are at high risk and cannot be treated with traditional surgical intervention. The procedure, performed in the cardiac catheterization laboratory, involves inserting a bioprosthetic valve, which is advanced over a stiff guide wire using a femoral arterial approach (Asgar et al., 2019).

Percutaneous Transluminal Balloon Valvuloplasty. An alternative treatment for some patients with valvular heart disease is the *percutaneous transluminal balloon valvuloplasty* (PTBV) procedure, in which the fused commissures are split open. PTBV is used for mitral, tricuspid, and pulmonic stenosis and less often for aortic stenosis. The procedure, performed in the cardiac catheterization laboratory, involves threading a balloon-tipped catheter from the femoral artery or vein to the stenotic valve so that the balloon may be inflated in an attempt to separate the valve leaflets. A single- or double-balloon technique may be used for the PTBV procedure. Currently, the use of a single Inoue balloon with hourglass configuration allows sequential inflation. This technique is most popular because it is easy, has good results, and has fewer complications (e.g., left ventricular perforation). The PTBV procedure is generally indicated for older patients and for patients who are poor surgery candidates. PTBV has fewer complications than valve replacement. The long-term results of PTBV are similar to those of surgical commissurotomy.

Surgical Therapy. The decision for surgical intervention is based on the clinical state of the patient. The type of surgery used for a particular patient depends on the valves involved, the valvular pathology, the severity of the disease, and the patient's clinical condition. All types of valve surgery are palliative, not curative, and patients will require lifelong health care. Valve repair is typically the surgical procedure of choice. It is often used in mitral or tricuspid valvular heart disease and has a lower operative mortality rate than replacement. Mitral *commissurotomy (valvulotomy)* is the procedure of choice for patients with pure mitral stenosis. The less precise closed method of commissurotomy has generally been replaced by the open method in Canada, the United States, and Western Europe. The direct vision, or open, procedure requires the use of cardiopulmonary bypass, removal of thrombi from the atrium, excision of the left atrial appendage, commissure incision, and, as indicated, separation of fused chordae, splitting of underlying papillary muscle, and debriding of calcification of the valve. In contrast, the closed procedure is usually performed with the aid of a transventricular dilator inserted through the apex of the left ventricle into the ostium of the mitral valve.

Open surgical *valvuloplasty* involves repairing the valve by suturing the torn leaflets, chordae tendineae, or papillary muscles. It is primarily used to treat mitral or tricuspid regurgitation. Valve repair avoids the risks of replacement but may not establish total valvular competence. *Minimally invasive valvuloplasty* surgery, or robotic mitral valve repair, using mini-sternotomy or parasternal approaches, has shown results comparable to those of the open procedure. It also decreases length of hospitalization, use of blood transfusions, and risk of infection; has a superior cosmetic result; and reduces postoperative atrial fibrillation (Suri et al., 2016).

Further repair or reconstruction of the valve may be necessary and can be achieved by annuloplasty, a procedure also used in cases of mitral or tricuspid regurgitation. *Annuloplasty* entails reconstruction of the annulus, with or without the aid of prosthetic rings.

INFORMATICS IN PRACTICE

Heart Surgery Video or CD

- To learn about a procedure, many patients prefer to watch a video or listen to a CD instead of reading a pamphlet. A video can be an effective tool for the nurse to use in teaching the patient facing heart surgery and the patient's caregiver what to expect before and after the procedure.
- The nurse should remember that the video or CD is not the teacher.
- Before providing the patient with the video or CD, the nurse should discuss with the patient what the video or CD will cover and encourage the patient and caregiver to write down questions or to note what they do not understand.
- After the patient and caregiver view or listen to the material, the nurse should be available to answer any questions they have. The nurse should also reinforce important information from the video or CD.

Prosthetic Valves. Valvular replacement may be required for treating mitral, aortic, tricuspid, and occasionally pulmonic valvular disease. This procedure is the surgical treatment of choice for combined aortic stenosis and AR.

A wide variety of prosthetic valves are available. Desirable valves are nonthrombogenic and durable and create minimal stenosis. Prosthetic valves are categorized as mechanical or biological (tissue) valves (Table 39.16 and Figure 39.10).

Mechanical valves are manufactured from artificial materials and consist of combinations of metal alloys, Pyrolite carbon, and Dacron. *Biological valves* are constructed from bovine, porcine, and human cardiac tissue and usually contain some artificial materials. Innovations in freezing and thawing techniques have enabled human grafts to be preserved for extensive periods while retaining viability. Mechanical prosthetic valves are more durable and last longer

than biological valves; however, they create an increased risk for thromboembolism, necessitating long-term anticoagulation therapy. The main complication of mechanical valves is hemorrhage from the use of anticoagulants. Biological valves do not require long-term anticoagulation therapy because of their low thrombogenicity, although anticoagulation therapy is recommended for 3 to 6 months postoperatively for these patients for prevention of stroke (Nishimura et al., 2017). However, they are less durable because of the tendency for early calcification, tissue degeneration, and stiffening of the leaflets. Risks with both types of prosthetic valves include paravalvular leaks and endocarditis.

Long-term anticoagulation therapy is recommended for all patients with mechanical valves and for those with biological valves and atrial fibrillation. Some patients with biological valves or annuloplasty with prosthetic rings may need

TABLE 39.16   TYPES OF CARDIAC PROSTHETIC AND TISSUE VALVES

Type	Description	Advantages	Disadvantages
Mechanical			
Caged-ball valve (Starr–Edwards, Magovern–Cromie)	Metal cage with several struts mounted on a circular ring; hollow metal or plastic ball (poppet) inside of cage	High durability (≤20 yr)	Possibility of blood clots forming on or around valve (thrombogenic) with risk for embolism Need for long-term anticoagulation therapy Very large
Tilting-disc valve (Lillehei–Kaster Therapy, Medtronic Hall)	Mobile, lens-shaped disc attached to a circular sewing ring by two offset transverse struts; Pyrolite carbon composition	Hemodynamic efficiency High durability Low thrombogenicity	Need for long-term anticoagulation
Bileaflet valve (St. Jude Medical, Edwards Duromedics, Carbomedics)	Two pivoting semicircular discs that open centrally, mounted directly onto a sewing ring	Compact Successful use in children and patients with small aortic roots	Possibility of thrombogenicity and embolism Need for long-term anticoagulation therapy
Biological			
Porcine heterograft (Carpentier–Edwards, Medtronic Hancock)	Harvested aortic valve of pig that is preserved in glutaraldehyde and mounted on specially designed sewing ring	Low thrombogenicity Need for anticoagulation therapy for only 3 mo after placement	Limited durability (failure rate increases sharply after 5–7 yr) Cumbersome structural design
Pericardial heterograft (Carpentier–Edwards, Ionescu–Shiley)	Three leaflets composed of pericardium from 16- to 18-mo-old calves that are preserved in glutaraldehyde and mounted on a Dacron-covered frame	Low thrombogenicity Need for only short-term anticoagulation therapy Less resistance to blood flow; useful in patients with small aortic roots Outstanding durability	Early valve failure secondary to calcification and degeneration
Homograft (cadaver valve)	Harvested aortic valve from human cadaver that is initially frozen until needed for valve replacement, and then thawed, trimmed, and sewn into place with special mounting material	Excellent hemodynamics No hemolysis and low risk for embolism Only rare need for anticoagulation therapy	Limited durability Not useful for mitral or tricuspid valve replacement

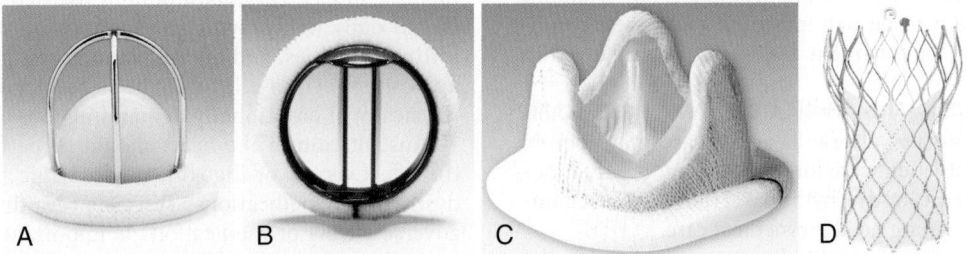

FIG. 39.10 Different types of prosthetic heart valves. **A,** Starr–Edwards caged ball valve. **B,** St. Jude bi-leaflet valve. **C,** Carpentier–Edwards porcine valve. **D,** CoreValve transcatheter aortic valve (CoreValve Evolut R). Source: *A to C,* Bonow, R. O., Mann, D. L., Zipes, D. P., et al (2012). *Braunwald's heart disease: A textbook of cardiovascular medicine* (9th ed.). Saunders; *D,* © Medtronic 2017.

anticoagulation therapy for the first few months after surgery, until the suture lines are covered by endothelial cells (endothelialized).

The choice of valves depends on many factors. For example, if a patient cannot take an anticoagulant (e.g., women of childbearing age), a biological valve may be considered. A mechanical valve may be best for a younger patient because it is more durable. For patients older than age 65, durability is less important than the risk for hemorrhage from anticoagulants.

NURSING MANAGEMENT VALVULAR DISORDERS

NURSING ASSESSMENT
Subjective and objective data should be obtained from patients with valvular disease and are presented in Table 39.17.

NURSING DIAGNOSES
Nursing diagnoses for the patient with valvular heart disease may include but are not limited to the following:
- *Decreased cardiac output* (resulting from valvular incompetence)
- *Excess fluid volume* resulting from *excessive fluid intake, excessive sodium intake* (fluid retention secondary to valvular-induced heart failure)
- *Reduced stamina* resulting from *imbalance between oxygen supply/demand*

Additional information on nursing diagnoses is presented in NCP 39.2, available on the Evolve website for this chapter.

PLANNING
The overall goals for the patient with valvular heart disease include (a) normal cardiac function, (b) improved activity tolerance, and (c) an understanding of the disease process and health maintenance measures.

NURSING IMPLEMENTATION
HEALTH PROMOTION. Diagnosing and treating streptococcal infections and providing prophylactic antibiotics for patients with a history of rheumatic fever are critical to preventing acquired rheumatic valvular disease. Patients at high risk for endocarditis and those with valvular prostheses must also be treated with prophylactic antibiotics (see Table 39.4).

Patients must adhere to recommended therapies. Individuals with a history of rheumatic fever, endocarditis, or congenital heart disease should know the symptoms suggestive of valvular heart disease so that early medical treatment may be obtained. The nurse's role is to educate individuals about their condition and the importance of adherence to prescribed therapies. Patient- and family-centred care is important. It is important for patients and caregivers to be well informed about their condition and the options for treatment and be actively involved in decision making.

ACUTE INTERVENTION AND AMBULATORY AND HOME CARE. Patients with progressive valvular heart disease may require hospitalization or outpatient care for management of HF, endocarditis, embolic disease, or dysrhythmias. HF is the most common reason for an ongoing need for medical care.

The role of the nurse is to implement and evaluate the effectiveness of therapeutic management. Activity should be designed after considering the patient's limitations. An appropriate exercise plan can increase cardiac tolerance. However,

---

TABLE 39.17   NURSING ASSESSMENT
Valvular Heart Disease

Subjective Data
Important Health Information

Past health history: Rheumatic fever, endocarditis, congenital defects, myocardial infarction, chest trauma, cardiomyopathy, syphilis, Marfan syndrome, staphylococcal or streptococcal infections, HIV infection, or compromised immune system

Medications
IV drug misuse

Symptoms
- Fatigue, generalized weakness, activity intolerance
- Palpitations, dizziness, fainting
- Dyspnea on exertion, cough, hemoptysis, orthopnea, paroxysmal nocturnal dyspnea
- Anginal or atypical chest pain

Objective Data
General
Fever

Integumentary
Diaphoresis, flushing, cyanosis, clubbing; peripheral edema

Respiratory
Crackles, wheezes, hoarseness

Cardiovascular
Abnormal heart sounds, including opening snaps, clicks, thrills, systolic and diastolic murmurs, S_3, and S_4; dysrhythmias, including premature atrial contraction, atrial fibrillation; tachycardia; ↑ or ↓ in pulse pressure; hypotension, water-hammer or thready peripheral pulses, brisk carotid pulses

Gastrointestinal
Ascites, hepatomegaly

Possible Diagnostic Findings
Cardiomegaly on chest radiograph; ECG abnormalities specific to involved valve; echocardiogram (valve abnormalities and chamber dilation); cardiac catheterization (abnormalities in valves, chamber pressures, gradients, cardiac output, and blood flow depending on involved valve)

ECG, electrocardiogram; *HIV,* human immunodeficiency virus; *IV,* intravenous; S_3, third heart sound; S_4, fourth heart sound.

---

activities that regularly produce fatigue and dyspnea should be restricted, and an explanation should be provided to the patient. Smoking cessation should be discussed and encouraged. Strenuous physical exercise should be avoided because damaged valves may not be able to handle the required increase in CO. Patients should be assisted in planning activities of daily living, with an emphasis on conserving energy, setting priorities, and taking planned rest periods. Referral to a vocational counsellor may be necessary for patients with a physically or emotionally demanding job.

Auscultation of the heart should be performed to monitor the effectiveness of digoxin, β-adrenergic blockers, and antidysrhythmic medications. Teaching regarding the actions and adverse effects of medications is important to achieve adherence. Patients must understand the importance of prophylactic antibiotic therapy to prevent IE (see Table 39.4). If the valve disease was caused by rheumatic fever, ongoing prophylaxis to prevent recurrence is necessary.

When valvular heart disease can no longer be managed medically, surgical intervention becomes necessary. Patients who are on anticoagulation therapy after surgery for valve replacement must have their international normalized ratio (INR) checked regularly (usually monthly) to assess the adequacy of therapy. The INR is a standardized system of reporting prothrombin time. INR values of 2.5 to 3.5 are therapeutic for patients with mechanical valves.

Patients must realize that valve surgery is not a cure and that regular follow-up examinations by the health care provider will be required. The nurse must also teach the patient about when to seek medical care. Any manifestations of infection or HF, any signs of bleeding, and any planned invasive or dental procedures require the patient to notify the health care provider. Finally, patients should be encouraged to wear medical alert identification (e.g., bracelet).

EVALUATION

The expected outcomes for a patient with valvular heart disease are addressed in NCP 39.2, available on the Evolve website for this chapter.

ETHICAL DILEMMAS

Do Not Resuscitate

Situation
A 68-year-old male has been admitted for a second mitral valve surgery and coronary artery bypass graft surgery. He did not adhere to the treatment plan following his original surgery 7 years ago. The nurse is worried about his future adherence to medication, diet, and exercise regimens. His kidneys are failing, and he is on dialysis, making him a high-risk surgical patient. The patient and caregivers want all possible treatment and refuse to discuss do-not-resuscitate (DNR) orders.

Important Points for Consideration
- Nonadherence to the treatment plan in the past does not always indicate the patient will not follow the plan of care in the future. Many circumstances related to nonadherence are outside the patient's control, such as finances, transportation, availability of assistance, and declining physical and mental capabilities.
- A competent patient can decide whether he wants continued treatment so as to be able to fight to live. This is even more important when family members support the patient's decision.
- Health care providers have an obligation to respect the patient's request for treatment unless there is no clear benefit to continued treatment. Patients' choices to continue or end treatment are based on their values and beliefs, which may not always coincide with those of the health care provider or team.
- DNR orders should reflect the patient's expressed wishes. These wishes can be expressed either through conversation, advance directives, or a surrogate decision maker.
- DNR orders should be re-evaluated periodically with the patient and family, especially before major diagnostic procedures or treatments.
- A nurse who does not agree with a patient's treatment choice should nevertheless respect the patient's choice and ask the patient to explain more about their situation and decision. The nurse should communicate the patient's choice to the health care team and a referral should be made to an ethics committee or similar group as appropriate.

Discussion Questions
1. What type of information should be provided to a patient and family in discussions about DNR orders? Who should provide this information?
2. What measures or strategies would be beneficial to assist the patient to better adhere to the treatment plan?
3. Who can initiate a referral to an ethics committee?

CARDIOMYOPATHY

Cardiomyopathy comprises a group of diseases that directly affect the structural or functional ability of the myocardium. A diagnosis of cardiomyopathy is made on the basis of the patient's clinical manifestations and noninvasive and invasive diagnostic procedures.

Cardiomyopathy can be classified as primary or secondary. *Primary cardiomyopathy* refers to those conditions in which the etiology of the heart disease is unknown (idiopathic). The heart muscle in this case is the only portion of the heart involved; other cardiac structures are unaffected. In *secondary cardiomyopathy*, the cause of the myocardial disease is known and is secondary to another disease process. Common causes of secondary cardiomyopathy are listed in Table 39.18. Each type has its own pathogenesis, clinical presentation, and treatment policies (Tables 39.19 and 39.20). Cardiomyopathies can lead to cardiomegaly and HF and are the leading reason for heart transplantation.

TABLE 39.18   CAUSES OF SECONDARY CARDIOMYOPATHY

Dilated
- Cardiotoxic agents—alcohol, cocaine, doxorubicin
- Genetic (autosomal dominant) or familial
- Hypertension
- Ischemia (coronary artery disease)
- Metabolic disorders
- Muscular dystrophy
- Myocarditis
- Pregnancy
- Valve disease

Hypertrophic
- Aortic stenosis
- Genetic (autosomal dominant)
- Hypertension

Restrictive
- Amyloidosis
- Endomyocardial fibrosis
- Neoplastic tumour
- Post–radiation therapy
- Sarcoidosis

TABLE 39.19   COMPARISON OF CARDIOMYOPATHIES

	Dilated	Hypertrophic	Restrictive
Major Manifestations	Fatigue, weakness, palpitations, dyspnea	Exertional dyspnea, fatigue, angina, syncope, palpitations	Dyspnea, fatigue
	Cardiomegaly: moderate to marked	Mild to moderate	Mild
Contractility	↓	↑ or ↓	Normal or ↓
Valvular Incompetence	Atrioventricular valves, particularly mitral	Mitral valve	Atrioventricular valves
Dysrhythmias	Sinoatrial tachycardia, atrial and ventricular dysrhythmias	Atrial and ventricular dysrhythmias	Atrial and ventricular dysrhythmias
Cardiac Output	↓	Normal or ↓	Normal or ↓
Outflow Tract Obstruction	None	↑	None

TABLE 39.20	INTERPROFESSIONAL CARE

Cardiomyopathy

Diagnostic	Interprofessional Therapy
• History and physical examination	• Treatment of underlying cause
• Electrocardiogram	• Medication therapy
• B-type natriuretic peptide (NT-ProBNP)	• Nitrates (except in HCM)
	• β-Adrenergic blockers
• Chest radiograph	• Antidysrhythmics
• Echocardiogram	• ACE inhibitors or angiotensin receptor blocker (ARB)
• Nuclear imaging studies	• Or angiotensin receptor-neprilysin inhibitor (ARNI)
• Cardiac catheterization	
• Endocardial biopsy	• Diuretics
	• Mineralocorticoid receptor antagonist (MRA)
	• Digitalis (except in HCM) unless used to treat atrial fibrillation)
	• Anticoagulants (if indicated)
	• Ventricular assist device
	• Cardiac resynchronization therapy
	• Implantable cardioverter–defibrillator
	• Surgical correction
	• Cardiac transplant

ACE, angiotensin-converting enzyme; *HCM*, hypertrophic cardiomyopathy.

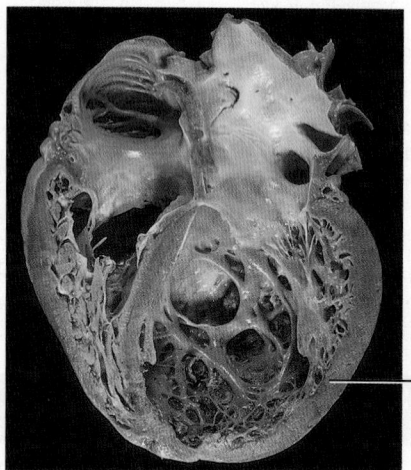

FIG. 39.11 Dilated cardiomyopathy. The dilated left ventricular wall has thinned, and the chamber size and volume are increased. Source: Kumar, V., Abbas, A. K., & Aster, J. (2013). *Robbins basic pathology* (9th ed., p. 399). Elsevier Saunders.

Left ventricular wall

DILATED CARDIOMYOPATHY

Etiology and Pathophysiology

Dilated cardiomyopathy (DCM) is the most common type of cardiomyopathy, with multiple etiologies. DCM is one of the most common causes of HF, with a genetic link in up to 35% of cases (Weintraub et al., 2017). DCM is characterized by a diffuse inflammation and rapid degeneration of myocardial fibres. These changes result in ventricular dilation, impairment of systolic function, atrial enlargement, and stasis of blood in the left ventricle. Cardiomegaly results from ventricular dilation (Figure 39.11) and causes contractile dysfunction in spite of an enlarged chamber size. In contrast to HF, the walls of the ventricles do not hypertrophy (Figure 39.12).

DCM often follows infectious myocarditis. Other common causes of DCM are listed in Table 39.18.

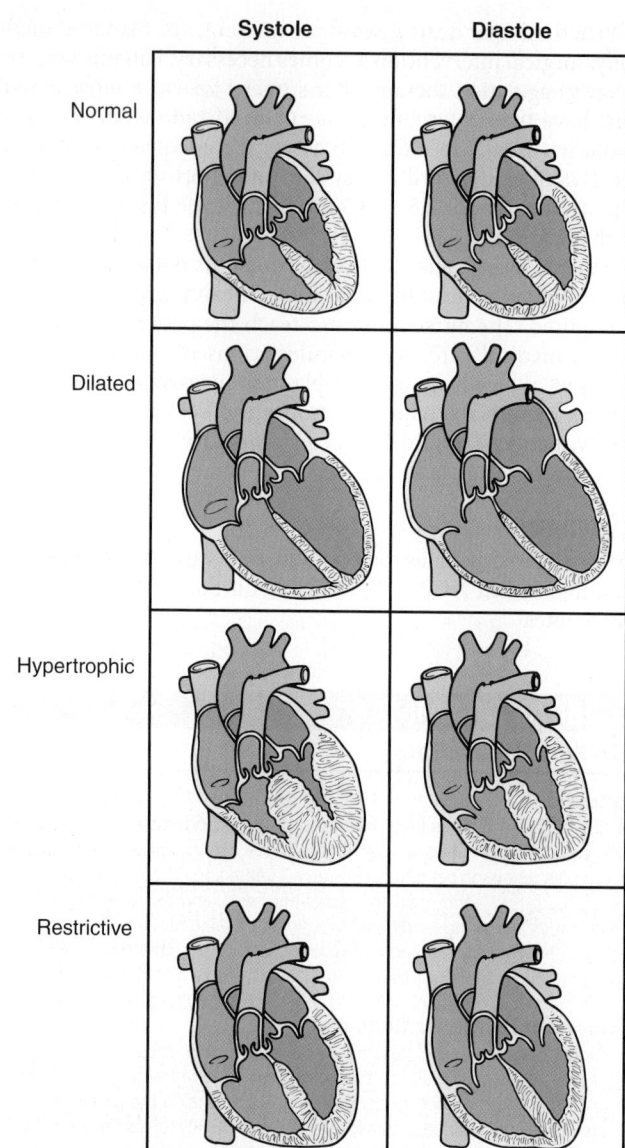

FIG. 39.12 Types of cardiomyopathies and the differences in ventricular diameter during systole and diastole, compared with a normal heart. Source: Adapted from Urden, L. D., Stacy, K. M., & Lough, M. E. (2014). *Critical care nursing: Diagnosis and management* (7th ed., p. 376). Mosby.

Clinical Manifestations

The signs and symptoms of DCM may develop acutely after an infectious process or insidiously over time. Most people eventually develop HF. Symptoms can include decreased exercise capacity, fatigue, dyspnea at rest, paroxysmal nocturnal dyspnea, and orthopnea. As the disease progresses, the patient may experience dry cough, palpitations, abdominal bloating, nausea, vomiting, and anorexia. Signs can include an irregular heart rate with an abnormal S_3 or S_4 or both, tachycardia or bradycardia, pulmonary crackles, edema, weak peripheral pulses, pallor, hepatomegaly, and jugular venous distension. Heart murmurs and dysrhythmias are common. Decreased blood flow through an enlarged heart promotes stasis and blood clot formation and may lead to systemic embolization.

Diagnostic Studies

The diagnosis of DCM is made on the basis of the patient's history and by ruling out other conditions that cause HF. Doppler echocardiography provides the basis for the diagnosis of DCM in the majority of patients and distinguishes DCM from other structural abnormalities. The chest radiograph may show cardiomegaly with signs of pulmonary venous hypertension as well as pleural effusion. The ECG may reveal tachycardia, bradycardia, and dysrhythmias with conduction disturbances. Laboratory studies may reveal elevated serum levels of B-type natriuretic peptide (BNP or NT-Pro-BNP) in the presence of HF.

Cardiac catheterization is done to confirm or rule out coronary artery disease, and multiple gated acquisition (MUGA) radionuclide angiocardiographies are done to determine ejection fraction (EF). EFs of less than 20% are associated with a 50% mortality within 1 year. EMB may be done at the time of the right-sided heart catheterization to detect viral antigens in myocardial tissue.

NURSING AND INTERPROFESSIONAL MANAGEMENT DILATED CARDIOMYOPATHY

Interventions focus on controlling HF by enhancing myocardial contractility and decreasing afterload. Treatment of patients with NYHA class IV, stage D HF is more palliative than curative. Several different types of medications are used to manage HF (see Chapter 37, Figure 37.6). Nitrates (e.g., nitroglycerin) and loop diuretics (e.g., furosemide [Lasix]) are used to decrease preload, and ACE inhibitors (e.g., captopril), ARBs, or an angiotensin-neprolysin inhibitor (ARNI) are used to reduce afterload. β-Adrenergic blockers (e.g., bisoprolol [Monocor]) and aldosterone antagonists (e.g., spironolactone [Aldactone]) are used to control the neurohormonal stimulation that occurs in HF. Digoxin is used to treat atrial fibrillation but must be used with caution because of increased susceptibility to digoxin toxicity in these patients. Other dysrhythmias are treated with antidysrhythmia medications (e.g., amiodarone) as indicated (see Chapter 38).

Medication and nutritional therapy and cardiac rehabilitation may help alleviate symptoms of HF as well as improve CO and quality of life. Patients with secondary DCM must be treated for the underlying disease process. For example, a patient with alcohol-related DCM must abstain from all alcohol intake. (See Chapter 37 for a complete discussion of HF.)

Unfortunately, DCM does not respond well to therapy, and patients may experience multiple episodes of HF. Patients may require admission to the hospital for aggressive diuresis when they decompensate.

Patients also may benefit from nonpharmacological therapies, such as cardiac resynchronization therapy (Ezekoitz et al., 2017) or a ventricular assist device (VAD), that may allow the heart to rest and recover from acute HF or be a bridge to heart transplantation. Patients with terminal end-stage cardiomyopathy may be considered for heart transplantation or destination therapy with a permanent or implantable VAD (see Chapter 37). Currently, approximately 50% of heart transplantations are performed for treatment of cardiomyopathy. Heart transplant recipients have a good prognosis for survival. However, donor hearts are difficult to obtain, and many patients with DCM die while awaiting heart transplantation.

Patients with DCM are very ill people with a grave prognosis who need expert nursing care. Patients' families must learn cardiopulmonary resuscitation (CPR) and know how to access emergency care. The nurse should include family members and other support systems when planning a patient's care.

Home health and hospice nursing can provide the patient and the family with the continuous assessments and therapeutic interventions that are required to maximize and maintain functional status or prepare for a peaceful death. Observing for signs and symptoms of worsening HF, dysrhythmias, and embolic formation is paramount in these patients, as is monitoring medication responsiveness. The goal of therapy is to keep the patient at an optimal level of function and out of the hospital.

HYPERTROPHIC CARDIOMYOPATHY

Etiology and Pathophysiology

Hypertrophic cardiomyopathy (HCM), formerly called *hypertrophic subaortic stenosis, asymmetrical septal hypertrophy (ASH),* or *hypertrophic obstructive cardiomyopathy (HOCM),* is asymmetrical left ventricular hypertrophy without ventricular dilation. (HOCM was a misleading term because one third of all patients with HCM have a nonobstructive left ventricular outflow tract [LVOT] at rest or with exertion.) In one form of the disease, the septum between the two ventricles becomes enlarged and obstructs the blood flow from the left ventricle. HCM can be idiopathic, although about one half of all cases have a genetic basis characterized by inappropriate myocardial hypertrophy (see Table 39.18). HCM occurs less commonly than DCM and is more common in men aged 30 to 40 years than in women. In one study, HCM occurred more frequently in young Black male athletes than in young White male athletes. The four main characteristics of HCM are (1) massive ventricular hypertrophy, (2) rapid, forceful contraction of the left ventricle, (3) impaired relaxation (diastolic dysfunction), and (4) obstruction of LVOT (not present in all patients). Ventricular hypertrophy is associated with a thickened intraventricular septum and ventricular wall (Figure 39.13). The end result is impaired ventricular filling as the ventricle becomes noncompliant and unable to relax. The primary defect of HCM is diastolic dysfunction from left ventricular stiffness. Decreased ventricular filling and obstruction to outflow can result in decreased CO, especially during

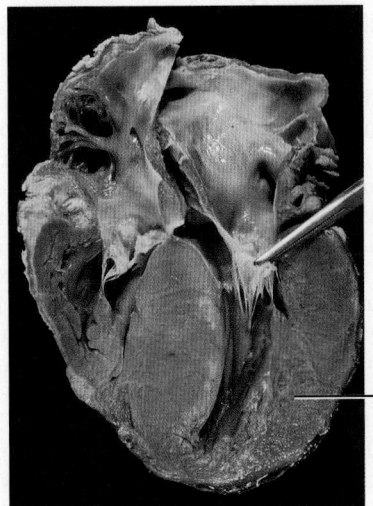

Left
ventricular
hypertrophy

FIG. 39.13 Hypertrophic cardiomyopathy. There is marked left ventricular hypertrophy, and the chamber size and volume are decreased. Source: Kumar, V., Abbas, A. K., & Aster, J. (2013). *Robbins basic pathology* (9th ed., p. 400). Elsevier Saunders.

exertion. HCM is the most common cause of SCD in otherwise healthy young people. It accounts for 3% of deaths in young competitive athletes (usually diagnosed in young adulthood) and is often seen in active, athletic individuals (Marian & Braunwald, 2017).

Clinical Manifestations

Patients with HCM may be asymptomatic or may have exertional dyspnea, fatigue, angina, and syncope. The most common symptom is dyspnea, which is caused by an elevated left ventricular diastolic pressure. Fatigue occurs because of the resultant decrease in CO and in exercise-induced flow obstruction. Angina can occur and is most often caused by the increased left ventricular muscle mass or compression of the small coronary arteries by the hypercontractile ventricular myocardium. The patient may also have syncope, especially during exertion. Syncope is most often caused by an increase in obstruction to aortic outflow during increased activity, resulting in decreased CO and cerebrovascular circulation. Syncope can also be caused by dysrhythmias. Common dysrhythmias include supraventricular tachycardia, atrial fibrillation, ventricular tachycardia, and ventricular fibrillation. Any of these dysrhythmias may lead to loss of consciousness or SCD (SCD is discussed in Chapter 36).

Diagnostic Studies

Clinical findings on examination may be unremarkable. However, on palpation of the chest, there may be a forced apical impulse that may be displaced laterally. Auscultation may reveal an S_4 and a systolic ejection murmur between the apex and the sternal border at the fourth intercostal space. ECG findings usually indicate ventricular hypertrophy, ST–T-wave abnormalities, prominent Q waves in the inferior or precordial leads, left-axis deviation, and ventricular and atrial dysrhythmias (see Chapter 38).

The echocardiogram is the primary diagnostic tool to confirm the classic feature of HCM, which is left ventricular hypertrophy. The echocardiogram may also demonstrate wall motion abnormalities and diastolic dysfunction. Cardiac catheterization may also be helpful in the diagnosis of HCM.

NURSING AND INTERPROFESSIONAL MANAGEMENT HYPERTROPHIC CARDIOMYOPATHY

Goals of intervention are to improve ventricular filling by reducing ventricular contractility and relieving LVOT obstruction. These can be accomplished with the use of β-adrenergic blockers, such as metoprolol (Lopressor), or calcium channel blockers, such as verapamil. Use of digitalis preparations is contraindicated unless they are used to treat atrial fibrillation. Antidysrhythmics, such as amiodarone or sotalol, are effective medications for dysrhythmias. However, their use has not been shown to prevent SCD. For patients at risk for SCD, the implantation of a cardioverter–defibrillator is recommended (see Chapter 38).

AV pacing can be beneficial for patients with HCM and LVOT obstruction. By pacing the ventricles from the apex of the right ventricle, septal depolarization occurs first, allowing the septum to move away from the left ventricular wall and reducing the degree of obstruction of the LVOT.

Some patients may be candidates for surgical treatment of their hypertrophied septum. The indications for surgery include severe symptoms refractory to therapy with marked obstruction to aortic outflow (>50 mm Hg) while at rest. The surgery is termed a *ventriculomyotomy and myectomy*. It involves incision of the hypertrophied septal muscle and resection of some of the hypertrophied ventricular muscle. Most patients have good symptomatic improvement and improved exercise tolerance after surgery.

An alternative, nonsurgical procedure to reduce symptoms and the LVOT obstruction is alcohol-induced percutaneous transluminal septal myocardial ablation (PTSMA). Through this procedure, alcohol is administered into the first septal artery branching off the left anterior descending artery, causing ischemia and septal wall MI. Ablation of the septal wall decreases the flow obstruction, and the patient's symptoms decrease. The procedure improves HF symptoms and exercise capacity about 3 months after ablation. Mortality rates for the procedure are approximately 1% depending on the age and condition of the patient. Information on long-term effects of PTSMA in treated patients is lacking because the procedure is still new. Potential complications of PTSMA include conduction disturbances (e.g., heart block) and MI beyond the intended septum.

Nursing interventions for HCM focus on relieving symptoms, observing for and preventing complications, and providing emotional and psychological support. Teaching should focus on helping patients adjust their lifestyle to avoid strenuous activity and dehydration. Any activity, such as competitive sports, that causes an increase in systemic vascular resistance (thus increasing the obstruction to forward flow) is dangerous and should be avoided. HCM patients who experience chest pain need to rest and elevate their feet to improve venous return to the heart. Vasodilators such as nitroglycerin may worsen the chest pain by decreasing venous return to the heart, which can further obstruct blood flow from the heart.

RESTRICTIVE CARDIOMYOPATHY

Etiology and Pathophysiology

Restrictive cardiomyopathy (RCM) is the least common of the cardiomyopathic conditions. It is a disease of the heart muscle that impairs diastolic filling and stretch (see Figure 39.12). Systolic function remains unaffected. Although the specific etiology of RCM is unknown, a number of pathological processes may be involved in its development. Myocardial fibrosis, hypertrophy, and infiltration produce stiffness of the ventricular wall with loss of ventricular compliance. Secondary causes of RCM include amyloidosis, endocardial fibrosis, sarcoidosis, fibrosis of different etiology, and radiation to the thorax. When amyloidosis is suspected, identification of ATTR cardiac amyloidosis should be pursued for the future possibility of tafamidis treatment (O'Meara et al., 2020). With RCM, the ventricles are resistant to filling and therefore demand high diastolic filling pressures to maintain CO.

Clinical Manifestations

Classic symptoms of RCM are fatigue, exercise intolerance, and dyspnea because the heart cannot increase CO by increasing the heart rate without further compromising ventricular filling. Additional symptoms may include angina, orthopnea, syncope, and palpitations. The patient may have signs of HF, including dyspnea, peripheral edema, ascites, hepatomegaly, and jugular venous distension.

Diagnostic Studies

The chest radiograph may be normal, or it may show cardiomegaly from right and left atrial enlargement. Pleural effusions and pulmonary congestion may be evident in patients with progression to HF. The ECG may reveal a mild tachycardia at rest. The most common dysrhythmias are supraventricular (atrial fibrillation) and AV block. Echocardiography may reveal a left ventricle that is of normal size with a thickened wall, slightly dilated right ventricle, and dilated atria. EMB, CT, and nuclear imaging may be helpful in the diagnosis.

NURSING AND INTERPROFESSIONAL MANAGEMENT RESTRICTIVE CARDIOMYOPATHY

Currently, no specific treatment for RCM exists. Interventions are aimed at improving diastolic filling and the underlying disease process. Treatment includes conventional therapy for HF and dysrhythmias. Heart transplantation may also be considered. Nursing care is similar to the care of a patient with HF. As in the treatment of patients with HCM, the patient should be taught to avoid situations that impair ventricular filling (e.g., strenuous activity, dehydration, and increases in systemic vascular resistance).

Nursing care of a patient with cardiomyopathy includes individualized teaching based on the patient's clinical manifestations. All patients with cardiomyopathy are at risk for IE from any procedure that may cause bacteremia and should be instructed on the need for prophylactic antibiotics (see Table 39.3). A general patient and caregiver teaching guide is presented in Table 39.21.

TABLE 39.21	PATIENT & CAREGIVER TEACHING GUIDE

Cardiomyopathy

The following information should be included in the teaching plan for a patient with cardiomyopathy and the patient's caregiver.

- Take all medications as prescribed and follow up with health care provider.
- Eat a low-sodium diet (if ordered) and read all product labels (food and over-the-counter medications) for sodium content.
- Unless fluids are restricted, drink six to eight glasses of water a day.
- Achieve and maintain a reasonable weight, and avoid large meals.
- Avoid using alcohol, caffeine, diet pills, and over-the-counter cold medicines that may contain stimulants.
- Balance activity and rest periods.
- Avoid doing heavy lifting or vigorous isometric exercises, and check with health care provider for exercise guidelines.
- Use stress-reduction activities: relaxation to relieve tension, guided imagery, diversional activities (see Chapter 8).
- Report to health care provider any signs of heart failure, including weight gain, edema, shortness of breath, and increased fatigue.
- Consider having family members learn CPR because of the potential for sudden cardiac arrest.
- Notify health care provider or dentist before undergoing any invasive medical or dental procedures since patients with cardiomyopathy are at risk for endocarditis (see Table 39.3).

CPR, cardiopulmonary resuscitation.

CASE STUDY

Valvular Heart Disease

Patient Profile
R. B. (pronouns he/him), 50 years old, is admitted to the hospital for valvular heart disease.

Subjective Data
- Reports history of IV drug use
- Prior and current regular alcohol intake of approximately 475 mL of whisky per day
- Complains of chest pain with minimal exertion
- Recently unemployed
- States being short of breath and cannot sleep lying flat
- States being tired and irritable all the time
- States cannot afford medications
- Smokes a pack of cigarettes a day

Objective Data
Physical Examination
- Third heart sound (S_3)
- Loud holosystolic murmur of MR
- Wears dentures (teeth removed due to periodontal disease)
- Vital signs: temperature 37.2°C; pulse 110, irregular; respirations 24; BP 104/58

Diagnostic Studies
- ECG shows atrial fibrillation and a rapid ventricular response.
- Chest radiograph reveals pulmonary congestion and cardiomegaly.
- Transesophageal echocardiography shows left atrial and ventricular hypertrophy and mitral and aortic regurgitation.

Discussion Questions
1. Identify the cause and course of R. B.'s disease based on his history and current examination.
2. Differentiate between mitral and aortic regurgitation.
3. What medical treatments or surgical procedures will R. B. probably require as his condition worsens?
4. **Priority decision:** On the basis of the assessment data provided, what are the priority nursing diagnoses?
5. **Priority decision:** Identify the priority nursing interventions for R. B.
6. **Evidence-informed practice:** R. B. asks why "blood thinners" are needed after the valves are replaced.

℮volve
Answers are available at http://evolve.elsevier.com/Canada/Lewis/medsurg.

REVIEW QUESTIONS

The number of the question corresponds to the same-numbered objective at the beginning of the chapter.

1. Assessment of an IV cocaine user with infective endocarditis should focus on which of the following signs and symptoms? *(Select all that apply.)*
   a. Retinal hemorrhages
   b. Splinter hemorrhages
   c. Presence of Osler's nodes
   d. Painless nodules over bony prominences
   e. Painless erythematous macules on the palms and soles

2. Which of the following are nursing assessment findings for acute pericarditis?
   a. Wheezing and dull precordial pain
   b. Bradycardia, tachypnea, and murmur
   c. Chest pain, dyspnea, and pericardial friction rub
   d. Respiratory stridor, dull chest pain, and abdominal discomfort

3. Which of the following at-risk individuals need prophylactic antibiotics to prevent IE?
   a. Those with a history of IE
   b. Those having a viral respiratory infection
   c. Those entering the third trimester of pregnancy
   d. Those exposed to human immunodeficiency virus (HIV)

4. A client is admitted with myocarditis. Which of the following clinical signs and symptoms might the nurse find while performing the initial assessment? *(Select all that apply.)*
   a. Angina
   b. Pleuritic chest pain
   c. Splinter hemorrhages
   d. Pericardial friction rub
   e. Presence of Osler's nodes

5. When teaching a client about the long-term consequences of rheumatic fever, what possibilities should the nurse discuss?
   a. Valvular heart disease
   b. Pulmonary hypertension
   c. Superior vena cava syndrome
   d. Hypertrophy of the right ventricle

6. A client with rheumatic fever should be taught about the need for which of the following?
   a. Regular exercise
   b. Antibiotic therapy
   c. A high-protein diet
   d. Anticoagulant therapy

7. What is a common cause of aortic valve stenosis in older people?
   a. Rheumatic fever
   b. Cardiomyopathy
   c. Congenital heart disease
   d. Acute infective endocarditis

8. Which of the following findings is indicative of left ventricular overload in a client with chronic aortic regurgitation?
   a. Dehydration and a pericardial friction rub
   b. An audible third heart sound and a mid-systolic murmur
   c. Exertional dyspnea and a diastolic high-pitched murmur
   d. An audible third heart sound and a pansystolic or holosystolic murmur

9. A client hospitalized with aortic stenosis has a nursing diagnosis of *reduced stamina* resulting from *imbalance between oxygen supply/demand*. Which of the following is an appropriate nursing intervention for this client?
   a. Monitoring electrocardiogram to assess cardiac output
   b. Maintaining client on bed rest to reduce tissue oxygen demands
   c. Progressively increasing activity to increase cardiac tolerance
   d. Using semi-Fowler's position to decrease venous return and increase respiratory excursion

10. What should the nurse caring for a client scheduled for a mitral valve replacement with a mechanical valve understand about this procedure?
    a. It is similar to a commissurotomy.
    b. It requires long-term anticoagulation therapy.
    c. It is the treatment of choice for an older client with a history of falling.
    d. It involves the insertion of a transventricular dilator into the opening of the valve.

11. Which of the following assessment findings would the nurse expect in a client with dilated cardiomyopathy?
    a. Dyspnea and fatigue
    b. Wheezing and epigastric pain
    c. Palpitations and left lower quadrant tenderness
    d. Excessive sputum and lower abdominal cramping

12. The nurse plans care for a client with dilated cardiomyopathy based on what knowledge?
    a. Family members may be at risk because of the infectious nature of the disease.
    b. Medical management of the disorder focuses on treatment of the underlying cause.
    c. The prognosis of the client is poor, and emotional support is a high priority of care.
    d. The condition may be successfully treated with surgical ventriculomyotomy and septal ablation.

1. a, b, c, e; 2. c; 3. a; 4. a, b, d; 5. a; 6. b; 7. a; 8. c; 9. c; 10. b; 11. a; 12. c.

ⓔvolve

For even more review questions, visit http://evolve.elsevier.com/Canada/Lewis/medsurg.

REFERENCES

Ammirati, E., Veronese, G., Cipriani, M., et al. (2018). Acute and fulminant myocarditis: A pragmatic clinical approach to diagnosis and treatment. *Current Cardiology Reports, 20*(11), 114. https://doi.org/10.1007/s11886-018-1054-z

Andreis, A., Imazio, M., & de Ferrari, G. M. (2019). Contemporary diagnosis and treatment of recurrent pericarditis. *Expert Review of Cardiovascular Therapy, 17*(11), 817–826. https://doi.org/10.1080/14779072.2019.1691916

Asgar, A. W., Ouzounian, M., Adams, C., et al. (2019). Canadian Cardiovascular Society position statement for transcatheter aortic valve implantation. *Canadian Journal of Cardiology, 35*(11), 1437–1448. https://doi.org/10.1016/j.cjca.2019.08.011

Cahill, T. J., Baddour, L. M., Habib, G., et al. (2017). Challenges in infective endocarditis. *Journal of American College of Cardiology, 69*(3), 325–344. https://doi.org/10.1016/j.jacc.2016.10.066

Dayer, M., & Thornhill, M. (2018). Is antibiotic prophylaxis to prevent infective endocarditis worthwhile? *Journal of Infection and Chemotherapy, 24*(1), 18–24. https://doi.org/10.1016/j.jiac.2017.10.006

Ezekowitz, J. A., O'Meara, E., McDonald, M. A., et al. (2017). 2017 Comprehensive update of the Canadian Cardiovascular Society guidelines for the management of heart failure. *Canadian Journal of Cardiology, 33*(11), 1342–1433. https://doi.org/10.1016/j.cjca.2017.08.022

Fardman, A., Charron, P., Imazio, M., et al. (2016). European guidelines on pericardial diseases. A focused review of novel aspects. *Current Cardiology Reports, 18*(46). https://doi.org/10.1007/s11186-016-072-1

Gewitz, M. H., Baltimore, R. S., Tani, L. Y., et al. (2015). Revision of the Jones criteria for the diagnosis of acute rheumatic fever in the era of Doppler echocardiography: A scientific statement from the American Heart Association. *Circulation, 131*(20), 1806–1818. https://doi.org/10.1161/CIR.0000000000000205. (Seminal).

Habib, G., Lancellotti, P., Antunes, M. J., et al. (2015). 2015 ESC guidelines for the management of infective endocarditis. *European Heart Journal, 36*(44), 3075–3128. https://doi.org/10.1093/eurheartj/ehv319

Heart and Stroke Foundation of Canada. (2021a). *Infective (bacterial) endocarditis.* https://www.heartandstroke.ca/heart/conditions/infective-endocarditis

Heart and Stroke Foundation of Canada. (2021b). *Rheumatic heart disease.* https://www.heartandstroke.ca/heart/conditions/rheumatic-heart-disease

Imazio, M., & Gaita, F. (2017). Acute and recurrent pericarditis. *Cardiology Clinics, 35*(4), 505–513. https://doi.org/10.1016/j.ccl.2017.07.004

Lung, B., & Kappetein, D. (2018). Introduction and general comments. In A. J. Camm, T. Lüscher, & G. Maurer (Eds.), ESC CardioMed (3rd ed.). Chapter 35.1 Valvular heart disease. Oxford University Press. https://oxfordmedicine.com/view/10.1093/med/9780198784906.001.0001/med-9780198784906-chapter-764

Marian, A. J., & Braunwald, E. (2017). Hypertrophic Cardiomyopathy: Genetics, pathogenesis, clinical manifestations, diagnosis and therapy. *Circulation Research, 121*(7), 749–770. https://doi.org/10.1161/CIRCRESAHA.117.311059

McNamara, N., Ibrahim, A., Satti, Z., et al. (2019). Acute pericarditis: a review of current diagnostic and management guidelines. *Future Cardiology, 15*(2), 119–126. https://doi.org/10.1080/14779072.2019.1691916

Nishimura, R. A., Otto, C. M., Bonow, R. O., et al. (2017). 2017 AHA/ACC focused update of the 2014 guideline for the management of valvular heart disease: A report of the American College of Cardiology/American Heart Association Task Force on Clinical Guidelines. *Circulation, 135*(25), e1135–e1195. https://doi.org/10.1161/CIR.0000000000000503

O'Meara, E., McDonald, M., Chan, M., et al. (2020). CCS/CHFS heart failure guidelines: Clinical trial update on functional mitral regurgitation, SGLT2 inhibitors, ARNI in HFPEF, and tafamidis in amyloidosis. *Canadian Journal of Cardiology, 36*(2), 159–169. https://doi.org/10.1016/j.cjca.2019.11.036

Otta, C.M., Nishimura, R.O., Carabello, B.A., et al. (2020). *2020 ACC/AHA Guideline for the Management of Patients with Valvular Heart Disease: Executive Summary: A Report of the American College of Cardiology/American Heart Association Join Committee on Clinical Practice Guidelines.* https://doi.org/10.1161/CIR.0000000000000932

Suri, R. M., Dearani, J. A., Mihaljevic, T., et al. (2016). Mitral valve repair using robotic technology: Safe, effective, and durable. *The Journal of Thoracic and Cardiovascular Surgery, 151*(6), 1450. https://doi.org/10.1016/j.jtcvs.2016.02.030

Vahanian, A. (2018). Mitral stenosis. In A. J. Camm, T. Lüscher, & G. Maurer (Eds.), *ESC CaradioMed* (3rd ed.). Oxford University Press. Chapter 35.5. Valvular heart disease. https://oxfordmedicine.com/view/10.1093/med/9780198784906.001.0001/med-9780198784906-chapter-768

Watkins, D. A., Beaton, A. Z., Carapetis, J. R., et al. (2018). Rheumatic heart disease worldwide: JACC scientific expert panel. *Journal of the American College of Cardiology, 72*(12), 1397–1416. https://doi.org/10.1016/j.jacc.2018.06.063

Weintraub, R. G., Semsarian, C., & MacDonald, P. (2017). Dilated cardiomyopathy. *The Lancet, 390*(10092), 400–414. https://doi.org/10.1016/S0140-6736(16)31713-5

Welch, T. D. (2018). Constrictive pericarditis: Diagnosis, management and clinical outcomes. *Heart, 104*(9), 725–731. https://doi.org/10.1136/heartjnl-2017-311683

Zuhlke, L. J., Beaton, A., Engel, M., et al. (2017). Group A streptococcus, acute rheumatic fever and rheumatic heart disease: Epidemiology and clinical considerations. *Current Treatment Options in Cardiovascular Medicine, 19*(2), 15. https://doi.org/10.1007/s11936-017-0513-y

RESOURCES

Resources for this chapter are listed in Chapter 36 and Chapter 37.

40

Nursing Management
Vascular Disorders

Wendy Bowles and Jane Tyerman
Originating US chapter by Kimberly Day

evolve WEBSITE

http://evolve.elsevier.com/Canada/Lewis/medsurg

- Review Questions (Online Only)
- Key Points
- Answer Guidelines for Case Study
- Student Case Studies
  - Abdominal Aortic Aneurysm
  - Chronic Peripheral Artery Disease

- Customizable Nursing Care Plans
  - Peripheral Arterial Disease of the Lower Extremities
  - Patient after Surgical Repair of the Aorta
- Conceptual Care Map Creator

- Audio Glossary
- Content Updates

LEARNING OBJECTIVES

1. Relate the etiology and pathophysiology of peripheral artery disease (PAD) to the major risk factors.
2. Describe the clinical manifestations and interprofessional and nursing management of the patient with PAD of the lower extremities.
3. Plan appropriate nursing and interprofessional management for the patient with acute arterial ischemic disorders of the lower extremities.
4. Describe the pathophysiology, clinical manifestations, and nursing and interprofessional management of the patient with thromboangiitis obliterans (Buerger's disease) and Raynaud's phenomenon.
5. Describe the pathophysiology, clinical manifestations, and interprofessional and nursing management of patients with different types of aortic aneurysms.
6. Select appropriate nursing interventions for a patient undergoing an aortic aneurysm repair.
7. Describe the pathophysiology, clinical manifestations, and interprofessional and nursing management of the patient with aortic dissection.
8. Evaluate the risk factors predisposing patients to develop superficial vein thrombosis or venous thromboembolism (VTE).
9. Distinguish between the clinical characteristics of superficial vein thrombosis and VTE.
10. Outline the interprofessional and nursing management of patients with superficial vein thrombosis and VTE.
11. Prioritize the key aspects of nursing management for the patient receiving anticoagulant therapy.
12. Relate the pathophysiology and clinical manifestations to the interprofessional care of patients with varicose veins, chronic venous insufficiency, and venous leg ulcers.

KEY TERMS

acute arterial ischemia
aneurysm
aortic dissection
chronic venous insufficiency (CVI)
critical limb ischemia
deep vein thrombosis (DVT)

embolus
intermittent claudication
peripheral artery disease (PAD)
post-thrombotic syndrome
Raynaud's phenomenon
superficial vein thrombosis (SVT)

thromboangiitis obliterans (TAO)
thrombus
varicose veins
venous thromboembolism (VTE)
Virchow's triad

Health challenges related to the vascular system include disorders of the arteries, veins, and lymphatic vessels. Arterial disorders are classified as aneurysmal, atherosclerotic, and non-atherosclerotic vascular diseases. Atherosclerotic vascular disease is divided into coronary, cerebral, peripheral, mesenteric, and renal artery disease. This chapter provides a discussion of peripheral artery disease (PAD), aortic aneurysm and dissection, and venous diseases.

PERIPHERAL ARTERY DISEASE

Peripheral artery disease (PAD) is a condition that involves thickening of the artery walls, which results in a progressive narrowing of the arteries of the upper and lower extremities. The risk of developing PAD increases with age. Individuals typically become symptomatic between ages 50 and 70 years. In people with diabetes mellitus, symptoms of PAD may occur at a much earlier age.

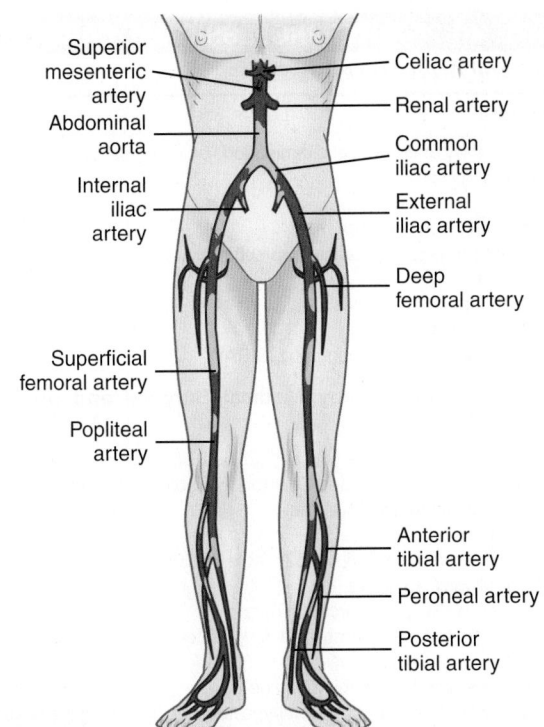

FIG. 40.1 Common anatomical locations (shown in yellow) of atherosclerotic lesions of the abdominal aorta and lower extremities.

PAD is associated with coronary artery disease (CAD) and its risk factors. Thus, PAD is a marker of more advanced systemic atherosclerosis. An estimated 800 000 Canadians have been diagnosed with PAD, with a higher proportion being Indigenous people because of the higher prevalence of risk factors such as diabetes, smoking, and kidney disease in this population (Bonneau et al., 2018).

PAD may affect the aortoiliac, femoral, popliteal, tibial, or peroneal arteries or any combination of these (Figure 40.1). The femoral popliteal area is the site most commonly affected in nondiabetic patients. Patients with diabetes mellitus tend to develop PAD in the arteries below the knee. In advanced PAD, occlusions are found at multiple levels.

ETIOLOGY AND PATHOPHYSIOLOGY OF PERIPHERAL ARTERY DISEASE

The leading cause of PAD is *atherosclerosis*, a gradual thickening of the *intima* (the innermost layer of the arterial wall) and the *media* (middle layer of the arterial wall). This results from cholesterol and lipids deposited within the vessel walls and leads to progressive narrowing of the artery lumen (see Figure 36.1). Atherosclerosis often affects certain segments of the arterial tree. These include the coronary (see Chapter 36), carotid (see Chapter 60), aorta, common iliac, superficial femoral, popliteal, and tibial and pedal arteries (see Figure 40.1). Clinical symptoms occur when vessels are 60 to 75% blocked. As stated earlier, PAD is also highly correlated with CAD (Ozkaramanli Gur et al., 2018).

Although the exact cause or causes of atherosclerosis are unknown, inflammation and endothelial injury play a major role (see Chapter 36). While PAD is systemic, it typically is most symptomatic in the aortoiliac system or the peripheral system, in the lower extremities.

Significant risk factors for PAD include tobacco use (most important), diabetes, uncontrolled hypertension, and hyperlipidemia. Other risk factors include family history, hypertriglyceridemia, increasing age, hyperhomocysteinemia, hyperuricemia, obesity, sedentary lifestyle, and stress (Kulezic et al., 2019). The TASC II guidelines describe the etiology, pathophysiology, and treatment more extensively, and while more recent work exists, these guidelines remain highly applicable to the understanding and treatment of PAD (Norgren et al., 2007).

PERIPHERAL ARTERY DISEASE

Clinical Manifestations

The severity of PAD depends on the site and extent of the obstruction and the amount of collateral circulation. The classic symptom of lower extremity PAD is intermittent claudication, an ischemic muscle ache or "leg attack" that is precipitated by exercise, resolves with rest, and is reproducible. The ischemic pain is a result of the accumulation of end products of anaerobic cellular metabolism, such as lactic acid. Once the patient stops exercising, the metabolites are cleared and the pain subsides. PAD of the aortoiliac arteries produces claudication in the buttocks and thighs, whereas calf claudication indicates femoral or popliteal artery involvement. Only about 10% of patients with PAD display the well-known symptom of intermittent claudication (Fereydooni et al., 2019).

The physical appearance of the limb provides important information about blood flow. The skin becomes thin, shiny, and taut, and hair loss occurs on the lower legs. In the presence of diabetes, foot architecture can be altered, including hammer toes and Charcot deformity. Pedal, popliteal, or femoral pulses are diminished or absent. The assessment of PAD also includes changes in colour, warmth, sensation, and movement (CWMS). These are part of the 6 P's used to assess acute arterial ischemia (discussed later in this chapter).

Paresthesia, manifested as numbness or tingling in the toes or feet, may result from nerve tissue ischemia. True peripheral neuropathy occurs more commonly in patients with diabetes (see Chapter 52) and in those with long-standing ischemia. Neuropathy can produce excruciating shooting or burning pain in the extremity, does not follow particular nerve roots, and may be present near ulcerated areas. Gradually diminishing perfusion to neurons obviates sensations of both pressure and deep pain. Thus, affected patients may not notice lower extremity injuries.

Pallor (blanching of the foot) develops with leg elevation (*elevation pallor*). In dark-skinned patients with pallor, normal brown skin appears to be yellow-brown, and normal black skin often appears to be ashen grey. Assessment of limb pallor in the dark-skinned patient requires observation of less pigmented areas such as the nailbeds or sole of the foot. Conversely, *reactive hyperemia* (redness of the foot) develops when the limb is in a dependent position (*dependent rubour;* Table 40.1). It is difficult to observe erythema in the dark-skinned patient, but the limb colour would be darker than other skin areas.

As PAD progresses and involves multiple arterial segments, continuous pain at rest develops. *Rest pain* most often occurs in the forefoot or toes and is aggravated by limb elevation; the blood flow is insufficient to meet basic metabolic requirements of the distal tissues. Rest pain occurs more often at night because cardiac output tends to drop during sleep and the limbs are at the level of the heart. Affected patients often try to partially relieve the pain by dangling their leg over the side of the

TABLE 40.1	COMPARISON OF PERIPHERAL ARTERY AND VENOUS DISEASE	
Characteristic	Peripheral Artery Disease	Venous Disease
Peripheral pulses	Decreased or absent	Present; may be difficult to palpate with edema
Capillary refill	>2 sec	<2 sec
Ankle–brachial index	≤0.95	>0.90
Edema	Absent unless leg is constantly in dependent position (advanced disease)	Lower leg edema
Hair	Loss of hair on legs, feet, toes	Hair may be present or absent
Ulcer location	Tips of toes, foot, or lateral malleolus	Near medial malleolus
Ulcer margin	Rounded, smooth, looks "punched out"	Irregularly shaped
Ulcer drainage	Minimal	Moderate to large amount
Ulcer tissue	Black eschar or pale pink granulation	Yellow slough or dark red, "ruddy" granulation
Pain	Intermittent claudication or rest pain in foot; ulcer may or may not be painful	Dull ache or sensation of heaviness in calf or thigh; ulcer often painful
Nails	Thickened; brittle; common fungal infections	Normal or thickened
Skin colour	Dependent rubour; elevation pallor; pale	Bronze-brown pigmentation (hemosiderin staining); varicose veins may be visible
Skin texture	Thin, shiny, taut	Skin thick, hardened, and indurated
Skin temperature	Cool, temperature gradient down the leg	Warm, no temperature gradient
(Stasis) Dermatitis	Rare	Frequent
Pruritus	Rare	Frequent

TABLE 40.2	INTERPROFESSIONAL CARE

Peripheral Artery Disease

Diagnostic

- Health history and physical examination, including palpation of peripheral pulses
- Ankle–brachial index (ABI)
- Segmental blood pressures
- Computed tomographic angiography (CTA)
- Angiography (invasive)
- Doppler ultrasound studies
- Duplex imaging
- Magnetic resonance angiography (MRA)

Interprofessional Therapy; Medical, Surgical, and Interventional Management

- Life style factors; achieve or maintain ideal body weight; dietary optimization (DASH diet; see Chapter 35, Table 35.7), increase physical activity (patient specific)
- Smoking cessation
- Proper foot care (see Chapter 52, Table 52.20)
- Regular physical exercise
- Structured walking or exercise program
- Wound care and management, in conjunction with other medical and revascularization modalities
- Medical therapy with antiplatelet agents
- Tight blood pressure control; antihypertensives including β blockers, thiazide diuretics, and calcium channel blockers and angiotensin-converting enzyme inhibitors (see Table 35.8)
- Treatment of hyperlipidemia (see Chapter 36, Table 36.5) and hypertriglyceridemia
- Tight glucose control in diabetic patients; antihyperglycemics; SGLT inhibitors, DPP-4 inhibitors and insulin; basal, intermediate, and short acting
- Surgical interventions, including endarterectomy, bypass grafting, extra-anatomical bypass, and amputation
- Endovascular interventions, including angioplasty, patch angioplasty (in conjunction with surgery), stenting
- Thrombolytic therapy (for acute ischemia only)
- Sympathectomy (for pain control)

bed or sleeping in a chair to allow gravity to maximize blood flow, which can manifest as dependent edema, not to be confused with peripheral edema secondary to heart failure.

Critical Limb Ischemia

Critical limb ischemia (CLI) is a condition characterized by chronic ischemic rest pain lasting more than 2 weeks, arterial leg ulcers, or gangrene of the leg as a result of PAD (Fereydooni et al., 2019). Patients with PAD who have diabetes, heart failure (HF), and a history of a stroke are at increased risk for CLI.

Complications

Lower extremity PAD progresses slowly. Prolonged ischemia leads to atrophy of the skin and underlying muscles. Because of the decreased arterial blood flow, even minor trauma to the legs and feet (e.g., blister from ill-fitting shoes) may result in delayed healing, wound infection, and tissue necrosis, especially in diabetic patients. Arterial (ischemic) ulcers most commonly occur over bony prominences on the toes, feet, and lower leg (see Table 40.1). Nonhealing arterial ulcers and gangrene are the most serious complications. Stages of PAD can be separated into classes 0 (asymptomatic) to 6 (major tissue loss, nonhealing ulcer above

midfoot) (Cronenwett & Johnston, 2014). Chronic rest pain, ulceration, or gangrene is characteristic of critical limb ischemia. Every attempt is made to save the limb, and surgical or endovascular revascularization is indicated. If a patient is not a candidate for revascularization, or if revascularization is not technically possible, medical treatment is indicated. PAD is highly associated with early mortality due to cardiovascular events.

Amputation may be needed if blood flow is not restored adequately or if severe infection occurs. If PAD has been present for an extended period, collateral circulation will develop and may prevent gangrene of the extremity, but typically collaterals cannot support the healing of an ulcer. Uncontrolled pain and severe, spreading infection are indicators that an amputation is required in individuals who are not candidates for revascularization. The rate of PAD-related lower-limb amputations among Indigenous people is three to five times higher than that for non-Indigenous populations. Indigenous people also have a higher mortality rate as a result of PAD (Bonneau et al., 2018).

Diagnostic Studies

Various tests are used to assess blood flow and outline the vascular system (Table 40.2). Doppler ultrasound with duplex imaging maps blood flow through the entire region of an artery. When palpation of a peripheral pulse proves inadequate for

TABLE 40.3	INTERPRETATION OF ANKLE–BRACHIAL INDEX RESULTS
Ankle–Brachial Index (ABI)	**Clinical Significance**
≥1.40	Noncompressible arteries
1.00–1.40	Normal ABI
0.95–0.99	Borderline ABI
≤0.95	Abnormal ABI
Classification of PAD Severity	
0.95–0.71	Mild PAD
0.71–0.41	Moderate PAD
≤40	Severe PAD

PAD, peripheral artery disease.

assessment because of severe PAD, Doppler ultrasound can be used to determine the degree of blood flow. A palpable pulse and a Doppler pulse are not equivalent, and the terms are not interchangeable.

Segmental blood pressures (BPs) are measured (with Doppler ultrasonography and a sphygmomanometer) at the thigh, below the knee, and at ankle level while the patient is supine in order to localize the area of stenosis. A drop in segmental BP of greater than 30 mm Hg suggests PAD.

The *ankle–brachial index* (ABI) is the mainstay of PAD assessment. It can be used to identify the presence as well as severity of PAD. It is also an independent screening tool for CAD (an ABI <0.9 is indicative of asymptomatic CAD). ABI is measured with a handheld Doppler probe or in a vascular lab. To calculate the ABI, the ankle systolic BPs are divided by the higher of the left and right brachial systolic BP. A normal ABI is 1.00 to 1.40 and indicates adequate BP in the extremities. An ABI between 0.95 and 0.99 is considered borderline, a value of 0.95 or less is abnormal, and values greater than 1.40 indicate noncompressible arteries (Table 40.3), which can occur in the setting of diabetes and advanced PAD. Calcified and stiff arteries in older patients and those with diabetes often show a falsely elevated ABI.

Computed tomographic angiography (CTA) is the most common modality used to delineate the location and extent of PAD. Image interpretation can be challenging as calcium cannot be extracted from the digital subtraction image. In addition, systemic contrast is used in order to make the vessels visible and can be contraindicated in patients with significant renal disease as it is excreted by the kidneys and can cause contrast-induced nephropathy. In such patients, magnetic resonance angiography (MRA) may be indicated, as less contrast is used. Both of these tests provide information on inflow and outflow vessels to plan for surgery (see Table 34.6). CTA should be used with caution in patients with renal insufficiency, diagnosed or not, as they may suffer from contrast-induced nephropathy post-CTA because of the effect of the contrast load on the kidneys.

Interprofessional Care
Table 40.2 summarizes the interprofessional care for a patient with PAD.

Risk Factor Modification. Patients with diabetes and atherosclerotic vascular disease such as CAD or PAD are at the highest risk for cardiovascular events such as myocardial infarction (MI), ischemic stroke, and cardiovascular disease–related death, also known as MACE (major adverse cardiovascular event). The clinical practice guidelines of the Diabetes Canada

Clinical Practice Guidelines Expert Committee (2018) stress the importance of lifestyle modifications such as achieving and maintaining a healthy body weight, regular physical activity, smoking cessation, optimal BP control, and optimal glycemic control (Houlden, 2018). Risk factors may be modified with medication therapy and lifestyle changes for the patient (see Tables 36.1 through 36.5). Tobacco cessation is essential in the management of patients with PAD to reduce the risk of cardiovascular disease–related events, PAD progression, and death. Tobacco cessation is a complex and difficult process with a high incidence of relapse. All patients with PAD should have access to comprehensive smoking cessation interventions, if needed (see the Resources at the end of Chapter 11).

Canadian lipid guidelines recommend aggressive management, with target levels for low-density lipoprotein (LDL) cholesterol being 2.0 mmol/L or less, total cholesterol, high-density lipoprotein (HDL) cholesterol ratio less than 4.0 mmol/L, and Apo B less than 0.8 g/L or non-HDL cholesterol less than 2.6 mmol/L. Although dietary change is also recommended, this alone is unlikely to achieve these goals. Research indicates that in patients with PAD, treatment with a statin (e.g., atorvastatin [Lipitor]) not only lowers cholesterol levels but also reduces risks of cardiovascular disease–related morbidity and mortality. If pharmacological treatment is started, a goal of greater than 50% reduction in LDL cholesterol or the above targets guides therapy (Reynolds et al., 2020). Table 36.5 lists medications used to lower cholesterol.

Hypertension is a major risk factor for PAD progression, as well as for other cardiovascular disease–related events. The Canadian Hypertension Education Program (2018) recommendations for the management of hypertension in patients with no comorbid conditions of diabetes, kidney disease, or end-organ damage include BP lower than 140/90 mm Hg. In patients with diabetes mellitus, BP lower than 130/80 mm Hg is recommended (Stone et al., 2018). Initial antihypertensive medication therapy includes thiazides, long-acting calcium channel blockers, angiotensin-converting enzyme (ACE) inhibitors, and angiotensin II receptor blockers (ARBs). Lifestyle changes are encouraged and include reducing dietary sodium and following the Dietary Approaches to Stop Hypertension (DASH) diet. (Hypertension is discussed in Chapter 35.)

Diabetes is also a well-known risk factor for PAD. Neuropathy is a predominant symptom, and neuropathy or loss of protective sensation is the leading cause of amputation, which is classified as a major adverse limb event (MALE). It is recommended that patients with diabetes maintain a glycosylated hemoglobin (hemoglobin A_{1c}) below 7.0% and less than 6.5% for those at high risk for MACE or MALE. (Diabetes mellitus is discussed in Chapter 52.) These patients should regularly check their sensation (using the LEAP Program; see Resources at the end of the chapter) with a health care provider.

Medication Therapy. ACE inhibitors (e.g., ramipril [Altace]) can reduce PAD symptoms. Antiplatelet agents are considered crucial for reducing the risks of cardiovascular disease–related events and death. Guidelines for oral antiplatelet therapy recommend acetylsalicylic acid (ASA). For patients who are ASA intolerant, clopidogrel (Plavix) is indicated. Combination antiplatelet therapy with ASA (Aspirin) and clopidogrel may be used by select high-risk patients. Anticoagulants, including both the older agents such as warfarin and the newer direct oral anticoagulants, are not recommended for the prevention of cardiovascular disease–related events in patients with PAD.

Two medications are available to treat intermittent claudication: cilostazol and pentoxifylline. Cilostazol, a phosphodiesterase inhibitor, inhibits platelet aggregation and increases vasodilation. Pentoxifylline, a xanthine derivative, improves the flexibility of red blood cells (RBCs) and white blood cells (WBCs) and decreases fibrinogen concentration, platelet adhesiveness, and blood viscosity. It is not as effective as cilostazol. Cilostazol is usually stopped within 3 months because of its adverse effects.

Exercise Therapy. The primary nonpharmacological treatment for intermittent claudication is tobacco cessation in combination with a formal, supervised exercise-training program. A supervised PAD rehabilitation program is an effective means of improving exercise performance. Such programs typically include moderate to vigorous exercise for 30 to 60 minutes a day, three to five times a week, for a minimum of 3 months. Walking is the most effective exercise for patients with PAD. Supervised, treadmill exercise training improves walking performance and quality of life in patients with PAD regardless of whether they have claudication (Khoury et al., 2019). A home exercise program is an alternative to a formal program. The nurse should encourage slow, progressive physical activity after a warm-up period. The patient is instructed to walk until the point of discomfort, stop and rest, and then resume walking until the discomfort recurs. An exercise therapy program should also be implemented in patients with PAD after surgical interventions (discussed later in this chapter).

Nutritional Therapy. Patients with PAD should be taught to adjust their dietary intake so that their body mass index is less than 25 kg/m² and their waist circumference is less than 101.6 cm (37 inches) for men and less than 89 cm (31.5 inches) for women (Warton et al., 2020). A diet high in fruits, vegetables, and whole grains and low in cholesterol, saturated fat, and salt is recommended. Dietary cholesterol intake should be less than 200 mg/day, saturated fat intake should be substantially reduced, and dietary sodium should be 2 g/day or less (see Chapter 37, Table 37.11).

Complementary and Alternative Therapies. A number of vitamin, mineral, dietary, and herbal supplements have been investigated in the treatment of intermittent claudication. Currently, data are insufficient to support the efficacy of supplemental fish oil, ginkgo biloba, L-arginine, or homocysteine-lowering vitamins (e.g., folate, vitamin B₆, cobalamin) in the treatment of claudication. Vitamin E is not recommended to treat claudication. Patients taking antiplatelet agents, nonsteroidal anti-inflammatory agents (NSAIDs) and anticoagulants should consult with their health care provider before taking any dietary or herbal supplements because of potential interactions and bleeding risks (see the Complementary & Alternative Therapies: Natural Health Products That May Affect Clotting box later in the chapter).

Interventional Radiological Catheter-Based Procedures. Interventional radiology catheter-based procedures are alternatives to open surgical approaches for treatment of PAD in the lower extremity. These procedures take place both in interventional radiology and operative suites. All of these procedures are similar to angiography in that they involve the insertion of a specialized catheter into the femoral artery. *Percutaneous transluminal angioplasty* (PTA) involves the use of a catheter that contains a cylindrical balloon at the tip. The end of the catheter is advanced to and crosses the narrowed (stenotic) area of the artery. When in position, the balloon is inflated, compressing

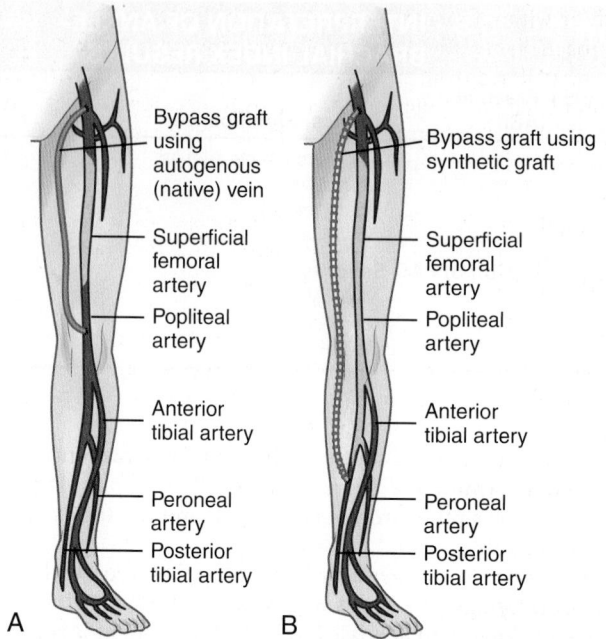

FIG. 40.2 A, Femoral–popliteal bypass graft around an occluded superficial femoral artery. **B,** Femoral–posterior tibial bypass graft around occluded superficial femoral, popliteal, and proximal tibial arteries.

the atherosclerotic intimal lining while also stretching the underlying media.

Stents, expandable metallic devices, are placed within the artery after the balloon angioplasty. The stent holds the artery open and can be used as a treatment for PAD as well as dissections that can spontaneously occur in the peripheral system or can be an adverse event associated with interventions for PAD (Stoner et al., 2016).

Atherectomy is the removal of the obstructing plaque. In directional atherectomy, a high-speed cutting disc built into the catheter end cuts long strips of the atheroma. In laser atherectomy, ultraviolet energy is used to break the molecular bonds of the atheroma to reduce the stenosis and is used in some cases to treat PAD.

Cryoplasty combines PTA and cold therapy. A specialized balloon is filled with liquid nitrous oxide, which changes to gas as it enters the balloon. Expansion of the gas results in cooling to –10°C (14°F). The cold temperature limits restenosis by reducing smooth muscle cell activity.

Surgical Interventions. Various surgical approaches can be used to improve blood flow in a stenotic or occluded artery. Several options for revascularization exist. When possible, peripheral artery bypass surgery is done with an autogenous (native) vein or synthetic graft material to bypass or detour blood around the lesion (Figure 40.2). Autogenous grafts can be either reversed or in situ. Saphenous vein is the most common composite as it is the superficial vein, thus preserving the deep system for venous return. PTA with stenting may also be done, in combination with bypass surgery.

Other surgical options include *endarterectomy* (opening the artery and removing the obstructing plaque) and *patch graft angioplasty* (opening the artery, removing plaque, and sewing a patch to the opening to widen the lumen, which can be vein, Dacron, or bovine pericardium).

Endovascular Interventions. PTA and stenting can be used alone or in combination with bypass surgery. Angioplasty with or without stenting has become an increasingly common approach, especially with an increasingly fragile patient population, as it avoids a more invasive approach and requires less wound healing. While the patency is not as long as with a full bypass, it is often long enough in this population as the life expectancy in older persons with PAD is typically less than 5 years.

Amputation may be required if tissue necrosis is extensive, if infectious gangrene or osteomyelitis (infection in the bone) develops, or if all major arteries in the limb are occluded, all of which preclude the possibility of successful reparative surgery (TASC et al., 2015). Every effort is made to preserve as much of the limb as possible so that the potential for rehabilitation is optimized. Implementation of an amputee mobility policy after surgery can increase functional mobility of patients with a lower limb amputation and maximize their rehabilitation potential. (Amputation is discussed in Chapter 65.)

🌿 COMPLEMENTARY & ALTERNATIVE THERAPIES
Natural Health Products That May Affect Clotting

Anticoagulant Effects
Increased
- Angelica, anise, bilberry, bromelain, celery, chamomile, devil's claw, dong quai, fenugreek, feverfew, garlic, ginger, *Ginkgo biloba,* goldenseal, horse chestnut, licorice root, lovage root, meadowsweet, motherwort, parsley, passionflower, red clover, rue, turmeric, willow bark

Decreased
- Coenzyme Q$_{10}$, ginseng, green tea, St. John's wort

Nursing Implications
- In general, these natural products should be used with caution or not at all by patients with bleeding or clotting disorders or those taking anticoagulant and antiplatelet medications. These patients should consult with a health care provider before using any of these natural products.
- These natural health products should be discontinued at least 2 to 3 weeks before surgery to avoid potential complications. If this is not possible, the herbal product in its original container should be brought to the health care provider or the surgery site so that the anaesthesia care provider knows exactly what the patient is taking.
- One common mechanism of these products is to inhibit platelet aggregation.
- Cannabinoids are the latest trend and are being used by many patients, especially when trying to manage pain. The effects on the vascular system are concerning and need to be a part of the health assessment (Alberta Rheumatology, 2021; Banerjee & McCormack, 2019).

NURSING MANAGEMENT
LOWER EXTREMITY PERIPHERAL ARTERY DISEASE AND CRITICAL LIMB ISCHEMIA

NURSING ASSESSMENT
Table 40.4 lists subjective and objective data that the nurse should obtain from a patient with PAD.

NURSING DIAGNOSES
Nursing diagnoses for a patient with PAD of the lower extremities (who has not undergone surgery) may include but are not limited to the following:
- *Inadequate peripheral tissue perfusion*
- *Reduced stamina*

TABLE 40.4 NURSING ASSESSMENT
Peripheral Artery Disease

Subjective Data
Important Health Information
Past health history: Diabetes mellitus, tobacco use, hypertension, hyperlipidemia, stoke, myocardial infarction, hypertriglyceridemia, hyperuricemia, impaired renal function, obesity; ↑ high-sensitivity C-reactive protein, homocysteine or lipoprotein (a) levels; positive family history; exposure to environmental smoke; sedentary lifestyle; stress, diet
High intake of sodium, saturated fat, and cholesterol; elevated hemoglobin A$_{1c}$ level
Exercise intolerance

Symptoms
- Intermittent claudication; buttock, thigh, or calf pain that is precipitated by exercise and that subsides with rest
- 6 P's (**p**allor, **p**ain, **p**aresthesia, **p**aralysis, **p**oikilothermia, **p**ulselessness); changes in colour, warmth, sensation, movement; numbness, tingling, sensation of cold in legs or feet; progressive loss of sensation and deep pain in extremities
- Rest pain; claudication that progresses to pain at rest; burning pain in feet and toes at rest
- Erectile dysfunction

Objective Data
Integumentary
Loss of hair on legs and feet; thick toenails; pallor with elevation; dependent rubour; thin, cool, shiny skin with muscle atrophy; skin breakdown and arterial ulcers, especially over bony areas; gangrene

Peripheral Vascular
Decreased or absent peripheral pulses; feet cool to touch; capillary refill >3 sec; possible presence of bruits at pulse sites

Neurological
Mobility or sensation impairment

Possible Diagnostic Findings
↓ Ankle–brachial index (ABI), arterial stenosis evident with duplex imaging, ↓ segmental limb pressures (Doppler ultrasound pressures combined with blood pressure measurements), CTA or traditional angiogram indicative of peripheral atherosclerosis

CTA, computed tomographic angiography.

- *Chronic pain* (ischemia, inflammation, and swelling)
- *Inadequate knowledge of treatment plan,* difficulty managing complex treatment regimen

Additional information on nursing diagnoses for the patient with PAD of the lower extremities is presented in Nursing Care Plan (NCP) 40.1, available on the Evolve website for this chapter.

PLANNING
Nursing care focuses on the priority problems of poor tissue perfusion and pain. The overall goals for a patient who has PAD include (a) adequate tissue perfusion; (b) relief of pain; (c) increased exercise tolerance; (d) intact, healthy skin on extremities; and (e) increased knowledge of the disease and treatment plan.

NURSING IMPLEMENTATION
HEALTH PROMOTION. The nurse needs to assess the patient for risk factors for cardiovascular disease and provide instructions on how to control these factors (see Chapter 36, Tables 36.1 and 36.2). The nurse should also teach diet modification to reduce the intake of cholesterol, saturated fat, and refined sugars, as well as proper care of the feet. The patient should be advised to

avoid of injury to the extremities. Patients with positive family histories of cardiac, diabetic, or vascular disease are encouraged to obtain regular follow-up care.

ACUTE INTERVENTION. After surgical or radiological intervention, the patient is moved to a recovery area for observation. The nurse checks the operative extremity every 15 minutes initially and then hourly for colour, temperature, sensation, movement, capillary refill, and presence of peripheral pulses or Doppler signals. If the nurse observes loss of palpable pulses or a change in the Doppler signal, or both, the health care provider or radiologist must be notified immediately and prompt intervention undertaken. ABI measurements may be ordered; the indexes should be higher than the patient's baseline and should remain stable if the bypass (or stent) remains patent. The nurse compares all assessment findings with the patient's baseline and with findings in the opposite limb. Many patients with PAD have a history of chronic ischemic rest pain and may have developed a tolerance to opioids. Therefore, aggressive pain management may be needed postoperatively, and most institutions utilize an acute pain service to aid in pain management.

After the patient leaves the recovery area, the nurse continues to monitor perfusion to the extremities and to assess for potential complications such as bleeding, hematoma, and graft failure. A dramatic increase in pain, loss of previously palpable pulses, pallor or cyanosis, decreasing ABIs, numbness or tingling, or a cold extremity suggests occlusion of the graft or stent. Hypotension in the postoperative period can also contribute to graft failure. The nurse must report these findings to the health care provider immediately.

The nurse should not place the patient in a knee-flexed position except for exercise. The patient should be turned and positioned frequently with pillows to avoid strain on the incision. On postoperative day 1, the nurse assists the patient out of bed several times daily. Short periods of different leg and body positions will not impair postoperative skin oxygen levels. The nurse needs to discourage prolonged sitting with leg dependency, since it may cause pain and edema, increase the risk of venous thrombosis, and place stress on the suture lines. If edema develops, the nurse can position the patient supine and elevate the edematous leg above heart level. On occasion, graduated compression stockings are used to help control leg edema. Walking even short distances is desirable. The use of a walker may be helpful, especially in frail older patients. Although graft patency and mortality rates are equivalent for men and women after lower extremity revascularization, women are more likely to develop wound complications than are men (Sharath et al., 2019).

Surgical site infection (SSI) after lower extremity revascularization is a serious complication. Careful postoperative assessment and wound care are important. SSIs are associated with early graft loss, reoperation, sepsis, and longer hospitalizations. In some cases, advanced wound care technologies including negative pressure therapy can be used (Sexton et al., 2020). If no complications are present, discharge from the hospital can be anticipated in 3 to 5 days.

AMBULATORY AND HOME CARE. The nurse should assess for risk factors for cardiovascular disease and be alert for opportunities to teach health promotion strategies to patients and their caregivers (see Chapters 4 and 36). Tobacco use in any form (including environmental smoke) is contraindicated. Nicotine exerts vasoconstrictive effects, and tobacco smoke impairs transport and cellular utilization of oxygen and increases blood viscosity and homocysteine levels. Continued tobacco use dramatically decreases the long-term patency rates of grafts and stents and increases the risk of an MI or stroke.

The nurse should encourage physical activity and a healthy diet and explain that it improves a number of risk factors for cardiovascular disease, including hypertension, hyperlipidemia, obesity, and glucose levels. Physical activity also improves peripheral circulation and increases walking distance (Sharath et al., 2019).

Foot care should be taught to all patients with PAD. Meticulous foot care is especially important in diabetic patients with PAD (see Table 52.20) as diabetic neuropathy increases these patients' susceptibility to traumatic injury and results in delay in seeking treatment.

Neuropathy, or the loss of protective sensation, is the leading cause of amputation; therefore, patients are instructed to inspect their legs and feet daily for changes in skin colour, sensation, warmth, and changes in bony structures such as hammer toes or pressure points and reduction in hair growth. The nurse should emphasize that patients must report any changes in these findings or the development of any ulceration or inflammation to their health care provider. Thick or overgrown toenails and calluses are potentially serious and require regular attention by a skilled health care provider (e.g., podiatrist). Patients with poor eyesight, back pain, obesity, or arthritis may need assistance with foot care. Patients are encouraged to wear clean, all-cotton or all-wool socks and comfortable shoes with rounded (not pointed) toes and soft insoles. Shoes should be laced loosely, and patients should break in new shoes gradually. Patients with diabetes are most at risk for peripheral neuropathy so should focus on appropriate footwear and nail care (Table 40.5).

▌EVALUATION

NCP 40.1, available on the Evolve website, addresses the expected outcomes for the patient with PAD of the lower extremities.

ACUTE ARTERIAL ISCHEMIC DISORDERS

Etiology and Pathophysiology

Acute arterial ischemia is a sudden interruption in the arterial blood supply to a tissue, organ, or extremity that, if left untreated, can result in tissue death. It is caused by embolism, thrombosis of a pre-existing atherosclerotic artery, or trauma. Embolization of a thrombus (clot) from the heart is the most frequent cause of acute arterial occlusion. Heart conditions in which thrombi can develop include infective endocarditis, mitral valve disease, atrial fibrillation, cardiomyopathies, and prosthetic heart valves. Noncardiac sources of emboli include aneurysms, ulcerated atherosclerotic plaque, and venous thrombi. Emboli can also develop as a result of recent endovascular procedures and, in rare cases, arteritis (Kalsi et al., 2017).

Thrombi that originate in the left side of the heart may dislodge and travel anywhere in the systemic circulation. The majority of emboli obstruct an artery of the lower extremity (e.g., iliofemoral, popliteal, tibial).

Arterial emboli tend to lodge at sites of arterial branching or in areas of atherosclerotic narrowing. An acute arterial occlusion causes the oxygen and blood supply distal to the embolus to decrease suddenly, producing ischemia. The

TABLE 40.5 PATIENT & CAREGIVER TEACHING GUIDE

Peripheral Artery Bypass Surgery

The following information should be included in the teaching plan for a patient undergoing peripheral revascularization procedures and the patient's caregiver:

1. Patients can reduce risk factors by stopping the use of tobacco products, by controlling blood pressure and blood glucose levels (if diabetic), by lowering cholesterol and triglyceride levels, by achieving and maintaining ideal body weight, and by exercising following a walking program.
2. Patients should be provided rationales, basic mechanism of action, and anticipated duration of medications such as antiplatelets, antihypertensives, anticholesterol therapy, and pain medication.
3. Diet: A healthy diet is essential to recovery. Patients should drink plenty of fluids, follow a well-balanced diet (e.g., foods high in protein, vitamins C and A, and zinc; high-fibre foods; fresh fruits and vegetables), eat fewer high-fat foods, and reduce salt intake.
4. Exercise: Patients should participate in a supervised exercise program, take a daily walk, or both. In the beginning, patients may take several short walks a day and rest between activities. Walking is gradually increased to 30–40 min/day, 3–5 days/wk. For patients who are unable to take part in a walking program other forms of exercise including an upper arm ergometer is helpful.
5. Foot care: Patients should care for their feet and legs; inspect feet and wash them daily; wear clean cotton or wool socks and well-fitting shoes; file toenails straight across; and avoid sitting with legs crossed, extreme hot and cold temperatures, and prolonged standing.
6. Postoperative: Routine postoperative wound care includes keeping the incision clean and dry; Steri-Strips (if present) should not be disturbed.
7. Wound healing: Patients should monitor for signs and symptoms of impaired healing and infection of the leg incision, and they should notify the health care provider if any of the following occur:
   - Prolonged drainage or pus from the incision
   - Increased redness, warmth, pain, or hardness along incision
   - Separation of wound edges
   - Body temperature greater than 37.8°C
8. Follow-up: Patients must keep all follow-up appointments with their health care provider.
9. Alarm symptoms: The health care provider should be notified if the patient experiences increased leg or foot pain or a change in the colour or temperature of the foot and leg.

amount of tissue and muscle at risk, degree of the ischemia, and extent of the symptoms depend on several factors, including (a) the location and size of the occlusion, (b) the occurrence of clot fragmentation with embolism to smaller vessels, (c) the degree of PAD already present, (d) the presence of collateral vessels around the acute obstruction, and (e) time to treatment (time = tissue).

Sudden local thrombosis may occur at the site of an atherosclerotic plaque. States of hypovolemia (e.g., resulting from shock), hyperviscosity (e.g., resulting from polycythemia), and hypercoagulability (e.g., resulting from cancer and chemotherapy, antiphospholipid syndrome, factor V Leiden disorder, or protein C or S disorder) predispose an individual to thrombotic arterial occlusion.

Traumatic injury to the extremity itself may cause partial or total occlusion or a cessation of perfusion secondary to an arterial injury or transection. Acute arterial occlusion may also develop as a result of arterial dissection spontaneously or as a result of iatrogenic arterial injury (e.g., after angiography).

Clinical Manifestations

Clinical manifestations of acute arterial ischemia include the "six P's": **p**ain, **p**allor, **p**aralysis, **p**ulselessness, **p**aresthesia, and **p**oikilothermia (adaptation of the limb to the environmental temperature, most often cool). Once an acute ischemic injury is revascularized, compartment syndrome is a real and present danger. In a cerebral artery this will manifest as increased intracranial pressure (Galyfos et al., 2017), and in the extremities compartment syndrome can be an emergent situation needing fasciotomy to relieve pressure to save the limb.

Complications

Without immediate intervention, ischemia may progress quickly to tissue necrosis and gangrene within a few hours. If the nurse detects these signs, the nurse should immediately notify the health care provider. Paralysis is a very late sign of acute arterial ischemia and signals the death of nerves supplying the extremity. Footdrop occurs as a result of nerve damage. Because nerve tissue is extremely sensitive to hypoxia, limb paralysis or ischemic neuropathy may be permanent even after revascularization.

Interprofessional Care

Early diagnosis and treatment are essential to keep the affected limb viable during acute arterial ischemia. Continuous intravenous (IV) unfractionated heparin is started to prevent thrombus enlargement and inhibit further embolization. In patients undergoing embolectomy, unfractionated heparin should be followed by long-term anticoagulation (see discussion of other anticoagulant options later in this chapter).

To restore blood flow, the embolus or thrombus is removed as soon as possible. Options for embolus or thrombus removal include percutaneous catheter-directed thrombolytic therapy, percutaneous mechanical thrombectomy with or without thrombolytic therapy, surgical thrombectomy, or surgical bypass. Catheter-directed intra-arterial thrombolytic therapy (e.g., tissue plasminogen activator) is recommended for patients with short-term (<14 days) thromboembolic disease. A percutaneous catheter is inserted into the femoral artery and threaded to the site of the clot, and the thrombolytic medication is infused. Thrombolytic agents work by directly dissolving the clot over a period of 24 to 48 hours. (Thrombolytic therapy is discussed in Chapter 36.) The catheter may act as a mechanical thrombectomy device; that is, it is also designed to remove or fragment the thrombus (Fimhaber, & Powell, 2019). Close monitoring is required to make sure the catheter does not move and the patient does not bleed from the site of the catheter insertion.

Surgical intervention is recommended for some patients (e.g., those with ischemia for more than 14 days when catheter-based interventions are not possible). Direct arteriotomy may be necessary to remove the clot. Surgical revascularization may be used in a patient with trauma (e.g., laceration of the artery) or with significant arterial occlusion or if interventional radiology is not available. Amputation is reserved for patients with ischemic rest pain and tissue loss, for whom limb salvage is not possible (i.e., delayed presentation). If the patient remains at risk for further embolization from a persistent source (e.g., chronic atrial fibrillation, cancer or other hypercoagulable state), long-term oral anticoagulation is recommended to prevent further acute arterial ischemic episodes (see Table 40.10 later in this chapter).

OTHER PERIPHERAL ARTERIAL DISORDERS

Thromboangiitis obliterans (TAO) (also known as *Buerger's disease*) is a nonatherosclerotic, segmental, recurrent inflammatory disorder of the small and medium-sized arteries and veins of the upper and lower extremities.

Etiology and Pathophysiology

In rare cases, systemic manifestations of the disease may involve cerebral, mesenteric, or coronary arteries. The disorder occurs predominantly in young men (<45 years) with a long history of tobacco or marihuana use (or both), but without other risk factors for cardiovascular disease (e.g., hypertension, hyperlipidemia, diabetes mellitus).

In TAO, an inflammatory process damages the blood vessel wall. Lymphocytes and giant cells infiltrate the vessel wall and fibroblasts proliferate. Ultimately, thrombosis and fibrosis occur in the vessel, causing tissue ischemia. Patients with TAO have a high rate of periodontitis and the presence of *Porphyromonas gingivalis* (a periodontal pathogen) in the occluded blood vessels. This suggests that bacterial infection plays a role in the pathogenesis of TAO.

Clinical Manifestations

The symptom complex of TAO often is confused with PAD and other inflammatory or autoimmune diseases (e.g., scleroderma). Most commonly, two or more limbs are involved and patients are often younger and commonly are smokers. Patients may have intermittent claudication of the feet, hands, or arms. As the disease progresses, rest pain and ischemic ulcerations develop. Other signs and symptoms may include colour and temperature changes of the limbs, paresthesia, superficial vein thrombosis, and cold sensitivity.

Diagnostics

There are no laboratory or diagnostic tests specific to TAO. Diagnosis is based on age at onset; history; clinical symptoms; involvement of distal vessels; presence of ischemic ulcerations; exclusion of diabetes mellitus, autoimmune disease, and thrombophilia (inherited tendency to clot); and other sources of emboli, such as atherosclerosis and aneurysm (Rivera-Chavarria & Brenes-Gutierrez, 2016).

Medical Therapy

The mainstay of treatment for TAO is the complete cessation of tobacco and marihuana use in any form. Use of nicotine replacement products is contraindicated. Conservative management includes the use of antibiotics to treat any infected ulcers and analgesics to manage the ischemic pain. Patients must avoid trauma to the extremities.

Surgical and Interventional Therapy

Surgical options include lumbar sympathectomy (transection of a nerve, ganglion, and/or plexus of the sympathetic nervous system), implanting of a spinal cord stimulator, microsurgical flap and omental transfer, bypass surgery, and stem cell therapy. Sympathectomy and a spinal cord stimulator can improve distal blood flow, reduce pain, and decrease the rate of amputation, but neither alters the inflammatory process. Bypass surgery typically is not an option because of the involvement of smaller, distal vessels. It may be used in select patients with severe ischemia. Stem cells can differentiate into specialized adult cells, with the potential to become any tissue in the human body. Stem cell therapy promotes ulcer healing, new blood vessel formation, and nerve cell regeneration (Cacione et al., 2018).

Painful ulcerations may necessitate finger or toe amputations. Amputation below the knee may be necessary in severe cases. The rate of amputation in patients who continue tobacco or marihuana use after diagnosis is much higher than that for the general population.

RAYNAUD'S PHENOMENON

Raynaud's phenomenon is an overarching term that encompasses Raynaud disease and Raynaud syndrome. In his original thesis, Maurice Raynaud described the ischemic mechanism but the nomenclature has been less than clear. These terms differentiate the two main etiological subsets of Raynaud's phenomenon: *Raynaud disease*, where there is no associated or underlying disorder, and *Raynaud syndrome*, where there is an episodic vasospastic disorder of small cutaneous arteries, most frequently involving the fingers and toes. Raynaud's phenomenon occurs primarily in young women (typically between 15 and 40 years of age) (Fábián et al., 2019). The exact etiology of Raynaud's phenomenon remains unknown. One theory is that the vasospasm results from an exaggerated response to sympathetic nervous system stimulation. Other contributing factors include occupation-related trauma and pressure to the fingertips, as noted in typists, pianists, and people who use handheld vibrating equipment. Exposure to heavy metals (e.g., lead) may also be a contributing factor.

Primary Raynaud's phenomenon, the more common form of the disease, is associated with significantly poorer physical and mental health–related quality of life. When symptoms occur in association with autoimmune diseases (e.g., rheumatoid arthritis, systemic lupus erythematosus), the disorder is called *secondary Raynaud's phenomenon*.

Clinical Manifestations

Raynaud's phenomenon is characterized by vasospasm-induced colour changes of the fingers, toes, ears, and nose (white, blue, and red). Decreased perfusion results in pallor (white). The digits then appear cyanotic (bluish-purple) (Figure 40.3). These changes are followed by rubour (redness), caused by the hyperemic response that occurs when perfusion is restored. The patient usually describes coldness and numbness in the vasoconstrictive phase, followed by throbbing, aching pain; tingling; and swelling in the hyperemic phase. An episode usually lasts only minutes but, in severe cases, may persist for several hours. Exposure to cold, emotional upset, tobacco use, and caffeine usually precipitate symptoms. After frequent, prolonged attacks, the skin may become thickened and the nails brittle. On occasion, complications include punctate (small hole) lesions of the fingertips and superficial gangrenous ulcers in advanced stages. Diagnosis is based on persistence of symptoms for at least 2 years. Patients should stop using all tobacco products and avoid using caffeine and other medications or drugs that have vasoconstrictive effects (e.g., amphetamines, cocaine, ergotamine, pseudoephedrine).

Patients with Raynaud's phenomenon often describe themselves as anxious or depressed, or both (Fábián et al., 2019). Biofeedback, relaxation training, and stress management may be useful, but research in this area is inconclusive. If these options are appropriate, the nurse should encourage patients to explore them. When a patient's episodes are severe and other therapies

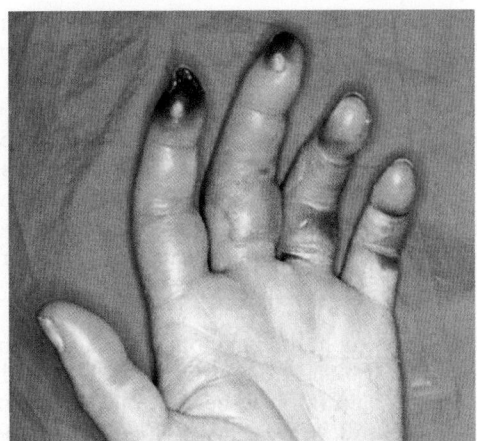

FIG. 40.3 Raynaud's phenomenon. Source: Kamal, A., & Brockelhurst, J. C. (1991). *Color atlas of geriatric medicine* (2nd ed.). Mosby–Year Book.

are ineffective, medication therapy is considered. Calcium channel blockers (e.g., diltiazem [Cardizem]) are the first-line medication therapy (Herrick & Wigley, 2020). Calcium channel blockers relax smooth muscles of the arterioles by blocking the influx of calcium into the cells, thus reducing the frequency and severity of vasospastic attacks.

Interventional Therapy

Sympathectomy is considered only in advanced cases. Patients with Raynaud's phenomenon should receive routine follow-up to monitor for development of connective tissue or autoimmune diseases because Raynaud's phenomenon may be an early sign of scleroderma.

Interprofessional Care

The primary focus of nursing management of Raynaud's phenomenon is patient education. Instructions should focus on preventing recurrent episodes. Patients should wear loose, warm clothing as protection from the cold, including gloves when using the refrigerator or freezer or when handling cold objects. At all times, patients should avoid temperature extremes. Immersing hands in warm water often decreases the vasospasm.

OTHER VASCULAR DISORDERS

There are several other vascular disorders that go beyond the scope of this chapter but can be of significant interest to the reader. These include nonspecific arteriopathies such as Takayasu's disease and connective tissue disorders, including Marfan syndrome and Ehlers-Danlos syndrome. Less common causes of vasculitis include Bechet's disease, polyarteritis nodosa, and Kawasaki's disease. Finally, uncommon causes of resistant hypertension and renovascular disease include fibromuscular dysplasia, aortic coarctation, and neurofibromatosis.

AORTIC ANEURYSMS

The aorta is the largest artery and supplies oxygen and blood to all vital organs. One of the most common conditions affecting the aorta is an aneurysm, a permanent, localized outpouching or dilation of the vessel wall (either congenital or acquired). Aneurysms occur in men more often than in women, and their

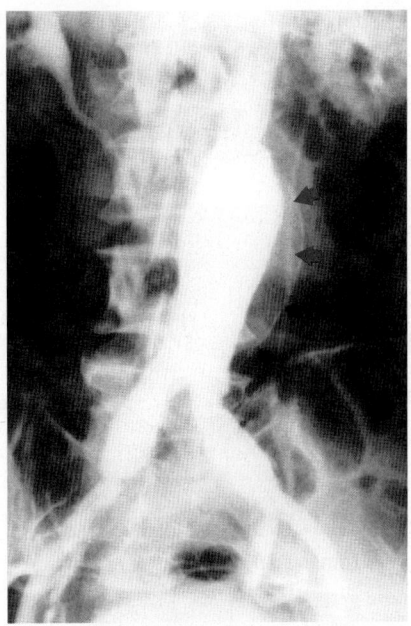

FIG. 40.4 Angiogram demonstrates a fusiform abdominal aortic aneurysm. Note calcification of the aortic wall *(arrows)* and extension of the aneurysm into the common iliac arteries. Source: Courtesy James O. Menzoian, Boston, MA.

incidence increases with age (Golledge, 2019). Peripheral artery aneurysms also develop but are less common.

Etiology and Pathophysiology

Aortic aneurysms may involve the aortic arch, thoracic aorta, abdominal aorta, or a combination. Most aneurysms, however, are found in the abdominal aorta below the level of the renal arteries (infrarenal). The growth rate of aneurysms is unpredictable, but the larger the aneurysm, the greater the risk of rupture. The dilated aortic wall becomes lined with thrombi that can embolize, leading to acute ischemic symptoms to distal (downstream) branches. Of true aortic aneurysms, 75% occur in the abdomen (Figure 40.4) and 25% in the thoracic aorta. Popliteal artery aneurysms rank third in frequency. Patients may have more than one aneurysm, in different locations.

Although various disorders are associated with aortic aneurysms, the primary cause may be classified as degenerative, congenital, mechanical, inflammatory, or infectious. The most common etiology of aneurysms of the aorta is atherosclerosis (Leone et al., 2020). Atherosclerotic plaques are deposited beneath the *intima* (the innermost layer of the arterial wall). This plaque formation is thought to cause degenerative changes in the *media* (middle layer of the arterial wall), leading to loss of elasticity, weakening, and eventual dilation of the aorta.

Male sex, age of 65 years or older, and tobacco use are the major risk factors for abdominal aortic aneurysms (AAAs) of atherosclerotic origin. Other risk factors include the presence of CAD or PAD, hypertension, and high cholesterol levels (Black & Burke, 2020). Studies have shown a strong genetic component in AAA development. The familial tendency is related to a number of congenital anomalies, including specific collagen defects (e.g., Ehlers-Danlos syndrome) and premature breakdown of vascular elastic tissue (Marfan syndrome). Less common causes of AAAs include penetrating or blunt trauma from motor vehicle collisions, inflammatory aortitis (e.g., Takayasu's or giant cell arteritis), and infectious aortitis (e.g., from syphilis or *Salmonella* or human immunodeficiency virus [HIV] infection).

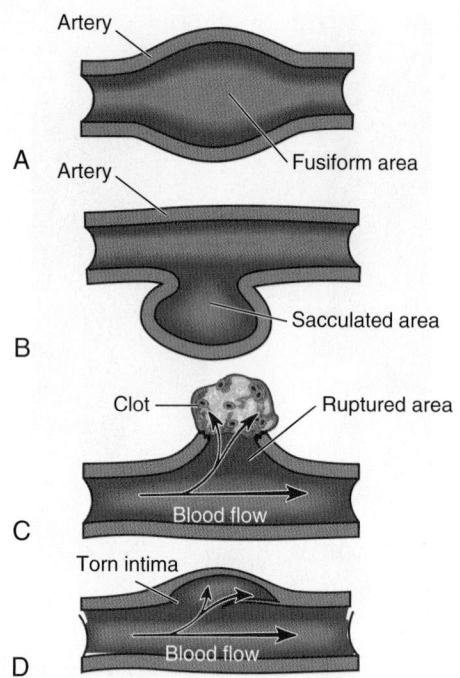

FIG. 40.5 A, True fusiform abdominal aortic aneurysm. **B,** True saccular aortic aneurysm. **C,** False aneurysm, or pseudoaneurysm. **D,** Aortic dissection.

Classification

Aneurysms are classified as true or false (Figure 40.5, *A* to *D*). A *true aneurysm* is one in which the wall of the artery forms the aneurysm, with at least one vessel layer still intact. True aneurysms can be further subdivided into fusiform and saccular dilations. A *fusiform aneurysm* is circumferential and relatively uniform in shape. A *saccular aneurysm* is pouchlike with a narrow neck connecting the bulge to one side of the arterial wall. Saccular aneurysms are more susceptible to rupture than fusiform.

A *false aneurysm,* or *pseudoaneurysm,* is not an aneurysm but a disruption of all layers of the arterial wall, resulting in bleeding that is contained by surrounding structures. False aneurysms may result from trauma or infection or occur after peripheral artery bypass graft surgery. They may also result from arterial leakage after removal of cannulas such as lower extremity arterial catheters and intra-aortic balloon pump devices.

Clinical Manifestations

Thoracic aortic aneurysms (TAAs) are often symptomatic. When present, symptoms include deep, diffuse chest pain extending to the interscapular area. Ascending aorta and aortic arch aneurysms can cause (1) angina from decreased blood flow to the coronary arteries; (2) transient ischemic attacks from decreased blood flow to the carotid arteries; and (3) coughing, shortness of breath, hoarseness, and/or difficulty swallowing from pressure on the laryngeal nerve. If the aneurysm presses on the superior vena cava, decreased venous return can result in jugular venous distention and edema of the face and arms.

AAAs are often asymptomatic and frequently detected on routine physical examination or when the patient is examined for an unrelated health issue (e.g., on abdominal radiographic examination, ultrasound study, CT scan). A pulsatile mass in the periumbilical area slightly to the left of the midline may be present. Bruits may be audible through a stethoscope placed over the aneurysm. These physical findings may be more difficult to detect in individuals with obesity and may be falsely identified in thin individuals.

Symptoms of an AAA may mimic pain associated with any abdominal or back disorder. Compression of nearby aortic autonomic structures and nerves may cause symptoms, such as back pain, epigastric discomfort, alteration in bowel elimination, and intermittent claudication. On occasion, embolization is caused by plaque released by an aneurysm, even a small one.

Complications

The most serious complication of thoracic and abdominal aneurysms is rupture. If blood from a rupture leaks into the retroperitoneal space, bleeding may be controlled by surrounding anatomical structures, preventing exsanguination and death. In such cases, many patients have severe back pain and may or may not have back or flank ecchymosis *(Grey Turner's sign)*. In cases in which blood from a rupture leaks into the thoracic or abdominal cavity, more than 90% of patients die from massive hemorrhage (Scott et al., 2020). Such a patient who reaches the hospital is in or is moving toward hypovolemic shock with tachycardia, hypotension, pale clammy skin, decreased urine output, altered level of consciousness, and abdominal tenderness. (Shock is discussed in Chapter 69.) In this situation, simultaneous resuscitation and immediate surgical or endovascular repair are necessary.

Diagnostic Studies

Chest X-rays are performed to reveal abnormal widening of the thoracic aorta, and abdominal X-rays may show calcification within the aortic wall. An ECG may rule out MI, since thoracic aneurysm or dissection symptoms can mimic angina. Echocardiography is used to assess the function of the aortic valve. Ultrasound is useful for aneurysm screening and monitoring aneurysm size. A CT scan is the most accurate test for determining the length and cross-sectional diameter and the presence of thrombus in the aneurysm (Forbes, n.d.). Three-dimensional CT scans can assist in determining what type of surgical repair should be done. Magnetic resonance imaging (MRI) also may be used to diagnose and assess the location and severity of aneurysms and is usually employed when contrast is contraindicated.

Angiography, or anatomical mapping of the aortic system by contrast imaging, provides information about the involvement of intestinal, renal, or distal vessels. Angiography is rarely used as a primary diagnostic unless as part of an endovascular repair. (Angiography is discussed in Chapter 34 and Table 34.6.)

Surgical Intervention

Before open surgical repair, the patient is hydrated, and any electrolyte, coagulation, and hematocrit abnormalities are corrected. If the aneurysm has ruptured, emergency intervention, either interventional or open, is required. With ruptured AAAs, the mortality rate is as high as 90%, although screening has been shown to have an effect on lowering the death rate (Galyfos et al., 2019).

The open aneurysm repair involves a large abdominal incision through which the surgeon (a) incises the diseased aortic segment, (b) removes any thrombus or plaque, (c) sutures a synthetic graft to the aorta proximal and distal to the aneurysm, and (d) sutures the native aortic wall around the graft to act as a protective cover (Figure 40.6). If the iliac arteries are also

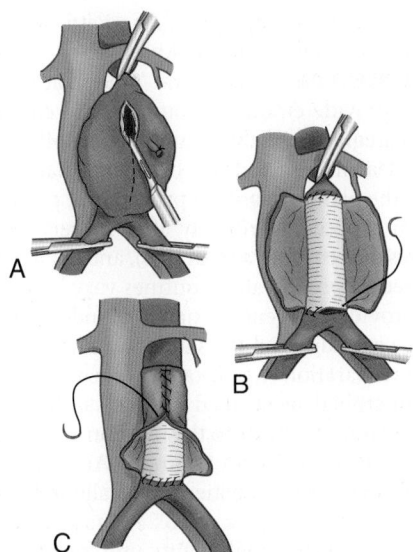

FIG. 40.6 Surgical repair of an abdominal aortic aneurysm. **A,** Incising the aneurysmal sac. **B,** Insertion of synthetic graft. **C,** Suturing native aortic wall over synthetic graft.

Renal artery

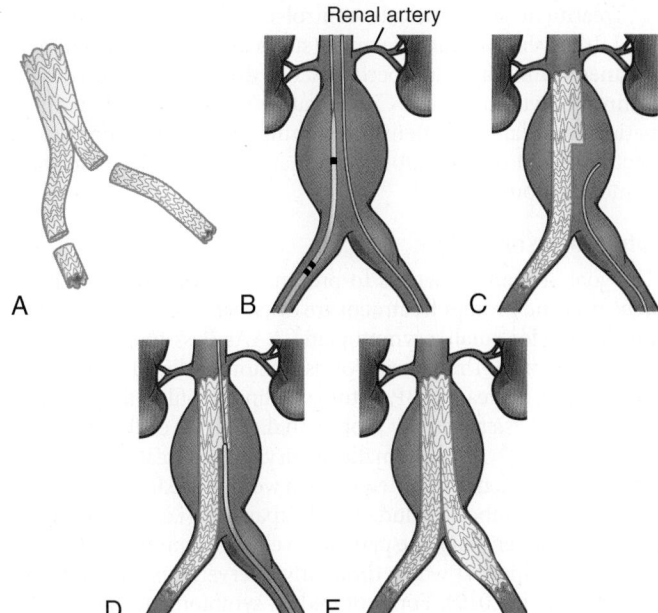

FIG. 40.7 Bifurcated (two-branched) endovascular stent grafting of an aneurysm. **A,** Insertion of a woven polyester tube (graft) covered by a tubular metal web (stent). **B,** The stent graft is inserted through a large blood vessel (e.g., femoral artery) by a delivery catheter. The catheter is positioned below the renal arteries in the area of the aneurysm. **C,** The stent graft is slowly released (deployed) into the blood vessel. When the stent comes in contact with the blood vessel, it expands to a preset size. **D,** A second stent graft can be inserted in the contralateral (opposite) vessel if necessary. **E,** Fully deployed bifurcated stent graft.

aneurysmal, a bifurcated graft replaces the entire diseased segment. With saccular aneurysms, it may be possible to excise only the bulbous lesion, the artery being repaired by primary closure (suturing the artery together) or by application of an autogenous or synthetic patch graft. *Autotransfusion,* in which the patient's own blood is recycled, reduces the need for blood transfusions (cell savers) during AAA surgery. (Autotransfusion is discussed in Chapter 33.)

All AAA resections necessitate aortic cross-clamping proximal and distal to the aneurysm. Most resections are performed in 30 to 45 minutes, after which time the clamps are removed and blood flow is restored. If the cross-clamp must be applied above the renal arteries, adequate renal perfusion after clamp removal should be ensured before the abdominal incision is closed. The risk of postoperative renal complications such as acute renal failure increases significantly when surgical repair of AAAs is above the level of the renal arteries. If the clamp is supraceliac, the risk of postoperative bowel complications such as ischemic bowel increases and should be monitored closely.

Endovascular Intervention

Minimally invasive endovascular aneurysm repair (EVAR) includes aortic, thoracic, and fenestrated grafts (EVAR, TEVAR, FEVAR). These are alternatives to open aneurysm repair and have replaced the open repair in most centres at this time, although research is ongoing regarding best outcomes in the long term. Endovascular approaches can also be part of a staged open/endo repair. Endovascular approaches involve the placement of a sutureless aortic graft into the abdominal aorta inside the aneurysm via the femoral artery. Grafts are made of various materials, such as a Dacron cylinder consisting of several components, which is supported with multiple rings of flexible wire and can be placed with each piece fitting into the next depending on size and location (Figure 40.7) based on detailed measurements obtained by CT (for scheduled repairs).

The main section of the graft is bifurcated and delivered through a femoral artery catheter. The second part of the graft is inserted through the opposite femoral artery. When all graft components are in place, they are released (deployed) against the vessel wall by balloon inflation (which creates a circumferential seal). The blood then flows through the endovascular graft, preventing further expansion of the aneurysm. Angiography is done afterward to check for any leaks and to confirm patency of all stent-graft components. The aneurysmal wall shrinks over time because the blood is diverted through the endograft. EVAR is less invasive than open aneurysm repair and requires a shorter hospital stay. EVAR also has fewer complications, such as paraplegia and death.

Complications of Open and Endovascular Repair. The most common complication of AAA repair is endoleak, the seepage of blood back into the old aneurysm. This may result from an inadequate seal at either graft end, a tear through the graft fabric, or leakage between overlapping graft segments. Repair may require coil embolization (insertion of beads) for hemostasis.

Other complications include aneurysm growth above or below the graft, aneurysm rupture, aortic dissection, bleeding, renal artery occlusion caused by stent migration, graft thrombosis, incisional site hematoma, and incisional infection. Patients undergoing EVAR need periodic imaging for the rest of their lives to monitor for an endoleak, document stability of the aneurysm sac, and determine the need for surgical intervention.

A potentially lethal complication in an emergency repair of a ruptured AAA is the development of intra-abdominal hypertension (IAH) with associated abdominal compartment syndrome. Persistent IAH reduces blood flow to the viscera. *Abdominal compartment syndrome* refers to the impaired organ perfusion caused by IAH and resulting multisystem organ failure. IAH is confirmed by measuring the patient's intra-abdominal pressure indirectly through a catheter and transducer system.

Treatment goals include control of situations that lead to IAH. Interventions include open (surgical) decompression, percutaneous drainage, and percutaneous drainage combined with a thrombolytic infusion. Conservative measures, such as intubation, ventilation, patient positioning, gastric decompression, cautious fluid resuscitation, pain management, and temporary hemofiltration, are used.

Interprofessional Care

The goal of management is to prevent aneurysm rupture. Early detection and prompt treatment are essential. Conservative medical therapy for small, asymptomatic AAAs (less than 5.4 cm) is the best practice. This consists of risk factor modification (ceasing tobacco use, decreasing BP, optimizing lipid profile, and gradually increasing physical activity [Forbes, n.d.; Galyfos et al., 2019; Rylski et al., 2017]). Asymptomatic aneurysms are treated in men at greater than 5.5 cm in diameter and in women at 5.0 cm. The caveats to these numbers include rapid expansion (i.e., >1-cm diameter increase per year), the patient develops symptoms, or the risk of rupture is high, at which time early intervention is undertaken (Galyfos et al., 2019). For ruptured or symptomatic aneurysms, early detection and prompt appropriate treatment are essential. A careful review of body systems is necessary to identify any comorbid conditions, especially of the lungs, heart, or kidneys, because they may influence the patient's risk for surgical complications. Conservative therapy of small, asymptomatic AAAs is the best practice. This consists of risk factor modification (ceasing tobacco use, decreasing BP, optimizing lipid profile) and annual monitoring of aneurysm size with ultrasonography, CT, or MRA.

NURSING MANAGEMENT
AORTIC ANEURYSMS

NURSING ASSESSMENT

Prior to an elective repair, the nurse should obtain a thorough history and perform a thorough physical assessment. Because aneurysmal and atherosclerosis are systemic diseases, the nurse should look for signs of coexisting cardiac, pulmonary, cerebral, and lower extremity vascular conditions. The patient is monitored for signs of aneurysm rupture, such as diaphoresis; pallor; weakness; tachycardia; hypotension; abdominal, back, groin, or periumbilical pain; changes in level of consciousness; or a pulsating abdominal mass.

Establishing baseline data is critical for comparison with later postoperative assessments; however, with most surgeries being done with same-day admissions, getting a baseline may more difficult. The nurse must pay special attention to the character and quality of the patient's peripheral pulses and renal and neurological status. Before surgery, the nurse should mark and document pedal pulse sites (dorsalis pedis and posterior tibial) and any skin lesions on the lower extremities.

PLANNING

The overall goals for a patient undergoing aortic surgery include (a) normal tissue perfusion, (b) intact motor and sensory function, and (c) no complications related to surgical repair, such as thrombosis, infection, or rupture, MACE or MALE.

NURSING IMPLEMENTATION

HEALTH PROMOTION. To promote overall health, the nurse encourages the patient to reduce risk factors for cardiovascular disease (see Table 36.2), including BP control, tobacco cessation (see Chapter 11), increasing physical activity, and maintaining normal body weight and serum lipid levels.

ACUTE INTERVENTION. During the preoperative period, the nurse should provide emotional support and education to the patient and caregiver and thoroughly assess all body systems. Preoperative teaching includes a brief explanation of the disease process, the planned surgical procedures, preoperative routines, what to expect immediately after surgery (e.g., recovery room, the presence of tubes and drains), and usual postoperative timelines. Specific preoperative routines vary by institution and health care provider. In general, patients undergoing scheduled aortic surgery are admitted for same-day surgery and may not have a bowel preparation (e.g., laxatives, enemas). Skin cleansing with an antimicrobial agent the day before surgery and IV antibiotics up to 30 minutes prior to the incision are standard preparation (American Association of Nursing Anaethetists, 2021).

After open aortic surgery, patients typically go to a critical care unit or specialized recovery for up to 24 hours for close monitoring and then typically to a high-acuity unit for a further 24 to 36 hours. When the patient arrives in the critical care unit, various devices are in place, including an endotracheal tube for mechanical ventilation; an arterial line; a central venous pressure (CVP) or pulmonary artery catheter; peripheral IV lines; an in-dwelling urinary catheter; and, depending on the approach and the surgeon's preference, a nasogastric tube. If the thorax is opened during surgery, chest tubes are in place. The patient needs continuous electrocardiographic and pulse oximetry monitoring. Pain medication is administered via epidural catheter or patient-controlled analgesia. In addition to the usual goals of care for a postoperative patient (e.g., maintaining BP, adequate respiratory function, fluid and electrolyte balance, and pain control; see Chapter 22), the nurse should monitor for potential complications related to the systems outlined above. The nurse should also monitor for and intervene to limit or treat dysrhythmias, hemodynamic instability, and neurological complications. See NCP 40.2, available on the Evolve website for this chapter, for care of the patient with an aneurysm repair or other aortic surgery. Administration of IV fluids and blood components (as indicated) is essential to maintain perfusion. CVP readings or pulmonary artery pressures and urinary output are monitored hourly in the immediate postoperative period to help assess the patient's hydration and perfusion status. Hypotension may be managed by administration of vasopressors and fluids, including colloids and crystalloids.

Severe hypertension must be prevented because it may cause undue stress on the arterial anastomoses, resulting in leakage of blood or rupture at the suture lines. Medication therapy with IV diuretics (e.g., furosemide [Lasix]) or IV antihypertensive agents (e.g., nitroprusside [Nipride], esmolol [Brevibloc], and labetalol [Trandate]) may be indicated.

The nurse should provide the same emotional and educational support as with an open procedure. The postoperative care and monitoring are focused primarily on prevention of cardiac and graft complications. Depending on the location of the aneurysm, this will dictate the systems most affected—that is, below or above the renal arteries, mesenteric arteries, or in the thoracic aorta. An adequate BP is important to maintain graft patency. Prolonged low BP may result in graft thrombosis. The nurse should give IV fluids and blood components as ordered to maintain adequate blood flow. The nurse also needs to monitor CVP or PA pressures and urine output hourly in the immediate postoperative period to assess the patient's hydration and perfusion status.

The patient must avoid severe hypertension, which may stress the arterial anastomoses, resulting in leakage of blood or rupture at the suture lines. Medication therapy with IV diuretics (e.g., furosemide) or IV antihypertensive agents (e.g., labetalol, metoprolol, hydralazine, sodium nitroprusside) may be indicated.

PERIOPERATIVE ADVANCED NURSING CARE FOR AORTIC ANEURYSMS

Cardiovascular Status. Myocardial ischemia or infarction may occur in the perioperative period because of decreased myocardial oxygen supply or increased myocardial oxygen demands. Cardiac dysrhythmias may occur because of electrolyte imbalances, hypoxemia, hypothermia, or myocardial ischemia. Nursing interventions include continuous electrocardiographic monitoring; frequent electrolyte and arterial blood gas determinations; administration of oxygen, IV antidysrhythmic and antihypertensive medications, and electrolytes as needed; adequate pain control; and resumption of cardiac medications.

Respiratory Status. In open procedures and with ruptures, because of the large amounts of blood products and fluid, risk of increased lung permeability, decreased lung compliance, and increased oxygen requirements are risks especially in patients with pre-existing pulmonary dysfunction. Prolonged cross-clamp time can lead to lower extremity ischemia, and potential release of inflammatory mediators can also contribute to respiratory failure. Monitoring oxygen saturations and other vital signs along with fluid status is part of postoperative care, with specifics depending on type of surgery, patient characteristics, and institutional norms.

Infection. A prosthetic vascular graft infection is a relatively rare but potentially life-threatening complication but is usually a delayed complication rather than in the initial period. Nursing interventions to prevent infection should include ensuring that the patient receives a broad-spectrum antibiotic as prescribed in the perioperative period (usually 24 hours unless complications arise). For other infections including access sites or that are respiratory, the nurse should assess body temperature regularly and report elevations promptly. Laboratory data should be monitored for an elevated WBC count, which may be the first indication of an infection. The nurse should ensure adequate nutrition and assess the surgical incision and access sites for signs of infection (e.g., redness, swelling, drainage). All IV, arterial, and CVP or pulmonary artery catheter insertion sites should be cared for with strict aseptic technique because they are ports of entry for bacteria. Meticulous perineal care for the patient with an in-dwelling urinary catheter is essential to minimize the risk of urinary tract infection, and early removal is recommended as long the patient is stable and does not need ongoing close monitoring. Surgical incisions must be kept clean and dry.

Gastrointestinal Status. After open abdominal aortic surgery, paralytic ileus may develop as a result of anaesthesia and the handling of the bowel during surgery. The intestines may become swollen and bruised, and peristalsis ceases for variable intervals. A retroperitoneal surgical approach can be used to decrease the risk of bowel complications but is usually reserved for the hostile abdomen.

A nasogastric tube may be placed during surgery and arranged with low, intermittent suction to decompress the stomach, prevent aspiration of stomach contents, and decrease pressure on suture lines. The nurse needs to record the amount and character of the nasogastric output. While the patient is NPO, oral care should be provided frequently. Ice chips or lozenges may be used to soothe a dry or irritated throat. The nurse should assess for bowel sounds; the passing of flatus signals returning bowel function and should be noted. Early ambulation should be encouraged because this promotes the return of bowel functioning. A paralytic ileus rarely lasts beyond the fourth postoperative day.

If the blood supply to the bowel is disrupted during surgery, temporary ischemia or infarction (leading to death) of intestinal tissue may result. Clinical manifestations of this rare but serious complication include absence of bowel sounds, fever, abdominal distension, diarrhea, and bloody stools. If bowel infarction occurs, immediate reoperation is necessary to restore blood flow, with probable resection of the infarcted bowel.

Neurological Status. For all aortic surgery, the nurse should monitor basic neurological function, including level of consciousness, pupil reaction, speech, and ability to move all limbs, as major surgery and the anaesthetic can evoke many complications. When the ascending aorta and aortic arch are involved, the nurse should assess the patient's level of consciousness, pupil size and response to light, facial symmetry, tongue position, speech, upper extremity movement, and quality of hand grasps. When the descending aorta is involved, neurovascular assessment of the lower extremities is important. The nurse must record all assessments and report changes from baseline to the health care provider immediately.

Peripheral Perfusion Status. The location of the aneurysm determines what type of peripheral perfusion assessment to do. The nurse should check and record all peripheral pulses hourly for several hours and then routinely, according to institutional policy. When the ascending aorta and aortic arch are involved, the nurse assesses the carotid, radial, and temporal artery pulses. For surgery of the descending aorta, the nurse assesses the femoral, popliteal, posterior tibial, and dorsalis pedis pulses (see Chapter 34, Figure 34.6).

When checking pulses, the nurse should mark the locations with a felt-tip pen so that other medical staff can locate them easily. In some cases, a Doppler may be needed to assess peripheral signals. The nurse needs to check colour, skin temperature, movement, and sensation (CWMS) as well as capillary refill time (see Chapter 34).

Sometimes, lower extremity pulses may be absent for a short time after surgery because of vasospasm and hypothermia. Decrease in or absence of the pulse accompanied by coolness, pallor, or mottling of the extremity or pain in the extremity may indicate embolization or graft occlusion. These findings must be reported to the health care provider immediately. Graft compromise necessitates reoperation or reintervention if identified early. In some patients, pulses may have been absent before surgery owing to coexistent PAD. It is essential to compare findings with those of the preoperative status to determine the cause of a decrease in or absence of pulse and the proper treatment.

Renal Perfusion Status. Postoperatively, the patient will have an in-dwelling urinary catheter. In the immediate postoperative period, for open repairs, the nurse records urine output hourly, and urinary output is maintained at 0.5 to 1 mL/kg/hr. The nurse needs to maintain accurate fluid intake and output and record daily weights until the patient resumes a regular diet. CVP and pulmonary artery pressures also provide important information about hydration status; these are monitored when the patient is in a critical care unit or high-acuity unit. The nurse evaluates renal function by monitoring daily blood urea nitrogen and serum creatinine levels. (For signs and symptoms of acute kidney injury, see Chapter 49.) Irreversible renal failure may occur after aortic surgery, particularly in individuals at high risk for complications (e.g., patients with hypotension, suprarenal or prolonged clamping during surgery, or pre-existing renal disease and diabetes). Renal perfusion can decrease as a result of embolization of the aortic thrombus or plaque to one or both renal arteries. This causes ischemia of one or both kidneys.

AMBULATORY AND HOME CARE. The nurse needs to instruct the patient and caregiver to increase activities gradually after the patient returns home. Fatigue, low mood, poor appetite, and irregular bowel habits are common after open surgery. The patient should avoid heavy lifting for 6 weeks after open surgery. Any redness, swelling, increased pain, drainage from incisions or percutaneous access sites, or fever greater than 37.8°C should be reported to a health care provider.

The patient and caregiver need to be taught to look for changes in colour or warmth of the extremities. Patients and caregivers can learn to palpate peripheral pulses to assess changes in their quality.

Sexual dysfunction in male patients is common after aortic surgery. A referral to a urologist and sexual health counsellor may be useful if erectile dysfunction occurs.

EVALUATION

Expected outcomes for the patient who undergoes aortic surgery include the following:

- Patent arterial graft with adequate distal perfusion and exclusion of aneurysm
- Adequate urine output (renal perfusion) and bowel function
- Absence of infection

AORTIC DISSECTION

Aortic dissection, often misnamed *dissecting aneurysm*, is not a type of aneurysm. Rather, dissection (tearing of the inner layer of the vessel) results from the creation of a false lumen (between the intima and the media) through which blood flows (see Figure 40.5, *D*). Classification is based on anatomical location (ascending versus descending aorta) and duration of onset (acute versus chronic). Type A dissection affects the ascending aorta and arch, requiring emergency surgery. Type B dissection begins in the descending aorta, allowing for potential conservative management. Dissections are also described as *acute* (first 14 days), *subacute* (14 to 90 days), or *chronic* (greater than 90 days), based on symptom onset (DeMartino et al., 2018).

Etiology and Pathophysiology

Nontraumatic aortic dissection is caused by weakened elastic fibres in the arterial wall. Chronic hypertension accelerates the degradation process. Aortic dissection is believed to arise from an intimal tear. Intimal tears typically occur in areas with the greatest rate of rise of BP—for example, immediately above the aortic valve and just distal to the left subclavian artery. As the heart contracts, each systolic pulsation causes increased pressure on the damaged area, which further increases the dissection. Extension of the dissection may cut off blood supply to critical areas such as the brain, kidneys, spinal cord, and extremities. The false lumen may remain patent, become thrombosed (clotted), rejoin the true lumen by way of a distal tear, or rupture.

Aortic dissection affects more men than women with ratios as high as 5:1 and occurs mostly in the sixth and seventh decades of life. Approximately half of all dissections in women younger

than 40 years occur during pregnancy. Hypertension is the most important risk factor for aortic dissection. Other predisposing factors include age, aortic diseases (e.g., aortitis, coarctation, arch hypoplasia), atherosclerosis, blunt trauma, tobacco use, cocaine or methamphetamine use, congenital heart disease (e.g., bicuspid aortic valve), connective tissue disorders (e.g., Marfan or Ehlers-Danlos syndrome), family history, history of heart surgery, and pregnancy.

Clinical Manifestations

About 80% of patients with an acute type A aortic dissection report an abrupt onset of severe anterior chest or back pain. Patients with acute type B aortic dissection are more likely to report pain in their back, abdomen, or legs. Pain location may overlap between type A and B dissections. The pain may be described as "sharp" and "worst ever," or as "tearing," "ripping," or "stabbing."

Dissection pain can be differentiated from MI pain, whose onset is more gradual and of increasing intensity. As the dissection progresses, pain may migrate. Older patients are less likely to have abrupt onset of chest or back pain (in their back, abdomen, or legs) and more likely to have hypotension and vague symptoms. Some patients have a painless aortic dissection, which emphasizes the importance of the physical examination.

If the aortic arch is involved, the patient may exhibit neurological deficits, such as altered level of consciousness, weakened or absence of carotid and temporal pulses, and dizziness or syncope. An ascending aortic dissection usually produces some degree of disruption in blood flow in the coronary arteries and aortic valve insufficiency. The patient may develop angina, MI, and a new high-pitched, diastolic heart murmur. If severe enough, these complications can result in left ventricular failure with the development of dyspnea, orthopnea, and pulmonary edema. When either subclavian artery is involved, radial, ulnar, and brachial pulse quality and BP readings may be different between the left and the right arms. As the dissection progresses down the aorta, the abdominal organs and lower extremities demonstrate evidence of decreased tissue perfusion.

Complications

A severe and life-threatening complication of an acute ascending aortic dissection is cardiac tamponade, which occurs when blood from the dissection leaks into the pericardial sac. Clinical manifestations of tamponade include hypotension, narrowed pulse pressure, jugular venous distension, muffled heart sounds, and pulsus paradoxus (see Chapter 39).

The aorta may rupture because it is weakened by the dissection. Hemorrhage may occur into the mediastinal, pleural, or abdominal cavities. Aortic rupture typically results in exsanguination and death. Dissection can lead to occlusion of the blood supply to vital organs. Symptoms of spinal cord ischemia range from weakness and decreased sensation to complete lower extremity paralysis. Renal ischemia can lead to renal failure. Manifestations of abdominal (mesenteric) ischemia include abdominal pain, decreased bowel sounds, altered bowel function, and bowel ischemia. Arteries to these organs may come off the true or false lumen, with the latter being more prone to impaired perfusion and an increase in complications.

Diagnostic Studies

Diagnostic studies to detect and classify (type A or B) aortic dissection are similar to those performed for suspected aneurysms

TABLE 40.6 INTERPROFESSIONAL CARE
Aortic Dissection

Diagnostic	Interprofessional Therapy
• Health history and physical examination • Chest radiography • CT scan angiography • Electrocardiography • Traditional angiography • Magnetic resonance angiography • Transesophageal echocardiography	• Bed rest • Blood transfusion (if necessary) • Pain relief with acetaminophen, neuroleptics, opioids (opioids are meant for acute vs. chronic pain control) **Medication Therapy (see Table 35.8)** • ACE inhibitors • IV β-blockers (e.g., esmolol [Brevibloc]) • IV calcium channel blockers • Sodium nitroprusside (Nipride) **Surgical and Interventional Therapy** • Surgical aortic resection and repair • Endovascular aortic dissection repair

ACE, angiotensin-converting enzyme; *CT,* computed tomography; *IV,* intravenous.

(Table 40.6). A chest radiograph may show a widening of the mediastinum and pleural effusion. Three-dimensional CT scanning, MRI, and transesophageal echocardiography are equally reliable for the diagnosis of acute aortic dissection. A CT scan or MRI can provide more detailed information on the presence and severity of the dissection. Transesophageal echocardiography is preferred in very unstable patients or those with contraindications to CT or MRI (e.g., those with metal implants, allergies to contrast material) (Fitzgibbon et al., 2018).

Conservative Therapy

A patient with an acute descending aortic dissection (Type B) without complications can be treated conservatively. Supportive treatment includes pain relief and BP control. Conservative treatment includes BP control with an aim usually less than 120 to 140 systolic, pain relief, heart rate control, and cardiovascular disease risk-factor modification.

Endovascular Intervention

Endovascular repair is a treatment option for acute Type B aortic dissections with complications (e.g., hemodynamic instability) and chronic Type B aortic dissection with complications (e.g., peripheral ischemia). Thoracic endovascular aortic repair (TEVAR) is similar to EVAR. Fewer postsurgical complications occur with TEVAR. However, TEVAR does not prevent the risk for renal failure, paraplegia, or stroke. A lumbar spinal drain may be inserted to help decrease or prevent neurological complications. If a lumbar drain is used, strict aseptic technique is essential to prevent infection.

Surgical Intervention

An acute Type A aortic dissection is a surgical emergency. Otherwise, surgery is indicated when medication therapy is ineffective or when complications (e.g., heart failure) occur. Open surgical repair is recommended for patients with a chronic dissection who have a connective tissue disorder or an aneurysm greater than 5.5 cm (Li et al., 2018).

The aorta is fragile after dissection. Surgery is delayed, when possible, to allow time for edema to decrease and to permit blood clotting in the false lumen. Surgery involves resection of the aortic segment with the intimal tear and replacement with a synthetic graft, to replace the site of the primary intimal tear

with Dacron graft and remove thrombus from the false lumen. Even with prompt surgical intervention, the in-hospital rate of mortality from acute aortic dissection remains high. Causes of in-hospital mortality include aortic rupture, mesenteric ischemia, sepsis, and multi-organ failure.

Interprofessional Care

Patients with acute aortic dissection are managed in the critical care unit. The initial goals of therapy for acute aortic dissection without complications are heart rate and BP control and pain management. Heart rate and BP control reduces stress on the aortic wall by reducing systolic BP and myocardial contractility (see Table 40.6). An IV β-adrenergic blocker is titrated to a target heart rate of 60 beats/minute or less. A calcium channel blocker can be used to lower heart rate if a β-adrenergic blocker is contraindicated. An IV angiotensin-converting enzyme inhibitor may also be used. Reducing the heart rate, BP, and myocardial contractility limits extension of the dissection. Morphine is the preferred analgesic because it decreases sympathetic nervous system stimulation and relieves pain. Supportive treatment for an acute aortic dissection serves as a bridge to surgery.

NURSING MANAGEMENT
AORTIC DISSECTION

Preoperatively, nursing management includes keeping the patient in bed in a semi-Fowler's position and maintaining a quiet environment. These measures help to keep the systolic BP at the lowest possible level that maintains vital organ perfusion (typically between 110 and 120 mm Hg); the desired outcome is to maintain a mean arterial pressure of greater than 65 mm Hg. In order to maintain the mean arterial pressure, the minimal diastolic pressure ought to be approximately 44 mm Hg. Opioids and sedatives are administered as ordered. Pain and anxiety must be managed because these symptoms can cause elevations in the heart rate and systolic BP.

Titrating IV antihypertensive agents requires careful supervision, including continuous electrocardiographic and intra-arterial BP monitoring (see Chapters 35 and 68). The nurse needs to monitor vital signs frequently, sometimes as often as every 2 to 3 minutes, until target BP is reached. The nurse must also observe for changes in peripheral pulses and signs of increasing pain, restlessness, and anxiety. Postoperative care is similar to that after aortic aneurysm repair (see the Nursing Management: Aortic Aneurysms section earlier in this chapter, and NCP 40.1 on the Evolve website).

In preparation for discharge, the nurse should focus on patient and caregiver teaching. All patients with a history of aortic dissection require long-term medical therapy to control BP. Patients need to understand that antihypertensive medications must be taken daily for the rest of their lives. β-Adrenergic blockers are used to control BP and decrease myocardial contractility. It is important that patients understand the medication regimen and potential adverse effects (e.g., dizziness, depression, fatigue, erectile dysfunction). The patient should be instructed to discuss any adverse effects with the health care provider before discontinuing the medication. Follow-up with regularly scheduled MRI or CT is essential. The most common cause of death in long-term survivors is aortic rupture from re-dissection or aneurysm formation. The nurse must instruct patients that, if the pain or other symptoms return, they should contact emergency medical services for immediate care.

VENOUS DISORDERS

PHLEBITIS

Phlebitis is the inflammation (e.g., redness, tenderness, warmth, mild edema) of a superficial vein without the presence of a thrombus (Chang & Peng, 2018). Risk factors are mechanical irritation from the catheter, infusion of irritating medications, and catheter location. Severe phlebitis is more likely to occur in areas of flexion (e.g., wrist and antecubital area). IV catheter insertion in this area should be avoided whenever possible.

Any peripheral IV catheter or midline catheter should be removed if there is any evidence of complication (e.g., phlebitis or infiltration). Phlebitis is rarely infectious and usually resolves quickly after catheter removal. If edema is present, the extremity can be elevated to promote reabsorption of fluid. Application of warm, moist heat and use of oral NSAIDs (e.g., ibuprofen) or topical NSAIDs (e.g., diclofenac gel) can relieve pain and inflammation. The rate of phlebitis in patients receiving IV therapy is widely variable but definitely rises the longer the IV remains in place, with rates higher than 50% after 5 days of insertion (Palese et al., 2016).

VENOUS THROMBOEMBOLISM

Venous thromboembolism (VTE), also known as *venous thrombosis,* is a condition in which a thrombus forms in association with inflammation of the vein. It is the most common disorder of the veins and is classified as either superficial or deep vein thrombosis. Superficial vein thrombosis (SVT) is the formation of a thrombus in a superficial vein, usually the greater or lesser saphenous vein. Deep vein thrombosis (DVT) is a disorder involving a thrombus in a deep vein, most commonly the iliac and femoral veins. VTE represents the spectrum of pathology from DVT to pulmonary embolism (Table 40.7). (Pulmonary embolism is discussed in Chapter 30.)

SVT is generally a benign disorder. However, patients with SVT are at risk for VTE and need workup including a vascular lab if any risk factors exist to rule this out. There is a risk for extension of the clot to deeper veins if the thrombus involves the superficial femoral vein or is near the saphenofemoral junction (Litwok et al., 2016).

Etiology and Pathophysiology

The three factors (called Virchow's triad) that cause venous thrombosis are (a) venous stasis, (b) damage of the endothelium (inner lining of the vein), and (c) hypercoagulability of the blood. The patient at risk for the development of venous thrombosis usually has conditions predisposing to these three disorders (Table 40.8).

Venous Stasis. Normal venous blood flow depends on the action of muscles in the extremities and the functional adequacy of venous valves, which allow unidirectional flow. *Venous stasis* occurs when the valves are dysfunctional or the muscles of the extremities are inactive. Venous stasis occurs more often in people who are obese or pregnant, have chronic heart failure or atrial fibrillation, have been on long trips without regular exercise (i.e., sitting for long periods), have a prolonged surgical procedure, or are immobile for long periods (e.g., with spinal cord injury, fractured hip, limb paralysis).

Endothelial Damage. Damage to the endothelium of the vein may be caused by direct (e.g., surgery, intravascular catheterization, trauma, fracture, burns) or indirect (chemotherapy, vasculitis, sepsis, hyperhomocysteinemia, diabetes) injury to the vessel. Damaged endothelium stimulates platelet activation and initiates the coagulation cascade. This results in decreased fibrinolytic capabilities and predisposes the patient to thrombus development.

Hypercoagulability of Blood. Blood hypercoagulability occurs in many hematological disorders, particularly polycythemia, severe anemias, malignancies (e.g., cancers of the breast, brain, pancreas, and gastrointestinal tract), nephrotic syndrome, antithrombin III deficiency, elevated lipoprotein (a) levels, elevated (clotting) factor VIII levels, hyperhomocysteinemia, and protein C or protein S deficiency (Rattan et al., 2015). A patient with sepsis is predisposed to hypercoagulability because of endotoxins that are released. Some medications (e.g., corticosteroids, estrogens) predispose a patient to thrombus formation.

Women of childbearing age who take estrogen-based oral contraceptives or who are pregnant, as well as postmenopausal women receiving oral hormone replacement therapy, are at increased risk for VTE. Women who use oral contraceptives and tobacco double their risk because of the vasoconstricting effects of nicotine. Smoking causes hypercoagulability by increasing plasma fibrinogen and homocysteine levels and activating the intrinsic coagulation pathway.

TABLE 40.7	COMPARISON OF SUPERFICIAL VEIN THROMBOSIS AND VENOUS THROMBOEMBOLISM	
Characteristic	**Superficial Vein Thrombosis**	**Venous Thromboembolism**
Usual location	Typically, superficial leg veins (e.g., varicosities); occasionally, superficial arm veins	Deep veins of arms (e.g., axillary, subclavian), legs (e.g., femoral), and pelvis (e.g., iliac or inferior or superior vena cava) and pulmonary system
Clinical findings	Tenderness, rubour, warmth, pain, inflammation and induration along the course of the superficial vein	Tenderness to pressure over involved vein, induration of overlying muscle, venous distension
	Vein appears as palpable cord.	Edema
	Edema rarely occurs.	Mild to moderate pain possible
		Deep rubour in area caused by venous congestion
		Systemic temperature possibly greater than 38°C
		Note: Some patients may have no obvious physical changes in the affected extremity.
Sequelae	If left untreated, clot may extend to deeper veins and VTE may occur.	Embolization to lungs (pulmonary embolism) may occur and may result in death.*
		Pulmonary hypertension and post-thrombotic syndrome with or without venous leg ulceration may develop.

IV, intravenous; *VTE,* venous thromboembolism.
*See Chapter 30 for clinical findings related to pulmonary embolism.

TABLE 40.8 RISK FACTORS FOR VENOUS THROMBOEMBOLISM

Venous Stasis	
• Advanced age	• Hyperhomocysteinemia
• Atrial fibrillation	• Malignancies (especially
• Bed rest	breast, brain, hepatic,
• Chronic heart failure	pancreatic, and
• Fractured leg or hip	gastrointestinal)
• Long trips without adequate	• Nephrotic syndrome
exercise	• Oral contraceptives, especially
• Obesity	in women >35 yr of age who
• Orthopedic surgery (especially	use tobacco
lower extremity)	• Polycythemia vera
• Pregnancy and postpartum period	• Pregnancy and postpartum
• Prolonged immobility	period
• Spinal cord injury or limb paralysis	• Protein C deficiency
• Stroke	• Protein S deficiency
• Varicose veins	• Sepsis
	• Severe anemia
Hypercoagulability of Blood	• Tobacco use
• Antiphospholipid antibody	
syndrome	**Endothelial Damage**
• Antithrombin III deficiency	• Abdominal and pelvic surgery
• Dehydration or malnutrition	(e.g., gynecological or
• Elevated (clotting) factor VIII or	urological surgery)
lipoprotein (a) level	• Caustic or hypertonic
• Erythropoiesis-stimulating	intravenous medications
medications (e.g., epoetin alfa	• Fractures of pelvis, hip, or leg
[Eprex])	• History of previous venous
• Factor V Leiden or prothrombin	thromboembolism (VTE)
gene mutation	• In-dwelling, peripherally
• High altitudes	inserted central vein catheter
• Hormone replacement therapy	• Intravenous drug misuse
	• Trauma

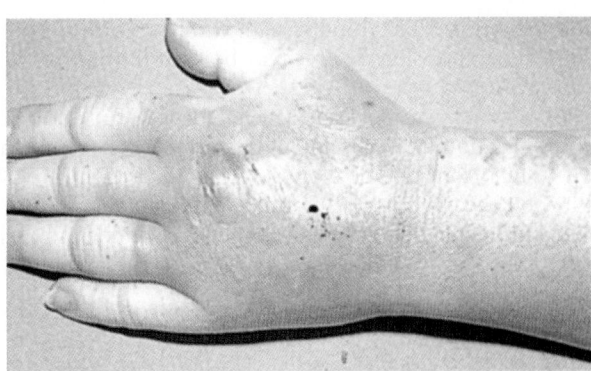

FIG. 40.8 Superficial vein thrombosis of the hand following intravenous therapy. Source: Grieg, J. D., & Garden, O. J. (1996). *Color atlas of surgical diagnosis.* Times Mirror International.

Pathophysiology involves localized platelet aggregation and fibrin which entrap RBCs, WBCs, and more platelets to form a thrombus. A frequent site of thrombus formation is the valve cusps of veins, where venous stasis occurs. As the thrombus enlarges, increased numbers of blood cells and fibrin collect behind it, producing a larger clot with a "tail" that eventually occludes the lumen of the vein.

If a thrombus only partially occludes the vein, endothelial cells cover the thrombus and stop the thrombotic process. If the thrombus does not become detached, it undergoes lysis or becomes firmly organized and adherent within 5 to 7 days. Organized thrombi may detach and result in emboli. Turbulence of blood flow is a major factor contributing to embolization. A thrombus can become an embolus that flows through the venous circulation to the heart and lodges in the pulmonary circulation, becoming a pulmonary embolism (see Chapter 30, Figure 30.11).

Superficial Vein Thrombosis

Clinical Manifestations. The patient with SVT may have a palpable, firm, subcutaneous cordlike vein (see Table 40.7). The area surrounding the vein may be tender to the touch, reddened, and warm (Figure 40.8). A mild systemic temperature elevation and leukocytosis may be present. Extremity edema may or may not occur. The most common cause of upper extremity SVT is vein trauma caused by cannulation of a vein or IV therapy. It is more likely to occur if the catheter is located in a small vein or is left in place for more than 48 hours or if the IV solutions administered are caustic or hyperosmolar.

Risk factors for SVT include increased age, pregnancy, obesity, malignancy, thrombophilia, estrogen therapy, recent sclerotherapy (e.g., treatment for varicose veins), long-distance travel, and a history of chronic venous insufficiency, SVT, or VTE (Musil et al., 2017). SVT also can occur in persons with endothelial alterations (e.g., TAO). It also may be unprovoked.

Interprofessional Care. The initial treatment of infusion-related SVT involves the immediate removal of the IV catheter. Ultrasound is used to confirm the diagnosis (clot 5 cm or larger) and to rule out clot extension to a deep vein (Bernardi & Camporese, 2018). If the superficial vein thrombosis affects a very short vein segment (less than 5 cm) and is not near the saphenofemoral junction, anticoagulants may not be needed and oral NSAIDs can ease symptoms. Other interventions include instructing the patient to wear graduated compression stockings or bandages, apply warm compresses, elevate the affected limb above the level of the heart, apply topical NSAIDs, and perform mild exercise, such as walking.

Deep Vein Thrombosis

Clinical Manifestations. Patients with lower extremity VTE may or may not have unilateral leg edema, pain, tenderness with palpation, dilated superficial veins, a sense of fullness in the thigh or the calf, paresthesias, warm skin, erythema, or a systemic temperature greater than 38°C (see Table 40.7). If the inferior vena cava is involved, the legs may be edematous and cyanotic. Diagnosis of an initial VTE is based on clinical assessment using risk scales such as Wells Rule, combined with D-dimer testing and duplex ultrasonography.

Complications. The most serious complications of VTE are pulmonary embolism, post-thrombotic syndrome (PTS), and phlegmasia cerulea dolens (described later in this chapter). Pulmonary embolism is a potentially life-threatening complication of VTE (see Chapter 30).

Post-thrombotic syndrome occurs in 20 to 50% of patients with VTE despite adequate anticoagulant therapy. Chronic venous hypertension is caused by vein wall and vein valve damage (from acute inflammation and thrombus reorganization), venous valve reflux, and persistent venous (outflow) obstruction. Symptoms include pain, aching, fatigue, heaviness, sensation of swelling, cramps, pruritus, tingling, itching, paresthesia, bursting pain with exercise, and venous claudication.

Clinical signs include persistent edema, increased pigmentation, eczema, secondary varicosities, hemosiderin staining, and *lipodermatosclerosis* (Figure 40.9). In advanced stages complications can include venous ulceration, usually located in the gaiter area of the calf, most commonly on the medial aspect.

Manifestations of PTS typically begin within 2 years of a VTE. Sequential compression devices may be used for patients with severe PTS.

Phlegmasia cerulea dolens (swollen, blue, painful leg), a very rare complication, may develop in the advanced stages of cancer. It results from one or more severe lower extremity VTEs that involve the major leg veins, causing near-total occlusion of venous outflow. Patients typically experience sudden, massive swelling, deep pain, and intense cyanosis of the extremity. If

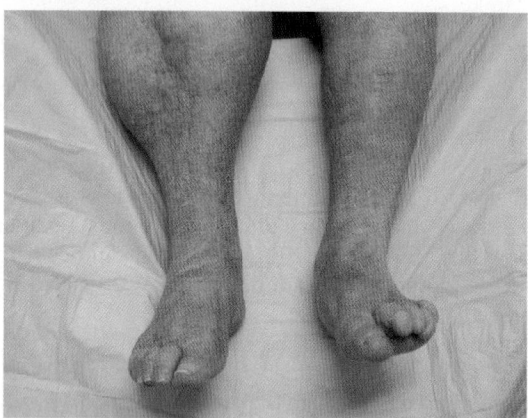

FIG. 40.9 Lipodermatosclerosis. Skin on lower leg becomes scarred, and the leg becomes tapered like an "inverted bottle." Hallmark signs of lipodermatosclerosis are leathery skin, brown discoloration, hyperpigmentation and hypopigmentation, and circumferential or near-circumferential scarring and shrinking of the extremity. Source: Etufugh, C. N., & Phillips, T. J. (2007). Venous ulcers. *Clinics in Dermatology, 25*(1), 125. doi:10.1016/j.clindermatol.2006.09.004.

untreated, the venous obstruction causes arterial occlusion and gangrene and necessitates amputation.

Diagnostic Studies. Table 40.9 lists the various diagnostic studies used to determine the site or location and extent of a VTE.

Interprofessional Care
Prevention and Prophylaxis of Venous Thromboembolism.
VTE prophylaxis is a core measure of quality health care in hospitalized patients undergoing surgery. In addition, it is recommended that hospitals have a formal, hospital-wide thromboprophylaxis policy that addresses VTE prevention on admission of all adult patients (Canadian Patient Safety Institute, 2017). While it is the health care provider who ultimately orders chemoprophylaxis, nursing care and use of nonpharmacological strategies have a great effect on VTE prophylaxis.

In patients at risk for VTE, both pharmacological and nonpharmacological interventions are used to prevent and treat VTE. Early and aggressive mobilization based on the patient's condition is the easiest and most cost-effective method to decrease VTE risk. Patients on bed rest need to change position every 2 hours. Unless it is contraindicated, the nurse should teach patients to flex and extend their feet, knees, and hips every 2 to 4 hours while awake. Patients who are able to get out of bed need to be in a chair for meals and ambulate at least four to six times per day as tolerated.

Graduated compression (antiembolism) stockings are a part of VTE prevention in hospitalized patients. When fitted and worn properly, these stockings increase venous blood flow velocity, prevent venous wall dilation, improve venous valve function, and stimulate endothelial fibrinolytic activity. Proper stocking

TABLE 40.9   DIAGNOSTIC STUDIES
Venous Thromboembolism*

Study	Description and Abnormal Findings
Blood Laboratory Studies	
ACT, aPTT, INR, bleeding time, Hb, Hct, platelet count	Alterations if patient has underlying blood dyscrasia (e.g., increased Hb and Hct in patient with polycythemia)
D-dimer (nonspecific)	Fragment of fibrin is formed as result of fibrin degradation and clot lysis. Elevated results suggest venous thromboembolism (VTE). *Normal results:* 3.0 mmol/L (<50 ng/mL)
Fibrin monomer complex	Forms when concentration of thrombin exceeds that of antithrombin. Presence is evidence of thrombus formation and suggests VTE. *Normal results:* <10 mg/dL (<10 mcg/mL)
Noninvasive Venous Studies	
Venous compression ultrasonography	Evaluation of deep femoral, popliteal, and posterior tibial veins *Normal finding:* Veins collapse with application of external pressure. *Abnormal finding:* Veins fail to collapse with application of external pressure; failure to collapse suggests a thrombus.
Duplex ultrasonography	Combination of compression ultrasonography with spectral and colour flow Doppler study. Veins are examined for respiratory variation, compressibility, and intraluminal filling defects to help determine location and extent of thrombus (most widely used test to diagnose VTE).
Invasive Venous Studies	
Computed tomography venography (CTV)	Spiral CT used to evaluate veins in the pelvis, thighs, and calves after injection of venous-phase contrast material; involves less contrast material than does traditional venography; may be performed simultaneously with CT angiography of pulmonary vessels for patients being evaluated for VTE
Magnetic resonance venography	MRI with specialized software to evaluate blood flow through veins; can be performed with or without contrast material; highly accurate for pelvic and proximal veins; less accurate for calf veins; can distinguish acute and chronic thrombus
Contrast venography (phlebography)	Radiographic determination of location and extent of clot with contrast media to outline filling defects; identifies the presence of collateral circulation; once the gold standard of invasive venous studies but currently rarely performed

ACT, activated clotting time; *aPTT,* activated partial thromboplastin time; *CT,* computed tomography; *Hb,* hemoglobin; *Hct,* hematocrit; *INR,* international normalized ratio; *MRI,* magnetic resonance imaging.
*See Table 30.25 for diagnostic studies for pulmonary embolism.

use means any toe hole is under the toes, the heel patch is over the heel, a thigh gusset is on the inner thigh (thigh length only), and there are no wrinkles. The stockings should not be rolled down, cut, or otherwise altered. If the stockings are not fitted and worn correctly, venous return is impeded. This can cause arterial ischemia, edema, skin breakdown, and VTE. Stockings are not recommended if the patient already has a VTE.

Sequential compression devices (SCDs) are inflatable garments wrapped around the legs that apply intermittent external pressure to the lower extremities. They are often used in combination with graduated compression stockings. The nurse needs to ensure correct fit by accurately measuring the extremities. SCDs will not provide effective VTE prophylaxis if they are not applied correctly, if the fit is incorrect, or if the patient does not wear the device continuously while at rest. VTE prevention is enhanced if SCDs are used along with anticoagulation.

Medication Therapy. Anticoagulants are used routinely for VTE prevention and treatment. The regimen depends on the patient's VTE risk. The goal of anticoagulant therapy for VTE prophylaxis is to prevent clot formation. The goals for treatment of a confirmed VTE are to prevent new clot development, prevent spread of the clot, and prevent embolization.

Three major classes of anticoagulants are available: (1) vitamin K antagonists, (2) thrombin inhibitors (both indirect and direct), and (3) factor Xa inhibitors (Burcham & Rosenthal, 2019; Table 40.10). Anticoagulant therapy does not dissolve the clot. Lysis of the clot begins spontaneously through the body's intrinsic fibrinolytic system (see Chapter 32).

Vitamin K Antagonists. The oral anticoagulant for long-term or extended anticoagulation is warfarin, a vitamin K antagonist. Warfarin inhibits activation of the vitamin K–dependent coagulation factors II, VII, IX, and X, as well as the anticoagulant proteins C and S (Barnes, & Renner, 2018). (Figure 32.4 displays the clotting pathways, and clotting factors are listed in Table 32.3.) Warfarin begins to take effect in 48 to 72 hours. It then takes several more days to achieve a maximum effect. Thus, an overlap of

TABLE 40.10 MEDICATION THERAPY

Anticoagulant Therapy

Anticoagulant	Medication	Route of Administration	Comments
Vitamin K antagonists	Warfarin (Coumadin)	PO	INR is used for monitoring therapeutic levels. Medications are administered at the same time each day. Variations of certain genes (e.g., *CYP2CP, VKORC1*) may influence response to the medication. *Antidote:* Vitamin K
Thrombin Inhibitors: Indirect			
Unfractionated heparin	Heparin sodium	Continuous IV Subcut	Therapeutic effects are measured at regular intervals by the aPTT or ACT. CBC is monitored at regular intervals. If administered subcutaneously, medication should be injected deep into subcutaneous tissue (preferably into the abdominal fatty tissue or above the iliac crest), inserting the entire length of the needle. Skinfold is held during injection but released before needle is removed. The nurse should not aspirate, not inject intramuscularly, and not rub site after injection. Sites should be rotated. *Antidote:* Protamine
Low-molecular-weight heparin (LMWH)	Enoxaparin Tinzaparin Dalteparin Nadroparin Enoxaparin Dalteparin	Subcut	Routine coagulation tests are typically not required. CBC is monitored at regular intervals. Air bubble should not be expelled before medication is administered subcutaneously. The nurse should follow remaining administration guidelines as described for unfractionated heparin. Dosage should be reduced in patients with renal impairment. Extreme caution should be used in patients with a history of HIT. *Antidote*: Protamine
Thrombin Inhibitors: Direct			
Hirudin derivatives	Lepirudin	IV or subcut IV	Therapeutic effect is measured by ACT or aPTT. Used in patients with HIT when anticoagulation is still required.
	Bivalirudin	IV or subcut	*Antidote:* None
Synthetic thrombin inhibitors	Argatroban	IV	Therapeutic effect is measured by aPTT. Used in patients at risk for or with HIT.
	Dabigatran	Subcut	*Antidote:* None
Factor Xa Inhibitors			
	Fondaparinux Rivaroxaban Apixaban	Subcut and IV PO	Routine coagulation tests are not required. CBC and creatinine are monitored at regular intervals. Air bubble should not be expelled before medication is administered. The nurse should follow remaining administration guidelines as described for unfractionated heparin. Approved for VTE prophylaxis and treatment. For patients undergoing surgery, initial dose should be given no earlier than 6 hr postoperatively. Should be administered with caution in older patients and in patients with impaired renal function. May cause thrombocytopenia. If uncontrollable bleeding occurs, treatment with recombinant factor VIIa may be effective. *Antidote:* None

ACT, activated clotting time; *aPTT,* activated partial thromboplastin time; *CBC,* complete blood count; *HIT,* heparin-induced thrombocytopenia; *INR,* international normalized ratio; *IV,* intravenous; *PO,* oral; *Subcut,* subcutaneous; *VTE,* venous thromboembolism.

a parenteral anticoagulant (e.g., unfractionated heparin or low-molecular-weight heparin [LMWH]) and warfarin typically is required for 5 days or until the international normalized ratio (INR) is greater than 2.0 for 24 hours. The level of anticoagulation is monitored daily with the INR. The INR is a standardized system of reporting prothrombin time (Table 40.11). The antidote for warfarin-related bleeding is vitamin K, prothrombin complex concentrate (human), or fresh-frozen plasma.

The nurse should carefully document the patient's medical history before warfarin therapy is started. Antiplatelet agents generally are not given with warfarin because they increase bleeding risk. Other medications that interact with warfarin include NSAIDs, phenytoin (Dilantin), barbiturates, and many vitamin, mineral, dietary, and herbal supplements (see the Complementary & Alternative Therapies: Natural Health Products That May Affect Clotting box). A diet that frequently varies in vitamin K intake (e.g., green leafy vegetables) can make it difficult to achieve and maintain a therapeutic INR level. Achieving and maintaining a therapeutic INR is challenging. This, along with the multiple medication interactions with warfarin and the increasingly broad indications for the newer anticoagulants, has made warfarin not necessarily the best choice. In the next section, the newer agents, their benefits, indications, and challenges are discussed (Kearon, 2019).

Thrombin Inhibitors. There are two major classes of indirect thrombin inhibitors: unfractionated heparin and LMWHs. Unfractionated heparin (e.g., heparin) affects both the intrinsic and common pathways of blood coagulation by way of the plasma antithrombin. Antithrombin inhibits thrombin-mediated conversion of fibrinogen to fibrin by affecting factors II (prothrombin), IX, X, XI, and XII (see Figure 32.4).

Heparin can be given subcutaneously for VTE prophylaxis, although this practice has largely been replaced by LWMHs or by continuous IV infusion for VTE treatment. When heparin is given intravenously, clotting status, as measured by activated partial thromboplastin time (aPTT), must be monitored frequently (see Table 40.11).

One serious adverse effect of heparin is *heparin-induced thrombocytopenia* (HIT). HIT is an immune reaction to heparin in which the platelet count diminishes severely and suddenly, along with a paradoxical increase in venous or arterial thrombosis. HIT is diagnosed by measurements for the presence of heparin antibodies in the blood. Treatment requires immediately stopping heparin therapy and, if further anticoagulation is required, using a nonheparin anticoagulant (Hasan et al., 2016). Another adverse effect of long-term heparin therapy is osteoporosis.

LMWHs (e.g., enoxaparin) are derived from unfractionated heparin. They have more predictable dose effects, a longer half-life, and fewer bleeding complications than unfractionated heparin. LMWHs also are less likely than heparin to cause HIT and osteoporosis. LMWHs typically do not necessitate anticoagulant monitoring and dose adjustment. Their anti-inflammatory properties may help prevent PTS and venous ulcer development. Protamine neutralizes the effect of LMWH.

Direct thrombin inhibitors are classified as hirudin derivatives or synthetic thrombin inhibitors. Hirudin is manufactured through recombinant DNA technology. It binds specifically with thrombin and directly inhibits its function without causing plasma protein and platelet interactions. Hirudin derivatives are administered by continuous IV infusion. Lepirudin is approved for prophylaxis or treatment of HIT, whereas bivalirudin is approved for patients with HIT who undergo percutaneous coronary angioplasty. Anticoagulant activity is monitored according to aPTT or activated clotting time (see Table 40.11). There is no antidote for hirudin derivatives if bleeding occurs.

Argatroban, a synthetic direct thrombin inhibitor, inhibits thrombin. It is used as an alternative to heparin for the prevention and treatment of HIT and for patients known to have or are at risk for HIT needing percutaneous coronary interventions. The effect of argatroban is not reversible. Its anticoagulant effect is monitored using aPTT or activated clotting time.

Dabigatran (Pradaxa), an oral direct thrombin inhibitor, is used for VTE prevention after elective joint replacement, for stroke prevention in nonvalvular atrial fibrillation, and as a treatment option for VTE. Idarucizumab (Praxbind) neutralizes the effect of dabigatran. Dabigatran has five major advantages compared to warfarin: rapid onset, no need to monitor anticoagulation, few medication–food interactions, lower risk for major bleeding, and predictable dose response.

Factor Xa Inhibitors. *Factor Xa inhibitors* inhibit factor Xa directly or indirectly, producing rapid anticoagulation. These include fondaparinux (Arixtra), rivaroxaban (Xarelto), and apixaban (Eliquis). All are used for both VTE prevention and treatment. Fondaparinux is given subcutaneously. It is contraindicated in patients with severe renal disease. Rivaroxaban and apixaban are oral medications. Coagulation monitoring or dose adjustment is not needed, although its anticoagulant activity can be measured with anti–factor Xa assays (see Table 40.11). If uncontrollable bleeding occurs, recombinant factor VIIa may be useful.

The COMPASS trial—the first in many years—has provided evidence for treatment of PAD with anticoagulation. For patients with concomitant CAD and PAD, treatment with rivaroxaban and ASA has been shown to prevent cardiovascular events, with fewer serious adverse effects, including major bleeding (Anand et al., 2019).

Anticoagulation Therapy for Prevention of Venous Thromboembolism. For VTE prevention in the hospitalized medical

TABLE 40.11	TESTS OF BLOOD COAGULATION		
Medications Monitored	**Normal Value**	**Therapeutic Value**	
International normalized ratio (INR) • Vitamin K antagonists (e.g., warfarin [Coumadin])	0.75–1.25	2–3 (for PAD)	
Activated partial thromboplastin time (aPTT) • Unfractionated heparin (e.g., heparin) • Hirudin derivatives (e.g., bivalirudin [Angiomax]) • Synthetic thrombin inhibitors (e.g., argatroban; dabigatran [Pradaxa])	25–35 sec	46–70 sec	
Activated clotting time (ACT) • Unfractionated heparin • Hirudin derivatives • Synthetic thrombin inhibitors Anti–factor Xa	70–20 sec*	>300 sec	
• Low-molecular-weight heparin (e.g., enoxaparin)	0 U/mL	U/mL	
• Factor Xa inhibitors (e.g., apixaban; rivaroxaban)	0 U/mL	No therapeutic level monitored for dosing	

PAD, peripheral artery disease.
*Varies based on type of system and test reagent or activator used.

patient at risk for thrombosis who is not bleeding, low-dose unfractionated heparin, LMWH, or fondaparinux is used. If the patient is at low VTE risk, medication prophylaxis is not needed. Patients with moderate VTE risk (e.g., general, gynecological, or urological surgery) should receive either unfractionated heparin or LMWH. Patients with high VTE risk (e.g., trauma) should receive unfractionated heparin or LMWH until discharge. Patients having abdominal or pelvic surgery for cancer or major orthopedic surgery (e.g., total knee or hip replacement) should receive VTE prophylaxis (Kearon, 2019).

Anticoagulant Therapy for Venous Thromboembolism Treatment. Patients with confirmed VTE should receive initial treatment with either LMWH, unfractionated heparin, or an oral factor Xa medication. Oral vitamin K antagonist therapy may be an option. A therapeutic INR is maintained between 2.0 and 3.0 if vitamin K antagonist therapy is used. Active treatment of VTE should continue for at least 3 months and may continue longer in some patients (Kaeron, 2019).

Patients with multiple comorbidities, complex medical issues, or a very large VTE usually are hospitalized for treatment. Parenteral administration of unfractionated heparin is the typical initial treatment. Depending on the presentation and home situation, patients may be safely and effectively managed as outpatients.

Thrombolytic Therapy for Venous Thromboembolism Treatment. Another treatment option for patients with a thrombus is catheter-directed administration of a thrombolytic medication (e.g., urokinase, tissue plasminogen activator). It dissolves the clot(s), reduces the acute symptoms, improves deep venous flow, reduces valvular reflux, and may help to decrease the incidence of PTS. Catheter-directed thrombolytic medications directly dissolve clots, reduce the acute symptoms, and decrease the incidence of postphlebitic vein complications. Additional catheter-based interventions, such as angioplasty, stents, or mechanical thrombectomy with a high-speed impeller to fragment the thrombus, can be used in conjunction with the thrombolytic medication. (Thrombolytic therapy is discussed in Chapter 36.)

Surgical and Interventional Therapy. Currently, most cases of VTE are managed medically, with some undergoing mechanical directed thrombectomy or thrombolysis. The use of surgical options is rare but does include open venous thrombectomy and inferior vena cava interruption. Venous thrombectomy involves the removal of a thrombus through an incision in the vein.

Vena cava interruption devices (e.g., inferior vena cava filters) can be inserted percutaneously through the right femoral or right internal jugular veins. The filter device is opened and the spokes penetrate the vessel walls (Figure 40.10). This results in "sieve-type" obstruction, allowing filtration of clots without interruption of blood flow. Complications after insertion of the device are rare but include air embolism, improper placement, migration of the filter, and perforation of the vena cava with retroperitoneal bleeding. Over time, venous congestion can occur from accumulation of trapped clots, requiring filter removal and replacement. A filter device is recommended with acute PE or proximal VTE of the leg in patients with active bleeding or if anticoagulant therapy is contraindicated.

Percutaneous endovascular interventional radiology procedures can be used along with catheter-directed thrombolytic therapy, especially for severely symptomatic patients with iliocaval or iliofemoral obstruction (Hattab et al., 2017). The interventional radiology procedures are like those used in the treatment of lower extremity PAD. The difference is accessing an occluded vein instead of an artery. Options include

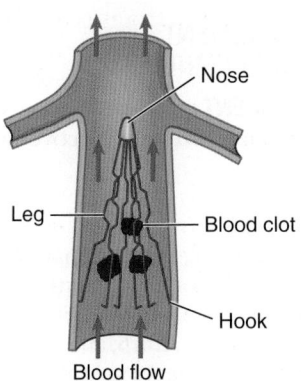

FIG. 40.10 Inferior vena caval interruption technique with a Greenfield stainless steel filter to prevent pulmonary embolism. As blood travels up the vena cava, clots are trapped in the filter.

mechanical thrombectomy, pharmacomechanical devices, and post-thrombus extraction, angioplasty, and/or stenting. Anticoagulation therapy is recommended after an iliofemoral interventional radiology procedure. Postprocedure nursing care focuses on (1) maintaining catheter systems (if continuous infusions); (2) monitoring for bleeding, embolization, and impaired perfusion; and (3) VTE prevention teaching (Hattab et al., 2017).

◨ EVIDENCE-INFORMED PRACTICE
Translating Research Into Practice

The nurse is caring for H. B. (pronouns she/her), 78 years old, who is being discharged with a prescription for enoxaparin (Lovenox) after a knee replacement. Her granddaughter will be her primary caregiver. Because arthritis limits dexterity in H. B.'s hands, the nurse is preparing to teach her granddaughter how to inject the medication. H. B.'s granddaughter tells the nurse that her grandmother is a modest woman and will not permit her abdomen to be exposed. She asks if the injection can be given in her arm.

Best Available Evidence	Clinician Expertise	Patient Preferences and Values
Enoxaparin (per the package literature) should be administered by deep subcutaneous injection in the abdomen. Injection sites should be rotated.	Some patients have told the nurse that they used alternate sites for injection of enoxaparin, specifically the thighs and upper arms. The nurse has no evidence about the efficacy of the medication when alternate sites are used.	H. B. states she does not want to expose herself to her granddaughter. The granddaughter expresses a desire to support her grandmother's need for modesty.

Decision and Action

The nurse discusses the importance of following the medication manufacturer's recommendations regarding site selection with H. B. and her granddaughter. The nurse further explains that there is no evidence on whether alternate sites are equally effective. H. B.'s granddaughter states that she is the only one available to do this and she needs to respect her grandmother's wishes. The nurse teaches the granddaughter how to inject enoxaparin in H. B.'s upper arms and to alternate the sites and arms. The nurse informs the health care provider of H. B.'s decision and documents the teaching and related conversation.

Reference for Evidence

Sanofi-Aventis (1993, revised 2019). *Product monograph: Lovenox.* https://products.sanofi.ca/en/lovenox.pdf

NURSING MANAGEMENT
VENOUS THROMBOEMBOLISM

NURSING ASSESSMENT

Table 40.12 lists the subjective and objective data to obtain from a patient with VTE.

NURSING DIAGNOSES

Nursing diagnoses and interprofessional issues for a patient with VTE include but are not limited to the following:

- *Acute pain* resulting from *physical injury agent* (venous congestion, impaired venous return, and inflammation)
- *Ineffective health maintenance* as a result of *insufficient resources* (lack of knowledge about disorder and its treatment)
- *Impaired skin integrity* resulting from *alteration in fluid volume* (altered peripheral tissue perfusion)
- *Risk for bleeding* related to *anticoagulant therapy*

PLANNING

The overall goals for VTE should be reviewed with and agreed on with the patient and include (a) pain relief, (b) decreased edema, (c) no skin ulceration, (d) no bleeding complications, and (e) no evidence of pulmonary embolism.

NURSING IMPLEMENTATION

ACUTE INTERVENTION. Nursing care for the patient with VTE is directed toward the prevention of emboli formation and the reduction of inflammation. The nurse needs to review with the patient any medications, vitamins, minerals, and dietary and natural health products being taken that may interfere with anticoagulation therapy (see the Complementary and Alternative Therapies: Natural Health Products That May Affect Clotting box). Depending on the anticoagulant ordered, the nurse should monitor INR, aPTT, activated clotting time, CBC, creatinine, hemoglobin, hematocrit, platelet levels, and liver enzyme levels. Platelet counts in patients receiving unfractionated heparin or LMWH should be monitored to assess for HIT. Doses of unfractionated heparin, warfarin, and direct thrombin inhibitors should be titrated on the basis of results of clotting studies and physician-established parameters. Dosages of direct thrombin inhibitors may need adjustment for patients with impaired renal or liver function. The nurse should always check the results of appropriate tests before initiating, administering, or adjusting anticoagulant therapy.

> **MEDICATION ALERT—Anticoagulant Therapy**
> - Patients should be instructed to avoid taking aspirin, NSAIDs, fish oil supplements, garlic supplements, ginkgo biloba, and certain antibiotics (e.g., sulfamethoxazole and trimethoprim).
> - Patients should be instructed to report bleeding: black or bloody stools, bleeding gums, bloody urine or sputum, coffee-ground or bloody vomit, excessive bruising, nosebleeds, and excessive menstrual bleeding.
> - The nurse should assess for signs of bleeding (e.g., hypotension, tachycardia, hematuria, melena, hematemesis, petechiae, ecchymosis).

The nurse needs to monitor for bleeding and reduce the risk of bleeding that may occur with anticoagulant therapy (Table 40.13). Bleeding is greater in persons receiving any anticoagulant with an active gastroduodenal ulcer, prior bleeding history, low platelet count, hepatic or renal failure, rheumatic disease, and cancer and in persons older than 85 years (Elsebai et al., 2019). Patients receiving warfarin with an INR of 5.0 or more are also at increased risk for bleeding. In the event of anticoagulation above target goals, the nurse should give reversal agents (e.g., protamine, vitamin K) or make dosage adjustments

TABLE 40.12   NURSING ASSESSMENT

Venous Thromboembolism

Subjective Data

Important Health Information

Past health history: Trauma to vein, intravascular catheter (e.g., peripherally inserted central catheter), varicose veins, pregnancy or recent childbirth, obesity, prolonged bed rest, irregular heartbeat (e.g., atrial fibrillation), COPD, HF, cancer, coagulation disorders and hypercoagulable states, systemic lupus erythematosus, MI, spinal cord injury, stroke, prolonged air travel, recent bone fracture, dehydration

Medications: Use of estrogens (including oral contraceptives, hormone replacement therapy), tamoxifen, corticosteroids, excessive amounts of vitamin E, IV use of illicit drugs

Surgery or other treatments: Any recent surgery, especially orthopedic, gynecological, gastric, or urological; previous surgery involving veins; central venous catheter

Symptoms

Pain in area on palpation or ambulation

Objective Data

General

Fever, anxiety, pain

Integumentary

Increased size of affected extremity in comparison with opposite extremity; taut, shiny, warm skin; erythematous skin; tenderness to palpation. Some patients may have no physical changes in the affected extremity.

Cardiovascular

Distension and warmth of superficial veins in affected area; edema and cyanosis of extremities, neck, back, and face (if superior vena cava involvement)

Possible Findings

Leukocytosis, abnormal coagulation, anemia or ↑ hematocrit and RBC count, ↑ D-dimer level, positive venous compression on duplex ultrasound study; positive findings on CTV, magnetic resonance venography, or contrast venography

COPD, chronic obstructive pulmonary disease; *CTV,* computed tomography venography; *HF,* heart failure; *IV,* intravenous; *MI,* myocardial infarction; *RBC,* red blood cell.

as ordered. In the event of major vitamin K antagonist–related bleeding, rapid treatment with four-factor prothrombin complex concentrate and IV vitamin K is recommended over fresh-frozen plasma.

> **SAFETY ALERT**
> - The nurse should observe and teach the patient to observe closely for the following events:
>   - Any overt or occult bleeding
>   - Epistaxis and bleeding gingivae
>   - Blood (visible or occult) in emesis, urine, stool, and sputum
>   - Oozing or visible bleeding from trauma site or surgical incision
>   - Excessive menstrual bleeding
> - The nurse should monitor vital signs for changes: decreased blood pressure, increased heart rate
> - Intramuscular injections should be avoided
> - The patient should be assessed for mental status changes, especially in the older patient, because they may indicate cerebral bleeding.

Early ambulation does not increase the short-term risk of a pulmonary embolism in patients with VTE. In addition, early exercise after VTE results in a more rapid decrease in edema and limb pain, fewer PTS symptoms, and better quality of life.

TABLE 40.13 NURSING INTERVENTIONS FOR PATIENTS RECEIVING ANTICOAGULANTS

Assessment
- Evaluating appropriate laboratory coagulation tests for target therapeutic levels, if appropriate
- Evaluating lower extremity for ecchymosis/hematoma development if intermittent compression device is used
- Evaluating platelet count for signs of heparin-induced thrombocytopenia (HIT)
- Examining urine and stool for overt signs of blood
- Inspecting skin frequently, especially under any splinting devices
- Monitoring vital signs as indicated
- Notifying the health care provider of any abnormalities in assessments, vital signs, or laboratory values
- Performing assessment of risk for falling per institutional policy and implementing safety measures as needed
- Performing assessments frequently to observe for signs and symptoms of bleeding (e.g., hypotension, tachycardia), clotting, or both

Injections
- Applying manual pressure for at least 10 min (or longer if needed) on venipuncture sites
- Avoiding intramuscular injections
- Minimizing venipunctures
- Using small-gauge needles for venipunctures unless ordered that therapy necessitates use of a larger gauge

Routine Care and Patient Education
- Administering stool softeners to avoid hard stools and straining
- Applying graduated compression stockings or sequential compression devices as ordered and with attention to proper size, application, and use
- Applying moisturizing lotion to skin
- Avoiding removal or disruption of established clots
- Avoiding restraints if possible; using only soft, padded restraints if needed
- Instructing patient not to forcefully blow nose
- Instructing patient to avoid restrictive clothing
- Instructing patient to use electric razors, not straight razors
- Instructing patient to use soft toothbrushes or foam swabs for oral care
- Limiting tape application; using paper tape as appropriate
- Lubricating tubes (e.g., suction catheter) adequately before insertion
- Performing physical care in a gentle manner
- Repositioning patient carefully at regular intervals
- Using humidified O_2 source
- Using support pads, mattresses, and therapeutic beds as indicated

TABLE 40.14 PATIENT & CAREGIVER TEACHING GUIDE

Anticoagulant Therapy

The following information should be included in the teaching plan for a patient receiving anticoagulant therapy and for the patient's caregiver.

1. Reasons for and basic mechanism of action of anticoagulant therapy and how long the anticipated therapy will last and availability of reversal agents or not
2. The need to take medication at same time each day (preferably in afternoon or evening)
3. Depending on medication prescribed, the need for frequent follow-up with blood tests to assess therapeutic effect of the medication and whether change in medication dosages is required
4. Adverse effects of medication therapy that necessitate medical attention:
   - Any bleeding that does not stop after a reasonable amount of time (usually 10–15 min)
   - Blood in urine or stool, or black, tarry stools
   - Chest pain, shortness of breath, palpitations (heart racing)
   - Cold, blue, or painful feet
   - Severe headaches or stomach pains
   - Unusual bleeding from gums, throat, skin, or nose, or heavy menstrual bleeding
   - Vomiting blood or coffee-ground emesis
   - Weakness, dizziness, mental status changes
5. Avoidance of any trauma or injury that might cause bleeding (e.g., vigorous brushing of teeth, contact sports, in-line roller skating, use of straight razor)
6. Avoidance of all ASA products unless prescribed by a specialist, or nonsteroidal anti-inflammatory drugs (NSAIDs)
7. Limiting alcohol intake: small to moderate amount (341 mL [12 oz] of beer, 118 mL [4 oz] of wine, or 30 mL [1 oz] of hard liquor per day)
8. Wearing a Medic Alert bracelet or necklace indicating what anticoagulant is being taken
9. Avoiding frequent changes in eating habits, such as dramatically increasing foods high in vitamin K (e.g., broccoli, spinach, kale, greens); avoiding supplemental vitamin K
10. Consulting with health care provider before beginning or discontinuing any medication, vitamin, mineral, or dietary or herbal supplement (see the Complementary and Alternative Therapies: Natural Health Products That May Affect Clotting box)
11. Informing all health care providers, including dentist, of anticoagulant therapy
12. The necessity of correct dosing; supervision may be required (e.g., patients experiencing confusion or cognitive impairment)

The nurse should emphasize to the patient and caregiver the importance of exercise and assist the patient to ambulate several times a day. For patients who have acute VTE with severe edema and limb pain, bed rest with limb elevation may initially be prescribed.

AMBULATORY AND HOME CARE. Discharge teaching is focused on modification of VTE risk factors, monitoring laboratory values, dietary and medication instructions, and guidelines for follow-up. Once the edema is resolved, the patient should be measured for custom-fit, graduated compression stockings. Stocking use (or sleeves in the case of an upper extremity VTE) is recommended for at least 1 to 2 years after a VTE to support the vein walls and valves and decrease swelling and pain and should be based on patient symptoms (Bernstein et al., 2016).

Patients should be instructed to stop smoking, to avoid using all nicotine products, and to avoid wearing constrictive clothing. Patients need to avoid standing or sitting in a motionless, leg-dependent position. Frequent knee flexion, ankle rotation, and active walking during long periods of sitting or standing, as on car or airplane trips, should be encouraged. For those at high risk for VTE who are planning a long trip, properly fitted, knee-high graduated compression stockings are recommended during travel to decrease edema and VTE risk. Aspirin or anticoagulant use is not suggested for long-distance travellers. The patient and caregiver should be taught about signs and symptoms of pulmonary embolism, such as sudden onset of dyspnea, tachypnea, and pleuritic chest pain. They should seek emergency medical care if these symptoms occur.

The patient and caregiver need thorough education regarding medication dosage, actions, and adverse effects; the need for routine blood tests; and what symptoms to report to the health care provider (Table 40.14). Devices are available for home monitoring of INR. Patients taking medications requiring injection, or their caregivers, should be taught how to administer the medication subcutaneously. Active or young patients need to avoid playing contact sports and activities with high risk for trauma (e.g., skiing). Older patients need to know to take safety precautions in order to prevent falls. The nurse must instruct the patient and caregiver to apply pressure for 10 to 15 minutes if bleeding occurs (e.g. nosebleeds). If the bleeding persists, they should contact emergency medical services.

A well-balanced diet, including calcium and vitamin E, is important because these affect coagulation. Patients taking warfarin should be taught to follow a consistent diet of foods containing vitamin K, to avoid taking any supplements containing vitamin K, and to avoid excessive amounts of vitamin E and alcohol. Proper hydration to prevent additional hypercoagulability of the blood, which may occur with dehydration, should be encouraged.

Patients who are overweight need to limit carbohydrates in their diet as well as total caloric intake and to increase physical activity to achieve and maintain their desired weight. A balanced program of rest and exercise also improves venous return. The nurse should assist the patient to develop an exercise program with an emphasis on exercises the patient can manage.

EVALUATION

The expected outcomes for the patient with VTE include the following:

- Manageable pain (measure by functional ability)
- Intact skin
- No signs of hemorrhage or occult bleeding
- No signs of respiratory distress

VARICOSE VEINS

Varicose veins, or *varicosities,* are dilated (3 mm or larger in diameter), tortuous subcutaneous veins most commonly found in the saphenous vein system. Varicosities may be small and innocuous or large and bulging. *Primary varicose veins* (idiopathic) are caused by a congenital weakness of the veins and are more common in women. *Secondary varicose veins* typically result from a previous VTE. Secondary varicose veins also may occur in the esophagus (esophageal varices), vulva, spermatic cords (varicoceles), and anorectal area (hemorrhoids), and as abnormal arteriovenous connections. Reticular veins are smaller varicose veins that appear flat, less tortuous, and bluishgreen. *Telangiectasias* (often referred to as *spider veins*) are very small, visible vessels (generally <1 mm in diameter) that appear bluish-black, purple, or red.

Etiology and Pathophysiology

Superficial veins in the lower extremities become dilated and tortuous in response to backward (retrograde) blood flow and increased venous pressure. Risk factors include a family history of chronic venous disease, weakness vein structure, female gender, tobacco use, increasing age, obesity, multiparity, history of VTE, venous obstruction resulting from extrinsic pressure by tumours, thrombophelia, phlebitis, previous leg injury, and occupations that require prolonged standing (Wittens et al., 2015).

In primary varicose veins, weak vein walls allow the vein valve ring to enlarge, so the leaflets no longer fit together properly (incompetent). Incompetent vein valves allow backward blood flow, particularly when the patient is standing. This results in increased venous pressure and further venous distention. High pressure in the superficial veins also can be caused by vein valve dysfunction in the deep veins or perforator veins (veins that perforate the deep fascia of muscles to connect the superficial veins to the deep veins).

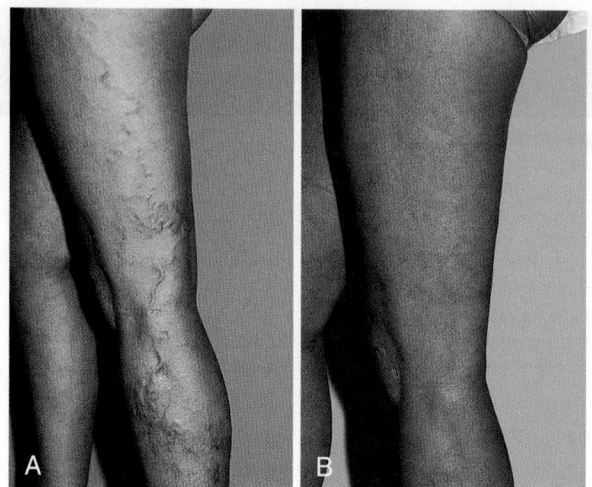

FIG. 40.11 A, Lateral aspect of varicose veins before treatment. **B,** Lateral aspect of varicose veins 2 years after initial treatment with sclerotherapy. Source: Goldman, M. P., Guex, J. J., & Weiss, R.A. (2011). *Sclerotherapy: Treatment of varicose and telangiectatic leg veins* (5th ed.). Mosby.

Clinical Manifestations and Complications

Discomfort from varicose veins varies among people and tends to be worse after episodes of SVT. Many patients are concerned about cosmetic disfigurement. The most common varicose vein symptom is a heavy, achy feeling or pain after prolonged standing, which is relieved by walking or limb elevation. Some patients feel pressure or experience an itchy, burning, or cramplike sensation in the affected leg. Swelling or nocturnal leg cramps also may occur.

Superficial venous thrombosis is the most frequent complication of varicose veins. It may occur spontaneously or after trauma, surgical procedures, or pregnancy. Rare complications include rupture of the varicose veins, resulting in external bleeding and skin ulcerations.

Diagnostic Studies

Superficial varicose veins can be diagnosed by appearance. Duplex ultrasonography is the gold standard to evaluate venous anatomy, valvular competence, and venous obstruction.

Invasive and Surgical Intervention. *Sclerotherapy* involves the direct IV injection of a substance that obliterates venous telangiectasias, reticular veins, and small, superficial varicose veins 5 mm or larger in diameter (Figure 40.11). Commonly used sclerosing agents include detergents (e.g., hypertonic saline), as well as other agents such as foams (e.g., polidocanol) and cyanoacrylate. Direct IV injection of a sclerosing agent induces inflammation and results in eventual thrombosis of the vein.

Potential complications include itching, pain, blistering, edema, hyperpigmentation, necrosis, and recurrence of varicosities, SVT, visual disturbances, and VTE. After injection, a thigh-high graduated compression stocking is worn or an elastic bandage is applied to the leg for several days to maintain pressure over the vein. Long-term compression therapy is advised to help prevent the development of further varicosities.

Other, more costly, but noninvasive options for the treatment of venous telangiectasias and varicose veins include laser therapy and radiofrequency ablation, indirect or direct. Laser therapy can be used in telangiectasias or in larger veins, including greater saphenous vein incompetence. Radiofrequency ablation, either direct or indirect, works by thermal destruction of venous tissues with the use of electrical energy in the form of high-frequency alternating current (Hamann et al., 2019). Potential complications of these therapies include pain, bruising, paresthesia, blistering, hyperpigmentation, and superficial erosions. These therapies can be used alone or in combination with saphenofemoral ligation or phlebectomy.

Surgical intervention is indicated for recurrent superficial venous thrombosis or symptoms that cannot be controlled with conservative therapy. The traditional surgical intervention involves ligation of the entire vein (usually the greater saphenous vein) and removal of its incompetent tributaries. An alternative but time-consuming technique is *ambulatory phlebectomy*. This involves pulling the varicosity through a "stab" incision followed by excision of the vein. Complications include bleeding, bruising, and infection.

Interprofessional Care

If venous insufficiency develops, interprofessional care involves rest with limb elevation, graduated compression stockings, and exercise, such as walking. Two herbal therapies, horse chestnut seed extract *(Aesculus hippocastanum)* and butcher's broom *(Ruscus aculeatus)*, have historically been available, but the agent with the best evidence to date is micronized purified flavonoid fraction (das Graças et al., 2018). These medications are most effective in the early stages. None of these medications have proven to be effective in late stages of chronic venous insufficiency. (See the Chronic Venous Insufficiency and Venous Leg Ulcers section later in this chapter.)

NURSING MANAGEMENT
VARICOSE VEINS

Prevention is a key factor related to varicose veins. The patient should be instructed to avoid risk factors (see previous section) and to walk daily.

After vein ligation surgery, the patient should be encouraged to practice deep breathing, which promotes venous return. It is important to check the extremities regularly for colour, movement, sensation, temperature, edema, and quality of pedal pulses. Postoperatively, the legs should be elevated 15 degrees to limit edema. Graduated compression stockings or bandages should be applied. They should be removed every 8 hours for short periods and then reapplied.

Long-term management of varicose veins is directed toward improving circulation appearance, relieving discomfort, and avoiding complications and ulceration. Varicosities can recur in other veins after surgery. Patients should be taught the proper use and care of custom-fitted graduated compression stockings. The patient should apply stockings in bed, before rising in the morning. The importance of periodic positioning of the legs above the heart should be stressed, along with weight management, frequent position changes, flexing and extending lower extremities to activate the calf muscle for venous return, and avoidance of prolonged sitting.

CHRONIC VENOUS INSUFFICIENCY AND VENOUS LEG ULCERS

Chronic (and acute) venous insufficiency (CVI), a common disorder in women and older persons, is a condition in which leg veins and valves fail to keep blood moving forward. This

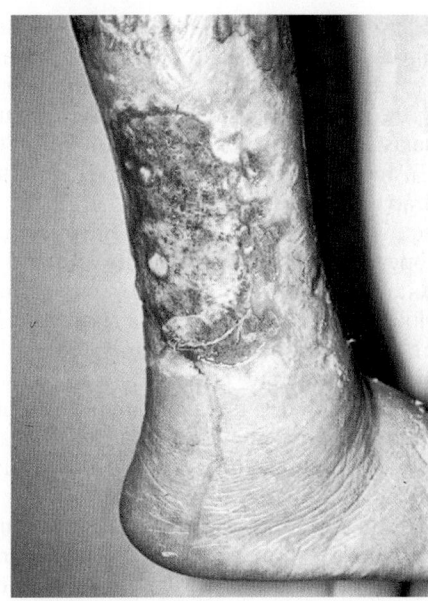

FIG. 40.12 Venous leg ulcer. Source: Kamal, A., & Brocklehurst, J. C. (1991). *Color atlas of geriatric medicine* (2nd ed.). Mosby–Year Book.

results in *ambulatory venous hypertension*. CVI can lead to *venous leg ulcers* (formerly called *venous stasis ulcers* or *varicose ulcers*) (Labropoulos, 2019). Although CVI and venous leg ulcers are not life-threatening diseases, they are painful and debilitating and impair quality of life. They are a common problem in older persons.

Etiology and Pathophysiology

Both long-standing primary varicose veins and PTS can progress to CVI. *Ambulatory venous hypertension* causes serous fluid and RBCs to leak from the capillaries and venules into the tissue. This causes edema and chronic inflammatory changes. Enzymes in the tissue eventually break down RBCs, causing the release of *hemosiderin,* which causes a brownish skin discoloration. Over time, fibrous tissue replaces the skin and subcutaneous tissue around the ankle. This results in thick, hardened, contracted skin. Although the causes of CVI are known, the exact pathophysiology of venous leg ulcers is unknown.

Clinical Manifestations and Complications

Advanced CVI causes hemosiderin staining and lipodermatosclerosis, which causes impaired skin perfusion and trapping of deleterious material within the subcuticular tissues. This leads to ulceration or prevents healing in the setting of a wound. Eczema, or "stasis dermatitis," is often present, and pruritus is a common complaint (see Table 40.1).

Venous ulcers classically are located above the medial malleolus (Figure 40.12). These ulcers are quite painful, particularly when in a dependent position. If untreated, the wound becomes wider and deeper, increasing the risk for infection.

Interprofessional Care

Compression is the cornerstone for CVI treatment, venous ulcer healing, and prevention of ulcer recurrence. A variety of options are available for compression therapy, including custom-fitted graduated compression stockings, short stretch bandages, and multilayer bandage systems, including a two-layer (Coban) and four-layer system (Profore) (Haesler, 2019). Other options include a Velcro wrap (CircAid), SCDs, and a paste bandage (Unna boot). Patients should be evaluated individually when choosing a compression method. Before instituting compression therapy, the nurse should assess the arterial status to make sure that coexistent PAD is not present. An ABI of 0.4 or less suggests PAD, and the patient should not have any type of compression therapy (Gerhard-Herman et al., 2017).

The nurse needs to discuss with the patient activity guidelines and proper limb positioning. Patients with CVI should be instructed to avoid standing or sitting for long periods, which decreases blood return from the lower extremities. Patients should also be informed to frequently elevate their legs above the level of the heart to reduce edema. The nurse can encourage patients to begin a daily walking program once an ulcer heals. The patient and caregiver should be instructed to avoid trauma to the limbs, and they should be taught proper foot and leg care to avoid more skin trauma.

Moist environment dressings are the basis of wound care. A variety of these dressings are available and include transparent film dressings, hydrocolloids, hydrogels, foams, calcium alginates, impregnated gauze, and combination dressings. When used in conjunction with compression, moist environment dressings are more effective than dry dressings in hastening the healing of venous leg ulcers. (Hydrocolloid and other dressings are discussed in Chapter 14, Table 14.11.)

The nutritional status of a patient with a venous ulcer needs to be evaluated. A balanced diet with adequate protein, calories, and micronutrients is essential for healing. Nutrients most important for healing include protein, vitamins A and C, and zinc. Foods high in protein (e.g., meat, beans, cheese, tofu), vitamin A (green leafy vegetables), vitamin C (citrus fruits, tomatoes, cantaloupe), and zinc (meat, seafood) must be provided. For patients with diabetes, maintaining normal blood glucose levels aids the healing process.

Although venous leg ulcers are colonized by bacteria, routine antibiotic therapy is not indicated. Signs of infection in a venous ulcer include change in quantity, colour, or odour of the drainage; presence of pus; erythema of the wound edges; change in sensation around the wound; warmth around the wound; increased local pain or edema, or both; dark-coloured granulation tissue; induration around the wound; delayed healing; and cellulitis. If signs of infection are present, a wound culture should be obtained as culture results guide antibiotic therapy. The usual treatment for infection is wound debridement, wound excision, and systemic antibiotics.

Medical Therapy. If the ulcer does not heal with conservative therapy, medication therapy should be considered. Micronized purified flavonoid fraction is recommended with compression to improve healing. Micronized purified flavonoid fraction acts on WBCs to decrease inflammation and edema and can play a role in early intervention for varicose veins (das Graças et al., 2018).

Alternative treatments include coverage with a split-thickness skin graft, cultured epithelial autograft, allograft, or bioengineered skin, although these are expensive solutions and, without ongoing compression, are not likely to offer a long-term solution. (Skin grafting is discussed in Chapter 27.) A recent treatment advanced is radiofrequency ablation, which is done directly under the ulcer bed to remove varicosities that are contributing to the ulceration. This treatment is still in development.

NURSING MANAGEMENT
CHRONIC VENOUS INSUFFICIENCY AND VENOUS LEG ULCERS

Long-term management of venous leg ulcers should focus on teaching the patient about self-care measures because the ulcers often recur. Patients with CVI have dry, flaky, itchy skin; thus, daily moisturizing can decrease itching and prevent skin cracking. Contact dermatitis may result from contact with sensitizing products, such as topical antimicrobial agents (e.g., gentamicin); additives in bandages or dressings (e.g., adhesives); ointments containing lanolin, alcohols, or benzocaine; and over-the-counter creams or lotions with fragrance or preservatives. The nurse needs to assess wounds for signs of infection with each dressing change.

CASE STUDY

Peripheral Artery Disease

Patient Profile
L. D. (pronouns he/him), 76 years old, is admitted to the hospital with rest pain in both legs and a nonhealing ulcer of the big toe on his right foot.

Subjective Data
- History of a myocardial infarction, stroke, hypertension, arthritis, and type 1 diabetes mellitus
- Underwent a left femoral–popliteal bypass 5 years ago
- Has a history of current tobacco use ½ to 1 pack a day
- Has been using insulin for 30 years
- Complains of sudden, intense increase in right foot pain for past 2 hr
- Has slept in recliner with right leg in dependent position for several months

Current Medications
- Furosemide (Lasix), 40 mg/day PO
- Ramipril 5 mg/day PO
- Aspart (NovoRapid) insulin with meals
- Glargine insulin (Lantus), 50 units daily subcutaneously
- Amlodipine 10 mg/ day PO
- ASA (Aspirin), 81 mg/day PO
- Fish oil daily (self-prescribed)

Objective Data
Physical Examination
- BP, 148/92 mm Hg; irregular apical heart rate, 90/min; respiratory rate, 22/min; temperature, 36.6°C
- Alert and oriented but anxious, no apparent physical or mental deficits from previous stroke
- Diminished right femoral pulse, popliteal signal detected only with use of a Doppler probe, posterior tibial signal detected with use of Doppler probe, and dorsalis pedis pulse absent (not palpable or auscultated with Doppler); left leg pulses are weakly palpable
- Right leg ABI: 0.20; left leg ABI: 0.68
- Has a 2-cm necrotic ulcer on tip of right big toe
- Has thickened toenails; shiny, thin skin on legs; and hair absent on both lower legs
- Right foot is very cool, pale, and mottled in colour with decreased sensation
- No peripheral edema is present

CASE STUDY

Peripheral Artery Disease—cont'd

- Bedside glucose measurement 16 mmol/L (last meal 4 hr before admission)

Discussion Questions
1. What are L. D.'s risk factors for peripheral artery disease (PAD)?
2. Differentiate L. D.'s signs and symptoms of chronic PAD from those of acute arterial ischemia.
3. Identify the possible cause or causes for the sudden, intense increase in right foot pain.
4. How would the nurse interpret L. D.'s ABI findings?
5. What additional diagnostic tests can be performed to assess the extent of L. D.'s PAD?
6. Given the physical examination data, what initial medications might the physician prescribe?

7. What treatment modalities are possible for L. D.?
8. *Priority decision:* What are the priority nursing responsibilities in caring for L. D.?
9. *Priority decision:* On the basis of the assessment data presented, what are the priority nursing diagnoses? Are there any interprofessional issues?
10. *Evidence-informed practice:* In patient education for L. D., what evidence-informed advice should the nurse give regarding the use of dietary supplements such as fish oil?

ⓔvolve

Answers are available at http://evolve.elsevier.com/Canada/Lewis/medsurg.

REVIEW QUESTIONS

The number of the question corresponds to the same-numbered objective at the beginning of the chapter.

1. A 50-year-old woman weighs 95 kg and has a history of tobacco use, high blood pressure, high sodium intake, and sedentary lifestyle. When an individualized care plan is developed for this client, which of the following risk factors related to PAD would the nurse determine need to be modified?
   a. Salt intake
   b. Sedentary lifestyle
   c. Tobacco use
   d. Excess weight

2. When teaching a patient about rest pain and PAD, what should the nurse explain as the cause of the pain?
   a. Vasospasm of cutaneous arteries in the feet
   b. Increase in retrograde venous perfusion of the lower legs
   c. Decrease in arterial blood flow to the nerves of the feet
   d. Decrease in arterial blood flow to the leg muscles during exercise

3. A client with infective endocarditis develops sudden left leg pain with pallor, paresthesia, and a loss of peripheral pulses. What should the nurse's initial action be?
   a. Elevate the leg to promote venous return.
   b. Start anticoagulant therapy with IV heparin.
   c. Notify the health care provider of the change in perfusion.
   d. Position the patient in reverse Trendelenburg position to promote perfusion.

4. Which clinical manifestations are seen in clients with both Buerger's disease and clients with Raynaud's phenomenon? *(Select all that apply.)*
   a. Intermittent low-grade fevers
   b. Sensitivity to cold temperatures
   c. Gangrenous ulcers on fingertips
   d. Colour changes of fingers and toes
   e. Episodes of superficial vein thrombosis

5. A client is admitted to the hospital with a diagnosis of abdominal aortic aneurysm. Which signs and symptoms would suggest that his aneurysm has ruptured?
   a. Sudden shortness of breath and hemoptysis
   b. Sudden, severe low back pain and bruising along his flank
   c. Gradually increasing substernal chest pain and diaphoresis
   d. Sudden, patchy blue mottling on feet and toes and rest pain

6. Which of the following are *priority* nursing measures 8 hours after an abdominal aortic aneurysm repair?
   a. Assessment of cranial nerves and mental status
   b. Administration of IV heparin and monitoring of aPTT
   c. Administration of IV fluids and monitoring of kidney function
   d. Elevation of the legs and application of graduated compression stockings

7. What is the *first* priority of interprofessional care of a client with a suspected acute aortic dissection?
   a. Reduce anxiety.
   b. Control blood pressure.
   c. Monitor for chest pain.
   d. Increase myocardial contractility.

8. Which of the following clients has the *highest* risk for venous thromboembolism (VTE)?
   a. A 62-year-old man with spider veins who is having arthroscopic knee surgery
   b. A 32-year-old woman who smokes, takes oral contraceptives, and is planning a trip to Europe
   c. A 26-year-old woman who is 3 days postpartum and received maintenance IV fluids for 12 hours during her labour
   d. An active 72-year-old man at home recovering from transurethral resection of the prostate for benign prostatic hyperplasia

9. Which clinical findings should the nurse expect in a person with an acute lower extremity VTE? *(Select all that apply.)*
   a. Pallor and coolness of foot and calf
   b. Mild to moderate calf pain and tenderness
   c. Grossly diminished or absent pedal pulses
   d. Unilateral edema and induration of the thigh
   e. Palpable cord along a superficial varicose vein

10. What treatment should the nurse anticipate for an otherwise healthy person with no significant comorbid conditions?
    a. IV argatroban while the person is an inpatient
    b. IV unfractionated heparin as an inpatient
    c. Subcutaneous unfractionated heparin as an outpatient
    d. Subcutaneous low-molecular-weight heparin as an outpatient

11. Which of the following is a *key* teaching instruction for the client who is receiving anticoagulant therapy?
    a. Monitor for and report any signs of bleeding.
    b. Do not take acetaminophen (Tylenol) for a headache.
    c. Decrease your dietary intake of foods containing vitamin K.
    d. Arrange to have blood drawn routinely to check medication levels.

12. The nurse is planning care and teaching for a patient with venous leg ulcers. Which is the *most* important client action in healing and control of this condition?
    a. Follow activity guidelines.
    b. Using moist environment dressings.
    c. Taking horse chestnut seed extract daily.
    d. Apply graduated compression stockings.

1. c; 2. c; 3. c; 4. b, c, d; 5. b; 6. c; 7. b; 8. b; 9. b, d; 10. d; 11. a; 12. d

ⓔvolve

For even more review questions, visit http://evolve.elsevier.com/Canada/Lewis/medsurg.

REFERENCES

Alberta Rheumatology. (2021). *Marijuana (cannabis)*. https://albertarheumatology.com/natural-health-products/marijuana-cannabis/

American Association of Nurse Anaesthetists. (2021). *Enhanced recovery after surgery*. https://www.aana.com/practice/clinical-practice-resources/enhanced-recovery-after-surgery

Anand, S. S., Eikelboom, J. W., Dyal, L., et al. (2019). Rivaroxaban plus aspirin versus aspirin in relation to vascular risk in the COMPASS trial. *Journal of the American College of Cardiology, 73*(25), 3271–3280. https://doi.org/10.1016/j.jacc.2019.02.079

Banerjee, S., & McCormack, S. (2019). *Medical cannabis for the treatment of chronic pain: A review of clinical effectiveness and guidelines*. CADTH. https://www.ncbi.nlm.nih.gov/books/NBK546424/pdf/Bookshelf_NBK546424.pdf

Barnes, G. D., & Renner, E. T. (2018). Anticoagulation in venous thromboembolism. In J. F. Lau, G. Barnes, & M. Streiff (Eds.), *Anticoagulation therapy* (pp. 297–323). Cham: Springer.

Bartholomew, J. R., & Evans, N. S. (2019). Travel-related thromboembolism. *Vascular Medicine, 24*(1), 93–95. https://doi.org/10.1177/1358863X18818323

Beckman, J. A. (2018). ABI: The goal line is in sight. *Vascular Medicine, 23*(2), 107–108. https://doi.org/10.1177/1358863X17749300

Bernardi, E., & Camporese, G. (2018). Diagnosis of deep-vein thrombosis. *Thrombosis Research, 163*, 201–206. https://doi.org/10.1016/j.thromres.2017.10.006

Bernstein, C. F., Kristianson, A., Akl, E. A., et al. (2016). Compression stockings for preventing the post-thrombotic syndrome in patients with deep vein thrombosis. *American Journal of Medicine, 129*(4), 447.e1–447.e20. https://doi.org/10.1016/j.amjmed.2015.11.031

Black, J. H., & Burke, C. R. (2020). Epidemiology, risk factors, pathogenesis, and natural history of thoracic aortic aneurysm. *UpToDate*. https://www.uptodate.com/contents/epidemiology-risk-factors-pathogenesis-and-natural-history-of-thoracic-aortic-aneurysm

Bonneau, C., Caron, N. R., Hussain, M. A., et al. (2018). Peripheral artery disease among Indigenous Canadians: What do we know? *Canadian Journal of Surgery, 61*(5), 305. https://doi.org/10.1503/cjs.013917

Burcham, J. R., & Rosenthal, L. D. (2019). *Lehne's pharmacology for nursing care* (10th ed.). Elsevier.

Cacione, D. G., do Carmo Novaes, F., & Moreno, D. H. (2018). Stem cell therapy for treatment of thromboangiitis obliterans (Buerger's disease). *Cochrane Database of Systematic Reviews, (10)*, Article No. CD012794. https://doi.org/10.1002/14651858.CD012794.pub2

Canadian Patient Safety Institute. (2017). *Venous thromboembolism (VTE) prevention: Getting started kit components*. https://era.library.ualberta.ca/items/4512216f-5a90-4ccf-bd13-6618ae9ade55/view/d597a2d5-2a20-4ba4-859a-f602bb4d6c0d/VTE%20GSK%20EN.pdf

Chang, W. P., & Peng, Y. X. (2018). Occurrence of phlebitis: A systematic review and meta-analysis. *Nursing Research, 67*(3), 252–260. https://doi.org/10.1097/NNR.0000000000000279

Cronenwett, J., Johnston, K. W. (Eds.), *Rutherford's vascular surgery* (8th ed.). Philadelphia: Saunders.

das Graças, C. M., Cyrino, F. Z., de Carvalho, J. J., et al. (2018). Protective effects of micronized purified flavonoid fraction (MPFF) on a novel experimental model of chronic venous hypertension. *European Journal of Vascular and Endovascular Surgery, 55*(5), 694–702. https://doi.org/10.1016/j.ejvs.2018.02.009

DeMartino, R., Sen, I., Huang, Y., et al. (2018). Population-based assessment of the incidence of aortic dissection, intramural hematoma, and penetrating ulcer, and its associated mortality from 1995 to 2015. *Circulation: Cardiovascular Quality and Outcomes, 11*(8), e004689.

Diabetes Canada Clinical Practice Guidelines Expert Committee. (2018). Diabetes Canada 2018 clinical practice guidelines for the prevention and management of diabetes in Canada. *Canadian Journal of Diabetes, 42*(Suppl 1), S1–S325. http://guidelines.diabetes.ca/cpg

Elsebaie, M. A., van Es, N., Langston, A., et al. (2019). Direct oral anticoagulants in patients with venous thromboembolism and thrombophilia: A systematic review and meta-analysis. *Journal of Thrombosis and Haemostasis, 17*(4), 645–656. https://doi.org/10.1111/jth.14398

Fábián, B., Fábián, A., Bugán, A., et al. (2019). Comparison of mental and physical health between patients with primary and secondary Raynaud's phenomenon category. *Journal of Psychosomatic Research, 116*, 6–9. https://doi.org/10.1016/j.jpsychores.2018.11.001

Fereydooni, A., Gorecka, J., & Dardik, A. (2019). Using the epidemiology of critical limb ischemia to estimate the number of patients amenable to endovascular therapy. *Vascular Medicine, 25*(1), 78–87. https://doi.org/10.1177/1358863X19878271.

Firnhaber, J. M., & Powell, C. S. (2019). Lower extremity peripheral artery disease: Diagnosis and treatment. *American Family Physician, 99*(6), 362–369.

Fitzgibbon, B., Jordan, F., Hynes, N., et al. (2018). Endovascular versus open surgical repair for complicated chronic type B aortic dissection. *Cochrane Database of Systematic Reviews, 4*, CD012992. https://doi.org/10.1002/14651858.CD012992

Forbes, T. (n.d.). *Abdominal aortic aneurysm (AAA)*. Canadian Society for Vascular Surgery. https://vascular.ca/Abdominal-Aortic-Aneurysms/

Galyfos, G., Sigala, F., Mpananis, K., et al. (2019). Small abdominal aortic aneurysms: Has anything changed so far? *Trends in Cardiovascular Medicine, 10*(23), 1–6. https://doi.org/10.1016/j.tcm.2019.11.006

Gerhard-Herman, M. D., Gornik, H. L., Barrett, C., et al. (2017). 2016 AHA/ACC guideline on the management of patients with lower extremity peripheral artery disease: Executive summary: a report of the American College of Cardiology/American Heart Association Task Force on Clinical Practice Guidelines. *Journal of the American College of Cardiology, 69*(11), 1465–1508.

Giustozzi, M., Franco, L., Vedovati, M. C., et al. (2019). Safety of direct oral anticoagulants versus traditional anticoagulants in venous thromboembolism. *Journal of Thrombosis and Thrombolysis, 48*(3), 439–453. https://doi.org/10.1007/s11239-019-01878-x

Golledge, J. (2019). Abdominal aortic aneurysm: Update on pathogenesis and medical treatments. *Nature Reviews Cardiology, 16*(4), 225–242. https://doi.org/10.1038/s41569-018-0114-9

Haesler, E. (2019). Evidence summary: Venous leg ulcers: Compression with short stretch (inelastic) bandages. *Wound Practice and Research, 27*(2), 134–136.

Hajibandeh, S., Hajibandeh, S., Shah, S., et al. (2017). Prognostic significance of ankle brachial pressure index: A systematic review and meta-analysis. *Vascular, 25*(2), 208–224. https://doi.org/10.1177/1708538116658392

Hamann, S. A. S., Timmer–de Mik, L., Fritschy, W. M., et al. (2019). Randomized clinical trial of endovenous laser ablation versus direct and indirect radiofrequency ablation for the treatment of great saphenous varicose veins. *British Journal of Surgery, 106*(8), 998–1004. https://doi.org/10.1002/bjs.11187

Hasan, M., Malalur, P., Agastya, M., et al. (2016). A high-value cost conscious approach to minimize heparin induced thrombocytopenia antibody (HITAb) testing using the 4T score. *Journal of Thrombosis and Thrombolysis, 42*(3), 441–446. https://doi.org/10.1007/s11239-016-1396-6

Hattab, Y., Küng, S., Fasanya, A., et al. (2017). Deep venous thrombosis of the upper and lower extremity. *Critical Care Nursing Quarterly, 40*(3), 230–236.

Herrick, A. L., & Wigley, F. M. (2020). Raynaud's phenomenon. *Best Practice & Research Clinical Rheumatology, 34*(1), 101474. https://doi.org/10.1016/j.berh.2019.101474

Houlden, R. (2018). 2018 Clinical practice guidelines: Introduction—Diabetes Canada clinical practice guidelines expert committee. *Canadian Journal of Diabetes, 42*(S1), S1–S5. https://doi.org/10.1016/j.jcjd.2017.10.001

Kalsi, R., Oates, C. P., Olson, S., et al. (2017). Lower extremity ischemia, an ominous complication after elective EVAR. *Journal of Vascular Surgery, 66*(2), E22.

Kearon, C. (2019). The American College of Chest Physicians score to assess the risk of bleeding during anticoagulation in patients with venous thromboembolism: More. *Journal of Thrombosis and Haemostasis, 17*(7), 1180–1182. https://doi.org/10.1111/jth.14459

Khan, N. (2015). Developments and risk analysis in anticoagulation. *British Journal of Cardiac Nursing, 10*(2), 66–73. https://doi.org/10.12968/bjca.2015.10.2.66

Khoury, S. R., Evans, N. S., & Ratchford, E. V. (2019). Exercise as medicine. *Vascular Medicine, 24*(4), 371–374. https://doi.org/10.1177/1358863X19850316

Kulezic, A., Bergwall, S., Fatemi, S., et al. (2019). Healthy diet and fiber intake are associated with decreased risk of incident symptomatic peripheral artery disease–A prospective cohort study. *Vascular Medicine, 24*(6), 511–518. https://doi.org/10.1177/1358863X19867393

Labropoulos, N. (2019). How does chronic venous disease progress from the first symptoms to the advanced stages? A review. *Advances in Therapy, 36*(1), 13–19.

Leone, O., Corsini, A., Pacini, D., et al. (2020). The complex interplay among atherosclerosis, inflammation, and degeneration in ascending thoracic aortic aneurysms. *The Journal of Thoracic and Cardiovascular Surgery, 160*(6), 1434–1443. https://doi.org/10.1016/j.jtcvs.2019.08.108

Li, F. R., Wu, X., Yuan, J., et al. (2018). Comparison of thoracic endovascular aortic repair, open surgery and best medical treatment for type B aortic dissection: A meta-analysis. *International Journal of Cardiology, 250*, 240–246. https://doi.org/10.1016/j.ijcard.2017.10.050

Musil, D., Kaletová, M., & Herman, J. (2017). Venous thromboembolism–prevalence and risk factors in chronic venous disease patients. *Phlebology, 32*(2), 135–140. https://doi.org/10.1177/0268355516633392

Norgren, L., Hiatt, W. R., Dormandy, J. A., et al. (2007). Inter-society consensus for the management of peripheral arterial disease (TASC II). *Journal of Vascular Surgery, 45*(1), S5–S67. https://doi.org/10.1016/j.jvs.2006.12.037

Ozkaramanli Gur, D., Guzel, S., Akyuz, A., et al. (2018). The role of novel cytokines in inflammation: Defining peripheral artery disease among patients with coronary artery disease. *Vascular Medicine, 23*(5), 428–436. https://doi.org/10.1177/1358863X18763096

Palese, A., Ambrosi, E., Fabris, F., et al. (2016). Nursing care as a predictor of phlebitis related to insertion of a peripheral venous cannula in emergency departments: Findings from a prospective study. *Journal of Hospital Infection, 92*(3), 280–286. https://doi.org/10.1016/j.jhin.2015.10.021

Rattan, R., Jones, K. M., & Namias, N. (2015). Management of lower extremity vascular injuries: State of the art. *Current Surgery Reports, 3*(11), 1–9. https://doi.org/10.1007/s40137-015-0118-x

Reynolds, K., Mues, K. E., Harrison, T. N., et al. (2019). Trends in statin utilization among adults with severe peripheral artery disease including critical limb ischemia in an integrated healthcare delivery system. *Vascular Medicine, 25*(1), 3–12 1358863X19871100.

Rylski, B., Pérez, M., Beyersdorf, F., et al. (2017). Acute non-A non-B aortic dissection: Incidence, treatment and outcome. *European Journal of Cardio-Thoracic Surgery, 52*(6), 1111–1117.

Scott, D. J., Steenberge, S. P., Bena, J. F., et al. (2020). Morphologic and operative evolution of open ruptured abdominal aortic aneurysm repair. *Annals of Vascular Surgery, 63*, 68–82. https://doi.org/10.1016/j.avsg.2019.08.098

Sexton, F., Healy, D., Keelan, S., et al. (2020). A systematic review and meta-analysis comparing the effectiveness of negative-pressure wound therapy to standard therapy in the prevention of complications after vascular surgery. *International Journal of Surgery, 76*, 94–100. https://doi.org/10.1016/j.ijsu.2020.02.037

Sharath, S. E., Lee, M., Kougias, P., et al. (2019). Delayed gratification and adherence to exercise among patients with claudication. *Vascular Medicine, 24*(6), 519–527. https://doi.org/10.1177/1358863X19865610

Stone, J. A., Houlden, R. L., Udell, J. A., et al. (2018). Cardiovascular protection in people with diabetes. *Canadian Journal of Diabetes, 42*, S162–S169. https://doi.org/10.1016/j.jcjd.2017.10.024

Stoner, M. C., Calligaro, K. D., Chaer, R. A., et al. (2016). Reporting standards of the Society for Vascular Surgery for endovascular treatment of chronic lower extremity peripheral artery disease. *Journal of Vascular Surgery, 64*(1), e1–e21. https://doi.org/10.1016/j.jvs.2016.03.420

TASC Steering Committee, Jaff, M. R., White, C. J., et al. An update on methods for revascularization and expansion of the TASC lesion classification to include below-the-knee arteries: A supplement to the Inter-Society Consensus for the Management of Peripheral Arterial Disease (TASC II). *Vascular Medicine, 20*(5), 465-478. https://doi.org/10.1177/1358863X15597877 (Seminal).

Wharton, S., Lau, D. C. W., Vallis, M., et al. (2020). Obesity in adults: A clinical practice guideline. *CMAJ, 192*(4), E875–E891. https://doi.org/10.1503/cmaj.191707

Wittens, C., Davies, A. H., Baekgaard, R., et al. (2015). Management of chronic venous disease: Clinical practice guidelines of the European Society for Vascular Surgery (ESVS). *European Journal of Vascular and Endovascular Surgery, 49*(6), 678–737. https://doi.org/10.1016/j.ejvs.2015.02.007

RESOURCES

Canadian Cardiovascular Society
https://ccs.ca/

Canadian Council of Cardiovascular Nurses
https://www.cccn.ca/

Canadian Patient Safety Institute—*Venous Thromboembolism: Introduction*
https://www.patientsafetyinstitute.ca/en/toolsResources/Hospital-Harm-Measure/Improvement-Resources/VTEOverview/Pages-/default.aspx

Canadian Society for Vascular Surgery
https://canadianvascular.ca

Canadian Society of Vascular Nursing
https://csvn.ca/

Heart and Stroke Foundation of Canada
https://www.heartandstroke.ca

Hypertension Canada
https://www.hypertension.ca

Health Resources and Services Administration—*Lower Extremity Amputation Prevention (LEAP) Program*
https://www.hrsa.gov/hansens-disease/leap

ⓔvolve

For additional Internet resources, see the website for this book at http://evolve.elsevier.com/Canada/Lewis/medsurg.

Conditions of Ingestion, Digestion, Absorption, and Elimination

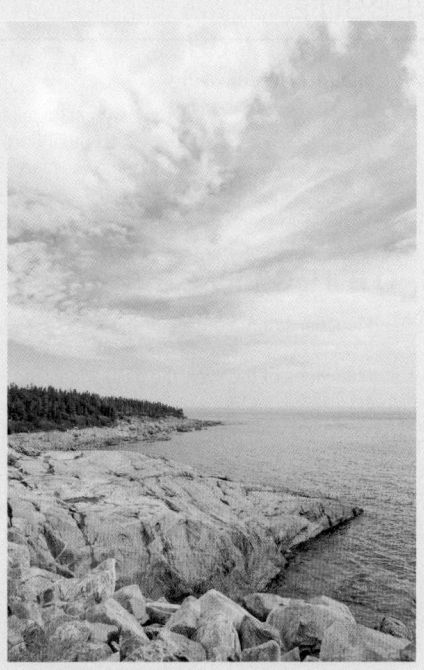

Source: © CanStock Photo / Pavels

41

Nursing Assessment

Gastrointestinal System

Myriam Breau
Originating US chapter by Kara Ann Ventura

⊖volve WEBSITE

http://evolve.elsevier.com/Canada/Lewis/medsurg

- Review Questions (Online Only)
- Key Points
- Answer Guidelines for Case Study
- Conceptual Care Map Creator
- Audio Glossary
- Supporting Media—Animations
  - Rectal Examination
- Content Updates

LEARNING OBJECTIVES

1. Describe the structures and functions of the organs of the gastrointestinal tract.
2. Describe the structures and functions of the liver, the gallbladder, the biliary tract, and the pancreas.
3. Differentiate between the processes of ingestion, digestion, absorption, and elimination.
4. Relate the age-related changes in the gastrointestinal system to differences in assessment findings.
5. Select the significant subjective and objective data related to the gastrointestinal system that should be obtained from a patient.
6. Describe the appropriate techniques used in the physical assessment of the gastrointestinal system.
7. Differentiate normal from abnormal findings of a physical assessment of the gastrointestinal system.
8. Describe the purpose, significance of results, and nursing responsibilities related to diagnostic studies of the gastrointestinal system.

KEY TERMS

absorption
bilirubin
defecation
deglutition
digestion
endoscopy

hematemesis
hepatocytes
ingestion
Kupffer cells
melena
pyrosis

steatorrhea
tenesmus
Valsalva manoeuvre
villi

The main function of the gastrointestinal (GI) system is to supply nutrients to body cells. This function is accomplished through the processes of *ingestion* (taking in food), *digestion* (breakdown of food), and *absorption* (transfer of food products into circulation). *Elimination* is the process of excreting the waste products of digestion.

The GI system (also called the *digestive system*) consists of the GI tract and its associated organs and glands. Included in the GI tract are the mouth, the esophagus, the stomach, the small intestine, the large intestine, the rectum, and the anus. The associated organs are the liver, the pancreas, and the gallbladder (Figure 41.1).

STRUCTURES AND FUNCTIONS OF THE GASTROINTESTINAL SYSTEM

The GI tract is a tube approximately 9 m long, extending from the mouth to the anus. The entire tract is composed of four common layers. From the inside to the outside, these layers are (1) *mucosa*, (2) *submucosa*, (3) *muscle*, and (4) *serosa* (see Figure 41.1). In the esophagus, the outer coat is fibrous tissue rather than serosa. The muscular coat consists of two layers: the *circular* (inner) and the *longitudinal* (outer).

The GI tract is innervated by the parasympathetic and the sympathetic branches of the autonomic nervous system. Each

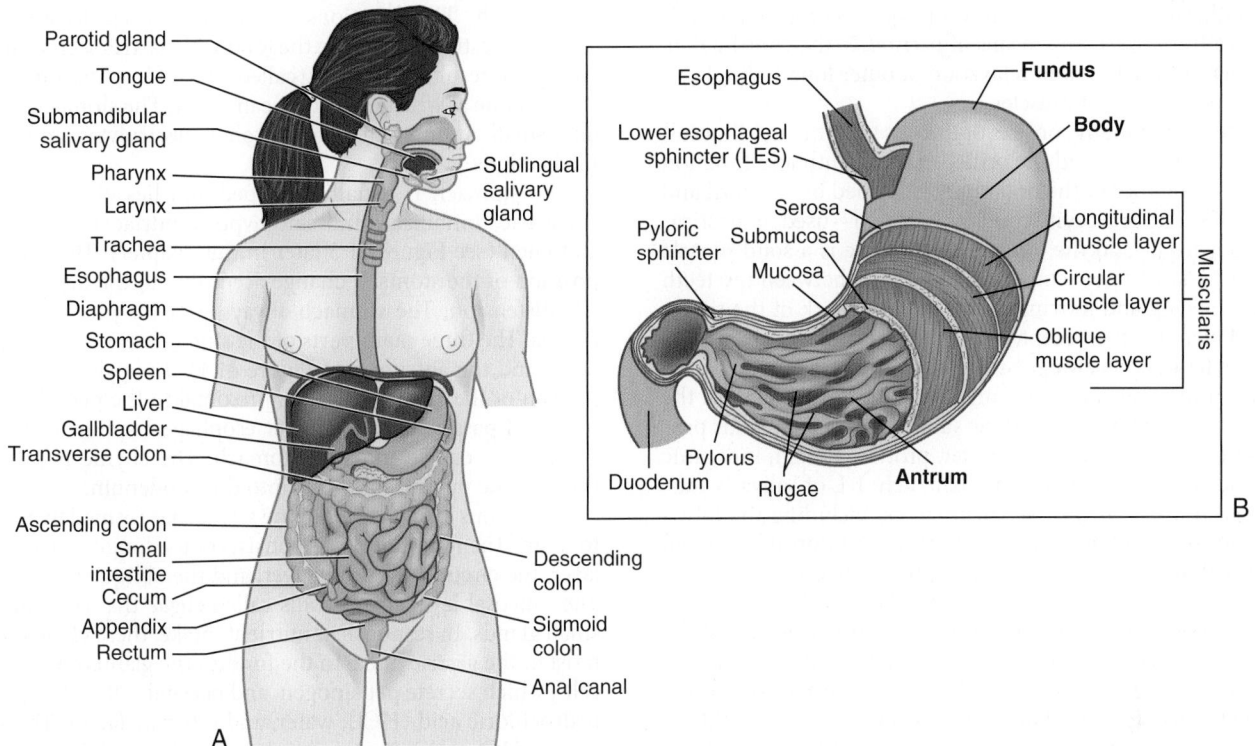

Parotid gland
Tongue
Submandibular salivary gland
Pharynx
Larynx
Trachea
Esophagus
Diaphragm
Stomach
Spleen
Liver
Gallbladder
Transverse colon

Ascending colon
Small intestine
Cecum
Appendix
Rectum

Sublingual salivary gland

Descending colon

Sigmoid colon

Anal canal

A

Esophagus
Lower esophageal sphincter (LES)
Pyloric sphincter
Serosa
Submucosa
Mucosa
Duodenum
Pylorus
Rugae
Antrum

Fundus
Body
Longitudinal muscle layer
Circular muscle layer
Oblique muscle layer
Muscularis

B

FIG. 41.1 Location of organs of the gastrointestinal system.

branch has its function on the GI tract. The parasympathetic system exerts both excitatory and inhibitory control over gastric and intestinal tone and mobility. The sympathetic nervous system exerts a predominantly inhibitory effect on GI muscle and provides a tonic inhibitory influence over mucosal secretion while, at the same time, regulating GI blood flow via neurally mediated vasoconstriction. Sensory information is relayed via both sympathetic and parasympathetic afferent fibres.

The GI tract and accessory organs receive approximately 25 to 30% of the cardiac output. Circulation in the GI system is unique in that venous blood that drains from the GI tract organs empties into the portal vein, which then perfuses the liver. The upper portion of the GI tract receives its blood supply from the splanchnic artery. The small intestine receives its blood supply from branches of the hepatic and superior mesenteric arteries. The large intestine receives its blood supply mainly from the superior and inferior mesenteric arteries. Because such a large percentage of the cardiac output is used to perfuse these organs, the GI tract is a major source from which blood flow can be diverted during exercise or stress.

The two types of movement of the GI tract are *mixing* (segmentation) and *propulsion* (peristalsis). The secretions of the GI system consist of enzymes and hormones for digestion, mucus to provide protection and lubrication, and water and electrolytes.

The abdominal organs are almost completely covered by the peritoneum, which secures the viscera within the abdomen. The peritoneum is divided into two section, the *parietal* peritoneum, which lines the abdominal cavity wall, and the *visceral* peritoneum, which covers the abdominal organs.

The *peritoneal cavity* is the potential space between the parietal and visceral layers. The two folds of the peritoneum are the *mesentery* and the *omentum*.

The primary functions of the GI system are (a) ingestion and propulsion (movement) of food; (b) secretion of mucus, water, and enzymes; (c) digestion; (d) absorption; and (e) elimination. Each part of the GI system performs different activities to accomplish these functions. Physical factors such as dietary intake, ingestion of alcohol and caffeine-containing products, cigarette smoking, and fatigue can affect GI function. Psychological and emotional factors such as stress and anxiety may also influence its functioning. Stress may be manifested as anorexia, nausea, epigastric and abdominal pain, or diarrhea. Physical and psychologically based conditions can exist independently or concurrently. Some organic diseases of the GI system, such as peptic ulcer disease and ulcerative colitis, may be aggravated by stress.

Ingestion and Propulsion of Food

Ingestion is the intake of food. The organs involved in the swallowing of food are the mouth, the pharynx, and the esophagus. A person's appetite or desire to ingest food is a significant factor in how much food is eaten. Multiple factors are involved in the control of appetite. An appetite centre is located in the hypothalamus. It is directly or indirectly stimulated by hypoglycemia, an empty stomach, decrease in body temperature, and input from higher brain centres. The hormone *ghrelin*, released from the stomach mucosa, plays a role in appetite stimulation. Another hormone, *leptin,* is involved in appetite suppression (see Chapter 43, Table 43.3). The sight, smell, and taste of food frequently stimulate appetite. Appetite may be inhibited by stomach distension, illness (especially accompanied by fever), hyperglycemia, nausea and vomiting, certain medications (e.g., amphetamines), and psychological factors, such as depression.

Swallowing (deglutition) is the mechanical component of ingestion. The organs involved in the swallowing of food are the mouth, the pharynx, and the esophagus. Swallowed food is moved to the stomach by means of *peristalsis*, the coordinated, sequential contraction and relaxation of outer longitudinal and inner circular layers of muscles.

Mouth. The mouth consists of the lips and the oral (buccal) cavity. The lips surround the orifice of the mouth and function in speech. The roof of the oral cavity is formed by the hard and soft palates. The oral cavity contains the teeth—used in mastication (chewing)—and the tongue. The tongue is a solid muscle mass and assists in chewing by keeping food between the teeth during chewing and moving the food to the back of the throat for swallowing. Taste receptors are found on the sides and the tip of the tongue. The tongue is also important in speech.

Within the oral cavity are three pairs of salivary glands: the parotid, the submaxillary, and the sublingual. These glands produce saliva, which consists of water, protein, mucin, inorganic salts, and salivary amylase. Approximately 1 L of saliva is produced each day. Saliva serves many roles, including the lubrication of food (enhance mastication), prevention of bacterial overgrowth in the oral cavity, and improved digestion.

Pharynx. The pharynx is a muscular-membranous tube that is divided into the nasopharynx, the oropharynx, and the laryngeal pharynx. The mucous membrane of the pharynx is continuous with the nasal cavity, the mouth, the auditory tubes, and the larynx. The oropharynx secretes mucus, which aids in swallowing. The epiglottis is a lid of fibrocartilage that closes over the larynx during swallowing. During ingestion, the oropharynx provides a route for the food from the mouth to the esophagus. When receptors in the oropharynx are stimulated by food or liquid, the swallowing reflex is initiated.

Esophagus. The esophagus is a hollow, muscular tube that receives food from the pharynx and moves it to the stomach by peristaltic contractions. It is 23 to 25 cm long and 2 cm in diameter. The esophagus is located in the thoracic cavity; it starts behind the trachea at the lower end of the pharynx and extends to the stomach. The upper one-third of the esophagus is composed of striated skeletal muscle, and the distal two-thirds are composed of smooth muscle.

With swallowing, the upper esophageal sphincter (cricopharyngeal muscle) relaxes, and a peristaltic wave moves the bolus into the esophagus. Between swallows, the esophagus is collapsed. It is structurally composed of four layers: the inner mucosa, submucosa, muscularis propria, and outermost adventitia. The muscular layers contract (peristalsis) and propel the food to the stomach. The lower esophageal sphincter (LES) at the distal end of the esophagus remains contracted except during swallowing, belching, or vomiting. The LES is an important barrier that prevents reflux of acidic gastric contents into the esophagus.

Digestion and Absorption

Mouth. Digestion involves both a mechanical process (mastication) and a chemical process. The process of digestion begins in the mouth, where the food is chewed, mechanically broken down, and mixed with saliva. Saliva is the first secretion involved, and its main function is to lubricate and soften the food mass, thus facilitating swallowing. Saliva contains amylase (ptyalin), which hydrolyzes starches to maltose. Salivary gland secretion is stimulated by chewing movements and the sight, smell, thought, and taste of food. Food is swallowed and passes into the esophagus, where peristaltic waves propel it to the stomach. No digestion or absorption occurs in the esophagus.

Stomach. The functions of the stomach are to store food, secrete digestive juices, mix the food with gastric secretions, and empty the resulting content (called *chyme*) into the small intestine at a rate at which digestion can occur. The stomach absorbs only small amounts of water, alcohol, electrolytes, and certain medications.

The stomach is usually J-shaped and lies obliquely in the epigastric, umbilical, and left hypochondriac regions of the abdomen (see Figure 41.5 later in this chapter). The shape and position of the stomach change according to the degree of gastric distension. The stomach always contains gastric fluid and mucus. The three main parts of the stomach are the fundus, the body, and the antrum (see Figure 41.1). The pylorus is a small portion of the antrum that lies proximal to the pyloric sphincter. Food passes from the lower esophageal sphincter through the cardiac orifice into the stomach. The chyme is propelled through the pyloric sphincter into the duodenum.

The serous (outer) layer of the stomach is formed by the peritoneum. The muscular layer consists of the longitudinal (outer) layer, the circular (middle) layer, and the oblique (inner) layer. The mucosal layer forms folds called *rugae* that contain many small glands. In response to nutrient intake, these glands secrete most of the gastric juice. In the fundus, the glands contain chief cells, which secrete pepsinogen, and parietal cells, which secrete hydrochloric acid (HCl), water, and intrinsic factor. The secretion of HCl makes gastric juice acidic. This acidic pH aids in the protection against ingested organisms. Intrinsic factor promotes cobalamin (vitamin B_{12}) absorption in the small intestine. Mucus is secreted by glands in the cardiac and pyloric areas.

Small Intestine. The two primary functions of the small intestine are digestion and absorption. The small intestine is a coiled tube approximately 5 to 6 m in length and from 2.5 to 2.8 cm in diameter, narrowing at the lower end. It extends from the pylorus to the ileocecal valve. The small intestine is composed of the duodenum, the jejunum, and the ileum. The ileocecal valve, which separates the small intestine from the large intestine, prevents reflux of large intestine contents into the small intestine.

The serous coat of the small intestine is formed by the peritoneum. The mucosa is thick, vascular, and glandular. Folds in the mucosa slow the passage of food and provide a greater surface area for digestion and absorption.

Physiology of Digestion. Digestion is the physical and chemical breakdown of food into absorbable substances. Digestion in the GI tract is facilitated by the timely movement of food through the various organs and the secretion of specific enzymes. These enzymes break down foodstuffs to particles of appropriate size for absorption (Table 41.1).

In the stomach, the digestion of proteins begins with the release of pepsinogen from chief cells. The acidic environment of the stomach results in the conversion of pepsinogen to its active form, pepsin. Pepsin begins the initial breakdown of proteins. In the stomach, digestion of starches and fats is minimal. The food is mixed with gastric secretions, which are under neural and hormonal control (Tables 41.2 and 41.3). The stomach also serves as a reservoir for food, which is slowly expelled into the small intestine. The length of time that food remains in the stomach depends on the composition of the food, but average meals remain from 3 to 4 hours.

Digestion is completed in the small intestine, where carbohydrates are hydrolyzed to monosaccharides, fats to glycerol and fatty acids, and proteins to amino acids. The presence of *chyme*,

TABLE 41.1 GASTROINTESTINAL SECRETIONS RELATED TO DIGESTION

Daily Amount (mL)	Secretions or Enzymes	Action
Salivary Glands		
1000–1500	Salivary amylase (ptyalin)	Initiation of starch digestion
Stomach		
2500	Pepsinogen	Protein digestion
	HCl	Activation of pepsinogen to pepsin
	Lipase	Fat digestion
	Intrinsic factor	Essential for absorption of cobalamin in the ileum
Small Intestine		
3000	Enterokinase	Activation of trypsinogen to trypsin
	Amylase	Carbohydrate digestion
	Peptidases	Protein digestion
	Aminopeptidase	Protein digestion
	Maltase	Maltose to two glucose molecules
	Sucrase	Sucrose to glucose and fructose
	Lactase	Lactose to glucose and galactose
	Lipase	Fat digestion
Pancreas		
700	Trypsinogen	Protein digestion
	Chymotrypsin	Protein digestion
	Amylase	Starch to disaccharides and trisaccharides
	Lipase	Fat digestion
Liver and Gallbladder		
700–1200	Bile	Emulsification of fats and aid in absorption of fatty acids and fat-soluble vitamins (A, D, E, and K)

HCl, hydrochloric acid.

TABLE 41.2 PHASES OF GASTRIC SECRETION

Phase	Stimulus to Secretion	Secretion
Cephalic (nervous)	Sight, smell, taste of food (before food enters stomach); initiated in the CNS and mediated by the vagus nerve	HCl, pepsinogen, mucus
Gastric (hormonal and nervous)	Food in antrum of stomach, vagal stimulation	Release of gastrin from antrum into circulation to stimulate gastric secretions and motility
Intestinal (hormonal)	Presence of acidic chyme (pH <2) in small intestine stimulates release of secretin, gastric inhibitory polypeptide, and cholecystokinin into circulation to decrease acid secretion	Chyme (pH >3) stimulates release of duodenal gastrin to increase acid secretion

CNS, central nervous system; *HCl*, hydrochloric acid.

Absorption is the transfer of the end products of digestion across the intestinal wall to the circulation. Absorption occurs through the villi, which are functional units present throughout the entire small intestine. The surface area of the small intestine is greatly increased by its circular folds, villi, and microvilli, allowing for the breakdown of nutrients to be absorbed. The movement of the villi enables the end products of digestion to come in contact with the absorbing membrane. They contain goblet cells that secrete mucus and epithelial cells that produce the intestinal digestive enzymes. The villi are surrounded by the crypts of Lieberkühn, which contain the multipotent stem cells for the other epithelial cell types. (Stem cells are discussed in Chapter 16.) Brunner's glands in the submucosa of the duodenum secrete mucus. Monosaccharides (from carbohydrates), fatty acids (from fats), amino acids (from proteins), water, electrolytes, and vitamins are absorbed.

Elimination

Large Intestine. The large intestine is a hollow, muscular tube approximately 1.5 to 2 m long and 5 cm in diameter. The four parts of the large intestine are (1) the cecum and the appendix, a narrow tube at the end of the cecum; (2) the colon (ascending colon on the right side, transverse colon across the abdomen, descending colon on the left side, and the sigmoid colon); (3) the rectum; and (4) the anus, the terminal portion of the large intestine (Figure 41.2).

The most important function of the large intestine is the absorption of water and electrolytes. It also forms feces and serves as a reservoir for the fecal mass until defecation occurs. Feces are composed of water, bacteria, food residue, unabsorbed GI secretions, and desquamated epithelial cells. The large intestine secretes mucus, which acts as a lubricant and protects the mucosa.

Microorganisms in the colon play an important role in metabolism of bile salts, estrogens, androgens, lipids, carbohydrates, various nitrogenous substances, and medications, as well as in protecting against infection. Intestinal bacteria

due to its chemical nature in the small intestine, stimulates motility and secretion. Secretions involved in digestion include enzymes from the pancreas, bile from the liver (see Table 41.1), and intestinal secretions from glands in the small intestine. Both secretion and motility are under neural and hormonal control.

When food enters the stomach and small intestine, hormones are released into the bloodstream (see Table 41.3). The hormone *secretin* stimulates the pancreas to secrete fluid with a high concentration of bicarbonate. This alkaline secretion enters the duodenum and neutralizes acid in the chyme. The duodenal mucosa also secretes mucus to protect against the HCl acid. In response to the presence of chyme, the hormone *cholecystokinin* (CCK), produced by the duodenal mucosa, enters the bloodstream and stimulates contraction of the gallbladder and relaxation of the sphincter of Oddi. These actions enable bile to flow from the common bile duct into the duodenum. Bile is necessary for the digestion of fats. CCK also stimulates the pancreas to synthesize and secrete enzymes for enzymatic digestion of carbohydrates, fats, and proteins.

Enzymes on the brush border of the microvilli complete the digestion process. These enzymes hydrolyze disaccharides to monosaccharides and peptides to amino acids for absorption.

TABLE 41.3	MAJOR HORMONES CONTROLLING GASTROINTESTINAL SECRETION AND MOTILITY		
Hormone	Source	Activating Stimuli	Function
Gastrin	Gastric and duodenal mucosa	Stomach distension, partially digested proteins in pylorus	Stimulates gastric acid secretion and motility; maintains lower esophageal sphincter tone
Secretin	Duodenal mucosa	Acid entering small intestine	Inhibits gastric motility and acid secretion; stimulates pancreatic bicarbonate secretion
Cholecystokinin	Duodenal mucosa	Fatty acids and amino acids in small intestine	Causes contraction of gallbladder and relaxation of sphincter of Oddi, allowing increased flow of bile into duodenum; stimulates release of pancreatic digestive enzymes
Gastric inhibitory peptide	Duodenal mucosa	Fatty acids and lipids in small intestine	Inhibits gastric acid secretion and gastric motility

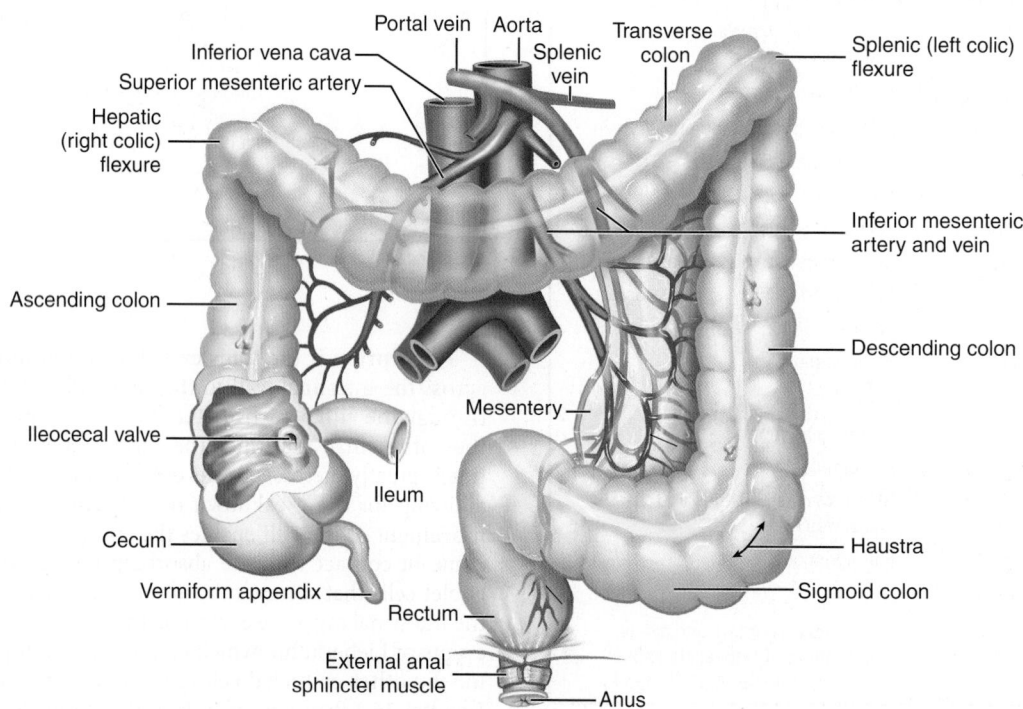

FIG. 41.2 Anatomical locations of the large intestine. Source: Patton, K. T., & Thibodeau, G. A. (2019). *Anatomy and physiology* (10th ed.). Mosby.

are responsible for the breakdown of proteins not digested or absorbed in the small intestine. These amino acids are deaminated by the bacteria, leaving ammonia, which is carried to the liver and converted to urea. Bacteria in the colon also synthesize vitamin K and some of the B vitamins. In addition, bacteria play a part in the production of flatus.

The movements of the large intestine are usually slow. When the circular muscles contract, they produce a kneading action termed *haustral churning*. Propulsive mass movement (peristalsis) also occurs. When food enters the stomach and the duodenum, the gastrocolic and duodenocolic reflexes are initiated, resulting in peristalsis in the colon. These reflexes are more active after the first daily meal and frequently result in bowel evacuation.

Defecation, the discharge of feces from the rectum, is a reflex action involving voluntary and involuntary control. Feces in the rectum stimulate sensory nerve endings that produce the urge to defecate. The reflex centre for defecation is in the sacral portion of the spinal cord (parasympathetic nerve fibres). These fibres produce contraction of the rectum and relaxation of the internal anal sphincter. Defecation is controlled voluntarily by relaxing the external anal sphincter when the urge to defecate is felt. An acceptable environment for defecation is usually necessary; otherwise the urge to defecate is suppressed. If defecation is suppressed over long periods, elimination difficulties can occur, such as constipation or stool impaction.

Defecation can be facilitated by appropriate positioning (sitting or squatting) or by the Valsalva manoeuvre. This manoeuvre involves contraction of the chest muscles on a closed glottis with simultaneous contraction of the abdominal muscles. These actions result in increased intra-abdominal pressure. The Valsalva manoeuvre may be contraindicated in patients with head injury, cardiac conditions, hemorrhoids, or liver cirrhosis with portal hypertension and in persons who have undergone recent eye or abdominal surgery.

Liver, Biliary Tract, and Pancreas

Liver. The liver is the largest internal organ in the body, weighing approximately 1 200 to 1 600 g in adults. It lies in the right hypochondriac and epigastric regions (see Figure 41.5) and is divided into right and left lobes (Figure 41.3). Glisson's capsule, which contains blood vessels, lymphatic vessels, and

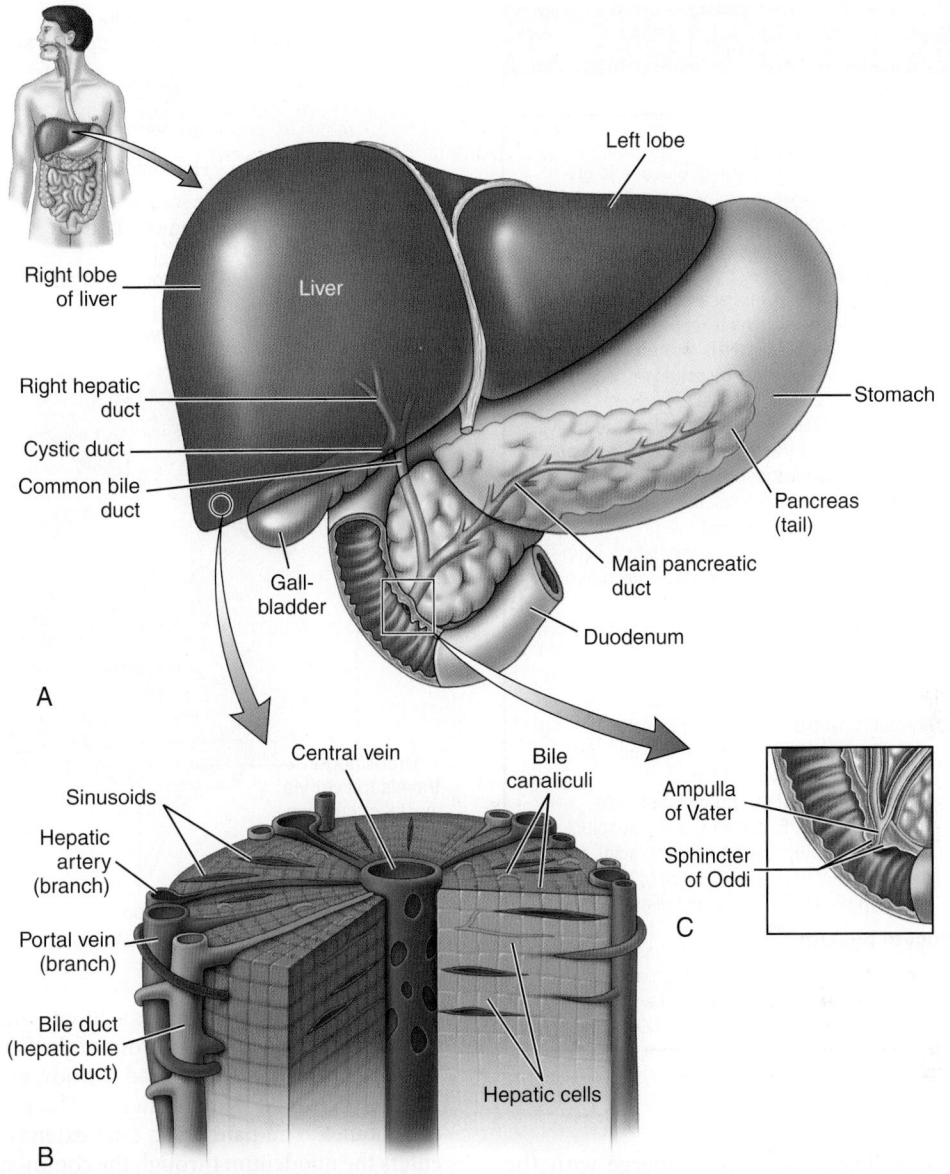

FIG. 41.3 A, Gross structure of the liver, gallbladder, pancreas, and duct system. **B,** Liver lobule. **C,** Entrance of the common bile duct into the duodenum.

nerves, covers the liver. Liver disease or swelling may cause this capsule to become distended, leading to pain and oozing of lymphatic fluid into the peritoneal space.

The functional units of the liver are lobules. The lobule consists of plates of specialized hepatic cells (**hepatocytes**) arranged around a central vein. The capillaries (sinusoids) are located between the plates of hepatocytes and are lined with **Kupffer cells**, which carry out phagocytic activity (removal of bacteria and toxins from the blood). Kupffer cells also ingest aged red blood cells, breaking down hemoglobin into heme and globin. The heme is further broken down into iron and bilirubin, which is secreted into the bile. Interlobular bile ducts form from bile capillaries *(canaliculi).* The hepatic cells secrete bile into the canaliculi.

The nerve supply to the liver is from the left vagus and the sympathetic celiac plexus. The liver receives both arterial and venous blood. About one-third of the blood supply comes from the hepatic artery (branch of the celiac artery), and two-thirds comes from the portal vein.

A large amount of blood is required for the liver to fulfill its metabolic functions. The portal (enterohepatic) circulatory system brings blood to the liver from the stomach, intestines, spleen, and pancreas. This blood enters the liver through the portal vein. The portal vein carries absorbed products of digestion directly to the liver. In the liver, the portal vein branches and comes into contact with each lobule. The blood in the sinusoids is a mixture of arterial and venous blood.

The liver functions in the manufacture, storage, transformation, and excretion of a number of substances involved in metabolism. The functions of the liver are numerous but can be classified into three main areas, as identified in Table 41.4.

Biliary Tract. The biliary tract consists of the gallbladder and the duct system. The gallbladder is a pear-shaped sac located below the liver. The function of the gallbladder is to concentrate and store bile. It can hold approximately 45 mL of bile.

Bile is produced by the hepatic cells and secreted into the biliary canaliculi of the lobules. Bile then drains into the interlobular bile ducts, which unite into the two main left

<table>
<tr><td colspan="2">**TABLE 41.4** **MAJOR FUNCTIONS OF THE LIVER**</td></tr>
</table>

Function	Description
Metabolic Functions	
Carbohydrate metabolism	Glycogenesis (conversion of glucose to glycogen), glycogenolysis (process of breaking down glycogen to glucose), gluconeogenesis (formation of glucose from amino acids and fatty acids)
Protein metabolism	Synthesis of nonessential amino acids, synthesis of plasma proteins (except γ-globulin), urea formation from NH_3 (NH_3 formed from deamination of amino acids by action of bacteria on proteins in colon)
Fat metabolism	Synthesis of lipoproteins, breakdown of triglycerides into fatty acids and glycerol, formation of ketone bodies, synthesis of fatty acids from amino acids and glucose, synthesis and breakdown of cholesterol
Detoxification	Inactivation of medications and harmful substances and excretion of their breakdown products
Steroid metabolism	Conjugation and excretion of gonadal and adrenal steroid hormones
Bile Synthesis	
Bile production	Formation of bile, containing bile salts, bile pigments (mainly bilirubin), and cholesterol
Bile excretion	Bile excretion by liver ($\cong$1 L/day)
Storage	Glucose in form of glycogen; fat-soluble vitamins (A, D, E, and K) and water-soluble vitamins (B_1, B_2, cobalamin, folic acid); fatty acids; minerals (iron and copper); amino acids in form of albumin and β-globulins
Mononuclear Phagocyte System	
Kupffer cells	Breakdown of old RBCs, WBCs, bacteria, and other particles; breakdown of hemoglobin from old RBCs to bilirubin and biliverdin

NH₃, ammonia; *RBC,* red blood cell; *WBC,* white blood cell.

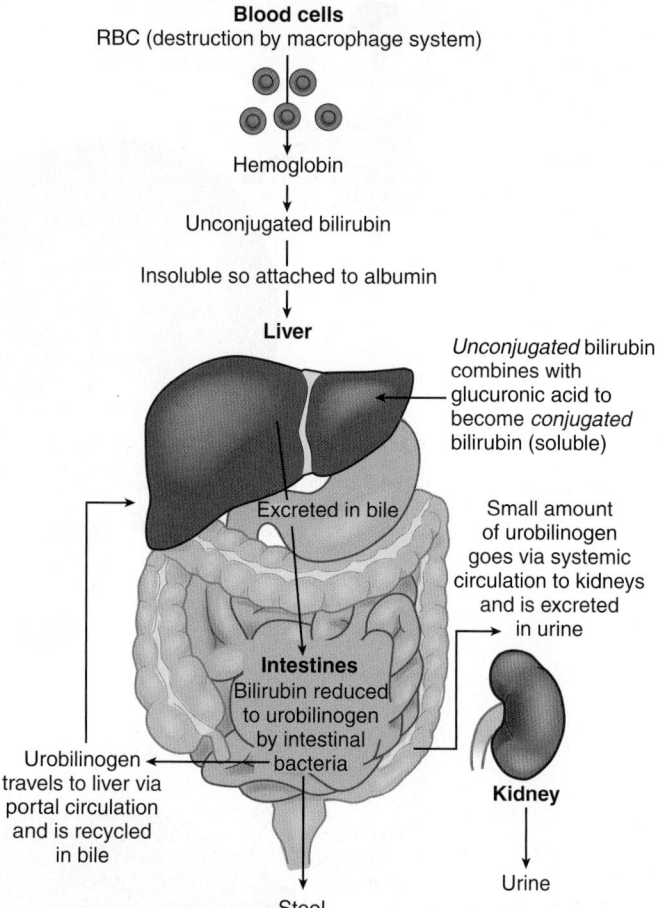

FIG. 41.4 Bilirubin metabolism and conjugation. *RBC,* red blood cell.

and right hepatic ducts. The hepatic ducts merge with the cystic duct from the gallbladder to form the common bile duct (see Figure 41.3). Most bile is stored and concentrated in the gallbladder. It is then released into the cystic duct and moves down the common bile duct to enter the duodenum at the ampulla of Vater. In the intestines, most of the bilirubin is reduced to stercobilinogen and urobilinogen by bacterial action. Stercobilinogen accounts for the brown colour of stool. A small amount of conjugated bilirubin is reabsorbed by the blood. Some urobilinogen is reabsorbed by the blood and returned to the liver through the portal circulation and excreted in the bile. An insignificant amount of urobilinogen is excreted in the urine.

Bilirubin Metabolism. Bilirubin, a pigment derived from the breakdown of aged red blood cells, is produced constantly (Figure 41.4). There are two forms of bilirubin. The unconjugated bilirubin is insoluble in water; it is bound to albumin for its transport to the liver. The conjugated bilirubin is the form that is conjugated with glucuronic acid in the liver. Conjugated bilirubin is water soluble and is excreted in bile. Bile also consists of water, cholesterol, bile salts, electrolytes, and phospholipids. Bile salts are needed for fat emulsification and digestion.

Pancreas. The pancreas is a 20-cm long, slender gland lying behind the stomach and in front of the first and second lumbar vertebrae. It consists of a head, a body, and a tail. The anterior surface is covered by peritoneum. The pancreas contains lobes and lobules. The pancreatic duct extends along the gland and enters the duodenum through the common bile duct (see Figure 41.3). The pancreas has both exocrine and endocrine functions. The exocrine function of the pancreas contributes to the process of digestion. Exocrine cells in the pancreas secrete pancreatic enzymes (see Table 41.1). The endocrine function occurs in the islets of Langerhans, whose β cells secrete insulin; α cells secrete glucagon; δ cells secrete somatostatin; and F cells secrete pancreatic polypeptide.

AGE-RELATED CONSIDERATIONS

EFFECTS OF AGING ON THE GASTROINTESTINAL SYSTEM

The process of aging causes changes in the functional ability of the GI system, although to a lesser extent than in other organ systems. Older persons, especially those older than 85, are at risk for decreased food intake as a result of financial, environmental, and social circumstances (Miller, 2018). Financial constraints can affect both the quality and quantity of food available. Gait speed and tolerance to food are elements to consider in the older person. Physiological age-related changes in the GI system and differences in assessment findings are presented in Table 41.5.

The tooth enamel and dentin wear down, making the teeth susceptible to caries. Periodontal disease can lead to the loss

TABLE 41.5 AGE-RELATED DIFFERENCES IN ASSESSMENT

Gastrointestinal System

Potential Changes	Differences in Assessment Findings
Mouth	
Periodontal disease	Red, swollen, bleeding gums; painful chewing; loose or sensitive teeth, abnormal shape and position of teeth; discoloration, or inflammation of the gingivae
Loss of teeth	Presence of dentures, difficulty chewing
Decreased sensitivity of taste buds, decreased sense of smell	Diminished sense of taste (especially saltiness and sweetness)
Decreased volume of saliva	Dry oral mucosa
Atrophy of gingival tissue	Poorly fitting dentures
Esophagus	
Decreased tone and motility	Reports of pyrosis (heartburn), dysphagia, eructation (belching); potential for hiatal hernia and aspiration
Stomach	
Atrophy of gastric mucosa, decreased blood flow	Food intolerances; signs of anemia as result of cobalamin malabsorption; slower gastric emptying
Small Intestine	
Slightly decreased secretion of most digestive enzymes, decreased motility	Reports of indigestion; slowed intestinal transit; delayed absorption of fat-soluble vitamins
Liver, Gallbladder, Pancreas	
Decreased size and lowered position	Easier palpation because lower border extends past costal margin
Decreased protein synthesis, decreased ability to regenerate cells	Decreased medication and hormone metabolism
Distension of pancreatic ducts, decreased lipase production, impairment of pancreatic reserve	Impaired fat absorption, decreased glucose tolerance
Large Intestine, Anus, Rectum	
Decreased anal sphincter tone and nerve supply to rectal area	Increased possibility of fecal incontinence
Decreased muscular tone, decreased motility	Flatulence, abdominal distension, relaxed perineal musculature
Increased transit time, decreased sensation to defecation	Constipation, fecal impaction

of teeth. Xerostomia (decreased saliva production), or "dry mouth," affects many older persons and may be associated with difficulty swallowing (dysphagia). Dysphagia is characterized by abnormal passage of food from the mouth to the stomach. It may involve oral, pharyngeal, or esophageal processes of swallowing. Dysphagia is more common in older persons because of inadequate chewing or insufficient lubrication. The number of taste buds decreases, the sense of smell diminishes, and salivary secretions lessen, all of which can lead to a decrease in appetite and make eating less pleasurable.

Age-related changes in the esophagus include delayed emptying caused by smooth muscle weakness and an incompetent lower esophageal sphincter (Miller, 2018). Motility of the

GI system decreases with age, but secretion and absorption are affected to a lesser extent. Many older people experience a decrease in HCl secretion (hypochlorhydria), delayed gastric emptying, and constipation. With chronic atrophic gastritis, the number of parietal cells decreases, and the amount of acid and intrinsic factor secreted is subsequently reduced. Intestinal absorption, motility, and blood flow decrease, thus hampering nutrient absorption.

Liver mass decreases after the age of 40 years, but results of liver function tests remain within normal ranges. Age-related enzyme changes in the liver decrease the liver's ability to metabolize medications and hormones. Blood flow to the liver decreases, which affects the efficiency of medication metabolism. The size of the pancreas is unaffected by aging, but it does undergo structural changes such as fibrosis, fatty acid deposits, and atrophy. Secretion of digestive enzymes decreases. Aging does not cause changes in the structure and function of the gallbladder and bile ducts, although the incidence of gallstones increases (Heuman, 2019).

Rectal muscle mass is reduced, and the anal sphincter weakens. Changes in the enteric nervous system, reduction in dietary fibre, and polypharmacy, along with reduced fluid intake and decreased physical activity, all contribute to constipation in older people.

ASSESSMENT OF THE GASTROINTESTINAL SYSTEM

Subjective Data

Important Health Information

Past Health History. Patients should be asked about changes in weight. Any unexplained weight loss or weight gain within the past 12 months should be explored. A history of chronic dieting and repeated weight loss and gain should also be documented. Usual patterns of elimination should be noted. Nutritional habits should be assessed per *Canada's Food Guide* (Health Canada, 2019). Recent travel should also be noted in relation to hepatitis exposure or parasitic infestation. Frequency of alcohol consumption and drugs use (e.g. tobacco, cannabis) should be assessed. Other functional health patterns, such as exercising and sleeping quality; acceptance of self; stress mechanisms; and cultural and religious beliefs should be assessed.

Detailed information should be gathered about the history or existence of the following conditions related to GI functioning: abdominal pain, nausea and vomiting, diarrhea, constipation, abdominal distension, jaundice, anemia, heartburn, dyspepsia, changes in appetite, hematemesis, food intolerance (including lactose) or allergies, dysphagia, indigestion, excessive gas, bloating, melena, hemorrhoids, and rectal bleeding. In addition, patients should be asked about the frequency of bowel movements, use of laxatives and antacids, and history or existence of diseases such as gastritis, hepatitis, colitis, gallbladder disease, peptic ulcer, or cancer; of hernias (especially hiatal hernias); or of infection with *Clostridium difficile*. (*C. difficile* is discussed in Chapter 45.)

Medications. The health history should include an assessment of the patient's past and current use of medications. This is a critical aspect of history taking because many medications may not only have an effect on the GI system but also be affected by abnormalities of the GI system and surrounding organs. The medication assessment should include information about the use of over-the-counter (OTC) medications, prescription medications, herbal products, nutritional supplements, and traditional medicines (see Chapter 12). Indigenous people may not disclose the use of traditional medicine for fear of judgement; hence it is important to build trust and practise culturally safe care to enhance the assessment findings. Many chemicals and drugs are potentially hepatotoxic (Table 41.6) and can result in significant harm to the patient unless their use is monitored closely. For example, chronic high doses of acetaminophen may be hepatotoxic. Nonsteroidal anti-inflammatory drugs (NSAIDs) (including acetylsalicylic acid [ASA; Aspirin]) may predispose patients to upper GI bleeding if not taken with caution with food or if a patient has severe liver disease. Antibiotics can cause changes in the normal bacterial composition in the GI tract that result in diarrhea. The nurse should ask patients about laxative or antacid use, including the type and the frequency.

Surgery or Other Treatments. Information should be obtained about hospitalizations for any conditions related to the GI system, particularly any abdominal or rectal surgery, including the year, the reason for surgery, the postoperative course, and any blood transfusions. Terms related to surgery of the GI system are listed in Table 41.7.

CASE STUDY

Patient Introduction

L. C. (pronouns he/him), 58 years old, is from Drury, Ontario. L.C.'s partner and family drove 50 kilometers to arrive at the hospital because of his deteriorating health. Arriving at the emergency department (ED), L.C. is doubled over in pain, grimacing and holding his abdomen with both arms, and presents to the triage nurse.

Critical Thinking

Throughout this assessment chapter, think about L. C. with the following questions in mind:
1. What are the possible causes for L. C.'s acute abdominal pain?
2. What would be the nurse's priority assessment?
3. What questions should the nurse ask L. C.?
4. What should be included in the physical assessment? What should the nurse be looking for?
5. What diagnostic studies might be ordered?

evolve
Answers are available at http://evolve.elsevier.com/Canada/Lewis/medsurg.

TABLE 41.6	POTENTIALLY HEPATOTOXIC MEDICATIONS AND CHEMICALS	
Dosage-Related	**Idiosyncratic/Rare**
Hepatotoxic Medications and Chemicals	
• Acetaminophen (Tylenol) • Isoniazid • Methotrexate	• Amiodarone • Alcohol • Amoxicillin-clavulanic acid (Clavulin 400) • Carbamazepine • Ketoconazole • Nonsteroidal anti-inflammatory drugs (NSAIDs) • Ramipril (Altace)
Hepatotoxic Medication Classes	
	• NSAIDs • Statins • Sulphonamides (sulpha) • Thiazolidinediones (glitazones)

Objective Data

In addition to collecting subjective data related to the patient's diet history and overall health (Table 41.8), objective data related to a nutritional assessment should be obtained. Examples of objective data include anthropometric measurements (height, weight, skinfold thickness), results of blood studies such as serum protein, albumin, and hemoglobin levels, as well as a physical examination.

Physical Examination. The physical examination should be performed in a well-lit room. The nurse needs to obtain consent prior to beginning the exam, as unwanted touching may trigger historical trauma—for example, abusive experiences among Indigenous people that attended residential schools.

TABLE 41.7	SURGICAL PROCEDURES INVOLVING THE GASTROINTESTINAL SYSTEM	
Surgical Procedure	**Description**
Antrectomy	Removal of antrum portion of stomach
Appendectomy	Removal of appendix
Cecostomy	Opening into cecum
Cholecystectomy	Removal of gallbladder
Cholecystostomy	Opening into gallbladder
Choledochojejunostomy	Opening between common bile duct and jejunum
Choledocholithotomy	Opening into common bile duct for removal of stones
Colectomy	Removal of colon
Colostomy	Opening into colon
Gastrectomy	Removal of stomach
Gastrostomy	Opening into stomach
Glossectomy	Removal of tongue
Hemiglossectomy	Removal of half of tongue
Ileostomy	Opening into ileum
Pyloroplasty	Enlargement and repair of pyloric sphincter area
Vagotomy	Resection of branch of vagus nerve

CASE STUDY

Subjective Data

A focused subjective assessment of L. C. reveals the following information:
- **History of current illness:** L. C. presents with intense abdominal pain without radiation. States he has had no appetite for the past several weeks, feels weak, and is easily fatigued. Denies exposure to chemicals. No recent travel outside of Canada. Rates pain as a 9 on a scale of 0–10. States pain comes and goes in waves. Prefers to lie still with his knees flexed and drawn into his abdomen. States he has had alternating episodes of constipation and diarrhea. Has noticed some bright red blood in stools. Has not had a bowel movement for 4 days.
- **Past medical history:** Negative history for medical or surgical conditions
- **Medications:** None
- **Functional assessment:** L. C. is 175 cm tall and weighs 64 kg (BMI: 20.9 kg/m²). States he has been losing weight over the past several months and does not have an appetite. No food allergies. Smokes approximately 1 pack of cigarettes/day for 20 yr. Drinks beer daily, typically three or four bottles per day.

See Case Study: Objective Data: Physical Examination and Case Study: Objective Data: Diagnostic Studies for more information on L. C.

Mouth

Inspection. The lips should be inspected for symmetry, colour, and size and for abnormalities such as pallor or cyanosis, cracking, ulcers, or fissures. The dorsum (top) of the tongue should have a thin white coating; the undersurface should be smooth. The nurse should observe for any lesions. Using a tongue blade, the nurse should inspect the buccal mucosa and note the colour, any areas of pigmentation, and any lesions. Dark-skinned individuals normally have patchy areas of pigmentation. When assessing the teeth and gums, the nurse should look for caries and signs of periodontal disease (see Table 41.5). Any distinctive breath odour should be noted.

The pharynx is inspected by tilting the patient's head back and depressing the tongue with a tongue blade. The tonsils, the uvula, the soft palate, and the anterior and posterior pillars should be observed. The uvula and the soft palate should rise and remain in the midline when the patient says "Ah."

Palpation. The nurse should palpate any suspect areas in the mouth such as ulcers, nodules, indurations, and areas of tenderness (see also Chapter 44 for information related to oral cancer). In older persons, particular attention should be given to the condition of the gums and the tongue, the fit and the condition of dentures (if present), the ability to swallow, and the presence of lesions. Dentures should be removed to allow for adequate visualization and palpation of the area.

Abdomen

Two anatomical systems are used to describe the surface of the abdomen. In one system, the abdomen is divided into four quadrants by a vertical line from the sternum to the pubic bone and by a perpendicular line across the abdomen at the umbilicus (Figure 41.5, A; Table 41.9). In the other system, the abdomen is divided into nine regions (see Figure 41.5, B), but only the epigastric, umbilical, and suprapubic or hypogastric regions are commonly addressed.

The patient should be in the supine position and as relaxed as possible. To help relax the abdominal muscles, the patient should slightly flex the knees, and the head of the bed should be raised slightly. The patient should have an empty bladder. The nurse's hands should be warm when the abdominal examination is performed, to avoid eliciting muscle guarding. The patient should be instructed to breathe slowly through the mouth.

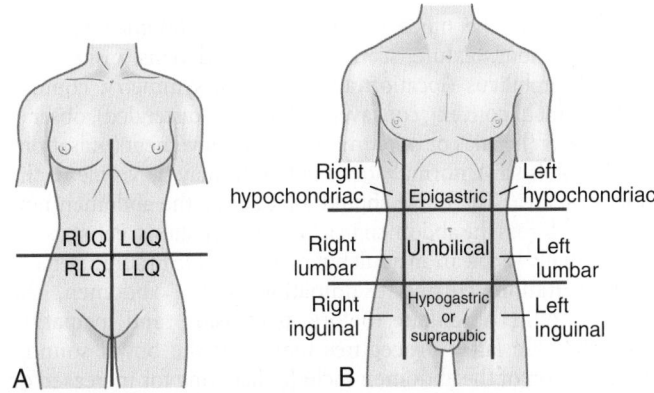

FIG. 41.5 A, Abdominal quadrants. **B,** Abdominal regions. *LLQ,* left lower quadrant; *LUQ,* left upper quadrant; *RLQ,* right lower quadrant; *RUQ,* right upper quadrant.

TABLE 41.8 HEALTH HISTORY

Gastrointestinal System: Questions for Obtaining Subjective Data

Appetite
- Any change in appetite?* Are you more or less hungry?
- Any change in weight?* Do your clothes still fit the same as they used to? How much weight have you gained or lost? Over what time frame? Is the change in weight intentional?

Dysphagia
- Any difficulties swallowing?* How long have you had this problem?

Food Intolerance or Allergies
- Are there any foods you cannot eat?* What happens when you do eat them (e.g., heartburn, gas, bloating, indigestion, allergic reaction)?

Abdominal Pain
- Do you have any abdominal pain?*
- Is the pain in one spot, or does it move around?
- How long have you had this pain?
- Does it come and go, or is it constant? Does it get worse before or after meals? When is the pain worst (e.g., position, stress, activity)?
- Can you describe how it feels (e.g., cramping, burning, stabbing, aching)?
- What brings on the pain (e.g., menstruation, stress, overeating, fatigue)?
- Do any other symptoms occur when you have the pain (e.g., nausea and vomiting, gas, rectal bleeding, frequent urination, vaginal or penile discharge)?*
- What works to relieve the pain (e.g., rest, heat, walking, change of position, medication)?

Nausea and Vomiting
- Any nausea or vomiting?* How much comes up?
- What colour is it? Is it bloody? Is there a particular odour?
- Do you have pain, diarrhea, fever, or chills at the same time as the nausea and vomiting?
- Does anyone else you have been in contact with over the past 24 hours have the same symptoms? Have you eaten any foods in the past 24 hours that you suspect may be the cause?

Bowel Habits
- How often do you have a bowel movement?
- Any recent changes in colour, consistency, or frequency?
- Any problems with diarrhea or constipation?
- Do you use laxatives or stool softeners? Which ones? How often?

Past History
- Any past difficulties with your digestive system (e.g., ulcer, gallbladder issues, hepatitis, appendicitis, colitis, hernia)?*
- Any surgical procedures on your abdomen?*
- Do you know the results of any tests that were done relating to your abdomen?*

Medications
- What medications are you currently taking?
- How much alcohol do you drink each day? When was your last alcoholic drink?
- Do you smoke? How many packs a day?

Nutrition Assessment
- Describe your usual daily food and fluid intake.

*If yes, describe.
Source: Based on Jarvis, C., Browne, A. J., MacDonald-Jenkins, J., et al. (Eds.). (2019). *Physical examination and health assessment* (3rd Canadian ed.). Elsevier Inc.

TABLE 41.9 ABDOMINAL STRUCTURES IN REGIONS OF ABDOMEN

Right Upper Quadrant	Left Upper Quadrant	Right Lower Quadrant	Left Lower Quadrant
• Liver and gallbladder • Pylorus • Duodenum • Head of pancreas • Right adrenal gland • Portion of right kidney • Hepatic flexure of colon • Portion of ascending and transverse colon	• Left lobe of liver • Spleen • Stomach • Body of pancreas • Left adrenal gland • Portion of left kidney • Splenic flexure of colon • Portion of transverse and descending colon	• Lower pole of right kidney • Cecum and appendix • Portion of ascending colon • Bladder (can be palpated only if distended) • Right ovary and salpinx • Uterus (can be palpated only if enlarged) • Right spermatic cord • Right ureter	• Lower pole of left kidney • Sigmoid flexure • Portion of descending colon • Bladder (can be palpated only if distended) • Left ovary and salpinx • Uterus (can be palpated only if enlarged) • Left spermatic cord • Left ureter

Inspection. The nurse should assess the abdomen for skin changes (colour, texture, scars, striae, dilated veins, rashes, and lesions), umbilicus (location and contour), symmetry, contour (flat, rounded [convex], concave, protuberant, distended), observable masses (hernias or other masses), and movement (pulsations and peristalsis). A normal aortic pulsation may be visible in the epigastric area. The nurse should look across the abdomen tangentially (across the abdomen in a line) for peristalsis. Peristalsis is not normally visible in an adult but may be visible in a thin person.

Auscultation. During examination of the abdomen, the nurse should auscultate before percussion and palpation because these latter procedures may alter the bowel sounds. Auscultation of the abdomen includes listening for increased or decreased bowel sounds and vascular sounds. The diaphragm of the stethoscope is used to auscultate bowel sounds because they are relatively high pitched. The bell of the stethoscope is used to detect lower-pitched sounds. Normal bowel sounds occur 5 to 35 times per minute and sound like high-pitched clicks or gurgles. Warming the stethoscope in the hands before auscultation helps prevent abdominal muscle contraction. The nurse should listen in the epigastrium and in all four quadrants (starting in the lower right quadrant going counterclockwise) for bowel sounds for 2 to 5 minutes. A perfectly "silent abdomen" is uncommon (Jarvis et al., 2019). The nurse normally listens for 1 minute in each location (quadrant and epigastrium). Most times, the nurse will find that the sounds are not absent but hypoactive or intermittent. The nurse notes the findings and precisely records the amount of time listened for each region.

The frequency and intensity of bowel sounds vary, depending on the phase of digestion. Normally, they sound relatively high pitched and gurgling. Loud gurgles indicate hyperperistalsis and are termed *borborygmi* (stomach growling). The bowel sounds are higher pitched (rushes and tinkling) when the intestines are under tension, such as in intestinal obstruction. The nurse should listen for decreased or absent bowel sounds. Terms used to describe bowel sounds include *present, absent, increased, decreased, high pitched, tinkling, gurgling,* and *rushing.* Normally, no aortic bruits should be heard. A bruit, best heard with the bell of the stethoscope, is a swishing or buzzing sound and indicates turbulent blood flow. Aortic bruit can be the consequence of an abdominal aortic aneurysm, mass, or major artery stenosis.

Percussion. The purpose of percussion of the abdomen is to determine the presence of fluid, distension, and masses. Sound waves vary according to the density of underlying tissues. The presence of air produces a higher-pitched, hollow sound, termed *tympany,* and the presence of fluid or masses produces a short, high-pitched sound with little resonance, termed *dullness.* The nurse should lightly percuss all four quadrants of the abdomen and assess the distribution of tympany and dullness. Tympany is the predominant percussion sound of the abdomen.

Dullness in the dependent parts of the abdomen may reflect ascites (see Table 41.11 later in the chapter). Percussion for *shifting dullness* is a test used to assess for ascites. With the person in the supine position, the nurse percusses from the top of the abdomen down the sides of the abdomen and marks the border between tympany and dullness. Then the person is turned onto their side and the nurse percusses from the upper side of the abdomen downward. The sound changes from tympany to dullness as the fluid level is reached (Jarvis et al., 2019).

To percuss the liver, the nurse should start below the umbilicus in the right midclavicular line and percuss lightly upward until dullness is heard, thus determining the lower border of liver dullness. After determining the lower border of the liver, the nurse should start at the nipple line in the right midclavicular line and percuss downward between ribs to the area of dullness, which indicates the upper border of the liver. The height or vertical space between the two areas should be measured to determine the size of the liver. The normal range of liver span is 6 to 12 cm, in correlation to the height of the person. A liver span greater than 12 cm may indicate liver enlargement.

Palpation. The nurse may perform light palpation. *Light palpation* is used to detect tenderness or cutaneous hypersensitivity, muscular resistance, masses, and swelling. It also helps patients to relax for deeper palpation. The nurse should keep fingers together and press gently with the pads of the fingertips, depressing the abdominal wall about 1 cm. Smooth movements should be used and all quadrants palpated (Figure 41.6, A). *Voluntary guarding* occurs when the person is ticklish, cold, or tense, and it occurs bilaterally. The nurse should help the person to relax because guarding interferes with deep palpation. *Deep palpation* is an advanced practice nursing skill and is used to delineate abdominal organs and masses (see Figure 41.6, B). The palmar surfaces of the fingers should be used to press more deeply. Again, all quadrants should be palpated. When palpating masses, the location, the size, the shape, and the presence of tenderness should be noted. The patient's facial expression should be observed during these manoeuvres because it will provide nonverbal cues of discomfort or pain.

An alternative method for deep abdominal palpation is the two-hand method (Figure 41.7, B). One hand is placed on top of the other. The fingers of the top hand apply pressure to the bottom hand. The fingers of the bottom hand feel for organs and masses. This method may be more effective with an obese abdomen.

The nurse can check any areas of concern for rebound tenderness by pressing in slowly and firmly over the painful site. The palpating fingers are withdrawn quickly. Pain on withdrawal of the fingers indicates peritoneal inflammation. Rebound tenderness may produce pain and severe muscle spasm; therefore, it should be performed at the end of the examination and only by an experienced practitioner. To palpate the liver, the nurse's left hand

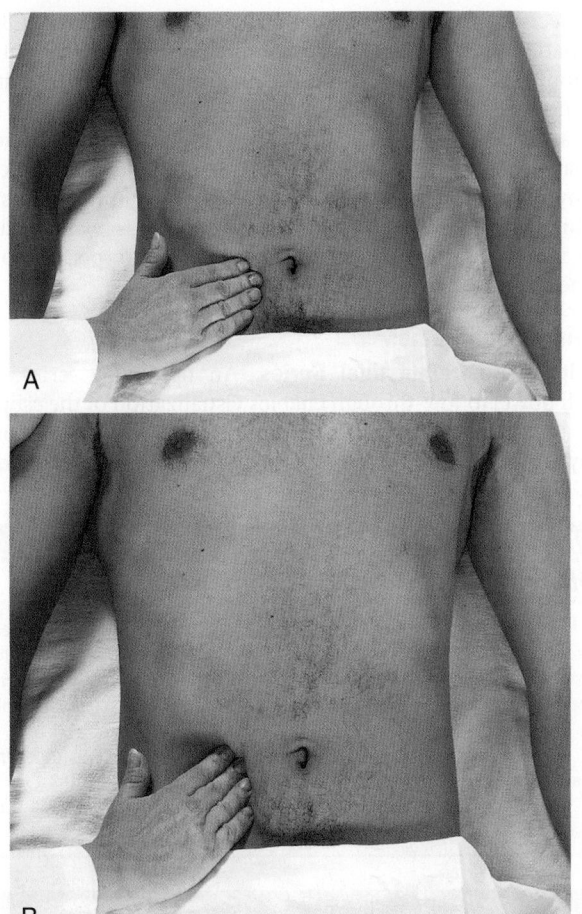

FIG. 41.6 Palpation of the abdomen. **A**, Technique for light palpation. **B**, Technique for deep palpation. Source: Jarvis, C., Browne, A. J., MacDonald-Jenkins, J., et al. (Eds.) (2019). *Physical examination and health assessment* (3rd Canadian ed., pp. 582 and 589). Elsevier Inc.

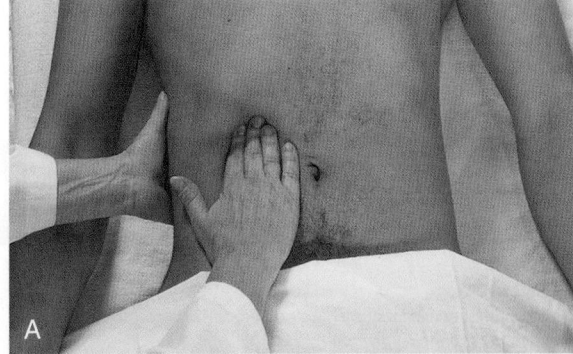

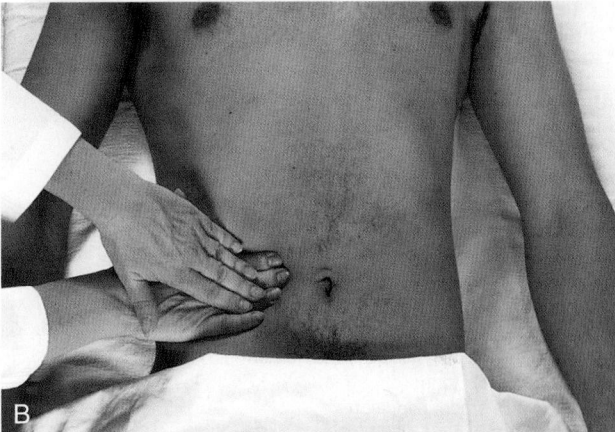

FIG. 41.7 Liver palpation. **A**, Technique with one hand under the patient. **B**, Alternative technique to palpate liver with fingers hooked over the costal region. Source: Jarvis, C., Browne, A. J., MacDonald-Jenkins, J., et al. (Eds.). (2019). *Physical examination and health assessment* (3rd Canadian ed., pp. 582 and 589). Elsevier Inc.

is placed beneath the supine patient to support the right eleventh and twelfth ribs (see Figure 41.7, *A*). The patient may relax on the nurse's hand. The nurse presses the left hand forward and places the right hand on the patient's right abdomen, lateral to the rectus muscle. The fingertips should be below the lower border of liver dullness and pointed toward the right costal margin. The nurse gently presses in and up. The patient should take a deep breath with the abdomen so that the liver drops and is in a better position to be palpated. The nurse should try to feel the liver edge as it comes down to the fingertips. During inspiration, the liver edge should feel firm, sharp, and smooth. The nurse then documents the description of the surface, contour, and any tenderness.

To palpate the spleen, the nurse moves to the left side of the patient. The nurse places the right hand under the patient and supports and presses the patient's left lower rib cage forward. The left hand is placed below the left costal margin and presses it in toward the spleen. The nurse should ask the patient to breathe deeply. The nurse's fingertips can feel the tip or edge of an enlarged spleen. The spleen is not normally palpable. If it is palpable, the nurse should not continue because manual compression of an enlarged spleen may cause it to rupture.

Rectum and Anus. The nurse should inspect the perianal and anal areas for colour, texture, lumps, rashes, scars, erythema, fissures, and external hemorrhoids. Any lumps or unusual areas should be palpated with a gloved hand.

For the digital examination of the rectum, the gloved, lubricated index finger is placed against the anus while the patient strains (Valsalva manoeuvre). Then, as the sphincter relaxes, the nurse inserts the gloved, lubricated finger. The finger is pointed toward the umbilicus. The nurse should try to get the patient to relax. The finger is inserted into the rectum as far as possible, and all surfaces are palpated. Nodules, tenderness, or any irregularities should be assessed. A sample of stool can be removed with the gloved finger and checked for occult blood. However, a single guaiac-based fecal occult blood test has limited sensitivity in detecting colorectal cancer.

Documentation of a normal physical assessment of the GI system is described in Table 41.10. Age-related differences in the GI system and differences in assessment findings are described in Table 41.5. Assessment abnormalities are listed in Table 41.11. A focused assessment is used to evaluate the status of previously identified GI disorders and to monitor for signs of new conditions (see Table 3.5). A focused assessment of the GI system is presented in the Focused Assessment box.

DIAGNOSTIC STUDIES OF THE GASTROINTESTINAL SYSTEM

Diagnostic studies provide objective data for monitoring the patient's condition and planning appropriate interventions. Table 41.12 lists common diagnostic studies of the GI system. A consent form is required for most diagnostic studies. The health care provider providing the procedure is responsible for the patient's consent and related explanations. However, nurses play an important role in educating patients about the procedures.

When preparing patients, the nurse must ask about any known allergies to medications or contrast media.

Many of the diagnostic procedures of the GI system necessitate measures to cleanse the GI tract, as well as the ingestion or injection of a contrast medium or a radiopaque tracer. Often, the patient undergoes a series of GI diagnostic tests. The patient is monitored closely to ensure adequate hydration and nutrition during the testing period. Some diagnostic studies of the GI system are especially difficult and uncomfortable for older persons. It may be necessary to individualize care and make adjustments. Many radiological studies use diatrizoate meglumine (Gastrografin) as a contrast medium. Gastrografin is water soluble and rapidly absorbed, so it is preferred when a perforation is suspected.

Radiological Studies

Upper Gastrointestinal Series. An upper GI series with small bowel follow-through enables visualization of the esophagus, the stomach, and the small intestine by means of fluoroscopy and radiographic examination. A barium swallow study is

---

TABLE 41.10 NORMAL FINDINGS IN PHYSICAL ASSESSMENT OF THE GASTROINTESTINAL SYSTEM

Mouth
- Moist, pink lips
- Moist, pink buccal mucosa and gingivae without plaques or lesions
- Teeth in good repair
- Protrusion of tongue in midline without deviation or fasciculations
- Pink uvula in midline, soft palate, tonsils, and posterior pharynx
- Smooth swallowing without coughing or gagging

Abdomen
- Flat without masses or scars
- No abdominal tenderness
- No bruises
- Bowel sounds in all quadrants
- Nonpalpable liver and spleen
- Liver 10 cm in right midclavicular line
- Generalized tympany

Anus
- Absence of lesions, fissures, and hemorrhoids
- Good sphincter tone
- Rectal walls smooth and soft
- No masses
- Stool soft, brown, and heme negative

CASE STUDY

Objective Data: Physical Examination

A focused assessment of L. C. reveals the following: BP 120/74, heart rate 110, respiratory rate 24, temp 38°C. Abdomen firm and slightly distended. High-pitched bowel sounds in upper quadrants. No bowel sounds auscultated in left lower quadrant. Mild abdominal palpation elicits pain.

As you continue to read this chapter, consider diagnostic studies that may be ordered for him.

See Case Study: Subjective Data and Case Study: Objective Data: Diagnostic Studies for more information on L. C.

TABLE 41.11 ASSESSMENT ABNORMALITIES

Gastrointestinal System

Finding	Description	Possible Etiology and Significance
Mouth		
Ulcer, plaque on lips or in mouth	Sore or lesion	Carcinoma, viral infections
Cheilosis	Softening, fissuring, and cracking of lips at angles of mouth	Riboflavin deficiency
Cheilitis	Inflammation of lips (usually lower) with fissuring, scaling, crusting	Often unknown
Geographic tongue	Scattered red, smooth (loss of papillae) areas on dorsum of tongue	Unknown
Smooth tongue	Red, slick appearance	Cobalamin deficiency
Leukoplakia	Thickened white patches	Premalignant lesion
Pyorrhea	Recessed gingivae, purulent pockets	Periodontitis
Herpes simplex	Benign vesicular lesion	Herpesvirus
Candidiasis	White, curdlike lesions surrounded by erythematous mucosa	*Candida albicans*
Glossitis	Reddened, ulcerated, swollen tongue	Exposure to streptococci, irritation, injury, vitamin B deficiencies, anemia
Acute marginal gingivitis	Friable, edematous, painful, bleeding gingivae	Irritation from ill-fitting dentures, calcium deposits on teeth, food impaction
Esophagus and Stomach		
Dysphagia	Difficulty swallowing, sensation of food sticking in esophagus	Esophageal conditions, cancer of esophagus
Hematemesis	Vomiting of blood	Esophageal varices, bleeding peptic ulcer (bleeding in upper GI tract)
Pyrosis	Heartburn, burning in epigastric or substernal area	Hiatal hernia, esophagitis, incompetent lower esophageal sphincter
Dyspepsia	Burning or indigestion	Peptic ulcer, gallbladder disease
Odynophagia	Painful swallowing	Cancer of esophagus, esophagitis
Eructation	Belching	Gallbladder disease
Nausea and vomiting	Feeling of impending vomiting, expulsion of gastric contents through mouth	GI infections, common manifestation of many GI diseases; stress, fear, and pathological conditions
Abdomen		
Distension	Excessive gas accumulation, enlarged abdomen; generalized tympany	Obstruction, paralytic ileus
Ascites	Accumulated fluid within abdominal cavity; eversion of umbilicus (usually)	Peritoneal inflammation, heart failure, metastatic carcinoma, cirrhosis

TABLE 41.11 ASSESSMENT ABNORMALITIES

Gastrointestinal System—cont'd

Finding	Description	Possible Etiology and Significance
Bruit	Humming or swishing sound heard through stethoscope over vessel	Partial arterial obstruction (narrowing of vessel), turbulent flow (aneurysm)
Hyper-resonance	Loud, tinkling rushes	Intestinal obstruction
Borborygmi	Audible waves of loud, gurgling abdominal sounds produced by hyperactive bowel	Hyperactive intestinal peristalsis; result of eating, inflammatory bowel disease, infectious enteritis, mesenteric ischemia
Reduced or absent bowel sounds	No auscultation of bowel sounds	Peritonitis, paralytic ileus, obstruction; hypoactive bowel sounds are normal immediately postoperatively
Absence of liver dullness	Tympany on percussion	Air from viscus (e.g., perforated ulcer)
Masses	Lump on palpation	Tumours, cysts
Rebound tenderness	Sudden pain when examiner's fingers are withdrawn quickly (Blumberg sign)	Peritoneal inflammation, appendicitis
Inspiratory arrest	Sharp pain stops inspiration when the liver is palpated during a deep breath (Murphy sign)	Cholecystitis
Nodular liver	Enlarged, hard liver with irregular edge or surface	Cirrhosis, carcinoma
Hepatomegaly	Enlargement of liver, liver edge >1–2 cm below costal margin	Metastatic carcinoma, hepatitis, venous congestion
Splenomegaly	Enlargement of spleen	Chronic leukemia, hemolytic states, portal hypertension, some infections
Hernia	Bulge or nodule in abdomen, usually appearing on straining	Inguinal (in inguinal canal), femoral (in femoral canal), umbilical (herniation of umbilicus), or incisional (defect in muscles after surgery)
Rectum and Anus		
Hemorrhoids	Thrombosed veins in rectum and anus (internal or external)	Portal hypertension, chronic constipation, prolonged sitting or standing, pregnancy
Mass	Firm, nodular edge	Tumour, carcinoma
Pilonidal cyst	Opening of sinus tract, cyst in midline just above coccyx	Probably congenital
Fissure	Ulceration in anal canal	Straining, irritation
Melena	Abnormal, black, tarry stool containing digested blood	Cancer, bleeding in upper GI tract from ulcers, varices
Tenesmus	Spasmodic contraction of the anal sphincter with pain and persistent desire to empty the bowel; painful and ineffective straining at stool	Ulcerative colitis, diarrhea secondary to GI infection such as food poisoning
Steatorrhea	Passage of large amounts of fat as a fatty, frothy, foul-smelling stool	Chronic pancreatitis, biliary obstruction, malabsorption difficulties (result of failure to digest and absorb fat)

GI, gastrointestinal.

FOCUSED ASSESSMENT

Gastrointestinal (GI) System

Use this checklist to make sure the key assessment steps have been done.

Subjective
Ask the patient about any of the following and note the responses:

Change or loss of appetite	Y	N
Abdominal pain	Y	N
Changes in stools; if so, check colour, consistency, frequency, for presence of blood and any other unexpected findings	Y	N
Nausea, vomiting	Y	N
Painful swallowing	Y	N

Objective: Diagnostic
Check the following laboratory results for critical values:

Endoscopy: colonoscopy, sigmoidoscopy, esophagogastroduodenoscopy ✓
Radiology: upper GI series, lower GI series ✓
Stool for occult blood or ova and parasites ✓
Liver function tests ✓

Objective: Physical Examination
Inspect

Skin for colour, lesions, scars, petechiae, and any other unexpected findings ✓
Abdominal contour for symmetry and distension ✓
Anus and rectum for intact skin, presence or absence of hemorrhoids ✓

Auscultate*

Bowel sounds ✓

Palpate

Abdominal quadrants with light touch ✓
Abdominal quadrants with deep technique ✓

*Note: Perform auscultation before palpation.

used to identify esophageal, stomach, and small intestine disorders such as esophageal strictures, varices, polyps, tumours, hiatal hernia, and foreign bodies, as well as peptic ulcers in the stomach or duodenum. The barium swallow study begins with the patient swallowing a thick barium solution (contrast medium). The patient then assumes different positions on the radiographic study examination table. The movement of the contrast medium through the upper GI tract is observed with fluoroscopy, and several radiographic images are obtained (see Table 41.12).

TABLE 41.12   **DIAGNOSTIC STUDIES**

Gastrointestinal (GI) System

Study	Description and Purpose	Nursing Responsibility
Radiology		
Upper GI series or barium swallow study	Fluoroscopic radiographic study using contrast medium Used to diagnose structural abnormalities of the esophagus, the stomach, and the duodenal bulb	Explain procedure to patient, including the need to drink contrast medium and to assume various positions on radiographic study examination table. Keep patient NPO for 8–12 hr before procedure. Instruct patient to avoid smoking after midnight the night before the study. After radiograph, take measures to prevent contrast medium impaction (fluids, laxatives). Warn patient that stool may be white for up to 72 hr after test.
Small bowel series	Fluoroscopic radiographic study using contrast medium Images are obtained q30 min until medium reaches terminal ileum.	Same as for upper GI series.
Lower GI series or barium enema study	Fluoroscopic radiographic examination of colon using contrast medium, which is administered rectally (enema) Double-contrast or air-contrast barium enema is the test of choice. Air is infused after thick barium flows through transverse colon. Endoscopic procedures have made necessity for this test less common than in the past.	The evening before the procedure, administer purgatives, laxatives, enemas, or a combination of these until colon is clear of stool. The patient is put on a clear liquid diet the evening before procedure. Keep patient NPO for 8 hr before test. Instruct patient about being given barium by enema. Explain that cramping and urge to defecate may occur during procedure and that patient may be placed in various positions on tilt table. After the procedure, administer fluids, laxatives, or suppositories to assist in expelling barium. Observe stool for passage of contrast medium.
Cholangiography		
Percutaneous transhepatic cholangiography (PTC)	Fluoroscopic radiographic study used to determine filling of hepatic and biliary ducts After local anaesthesia is induced and with monitored anaesthesia care (formerly called *conscious sedation*), the liver is entered with a long needle (under fluoroscopy), the bile duct is entered, bile withdrawn, and radiopaque contrast medium is injected. IV antibiotics are administered prophylactically.	Observe patient for signs of hemorrhage, bile leakage, and infection. Assess patient's medications for possible contraindications, precautions, or complications with the use of contrast medium.
Surgical cholangiography	Study performed during surgery on biliary structures, such as gallbladder Contrast medium is injected into common bile duct.	Explain to patient that anaesthetic and contrast medium will be used. Assess patient's medications for possible contraindications, precautions, or complications with the use of contrast medium.
Magnetic resonance cholangiopancreatography (MRCP)	MRI technology used to obtain images of biliary and pancreatic ducts	Explain procedure to patient. It is contraindicated in a patient with metal implants (e.g., pacemaker) or who is pregnant.
Ultrasonography	Nonradiographic study used to show the size and configuration of organs Noninvasive procedure in which high-frequency sound (ultrasound) waves are passed into body structures and recorded as they are reflected (bounded)	
Abdominal ultrasonography	Ultrasound study used to detect abdominal masses (tumours and cysts), biliary and liver disease, gallstones A conductive gel (lubricant jelly) is applied to the skin and a transducer is placed on the area.	Keep patient NPO for 8–12 hr before procedure. Air or gas can reduce quality of images. Food intake can cause gallbladder contraction, resulting in suboptimal study results.
Endoscopic ultrasonography (EUS)	Ultrasound study using a small transducer installed on tip of endoscope Because EUS transducer gets close to the organs being examined, images obtained are often more accurate and detailed than images provided by traditional ultrasonography. Detects and helps stage esophageal, gastric, rectal, biliary, and pancreatic tumours and abnormalities Also used to guide fine-needle aspiration to diagnose cancer or dysplasia	Same as for esophagogastroduodenoscopy.

TABLE 41.12	**DIAGNOSTIC STUDIES**	
Gastrointestinal (GI) System—cont'd		
Study	**Description and Purpose**	**Nursing Responsibility**
Nuclear Imaging Scans (scintigraphy)	Radionuclide studies used to show size, shape, and position of organ Functional disorders and structural defects may be identified. Radionuclide (radioactive isotope) is injected IV, and a counter (scanning) device picks up radioactive emission, which is recorded on paper. Only tracer doses of radioactive isotopes are used.	Tell patient that substance to be ingested contains only traces of radioactivity and poses little to no danger. Schedule no more than one radionuclide test per day. Explain to patient the need to lie flat during the scan.
Gastric emptying studies	Radionuclide studies used to assess ability of stomach to empty solids or liquids in patients with emptying disorders resulting from peptic ulcer, ulcer surgery, diabetes, gastric malignancies, or functional disorders • Solid-emptying study: cooked egg white containing ^{99m}Tc is eaten. • Liquid-emptying study: orange juice with ^{99m}Tc is swallowed. Sequential images from gamma camera are recorded q2min for up to 60 min.	Same as for nuclear imaging scans.
Hepatobiliary (HIDA) scintigraphy	Radionuclide study used to identify obstructions of bile ducts (e.g., gallstones, tumours), diseases of gallbladder, and bile leaks Patient is given ^{99m}Tc IV and positioned under camera to record distribution of tracer in the liver, biliary tree, gallbladder, and proximal small bowel.	Same as for nuclear imaging scans.
Scintigraphy of GI bleeding	Radionuclide study used to reveal exact site of active GI blood loss Patient is given ^{99m}Tc-labelled sulphur colloid or patient's own red blood cells (RBCs) labelled with ^{99m}Tc, and images of the abdomen are obtained at intermittent intervals.	Same as for nuclear imaging scans.
Scanning and Imaging		
Computed tomographic (CT) scan	Noninvasive radiological examination allows exposures at different depths Used to detect biliary tract, liver, and pancreatic disorders Use of oral and IV contrast media accentuates density differences	Explain procedures to patient. Determine sensitivity to iodine if contrast material is used.
Magnetic resonance imaging (MRI)	Noninvasive procedure using radiofrequency waves and a magnetic field Used to detect hepatobiliary disease, hepatic lesions, and sources of GI bleeding and to stage colorectal cancer IV contrast medium (gadolinium) may be used.	Explain procedure to patient. MRI is contraindicated in patients with metal implants (e.g., pacemaker) or who are pregnant.
Virtual colonoscopy	Combines CT scanning or MRI with computer virtual reality software to detect colon and bowel diseases and conditions, including polyps, colorectal cancer, diverticulosis, and lower GI bleeding Air is introduced via a tube placed in the rectum to enlarge the colon to enhance visualization. Images are obtained while patient is on back and stomach. Images are combined on a computer to form two- and three-dimensional images, which are viewed on monitor.	Bowel preparation is similar to that for colonoscopy (see below under "Endoscopy"). Unlike conventional colonoscopy, virtual colonoscopy necessitates no sedatives and no endoscope. The procedure takes about 15–20 min.
Endoscopy		
Esophagogastroduo-denoscopy (EGD)	Enables direct visualization of mucosal lining of esophagus, stomach, and duodenum with flexible endoscope Video imaging may be used to visualize stomach motility. Inflammations, ulcerations, tumours, varices, or Mallory–Weiss tear may be detected. Biopsy samples may be obtained, and varices can be treated with band ligation or sclerotherapy.	Before the procedure: Keep patient on NPO status for 8 hr. Make sure signed consent is obtained. Give preoperative medication if ordered. Explain to patient that local anaesthetic may be sprayed on the throat before insertion of endoscope and that patient will be sedated during the procedure. After the procedure: Keep patient NPO until gag reflex returns (usually 2–4 hr); gently tickle back of patient's throat to determine return of reflex. Instruct patient to use warm saline gargles for relief of sore throat. Check temperature q15–30 min for 1–2 hr (sudden temperature spike is sign of perforation).

Continued

Study	Description and Purpose	Nursing Responsibility
Colonoscopy	Enables direct visualization of entire colon up to ileocecal valve with flexible fibre-optic endoscope The patient's position is changed frequently during the procedure to assist with advancement of the endoscope to the cecum. Used to detect and diagnose inflammatory bowel disease, polyps, tumours, and diverticulosis and to dilate strictures The procedure allows for removal of colonic polyps without laparotomy.	Before the procedure: Bowel preparation is completed. Procedure varies with physician preference. For example, patient may be kept on clear fluids 1–2 days before procedure, and cathartic or enema (or both) administered the night before. An alternative is to give 4.5 L (1 gal) of polyethylene glycol (Co-lyte) the evening before (8-oz glass q10min). Purgatives such as PICO-SALAX may be administered. Explain to patient that a flexible endoscope will be inserted while patient is in a side-lying position and that a sedative will be given. After procedure: Be aware that patient may experience abdominal cramps caused by stimulation of peristalsis because bowel is constantly inflated with air during procedure. Observe for rectal bleeding and signs of perforation (e.g., malaise, abdominal distension, tenesmus). Check vital signs.
Capsule endoscopy	Study most commonly used to visualize small intestine and diagnose diseases such as Crohn's disease, small bowel tumours, celiac disease, and malabsorption syndrome and to identify sources of possible GI bleeding in areas not accessible by upper endoscopy or colonoscopy The patient swallows a capsule (approximately the size of a large vitamin) with a camera that provides endoscopic observation of GI tract (see Figure 41.10); the camera takes >50 000 images during an 8-hr examination. The capsule relays images to a monitoring device that patient wears on a belt. After examination, images are downloaded to a workstation. Not used in patients with suspected intestinal strictures	Dietary preparation is similar to that for colonoscopy. The video capsule is swallowed, and the patient is usually kept NPO until 4–6 hr later. The procedure is comfortable for most patients. Eight hours after swallowing the capsule, the patient returns to have the monitoring device removed. Peristalsis causes passage of the disposable capsule with a bowel movement.
Sigmoidoscopy	Enables direct visualization of rectum and sigmoid colon with lighted flexible endoscope Sometimes a special table is used to tilt patient into knee–chest position. Used to detect tumours, polyps, inflammatory and infectious diseases, fissures, hemorrhoids	Administer enemas the evening before and morning of procedure. Make sure signed consent is obtained. Patient may have clear liquids the day before, or no dietary restrictions may be necessary. Explain to patient knee–chest position (unless patient is older person or very ill), the need to take deep breaths during insertion of scope, and possible urge to defecate as scope is passed. Encourage patient to relax and let abdomen go limp. Observe for rectal bleeding after polypectomy or biopsy.
Endoscopic retrograde cholangio-pancreatography (ERCP)	Endoscopic technique enables direct visualization of structures. A fibre-optic endoscope (using fluoroscopy) is inserted through the oral cavity into the descending duodenum, and then common bile and pancreatic ducts are cannulated. Contrast medium is then injected into ducts. The technique can also be used to retrieve a gallstone from the distal common bile duct, dilate strictures, obtain biopsy of tumours, or diagnose pseudocysts.	Before the procedure, explain procedure to patient, including patient's role. Keep patient NPO for 8 hr before procedure. Make sure signed consent is obtained. Administer sedative immediately before and during procedure. Administer antibiotics if ordered. After the procedure, check vital signs. Check for signs of perforation or infection. Be aware that ERCP-induced pancreatitis is the most common complication; this complication manifests as abdominal pain, nausea, and vomiting. Check for return of gag reflex.
Endoscopic ultra-sonography	Combined use of endoscopy and ultrasonography with the use of an ultrasound transducer attached to an endoscope Enables visualization of esophagus, stomach, intestine, liver, pancreas, and gallbladder	Similar to that for esophagogastroduodenoscopy.
Laparoscopy (peritoneoscopy)	Enables visualization of peritoneal cavity and contents with laparoscope Biopsy specimen may be obtained. Performed with patient under general anaesthesia in operating room Double-puncture peritoneoscopy enables better visualization of abdominal cavity, especially liver. Can eliminate need for exploratory laparotomy in many patients	Keep patient on NPO status for 8 hr before study. Make sure signed consent is obtained. Administer preoperative sedative. Ensure that bladder and bowel are emptied. Inform patient that local anaesthetic is used before laparoscope insertion. Observe for possible complications of bleeding and bowel perforation after the procedure.
Blood Studies		
Amylase	Measures secretion of amylase by pancreas Is important in diagnosing acute pancreatitis Level peaks in 24 hr and then drops to normal in 48–72 hr Depending on method, reference range is 100–300 U/L (60–120 SU/dL)	Obtain blood sample in acute attack of pancreatitis. Explain procedure to patient.

TABLE 41.12 DIAGNOSTIC STUDIES
Gastrointestinal (GI) System—cont'd

Study	Description and Purpose	Nursing Responsibility
Lipase	Measures secretion of lipase by pancreas. Level stays elevated longer than that of serum amylase Reference range is <160 U/L	Explain procedure to patient.
Gastrin	Measures secretion of gastrin by the cells of the antrum of the stomach and by the pancreatic islets of Langerhans Reference interval: 0–180 ng/L (0–180 pg/mL) during fasting	Explain procedure to patient.
Liver Biopsy	Percutaneous procedure in which needle is inserted between sixth and seventh or between eighth and ninth intercostal spaces on the right side to obtain specimen of hepatic tissue Often performed under ultrasound or CT guidance	Before procedure, check patient's coagulation status (prothrombin time, clotting or bleeding time). Ensure that patient's blood is typed and crossmatched. Measure vital signs as baseline data. Explain holding of breath after expiration when needle is inserted. Make sure signed consent is obtained. After procedure, check vital signs to detect internal bleeding q15min × 2, q30min × 4, q1hr × 4. Keep patient lying on right side for a minimum of 2 hr to splint puncture site. Keep patient in bed in flat position for 12–14 hr. Assess patient for complications such as bile peritonitis, shock, and pneumothorax.
Fecal Tests		
Fecal immunochemical test	Tests for the presence of blood in stool Possible indicator of colorectal cancer	Explain procedure and indication to patient. There are no medical or dietary restrictions.
Fecal analysis	Form, consistency, and colour of fecal sample are noted Specimen examined for mucus, blood, pus, parasites, and fat content Fecal occult blood test (FOBT): guaiac test, Hemoccult, Hemoccult II, Hemoccult-SENSA, Hematest are performed Single DNA test (PreGen-Plus) is a panel of DNA markers used to detect and monitor colorectal cancer.	Observe patient's stools. Collect stool specimens. Check stools for blood. Keep diet free of red meat for 24–48 hr before occult blood test.
Stool culture	Tests for presence of bacteria, including *Clostridium difficile*	Collect stool specimen.

GI, gastrointestinal; *IV*, intravenously; *ng/L*, nanograms per litre; *NPO*, nothing by mouth; *pg/mL*, pictograms per millilitre; *RBCs*, red blood cells; *SU*, Somogyi units; *99mTc*, technetium-99m; *U/L*, units per litre; *WBCs*, white blood cells.

Lower Gastrointestinal Series. The purpose of a lower GI series (barium enema radiograph) is to observe by means of fluoroscopy the filling of the colon with contrast medium and to observe by radiograph the filled colon. This procedure helps identify polyps, tumours, and other lesions in the colon. The patient is administered an enema of contrast medium. The air-contrast barium enema provides better visualization of inflammatory bowel disease, polyps, tumours, and gallstones (Figure 41.8). Because the patient must retain the barium, this study is not tolerated well by patients who are older or immobile.

Abdominal Ultrasonography. Ultrasonography is a noninvasive, nonradiographic approach used to show the size and the configuration of organs. It is the diagnostic procedure of choice for detecting cholelithiasis (gallstones). Ultrasonography is also used for detecting appendicitis, acute cholecystitis, and other changes in abdominal organs (see Table 41.12).

Endoscopy

Endoscopy is the direct visualization of a body structure through a lighted fibre-optic instrument (endoscope). The GI structures that can be examined through endoscopy include the esophagus, the stomach, the duodenum, the colon, and, with the aid of fluoroscopy and radiographs, the pancreas and the biliary tree. The pancreatic, hepatic, and common bile ducts can be visualized with side-viewing flexible endoscopes. This procedure is called *endoscopic retrograde cholangiopancreatography* (ERCP) and is illustrated in Figure 41.9.

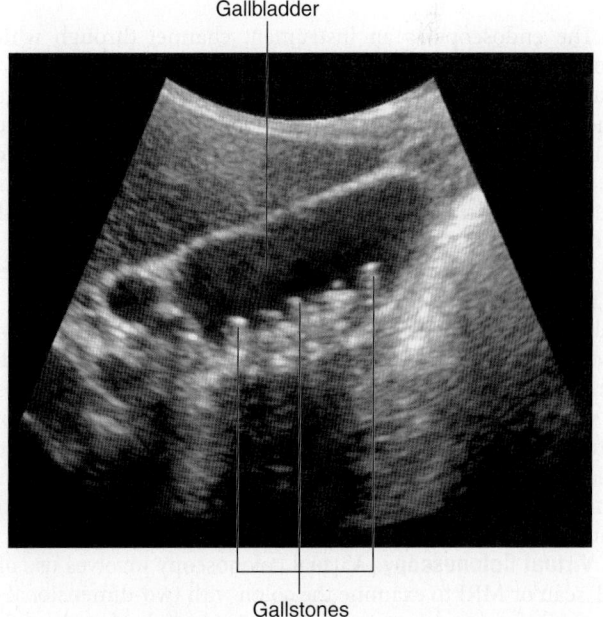

FIG. 41.8 Radiography image of gallbladder, showing multiple gallstones. Source: Drake, R.L., Vogl, W., & Mitchell, A. W. M. (2015). *Gray's anatomy for students* (3rd ed., p, 326). Churchill Livingstone.

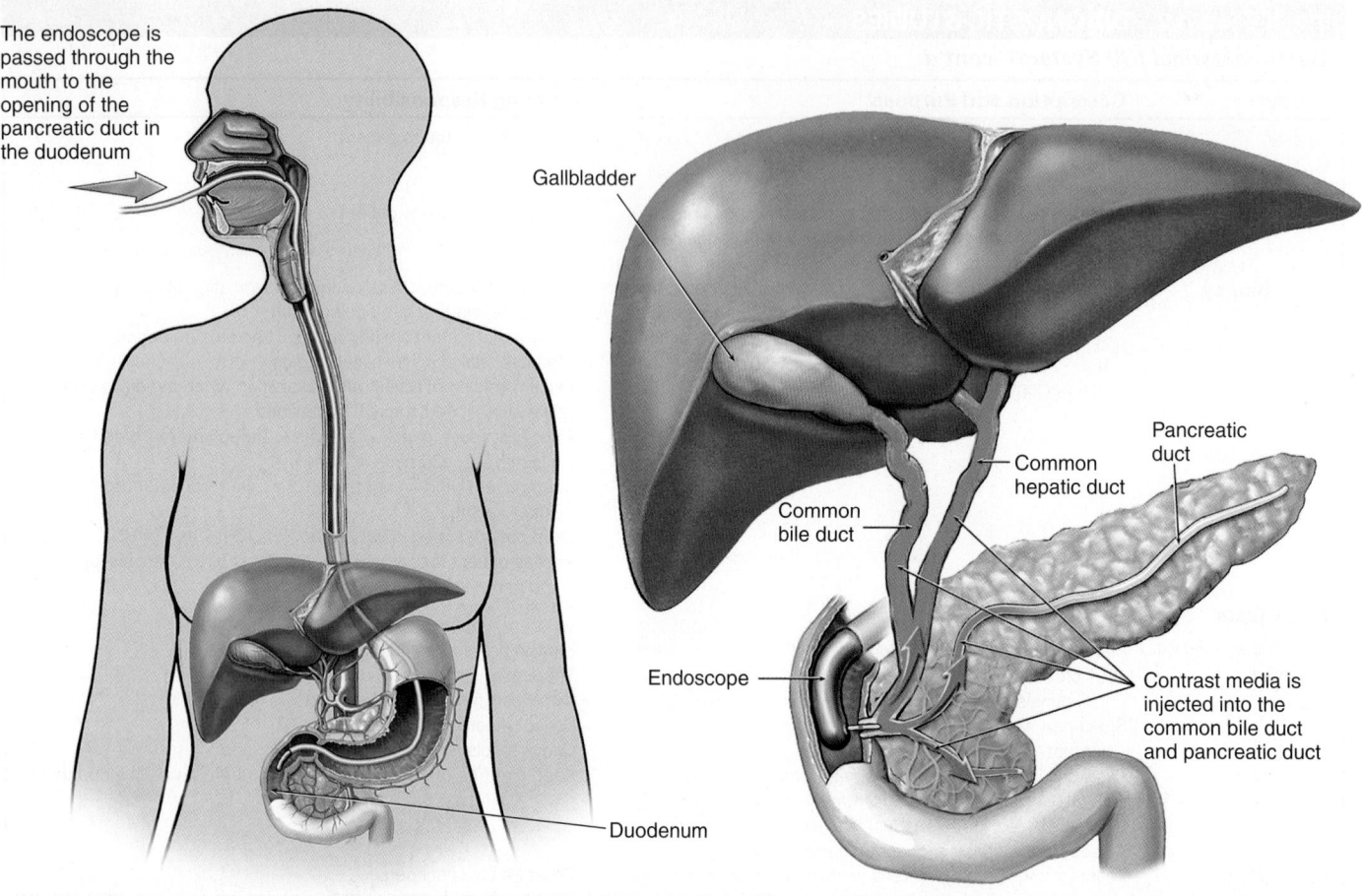

The endoscope is passed through the mouth to the opening of the pancreatic duct in the duodenum

Gallbladder

Pancreatic duct

Common hepatic duct

Common bile duct

Endoscope

Contrast media is injected into the common bile duct and pancreatic duct

Duodenum

FIG. 41.9 Endoscopic retrograde cholangiopancreatography. Source: Nucleus Medical Media Inc./Alamy Stock Photo.

The endoscope is an instrument channel through which biopsy forceps and cytology brushes may be passed. Cameras may be attached to take video recordings and still pictures. Endoscopy of the GI tract is often performed in combination with biopsy and cytological studies. The major complication of GI endoscopy is perforation through the structure being viewed. The incidence of this complication is decreased with the use of the flexible fibre-optic endoscopes.

For all endoscopic procedures, informed written consent is required. Specific endoscopy procedures are discussed in Table 41.12. In addition to diagnostic procedures, many invasive and therapeutic procedures may be performed with endoscopes. These include procedures such as polypectomy, sclerosis of varices, laser treatment, cauterization of bleeding sites, papillotomy, removal of stones in the common bile duct, and balloon dilations. For many endoscopic procedures, patients require intravenous short-acting sedatives. The nurse monitors the patient's level of comfort.

Virtual Colonoscopy. Virtual colonoscopy involves use of a CT scan or MRI to examine the colon with two-dimensional or three-dimensional images of the entire bowel, after the colon has been cleansed (enema). The procedure is less invasive than an endoscopy, and no sedation is required. It is a useful procedure for detecting polyps or cancer in the large intestine. *Polyps* are growths that arise from the inner lining of the intestine (see Table 41.12).

Endoscopic Ultrasonography. Endoscopic ultrasound (EUS) is a relatively new endoscopic technique that provides highly accurate images of the esophagus, GI tract, pancreas, and liver. EUS provides high-resolution imaging of the GI tract because of its unique ability to differentiate the histological layers of the GI tract wall. It is most often used for preoperative staging of esophageal, gastric, pancreatic, and colorectal cancers. It can also be used to detect gallstones.

Capsule Endoscopy. In capsule endoscopy, the patient swallows a capsule containing a disposable video camera (Figure 41.10). As the video camera passes through the intestine, images are transmitted by radiofrequency. This procedure is useful in visualization of the portion of the small bowel that is not within reach of standard upper and lower endoscopy. It allows more access to the small bowel for patients with an obscure source of GI bleeding. This technology may be helpful in discovering the cause of GI bleeding when results of standard upper endoscopy and colonoscopy are normal.

Liver Biopsy

A liver biopsy is performed when hepatic tissue is needed to establish a diagnosis such as fibrosis, cirrhosis, hepatitis, and neoplasms. It may also be used for monitoring the progress of liver disease. Liver biopsy may be performed as an open or closed procedure. The *open method* involves making an incision and removing a wedge of tissue. It is performed in the operating room, often concurrently with another surgical procedure, with the patient under general anaesthesia. The *closed*, or *needle, biopsy* is a percutaneous procedure in which the site is infiltrated with a local anaesthetic and a needle is inserted between the sixth and seventh or between the eighth and ninth intercostal spaces on the right side. The patient lies supine with the right arm over the head. The patient should be instructed to exhale fully and not breathe while the needle is inserted (see Table 41.12). It is important to perform a nursing assessment before and after a liver biopsy to prevent complications (e.g., hemorrhage, infection).

CASE STUDY

Objective Data: Diagnostic Studies

The ED health care provider performs a rectal examination and finds a palpable mass. The following diagnostic tests are ordered:
- CBC
- Electrolytes
- Liver function tests
- Urinalysis
- CT scan of the abdomen
- Colonoscopy

The CBC reveals an Hb of 68 mmol/L and an Hct of 20%. The white blood cell count is normal. The electrolytes, liver function tests, and urinalysis are within normal limits. The CT scan reveals pockets of gas and fluid in the ascending colon and two medium-sized tumours in the transverse colon.

See Case Study: Subjective Data and Case Study: Objective Data: Physical Examination for more information on L. C.

Liver Function Studies

Liver function tests are usually described separately from other GI diagnostic studies. Liver function tests are laboratory (blood) studies that reflect hepatic disease. Table 41.13 lists some common liver function tests.

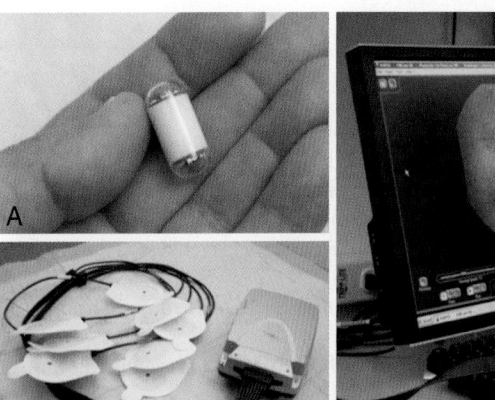

FIG. 41.10 Capsule endoscopy. **A,** The pill-sized video capsule has its own camera and light source. **B,** As it travels through the GI tract, it sends messages through sensing electrodes placed on the chest and abdomen to a data recorder worn on a waist belt. **C,** After the test, the images are viewed on a computer. Source: Dye, C. E., Gaffney, R. R., Dykes, T. M., et al. (2012). Endoscopic and radiographic evaluation of the small bowel in 2012. *The American Journal of Medicine, 125*(12), 1228.e1–1288.e12.

TABLE 41.13 DIAGNOSTIC STUDIES

Liver Function Tests

Test	Description and Purpose	Test	Description and Purpose
Bile Formation and Excretion		**Hemostatic Functions**	
Serum bilirubin	Measurement of ability of liver to conjugate and excrete bilirubin; enables differentiation between unconjugated (indirect) and conjugated (direct) bilirubin in plasma	Prothrombin	Determination of prothrombin activity Reference range: 11–12.5 sec
• Total	Measurement of direct and indirect total bilirubin Reference range: 5.1–17 mcmol/L	Vitamin K	Essential cofactor for many clotting factors Reference range: 0.22–4.88 nmol/L
• Direct	Measurement of conjugated bilirubin; level is elevated in obstructive jaundice Reference range: 1.7–5.1 mcmol/L	**Serum Enzyme Tests**	
• Indirect	Measurement of unconjugated bilirubin; level is elevated in hepatocellular (hepatitis, cirrhosis, neoplasm or hepatic congestion) and hemolytic conditions Reference range: 3.4–12 mcmol/L	Alkaline phosphatase (ALP)	Origination in bone and liver; serum level elevated when excretion is impaired as a result of obstruction in the biliary tract Reference range: 35–120 U/L
Urinary bilirubin	Measurement of urinary excretion of conjugated bilirubin Normal finding: 0–0.034 mcmol/L (negative)	Aspartate aminotransferase (AST)	Serum level elevated in liver damage and inflammation Reference range: 0–35 U/L Women's values are slightly lower than men's
Protein Metabolism		Alanine aminotransferase (ALT)	Serum level elevated in liver damage and inflammation Reference range: 4–36 U/L
Serum protein levels	Measurement of serum proteins manufactured by the liver Albumin (A) reference range: 35–50 g/L; globulin (G) reference range: 23–34 g/L; total protein reference range: 64–83 g/L Normal A/G ratio: 1.5:1–2.5:1	γ-Glutamyl transpeptidase (GGT)	Present in biliary tract (not in skeletal muscle or cardiac tissue); serum level elevated in hepatitis and alcoholic liver disease; more sensitive for detecting biliary obstruction, cholangitis, or cholecystitis than ALP Reference range: 8–38 IU/L
α-Fetoprotein	Tumour marker, especially for hepatic cancer Reference range: <40 mcg/L	**Lipid Metabolism**	
Ammonia	Conversion of ammonia to urea normally occurs in the liver; elevated ammonia level can result in hepatic encephalopathy secondary to liver cirrhosis Reference range: 6–47 mcmol/L	Serum cholesterol	Synthesis and excretion by liver; serum level elevated in biliary obstruction, lowered in extensive liver disease and malnutrition Reference range: <5.0 mmol/L, age dependent HDL reference range: >1.55 mmol/L LDL reference range: <2.59 mmol/L

HDL, high-density lipoprotein; *IU/L,* international units per litre; *LDL,* low-density lipoprotein; *U/L,* units per litre.

REVIEW QUESTIONS

The number of the question corresponds to the same-numbered objective at the beginning of the chapter.

1. A client is admitted to the hospital with a diagnosis of diarrhea with dehydration. The nurse recognizes that increased peristalsis resulting in diarrhea can be related to which of the following mechanisms?
   a. Sympathetic inhibition
   b. Mixing and propulsion
   c. Sympathetic stimulation
   d. Parasympathetic stimulation

2. A client has an elevated blood level of indirect (unconjugated) bilirubin. Which of the following might cause this finding?
   a. The gallbladder is unable to contract to release stored bile.
   b. Bilirubin is not being conjugated and excreted into the bile by the liver.
   c. The Kupffer cells in the liver are unable to remove bilirubin from the blood.
   d. There is an obstruction in the biliary tract preventing flow of bile into the small intestine.

3. Which of the following normally protects the bowel from the acidity of gastric contents as they move into the small intestine?
   a. Inhibition of secretin release
   b. Release of bicarbonate by the pancreas
   c. Release of pancreatic digestive enzymes
   d. Release of gastrin by the duodenal mucosa

4. An 80-year-old client states that although a lot of salt is added to the food consumed, it still does not have much flavour. Which of the following factors related to aging would account for this finding?
   a. This finding is not an age-related change.
   b. Loss of taste buds, especially for sweetness and saltiness
   c. Some loss of taste sensation but no difficulty chewing food
   d. Loss of the sense of taste because the ability to smell is decreased

5. Which of the following questions is appropriate to initiate a GI assessment?
   a. "What is your usual bowel elimination pattern?"
   b. "What percentage of your income is spent on food?"
   c. "Have you travelled to a foreign country in the past year?"
   d. "Does stress give you diarrhea?"

6. Which of the following is appropriate for the nurse to undertake during an examination of the abdomen?
   a. Position the client in the supine position with the bed flat and knees straight.
   b. Listen in the epigastrium and all four quadrants for 2 to 5 minutes for bowel sounds.
   c. Use the following order of techniques: inspection, palpation, percussion, auscultation.
   d. Describe bowel sounds as absent if no sound is heard in the lower right quadrant after 2 minutes.

7. A client is admitted for appendicitis and surgery is scheduled to take place in 4 hours. The client is vomiting and indicates an increase in abdominal pain. The nurse noted a distended abdomen and diminished bowel sounds upon assessment. Which of the following is the most appropriate nursing intervention?
   a. Administer analgesic
   b. Notify the primary health care provider
   c. Call the operating room to perform surgery as soon as possible
   d. Reposition the patient and apply a heating pad to the client's abdomen

8. Which of the following is correct in preparing a client for a colonoscopy?
   a. A signed consent form is not necessary.
   b. Sedation may be used during the procedure.
   c. Only one cleansing enema is necessary for preparation.
   d. A light meal should be eaten the day before the procedure.

1. d; 2. b; 3. b; 4. b; 5. a; 6. b; 7. b; 8. b.

For even more review questions, visit http://evolve.elsevier.com/Canada/Lewis/medsurg.

REFERENCES

Health Canada. (2019). *Canada's dietary guidelines for health professionals and policy makers.* Author.

Heuman, D. M., Anastasios, A. M., & Allen, J. (2019). *Gallstones (cholelithiasis).* Medscape. https://emedicine.medscape.com/article/175667-overview#a5

Jarvis, C., Browne, A. J., MacDonald-Jenkins, J., et al. (Eds.). (2019). *Physical examination & health assessment* (3rd Canadian ed.). Elsevier Inc.

Miller, C. A. (2018). *Nursing for wellness in older adults* (8th ed.). Wolters Kluwer Health Lippincott, Williams & Wilkins.

RESOURCES

Resources for this chapter are listed in Chapters 42, 44, 45, and 46.

Nursing Management
Nutritional Conditions

Ellen Vogel, Christina Vaillancourt, and Andrea Miller
Originating US chapter by Mariann M. Harding

⊖volve WEBSITE

http://evolve.elsevier.com/Canada/Lewis/medsurg

- Review Questions (Online Only)
- Key Points
- Answer Guidelines for Case Study
- Customizable Nursing Care Plans
  - Enteral Nutrition
  - Parenteral Nutrition
- Conceptual Care Map Creator
- Audio Glossary
- Content Updates

LEARNING OBJECTIVES

1. Relate the essential components of a well-balanced diet to their impact on health outcomes.
2. Explain the impact that food insecurity has on the health of individuals.
3. Describe the common etiological factors, clinical manifestations, and interprofessional management of malnutrition.
4. Describe the components of a nutritional assessment.
5. Explain the indications for, complications of, and nursing management principles related to the use of enteral nutrition.
6. Explain the indications for, complications of, and nursing management related to the use of parenteral nutrition.
7. Describe the etiological factors, clinical manifestations, and nursing management of eating disorders.

KEY TERMS

anorexia nervosa
bulimia nervosa
enteral nutrition (EN)
food security

malabsorption syndrome
malnutrition
nutrition
optimal nutritional status

overnutrition
parenteral nutrition (PN)
protein–calorie malnutrition (PCM)
undernutrition

This chapter focuses on health conditions related to nutrition. A review of healthy nutrition provides a basis for evaluating nutritional status. Malnutrition, eating disorders, and types of supplemental nutrition, including enteral and parenteral nutrition, are discussed.

NUTRITIONAL CONDITIONS

As one of the fundamental requirements for sustaining life, eating is a highly symbolic and culturally meaningful act. It is unusual to hear a newscast that does not have several stories relating to the food we eat. Newspapers and bestseller lists frequently highlight nutrition- and food-related books, illustrating the importance of food and eating to all people. Nutrition is also inextricably linked to the development of and the recovery from illness.

Nurses, as the first point of contact for patients, frequently initiate patient referrals to dietitians employed in a range of settings (e.g., acute care, long-term care, community, private practice). Thus, knowledge and skills in nutrition and nutritional screening are essential to effective patient care. Dietitians and nurses often collaborate in the development and implementation of nutritional care plans.

Dietitians, as part of the interprofessional team, provide expertise in assessment of the nutritional status of individuals throughout the life cycle and in the development of nutritional care plans for wide-ranging health concerns. Dietitians have extensive knowledge of the biochemical and nutritional components of foods and how these influence metabolic and physiological processes. Importantly, dietitians understand the feeding environment and underlying psychosocial, economic, and health determinants that influence food intake at individual, family, and societal levels (Dietitians of Canada, 2021a). In Canada, dietitians are accountable to provincial regulatory bodies for the highest standards of education and ethics. Currently, professions such as Registered Holistic Nutritionist and those equivalent to Registered Dietitian, as well as the individuals in these roles, are not provincially regulated (Dietitians of Canada, 2021b).

Nutrition is the process by which the body uses food for energy, growth, maintenance, and repair of body tissues. *Nutritional status* can be viewed as a continuum from undernutrition to optimal nutrition to overnutrition. Any alteration in the process of nutrient intake or use can potentially cause nutritional challenges. Nutritional conditions can occur in all age groups, cultures, ethnic groups, and socioeconomic classes and across all educational levels. Attitudes toward the importance of food and eating habits are established early. Cultural or religious preferences and requirements are frequently reflected in dietary intakes.

Food insecurity, or inadequate access to foods due to financial constraints, is a growing public health concern in Canada, with one in eight households experiencing some level of food insecurity. Many low-income families have to decide between paying rent or buying food (Kramer et al., 2019). Food insecurity is associated with a higher incidence of chronic conditions (e.g., diabetes mellitus, iron-deficient anemia), mental health disorders, and suboptimal management of these disorders (Davison et al., 2017).

Men and colleagues (2020), using a population-based sample of Canadian adults, found a graded positive association between household food insecurity and premature mortality. With the exception of cancers, severe food insecurity predicted higher mortality across all causes of death. Adults who died prematurely and self-reported severe food insecurity died at an age 9 years earlier than their food-secure counterparts.

National data compare the number of individuals living in food-insecure households and the number of individuals assisted by food banks in 2015–16. The results show that the most severely food-insecure households did not report accessing a food bank. Rather, food bank use was one of the least common coping strategies employed by severely food-insecure households (University of Toronto, 2020). Most food-insecure individuals do not see food banks as a solution. While offering short-term relief, other policy-focused options are necessary including increasing economic resources for low income Canadians to reduce food insecurity (McIntyre et al., 2016).

Many Indigenous communities face challenges associated with extremely high rates of food insecurity. Overall, almost half of all First Nations communities have difficulty accessing food, and families with young children are particularly at risk. Across Canada, food costs are higher in communities more than 50 km outside major urban centres, with even higher costs in "fly-in" First Nations communities (Chan et al., 2019).

Currently, there is much interest in understanding the link between nutrition and the onset of chronic diseases. Numerous reports have shown that a significant portion of morbidity and mortality among Canadians is related to chronic diseases. Forty-four percent of adults 20 years of age and older have at least 1 of 10 common chronic health conditions (Public Health Agency of Canada, 2019). In First Nations communities the health of many adults is at risk because of very high rates of smoking and obesity (double the obesity rate among non-Indigenous Canadians), and one fifth of the adult population is diagnosed with type 2 diabetes mellitus (more than double the national average) (Chan et al., 2019). Inadequate nutrition is a key preventable risk factor for many of the chronic diseases that influence morbidity, disability, and premature death in Canada.

Internationally, Canada's health care spending is among the highest in the world, representing approximately 11% of the gross domestic product in 2019 (Canadian Institute for Health Information, 2021). Canadian costs associated with poor diet quality reach upwards of $13.8 billion per year (Lieffers et al., 2018).

HEALTHY NUTRITION

Undernutrition occurs when nutritional reserves become depleted or when nutrient intake is inadequate to meet daily requirements or metabolic demands. Undernutrition affects vulnerable groups, including infants, children, pregnant women, new immigrants, individuals living in rural or remote communities, individuals with low incomes, hospitalized people, and older persons. Undernutrition increases the risk for impaired growth and development, lowers resistance to infection and disease, delays wound healing, results in longer hospital stays, and increases health-related expenses.

Optimal nutritional status is achieved when nutrients consumed meet daily requirements and metabolic demands, including any increased demands related to growth, pregnancy, or illness. Individuals with optimal nutritional status have a lower risk of developing chronic diseases and generally live longer than those with a chronic illness.

Overnutrition results from the consumption of nutrients—most frequently, calories, sodium, and fat—in excess of requirements. A major nutritional problem today, overnutrition results in the development of chronic diseases, including obesity, some cancers, and type 2 diabetes. Over the past three decades, the prevalence of obesity has increased three-fold in Canada. Severe obesity has increased more than four-fold and, in 2016, affected an estimated 1.9 million Canadian adults (Wharton et al., 2020). Individuals with obesity experience persistent weight bias and stigma, which contributes to increased morbidity and mortality. The Canadian Adult Obesity Clinical Practice Guidelines provide an evidence-informed and experience-based, patient-centred framework for health care providers, patients, and policymakers. The guidelines are the first comprehensive update in Canadian obesity guidelines since 2007 and the most extensive review of published evidence in obesity worldwide. This guideline reflects advances in the epidemiology, social determinants, pathophysiology, assessment, prevention, and treatment of obesity and shifts the focus of obesity management toward improving patient-centred health outcomes, rather than on weight loss alone (Wharton et al., 2020).

The nutrients required to optimize health over a lifetime are the same for all healthy individuals; however, the amount required of each nutrient differs according to one's stage of the life cycle. Nutritional needs can be viewed as a continuum across the lifespan: They change as individuals grow, age, and respond to variations in their environment, physical activity, and health. Optimal nutrition is essential for maintaining overall health and well-being and preventing chronic conditions.

Optimal nutrition in the absence of any underlying disease process results from the ingestion of a balanced diet.

Canada's Food Guide provides Canadians with recommendations for healthy eating (Health Canada, 2021a) (Figure 42.1). The guide is based on current nutritional science and promotes healthy eating and overall nutritional well-being, in addition to supporting improvements to the Canadian food environment.

Canada's *Food Guide* is meant to be used by healthy Canadians to plan a healthy diet; it is flexible and can be adapted to include combination foods and ethnically diverse foods that reflect the country's multicultural profile. In addition to English and French, the guide is available in 29 other languages, including eight traditional First Nations languages (Health Canada, 2019b).

The current version of Canada's *Food Guide* provides a visual representation of recommended portions of food,

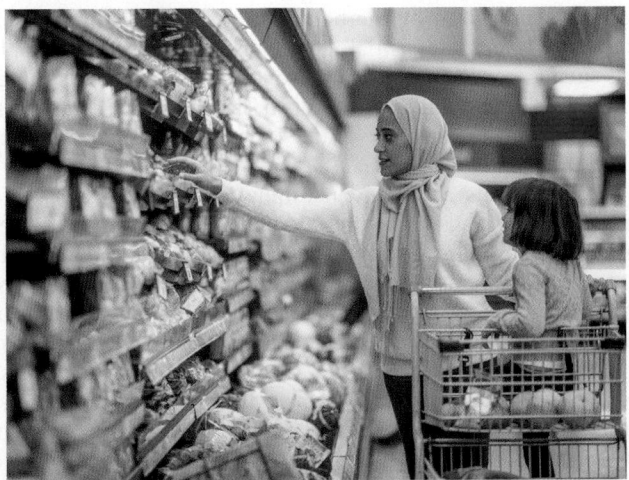

FIG. 42.1 Optimal nutrition in the absence of any underlying disease process results from the ingestion of a balanced diet. Source: iStock.com/Fat-Camera.

rather than prescriptive food servings. The *Food Guide* encourages that half the plate be made up of vegetables and fruit; one quarter, whole grains; and one quarter, protein-rich foods, including plant- and animal-based protein sources, as well as calcium-rich foods, milk, cheese, and yogourt. Although in the current version of *Canada's Food Guide* no food group specific to milk and dairy products is listed, no less importance should be applied to encourage Canadians to meet the recommended nutrient requirements for calcium and vitamin D (Health Canada, 2020b). The *Food Guide* also includes guidelines for healthy food choices, healthy eating habits, recipes, tips for meal planning and eating out, nutrition strategies for different ages and stages of the lifecycle, and resources for both consumers and professionals (Health Canada, 2021a).

Canada's Food Guide was developed in accordance with the daily dietary reference intake (DRI) requirements, a comprehensive set of nutrient reference values for healthy populations (Table 42.1). There is a DRI set for each nutrient. These nutrient reference values are intended to help individuals optimize their health, prevent disease, and avoid overconsumption of any single nutrient. The reference values include the estimated average requirement (EAR), the recommended dietary allowance (RDA), the adequate intake (AI), and the tolerable upper limit (UL) (Institute of Medicine, 2005). The DRI values are designed to maintain health and prevent disease, not to restore health. Nutrient needs may exceed DRIs during times of acute stress or chronic illness.

In recent years, there has been considerable interest in vitamin and mineral supplementation as a means of prevention and treatment of acute and chronic diseases. Although evidence suggests that some nutrients are beneficial to health, it is essential to exercise caution when recommending supplementation. Exceeding the UL can increase a person's risk of nutrient toxicity. As well, the consumption of high levels of one vitamin or mineral may interfere with the absorption of another. For example, ingestion of high levels of zinc can interfere with the

TABLE 42.1	RECOMMENDED DAILY VITAMIN INTAKE AND MANIFESTATIONS OF DEFICIENCIES	
Vitamin	**Dietary Reference Intake**	**Manifestations of Deficiencies**
A (retinol)	*Men: 900 mcg/retinol equivalents** *Women: 700 mcg/retinol equivalents*	Dry, scaly skin; increased susceptibility to infection; night blindness; anorexia; eye irritation; keratinization of respiratory and GI mucosa; bladder stones; anemia; restricted growth
D	*Adults age 19–70: 600 IU* *Adults age >70: 800 IU*	Muscular weakness, excessive sweating, diarrhea, and other GI disturbances, bone pain, active or healed rickets, osteomalacia
E	*Adults: 15 mg*	Neurological deficits
K	*Men: 120 mcg* *Women: 90 mcg*	Defective blood coagulation
B₁ (thiamine)	*Men: 1.2 mg* *Women: 1.1 mg*	Anorexia, fatigue, nervous irritability, constipation, paresthesias, insomnia
B₆ (pyridoxine)	*Men age 19–50: 1.3–1.7 mg* *Men age >51: 1.7 mg* *Women age 19–50: 1.3–1.5 mg* *Women age >51: 1.5 mg*	Seizures, dermatitis, anemia, neuropathy with motor weakness, anorexia
B₁₂ (cobalamin)	*Adults: 2–4 mcg*	Megaloblastic anemia, anorexia, glossitis, sore mouth and tongue, pallor, neurological conditions such as depression and dizziness, weight loss, nausea, constipation
C	*Men: 90 mg* *Women: 75 mg*	Bleeding gums; loose teeth; easy bruising; poor wound healing; scurvy; dry, itchy skin
Folate (folic acid)	*Adults: 400 mcg*	Impaired cell division and protein synthesis, megaloblastic anemia, anorexia, fatigue, sore tongue, diarrhea, forgetfulness

GI, gastrointestinal; *IU,* international units.
*1 retinol equivalent = 10 international units vitamin A activity from β-carotene or 3.33 international units vitamin A activity from retinol.

absorption of calcium; ingestion of high levels of vitamin C enhances the absorption of iron, which can lead to iron toxicity. To avoid harmful adverse effects, patients should be encouraged to discuss vitamin and mineral supplementation with their dietitian, pharmacist, and health care provider before using such supplements.

Major Nutrients

The major nutritional constituents of foods are carbohydrates (and fibre), fats, proteins, vitamins, minerals, and water. Carbohydrates, fats, and proteins provide energy. Vitamins, minerals, and water do not provide energy; some serve as structure (e.g., calcium in bones), and all assist in body processes such as food digestion, muscle movement, waste disposal, growth of new tissues (e.g., wound healing), and energy production (from carbohydrates, proteins, and fats). An individual's daily calorie requirements are influenced by body composition, age, gender, and physical activity. Adjustments in caloric intake are necessary when there are changes in a person's health status and daily activity level. An average adult requires an estimated 20 to 35 kcal/kg of body weight per day; amounts lean toward the higher end if the person is critically ill or very active and the lower end if the person is sedentary (American Society of Parenteral and Enteral Nutrition, 2016). (*Kilocalorie* is the correct unit to designate caloric intake and expenditure; however, *calorie* is the term more commonly used.)

Carbohydrates, the body's primary source of energy, yield approximately 4 kcal/g. Carbohydrates are classified as simple or complex. *Simple* carbohydrates include *monosaccharides* (e.g., glucose and fructose), found in fruits and honey, and *disaccharides* (e.g., sucrose, maltose, and lactose), found in foods such as table sugar, milk, and dairy products. Diets high in sugar (natural and processed) are associated with a higher risk of dental decay, weight gain, overweight, obesity, and type 2 diabetes (Health Canada (2021a). Canada's Dietary Reference Guidelines recommend reducing intake of added sugars (defined as "all sugars added to foods and beverages during processing or preparation") and free sugars (defined as "added sugars as well as sugars naturally present in honey, syrups, fruit juices, and fruit juice concentrates") (Health Canada, 2021a). *Complex* carbohydrates, or *polysaccharides*, include starches such as cereal grains, potatoes, and legumes. Carbohydrates are the chief protein-sparing ingredients in a nutritionally sound diet. Dietary reference intake recommendations for carbohydrates for healthy adults are that they get 45 to 65% of their total calories from carbohydrate food sources, especially foods rich in complex carbohydrates and fibre (Institute of Medicine, 2005).

Fibre is the indigestible part of plant foods. Diets rich in fibre are associated with improved blood cholesterol and blood glucose levels, healthy bowel function, and healthy body weight (Table 42.2).

Fats are stored in adipose tissue and the abdominal cavity. Besides being a major source of energy, fats act as insulation, which reduces the loss of body heat in cold environments and provides padding and protection for vital organs. Fats also act as carriers of essential fatty acids (linoleic and alpha-linolenic) and fat-soluble vitamins (A, D, E, and K). Fats provide a feeling of satiety after eating. A healthy diet containing 25 to 35% of total calories from fat is recommended for healthy adults. *Canada's Food Guide* recommends that most fat choices be unsaturated

TABLE 42.2   DIETARY REFERENCE INTAKE (DRI) FOR FIBRE

	Grams of Fibre per Day
Men 19–50 years of age	38
Men ≥51 years of age	30
Women 19–50 years of age	25
Women ≥51 years of age	21

fat and that saturated fat intake be minimized, to decrease the risk of heart disease (Health Canada, 2021b). One gram of fat yields nine calories.

Dietary fat is composed of four types of fatty acids: polyunsaturated, monounsaturated, saturated, and trans fats. Monounsaturated and polyunsaturated fats lower the risk of heart disease. *Polyunsaturated* fats, including omega-3 and omega-6 fats, are essential to good health. These fatty acids are not synthesized by the body and must be obtained from the diet. Omega-6 essential fatty acids are found in vegetable oils such as corn, sunflower, and soybean oils; primary sources of omega-3 fatty acids are fatty fish, flaxseed, and some nuts. *Monounsaturated* fats are found in vegetable oils, including olive and canola oils.

Saturated fats are found naturally in both vegetable- and animal-based foods, including coconut and palm oil and butter and full-fat animal-milk products. *Trans* fats are found naturally in some animal-based foods. Health Canada banned the use of trans fat, in the form of partially hydrogenated oils, in foods in 2018 (Health Canada, 2019a).

Saturated and trans fats increase the risk for heart disease because they raise serum low-density lipoprotein (LDL) cholesterol levels ("bad" cholesterol) (Health Canada, 2021b; Leech, 2018). Trans fats are particularly dangerous because they also reduce levels of high-density lipoprotein (HDL) cholesterol ("good" cholesterol) (Leech, 2018).

Proteins, another essential component of a well-balanced diet, can be obtained from both animal and plant sources. Proteins are vital for tissue growth, repair, and maintenance; body regulatory functions; and energy production. Ideally, proteins provide 10 to 35% of daily caloric needs. The recommended daily intake (RDI) for protein is 0.8 to 1 g/kg of body weight. One gram of protein yields four calories. Proteins are complex nitrogenous organic compounds, of which amino acids are the fundamental units of structure. The 22 amino acids can be classified as *essential* and *nonessential*. The body is capable of synthesizing nonessential amino acids if an adequate supply of protein is available. The nine essential amino acids must be provided through dietary sources. Protein sources containing all the essential amino acids are considered to be high-quality proteins that are easier to digest. Animal-based proteins are easier to digest and contain all essential amino acids as compared to plant-based proteins (Berrazaga et al., 2019). Healthy eating guidelines encourage the regular consumption of plant-based proteins such as legumes, nuts, seeds, and tofu (Health Canada, 2021a).

Grain products also contribute to protein intake. Plant-based proteins such as legumes and grains lack one or more of the essential amino acids and are more difficult to digest. These types of proteins are called *incomplete proteins*. The digestion difficulty can be overcome by combining high-protein

TABLE 42.3	GOOD SOURCES OF PROTEIN
Complete Proteins	**Incomplete Proteins**
• Eggs • Fish • Dairy products (e.g., cheese) • Meats • Poultry	• Grains (e.g., corn) • Legumes (e.g., navy beans, soybeans, peas) • Nuts (e.g., peanuts) • Seeds (e.g., sesame seeds, sunflower seeds)

TABLE 42.4	MAJOR MINERALS AND TRACE ELEMENTS
Major Minerals	**Trace Elements**
• Calcium • Chloride • Magnesium • Phosphorus • Potassium • Sodium • Sulphur	• Chromium • Copper • Fluoride • Iodine • Iron • Manganese • Molybdenum • Selenium • Zinc

plant-based foods. This concept is called *mutual supplementation*. Mutual supplementation is the strategy of combining two incomplete protein sources so that the amino acids in one food compensate for the missing ones in the other food. See Table 42.3 for a list of good sources of protein.

Vitamins are organic compounds required in small amounts for normal metabolism. Vitamins function primarily in enzyme reactions that facilitate the metabolism of amino acids, fats, and carbohydrates. Vitamins are divided into two categories: *water-soluble* vitamins (vitamin C and the B-complex vitamins) and *fat-soluble* vitamins (vitamins A, D, E, and K). Vitamin D in particular has received widespread attention because of a growing body of evidence that suggests it may have a beneficial effect on some types of cancer, especially colorectal cancer, and on other immune-related diseases (Canadian Cancer Society, 2021). Since the body stores fat-soluble vitamins, consuming too much of them can result in toxicity. Upper limits have been established for vitamins A, D, and E.

Mineral salts (e.g., magnesium, iron, calcium) make up approximately 4% of total body weight. Minerals present in minute amounts are referred to as *trace elements*. Minerals required in amounts greater than 100 mg/day are called *major minerals*. Minerals are necessary to build tissues, regulate body fluids, and assist in various body functions. Some minerals are stored and can be toxic if taken in excess amounts. The daily requirement for minerals varies greatly, from a few micrograms of trace minerals to 1 g or more of the major minerals, such as calcium, phosphorus, and sodium. Table 42.4 lists the major minerals and trace elements. A well-balanced diet based on *Canada's Food Guide* will typically meet the daily requirements for minerals.

Vegetarian Diet

The common element among all vegetarians is the exclusion of meat, poultry, game, fish, shellfish or crustaceans, and meat by-products from the diet. Vegetarians base their diet on convictions founded in religious or cultural beliefs, respect for all living beings, ethical–ecological ideals, economics, or food preferences. *Vegans* eat only plant-based food, whereas *lacto-ovo-vegetarians* eat plant-based foods as well as animal-based milk products and eggs.

Vegetarians can be at risk for vitamin, mineral, or protein deficiencies unless their diets are well planned. Plant-based protein sources, although of a lesser quality than that of animal origin, fulfill most of the protein requirements in a vegetarian diet. Combinations of vegetable-protein foods (e.g., rice and kidney beans) can increase digestibility and nutritional quality. Lacto-ovo-vegetarians can obtain protein from milk products and eggs. Plant-based milk alternatives, including soy milk and nut-based milks, are fortified with calcium and vitamin D. Soy milk is a reliable source of protein, while nut-based milks contain almost no protein. Many palatable meat analogue products

TABLE 42.5	NUTRITIONAL THERAPY

Foods High in Iron

These foods provide 25–39% of the dietary reference intake (DRI) of iron.

Food	Serving Size
Breads, Cereals, and Grain Products	
Farina, regular or quick-cooked (enriched)	160 mL (⅔ cup)
Oatmeal, instant, fortified, prepared (enriched)	160 mL (⅔ cup)
Ready-to-eat cereals, fortified (enriched)	30 g (1 oz.)
Meat, Poultry, Fish, and Alternatives	
Beef liver, braised	90 g (3 oz.)
Pork liver, braised	90 g (3 oz.)
Chicken or turkey liver, braised	125 mL (½ cup), diced
Clams: steamed, boiled, or canned (drained)	90 g (3oz.)
Oysters: baked, broiled, steamed, or canned (undrained)	90 g (3oz.)
Soybeans, cooked	125 mL (½ cup)

are now available for individuals following a vegetarian diet, but as with all food choices, it is important to read food labels to avoid foods high in added sodium and sugar.

The primary risk for nutrient deficiency in a strict vegan is the lack of cobalamin (vitamin B$_{12}$). Vegans not taking cobalamin supplements or consuming foods fortified with cobalamin are susceptible to the development of megaloblastic anemia and the neurological signs of cobalamin deficiency. Strict vegetarians and lacto-ovo-vegetarians are also at risk for iron deficiency. Non-heme iron found in plant-based foods such as legumes, dark-green leafy vegetables, iron-fortified cereals, and whole grains and cereals is less well absorbed than the heme-based iron found in animal foods. Table 42.5 lists examples of foods high in iron. Consuming foods rich in vitamin C (e.g., citrus fruits, tomatoes, potatoes, peppers, and strawberries) will enhance the absorption of non-heme iron from plant-based iron-rich foods.

CULTURALLY COMPETENT CARE

Culture is a determinant of health (Earle, 2011). People's unique cultural heritages may affect their eating customs and nutritional status. Each culture has its own beliefs and behaviours related to food and the role that food plays in the etiology and treatment of disease. In addition, culture and religion can influence what food is considered edible, as well as how it is prepared and when it is eaten. It is important to consider cultural, religious, and ethnic influences when assessing a patient's nutritional status and suggesting interventions requiring dietary changes. It is also important that the nurse avoid *cultural stereotyping* by making assumptions or generalizations about diet based on an individual's cultural background, as culture is not homogeneous. Indigenous people in Canada have undergone a significant nutritional transition whereby traditional diets have been replaced with foods and eating patterns associated with increased risk of chronic disease (Earle, 2011). Evidence is emerging that shows intakes of traditional foods are beneficial both from a nutritional and mental health perspective. Studies have noted that First Nations, Dene, Métis, and Inuit peoples in the Arctic have higher intakes of riboflavin, iron, zinc, copper, magnesium, manganese, phosphorus, potassium, selenium, and vitamins A, D, E, and B_6 when they eat traditional foods than when traditional foods are not consumed (Earle, 2011). Additionally, the activities associated with traditional diets promote the practice of cultural values, community and social cohesion, and the passing down of cultural traditions (Earle, 2011).

MALNUTRITION

Malnutrition is a deficit, excess, or imbalance of the essential components of a balanced diet. Malnutrition can refer to alterations in *macronutrients* (carbohydrates, proteins, and fat) or *micronutrients* (electrolytes, minerals, and vitamins). The terms *undernutrition* and *overnutrition* are also used to describe malnutrition.

Undernutrition affects body tissues, functional ability, and overall health (Allard et al., 2015). Undernutrition does exist in Canada, where income-related food insecurity is increasingly acknowledged as a key social determinant of health. Malnutrition is a problem in both developing and developed countries and across the continuum of care (community, hospital, long-term care). The prevalence of malnutrition in Canadian hospitals has been reported to be 15 to 75% (Allard et al., 2015).

Etiology of Malnutrition

Several terms describe the types and causes of adult malnutrition. **Protein–calorie malnutrition (PCM)** is the most common form of undernutrition. The following etiology-based terms are preferred for use in clinical practice settings, as they indicate the interaction and importance of inflammation on nutritional status (White et al., 2012).

- *Starvation-related malnutrition*, or primary PCM, occurs when nutritional needs are not met (Figure 42.2). In primary PCM, there is chronic starvation without inflammation (e.g., anorexia nervosa).
- *Chronic disease–related malnutrition*, or secondary PCM, is associated with conditions that have sustained mild to moderate inflammation. It occurs when dietary intake does not meet tissue needs because of disease, although it would under normal conditions. Examples of conditions associated with this type of malnutrition include organ failure, cancer, rheumatoid arthritis, obesity, and metabolic syndrome.
- *Acute disease– or injury-related malnutrition* is associated with acute disease or injury states with a marked inflammatory response (e.g., major infection, burns, trauma, surgery).

Many factors contribute to the development of malnutrition, including socioeconomic factors, physical illnesses, incomplete diets, food–medication interactions, and psychological illnesses

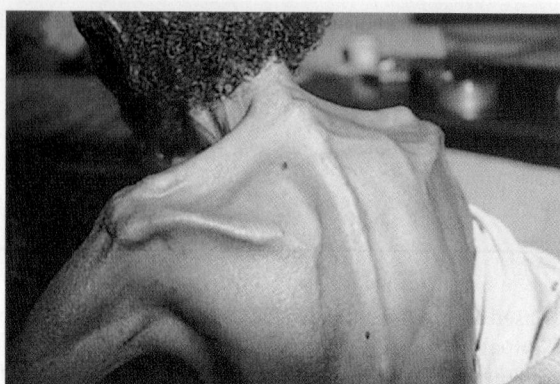

FIG. 42.2 Patient with malnutrition. Source: Morgan, S. L., & Weiniser, R. (1998). *Fundamentals of clinical nutrition* (2nd ed.). Mosby.

TABLE 42.6	CONDITIONS THAT INCREASE THE RISK FOR MALNUTRITION

- Alcohol use disorder
- Decreased mobility that limits access to food or its preparation
- Dementia
- Depression
- Medications with antinutrient or catabolic properties, such as corticosteroids and oral antibiotics
- Excessive dieting to lose weight
- Need for nutrients because of hypermetabolism or stresses such as infection, burns, trauma, or fever
- No oral intake, receiving standard intravenous solutions (e.g., 5% dextrose), or both for 5 days
- Nutrient losses from malabsorption, dialysis, fistulas, or wounds
- Swallowing disorders (e.g., neurological conditions, head and neck cancer, stroke)

such as eating disorders. Table 42.6 lists conditions that increase the risk of malnutrition.

Socioeconomic Factors. At every stage of the life cycle, health is directly or indirectly influenced by key determinants of health such as education and literacy, income and social status, employment and working conditions, and social environments (Health Canada, 2020a). Although the health of Canadians is considered to be very good by international standards, a number of factors influence overall quality of life, including the aging of the population; increasing survival rates for potentially fatal conditions; and changes in behaviours related to eating, physical activity, and the use of substances such as drugs, tobacco, and alcohol.

Food security is defined as "a situation that exists when all people, at all times, have physical, social and economic access to sufficient, safe and nutritious food that meets their dietary needs and food preferences for an active and healthy life" (Food and Agriculture Organization of the United Nations et al., 2018, p. 159). Individuals or families with limited financial resources may have *food insecurity* (inadequate access). Food insecurity is problematic, as it affects the overall quality (i.e., nutritional value) and quantity of food that is available. Families with food insecurity often choose less expensive "filling" foods, which are more energy-dense (high fat) and less nutritious. This type of diet increases the risk of nutrient deficiencies.

Older people on a fixed income may have an added burden of deciding whether to pay for medications or to buy food. Nurses and dietitians need to screen for food security concerns when completing patient assessments, and when concerned, appropriate referrals to community assistance programs should be made. Additionally, the nurse and the dietitian can assist patients in selecting foods that meet nutritional requirements while staying within their limited resources.

Physical Illnesses. Regardless of the illness, an individual who is ill has increased nutritional needs. Pathological conditions are frequently aggravated by undernutrition, and an existing nutrient deficiency is likely to become more severe during illness. Malnutrition is a common consequence of illness, surgery, injury, or hospitalization. Hospitalized patients, especially older persons, are at risk of becoming malnourished. Prolonged illness, major surgery, sepsis, draining wounds, burns, hemorrhage, fractures, and immobilization can all contribute to malnutrition.

Anorexia, nausea, vomiting, diarrhea, abdominal distension, and cramping may accompany diseases of the gastrointestinal (GI) system. Any combination of these symptoms interferes with usual food consumption and metabolism. Whereas *anorexia* is a loss of normal appetite and may occur as a result of physical or mental illness, *cachexia* refers to a wasting syndrome that causes weakness and loss of weight, fat, and muscle. Cachexia is a major cause of morbidity and mortality in patients with cancer or other serious long-term illnesses such as chronic obstructive pulmonary disease (COPD).

Fever accompanies many illnesses, injuries, and infections, with a concomitant increase in the body's basal metabolic rate (BMR) and nitrogen loss. Each degree of temperature increase on the Celsius scale raises the BMR by about 13%. Without an increase in caloric intake, the body uses protein stores to supply calories and protein depletion develops. After the body temperature returns to normal, the rate of protein breakdown and resynthesis may be increased for several weeks.

It is important to consider the nutritional requirements of a patient who is not overtly ill but is undergoing diagnostic studies. This patient may be nutritionally fit on entering the hospital but can become malnourished because of the dietary restrictions and missed meals imposed by multiple diagnostic studies.

Malabsorption syndrome is the impaired absorption of nutrients from the GI tract. Decreases in digestive enzymes or in bowel surface area can quickly lead to a deficiency state. Many medications have undesirable GI adverse effects and alter normal digestive and absorptive processes. Antibiotic use appears to modify the intestinal microbiome in the normal state. Research suggests that the microbiome likely plays a critical role in the healthy human immune system and metabolism (Lazar et al., 2018).

Use of Probiotics. The Food and Agriculture Organization of the United Nations and the World Health Organization define probiotics as "living microorganisms, which when administered in adequate amounts confer health benefits on the host" (National Centre for Complementary and Integrative Health, 2019). Research suggests that changes in the gut microbiota may increase a person's predisposition to certain diseases (Zhang et al., 2015). Dietary nutrients may be converted into metabolites by intestinal microbes that serve as biologically active molecules, which affect regulatory functions in the host. Probiotics may restore the composition of the gut microbiome and introduce beneficial functions to gut microbial communities, resulting in amelioration or prevention of gut inflammation (Kim et al., 2019).

Incomplete Diets. Most vitamin deficiencies are rare in most developed countries. When present, vitamin deficiencies may involve several vitamins. When vitamin imbalances occur because of incomplete diets, they are often found among people with a pattern of alcohol or drug use; people who are food insecure, chronically ill, or receiving cancer treatment; and individuals who maintain nutritionally inadequate dietary practices. People who have had GI surgery may be at risk for vitamin deficiencies related to decreased nutrient absorption. For example, resection of the terminal ileum poses a risk for deficiencies of fat-soluble vitamins. After a gastrectomy, patients require cobalamin (vitamin B_{12}) supplementation. Individuals following fad or restrictive diets or those with poorly planned vegetarian diets are also at risk.

Clinical manifestations of vitamin imbalances are often exhibited as neurological manifestations. In the growing child, the central nervous system (CNS) is primarily involved, whereas the peripheral nervous system is most often affected in adults. The recommended DRIs and manifestations of deficiencies are presented in Table 42.1.

Medication–Nutrient Interactions. A *medication–nutrient interaction* occurs when a medication affects the use of nutrients in the body. Many medications may interact with food or beverages. Potential adverse interactions include incompatibilities, altered medication effectiveness, and impaired nutritional status. For example, many medications produce adverse effects such as changes in taste, changes in appetite, and nausea. Grapefruit juice can increase the absorption of some medications, enhancing their effect. Individuals taking thyroid replacement hormone (e.g., levothyroxine [Synthroid]) have been instructed to avoid taking milk products, antacids, or iron preparations within 1 hour of taking their medication.

Medication–nutrient interactions can also occur with over-the-counter medications and herbal and dietary supplements. The role of the interdisciplinary team is to monitor and prevent these potential interactions for patients while in the hospital and after discharge.

Eating Disorders. Eating disorders are complex psychiatric disorders strongly associated with other mental illnesses, such as mood, personality, and anxiety disorders. Society's promotion of an ideal body image has also been implicated. Eating disorders have the highest mortality rate of any mental illness. According to the National Initiative for Eating Disorders (NIED) (2018), approximately 1 million Canadians meet the diagnostic criteria for an eating disorder, with an even larger number of individuals reporting symptoms that are seriously debilitating but insufficient for diagnosis. Younger Canadians engage in dieting behaviours that may put them at risk of developing an eating disorder or other health-related conditions (NIED, 2018). Eating disorders involve a serious disturbance in eating behaviour, in addition to disturbances in perception of body size and shape. There is a growing recognition that eating disorders are not exclusively experienced by women, with up to 20% of patients with an eating disorder identifying as male (Kinnaird, 2019). It is important to approach treatment on a person-centred basis to avoid gender-based bias.

The *female athlete triad* is a syndrome in which eating disorders, amenorrhea, and osteoporosis are present (Gottschlich, 2017). The triad is seen in females participating in sports that emphasize leanness and low body weight. It is important to note that eating disorders routinely go undetected in clinical settings. Although anorexia nervosa often presents with emaciation, other clinically significant eating disorders can present without any physical signs or laboratory abnormalities. Clinical detection may rely on a patient's willingness and ability to share information about body and weight concerns and food-related behaviours. Restriction of food intake by an individual with obesity may be a risk factor and a comorbidity for eating disorders. Assumptions about body weight should not preclude screening for disordered eating behaviours (Nicholls & Becker, 2020).

Anorexia Nervosa. Anorexia nervosa is a serious, often chronic, and life-threatening eating disorder characterized by self-imposed weight loss, endocrine dysfunction, and a distorted psychopathological attitude toward weight and eating (National Eating Disorder Information Centre [NEDIC], 2021a). It manifests clinically as abnormal weight loss, deliberate self-starvation, intense fear of gaining weight or becoming fat, lanugo (soft, downy hair covering the body except the palms and soles), refusal to eat, continuous dieting, hair loss, sensitivity to cold, compulsive exercising, absent or irregular menstruation, dry skin, and constipation. Diagnostic studies often show iron-deficiency anemia and an elevated serum urea (nitrogen) level that reflects marked intravascular volume depletion and prerenal azotemia. A lack of potassium in the diet and loss of potassium in the urine lead to potassium deficiency resulting in muscle weakness, cardiac dysrhythmias, and renal failure. If the eating pattern continues for a prolonged time, body wasting with signs of severe malnutrition becomes evident, and death may be imminent.

🔍 EVIDENCE-INFORMED PRACTICE

Research Highlight

What Is the Efficacy of Family Therapy Approaches for Anorexia Nervosa?

Clinical Question
In persons with anorexia nervosa (P), is family therapy (I) effective in the treatment of anorexia nervosa (O)?

Synthesis of Best Available Evidence
- Systematic review of randomized controlled trials (RCTs)
- Twenty-five RCTs of persons with a primary clinical diagnosis of anorexia nervosa. Sixteen studies were of adolescents, eight studies were of adults, and one study included both. Most trials investigated family-based therapies. The main outcome measure was remission, and secondary outcome measures were weight, eating disorder psychopathology, dropouts, relapse, or family functioning measures.
- There was no indication that the age group studies had any impact on the overall treatment effect.

Conclusions
- There is evidence to suggest that family therapy approaches may be more effective than any other type of intervention, but evidence was insufficient to determine whether one type of family therapy approach is more effective than others.

Implications for Nursing Practice
- Why is it important for health care providers to facilitate alternative methods of treatment that embrace family therapy and family-centred care?

Reference for Evidence
Fisher, C., Skocic, S., Rutherford, K., et al. (2019). Family therapy approaches for anorexia nervosa. *Cochrane Database of Systematic Reviews, 5,* CD004780. https://doi.org/10.1002/14651858.CD004780.pub4.
P, patient population of interest; *I,* intervention or area of interest; *O,* outcome(s) of interest (see Chapter 1).

Multidisciplinary treatment involving health care providers competent in treatment of eating disorders must involve a combination of nutritional support and psychiatric care. Although most of the treatment for eating disorders is provided in the community, hospitalization may be necessary for patients with severe physical or metabolic complications that cannot be managed in an outpatient setting. Nutritional replenishment must be closely supervised to ensure consistent and ongoing weight gain. Refeeding syndrome (discussed later in the chapter) is a rare but serious complication of refeeding programs. The use of enteral or parenteral feedings may be necessary. Improved nutrition is not a cure for anorexia nervosa; the underlying psychiatric problem must be identified and addressed.

Bulimia Nervosa. Bulimia nervosa is an eating disorder characterized by periods of food restriction, followed by binge eating, with recurrent compensatory behaviours such as purging or restriction, accompanied by feelings of loss of control and a persistent concern with body image (NEDIC, 2021b). Individuals with bulimia nervosa often fall within a *normal* weight range, but weight may fluctuate with bingeing and purging. They may use diet drugs, laxatives, or diuretics, or they may exercise excessively. Warning signs of frequent vomiting include macerated knuckles, swollen salivary glands, broken blood vessels in the eyes, and dental problems. Abnormal laboratory parameters, including hypokalemia, metabolic alkalosis, and elevated serum amylase, may occur with frequent vomiting (Westmoreland et al., 2016).

Causes of bulimia remain unclear. Substance abuse, anxiety, affective disorders, and personality disturbances have been reported among persons with bulimia. Patients with bulimia often go to great lengths to conceal abnormal eating habits. As the behaviour persists, many problems associated with the condition become increasingly hard for patients to deal with effectively.

Treatment for bulimia requires a combination of psychological counselling and nutrition therapy. Support groups such as the National Eating Disorder Information Centre (NEDIC) (see the Resources at the end of this chapter) are helpful to those affected by these disorders. The therapeutic relationship between the patient and care providers is essential in the care and management of eating disorders. Care providers must be competent in eating disorder treatment, to ensure that appropriate and safe treatment and follow-up are provided.

Pathophysiology of Starvation

Knowledge of the pathophysiology of the starvation process is useful in understanding the physiological changes that occur in PCM. Initially, the body selectively uses carbohydrates (glycogen) rather than fat and protein to meet metabolic needs. These carbohydrate stores, found in the liver and muscles, are minimal and may be depleted within 18 hours. During this early phase of starvation, the only use of protein is in its obligatory participation in cellular metabolism. However, once carbohydrate stores are depleted, protein begins to be converted to glucose for energy. The resulting available plasma glucose allows the metabolic processes to continue. As the body uses amino acids for energy, a negative nitrogen balance (greater nitrogen excretion) occurs. However, within 5 to 9 days, body fat is fully mobilized to supply much of the needed energy.

In prolonged starvation, up to 97% of calories are provided by fat, and protein is conserved. Once fat stores are depleted (approximately 4 to 6 weeks), protein, including that from internal organs and plasma, can no longer be spared and rapidly decreases, as it is the only remaining source of energy.

If malnourished patients have surgery, experience bodily trauma, or have an infection, the stress response, with a concomitant increase in energy expenditure, is superimposed on the starvation response, resulting in an increase in the metabolic rate and a subsequent increase in energy requirements. Protein stores are no longer spared and are used with increasing frequency to meet the demands of the increased metabolic needs.

As protein depletion continues, liver function becomes impaired, and synthesis of protein decreases. As a result of this decrease, the plasma oncotic pressure decreases, and body fluids shift from the vascular space into the interstitial compartment. As protein ingestion decreases and body stores are depleted, albumin eventually leaks into the interstitial space along with the fluid. Edema becomes clinically observable, and when present in the face and the legs of a patient, it often masks underlying wasting of muscle.

With the shift of fluids to the interstitial space, ions also move. Sodium (a predominant extracellular ion) is found in increased amounts within the cell, and potassium (a predominant intracellular ion) and magnesium shift to the extracellular space. The sodium–potassium exchange pump has high energy needs, using 20 to 50% of all calories ingested. When the diet is extremely deficient in calories and essential proteins, the pump will fail, leaving sodium inside the cell (along with water), and the cell will expand, resulting in edema.

The liver is the organ that loses the most mass during protein deprivation. It gradually becomes infiltrated with fat, secondary to decreased synthesis of lipoproteins. Immediate intervention is required, or death will rapidly ensue.

Clinical Manifestations

The clinical manifestations of malnutrition range from mild to emaciation and death. The most obvious signs on physical examination are apparent in the skin (dry and scaly skin, brittle nails, rashes, hair loss), mouth (crusting and ulceration, changes in tongue), muscles (decreased mass and weakness), and CNS (mental changes such as confusion, irritability). The speed at which malnutrition develops depends on the quantity and quality of the protein intake, caloric value, illness, and the person's age.

The manifestations of malnutrition result from numerous interactions at the cellular level. As protein intake declines, the muscles (which are the largest store of protein in the body) become wasted and flabby. This wasting away leads to weakness and fatigability. Decreased protein is available for tissue repair, causing delayed wound healing. The person becomes more susceptible to infections. Both humoral and cell-mediated immunity are deficient. Leukocytes in the peripheral blood decrease. Many malnourished people are anemic, generally because of nutritional deficiencies in iron and folic acid (necessary building blocks for red blood cells).

NURSING AND INTERPROFESSIONAL MANAGEMENT MALNUTRITION

NURSING ASSESSMENT

Regardless of setting, the nurse must be aware of the nutritional status of the patient. The nurse is often the first-line health care provider for a patient. The patient's height, weight, and diet history are important components of all assessments. Nutritional status may well be a major factor in the outcome of, and perhaps the underlying reason for, many illnesses.

Nutrition screening, the first step in assessing nutritional status, can be completed in any setting (e.g., clinic, home, hospital, long-term care facilities). Based on readily obtained data, nutrition screening is an efficient way to identify individuals at nutrition risk, including those who have experienced unintentional weight loss, inadequate food intake, or recent illness. Results of nutrition screening are used to determine whether a more detailed nutrition assessment is necessary (Table 42.7). A variety of valid tools, such as the Canadian Nutrition Screening Tool (CNST), is available for screening different populations (Figure 42.3).

ASSESSMENT OF NUTRITIONAL INTAKE. Individuals identified as being at nutritional risk during screening should be referred, when possible, to a dietitian to undergo a *comprehensive nutritional assessment*, which includes evaluation of dietary history and clinical information, physical examination, and anthropometric measures.

Various methods for collecting current dietary intake information are available, including the 24-hour recall, food frequency questionnaire, and food diary. Documentation of nutritional intake for hospitalized patients can best be achieved through calorie counts of nutrients consumed or infused.

The 24-Hour Recall. The most common method of obtaining information about dietary intake is the *24-hour recall*. The individual or family member is asked to recall everything eaten within the past 24 hours. It is important to be aware of potential information gaps when this method is used: (a) the individual or family member may not be able to recall type or amount of food eaten; (b) intake within the past 24 hours may be atypical of usual intake; (c) the individual or family member may alter the truth for a variety of reasons; and (d) snack items and use of added fat, sugar or salt, and condiments may be underreported.

The Food Frequency Questionnaire. To counter some of the challenges inherent in the 24-hour recall method, a *food frequency questionnaire* may also be completed. Information is collected regarding how many times per day, week, or month an individual eats particular foods. The food frequency questionnaire does not quantify the amount of food eaten, and, like the 24-hour recall, it relies on the individual's or family member's memory.

The Food Diary. Food diaries require the individual or family member to write down everything consumed for a certain period of time. Three days—2 working and 1 nonworking day—are customarily used. A food diary is most accurate if the individual is instructed to record information immediately after eating. Potential challenges with the food diary include (a) nonadherence, (b) inaccurate recording, (c) atypical intake on the recording days, and (d) conscious alteration of diet during the recording period.

Direct Observation. *Direct observation* of the feeding and eating process can lead to detection of problems not readily identified through standard nutrition interviews. For example, observing the typical feeding techniques used by a parent or caregiver and the interaction between the individual and the caregiver can be of value when assessing failure to thrive in children or unintentional weight loss in older persons. Observation of food intake may also identify any problems with chewing or swallowing.

TABLE 42.7   NURSING ASSESSMENT
Malnutrition

Subjective Data
Important Health Information

Current health: ↑ or ↓ weight, weight problems; ↑ or ↓ appetite, typical dietary intake; food preferences and aversions; food allergies or intolerances; ill-fitting or absent dentures; dry mouth, difficulty in chewing or swallowing; bloating or gas; ↑ sensitivity to cold; delayed wound healing; constipation, diarrhea, nocturia, decreased urinary output

Past health history: Severe burns, major trauma, hemorrhage, draining wounds, bone fractures with prolonged immobility, chronic renal or liver disease, cancer, malabsorption syndrome, GI obstruction, infectious diseases (e.g., TB, AIDS), acute (e.g., trauma, sepsis) or chronic (e.g., rheumatoid arthritis) inflammatory condition

Medications: Corticosteroids, chemotherapeutic agents, diet pills

Surgery or other treatments: Recent surgery, radiation

Functional assessment: ↑ or ↓ activity patterns; weakness, fatigue, ↓ endurance; alcohol or drug misuse; change in family (e.g., loss of a spouse); financial resources

Objective Data
General

Listless, cachectic; underweight for height

Integumentary

Dry, brittle, sparse hair with colour changes and lack of lustre, alopecia; dry, scaly lips, fever blisters, angular crusts and lesions at corners of mouth (cheilosis); brittle, ridged nails; ↓ tone and elasticity of skin; cool, rough, dry, scaly skin with brown-grey pigment changes; reddened, scaly dermatitis, scrotal dermatitis; slight cyanosis; peripheral edema

Eyes

Pale or red conjunctivae, grey keratinized epithelium on conjunctiva (Bitot's spots); dryness and dull appearance of conjunctiva and cornea, soft cornea; blood vessel growth in cornea; redness and fissuring of eyelid corners

Respiratory

↓ respiratory rate, ↓ vital capacity, crackles, weak cough

Cardiovascular

↑ or ↓ heart rate, ↓ BP, dysrhythmias

Gastrointestinal (GI)

Swollen, smooth, raw, beefy red tongue (glossitis), hypertrophic or atrophic papillae; dental caries, absent or loose teeth, discoloured tooth enamel; spongy, pale, receded gums with a tendency to bleed easily, periodontal disease; ulcerations, white patches or plaques, redness, swelling of oral mucosa; distended, tympanic abdomen; ascites, hepatomegaly, ↓ bowel sounds; steatorrhea

Neurological

Decreased or loss of reflexes, tremor; inattention, irritability, confusion, syncope

Musculoskeletal

↓ muscle mass with poor tone, "wasted" appearance; bow legs, knock knees, beaded ribs, chest deformity, prominent bony structures

Possible Diagnostic Findings

↓ hemoglobin and hematocrit; ↓ MCV, MCH, or MCHC (iron deficiency); ↑ MCV or MCH (folic acid or cobalamin deficiency); altered serum electrolyte levels, especially hyperkalemia; ↓ BUN (serum urea [nitrogen]) and creatinine; ↓ serum albumin, transferrin, and prealbumin; ↓ lymphocytes; ↑ liver enzymes; ↓ serum vitamin levels

AIDS, acquired immune deficiency syndrome; *BP,* blood pressure; *BUN,* blood urea nitrogen; *GI,* gastrointestinal; *MCH,* mean corpuscular hemoglobin; *MCHC,* mean corpuscular hemoglobin concentration; *MCV,* mean corpuscular volume; *TB,* tuberculosis.

	Date:		Date:	
	Admission		**Rescreening**	
Ask the patient the following questions*	Yes	No	Yes	No
Have you lost weight in the past 6 months **WITHOUT TRYING** to lose this weight? If the patient reports a weight loss but gained it back, consider it as NO weight loss.				
Have you been eating less than usual **FOR MORE THAN A WEEK**?				
Two "YES" answers indicate nutrition risk				

* If the patient is unable to answer the questions, a knowledgeable informant can be used to obtain the information. If the patient is uncertain regarding weight loss, ask if clothing is now fitting more loosely.

FIG. 42.3 Canadian Nutrition Screening Tool (CNST). Source: Canadian Malnutrition Task Force. (March 2014). *Canadian nutrition screening tool.* http://nutritioncareincanada.ca/sites/default/uploads/files/CNST.pdf

ASSESSING HEIGHT AND WEIGHT. Obtaining accurate height and weight measurements is critical. When possible, the nurse should measure the patient's actual height rather than using self-reported data. For patients confined to a bed, a Luft ruler is used as an alternative to standing height.

When assessing weight, the nurse obtains a detailed weight history, noting weight changes over the previous 6 months. The nurse should ask whether weight changes were intentional or unintentional and the period over which changes took place. Whether the weight change was intentional or not is a critical indicator for further assessment, especially in older persons (Park et al., 2018). If involuntary weight loss exceeds 10% of the usual body weight, the reason needs to be determined. All patients should be assessed for unintentional weight loss, including patients assessed as obese, as latent malnutrition may be present despite excess body weight.

NURSING DIAGNOSES

Nursing diagnoses for the patient with malnutrition include but are not limited to the following:

- *Inadequate nutrition* resulting from *insufficient dietary intake* (decreased access, ingestion, digestion, or absorption of food)
- *Decrease in self- feeding ability* resulting from *fatigue, weakness, discomfort*
- *Inadequate fluid volume* resulting from *insufficient fluid intake* (access to or absorption of fluids)
- *Potential for impaired skin integrity* resulting from *inadequate nutrition*
- *Reduced health maintenance* resulting from *ineffective coping strategies, insufficient resources*

PLANNING

The overall goals are that the patient with malnutrition will (a) achieve weight gain, (b) consume appropriate energy (calories) and protein (with a diet individualized for the patient), and (c) have no adverse consequences related to malnutrition or nutrition therapies.

NURSING IMPLEMENTATION

HEALTH PROMOTION. Nurses are in an ideal position to teach and reinforce healthy eating habits with individuals throughout the lifespan. Nurses often collaborate with interprofessional health care team members (e.g., dietitians, social workers, physicians) in the nutritional assessment and health education of patients. They may use or refer patients to free local nutrition resources (see the Resources at the end of this chapter).

As part of the interprofessional team, the nurse can support a patient in improving their health status by reinforcing healthy eating habits throughout the lifespan. Nurses can help patients find reliable Internet-based resources that provide evidence-informed food and nutrition recommendations. Nurses can also encourage healthy eating by providing links to *Canada's Food Guide* and encouraging patients to read food labels. Nutrition labelling is mandatory on most prepackaged foods. The Nutrition Facts table (Figure 42.4) provides information on serving size, calories, core nutrients and % daily values (% DV). The % DV can be used as a guide to show you if the serving of stated size has a little or a lot of a nutrient. This information allows for the comparison of food products to help make informed food choices.

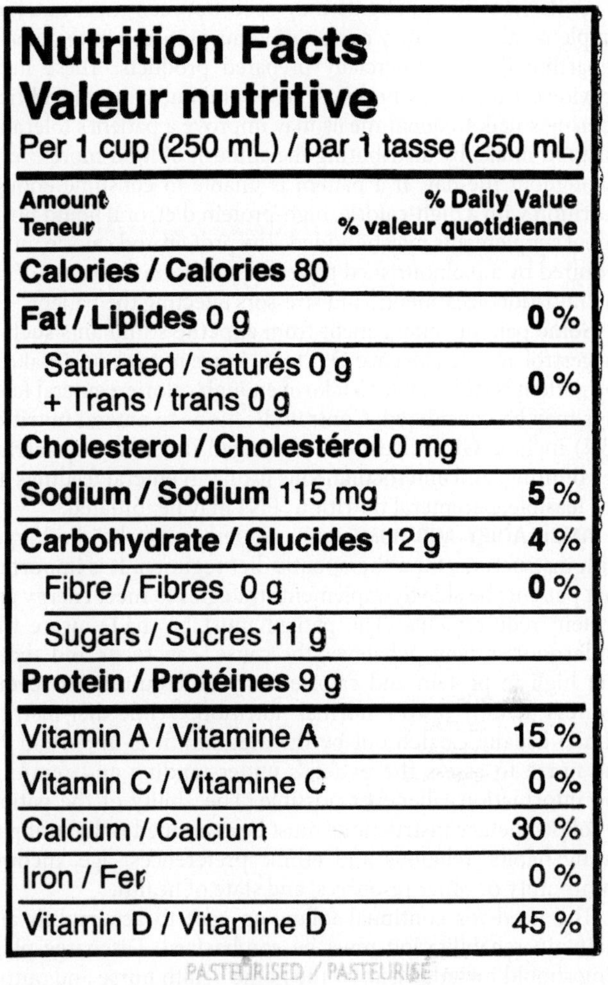

Nutrition Facts Valeur nutritive Per 1 cup (250 mL) / par 1 tasse (250 mL)	
Amount Teneur	% Daily Value % valeur quotidienne
Calories / Calories 80	
Fat / Lipides 0 g	0 %
Saturated / saturés 0 g + Trans / trans 0 g	0 %
Cholesterol / Cholestérol 0 mg	
Sodium / Sodium 115 mg	5 %
Carbohydrate / Glucides 12 g	4 %
Fibre / Fibres 0 g	0 %
Sugars / Sucres 11 g	
Protein / Protéines 9 g	
Vitamin A / Vitamine A	15 %
Vitamin C / Vitamine C	0 %
Calcium / Calcium	30 %
Iron / Fer	0 %
Vitamin D / Vitamine D	45 %

PASTEURISED / PASTEURISÉ

FIG. 42.4 Nutrition Facts table. More information on using food labels to make informed choices is available at https://food-guide.canada.ca. Source: iStock.com/Jamesmcq24.

ACUTE INTERVENTION. Nurses collaborate with the dietitian to identify nutrition risk and implement appropriate interventions to meet the patient's nutritional needs. The patient's nutritional state, including risk factors for malnutrition, should be assessed during the nurse's physical evaluation.

With increased stress, such as surgery, severe trauma, and sepsis, the patient needs more calories and protein. Wound healing requires increased protein synthesis. The patient who is malnourished or is at risk for malnutrition and is undergoing major surgery needs several weeks of increased protein and calorie intake preoperatively to promote healing and replenish body stores postoperatively. When fever is present, the metabolic rate increases and nitrogen loss accelerates. Despite the return of body temperature to normal, the rate of protein breakdown and resynthesis may be accelerated for several weeks.

A patient's weight and height should be recorded on admission and the weight routinely assessed and documented throughout a hospital stay. To ensure accuracy, the nurse should weigh the patient at the same time each day, on the same scale, with the same type or amount of clothing, and with an empty bladder. Patients and caregivers should be taught the importance of good nutrition and the reason for recording their daily weight, intake, and output.

Before discharge, the patient and caregiver need to be taught the importance of good nutrition and strategies to monitor nutrition risk at home. Rapid weight gain or loss are usually the result of shifts in fluid balance. In conjunction with accurate recording of food and fluid intake, the body weight provides a clearer picture of the patient's fluid and nutritional state.

If the patient is able to take food by mouth, obtaining a daily calorie count and food diary can help ensure an accurate record of food intake. The nurse and the dietitian can assist the patient and family in selecting high-calorie and high-protein foods (unless medically contraindicated). Offering foods preferred by the patient enhances intake, so the family should be encouraged to bring the patient's favourite foods from home.

The environment should be conducive to eating: quiet, with the bedside table cleared of clutter and set at the appropriate height, and urinals, bedpans, and emesis basins placed out of sight. The patient should be offered oral hygiene and hand hygiene and assisted into a comfortable position. If the patient needs help, the nurse should open cartons and packages. Nonurgent care should be performed before or after mealtime to avoid unnecessary interruptions.

Undernourished patients may need between-meal nutrition supplements. These may consist of items prepared in the dietary department or commercially prepared products. These items provide extra calories, proteins, fluids, and nutrients. In addition, offering small, frequent meals may improve a patient's tolerance for food intake by distributing the amount of food more evenly throughout the day. If a patient is unable to consume enough nutrition with a high-calorie, high-protein diet, oral liquid nutritional supplements may be added. The protein and calorie intake required by a malnourished patient depends on the cause of the malnutrition, treatments, and stressors affecting the patient.

Some patients may benefit from appetite stimulants such as megestrol acetate (Megace OS) to improve nutritional intake. If the patient is still unable to take in enough calories, enteral feedings may be considered. Contraindications to enteral nutrition (EN) include GI obstruction, prolonged ileus, severe diarrhea or vomiting, and enterocutaneous fistula. If enteral feedings are not feasible, parenteral nutrition (PN) may be initiated.

AMBULATORY AND HOME CARE. Patients may be discharged with instructions for a therapeutic diet regimen. It is important that patients be able to implement strategies to meet energy and protein requirements. The patient must be made aware that undernourishment, whatever the cause, can recur and that a diet high in protein and calories may be required for several months to fully restore normal nutrition. While diet instruction is usually carried out by the dietitian, it is important for the nurse to assess the patient's understanding and reinforce the information whenever possible. The ability of the patient to follow dietary instructions must be examined in light of past eating habits, religious and ethnic preferences, age, income, community or other resources, and state of health.

The need for continual follow-up care to accomplish and maintain rehabilitation must be emphasized. Discharge planning should include visits by the home health nurse and outpatient dietitian referrals.

EVALUATION

The following are expected outcomes for a patient recovering from decreased nutrition status:
- The patient will achieve and maintain optimal body weight.
- The patient will consume a well-balanced diet.
- The patient will experience no adverse outcomes related to malnutrition.
- The patient will maintain optimal physical functioning.

AGE-RELATED CONSIDERATIONS

MALNUTRITION

Older persons are particularly vulnerable to malnutrition, which increases frequency of hospitalization and care costs. Older hospitalized patients with malnutrition are more likely to have longer hospital stays, pressure injuries, infections, and increased morbidity and mortality (Avelino-Silva & Jaluul, 2017). (Pressure injuries are discussed in Chapter 14.) Older people commonly report a decreased appetite, problems with chewing or swallowing, inadequate nutrient intake, and consumption of only one meal per day. Being on a limited income may play a role in the number of meals eaten per day or the dietary quality of meals. Social isolation is a concern for many older people. Those who live alone may lose their desire to cook and often report a decrease in appetite. Some older persons may have functional limitations that affect their ability to purchase

TABLE 42.8   AGE-RELATED DIFFERENCES IN ASSESSMENT

Factors Affecting Nutritional Intake in Older Persons

Physical Factors
- Age
- Anorexia
- Decreased number of taste buds
- Dental problems
- Food intolerances
- Health status
- Physical disability
- Prescribed diets
- Prescribed or over-the-counter medications

Psychosocial Factors
- Importance of food in the past
- Loneliness or loss
- Mental awareness
- Social isolation

Socioeconomic Factors
- Availability of desired foods
- Availability of transportation to food stores
- Available time for food preparation and eating
- Education level and nutritional knowledge
- Financial status
- Food restrictions (intentional or unintentional)
- Lack of food preparation equipment

and prepare food. Furthermore, older people may lack access to transportation to buy food. For a complete list of factors affecting nutritional intake of older persons, see Table 42.8.

Chronic illnesses associated with aging can also affect nutritional status. For example, depression and dysphagia can affect intake. Poor oral health from cavities, gum disease, and missing teeth as well as xerostomia (dry mouth) can impair the older person's ability to lubricate, masticate, and swallow food (Hengeveld et al., 2018). Medications (e.g., antidepressants, antihypertensives, bronchodilators) can cause dry mouth, alter the taste of food, or decrease appetite.

Physiological changes associated with aging include a decrease in lean body mass and redistribution of fat around internal organs, which can decrease energy requirements. Sarcopenia (loss of lean body mass with aging) affects muscle strength and function (Cruz-Jentoft & Sayer, 2019). Older persons on bed rest or prolonged inactivity lose proportionately more lean body mass than younger adults (Bilo et al., 2017). Changes in smell and taste perception (due to medications, nutrient deficiencies, or taste-bud atrophy) can also alter food intake and nutritional status.

Lifestyle changes such as retirement or relocation to assisted living can have a significant impact on the eating habits of older people. Factors including ethnic background, previous dietary practices, food preferences, knowledge of healthy eating, food availability, accessibility of safe food storage and cooking, transportation, and health status should all be assessed in older persons. Problems related to any or all of these areas can alert the nurse to the possibility of risk for inadequate nutrition. For older patients living in long-term care facilities, eating with others, having the freedom to choose the menu and one's table companions, having appropriate feeding assistance available, and enjoying a calm atmosphere can contribute to residents' experiencing more pleasure and improving nutrient intake.

Some of the physiological changes associated with aging affect the nutritional status of older persons. The following changes are important:

1. Changes in the oral cavity (e.g., change in bite surfaces of the teeth, periodontal disease, drying of the mucous membranes of the mouth and tongue, poorly fitting dentures, decreased muscle strength for chewing, decreased number of taste buds, decreased saliva production)
2. Changes in digestion and motility (e.g., decreased absorption of cobalamin, vitamin A, and folic acid and decreased GI motility)
3. Changes in the endocrine system (e.g., decreased tolerance to glucose)
4. Changes in the musculoskeletal system (e.g., decreased bone density, degenerative joint changes)
5. Decrease in vision and hearing (e.g., procurement and preparation of food are more difficult)

Some illnesses that are more prevalent in the older population are diet related. These include atherosclerosis, osteoporosis, diabetes mellitus, dementia, some forms of cancer, and diverticulosis. Multiple medications are often required to treat these and other common chronic illnesses of older patients, and many of these medications have an adverse effect on the appetite, increasing nutrition risk.

Daily requirements for healthy older persons to maintain weight include 30 kcal/kg of usual body weight and 0.8 to 1 g/kg of usual body weight of protein per day. Requirements may differ among individuals, depending on the degree of malnutrition and physiological stress. To prevent loss of muscle mass and maintain function, older people should consume high-quality protein at each meal (Cruz-Jentoft & Sayer, 2019). Older persons are encouraged to take a vitamin D supplement containing at least 800 IU daily (Osteoporosis Canada, 2021).

Malnutrition can occur in an older person independent of changes in weight and energy requirements. Special strategies, such as adaptive devices (e.g., large-handled eating utensils), often are helpful in increasing dietary intake. Some older people may require nutritional support therapies until their strength and general health improve. Before starting any nutritional support therapy (e.g., EN or PN), the nurse should review the older person's advance directives regarding the use of artificial nutrition and hydration.

Malnourished or nutritionally at-risk older persons are vulnerable when discharged from the hospital. Older people may not be able to shop for or prepare foods during their initial recovery period. The nurse should consult with the interprofessional team to ensure that the older person has access to healthy food options and is able to prepare food upon discharge. Some communities offer community nutrition programs for older people as well as home-delivered meal programs such as Meals on Wheels. However, these programs alone may not be able to fully support older persons in accessing adequate nutritious food. It is not uncommon for older people to access food banks.

Dysphagia

Dysphagia, or difficulty in swallowing, is a symptom of disease or dysfunction and can result from several medical conditions. Among adults, the prevalence of dysphagia ranges from 12 to 13% in acute-care facilities and up to 60% in long-term care facilities (Touhy et al., 2018). Dysphagia increases the risk for malnutrition, dehydration, choking episodes, aspiration, chest infections or pneumonia, and death. In addition, it can cause

TABLE 42.9	INDICATORS OF DYSPHAGIA

Obvious Indicators of Dysphagia
- Difficult, painful chewing or swallowing
- Regurgitation of undigested food
- Difficulty controlling food or liquid in the mouth
- Drooling
- Hoarse voice
- Coughing or choking before, during, or after swallowing
- Globus sensation (lump in the throat)
- Nasal regurgitation
- Feeling of obstruction
- Unintentional weight loss—for example, in people with dementia

Less Obvious Indicators of Dysphagia
- Change in respiration pattern
- Unexplained temperature spikes
- Wet voice quality
- Tongue fasciculation (may indicate motor neuron disease)
- Xerostomia
- Heartburn
- Change in eating—for example, eating slowly or avoiding social occasions
- Frequent throat clearing
- Recurrent chest infections
- Atypical chest pain

Source: University of Maryland Medical Centre. (2016). *Dysphagia.* http://www.umm.edu/health/medical/altmed/condition/dysphagia

psychosocial problems, such as social isolation and embarrassment, which may reduce quality of life (Dietitians of Canada, 2015).

Nurses must carefully assess all patients for signs of dysphagia (Table 42.9) and refer any patients with suspected symptoms for a swallowing assessment by a speech–language pathologist or a registered dietitian trained to perform swallowing assessments. Screening tools such as the TOR-BSST can be used to identify patients at high risk for dysphagia (Martino et al., 2009). A swallowing assessment can help in identifying patients at risk for aspiration, including the location of the swallowing problem and which food consistencies are safest. The speech–language pathologist may also determine swallowing exercises, appropriate head positioning, and swallowing techniques.

The goal of nutrition intervention in dysphagia management should be to minimize weight loss (through adequate energy and protein intakes) and maintain hydration. Diet texture and fluid consistency modifications may be required for patient safety. The National Dysphagia Diet, developed by dietitians, speech–language pathologists, and food scientists, has served to standardize the nutrition care for individuals with dysphagia (DeBruyne & Pinna, 2020). Food texture may be modified with the addition of sauces or gravies and through mechanical alteration such as mincing or puréeing. The consistency of beverages may also be modified using thickening agents. Thickened fluids range in consistency from nectar-like to honey-like to pudding-like consistency.

SPECIALIZED NUTRITION SUPPORT

Oral Nutrition

If patients are unable to maintain or achieve adequate nutritional status, nutrition support may be necessary. High-calorie, high protein oral nutrition supplements can help improve the nutritional status of older persons. These supplements should not be used as meal replacements, but between meals as snacks.

Research Highlight

Does Nutritional Support Improve Outcomes in Hospitalized Adults at Nutritional Risk?
Clinical Question
In older persons (P), what is the effect of nutritional support (I) on adverse events, quality of life, and mortality (O)?

Best Available Evidence
- Meta-analysis of randomized controlled trials (RCTs)

Critical Appraisal and Synthesis of Evidence
- Two-hundred forty-four RCTs (*n* = 28 619) of hospitalized older persons (65 yr and older) with various diseases. Experimental interventions were parenteral nutrition, enteral nutrition, oral nutrition support, general nutrition support, and fortified food support. Control interventions were treatment as usual, no intervention, and placebo. In 204/244 trials, the intervention lasted 3 or more days.
- Outcomes included adverse event, quality of life, and mortality.
- Results showed that enteral nutrition may reduce serious adverse events, but there was no beneficial effect of oral nutrition support or parental support on mortality and serious adverse events. There was insufficient evidence to confirm or reject an association between nutritional support interventions and quality of life.
- There is some evidence to support an increase in weight with nutrition support for hospitalized adults at nutritional risk.

Conclusion
- Enteral nutrition support in older persons at nutritional risk was associated with a decrease in serious adverse events; however, the effect of other nutritional supports in relation to adverse events, quality of life, and mortality requires more research.

Implications for Nursing Practice
- The nurse should collaborate with the interprofessional team to complete a thorough assessment of the hospitalized older person who is at nutritional risk to assess the patient's situation and capacity to receive nutritional support.
- The nurse should assess the use of enteral nutrition support for older patients in hospital who are at nutritional risk.

Reference for Evidence
Feinberg, J., Nielsen, E., Korang, S., et al. (2017). Nutrition support in hospitalized adults at nutritional risk. *Cochrane Database of Systematic Reviews, 5*, CD011598. https://doi.org/10.1002/14651858.CD011598.pub2.
P, patient population of interest; *I,* intervention or area of interest; *O,* outcomes of interest (see Chapter 1).

In some hospitals and long-term care facilities, these beverages are used instead of water with oral medication administration to increase energy or protein intake (often referred to as *Med Pass*).

For patients who are unable to consume adequate nutrition orally with a high-calorie, high-protein diet (food and supplements), nutrition support such as EN (also called *tube feeding*) may be considered. If EN is not feasible, PN may be considered. For a decision-making plan related to nutrition support, see the algorithm in Figure 42.5.

Enteral Nutrition

Enteral nutrition (EN), also known as *tube feeding*, is nutrition (e.g., a nutritionally balanced liquefied food or formula) delivered through the GI tract distal to the oral cavity via a tube, catheter, or stoma. EN may be ordered for the patient who has a functioning GI tract but is unable to take any or enough oral nourishment.

Indications for EN may include anorexia, orofacial fractures, head and neck cancer, neurological or psychiatric conditions that prevent oral intake, extensive burns, critical illness, mechanical ventilation, and chemotherapy or radiation therapy. EN is considered to be more easily administered, safer, more physiologically efficient, and less expensive than PN. EN is used to provide nutrients by way of the GI tract either alone or as a supplement to oral nutrition or PN.

There is a wide variety of enteral formulas. Formula concentration, flavour, osmolality, and amounts of protein, sodium, and fat vary. There are special formulas for patients with diabetes and with liver, kidney, or lung disease. Most enteral formulas are lactose free. Most standard formulas provide between 1 and 1.5 kcal/mL; high-energy formulas provide 2 kcal/mL. The more calorically dense the formula, the less water it contains. The number and size of particles in the formula determine its osmolality. The more hydrolyzed or broken down the nutrients, the greater the osmolality.

Common EN delivery options are continuous or cyclical infusion by pump, intermittent infusion by gravity, or by bolus with a syringe. Continuous infusion is used most often with critically ill patients. Intermittent (bolus) feeding may be preferred as the patient improves or is discharged home on a tube-feeding regimen (Cardon-Thomas et al., 2017).

A nasogastric (NG) tube is commonly used for short-term feeding (<4 weeks). If EN is required for an extended period of time, other means of feeding may be used, such as an esophagostomy tube, a gastrostomy tube, or a jejunostomy tube, that delivers nutrients directly into the jejunum. Transpyloric (nasointestinal) tube placement or placement into the jejunum is used when physiological conditions warrant feeding the patient below the pyloric sphincter. Figure 42.6 shows the locations of commonly used enteral feeding tubes.

Orogastric, Nasogastric, and Nasointestinal Tubes. Polyurethane or silicone feeding tubes are long, small in diameter, soft, and flexible, thereby decreasing the risk for mucosal damage from prolonged placement. Polyurethane and silicone tubes are radiopaque, making their position readily identified by radiograph. Placement into the small intestine decreases the likelihood of regurgitation of contents into the esophagus and subsequent aspiration (Cardon-Thomas et al., 2017). With the use of a stylet, these tubes can be placed in a comatose patient because the ability to swallow is not essential during insertion.

Although the smaller feeding tubes (12–8 French) have advantages over wider-lumen tubes (≥14 French), such as the standard decompression NG tube, there are some disadvantages. Because of the small diameter, these tubes are more easily occluded and it can be more problematic to check for gastric residual volumes. They are particularly prone to obstruction when oral medications have not been thoroughly crushed and dissolved in water before administration. Failure to flush the tubing after both medication administration and residual volume determinations can result in tube clogging. Clogging of the tube may necessitate removal and insertion of a new tube, adding to cost and patient discomfort.

Gastrostomy and Jejunostomy Tubes. A gastrostomy tube may be used for a patient who requires EN over an extended period of time (>4–6 weeks) (Figure 42.7).

Gastrostomy tubes can be placed surgically, radiologically, or endoscopically. The placement of a percutaneous endoscopic gastrostomy (PEG) tube is shown in Figure 42.8. The patient must have an intact, unobstructed GI tract, and the esophageal lumen must be wide enough to pass the endoscope for PEG

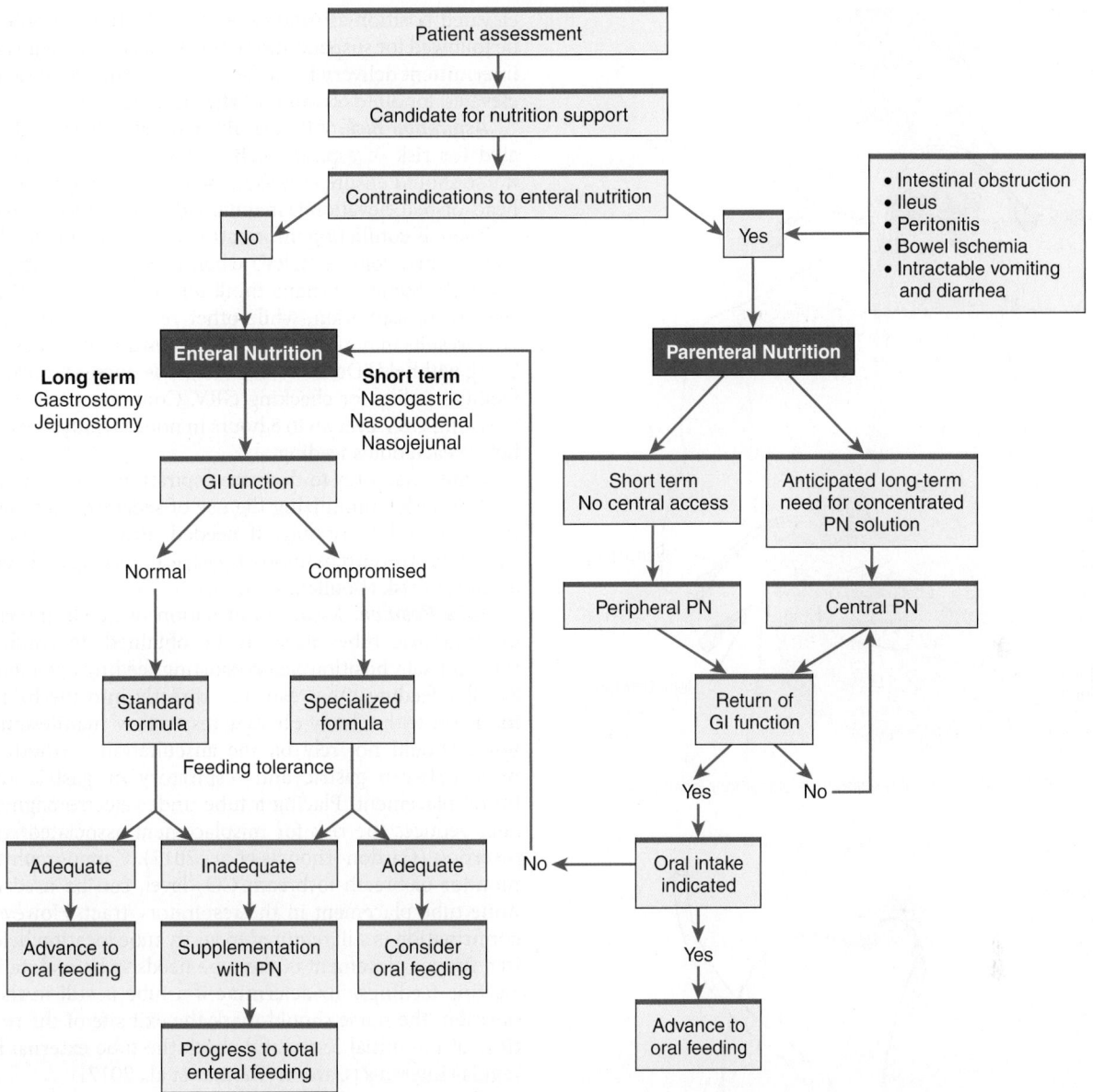

FIG. 42.5 Nutrition support algorithm. *GI,* gastrointestinal, *PN,* parenteral nutrition. Source: Adapted from Ukleja, A., Freeman, K. L., Gilbert, K., ASPEN Board of Directors. (2010). Standards for nutrition support: Adult hospitalized patients. *Nutrition in Clinical Practice 25,* 403.

tube placement. A PEG tube and a radiologically placed gastrostomy tube have several advantages. These procedures have fewer risks than surgical placement. They require IV sedation and local anaesthesia, a technique that can be done at a lower cost. IV antibiotics are given before the procedure.

For the patient with chronic reflux, a jejunostomy tube with continuous feedings may be appropriate to reduce the risk for aspiration (Bankhead et al., 2009). Jejunostomy tubes are placed either endoscopically or with open or laparoscopic surgery. Combination gastrojejunostomy (GJ) tubes allow for simultaneous gastric decompression and small bowel feeding. When a patient has a GJ tube, it is important to know which port is the gastric and which is the jejunal.

Enteral feedings can be started within 24 to 48 hours after surgical placement of a gastrostomy or jejunostomy tube, without waiting for flatus or a bowel movement. Most PEG tube feeding can start within 2 hours of insertion, although institutional

policies may vary (Cardon-Thomas et al., 2017). The feeding tube is either premarked or marked at the skin insertion site. At regular intervals, the tube insertion length should be rechecked. The tube is most often connected to a pump for continuous feeding.

Enteral Nutrition and Safety. Nurses play a critical role in ensuring that tube feedings are administered safely. Aspiration and dislodged tubes are two important safety concerns. Nursing management of tube feedings is addressed in Table 42.10.

Accidental tube removal can result in delayed feedings and potential discomfort because of tube replacement. The management of common complications in patients receiving tube feedings is presented in Table 42.11. See Nursing Care Plan (NCP) 42.1 for the patient receiving enteral nutrition, available on the Evolve website.

Specific care and teaching related to feeding tubes and enteral nutrition are summarized in the following sections. It is important to teach the patient and caregiver how to care for the feeding tube and how to properly administer enteral nutrition.

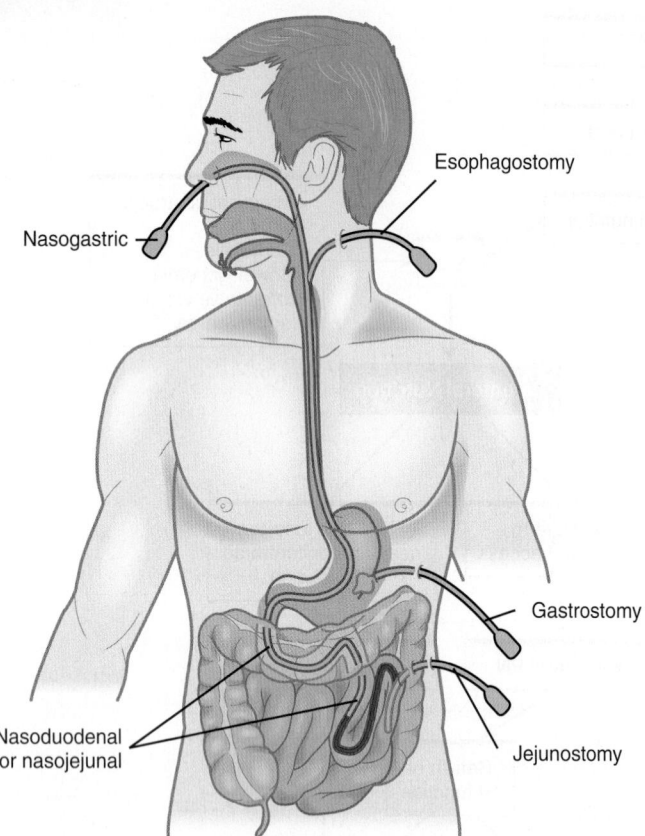

FIG. 42.6 Common enteral feeding tube placement locations.

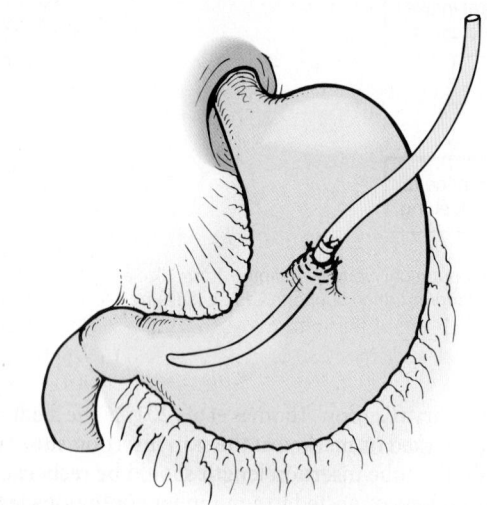

FIG. 42.7 Placement of a gastrostomy tube. Source: Redrawn from Mahan, L. K., & Arlin, M. (1992). *Krause's food, nutrition, and diet therapy* (8th ed.). Saunders.

Patient Position. Proper patient positioning decreases the risk for aspiration. To prevent aspiration, the nurse should elevate the head of the bed to a minimum of 30 degrees, but preferably 45 degrees (Cardon-Thomas et al., 2017). If the patient does not tolerate a backrest elevation, the reverse Trendelenburg position should be used to elevate the head of the bed unless contraindicated. If the head of the bed needs to be lowered for a procedure, the patient should be returned to an

elevated position as soon as possible. Institution policy should be followed for suspending feeding while the patient is supine. If intermittent delivery is used, the head of the bed should remain elevated for 30 to 60 minutes after feeding.

Aspiration Risk. All enterally fed patients should be evaluated for risk of aspiration. Before starting tube feedings, the nurse should ensure that the tube is in the proper position and head-of-bed elevation is maintained as described above.

There is conflicting information about whether to check gastric residual volume (GRV) when delivering feedings into the stomach. Some clinicians think an increase in GRV increases the risk of aspiration, while other research demonstrates that GRV results in nutritional goals not being met because feeds are being withheld (Deane et al., 2007). The nurse should follow the facility's policy for checking GRV. Common protocols call for checking GRV every 6 to 8 hours in noncritically ill patients and before each bolus feeding.

Other measures to decrease aspiration risk include feeding continuously, minimizing the use of sedation, and performing frequent oral suctioning, if needed. Promotility medications such as erythromycin improve gastric emptying and may reduce aspiration risk (Boullata et al., 2017).

Tube Position. X-ray confirmation of newly inserted nasal or orogastric tubes needs to be obtained, to confirm accurate and safe position before starting feedings or medications. Smaller feeding tubes can pass directly into the bronchus on insertion without any obvious respiratory manifestations. The nurse should not rely on the auscultation method to determine between gastric and respiratory or gastric and small bowel placement. Placing a tube under electromagnetic guidance reduces the risk for misplacement associated with blind insertion (Cardon-Thomas et al., 2017). Capnography, a direct monitor of breath-to-breath CO_2 level, can be used to determine tube placement in the respiratory tract. However, X-ray confirmation is still required to verify tube location before feeding. Proper placement of the tube needs to be maintained after starting feedings. To determine if a tube is still in the correct position, the nurse should mark the exit site of the tube at the time of the initial X-ray and check the tube external length at regular intervals (Cardon-Thomas et al., 2017).

The nurse may consider applying a nasal bridle on patients who try to pull out a tube or for whom taping the nose is difficult. A small-bowel tube may dislocate upward into the stomach, or the tube's tip can dislocate upward into the esophagus. If a significant increase in the external length is seen, other bedside tests can be used to help determine whether the tube has become dislocated. These measures include assessing aspirate colour and pH. Because each of these measures has limitations, placement should be confirmed by more than one test. When checking GVR, the nurse needs to watch for unexpected changes in volume. An increase in GVR may indicate the displacement of a small intestine tube into the stomach (Boullata et al., 2017).

Site Care. Skin care around gastrostomy and jejunostomy tube sites is important because the action of digestive juices irritates the skin. The skin around the feeding tube should be assessed daily for signs of redness and maceration. The nurse needs to monitor bumper tension and routinely check for pressure injury.

To keep the skin clean and dry, the nurse should initially rinse it with sterile water, dry it, and apply a dressing until the site is healed. After that, the site can be washed with mild soap

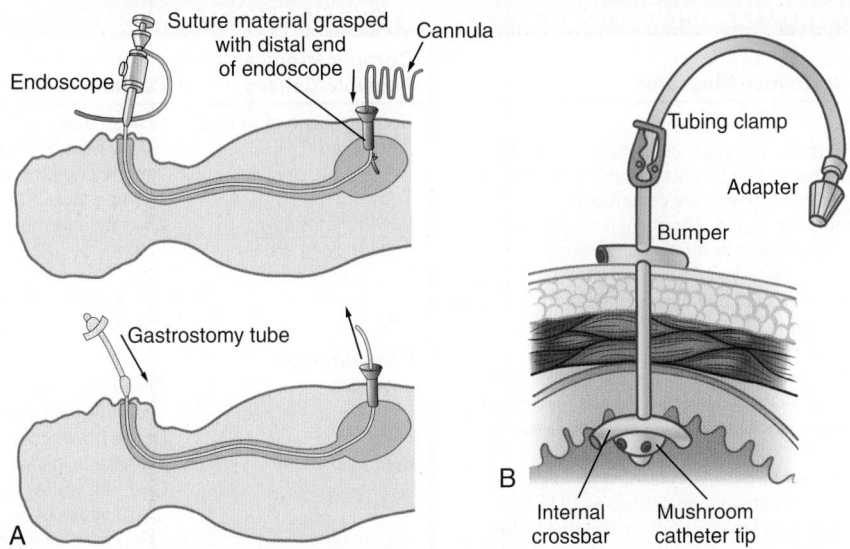

Endoscope
Suture material grasped with distal end of endoscope
Cannula

Gastrostomy tube

A

Tubing clamp
Adapter
Bumper

B
Internal crossbar
Mushroom catheter tip

FIG. 42.8 Percutaneous endoscopic gastrostomy. **A,** Gastrostomy tube placement via percutaneous endoscopy. Using endoscopy, a gastrostomy tube is inserted through the esophagus into the stomach and then pulled through a stab wound made in the abdominal wall. **B,** A retention disc and bumper secure the tube.

TABLE 42.10 NURSING MANAGEMENT

Feeding Tubes

1. The nurse should check tube placement before feeding and before each medication administration.
2. GI contractility factors should be evaluated when initiating EN, assess for bowel sounds; overt signs of contractility should not be required prior to initiation of EN.
3. Liquid medications should be used rather than pills, as appropriate.
   - Viscous liquid medications should be diluted.
   - The nurse should confirm whether medications are intended to be taken with meals.
   - Medications should not be added to enteral feeding formula.
4. If it is necessary to use tablets, they should be crushed to a fine powder and dissolved in 30 to 60 mL of water to prevent clogging feeding tubes.
5. General principles of tube feeding (e.g., bed elevation, checking gastric residual volume, and flushing tube with water) must be followed.
6. The nurse should assess regularly for complications (e.g., aspiration, diarrhea, abdominal distension, hyperglycemia, constipation, and fecal impaction).
7. The nurse must collaborate with the interprofessional health care team as required.

EN, enteral nutrition; *GI,* gastrointestinal.

and water. A protective ointment (zinc oxide, petroleum gauze) or a skin barrier may be used on the skin around the tube. If the skin is irritated, the nurse should consider using other types of drain or tube pouches. A wound, ostomy, and continence nurse can provide assistance if issues arise.

Tube Patency. All enteral feeding tubes require routine flushing. They should be flushed with 30 mL of warm tap water every 4 hours during continuous feedings or before and after each intermittent feeding. Sterile water should be used in immunocompromised and critically ill patients. Tubes must be flushed between each medication and after all medications are given. Where possible, the nurse should try to only use liquid medications. Clogged tubes should be flushed with warm water, using a back-and-forth motion. If unsuccessful, a pancreatic enzyme solution or a mechanical device for clearing feeding tubes may

be used (Cardon-Thomas et al., 2017). The nurse needs to follow facility policy for flushing a clogged feeding tube.

Misconnection. An *enteral feeding misconnection* is an inadvertent connection between an enteral feeding system and a nonenteral system such as an IV line, a peritoneal dialysis catheter, or a tracheostomy tube cuff. With an enteral feeding misconnection, nutritional formula intended for administration into the GI tract is administered via the wrong route, resulting in serious and potentially life-threatening consequences. Nursing interventions aimed at decreasing the risk for enteral feeding misconnections are found in Table 42.12. (See also NCP 42.1, available on the Evolve website, for patients receiving EN.)

AGE-RELATED CONSIDERATIONS

ENTERAL FEEDS

EN feeding strategies are used in older patients to improve nutritional status. Because of physiological changes associated with aging, older persons are more vulnerable to complications associated with nutritional interventions, especially fluid and electrolyte imbalances. Complications such as diarrhea can leave the patient dehydrated. Decreased thirst perception or impaired cognitive function can decrease the patient's ability to seek additional fluids.

With aging comes an increased risk for glucose intolerance. As a result, older patients may be more susceptible to hyperglycemia in response to the high carbohydrate load of some EN formulas. Older people with compromised cardiovascular function (e.g., heart failure) will have a decreased ability to handle large volumes of formula. If this happens, the patient may need a more concentrated formula (2.0 kcal/mL). Older persons have an increased risk for aspiration caused by gastroesophageal reflux disease (GERD), delayed gastric emptying, hiatal hernia, or diminished gag reflex. Physical mobility, fine motor movement, and visual system changes associated with aging may contribute to difficulties in managing EN in the home setting.

Parenteral Nutrition

Parenteral nutrition (PN) refers to the administration of nutrients by a route other than the GI tract (e.g., the bloodstream).

TABLE 42.11   COMMON COMPLICATIONS IN PATIENTS RECEIVING TUBE FEEDINGS

Complications and Possible Causes	Corrective Measures	Complications and Possible Causes	Corrective Measures
Vomiting and Aspiration		Contamination of formula or tubing	Change tubing q24h.
Improper tube placement	Replace tube in proper position and check tube position before beginning feeding and q8h if feedings are continuous.		Follow manufacturer's guidelines for maximum length of time formula can be at room temperature.
Delayed gastric emptying, increased residual volume	Hold feeding for 1 hr; then, if residual volume is less than before, resume feeding.	Low-fibre formula	Change to formula with more fibre.
		Tube moving distally	Properly secure tube before beginning feeding.
Aspiration risk	Keep head of bed elevated to 30- to 45-degree angle.		Check tube position before each feeding or at least q24h if feedings are continuous.
	Have patient sit up on side of bed or in a chair. Encourage ambulation unless contraindicated.	**Constipation**	
Contamination of formula	Refrigerate unused formula and record date opened; discard outdated formula every 24 hr.	Low fibre	Consult health care provider for change in formula to one with higher fibre content. Obtain bowel routine order.
	Discard formula left standing for longer than manufacturer's guidelines: 8–12 hr for ready-to-feed formulas (cans) or 4 hr for reconstituted formula or closed system as per manufacturer's guidelines.	Poor fluid intake	Increase fluid intake if not contraindicated. Give free water, as well as formula, to a total fluid intake of 30 mL/kg body weight.
		Medications	Check for medications that may be constipating.
		Impaction	Perform rectal examinations to check for and manually remove feces if present.
Diarrhea		**Dehydration**	
Feeding too fast, hypertonic formula, or medications	Evaluate number and volume of stools (if greater than three to five per day or >500 mL), consider patient's medical history, and assess abdomen for distension or pain.	Excessive diarrhea, vomiting	Decrease rate of or change formula.
			Check medications that patient is receiving, especially antibiotics.
	Contact health care provider, consider medications, and rule out infection (*Clostridium difficile*).		Take care to prevent bacterial contamination of formula and equipment.
	Decrease rate of feeding.	Poor fluid intake	Increase intake, if appropriate, and check amount and number of feedings.
	Change to continuous drip feedings.	High-protein formula	Change formula.
	Check for medications that may cause diarrhea (e.g., antibiotics).	Hyperosmotic diuresis	Check blood glucose levels frequently. Change formula.

PN is used when the GI tract cannot be used for the ingestion, digestion, and absorption of essential nutrients. PN is a relatively safe method of providing complete nutritional support.

PN is customized to meet the needs of each patient. The composition is reformulated as the patient's condition changes. The nurse must collaborate with the interprofessional team in delivering PN to the patient.

Composition. Commercially prepared PN base solutions are available. These solutions contain dextrose and protein in the form of amino acids. The pharmacy adds prescribed electrolytes (e.g., sodium, potassium, chloride, calcium, magnesium, and phosphate), vitamins, and trace elements (e.g., zinc, copper, chromium, and manganese) to meet the patient's needs. A three-in-one or total nutrient admixture containing an IV fat emulsion (lipids), dextrose, and amino acids is widely used. Premixed PN solutions are relatively new and require manipulation of the dextrose and amino acids prior to use. Standard electrolytes are available in premixed solutions and multivitamins are added prior to use (Mehta et al., 2017). Table 42.13 lists common indications for the use of PN. NCP 42.2, available on the Evolve website, presents nursing diagnoses and care for patients undergoing parenteral nutrition.

Calories. Calories in PN are supplied primarily by carbohydrates in the form of dextrose and by fat in the form of fat emulsion. The administration of between 100 and 150 g of dextrose (1 g provides ≈3.4 kcal, in contrast to oral carbohydrates, which provide 4 kcal) has a protein-sparing effect. Providing adequate nonprotein calories in the form of glucose and fat allows the use of amino acids for wound healing and not for energy. However, overfeeding can lead to metabolic complications. To minimize these problems, an energy intake of 25 to 35 kcal/kg/day in a nonobese patient is often recommended.

Fat-emulsion solutions of 10%, 20%, and 30% are available. Fat emulsions provide approximately 1 kcal/mL (10% solution) or 2 kcal/mL (20% solution). Fat emulsions primarily contain soybean or safflower triglycerides with egg phospholipids added as an emulsifier. They provide a large number of calories in a relatively small amount of fluid. This is beneficial when the patient is at risk for fluid overload.

IV fat emulsions should provide up to 30% of total calories. Most stable patients receive 1 g/kg/day, and the maximum daily lipid dose is 2.5 g/kg. Critically ill patients may not tolerate this dose and may receive less than 1 g/kg/day. Serum triglyceride levels are determined at the beginning of PN and then monitored closely after that. IV fat emulsions administered separately should be administered over a course of 12 hours, and infusion rates should not exceed 0.5 mL/kg/hour (Mehta et al., 2017)

Nausea, vomiting, and elevated temperature may occur, especially when lipids are infused quickly. Fat emulsions are contraindicated in the patient with a disturbance in fat metabolism, such as hyperlipidemia. They are used with caution in the patient at risk for fat embolism (e.g., fractured femur) and the patient with an allergy to eggs or soybeans. Lipid emulsions are also used with caution in patients with pancreatitis, bleeding disorders, liver failure, or respiratory disease.

TABLE 42.12 NURSING MANAGEMENT

Decrease Risk for Enteral Feeding Misconnections

To decrease the risk for enteral feeding misconnections, the nurse should do the following:

1. Teach visitors and nonclinical staff to notify a nurse if an enteral feeding line becomes disconnected.
2. Instruct visitors and nonclinical staff not to reconnect enteral feeding lines.
3. Never modify or adapt IV or feeding devices, because doing so may compromise the safety features incorporated into their design.
4. When making a reconnection, routinely trace lines back to their origins and then ensure that they are secure.
5. Never force connections if the device parts do not seem to fit properly. Ill-fitting pieces indicate a problem.
6. When a patient arrives on a new unit or in a new setting, or during shift-to-shift hand-off, recheck connections and trace all tubes.
7. Route tubes and catheters that have different purposes in distinct and standardized directions (e.g., IV lines should be routed toward the patient's head, enteral lines should be routed toward the feet).
8. Package together all parts needed for enteral feeding and reduce the availability of additional adapters and connectors so as to minimize the presence of dissimilar tubes or catheters that could be improperly connected.
9. Label or colour-code feeding tubes and connectors and educate staff about the labelling or colour-coding process in the institution's enteral feeding system.
10. Always identify and confirm the solution's label, because a three-in-one parenteral nutrition solution can appear similar to an enteral nutrition formulation bag. The bags should be labelled with large, bold statements, such as "WARNING! For Enteral Use Only—NOT for IV Use."
11. Make all connections under proper lighting conditions.
12. Follow the facility's protocol for reporting adverse events and near misses.

IV, intravenous.

Source: Reprinted from *The Joint Commission Journal on Quality and Patient Safety*, 34(5), Peggi Guenter, Rodney W. Hicks, Debora Simmons, Jay Crowley, Stephanie Joseph, Richard Croteau, Cathie Gosnell, Nancy G. Pratt, Timothy W. Vanderveen, Enteral feeding misconnections: A consortium position statement, pp. 289–290, Copyright 2008, with permission from Elsevier.

TABLE 42.13 COMMON INDICATIONS FOR PARENTERAL NUTRITION*

- Chronic severe diarrhea and vomiting
- Complicated surgery or trauma
- Gastrointestinal obstruction
- Gastrointestinal tract anomalies and fistulas
- Intractable diarrhea
- Severe anorexia nervosa
- Severe malabsorption
- Short bowel syndrome

*This list is not all-inclusive.

Protein. A healthy person of average body size needs approximately 45 to 65 g (0.8–1 g/kg/day) of protein daily. Protein should be provided at the rate of 1 to 1.5 g/kg/day, depending on the patient's needs. In a nutritionally depleted patient who is also under the stress of illness or surgery, protein requirements can exceed 150 g/day (1.5 to 2 g/kg/day) to ensure positive nitrogen balance. Burn patients, who are often on PN, EN, and oral food, may need upward of 2 g/kg/day (Guenter et al., 2018). Protein needs may be lower than 1 g/kg/day and restricted in individuals with end-stage renal disease who are not on dialysis.

Electrolytes. The exact amount of electrolytes needed depends on the patient's health condition and serum electrolyte

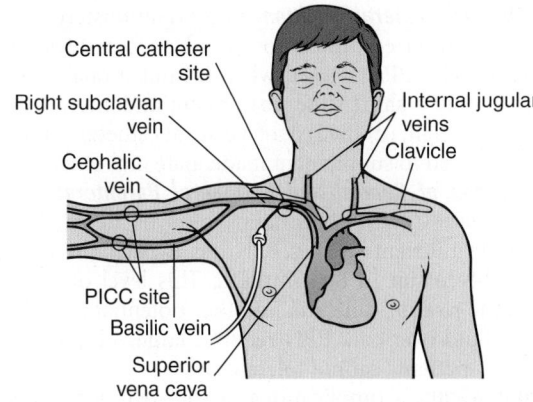

FIG. 42.9 Placement of a catheter for central parenteral nutrition using the subclavian vein. Peripherally inserted central catheters (PICCs) are inserted using the basilic or the cephalic vein. Source: Redrawn from Mahan, L. K., & Arlin, M. (1992). *Krause's food, nutrition, and diet therapy* (8th ed.). Saunders.

levels. The assessment of individual requirements should take place at the beginning of therapy and then several times a week as the treatment progresses. The following are ranges for average daily electrolyte requirements for adult patients without renal or hepatic impairment (Ayers et al., 2014):

Sodium: 1 to 2 mmol/kg/day
Potassium: 1 to 2 mmol/kg/day
Chloride: as needed to maintain acid–base balance
Magnesium: 8 to 20 mmol/day
Calcium: 10 to 15 mmol/day
Phosphate: 20 to 40 mmol/day

Requirements for electrolytes depends on the patient's health condition and electrolyte levels as determined by blood testing.

Trace Elements and Vitamins. Zinc, copper, chromium, manganese, selenium, and chromium supplements may be added according to the patient's condition and needs. Levels of these elements are monitored in the patient receiving PN. The health care provider may order additional amounts of these elements to be added to the solutions, according to the patient's requirements.

The daily addition of a multivitamin preparation to the PN generally meets the vitamin requirements.

Methods of Administration. PN may be administered as central parenteral nutrition (CPN) or peripheral parenteral nutrition (PPN). Both CPN and PPN are used in patients who are not candidates for EN.

Central Parenteral Nutrition. CPN is indicated when long-term support is necessary or when the patient has high protein and energy requirements. CPN is administered through a central venous catheter or a peripherally inserted central catheter (PICC) whose tip lies in the superior vena cava (see Chapter 19). CPN solutions are hypertonic, measuring at least 1 600 mmol/L. The high glucose content ranges from 20 to 50%. CPN must be infused in a large central vein so that rapid dilution can occur. The use of a peripheral vein for hypertonic CPN solutions would cause irritation and thrombophlebitis.

CPN may be given through a central venous catheter that originates at the subclavian or jugular vein and whose tip lies in the superior vena cava (Figure 42.9). It can also be given using a PICC that is placed into the basilic or cephalic vein and then advanced into the distal end of the superior vena cava (see Figure 19.19).

Peripheral Parenteral Nutrition. PPN is administered through a peripherally inserted catheter or vascular access device, which uses a large vein. PPN is used when (a) nutritional support is needed for only a short time, (b) protein and energy requirements are not high, (c) the risk of a central catheter is too great, or (d) PN is used to supplement inadequate oral intake.

Comparison of Central and Peripheral Parenteral Nutrition. Compared with CPN, PPN contains fewer nutrients. Although having fewer nutrients makes PPN less hypertonic, it still has an osmolality of up to 800 mmol/L. This level of osmolality increases the risk for phlebitis. Another potential complication of PPN is fluid overload. PPN requires large volumes of fluid, which many patients cannot tolerate.

Complications. Complications associated with PN are related either to the catheter or to the PN infusion itself (Table 42.14). Refeeding syndrome is characterized by fluid retention and electrolyte imbalances (hypophosphatemia, hypokalemia, hypomagnesemia). Hypophosphatemia is the hallmark of refeeding syndrome and is associated with serious outcomes, including cardiac dysrhythmias, respiratory arrest, and neurological disturbances (e.g., paresthesias). Conditions that predispose patients to refeeding syndrome include long-standing malnutrition states, such as alcohol use disorder, vomiting and diarrhea, chemotherapy, and major surgery. Refeeding syndrome can occur any time a malnourished patient starts aggressive nutritional support.

NURSING MANAGEMENT PARENTERAL NUTRITION

HOME NUTRITION SUPPORT

Home PN or EN is an accepted mode of nutritional therapy for individuals who do not require hospitalization but require continued nutrition support. Some patients have been successfully treated at home for many months and even years. It is important

TABLE 42.14	COMPLICATIONS OF PARENTERAL NUTRITION

Infection
- Fungal
- Gram-positive bacteria
- Gram-negative bacteria

Metabolic
- Hyperglycemia; hypoglycemia; and hyperosmolar, hyperglycemic state
- Altered renal function (prerenal azotemia)
- Essential fatty acid deficiency
- Electrolyte and vitamin excesses and deficiencies
- Trace mineral deficiencies
- Hyperlipidemia
- Liver dysfunction
- Refeeding syndrome

Catheter-Related Problems
- Air embolus
- Pneumothorax, hemothorax, and hydrothorax
- Hemorrhage
- Dislodgement, occlusion
- Thrombosis of great vein
- Phlebitis

for the nurse to educate the patient or caregiver about catheter or tube care, proper technique in mixing and handling of the solutions and tubing, and adverse effects and complications.

Home nutritional therapies are expensive, and specific criteria must be met for these expenses to be reimbursed by federal, provincial, territorial, or private health insurance programs. The discharge planning team needs to be involved early in the admission to help plan for discharge. Home nutrition support may also be a burden on the patient and caregivers and may affect their quality of life.

CASE STUDY

Undernutrition

Patient Profile

M. S. (pronouns she/her), 70 years old, is 162.5 cm tall and weighs 45.4 kg. She was recently admitted to the medical unit at a regional hospital.

Subjective Data

- Reports 13.5-kg weight loss during past 2 months
- Has recently had a thrombotic stroke with hemiparesis and dysphagia
- Has a history of rheumatoid arthritis
- Has had nothing by mouth for the past 24 hours and just started enteral nutrition via a PEG tube
- Lives with her daughter, who is at her bedside

Objective Data

Physical Examination

- Has left-sided weakness
- Blood pressure is 150/90 mm Hg
- A PEG tube was recently placed

Laboratory Results

- Serum albumin 29 g/L
- Prealbumin 1.1 g/L

Discussion Questions

1. What are M. S.'s risk factors for malnutrition?
2. Are there any concerns regarding her current weight and recent weight history?
3. What factors increase M. S.'s risk for developing dysphagia and malnutrition?
4. What should the nurse include in a successful weight-restoration plan for M. S.?
5. What possible complications of enteral nutrition could M. S. be at risk for developing?
6. ***Priority decision:*** What is the priority of the nursing care for M. S.?
7. ***Priority decision:*** Based on the assessment data presented, what are the priority nutrition-related concerns and the issues that the interprofessional team could collaborate on to improve M. S.'s nutritional status?
8. ***Evidence-informed practice:*** M. S.'s daughter tells the nurse that her mother's abdomen appears bloated, and she wonders if she should massage it. What is the most appropriate response?

evolve

Answers are available at http://evolve.elsevier.com/Canada/Lewis/medsurg.

REVIEW QUESTIONS

The number of the question corresponds to the same-numbered objective at the beginning of the chapter.

1. According to *Canada's Food Guide*, which proportion of foods is consistent on a plate?
   a. 50% whole grains, 25% vegetables and fruits, 25% protein-rich food
   b. 50% vegetables and fruits, 25% whole grains, 25% dairy products
   c. 50% vegetables and fruits, 25% protein-rich foods, 25% whole grains
   d. 25% protein-rich foods, 25% vegetables and fruits, 25% dairy products, 25% whole grains

2. Food insecurity places an individual at risk for poor health outcomes. Which of the following conditions are food-insecure individuals more at risk for than their food-secure counterparts? *(Select all that apply.)*
   a. Hypertension
   b. Diabetes mellitus
   c. Glaucoma
   d. Iron-deficient anemia
   e. Depression

3. During starvation, in what order does the body obtain substrate for energy?
   a. Glycogen, skeletal protein, fat, visceral protein
   b. Visceral protein, fat stores, glycogen
   c. Fat stores, skeletal protein, visceral protein
   d. Liver protein, muscle protein, visceral protein

4. For which type of client is a complete nutritional assessment important? *(Select all that apply.)*
   a. A client with recent, unintentional weight loss
   b. A client experiencing frequent nocturia
   c. A client who reports a 5-year history of constipation
   d. A client who reports an unintentional weight loss of 3 kg in 2 months

5. What is one advantage of a percutaneous endoscopic gastrostomy (PEG) tube placement relative to nasogastric (NG) feedings for the client receiving long-term enteral nutrition?
   a. It increases client comfort.
   b. It eliminates the risk for aspiration.
   c. Feedings can be initiated before bowel sounds are present.
   d. More calories can be delivered than with NG feeding.

6. A client is receiving peripheral parenteral nutrition. The PN solution is completed before the new solution arrives on the unit. What should the nurse administer?
   a. 20% intralipids
   b. 5% dextrose solution
   c. 5% Ringer's lactate solution
   d. 0.45% normal saline solution

7. A client with anorexia nervosa shows signs of malnutrition. During initial refeeding, what does the nurse carefully assess the client for?
   a. Hyperkalemia
   b. Hypoglycemia
   c. Hypercalcemia
   d. Hypophosphatemia

1. b; 2, a, b, d, e; 3, a; 4, a, d; 5. c; 6. b; 7. a.

ⓔvolve

For even more review questions, visit http://evolve.elsevier.com/Canada/Lewis/medsurg.

REFERENCES

Allard, J. P., Keller, H., Jeejeebhoy, K. N., et al. (2015). Malnutrition at hospital admission—Contributors and effect on length of stay: A prospective cohort study from the Canadian malnutrition Task Force. *Journal of Parenteral and Enteral Nutrition, 40*(4), 487–497. https://doi.org/10.1177/0148607114567902

American Society for Parenteral and Enteral Nutrition. (2016). Guidelines for the provision and assessment of nutrition support therapy in the adult critically ill patient. *Journal of Parenteral and Enteral Nutrition, 40*(2), 159–211. https://doi.org/10.1177/0148607115621863

Avelino-Silva, T., & Jaluul, O. (2017). Malnutrition in hospitalized older patients: Management strategies to improve patient care and clinical outcomes. *International Journal of Gerontology, 11*(2), 56–61. https://doi.org/10.1016/j.ijge.2016.11.002

Ayers, P., Holcombe, B., Plogsted, S., et al. (2014). *ASPEN parental nutrition handbook* (2nd ed.). ASPEN.

Bankhead, R., Boullata, J., Brantley, S., et al. (2009). A.S.P.E.N. enteral nutrition practice recommendations. *Journal of Enteral and Parenteral Nutrition, 33*(2), 122–167. https://doi.org/10.1177/0148607108330314. (Seminal).

Berrazaga, I., Micard, V., Gueugneau, M., et al. (2019). The role of the anabolic properties of plant- versus animal-based protein sources in supporting muscle mass maintenance: A critical review. *Nutrients, 11*(8), 1825. https://doi.org/10.3390/nu11081825

Bilo, G., Pišot, R., Mazzucco, S., et al. (2017). Anabolic resistance assessed by oral stale isotope ingestion following bed rest in young and older adult volunteers: Relationships with changes in muscle mass. *Journal of Clinical Nutrition, 36,* 1420–1426. https://doi.org/10.1016/j.clnu.2016.09.019

Boullata, J. I., Carrera, A. L., Harvey, L., et al. (2017). ASPEN safe practices for enteral nutrition therapy. *Journal of Parental and Enteral Nutrition, 41*(1), 15–103. https://doi.org/10.1177/0148607116673053

Canadian Cancer Society. (2021). *Eating well extras to consider: Should I take a vitamin D supplement?* https://www.cancer.ca/en/prevention-and-screening/reduce-cancer-risk/make-healthy-choices/eat-well/should-i-take-a-vitamin-d-supplement/?region=on

Canadian Institute for Health Information (CIHI). (2021). *Health spending.* https://www.cihi.ca/en/health-spending

Cardon-Thomas, D. K., Riviere, T., Tieges, Z., et al. (2017). Dietary protein in older adults: Adequate daily intake but potential for improved distribution. *Nutrients, 9*(3), 184. https://doi.org/10.3390/nu9030184

Chan, L., Maleeka, B., Tonio, S., et al. (2019). *FNFNES final report for eight Assembly of First Nations Regions. Draft comprehensive technical report.* Assembly of First Nations, University of Ottawa, Universite de Montreal. http://www.fnfnes.ca/docs/CRA/FNFNES_draft_technical_report_Nov_2__2019.pdf

Cruz-Jentoft, A., & Sayer, A. (2019). Sarcopenia. *The Lancet, 393*(10191), 2636–2646. https://doi.org/10.1016/S0140-6736(19)31138-9

Davison, K. M., Gondara, L., & Kaplan, B. J. (2017). Food insecurity, poor diet quality, and suboptimal intakes of folate and iron are independently associated with perceived mental health in Canadian adults. *Nutrients, 9*(3), 274. https://doi.org/10.3390/nu9030274

Deane, A., Chapman, M. J., Fraser, R. J., et al. (2007). Mechanisms underlying feed intolerance in the critically ill: Implications for treatment. *World Journal of Gastroenterology, 13*(29), 3909–3917. https://doi.org/10.3748/wjg.v13.i29.3909

DeBruyne, L. K., & Pinna, K. (2020). *Nutrition & diet therapy* (10th ed.). Centage.

Dietitians of Canada. (2015). *Defining the role of the dietitian in dysphagia assessment and management.* https://www.dietitians.ca/DietitiansOfCanada/media/Documents/Resources/Dysphagia-Role-Paper-2015.pdf

Dietitians of Canada. (2021a). *Learn about dietitians.* https://www.dietitians.ca/About/Learn-About-Dietitians

Dietitians of Canada. (2021b). *The difference between a dietitian and a nutritionist.* https://www.dietitians.ca/About/Learn-About-Dietitians/The-difference-between-a-dietitian-and-nutritionis

Earle, L. (2011). *Traditional Aboriginal diets and health.* https://www.ccnsa-nccah.ca/docs/emerging/FS-TraditionalDietsHealth-Earle-EN.pdf

Food and Agriculture Organization of the United Nations, International Fund for Agriculture Development, UNICEF, World Food Program, and World Health Organization. (2018). *The state of food security and nutrition in the world. Building climate resilience for food security and nutrition.* https://www.fao.org/3/i9553en/i9553en.pdf

Gottschlich, L. (2017). Female athlete triad. *Medscape,* ART. 89260. https://emedicine.medscape.com/article/89260-overview

Guenter, P., Worthington, P., Ayers, R., et al. (2018). Standardized competencies for parenteral nutrition administration: The ASPEN model. *Nutrition in Clinical Practice, 33*(2), 295–304. https://doi.org/10.1002/ncp.10055

Health Canada. (2019a). *Fats.* https://www.canada.ca/en/health-canada/services/nutrients/fats.html

Health Canada. (2019b). *Food guide snapshot—other languages.* https://www.canada.ca/en/health-canada/services/canada-food-guide/resources/snapshot/languages.html

Health Canada. (2020a). *Social determinates of health and health inequalities.* https://www.canada.ca/en/public-health/services/health-promotion/population-health/what-determines-health.html

Health Canada. (2020b). *Vitamin D and calcium: Updated dietary reference intakes.* https://www.canada.ca/en/health-canada/services/food-nutrition/healthy-eating/vitamins-minerals/vitamin-calcium-updated-dietary-reference-intakes-nutrition.html#a2

Health Canada. (2021a). *Canada's food guide.* https://food-guide.canada.ca/en/

Health Canada. (2021b). *Choose foods with healthy fats.* https://food-guide.canada.ca/en/healthy-eating-recommendations/make-it-a-habit-to-eat-vegetables-fruit-whole-grains-and-protein-foods/choosing-foods-with-healthy-fats/

Hengeveld, L. M., Wijnhoven, H. A., Olthof, M. R., et al. (2018). Prospective associations of poor diet quality with long-term incidence of protein-energy malnutrition in community-dwelling older adults: The health, aging and body composition study. *American Journal of Clinical Nutrition, 107*(2), 155–164. https://doi.org/10.1093/ajcn/nqx020

Institute of Medicine. (2005). *Dietary reference intakes for energy, carbohydrate, fat, fatty acids, cholesterol, protein and amino acids.* National Academies Press. https://doi.org/10.17226/10490. (Seminal).

Kim, S., Guevarra, R., Kim, Y., et al. (2019). Role of probiotics in human gut microbiome-associated diseases. *Journal of Microbiology and Biotechnology, 29*(9), 1335–1340. https://doi.org/10.4014/jmb.1906.06064

Kinnaird, E., Norton, C., Pimblett, C., et al. (2019). "There's nothing there for guys". Do men with eating disorders want treatment adaptations? A qualitative study. *Eating and Weight Disorders, 24*(5), 845–852. https://doi.org/10.1007/s40519-019-00770-0

Kramer, D., Ferguson, R., & Reynolds, J. (2019). *Sustainable consumption for all: Improving the accessibility of sustainably produced foods in Canada. Food Secure Canada research report.* https://foodsecurecanada.org/sites/foodsecurecanada.org/files/attached_files/research_report_sustainable_consumption_for_all_fsc_may_2019.pdf

Lazar, V., Ditu, L. M., Pircalabioru, G. G., et al. (2018). Aspects of gut microbiota and immune system interactions in infectious diseases, immunopathology, and cancer. *Frontiers in Immunology, 9,* 1830. https://doi.org/10.3389/fimmu.2018.01830

Leech, J. (2018). *What are trans fats and why are they bad for me? Healthline.* https://www.healthline.com/nutrition/why-trans-fats-are-bad

Lieffers, J. R. L., Ekwaru, J. P., Ohinmaa, A., et al. (2018). The economic burden of not meeting food recommendations in Canada: The cost of doing nothing. *PLoS One, 13*(4), e0196333. https://doi.org/10.1371/journal.pone.0196333

Martino, R., Silver, F., Teasell, R., et al. (2008). The Toronto bedside swallowing screening test. *Stroke, 40,* 555–561. https://doi.org/10.1161/STROKEAHA.107.510370

McIntyre, L., Dutton, D. J., Kwok, C., et al. (2016). Reduction of food insecurity among low-income Canadian seniors as a likely impact of a guaranteed annual income. *Canadian Public Policy, 42*(3), 274–286. https://doi.org/10.3138/cpp.2015-069

Mehta, N. M., Skillman, H. E., Irving, S. Y., et al. (2017). Guidelines for the provision and assessment of nutrition support therapy in the pediatric critically ill patient: Society of Critical Care Medicine and A.S.P.E.N. *Journal of Parenteral and Enteral Nutrition, 41*(5), 706–742. https://doi.org/10.1177/0148607117711387

Men, F., Gundersen, C., Urquia, M. L., et al. (2020). Association between household food insecurity and mortality in Canada: A population-based retrospective cohort study. *Canadian Medical Association Journal, 192*(3), E53–E60. https://doi.org/10.1503/cmaj.190385. https://doi.org/10.1503/cmaj.190385

National Centre for Complementary and Integrative Health. (2019). *Probiotics: What you need to know.* https://nccih.nih.gov/health/probiotics/introduction.htm

National Eating Disorder Information Centre (NEDIC). (2021a). *Anorexia nervosa.* https://nedic.ca/eating-disorders-treatment/anorexia-nervosa/

National Eating Disorder Information Centre (NEDIC). (2021b). *Bulimia nervosa.* https://nedic.ca/eating-disorders-treatment/bulimia-nervosa/

National Initiative for Eating Disorders (NIED). (2018). *About eating disorders in Canada.* https://nied.ca/about-eating-disorders-in-canada/

Nicholls, D., & Becker, A. (2020). Food for thought: Bringing eating disorders out of the shadows. *British Journal of Psychology, 216*, 67–68. https://doi.org/10.1192/bjp.2019.179

Osteoporosis Canada. (2021). *Vitamin D.* https://osteoporosis.ca/vitamin-d/

Park, S. Y., Wilkens, L. R., Maskarinec, G., et al. (2018). Weight change in older adults and mortality: The multiethnic cohort study. *International Journal of Obesity, 42*(2), 205–212. https://doi.org/10.1038/ijo.2017.188

Public Health Agency of Canada. (2019). *Prevalence of chronic diseases among Canadian adults.* https://www.canada.ca/en/public-health/services/chronic-diseases/prevalence-canadian-adults-infographic-2019.html

Touhy, T., Jett, K., Boscart, V., et al. (2018). *Ebersole and Hess' gerontological nursing and healthy aging in Canada* (2nd Canadian ed.). Elsevier.

University of Toronto. (2020). *PROOF, fact sheet; Relationship between food banks and food insecurity in Canada.* https://proof.utoronto.ca/wp-content/uploads/2019/11/PROOF_FACTSHEET_Foodbanks-112019.pdf

Westmoreland, P., Krantz, M., & Mehler, P. (2016). Medical complications of anorexia nervosa and bulimia. *The American Journal of Medicine, 129*(1), 30–37. https://doi.org/10.1016/j.amjmed.2015.06.031

Wharton, S., Lau, D., Vallis, M., et al. (2020). Obesity in adults: A clinical practice guideline. *Canadian Medical Association Journal, 192*(31), E875–E891. https://doi.org/10.1503/cmaj.191707

White, J. V., Guenter, P., Jensen, G., et al. (2012). Consensus statement of the Academy of nutrition and Dietetics/American society for parenteral and enteral nutrition: Characteristics recommended for the identification and documentation of adult malnutrition (undernutrition). *Journal of the Academy of Nutrition and Dietetics, 112*(11), 730–738. https://doi.org/10.1016/j.jand.2012.03.012

Zhang, Y. J., Li, S., Gan, R. Y., et al. (2015). Impacts of gut bacteria on human health and diseases. *International Journal of Molecular Sciences, 16*(4), 7493–7519. https://doi.org/10.3390/ijms16047493

RESOURCES

Canadian Malnutrition Task Force
https://nutritioncareincanada.ca
Canadian Mental Health Association
https://www.cmha.ca
Canadian Nutrition Society
https://www.cns-scn.ca
Canadian Vascular Access Association
https://cvaa.info
Diabetes Canada
http://www.guidelines.diabetes.ca
Dietitians of Canada
https://www.dietitians.ca

Eat Smart Meet Smart (Saskatchewan)
https://www.saskatchewan.ca/residents/health/wellness-and-prevention/nutrition-and-exercise/eat-smart-meet-smart
Government of Canada—*Canada's Food Guide*
https://food-guide.canada.ca/en/
Government of Canada—*Dietary Reference Intakes Tables*
https://www.canada.ca/en/health-canada/services/food-nutrition/healthy-eating/dietary-reference-intakes/tables.html
Government of Canada—*Health*
https://www.canada.ca/en/services/health.html
Health Canada: *Interactive Nutrition Facts Table*
https://www.canada.ca/en/health-canada/services/understanding-food-labels/nutrition-facts-tables.html#a4
Health Canada: *Therapeutic Products Directorate*
https://www.canada.ca/en/health-canada/corporate/about-health-canada/branches-agencies/health-products-food-branch/therapeutic-products-directorate.html
Healthy Families BC: *Healthy Eating*
https://www.healthyfamiliesbc.ca/work/healthy-eating
Healthy Nutrition (New Brunswick)
https://www2.gnb.ca/content/gnb/en/departments/ocmoh/healthy_people/content/HealthyNutrition.html
Heart and Stroke Foundation of Canada
https://www.heartandstroke.ca
National Eating Disorder Information Centre
https://www.nedic.ca
Public Health Agency of Canada
https://www.phac-aspc.gc.ca
UnlockFood.ca (formally EatRight Ontario)
https://www.unlockfood.ca/en/default.aspx

Academy for Eating Disorders
https://www.aedweb.org
American Society for Parenteral and Enteral Nutrition (ASPEN)
https://www.nutritioncare.org
Critical Care Nutrition
https://www.criticalcarenutrition.com
European Society for Parenteral and Enteral Nutrition and Metabolism (ESPEN)
https://www.espen.org
National Association of Anorexia Nervosa and Associated Disorders (ANAD)
https://www.anad.org
Oley Foundation
http://www.oley.org

evolve

For additional Internet resources, see the website for this book at http://evolve.elsevier.com/Canada/Lewis/medsurg.

Nursing Management

Obesity

Carol A. Kuzio and Jean Jacque E. Lovely
Originating US chapter by Mariann M. Harding

⊖volve WEBSITE

http://evolve.elsevier.com/Canada/Lewis/medsurg

- Review Questions (Online Only)
- Key Points
- Answer Guidelines for Case Study

- Student Case Study
  - Obesity and Osteoarthritis
- Conceptual Care Map Creator

- Audio Glossary
- Content Updates

LEARNING OBJECTIVES

1. Discuss the epidemiology and etiology of obesity.
2. Describe the classification systems for determining a person's body size and associated health risks.
3. Explain the health risks associated with obesity.
4. Discuss nutritional, physical activity, and behaviour-modification therapies for patients who have obesity.
5. Describe the different bariatric surgical procedures used to treat obesity.

6. Describe the nursing management related to conservative and surgical therapies for obesity.
7. Describe the etiology and the clinical manifestations of metabolic syndrome and the nursing and interprofessional management of patients with metabolic syndrome.

KEY TERMS

bariatric surgery
body mass index (BMI)
lipectomy

metabolic syndrome
morbidly obese
obese

obesity
overweight
waist-to-hip ratio (WHR)

OBESITY

Obesity is a complex, chronic, multifactorial disease that develops from the interaction between genetics and the environment. It manifests as an abnormal increase in the proportion of fat cells in the body. Weight gain in which the body is moving toward an overweight or obese state is characterized predominantly by adipocyte hypertrophy and hyperplasia. Through this process, adipocytes can increase their volume several thousand times to accommodate large increases in lipid storage. In addition, preadipocytes are triggered to become adipocytes. This process occurs primarily in the visceral (intra-abdominal) and subcutaneous tissues of the body. Recognizing the significance of the characteristics of adiposity, including total amount, distribution, and function of the adipose tissue in the development of comorbid conditions, there is recent movement toward coining *obesity* as an adiposity-based, chronic disease (Mechanick et al., 2017).

Overweight and obesity result from a complex interaction of genetic, nutritional, physiological, psychological, behavioural, environmental, and social factors that create an imbalance between energy intake and energy expenditure. Obesity is not a condition resulting from a lack of willpower and self-control but, instead, is a pervasive, progressive, and serious chronic condition that is strongly associated with a variety of comorbid conditions and that has a major effect on the physical, mental, social, cultural, and economic health of those affected (Williams et al., 2015). Interventions to address obesity must account for the complexity and progressive nature of the chronic condition and promote appropriate lifelong management, which often necessitates sustained contact and support from trained health care providers (Bomberg et al., 2019).

Classifications of Body Weight and Obesity

The degree to which a patient is classified as having underweight, normal weight, overweight, or obesity is assessed with the use of a body mass index (BMI) chart (Figure 43.1). BMI is calculated by dividing weight (in kilograms) by height (in metres squared). Research studies in large groups of people have shown that the BMI can be classified into ranges associated with health risk (Table 43.1). Individuals with a BMI of 25 to 29.9 kg/m² are classified as having overweight, those with a BMI of 30 to 34.9 kg/m² are classified as having class 1 obesity, those with a BMI of 35 to 39.9 are classified as having class 2 obesity, and those with a BMI of 40 kg/m² or greater are classified as having class 3 obesity. BMI should be considered an indicator but not a definitive determinant of health risk as it does not take into consideration whether the weight consists of muscle or fat.

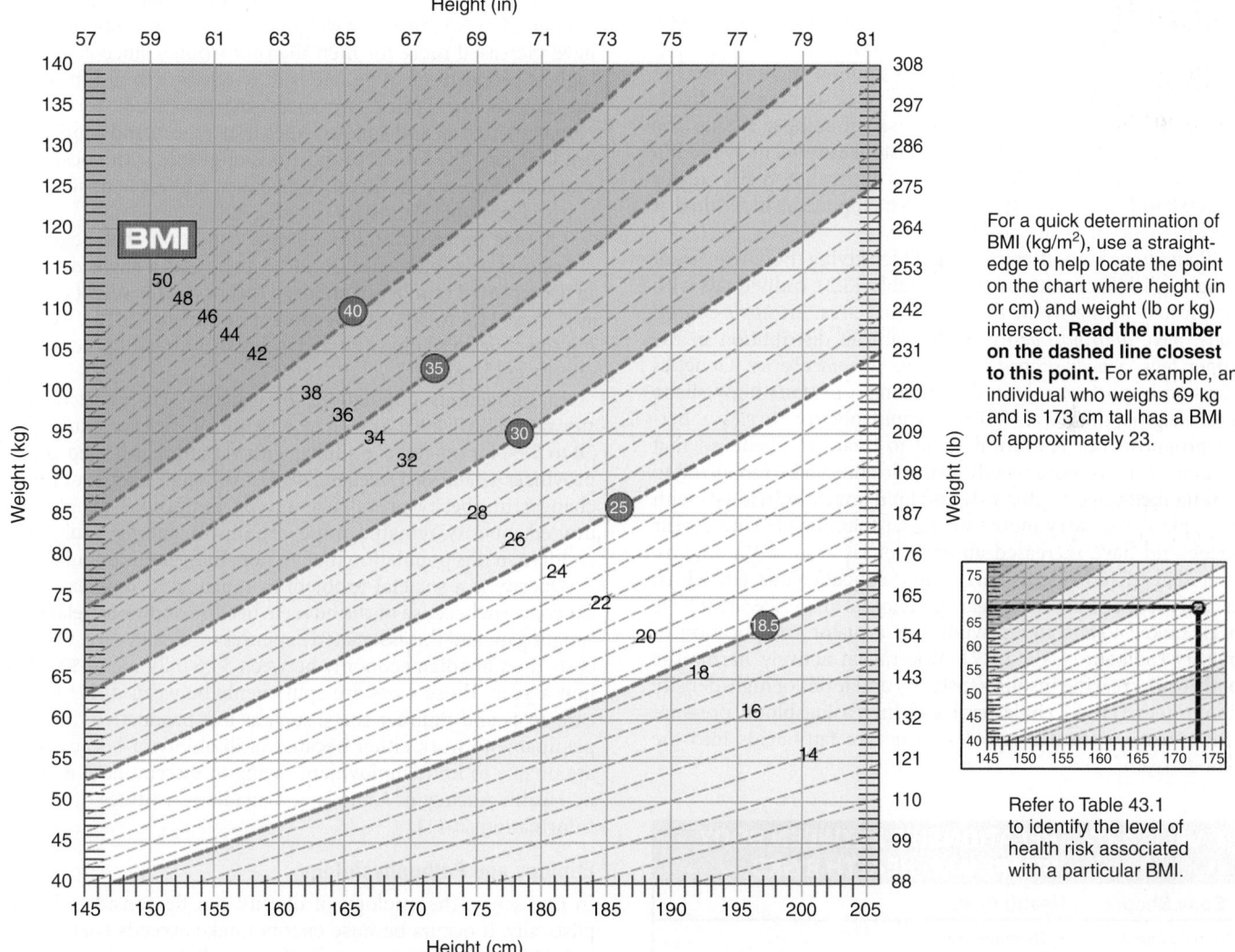

For a quick determination of BMI (kg/m²), use a straight-edge to help locate the point on the chart where height (in or cm) and weight (lb or kg) intersect. **Read the number on the dashed line closest to this point.** For example, an individual who weighs 69 kg and is 173 cm tall has a BMI of approximately 23.

Refer to Table 43.1 to identify the level of health risk associated with a particular BMI.

FIG. 43.1 Body mass index chart. Source: Health Canada. (2003). *Canadian guidelines for body weight classification in adults* (Cat. no. H49-179/2003E). Author. http://www.hc-sc.gc.ca/fn-an/alt_formats/hpfb-dgpsa/pdf/nutrition/cg_quick_ref-ldc_rapide_ref-eng.pdf

TABLE 43.1 CLASSIFICATION OF OVERWEIGHT AND OBESITY

	BMI (kg/m²)	Obesity Class	Disease Risk Based on Waist Circumference*	
			Men ≤102 cm Women ≤89 cm	Men >102 cm Women >89 cm
Underweight	<18.5	—	—	—
Normal†	18.5–24.9	—	—	—
Overweight	25.0–29.9	—	Increased	High
Obese	30.0–34.9	Class I	High	Very high
	35.0–39.9	Class II	Very high	Very high
Morbidly obese	≥40.0	Class III	Extremely high	Extremely high

BMI, body mass index.
*Disease risk for type 2 diabetes, hypertension, and cardiovascular disease.
†Increased waist circumference can also be a marker for increased risk in persons of normal weight.
Source: Adapted from National Heart, Lung, and Blood Institute. (n.d.). *Classification of overweight and obesity by BMI, waist circumference, and associated disease risks.* http://www.nhlbi.nih.gov/health/public/heart/obesity/lose_wt/bmi_dis.htm

As such, BMI is not used for highly muscular people, very lean body builds, pregnant women, older persons, or young children (Health Canada, 2019).

Waist circumference is another way to assess and classify a person's health risk associated with weight (see Table 43.1). Health risks increase with a waist circumference greater than 101.6 cm in men and greater than 88.9 cm in women (Ford et al., 2014). People who have visceral fat with truncal obesity are at an increased risk for cardiovascular disease and metabolic syndrome (discussed later in this chapter).

The waist-to-hip ratio (WHR) is another method used to assess obesity. This ratio is a method of describing the distribution of both subcutaneous and visceral adipose tissue. The ratio is calculated by dividing the waist measurement by the hip measurement. A WHR less than 0.8 is optimal. A WHR greater than 0.8 indicates more truncal fat, which puts the individual at a greater risk for health complications.

Body shape is another method of identifying those who are at a higher risk for health problems (Table 43.2). Individuals with fat located primarily in the abdominal area, an *apple-shaped body,* have *android obesity.* Those with fat distribution in the upper legs, a *pear-shaped body,* have *gynoid obesity.* Genetics plays an important role in determining a person's body shape and weight (Goodarzi, 2018). Gynoid obesity carries a better prognosis but is more difficult to treat. It is believed that abdominal fat is more readily available and can be mobilized to maintain elevated triglyceride and lipid levels. Individuals with an apple shape carry more visceral fat than people with a pear shape and have increased amounts of fat around the organs. Pear-shaped individuals carry more subcutaneous fat, which causes more cellulite to appear. Abdominal and visceral fat have been linked to metabolic syndrome, a major complication of obesity (Shibata et al., 2017). Visceral fat actively harms the body by decreasing insulin sensitivity and levels of high-density lipoprotein (HDL) cholesterol and increasing blood pressure (BP). Visceral fat also releases more free fatty acids into the bloodstream.

TABLE 43.2	RELATIONSHIP BETWEEN BODY SHAPE AND HEALTH RISKS
Body Shape	**Health Risks**
Gynoid (pear)	• Osteoporosis • Varicose veins • Cellulite • Subcutaneous fat traps and stores of dietary fat • Trapped fatty acids stored as triglycerides

Android (apple)	• Heart disease
	• Diabetes mellitus
	• Breast cancer
	• Endometrial cancer
	• Visceral fat more active, causing:
	  • ↓ insulin sensitivity
	  • ↑ triglycerides
	  • ↓ HDL cholesterol
	  • ↑ BP
	  • ↑ free fatty acid release into blood

BP, blood pressure; *HDL,* high-density lipoprotein.

Epidemiology of Obesity

In developed and developing countries, obesity has reached epidemic proportions. The prevalence of overweight and obesity among Canadians has approximately doubled since the early 1980s. In 2018, just over 63% of Canadians over age 18 years self-reported having overweight or obesity, with one in four adult Canadians (26.8%) being classified as having obesity (Statistics Canada, 2019). In general, more men (69.4%) than women (57.6%) have overweight or obesity, and obesity rates have increased more for men than for women since 2003. The highest proportions of people with obesity are found in Atlantic Canada, the Prairie provinces, the Northwest Territories, Nunavut, Yukon, and smaller cities in northern and southwestern Ontario. The lowest proportions of people with obesity are found in Toronto, Montreal, Vancouver, and areas of southern British Columbia (Statistics Canada, 2019).

Obesity in adulthood is often a condition that begins in childhood or adolescence. In 2017, there was a slight decrease in the reported number of children that have overweight or obesity, from 31.5 to 30% (Government of Canada, 2018). Reversing the childhood obesity crisis is key to addressing the overall obesity epidemic.

In Indigenous populations in Canada, self-reported obesity rates (BMI ≥30) are 21 to 42% for off-reserve adults and 30 to 51% for on-reserve adults, with variation indicated across provinces (Batal & Decelles, 2019). Although data examining changes in obesity prevalence among Indigenous peoples are limited, obesity remains more prominent among adults and children in this population than in non-Indigenous populations.

Obesity is a societal problem as much as a complex medical concern, because of the adverse health conditions related to weight gain and the associated expenses for health care. Obesity costs the Canadian economy between $4.6 billion and $7.1 billion a year. Those costs are split evenly between direct health care costs and indirect costs, such as lost productivity of people unable to work either because of disability or because they are unable to find employment owing to discrimination (Public Health Agency of Canada & Canadian Institutes of Health Information, 2011).

Etiology and Pathophysiology

In one sense, the etiology of obesity can be considered simplistically. It occurs because energy intake exceeds energy output. However, the processes leading to obesity are much more complex and still undergoing investigation. The causes of obesity involve significant genetic–biological susceptibility factors that are highly influenced by environmental and psychosocial factors.

Genetic–Biological Basis. A genetic predisposition to obesity may be present in as many as 70% of those with obesity (Albuquerque et al., 2017). While genetic factors do not totally account for the etiology of obesity (Ellis et al., 2018), a number of genes have been linked to obesity. Genes actually may influence how calories are stored and energy released. "Energy-thrifty" genes, once protective against long periods when food was not available, are now maladaptive in societies in which food availability is no longer a primary issue. Genes may be responsible for why two individuals living in the same environment can vary considerably in body size.

A strong link exists between a gene known as *FTO* (fat mass and obesity-associated gene) and a person's BMI. Variants of this gene may explain why some people become overweight whereas others do not. People with two copies of a certain allele at the *FTO* gene weigh more and have a greater risk for obesity than those who do not have the risk allele (Tung et al., 2014). More research is needed to better understand the role of genes in obesity.

Regulation of eating behaviour, energy metabolism, and body fat metabolism are controlled by signals from the periphery that act on the hypothalamus (Figure 43.2). Appetite is influenced by many factors that are integrated by the brain, most importantly within the hypothalamus. Input to the hypothalamus is received from the periphery from many different hormones and peptides (Table 43.3). Interaction of these hormones and peptides at the level of the hypothalamus may be an important determinant in factors contributing to obesity.

Adipocytes are not just a storage unit for triglycerides; they are also endocrine cells known to produce at least 100 different proteins. These proteins are secreted as enzymes, adipokines, growth factors, and hormones that contribute to the development of insulin resistance and atherosclerosis.

Environmental Factors. Environmental factors play an important role in obesity. In today's culture, there is greater access to food, particularly prepackaged and fast foods, as well as soft drinks, which may have poor nutritional quality. Portion size of meals has also increased (Table 43.4). As well, eating outside of the home impedes the ability to control the composition and quality of food.

Lack of physical activity is another factor that contributes to weight gain and obesity. The amount of physical activity people engage in has decreased, both in the workplace and at home. With increases in technology and labour-saving devices, Canadians are expending less energy in their everyday lives. Numerous initiatives have been enacted in Canada to address inactivity and resultant obesity throughout the lifespan, such as ParticipACTION (see the Resources at the end of the chapter), but further measures are needed.

Socioeconomic status can affect obesity in a variety of indirect ways. People with low incomes may buy food that is less expensive and also often has poorer nutritional quality and greater caloric content. For example, prepackaged foods are purchased rather than fresh meats and produce. This population may also live in environments with limited access to recreation

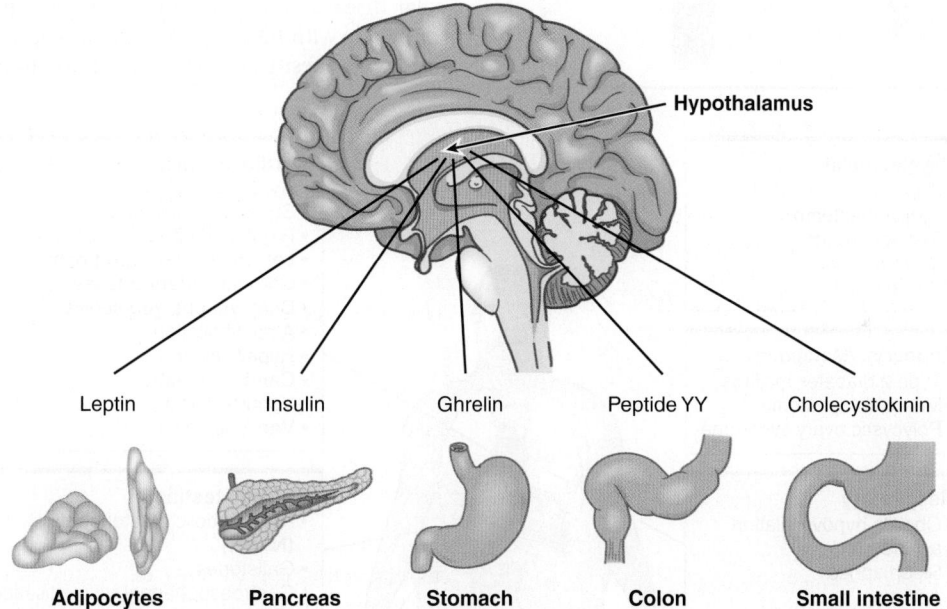

FIG. 43.2 Some of the common hormones and peptides that interact with the hypothalamus to control and influence eating patterns, metabolic activities, and digestion. Obesity causes a disruption in this balance (see Table 43.3).

TABLE 43.3	HORMONES AND PEPTIDES IN OBESITY		
Hormone or Peptide	**Where Produced**	**Normal Function**	**Alteration in Obesity**
Leptin	Adipocytes	Suppresses appetite and hunger Regulates eating behaviour	Obesity is associated with high leptin levels, and when leptin levels are high, leptin resistance develops; thus people who are obese may lose the effect of appetite suppression.
Insulin	Pancreas	Decreases appetite	Circulating levels are frequently high.
Ghrelin	Stomach (primarily)	Stimulates appetite ↑ after food deprivation ↓ in response to the presence of food in the stomach	Normal postprandial decline does not occur; increased appetite and overeating may result.
Peptide YY	Descending colon and rectum	Inhibits appetite by slowing GI motility and gastric emptying	Circulating levels are decreased; release is decreased after eating.
Cholecystokinin	Duodenum Jejunum	Inhibits gastric emptying and sends satiety signals to hypothalamus	Its role is unknown.

GI, gastrointestinal.

TABLE 43.4 PORTION SIZES
Past Versus Present

Food	20 Years Ago	Today
Turkey sandwich	320 cal	820 cal
Bagel	7.6 cm diameter: 140 cal	15.2 cm diameter: 350 cal
Cheeseburger	333 cal	590 cal
Soft drink	237 mL: 105 cal	591 mL: 250 cal

areas (e.g., playgrounds, walking tracks, tennis courts, swimming pools). The cost of gym memberships may also be prohibitive, preventing this venue for physical activity.

Psychosocial Factors. People use food for many reasons beyond nutritional maintenance. Many food associations begin in childhood, such as using food for comfort and reward. Furthermore, when overeating begins in childhood and continues into adulthood, a person's ability to sense fullness, or *satiety,* is compromised. Whether the desire to eat is triggered by specific foods or by the availability of a wide variety, some people consume food beyond their body's needs. The social component of eating occurs because of the association of food with pleasure. Food has become the central focus of most social events and celebrations. All of these factors must be included when considering the etiology and treatment of obesity.

Health Risks Associated With Obesity

Many health problems are more prevalent among people with obesity (Figure 43.3). The mortality rate rises as the rate of obesity increases, especially when obesity is associated with visceral fat. Among people with a BMI of 30 kg/m² or higher, the mortality rates from all causes—especially from cardiovascular disease—are generally 50 to 100% higher than the rates for people with BMIs in the normal range. The number of years lived with obesity also has a direct link to the risk for mortality

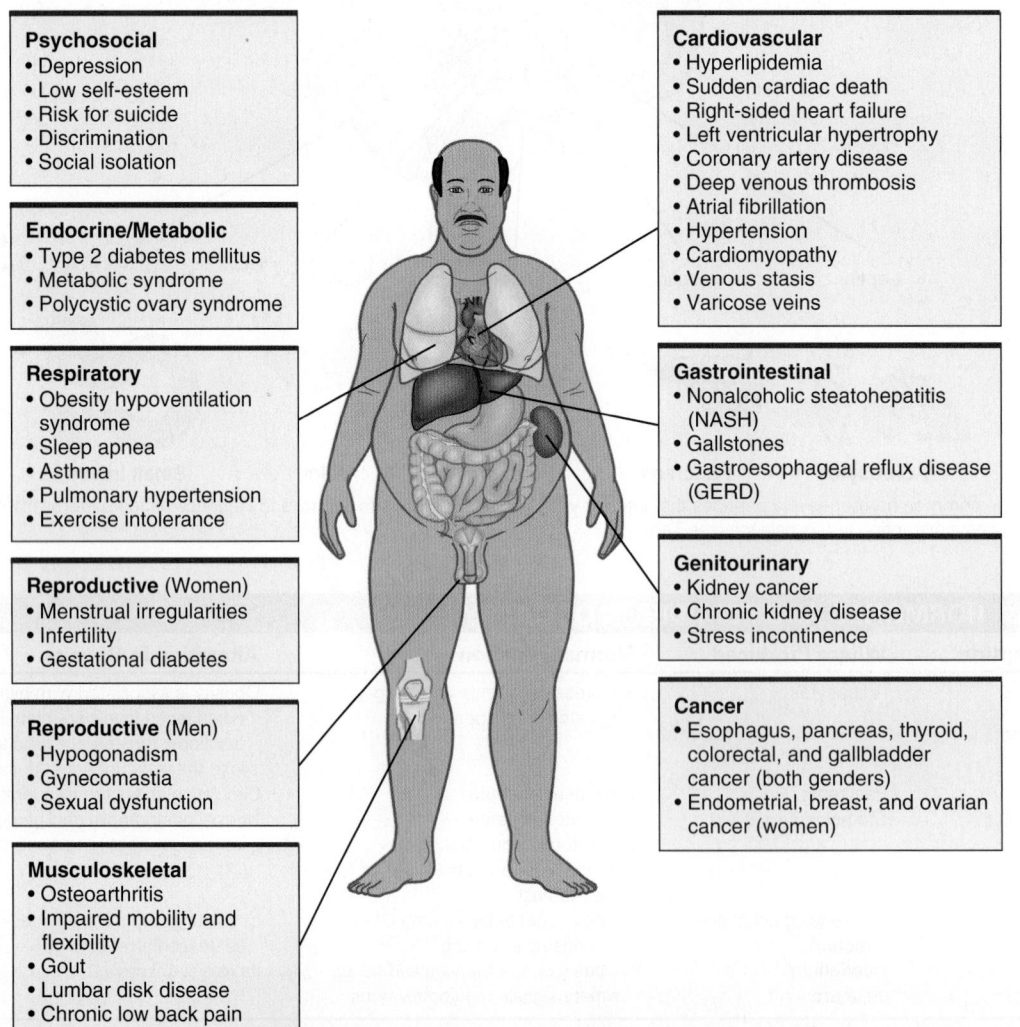

FIG. 43.3 Health risks associated with obesity.

TABLE 43.5	DIAGNOSTIC CRITERIA FOR METABOLIC SYNDROME*
Measurement	**Categorical Cutoff Point**
Waist circumference	Men: ≥102 cm
	Women: ≥88 cm
Triglyceride levels	≥1.7 mmol/L
	or
	Medication treatment for elevated triglyceride levels
HDL cholesterol level	Men: <1.0 mmol/L
	Women: <1.3 mmol/L
	or
	Medication treatment for reduced HDL cholesterol level
BP	≥130 mm Hg systolic
	or
	≥85 mm Hg diastolic
	or
	Medication treatment for hypertension
Fasting glucose level	≥5.6 mmol/L
	or
	Medication treatment for elevated glucose level

BP, blood pressure; *HDL*, high-density lipoprotein.
*At least three of the five measures must exceed the cutoff level for a diagnosis of metabolic syndrome.
Source: Alberti, K. G., Eckel, R. H., Grundy, S. M., et al. (2009). Joint scientific statement: Harmonizing the metabolic syndrome: A joint interim statement of the International Diabetes Federation Task Force on Epidemiology and Prevention; National Heart, Lung, and Blood Institute; American Heart Association; World Heart Federation; International Atherosclerosis Society; and International Association for the Study of Obesity. *Circulation, 120*, 1640–1645.

(Chen et al., 2019). In addition to these health risks, patients with obesity tend to have a reduced quality of life. Fortunately, most of these conditions can improve with weight loss. A loss of 5 to 10% of excess body weight can significantly improve obesity-related comorbid conditions (Fruh, 2017).

METABOLIC SYNDROME

Metabolic syndrome—also known as *syndrome X*, *insulin resistance syndrome*, and *dysmetabolic syndrome*—is a collection of risk factors that increase an individual's chance of developing cardiovascular disease and diabetes mellitus. Metabolic syndrome is diagnosed if an individual has three or more of the conditions listed in Table 43.5.

Etiology and Pathophysiology

The main underlying risk factor for metabolic syndrome is insulin resistance related to excessive visceral fat (Figure 43.4). Insulin resistance is the decreased ability of the body's cells to respond to the actions of insulin. To compensate, the pancreas secretes more insulin, which results in hyperinsulinemia.

Other characteristics associated with metabolic syndrome include hypertension, increased risk of clotting, and abnormalities in cholesterol levels. The net effect of these conditions is an increased prevalence of coronary artery disease.

NURSING AND INTERPROFESSIONAL MANAGEMENT METABOLIC SYNDROME

Lifestyle therapies are the first-line interventions to reduce the risk factors for metabolic syndrome. Interventions focus on reducing the major risk factors of cardiovascular disease:

PATHOPHYSIOLOGY MAP

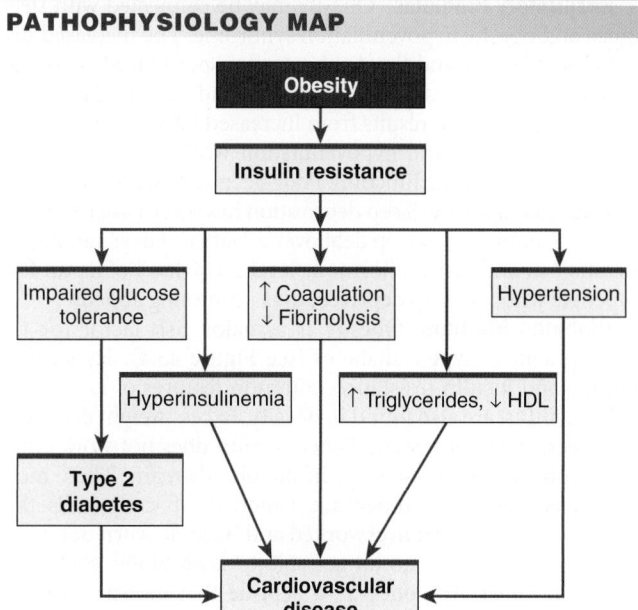

FIG. 43.4 Relationships among insulin resistance, obesity, diabetes mellitus, and cardiovascular disease. *HDL*, high-density lipoprotein.

lowering low-density lipoprotein (LDL) cholesterol level, quitting smoking, lowering BP, and reducing glucose levels. For long-term reduction of risk, weight should be decreased, physical activity increased, and healthy dietary habits established.

Nurses can assist patients by providing information on healthy eating, physical activity, and positive lifestyle changes. Weight reduction and maintenance of a lower weight should be the first priority in patients with abdominal obesity and metabolic syndrome.

Because a sedentary lifestyle contributes to metabolic syndrome, increasing regular physical activity reduces a patient's risk factors. In addition to assisting in weight reduction, regular physical activity has been found to decrease the triglyceride level and increase the HDL cholesterol level in patients with metabolic syndrome.

Patients who are unable to reduce their risk factors with lifestyle therapies alone and those at high risk for a coronary event or diabetes may be considered for medication therapy. Although there is no medication for metabolic syndrome, cholesterol-lowering medication and antihypertensives can be used. Metformin (Glucophage) has also been used to prevent or delay type 2 diabetes by lowering glucose levels and enhancing the cells' sensitivity to insulin.

Cardiovascular Problems. Obesity is a significant risk factor for predicting cardiovascular disease and stroke in both men and women. The WHR is the best predictor of these risks. Obesity, especially android obesity, is connected with increased levels of LDLs and triglycerides and decreased levels of HDLs (Bjornson et al., 2017). Obesity is also associated with hypertension. Hypertension can occur because of increased circulating blood volume, abnormal vasoconstriction, decreased vascular relaxation, and increased cardiac output with an accompanying increased risk for sleep apnea. Excess body fat can lead to chronic inflammation throughout the body, especially in blood vessels, thus increasing the risk for heart disease. Measurement of BP in a patient with obesity may require the use of a larger cuff size to ensure accuracy.

Respiratory Problems. Obesity may be connected with sleep apnea and obesity hypoventilation syndrome. The increased distribution of fat around the diaphragm causes reduced chest wall compliance, increased work of breathing, and decreased total lung capacity. Sleep apnea results from increased fat around the neck, leading to snoring and hypoventilation while sleeping. Weight loss can improve lung function. Poor sleep and sleep deprivation may increase appetite. Sleep deprivation has been associated with obesity. Building up a sleep debt over a matter of days can impair metabolism and disrupt hormone levels. The level of leptin falls in people who are sleep deprived, thus promoting appetite.

Diabetes Mellitus. Obesity is a major risk factor for the development of type 2 diabetes (see Figure 43.4). Hyperinsulinemia and insulin resistance, common features of type 2 diabetes mellitus, are also found in obesity. Excess weight decreases the effectiveness of insulin. When insulin does not work effectively, too much glucose stays in the bloodstream. Thus, more insulin is made to compensate. Pancreatic β cells (cells that make insulin) may get overworked and become worn out. Over time, the pancreas is no longer able to keep blood glucose in a normal range. Adiponectin, a peptide that increases insulin sensitivity, is decreased in people with obesity. Obesity complicates the management of type 2 diabetes mellitus by increasing insulin resistance and glucose intolerance. These factors make medication treatment for diabetes mellitus less effective.

Musculoskeletal Problems. Obesity is correlated with an increased incidence of osteoarthritis as a result of stress put on weight-bearing joints. Increased body fat also triggers inflammatory mediators and contributes to deterioration of cartilage. Hyperuricemia and gout are often found in people with obesity and in those who have metabolic syndrome.

Gastrointestinal and Liver Problems. Gastroesophageal reflux disease (GERD; also called *acid reflux*) and gallstones are prevalent among people with obesity. Gallstones occur when bile becomes supersaturated with cholesterol. Nonalcoholic steatohepatitis (NASH) is more common in people with obesity. In people with NASH, lipids are deposited in the liver, resulting in a fatty liver. NASH is associated with increased production of hepatic glucose and can eventually progress to cirrhosis and be fatal. Weight loss can improve symptoms associated with NASH.

Cancer. Overweight and obesity not only increase the risk for cardiovascular disease and type 2 diabetes mellitus but also are now known risk factors for a variety of cancer types (Avgerinoset et al., 2019; Lorenzo et al., 2019). The risk for breast, endometrial, ovarian, and cervical cancer is increased in women with obesity, possibly because of the increased estrogen levels (estrogen is stored in fat cells) associated with obesity in postmenopausal women. Colorectal cancer has been linked to hyperinsulinemia. Increased waist circumference and WHR, indicators of abdominal obesity, are associated with increased risk for colon cancer in both men and women. Esophageal cancer may be related to acid reflux caused by abdominal obesity. Several hormones and factors often present in obese states increase the risk for cancer. For example, insulin, a powerful cellular growth factor, is increased in obesity. The resulting hyperinsulinemia may affect cancer cells. Adipokines from fat cells may stimulate or inhibit cell growth. For example, leptin, which is increased in people with obesity, promotes cell proliferation.

Psychosocial Issues. The impact of obesity extends beyond physical changes and often affects the individual's emotional well-being. Clear and consistent stigmatization of people with obesity and, in some cases, discrimination occur in three important areas of living: employment, education, and health care. In addition to coping with the negative social impact, many people with obesity have low self-esteem, withdraw from social interaction, and can experience major depression and anxiety (Amiri & Behnezhad, 2019; Rotenberg, 2017).

NURSING AND CONSERVATIVE INTERPROFESSIONAL MANAGEMENT
PATIENTS WITH OBESITY

NURSING ASSESSMENT

The nurse plays a major role in the planning and management of care for patients with obesity. Information that can assist nurses in understanding patients with obesity and provide a basis for intervention is presented in Table 43.6. Because many individuals with obesity have experienced weight bias in the past, nurses should be aware of their own perceptions and beliefs about obesity and ensure that their approach and actions are free of any possible interpretation of continued insensitivity (Ramos-Salas et al., 2017). By being sensitive when asking specific and leading questions, nurses can often obtain information that patients may otherwise withhold out of embarrassment or shyness (Table 43.7). Nurses must provide acceptable reasons for asking personally intrusive questions, respond to patients' concerns about diagnostic tests, and interpret test outcomes. A patient's answers to questions must be treated with respect, understanding, and a nonjudgemental attitude. Knowledge regarding assessment and stepwise management for the treatment of obesity can help nurses and interprofessional team members guide patients and their families through weight loss interventions.

The health care provider should determine whether any physical conditions are present that may be causing or contributing to obesity. This determination requires a thorough history and physical examination. When obtaining the history, the nurse needs to explore genetic and endocrine factors such as hypothyroidism, hypothalamic tumours, Cushing's syndrome, hypogonadism in men, and polycystic ovary disease in women. Laboratory tests of liver function, fasting glucose level, and lipid panel (triglyceride level and LDL and HDL cholesterol levels) assist in evaluating the cause and effects of obesity.

As part of the initial nursing history and physical examination, each body system should be examined, with particular attention given to the organ system in which the patient has expressed a problem or concern. Measurements may include waist circumference, height (without shoes), and weight (in a private location and in a gown, if possible) to calculate BMI. The nurse needs to have the right equipment to take these measurements and to provide appropriately sized chairs, examination tables, and scales that can accommodate a person with obesity. Specific documentation of these measurements assists the health care provider with a more in-depth history and physical examination.

NURSING DIAGNOSES

Nursing diagnoses for the patient with obesity include but are not limited to the following:

- *Inadequate breathing pattern* resulting from *obesity* (decreased lung expansion)
- *Obesity* resulting from *energy expenditure below energy intake based on standard assessment*
- *Reduced skin integrity* resulting from *moisture, pressure over bony prominence*

TABLE 43.6 NURSING ASSESSMENT

Patient With Obesity

Subjective Data

Important Health Information

Past health history: Time of obesity onset; diseases related to metabolism and obesity (e.g., hypertension, cardiovascular conditions, stroke, cancer, chronic joint pain, respiratory conditions, diabetes mellitus, cholelithiasis, metabolic syndrome); family history of obesity; history of weight gain and loss

Medications: Prescription and over-the-counter (including supplements and herbal products)

Surgery or other treatments: Prior bariatric surgery, other weight-reduction procedures, or other major surgical procedures related to risk factors precipitated by obesity

Medical History

- Comorbid conditions (time since diagnosis, current treatment, and current symptoms)
- Drowsiness, somnolence; dyspnea on exertion, orthopnea, paroxysmal nocturnal dyspnea
- History or symptoms of mental illness (feelings of depression, guilt, rejection, isolation)
- Psychosocial history (income, housing, supports)
- Menstrual irregularity, heavy menstrual flow in women, infertility
- Altered sexual activity or function
- Barriers to performing activities of daily living
- Nutritional status

Objective Data

General

BMI ≥30 kg/m²; waist circumference: woman, >88 cm; man, >102 cm

Respiratory

Increased work in breathing; wheezing; rapid, shallow breathing, sleep apnea, neck circumference (<42 cm = low risk)

Cardiovascular

Hypertension, tachycardia, dysrhythmias, hyperlipidemia

Musculoskeletal

Decreased joint mobility and flexibility; knee, hip, and low back pain

Reproductive

Menstrual irregularities and infertility in women; gynecomastia and hypogonadism in men

Possible Findings

Elevated levels of serum glucose, cholesterol, triglycerides, and A_{1c}; chest radiograph demonstrating an enlarged heart; ECG tracing showing dysrhythmia; abnormal results of liver function tests, radiograph evidence of osteoarthritis

BMI, body mass index; *ECG,* electrocardiogram.

- *Reduced self-esteem* resulting from *cultural incongruence, inadequate respect from others, inadequate belonging*
- *Reduced physical mobility* resulting from *BMI greater than seventy-fifth percentile appropriate for age and gender*
- *Disrupted body image* resulting from *alteration in self-perception*

PLANNING

The overall goals are that the patient with obesity will (a) modify their eating patterns, (b) participate in a program of regular physical activity, (c) achieve weight maintenance (stop historic pattern of continued weight gain over time) or achieve weight loss to a specified level, (d) maintain weight loss at a specified level, and (e) minimize or prevent health problems related to obesity.

TABLE 43.7 ASSESSING A PATIENT WITH OBESITY

When assessing a patient with obesity, the nurse should consider asking several different types of questions, such as the following:

- What is the patient's history with weight gain and weight loss?
- Is the patient interested in losing weight or managing weight differently?
- What does the patient think contributes to their weight?
- What barriers does the patient feel impede weight loss efforts?
- What does food mean to the patient? How does the patient use food (e.g., to relieve stress, provide comfort)?
- Is the patient's food intake influenced by hunger?
- Are other family members overweight?
- Are there environmental or genetic factors influencing the weight gain?

NURSING IMPLEMENTATION

Obesity is one of the most challenging health care problems. For most patients, successful weight management will require lifelong efforts. The nurse, working closely with the other members of the health care team, plays a major role in the planning and management of the care of a patient with obesity. As stated earlier, to be effective, nurses must be aware of their own perceptions of and beliefs about obesity and obesity interventions. Although health care for patients with obesity has inherently greater demands, health care providers often fail to address these needs, and people with obesity underutilize health care opportunities available to them. In addition, health care providers may be reluctant to counsel patients about obesity, often citing a lack of time during appointments, lack of professional reward for weight management, lack of reimbursement for weight management services, and a lack of knowledge of or faith in the effectiveness of weight management interventions. If a health care provider associates obesity with lack of willpower and with overindulgence, patients can experience weight bias and stigma in the health care setting. Nurses are in a pivotal position to help people with overweight and obesity manage negative experiences and educate other health care providers to reduce or eliminate their bias.

Despite knowing benefits of weight loss, most people find the process of losing weight tough. Achieving an "ideal" BMI is not necessary and may not be a realistic goal. Modest weight loss of even 3 to 5% of starting weight can have clinical benefits, and additional weight loss can produce greater benefits (Acosta et al., 2017). In general, the average weight loss program (excluding bariatric surgery) results in a 10% reduction of body weight. This average should not be considered a failure since it is associated with significant health benefits.

Exploring a person's motivation for weight loss is essential for overall success. Using principles from motivational interviewing (see Chapter 4), the nurse can help patients understand their desire to lose weight and gain confidence in achieving weight loss. Focusing on the reasons for wanting to lose weight may help patients develop strategies for a weight management program. Any supervised plan of care must be directed at two different processes: (1) successful weight loss, which requires a short-term energy deficit, and (2) successful weight maintenance, which requires long-term behavior changes. A holistic approach for weight management must be used that includes medical nutritional therapy, physical activity, behavioural and psychological interventions, and, for some individuals, pharmacotherapy or surgical intervention. Combining more than one aspect supports more effective weight loss and weight maintenance efforts. While teaching patients, the nurse should stress healthy eating habits and adequate physical activity as lifestyle patterns to develop and maintain.

Obesity Canada's (Canadian Obesity Network, 2011) 5A's of Obesity Management (Figure 43.5) was designed as a five-step framework to assist health care providers in supporting patients with obesity treatment. This method emphasizes that obesity is a chronic disease and requires long-term treatment. Even with a comprehensive action plan, there is a high rate of weight regain among people in all age groups, which is discouraging considering the amount of time and effort expended in the process of attempting to lose weight. For successful management of obesity, it should be viewed as a chronic condition that requires day-to-day attention to support losing weight and maintaining weight loss and the other health benefits achieved through treatment.

MEDICAL NUTRITIONAL THERAPY. Nutrition interventions should be developed with a qualified and experienced health care provider, preferably a registered dietitian (Early & Stanley, 2018). Diets may be classified as low-calorie (800–1 200 kcal/day) or very-low-calorie (less than 800 kcal/day). Although the example of a low-calorie diet presented in Table 43.8 can be used, it is important for the nurse to be aware that dietitians work with patients to develop a safe, individualized plan that ensures nutritional needs are met and aligns with the patient's values, preferences, and treatment goals (Brown et al., 2020).

Individuals on low-calorie and very-low-calorie diets require professional monitoring because the severe energy restriction places them at risk for deficiency of multiple nutrients. A diet that includes adequate amounts of fruits and vegetables provides fibre to support the prevention of constipation and to meet daily vitamin A and vitamin C requirements. Lean meat, fish, and eggs can provide sufficient protein and B-complex vitamins.

Most people with overweight or obesity have at some time attempted to lose weight. Some have had limited and temporary success, and others have met only with failure. Many individuals attempt weight loss by trying a least one of the many fad diets that offer the enticement of quick weight loss with little effort. Often fad diets advocate for the elimination of one or more categories of foods (e.g., carbohydrates) and should not be followed. Low-carbohydrate diets, for example, do produce a rapid weight loss, but they also may not allow for adequate amounts of fibre, vitamins, and minerals. Fad diets are difficult to maintain in the long term because of their restrictive nature.

Assessing and supporting readiness for change and patient motivation are essential steps in successful weight management interventions. The nurse can assist by helping the patient track eating patterns with a food journal. Setting realistic and healthy goals must be mutually agreed on at the outset. A weekly check of body weight is a good method of monitoring progress. Daily weighing is not recommended because of the frequent fluctuations resulting from retained water (including urine) and elimination of feces. The patient should be instructed to record their weight at the same time of the day, wearing the same type of clothing.

There is no firm agreement on the number of meals to be eaten when reducing caloric intake. Some advocate several small meals per day because the body's metabolic rate is temporarily increased immediately after eating. However, when several small meals are ingested per day, more calories may be

---

TABLE 43.8   NUTRITIONAL THERAPY

Sample 1 200-Calorie Weight Reduction Diet*

General Principles

1. Eat regularly. Do not skip meals.
2. Measure foods to determine the correct portion size.
3. Avoid concentrated sweets, such as sugar, candy, honey, pies, cakes, cookies, and regular soft drinks.
4. Reduce fat intake by baking, broiling, or steaming foods.
5. Maintain a regular physical activity program for successful weight loss.

Meal	Menu Plan
Breakfast	30 g (¾ cup) dry cereal (unsweetened) 1 small banana 250 mL (1 cup) non-fat milk Coffee, black, unsweetened
Lunch	Beef and cheese enchiladas (made with 35 g cheese and 57 g lean ground beef) 2 corn tortillas with shredded lettuce 10 mL (2 tsp) chili sauce 175 g (1 cup) sliced tomatoes and cucumbers 30 mL (1 tbsp) low-fat salad dressing 90 g (approx 12) grapes 500 mL (2 cups) water
Dinner	75 g baked chicken breast (no skin) 5 mL (1 tsp) margarine 350 g (2 cups) tossed salad and 30 mL (1 tbsp) low-fat salad dressing 90 g (½ cup) strawberries 90 g (½ cup) whole grain rice 250 mL (1 cup) nonfat milk

*For 1 500 calories, add one meat and alternative serving and two vegetable and fruit servings, and include one serving of the daily recommended oil and fats. For 1 800 calories, add one grain product serving, one milk and alternative, two meat and alternative servings, two vegetable and fruit servings, and an additional serving of oil and fats.

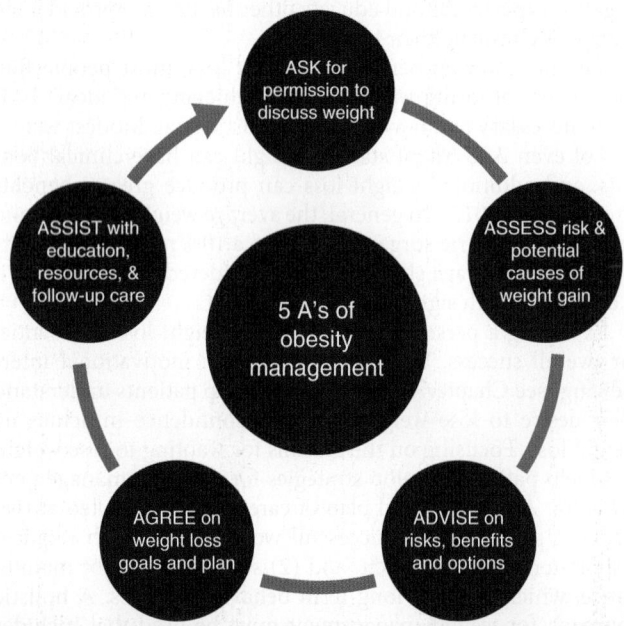

FIG. 43.5 Obesity Canada's 5As of obesity management. Source: © 2011 Canadian Obesity Network. All rights reserved. https://obesitycanada.ca/wp-content/uploads/2018/02/Practitioner_Guide_Personal_Use.pdf

consumed. The patient should be provided education regarding portion sizes to achieve nutritional goals.

Portion sizes have increased considerably (see Table 43.4) over the last 40 years. Food portions can be weighed on a scale, or everyday objects can be used as a visual cue to determine portion sizes; for example, the size of a woman's fist or a baseball is equivalent to one serving of vegetables or fruit. A serving of meat is about the size of an adult's palm or a deck of cards. A serving of cheese is about the size of a thumb or six dice (see the Alberta Health Services website listed in the Resources section at the end of this chapter for a sample patient teaching tool). A test on portion sizes is also available online (see the Resources at the end of this chapter). A food journal is an important tool for understanding eating habits, bringing awareness to the patient regarding actual food consumed, and informed goal setting.

Canada's Food Guide, updated in 2019, focuses on choosing healthy foods, limiting intake of processed foods, making water one's drink of choice, using food labels to make wise food choices, and being aware of marketing influences (Government of Canada, 2020). Patients can be further assisted in understanding and exercising good portion control and choosing appropriate proportions from each of the food groups by learning how portions fit on a plate to make up a healthy meal. Half of the plate should be vegetables and fruit; one quarter, whole grains; and one quarter, protein-rich foods, including plant- and animal-based protein sources, as well as calcium-rich foods, milk, cheese, and yogourt (Health Canada, 2021). For further details see Chapter 42.

PHYSICAL ACTIVITY. Physical activity is an essential part of a weight management program. Current recommendations state that, to achieve health benefits, people aged 18 to 64 should accumulate at least 150 minutes of moderate to vigorous aerobic activity per week, in bouts of at least 10 minutes or more (Canadian Society for Exercise Physiology, 2021). There is no evidence that increased activity promotes an increase in appetite or leads to dietary excess. In fact, physical activity frequently has the opposite effect. The addition of physical activity produces more weight loss than does dieting alone. Increasing physical activity has a favourable effect on body fat distribution with a reduction in WHR. Physical activity is especially important in maintaining weight loss in people with overweight and obesity.

The nurse and the patient should explore possible ways to increase physical activity in daily routines. It may be as simple as parking farther from a patient's place of employment or taking the stairs rather than the elevator. The patient should be encouraged to wear a fitness tracker to track daily activity, with a goal of 10 000 steps a day (Bray et al., 2016). However, initial success may be walking a third of the recommended steps, with incremental increases over time.

Walking, swimming, and cycling are sensible forms of physical activity and have long-term benefits. Engaging in weekend exercise only or in spurts of strenuous activity is not advantageous and can actually be dangerous. When large muscles are involved in the physical activity program, a primary benefit is cardiovascular conditioning. Individuals with overweight who are active and fit have lower rates of morbidity and mortality than individuals with overweight who are sedentary and unfit. Therefore, physical activity is of benefit to people with overweight, even if it does not make them lean.

An increased physical activity program offers many psychological benefits. Patients can achieve reduction in tension and stress, better quality sleep and rest, increased stamina and energy, improved self-concept and self-confidence, better attitudes toward work and play, and increased optimism about the future.

BEHAVIOUR MODIFICATION. Most behaviour-modification programs de-emphasize the diet and focus on how and when the person eats. Ideally, behavior intervention should begin with counselling sessions with a trained interventionist. People who have undergone behaviour therapy are more successful in maintaining their losses over an extended time than are those who do not participate in such training (Lv et al., 2017).

Common behavioural techniques included in weight management interventions are (a) self-monitoring, (b) stimulus control, and (c) rewards. *Self-monitoring* may involve the person keeping a record of what and when foods are eaten, as well as how the person was feeling when the foods were consumed. *Stimulus control* is aimed at separating events that trigger eating from the act of eating. For example, if the patient overeats while watching television, limiting eating to a certain area (e.g., kitchen table) can be an effective way to weaken the link between eating and television watching. The more often the person does not eat in front of the television, the less likely television watching will trigger overeating. *Rewards* may be used as incentive for weight loss. Short- and long-term goals are useful benchmarks for earning rewards. It is important that the reward for a specified weight loss not be associated with food, such as dinner out or a favourite treat. Reward items do not have to have a monetary component. For example, time for a hot bath or an hour of pleasure reading would be an enjoyable reward for many people.

People may participate in group or individual sessions or both as they work toward their goals.

SUPPORT GROUPS. Patients may benefit from joining a support group that includes professional counselling or trained facilitation. Many self-help groups are available to people who want to learn more about successful obesity management and who like the support of others who have the same issues and similar experiences. Take Off Pounds Sensibly (TOPS) is the oldest nonprofit organization of this type in the world. Behaviour modification is an integral part of the program, along with nutrition education. Weight Watchers (WW) International, Inc. is one of the most successful commercial weight-reduction enterprises (Alfaris et al., 2016).

Commercial weight-reduction centres have proliferated across the nation. Although behaviour-modification training is often incorporated within these programs, they are often costly, and the cost may be prohibitive for people with limited financial resources. In addition, many of these programs offer special prepackaged foods and supplements that must be purchased as part of the weight-reduction plan. Only these prescribed foods and drinks are to be consumed until an agreed-on amount of weight is lost. The patient is often encouraged to buy the same type of foods for the maintenance phase of the program, which lasts from 6 months to 1 year. This is problematic for reasons beyond just the associated costs. Obesity, as with all chronic diseases, resumes its course when the intervention stops. Patients are often frustrated to find that the weight they lost is regained once they stop participating in the commercial program.

Many places of employment have started wellness programs for their employees. The rationale for such programs is that better health repays the cost of the programs through improved work performance, decreased absenteeism, and, eventually, less hospitalization.

MEDICATION THERAPY

Medications can be used as part of an obesity treatment plan in conjunction with nutrition therapy, physical activity, and behaviour-modification therapies. Pharmacotherapy should be reserved for patients with a BMI ≥ 27 kg/m^2 who have existing comorbid conditions (e.g., hypertension, dyslipidemia, coronary artery disease, type 2 diabetes mellitus, and sleep apnea) and for those with a BMI ≥ 30 kg/m^2.

Pharmacotherapy does not cure obesity, and the patient must understand that without sustained nutritional, physical-activity, and behavioural changes, weight will be regained when medication therapy is stopped. Supervised long-term medication therapy with safe compounds can contribute to weight management as well as weight loss. As with any pharmacological treatment, there can be adverse effects. Careful evaluation for the presence of other medical conditions can help determine which medications, if any, would be advisable for a given patient.

The role of the nurse in relation to pharmacotherapy should centre on teaching the patient about proper administration and adverse effects and how the medication fits into the larger weight management plan. Modifying the dosage without consulting a health care provider can have detrimental effects. The purchase of over-the-counter diet aids should be discouraged unless recommended by a health care provider.

Orlistat (Xenical)

Orlistat (Xenical) was developed for weight loss and maintenance and works by blocking fat breakdown and absorption in the intestine. It inhibits the action of intestinal lipases. The undigested fat is excreted in the feces. Although this medication has a high safety profile, levels of some fat-soluble vitamins may decrease, and those vitamins may have to be supplemented. Orlistat is associated with leakage of stool, flatulence, diarrhea, and abdominal bloating, which is accentuated if a high-fat diet is consumed. These adverse effects limit its acceptance as a weight loss tool (CHEPLAPHARM, 2017).

Liraglutide (Saxenda)

Liraglutide (Saxenda) is an injectable medication used for weight management. It works by blocking GLP1 (glucagon-like peptide). Normally, liraglutide is used for the treatment of type 2 diabetes, but higher doses have been found to help with weight loss in patients following a calorie-reduced diet and a physical activity regimen (Pi-Sunyer et al., 2015). Health Canada approved the use of liraglutide (Saxenda) for weight management in patients with BMI >27 kg/m^2 and one or more health-related comorbidities or with a BMI >30 kg/m^2. Adverse effects of liraglutide include nausea and diarrhea as well as increased risk for pancreatitis and gallbladder disease (Novo Nordisk, 2016).

Naltrexone HCL/ Bupropion HCL (Contrave®)

Naltrexone HCL/bupropion HCL (Contrave®) is approved for use in individuals with a BMI >27 kg/m^2 and one or more health-related comorbidities or a BMI of >30 kg/m^2. Contrave® combines low doses of naltrexone, a medication commonly used to manage alcohol and opioid dependency, and bupropion, an atypical antidepressant that is also prescribed for smoking cessation. These medicines work on two separate areas of the brain that are involved in controlling eating (hunger and cravings). Adverse effects include increased suicidal thoughts or actions, seizures, risk of sudden opioid withdrawal or overdose, increased heart rate and BP, and risk for liver damage or hepatitis (Valeant Canada, 2018).

BARIATRIC SURGICAL THERAPY

Bariatric surgery is an invasive procedure used to treat morbid obesity. Bariatric surgery is currently the only treatment that has been found to help sustain weight loss in individuals who have severe obesity (Gadde et al., 2018). The majority of patients who undergo bariatric surgery have successfully improved their overall quality of life. In addition to losing weight, outcomes include improved glucose control with improvement or reversal of diabetes, normalization of BP, decreased total cholesterol and triglycerides, decreased GERD, and decreased sleep apnea (Adams et al., 2017).

Criteria guidelines for bariatric surgery include having a BMI of 40 kg/m^2 or higher or a BMI of 35 kg/m^2 or higher plus one or more obesity-related comorbid conditions (e.g., hypertension, type 2 diabetes mellitus, heart failure, or sleep apnea). Adults who meet this criteria should also have a documented history of conventional weight loss attempts that have been unsuccessful over time and a demonstrated history of accountability and responsibility marked by attending appointments regularly, practicing self-monitoring, completing laboratory tests, regularly taking medications, and making time for healthy eating and activity. The patient must have full understanding of the benefits and limitations of a surgical procedure to assist with the management of obesity, and the risk of the surgical procedure must be lower than the risks of not providing the treatment. Table 43.9 provides exclusion criteria for bariatric surgery.

Although overall mortality is very low, several complications can arise from surgery. Therefore, having surgery is carefully considered. Candidates for surgery must be screened for psychological, physical, and behavioural conditions that have been associated with poor surgical outcomes. These include untreated depression, binge eating disorders, and drug and alcohol misuse that may interfere with a commitment to lifelong behavioral changes. Other contraindications to surgery include an inability to follow nutritional recommendations or illnesses that are known to reduce life expectancy and are not likely to improve with weight reduction. These include advanced cancer; end-stage kidney, liver, and cardiopulmonary disease; and severe coagulopathy. Bariatric surgeries fall into one of three broad categories: restrictive, malabsorptive, or a combination of malabsorptive and restrictive (Table 43.10 and Figure 43.6). In *restrictive* procedures, the stomach is reduced in size (less food eaten), and in *malabsorptive* procedures, the length of the small intestine is decreased (less food absorbed).

Restrictive Surgeries

Restrictive bariatric surgery reduces either the size of the stomach, which causes the patient to feel full more quickly, or the amount allowed to enter the stomach. The stomach and the intestine digest and absorb food normally when restrictive gastrointestinal surgery is performed. Because digestion is not altered, the risk for anemia or cobalamin deficiency is low. The most common restrictive surgeries include adjustable gastric banding and vertical sleeve gastrectomy.

TABLE 43.9 EXCLUSION CRITERIA FOR BARIATRIC SURGERY

Patients *who are* or *who have* any of the following characteristics should not be offered bariatric surgery:

- BMI <35 kg/m²
- Age <18 yr or >65 yr
- A medical condition that makes surgery too risky
- Clinically significant or unstable mental health concerns
- An unrealistic postsurgical target weight
- Unrealistic expectations of a surgical procedure
- Not tried or optimized lifestyle or medical treatments
- A history of poor adherence to lifestyle, medical, or mental health interventions
- Pregnant, lactating, or plan for pregnancy within 2 yr of potential surgical treatment
- Lack of safe access to abdominal cavity or gastrointestinal tract
- Smokers (All smokers, regardless of their weight status, should quit smoking for at least 8 weeks before surgery as a goal of risk-factor management. All patients should be encouraged to remain nonsmokers or participate in smoking cessation programs.)

BMI, body mass index.
Source: Data from National Institutes of Health; National Heart, Lung, and Blood Institute; National Institute of Diabetes and Digestive and Kidney Diseases. (1998). *Clinical guidelines on the identification, evaluation, and treatment of overweight and obesity in adults. The evidence report.* National Institutes of Health. https://www.nhlbi.nih.gov/guidelines/obesity/ob_gdlns.pdf; and Mechanick, J. I., Kushner, R. F., Sugerman, H. J., et al. (2009). American Association of Clinical Endocrinologists, The Obesity Society, and American Society for Metabolic & Bariatric Surgery medical guidelines for the clinical practice for the perioperative nutritional, metabolic and nonsurgical support of the bariatric surgery patient. *Obesity, 17*(Suppl 1), S1–S70, v.

Adjustable Gastric Banding. With adjustable gastric banding, the stomach size is limited by an inflatable band placed around the fundus of the stomach. The band is connected to a subcutaneous port and can be inflated or deflated (by fluid injection in the health care provider's office) to change the stoma size to meet the patient's needs as weight is lost. The procedure can be done laparoscopically and can be modified or reversed after the initial procedure. Adjustable gastric banding is the preferred option for patients who are at surgical risk because it is a less invasive approach. Because it is restrictive only, patients must closely adhere to their nutritional plan to lose weight and avoid weight regain.

Vertical Sleeve Gastrectomy. In the vertical sleeve gastrectomy, about 75% of the stomach is removed, leaving a sleeve-shaped stomach. Although the stomach is drastically reduced in size, its function is preserved. Removing most of the stomach results in changes in hormones that stimulate hunger, such as ghrelin (Dimitriadis et al., 2017). The vertical sleeve gastrectomy cannot be reversed. The patient will need to follow a vitamin and mineral regimen after surgery.

Malabsorptive Surgery

In malabsorptive surgery to reduce weight, the surgeon bypasses various lengths of the small intestine so that less food is absorbed.

Biliopancreatic Diversion. Biliopancreatic diversion (BPD) involves removing approximately 75% of the stomach to produce both restriction of food intake and reduction of acid

TABLE 43.10 SURGICAL INTERVENTIONS FOR MORBID OBESITY*

Procedure	Anatomical Changes	Advantages	Complications
Restrictive Surgery			
Adjustable gastric banding (AGB) (Lap-Band, Realize band)	Band encircles the stomach, creating a stoma and a gastric pouch with 10- to 15-mL capacity	Food digestion occurs through normal process Band can be adjusted to ↑ or ↓ restriction Surgery can be reversed Absence of dumping syndrome Lack of malabsorption	Low complication rate Some nausea and vomiting initially Problems with adjustment device Band may slip or erode into stomach wall Gastric perforation
Vertical sleeve gastrectomy	About 85% of stomach removed, leaving a sleeve-shaped stomach with 60- to 150-mL capacity	Function of stomach preserved No bypass of intestine Avoids complications of obstruction, anemia, vitamin deficiencies	Possible limitation to weight loss Leakage related to stapling
Malabsorptive Surgery			
Biliopancreatic diversion (BPD) with or without duodenal switch	70% of the stomach removed horizontally Anastomosis between the stomach and the intestine Decreases the amount of small intestine available for nutrient absorption Duodenal switch cuts the stomach vertically so stomach is shaped like a tube	Increased amount of food intake Less food intolerance Greater long-term weight loss Rapid weight loss	Abdominal bloating, diarrhea, and foul-smelling gas (steatorrhea) Three or four loose bowel movements a day Malabsorption of fat-soluble vitamins Iron deficiency Protein-calorie malnutrition† Dumping syndrome†
Combination of Restrictive and Malabsorptive Surgery			
Roux-en-Y gastric bypass (RYGB)	Restrictive surgery on stomach, creating small gastric pouch connected to jejunum Remaining stomach and first segment of small intestine are bypassed	Better weight loss results than with gastric restrictive procedures Lower incidence of malnutrition and diarrhea Rapid improvement of weight-related comorbidities	Leak at site of anastomosis Anemia: iron deficiency, cobalamin deficiency, folic acid deficiency Calcium deficiency Dumping syndrome

*See Figure 43.6.
†Less common with duodenal switch.

output. The remaining portion of the stomach is connected to the lower portion of the small intestine. Nutrients pass without being digested. The patient loses weight because most of the calories and nutrients are routed into the colon, where they are not absorbed.

This procedure can increase the risk for gallstone formation and may necessitate removal of the gallbladder. Patients should be aware of the possibilities of intestinal irritation and ulcers. Other risks from BPD include abdominal bloating and foul-smelling stool or gas. During the period when the intestines adjust, bowel movements can be very liquid and frequent. This condition may lessen over time, but it may be a lifelong condition. Patients should also monitor their protein, iron, and cobalamin intake to ensure that they do not develop malnutrition or anemia. Supplements and vitamins should be taken to offset these risks.

Biliopancreatic Diversion With Duodenal Switch. A variation of the BPD procedure involves a duodenal switch in which the surgeon leaves intact a larger portion of the stomach, as well as a small part of the duodenum. This procedure also enables sparing of the pyloric valve, which helps prevent dumping syndrome.

Combination of Restrictive and Malabsorptive Surgery

Roux-en-Y Gastric Bypass. The Roux-en-Y gastric bypass procedure is a combination of restrictive and malabsorptive surgery. Complication rates with this procedure are low, patient tolerance is excellent, and the procedure has proved to sustain long-term weight loss. Because of this, the Roux-en-Y gastric bypass procedure is the bariatric surgery most commonly performed. In this procedure, the stomach size is decreased with a gastric pouch anastomosis that empties directly into the jejunum. This surgery can be performed through an open abdominal incision or through laparoscopy. Variations of this procedure include (a) stapling the stomach without transection to create a small gastric pouch (capacity of 20–30 mL), (b) creating an upper and a lower gastric pouch that are totally disconnected from each other, and (c) creating an upper gastric pouch and completely removing the lower pouch. After the procedure, food bypasses 90% of the stomach, the duodenum, and a small segment of jejunum.

A complication of this procedure is *dumping syndrome,* in which gastric contents empty too rapidly into the small intestine, overwhelming its ability to digest nutrients (see Chapter 44).

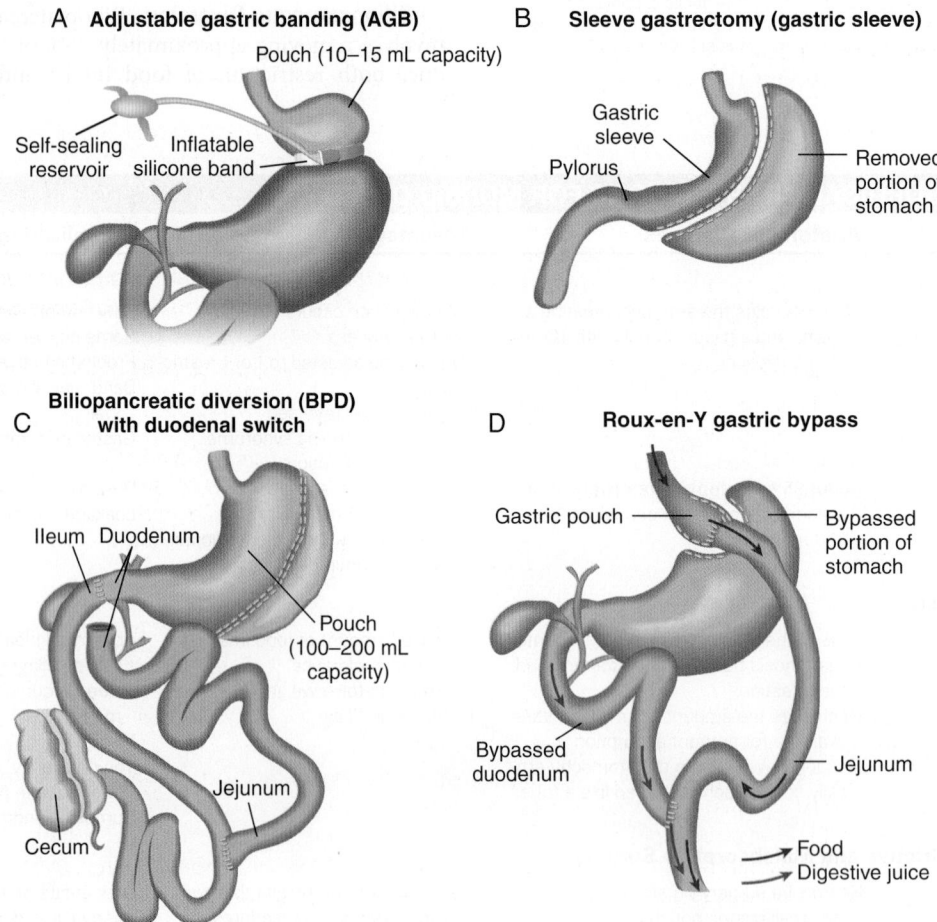

FIG. 43.6 Bariatric surgical procedures. **A,** Adjustable gastric banding involves the use of a band to create a gastric pouch. **B,** Vertical sleeve gastrectomy involves creating a sleeve-shaped stomach by removing approximately 85% of the stomach. **C,** Biliopancreatic diversion with duodenal switch procedure involves creating an anastomosis between the stomach and intestine. **D,** Roux-en-Y gastric bypass procedure involves constructing a gastric pouch whose outlet is a Y-shaped limb of small intestine.

Symptoms can include vomiting, nausea, weakness, sweating, faintness, and, on occasion, diarrhea. To avoid dumping syndrome, patients are discouraged from eating sugary foods after surgery. Because sections of the small intestine are bypassed, poor absorption of iron can cause iron-deficiency anemia. The patient needs to take a multivitamin with iron and calcium supplements. Chronic anemia caused by cobalamin deficiency may also occur. This problem usually can be managed with cobalamin injections or intranasal cobalamin preparations.

Cosmetic Surgical Therapy

Lipectomy. Lipectomy (adipectomy) is performed to remove unsightly loose folds of adipose tissue for cosmetic reasons. In some patients, up to 15% of the total fat cells can be removed from the breasts, the abdomen, and the lumbar and femoral areas. There is no evidence that adipose tissue regenerates at the surgical sites. However, it must be emphasized to the patient that surgical removal does not prevent obesity from recurring, especially if lifetime eating habits remain the same. Although body image and self-esteem may be enhanced by such procedures, these operations are not without complications. In patients with obesity, the effects of anaesthetics can be dangerous, and wound healing has the potential to be poor. It is more useful for the majority of patients contemplating a lipectomy to be instructed in preventive health measures, such as slow weight reduction to maintain and preserve tissue integrity, the value of physical activity, and behaviour-modification techniques.

Liposuction. Another surgical procedure is *liposuction,* or suction-assisted lipectomy. The current use is for cosmetic purposes and not for weight reduction. This surgical intervention helps improve facial appearance and body contours. A good candidate for this type of surgery is a person who has achieved weight reduction but has excess fat under the chin, along the jawline, in the nasolabial folds, over the abdomen, or around the waist and upper thighs. A long, hollow, stainless steel cannula is inserted through a small incision over the fatty tissue to be suctioned. The purpose of this type of surgery is to improve body appearance, thereby enhancing body image and self-concept. It is not usually recommended for older patients because the skin is less elastic and does not accommodate the new underlying shape.

NURSING MANAGEMENT
PERIOPERATIVE CARE OF THE PATIENT WITH OBESITY

NURSING IMPLEMENTATION

PERIOPERATIVE CARE. Patients with a BMI greater than 35 kg/m^2 may have other comorbid conditions related to obesity that increase their surgical risk factors and affect their care before, during, and after surgery. This section discusses general nursing considerations for the care of patients with obesity who are having surgery. (General care of patients before, during, and after surgery is discussed in Chapters 20 to 22).

PREOPERATIVE CARE. There are special care considerations for patients with obesity admitted to the hospital for surgical treatment, especially those who have morbid obesity. Before surgery, it is important to conduct a preoperative interview with the patient to obtain past and current health information and to ensure that the patient understands the surgical procedure that they are scheduled to undergo. If the patient has a disease other than obesity, care may need to be coordinated with the interprofessional team.

Every effort should be made to ensure the patient's dignity and privacy before admission. To eliminate embarrassment for the patient and frustration for the staff, a plan should be in place before the patient's arrival to ensure the unit is able to meet particular needs. Appropriate-size hospital gowns, beds that accommodate an increased body size, and necessary patient transfer equipment should be available. An oversized BP cuff should be available and placed in the patient's room. The nurse should consider how the patient will be weighed and transported throughout the hospital. A wheelchair with removable arms that is large enough to safely accommodate the patient and pass easily through doorways should be available. A single-bed room may be necessary for the privacy of the patient and to accommodate the bed and sitting arrangements (Alberta Health Services, 2021). A strongly reinforced trapeze bar should be placed over the bed to facilitate movement and positioning. Bathing, turning, and ambulating the patient may require additional staff, and a plan to meet this need should be in place before the patient's admission.

Obesity can cause a patient's breathing to become shallow and rapid. The extra adipose tissue in the chest and the abdomen compresses the diaphragmatic, thoracic, and abdominal structures. This compression restricts the chest's ability to expand, causing the lungs to not work as efficiently as they would otherwise. Thus, the patient retains more carbon dioxide. In addition, less oxygen is delivered to the lungs, resulting in hypoxemia, pulmonary hypertension, and polycythemia. The patient should be instructed in the proper coughing technique, deep breathing, and methods of turning and positioning to prevent pulmonary complications after surgery. The nurse should introduce the use of spirometry before surgery. Use of the spirometer helps prevent and alleviate postoperative lung congestion. Practising these strategies preoperatively can aid the patient in performing them correctly after surgery. Furthermore, if the patient uses a continuous positive airway pressure (CPAP) device at home for sleep apnea (see Chapter 9), arrangements should be made for use of a CPAP machine while the patient is in the hospital (see Chapter 68).

Obtaining venous access may also be complicated by excess adipose tissue. An assistant may be needed to help. If a patient has pitting edema or excess adipose tissue, the nurse should firmly, with pressure, hold a finger over the spot. The nurse may also want to mark the spot of injection with a sterile skin marker once a vein is found. Edema can become worse if the nurse chooses to anchor the catheter by taping the arm. This action can further impede venous return, causing venous stasis, pooling of intravenous fluids, extravasation, or infiltration. The nurse may also want to use multiple tourniquets to distend veins and hold back excess tissue. To avoid aggravating the edema, the tourniquet should be removed as soon as it is no longer needed. The nurse may also need a longer catheter (longer than 2.5 cm) to traverse overlying tissue. The cannula must reach far enough into the vein to ensure that it does not become dislodged or cause infiltration.

Special Considerations for Bariatric Surgery. The hospital experience will depend on the type of procedure and the surgical approach. The nurse should prepare the patient before surgery for the possibility of returning to the room with one or more of the following: urinary catheter, intravenous catheter, and compression stockings. The nurse should emphasize that vital signs will be checked and general assessment conducted frequently to monitor for immediate complications. Furthermore, the patient will be assisted with ambulation soon after surgery and encouraged to do deep-breathing exercises to prevent pulmonary complications. Liquids will be started soon after surgery but only after the patient is fully awake and no anastomotic leaks are found.

POSTOPERATIVE CARE. The initial postoperative care focuses on careful assessment and immediate intervention for cardiopulmonary complications, thrombus formation, anastomotic leaks, and electrolyte imbalances. The transfer of the patient from surgery may require additional staff members. During the transfer, the patient's airway should remain stabilized, and pain should be managed at a tolerable level. The head of the bed should be maintained at a 35- to 40-degree angle to reduce abdominal pressure and increase tidal flow (Thorell et al., 2016).

The nursing team should closely monitor for rapid oxygen desaturation. The body stores anaesthetic agents in adipose tissue; thus, the patient with excess adipose tissue is at risk for resedation. As adipose cells release anaesthetic back into the bloodstream, the patient may become sedated after surgery. If this happens, the nursing care team should be prepared to perform a head-tilt or jaw-thrust manoeuvre and keep the patient's oral and nasal airways opened. Early ambulation is essential for the postoperative bariatric patient. Preoperative teaching facilitates the patient's cooperation with what will be an uncomfortable activity. The patient should be informed that typically the evening after surgery, they will be assisted to walk and then be ambulated at least three or four times each day. The dangers of thrombophlebitis and the measures to counteract its development are a routine part of preoperative care. The patient should know that sequential compression devices or elastic compression stockings will be applied to the legs and that active and passive range-of-motion exercises will be a frequent part of daily care (Thorell et al., 2016). Antithrombotic medication may be ordered to help prevent blood clots.

Special Considerations for Bariatric Surgery. The nurse must be diligent in assessing pain and be aware that pain could be caused by an anastomotic leak rather than typical surgical pain. Pain medications should be given as frequently as necessary during the immediate postoperative period (first 24 hours). Depending on the size of the patient and the amount of pain experienced, the patient may not be able to assist the nurse in turning. Additional staff may be needed to help turn the patient safely. Abdominal wounds must be observed frequently for the amount and type of drainage, condition of the sutures, and signs of infection. The nurse must protect the incision against undue straining that accompanies turning and coughing. Wound dehiscence and impaired wound healing are potential problems for patients with obesity. Monitoring the vital signs assists in identifying complications such as infection or anastomotic leak.

Skin care should be performed several times each shift. Perspiration may be excessive at times. Skin folds should be kept clean and dry to prevent skin breakdown. For the patient who has an in-dwelling catheter, perineal care is important to prevent urinary tract infection.

During the immediate postoperative period (first 24 hours), the patient is given water and sugar-free clear liquid as soon as the patient is fully awake and there is no evidence of any anastomotic leaks. The nurse should begin with 15-mL increments every 10 to 15 minutes. The patient should be taught to avoid gulping fluids or drinking with a straw to reduce the incidence of air swallowing.

AMBULATORY AND HOME CARE

Special Considerations for Bariatric Surgery. The patient who has undergone major surgical treatment for obesity has been unsuccessful in the past following or maintaining a prescribed diet. Now the patient must reduce oral intake because of the anatomic changes from the surgical procedure. The patient must clearly understand the nutritional plan. A dietitian is usually part of the interprofessional team and helps the patient with the transition to the new nutritional plan. Patients usually are discharged on a full-liquid diet. Within 10 to 14 days after surgery, depending on tolerance, the patient may begin a pureed or soft-foods diet with vitamin supplementation. Most patients are able to transition to solid foods 4 to 6 weeks after surgery (Dagan et al., 2017). Patients may require a protein supplement once or twice a day for the first few months after surgery to meet their protein needs. Patients should not consume fluids with meals. Fluids and foods high in carbohydrate tend to promote symptoms of dumping syndrome. Calorie-dense foods should be avoided to permit more nutritionally sound food to be consumed. The patient should be taught to eat slowly and stop eating when feeling full. Weight loss is considerable during the first 6 to 12 months. Although behaviour modification is not necessarily an intended outcome with these surgical procedures, it becomes an unexpected secondary gain. For example, a person who has had bariatric surgery cannot overeat or binge eat without consequences (e.g., vomiting, abdominal pain).

The nurse needs to stress the importance of long-term follow-up care, in part because of potential complications. Patients should be taught to inform the health care provider of any changes in their physical or emotional condition. Nutritional deficiencies can occur after bariatric surgery, including anemia, vitamin deficiencies, and diarrhea. Patients should take multivitamins with folate, calcium, vitamin D, iron, and vitamin B_{12} for life (Cooley, 2017). Peptic ulcer formation, dumping syndrome, and small bowel obstruction may be seen late in the recovery and rehabilitation stage (see the Evidence-Informed Practice box).

By 6 to 8 months after surgery, considerable weight loss will have occurred, and patients are able to see clearly how much their appearance has changed. Massive weight loss often leaves the patient with large quantities of loose skin that can cause issues related to altered body image. Reconstructive surgery at least 1 full year after the initial surgery may alleviate this situation. Reduction of breasts, upper arms, thighs, and excess abdominal skin folds are possible solutions. Discussion of this possible outcome with the patient before surgery and again during the rehabilitation phase of recovery can help facilitate the patient's adjustment to a new body image and social reintegration.

EVIDENCE-INFORMED PRACTICE
Translating Research Into Practice

W. G. (pronouns he/him) is a 35-year-old patient weighing 166.4 kg with a BMI of 54.3 kg/m². He underwent gastric bypass surgery and is now ready for discharge. The bariatric program at the hospital recommends attendance at support groups after surgery. W. G. informs the nurse that he does not feel comfortable in group settings and will not be attending these meetings.

Best Available Evidence	Clinician Expertise	Patient Preferences and Values
Patients attending psychotherapeutic interventions or support groups in combination with bariatric surgery experience greater weight loss results than patients treated with only bariatric surgery.	The nurse has heard from several former bariatric patients who have maintained their weight loss after surgery and attributed this success, in part, to their participation in the support group offered at the facility.	Patient does not feel comfortable in group settings.

Decision and Action

The nurse explores W. G.'s feelings about groups and shares the reports from former patients with him. He continues to be firm about his unwillingness to attend any support groups. The nurse discusses with him that it is his decision and assures him that his progress will be monitored. The nurse also gently reminds him that he can change his decision at any time. The health care provider is informed of the patient's choice.

Reference for Evidence

Wnuk, S., Gougeon, L., & Basterfield, A. (2018). Support groups for severe obesity. In S. Cassin, R. Hawa, & S. Sockalingam (Eds.), *Psychological care in severe obesity: A practical and integrated approach.* Cambridge University Press.

EVALUATION

The following outcomes are expected for patients with obesity after surgery:
- The patient will experience long-term weight loss.
- The patient will experience improvement in obesity-related comorbid conditions.
- The patient will integrate healthy practices into daily routines.
- The patient will monitor for adverse effects of surgical therapy.
- The patient will have an improved self-image.

AGE-RELATED CONSIDERATIONS
OBESITY IN OLDER PERSONS

The prevalence of obesity is increasing in all age groups, including older people (Statistics Canada, 2019). The number of older persons with obesity has risen markedly because of both an increase in the total number of older people and an increase in the percentage of people with obesity. Obesity is more common in older women than in older men. A decrease in energy expenditure is an important contributor to a gradual increase in body fat with increasing age.

Obesity in older persons can exacerbate age-related declines in physical function and lead to frailty and disability. Excess body weight places more demands on arthritic joints; mechanical strain on weight-bearing joints can lead to premature immobility. Older persons may find that excess intra-abdominal weight causes urinary incontinence. Excess weight may also contribute to hypoventilation and sleep apnea. Obesity is associated with a shortened lifespan: Individuals with obesity live 6 to 7 years less than do people of normal weight.

Obesity affects quality of life for older people. Weight loss can improve their quality of life and physical function and lessen obesity-related health complications. The same therapeutic approaches to obesity discussed earlier also apply to older people.

CASE STUDY
Obesity

Patient Profile
S. R. (pronouns she/her) is 60 years old.

Subjective Data
- Reports gradual weight gain of 30 kg during past 40 years
- Spends most free time watching television
- Reports health problems related to type 2 diabetes mellitus, shortness of breath, hypertension, chest pressure, and osteoarthritis
- Underwent knee replacement surgery at age 56 for osteoarthritis

Objective Data
Physical Examination
- Height: 162.5 cm; weight: 105 kg
- Has obese, nontender, soft abdomen
- Blood pressure: 160/100 mm Hg

Laboratory Results
- Fasting blood glucose level: 13.9 mmol/L
- Total cholesterol level: 5.3 mmol/L
- Triglyceride level: 3.36 mmol/L
- HDL cholesterol level: 0.8 mmol/L

Discussion Questions
1. What are S. R.'s risk factors for obesity?
2. What is her estimated BMI?
3. Of the possible complications of obesity, which ones does S. R. have? Why did she develop them?
4. *Priority decision:* How would the nurse assist S. R. in designing a successful program for weight loss and weight management?
5. What are S. R.'s risk factors for metabolic syndrome?
6. Is S. R. a candidate for surgical intervention for obesity? If so, why? If not, why not?
7. *Priority decision:* On the basis of the assessment data presented, what are the priority nursing diagnoses? Are there any interprofessional issues?

ℓvolve
Answers are available at http://evolve.elsevier.com/Canada/Lewis/medsurg.

REVIEW QUESTIONS

The number of the question corresponds to the same-numbered objective at the beginning of the chapter.

1. Which of the following statements best describes the etiology of obesity?
   a. Obesity results primarily from a genetic predisposition.
   b. Psychosocial factors can override the effects of genetics in the etiology of obesity.
   c. Obesity is the result of complex interactions between genetic and environmental factors.
   d. Genetic factors are more important than environmental factors in the etiology of obesity.

2. Which obesity classification is *most* often associated with cardiovascular health problems?
   a. Obesity class 1
   b. Obesity class 2
   c. Gynoid fat distribution
   d. Android fat distribution

3. Health risks associated with obesity include which of the following? *(Select all that apply.)*
   a. Colorectal cancer
   b. Rheumatoid arthritis
   c. Polycystic ovary disease
   d. Nonalcoholic steatohepatitis
   e. Systemic lupus erythematosus

4. What is the best nutritional therapy for a person with obesity?
   a. Low-carbohydrate diet
   b. High-protein diet
   c. Low-sugar diet
   d. Foods from the basic food groups

5. Which bariatric surgical procedure involves creating a stoma and gastric pouch that is reversible and does not involve malabsorption?
   a. Sleeve gastrectomy
   b. Biliopancreatic diversion
   c. Roux-en-Y gastric bypass
   d. Adjustable gastric banding

6. A client with obesity has undergone Roux-en-Y gastric bypass surgery. In planning postoperative care, what should the nurse anticipate?
   a. The client may have severe diarrhea early in the postoperative period.
   b. The client will not be allowed to ambulate for 1 to 2 days postoperatively.
   c. The client will require nasogastric suctioning until healing of the incision occurs.
   d. The client may have only liquids orally, and in very limited amounts, during the early postoperative period.

7. Which of the following criteria must be met for a diagnosis of metabolic syndrome? *(Select all that apply.)*
   a. Hypertension
   b. Elevated triglyceride levels
   c. Elevated plasma glucose level
   d. Increased waist circumference
   e. Decreased LDL levels

1. c; 2. d; 3. a, c, d; 4. d; 5. d; 6. d; 7. a, b, c, d.

ⓔvolve

For even more review questions, visit http://evolve.elsevier.com/Canada/Lewis/medsurg.

REFERENCES

Adams, T. D., Davidson, L. E., Litwin, S. E., et al. (2017). Weight and metabolic outcomes 12 years after gastric bypass. *New England Journal of Medicine, 377*, 1143–1155. https://doi.org/10.1056/NEJMoa1700459

Alberta Health Services. (2021). *Guidelines for in-hospital care of the patient with bariatric care needs.* https://www.albertahealthservices.ca/assets/about/scn/ahs-scn-don-guidelines-for-hospitalized-patients-bariatric-needs.pdf

Albuquerque, D., Nóbrega, C., Manco, L., et al. (2017). The contribution of genetics and environment to obesity. *British Medical Bulletin, 123*(1), 159–173. https://doi.org/10.1093/bmb/ldx022

Alfaris, N., Minnick, A., Hong, P., et al. (2016). A review of commercial and proprietary weight loss programs. In J. Mechanik, & R. Kushner (Eds.), *Lifestyle medicine: A manual for clinical practice.* Springer.

Amiri, S., & Behnezhad, S. (2019). Obesity and anxiety symptoms: A systematic review and meta-analysis. *Neuropsychiatry, 33*, 72–89. https://doi.org/10.1007/s40211-019-0302-9

Avgerinos, K. I., Spyrou, N., Mantzoros, C. S., et al. (2019). Obesity and cancer risk: Emerging biological mechanisms and perspectives. *Metabolism, 92*, 121–135. https://doi.org/10.1016/j.metabol.2018.11.001

Batal, M., & Decelles, S. (2019). A scoping review of obesity among Indigenous peoples in Canada. *Journal of Obesity.* https://doi.org/10.1155/2019/9741090

Björnson, E., Adiels, M., Taskinen, M. R., et al. (2017). Kinetics of plasma triglycerides in abdominal obesity. *Current Opinion in Lipidology, 28*(1), 11–18. https://doi.org/10.1097/MOL.0000000000000375

Bomberg, E. M., Ryder, J. R., Brundage, R. C., et al. (2019). Precision medicine in adult and pediatric obesity: A clinical perspective. *Therapeutic Advances in Endocrinology and Metabolism, 10*, 1–25 doi:10.177/2042018819863022.

Bray, G. A., Frühbeck, G., Ryan, D. H., et al. (2016). Management of obesity. *Lancet, 387*(10031), 1947–1956. https://doi.org/10.1016/S0140-6736(16)00271-3

Brown, J., Clarke, C., Johnson Stoklossa, C., et al. (2020). *Canadian adult obesity clinical practice guidelines: Medical nutrition therapy in obesity management.* https://obesitycanada.ca/guidelines/nutrition

Canadian Obesity Network. (2011). *5As of obesity management.* Obesity Canada. https://obesitycanada.ca/wp-content/uploads/2018/02/Practitioner_Guide_Personal_Use.pdf

Canadian Society for Exercise Physiology. (2021). *Canadian 24-hour movement guidelines: An integration of physical activity, sedentary behaviour, and sleep.* https://csepguidelines.ca

Chen, C., Ye, Y., Zhang, Y., et al. (2019). Weight change across adulthood in relation to all cause and cause specific mortality: Prospective cohort study. *BMJ*, l5584. https://doi.org/10.1136/bmj.l5584

CHEPLAPHARM. (2017). *Product monograph. Xenical®.* https://pdf.hres.ca/dpd_pm/00041463.PDF

Cooley, M. (2017). Preventing long-term poor outcomes in the bariatric patient postoperatively. *Dimensions of Critical Care Nursing, 36*(1), 30–35. https://doi.org/10.1097/DCC.0000000000000223

Dagan, S. S., Goldenshluger, A., Globus, I., et al. (2017). Nutritional recommendations for adult bariatric surgery patients. *Advances in Nutrition, 8*(2), 382–394. https://doi.org/10.3945/an.116.014258

Dimitriadis, G. K., Randeva, M. S., & Miras, A. D. (2017). Potential hormone mechanisms of bariatric surgery. *Current Obesity Reports, 6*, 253–265. https://doi.org/10.1007/s13679-017-0276-5

Early, K., & Stanley, K. (2018). Position of the Academy of Nutrition and Dietetics: The role of medical nutrition therapy and registered dietitian nutritionists in the prevention and treatment of prediabetes and type 2 diabetes. *Journal of the Academy of Nutrition and Dietetics, 118*(2), 343–353. https://doi.org/10.1016/j.jand.2017.11.021

Ellis, L. J., Demaio, A., & Farpour-Lambert, N. (2018). Diet, genes, and obesity. *BMJ, 360*, k7. https://doi.org/10.1136/bmj.k7

Ford, E. S., Maynard, L. M., & Li, C. (2014). Trends in mean waist circumference and abdominal obesity among US adults, 1999–2012. *Journal of the American Medical Association, 312*(11), 1151–1153. https://doi.org/10.1001/jama.2014.8362

Fruh, S. (2017). Obesity: Risk factors, complications, and strategies for sustainable long-term weight management. *Journal of the American Association of Nurse Practitioners, 29*(S1), S3–S14. https://doi.org/10.1002/2327-6924.12510

Gadde, K. M., Martin, C. K., Berthoud, H. R., et al. (2018). Obesity: Pathophysiology and management. *Journal of the American College of Cardiology, 71*(1), 69–84. https://doi.org/10.1016/j.jacc.2017.11.011

Goodarzi, M. O. (2018). Genetics of obesity: What genetic association studies have taught us about the biology of obesity and its complications. *The Lancet Diabetes & Endocrinology, 6*(3), 223–236. https://doi.org/10.1016/S2213-8587(17)30200-0

Government of Canada. (2018). *Tackling obesity in Canada: Childhood obesity and excess weight rates in Canada.* https://www.canada.ca/en/public-health/services/publications/healthy-living/obesity-excess-weight-rates-canadian-children.html

Government of Canada. (2020). *Healthy food choices.* https://food-guide.canada.ca/en/healthy-food-choices/

Health Canada. (2019). *Canadian guidelines for body weight classification in adults.* https://www.canada.ca/en/health-canada/services/food-nutrition/healthy-eating/healthy-weights/canadian-guidelines-body-weight-classification-adults/questions-answers-public.html

Health Canada. (2021). *Canada's Food Guide.* https://food-guide.canada.ca/en/

Lorenzo, A. D., Gratteri, S., Gualtieri, P., et al. (2019). Why primary obesity is a disease? *Journal of Translational Medicine, 17*(1), 169. https://doi.org/10.1186/s12967-019-1919-y

Lv, N., Azar, K. M., Rosas, L. G., et al. (2017). Behavioral lifestyle interventions for moderate and severe obesity: A systematic review. *Preventive Medicine, 100*, 180–193. https://doi.org/10.1016/j.ypmed.2017.04.022

Mechanick, J. L., Hurley, D. L., & Garvey, W. T. (2017). Adiposity-based chronic disease as a new diagnostic term: The American Association of Clinical Endocrinologists and American College of Endocrinology position statement. *AACE Endocrinology Practice, 23*(3), 372–378. https://doi.org/10.4158/EP161688.PS

Novo Nordisk. (2016). *Saxenda.* https://www.saxenda.com

Pi-Sunyer, X., Astrup, A., Fujioka, K., et al. (2015). A randomized, controlled trial of 3.0 mg of liraglutide in weight management. *The New England Journal of Medicine, 373*(1), 11–22. https://doi.org/10.1056/NEJMoa1411892

Public Health Agency of Canada & Canadian Institutes of Health Information. (2011). *Obesity in Canada.* https://secure.cihi.ca/free_products/Obesity_in_canada_2011_en.pdf

Ramos-Salas, X., Alberga, A. S., Cameron, E., et al. (2017). Adding weight bias and discrimination: Moving beyond raising awareness to creating change. *Obesity Review, 18*(11), 1323–1335.

Rotenberg, K. J., Bharathi, C., Davies, H., et al. (2017). Obesity and the social withdrawal syndrome. *Eating Behaviors, 26*, 167–170. https://doi.org/10.1016/j.eatbeh.2017.03.006

Shibata, R., Ouchi, N., Ohashi, K., et al. (2017). The role of adipokines in cardiovascular disease. *Journal of Cardiology, 70*(4), 329–334. https://doi.org/10.1016/j.jjcc.2017.02.006

Statistics Canada. (2019). *Overweight and obese adults, 2018.* https://www150.statcan.gc.ca/n1/en/pub/82-625-x/2019001/article/00005-eng.pdf%3Fst%3DOBRuwojR

Thorell, A., MacCormick, A. D., Awad, S., et al. (2016). Guidelines for perioperative care in bariatric surgery: Enhanced Recovery After Surgery (ERAS) Society recommendations. *World Journal of Surgery, 40*, 2065–2083. https://doi.org/10.1007/s00268-016-3492-3

Tung, Y. L., Yeo, G. S., O'Rahilly, S., et al. (2014). Obesity and FTO: Changing focus at a complex locus. *Cell Metabolism, 20*(5), 710–718. https://doi.org/10.1016/j.cmet.2014.09.010

Valeant Canada. (2018). *Product monograph. Contrave®.* https://pdf.hres.ca/dpd_pm/00043849.PDF

Williams, E. P., Mesidor, M., Winters, K., et al. (2015). Overweight and obesity: Prevalence, consequences, and causes of a growing public health problem. *Current Obesity Reports, 4*(3), 363–370. https://doi.org/10.1007/s13679-015-0169-4

RESOURCES

Alberta Health Services—*Healthy Eating Starts Here: Know Your Portions*
https://www.albertahealthservices.ca/nutrition/page5623.aspx
Canadian Association of Bariatric Physicians and Surgeons
https://www.cabps.ca
Canadian Cancer Society: Research
https://www.cancer.ca/Research.aspx
Canadian Guidelines for Body Weight Classification in Adults
https://www.hc-sc.gc.ca/fn-an/alt_formats/hpfb-dgpsa/pdf/nutrition/cg_quick_ref-ldc_rapide_ref-eng.pdf
Canadian Institutes of Health Research: Institute of Nutrition, Metabolism & Diabetes (INMD)
https://www.cihr-irsc.gc.ca/e/13521.html
Canadian Society for Exercise Physiology
https://www.csep.ca/home
Canadian 24-Hour Movement Guidelines
https://csepguidelines.ca/
Dietitians of Canada
https://www.dietitians.ca
Health Canada
https://www.hc-sc.gc.ca
National Eating Disorder Information Centre
https://www.nedic.ca

Obesity Canada
  https://www.obesitynetwork.ca
Public Health Agency of Canada—*Being Active*
  http://www.phac-aspc.gc.ca/pau-uap/paguide/index.html

Academy for Eating Disorders
  https://www.aedweb.org
National Eating Disorders Association
  https://www.nationaleatingdisorders.org
National Heart, Lung, and Blood Institute—**Portion Distortion**
  https://www.nhlbi.nih.gov/health/educational/wecan/eat-right/portion-distortion.htm

Overeaters Anonymous
  https://oa.org
Take Off Pounds Sensibly (TOPS)
  https://www.tops.org
Weight Watchers International, Inc.
  https://www.weightwatchers.com

evolve

For additional Internet resources, see the website for this book at http://evolve.elsevier.com/Canada/Lewis/medsurg.

Nursing Management
Upper Gastrointestinal Conditions

Denise Delorey
Originating US chapter by Kara Ann Ventura

⊖volve WEBSITE

http://evolve.elsevier.com/Canada/Lewis/medsurg

- Review Questions (Online Only)
- Key Points
- Answer Guidelines for Case Study
- Student Case Studies

- Patient with Oral Cancer
- Patient with Peptic Ulcer Disease
- Customizable Nursing Care Plans
- Nausea and Vomiting

- Peptic Ulcer Disease
- Conceptual Care Map Creator
- Audio Glossary
- Content Updates

LEARNING OBJECTIVES

1. Describe the etiology, complications, interprofessional care, and nursing management of nausea and vomiting.
2. Describe the etiology, clinical manifestations, and treatment of common oral inflammations and infections.
3. Describe the etiology, clinical manifestations, complications, interprofessional care, and nursing management of oral cancer.
4. Explain the types, pathophysiology, clinical manifestations, complications, and interprofessional care, including surgical therapy, and nursing management of gastroesophageal reflux disease and hiatal hernia.
5. Describe the pathophysiology, clinical manifestations, complications, and interprofessional care of esophageal cancer, diverticula, achalasia, and esophageal strictures.

6. Differentiate between acute and chronic gastritis, including the etiology, pathophysiology, interprofessional care, and nursing management.
7. Explain the common etiology, clinical manifestations, interprofessional care, and nursing management of upper gastrointestinal bleeding.
8. Compare and contrast gastric and duodenal ulcers, including their etiology and pathophysiology, clinical manifestations, complications, interprofessional care, and nursing management.
9. Describe the clinical manifestations, interprofessional care, and nursing management of gastric cancer.
10. Identify the common types of food poisoning and the nursing responsibilities related to food poisoning.

KEY TERMS

achalasia
Barrett's esophagus
dysphagia
esophageal cancer
esophageal diverticula
esophagitis

gastric cancer
gastritis
gastroesophageal reflux disease (GERD)
hiatal hernia
leukoplakia
Mallory-Weiss tear

nausea
peptic ulcer disease (PUD)
physiological stress ulcer
vomiting

NAUSEA AND VOMITING

Nausea and vomiting are the most common manifestations of gastrointestinal (GI) diseases. Nausea is a feeling of discomfort in the epigastrium with a conscious desire to vomit. Vomiting is the forceful ejection of partially digested food and secretions *(emesis)* from the upper GI tract. Vomiting is a complex act that requires the coordinated activities of several structures: closure of the glottis, deep inspiration with contraction of the diaphragm in the inspiratory position, closure of the pylorus, relaxation of the stomach and lower esophageal sphincter (LES), and contraction of the abdominal muscles with increasing intra-abdominal pressure. These simultaneous activities force the stomach contents up through the esophagus, into the pharynx, and out the mouth. Although nausea and vomiting can occur independently, they are usually closely related and usually treated as one condition.

Etiology and Pathophysiology

Nausea and vomiting occur in a wide variety of GI disorders, as well as in conditions that are unrelated to GI disease. Such conditions include pregnancy, infectious diseases, central nervous system (CNS) disorders (e.g., meningitis, CNS tumour), cardiovascular disease (e.g., myocardial infarction, heart failure), metabolic disorders (e.g., Addison's disease, uremia), adverse effects of medications (e.g., opioids digitalis), allergies, and psychological factors (e.g., stress, fear).

In general, nausea occurs before vomiting and is characterized by contraction of the duodenum and by slowing of gastric motility and emptying. A single episode of nausea accompanied by vomiting may not be significant. However, if vomiting occurs several times, it is important that the cause be identified.

A vomiting centre in the brainstem coordinates the multiple components involved in emesis. This centre receives input from various stimuli. Neural impulses reach the vomiting centre via afferent pathways through branches of the autonomic nervous system. Visceral receptors for these afferent fibres are located in the GI tract, the kidneys, the heart, and the uterus. When stimulated, these receptors relay information to the vomiting centre, which then initiates the vomiting reflex (Figure 44.1).

In addition, the chemoreceptor trigger zone (CTZ), located on the floor of the fourth ventricle in the brain, responds to chemical stimuli of medications and toxins. The CTZ also plays a role in emesis when it is caused by labyrinthine stimulation (e.g., motion sickness). Once stimulated, the CTZ transmits impulses directly to the vomiting centre.

Vomiting also can occur when the GI tract becomes overly irritated, excited, or distended. It can be a protective mechanism to rid the body of spoiled or irritating foods and liquids. Immediately before the act of vomiting, the person becomes aware of the need to vomit. The autonomic nervous system is activated, resulting in both parasympathetic and sympathetic nervous system stimulation. Sympathetic activation produces tachycardia, tachypnea, and diaphoresis. Parasympathetic stimulation causes relaxation of the lower esophageal (cardiac) sphincter, an increase in gastric motility, and a pronounced increase in salivation. These manifestations are experienced immediately before emesis.

Clinical Manifestations

Nausea is a subjective symptom. *Anorexia* (lack of appetite) usually accompanies nausea and is brought on by unpleasant stimulation involving any of the five senses. When nausea and vomiting are prolonged, dehydration can develop rapidly. In addition to water, essential electrolytes (e.g., potassium, sodium, chloride, hydrogen) are also lost. As vomiting persists, the patient may suffer severe electrolyte imbalances, loss of extracellular fluid volume, decreased plasma volume, and eventually circulatory failure. Metabolic alkalosis can result from loss of gastric hydrochloric acid (HCl). Metabolic acidosis can occur because of the loss of bicarbonate when contents from the small intestine are vomited. However, metabolic acidosis is a less common result of severe vomiting than is metabolic alkalosis. Weight loss resulting from fluid loss is evident in a short time when vomiting is severe.

The threat of pulmonary aspiration is a concern when vomiting occurs in a patient who is an older person, is unconscious, or has other conditions that impair the gag reflex. A patient who cannot adequately manage self-care should be put in a semi-Fowler's or side-lying position to prevent aspiration.

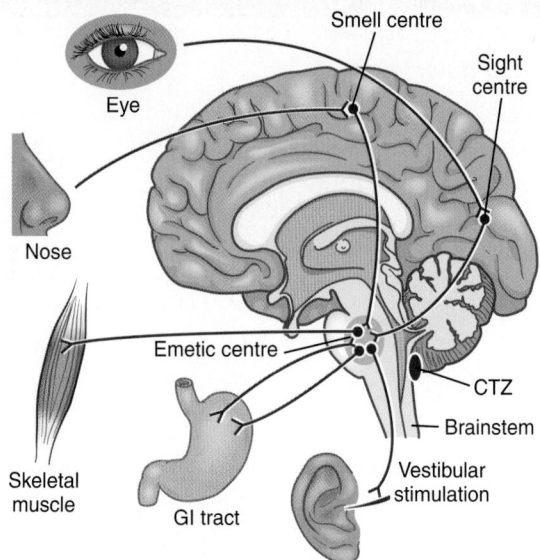

FIG. 44.1 Stimuli involved in the act of vomiting. *CTZ,* chemoreceptor trigger zone; *GI,* gastrointestinal. Source: Modified from McKenry, L., Tessier, E., & Hogan, M. (2006). *Mosby's pharmacology in nursing* (22nd ed.). Mosby.

Interprofessional Care

The goals of interprofessional care are to determine and treat the underlying cause of the nausea and vomiting and to provide symptomatic relief. Determining the cause is often difficult because nausea and vomiting are manifestations of many conditions of the GI tract and of disorders of other body systems. An interprofessional approach to management of patients, involving nurse practitioners, nurses, pharmacists, dietitians, and social workers, should be considered.

The history must include important information regarding times when the vomiting occurs, precipitating factors, and a description of the contents of the vomitus or emesis. There are sex-related differences in risk for nausea and vomiting associated with both surgical procedures and motion sickness. Women are more likely than men to experience nausea and vomiting (Halpin & Huckabay, 2019). In all patients, vomiting, regurgitation, and projectile vomiting must be differentiated. *Regurgitation* is a process in which partially digested food is slowly brought up from the stomach. Retching or vomiting seldom precedes it. *Projectile vomiting* is a very forceful expulsion of stomach contents without nausea and is a characteristic of increased intracranial pressure.

The presence of fecal odour and bile after prolonged vomiting indicates intestinal obstruction below the level of the pylorus. The presence of bile in the emesis may suggest obstruction below the ampulla of Vater or bile reflux gastritis. The presence of partially digested food several hours after a meal is indicative of gastric outlet obstruction or delay in gastric emptying.

The colour of the emesis aids in determining the presence and the source of bleeding. Vomitus with a "coffee grounds" appearance is associated with bleeding in the stomach, where blood changes to dark brown as a result of its interaction with gastric acid. Bright red blood indicates active bleeding, which is suggestive of a tear in the mucosal lining of the lower esophagus or the fundus of stomach, bleeding gastric or duodenal ulcer or neoplasm, or bleeding esophageal varices.

Medication Therapy. The choice of medications in the treatment of nausea and vomiting depends on the cause of the

TABLE 44.1 MEDICATION THERAPY
Nausea and Vomiting

Classification	Medication
Dopamine antagonists	• Domperidone (Motilium) • Haloperidol (Haldol) • Metoclopramide
Antihistamine	• Cyclizine • Dimenhydrinate (Gravol) • Diphenhydramine (Benadryl)
Serotonin antagonist	• Dolasetron (Anzemet) • Granisetron (Kytril) • Ondansetron (Zofran)
Antimuscarinic (anticholinergic)	• Scopolamine (hyoscine)
Phenothiazine	• Chlorpromazine (Largactil) • Prochlorperazine (Stemetil) • Promethazine (Phenergan)
Benzodiazepine	• Clonazepam (Clonapam) • Diazepam (Valium) • Lorazepam (Ativan)
Others	• Aprepitant (Emend) • Corticosteroids • Dexamethasone (Decadron)

problem. Many different medications can be used (Table 44.1). Because the cause cannot always be readily determined, medications must be administered with caution. Treatment with antiemetics prior to diagnosis may mask the underlying disease process and delay diagnosis and treatment. Many of the antiemetic medications act on the CNS at the level of the CTZ. In general, they block the neurochemicals that appear to trigger nausea and vomiting.

Many medications that control nausea and vomiting—antimuscarinics, antihistamines, and phenothiazines—have anticholinergic actions, and their use is contraindicated in patients with glaucoma, prostatic hyperplasia, pyloric or bladder neck obstruction, or biliary obstruction. They share many common adverse effects, which include dry mouth, hypotension, sedative effects, rashes, and GI disturbances such as constipation. Consultation with a pharmacist may be indicated before these medications are administered to a patient with multiple medical conditions.

Metoclopramide and domperidone (Motilium) act both centrally and peripherally on dopamine receptors. Peripherally, they enhance the release of acetylcholine, which results in increased gastric emptying. Because of this effect, these medications are considered prokinetics. However, about 10 to 20% of patients taking metoclopramide experience adverse CNS effects ranging from anxiety to hallucinations. Extrapyramidal adverse effects, including tremor and dyskinesias similar to those of Parkinson's disease, may also occur. Domperidone does not cross the blood–brain barrier and thus produces fewer adverse effects than does metoclopramide.

MEDICATION ALERT—Metoclopramide
• Chronic use or high doses of metoclopramide carry the risk of tardive dyskinesia.
• Tardive dyskinesia is a neurological condition characterized by involuntary and repetitive movements of the body (e.g., extremity movements, lip smacking).
• With discontinuation of the medication, the tardive dyskinesia persists.

Antagonists to specific serotonin (5-HT) receptors have been found to act both centrally and peripherally to reduce nausea and vomiting. In particular, antagonists to the 5-HT3 receptor are effective in reducing cancer chemotherapy–induced

vomiting, vomiting caused by total body irradiation, GI motility disturbances, carcinoid syndrome, and nausea and vomiting related to migraine headache and anxiety. Serotonin antagonists, including ondansetron (Zofran), granisetron (Kytril), and dolasetron (Anzemet), act both centrally in the vomiting centre and peripherally to enhance gastric emptying.

Dexamethasone is used in the management of cancer chemotherapy–induced emesis, usually in combination with other antiemetics. Dexamethasone alone or in combination with ondansetron reduces both acute and delayed chemotherapy-induced nausea and vomiting. Aprepitant (Emend), a substance P/neurokinin-1 receptor antagonist, is used for the prevention of chemotherapy-induced nausea and vomiting, as well as prevention of postoperative nausea and vomiting. Benzodiazepines have no direct antiemetic effect but may be useful as adjunct therapy in the treatment of chemotherapy-induced nausea and vomiting.

Nutritional Therapy. Patients with severe vomiting require intravenous (IV) fluid therapy with electrolyte and glucose replacement until they are able to tolerate oral intake. In some cases, a nasogastric (NG) tube and suction are used to decompress the stomach. Keeping the stomach empty reduces the stimulus to vomit. The NG tube should be stabilized to eliminate its movement in the nose and back of the throat because this can stimulate nausea and vomiting.

Once the symptoms have subsided, oral nourishment is started with clear liquids. Extremely hot or cold liquids are not usually well tolerated. Warm tea and room-temperature flat soda are more easily tolerated. The addition of dry toast or crackers may alleviate the feeling of nausea and help prevent vomiting. Water is the initial fluid of choice for rehydration by mouth.

As the patient's condition improves, a diet high in carbohydrates and low in fatty foods should be provided. Items such as a baked potato, plain gelatin, cereal with milk and sugar, and hard candy may be added. Foods that are known to be poorly tolerated include coffee, spicy foods, and highly acidic foods. Food should be eaten slowly and in small amounts to prevent overdistension of the stomach. When solid foods have been reintroduced, fluids should be taken between meals rather than with meals. It is advised that the patient avoid physical activity and sit upright for approximately 1 hour after meals. A dietitian may be consulted about appropriate foods that will maintain nutritional health and are well tolerated by the patient during the recovery process.

🌿 COMPLEMENTARY & ALTERNATIVE THERAPIES
Ginger

Scientific Evidence
• May be effective for nausea and vomiting in pregnancy when used at recommended doses for short periods
• May help chemotherapy-induced nausea and vomiting if used with antiemetic medications
• Some patients use herbs such as ginger and peppermint oil for nausea and vomiting. Breathing exercises, massage, changing body position, self-hypnosis, guided imagery, biofeedback, music therapy, or exercise may be helpful for some patients (Canadian Cancer Association, 2021c).

Nursing Implications
• Few adverse effects reported with short-term use
• May interact with anticoagulants and increase risk for bleeding
• Use with caution in people with gallbladder disease

Source: https://www.nccih.nih.gov/health/ginger.

TABLE 44.2   NURSING ASSESSMENT
Nausea and Vomiting

Subjective Data
Important Health Information
Past health history: GI disorders, chronic indigestion, food allergies, pregnancy, infection, CNS disorders, recent travel, bulimia, metabolic disorders, cancer, cardiovascular disease, renal disease
Medications: Use of antiemetics, digitalis, opioids, ferrous sulphate, ASA (Aspirin), aminophylline, alcohol, antibiotics; general anaesthetic; chemotherapy
Surgery or other treatments: Recent surgery

Symptoms
- Emesis, dry heaves, dry mouth, anorexia, weight loss
- Weakness, fatigue
- Abdominal tenderness or pain

Objective Data
General
Lethargy, sunken eyeballs

Integumentary
Pallor, dry mucous membranes, poor skin turgor

Gastrointestinal
Amount, frequency, character (e.g., projectile), content (undigested food, blood, bile, feces), and colour of vomitus (red, "coffee grounds," green-yellow)

Urinary
Decreased output, concentrated urine

Possible Findings
Altered serum electrolyte levels (especially hypokalemia), metabolic alkalosis, abnormal upper GI findings on endoscopy or abdominal radiographs

ASA, acetylsalicylic acid; *CNS,* central nervous system; *GI,* gastrointestinal.

NURSING MANAGEMENT
NAUSEA AND VOMITING

NURSING ASSESSMENT

Each patient with a history of prolonged and persistent nausea or vomiting requires a thorough nursing assessment before a specific plan of care is developed. Although the conditions associated with nausea and vomiting are numerous, the nurse should have a basic understanding of the more common conditions and should be able to identify a patient who is at high risk of complications from nausea and vomiting. Knowledge of the physiological mechanisms involved in nausea and vomiting and demonstration of a genuine regard for the patient are essential. Table 44.2 lists subjective and objective data that should be obtained from a patient with nausea and vomiting, regardless of the underlying cause.

NURSING DIAGNOSES

Nursing diagnoses for the patient with nausea and vomiting may include but are not limited to the following:

- *Nausea* resulting from *noxious environmental stimuli, noxious taste, unpleasant visual stimuli*
- *Disrupted fluid and electrolyte balance* resulting from *insufficient fluid intake (prolonged vomiting)*
- *Inadequate nutrition* resulting from *insufficient dietary intake* (nausea and vomiting)

Additional information on nursing diagnoses is presented in Nursing Care Plan (NCP) 44.1, available on the Evolve website.

PLANNING

The overall goals are that the patient with nausea and vomiting will (a) experience minimal or no nausea and vomiting, (b) have normal electrolyte levels and hydration status, and (c) return to a normal pattern of fluid balance and nutrient intake.

NURSING IMPLEMENTATION

ACUTE INTERVENTION. The majority of individuals with nausea and vomiting can be managed at home. However, when nausea and vomiting persist regardless of home treatment strategies, hospitalization may be necessary for diagnosis of the underlying health problem. Until a diagnosis is confirmed, the patient is kept on nothing-by-mouth (NPO) status and given IV fluids. An NG tube connected to suction may be necessary for a patient with persistent vomiting and for a patient in whom the possible diagnosis may be bowel obstruction or paralytic ileus.

With prolonged vomiting, there is a probability of dehydration and of acid–base and electrolyte imbalances. The nurse plans care that includes accurate recording of intake and output, monitoring of vital signs, assessment for signs of dehydration, proper patient positioning to prevent possible aspiration by a susceptible patient, and observing for changes in the patient's general physical comfort and mentation. The nurse needs to take responsibility for providing physical and emotional support; maintaining a quiet, odour-free environment; and giving explanations regarding any diagnostic tests or procedures performed.

Patients who are hospitalized for other health problems may be prone to episodes of nausea and vomiting. These individuals include patients who are recovering immediately after surgery from the effects of the procedure, anaesthesia, and pain. Nausea and vomiting are common adverse effects in patients with cancer who are receiving chemotherapeutic agents. (Nursing care of patients with cancer is discussed in Chapter 18 and in NCP 18.2, available on the Evolve website.)

AMBULATORY AND HOME CARE. The patient and caregiver may need instructions on (a) how to successfully manage the unpleasant sensations of nausea, (b) methods of preventing nausea and vomiting, and (c) strategies to maintain fluid and nutritional intake. The occurrence of nausea or vomiting may be minimized if measures are taken to keep the immediate environment quiet, free of noxious odours, and well ventilated. Sudden changes of position and unnecessary activity should be avoided. Use of relaxation techniques, acupressure, frequent rest periods, and diversional tactics can help prevent nausea and vomiting and facilitate a more rapid recovery from their effects. Cleansing the person's face and the hands with a cool washcloth and providing mouth care between episodes increase the person's comfort level. When the symptoms occur, all foods and medications should be stopped until the acute phase is past.

If a medication is suspected as the cause of nausea, the medication should be administered with food, if appropriate. If nausea is severe or prolonged, the health care provider should be notified so that either the dosage can be altered or a different medication can be prescribed. The patient should be reminded that stopping a prescribed medication without consulting the health care provider may eliminate the immediate cause of the nausea and vomiting but may also have detrimental effects on health or the disease state.

When food is identified as the precipitating cause of nausea and vomiting, the nurse should help the patient solve the problem. What food was it? When was it eaten? Has this food caused problems in the past? Is anyone else in the family sick?

When the patient believes some foods and fluids can be tolerated, the nurse might suggest that it would be helpful to begin with clear liquids or warm beverages, sports drinks, tea or broth, dry crackers or toast, and then plain gelatin. Bland foods, such as pasta, rice, and cooked chicken, are generally well tolerated in small amounts. An antiemetic medication should be taken only if prescribed by the health care provider. Patients should be asked to describe use of any medications other than those prescribed by their health care provider, such as over-the-counter (OTC), herbal, or traditional medications. It is important for the nurse to validate the appropriate use of Indigenous traditional medications, to prevent interactions with medications they may receive in the health care setting.

EVALUATION

The following are expected outcomes for the patient with nausea and vomiting:

- The patient will be comfortable with minimal or no nausea and vomiting.
- The patient will maintain body weight.
- The patient's electrolyte levels will be within normal range.
- The patient will be able to maintain adequate intake of fluids and nutrients.
- The patient will maintain normal urine volume.

AGE-RELATED CONSIDERATIONS

NAUSEA AND VOMITING

Older patients experiencing nausea and vomiting require careful assessment and monitoring, particularly during periods of fluid loss and subsequent rehydration therapy. Older persons are more likely to have cardiac or renal insufficiency, which increases their risk for life-threatening fluid and electrolyte imbalances. In addition, excessive replacement of fluid and electrolytes may result in adverse consequences for an older person who has heart failure or renal disease. Moreover, older people with a decreased level of consciousness may be at high risk for aspiration of vomitus. Close monitoring of the patient's physical status and level of consciousness during episodes of vomiting must be a primary concern for the nurse.

In addition, older persons are particularly susceptible to the CNS adverse effects of antiemetic medications; these medications may produce confusion and increase risk of falls. Dosages should be reduced and efficacy closely evaluated. Safety precautions also should be instituted for these patients.

FOODBORNE ILLNESS

Foodborne illness and *food poisoning* are nonspecific terms that describe acute GI symptoms such as nausea, vomiting, diarrhea, and colicky abdominal pain caused by the intake of contaminated food. Food most commonly causes illness if it is contaminated with microorganisms or their products. The GI tract is frequently the portal of entry for the microorganisms. The epidemiology of foodborne illness is changing; there are new organisms and many have spread worldwide. The two main types of food poisoning are (1) acute gastroenteritis from bacteria and (2) neurological symptoms from botulism. Bacteria account for most foodborne illnesses. Raw foods that have become contaminated during growing, harvesting, processing, storing, shipping, or final preparation are the most common source. When food is uncooked and left out for more than 2 hours at room temperature, bacteria can multiply quickly. The most common bacterial causes of food poisoning are listed in Table 44.3.

Poisonous chemicals, such as mercury, arsenic, zinc, and potassium chlorate, may contaminate foods. Poisoning can also occur from ingestion of poisonous plants (e.g., certain mushroom species).

Prevention of food poisoning is the focus of interventions. Teaching should include correct food preparation and cleanliness, adequate cooking, and refrigeration. If the patient is hospitalized, care focuses on correction of fluid and electrolyte imbalance from diarrhea and vomiting. With botulism, additional assessment and care relative to neurological symptoms are indicated (see Chapter 63).

Escherichia coli O157:H7 Poisoning

Escherichia coli O157:H7 causes hemorrhagic colitis and kidney failure, and in young children and older persons, *E. coli* O157:H7 infection can be life-threatening (Centers for Disease Control and Prevention, 2015). *E. coli* O157:H7 is found primarily in undercooked meats, particularly poultry and hamburger. *E. coli* outbreaks have also been observed with contaminated leafy vegetables, fruits, and nuts. Person-to-person contact in families, long-term care facilities, and child care centres is also an important mode of transmission. Infection can occur after drinking raw milk, unpasteurized juice, or contaminated fruit juices and after swimming in or drinking sewage-contaminated water.

Most strains of *E. coli* are harmless and live in the intestines of healthy humans and animals. *E. coli* O157:H7 produces a powerful toxin and can cause severe illness. The clinical manifestations of *E. coli* O157:H7 infection include diarrhea and abdominal cramping pain for 2 to 8 days (on average, 3–4 days) after the organism is swallowed. The diarrhea is variable, ranging from mild to bloody, starting as watery and progressing to bloody. Systemic complications, including hemolytic uremia and thrombocytopenic purpura, and even death can occur.

Infection with *E. coli* O157:H7 is diagnosed when the bacteria are detected in the stool. All people who suddenly have diarrhea with blood should get their stool tested (stool culture) for *E. coli* O157:H7.

Treatment involves supportive care to maintain blood volume. The use of antibiotics remains controversial. Most affected people recover without receiving antibiotics or other specific treatment. Patients should avoid using antidiarrheal agents, such as loperamide (Imodium). Other therapies may include dialysis and plasmapheresis.

In approximately 2 to 7% of infections, particularly in young children and older people, hemolytic uremic syndrome (HUS) occurs, in which the red blood cells (RBCs) are destroyed and kidney function fails. HUS is a life-threatening condition, and approximately 3 to 5% of patients with HUS die. About one third of people with HUS have abnormal kidney function many years after its onset, and a few require long-term dialysis. Additional long-term complications of HUS include hypertension, seizures, blindness, and paralysis.

ORAL INFLAMMATIONS AND INFECTIONS

Oral infections and inflammations may be manifestations of specific mouth diseases, or they may occur in the presence of some systemic diseases such as leukemia or vitamin deficiency. Oral inflammations and infections can severely impair the ingestion of food and fluids. Common inflammations and

TABLE 44.3	BACTERIAL FOOD POISONING				
Causative Agent	Sources	Onset of Symptoms	Clinical Manifestations	Treatment	Prevention
Staphylococcal Toxin from *Staphylococcus aureus*	Meat, bakery products, cream fillings, salad dressings, milk; skin and respiratory tract of food handlers	30 min–7 hr	Vomiting, nausea, abdominal cramping, diarrhea	Symptomatic, fluid and electrolyte replacement, antiemetics	Immediate refrigeration of foods, monitoring of food handlers
Clostridial *Clostridium perfringens*	Meat or poultry dishes cooked at lower temperature (stew or pot pie), rewarmed meat dishes, gravies, improperly canned vegetables	8–24 hr	Diarrhea, nausea, abdominal cramps, vomiting (rare); midepigastrium pain	Symptomatic, fluid replacement	Correct preparation of meat dishes, serving of food immediately after cooking, or rapid cooling of food
***Salmonella* Organisms** *Salmonella typhimurium* (grows in gut)	Improperly cooked poultry, pork, beef, lamb, and eggs	8 hr to several days	Nausea and vomiting, diarrhea, abdominal cramps, fever and chills	Symptomatic, fluid and electrolyte replacement	Correct preparation of food
Botulism Toxin from *Clostridium botulinum*; ingested toxin is absorbed from gut and blocks acetylcholine at neuromuscular junction	Improperly canned or preserved food, home-preserved vegetables, preserved fruits and fish, canned commercial products	12–36 hr	GI symptoms: nausea, vomiting, abdominal pain, constipation, distension. Central nervous system symptoms: headache, dizziness, muscular incoordination, weakness, inability to talk or swallow, diplopia, breathing difficulties, paralysis, delirium, coma	Maintenance of ventilation, polyvalent antitoxin, guanidine HCl (enhances acetylcholine release)	Correct processing of canned foods, discarding suspect canned goods
Escherichia coli *E. coli* serotype O157:H7	Contaminated beef, pork, milk, cheese, fish, prepackaged cookie dough	Varies by strain: 8 hr–1 wk	Bloody stools, hemolytic uremic syndrome, abdominal cramping, profuse diarrhea	Symptomatic, fluid and electrolyte replacement	Correct preparation of food
***Listeria* Organisms** Gram-positive rod-shaped bacterium	Most cases associated with ingesting contaminated dairy products, poultry, and meat	1–90 days	In immunocompetent host: fever, diarrhea. Immunocompromised host (pregnant women, older persons, immunocompromised persons at greatest risk): meningitis ± septicemia	Ampicillin and trimethoprim-sulphamethoxazole or erythromycin	Pasteurization, proper washing, refrigeration, and cooking of foods potentially contaminated with animal manure or sewage

GI, gastrointestinal; *HCl*, hydrochloric acid.

infections of the oral cavity are listed in Table 44.4. Patients who are immunosuppressed (e.g., those with acquired immune deficiency syndrome [AIDS] and those receiving chemotherapy) are most susceptible to oral infections. Patients receiving corticosteroid inhalant treatment for asthma are at risk for oral infections, especially candidiasis.

Oral infections may predispose a person to infections in other body organs. For example, the oral cavity can be considered a potential reservoir for respiratory pathogens. Oral pathogens have also been associated with heart disease.

An important element in reducing the incidence of oral infections and inflammation is good oral hygiene. Management of oral infections and inflammation is focused on identification of the cause, elimination of infection, provision of comfort measures, and maintenance of nutritional intake.

There are reported high rates of dental decay in Indigenous children in Canada, disproportionately affecting disadvantaged Canadian Indigenous communities (Baghdadi, 2016). Many Indigenous children have high rates of dental caries due to poverty, which is associated with lack of access to oral health care and poor diet, and exposure to cigarette smoke (Baghdadi, 2016).

ORAL CANCER

Oral (or oropharyngeal) cancer may occur on the lips or anywhere within the mouth (e.g., tongue, floor of the mouth, buccal mucosa, hard palate, soft palate, pharyngeal walls, tonsils). It is estimated that 5 300 new cases of oral cancer were diagnosed in Canada in 2019, and that 1 450 persons would die from the

TABLE 44.4	INFECTIONS AND INFLAMMATION OF THE MOUTH		
Condition	**Etiology**	**Clinical Manifestations**	**Treatment**
Gingivitis	Neglected oral hygiene, malocclusion, missing or irregular teeth, faulty dentistry, eating of soft rather than fibrous foods	Inflamed gingivae and interdental papillae; bleeding during toothbrushing; development of pus; formation of abscess with loosening of teeth (periodontitis)	Prevention through health teaching, dental care, gingival massage, professional cleaning of teeth, fibrous foods, conscientious brushing habits with flossing
Vincent's infection (acute necrotizing ulcerative gingivitis, trench mouth)	Fusiform bacteria; Vincent's spirochetes; predisposing factors of stress, excessive fatigue, poor oral hygiene, nutritional deficiencies (vitamins B and C)	Painful, bleeding gingivae; eroding necrotic lesions of interdental papillae; ulcerations that bleed; increased saliva with metallic taste; fetid mouth odour; anorexia, fever, and general malaise	Rest (physical and mental); avoidance of smoking and alcoholic beverages; soft, nutritious diet; correct oral hygiene habits; topical applications of antibiotics; mouth rinses with hydrogen peroxide and saline solutions
Oral candidiasis (moniliasis or thrush)	*Candida albicans* (a yeastlike fungus), debilitation, prolonged high-dose antibiotic or corticosteroid therapy	Pearly, bluish-white "milk-curd" membranous lesions on mucosa of mouth and larynx; sore mouth; yeasty halitosis	Nystatin suspension or fluconazole as oral therapy, good oral hygiene
Herpes simplex (cold sore, fever blister)	Herpes simplex virus type 1 or 2; factors predisposing to upper respiratory infections, excessive exposure to sunlight, food allergies, emotional tension, onset of menstruation	Lip lesions, mouth lesions, vesicle formation (single or clustered); shallow, painful ulcers	Spirits of camphor, corticosteroid cream, mild antiseptic mouthwash, viscous lidocaine; removal or control of predisposing factors, antiviral agents (e.g., acyclovir [Zovirax])
Aphthous stomatitis (canker sore)	Recurrent and chronic form of infection secondary to systemic disease, trauma, stress, or unknown causes	Ulcers of mouth and lips, causing extreme pain; ulcers surrounded by erythematous base	Corticosteroids (topical or systemic), tetracycline oral suspension
Parotitis (inflammation of parotid gland, surgical mumps)	Usually *Staphylococcus* species, occasionally *Streptococcus* species, debilitation and dehydration with poor oral hygiene, NPO status for an extended time	Pain and swelling in area of gland and ear, absence of salivation, purulent exudate from gland, erythema, ulcers	Antibiotics, mouthwashes, warm compresses; preventive measures such as chewing gum, sucking on hard candy, adequate fluid intake
Stomatitis (inflammation of mouth)	Trauma; pathogens; irritants (tobacco, alcohol); renal, liver, and hematological diseases; adverse effect of many cancer chemotherapy medications and irradiation	Excessive salivation, halitosis, sore mouth	Removal or treatment of cause, oral hygiene with soothing solutions, topical medications; soft, bland diet

NPO, nothing by mouth.

disease (Canadian Cancer Society's Advisory Committee on Cancer Statistics, 2019). Oral cancer is more common after 45 years of age, and it is more common in men than in women (male-to-female ratio, 2:1). Squamous cell carcinoma is the most common oral malignant tumour (95% of cases of oral cancer). Mortality rates have been decreasing since the early 1980s. The rate of 5-year survival for all stages of cancer of the oral cavity and pharynx combined is 63%.

Most of the oral malignant lesions occur on the lower lip. Other common sites are the lateral border and undersurface of the tongue, the labial commissure, and the buccal mucosa. Carcinoma of the lip has the most favourable prognosis of any of the oral tumours, probably because lip lesions are more apparent to the patient than other oral lesions and are usually diagnosed earlier.

Etiology and Pathophysiology

Although the definitive cause of oral cancer is unknown, there are a number of predisposing factors (Table 44.5). Factors that influence the development of oral cancer include tobacco use (e.g., cigar, cigarette, pipe, snuff), excessive alcohol intake, human papillomavirus infection, chewing betel quid or areca nut, precancerous conditions of the oral cavity (e.g., leukoplakia), and a family history of squamous cell carcinoma. A history of tobacco and alcohol use, in the past or currently, is the most significant etiological factor in oral cancer. Constant

overexposure to ultraviolet radiation from the sun is also a factor in the development of cancer of the lip. Irritation from the pipe stem resting on the lip is a risk factor among pipe smokers.

Clinical Manifestations

The common manifestations of oral cancer are leukoplakia, erythroplakia, ulcerations, a sore that bleeds easily and does not heal, and a rough area (felt with the tongue). Leukoplakia, called "white patch" or "smoker's patch," is often considered a precancerous lesion; approximately 3 to 17.5% of these lesions actually transform into malignant cells within 15 years. Leukoplakia is a whitish patch on the mucosa of the mouth or the tongue that results from chronic irritation, especially from smoking. The patch becomes *keratinized* (hard and leathery) and is sometimes described as *hyperkeratosis. Erythroplasia* (erythroplakia), which is seen as a red, velvety patch on the mouth or tongue, is also considered a precancerous lesion. Areas of erythroplakia have a 51% chance of becoming malignant. Later symptoms of oral cancer are pain, dysphagia (difficulty swallowing), and difficulty in moving the jaw (e.g., chewing and speaking).

Cancer of the lip usually appears as an indurated, painless ulcer on the lip. The first sign of carcinoma of the tongue is an ulcer or area of thickening. Soreness or pain of the tongue may occur, especially when hot or highly seasoned foods are eaten. Cancerous lesions are most likely to develop in the proximal half of the tongue. Some patients experience limitation of movement

TABLE 44.5   TYPES AND CHARACTERISTICS OF ORAL CANCER

Location	Predisposing Factors	Clinical Manifestations	Treatment
Lip	Constant overexposure to sun, ruddy and fair complexions, recurrent herpetic lesions, irritation from pipe stem, syphilis, immunosuppression	Indurated, painless ulcer	Surgical excision, radiation therapy
Tongue	Tobacco, alcohol, chronic irritation, syphilis	Ulcer or area of thickening; soreness or pain; increased salivation, slurred speech, dysphagia, toothache, earache (later signs)	Surgery (hemiglossectomy or glossectomy), radiation therapy
Oral cavity	Poor oral hygiene, tobacco usage (pipe and cigar smoking, snuff, chewing tobacco), chewing betel nut, chronic alcohol intake, chronic irritation (jagged tooth, ill-fitting prosthesis, chemical or mechanical irritants), exposure to HPV	Leukoplakia; erythroplakia; ulcerations; sore spot; rough area; pain, dysphagia, difficulty in chewing and speaking (later signs)	Surgery (mandibulectomy, radical neck dissection, resections of buccal mucosa), internal and external radiation therapy

HPV, human papillomavirus.

TABLE 44.6   INTERPROFESSIONAL CARE

Oral Cancer

Diagnostic	Interprofessional Therapy*

• History and physical examination
• Biopsy
• Oral exfoliative cytological study
• Radiographs, CT, and MRI
	• Surgery
	  • Surgical excision of the tumour
	  • Radical neck dissection
	• Radiation therapy (internal or external)
	• Combined surgical resection with radiation therapy
	• Chemotherapy

CT, computed tomography; *MRI*, magnetic resonance imaging.
*Any of these approaches may be used, depending on the primary lesion and the extent of metastasis.

of the tongue. Later symptoms of cancer of the tongue include increased salivation, slurred speech, dysphagia, toothache, and earache. Approximately 30% of patients with oral cancer have an asymptomatic neck mass.

Diagnostic Studies

Endoscopic examination in combination with biopsy of the suspected lesion with cytological examination is the best definitive diagnostic study for oral cancer. Oral exfoliative cytological study involves scraping the suspect lesion and spreading this scraping on a slide. In contrast to biopsy, a negative result of a cytological smear does not reliably rule out the possibility of a malignant condition, but it may be used as an initial screening test. The definitive diagnosis of cancer is based on biopsy and histological findings. Once cancer is diagnosed, radiographs, computed tomography (CT), and magnetic resonance imaging (MRI) are useful in the staging of oral cancer (Canadian Cancer Society, 2021b).

Interprofessional Care

Interprofessional care of patients with oral carcinoma usually consists of surgery, radiation therapy, chemotherapy, nutritional therapy, or a combination of these treatments (Table 44.6).

Surgical Therapy. Surgery remains the most effective treatment, especially for removing the central core of the tumour. Various surgical procedures may be performed, depending on the location and the extent of the tumour. Many of the operations are radical procedures involving extensive resections.

Some examples are partial *mandibulectomy* (removal of the mandible), *hemiglossectomy* (removal of half of the tongue), *glossectomy* (removal of the tongue), resections of the buccal mucosa and the floor of the mouth, and radical neck dissection. Composite resections, which are combinations of the various surgical procedures, may be performed.

Because cancers of the oral cavity metastasize early to the cervical lymph nodes, a radical neck dissection is commonly performed. It includes wide excision of the involved primary lesion with removal of the regional lymph nodes, the deep cervical lymph nodes, and their lymphatic channels. In addition, the following structures may also be removed or transected (depending on the extent of the primary lesion): sternocleidomastoid muscle and other closely associated muscles, internal jugular vein, mandible, submaxillary gland, part of the thyroid and parathyroid glands, and spinal accessory nerve. A tracheostomy is commonly performed along with the radical neck dissection. Drainage tubes are inserted into the surgical area and connected to the suction device to remove fluid and blood.

Nonsurgical Therapy. Chemotherapy and radiation therapy are used together when the lesions are more advanced, involve several structures of the oral cavity, or have metastasized. Chemotherapy may also be used when surgery and radiation therapy fail or as the initial therapy for smaller tumours (see Chapter 18).

Palliative treatment may be the best management when the prognosis is poor, the cancer is inoperable, or the patient decides against surgery. The aim of palliation is to treat the symptoms and make the patient more comfortable. If it becomes difficult for the patient to swallow, a gastrostomy may be performed to allow for adequate nutritional intake. (Gastrostomy is discussed in Chapter 42.) Analgesic medication should be given freely to such patients. Frequent suctioning of the oral cavity becomes necessary when swallowing becomes difficult. (Other nursing measures for terminally ill patients are discussed in Chapter 13.)

Nutritional Therapy. Because of depression, alcoholism, or presurgery radiation treatment, patients may be malnourished even before surgery. After radical neck surgery, the patient may be unable to take in nutrients through the normal route of ingestion because of swelling, location of sutures, or difficulty with swallowing. Parenteral fluids are given for the first 24 to 48 hours. After this time, tube feedings are usually given via an NG tube or a nasointestinal tube that was placed during surgery. Sometimes a temporary feeding gastrostomy may be used. (NG and gastrostomy feedings are described in Chapter 42.) Cervical esophagostomy and pharyngostomy have also been used. The nurse must observe for tolerance of the feedings and (in consultation with a dietitian) adjust the amount, the time, and the formula if nausea, vomiting, diarrhea, or distension occurs. The patient should be instructed about the tube feedings. When the patient can swallow, small amounts of water are given. Close observation for choking is essential. Suctioning may be necessary to prevent aspiration.

NURSING MANAGEMENT
ORAL CANCER

NURSING ASSESSMENT

Subjective and objective data that should be obtained from a patient with oral cancer are listed in Table 44.7.

NURSING DIAGNOSES

Nursing diagnoses for patients with oral cancer may include but are not limited to the following:

- *Inadequate nutrition* resulting from *insufficient dietary intake* (oral pain, difficulty chewing and swallowing, surgical resection, and radiation treatment)
- *Chronic pain* resulting from *injury agent* (tumour, surgery, or radiation treatment)
- *Anxiety* resulting from *stressors, threat of death, threat to current status* (diagnosis of cancer, potential for disfiguring surgery)
- *Potential for airway obstruction* resulting from *injury agent* (tumour, surgery, or radiation treatment).

TABLE 44.7 NURSING ASSESSMENT

Oral Cancer

Subjective Data

Important Health Information

Current health history: Use of alcohol or tobacco, pipe smoking, poor oral hygiene

Past health history: Recurrent oral herpetic lesions, syphilis, exposure to sunlight, HPV infection or vaccination

Medications: Immunosuppressants

Surgery or other treatments: Removal of prior tumours or lesions

Symptoms

- Reduced oral intake, weight loss, difficulty in chewing or swallowing food; increased salivation; intolerance to certain foods or temperatures of food
- Mouth or tongue soreness or pain, toothache, earache, neck stiffness, difficulty speaking

Objective Data

Integumentary

Indurated, painless ulcer on lip; painless neck mass

Gastrointestinal

Areas of thickening or roughness, ulcers, leukoplakia, or erythroplakia on the tongue or the oral mucosa; limited movement of the tongue; increased salivation, drooling; slurred speech; poor oral hygiene, foul breath odour

Possible Findings

Positive result of exfoliative cytological smear (microscopic examination of cells removed by scraping); positive biopsy findings

HPV, human papillomavirus.

PLANNING

The overall goals are that the patient with carcinoma of the oral cavity will (a) have a patent airway, (b) be able to communicate, (c) have adequate nutritional intake to promote wound healing, and (d) have relief of pain and discomfort.

NURSING IMPLEMENTATION

HEALTH PROMOTION. The nurse has a significant role in the prevention, early detection, and treatment of oral cancer. The nurse must provide the patient with information regarding predisposing factors, such as constant overexposure to the sun, tobacco, and other irritants, such as chewing betel nuts. Smoking and long-term use of smokeless tobacco are the major risk factors for oral cancer. A patient identified as a smoker should be informed about smoking cessation programs available in the community. (Smoking cessation is discussed in Chapter 11. See also the link to the CAN-ADAPTT *Canadian Smoking Cessation Clinical Practice Guideline* in the Resources at the end of this chapter.)

It is important that adolescents and teenagers be informed about the danger of using snuff, chewing tobacco, e-cigarettes, and other vaping products. In addition, oral cancers have an increased chance of recurrence if risk factors are not reduced. The nurse should also teach correct oral hygiene and dental care and encourage the patient to seek preventive dental care. Risk factors should be identified. Because early detection of oral cancer is important, the patient should be taught to examine the mouth and to recognize danger signals of oral cancer. If any of these signals are present, the patient should be instructed to visit a health care provider. Danger signals include unexplained pain or soreness in the mouth, unusual bleeding from the oral cavity, dysphagia, and swelling or a lump in the neck.

Any individual with an ulcerative lesion that does not heal within 2 to 3 weeks should be referred to a health care provider, and a biopsy of the lesion should probably be performed. The nurse should inspect the patient's oral cavity to detect suspect lesions.

ACUTE INTERVENTION. Preoperative care for a patient who is to undergo a radical neck dissection involves consideration of the patient's physical and psychosocial needs. Physical preparation is the same as for any major surgery, with special emphasis on oral hygiene. Alcohol intake should be assessed thoroughly, and measures should be implemented early to assess and treat withdrawal if it is a concern. Explanations and emotional support are of special significance and should include postoperative measures relating to communication and feeding. The surgical procedure should be explained to the patient, and the nurse needs to make sure that the patient understands the information. (Radical neck dissection and related nursing management are discussed in Chapter 29 and in NCP 29.2, available on the Evolve website.)

EVALUATION

The following are expected outcomes for the patient with oral cancer:

- The patient will have no respiratory complications.
- The patient will be able to communicate.
- The patient will participate in regular follow-up examinations.
- The patient will maintain adequate nutritional intake to promote wound healing and overall health.
- The patient will experience minimal pain and discomfort with eating, drinking, and talking.

ESOPHAGEAL DISORDERS

GASTROESOPHAGEAL REFLUX DISEASE

Etiology and Pathophysiology

Gastroesophageal reflux disease (GERD) is not a disease but a syndrome. *GERD* is defined as any clinically significant symptomatic condition or histopathological alteration presumed to be secondary to reflux of gastric contents into the lower esophagus. In Canada, GERD is the most prevalent acid-related disorder; approximately 13 to 29% of Canadians will experience reoccurring GERD symptoms (Canadian Society of Intestinal Research, 2021).

There is no single cause of GERD; several factors or a combination of factors can be involved (Figure 44.2). It results when the defences of the lower esophagus are overwhelmed by the reflux of stomach acidic contents into the esophagus. Predisposing conditions include hiatal hernia, incompetent LES, decreased esophageal clearance (ability to clear liquids or food from the esophagus into the stomach) as a result of impaired esophageal motility, and decreased gastric emptying. The acidic gastric secretions that are regurgitated up into the lower esophagus result in esophageal irritation and inflammation (esophagitis). In addition, the presence of the gastric enzyme pepsin, intestinal enzymes (e.g., trypsin), and bile salts is corrosive to the esophageal mucosa. The degree of inflammation depends on the amount and composition of gastric reflux and on the ability of the esophagus's mucosal defence mechanisms to clear the acidic contents.

One of the primary factors in GERD is incompetence of the LES. The LES opens to allow food to pass into the stomach and quickly closes. An incompetent LES fails to close, resulting in a backflow of stomach contents into the esophagus when the patient is supine or has an increase in intra-abdominal pressure. Decreases in LES pressure can be caused by certain foods (e.g., caffeine, chocolate) and medications (e.g., anticholinergics). A common cause of GERD is a hiatal hernia, which is discussed in the next section.

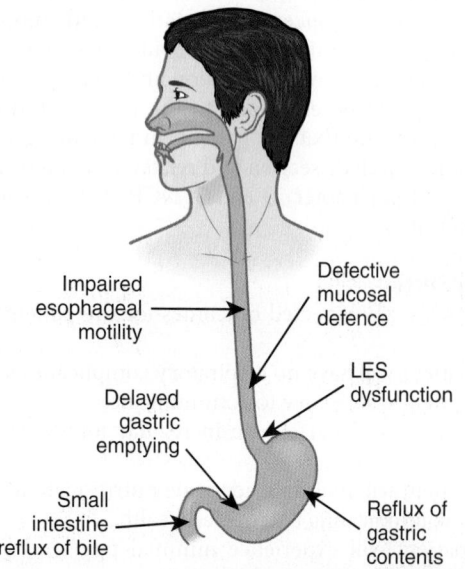

FIG. 44.2 Factors involved in the pathogenesis of gastroesophageal reflux disease (GERD). *LES,* lower esophageal sphincter.

Clinical Manifestations

The symptoms of GERD vary from individual to individual, but the diagnosis can usually be made on the basis of history and physical examination. Heartburn *(pyrosis)* from gastroesophageal reflux is the most common clinical manifestation. It is caused by irritation of the esophagus by the gastric secretions. Heartburn is described as a burning, tight sensation that is felt intermittently beneath the lower sternum and spreads upward to the throat or the jaw. Approximately once a week, the majority of patients with GERD have mild symptoms, including heartburn after a meal, with no evidence of mucosal damage.

Heartburn may occur after ingestion of food or medications that decrease the LES pressure or are directly irritating to the esophageal mucosa (Table 44.8). An individual with GERD may also report respiratory symptoms, including wheezing, coughing, and dyspnea. Otolaryngological symptoms include hoarseness, sore throat, a globus sensation (sensation of a lump in the throat), and choking. *Regurgitation* (effortless return of food or gastric contents from the stomach into the esophagus or mouth) is a fairly common manifestation of GERD. It is often described as hot, bitter, or sour liquid coming into the throat or mouth. Gastric symptoms—including early satiety, bloating after a meal, nausea, and vomiting—are related to delayed gastric emptying. Symptoms that would prompt endoscopic evaluation include dysphagia (solid food, progressive), odynophagia (painful swallowing), bleeding and subsequent anemia, weight loss, and persistent vomiting. Further investigation is indicated if suspected GERD symptoms are actually cardiac in origin. GERD-induced chest pain is similar to angina pain and the two are often confused (Chen et al., 2016).

Complications

Complications of GERD are related to the direct local effects of gastric acid on the esophageal mucosa. **Esophagitis** (inflammation of the esophagus) is a frequent complication of GERD. Other risk factors for esophagitis include hiatal hernia, chemical irritation from lye, and physical irritants such as smoking, cold or hot liquids, and excessive alcoholic intake. Trauma to the esophagus may also produce inflammation. The appearance of esophagitis with esophageal ulcerations is shown in Figure 44.3.

Repeated exposure may cause scar tissue formation and decreased distensibility of the esophagus *(esophageal stricture).* This may result in dysphagia.

Another complication of GERD is **Barrett's esophagus** (esophageal metaplasia). Barrett's esophagus is considered a precancerous lesion and increases the risk for esophageal

TABLE 44.8	COMMON FOODS AND MEDICATIONS AFFECTING LOWER ESOPHAGEAL SPHINCTER PRESSURE	
Increase Pressure	• Tea, coffee (caffeine)	
• Bethanechol (Duvoid)	• Medications	
• Metoclopramide	• Anticholinergics	
	• β-Adrenergic blockers	
Decrease Pressure	• Calcium channel blockers	
• Alcohol	• Diazepam (Valium)	
• Chocolate (theobromine)	• Morphine sulphate	
• Fatty foods	• Nitrates	
• Nicotine	• Progesterone	
• Peppermint, spearmint	• Theophylline	

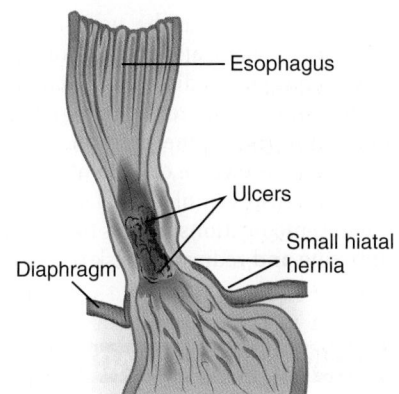

FIG. 44.3 Esophagitis with esophageal ulcerations.

cancer. In Barrett's esophagus, the normal squamous epithelium of the esophagus is replaced with columnar epithelium. These cell changes are thought to be related to chronic reflux esophagitis. Signs and symptoms of Barrett's esophagus can range from none to mild to bleeding and perforation. Given the increased risk of adenocarcinoma in patients with Barrett's esophagus, recommendations for endoscopic and biopsy screening are determined by the presence and grade of dysplasia within the segment of Barrett's esophagus (BC Cancer Agency, 2021b).

Respiratory complications of GERD include bronchospasm, laryngospasm, and cricopharyngeal spasm. These complications are caused by irritation of the upper airway by gastric secretions. With GERD, there is also the potential for pneumonia as a result of aspiration of gastric contents into the respiratory system. Dental erosion, especially in the posterior teeth, may result from acid reflux into the mouth.

Diagnostic Studies

Diagnostic studies are performed to determine the cause of the GERD, such as hiatal hernia (Table 44.9). Barium swallow studies may be done to determine whether there is protrusion of the upper part of the stomach (called the *gastric fundus*). Endoscopy is useful in assessing the competence of the LES and the extent of inflammation (if present), potential scarring, and strictures (Canadian Society of Intestinal Research, 2021). Biopsy and cytological specimens can be obtained to differentiate carcinoma of the stomach or esophagus from Barrett's esophagus. Esophageal manometric studies can be performed to measure pressure in the esophagus, as well as in the LES. The pH may be determined with the use of specially designed probes in the laboratory or ambulatory monitoring systems, which may demonstrate the presence of acid in the normally alkaline esophagus. Radionuclide tests may also be performed to detect reflux of gastric contents and the rate of esophageal clearance.

Interprofessional Care

Most cases of GERD can be successfully managed by lifestyle modifications and medication therapy. These are long-term approaches requiring an interprofessional approach to patient education and adherence to therapeutic regimens. When these therapies are ineffective, surgery is an option (see Table 44.9).

Lifestyle Modifications. Patients with GERD are taught to avoid factors that aggravate symptoms. Particular attention is given to diet and medications that may affect the LES, acid

TABLE 44.9 INTERPROFESSIONAL CARE
GERD and Hiatal Hernia

Diagnostic Assessment
- History and physical examination
- Upper GI endoscopy with biopsy and cytological analysis
- Esophagram (barium swallow)
- Motility (manometry) studies
- pH monitoring (laboratory or 24-hr ambulatory)
- Radionuclide studies

Management
Conservative
- Elevate head of bed on 10- to 15-cm locks
- Avoid intake of reflux-inducing foods (fatty foods, chocolate, peppermint)
- Avoid alcohol use
- Reduce or avoid intake of acidic pH beverages (colas, red wine, orange juice)

Medication Therapy
- PPIs
- H_2 receptor blockers*
- Antacids
- Prokinetic medication therapy*

Surgical Therapy
- Nissen fundoplication
- Toupet fundoplication

Endoscopic Therapy
- Intraluminal valvuloplasty
- Radiofrequency ablation

*See Table 44.10.
PPI, proton pump inhibitor.

secretion, or gastric emptying. Patients with overweight or obesity are encouraged to lose weight. Patients who smoke are encouraged to stop smoking.

Nutritional Therapy. Diet does not cause GERD, but food can aggravate symptoms. No specific diet is necessary, but foods that cause reflux should be avoided. Fatty foods stimulate the release of cholecystokinin, a hormone from the duodenum that decreases LES pressure. High-fat foods also decrease the rate of gastric emptying. Foods that decrease LES pressure, such as chocolate, peppermint, and caffeinated beverages (coffee, cola, and tea; see Table 44.8), should be avoided because they are conducive to reflux. Milk products should be avoided, especially at bedtime, because milk increases gastric acid secretion. To prevent overdistension of the stomach, small, frequent meals are advised. The patient should avoid having late-evening meals and nocturnal snacking. Fluids should be taken between rather than with meals to reduce gastric distension. Certain foods (e.g., tomato-based products, orange juice) may irritate the acid-sensitive esophagus and may have to be avoided. To reduce intra-abdominal pressure, weight reduction is recommended if the patient is overweight. Referral to dietitian can be beneficial to aid in meal planning and weight reduction, as required.

Medication Therapy. Medication therapy for GERD is focused on improving LES function, increasing esophageal clearance, decreasing the volume and acidity of reflux, and protecting the esophageal mucosa (Table 44.10). There are two approaches to medication therapy. In the "step-up" approach, therapy starts with antacids and OTC histamine (H_2)-receptor (H_2R) blockers, then prescription H_2R blockers, and finally,

TABLE 44.10 MEDICATION THERAPY
Gastroesophageal Reflux Disease (GERD)

Mechanism of Action	Examples
Increase Lower Esophageal Sphincter Pressure	
Cholinergic	Bethanechol (Duvoid)
Promotility	
Prokinetic	Metoclopramide
Acid-Neutralizing	
Antacids	Aluminum hydroxide and magnesium hydroxide (Maalox, Mylanta)
Antisecretory	
H_2-receptor blockers	Famotidine (Pepcid)
	Nizatidine (Axid)
	Ranitidine (Zantac)
Proton pump inhibitors	Esomeprazole (Nexium)
	Dexlansoprazole (Dexilant)
	Lansoprazole (Prevacid)
	Omeprazole (Losec)
	Pantoprazole (Pantoloc)
	Rabeprazole (Pariet)
Cytoprotective	
Alginic acid-antacid	Aluminum hydroxide + magnesium trisilicate (Gaviscon)
Acid-protective	Sucralfate

proton pump inhibitors (PPIs) are included. The "step-down" approach involves starting with a PPI and, over time, titrating down to prescription H_2R blockers and, finally, to OTC H_2R blockers and antacids.

Antacids produce quick but short-lived relief of heartburn. They act by neutralizing HCl. They should be taken 1 to 3 hours after meals and at bedtime. OTC antacids with or without alginic acid (e.g., Gaviscon) may be useful in patients with mild, intermittent heartburn. The alginic acid reacts with sodium bicarbonate and forms a viscous solution that floats to the surface of the gastric contents and coats the esophagus, acting as a mechanical barrier to reflux. However, in patients with moderate to severe or frequent symptoms, or in patients with documented esophagitis, these regimens are not effective in relieving symptoms or healing erosive lesions.

Antisecretory agents decrease the secretion of HCl by the stomach. H_2R blockers (e.g., ranitidine [Zantac]) are available in OTC and prescription formulations. Some formulations include combinations of H_2R blockers and antacids; for example, Pepcid Complete includes famotidine, calcium carbonate, and magnesium hydroxide. In prescription-strength doses, H_2R blockers reduce symptoms and promote esophageal healing in approximately 50% of patients. Many patients experience relapse (i.e., GERD symptoms return) with discontinuation of the medication.

PPIs also decrease stomach HCl secretion. These medications act by inhibiting the proton pump mechanism responsible for the secretion of hydrogen ions (H^+). PPIs promote esophageal healing in approximately 80 to 90% of patients but are more expensive than H_2R blockers. PPIs may also be beneficial in decreasing the incidence of esophageal strictures, a complication of chronic GERD. Long-term use of PPIs has been associated with increased risk for fractures of hip, wrist, and spine; increased risk of infection with *Clostridium difficile* in hospitalized patients; and pneumonia (Nehra et al., 2018).

Another medication that may be used to treat GERD is sucralfate, an antiulcer medication used for its cytoprotective properties. Cholinergic medications, such as bethanechol (Duvoid), may be used to increase LES pressure, improve esophageal emptying in the supine position, and increase gastric emptying. However, the value of current cholinergic agents is limited because they also stimulate HCl secretion. Prokinetic (motility-enhancing) medications such as metoclopramide promote gastric emptying and reduce the risk of gastric acid reflux (see Table 44.10).

EVIDENCE-INFORMED PRACTICE
Research Highlight

Are Proton Pump Inhibitors Associated With Improved Symptoms of Dyspepsia?
Clinical Question
Among patients with dyspepsia (P), does the use of proton pump inhibitor (PPI) medications (I) improve symptoms of dyspepsia and improve quality of life (O)?

Best Available Evidence
Systematic review of randomized controlled trials (RCTs)

Critical Appraisal and Synthesis of Evidence
- 25 RCTs ($N = 8\,453$ participants) examining the effects of PPIs versus placebo, H_2RAs, or prokinetics for improvement in symptoms of dyspepsia and quality of life.

Conclusion
- There is moderate evidence to support PPI use being more effective in relieving symptoms of dyspepsia than placebo.
- There was no evidence to support an association between the use of PPIs and quality of life.

Implications for Nursing Practice
- Collaborate with the interprofessional team to advocate for patients experiencing dyspepsia to institute use of PPIs.

References for Evidence
Janarthanan, S., Ditah, I., Adler, D. G., et al. (2012). Clostridium difficile–associated diarrhea and proton pump inhibitor therapy: A meta-analysis. *American Journal of Gastroenterology, 107*(7), 1001–1010. https://doi.org/10.1038/ajg.2012.179
Pinto-Sanchez, M., Yuan, Y., Hassan, A., et al. (2017). Proton pump inhibitors for functional dyspepsia. *Cochrane Database of Systematic Reviews, 2017*(11), CD011194. https://doi.org/10.1002/14651858.CD011194.pub3.
H_2RAs, H_2 receptor antagonists; *P*, patient population of interest; *I*, intervention or area of interest; *O*, outcomes of interest (see Chapter 1).

Surgical Therapy. Surgical therapy (antireflux surgery) may be necessary if long-term conservative therapy fails, in the presence of a hiatal hernia, or in the presence of complications, such as esophageal stricture and stenosis (narrowing), chronic esophagitis, and bleeding. Many surgical procedures are performed laparoscopically. The objective of surgical interventions for GERD is to reduce reflux of gastric contents by enhancing the integrity of the LES. Surgical interventions for GERD are called *antireflux procedures*. In these procedures, the fundus of the stomach is wrapped around the lower portion of the esophagus in varying positions.

A diagram of the Nissen fundoplication is shown in Figure 44.4. Laparoscopically performed Nissen and Toupet fundoplications have become the standard antireflux surgical procedures. The use of laparoscopic antireflux surgery for GERD has

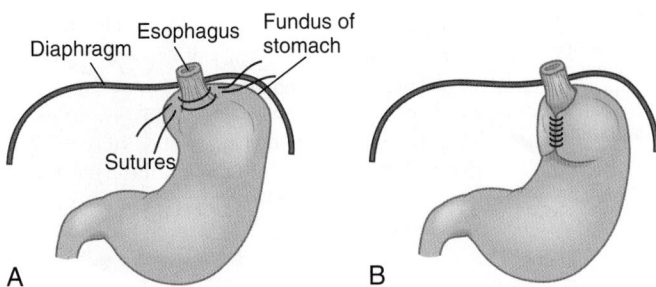

FIG. 44.4 Nissen fundoplication for repair of hiatal hernia. **A,** The fundus of the stomach is wrapped around the distal esophagus. **B,** The fundus is then sutured to itself. Source: Modified from Doughty, D. B., & Jackson, D. B. (1993). *Mosby's clinical nursing series: Gastrointestinal disorders.* Mosby.

many advantages compared to the open approach, including decreased mortality, decreased length of hospital stay, decrease in respiratory complications, and a faster recovery (Buckley, 2020).

Endoscopic Therapy. Alternatives to surgical therapy include endoscopic mucosal resection, photodynamic therapy, cryotherapy, and radiofrequency ablation (an image-guided technique that kills cells through heating). For patients with high-grade dysplasia, endoscopic mucosal resection can also be used as a diagnostic test to obtain biopsy samples.

NURSING MANAGEMENT
GASTROESOPHAGEAL REFLUX DISEASE

Patients with GERD must avoid practices and other factors that cause reflux. A patient teaching guide is provided in Table 44.11. Patients who smoke should stop. Smoking causes an almost immediate drop in LES pressure and decreases the ability to clear acid from the esophagus. Patients may need to be referred to other members of the health care team or to community resources for assistance in stopping smoking. (See Chapter 11 for additional information related to smoking cessation.) Substances that decrease LES pressure and tone should be avoided (see Table 44.8). If stress seems to cause symptoms, measures to cope with stress should be discussed. (See Chapter 8 for stress management techniques.) The patient should also be taught possible adverse effects of medications.

Nursing care for the patient who is having acute symptoms consists mainly of encouraging the patient to follow the necessary regimen, as described in Table 44.11. The patient may be taking medications to relieve heartburn, so the nurse must both observe for adverse effects and evaluate the medications' effectiveness. Even when symptoms are brought under control, the patient may need to continue taking the medications because the underlying health problem is still present. Because of the link between GERD and metaplastic changes in the lower esophagus (Barrett's esophagus), patients are instructed to see their health care provider if symptoms persist.

The nurse must observe for and instruct the patient about adverse effects of the medications being taken. H_2R blockers and PPIs are being prescribed less frequently because of increasing evidence of negative long-term effects with continued use. Antacids have minimal adverse effects; those that contain calcium and aluminum tend to cause constipation, whereas those that contain magnesium tend to cause diarrhea. Several of the antacids are combinations of calcium, aluminum, and magnesium designed to minimize these adverse effects. If

TABLE 44.11	**PATIENT & CAREGIVER TEACHING GUIDE**

Prevention of Gastroesophageal Reflux Disease

The following guidelines should be included when teaching the patient and caregiver about prevention of gastroesophageal reflux disease. The nurse should:
1. Explain the rationale for a high-protein, low-fat diet. If the patient is overweight or obese, the need for weight loss should be discussed.
2. Encourage the patient to eat small, frequent meals to prevent gastric distension.
3. Explain the rationale for avoiding alcohol use, smoking (which causes an almost immediate, marked decrease in LES pressure), and drinking beverages that contain caffeine.
4. Teach the patient not to lie down for 2–3 hr after eating, not to wear tight clothing around the waist, and not to bend over (especially after eating).
5. Encourage the patient to sleep with the head of the bed elevated 30 degrees (gravity fosters esophageal emptying).
6. Teach information regarding medications, including the rationale for their use and common adverse effects.
7. Discuss strategies for weight reduction, if appropriate.
8. Encourage the patient and caregiver to share concerns about lifestyle changes and living with a chronic condition.

LES, lower esophageal sphincter.

the patient is taking bethanechol (Duvoid), adverse effects to observe for include urinary urgency, increased salivation, and abdominal cramping with diarrhea, nausea, vomiting, and hypotension. Such adverse effects often limit the effectiveness of cholinergic agents in the treatment of GERD. Adverse effects of metoclopramide include restlessness, anxiety, insomnia, and hallucinations. Adverse effects of sucralfate include drowsiness, dizziness, nausea, vomiting, constipation, urticaria, and other types of rash.

Postoperative care focuses on concerns related to prevention of respiratory complications, maintenance of fluid and electrolyte balance, and prevention of infection. If a thoracic approach is used, a chest tube is inserted. Assessment and management related to closed chest drainage are important (see Chapter 30).

If an open abdominal incision is used, respiratory complications can occur in a patient because it is a high abdominal incision. Respiratory assessment should include respiratory rate and rhythm, pulse rate and rhythm, and signs of pneumothorax (e.g., dyspnea, chest pain, cyanosis). Deep breathing is essential to fully expand the lungs.

The patient receives IV fluids and electrolytes until the return of peristalsis. Care should be taken to maintain patency of the NG tube (if present) to prevent the need to reinsert the tube. It is dangerous to attempt to replace the tube because the surgical repair can be perforated. Immediately after the surgical procedure, the patient cannot voluntarily vomit or belch and thus may experience bloating and abdominal discomfort. When peristalsis returns, only fluids are given initially. Solids are added gradually so that the stomach is not overdistended. The nurse must maintain an accurate recording of intake and output and observe for fluid and electrolyte imbalances (see Chapter 19). (Care of the patient after a laparotomy procedure is described in Chapter 45 and NCP 45.2, available on the Evolve website.)

After surgical therapy, there should be no symptoms of gastric reflux. However, the recurrence rate may range from 10 to 30% over a 20-year period after surgery. The patient should be instructed to report symptoms such as heartburn and regurgitation. Such symptoms may be temporary and resolve with time.

The patient should report persistent dysphagia, sense of epigastric fullness, and bloating. A normal diet is gradually resumed. The patient should avoid eating foods that are gas forming and should try to prevent gastric distension. Food should be chewed thoroughly.

HIATAL HERNIA

Hiatal hernia is herniation of a portion of the stomach into the esophagus through an opening (hiatus) in the diaphragm. It is also referred to as *diaphragmatic hernia* and *esophageal hernia*. The incidence of hiatal hernia is difficult to determine. However, it is the most common abnormality found on radiographic examination of the upper GI tract. Hiatal hernias are common in older people and are more common in women than in men.

Types

Hiatal hernias are classified into the following two types (Figure 44.5):
1. *Sliding:* The junction of the stomach and the esophagus is above the hiatus of the diaphragm, and a part of the stomach slides through the hiatal opening in the diaphragm. The stomach "slides" into the thoracic cavity when the patient is supine and usually goes back into the abdominal cavity when the patient is standing upright. This is the most common type of hiatal hernia.
2. *Paraesophageal* or *rolling:* The esophagogastric junction remains in the normal position, but the fundus and the greater curvature of the stomach roll up through the diaphragm, forming a pocket alongside the esophagus.

Etiology and Pathophysiology

Many factors contribute to the development of hiatal hernia. Structural changes, such as weakening of the muscles in the diaphragm around the esophagogastric opening, are usually contributing factors. Factors that increase intra-abdominal pressure, including obesity, pregnancy, ascites, tumours, tight corsets, intense physical exertion, and heavy lifting on a continual basis, may also predispose to development of a hiatal hernia. Other predisposing factors are increased age, trauma, poor nutrition, and a forced recumbent position, as when a prolonged illness confines the person to bed. In some cases, congenital weakness is a contributing factor.

Clinical Manifestations

Hiatal hernia may be asymptomatic. The signs and symptoms of hiatal hernia, when present, are similar to those described for GERD. Heartburn, especially after a meal or after lying supine, is a common symptom. Affected patients may report dysphagia. Frequently, the symptoms of hiatal hernia mimic those of gallbladder disease, peptic ulcer disease (PUD), and angina. Reflux and discomfort are also associated with position, occurring soon or several hours after the person lies down. Bending over may cause a severe burning pain, which is usually relieved by sitting or standing. Other common precipitating factors of pain include consumption of large meals and alcohol and smoking. Nocturnal symptoms of heartburn are common, especially if the person has eaten before going to sleep.

Complications

Complications that may occur with hiatal hernia include GERD, hemorrhage from erosion, stenosis (narrowing of the

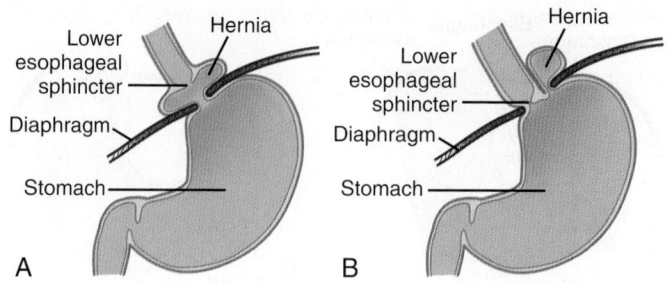

FIG. 44.5 **A,** Sliding hiatal hernia. **B,** Paraesophageal (rolling) hiatal hernia.

esophagus), ulcerations of the herniated portion of the stomach, strangulation of the hernia, and regurgitation with tracheal aspiration.

Diagnostic Studies

A barium swallow study is an important diagnostic measure that may reveal the protrusion of gastric mucosa through the esophageal hiatus in a patient with hiatal hernia. Endoscopic visualization of the lower esophagus provides information on the degree of mucosal inflammation or other abnormalities. Other tests are similar to those described in Table 44.9.

NURSING AND INTERPROFESSIONAL MANAGEMENT HIATAL HERNIA

CONSERVATIVE THERAPY

Conservative therapy for hiatal hernia is similar to that described for GERD, including lifestyle modifications (e.g., reduction of intra-abdominal pressure by not wearing constricting garments, avoiding lifting and straining, eliminating use of alcohol and smoking, elevating the head of the bed) and the use of antacids and antisecretory agents (i.e., PPIs, H_2R blockers). Elevation of the head of the bed on 10- to 15-cm blocks assists gravity in maintaining the stomach in the abdominal cavity and also helps prevent reflux and tracheal aspiration. If the patient is overweight, the patient should be encouraged to lose weight.

SURGICAL THERAPY

The objective of surgical interventions for hiatal hernia is to reduce reflux by enhancing the integrity of the LES. There are four slightly varied procedures: the Nissen fundoplication, the Toupet fundoplication or technique, the Hill gastropexy, and the Belsey fundoplication. These surgical procedures are all variations of fundoplication, which involves wrapping the fundus of the stomach around the lower portion of the esophagus in varying positions. These procedures reduce the hernia, help maintain an acceptable LES pressure, and prevent movement of the gastroesophageal junction. The Nissen fundoplication is illustrated in Figure 44.4. As with GERD, laparoscopically performed Nissen and Toupet techniques have become the standard antireflux surgeries for hiatal hernia (Buckley, 2020). A thoracic or open abdominal approach may also be used in selected cases.

AGE-RELATED CONSIDERATIONS

GASTROESOPHAGEAL REFLUX DISEASE AND HIATAL HERNIA

Both the incidence of GERD and that of hiatal hernia increase with age. They are associated with weakening of the diaphragm, obesity, kyphosis, and use of corsets or other factors that increase intra-abdominal pressure. In some older persons, hiatal hernia is asymptomatic. The first indications may include esophageal bleeding secondary to esophagitis or respiratory complications (e.g., aspiration pneumonia) related to aspiration of gastric contents. The LES may become less competent with aging in some individuals.

The clinical course and the management of GERD and hiatal hernia in older people are similar to those for the younger adult. With the increased use of laparoscopic procedures, surgical risks have been reduced. However, an older person with cardiovascular and pulmonary conditions may not be a good candidate for surgical intervention. In addition, changes in lifestyle, including elimination of dietary factors such as caffeine-containing beverages and chocolate, and elevating the head of the bed on blocks, may be more difficult for the older person.

ESOPHAGEAL CANCER

Esophageal cancer is a rare, malignant neoplasm of the esophagus. There are two main types: squamous cell carcinoma and adenocarcinoma. Adenocarcinomas arise from the glands lining the esophagus and resemble cancers of the stomach and the small intestine, whereas squamous cell carcinoma starts in the squamous cells that line the esophagus. The incidence of esophageal cancer increases with age. Cancer of the esophagus occurs in three times as many men as women, and the rate has remained relatively stable since the mid-1980s. However, the incidence of one type of esophageal cancer, esophageal adenocarcinoma, rose by 1.9% per year from 1998 to 2016 in Ontario, Canada (Cancer Care Ontario, 2019). This increase is attributed to the rising rates of obesity, which contributes to the development of GERD. It is estimated that 2 300 new cases of esophageal cancer were diagnosed in Canada in 2019 (Canadian Cancer Society's Advisory Committee on Cancer Statistics, 2019). The rate of 5-year survival is 14% despite multimodal treatment options.

Etiology and Pathophysiology

The cause of esophageal cancer is unknown. Important risk factors are smoking and excessive alcohol intake, chewing betel quid, GERD, tylosis, achalasia, Plummer-Vinson syndrome, chemical injury to the esophagus, exposure to ionizing radiation, and a personal history of oral cancer or a family history of esophageal cancer (Canadian Cancer Society, 2021d). One risk factor for esophageal adenocarcinoma is Barrett's esophagus. (Barrett's esophagus is described in the earlier Complications section under Gastroesophageal Reflux Disease.)

The majority of esophageal tumours are located in the middle and lower portions of the esophagus. The malignant tumour usually appears as an ulcerated lesion and has often advanced by the time the patient experiences symptoms. The tumour may penetrate the muscular layer and even extend outside the wall of the esophagus. Obstruction of the esophagus occurs in the later stages.

Clinical Manifestations

The onset of symptoms is usually late in relation to the extent of the tumour. Progressive dysphagia is the most common symptom and may be expressed as a substernal feeling as if food is not passing (globus sensation). Initially, the dysphagia occurs only with meat, then with soft foods, and eventually with liquids.

Pain develops late in the course of the disease and is described as occurring in the substernal, epigastric, or back areas and

usually increases with swallowing. The pain may radiate to the neck, the jaw, the ears, and the shoulders. If the tumour is in the upper third of the esophagus, symptoms such as sore throat, choking, and hoarseness may occur. Weight loss is fairly common. When esophageal stenosis is severe, regurgitation of blood-flecked esophageal contents is common.

Complications

Hemorrhage may occur if the cancer erodes through the esophagus and into the aorta. Esophageal perforation with fistula formation into the lung or the trachea sometimes develops. The tumour may enlarge enough to cause esophageal obstruction. Metastases spread via the lymph system, the liver and the lungs being common sites of metastasis.

Diagnostic Studies

A barium swallow study with fluoroscopy may demonstrate a narrowing of the esophagus at the site of the tumour (Table 44.12). Sometimes a crater is visible. Endoscopy with biopsy is necessary to make a definitive diagnosis of carcinoma by identification of malignant cells. Endoscopic ultrasonography is an important tool used to stage esophageal cancer. A bronchoscopic examination may be performed to detect malignant involvement of the lung. CT and MRI are also used to assess the extent of the disease.

Interprofessional Care

The treatment of esophageal cancer depends on the location of the tumour and whether invasion or metastasis has occurred (see Table 44.12). Esophageal cancer has a poor prognosis, mainly because it is not usually diagnosed until the disease is advanced. Treatment involves an interprofessional team approach. The best results may be obtained with a combination of surgery, chemotherapy, and radiation.

The types of surgical procedures that can be performed are (a) removal of part or all of the esophagus (*esophagectomy*) with use of a Dacron graft to replace the resected part, (b) resection of a portion of the esophagus and anastomosis of the remaining portion to the stomach (*esophagogastrostomy*), and (c) resection of a portion of the esophagus and anastomosis of a segment of colon to the remaining portion (*esophagoenterostomy*). The surgical approaches may be thoracic or both abdominal and thoracic. In comparison with the other procedures, minimally invasive esophagectomy (laparoscopic vagal nerve–sparing surgery) has the advantages of smaller incisions, shorter hospital stays, and fewer pulmonary complications. Overall outcomes

TABLE 44.12 **INTERPROFESSIONAL CARE**

Esophageal Cancer

Diagnostic Studies	Interprofessional Therapy
• History and physical examination	• Surgical resection
• Barium swallow study	• Esophagectomy
• Bronchoscopy	• Esophagogastrostomy
• CT, MRI	• Esophagoenterostomy
• Endoscopic ultrasonography	• Gastrostomy
• Endoscopy of esophagus with biopsy	• Chemotherapy
	• Dilation
	• Laser therapy
	• Palliative therapy
	• Radiation
	• Stent or prosthesis

CT, computed tomography; *MRI,* magnetic resonance imaging.

appear to be similar to those with open resection of the esophagus. Chemotherapy in combination with radiation treatment before or after surgery is currently used (BC Cancer Agency, 2021a); current treatment regimens can be found through the Canadian Cancer Society. If the tumour is in the cervical section (upper third) of the esophagus, radiation treatment is usually indicated. A tumour in the lower third of the esophagus is usually resected surgically.

Palliative therapy consists of restoration of the swallowing function and maintenance of nutrition and hydration. Dilation, stent placement, or both can relieve obstruction. Dilation is accomplished with various types of dilators (e.g., Celestin's tube). Dilation often relieves dysphagia and allows for improved nutrition. Placement of a stent or prosthesis may help when dilation is no longer effective. The prostheses are composed of silicone rubber or nylon-reinforced latex tubes with distal and proximal collars. The prosthesis is placed in the esophagus so that food and fluids can pass through the stenotic segment of the esophagus. The prosthesis can be placed endoscopically.

Endoscopic laser therapy or vaporization of the tumour may be used in combination with dilation. Obstruction recurs as the tumour grows, but laser therapy can be repeated. Sometimes these procedures are combined with radiation therapy. Other measures for palliation include gastrostomy or esophagostomy tube placements for nutritional support and pain management.

Nutritional Therapy. After esophageal surgery, parenteral fluids are given. When fluids are allowed, 30 to 60 mL of water is given hourly, with gradual progression to small, frequent bland meals. The patient should be in an upright position to prevent regurgitation of the fluid. The patient is observed for signs of intolerance to the feeding or leakage of the feeding into the mediastinum. Symptoms that indicate leakage are pain, increased temperature, and dyspnea. Symptoms of food intolerance include vomiting and abdominal distension. A gastrostomy may be performed for the purpose of feeding the patient. (Gastrostomy and tube feedings are discussed in Chapter 42.) Referral to a dietitian and speech language pathologist may be indicated to enhance nutrition therapy.

NURSING MANAGEMENT
ESOPHAGEAL CANCER

NURSING ASSESSMENT

The patient should be asked about any history of GERD, hiatal hernia, achalasia, or Barrett's esophagus. The patient is also questioned regarding tobacco and alcohol use. The patient should be assessed for progressive dysphagia and *odynophagia* (burning, squeezing pain during swallowing). The nurse should ask the patient about the types of substances ingested that cause dysphagia, such as meat, soft foods, and liquids. The patient is also assessed for pain (substernal, epigastric, or back areas), choking, heartburn, hoarseness, cough, anorexia, weight loss, and regurgitation (sometimes bloody).

NURSING DIAGNOSES

Nursing diagnoses for the patient with esophageal cancer include but are not limited to the following:

- *Chronic pain* resulting from *injury agent* (compression of tumour on surrounding tissues)
- *Inadequate nutrition* resulting from *insufficient dietary intake* (dysphagia, odynophagia, weakness)
- *Potential for aspiration* resulting from *decrease in gastrointestinal motility* (difficulty swallowing and regurgitation)
- *Anxiety* resulting from *threat to current status, threat of death*

PLANNING

The overall goals are that the patient with esophageal cancer will (a) have relief of symptoms, including pain and dysphagia; (b) achieve optimal nutritional intake; (c) understand the prognosis of the disease; and (d) experience the best possible quality of life during disease progression.

NURSING IMPLEMENTATION

HEALTH PROMOTION. Patients with diagnosed GERD and hiatal hernia need to be counselled regarding regular follow-up evaluation. Health counselling should focus on elimination of smoking and excessive alcohol intake, as well as other risk factors for GERD. Maintenance of good oral hygiene and dietary habits (intake of fresh fruits and vegetables) may also be helpful.

Patients with Barrett's esophagus need to be monitored because this is considered a premalignant condition. Early diagnosis of esophageal tumours is important but difficult because the onset of symptoms is usually late in the course of the disease. Patients are encouraged to seek medical attention for any esophageal issues, especially dysphagia. Patients who are at risk for esophageal adenocarcinoma, such as those with evidence of Barrett's esophagus and a diagnosis of achalasia (discussed later in the Other Esophageal Disorders section), may need regular endoscopic screening with biopsy and cytological study.

ACUTE INTERVENTION

Preoperative Care. In addition to general preoperative teaching and preparation, particular attention to the patient's nutritional needs and oral care is important. Many patients are inadequately nourished because of the inability to ingest sufficient amounts of food and fluids before surgery. A high-calorie, high-protein diet is recommended. It may have to be in liquid form. Some patients may need IV fluid replacement or parenteral nutrition. The patient and the family are instructed in how to keep an intake and output record and how to assess for signs of fluid and electrolyte imbalance. Some treatment protocols necessitate preoperative radiation treatment and chemotherapy.

Meticulous oral care is essential. The mouth, including tongue, gingivae, and teeth or dentures, must be cleaned thoroughly. Milk of magnesia with mineral oil may be used to remove any crusting that has formed. A mixture of mouthwash (nonalcohol), ice, and water makes a refreshing rinse for the patient.

Teaching should include information about chest tubes (if a thoracic approach is used), IV lines, NG tubes, gastrostomy feeding, turning, coughing, and deep breathing. (General preoperative care is presented in Chapter 20.)

Postoperative Care. After surgery for esophageal cancer, most patients have an NG tube in place, and there may be bloody drainage for 8 to 12 hours. The drainage gradually changes to greenish yellow. Assessment of the drainage, maintenance of the tube, and oral and nasal care are nursing responsibilities. The nurse should not reposition or reinsert the NG tube without consulting with the surgeon.

Because of the location of the incision and the general condition of the patient, special emphasis must be placed on prevention of respiratory complications. Turning and deep breathing should be done every 2 hours. Use of an incentive spirometer helps to prevent respiratory complications.

The patient should be positioned in a semi-Fowler's or Fowler's position to prevent reflux and aspiration of gastric secretions. When the patient can drink fluids or eat, the upright position should be maintained for at least 2 hours after eating in order to assist the movement of food through the GI tract.

AMBULATORY AND HOME CARE. Many patients require long-term follow-up care after surgery for esophageal cancer. Patients may undergo chemotherapy and radiation treatment after surgery. These patients need encouragement and assistance in maintaining adequate nutrition. A permanent feeding gastrostomy may be necessary. Most of these patients have fears and anxieties about a diagnosis of cancer. The nurse should know what the health care provider has told the patient regarding the prognosis and provide appropriate counselling.

Referral to a home health nurse may be necessary for continued care of the patient (e.g., gastrostomy teaching, follow-up wound care). (See Chapter 13 for management of terminally ill patients, and Chapter 18 for that of patients with cancer.)

EVALUATION

The following are expected outcomes for the patient with esophageal cancer:
- The patient will maintain a patent airway.
- The patient will have relief of pain.
- The patient will be able to swallow comfortably.
- The patient will consume adequate nutritional intake.
- The patient will understand the prognosis of the disease.
- The patient will experience the best possible quality of life during disease progression.

OTHER ESOPHAGEAL DISORDERS

Eosinophilic Esophagitis

Eosinophilic esophagitis is characterized by swelling of the esophagus caused by an infiltration of *eosinophils*. Many people with this condition have a personal or family history of other allergic diseases. The most common food triggers are milk, egg, wheat, rye, and beef. Environmental allergens—such as pollens, moulds, and cat, dog, and dust mite allergens—may be involved in the development of eosinophilic esophagitis.

Clinical manifestations include severe heartburn, difficulty swallowing, food impaction in the esophagus, nausea, vomiting, and weight loss. The diagnosis is based on the symptoms and biopsy findings of eosinophils infiltrating the esophageal tissue obtained from endoscopy.

Allergy skin testing is used to help determine the person's allergens. A trial of avoidance of the foods to which the person's allergy test results are positive is the initial form of treatment for eosinophilic esophagitis. A variety of treatment approaches, including acid suppression, corticosteroids, and endoscopic dilation, can be used alone or in combination.

Corticosteroids are frequently used to treat eosinophilic esophagitis when avoidance of allergic triggers does not relieve symptoms. Corticosteroids may be used orally (prednisone) or as a topical therapy, such as fluticasone (Flovent) or budesonide, in liquid form. In eosinophilic esophagitis, they are swallowed, resulting in delivery of the medication directly to the esophagus.

Esophageal Diverticula

Esophageal diverticula are saclike outpouchings of one or more layers of the esophagus. They occur in three main areas: (1) above the upper esophageal sphincter (*Zenker's diverticulum*),

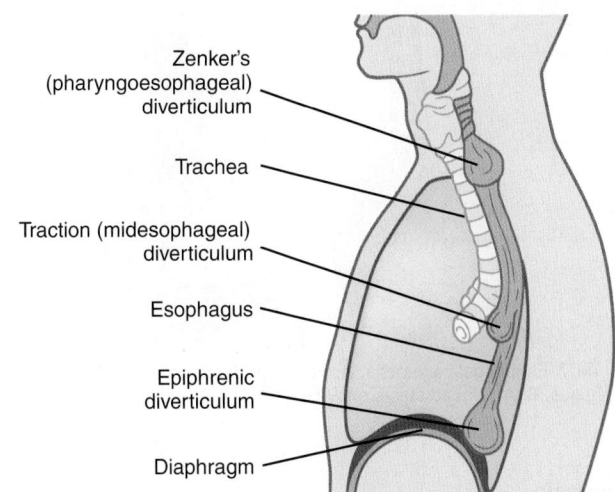

FIG. 44.6 Possible sites for the occurrence of esophageal diverticula. These hollow outpouchings may occur just above the upper esophageal sphincter (Zenker's, the most common type of diverticulum), near the midpoint of the esophagus (traction), and just above the lower esophageal sphincter (epiphrenic). Source: Modified from Price, S. A., & Wilson, L. M. (2003). *Pathophysiology: Clinical concepts of disease processes* (6th ed.). Mosby.

which is the most common location; (2) near the esophageal midpoint (*traction diverticulum*); and (3) above the LES (*epiphrenic diverticulum*) (Figure 44.6). Pharyngeal pouches (Zenker's diverticula) occur most commonly in older persons (age >70 years), and typical symptoms include dysphagia, regurgitation, chronic cough, aspiration, and weight loss. Traction diverticulum may not cause signs and symptoms. However, many affected patients report a sour taste in the mouth and halitosis (foul smelling breath) caused by the decomposition of stagnant food in the diverticulum. Complications include malnutrition, aspiration, and perforation. A diagnosis is easily established by barium studies.

Treatment for diverticula is not required unless nutrition becomes impaired. Some patients find they can empty the pocket of food that collects by applying pressure at a point on the neck. The diet may have to be limited to foods that pass more readily (e.g., blenderized foods). When nutrition becomes impaired, surgical treatment is required. Surgical treatment is via an endoscopic or external cervical approach and should include a cricopharyngeal myotomy. Open approaches have been associated with significant morbidity because the majority of affected patients are older people, many of whom have general medical conditions.

Esophageal Strictures

The most common cause of esophageal strictures (narrowing) is chronic GERD. The ingestion of strong acids or alkalis, external beam radiation, and surgical anastomosis can also lead to the development of strictures. In addition, trauma such as throat lacerations and gunshot wounds may lead to strictures as a result of scar formation (collagen deposition) from healing. The strictures usually develop over a long period of time. Strictures can be dilated endoscopically with *bougies* (dilating instruments). Another technique is balloon dilation, which is done under endoscopic guidance and does not require fluoroscopy. Surgical excision with anastomosis is sometimes necessary. The patient may have a temporary or permanent gastrostomy.

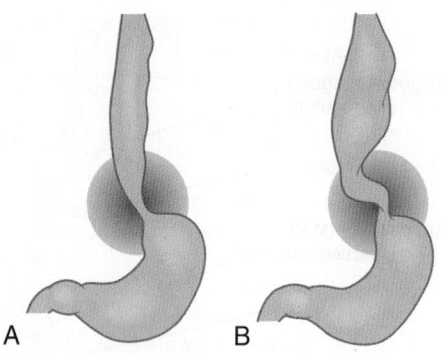

FIG. 44.7 Esophageal achalasia. **A,** Early stage, showing tapering of lower esophagus. **B,** Advanced stage, showing dilated, tortuous esophagus.

Achalasia

Achalasia is the absence of peristalsis of the lower two thirds (smooth muscle) of the esophagus. Pressure in the LES is increased, and relaxation of the LES is incomplete. Obstruction of the esophagus at or near the diaphragm occurs. Food and fluid accumulate in the lower esophagus. The result of this condition is dilation of the lower esophagus (Figure 44.7). The altered peristalsis is a result of impairment of the neurons that innervate the lower esophagus. There is a selective loss of inhibitory neurons, which results in unopposed excitation of the LES. Achalasia affects people of all ages and both sexes. The course of the disease is chronic.

Dysphagia (difficulty swallowing) is the most common symptom and occurs with both liquids and solids. Patients may report a globus sensation. Substernal chest pain (similar to the pain of angina) occurs during or immediately after a meal. *Halitosis* and the inability to eructate (belch) are other symptoms. Another common symptom is regurgitation of sour-tasting food and liquids, especially when the patient is in a horizontal position. Patients with achalasia also report symptoms (e.g., heartburn) of GERD. Weight loss is typical.

Diagnosis usually involves manometric studies of the lower esophagus, endoscopy, or both. The exact cause of achalasia is not known, thus treatment is focused on symptom management. Treatment consists of dilation, surgery, and use of medications. All of these therapies are directed at relieving the stasis caused by the increased LES pressure, the nonrelaxing LES, and the aperistaltic esophagus. Treatment of symptoms consists of a semisoft bland diet, eating slowly and drinking fluid with meals, and sleeping with the head elevated.

Medication therapy is used to manage early achalasia when there is no significant esophageal dilation. Medication therapy is used as a short-term measure and is considered an alternative only in patients unable to undergo pneumatic dilation or surgery. Endoscopic injection of botulinum toxin (Botox) into the LES can be offered for initial relief of symptoms, but the effects are short term, and symptoms are likely to recur within 1 year. It works by inhibiting the release of acetylcholine from nerve endings, thereby promoting relaxation of the smooth muscle. This treatment does not carry the risk of perforation that can occur with pneumatic dilation. Repeated injections are required, or the patient must be switched to another therapy. However, there may be subsets of patients, such as older patients or those with multiple medical conditions, who are poor candidates for more invasive procedures, for whom botulinum toxin injection is the preferred approach. Other classes of medications used in

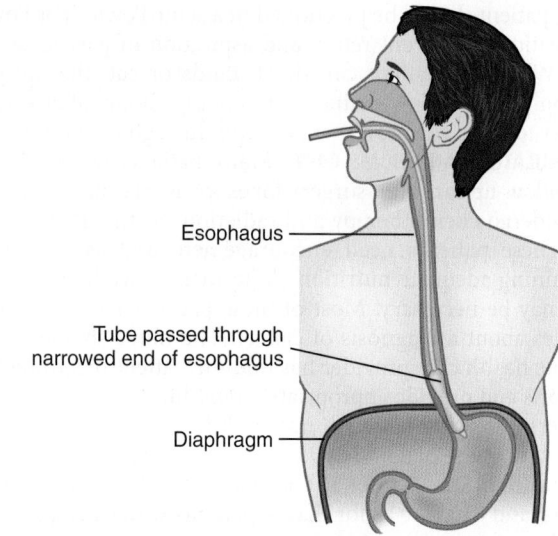

FIG. 44.8 Pneumatic dilation attempts to treat achalasia by maintaining an adequate lumen and decreasing lower esophageal sphincter tone. Source: Modified from Price, S. A., & Wilson, L. M. (2003). *Pathophysiology: Clinical concepts of disease processes* (6th ed.). Mosby.

the management of achalasia include anticholinergics, calcium channel blockers, and long-acting nitrates, which act by relaxing the smooth muscle.

Esophageal dilation *(bougienage)* is an effective treatment measure for many patients. The LES is usually pneumatically dilated with a balloon-tipped dilator passed orally. A variety of different dilators are available for this procedure. All of them depend on forcible expansion of a balloon in the LES (Figure 44.8). The forceful dilation does not restore normal esophageal motility, but it does provide for emptying of the esophagus into the stomach.

Surgical intervention may become necessary. An esophagomyotomy may be performed. In this procedure, the muscle fibres that enclose the narrowed area of the esophagus are divided. This allows the mucosa to pouch out through the division in the muscle layer so that food can be swallowed without obstruction.

A similar procedure is the Heller myotomy (cardiomyotomy), which disrupts the LES and reduces LES pressure. An antireflux procedure is often performed with the myotomy. The Heller myotomy can be done laparoscopically, which reduces the potential for postoperative complications.

Esophageal Varices

Esophageal varices are veins in the lower portion of the esophagus that become dilated and tortuous as a result of portal hypertension. Esophageal varices are a common complication of liver cirrhosis and are discussed further in Chapter 46.

DISORDERS OF THE STOMACH AND UPPER SMALL INTESTINE

GASTRITIS

Types

Gastritis, an inflammation of the gastric mucosa, is one of the most common conditions affecting the stomach. Gastritis may be acute or chronic and may be diffuse or localized. Chronic

TABLE 44.13 CAUSES OF GASTRITIS

Medications	Pathophysiological Conditions
• Acetylsalicylic acid (ASA; Aspirin)	• Burns
• Corticosteroid medications	• Crohn's disease
• Nonsteroidal anti-inflammatory medications	• Large hiatal hernia
	• Physiological stress
Diet	• Reflux of bile and pancreatic secretions
• Alcohol	• Renal failure (uremia)
• Spicy, irritating food	• Sepsis
	• Shock
Microorganisms	**Other Factors**
• *Helicobacter pylori*	• Endoscopic procedures
• *Salmonella* organisms	• Nasogastric suction
• *Staphylococcus* organisms	• Psychological stress
Environmental Factors	
• Radiation	
• Smoking	

gastritis has been further divided into three subtypes: (1) *autoimmune,* which involves the body and the fundus of the stomach; (2) *diffuse antral,* which affects primarily the antrum; and (3) *multifocal,* which is diffuse throughout the stomach. The causes of gastritis and its relationship to other gastric disorders, such as *Helicobacter pylori* infection and gastric cancer, are the focus of ongoing research.

Etiology and Pathophysiology

Gastritis occurs as the result of a breakdown in the normal gastric mucosal barrier. This mucosal barrier normally protects the stomach tissue from autodigestion by HCl and the proteolytic enzyme pepsin. When the barrier is broken, HCl can diffuse back into the mucosa. The backward diffusion of acid results in tissue edema, disruption of capillary walls with loss of plasma into the gastric lumen, and possibly hemorrhage.

Causes of gastritis are listed in Table 44.13. Nonsteroidal anti-inflammatory drugs (NSAIDs), digitalis, and corticosteroids cause irritation of the gastric mucosa by inhibiting the synthesis of prostaglandins, which serves as a protection to the gastric mucosa. NSAID-related gastritis is associated with many of the older commonly used medications, such as naproxen (Naprosyn), diclofenac (Voltaren), and ibuprofen (Motrin, Advil). Use of cyclo-oxygenase-2 (COX-2) inhibitors has been associated with fewer GI adverse effects than the nonselective use of NSAIDs.

Large intake of alcoholic beverages can cause acute damage to the gastric mucosa. Prolonged damage induced by repeated alcohol misuse can result in chronic gastritis. Eating large quantities of spicy, irritating foods and metabolic conditions such as uremia can also cause acute gastritis.

An important causative factor in chronic gastritis is *H. pylori* infection. *H. pylori*–associated gastritis is a common health problem in adults, many of whom do not have symptoms of gastritis. It is currently thought that *H. pylori* infection is acquired in childhood. For reasons not clearly understood, *H. pylori* is capable of promoting the breakdown of the gastric mucosal barrier, given certain "triggers" or conditions. *H. pylori* has been linked to gastric cancer and mucosa-associated lymphoid tissue (MALT) lymphoma of the stomach. (The role of *H. pylori* in ulcer development is discussed in greater detail later in the Duodenal Ulcers section.)

Autoimmune atrophic gastritis is a form of chronic gastritis that affects both the fundus and the body of the stomach and is associated with an increased risk of gastric cancer. Approximately 30% of patients with *H. pylori* infection are found to have antigastric antibodies as well. Thus, there may be a link between the host's response to the presence of *H. pylori* and the development of autoimmune chronic gastritis.

Although not as common, infections with bacteria, viruses, and fungi, including *Mycobacterium,* cytomegalovirus, and *Treponema pallidum,* are associated with chronic gastritis. Gastritis can result from reflux of bile salts from the duodenum into the stomach following surgical procedures such as gastroduodenostomy and gastrojejunostomy and with prolonged vomiting. In addition, intense emotional responses and CNS lesions may produce inflammation of the mucosal lining as a result of hypersecretion of HCl.

Hypochlorhydria (decreased acid secretion) or *achlorhydria* (lack of acid secretion) occurs as progressive gastric mucosal atrophy and the gastric chief and parietal cells die.

Clinical Manifestations

The symptoms of acute gastritis include anorexia, nausea and vomiting, epigastric tenderness, and a feeling of fullness. Hemorrhage is commonly associated with alcohol misuse and at times may be the only symptom. Acute gastritis is self-limiting, lasting from a few hours to a few days, and the mucosa is expected to heal completely.

The manifestations of chronic gastritis are similar to those described for acute gastritis. Some affected patients have no symptoms directly associated with the gastric lesion. However, when the acid-secreting cells are lost or do not function as a result of atrophy, the source of *intrinsic factor* is also lost. The loss of intrinsic factor, a substance secreted by the gastric mucosa that is essential for the absorption of cobalamin (vitamin B_{12}, which is essential for the growth and maturation of RBCs) in the terminal ileum, ultimately results in cobalamin deficiency. Over time, the body's storage of cobalamin in the liver is depleted and a deficiency state exists. Lack of this important vitamin results in the development of anemia and neurological complications. (Cobalamin deficiency anemia is discussed in Chapter 33.)

Diagnostic Studies

Diagnosis of acute gastritis is most often based on a history of drug and alcohol use. The diagnosis of chronic gastritis may be delayed or completely missed because the symptoms are nonspecific. Endoscopic examination with biopsy is necessary to obtain a definitive diagnosis. Breath, urine, serum, stool, and gastric tissue biopsy tests are available for the determination of *H. pylori*. These tests are described later in this chapter in the Diagnostic Studies section under Peptic Ulcer Disease. Radiological studies are not helpful because the superficial mucosa is generally involved, and changes are not clearly visible on radiographs. A complete blood cell count (CBC) may demonstrate the presence of anemia that results from blood loss or lack of intrinsic factor. Stools are tested for the presence of occult blood. A gastric analysis, although currently not used as much, demonstrates the amount of HCl present; achlorhydria is a common sign of severe atrophic gastritis. Serum tests for antibodies to parietal cells and intrinsic factor may be performed. Tissue biopsy with cytological examination is necessary to rule out gastric carcinoma.

NURSING AND INTERPROFESSIONAL MANAGEMENT GASTRITIS

ACUTE GASTRITIS

Eliminating the cause and preventing or avoiding it in the future are generally all that is needed to treat acute gastritis. The plan of care is supportive and similar to that described for nausea and vomiting. If vomiting accompanies acute gastritis, bed rest, NPO status, and IV fluids may be prescribed. Dehydration can occur rapidly in patients with acute gastritis with vomiting. Fluids and electrolytes lost through vomiting and occasionally diarrhea are replaced. Antiemetics are given for nausea and vomiting (see Table 44.1). In severe cases of acute gastritis, an NG tube may be used, either for lavage of the precipitating agent from the stomach or in conjunction with suction to keep the stomach empty and free of noxious stimuli. Clear liquids are resumed when acute symptoms have subsided, with gradual reintroduction of solid, bland foods.

If hemorrhage is considered likely, vital signs must be checked frequently and the vomitus tested for blood. All of the management strategies discussed later in the Upper Gastrointestinal Bleeding section also apply to severe gastritis.

Medication therapy is focused on reducing irritation of the gastric mucosa and providing relief of symptoms. Antacids are beneficial in the relief of abdominal discomfort by raising intragastric pH to above 6. H_2R blockers or PPIs may be used to reduce gastric HCl secretion. The nurse must have knowledge of the action and the therapeutic effects of PPIs and H_2R blockers to teach the patient and to monitor the effects of the medications.

CHRONIC GASTRITIS

The treatment of chronic gastritis focuses on evaluating and eliminating the specific cause (e.g., cessation of alcohol intake, abstinence from drugs, *H. pylori* eradication). Currently, antibiotic and antisecretory agent combinations are used to eradicate infection with *H. pylori* (Table 44.14). For patients with pernicious anemia, oral or parenteral administration of cobalamin is needed (see Chapter 33). Discussion of the continued need for this essential vitamin must be included in the plan of care.

The patient undergoing treatment for chronic gastritis may have to adapt to many lifestyle changes and adhere strictly to a medication regimen. A nonirritating diet consisting of six small meals a day and the use of an antacid after meals may help provide relief from symptoms. Smoking is contraindicated. An interprofessional team approach in which the health care provider, the nurse, the dietitian, and the pharmacist provide consistent information and support may increase the patient's success in making these alterations. Because the incidence of gastric cancer is higher among patients who have a history of chronic gastritis, especially atrophic gastritis, close medical follow-up should be emphasized.

GASTRIC CANCER

Gastric cancer (also called *stomach cancer*) is an adenocarcinoma of the stomach wall (Figure 44.9). It is the third most frequent cause of cancer death worldwide (Rawla & Barsouk, 2019). Although less common in Canada, it is estimated that 4 100 new gastric cancer cases were diagnosed in 2019 (Canadian Cancer Society, 2021f). In 2015, it was estimated 1 in 74 males and 1 in 142 females would develop gastric cancer (Canadian

TABLE 44.14	MEDICATION THERAPY	
Helicobacter pylori *Infection*		
Treatment	**Duration**	**Eradication Rate**
Triple-Medication Therapy (Recommended as First-Line Therapy)		
Proton pump inhibitor* Amoxicillin Clarithromycin (Biaxin)	7–14 days	>70–85%
Quadruple Therapy Proton pump inhibitor* Bismuth subsalicylate Tetracycline Metronidazole (Flagyl)	10–14 days	85%

*See Table 44.10.

Cancer Society's Advisory Committee on Cancer Statistics, 2019). The prevalence in males increases with age over 50 years. Younger Indigenous populations are disproportionately affected by gastric cancer in northern Canada (Colquhoun et al., 2019). Gastric cancer is typically at an advanced stage when diagnosed and is not usually amenable to surgical resection. The disease is confined to the stomach in only 10 to 20% of affected patients. The rate of 5-year survival is 25%.

Etiology and Pathophysiology

Many factors have been implicated in the development of gastric cancer: *H. pylori* infection; smoking; family history of gastric cancer; inherited conditions (e.g., hereditary diffuse gastric cancer); certain stomach conditions, including gastritis; previous stomach surgery; infection with the Epstein-Barr virus; exposure to ionizing radiation; and type A blood (Canadian Cancer Society, 2021e).

Gastric carcinogenesis probably begins with a nonspecific mucosal injury secondary to aging, autoimmunity, or repeated exposure to irritants such as bile, anti-inflammatory agents, or alcohol. Nutritional or other undetermined genetic deficiencies may impede mucosal repair, which results in chronic gastritis and subsequent proliferation of *H. pylori*. Infection with *H. pylori*, especially at an early age, is considered a definite risk factor for gastric cancer. It is possible that *H. pylori* and resulting metabolic changes can induce a sequence of transitions from dysplasia to carcinoma in situ. Individuals with MALT lymphoma are at higher risk for gastric cancer.

Other predisposing factors associated with a high incidence of gastric cancer are atrophic gastritis, pernicious anemia, adenomatous polyps, hyperplastic polyps, and achlorhydria. The relationship between chronic gastric ulcers and the development of gastric cancer is still not completely understood. Malignant transformation of a benign chronic ulcer does occur but accounts for fewer than 5% of all gastric cancers. It is known that people with achlorhydria or pernicious anemia are more likely to develop gastric cancer than are people with normal gastric acid production.

Gastric cancers often spread to adjacent organs before any distressing symptoms occur. The tumour may grow to large dimensions without obstructing the lumen of the stomach, simply because the lumen itself is so large. The interval from onset of symptoms to consultation with a health care provider may be as long as 6 months. This long delay is largely attributed to

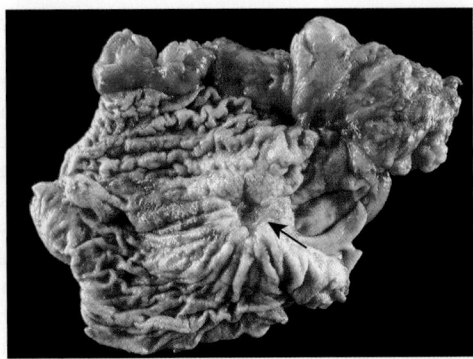

FIG. 44.9 Gastric cancer. Gross photograph shows an ill-defined, excavated central ulcer surrounded by irregular, heaped-up borders. Source: Kumar, V., Abbas, A. K., Fausto, N., et al. (2010). *Robbins and Cotran pathologic basis of disease* (8th ed.). Saunders.

TABLE 44.15 **INTERPROFESSIONAL CARE**	
Gastric Cancer	
Diagnostic Studies	**Interprofessional Therapy**
• History and physical examination	*Surgical Therapy*
• α-Fetoprotein measurement	• Subtotal gastrectomy: Billroth I or II procedure
• Carbohydrate antigen (CA-) 19-9, CA-125, CA 72-4 assessments	• Total gastrectomy with esophagojejunostomy
• Carcinoembryonic antigen (CEA) assessment	*Adjuvant Therapy*
• Complete blood cell count	• Radiation therapy
• Endoscopic ultrasonography	• Chemotherapy
• Endoscopy and biopsy	• Combination radiation therapy and chemotherapy
• Exfoliative cytological study	
• Liver enzyme measurements	
• Serum amylase measurement	
• Stool examination	
• Tumour marker assessment	
• Upper GI barium study	
• Urinalysis	

GI, gastrointestinal.

nonspecific symptoms of vague, intermittent abdominal distress that are often seen in healthy persons due dietary indiscretions, nervous tension, and anxiety.

Gastric cancer can occur in any portion of the stomach. Tumours located at the cardia and the fundus are associated with a poor prognosis. These tumours typically infiltrate rapidly to the surrounding tissue, regional lymph nodes, and liver. Patients with tumour growth along the lesser curvature have a better survival rate. Adenocarcinomas account for more than 95% of the cancers, and sarcomas (comprising lymphomas and leiomyomas) make up the rest.

The tumour growth is insidious and follows a pattern of continuous infiltration. Gastric cancer may spread by direct extension along the mucosal surface and infiltrate through the stomach wall. The rich lymphatic plexuses in the stomach facilitate distant metastasis. Seeding of tumour cells into the peritoneal cavity may occur late in the course of the disease.

Clinical Manifestations

The clinical manifestations exhibited by persons with gastric cancer can be categorized by signs and symptoms of anemia, PUD, or indigestion. Anemia is a common occurrence with gastric cancer. It is caused by chronic blood loss that occurs as the lesion erodes through the mucosa or as a direct result of pernicious anemia, which develops when intrinsic factor is lost. The affected person appears pale and weak and reports fatigue, weakness, dizziness, and, in extreme cases, shortness of breath. The stool specimen may be positive for occult blood.

The symptoms of gastric cancer are sometimes identical to those of PUD. The pain and discomfort may be alleviated by belching and by the use of antacids, antisecretory agents, and diet modifications. Manifestations related to indigestion include a vague feeling of epigastric fullness with sense of early satiety after meals. Weight loss, dysphagia, and constipation frequently accompany epigastric distress. When nausea, vomiting, and hematemesis occur, they may indicate gastric outlet obstruction or may be a warning of impending hemorrhage.

With more advanced disease, the physical examination may reveal that the patient is pale and lethargic if anemia is present. When the appetite has been poor and weight loss has been considerable, the patient may appear cachectic. A mass may be detected beneath the abdominal wall and is seen to move with each inspiration. On palpation, the mass may be felt in the epigastrium. Masses that are predominantly in the antrum of the stomach are generally found to the left of the midline. Masses

located to the right of midline usually tend to be metastases to the liver or indicate involvement of the perigastric lymph nodes. Supraclavicular lymph nodes that are hard and enlarged and located on the left side are suggestive of metastasis via the thoracic duct from the stomach lesion. The presence of ascites is a poor prognostic sign.

Diagnostic Studies

The diagnostic studies for gastric cancer are presented in Table 44.15.

Endoscopic examination of the stomach remains the best diagnostic tool. Lesions that go undetected on the radiograph can be viewed more easily and a biopsy performed when endoscopy is used. The stomach can be distended with air during the procedure so that the mucosal folds can be stretched. Fixation of the mucosa is indicative of malignancy.

Upper GI barium studies may demonstrate alterations in gastric contractility and emptying but do not always reveal small lesions of the cardia and fundus.

Blood chemistry studies assist in the determination of anemia and its severity. Elevations in liver enzymes and serum amylase levels may indicate liver and pancreatic involvement. Stool examination provides evidence of occult or gross bleeding.

Several tumour markers are often present in patients with gastric cancer (see Table 44.15). Serum tests for these markers are commonly performed before surgery for this disease. Serum markers are not used as the only diagnostic tools for gastric cancer because elevations may be related to other factors such as smoking and the presence of benign lesions. (Carcinoembryonic antigen and other tumour markers are discussed in Chapter 18.)

Interprofessional Care

When the diagnosis of gastric cancer has been confirmed, the treatment of choice is surgical removal of the tumour. An interprofessional approach to preoperative management of the patient with gastric cancer focuses on the correction of nutritional deficits, treatment of anemia, and replacement of blood volume.

Transfusions of packed RBCs correct the anemia. If a gastric lesion has been located at or near the pylorus and is causing gastric outlet obstruction, gastric decompression may be necessary before surgery. When the tumour has extended into the transverse colon, and if partial colon resection is also required, special preparation of the bowel is necessary. This preparation may include a low-residue diet, enemas to cleanse the bowel, and the use of antibiotics to reduce the intestinal bacteria. Correction of malnutrition is important before the planned surgery Malnutrition is associated with increased rates of postoperative complications and mortality.

Surgical Therapy. The surgical intervention used in the treatment of gastric cancer may be the same surgical procedures used for PUD. The location and the extent of the lesion, the patient's physical condition, and the preference of the surgeon determine the specific surgery employed. When metastasis is widespread at the time of diagnosis, surgical intervention may be only palliative.

The surgical aim is to remove the tumour by resecting as much of the stomach as necessary and a margin of normal tissue. When the lesion is located in the cardia or high in the fundus, a total gastrectomy with esophagojejunostomy is performed. This combination of procedures involves anastomosis of the lower end of the esophagus to the jejunum (Figure 44.10). Lesions located in the antrum or the pyloric region are generally treated in either a Billroth I or a Billroth II procedure. When the tumour has metastasized to adjacent organs, such as the spleen, ovaries, or bowel, the surgical procedures must be modified and extended as necessary.

The chance of a complete cure by surgical means is decreased considerably when the lymph nodes are involved. Survival is shortened when organs adjacent to the stomach show evidence of invasion at the time of surgery.

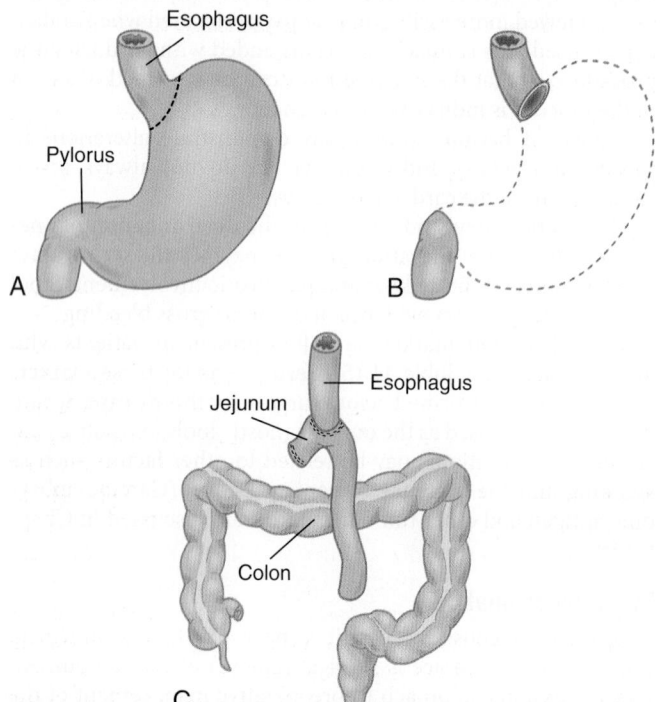

FIG. 44.10 Total gastrectomy for gastric cancer. **A,** Normal anatomical structure of the stomach. **B,** Removal of the stomach (total gastrectomy). **C,** Anastomosis of the esophagus with the jejunum (esophagojejunostomy).

Adjuvant Therapy. Surgery is the only definitive means of achieving a cure. However, when the patient cannot physically withstand a surgical procedure or when surgical cure is not feasible, radiation therapy or chemotherapy alone or in combination may be used. Neither radiation therapy nor chemotherapeutic agents have been very successful when used as the primary mode of treatment. Because the radiosensitivity of gastric cancers is low, radiation therapy has proved to be of little value. When it is used as a palliative measure, the tumour mass can be decreased, with temporary relief of the cardia or pyloric obstruction.

The combination of chemotherapy and radiation therapy is now being used for patients who are at high risk for disease recurrence after surgery. Single-agent chemotherapy for gastric cancer has traditionally been of little value. Agents that have been identified as having some effect on gastric cancer are a combination of 5-fluorouracil and cisplatin (Canadian Cancer Society, 2021a). The combination of radiation therapy with chemotherapy involving 5-fluorouracil and leucovorin after surgical resection increases survival. Additional therapies, including intraperitoneal administration of chemotherapeutic agents, are undergoing evaluation. The role of biological therapy is still under investigation for use in gastric cancer. (These therapies are discussed in Chapter 18.)

NURSING MANAGEMENT
GASTRIC CANCER

NURSING ASSESSMENT

The assessment of a person with possible gastric cancer is similar to that done for PUD (see Table 44.25 later in the chapter). Important information that should be obtained from the patient and the family include data from a nutritional assessment, a psychosocial history, the patient's perceptions of the health problem and the need for hospitalization, and the physical examination of the patient.

The nutritional assessment must elicit information regarding appetite and changes in eating patterns over the previous 6 months. It is necessary to determine the patient's normal weight and any changes that may have occurred in the preceding few months. Unexplained weight loss is common in many types of cancer before diagnosis. A history of vague symptoms of dyspepsia, early satiety, feeling full after consuming even a small amount of food, or symptoms of gas pain should help the nurse differentiate these typical gastric cancer symptoms from those of peptic ulcer. The nurse should determine whether pain is present, where and when it occurs, and how it is relieved. When the pain has been controlled with ingestion of foods, fluids, or antacids for a time but now continues or worsens regardless of interventions, gastric cancer may be the underlying cause.

Psychosocial and demographic data include the patient's age, present or previous occupation, and financial status. Gastric cancer can occur at any age, but the risk increases with age. The majority of new cases occur in people older than 65. A family history of cancer, especially gastric cancer, confers a greater than normal risk.

It is important to determine the patient's personal perception of the health problem and method of coping with hospitalization, diagnostic tests, and procedures. The possibility of a diagnosis of cancer and a treatment regimen that may include surgery, chemotherapy, or radiation treatment is predictive of a prolonged stressful period and a possibly fatal outcome. Therefore, it is important for the nurse to support the patient and the family if tests result in an unfavourable diagnosis and complex treatment interventions are planned. If surgery is probable, the nurse should assess what the patient expects from surgery (cure or palliation) and how that patient has responded to any previous surgical procedures.

A complete physical examination should include determining the patient's current functional abilities, the presence of other health conditions, and an estimate of how well the patient may respond to therapy. Cachexia may be evident if the nutritional state has been compromised for an extended time. A malnourished patient does not respond well to chemotherapy or radiation therapy and is a poor candidate for surgery.

NURSING DIAGNOSES

Nursing diagnoses for the patient with gastric cancer include but are not limited to the following:

- *Inadequate nutrition* resulting from *insufficient dietary intake* (inability to ingest, digest, or absorb nutrients)
- *Acute pain* resulting from *biological injury agent* (underlying disease process)
- *Anxiety* resulting from *threat to current status, threat of death*

PLANNING

The overall goals are that the patient with gastric cancer will (a) experience minimal discomfort, (b) achieve optimal nutritional status, and (c) maintain a degree of spiritual and psychological well-being appropriate to the disease stage.

NURSING IMPLEMENTATION

HEALTH PROMOTION. The nursing role in the prevention and early detection of cancer of the stomach is focused primarily on identification of the patient at risk because of specific disorders such as pernicious anemia and achlorhydria. The nurse should be aware of symptoms associated with gastric cancer, its pattern of spread, and the significant findings on physical examination. The nurse should understand that the cure rate is often quite dismal because symptoms do not arise until late in the course of the disease process, are vague, and often mimic other conditions, such as PUD.

The nurse must be alert to symptoms suggesting gastric cancer, such as loss of appetite, weight loss, fatigue, and persistent gastric distress. If any of these manifestations are present, medical attention should be obtained and the necessary diagnostic tests performed.

In addition, any patient with a positive family history of gastric cancer should be encouraged to undergo diagnostic evaluation if manifestations of anemia, peptic ulcer, or vague epigastric distress are present. It is important that the nurse recognize the possibility of gastric cancer in a patient in whom 3 weeks of prescribed therapy for peptic ulcer fails to provide relief.

ACUTE INTERVENTION

Preoperative Care. When the diagnostic tests confirm the presence of a malignancy, patients and their families generally react with shock, disbelief, and depression, regardless of how thoroughly they may have been prepared for this possible outcome. Throughout this period, the nurse needs to give emotional and physical support, provide information, clarify test results, and maintain a positive attitude with respect to the patient's immediate recovery and long-term survival.

On admission to hospital, the patient may be in poor physical condition. Surgery may have to be delayed while the patient's physical health is improved to be able to withstand the strain of a major operation. A positive nutritional state enhances wound healing, as well as the ability to withstand infection and other possible postoperative complications. Often, the patient is better able to tolerate several small meals a day than three regular meals. The diet may be supplemented by a variety of commercial liquid supplements (see Chapter 42) and vitamins. The nurse may be challenged to find innovative ways of encouraging the patient to eat when lack of appetite and state of mind make eating difficult and unrewarding. Enlisting the family's assistance with meals and encouraging intake may be beneficial. If the patient is unable to ingest oral feedings, it may be necessary to provide nutritional needs with tube feedings or parenteral nutrition.

If needed, blood replacement and fluid volume restoration may be carried out in the preoperative period. Because anemia is usually present, packed RBCs may be administered. Close observation for reactions to the transfusions is important. The hemoglobin and hematocrit levels provide information on the progress of therapy.

The preoperative teaching plan before gastric surgery for cancer is much the same as that for peptic ulcer surgery (see Interprofessional Care: Surgical Therapy for Peptic Ulcer Disease section under Peptic Ulcer Disease).

Postoperative Care. Postoperative care of the patient with gastric cancer is similar to that after a Billroth I or II procedure (see Interprofessional Care: Surgical Therapy for Peptic Ulcer Disease section under Peptic Ulcer Disease). When the surgical intervention has involved a total gastrectomy, the plan of care is somewhat different. The operation performed usually requires resection of some of the lower esophagus along with the removal of the entire stomach and anastomosis of the esophagus to the jejunum. The chest cavity must be entered, and drainage is accomplished by the insertion of chest tubes. (Chest surgery and drainage tubes are discussed in Chapter 30.) After total gastrectomy, the NG tube does not drain a large quantity of secretions because removal of the stomach has eliminated the reservoir capacity. The NG tube is removed after several days, when intestinal peristalsis has resumed. Small amounts of clear fluid may then be started. The patient requires close observation for signs of leakage of the fluids at the anastomosis, as evidenced by an elevation in body temperature and increasing dyspnea. When fluids are well tolerated without distress, the amount may be increased and some solid foods added.

As a consequence of a total gastrectomy, patients experience the symptoms of dumping syndrome (see Dumping Syndrome) Unfortunately, weight loss is very common among such patients, and poor nutritional intake often contributes to this. Postoperative wound healing may be impaired because of inadequate dietary intake, requiring parenteral or oral replacement of vitamins C, D, and K; the B-complex vitamins; and cobalamin. Because these vitamins (with the exception of cobalamin) are absorbed primarily in the upper part of the small intestine, they must be replaced because the duodenum has been bypassed in the surgical procedure.

Postoperative care after a Billroth I or II operative procedure should be the same as that after peptic ulcer surgery. Patients who have undergone these procedures are also subject to the same type of postgastrectomy complications, such as dumping syndrome and postprandial hypoglycemia.

Patients with advanced malignant disease can be offered only palliative treatment. When chemotherapy is prescribed, the nurse must have current information regarding the action and adverse effects of the drugs. Patients should be made aware of the potential benefits and hazards that can result from the chemotherapy. Radiation therapy can be used as an adjuvant to surgery or for palliation. In general, patients are quite fearful of radiation therapy and may have many misconceptions regarding its value and dangers. To reassure the patient and ensure completion of the designated number of treatments, the nurse must provide detailed instruction. Because most therapy is completed on an outpatient basis, the nurse should assess each patient's knowledge of radiation therapy, care of the skin, the need for good nutrition and fluid intake during therapy, and the appropriate use of antiemetic medications. (Specific care of patients receiving chemotherapy and radiation therapy is discussed in Chapter 18 and in NCP 18.1 and NCP 18.2, available on the Evolve website.)

AMBULATORY AND HOME CARE. Before the patient is discharged, the need for teaching should be reviewed. Most dietary measures useful after peptic ulcer surgery are applicable after surgery for gastric cancer. Plans should be made for the relief of pain, including comfort measures and the judicious use of analgesics. Wound care, if needed, must be taught to the primary caregiver in the home situation. Dressings, special equipment, or special services may be required for the patient's continued care at home. A list of community agencies that are available for assistance can be provided before the patient goes home. The services of the Canadian Cancer Society are especially helpful.

When chemotherapy or radiation therapy is to be continued after discharge, a referral for a home health nurse may be beneficial. The home health nurse can assist with recovery, determine the degree of patient adherence, and be an empathetic health care provider with whom the patient can consult.

Long-term follow-up must be stressed. The patient must be encouraged to adhere to the prescribed dietary and medication regimens, to keep appointments for chemotherapy administration or radiation treatments, and to keep the health care provider informed of changes in physical condition. (Long-term management of patients with cancer is discussed in Chapter 18.)

EVALUATION

Expected outcomes are the following for the patient with gastric cancer:

- The patient will experience no or minimal discomfort, pain, or nausea.
- The patient will achieve optimal nutritional status.
- The patient will maintain a degree of psychological well-being appropriate to the disease stage.

UPPER GASTROINTESTINAL BLEEDING

Upper GI bleeding represents a significant clinical and societal burden because of the associated morbidity, mortality, and financial implications. Despite advances in critical care, hemodynamic monitoring, and endoscopy, there has been little change in the mortality rate for upper GI bleeding, which has remained approximately 6 to 10% since the 1960s. This is partly because the incidence of upper GI bleeding is higher among older persons, men, and individuals in lower socioeconomic groups (Kurian & Lobo, 2015).

Etiology and Pathophysiology

Although the most serious loss of blood from the upper GI tract is characterized by a sudden onset, insidious occult bleeding can also be a major concern. The severity of bleeding depends on whether the origin is venous, capillary, or arterial. (Types of upper GI bleeding are listed in Table 44.16.) Bleeding from an arterial source is profuse, and the blood is bright red. The bright red colour indicates that the blood has not been in contact with the stomach's acid secretions. In contrast, "coffee grounds" vomitus indicates that the blood and other contents have been in the stomach for some time and have been changed by contact with gastric secretions. A massive upper GI hemorrhage is generally defined as a loss of more than 1 500 mL of blood or of 25% of intravascular blood volume. *Melena* (black, tarry stools) indicates slow bleeding from an upper GI source. The longer the passage of blood through the intestines, the darker the colour of the stool as a result of the degradation of hemoglobin and the release of iron.

Discovering the cause of the bleeding is not always an easy task. A variety of areas in the GI tract may be involved, and there may be many different reasons for the blood loss. Table 44.17 lists the common causes of upper GI bleeding. Although systemic diseases (e.g., leukemia, blood dyscrasias) that interfere with normal blood clotting must be considered whenever upper GI bleeding occurs, the most common sites are the esophagus, stomach, and duodenum.

Esophageal Origin. Bleeding from an esophageal source is probably the result of chronic esophagitis, a Mallory–Weiss tear, or esophageal varices. Chronic esophagitis can be caused by the ingestion of chemicals, including medications irritating to the mucosa. Alcohol and smoking are known irritants of the esophageal mucosa. GERD with or without a hiatal hernia can lead to chronic irritation and erosion. A Mallory–Weiss tear is usually caused by severe retching and vomiting. This tear occurs in the esophageal mucosa at the junction of the esophagus and the stomach and results in severe bleeding.

TABLE 44.16	**TYPES OF UPPER GASTROINTESTINAL BLEEDING**	
Type	**Clinical Manifestations**
Obvious bleeding	
• Hematemesis	Bloody vomitus appearing as fresh, bright red blood or having "coffee grounds" appearance (dark, grainy digested blood)
• Melena	Black, tarry stools (often foul smelling) caused by digestion of blood in the gastrointestinal tract; the discoloration is caused by the presence of iron
Occult bleeding	Small amounts of blood in gastric secretions, vomitus, or stools not apparent by appearance; detectable by guaiac test

TABLE 44.17	**COMMON CAUSES OF UPPER GASTROINTESTINAL BLEEDING**
Medication-Induced	**Stomach and Duodenum**
• Corticosteroids	• Gastric cancer
• Nonsteroidal anti-inflammatory medications	• Hemorrhagic gastritis
	• Peptic ulcer disease
• Salicylates	• Polyps
	• Stress-related mucosal disease
Esophagus	
• Esophageal varices	**Systemic Diseases**
• Esophagitis	• Blood dyscrasias (e.g., leukemia, aplastic anemia)
• Mallory–Weiss tear	• Liver failure (cirrhosis)
	• Renal failure (uremia)

Esophageal varices are usually secondary to cirrhosis of the liver. Anything that may increase the pressure (e.g., coughing, sneezing, trauma) or cause mechanical irritation (e.g., vomiting, irritation, erosion) may result in sudden, massive bleeding. (Esophageal varices are discussed in Chapter 46.)

Stomach and Duodenal Origin. PUD is responsible for 27% to 40% of cases of upper GI bleeding (Upchurch, 2021). Erosion of a blood vessel by an ulcer located in the stomach or duodenum must always be considered as a possible cause of upper GI bleeding. A gastric ulcer may penetrate the left gastric artery, and a duodenal ulcer may penetrate the superior pancreatico-duodenal artery.

Acute gastritis produced by ingestion of drugs or alcohol or the reflux of bile from the small intestine can result in bleeding. Medications, either prescribed by the health care provider or OTC, are a major cause of upper GI bleeding. For example, a patient who regularly takes ASA (Aspirin) or ASA-containing compounds may be at risk for bleeding episodes. ASA (Aspirin), NSAIDs (e.g., ibuprofen), and corticosteroids can cause irritation and disruption of the gastric mucosal barrier. ASA-containing products are sold without prescriptions as OTC medications. A thorough history of all commonly used medications is therefore necessary whenever upper GI bleeding is suspected.

Stress-related mucosal disease (SRMD), also called *physiological stress ulcers,* occurs in patients who have sustained severe burns or trauma or had major surgery. In SRMD, there is either diffuse superficial mucosal injury or discrete deeper ulcers in the fundus and body portions of the stomach (Figure 44.11). Those patients at higher risk for developing SRMD include patients with coagulopathy, sepsis, hepatic failure, renal failure, burns, head trauma, a history of GI bleed, and multiorgan failure; those on mechanical ventilation greater than 48 hours; and those using vasopressors or high-dose systemic corticosteroids (Siddiqui et al., 2021).

Emergency Assessment and Management

In approximately 80 to 85% of patients who have massive upper GI hemorrhage, the bleeding stops spontaneously; however, the cause must be identified and treatment initiated immediately. Although a complete history of events leading to the bleeding episode is important in discovering the cause of the blood loss, its documentation should be deferred until emergency care has been initiated. The immediate physical examination must

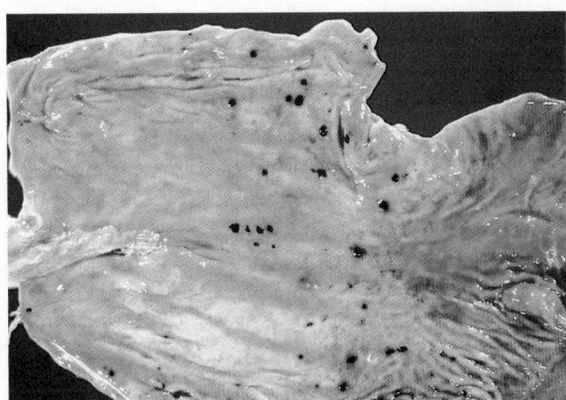

FIG 44.11 Multiple stress ulcers of the stomach, highlighted by dark digested blood on their surfaces. Source: Kumar, V., Abbas, A. K., & Fausto, N. (2005). *Robbins and Cotran pathologic basis of disease* (7th ed.). Saunders.

include a systematic evaluation of the patient's condition with emphasis on blood pressure, rate and character of pulse, peripheral perfusion with capillary refill, and observation for the presence or absence of neck vein distension. Vital signs should be monitored every 15 to 30 minutes. Signs and symptoms of shock must be evaluated, and treatment should be started as soon as possible if it occurs (see Chapter 69). The patient's respiratory status is carefully assessed, along with a thorough abdominal examination. The presence or absence of bowel sounds should be assessed and noted. A tense, rigid, boardlike abdomen may indicate the presence of a perforation and peritonitis.

Once the immediate interventions have begun, the patient or the family should answer the following questions: Does the patient have a history of previous bleeding episodes? Has weight loss been a recent problem? Has the patient received blood transfusions in the past, and were there any transfusion reactions? Does the patient have a religious preference that prohibits the use of blood or blood products? Does the patient have any other illnesses that may contribute to bleeding or interfere with treatment (e.g., heart failure, diabetes mellitus)?

Laboratory studies are ordered, including a CBC; prothrombin time measurement; measurements of blood urea nitrogen (BUN), serum electrolytes, blood glucose, liver enzymes, and arterial blood gases; and a type and crossmatch for possible blood transfusions. Vomitus and stools can be tested for the presence of gross and occult blood. A urinalysis provides information on the presence of blood in the urine, and the specific gravity gives an immediate indication of the patient's hydration status.

IV lines, preferably two, with a 16- or 18-gauge needle, should be established for fluid and blood replacement. The type and amount of fluids infused are dictated by physical and laboratory findings. It is generally best to begin with an isotonic crystalloid solution (e.g., lactated Ringer's solution). Whole blood, packed RBCs, and fresh-frozen plasma may be used to replace lost volume in massive hemorrhage. Because of the potential for fluid overload and immunological reactions, packed RBCs are often preferred over whole blood. (The use of blood transfusions is discussed in Chapter 33.) The hemoglobin and hematocrit values are not of immediate assistance in estimating the degree of blood loss, but they provide a baseline for guiding further treatment. The initial hematocrit may be normal and may not reflect the loss until 4 to 6 hours after fluid replacement has taken place because initially the loss of plasma and RBCs is equal. When upper GI bleeding is less profuse, infusion of isotonic saline solution followed by packed RBCs helps restore the hematocrit more quickly and does not create complications related to fluid volume overload. The use of supplemental oxygen may help increase blood oxygen saturation.

For most patients with profuse bleeding, an in-dwelling urinary catheter is inserted so that urine volume can be accurately assessed every hour. A central venous pressure line may be inserted so that the patient's fluid volume status can be monitored easily. Empirical PPI therapy with high-dose bolus and subsequent infusion is often started before endoscopy.

Diagnostic Studies

Endoscopic procedures enable health care providers to identify sources of GI bleeding through direct visualization. For example, the site of bleeding from severe gastritis, an esophageal varix, a gastric or duodenal ulcer, or angiodysplasia can be determined easily and treated effectively. The endoscope is designed to facilitate the passing of various instruments, sclerosing medications, and probes to control and stop GI bleeding. In addition to using endoscopic procedures to stop bleeding, these procedures also allow direct visualization of the bleeding site. Angiography is used in diagnosing upper GI bleeding only when endoscopy cannot be done. It is an invasive procedure for which preparation and setup time are required, and it may not be appropriate for a patient at high risk for complications and whose condition is unstable. In this procedure, a catheter is placed into the left gastric or superior mesenteric artery and advanced until the site of bleeding is discovered.

Interprofessional Care

Endoscopic Therapy. Endoscopic hemostasis is used to identify and stop bleeding. Endoscopy performed within the first 24 hours of bleeding is important for diagnosis and determining the need for surgical or radiological intervention.

The goal of endoscopic hemostasis is coagulation or thrombosis in the bleeding vessel. Several techniques are used, including (a) thermal (heat) probe, (b) multipolar and bipolar electrocoagulation probe, (c) argon plasma coagulation (APC), and (d) neodymium:yttrium–aluminum–garnet (Nd:YAG) laser. Multipolar electrocoagulation and thermal probe are the two most commonly used procedures. The heat probe causes tissue coagulation by directly applying a heating element to the bleeding site. Argon plasma coagulation is a noncontact method in which monopolar current is delivered to tissue. For variceal bleeding, other strategies include variceal ligation, injection sclerotherapy, and balloon tamponade.

Surgical Therapy. Surgical intervention is indicated when bleeding continues despite the therapy provided and when the site of the bleeding has been identified. The site of the hemorrhage determines the choice of operation. In addition, the surgeon must consider the age of the patient because mortality rates are considerably higher among patients older than 60 years.

Medication Therapy. During the acute phase, medications are used to decrease bleeding, decrease HCl secretion, and neutralize the HCl that is present. Medication therapy to decrease bleeding is administered during endoscopy. Injection therapy with epinephrine (1:10 000 dilution) is effective for acute

hemostasis. These agents produce tissue edema and, ultimately, pressure on the source of bleeding. To prevent rebleeding, injection therapy is often combined with other therapies (e.g., thermocoagulation or laser treatment). A *sclerosant* (an agent that produces inflammation and results in fibrosis of the tissues) such as ethanolamine may be used, especially if the cause of bleeding is esophageal varices.

Antidiuretic hormone, a chemical released from the posterior pituitary, can be used for the management of variceal bleeding because it promotes vasoconstriction. It is used to treat upper GI bleeding in patients whose bleeding does not respond to other therapies and who are poor candidates for surgery. It is administered systemically through a vein or intra-arterially at the local site of actual bleeding. Adverse effects of intravenously administered vasopressin include decreased myocardial contractility and decreased coronary blood flow. The patient undergoing vasopressin therapy must be closely monitored for its myocardial, visceral, and peripheral ischemic adverse effects. Vasopressin should be used with caution in patients with a known history of vascular disease.

Efforts are made to reduce acid secretion because the acidic environment can alter platelet function and interfere with clot stabilization. H_2R blockers (e.g., ranitidine [Zantac]) or PPIs (e.g., pantoprazole [Pantoloc]) are administered intravenously to decrease acid secretion. Table 44.18 reviews the mechanism of action of H_2R blockers and PPIs. Although these medications have no proven ability to control active bleeding, they have become part of standard treatment protocols.

In patients with upper GI bleeding, early administration of the somatostatin analogue octreotide (Sandostatin) may be used. The medication reduces splanchnic blood flow, as well as acid secretion. This medication is given in IV boluses up to 5 to 6 days after the onset of bleeding.

Antacids have long been known to neutralize HCl and continue to be used as an adjunct therapy for PUD. Because antacids neutralize HCl and increase the pH of gastric contents to above 5, the conversion of pepsinogen to its active form, pepsin, is inhibited. The most frequently used antacid preparations are magnesium hydroxide, magnesium trisilicate, aluminum hydroxide, calcium carbonate, and sodium bicarbonate (see Table 44.23 later in this chapter). Aluminum hydroxide

TABLE 44.18   MEDICATION THERAPY

Gastrointestinal Bleeding

Medication	Source of Gastrointestinal Bleeding	Mechanism of Action
Antacids*	Duodenal ulcer, gastric ulcer, acute gastritis (corrosive, erosive, and hemorrhagic)	Neutralize acid and maintain gastric pH >5.5; elevated pH inhibits activation of pepsinogen
H_2-receptor blockers: cimetidine, famotidine (Pepcid), nizatidine (Axid), ranitidine (Zantac)	Duodenal ulcer, gastric ulcer, esophagitis, acute gastritis (especially hemorrhagic)	Inhibit action of histamine at H_2 receptors on parietal cells and decrease HCl secretion
Proton pump inhibitors: omeprazole (Losec), esomeprazole (Nexium), lansoprazole (Prevacid), pantoprazole (Pantoloc)	—	Inhibit the cellular pump, which is necessary for secretion of HCl
Vasopressin	Acute gastritis (corrosive, erosive, and hemorrhagic), esophageal varices	Causes vasoconstriction and increases smooth muscle activity of the GI tract; reduces pressure in the portal circulation and arrests bleeding
Octreotide (Sandostatin)	Upper gastrointestinal bleeding, esophageal varices	Somatostatin analogue that decreases splanchnic blood flow; decreases HCl secretion via decrease in release of gastrin

*See Table 44.23.

GI, gastrointestinal; *HCl*, hydrochloric acid.

and magnesium trisilicate are the most useful because they are nonabsorbable. Calcium carbonate and sodium bicarbonate are absorbable, and prolonged use can lead to systemic alkalosis.

NURSING MANAGEMENT
UPPER GASTROINTESTINAL BLEEDING

NURSING ASSESSMENT

As the nurse begins care of a patient admitted with upper GI bleeding, a thorough and accurate nursing assessment is an essential first step. Subjective and objective data that should be obtained from the patient or significant others are listed in Table 44.19.

The patient experiencing upper GI bleeding may not be able to provide specific information about the cause of the bleeding until their immediate physical needs are met. An immediate nursing assessment is performed while the patient is being prepared for initial treatment. The assessment includes the patient's level of consciousness, vital signs, appearance of neck veins,

---

TABLE 44.19 NURSING ASSESSMENT

Upper Gastrointestinal Bleeding

Subjective Data

Important Health Information

Past health history: Precipitating events before bleeding episode, previous bleeding episodes and treatment, peptic ulcer disease, esophageal varices, esophagitis, acute and chronic gastritis, stress-related mucosal disease; family history of bleeding; history of smoking or heavy alcohol use

Medications: Use of ASA (Aspirin), nonsteroidal anti-inflammatory medications, corticosteroids, anticoagulants

Symptoms
- Nausea, vomiting, weight loss; thirst
- Diarrhea; black, tarry stools; decreased urinary output; sweating
- Weakness, dizziness, fainting
- Epigastric pain, abdominal cramps

Objective Data

General

Fever

Integumentary

Clammy, cool, pale skin; pale mucous membranes, nail beds, and conjunctivae; spider angiomas; jaundice; peripheral edema

Respiratory

Rapid, shallow respirations

Cardiovascular

Tachycardia, weak pulse, orthostatic hypotension, slow capillary refill

Gastrointestinal

Red or "coffee grounds" vomitus; tense, rigid abdomen, ascites; hypoactive or hyperactive bowel sounds; black, tarry stools

Urinary

Decreased urinary output, concentrated urine

Neurological

Agitation, restlessness; decreasing level of consciousness

Possible Findings
- ↓ Hematocrit and hemoglobin; hematuria; guaiac-positive stools, emesis, or gastric aspirate
- ↓ levels of clotting factors; ↑ liver enzymes; abnormal results of upper GI studies or endoscopy

ASA, acetylsalicylic acid; *GI,* gastrointestinal.

---

skin colour, and capillary refill. The abdomen is assessed for guarding and peristalsis. Immediate determination of vital signs should indicate whether the patient is in shock from blood loss and also provide a baseline blood pressure and pulse by which to monitor the progress of treatment. Signs and symptoms of hypovolemic shock include low blood pressure; rapid, weak pulse; increased thirst; cold, clammy skin; and restlessness. Vital signs are monitored every 15 to 30 minutes, and the health care provider should be informed of any significant changes.

NURSING DIAGNOSES

Nursing diagnoses for the patient with upper GI bleeding include but are not limited to the following:
- *Potential decreased cardiac output* resulting from *loss of blood*
- *Dehydration* resulting from *insufficient fluid intake, excessive fluid loss through abnormal route* (acute loss of blood and gastric secretions)
- *Reduced peripheral tissue perfusion* resulting from *insufficient fluid intake, excessive fluid loss through abnormal route* (loss of circulatory volume)
- *Anxiety* resulting from *threat to current status, threat of death*

PLANNING

The overall goals are that the patient with upper GI bleeding will (a) have no further GI bleeding, (b) have the cause of the bleeding identified and treated, (c) experience a return to a normal hemodynamic state, (d) experience minimal or no symptoms of pain or anxiety, and (e) be able to verbalize causative and preventive measures.

NURSING IMPLEMENTATION

HEALTH PROMOTION. Although not all cases of upper GI bleeding can be anticipated and prevented, the nurse shares responsibility with the health care provider in trying to identify the patient who is at high risk. Patients with a history of chronic gastritis or PUD should always be considered in the high-risk category because of the increased incidence of bleeding associated with chronic irritation or chronic ulcers. Patients who have had one major bleeding episode are more likely than others to have a repeat episode. Patients are instructed to avoid gastric irritants such as alcohol and smoking, to prevent or decrease stress-inducing situations at home or at work, and to take only prescribed medications. OTC medications can be harmful because they may contain ingredients (e.g., ASA [Aspirin]) that have potentially irritating effects on the mucosa.

Patients who require regular administration of ulcerogenic medications, such as ASA (Aspirin), corticosteroids, or NSAIDs, need instruction regarding the potential adverse effects that these medications may have on the GI mucosa. These medications are to be avoided if at all possible. However, if ASA (Aspirin) must be prescribed, enteric-coated tablets can be substituted for regular tablets. Taking the medications with meals or snacks lessens the potential irritating effects. For patients who must take NSAIDs, a change to a preparation with less GI toxicity may be considered. COX-2 inhibitors (e.g., celecoxib [Celebrex]) have less of an effect on the production of tissue prostaglandins and are associated with fewer GI adverse effects, although cardiac risks are associated with COX-2 inhibitors. The coadministration of an NSAID with a PPI can reduce bleeding risk. For the patient at risk for gastric ulcers because of NSAID use, misoprostol may also be prescribed. This prostaglandin analogue inhibits acid secretion and reduces the incidence of upper GI bleeding episodes associated with NSAID use. However, the medication has several important adverse effects, including uterine cramping in women and diarrhea. Because of its effects on the uterus, its use is contraindicated in women of childbearing age.

When the nurse is working with a patient who has a history of liver cirrhosis with esophageal varices, the instructions must be specific about the importance of avoiding known irritants, such as alcohol and smoking. The prompt treatment of an upper respiratory tract infection should be stressed. Severe coughing or sneezing can create increased pressure on the already fragile varices and may result in massive hemorrhage.

Patients who are known to have blood dyscrasias (e.g., aplastic anemia) or liver dysfunction or who are taking cancer chemotherapeutic drugs have a potential for a bleeding disorder because of altered hemostasis caused by a decrease in clotting factors and platelets. When such patients also have a history of ulcer disease, gastritis, varices, or drug and alcohol misuse, they should be carefully instructed regarding their disease process and drugs, and they should be closely observed for bleeding.

ACUTE INTERVENTION. Patients should be approached in a calm and assured manner to help decrease their level of anxiety. Caution should be used before sedatives are administered as this may mask important symptoms for diagnosis (e.g., restlessness is a warning sign of shock).

Once an infusion has been started, the IV line must be maintained for fluid or blood replacement. An accurate intake and output record is essential so that the patient's hydration status can be assessed. Urine output should be measured hourly. A rate of at least 0.5 mL/kg/hr indicates adequate renal perfusion. Lesser amounts may indicate renal insufficiency secondary to loss of blood volume. Specific gravity readings consistently greater than 1.030 (normal is 1.005–1.030) indicate that the urine is extremely concentrated and that the blood volume is probably low. The health care provider must be kept informed of these important parameters so that the IV solutions can be increased or decreased accordingly. If a patient has a central venous pressure line in place, readings should be recorded every 1 to 2 hours. Hemodynamic monitoring provides an accurate and quick assessment of blood flow and pressure within the cardiovascular system (see Chapter 68).

Older patients and patients with a history of cardiovascular conditions should be observed closely for signs of fluid overload. However, the threat of volume overload and pulmonary edema is a constant concern in all patients who are receiving large amounts of IV fluids within a short time. Therefore, auscultation of breath sounds and close observation of respiratory effort are important measures. Electrocardiographic monitoring can also be used to evaluate cardiac function.

Foods such as beets or even swallowed mouthwash can give vomitus a bloody appearance. Unless the contents of the vomitus are checked for occult blood, recorded observations gleaned from appearance alone may be false. Swallowed blood from a nosebleed must also be accurately noted to avoid misdiagnosis of an upper GI bleeding episode. When an NG tube is inserted, the nurse must pay special attention to keeping it in proper position and observing the aspirate for blood.

The nurse caring for a patient with upper GI bleeding should be well informed as to what constitutes blood in the stools. Black, tarry stools are not usually associated with a brisk hemorrhage but are indicative of the presence of bleeding of prolonged duration. Bright red blood in the stool is usually from a source in the lower bowel. (Lower GI bleeding is discussed in Chapter 45.) Menses and bleeding hemorrhoids should be ruled out as possible sources of blood in the stools. When vomitus contains blood but the stool contains no gross or occult blood, the hemorrhage is considered to have been of short duration.

By monitoring results of the patient's laboratory studies, the nurse can estimate the effectiveness of therapy. The hemoglobin and hematocrit are usually evaluated about every 4 to 6 hours if the patient is actively bleeding. At first, the hematocrit level may not accurately reflect the amount of blood lost or the amount of blood replaced and will appear falsely high or low. The patient's BUN level is assessed. It is generally elevated with a significant hemorrhage because blood proteins are broken down by bacteria in the GI tract. However, renal disease may also result in an elevated BUN level. Many patients receive oxygen by mask or nasally to ensure that the circulating blood has an adequate oxygen content.

When oral nourishment is begun, the patient is observed for symptoms of nausea and vomiting and a recurrence of bleeding. Feedings initially consisting of clear fluids are given hourly until tolerance is determined. These feedings help neutralize the gastric secretions and assist in the mucosal repair. Foods are then introduced gradually if the patient exhibits no signs of discomfort. Consultation with a dietitian can ensure the introduction of appropriate foods and support for the patient's nutrition.

The patient in whom hemorrhage was the result of chronic alcohol misuse requires close observation for the beginning of delirium tremens as withdrawal from alcohol takes place. Symptoms indicating the beginning of delirium tremens are agitation, uncontrolled shaking, sweating, and vivid hallucinations. (Alcohol withdrawal is discussed in Chapter 11.)

AMBULATORY AND HOME CARE. Patients and caregivers must be taught how to avoid future bleeding episodes. Ulcer disease, drug or alcohol misuse, and liver and respiratory diseases can all result in upper GI bleeding. Patients and caregivers must be made aware of the consequences of nonadherence to diet and medication therapy. It must be emphasized that no medications (especially ASA [Aspirin] and NSAIDs) other than those prescribed by the health care provider should be taken. With the assistance of programs for smoking or alcohol cessation or rehabilitation, smoking and alcohol use should be eliminated because they are sources of irritation and interfere with tissue repair. The need for long-term follow-up care may be necessary because of the possibility of another bleeding episode. The patient and their family should be instructed on what to do if an acute hemorrhage occurs in the future.

EVALUATION

The following are expected outcomes for the patient with upper GI bleeding:

- The patient will have no upper GI bleeding.
- The patient will maintain normal fluid volume.
- The patient will experience a return to a normal hemodynamic state.
- The patient will experience absence of or tolerable levels of pain and will be comfortable.
- The patient will understand potential etiological factors and make appropriate lifestyle modifications.

PEPTIC ULCER DISEASE

Peptic ulcer disease (PUD) is a condition characterized by erosion of the GI mucosa that results from the digestive action of

HCl and pepsin. Any portion of the GI tract that comes into contact with gastric secretions is susceptible to ulcer development, including the lower esophagus, stomach, duodenum, and margin of gastrojejunal anastomosis after surgical procedures.

Types

Peptic ulcers can be classified as acute or chronic, depending on the degree and duration of mucosal involvement (Figure 44.12), and as gastric or duodenal, according to the location. Acute ulcers (see Figure 44.12) are characterized by superficial erosion and minimal inflammation. They are of short duration and resolve quickly when the cause is identified and removed. Chronic ulcers (Figure 44.13) are of long duration, eroding through the muscular wall with the formation of fibrous tissue. They are present continuously for many months or intermittently throughout the lifetime. Chronic ulcers are at least four times as common as acute ulcers.

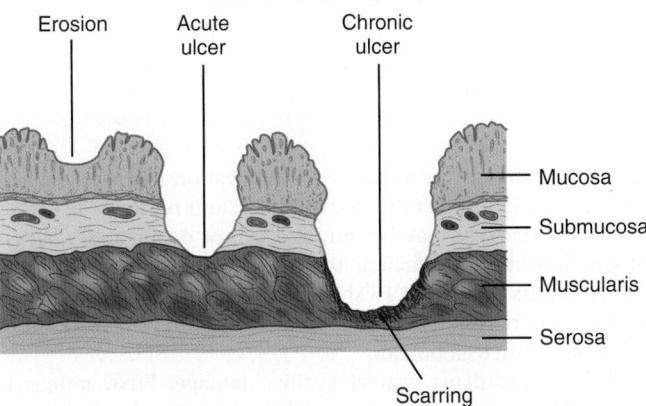

FIG. 44.12 Peptic ulcers, including an erosion, an acute ulcer, and a chronic ulcer. Both the acute and the chronic ulcers may penetrate the entire wall of the stomach. Source: Modified from Price, S. A., & Wilson, L. M. (2003). *Pathophysiology: Clinical concepts of disease processes* (6th ed., p. 331). Mosby.

Gastric and duodenal ulcers, although defined as peptic ulcers, have different causes and incidences (Table 44.20). In general, treatment is similar for all types of ulcers.

Etiology and Pathophysiology

Peptic ulcers develop only in the presence of an acidic environment. In typical cases, a person with a gastric ulcer has normal to less-than-normal gastric acidity in comparison with the person with a duodenal ulcer. However, some intraluminal acid does seem to be essential for a gastric ulcer to occur.

Pepsinogen, the precursor of pepsin, is activated to pepsin in the presence of HCl and a pH of 2 to 3. The HCl secreted by the parietal cells has a pH of 0.8. After HCl mixes with the stomach contents, the pH reaches 2 to 3, a range of acidity highly favourable for pepsin activity. When the stomach acid level is neutralized by the presence of food or antacids, or acid secretion is blocked by medications, the pH is increased to 3.5 or more. At a pH of 3.5 or more, pepsin has little or no proteolytic activity.

The stomach is normally protected from autodigestion by the gastric mucosal barrier. The GI tract has a high rate of cell turnover, and the surface mucosa of the stomach is renewed about every 3 days. As a result of this high turnover rate, the mucosa can continually repair itself except in extreme instances, when

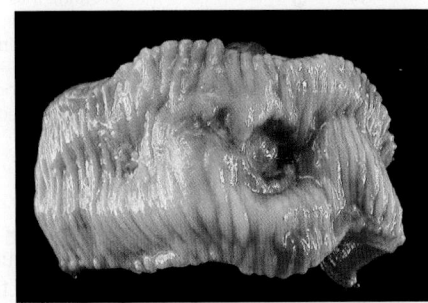

FIG. 44.13 Peptic ulcer of the duodenum. Source: Kumar, V., Abbas, A. K., Fausto, N., et al. (2010). *Robbins and Cotran pathologic basis of disease* (8th ed.). Saunders.

TABLE 44.20 COMPARISON OF GASTRIC AND DUODENAL ULCERS

Characteristic	Gastric Ulcers	Duodenal Ulcers
Lesion	Superficial; smooth margins; round, oval, or cone shaped	Penetrating (associated with deformity of duodenal bulb from healing of recurrent ulcers)
Location of lesion	Predominantly in the antrum; also in body and fundus of stomach	First 1–2 cm of duodenum
Gastric secretion	Normal to decreased	Increased
Incidence	• Greater in women	• Greater in men, but increasing in women, especially postmenopausal
	• Peak age, 50–60 yr	• Peak age, 35–45 yr
	• Increased with smoking, drug, and alcohol use	• Increased with smoking, drug, and alcohol use
	• More common among persons of lower socioeconomic status and in unskilled labourers	• Associated with psychological stress
	• Increased with incompetent pyloric sphincter and bile reflux	• Associated with other diseases (e.g., chronic obstructive pulmonary disease, pancreatic disease, hyperparathyroidism, Zollinger–Ellison syndrome, chronic renal failure)
	• Increased with stress ulcers after severe burns, head trauma, and major surgery	
Clinical manifestations	• Burning or gaseous pressure in high left epigastrium and back and upper abdomen	• Pain 2–4 hr after meals and midmorning, midafternoon, middle of night; pain is periodic and episodic
	• Burning, cramping, pressure-like pain across midepigastrium and upper abdomen; back pain with posterior ulcers	• Pain relief with antacids and food; occasional nausea and vomiting
	• Pain 1–2 hr after meals; if penetrating ulcer, aggravation of discomfort with food	
	• Occasional nausea and vomiting, weight loss	
Recurrence rate	High	High
Complications	Hemorrhage, perforation, outlet obstruction, intractability	Hemorrhage, perforation, obstruction

PATHOPHYSIOLOGY MAP

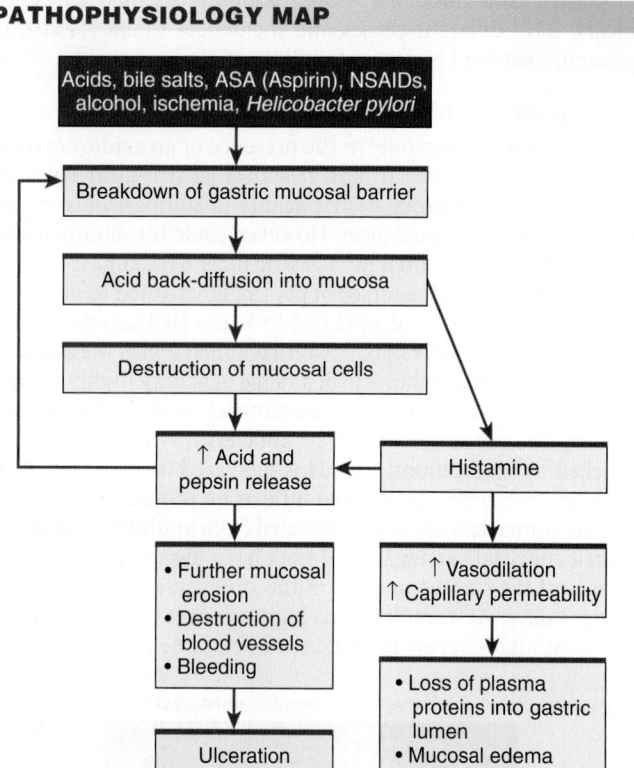

FIG. 44.14 Disruption of gastric mucosa and pathophysiological consequences of backwards diffusion of acids. *ASA,* acetylsalicylic acid; *NSAIDs,* nonsteroidal anti-inflammatory drugs.

PATHOPHYSIOLOGY MAP

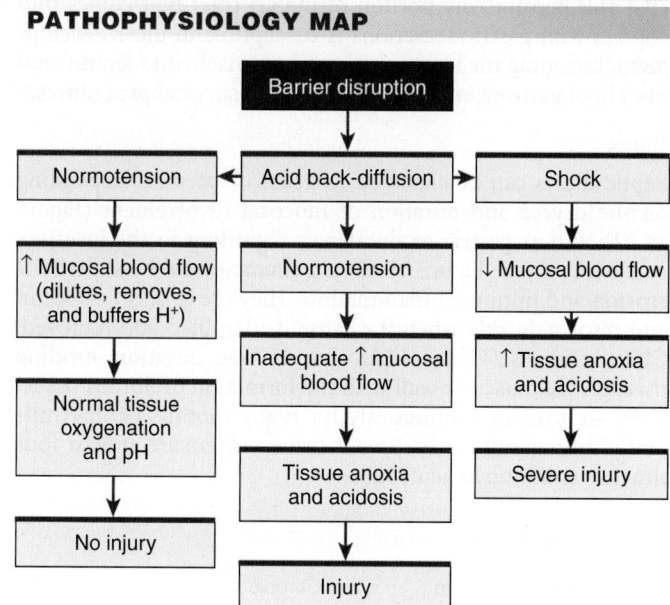

FIG. 44.15 Relationship between mucosal blood flow and disruption of the gastric mucosal barrier.

the cell breakdown rate surpasses the cell renewal rate. Normally, water, electrolytes, and water-soluble substances (e.g., glucose) can easily pass through the barrier. However, the mucosal barrier prevents the backwards diffusion of acid from the gastric lumen through the mucosal layers to the underlying tissue.

Under specific circumstances, the mucosal barrier can be impaired, and backwards diffusion of acid can occur (Figure 44.14). When the barrier is broken, HCl freely enters the mucosa and injury to the tissues occurs. This results in cellular destruction and inflammation. Histamine is released from the damaged mucosa, resulting in vasodilation and increased capillary permeability. The released histamine is then capable of stimulating further secretion of acid and pepsin.

As described in the Gastritis section, a variety of agents are known to destroy the mucosal barrier. By generating ammonia in the mucous layer, *H. pylori* may create a condition of chronic inflammation, rendering the mucosa especially vulnerable to other noxious substances. Ulcerogenic medications, such as ASA (Aspirin) and NSAIDs, inhibit synthesis of prostaglandins and cause abnormal permeability of the mucosal barrier. Corticosteroids have the ability to decrease the rate of mucosal cell renewal and thereby decrease its protective effects. Lipid-soluble cytotoxic medications can pass through the barrier and destroy it.

When the mucosal barrier is disrupted, there is a compensatory increase in blood flow (Figure 44.15). This phenomenon can occur in several ways. Prostaglandin-like substances and histamine act as vasodilators, thus increasing capillary blood flow. As blood flow increases within the affected mucosa, H+ are rapidly removed from the area, buffers are delivered to help neutralize the H+ present, nutrients necessary for cell function

arrive, and the rate of mucosal cell replication increases. When the increase is sufficient to dilute, buffer, and remove the excess H+, tissue damage may be minimal or not occur at all. When blood flow is not sufficient to carry out these events, tissue injury results. Figure 44.15 shows a representation of the interrelationship between the mucosal blood flow and disruption of the gastric mucosal barrier.

Two mechanisms protect against damage. First, mucus is secreted by superficial mucous cells and forms a layer that can entrap or slow the diffusion of H+ across the mucosal barrier in the stomach. Second, bicarbonate is secreted by the gastric and duodenal mucosa, and this helps neutralize HCl in the lumen of the GI tract.

Increased vagal nerve stimulation from a variety of causes (e.g., emotions) results in hypersecretion of HCl. Increased concentrations of HCl can alter the mucosal barrier. Duodenal ulcers are associated with high acid content. It has been suggested that the continual response of the parietal cells to maximal stimulation results in hyperplasia of the cells.

Gastric Ulcers. Although gastric ulcers can occur in any portion of the stomach, they are most commonly found on the lesser curvature close to the antral junction. Gastric ulcers are less common than duodenal ulcers. Gastric ulcers are more prevalent among women and in older persons. The rate of mortality from gastric ulcers is greater than that from duodenal ulcers because the incidence of gastric ulcers peaks in persons older than 50 years. Persons from a lower socioeconomic class and manual or unskilled workers are more prone to gastric ulcers.

Although gastric ulcers are characterized by normal to low secretion of gastric acid, the backwards diffusion of acid is greater with chronic gastric ulcers than with duodenal ulcers or in the healthy person. Therefore, the critical pathological process in gastric ulcer formation may not be the amount of acid that is secreted but the amount that is able to penetrate the mucosal barrier.

Gastric ulcers have also been attributed to various factors that can lead to acute episodes or to chronic involvement. The role of *H. pylori* in ulcer development is discussed in the following Duodenal Ulcers section. It is thought that destruction of the gastric mucosa by noxious agents such as drugs or smoking may be enhanced by the presence of *H. pylori,* which further promotes gastric mucosal destruction.

Medications can cause acute gastric ulcers and, in some cases, lead to the development of chronic ulcers. The medications most often implicated include ASA (Aspirin), corticosteroids, NSAIDs (e.g., ibuprofen), and reserpine (Serpasil) (not commercially available in Canada). It is estimated that 1 to 3% of patients taking NSAIDs for 1 year experience serious GI complications, including gastritis, gastric ulcer, upper GI hemorrhage, or ulcer perforation. Other known causes of gastric ulcer formation are chronic alcohol misuse, chronic gastritis, and bile reflux gastritis that results from an incompetent pyloric sphincter. Cigarette smoking is positively linked with gastric ulcers. Nicotine seems to enhance reflux of duodenal contents into the antrum of the stomach. The ingestion of hot, rough, or spicy foods has been suggested as a cause, but there is no evidence to substantiate this claim.

Duodenal Ulcers. Duodenal ulcers account for about 80% of all peptic ulcers. Although duodenal ulcers still affect more men than women, the incidence of duodenal ulcers has followed a downward trend among men and steadily increased among women. The explanation for this change has not been clearly identified. Duodenal ulcers may occur at any age, but the incidence is especially high between the ages of 35 and 45 years. Duodenal ulcers can develop in anyone, regardless of occupation or socioeconomic group.

The development of duodenal ulcers is associated with high HCl secretion. Several diseases have been identified with a high risk of duodenal ulcer development, including chronic obstructive pulmonary disease, cirrhosis of the liver, chronic pancreatitis, hyperparathyroidism, chronic renal failure, and Zollinger–Ellison syndrome. (*Zollinger–Ellison syndrome* is a rare condition characterized by severe peptic ulceration, gastric acid hypersecretion, elevated serum gastrin levels, and gastrinoma of the pancreas or the duodenum.) The treatments used for these conditions may also promote ulcer development. Alcohol ingestion and heavy smoking habits are also associated with duodenal ulcer formation, as both are known stimulants of acid secretion.

Although many factors are thought to contribute to the formation of duodenal ulcers, *H. pylori* has been identified as playing a key role. *H. pylori* is found in approximately 90 to 95% of patients with duodenal ulcers. However, a clear-cut direct causal relationship between *H. pylori* and duodenal ulcer formation has not yet been proved. Not all individuals with evidence of *H. pylori* go on to develop ulcers, which suggests that additional factors are needed to produce these conditions. *H. pylori* survives in the human upper GI tract for a long time because of its ability to move in mucus and attach to mucosal cells. In addition, it secretes a substance called *urease,* which buffers the area around the bacterium and protects it from destruction in an acidic environment.

Infection with *H. pylori* is most common in underdeveloped countries and among persons of low socioeconomic status. Although the routes of transmission are largely unknown, it is thought that infection occurs during childhood via transmission from family members to the child, possibly through a fecal–oral route, an oral–oral route, or both. In Canada and the United States, persons born before 1940 have a significantly higher risk of carrying *H. pylori* than do younger persons. This enhanced prevalence in older persons has been attributed to the presence of crowded living conditions and poor sanitation practices, which were more common in the first half of the twentieth century.

Research into a genetic cause for ulcers has shown that some members of the same family are more prone than others to develop gastric or duodenal ulcers. Supporting a genetic etiology is the fact that persons with blood group O have an increased incidence of duodenal ulcers. Evidence is not complete, however, and the ulcer development could just as well be the result of sharing the same environment.

Stress-Related Mucosal Disease. *Stress-related mucosal disease* (SRMD) is a condition of acute ulcers that develop after a major physiological insult such as trauma or surgery. A physiological stress ulcer is a form of erosive gastritis. It is believed that the gastric mucosa of the body of the stomach undergoes a period of transient ischemia in association with hypotension, severe injury, extensive burns, and complicated surgery. The ischemia is caused by decreased capillary blood flow or shunting of blood away from the GI tract so that blood flow bypasses the gastric mucosa. This occurs as a compensatory mechanism in hypotension or shock. The decrease in blood flow produces an imbalance between the destructive properties of HCl and pepsin and the protective factors of the stomach's mucosal barrier, especially in the fundic portion, and this imbalance results in ulceration. Multiple superficial erosions result, which may bleed. Risk factors for development of stress ulcer bleeding are respiratory failure and coagulopathy. Patients with these conditions should receive prophylaxis with antisecretory agents. Stress gastritis is diagnosed with endoscopy, and treatment is with aggressive reduction of gastric acid secretions by means of H_2R blockers or PPIs.

Clinical Manifestations

It is common for patients with gastric or duodenal ulcers to have no pain or other symptoms. The gastric and duodenal mucosae are not rich in sensory pain fibres, which may account for this phenomenon. When pain does occur with duodenal ulcer, it is described as "burning" or "cramplike," and it is most often located in the midepigastric region beneath the xiphoid process. In contrast, the pain associated with gastric ulcers is located high in the epigastrium; it occurs spontaneously about 1 to 2 hours after meals and is described as "burning" or "gaseous." The pain can occur when the stomach is empty or when food has been ingested. If the ulcer has eroded through the gastric mucosa, food tends to aggravate rather than alleviate the pain. Some persons do not experience any pain even when the ulcer is identified through a serious complication such as hemorrhage or perforation.

Ulcers located on the posterior aspect of the duodenum can be manifested by back pain. The pain usually occurs 2 to 4 hours after meals. It is relieved by antacids alone or in combination with an H_2R blocker or PPI and sometimes by foods that neutralize and dilute the HCl. A characteristic of duodenal ulcer is its tendency to occur continuously for a few weeks or months and then disappear for a time, only to recur some months later.

Complications

The three major complications of chronic PUD are hemorrhage, perforation, and gastric outlet obstruction. All are considered emergency situations and are initially treated conservatively. However, surgery may become necessary at any time during the course of the therapy.

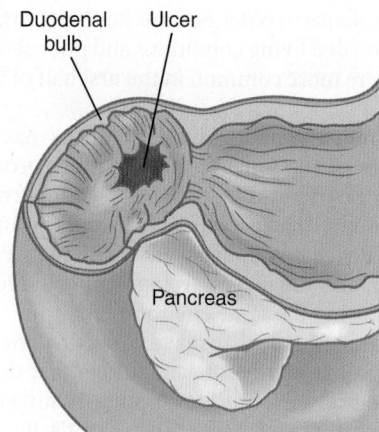

Duodenal bulb   Ulcer

Pancreas

FIG. 44.16 Duodenal ulcer of the posterior wall penetrating into the head of the pancreas, resulting in walled-off perforation.

Hemorrhage. Hemorrhage is the most common complication of PUD. It develops as a result of erosion of the granulation tissue at the base of the ulcer during healing or erosion of the ulcer through a major blood vessel. Duodenal ulcers account for a greater percentage of upper GI bleeding episodes than do gastric ulcers.

Perforation. Perforation of an ulcer is considered the most lethal complication of peptic ulcer. Perforation is common in large penetrating duodenal ulcers that have not healed and are located on the posterior mucosal wall (Figure 44.16). Perforated gastric ulcers are most often located on the lesser curvature of the stomach. Even though duodenal ulcers are more prevalent and perforate more frequently, mortality rates associated with perforation of gastric ulcers are higher.

Perforation of a peptic ulcer occurs when the ulcer penetrates the serosal surface, with spillage of either gastric or duodenal contents into the peritoneal cavity. The size of the perforation is directly proportional to the length of time the patient has had the ulcer: the larger the perforation, the longer the history of the ulcer. Small perforations seal themselves and result in a cessation of symptoms; larger perforations necessitate immediate surgical closure. Spontaneous sealing occurs as a result of large amounts of fibrin being produced in response to the perforation. This leads to fibrinous fusion of the duodenum or the gastric curvature to adjacent tissue, mainly the liver.

The clinical manifestations of perforation are characterized by their sudden and dramatic onset. The patient experiences sudden, severe upper abdominal pain that quickly spreads throughout the abdomen. The visceral and parietal layers of the peritoneum have an abundance of pain receptors, which contributes to the abruptness and intensity of the pain experienced. There may be shoulder pain if the spillage causes irritation to the phrenic nerve. The abdominal muscles contract, appearing rigid and boardlike as they attempt to protect the abdomen from further injury. The patient's respirations become shallow and rapid. Bowel sounds are usually absent. Nausea and vomiting may occur but are generally absent. Many affected patients report a history of ulcer disease or recent symptoms of indigestion.

The contents entering the peritoneal cavity from the stomach or the duodenum contain a variety of ingredients that include air, saliva, food particles, HCl, pepsin, bacteria, bile, and pancreatic fluid and enzymes. Bacterial peritonitis may occur within 6 to 12 hours. The intensity of the peritonitis is proportional to the amount and the duration of the spillage through the

perforation. It is difficult to determine from the sudden onset of symptoms whether gastric or duodenal ulcer is the cause because the clinical characteristics of intestinal perforation are the same (see Chapter 45).

Gastric Outlet Obstruction. Ulcers located in the antrum and the prepyloric and pyloric areas of the stomach and the duodenum can predispose to gastric outlet obstruction. In the early phase of obstruction (often referred to as the *compensated phase*), gastric emptying is normal to near normal. Over time, the increase in contractile force needed to empty the stomach results in hypertrophy of the stomach wall. After long-standing obstruction, the stomach enters the decompensated phase, which results in dilation and atony. The obstruction is not totally the result of fibrous scar tissue because active ulcer formation is associated with edema, inflammation, and pylorospasm, all of which contribute to the narrowing of the pylorus.

Patients with gastric outlet obstruction generally have a long history of ulcer pain. Ulcer-like pain of short duration or complete absence of pain is more indicative of a malignant obstruction. The pain progresses to a more generalized upper abdominal discomfort that becomes worse toward the end of the day as the stomach fills and dilates. Relief may be obtained by belching or by self-induced vomiting. Involuntary vomiting is common and often projectile. The vomitus contains food particles that were ingested many hours or even a day or two before the vomiting episode. There is often an offensive odour if the contents have been dormant in the stomach for a time. Affected patients who vomit frequently are anorexic, with evident weight loss, and report thirst and an unpleasant taste in the mouth.

Patients with gastric outlet obstruction may have a swelling in the upper abdomen that indicates dilation of the stomach. Peristalsis is loud, and visible peristaltic waves are often observed passing across the abdomen from left to right. If the stomach is grossly dilated, it is possible to palpate it as well.

Diagnostic Studies

The diagnostic measures used to determine the presence and location of a peptic ulcer are similar to those used for acute upper GI bleeding. Endoscopy is the procedure most often used because of the manoeuvrability of fibre-optic endoscopes for viewing the entire gastric and duodenal mucosa (Figure 44.17). This procedure can also be used to determine the degree of ulcer healing after treatment. During endoscopy, tissue specimens can be obtained for identification of *H. pylori* and to rule out gastric cancer.

Currently, several diagnostic tests are available to confirm *H. pylori* infection. These are classified as noninvasive and invasive. *Noninvasive tests* include serum or whole blood antibody tests, particularly immunoglobulin G (IgG). However, because of the length of time that IgG levels remain elevated in the blood after the infection, the serological tests do not help distinguish active from recently treated disease. The urea breath test can be used to determine the presence of active infection. Urea is a by-product of the metabolism of *H. pylori* bacteria. A stool antigen test can identify the immune response to fight *H. pylori*. *Invasive tests* involve biopsy of the stomach and include the rapid urease test and tests of other histological markers of infection. These tests have greater sensitivity and specificity but involve an endoscopic procedure.

Barium studies are of benefit in the diagnosis of gastric outlet obstruction. Barium normally should pass from the stomach within 2 hours, but with gastric outlet obstruction, 50% of the barium remains on follow-up films up to 6 hours later.

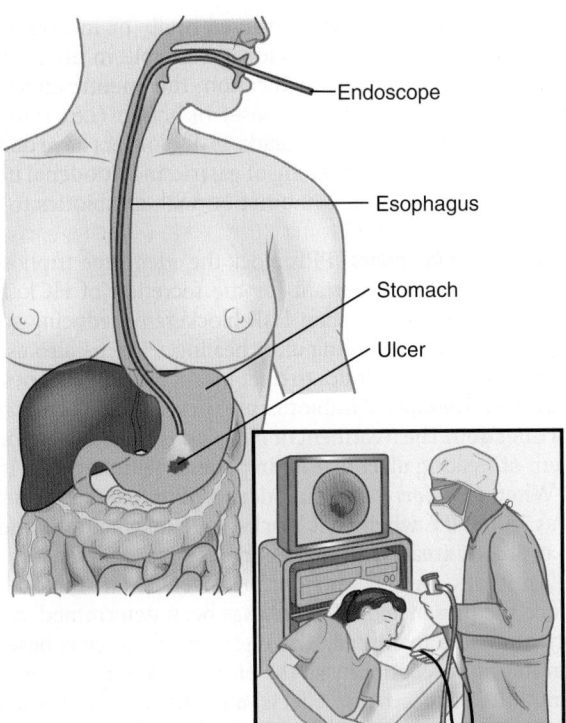

- Endoscope
- Esophagus
- Stomach
- Ulcer

FIG. 44.17 Esophagogastroduodenoscopy (EGD) enables the examiner to directly visualize the mucosal lining of the stomach with a flexible endoscope. Ulcers or tumours can be directly visualized and biopsy samples taken.

TABLE 44.21 **INTERPROFESSIONAL CARE**
Peptic Ulcer Disease

Diagnostic	**Acute Exacerbation Without Complications**
• History and physical examination	• Adequate rest
• Complete blood cell count	• Cessation of smoking
• *Helicobacter pylori* testing of breath, urine, blood, tissue	• IV fluid replacement
• Liver enzyme measurements	• NPO
• Serum electrolyte measurements	• Medication therapy
• Upper GI endoscopy with biopsy	• Antacids
• Urinalysis	• Anticholinergics
	• H₂-receptor blockers
	• Proton pump inhibitors
	• Sedatives
Interprofessional Therapy Conservative Therapy	**Acute Exacerbation With Complications (Hemorrhage, Perforation, Obstruction)**
• Adequate rest	• Bed rest
• Bland diet (six small meals a day)	• Blood transfusions
• Cessation of smoking	• IV fluid replacement (lactated Ringer's solution)
• Medication therapy	• NG suction
• Antacids (see Table 44.23)	• NPO
• Antibiotics for *H. pylori* infection (see Table 44.14)	• Stomach lavage (possible)
• Anticholinergics	**Surgical Therapy**
• Cytoprotective medications	• Billroth I and II procedures
• H₂-receptor blockers (see Table 44.22)	• Gastric outlet obstruction: pyloroplasty and vagotomy
• Proton pump inhibitors (see Table 44.22)	• Perforation: simple closure with omentum graft
• Stress reduction	• Ulcers: removal or reduction
	• Vagotomy and pyloroplasty

GI, gastrointestinal; *IV*, intravenous; *NG*, nasogastric; *NPO*, nothing by mouth.

Gastric analysis has questionable value in the diagnosis of PUD because, in many patients, gastric secretions are normal in amount and composition. However, it can provide important data for (a) identifying a possible gastrinoma (Zollinger–Ellison syndrome), (b) determining the degree of gastric hyperacidity, and (c) evaluating the results of therapy such as vagotomy and antisecretory medication therapy. The gastric analysis procedure is described in Chapter 41.

Laboratory analyses, including a CBC, urinalysis, liver enzyme studies, serum amylase determination, and stool examination, should be performed. A CBC may indicate the presence of anemia secondary to bleeding from the ulcer. Liver enzyme studies help determine any liver conditions, such as cirrhosis, that may complicate the treatment of the ulcer. A serum amylase determination frequently provides information on pancreatic function in patients in whom posterior penetration of the pancreas is suspected.

Interprofessional Care: Conservative Therapy

When the patient's clinical manifestations and health history suggest the diagnosis of PUD and diagnostic studies confirm it, a medical regimen is instituted (Table 44.21). This regimen will require a interprofessional team approach. The regimen consists of adequate rest, dietary modifications, medication therapy, cessation of smoking, and long-term follow-up care. The aim of the treatment program is to decrease the degree of gastric acidity, enhance mucosal defense mechanisms, and minimize the harmful effects on the mucosa.

Patients are generally treated in ambulatory care clinics. Pain disappears after 3 to 6 days, but ulcer healing is much slower. Complete healing may take 3 to 9 weeks, depending on ulcer size and the treatment regimen employed. Healing of the ulcer should be assessed by means of radiographic or endoscopic examination. Endoscopic examination is the only accurate

method by which to monitor ulcer healing; follow-up examinations are performed 3 to 6 months after diagnosis and treatment.

Adequate rest, both physical and emotional, is important in the treatment process. A quiet, calm environment at home or on the job is not easy to achieve, and some modifications in the patient's daily routine may be needed. The elimination or reduction of stressors helps decrease the stimulus for overproduction of HCl. Moderation in daily activity is essential.

As mentioned previously, smoking has an irritating effect on the mucosa, increases gastric motility, and delays mucosal healing. It should be eliminated completely or drastically reduced. The combination of adequate rest and abstinence from smoking accelerates ulcer healing.

Medication Therapy. Medications are a vital part of therapy and a referral to pharmacist may be warranted. The patient must be well informed about each medication prescribed, why it is ordered, and the expected benefits. Strict adherence to the prescribed regimen of medications is important. Medication therapy includes the use of antacids, H₂R blockers, PPIs, antibiotics, anticholinergics, and cytoprotective therapy (Tables 44.22, 44.23, and 44.24).

Because recurrence of peptic ulcer is frequent, interruption or discontinuation of therapy can have detrimental results. The patient must be encouraged to adhere to therapy and continue with follow-up care for at least 1 year. If changes in lifestyle are part of the prescribed therapy, they should be maintained. Antacids, H₂R blockers, and PPIs may be stopped after the ulcer has healed or may be prescribed in the form of low-dose maintenance therapy. No other medications, unless prescribed by the

TABLE 44.22 MEDICATION THERAPY

Peptic Ulcer Disease

Antisecretory	Cytoprotective
• H$_2$-receptor blockers	• Sucralfate bismuth subsalicylate (Pepto-Bismol)
• Famotidine (Pepcid)	
• Nizatidine (Axid)	**Neutralizing**
• Ranitidine (Zantac)	• Antacids*
• Proton pump inhibitors	
• Dexlansoprazole (Dexilant)	**Antibiotics for *Helicobacter pylori* Infection**
• Esomeprazole (Nexium)	• Amoxicillin
• Lansoprazole (Prevacid)	• Clarithromycin (Biaxin)
• Omeprazole (Losec)	• Metronidazole (Flagyl)
• Pantoprazole (Pantoloc)	• Tetracycline
• Anticholinergics	
	Others
Antisecretory and Cytoprotective	• Tricyclic antidepressants
• Misoprostol	• Doxepin (Sinequan)
	• Imipramine

*See Table 44.23.

TABLE 44.23 MEDICATION THERAPY

Antacid Preparations

Ingredient	Trade Name
Single substance	
• Aluminum carbonate	Basaljel
• Aluminum hydroxide gel tablets	Amphojel
• Aluminum phosphate	Phosphalugel
• Calcium carbonate	Alka-2, Tums
• Dihydroxyaluminum sodium carbonate	Rolaids
• Magaldrate	Riopan
• Magnesium hydroxide	Milk of magnesia
• Sodium bicarbonate	Alka-Seltzer
Mixtures of aluminum hydroxide and magnesium salts	Gaviscon, Maalox/Diovol

TABLE 44.24 MEDICATION THERAPY

Adverse Effects of Antacid Therapy

Antacid	Reactions
Aluminum hydroxide gels	Constipation, phosphorus depletion with chronic use
Calcium carbonate	Constipation or diarrhea, hypercalcemia, milk-alkali syndrome, renal calculi
Magnesium preparations	Diarrhea, hypermagnesemia
Sodium preparations	Milk–alkali syndrome if used with large amounts of calcium; used with caution in patients with sodium restrictions

health care provider, should be taken because they may have an ulcerogenic effect. Finally, the patient and the family should be told what to do in the event that pain and discomfort recur or blood is noted in the vomitus or stools.

Histamine-2 Receptor Blockers. H$_2$-receptor blockers, also called *H2R blockers*, are frequently used in the management of PUD. These medications block the action of histamine on the H$_2$Rs and thus reduce HCl secretion. This decreases the conversion of pepsinogen to pepsin and accelerates ulcer healing. (Antihistamine medications used to treat allergies are H$_1$R blockers and have no effect on gastric acid secretion.)

H$_2$R blockers may be administered orally or intravenously; however, only ranitidine (Zantac) is available in an IV form. Depending on the specific medication, therapeutic effects last up to 12 hours. However, the onset of action (i.e., symptom relief) is longer than that of antacids. H$_2$R blockers have demonstrated capabilities in the healing of gastric and duodenal ulcers. H$_2$R blockers are used in combination with antibiotics to treat ulcers related to *H. pylori*.

Proton Pump Inhibitors. PPIs block the adenosine triphosphatase enzyme that is important for the secretion of HCl. These agents are more effective than H$_2$R blockers in reducing gastric acid secretion and promoting ulcer healing. PPIs are also used in combination with antibiotics to treat ulcers caused by *H. pylori*.

Antibiotic Therapy. Antibiotics are prescribed to eradicate *H. pylori* infection. The treatment of *H. pylori* is the most important element of treating ulcer disease in patients with *H. pylori* infection. When *H. pylori* is present, ulcer recurrence rates can be as high as 75 to 90% when H$_2$R blockers are taken alone, whereas with antibiotic treatment, the recurrence rate may be less than 10%. Antibiotic therapy for *H. pylori* is detailed in Table 44.14.

Once the presence of *H. pylori* has been determined, antibiotic treatment is instituted. The regimen of choice is based on the antibiotic susceptibility of the *H. pylori* organism, allergies, patient adherence, adverse effects, and costs. Most medication regimens involve treatment for 7 to 14 days (Rx Files Academic Detailing Program, 2017).

Antacids. Antacids are used as adjunct therapy for PUD. They increase gastric pH by neutralizing the acid. As a result, the acid content of chyme reaching the duodenum is reduced. In addition, some antacids, such as aluminum hydroxide, can bind to bile salts, thus decreasing the detrimental effects of bile on the gastric mucosa. Patients who are vulnerable to SRMD may be treated prophylactically with antacids along with an antisecretory agent.

Antacids consist of systemic and nonsystemic types. *Systemic antacids,* such as sodium bicarbonate, are extremely soluble and are absorbed into the circulation. Their long-term use can lead to systemic alkalosis; therefore, they are rarely used in ulcer treatment. The *nonsystemic antacids* are insoluble and poorly absorbed. The common commercial nonsystemic antacids consist of magnesium hydroxide or aluminum hydroxide as single preparations or in various combinations (see Table 44.23). The antacid preparation may be in liquid or tablet form. The neutralizing effects of antacids taken on an empty stomach last only 20 to 30 minutes because they are quickly evacuated. When antacids are taken after meals, the effects may last as long as 3 to 4 hours. With therapy regimens that call for frequent administration (e.g., hourly), adherence is often poor.

The type and dosage of the antacid prescribed depends on adverse effects (see Table 44.24), as well as potential medication interactions. Preparations with high sodium content should be administered with caution in older people and in patients with liver cirrhosis, hypertension, heart failure, or renal disease. Magnesium preparations should not be prescribed for patients with renal failure because of the risk of magnesium toxicity. The most frequent adverse effect experienced with magnesium antacids is diarrhea. Aluminum hydroxide causes constipation. An antacid combination of aluminum and magnesium salts seems to lessen the adverse effects of both.

Antacids have the capacity to interact unfavourably with some medications. They can enhance the absorption of medications such as dicumarol and amphetamines. The action of digitalis preparations can be potentiated when taken in combination with calcium or magnesium antacids. Also, antacids may decrease the absorption rates of prescribed medications, such as tetracycline. Therefore, it is important to inform the health care provider of any medications that the patient is taking before antacid therapy is begun.

Anticholinergic Medications. Anticholinergic medications (e.g., scopolamine [hyoscine]) are only occasionally ordered in the treatment of PUD. These medications decrease cholinergic (vagal) stimulation of HCl secretion. Opinion is divided with regard to their efficacy in preventing recurrences and their therapeutic effectiveness in alleviating symptoms and preventing complications. Because of their tendency to decrease gastric motility, they should not be used for gastric ulcers in which stasis of secretions increases the patient's pain and discomfort. Anticholinergics are associated with a number of adverse effects, such as dry mouth and skin, flushing, thirst, tachycardia, dilated pupils, blurred vision, and urine retention. Anticholinergics must be prescribed with caution in patients with narrow-angle glaucoma, benign prostatic hyperplasia, and gastric outlet obstruction.

Cytoprotective Medication Therapy. Sucralfate is used for the short-term treatment of ulcers. It has proved to be cytoprotective of the esophagus, the stomach, and the duodenum. Its ability to accelerate ulcer healing is thought to be a result of the formation of an ulcer-adherent complex covering the ulcer and thereby protecting it from erosion caused by pepsin, acid, and bile salts. Sucralfate does not have acid-neutralizing capabilities. Its action is most effective at a low pH, and it should be given at least 30 minutes before or after an antacid. Adverse effects are minimal. However, it does bind with digoxin, warfarin (Coumadin), phenytoin (Dilantin), and tetracycline, which reduces the bioavailability of these medications.

Misoprostol is a synthetic prostaglandin analogue. It has protective and some antisecretory effects on gastric mucosa. It is used for the prevention of gastric ulcers induced by NSAIDs and ASA (Aspirin). A major advantage of misoprostol is that it does not interfere with the therapeutic effects of ASA (Aspirin) and NSAIDs. Persons who require ongoing NSAID therapy, such as those with osteoarthritis, may benefit from the use of misoprostol. All NSAIDs, even COX-2 inhibitors, impair ulcer healing.

Other Medications. Tricyclic antidepressants (e.g., imipramine, doxepin [Sinequan]) and serotonin reuptake inhibitors may be prescribed for patients with ulcer disease. Antidepressants may contribute to overall pain relief through their effects on pain transmission by afferent fibres. In addition, tricyclic antidepressants have, to varying degrees, some anticholinergic properties, which result in reduced acid secretion. Selective serotonin reuptake inhibitors are associated with a slight increase in risk of upper GI bleeding.

Nutritional Therapy. Dietary modifications may be necessary so that foods and beverages irritating to the patient can be avoided or eliminated from the diet. Intake of alcohol and caffeine-containing products should be avoided because of their irritating effects.

Dietary instructions should include a sample diet with a list of foods that usually cause distress and should be eliminated from the diet; referral to a dietitian may also benefit the patient. Foods known to irritate the gastric mucosa include hot, spicy foods and pepper, alcohol, carbonated beverages, tea, coffee, and broth (meat extract). These foods also have limited buffering ability in addition to stimulating gastric acid secretion.

Foods high in roughage, such as raw fruit, salads, and vegetables, may irritate an inflamed mucosa. If these foods are well chewed, this seems to be less of a problem.

Protein is considered the best neutralizing food, but it also stimulates gastric secretions. Carbohydrates and fats are the least stimulating to HCl secretion, but they do not neutralize acid well. The patient must determine a suitable combination of these essential nutrients that does not cause undue distress.

Milk is no longer recommended as a dietary aid to reduce pain associated with PUD because of the buffering effect and the significant acid secretion it may cause (Vomero & Colpo, 2014).

Therapy Related to Complications of Peptic Ulcer Disease

Acute Exacerbation. An acute exacerbation of peptic ulcer can usually be treated with the same regimen used for conservative therapy. However, the situation is considered more serious because of the possible complications of perforation, hemorrhage, and gastric outlet obstruction.

Bleeding, increased pain and discomfort, and nausea and vomiting frequently accompany an acute exacerbation. If the patient experiences recurrent vomiting or gastric outlet obstruction, an NG tube may be placed into the stomach with intermittent suction for about 24 to 48 hours.

If the patient has a history of an incompetent pyloric sphincter that allows reflux of duodenal contents into the stomach, an NG tube is used to remove intestinal contents from the stomach. This period of stomach rest eliminates any causative factors that may have precipitated the acute exacerbation and enables the resolution of edema and inflammation of the mucosa. Fluids and electrolytes are replaced by IV infusion until the patient is able to tolerate oral feedings without distress.

Management is similar to that described for upper GI bleeding. Blood or blood products may be administered. Careful monitoring of vital signs, intake and output, laboratory study results, and signs of impending shock is important during an acute episode.

Endoscopic evaluation is performed to reveal the degree of inflammation or bleeding, as well as the ulcer location. It is important to ascertain the presence of a prepyloric or pyloric ulcer that can cause gastric outlet obstruction. When endoscopic examination reveals no major concerns and the patient's physical condition stabilizes, the plan of care for the patient should follow the same regimen of diet, activity, and medications used in conservative therapy. A 5-year follow-up program is recommended after acute exacerbation. An increase in the healing rate is achieved after conservative treatment, but the treatment plan cannot prevent the scar formation that can result in gastric outlet obstruction.

Perforation. The immediate focus of management of a patient with a perforation is to stop the spillage of gastric or duodenal contents into the peritoneal cavity and restore blood volume. An NG tube is inserted into the stomach to provide continuous aspiration and gastric decompression to halt spillage through the perforation. Although duodenal aspiration is not achieved as promptly, placement of the tube as near to the perforation site as possible facilitates decompression.

Circulating blood volume must be replaced with lactated Ringer's and albumin solutions. These solutions substitute for the fluids lost from the vascular and interstitial space as the peritonitis develops. Blood replacement in the form of packed RBCs may be necessary. A central venous pressure line and an in-dwelling urinary catheter, unless contraindicated, should be inserted and monitored hourly. Broad-spectrum antibiotic therapy should be started immediately to treat bacterial peritonitis. Administration of pain medications provides comfort.

The operative procedure involving the least risk to the patient is simple oversewing of the perforation and reinforcement of the area with a graft of omentum. The excess gastric contents are suctioned from the peritoneal cavity during the surgical procedure. There is controversy over whether more definitive surgical treatment of a perforated ulcer achieves better results than does simple closure. Other types of surgical procedures depend on the location of the peptic ulcer and the surgeon's preference. If cure of the ulcer is the ultimate goal, the surgical procedures may include gastric resection or vagotomy and pyloroplasty.

Gastric Outlet Obstruction. The aim of therapy for obstruction is to decompress the stomach, correct any existing fluid and electrolyte imbalances, and improve the patient's general state of health. An NG tube is inserted into the stomach and attached to continuous suction to remove excess fluids and undigested food particles. With continuous decompression for several days, the stomach has the opportunity to regain its normal muscle tone, the ulcer can begin healing, and the inflammation and edema will subside.

The tube is clamped after several days of suction, and gastric residue is measured periodically. The frequency and amount of time the tube remains clamped are proportional to the amount of aspirate obtained and the comfort level of the patient. A method commonly followed is to clamp the tube overnight for approximately 8 to 12 hours and to measure the gastric residue in the morning. When the aspirate falls below 200 mL, it is considered to be within a normal range, and the patient can begin oral intake of clear liquids. Initially, oral fluids are begun at 30 mL/hr and then gradually increased in amount. The patient must be watched carefully for signs of distress or vomiting. As the amount of gastric residue decreases, solid foods are added and the tube is removed.

IV fluids and electrolytes are administered according to the degree of dehydration, vomiting, and electrolyte imbalance indicated by laboratory studies. Pain relief results from the decompression measures, and analgesics are usually not necessary. Antacids and antisecretory medication therapy (i.e., H_2R blockers, PPIs) are an integral part of treatment if the obstruction has been determined on endoscopic examination to be the result of an active ulcer. Pyloric obstruction may be treated nonsurgically by balloon dilations performed through the endoscope. Surgical intervention may be necessary to remove scar tissue.

NURSING MANAGEMENT PEPTIC ULCER DISEASE

NURSING ASSESSMENT

Subjective and objective data that should be obtained from a patient with PUD are presented in Table 44.25.

NURSING DIAGNOSES

Nursing diagnoses related to PUD may include but are not limited to the following.
- *Acute pain* resulting from *biological injury agent* (increased gastric secretions)
- *Potential for nonadherence* resulting from *insufficient knowledge of therapeutic regimen*
- *Nausea* resulting from *anxiety, fear, gastrointestinal irritation*

TABLE 44.25   **NURSING ASSESSMENT**
Peptic Ulcer Disease
Subjective Data
Important Health Information
Current health history: Chronic alcohol misuse, smoking, caffeine use
Past health history: Chronic kidney disease, pancreatic disease, chronic obstructive pulmonary disease, serious illness or trauma, hyperparathyroidism, cirrhosis of the liver, Zollinger–Ellison syndrome; family history of peptic ulcer disease
Medications: Use of acetylsalicylic acid (ASA: Aspirin), corticosteroids, nonsteroidal anti-inflammatory medications
Surgery or other treatments: Complicated or prolonged surgery
Symptoms
• Black, tarry stools
• Common: burning midepigastric or back pain occurring 2–4 hr after meals and relieved by food (duodenal ulcers), nocturnal pain; high epigastric pain occurring 1–2 hr after meals (gastric ulcers); pain may be precipitated or aggravated by food
• Weight loss, anorexia; nausea and vomiting, hematemesis; dyspepsia, heartburn, belching
Objective Data
General
Anxiety, irritability
Gastrointestinal
Epigastric tenderness
Possible Findings
Anemia; guaiac-positive stools; positive blood, urine, breath, or stool tests for *Helicobacter pylori*; abnormalities revealed by upper gastrointestinal endoscopic and barium studies

Additional information on nursing diagnoses for the patient with PUD is presented in NCP 44.2, available on the Evolve website.

PLANNING

Overall goals are that the patient with PUD will (a) adhere to the prescribed therapeutic regimen, (b) experience a reduction in or absence of discomfort related to PUD, (c) exhibit no signs of GI complications related to the ulcerative process, (d) have complete healing of the peptic ulcer, and (e) make appropriate lifestyle changes to prevent recurrence.

NURSING IMPLEMENTATION

HEALTH PROMOTION. Nurses must be involved in identifying patients at risk for ulcer development. Early detection and treatment of ulcers are important aspects of reducing morbidity associated with ulcers. Patients with PUD who are taking ulcerogenic medications such as ASA (Aspirin) and NSAIDs are at risk for ulcer development. Patients need to be encouraged to take these medications with food. Patients should be taught to report symptoms related to gastric irritation, including epigastric pain, to their health care provider.

ACUTE INTERVENTION. During the acute exacerbation of an ulcer, patients generally report increased pain and nausea and vomiting, and some may have evidence of bleeding. Initially, many patients attempt to cope with the symptoms at home before seeking medical assistance.

During this acute phase, the patient may be maintained on NPO status for a few days, an NG tube is inserted and connected to intermittent suction, and fluids are replaced intravenously.

The rationale for this therapy must be conveyed to the anxious patient and caregiver. They must understand that the advantages far outweigh any temporary discomfort imposed by the presence of the tube. Regular mouth care alleviates the dry mouth. Cleansing and lubrication of the nares facilitates breathing and decreases soreness. When the stomach is kept empty of gastric secretions, the ulcer pain diminishes and ulcer healing begins. Usually, this form of intervention is effective.

Because the patient is on NPO status, IV fluids are ordered. The type and amount administered are directly related to the fluid lost, the manifestations exhibited by the patient, and the results of the hemoglobin, hematocrit, and electrolyte determinations. The nurse should be aware of any other current health problems that could be adversely affected by the type of fluid used or the rate of the infusion. Repeated monitoring of these parameters provides information on the hydration status and the effectiveness of treatment. Vital signs are initially measured at least hourly so that shock can be detected and treated.

Physical and emotional rest are conducive to ulcer healing. The patient's immediate environment should be quiet and restful. The use of a mild sedative or tranquilizer has beneficial effects when the patient is anxious and apprehensive. The nurse must use good judgement before sedating a person who is becoming increasingly restless. There is a danger that the medication will mask the signs of shock secondary to upper GI bleeding.

If the patient's condition improves without progression of symptoms (e.g., increased pain, vomiting, and hemorrhage), the regimen outlined for conservative therapy is followed. However, complications such as hemorrhage, perforation, and obstruction can occur.

Hemorrhage. Changes in vital signs and an increase in the amount and redness of the aspirate often signal massive upper GI bleeding. When there is an increased amount of blood in the gastric contents, the patient's pain is often decreased because the blood helps to neutralize the acidic gastric contents. It is important to maintain the patency of the NG tube so that blood clots do not obstruct the tube. If the tube becomes blocked, the patient can develop abdominal distension. Interventions are used that are similar to those described for upper GI bleeding in the section Nursing Management: Upper Gastrointestinal Bleeding. The nurse must monitor the results of the hemoglobin and hematocrit determinations.

Perforation. When there is sudden, severe abdominal pain unrelated in intensity and location to the pain that brought the patient to the hospital, the nurse must recognize the possibility of ulcer perforation. When any patient with an ulcer, particularly a chronic duodenal ulcer, demonstrates these manifestations, perforation should be suspected and the health care provider notified immediately.

Patients with perforation demonstrate a rigid, boardlike abdomen; have severe generalized abdominal and shoulder pain; draw up their knees; and have shallow, grunting respirations. The bowel sounds that may have been previously normal or hyperactive may diminish and disappear.

Vital signs are important parameters and should be promptly recorded every 15 to 30 minutes. The nurse should temporarily stop all oral or NG medications and feedings until the health care provider can be notified and a definitive diagnosis made. If perforation has taken place, anything taken internally can add to the spillage into the peritoneal cavity and increase discomfort. If IV fluids are being administered at the time of the perforation, the rate should be maintained or increased to replace the depleted plasma volume.

When perforation is confirmed, antibiotic therapy is usually started, and careful observation for allergic reactions must be made. When the perforation fails to seal spontaneously, surgical closure is necessary and is performed as soon as possible. There is often little time to prepare the patient and caregiver thoroughly for the surgical intervention, but some instructions can be conveyed while the immediate therapy is begun. If major reconstructive surgery is anticipated, the patient and caregiver may question the need when the issue is only a small hole.

Gastric Outlet Obstruction. Gastric outlet obstruction can occur at any time and is most likely to occur in patients in whom the ulcer is located close to the pylorus. Because the onset of symptoms is usually gradual, the condition is not generally as serious an emergency as hemorrhage or perforation. Relief of symptoms may be achieved by constant NG aspiration of stomach contents. This allows edema and inflammation to subside and then enables normal flow of gastric contents through the pylorus.

Obstruction can also occur during the treatment of an acute episode of peptic ulcer exacerbation. If these symptoms are experienced while the patient is still on NPO status, the patency of the NG tube should be investigated. Regular irrigation of the tube with a saline solution facilitates proper functioning. It may be helpful to reposition the patient from side to side so that the tube tip is not constantly lying against the mucosal surface.

When oral feedings have been resumed and symptoms of obstruction are observed, the health care provider should be promptly informed. In general, all that is necessary to treat the obstruction is to resume gastric aspiration so that the edema and inflammation resulting from the acute episode have time to resolve. IV fluids with electrolyte replacement keep the patient hydrated during this period. The NG tube can be clamped, and gastric fluids can be aspirated to check for retention. It is important to maintain accurate intake and output records, especially of the gastric aspirate. The patient should be kept aware of why these symptoms are being experienced. In some instances in which treatment is not successful, surgery may be performed after the acute phase has passed.

AMBULATORY AND HOME CARE. Patients in whom PUD has been diagnosed have specific needs that must be met to prevent and avoid recurrence or complications. General instructions should cover aspects of the disease process itself, medications, possible changes in lifestyle (including diet), and regular follow-up care. Table 44.26 provides a patient and caregiver teaching guide for patients with PUD.

Knowing the cause of the ulcer and understanding the disease process may motivate a patient to become more involved in self-care and to adhere to the therapy regimen. The patient must understand the dietary modifications and why they are important for recovery and health maintenance. The nurse and the dietitian should obtain a dietary history from the patient and plan for ways that dietary modifications can be easily incorporated into the patient's home and work setting. The patient who is following a diet prescribed for another illness needs to know how to balance the two so that neither condition is harmed by dietary interventions.

Patients do not always give the health care provider accurate information regarding habitual use of alcohol or cigarettes. The nurse should provide useful information about the detrimental

TABLE 44.26	PATIENT & CAREGIVER TEACHING GUIDE

Peptic Ulcer Disease

The following guidelines should be included when teaching the patient and caregiver about peptic ulcer disease. The nurse should:

1. Describe dietary modifications, including avoidance of foods that cause epigastric distress. These foods may include black pepper, spicy foods, and acidic foods. Carbonated beverages and caffeine should also be avoided.
2. Explain the rationale for avoiding cigarettes. In addition to promoting ulcer development, smoking delays ulcer healing.
3. Emphasize the need to reduce or eliminate alcohol ingestion.
4. Explain the rationale for avoiding OTC medications unless approved by the patient's health care provider. Many preparations contain ingredients, such as ASA (Aspirin), that should not be taken unless approved by the health care provider. The patient should check with the health care provider regarding the use of nonsteroidal anti-inflammatory medications.
5. Explain the rationale for not interchanging brands of antacids and H_2-receptor blockers that can be purchased OTC without checking with the health care provider. Doing so can lead to harmful adverse effects.
6. Emphasize the need to take all medications as prescribed, including both antisecretory and antibiotic medications. Failure to take medications as prescribed can result in relapse.
7. Explain the importance of reporting any of the following:
   - Bloody emesis or tarry stools
   - Increase in epigastric pain
   - Increased nausea or vomiting
8. Describe the relationship between symptoms and stress. Stress-reducing activities and relaxation strategies are encouraged.
9. Encourage patient and caregiver to share concerns about lifestyle changes and living with a chronic illness.

ASA, acetylsalicylic acid; *OTC*, over-the-counter.

effects of alcohol and cigarettes on ulcer disease and ulcer healing and provide resources on cessation and rehabilitation programs.

The nurse should teach the patient about their prescribed medications, including their actions, adverse effects, and inherent dangers if omitted for any reason. The patient should know why OTC medications (e.g., ASA [Aspirin]) should not be taken unless approved by the health care provider. Because antacids and some H_2R blockers may be purchased without a prescription, the patient must be informed that interchanging brands without checking with the health care provider or nurse can lead to harmful adverse effects.

Efforts should be made to obtain more information about the patient's psychosocial status. Knowledge of lifestyle, occupation, and coping behaviours can be helpful in developing the plan of care. The patient may be reluctant to talk about personal subjects, the stress experienced at home or on the job, the usual methods of coping, or dependence on drugs or alcohol. Unfortunately, the patient often does not recognize the relationship between lifestyle or occupation and ulcer disease. It is important to listen for subtle clues from the patient's statements and to observe for behaviours that broaden the database of what is known about the patient.

The need for long-term follow-up care must be stressed. Because successful treatment is frequently followed by a recurrence of the ulcer disease, patients should be encouraged to seek immediate intervention if symptoms of the disease come back. Patients who have recurrence of ulcer disease after initial healing must learn to live with a disease that is chronic. They may be

angry and frustrated, especially if the prescribed mode of therapy has been faithfully followed and yet has failed to prevent the recurrence or extension of the disease process.

Unfortunately, many patients do not adhere to the plan of care originally designed and they experience repeated exacerbations. Patients quickly learn that they often experience no discomfort when they omit prescribed medications or indulge in occasional dietary indiscretions. Consequently, they may make no or little alteration in lifestyle. After an acute exacerbation, the patient is often more amenable to following the plan of care and open to suggestions for changes in lifestyle. Changes, such as smoking cessation and alcohol abstinence, are difficult for many people, and the idea of making these changes may be met with resistance. The patient may fare better from a reduction in their use of these substances rather than from total elimination. Although alcohol and smoking are known to interfere with ulcer healing, they frequently serve as coping mechanisms. From the patient's point of view, the distress caused by their total elimination may outweigh the benefits to be gained from abstention. The goal, however, should always be total cessation. A patient with chronic ulcers must be aware of the complications that may result from the disease, the clinical manifestations indicating their presence, and what to do about them until they can see a health care provider.

EVALUATION

Expected outcomes for the patient with PUD are addressed in NCP 44.2 on the Evolve website.

Interprofessional Care: Surgical Therapy for Peptic Ulcer Disease

Because of the use of antisecretory and antibiotic agents, surgery for PUD is uncommon. Surgery is performed on patients with complications that are unresponsive to medical management or who have concerns about gastric cancer. Care of the patient undergoing surgical procedure and postoperative care requires an interprofessional team approach.

A variety of surgical procedures are used to treat ulcer disease. They usually involve a partial gastrectomy, vagotomy, or pyloroplasty. Partial gastrectomy with removal of the distal two thirds of the stomach and anastomosis of the gastric stump to the duodenum is called a *gastroduodenostomy*, or *Billroth I* operation (Figure 44.18). Partial gastrectomy with removal of the distal two thirds of the stomach and anastomosis of the gastric stump to the jejunum is called a *gastrojejunostomy*, or *Billroth II* operation. In both procedures, the antrum and the pylorus are removed. Because the duodenum is bypassed, the Billroth II operation is the preferred surgical procedure to prevent recurrence of duodenal ulcers.

Vagotomy is the severing of the vagus nerve, either totally (truncal) or selectively at some point in its innervation to the stomach. In a truncal vagotomy, both the anterior and the posterior trunks are severed. *Selective vagotomy* consists of cutting the nerve at a particular branch of the vagus nerve, resulting in denervation of only a portion of the stomach, such as the antrum or the parietal cell mass.

Pyloroplasty consists of surgical enlargement of the pyloric sphincter to facilitate the easy passage of contents from the stomach. It is most commonly done after vagotomy or to enlarge an opening that has been constricted from scar tissue. A vagotomy decreases gastric motility and, subsequently, gastric emptying. A pyloroplasty accompanying vagotomy increases gastric emptying.

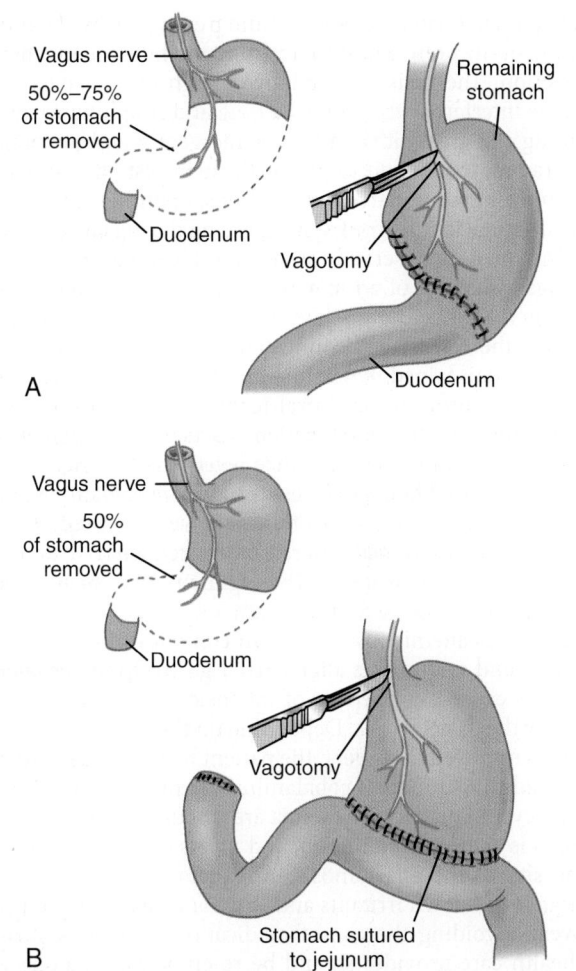

A

B

FIG. 44.18 **A,** Billroth I procedure (subtotal gastric resection with gastroduodenostomy anastomosis). **B,** Billroth II procedure (subtotal gastric resection with gastrojejunostomy anastomosis).

Postoperative Complications. The most common postoperative complications from peptic ulcer surgery are dumping syndrome, postprandial hypoglycemia, and bile reflux gastritis.

Dumping Syndrome. Dumping syndrome, in which patients experience vagal symptoms after a meal, such as generalized weakness or dizziness, is the direct result of surgical removal of a large portion of the stomach and the pyloric sphincter. These changes drastically reduce the reservoir capacity of the stomach. Although dumping syndrome is more commonly experienced after a Billroth II procedure, it can occur after any gastric reconstruction and vagotomy.

Dumping syndrome is associated with meals having a hyperosmolar composition. Normally, gastric chyme enters the small intestine in small amounts, and shifts in fluid from the extracellular space are minimal. After surgery, however, the stomach no longer has control over the amount of gastric chyme entering the small intestine. Consequently, a large bolus of hypertonic fluid enters the intestine and results in fluid being drawn into the bowel lumen. This creates a decrease in plasma volume. A secondary consequence of this fluid shift is distension of the bowel lumen, which stimulates intestinal motility and the urge to defecate.

Approximately one-third to one-half of patients experience dumping syndrome after peptic ulcer surgery. The onset of symptoms occurs at the end of a meal or within 15 to 30 minutes after eating. The patient usually describes feelings of generalized

weakness, sweating, palpitations, and dizziness. These symptoms are attributed to the sudden decrease in plasma volume. The patient reports abdominal cramps, borborygmi (audible abdominal sounds produced by hyperactive intestinal peristalsis), and the urge to defecate. These manifestations usually last for no longer than an hour after meals.

Postprandial Hypoglycemia. Postprandial hypoglycemia is considered a variant of the dumping syndrome because it is the result of uncontrolled gastric emptying of a bolus of fluid high in carbohydrate into the small intestine. The bolus of concentrated carbohydrate results in hyperglycemia and the release of excessive amounts of insulin into the circulation. A secondary hypoglycemia then occurs, with symptoms appearing about 2 hours after meals. The symptoms experienced are those observed in any hypoglycemic reaction and include sweating, weakness, mental confusion, palpitations, tachycardia, and anxiety.

Bile Reflux Gastritis. Gastric surgery that involves the pylorus, either reconstruction or removal, can result in reflux alkaline gastritis. Prolonged contact with bile, especially bile salts, causes damage to the gastric mucosa. Chronic gastritis of this form may result in the backwards diffusion of H^+ through the gastric mucosa. Paradoxically, peptic ulcer may recur after surgical treatment that was intended as a cure.

The symptoms associated with reflux alkaline gastritis are continuous epigastric distress that increases after meals. Vomiting relieves the distress, but only temporarily. The administration of cholestyramine, either before or with meals, has met with success. Cholestyramine binds with the bile salts that are the source of irritation in this condition. Aluminum hydroxide antacids have also been used in the treatment of this condition.

Nutritional Therapy. Discharge planning and instruction should be started as soon as the immediate postoperative period is successfully passed. Dietary instructions may be given by the dietitian and reinforced by the nursing staff. Because the stomach's reservoir has been greatly diminished after gastric resection, the meal size must be reduced accordingly. The patient should be advised to stop drinking fluids with meals. Dry foods with a low-carbohydrate content and moderate protein and fat content are better tolerated initially. These dietary changes, with the incorporation of a short rest period after each meal, reduce the likelihood of dumping syndrome. Reassurance that following these dietary measures will result in cessation of these symptoms within a few months is essential for long-term adherence to instructions.

Postprandial hypoglycemic reaction can be avoided if these dietary instructions are followed. The immediate ingestion of sugared fluids or candy relieves the hypoglycemic symptoms. The treatment of this type of hypoglycemia is similar to that of dumping syndrome (Table 44.27). To avoid similar occurrences, the patient should be instructed to limit the amount of sugar consumed with each meal and to eat small, frequent meals with moderate amounts of protein and fat. Although only a small percentage of patients experience bile reflux gastritis, all patients must be cautioned to notify the health care provider of any continuous epigastric distress after meals that is similar to that felt before surgery.

NURSING MANAGEMENT
SURGICAL THERAPY FOR PEPTIC ULCER DISEASE

PREOPERATIVE CARE

Preoperative care focuses on educating the patient on the procedure and expected outcomes to ensure the patient can make

---

TABLE 44.27 NUTRITIONAL THERAPY

Postgastrectomy Dumping Syndrome

Purpose

To slow the rapid passage of food into the intestine; to control symptoms of the dumping syndrome (dizziness, sense of fullness, diarrhea, tachycardia), which sometimes occur after a partial or total gastrectomy

Diet Principles

1. Meals are divided into six small feedings to avoid overloading intestines at mealtimes.
2. Fluids should not be taken with meals but at least 30–45 min before or after meals; this helps prevent distension or a feeling of fullness.
3. Concentrated sweets (e.g., honey, sugar, jelly, jam, candies, sweet pastries, sweetened fruit) are avoided because they sometimes cause dizziness, diarrhea, and a sense of fullness.
4. Protein and fats are increased to promote rebuilding of body tissues and to meet energy needs. Meat, cheese, eggs, and milk products are specific foods to increase in the diet.
5. The amount of time these restrictions should be followed varies. The health care provider decides the proper amount of time to remain on this prescribed diet according to the patient's clinical condition and progress.

---

an informed decision. It is important for the nurse to implement a preoperative teaching plan about the procedure and expectations following surgery, such as comfort measures, pain relief, coughing and breathing exercises, use of an NG tube, and IV fluid administration (see Chapter 20).

POSTOPERATIVE CARE

Care of the patient after major abdominal surgery is similar to the postoperative care after abdominal laparotomy (see Chapter 45 and NCP 45.2). An NG tube is used to decompress the remaining portion of the stomach to decrease pressure on the suture line and to allow for resolution of edema and inflammation resulting from surgical trauma.

The gastric aspirate must be carefully observed for colour, amount, and odour during the immediate postoperative period. The colour of the aspirate is expected to be bright red at first, with a gradual darkening within the first 24 hours after surgery. Normally, the colour changes to yellow-green within 36 to 48 hours. If the tube becomes clogged during this period, the health care provider may order periodic gentle irrigations with normal saline solution. It is essential that the NG suction is working and that the tube remains patent so that accumulated gastric secretions do not put a strain on the anastomosis. Such a strain can lead to distension of the remaining portion of the stomach and result in (a) rupture of the sutures, (b) leakage of gastric contents into the peritoneal cavity, (c) hemorrhage, and (d) possible abscess formation. If the tube must be replaced or repositioned, the health care provider must be called to perform this task because of the danger of perforating the gastric mucosa or disrupting the suture line.

The nurse observes the patient for signs of decreased peristalsis and lower abdominal discomfort that may indicate impending intestinal obstruction. Accurate intake and output records must be kept. Vital signs are monitored and recorded every 4 hours.

The patient is kept comfortable and free of pain by the administration of the prescribed medications and by frequent changes in position. The incision is relatively high in the epigastrium and may interfere with deep-breathing and coughing measures. Splinting the area with a pillow while gently and persistently encouraging the patient to put forth their best efforts possible helps prevent pulmonary complications. Splinting also protects the abdominal suture line from rupturing during coughing. The dressing must be observed for signs of bleeding or odour and drainage indicative of an infection. Ambulation is encouraged and is increased daily.

While the NG tube is connected to suction equipment, IV therapy is maintained. Potassium and vitamin supplements are added to the infusion until oral feedings are resumed. Before the NG tube is removed, the patient starts oral feedings of clear liquids to determine the tolerance level. The stomach is aspirated within 1 or 2 hours to assess the amount remaining and its colour and consistency. When fluids are well tolerated, the tube is removed, and fluids are increased in frequency with a slow progression to regular foods. The regimen of six small meals a day is begun.

Pernicious anemia is a long-term complication of total gastrectomy and may occur after partial gastrectomy. Pernicious anemia is caused by the loss of intrinsic factor, which is produced by the parietal cells. Depending on the amount of parietal cell mass removed in surgery, the patient may eventually require regular administration of cobalamin (vitamin B_{12}). (Cobalamin deficiency and pernicious anemia are discussed in Chapter 33.)

PUD is a chronic condition, and ulcers can recur, especially at the site of the anastomosis. Adequate rest, nutrition, and avoidance of known irritants and stressors are keys to complete recovery. Avoiding the use of medications not prescribed by the health care provider should be re-emphasized, along with restrictions on smoking and alcohol use. If the patient is willing to make these kinds of adjustments in their lifestyle, rehabilitation is more likely to be successful.

AGE-RELATED CONSIDERATIONS

PEPTIC ULCER DISEASE

The incidence of peptic ulcers and, in particular, gastric ulcers in patients older than 60 years is increasing. This incidence is related to the increased use of NSAIDs. In older persons, pain may not be the first symptom associated with an ulcer. For some patients, the first manifestation may be frank gastric bleeding (e.g., hematemesis, melena) or a decrease in hematocrit. The rates of morbidity and mortality associated with gastric ulcers are higher in older people than in younger adults because of concomitant health problems (e.g., cardiovascular, pulmonary) and a decreased ability to withstand hypovolemia.

The treatment and management of ulcers in older persons are similar to that in younger adults. An emphasis is placed on prevention of both gastritis and peptic ulcers. This includes teaching patients to take NSAIDs and other gastric-irritating medications with food, milk, or antacids. Patients may be treated with antisecretory agents (i.e., PPIs or H_2R blockers). They should be instructed to avoid irritating substances, such as alcohol and smoking, and to report abdominal pain or discomfort to the health care provider.

CASE STUDY

Hiatal Hernia

Patient Profile
I. C. (pronouns she/her), a 45-year-old elementary school teacher, has had a sliding hiatal hernia for 10 years. She is admitted to the hospital for a hiatal hernia repair.

Subjective Data
- Reports increasing heartburn, especially at night
- Is currently on a bland diet and taking antacids
- Reports substernal pain and heartburn
- Reports some problems with regurgitation

Objective Data
Physical Examination
- 157 cm tall and weighs 88 kg

Diagnostic Study
- Barium swallow study and an endoscopy revealed a large sliding hiatal hernia.

Interprofessional Care
- The patient underwent a Nissen fundoplication through a laparoscopic approach.

Discussion Questions
1. Explain the pathophysiology of a hiatal hernia. What is the difference between a sliding and a paraesophageal hiatal hernia?
2. What are the characteristic symptoms of a hiatal hernia? Which of these did I. C. have?
3. Describe a Nissen fundoplication procedure. What is the objective of this surgical procedure? Why was a laparoscopic approach used?
4. What are potential postoperative complications, and what nursing measures prevent them?
5. What should be included in a teaching plan for I. C.?
6. **Priority decision:** On the basis of the assessment data presented, what are the priority nursing diagnoses? Are there any interprofessional issues?

evolve

Answers are available at http://evolve.elsevier.com/Canada/Lewis/medsurg.

REVIEW QUESTIONS

The number of the question corresponds to the same-numbered objective at the beginning of the chapter.

1. The daughter of a client calls to tell the nurse that her 85-year-old mother has been nauseated all day and has vomited twice. Before the nurse hangs up and telephones the health care provider to communicate the assessment data, what does the nurse instruct the client's daughter to do?
   a. Administer antispasmodic medications and observe skin turgor.
   b. Give her mother sips of water and elevate the head of her bed to prevent aspiration.
   c. Offer her mother a high-protein liquid supplement to drink to maintain her nutritional needs.
   d. Offer her mother large quantities of Gatorade to drink because older persons are at risk for sodium depletion.

2. The nurse explains to a patient with Vincent's infection that treatment will include which of the following?
   a. Smallpox vaccinations
   b. Viscous lidocaine rinses
   c. Amphotericin B suspension
   d. Topical application of antibiotics

3. The nurse is involved in health promotion related to oral cancer. Which behaviours are included in the teaching of adolescents with regard to behaviours that put them at risk for oral cancer? *(Select all that apply.)*
   a. Avoiding use of perfumed lip gloss
   b. Discouraging use of chewing gum
   c. Avoiding use of smokeless tobacco
   d. Discouraging drinking of carbonated beverages
   e. Avoiding excessive alcohol consumption

4. What information is included when the nurse is explaining gastroesophageal reflux disease (GERD) to a client with GERD?
   a. Results in acid erosion and ulceration of the esophagus caused by frequent vomiting
   b. Will require surgical wrapping or repair of the pyloric sphincter to control the symptoms
   c. Is the protrusion of a portion of the stomach into the esophagus through an opening in the diaphragm
   d. Often involves relaxation of the lower esophageal sphincter, allowing stomach contents to back up into the esophagus

5. A client who has undergone an esophagectomy for esophageal cancer develops increasing pain, fever, and dyspnea when a full liquid diet is started postoperatively. What are these symptoms most indicative of?
   a. An intolerance to the feedings
   b. Extension of the tumour into the aorta
   c. Leakage of fluid or foods into the mediastinum
   d. Esophageal perforation with fistula formation into the lung

6. The pernicious anemia that may accompany gastritis is caused by which of the following?
   a. Chronic autoimmune destruction of cobalamin stores in the body
   b. Progressive gastric atrophy from chronic breakage in the mucosal barrier and blood loss
   c. A lack of intrinsic factor normally produced by acid-secreting cells of the gastric mucosa
   d. Hyperchlorhydria resulting from an increase in acid-secreting parietal cells and degradation of red blood cells

7. For the client being discharged after an acute episode of gastrointestinal (GI) bleeding, what information would the nurse's teaching plan include?
   a. Take only medications prescribed by the health care provider.
   b. Avoid taking ASA (Aspirin) with acidic beverages such as orange juice.
   c. Take all medications 1 hour before mealtime to prevent further bleeding.
   d. Read all over-the-counter (OTC) medication labels to avoid those containing stearic acid and calcium.

8. The nurse is teaching the client and her family about possible causes of peptic ulcers. How does the nurse explain ulcer formation?
   a. Caused by a stressful lifestyle and other acid-producing factors such as *Helicobacter pylori*
   b. Inherited within families and reinforced by bacterial spread of *Staphylococcus aureus* in childhood
   c. Promoted by factors that tend to cause oversecretion of acid, such as excess dietary fats, smoking, and *H. pylori*
   d. Promoted by a combination of possible factors that may result in erosion of the gastric mucosa, including certain medications and alcohol

9. What information should be included in an optimal teaching plan for an outpatient with gastric cancer who is receiving radiation therapy?
   a. Cancer support groups, alopecia, and stomatitis
   b. Avitaminosis, ostomy care, and community resources
   c. Prosthetic devices, skin conductance, and grief counselling
   d. Wound and skin care, nutrition, medications, and community resources

10. Several clients are seen at an urgent care centre with symptoms of nausea, vomiting, and diarrhea that began 2 hours ago while they were attending a large family reunion potluck dinner. What kinds of foods that were ingested should the nurse question the patients specifically about? *(Select all that apply.)*
    a. Beef
    b. Meat and milk
    c. Poultry and eggs
    d. Home-preserved vegetables
    e. Potato salad

1. b; 2. d; 3. c; 4. d; 5. c; 6. c; 7. a; 8. d; 9. d; 10. b, e.

For even more review questions, visit http://evolve.elsevier.com/Canada/Lewis/medsurg.

REFERENCES

Almond, L. M., & Barr, H. (2014). Management controversies in Barrett's esophagus. *Journal of Gastroenterology, 49*(2), 195–205. https://doi.org/10.1007/s00535-013-0816-z

Baghdadi, Z. D. (2016). Early childhood caries and Indigenous children in Canada: Prevalence, risk factors, and prevention strategies. *Journal of International Oral Health, 8*(7), 830–837. https://doi.org/10.2047/jioh-08-07-17

BC Cancer Agency. (2021a). *Chemotherapy protocols: Gastrointestinal.* http://www.bccancer.bc.ca/health-professionals/clinical-resources/chemotherapy-protocols/gastrointestinal#Esophaghus

BC Cancer Agency. (2021b). *Esophageal and esophagogastric junction—Screening.* http://www.bccancer.bc.ca/books/esophageal-and-esophagogastric-junction/1-screening

Buckley, F. P. (2020). *Laparoscopic Nissen fundoplication.* https://emedicine.medscape.com/article/1892517-overview

Canadian Cancer Society. (2021a). *Chemotherapy for stomach cancer.* http://www.cancer.ca/en/cancer-information/cancer-type/stomach/treatment/chemotherapy/?region=on

Canadian Cancer Society. (2021b). *Diagnosis of oral cancer.* https://cancer.ca/en/cancer-information/cancer-types/oral/diagnosis

Canadian Cancer Society. (2021c). *Nausea and vomiting.* http://www.cancer.ca/en/cancer-information/diagnosis-and-treatment/managing-side-effects/nausea-and-vomiting/?region=on

Canadian Cancer Society. (2021d). *Risk factors for esophageal cancer.* https://cancer.ca/en/cancer-information/cancer-types/esophageal/risks

Canadian Cancer Society. (2021e). *Risks for stomach cancer.* https://www.cancer.ca/en/cancer-information/cancer-type/stomach/risks/?region=on

Canadian Cancer Society. (2021f). *Stomach cancer statistics.* https://www.cancer.ca/en/cancer-information/cancer-type/stomach/statistics/?region=on

Canadian Cancer Society's Advisory Committee on Cancer Statistics. (2019). *Canadian cancer statistics 2019.* https://cdn.cancer.ca/-/media/files/research/cancer-statistics/2019-statistics/canadian-cancer-statistics-2019-en.pdf

Canadian Society of Intestinal Research. (2021). *Gastroesophageal reflux disease (GERD).* https://badgut.org/information-centre/a-z-digestive-topics/gerd/

Cancer Care Ontario. (2019). *Ontario cancer facts: Incidence of esophageal adenocarcinoma continues to rise.* https://www.cancercareontario.ca/en/cancer-facts/incidence-esophageal-adenocarcinoma-continues-rise

Centers for Disease Control and Prevention. (2015). *E. coli (Escherichia coli).* https://www.cdc.gov/ecoli/general/index.html

Chen, C. H., Lin, C. L., & Kao, C. H. (2016). Association between gastroesophageal reflux disease and coronary heart disease: A nationwide population-based analysis. *Medicine, 95*(27), e4089. https://doi.org/10.1097/MD.0000000000004089

Colquhoun, A., Hannah, H., Corriveau, A., et al. (2019). Gastric cancer in northern Canadian populations: A focus on cardia and non-cardia subsites. *Cancers, 11*(4), 534. https://doi.org/10.3390/cancers11040534

Halpin, A., & Huckabay, L. (2019). Benefits of nausea vomiting scales in practice—a research study. *EC Emergency Medicine and Critical Care, 3*(11), 1–11.

Jaynes, M., & Kumar, A. B. (2018). The risks of long-term use of proton pump inhibitors: A critical review. *Therapeutic Advances in Drug Safety, 10.* https://doi.org/10.1177/2042098618809927

Kovac, A. (2013). Update on the management of postoperative nausea and vomiting. *Drugs, 73*(14), 1525–1547. https://doi.org/10.1007/s40265-013-0110-7

Kurian, M., & Lobo, A. (2015). Acute upper gastrointestinal bleeding. *Clinical Medicine, 15*(5), 481–485. https://doi.org/10.7861/clinmedicine.15-5-481

Nehra, A. K., Alexander, J. A., Loftus, C. G., et al. (2018). Proton pump inhibitors: Review of emerging concerns. *Mayo Clinic Proceedings, 93,* 240–246. https://doi.org/10.1016/j.mayocp.2017.10.022

Rawla, P., & Barsouk, A. (2019). Epidemiology of gastric cancer: Global trends, risk factors and prevention. *Przegląd Gastroenterologiczny, 14*(1), 26–38. https://doi.org/10.5114/pg.2018.80001

Rx Files Academic Detailing Program. (2014). *Rx files: Drug comparison charts*. Saskatoon Health Region.

Siddiqui, A. H., Farooq, U., & Siddiqui, F. (2021). *Curling ulcer*. StatPearls Publishing. https://www.ncbi.nlm.nih.gov/books/NBK482347

Upchurch, B. (2021). *What is the role of peptic ulcer disease in the etiology of upper gastrointestinal bleeding (UGIB)?* https://www.medscape.com/answers/187857-193365/what-is-the-role-of-peptic-ulcer-disease-in-the-etiology-of-upper-gastrointestinal-bleeding-ugib

Vomero, N. D., & Colpo, E. (2014). Nutritional care in peptic ulcer. *Brazilian Archives of Digestive Surgery, 27*(4), 298–302. https://doi.org/10.1590/S0102-67202014000400017

RESOURCES

CAN-ADAPTT Canadian Smoking Cessation Clinical Practice Guideline
https://www.nicotinedependenceclinic.com/en/canadaptt/PublishingImages/Pages/CAN-ADAPTT-Guidelines/CAN-ADAPTT%20Canadian%20Smoking%20Cessation%20Guideline_website.pdf

Canadian Association of Gastroenterology
https://www.cag-acg.org

Canadian Cancer Society
https://www.cancer.ca

Canadian Society of Gastroenterology Nurses and Associates
https://csgna.com

Canadian Society of Intestinal Research
https://www.badgut.org/

evolve

For additional Internet resources, see the website for this book at http://evolve.elsevier.com/Canada/Lewis/medsurg.

Nursing Management
Lower Gastrointestinal Conditions

Denise Delorey
Originating US chapter by Mariann M. Harding

evolve WEBSITE

http://evolve.elsevier.com/Canada/Lewis/medsurg

- Review Questions (Online Only)
- Key Points
- Answer Guidelines for Case Study
- Student Case Study
  - Ulcerative Colitis

- Customizable Nursing Care Plans
  - Acute Infectious Diarrhea
  - Colostomy/Ileostomy
  - Inflammatory Bowel Disease
  - Laparotomy

- Conceptual Care Map Creator
- Audio Glossary
- Content Updates

LEARNING OBJECTIVES

1. Explain the common etiologies of and the interprofessional care and nursing management of patients with diarrhea, constipation, and fecal incontinence.
2. Describe the common causes of acute abdominal pain and nursing management of the patient who has undergone an exploratory laparotomy.
3. Describe the interprofessional care and nursing management of patients with acute appendicitis, peritonitis, and gastroenteritis.
4. Compare and contrast ulcerative colitis and Crohn's disease, including their pathophysiology, clinical manifestations, complications, interprofessional care, and nursing management.
5. Differentiate among mechanical, neurogenic, and vascular bowel obstructions, including their causes and associated interprofessional care and nursing management.

6. Describe the clinical manifestations and interprofessional management of colorectal cancer.
7. Explain the anatomical and physiological changes and nursing management of the patient with an ileostomy and the patient with a colostomy.
8. Differentiate between diverticulosis and diverticulitis, including their clinical manifestations and associated interprofessional care and nursing management.
9. Compare and contrast the types of hernias, including etiology and surgical and nursing management.
10. Describe the types of malabsorption syndrome and their interprofessional care.
11. Describe the types and clinical manifestations of anorectal conditions and the interprofessional care and nursing management of patients with these conditions.

KEY TERMS

anal fissure
anal fistula
appendicitis
celiac disease
colorectal cancer
constipation
Crohn's disease
diarrhea

diverticulum
fecal impaction
fecal incontinence
gastroenteritis
hemorrhoids
hernia
inflammatory bowel disease (IBD)
intestinal obstruction

irritable bowel syndrome (IBS)
lactase deficiency
ostomy
peritonitis
pilonidal sinus
pseudo-obstruction
short bowel syndrome (SBS)
ulcerative colitis (UC)

DIARRHEA

Diarrhea—the frequent passage of loose, watery stools—is not a disease but a symptom. The term *diarrhea* may mean different things to different patients. It is commonly used to denote an increase in stool frequency or volume and an increase in the looseness of stool.

Etiology and Pathophysiology

Causes of diarrhea can be divided into general classifications of decreased fluid absorption, increased fluid secretion, motility disturbances, or a combination of these (Table 45.1). Causes of acute infectious diarrhea are listed in Table 45.2.

Ingestion of infectious organisms is the primary cause of acute diarrhea. Viruses cause most cases of infectious diarrhea.

Although viral infections can be deadly, they are usually short-lived (48 hours) and mild. Therefore, most patients rarely seek treatment.

Infectious organisms attack the intestines in different ways. Some organisms (e.g., rotavirus A, norovirus, *Giardiasis lamblia*) alter secretion or absorption (or both) of the enterocytes of the small intestine without causing inflammation. Other organisms (e.g., *Clostridioides difficile*, also known as *Clostridium difficile*) impair absorption by destroying cells, cause inflammation in the colon, and produce toxins that also cause damage.

Organisms enter the body in contaminated food (e.g., *Salmonella* organisms in undercooked eggs and chicken) or contaminated drinking water (e.g., *G. lamblia* in contaminated lakes or pools). Travellers often get diarrhea, especially if they travel to countries with poorer sanitation than their own. An infection can also be transmitted from one individual to another via the fecal–oral route. For example, adult day care workers can transmit infection from one resident to another if they do not wash their hands thoroughly after changing soiled linen.

An individual's susceptibility to pathogenic organisms is influenced by age, gastric acidity, intestinal microflora, and immunocompetence. Older people are most likely to suffer life-threatening diarrhea. Since stomach acid kills ingested pathogens, medications designed to decrease stomach acid (e.g., proton pump inhibitors) will promote the growth of gastrointestinal (GI) microflora, alter the GI microbiome, and weaken the immune system (Vilcu et al., 2019).

The healthy human colon contains short-chain fatty acids and bacteria such as *Escherichia coli*. These organisms aid in fermentation and provide a microbial barrier against pathogenic bacteria. Antibiotics kill off the normal flora, making the individual more susceptible to pathogenic organisms. For example, patients receiving broad-spectrum antibiotics (e.g., clindamycin, cephalosporins, fluoroquinolones) are susceptible to pathogenic strains of *C. difficile*. *C. difficile* is the most serious antibiotic-associated diarrhea and is becoming more prevalent. Probiotics, in particular *Saccharomyces boulardii* and *Lactobacillus*, have been shown to be beneficial and safe to use in preventing antibiotic-induced diarrhea in some patients (Blaabjerg et al., 2017).

People who are immunocompromised because of disease (e.g., human immunodeficiency virus [HIV]) or immunosuppressive medications are susceptible to GI tract infection.

Not all diarrhea is due to infection. For example, medications and specific food intolerances can cause diarrhea. Also, large amounts of undigested carbohydrate in the bowel produce an osmotic diarrhea that promotes rapid transit and prevents absorption of fluid and electrolytes. Lactose intolerance and

TABLE 45.1 CAUSES OF DIARRHEA

Decreased Fluid Absorption
- Oral intake of poorly absorbable solutes (e.g., laxatives)
- Maldigestion and malabsorption
- Mucosal damage: celiac disease, inflammatory bowel disease, radiation injury, ischemic bowel
- Pancreatic insufficiency (e.g., cystic fibrosis)
- Intestinal enzyme deficiencies (e.g., lactase)
- Bile salt deficiency
- Decreased surface area (e.g., intestinal resection, short gut syndrome)

Increased Fluid Secretion
- Infectious: bacterial endotoxins (e.g., cholera, *Escherichia coli*, *Shigella*, *Salmonella*, *Staphylococcus*, *Clostridium difficile*), viral agents (e.g., rotavirus), and parasitic agents (e.g., *Giardia lamblia*)
- Medications: laxatives, antibiotics, suspensions, or elixirs containing sorbitol
- Foods: candy, gum, and mints containing sorbitol
- Hormonal: vasoactive intestinal polypeptide secretion from adenoma of the pancreas; gastrin secretion caused by Zollinger–Ellison syndrome; calcitonin secretion from carcinoma of the thyroid
- Tumour: villous adenoma

Motility Disturbances
- Irritable bowel syndrome: ↑ visceral sensitivity and transit
- Diabetic enteropathy: ↑ transit secondary to autonomic neuropathy
- Gastrectomy: ↑ transit as a result of dumping syndrome

TABLE 45.2 CAUSES OF ACUTE INFECTIOUS DIARRHEA

	Onset	Duration	Symptoms and Signs
Viral			
Rotavirus	18–24 hr	3–8 days	Fever, vomiting, and profuse watery diarrhea
Norwalk virus	18–24 hr	24–48 hr	Nausea, vomiting, diarrhea, stomach cramping
Bacterial			
Escherichia coli	4–24 hr	3–4 days	Four or five loose stools per day, nausea, malaise, low-grade fever
Enterohemorrhagic *E. coli* (O157:H7)	4–24 hr	4–9 days	Bloody diarrhea, severe cramping, fever
Shigella	24 hr	7 days	Watery stools containing blood and mucus; tenesmus, urgency, severe cramping, fever
Salmonella	6–48 hr	2–5 days	Watery diarrhea, nausea, vomiting, abdominal cramps, fever
Campylobacter species	24 hr	<7 days	Profuse, watery diarrhea; malaise, nausea, abdominal cramps, low-grade fever
Clostridium perfringens	8–12 hr	24 hr	Watery diarrhea, abdominal cramps, vomiting
Clostridium difficile	4–9 days after start of antibiotics	24 hr	Associated with antibiotic treatment; symptoms range from mild, watery diarrhea to severe abdominal pain, fever, leukocytosis, leukocytes in stool
Parasitic			
Giardia lamblia	1–3 wk	Few days to 3 months	Sudden onset; malodorous, explosive, watery diarrhea; flatulence, epigastric pain and cramping, nausea
Entamoeba histolytica	4 days	Weeks to months	Frequent soft stools with blood and mucus (in severe cases, watery stools), flatulence, distension, abdominal cramps, fever, leukocytes in stool
Cryptosporidium	2–10 days	1–6 months	Watery diarrhea, nausea, vomiting, abdominal cramps, weight loss in AIDS

AIDS, acquired immune deficiency syndrome.

certain laxatives (e.g., lactulose, sodium phosphate, magnesium citrate) produce an osmotic diarrhea. Bile salts and undigested fats also lead to excessive fluid secretion in the GI tract. The diarrhea from celiac disease and short bowel syndrome results from malabsorption in the small intestine.

Clinical Manifestations

Diarrhea may be acute or chronic. Acute diarrhea most commonly results from infection. Bacterial or viral infection of the intestine may result in explosive watery diarrhea, tenesmus (spasmodic contraction of the anal sphincter, with pain and persistent desire to defecate), and cramping abdominal pain. Perianal skin irritation may also develop. Systemic manifestations include fever, nausea, vomiting, and malaise. Leukocytes, blood, and mucus may be present in the stool, depending on the causative agent (see Table 45.2). Acute diarrhea is often self-limiting in the adult. Symptoms continue until the irritant or the causative agent is excreted. The mucous membrane lining of the GI tract is composed of epithelial cells, which regenerate following the inflammatory response.

Diarrhea is considered chronic when it persists for at least 2 weeks or when it subsides and returns more than 2 to 4 weeks after the initial episode. Severe diarrhea may be debilitating and life-threatening. A patient may have severe dehydration (water and sodium loss) and electrolyte disturbances (e.g., hypokalemia). Malabsorption and malnutrition are also sequelae of chronic diarrhea. Throughout the world, diarrhea is one of the major causes of death.

Diagnostic Studies

Accurate diagnosis and management of diarrhea require a thorough history, physical examination, and when indicated, laboratory tests. A thorough history, including history of travel, medication use, diet and food allergies, previous surgery and adjunctive therapies, interpersonal contacts, and family history, should be obtained. Blood tests may identify anemia, elevated white blood cell (WBC) count, iron and folate deficiencies, elevated liver enzyme levels, and electrolyte disturbances. Stools may be examined for the presence of blood, mucus, WBCs, and ova and parasites. Stool cultures help in identifying infectious organisms.

In a patient with chronic diarrhea, measurement of stool electrolytes, pH, and osmolality may help determine whether the diarrhea is related to decreased fluid absorption or increased fluid secretion (secretory diarrhea). Measurement of stool fat and undigested muscle fibre may indicate fat and protein malabsorption conditions, including pancreatic insufficiency. Elevated serum levels of GI hormones such as vasoactive intestinal polypeptide and gastrin may be present in some patients with secretory diarrhea. Endoscopy may be used to examine the mucosa and to obtain specimens via biopsy for examination. Upper and lower radiographic studies with barium contrast may be helpful in detecting mucosal disease as well as structural abnormalities.

Interprofessional Care

The treatment of diarrhea is based on the cause and is aimed at replacing fluid and electrolytes and decreasing the number, volume, and frequency of stools. Oral solutions containing glucose and electrolytes (e.g., Pedialyte) may be sufficient to replace losses from mild diarrhea. In situations of severe diarrhea, parenteral administration of fluids, electrolytes, vitamins, and nutrition is warranted.

TABLE 45.3 MEDICATION THERAPY
Antidiarrheal Medications

Type	Mechanism of Action	Examples
Demulcent	Soothes, coats, and protects mucous membranes	Bismuth subsalicylate* (Pepto-Bismol); calcium polycarbophil
Anticholinergic (combination products)	Inhibits GI motility	Diphenoxylate with atropine sulphate (Lomotil), loperamide (Imodium)†‡
Antisecretory	Decreases intestinal secretion	Octreotide (Sandostatin), a synthetic analogue of somatostatin
Opioid	Decreases CNS stimulation of GI tract motility and secretion; directly inhibits GI motility	Codeine
Probiotics	Alters balance of intestinal flora	*Saccharomyces, Lactobacillus*

CNS, central nervous system; *GI*, gastrointestinal.
*Also inhibits bacterial activity.
†Also absorbent, which contributes to adhesiveness of the stool.
‡Has cholinergic and noncholinergic actions.

Once the cause of the diarrhea has been determined, pharmacological agents may be given to coat and protect mucous membranes, absorb irritating substances, inhibit GI motility, decrease intestinal secretions, and decrease central nervous system stimulation of the GI tract (Table 45.3). Patients with infectious diarrhea are not given antidiarrheal agents because of the potential of prolonging exposure to the infectious agent. Regardless of the cause of diarrhea, antidiarrheal medications should not be given for a prolonged period of time. Antibiotics are reserved for treating specific bacterial organisms. Antibiotics can cause diarrhea by altering the normal bowel flora. Patients receiving antibiotics (e.g., clindamycin) are susceptible to *C. difficile* infection.

C. difficile is a bacterium that causes diarrhea and inflammation of the colon (*colitis*) (Centers for Disease Control and Prevention, 2021). This bacterium has been found to be present in normal bowel flora as well as in the genitourinary tract, in abdominal wounds, and on the skin of hospital workers. Patients entering hospitals may already be colonized with *C. difficile*. Generally, healthy people are not usually vulnerable to the organism. Prolonged antibiotic therapy, cytotoxic chemotherapy, and advanced age are risk factors that may affect the bowel's resistance to colonization or its ability to suppress competing organisms, thus enhancing the growth of *C. difficile*. *C. difficile* is the most common cause of infectious diarrhea in the developed world and one of the most common infections in both hospitals and long-term care facilities in Canada. Health care workers should follow infection control precautions to prevent transmission of *C. difficile* from patient to patient (Table 45.4). Symptoms of *C. difficile* include watery diarrhea with or without blood (at least three bowel movements per day for 2 or more days), fever, loss of appetite, nausea, and abdominal pain or tenderness.

Laboratory confirmation may be made on the basis of a single, unpreserved stool sample. Metronidazole (Flagyl) is the first-line therapy for this infection, followed by vancomycin. Although vancomycin and fidaxomicin have been found to be

TABLE 45.4 HAND HYGIENE TO PREVENT HEALTH CARE–ASSOCIATED INFECTIONS

The Five Moments for Hand Hygiene in Health Care
1. BEFORE touching a patient
2. BEFORE clean/aseptic procedures
3. AFTER body fluid exposure/risk
4. AFTER touching a patient–patient
5. AFTER touching a patient environment contact

Source: World Health Organization. (2020). *My 5 moments for hand hygiene.* https://www.who.int/campaigns/world-hand-hygiene-day

TABLE 45.5 NURSING ASSESSMENT

Diarrhea

Subjective Data
Important Health Information
Past health history: Recent travel, infections, stress; diverticulitis or malabsorption; metabolic disorders; inflammatory bowel disease; irritable bowel syndrome; chronic laxative abuse
Medications: Use of laxatives, magnesium-containing antacids, sorbitol-containing suspensions or elixirs, antibiotics, methyldopa, digitalis, colchicine; OTC antidiarrheal medications
Surgery or other treatments: Stomach or bowel surgery, radiation

Symptoms
- Malaise
- Food intolerances; anorexia, nausea, vomiting; weight loss; thirst
- Increased stool frequency, volume, and looseness; change in colour and character of stools; steatorrhea, abdominal bloating; decreased urinary output
- Abdominal tenderness, abdominal pain and cramping; tenesmus

Objective Data
General
Lethargy, sunken eyeballs, fever, malnutrition

Integumentary
Pallor, dry mucous membranes, poor skin turgor, perianal irritation

Gastrointestinal
Frequent soft to liquid stools that may alternate with constipation; altered stool colour; abdominal distension, hyperactive bowel sounds; presence of pus, blood, mucus, or fat in stools; fecal impaction

Urinary Tract
Decreased output, concentrated urine

Possible Findings
Abnormal serum electrolyte levels; anemia; leukocytosis; eosinophilia; hypoalbuminemia; positive stool cultures; presence of ova, parasites, leukocytes, blood, or fat in stool; abnormal sigmoidoscopic or colonoscopic findings; abnormal lower GI series (barium enema study)

GI, gastrointestinal; *OTC,* over-the-counter.

more effective than metronidazole, the difference in effectiveness was minimal and did not outweigh the cost savings of metronidazole (Nelson et al., 2017).

NURSING MANAGEMENT ACUTE INFECTIOUS DIARRHEA

NURSING ASSESSMENT

Nursing assessment should begin with a thorough history and physical examination (Table 45.5). The patient should be asked to describe the stool pattern and associated symptoms. Questions should focus on duration of diarrhea and frequency, character, and consistency of stool. A medication history should include use of antibiotics, laxatives, and other medications known to cause diarrhea. Recent travel, stress, and health and family illnesses should be discussed. Dietary history should include questions about eating habits, appetite, and food intolerances, especially milk and dairy products, as well as food preparation practices.

Physical examination begins with obtaining vital signs, height, and weight. The patient's skin should be inspected for decreased turgor, dryness, and areas of breakdown. The abdomen should be inspected for distension, auscultated for bowel sounds, and palpated for tenderness.

NURSING DIAGNOSES

Nursing diagnoses for the patient with acute infectious diarrhea may include but are not limited to the following:
- *Diarrhea* resulting from *infection*
- *Dehydration* resulting from *insufficient fluid intake, excessive fluid loss through abnormal route*

For additional information on nursing diagnoses for diarrhea, see those presented in Nursing Care Plan (NCP) 45.1, available on the Evolve website.

PLANNING

The overall goals are that the patient with diarrhea will (1) not transmit the microorganism causing the infectious diarrhea, (2) cease having diarrhea and resume normal bowel patterns, (3) have normal fluid and electrolyte and acid–base balance, (4) have normal nutritional intake, and (5) have no perianal skin breakdown.

NURSING IMPLEMENTATION

Adherence to appropriate infection control practices and precautions (see Chapter 17, Table 17.8) is important, and all cases of acute diarrhea should be considered infectious until the cause is determined. The use of precautions is effective in reducing the spread of infectious diarrhea.

Hand hygiene is the most important measure in preventing the transfer of microorganisms. Hands should be washed before and after contact with each patient and when body fluids of any kind are handled. The patient should be taught the principles of hygiene, infection control practices and precautions, and the potential dangers of an illness that is infectious to themselves and others. Family and visitors should also be advised of precautions. Proper handling, cooking, and storage of food should be discussed with the patient suspected of having infectious diarrhea.

Best practice guidelines for the management of *C. difficile* (see the Resources at the end of this chapter) state that all patients suspected of having *C. difficile* should be placed in a single room with dedicated toileting facilities such as a private bathroom or individual commode chair. When the number of patients with *C. difficile* exceeds the institution's single-room capacity, those patients with confirmed *C. difficile* may share a room. For patients in multi-bed rooms, the following precautions should be observed:
1. Signage indicating the precautions to be used should be visibly displayed.
2. An isolation cart should be easily accessible.
3. A laundry hamper should be placed as close to the patient's bed space as possible.
4. A commode chair should be dedicated for the patient's use.

Signage indicating that contact precautions are to be used should be posted on the door of any room of a patient with suspected or confirmed *C. difficile.* The nurse should ensure that appropriate environmental cleaning is taking place, including twice-daily cleaning with a hospital-grade disinfectant, that is approved by Health Canada to kill *C. difficile* spores, of all horizontal surfaces in the room and all items within reach of patients with suspected or confirmed *C. difficile.* Visitors should receive instruction from the nurse regarding the nature of *C. difficile* and the importance of hand hygiene and how to properly carry it out. Use of soap and warm water is recommended because alcohol-based hand sanitizers do not effectively destroy *C. difficile* spores. If a visitor is providing care for a patient or having significant contact with the patient's immediate environment, the visitor should wear gloves and a gown. The visitor should also receive instruction from the nurse on the correct use of personal protective equipment and be instructed not to use the patient's toilet or go into other patients' rooms. Chapter 17 discusses contact precautions.

Meticulous perianal skin care is important to implement for patients with diarrhea in order to avoid skin breakdown. Products that could cause harm (e.g., anal scented wipes, steroid ointments) in the perianal area should not be used, as contact dermatitis is associated with delayed symptom improvement (Chang, 2016). The nurse should educate the patient about proper perianal care after elimination. The nurse needs to monitor the patient's fluid and electrolyte status (see Chapter 19) and implement measures to support healthy nutrition.

CONSTIPATION

Constipation is a decrease in frequency of bowel movements from what is usual for the individual; the presence of hard, difficult-to-pass stools; a decrease in stool volume; retention of feces in the rectum; or some combination of these conditions. Because individuals vary, it is important to compare current symptoms with the patient's usual pattern of elimination. It is also important to remember that changes in bowel habits may indicate bowel obstruction produced by an underlying disease process, such as a tumour.

Etiology and Pathophysiology

Constipation may be caused by insufficient dietary fibre, inadequate fluid intake, medications, and lack of exercise. If proper preventive measures are subsequently taken, constipation should not recur. Constipation may also occur as a result of behaviours related to sociocultural beliefs, environmental constraints, ignoring the urge to defecate, chronic laxative abuse, and multiple organic causes. Changes in diet, mealtime, or daily routines are a few environmental factors that may cause constipation. Depression and stress can also result in constipation.

Some patients believe that they are constipated if they do not have a daily bowel movement. This can result in chronic laxative use and subsequent cathartic colon syndrome. In this condition, the colon becomes dilated and *atonic* (lacking muscle tone).

Ignoring the urge to defecate for a time causes the muscles and mucosa in the rectal area to become insensitive to the presence of feces. In addition, the prolonged retention of feces in the rectum results in drying of the stool because of the absorption of water. The harder and drier the feces, the more difficult they are to expel.

TABLE 45.6	CLINICAL MANIFESTATIONS OF CONSTIPATION
• Abdominal distension or bloating	• Increased rectal pressure
• Abdominal pain	• Nausea
• Anorexia	• Palpable mass
• Decreased frequency of bowel movements	• Stone- or rock-shaped stool (fecalith)
• Hard, dry stool	• Stool with blood
• Headache	• Straining
• Increased flatulence	• Tenesmus

Clinical Manifestations

The clinical presentation of constipation may vary from a chronic discomfort to an acute event mimicking an "acute abdomen." Other clinical manifestations are presented in Table 45.6. Hemorrhoids, or dilated hemorrhoidal veins or varicosities, are the most common complication of chronic constipation. They result from venous engorgement caused by repeated executions of the Valsalva manoeuvre (straining) and venous compression from hard, impacted stool. (Hemorrhoids are further discussed later in this chapter, in the section on anorectal conditions.)

The Valsalva manoeuvre involves contraction of the chest muscles on a closed glottis with simultaneous contraction of the abdominal muscles; it is used during straining to pass a hardened stool and may cause serious conditions in patients with heart failure, cerebral edema, hypertension, and coronary artery disease. During straining, the patient takes a deep inspiration, the breath is held, and the glottis closes and traps the air. Simultaneously with the contraction of the chest muscles against the closed airway, the abdominal muscles contract and try to push against the colon. Increases in intra-abdominal pressure and intrathoracic pressure occur, reducing venous return to the heart. The heart slows (bradycardia) temporarily, cardiac output is decreased, and there is a transient drop in arterial pressure. When the patient relaxes, there is decreased thoracic pressure and a sudden flow of blood into the heart, causing distension and an increase in heart rate. Immediately, arterial pressure rises momentarily. These changes may be fatal for the patient who cannot compensate for sudden overload of blood flow returning to the heart.

Constipation may contribute to diverticulosis. Diverticula are thought to be caused by increased intraluminal pressure and decreased intestinal compliance. Diverticulosis and diverticulitis are described later in this chapter.

In the presence of *obstipation,* or fecal impaction secondary to constipation, colonic perforation may occur. Perforation, which is life-threatening and can lead to peritonitis, causes abdominal pain, nausea, vomiting, fever, and an elevated WBC count. An abdominal radiograph shows the presence of free air, which is diagnostic of perforation. Anal fissures and rectal mucosal ulcers may also occur as a result of stool stasis or straining.

Diagnostic Studies and Interprofessional Care

A thorough history and physical examination should be performed to determine the underlying cause of constipation and initiate treatment. Abdominal radiographs, barium enema, colonoscopy, sigmoidoscopy, and anorectal manometry may be helpful in the diagnosis. Many cases of constipation can be managed with diet therapy, including increased intake of

TABLE 45.7   MEDICATION THERAPY

Cathartic Agents

Category	Mechanisms of Action	Example	Onset of Action	Comments
Bulk-forming	Absorb water; increase bulk-stimulating peristalsis	Psyllium: Metamucil	Usually within 24 hr	Must be taken with adequate fluids; can increase gas; contraindicated in patients with possible obstruction or known strictures
Stool softeners and lubricants	Lubricate intestinal tract and soften feces, making hard stools easier to pass; do not affect peristalsis	Mineral oil, docusate calcium, docusate sodium (Colace)	Softeners up to 72 hr; lubricants up to 8 hr	Can block absorption of fat-soluble vitamins A, D, E, and K
Saline and osmotic solutions	Cause retention of fluid in intestinal lumen due to osmotic effect	Magnesium salts: magnesium citrate, magnesium hydroxide (milk of magnesia) Sodium phosphates: Fleet enema, Fleet Phospho-Soda oral solution Lactulose Polyethylene glycol saline solutions: PegLyte, GoLYTELY, Colyte	15 min–3 hr	Magnesium-containing products may cause hypermagnesemia in patients with renal insufficiency; sodium phosphate products may cause electrolyte imbalances in patients with renal insufficiency (increased sodium, increased phosphate, decreased calcium)
Stimulants	Increase peristalsis by irritating colon wall and stimulating enteric nerves	Anthraquinone medications: cascara sagrada, senna (Senokot) bisacodyl (Dulcolax)	Usually within 12 hr	Can cause melanosis coli (brown or black pigmentation of colon); are most widely abused laxatives; should not be used in patients with impaction or obstipation
Selective chloride channel activator	Increases intestinal fluid secretion and motility	Lubiprostone (Amitiza)	Usually within 24 hr	Used in the treatment of idiopathic constipation and irritable bowel syndrome with constipation (women only) Contraindicated in patients with history of mechanical GI obstruction
Intestinal secretagogue	Increases fluid secretion and accelerates intestinal transit	Linaclotide (Constella)	Usually within 24 hr	Used in the treatment of idiopathic constipation and irritable bowel syndrome with constipation (men and women)

fibre and fluids, and an exercise program. A dietitian can be consulted to review dietary influences. Laxatives (Table 45.7) should be used with caution because with chronic overuse, they may contribute to ongoing constipation. A stepwise approach for laxative use that progresses from bulk-forming fibre preparations to stimulants is recommended, depending on the acuteness of the constipation episode. Enemas are fast-acting and are beneficial in the immediate treatment of constipation, but their use for long-term treatment of constipation should be limited. Soapsuds enemas should be avoided because they may lead to inflammation of colonic mucosa. Excessive hypotonic enemas with tap water can cause intravascular fluid volume excess, and sodium phosphate enemas have been associated with electrolyte imbalances. Oil-retention enemas may be used to soften fecal impactions. Biofeedback therapy may benefit patients who are constipated as a result of *anismus* (uncoordinated contraction of the anal sphincter during straining). Methylnaltrexone (Relistor) is a peripheral μ-opiate receptor antagonist that decreases constipation caused by opioid use. The medication is administered subcutaneously. This agent does not block the analgesic effects (Salix Pharmaceuticals, 2018).

Nurses must educate patients in whom the perception of constipation is related to beliefs and misinformation about bowel function. Appropriate information on normal bowel function must be given and discussed along with information on the adverse consequences of excessive use of laxatives and enemas.

A patient with severe constipation related to bowel motility or mechanical disorders may require more intensive treatment.

Diagnostic studies such as anorectal manometry, GI tract transit studies, and sigmoidoscopic rectal biopsies should be performed before treatment.

Nutritional Therapy. Diet is an important factor in the prevention of constipation. Many patients experience an improvement in their symptoms when they simply increase their intake of dietary fiber and fluids. Dietary fiber is found in two forms: insoluble and soluble in water. Both are contained in most foods, but some foods are higher in soluble fibre (Table 45.8).

Insoluble fibre, which is found in higher concentrations in whole wheat and bran, remains essentially unchanged by the time it reaches the colon. Soluble fibers form gel-like substances that add viscosity to the digested contents, causing decreased gastric emptying and increased transit in the small intestine. When these fibres ferment and form gas, the gas increases stool bulk, promoting defecation and sequestering fluid, which softens stools. Soluble fibre is found in oat bran, fruits, vegetables, and psyllium. Patients should be informed that fibre will increase gas production initially but that this effect decreases with time.

The diet should also include a fluid intake of at least 3 000 mL/day, unless contraindicated by cardiac or renal disease. Increasing fiber intake without increasing fluids may predispose the patient to worsening constipation, impaction, or obstruction. The nurse should consult a dietitian to help with patient food preferences and access. The patient's understanding of the diet and the importance of dietary fibre is important for ensuring compliance.

TABLE 45.8 NUTRITIONAL THERAPY
High-Fibre Foods*

	Fibre per Serving (g)	Size of Serving	Calories of Serving
Vegetables			
Asparagus	3.5	½ cup	18
Beans			
• Navy	8.4	½ cup	80
• Kidney	9.7	½ cup	94
• Lima	8.3	½ cup	63
• Pinto	8.9	½ cup	78
• String	2.1	½ cup	18
Broccoli	3.5	½ cup	18
Carrots, raw	1.8	½ cup	15
Corn	2.6	½ medium ear	72
Peas, canned	6.7	½ cup	63
Potatoes			
• Baked	1.9	½ medium	72
• Sweet	2.1	½ medium	79
Squash, acorn	7.0	1 cup	82
Tomato, raw	1.5	1 small	18
Fruits			
Apple	2.0	½ large	42
Banana	1.5	½ medium	48
Blackberries	6.7	¾ cup	40
Orange	1.6	1 small	35
Peach	2.3	1 medium	38
Pear	2.0	½ medium	44
Raspberries	9.2	1 cup	42
Strawberries	3.1	1 cup	45
Grain Products			
Bread			
• Rye	0.8	1 slice	62
• White	0.7	1 slice	64
• Whole wheat	1.3	1 slice	59
Cereal			
• All-Bran (100%)	8.4	⅓ cup	70
• Corn Flakes	2.6	¾ cup	70
• Shredded Wheat	2.8	1 biscuit	70
Crackers, graham	1.4	2 squares	53
Popcorn	3.0	3 cups	62
Rice			
• Brown	1.6	⅓ cup	72
• White	0.5	⅓ cup	76

*Recommended for patients with diverticulosis, irritable bowel syndrome, constipation, hemorrhoids, atherosclerosis, dyslipidemia, and diabetes mellitus.

NURSING MANAGEMENT CONSTIPATION

NURSING ASSESSMENT
Subjective and objective data that should be obtained from a patient with constipation are presented in Table 45.9.

NURSING DIAGNOSES
Nursing diagnoses for the patient with constipation can include but are not limited to the following:
• *Constipation* resulting from *decrease in gastrointestinal motility, dehydration*

PLANNING
The overall goals are that the patient with constipation will (1) increase dietary intake of fibre and fluids; (2) have the passage of soft, formed stools; and (3) not have any complications, such as bleeding hemorrhoids.

TABLE 45.9 NURSING ASSESSMENT
Constipation

Subjective Data
Important Health Information
Current health history: Chronic laxative or enema abuse; rigid beliefs regarding bowel routine; changes in diet or mealtime; inadequate fibre and fluid intake; immobility; change in daily activity routines; sedentary lifestyle
Past health history: Colorectal disease, neurological dysfunction, bowel obstruction, environmental changes, cancer, irritable bowel syndrome; history of chronic laxative or enema abuse
Medications: Use of aluminum and calcium antacids, anticholinergics, antidepressants, antihistamines, antipsychotics, diuretics, opioids, iron, laxatives, enemas

Symptoms
• Malaise
• Anorexia, nausea
• Hard, difficult-to-pass stool, decrease in frequency and amount of stools; flatus, abdominal distension; tenesmus, rectal pressure; fecal incontinence (if impacted)
• Dizziness, headache, anorectal pain; abdominal pain on defecation

Objective Data
General
Lethargy

Integumentary
Anorectal fissures, hemorrhoids

Gastrointestinal
Abdominal distension; hypoactive or absent bowel sounds; palpable abdominal mass, usually in LLQ; fecal impaction; small, hard, dry stool; stool streaked with blood

Possible Findings
Positive FOB; abdominal radiograph demonstrating stool in lower colon

FOB, fecal occult blood test; *LLQ,* left lower quadrant.

NURSING IMPLEMENTATION
Nursing management should be based on the patient's symptoms (see Table 45.6) and the assessment of the patient (see Table 45.9). An important role of the nurse is teaching the patient the importance of dietary measures to prevent constipation. A patient and caregiver teaching guide for constipation is presented in Table 45.10. Additional constipation guidelines are readily available, including those developed by the Registered Nurses' Association of Ontario (RNAO, 2011). Emphasis should be placed on maintenance of a high-fibre diet, increased fluid intake, and a regular exercise program. The patient should be taught to (1) establish a regular meal pattern, (2) maintain a regular time to defecate, and (3) avoid suppressing the urge to defecate. In many people, the urge to defecate occurs after breakfast because of the stimulation of the gastrocolic reflex. The patient should be discouraged from using laxatives and enemas to achieve and maintain fecal elimination.

Proper position is important when defecating. For a patient in bed, the bedpan should be placed and the head of the bed should be elevated as high as the patient can tolerate. For the person who can sit on a toilet, a footstool may be placed in front of the toilet. Placing the feet on the footstool promotes flexion of the hips, which assists in defecation. For patients requiring commodes, tilt commodes may provide proper positioning.

The patient with poor muscle tone should be assessed by a physiotherapist for abdominal muscle strength and taught to

TABLE 45.10	**PATIENT & CAREGIVER TEACHING GUIDE**

Constipation

The following guidelines should be included when teaching the patient and caregiver(s) about constipation.

1. Eat dietary fibre.
   Eat 20 to 30 g of fibre per day. Gradually, over 1 to 2 weeks, increase the amount of fibre eaten. Fibre softens hard stools and adds bulk to stool, promoting evacuation.
   - Foods high in fibre: raw vegetables and fruits, beans, breakfast cereals (All-Bran, oatmeal)
   - Fibre supplements: Metamucil, Citrucel, FiberCon
2. Drink fluids.
   Drink 3 L/day. Drink water or fruit juices; avoid large volumes of caffeinated coffee, tea, and cola. Fluids soften hard stools; caffeine promotes fluid loss through urination.
3. Exercise regularly.
   Walk, swim, or bike at least three times per week. Contract and relax abdominal muscles when standing or by doing sit-ups to strengthen muscles and prevent straining. Exercise stimulates bowel motility and moves stool through the intestine.
4. Establish a regular time to defecate.
   First thing in the morning or after the first meal of the day is a good time because people often have the urge to defecate at this time.
5. Do not delay defecation.
   Respond to the urge to have a bowel movement as soon as possible. Persistently delaying defecation results in hard stools and a decreased "urge" to defecate. More water is absorbed from stool by the intestine over time. The intestine becomes less sensitive to the presence of stool in the rectum.
6. Record your bowel elimination pattern.
   Record bowel movements on a calendar. Regular monitoring of bowel movement will assist in early identification of a health problem.
7. Avoid use of laxatives and enemas.
   Do not overuse laxatives and enemas. They may actually promote constipation because the normal motility of the bowel is interrupted and bowel habituation cannot occur.

TABLE 45.11	**CAUSES OF FECAL INCONTINENCE**

Traumatic
- Anorectal surgery
- Fistulectomy
- Hemorrhoidectomy
- Abdominal surgery (e.g., nerve injury)
- Traumatic injuries (e.g., gunshot wounds, impalements, foreign body insertion)
- Traumatic childbirth
- Sexual abuse
- Anal intercourse

Neurological
- Degenerative diseases
- Dementia
- Diabetes mellitus (secondary to neuropathic changes)
- Multiple sclerosis
- Spinal cord injuries
- Spinal cord tumour
- Stroke

Inflammatory
- Infection
- Radiation
- Inflammatory bowel disease

Other
- Diarrhea
- Fecal impaction
- Loss of rectal elasticity

Pelvic Floor Dysfunction
- Medications
- Rectal prolapse

Functional
- Physical or mobility impairments affecting toileting ability

contract the abdominal muscles several times a day. Sit-ups and straight leg raises can also be used to improve abdominal muscle tone.

FECAL INCONTINENCE

Etiology and Pathophysiology

Fecal incontinence, or the involuntary passage of stool, may result from multiple causes (Table 45.11). It is important to understand normal fecal continence to understand fecal incontinence. Normally, fecal contents pass from the sigmoid colon into the rectum, causing rectal distension. Sensory (stretch) receptors in the muscles surrounding the rectum provide the sensation of rectal filling. This causes a reflex relaxation of the internal anal sphincter and contraction of the external anal sphincter. Sensory receptors in the epithelium of the anal canal can usually distinguish among solid, liquid, and gas. The combination of contraction of the abdominal muscles, relaxation of the pelvic muscles, squatting (which straightens the anorectal angle), and voluntary relaxation of the external anal sphincter allows for elimination of feces. Therefore, motor (contraction of muscles) or sensory (ability to perceive presence of stool or to experience the urge to defecate) disorders or their combination can result in fecal incontinence. In addition, fecal incontinence can be secondary to fecal impaction, which is an accumulation

of hardened feces in the rectum or the sigmoid colon that the individual is unable to move. Fecal incontinence caused by fecal impaction is a common concern in older persons.

Diagnostic Studies and Interprofessional Care

The diagnosis and effective management of fecal incontinence require a thorough health history and physical examination, with appropriate diagnostic studies. In all cases, a rectal examination should be performed, followed by examination with a flexible sigmoidoscope. Fecal impaction, internal prolapse, increased perineal descent, and rectocele may be identified by rectal examination. If the impaction is higher in the colon, an abdominal radiograph may be helpful. Flexible sigmoidoscopy may identify inflammation, tumours, fissures, and other sigmoid–rectal pathological conditions. Other studies may include barium enema, colonoscopy, endorectal ultrasound, and anorectal manometry.

Treatment of incontinence depends on the cause. If fecal incontinence is resulting from noninfectious diarrhea, dietary changes may be advised, and antidiarrheal agents may be prescribed. In contrast, the management of rectoceles (a defect of the recto-vaginal septum) may include teaching the patient exercises to strengthen the muscles of the pelvic floor (Kegel exercises), insertion of a vaginal pessary, and in some cases, surgery.

Fecal impaction usually resolves after manual disimpaction and use of lubricants and cleansing enemas. To prevent recurrence, a high-fibre diet (see Table 45.8), along with increased fluid intake, should be given unless contraindicated. Dietary fibre supplements or bulk-forming laxatives (e.g., psyllium) can improve continence by increasing stool bulk, firming consistency, and promoting sensation of rectal filling. Protection of perianal skin and the use of appropriate fecal containment devices (e.g., perianal pouches or adult briefs) will help to protect skin and promote patient comfort and dignity.

Biofeedback therapy may be an option for the patient. This therapy uses visual and verbal feedback to improve anorectal sensory function, to increase strength of pelvic floor and improve pelvic coordination (Parker et al., 2019). Biofeedback training requires adequate mental status and motivation to learn. It is a safe, painless, and inexpensive treatment for fecal incontinence. (Biofeedback is discussed further in Chapter 12.)

Surgery (e.g., sphincter repair procedures, diverting ostomy) should be considered only when conservative treatment fails.

NURSING MANAGEMENT
FECAL INCONTINENCE

NURSING ASSESSMENT

Fecal incontinence is not only an embarrassment to the patient but also a potential hazard to the patient's normal skin integrity. An assessment of the patient's general condition is necessary to identify the best alternative for managing the patient with fecal incontinence. The health care provider should identify normal bowel habits and current symptoms, including stool frequency and consistency. Information about the passage of blood or mucus, pain during defecation, and a feeling of incomplete evacuation is required. The health care provider determines whether the patient has defecation urgency and is aware of leaking stool. It should be determined whether there is coexisting urinary incontinence.

Assessment should also include history of multiple or traumatic childbirths, previous anorectal surgery, and injury. A neurological assessment that includes evaluation of mental status can be helpful in identifying the most effective treatment for the patient.

NURSING DIAGNOSES

Nursing diagnoses for the patient with fecal incontinence include but are not limited to the following:

- *Bowel incontinence* resulting from *generalized decline in muscle tone* (dysfunctional rectal sphincter)
- *Toileting self-care deficit* resulting from *reduced ability to transfer, impaired mobility*
- *Potential for falls* resulting from *diarrhea, incontinence*
- *Potential for situational low self-esteem* resulting from *decrease in control over environment* (inability to control bowel movements, hospital isolation protocols)
- *Potential for reduced skin integrity* resulting from *excretions* (incontinence of stool)
- *Potential for social isolation* resulting from *social behaviour incongruent with norms* (bowel incontinence)

PLANNING

The overall goals are that the patient with fecal incontinence will (1) have normal bowel control, (2) maintain perianal skin integrity, and (3) not suffer any self-esteem issues resulting from problems with bowel control.

NURSING IMPLEMENTATION

Before starting interventions, it is important to collaborate with the patient. The nurse should inquire whether they have experienced this condition before and, if so, what strategies were helpful. If appropriate, prevention and treatment of fecal incontinence may be managed by implementing a bowel training program. Bowel training is effective for many patients because, once the bowel is empty, the rectum does not fill until the next day. The lack of stool in the rectum reduces the likelihood of incontinence. The patient should be assisted to a commode or bathroom at a regular time daily to assist with re-establishment of

bowel regularity. A good time to establish this pattern is within 30 minutes after breakfast. Most individuals experience an urge to defecate following the first meal of the day because of the gastrocolic reflex. If the usual bowel habits differ from this pattern, efforts should be made to adhere to the patient's individual timing. Patients are at potential for injury due to falls resulting from their inability to control bowel evacuation and attempting to reach a bathroom in time. Safety measures should be implemented to prevent these situations. Best practice guidelines on the prevention of falls are available from the RNAO (2017).

If these techniques are ineffective in re-establishing bowel regularity, a bisacodyl (Dulcolax) or glycerin suppository or a small phosphate enema may be administered 15 to 30 minutes before the usual evacuation time. These preparations stimulate the anorectal reflex and often can be discontinued when a regular pattern is re-established.

Maintenance of skin integrity is important, especially in patients who are bedridden or older persons. Nursing management may necessitate the use of fecal containment devices, incontinence briefs, and meticulous skin care. Rectal tubes and catheters are usually not recommended because their use for an extended period may decrease responsiveness of the rectal sphincter and cause ulceration or perforation of the rectal mucosa. Use of incontinence briefs may be helpful in maintaining skin integrity if changed frequently. Meticulous cleaning after each stool is required. Gentle washing, rinsing, thorough drying, and application of a protective barrier cream with each bowel movement are essential to the maintenance of skin integrity. The skin should also be monitored for the development of yeast or fungal infections.

Perianal pouching is an alternative in the management of fecal incontinence. These are pouches similar in appearance to one-piece ostomy pouches that are designed to be applied over the anus, allowing for the collection of stool. In addition to collecting stool, pouching provides skin protection, odour control, fecal containment, comfort, and dignity. Odour is a common concern to patients; in addition to using pouching, deodorant sprays and room deodorizers may be used. For the patient who is ambulatory, a regular chair or special tilt commode wheelchair may be used. Regardless of the patient's mobility, the nurse must make sure that the skin is clean and intact and the odour is controlled.

ACUTE ABDOMINAL PAIN

Etiology and Pathophysiology and Clinical Manifestations

The causes of an acute onset of abdominal pain ("acute abdomen") are varied and can include conditions related to inflammation, peritonitis, obstruction, and internal bleeding (Table 45.12). The patient may experience abdominal tenderness, nausea, vomiting, diarrhea, constipation, flatulence, fatigue, fever, and abdominal distension.

Diagnostic Studies and Interprofessional Management

Many disorders must be ruled out before a diagnosis is confirmed, requiring an interprofessional team approach. Diagnosis begins with a complete history and physical examination. Physical examination should include a rectal and pelvic examination. A complete blood cell count (CBC), urinalysis, an abdominal radiographic examination, and an electrocardiogram (ECG) are done initially. In women of childbearing age who have acute abdominal pain, pregnancy tests should be performed to rule out ectopic pregnancy. The findings of these studies may provide some information about the cause of the acute abdomen.

Emergency management of the patient with acute abdominal pain is presented in Table 45.13. The goal of management is to stabilize the patient's condition and to identify and treat the cause. When the patient is seen with an acute condition in the abdomen, the health care provider attempts to make a differential diagnosis because some causes of abdominal pain do not necessitate surgery (see Table 45.12). It was previously thought that pain medication should be withheld because analgesics might obscure progression of clinical manifestations and impede diagnosis. In fact, appropriate pain management that does not result in altered consciousness can decrease diffuse pain and abdominal rigidity and help localize the pain, leading to earlier diagnosis and treatment.

In addition to being a therapeutic measure, surgery can also be diagnostic. Operative exploration is done, usually after a careful examination, a review of patient status, and a review of diagnostic test results. Surgical exploration may be done laparoscopically or through an open midline abdominal wound (laparotomy). Direct examination may aid in identifying the cause of the pain and allow for completion of the definitive procedure.

TABLE 45.12	CAUSES OF ACUTE ABDOMINAL PAIN
• Abdominal penetrating trauma	• Mesenteric adenitis
• Acute ischemic bowel injury	• Pancreatitis
• Appendicitis	• Pelvic inflammatory disease
• Blunt abdominal trauma	• Peptic ulcer
• Bowel obstruction with perforation or necrosis	• Perforated gastrointestinal malignancy
• Cholecystitis	• Peritonitis
• Crohn's disease	• Postcolonoscopy bowel perforation
• Diverticulitis ± peritonitis	• Ruptured abdominal aneurysm
• Foreign body perforation	• Ruptured ectopic pregnancy
• Gastritis	• Ruptured ovarian cyst
• Gastroenteritis	• Ulcerative colitis ± toxic megacolon
• Incarcerated or strangulated hernias	• Uterine rupture
	• Volvulus

NURSING MANAGEMENT
ACUTE ABDOMINAL PAIN

NURSING ASSESSMENT

Vital signs, including blood pressure and pulse rate, should be taken immediately to determine hypovolemic changes. An elevated temperature may indicate an inflammatory or infectious process. The abdomen should be inspected for distension, masses, abnormal pulsation, rashes, scars, and pigmentation changes. Bowel sounds should be auscultated. Bowel sounds that are diminished, absent, or hyperactive in a quadrant may indicate a complete bowel obstruction, acute peritonitis, or paralytic ileus. Palpation should be gentle.

A thorough assessment of the patient's symptoms should be made to determine onset, location, intensity, duration, frequency, and character of pain. The nurse should determine

TABLE 45.13	EMERGENCY MANAGEMENT	

Acute Abdominal Pain

Etiology	Assessment Findings	Interventions
Inflammation • Appendicitis • Cholecystitis • Crohn's disease • Diverticulitis • Gastritis • Pancreatitis • Ulcerative colitis	**Abdominal and Gastrointestinal Findings** • Diffuse, localized, dull, burning, or sharp abdominal pain or tenderness • Rebound tenderness and guarding • Abdominal distension • Abdominal rigidity • Nausea and vomiting • Diarrhea • Hematemesis • Melena	**Initial** • Ensure patent airway. • Administer oxygen via nasal cannula or nonrebreather mask if O_2 saturation <94%. • Establish IV access with large-bore catheter and infuse warm normal saline or lactated Ringer's solution. Insert additional large-bore catheter if shock is present, as ordered. • Obtain blood for CBC and serum electrolytes assessment. • Consider ECG.
Vascular Conditions • Ruptured aortic aneurysm • Mesenteric vascular occlusion or ischemia	**Hypovolemic Shock** • ↓ Blood pressure • ↓ Pulse pressure • Tachycardia • Cool, clammy skin • ↓ Level of consciousness	• Anticipate order for amylase level, pregnancy tests, clotting studies, and type and crossmatch as appropriate. • Insert indwelling urinary catheter. • Obtain urine R&M, C&S. • Insert NG tube as needed. • Keep patient on NPO status. • Assess bowel sound characteristics.
Gynecological Conditions • Pelvic inflammatory disease • Ruptured ectopic pregnancy • Ruptured ovarian cyst		**Ongoing Monitoring** • Monitor vital signs, level of consciousness, O_2 saturation, and intake–output.
Infectious Diseases • Giardiasis • Salmonellosis		• Assess pain characteristics. • Assess amount and character of emesis. • Anticipate diagnostic tests.
Other • Obstruction or perforation of abdominal organ • Gastrointestinal bleeding • Trauma		• Anticipate surgical intervention. • Maintain NPO status.

CBC, complete blood cell count; *C&S*, culture and sensitivity; *ECG*, electrocardiogram; *IV*, intravenous; *NG*, nasogastric; *NPO*, nothing by mouth; *R&M*, routine and microscopic.

whether the pain has spread or moved to new locations (quadrants) as well as what makes the pain worse or better. It should also be determined whether the pain is associated with other symptoms, such as nausea, vomiting, changes in bowel and bladder habits, or vaginal discharge in women. Assessment of vomiting should include amount, colour, consistency, and odour of the vomitus. Bowel patterns and habits should also be assessed carefully.

NURSING DIAGNOSES

Nursing diagnoses for the patient with acute abdominal pain include but are not limited to the following:

- *Acute pain* resulting from *biological injury agent* (inflammation of the peritoneum, abdominal distension)
- *Potential for inadequate fluid volume* resulting from *insufficient fluid intake* (inflammation or infection)
- *Anxiety* resulting from *threat to current status, threat of death*

PLANNING

The overall goals are that the patient with acute abdominal pain will have (1) resolution of the underlying process, (2) relief of abdominal pain, (3) freedom from complications (especially hypovolemic shock), and (4) normal nutritional status.

NURSING IMPLEMENTATION

Nursing interventions are based on the diagnosis and medical or surgical management of the patient. General care for the patient involves management of fluid and electrolyte imbalances, pain, and anxiety.

ACUTE INTERVENTION

Preoperative Care. Emergency preparation of the patient with acute abdominal pain is usually limited to a CBC, typing and crossmatching of blood, and clotting studies. Catheterization, administration of medications (e.g., antibiotics), and the passage of a nasogastric (NG) tube may be done in the emergency department or operating room. (General care of the preoperative patient is discussed in Chapter 20.)

Postoperative Care. Postoperative care depends on the type of surgical procedure performed. The increased use of laparoscopic procedures has reduced the risk for potential postoperative complications related to wound care and altered GI motility. These newer procedures generally result in shorter hospital stays. A general NCP for the postoperative patient is available on the Evolve website for Chapter 22. Nursing care for the patient following a laparotomy is presented in NCP 45.2, also on the Evolve website.

An NG tube may or may not be present in the patient returning from surgery. If present, the NG tube is connected to suction as ordered. The purpose of the NG tube is to empty the stomach of secretions and gas to prevent gastric distension. GI peristaltic activity is often impaired because of the manipulative procedures of the surgery and anaesthesia.

If the upper GI tract has been entered, drainage from the NG tube may be dark brown to dark red for the first 12 hours. Later, it should be light yellowish-brown, or it may have a greenish tinge because of the presence of bile. If a dark red colour continues or if bright red blood is observed, the health care provider should be notified at once of the possibility of hemorrhage. The "coffee grounds" appearance of the drainage is due to the presence of small amounts of blood that have been chemically altered by gastric secretions.

The NG tube needs to be checked regularly for patency. The tube may become obstructed with mucus, sediment, or blood clots. An order is usually written to irrigate the tube with 20 to 30 mL of tap or sterile water or normal saline solution if needed. An accurate record of intake and output, including emesis and gastric drainage, is essential. The nurse needs to assess serum electrolyte values and acid–base balance because prolonged gastric suctioning can result in loss of sodium, chloride, potassium, water, and hydrochloric acid.

The NG tube is removed when intestinal peristalsis returns, usually 24 to 72 hours after surgery. Motility of the stomach normally returns within 24 to 48 hours. Motility of the small intestine usually resumes within 12 to 24 hours, whereas return of large intestine motility may take as long as 3 to 5 days. Peristaltic activity can be assessed by auscultation for bowel sounds.

Mouth care and nasal care are essential. The patient tends to breathe through the mouth while the NG tube is in place. In addition, increased nasal secretions and crusting result from mechanical stimulation of the NG tube.

Parenteral fluids are administered to provide the patient with fluids and electrolytes until bowel sounds return. Ice chips may be ordered because they aid in the flow of saliva and prevent a dry mouth and sore throat. When bowel sounds return, fluids and food are increased gradually. Nausea and vomiting are not uncommon after abdominal surgery and are often self-limiting. Observation is important in determining the cause. Antiemetics such as dimenhydrinate (Gravol), ondansetron (Zofran), or metoclopramide may be ordered.

Abdominal distension and gas pains are also common after surgery, as a result of swallowed air and impaired peristalsis resulting from immobility, manipulation of abdominal contents during surgery, and adverse effects of anaesthesia. The health care provider should be informed of abdominal distension and rigidity and worsening abdominal pain. Gradually, as intestinal activity increases, distension and gas pains should decrease.

CARE OF NASOGASTRIC AND NASOINTESTINAL TUBES.
Nurses may be instructed to insert NG tubes. Insertion is easier if the patient relaxes, takes deep breaths, and swallows when instructed. Once the tube is in place, it is extremely important to (1) confirm placement of the tube (e.g., by aspiration of gastric contents), (2) ensure the tube is properly secured to prevent dislodgement, and (3) provide appropriate nasal and mouth care. When an NG tube is in place, the patient breathes through the mouth, drying the mouth and lips. The nurse should encourage and assist the patient to brush their teeth frequently. Mouthwash and water for the patient to use in rinsing the mouth and petroleum jelly (if the patient is not on oxygen) or water-soluble lubricant for the lips should be provided at the bedside.

The patient's nose should be assessed for signs of irritation from the NG tube. This area should be cleaned and dried daily with application of a water-soluble lubricant and resecuring the tube with tape or a securement device (e.g., the Dale NasoGastric Tube Holder, Hollister feeding tube attachment device). NG tubes should be checked every 4 hours for patency. Characteristics of NG losses may differ depending on the underlying reason for tube placement. Pale yellow to dark green bile drainage is more likely after abdominal surgery, whereas odoriferous, thick drainage with food particles may be seen with bowel obstructions. Hemolyzed sanguineous drainage (often called "coffee grounds" because of its dark brown, granular appearance) or fresh sanguineous drainage should be reported immediately to the physician or surgeon. The volume of NG losses should also be monitored. Excessive losses (>500–1 000 mL/24 hr) may have to be replaced with intravenous (IV) fluids and electrolytes to maintain adequate hydration. Generally, NG tubes can be removed once normal bowel function returns (passing of gas and stool) and the patient is no longer vomiting.

AMBULATORY AND HOME CARE. Preparation for discharge begins when the patient returns from the operating room. Instructions to the patient and family should include any modifications in activity, care of the incision, diet, and medication therapy. Small, frequent meals high in calories should be taken initially, with a gradually increased intake of food as tolerated.

Normal activities should be resumed gradually. Some activity restrictions may be required for 6 to 8 weeks. The patient should be aware of possible complications after surgery and should notify the health care provider immediately if vomiting, fever, pain, weight loss, incisional drainage, or changes in bowel function occur.

EVALUATION

The expected outcomes are that the patient with acute abdominal pain will have (1) resolution of the cause of the acute abdominal pain; (2) relief of abdominal pain and discomfort; (3) freedom from complications (especially hypovolemic shock and septicemia); and (4) normal fluid, electrolyte, and nutritional status.

ABDOMINAL TRAUMA

Etiology and Pathophysiology

Injuries to the abdominal area occur most often as a result of blunt trauma (e.g., motor vehicle accident) or penetration injuries, primarily gunshot wounds or stab wounds to the abdomen.

Blunt trauma is most common. For Indigenous Canadians, the number intentional injuries is four times higher than for other Canadians (George et al., 2017). Regardless of whether it is a blunt or penetration injury, the result is often the same: damage to or alteration of the internal organs.

Common injuries of the abdomen include lacerated liver, ruptured spleen, pancreatic trauma, mesenteric artery tears, diaphragmatic rupture, urinary bladder rupture, great vessel tears, renal injury, and stomach or intestinal rupture. These injuries may result in massive blood loss and hypovolemic shock. Surgery must be performed as early as possible to repair the damaged organs and to stop the bleeding. Common sequelae of intra-abdominal trauma are peritonitis and sepsis, particularly when the bowel is perforated.

Clinical Manifestations

Clinical manifestations of abdominal trauma are (1) guarding and splinting of the abdominal wall; (2) a hard, distended abdomen (which may indicate intra-abdominal bleeding); (3) decreased or absent bowel sounds; (4) contusions, abrasions, or bruising over the flanks or the abdomen; (5) severe abdominal pain; (6) pain over the scapula caused by irritation of the phrenic nerve by free blood in the abdomen; (7) hematemesis or hematuria; and (8) signs of hypovolemic shock (Table 45.14). An ecchymotic discoloration around the umbilicus (Cullen's sign) and ecchymosis or discoloration of the flanks (Grey Turner sign) can indicate intra-abdominal or retroperitoneal hemorrhage.

Intra-abdominal injuries can also be associated with low rib fractures, fractured femur, fractured pelvis, and thoracic injury. If any of these injuries are present, the patient should be observed for abdominal trauma.

✚ TABLE 45.14 EMERGENCY MANAGEMENT

Abdominal Trauma

Etiology	Assessment Findings	Interventions
Blunt	**Hypovolemic Shock**	**Initial**
• Falls	• ↓ Level of consciousness	• Ensure patent airway.
• Motor vehicle collisions	• Tachypnea	• Administer O$_2$ via face mask.
• Pedestrian accidents	• Tachycardia	• Control external bleeding with direct pressure or sterile
• Assault with blunt object	• ↓ Blood pressure	pressure dressing.
• Crush injuries	• ↓ Pulse pressure	• Establish IV access with two large-bore catheters, and infuse
• Explosions		warm normal saline or lactated Ringer's solution.
	Surface Findings	• Obtain blood for type and crossmatch and CBC.
Penetrating	• Abrasions or ecchymoses on	• Remove clothing.
• Knife	abdominal wall, flank, or perineum	• Stabilize impaled objects with bulky dressing—do not remove.
• Gunshot wounds	• Open wounds: lacerations, eviscerations,	• Cover protruding organs or tissue with sterile, saline dressing.
• Other missiles	puncture wounds, gunshot wounds	• Insert in-dwelling urinary catheter if there is no blood at the
	• Impaled object	meatus, pelvic fracture, or boggy prostate.
	• Healed incisions or old scars	• Obtain urine for urinalysis.
		• Insert NG tube if no evidence of facial or neck trauma.
	Abdominal and Gastrointestinal	• Anticipate diagnostic peritoneal lavage.
	Findings	
	• Nausea and vomiting	**Ongoing Monitoring**
	• Bloody urine	• Monitor vital signs, level of consciousness, O$_2$ saturation, and
	• Abdominal pain	urine output.
	• Abdominal distension	• Maintain patient warmth using blankets, warm IV fluids
	• Abdominal rigidity	(40–45°C), or warm humidified oxygen.
	• Guarding	
	• Rebound tenderness	
	• Pain with radiation to shoulder and back	

CBC, complete blood cell count; *IV*, intravenous; *NG*, nasogastric.

Diagnostic Studies

Specific diagnostic procedures include CBC, urinalysis, radiographs of the abdomen and the chest, high-resolution computed tomographic (CT) scan, and abdominal ultrasound. With the availability of emergency department ultrasound and CT, peritoneal lavage is rarely performed as a diagnostic tool and is contraindicated in pregnant women or patients with pelvic fractures. If performed, the fluid is observed for gross abnormalities—such as the presence of blood, bile, feces, or food fibres—and is sent to the laboratory for microscopic evaluation.

NURSING AND INTERPROFESSIONAL MANAGEMENT ABDOMINAL TRAUMA

Emergency management of abdominal trauma involves an interprofessional team approach and focuses on establishing a patent airway and adequate breathing, fluid replacement, and prevention of hypovolemic shock (see Table 45.14). IV lines are inserted, and volume expanders or blood is given if the patient is hypotensive. An NG tube is inserted to decompress the stomach and prevent the aspiration of vomitus.

Regardless of the mechanism of injury, physical evidence of abdominal trauma in a patient who is hemodynamically unstable mandates immediate laparotomy. In other cases, the indications for laparotomy must be correlated with the mechanism of injury. For example, if an individual has a gunshot wound or impaled object, surgery is usually indicated. An impaled object should never be removed until skilled surgical care is available. Removal may cause further injury and bleeding. If surgery is performed, the postoperative nursing care is similar to the care of the patient after laparotomy (see NCP 45.2, available on the Evolve website).

CHRONIC ABDOMINAL PAIN

Chronic abdominal pain may originate from abdominal structures or may be referred from a site with the same or a similar nerve supply. Some common causes are irritable bowel syndrome, peptic ulcer disease, diverticulitis, chronic pancreatitis, hepatitis, cholecystitis, pelvic inflammatory disease, and vascular insufficiency.

Diagnosis of the cause of chronic abdominal pain presents a challenge. Assessment should begin with a thorough history and identification of the specific pain pattern. Character and severity of pain and its location, duration, and onset should be determined. The assessment should also include the relationship of pain to meals, defecation, and activity and factors that increase or decrease the pain. Chronic abdominal pain can be described as dull, aching, or diffuse.

Endoscopy, CT scans, magnetic resonance imaging (MRI), laparoscopy, and radiological barium studies have decreased the need for exploratory laparotomy. Treatment for chronic abdominal pain is comprehensive and directed toward palliation of symptoms using appropriate medications, such as analgesics and antiemetics, as well as psychological or behavioural therapies (e.g., relaxation therapies).

IRRITABLE BOWEL SYNDROME

Irritable bowel syndrome (IBS) is a chronic functional disorder characterized by intermittent and recurrent abdominal pain associated with an alteration in bowel function (diarrhea or constipation, or both). Other symptoms commonly found include abdominal distension, excessive flatulence, bloating, urge to defecate, urgency, and sensation of incomplete evacuation. IBS is a common condition affecting approximately 5 million Canadians (Canadian Society of Intestinal Research, 2021c). Numerous factors have been identified that precipitate IBS symptoms, including neurological hypersensitivity within the GI (enteric) nerves, physical or emotional stress (or both), dietary issues such as food allergies or sensitivities, antibiotic use, GI infection, bile acid malabsorption, chronic alcohol misuse, abnormalities in GI secretions or digestive muscle contractions *(peristalsis)* (or both), and acute infection or inflammation of the intestine *(enteritis)* such as with travellers' diarrhea (Canadian Society of Intestinal Research, 2021c). IBS is not a psychological disorder, although stress, depression, panic, or anxiety may aggravate bowel symptoms.

The key to accurate diagnosis is a thorough history and physical examination. Emphasis should be placed on symptoms, past health history (including psychosocial aspects such as physical or sexual abuse), family history, and medication and dietary history. Diagnostic tests should be used to rule out more serious life-threatening disorders with symptoms similar to those of IBS, such as colorectal cancer, peptic ulcer disease, inflammatory bowel disease (IBD), and malabsorption disorders. Symptom-based criteria for IBS have been standardized and are referred to as the Rome IV criteria. The Rome IV criteria include abdominal pain once per week for at least 3 months on average that has at least two of the following characteristics: (1) pain related to defecation, (2) pain associated with a change in stool frequency, or (3) pain associated with a change in stool form (appearance) (Schmulson & Drossman, 2017).

Management of IBS is challenging for both the patient and the interprofessional team, requiring a positive therapeutic relationship combined with support and patient education. The team may include specialist nurses, dietitians, psychologists, or social workers who can improve or maintain the patient's quality of life through symptom management.

The health care provider should encourage the patient to verbalize their concerns and anxiety. A diet containing at least 20 g/day of dietary fibre should be initiated, as well as increasing fluid intake (see Table 45.8). This may also include the addition of psyllium-containing products (e.g., Metamucil).

The patient whose primary symptoms are abdominal distension and increased flatulence should be advised to eliminate common gas-producing foods such as broccoli and cabbage from the diet and to use lactose-free products if there is lactose intolerance. Various medications are available, and choice will depend on whether the patient has diarrhea or constipation. Other therapies include relaxation and stress management techniques, antidepressants, acupuncture, and herbal therapy, although no single therapy has been found to be effective for all patients. Patients should be referred to a dietitian to review dietary practices. Maintaining a healthy diet according to *Canada's Food Guide* (see Chapter 42) should be encouraged.

INFLAMMATORY DISORDERS

APPENDICITIS

Appendicitis is an inflammation of the appendix, a narrow, blind tube that extends from the inferior part of the cecum. Appendicitis occurs in approximately 8% of the world's population. It can occur at any age but occurs most often between 10 and 20 years of age (Baird et al., 2017).

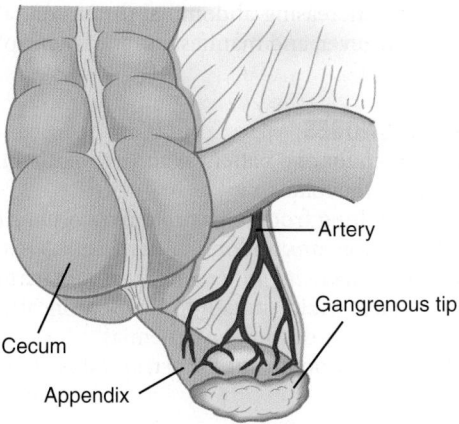

FIG. 45.1 In appendicitis, the blood supply of the appendix is impaired by inflammation and bacterial infection in the wall of the appendix, which may result in gangrene.

Etiology and Pathophysiology

The most common causes of appendicitis are occlusion of the appendiceal lumen by a *fecalith* (accumulated feces) (Figure 45.1) and intramural thickening caused by hypergrowth of lymphoid tissue. Obstruction results in edema, venous engorgement, and invasion by bacteria, which can lead to gangrene and perforation.

Clinical Manifestations

Appendicitis typically begins with periumbilical pain, followed by anorexia, nausea, and vomiting. The pain is persistent and continuous, eventually shifting to the right lower quadrant and localizing at the McBurney point (located halfway between the umbilicus and the right iliac crest). The iliopsoas and obturator tests may further support a diagnosis of appendicitis. Further assessment of the patient reveals localized tenderness, rebound tenderness (Blumberg sign), and muscle guarding. The patient usually prefers to lie still, often with the right leg flexed. Low-grade fever may or may not be present, and coughing aggravates pain. Older persons may report less severe pain, slight fever, and discomfort in the right iliac fossa. The Rovsing sign may be elicited by palpation of the left lower quadrant, causing pain to be felt in the right lower quadrant. Complications of acute appendicitis are perforation, peritonitis, and abscesses.

Diagnostic Studies and Interprofessional Care

Examination of the patient includes a complete history and physical examination (particularly palpation of the abdomen) and a differential WBC count. A urinalysis may be done to rule out genitourinary conditions that mimic the manifestations of appendicitis. CT is the preferred diagnostic procedure, but ultrasound is also used.

The treatment of appendicitis may include surgical removal (appendectomy) if the inflammation is localized. If the appendix has ruptured and there is evidence of peritonitis or an abscess, conservative treatment, consisting of antibiotic therapy and parenteral fluids, may be used to prevent sepsis and dehydration for 6 to 8 hours before an appendectomy is performed.

NURSING MANAGEMENT APPENDICITIS

The patient with abdominal pain is encouraged to see a health care provider and to avoid self-treatment, particularly with laxatives and enemas. The increased peristalsis from these may cause perforation of the appendix. Until the patient is seen by a health care provider, nothing should be taken by mouth (NPO) to ensure that the stomach is empty in the event that surgery is needed. Local application of heat is never used because it may cause the appendix to rupture. In addition, the patient should be observed for evidence of peritonitis. Usually, surgery is performed as soon as a diagnosis is made.

Postoperative nursing management is similar to postoperative care of the patient after laparotomy (see NCP 45.2 on the Evolve website). Ambulation begins the day of surgery or the first postoperative day. The diet is advanced as tolerated. The patient is usually discharged on the first or second postoperative day, and normal activities are resumed 2 to 3 weeks after surgery.

PERITONITIS

Etiology and Pathophysiology

Peritonitis results from a localized or generalized inflammatory process of the peritoneum. Causes of peritonitis are listed in Table 45.15. Peritonitis may appear in acute and chronic forms; trauma or rupture of an organ containing chemical irritants or bacteria (which are released into the peritoneal cavity) may cause it. Examples of a chemical peritonitis include peptic ulcer perforation and ruptured ectopic pregnancy. A chemical peritonitis is commonly followed by bacterial invasion. Bacterial peritonitis can be caused by a traumatic injury (e.g., gunshot wound, ruptured appendix), or it can be secondary to other diseases or conditions (e.g., pancreatitis, peritoneal dialysis).

The response of the peritoneum to the leakage of GI contents is to attempt to localize the offending agent by "walling it off" by exuding fibrin-containing fluids and swelling. Adhesions may form. These adhesions may reduce or disappear when the infection is eliminated. Normally, peritoneal injuries heal without formation of adhesions unless other factors—such as infection, ischemia, or foreign substances—are present.

Clinical Manifestations

Abdominal pain is the most common symptom of peritonitis. A universal sign of peritonitis is tenderness over the involved area. Rebound tenderness, muscular rigidity, and spasm are other major signs of irritation of the peritoneum. Abdominal distension or ascites, fever, tachycardia, tachypnea, nausea, vomiting, and altered bowel habits may also be present. These manifestations vary depending on severity and acuteness of the underlying cause. Complications of peritonitis include sepsis, septic shock, intra-abdominal abscess formation, paralytic ileus, and organ failure.

Diagnostic Studies

A CBC is done to determine elevations in WBC count and hemoconcentration (Table 45.16). Peritoneal aspiration may be performed and the fluid analyzed for blood, bile, pus, bacteria, fungus, and amylase content. A radiograph of the abdomen may show dilated loops of bowel consistent with paralytic ileus, free air if perforation has occurred, or air–fluid levels if an obstruction is present. Ultrasound and CT scans may be used to identify the presence of ascites and abscesses. *Peritoneoscopy* (an endoscope is placed through a stab wound in the abdomen to

TABLE 45.15   CAUSES OF PERITONITIS

Primary	Secondary
• Bloodborne organisms	• Appendicitis with rupture
• Genital tract organisms	• Blunt or penetrating trauma to
• Cirrhosis with ascites	abdominal organs
• GI tract organisms	• Diverticulitis with rupture
	• Ischemic bowel disorders
	• Obstruction in the GI tract
	• Pancreatitis
	• Perforated peptic ulcer
	• Peritoneal dialysis
	• Postoperative anastomotic leak

GI, gastrointestinal.

TABLE 45.16   INTERPROFESSIONAL CARE

Peritonitis

Diagnostic	Postoperative
• History and physical examination	• NPO status
• CBC	• NG tube to suction
• Serum electrolytes	• Semi-Fowler's position
• Abdominal radiographic	• IV fluids with electrolyte
examination	replacement
• Abdominal paracentesis and	• Nutritional support as needed
culture of fluid	• Antibiotic therapy
• CT scan or ultrasound	• Blood transfusions as needed
• Peritoneoscopy	• Sedatives and opioids

Interprofessional Therapy
Preoperative or Nonoperative
• NPO status
• Oxygen support
• Fluid replacement
• Antibiotic therapy
• NG suction
• Analgesics
• Preparation for surgery to include
  the above and nutritional support

CBC, complete blood cell count; *CT*, computed tomographic (scan); *IV*, intravenous; *NG*, nasogastric; *NPO*, nothing by mouth.

inspect the peritoneum) may be helpful in the patient without ascites. Direct examination of the peritoneum can be obtained along with biopsy specimens for diagnosis.

Interprofessional Care

The goals of the management of peritonitis are to identify and treat the cause, eliminate infection, and prevent complications. Patients with milder cases of peritonitis or those who are poor surgical risks may be managed nonsurgically. Treatment consists of antibiotics, NG suction, analgesics, and IV fluid administration. Patients who require surgery need preoperative preparation as previously described. These patients may be placed on parenteral nutrition (PN) because of increased nutritional requirements. (PN, formerly called *total parenteral nutrition* [TPN], is discussed in Chapter 42.)

NURSING MANAGEMENT
PERITONITIS

NURSING ASSESSMENT

Assessment of the patient's pain, including the location, is important and may help in determining the cause of peritonitis. The patient should be assessed for the presence and the quality

of bowel sounds, increasing abdominal distension, abdominal guarding, nausea, fever, and manifestations of hypovolemic and septic shock.

NURSING DIAGNOSES

Nursing diagnoses for the patient with peritonitis include but are not limited to the following:
• *Acute pain* resulting from *biological injury agent* (inflammation of the peritoneum, abdominal distension)
• *Potential for inadequate fluid volume* resulting from *insufficient fluid intake* (fluid shifts into the peritoneal cavity secondary to trauma, infection or ischemia)
• *Anxiety* resulting from *threat to current status, threat of death*

PLANNING

The overall goals for the patient with peritonitis are for (1) resolution of inflammation, (2) relief of abdominal pain, (3) freedom from complications, and (4) normal nutritional status.

NURSING IMPLEMENTATION

The patient with peritonitis is extremely ill and needs skilled supportive care. The patient is monitored for signs of sepsis, pain, and response to analgesic therapy. The patient may be positioned with knees flexed to increase comfort. The nurse should provide rest and a quiet environment.

Accurate monitoring of fluid intake and output and electrolyte status is necessary to determine replacement therapy. Vital signs are monitored frequently. Antiemetics may be administered to decrease nausea and vomiting and further fluid losses. The patient is on NPO status and may have an NG tube in place to decrease gastric distension.

If the patient has an open surgical procedure, drains are inserted to remove purulent drainage and excessive fluid. Postoperative care of the patient is similar to the care of the patient with an exploratory laparotomy (see NCP 45.2, on the Evolve website).

GASTROENTERITIS

Gastroenteritis is an inflammation of the mucosa of the stomach and the small intestine. Clinical manifestations include nausea, vomiting, diarrhea, abdominal cramping, and distension. Fever, increased WBC counts, and blood or mucus in the stool may be present. Causative agents are varied (see Table 45.2). Most cases are self-limiting and do not require hospitalization. However, older patients and patients who are chronically ill may be unable to consume sufficient fluids orally to compensate for fluid loss. Until vomiting has ceased, the patient should be on NPO status. If dehydration has occurred, IV replacement of fluids may be necessary. As soon as tolerated, oral fluids containing glucose and electrolytes should be given. If the causative agent is identified, appropriate pharmacological therapy is initiated.

NURSING MANAGEMENT
GASTROENTERITIS

Accurate monitoring of intake and output is important for successful replacement of lost fluid. Strict medical asepsis and infection control precautions should be instituted when indicated. The patient should be instructed in the importance of proper food handling and preparation of food to prevent infections such as salmonellosis and botulism (see Chapter 44, Table 44.3).

Symptomatic nursing care is given for nausea, vomiting, and diarrhea. The importance of rest and increased fluid intake should be stressed. The nurse should assess reports of pain, vomiting, and diarrhea because often gastroenteritis is confused with appendicitis. To allay the patient's apprehension, the nurse should explain that gastroenteritis usually runs an acute course with no sequelae.

INFLAMMATORY BOWEL DISEASE

Inflammatory bowel disease (IBD) is an autoimmune disease that currently refers to two disorders of the GI tract (Crohn's disease and ulcerative colitis [UC]) characterized by idiopathic inflammation and ulceration. Etiology is based on three characteristics: (1) genetics, (2) altered dysregulated immune response, and (3) altered response to gut microorganisms. The primary trigger is unknown; however, environmental characteristics such as smoking and a diet high in animal protein increase risk of IBD (Rowe 2020). Both UC and Crohn's disease commonly occur during the teenage years and early adulthood, but both have a second peak from ages 50 to 70. Both are more prevalent in industrialized regions of the world. Epidemiological studies show a higher incidence of IBD in White people (particularly those of Jewish descent) (see the Determinants of Health box) and in family members (especially monozygotic compared with dizygotic twins). For both conditions, the clinical manifestations are varied, with unpredictable periods of remission interspersed with episodes of acute inflammation (Figure 45.2). Both diseases can be debilitating. In Canada, 7 out of 1 000 people currently have IBD (Benchimol et al., 2019). Many patients with IBD are treated with immunosuppressant medications and may be at a higher risk of infection (see treatment for specific IBD conditions).

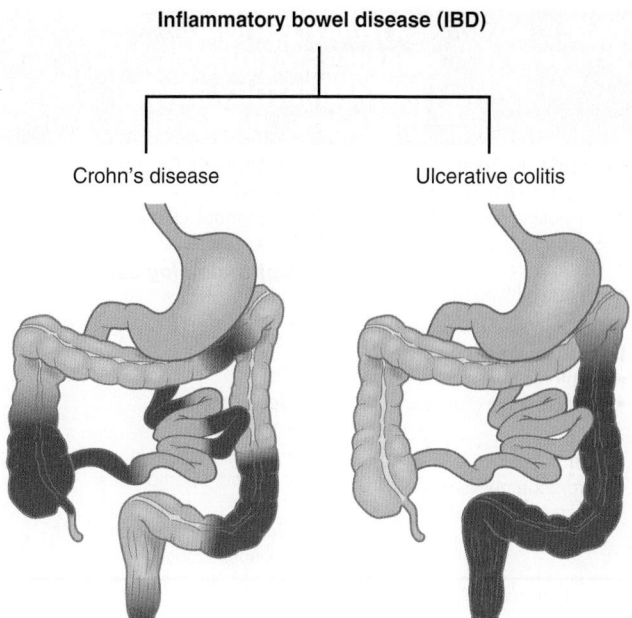

Inflammatory bowel disease (IBD)

Crohn's disease   Ulcerative colitis

FIG. 45.2 Comparison of distribution patterns of Crohn's disease and ulcerative colitis.

ULCERATIVE COLITIS

Ulcerative colitis (UC) is a chronic IBD characterized by inflammation and ulceration of the rectum and the colon. It may occur at any age but peaks between the ages of 15 and 45 years. UC equally affects both sexes (Crohn's & Colitis Canada, 2019b).

Etiology and Pathophysiology

The inflammation of UC is diffuse and involves the mucosa and the submucosa, with alternate periods of exacerbations and remissions (see Table 45.22 later in the chapter). The disease begins in the rectum and spreads proximally along the colon in a continuous fashion.

The mucosa of the rectum and the colon is hyperemic and edematous in the affected area. Multiple abscesses develop in the crypts of Lieberkühn (intestinal glands). As the disease advances, the abscesses break through the crypts into the submucosa, leaving ulcerations. These ulcerations also destroy the mucosal epithelium, causing bleeding and diarrhea. Losses of fluid and electrolytes occur because of the decreased mucosal surface area for absorption. Breakdown of cells results in protein loss through the stool. Areas of inflamed mucosa can form *pseudopolyps*—tongue-like projections into the bowel lumen. Granulation tissue develops, and the mucosa musculature becomes thickened, shortening the colon.

Although the precipitating factors involved in UC are poorly understood, it is clear that the disease onset involves an inflammatory response. Specific proinflammatory cytokines such as tumour necrosis factor–alpha (TNF-α) have been implicated in promoting this inflammatory response.

Clinical Manifestations

UC may appear as an acute fulminating crisis or, more commonly, as a chronic disorder with mild to severe, acute exacerbations that occur at unpredictable intervals over many years. The major symptoms of UC are bloody diarrhea and abdominal pain. Pain may vary from the mild lower abdominal cramping

TABLE 45.17 EXTRAINTESTINAL MANIFESTATIONS OF INFLAMMATORY BOWEL DISEASE

Musculoskeletal
- Peripheral arthritis (colitic)
- Ankylosing spondylitis
- Sacroiliitis
- Osteoporosis
- Finger clubbing

Dermatological
- Erythema nodosum
- Pyoderma gangrenosum

Other
- Thromboembolism
- *Clostridium difficile*

Metastatic Crohn's Disease
Mouth
- Aphthous ulcers (stomatitis)

Ophthalmological
- Conjunctivitis
- Uveitis
- Episcleritis

Hepatobiliary
- Gallstones
- Primary sclerosing cholangitis
- Portal vein thrombosis

Genitourinary
- Kidney stones

TABLE 45.18 INTERPROFESSIONAL CARE

Ulcerative Colitis

Diagnostic
- History and physical examination
- Colonoscopy
- Sigmoidoscopy
- Barium enema
- CBC, ESR, electrolytes, BUN,* creatinine, albumin
- Culture and sensitivity testing of stool (including *Clostridium difficile*)
- Stool for occult blood

Interprofessional Therapy
Mild and Moderate Disease
- Nutritional support (low-residue diet and no dairy products)
- Antimicrobial therapy†
- 5-Aminosalicylates†
- Corticosteroids†
- Antidiarrheal agents†

Severe (Fulminant) Disease
- IV fluids with electrolytes
- Blood transfusions
- NPO status
- Nutritional support (parenteral therapy)
- Antimicrobial therapy†
- Immunosuppressants†
- Immunomodulators†
- Corticosteroids†
- Surgery if no improvement

BUN, blood urea nitrogen; *CBC,* complete blood cell count; *ESR,* erythrocyte sedimentation rate; *IV,* intravenous; *NPO,* nothing by mouth.
*Serum urea (nitrogen).
†See Table 45.19.

associated with diarrhea to the severe, constant abdominal pain that may be associated with toxic megacolon and acute perforations. With mild disease, diarrhea may consist of one or two semiformed stools, containing small amounts of blood, per day. The patient may have no other systemic manifestations. In moderate UC, there is increased stool output (four to five stools per day), increased bleeding, and systemic symptoms (e.g., fever, malaise, anorexia). In severe cases, diarrhea is bloody, contains mucus, and occurs 10 to 20 times a day. In addition, fever, weight loss greater than 10% of total body weight, anemia, tachycardia, and dehydration are present.

Complications

Complications of UC may be classified into those that are intestinal and those that are extraintestinal. *Intestinal* complications of UC include hemorrhage, perforation, toxic megacolon, and colonic dilation. Hemorrhage is a result of inflamed, ulcerated mucosa and is usually controlled with conservative medical therapy. Massive hemorrhage is unusual and requires emergency surgery. *Toxic megacolon* (extensive dilation and paralysis of the colon), bleeding, and fulminant colitis are the most common complications associated with UC. Colonic dilation, most often in the transverse colon, occurs as a result of severe acute inflammation of the entire colon wall. Perforation is most often associated with toxic megacolon but may occur alone. Most cases of perforation occur in the left side of the colon. A patient who has had UC for more than 10 years is at greater risk for colorectal cancer; the risk for cancer depends on age at onset, duration, and extent of disease. The patient should be regularly screened with colonoscopy.

Extraintestinal manifestations of the disease may be directly related to the colitis, or they may be nonspecific complications mediated by a disturbance in the immune system (Table 45.17). Colitis-related complications are associated with active inflammation and may respond to treatment of the underlying bowel disease. These manifestations can involve the joints, the skin, the mouth, and the eyes as well as disturbances of the hematological system, including anemia, leukocytosis, and thrombocytosis. Skin lesions such as erythema nodosum and pyoderma gangrenosum are among the most frequently seen extraintestinal manifestations. Uveitis is the most common eye complication (Crohn's and Colitis Canada, 2019a).

Diagnostic Studies

Several studies are appropriate for the diagnosis of UC (Table 45.18). Blood studies include a CBC, serum electrolytes, and serum protein levels to establish hydration and nutritional status. In addition, the CBC may identify iron-deficiency anemia related to malabsorption of iron through the GI tract or blood loss. The stool should be examined for blood, pus, and mucus. Stool cultures should be obtained to rule out infectious causes of inflammation. Nursing assessment should include discussion regarding the impact of symptoms on quality of life and ability to maintain activities of daily living (ADLs) and to attend work. This discussion often sets the stage for consideration of surgery if conservative medical treatment fails.

Imaging studies include double-contrast barium enema, small bowel series (small bowel follow-through), transabdominal ultrasound, CT, and MRI. Examinations with a sigmoidoscope and a colonoscope enable direct examination of the mucosa of the lower GI tract. Using a sigmoidoscope, the health care provider can view the rectum, the sigmoid colon, and the distal descending colon. The colonoscope allows for examination of the entire large intestine. The extent of inflammation, ulcerations, pseudopolyps, strictures, and lesions may be identified. Biopsy specimens should be taken for definitive diagnosis. Scopes should not be used when the rectum and the colon are severely inflamed, because of the risk for perforation.

Interprofessional Care

The interprofessional team strives to meet the following goals of treatment: (1) rest the bowel, (2) control the inflammation, (3) manage fluids and nutrition, (4) manage patient stress, (5) provide education about the disease and treatment, and (6) provide symptomatic relief. The mainstays of medication therapy are sulphasalazine (Salazopyrin) and corticosteroids. Hospitalization is indicated if the patient's condition fails to respond to corticosteroid therapy or if complications are suspected.

TABLE 45.19 MEDICATION THERAPY
Inflammatory Bowel Disease

Category	Action	Examples
Antimicrobial	Prevent or treat secondary infection	Metronidazole (Flagyl), ciprofloxacin (Cipro)
5-Aminosalicylates (5-ASA)	Decrease GI inflammation*	*Systemic:* sulphasalazine (Salazopyrin), mesalazine (Asacol, Pentasa), olsalazine (Dipentum) *Rectal suppository:* mesalazine (Salofalk)
Corticosteroids	Decrease inflammation	*Systemic:* corticosteroids (cortisone, prednisone, budesonide) *Enemas:* hydrocortisone (Cortenema), budesonide (Entocort) *Rectal foam:* hydrocortisone (Cortifoam)
Antidiarrheal	Decrease GI motility†	Diphenoxylate (Lomotil), loperamide (Imodium)
Immunosuppressants	Suppress immune response	Azathioprine (Imuran), cyclosporine (Neoral)
Immunomodulators	Inhibit the cytokine tumour necrosis factor–alpha (TNF-α)	Infliximab (Remicade), adalimumab (Humira)
Hematinics and vitamins	Correct iron deficiency anemia and promote healing	*Oral iron:* ferrous sulphate, ferrous gluconate *Iron injection:* iron dextran (DexIron), iron sucrose (Venofer)

GI, gastrointestinal.
*Mechanism of action unknown, possibly antimicrobial as well as anti-inflammatory.
†Used with caution during severe disease because of potential to produce toxic megacolon.

Medication Therapy. Medication therapy is an extremely important aspect of treatment (Table 45.19). The principal medication used is sulphasalazine (Salazopyrin), a combination of sulphapyridine and 5-aminosalicylic acid (5-ASA). It is effective in the maintenance of clinical remission and in the treatment of mild to moderately severe disease episodes. After remission is obtained, therapy is continued, with a gradual reduction over several months. The maintenance dose is usually continued for at least 1 year.

> **MEDICATION ALERT—Sulphasalazine (Salazopyrin)**
> - It may cause yellowish-orange discoloration of skin and urine.
> - Patient should avoid exposure to sunlight and ultraviolet light until photosensitivity is determined.

During active disease, 5-ASA (the active form of sulphasalazine) and corticosteroid enemas are effective in the treatment of left-sided UC and proctitis. Topical salicylate therapy is the treatment of choice in patients with localized disease. 5-ASA (mesalazine) can also be administered orally. The acrylic-coated tablets provide delivery of the medication more distally in the intestine.

Corticosteroids are of proven benefit in the management of active UC. Oral prednisone or prednisolone is effective in treatment of mild to moderate disease without systemic manifestations. If remission is not achieved, the patient requires hospitalization and IV corticosteroid therapy. The patient is placed on a regimen of bowel rest; fluids and electrolytes are administered intravenously. For *proctitis* (inflammation of the rectum and the anus), hydrocortisone enemas, rectal foams, or suppositories can be effective in the treatment of inflammation. Rectal foams are usually administered in 5-mL volumes, and patients can generally administer this themselves. Enemas are the preferred choice if the disease spreads beyond the rectum. Retention enemas have been shown to deliver medications into the descending colon and beyond in patients with active disease. Patients taking corticosteroids need to be monitored for common adverse effects such as Cushing's syndrome, hypertension, hirsutism, and mood swings.

Immunosuppressive medications (e.g., cyclosporin) have been used in severe cases of UC, when a patient's condition has failed to respond to any of the usual medications and before surgery is considered. Adverse effects of cyclosporin include renal dysfunction, hypertension, headache, and muscle cramps. Regular cyclosporin trough levels should be determined to ensure proper dosing of this medication. Therapeutic response to IV cyclosporin usually allows for conversion to an oral preparation for long-term therapy. Anti–TNF-α blocking agents (e.g., infliximab [Remicade]) were previously considered for use more with Crohn's disease; they are now also considered valuable in the management of moderate to severe refractory UC (Janssen, 2017).

Surgical Therapy. Approximately 80 to 85% of patients with UC go into remission with conservative therapy and nursing management, but 15 to 20% of patients require surgery. Surgery is indicated if (1) the patient fails to respond to treatment; (2) exacerbations are frequent and debilitating; (3) massive bleeding, perforation, strictures, or obstruction occurs; (4) there are tissue changes that suggest that dysplasia is occurring; or (5) carcinoma develops.

Surgical procedures used to treat chronic UC include (1) total proctocolectomy with permanent ileostomy and (2) total proctocolectomy with ileoanal reservoir.

Total Proctocolectomy With Permanent Ileostomy. Total proctocolectomy with a permanent ileostomy is a one-stage operation involving removal of the colon, the rectum, and the anus, with closure of the anus. The end of the terminal ileum is brought out through the abdominal wall and forms a stoma, or ostomy. The stoma is usually placed in the right lower quadrant within the rectus muscle.

Total Proctocolectomy With Ileoanal Reservoir. A more widely performed procedure involves total proctocolectomy with the formation of an ileal reservoir and anal anastomosis (Figure 45.3). The ileoanal reservoir surgical procedure is usually a staged approach, encompassing a combination of one to three procedures, performed approximately 12 weeks apart. The initial procedure generally includes a colectomy with temporary end ileostomy and a possible mucous fistula. The second surgery involves a takedown of the ileostomy and mucous fistula, resection of the rectal stump to just above the anal sphincters, and formation of the ileal reservoir and subsequent anastomosis to the anus, with a diverting temporary loop ileostomy (to protect the reservoir during healing). The final, third surgery involves a takedown of the loop ileostomy, which functionalizes the reservoir. Depending on the preoperative health of the patient, these staged surgeries may be combined into a two-stage procedure or a single operation. Adaptation to the reservoir occurs over the next 3 to 6 months, which usually results in a bowel movement frequency of four to eight pasty stools per day and good daytime continence.

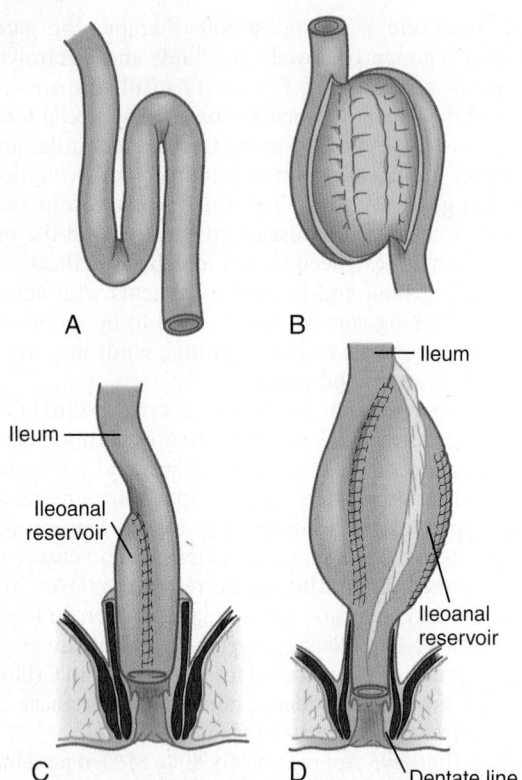

FIG. 45.3 Ileoanal reservoir. **A,** Formation of a reservoir. **B,** Posterior suture lines completed. **C,** J-shaped configuration for an ileoanal reservoir. **D,** S-shaped configuration for an ileoanal reservoir.

Patient selection includes absence of colorectal cancer, small intestine free of disease (e.g., Crohn's disease), competent anorectal sphincter, and physical status adequate to permit lengthy surgery. In addition, the patient needs to be motivated and capable of understanding self-care instructions.

Postoperative Care. Postoperative care following surgical procedures to treat UC includes routine observations used for patients who have had abdominal surgery. Stoma viability, mucocutaneous border (the area where the mucous membrane of the bowel is sutured to the skin), and peristomal skin integrity must be monitored. Because a more proximal portion of the bowel is used to create the diverting loop ileostomy in the second stage, stomal output may be as high as 1500 to 2000 mL/24 hr. Intravenous fluid support is important, including replacements for excessive ileostomy losses (>1200 mL/24 hr). The patient must be observed for signs of hemorrhage, abdominal abscesses, small bowel obstruction, dehydration, and other related complications. If an NG tube is used, it will be removed when bowel function returns. Drainage of serosanguineous fluid from the abdominal drain site may vary from 100 to 150 mL/24 hr. The drain is usually removed within 3 to 4 days of surgery. The urinary catheter is removed 2 to 4 days after surgery. Systemic antibiotics are discontinued within 24 hours of the operation, and corticosteroids, if used, are tapered.

Transient incontinence of mucus from the reservoir is a result of intraoperative manipulation of the anal canal and the effects of some medications (opioids, sedatives). The patient should be reassured before and after the operation regarding this potential but transient problem. Kegel exercises may be recommended several weeks postoperatively to strengthen the pelvic floor and the sphincter muscles. They are not recommended in the immediate postoperative period. Perianal skin care must

be implemented with the first bowel movement to protect the epidermis from frequent pericare and stool irritation. The patient should be instructed to gently rinse the skin with water or a spray cleanser with a surfactant and dry thoroughly. A barrier cream should be used, and a perineal pad may be required.

The most frequent type of ileostomy that is constructed is a loop. This can present as a pouching challenge because the os (opening) may tilt down and drain inferiorly such that stool causes irritation to the surrounding skin. An enterostomal therapy (ET) nurse, who specializes in ostomy care, will help with these challenging issues. Self-care instructions should be taught and reviewed, and written information with discharge supplies should be provided before discharge. Stoma care is presented later in this chapter (see Nursing Management: Ostomy Surgery).

Nutritional Therapy. An important component in the treatment of UC is diet. The dietitian is an important member of the team and should be consulted regarding dietary recommendations. The goals of diet management are to provide adequate nutrition without exacerbating symptoms, to correct and prevent malnutrition, to replace fluid and electrolyte losses, and to prevent weight loss. The diet for each patient must be individualized.

Traditionally, during the acute phase, the patient may be on NPO status. When food is permitted, a high-calorie, high-protein, low-residue diet with vitamin and iron supplements is frequently prescribed. (A low-residue diet is presented in Table 45.20.) Special dietary restrictions are not usually necessary. Some health care providers allow the patient to eat anything that does not cause symptoms. Cold foods, high-residue foods (e.g., whole wheat bread, cereal with bran, nuts, raw fruit), and smoking increase GI motility and should be avoided. Fish oil preparations have been evaluated for their ability to reduce inflammation in active UC. However, their palatability is low.

Often, enteral supplements and PN are necessary. Patients with systemic manifestations, significant fluid and electrolyte losses, or malabsorption may need PN or enteral feedings, such as elemental diets. Elemental diets are high in calories and nutrients, lactose free, and absorbed in the proximal small intestine.

PN allows for a positive nitrogen balance. Vitamins, minerals, electrolytes, and other important nutrients (e.g., glucose, amino acids) can be administered to promote healing and correct nutritional deficiencies. (PN is discussed in Chapter 42.)

Supplemental iron (ferrous sulphate or ferrous gluconate) may be necessary to prevent or treat iron-deficiency anemia resulting from chronic blood loss. Parenteral iron may be needed for patients who cannot tolerate oral iron. Iron dextran (DexIron) administered intravenously may be necessary if anemia is severe. In patients receiving long-term sulphasalazine therapy, folic acid deficiency may develop, and supplementation may be necessary. Potassium supplements may be necessary if corticosteroid therapy is used because retention of sodium and loss of potassium can result in hypokalemia and subsequent toxic megacolon. Zinc deficiency can result from severe or chronic diarrhea, and supplementation may be necessary.

NURSING MANAGEMENT
ULCERATIVE COLITIS

NURSING ASSESSMENT

Subjective and objective data that should be obtained from a patient with UC are presented in Table 45.21.

TABLE 45.20 NUTRITIONAL THERAPY
Low-Residue Diet

Purpose

A low-residue diet provides foods low in fibre, which will result in a reduced amount of fecal material in the lower intestinal tract.

General Principles

1. This diet eliminates foods that are indigestible or stimulating to the intestinal tract to reduce the amount of residue in the colon. Foods should be included or excluded according to the following list.
2. Hot and cold foods should be eaten slowly.
3. Milk products are limited to 2 cups daily. For a more restricted-residue diet, milk should be eliminated.

Food	Foods Included	Foods Excluded
Beverages	Carbonated drinks, coffee, tea, cocoa, strained fruit juices	Alcohol, fruit juices with pulp
Bread	White bread, rolls, rusks, melba toast, crackers	Bread and crackers containing whole grain flour or bran; any hot breads such as biscuits, muffins, waffles, or pancakes
Cereals	Cooked, refined, or strained cereals: cream of wheat, cream of rice, farina, grits, dry cereals without bran; noodles; spaghetti; macaroni	Whole grain cereals; cereals containing bran, nuts, and raisins; Shredded Wheat
Meat	Lean, tender ground beef, lamb, pork, veal, or fish, broiled, stewed, or baked; canned tuna or salmon; shellfish; crisp bacon, chicken or turkey without skin, liver; creamy peanut butter	Fried, smoked, pickled, or cured meats; highly seasoned ham; fried fish; luncheon meats
Egg	All but fried	Fried or uncooked eggs
Cheese	Milk, cheese (aged cheddar), cottage cheese	All other cheeses
Milk	Limit to 1–2 cups (if tolerated), including that used in cooking; plain yogurt	Fruit yogurt
Fats	Butter, margarine, cream, oil, crisp bacon, mayonnaise, plain gravy, creamy peanut butter	Any other; rich or spiced gravies
Soup	Cream and vegetable soups made from foods allowed and with quantity of milk allowed, bouillon, broth; strained vegetable juices	Cream and vegetable soups made from foods not allowed (peas and dried beans)
Vegetables	Cooked or canned vegetables; strained vegetables; potatoes without skins; vegetable juices	Raw vegetables, all vegetables not strained, dried beans, peas, and legumes
Fruits	Strained fruit juices, cooked or canned fruits; ripe bananas, applesauce, pears, peaches, peeled apricots, Napoleon cherries, baked apple (no skin)	Raw fruits, fruits with skins, seeds
Desserts	Plain desserts (custards and puddings, plain ice cream for milk allowance), sherbet, plain gelatin desserts, angel food cake, sponge cake, plain butter cake, plain cookies	Nuts, coconut, raisins, rich desserts (pies, rich cakes, cobblers)
Condiments	Allspice, cinnamon, mace, paprika, salt, ground thyme, sugar, vinegar, lemon juice	All others

TABLE 45.21 NURSING ASSESSMENT
Ulcerative Colitis

Subjective Data
Important Health Information
- *Past health history:* Infection; autoimmune disorders; family history of inflammatory bowel disease
- *Medications:* Use of antidiarrheal medications, steroids, other immunosuppressives; herbal, homeopathic, or naturopathic remedies

Symptoms
- Fatigue, malaise
- Nausea, vomiting, anorexia; weight loss; dietary intolerances
- Frequent bloody stools containing mucus and pus
- Lower abdominal pain (worse before defecating), cramping, tenesmus

Objective Data
General
Intermittent fever; emaciated appearance

Integumentary
Pale skin with poor turgor, dry mucous membranes; rash, nodules (on lower legs), or blisters; anorectal irritation

Gastrointestinal
Abdominal distension, hyperactive bowel sounds, abdominal cramps

Cardiovascular
Tachycardia, hypotension (including postural)

Possible Findings
Anemia; leukocytosis; electrolyte imbalance; hypoalbuminemia; vitamin and trace metal deficiencies; abnormal sigmoidoscopic, colonoscopic, and barium enema findings

NURSING DIAGNOSES

Nursing diagnoses for the patient with UC include but are not limited to the following:

- *Diarrhea* resulting from *increase in stress level* (bowel inflammation and intestinal hyperactivity)
- *Inadequate nutrition* resulting from *insufficient dietary intake* (decreased absorption, increased nutrient loss through diarrhea)
- *Inadequate coping* resulting from *insufficient sense of control, inadequate confidence in ability to deal with situation*

For additional information on nursing diagnoses on IBD, see NCP 45.3, available on the Evolve website.

PLANNING

The overall goals are that the patient with UC will (1) respond to medical management, (2) maintain normal fluid and electrolyte balance, (3) be free from pain or discomfort, (4) participate in medical and surgical management, and (5) maintain nutritional balance.

NURSING IMPLEMENTATION

During the acute phase, attention is focused on hemodynamic stability, pain control, fluid and electrolyte balance, and nutritional support. Accurate intake and output records must be maintained. The number and characteristics of stools are monitored. Nursing care of the patient with UC is directed toward implementing an intensive therapeutic and supportive program (see NCP 45.3). It is important for the nurse to establish a good working relationship with the patient and encourage them to talk about their concerns and their daily activities.

An explanation of all procedures and treatment is necessary and may allay some apprehension.

Psychosocial support may be indicated if the patient is experiencing emotional challenges, but the nurse must recognize that the patient's behaviour may result from factors other than emotional ones. Any person who has 10 to 20 bowel movements a day and has rectal discomfort may be anxious, frustrated, discouraged, and depressed. Along with other team members, the nurse can assist the patient to accept the chronic condition and to have an optimistic view with the possibility of cure after surgery. The nurse may find that the inadequate coping mechanisms in the patient with UC are due to early onset of the disease (often at 10–15 years of age), which may have interfered with usual growth, development, and maturation.

Restricted physical activity and possibly bed rest may be ordered if the patient has a severe exacerbation. Nursing interventions to prevent complications of immobility should be instituted. Teaching related to treatment, medications, diet, diagnostic tests, and the disease and its management is important.

Rest is important in the management of UC. Patients may lose much sleep because of frequent episodes of diarrhea and abdominal pain. Nutritional deficiencies and anemia leave the patient feeling weak and listless. Activities should be scheduled around rest periods. Nurses can provide physical and emotional support to the patient during acute exacerbations.

Until diarrhea is controlled, the patient must be kept clean, dry, and free of odour. Facilitating management of bowel movements, including close proximity to a bathroom or a bedside commode, is helpful. A deodorizer should be placed in the room. Antidiarrheal agents should be administered as ordered. If the patient has continuous diarrhea, the ET nurse may have helpful suggestions to address this. Meticulous perianal skin care using plain water or a skin cleanser (no harsh soap) is necessary to treat and prevent skin breakdown. Use of skin barrier creams may help to protect perianal skin.

EVALUATION

The expected outcomes for the patient with UC are presented in NCP 45.3, available on the Evolve website.

CROHN'S DISEASE

Crohn's disease is a chronic IBD of unknown origin that can affect any part of the GI tract from the mouth to the anus. Crohn's disease occurs most often between the ages of 15 and 30 years. When it occurs in older persons, the morbidity and mortality rates are higher because of other chronic conditions that may be present. Both sexes are affected, with a slightly higher incidence in women. Similar to UC, it occurs more often in Jewish and upper–middle-class urban populations. Canada may have one of the highest incidence rates of both Crohn's disease and UC in the world.

Etiology and Pathophysiology

While the cause of Crohn's disease is undetermined, considerable research suggests interactions among environmental factors, intestinal microorganisms, immune dysregulation, and genetic predisposition (Canadian Society of Intestinal Research, 2021b). Recently, the first gene associated with Crohn's disease, the *NOD2* gene, was identified. Research is ongoing to understand how defects in the *NOD2* gene lead to Crohn's disease and

to find the other genes that cause IBD. Crohn's disease can affect any part of the GI tract but is most often seen in the terminal ileum and the colon. Approximately 5% of patients with Crohn's disease have ileojejunitis. Involvement of the esophagus, the stomach, or the duodenum is uncommon. The inflammation involves all layers of the bowel wall (i.e., it is transmural). Areas of involvement are usually discontinuous *skip lesions,* with segments of normal bowel occurring between diseased portions (Table 45.22). Typically, ulcerations are deep and longitudinal and penetrate between islands of inflamed edematous mucosa, causing the classic cobblestone appearance. Thickening of the bowel wall occurs, as well as narrowing of the lumen with stricture development. Abscesses or fistula tracts that communicate

TABLE 45.22	COMPARISON OF ULCERATIVE COLITIS AND CROHN'S DISEASE	
Characteristic	**Ulcerative Colitis**	**Crohn's Disease**
Clinical		
Usual age at onset	Teens to mid-30s	Teens to mid-30s
Diarrhea	Common	Common
Abdominal cramping pain	Common	Common
Fever (intermittent)	During acute episodes	Common
Weight loss	Rare	Severe
Rectal bleeding	Common	Fairly common
Tenesmus	Severe	Infrequent
Malabsorption and nutritional deficiencies	Minimal incidence	Common
Pathological		
Location	Starts distally in the rectum and spreads proximally in a continuous fashion up the colon	Can occur anywhere along GI tract from mouth to anus, with characteristic skip lesions; most frequent site is terminal ileum
Distribution	Continuous	Segmental (skip lesions)
Depth of involvement	Mucosa and submucosa	Entire thickness of bowel wall (transmural)
Granulomas	Occasional	Common
Cobblestoning of mucosa	Rare	Common
Pseudopolyps	Common	Rare
Small bowel involvement	Minimal (backwash ileitis)	Common
Complications		
Fistulas	Rare	Common
Strictures	Occasional	Common
Anal abscesses	Rare	Common
Perforation	Common	Common
Toxic megacolon	Common	Rare
Carcinoma	Increased incidence after 10 yr of disease	Slightly greater than general population
Recurrence after surgery	Cure with proctocolectomy	40–60% or more recurrence after segmental resections of small or large intestine

GI, gastrointestinal.

with other loops of bowel, the skin, the bladder, the rectum, or the vagina may develop. Histologically, granulomas (chronic inflammatory lesions) are present in 50% of patients and may be located in any layer of the bowel wall.

Clinical Manifestations

The manifestations of Crohn's disease depend largely on the anatomical site of involvement, the extent of the disease process, and the presence or absence of complications. The onset of Crohn's disease is usually insidious, with nonspecific symptoms such as diarrhea, fatigue, abdominal pain, weight loss, and fever. Early diagnosis may be more difficult than for UC. The principal manifestations of Crohn's disease are diarrhea and abdominal pain. Diarrhea is usually nonbloody and is a result of the inflammatory process or malabsorption. Pain may be severe and intermittent or constant, depending on the cause. Other manifestations include abdominal cramping and tenderness, abdominal distension, fever, and fatigue. Similar to UC, extraintestinal complications may be directly related to the GI inflammation and small intestinal pathological conditions (malabsorption), or they may be nonspecific complications mediated by a disturbance in the immune system. Extraintestinal manifestations, such as arthritis and finger clubbing, may precede the onset of bowel disease. As the disease progresses, there is weight loss, malnutrition, dehydration, electrolyte imbalances, anemia, increased peristalsis, pain around the umbilicus and right lower quadrant, and possible perianal disease.

Crohn's disease is a chronic disorder with unpredictable periods of recurrence and remission. Attacks are intermittent, usually recurring over a period of several weeks to months.

Complications

Complications, both GI and extraintestinal, are common in Crohn's disease. Scar tissue from the inflammation and ulceration narrows the lumen of the intestine and may cause strictures and obstruction, a frequent complication. Fistulas are a cardinal feature and may develop between segments of bowel. Cutaneous fistulas, common in the perianal area, and rectovaginal fistulas also occur. Fistulas communicating with the urinary tract may cause urinary tract infections. Inflammation of the intestines may involve all layers, predisposing the patient to perforation and the formation of intra-abdominal abscesses and peritonitis (Carvalho et al., 2018).

Impaired absorption causing various nutritional abnormalities may occur as a result of damage to areas of the intestinal mucosa. Fat malabsorption causes a deficiency in the fat-soluble vitamins (A, D, E, and K). The patient may have an intolerance to gluten (a protein found in barley, rye, and wheat).

Systemic complications are similar to those of UC and include arthritis, liver disease, cholelithiasis (especially with ileal involvement), ankylosing spondylitis, pyoderma gangrenosum, erythema nodosum, and uveitis. Renal disorders are common, especially nephrolithiasis (kidney stones) secondary to increased oxalate absorption.

Diagnostic Studies

Diagnosis of Crohn's disease can be made with a thorough history and physical examination, to establish clinical signs and symptoms; barium studies; and endoscopy with biopsy (Table 45.23). Laboratory studies may determine electrolyte disturbances and the presence of anemia. Barium studies are useful in determining the location and extent of the disease and

TABLE 45.23	**INTERPROFESSIONAL CARE**
Crohn's Disease	
Diagnostic	**Interprofessional Therapy**
• History and physical examination • CBC, ESR • Serum chemistries • Testing of stool for occult blood • Radiological studies with barium contrast • Sigmoidoscopy and colonoscopy with biopsy	• High-calorie, high-vitamin, high-protein, low-residue, dairy-free diet • Antimicrobial agents* • Corticosteroid medications* • Immunosuppressants* • Immunomodulators* • Supplementary PN • Elemental diet • Physical and emotional rest • Surgery†

CBC, complete blood cell count; *ESR*, erythrocyte sedimentation rate; *PN*, parenteral nutrition.
*See Table 45.19.
†See Table 45.24.

may reveal classic findings, such as stricture formations in the ileum (string sign), cobblestoning of the mucosa, fistulas, and areas of abnormal and normal mucosa. Endoscopic studies, such as colonoscopy and sigmoidoscopy, are useful in detecting such early mucosal changes as patchy inflammation, small ulcerations, and skip areas that may not be seen radiologically. Biopsies may be performed to determine the presence of granulomas. Barium studies are performed to determine the degree of ileal involvement. Upper GI barium studies are done to diagnose upper gastroduodenal disease. Because an endoscope can enter only the distal ileum, capsule endoscopy may be used in the diagnosis of small intestine disease. Capsule endoscopy is a useful diagnostic test, but the high cost of the procedure limits its use (Canadian Society of Intestinal Research, 2021a).

Interprofessional Care

The goal of interprofessional care is to control the inflammatory process, relieve symptoms, correct metabolic and nutritional disorders, and promote healing. Medication therapy and nutritional support are the mainstays of treatment.

Medication Therapy. Medication therapy for Crohn's disease is presented in Table 45.19. Sulphasalazine (Salazopyrin) is effective when the disease involves the large intestine but is much less effective when only the small intestine is involved. Corticosteroid therapy is effective in reducing inflammation and suppressing disease. The dosage and the route of administration depend on the severity of the illness and the area involved. Once clinical symptoms subside, the dosage should be tapered. Immunosuppressive agents (azathioprine) may be tried if repeated trials with corticosteroids fail. Patients require close monitoring because of the serious adverse effects of these medications. Metronidazole (Flagyl) is useful in treating Crohn's disease of the perianal area. Marked exacerbations have been reported when the medication is stopped. In patients with Crohn's disease in remission, fish oil preparations have been evaluated for their ability to prevent recurrence of inflammation; however, their palatability is low.

Biological medication therapies of Crohn's disease include monoclonal antibodies to TNF-α (infliximab [Remicade], adalimumab [Humira]), α4β7 integrin blockers (vedolizumab [Entyvio]), and a leukocyte adhesion molecule (natalizumab [Tysabri]). Infliximab has been shown to reduce the degree of inflammation in patients who are refractory to other

TABLE 45.24	INDICATIONS FOR SURGICAL THERAPY FOR CROHN'S DISEASE

- Drainage of abdominal abscess
- Failure to respond to conservative therapy
- Fistulas
- Inability to decrease corticosteroids
- Intestinal obstruction
- Massive hemorrhage
- Perforation
- Secondary hydronephrosis
- Severe anorectal disease
- Suspicion of carcinoma

medication therapies. However, not all patients with Crohn's disease respond to infliximab.

Nutritional Therapy. Elemental diets and PN may be used in patients with Crohn's disease (see Chapter 42). PN may be given to patients with severe disease, small bowel fistulas, or short bowel syndrome (described later in this chapter). It is given before and after surgery to promote wound healing, reduce complications, and hasten recovery. The elemental diet provides a high-calorie, high-nitrogen, fat-free, no-residue substrate that is absorbed in the proximal small bowel. This diet can be given to most patients with Crohn's disease, even during acute exacerbations.

The diet should otherwise be low in residue, roughage, and fat but high in calories and protein. It may be difficult to maintain adequate absorption during periods of disease exacerbation and even during periods of remission. Milk and milk products may have to be excluded from the diet. Lactose, the primary disaccharide found in milk, may not be adequately digested because of the inability of the damaged intestinal mucosa to produce sufficient amounts of lactase. High-fat diets are poorly tolerated because of the loss of absorbing mucosa and altered bile salt metabolism and absorption.

Vitamin deficiencies may develop as a result of malabsorption. Cobalamin (vitamin B_{12}) injections every month may be needed because of the inability of the terminal ileum (if affected) to absorb this vitamin.

Surgical Therapy. Surgery is used in patients with severe symptoms that are unresponsive to therapy and in patients with life-threatening complications. The majority of patients with Crohn's disease eventually require surgery at least once in the course of their disease. Indications for surgery are outlined in Table 45.24. Unlike UC, Crohn's disease is not cured by surgery. The recurrence rate after surgery is high. The surgical procedure depends on the affected area and the condition of the patient. Conservative intestinal resection with anastomosis of healthy bowel is the procedure of choice.

NURSING MANAGEMENT CROHN'S DISEASE

Care of patients with Crohn's disease is similar to that of patients with UC (see NCP 45.3, available on the Evolve website). As the patient's condition improves, the nurse should allow for more self-care, provide frequent rest periods, and advise the patient of the importance of rest and avoidance or control of emotional stress. This may be difficult for the patient when told the nature of the disease and the limitations of the treatment. Patients who have perianal fistulas or abscesses may need special skin care. Postoperative care should be the same as for laparotomy.

In the majority of patients with Crohn's disease, the course is chronic and intermittent. The patient and family may need

help in setting realistic short- and long-term goals. Teaching should include (1) the importance of rest and diet management, (2) perianal care, (3) action and adverse effects of medications, (4) symptoms of recurrence of disease, (5) when to seek medical care, and (6) use of stress-management techniques.

AGE-RELATED CONSIDERATIONS

INFLAMMATORY BOWEL DISEASE
Although IBDs (i.e., UC and Crohn's disease) are considered diseases of young adults, a second peak in the distribution of these inflammatory conditions occurs around the ages of 50 to 70 years. The pathogenesis, natural history, and clinical course of UC and Crohn's disease in older persons are similar to those observed in younger patients. However, the distribution of the inflammation appears to be somewhat different. In older patients with UC, the distal colon is usually involved (proctitis). In older persons with Crohn's disease, the colon rather than the small intestine tends to be involved. There is less recurrence of Crohn's disease in older persons treated with surgical resection. The degree of inflammation associated with both conditions tends to be less in older patients than in younger patients.

Interprofessional care of older patients with one of these conditions is similar to care of younger patients. However, because of increased risk for cardiovascular and pulmonary complications, older people tend to have increased morbidity associated with surgical procedures.

In addition to Crohn's disease and UC, older persons are also vulnerable to inflammation of the colon (colitis) from medication use and systemic vascular disease. Medications such as nonsteroidal anti-inflammatory drugs (NSAIDs), digitalis, vasopressin, estrogen, and allopurinol (Zyloprim) have been associated with development of colitis in older patients. Colitis may also be secondary to ischemic bowel disease related to atherosclerosis and heart failure.

Inflammation of the colon as a result of Crohn's disease or UC results in diarrhea, which may be bloody. The loss of fluid and electrolytes and, possibly, blood may leave older people more vulnerable to conditions related to volume depletion and dehydration. This may be particularly problematic in patients with diminished renal and cardiovascular function. Thus, nursing management is focused on careful assessment of fluid and electrolyte status and evaluation of the replacement therapies.

MALABSORPTION SYNDROME

Malabsorption results from impaired absorption of fats, carbohydrates, proteins, minerals, and vitamins. The stomach, small intestine, liver, and pancreas regulate normal digestion and absorption. Digestive enzymes ordinarily break down nutrients so that absorption can take place through the intestinal mucosa and nutrients can get into the bloodstream. If there is an interruption in this process at any point, malabsorption may occur. Several factors can cause malabsorption (Table 45.25). They can be classified into malabsorption caused by (1) biochemical or enzyme deficiencies, (2) bacterial proliferation, (3) disruption of small intestine mucosa, (4) disturbed lymphatic and vascular circulation, or (5) surface area loss. Lactose intolerance is the most common malabsorption disorder, followed by IBD, celiac disease, tropical sprue, and cystic fibrosis.

The most common clinical manifestation of malabsorption is *steatorrhea*, which is the passage of large amounts of fat as

TABLE 45.25	COMMON CAUSES OF MALABSORPTION

Biochemical or Enzyme Deficiencies	**Disturbed Lymphatic and Vascular Circulation**
• Lactase deficiency	• Lymphoma
• Biliary tract obstruction	• Ischemia
• Pancreatic insufficiency	• Lymphangiectasia
• Cystic fibrosis	• Heart failure
• Chronic pancreatitis	
• Zollinger–Ellison syndrome	**Surface Area Loss**
	• Billroth II gastrectomy
Bacterial Proliferation	• Gastrojejunal bypass surgery for obesity
• Tropical sprue	• Short bowel syndrome
• Parasitic infection	• Distal ileal resection, disease, or bypass
Small Intestinal Mucosal Disruption	
• Celiac disease	
• Whipple's disease	
• Crohn's disease	

bulky, fatty, frothy, foul-smelling, yellow-grey, greasy stools with putty-like consistency that float in water and are difficult to flush (Table 45.26).

Tests used to determine the cause of malabsorption include qualitative examination of stool for fat (e.g., Sudan III stain), a 72-hour stool collection for quantitative measurement of fecal fat, serological testing for celiac disease, and fecal elastase testing to determine if there is pancreatic insufficiency. Other diagnostic studies include CT and endoscopy to obtain a small bowel biopsy specimen for diagnosis. A small bowel barium enema is performed to identify abnormal mucosal patterns. Capsule endoscopy can be used to assess the small intestine for alterations in mucosal integrity and inflammation.

Tests for carbohydrate malabsorption include the D-xylose test and the lactose tolerance test. Laboratory studies that are frequently ordered include a CBC, measurement of prothrombin time (to see if vitamin K absorption is adequate), serum vitamin A and carotene levels, serum electrolytes, cholesterol, and calcium.

CELIAC DISEASE

Celiac disease is a unique autoimmune disease in individuals with a genetic background of *HLA-DQ2/DQ8* positivity and non-HLA genes, characterized by damage to the small intestinal mucosa from the ingestion of wheat, barley, and rye (Caio et al., 2019). It is relatively common, occurs at all ages, and has a wide variety of symptoms. Celiac disease is most common in people of European ancestry, and it is estimated that approximately 1 in every 100 people in Canada is affected by celiac disease (Canadian Celiac Professional Advisory Council, 2016).

Etiology and Pathophysiology

Three factors necessary for developing celiac disease are genetic predisposition, gluten ingestion, and an immune-mediated response. As with other autoimmune diseases, the tissue destruction that occurs with celiac disease is the result of chronic inflammation. Inflammation is activated by the ingestion of gluten found in wheat, rye, and barley. Gluten contains specific peptides called *prolamines*. In genetically susceptible

TABLE 45.26	CLINICAL MANIFESTATIONS OF MALABSORPTION

Clinical Manifestations	Pathophysiology
Gastrointestinal	
Weight loss	Malabsorption of fat, carbohydrates, and protein leading to loss of calories; marked reduction in caloric intake or increased use of calories
Diarrhea	Impaired absorption of water, sodium, fatty acids, bile, or carbohydrates
Flatulence	Bacterial fermentation of unabsorbed carbohydrates
Steatorrhea	Undigested and unabsorbed fat
Glossitis, cheilosis, stomatitis	Deficiency of iron, riboflavin, cobalamin, folic acid, and other vitamins
Hematological	
Anemia	Impaired absorption of iron, cobalamin, and folic acid
Hemorrhagic tendency	Vitamin C deficiency
	Vitamin K deficiency inhibiting production of clotting factors II, VII, IX, and X
Musculoskeletal	
Bone pain	Osteoporosis from impaired calcium absorption
	Osteomalacia secondary to hypocalcemia, hypophosphatemia, inadequate vitamin D
Tetany	Hypocalcemia, hypomagnesemia
Weakness, muscle cramps	Anemia, electrolyte depletion (especially potassium)
Muscle wasting	Protein malabsorption
Neurological	
Altered mental status	Dehydration
Paresthesias	Cobalamin deficiency
Peripheral neuropathy	Cobalamin deficiency
Night blindness	Thiamine deficiency, vitamin A deficiency
Integumentary	
Bruising	Vitamin K deficiency
Dermatitis	Fatty acid deficiency, zinc deficiency, niacin and other vitamin deficiencies
Brittle nails	Iron deficiency
Hair thinning and loss	Protein deficiency
Cardiovascular	
Hypotension	Dehydration
Tachycardia	Hypovolemia, anemia
Peripheral edema	Protein malabsorption, protein loss in diarrhea

individuals, partial digestion of gluten releases prolamine peptides, which are absorbed into the lamina propria in the intestinal submucosa.

Once in the lamina propria, peptides bind to human leukocyte antigen (HLA)-DQ2 and HLA-DQ8 (or both) and activate an inflammatory response. Additionally, a loss of intestinal barrier function and an inappropriate adaptive immune response can result in damage to the microvilli and brush border of the small intestine, decreasing the amount of surface area available for nutrient absorption (Caio et al., 2019). Damage is most severe in the duodenum, probably related to the greater exposure to gluten. The intestinal damage decreases distal to the duodenum. The inflammation continues until gluten ingestion ceases.

Clinical Manifestations

Classic signs of celiac disease include foul-smelling diarrhea, steatorrhea, flatulence, abdominal distension, and symptoms of malnutrition. Some people have no obvious GI symptoms and may have atypical symptoms, such as decreased bone density and osteoporosis, dental enamel hypoplasia, iron and folate deficiencies, peripheral neuropathy, and reproductive conditions (Canadian Celiac Association, 2016a). A pruritic, vesicular skin lesion, called *dermatitis herpetiformis*, is sometimes present and occurs as a rash on the buttocks, scalp, face, elbows, and knees. Celiac disease is also associated with autoimmune diseases, particularly rheumatoid arthritis, type 1 diabetes mellitus, and thyroid disease. Protein, fat, and carbohydrate absorption is affected, leading to poor growth, weight loss, muscle wasting, and other signs of malnutrition. Abnormal folate, iron, and cobalamin levels can occur. Iron-deficiency anemia is one of the most common manifestations of celiac disease. Patients may exhibit lactose intolerance and should eliminate lactose-containing products from their diet until the disease is under control. Inadequate calcium intake and vitamin D absorption can lead to decreased bone density and osteoporosis. Poor nutrition can lead to reproductive disorders.

Diagnostic Studies and Interprofessional Care

Celiac disease is confirmed when (1) there is histological evidence of the disease following biopsy from the small intestine, and (2) the symptoms and histological evidence disappear when the person eats a gluten-free diet (Canadian Celiac Association, 2016b). Diagnostic testing must be done before the person is placed on a gluten-free diet because the diet will alter the results. Biopsies show flattened mucosa and noticeable losses of villi. Celiac disease should be ruled out during a diagnostic workup of IBS because the symptoms are similar. Many people spend years seeking treatment for nonspecific symptoms before celiac disease is diagnosed (thus the large number of people who are diagnosed in adulthood). Treatment with a gluten-free diet halts the disease process. Most patients recover completely within 3 to 6 months of treatment, but they need to maintain a gluten-free diet for life. Wheat, barley, oats, and rye products must be avoided. Although pure oats do not contain gluten, oat products can become contaminated with wheat, rye, and barley during the milling process. Gluten is also found in some medications and in many food additives, preservatives, and stabilizers. A combination of corticosteroids and a gluten-free diet is used to treat individuals who do not respond to the gluten-free diet alone. If the disease is untreated, chronic inflammation and hyperplasia continue. Individuals with celiac disease have an increased risk for non-Hodgkin's lymphoma and GI cancers.

LACTASE DEFICIENCY

Lactase deficiency is a condition in which the lactase enzyme is deficient or absent. *Lactase* is the enzyme that breaks down lactose into two simple sugars—glucose and galactose. Although primary lactase deficiency seems to be hereditary, milk intolerance may not become clinically evident until late adolescence or early adulthood. About 5% of the adult population has primary lactase deficiency. The highest incidence in Canada is found in people who are Black or Indigenous or of Latin American, Asian, or Jewish descent. Often, acquired lactase deficiency is seen in conjunction with other GI diseases in which the mucosa has been damaged, including UC, Crohn's disease, gastroenteritis, and celiac disease.

Clinical Manifestations

The symptoms of lactose intolerance include bloating, flatulence, crampy abdominal pain, and diarrhea. They may occur within a half hour to several hours after drinking a glass of milk or ingesting a milk product. The diarrhea of lactose intolerance results from fluid secretion into the small intestine, a response to the osmotic action of undigested lactose.

NURSING AND INTERPROFESSIONAL MANAGEMENT LACTASE DEFICIENCY

Many people who are lactose-intolerant are aware of their milk intolerance and avoid intake of milk. A lactose intolerance test can be done to rule out milk allergies. The patient is given 50 g of lactose orally. Blood samples are drawn before the consumption of lactose and at 15-, 30-, 60-, and 90-minute intervals thereafter. Failure of the blood glucose level to increase more than 20 mg/dL is suggestive of lactase deficiency. Results of the hydrogen breath test after ingestion of lactose are abnormal.

Treatment consists of eliminating lactose from the diet by avoiding intake of milk and milk products. A lactose-free diet is given initially and is gradually advanced to a low-lactose diet, as tolerated by the patient. Many people who are lactose-intolerant may not exhibit symptoms if lactose is taken in small amounts. In some people, lactose may be tolerated better if taken with meals.

The patient needs to be aware that milk, ice cream, cottage cheese, and cheese have a high lactose content. If the milk has been fermented (e.g., cultured buttermilk, yogourt, sour cream), the patient with low lactase levels may tolerate it better.

Lactase enzyme (Lactaid) is available commercially as an over-the-counter (OTC) product. It is mixed with milk and breaks down the lactose before the milk is ingested. Lactase tablets can also be taken with the ingestion of other dairy products. Since decreased or no intake of milk and milk products can lead to calcium deficiency, supplements may be necessary to prevent osteoporosis.

SHORT BOWEL SYNDROME

Short bowel syndrome (SBS) results from extensive resection of the small intestine. Rapid intestinal transit, impaired digestive and absorption processes, and fluid and electrolyte losses characterize the syndrome. In adults, extensive resection of the small intestine may be necessary for bowel infarction because of vascular thrombosis or insufficiency, abdominal trauma, cancer, radiation enteritis, or Crohn's disease.

Clinical Manifestations

The predominant manifestations of SBS are diarrhea, steatorrhea, and weight loss. There may be signs of malnutrition and multiple vitamin and mineral deficiencies (e.g., cobalamin and zinc deficiency, hypocalcemia). The patient may develop lactase deficiency and bacterial overgrowth. Oxalate kidney stones may form from increased colonic absorption of oxalate.

Interprofessional Care

The overall goals of interprofessional care are that the patient with SBS will have fluid and electrolyte balance, normal

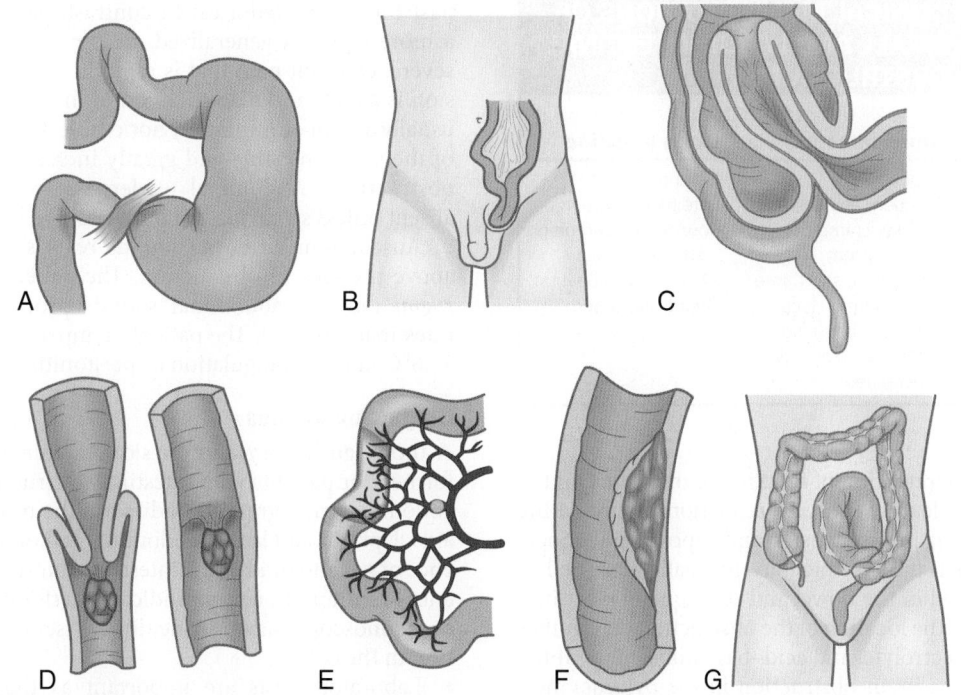

FIG. 45.4 Bowel obstructions. **A,** Adhesions. **B,** Strangulated inguinal hernia. **C,** Ileocecal intussusception. **D,** Intussusception from polyps. **E,** Mesenteric occlusion. **F,** Neoplasm. **G,** Volvulus of the sigmoid colon.

nutritional status, and control over diarrhea. In the period immediately following massive bowel resection, patients receive PN to replace fluid, electrolyte, and nutrient losses. Hypersecretion of gastric acid, for which the cause is unknown, is reduced by proton pump inhibitors (e.g., omeprazole [Losec]).

The patient with SBS is encouraged to eat at least six to eight meals per day to increase the overall time food is present in and in contact with the intestine. Oral intake can be supplemented with elemental nutrient formulas and tube feeding during the night. For patients with severe malabsorption, PN may be reinstituted. Oral supplements of calcium, zinc, and multivitamins are typically recommended. Opioid antidiarrheal medications are the most effective in decreasing intestinal motility (see Table 45.3).

INTESTINAL OBSTRUCTION

Intestinal obstruction occurs when a partial or complete obstruction of the intestine prevents intestinal contents from passing through the GI tract; it requires prompt treatment. The causes of intestinal obstruction can be classified as mechanical or nonmechanical.

Types of Intestinal Obstruction

Mechanical. *Mechanical obstruction* (caused by an object) may be caused by an occlusion of the lumen of the intestinal tract (Figure 45.4). Most intestinal obstructions occur in the small intestine and are usually due to adhesions, which can develop after abdominal surgery. Obstruction can occur within days of surgery or years later. Carcinoma is the most common cause of large bowel obstruction, followed by volvulus and diverticular disease.

Nonmechanical. A *nonmechanical obstruction* (caused by paralysis) may result from a neuromuscular or vascular disorder.

Paralytic (adynamic) ileus is an impairment of intestinal motility (ileus that persists for more than 2 to 3 days) and is the most common form of nonmechanical obstruction. It can occur after any abdominal surgery. Other causes of paralytic ileus include peritonitis, inflammatory responses (e.g., acute pancreatitis, acute appendicitis), electrolyte abnormalities, and thoracic or lumbar spinal fractures.

Pseudo-obstruction is an apparent mechanical obstruction of the intestine without demonstration of obstruction by radiological methods. Collagen vascular diseases and neurological and endocrine disorders may cause pseudo-obstruction, but mostly it is found to be idiopathic.

Vascular obstructions are rare and are due to an interference with the blood supply to a portion of the intestines. The most common causes are emboli and atherosclerosis of the mesenteric arteries. The celiac, inferior, and superior mesenteric arteries supply blood to the bowel. Emboli may originate from thrombi in patients with chronic atrial fibrillation, diseased heart valves, and prosthetic valves. Venous thrombosis may be seen in low–blood flow states, such as heart failure and shock.

Etiology and Pathophysiology

Normally, 6 to 8 L of fluid enters the small bowel daily. Most of the fluid is absorbed before it reaches the colon. Approximately 75% of intestinal gas is swallowed air. Bacterial metabolism produces methane and hydrogen gases. Fluid, gas, and intestinal contents accumulate proximal to the intestinal obstruction. This causes distension, and the distal bowel may collapse. The distension reduces the absorption of fluids and stimulates intestinal secretions. As the fluid increases, so does the pressure in the lumen of the bowel. The increased pressure leads to an increase in capillary permeability and extravasation of fluids and electrolytes into the peritoneal cavity. Edema, congestion, and necrosis from impaired blood supply as well as possible rupture of the

TABLE 45.27	**CLINICAL MANIFESTATIONS OF SMALL AND LARGE INTESTINAL OBSTRUCTIONS**	
Clinical Manifestations	**Small Intestine**	**Large Intestine**
Onset	Rapid	Gradual
Vomiting	Frequent and copious	Late manifestation
Pain	Colicky, cramplike, intermittent	Low-grade, cramping abdominal pain
Bowel movement	Feces for a short time	Absolute constipation
Abdominal distension	Dependent on location of obstruction, minimal to greatly increased	Greatly increased

bowel may occur. The retention of fluid in the intestine and the peritoneal cavity can lead to a severe reduction in circulating blood volume, resulting in hypotension and hypovolemic shock.

The electrolyte-rich fluids, which are normally absorbed in the bowel, are retained in the bowel and subsequently lost into the peritoneal cavity. The location of the obstruction determines the extent of fluid, electrolyte, and acid–base imbalances. If the obstruction is high, as in an obstruction in the pylorus, metabolic alkalosis may result from the loss of hydrochloric acid from the stomach through vomiting or NG intubation.

When the obstruction is located in the small bowel, dehydration occurs rapidly. Dehydration and electrolyte imbalances do not occur early in large bowel obstruction. If the obstruction is below the proximal colon, most GI fluids have been absorbed before reaching the point of the obstruction. Solid fecal material accumulates until symptoms of discomfort appear. Reverse peristalsis may cause vomiting of fecal material very late in the bowel obstruction.

Simple obstructions of the intestine involve blockage of the lumen in one spot. A closed-loop obstruction occurs when the lumen is blocked in two different spots (e.g., volvulus). This results in an isolated segment of bowel and obstruction proximal to that segment. Strangulation and gangrene are likely to develop if treatment is not immediate. A strangulated obstruction occurs when the circulation to the obstructed intestine is impaired. This is the most dangerous form of obstruction because it may lead to necrosis of the intestine (incarcerated). Volvulus, hernias, or adhesions are the most common causes.

Clinical Manifestations

The clinical manifestations of intestinal obstruction vary, depending on the location of the obstruction, and include nausea, vomiting, abdominal pain, distension, inability to pass flatus, and obstipation (Table 45.27). Obstruction located high in the small intestine produces rapid-onset, sometimes projectile vomiting with bile-containing vomitus. Vomiting from more distal obstructions of the small intestine is more gradual in onset. The vomitus may be orange-brown and foul smelling because of bacterial overgrowth. Vomiting may be entirely absent in large bowel obstruction if the ileocecal valve is competent; otherwise, the patient may eventually vomit fecal material.

Vomiting usually relieves abdominal pain in high intestinal obstructions. Persistent, colicky abdominal pain is seen with lower intestinal obstruction. A characteristic sign of mechanical obstruction is pain that comes and goes in waves. This is caused by intestinal peristalsis working to move bowel contents past the obstructed area. In contrast, paralytic ileus produces a more constant generalized discomfort. Strangulation causes severe, constant pain that is rapid in onset. Abdominal distension is a common manifestation of intestinal obstructions. It is usually absent or minimally noticeable in proximal obstructions of the small intestine and greatly increased in lower intestinal obstructions. Abdominal tenderness and rigidity are usually absent unless strangulation or peritonitis has occurred.

Auscultation of bowel sounds reveals high-pitched sounds above the area of obstruction. The patient often notes *borborygmi* (audible abdominal sounds produced by hyperactive intestinal motility). The patient's temperature rarely rises above 37.8°C unless strangulation or peritonitis has occurred.

Diagnostic Studies

A thorough history and physical examination should be performed for patients with intestinal obstruction. A CT scan and abdominal radiographic studies are the most useful diagnostic aids. Upright and lateral abdominal radiographs show the presence of gas and fluid in the intestines (air–fluid levels). The presence of intraperitoneal air indicates perforation. Sigmoidoscopy or colonoscopy may provide direct visualization of an obstruction in the colon.

Laboratory tests are important as they provide essential information for diagnosis. A CBC and serum electrolyte, amylase, and blood urea nitrogen (BUN) tests should be performed. An elevated WBC count may indicate strangulation or perforation; elevated hematocrit values may reflect hemoconcentration. Decreased hemoglobin and hematocrit values may indicate bleeding from a neoplasm or strangulation with necrosis. Serum electrolytes should be monitored to assess the patient's fluid and electrolyte balance. Serum sodium, potassium, and chloride concentrations are decreased in small bowel obstruction. The BUN value may be increased because of dehydration. The stool should be checked for occult blood.

Interprofessional Care

Treatment for intestinal obstruction is directed toward decompression of the intestine by removal of gas and fluid, correction and maintenance of fluid and electrolyte balance, and relief or removal of the obstruction. NG tubes may be used to decompress the bowel. NG tubes may be inserted before surgery to empty the stomach and relieve distension. NG or venting percutaneous tubes are effective in the treatment of patients with neurogenic obstruction who do not require surgery.

Sigmoidoscopy may successfully reduce a sigmoid volvulus. Colon-decompression catheters may be passed through partially obstructed areas via a colonoscope to decompress the bowel before surgery.

IV infusions that contain normal saline solution and potassium should be given to maintain fluid and electrolyte balance. PN may be necessary in some cases to correct nutritional deficiencies, improve the patient's nutritional status before surgery, and promote postoperative healing.

Most mechanical obstructions are treated surgically. Surgery may involve resecting the obstructed segment of bowel and anastomosing the remaining healthy bowel. Partial or total colectomy, colostomy, or ileostomy may be required when extensive obstruction or necrosis is present. Occasionally, obstructions can be removed nonsurgically. A colonoscope can be used to remove polyps, dilate strictures, and remove and destroy tumours with a laser.

NURSING MANAGEMENT INTESTINAL OBSTRUCTION

NURSING ASSESSMENT

Intestinal obstruction is a potentially life-threatening condition. Nursing assessment must begin with a detailed patient history and physical examination. The type and the location of obstruction usually cause characteristic symptoms. The nurse should determine the location, duration, intensity, and frequency of abdominal pain and whether abdominal tenderness or rigidity is present. For vomiting, the onset, frequency, colour, odour, and amount of vomitus should be recorded. Bowel function, including passage of flatus, should be determined. The nurse auscultates for bowel sounds and documents the character and the location; inspects the abdomen for scars, palpable masses, and distension; and observes for muscle guarding and tenderness.

NURSING DIAGNOSES

Nursing diagnoses for patients with intestinal obstructions include but are not limited to the following:

- *Acute pain* resulting from *biological injury agent* (abdominal distension and increased peristalsis)
- *Dehydration* resulting from *insufficient fluid intake* (decrease in intestinal fluid absorption, third space fluid shifts, NG suction)

PLANNING

The overall goals are that the patient with an intestinal obstruction will have (1) relief of the obstruction and return to normal bowel function, (2) minimal to no discomfort, (3) normal fluid and electrolyte status, and (4) maintenance of adequate nutrition.

NURSING IMPLEMENTATION

The patient should be monitored closely for signs of dehydration and electrolyte imbalance. A strict intake and output record should be maintained. IV fluids should be administered as ordered. Serum electrolyte levels should be monitored. A patient with a high obstruction is more likely to have metabolic alkalosis; a patient with a low obstruction is at greater risk for metabolic acidosis. The patient is often restless and constantly changes position to relieve the pain. The nurse should provide comfort measures, promote a restful environment, and keep distractions and visitors to a minimum. Nursing care of the patient after surgery for an intestinal obstruction is similar to care of a patient after a laparotomy (see NCP 45.2, available on the Evolve website).

POLYPS OF THE LARGE INTESTINE

Colonic polyps arise from the mucosal surface of the colon and project into the lumen. They may be *sessile* (flat, broad based, and attached directly to the intestinal wall) or *pedunculated* (attached to the intestinal wall by a stalk). Polyps tend to be sessile when small and become pedunculated as they enlarge, especially if they are in the left or descending colon (Figure 45.5). They may be found anywhere in the large intestine but are most commonly found in the rectosigmoid area. Although most polyps are asymptomatic, rectal bleeding or occult blood in the stool are the most common manifestations.

Types of Polyps

The most common types of polyp are hyperplastic and adenomatous. *Hyperplastic polyps* originate from the epithelium and are non-neoplastic growths. They rarely grow larger than 5 mm and never cause clinical symptoms. Other benign (non-neoplastic)

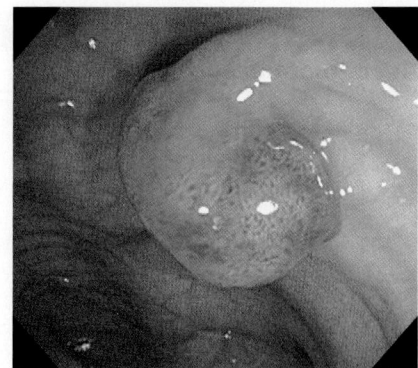

FIG. 45.5 Endoscopic image of a pedunculated polyp in the descending colon. Source: David Musher/Science Source.

TABLE 45.28 TYPES OF POLYPS OF THE LARGE INTESTINE

Neoplastic	Non-Neoplastic
• Epithelial polyps (adenomatous)	• Epithelial polyps (hyperplastic)
• Tubular adenoma	• Hereditary polyposis syndromes
• Tubular villous adenoma	• Familial juvenile polyposis
• Villous adenoma	• Inflammatory polyps
• Hereditary polyposis syndromes (adenomatous polyposis syndrome)	• Pseudopolyps
• Familial adenomatous polyposis (FAP)	• Benign lymphoid polyps
	• Submucosal
	• Lipomas
	• Leiomyomas
	• Fibromas

polyps include inflammatory polyps, lipomas, and juvenile polyps (Table 45.28).

Adenomatous polyps are characterized by neoplastic changes in the epithelium. They are closely linked to colorectal adenocarcinoma. Structurally, there are three types, with tubular adenomas being the most prevalent. The risk for cancer in the polyp increases with polyp size and villous structure. Villous adenomas have a higher risk of turning cancerous than do tubular adenomas. Removing adenomatous polyps decreases the occurrence of colorectal cancer.

Although there are several polyposis syndromes, they are relatively rare. Of these, *familial adenomatous polyposis* (FAP) is the most common (see the Genetics in Clinical Practice box). This disorder is characterized by multiple polyps that at times number in the thousands and that are located in the large intestine and sometimes in other areas of the GI tract. Patients with a history of FAP have a lifetime risk of developing colorectal cancer that approaches 100%. They also develop cancer at an earlier age (i.e., <40 years of age) than patients with non-FAP colorectal cancer. For children of patients with FAP, screening must be initiated at puberty and then conducted annually. These children have a 50% risk of developing FAP. When there is indication of disease, total colectomy with ileostomy is the treatment of choice. Patients with FAP are also at risk for cancers of the thyroid, small bowel, liver, and brain, so lifetime cancer surveillance is essential (Suhaimi et al., 2015).

Diagnostic Studies and Interprofessional Care

Barium enema, sigmoidoscopy, colonoscopy, and CT/MRI colonography (virtual colonoscopy) are used to diagnose polyps. All polyps are considered abnormal and should be removed. In patients whose polyps are identified through barium enema, removal (polypectomy) should be done through a colonoscope or a sigmoidoscope. If the polyp is not removable, a biopsy

GENETICS IN CLINICAL PRACTICE
Familial Adenomatous Polyposis (FAP)

Genetic Basis
- Autosomal dominant disorder
- Mutation in *APC* gene located on chromosome 5

Incidence
- 1 in 5 000–7 500 people
- Men and women affected equally

Genetic Testing
- DNA testing available to detect *APC* gene mutation

Clinical Implications
- FAP is characterized by the presence of colorectal polyps (usually >1 000).
- Polyps are not present at birth but appear during adolescence and early adulthood.
- FAP accounts for at least 1% of all colorectal cancers.
- If untreated, FAP almost always results in the development of colon cancer before the age of 40 years.
- With FAP, there is also increased incidence of gastric and small intestinal polyps.
- Many deaths related to FAP could be prevented with early and aggressive monitoring and treatment, including frequent colonoscopies and total colectomy.
- Individuals with a family history of FAP could benefit from genetic counselling and teaching.

APC, adenomatous polyposis coli; *FAP*, familial adenomatous polyposis.

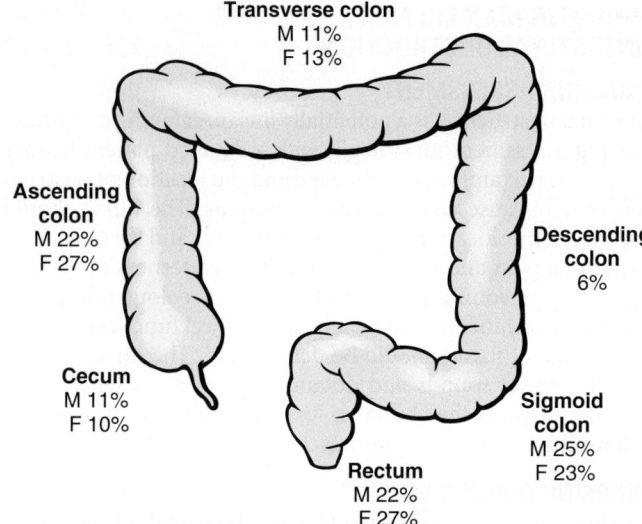

FIG. 45.6 Incidence of colorectal cancer. Approximately one half of all colon cancers occur in the rectosigmoid area. Percentages are listed for males *(M)* and females *(F)*.

TABLE 45.29	RISK FACTORS FOR COLORECTAL CANCER

- Age >50 years
- Alcohol (over 4 drinks per week)
- Chronic inflammatory bowel disease
- Cigarette smoking
- Colorectal polyps
- Familial adenomatous polyposis (FAP)
- Family history of colorectal cancer or adenomas
- History of ovarian, endometrial, or breast cancer (women)
- Increased consumption of red meat
- Obesity
- Previous history of colorectal cancer

specimen should be taken for tissue examination. Surgery is not indicated unless carcinoma is present or certain cases of polyposis syndromes warrant it. The patient should be observed for rectal bleeding, fever, severe abdominal pain, and abdominal distension, which may indicate hemorrhage or perforation.

COLORECTAL CANCER

Colorectal cancer (a malignant disease of the colon, the rectum, or both) is the second-most common cause of cancer death in Canada. In 2019, it was estimated that there were 24 800 new cases of colorectal cancer diagnosed in Canada, and that 9 600 people died from it (Canadian Cancer Society, 2021a).

The incidence of colorectal cancer at specific sites varies (Figure 45.6). In both sexes, the incidence of right colon cancers has increased, and cancers in the rectum have decreased. The highest percentages of colorectal cancers in Canada are currently located in the rectum, the ascending colon, and the sigmoid colon. Approximately 20% of colorectal cancers are within reach of the examining finger, and 50% are within reach of the sigmoidoscope.

Etiology and Pathophysiology

Risk factors for colorectal cancer include a diet high in red or processed meat; obesity; physical inactivity; alcohol use; long-term smoking, and low intake of fruits and vegetables. Groups at high risk for colorectal cancer have been identified (Table 45.29), and genetic conditions such as FAP and a history of IBD place an individual at risk for colorectal cancer. About one third of cases of colorectal cancer occur in patients with a family history of colorectal cancer. (See the two Genetics in Clinical Practice boxes in this chapter.) The risk for development in the general population increases slightly after the age of 50 years and then rises rapidly in the following decades regardless of gender.

GENETICS IN CLINICAL PRACTICE
Hereditary Nonpolyposis Colorectal Cancer

Genetic Basis
- Autosomal dominant disorder
- Mutations in *MSH2, MLH1, MSH6, PMS2* genes
- Mutations in genes that error-check DNA (repair genes)

Incidence
- 1 in 500–2 000 people

Genetic Testing
- DNA testing available

Clinical Implications
- HNPCC accounts for 5% of all colorectal cancers.
- Individuals with gene mutation have an 80–90% lifetime risk of developing colorectal cancer.
- The average age of diagnosis is in the mid-40s.
- Cancer arises from single colorectal lesion in the absence of polyposis.
- Cancers tend to occur on the right side of the colon.
- HNPCC is less aggressive and is associated with longer survival rates than colon cancers that develop without known risk factors.
- People with gene mutations are at high risk of developing other cancers, including uterine, ovarian, ureter, pancreas, stomach, and small intestinal cancer.
- Individuals with known gene mutations should be monitored with colonoscopy every year.
- Examination by pelvic ultrasound and endometrial biopsy should also be considered for women.

HNPCC, hereditary nonpolyposis colorectal cancer.

Adenocarcinoma is the most common type of colorectal cancer. Most colorectal cancers begin as adenomatous polyps that arise from the mucosa lining the lumen of the colon and the rectum. As it grows, the cancer progresses down from the tip of the polyp through the body and stalk. It becomes invasive and penetrates the muscularis mucosae. Once through the muscularis mucosae, tumour cells gain access to the regional lymph nodes and the vascular system and can spread to distant sites. The most common sites of metastasis are the regional lymph nodes, liver, lungs, and peritoneum. Because venous blood leaving the colon and rectum flows through the portal vein and inferior rectal vein, the liver and lung are common sites of metastasis. The cancer spreads from the liver to other sites, including the lungs, bones, and brain. The cancer can also spread directly into adjacent structures. The growing tumour can obstruct the bowel. Other complications include bleeding, perforation, peritonitis, and fistula formation.

Clinical Manifestations

Clinical manifestations of colorectal cancer are usually nonspecific or do not appear until the disease is advanced. Rectal bleeding is the most common symptom of colorectal cancer but it may not be visible to the naked eye. Other commonly seen manifestations include alternating constipation and diarrhea, abdominal cramps, gas or bloating, change in stool calibre (narrow, ribbon-like), loss of appetite, early satiety, weight loss, lethargy, and sensation of incomplete evacuation (Figure 45.7) (Colorectal Cancer Association of Canada, 2021a).

Iron-deficiency anemia and occult bleeding dictate further investigation. Because of increased emphasis on screening practices, colon cancer is now often detected during screening procedures. However, there are barriers to adequate colorectal cancer screening for Indigenous Canadians. For example, access to culturally competent health service is lacking, in particular access to Indigenous health providers, and long-standing mistrust of Western medicine and health staff exists (D'Onise et al., 2020).

Diagnostic Studies

A thorough history, with close attention to family history, should be obtained, and a physical examination should be performed (Table 45.30). The digital rectal examination is the most important aspect of the physical examination because many rectal cancers are within reach of the finger. In the asymptomatic person who is between 50 and 74 years with no risk factors (other than age), a *fecal occult blood test* (FOBT) or *fecal immunochemical test* (FIT) should be done every 2 years. Follow-up for a positive test should include a colonoscopy or flexible sigmoidoscopy. A colonoscopy is not usually recommended as a routine screening test for people who don't have a high risk for colorectal cancer. FOBTs have been used for more than 30 years to screen for colorectal cancer and continue to be widely used in North America. Patients need to be taught to abstain from eating red meat and using acetylsalicylic acid (ASA; Aspirin) and NSAIDs (if medically safe) before testing, to avoid false-positive results. The FIT uses antibodies to detect human hemoglobin protein in the stool. It is performed in much the same way as the FOBT but there are no medication or dietary restrictions. The Septin9 blood test is another screening tool for colorectal cancer. It is used to detect the presence of methylated Septin9 DNA, which is correlated with an increased risk for colorectal cancer (Xie et al., 2018).

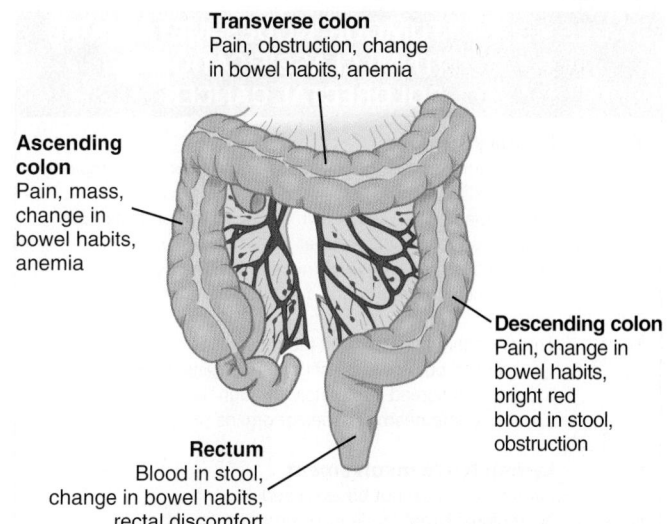

FIG. 45.7 Signs and symptoms of colorectal cancer by location of primary lesion. Source: Modified from McCance, K. L., & Huether, S. E. (2010). *Pathophysiology: The biologic basis for disease in adults and children* (6th ed., p. 1502). Mosby.

TABLE 45.30 INTERPROFESSIONAL CARE

Colorectal Cancer

Diagnostic	Interprofessional Therapy
• History and physical examination • Digital rectal examination • Sigmoidoscopy • Colonoscopy • Barium enema • CBC • Liver function tests • Testing of stool for occult blood • Carcinoembryonic antigen (CEA) test • CT scan of abdomen • Ultrasound (including endorectal) • MRI	• Surgery • Right hemicolectomy • Left hemicolectomy • Abdominal–perineal resection • Laparoscopic colectomy • Radiation • Chemotherapy

CBC, complete blood cell count; *CT,* computed tomographic (scan); *MRI,* magnetic resonance imaging.

Colonoscopy is the procedure of choice. Synchronous lesions may be present at other sites in the colon, and tissue diagnosis may be made by biopsy during the procedure. Other procedures include endorectal ultrasonography and CT colonography (virtual colonoscopy) to localize the lesion and determine its size or the presence of metastases.

Laboratory studies should include a CBC to check for anemia, clotting studies, and liver function tests. A CT scan of the abdomen may be helpful in detecting liver metastases, retroperitoneal and pelvic disease, and depth of penetration of the tumour into the bowel wall. A CT scan should be done before surgery. Liver function tests are performed to determine the presence of liver metastases.

A carcinoembryonic antigen (CEA) test is often performed, although it is not specific for colorectal cancer. A normal level of CEA does not exclude the possibility of a malignant condition. This test is used most effectively in following the progress of a patient after surgery. Return to normal of a previously elevated CEA indicates successful removal of the tumour. In contrast, postoperative CEA levels that are persistently elevated or that increase suggest the presence of residual tumour or tumour spread.

TABLE 45.31	**TUMOUR–NODES–METASTASIS (TNM) CLASSIFICATION OF COLORECTAL CANCER**		
T	**Primary Tumour**		
T_x	Primary tumour cannot be assessed because of incomplete information.		
T_{is}	Carcinoma in situ. Cancer is in earliest stage and has not grown beyond mucosa layer.		
T_1	Tumour has grown beyond mucosa into the submucosa.		
T_2	Tumour has grown through submucosa into muscularis propria.		
T_3	Tumour has grown through the muscularis propria into the subserosa but not to neighbouring organs or tissues.		
T_4	Tumour has spread completely through the colon or rectal wall and into nearby tissues or organs.		
N	**Lymph Node Involvement**		
N_x	Lymph nodes cannot be assessed.		
N_0	No regional lymph node involvement is found.		
N_1	Cancer is found in one to three nearby lymph nodes.		
N_2	Cancer is found in four or more nearby lymph nodes.		
M	**Metastasis**		
M_x	Presence of distant metastasis cannot be assessed.		
M_0	No distant metastasis is seen.		
M_1	Distant metastasis is present.		
Stage	**TNM**		
0	T_{is}	N_0	M_0
IA	T_1	N_0	M_0
IB	T_2	N_0	M_0
II	T_1	N_2	M_0
	T_2	N_1	M_0
	T_3	N_0	M_0
IIIA	T_2	N_2	M_0
	T_3	N_{1-2}	M_0
IIIB	T_4	N_{0-1}	M_0
IV	T_4	N_2	M_0
	T_{1-4}	N_{0-2}	M_1

Interprofessional Care

Prognosis and treatment correlate with pathological staging of the disease. Several methods of staging are available, with the TNM (tumour–nodes–metastasis) system (Table 45.31) being the most widely used. It describes a patient's cancer on the basis of degree of invasion of the primary tumour, lymph node involvement, and presence of metastasis. The stage at diagnosis is key in determining prognosis and appropriate treatment.

Several noninvasive procedures may be performed through a colonoscope to effectively treat certain types of colorectal cancer. Endoscopic polypectomy is a highly effective and safe procedure. Adequate treatment can be obtained if the resected margin of the polyp is free of cancer, the cancer is well differentiated, and there is no apparent lymphatic or blood vessel involvement. Laser therapy may be used to ablate nonresectable tumours. This is usually used only as palliative therapy in patients with obstructive symptoms.

Surgical Therapy. The location and the extent of the cancer determine the type of surgery performed. Success of surgery depends on resection of the tumour with an adequate margin of healthy bowel and resection of the regional lymph nodes.

Right hemicolectomy is performed when the cancer is located in the cecum, the ascending colon, the hepatic flexure, or the transverse colon to the right of the middle colic artery.

A portion of the terminal ileum, the ileocecal valve, and the appendix are removed, and an ileotransverse anastomosis is performed. A left hemicolectomy involves resection of the left transverse colon, the splenic flexure, the descending colon, the sigmoid colon, and the upper portion of the rectum.

Clear margins are most difficult to obtain with rectal carcinoma. Location of the rectal lesion determines the surgical procedure to be performed. There must be enough rectum left to ensure a secure anastomosis and preservation of anal sphincter function, or an abdominal–perineal resection is indicated. Abdominal–perineal resection is most often performed when the cancer is located within 5 cm of the anus, although ultra-low anterior resections can be performed (within 1 to 2 cm of the anus) by skilled surgeons.

In the abdominal–perineal resection, an abdominal incision is made, and the proximal sigmoid is brought through the abdominal wall as a permanent colostomy. The distal sigmoid, rectum, and anus are removed through a perineal incision. The perineal wound may be primarily closed with a drain or left open with appropriate dressings to allow healing by secondary intention. Complications that can occur are delayed wound healing, hemorrhage, persistent perineal sinus tracts, infections, and urinary tract and sexual dysfunctions.

Low anterior resection may be indicated for tumours of the rectosigmoid and the mid-to-upper rectum. The use of end-to-end anastomosis (EEA) staplers has enabled lower and more secure anastomoses. The stapler is passed through the anus, where the colon is stapled to the rectum. This technique has made it possible to resect lesions to a point as low as 1 to 2 cm from the anus.

Sphincter-sparing procedures are being performed on patients who are a poor operative risk and on patients with early disease. The number of these procedures may increase with continued early detection and surveillance. In these procedures, a local resection is performed, and the anal sphincters are left intact.

Laparoscopic colectomy may be an option in earlier-stage cancers. Potential benefits are faster return of bowel function, fewer incisional infections, shortened hospital stay, and improved cosmetic appearance (Colorectal Cancer Association of Canada, 2021b).

Chemotherapy and Radiation Therapy. Chemotherapy is recommended when a patient has positive lymph nodes at the time of surgery or has metastatic disease. Chemotherapy is used both as an adjuvant therapy following colon resection and as primary treatment for nonresectable colorectal cancer. Various chemotherapy agents, including capecitabine (Xeloda), fluorouracil (Efudex), folinic acid (leucovorin), and other medications are used, with medication choice being based on the stage of the disease (Colorectal Cancer Association of Canada, 2021c).

Radiation may be used preoperatively as an adjuvant to colon resection and chemotherapy or as a palliative measure for patients with advanced lesions. As a palliative measure, its primary objective is to reduce tumour size and provide symptomatic relief. (For a discussion of radiation therapy, see Chapter 18.)

NURSING MANAGEMENT COLORECTAL CANCER

NURSING ASSESSMENT

Subjective and objective data that should be obtained from a patient with colorectal cancer are presented in Table 45.32.

TABLE 45.32 NURSING ASSESSMENT
Colorectal Cancer

Subjective Data
Important Health Information
Past health history: Previous breast or ovarian cancer, familial adenomatous polyposis (FAP), callous adenoma, adenomatous polyps, inflammatory bowel disease; family history of colorectal, breast, or ovarian cancer
Medications: Use of any medication affecting bowel function (e.g., cathartics, antidiarrheal agents)

Symptoms
- Weakness, fatigue
- Anorexia, weight loss; nausea and vomiting
- Change in bowel habits; alternating diarrhea and constipation, defecation urgency; rectal bleeding; mucoid stools; black, tarry stools; increased flatus, decrease in stool calibre; feelings of incomplete evacuation
- Abdominal and low back pain, tenesmus

Objective Data
General
Pallor, cachexia, lymphadenopathy (later signs)

Gastrointestinal
Palpable abdominal mass (late sign), distension, ascites, and hepatomegaly (liver metastasis)

Possible Findings
Anemia; positive fecal occult blood; palpable mass on digital rectal examination; positive sigmoidoscopy, colonoscopy, barium enema, or CT scan; positive biopsy

CT, computed tomographic (scan).

NURSING DIAGNOSES

Nursing diagnoses for the patient with cancer of the colon or the rectum include but are not limited to the following:
- *Constipation* resulting from *decrease in gastrointestinal motility*
- *Anxiety* resulting from *threat to current status, threat of death*
- *Inadequate coping* resulting from *inadequate opportunity to prepare for stressor, insufficient sense of control* (diagnosis of cancer, adverse effects of treatment)

PLANNING

The overall goals are that the patient with colorectal cancer will have (1) appropriate treatment (removal of tumour, adjunctive therapy), (2) normal bowel elimination patterns, (3) quality of life appropriate to disease prognosis, (4) relief of pain, and (5) feelings of comfort and well-being.

NURSING IMPLEMENTATION

HEALTH PROMOTION. The current recommendations from the Canadian Cancer Society, 2021b) for colorectal cancer screening in patients who are between 50 and 74 years and not at high risk include FOBT or FIT performed every 2 years. People over age 74 years should discuss an individual screening plan with their health care provider. Positive findings should be followed with flexible sigmoidoscopy, colonoscopy, or double-contrast barium enema. Screening for high-risk patients should begin before age 50, usually beginning with colonoscopy and continuing at more frequent intervals that vary according to risk factors (Canadian Cancer Society, 2021b).

A number of epidemiology studies have reported that use of NSAIDs (e.g., ibuprofen [Advil]) or long-term use of ASA (Aspirin) may reduce the development of adenomatous colorectal polyps and reduce the risk for colorectal cancer (Friis et al., 2015).

ACUTE INTERVENTION

Preoperative Care. Acute nursing care for the patient with a colon resection is similar to the care of the patient having a laparotomy (see NCP 45.2, available on the Evolve website). In addition to general preoperative teaching and ostomy care instructions, the patient undergoing abdominal–perineal resection should be informed of the extent of the surgical procedure and the potential for sexual dysfunction after surgery. Comfortable positioning may be difficult with either an open or a closed perineal wound. Side-to-side positioning in bed and the use of pressure-reducing support surfaces for the bed and chair may be helpful. Doughnut cushions should not be used because these delay wound healing. The patient may experience phantom rectal sensation because the sympathetic nerves responsible for rectal control are not severed during the surgery. The nurse must be astute in distinguishing phantom sensations from perineal abscess pain.

Postoperative Care. After an abdominal–perineal resection, there are two wounds, and a stoma is surgically constructed in the left lower quadrant. There is an abdominal incision through which the colon is resected, and an incision is made in the perineum. The management of a perineal incision differs according to the type of wound. Different approaches may be taken with the perineal wound: (1) packing of the entire open wound or (2) primary closure of the perineal wound with closed-suction drainage of the pelvic cavity. The type of management of the perineal wound is individualized. The open and packed method is used in patients with extensive bleeding in the perineal wound or when there are concerns about local wound infection. A Jackson-Pratt or a Hemovac suction device placed through the buttocks into the pelvic cavity is commonly used to provide drainage of the operative site during the early postoperative period.

A patient who has open and packed wounds requires meticulous postoperative care. During the immediate postoperative period, the perineal dressing may quickly become saturated with serosanguineous drainage. Proper containment of the drainage with appropriate topical dressings such as calcium alginates or hydrofibres will assist in management of the wound. All drainage is carefully assessed for amount, colour, and consistency.

The nurse should examine the wound regularly and record bleeding, excessive drainage, and unusual odour. The perineal wound is usually irrigated with a normal saline solution when the dressings are changed. Topical dressing selection should be made applying wound care principles: reduce bacterial burden, facilitate moist wound healing, contain drainage, and protect periwound skin. Negative-pressure therapy may be an option to enhance wound healing. Aseptic technique is always used.

When the perineal wound is closed, the drains are left in place for approximately 3 to 5 days. During this time, the drainage is examined and observations recorded. The area around the drains is observed for signs of inflammation and is kept clean and dry. The nurse should observe for signs of induration, erythema, purulent drainage around the suture line, fever, and elevated WBC count. Perineal wound closure may be done with removable or dissolvable sutures. If removable sutures are used, these are generally left in place for 2 to 3 weeks.

If the patient reports pain and itching in and around the wound, the nurse should carefully inspect the wound for signs of local infection, maceration from wound drainage, or yeast. Use of a pressure-reducing chair cushion provides comfort when sitting, and side-to-side positioning in bed will help with comfort.

Sexual dysfunction is a possible complication of an abdominal–perineal resection and should be addressed in the plan of care. Although the effect of the procedure depends on the extent of pelvic dissection, the surgeon must inform the patient of the risk preoperatively. The nurse should understand that erection, ejaculation, and orgasm involve different nerve pathways and that a dysfunction of one does not mean total sexual dysfunction. The ET nurse is an important member of the team and can often provide factual information concerning sexual dysfunction and management options.

AMBULATORY AND HOME CARE. Psychological support for the patient and family is important. The relative 5-year survival rate for patients with colorectal cancer is 64%. This presents a challenge for the patient and health care providers because of the often painful, debilitating, and demoralizing manifestations produced by the recurrent disease and the lack of any effective palliative therapy. Chemotherapy may be used as an adjuvant measure for the patient with evidence of local or distant metastasis. (The special needs of the patient with cancer are discussed in Chapter 18.)

The open perineal wound may not be completely healed before discharge. After discharge, the health care provider, home health nurse, and ET nurse usually see the patient. The wound should be regularly assessed to determine progress and to manage its ideal topical dressing. Clipping the buttock hair close to the perineal wound will aid in dressing adherence and prevent wound bed irritation from long hairs. The nurse should report persistent drainage or prolonged wound healing because it may also indicate the presence of a foreign body, fistula, or rectal tissue not removed during surgery. The patient and family may need to be taught assessment and management of the wound. The patient and family should also be made aware of all community services available for assistance.

Patients with colostomies need to know how to care for them. Even when patients do not have stomas, they may experience diarrhea, constipation, incontinence, or difficulty passing stool, depending on the section of the colon removed and the surgical procedure performed. Patients need to know about diet, incontinence products, and strategies for managing bloating, diarrhea, and bowel evacuation. Often a combination of dietary changes and medications is used to control diarrhea and constipation.

Patients with sphincter-sparing surgery frequently experience diarrhea and incontinence of feces and gas. They often need antidiarrheal medications or bulking agents to control the diarrhea but may overuse them and become constipated. Consultation with a dietitian can help patients and caregivers understand how to choose foods that are less likely to cause diarrhea and odour and help them discover which foods are problematic for them.

EVALUATION

The following are expected outcomes for the patient with colorectal cancer:
- The patient will have regular bowel elimination patterns.
- The patient will have relief of pain.
- The patient will have balanced nutritional intake.
- The patient will have quality of life appropriate to disease prognosis.
- The patient will have feelings of comfort and well-being.

OSTOMY SURGERY

Types

The creation of an *ostomy* is a surgical procedure in which an opening is made to allow passage of urine from the bladder, or intestinal contents from the bowel, to an incision or stoma surgically created in the wall of the abdomen. In the context of intestinal reconstruction, the bowel is brought through an opening in the abdominal wall. The edges of the bowel are sutured to the surrounding skin, exposing the inner lining of the bowel (mucosa); this opening is the stoma. Bowel excretion will now occur through the stoma. The stoma may be permanent or temporary, depending on the underlying reason for the surgery.

When the ileum is brought through the abdominal wall, it is called an *ileostomy* (Figure 45.8). It is commonly used in surgical treatment of UC, Crohn's disease, and FAP and may be used to temporarily protect distal anastomoses, such as in a low anterior resection.

In a *colostomy* the colon is brought through the abdominal wall. *Colostomy* is a generic term and may be used to describe any part of the colon (large intestine) that is brought to the surface. Locations for colostomies are shown in Figure 45.8. A temporary colostomy may be created as an emergency measure following bowel obstruction (e.g., malignant tumour), abdominal trauma (e.g., gunshot wound), or a perforated diverticulum. A loop colostomy (Figure 45.9) and double-barrelled colostomy (see Figure 45.8) may be created as temporary colostomies, but

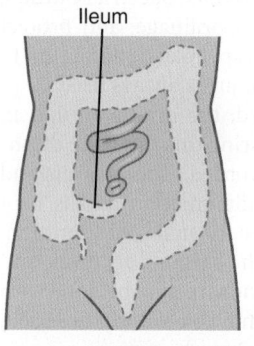
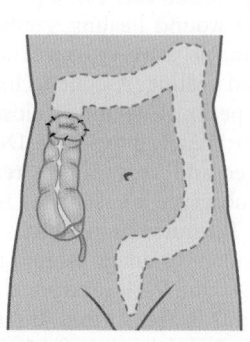
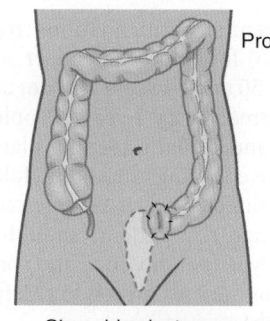
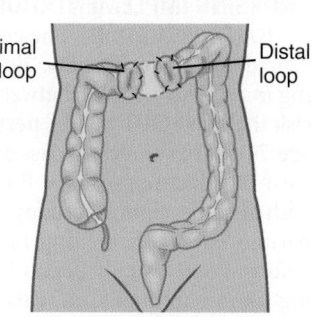

Ileostomy | Ascending colostomy | Descending colostomy | Sigmoid colostomy single-barrelled | Transverse colostomy double-barrelled

FIG. 45.8 Types of ostomies.

they may be permanent if the reason for surgery is palliation for obstructing cancer. A comparison of colostomies and ileostomy is shown in Table 45.33.

SURGICAL THERAPY

End Stoma. An *end stoma* is surgically constructed by dividing the bowel and bringing out the proximal end as a single stoma. The distal portion of the GI tract is either surgically removed or the distal segment is oversewn and left in the abdominal cavity with its mesentery intact. An end colostomy or ileostomy is then constructed. When the distal bowel is oversewn rather than removed, the result of the procedure is known as a *Hartmann pouch* (Figure 45.10). If the distal bowel is removed, the stoma is permanent; if the distal bowel remains intact and oversewn, the potential exists for the bowel to be reanastomosed and the stoma to be closed (referred to as a *takedown*).

Loop Stoma. A *loop stoma* is constructed by bringing a loop of bowel to the abdominal surface and then opening the anterior wall of the bowel to provide fecal diversion. This results in one stoma with a proximal and distal opening as well as an intact posterior wall that separates the two openings. The loop of bowel may be supported by a plastic rod for 3 to 7 days after surgery to prevent it from slipping back into the abdominal cavity (see Figure 45.9). A loop stoma is usually temporary.

Double-Barrelled Stoma. When the bowel is divided, both the proximal and the distal ends are brought through the abdominal wall as two separate stomas (see Figure 45.8). The proximal one is the functioning stoma; the distal stoma is referred to as the *mucous fistula*. The double-barrelled stoma is usually temporary.

Ileoanal Reservoir. As described in the section on UC earlier in this chapter, this procedure involves total colectomy and ileoanal anastomosis, with the formation of an ileoanal reservoir (see Figure 45.3).

NURSING MANAGEMENT
OSTOMY SURGERY

PREOPERATIVE CARE

It is important to review the information the patient has received from the health care provider. The patient and the family should understand the extent of surgery, the type of stoma, and its care. The family and the patient usually have many questions concerning the procedures. If available, an ET nurse should visit with the patient and the family as an ET nurse has additional education and training in the care and management of individuals with ostomies and can address their questions. The nurse or the ET nurse must determine the patient's ability to perform self-care, identify support systems, and determine potential adverse factors that could be modified to facilitate learning during rehabilitation.

Preoperative assessment must be comprehensive and include physical, psychological, social, cultural, and educational components. Assessment is ongoing, including of both the patient and the family. Psychological preparation and support are very important. Trained visitors from ostomy support groups may provide reassurance and guidance for the patient and family. The patient and family have the opportunity to see a person who

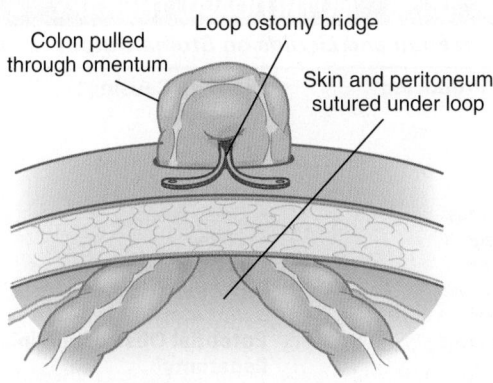

FIG. 45.9 Loop colostomy.

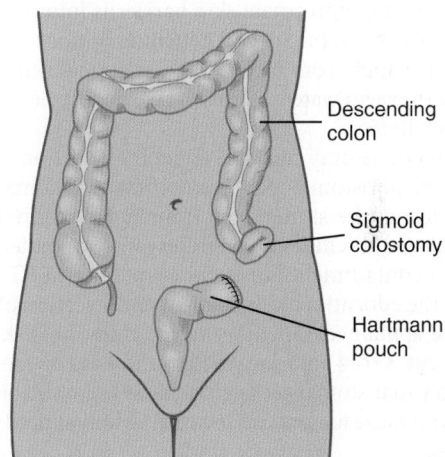

FIG. 45.10 Sigmoid colostomy. Distal bowel is oversewn and left in place to create a Hartmann pouch.

TABLE 45.33 COMPARISON OF COLOSTOMIES AND ILEOSTOMY

	Colostomy		Ileostomy
	Transverse	**Sigmoid**	
Stool consistency	Semiliquid to semiformed	Formed	Liquid to pasty
Fluid requirement	Possibly increased	No change	Increased
Bowel regulation	No	Yes (if there is a history of a regular bowel pattern)	No
Pouch and skin barriers	Yes	Dependent on regulation	Yes
Irrigation	No	Possible every 24–48 hr (if patient meets criteria)	No
Indications for surgery	Palliation for distal, nonoperable obstructing cancers; trauma	Cancer of the rectum or rectosigmoid area; perforated diverticulitis; trauma; invading gynecological cancers	Ulcerative colitis, Crohn's disease, diseased or injured colon, birth defect, familial adenomatous polyposis; trauma; cancer; ischemic colitis

has adjusted well and who has experienced some of the same feelings and concerns.

The ET nurse marks the stoma site before surgery. An improperly placed stoma complicates rehabilitation by increasing patient dependency on nursing support and increasing time, frequency, and expense of pouch change routine. It can also contribute to skin irritation and poor adaptation. Stomas should be placed within the rectus muscle, on the superior aspect of a skinfold, within the patient's visual field, above or below the beltline, and away from obvious creases and folds.

Bowel preparation before surgery may be required. Orally administered osmotic lavages (e.g., GoLYTELY) have shortened the classic 72-hour preparation with clear liquids, cathartics, and enemas. Preoperative IV antibiotics are given.

COLOSTOMY CARE

Postoperative nursing care should focus on assessing the stoma, protecting the skin and the stoma, selecting the pouch, providing patient education on ostomy self-care, and assisting the patient to adapt psychologically to a changed body. Nursing care for the patient with a colostomy is presented in NCP 45.4, available on the Evolve website.

The stoma should be pink or red. A dusky purple stoma indicates ischemia, and a brown-black stoma indicates necrosis. The nurse should assess and document stoma colour every 4 to 8 hours for the first 72 hours after surgery, when necrosis is more likely to occur. There is initial mild to moderate swelling of the stoma, which will settle 4 to 6 weeks after surgery (Table 45.34). Application of an appropriate skin barrier is important to protect the peristomal skin. Several pouching options are available from ostomy supply companies. The peristomal skin should be cleansed with warm water and dried thoroughly before the new barrier is applied.

Principles of ostomy care and pouching selection include (1) protection of peristomal skin from effluent, trauma, or both; (2) protection of the stoma from trauma; (3) secured containment of odour and effluent; (4) preservation of patient dignity; and (5) cost containment of pouching system. An ET nurse can assist with the education of the patient and selection of the most appropriate appliance. Openings to the traditional skin barrier should be cut 3 to 4 mm larger than the base of the stoma to allow for normal stomal peristalsis. Newer, mouldable barriers eliminate the need for precise measuring and simplify the care for patients.

The volume, colour, and consistency of the drainage are recorded. Each time the pouch is changed, the condition of the skin and stoma are observed. If any abnormalities are noted (rash, blisters, ulcers), an ET nurse should be consulted for assessment and management.

A colostomy in the transverse colon has semiliquid to pasty stools and moderate to large volumes of flatus. A colostomy in the sigmoid or the descending colon has semiformed or formed stools and can sometimes be regulated by the irrigation method. Patients may choose to use drainable, closed-end pouches or pouch liners to manage the stool. Currently available are flushable pouch liners, which increase the life of the ostomy bag and are convenient to use.

For most patients with colostomies there are few, if any, dietary restrictions. A well-balanced diet and adequate fluid intake are important. The patient's medical and surgical history must be considered when individualizing dietary instructions. Table 45.35 lists foods and their effects on stoma output.

TABLE 45.34	POSTOPERATIVE CHARACTERISTICS OF STOMA
Characteristic	**Description or Cause**
Colour*	
Pink, rose to brick red	Viable stoma mucosa
Pale pink	May indicate anemia
Blanching, dark red to purple	May indicate inadequate blood supply to the stoma, low flow state, excessive tension on the bowel mesentery at the time of construction, or venous congestion; usually occurs in first 72 hr after surgery
Edema†	
Mild to moderate edema	Normal in the initial postoperative period
	Trauma to the stoma
	Any medical condition that results in edema
Moderate to severe edema	Obstruction proximal to the stoma
Bleeding	
Small amount	Oozing from the stomal mucosa when touched or cleansed is normal because of its vascularity
Moderate to large amount‡	Moderate to large amount of bleeding from stomal mucosa could indicate coagulation factor deficiency; trauma to the stoma
	Moderate to large amount of bleeding from intestinal stoma could indicate lower gastro-intestinal bleeding

*Sustained colour changes must be reported to the surgeon.
†Closely observe, monitor, and report to the surgeon.
‡Report moderate to large amounts of bleeding to the surgeon.

TABLE 45.35	NUTRITIONAL THERAPY

Effects of Food and Liquids on Stoma Output

Odour Producing*	**Diarrhea Causing***
• Eggs	• Alcohol
• Garlic	• Beer
• Onions	• Cabbage family
• Fish	• Spinach
• Asparagus	• Green beans
• Cabbage	• Coffee
• Broccoli	• Spicy foods
• Cauliflower	• Fruits and vegetables (raw)
• Alcohol	
• Spicy foods	**Potential Obstruction in Ileostomy†**
	• Nuts
Gas Forming*	• Raisins
• Beans and legumes	• Popcorn
• Cabbage family	• Seeds
• Onions	• Fruits and vegetables (raw)
• Beer	
• Carbonated beverages	
• Cheeses (strong)	
• Asian vegetables	

*The effect of food on stoma output is individual. Patients are not discouraged from eating the above-listed foods and beverages.
†Patients are encouraged to chew high-roughage food well or cook the foods and limit the amounts in the initial postoperative period (4–6 wk after surgery) and to drink increased amounts of fluids.

COLOSTOMY IRRIGATIONS. Colostomy irrigations can be used to regulate bowel function, treat constipation, or prepare the bowel for surgery. When done to achieve a regular bowel pattern, the irrigations habituate the bowel to function at a specific time every day or every other day. If control is achieved, there should be little or no spillage between irrigations. The patient who establishes regularity may need to wear only a pad or small pouch over the stoma. Not all patients can be managed with irrigations. An ET nurse can help to assess whether this is an appropriate management technique. The patient who is not eligible for irrigations or chooses not to establish regularity by irrigations must wear a pouch at all times.

All equipment should be assembled before irrigation. Usually, a commercially obtained irrigation set has all the equipment needed. The nurse should encourage the patient to watch the procedure and should explain each step to the patient. The cone tip on the tubing controls the depth of insertion and prevents the water from prematurely coming out from the stoma. If resistance is met, force should not be used because perforation of the intestine can result. However, this occurrence is unlikely when using a stoma cone. A hard plastic catheter is not recommended because of the risk for intestinal perforation. The procedure should not be rushed; the patient should feel relaxed. The patient or a family member must be instructed in the procedure and must be able to demonstrate the ability to irrigate before doing so independently. This can be done in the outpatient setting. Habituation of the bowel takes 3 to 6 weeks.

The patient should be able to perform a pouch change, care for skin and stoma, control odour, and identify signs and symptoms of complications. The patient should know the importance of fluids and food in the diet, have access to community resources, and know when to seek medical care. Home care and outpatient follow-up by an ET nurse are highly recommended. Patients should be discharged with written instructions for pouch change, teaching literature relevant to the type of stoma they have, a list and samples of products they use, a list of product retailers (including names and phone numbers), outpatient follow-up appointments with the surgeon and the ET nurse, and the phone numbers of the surgeon and the nurse. The patient and caregiver teaching guidelines are included in Table 45.36.

ILEOSTOMY CARE

Care of the ileostomy is presented in NCP 45.4, available on the Evolve website. Ileostomy stomal protrusion of at least 2 cm makes care easier. When the stoma is flat, stool can undermine the seal and cause altered skin integrity. Stomal function is frequent, and the stool is extremely irritating to the skin. Regularity cannot be established, so a pouch must be worn at all times. An open-ended, drainable pouch is worn by the patient so that effluent can be emptied when the pouch is one-third full. Usually, the drainable pouch is worn for 4 to 7 days before being changed, as long as leakage does not occur under the pouching system. If pouch leakage occurs, the pouch should be promptly removed, the skin should be cleansed, and a new pouching system applied. Frequent leaks of the appliance warrant assessment of appropriateness of the pouching by an ET nurse. A transparent pouch may be used in the initial postoperative period to facilitate assessment of stoma viability and stoma function, but opaque pouches for discharge and home enhance aesthetics.

Immediately after surgery, intake and output must be accurately monitored. The patient should be observed for signs and symptoms of fluid and electrolyte imbalance, particularly potassium, sodium, and fluid deficits. In the first 24 to 48 hours after surgery, the amount of drainage from the stoma may be negligible. A person with an ileostomy has lost the absorptive functions provided by the colon as well as the delay feature provided by the ileocecal valve. Once peristalsis returns, the patient

---

TABLE 45.36 PATIENT & CAREGIVER TEACHING GUIDE

Ostomy Self-Care

The following guidelines should be included when teaching the patient and caregiver about ostomy care. The nurse should:

1. Explain the following principles of ostomy care:
   - Routinely change appliances, cleanse skin, and inspect stoma and skin.
   - Empty pouch before it is one-third full.
   - Use deodorants as needed.
   - The nurse should explain how to contact the enterostomal therapy nurse.
   - The nurse should explain how to obtain additional supplies or accessories.
   - Ensure access to home health services.
2. Identify a well-balanced diet and dietary supplements if necessary to prevent nutritional deficiencies, and teach the following dietary and fluid intake guidelines:
   - Identify foods to reduce diarrhea, gas, or obstruction (with ileostomy).
   - Identify foods to reduce constipation and gas (with colostomy).
   - Drink at least 1 500–3 000 mL/day of fluid to prevent dehydration (unless contraindicated).
   - Increase fluid intake during hot weather, excessive perspiration, or diarrhea to replace losses and prevent dehydration.
   - Get to know the signs and symptoms of dehydration and when to seek help from a health care provider.
   - Contact a registered dietitian with any questions.
3. Describe potential resources to assist with emotional and psychological adjustment, and teach the patient to:
   - Identify people available to provide emotional support.
   - Identify community resources for psychosocial support.
   - Contact local ostomy support groups for information or peer support.
4. Explain the importance of follow-up care and reporting any signs and symptoms of the following:
   - Fluid and electrolyte deficits (dehydration)
   - Fever
   - Diarrhea
   - Constipation
   - Other stoma complications, including a change in appearance of the stoma or its function, a change in the peristomal skin, tenderness, erythema, or pain

---

may experience a period of high-volume bilious output of 1 200 to 1 800 mL/day. Later, the amount can average 800 mL daily because the proximal small bowel adapts and absorbs more fluid. If the small bowel has been shortened as a result of surgical resections, the drainage from the ileostomy may be greater. The patient must understand the importance of maintaining fluid and electrolyte balance. A dietitian can be helpful in assessing and determining patient food and fluid requirements.

The patient should be instructed to drink at least 1.5 to 2 L of fluid daily; more may be necessary when diarrhea occurs and when perspiration is increased. Diarrhea from an ileostomy can produce dehydration and acidosis from the loss of bicarbonate. The patient may require brief hospitalization for IV fluid rehydration if large volumes of diarrhea occur.

Usually a low-residue diet is ordered initially. Insoluble fibre–containing foods are reintroduced gradually. Later, there are few dietary restrictions. It is important that the patient limit the amount of high-roughage foods (e.g., popcorn), chew them well, and accompany their intake with fluids. The goal for the patient is a return to a normal, presurgical diet.

The stoma may bleed easily when it is touched or cleansed because it has a high vascular supply. The patient should be informed that minimal oozing of blood is normal. If the terminal ileum has been removed, the patient may need cobalamin (vitamin B$_{12}$) supplementation.

ADAPTATION TO AN OSTOMY

Adaptation to the ostomy is a gradual process. The patient experiences a grief reaction to the loss of a body part and an alteration in body image, thus psychological support during the grieving process is needed. Each person uses different coping mechanisms; the adjustment period for the person depends on the individual. There are many concerns, including body image, sexual activity, family responsibilities, and changes in lifestyle. The patient may become resentful and have fears of odour or leakage. Supportive measures by nurses include helping the patient acquire knowledge, providing or recommending support services, and identifying coping mechanisms that are effective. The nurse can provide support by responding to the physiological needs of stoma care and psychosocial needs related to self-esteem.

Gradual involvement of the patient in self-care of the ostomy should be encouraged. Although initial visualization of the stoma and participation in care is distressing, supportive teaching from the nurse will enhance the patient's confidence and independence in care. Teaching at the appropriate time is an important part of the care and can contribute to a smooth adjustment process.

Gradual resumption of activities of daily living can occur within 2 to 3 weeks. Heavy lifting, physical exertion, and participation in sports should be avoided for 6 to 8 weeks. The patient's physical condition determines when sexual activity may be resumed. Bathing and swimming are not prohibited. Patients should be referred to the Ostomy Canada Society for information and support (https://www.ostomycanada.ca).

SEXUAL DYSFUNCTION AFTER OSTOMY SURGERY

Discussion of sexuality and sexual function must be incorporated in the plan of care. The nurse can help the patient understand that sexual function or sexual activity may be affected but that sexuality does not have to be altered.

Pelvic surgery can disrupt nerve and vascular supply to the genitals. Radiation, chemotherapy, and medications can also alter sexual function. Hormones and overall physical health of the patient influence desire. Certain pain medications and antiemetics can lower libido. Generalized fatigue caused by illness can also influence desire. By communicating this information to patients, they can plan sexual activity around a medication schedule and energy levels. Any pelvic surgery that removes the rectum has the potential of damaging the parasympathetic nerve plexus. Erection in men depends on the parasympathetic nerves that control blood flow and vascular supply to the pelvis and the pudendal nerves that transmit sensory responses from the genital area. Nerve-sparing surgical techniques are used when possible to preserve sexual function. Radiation therapy to the pelvis can reduce blood vascularity to the pelvis by causing scarring in the small blood vessels. Pelvic surgery usually does not affect a woman's arousal unless part of or the entire vagina is removed. Radiation therapy can affect vaginal expansion and lubrication.

Muscular contraction and the genital pleasure that occur during orgasm are not disrupted by pelvic surgery. If the sympathetic nerves in the presacral area are damaged, the male mechanism of emission can be disrupted. This can occur with

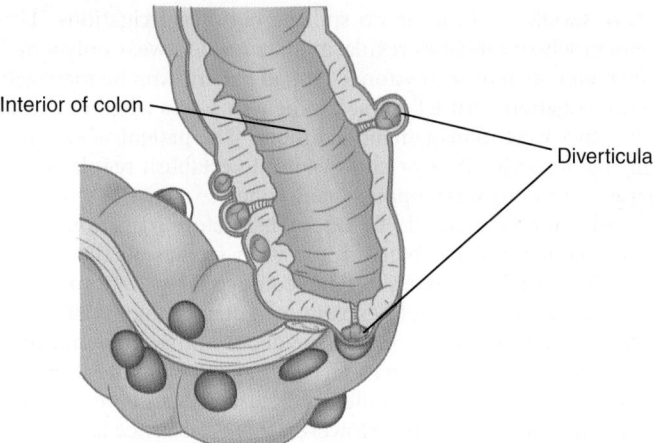

FIG. 45.11 Diverticula are outpouchings of the colon. When they become inflamed, the condition is diverticulitis. The inflammatory process can spread to the surrounding area in the intestine.

an abdominal–perineal resection. Orgasms can occur in both men and women who have had stoma surgery, although other aspects of the sexual response may be affected.

The psychological impact of the stoma and how it affects the patient's body image and self-esteem must be discussed. Emotional factors can contribute to sexual issues. A life-threatening illness can override concerns about sexual function. The nurse can assist a patient to identify ways of coping with depression and anxiety resulting from illness, surgery, or postoperative complications.

The social impact of the stoma is interrelated with its psychological, physical, and sexual aspects. Concerns of people with stomas include the ability to resume sexual activity, altering clothing styles, the effect on daily activities, sleeping while wearing a pouch, passing gas, the presence of odour, cleanliness, and deciding when or whether to tell others about the stoma. The fear of rejection from a partner or the fear that others will not find them desirable as a sexual partner can be a concern. The nurse should encourage open communication about feelings and should realize that the patient needs time to adjust to the pouch and to body changes before feeling secure in their sexual functioning.

Pregnancy is possible with an ostomy. As the abdomen expands in the second and third trimesters, the stoma may retract and alternate pouching may be required. A woman with an ostomy who becomes pregnant should have regular medical care and assessment by an ET nurse.

DIVERTICULOSIS AND DIVERTICULITIS

A **diverticulum** is an outpouching of the mucosa through the circular smooth muscle of the intestinal wall. Diverticula may occur at any point within the GI tract but are most commonly found in the sigmoid colon. Clinically, diverticular disease occurs in two forms: diverticulosis and diverticulitis. With *diverticulosis*, multiple noninflamed diverticula are present; the patient is most often free of symptoms or may have alternating periods of constipation and diarrhea. In *diverticulitis*, inflammation of the diverticula occurs (Figure 45.11).

Etiology and Pathophysiology

Diverticular disease is a common GI disorder that affects over 50% of Canadians over the age of 80 (Canadian Digestive Health

Foundation, 2021). It affects men and women equally, but men seem to have a higher rate of complications. Most people with diverticular disease are asymptomatic and are unaware that they have the disease.

There is no known cause of diverticular disease, but deficiency in dietary fibre has been associated with it. The disease is more prevalent in Western populations that consume diets low in fibre and high in refined carbohydrates.

When diverticula form, the smooth muscle of the colon wall becomes thickened. Lack of dietary fibre slows transit time, and more water is absorbed from the stool, making its passage through the lumen more difficult. Decreased bulk of the stool, combined with a more acutely narrowed lumen in the sigmoid colon, causes high intraluminal pressures. These factors are believed to contribute to the formation of diverticula.

The cause of diverticulitis is related to the retention of stool and bacteria in the diverticulum, forming a hardened mass called a *fecalith*. This occurrence causes inflammation and usually small perforations. Inflammation of the diverticulum spreads to the surrounding tissues (Figure 45.12), causing it to become edematous. Abscesses may form, or complete perforation with peritonitis may occur.

Clinical Manifestations

The majority of patients with diverticulosis have no symptoms. Those with symptoms typically have crampy abdominal pain located in the left lower quadrant that is usually relieved by passage of flatus or bowel movement. Alternating constipation and diarrhea may be present.

In patients with diverticulitis, abdominal pain is localized over the involved area of the colon. A tender left lower quadrant mass may be felt on palpation of the abdomen. Fever, chills, nausea, anorexia, and elevated WBC count may be present. Older persons with diverticulitis are frequently afebrile, with a normal WBC count and little, if any, abdominal tenderness.

Complications of diverticulitis include perforation with peritonitis, abscess and fistula formation, bowel obstruction, ureteral obstruction, and bleeding. Diverticular bleeding is the most common cause of lower GI bleeding. Bleeding usually stops spontaneously.

Diagnostic Studies

A CT scan with oral contrast is the test of choice for diverticulitis. A CBC, urinalysis, and FOBT should be performed (Table 45.37). A barium enema is used to determine narrowing or obstruction of the colonic lumen. A colonoscopy may be performed to rule out possible hidden polyps or lesions. A patient with acute diverticulitis should not have a barium enema or colonoscopy because of the possibility of perforation and peritonitis.

NURSING AND INTERPROFESSIONAL MANAGEMENT DIVERTICULOSIS AND DIVERTICULITIS

Using an interprofessional team approach, uncomplicated diverticular disease is treated with a high-fibre diet (see Table 45.8) and bulk laxatives, such as psyllium hydrophilic mucilloid (Metamucil). In acute diverticulitis, the goal of treatment is to allow the colon to rest and the inflammation to subside. The patient is kept on NPO status with parenteral fluids for hydration. The patient should be observed for signs of possible peritonitis. In acute diverticulitis, broad-spectrum antibiotic therapy is required. The temperature and the WBC count are monitored.

PATHOPHYSIOLOGY MAP

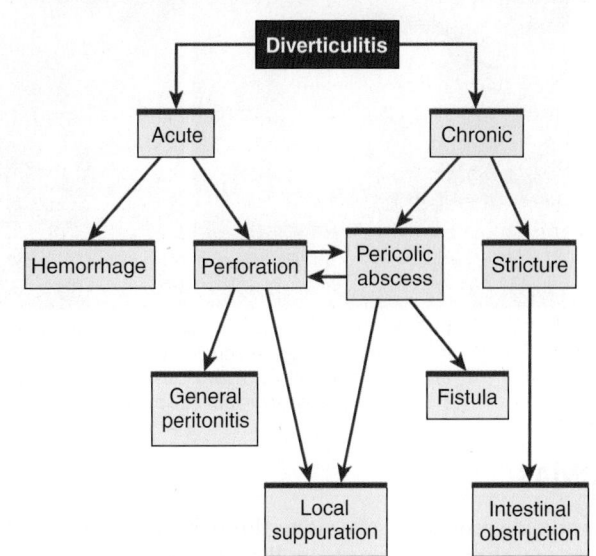

FIG. 45.12 Complications of diverticulitis.

TABLE 45.37 INTERPROFESSIONAL CARE
Diverticulosis and Diverticulitis

Diagnostic	Interprofessional Therapy
• History and physical examination • Testing of stool for occult blood • Barium enema • Sigmoidoscopy • Colonoscopy • CBC • CT scan with contrast • Urinalysis • Blood culture • Abdominal radiograph • Chest radiograph	**Ambulatory and Home Care** • High-fiber diet (during nonsymptomatic periods) • Dietary fiber supplements (during nonsymptomatic periods) • Stool softeners • Clear liquid diet • Oral antibiotics • Bulk laxatives • Weight reduction (if overweight) **Acute Care: Diverticulitis** • IV antibiotics • NPO status • IV fluids • Possible colon resection for perforation, obstruction, or hemorrhage • Bed rest

CBC, complete blood cell count; *CT,* computed tomographic (scan); *IV,* intravenous; *NPO,* nothing by mouth.

When the acute attack subsides, oral fluids are allowed, progressing to a semisolid diet. At this stage, the patient should be observed for a recurrent attack. If the patient has a bowel resection or colostomy, the nursing care is the same as for these procedures.

Surgical intervention is necessary to drain abscesses and to resect an obstructing inflammatory mass or perforated segment. The usual surgical procedures involve resection of the involved colon with a temporary diverting colostomy. The bowel is reanastomosed after the colon has healed.

The patient should be provided with a full explanation of the condition. Consultation with a dietitian regarding high-fibre diets is recommended.

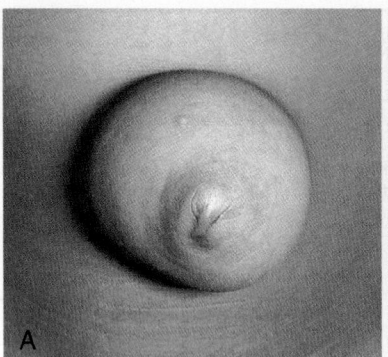 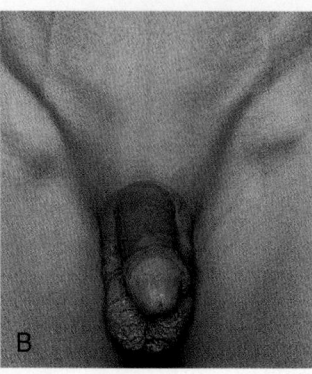 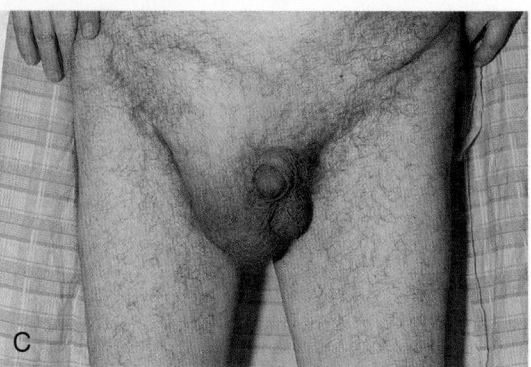

FIG. 45.13 Types of hernias. **A,** Umbilical hernia. **B,** Femoral hernias (note swelling below the inguinal ligaments). **C,** Indirect inguinal hernia. Source: *A* and *B*, from Zitelli, B. J., McIntire, S. C., & Nowalk, A. J. (2012). *Zitelli and Davis' atlas of pediatric physical diagnosis* (6th ed.). Saunders; *C*, from Swartz, M. H. (2010). *Textbook of physical diagnosis: History and examination* (6th ed., p. 545). Saunders.

HERNIAS

A hernia is a protrusion of a viscus through an abnormal opening or a weakened area in the wall of the cavity in which it is normally contained. If the hernia can be placed back into the abdominal cavity, it is known as *reducible*. The hernia can be reduced by manipulation, or reduction can occur spontaneously when the person lies down. If the hernia cannot be placed back into the abdominal cavity, it is known as *irreducible* or incarcerated, and the intestinal flow may be obstructed. When the hernia is irreducible and the intestinal flow and blood supply are obstructed, the hernia is *strangulated*. The result is an acute intestinal obstruction and ischemia, necessitating surgery.

Types

The *inguinal hernia* is the most common type of hernia and occurs at the point of weakness in the abdominal wall where the spermatic cord emerges in men and the round ligament in women (Figure 45.13). When the protrusion escapes through the inguinal ring and follows the spermatic cord or the round ligament, it is termed an *indirect* hernia. When it escapes through the posterior inguinal wall, it is a *direct* hernia. An inguinal hernia is more common in men.

A *femoral hernia* occurs when there is a protrusion through the femoral ring into the femoral canal. It occurs below the inguinal (Poupart) ligament as a bulge. It becomes strangulated easily and occurs more often in women. The umbilical hernia occurs when the rectus muscle is weak or the umbilical opening fails to close after birth.

Ventral, or *incisional*, *hernia* is caused by weakness of the abdominal wall at the site of a previous incision. It is found most commonly in patients with obesity, who have had multiple surgical procedures in the same area, and who have had inadequate wound healing because of poor nutrition or infection.

Clinical Manifestations

Commonly, a hernia occurs over the involved area when the patient stands or strains. Severe pain is caused if the hernia becomes strangulated. In this situation, the clinical manifestations of a bowel obstruction, such as vomiting, crampy abdominal pain, and distension, are found.

NURSING AND INTERPROFESSIONAL MANAGEMENT HERNIAS

Diagnosis is based on history and physical examination findings. Surgery is the treatment of choice for hernias to prevent the possible complication of strangulation. The surgical repair of a hernia is known as a *herniorrhaphy*. The reinforcement of the weakened area with fascia or mesh is known as a *hernioplasty*. When there is strangulation, necrosis and gangrene may develop if immediate care is not given. A bowel resection of the involved area or a temporary ostomy may be needed to treat a strangulated hernia.

Some patients with inguinal hernias wear a truss, a firm pad placed over the hernia and held in place with a belt. The truss is worn to keep the hernia from protruding. The truss should be applied when the hernia is reduced. If the hernia cannot be reduced, the truss should not be used. If a patient wears a truss, the nurse should check for skin irritation caused by the continual rubbing and pressure of the truss.

After an inguinal hernia repair, the patient may have difficulty voiding; thus, the nurse should observe for a distended bladder. An accurate intake and output record is important. Scrotal edema is a painful complication after an inguinal hernia repair. A scrotal support may help relieve discomfort. Coughing is not encouraged, but the patient should practise deep breathing and turn frequently. If the patient needs to cough or sneeze, the incision should be splinted during these functions. After discharge, the patient may be restricted from heavy lifting or activities for 6 to 8 weeks. Some surgeons do not put any limitations on physical activities.

ANORECTAL CONDITIONS

HEMORRHOIDS

Hemorrhoids are varicosities in the lower rectum or the anus caused by congestion in the veins of the hemorrhoidal plexus. They may be *internal* (occurring above the internal sphincter) or *external* (occurring outside the external sphincter) (Figures 45.14 and 45.15). Symptoms of hemorrhoids, including bleeding, pruritus, prolapse, and pain, are common in all age groups. In affected people, hemorrhoids appear periodically, depending on the amount of anorectal pressure.

Etiology and Pathophysiology

Hemorrhoids are thought to develop as a result of shearing forces during defecation. This force damages supporting muscles. When supporting tissues in the anal canal weaken, usually as a result of straining at defecation, venules become dilated. In addition, blood flow through the veins of the hemorrhoidal plexus is impaired. An intravascular clot in the venule results in

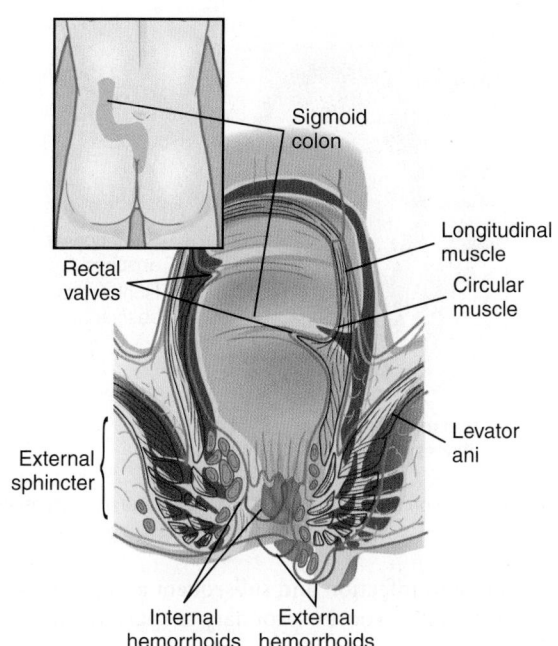

FIG. 45.14 Anatomical structures of the rectum and the anus with external and internal hemorrhoids.

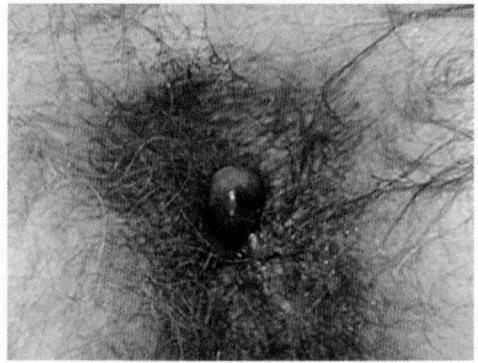

FIG. 45.15 Thrombosed external hemorrhoids. Source: Townsend, C. M., Beauchamp, R. D., Evers, B. M., et al. (Eds.). (2012). *Sabiston textbook of surgery: The biological basis of modern surgical practice* (19th ed.). Elsevier.

a thrombosed external hemorrhoid. They are the most common cause of bleeding with defecation. The amount of blood lost at one time may be small but may lead to iron-deficiency anemia over time.

Hemorrhoids may be precipitated by many factors, including pregnancy, prolonged constipation, straining in an effort to defecate, heavy lifting, prolonged standing and sitting, and portal hypertension (as found in cirrhosis).

Clinical Manifestations

The patient with internal hemorrhoids may be asymptomatic. However, when internal hemorrhoids become constricted, the patient will report pain. Internal hemorrhoids can bleed, resulting in blood on toilet paper after defecation or blood on the outside of stool. The patient may report a chronic, dull, aching discomfort, particularly when the hemorrhoids have prolapsed.

External hemorrhoids are reddish blue and may or may not bleed or cause pain unless a vein ruptures. If the blood clots in external hemorrhoids, they become inflamed and painful and are said to be thrombosed. External hemorrhoids cause intermittent pain, pain on palpation, itching, and burning. Patients also report bleeding associated with defecation. Constipation or diarrhea can aggravate these symptoms.

Diagnostic Studies and Interprofessional Care

Internal hemorrhoids are diagnosed by digital examination, anoscopy, or sigmoidoscopy. External hemorrhoids can be diagnosed by visual inspection and digital examination. Therapy should be directed toward the causes and the patient's symptoms. A high-fibre diet and increased fluid intake prevent constipation and reduce straining, which allows engorgement of the veins to subside. Ointments, creams, suppositories, and impregnated pads that contain anti-inflammatory agents (e.g., hydrocortisone), or astringents and anaesthetics (e.g., witch hazel, benzocaine) may be used to shrink the mucous membranes and relieve discomfort. Stool softeners may be ordered to keep the stools soft; sitz baths may be ordered to relieve pain.

Surgical excision and clot removal are generally recommended for thrombosed external hemorrhoids. For internal hemorrhoids, one of four nonsurgical approaches can be used. The first is *band ligation*. Through an anoscope, the hemorrhoid is identified and then ligated with a rubber band. The constrictive effect impairs circulation, and the tissue becomes necrotic, separates, and sloughs off. There is some local discomfort with this procedure, but no anaesthetic is required. *Infrared coagulation* can be used to treat bleeding internal hemorrhoids. In this procedure, either infrared or electrical current reduces local inflammation. *Cryotherapy* involves rapid freezing of the hemorrhoid. Because this method can result in acute pain, it is used less often. Finally, *laser treatment* can be used to treat internal hemorrhoids. This procedure involves expensive equipment and tends to be more costly than band ligation and coagulation therapies.

A *hemorrhoidectomy* is the surgical excision of hemorrhoids. Surgery is indicated when there is prolapse, excessive pain or bleeding, or large hemorrhoids. In general, hemorrhoidectomy is reserved for patients with severe symptoms related to multiple thrombosed hemorrhoids or marked protrusion. Surgical removal may be done by cautery, clamp, or excision. One surgical approach is to leave the area open so that healing takes place by secondary intention. In another approach, the hemorrhoids are removed, the tissue is sutured, and healing takes place by primary-intention wound healing.

NURSING MANAGEMENT HEMORRHOIDS

Conservative nursing management for the patient with hemorrhoids includes teaching measures regarding prevention of constipation, avoidance of prolonged standing or sitting, proper use of OTC medications available for hemorrhoidal symptoms, and the need to seek medical care for severe symptoms of hemorrhoids (e.g., excessive pain and bleeding, prolapsed hemorrhoids) when necessary. Sitz baths (15–20 minutes), two to three times each day for 7 to 10 days, may be helpful to reduce the discomfort and swelling associated with hemorrhoids.

Pain caused by sphincter spasm is a common symptom after a hemorrhoidectomy. The nurse must be aware that, although the procedure is minor, the pain is severe. Opioids are usually given initially. Sitz baths are started 1 to 2 days after surgery. A warm sitz bath provides comfort and keeps the anal area clean. The patient should be monitored for weakness or fainting following surgery.

Packing may be inserted into the rectum to absorb drainage. A T-binder may hold the dressing in place. If packing is inserted, it usually is removed on the first or second postoperative day. The nurse should assess for rectal bleeding. The patient may be embarrassed when the dressing is changed, and privacy should be provided. The patient usually dreads the first bowel movement and often resists the urge to defecate. Pain medication may be given before the bowel movement to reduce discomfort.

A stool softener such as docusate (Colace) is usually ordered for the first few postoperative days. If the patient does not have a bowel movement within 2 to 3 days, other oral laxatives may be given.

Patients are taught the importance of diet, care of the anal area, symptoms of complications (especially bleeding), and avoidance of constipation and straining. Sitz baths are recommended for 1 to 2 weeks. The health care provider may order a stool softener to be taken for a time. Hemorrhoids may recur. Occasionally, anal strictures develop and dilation is necessary. Regular checkups are important in the prevention of any further health problems.

ANAL FISSURE

An **anal fissure** is a skin ulcer or a crack in the lining of the anal wall that is caused by trauma, local infection, or inflammation. Fissures are considered either primary or secondary, based on their etiology. *Primary fissures* usually occur as a result of local trauma associated with defecation or anal intercourse. When there is high pressure in the internal anal sphincter, it can result in ischemia, which can lead to fissuring. Thus, sexual practices and conditions that promote constipation are likely to be associated with fissure development. *Secondary fissures* are caused by a variety of conditions, including IBD, prior anal surgery, infection (syphilis, tuberculosis, chlamydia, gonorrhea, herpes simplex virus), and HIV infection.

The most common clinical manifestations are painful spasms of the anal sphincter and severe, burning pain during defecation. Some bleeding may occur, and constipation results because of fear of pain associated with bowel movements.

Anal fissures are diagnosed through physical examination. Treatment of anal fissures is directed at correcting the underlying conditions, such as hard stools. Most acute fissures require 2 to 4 weeks to heal. Conservative treatment consists of bowel regulation with mineral oil and stool softeners. Warm sitz baths (15–20 minutes, three times a day) and anal anaesthetic suppositories (Anusol) are also ordered. Topical preparations, including nitrates and calcium channel blockers, are used to decrease rectal and anal pressure to allow the fissure to heal without sphincter damage. Local injections of botulinum toxin are also used to decrease rectal and anal pressure and are most effective when combined with nitrates.

For chronic fissures, other invasive procedures may be needed. These include coagulation therapy or surgical treatment (sphincterotomy). Surgical treatment involves excision of the fissure. Postoperative nursing care is the same as the care for the patient who has had a hemorrhoidectomy.

ANORECTAL ABSCESS

Anorectal abscesses are undrained collections of perianal pus (Figure 45.16). They are the result of obstruction of the anal

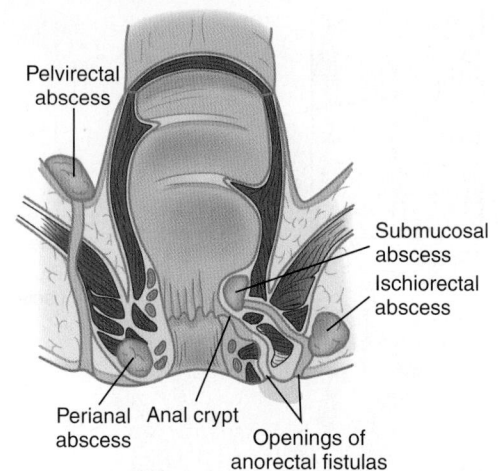

FIG. 45.16 Common sites of anorectal abscesses and fistula formation.

glands, leading to infection and subsequent abscess formation. Abscess formation can occur secondary to anal fissures, trauma, or IBD.

The most common causative organisms are *Escherichia coli*, staphylococci, and streptococci. Clinical manifestations include local pain and swelling, foul-smelling drainage, tenderness, and elevated temperature. Sepsis can occur as a complication. Anorectal abscesses are diagnosed by rectal examination.

Surgical therapy consists of drainage of abscesses. The wound will be left open and allowed to heal by secondary intention. Topical dressing selection is determined on the basis of wound care principles (maintain moist wound environment, manage bacterial burden, protect from further trauma). Care must be taken to avoid soiling the dressing during urination or defecation. A low-residue diet is given. Discharge teaching should include access to home health care, wound care, the importance of sitz baths, thorough cleaning after bowel movements, and follow-up visits to a health care provider.

ANAL FISTULA

An **anal fistula** is an abnormal tunnel leading out from the anus or the rectum. It may extend to the outside of the skin, the vagina, or the buttocks. Anal fistulas are a complication of Crohn's disease (occurring in the perianal area). This condition often precedes an anorectal abscess.

Feces enter the fistula and may cause a localized infection. There may be persistent, blood-stained, purulent discharge or stool leakage from the fistula. The patient may need to use dressings to contain the drainage and protect perifistular skin.

Surgical therapy may involve a fistulotomy or a fistulectomy. In a *fistulotomy*, the fistula is opened and healthy tissue is allowed to granulate. A *fistulectomy* is an excision of the entire fistulous tract. Appropriate topical therapy is used, and the wound is allowed to heal by secondary intention. In severe cases of perianal disease caused by Crohn's disease, a diverting loop ileostomy may be required to manage the fistulas. Care is the same as that given after a hemorrhoidectomy.

ANAL CANCER

Anal cancer is uncommon in the general population, but the incidence is increasing. Human papillomavirus (HPV) is associated with about 80% of the cases of anal cancer. Risk factors include having many sexual partners, genital warts (which are caused by HPV), smoking, receptive anal sex, and HIV infection.

Most frequently, the initial symptom is rectal bleeding. Other symptoms include rectal pain and sensation of a rectal mass. Some patients have no symptoms, which leads to delayed diagnosis and treatment.

It is especially important to screen high-risk individuals. A swab of the anal mucosa can be obtained during a digital rectal examination. Identification of cell changes (e.g., dysplasia, neoplasia) can be determined. High-resolution anoscopy allows for visualization of the mucosa and biopsy. An endo-anal (endorectal) ultrasound may also be done.

The use of condoms to reduce the transmission of HPV is recommended. The HPV vaccine Gardasil is used for the prevention of anal cancer and associated precancerous lesions caused by HPV types 6, 11, 16, and 18. Another HPV vaccine, Cervarix, may also be useful in the prevention of HPV-associated anal cancer. After vaccination with HPV vaccine, patients at risk need to continue their recommended screening program.

Treatment of anal cancer depends on the size and depth of the lesions. Topical therapy with bichloroacetic or trichloroacetic acid may be used to kill the HPV virus. Imiquimod (Aldara), an immunomodulator, is also used as a topical agent. Therapy also includes surgery, radiation, and chemotherapy.

PILONIDAL SINUS

A pilonidal sinus is a small tract under the skin between the buttocks in the sacrococcygeal area. It is thought to be of congenital origin. It may have several openings and is lined with epithelium and hair, thus given the name *pilonidal* ("a nest of hair").

The skin in the sacrococcygeal region is moist, and the movement of the buttocks causes the short, wiry hair to penetrate the skin. The irritated skin becomes infected and forms a pilonidal cyst or abscess. There are no symptoms unless there is an infection. If it becomes infected, the patient experiences pain and swelling at the base of the spine, and there may be spontaneous drainage of pus.

The formed abscess requires incision and drainage. The wound may be primarily closed or left open to heal by secondary intention. The wound is packed with appropriate topical therapeutic material. The wounds are often very painful, and the patient may require premedication before dressing changes. The patient is usually more comfortable lying on their abdomen or side. Sitting for prolonged periods of time may be difficult. Activities that contribute to shear in the area (running, sports, long walks) should be avoided until the wound heals. Because the area is poorly vascularized, healing of open pilonidal wounds may be prolonged. Ensuring that surrounding hair is clipped and kept out of the wound bed is imperative. Unfortunately, despite excision of the tract, pilonidal cysts or abscesses may reoccur.

CASE STUDY

Colorectal Cancer

Patient Profile

L. C. (pronouns he/him), 58 years old, is from Drury, Ontario. L.C. and his partner drove 50 kilometres to seek hospital care because of his deteriorating health (see the Case Study in Chapter 41).

Subjective Data

See the Case Study in Chapter 41.

Objective Data
Physical Examination

See the Case Study in Chapter 41.

Laboratory Tests
- CT scan and colonoscopy show two medium-sized tumours in the transverse colon.

Interprofessional Care
Surgical Procedure
- Transverse hemicolectomy is performed and lymph node biopsies are taken.
- Pathology results indicate that the adenocarcinoma tumour has invaded the muscle wall of the colon, and two out of five lymph nodes are positive for cancer.

Postoperative
- Feels like his life has ended and does not want to leave hospital
- States that there is no one to help with care at home and is far away from the hospital

Follow-Up Treatment
- Scheduled for outpatient chemotherapy

Discussion Questions

1. What are the signs and symptoms of colorectal cancer that L. C. has manifested (see the Case Study in Chapter 41)?
2. What types of diagnostic information are available from a colonoscopy versus a sigmoidoscopy?
3. What stage of colorectal cancer does L. C. most likely have? What treatment is recommended for this stage of colorectal cancer?
4. How could the nurse provide emotional support to L. C. and his partner?
5. What is a culturally sensitive way for the nurse to support L. C. and his partner in making decisions about continued health care?
6. *Priority decision:* Based on the assessment data, what are the priority nursing diagnoses? Are there any interprofessional issues?
7. *Priority decision:* What are the priority nursing interventions for L. C. at this stage of illness?
8. *Evidence-informed practice:* L. C. had not had a previous colonoscopy. He is worried that other family members may have colon cancer. What information can the nurse provide about the recommendations for colorectal cancer screening?

@volve

Answers available at http://evolve.elsevier.com/Canada/Lewis/medsurg.

REVIEW QUESTIONS

The number of the question corresponds to the same-numbered outcome at the beginning of the chapter.

1. The appropriate interprofessional therapy for the client with acute diarrhea caused by a viral infection is to do which of the following?
   a. Increase fluid intake.
   b. Administer an antibiotic.
   c. Administer antimotility medications.
   d. Quarantine the client to prevent spread of the virus.

2. When a 35-year-old female client is admitted to the emergency department with acute abdominal pain, which possible diagnosis should the nurse consider that may be the cause of her pain? *(Select all that apply.)*
   a. Gastroenteritis
   b. Ectopic pregnancy
   c. Gastrointestinal bleeding
   d. Irritable bowel syndrome
   e. Inflammatory bowel disease

3. Assessment findings suggestive of peritonitis include which of the following?
   a. Rebound abdominal pain
   b. A soft, distended abdomen
   c. Dull, continuous abdominal pain
   d. Restlessness

4. In planning care for the client with Crohn's disease, the nurse recognizes which major factor about Crohn's disease that differentiates it from ulcerative colitis?
   a. It frequently results in toxic megacolon.
   b. It causes fewer nutritional deficiencies than ulcerative colitis.
   c. It often recurs after surgery, whereas ulcerative colitis is curable with a colectomy.
   d. It is manifested by rectal bleeding and anemia more frequently than ulcerative colitis is.

5. The nurse performs a detailed assessment of the abdomen of a client with a possible bowel obstruction, knowing that which of the following are manifestations of an obstruction in the large intestine? *(Select all that apply.)*
   a. Persistent abdominal pain
   b. Marked abdominal distension
   c. Diarrhea that is loose or liquid
   d. Colicky, severe, intermittent pain
   e. Profuse vomiting that relieves abdominal pain

6. A client with stage I colorectal cancer is scheduled for surgery. Teaching for this client would include an explanation of which of the following?
   a. That chemotherapy will begin after recovery from the surgery
   b. That both chemotherapy and radiation can be used as palliative treatments
   c. That follow-up colonoscopies will be needed to ensure that the cancer does not recur
   d. That a wound nurse, ostomy nurse, and continence nurse will visit to identify an abdominal site for the ostomy

7. The nurse explains to the client undergoing ostomy surgery that the procedure that maintains the most normal functioning of the bowel is which of the following?
   a. A sigmoid colostomy
   b. A transverse colostomy
   c. A descending colostomy
   d. An ascending colostomy

8. In contrast to the client with diverticulitis, which of the following is true for the client with diverticulosis?
   a. Has rectal bleeding
   b. Often has no symptoms
   c. Has localized cramping pain
   d. Frequently develops peritonitis

9. Which of the following is a nursing intervention that is most appropriate to decrease postoperative edema and pain after an inguinal herniorrhaphy?
   a. Applying a truss to the hernia site
   b. Allowing the client to stand to void
   c. Supporting the incision during coughing
   d. Applying a scrotal support with ice bag

10. The nurse determines that the goals of dietary teaching have been met when the client with celiac disease selects which of the following from the menu?
    a. Scrambled eggs and sausage
    b. Buckwheat pancakes with syrup
    c. Oatmeal, skim milk, and orange juice
    d. Yogourt, strawberries, and rye toast with butter

11. What should a client be taught after a hemorrhoidectomy?
    a. Take mineral oil before bedtime.
    b. Eat a low-fibre diet to rest the colon.
    c. Administer oil-retention enema to empty the colon.
    d. Use prescribed pain medication before a bowel movement.

1. a; 2, a, b, c, d, e; 3, a; 4, c; 5, a, b; 6, c; 7, a; 8, b; 9, d; 10, a; 11, d.

⟳volve

For even more review questions, visit http://evolve.elsevier.com/Canada/Lewis/medsurg.

REFERENCES

Baird, D. L. H., Constantinos, S., Christos, K., et al. (2017). Acute appendicitis. *BMJ, 357*, j1703. https://doi.org/10.1136/bmj.j1703

Benchimol, E. I., Charles, N., Bernstein, C. N., et al. (2019). The impact of inflammatory bowel disease in Canada 2018: A scientific report from the Canadian Gastro-Intestinal Epidemiology Consortium to Crohn's and Colitis Canada. *Journal of the Canadian Association of Gastroenterology, 2*(Suppl 1), S1–S5. https://doi.org/10.1093/jcag/gwy052

Blaabjerg, S., Artzi, D. M., & Aabenhus, R. (2017). Probiotics for the prevention of antibiotic-associated diarrhea in outpatients—A systematic review and meta-analysis. *Antibiotics (Basel, Switzerland), 6*(4), 21. https://doi.org/10.3390/antibiotics6040021

Caio, G., Volta, U., Sapone, A., et al. (2019). Celiac disease: A comprehensive current review. *BMC Medicine, 17*, 142. https://doi.org/10.1186/s12916-019-1380-z

Canadian Cancer Society. (2021a). *Colorectal cancer statistics.* https://cancer.ca/en/cancer-information/cancer-types/colorectal/statistics

Canadian Cancer Society. (2021b). *Screening for colorectal cancer.* https://www.cancer.ca/en/cancer-information/cancer-type/colorectal/screening/?region=on

Canadian Celiac Association. (2016a). *Celiac disease.* https://www.celiac.ca/gluten-related-disorders/celiac-disease

Canadian Celiac Association. (2016b). *Screening and diagnosis of celiac disease.* https://www.celiac.ca/healthcare-professionals/diagnosis/

Canadian Celiac Professional Advisory Council. (2016). *A resource for health care professionals screening and diagnosis of celiac disease.* https://www.celiac.ca/wp-content/uploads/2019/07/Diagnosis-Fact-Sheet-2019-1.pdf

Canadian Digestive Health Foundation. (2021). *Statistics: Diverticular disease: Statistics.* https://cdhf.ca/digestive-disorders/diverticular-disease/statistics/

Canadian Society of Intestinal Research. (2021a). *Capsule endoscopy.* https://badgut.org/information-centre/a-z-digestive-topics/capsule-endoscopy/

Canadian Society of Intestinal Research. (2021b). *Crohn's disease.* https://badgut.org/information-centre/a-z-digestive-topics/crohns-disease/

Canadian Society of Intestinal Research. (2021c). *Irritable bowel syndrome (IBS).* https://badgut.org/information-centre/a-z-digestive-topics/ibs/

Carvalho, A., Esberard, B., & Moreira, A. (2018). Current management of spontaneous intra-abdominal abscess in Crohn's disease. *Journal of Coloproctology, 38*(2), 158–163. https://doi.org/10.1016/j.jcol.2016.05.003

Centers for Disease Control and Prevention. (2021). *Clostridioides difficile.* https://www.cdc.gov/cdiff/index.html

Chang, J. (2016). Anal health care basics. *The Permanente Journal, 20*(4), 15–222. https://doi.org/10.7812/TPP/15-222

Colorectal Cancer Association of Canada. (2021a). *Colorectal cancer symptoms.* https://www.colorectalcancercanada.com/colorectal-cancer/colorectal-cancer-symptoms/

Colorectal Cancer Association of Canada. (2021b). *Colorectal cancer treatment options in Canada.* https://www.colorectalcancercanada.com/colorectal-cancer/treatment/

Crohn's and Colitis Canada. (2019a). *Complications and extraintestinal manifestations.* https://crohnsandcolitis.ca/Living-with-Crohn-s-colitis/Complications

Crohn's and Colitis Canada. (2019b). *What are Crohn's and colitis?.* https://crohnsandcolitis.ca/About-Crohn-s-Colitis/What-are-Crohns-and-Colitis

D'Onise, K., Iacobini, E. T., & Tanuto, K. J. (2020). Colorectal cancer screening using faecal occult blood tests for Indigenous adults: A systematic literature review of barriers, enablers and implemented strategies. *Preventive Medicine, 134*, 1p. https://doi.org/10.1016/j.ypmed.2020.106018

Friis, S., Riis, A. H., Erichsen, R., et al. (2015). Low-dose Aspirin or nonsteroidal anti-inflammatory drug use and colorectal cancer risk: A population-based, case-control study. *Annals of Internal Medicine, 163*(5), 347–355. https://doi.org/10.7326/M15-0039

George, M. A., Jin, A., Brussoni, M., et al. (2017). Intentional injury among the Indigenous and total populations in British Columbia, Canada: Trends over time and ecological analyses of risk. *International Journal for Equity in Health, 16*, 141. https://doi.org/10.1186/s12939-017-0629-4

Janssen. (2017). *Product monograph. Remicade®.* https://crohnsandcolitis.ca/Crohns_and_Colitis/images/living-with-crohns-colitis/REMICADE-MONOGRAPH.PDF

Nelson, R. L., Suda, K. J., & Evans, C. T. (2017). Antibiotic treatment for *Clostridium difficile*–associated diarrhea in adults. *Cochrane Database of Systematic Reviews, 3.* Art. No. CD004610. https://doi.org/10.1002/14651858.CD004610.pub5

Parker, C. H., Henry, S., & Liu, L. W. (2019). Efficacy of biofeedback therapy in clinical practice for the management of chronic constipation and fecal incontinence. *Journal of the Canadian Association of Gastroenterology, 2*(3), 126–131. https://doi.org/10.1093/jcag/gwy036

Registered Nurses' Association of Ontario (RNAO). (2011). *Prevention of constipation in the older adult population.* http://rnao.ca/sites/rnao-ca/files/Constipation_supplement_2011.pdf

Registered Nurses' Association of Ontario (RNAO). (2017). *Prevention of falls and fall injuries in the older adult* (4th ed.). https://rnao.ca/bpg/guidelines/prevention-falls-and-fall-injuries

Rowe, W. A. (2020). What is the global prevalence of inflammatory bowel disease (IBD)? https://www.medscape.com/answers/179037-54870/what-is-the-global-prevalence-of-inflammatory-bowel-disease-ibd

Salix Pharmaceuticals. (2018). *Product monograph. Relistor®.* https://pdf.hres.ca/dpd_pm/00046609.PDF

Schmulson, M. J., & Drossman, D. A. (2017). What is new in Rome IV. *Journal of Neurogastroenterology and Motility, 23*(2), 151–163. https://doi.org/10.5056/jnm16214

Suhaimi, S. N. A., Nazri, N., Latar, N. H. M., et al. (2015). Familial adenomatous polyposis–associated papillary thyroid cancer. *Malaysian Journal of Medical Sciences, 22*(4), 69–72.

Vilcu, A., Sabatte, L., Blanchon, T., et al. (2019). Association between acute gastroenteritis and continuous use of proton pump inhibitors during winter periods of highest circulation of enteric viruses. *JAMA Netw Open, 2*(11), e1916205. https://doi.org/10.1001/jamanetworkopen.2019.16205

Xie, L., Jiang, X., Li, Q., et al. (2018). Diagnostic value of methylated *Septin9* for colorectal cancer detection. *Frontiers in Oncology, 8*, 247.

RESOURCES

Canadian Association of Gastroenterology
https://www.cag-acg.org
Canadian Cancer Society
https://www.cancer.ca
Canadian Celiac Association
https://www.celiac.ca/
Canadian Society of Gastroenterology Nurses and Associates
https://www.csgna.com
Canadian Society of Intestinal Research
https://www.badgut.com
Colorectal Cancer Canada
https://www.colorectalcancercanada.com
Crohn's and Colitis Canada
https://www.crohnsandcolitis.ca
Nurses Specialized in Wound, Ostomy and Continence Canada
https://www.nswoc.ca/

evolve

For additional Internet resources, see the website for this book at http://evolve.elsevier.com/Canada/Lewis/medsurg.

CHAPTER

46

Nursing Management

Liver, Pancreas, and Biliary Tract Conditions

Colina Yim and Elizabeth Lee
Originating US chapter by Mary C. Olson

evolve WEBSITE

http://evolve.elsevier.com/Canada/Lewis/medsurg

- Review Questions (Online Only)
- Key Points
- Answer Guidelines for Case Study
- Student Case Studies
  - Acute Pancreatitis and Septic Shock
  - Cholelithiasis and Cholecystitis
  - Hepatitis

- Customizable Nursing Care Plans
  - Acute Viral Hepatitis
  - Advanced Cirrhosis
  - Acute Pancreatitis

- Conceptual Care Map Creator
- Conceptual Care Map for Textbook Case Study
- Audio Glossary
- Content Updates

LEARNING OBJECTIVES

1. Differentiate among the types of viral hepatitis, including their pathophysiology, clinical manifestations, and complications and the interprofessional care of patients with viral hepatitis A, B, and C.
2. Describe the nursing management, including health promotion, of patients with viral hepatitis.
3. Describe the cause and clinical manifestations of and interprofessional care of patients with nonalcoholic fatty liver disease.
4. Explain the etiology, pathophysiology, clinical manifestations, and complications of cirrhosis and the interprofessional care and nursing management of patients with cirrhosis.
5. Describe the clinical manifestations and management of hepatocellular carcinoma.
6. Differentiate between acute and chronic pancreatitis with regard to pathophysiology, clinical manifestations, complications, interprofessional care, and nursing management.
7. Explain the clinical manifestations, interprofessional care, and nursing management of patients with pancreatic cancer.
8. Explain the pathophysiology, clinical manifestations, and complications of gallbladder disorders and the interprofessional care, including surgical therapy, of patients with these disorders.
9. Describe the nursing management of patients undergoing surgical treatment of cholecystitis and cholelithiasis.

KEY TERMS

acute liver failure
acute pancreatitis
alcohol-associated liver disease (ALD)
ascites
asterixis
cholecystitis
cholelithiasis
chronic pancreatitis

cirrhosis
esophageal varices
fetor hepaticus
fulminant hepatitis
hepatic encephalopathy
hepatitis
hepatorenal syndrome (HRS)
jaundice

nonalcoholic fatty liver disease (NAFLD)
nonalcoholic steatohepatitis (NASH)
paracentesis
portal hypertension
pseudocyst
spider angiomas

The liver, the pancreas, and the biliary tract are critical organs that are responsible for many functions vital to life. Nursing management of patients with liver, pancreatic, and gallbladder disorders is the focus of this chapter. Viral hepatitis, cirrhosis, acute pancreatitis, cholecystitis, and cholelithiasis are described in detail.

DISORDERS OF THE LIVER

VIRAL HEPATITIS

Hepatitis is a broad term meaning inflammation of the liver. It is most often caused by viral infection, although there are other possible causes such as alcoholic hepatitis and autoimmune hepatitis.

At least five types of hepatitis virus (A, B, C, D, E) have been identified to date. The first three types (A, B, C) are responsible for 90% of acute hepatitis cases in Canada (Health Canada, 2021). Other viruses—such as cytomegalovirus, Epstein-Barr virus, herpesvirus, coxsackievirus, and rubella virus—may cause hepatitis, but the liver is usually not the primary infected organ.

Viral hepatitis is a major public health concern. Confirmed cases are reportable to the National Notifiable Disease Reporting System of Health Canada. The major characteristics of the hepatitis viruses are presented in Table 46.1. Each type of viral hepatitis is discussed in detail later in this chapter.

TABLE 46.1   CHARACTERISTICS OF HEPATITIS VIRUSES

Incubation Period and Mode of Transmission	Sources of Infection	Infectivity
Hepatitis A Virus (HAV) *Incubation:* 15–50 days (average 28) Fecal–oral (primarily fecal contamination and oral ingestion)	• Contaminated food, milk, water, shellfish • Crowded conditions (e.g., day care center, long-term care facility) • Persons with subclinical infections, infected food handlers, sexual contact, IV drug users • Inadequate personal hygiene • Poor sanitation	• Most infectious during 2 wk before onset of symptoms • Infectious until 1–2 wk after the start of symptoms
Hepatitis B Virus (HBV) *Incubation:* 115–180 days (average 56–96) Percutaneous (parenteral) or mucosal exposure to blood or blood products Sexual contact Perinatal transmission	• Contaminated needles, syringes, and blood products • HBV-infected mother (perinatal transmission) • Sexual activity with infected partners. Asymptomatic carriers • Tattoos or body piercing with contaminated needles	• Before and after symptoms appear • Infectious for months • Carriers continue to be infectious for life
Hepatitis C Virus (HCV) *Incubation:* 14–180 days (average 56) Percutaneous (parenteral) or mucosal exposure to blood or blood products High-risk sexual contact Perinatal contact	• Blood and blood products • Needles and syringes • Sexual activity with infected partners, low risk	• 1–2 wk before symptoms appear • Continues during clinical course • 75–85% go on to develop chronic hepatitis C and remain infectious
Hepatitis D Virus (HDV) *Incubation:* 2–26 wk HBV must precede HDV Chronic carriers of HBV are always at risk	• Same as HBV • Can cause infection only when HBV is present	• Blood infectious at all stages of HDV infection
Hepatitis E Virus (HEV) *Incubation:* 15–64 days (average 26–42 days) Fecal–oral route Outbreaks associated with contaminated water supply in developing countries	• Contaminated water, poor sanitation • Found in Asia, Africa, and Mexico • Not common	• Not known • May be similar to HAV

IV, intravenous.

DETERMINANTS OF HEALTH

Hepatitis C Virus (HCV) Infection

Culture and Ethnicity
• The prevalence of hepatitis C infection among Indigenous people, especially women and youth, is nearly five times higher than in the non-Indigenous Canadian-born population.*
• Thirty-five percent of individuals infected with hepatitis C were born outside Canada.

Personal Health Practices and Coping Skills
• Given their tendency to engage in high-risk behaviours, prison inmates are at greater risk for HCV exposure than the general Canadian population is.†
• People who inject drugs (PWIDs) and share drug preparation equipment are at risk for new hepatitis C infections.*
• Up to 43% of new hepatitis C infections occur among the PWID population.*‡

Age and Gender
• People born between 1945 and 1975 (baby boomers) account for over 60% of hepatitis C infections in Canada.*
• Gay men, bisexual men, and transgender persons are disproportionately affected by sexually transmitted blood-borne diseases, including viral hepatitis B and C.**

References
*Canadian Network on Hepatitis C (CanHepC). (2019). *Blueprint to inform hepatitis C elimination efforts in Canada.* https://www.canhepc.ca/sites/default/files/media/documents/blueprint_hcv_2019_05.pdf
†Kouyoumdjian, F. G., & McIsaac, K. E. (2015). Persons in correctional facilities in Canada: A key population for hepatitis C prevention and control. *Canadian Journal of Public Health, 106*(6), E454. https://doi.org/10.17269/cjph.106.5132
‡Government of Canada. (2018). *Canadian communicable disease report, 44*(7/8). https://www.canada.ca/en/public-health/services/reports-publications/canada-communicable-disease-report-ccdr/monthly-issue/2018-44/issue-7-8-july-5-2018/article-7-hepatitis-c-canada-2018-infographic.html
**Government of Canada. (2018). *Reducing the health impact of sexually transmitted and blood-borne infections in Canada by 2030: A Pan-Canadian STBBI framework for action.* https://www.canada.ca/en/public-health/services/infectious-diseases/sexual-health-sexually-transmitted-infections/reports-publications/sexually-transmitted-blood-borne-infections-action-framework.html.

Pathophysiological Features

Liver. The pathophysiological changes in the various types of viral hepatitis are similar. Hepatitis involves widespread inflammation of liver tissue. In viral hepatitis, hepatocytes (liver cells) are the targets of destruction by the virus through either direct action of the virus (as in hepatitis C infection) or through a cell-mediated immune response to the virus (as in hepatitis B infection).

During an acute viral hepatitis infection, large numbers of infected hepatocytes are destroyed, leading to liver cell necrosis (death). Liver injuries affect normal liver functions, including protein metabolism, blood coagulation, and bile production, causing *cholestasis* (impaired flow of bile). After resolution of an acute infection, liver cells can normally regenerate through cellular replication, and if no complications occur, they should resume their normal function. If liver cell loss is massive, cellular repair may not be possible.

Chronic viral hepatitis infections can be insidious and silent with no symptoms until the destructions of hepatocytes become so severe that liver synthetic functions are compromised. Chronic liver inflammation will also lead to development of scar tissues (fibrosis), which over decades can progress to cirrhosis and liver failure. (Cirrhosis is discussed later in this chapter.)

Systemic Effects. In the early phases of viral hepatitis infections, the antigen–antibody complexes between the virus and its corresponding antibody form a circulating immune complex. The circulating immune complexes activate the complement system (see Chapter 16). The clinical manifestations of this activation may include rash, angioedema, arthritis, fever, and malaise. *Cryoglobulinemia* (presence of abnormal proteins in the blood), glomerulonephritis, and vasculitis have also been found secondary to immune complex activation.

Clinical Manifestations

The clinical manifestations of viral hepatitis can be classified into acute and chronic hepatitis (Table 46.2).

Acute Phase. Many individuals with acute hepatitis have no symptoms and are unaware of the infection. As a result, many acute infections are often not diagnosed. Clinical symptoms in acute infections, if present, are similar across all types of hepatitis viruses. Symptoms may include anorexia, nausea, vomiting, malaise, fatigue, headache, low-grade fever, arthralgias, skin rashes, and right upper quadrant discomfort. The infected person may find food or alcohol repugnant and, if a smoker, may develop a distaste for cigarettes. Physical examination may reveal hepatomegaly, lymphadenopathy, and sometimes splenomegaly. The acute phase is the period of maximal infectivity.

Jaundice, a yellowish discoloration of the sclera and body tissues, results when the concentration of bilirubin in the blood becomes abnormally increased (Figure 46.1). The acute phase may be *icteric* (jaundice) or *anicteric* (no jaundice). Jaundice occurs when the bilirubin metabolism changes or when the bile flow in the hepatic or biliary systems is obstructed. The types of jaundice are described in Table 46.3. The urine may appear darker because excess bilirubin is being excreted by the kidneys. If conjugated bilirubin cannot pass into the intestines from the liver because of obstruction or inflammation of the bile ducts, the stools become light or clay coloured. Pruritus sometimes accompanies jaundice and occurs as a result of the accumulation of bile salts beneath the skin.

TABLE 46.2	CLINICAL MANIFESTATIONS OF HEPATITIS
Acute	**Chronic**
• Altered taste and smell	• Fatigue
• Anorexia	• Hepatomegaly
• Arthralgias	• Malaise
• Dark urine	• Myalgia and arthralgia
• Fatigue	• Easy bruising
• Low-grade fever	• Palmar erythema
• Headache	• Spider angiomas
• Hepatomegaly	• Splenomegaly
• Jaundice	
• Clay-coloured stools	
• Malaise	
• Nausea, vomiting	
• Pruritus	
• Right upper quadrant tenderness	
• Splenomegaly	
• Weight loss	

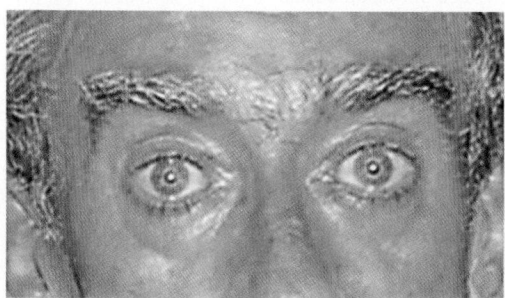

FIG. 46.1 Patient with jaundice. Source: Butcher, G. P. (2004). *Gastroenterology: An illustrated colour text.* Churchill Livingstone.

The convalescent phase begins as jaundice is fading and lasts from weeks to months; the average is 2 to 4 months. During this period, the patient's major symptoms are malaise and easy fatigability. Hepatomegaly remains for several weeks, but splenomegaly usually subsides. The overall mortality rate for acute viral hepatitis is less than 1%.

Chronic Phase. The disappearance of jaundice may not mean resolution of the virus infection. Many hepatitis B and C infections result in chronic, lifelong disease, whereas almost all cases of acute hepatitis A resolve with no progression to a chronic state. Although most patients with chronic viral hepatitis B or C have no symptoms, others may have malaise, fatigue, myalgias, arthralgias, and hepatomegaly (see Table 46.2). Chronic hepatitis B and C can further progress to severe scarring of the liver (cirrhosis), hepatocellular carcinoma (HCC), and liver failure if left untreated.

Complications

Fulminant hepatitis is an uncommon acute clinical syndrome that results in severe impairment or necrosis of liver cells and potential liver failure. It may develop in hepatitis B and hepatitis D co-infection. Liver failure usually causes death unless liver transplantation is performed. (Fulminant hepatitis is discussed further later in this chapter.)

Diagnostic Studies

Viral Serological Tests. The only definitive way to distinguish among the various types of viral hepatitis is by the

TABLE 46.3	CLASSIFICATION OF JAUNDICE		
	Prehepatic Jaundice	**Hepatic Jaundice**	**Posthepatic (Obstructive) Jaundice**
Description	• Results when excess unconjugated bilirubin in circulation is produced faster than the liver can conjugate it for excretion • Most commonly due to increased hemolysis, i.e., increased breakdown of RBCs, which produces an increased amount of unconjugated bilirubin in blood	• Results from a change in liver's ability to take up bilirubin from blood or to conjugate or excrete it • Liver cell injuries lead to bilirubin leak and thus raise the conjugated bilirubin levels • In severe liver injuries, both conjugated and unconjugated bilirubin are elevated	• Results from decreased or obstructed flow of bile through liver or biliary duct system • Obstruction may occur in intrahepatic or extrahepatic bile ducts • Intrahepatic obstructions are due to swelling or fibrosis of the liver's canaliculi and bile ducts
Common causes	• Sickle cell disease, thalassemia major, blood transfusion reactions	• Cirrhosis, alcoholic hepatitis, drug-induced hepatitis, liver cancer	• Cirrhosis, hepatitis, liver cancer • Common bile duct obstruction from stone(s), biliary strictures, pancreatic cancer, sclerosing cholangitis
Diagnostic Findings ***Serum Bilirubin***			
Unconjugated (indirect)	↑	↑	Normal
Conjugated (direct)	Normal	↑	↑
Urine Bilirubin	Negative	↑	↑
Urobilinogen			
Stool	↑	Normal, ↓	↓
Urine	↑	Normal, ↑	↓

RBC, red blood cells.

presence of specific serological markers (i.e., antigens and antibodies). The serological markers and their interpretations for each type of viral hepatitis are explained under the headings of the particular viruses.

Serum Liver Enzymes. Serum liver enzyme tests cannot differentiate one type of hepatitis from another, but they are helpful in determining whether it is related to liver cell injury or bile duct abnormalities. Aspartate aminotransferase (AST) and alanine aminotransferase (ALT) are liver enzymes whose abnormal levels indicate liver cell injury. In severe acute viral hepatitis, the levels can be markedly increased to more than 1 000 U/L. Elevated levels of alkaline phosphatase (ALP) and γ-glutamyl transpeptidase (GGT) are usually associated with bile duct injuries, but these levels can rise to a lesser extent in viral hepatitis infections.

Liver Function Tests. The term *liver function tests* has often been used broadly to include liver enzyme measurements. In hepatology specialty, liver function tests that more accurately reflect liver function are serum albumin, serum bilirubin, and prothrombin time (PT), which is standardized to the international normalized ratio (INR). In mild cases of viral hepatitis, serum albumin, serum bilirubin, and INR remain normal. When jaundice is detectable on physical examination, the serum bilirubin level is usually at least twice the normal upper limit (>34 mcmol/L). Deteriorating liver function is demonstrated by increased INR and serum bilirubin and decreased serum albumin.

Liver Biopsy. A liver biopsy is done in acute hepatitis only if the diagnosis is uncertain. In chronic hepatitis, a liver biopsy, where liver cells are examined histologically, is useful in determining the degree of inflammation and the stage of fibrosis (scar tissues). Liver biopsy, however, is invasive, and complications such as bleeding can occur. In patients with a bleeding disorder or severe coagulopathy, a transjugular liver biopsy is an option, where liver tissue is accessed via the transjugular vein under the ultrasound guidance.

Noninvasive Assessment. Techniques for noninvasive assessment of liver fibrosis are increasingly used to replace the need for liver biopsy. One commonly used technique is transient elastography (e.g., FibroScan®). Transient elastography is an ultrasound-based technique used to measure how fast the pressure wave propagates within the liver, providing measurements that predict the degree of fibrosis in the liver.

Hepatitis A

Hepatitis A is not commonly diagnosed in Canada, with an annual average of about 236 cases (Government of Canada, 2018). Worldwide, it can occur as sporadic outbreaks or epidemics (Ontario Ministry of Health and Long-term Care, 2019). In developing countries, hepatitis A infection is nearly universal during childhood.

Hepatitis A is typically an acute self-limiting infection. It is caused by the hepatitis A virus (HAV), which is a ribonucleic acid (RNA) virus. The virus is found in feces 2 weeks or more before the onset of symptoms and up to 1 week after the onset of jaundice (Figure 46.2). The detection of anti-HAV immunoglobulin M (IgM) indicates acute hepatitis. A positive anti-HAV immunoglobulin G (IgG) indicates a past infection or an immune response as a result of vaccination. The presence of antibody provides lifelong immunity (Table 46.4).

HAV is transmitted primarily through the fecal–oral route (by ingesting contaminated foods or water) and rarely parenterally. Poor hygiene, improper handling of food, crowded situations, and poor sanitary conditions are related factors. Foodborne hepatitis A outbreaks usually result from contamination of food during preparation by an infected food handler. The risk for transmission is highest before clinical symptoms are apparent.

Clinical Manifestations. Hepatitis A usually causes acute symptoms (see Table 46.2) in adults but not in younger children. Fewer than 10% of affected children younger than 6 years of age develop jaundice. Recovery usually takes 4 to 6 weeks,

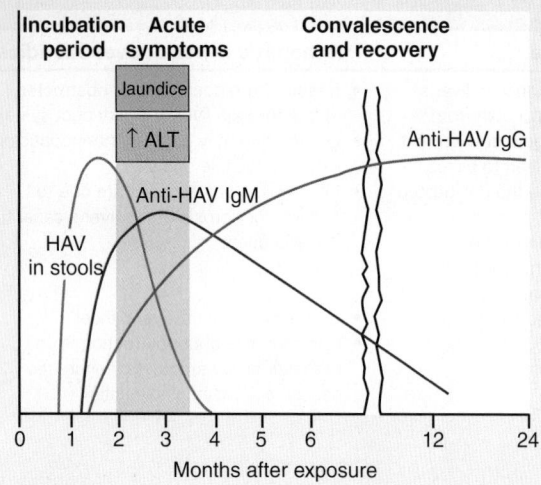

FIG. 46.2 Course of infection with hepatitis A virus (HAV). *ALT,* alanine aminotransferase; *anti-HAV IgG,* immunoglobulin G class antibody to hepatitis A virus; *anti-HAV IgM,* immunoglobulin M class antibody to hepatitis A virus. Source: McCance, K. L., & Huether, S. E. (2010). *Pathophysiology: The biologic basis for disease in adults and children* (6th ed., p. 1488). Mosby.

TABLE 46.4	SEROLOGY TESTS FOR HAV INFECTION
Tests	**Significance of a Positive Finding**
Anti-HAV IgM (antibody to HAV, immunoglobulin M)	Acute infection
Anti-HAV IgG (antibody to HAV, immunoglobulin G)	Long-term immunity, due to either a past infection or vaccination

HAV, hepatitis A virus.

but it may take months. Hepatitis A does not lead to chronicity and rarely causes fulminant hepatic failure. There is no specific treatment for hepatitis A. Hospitalization is normally unnecessary unless the patient is severely dehydrated. Management is focused on relief of symptoms. Recovery from HAV infection confers lifelong immunity against the virus.

Hepatitis B

Hepatitis B is a vaccine-preventable infectious disease. Worldwide, 257 million people are chronically infected. In Canada, the overall prevalence of the infection has declined with the availability of vaccination in Canadian-born people (Coffin et al., 2019). Because of the heterogeneity of the Canadian population, immigrants, particularly those from regions highly endemic for hepatitis B, constitute the largest group of carriers of chronic hepatitis B.

Hepatitis B virus (HBV) is a deoxyribonucleic acid (DNA) virus that is far more infectious than the human immunodeficiency virus (HIV). It can live outside a human body for up to 7 days. HBV expresses a few viral proteins or antigens that can be measured in blood. The three serology tests to screen for hepatitis B among the at-risk groups are hepatitis B surface antigen (HBsAg), antibody to hepatitis B surface antigen (anti-HBs), and antibody to hepatitis B core antigen (anti-HBc). The different serological markers of hepatitis B and their significance are explained in Table 46.5.

TABLE 46.5	SEROLOGY TESTS FOR HBV INFECTION
Test	**Significance of a Positive Finding**
HBsAg (hepatitis B surface antigen)	Infection; persistence of positive result >6 mo indicates chronic infection
Anti-HBs (antibody to hepatitis B surface antigen)	Immunity; produced with recovery from past infection or from vaccination
HBeAg (hepatitis B e antigen)	High virus activity and high degree of infectiousness
Anti-HBe (antibody to hepatitis B e antigen)	Associated with lower rate of virus replication and less infectivity in general
Anti-HBc total (total antibody to hepatitis B core antigen)	Past or ongoing infection; does not appear after vaccination
Anti-HBc IgM (IgM class antibody to hepatitis B core antigen)	Acute infection

HBV, hepatitis B virus; *IgM,* immunoglobulin M.

HBV can be transmitted in several ways: (a) perinatally from infected mothers to their infants, the most common route of transmission in high-endemic regions such as Asia and the Pan-Pacific; (b) percutaneously (e.g., intravenous [IV] drug use, accidental needle-stick punctures, tattoos); (c) sexually; or (d) horizontally by permucosal exposure to infectious blood, blood products, or other body fluids (e.g., semen, vaginal secretions). Kissing, hugging, sharing food, and casual contacts with infected individuals is not known to transmit HBV infection.

In people with HBV, HBsAg has been detected in almost every bodily fluid. Infected semen and saliva contain much lower concentrations of HBV than does blood, and the risk of virus transmission via these secretions is very low. There is no evidence that urine, feces, tears, and sweat are infective.

All infants born to HBV-infected mothers must receive the first dose of vaccination and immune globulins within 12 hours of birth. Breastfeeding is safe and not a risk factor for mother-to-child transmission as long as the infant receives immunoprophylaxis at birth (Society for Maternal-Fetal Medicine et al., 2016). All breastfeeding mothers should take good care of their nipples to avoid cracking and bleeding.

At-risk groups that should be screened for hepatitis B include those who were born in regions where HBV is common; household contacts with HBV carriers; injection or inhalation drug users; sexual partners of HBV carriers; persons with multiple sexual partners; inmates; pregnant women; persons with chronic liver disease; and persons needing immunosuppressive therapy (Coffin et al., 2018).

Acute Hepatitis B. Acutely infected newborns and young children born to mothers with hepatitis B mostly have no symptoms. The course of an acute HBV infection that spontaneously resolves is shown in Figure 46.3. After an acute infection, up to 90% of newborns who contract HBV at birth become chronically infected. In contrast, more than 95% of adults can clear the HBV infection except for those who are immunocompromised, such as those with HIV co-infection. Children under age 6 years with HBV have a 30 to 50% risk of it developing into a chronic infection (Coffin et al., 2018). Management of acute hepatitis B focuses on relief of symptoms and counselling to prevent virus transmission, including contact tracing. The need for antiviral treatment should be individually assessed.

Chronic Hepatitis B. The course of a chronic hepatitis B infection in persons who were infected at a young age is highly variable and rather complex (Figure 46.4). It is classified into four phases, with recent changes of terminology according to hepatitis B e antigen (HBeAg) status:

1. HBeAg-positive chronic infection (previously known as *immune tolerant*) phase. It is characterized by a high level of virus replication (HBV DNA or viral load) in the blood but no or minimal hepatic inflammation. Affected individuals are HBeAg positive but have normal ALT levels (<40 IU/mL) because of the lack of immune response to the virus.

2. HBeAg-positive chronic hepatitis (previously known as *immune clearance or active*) phase. Liver inflammation in this phase can be intermittent with varying degrees of inflammatory activity. HBV DNA is high. Liver enzyme levels are abnormal because the immune response against the virus has begun.

3. HBeAg-negative chronic infection (previously known as *inactive carrier*) phase. Viral load in this phase is low or undetectable. There is no inflammatory activity in the liver, so liver enzyme levels are normal.

4. HBeAg-negative chronic hepatitis (previously known as *reactivation*) phase. Affected persons develop a high viral load and abnormal liver enzyme levels, signaling reactivation of HBV infection.

Chronic hepatitis B can progress to cirrhosis and end-stage liver disease in 20 to 25% of individuals. The incidence of HCC in persons with cirrhosis is about 2 to 3%. Every year, about 1% of patients become cleared of HBsAg.

Medication Therapy. Medication therapy for chronic hepatitis B includes oral antiviral agents and pegylated-interferon alfa (PEG-IFN alfa). The aim of therapy is to suppress viral load, normalize liver enzymes, and slow the rate of disease progression. The long-term goals are to prevent cirrhosis, liver failure, and HCC (Coffin et al., 2018).

Pegylated-Interferon Alfa. Interferons have both antiviral and immunomodulatory activities. Pegylated-IFN alfa is a long-acting weekly subcutaneous injection. In Canada, it is used only in a very small proportion of infected individuals because of its many significant adverse effects. These adverse events are dosage related and tend to decrease in severity with continued treatment. For patients receiving IFN, blood cell counts and liver enzyme levels should be measured.

Nucleos(t)ide Analogues. Oral nucleoside and nucleotide analogues (NAs) are the mainstay of treatment for chronic hepatitis B. These medications inhibit viral DNA replication by mimicking normal DNA building blocks. Once they become incorporated into the hepatitis B virus DNA, they stop the DNA reproduction and are thus able to lower the amount of virus in the blood.

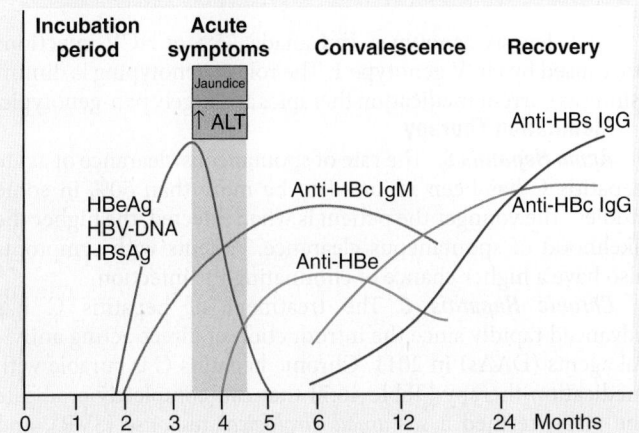

FIG. 46.3 Course of a resolved hepatitis B (HBV) infection. *ALT,* alanine aminotransferase; *anti-HBc,* antibody to hepatitis B core antigen; *anti-HBe,* antibody to HBeAg; *anti-HBs,* antibody to HBsAg; *HBeAg,* hepatitis B e antigen; *HBsAg,* hepatitis B surface antigen; *HBV,* hepatitis B virus; *IgG,* immunoglobulin G; *IgM,* immunoglobulin M. Source: McCance, K. L., & Huether, S. E. (2014). *Pathophysiology: The biologic basis for disease in adults and children* (7th ed., p. 1458). Mosby.

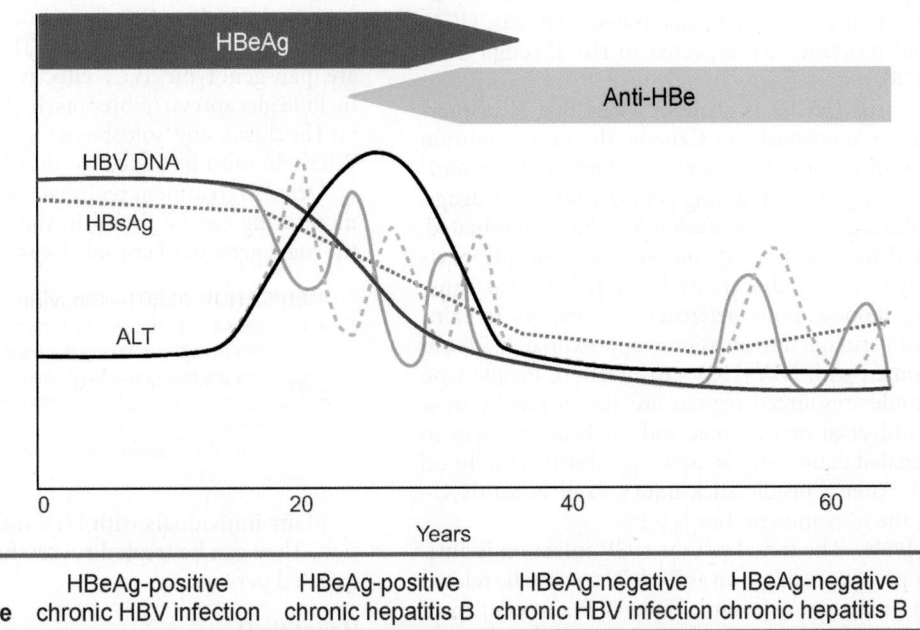

FIG. 46.4 Phases of chronic hepatitis B infection. *ALT,* alanine aminotransferase; *anti-HBe,* antibody to HBeAg; *HBeAg,* hepatitis B e antigen; *HBsAg,* hepatitis B surface antigen; *HBV,* hepatitis B virus. Source: European Association for the Study of the Liver. (2017). EASL 2017 clinical practice guidelines on the management of hepatitis B virus infection. *Journal of Hepatology, 67,* 370–398.

Current commonly used NAs in Canada include lamivudine (Heptovir), entecavir (Baraclude), tenofovir disoproxil fumarate (Viread), and tenofovir alafenamide (Vemlidy). Entecavir and tenofovir are the first-line medications of choice because of their high antiviral potency and low medication resistance risk. Lamivudine is used mainly as prophylaxis for immunosuppressed HBsAg-positive patients to avoid hepatitis B reactivation. Tenofovir alafenamide, a novel product of tenofovir, has similar clinical efficacy to that of tenofovir but less renal toxicity, as demonstrated in clinical studies. These medications are given when there is evidence of active viral replication. Entecavir should not be taken by women who are pregnant.

Most patients with HBV infection require long-term treatment. If these medications are discontinued for any reason, liver function and liver enzymes must be monitored closely for several months. Acute, severe exacerbations of hepatitis B have been reported after discontinuation of medications (Liem et al., 2019).

MEDICATION ALERT—Tenofovir Disoproxil Fumarate (Viread)
- This medication can cause nephrotoxicity, although it is uncommon (1.2%).
- Serum creatinine levels should be monitored, especially in patients at risk, including those with pre-existing renal disease and those taking nephrotoxic medications (e.g., cyclosporine, aminoglycoside, vancomycin).

MEDICATION ALERT—Entecavir
- This medication should not be taken by pregnant women because of the potential teratogenic effects.

Hepatitis C

An estimated 252 000 Canadians have been chronically infected with hepatitis C (Myers et al., 2015). The birth cohort of 1945–1975 has the highest prevalence. A large proportion of these individuals remain undiagnosed because of the asymptomatic nature and the slow progression of the infection (Shah et al., 2018). Although the overall prevalence of chronic hepatitis C is declining, its complications are increasing because of aging of the infected population and progression of the disease. Modelling data suggest that cases of decompensated cirrhosis, HCC, and liver-related mortality are expected to rise through 2035 (Shah et al., 2018).

Hepatitis C virus (HCV) is an RNA virus that is primarily transmitted percutaneously. In Canada, the most common mode of HCV transmission is through the sharing of contaminated needles and equipment among people who inject drugs. Transmission during blood transfusion has been eliminated. High-risk sexual behaviour (unprotected sex, multiple partners) is associated with a higher transmission risk. Sexual transmission among monogamous heterosexual partners remains rare. The risk for perinatal transmission is approximately 5% but is higher in women with HIV–HCV co-infection. People who were born in under-resourced regions are also at risk because of the lack of universal precautions, and medical practices in which contaminated equipment is used (e.g., during childhood immunization). After a needle-stick injury from hepatitis C–positive blood, the transmission rate is 0.1%.

Diagnostic Tests.
The initial test for HCV infection is antibody testing. A positive result of an anti-HCV test can be related to either a past or current exposure (Table 46.6). To confirm if disease is active or not, HCV RNA (the presence of replicating HCV) should be tested. In persons who cleared HCV infection, HCV RNA will be negative, but anti-HCV remains positive.

TABLE 46.6	SEROLOGY TESTS FOR HCV INFECTION
Test	**Significance**
Anti-HCV (antibody to hepatitis C virus)	Positive result indicates either past or current infection An initial screening test for HCV
HCV RNA	Quantitative result indicates ongoing viral replication, also referred to as *viral load*

HCV, hepatitis C virus; *RNA,* ribonucleic acid.

HCV RNA detection is particularly useful in immunocompromised patients (e.g., patients with HIV) who have active disease but whose anti-HCV is negative because antibody production is very low (below the detection level of the antibody tests).

HCV has six genotypes. In Canada, 75% of HCV infections are caused by HCV genotype 1. The role of genotyping is diminishing as current medication therapies are largely pan-genotypic.

Medication Therapy

Acute Hepatitis C. The rate of spontaneous clearance of acute hepatitis C has been reported to be more than 50% in some studies. The younger the patient is when infected, the higher the likelihood of spontaneous clearance. Patients with symptoms also have a higher chance of eliminating the infection.

Chronic Hepatitis C. The treatment of hepatitis C has advanced rapidly since the introduction of direct-acting antiviral agents (DAAs) in 2011. Chronic hepatitis C is curable with medication therapy (Table 46.7) that can completely eradicate the virus, termed a *sustained virological response* (SVR), and thus prevent HCV-related complications. The all-oral DAA therapy is a major breakthrough in the field of viral hepatitis. They have only a few common adverse effects, including headaches and fatigue. There is no medical justification to restrict therapy, except in persons with severely decompensated liver disease. As such, all individuals with chronic HCV infections should be considered for treatment. Current Health Canada–approved DAA antiviral regimens include genotype-specific and pan-genotypic formulas. The commonly used regimens are pan-genotypic (i.e., effective against all genotypes) and include glecaprevir/pibrentasvir (Maviret), sofosbuvir/velpatasvir (Epclusa), and sofosbuvir/velpatasvir/voxilaprevir (Vosevi). Ribavirin must be added to certain regimens (see Table 46.7).

Detailed treatment regimens, dosing schedule, duration, and monitoring can be found in the 2018 Canadian guidelines on the management of chronic hepatitis C (Shah et al., 2018).

MEDICATION ALERT—Ribavirin
- May cause birth defects. During treatment, pregnancy must be avoided, both by women taking the medication and by women whose male partners are taking the medication.
- May cause anemia. Hemoglobin must be closely monitored during treatment.
- Must be used in combination with a DAA. It is not effective when used alone.

Many individuals with HIV infection also have HCV infection. They can be treated successfully the same as HCV mono-infected persons.

Hepatitis D

Hepatitis D virus (HDV), also called *delta virus,* is a defective single-stranded RNA virus that cannot survive on its own and

TABLE 46.7	HEPATITIS C DIRECT-ACTING ANTIVIRAL (DAA) REGIMEN IN CANADA	
Medications	**Genotype**	**Treatment Duration (wk)**
Genotype-Specific Regimens		
Elbasvir/grazoprevir (Zepatier)	1, 4	12–16
Ledipasvir/sofosbuvir (Harvoni)	1, 4, 5, 6	8–24
Paritaprevir/ritonavir/ombitasvir + dasabuvir (Holkira-pak)	1, 1b	8–24
Paritaprevir/ritonavir/ombitasvir (Technivie)	4	12
Sofosbuvir + daclatasvir (Sovaldi + Daklinza)	1, 3	12–24
Pan-genotypic Regimens		
Glecaprevir/pibrentasvir (Maviret)	1–6	8–16
Sofosbuvir/velpatasvir (Epclusa)	1–6	12
Sofosbuvir/velpatasvir/voxilaprevir (Vosevi)	1–6	12

requires HBV to replicate. Although the prevalence of HDV in Canada is extremely low, people who are at risk for HBV infection (e.g., people who use injection drugs) should also be screened for HDV.

HDV can be acquired at the same time as HBV (co-infection) or at a later time in an existing HBV infection (superinfection). HBV–HDV co-infection can cause fulminant hepatitis and more severe disease than HBV infection alone. A positive anti-HDV (hepatitis D antibody) test indicates exposure to HDV, whereas HDV RNA confirms active disease. Currently in Canada, HDV RNA testing can be performed only in government-approved laboratories.

HDV, similar to HBV, is transmitted percutaneously. HDV is rarely acquired through sexual transmission. The symptoms of acute infection are the same as those of other viral hepatitis infection. People at risk for HDV infection are only those at risk for HBV. No vaccine for HDV is available; however, vaccination against HBV reduces risk for HDV co-infection. Treatment of HDV infection is with IFN alfa. However, response rates are poor (<30%), and relapse is common.

Hepatitis E

Like hepatitis A, the hepatitis E virus (HEV) is an RNA virus transmitted via the fecal–oral route, most commonly through drinking contaminated water. Infection with HEV, initially thought to occur primarily in developing countries, has been reported in increasing numbers in Europe and North America as a zoonotic disease. A large data set on Canadian blood donors found that HEV prevalence in Canada remains rare (Fearon et al., 2017). HEV infection causes acute self-limiting hepatitis. Pregnant women, however, are at risk for more severe disease. In immunosuppressed persons, hepatitis E may progress to a chronic infection and even cirrhosis. An acute diagnosis is confirmed through detection of IgM anti-HEV antibodies.

Table 46.8 shows the interprofessional care for viral hepatitis.

NURSING MANAGEMENT VIRAL HEPATITIS

NURSING ASSESSMENT

Subjective and objective data that should be obtained from a person with hepatitis are presented in Table 46.9.

TABLE 46.8	INTERPROFESSIONAL CARE

Viral Hepatitis

Diagnostic
- History and physical examination
- Liver enzyme measurements
- Alanine aminotransferase (ALT)
- Aspartate aminotransferase (AST)
- Liver function tests
- Albumin, bilirubin, INR
- Hepatitis tests
  - Hepatitis A: anti-HAV IgM, anti-HAV IgG
  - Hepatitis B: HBsAg, anti-HBs, anti-HBc IgM or total, HBV DNA
  - Hepatitis C: anti-HCV, HCV RNA, genotyping
  - Hepatitis D: anti-HDV
  - Hepatitis E: anti-HEV

Interprofessional Therapy
Acute and Chronic
- Well-balanced diet
- Vitamin supplements if needed
- Rest (degree of strictness varies)
- Avoid using alcohol and hepatotoxic medications

Chronic HBV
- Pegylated-interferon alfa therapy (sparingly used in Canada)
- Commonly used oral antiviral agents
- Entecavir, tenofovir, tenofovir alafenamide (Vemlidy)

Chronic HCV
- Genotype-specific regimens: Pan-genotypic regimens: glecaprevir/pibrentasvir (Maviret), sofosbuvir/velpatasvir (Epclusa), and sofosbuvir/velpatasvir/voxilaprevir (Vosevi)

Anti-HBc, antibody to hepatitis B core antigen; *anti-HBs*, antibody to surface antigen; *DNA*, deoxyribonucleic acid; *HAV*, hepatitis A virus; *HBsAg*, hepatitis B surface antigen; *HBV*, hepatitis B virus; *HCV*, hepatitis C virus; *HDV*, hepatitis D virus; *IgG*, immunoglobulin G; *IgM*, immunoglobulin M; *IFN*, interferon; *INR*, international normalized ratio; *RNA*, ribonucleic acid.

NURSING DIAGNOSES

Nursing diagnoses for the patient with hepatitis may include but are not limited to the following:
- *Inadequate nutrition* resulting from *insufficient dietary intake* (anorexia and nausea)
- *Reduced stamina* resulting from *physical deconditioning* (fatigue and weakness)
- *Potential for impaired liver function* (bleeding resulting from viral infection)

Additional information on nursing diagnoses for the patient with hepatitis is presented in Nursing Care Plan (NCP) 46.1, available on the Evolve website.

PLANNING

The overall goals are that the patient with viral hepatitis will (a) have relief of discomfort, (b) be able to resume their usual activities, and (c) experience a return to normal liver function without complications.

NURSING IMPLEMENTATION

HEALTH PROMOTION. Viral hepatitis is a public health problem. The nurse has a significant role in the prevention and control of this infectious disease. It is helpful for the nurse to understand the epidemiology of the different types of viral hepatitis, including risk factors for acquisition, when considering appropriate control measures.

TABLE 46.9   NURSING ASSESSMENT
Viral Hepatitis

Subjective Data

Important Health Information

Past health history: Family history of or exposure to person infected with viral hepatitis; exposure to benzene, carbon tetrachloride or other hepatotoxic agents; recent travel; ingestion of contaminated food or water; exposure to contaminated needles, including medical or dental equipment; hemodialysis; blood or blood product transfusions; organ transplantation; misuse of alcohol; previous injection drug use; previous illegal substance use; smoking history; high-risk sexual behaviour; exposure as health care worker; chronic care institution resident; incarceration

Medications: Use and misuse of acetaminophen, new prescriptions, over-the-counter or herbal medications or supplements

Symptoms

- Weight loss, anorexia and vomiting
- Malaise; taste change
- Skin rashes or hives, pruritus
- Right upper quadrant pain and tenderness
- Jaundice, dark urine; clay-coloured stools
- Fatigue, arthralgias, myalgias

Objective Data

General

Low-grade fever, lethargy, lymphadenopathy

Integumentary

Rash, other skin changes, jaundice, icteric sclera, interferon injection sites

Gastrointestinal

Hepatomegaly, splenomegaly

Possible Diagnostic Findings

Elevated liver enzyme levels; ↑ serum bilirubin, hypoalbuminemia, anemia, bilirubin in urine, and ↑ urobilinogen; prolonged prothrombin time (INR); positive test results for hepatitis, including anti-HAV IgM, anti-HAV IgG, HBsAg, anti-HBc IgM, HBV DNA, anti-HCV, HCV RNA, and anti-HDV; abnormal findings on radiological imaging

DNA, deoxyribonucleic acid; *HAV,* hepatitis A virus; *HBc,* hepatitis B core antigen; *HBeAg,* hepatitis B e antigen; *HBsAg,* hepatitis B surface antigen; *HBV,* hepatitis B virus; *HCV,* hepatitis C virus; *HDV,* hepatitis D virus; *IgG,* immunoglobulin G; *IgM,* immunoglobulin M; *INR,* international normalized ratio; *RNA,* ribonucleic acid.

TABLE 46.10   VIRAL HEPATITIS
Health Promotion and Preventive Measures

Hepatitis A

General Measures

- Good hand hygiene
- Proper personal hygiene
- Environmental sanitation
- Control and screening (signs, symptoms) of food handlers
- Serological screening
- Active immunization for people in at-risk groups

Use of Immune Globulin

- Early administration (1–2 wk after exposure) to those exposed
- Prophylaxis for travellers to areas where hepatitis A is common if they have not previously received HAV vaccine

Special Considerations for Health Care Providers

- Wash hands after contact with an affected patient or after removal of gloves
- Use infection-control precautions

Hepatitis B and C Percutaneous/Vertical Transmission

- Screening of donated blood
- Hepatitis B: HBsAg
- Hepatitis C: anti-HCV
- Screening of pregnant women
- Use of disposable needles and syringes

Sexual Transmission

- Acute exposure: HBIG administration to sexual partner of HBsAg-positive person
- Administration of HBV vaccine series to uninfected sexual partners
- Use of condoms for sexual intercourse

General Measures

- Good hand hygiene
- Avoid sharing toothbrushes and razors
- HBIG administration for one-time exposure (needle-stick, contact of mucous membranes with infectious material)
- Active immunization: HBV vaccine

Special Considerations for Health Care Providers

- Use infection-control precautions
- Handle all patients' blood as potentially infectious
- Dispose of syringes and needles properly
- Use needleless IV access devices when available

HAV, hepatitis A virus; *HBIG,* hepatitis B immunoglobulin; *HBsAg,* hepatitis B surface antigen; *HBV,* hepatitis B virus; *HCV,* hepatitis C virus; *IV,* intravenous.

Hepatitis A. HAV is usually the cause of outbreaks of viral hepatitis. Preventive measures include personal and environmental hygiene and health education to promote good sanitation. Careful handwashing, especially after bowel movements and before eating, is probably the most important precaution. Both hepatitis A vaccine and immune globulin are administered for prevention. (See Table 46.10 for more information on hepatitis A health promotion and prevention.)

Vaccination, or active immunization, is an effective means of controlling hepatitis A and the best protection against HAV infection. Canada currently does not have a universal HAV immunization program. Adults at risk are advised to receive the vaccine as pre-exposure prophylaxis. These include people who travel to HAV-endemic regions, users of illicit drugs, men who have sex with men, persons with chronic liver disease, persons with clotting factor disorders (e.g., hemophilia), and residents of communities where hepatitis A is highly endemic (Public Health Agency of Canada [PHAC], 2021b).

The HAV vaccine is inactivated hepatitis A virus and is currently available in several forms, including Avaxim, Havrix, and Twinrix. Vaccines are available in both adult and pediatric doses. Primary immunization consists of a single dose administered intramuscularly in the deltoid muscle. A booster dose is given 6 to 36 months later, depending on the product, to ensure long-term protection (PHAC, 2021a). The primary immunization provides immunity within 30 days after a single dose in more than 95% of those vaccinated. The adverse effects of the vaccine are mild and are usually limited to soreness and redness at the injection site.

Hepatitis A immunoglobulin can be administered either before or after exposure. Immunoglobulin provides temporary (6 to 8 weeks) passive immunity and is effective for preventing hepatitis A if given within 1 to 2 weeks after exposure. Immunoglobulin is recommended for individuals without anti-HAV antibodies who are exposed to hepatitis A by close contact (e.g., household, day care centre) with people who have HAV or through foodborne exposure. Although immunoglobulin may not prevent infection in all persons, it may modify the illness to a subclinical infection. It may also be administered as a prophylactic measure for travellers to countries that have a high incidence of hepatitis A.

The patient with acute hepatitis A is hospitalized only when symptoms are severe. Isolation is generally not required for hepatitis A; however, infection-control precautions must be used (see Chapter 17, Table 17.8). A private room is indicated if the patient is incontinent of stool or has inadequate personal hygiene.

Hepatitis B. The best way to reduce HBV infection is to identify persons at risk, screen them for HBV, and vaccinate those who are not infected (see Table 46.10). The nurse must be aware of which individuals are at risk for contracting hepatitis B and teach them ways to reduce risks of transmission.

Hepatitis B vaccine is the most effective means of prevention. Since the late 1990s, universal immunization against HBV has been part of the vaccine programs offered by all provinces and territories in Canada. Although different jurisdictions offer the vaccines for people of different ages, the HBV vaccine programs ensure that every child is vaccinated by the end of high school. It is also important to vaccinate adults in at-risk groups, including people who use injection or inhalation drugs, those who live with or have sexual contact with hepatitis B carriers, persons with chronic liver disease, people with hemophilia, persons with chronic renal disease or undergoing dialysis, individuals infected with HIV, and health care providers (PHAC, 2021a).

Hepatitis B vaccine is produced through recombinant DNA technology. The approved vaccines include Engerix-B, Recombivax, and Twinrix. These are given usually in a series of three injections in the deltoid muscle. The second dose is administered within 1 month of the first one, and the third one within 6 months of the first, depending on the product. The hepatitis B–containing combination vaccine, Infanrix hexa, also contains diphtheria, tetanus toxoids, pertussis, poliomyelitis, and *Haemophilus influenzae* type b (DTap-HB-IPV-Hib) vaccine and is given at 2, 4, 6, and 12 to 23 months of age. Hepatitis B vaccine is more than 95% effective. Successful vaccination should result in anti-HBs titres of 10 IU/mL or greater. Boosters (additional doses) to increase the antibody levels are generally not recommended. Only minor adverse reactions have been reported with vaccination, including transient fever and soreness at the injection site. The vaccine is not contraindicated during pregnancy.

For postexposure prophylaxis, the vaccine and hepatitis B immune globulin (HBIG) are administered. HBIG contains antibodies to HBV and confers temporary passive immunity. It is prepared from plasma of donors with a high titre of anti-HBs. HBIG is recommended for postexposure prophylaxis in cases of needle-stick, mucous membrane contact, or sexual exposure. It should be given after exposure, preferably within 24 hours. The vaccine series should also be started. Infants born to HBV-infected mothers must receive the first dose of HBV vaccine and HBIG within 12 hours of birth for maximal protection.

Preventive measures should also include teaching individuals at high risk of contracting HBV how to reduce risks. Good hygienic practices, including handwashing and using gloves when expecting contact with blood, are important. HBV-infected individuals should not share razors, toothbrushes, and other personal items. Safer sex practices, such as use of condoms and vaccination of the person's sexual partner, should also be taught.

Hepatitis C. No vaccine is currently available for hepatitis C. The primary measures to prevent HCV transmission include screening of blood, organ, and tissue donors; using infection-control precautions; and modifying high-risk behaviour. As with HBV prevention, the nurse should identify individuals at high risk for contracting HCV and teach ways to reduce risks. Individuals at risk include those who use injection drugs (or have used them in the past, even once or many years ago), people who received blood or blood products before 1992, patients who are or have been undergoing hemodialysis, workers in hemodialysis units and laboratories in which blood is handled, people with multiple sexual partners, prisoners, and sexual partners of individuals with HCV infection. Because of the number of people with hepatitis C who have not been diagnosed, birth-cohort screening (1945–1975) regardless of risk factor status is cost-effective (Shah et al., 2018).

Currently, the Public Health Agency of Canada does not recommend immune globulin for postexposure prophylaxis (e.g., needle-stick exposure from an infected person) for HCV infection. After an acute exposure (e.g., through needle-stick), baseline anti-HCV and ALT levels should be measured in both the person already infected (i.e., the source) and the person exposed to HCV. Follow-up testing for anti-HCV and ALT activity should be performed 4 to 6 months later. If the source is someone with known HCV infection, HCV RNA should be measured 2 weeks later to confirm viral transmission.

As with hepatitis B prevention, the use of universal precautions is important. The use of a condom is advised for sexual intercourse with an individual with HCV, and razors, toothbrushes, and other personal items should not be shared. Health promotion and preventive measures for hepatitis A, B, and C are summarized in Table 46.10.

ACUTE CARE INTERVENTION. In patients with acute hepatitis, the nurse assesses for jaundice. In light-skinned people, jaundice is usually observed first in the sclera of the eyes and later in the skin. In dark-skinned people, jaundice is observed in the hard palate of the mouth and the inner canthus of the eyes. The urine may be dark brown or brownish-red because of the presence of bilirubin. Comfort measures should be used to relieve fatigue, weakness, headache, and arthralgias (see NCP 46.1, available on the Evolve website).

Ensuring that the patient receives adequate nutrition can be a challenge. Anorexia and a distaste for food can cause nutritional concerns. Dietary assessment should be performed. Small, frequent meals may be preferable to three large ones and may help prevent nausea. Measures to stimulate the appetite—such as mouth care, antiemetics, and attractively served meals in pleasant surroundings—should be included in the nursing care plan. Carbonated beverages, ginger, and avoidance of very hot or very cold foods may help counteract the symptom of nausea. Adequate hydration is important.

Patients with symptomatic acute viral hepatitis have fatigue and decreased energy. Rest is important to help conserve energy and to promote hepatocyte regeneration. The nurse should help the patient space activities both to conserve energy and to avoid overexertion; assess the patient's response to the rest and activity plan; and modify it as needed based on symptoms and liver function tests.

AMBULATORY AND HOME CARE. Most individuals with viral hepatitis are cared for at home. The nurse needs to assess patients' knowledge of nutrition and provide the necessary dietary teaching. Rest and adequate nutrition are important for those with impaired liver synthetic functions. Patients should be cautioned about overexertion and the need to follow the health care provider's advice about when to return to work. Patients and their families should be taught how to prevent transmission among household members and what symptoms should be reported to the health care provider. Signs and symptoms of worsening liver function include bleeding tendencies (caused by increased INR), abdominal swelling (from ascites), vomiting of blood or tarry stools (caused by varices bleeding), and confusion (caused by encephalopathy). Patients should be instructed to have regular follow-up for at least 1 year after the diagnosis of acute viral hepatitis. Those who are unable to resolve the acute infection and become chronic HBV or HCV carriers should be assessed for the need of a referral to a hepatologist, if it has not already been done. All patients with chronic HBV or HCV infection should avoid excessive use of alcohol, to prevent acceleration of disease progression. Individuals who remain positive for HBsAg or anti-HCV positive should not donate blood, semen, or organs.

EVALUATION

Expected outcomes for the patient with viral hepatitis are addressed in NCP 46.1, available on the Evolve website.

NONALCOHOLIC FATTY LIVER DISEASE AND NONALCOHOLIC STEATOHEPATITIS

Nonalcoholic fatty liver disease (NAFLD) refers to a spectrum of disease that ranges from simple fatty liver (steatosis) that causes no hepatic inflammation, to nonalcoholic steatohepatitis (NASH), to severe liver scarring (cirrhosis). This spectrum of liver disease occurs in people who drink little or no alcohol. NAFLD is characterized by the accumulation of fat in liver cells. When this fat buildup causes inflammation and liver cell injury resulting in fibrosis, it will turn into NASH. NASH can only be diagnosed histologically (through a liver biopsy) with liver cell ballooning and Mallory bodies. NASH can progress and cause cirrhosis, which can lead to liver cancer and liver failure. When the liver fails, liver transplantation is the only available treatment alternative.

Causes

NAFLD is a growing concern around the globe. The most common cause of fatty liver disease is obesity. Worldwide, obesity has almost tripled since 1975 (World Health Organization [WHO], 2021). According to Statistics Canada (2019), 27% of Canadians have obesity and 34% are overweight. Although obesity is also increasing among the Canadian First Nations population, the prevalence of NAFLD appears to be similar to that of non–First Nations patients (Uhanova et al., 2016). Obesity is linked to many chronic diseases, fatty liver disease being one of them. About 75% of people with obesity are at risk of developing simple fatty liver and, of those, up to 25% are at risk of developing fatty liver with inflammation (i.e., NASH). NAFLD also occurs in patients with metabolic syndrome.

Clinical Manifestations and Diagnostic Studies

NAFLD is usually diagnosed during routine medical checkup or during evaluation of other health conditions such as hypertension, diabetes, hyperlipidemia, and obesity (metabolic syndrome). Elevations in liver enzyme levels (ALT, AST) are often

the first signs of NAFLD. However, such elevations may be associated with other liver disorders.

Most patients with NAFLD have no symptoms. Symptoms, if present, are nonspecific and may include fatigue, malaise, and vague pain in the right upper abdominal quadrant. Enlarged liver (hepatomegaly) and enlarged spleen (splenomegaly) may be detected on first examination of the patient. A small number of patients are only diagnosed when they exhibit signs of serious liver disease (e.g., ascites, variceal hemorrhage). Definitive diagnosis is by liver biopsy. Ultrasonography and computed tomography (CT) are also used to diagnose NAFLD.

Interprofessional Care

Patients with NAFLD who are older, have obesity, or have diabetes mellitus are at risk for advanced liver disease. Currently, there is no approved medication. Therapy is directed at reduction of risk factors, including treatment of diabetes, reduction in body weight, and elimination of harmful medications. Lifestyle counselling interventions that focus on physical activities and eating behaviours have enabled significant improvement for patients with liver dysfunction.

Health promotion and patient education about fatty liver for people at all ages are important in preventing the development of NAFLD. Ways to prevent fatty liver include maintaining a healthy body mass index (BMI) (≤25 BMI), avoiding increased abdominal fat (for men, keeping waist circumference <102 cm; for women, <88 cm), eating a heart-healthy diet, exercising at least three times weekly, limiting alcohol to no more than two drinks at a time, taking only medications that are needed, and following health care providers' recommendations.

While there are no approved medications for NAFLD at present, many therapeutic agents are currently being investigated within the context of clinical trials.

ALCOHOL-ASSOCIATED LIVER DISEASE (ALD)

Alcohol consumption is a frequent cause of acute and chronic liver disease. Alcohol-associated liver disease (ALD) presents a spectrum of liver injury as a result of alcohol use, ranging from simple liver fat (steatosis) to alcohol-associated steatohepatitis, alcoholic hepatitis, and alcohol-associated cirrhosis. Progression of the disease depends on continued heavy alcohol use and other cofactors, including female sex, genetic susceptibility, diet, and comorbid liver disease such as hepatitis C (Crabb et al., 2020).

Alcohol-associated steatosis usually presents with no symptoms. Mild elevation of AST and GGT are probably the best indicators of recent excessive alcohol intake. As disease progresses, symptoms associated with ALD may include abdominal pain, tiredness, peripheral neuropathy, muscle loss, and odour of alcohol on the breath.

Alcoholic hepatitis is a syndrome of hepatomegaly, jaundice, elevation in liver enzyme levels (AST, ALT, ALP) and bilirubin, low-grade fever, and possibly ascites and prolonged INR. These symptoms may improve if alcohol intake stops.

Many patients are often unaware of the liver damage caused by their alcohol overuse and they are diagnosed only when complications of cirrhosis occur. Even at the advanced stage of cirrhosis, abstinence can result in significant reversal of liver disease in some patients. If liver function does not recover after abstaining from alcohol for several months or longer, liver transplantation may be considered.

Drug-Induced Liver Injury (DILI)

Drug-induced liver injury (DILI) refers to liver injury induced by both prescription or nonprescription medications, including health products, dietary and herbal supplements, Chinese medicines, and natural medicines. It is one of the most common and severe drug reactions causing jaundice, acute liver failure, and even death (Yu et al., 2017). The pattern of injury depends on the medication causing the reaction. The main cause of DILI is antimicrobial agents, particularly amoxicillin-clavulanate, and the most common medication causing acute liver failure is acetaminophen.

The LiverTox website (http://www.livertox.nih.gov) provides up-to-date information on over 400 types of common medications that can cause hepatotoxicity.

> **MEDICATION ALERT—Acetaminophen (Tylenol)**
> - It is safe if taken at recommended levels and not combined with alcohol.
> - It is also present in a variety of pain relievers, fever reducers, and cough medicines as a somewhat "hidden" ingredient; thus patients taking several medications may not realize that they are taking a higher amount of acetaminophen, and overdose may occur.
> - Its toxic effects are dose related. Ingestion of more than 10 g/day leads to acute liver failure.
> - Combining the medication with alcohol increases risk for liver injury.

The pathophysiological changes in the liver and the clinical manifestations of toxic and drug-induced hepatitis are similar to those of viral hepatitis. The usual presenting clinical findings are anorexia, nausea, vomiting, hepatomegaly, splenomegaly, and abnormal results of liver function studies. Treatment is largely supportive, as in acute viral hepatitis. Recovery may be rapid if the hepatotoxin is identified and removed. Liver transplantation may be necessary in patients with severe liver injuries.

AUTOIMMUNE AND GENETIC LIVER DISEASES

Autoimmune Hepatitis

Autoimmune hepatitis (AIH) can be presented as an acute or chronic inflammatory disorder of the liver that occurs when the body's immune system attacks its own liver cells. While the cause is unknown, its occurrence may be related to genetic and environmental factors or to drug, virus, or toxin exposure that triggers the activation of the immune system. However, the immune system remains activated after the trigger is removed. AIH affects all ages, both genders, and all ethnicities, although the majority of affected persons are female adults (Mack et al., 2020). Many patients have other autoimmune diseases, such as celiac disease or hypothyroidism.

The course of AIH is variable. Some patients have no symptoms, whereas others have an acute presentation with symptoms similar to those of acute viral hepatitis. Most patients develop chronic hepatitis. Symptoms include fatigue, arthralgia, abdominal pain, and occasionally jaundice. Diagnosis is usually based on the presence of antinuclear antibodies (ANA) and anti–smooth muscle antibodies (SMA), high levels of serum IgG, and elevated liver enzymes. Liver cancer develops in approximately 6% of patients with AIH.

The recommended treatment for active AIH is prednisone or in combination with azathioprine (Imuran). If these drugs are not effective, other immunosuppressive therapies (e.g., cyclosporine, tacrolimus [Prograf], or mycophenolate mofetil [CellCept]) are options. Many patients who stop treatment experience relapse; therefore, treatment is usually lifelong to maintain remission. The most common cause of relapse is failure to adhere to the treatment regimen. Patients who do adhere and respond do not have a shortened life expectancy. However, liver transplantation is indicated for those with liver failure.

Wilson Disease

Wilson disease is an autosomal recessive gene disorder of copper transport that affects mainly the liver but also the brain, eyes, and kidneys. When the process of excreting excess dietary copper in the biliary system is impaired, copper will become accumulated in the liver. Mutations in the affected gene, *ATP7*, lead to decreased biliary excretion of copper. The increased storage of copper in the liver can cause progressive liver injury and cirrhosis. Wilson disease has an average worldwide prevalence of about 30 per million population. It occurs more often in children and young adults than in older individuals. First-degree relatives of patients with Wilson disease must be screened for the disease (Palumbo & Schilsky, 2019).

The hallmark of Wilson disease is corneal Kayser–Fleischer rings, which are brownish-red rings seen in the cornea near the limbus. However, the absence of Kayser-Fleischer rings does not exclude the diagnosis. In addition to liver disease, many affected patients also have neurological dysfunction, including movement disorders (tremor, involuntary movements), drooling, dysarthria, rigid dystonia, seizures, migraine headaches, and insomnia.

Diagnosis is based on clinical findings, including the corneal rings and neurological symptoms. Serum ALT and AST levels are elevated, serum ceruloplasmin levels are extremely low, and urinary copper excretion levels are increased. Markedly elevated copper concentrations from liver biopsy samples are present.

The recommended initial treatment of symptomatic patients or those with active disease is with chelating agents, such as D-penicillamine or trientine, that promote excretion of urinary copper. After adequate treatment with a chelating agent, patients with stable disease may be continued on a lower dose of a chelator or switch to treatment with zinc. Zinc interferes with copper absorption and is better tolerated long term with few adverse effects. Patients should avoid eating foods with very high concentrations of copper, such as shellfish, nuts, chocolate, and organ meats. Use of copper cookware and containers should also be avoided. Treatment of Wilson disease is lifelong. A low-copper diet combined with treatment is recommended. Liver transplantation may be necessary for acute liver failure or for treatment failure.

Hereditary Hemochromatosis

Hereditary hemochromatosis is a genetic disorder that affects the liver, heart, pancreas, and endocrine system. It is an inherited condition that is related to mutation in the *HFE* gene, causing an increase and inappropriate absorption of dietary iron. Prolonged increased iron absorption can lead to complications such as cirrhosis, HCC, diabetes, and heart disease. (Hemochromatosis is discussed further in Chapter 33.)

Primary Biliary Cholangitis

Primary biliary cholangitis (PBC), formerly known as *primary biliary cirrhosis* (Beuers et al., 2015), is a chronic and slowly progressive disease of the small bile ducts of the liver. A T cell–mediated attack on the small bile duct epithelial cells results in loss of bile ducts and ultimately in *cholestasis* (blockage of bile flow). Over time, the chronic destruction and inflammation of the bile ducts lead to liver fibrosis and cirrhosis. Although the etiology of PBC is not completely understood, it appears that both genetic and environmental factors such as chemical exposure and infection may play a role.

Most patients diagnosed with PBC are middle-aged women. The disease is associated with three major autoimmune disorders: Sjogren's syndrome, CREST (**c**alcinosis, **R**aynaud's disease, **e**sophageal dysfunction, **s**clerodactyly, and **t**elangiectasias), and scleroderma (Lindor et al., 2019).

In the early stages, patients may have no symptoms. The major symptoms of PBC are fatigue and generalized pruritus (itching). Patients with more advanced disease have more symptoms, including hepatomegaly and hyperpigmentation of the skin. Jaundice is a sign of late-stage disease. Osteoporosis is also found in a significant number of patients with PBC. They may also have signs of fat malabsorption, including low levels of fat-soluble vitamins, which occur because of decreased bile secretion. Levels of serum ALP, antimitochondrial antibodies (AMA), ANA, and serum lipid levels are also elevated in patients with PBC. Histological evidence of disease is found on liver biopsy.

The goals of treatment are suppression of ongoing liver damage, prevention of complications, and symptom management. The approved drugs for treatment of PBC in Canada are ursodeoxycholic acid (UDCA) and obeticholic acid (Ocaliva). Ocaliva is a newer agent indicated for use in combination with UDCA when there is inadequate response to UDCA alone, or as monotherapy for those who cannot tolerate UDCA. Other management focuses on malabsorption, skin disorders such as pruritus and xanthomas (cholesterol deposits in the skin), hyperlipidemia, vitamin deficiencies, anemia, and fatigue. Cholestyramine is used to treat pruritus. Patients are monitored for progression to cirrhosis. Liver transplantation is a treatment option for end-stage liver disease in patients with PBC.

Primary Sclerosing Cholangitis

Primary sclerosing cholangitis (PSC) is a disease of unknown etiology, characterized by chronic inflammation, fibrosis, and strictures (narrowing) of the medium and large bile ducts inside and outside of the liver. The majority of patients with PSC also have ulcerative colitis. Complications of PSC can include cholangitis, cholestasis with jaundice, cholangiocarcinoma (bile duct cancer), and cirrhosis.

Medication therapy with ursodial has not been beneficial. Treatment is directed at reducing the incidence of biliary complications and at screening for bile duct and colorectal cancer, which is related to the high incidence of ulcerative colitis. Patients with advanced liver disease may require liver transplantation.

CIRRHOSIS OF THE LIVER

Cirrhosis is a condition (not a disease) that results from chronic liver inflammation from any etiology. Cirrhosis is characterized by extensive fibrosis (scar tissue) and regenerative nodules that occur from the liver's attempt to repair itself, leading to permanent distortion in the liver architecture (Figure 46.5). Fibrosis occurs when the liver cells attempt to regenerate after liver injuries but the regenerative process is disorganized. The overgrowth of new and fibrous connective tissue distorts the normal lobular structure, resulting in lobules of irregular size and shape with impeded blood flow. Eventually, irregular and disorganized

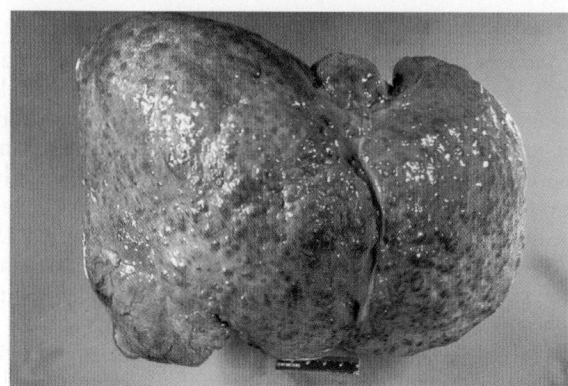

FIG. 46.5 Cirrhosis that developed secondary to alcoholism. The characteristic diffuse nodularity of the surface is caused by the combination of regeneration and scarring of the liver. Source: Kumar, V., Abbas, A. K., Fausto, J. N., et al. (2010). *Robbins and Cotran pathologic basis of disease* (8th ed., p. 858). W. B. Saunders.

regeneration, leading to impaired perfusion due to architectural distortion at the cellular level, results in impaired liver synthetic function. Cirrhosis is the final stage of chronic liver disease.

Cirrhosis is a significant cause of morbidity and mortality. It is ranked as the eleventh leading cause of death in Canadians (Statistics Canada, 2021a); the incidence has increased over the past two decades (1997–2016) and more so in younger birth cohorts born in 1980 and in 1990 compared with a person of the same age born in 1951. The increase in incidence of cirrhosis has been greater in women than in men (Flemming et al., 2019).

Etiology

Any chronic liver disease—including chronic viral hepatitis, NAFLD, ALD, and autoimmune liver diseases (AIH, PBC, PSC) can cause cirrhosis. These diseases are all described earlier in this chapter. However, excessive alcohol ingestion remains one of the most common causes of cirrhosis. Alcohol has a direct hepatotoxic effect, and it causes cell necrosis and fatty infiltration in the liver. In patients with alcohol-associated liver disease, controversy exists as to the degree to which malnutrition adds to the damage caused by the alcohol itself. Some cases of nutrition-related cirrhosis have resulted from extreme dieting, malabsorption, and obesity. Environmental factors and genetic disposition may lead to the development of cirrhosis, regardless of dietary or alcohol intake.

Approximately 20% of patients with chronic hepatitis C and 25% of those with chronic hepatitis B develop cirrhosis. Chronic inflammation and cell necrosis can result in progressive fibrosis and cirrhosis. Chronic hepatitis combined with alcohol use has a synergistic effect in accelerating liver damage.

Cardiac cirrhosis includes a spectrum of hepatic conditions that result from long-standing, severe, right-sided heart failure. It causes hepatic venous congestion, parenchymal damage, necrosis of liver cells, and fibrosis over time. Treatment is aimed at managing the patient's underlying heart failure.

Clinical Manifestations

Cirrhosis can be classified as *compensated* or *decompensated*. In compensated cirrhosis, the liver is able to continue to function normally despite severe hepatic cell injury and architectural distortion of the liver. Blood tests reflecting liver synthetic function—which include serum albumin level, bilirubin level, PT, and INR—are normal. In decompensated cirrhosis, these blood

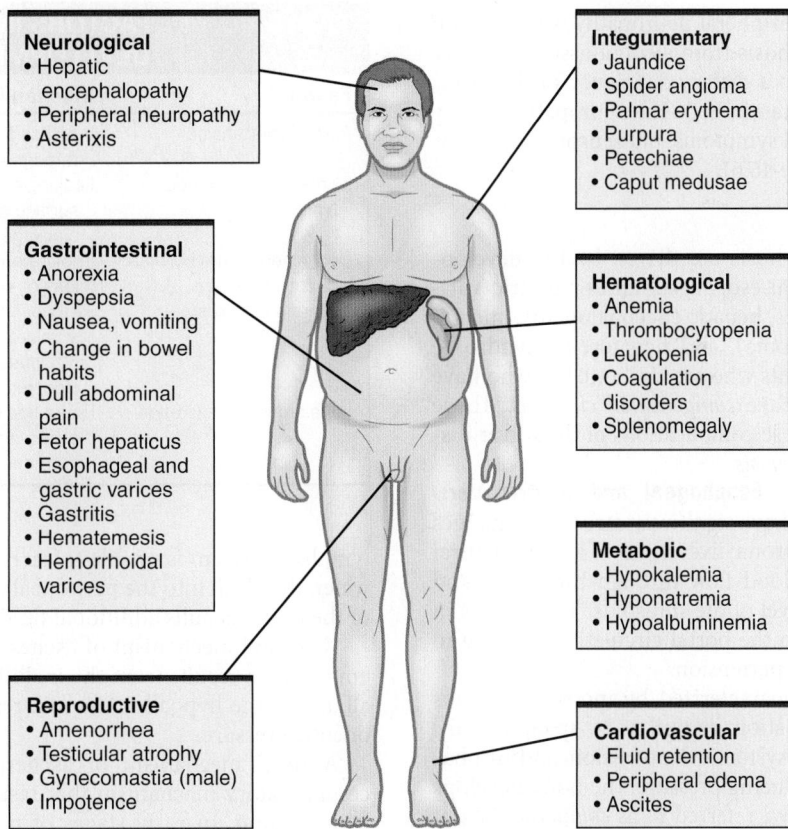

Neurological
• Hepatic encephalopathy
• Peripheral neuropathy
• Asterixis

Gastrointestinal
• Anorexia
• Dyspepsia
• Nausea, vomiting
• Change in bowel habits
• Dull abdominal pain
• Fetor hepaticus
• Esophageal and gastric varices
• Gastritis
• Hematemesis
• Hemorrhoidal varices

Reproductive
• Amenorrhea
• Testicular atrophy
• Gynecomastia (male)
• Impotence

Integumentary
• Jaundice
• Spider angioma
• Palmar erythema
• Purpura
• Petechiae
• Caput medusae

Hematological
• Anemia
• Thrombocytopenia
• Leukopenia
• Coagulation disorders
• Splenomegaly

Metabolic
• Hypokalemia
• Hyponatremia
• Hypoalbuminemia

Cardiovascular
• Fluid retention
• Peripheral edema
• Ascites

FIG. 46.6 Systemic clinical manifestations of advanced liver cirrhosis.

tests will become abnormal, and are associated with clinical symptoms and complications that will be detailed in the following section.

The onset of cirrhosis is a gradual process over time. As such, most patients with compensated cirrhosis will unlikely have specific physical symptoms. Some patients may experience abdominal pain, described as a dull, heavy feeling in the right upper quadrant or epigastrium. The pain may be caused by swelling and stretching of the liver capsule, spasm of the biliary ducts, intermittent vascular spasm, or a combination of these. Other early clinical manifestations are nonspecific, including anorexia, dyspepsia, nausea and vomiting, weakness, muscle loss, fatigue, slight weight loss, hepatomegaly or shrunken liver (depending on disease process), and splenomegaly. In decompensated cirrhosis, patients present with overt clinical manifestations.

Manifestations of Decompensated Cirrhosis. Late symptoms result from the complications of portal hypertension and liver failure. Jaundice, peripheral edema, and ascites develop gradually as the liver's synthetic function deteriorates. Other late symptoms include skin lesions, hematological disorders, endocrine disturbances, and peripheral neuropathies (Figure 46.6). In the advanced stages, the liver becomes small and nodular and feels firm on palpation.

Jaundice. Jaundice occurs as a result of the liver's decreased ability to excrete conjugated bilirubin (hepatic jaundice). The jaundice may be minimal or severe, depending on the degree of liver damage. If obstruction of the biliary tract occurs, obstructive jaundice may also occur and is usually accompanied by pruritus. The pruritus is caused by an accumulation of bile salts underneath the skin.

Skin Lesions. Various skin manifestations are commonly seen in cirrhosis. Spider angiomas (*telangiectasia* or *spider*

nevi) are small, dilated blood vessels with a bright-red centre and spider-like branches. They occur on the nose, cheeks, upper trunk, neck, and shoulders. *Palmar erythema* (a red area that blanches with pressure) appears on the palms of the hands. Both of these abnormalities are attributed to an increase in circulating estrogen as a result of the damaged liver's inability to metabolize steroid hormones.

Hematological Conditions. Hematological conditions include thrombocytopenia, leukopenia, anemia, and coagulation disorders. Thrombocytopenia is the strongest indicator of cirrhosis. Major mechanisms for thrombocytopenia in liver cirrhosis are (a) platelet sequestration in the spleen and (b) decreased production of thrombopoietin in the liver (Moore, 2019). Anemia can result from inadequate red blood cell production and survival, poor diet, poor absorption of folic acid, and bleeding from varices.

The coagulation disorders result from the liver's inability to produce prothrombin and other factors essential for blood clotting. Manifestations of coagulation conditions (bleeding tendencies) include epistaxis, purpura, petechiae, easy bruising, gingival bleeding, and dysmenorrhea.

Endocrine Disturbances. Normally, the liver metabolizes hormones including adrenocortical hormones, estrogen, and testosterone. When the damaged liver is unable to do so, various manifestations occur. In men, gynecomastia, loss of axillary and pubic hair, testicular atrophy, and impotence with loss of libido may occur as a result of estrogen accumulation. Younger women with cirrhosis may develop amenorrhea, and older women may have vaginal bleeding. The liver fails to metabolize aldosterone properly, which can lead to hyperaldosteronism with subsequent sodium retention, water retention, and potassium loss.

Peripheral Neuropathy. Peripheral neuropathy is a common finding in patients with cirrhosis from alcohol-associated liver disease. It is probably due to a dietary deficiency of thiamine, folic acid, and cobalamin (vitamin B_{12}). The neuropathy usually results in mixed neurological symptoms, but sensory symptoms may predominate (see Figure 46.6).

Complications

Major complications of cirrhosis are driven by the development of portal hypertension: esophageal and/or gastric varices, peripheral edema, ascites, hepatic encephalopathy (mental status changes, including coma), and hepatorenal syndrome (D'Amico et al., 2018). Patients who are cirrhotic but who have no obvious complications have *compensated cirrhosis.* Those who have one or more of these complications of their liver disease have *decompensated cirrhosis.*

Portal Hypertension and Esophageal and Gastric Varices. Patients with cirrhosis have significant structural changes in the liver resulting from chronic liver injury. These structural changes lead to impaired blood flow through the portal and hepatic veins down to the level of the sinusoids. This results in increased venous pressure to the portal circulation, leading to the development of portal hypertension.

Portal hypertension is characterized by increased venous pressure in the portal circulation, as well as by splenomegaly, large collateral veins, ascites, systemic hypotension, and esophageal varices. As a way of reducing pressure, the body develops alternate circulatory pathways, referred to as *collateral circulation.* The collateral channels often form in the lower esophagus (the anastomosis of the left gastric vein and the azygos veins), anterior abdominal wall, parietal peritoneum, and rectum. Varicosities may develop in areas where the collateral and systemic circulations communicate, resulting in esophageal and gastric varices, *caput medusae* (ring of varices around the umbilicus), and hemorrhoids (Garcia-Tsao et al., 2017).

Esophageal varices are complexes of tortuous veins located at the lower end of the esophagus. *Gastric varices* are located in the fundus (upper part of the stomach). These varices are fragile and do not tolerate high pressure so they can bleed easily. Large varices are more likely to bleed. Esophageal varices can cause variceal hemorrhages with a 5-year mortality of 20%. The patient may present with melena or hematemesis. Ruptured esophageal varices are the most life-threatening complication of cirrhosis and considered a medical emergency.

Peripheral Edema and Ascites. Peripheral edema sometimes precedes ascites, but in some patients, its development coincides with or occurs after ascites. Edema is caused by decreased colloidal oncotic pressure as a result of impaired liver synthesis of albumin and by increased portacaval pressure from portal hypertension. Peripheral edema manifests as ankle and presacral edema.

Ascites is the accumulation of serous fluid in the peritoneal or the abdominal cavity. It is a common manifestation of decompensated cirrhosis. Development of fluid retention in the setting of cirrhosis is an important landmark in the natural history of chronic liver disease: approximately 15% of patients with ascites succumb in 1 year and 44% succumb in 5 years.

Several mechanisms lead to ascites (Table 46.11). One mechanism of ascites occurs with the development of portal hypertension from cirrhosis. Increased portal pressures cause proteins to shift from the blood vessels via the larger pores of the sinusoids (capillaries) into the lymphatic space (Figure 46.7). When the

TABLE 46.11	FACTORS INVOLVED IN THE DEVELOPMENT OF ASCITES
Factor	**Mechanism**
Portal hypertension	Increase in resistance of blood flow through liver
Increased flow of hepatic lymph	Leaking of protein-rich lymph from surface of cirrhotic liver; intrahepatic blockage of lymph channels
Decreased serum colloidal oncotic pressure	Impairment of liver synthesis of albumin; loss of albumin into peritoneal cavity
Hyperaldosteronism	Increase in aldosterone secretion, stimulated by decreased renal blood flow; decreased liver metabolism of aldosterone
Impaired water excretion	Reduction in renal vascular flow and excessive serum levels of antidiuretic hormone

lymphatic system is unable to carry off the excess proteins and water, they leak into the peritoneal cavity. The osmotic pressure of the proteins pulls additional fluid into the peritoneal cavity.

A second mechanism of ascites formation is hypoalbuminemia, which results from the inability of the liver to synthesize albumin. The hypoalbuminemia results in decreased colloidal oncotic pressure.

A third mechanism of ascites, hyperaldosteronism, is a compensatory mechanism that results from progressive portal hypertension. In early stages of portal hypertension, there is moderate splanchnic arterial vasodilation, which is compensated by an increase in cardiac output, thus permitting arterial pressure and effective arterial blood volume to remain normal. However, in advanced stages of cirrhosis, the reduction in systemic vascular resistance is marked and cannot be compensated further by increases in cardiac output. This results in underfilling of the arterial circulation and an overall reduction of cardiac output. As such, arterial pressure must be maintained by the continued activation of vasoconstrictor systems, including the renin–angiotensin–aldosterone system (RAAS), the sympathetic nervous system, and a nonosmotic hypersecretion of arginine vasopressin (antidiuretic hormone). These systems help maintain effective arterial blood volume and arterial pressure; however, both have important effects on kidney function, particularly sodium and fluid retention leading to clinical manifestations, including abdominal distension due to ascites and edema (Figure 46.8). If the ascites is severe, the umbilicus may be everted. Abdominal striae with distended abdominal wall veins may be present. Urinary output is decreased, and signs of dehydration (e.g., dry tongue and skin, sunken eyeballs, muscle weakness) are manifested.

Hepatic Encephalopathy. Hepatic encephalopathy is a neuropsychiatric manifestation of advanced liver disease. The pathogenesis of hepatic encephalopathy is multifactorial and includes the neurotoxic effects of ammonia, abnormal neurotransmission, astrocyte swelling, and inflammatory cytokines. A major source of ammonia is the bacterial and enzymatic deamination of amino acids in the intestines. The ammonia that results from this deamination process normally goes to the liver via the portal circulation and is converted to urea, which is then excreted by the kidneys. When the blood is shunted past the liver via the collateral vessels, or when the liver is unable to convert ammonia to urea, ammonia levels in the systemic circulation rise. The ammonia crosses the blood–brain barrier

PATHOPHYSIOLOGY MAP

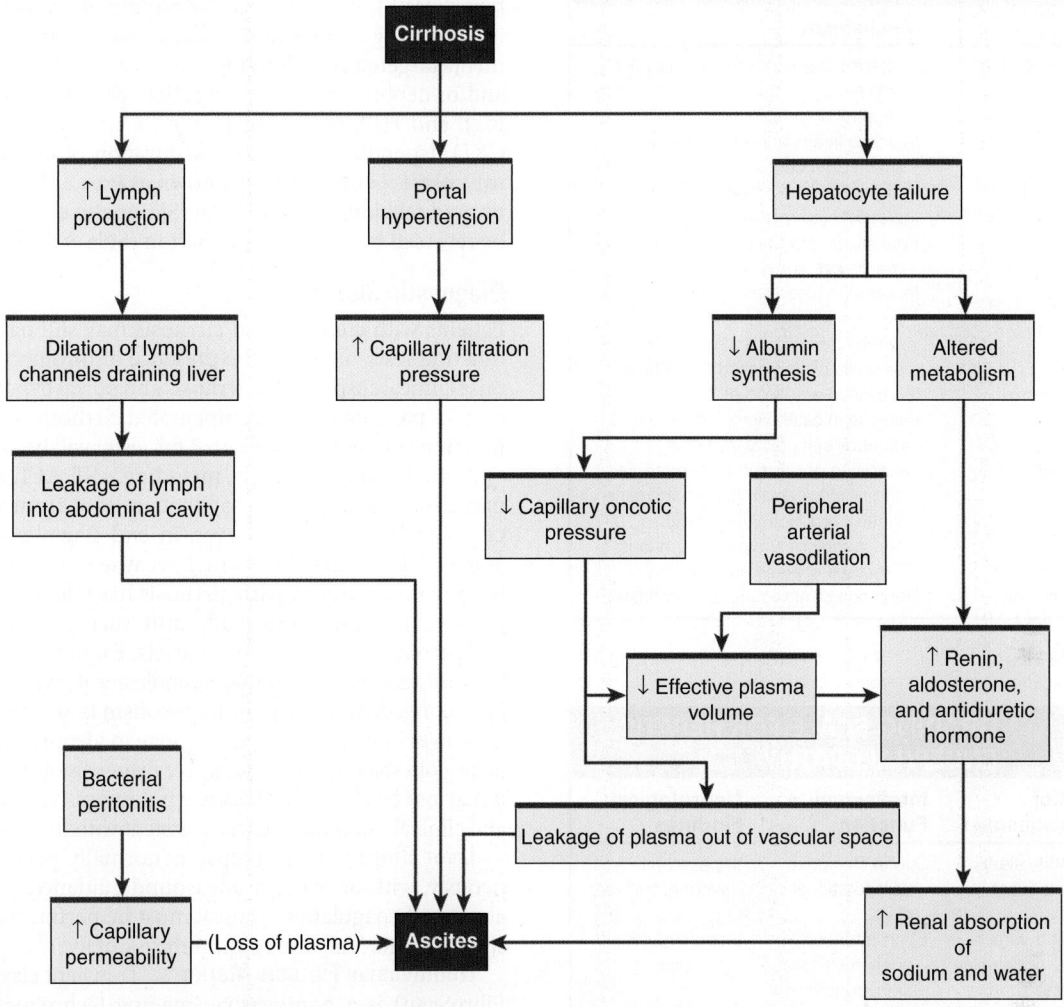

FIG. 46.7 Mechanisms for development of ascites. Source: Adapted from McCance, K. L., & Huether, S. E. (2014). *Pathophysiology: The biologic basis for disease in adults and children* (7th ed., p. 1454). Mosby.

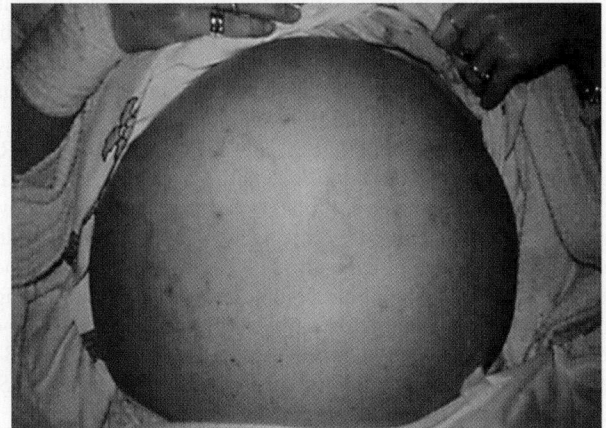

FIG. 46.8 Gross ascites. Source: Butcher, G. P. (2004). *Gastroenterology: An illustrated colour text*. Churchill Livingstone.

and produces neurological toxic manifestations. Factors that increase ammonia in circulation may precipitate hepatic encephalopathy (Table 46.12). Hepatic encephalopathy can also occur after placement of a transjugular intrahepatic portosystemic shunt (TIPS), which is used to treat portal hypertension (Novelli, 2017).

Clinical manifestations of encephalopathy include changes in neurological and mental responsiveness; impaired consciousness; inappropriate behaviour; concentration difficulties; and fluctuating levels of consciousness, ranging from sleep disturbances to lethargy to deep coma. Changes may occur suddenly because of an increase in ammonia in response to bleeding varices, or they may occur gradually as blood ammonia levels slowly increase. A grading system is used to classify the stages of hepatic encephalopathy (Table 46.13).

A characteristic manifestation of hepatic encephalopathy that is graded 1 or higher is asterixis (flapping tremors) involving the arms and hands. When asked to stretch out the arms and hands, the patient is unable to hold this position, and the hands exhibit a series of rapid flexion and extension movements.

Other clinical manifestations include impairments in writing—difficulty in moving the pen or pencil from left to right and *constructional apraxia* (the inability to construct simple figures). Other signs include hyperventilation, hypothermia, and grimacing and grasping reflexes.

Fetor hepaticus can also occur as an accumulation from the accumulation of digestive by-products that the liver is unable to degrade. It is characterized by a musty, sweet odour of the patient's breath.

TABLE 46.12	FACTORS PRECIPITATING HEPATIC ENCEPHALOPATHY
Factor	**Mechanism**
Cerebral depressants (e.g., opioids)	Decrease in drug metabolism by liver, which causes higher drug levels and cerebral depression
Constipation	Increase in ammonia from bacterial action on feces
Dehydration	Potentiation of ammonia toxicity
GI hemorrhage	Increase in ammonia in GI tract
Hypokalemia	Potassium ions are needed by brain to metabolize ammonia
Hypovolemia	Increase in blood ammonia, caused by hepatic hypoxia; impairment of cerebral, hepatic, and renal function because of decreased blood flow
Increased metabolism	Increase in workload of liver
Infection	Increase in catabolism; increase in cerebral sensitivity to toxins
Metabolic alkalosis	Facilitation of transport of ammonia across blood–brain barrier; increase in renal production of ammonia
Paracentesis	Loss of sodium and potassium ions; decrease in blood volume
Uremia (kidney failure)	Retention of nitrogenous metabolites

GI, gastrointestinal.

TABLE 46.13	GRADING SCALE FOR HEPATIC ENCEPHALOPATHY		
Grade	**Level of Consciousness**	**Intellectual Function**	**Neurological Findings**
0	Insomnia, sleep disturbances	Subtle change in computational skills	Impaired handwriting, tremor
1	Lack of awareness, personality change	Short attention span, mild confusion, depression	Incoordination, asterixis
2	Lethargy, drowsiness, inappropriate behaviour	Disorientation	Asterixis, abnormal reflexes
3	Asleep, rousable	Loss of meaningful conversation, marked confusion, incomprehensible speech	Asterixis, abnormal reflexes
4	Not rousable	Absent	Decerebrate May be responsive to painful stimuli

Hepatorenal Syndrome. Hepatorenal syndrome (HRS) is a serious complication of decompensated cirrhosis. It is a unique form of renal failure that develops in patients with cirrhosis, in the absence of precipitating factors (e.g., shock, no current or recent use of nephrotoxic drugs), structural kidney injury (absence of both proteinuria and hematuria), and normal findings of renal ultrasound. The etiology is complex, but the generally accepted theory is that HRS is of circulatory origin and occurs as a consequence of reduction in renal blood flow and glomerular filtration rate (GFR) secondary to marked arterial vasodilation in the splanchnic circulation. This leads to a reduction of effective arterial blood volume and arterial pressure with compensatory activation of vasoconstrictor systems,

particularly the sympathetic nervous system and RAAS. HRS occurs in two different forms: HRS-AKI (formerly known as type 1 HRS), characterized by rapidly progressive renal failure in the setting of multiorgan failure that is unresponsive to treatments targeted at underlying causes (e.g., hypovolemia, diuretics and/or nephrotoxic drugs, infection, gastrointestinal [GI] bleeding), and HRS-NAKI (further split into HRS-AKD and HRS-CKD depending on period of duration of estimated GFR <60 mL/min/1.73 m^2; formerly known as type 2 HRS), characterized by gradual kidney dysfunction (Simonetto et al., 2020). HRS can be reversed by liver transplantation (Sola & Gines, 2010).

Diagnostic Studies

Patients with compensated cirrhosis may still have normal liver function tests, although the presence of thrombocytopenia does raise clinical suspicion of cirrhosis and portal hypertension. However, in patients with decompensated cirrhosis, most of the liver function studies (see Table 46.8 for tests) will become abnormal.

Initially, enzymes levels, including AST, ALT, ALP, and GGT, may be elevated because of their release from damaged liver cells and bile ducts. However, in end-stage liver disease, AST and ALT levels may be normal because of the death and loss of hepatocytes. Patients with cirrhosis have decreased total serum protein, decreased serum albumin, increased serum bilirubin, and increased serum globulin levels. Fat metabolism abnormalities are reflected by decreased cholesterol levels. The PT or INR is prolonged, and bilirubin metabolism is altered.

A liver biopsy, which may be done to identify liver cell changes, is the gold standard for a definitive diagnosis of cirrhosis, although it may not be clinically necessary if noninvasive markers, imaging, and clinical examination are consistent with findings of cirrhosis.

Liver Biopsy. Liver biopsy is normally performed percutaneously, with or without ultrasound guidance. In patients with abnormal coagulation, biopsy must be performed via the transjugular vein. The most common risk of liver biopsy is bleeding.

Noninvasive Fibrosis Markers. Transient elastography (e.g., FibroScan) is a noninvasive imaging technique by which the degree of hepatic fibrosis is measured. Its use in Canada was approved in 2010. It is an ultrasound-based imaging technique for detecting liver stiffness, which is generally correlative with the degree of liver fibrosis. It has been validated for use in different types of liver disease. It has excellent diagnostic accuracy for the diagnosis of cirrhosis, regardless of the underlying cause or causes of the liver disease (Wilder & Patel, 2014).

Models of serum markers (e.g., FibroTest, FIB-4, and APRI) are noninvasive indices used for predicting liver fibrosis and cirrhosis using blood samples. FibroTest is used in Canada; however, its use may be limited by testing availability. In this model, five parameters are used (bilirubin, GGT, haptoglobin, apolipoprotein, and α_2-macroglobulin), in addition to the patient's age and sex, to calculate a fibrosis score for predicting the degree of liver fibrosis. The latter two models are more widely used: FIB-4 uses age, AST, platelets, and ALT in its model; APRI uses AST and platelets only (Lin et al., 2011).

Interprofessional Care in Advanced Cirrhosis of the Liver

The goal of therapy for patients with cirrhosis is to slow the disease progression by treating the etiology and to prevent and manage symptoms associated with liver decompensation. Interprofessional care measures are listed in Table 46.14. Management of specific complications related to decompensated cirrhosis is described next.

TABLE 46.14 INTERPROFESSIONAL CARE
Advanced Cirrhosis of the Liver

Diagnostic
- History and physical examination
- CBC
- Computed tomography
- Endoscopy (esophagogastroduodenoscopy)
- Liver biopsy (if indicated)
- Liver enzyme measurements (AST, ALT, ALP, GGT)
- Liver function studies (albumin, bilirubin, INR)
- Liver stiffness measurement (FibroScan)
- Liver ultrasonography
- Magnetic resonance imaging
- Serum electrolyte measurements
- Serum fibrosis markers (FibroTest)

Interprofessional Therapy
Conservative Therapy
- Avoidance of alcohol, acetylsalicylic acid (Aspirin), sedatives, and nonsteroidal anti-inflammatory medications
- Rest (in decompensated cirrhosis)

Ascites
- Diuretics
- Low-sodium diet
- Paracentesis (if indicated)
- TIPS

Esophageal and Gastric Varices
- Balloon tamponade
- Drugs
- Nonselective β-blockers (e.g., nadolol)
- Octreotide (Sandostatin)
- Vasopressin
- Endoscopic sclerotherapy or band ligation
- TIPS

Hepatic Encephalopathy
- Antibiotics (rifaximin [Zaxine])
- Lactulose

ALP, alkaline phosphatase; *ALT*, alanine aminotransferase; *AST*, aspartate aminotransferase; *CBC*, complete blood cell count; *GGT*, γ-glutamyl transpeptidase; *INR*, international normalized ratio; *TIPS*, transjugular intrahepatic portosystemic shunt.

Ascites. Management is focused on sodium restriction, diuretics, and fluid removal. Affected patients are encouraged to limit sodium intake to 2 g (88 mmol) per day. More stringent sodium restriction is no longer recommended because it can result in reduced nutritional intake and subsequent malnutrition concerns. Fluid restriction is usually not necessary unless severe hyponatremia develops. Fluid and electrolyte balance should be accurately assessed and controlled. Albumin infusions are used to help maintain intravascular volume and adequate urinary output by increasing plasma colloid oncotic pressure.

Diuretic therapy is an important part of current medical management, alongside dietary sodium restriction, to increase renal sodium excretion. The aim of the treatment is to achieve a natriuresis higher than sodium intake that causes negative sodium and fluid balance with weight loss and reduction in extracellular fluid volume. The diuretics of choice are aldosterone antagonists because of the increased aldosterone secretion in cirrhosis. Combination therapy with loop diuretics (most commonly used is furosemide) alongside aldosterone antagonists is generally more effective in diuresis and maintaining electrolyte

balances (since aldosterone antagonists are potassium sparing) as these drugs work at multiple sites of the nephron. Spironolactone is usually the aldosterone antagonist of choice and is very effective. Other aldosterone antagonists include amiloride and triamterene, although triamterene is not used commonly. Hydrochlorothiazide is rarely administered because it is not as potent as the loop diuretics.

Paracentesis is a sterile procedure in which a catheter is used to withdraw fluid from the abdominal cavity. This procedure can be used to diagnose a medical condition, rule out infection in the fluid (spontaneous bacterial peritonitis), or relieve pain, pressure, or difficulty breathing. However, it is generally indicated only when the diuretic therapy fails and to relieve symptoms such as abdominal pain or difficulty breathing (i.e., therapeutic paracentesis), although it can also be done diagnostically at index presentation to determine the etiology for ascites (i.e., diagnostic paracentesis). The relief provided by therapeutic paracentesis is only temporary because the fluid reaccumulates. In-dwelling catheters such as PleurX catheter drainage systems are put in place to provide symptomatic relief (i.e., palliation) at home for end-stage liver disease.

A TIPS procedure can be considered for management of ascites in individuals with portal hypertension whose condition does not respond to diuretics. This procedure will be discussed later in this chapter.

Esophageal and Gastric Varices. The main therapeutic goal for esophageal and gastric varices is to prevent bleeding. All patients with cirrhosis should have an upper endoscopy (esophagogastroduodenoscopy) to screen for varices (Boregowda et al., 2019). Risk factors for esophageal bleeding include variceal size (the largest varices are at highest risk of bleeding), decreased wall thickness, and degree of liver dysfunction (associated with increased portal hypertension). Patients who have esophageal varices should avoid ingesting alcohol, acetylsalicylic acid (ASA; Aspirin), and nonsteroidal anti-inflammatory drugs (NSAIDs). For patients who have esophageal varices that have not bled, primary bleeding prophylaxis with nonselective β-blockers (e.g., propranolol, nadolol, carvedilol) has been shown to reduce the risk of bleeding as well as the number of bleeding-related deaths. Nonselective β-blockers reduce portal venous pressure by decreasing cardiac output and possibly by constricting splanchnic vessels.

When variceal bleeding occurs, the first step is to stabilize the patient and manage the airway. IV therapy is initiated and may include administration of blood products. Care then moves toward stopping the bleeding, identifying the source or sources, and applying interventions to prevent further bleeding. Variceal bleeding is diagnosed on endoscopic examination. A combination of drug therapy and endoscopic therapy is more successful in preventing rebleeding than each therapy alone.

Medication therapy may include octreotide (Sandostatin) or vasopressin. Both therapies produce vasoconstriction of the splanchnic arterial bed, decrease portal blood flow, and decrease portal hypertension. Octreotide is used more often because it has fewer adverse effects than vasopressin. Because of vasopressin's adverse effects (including decreased coronary blood flow and heart rate and increased blood pressure), nitroglycerin is often administered in combination with vasopressin for reducing the detrimental effects of the vasopressin while enhancing its beneficial effect. Vasopressin should be avoided or administered with caution in older persons because of the risk of cardiac ischemia.

Endoscopic therapies include sclerotherapy and ligation of varices. Endoscopic sclerotherapy involves injecting a sclerosing agent into the varices to thrombose and obliterate the distended veins. Endoscopic ligation or banding of the varices is performed by placing a small rubber band (elastic O-ring) around the base of the varix. Endoscopic ligation is as effective as endoscopic sclerotherapy with fewer complications.

Balloon tamponade is an option when endoscopy does not control acute esophageal or gastric variceal hemorrhage, usually as a last resort in an emergent clinical situation. Balloon tamponade controls the hemorrhage by mechanical compression of the varices. Balloon tamponade is typically completed in the critical care unit setting as the patient requires close monitoring; the patient is typically intubated prior to insertion of a balloon tamponade. Several types of tubes are available. The Sengstaken-Blakemore tube (Figure 46.9) has two balloons, gastric and esophageal, with three lumens: one for the gastric balloon, one for the esophageal balloon, and one for gastric aspiration. When inflated, the gastric and esophageal balloons put mechanical compression on the varices. The gastric balloon anchors the tube in position and also applies pressure to any bleeding gastric varices. Two other types of balloons are the Minnesota tube (a modified Sengstaken-Blakemore tube with an esophageal suction port above the esophageal balloon) and the Linton-Nachlas tube.

SAFETY ALERT—Balloon Tamponade
- Label each lumen to avoid confusion.
- Secure the tube to prevent movement of the tube that could result in occlusion of the airway.
- Deflate balloons for 5 minutes every 8 to 12 hr per facility policy to prevent tissue necrosis.

Supportive measures during an acute variceal bleed include administration of fresh-frozen plasma and packed red blood cells, vitamin K, and proton pump inhibitors. Lactulose may be administered to prevent hepatic encephalopathy from breakdown of blood and the release of ammonia in the intestine. Antibiotics such as norfloxacin are given prophylactically because of the risk of bacterial translocation into the peritoneal cavity, causing spontaneous bacterial peritonitis.

Because of the high incidence of recurrent bleeding and the mortality risk with each bleeding episode, continued therapy is necessary. Long-term management of patients who have had an episode of bleeding includes the use of nonselective β-blockers, repeated endoscopic ligation, and portosystemic shunts.

Shunting Procedures. Surgical and nonsurgical methods of shunting blood away from the esophageal varices are available. Shunting procedures tend to be used more after a second major bleeding episode than after an initial bleeding episode. TIPS, an interventional radiological technique in which the hypertensive portal vein is connected with a normotensive hepatic vein by a coated stent (shunt), helps redirect portal flow, leading to significant overall reduction, and even normalization, of portal pressure (Figure 46.10).

Achieving an overall reduction in portal pressures can control variceal bleeding and, as noted previously, can also be used for management of refractory or diuretic-intolerant ascites. In individuals with functional TIPS, the need for other therapies for portal hypertension (nonselective β-blockers, variceal ligation) could be eliminated. This procedure does not interfere with future liver transplantation. Limitations of the TIPS procedure include the increased risk for hepatic encephalopathy and stenosis of the stent. TIPS is contraindicated in patients with

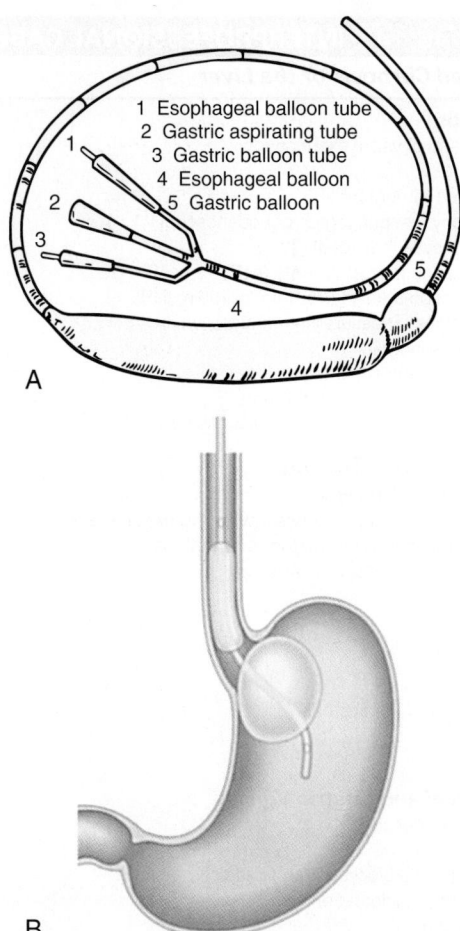

1 Esophageal balloon tube
2 Gastric aspirating tube
3 Gastric balloon tube
4 Esophageal balloon
5 Gastric balloon

FIG. 46.9 A, Diagram of Sengstaken–Blakemore tube. **B,** Diagram of tube inserted into esophagus and stomach.

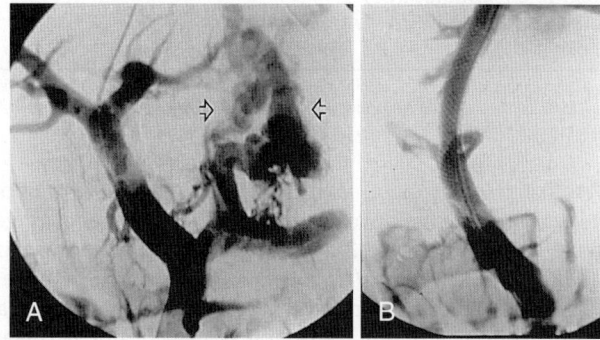

FIG. 46.10 Total portal diversion after insertion of a transjugular intrahepatic portosystemic shunt (TIPS). **A,** Portal venogram before TIPS insertion shows filling of large esophageal varices *(arrows).* **B,** After TIPS insertion, flow to varices is eliminated. The direction of intrahepatic portal vein flow is now reversed, toward the TIPS. Source: Reprinted from *Journal of Vascular Surgery,* Volume 16(2), Jeanne M. LaBerge, Ernest J. Ring, John R. Lake, Linda D. Ferrell, Margaret M. Doherty, Roy L. Gordon, John P. Roberts, Marc Y. Peltzer, Nancy L. Ascher, "Transjugular intrahepatic portosystemic shunts: Preliminary results in 25 patients," pp. 258–267, Copyright 1992, with permission from Elsevier.

advanced age (typically over age 65 years), cardiac dysfunction, severe hepatic encephalopathy, severe hepatorenal syndrome, HCC (relative contraindication dependent on imaging) and significant portal vein thrombosis (relative contraindication dependent on imaging). Various surgical shunting procedures are no longer in common use but may be used to decrease portal

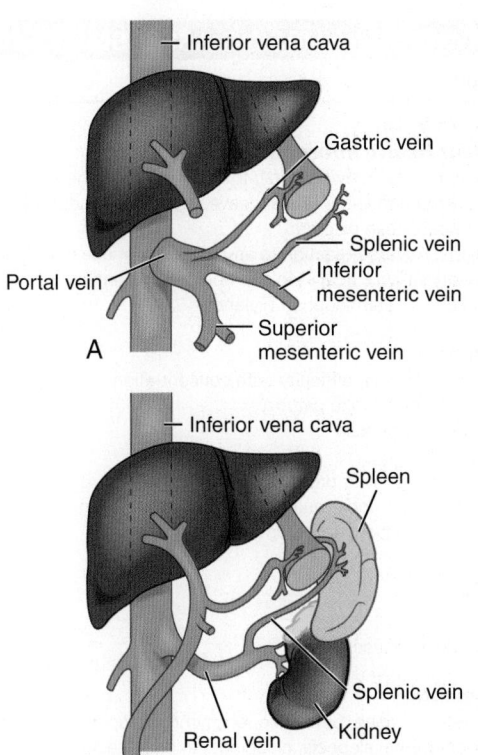

FIG. 46.11 Portosystemic shunts. **A,** Portacaval shunt. The portal vein is anastomosed to the inferior vena cava, diverting blood from the portal vein to the systemic circulation. **B,** Distal splenorenal shunt. The splenic vein is anastomosed to the renal vein. The portal venous flow remains intact, and esophageal varices are selectively decompressed (by decompression of the short gastric veins). The spleen conducts blood from the high pressure of the esophageal and gastric varices to the low-pressure renal vein.

TABLE 46.15	**MEDICATION THERAPY**
Advanced Cirrhosis	
Medication	**Mechanism of Action**
Diuretics	
• Spironolactone (Aldactone)	Blocking action of aldosterone; potassium sparing
• Amiloride (Apo-Amilzide)	Inhibition of reabsorption of sodium and secretion of potassium
• Furosemide (Lasix)	Rapid action on distal tubule and loop of Henle to prevent reabsorption of sodium and water
• Triamterene (Teva-Triamterene)	Inhibition of reabsorption of sodium and secretion of potassium
• Lactulose	Acidification of feces in bowel and trapping of ammonia, causing its elimination in feces
Propranolol (Inderal) or nadolol	Reduction of portal venous pressure
Proton pump inhibitors (e.g., pantoprazole [Pantoloc])	Decrease in gastric acidity
Rifaximin (Zaxine)	Decrease in bacterial flora, decrease in formation of ammonia
Neomycin sulphate	
Vasopressin	Hemostasis and control of bleeding in esophageal varices; constriction of splanchnic arterial bed
Octreotide (Sandostatin)	
Vitamin K	Correction of clotting abnormalities

hypertension by diverting some of the portal blood flow and simultaneously allowing adequate liver perfusion. The surgical shunts still in use are the portacaval shunt and the distal splenorenal shunt (Figure 46.11). Surgical shunts are more likely to be used in emergency situations. Although a prophylactic portacaval shunt decreases bleeding episodes, it does not prolong life. Patients can develop hepatic encephalopathy as a result of the diversion of the ammonia past the liver and into the systemic circulation.

Hepatic Encephalopathy. The goal of management of hepatic encephalopathy is the reduction of ammonia formation. Ammonia formation in the intestines is reduced with lactulose, a medication that traps the ammonia in the gut. The laxative effect of lactulose expels the ammonia from the colon. It is usually administered orally to prevent encephalopathy but can be given as an enema or via a nasogastric (NG) tube.

Antibiotics such as rifaximin (Zaxine) may also be given concomitantly in patients whose condition does not respond to lactulose alone. The use of rifaximin can reduce production of ammonia-producing bacteria to decrease overall ammonia burden to reduce recurrent hepatic encephalopathy. Regular and frequent bowel movements are necessary to minimize the ammonia buildup, so a regular bowel regimen should be reinforced.

Prevention of recurrent hepatic encephalopathy also involves treatment of precipitating causes (see Table 46.12). The most common precipitating factors include GI bleeding, infections, electrolyte disorders, acid–base imbalances, constipation, and lactulose nonadherence or under-dosing.

Medication Therapy. There is no specific medication therapy for cirrhosis. However, a number of medications are used to treat symptoms and complications of advanced liver disease (Table 46.15).

Nutritional Therapy. The diet for a patient with cirrhosis without complications is high in calories (3 000 kcal/day, target protein intake 1.2 g to 1.5 g/kg/day) with high carbohydrate content and moderate to low levels of fat (Tandon et al., 2018). Protein restriction may be appropriate in some patients immediately after a severe flare of symptoms (i.e., episodic hepatic encephalopathy). However, protein restriction is rarely justified in patients with cirrhosis and persistent hepatic encephalopathy. Indeed, malnutrition is a more serious clinical concern than hepatic encephalopathy for many of these patients. In fact, malnutrition has been seen to be a driver for index and recurrent episodes of hepatic encephalopathy.

Many patients with alcohol-related cirrhosis have malnutrition. Enteral formulas containing protein from branched-chain amino acids (e.g., beef, chicken, whey, soy, or tuna) that are metabolized by the muscles may be required. These formulas provide protein that is more easily metabolized by the liver. Parenteral nutrition or enteral tube feedings may be considered, particularly for patients who are being hospitalized and may be NPO for clinical procedures.

Patients with ascites and edema require a no-added-sodium diet (target sodium intake 2 g [88 mmol]/day). The degree of sodium restriction depends on the patient's condition. Education of the patient and caregiver(s) around identification of sodium-containing foods and reading food labels is important and helpful. Table salt is a common, well-known source of sodium; however, there are less obvious common sources, including baking soda and baking powder. Other foods high in sodium content include canned soups and vegetables, salted snacks (e.g., potato chips), nuts, smoked meats and fish, crackers, breads, olives, pickles, ketchup, and beer. Sodium is also present in many over-the-counter medications (e.g., antacids), although most antacids have lower sodium content now than they did in the past. Carbonated beverages tend to be high in sodium, but low-sodium and sodium-free carbonated drinks are also available. Suggestions about how to make the diet more palatable should be offered—for example, seasonings such as garlic, onion, lemon juice, and low-sodium herbs and spice rubs. Salt substitutes are discouraged as they often contain potassium chloride and could precipitate electrolyte imbalances. Collaboration with a registered dietitian about dietary strategies in cirrhosis management is encouraged.

NURSING MANAGEMENT
CIRRHOSIS

NURSING ASSESSMENT

Subjective and objective data that should be obtained from an individual with cirrhosis are presented in Table 46.16.

NURSING DIAGNOSES

Nursing diagnoses for the patient with advanced cirrhosis include but are not limited to the following:

- *Inadequate nutrition* resulting from *insufficient dietary intake* (anorexia, nausea, impaired protein synthesis, utilization and storage of nutrients)
- *Reduced tissue integrity* resulting from *moisture, pressure over bony prominence* (peripheral edema, ascites, cachexia, pruritus)
- *Excess fluid volume* resulting from *compensatory regulatory mechanisms* (portal hypertension and hyperaldosteronism)
- *Inadequate health maintenance* resulting from *ineffective coping strategies* (alcohol use)

Additional information on nursing diagnoses for the patient with cirrhosis is presented in NCP 46.2, available on the Evolve website.

PLANNING

The overall goals are that the patient with cirrhosis will (a) have relief of discomfort, (b) have minimal to no complications (ascites, varices, hepatic encephalopathy), and (c) maintain a lifestyle as close to their usual one as possible.

NURSING IMPLEMENTATION

HEALTH PROMOTION. The common causes of cirrhosis are alcohol, viral hepatitis, biliary obstruction, metabolic disease, and right-sided heart failure. Prevention and early treatment of cirrhosis must focus on eliminating the primary cause. Alcohol use disorder must be addressed through pharmacological and nonpharmacological interventions, as well as concurrent disorders. Patients should be urged to avoid alcohol ingestion, and concurrent strategies aimed at relapse prevention should be supported. Adequate nutrition, especially for persons at risk for cirrhosis, is essential to prevent muscle loss. Acute and chronic viral hepatitis must be identified and treated early so that it does not progress to cirrhosis or liver failure. Biliary disease should be treated to avoid biliary obstruction and infection. Right-sided heart failure should be targeted and optimized to prevent hepatic congestion.

ACUTE INTERVENTION. Nursing care for the patient with advanced cirrhosis focuses on conserving the patient's strength while maintaining muscle strength and tone (see NCP 46.2). Patients should be provided rest periods for recovery but be

TABLE 46.16 NURSING ASSESSMENT
Cirrhosis

Subjective Data
Important Health Information
Past health history: Previous viral, toxic, or idiopathic hepatitis; chronic biliary obstruction and infection; severe right-sided heart failure; chronic alcohol use disorder
Medications: Adverse reaction to any medication; use of anticoagulants, acetylsalicylic acid (Aspirin), nonsteroidal anti-inflammatory medications, acetaminophen (Tylenol)

Symptoms
- Weakness, fatigue, difficulty with concentration
- Change in sleep–wake pattern
- Anorexia, muscle loss
- Gum bleeding
- Yellow sclera or skin; pruritus; easy bruising
- Dull pain in right upper quadrant or epigastric region
- Erectile dysfunction; amenorrhea

Objective Data
General
Fever, cachexia, muscle wasting

Integumentary
Icteric sclera, jaundice, petechiae, ecchymoses, spider angiomas, palmar erythema, alopecia, clubbing, peripheral edema

Respiratory
Shallow, rapid respirations, epistaxis

Gastrointestinal
Abdominal distension, ascites, distended abdominal wall veins, palpable liver and spleen, foul-smelling breath; hematemesis; black, tarry stools; hemorrhoids, fetor hepaticus

Neurological
Confusion, asterixis

Reproductive
Gynecomastia and testicular atrophy (men), erectile dysfunction (men), loss of libido (men and women), amenorrhea or heavy menstrual bleeding (women)

Possible Findings
Anemia, thrombocytopenia; leukopenia; ↓ serum albumin level; abnormal liver function studies; ↑ INR and bilirubin levels; abnormal abdominal ultrasound or MRI results

INR, international normalized ratio; *MRI,* magnetic resonance imaging.

encouraged to engage in activities as tolerated. The nurse should modify the patient's activity and rest schedule according to signs of clinical improvement.

Anorexia, nausea and vomiting, pressure from ascites, and poor eating habits all interfere with maintaining adequate nutrition. Oral hygiene before meals may improve the patient's taste sensation. Between-meal snacks should be available at times when food is best tolerated, and small, frequent meals should be encouraged, as well as a night-time snack. Preferred foods should be offered whenever available, as it will encourage the patient to eat more and frequently. The nurse should explain to the patient and caregivers the reasons for any dietary restrictions, along with relevant education.

Nursing assessment and care should include the patient's physiological response to cirrhosis. If jaundice is present, the nurse should document where it is observed—sclera, skin, or hard palate. If the jaundice is accompanied by pruritus, cholestyramine, hydroxyzine, gabapentin, or rifampin may help. Other measures to help alleviate pruritus include baking soda baths, moisturizing bath oils and lotions, soft or old linens, and control of temperature (to avoid extremes of hot and cold). The patient's nails should be kept short and clean.

The colour of the urine and stools should be noted. When jaundice is present, the urine is often dark brown and foamy when shaken. The stool is grey or tan.

Edema and ascites require frequent nursing assessment and interventions. Accurate calculation and recording of intake and output, daily weight, and measurement of extremities and abdominal girth help in ongoing assessment of the location and extent of the edema.

The patient should be asked about dyspnea during rest and exertion and orthopnea to provide a sense of their tolerance to their current fluid status. Dyspnea is a frequent symptom for patients with ascites, which can often lead to pleural effusion. A semi-Fowler's or Fowler's position allows for maximal respiratory efficiency. Pillows can be used to support the arms and chest and may increase the patient's comfort and ability to breathe.

When paracentesis is required, the patient should void immediately before the procedure to prevent puncture of the bladder. After the procedure, the nurse should monitor vital signs for hypovolemia and check the dressing for bleeding and leakage from the puncture site.

Meticulous skin care is essential because edematous tissues are prone to breakdown. An alternating–air pressure mattress or other special mattress should be used, if possible. A turning schedule (minimum of every 2 hours) must be adhered to strictly. The patient's abdomen should be supported with pillows. If the abdomen is taut, cleansing must be done very gently. Patients with ascites tend to move very little because of the abdominal discomfort and dyspnea; range-of-motion, deep-breathing, and coughing exercises are helpful in preventing respiratory difficulties. The lower extremities may be elevated. If scrotal edema is present, a scrotal support provides some comfort.

When the patient is taking diuretics, the nurse needs to monitor serum levels of sodium, potassium, chloride, bicarbonate, and creatinine, especially with any changes in the diuretic dosage. The nurse should observe for signs of fluid and electrolyte imbalance. Hypokalemia may be manifested by cardiac dysrhythmias, hypotension, tachycardia, and generalized muscle weakness. Hyponatremia from water excess is manifested by muscle cramping, weakness, lethargy, and confusion.

Observations and nursing care in relation to hematological disorders (bleeding tendencies, anemia, increased susceptibility to infection) are the same as for patients with advanced liver disease (see NCP 46.2 on the Evolve website).

The nurse should also assess a patient's response to altered body image resulting from jaundice, spider angiomas, palmar erythema, ascites, and gynecomastia. The patient may experience anxiety and embarrassment regarding these changes. The nurse should explain these phenomena and be a supportive listener. Nursing care with concern and warmth can help the patient maintain self-esteem.

Bleeding Varices. If the patient has esophageal or gastric varices, the nurse should observe for signs of bleeding from the varices, such as hematemesis and melena. If hematemesis occurs, the nurse must call the health care provider and be ready to assist with treatment and procedures used to control the bleeding. The nurse should anticipate that the patient may be admitted to a critical care unit. The patient's airway must be maintained.

To stop the bleeding, the physician may perform sclerotherapy or ligation procedures. Balloon tamponade may be used in cases of refractory bleeding that is unresponsive to sclerotherapy or band ligation. When balloon tamponade is used, the initial nursing task is to explain to the patient and caregiver(s) the use of the tube and how it will be inserted. The balloons should be checked for patency. It is usually the physician's responsibility to insert the tube via the nose or the mouth (see Figure 46.9). Then the gastric balloon is inflated with approximately 250 mL of air, and the tube is retracted until resistance (gastroesophageal junction) is felt. The tube is secured by placing a piece of sponge or foam rubber at the nostrils (nasal cuff). For continued bleeding, the esophageal balloon is then inflated. A sphygmomanometer is used to measure and maintain the desired pressure at 20 to 40 mm Hg. The positions of the balloons are verified with radiography.

Nursing care includes monitoring for complications of rupture or erosion of the esophagus, regurgitation and aspiration of gastric contents, and occlusion of the airway by the balloon. If the gastric balloon breaks or is deflated, the esophageal balloon will slip upward, obstructing the airway and causing asphyxiation. If this happens, the nurse must cut the tube or deflate the esophageal balloon; thus scissors should be kept at the patient's bedside. Regurgitation is minimized by oral and pharyngeal suctioning and by keeping the patient in a semi-Fowler's position.

The patient is unable to swallow saliva because the esophagus is occluded by the inflated esophageal balloon. The patient should be encouraged to expectorate, and an emesis basin and tissues should be provided. Frequent oral and nasal care provides relief from the taste of blood and irritation from mouth breathing.

Hepatic Encephalopathy. The focus of nursing care of the patient with hepatic encephalopathy is on maintaining a safe environment, sustaining life, and assisting with measures to reduce episodes of drowsiness and disorientation. The nurse should assess (a) the patient's level of responsiveness (e.g., reflexes, pupillary reactions, orientation), (b) sensory and motor abnormalities (e.g., hyperreflexia, asterixis, motor coordination), (c) fluid and electrolyte imbalances, (d) acid–base imbalances, and (e) the effect of treatment measures.

Assessment of neurological status should be performed at least every 2 hours and should include an exact description of the patient's behaviour. The care of the patient with neurological conditions is based on the severity of the encephalopathy.

Targeting and treating precipitating factors can prevent recurrent episodes of hepatic encephalopathy. Constipation, which is a common precipitating factor for encephalopathy, should be prevented. Drugs, laxatives, and enemas for treating constipation should be given as ordered. Alertness and level of consciousness should be assessed when considering the optimal daily dosing of lactulose. Generally, lactulose dosing should be titrated to approximately two to three soft stools per day, and regular assessment in the number of bowel movements should be completed to avoid constipation or diarrhea, since excessive fluid and electrolyte losses could also precipitate hepatic encephalopathy. Education should be provided to the patient and caregivers regarding the importance of adhering to daily lactulose therapy. If lactulose needs to be titrated beyond two to three soft stools per day in order to prevent recurrent hepatic

TABLE 46.17   PATIENT & CAREGIVER TEACHING GUIDE

Cirrhosis in Ambulatory and Home Care Setting

The following guidelines should be included when teaching the patient and caregiver. The nurse should:

1. Explain the importance of continuous medical care with the goal of prolonging survival and avoiding disease complications.
2. Teach about the symptoms of complications (e.g., coffee-ground emesis, black tarry stools, confusion) and when to seek medical attention to enable prompt treatment of complications.
3. Teach about the importance of a low-sodium diet and how to make food more palatable by using herbs and spices.
4. Teach patient to avoid certain drugs:
   - ASA (Aspirin): increases risk of bleeding
   - NSAIDs: increase risk of bleeding, edema
   - ASA, NSAIDs, aminoglycoside: increase risk of renal impairment
   - ACE inhibitors: increase risk for decreased GFR
   - Sleeping pills, sedatives, and cough syrups that contain opioids may cause confusion
5. Encourage complete abstinence from alcohol because alcohol use can further injure the liver.
6. Teach patient to seek medical attention promptly for any type of infections to avoid complications.
7. Teach patient to avoid heavy lifting (e.g., Valsalva manoeuvre), which increases portal pressure and heightens risk of hemorrhage.
8. Encourage patient to receive hepatitis A and B vaccine, if the patient is not immune, to prevent risk for fulminant hepatitis when exposed to these viruses.
9. Ensure that patient undergoes ultrasound surveillance every 6 months for early detection of liver cancer.

ACE, angiotensin-converting enzyme; *ASA,* acetylsalicylic acid; *NSAIDs,* nonsteroidal anti-inflammatory drugs.

encephalopathy, rifaximin should be added as combination therapy for treatment of hepatic encephalopathy. GI bleeding and infections can cause recurrent encephalopathy and should be identified and communicated to the health care provider in a timely manner in order to facilitate appropriate medical intervention. Careful medication reconciliation can also help identify pharmacological precipitants for hepatic encephalopathy.

AMBULATORY AND HOME CARE. The patient with advanced cirrhosis may face a prolonged disease course and the possibility of serious, life-threatening conditions and complications. The patient and caregivers need to understand the importance of continuous health care and medical supervision and ways to reduce mortality risk (Table 46.17).

Patients with cirrhosis should receive vaccination for hepatitis A and B if they are not already immune. Infection with these viruses in patients with cirrhosis can lead to fulminant hepatitis. Patients should avoid using ASA, NSAIDs, and aminoglycosides, which can cause bleeding, edema, and renal complications. Patients should also avoid using sleeping pills or sedatives that contain codeine because they can lead to encephalopathy. Abstinence from alcohol is important to maintain and results in improvement in health for most patients. A low-sodium diet should be followed at home. Patients with cirrhosis have higher risks for infection and surgical complications; thus any infections must be promptly treated, and surgical procedures that necessitate general anaesthesia must first be discussed with the liver specialist. Patients with cirrhosis are at increased risk for HCC compared to that of the general population. The current recommendation is hepatoma surveillance with abdominal ultrasonography every 6 months. HCC, when small, can be treated with therapies aimed at curative intent.

Cirrhosis is a chronic condition. The patient is affected not only physically but also psychologically, socially, and economically. Major lifestyle changes may be required, especially if alcohol use is the primary cause. The nurse should provide information regarding community support programs and rapid access addiction medicine (RAAM) clinics for pharmacological and nonpharmacological help with alcohol use disorder. Other health teaching should include information about signs of liver decompensation, such as black stools and abdominal swelling, and advice on where to seek further medical attention. Counselling information regarding sexual concerns may be needed. The emphasis of home care for patients with cirrhosis should focus on helping patients maintain the highest level of wellness possible and initiate and maintain necessary lifestyle changes.

EVALUATION

Expected outcomes for patients with advanced cirrhosis are addressed in NCP 46.2, available on the Evolve website.

ACUTE LIVER FAILURE

Acute liver failure is a clinical condition characterized by rapid deterioration of liver function resulting in encephalopathy and coagulopathy in persons with no known history of liver disease. It is a broad term that encompasses *fulminant hepatic failure,* which describes development of encephalopathy within 8 weeks of the onset of the illness. In general, the disease runs its course over 8 weeks, but it can last as long as 26 weeks. Depending on the cause, survival rates range from 10 to 40% with intensive support.

The most common cause of acute liver failure is medications, usually acetaminophen, in combination with alcohol (Sood, 2019). People with alcohol use disorder are particularly susceptible to the detrimental effects of acetaminophen on the liver. Other medications that can cause acute liver failure include isoniazid, antibiotics, sulpha-containing medications, and anticonvulsants. Drugs can cause liver cell failure by disrupting essential intracellular processes or causing an accumulation of toxic metabolic products. Mushroom poisoning is also associated with fulminant liver failure. The majority of mushroom poisonings occur with *Amanita phalloides* (also known as "death cap").

Other causes of acute liver failure include viral hepatitis, especially HBV. Hepatic failure may occur rarely with HAV infection. Acute thrombosis of the hepatic veins (Budd Chiari syndrome) should also be considered.

Clinical Manifestations and Diagnostic Studies

Manifestations of acute liver failure include jaundice, coagulation abnormalities, and encephalopathy; changes in cognitive function are the first clinical sign. Patients with acute liver failure are susceptible to a wide variety of complications, including cerebral edema, renal failure, hypoglycemia, metabolic acidosis, sepsis, and multiorgan failure.

Acute liver failure is identified in most patients by abnormalities in laboratory values and clinical manifestations resulting from hepatic necrosis and fibrosis. Most often, serum bilirubin levels are elevated and the PT is prolonged. Liver enzyme levels (AST, ALT) are often markedly elevated. Additional laboratory tests include blood chemistry evaluation (especially glucose because hypoglycemia may be present and require correction); complete blood cell counts (CBCs); acetaminophen level; screening for other drugs and toxins; viral hepatitis serology (especially for HAV, HBV, and HEV); and measurements of serum ceruloplasmin (enzyme synthesized in liver) levels, α_1-antitrypsin levels, iron levels, immunoglobulins, and autoantibodies (ANA and anti-SMA). Plasma ammonia levels may also be measured.

Liver biopsy may be performed via the transjugular route because of coagulopathy, or when conditions such as autoimmune hepatitis, metastatic liver disease, or infiltrative liver disease (e.g., lymphoma) are suspected. In addition, ultrasonography with Doppler, CT, or magnetic resonance imaging (MRI) is helpful in providing information about the liver size and contour, presence of ascites, presence of tumours, and patency of the blood vessels.

NURSING AND INTERPROFESSIONAL MANAGEMENT ACUTE LIVER FAILURE

Since acute liver failure may progress rapidly, with hour-by-hour changes in consciousness, early transfer to the critical care unit is preferred once the diagnosis is made. Planning for transfer to a transplantation centre should begin for patients with grade 1 or 2 encephalopathy because the condition may worsen rapidly. Early transfer is important because the risks involved with patient transport may increase or even preclude transfer once grade 3 or 4 encephalopathy develops (see Table 46.13).

Liver transplantation is the treatment of choice for acute liver failure. Cerebral edema, cerebellar herniation, and brainstem compression are the most common causes of death, thus frequent monitoring of the patient's cognitive status is paramount. (Treatment of cerebral edema is described in Chapter 59.)

Renal failure is a frequent complication in patients with liver failure and may be caused by dehydration, hepatorenal syndrome, or acute tubular necrosis. The probability of renal failure may be even greater with acetaminophen overdose or other toxins, in which direct renal toxicity occurs. Although few patients die of renal failure alone, it often contributes to mortality risk and may worsen the prognosis.

The nurse should protect a patient's renal function by maintaining adequate fluid balance, avoiding use of nephrotoxic agents (e.g., aminoglycosides, NSAIDs), and promptly identifying and treating infection.

Monitoring and management of hemodynamic and renal function, as well as glucose, electrolytes, and acid–base status, are critical. The nurse needs to conduct frequent neurological evaluations for signs of increased intracranial pressure. The patient is positioned with the head elevated at 30 degrees. The nurse should avoid causing excessive patient stimulation. Manoeuvres that cause straining or Valsalva-like movements may increase intracranial pressure. The use of any sedatives should be avoided because of their effects on mental status, as well as the use of benzodiazepines because of the increased risk of encephalopathy.

The nurse needs to check the patient's mental status frequently if the level of consciousness declines. To minimize agitation, the patient's environment should be kept quiet. Additional measures include padding bedrails to avoid injury from possible seizures, observing the patient closely to avoid injuries, monitoring intake and output for renal function, and providing good skin and oral care to avoid skin breakdown and infection.

Alterations in level of consciousness may compromise nutritional intake. Factors such as coagulation disorders may influence whether enteral nutrition is initiated. An NG tube may irritate the nasal and esophageal mucosa and thus cause bleeding.

HEPATOCELLULAR CARCINOMA

Hepatocellular carcinoma (HCC), the primary liver cancer, is the fourth most common cause of cancer-related death in the world (Villanueva, 2019). The World Health Organization predicts that more than 1 million patients will die from liver cancer in 2030. HCC is rarely seen in patients without liver disease and is twice as common in men as in women (Villanueva, 2019).

Approximately 80 to 90% of people with HCC have cirrhosis of the liver. Cirrhosis is therefore a major risk factor regardless of the cause of cirrhosis. In North America, chronic HCV infection is the major underlying cause of HCC. Among those with chronic HBV infection, the risk for HCC is further increased if they are male, are older, have a family history of HCC, or are infected with HBV genotype C. NAFLD is also a well-established risk factor for HCC, although to a lesser extent than HBV and HCV infections (Marrero et al., 2018).

In primary liver cancer, lesions may be singular or numerous and nodular or diffusely spread over the entire liver. Some tumours infiltrate other organs, such as the gallbladder, or move to the peritoneum or the diaphragm. Primary liver cancer often metastasizes to the lung.

Metastatic cancer to the liver is more common than primary liver cancer. The liver is a common site of metastatic growth because of its high rate of blood flow and extensive capillary network. Cancer cells in other parts of the body are commonly carried to the liver via the portal circulation (Figure 46.12).

Clinical Manifestations and Diagnostic Studies

The manifestations of early liver cancer can be absent or subtle. Diagnosing small liver cancers in the presence of cirrhosis is sometimes a challenge when the liver is nodular and severely scarred. Clinical manifestations in progressive untreated liver cancer include weight loss, epigastric or right upper quadrant pain, anorexia, nausea and vomiting, weakness, and jaundice. Ascites, peripheral edema, encephalopathy, and variceal bleeding can occur in the setting of decompensated liver disease. A hemorrhagic tumour can cause blood clots to form, leading to pulmonary emboli as a complication.

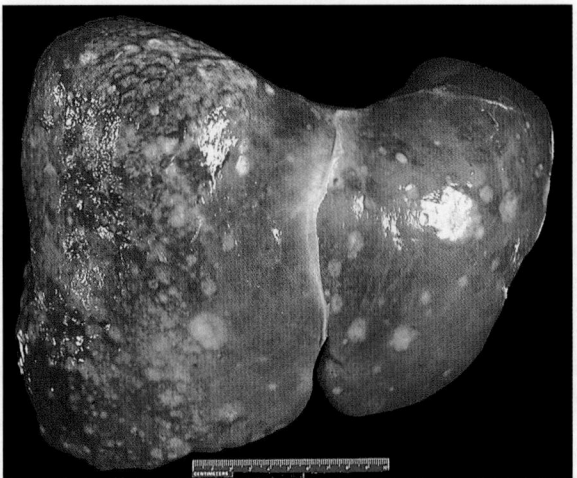

FIG. 46.12 Multiple hepatic metastases from a primary colon cancer. Source: Kumar, V., Abbas, A. K., & Fausto, N. (2005). *Robbins and Cotran pathologic basis of disease* (7th ed.). W. B. Saunders.

In Canada, ultrasound is generally used for HCC screening and identification of suspicious nodules. Diagnostic imaging for HCC includes contrast-enhanced ultrasound, quadriphasic CT, and MRI. An ultrasound-guided percutaneous biopsy may be performed when the results of diagnostic imaging studies are inconclusive or tissue is needed to guide treatment. Risks of biopsy include bleeding and potential tumour cell seeding along the needle tract. Serum α-fetoprotein (AFP) levels are elevated in approximately 60% of patients with HCC. The level of elevation may not correlate with clinical staging of HCC. (α-Fetoprotein is discussed in Chapter 18.)

NURSING AND INTERPROFESSIONAL MANAGEMENT LIVER CANCER

Treatment of liver cancer depends primarily on the stage of cancer: number, size, and location of tumours; involvement of any blood vessels; patient age and overall health; and extent of underlying liver disease. When diagnosed at its earliest stages, therapies with curative intent (surgical liver resection, radiofrequency ablation [RFA], liver transplantation) can be considered by the interprofessional health care team in collaboration with the patient and their family.

Surgical liver resection (partial hepatectomy) is performed when there is no evidence of invasion of hepatic blood vessels. Hepatectomy offers the best chance for cure of liver cancer. However, only about 15% of people have enough healthy liver tissue for this to be an option. Underlying cirrhosis and portal hypertension often compromise liver function and may cause liver failure after surgery.

RFA has become the most frequently used modality for treating tumours that are less than 2 cm in diameter, with preserved liver synthetic function. The overall survival rates are 98.2%, 86.2%, and 79.0% at 1, 3, and 5 years for those with HCC tumours less than 2 cm, versus 93.3%, 86.2%, and 79.0% for those with HCC tumours measuring 2 to 3 cm; however, the 5-year recurrence rates were as high as 75% (Doyle, 2019). In RFA, a thin needle is inserted into the core of the tumour. Electrical energy is then used to create heat in a specific location for a limited time. The end result is destruction of tumour cells. Complications are uncommon but can include infection, bleeding, dysrhythmias, and skin burn.

For those patients who have early-stage liver cancer and impaired liver function, liver transplantation offers a good prognosis.

For patients with multifocal HCC or intermediate-stage liver cancer, transarterial chemoembolization (TACE) or transarterial radioembolization (TARE) are minimally invasive procedures performed by interventional radiologists. A catheter is placed via the femoral artery or radial artery and advanced to the arterial blood supply of the tumours, and an embolic agent is administered, mixed with one or more chemotherapeutic agents. TACE works by shutting off the blood supply to the tumours and exposing liver tumour cells to the chemotherapy agent. TARE destroys the tumour(s) by slowly releasing radioactive material directly to the tumour. A postembolization syndrome of fever and abdominal pain related to liver ischemia occurs in up to 50% of patients receiving chemoembolization. It can take up to 3 months to determine the response to therapy.

In patients with advanced HCC (large inoperable tumours, elevated AFP unable to be down-staged for liver transplantation, metastatic disease with or without vascular invasion),

systemic therapy can be considered. Sorafenib (Nexavar), a targeted therapy, is an oral therapy that can block certain proteins (kinases) that play a role in tumour growth and cancer progression. It has many adverse effects, including rash on the hands and feet, diarrhea, and fatigue. Newer Health Canada–approved therapies include regorafenib, a small-molecule multikinase inhibitor, used as a second-line agent in patients with tumour progression on sorafenib, and nivolumab, an anti-PD-1 monoclonal antibody, also being used as a second-line agent. Treatment of multifocal HCC that is unresectable is an emerging field, with numerous clinical trials for other therapies currently in progress.

Nurses play a very important role in health promotion and health teaching for prevention of HCC. HBV vaccination for people at high risk for HBV infection can drastically reduce the occurrence of liver cancer. Early treatment for chronic hepatitis B and C viral infections before the establishment of cirrhosis also helps decrease risk for liver cancer. For patients at risk of developing HCC (e.g., those with cirrhosis), cancer surveillance with ultrasound every 6 months is the recommended clinical practice as small cancers are potentially curable (Villanueva, 2019).

The prognosis for patients with liver cancer depends on how early the tumour is detected; thus improved early screening and surveillance programs for those with chronic hepatitis and/or cirrhosis are paramount. Liver cancer, when untreated, often progresses rapidly, with patients having complications from the advancing cancer and declining liver function. Nursing interventions for patients with liver cancer focus on keeping patients as comfortable as possible. (See Chapter 18 for care of patients with cancer.)

LIVER TRANSPLANTATION

Canada's first liver transplantation was performed in Montreal in 1970. In 2018, 533 liver transplantations were performed in Canada (Canadian Institute for Health Information [CIHI], 2019).

Liver transplantation has become an acceptable therapeutic option for many people with end-stage liver disease or localized and recurrent HCC. It improves overall health and quality of life. Liver transplantation is contraindicated in patients with widespread malignant disease. Among index liver transplant recipients from deceased donors, 5-year survival rates were 87.7% (CIHI, 2019).

Liver transplant candidates undergo a rigorous pretransplantation assessment to confirm the diagnosis of end-stage liver disease and to assess for other comorbid conditions (e.g., cardiovascular disease, lung disease, chronic kidney disease) that may affect the patient's surgical outcome. The evaluation includes physical examination, laboratory tests (CBC, liver function tests), cardiac and pulmonary evaluations, endoscopy, CT scan, and psychological testing. Contraindications for liver transplantation include severe extrahepatic disease, advanced HCC beyond inclusion criteria, recent history of other malignancy, ongoing drug or alcohol use, and inability to comprehend or adhere to the rigorous post-transplantation course.

Liver transplantation is performed using either a deceased- (cadaveric) or living-donor liver. (See Chapter 49 for a general discussion of organ transplants.) For living-donor liver transplantation, a living person donates a portion of their liver to the intended recipient. However, live liver donation poses potential risks to the donor, including biliary disorders, hepatic artery thrombosis, wound infection, postoperative ileus, and pneumothorax.

Postoperative complications of liver transplantation include bleeding, infection, and rejection. Immunosuppressive therapy generally involves a combination of corticosteroids, a calcineurin inhibitor (e.g., cyclosporine, tacrolimus), and an antiproliferative agent (e.g., azathioprine). The mechanism of action and adverse effects of cyclosporine are discussed in Chapter 16 and Table 16.16. Other immunosuppressants used include mycophenolate mofetil (CellCept), azathioprine (Imuran), corticosteroids, and sirolimus (Rapamune) (see Chapter 16, Table 16.16). The interleukin-2 receptor antagonist basiliximab (Simulect) and polyclonal antilymphocyte antibodies, such as thymoglobulin, may be administered to patients at high risk for complications.

About 80% of patients live more than 5 years after liver transplant. Long-term survival depends on the cause of liver failure (e.g., localized HCC, chronic hepatitis B or C, biliary disease). Patients with liver disease from hepatitis B or C often have reinfection of the transplanted liver. For patients with hepatitis B, treatment after surgery with IV HBIG and a nucleoside or nucleotide analogue used to treat HBV infection (e.g., lamivudine, entecavir, or tenofovir) has reduced rates of reinfection of the transplanted liver. For patients with HCV, treatment with the new DAAs that can cure HCV infection has provided the opportunity to use HCV-positive liver grafts. The need for liver transplantation may decrease in the HCV population. Research is ongoing to decide if DAAs should be started before or after transplant.

The patient who has undergone liver transplantation requires highly skilled nursing care, either in the critical care unit or other specialized unit. Postoperative nursing care includes assessing neurological status; monitoring for signs of hemorrhage; preventing pulmonary complications; measuring electrolyte levels and urine output; and monitoring for manifestations of infection and rejection. Common respiratory conditions are pneumonia, atelectasis, and pleural effusions. To prevent these complications, the nurse needs to encourage the patient to cough, deep breathe, use incentive spirometry, and frequently reposition. The nurse should measure the drainage from the Jackson-Pratt drain, NG tube, and T tube and note the colour and consistency of the drainage at regular intervals.

Monitoring for infection is a critical aspect of nursing care after liver transplantation because infection is the most common cause of mortality and morbidity. Infections can be viral, fungal, or bacterial. Fever may be the only sign of infection. Nutrition, physiotherapy, and patient education focused on medication regimens, signs and symptoms of infection, and lifestyle practices are all key to lifelong success in transplant recipients. Emotional support for the patient and family is also essential for successful transplantation outcomes.

AGE-RELATED CONSIDERATIONS

LIVER DISEASE IN OLDER PERSONS
The incidence of liver disease increases with age. With aging, the liver size decreases, medication metabolism slows, and hepatobiliary function is altered. The liver has a decreased capacity to respond to injury and has less regenerative ability (Kamimura et al., 2019). As well, transplanted livers take longer to regenerate in older persons than in younger adults.

Older patients are particularly vulnerable to medication-induced liver injury. This vulnerability is due to several factors, including decline in body weight and increased use of prescription and over-the-counter medications, which can lead to medication interactions and potential medication toxicity. Age-related decreases in liver function caused by decreased liver blood flow and enzyme activity result in decreased medication metabolism and a decreased ability to recover from drug-induced liver injury.

A growing number of older people have chronic hepatitis C infection and resulting cirrhosis. The presence of HCV infection and elevated liver enzyme levels are often found during a routine health assessment. Because older persons have more comorbid conditions, liver transplantation may not be possible if liver decompensation has occurred.

Lifetime health behaviours may also influence the development of chronic liver disease in the older person. Chronic alcohol use and metabolic disease can contribute to cirrhosis, NASH, and liver failure. Older people with comorbid cardiovascular and pulmonary diseases are less able to tolerate variceal bleeding. In older persons with liver disease, hepatic encephalopathy may be misdiagnosed as dementia and overlooked as a treatable differential.

DISORDERS OF THE PANCREAS

ACUTE PANCREATITIS

Acute pancreatitis is an acute inflammation of the pancreas. Spillage of pancreatic enzymes into surrounding pancreatic tissue causes autodigestion and severe pain. The degree of inflammation varies from mild edema to severe hemorrhagic necrosis. Acute pancreatitis is most common in middle-aged men and women.

Etiology and Pathophysiology
Many factors can cause injury to the pancreas. In Canada, the most common cause is gallbladder disease (gallstones), followed by alcohol use disorder. Acute pancreatitis attacks are also associated with hypertriglyceridemia (serum triglyceride level >11 mmol/L). Less common causes include trauma (postsurgical, abdominal), viral infections, penetrating duodenal ulcer, cysts, abscesses, cystic fibrosis, medications, metabolic disorders (hyperparathyroidism, renal failure), and vascular disease. Pancreatitis may occur after surgical procedures on the pancreas, stomach, duodenum, or biliary tract. Pancreatitis can also develop following endoscopic retrograde cholangiopancreatography (ERCP). In some cases, the cause is unknown (idiopathic).

The most common pathogenic mechanism is autodigestion of the pancreas (Figure 46.13). Injury to pancreatic cells or activation of the pancreatic enzymes is caused in the pancreas rather than in the intestine. The activation of pancreatic enzymes may be due to reflux of bile acids into the pancreatic ducts through an open or distended sphincter of Oddi. This reflux may result from blockage created by gallstones. Obstruction of a pancreatic duct results in pancreatic ischemia.

Trypsinogen is an inactive proteolytic enzyme produced by the pancreas. It is released into the small intestine via the pancreatic duct. In the intestine, it is activated to trypsin by enterokinase. Normally, trypsin inhibitors in the pancreas and

PATHOPHYSIOLOGY MAP

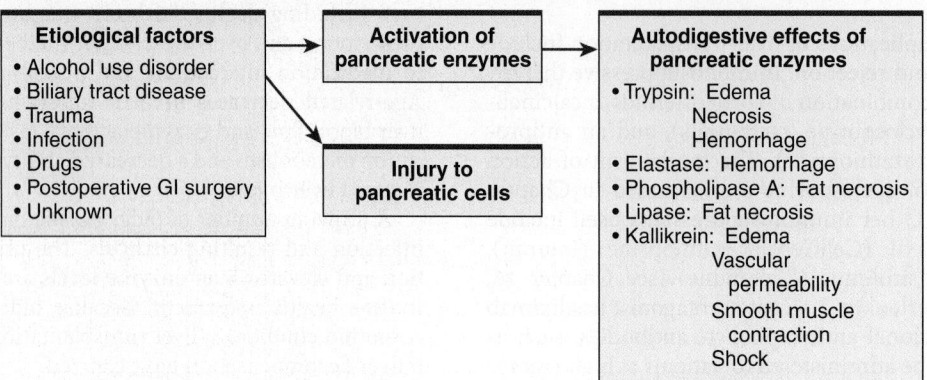

FIG. 46.13 Pathogenic process of acute pancreatitis. *GI*, gastrointestinal.

the plasma bind and inactivate any trypsin that is inadvertently produced. In pancreatitis, activated trypsin is present in the pancreas and can digest the pancreas and produce bleeding.

It is not entirely clear how chronic alcohol use causes acute pancreatitis. It is thought that alcohol increases the production of digestive enzymes in the pancreas. However, because only 5 to 10% of people with alcohol use disorder develop pancreatitis, it is believed that other factors such as environment (high-fat diet, smoking) and genetics also contribute to the cause.

The pathophysiological involvement of acute pancreatitis ranges from mild (*edematous* or *interstitial pancreatitis*) to severe (*necrotizing pancreatitis;* Figure 46.14). In mild pancreatitis, the functions of the gland return to normal upon recovery. In severe pancreatitis, approximately half of patients have a permanent decrease in endocrine and exocrine function. Such patients are also at risk of developing pancreatic necrosis, organ failure, septic complications, or a combination of these, all of which are associated with higher mortality rates (Hines & Pandol, 2019).

Clinical Manifestations

Abdominal pain is the main symptom of acute pancreatitis. The pain is caused by distension of the pancreas, peritoneal irritation, and obstruction of the biliary tract.

The pain is usually located in the left upper quadrant, but it may be in the midepigastrium. It commonly radiates to the back because of the retroperitoneal location of the pancreas. The pain has a sudden onset and is described as severe, deep, piercing, and continuous or steady. It is aggravated by eating and frequently occurs when the patient is recumbent. It is not relieved by vomiting. The pain may be accompanied by flushing, cyanosis, and dyspnea. The patient may assume various positions involving flexion of the spine in an attempt to relieve the severe pain.

Other manifestations of acute pancreatitis include nausea and vomiting, low-grade fever, leukocytosis, hypotension, tachycardia, and jaundice. Abdominal tenderness with muscle guarding is common. Bowel sounds may be decreased or absent. Paralytic ileus may occur and causes marked abdominal distension. The lungs are frequently involved, with crackles present. Intravascular damage from circulating trypsin may cause areas of cyanosis or greenish to yellow-brown discoloration of the abdominal wall. Other areas of ecchymoses are the flanks (*Grey Turner's spots* or *sign,* a bluish flank discoloration) and the periumbilical

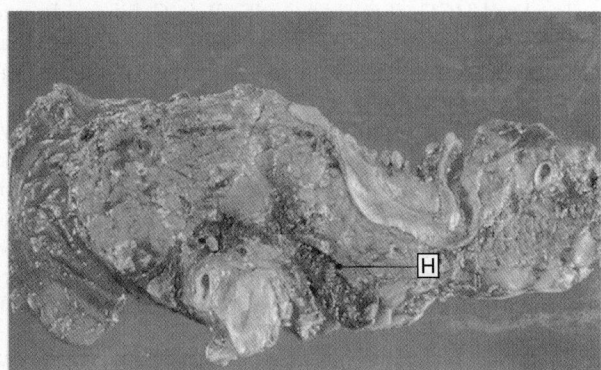

FIG. 46.14 In acute pancreatitis, the pancreas appears edematous and is commonly hemorrhagic (*H*). Source: Stevens, A., & Lowe, J. (2000). *Pathology: Illustrated review in colour* (2nd ed.). Mosby.

area (*Cullen's sign,* a bluish periumbilical discoloration). These ecchymoses may occur in severe cases as a result of seepage of blood-stained exudate from the pancreas.

Shock is possible as a result of hemorrhage into the pancreas, toxemia from the activated pancreatic enzymes, or hypovolemia due to massive fluid shifts into the retroperitoneal space.

Complications

The severity of the disease varies according to the extent of pancreatic destruction. Some patients recover completely, some have recurring attacks, and some develop chronic pancreatitis. Acute pancreatitis can be life-threatening.

Two significant local complications of acute pancreatitis are pseudocyst and abscess. A pancreatic **pseudocyst** is an accumulation of fluid, pancreatic enzymes, tissue debris, and inflammatory exudates surround by a wall next to the pancreas. Clinical manifestations of pseudocyst are abdominal pain, palpable epigastric mass, nausea, vomiting, and anorexia. The serum amylase level frequently remains elevated. These cysts usually resolve spontaneously within a few weeks, but they may perforate, causing peritonitis, or they may rupture into the stomach or duodenum. Treatment consists of an internal drainage procedure with an anastomosis between the pancreatic duct and the jejunum.

When a pseudocyst gets infected, a *pancreatic abscess* results from extensive necrosis in the pancreas. It may rupture or perforate into adjacent organs. Manifestations of an abscess include upper abdominal pain, abdominal mass, high fever, and leukocytosis. Pancreatic abscesses need prompt surgical drainage to prevent sepsis.

The main systemic complications of acute pancreatitis are cardiovascular and pulmonary (hypotension, tachycardia, pleural effusion, atelectasis, and pneumonia, acute respiratory distress syndrome). The pulmonary complications are likely caused by the passage of exudate containing pancreatic enzymes from the peritoneal cavity through transdiaphragmatic lymph channels. Enzyme-induced inflammation of the diaphragm reduces diaphragm movement, which leads to atelectasis. Trypsin can activate prothrombin and plasminogen, increasing the patient's risk for intravascular thrombi, pulmonary emboli, and disseminated intravascular coagulation. Hypocalcemia is a sign of severe disease, caused in part by the combining of calcium and fatty acids during fat necrosis. The exact mechanisms of how or why hypocalcemia occurs are not well understood.

Diagnostic Studies

The primary diagnostic tests for acute pancreatitis are serum amylase and lipase. The serum amylase level is usually elevated early and remains so for 24 to 72 hours. The serum lipase level is elevated in acute pancreatitis and is an important test because other disorders (e.g. mumps, renal transplantation, and cerebral trauma) may increase serum amylase levels. Other abnormal findings include an increase in liver enzymes, triglycerides, glucose, and bilirubin and a decrease in calcium.

Diagnostic evaluation of acute pancreatitis is directed at determining the cause. An abdominal ultrasound, radiograph, or CT scan can be used to identify pancreatic conditions. Contrast-enhanced CT and magnetic resonance cholangiopancreatography (MRCP) are used for detecting pancreatitis-related complications such as pseudocysts and abscesses. MRCP often replaces the use of ERCP, which itself can cause acute pancreatitis.

Interprofessional Care

Objectives of interprofessional care for acute pancreatitis include (a) relief of pain; (b) prevention or alleviation of shock; (c) reduction of pancreatic secretions; (d) control of fluid and electrolyte imbalance; (e) prevention or treatment of infections; and (f) removal of the precipitating cause, if possible (Table 46.18).

Conservative Therapy. Treatment is primarily focused on supportive care, including aggressive hydration, pain management, management of metabolic complications, and minimization of pancreatic stimulation. Relief and control of pain are very important. IV opioid analgesics may be administered. Pain medications may be combined with an antispasmodic agent. However, atropine-like medications should be avoided when paralytic ileus is present because they may decrease GI motility and further contribute to the problem. Other medications that relax smooth muscles (spasmolytics), such as nitroglycerin or papaverine, may be used.

If shock is present, plasma or plasma volume expanders such as dextran or albumin may be given. Fluid and electrolyte imbalances are corrected with lactated Ringer's solution or other crystalloids. Central venous pressure readings can help with determining fluid status and fluid replacement requirements. Vasoactive drugs may be needed to increase systemic vascular resistance in patients with septic shock.

Pancreatic enzyme secretion must be reduced or suppressed in order to decrease stimulation of the pancreas and allow it

TABLE 46.18 **INTERPROFESSIONAL CARE**	
Acute Pancreatitis	
Diagnostic	**Interprofessional Therapy**
• History and physical examination • Abdominal ultrasound • Blood glucose • Chest radiograph • Contrast-enhanced CT • Endoscopic ultrasound • ERCP • Flat-plate radiograph of the abdomen • MRCP • Serum amylase • Serum calcium • Serum lipase • Triglycerides	• Albumin (if shock is present) • Antibiotics (if necrotizing pancreatitis is present) • IV calcium gluconate, 10% (if tetany is present) • Lactated Ringer's solution • NPO with NG tube to suction • Pain medication (e.g., morphine) • Proton pump inhibitors (e.g., omeprazole [Losec])

CT, computed tomography; *ERCP*, endoscopic retrograde cholangiopancreatography; *IV*, intravenous; *MRCP*, magnetic resonance cholangiopancreatography; *NG*, nasogastric; *NPO*, nothing by mouth.

to rest. Suppression of pancreatic secretion is accomplished by keeping the patient on nothing-by-mouth (NPO) status and by using NG suction to reduce vomiting and gastric distension and to prevent gastric acidic contents from entering the duodenum. Certain medications may also be administered for this purpose (Table 46.19). With resolution of the pancreatitis, the patient resumes oral intake. For the patient with severe acute pancreatitis who does not resume oral intake, enteral nutrition support may be initiated.

The inflamed and necrotic pancreatic tissue is a good medium for bacterial growth. In patients with acute necrotizing pancreatitis, infection is the leading cause of morbidity and mortality. Therefore, it is important to prevent infections. Patient should be monitored closely so that antibiotic therapy can be started early if necrosis and infection occur.

Interventional Therapy. When the acute pancreatitis is related to gallstones, urgent ERCP and endoscopic sphincterotomy (severing of the muscle layers of the sphincter of Oddi) may be performed. Laparoscopic cholecystectomy may follow ERCP to reduce the potential for recurrence. Surgical intervention may also be indicated when the diagnosis is uncertain and for patients whose condition does not respond to conservative therapy. Patients with severe acute pancreatitis may require drainage of necrotic fluid collections. Drainage can be accomplished either surgically under CT guidance or endoscopically. A pseudocyst can be drained percutaneously, and a drainage tube is left in place.

Medication Therapy. Several different medications are used to treat symptoms associated with pancreatitis (see Table 46.19). Currently, there are no medications that cure pancreatitis.

Nutritional Therapy. Initially, patients with acute pancreatitis are kept on NPO status to reduce pancreatic secretion. In cases of moderate to severe pancreatitis, the patient may require enteral feeding via a jejunal feeding tube. When food is allowed, small, frequent feedings are given. The diet is usually high in carbohydrate content because that is the least stimulating to the exocrine portion of the pancreas. Intolerance to oral foods should be suspected if a patient reports pain, has increasing abdominal girth, or has elevated amylase and lipase levels. The patient needs to abstain from using alcohol. Supplemental fat-soluble vitamins may be administered (see Chapter 42).

TABLE 46.19   MEDICATION THERAPY
Acute and Chronic Pancreatitis

Medication	Mechanism of Action or Rationale
Acute Pancreatitis	
Antacids	Neutralization of gastric HCl secretion and subsequent decrease in secretin, which stimulates production and secretion of pancreatic secretions
Antispasmodics (e.g., dicyclomine [Bentylol])*	Decrease of vagal stimulation, motility, and pancreatic outflow (through inhibition of volume and concentration of bicarbonate and enzymatic secretion)
Carbonic anhydrase inhibitor (acetazolamide)	Reduction in volume and bicarbonate concentration of pancreatic secretion
Morphine, meperidine (Demerol)	Relief of pain
Nitroglycerin or papaverine	Relaxation of smooth muscles and relief of pain
Proton pump inhibitors (omeprazole [Losec])	Decrease in HCl secretion (HCl stimulates pancreatic activity)
Chronic Pancreatitis	
Insulin	Treatment for diabetes mellitus, if it occurs, or for hyperglycemia
Pancreatin, pancrelipase	Replacement therapy for pancreatic enzymes

HCl, hydrochloric acid.
*Contraindicated in patients with paralytic ileus.

NURSING MANAGEMENT
ACUTE PANCREATITIS

NURSING ASSESSMENT
Subjective and objective data that should be obtained from a person with acute pancreatitis are presented in Table 46.20.

NURSING DIAGNOSES
Nursing diagnoses for patients with acute pancreatitis may include but are not limited to the following:
- *Acute pain* resulting from *physiological injury* (distention of pancreas, peritoneal irritation, obstruction of biliary tract)
- *Reduced fluid volume* resulting from *insufficient fluid intake and septic shock* (vomiting, restricted oral intake, fluid shift into the retroperitoneal space)
- *Inadequate nutrition* resulting from *insufficient dietary intake* (anorexia, dietary restrictions, nausea)
- *Potential for inadequate health management* resulting from *insufficient knowledge of therapeutic regime*
- *Disrupted electrolyte balance* resulting from *physiological injury and fluid status*

Additional information on nursing diagnoses for the patient with pancreatitis is presented in NCP 46.3, available on the Evolve website for this chapter.

PLANNING
The overall goals are that patients with acute pancreatitis will have (a) relief of pain, (b) normal fluid and electrolyte balance, (c) minimal to no complications, and (d) no recurrent attacks.

NURSING IMPLEMENTATION
HEALTH PROMOTION. Health promotion is focused on the assessment of the predisposing and etiological factors of pancreatitis and on encouragement of early intervention to prevent

TABLE 46.20   NURSING ASSESSMENT
Acute Pancreatitis

Subjective Data
Important Health Information
Past health history: Biliary tract disease, alcohol use, abdominal trauma, duodenal ulcers, infection, metabolic disorders
Medications: Thiazides, anti-inflammatory medications
Surgery or other treatments: Surgical procedures on the pancreas, stomach, duodenum, or biliary tract; ERCP

Symptoms
- Dyspnea
- Nausea, vomiting, or both; anorexia
- Severe abdominal pain that may radiate to the back and is aggravated by food, alcohol, or both
- Weakness or lassitude

Objective Data
General
Restlessness, anxiety, low-grade fever

Integumentary
Flushing, diaphoresis, discoloration of abdomen and flanks, cyanosis, jaundice; decreased skin turgor; dry mucous membranes

Respiratory
Tachypnea, basilar crackles

Cardiovascular
Tachycardia, hypotension

Gastrointestinal
Abdominal distension, tenderness, and muscle guarding; diminished bowel sounds

Possible Findings
↑ Serum amylase and lipase levels, leukocytosis, hyperglycemia, dyslipidemia, hypocalcemia, abnormal findings on ultrasound and CT scan of pancreas, abnormal findings on ERCP or MRCP

CT, computed tomographic; ERCP, endoscopic retrograde cholangiopancreatography; MRCP, magnetic resonance cholangiopancreatography.

occurrence of acute pancreatitis. The patient should be advised to eliminate alcohol intake, especially if there have been any previous episodes of pancreatitis. Attacks of pancreatitis become milder or disappear when alcohol use is discontinued.

ACUTE INTERVENTION. During the acute phase, it is important to monitor vital signs. Hemodynamic stability may be compromised by hypotension, fever, and tachypnea. A vital part of the nursing care plan for patients with acute pancreatitis is monitoring for signs of shock, electrolyte imbalances, and response to IV fluids. Frequent vomiting, along with gastric suction, may cause electrolyte levels to decrease. Respiratory failure may develop in patients with severe acute pancreatitis. It is important to assess respiratory function (e.g., lung sounds, oxygen saturation levels). If acute respiratory distress syndrome develops, the patient may require intubation and mechanical ventilatory support. Because hypocalcemia can also occur, the nurse must observe for symptoms of tetany, such as jerking, irritability, and muscular twitching. Numbness or tingling around the lips and in the fingers is an early indicator of hypocalcemia. The patient should be assessed for a positive Chvostek's or Trousseau's sign (see Chapter 19). Calcium gluconate (as prescribed) should be given to treat symptomatic hypocalcemia. In addition, hypomagnesemia may develop, necessitating the observation of serum magnesium levels.

Because abdominal pain is a primary symptom of pancreatitis, a major focus of nursing care is pain relief (see NCP 46.3). Pain and restlessness can increase the metabolic rate and contribute to hemodynamic instability. Opioids may be used for pain relief. The nurse should assess and document the duration of pain relief. Comfortable positioning, frequent changes in position, and relief of nausea and vomiting can help reduce the restlessness that usually accompanies the pain. Assuming positions that flex the trunk and draw the knees up to the abdomen may decrease pain. A side-lying position with the head elevated 45 degrees decreases tension on the abdomen and may help ease the pain.

Nursing measures for the patient who is kept NPO or has an NG tube should include frequent oral and nasal care to relieve the dryness of the mouth and nose. Oral care is essential to prevent parotitis. If the patient is taking anticholinergics to decrease GI secretions, oral mucosa will be extremely dry. If patients are taking antacids to neutralize gastric acid secretions, they should be sipped slowly or administered through the NG tube.

The patient with acute pancreatitis is susceptible to infections. The nurse should monitor for fever and other manifestations of infection. Respiratory infections are common because the retroperitoneal fluid raises the diaphragm, which causes the patient to take shallow, guarded abdominal breaths. Measures to prevent respiratory tract infections include frequent turning, coughing, deep breathing, and assuming a semi-Fowler's position. Other important assessments are for signs of paralytic ileus, renal failure, and mental changes. The blood glucose level should be monitored to assess damage to the β cells of the islets of Langerhans in the pancreas.

After pancreatic surgery, the patient may require special wound care for an anastomotic leak or a fistula. To prevent skin irritation, measures such as skin barriers (Stomahesive or Karaya paste), pouching, and drains should be used. In addition to protecting the skin, pouching also provides a more accurate determination of fluid and electrolyte losses and increases patient comfort.

AMBULATORY AND HOME CARE. After acute pancreatitis, most patients may need home care follow-up. Physiotherapy may be needed if the patient has lost physical reserve and muscle strength. Patient counselling should include that directed toward alcohol abstinence and cigarette smoking cessation. Counselling regarding abstinence from alcohol can prevent future attacks of acute pancreatitis and development of chronic pancreatitis. Because nicotine can stimulate the pancreatic enzyme secretions, smoking should be avoided. Counselling recommendations and strategies for smoking cessation, including resources, can be referenced from the *Integrating Smoking Cessation Into Daily Nursing Practice* best practice guideline by the Registered Nurses' Association of Ontario (RNAO), listed in the Resources at the end of this chapter.

Dietary teaching should include restriction of fats because they stimulate the secretion of cholecystokinin, which then stimulates the pancreas. Carbohydrates are less stimulating to the pancreas. The patient should be advised to avoid crash-and-binge dieting because these diets can precipitate attacks. The patient and the caregivers should be taught the symptoms of infection, diabetes, and steatorrhea (foul-smelling, fatty stools). These changes indicate possible ongoing destruction of pancreatic tissue and pancreatic insufficiency. The patient may require exogenous enzyme supplementation.

EVALUATION

Expected outcomes for patients with acute pancreatitis are presented in NCP 46.3, available on the Evolve website.

CHRONIC PANCREATITIS

Chronic pancreatitis is a continuous, prolonged inflammatory and fibrosing process of the pancreas. The pancreas is progressively destroyed as it is replaced with fibrotic tissues. Strictures and calcifications may also occur in the pancreas.

Etiology and Pathophysiology

In Western countries, 70% of cases of chronic pancreatitis are associated with alcohol use disorder. However, not all people who overuse alcohol develop chronic pancreatitis, which suggests that affected people have cofactors that predispose them to the direct toxic effect of the alcohol on the pancreas. In some patients, an identifiable cause may not be found (*idiopathic pancreatitis*). Chronic pancreatitis may follow acute pancreatitis, but it may also occur in the absence of any history of acute episodes.

Chronic pancreatitis can be classified as obstructive and nonobstructive. In *nonobstructive* pancreatitis, there is inflammation and sclerosis, mainly in the head of the pancreas and around the pancreatic duct. The ducts are obstructed with protein precipitates. These precipitates block the pancreatic duct and eventually calcify. This process is followed by fibrosis and glandular atrophy. Pseudocysts and abscesses commonly develop. Alcohol use disorder is the most common cause of nonobstructive calcifying pancreatitis.

Obstructive pancreatitis is associated with biliary disease. The most common cause is inflammation of the sphincter of Oddi associated with cholelithiasis. Cancer of the ampulla of Vater, the duodenum, or the pancreas can also cause this type of chronic pancreatitis.

Clinical Manifestations

As with acute pancreatitis, a major manifestation of chronic pancreatitis is abdominal pain. The patient may have episodes of acute pain, but it usually is chronic (recurrent attacks at intervals of months or years). The attacks may become more and more frequent until they are almost constant, or they may diminish as pancreatic fibrosis develops. The pain is located in the same areas as in acute pancreatitis but is usually described as a heavy, gnawing feeling or sometimes as burning and cramplike. The pain is not relieved by food or antacids.

Other clinical manifestations are symptoms of pancreatic insufficiency, including malabsorption with weight loss, constipation, mild jaundice with dark urine, steatorrhea, and diabetes. The steatorrhea may become severe, with voluminous, foul-smelling, fatty stools. Urine and stool may be frothy. Some abdominal tenderness may be present. Chronic pancreatitis is also associated with a variety of complications, including pseudocyst formation, bile duct or duodenal obstruction, diabetes, pancreatic ascites or pleural effusion, splenic vein thrombosis, pseudoaneurysms, and pancreatic cancer.

Diagnostic Studies

The diagnosis is based on the patient's signs and symptoms, laboratory studies, and imaging. In chronic pancreatitis, the levels of serum amylase and lipase may be elevated slightly or not at all, depending on the degree of pancreatic fibrosis. Serum bilirubin and ALP levels may be increased. There is usually mild leukocytosis and a high sedimentation rate.

ERCP can be used to visualize the pancreatic and common bile ducts. Imaging studies, such as CT, MRI, MRCP, abdominal ultrasound, and EUS, can show a variety of changes, including calcifications, ductal dilation, pseudocysts, and enlargement of the pancreas.

Stool samples are examined for fecal fat content. Deficiencies of fat-soluble vitamins and cobalamin, glucose intolerance, and possibly diabetes may also be found in patients with chronic pancreatitis. The secretin stimulation test can be used to help assess pancreatic function, although it is not widely used.

Interprofessional Care

When a patient with chronic pancreatitis experiences an acute attack, the therapy is identical to that for acute pancreatitis. At other times, the focus is on prevention of further attacks, relief of pain, and control of pancreatic exocrine and endocrine insufficiency. Sometimes, doses of analgesics must be large and frequent to relieve the pain.

Diet, pancreatic enzyme replacement, and control of diabetes are measures used to control the pancreatic insufficiency. Small, bland, frequent meals that are low in fat content are recommended to decrease pancreatic stimulation. The patient is strongly encouraged to eliminate alcohol from the diet. If the patient is dependent on alcohol, the patient should be referred to other resources as needed. Smoking should be stopped as it is associated with accelerated progression of chronic pancreatitis.

Pancreatic enzyme products (e.g., pancreatin and pancrelipase) containing amylase, lipase, and trypsin are administered to replace the deficient pancreatic enzymes. They are usually enteric coated to prevent their breakdown or inactivation by gastric hydrochloric acid. Bile salts are sometimes administered to facilitate the absorption of the fat-soluble vitamins (A, D, E, and K) and to prevent further fat loss. If diabetes develops, it is controlled with insulin or oral hypoglycemic agents. Acid-neutralizing (e.g., antacids) and acid-inhibiting drugs (e.g., proton pump inhibitors) may be administered to decrease hydrochloric acid levels, but they have little overall effect on the outcome of the disease.

When biliary disease is present or if obstruction or pseudocyst develops, surgery may be indicated. Surgical procedures can divert bile flow or relieve ductal obstruction. A choledochojejunostomy diverts bile around the ampulla of Vater, where spasm or hypertrophy of the sphincter may be present. In this procedure, the common bile duct is anastomosed into the jejunum. Another type of surgical diverting procedure is the Roux-en-Y pancreatojejunostomy, in which the pancreatic duct is opened and an anastomosis is made with the jejunum. Pancreatic drainage procedures relieve ductal obstruction. Pancreatic drainage procedures can relieve ductal obstruction and are often done with ERCP. Some patients may have an ERCP with sphincterotomy and/or stent placement at the site of obstruction. These patients require follow-up ERCP to either exchange or remove the stent.

NURSING MANAGEMENT
CHRONIC PANCREATITIS

Clinical management during acute or chronic pancreatitis is primarily focused on clinical stabilization. The focus of nursing management in chronic pancreatitis is on chronic care and health promotion. Patients must be instructed to take measures to prevent recurrent acute episodes. Dietary control, along with adherence to pancreatic enzyme treatment regimens, is essential. The pancreatic enzymes are taken with meals or snacks. Patients' stools should be examined for steatorrhea to help determine the effectiveness of the enzyme treatment. Patients and caregivers must be given clear instructions on stool assessment.

If diabetes mellitus has developed, patients need instruction in testing of blood glucose levels and medications (see Chapter 52). Patients who are taking anti-secretory agents must take them as ordered to control gastric acidity.

Alcohol consumption should be avoided. Patients who have developed a dependence on alcohol may need referral to other agencies or resources to help with alcohol cessation and relapse prevention (see Chapter 11).

PANCREATIC CANCER

Pancreatic cancer has a high mortality rate. In Canada, it was estimated that in 2019, 6 000 Canadians were diagnosed with pancreatic cancer and 5 300 died from this disease (Canadian Cancer Society, 2021). Pancreatic cancer affects older people; the incidence peaks among those 65 to 75 years of age. The prognosis of pancreatic cancer is poor. The majority of patients die within 5 to 12 months of the initial diagnosis, and the overall 5-year survival rate is about 9%.

Etiology and Pathophysiology

The cause of pancreatic cancer remains unknown. Risk factors for pancreatic cancer include chronic pancreatitis, diabetes, age, cigarette smoking, family history of pancreatic cancer, high-fat diet, and exposure to chemicals, such as benzidine. Cigarette smoking is the most established environmental risk factor for pancreatic cancer (Canadian Cancer Society, 2021). Active smokers are twice as likely as nonsmokers to develop pancreatic cancer. The risk is related to both duration and number of cigarettes smoked.

Most pancreatic tumours are adenocarcinomas originating from the epithelium of the ductal system. More than half the tumours occur in the head of the pancreas. As the tumour grows, the common bile duct becomes obstructed, and obstructive jaundice develops. Tumours starting in the body or the tail often do not produce symptoms until their growth is advanced. The majority of cancers have metastasized at the time of diagnosis. Metastases to the lymph nodes are common.

Clinical Manifestations

Common manifestations of pancreatic cancer include abdominal pain (dull, aching), anorexia, nausea, and rapid and progressive weight loss. Jaundice occurs when the cancer is in the head of the pancreas because of the ductal obstruction. Pruritus may accompany obstructive jaundice.

Pain is common and is related to the location of malignancy. Extreme, unrelenting pain is related to extension of the cancer into the retroperitoneal tissues and nerve plexuses. The pain is frequently located in the upper abdomen or the left hypochondrium and often radiates to the back. Its onset is commonly related to eating, and it also occurs at night. Weight loss results from poor digestion and absorption caused by lack of digestive enzymes from the pancreas.

Diagnostic Studies

Endoscopic ultrasonography (EUS), CT, ERCP, MRI, and MRCP are the most commonly used imaging techniques for diagnosing pancreatic diseases, including cancer. EUS involves imaging the pancreas with the use of an endoscope positioned in the stomach and duodenum. It also allows for fine-needle aspiration of the tumour. A CT scan is often the initial study and provides information on metastasis and vascular involvement. ERCP enables visualization of the pancreatic duct and the biliary system. When ERCP is used, pancreatic secretions and tissue can be collected for analysis of different tumour markers. MRI and MRCP can also be used for diagnosing and staging the cancer.

Tumour markers are used both for establishing the diagnosis of pancreatic adenocarcinoma and for monitoring the response to treatment. Cancer-associated antigen (CA-19-9) is elevated in pancreatic cancer and is the most commonly used tumour marker.

Interprofessional Care

Surgery is the most effective treatment for cancer of the pancreas. Only 15 to 20% of affected patients have resectable tumours. The type of surgery depends on the size and location of the tumour. Pancreatic head tumours require a classic surgical procedure called a *radical pancreaticoduodenectomy*, or *Whipple procedure* (Figure 46.15). The proximal pancreas (proximal pancreatectomy), along with duodenum (duodenectomy), distal segment of the common bile duct, and distal part of the stomach (partial gastrectomy) are removed together, followed by a surgical anastomosis of the pancreatic duct, common bile duct, and stomach to the jejunum. Pancreatic body and/or tail tumours require a distal pancreatectomy procedure. A total pancreatectomy can also be considered. However, this requires pancreatic enzyme replacements and ongoing diabetes management with exogenous insulin. Common postsurgical complications include delayed gastric emptying and pancreatic anastomotic leaks.

If the pancreatic tumour cannot be removed surgically, palliative measures, such as a cholecystojejunostomy to relieve biliary obstruction and/or endoscopically placed biliary stents, can be used. Other palliative measures include radiation therapy, which can be effective for pain relief. External radiation is most common, but implantation of internal radiation seeds into the tumour have been used.

The role of chemotherapy in pancreatic cancer continues to be limited. Commonly used chemotherapeutic agents include 5-fluorouracil; Nab-Paclitaxel; gemcitabine, and/or combination therapy with folinic acid, fluorouracil, oxaliplatin (FOLFOX). Erlotinib is the only currently approved targeted therapy and is used in combination with gemcitabine.

NURSING MANAGEMENT
PANCREATIC CANCER

Because patients with pancreatic cancer have many of the same challenges as patients with pancreatitis, nursing care includes many of the same measures (see NCP 46.3, available on the Evolve website for this chapter). The nurse should provide symptomatic and supportive nursing care and administer analgesics and comfort measures to relieve pain. Psychological support to both the patient and the family is essential, especially during times of anxiety or depression.

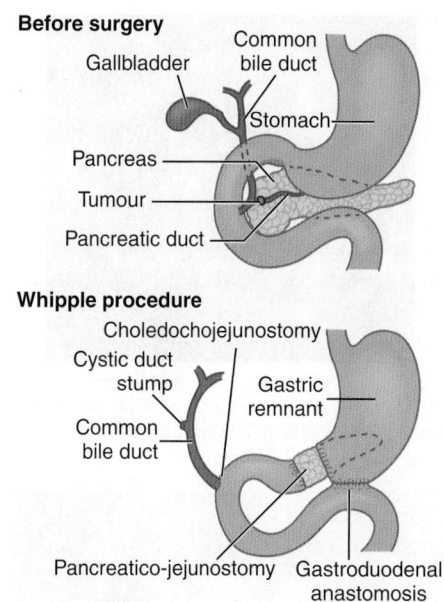

FIG. 46.15 Whipple procedure, or radical pancreaticoduodenectomy. This surgical procedure involves resection of the proximal pancreas, adjoining duodenum, distal portion of the stomach, and distal segment of the common bile duct, and the removal of the gallbladder. An anastomosis of the pancreatic duct, common bile duct, and stomach to the jejunum is created.

Adequate nutrition is an important part of the nursing care plan. Frequent and supplemental feedings may be necessary. Measures to stimulate the appetite and to overcome anorexia, nausea, and vomiting should be considered as part of the nursing care plan. If a patient is undergoing radiation therapy, the nurse should observe for adverse reactions, such as anorexia, nausea, vomiting, and skin irritation. The prognosis for patients with pancreatic cancer is poor. A significant component of the nursing care is helping the patient and caregiver(s) cope with the diagnosis and prognosis.

DISORDERS OF THE BILIARY TRACT

CHOLELITHIASIS AND CHOLECYSTITIS

The most common disorder of the biliary system is cholelithiasis (stones in the gallbladder) (Figures 46.16 and 46.17). The stones may be lodged in the neck of the gallbladder or in the cystic duct. Cholecystitis (inflammation of the gallbladder) is usually associated with cholelithiasis. Cholecystitis may be acute or chronic.

Cholelithiasis occurs in 10 to 15% of adults in developed countries. The prevalence is highest in Indigenous populations, affecting approximately 64% of women and 30% of men in certain communities (Stinton & Shaffer, 2012). *Cholecystectomy* (removal of the gallbladder) ranks among the most common surgical procedures. Although gallstones are common, more than 80% of affected patients have no symptoms. The incidence of cholelithiasis is higher in women, particularly multiparous women, and in people older than 40 years. Postmenopausal women on estrogen replacement therapy and younger women on oral contraceptives are at increased risk for gallbladder disease, with the postmenopausal women being at greater risk than the younger women. Oral contraceptives impede bile flow and increase cholesterol saturation. Other factors that increase the

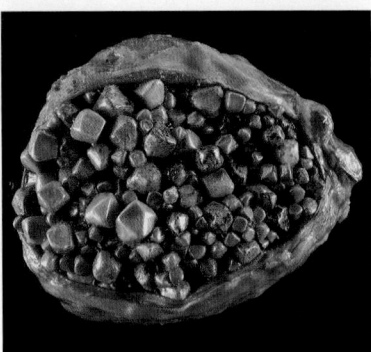

FIG. 46.16 Cholesterol gallstones in a gallbladder that was removed. Source: Kumar, V., Abbas, A. K., Aster, J. C., et al. (2010). *Robbins and Cotran pathologic basis of disease* (8th ed.). W. B. Saunders.

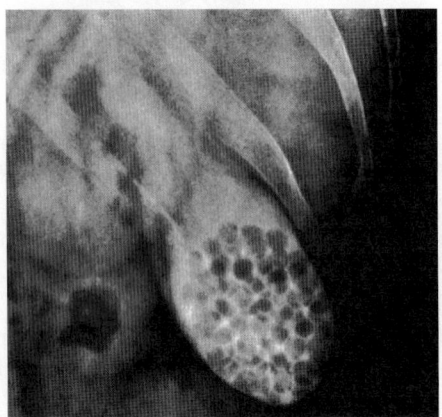

FIG. 46.17 Radiograph of a gallbladder with gallstones.

TABLE 46.21	CLINICAL MANIFESTATIONS CAUSED BY OBSTRUCTED BILE FLOW
Clinical Manifestation	**Etiology**
Bleeding tendencies	Lack of or decreased absorption of vitamin K, resulting in decreased production of prothrombin
Clay-coloured stools	Blockage of flow of bile salts out of the liver
Dark amber urine, which foams when shaken	Soluble bilirubin in urine
Intolerance of fatty foods (nausea, sensation of fullness, anorexia)	No bile in small intestine for fat digestion
No urobilinogen in urine	No bilirubin reaching small intestine to be converted to urobilinogen
Obstructive jaundice	No bile flow into duodenum
Pruritus	Deposition of bile salts in skin tissues
Steatorrhea	No bile salts in duodenum, preventing fat emulsion and digestion

occurrence of gallbladder disease are a sedentary lifestyle, a familial tendency, and obesity. Obesity causes increased secretion of cholesterol in bile.

Etiology and Pathophysiology

Cholelithiasis. The cause of gallstones is unknown. Gallstones develop when the balance that keeps cholesterol, bile salts, and calcium in solution is changed so that these substances precipitate. Conditions that upset this balance include infection and changes in cholesterol metabolism. In patients with gallstones, the bile secreted by the liver is supersaturated with cholesterol (lithogenic bile). The bile in the gallbladder then becomes supersaturated with cholesterol and precipitation of cholesterol occurs in the gallbladder. Other components of bile that precipitate into stones are bile salts, bilirubin, calcium, and protein. Cholesterol gallstones account for 90% of all gallstones. Risk factors for developing cholesterol gallstones can be genetic, dietary, and medication related.

Black pigment gallstones account for 2% of gallstones; they consist of polymerized calcium bilirubinate. Patients with hemolytic anemia, cirrhosis, and ileal diseases are at highest risk for developing black pigment stones.

Brown pigment gallstones are infrequent and usually form in the bile ducts as a result of stasis of bile and infection. These stones consist of unconjugated bilirubin and calcium salts. People at risk include those with duodenal diverticula, bile duct strictures, or parasitic diseases.

The stones may remain in the gallbladder or migrate to the cystic duct or to the common bile duct. They cause pain as they

pass through the ducts, and they may lodge in the ducts and cause an obstruction. Small stones are more likely to move into a duct and cause obstruction. Table 46.21 lists the changes and manifestations that occur when the stones obstruct the common bile duct. If the blockage occurs in the cystic duct, the bile can continue to flow into the duodenum directly from the liver. However, when the bile in the gallbladder cannot escape, this stasis of bile may lead to cholecystitis.

Cholecystitis. Cholecystitis is most often associated with obstruction caused by gallstones or biliary sludge. Cholecystitis in the absence of obstruction *(acalculous cholecystitis)* occurs most commonly in older persons and in patients who are critically ill. Acalculous cholecystitis can also occur as a result of prolonged immobility and fasting, prolonged parenteral nutrition, and diabetes. Other risk factors for acalculous cholecystitis include adhesions, cancer, anaesthesia, and opioids. Once acalculous cholecystitis is present, secondary infection with enteric pathogens (e.g., *Escherichia coli*, *Streptococcus*, *Pseudomonas*, and *Salmonellae*) can occur. In severe cases, the gallbladder can perforate.

Inflammation is the major pathophysiological condition. The inflammation may be confined to the mucous lining, or it may involve the entire wall of the gallbladder. During an acute attack of cholecystitis, the gallbladder is edematous and hyperemic, and it may be distended with bile or pus. The cystic duct is also involved and may become occluded. The wall of the gallbladder becomes scarred after an acute attack. Functioning decreases if large amounts of tissue become fibrotic.

Clinical Manifestations

Cholelithiasis may produce severe symptoms or none at all *(silent cholelithiasis)*. The severity of symptoms depends on whether the stones are stationary or mobile and whether obstruction is present. When a stone is lodged in the ducts or when stones are moving through the ducts, spasms may result. The gallbladder spasms occur in response to the stone. The spasms sometimes produce severe pain, which is termed *biliary colic*, even though the pain is rarely colicky; it is more often steady. The pain can be excruciating and accompanied by tachycardia, diaphoresis, and prostration. The severe pain may last up to an hour, and when it subsides there is residual tenderness in the right upper quadrant. The attacks of pain frequently occur 3 to 6 hours after a high-fat meal or when the patient lies down. When total obstruction occurs, symptoms related to bile duct blockage manifest (see Table 46.21). Patients with upper abdominal pain and the 5 F's for risk factors (**f**emale, **f**at, **f**ertile, **f**latulence, and **f**orty) are likely to have cholelithiasis (Cao et al., 2020).

Manifestations of cholecystitis vary from indigestion to moderate to severe pain, fever, and jaundice. Initial symptoms of acute cholecystitis include indigestion and acute pain and tenderness in the right upper quadrant, which may be referred to the right shoulder and scapula. The pain may be acute and be accompanied by nausea and vomiting, restlessness, and diaphoresis. Manifestations of inflammation include leukocytosis and fever. Physical findings include a positive Murphy sign, a manoeuvre that elicits a painful response when the right subcostal region is palpated. The manoeuvre may cause a sudden stop of inspiration as the inflamed gallbladder reaches the examiner's fingers (*inspiratory arrest*). Symptoms of chronic cholecystitis include fat intolerance, dyspepsia, heartburn, and flatulence.

Complications

Complications of cholelithiasis and cholecystitis include gangrenous cholecystitis, subphrenic abscess, acute pancreatitis, *cholangitis* (inflammation of bile ducts), biliary cirrhosis, fistulas, and rupture of the gallbladder, which can cause bile peritonitis. In older patients and those with diabetes, gangrenous cholecystitis and bile peritonitis are the most common complications of cholecystitis. *Choledocholithiasis* (stone in the common bile duct) may occur, producing symptoms of obstruction.

Diagnostic Studies

Ultrasound is often used to diagnose gallstones. It is especially useful for patients who are allergic to contrast medium and may have renal insufficiency. ERCP allows for visualization of the gallbladder, the cystic duct, the common hepatic duct, and the common bile duct. Bile samples taken during ERCP are sent for culture to identify possibly infecting organisms. Laboratory tests may reveal fluctuating elevated liver enzymes, such as ALP, ALT, and AST. The white blood cell (WBC) count is increased as a result of inflammation. Both the direct and indirect bilirubin levels are elevated, as is the urinary bilirubin level if an obstructive process is present. If the common bile duct is obstructed, no bilirubin reaches the small intestine to be converted to urobilinogen. The serum amylase and lipase are increased if the pancreas is involved.

Interprofessional Care

Once gallstones become symptomatic, definitive surgical intervention with cholecystectomy is usually indicated. However, in some cases, conservative therapy may be considered; age and associated comorbidities are all factors in determining surgical risk.

Conservative Therapy

Cholelithiasis. The treatment of gallstones depends on the stage of the disease. Bile acids (cholesterol solvents) such as ursodeoxycholic acid (UDCA) are administered to dissolve stones. However, the gallstones may recur. Gallstones are not usually treated with medications because of the high use and success of laparoscopic cholecystectomy.

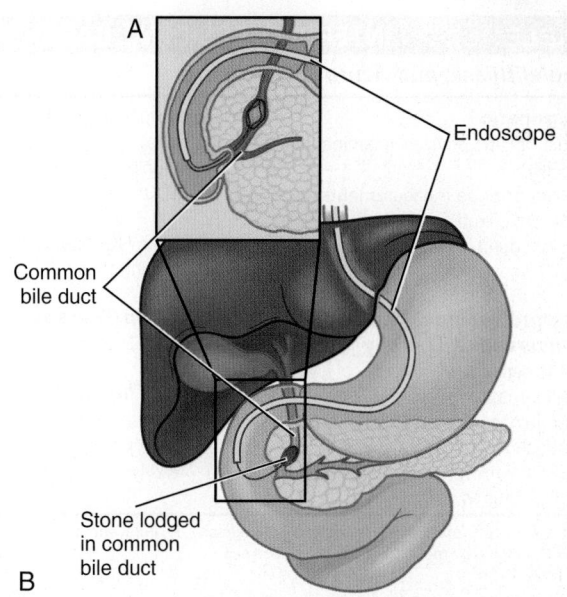

FIG. 46.18 Standard endoscopic retrograde cholangiopancreatography (ERCP). **A,** During endoscopic sphincterotomy, an endoscope is advanced through the mouth and stomach until its tip sits in the duodenum opposite the common bile duct. **B,** After widening the duct mouth by incising the sphincter muscle, the physician advances a basket attachment into the duct and snags the stone.

Standard ERCP clears stones from the common bile duct in approximately 90% of patients (Figure 46.18). This procedure allows for visualization of the biliary system, placement of stents, and sphincterotomy (papillotomy) if warranted. In this procedure, the endoscope is passed through the duodenum. With an electrodiathermy knife attached to the endoscope, the sphincter of Oddi is widened (sphincterotomy). A basket is used to retrieve the stone. The stone may be removed in the basket, but more commonly it is left in the duodenum and will be passed naturally in the stool.

Extracorporeal shock-wave lithotripsy (ESWL) is another nonsurgical treatment for gallstones. In ESWL, a lithotripter uses high-energy shock waves to disintegrate gallstones once they have been located by ultrasound. It usually takes 1 to 2 hours to disintegrate the stones. After they are broken up, the fragments pass through the common bile duct and into the small intestine. Usually ESWL and oral dissolution therapy are used together.

Cholecystitis. During an acute episode of cholecystitis, the focus of treatment is on pain control, source control of possible infection with antibiotics, and maintenance of fluid and electrolyte balance (Table 46.22). If nausea and vomiting are severe, an NG tube may be inserted, and gastric decompression may be used to prevent further gallbladder stimulation. Anticholinergics are administered to decrease secretion and counteract smooth muscle spasms. Analgesics are given for pain relief.

Surgical Therapy. Laparoscopic cholecystectomy is the treatment of choice for symptomatic cholelithiasis. Approximately 92% of all cholecystectomies are performed laparoscopically. In this procedure, the gallbladder is removed through one to four small punctures in the abdomen. A 1-cm puncture is made slightly above the umbilicus, and the surgeon inflates the abdominal cavity with 3 to 4 L of CO_2 to improve visibility. A laparoscope that has a camera attached is inserted into the abdomen. Two additional punctures made just below the ribs

TABLE 46.22 INTERPROFESSIONAL CARE

Cholelithiasis and Acute Cholecystitis

Diagnostic
- History and physical examination
- ERCP
- Liver enzyme measurements
- Serum bilirubin
- Ultrasound
- WBC count

- Extracorporeal shock-wave lithotripsy
- Fat-soluble vitamins (A, D, E, and K)
- IV fluids
- NPO with NG tube, later progressing to low-fat diet

Interprofessional Therapy
Conservative Therapy
- Analgesics
- Antiemetics
- Antibiotics (for secondary infection)
- Anticholinergics (antispasmodics)
- ERCP with sphincterotomy (papillotomy)

Dissolution Therapy
- Ursodeoxycholic acid

Surgical Therapy*
- Incisional cholecystectomy
- Laparoscopic cholecystectomy

ERCP, endoscopic retrograde cholangiopancreatography; *IV*, intravenous; *NG*, nasogastric; *NPO*, nothing by mouth; *WBC*, white blood cell.
*See Table 46.24.

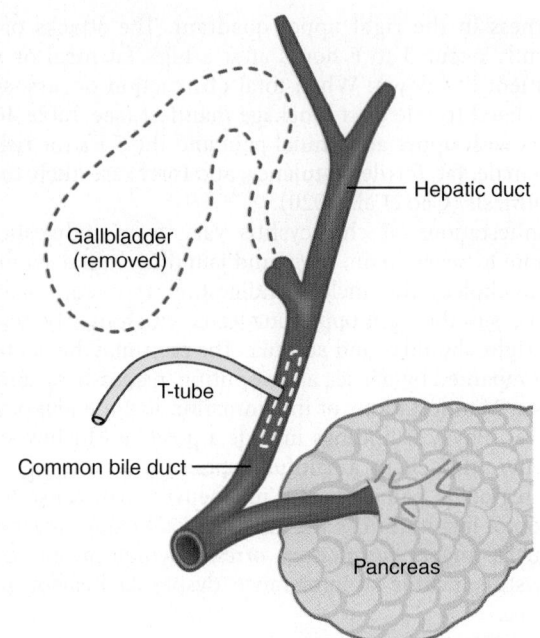

FIG. 46.19 Placement of T-tube during cholecystectomy. *Dotted lines* indicate parts removed.

are used for insertion of grasping forceps. A dissection laser is inserted into the fourth puncture. (The incision sites may vary.) Using closed-circuit monitors to view the abdominal cavity, the surgeon retracts and dissects the gallbladder and removes it with grasping forceps.

This procedure is relatively minor and entails few complications. Most patients have minimal postoperative pain and are discharged the day of or the day after surgery. In most cases, patients are able to resume normal activities and return to work within 1 week. The main complication is injury to the common bile duct. The few contraindications to laparoscopic cholecystectomy include peritonitis, cholangitis, gangrene or perforation of the gallbladder, portal hypertension, and serious bleeding disorders.

On select patients, an incisional (open) cholecystectomy may be performed. This procedure involves removal of the gallbladder through a right subcostal incision. A T-tube is inserted into the common bile duct during surgery when a common bile duct exploration is part of the surgical procedure (Figure 46.19). This ensures patency of the duct until the edema produced by the trauma of exploring and probing the duct has subsided. It also allows the excess bile to drain while the small intestine is adjusting to receiving a continuous flow of bile.

Transhepatic Biliary Catheter. The transhepatic biliary catheter can be used preoperatively in biliary obstruction and in hepatic dysfunction secondary to obstructive jaundice. It can also be inserted for palliative care when inoperable liver, pancreatic duct, or bile duct cancer obstructs bile flow. Under fluoroscopic guidance, the catheter is percutaneously inserted across the liver parenchyma into the common bile duct and duodenum. It decompresses obstructed extrahepatic bile ducts so that bile can flow freely. After insertion, the catheter is connected to a drainage bag. The skin around the catheter insertion site has to be cleansed daily with an antiseptic. It is important to observe for bile leakage at the insertion site. Depending on the reason for the catheter, the patient may be discharged with it in place.

Medication Therapy. The most common medications used in the treatment of gallbladder disease are analgesics, anticholinergics (antispasmodics), fat-soluble vitamins, and bile salts. Opioid analgesics may be administered for pain management.

Anticholinergics such as atropine and other antispasmodics may be administered to relax the smooth muscle and decrease ductal tone. If a patient has chronic gallbladder disease or any biliary tract obstruction, fat-soluble vitamins (A, D, E, and K) may be replaced. Bile salts may be administered to facilitate digestion and vitamin absorption. For pruritus, cholestyramine may provide relief. Cholestyramine is a resin that binds bile salts in the intestine, increasing their excretion in the feces. It comes in powder form and should be mixed with milk or juice. Adverse effects include nausea, vomiting, diarrhea or constipation, and skin reactions. Cholestyramine can bind with other medications, so appropriate spacing of medication administration times needs to be considered.

Nutritional Therapy. Many patients have fewer difficulties if they eat smaller, more frequent meals, with some fat at each meal to promote gallbladder emptying. With obesity, a reduced-calorie diet is indicated. The diet should be low in saturated fats (e.g., butter, shortening) and high in fibre and calcium. Rapid weight loss should be avoided because it can promote gallstone formation.

After a laparoscopic cholecystectomy, the patient should have liquids for the rest of the day and eat light meals for a few days. If an incisional cholecystectomy is performed, the patient may progress from liquids to a bland diet once bowel sounds and flatulence have returned. The amount of fat in the postoperative diet depends on the patient's tolerance of fat. A low-fat diet may be helpful if the flow of bile is reduced (usually only in the early postoperative period) or if the patient is overweight. Some patients need to restrict fats for 4 to 6 weeks. Otherwise, no special dietary instructions are needed other than to eat nutritious meals and avoid excess fat intake.

NURSING MANAGEMENT GALLBLADDER DISEASE

NURSING ASSESSMENT

Subjective and objective data that should be obtained from a person with gallbladder disease are presented in Table 46.23.

TABLE 46.23 NURSING ASSESSMENT
Cholecystitis or Cholelithiasis

Subjective Data
Important Health Information
Past health history: Obesity, multiparity, infection, cancer, extensive fasting, pregnancy; positive family history; sedentary lifestyle
Medications: Estrogen or oral contraceptives
Surgery or other treatments: Previous abdominal surgery

Symptoms
- Clay-coloured stools, steatorrhea, flatulence; dark urine
- Moderate to severe pain in right upper quadrant that may radiate to the back or scapula
- Positive Murphy sign
- Pruritus
- Weight loss, anorexia; indigestion, fat intolerance, nausea and vomiting, dyspepsia; chills

Objective Data
General
Fever, restlessness

Integumentary
Jaundice, icteric sclera; diaphoresis

Respiratory
Tachypnea, splinting during respirations

Cardiovascular
Tachycardia

Gastrointestinal
Palpable gallbladder, abdominal guarding and distension

Possible Findings
↑ Serum liver enzymes and bilirubin; absence of urobilinogen in urine; ↑ urinary bilirubin; leukocytosis; abnormal ultrasound findings

NURSING DIAGNOSES
Nursing diagnoses for patients with gallbladder disease treated surgically include but are not limited to the following:
- *Acute pain* resulting from *physical injury agent* (surgical procedure)
- *Inadequate health management* resulting from *insufficient resources* (lack of knowledge of diet and postoperative management)

PLANNING
The overall goals are that the patient with gallbladder disease will have (a) relief of pain and discomfort, (b) no complications postoperatively, and (c) no recurrent attacks of cholecystitis or cholelithiasis.

NURSING IMPLEMENTATION
HEALTH PROMOTION. The nurse should recognize the predisposing factors for gallbladder disease in general health screening. Patients at risk should be taught the initial clinical manifestations and be instructed to seek medical attention if these manifestations occur. Patients with chronic cholecystitis do not have acute symptoms and may not seek help until jaundice and biliary obstruction occur. Earlier detection in these patients is beneficial so that the condition can be managed with lifestyle modifications (e.g., a low-fat diet).

ACUTE INTERVENTION. Nursing objectives for the patient undergoing conservative therapy include managing pain, relieving nausea and vomiting, providing comfort and emotional support, maintaining fluid and electrolyte balance, maintaining nutrition, making accurate assessments of effectiveness of treatment, and observing for complications.

Many patients with acute cholecystitis or cholelithiasis have severe pain. The medications ordered to relieve the pain should be administered as required by patients and before the pain becomes more severe. Ongoing assessment of quality of pain and efficacy of pain control is required. Adverse effects of using analgesics should be monitored. Nursing comfort measures, such as a clean bed, comfortable positioning, and oral care, are appropriate.

For patients who have severe nausea and vomiting, insertion of an NG tube and gastric decompression may be necessary. Eliminating food and fluid intake can prevent further stimulation of the gallbladder. Oral hygiene, care of nares, accurate intake and output measurements, and maintenance of suction should be a part of the nursing care plan. For patients with less severe nausea and vomiting, antiemetics are usually adequate. When a patient is vomiting, comfort measures such as frequent mouth rinses should be provided. Any vomitus should be removed immediately from the patient's view.

If pruritus occurs with jaundice, measures to relieve itching include baking soda or oatmeal baths; lotions, such as those containing calamine; antihistamines; soft, old linen; and control of the temperature (not too hot and not too cold). The patient's nails should be kept short and clean. Patients should be taught to rub with their knuckles rather than scratch with their nails when they cannot resist scratching.

Ongoing assessment includes progression of symptoms and development of complications of biliary obstruction. Clinical signs to monitor include jaundice; clay-coloured stools; dark, foamy urine; steatorrhea; fever; and increased WBC count.

When symptoms of biliary obstruction are present (see Table 46.21), bleeding may result of decreased prothrombin production by the liver. Common sites to observe for bleeding are the mucous membranes of the mouth, the nose, the gingivae, and injection sites. When administering injections, a small-gauge needle is used and gentle pressure applied after the injection. The nurse should know the patient's PT and use this as a guide in the assessment process.

Assessment for infections includes monitoring of vital signs. Clinical symptoms including fever with chills, right upper quadrant pain, and jaundice may indicate choledocholithiasis. Nursing care of the patient after ERCP with papillotomy includes assessment to detect complications such as pancreatitis, perforation, infection, and bleeding. Abdominal pain, fever, and rising amylase and lipase may indicate pancreatitis. The patient should rest for several hours and ingest nothing by mouth until the gag reflex returns.

Postoperative Care. Postoperative nursing care after a laparoscopic cholecystectomy includes monitoring for complications such as bleeding, making the patient comfortable, and preparing the patient for discharge. A common postoperative condition is referred pain to the shoulder because of the carbon dioxide that is used to inflate the abdominal cavity during surgery. Carbon dioxide may not be released or absorbed by the body. The carbon dioxide can irritate the phrenic nerve and the diaphragm, causing some difficulty in breathing. Placing the patient in a Sims' position (on their left side with right knee flexed) helps move the gas pocket away from the diaphragm. Deep breathing

TABLE 46.24 PATIENT & CAREGIVER TEACHING GUIDE

Laparoscopic Cholecystectomy: Postoperative Care

The following guidelines should be included when teaching the patient and caregiver about postoperative care following laparoscopic cholecystectomy.
1. Remove the bandages on the puncture site the day after surgery, and bathe or shower.
2. Notify the surgeon of any of the following signs and symptoms:
   - Redness; swelling; bile-coloured drainage or pus from any incision
   - Severe abdominal pain, nausea, vomiting, fever, chills
3. Resume normal activities gradually.
4. Return to work within 1 week of surgery if no complications ensue.
5. Resume normal diet; a low-fat diet, however, is usually better tolerated for several weeks after surgery.

and early ambulation should be encouraged. Severe pain can be relieved by opioid analgesics. The patient is allowed clear liquids and can walk to the bathroom to void. Many patients go home the same day as the procedure.

Postoperative nursing care for incisional cholecystectomy is the same as general postoperative nursing care (see Chapter 22). The goal is to prevent postoperative complications. If the patient has a T-tube (see Figure 46.19), the nursing care plan should focus on maintaining bile drainage and observing for the T-tube functioning and drainage. The T-tube is connected to a closed gravity drainage system. If the Penrose or Jackson-Pratt drain or the T-tube is draining large amounts, a sterile pouching system should be used to protect the skin.

AMBULATORY AND HOME CARE. For patients who have conservative therapy, long-term nursing management depends on symptoms and on whether surgical intervention is planned. Dietary teaching is usually necessary. The food should be low in fat. A weight-reduction program should be recommended for patients with obesity. Patients may need to take fat-soluble vitamin supplements. The nurse should instruct patients about symptoms that indicate obstruction (stool and urine changes, jaundice, and pruritus). The nurse should also explain the importance of continued follow-up care. Patients who undergo a laparoscopic cholecystectomy are discharged soon after the surgery; therefore, home care is important. Teaching is essential; a teaching guide is presented in Table 46.24.

After an incisional cholecystectomy, the patient is usually discharged in 2 to 3 days. The patient must avoid heavy lifting for

4 to 6 weeks. Usual sexual activities, including intercourse, can be resumed as soon as the patient feels ready, unless the health care provider instructs otherwise. If the patient is required to remain on a low-fat diet for 4 to 6 weeks, a dietary teaching plan is necessary. A weight-reduction program may be helpful if the patient is overweight. Most patients tolerate a regular diet with no difficulties but should avoid excessive fats.

EVALUATION

The overall expected outcomes are that the patient with gallbladder disease will (a) be comfortable and free of pain and (b) will verbalize understanding of activity level and dietary restrictions.

GALLBLADDER CANCER

In 2017, the incidence rate of primary gallbladder cancer in Canada was 1.5 per 100 000 individuals (Statistics Canada, 2021b). The majority of gallbladder carcinomas are adenocarcinomas. A relationship exists between cancer of the gallbladder and chronic cholecystitis and cholelithiasis. The early symptoms of carcinoma of the gallbladder are nonspecific and similar to those of chronic cholecystitis and cholelithiasis, which makes diagnosis difficult. Later symptoms are usually those of biliary obstruction.

Diagnosis and staging of gallbladder cancer are done using EUS, abdominal ultrasound, CT, MRI, and/or MRCP. Unfortunately, gallbladder cancer often is not detected until the disease is advanced. When it is found early, surgery can be curative. Several factors influence successful surgical outcomes, including the depth of cancer invasion, extent of liver involvement, presence of venous or lymphatic invasion, and lymph node metastasis. Extended cholecystectomy with lymph node dissection has improved the outcomes for patients with gallbladder cancer.

When surgery is not an option, endoscopic stenting of the biliary tract can reduce complications related to obstructive symptoms. Adjuvant therapies, including radiation therapy and chemotherapy, may be used, depending on the disease state. Overall, cancer of the gallbladder has a poor prognosis.

Nursing management involves supportive care with special attention to nutrition, hydration, skin care, and pain relief. Nursing care measures used for patients with cholecystitis and cholelithiasis and nursing care measures for patients with cancer (see Chapter 18) are appropriate.

CASE STUDY

Cirrhosis of the Liver

Patient Profile
A. B. (pronouns he/him), 55 years old, was admitted with a diagnosis of an upper GI bleed secondary to cirrhosis of the liver.

Subjective Data
- Has been vomiting for 2 days, noticed blood in the toilet when vomiting
- Was diagnosed with cirrhosis 10 years ago
- Had a blood transfusion 25 years ago after a car accident
- Acknowledges drinking heavily for more than 30 years
- Complains of anorexia, nausea, and abdominal discomfort

Objective Data
Physical Examination
- Is thin and malnourished
- Has moderate ascites
- Has jaundice of sclera and skin
- Has 4+ pitting edema of the lower extremities
- Has palpable liver and spleen

Laboratory Values
- Total bilirubin: 150 mcmol/L
- Albumin: 26 g/L
- AST: 210 U/L
- ALT: 85U/L

CASE STUDY

Cirrhosis of the Liver—cont'd

- Hb 60 g/L and Hct of 20%
- Platelet count: 75 × 10⁹/L
- INR: 2.1
- Anti-HCV (antibody to hepatitis C) positive and HCV RNA negative
- HBsAg (hepatitis B surface antigen) negative and anti-HBs (antibody to hepatitis B surface antigen) positive

Discussion Questions

1. What are the possible causes of cirrhosis? What is the most likely etiology responsible for A. B.'s cirrhosis?
2. Describe the pathophysiological changes that occur in the liver as cirrhosis develops.
3. List his clinical manifestations of liver failure. For each manifestation, explain the pathophysiological basis.

4. Explain the significance of the results of A. B.'s laboratory values.
5. If he begins to manifest signs and symptoms of hepatic encephalopathy, what would the nurse monitor? What measures should be instituted to control or decrease encephalopathy?
6. A. B. was being closely observed for the possibility of GI bleeding. Why is this considered a possible complication?
7. ***Priority decision:*** On the basis of the assessment data presented, what are the nursing diagnoses? Are there any interprofessional issues?
8. ***Priority decision:*** What are the priority nursing interventions for the patient at this stage of illness?

⊖volve
Answers are available on http://evolve.elsevier.com/Canada/Lewis/medsurg

REVIEW QUESTIONS

The number of the question corresponds to the same-numbered objective at the beginning of the chapter.

1. A client with hepatitis A is in the acute phase. Which of the following should be considered in the nurse's plan of care?
   a. Pruritus is a common condition with jaundice in this phase.
   b. The client is most likely to transmit the disease during this phase.
   c. Gastrointestinal symptoms are not as severe in hepatitis A as they are in hepatitis B.
   d. Extrahepatic manifestations of glomerulonephritis and polyarteritis are common in this phase.

2. A client with acute hepatitis B is being discharged in 2 days. Which of the following instructions should the nurse include in the discharge teaching plan?
   a. Resume alcohol as soon as he is symptom free.
   b. Use a condom during sexual intercourse.
   c. Have family members get an injection of immune globulin.
   d. Follow a low-protein, moderate-carbohydrate, moderate-fat diet.

3. A client has been told that she has elevated liver enzyme caused by NAFLD. Which of the following instructions should the nurse's teaching plan include?
   a. Have genetic testing performed.
   b. Follow a heart-healthy diet and a regular exercise program.
   c. Lose weight quickly within the next 4 weeks.
   d. Avoid using alcohol until the liver enzyme levels return to normal.

4. A client with advanced cirrhosis asks the nurse why his abdomen is so swollen. The nurse's response is based on knowledge of which of the following?
   a. A lack of clotting factors promotes the collection of blood in the abdominal cavity.
   b. Portal hypertension and hypoalbuminemia cause a fluid shift into the peritoneal space.
   c. Decreased peristalsis in the gastrointestinal tract contributes to gas formation and distension of the bowel.
   d. Bile salts in the blood irritate the peritoneal membranes, causing edema and pocketing of fluid.

5. In caring for a client with hepatocellular carcinoma, which of the following should the nurse perform?
   a. Focus primarily on symptomatic and comfort measures.
   b. Reassure the client that chemotherapy offers a good prognosis for recovery.

   c. Promote the client's confidence that surgical excision of the tumour will be successful.
   d. Provide information necessary for the client to make decisions regarding liver transplantation.

6. Nursing management of a client with acute pancreatitis includes which of the following? *(Select all that apply.)*
   a. Checking for signs of hypocalcemia
   b. Observing stools for signs of steatorrhea
   c. Providing a diet low in carbohydrates with moderate fat
   d. Giving insulin based on a sliding scale
   e. Monitoring for infection, particularly respiratory tract infection

7. A client with pancreatic cancer is admitted to the hospital for evaluation for treatment. The client asks the nurse to describe Whipple procedure, which the surgeon has planned. Which of the following would the nurse include in the explanation to the client?
   a. Creation of a bypass around the obstruction caused by the tumour by joining the gallbladder to the jejunum
   b. Resection of the entire pancreas and the distal portion of the stomach, with anastomosis of the common bile duct and the stomach into the duodenum
   c. Removal of part of the pancreas, part of the stomach, the duodenum, and the gallbladder, with joining of the pancreatic duct, the common bile duct, and the stomach to the jejunum
   d. Radical removal of pancreas, duodenum, and spleen, and attachment of the stomach to the jejunum, which requires oral supplementation of pancreatic digestive enzymes and insulin replacement therapy

8. The nursing management of a client with cholecystitis in association with cholelithiasis should include which of the following?
   a. Recommendation of a diet low in saturated fat
   b. Information that gallstones once removed tend not to recur
   c. Avoidance of morphine in the management of pain
   d. Treatment with oral bile salts that dissolve gallstones

9. What information should be included in teaching about home management after a laparoscopic cholecystectomy?
   a. Keep the bandages on the puncture sites for 48 hours.
   b. Report any bile-coloured drainage or pus from any incision.
   c. Use over-the-counter antiemetics if nausea and vomiting occur.
   d. Empty and measure the contents of the bile bag from the T-tube every day.

1. b; 2. b; 3. b; 4. b; 5. a; 6. a, e; 7. c; 8. a; 9. b.

Ⓔvolve

For even more review questions, visit http://evolve.elsevier.com/
Canada/Lewis/medsurg.

REFERENCES

Beuers, U., Gershwin, M. E., Gish, R. G., et al. (2015). Changing
nomenclature for PBC: From "cirrhosis" to "cholangitis". *Gastroenterology*, 149(6), 1627–1629. https://doi.org/10.1053/j.gastro.2015.08.031

Boregowda, U., Umapathy, C., Halim, N., et al. (2019). Update on the
management of gastrointestinal varices. *World Journal of Gastrointestinal Pharmacology and Therapeutics*, 10(1), 1–21. https://doi.org/10.4292/wjgpt.v10.i1.1

Canadian Cancer Society. (2021). *What is pancreatic cancer?*.
https://www.cancer.ca/en/cancer-information/cancertype/pancreatic/pancreatic-cancer/?region=on

Canadian Institute for Health Information (CIHI). (2019). *Annual
statistics on organ replacement in Canada: Dialysis, transplantation
and donation, 2009 to 2018*. https://www.cihi.ca/sites/default/files/
document/corr-snapshot-2019-en.pdf

Cao, Z., Wei, J., Zhang, N., et al. (2020). Risk factors of systematic biliary complications in patients with gallbladder stones. *Irish Journal
of Medical Science*, 189(3), 943–947. https://doi.org/10.1007/
s11845-019-02161-x

Coffin, C. S., Fung, S. K., Alvarez, F., et al. (2018). Management of
hepatitis B virus infection: 2018 guidelines from the Canadian
Association for the Study of the Liver and Association of Medical
Microbiology and Infectious Disease Canada. *Canadian Liver Journal*, 1(4), 156–217. https://doi.org/10.3138/canlivj.2018-0008

Coffin, C. S., Ramji, A., Cooper, C. L., et al. (2019). Epidemiologic
and clinical features of chronic hepatitis B virus infection in 8
Canadian provinces: A descriptive study by the Canadian HBV
network. *CMAJ Open*, 7(4), E610–E617. https://doi.org/10.9778/
cmajo.20190103

Crabb, D. W., Im, G. Y., Szabo, G., et al. (2020). Practice guidance
from the American Association for the Study of Liver Disease.
Hepatology, 71(1), 306–333. https://doi.org/10.1002/hep.30866

D'Amico, G., Morabito, A., D'Amico, M., et al. (2018). Clinical states
of cirrhosis and competing risks. *Journal of Hepatology*, 68(3),
563–576. https://doi.org/10.1016/j.jhep.2017.10.020

Doyle, A., Gorgen, A., Muaddi, H., et al. (2019). Outcomes of radiofrequency ablation as first-line therapy for hepatocellular carcinoma less than 3 cm in potentially transplantable patients. *Journal
of Hepatology*, 70, 866–873.

Fearon, M. A., O'Brien, F. S., Delae, G., et al. (2017). Hepatitis E in
Canadian blood donors. *Transfusion*, 57(6), 1420–1425. https://
doi.org/10.1111/trf.14089

Flemming, J. A., Dewit, Y., Mah, J. M., et al. (2019). Incidence of
cirrhosis in young birth cohorts in Canada from 1997 to 2016: A
retrospective population-based study. *The Lancet Gastroenterology & Hepatology*, 4(3), 217–226. https://doi.org/10.1016/S2468-1253(18)30339-X

Garcia-Tsao, G., Abraldes, J. G., Berzigotta, A., et al. (2017). Portal hypertensive bleeding in cirrhosis: Risk stratifications, diagnosis, and
management: 2016 practice guidance by the American Association
for the Study of Liver Diseases. *Hepatology*, 65(1), 310–335.

Government of Canada. (2018). *Surveillance of hepatitis A*. https://www.
canada.ca/en/public-health/services/diseases/hepatitis-a/surveillance.
html

Health Canada. (2021). *Hepatitis*. https://www.canada.ca/en/healthcanada/services/health-concerns/diseases-conditions/hepatitis.html

Hines, O., & Pandol, S. (2019). Clinical review. Management of severe
acute pancreatitis. *British Medical Journal*, 367, I6227. https://doi.
org/10.1136/bmj.l6227

Kamimura, K., Sakamaki, A., Kamimura, H., et al. (2019). Considerations of elderly factors to manage the complication of liver cirrhosis in elderly patients. *World Journal of Gastroenterology*, 25(15),
1817–1827. https://doi.org/10.3748/wjg.v25.i15.1817

Liem, K. S., Fung, S., Wong, D. K., et al. (2019). Limited sustained
response after stopping nucleos(t)ide analogues in patients with
chronic hepatitis B: Results from a randomized controlled trial
(Toronto STOP study). *Gut*, 68(12), 2206–2213. https://doi.
org/10.1136/gutjnl-2019-318981

Lin, Z. H., Xin, Y. N., Dong, Q. J., et al. (2011). Performance of the
aspartate aminotransferase-to-platelet ratio index for the staging of
hepatitis C–related fibrosis: An updated meta-analysis. *Hepatology*,
53(3), 726–736.

Lindor, K. D., Bowlus, C. L., Boyer, J., et ai. (2019). Primary biliary
cholangitis: 2018 practice guidance from the American Association for the Study of Liver Disease. *Hepatology*, 69(1), 394–419.
https://doi.org/10.1002/hep.30145

Mack, C. L., Adams, D., Assis, D. N., et al. (2020). Diagnosis and
management of autoimmune hepatitis in adults and children: 2019
practice guidelines from the American Association for the Study of
Liver Disease. *Hepatology*, 72(2), 671–722. https://doi.org/10.1002/
hep.31065

Marrero, J. A., Kulik, L. M., Sirlin, C. B., et al. (2018). Diagnosis, staging, and management of hepatocellular carcinoma: 2018 practice
guidance by the American Association for the Study of Liver
Diseases. *Hepatology*, 68(2), 723–750.

Moore, A. H. (2019). Thrombocytopenia in cirrhosis: A review of
pathophysiology and management options. *Clinical Liver Disease*,
14(5), 183–186.

Myers, R. P., Shah, H., Burak, K. W., et al. (2015). An update on the
management of chronic hepatitis C: 2015 Consensus guidelines
from the Canadian Association for the Study of the Liver. *Canadian Journal of Gastroenterology Hepatology*, 29(1), 19–34. https://
doi.org/10.1155/2015/692408

Novelli, P. (2017). *Transjugular intrahepatic portosystemic shunt in
radiology*. Medscape. https://emedicine.medscape.com/artic
le/420343-overview#a6

Ontario Ministry of Health and Long-term Care. (2019). *Infectious
diseases protocol. Appendix A: Disease specific chapter on hepatitis
A*. http://www.health.gov.on.ca/en/pro/programs/publichealth/oph
_standards/docs/hep_a_chapter.pdf

Palumbo, C. S., & Schilsky, M. L. (2019). Clinical practice guidelines
in Wilson disease. *Annals of Translational Medicine*, 7(Suppl 2),
S65. https://doi.org/10.21037/atm.2018.12.53

Public Health Agency of Canada (PHAC). (2021a). *Canadian immunization guide: Part 4—Active vaccines*.
https://www.canada.ca/en/public-health/services/publica
tions/healthy-living/canadian-immunization-guide-part-
-4-active-vaccines.html

Public Health Agency of Canada (PHAC). (2021b). *For health
professionals: Hepatitis A*. https://www.canada.ca/en/publichealth/services/diseases/hepatitis-a/for-health-professionals.html

Shah, H., Bilodeau, M., Burak, K. W., et al. (2018). The management
of chronic hepatitis C: 2018 guideline update from the Canadian
Association for the Study of the Liver. *Canadian Medical Association
Journal*, 190(22), 677–687. https://doi.org/10.1503/cmaj.170453

Simonetto, D., Gines, P., & Kamath, P. (2020). Hepatorenal syndrome:
Pathophysiology, diagnosis and management. *British Medical Journal*, 370, m2687. https://doi.org/10.1136/bmj.m2687

Society for Maternal-Fetal Medicine, Dionne-Odom, J., Tita, A. T. N., et al. (2016). #38: Hepatitis B in pregnancy screening, treatment, and prevention of vertical transmission. *American Journal of Obstetric and Gynecology, 214*(1), 6–14. https://doi.org/10.1016/j.ajog.2015.09.100

Sola, E., & Gines, P. (2010). Renal and circulatory dysfunction in cirrhosis: Current management and future perspectives. *Journal of Hepatology, 53*, 1135–1145.

Sood, G. (2019). *Acute liver failure.* Medscape. https://emedicine.medscape.com/article/177354-overview#a5

Statistics Canada. (2019). *Obesity in Canadian adults, 2016, 2017.* https://www150.statcan.gc.ca/n1/pub/11-627-m/11-627-m2018033-eng.htm

Statistics Canada. (2021a). *Leading causes of death, total population, by age group and sex, Canada. Table 13-10-0394-01 (formerly CAN-SIM database Table 102-0561).* http://www5.statcan.gc.ca/cansim/a05?lang=eng&id=1020561

Statistics Canada. (2021b). *Number of rates of new cases of primary cancer, by cancer type, age group and sex.* Table 13-10-0111-01 https://www150.statcan.gc.ca/t1/tbl1/en/tv.action?pid=1310011101

Tandon, P., DenHeyer, V., Ismond, K. P., et al. (2018). *The nutrition in cirrhosis guide.* University of Alberta, 1–40.

Uhanova, J., Minuk, G., Lopez Ficher, F., et al. (2016). Non-alcoholic fatty liver disease in Canadian First Nations and non-First Nations patients. *Canadian Journal of Gastroenterology and Hepatology.* Article ID 6420408. https://doi.org/10.1155/2016/6420408.

Villanueva, A. (2019). Hepatocellular carcinoma. *New England Journal of Medicine, 380*, 1450–1462. https://doi.org/10.1056/NE-JMra1713263

Wilder, J., & Patel, K. (2014). The clinical utility of FibroScan® as a noninvasive diagnostic test for liver disease. *Medical Devices (Auckland, NZ), 7*, 107. https://doi.org/10.2147/MDER.S46943

World Health Organization (WHO). (2021). *Obesity and over-weight fact sheet.* https://www.who.int/news-room/fact-sheets/detail/obesity-and-overweight

Yu, Y., Mao, Y., Chen, C., et al. (2017). CAH guidelines for the diagnosis and treatment of drug-induced liver injury. *Hepatology International, 11*(3), 221–241. https://doi.org/10.1007/s12072-017-9793-2

RESOURCES

BC Centre for Disease Control
http://www.bccdc.ca
Canadian Association for the Study of the Liver
https://hepatology.ca/
Canadian Association of Gastroenterology
https://www.cag-acg.org
Canadian Hemophilia Society
https://www.hemophilia.ca
Canadian Liver Foundation
https://www.liver.ca
Hepatitis C Information for Immigrants and Newcomers
http://www.hepcinfo.ca
Hepatitis Central—Hepatitis C Support Groups
https://www.hepatitis-central.com/hcv/support/canada/toc.html
Public Health Agency of Canada
http://www.phac-aspc.gc.ca/index-eng.php
Registered Nurses' Association of Ontario—*Integrating Smoking Cessation Into Daily Nursing Practice*
http://rnao.ca/sites/rnao-ca/files/Integrating_Smoking_Cessation_into_Daily_Nursing_Practice.pdf

evolve

For additional Internet resources, see the website for this book at http://evolve.elsevier.com/Canada/Lewis/medsurg.

Conditions of Urinary Function

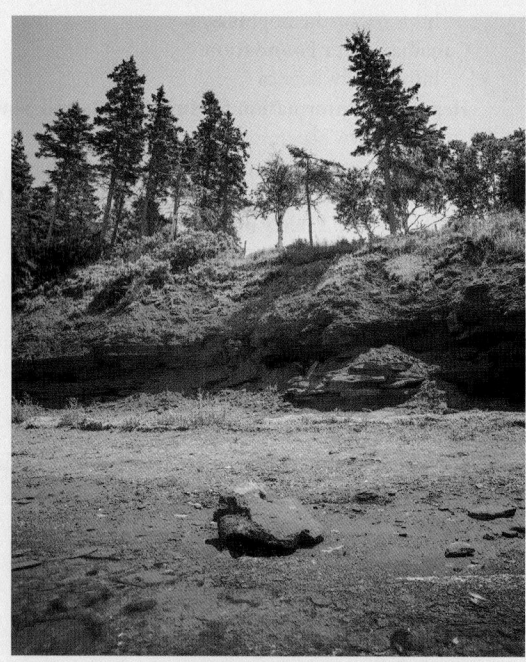

Source: © CanStock Photo / Elenathewise

Nursing Assessment
Urinary System

Kathleen Rodger and Lynn Jansen
Originating US chapter by Teresa Turnbull

evolve WEBSITE

LEARNING OBJECTIVES

1. Describe the anatomical location and functions of the kidneys, the ureters, the bladder, and the urethra.
2. Explain the physiological events involved in the formation and passage of urine, from glomerular filtration to voiding.
3. Identify relevant subjective patient information and objective data that should be collected to determine health history, health status, and clinical manifestations of patients with urinary disorders.
4. Describe age-related changes in the urinary system.
5. Describe the appropriate techniques used in the physical assessment of the urinary system.
6. Differentiate normal from common abnormal findings of a physical assessment of the urinary system.
7. Describe the range of tests performed in the analysis of urine.
8. Describe the normal physical and chemical characteristics of urine.

KEY TERMS

costovertebral angle
creatinine
cystometrography
cystoscopy

glomerular filtration rate (GFR)
glomerulus intravenous pyelography (IVP)
nephron
renal arteriography

renal biopsy
retrograde pyelography
urinalysis
urodynamics testing

"Bones can break, muscles can atrophy, glands can loaf, even the brain can go to sleep without immediate danger to survival. But should the kidneys fail ... neither bone, muscle, gland, nor brain could carry on" (Smith, 1953). This statement underlines the importance of kidneys to our lives. Adequate functioning of the kidneys is essential to the maintenance of a healthy body. If the kidneys fail completely and treatment is not given, death is inevitable.

The primary functions of the kidneys are to (a) filter waste products from the bloodstream, (b) maintain fluid and electrolyte and acid–base balance in the body, and (c) excrete metabolic waste products. The two kidneys perform the primary physiological functions. Secondary functions of the kidneys are to regulate (a) blood pressure, (b) bone density, and (c) erythropoiesis. The kidneys are connected to two narrow tubules, the ureters, which reabsorb 99% of filtered products and transport urine from the kidney to the bladder. Urine then flows from the bladder and out of the body through the urethra (Figure 47.1).

STRUCTURES AND FUNCTIONS OF THE URINARY SYSTEM

Kidneys

Macrostructure. The paired kidneys are bean-shaped organs that are *retroperitoneal* (behind the peritoneum), on either side of the vertebral column at about the level of the twelfth thoracic (T12) vertebra to the third lumbar (L3) vertebra. Each kidney weighs 115 to 175 g and is about 12 cm long. With the liver above it, the right kidney is at the level of the twelfth rib, lower than the left kidney. The adrenal gland lies on top of each kidney.

Each kidney is surrounded by a considerable amount of fat and connective tissue that serve to support and maintain its

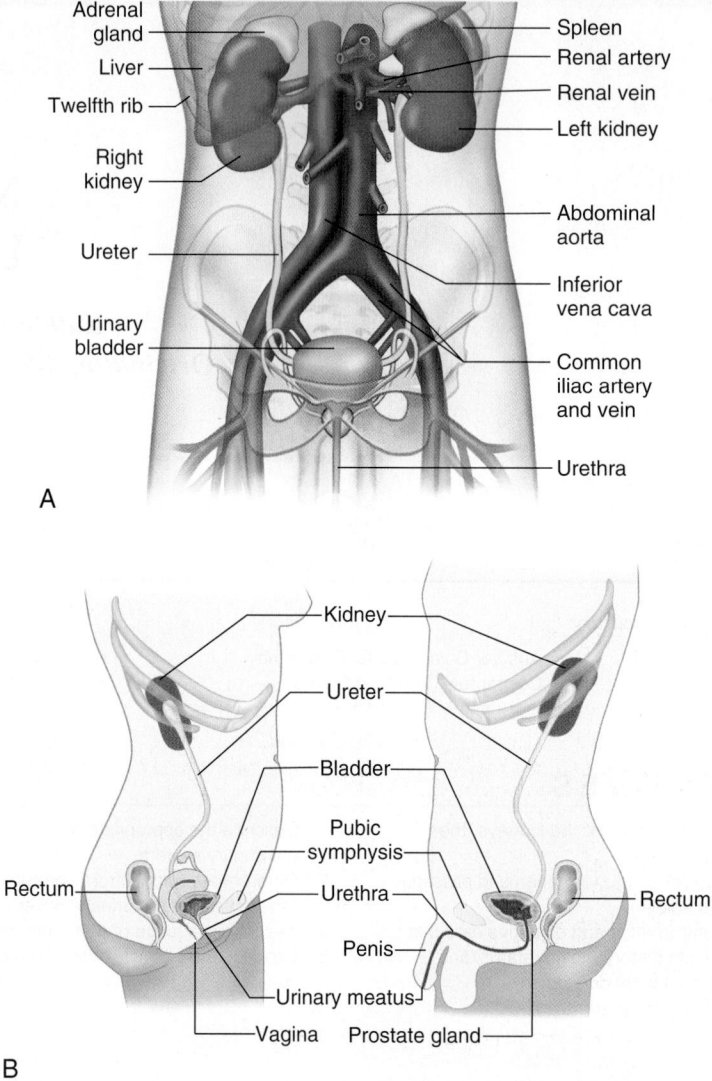

FIG. 47.1 Illustrations of organs of the urinary system. **A,** Upper urinary tract in relation to other anatomical structures. **B,** Male urethra in relation to other pelvic structures and female urethra in relation to other pelvic structures. Source: Patton, K. T., & Thibodeau, G. A., (2015). *Anatomy and physiology* (9th ed., p. 969, Figure 42-4). Mosby. Copyright Elsevier 2015.

position. The surface of the kidney is covered by a thin, smooth layer of fibrous membrane called the *capsule*. These structures protect the kidney and serve as a shock absorber should the kidney be subjected to a sudden force from a blunt object striking the abdomen or back. The *hilus* on the medial side of the kidney serves as the entry site for the renal artery and nerves, as well as the exit site for the renal vein and the ureter.

On a longitudinal section of the kidney (Figure 47.2), the parenchyma (actual tissue) of the kidney can be visualized. The outer layer is termed the *cortex*, and the inner layer is called the *medulla*. The medulla consists of a number of pyramids. The apices of these pyramids are called *papillae*, and urine passes through the papillae to enter the *calyces*. The minor calyces widen and merge to form major calyces, which form a funnel-shaped sac called the *renal pelvis*. The minor and major calyces transport urine to the renal pelvis in preparation for transportation to the bladder via the ureter. The renal pelvis can store a small volume of urine (3 to 5 mL).

Microstructure. The functional unit of the kidney is the **nephron**. Each kidney has about 1 million nephrons. A nephron is composed of a glomerulus, Bowman capsule, and the tubular system. The tubular system consists of the proximal convoluted tubule, the loop of Henle, and the distal convoluted tubule (Figure 47.3). The glomeruli, Bowman capsule, the proximal tubule, and the distal tubule are located in the cortex of the kidney. The loop of Henle and the collecting ducts are located in the medulla (Figure 47.4; see also Figure 47.2). Several nephrons converge into a collecting duct, which eventually merges into a pyramid and empties via the papilla into a minor calyx (see Figures 47.2 and 47.4).

Blood Supply. A blood supply of about 1 200 mL/min, which is 20 to 25% of total cardiac output, flows to the two kidneys. Blood reaches the kidneys via the renal artery, which arises from the aorta and enters the kidney through the hilus. The renal artery divides into secondary branches and then into still smaller branches, each of which eventually forms an afferent arteriole. The afferent arteriole divides into a capillary network termed the *glomerulus*. The capillaries of the glomerulus eventually unite in the efferent arteriole (Figure 47.5). This arteriole splits to form a capillary network called the *peritubular*

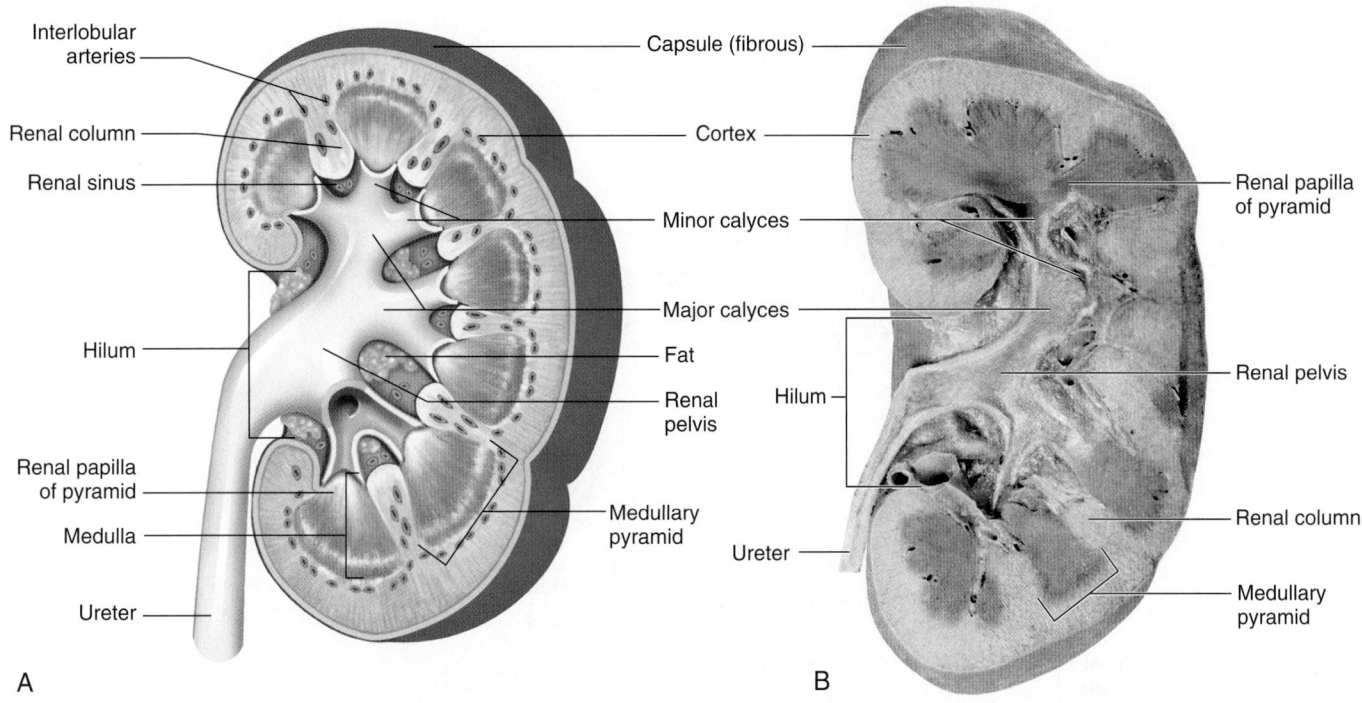

FIG. 47.2 Illustration of a longitudinal section of the kidney. Source: Patton, K. T., & Thibodeau, G. A., (2015). *Anatomy and physiology* (9th ed., p. 968, Figure 42-2). Mosby. Copyright Elsevier 2015. *A,* Adapted from Brundage DJ: *Renal disorders, Mosby's clinical nursing series*, 1992, Mosby.

capillaries, which, as the name suggests, surround the tubular system. All peritubular capillaries eventually drain into the venous system. The renal vein empties into the inferior vena cava.

Physiology of Urine Formation. The process of urine formation is extremely complex. It represents the outcome of a multistep process of filtration, reabsorption, secretion, and excretion of water, electrolytes, and metabolic waste products. Although urine formation is the result of this process, the primary function of the kidneys is to filter the blood and maintain the body's internal homeostasis.

Glomerular Function. Urine formation starts at the glomerulus, where blood is filtered. The **glomerulus**, a capillary network within the kidneys that comprises up to 50 capillaries, is a semipermeable membrane and so allows for filtration (see Figure 47.3). The hydrostatic pressure of the blood within the glomerular capillaries causes a portion of blood to be filtered across the semipermeable membrane into Bowmans capsule, where the filtered portion of the blood, called the *glomerular filtrate,* begins to pass down to the tubule. Filtration is more rapid in the glomerulus than in ordinary tissue capillaries because of the permeability of the glomerular membrane. The ultrafiltrate is similar in composition to plasma except that it lacks blood cells, platelets, and large plasma proteins. Under normal conditions, the capillary pores are too small to allow the loss of these large blood components. Capillary permeability is increased in many renal diseases, enabling plasma proteins to pass into the urine.

The amount of blood filtered by the glomeruli in a given time is termed the **glomerular filtration rate (GFR)**. The normal GFR is about 125 mL/min (Huether & El-Hussein, 2018). However, on average, only 1 mL is excreted as urine per minute because the peritubular capillary network reabsorbs most glomerular filtrate before it reaches the end of the collecting duct.

TABLE 47.1	**FUNCTIONS OF THE SEGMENTS OF THE NEPHRON**
Component	**Function**
Glomerulus	Selective filtration of water and solutes from the blood
Proximal tubule	Reabsorption of 80% of electrolytes and water; reabsorption of all glucose and amino acids; reabsorption of HCO_3^-; secretion of H^+ and creatinine
Loop of Henle	Reabsorption of Na^+ and Cl^- in ascending limb; reabsorption of water in descending loop; concentration of filtrate
Distal tubule	Secretion of K^+, H^+, and ammonia; reabsorption of water (regulated by ADH); reabsorption of HCO_3^-; regulation of Ca^{2+} and PO_4^{2-} by parathyroid hormone, regulation of Na^+ and K^+ by aldosterone
Collecting duct	Reabsorption of water (ADH required)

ADH, antidiuretic hormone; Ca^{2+}, calcium; Cl^-, chloride; H^+, hydrogen; HCO_3^-, bicarbonate; K^+, potassium; Na^+, sodium; PO_4^{2-}, phosphate.

Tubular Function. Because the glomerular membrane is a selective filtration membrane that filters primarily by size, provision is made for the reabsorption of essential materials and the excretion of nonessential ones (Table 47.1).

In the proximal convoluted tubule, about 80% of the electrolytes are reabsorbed. Normally, all the glucose, amino acids, and small proteins are reabsorbed. For the most part, reabsorption occurs by active transport. Hydrogen ions (H^+) and creatinine are secreted into the filtrate (Huether & El-Hussein, 2018).

The loop of Henle is important in conserving water and thus concentrating the filtrate. Reabsorption continues in the loop of Henle. The descending loop is permeable to water and moderately permeable to sodium, urea, and other solutes. In the ascending limb, chloride ions (Cl^-) are actively reabsorbed,

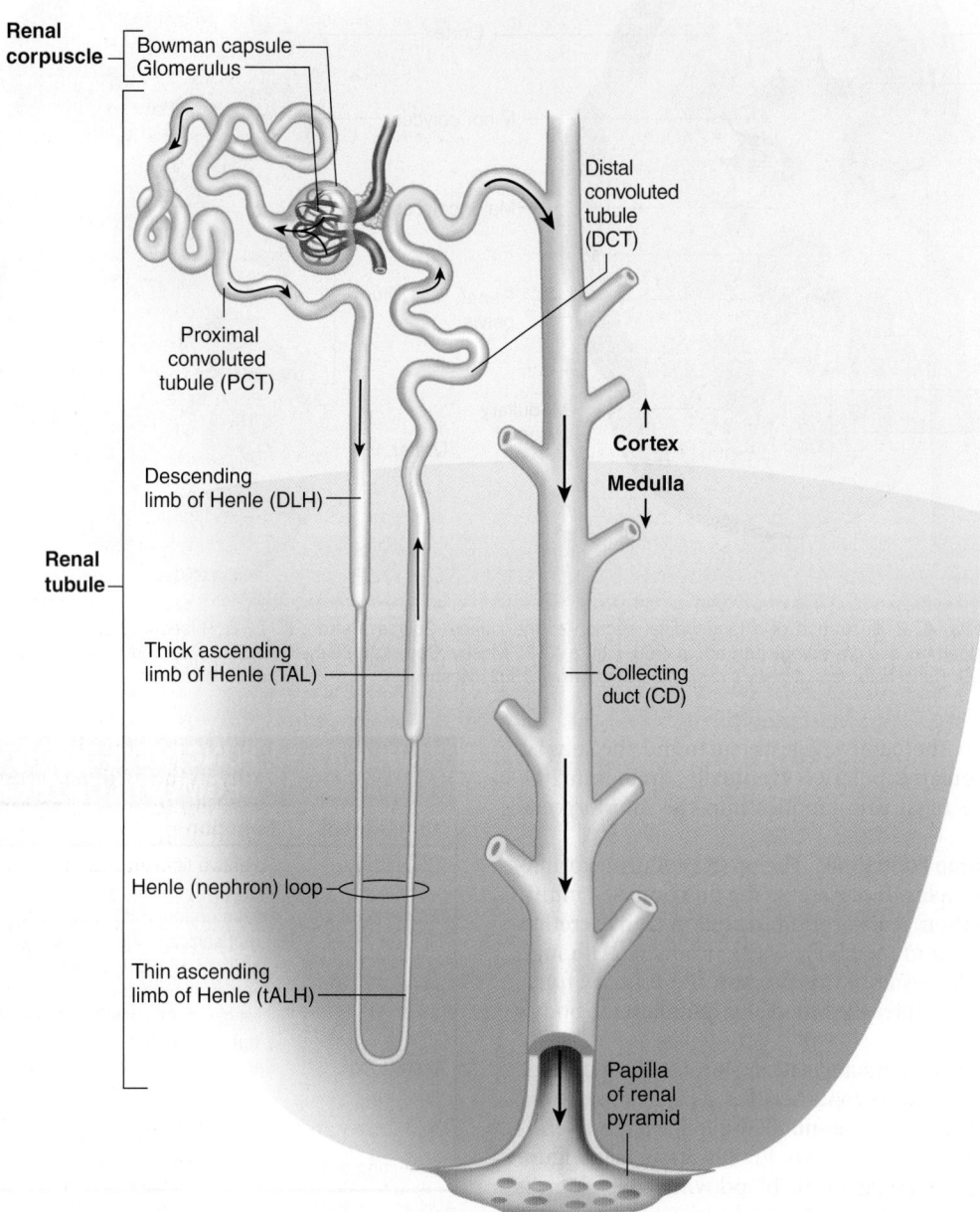

Renal corpuscle — Bowman capsule
Glomerulus

Distal convoluted tubule (DCT)

Proximal convoluted tubule (PCT)

Cortex

Medulla

Renal tubule

Descending limb of Henle (DLH)

Thick ascending limb of Henle (TAL)

Collecting duct (CD)

Henle (nephron) loop

Thin ascending limb of Henle (tALH)

Papilla of renal pyramid

FIG. 47.3 The nephron is the basic functional unit of the kidney. This illustration of a single nephron unit also shows the surrounding blood vessels. Source: Patton, K. T., & Thibodeau, G. A., (2015). *Anatomy and physiology* (9th ed., p. 971, Figure 42-10). Mosby. Copyright Elsevier 2015. Adapted from Brundage, D. J. (2991). *Renal disorders, Mosby's clinical nursing series.* Mosby.

followed passively by sodium ions (Na+). About 25% of the filtered sodium is reabsorbed in the ascending limb.

Two important functions of the distal convoluted tubules are final regulation of water balance and acid–base balance (Huether & El-Hussein, 2018). Antidiuretic hormone (ADH), released by the posterior portion of the pituitary gland, is required for water reabsorption. The stimuli for ADH release are increased serum osmolality and decreased blood volume. ADH makes the distal convoluted tubules and the collecting ducts more permeable to water, allowing it to be reabsorbed into the peritubular capillaries and to be eventually returned

to circulation. In the absence of ADH, the tubules are practically impermeable to water, and any water in the tubules leaves the body as urine.

In the presence of aldosterone (released from the adrenal cortex) acting on the distal tubule, reabsorption of Na+ and water occurs. In exchange, potassium ions (K+) are excreted. The secretion of aldosterone is influenced by both circulating blood volume and plasma concentrations of Na+ and K+.

Acid–base regulation involves reabsorbing and conserving most of the bicarbonate (HCO$_3^-$) and secreting excess H+. The distal tubule functions in different ways to maintain the pH of

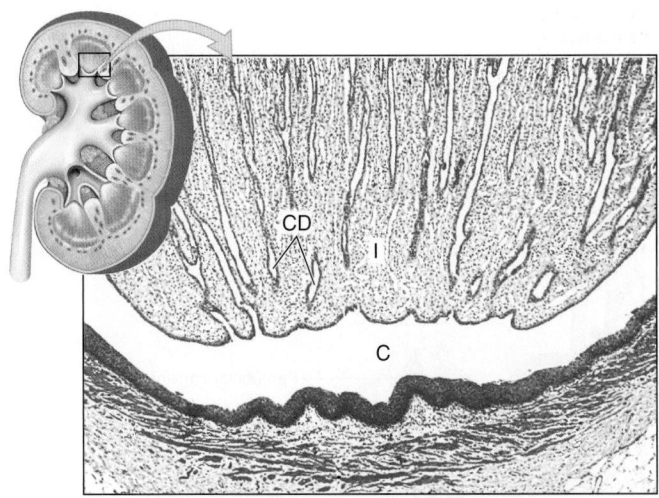

FIG. 47.4 Illustration of collecting ducts *(CD)* seen opening into a calyx *(C)* at the papillary tip. The interstitial tissue *(I)* includes some loops of Henle. Source: Patton, K. T., & Thibodeau, G. A. (2013). *Anatomy and physiology* (8th ed., p. 980, Figure 31-16). Mosby.

extracellular fluid (ECF) volume within a range of 7.35 to 7.45 (see Chapter 19).

Atrial natriuretic factor (ANF) is a hormone secreted from cells in the right atrium when right atrial blood pressure increases. ANF inhibits the secretion and effect of ADH and results in a large volume of dilute urine.

Parathyroid hormone is released from the parathyroid gland in response to low serum calcium levels. It causes increased tubular reabsorption of calcium ions (Ca^{2+}) and decreased tubular reabsorption of phosphate ions (PO_4^{2-}). Therefore, serum Ca^{2+} levels are increased.

The basic function of nephrons is to cleanse or clear blood plasma of unnecessary substances. After the glomerulus has filtered the blood, the tubules separate the portions of tubular fluid that are useful to the body from those that are not. The necessary portions are returned to the blood, and the unnecessary portions pass into urine as waste.

Other Functions of the Kidney. In addition to their function of regulating the volume and the composition of ECF, the kidneys have other vital functions, including the production of erythropoietin, activation of vitamin D, and production and secretion of renin.

Production of Erythropoietin. Erythropoietin is a hormone produced by the kidney and released in response to hypoxia and decreased renal blood flow. Erythropoietin stimulates the production of red blood cells (RBCs) in the bone marrow. A deficiency of erythropoietin in renal failure leads to anemia.

Activation of Vitamin D. Vitamin D is a hormone that can be obtained in the diet or synthesized by the action of ultraviolet radiation on cholesterol in the skin. These forms of vitamin D are inactive and require two more steps to become metabolically active. The first step in activation occurs in the liver; the second step occurs in the kidneys. Active vitamin D is essential for the absorption of calcium from the gastrointestinal (GI) tract. The patient with kidney failure (also called *renal failure*) has a deficiency of the active metabolite of vitamin D, which manifests as problems of altered calcium and phosphate balance.

Production and Secretion of Renin. Renin, an enzyme, is important in the regulation of blood pressure and is the first step in the (renin–angiotensin–aldosterone (RAA) pathway. Renin is released from the *juxtaglomerular apparatus* of the nephron (Figure 47.6) in response to decreased arterial blood pressure, renal ischemia, ECF depletion, increased norepinephrine, and increased urinary Na^+ concentration. Renin catalyzes the splitting of the plasma protein angiotensinogen (from the liver) into angiotensin I, which is subsequently converted to angiotensin II by a converting enzyme made in the lungs. Angiotensin II stimulates the release of aldosterone from the adrenal cortex, which causes retention of Na^+ and water, leading to an increase in ECF. Angiotensin II also causes increases in peripheral vasoconstriction. The increases in ECF and vasoconstriction cause an elevation in blood pressure, which inhibits renin release. Excessive renin production caused by impaired renal perfusion may be a contributing factor in hypertension (see Chapters 35 and 49).

ANF acts directly on the medullary collecting ducts and indirectly on other tubular segments (by inhibiting several steps in the RAA pathway) to inhibit sodium reabsorption. It inhibits secretion of renin and aldosterone and causes an increase in GFR (through its effects on the renal arterioles), all of which increase excretion of sodium and water. Angiotensin converting enzyme (ACE) inhibitors and angiotensin receptor blockers (ARBs) are commonly used medications to help control blood pressure in patients with hypertension and cardiovascular disease. Since the mechanism of action works directly on RAA pathway, these medications can potentially cause adverse effects that can directly affect kidney function, such as proteinuria, increased serum creatinine, nephrotic syndrome, and renal failure (McCance & Huether, 2019).

Prostaglandins (PGs) are important regulators of cellular function. In the kidney, PG synthesis (primarily PGE_2 and PGI_2) occurs primarily in the medulla. These PGs have a vasodilating action in addition to increasing renal blood flow and promoting Na^+ excretion. They also counteract the vasoconstrictor effect of substances such as angiotensin and norepinephrine. Renal PGs may have a systemic effect in lowering blood pressure by decreasing systemic vascular resistance (McCance & Huether, 2019). In addition, they are associated with hypertension that develops in renal failure. When there is a loss of functioning tissue, these renal vasodilators are also lost (see Chapter 49).

Ureters

The *ureters* are tubes approximately 25 to 35 cm long and 2 to 8 mm in diameter that carry urine from the renal pelvis to the bladder (see Figure 47.1). The narrow area where the ureter joins the renal pelvis is termed the *ureteropelvic junction*. After coursing down along the psoas muscle, the ureter crosses over the pelvic brim and the iliac artery and inserts into the base of the bladder at the *ureterovesical junction* (UVJ). The ureteral lumen is narrowest at these junctions; consequently, they are often the sites of urinary stone (calculus) obstruction. Because the lumen of the ureter is narrow, it can be easily occluded internally (e.g., by calculi) or externally (e.g., by tumours, adhesions, or inflammation).

Sympathetic and parasympathetic nerves, along with the vascular supply, surround the mucosal lining of the ureter. Circular and longitudinal smooth muscle fibres are arranged in a mesh-like outer layer and contract to promote the peristaltic one-way flow of urine. These muscle contractions can be affected by distension as well as by neurological, endocrine, and pharmacological factors. Stimulation of these nerves during passage of a stone or clot may cause acute, severe pain, termed *renal colic*.

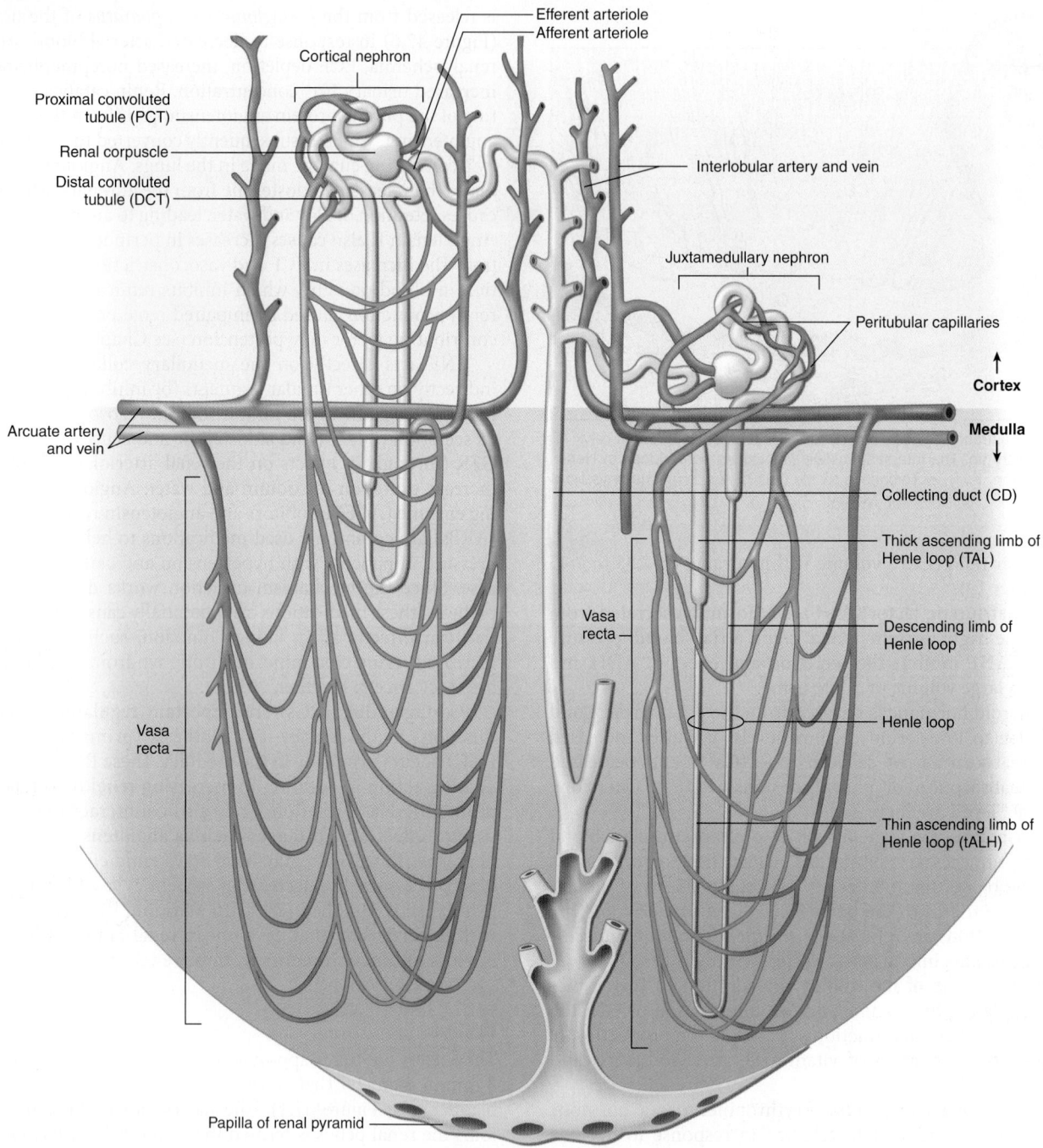

Efferent arteriole
Afferent arteriole
Cortical nephron
Proximal convoluted tubule (PCT)
Renal corpuscle
Distal convoluted tubule (DCT)
Interlobular artery and vein
Juxtamedullary nephron
Peritubular capillaries
Cortex
Medulla
Arcuate artery and vein
Collecting duct (CD)
Thick ascending limb of Henle loop (TAL)
Vasa recta
Descending limb of Henle loop
Vasa recta
Henle loop
Thin ascending limb of Henle loop (tALH)
Papilla of renal pyramid

FIG. 47.5 Blood supply of nephrons. In this illustration, two types of nephrons (cortical and juxtaglomerular) are shown surrounded by the peritubular blood supply. Source: Patton, K. T., & Thibodeau, G. A. (2013). *Anatomy and physiology* (8th ed., p. 981, Figure 31-17). Mosby.

Because the renal pelvis holds only 3 to 5 mL of urine, kidney damage can result from a backflow of more than that amount of urine. The UVJ relies on the ureter's angle of bladder penetration and muscle fibre attachments with the bladder to prevent the backflow of urine (reflux) and ascending infection. The distal ureter entering the bladder has more longitudinal muscle fibres than the upper ureter. This segment enters the bladder laterally at its base, courses along obliquely through the bladder wall for about 1.5 cm, and intermingles with muscle fibres of the bladder base. Circular and longitudinal bladder muscle fibres adjacent to the embedded ureter help secure it. When bladder pressure rises (e.g., during voiding or coughing), muscle fibres

that the ureter shares with the bladder base contract first to help promote urethral lumen closure. The bladder then contracts against its base to further close the UVJ and prevent urine from moving back through the junction.

Bladder

The urinary bladder is a distensible organ positioned behind the symphysis pubis and is anterior to the vagina and the rectum. (Figure 47.7 shows the male urinary bladder.) Its primary functions are to serve as a reservoir for urine and to help the body eliminate waste products. Normal adult urine output is approximately 1 500 mL/day, which varies with food and fluid intake. The

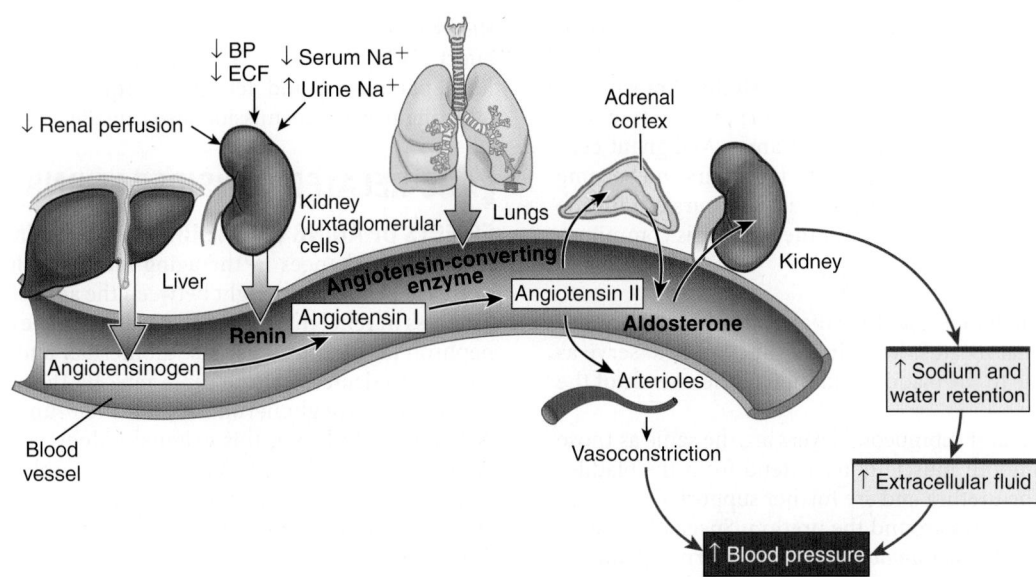

FIG. 47.6 Renin–angiotensin–aldosterone system. *BP*, blood pressure; *ECF*, extracellular fluid. Source: Adapted from Herlihy, B. (2014). *The human body in health and illness* (5th ed., p. 466, Figure 24-3). W. B. Saunders.

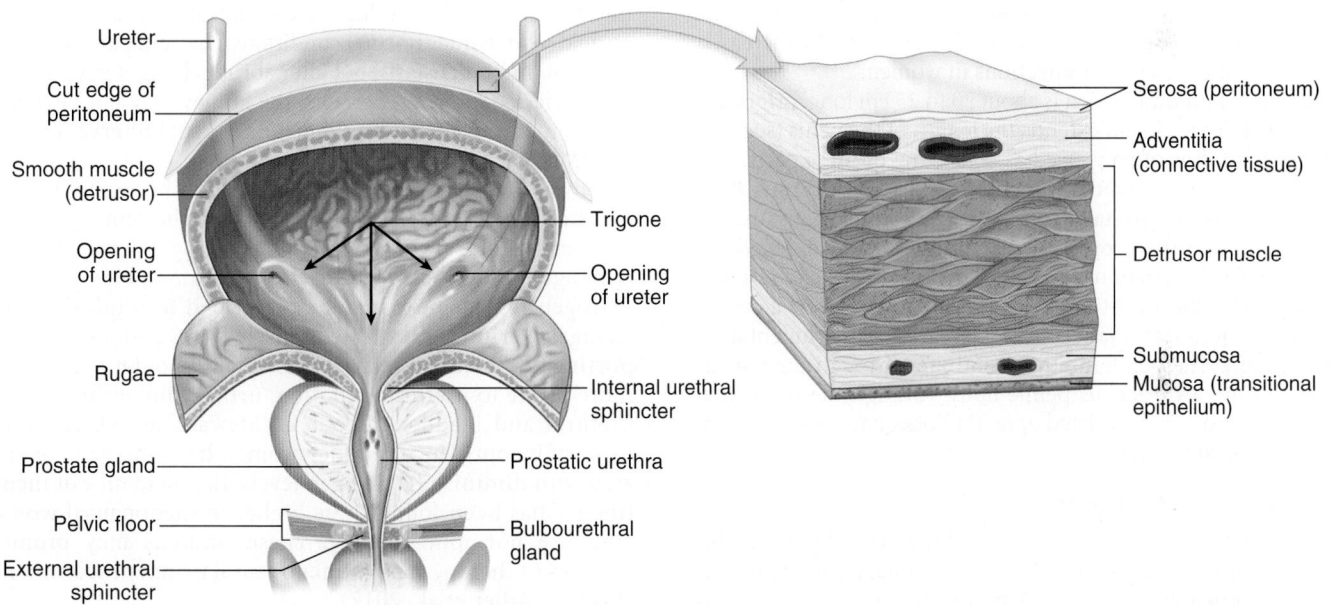

FIG. 47.7 Illustration of the male urinary bladder. Source: Patton, K. T., & Thibodeau, G. A. (2013). *Anatomy and physiology* (8th ed., p. 974, Figure 31-5). Mosby.

volume of urine produced at night is less than half of that formed during the day because of hormonal influences (e.g., ADH). This diurnal pattern of urination is normal. Most people urinate five to six times during the day and only occasionally at night.

The triangular area formed by the two ureteral openings and the bladder neck at the base of the bladder is the *trigone*. It is affixed to the pelvis by many ligaments, and it does not change its shape during bladder filling or emptying. The bladder muscle, the *detrusor,* is composed of layers of intertwined smooth muscle fibres and is capable of considerable distension during bladder filling and contraction during emptying. It is affixed to the abdominal wall by an umbilical ligament. As the bladder fills, it rises toward the umbilicus. The dome, anterior, and lateral aspects of the bladder expand and contract. When the bladder is empty, it appears as multiple folds within the pelvis.

On average, 200 to 250 mL of urine in the bladder causes moderate distension and the urge to urinate. When the quantity of urine reaches about 400 to 600 mL, the person feels uncomfortable. Bladder capacity varies with the individual, usually ranging from 600 to 1 000 mL. Evacuation of urine is termed *urination, micturition,* or *voiding.*

The lining of the bladder is identical to that of the renal pelvis, the ureter, and the bladder neck. It is called *transitional cell epithelium* or *urothelium* and is unique to the urinary tract. Transitional cell epithelium is resistant to absorption of urine. Therefore, urinary wastes produced by the kidneys do not leak out of the urinary system after they leave the kidneys. Microscopically, transitional cell epithelium is several cells deep. These cells stretch out in the bladder so that the epithelium is only a few cells deep as it accommodates filling. As the bladder empties, the epithelium resumes its multicellular layer formation.

Because the linings of these organs are similar, transitional cell tumours that occur in one section of the urinary tract can easily metastasize to other urinary tract areas. Malignant cells may move down from upper urinary tract tumours and become established in the bladder, or large bladder tumours can invade the ureter. Tumour recurrence within the bladder is common.

Urethra

The *urethra* is a small muscular tube that leads from the bladder neck to the external meatus. Its primary function is to serve as a conduit for urine to the bladder and then to the outside of the body.

The urothelium and submucosal layers are the same as those of the bladder. Smooth muscle fibres extend from the bladder neck down into the urethra and are further supported by circular smooth muscle fibres around the urethra. Special C-shaped striated muscle fibres (the *rhabdosphincter* or *external sphincter*) surround a portion of the urethra and, when bladder pressure increases, voluntarily contract and prevent leaking.

The female urethra is 3 to 5 cm long and lies behind the symphysis pubis but anterior to the vagina (see Figure 47.1, *B*). The rhabdosphincter encircles the middle third of the urethra. The shortness of the urethra is a contributing factor to the increased incidence of urinary tract infections in women.

The male urethra, which is about 20 to 25 cm long, originates at the bladder neck and extends the length of the penis (see Figure 47.1, *B*). It is often viewed as consisting of three parts. The prostatic urethra extends from the bladder neck through the prostate to the urogenital diaphragm. The membranous urethra passes through the urogenital diaphragm. The rhabdosphincter encircles this portion. Because of the concentrated muscular support, this short portion is not very expandable. As a consequence, stricture formation in this area after instrumentation is common. The penile urethra continues through the corpus spongiosum, a cavernous penile body, through the urogenital diaphragm to a distal dilated area, the fossa navicularis, before terminating at the meatus.

Urethrovesical Unit Function

Together, the bladder, the urethra, and the pelvic floor muscles form the *urethrovesical unit.* Normal voluntary control of this unit is defined as *continence.* Various areas of the brain send stimulating and inhibiting impulses to the thoracolumbar (T11–L2) and sacral (S2–S4) areas of the spinal cord to control voiding. Distension of the bladder stimulates stretch receptors within the bladder wall. Impulses are transmitted to the sacral spinal cord and then to the brain, causing a desire to urinate. If the time is not appropriate for voiding, inhibitor impulses in the brain are stimulated and transmitted back to the thoracolumbar and sacral nerves innervating the bladder. In a coordinated manner, the detrusor accommodates to the pressure (does not contract), while the sphincter and pelvic floor muscles tighten to resist bladder pressure. If the time is appropriate for voiding, cerebral inhibition is voluntarily suppressed, and impulses are transmitted via the spinal cord for the bladder neck, the sphincter, and the pelvic floor muscles to relax and for the bladder to contract. The sphincter closes, and the detrusor muscle relaxes when the bladder is empty.

Any disease or trauma that affects function of the brain, the spinal cord, or the nerves that directly innervate the bladder,

the bladder neck, the external sphincter, or the pelvic floor can affect bladder function. These conditions include diabetes mellitus, paraplegia, and tetraplegia (quadriplegia). Medications affecting nerve transmission also can affect bladder function.

AGE-RELATED CONSIDERATIONS

EFFECTS OF AGING ON THE URINARY SYSTEM

Anatomical changes in the aging kidney include a 20 to 30% decrease in size and weight between the ages of 30 and 90 years. This loss in renal mass is predominantly in the cortex. The aging nephron fails as a unit because glomerular and tubular function appears to decrease at the same rate. By the seventh decade of life, 30 to 50% of glomeruli have lost their function (Denic et al., 2017). Despite losing this original kidney volume, older individuals maintain body fluid homeostasis unless they encounter diseases or other physiological stressors.

Blood flow to and within the kidneys also decreases with age. There is no evidence, however, that atherosclerotic vascular disease is primarily responsible for the age-related changes in the kidneys.

Physiological changes in the aging kidney include a decrease in renal blood flow, a decrease in GFR, and decreases in the abilities to conserve Na$^+$, dilute or concentrate urine, and excrete an acid load. Under normal conditions, the aging kidney is able to maintain homeostasis, but after abrupt changes in blood volume, acid load, or other insults, the kidney may not be able to function effectively because much of its renal reserve has been lost (McCance & Huether, 2019).

Physiological changes also occur in the aging bladder and urethra. Estrogen receptors exist in the female urethra, bladder, vagina, and pelvic floor. As estrogen levels decrease with age, tissues become less elastic, thin, and less vascular. Estrogen replacement may be prescribed to minimize these changes. Periurethral striated muscle fibres and muscles supporting the bladder relax. Consequently, older women are more prone to urethral irritation, urinary incontinence, and urethral and bladder infections (Stewart, 2018). Although urinary incontinence in older women has long been associated with diminished estrogen levels, the incidence of incontinence has been found to be higher in menopausal women who use hormone therapy. These findings may promote changes in therapy for postmenopausal urinary incontinence (Bodner-Adler et al., 2017).

Approximately one third of older women suffer from urinary tract infections each year. In a qualitative descriptive study it was found that these women struggled with activities of daily life and felt unwell and restricted when the urinary tract infection was acute. Many of these women were identified as having other health conditions and were frail and thus vulnerable to disease. It is thus important to adapt supportive nursing strategies to both assess for and prevent urinary tract infections in this population (Aoki et al., 2017).

Men's prostates enlarge as they age, and because the prostate surrounds the proximal urethra, increasing prostate size may affect urinary patterns in men, causing hesitancy, retention, slow stream, and bladder infections. Constipation, a condition often experienced by older people, can also affect urination. Partial urethral obstruction may occur because of the rectum's close proximity to the urethra (Spencer et al., 2017).

A summary of age-related changes in the urinary system and differences in assessment findings is presented in Table 47.2.

TABLE 47.2 AGE-RELATED DIFFERENCES
Urinary System

Changes	Differences in Assessment Findings
Kidney	
↓ Amount of renal tissue	Less palpable
↓ Number of nephrons and renal blood vessels; thickened basement membrane of Bowman capsule and glomeruli	↓ Creatinine clearance, ↑ BUN level
↓ Function of loop of Henle and tubules	Alterations in medication excretion; nocturia; loss of normal diurnal excretory pattern because of ↓ ability to concentrate urine; less concentrated urine
Ureter, Bladder, and Urethra	
↓ Elasticity and muscle tone	Palpable bladder after urination because of retention
Weakening of urinary sphincter	Stress incontinence (especially during Valsalva manoeuvre), dribbling of urine after urination
↓ Bladder capacity and sensory receptors	Frequency, urgency, nocturia, overflow incontinence
Estrogen deficiency, leading to thinning and dryness of vaginal tissue	Stress or overactive bladder, dysuria
↑ Prevalence of unstable bladder contractions	Overactive bladder
Prostatic enlargement	Hesitancy, frequency, urgency, nocturia, straining to urinate, retention, dribbling

BUN, blood urea nitrogen.

TABLE 47.3 POTENTIALLY NEPHROTOXIC AGENTS

Antibiotics	Other Agents
• Amikacin	• Anaesthetics
• Amphotericin B	• Acetylsalicylic acid (ASA; Aspirin)
• Bacitracin	• Captopril
• Cephalosporins	• Cimetidine
• Gentamicin	• Cisplatin
• Neomycin	• Cocaine
• Polymyxin B	• Contrast medium
• Streptomycin	• Cyclosporin (Neoral, Sandimmune)
• Sulphonamides	• Ethylene glycol
• Tobramycin	• Gold
• Vancomycin	• Heavy metals
	• Heroin
	• Lithium
	• Methotrexate
	• Nonsteroidal anti-inflammatory medications (e.g., ibuprofen, indomethacin, naproxen)
	• Quinine
	• Rifampin
	• Salicylate (large quantities)

ASSESSMENT OF THE URINARY SYSTEM

Subjective Data

Important Health Information

Past Health History. The patient should be questioned about the presence or history of diseases that are known to be related to renal or other urological conditions. Some of these diseases are hypertension, diabetes mellitus, gout and other metabolic conditions, connective tissue disorders (e.g., systemic lupus erythematosus, systemic sclerosis [scleroderma]), skin or upper respiratory infections of streptococcal origin, tuberculosis, viral hepatitis, congenital disorders, neurological conditions (e.g., stroke, back injury), and trauma. Specific urinary conditions, such as cancer, infections, benign prostatic hyperplasia, and calculi, should be noted.

Medications. An assessment of the patient's current and past use of medications is important. This list should include over-the-counter medications, prescription medications, and herbs. Medications affect the urinary tract in several ways. Many medications are known to be nephrotoxic (Table 47.3). Certain medications may alter the quantity and character of urine output (e.g., diuretics). Numerous medications, such as nitrofurantoin, change urine colour. Anticoagulants may cause hematuria. Many antidepressants, calcium channel blockers, antihistamines, and medications used to treat neurological and musculoskeletal disorders affect the ability of the bladder or the sphincter to contract or relax normally.

Surgery and Other Treatments. The patient should also be questioned about any previous hospitalizations related to renal or urological diseases, and women should be asked about all urinary issues during past pregnancies. The duration, the severity, and the patient's perception of any health problem and its treatment should be sought. Past surgical procedures, particularly pelvic surgery, and urinary tract instrumentation should be documented. Information should be obtained from the patient about any radiation or chemotherapy treatment for cancer.

Key Questions. Nurses must convey sensitivity and understanding while asking urinary health assessment questions, to maintain the patient's physical and emotional comfort. Key questions to ask a patient with health problems related to the urinary system are listed in Table 47.4.

Health History. The nurse should ask about the patient's general health, particularly when disease affecting the kidneys is suspected. Sometimes responses such as "feeling tired all the time," changes in weight or appetite, excess thirst, fluid retention, and reports of headache, pruritus, or blurred vision may be related to abnormal kidney function. Similarly, in older patients, malaise and nonlocalized abdominal discomfort may be the only symptoms of a urinary tract infection (Wagner et al., 2019).

An occupational history should be taken. Exposure to certain chemicals can affect the kidneys and the urinary tract system. Phenol and ethylene glycol are examples of nephrotoxic chemicals. Aromatic amines and certain organic chemicals may increase the risk for bladder cancers. Textile workers, painters, hairdressers, and industrial workers have a higher incidence of bladder tumours.

A smoking history should be obtained. Cigarette smoking is a major factor in the risk for bladder cancer. Bladder tumours occur four times more frequently in cigarette smokers than in nonsmokers.

Places where a patient has lived may affect the incidence and prevalence of renal disease. Higher mineral content of the soil and water may be a contributing factor. People living in Middle Eastern countries or Africa can acquire certain parasites that can cause cystitis or bladder cancer.

A family history of certain renal or urological conditions increases the likelihood that similar conditions will occur in the patient. The nurse should ask about family members who have

TABLE 47.4   HEALTH HISTORY
Urinary System: Questions for Obtaining Subjective Data

Health History
- How is your energy level compared to how it was a year ago?
- Have you ever smoked? If yes, how many packs per day?
- What occupations or work positions have you held?
- Do you have any history of kidney disease, kidney stones, or urinary tract infections?*
- Have you had any tests or surgical procedures on your kidney, bladder, or [in men] prostate?*
- Do certain activities aggravate any urinary conditions you might have?*
- Have urinary problems caused you to alter or stop any activity or exercise?*
- How do you move or get to the bathroom?*
- What medications are you currently taking?*
- Do you take vitamin or mineral supplements?*

Nutritional Assessment
- How much and what kinds of fluids do you drink daily? Describe when fluid intake occurs over a day.
- Do you drink coffee? Colas? Alcohol? How often? How much?
- Do you eat chocolate? How often? How much?
- Do you spice your food heavily?*

Elimination Assessment
- Do you ever have difficulty holding your urine (water) long enough to get to the toilet? (or) How long can you hold your urine after you first feel the need to go to the bathroom?
- Do you ever leak urine? If so, what causes urine leakage? Do you leak when you cough or sneeze, laugh, walk, run, or lift a heavy object? Do you leak when you touch a doorknob or attempt to open the bathroom door or if you are unable to reach a toilet right away? When did the leaking begin?
- What have you done to manage leaking? (Have you cut down on the amount of fluids that you drink? Do you empty your bladder as a precautionary measure?)
- Are there certain things that make the problem worse or better?
- Does it happen all of the time, or just at certain times?
- Are you able to sit through a 2-hour meeting or ride in a car for 2 hours without urinating?
- Do you ever leak urine at night? If so, how often and how much do you leak? (If the response is affirmative, the nurse should try to differentiate between this symptom and the habit of going to the bathroom after waking up for some other reason.)
- Do you ever find that you have leaked without awareness of doing so?
- Do you use special devices or supplies for urine elimination or control? If so, (a) What types of devices or supplies do you use? (b) How often do you use these devices or supplies? (c) How many of these devices or supplies do you use on a daily basis?

- Immediately after urinating (passing your water), does it feel as if you have not emptied your bladder completely? Do you experience any hesitancy and straining? A weakened force of stream? Any dribbling?
- Do you have to exert pressure during urination to feel as if your bladder is being completely emptied?
- [Men] When you urinate (pass water), do you have any difficulty starting the stream or keeping the stream going?
- Do you ever notice blood in your urine?* If so, at what point in the urination does it occur?
- How often do you move your bowels? Do you ever experience constipation (hardened stools that are difficult to pass or a sensation that you are unable to completely evacuate your bowels)?

Activity Assessment
- Have you changed any of your activities because you need to stay near a toilet?
- Do you avoid going to certain places because of difficulty holding your urine (water)?

Pain Assessment
- Do you ever have pain when you urinate?* If so, where is the pain?
- [Women] Do you feel any pressure in your pelvic area?

Self-Concept Assessment
- How does the urinary problem make you feel about yourself?
- Have you been perceiving your body differently since the urinary problem developed?
- Does the urinary problem interfere with your relationships with family or friends?*
- Has the urinary problem caused a change in your job status or affected your ability to carry out job-related responsibilities?*

Sexuality Assessment
- Has the urinary problem caused any change in your sexual pleasure or performance?*
- Do you ever notice any blood or red-tinged urine when you urinate after intercourse?

Coping Assessment
- Have you ever sought help or talked to a health care provider about this condition?
- Do you feel able to manage the issues associated with your urinary problem? If not, explain.
- What strategies are you using to cope with your urinary problem?

*If yes, describe.
Source: Adapted from Jarvis, C., & Browne, A. J. (2019). Critical thinking and evidence-informed assessment. In C. Jarvis, P. Thomas, A. J. Browne, J. MacDonald-Jenkins, & M. Luctkar-Flude (Eds.), *Physical examination and health assessment* (3rd Canadian ed.). Elsevier.

had any of the diseases referred to in the past health history, as well as polycystic renal disease and congenital urinary tract abnormalities such as Alport syndrome (congenital nephritis).

Nutritional Assessment. The usual quantity and types of fluid that a patient drinks are important factors in relation to urinary tract disease. Dehydration may contribute to urinary infections, calculi formation, and renal failure. Large intake of particular foods, such as dairy products or foods high in proteins, may also lead to calculi formation. Asparagus may cause the urine to smell musty, and redness of urine caused by beet ingestion may be mistaken for blood. Coffee, alcohol, carbonated beverages,

or spicy foods often aggravate urinary inflammatory diseases. An unexplained weight gain may be the result of fluid retention secondary to a renal condition. Anorexia, nausea, and vomiting can dramatically affect fluid status and require careful assessment. Information on vitamin and mineral supplements and herbal therapies should be obtained. The patient may not think of these supplements and therapies when listing over-the-counter medications; supplements are often considered part of nutritional intake.

Elimination Assessment. Questions about urine elimination patterns are the cornerstone of the health history in patients with a lower urinary tract disorder. This line of inquiry begins with a question about how patients manage urine elimination. The majority of patients eliminate urine by spontaneous voiding, and they should be asked about daytime (diurnal) voiding frequency and the frequency of nocturia. Patients should also be queried about additional bothersome lower urinary tract symptoms, including urgency, incontinence, or urinary retention. Table 47.5 lists some of the common clinical manifestations of urinary tract disorders. Changes in the colour and the appearance of urine are often significant and should be evaluated. If blood is visible in the urine, it should be determined whether it occurs at the beginning, throughout, or at the end of urination.

Bowel function should also be investigated. Problems with fecal incontinence may signal neurological causes of bladder conditions because of shared nerve pathways. Constipation and fecal impaction can partially obstruct the urethra, causing inadequate bladder emptying, overflow incontinence, and infection.

The nurse should find out patients' methods of handling a urinary problem. A patient may already be using a catheter or collection device. Sometimes a patient has to assume a particular position to urinate or must perform such manoeuvres as pressing on the lower abdomen (Credé method), straining (Valsalva manoeuvre), or stretching the rectum to empty the bladder.

Activity Assessment. The patient's level of activity should be assessed. A sedentary person is more likely than an active individual to have stasis of urine, which can predispose to infection and calculi. Demineralization of bones in a person with limited physical activity causes increased urine calcium precipitation.

An active person may find that increasing activity aggravates a urinary problem. A patient who has had prostate surgery or who has weakened pelvic floor muscles may leak urine when attempting particular activities such as running. Some men may develop chronic inflammatory prostatitis or epididymitis after heavy lifting or long-distance driving.

Nocturia is a common and a particularly bothersome lower urinary tract symptom that often leads to sleep deprivation, daytime sleepiness, and fatigue. It occurs in multiple disorders affecting the lower urinary tract, including urinary incontinence, urinary retention, and interstitial cystitis. Nocturia also may be attributable to polyuria from renal disease, poorly controlled diabetes mellitus, alcoholism, excessive fluid intake, or obstructive sleep apnea. When the nurse asks the patient about nocturia, it is helpful to determine whether the desire to urinate is what causes the patient to arise from sleep or whether pain or some other symptom interrupts sleep and the person urinates as a matter of habit before returning to bed. Up to one episode of nocturia is considered normal in younger adults, and up to two episodes are considered acceptable among adults age 65 years or older. Sleep disturbances associated with a urinary disorder should be documented. Older persons may awaken several times during the night to urinate and may need to be assured that this may be normal. However, a complete assessment should be made to rule out any health concern.

Pain Assessment. Pain is a frequent symptom of urinary tract disease. Types of pain associated with renal and urological conditions include dysuria, groin pain, costovertebral pain, and suprapubic pain. If pain is present, the location, the character, and the duration should be assessed. The absence of pain when

TABLE 47.5	**CLINICAL MANIFESTATIONS OF DISORDERS OF THE URINARY SYSTEM**

Urinary System Symptoms
General Manifestations
- Anorexia
- Blurred vision
- Chills
- Change in body weight
- Change in mentation
- Excess thirst
- Fatigue
- Headaches
- Hypertension
- Itching
- Nausea and vomiting

Pain
- Dysuria
- Flank or costovertebral angle
- Groin
- Suprapubic

Changes in Patterns of Urination
- Change in stream
- Dribbling
- Dysuria
- Frequency
- Hesitancy of stream

- Incontinence
- Nocturia
- Overactive bladder
- Retention
- Stress incontinence
- Urgency

Changes in Urine Output
- Anuria
- Oliguria
- Polyuria

Changes in Urine Composition
- Colour (red, brown, yellowish-green)
- Increased concentration
- Dilution
- Hematuria
- Pyuria

Edema
- Anasarca
- Ankle
- Ascites
- Facial (periorbital)
- Sacral

CASE STUDY

Patient Introduction

A. M. (pronouns he/him), 28 years old, comes to the emergency department (ED) in acute distress with complaints of severe abdominal pain. His pain began about 6 hours ago after he finished a 16-kilometre marathon training run. A. M. says that the pain has steadily increased and is accompanied by nausea and dark, smoky-coloured urine.

Critical Thinking
Throughout this assessment chapter, think about A. M.'s symptoms with the following questions in mind:
1. What are the possible causes of A. M.'s abdominal pain, nausea, and urine colour?
2. What would be the priority assessment of A. M.?
3. What questions should be asked of A. M.?
4. What should be included in the physical assessment? What should be looked for?
5. What diagnostic studies should be ordered?

A. M.'s medical condition will be followed throughout this assessment chapter. See Case Study: Subjective Data, Case Study: Objective Data: Physical Examination, and Case Study: Objective Data: Diagnostic Studies for more information on A. M.

*e*volve
Answers available at http://evolve.elsevier.com/Lewis/medsurg.

other urinary symptoms exist is also significant. Many urinary tract tumours are painless in the early stages.

Self-Concept Assessment. Conditions associated with the urinary system—such as incontinence, urinary diversion procedures, and chronic fatigue—can result in loss of self-esteem and a negative body image. Sensitive questioning may elicit cues to challenges in this area.

Relationship and Sexuality Assessment. Urinary conditions can affect many aspects of a person's life, including the ability to work and relationships with others. These factors have important implications for future treatment and management. The nurse must be alert to cues from the patient.

Urinary system conditions may be serious enough to cause problems in job-related and social situations. Chronic dialysis therapy often makes regular employment or full-time home-making difficult. Also, concurrent poor health and negative body image can seriously alter existing roles. The nurse should assess this area to plan appropriate interventions.

The nurse should ask about the effect of a renal or urological condition on the patient's sexual patterns and satisfaction. Issues related to personal hygiene and fatigue can seriously affect a sexual relationship. Although urinary incontinence is not directly associated with sexual dysfunction, it often has a devastating effect on self-esteem and on social and intimate relationships. Counselling of both the patient and the partner may be indicated.

Objective Data

Physical Examination

Inspection. The nurse should assess for changes in the following:

Skin: Pallor, yellow-grey cast, excoriations, changes in turgor, bruises, texture (e.g., rough, dry skin)

Mouth: Stomatitis, ammonia breath odour

Face and extremities: Generalized edema, peripheral edema, bladder distension, masses, enlarged kidneys

Abdomen: Skin changes described earlier, as well as striae, abdominal contour for midline mass in lower abdomen (may indicate urinary retention) or unilateral mass (occasionally observed in adults, indicating enlargement of one or both kidneys from large tumour or polycystic kidney)

Weight: Weight gain secondary to edema; weight loss and muscle wasting in renal failure

General state of health: Fatigue, lethargy, and diminished alertness

Palpation. The kidneys are posterior organs protected by the abdominal organs, the ribs, and the heavy back muscles. A landmark useful in locating the kidneys is the costovertebral angle (CVA) formed by the rib cage and the vertebral column. The normal-sized left kidney is rarely palpable because the spleen lies directly on top of it. On occasion, the lower pole of the right kidney is palpable.

To palpate the right kidney, the examiner's left hand is placed behind and supports the patient's right side between the rib cage and the iliac crest (Figure 47.8). The patient's right flank is elevated with the examiner's left hand, and the examiner's right hand is used to palpate deeply for the patient's right kidney. The lower pole of the right kidney may feel like a smooth, rounded mass that descends on inspiration. If the kidney is palpable, its size, contour, and tenderness should be noted. Kidney enlargement is suggestive of neoplasm or other serious renal pathological conditions.

The urinary bladder is normally not palpable unless it is distended with urine. If the bladder is full, it may feel like a smooth, round, firm organ and is sensitive to palpation.

Percussion. Tenderness in the flank area may be detected by fist percussion. This technique is performed by striking the fist (kidney punch) of one hand against the dorsal surface of the other hand, which is placed flat on the patient along the posterior CVA margin. Normally, a firm blow in the flank area should not elicit pain. Tenderness and pain at the CVA may indicate a kidney infection or polycystic kidney disease.

Normally, a bladder is not percussible until it contains at least 150 mL of urine. If the bladder is full, dullness is heard above the symphysis pubis. A distended bladder may be percussed as high as the umbilicus.

Auscultation. The diaphragm of the stethoscope may be used to auscultate over both CVAs and in the upper abdominal quadrants. With this technique, the abdominal aorta and the renal arteries are auscultated for a bruit (an abnormal murmur), which indicates impaired blood flow to the kidneys.

Table 47.6 lists the normal physical assessment findings in the urinary system. Table 47.7 lists common assessment abnormalities of the urinary system. Variations in assessment findings may be normal in older persons. Table 47.2 shows the age-related changes in the urinary system and differences in assessment findings. The nurse should use a focused assessment to evaluate the status of previously identified urinary system conditions and to monitor for signs of new ones. A focused assessment of the urinary system is presented in the Focused Assessment: Urinary System box.

DIAGNOSTIC STUDIES

Table 47.8 lists and describes diagnostic tests common to the urinary system. It is important to conduct appropriate diagnostic tests to locate, understand, and manage urinary conditions.

CASE STUDY

Subjective Data

A focused subjective assessment of A. M. revealed the following information.

Past medical history: History of one isolated incidence of possible gout 6 years ago. Stopped drinking alcohol with no further occurrence. Appendectomy 12 years ago.

Medications: None.

Overall health management: A. M. states he is usually healthy. He does not smoke or drink alcohol. A. M. believes in the ability to monitor himself and maintain a healthy lifestyle. He has never experienced this type of pain before. Describes the pain as being sharp and colicky (coming in waves). Rates the pain as 9 on a scale of 0 to 10.

Functional Assessment

Nutrition and metabolic history: A. M. is currently on a high-protein diet while training for the marathon. He eats a lot of chicken, beef, and seafood. A. M. drinks milk-based protein shakes and water after exercising but admits he may not drink enough to replace fluid loss in perspiration. A. M. drinks coffee for energy but denies eating chocolate or other sweets or drinking sodas.

Elimination: A. M. denies any history of difficulty or pain on urination. No identified constipation or diarrhea. This is the first time he has ever noticed a change in his urine colour.

Self-care history: A. M. is proud of his ability to exercise and run without difficulty.

Coping and stress management: A. M. is worried that this pain may interfere with current marathon training.

See Case Study: Patient Introduction, Case Study: Objective Data: Physical Examination, and Case Study: Objective Data: Diagnostic Studies for more information on A. M.

The accuracy of the results is influenced by (a) adherence to the proper procedures related to the study and (b) cooperation of the patient in restricting fluids, collecting urine specimens, lying quietly on the examination table, and following other instructions.

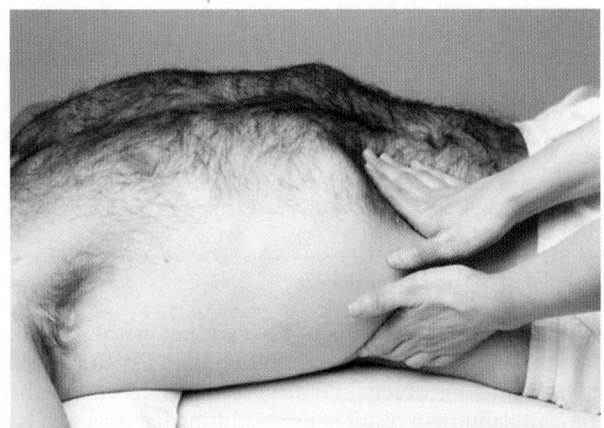

FIG. 47.8 Palpating the right kidney. Source: From Brundage, D. J. (1992). *Renal disorders*. Mosby.

TABLE 47.6   EVIDENCE OF NORMAL PHYSICAL FINDINGS

- No costovertebral angle tenderness
- Nonpalpable kidney and bladder
- No palpable masses

For many radiological investigations, a bowel preparation must be used the evening before the study in order to clear the lower GI tract of feces and flatus. Because the kidneys lie in a retroperitoneal location, the contents of the colon may obstruct visualization of the urinary tract. If a bowel preparation is not properly performed, a test may be unsuccessful and must be rescheduled. Commonly used bowel preparations include enemas, castor oil, magnesium citrate, and bisacodyl (Dulcolax) tablets or suppositories. Some bowel preparations, such as magnesium citrate and Fleet enema, are contraindicated for use in patients with renal failure—magnesium cannot be excreted by patients with renal failure (see Chapter 49).

When a patient has repeated diagnostic studies on consecutive days, it is important to prevent dehydration. It is not uncommon for a patient to take nothing by mouth (NPO) after midnight, spend all morning in the radiology department, be too tired to eat, sleep all afternoon, and be on NPO status after midnight again because of studies scheduled for the next day. Severe dehydration, especially in a patient who is diabetic or debilitated, or in an older patient, may lead to acute renal failure. The nurse is responsible for ensuring that a patient undergoing diagnostic studies is properly hydrated and given adequate nourishment between studies. The nurse should also check with the health care provider regarding the insulin dose for patients with diabetes who are NPO.

Analysis of Urine

Urinalysis. In evaluating disorders of the urinary tract, one of the first studies performed is a urinalysis (Table 47.9;

TABLE 47.7   ASSESSMENT ABNORMALITIES
Urinary System

Finding	Description	Possible Etiology and Significance
Anuria	Technically no urination (24-hr urine output of <100 mL)	Acute renal failure, end-stage renal disease, bilateral ureteral obstruction
Burning on urination	Stinging pain in urethral area	Urethral irritation, urinary tract infection
Dysuria	Painful or difficult urination	Sign of urinary tract infection, interstitial cystitis, and a wide variety of pathological conditions
Enuresis	Involuntary nocturnal urinating	Symptom of lower urinary tract disorder
Frequency	Increased incidence of urinating	Acutely inflamed bladder, retention with overflow, excess fluid intake
Hematuria	Blood in the urine	Cancer of genitourinary tract, blood dyscrasias, renal disease, urinary tract infection, stones in kidney or ureter, medications (anticoagulants)
Hesitancy	Delay or difficulty in initiating urination	Partial urethral obstruction
Incontinence	Inability to voluntarily control discharge of urine	Neurogenic bladder, bladder infection, injury to external sphincter
Nocturia	Frequency of urination at night	Renal disease with impaired concentrating ability, bladder obstruction, heart failure, diabetes mellitus. May occur after renal transplantation
Oliguria	Diminished amount of urine in a given time (24-hr urine output of 100–400 mL)	Severe dehydration, shock, transfusion reaction, kidney disease, end-stage renal disease
Pain	Presence of pain over suprapubic area (related to bladder), urethral pain (irritation of bladder neck), flank (CVA) pain	Infection, urinary retention, foreign body in urinary tract, urethritis, pyelonephritis, renal colic or stones
Pneumaturia	Passage of urine containing gas	Fistula connections between bowel and bladder, gas-forming urinary tract infections
Polyuria	Large volume of urine in a given time	Diabetes mellitus, diabetes insipidus, chronic renal failure, diuretics, excess fluid intake
Retention	Inability to urinate, even though bladder contains excessive amount of urine	Urethral stricture or obstruction; neurogenic bladder; postanaesthesia status. May occur after pelvic surgery, childbirth, catheter removal
Stress incontinence	Involuntary urination with increased pressure (sneezing or coughing)	Weakness of sphincter control
Urgency	Strong desire to urinate	Inflammatory lesions in bladder or urethra, acute bacterial infections

CVA, costovertebral angle.

FOCUSED ASSESSMENT
Urinary System

Use this checklist to ensure that the key assessment steps have been performed.

Subjective

Ask the patient about experiencing any of the following, and note responses.

Painful urination	Y	N
Changes in colour or clarity of urine (blood, cloudy)	Y	N
Change in characteristics of urination (diminished, excessive)	Y	N
Difficulties with frequent nighttime urination (nocturia)	Y	N

Objective: Diagnostic

Check the following laboratory results for critical values.

Blood urea nitrogen	✓
Serum creatinine	✓
Urinalysis	✓
Urine culture and sensitivity	✓

Objective: Physical Examination
Inspect

Abdomen	✓
Urinary meatus for inflammation or discharge	✓

Palpate

Abdomen for bladder distention, masses, or tenderness	✓

Percuss

Costovertebral angle for tenderness	✓

Auscultate

Renal arteries for bruits	✓

CASE STUDY
Objective Data: Physical Examination

A focused assessment of A. M. revealed the following information.

A. M. is lying on the ED stretcher with his knees bent and drawn to the abdominal area. He appears restless and keeps moving from back to side in an effort to reduce his discomfort. Vital signs as follows: BP 156/70, apical pulse 108, respiratory rate 24, temperature 37.4°C, O_2 saturation 96% on room air. Awake, alert, and oriented ×3. Lungs clear to auscultation. Apical pulse regular. Abdomen nondistended with + bowel sounds in all four quadrants. No rebound tenderness. Positive costovertebral tenderness. Voiding small amounts of dark, smoky urine.

As you continue to read this chapter, consider which diagnostic studies would likely be performed for A. M.

See Case Study: Patient Introduction, Case Study: Subjective Data, and Case Study: Objective Data: Diagnostic Studies for more information on A. M.

CASE STUDY
Objective Data: Diagnostic Studies

The health care provider orders the following initial diagnostic studies for A. M.:
- CBC, basic metabolic panel (electrolytes, BUN, creatinine)
- Urinalysis, culture if indicated
- Renal ultrasound

Although A. M.'s laboratory results are all within normal limits, the renal ultrasound identifies calculi in the left ureter. There is currently no hydronephrosis. The health care provider prescribes parenteral opioids for pain management and admits A. M. to a medical unit for further observation.

See Case Study: Patient Introduction, Case Study: Subjective Data, and Case Study: Objective Data: Physical Examination for more information on A. M.

see Table 47.8). This test is a general examination of urine for routine and microscopic findings and may establish baseline information, provide information about possible abnormalities, indicate what further studies need to be done, and supply information on the progression of a diagnosed disorder.

For a routine urinalysis, a specimen may be collected at any time of the day. However, it is best to obtain the first specimen urinated in the morning. This concentrated specimen is more likely to contain abnormal constituents if they are present in the urine. The specimen should be examined within 1 hour of urination. If it is not, bacteria multiply rapidly, RBCs hemolyze, casts (moulds of renal tubules) disintegrate, and the urine becomes alkaline as a result of urea-splitting bacteria. If it is not possible to send the specimen to the laboratory immediately, it should be refrigerated. However, to obtain the best results, the nurse should coordinate specimen collection with routine laboratory hours.

Multiple reagent strips (also called *urine dipsticks*) are commonly used by laboratories and in outpatient settings to provide chemical analysis of urine, along with a microscopic interpretation. The results of a urinalysis usually include a description of the appearance, specific gravity (mass and density), and pH of the urine; glucose, ketones, and protein in the urine; and a microscopic examination of urine sediment for white blood cells (WBCs), RBCs, crystals, and casts (see Table 47.9).

Composite Urine Collections. Composite urine specimens are collected over a period that may range from 2 to 24 hours. The purpose of a composite specimen is to examine or measure specific components, such as electrolytes, glucose, protein, 17-ketosteroids, catecholamines, creatinine, and minerals. These specimens may have to be refrigerated, or preservatives may have to be added to the container used for collecting urine.

For collection of a composite urine specimen, the patient is instructed to urinate and discard this first urine specimen. This time is noted as the start of the test. All urine from subsequent urinations is saved in a container for the designated period. Finally, at the end of the period, the patient is asked to urinate, and this urine sample is added to the container. Incomplete collections do not provide valid results. Reminding the patient to save all urine during the study period is critical.

Creatinine Clearance. One of the most common composite indicators used to analyze urinary system disorders is creatinine clearance. Creatinine is a waste product produced by protein breakdown (primarily body muscle mass). Urinary excretion of creatinine is a measure of the amount of active muscle tissue in the body, not of body weight; therefore, people with larger muscle mass have higher values. Because almost all creatinine in the blood is normally excreted by the kidneys, creatinine clearance is the most accurate indicator of renal function. The result of a creatinine clearance test closely approximates that of the GFR (National Kidney Foundation, n.d.). A blood specimen for serum creatinine determination should be obtained during the period of urine collection.

TABLE 47.8   DIAGNOSTIC STUDIES

Urinary System

Study	Description and Purpose	Nursing Responsibility
Urine Tests		
Urinalysis	This is a general examination of urine for routine and microscopic evaluation, to establish baseline information or provide data to establish a tentative diagnosis and determine whether further tests are to be ordered (see Table 47.9).	Usually the first urinated morning specimen is required, but it may not be appropriate for all diagnostic purposes. Ensure that the specimen is examined within 1 hr of urinating. Wash patient's perineal area if soiled with menses or fecal material.
Creatinine clearance	Creatinine is a waste product of protein breakdown (primarily body muscle mass). Clearance of creatinine by the kidney approximates the GFR. Normal creatinine clearance varies with age and is approximately 20% higher in men than in women. Normal finding is 1.42–2.25 mL/sec (85–135 mL/min).	Collect 24-hr urine specimen. Discard sample from first urination when test is started. Save urine from all subsequent urinations for 24 hr. Instruct patient to urinate at end of 24 hr and add that specimen to collection. Ensure that serum creatinine clearance is determined during 24-hr period.
Urine for culture and sensitivity (C&S) ("clean catch," "midstream")	This test is performed to confirm suspected urinary tract infection and identify causative organisms. Normally, the bladder is sterile, but the urethra contains bacteria and a few WBCs. If the specimen is properly collected, stored, and handled, the following can be expected: <10 000 organisms/mL usually indicates no infection; 10 000–100 000/mL is usually not diagnostic and the test may have to be repeated; and >100 000/mL indicates infection.	Use a sterile container for collection of urine. Touch only outside of the container. For women, separate labia with one hand and clean meatus with the other hand, using at least three sponges (saturated with cleansing solution) in a front-to-back motion. For men, retract foreskin (if present) and cleanse glans with at least three cleansing sponges (saturated with cleansing solution). After cleaning, instruct patient to start urinating and then continue voiding in sterile container. (The initial voided urine flushes out most contaminants in the urethra and the perineal area.) Catheterization may be needed if the patient is unable to do this procedure.
Concentration test	Study is an evaluation of renal concentration ability. Concentration is measured from specific gravity readings. Normal finding is 1.020–1.035.	Instruct patient to fast after a given time in the evening (in usual procedure). Collect three urine specimens at hourly intervals in the morning.
Residual urine	This test is a determination of amount of urine left in bladder after urination. The finding may be abnormal in patients who have difficulties with bladder enervation, sphincter impairment, BPH, equine syndrome (nerve compression), or urethral strictures. Normal finding is ≤50 mL urine (increases with age).	If a residual urine test is ordered, catheterize patient immediately after patient urinates, or use bladder ultrasonography equipment, including a portable scanner. If a large amount of residual urine is obtained, the health care provider may order the catheter to be left in the bladder.
Protein dipstick determination (Albustix, Combistix)	This test detects protein (primarily albumin) in urine. Normal finding is grade 0 to trace amounts.	Dip end of stick in urine, and read result by comparison with colour chart on the label as directed. Grading is from 0 to 4+. Interpret with caution. A positive result may not indicate significant proteinuria; some medications may produce false-positive readings.
Quantitative test for protein	A 12- or 24-hr collection yields a more accurate indication of the amount of protein in urine. Persistent proteinuria usually indicates glomerular renal disease. Normal finding is <0.15 g/24 hr (<150 mg/24 hr), and protein consists mainly of albumin.	Perform 12- or 24-hr urine collection.
Urine cytology	This test is used to identify changes in cellular structure indicative of malignancy, especially bladder cancer.	Obtain urine and send immediately to the laboratory. The first morning specimen should not be used.
Blood Tests		
Bicarbonate (HCO_3^-)	Most patients in renal failure have metabolic acidosis and low serum HCO_3^- levels. Normal finding is 21–28 mmol/L.	Explain the test and watch for postpuncture bleeding.
Blood urea nitrogen (BUN)	This test is most commonly used to identify presence of renal conditions. Concentration of urea in blood is regulated by the rate at which the kidney excretes urea. Normal finding is 3.6–7.1 mmol/L.	When interpreting BUN, the nurse should be aware that nonrenal factors (e.g., rapid cell destruction from infections, fever, GI bleeding, trauma, athletic activity and excessive muscle breakdown, corticosteroid therapy) may cause an increase in BUN level. A low BUN level could result from overhydration or advanced liver disease.
Creatinine	This study is more reliable than BUN as a determinant of renal function. Creatinine is an end product of muscle and protein metabolism and is liberated at a constant rate. Normal values: 53–106 mcmol/L for men, 44–97 mcmol/L for women. Normal finding is 44–133 mcmol/L.	Explain the test and watch for postpuncture bleeding.
Glomerular filtration rate (GFR)	Normal finding is about 125 mL/min.	
Urea-to-creatinine ratio	Normal finding is 10:1.	—
Calcium (Ca^{2+})	Calcium is the main mineral in bone and aids in muscle contraction, neurotransmission, and clotting. In renal disease, decreased reabsorption of Ca^{2+} leads to renal osteodystrophy. Normal calcium levels in adults range from 2.25 to 2.75 mmol/L.	Explain the test and watch for postpuncture bleeding.

Continued

TABLE 47.8 **DIAGNOSTIC STUDIES**
Urinary System—cont'd

Study	Description and Purpose	Nursing Responsibility
Potassium (K⁺)	Kidneys are responsible for excreting the majority of the body's potassium. In renal disease, K⁺ determinations are critical because K⁺ is one of the first electrolytes whose levels become abnormal. Highly elevated K⁺ levels (>6 mmol/L) can lead to muscle weakness and cardiac dysrhythmias. Normal values are 3.5–5 mmol/L.	Explain the test and watch for postpuncture bleeding.
Phosphorus	Phosphorus balance is inversely related to Ca^{2+} balance. In renal disease, phosphorus levels are elevated because the kidney is the primary excretory organ. Normal values are 0.97–1.45 mmol/L.	Explain the test and watch for postpuncture bleeding.
Sodium (Na⁺)	Sodium is the main extracellular electrolyte determining blood volume. Values usually stay within normal range until late stages of renal failure. Normal finding is 135–145 mmol/L.	Explain the test and watch for postpuncture bleeding.
Uric acid	This study is used as a screening test primarily for disorders of purine metabolism but can indicate kidney disease as well. Values depend on renal function and rate of purine metabolism and dietary intake of food rich in purines. Normal findings are 160–430 mcmol/L for women and 340–501 mcmol/L for men.	Explain the test and watch for postpuncture bleeding.

Radiological Procedures

Study	Description and Purpose	Nursing Responsibility
Kidneys, ureters, bladder (KUB)	This study involves radiographic examination of the abdomen and pelvis and delineates size, shape, and position of kidneys.	Perform bowel preparation (if ordered).
Intravenous pyelography (IVP)	Radiographic examination visualizes the urinary tract after IV injection of contrast material.	Assess renal function. If BUN and creatinine levels are elevated, use of contrast dye in diagnostic procedure may not be safe. The evening before the procedure, administer cathartic or enema to empty the colon of feces and gas. Keep patient on NPO status 8 hr before procedure. Before the procedure, assess patient for iodine sensitivity to avoid anaphylactic reaction. Inform patient that the procedure involves lying on a table and having serial radiographs taken. After the procedure, encourage oral intake of fluids (if permitted) to flush out contrast material.
Nephrotomography	Radiograph is performed with rotating tubes. This test delineates segments of the kidney at different levels. Multiple exposures are obtained to visualize specific sections of the kidney after IV injection of contrast material.	Explain the procedure and prepare patient as for IVP.
Retrograde pyelography	Radiograph of urinary tract is performed after injection of contrast material into kidneys. A cystoscope is inserted, and ureteral catheters are inserted through it into the renal pelvis. Contrast material is injected through the catheters.	Prepare patient as for IVP. Inform patient that pain may be experienced from distension of pelvis and discomfort from cystoscope. Inform patient that anaesthetic may be administered for procedure.
Renal arteriography (angiography)	This study helps visualize renal blood vessels. Contrast material is injected into the renal artery via a catheter inserted into the femoral artery.	Prepare patient the evening before the procedure by administering cathartic or enema. Before injection of contrast material, test for iodine sensitivity. After the procedure, check insertion site for bleeding, and measure peripheral pulses in involved leg every 30–60 min to detect occluded blood flow, if any.
Renal ultrasonography	A small external ultrasound probe is placed on patient's skin. Conductive gel is applied to the skin. Noninvasive procedure involves passing sound waves into body structures and recording images as the waves are reflected back. Computer software interprets tissue density on the basis of sound waves and displays it in picture form. This study is most valuable in detection of renal or perirenal masses and in differential diagnosis of renal cysts, solid masses, and identification of obstructions. It can be used safely in patients with renal failure.	Explain procedure to patient.
Computed tomography (CT)	This study provides excellent visualization of the kidneys. Kidney size can be evaluated; tumours, abscesses, suprarenal masses (e.g., adrenal tumours, pheochromocytomas), and obstructions can be detected. The advantage of CT over ultrasonography is its ability to distinguish subtle differences in density. Use of IV-administered contrast medium during CT accentuates density of renal tissue and helps differentiate masses.	Explain procedure to patient and ask patient about iodine sensitivity before injection of contrast material.

TABLE 47.8   DIAGNOSTIC STUDIES
Urinary System—cont'd

Study	Description and Purpose	Nursing Responsibility
Magnetic resonance imaging (MRI)	Computer-generated images rely on radiofrequency waves and alteration in magnetic field. MRI is useful for visualization of kidneys. It has not been proved useful for detecting urinary calculi or calcified tumours.	Explain procedure to patient. Have patient remove all metal objects. Patients with a history of claustrophobia may need to be sedated.
Cystography	The purpose of this study is to visualize the bladder and evaluate vesicoureteral reflux. Contrast material is instilled into the bladder via a cystoscope or catheter.	Explain procedure to patient. If procedure is performed via cystoscope, follow nursing care related to cystoscopy.
Renal Radionuclide Imaging		
Renal scan	The purpose of the scan is to show blood flow, glomerular filtration, tubular function, and excretion. Radioactive isotopes are injected by IV route. Radiation detector probes are placed over the kidney, and a scintillation counter monitors radioactive material in kidney. Radioisotope distribution in kidney is scanned and mapped. This test is useful in showing location, size, and shape of the kidney and, in general, assessing blood perfusion and the kidney's ability to secrete urine. Abscesses, cysts, and tumours may appear as cold spots because of presence of nonfunctioning tissue.	Scan requires no dietary or activity restriction. Inform patient that no pain or discomfort should be felt during test.
Surgical Study		
Renal biopsy	The purpose of this study is to obtain renal tissue for examination to determine type of renal disease or to monitor progress of renal disease. This technique is usually performed percutaneously (skin biopsy) through needle insertion into the lower lobe of the kidney. It can be guided by CT or ultrasonography.	Before the procedure, ascertain coagulation status through patient's history, medication history, CBC, hematocrit, prothrombin time, and bleeding and clotting times. Type and crossmatch for blood. Ensure consent form is signed. After the procedure, apply pressure dressing to biopsy site and check frequently for bleeding. Measure vital signs frequently. Observe urine for gross bleeding. Determine microscopic bleeding by use of dipstick. Assess patient for flank pain. Monitor hematocrit levels.
Endoscopy		
Cystoscopy	This study involves use of tubular lighted cystoscope to inspect bladder. Lithotomy position is used. The study may be performed while patient receives local or general anaesthesia, depending on needs and condition of the patient.	Before the procedure, force fluids or administer IV fluids if general anaesthesia is to be used. Ensure that consent form is signed. Explain procedure to patient. Administer preoperative medication. After the procedure, explain that burning on urination, pink-tinged urine, and urinary frequency are expected effects after cystoscopy. Do not let patient walk alone immediately after procedure because orthostatic hypotension may occur. Offer warm sitz baths, heat, and mild analgesics to relieve discomfort.
Urodynamics Testing		
Cystometrography	The purpose of the study is to evaluate bladder tone, sensations of filling, and bladder (detrusor) stability. The study involves insertion of a catheter and instillation of water or saline solution into the bladder. Measurements of pressure exerted against the bladder wall are recorded.	Explain procedure to patient and observe patient for manifestations of urinary infection after procedure.

BPH, benign prostatic hyperplasia; *CBC*, complete blood cell count; *GFR*, glomerular filtration rate; *eGFR*, estimated glomerular filtration rate; *GI*, gastrointestinal; *IV*, intravenous; *NPO*, nothing by mouth; *WBC*, white blood cell.

Creatinine levels remain remarkably constant for each person because they are not significantly affected by protein ingestion, muscular exercise, water intake, or rate of urine production. Normal creatinine clearance values range from 1.42 to 2.25 mL/sec (85–135 mL/min). After age 40, the creatinine clearance rate decreases at a rate of about 1 mL/min/yr.

Urine Cytology. Urine can be checked for abnormal cellular structures that occur with bladder cancer. Specimens may be obtained from voiding, catheterization, or bladder irrigation (bladder washing). The first morning's voided specimen should not be used because epithelial cells may change in appearance in urine held in the bladder overnight. As with urinalysis, the specimen should be fresh or brought to the laboratory within the hour. An alcohol-based fixative is then added to preserve the cellular structure. Urine cytological study is used for detection and monitoring the prognosis of bladder cancer.

Radiological Studies
Diagnostic urine studies are summarized in Table 47.8.

TABLE 47.9	**URINALYSIS FINDINGS**	
Evaluation	**Normal Finding**	**Abnormal Findings and Significance**
Colour	Amber yellow	Dark, smoky colour suggests hematuria. Yellow-brown to olive green indicates excessive bilirubin. Cloudiness of freshly voided urine indicates infection. Colourless urine indicates excessive fluid intake, renal disease, or diabetes insipidus.
Smell	Aromatic	After urine has been standing, its smell becomes more ammonia-like. In urinary tract infections, urine smells unpleasant.
Protein	<0.15 g/day	Persistent proteinuria is characteristic of acute and chronic renal disease, especially involving glomeruli. In absence of disease, a positive reading may be caused by high-protein diet, strenuous exercise, dehydration, fever, or emotional stress. Vaginal secretions may contaminate the urine specimen and produce a positive reading.
Glucose	None	Glycosuria indicates diabetes mellitus or low renal threshold for glucose reabsorption (if blood glucose level is normal). Small amounts may be found after glucose loading (e.g., glucose tolerance test).
Ketones	None	Altered carbohydrate and fat metabolism indicates diabetes mellitus and starvation. Findings can also occur in dehydration, vomiting, and severe diarrhea.
Bilirubin	None	Bilirubinuria is as significant as jaundice in detection of liver disorders. Bilirubin may appear in urine before jaundice becomes visible or may be present in persons with hepatic disorders who do not have recognizable jaundice.*
Specific gravity	1.005–1.030 Maximum concentrating ability of kidney (1.025–1.030)	*Low:* dilute urine and possibly excessive diuresis *High:* dehydration *Fixed at about 1.010:* kidneys are unable to concentrate urine, which suggests that kidneys are progressing to end-stage renal disease
Osmolality (random specimen)	50–1 200 mmol/kg	Measurement of osmolality is more accurate than measurement of specific gravity for determining diluting and concentrating ability of kidneys. Deviations from normal indicate tubular dysfunction. Findings indicate whether kidney has lost ability to concentrate or dilute urine. (Not part of routine urinalysis)
pH	4.6–8.0 (average, 6.0)	A pH >8.0 may be the result of standing of urine or urinary tract infection because bacteria decompose urea to form ammonia. A pH <4.0 may indicate respiratory or metabolic acidosis.
RBC	0–4/hpf	Bleeding in the urinary tract is caused by calculi, cystitis, neoplasm, glomerulonephritis, tuberculosis, kidney biopsy, or trauma.
WBC	0–5/hpf	Increased number of WBCs in urine (pyuria) indicates urinary tract infection or inflammation.
Casts	None; occasional hyaline casts	Casts are moulds of the renal tubules and may contain protein, WBCs, RBCs, or bacteria. Noncellular casts are hyaline in appearance, and a few may be found in normal urine. Casts indicate renal dysfunction or upper urinary tract infection.
Culture for organisms	No organisms in bladder; count of <10^5 CFU/L organisms/mL is result of normal urethral flora	Bacteria counts >10^8 CFU/L indicate urinary tract infection. Organisms most commonly found in urinary tract infections are *Escherichia coli*, enterococci, *Klebsiella* species, *Proteus* species, and streptococci.

CFU, colony-forming unit; *hpf*, high-powered field (or what can be seen in one view of the slide through the microscope); *RBC*, red blood cells; *WBC*, white blood cells.
*See Chapter 46 for further discussion.

Kidney, Ureter, and Bladder Radiography. The kidney, ureter, and bladder (KUB) radiograph is an abdominal view obtained without use of a contrast medium to show the renal outline, the psoas shadow, and the full bladder. Radiopaque stones and foreign bodies can be seen on this radiograph. The form, size, and position of the kidneys can also be seen. Abscesses, tumours, and cysts may distort anatomical relationships on the KUB image. Sometimes nephrotomography (sectional views that focus on a single plane of the kidney) is ordered at the same time as the KUB study to maximize visualization of the kidneys.

Intravenous Pyelography. Intravenous pyelography (IVP), or excretory urography, enables visualization of the urinary tract. The presence, position, size, and shape of the kidneys, the ureters, and the bladder can be evaluated. Cysts, tumours, lesions, and obstructions cause a distortion in the normal appearance of these structures.

The procedure consists of injecting an IV dose of contrast material, which circulates in the blood and is excreted by the kidneys into the urine. As with all contrast studies, possible iodine and shellfish allergies should be determined before the study. During injection, the patient may experience sensations of warmth, facial flushing, and a salty taste. After injection,

radiographs are taken sequentially. The sequencing of images is planned so that contrast excretion can be followed from the cortex of the kidney to the bladder. The presence of bladder atony or outlet obstruction also can be detected by an image obtained after urination, which shows the residual volume of urine in the bladder.

Patients with significantly decreased renal function should not undergo IVP because the contrast material is not properly excreted by the kidneys. Contrast medium can also be nephrotoxic and can worsen renal function.

Retrograde Pyelography. Retrograde pyelography is the radiographic visualization of the kidneys, the ureter, and the bladder after direct injection of contrast material into the kidney via a ureteral catheter introduced through a cystoscope. It may be performed if the urinary tract cannot be visualized using IVP or if the patient is allergic to IV contrast material or has decreased renal function. The risks associated with retrograde pyelography are similar to those related to cystoscopy, including the risk for infection and the use of anaesthetics.

Antegrade Pyelography. Antegrade pyelography is performed to evaluate the upper urinary tract when the patient has an allergy to contrast media, when renal function is decreased, or when abnormalities prevent passage of a ureteral catheter. Contrast media may be injected percutaneously into the renal pelvis or via a nephrostomy tube that is already in place (this method is also called *nephrostography*) when tube function or ureteral integrity must be determined after trauma or surgery. Complications of antegrade pyelography include hematuria, infection, and hematoma.

Renal Ultrasonography. Renal ultrasonography involves use of high-frequency sound waves to image the kidneys, the ureter, and the bladder. Because radiation exposure is avoided, a number of images can be obtained, and studies can be repeated over a brief period. Images can be obtained with the patient in both the prone and the supine positions. A bowel preparation is not required for renal ultrasonography.

Computed Tomography. Computed tomographic (CT) scanning of the abdomen and the pelvis may be performed to detect tumours and possible metastases. A CT can differentiate these from cysts or abscesses. Contrast material may be used to help visualize urinary structures more clearly in the computer-generated images. The patient is instructed to lie very still during the procedure while the machine takes precise transaxial images. Sedation may be required if the patient is unable to remain still.

Renal Arteriography. The purpose of renal arteriography (angiography) is to visualize the renal blood vessels. In this radiological study, contrast material is injected into the renal artery via a catheter inserted into the femoral artery. The findings in arteriography can assist in diagnosing renal artery stenosis (Figure 47.9), additional or missing renal blood vessels, and renovascular hypertension and can assist in differentiating between a renal cyst and a renal tumour. Renal arteriography is also included in the workup of a potential renal transplant donor.

The patient is given a local anaesthetic at the site of catheter insertion. Usually, a catheter is inserted into the femoral artery and passed up the aorta to the level of the renal arteries (Figure 47.10). Contrast media is then injected to outline the renal blood supply, and radiographic images are taken.

The patient may experience a transient warm feeling along the course of the blood vessel when the contrast material is injected. After the catheter is removed, a pressure dressing is placed over the femoral injection site. It is important to observe the site for bleeding. Usually, bed rest with the affected leg kept straight is prescribed. Peripheral pulses in the involved leg should be measured at least every 30 to 60 minutes to detect occlusion of blood flow caused by a thrombus, if any. Complications that may result from renal arteriography include thrombus, embolus, local inflammation, and hematoma. Patients with baseline renal insufficiency may experience a decrease in renal function secondary to the nephrotoxic contrast material.

Cystography. The purpose of cystography is to outline and visualize the bladder and evaluate the UVJ for reflux. In addition to suspected vesicoureteral reflux, indications for cystography include a neurogenic bladder and recurrent urinary tract infections. Cystography can also delineate abnormalities of the bladder, such as diverticula, calculi, and tumours. In this procedure, a contrast material is instilled via a cystoscope or catheter into the bladder.

Voiding cystourethrography (VCUG) is a voiding study of the bladder opening (bladder neck) and urethra. The bladder is filled with contrast material. During urination, images are

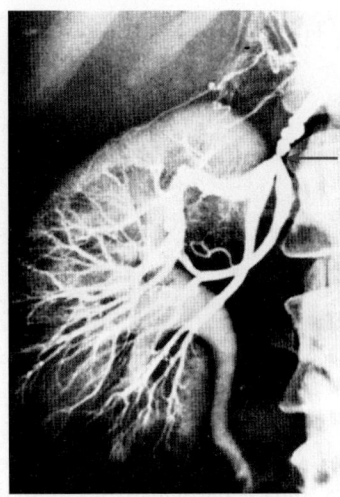

FIG. 47.9 Renal arteriogram showing stenosis *(arrow)* of the right renal artery. Source: Brundage, D. J. (1992). *Renal disorders*. Mosby.

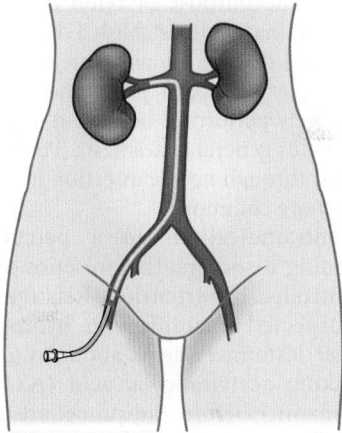

FIG. 47.10 Diagram of catheter insertion for renal arteriography.

obtained to visualize the bladder and the urethra. After urination, another image is obtained to assess for residual urine. VCUG can be used to detect abnormalities of the lower urinary tract, urethral stenosis, bladder neck obstruction, and prostatic enlargement (Rosier et al., 2017).

Urethrography. Urethrography is similar to cystography. Contrast material is injected in a retrograde manner into the urethra to identify strictures, diverticula, or other urethral pathological conditions. When urethral trauma is suspected, urethrography is performed before catheterization.

Loopography. Loopography is used to detect obstructions, anastomotic leaks, stones, reflux, and other uropathological features when a patient has a urinary pouch or ileal conduit. Because urinary diversions are created with sections of bowel, contrast absorption is a risk. The patient should be closely monitored for reactions to the contrast media.

Renal Radionuclide Imaging. Renal scans involving the use of radionuclides are useful in evaluating the anatomical structures, perfusion, and function of the kidneys. The results reveal the difference between the two kidneys with regard to blood flow, tubular function, and excretion. A normal scan shows symmetrical functioning of both kidneys. Normally, the distribution of activity is recorded throughout the kidneys. A lesion (e.g., a tumour) is indicated by the absence of radioactivity in

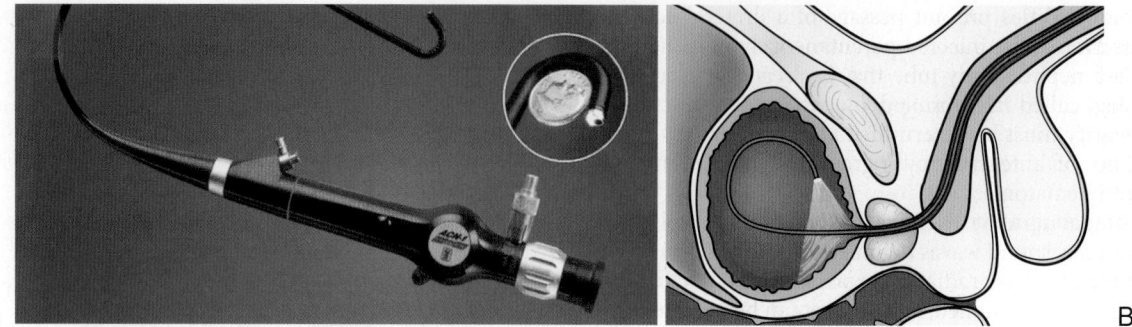

FIG. 47.11 Cystoscopic examination of the bladder. **A,** Flexible cystonephroscope. **B,** Illustration of nephroscope inserted into male bladder. Source: Courtesy Circon Corp., Santa Barbara, California.

the involved area and the appearance of the resultant defect on the scan. This study is particularly useful in detecting renal vascular disease, acute renal failure, and upper urinary tract obstruction. It is also useful in monitoring the function of a transplanted kidney.

Renal Biopsy. The purpose of renal biopsy is to obtain renal tissue for examination to establish a diagnosis or to monitor progress of renal disease. Biopsy material can be obtained through open biopsy or closed percutaneous needle biopsy. Open biopsy is rarely performed because it is a surgical procedure that necessitates general anaesthesia. Percutaneous needle biopsy, conducted through needle insertion into the lower lobe of the kidney, is more common.

Absolute contraindications to a percutaneous renal biopsy are bleeding disorders, the presence of a single kidney, and uncontrolled hypertension. Relative contraindications include suspected renal infection, hydronephrosis, and possible vascular lesions. Patients about to undergo biopsy should stop taking acetylsalicylic acid (ASA; Aspirin) or warfarin (Coumadin) before the procedure as advised by their physicians.

In this procedure, the patient lies prone with a pillow or sandbag to elevate the abdomen and the kidneys. The position of the kidney is marked on the body, under guidance with CT, IVP, or ultrasonography. Local anaesthetic is used, and a biopsy needle is inserted into the kidney just below the twelfth rib. The patient is instructed to hold their breath while the biopsy specimen is being taken.

After the procedure, a pressure dressing is applied, and the patient is kept prone for 30 to 60 minutes. Usually bed rest is prescribed for 24 hours. Vital signs should be measured every 5 to 10 minutes during the first hour and then, if no health problems are noted, with decreasing frequency. The biopsy site should be inspected frequently for bleeding. Serial urine specimens should be assessed for gross and microscopic hematuria. A dipstick can be used to test for bleeding, even when hematuria is not obvious. The physician may order all urine sent for laboratory analysis to detect possible hematuria. The patient should be assessed for flank pain, hypotension, decreasing hematocrit, and temperature elevation and should also be observed for chills, urinary frequency, and dysuria.

Complications of a renal biopsy include renal hemorrhage, hematoma, and infection. Even if no complications occur, the patient should be instructed to avoid lifting heavy objects for 5 to 7 days after the procedure. The patient should be instructed not to take any anticoagulant medications until permission is given by the physician who performed the biopsy.

Endoscopy

Cystoscopy. Cystoscopy is a radiological bladder procedure in which contrast material is instilled into the bladder. The main purpose is to inspect the interior of the bladder and evaluate the vesicoureteral reflux with a tubular lighted endoscope called a *cystoscope* (Figure 47.11). Cystoscopes can be used to insert ureteral catheters, remove calculi, obtain biopsy specimens of bladder lesions, and treat bleeding lesions. In most cases, bladder disorders can be determined by cystoscopic examination.

Cystoscopy is usually performed in a cystoscopy room in the radiology department, in a urology clinic, or in the operating room. Most of the pain associated with cystoscopy results from spasms and contractions of bladder and sphincter. Some of the bladder and sphincter spasms may be alleviated if the patient uses relaxation and deep breathing. A local anaesthetic is instilled into the urethra before cystoscope insertion. During the examination, saline solution is instilled slowly to distend the bladder. This improves visualization but causes an urge to urinate.

After the procedure, the patient can expect to have some burning on urination, blood-tinged urine, and urinary frequency from the irritation of cystoscope insertion and manipulation. The nurse should observe for bright red bleeding, which is not normal. After the procedure, the nurse is responsible for keeping the patient well hydrated, administering mild analgesics, providing sitz baths (a warm, shallow bath to cleanse the perineum), and applying heat to decrease the patient's discomfort. Complications that may result from cystoscopy include urinary retention, urinary tract hemorrhage, bladder infection, and perforation of the bladder.

Urodynamics Testing

Urodynamics testing is a set of studies designed to measure urinary tract function. Urodynamic tests entail study of the storage of urine within the bladder and the flow of urine through the urinary tract to the outside of the body. A combination of techniques may be used to provide a detailed assessment of urinary incontinence.

Urinary Flow Study. The *urinary flow study (uroflow)* entails measurement of urine volume in a single voiding, expelled in a specified time and expressed in millilitres per second. As the patient voids, the stream pattern is depicted graphically on a printout.

The patient is asked to start the test with a reasonably full bladder, urinate into a special container, and try to empty the bladder completely. The container generates a graph in which flow rate is compared to time. This test is used to (a) assess the degree of outflow obstruction caused by such conditions as benign prostatic hyperplasia or stricture, (b) assess bladder or sphincter dysfunction effects on voiding such as occurs with neuropathological conditions, and (c) evaluate the effects of treatment for lower urinary tract conditions. Residual urine volume should be measured immediately after a urinary flow study to help identify the degree of chronic urinary retention that is often associated with abnormal flow patterns.

A normal maximum flow rate is about 20 to 25 mL/sec for men and about 25 to 30 mL/sec for women. However, the volume voided and the patient's age can affect the flow rate; thus variations are normal and common. Graphic displays can illustrate straining and intermittent flow patterns or other abnormal voiding disorders.

Cystometrography. Cystometrography is an evaluation of the compliance (elastic property) and stability of the detrusor muscle of the bladder, as well as bladder tone, sensations of filling, and bladder (detrusor) instability. It is a measurement of intravesical pressure during the course of bladder filling. Usually, it is ordered if a patient has incontinence or neurogenic bladder. The procedure consists of insertion of a specially designed catheter while the patient is in a supine position. If abdominal pressure is also to be measured, a second tube is inserted into the rectum or the vagina. This tube is typically attached to a small, fluid-filled balloon to allow pressure recording. Saline or sterile water for irrigation, or contrast used for cystography, is infused into the bladder, and pressures are measured. During the infusion, the patient is asked about sensations of bladder filling, usually including the first urge to urinate, a strong urge to urinate, and perception of bladder fullness.

Sphincter Electromyography. In electromyography (EMG), the electrical activity created when the nervous system stimulates motor units within a muscle is recorded. Through the placement of needles, percutaneous wires, or patches near the urethra, the pelvic floor muscle activity can be assessed. During filling cystometrography, sphincter EMG is used to identify voluntary pelvic floor muscle contractions and the response of these muscles to bladder filling, coughing, and other provocative manoeuvres.

Voiding Pressure Flow Study. The voiding pressure flow study combines a urinary flow rate, cystometric pressures (intravesical, abdominal, and detrusor pressures), and a sphincter EMG for detailed evaluation of micturition. It is completed by assisting the patient to a specialized toilet and allowing them to urinate while the various pressure tubes and EMG apparatus remain in place.

Video-Urodynamics Testing. Video-urodynamics testing is a combination of the filling cystometrography, sphincter EMG, or urinary flow study (or both of the latter tests) with anatomical imaging of the lower urinary tract, typically via fluoroscopy. This combination is used in selected cases to identify an obstructive lesion and characterize anatomical changes in the bladder and lower urinary tract.

Radionuclide Cystography

Radionuclide cystography is used to detect and grade vesicoureteral reflux. Similar to VCUG, a small dose of radioisotope tracer is instilled into the bladder via urethral catheter. The procedure is more sensitive than VCUG, and the radiation dose is one-thousandth that used in VCUG.

Whitaker Test. Whitaker test is used to measure the pressure differential between the renal pelvis and the bladder. The presence of a ureteral obstruction can be assessed. Percutaneous access to the renal pelvis is achieved by placement of a catheter in the renal pelvis. A catheter is also placed in the bladder. Fluid is perfused through the percutaneous tube or needle at a rate of 10 mL/min. Pressure data are then collected. These pressure measurements are studied in combination with fluoroscopic imaging to identify the level of obstruction.

◾ REVIEW QUESTIONS

The number of the question corresponds to the same-numbered objective at the beginning of the chapter.

1. Which of the following is affected by a renal stone in the pelvis of the kidney?
   a. The structural support of the kidney
   b. Regulation of the concentration of urine
   c. The entry and exit of blood vessels at the kidney
   d. Collection and drainage of urine from the kidney

2. A client with renal disease has oliguria and a creatinine clearance rate of 40 mL/min. Which of the following functions of the kidney is most directly implicated in these abnormal findings?
   a. Tubular secretion
   b. Glomerular filtration
   c. Capillary permeability
   d. Concentration of filtrate

3. Which of the following conditions might place a client at risk for urinary calculi?
   a. Adrenal insufficiency
   b. Serotonin deficiency
   c. Hyperaldosteronism
   d. Hyperparathyroidism

4. Which of the following are normal changes associated with aging of the urinary system that the nurse would assess in an older person?
   a. Decreased levels of blood urea nitrogen
   b. Postvoiding residual urine
   c. Increased bladder capacity
   d. More easily palpable kidneys

5. Which of the following does the nurse undertake during physical assessment of the urinary system?
   a. Percussion of the flank area with a firm blow
   b. Palpation of an empty bladder as a small nodule
   c. Prone positioning of the client to palpate the kidneys
   d. Auscultation to determine the level of urine in the bladder

6. Identify the normal urinary system physical assessment findings. *(Select all that apply.)*
   a. Nonpalpable left kidney
   b. Auscultation of renal artery bruit
   c. CVA tenderness elicited by a kidney punch
   d. No CVA tenderness elicited by a kidney punch
   e. Palpable bladder to the level of the symphysis pubis

7. Which of the following is an important nursing responsibility after IVP?
   a. Assessment of the client for flank pain
   b. Encouragement of extra oral fluid intake
   c. Observation of urine for remaining contrast material
   d. Encouragement of ambulation 2 to 3 hours after the study
8. Which of the following would the nurse expect to find on reading the urinalysis results of a dehydrated client?
   a. A pH of 8.4
   b. RBC measurement of 4 per high-powered field
   c. Colour and appearance: yellow, cloudy
   d. Specific gravity of 1.035

1. d; 2. b; 3. d; 4. b; 5. a; 6. a; 7. b; 8. d.

⊜volve

For even more review questions, visit http://evolve.elsevier.com/Canada/Lewis/medsurg.

REFERENCES

Aoki, Y., Brown, H. W., Brubaker, L., et al. (2017). Urinary incontinence in women. *Nature Reviews Disease Primers*, 3(1), 1–20. https://doi.org/10.1038/nrdp.2017.42

Bodner-Adler, B., Bodner, K., Kimberger, O., et al. (2017). Role of serum steroid hormones in women with stress urinary incontinence: A case–control study. *BJU International*, 120(3), 416–421. https://doi.org/10.1111/bju.13902

Denic, A., Lieske, J. C., Chakkera, H. A., et al. (2017). The substantial loss of nephrons in healthy human kidneys with aging. *Journal of the American Society of Nephrology*, 28(1), 313–320. https:// doi.org/10.1681/ASN.2016020154

Huether, S. E., & El-Hussein, M. (2018). Structure and function of the renal and urological systems. In M. El-Hussein, K. Power-Keen, S. Zettel, et al. (Eds.), *Understanding pathophysiology* (1st Canadian ed., pp. 741–756). Elsevier.

McCance, K. L., & Huether, S. E. (2019). *Pathophysiology: The biologic basis for disease in adults and children* (8th ed.). Elsevier.

National Kidney Foundation. (n.d.). *Frequently asked questions about GFR estimates.* https://www.kidney.org/sites/default/files/docs/12-10-4004_abe_faqs_aboutgfrrev1b_singleb.pdf

Rosier, P., Schaefer, W., Lose, G., et al. (2017). International Continence Society good urodynamic practices and terms 2016: Urodynamics, uroflowmetry, cystometry, and pressure-flow study. *Neurourology and Urodynamics*, 36(5), 1243–1260. https://doi.org/10.1002/nau.23124

Smith, H. W. (1953). *Fish to philosopher*. Little, Brown. (Seminal).

Spencer, M., McManus, K., & Sabourin, J. (2017). Incontinence in older adults: The role of the geriatric multidisciplinary team. *BCMJ*, 59(2), 99–105.

Stewart, E. (2018). Assessment and management of urinary incontinence in women. *Nursing Standard*, 33(2), 75–81. https://doi.org/10.7748/ns.2018.e11148

Wagner, K., Hardin-Pierce, M., Welsh, D., et al. (2019). *High acuity nursing* (7th ed.). Pearson.

RESOURCES

Resources for this chapter are listed in Chapters 48 and 49.

Nursing Management
Renal and Urological Conditions

Kathleen Rodger and Lynn Jansen
Originating US chapter by Cynthia Ann Smith

evolve WEBSITE

http://evolve.elsevier.com/Canada/Lewis/medsurg

- Review Questions (Online Only)
- Key Points
- Answer Guidelines for Case Study
- Student Case Studies
  - Bladder Cancer and Urinary Diversion
  - Glomerulo-Nephritis and Acute Kidney Injury

- Customizable Nursing Care Plans
  - Acute Renal Lithiasis
  - Ileal Conduit
  - Urinary Tract Infection

- Conceptual Care Map Creator
- Audio Glossary
- Content Updates

LEARNING OBJECTIVES

1. Describe the pathophysiology and clinical manifestations of and interprofessional care and medication therapy for cystitis, urethritis, and pyelonephritis.
2. Explain the nursing management of urinary tract infections.
3. Describe the immunological mechanisms involved in glomerulonephritis.
4. Explain the clinical manifestations and the nursing and interprofessional management of acute poststreptococcal glomerulonephritis, Goodpasture's syndrome, and chronic glomerulonephritis.
5. Describe the common causes, clinical manifestations, and nursing management of nephrotic syndrome and interprofessional care of patients with nephrotic syndrome.
6. Compare and contrast the etiology, clinical manifestations, and interprofessional and nursing management of various types of urinary calculi.
7. Explain the common causes and management of renal trauma, renal vascular conditions, and hereditary renal disorders.
8. Describe the mechanisms of renal involvement in metabolic and connective tissue disorders.
9. Describe the clinical manifestations of kidney and bladder cancers and the interprofessional care for patients with these cancers.
10. Describe the common causes and management of bladder dysfunctions.
11. Differentiate among ureteral, suprapubic, nephrostomy, and urethral catheters with regard to indications for use and nursing responsibilities.
12. Explain the nursing and interprofessional management of the patient undergoing nephrectomy or urinary diversion surgery.

KEY TERMS

calculus
cystitis
glomerulonephritis
Goodpasture's syndrome
hydronephrosis
hydroureter
ileal conduit

interstitial cystitis (IC)
lithotripsy
nephrolithiasis
nephrosclerosis
nephrotic syndrome
polycystic kidney disease (PKD)
pyelonephritis

renal artery stenosis
renal vein thrombosis
stricture
urethritis
urinary incontinence (UI)
urinary retention

Renal and urological disorders encompass a wide spectrum of clinical conditions. The diverse causes of these disorders may involve infectious, immunological, obstructive, metabolic, collagen-related, and vascular, traumatic, congenital, neoplastic, and neurological mechanisms. This chapter discusses specific disorders of the kidneys, ureters, bladder, and urethra. Acute kidney injury and chronic kidney disease are discussed in Chapter 49. Female reproductive conditions are discussed in Chapter 56. Male reproductive conditions are discussed in Chapter 57.

INFECTIOUS AND INFLAMMATORY DISORDERS OF THE URINARY SYSTEM

URINARY TRACT INFECTION

Urinary tract infections (UTIs) are the second most common bacterial disease and the most common bacterial infection in women. In the older population, the prevalence of UTI varies from 30 to 50% in women and 25 to 40% in men. In some

TABLE 48.1	COMMON MICRO-ORGANISMS CAUSING URINARY TRACT INFECTIONS

- *Escherichia coli**
- *Candida*
- *Enterobacter*
- *Enterococcus*
- *Klebsiella*
- *Proteus*
- *Pseudomonas*
- *Serratia*
- *Staphylococcus*

*Causes about 80% of infections in persons who do not have urinary tract structural abnormalities or calculi.

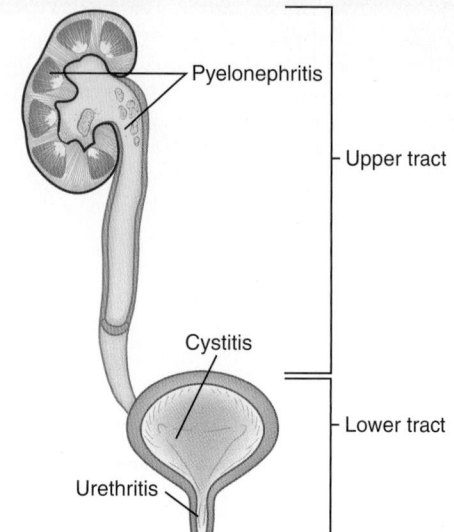

FIG. 48.1 Sites of infectious processes in the urinary tract.

cases, patients who develop Gram-negative bacteremia die, and one third of these cases are caused by bacterial infections originating in the urinary tract (National Institute of Diabetes and Digestive and Kidney Diseases [NIDDK], 2017).

Inflammation of the urinary tract may be attributable to a variety of disorders, but bacterial infection is by far the most common. In the majority of healthy persons, the bladder and its contents are free from bacteria. Nevertheless, a number of otherwise healthy individuals, including many younger and older women as well as men, have some bacteria colonizing the bladder. This condition is called *asymptomatic bacteriuria* and does not warrant treatment. In contrast, an infection of the urinary system is diagnosed when bacterial invasion of the urinary tract occurs. Bacterial counts of 10^5 colony-forming units per millilitre (CFU/mL) or higher typically indicate a clinically significant UTI. However, counts as low as 10^2 to 10^3 CFU/mL in a person with signs and symptoms are indicative of UTI.

Escherichia coli (E. coli) (Table 48.1) is the most common pathogen leading to a UTI. Although fungal and parasitic infections may also cause UTIs, they are uncommon. UTIs from these causes are sometimes observed in immunosuppressed patients, patients with diabetes mellitus, or patients who have undergone multiple courses of antibiotic therapy. They also may be seen in persons living in or having travelled to certain developing countries. Recurrent UTIs are one of the most common bacterial infections in women. Increased antibiotic resistance may be making treatment and prevention of UTIs difficult (Geerlings, 2017).

Classification

Several classification systems can be used for UTIs (Geerlings, 2017). For example, a UTI can be broadly classified as an *upper* or a *lower* UTI according to its location within the urinary system (Figure 48.1). Infection of the upper urinary tract (involving the renal parenchyma, renal pelvis, and ureters) typically causes fever, chills, and flank pain, whereas a UTI confined to the lower urinary tract does not usually have systemic manifestations. Specific terms are used to further delineate the location of a UTI or inflammation. For example, pyelonephritis implies inflammation (usually caused by infection) of the renal parenchyma and the collecting system. Cystitis indicates an inflammatory condition of the urinary bladder, characterized by pain, urgency and frequency of urination, and hematuria. Urethritis means inflammation of the urethra.

Classifying a UTI as complicated or uncomplicated is also useful. *Uncomplicated infections* are those that occur in an otherwise normal urinary tract (Geerlings, 2017). *Complicated*

infections include those that occur concurrently with obstruction, stones, or catheters; those that occur in patients with existing diabetes or neurological diseases; and recurrent infections. Patients with a complicated infection are at risk for renal damage.

UTIs can also be classified according to their natural history. An *initial infection* (sometimes called a *first* or an *isolated infection*) refers to an uncomplicated UTI in a person who has never had an infection or who experiences one that is remote from any previous UTI (usually separated by a period of years). In contrast, a *recurrent UTI* is a reinfection in a person who experienced a previous infection that was successfully eradicated. A recurrent UTI that occurs because the original infection was not adequately eradicated is classified as unresolved bacteriuria or bacterial persistence. *Unresolved bacteriuria* occurs when bacteria are initially resistant to the antibiotic used to treat an infection, when the antibiotic agent fails to achieve adequate concentrations in the urine or the bloodstream to kill bacteria, or when the antibiotic is discontinued before the underlying bacteriuria is completely eradicated. *Bacterial persistence* also may occur when bacteria develop resistance to the antibiotic agent selected for treatment or when a foreign body in the urinary system serves as a harbour or anchor allowing bacteria to survive despite appropriate therapy.

Etiology and Pathophysiology

The urinary tract above the urethra is normally sterile. Several physiological and mechanical defence mechanisms assist in maintaining sterility and preventing UTIs. These defences include normal voiding with complete emptying of the bladder, normal antibacterial capability of the bladder mucosa and urine, ureterovesical junction (UVJ) competence, and peristaltic activity that propels urine toward the bladder. An alteration in any of these defence mechanisms increases the risk of contracting a UTI. Table 48.2 lists predisposing factors to UTIs.

The organisms that usually cause UTIs are introduced via the ascending route from the urethra. Other, less common routes are via the bloodstream or the lymphatic system. Most infections are caused by Gram-negative bacilli normally found in

TABLE 48.2 PREDISPOSING FACTORS TO URINARY TRACT INFECTIONS

Factors Increasing Urinary Stasis
- Extrinsic obstruction (tumour, fibrosis compressing urinary tract)
- Intrinsic obstruction (stone, tumour of urinary tract)
- Urinary retention (including neurogenic bladder and low bladder-wall compliance)

Foreign Bodies
- In-dwelling catheter
- Ureteral stent (proximity of urethral and anal orifices)
- Urinary calculi

Anatomical Factors
- Congenital defects leading to obstruction or urinary stasis
- Fistula (abnormal opening) exposing urinary stream to skin, vagina, or fecal stream
- Shorter female urethra (proximity of urethral and anal orifices)

Factors Compromising Immune Response
- Diabetes mellitus
- Human immunodeficiency virus infection

Functional Disorders
- Constipation
- Voiding dysfunction with detrusor sphincter dyssynergia

TABLE 48.3 LOWER URINARY TRACT SYMPTOMS

Emptying Symptoms
- Dysuria—difficulty voiding
- Hesitancy—difficulty starting the urine stream, resulting in a delay between initiation of urination by relaxation of the urethral sphincter and the actual start of the urine stream
- Intermittency—interruption of the urinary stream while voiding
- Pain on urination
- Postvoid dribbling—urine loss after completion of voiding
- Urinary retention or incomplete emptying—inability to empty urine from the bladder, which can be caused by atonic bladder or obstruction of the urethra; can be acute or chronic
- Weak urinary stream

Storage Symptoms
- Incontinence—involuntary or unwanted loss or leakage of urine
- Nocturia—waking up two or more times at night because of the need or urge to void
- Nocturnal enuresis—loss of urine during sleep; called *bedwetting* in children
- Urgency—a sudden, strong, or intense desire to void immediately, usually accompanied by frequency
- Urinary frequency—an abnormally frequent (usually eight times in a 24-hr period) desire to void, often of only small quantities (e.g., <200 mL)

the gastrointestinal (GI) tract, although Gram-positive organisms such as streptococci, enterococci, and *Staphylococcus saprophyticus* can also cause urinary infections. A common factor contributing to ascending infection is urological instrumentation (e.g., catheterization, cystoscopic examinations). Instrumentation allows bacteria that are normally present at the opening of the urethra to enter the urethra or the bladder. Sexual intercourse promotes "milking" of bacteria from the vagina and the perineum and may cause minor urethral trauma that predisposes women to UTIs.

Rarely do UTIs result from a hematogenous route, where bloodborne bacteria secondarily invade the kidneys, the ureters, or the bladder from elsewhere in the body. For a kidney infection to occur from hematogenous transmission, there must be prior injury to the urinary tract, such as obstruction of a ureter, damage caused by stones, or renal scars.

An important source of UTIs is health care–acquired, or health care–associated, infection. The cause of health care–associated infection is often *E. coli* and, less frequently, *Pseudomonas* organisms. Urological instrumentation, particularly with an in-dwelling urinary catheter, is the most common predisposing factor.

Clinical Manifestations

Bothersome lower urinary tract symptoms (LUTS) are seen in UTIs of the upper urinary tracts as well as those confined to the lower tract. These symptoms are related to either bladder storage or bladder emptying. These symptoms are defined in Table 48.3. Symptoms include dysuria, frequency of urination (greater than every 2 hours), urgency, and suprapubic discomfort or pressure. The urine may contain grossly visible blood (hematuria) or sediment, giving it a cloudy appearance. Flank pain, chills, and the presence of a fever indicate an infection involving the upper urinary tract (pyelonephritis).

The symptoms that are commonly characteristic of a UTI are often absent in older persons. Older people tend to experience nonlocalized abdominal discomfort rather than dysuria and suprapubic pain (Froom & Shimoni, 2018). In addition, older persons may have cognitive impairment or delirium and therefore be unaware of any symptoms. Older people are also less likely to experience a fever with infection of the upper urinary tract. Patients older than age 80 years may experience a slight decline in temperature. People with significant bacteriuria may have no symptoms or may have nonspecific symptoms such as fatigue or anorexia.

Multiple factors may produce bothersome LUTS like those that can accompany a UTI. For example, patients with bladder tumours or those receiving intravesical chemotherapy or pelvic radiation usually experience urinary frequency, urgency, and dysuria. Interstitial cystitis, discussed later in this chapter, is a chronic inflammatory condition of unknown etiology also producing bothersome urinary symptoms that sometimes cause it to be confused with a UTI.

Diagnostic Studies

Dipstick urinalysis should be obtained initially to identify the presence of nitrites (indicating bacteriuria), white blood cells (WBCs), and leukocyte esterase (an enzyme present in WBCs). These findings can be confirmed by microscopic urinalysis. Following confirmation of bacteriuria and pyuria, a urine culture may be obtained. A urine culture is indicated in complicated or health care–associated UTIs, persistent bacteria, or frequently recurring UTIs (more than two to three episodes per year). Urine also may be cultured when the infection is unresponsive to empirical therapy or the diagnosis is questionable. A voided midstream technique yielding a clean-catch urine sample is preferred for obtaining a urine culture in most circumstances. (See Chapter 47, Table 47.8 for a description of this technique.) However, a specimen obtained by catheterization or suprapubic needle aspiration provides more accurate results and may be necessary when an adequate clean-catch specimen cannot be readily obtained.

A urine culture is accompanied by *sensitivity testing* to determine the bacteria's susceptibility to a variety of antibiotic medications. The results of this test assist the health care provider in selecting an antibiotic known to be capable of destroying the bacterial strain producing a UTI in a specific patient.

Imaging studies of the urinary tract are indicated in select cases. For example, an intravenous pyelogram (IVP) or abdominal computed tomographic (CT) scan may be obtained when obstruction of the urinary system is suspected of causing a UTI.

Interprofessional Care and Medication Therapy

Once a UTI has been diagnosed, appropriate antimicrobial therapy is initiated. An antibiotic may be selected on the basis of the health care provider's best judgement (empirical therapy) or the results of sensitivity testing. The interprofessional care and medication therapy of cystitis are summarized in Table 48.4. Uncomplicated cystitis can be treated by a short-term course of antibiotics, typically for 1 to 3 days. In contrast, complicated UTIs require longer-term treatment, lasting 7 to 14 days or even longer (Geerlings, 2017).

Trimethoprim–sulphamethoxazole (TMP-SMX) or nitrofurantoin is often used empirically to treat uncomplicated or initial UTIs. TMP-SMX has the advantages of being relatively inexpensive and being taken only twice daily. Nitrofurantoin is normally given three to four times daily, but a long-acting preparation (MacroBid) is available that is taken twice daily. Ampicillin or amoxicillin is not frequently selected when empirically treating an uncomplicated UTI because these antibiotics must be administered three to four times daily. In addition to these medications, the fluoroquinolones (including ciprofloxacin [Cipro], levofloxacin, and norfloxacin) may be used to treat complicated UTIs (Chu & Lowder, 2018). *Prophylactic*, or *suppressive*, *antibiotics* are sometimes administered to patients who experience repeated UTIs.

TABLE 48.4 INTERPROFESSIONAL CARE
Urinary Tract Infection

Diagnostic
- History and physical examination
- Imaging studies of urinary tract (e.g., IVP, cystoscopy) (if indicated)
- Urinalysis
- Urine for culture and sensitivity (if indicated)

Interprofessional Therapy
Uncomplicated UTI
- Adequate fluid intake
- Antibiotic: 1- to 3-day treatment regimen
  - Nitrofurantoin (MacroBid)
  - Trimethoprim–sulphamethoxazole (Septra)
- Counselling about risk for recurrence and reduction of risk factors

Recurrent, Uncomplicated UTI
- Repeated urinalysis and consideration of need for urine culture and sensitivity testing
- Antibiotic: 3- to 5-day treatment regimen
  - Nitrofurantoin (MacroBid)
  - Sensitivity-guided antibiotic (ampicillin, amoxicillin, first-generation cephalosporin, fluoroquinolone)
  - Trimethoprim–sulphamethoxazole (Septra)
- Consideration of 3- to 6-mo trial of suppressive antibiotics
- Adequate fluid intake
- Counselling about risk for recurrence and reduction of risk factors
- Imaging study of urinary tract in select cases

IVP, intravenous pyelogram; *UTI*, urinary tract infection.

MEDICATION ALERT—Nitrofurantoin (Macrobid)
- Avoid sunlight. Use sunscreen and wear protective clothing.
- Notify the health care provider immediately if fever, chills, cough, chest pain, dyspnea, rash, or numbness or tingling of fingers or toes develops.

A low dose of TMP-SMX, nitrofurantoin, or another antibiotic, such as ciprofloxacin, may be administered on a daily basis in an attempt to prevent recurring UTIs, or a single dose may be taken before an event likely to provoke a UTI, such as intercourse. However, although suppressive therapy is often effective on a short-term basis, this strategy is limited because of the risk for antibiotic resistance, ultimately leading to breakthrough infections with increasingly virulent pathogens.

NURSING MANAGEMENT
URINARY TRACT INFECTION

NURSING ASSESSMENT
Subjective and objective data that should be obtained from a patient with a UTI are presented in Table 48.5.

NURSING DIAGNOSES
Nursing diagnoses for the patient with a UTI may include but are not limited to the following:
- *Inadequate urinary elimination* resulting from *multiple causality* (effects of UTI)
- *Readiness for enhanced health management* as evidenced by *expressed desire to enhance management of risk factors*

Additional information on nursing diagnoses for the patient with a UTI is presented in Nursing Care Plan (NCP) 48.1, available on the Evolve website.

TABLE 48.5 NURSING ASSESSMENT
Urinary Tract Infection

Subjective Data
Important Health Information
Past health history: Previous UTIs; urinary calculi, stasis, reflux, strictures, or retention; neurogenic bladder; pregnancy; prostatic hyperplasia; sexually transmitted infection; bladder cancer
Medications: Use of antibiotics, anticholinergics, antispasmodics
Surgery or other treatments: Recent urological instrumentation (catheterization, cystoscopy, surgery)

Symptoms
- Lassitude, malaise
- Nausea, vomiting, and anorexia; chills
- Suprapubic or low back pain, pressure in bladder area, costovertebral tenderness; bladder spasms, dysuria, burning on urination, sense of incomplete emptying
- Urinary frequency, urgency, hesitancy; nocturia

Objective Data
General
Fever

Urinary
Hematuria; cloudy, foul-smelling urine; tender, enlarged kidney

Possible Findings
Leukocytosis; urinalysis positive for bacteria, pyuria, RBCs, and WBCs; positive urine culture; IVP, CT scan, ultrasound, voiding cystourethrogram and cystoscopy demonstrating abnormalities of urinary tract

CT, computed tomography; *IVP*, intravenous pyelogram; *RBCs*, red blood cells; *UTI*, urinary tract infection; *WBCs*, white blood cells.

PLANNING

The overall goals are (a) that the patient with a UTI will have relief from bothersome LUTS, (b) prevention of upper urinary tract involvement, and (c) prevention of recurrence.

NURSING IMPLEMENTATION

HEALTH PROMOTION. Health promotion measures include recognizing individuals who are at risk for a UTI. Debilitated persons, older persons, patients with underlying diseases (e.g., cancer, human immunodeficiency virus [HIV], or diabetes mellitus) that compromise host immune responses, and patients treated with immunosuppressive medications or corticosteroids are at high risk for UTIs. Especially for these individuals, health promotion activities can help decrease the frequency of infections and promote early detection of infection. Health promotion activities include educating the patient about preventive measures, such as (a) emptying the bladder regularly and completely, (b) evacuating the bowel regularly, (c) wiping the perineal area from front to back after urination and defecation, and (d) drinking an adequate amount of liquid each day. The recommended daily liquid intake for the ambulatory adult is approximately 33 mL/kg of body weight per day. Thus, a 70-kg person would require 2 310 mL each day. The person will obtain approximately 20% of this fluid from food, leaving 1 848 mL, or nearly eight 236-mL glasses of fluid, to be obtained by drinking.

Although daily intake of cranberry juice or cranberry capsules or powders have been and continue to be purported to assist in treating or preventing UTIs, there is currently no conclusive evidence to support advocating this treatment. Findings from current studies are disparate, reducing the likelihood that these treatments are worthwhile (Liska et al., 2016; Nicolle, 2016).

The nurse can play a major role in the prevention of health care–associated infections. Avoidance of unnecessary catheterization and early removal of in-dwelling catheters are the most effective means of reducing health care–associated UTIs. All patients undergoing instrumentation of the urinary tract are at risk of developing a health care–associated UTI. Aseptic technique must always be followed during these procedures. Performing hand hygiene before and after contact with each patient and wearing gloves for care involving the urinary system are especially important. When a catheter has been inserted, special measures must be employed, as explained in the section on urethral catheterization later in this chapter.

Routine and thorough perineal hygiene is important for all hospitalized patients, especially when a bedpan is used. Answering the call light quickly or offering the bedpan or urinal at frequent intervals to a bedridden patient should reduce the number of incontinent episodes.

ACUTE INTERVENTION. Acute intervention for a patient with a UTI includes ensuring adequate fluid intake if it is not contraindicated. It is sometimes difficult to convince a patient of maintaining an adequate fluid intake because they may think it will worsen the discomfort and frequency associated with a UTI. The patient needs to be taught that fluids will increase frequency of urination at first but will also dilute the urine, making the bladder less irritable. Fluids will help flush out bacteria before they have a chance to colonize in the bladder. Intake of alcohol, caffeine, some citrus juices, chocolate, and highly spiced foods or beverages should be avoided because they are potential bladder irritants. Water is the fluid of choice.

Local application of heat to the suprapubic area or lower back may relieve the discomfort associated with a UTI. The patient can be advised to apply a heating pad (turned to its lowest setting) to these areas. A warm shower can also be effective in providing temporary relief. The patient should be instructed about the prescribed medication therapy, including adverse effects. The nurse should emphasize the importance of taking the full course of antibiotics. Often patients stop antibiotic therapy once symptoms disappear. This practice can lead to inadequate treatment and recurrence of infection or to bacterial resistance to antibiotics. Sometimes a second medication or a reduced dose of medication is ordered after the initial course, to suppress bacterial growth in certain patients susceptible to recurrent UTIs. The patient should be advised to watch for any changes in the colour or the consistency of the urine and for a decrease in or cessation of symptoms as a sign of the effectiveness of therapy. The patient should be counselled that persistence of bothersome LUTS beyond the antibiotic treatment course or the onset of flank pain or fever should be reported promptly to a health care provider.

AMBULATORY AND HOME CARE. The nurse's responsibility in ambulatory and home care settings is to work with the patient to promote understanding about the need for ongoing care (Table 48.6).

The patient must understand the need for follow-up care with urine culture to determine if the infection has been adequately treated. Recurrent symptoms caused by bacterial persistence or inadequate treatment typically occur within 1 to 2 weeks after completion of therapy. If the patient has been adherent, a relapse indicates the need for further evaluation.

EVALUATION

The expected outcomes for the patient with a UTI are presented in NCP 48.1, available on the Evolve website.

TABLE 48.6 PATIENT & CAREGIVER TEACHING GUIDE

Urinary Tract Infection

The following information should be included when teaching the patient and caregiver about UTI to prevent recurrence:
1. The patient must take all antibiotics as prescribed. Symptoms may improve after 1 to 2 days of therapy, but organisms may still be present.
2. The patient must be instructed about appropriate hygiene, including the following:
   a. Careful cleansing of perineal region
   b. Wiping from front to back after urinating
   c. Cleansing with soap and water after each bowel movement
3. The patient should be taught about the importance of emptying the bladder before and after intercourse, which may help flush out bacteria introduced during intercourse. The patient should wash the genital area with warm water before having sex.
4. The patient should be advised to urinate regularly, approximately q2–4 hr during the day.
5. The patient should be advised about how to maintain adequate fluid intake (33 mL [1 oz] per kilogram of body weight per day).
6. The patient should understand why harsh soaps, bubble baths, powders, and sprays should not be applied in the perineal area.
7. The patient should be advised to report symptoms or signs of recurrent UTI (e.g., cloudy urine, pain on urination, urgency, frequency).

UTI, urinary tract infection.

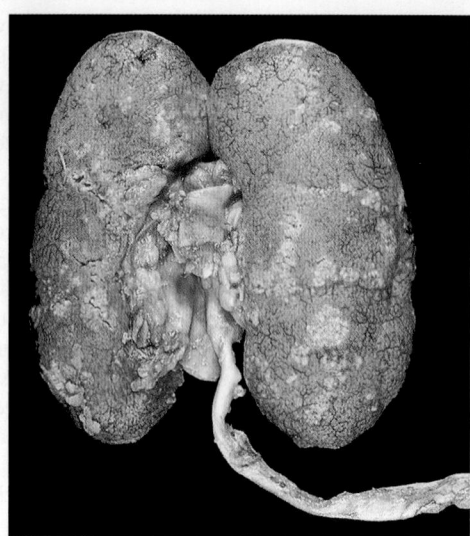

FIG. 48.2 Acute pyelonephritis. Cortical surface shows greyish-white areas of inflammation and abscess formation. Source: Kumar, V., Abbas, A. K., & Aster, J. (2015). *Robbins and Cotran pathologic basis of disease* (9th ed., p. 931, Figure 20-27). Saunders.

ACUTE PYELONEPHRITIS

Etiology and Pathophysiology

Pyelonephritis is an inflammation of the renal pelvis and kidney (Figure 48.2). The most common cause is bacterial infection, particularly Gram-negative organisms such as *E. coli*, but fungi, protozoa, or viruses sometimes infect the kidney (Johnson & Russo, 2018).

Urosepsis is a systemic infection arising from a urological source. Its prompt diagnosis and effective treatment are critical because, unless promptly eradicated, it leads to septic shock and death in 15% of cases. Septic shock is the outcome of unresolved bacteremia involving a Gram-negative organism. (Septic shock is discussed in Chapter 69.)

Pyelonephritis usually begins with colonization and infection of the lower urinary tract via the ascending urethral route. Bacteria normally found in the intestinal tract, such as *E. coli*, *Proteus*, *Klebsiella*, or *Enterobacter* species, frequently cause pyelonephritis. A pre-existing factor is often present, such as *vesicoureteral reflux* (retrograde or backward movement of urine from lower to upper urinary tract) or dysfunction of lower urinary tract function, such as obstruction from benign prostatic hyperplasia (BPH), a stricture, or a urinary stone.

Acute pyelonephritis commonly starts in the renal medulla and spreads to the adjacent cortex. Recurring episodes of pyelonephritis, especially in the presence of obstructive abnormalities, can lead to a scarred, poorly functioning kidney and a condition called *chronic pyelonephritis.*

Clinical Manifestations and Diagnostic Studies

The clinical manifestations of acute pyelonephritis vary from mild fatigue to the sudden onset of chills, fever, vomiting, malaise, flank pain, and the bothersome LUTS characteristic of cystitis. *Costovertebral tenderness* is typically present on the affected side. The clinical manifestations usually subside within a few days, even without specific therapy, but bacteriuria and pyuria usually persist.

Urinalysis shows pyuria, bacteriuria, and varying degrees of hematuria. WBC casts may be found in the urine, indicating involvement of the renal parenchyma. A complete blood cell count (CBC) will indicate leukocytosis and a shift to the left with an increase in immature neutrophils (bands). Urine cultures must be obtained when pyelonephritis is suspected. In patients with more severe illness who are hospitalized, blood cultures are also obtained.

Imaging studies, such as an IVP or CT scan, requiring intravenous injection of contrast materials, are usually not obtained in the early stages of pyelonephritis so as to prevent the possible spread of infection. Alternatively, ultrasonography of the urinary system may be obtained to identify anatomical abnormalities or the presence of an obstructing stone and reduce the need for catheterization. Imaging studies are also used to assess for complications of pyelonephritis such as impaired renal function, scarring, chronic pyelonephritis, or abscesses.

Urosepsis is characterized by bacteriuria and bacteremia (presence of bacteria in blood). If bacteremia is a possibility, close observation and monitoring of vital signs are essential. Prompt recognition and treatment of septic shock may prevent irreversible damage or death.

Interprofessional Care and Medication Therapy

The diagnostic tests and interprofessional therapy of acute pyelonephritis are summarized in Table 48.7. Patients with severe infections or complicating factors, such as nausea and vomiting with dehydration, require hospital admission.

Patients with mild symptoms may be treated on an outpatient basis with antibiotics for 14 to 21 days (see Table 48.7). Parenteral antibiotics are often given initially in the hospital to rapidly establish high serum and urinary medication levels. When initial treatment resolves acute symptoms and the patient is able to tolerate oral fluids and medications, the person may be discharged on a regimen of oral antibiotics for an additional 14 to 21 days. Symptoms and signs typically improve or resolve within 48 to 72 hours after starting therapy. Symptoms that do not resolve within this time frame may indicate the development of complications (Johnson & Russo, 2018).

Reinfections may be treated as individual episodes of disease or managed with long-term antibiotic therapy. The effectiveness of therapy is evaluated in accordance with the presence or absence of bacterial growth on a urine culture. Relapses are not common, but if they occur they could signal other complications or disease.

NURSING MANAGEMENT
ACUTE PYELONEPHRITIS

NURSING ASSESSMENT

Subjective and objective data that should be obtained from a patient with pyelonephritis are presented in Table 48.5.

NURSING DIAGNOSES

Nursing diagnoses for a patient with pyelonephritis include but are not limited to those for a patient with a UTI (see NCP 48.1).

PLANNING

The overall goals are that the patient with pyelonephritis will have (a) relief of pain, (b) normal body temperature, (c) no complications, (d) normal renal function, and (e) no recurrence of symptoms.

NURSING IMPLEMENTATION

HEALTH PROMOTION. Health promotion and maintenance measures are similar to those for cystitis (see Nursing Management: Urinary Tract Infection, earlier in this chapter). In

TABLE 48.7 INTERPROFESSIONAL CARE

Acute Pyelonephritis

Diagnostic
- History and physical examination
- Blood culture (if bacteremia is suspected)
- CBC count with WBC differential
- Palpation for flank pain
- Ultrasound (initially), IVP, VCUG, radionuclide imaging, CT scan
- Urinalysis
- Urine for culture and sensitivity

Interprofessional Therapy
Mild Symptoms
- Adequate fluid intake
- Follow-up urine culture and imaging studies
- Nonsteroidal anti-inflammatory medications or antipyretic medications
- Outpatient management or short hospitalization for IV antibiotics:
  - Empirically selected broad-spectrum antibiotics (ampicillin, vancomycin) combined with an aminoglycoside (e.g., tobramycin, gentamicin)
  - Switch to sensitivity-guided therapy (when results available) for 14–21 days
  - Trimethoprim–sulphamethoxazole (Septra)
  - Fluoroquinolones (e.g., ciprofloxacin [Cipro], norfloxacin)

Severe Symptoms
- Adequate fluid intake (initially parenteral; switched to oral fluids as nausea, vomiting, and dehydration subside)
- Hospitalization
- Nonsteroidal anti-inflammatory or antipyretic medications to reverse fever and relieve discomfort
- Parenteral antibiotics:
  - Empirically selected broad-spectrum antibiotics (e.g., ampicillin, vancomycin) combined with an aminoglycoside (e.g., tobramycin, gentamicin)
  - Switch to sensitivity-guided antibiotic therapy when results of urine and blood cultures are available
- Oral antibiotics when patient tolerates oral intake; administer for 7–21 days
- Urinary analgesics (e.g., to relieve bothersome lower urinary tract symptoms)
- Follow-up urine culture and imaging studies

CBC, complete blood count; *CT*, computed tomography; *IV*, intravenous; *IVP*, intravenous pyelogram; *VCUG*, voiding cystourethrogram; *WBC*, white blood cell.

addition, it is important that patients receive early treatment for cystitis to prevent ascending infections. The need for regular medical care should be stressed to patients with structural abnormalities of the urinary tract because these patients are at high risk for infection.

ACUTE INTERVENTION AND HOME CARE. Nursing interventions vary depending on the severity of symptoms. Interventions include teaching and working with the patient to promote understanding about the disease process with emphasis on (a) the need to continue medications as prescribed, (b) the need for a follow-up urine culture to ensure proper management, and (c) identification of risk for recurrence or relapse (see Table 48.5 and NCP 48.1). In addition to antibiotic therapy, patients should be encouraged to drink at least eight glasses of fluid every day, even after the infection has been treated. Rest is often indicated to increase patient comfort. Patients with frequent relapses or reinfections may be treated with long-term, low-dose antibiotics. Understanding the rationale for therapy

is important to enhance patient application of knowledge for disease management.

EVALUATION
The expected outcomes for patients with pyelonephritis are presented in NCP 48.1, available on the Evolve website.

CHRONIC PYELONEPHRITIS

Chronic pyelonephritis is a term used to describe a kidney that has become shrunken and has lost function owing to scarring or fibrosis. It usually occurs as the outcome of recurring infections involving the upper urinary tract. However, it also may occur in the absence of an existing infection and a recent or remote history of UTIs. Alternative terms used to describe this condition include *interstitial nephritis, chronic atrophic pyelonephritis,* or *reflux nephropathy* (when scarring occurs in the presence of vesicoureteral reflux).

Chronic pyelonephritis is diagnosed by radiological imaging and histological testing rather than assessment of clinical features. Imaging studies reveal a small, contracted kidney with a thinned parenchyma. The collecting system may be small or hydronephrotic. Pathological analysis indicates loss of functioning nephrons, infiltration of the parenchyma with inflammatory cells, and fibrosis.

The level of renal function in chronic pyelonephritis varies, depending on whether one or both kidneys are affected, the magnitude of scarring, and the presence of coexisting infection. Chronic pyelonephritis often progresses to end-stage renal disease when both kidneys are involved, even if the underlying infection is successfully eradicated. (Nursing and interprofessional management of patients with chronic kidney disease are discussed in Chapter 49).

URETHRITIS

Urethritis is an inflammation of the urethra. Causes of urethritis include a bacterial or viral infection, *Trichomonas* and monilial infection (especially in women), chlamydia, and gonorrhea (especially in men). In men, urethritis usually arises from sexual transmission; purulent discharge usually indicates a gonococcal urethritis, whereas a clear discharge typically signifies a nongonococcal urethritis. (Sexually transmitted infections are discussed in Chapter 55.) Urethritis also produces bothersome LUTS, including dysuria and frequent urination, similar to those seen with cystitis.

Urethritis is difficult to diagnose in women, as urethral discharge may not be present. Cultures on split urine collections (taken at beginning of urine flow and then midstream) or any urethral discharge may confirm a diagnosis of urethral infection.

Treatment is based on identifying and treating the cause and providing symptomatic relief. Sulphamethoxazole with trimethoprim or nitrofurantoin are examples of medications used for bacterial infections. Metronidazole (Flagyl) and clotrimazole may be used for treating *Trichomonas*. Medications such as fluconazole (Diflucan) may be prescribed for monilial infections. In chlamydial infections, doxycycline may be used. Urethritis in women with negative urine cultures and no pyuria does not usually respond to antibiotics. Hot sitz baths may temporarily relieve symptoms. Patients should be instructed to avoid the use of vaginal deodorant sprays, to properly cleanse the perineal area after bowel movements and urination, and to avoid intercourse until symptoms subside. Patients with sexually transmitted urethritis should be instructed to refer their sex partners for evaluation and testing if they had sexual contact in the 60 days preceding onset of symptoms or diagnosis.

URETHRAL DIVERTICULA

Urethral diverticula are the result of obstruction and subsequent rupture of the periurethral glands into the urethral lumen with epithelialization (regrowth of tissue) over the opening of the resulting periurethral cavity (Urology Care Foundation, 2021). Urethral diverticula are much more common in females than in males, with an incidence in women of 1 to 5%. Urethral diverticula occur mostly in the area of the periurethral glands. These glands are found along the entire length of the urethra, with the majority draining into the distal third of the urethra; Skene glands are the largest and most distal. A person may have more than one diverticulum, caused by urethral trauma from childbearing, urethral instrumentation, dilation or infection with gonococcal organisms, or normal vaginal flora. Urethral diverticula present some of the more challenging diagnostic and reconstructive cases in urology.

Symptoms include dysuria, postvoid dribbling, frequent urination (more than every 2 hours), urgency, suprapubic discomfort or pressure, dyspareunia, a feeling of incomplete bladder emptying, and urinary incontinence. As well, the urine may contain gross hematuria or sediment, giving it a cloudy appearance. However, one in four women have no symptoms. An anterior vaginal wall mass may be noted on physical examination, which, upon palpation, may be quite tender and express purulent discharge through the urethra. Radiographic studies such as voiding cystourethrography (VCUG) should be used to confirm the diagnosis. Additional studies include ultrasound and magnetic resonance imaging (MRI) to determine the size of the diverticulum in relation to the urethral lumen.

Surgical options include transurethral incision of the diverticular neck, marsupialization (creation of a permanent opening) of the diverticular sac into the vagina (often referred to as a *Spence procedure*), and surgical excision. Surgical excision of a urethral diverticulum should be performed with caution because the diverticular sac may be adherent to the adjacent urethral lumen, and careless excision of the sac may result in a large urethral defect requiring construction of a neourethra (new urethra). Other important considerations during surgery include identification and closure of the diverticular neck, complete removal of the mucosal lining of the diverticular sac to prevent recurrence, and a multiple-layered closure to prevent postoperative urethrovaginal fistula formation. A complication of the surgery may be stress urinary incontinence.

INTERSTITIAL CYSTITIS

Interstitial cystitis (IC) is a chronic, painful inflammatory disease of the bladder characterized by symptoms of urgency, frequency, and pain in the bladder, pelvis, or both. IC is often called *bladder pain syndrome* or *painful bladder syndrome* (PBS). The term *IC/PBS* refers to cases of urinary pain that cannot be attributed to other causes, such as UTI or urinary stones.

The cause of IC/PBS is unknown. It is likely multifactorial. Possible causes include neurogenic hypersensitivity of the lower urinary tract, changes in mast cells in the muscle and/or mucosal layers of the bladder, infection with an unusual organism (e.g., slow-growing virus), or production of a toxic substance in the urine. Many patients suffering from IC/PBS are older and with symptoms pointing to the presence of an inflammatory component causing urinary frequency, pelvic pain, and pelvic pressure (Han et al., 2018).

The two primary clinical manifestations that characterize IC are pain and bothersome LUTS (e.g., frequency, urgency). The pain associated with IC is usually located in the suprapubic area but may involve the vagina, labia, or entire perineal region. It varies from moderate to severe in intensity and is exacerbated by bladder filling, postponing urination, physical exertion, pressure against the suprapubic area, dietary intake of certain foods, and emotional distress. The pain is transiently relieved by urination. Bothersome LUTS are very similar to those of a UTI, and the condition is often misdiagnosed as a recurring or chronic UTI. The pain and voiding symptoms produced by IC remit and exacerbate over time. Some patients experience an onset of symptoms that disappear altogether after a period of weeks to months, whereas others have persistent symptoms over a period of months to years.

IC is a diagnosis of exclusion. The condition is suspected whenever a patient experiences symptoms of a UTI despite the absence of bacteriuria, pyuria, or a positive urine culture. A careful history and physical examination are necessary to exclude a variety of disorders that may produce somewhat similar symptoms, such as UTI or endometriosis. This evaluation must include at least one negative urine culture during a period of active symptoms. Cystoscopic examination may show a small bladder capacity and superficial ulcerations with bladder filling called *glomerulations*, but these findings are frequently absent and are not unique to IC. Criteria for diagnosing IC are presented in Table 48.8.

Interprofessional Care and Medication Therapy

Because the etiology of IC is unknown, no single treatment has been identified that consistently reverses or relieves symptoms. Various therapies have been effective in alleviating or relieving uncomfortable symptoms in most patients (Syed & Illchak, 2017). Dietary and lifestyle alterations are used to relieve pain and diminish voiding frequency and nocturia. Dietary

TABLE 48.8	CLINICAL CRITERIA FOR THE DIAGNOSIS OF INTERSTITIAL CYSTITIS

Inclusion Criteria
- Bothersome urinary urgency
- Cystoscopic evidence of ulcerations or glomerulations (not specific to interstitial cystitis)
- Pain with bladder filling or postponing urination
- Small bladder capacity on urodynamic testing

Exclusion Criteria
- Active genital herpes
- Bladder capacity >350 mL on urodynamic testing
- Bladder tumour
- Daytime voiding frequency (eight or more times per day)
- History of chemotherapy, particularly if treated with cyclophosphamide (Procytox)
- History of pelvic irradiation
- Overactive bladder contractions on urodynamic testing
- Tubercular cystitis

alterations include elimination of foods and beverages likely to exacerbate the symptoms. Eating a diet low in acidic foods and avoiding consumption of beverages such as coffee, tea, and carbonated and alcoholic drinks can be helpful in reducing IC symptoms (Han et al., 2018). Patients may be advised that an over-the-counter dietary supplement called *calcium glycerophosphate* alkalinizes the urine and can provide relief from the irritating effects of certain foods. This agent may be particularly helpful when dining away from home where the patient has less control over the preparation of foods.

A number of tricyclic antidepressants, including amitriptyline (Elavil) and doxepin, are used to reduce the burning pain and urinary frequency. Pentosan (Elmiron) is a medication used to enhance the protective effects of the glycosaminoglycan layer of the bladder. It is thought to relieve pain associated with IC by reducing the irritating effects of urine on the bladder wall. Medications that may provide modest relief from IC symptoms include nifedipine, which is a calcium channel blocker. Although these medications are effective over time (weeks to months), they do not provide the immediate relief that may be needed when a patient experiences an acute exacerbation of symptoms. For this relief, a short course of opioid analgesics may be given.

Several medications may be instilled directly into the bladder through a small catheter. Dimethyl sulphoxide probably acts by desensitizing pain receptors in the bladder wall. Heparin and hyaluronic acid also may be instilled into the bladder to relieve IC symptoms. Like pentosan, they are thought to enhance the protective properties of the glycosaminoglycan layer of the bladder. These medications are often administered with lidocaine, which rapidly desensitizes the bladder wall, rendering the patient better able to tolerate instillation of additional heparin or hyaluronic acid and providing transient relief from pain. The bacille Calmette–Guérin (BCG) vaccine, an attenuated form of *Mycobacterium bovis* administered intravesically, is now in clinical trials. The mechanism of action of BCG is unclear, but it may alleviate a possible autoimmune disorder provoking the chronic inflammation characteristic of the disorder.

Distension of the bladder during endoscopic examination relieves IC-related pain and voiding frequency, probably by temporarily disrupting sensory nerve endings in the bladder wall. Several surgical procedures have been used in an attempt to relieve severe, debilitating pain. Urinary diversion, the surgical removal of the bladder and rerouting flow of urine to an ostomy on the abdomen, is an approach that can be used when other measures fail. Unfortunately, some patients have reported pain within the urinary diversion, possibly indicating that components of the urine may contribute to IC in certain cases.

Other therapies used to relieve symptoms of IC include trigger point injections, neuromodulation, and cognitive behavioural therapy. Implementing pelvic floor physiotherapy has demonstrated positive benefits (Han et al., 2018).

NURSING MANAGEMENT INTERSTITIAL CYSTITIS

Assessment focuses on characterization of the pain associated with IC. The patient is asked about specific dietary or lifestyle factors known to exacerbate or alleviate pain and about the intensity of the pain. Objective data collection includes a bladder log or voiding diary kept over a period of at least 3 days to determine diurnal voiding frequency and patterns of nocturia. A simultaneous pain record may be useful.

Reassurance that IC is a real condition experienced by others and that it can be effectively treated may relieve the anxiety, anger, guilt, and frustration related to experiences of chronic pain and voiding dysfunction in the absence of a clear-cut diagnosis and treatment strategy.

A UTI may occur during the course of IC management. A UTI is likely to produce an acute exacerbation of bothersome LUTS and urinary frequency as well as dysuria (not typically associated with IC) and odorous urine, possibly with hematuria.

Broad dietary restrictions are often necessary to control IC-related pain. Patients must be given instruction about the need to maintain good nutrition. Specifically, they may be advised to take a multivitamin containing no more than the recommended dietary allowance for essential vitamins and to avoid high-potency vitamins, because these formulations may irritate the bladder. Patients are also advised to obtain information, including recipes and menus for a well-balanced diet specifically designed to avoid bladder-irritating foods and beverages, from support organizations such as the Women's College Hospital in Toronto and the Interstitial Cystitis Association in the United States (see the Resources at the end of this chapter). Elimination of a variety of foods and beverages from the diet that are likely to irritate the bladder typically provides modest to profound relief from symptoms. Typical bladder irritants include caffeine, alcohol, citrus products, aged cheeses, nuts, foods containing vinegar, curries or hot peppers, and foods or beverages likely to lower urinary pH. In addition, the patient should be taught to self-manage the use of calcium glycerophosphate or pantoprazole (Pantoloc). The patient is advised to avoid clothing that creates suprapubic pressure, including pants with tight belts or restrictive waistlines.

Written educational materials concerning diet, coping with the need for frequent urination, and strategies for coping with the emotional burden of IC are available from the Interstitial Cystitis Association. Providing such materials affords an excellent opportunity for the nurse to introduce the patient to this patient advocacy group.

RENAL TUBERCULOSIS

Renal tuberculosis (TB) is rarely a primary lesion. It is usually secondary to TB of the lung. In a small percentage of patients with pulmonary TB, the tubercle bacilli reach the kidneys via the bloodstream. Onset occurs 5 to 8 years after the primary infection. The patient is often asymptomatic when the kidney is initially infiltrated with bacilli. Sometimes, the patient experiences fatigue and develops a low-grade fever. As the lesions ulcerate, infection descends to the bladder, and the patient experiences frequent urination, burning on voiding, and epididymitis (in men). Symptoms of a UTI are the first sign in the majority of patients with renal TB. Renal lesions may calcify as they heal. Infrequently, renal colic, lumbar and iliac pain, and hematuria may be present. A diagnosis is based on localization of tubercle bacilli in the urine and on IVP findings.

Long-term complications of renal TB depend on the duration of the disease before treatment. The renal parenchyma become scarred and ureteral strictures develop. The earlier treatment is initiated, the less likely renal failure is to develop. Reduced bladder volume may be irreversible in advanced disease. The patient may require long-term urological follow-up. (Nursing and interprofessional management for the patient with TB are discussed in Chapter 30.)

IMMUNOLOGICAL DISORDERS OF THE KIDNEY

GLOMERULONEPHRITIS

Immunological processes involving the urinary tract predominantly affect the renal glomerulus. The disease process results in glomerulonephritis, an immune-related inflammation of the glomeruli characterized by proteinuria, hematuria, decreased urine production, and edema. The condition affects both kidneys equally. Although the glomerulus is the primary site of inflammation, tubular, interstitial, and vascular changes also occur. Glomerulonephritis is divided into a number of classifications, which may describe (a) the extent of damage (diffuse or focal), (b) the initial cause of the disorder (e.g., systemic lupus erythematosus, systemic sclerosis [scleroderma], streptococcal infection), or (c) the extent of changes (minimal or widespread).

Clinical Manifestations

Clinical manifestations of glomerulonephritis include varying degrees of hematuria (ranging from microscopic to gross) and urinary excretion of various formed elements, including red blood cells (RBCs), WBCs, and casts. Proteinuria and elevated serum urea (blood urea nitrogen [BUN]) and serum creatinine levels are other manifestations. In most cases, recovery from the acute illness is complete. However, if progressive involvement occurs, the result is destruction of renal tissue and marked renal insufficiency.

A patient's history provides important information related to glomerulonephritis. It is necessary to assess exposure to medications, immunizations, microbial infections, and viral infections such as hepatitis. It is also important to evaluate the patient for more generalized conditions involving immune disorders, such as systemic lupus erythematosus and systemic sclerosis.

ACUTE POSTSTREPTOCOCCAL GLOMERULONEPHRITIS

Acute poststreptococcal glomerulonephritis (APSGN) is most common in children and young adults, but all age groups can be affected. APSGN develops 5 to 21 days after an infection of the pharynx or the skin (e.g., streptococcal sore throat, impetigo) by certain nephrotoxic strains of group A β-hemolytic streptococci. The patient produces antibodies to the streptococcal antigen. Although the specific mechanism is not known, the antigen–antibody complexes are deposited in the glomeruli and activate complement, which causes an inflammatory reaction to the injury. (Complement activation is discussed in Chapter 14.) The response to the injury is also a decrease in the filtration of metabolic waste products from the blood and an increase in the permeability of the glomerulus to larger protein molecules.

Clinical Manifestations and Complications

The clinical manifestations of APSGN appear as a variety of signs and symptoms, which may include generalized body edema, hypertension, oliguria, hematuria with a smoky or rusty appearance, and proteinuria. Fluid retention occurs as a result of decreased glomerular filtration. The edema appears initially in low-pressure tissues, such as around the eyes (periorbital edema), but later progresses to involve the total body as ascites or peripheral edema in the legs. Smoky urine indicates bleeding in the upper urinary tract. The degree of proteinuria varies with the severity of the glomerulonephropathy. Hypertension

primarily results from increased extracellular fluid volume. Patients with APSGN may have abdominal or flank pain. Some, however, will have no symptoms, and the condition is found on routine urinalysis.

More than 95% of patients with APSGN recover completely or improve rapidly with conservative management.

Diagnostic Studies

The diagnosis of APSGN is based on a complete history and physical examination and laboratory studies (Table 48.9) to determine the presence or history of a group A β-hemolytic streptococcus in a throat or skin lesion. An immune response to the streptococcus is often demonstrated by assessment of antistreptolysin O titres. The finding of decreased complement components (especially C3 and CH50) indicates an immune-mediated response. A renal biopsy may be performed to confirm the presence of the disease.

Dipstick and urine sediment microscopy will reveal the presence of erythrocytes in significant numbers. Erythrocyte casts are highly suggestive of acute glomerulonephritis. Proteinuria may range from mild to severe. Screening blood tests include BUN and serum creatinine to assess the extent of renal impairment.

NURSING AND INTERPROFESSIONAL MANAGEMENT ACUTE POSTSTREPTOCOCCAL GLOMERULONEPHRITIS

The management of APSGN focuses on symptomatic relief (see Table 48.9). Rest is recommended until the signs of glomerular inflammation (proteinuria, hematuria) and hypertension subside. Edema is treated by restricting sodium and fluid intake and by administering diuretics. Severe hypertension is treated with antihypertensive medications. Dietary protein intake may be restricted if there is evidence of an increase in nitrogenous wastes (e.g., elevated BUN). The restriction varies with the degree of proteinuria. (Low-protein, low-sodium, fluid-restricted diets are discussed in Chapter 49.) Antibiotics should be given only if the streptococcal infection is still present. Corticosteroids and cytotoxic medications have not been shown to be of value.

One of the most important ways to prevent the development of APSGN is to encourage early diagnosis and treatment of a sore throat and skin lesions. If streptococci are found in the

TABLE 48.9   INTERPROFESSIONAL CARE
Acute Glomerulonephritis

Diagnostic
- History and physical examination
- BUN, serum creatinine, and albumin
- CBC
- Complement levels and ASO titre
- Renal biopsy (if indicated)
- Urinalysis

Interprofessional Therapy
- Adjustment of dietary protein intake to level of proteinuria and uremia
- Antihypertensive therapy
- Diuretics
- Rest
- Sodium and fluid restriction

ASO, antistreptolysin O; *BUN,* blood urea nitrogen; *CBC,* complete blood cell count.

culture, treatment with appropriate antibiotic therapy (usually penicillin) is essential. The patient must be encouraged to take the full course of antibiotics to ensure that the bacteria have been eradicated. Good personal hygiene is an important factor in preventing the spread of cutaneous streptococcal infections. (The Kidney Foundation of Canada website [see the Resources at the end of this chapter] provides information on the management of kidney disease and support groups.)

GOODPASTURE'S SYNDROME

Goodpasture's syndrome is an autoimmune disease characterized by the presence of antibodies circulating against the glomerular and alveolar basement membranes. Damage to the kidneys and lungs results when binding of the antibody causes an inflammatory reaction mediated by complement activation.

Goodpasture's syndrome is a rare disease that is seen mostly in young male smokers. The clinical manifestations include hemoptysis, pulmonary insufficiency, crackles, wheezes, renal involvement with hematuria and renal failure, weakness, pallor, and anemia. Pulmonary hemorrhage usually occurs and may precede glomerular abnormalities by weeks or months. Abnormal diagnostic findings include low hematocrit and hemoglobin levels, elevated BUN and serum creatinine levels, hematuria, and proteinuria. Circulating serum anti–glomerular basement membrane (anti-GBM) antibodies parallel the activity of the renal disease and are diagnostic of this syndrome.

NURSING AND INTERPROFESSIONAL MANAGEMENT GOODPASTURE'S SYNDROME

Until recently, the prognosis for patients with Goodpasture's syndrome was poor. However, with the development of immunosuppressive therapy and advances in transplantation techniques, the outlook has improved. Management consists of corticosteroids, immunosuppressive medications (e.g., cyclophosphamide [Procytox], azathioprine [Imuran]), plasmapheresis (see Chapter 16), and dialysis.

Nursing management appropriate for a critically ill patient who is experiencing symptoms of acute kidney injury and respiratory distress is instituted. Death is often secondary to hemorrhage in the lungs and respiratory failure. (Nursing interventions for a patient in acute kidney injury are discussed in Chapter 49, and nursing interventions for a patient with respiratory failure are discussed in Chapter 70).

RAPIDLY PROGRESSIVE GLOMERULONEPHRITIS

Rapidly progressive glomerulonephritis (RPGN) is glomerular disease associated with rapid, progressive loss of renal function over days to weeks. Renal failure may occur within weeks to months, in contrast to chronic glomerulonephritis, in which it develops insidiously and progresses over many years. The manifestations of RPGN are hypertension, edema, proteinuria, hematuria, and RBC casts.

RPGN can occur in a variety of situations: (a) as a complication of inflammatory or infectious disease (e.g., APSGN), (b) as a complication of a multisystemic disease (e.g., systemic lupus erythematosus, Goodpasture's syndrome), (c) as an idiopathic disease, or (d) in association with the use of certain medications (e.g., penicillamine).

Treatment is directed toward correction of fluid overload, hypertension, uremia, and inflammatory injury to the kidney. Treatment includes corticosteroids, cytotoxic agents, and plasmapheresis. Dialysis therapy and transplantation are used as maintenance therapy for the patient with RPGN. Following renal transplantation, RPGN may recur.

CHRONIC GLOMERULONEPHRITIS

Chronic glomerulonephritis is a syndrome that reflects the end stage of glomerular inflammatory disease. Most types of glomerulonephritis and nephrotic syndrome can eventually lead to chronic glomerulonephritis. The syndrome is characterized by proteinuria, hematuria, and the slow development of uremic syndrome as a result of decreasing renal function. Chronic glomerulonephritis does not usually follow an acute course; it progresses insidiously toward renal failure over a few to as many as 30 years.

Chronic glomerulonephritis is often found coincidentally as an abnormality on a urinalysis or when elevated blood pressure is detected. It is common to find that the patient has no recollection or history of acute nephritis or any renal disorders. A renal biopsy may be performed to determine the exact cause and nature of the glomerulonephritis. However, ultrasound and CT scanning are generally preferred as diagnostic measures.

Treatment is supportive and symptomatic. Hypertension and UTIs should be treated vigorously. Protein and phosphate restrictions may slow the rate of progression of kidney disease. (Management of chronic kidney disease is discussed in Chapter 49).

NEPHROTIC SYNDROME

Etiology and Clinical Manifestations

Nephrotic syndrome describes a clinical course that can be associated with a number of disease conditions. Some of the more common causes of nephrotic syndrome are listed in Table 48.10. In adults, about one third of patients with nephrotic syndrome will have a systemic disease such as diabetes or systemic lupus erythematosus (Semwal, 2020).

The characteristic manifestations include peripheral edema, massive proteinuria, dyslipidemia, and hypoalbuminemia. Characteristic blood chemistries include decreased serum albumin, decreased total serum protein, and elevated serum cholesterol. The increased glomerular membrane permeability found in nephrotic syndrome is responsible for the massive excretion of protein in the urine. This excretion results in decreased serum protein and subsequent edema formation. Ascites and anasarca (extreme generalized edema) develop if there is severe hypoalbuminemia.

The diminished plasma oncotic pressure from the decreased serum proteins stimulates hepatic lipoprotein synthesis, which results in dyslipidemia. Initially, cholesterol and low-density lipoproteins are elevated. Later, the triglyceride level also increases. Fat bodies (fatty casts) commonly appear in the urine.

Immune responses, both humoral and cellular, are altered in nephrotic syndrome. As a result, infection is an important cause of morbidity and mortality. Calcium and skeletal abnormalities may occur, including hypocalcemia, blunted calcemic response to parathyroid hormone, hyperparathyroidism, and osteomalacia.

TABLE 48.10	CAUSES OF NEPHROTIC SYNDROME

Primary Glomerular Disease
- Primary nephrotic syndrome
- Focal glomerulonephritis
- Inherited nephrotic disease

Extrarenal Causes
Multisystem Disease
- Amyloidosis
- Diabetes mellitus
- Systemic lupus erythematosus

Infections
- Bacterial (streptococcal, syphilis)
- Protozoal (malaria)
- Viral (hepatitis, human immunodeficiency virus infection)

Neoplasms
- Hodgkin's disease
- Leukemias
- Solid tumours of lungs, colon, stomach, breast

Drugs and Medications
- Captopril
- Heroin
- Nonsteroidal anti-inflammatory medications
- Penicillamine

Allergens (e.g., bee sting, pollen)

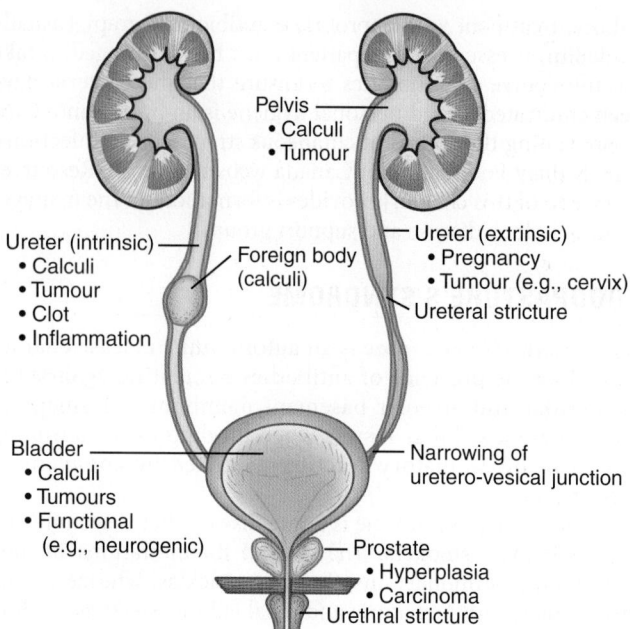

FIG. 48.3 Common causes of urinary tract obstruction.

With nephrotic proteinuria, loss of clotting factors can result in a relative hypercoagulable state. Hypercoagulability with thromboembolism is potentially the most serious complication of nephrotic syndrome. In nephrotic syndrome, formation of renal vein thrombi vein may be caused from the loss of fluid across the glomerulus. This hemoconcentration in postglomerular circulation is worsened by diuretic therapy, which then may promote thrombus formation in patients who are already hypercoagulable. Pulmonary emboli occur in about 40% of nephrotic patients with thrombosis.

Interprofessional Care

Treatment of nephrotic syndrome is symptomatic. The goals are to relieve edema and cure or control the primary disease. Management of the edema includes the cautious use of angiotensin-converting enzyme inhibitors, nonsteroidal anti-inflammatory medications, and a low-sodium (2–3 g/day), low- to moderate-protein (0.5–0.6 g/kg of body weight per day) diet. Dietary salt restriction is key to managing edema. In some individuals, thiazide or loop diuretics may be needed (Sinnakirouchenan, 2020). If urine protein loss exceeds 10 g/24 hr, additional dietary protein may be needed.

The treatment of dyslipidemia is often unsuccessful. However, treatment with lipid-lowering agents, such as colestipol (Colestid) and lovastatin, may result in moderate decreases in serum cholesterol levels. If thrombosis is detected, anticoagulant therapy may be necessary for up to 6 months.

Corticosteroids and cyclophosphamide (Procytox) may be used to treat severe cases of nephrotic syndrome. Management of diabetes and treatment of edema are the only measures used for nephrotic syndrome related to diabetes.

NURSING MANAGEMENT NEPHROTIC SYNDROME

A major nursing intervention for patients with nephrotic syndrome is related to edema. It is important to assess the edema by weighing the patient daily, accurately recording intake and output, and measuring abdominal girth or extremity size. Comparing this information daily provides the nurse with a tool for assessing the effectiveness of treatment. The edematous skin must be cleaned carefully. Trauma should be avoided, and the effectiveness of diuretic therapy must be monitored.

Patients with nephrotic syndrome have the potential to become malnourished or anorexic from the excessive loss of protein in the urine. Maintaining a low- to moderate-protein diet that is also low in sodium is not always easy. Serving small, frequent meals in a pleasant setting may encourage better dietary intake.

Because these patients are susceptible to infection, measures should be taken to avoid exposure to persons with known infections. People with nephrotic syndrome are often self-conscious about an edematous appearance and need support in coping with an altered body image.

OBSTRUCTIVE UROPATHIES

Urinary obstruction refers to any anatomical or functional condition that blocks or impedes the flow of urine (Figure 48.3). It may be congenital or acquired. Obstruction may be the result of (a) intrinsic causes such as anomalies, diverticula, tumours, or benign growth within the urinary tract; (b) extrinsic causes such as tumours, adhesions, retroperitoneal fibrosis, or prolapsed adjacent organs; or (c) functional causes as a result of neurological or psychogenic factors. Some common intrinsic obstructions are narrowing of the ureteropelvic junction (UPJ), bladder neck contracture, BPH, urethral stricture, and urethral meatal stenosis. Common extrinsic causes include pelvic and abdominal tumours or a prolapsed uterus. Examples of functional causes are neurogenic bladder and vesicosphincter dyssynergia (disturbance in muscle coordination) after spinal cord injury.

Damage from urinary tract obstruction affects the system above the level of the obstruction. The severity of these effects depends on location, duration of obstruction, amount of pressure or dilation, presence of urinary stasis, and the presence of infection. Infection increases the risk of irreversible damage.

Although obstruction distal to the prostate in men or the bladder neck in women causes mucosal scarring and a slower stream, it rarely results in major obstructive uropathy because the urethral wall pressure is less than that of the bladder neck and bladder. Urethral obstruction may contribute to outlet resistance and cause lower or upper urinary tract damage when other obstructive or dysfunctional factors are also present. For example, there is an increased risk for compromised renal function in a patient with a spinal cord injury with vesicosphincter dyssynergia.

When obstruction occurs at the level of the bladder neck or the prostate, significant bladder changes can occur. Detrusor muscle fibres hypertrophy (increase in size) to contract harder-to-push urine out a narrower pathway. Over a long period, the detrusor loses its ability to compensate for this resistance. Muscle bundles separate and become less compliant; this separation is called *trabeculation*. Trabeculation is caused by the deposition of collagen in the bladder wall that separates the smooth muscle fascicles. Trabeculation may hasten the decompensation of the detrusor. The areas between these muscle bundles are called *cellules*. Because these areas have no muscle support, the bladder mucosa can herniate between detrusor muscle bundles, forming sacs that drain poorly, called *diverticula*. The amount of residual urine in a noncompensating bladder can be very high.

Pressure increases during bladder filling or storage and can be transmitted to the ureter when *bladder outlet obstruction* is present. This pressure overcomes the normal peristaltic pressure and leads to *reflux* (a backflow of urine), which in turn causes ureteral dilation, kinking, and tortuosity; hydroureter (dilation of the renal pelvis); *vesicoureteral reflux* (backflow or backward movement of urine from the lower to upper urinary tracts); and hydronephrosis (dilation or enlargement of the renal pelvis and the calyces; Figure 48.4) and consequent chronic pyelonephritis and renal atrophy. If only one kidney is obstructed, the other kidney may try to compensate by hypertrophy, but the ureter will not be dilated on this contralateral side.

Partial obstruction may occur in the ureter or at the UPJ. If the pressure remains low or moderate, the kidney may continue to dilate with no noticeable loss of function. There is an increased risk of pyelonephritis because of urinary stasis and reflux. If only one kidney is involved and the other kidney is functioning, the patient may be free of symptoms. If both kidneys or only one functioning kidney is involved (e.g., if the patient has only one kidney), alterations in renal function (e.g., increased BUN or serum creatinine levels) are found. If the obstruction progresses, oliguria or anuria develops. Often, episodes of oliguria are followed by polyuria if the obstruction is a stone that becomes dislodged. Treatment calls for location and relief of the blockage. This can include insertion of a tube (e.g., urethral or ureteral), surgical correction of the disease process, or diversion of the urinary stream above the level of blockage.

URINARY TRACT CALCULI

One in 10 Canadians will have a kidney stone at some point in life (Canadian Kidney Foundation, 2020). Many of these

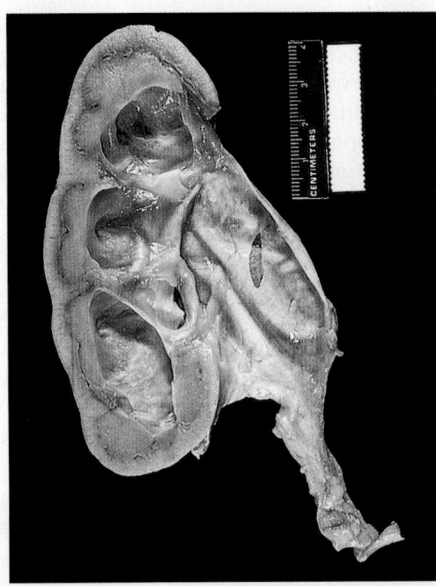

FIG. 48.4 Hydronephrosis of the kidney with marked dilation of the pelvis and the calyces and thinning of the renal parenchyma. Source: Kumar, V., Abbas, A. K.., & Aster, J. (2015). *Robbins and Cotran pathologic basis of disease* (9th ed., p. 950, Figure 20-48). Saunders.

people require hospitalization. In Canada, the incidence of kidney stones is highest in the East and decreases toward the West. Except for struvite (magnesium–ammonium phosphate) stones associated with UTI, stone disorders are more common in men than in women (Flannigan & Battison, 2018).

The majority of patients with stones are between 20 and 55 years of age. The incidence is also higher in persons with a family history of stone formation. Recurrence of stones can affect up to 50% of patients. There is seasonal variation, with stone formation occurring more often in the summer months in Canada, thus supporting the role of dehydration in this process. Stone formation in the kidney seems to increase in incidence as countries become more industrialized, whereas the incidence of bladder stones decreases.

Etiology and Pathophysiology

Many factors affect the incidence and the type of stone formation, including metabolic, dietary, genetic, climatic, lifestyle, and occupational influences (Table 48.11). Various theories have been proposed to explain the formation of stones in the urinary tract; however, no single theory can account for stone formation in all cases. Crystals, when in a supersaturated concentration, can precipitate and unite to form a stone. Keeping urine dilute and free flowing reduces the risk for recurrent stone formation in many individuals. It is known that a *mucoprotein* (the matrix for the stone) is formed in the kidney that forms stones. Urinary pH, solute load, and inhibitors in the urine affect the formation of stones. The lower the pH is, the less soluble uric acid and cystine are. The higher the pH, the less soluble calcium and phosphate are.

Other important factors in the development of stones include obstruction with urinary stasis and urinary infection with urea-splitting bacteria (e.g., *Proteus, Klebsiella, Pseudomonas*, and some species of staphylococci). These bacteria cause the urine to become alkaline and contribute to the formation of struvite (magnesium–ammonium phosphate) stones (Flannigan & Battison, 2018).

Infected stones, when they are entrapped in the kidney, may assume a staghorn configuration as they enlarge (Figure 48.5). Infected stones are frequent in patients with an external urinary diversion, long-term in-dwelling catheter, neurogenic bladder, or urinary retention. Genetic factors may also contribute to urine stone formation. Cystinuria is an autosomal recessive disorder in which there is a marked increased excretion of cystine.

Types

A **calculus** is an abnormal stone formed in body tissues by an accumulation of mineral salts. The term *calculus* refers to the stone, and *lithiasis* refers to stone formation (**nephrolithiasis** thus indicates the formation of stones in the urinary tract). The five major categories of stones are (a) calcium phosphate, (b) calcium oxalate, (c) uric acid, (d) cystine, and (e) struvite

TABLE 48.11	RISK FACTORS FOR THE DEVELOPMENT OF URINARY TRACT CALCULI

Metabolic
- Abnormalities that result in increased urine levels of calcium, oxaluric acid, uric acid, or citric acid

Climate
- Saunas, hot yoga, heavy exercise, and warm weather cause increased fluid loss through sweating causing low urine volume, and increased solute concentration in urine

Diet
- Food high in oxalate (i.e. peanuts, rhubarb, spinach, beets, chocolate, sweet potatoes)
- Large intake of calcium* and oxalate
- Large intake of dietary proteins (red meat, organ meats, shellfish) that increase uric acid excretion
- Alcohol increases uric acid levels
- Low fluid intake that increases urinary concentration

*It is important to eat and drink calcium and oxalate-rich foods together during a meal. In doing so, oxalate and calcium are more likely to bind to one another in the stomach and intestines before the kidneys begin processing, making it less likely that kidney stones will form (National Kidney Foundation, 2019).
Source: National Kidney Foundation (2019). *Kidney stone diet plan and prevention.* https://www.kidney.org/atoz/content/diet

(magnesium–ammonium phosphate) (Table 48.12). Stone composition may be mixed, although calcium stones are the most common. Calculi can be found in various locations in the urinary tract.

Clinical Manifestations

Urinary stones cause clinical manifestations when they obstruct urinary flow. Common sites of complete obstruction are at the UPJ (the point where the ureter crosses the iliac vessels) and the UVJ. Symptoms include abdominal or flank pain (usually severe), hematuria, and renal colic. The pain may be associated with nausea and vomiting. The type of pain is determined by the location of the stone. If the stone is nonobstructing, pain may be absent. If the obstruction is in a calyx or at the UPJ, the patient may experience dull costovertebral flank pain or even colic. Pain resulting from the passage of a calculus down the ureter is intense and colicky. The patient may be in mild shock with cool, moist skin. As a stone nears the UVJ, pain will be felt in the lateral flank and sometimes down into the testicles, the labia, or the groin. Other clinical manifestations include the presence of urinary infection accompanied by fever, vomiting, nausea, and chills.

Diagnostic Studies

Diagnostic studies useful in the evaluation and management of renal lithiasis include urinalysis, urine culture, IVP, retrograde pyelogram, ultrasound, and cystoscopy. A plain film of the abdomen and renal ultrasound will identify larger, radiopaque stones. An IVP or retrograde pyelogram is used to localize the degree and the site of obstruction or to confirm the presence of a radiolucent stone, such as a uric acid or cystine calculus (see Figure 48.5, *B*). Ultrasonography can be used to identify a radiopaque or radiolucent calculus in the renal pelvis, the calyx, or the proximal ureter; it is less useful when attempting to locate stones trapped in the midureter. A CT scan may be used to differentiate a nonopaque stone from a tumour.

Retrieval and analysis of the stones are important in the diagnosis of the underlying health problem contributing to stone formation. The patient's BUN, glomerular filtration rate (GFR), and serum creatinine levels are also measured to assess renal

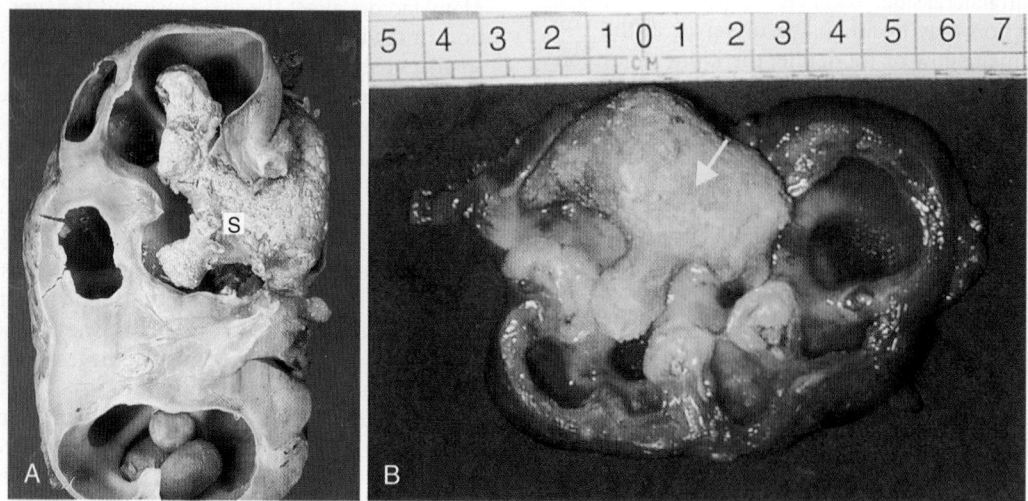

FIG. 48.5 A, Renal staghorn calculus. A large calculus fills the renal pelvis, shaped to its contours and resembling the horn of a stag *(S).* **B,** Embedded staghorn calculus *(yellow arrow)* in a hydronephrotic, infected, nonfunctioning kidney. Sources: *A,* Stevens, A., Lowe, J., & Scott, I. (2009). *Core pathology: Illustrated review in color* (3rd ed.). Mosby; *B,* Bullock, N., Doble, A., Turner, W., et al. (2008). *Urology: An illustrated colour text.* Churchill Livingstone.

TABLE 48.12   TYPES OF URINARY TRACT CALCULI

Urinary Stone	Incidence (%)	Characteristics	Predisposing Factors	Therapeutic Measures
Calcium oxalate*	35–40	Small, often possible to get trapped in ureter; more frequent in men than in women	Idiopathic hypercalciuria; hyperoxaluria; family history; independent of urinary pH	Increase hydration. Reduce dietary oxalate.† Give thiazide diuretics. Give cellulose phosphate to chelate calcium and prevent GI absorption. Give potassium citrate to maintain alkaline urine. Give cholestyramine to bind oxalate. Give calcium lactate to precipitate oxalate in GI tract.
Calcium phosphate	8–10	Mixed stones (typically); occur with struvite or oxalate stones	Alkaline urine, primary hyperparathyroidism	Treat underlying causes and other stones.
Struvite ($MgNH_4PO_4$)	10–15	Three to four times more common in women than men; always in association with urinary tract infections; large staghorn type (usually)‡	Urinary tract infections (usually *Proteus* organisms)	Administer antimicrobial agents, acetohydroxamic acid (Lithostat). Use surgical intervention to remove stone. Take measures to acidify urine.
Uric acid	5–8	Predominant in men, high incidence in Jewish men	Gout; acidic urine; inherited condition	Reduce urinary concentration of uric acid. Alkalinize urine with potassium citrate. Administer allopurinol. Reduce dietary purines.†
Cystine	1–2	Genetic autosomal recessive defect, defective absorption of cystine in GI tract and kidney, excess concentrations causing stone formation	Acidic urine	Increase hydration. Give penicillamine and tiopronin to prevent cystine crystallization. Give potassium citrate to maintain alkaline urine.

GI, gastrointestinal.
*Calcium stones can exist as calcium oxalate, calcium phosphate, or a mixture of both. Calcium stones account for the majority of all stones.
†See Table 48.13.
‡See Figures 48.5 and 48.6.

function. A careful history, including previous stone formation, prescribed and over-the-counter medications and dietary supplements, and family history of urinary calculi, is useful. Measurement of urine pH can aid in the diagnosis of struvite stones and renal tubular acidosis (tendency to alkaline pH) and uric acid stones (tendency to acidic pH).

Interprofessional Care

Evaluation and management of patients with renal lithiasis consist of two concurrent approaches. The first approach is directed toward management of the acute attack. This involves treating the symptoms of pain, infection, or obstruction as indicated for the individual patient. Opioids are typically required at frequent intervals for relief of renal colic pain. Many stones pass spontaneously. However, stones larger than 4 mm are unlikely to pass through the ureter. The second approach is directed toward evaluation of the cause of the stone formation and the prevention of further development of stones. Information to be obtained from the patient includes family history of stone formation, geographic residence, nutritional assessment including the intake of vitamins A and D, activity pattern (active or sedentary), history of periods of prolonged illness with immobilization or dehydration, and any history of disease or surgery involving the GI or genitourinary tract.

Therapy for people who are active stone formers requires a concerted management approach, with primary emphasis on teaching and on developing a therapeutic regimen that the patient can manage. Adequate hydration, dietary sodium restrictions, dietary changes (Table 48.13), and the use of medications can keep urinary stone formation to a minimum. The medications prescribed depend on the specific condition underlying stone formation. These medications prevent stone formation in various ways, including altering urine pH, preventing excessive urinary excretion of a substance, or correcting a primary disease (e.g., hyperparathyroidism).

TABLE 48.13   NUTRITIONAL THERAPY
Urinary Tract Calculi

Depending on the type of calculi, the diet should be modified to decrease foods that are high in the substance that is the cause of the calculi. Listed below are foods that are moderate or high in purine, calcium, or oxalate content.

Purine
- *High:* Sardines, herring, mussels, liver, kidney, goose, venison, meat soups, sweetbreads
- *Moderate:* Chicken, salmon, crab, veal, mutton, bacon, pork, beef, ham

Calcium
- Milk, cheese, ice cream, yogourt, sauces containing milk; all beans (except green beans), lentils; fish with fine bones (e.g., sardines, kippers, herring, salmon); dried fruits, nuts; chocolate, cocoa, Ovaltine

Oxalate
- Spinach, rhubarb, asparagus, cabbage, tomatoes, beets, nuts, celery, parsley, runner beans; chocolate, cocoa, instant coffee, Ovaltine, tea; Worcestershire sauce

Treatment of struvite stones calls for control of infection, which may be difficult if the stone remains in place. In addition to antibiotics, acetohydroxamic acid (Lithostat) may be used in the treatment of kidney infections that result in the continual formation of struvite stones. Acetohydroxamic acid (Lithostat), a urease inhibitor of the chemical action caused by the persistent bacteria, can be used effectively to retard struvite stone formation. This medication is available in Canada through the Special Access Drug Program at Health Canada. If the infection cannot be controlled, the stone may have to be removed surgically.

Indications for endourological, lithotripsy, or open surgical stone removal include the following:

- Stones too large for spontaneous passage
- Stones associated with bacteriuria or symptomatic infection
- Stones causing impaired renal function
- Stones causing persistent pain, nausea, or ileus
- Inability of the patient to be treated medically
- Patient having one kidney

Endourological Procedures. To remove a small stone located in the bladder, a cystoscopy is done. For large stones (Figure 48.6), a *cystolitholapaxy* is done. In this procedure, large stones are broken up with an instrument called a *lithotrite* (stone crusher). The bladder is then irrigated and the crushed stones are washed out. A *cystoscopic lithotripsy* uses an ultrasonic lithotrite to pulverize stones. Complications associated with these cystoscopic procedures include hemorrhage, retained stone fragments, and infection.

Flexible *ureteroscopes,* inserted via a cystoscope, can be used to remove stones from the renal pelvis and the upper urinary tract. Ultrasonic, laser, or electrohydraulic lithotripsy can be used in conjunction with the ureteroscope to pulverize and break the stone into fragments.

In *percutaneous nephrolithotomy,* a nephroscope is inserted through a sinus tract from the skin into the kidney pelvis. Stones can be fragmented using ultrasound, electrohydraulic, or laser lithotripsy. The stone fragments are removed and the pelvis is irrigated. A percutaneous nephrostomy tube is usually left in place to ensure that the ureter is not obstructed. Complications include bleeding, injury to adjacent structures, and infection.

Lithotripsy. Lithotripsy involves the use of sound waves to break renal stones into small particles that can be eliminated from the urinary tract. Lithotripsy techniques include percutaneous ultrasonic lithotripsy, electrohydraulic lithotripsy, laser lithotripsy, and extracorporeal shock-wave lithotripsy (Elmansy & Lingeman, 2016). Extracorporeal shock-wave lithotripsy and laser lithotripsy are the most common techniques used.

In *percutaneous ultrasonic lithotripsy,* an ultrasonic probe is placed in the renal pelvis via a percutaneous nephroscope (inserted through a small incision in the flank) and is positioned against the stone. The patient is given general or spinal anaesthesia for this procedure. The probe produces ultrasonic waves, which break the stone into sand-like particles. Percutaneous lithotripsy is not often used as a primary approach to a renal or upper ureteral stone unless the stone is large and other lithotripsy procedures have failed.

The *electrohydraulic lithotripsy* probe is also placed directly on a stone, but it breaks the stone into small fragments that are removed by forceps or suction. A continuous saline irrigation flushes out the stone particles, and all outflow drainage is strained so that the particles can be analyzed. Forceps or basket extraction can also be used to remove the calculi. Complications with this procedure are rare but include hemorrhage, sepsis, and abscess formation. Postoperatively, the patient usually experiences moderate to severe colicky pain. The first few voids are bright red; as the bleeding subsides, the urine becomes dark red or turns a smoky colour. Antibiotics are usually given for 2 weeks to reduce the risk for infection.

Laser lithotripsy probes are used to fragment lower ureteral and large bladder stones. A holmium laser medium is preferred; it fragments stones but does not injure the surrounding tissue.

In *extracorporeal shock-wave lithotripsy,* a noninvasive procedure, the patient is anaesthetized (spinal or general) and placed in a water bath. Anaesthesia is necessary to keep the patient very still during the procedure. Some of the newer-generation lithotripters do not require submersion and use other means of initiating shock waves.

Fluoroscopy or ultrasound is used to focus the lithotripter on the affected kidney, and a high-voltage spark generator produces high-energy acoustic shock waves that shatter the stone without damaging the surrounding tissues. The stone is broken into fine sand, which is excreted into the patient's urine within a few days after the procedure.

Hematuria is common after lithotripsy procedures. A self-retaining ureteral stent is often placed after the procedure to promote passage of sand from the fragmented stone and to prevent obstruction caused by its buildup in the ureter. The stent is removed 1 to 2 weeks after lithotripsy. A primary advantage of these techniques compared with open surgery is the decrease in length of hospitalization and the patient's earlier return to normal activities. Additional treatment may be necessary, especially if a stone is large and in the midureter or the distal ureter.

Surgical Therapy. A small group of select patients need open surgical procedures, such as patients with morbid obesity or those with complex abnormalities in the calyces or at the UPJ. The type of open surgery performed depends on the location of the stone. A *nephrolithotomy* is an incision into the

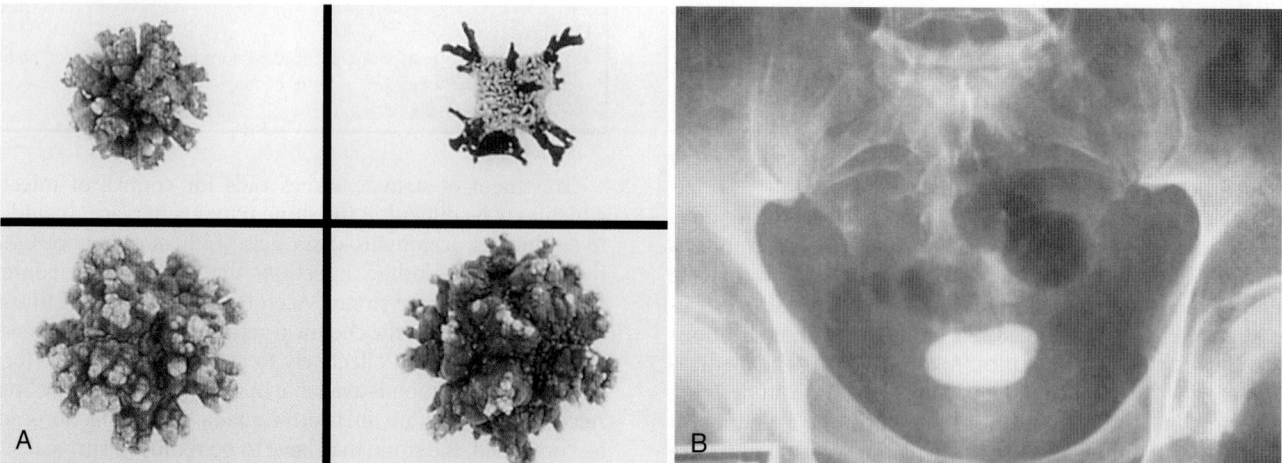

FIG. 48.6 A, Calcium oxalate stones. **B,** Plain abdominal radiograph shows a large bladder calculus. Source: Bullock, N., Doble, A., Turner, W., et al. (2008). *Urology: An illustrated colour text.* Churchill Livingstone.

kidney to remove a stone. A *pyelolithotomy* is an incision into the renal pelvis to remove a stone. If the stone is located in the ureter, a *ureterolithotomy* is performed. A *cystotomy* may be indicated for bladder calculi. For open surgery on the kidney or ureter, a flank incision directly below the diaphragm and across the side is usually the preferred surgical approach. The most common complication following these surgical procedures is hemorrhage.

Nutritional Therapy. Patients with an obstructing stone should be advised to drink adequate fluids to avoid dehydration. Forcing fluids is avoided because this strategy has not proved effective in assisting patients to spontaneously "pass" (excrete) the stone via the urine. In addition, forcing fluids may exacerbate the colic associated with this episode.

After an episode of urolithiasis, however, a high fluid intake (≈3 000 mL/day) is recommended to produce a urine output of at least 2 L/day. High urine output prevents supersaturation of minerals (i.e., dilutes the concentration) and promotes excretion of minerals within the urine, thus preventing stone formation. Increasing the fluid intake is especially important for patients who are active in sports, live in a dry climate, perform physical exercise, have a family history of stone formation, or work in an occupation that requires outdoor labour or a great deal of physical activity that can lead to dehydration. Water is the preferred fluid; consumption of sodas should be limited because high intake of these beverages tends to increase rather than diminish the risk for recurring urinary calculi. Intake of sugarless lemonade or of fluids containing high natural citrate have been shown to have a preventative effect on the formation of renal stones (National Kidney Foundation, 2019).

Dietary intervention may be important in the management of urolithiasis. In the past, calcium intake was routinely restricted for patients with kidney stones. However, more recent research suggests that a high dietary calcium intake, which was previously thought to contribute to kidney stones, may actually lower the risk, by reducing the urinary excretion of oxalate, a common factor in many stones (National Kidney Foundation, 2019). Initial nutritional management should include limiting oxalate-rich foods and thereby reducing oxalate excretion. Foods high in calcium, oxalate, and purines are presented in Table 48.13.

NURSING MANAGEMENT
RENAL CALCULI

NURSING ASSESSMENT

Subjective and objective data that should be obtained from a patient with urinary tract lithiasis are presented in Table 48.14.

NURSING DIAGNOSES

Nursing diagnoses for the patient with urinary tract lithiasis include but are not limited to the following:

- *Inadequate urinary elimination* resulting from *multiple causality* (trauma or obstruction)
- *Acute pain* resulting from *physical injury agent, biological injury agent* (effects of stones)
- *Inadequate knowledge* resulting from *insufficient information* (unfamiliarity with information resources, lack of experience with urinary stones)

Additional information on nursing diagnoses for the patient with urinary tract lithiasis is presented in NCP 48.2, available on the Evolve website.

PLANNING

The overall goals are that the patient with urinary tract calculi will have (a) relief of pain, (b) no urinary tract obstruction, and (c) an understanding of measures to prevent further recurrence of stones.

NURSING IMPLEMENTATION

A program to prevent stone recurrence always includes adequate fluid intake to produce a urine output of approximately 2 L/day. The nurse should consult with the health care provider on recommendations for fluid intake in a given patient. A modestly active, ambulatory patient would be required to drink about 2 000 to 2 200 mL/day with the residual 20 to 30% of fluids gained through consumption of foods. The volume of necessary fluids will be higher in the highly active patient who works outdoors or who regularly engages in demanding athletic activities. In contrast, fluid intake will be less for the very sedentary or immobile person. Preventive measures for the person who is on bed rest or is relatively immobile for a prolonged time include maintaining an adequate fluid intake, turning the patient every

---

TABLE 48.14   NURSING ASSESSMENT

Urinary Tract Calculi

Subjective Data

Important Health Information

Current health history: Dietary intake of purines, calcium, oxalates, phosphates; fluid intake

Past health history: Recent or chronic UTI; bed rest or sedentary lifestyle; immobilization; previous urinary tract stones, obstruction, or kidney disease with urinary stasis; gout; prostatic hyperplasia; hyperparathyroidism; family history of renal calculi

Medications: Prior use of medication for prevention of stones or treatment of UTI; allopurinol, analgesics

Surgery or other treatments: External urinary diversion, long-term indwelling urinary catheter

Symptoms

- Acute, severe, colicky pain in flank, back, abdomen, groin, or genitalia; burning on urination, dysuria, anxiety
- Decreased urinary output, urinary urgency, urinary frequency, feeling of bladder fullness
- Nausea, vomiting; chills

Objective Data

General

Guarding, fever

Integumentary

Warm, flushed skin or pallor with cool, moist skin (mild shock)

Gastrointestinal

Abdominal distension, absence of bowel sounds

Urinary

Oliguria, hematuria, tenderness on palpation of renal areas, passage of stone or stones

Possible Findings

↑ Serum urea (BUN) and serum creatinine levels; RBCs, WBCs, pyuria, crystals, casts, minerals, bacteria on urinalysis; ↑ uric acid, calcium, phosphorus, oxalate, or cystine values on 24-hr urine sample; calculi or anatomical changes on IVP or KUB radiographic study; direct visualization of obstruction on cystoureteroscopy

BUN, blood urea nitrogen; *IVP,* intravenous pyelogram; *KUB,* kidneys, ureters, bladder; *RBCs,* red blood cells; *UTI,* urinary tract infection; *WBCs,* white blood cells.

2 hours, and helping the patient to sit or stand, if possible, to maximize urinary flow.

Additional preventive measures focus on reducing metabolic or secondary risk factors. For example, dietary restriction of purines may be helpful to patients at risk for developing uric acid stones. Reduced intake of oxalates may be indicated for patients with recurring calcium oxalate calculi. Patients need to be taught about dosage, scheduling, and potential adverse effects of medications used to reduce the risk for stone formation. Select patients may be taught to self-monitor urinary pH or be asked to measure urinary output.

Pain management and patient comfort are primary nursing responsibilities when managing an obstructing stone and renal colic (see NCP 48.2). It is important to ensure that the patient retrieves any spontaneously passed stones. All urine voided by the patient should be strained through gauze or a special urine strainer in an effort to detect the stone. The high fluid intake necessary for stone prevention is suspended, but consumption should be adequate to meet daily needs and prevent dehydration. Ambulation is generally encouraged, to promote movement of the stone from the upper to the lower urinary tract, but the patient should not walk unattended when experiencing acute colic, particularly if opioid analgesics are being used.

EVALUATION

The expected outcomes for the patient with urinary calculi are presented in NCP 48.2, available on the Evolve website.

STRICTURES

A stricture is an abnormal temporary or permanent narrowing of the lumen of a hollow organ—in this context, of the ureter or the urethra.

Ureteral Strictures

Ureteral strictures can affect the entire length of the ureter, from the UPJ to the UVJ. These strictures are usually an unintended result of surgical intervention, usually secondary to adhesions or scar formation. Depending on its severity, ureteral obstruction can threaten the function of the kidney. Clinical manifestations of a ureteral stricture include mild to moderate colic; this pain may be of moderate to severe intensity if the patient consumes a large volume of fluids (alcohol, in particular) over a brief period. Infection is unusual unless a calculus or foreign object such as a stent or nephrostomy tube is present.

The discomfort and obstruction of a ureteral stricture may be temporarily bypassed by placing a stent under endoscopic control or by diverting urinary flow via a nephrostomy tube inserted into the renal pelvis of the affected kidney. Definitive correction requires dilation with a balloon or catheter. If the stricture is severe or recurs after initial balloon or catheter dilation, it may be incised under endoscopic control *(endoureterotomy)*. In select cases, an open surgical approach may be required to excise the stenotic area and reanastomose the ureter to the contralateral ureter *(ureteroureterostomy)* or to the renal pelvis. Alternatively, distal ureteral strictures may be managed by a *ureteroneocystostomy* (reimplantation of the ureter into the bladder wall).

Urethral Stricture

A *urethral stricture* is the result of fibrosis or inflammation of the urethral lumen (Urology Care Foundation, 2021). Causes of urethral strictures include trauma, urethritis (particularly following gonococcal infection), and a congenital defect in the canalization of the urethra; causes can also be iatrogenic (following surgical intervention). Once the process of inflammation and fibrosis begins, the lumen of the urethra narrows, and its compliance (ability to close or open in response to bladder filling or micturition) is compromised. Meatal stenosis, a narrowing of the urethral opening, is also common.

Clinical manifestations associated with a urethral stricture include a diminished force of the urinary stream, spraying, or a split urine stream. The patient may report feelings of incomplete bladder emptying with urinary frequency and nocturia. Moderate to severe obstruction of the bladder outlet may lead to acute urinary retention. The patient may report a history of urethritis, difficulty with placement of a urinary catheter, or trauma involving the penis or the perineum. However, many patients are unable to recall any such events, thus leading to a diagnosis of an idiopathic stricture. A history of a UTI is not uncommon, particularly if the stricture involves the distal urethra.

Initial management of a stricture may be based on dilation. A metal instrument (urethral sound) or a series of progressively enlarging stents can be placed into the urethra (filiforms and followers) to expand its lumen in a stepwise fashion. Although this procedure may be initially successful, recurring stenosis is frequent. Recurrences may be managed by teaching the patient to repeatedly dilate the urethra by self-catheterization every few days. Alternatively, an endoscopic or open surgical procedure may provide a more durable solution to an obstructive urethral stricture. Shorter strictures may be managed by resection of the fibrotic area with primary reanastomosis. Longer strictures may require autotransplantation of a substitute segment such as a skin flap.

RENAL TRAUMA

A rise in the incidence of traumatic renal injuries is related to an increase in the mechanization and speed of transportation and to the increase in violent crimes and injuries (da Costa et al., 2016). Blunt trauma is the most common cause of such injuries. Injury to the kidney should be considered in cases of multiple injuries, sports injuries, traffic accidents, and falls. It is especially likely when the patient injures the abdomen, the flank, or the back. Penetrating injuries may result from violent encounters (e.g., gunshot or stabbing incidents) or may be of iatrogenic origin.

Clinical findings include a history of trauma to the area of the kidneys. Gross or microscopic hematuria may be present. Diagnostic studies include urinalysis, IVP with cystography, ultrasound, CT scan, or MRI evaluation. Renal arteriography may also be used. Both the injured kidney and the uninvolved kidney should be evaluated to provide information for further management.

The severity of renal trauma depends on the extent of the injury. Treatments range from bed rest, fluids, and analgesia to surgical exploration and repair or nephrectomy.

Nursing interventions vary with the type and the extent of associated injuries. Specific interventions related to renal trauma include ensuring increased fluid intake, providing comfort measures, monitoring for shock (e.g., penetrating injury), monitoring intake and output, observing for hematuria, determining the presence of myoglobinuria, assessing the cardiovascular status, and monitoring the use of potentially nephrotoxic antibiotics.

RENAL VASCULAR CONDITIONS

Vascular conditions involving the kidney include (a) nephrosclerosis, (b) renal artery stenosis, and (c) renal vein thrombosis.

NEPHROSCLEROSIS

Nephrosclerosis is sclerosis of the small arteries and arterioles of the kidney, resulting in renal tissue destruction. The decreased blood flow results in patchy necrosis of the renal parenchyma. Ischemic necrosis and destruction of glomeruli with subsequent fibrosis also occur.

Benign nephrosclerosis usually occurs in adults 30 to 50 years of age. It is caused by vascular changes resulting from hypertension and from the process of atherosclerosis. Atherosclerotic vascular changes account for most of the loss of renal function associated with aging. There is a direct relation between the degree of nephrosclerosis and the severity of hypertension. The patient with benign nephrosclerosis may have normal renal function in the early stages. The only detectable abnormality may be hypertension.

Accelerated nephrosclerosis, or *malignant nephrosclerosis,* is associated with malignant hypertension, a complication of hypertension characterized by a sharp increase in blood pressure with a diastolic pressure greater than 130 mm Hg (Sangle, 2020). The patient is usually a young adult, with a male-to-female predominance of 2:1. Renal insufficiency progresses rapidly.

Treatment for benign nephrosclerosis is the same as that for essential hypertension (see Chapter 35). Malignant nephrosclerosis is treated with aggressive antihypertensive therapy (see Chapter 35). The availability and use of antihypertensives have improved the prognosis for patients with benign and malignant nephrosclerosis. Renal dysfunction and renal failure (in some persons) constitute two of the major complications of hypertension. The prognosis for patients with malignant hypertension is poor, with the major cause of death being related to renal failure.

Diabetic patients who have renal complications such as diabetic nephropathy often suffer progressive impairment of renal function (see Chapter 52).

RENAL ARTERY STENOSIS

Renal artery stenosis, a partial occlusion of one or both renal arteries and their major branches, is a major cause of abrupt-onset hypertension. It can be caused by atherosclerotic narrowing or fibromuscular hyperplasia. Renal artery stenosis accounts for 1 to 2% of all cases of hypertension.

When hypertension develops rather abruptly, renal artery stenosis should be considered as a possible cause, especially in patients younger than 30 or older than 50 years and in patients with no familial history of hypertension. This contrasts with the age distribution for essential hypertension, which peaks between 30 and 50 years of age. A renal arteriogram is the best diagnostic tool for identifying renal artery stenosis.

The goals of therapy are control of blood pressure and restoration of perfusion to the kidney. Percutaneous transluminal renal angioplasty is the procedure of choice, especially in older patients who are poor surgical risks. Surgical revascularization of the kidney is indicated when blood flow is decreased enough to cause renal ischemia or when evidence indicates that renovascular hypertension is present and might be resolved by surgical intervention. The surgical procedure usually involves anastomoses between the kidney and another major artery, usually the splenic artery or the aorta. In select cases of unilateral renal involvement with high renin production, unilateral nephrectomy may be indicated.

RENAL VEIN THROMBOSIS

Renal vein thrombosis, an embolus occurring in the renal vein, may occur unilaterally or bilaterally. Trauma, extrinsic compression (e.g., tumour, aortic aneurysm), renal cell carcinoma, pregnancy, contraceptive use, and nephrotic syndrome are associated with renal vein thrombosis.

Symptoms include flank pain, hematuria, or fever or nephrotic syndrome. Anticoagulation is important in treatment because there is a high incidence of pulmonary emboli. Corticosteroids may be used for patients with nephrosis. Surgical thrombectomy may be performed instead of or along with anticoagulation.

HEREDITARY RENAL DISEASES

Hereditary renal diseases involve developmental abnormalities of the renal parenchyma. These abnormalities are either isolated or part of more complex malformation syndromes. The majority of inherited structural abnormalities are cystic. However, cysts may also develop as a result of obstructive uropathies, metabolic derangements, or neurological diseases. Cysts may be evaluated to rule out any tumour content.

POLYCYSTIC KIDNEY DISEASE

Polycystic kidney disease (PKD) is one of the most common genetic diseases in Canada. It may first become apparent in either childhood or adulthood. It involves both kidneys and occurs in both men and women. The cortex and the medulla are filled with thin-walled cysts that are several millimetres to several centimetres in diameter (Figure 48.7). The cysts enlarge and destroy surrounding tissue by compression. They are filled with fluid and may contain blood or pus.

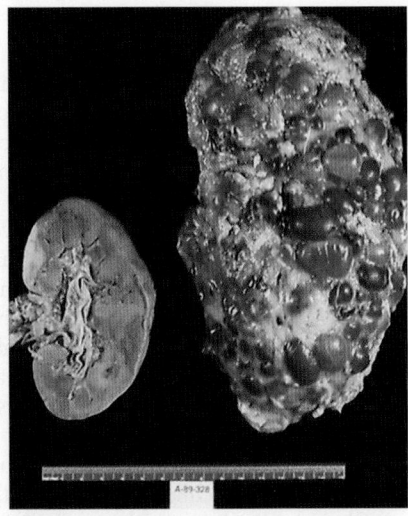

FIG. 48.7 Comparison of polycystic kidney with normal kidney. Source: Brundage, D. J. (1992). *Renal disorders.* Mosby.

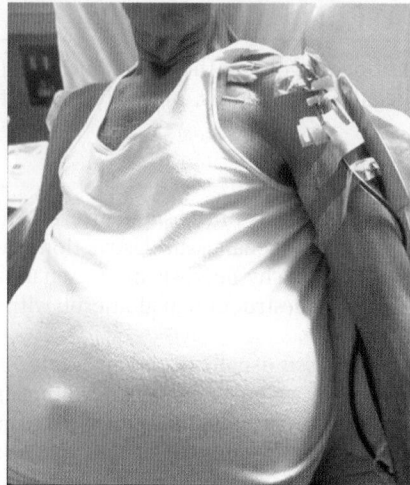

FIG. 48.8 Man with an 11-kg polycystic kidney. Source: Lemmi, F. O., & Lemmi, C. A. E. (2000). *Physical assessment findings* (CD-ROM). Saunders.

There are two forms of hereditary polycystic renal disease. The adult form of PKD is an autosomal dominant disorder. It is latent for many years and is usually evidenced between the ages of 30 and 40 years. However, PKD has also been found in newborns. The childhood form of PKD is a rare autosomal recessive disorder that is often rapidly progressive (see the Genetics in Clinical Practice box).

Clinical Manifestations

In the patient with PKD (Figure 48.8), symptoms appear when the cysts begin to enlarge. A common early symptom of adult PKD is abdominal or flank pain, which is steady and dull or abrupt in onset as well as episodic and colicky. This pain is often caused by bleeding into the cysts. On physical examination, palpable bilateral enlarged kidneys are often found. Other clinical manifestations include hematuria (from rupture of cysts), UTI, and hypertension.

Diagnosis is based on clinical manifestations, family history, IVP, ultrasound, or CT scan. Usually, the disease progresses to end-stage renal failure, although some individuals have relatively mild disease and die from unrelated health conditions. Loss of kidney function to the point of end-stage renal disease occurs by age 60 in 50% of patients (National Kidney Foundation, 2018).

Interprofessional Care

There is no specific treatment for PKD. A major aim of treatment is to prevent infections of the urinary tract or to treat them with appropriate antibiotics if they occur. Nephrectomy may be necessary if pain, bleeding, or infection becomes a chronic, serious condition.

When the patient begins to experience progressive renal failure, the interventions are determined by the remaining renal function. Nursing measures are those used for management of end-stage renal disease (see Chapter 49). They include diet modification, fluid restriction, medications (e.g., antihypertensives), assisting the patient to accept the chronic disease process, and assisting the patient and family to cope with physical, socioeconomic, and emotional reactions to the disease.

Patients with adult PKD often have children by the time the disease is diagnosed. Each child of a parent with PKD has a 50% chance of having the disease. Patients will need appropriate counselling regarding plans for having more children. In addition, genetic counselling resources should be provided for the children.

MEDULLARY CYSTIC DISEASE

Medullary cystic disease is a hereditary disorder that occurs in two forms. The *autosomal recessive form* is associated with renal failure before age 20 years; the *autosomal dominant form* is associated with renal failure after age 20. Most cysts are located in the medulla. The kidneys are asymmetrical, are significantly scarred, and have defects in their concentration ability. Polyuria, progressive renal failure, severe anemia, metabolic acidosis, and poor sodium conservation are common. Hypertension in patients with this disease can be a terminal event. Genetic counselling may be helpful in family planning. Treatment measures are those related to end-stage renal disease (see Chapter 49).

ALPORT SYNDROME

Alport syndrome is also known as *chronic hereditary nephritis*. Two forms of the disease exist: (a) classic Alport syndrome, which is inherited as a sex-linked disorder with hematuria, sensorineural deafness, and deformities of the anterior surface of the lens, and (b) nonclassic Alport syndrome, which is inherited as an autosomal trait that causes hematuria but not deafness or lens deformities (National Library of Medicine, 2020). The disease affects males earlier and more severely than females and is often diagnosed in the first decade of life. The basic defect is altered synthesis of the GBM, and patients most commonly have hematuria and progressive uremia. Treatment is supportive, although the disease will not recur after kidney transplantation. Corticosteroids and cytotoxic medications are not effective.

RENAL INVOLVEMENT IN METABOLIC AND CONNECTIVE TISSUE DISEASES

Various metabolic and connective tissue disease processes may have an effect on renal function. The pathophysiological effects on the renal parenchyma are not always specific to each process. The clinical course of renal involvement is that of chronic progressive nephropathy, which can result in uremia and death. Management includes treatment of the primary disorder along with symptomatic relief of renal involvement. If renal involvement progresses to end-stage renal disease, management includes dialysis or transplantation (see Chapter 49). Nursing interventions include teaching the patient about the primary disease process, the renal involvement, and the resulting need to adhere to dietary and fluid restrictions and medication regimens.

In Canada, diabetic nephropathy is the primary cause of end-stage renal failure (Bril et al., 2018). Diabetes mellitus may affect the kidneys in several ways. Microangiopathic changes in diabetes consist of diffuse glomerulosclerosis, involving thickening of the GBM, and nodular glomerulosclerosis (Kimmelstiel–Wilson syndrome), which is characterized by nodular lesions. Nodular glomerulosclerosis is reasonably specific for type 1 diabetes mellitus. Patients with diabetes who are prone to glomerulonephropathy (i.e., the presence of trace proteinuria or retinopathy) require careful monitoring of glucose levels and insulin requirements. (Diabetes mellitus is discussed in Chapter 52.)

Gout is a syndrome of acute attacks of arthritis caused by hyperuricemia (see Chapter 67). Monosodium urate crystals deposited in joints are responsible for the syndrome. Renal disease may develop as a result of damage caused by deposition of uric acid crystals in the renal interstitium and the tubules.

Amyloidosis is a group of disorders evidenced by impaired organ function from the infiltration of tissues with a hyaline substance (amyloid). The hyaline consists largely of protein. Kidney involvement is common in amyloidosis. Proteinuria is often the first clinical manifestation.

Systemic lupus erythematosus is a connective tissue disorder characterized by the involvement of several tissues and organs, particularly the joints, the skin, and the kidneys. (Systemic lupus erythematosus is discussed in Chapter 67.) Clinical manifestations of lupus nephritis are similar to those of other forms of glomerulonephritis. Renal failure frequently occurs in systemic lupus erythematosus and has a poor prognosis.

Systemic sclerosis (scleroderma) is a disease of unknown etiology characterized by widespread alterations of connective tissue and vascular lesions in many organs (see Chapter 67). In the kidney, vascular lesions are associated with fibrosis. An immune complex mechanism has been postulated as a possible etiological factor. The severity of renal involvement varies. Patients who develop severe renal lesions have a poor prognosis.

URINARY TRACT TUMOURS

KIDNEY CANCER

The incidence of kidney cancer in Canada is rising. In 2019, an estimated 72 000 Canadians were diagnosed with kidney cancer and 1 900 Canadians died from it, with a lifetime probability of 1.5% for developing kidney and renal pelvis cancer (Canadian Cancer Society, 2019). Tumours arising from both areas may be benign or malignant. However, malignant tumours are more frequent. Adenocarcinoma (renal cell carcinoma) is the most common type. Adenocarcinoma occurs twice as often in men as in women and is typically discovered when the person is 50 to 70 years old. Cigarette smoking is the most significant risk factor for the development of adenocarcinoma (Canadian Cancer Society, 2019). Other risk factors are obesity, the use of

phenacetin-containing analgesics, and exposure to asbestos, cadmium, and gasoline.

There are no characteristic early symptoms. Generalized symptoms of weight loss, weakness, and anemia are the earliest manifestations. The classic manifestations of gross hematuria, flank pain, and a palpable mass are those of advanced disease. The most common sites of metastases include the lungs, liver, and long bones. Local extension of kidney cancer into the renal vein and the vena cava is common (Figure 48.9). Renal cystic disease and renal-associated carcinomas may develop in patients with end-stage renal disease who are receiving maintenance renal dialysis (see Chapter 49).

Several studies are used to diagnose kidney cancer. IVP with nephrotomography is the primary examination by which most masses are detected and evaluated. Ultrasounds have improved the ability to differentiate between a tumour and a cyst. Angiography, percutaneous needle aspiration, CT, and MRI are also used in the diagnosis of renal tumours. Small renal tumours are found earlier because of the increased use of CT scans and MRI. Radionuclide isotope scanning is used to detect metastases. Robson's system of staging renal carcinoma is presented in Table 48.15.

The treatment of choice is a radical nephrectomy, which is the removal of the kidney, the adrenal gland, the surrounding

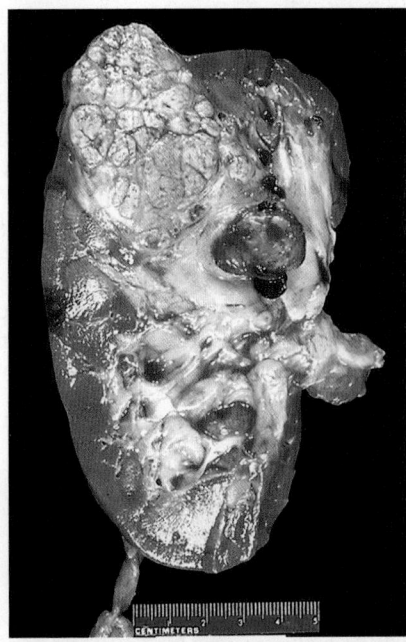

FIG. 48.9 Adenocarcinoma. Cross-section shows yellowish cancer in one pole of the kidney. The tumour also involves the dilated thrombosed renal vein. Source: Kumar, V., Abbas, A. K., & Aster, J. (2015). *Robbins and Cotran pathologic basis of disease* (9th ed., p. 954, Figure 20-51). Saunders.

TABLE 48.15	ROBSON'S SYSTEM OF STAGING RENAL CARCINOMA	
Stage	**Description**
I	Limitation to renal capsule
II	Spreading to perirenal fat but confined within fascia; includes metastasis to adrenal gland
III	Regional lymph node involvement, tumour thrombus in renal vein or vena cava, involvement of renal vein or vena cava
IV	Presence of distant metastases

fascia, part of the ureter, and the draining lymph nodes. Radiation therapy is used palliatively in inoperable cases and when there are metastases to bone or lungs.

Chemotherapy using 5-fluorouracil (5-FU) and gemcitabine is used to treat metastatic disease. However, renal cell carcinoma is refractory to most chemotherapy medications. Biological therapy, including interferon-alfa (IFN-alfa) and interleukin-2 (IL-2), is most promising in the treatment of metastatic disease (Jiang et al., 2016). Adverse effects of IL-2 include capillary leakage syndrome, fever, chills, fatigue, and hypotension.

The 5-year survival rate of patients with early-stage kidney cancer is 60 to 70% after undergoing radical nephrectomy. The 5-year survival rate for patients with metastatic disease is only 3 to 10%. However, patients with metastatic disease often remain stable for a prolonged period (Ali, 2019).

BLADDER CANCER

In 2019, an estimated 11 800 Canadians were diagnosed with bladder cancer and 2 500 Canadians died from it (Canadian Cancer Society, 2019). Bladder cancer is the sixth most common type of cancer diagnosed in Canadians. The most frequent malignant tumour of the urinary tract is transitional cell carcinoma of the bladder. Most bladder tumours are papillomatous growths within the bladder (Figure 48.10). Cancer of the bladder is most common between the ages of 60 and 70 years and is at least three times more common in men than in women. Risk factors for bladder cancer include cigarette smoking, exposure to dyes used in the rubber and cable industries, and chronic use of phenacetin-containing analgesics (Canadian Cancer Society, 2021). Women treated with radiation for cervical cancer and patients receiving cyclophosphamide (Procytox) also have increased risk, but the reason for this is unknown.

Individuals with chronic, recurrent stones (often bladder) and chronic lower urinary infections have an increased risk for squamous cell cancer of the bladder. Patients with in-dwelling catheters for long periods can develop these chronic conditions.

Clinical Manifestations and Diagnostic Studies

Gross, painless hematuria (chronic or intermittent) is the most common clinical finding. Bladder irritability with dysuria, urinary frequency, and urinary urgency may also occur. When cancer is suspected, urine specimens for cytology can be obtained to determine the presence of neoplastic or atypical cells. Exfoliated cells from the epithelial surface of the bladder can readily be detected in voided specimens. Other recently developed urine tests are used to assess for specific factors associated with bladder cancer, such as bladder tumour antigens. Bladder cancers can be detected using IVP, ultrasound, CT, or MRI. However, the presence of cancer is confirmed by cystoscopy and biopsy.

The depth of invasion of the bladder wall and surrounding tissue determines the clinical staging of carcinoma of the bladder. The Jewett–Strong–Marshall classification system broadly classifies bladder cancer as superficial (carcinoma in situ, O, A), invasive (B_1, B_2, C), or metastatic (D_1–D_4) disease. Pathological grading systems are also used to classify the malignant potential of tumour cells, indicating a scale ranging from well-differentiated to anaplastic categories. Low-stage, low-grade bladder cancers are the most responsive cancers to treatment and are more easily cured.

NURSING AND INTERPROFESSIONAL MANAGEMENT BLADDER CANCER

Interprofessional care of the patient with bladder cancer is outlined in Table 48.16.

SURGICAL THERAPY

Surgical therapies include a variety of procedures. *Transurethral resection with fulguration* (electrocautery) is used for the diagnosis and treatment of superficial lesions with a low recurrence rate. This procedure is also used to control bleeding in the patient who is a poor operative risk or who has advanced

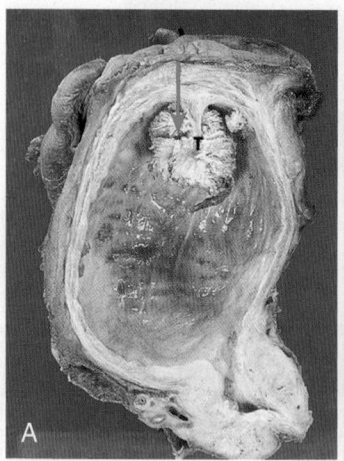 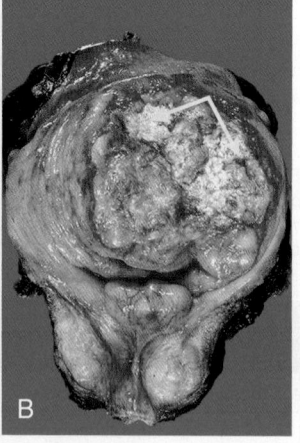

FIG. 48.10 A, A papillary transitional cell carcinoma is seen arising from the dome of the bladder as a cauliflower-like lesion. **B,** Opened bladder shows a bladder cancer at an advanced stage. The yellow areas represent ulcerations and necrosis. Source: *A,* Stevens, A., & Lowe, J. (2000). *Pathology: Illustrated review in color* (2nd ed.). Mosby; *B,* Kumar, V., Abbas, A. K., & Aster, J. (2015). *Robbins and Cotran pathologic basis of disease* (9th ed., p. 967, Figure 21-12). Saunders.

TABLE 48.16   **INTERPROFESSIONAL CARE**
Bladder Cancer

Diagnostic
- History and physical examination
- CT scan
- Cystoscopy with biopsy
- Cytology studies
- Intravenous pyelogram
- Ultrasound
- Urinalysis

Interprofessional Therapy
- Surgical treatment
  - Laser photocoagulation
  - Open loop resection or fulguration
  - Radical cystectomy
  - Segmental cystectomy
  - Transurethral resection with fulguration

- Radiation
- Intravesical immunotherapy
  - Bacille Calmette–Guérin
  - Interferon-alfa
- Intravesical chemotherapy
  - Doxorubicin
  - Mitomycin
  - Thiotepa
- Systemic chemotherapy

CT, computed tomography.

tumours. With this technique, the tumour mass is excised by means of a blade inserted through the cystoscope. The remaining portions of the tumour are cauterized.

A second technique, *laser photocoagulation,* is also used to treat superficial bladder cancers. This procedure can be repeated a number of times to manage recurrences. The advantages of laser treatment include bloodless destruction of the lesion, minimal risk for perforation, and lack of need for a urinary catheter. The primary disadvantage is that, owing to destruction of the tumour, pathological evaluation for grading and staging cannot be completed.

A third technique used is *open loop resection* (snaring of polyp types of lesion) *with fulguration.* It is used for the control of bleeding, for large superficial tumours, and for multiple lesions. Treatment of large lesions entails a segmental resection of the bladder (*segmental cystectomy*).

Postoperative instructions for patients undergoing any of these procedures includes drinking a large volume of fluid each day for the first week following the procedure and avoiding intake of alcoholic beverages. Patients are taught to self-monitor their urine. It is anticipated to be pink during the first several days after the procedure, but it should not be bright red or contain blood clots. Approximately 7 to 10 days following tumour resection or ablation, the patient may observe dark-red or rust-coloured flecks in the urine. These are anticipated and represent scabs from the healing tumour resection sites. Opioid analgesics may be required for a brief period after the procedure, along with stool softeners. Patients can be encouraged to take a 15- to 20-minute sitz bath two or three times a day to promote muscle relaxation and to reduce the risk for urinary retention. The nurse should also help the patient and family cope with fears about cancer, surgery, and effects on sexuality and should emphasize the importance of regular follow-up care. Frequent routine cystoscopies are required.

When the tumour is invasive or when it involves the *trigone* (the area where the ureters insert into the bladder) and the patient is free from metastasis beyond the pelvic area, a partial or radical cystectomy with urinary diversion is the treatment of choice (see the section on urinary diversion later in the chapter). A *partial cystectomy* includes resection of that portion of the bladder wall containing the tumour, along with a margin of normal tissue. A *radical cystectomy* involves removal of the bladder, the prostate, and the seminal vesicles in men, and the bladder, the uterus, the cervix, the urethra, and the ovaries in women (Chang et al., 2017).

RADIATION THERAPY AND CHEMOTHERAPY

Radiation therapy is used with cystectomy or as the primary therapy when the cancer is inoperable or when surgery is refused. Increasingly, radiation therapy is being combined with systemic chemotherapy. Sometimes, combination systemic chemotherapy is used for bladder cancer, usually preoperatively or before radiation therapy, or is used to treat distant metastases. Chemotherapy agents used in treating invasive bladder cancer include cisplatin, vinblastine, and methotrexate.

INTRAVESICAL THERAPY

Chemotherapy with local instillation of chemotherapeutic or immune-stimulating agents can be delivered directly into the bladder by a urethral catheter. Policies vary, but intravesical therapy is usually initiated at weekly intervals for 6 to 12 weeks. The chemotherapeutic agents are instilled directly into the patient's bladder and retained for about 2 hours. The patient's

position may be changed every 15 minutes for maximum contact in all areas of the bladder, especially if the tumour occurred on the bladder dome. The use of maintenance therapy after the initial induction regimen may be beneficial.

BCG, a weakened strain of *Mycobacterium bovis,* is the treatment of choice for carcinoma in situ. BCG stimulates the immune system rather than acting directly on cancer cells in the bladder. When BCG alone fails, IFN-alfa may be used in addition to BCG. Other treatments that can be used when BCG fails include thiotepa, an alkylating agent.

Most patients have irritation upon voiding and hemorrhagic cystitis following intravesical therapy. Thiotepa, when absorbed into circulation from the bladder wall, can significantly reduce WBC and platelet counts in some individuals. BCG may cause flulike symptoms, hematuria, or systemic infection. Other adverse effects usually associated with chemotherapy, such as nausea, vomiting, and hair loss, are not experienced with intravesical chemotherapy.

Nursing responsibilities include encouraging the patient to increase their daily fluid intake and to quit smoking, assessing the patient for secondary UTI, and stressing the need for routine urological follow-up. The patient may have fears or concerns about sexual activity or bladder function that will have to be addressed.

URINARY INCONTINENCE AND RETENTION

Urinary incontinence (UI) is an uncontrolled loss of urine that is of sufficient magnitude to be a problem for a person. Approximately 3.3 million Canadians experience incontinence, including 10% of children 6 years of age and up, 25% of women middle-aged and older, and 15% of men aged 60 years and older (Canadian Continence Foundation, 2021). Among younger adults, more women than men are affected by UI. Although UI has traditionally been viewed as a social or hygienic problem, it is now known to affect quality of life as well as contribute to morbidity in older persons. (UI is not a natural consequence of aging.)

Causes of UI may be transient (e.g., caused by confusion or depression, infection, medications, restricted mobility, or stool impaction). Acquired disorders are described in Table 48.17. Patients may have more than one type of incontinence and may not disclose UI symptoms because of associated stigma.

Urinary retention is the inability to empty the bladder despite micturition or the accumulation of urine in the bladder because of the inability to urinate. It may be associated with dribbling urinary leakage, called *overflow UI. Acute urinary retention* is the total inability to pass urine via micturition; it is a medical emergency. *Chronic urinary retention* is defined as incomplete bladder emptying despite urination. Postvoid residual volumes in patients with chronic urinary retention vary widely; values of 150 to 200 mL or higher generally necessitate further evaluation. Smaller volumes may justify evaluation when they produce LUTS or occur in a context of recurring UTIs. Urinary retention is caused by two different dysfunctions of the urinary system: bladder outlet obstruction and deficient detrusor contraction strength. Obstruction leads to urinary retention when the blockage prevents bladder evacuation of its contents despite a detrusor contraction. A common cause of obstruction in men is an enlarged prostate. Urinary retention also results when the detrusor muscle no longer has the strength to contract with enough force or for long enough to completely empty the bladder.

TABLE 48.17   ACQUIRED DISORDERS CAUSING URINARY INCONTINENCE

Type and Description	Causes	Treatment
Stress Incontinence* Sudden increase in intra-abdominal pressure causes involuntary passage of urine. It can occur during coughing, heavy lifting, straining, or laughing.	*Females:* Condition is found most commonly in women with relaxed pelvic musculature (frequently from obstetrical complications or multiple pregnancies). Structures of the female urethra atrophy when estrogen decreases. *Males:* Prostate surgery for benign prostatic hyperplasia or prostatic carcinoma.	Perineal muscle exercises (e.g., Kegel exercises), weight loss if patient is obese, insertion of vaginal pessary, estrogen (vaginal creams, tablets, or vaginal ring) Condom catheters or penile clamp, surgery Urethral inserts, patches, or bladder neck support devices to correct underlying condition
Urge Incontinence* Condition occurs randomly when involuntary urination is preceded by warning a few seconds to a few minutes in advance. Leakage is periodic but frequent. Nocturnal frequency and incontinence are common. Condition may appear with varying severity during psychological stress.	Condition is caused by uncontrolled contraction or overactivity of detrusor muscle. Bladder escapes central inhibition and contracts reflexively. Conditions include central nervous system disorders (e.g., cerebrovascular disease, Alzheimer's disease, brain tumour, Parkinson's disease), bladder disorders (e.g., carcinoma in situ, radiation effects, interstitial cystitis), interference with spinal inhibitory pathways (e.g., malignant growth in spinal cord, spondylosis), and bladder outlet obstruction, as well as conditions of unknown etiology.	Treatment of underlying cause, instruction to have patient urinate more frequently or on time schedule, anticholinergic medications (e.g., imipramine) at bedtime, calcium channel blockers, condom catheters, vaginal estrogen
Overflow Incontinence Pressure of urine in overfull bladder overcomes sphincter control. Urination may also occur frequently in small amounts during the night. Bladder remains distended and is usually palpable.	Disorder is caused by outlet obstruction (prostatic hyperplasia, bladder neck obstruction, urethral stricture) or by underactive detrusor muscle caused by myogenic or neurogenic factors (e.g., herniated disk, diabetic neuropathy). It may also occur after anaesthesia and surgery (especially procedures such as hemorrhoidectomy, herniorrhaphy, cystoscopy). Neurogenic bladder (flaccid type) is another cause.	Urinary catheterization to decompress bladder, implementation of Credé or Valsalva manoeuvre, α-adrenergic blocker (e.g., prazosin) to decrease outlet resistance, bethanechol (Duvoid) to enhance bladder contractions, intermittent catheterization, surgery to correct underlying health problem
Reflex Incontinence No warning or stress precedes periodic involuntary urination. Urination is frequent, is moderate in volume, and occurs equally during the day and night.	Spinal cord lesion above S2 interferes with central nervous system inhibition. Disorder results in detrusor hyper-reflexia and interferes with pathways coordinating detrusor contraction and sphincter relaxation.	Treatment of underlying cause, bladder decompression to prevent ureteral reflux and hydronephrosis, intermittent self-catheterization, α-adrenergic blocker (e.g., prazosin) to relax internal sphincter, diazepam or baclofen to relax external sphincter, prophylactic antibiotics, surgical sphincterotomy
Incontinence After Trauma or Surgery Vesicovaginal or urethrovaginal fistula may occur in women. Alteration in continence control in men involves proximal urethral sphincter (bladder neck and prostatic urethra) and distal urethral sphincter (external striated muscle).	Fistulas may occur during pregnancy, after delivery of baby, as a result of hysterectomy or invasive cancer of cervix, or after radiation therapy. Incontinence is found as postoperative complication after transurethral, perineal, or retropubic prostatectomy.	Surgery to correct fistula, urinary diversion surgery to bypass urethra and bladder, external condom catheter, penile clamp, placement of artificial implantable sphincter
Functional Incontinence Loss of urine resulting from patient mobility or environmental factors.	Older people often have health problems that affect balance and mobility.	Modifications of environment or care plan that facilitate regular, easy access to toilet and promote patient safety (e.g., better lighting, ambulatory assistance equipment, clothing alterations, timed voiding, different toileting equipment)

*Patients can have a combination of stress and urge incontinence that is referred to as *mixed incontinence*.

Common causes of deficient detrusor muscle contraction strength are neurological diseases affecting sacral segments 2, 3, and 4; long-standing diabetes mellitus; overdistension; chronic alcoholism; and medications (e.g., anticholinergic medications).

NURSING MANAGEMENT
URINARY INCONTINENCE

Nurses' relational care approaches through listening to patients' questions and valuing patients' knowledge about UI are required to address socioemotional well-being and promote application of UI management techniques. The majority of UI symptoms can be managed conservatively with the following interventions: hydration; reduction in consumption of caffeine and alcohol (bladder irritants); smoking cessation (smoking increases the risk of stress incontinence); and constipation management, which includes adequate fluid intake, increase in dietary fibre, light exercise, and judicious use of stool softeners. (The management of constipation is discussed in Chapter 45). As well, continence strategies can assist in preventing falls and fall-related injuries in older persons (Duong et al., 2019) and in monitoring for skin breakdown due to incontinence.

Habit training or prompted toileting is useful for patients with urge, mixed, and functional UI. Habit training involves using the results of a voiding diary or bladder log to determine patterns of daytime voiding frequency. A goal is then established for voiding frequency, usually ranging from 2 to 3 hours. Voiding is scheduled rigidly during waking hours according to the baseline urinary frequency identified on the bladder log. At night, the person is advised to urinate as normal if awakened from sleep with the desire to void. Habit training may be combined with pelvic muscle training, focusing on techniques such as urge suppression. Prompted toileting is indicated for patients with altered cognitive function and functional UI (usually coexisting with urge UI). Specifically, caregivers are taught to remind the patient to toilet on a regular basis (usually every 2–3 hours), and the patient is assisted to the toilet and given praise for successful toileting. A trial of prompted toileting, in conjunction with a urological evaluation, is used to predict the ultimate success of such a program.

In the hospital, nursing management includes maximizing toilet access and promoting privacy when offering the urinal or bedpan or assisting the patient to the bathroom every 2 to 3 hours or at scheduled times.

When attempting to manage UI, many women use feminine hygiene pads, and many men and women use household products such as rags, paper towels, or folded toilet tissue. None of these products is adequately designed to wick urine away from the skin, prevent soiling of clothing, and reduce or eliminate odour. The nurse should share information on products specifically designed to contain urine. For example, patients with mild to moderate UI often benefit from incontinence pads containing a material specifically designed to absorb many times its weight in water. Patients with higher-volume urine loss or those with double urinary and fecal incontinence may benefit from disposable or reusable incontinence briefs or pad–pant systems.

Diagnostic Studies

The basic evaluation for UI and urinary retention includes a focused history, physical assessment, and a bladder log or voiding record whenever possible. Information should be obtained regarding the onset of UI, factors that provoke urinary leakage, and associated conditions. The nurse should pay special attention to factors known to produce transient UI, particularly when a relatively sudden onset of urine loss is reported. The physical examination begins with an assessment of general health and functional issues associated with urinary function, including mobility, dexterity, and cognitive function. A pelvic examination includes careful inspection of the perineal skin for signs of erosion or rashes related to UI. Local innervation and pelvic muscle strength should also be evaluated. Whenever possible, the patient is asked to keep a bladder log or voiding diary documenting the timing of urinations, episodes of urinary leakage, and frequency

of nocturia for a period of 1 to 7 days. This record can be kept by nursing staff if the person is in an inpatient facility.

The urinalysis is used to identify possible factors contributing to transient UI or urinary retention (e.g., urinary infection, diabetes mellitus). A postvoid residual urine must be measured in the patient undergoing evaluation for urinary retention and UI. The postvoid residual volume is obtained by asking the patient to urinate, followed by catheterization within a relatively brief period (preferably 5–10 min). Alternatively, a bladder scan device can be used to estimate the residual volume. Although less accurate than the catheterized residual measurement, this technique avoids catheterization with its associated discomfort and risk for UTI. Urodynamic testing is indicated in select cases of UI and urinary retention (Taithongchai et al., 2019). Imaging studies of the upper urinary tract (e.g., CT scanning, ultrasound, IVP) are obtained when retention or UI is associated with UTIs or when there is evidence of upper urinary tract involvement.

Interprofessional Care: Urinary Incontinence

An estimated 80% of incontinence can be cured or significantly improved. Transient, reversible factors are corrected initially, followed by management of established UI (see Table 48.17). In general, less invasive treatments are attempted before more invasive methods (e.g., surgery) are used. Nevertheless, the choice of initial treatment is highly individualized and based on patient preference, the type and severity of UI, and associated anatomical defects.

Several therapies may be employed to improve urinary continence. These interventions are outlined in Table 48.18. Pelvic muscle training (Kegel exercises) is used to manage stress, urge, or mixed UI (Table 48.19). Biofeedback is used to assist the patient to identify, isolate, contract, and relax the pelvic muscles (see the Complementary & Alternative Therapies box). Strength training is used to improve the efficiency of the sphincter. Neuromuscular education is used to teach patients how and when to contract the pelvic floor muscles to maximize continence. Bladder training or habit training involves rigidly scheduled toileting intervals designed to enhance bladder capacity and reduce the frequency and volume of urine loss. *Prompted toileting* is a behavioural technique used in patients with functional UI. In this case, patients with impaired cognitive function are regularly reminded to urinate, assisted to the toilet, and offered praise for successful toileting.

🌿 COMPLEMENTARY & ALTERNATIVE THERAPIES
Biofeedback for Urinary Incontinence in Women

Clinical Uses
Kegel exercises help to strengthen the pelvic floor muscles. Biofeedback helps to isolate muscle groups in the pelvis.

Effects
Sensors for biofeedback are placed in the vagina or on the skin outside of the vagina. These sensors measure electrical signals produced when muscles contract. Biofeedback training develops an awareness of and control of the pelvic floor muscles.

Nursing Implications
If done correctly, pelvic floor muscle exercise is effective treatment for mild to moderate UI and other conditions related to pelvic floor muscle weakness. Unfortunately, many women do not do these exercises correctly. Biofeedback is a tool that can be used to ensure that these exercises are done correctly. Most supplementary insurance plans cover the cost of biofeedback.

TABLE 48.18 INTERVENTIONS FOR URINARY INCONTINENCE

Intervention	Description
Lifestyle Modifications	Self-management strategies to reduce or eliminate risk factors, including the following: • Smoking cessation • Weight reduction • Good bowel regimen • Reduction of bladder irritants such as caffeine • Fluid modifications for those with urge incontinence
Scheduling Voiding Regimens	
• Timed voiding	Toileting on a fixed schedule (typically q2–3h during waking hours)
• Habit retraining	Scheduled toileting with adjustments of voiding intervals (longer or shorter) based on the individual's voiding pattern
• Prompted voiding	Scheduled toileting that requires prompts to void from a caregiver (typically q3h); used in conjunction with operant conditioning techniques for rewarding individuals for maintaining continence and appropriate toileting
• Bladder retraining and urge-suppression strategies	Scheduled toileting with progressive voiding intervals; includes teaching of urge-control strategies using relaxation and distraction techniques, self-monitoring, use of reinforcement techniques, and other strategies such as conscious contraction of pelvic floor muscles
Pelvic Floor Muscle Rehabilitation	
• Pelvic floor muscle (Kegel) exercises or training	See Table 48.19
• Vaginal weight training	Active retention of increasing vaginal weights at least twice a day; typically used in combination with pelvic floor muscle exercises
• Biofeedback	See Complementary & Alternative Therapies box
• Electrical stimulation	Application of low-voltage electric current to sacral and pudendal afferent fibres through vaginal, anal, or surface electrodes; used to inhibit bladder overactivity and improve awareness, contractility, and efficiency of pelvic muscle contraction
Anti-Incontinence Devices	
• Intravaginal support devices (pessaries and bladder neck support prostheses)	Devices to support bladder neck, relieve minor pelvic organ prolapse, and change pressure transmission to the urethra
• Transvaginal sling device	Prevents involuntary release of urine through urethral support
• Intraurethral occlusive device (urethral plug)	Single-use device that is worn in the urethra to provide mechanical obstruction to prevent urine leakage; removed for voiding
• Penile compression device	Mechanical fixed compression applied to the penis to prevent any flow or leakage via the urethra; must be released hourly to void
Containment Devices	
• External collection devices	External catheter (condom) systems (i.e., penile sheaths) direct urine into a drainage bag; most commonly used by men
• Absorbent products	Variety of reusable and disposable pads and pant systems

Electrical stimulation of the pelvic floor muscles relies on very-low-voltage and low-frequency pulses to stimulate muscle contraction and diminish overactive bladder contractions. It can be used as monotherapy for the treatment of urge or mixed UI or in conjunction with pelvic muscle training in the management of stress UI. Minimally invasive electrical stimulation involves use of a transvaginal or transrectal probe, or a device can be surgically implanted near the pelvic nerve roots.

Medication Therapy. Medication therapy varies according to the UI type (Table 48.20). Medications have a very limited role in the management of stress UI. α-Adrenergic agonists can be used to increase urethral resistance at the level of the sphincter mechanism. Unfortunately, they exert a limited beneficial effect, and they are associated with adverse effects, including exacerbation of hypertension and tachycardia. Medications play a more central role in the management of urge or reflex UI. Antimuscarinic (also called *anticholinergic* or *antispasmodic*) medications relax the bladder muscle and inhibit overactive detrusor contractions. Two preparations, long-acting tolterodine (Detrol

LA) and oxybutynin in a releasing capsule (Ditropan XL), are preferred because of their efficacy and the modest incidence of their adverse effects compared with older antimuscarinic agents.

> **MEDICATION ALERT—Tolterodine (Detrol)**
> • Overdosage can result in severe anticholinergic effects.
> • These effects include GI cramping, diaphoresis, blurred vision, and urinary urgency.

Surgical Therapy. Surgical techniques also vary according to the type of UI. The Marshall–Marchetti–Krantz procedure involves suspending the urethra and the bladder neck by suturing the anterior vaginal wall on each side to the periosteum of the pubic bones and the lower rectum through an abdominal incision. The Pereyra procedure and subsequent modifications involve suspending the tissues adjacent to the bladder neck to the abdominal fascia, mainly through a transvaginal approach. Placement of a suburethral sling, using autologous fascia, cadaveric fascia, or synthetic material, can also correct stress UI in women. An artificial urethral sphincter can be used in women or men with intrinsic sphincter deficiency

TABLE 48.19 PATIENT & CAREGIVER TEACHING GUIDE

Pelvic Floor Muscle (or Kegel) Exercises

What Is the Pelvic Floor Muscle?

Your pelvic floor muscle provides support for your bladder and rectum and, in women, the vagina and the uterus. If it weakens or is damaged, it cannot support these organs and their position can change. This causes problems with the normal bladder and rectal function. If you have a weak pelvic floor muscle, you might want to do special exercises to make the muscle stronger, prevent unwanted urine leakage, and lessen urinary urgency.

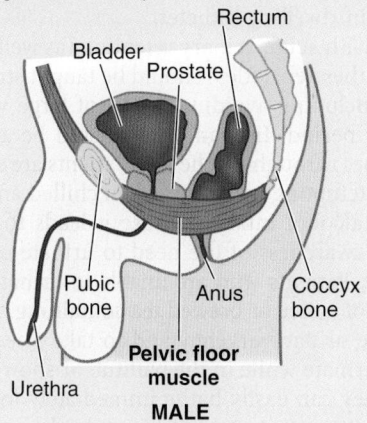
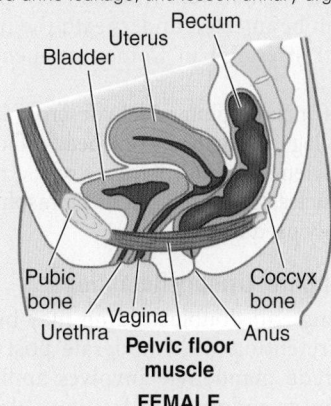

Finding the Pelvic Floor Muscle

Without tensing the muscles of your leg, buttocks, or abdomen, imagine that you are trying to control the passing of gas or pinching off a stool. Or imagine you are in an elevator full of people and you feel the urge to pass gas. What do you do? You tighten or pull in the ring of muscle around your rectum—your pelvic floor muscle. You should feel a lifting sensation in the area around the vagina or a pulling in of your rectum.

How to Do the Exercises

There are two different kinds of exercises—short squeezes and long squeezes.
1. To do the *short squeezes,* tighten your pelvic floor muscle quickly, squeeze hard for 2 sec, and then relax the muscle. Also, when you have strong urinary urges, try to tighten your pelvic floor muscle quickly and hard several times in a row until the urge passes.
2. To do the long squeezes, tighten the muscle for 5–10 sec before you relax. Do both of these exercises 40–50 times each day.

When to Do These Exercises

You can do these exercises anytime and anywhere. You can do these exercises in any position, but sitting or lying down may be the easiest.

How Long Does It Take Before You Notice a Change?

After 4–6 wk of doing these exercises, you should start to see less urine leakage and urinary urgency.

Source: Courtesy Diane Newman.

TABLE 48.20 MEDICATION THERAPY

*Voiding Dysfunction**

Medication Class and Mechanism of Action	Medication	Medication Class and Mechanism of Action	Medication
Muscarinic Receptor Antagonists and Anticholinergics Reduce overactive bladder contractions in urge urinary incontinence and overactive bladder	• Oxybutynin (Ditropan XL, Oxytrol transdermal system) • Tolterodine (Detrol, Detrol LA) • Dicyclomine (Bentylol)	**Tricyclic Antidepressants** Reduce sensory urgency and burning pain of interstitial cystitis Reduce overactive bladder contractions	• Imipramine • Amitriptyline (Elavil)
α-Adrenergic Antagonists Reduce urethral sphincter resistance to urinary outflow	• Doxazosin (Cardura) • Terazosin • Tamsulosin (Flomax CR)	**Calcium Channel Blockers** Reduce smooth muscle contraction strength May reduce burning pain of interstitial cystitis	• Nifedipine (Adalat) • Diltiazem • Verapamil (Isoptin)
5α-Reductase Inhibitors Androgen suppression that results in epithelial atrophy and a decrease in total prostate size	• Finasteride (Proscar)	**Hormone Therapy** Local application reduces urethral irritation and increases host defences against UTI	• Estrogen cream (Premarin, Estrace) • Estrogen vaginal ring (Estring) • Estrogen vaginal tablets (Vagifem)

UTI, urinary tract infection.
*The type of medication therapy depends on the type of incontinence.

and severe stress UI. Bolsters can also be implanted in men with stress UI to increase urethral resistance. This procedure is technically similar to the suburethral sling surgery often performed in women. A tension-free synthetic vaginal tape also can be used to treat stress UI. This transvaginal sling-like material is placed under the midurethra through incisions in the abdominal and vaginal wall. Alternatively, one of several bulking agents can be injected underneath the mucosa of the urethra to correct stress UI in women or men (Downey & Inman, 2019).

Bulking agents include glutaraldehyde cross-linked bovine collagen (GAX collagen), small silicone beads (Durasphere), or polytetrafluoroethylene (Teflon). Because of the risk of migration of Teflon particles, GAX collagen or Durasphere injections are most commonly used today.

Interprofessional Care: Urinary Retention

Scheduled toileting and double voiding may be effective in chronic urinary retention with moderate postvoid residual volumes. The Crede manoeuvre involves applying manual pressure to the lower abdomen to facilitate bladder emptying. For acute or chronic urinary retention, intermittent catheterization may be required. It allows the patient to remain free of an in-dwelling catheter with its associated risk of UTI and urethral irritation. However, an in-dwelling catheter is used when urethral obstruction renders intermittent catheterization uncomfortable or unfeasible, or when a patient is unwilling or unable to perform intermittent catheterization.

Medication Therapy. Several medications may be administered to promote bladder evacuation. For patients with obstruction at the level of the bladder neck, an α-adrenergic blocker may be prescribed. These medications relax the smooth muscle of the bladder neck, the prostatic urethra, and possibly the dually innervated rhabdosphincter, diminishing urethral resistance. Examples of α-adrenergic blocking agents are listed in Table 48.20. α-Adrenergic blocking medications are indicated for use in patients with BPH, bladder neck dyssynergia, or detrusor sphincter dyssynergia. Finasteride (Proscar) is a 5α-reductase enzyme inhibitor that reduces prostate size by inhibiting the conversion of testosterone to dihydrotestosterone. Finasteride is also useful for the hematuria that occasionally complicates symptomatic BPH in older men. Bethanechol chloride (Duvoid) is sometimes prescribed to promote contractility in the weakened detrusor muscle (Downey & Inman, 2019).

Surgical Therapy. Surgical interventions are often useful when managing urinary retention caused by obstruction. Transurethral or open surgical techniques are used in select patients to treat benign or malignant prostatic enlargement, bladder neck contracture, urethral strictures, or dyssynergia of the bladder neck. Pelvic reconstruction using an abdominal or transvaginal approach can be used to correct bladder outlet obstruction in women with severe pelvic organ prolapse.

Unfortunately, surgery plays little role in the management of urinary retention caused by deficient detrusor contraction strength. Attempts to create a bladder stimulator (implanted device capable of stimulating micturition) have proved largely unsuccessful because of the difficulty in achieving a coordinated detrusor contraction associated with pelvic muscle and striated sphincter relaxation.

NURSING MANAGEMENT URINARY RETENTION

Acute urinary retention is a medical emergency that requires prompt recognition and bladder drainage. The nurse should insert a catheter (as prescribed) unless otherwise directed. A catheter with a retention balloon is used in anticipation of the need for an in-dwelling catheter.

Patients with acute urinary retention (as well as patients predisposed to these episodes) should be taught strategies to minimize risk, including avoiding intake of large volumes of fluid over a brief period. Instead, they should be advised to drink small volumes throughout the day. Patients are advised to warm up before attempting urination when chilled and to avoid large volumes of alcohol intake because it leads to polyuria and a diminished awareness of the need to urinate until the bladder is distended. Patients who are unable to urinate are advised to drink a cup of coffee or brewed tea containing caffeine to create or maximize urinary urgency and to take a warm shower and attempt to urinate while in the bathtub or shower, with reassurance that they can easily bathe immediately following bladder evacuation. If these strategies do not lead to successful urination, patients are advised to seek immediate care.

Patients with chronic urinary retention may manage this condition by using behavioural methods, insertion of in-dwelling catheter or intermittent catheterization (Table 48.21) or surgery, or taking medications (NIDDK, 2019). Scheduled toileting and double voiding are the primary behavioural interventions used for chronic retention. Scheduled toileting is used to reduce rather than expand bladder capacity. In this case, patients are asked to void every 3 to 4 hours regardless of the desire to urinate. This intervention is particularly useful for patients with chronic overdistension, diabetes mellitus, or chronic alcohol use, who may have a large bladder capacity and diminished or delayed sensations of bladder filling and urgency. Double voiding is an attempt to maximize bladder evacuation. The patient is asked to urinate, sit on the toilet for 3 to 4 minutes, and urinate again before exiting the bathroom.

INSTRUMENTATION

Reasons for short-term urinary catheterization are listed in Table 48.21. Two reasons that are not valid indications for catheterization are (1) routine acquisition of a urine specimen for laboratory analysis and (2) convenience of the nursing staff or the patient's family. The risks for health care–associated infections are too high to allow catheterization of a patient for the convenience of health care providers or family members. Catheterization to obtain sterile urine specimens may occasionally be indicated when patients have a history of complicated urinary infection. These specimens have to be as free of contaminants as possible. A catheter should be the final means of providing the patient with a dry environment for prevention of skin breakdown and protection of dressings or skin lesions.

Urinary catheterization is used when indicated in the management of hospitalized patients. However, it is not without serious risks. The urinary tract is the most common site of health care–associated infections. Urinary catheterization is a major cause of UTIs. Strict aseptic technique is mandatory when a urinary catheter is inserted. After insertion, maintenance and protection of the closed drainage system are major nursing responsibilities. Irrigation of the catheter should not be routinely performed.

TABLE 48.21   INDICATIONS FOR URINARY CATHETERIZATION

In-Dwelling Catheter
- Accurate measurement of urinary output in critically ill patient
- Bladder decompression preoperatively and operatively for lower abdominal or pelvic surgery
- Facilitation of surgical repair of urethra and surrounding structures
- Measurement of residual urine after urination (referred to as postvoid residual [PVR]) if portable ultrasound not available
- Relief of urinary retention caused by lower urinary tract obstruction, paralysis, or inability to void
- Splinting of ureters or urethra to facilitate healing after surgery or other trauma in area
- Terminal illness or severe impairment that makes positioning or clothing changes uncomfortable or that is associated with intractable pain
- Urine contamination of stage 3 or 4 pressure injuries that has impeded healing, despite appropriate personal care for the incontinence

Straight (In-and-Out) Catheter
- Collection of sterile urine sample in select situations
- Instillation of medications into bladder
- Study of anatomical structures of urinary system
- Urodynamic testing

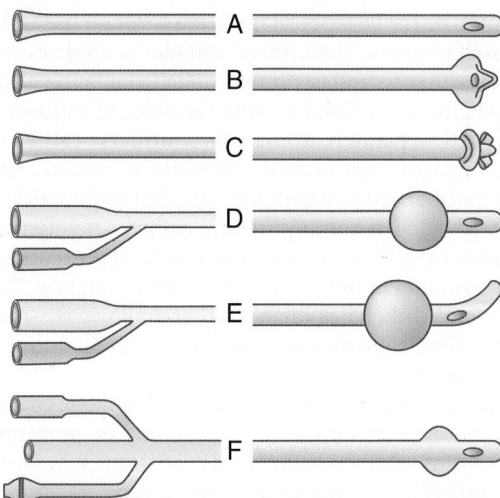

FIG. 48.11 Different types of commonly used catheters. **A,** Simple urethral catheter. **B,** Mushroom or Pezzar (can be used for suprapubic catheterization). **C,** Winged-tip or Malecot catheter. **D,** In-dwelling with inflated balloon. **E,** In-dwelling with coudé tip or Tiemann tip. **F,** Three-way in-dwelling (the third lumen is used for irrigation of the bladder).

While a patient has a catheter in place, nursing actions should include maintaining patency of the catheter, managing fluid intake, providing for the comfort and safety of the patient, and preventing infection. Attention should be given to the psychological implications of urinary drainage. Patient concerns can include embarrassment related to exposure of the body, an altered body image, and fear concerning the care of the catheter, which results in increased dependency.

Catheters vary in construction materials, tip shape (Figure 48.11), and size of the lumen. Catheters are sized according to the French scale. Each French unit equals 0.33 mm of diameter. The diameter measured is the internal diameter of the catheter. The size used varies with the size of the individual and the purpose for catheterization. In women, urethral catheter sizes 12 to 14F (smaller diameter) are the most common; in men, sizes 14 to 16F (larger diameter) are used. The primary issue resulting from too large a catheter is tissue erosion secondary to excessive pressure on the meatus or the urethra. Four routes are used for urinary tract catheterization: urethral, ureteral, suprapubic, and via a nephrostomy tube.

Urethral Catheterization

The most common route of catheterization is through the external meatus into the urethra, past the internal sphincter, and into the bladder. Principles that should be considered in the management of patients with a urethral catheter include the following:
- Catheterized patients, particularly those who are ambulatory, should receive appropriate instruction regarding catheter care.
- A sterile, closed drainage system should always be used in short-term catheterization. The distal urinary catheter and the proximal drainage tube should not be disconnected except for necessary catheter irrigation. The catheter should be taped to the leg. Unobstructed downhill flow must be maintained. The collecting bag should be emptied regularly and kept below the level of the bladder. A poorly functioning

catheter should be replaced. A leg bag should not be used for patients in a hospital setting on a short-term basis because the risk for bacterial infection is great when the catheter is disconnected and the drainage bags are exchanged.
- Perineal care (one to two times per day and when necessary) should include cleaning of the meatus–catheter junction with soap and water. Following this, an antimicrobial ointment may be applied. Lotion or powder should not be used near the catheter. The catheter should be properly secured to the leg to prevent movement and urethral traction.
- Sterile technique must be used whenever the collecting system is opened. Catheter irrigation is performed only when obstruction or blood clots are suspected or, in the case of long-term catheterization, to reduce sediment buildup. If frequent irrigations are necessary in short-term catheterization for catheter patency, a triple-lumen catheter may be preferable, permitting continuous irrigations within a closed system. Small volumes of urine for culture can be aspirated from the distal catheter by means of a sterile syringe and a 21-gauge needle after the drainage tubing is clamped. The puncture site must first be prepared with a tincture of iodine or alcohol solution. Many drainage systems are now equipped with a sampling port. Silicone or plastic catheters do not self-seal. Urine for chemical analysis (e.g., electrolytes) can be obtained from the drainage bag.
- When a patient is catheterized for less than 2 weeks, routine catheter change is not necessary. For long-term use of an in-dwelling catheter, regular replacement is necessary. With long-term use of a catheter, a leg bag may be used. If the collection bag is reused, it should be washed with soap and water and rinsed thoroughly. When not reused immediately, it should be filled with 0.5 cup of vinegar and drained. The vinegar is effective against Pseudomonas and other organisms and eliminates odours.

Ureteral Catheters

The ureteral catheter is placed through the ureters into the renal pelvis. The catheter is inserted either (a) by being threaded up the urethra and bladder to the ureters under cystoscopic observation or (b) by surgical insertion through the abdominal wall into the ureters. The ureteral catheter is used after surgery to splint the ureters and to prevent them from being obstructed by edema. The urine volume from the ureteral catheter should be recorded separately from other urinary catheters. The patient is usually kept on bed rest while a ureteral catheter is in place until specific orders indicate that ambulation is permissible. The self-retaining ureteral catheter is often inserted after a lithotripsy procedure or when ureteral obstruction from adjacent tumours or fibrosis threatens renal function. The double-J ureteral catheter is often used and allows the patient to ambulate. One end coils up in the kidney pelvis, and the other coils in the bladder.

The placement of the ureteral catheter should be checked frequently, and tension on the catheter should be prevented. The catheter drains urine from the renal pelvis, which has a capacity of 3 to 5 mL. If the volume of urine in the renal pelvis increases, the additional pressure will cause tissue damage to the pelvis. Therefore, the ureteral catheter should not be clamped. If the health care provider orders irrigation of the ureteral catheter, strict aseptic technique is required. If output is decreased, the health care provider should be notified immediately. Drainage should be checked often (at least every 1–2 hours). It is normal for some urine to drain around the ureteral catheter into the bladder. Accurate recording of urine output from both the ureters and the urethral catheter is essential. Sometimes, a ureteral catheter may be used as a stent and is not expected to drain. It is important to check with the health care provider as to the type of catheter and what to expect.

Suprapubic Catheters

Suprapubic catheterization is the simplest and oldest method of urinary diversion. The two methods of insertion of a suprapubic catheter into the bladder are (a) through a small incision in the abdominal wall and (b) by the use of a trocar. A suprapubic catheter is placed while the patient is under general anaesthesia for another surgical procedure or at the bedside with a local anaesthetic. The catheter may be sutured into place. Nursing responsibilities include taping the catheter to prevent dislodgement. The care of the tube and catheter is similar to that of the urethral catheter. A pectin-based skin barrier (e.g., Stomahesive) is effective around the insertion site in protecting the skin from breakdown.

The suprapubic catheter is used in temporary situations such as bladder, prostate, and urethral surgery. The suprapubic catheter is also used long term in select patients (e.g., a male patient with tetraplegia [quadriplegia] who tends to form penoscrotal fistulas).

A suprapubic catheter is prone to poor drainage because of mechanical obstruction of the catheter tip by the bladder wall, sediment, and clots. Nursing interventions to ensure patency of the tube include (a) preventing tube kinking by coiling the excess tubing and maintaining gravity drainage, and (b) having the patient turn from side to side. If these measures are not effective, the catheter is irrigated with sterile technique after a physician's order has been obtained.

If the patient experiences bladder spasms that are difficult to control, urinary leakage may result. Oxybutynin (Ditropan XL) or other oral antispasmodics or belladonna and opium (B&O) suppositories may be prescribed to decrease bladder spasms.

Nephrostomy Tubes

The nephrostomy tube (catheter) is inserted on a temporary basis to preserve renal function when a complete obstruction of the ureter is present. It is inserted directly into the pelvis of the kidney and attached to connecting tubing for closed drainage. The principle is the same as with the ureteral catheter—that is, the catheter should never be kinked, lain or leaned on, or clamped. If the patient reports excessive pain in the area or if there is excessive drainage around the tube, the catheter should be checked for patency. If irrigation is ordered, strict aseptic technique is required. No more than 5 mL of sterile saline solution is gently instilled at one time, to prevent overdistension of the kidney pelvis and renal damage. Infection and secondary stone formation are complications associated with the insertion of a nephrostomy tube.

Intermittent Catheterization

Clean intermittent catheterization is now considered the gold standard for urinary retention and an increasingly common approach particularly in conditions characterized by neurogenic bladder (e.g., spinal cord injuries, chronic neurological diseases) or bladder outlet obstruction in men. Clean intermittent self-catheterization is a manageable alternative to in-dwelling catheterization and has reduced the complications associated with in-dwelling catheters (Weynants et al., 2017). This type of catheterization may also be used in the oliguric and anuric phases of acute kidney injury to reduce the possibility of infection from an in-dwelling catheter. Intermittent catheterization is also used postoperatively, often after a surgical procedure for female incontinence or after radioactive seed implantation into the prostate for cancer. The main goal of intermittent catheterization is to prevent urinary retention, stasis, and compromised blood supply to the bladder caused by prolonged pressure.

The technique consists of inserting a urethral catheter into the bladder every 3 to 5 hours. Some patients do intermittent catheterization only once or twice a day to measure residual urine and to ensure an empty bladder. Patients should be instructed to wash and rinse the catheter and their hands with soap and water before and after catheterization. Water-soluble lubricant is necessary for men and may make catheterization more comfortable for women. The catheter may be inserted by the patient or the health care provider. Once the bladder is emptied, the catheter is removed. The catheter can be dried and placed in a carrying pouch or purse or folded in a paper towel until it is next needed. The same catheter can be used for weeks at a time. In general, patients should change the catheter every 2 to 4 weeks.

In the hospital, sterile technique is used. For home care, a clean technique that includes good handwashing with soap and water is used. There has been no significant increase in infection with the use of an appropriate clean technique as compared with sterile technique. Community patients who are candidates for clean intermittent self-catheterization need personal instruction and support to become comfortable with the procedure. Patients need to demonstrate the desire, motivation, and manual dexterity required to manage the procedure, and they need to commit to assimilating it into regular activities of daily living. They may feel anxious about performing such an intimate and possibly uncomfortable procedure. The nurse may need to balance the risks versus benefits of implementing the self-catheterization procedure for the patient. Instructing the patient to learn the proper clean procedure, in a logical step-by-step fashion, is recommended to support patients so that they can achieve independence (Weynants et al., 2017). The patient is taught to observe for signs of UTI so that treatment can be instituted early. If indicated, some patients are placed on a regimen of prophylactic antibiotics.

SURGERY OF THE URINARY TRACT

RENAL AND URETERAL SURGERY

The most common indications for nephrectomy are a renal tumour, polycystic kidneys that are bleeding or severely infected, massive traumatic injury to the kidney, and the elective removal of a kidney from a donor. Surgery involving the ureters and the kidneys is most commonly performed to remove calculi that become obstructive, correct congenital anomalies, and divert urine when necessary.

Preoperative Management

The basic needs of the patient undergoing renal and ureteral surgery are similar to those of any patient who experiences surgery (see Chapters 20 through 22). In addition, it is especially important preoperatively to ensure adequate fluid intake and a normal electrolyte balance. The patient should be told that there will probably be a flank incision on the affected side and that surgery will require a hyperextended, side-lying position. This position frequently causes the patient to experience muscle aches after surgery. If a nephrectomy is planned, the patient must be assured that one working kidney is sufficient to maintain normal renal function.

Postoperative Management

Specific postoperative needs of a patient are related to urine output, respiratory status, and abdominal distension.

Urine Output. In the immediate postoperative period, urine output should be determined at least every 1 to 2 hours. Drainage from various catheters should be recorded separately. The catheter or tube should not be clamped or irrigated without a specific order. The total urine output should be at least 0.5 mL/kg/hr. Peak flow rates can be measured with a urometer. It is also important to assess for urine drainage on the dressing and to estimate the amount. Daily weighing of the patient is important. The same scale should be used and properly balanced, and the patient should wear similar clothing and dressings each time.

It is important to observe and monitor the colour and the consistency of urine. Urine with increased amounts of mucus, blood, or sediment may occlude the drainage tubing or catheter.

Respiratory Status. Renal surgery is often performed through a flank incision just below the diaphragm and often involves removal of the twelfth rib. Postoperatively, it is important to ensure adequate ventilation. The patient is often reluctant to turn, cough, and deep breathe because of the incisional pain. Adequate pain medication should be given to ensure the patient's comfort and ability to perform coughing and deep-breathing exercises. Frequently, additional respiratory devices such as an incentive spirometer are used every 2 hours while the patient is awake. In addition, early and frequent ambulation assists in maintaining adequate respiratory function.

Abdominal Distension. Abdominal distension is present to some degree in most patients who have had surgery on their kidneys or ureters. It is most commonly the result of paralytic ileus caused by manipulation and compression of the bowel during surgery. Oral intake is restricted until bowel sounds are present (usually 24–48 hr after surgery). Intravenous fluids are given until the patient can take oral fluids. Progression to a regular diet follows.

Laparoscopic Nephrectomy

Laparoscopic nephrectomy can be performed in select situations to remove a diseased kidney. It can also be used to obtain a kidney from a living donor to be transplanted into a person with end-stage renal disease. In contrast to the open incision of about 18 cm required in a conventional nephrectomy, a laparoscopic nephrectomy is performed using five puncture sites. One incision is to view the kidney and another is to dissect it. The laparoscope contains a miniature camera so that the surgeons can watch what they are doing on a video monitor. Once dissected, the kidney is manoeuvred into a nylon impermeable sack, and its contents can then be safely removed from the patient. Compared with conventional nephrectomy, the laparoscopic approach is less painful and requires no sutures or staples, involves a shorter hospital stay, and has a much faster recovery.

URINARY DIVERSION

Urinary diversion may be performed with and without cystectomy. Urinary diversion procedures are performed to treat cancer of the bladder, neurogenic bladder, congenital anomalies, strictures, trauma to the bladder, and chronic infections with deterioration of renal function. Numerous urinary diversion techniques and bladder substitutes are possible, including an incontinent urinary diversion, continent urinary diversion catheterized by patient, or an orthotopic bladder so that the patient voids urethrally (NIDDK, 2020). Types of these surgical procedures are presented in Table 48.22 and Figure 48.12.

NCP 48.3, regarding care of patients with an ileal conduit, identifies key nursing diagnoses that apply to caring for patients with a nephrectomy pertaining to (a) management of anxiety related to lack of knowledge regarding a major surgical procedure; (b) knowledge deficits about preoperative, operative, and postoperative procedures; (c) risks for infection related to the surgical procedure; and (d) deficient fluid volume.

Incontinent Urinary Diversion

Incontinent urinary diversion is diversion to the skin, requiring an appliance. The simplest form is the cutaneous ureterostomy, but scarring and strictures of the ureter have led to the use of ileal or colonic conduits. The most commonly performed incontinent urinary diversion procedure is the **ileal conduit** (ileal loop). In this procedure, a 15- to 20-cm segment of the ileum is converted into a conduit for urinary drainage. The colon (colon conduit) can be used instead of the ileum. The ureters are anastomosed into one end of the conduit, and the other end of the bowel is brought out through the abdominal wall to form a stoma (Figure 48.13). Although the segment of bowel remains supported by the mesentery, it is completely isolated from the intestinal tract. The bowel is anastomosed and continues to function normally. Because there is no valve and no voluntary control over the stoma, drops of urine flow from the stoma every few seconds, requiring the use of a permanent external collecting device. The visible stoma and the need for

TABLE 48.22	TYPES OF URINARY DIVERSION SURGERY REQUIRING COLLECTION DEVICES		
Description	Advantages	Disadvantages	Special Considerations
Ileal Conduit ureters are implanted into part of ileum or colon that has been resected from intestinal tract. Abdominal stoma is created.	Relatively good urine flow with few physiological alterations	External appliance necessary to continually collect urine	Surgical procedure is more complex. Postoperative complications may be increased. Reabsorption of urea by ileum occurs. Meticulous attention is necessary to care for stoma and collecting device.
Cutaneous Ureterostomy Ureters are excised from bladder and brought through abdominal wall, and stoma is created. Ureteral stomas may be created from both ureters, or ureters may be brought together and one stoma created.	No need for major surgery as required with ileal conduit	External appliance necessary because of continuous urine drainage; possibility of stricture or stenosis of small stoma	Periodic catheterizations may be required to dilate stomas to maintain patency.
Nephrostomy Catheter is inserted into pelvis of kidney. Procedure may be done to one or both kidneys and may be temporary or permanent. It is most frequently done in advanced disease as palliative procedure.	No need for major surgery	High risk for renal infection; predisposition to calculus formation from catheter	Nephrostomy tube may have to be changed every month. Catheter must never be clamped.

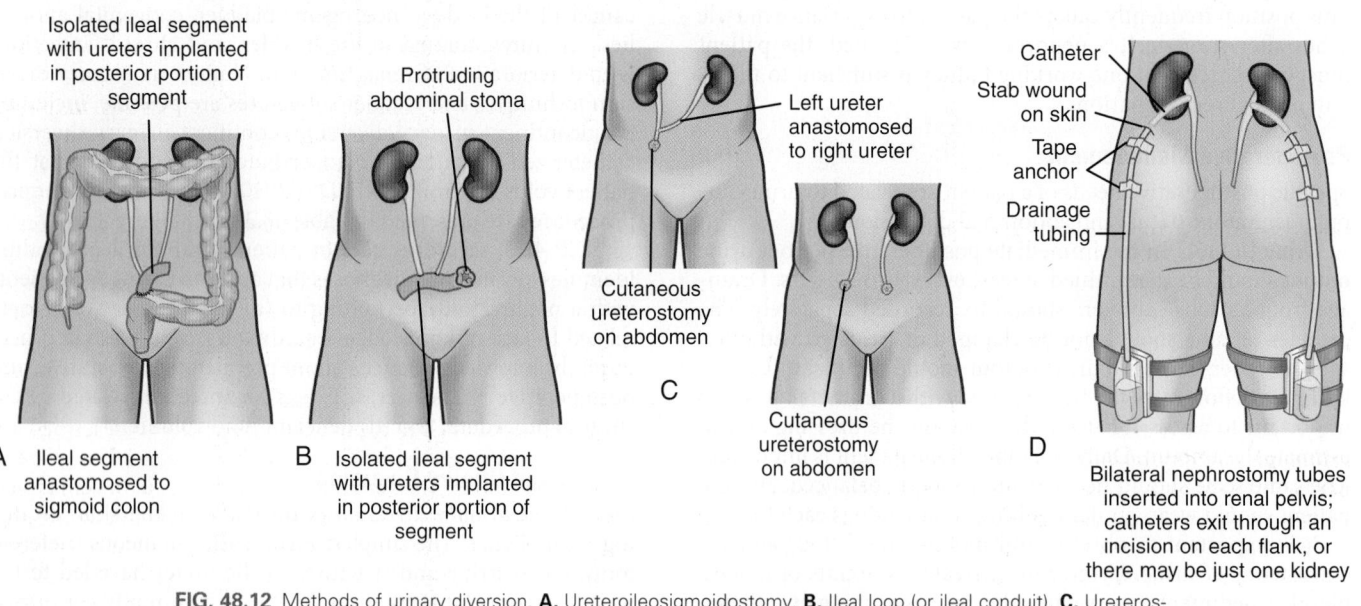

FIG. 48.12 Methods of urinary diversion. **A,** Ureteroileosigmoidostomy. **B,** Ileal loop (or ileal conduit). **C,** Ureterostomy (transcutaneous ureterostomy and bilateral cutaneous ureterostomies). **D,** Nephrostomy.

external collection devices are obvious disadvantages of this procedure. The lifelong care and managing the stoma and collection devices may be psychologically difficult. These challenges have led to an increasing use of continent diversions and orthotopic bladder substitutes.

Continent Urinary Diversions

A *continent urinary diversion* is an intra-abdominal urinary reservoir that is catheterizable or has an outlet controlled by the anal sphincter. Continent diversions are internal pouches created similarly to the ileal conduit. Reservoirs have been constructed from the ileum, ileocecal segment, or colon. Large segments of bowel are altered to prevent peristaltic action. A continence mechanism is formed between this large, low-pressure reservoir and the stoma by intussuscepting a portion of bowel. In this way, a patient does not leak involuntarily. The patient with a continent reservoir needs to self-catheterize every 4 to 6 hours but does not need to wear external attachments. Examples of continent diversions are the Kock (Figure 48.14), Mainz, Indiana, and Florida pouches. A main difference between these diversions is the segment of bowel used. For example, the Indiana pouch uses the right colon as a

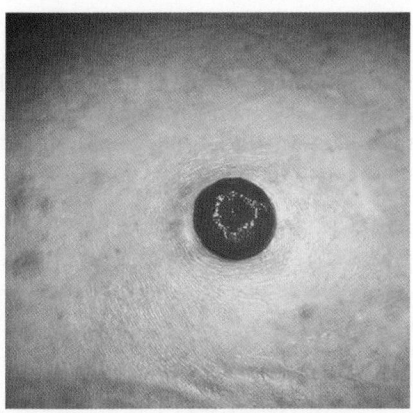

FIG. 48.13 Ideal urinary stoma. It is symmetrical, has no skin breakdown, and protrudes about 1.5 cm. The mucosa is a healthy red, and the configuration is flat when the patient is upright and supine. Source: Courtesy Lynda Brubacher, Virginia Mason Hospital, Seattle, WA.

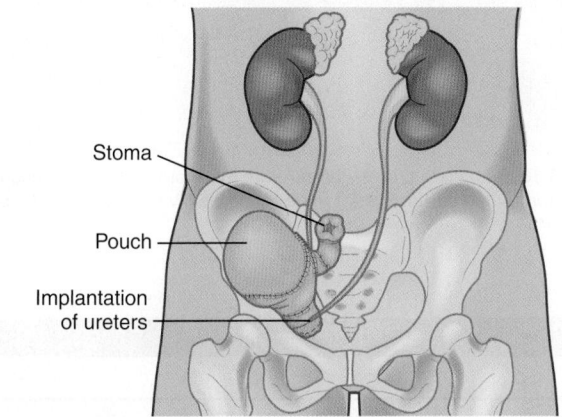

FIG. 48.14 Creation of a Kock pouch with implantation of ureters into one intussuscepted portion of the pouch and creation of a stoma with the other intussuscepted portion.

reservoir and has become a popular form of continent urinary diversion.

Orthotopic Bladder Substitution

Orthotopic bladder substitutes can be derived from various segments of the intestines. An isolated segment of the distal ileum is often preferred. Various procedures include the hemi-Kock pouch, Studer pouch, and the ileal W-neobladder. In these procedures, the bowel is surgically reshaped to become a neobladder. The ureters and urethra are sutured into the neobladder. Orthotopic bladder reconstruction has become a more viable option for both men and women if cancer does not involve the bladder neck or urethra (Qu & Lawrentschuk, 2019). The advantage of orthotopic bladder substitution is that it allows for natural micturition. Incontinence is a possible adverse effect with this technique, and intermittent catheterization may be required.

NURSING MANAGEMENT URINARY DIVERSION

PREOPERATIVE MANAGEMENT

Patients awaiting cystectomy and urinary diversion must be given a great deal of information. The nurse must assess their ability and readiness to learn before initiating a teaching program. If a patient is not ready to learn the information required, the teaching plan should be adjusted. The patient's anxiety and fear may be decreased by receiving pertinent information. However, their anxiety and fear may also interfere with learning. The patient's family and caregivers should be involved in the teaching process. A discussion of the social aspects of living with a stoma (including clothing, changes in body image and sexuality, exercise, and odour) provides the patient with facts that may allay some of their fears. Patients who will have a continent diversion must be taught to catheterize and irrigate the pouch and be able to adhere to a strict catheterization schedule. Patients with an orthotopic neobladder may have difficulties with incontinence. Concerns about the effect on sexual activities should also be discussed. The ostomate or enterostomal therapy nurse should be involved in the preoperative phase of the patient's care. Additional interventions are presented in NCP 48.3, available on the Evolve website.

POSTOPERATIVE MANAGEMENT

Nursing interventions during the postoperative period (see NCP 48.3 for care after an ileal conduit) should be planned to prevent surgical complications, such as postoperative atelectasis and shock (see Chapter 22). The incidence of thrombophlebitis increases after pelvic surgery. With removal of part of the bowel, the incidence of paralytic ileus and small bowel obstruction increases, the patient is kept on nothing-by-mouth status, and a nasogastric tube needs to be in place for 3 to 5 days.

Specific attention should be given to preventing injury to the stoma and maintaining urine output. Mucus is present in the urine because it is secreted by the intestines as a result of the irritating effect of the urine. Patients should be told that this is a normal occurrence. A high fluid intake is encouraged to "flush" the ileal conduit or continent diversion.

When an ileal conduit is created, the skin around the stoma requires meticulous care. Alkaline encrustations with dermatitis may occur when alkaline urine comes in contact with exposed skin (Figure 48.15). Other common peristomal skin conditions include yeast infections, product allergies, and shearing-effect excoriations. Changing appliances (pouches) is described in Table 48.23. A properly fitting appliance is essential to prevent skin complications. The appliance should be about 0.2 cm larger than the stoma. It is normal for the stoma to shrink within the first few weeks after surgery. The urine is kept acidic to prevent alkaline encrustations.

Acceptance of the surgery and of alterations in body image is needed to ensure the patient's best adjustment. Concerns of the patient include fear that the stoma will be offensive to others and will interfere with sexual, personal, professional, and recreational activities. The patient should know that few activities, if any, will be restricted as a result of the urinary diversion.

Discharge planning after an ileal conduit includes teaching the patient symptoms of obstruction or infection and care of the ostomy. The patient with an ileal conduit is fitted for a permanent appliance 7 to 10 days after surgery and may need to be refitted at a later time, depending on the degree of stoma shrinkage. Appliances are made of a variety of products, including natural and synthetic rubbers, plastics, and metals. Most appliances have a faceplate that adheres to the skin, a collecting pouch, and an opening to drain the pouch. The faceplate may be secured to the skin with glues, adhesives, or adhering synthetic wafers. Some appliances do not require adhesives, but their design relies on pressure to keep the pouch in place. If improperly fitted or applied, the faceplate may cause skin injuries (Figure 48.16). A bag may be used for night drainage. The patient

needs information on where to purchase supplies, emergency telephone numbers, location of ostomy support groups, and follow-up visits with an enterostomal therapist. Follow-up with a health care provider is imperative for monitoring and correcting homeostatic abnormalities and to prevent complications and renal function deterioration.

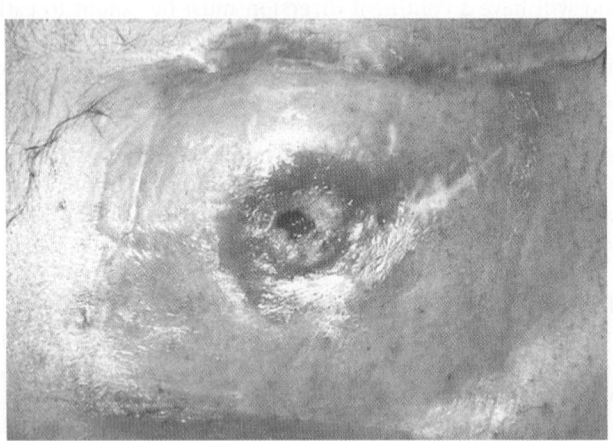

FIG. 48.15 Ammonia salt encrustation secondary to alkaline urine. Source: Courtesy Lynda Brubacher, Virginia Mason Hospital, Seattle, WA.

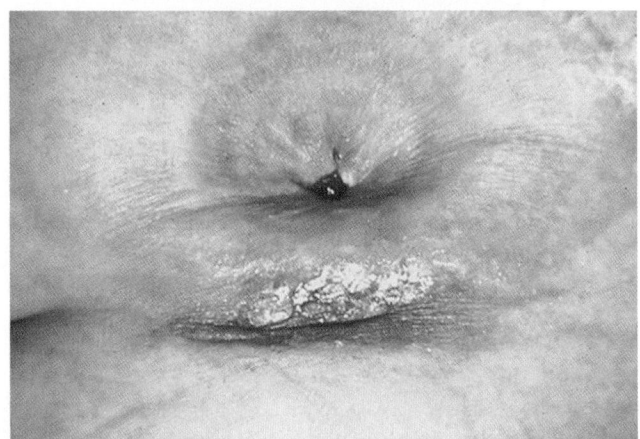

FIG. 48.16 Retracted urinary stoma with pressure sore from faceplate above stoma. Source: Courtesy Lynda Brubacher, Virginia Mason Hospital, Seattle, WA.

TABLE 48.23 PATIENT & CAREGIVER TEACHING GUIDE

Changing Ileal Conduit Appliances

Temporary Appliance
1. Cut hole in pouch to fit over stoma (pouch 3.2 mm [1/8 inch] larger than stoma).
2. Remove old pouch.
3. Clean area gently, and remove old adhesive.
4. Wash area with warm water.
5. Place wick (rolled-up 4 × 4–inch) over stoma to keep area dry during rest of procedure.
6. Dry skin around stoma.
7. Apply a prescribed skin protectant around stoma to area where pouch will be placed.
8. Apply pouch by first smoothing its edges toward side and lower portion of body.
9. Remove wick and complete application of bag.
10. For a patient who is usually in bed: Apply bag so that it lies toward side of body.
11. For a patient who is ambulatory: Apply bag so that it lies vertically.
12. Connect drainage tubing to pouch.
13. Keep drainage pouch on same side of bed as stoma.

Permanent Appliance*
1. Keep appliance in place for 2–14 days.
2. Change appliance when fluid intake has been restricted for several hours.
3. Sit or stand in front of mirror.
4. Moisten edge of faceplate with adhesive solvent and gently remove.
5. Clean skin with adhesive solvent.
6. Wash skin with warm water. (Patient may shower.)
7. Dry skin and inspect.
8. Place wick (rolled-up 4 × 4–inch) over stoma to keep skin free of urine.
9. Apply skin cement to faceplate and skin.
10. Place appliance over stoma.
11. Wash removed appliance with soap and lukewarm water; soak in distilled vinegar; rinse with lukewarm water and air dry.

*Many disposable appliances with self-adhesive backing are used as permanent appliances.

CASE STUDY

Urinary Tract Infection

Patient Profile

M. G. (pronouns she/her), a 28-year-old with diabetes, was seen in the nurse practitioner's office for a history of painful, frequent urination.

Subjective Data

- Has had history of painful, frequent urination with passage of small volumes of urine for 3 days
- Has had intermittent fever, chills, and back pain during these 3 days
- Was frightened when saw blood in urine
- Is anxious because her father died of kidney cancer
- Has a history of recurrent UTIs

Objective Data
Physical Examination

- Reports bilateral flank pain and abdominal tenderness to palpation
- Temperature is 38°C

Diagnostic Study

- Urinalysis: pyuria and hematuria

Discussion Questions

1. What are the most common organisms that cause UTIs?
2. What factors predispose a patient to a UTI?
3. What is the difference between upper and lower UTIs?
4. **Priority decision:** What are the priority nursing interventions that will help M. G. manage her symptoms?
5. What can the nurse do to help M. G. prevent another UTI?
6. Why might M.G. be having recurrent bouts of UTIs? What other diagnostic tests may be indicated?
7. **Priority decision:** Based on the data presented, write one or more appropriate nursing diagnoses. Are there any interprofessional issues?

ⓔvolve

Answers are available on http://evolve.elsevier.com/Canada/Lewis/medsurg.

REVIEW QUESTIONS

The number of the question corresponds to the same-numbered objective at the beginning of the chapter.

1. Organisms that cause pyelonephritis most commonly reach the kidneys through which means?
   a. The bloodstream
   b. The lymphatic system
   c. A descending infection
   d. An ascending infection

2. What should the nurse teach the female client who has frequent urinary tract infections (UTIs)?
   a. Urinate after sexual intercourse.
   b. Take tub baths with bubble bath.
   c. Take prophylactic sulphonamides for the rest of her life.
   d. Restrict fluid intake to prevent the need for frequent voiding.

3. Which of the following immunological mechanisms are involved in glomerulonephritis?
   a. Tubular blocking by precipitates of bacteria and antibody reactions
   b. Deposition of immune complexes and complement along the glomerular basement membrane (GBM)
   c. Thickening of the GBM from autoimmune microangiopathic changes
   d. Destruction of glomeruli by proteolytic enzymes contained in the GBM

4. What is one of the most important roles of the nurse regarding acute poststreptococcal glomerulonephritis (APSGN)?
   a. To promote early diagnosis and treatment of sore throats and skin lesions
   b. To encourage clients to request antibiotic therapy for all upper respiratory infections
   c. To teach clients with APSGN that long-term prophylactic antibiotic therapy is necessary to prevent recurrence
   d. To monitor clients for respiratory symptoms that indicate that the disease is affecting the alveolar basement membrane

5. Why does edema occur in nephrotic syndrome?
   a. Decreased aldosterone secretion from adrenal insufficiency
   b. Increased hydrostatic pressure caused by sodium retention
   c. Increased fluid retention caused by decreased glomerular filtration
   d. Decreased colloidal osmotic pressure caused by loss of serum albumin

6. A client is admitted to the hospital with severe renal colic caused by renal lithiasis. What is the nurse's first priority in management of the client?
   a. To administer opioids as prescribed
   b. To obtain supplies for straining all urine
   c. To encourage fluid intake of 3 to 4 L/day
   d. To keep the client on nothing-by-mouth status in preparation for surgery

7. In which of the following conditions should the nurse recommend genetic counselling for the client's children?
   a. Nephrotic syndrome
   b. Chronic pyelonephritis
   c. Malignant nephrosclerosis
   d. Adult-onset polycystic renal disease

8. The nurse instructs a client with diabetes to maintain careful control of his blood glucose levels related to which disease-related complication?
   a. Uric acid calculi and nephrolithiasis
   b. Renal sugar-crystal calculi and cysts
   c. Lipid deposits in the glomeruli and the nephrons
   d. Thickening of the GBM and glomerulosclerosis

9. Which of the following conditions would the nurse identify as a risk factor for kidney and bladder cancers? *(Select all that apply.)*
   a. Acetylsalicylic acid (ASA: Aspirin) use
   b. Tobacco use
   c. Chronic alcohol misuse
   d. Use of artificial sweeteners
   e. Chronic use of phenacetin-containing analgesics

10. Which nursing interventions are most important in order to increase bladder control in a client with urinary incontinence? *(Select all that apply.)*
    a. Restricting fluids to diminish the risk for urinary leakage
    b. Counselling the client to maintain a regular voiding schedule
    c. Clamping and releasing a catheter to increase bladder tone
    d. Teaching the client biofeedback mechanisms to suppress the urge to void

11. A client with a ureterolithotomy returns from surgery with a nephrostomy tube in place. What is the priority nursing action related to caring for this client?
   a. Encouraging the client to drink fruit juices and milk
   b. Encouraging intake of fluids of at least 2 to 3 L/day after nausea has subsided
   c. Notifying the health care provider if nephrostomy tube drainage is more than 30 mL/hr
   d. Irrigating the nephrostomy tube with 10 mL of normal saline solution as needed

12. A client has had a cystectomy and ileal conduit diversion performed. Four days postoperatively, mucous shreds are seen in the drainage bag. Which action should the nurse undertake?
   a. Notify the health care provider.
   b. Notify the charge nurse.
   c. Irrigate the drainage tube.
   d. Chart it as a normal observation.

1. d; 2. a; 3. b; 4. a; 5. d; 6. a; 7. d; 8. d; 9. b; 10. a, b; 11. b; 12. d.

Ⓔvolve

For even more review questions, visit http://evolve.elsevier.com/Canada/Lewis/medsurg.

REFERENCES

Ali, M. (2019). Renal cell carcinoma. *Journal of Saidu Medical College*, 9(1), 147–150.

Bril, V., Breiner, A., Perkins, B. A., et al. (2018). Neuropathy. *Canadian Journal of Diabetes*, 42(Suppl 1), S217–S221. https://doi.org/10.1016/j.jcjd.2017.10.028

Canadian Cancer Society. (2019). *Canadian cancer statistics 2019*. https://cdn.cancer.ca/-/media/files/research/cancer-statistics/2020-statistics/canadian-cancer-statistics/res-cancerstatistics-canadiancancerstatistics-2019-.en.pdf?rev=82dc3652fe3648988b9174ad4b397a24&hash=6D3186DF3AC76787C58EE95D1712033C&_ga=2.127115919.340386808.1635781328-193814398-1.1623777465

Canadian Cancer Society. (2021). *Risk factors for bladder cancer*. https://www.cancer.ca/en/cancer-information/cancer-type/bladder/risks/?region=on

Canadian Continence Foundation. (2021). What is urinary incontinence? http://www.canadiancontinence.ca/EN/what-is-urinary-incontinence.php

Canadian Kidney Foundation. (2020). *Claudin function in kidney development and disease*. https://kidney.ca/Research/Supported-Research/QC/The-role-of-dendritic-cells-and-follicular-hel-(8

Chang, S. S., Bochner, B. H., Chou, R., et al. (2017). Treatment of nonmetastatic muscle-invasive bladder cancer: American Urological Association/American Society of Clinical Oncology/American Society for Radiation Oncology/Society of Urologic Oncology clinical practice guideline summary. *Journal of Oncology Practice*, 13(9), 621–625. https://doi.org/10.1200/JOP.2017.024919

Chu, C. M., & Lowder, J. L. (2018). Diagnoses and treatment of urinary tract infections across age groups. *American Journal of Obstetrics and Gynecology*, 219(1), 40–51. https://doi.org/10.1016/j.ajog.2017.12.231

da Costa, I. A., Amend, B., Stenzl, A., et al. (2016). Contemporary management of acute kidney trauma. *Journal of Acute Disease*, 5(1), 29–36. https://doi.org/10.1016/j.joad.2015.08.003

Downey, A., & Inman, R. D. (2019). Recent advances in surgical management of urinary incontinence. *F1000 Research*, 8, 1294. https://doi.org/10.12688/f1000research.16356.1

Duong, E., Al Hamarneh, Y. N., Tsuyuki, R. T., et al. (2019). Case finding for urinary incontinence and falls in older adults at community pharmacies. *Canadian Pharmacists Journal/Revue des Pharmaciens du Canada*, 152(4), 228–233. https://doi.org/10.1177/1715163519852378

Elmansy, H. E., & Lingeman, J. E. (2016). Recent advances in lithotripsy technology and treatment strategies. *International Journal of Surgery*, 36, 676–680. https://doi.org/10.1016/j.ijsu.2016.11.097

Flannigan, R. K., Battison, A., De, S., et al. (2018). Evaluating factors that dictate struvite stone composition: A multi-institutional clinical experience from the EDGE Research Consortium. *Canadian Urological Association Journal*, 12(4), 131–136. https://doi.org/10.5489/cuaj.4804

Froom, P., & Shimoni, Z. (2018). The uncertainties of the diagnosis and treatment of a suspected urinary tract infection in elderly hospitalized patients. *Expert Review of Anti-infective Therapy*, 16(10), 763–770. https://doi.org/10.1080/14787210.2018.1523006

Geerlings, S. E. (2017). Clinical presentations and epidemiology of urinary tract infections. *Urinary tract infections: Molecular pathogenesis and clinical management*, 27–40. https://doi.org/10.1128/9781555817404.ch2

Han, E., Nyugen, L., Sirls, L., et al. (2018). Current best practice management of interstitial cystitis/bladder pain syndrome. *Therapeutic Advances in Urology*, 10(7), 197–211. https://doi.org/10.1177/1756287218761574

Jiang, T., Zhou, C., & Ren, S. (2016). Role of IL-2 in cancer immunotherapy. *Oncoimmunology*, 5(6), e1163462. https://doi.org/1080/2162402X.2016.1163462

Johnson, J., & Russo, T. A. (2018). Acute pyelonephritis in adults. *The New England Journal of Medicine*, 378(1), 48–59. https://doi.org/10.1056/NEJMcp1702758

Liska, D., Kern, H. J., & Maki, K. C. (2016). Cranberries and urinary tract infections: How can the same evidence lead to conflicting advice? *Journal of Advanced Nutrition*, 7(3), 498–506. https://doi.org/10.3945/an115011197

National Institute of Diabetes and Digestive and Kidney Diseases (NIDDK). (2017). *Bladder infection (urinary tract infection—UTI) in adults*. https://www.niddk.nih.gov/health-information/urologic-diseases/bladder-infection-uti-in-adults

National Institute of Diabetes and Digestive and Kidney Diseases (NIDDK). (2019). *Treatment of urinary retention*. https://www.niddk.nih.gov/health-information/urologic-diseases/urinary-retention/treatment

National Institute of Diabetes and Digestive and Kidney Diseases (NIDDK). (2020). *Urinary diversion*. https://www.niddk.nih.gov/health-information/urologic-diseases/urinary-diversion

National Kidney Foundation. (2018). *Polycystic kidney disease*. https://www.kidney.org/atoz/content/polycystic

National Kidney Foundation. (2019). *Kidney stone diet plan and prevention*. https://www.kidney.org/atoz/content/diet

National Library of Medicine. (2020). *Alport syndrome*. https://ghr.nlm.nih.gov/condition/alport-syndrome

Nicolle, L. E. (2016). Cranberry for prevention of urinary tract infection? Time to move on. *JAMA: Journal of the American*

Medical Association, 316(18), 1873–1874. https://doi:10.1001/ja ma.2016.16140

Qu, L. G., & Lawrentschuk, N. (2019). Orthotopic neobladder reconstruction: Patient selection and perspectives. *Research and Reports in Urology, 11*, 333–341. https://doi.org/10.2147/RRU. S181473

Sangle, N. (2020). *Malignant hypertension and accelerated nephroscle-rosis.* https://www.pathologyoutlines.com/topic/kidneymalignant hyper.html

Semwal, M. (2020). A review on nephrotic syndrome with their causes, complications and epidemiology. *Asian Pacific Journal of Nursing and Health Sciences, 3*(1), 12–15.

Sinnakirouchenan, R. (2020). What is the role of kidney function test-ing in the diagnosis of nephrotic syndrome? *Medscape.* http://eme dicine.medscape.com/article/244631-overview

Syed, L. J., & Illchak, D. L. Bladder pain syndrome in females. *The Journal for Nurse Practitioners 13*(4), 291–295. http://doi.org/10.10 16/j.nurpra.2016.11.025

Taithongchai, A., Sultan, A. H., & Thakar, R. (2019). A guide to indi-cations, components and interpretation of urodynamic investiga-tions. *The Obstetrician & Gynaecologist, 21*, 193–202. https://doi. org/10.1111/tog.12575-

Urology Care Foundation. (2021). What is urethral diverticulum? http://www.urologyhealth.org/urologic-conditions/urethral-diverticulum

Weynants, L., Hervé, F., Decalf, V., et al. (2017). Clean intermittent self-catheterization as a treatment modality for urinary retention: Perceptions of urologists. *International Neurourology Journal, 21*(3), 189.

RESOURCES

Canadian Association of Nephrology Nurses and Technologists
https://cannt.ca
Canadian Urological Association
https://www.cua.org

Cancer Care Ontario—*Guidelines and Advice*
https://www.cancercareontario.ca/en/guidelines-advice
Interstitial Cystitis Network: Canada IC, Bladder & Pelvic Pain Support Groups
https://www.ic-network.com/ic-support-center/canada-ic-bladder-pelvic-pain-support-groups/?
Kidney Foundation of Canada
https://www.kidney.ca/
Kidney Foundation of Canada—*Resources*
https://kidney.ca/Support/Resources/
Ostomy Canada Society
https://www.ostomycanada.ca
Registered Nurses' Association of Ontario Best Practice Guidelines
https://rnao.ca/bpg/guidelines/resources/continence/self-learning
Women's College Hospital—*Interstitial Cystitis*
https://www.womenshealthmatters.ca/health-centres/pelvic-health/interstitial-cystitis
Women's College Hospital—*Interstitial Cystitis: Coping*
https://www.womenshealthmatters.ca/health-centres/pelvic-health/interstitial-cystitis/coping

American Cancer Society
https://www.cancer.org
American Urological Association—**Bladder Health**
https://www.auanet.org/advocacy/advocacy-by-topic/bladder-health
International Continence Society (ICS)
https://www.ics.org
Interstitial Cystitis Association
https://www.ichelp.org/
Wound, Ostomy and Continence Nurses Society
https://www.wocn.org

evolve
For additional Internet resources, see the website for this book at http://evolve.elsevier.com/Canada/Lewis/medsurg.

49

Nursing Management

Acute Kidney Injury and Chronic Kidney Disease

Debbie Rickeard
Originating US chapter by Ann Crawford

℮volve WEBSITE

http://evolve.elsevier.com/Canada/Lewis/medsurg

- Review Questions (Online only)
- Key Points
- Answer Guidelines for Case Study

- Student Case Studies
  - Kidney Transplant
  - Glomerulonephritis and Acute Kidney Injury

- Customizable Nursing Care Plan
  - Chronic Kidney Disease in Stage 4
- Conceptual Care Map Creator
- Audio Glossary
- Content Updates

LEARNING OBJECTIVES

1. Differentiate between acute kidney injury and chronic kidney disease.
2. Identify criteria used in the classification of acute kidney injury using the acronym RIFLE (**r**isk, **i**njury, **f**ailure, **l**oss, **e**nd-stage kidney disease).
3. Describe the clinical course of acute kidney injury.
4. Explain the interprofessional care and nursing management of a patient with acute kidney injury.
5. Define chronic kidney disease and delineate the five stages of chronic kidney disease based on the glomerular filtration rate.
6. Identify risk factors that contribute to the development of chronic kidney disease.
7. Summarize the significance of cardiovascular disease in individuals with chronic kidney disease.
8. Explain the interprofessional care and related nursing management of the patient with chronic kidney disease.
9. Differentiate among renal replacement therapies for individuals with chronic kidney disease.
10. Discuss the role of the nurse in the management of individuals who receive a renal transplant.

KEY TERMS

acute kidney injury (AKI)
acute renal failure (ARF)
acute tubular necrosis (ATN)
arteriovenous fistula (AVF)
arteriovenous graft (AVG)
automated peritoneal dialysis (APD)
azotemia
chronic kidney disease (CKD)

chronic kidney disease–mineral and bone
  disorder (CKD–MBD)
continuous ambulatory peritoneal dialysis
  (CAPD)
continuous renal replacement therapy
  (CRRT)
dialysis
end-stage renal disease (ESRD)

hemodialysis (HD)
oliguria
paired organ donation
peritoneal dialysis (PD)
renal osteodystrophy
renal replacement therapy (RRT)
uremia

Kidney disease may cause the partial or complete impairment of kidney function. It results in an inability to excrete metabolic waste products and water, as well as functional disturbances of all body systems. This impairment may be acute or chronic in nature (Table 49.1). Acute kidney injury (AKI) has a rapid onset. Chronic kidney disease (CKD) usually develops slowly over months to years. If CKD progresses to stage 5 (worst functioning), **renal replacement therapy (RRT)** (dialysis or transplantation) is necessary for long-term survival. Early CKD care focuses on prevention and delaying progression of disease and

educating patients about treatment options for RRT so that they can make an informed decision when the time comes. As with other chronic illnesses in Canada, CKD is much more common in the older population. Between 2003 and 2013, the number of Canadians aged 45 to 64 with CKD increased by 46%, while Canadians 65 and older saw a 66% increase. During the same time period, the number of Canadians aged 45 and older with diabetes also increased by more than 60% (Canadian Institute for Health Information [CIHI], 2019). By the end of 2018, 40 289 Canadians (excluding Quebec) were being treated for end-stage

TABLE 49.1	COMPARISON OF ACUTE KIDNEY INJURY AND CHRONIC KIDNEY DISEASE	
	Acute Kidney Injury	**Chronic Kidney Disease**
Onset	Sudden	Gradual, often over many years
Most common cause	Acute tubular necrosis	Diabetic nephropathy
Diagnostic criteria	Acute reduction in urine output, elevation in serum creatinine, or both	GFR <60 mL/min/1.73 m² for >3 mo, kidney damage >3 mo, or both
Reversibility	Potentially	Progressive and irreversible
Mortality	High (~60%)	19–24% (patients on dialysis)
Primary cause of death	Infection	Cardiovascular disease

GFR, glomerular filtration rate.
Source: Kellum, J., Bellomo, R., & Ronco, C. (2008). Definition and classification of acute kidney injury. *Nephron Clinical Practice, 109*(4), 182–187. https://doi.org/10.1159/000142926; and U.S. Renal Data System. (2008). USRDS 2008 annual data report: Atlas of end-stage renal disease. National Institute of Diabetes and Digestive and Kidney Diseases.

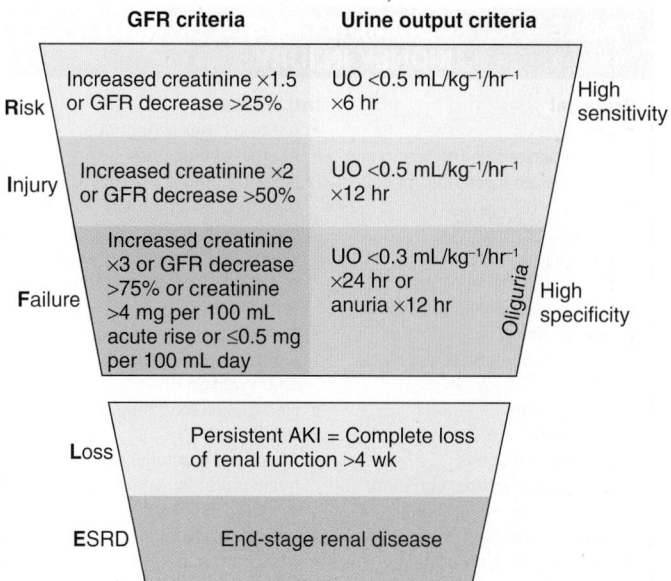

FIG. 49.1 RIFLE (**r**isk, **i**njury, **f**ailure, **l**oss, **e**nd-stage kidney disease) criteria. *AKI*, acute kidney injury; *ESRD*, end-stage renal disease; *GFR*, glomerular filtration rate; *UO*, urine output. Source: Williams, L. (2014). Take aim at acute kidney injury with RIFLE criteria. *Nursing, 44*(7), 50–55. doi:10.1097/01.NURSE.0000445730.84886.88

kidney disease, which is an increase of 35% from 2009. Of these patients, 42.2% had a functioning kidney transplant, and 57.8% were receiving some form of dialysis (CIHI, 2019).

ACUTE KIDNEY INJURY

Acute kidney injury (AKI), previously known as **acute renal failure (ARF)**, is a more inclusive term encompassing a broader subset of patients with varying degrees of kidney injury (Coelho et al., 2017). AKI is characterized by an abrupt decline in kidney function, leading to a rise in serum creatinine or a reduction in urine output, or both (Coelho et al., 2017). The severity of dysfunction can range from a small increase in serum creatinine or reduction in urine output to the development of **azotemia** (an accumulation of nitrogen waste products [urea nitrogen, creatinine] in the blood).

Although AKI is potentially reversible, despite advances in its treatment, the mortality rate is high (Bonfield, 2018). Usually, AKI affects people with other life-threatening conditions. Most commonly, AKI follows severe, prolonged hypotension or hypovolemia or exposure to a nephrotoxic agent.

The ARF associated with AKI usually develops over hours or days, with progressive elevations of blood urea nitrogen (BUN), creatinine, and potassium, with or without oliguria. Severe AKI develops in over 60% of critical care unit (CCU) patients, with mortality rates of 70 to 80%.

One of the most commonly used classification systems for AKI uses serum creatinine, glomerular filtration rate (GFR), and urine output to identify **r**isk, **i**njury, **f**ailure, **l**oss, and **e**nd-stage kidney disease (the RIFLE criteria) (Figure 49.1). The criteria for evaluating AKI have been found to correlate with outcome and are a good predictor of mortality in hospitalized patients.

Etiology and Pathophysiology

AKI is a complex disorder, with many etiological factors and varied clinical manifestations that range from minimal elevation in serum creatinine to anuric renal failure (Mercado et al.,

2019; Ülger, 2018). The causes leading to AKI with renal failure are divided into prerenal, intrarenal (or intrinsic), and postrenal categories (Table 49.2).

Prerenal causes of AKI are factors external to the kidneys. These factors reduce systemic circulation, causing a reduction in renal blood flow and lead to decreased glomerular perfusion and filtration. Although renal tubular and glomerular function is preserved, glomerular filtration is reduced as a result of decreased perfusion. Hypovolemia, decreased cardiac output, decreased peripheral vascular resistance, and vascular obstruction can all decrease the effective circulating volume of the blood. With a decrease in circulating blood volume, autoregulatory mechanisms that increase angiotensin II, aldosterone, norepinephrine, and antidiuretic hormone work to preserve blood flow to essential organs. Prerenal azotemia results in a reduction in the excretion of sodium (<20 mmol/L), increased salt and water retention, and decreased urine output.

Prerenal AKI can also be caused by vasoactive medications such as angiotensin-converting enzyme (ACE) inhibitors, angiotensin receptor blockers (ARBs), epinephrine, and large doses of dopamine that cause intrarenal vasoconstriction leading to hypoperfusion of the glomeruli (Mercado et al., 2019). AKI associated with prerenal causes is usually reversible. If the course of prerenal failure is prolonged, intrarenal damage may ensue, usually resulting in acute tubular necrosis.

Intrarenal causes include conditions that cause direct damage to the renal tissue (parenchyma), resulting in impaired nephron function. Intrarenal causes of AKI are usually due to prolonged ischemia or the presence of nephrotoxins, hemoglobin released from hemolyzed red blood cells (RBCs), or myoglobin released from necrotic muscle cells. Nephrotoxins can cause obstruction of intrarenal structures by crystallization or by actually damaging the epithelial cells of the tubules. Hemoglobin and myoglobin block the tubules and cause renal vasoconstriction. Primary renal diseases such as acute glomerulonephritis and systemic lupus erythematosus may also cause AKI.

TABLE 49.2   COMMON CAUSES OF ACUTE KIDNEY INJURY

Prerenal	Intrarenal
• Anaphylaxis	• Acute glomerulonephritis
• Antihypertensive medications	• Allergies (antibiotics [sulphonamides, rifampin], nonsteroidal anti-inflammatory drugs, ACE inhibitors)
• Bilateral renal vein thrombosis	
• Burns	
• Cardiac dysrhythmias	• Chemical exposure (ethylene glycol, lead, arsenic, carbon tetrachloride)
• Cardiogenic shock	
• Decreased cardiac output	
• Decreased peripheral vascular resistance	• Medications (aminoglycosides [gentamicin, amikacin], amphotericin B)
• Decreased renovascular blood flow	
• Dehydration	• Hemolytic blood transfusion reaction
• Embolism	
• Excessive diuresis	• Infections (bacterial [acute pyelonephritis], viral [CMV], fungal [candidiasis])
• GI losses (diarrhea, vomiting)	
• Heart failure	
• Hemorrhage	• Interstitial nephritis
• Hepatorenal syndrome	• Malignant hypertension
• Hypoalbuminemia	• Nephrotoxic injury
• Hypovolemia	• Prolonged prerenal ischemia
• Myocardial infarction	• Radiocontrast agents
• Neurological injury	• Severe crush injury
• Pericardial tamponade	• Systemic lupus erythematosus
• Pulmonary edema	• Thrombotic disorders
• Renal artery thrombosis	• Toxemia of pregnancy
• Septic shock	
• Valvular heart disease	**Postrenal**
	• Benign prostatic hyperplasia
	• Calculi formation
	• Cancer (bladder, prostate, cervical, colorectal)
	• Neuromuscular disorders
	• Spinal cord disease
	• Strictures
	• Trauma (back, pelvis, perineum)

ACE, angiotensin-converting enzyme; *CMV*, cytomegalovirus; *GI*, gastrointestinal.

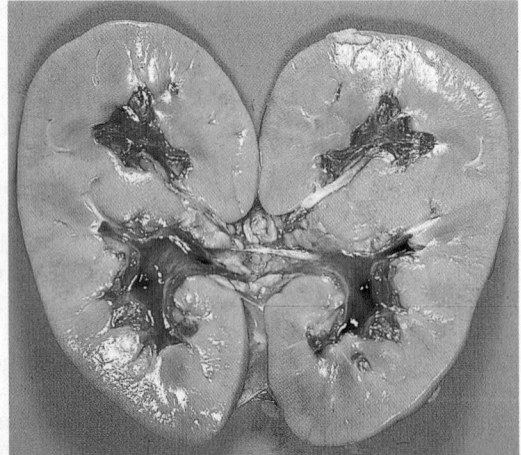

FIG. 49.2 Acute tubular necrosis. In acute tubular necrosis, the kidneys are swollen and pale. Source: Stevens, A., & Lowe, J. (2000). *Pathology: Illustrated review in color* (2nd ed.). Mosby.

Acute tubular necrosis (ATN) is the most common intrarenal cause of AKI and is primarily the result of ischemia, nephrotoxins, or sepsis (Figure 49.2). Severe renal ischemia causes a disruption in the basement membrane and patchy destruction of the tubular epithelium. Nephrotoxic agents cause necrosis of tubular epithelial cells, which slough off and plug the tubules. ATN is potentially reversible if the basement membrane is not destroyed and the tubular epithelium regenerates.

Possible pathological processes involved in ATN include the following:

1. Hypovolemia and decreased renal blood flow stimulate renin release, which activates the renin–angiotensin–aldosterone system (see Chapter 47, Figure 47.6) and results in constriction of the peripheral arteries and the renal afferent arterioles. With decreased renal blood flow, there is decreased glomerular capillary pressure and GFR as well as tubular dysfunction and, ultimately, oliguria.
2. Ischemia alters glomerular epithelial cells and decreases glomerular capillary permeability. This reduces the GFR, which significantly reduces blood flow and leads to tubular dysfunction.
3. When tubules are damaged, interstitial edema occurs, and necrotic epithelial cells accumulate in the tubules. The debris lowers the GFR by obstructing the tubules and increasing intratubular pressure.
4. Glomerular filtrate leaks back into plasma through holes in the damaged tubular membranes, which decreases intratubular fluid flow.

Postrenal causes of AKI involve mechanical obstruction of urinary outflow. As the flow of urine is obstructed, urine refluxes into the renal pelvis, impairing kidney function. The most common causes are benign prostatic hyperplasia, prostate cancer, calculi, trauma, and extrarenal tumours. Postrenal AKI is almost always treatable if identified before permanent kidney damage occurs.

Clinical Manifestations

Prerenal or postrenal AKI that has not caused intrarenal damage usually resolves quickly with correction of the cause. However, if parenchymal damage has occurred from either cause, or from intrarenal causes, ATN results or the course of AKI is prolonged. Clinically, ATN progresses through three phases: initiation, maintenance, and recovery (Benett, 2020). In some situations, the patient does not recover from AKI, and CKD results.

Initiation Phase. The initiation phase of ATN is characterized by an increase in serum creatinine and BUN and a decrease in urine output (Harrois et al., 2017).

Maintenance Phase. The maintenance phase of ATN may last from days to weeks. During this phase, patients may be anuric, oliguric, or nonoliguric. In patients who are nonoliguric, a dilute urine (low specific gravity) is made, but uremic toxins are not removed. The oliguric phase usually lasts 10 to 14 days, but it can last for months in some cases. The longer the oliguric phase lasts, the poorer the prognosis for recovery of complete renal function.

The manifestations of the oliguric phase are changes in urinary output, fluid and electrolyte abnormalities, and uremia. (For a definition of *uremia*, see discussion of the clinical manifestations of CKD, later in this chapter.) The nurse must be alert for the signs and symptoms of these changes.

Urinary Changes. The most common initial manifestation of ATN is **oliguria**, in which urine output generally decreases to less than 400 mL/24 hr. If ATN is caused by ischemia, oliguria will occur within 24 hours. If ATN is caused by nephrotoxic medications, the onset may be delayed for as long as a week. The duration of the oliguric phase is generally 10 to 14 days, but it can last months in some cases.

Oliguria associated with ATN is characterized by urine with a normal specific gravity (1.010) and a high sodium concentration (>40 mmol/L), and urine osmolality at about 300 mmol/kg, indicating that the injured tubules cannot respond to autoregulatory mechanisms. The urine sediment may show RBCs and white blood cells (WBCs), casts, and proteinuria. The casts are formed from mucoprotein impressions of the necrotic renal tubular epithelial cells, which detach or slough into the tubules.

Fluid Volume Excess. When urinary output decreases, fluid retention occurs. The severity of the symptoms depends on the extent of the fluid overload. The neck veins may become distended with a bounding pulse. Edema and hypertension may develop. Fluid overload can eventually lead to heart failure, pulmonary edema, and pericardial and pleural effusions.

Metabolic Acidosis. In renal failure, the kidneys cannot synthesize ammonia, which is needed for hydrogen ion excretion or to excrete acid products of metabolism. The serum bicarbonate level decreases because bicarbonate is used up in buffering hydrogen ions. In addition, defective reabsorption and regeneration of bicarbonate occurs. The patient may develop Kussmaul's respirations (rapid, deep respirations) to increase the excretion of carbon dioxide. Lethargy and changes in level of consciousness will occur if treatment is not started.

Sodium Balance. Damaged tubules cannot conserve sodium. Consequently, the urinary excretion of sodium may increase, resulting in normal or below-normal levels of serum sodium. Excessive intake of sodium should be avoided because it can lead to volume expansion, hypertension, and heart failure. Uncontrolled hyponatremia or water excess can lead to cerebral edema. The sodium level is also affected by the retention of fluid resulting in dilutional hyponatremia.

Potassium Excess. Hyperkalemia is a common, life-threatening complication seen in patients with oliguria. Serum potassium levels increase because the normal ability of the kidneys to regulate and excrete potassium is impaired. Hyperkalemia associated with AKI may be precipitated by a number of causes. Massive tissue trauma may result in the release of additional potassium into the extracellular fluid by the damaged cells. Bleeding and blood transfusions may cause cellular destruction, releasing more potassium into the extracellular fluid. Acidosis worsens hyperkalemia as hydrogen ions enter the cells and potassium is driven out of the cells into the extracellular fluid.

Most often, patients with hyperkalemia are asymptomatic. Some patients may experience weakness with severe hyperkalemia. Severe hyperkalemia requires immediate treatment as this may lead to lethal cardiac arrhythmias. Before clinical signs of hyperkalemia are apparent, the electrocardiogram (ECG) will show tall, peaked T waves; widening of the QRS complex; and ST depression. Progressive changes in the ECG that are related to increasing potassium levels are depicted in Chapter 19, Figure 19.14. Because cardiac muscle is very intolerant of acute increases in potassium, treatment is essential when hyperkalemia develops (Table 49.3 lists electrolyte changes during phases of AKI).

Hematological Disorders. Several hematological disorders are seen in connection with AKI. Anemia occurs because renal failure results in impaired erythropoietin production. Uremia decreases platelet adhesiveness and can lead to bleeding from multiple sources (e.g., intestines, brain). WBCs are also altered, causing immunodeficiency. This leaves the patient susceptible to numerous systemic and local infections. Infection (sepsis) in

TABLE 49.3	PHASES AND LABORATORY FINDINGS IN ACUTE KIDNEY INJURY
Oliguric phase	• Elevated BUN and creatinine • Decreased creatinine clearance • Decreased glomerular filtration rate • Hyperkalemia • Hypocalcemia • Hyperphosphatemia • Normal or low sodium levels
Diuretic phase	• Continued decline in BUN and creatinine • Continued decline in creatinine clearance and glomerular filtration rate • Hypokalemia • Hyponatremia • Hypovolemia
Recovery phase	• Increased glomerular filtration rate • Stabilizing or decreasing of the BUN and creatinine levels

BUN, blood urea nitrogen.

combination with AKI is associated with double the mortality rate, and half of the survivors suffer permanent kidney damage or chronic kidney disease (Skube et al., 2018).

Calcium Deficit and Phosphate Excess. Activated vitamin D must be present for calcium absorption from the gastrointestinal (GI) tract to occur. Only functioning kidneys can activate vitamin D. Thus, in the presence of kidney failure, GI absorption of calcium decreases, and a low serum calcium level results. When hypocalcemia occurs, the parathyroid gland secretes parathyroid hormone (PTH), which stimulates bone demineralization and causes calcium to be released from the bones. Phosphate is released as well, leading to hyperphosphatemia, which is worsened by the decreased excretion of phosphate by the kidneys. Normally, plasma calcium is found ionized or free (physiologically active form) or bound to protein. In the acidotic state associated with renal failure, more calcium is in the ionized form. Although it is unusual for hypocalcemia to be symptomatic in renal failure, an ionized calcium level that decreases significantly can lead to tetany.

Waste Product Accumulation. The kidneys are the primary excretory organs for urea, an end product of protein metabolism, and creatinine, an end product of endogenous muscle metabolism. The BUN and creatinine levels are elevated in kidney failure. An elevated BUN level must be interpreted with caution because dehydration, corticosteroids, catabolism resulting from infections, fever, severe injury, and GI bleeding can also elevate BUN. The best serum indicator of renal failure is creatinine because it is not significantly altered by other factors. Measuring creatinine clearance by using radioactive tracer (inulin) is the most accurate method for assessing renal function, but it is expensive and impractical. Clinically, the recommended method to evaluate kidney function is with an estimated glomerular filtration rate (eGFR) (Ptáčník et al., 2019).

Neurological Disorders. Neurological changes can occur as nitrogenous waste products accumulate in the brain and other nervous tissue. The symptoms can be as mild as fatigue and difficulty concentrating or can escalate to seizures, stupor, and coma. Eventually, all body systems become involved in the acute uremic syndrome. The extrarenal manifestations are generally similar to those found in the patient with chronic uremia (see the discussion of CKD later in this chapter).

Recovery Phase. The recovery phase of AKI is marked by a return of BUN, creatinine, and GFR toward normal ranges (Ptáčník et al., 2019). During this phase, patients may experience a diuretic phase that can result in fluid and electrolyte abnormalities. The diuretic phase begins with a gradual increase in daily urine output to 1 to 3 L per day, but it may reach 3 to 5 L or more per day. Although urine output increases, the nephrons are still not fully functional. The high urine volume is caused by osmotic diuresis from the high urea concentration in the glomerular filtrate and the inability of the tubules to concentrate the urine. In this phase, the kidneys have recovered their ability to excrete wastes but not to concentrate the urine. Hypovolemia and hypotension can occur from massive fluid losses. Because of the large losses of fluid and electrolytes, the patient must be monitored for hyponatremia, hypokalemia, and dehydration. The diuretic phase may last 1 to 3 weeks. Near the end of this phase, the patient's acid–base, electrolyte, and waste product (BUN, creatinine) values begin to normalize. Although the major improvements occur in the first 1 to 2 weeks of this phase, renal function may take up to 12 months to stabilize.

The outcome of AKI is influenced by the patient's overall health, the severity of renal failure, and the number and type of complications. Some individuals do not recover and progress to CKD. The older patient is less likely to recover full kidney function than the younger patient. Among the individuals who recover, the majority achieve clinically normal kidney function with no complications (e.g., hypertension).

Diagnostic Studies

Urinalysis is an important diagnostic test. Urine sediment containing abundant cells, casts, or proteins suggests intrarenal disorders. The urine osmolality, sodium content, and specific gravity help to differentiate the types of AKI. Urine sediment may be normal in both prerenal and postrenal AKI. Hematuria, pyuria, and crystals may be seen with postrenal AKI.

To establish a diagnosis of AKI, other testing may be required. A renal ultrasound is often the first test done and provides information about anatomy and function. Ultrasound does not require the use of nephrotoxic contrast agents. A renal scan can be used to assess renal blood flow and the integrity of the collecting system. A computed tomographic (CT) scan can identify lesions and masses as well as obstruction, but exposure to radiation is higher and it may involve contrast that can be nephrotoxic. Magnetic resonance imaging (MRI) and magnetic resonance angiography (MRA) are not recommended—gadolinium, a contrast medium used with MRI and MRA, has been associated with the development of *nephrogenic systemic fibrosis* in patients with compromised renal function.

Interprofessional Care

Because AKI is potentially reversible, the primary goals of treatment are to eliminate the cause, manage the signs and symptoms, and prevent complications while the kidneys recover (Table 49.4). The first step is to determine whether there is sufficient intravascular volume and cardiac output to ensure adequate perfusion of the kidneys. Crystalloids are used to provide adequate perfusion of kidneys. Diuretic therapy is often administered along with crystalloids to prevent fluid overload if the patient is not oliguric. Diuretic therapy usually includes loop diuretics (e.g., furosemide [Lasix]) or an osmotic diuretic (e.g., mannitol). If AKI is already established, forcing fluids and diuretics will not be effective and may, in fact, be harmful. Medical management without RRT may

TABLE 49.4	INTERPROFESSIONAL CARE
Acute Kidney Injury	
Diagnostic	**Interprofessional Therapy**

• History and physical examination
• Identification of precipitating cause
• Serum creatinine and BUN levels
• Serum electrolytes
• Urinalysis
• Renal ultrasound
• Renal scan (as indicated)
• CT scan (as indicated and without contrast if possible)
• Retrograde pyelogram (as indicated)
	• Treatment of precipitating cause
	• Fluid restriction (allowance = 600 mL + previous 24-hr fluid loss)
	• Nutritional therapy
	  • Adequate protein intake (0.6–2 g/kg/day), depending on degree of catabolism
	  • Potassium restriction
	  • Phosphate restriction
	  • Sodium restriction
	  • Measures to lower potassium (if elevated)*
	  • Calcium supplements or phosphate-binding agents
	  • Parenteral nutrition (if indicated)†
	  • Enteral nutrition (if indicated)†
	• Initiation of renal replacement therapy (if necessary)

BUN, blood urea nitrogen; *CT*, computed tomographic.
*See Table 49.5.
†Renal formulations of these two forms of nutrition are available.

be all that is necessary until renal function improves. The general trend is to initiate early and frequent RRT to minimize symptoms and prevent complications.

Fluid intake must be closely monitored during the oliguric phase. The general rule for calculating the permitted fluid intake is to add all losses of the previous 24 hours (e.g., urine, diarrhea, emesis, blood) plus 600 mL for insensible losses (e.g., respiration, diaphoresis). For example, if a patient excreted 300 mL of urine on Tuesday with no other losses, the fluid intake on Wednesday would be restricted to 900 mL.

Hyperkalemia is one of the most serious complications of AKI because it can cause life-threatening cardiac dysrhythmias. The various therapies used to treat elevated potassium levels are listed in Table 49.5. Both insulin and salbutamol temporarily shift potassium into the cells, but it eventually shifts back out. Calcium gluconate raises the threshold at which dysrhythmias will occur, serving to temporarily stabilize the myocardium. Only cation exchange resins, such as sodium polystyrene sulphonate (Kayexalate) or calcium resonium, and dialysis actually remove potassium from the body. Sodium polystyrene sulphonate should not be given, or mixed with sorbitol, to patients who do not have normal bowel function because of associated bowel necrosis.

The most common indications for RRT in AKI include (1) volume overload resulting in compromised cardiac or pulmonary status, or both; (2) elevated potassium levels; (3) metabolic acidosis (serum bicarbonate level <15 mmol/L); (4) BUN level greater than 43 mmol/L; (5) significant change in mental status; and (6) pericarditis, pericardial effusion, or cardiac tamponade. Although laboratory values provide rough parameters, the best guide to treatment is good clinical assessment.

If RRT is required, many options are available, but there is no consensus regarding the best approach. Even though peritoneal dialysis (PD) is considered a viable option for RRT, it is rarely used. Intermittent hemodialysis (HD) (e.g., at intervals of 4 hours, either daily or every other day, or three to four times per week) and continuous renal replacement therapy (CRRT) have

TABLE 49.5 TREATMENT OF HYPERKALEMIA

Stabilize Myocardium

- If the ECG shows hyperkalemia-related abnormalities, *calcium gluconate IV* is given. Calcium raises the threshold potential, thus counteracting the toxic effect of potassium on the myocardium, which can induce life-threatening dysrhythmias.

Shift Potassium Into Cells

- *Regular IV insulin administration* causes potassium to move into cells. Glucose is given concurrently to prevent hypoglycemia. When effects of insulin diminish, potassium shifts back out of cells.
- *Salbutamol* will also temporarily shift potassium back into cells.
- *Sodium bicarbonate* can correct acidosis and causes shift of potassium into cells.

Enhance Potassium Removal

- *Cation exchange resins* such as *sodium polystyrene sulphonate (Kayexalate)* are administered by mouth or retention enema. When resin is in the bowel, potassium is exchanged for sodium. Therapy removes 1 mmol of potassium/g of medication. *Calcium resonium* is another such resin.
- Sodium zirconium cyclosilicate (ZS-9) captures potassium in the GI tract and the potassium is excreted in the stool.
- Patiromer binds with potassium in the lumen of the GI tract and is able to increase fecal potassium excretion
- Loop diuretics such as *furosemide* can increase potassium excretion in the urine if the patient has any urine output.
- *Dialysis*, particularly *hemodialysis*, can bring potassium levels to normal within 30 min to 2 hr.

Long-Term Treatment

- *Restrict intake of dietary potassium* to 40 mmol/day and avoid potassium-containing salt substitutes.
- Limit or discontinue medications that can precipitate or exacerbate hyperkalemia such as ACE inhibitors, ARBs, and potassium-sparing diuretics.

ACE, angiotensin-converting enzyme; *ARBs*, angiotensin receptor blockers; *ECG*, electrocardiogram; *IV*, intravenous.

both been used effectively. CRRT is provided continuously over approximately 24 hours and has much slower blood flow rates than intermittent HD. HD is the method of choice when rapid changes are required in a short time. It is technically more complicated because specialized staff and equipment are required. It also requires anticoagulation to prevent the patient's blood from clotting when it contacts the foreign material in the dialysis circuit. Rapid fluid shifts during HD may cause hypotension. RRT, PD, HD, and CRRT are discussed later in this chapter.

Nutritional Therapy. The challenge of nutritional management in AKI is to provide adequate calories to prevent catabolism despite the restrictions required, to prevent electrolyte and fluid disorders and azotemia. Adequate energy should be provided from carbohydrate and fat sources to prevent ketosis from endogenous fat breakdown and gluconeogenesis from muscle-protein breakdown. The daily caloric intake for patients with AKI should be about 25 to 35 kcal/kg, based on estimated metabolic stress and protein energy requirements (Góes & Balbi, 2018). Protein dosage varies from 1.5 to 2.5 g/kg/day, depending on the stage of AKI and whether or not RRT is required. Given the complexity of the patient's nutritional needs, a renal dietitian should be consulted.

Potassium and sodium are regulated in accordance with plasma levels. Sodium is restricted as needed to prevent edema, hypertension, and heart failure. Hyperphosphatemia, hypocalcemia, and hypermagnesemia are common and must be monitored and regulated. Dietary fat intake is increased so that the patient receives at least 30 to 40% of total calories from fat. Fat-emulsion intravenous (IV) infusions can also be given as a nutritional supplement and provide a good source of non-protein calories (see Chapter 42). If a patient cannot maintain adequate oral intake, enteral nutrition is the preferred route for nutritional support (see Chapter 42). When the GI tract is not functional, parenteral nutrition (PN) is necessary for the provision of adequate nutrition. The patient treated with PN may need daily HD or CRRT to remove the excess fluid. Concentrated PN formulas are available to minimize fluid volume.

NURSING MANAGEMENT ACUTE KIDNEY INJURY

NURSING ASSESSMENT

An assessment of the patient with AKI includes the specific areas presented in Table 49.6. It is important to monitor the vital signs and intake and output. The urine should be examined for colour, specific gravity, glucose, protein, blood, and sediment. The patient's general appearance should be assessed, including skin colour, peripheral edema, neck vein distension, and bruises.

If the patient is receiving RRT, the access site should be observed for signs of inflammation. The patient's mental status and level of consciousness need to be evaluated. The nurse should examine the oral mucosa for dryness and inflammation and auscultate the lung fields for crackles and wheezes or diminished breath sounds. The nurse must also monitor the heart for the presence of a third heart sound (S_3 or gallop), murmurs, or a pericardial friction rub. ECG readings are assessed for the presence of dysrhythmias, and laboratory values and diagnostic test results are reviewed. All of the previous data are essential for developing an interprofessional plan of care.

NURSING DIAGNOSES

Nursing diagnoses and potential complications for the patient with AKI include but are not limited to the following:

- *Potential for* infection as evidenced by *alteration in skin integrity* (invasive lines)
- *Excess fluid volume* resulting from *excessive fluid intake* (kidney injury and fluid retention)
- *Fatigue* resulting from *malnutrition, physical deconditioning* (anemia, metabolic acidosis, uremic toxins)
- *Anxiety* resulting from *threat to current status, threat of death* (disease processes, therapeutic interventions, uncertainty of prognosis)
- Potential complication: dysrhythmias resulting from electrolyte imbalances

PLANNING

The overall goals for the patient with AKI are to (1) completely recover without any loss of kidney function, (2) maintain normal fluid and electrolyte balance, (3) have decreased anxiety, and (4) understand and adhere to the treatment plan and follow-up care.

NURSING IMPLEMENTATION

HEALTH PROMOTION. Prevention of AKI is essential because of the high mortality rate associated with it. Prevention efforts are primarily directed toward identifying and monitoring high-risk populations, controlling intake of nephrotoxic medications and

TABLE 49.6	MANIFESTATIONS OF ACUTE KIDNEY INJURY
Body System	**Clinical Manifestations**
Urinary	Casts ↓ Osmolality Proteinuria ↓ Specific gravity Urinary output ↑ Urinary sodium
Cardiovascular	Dysrhythmias Heart failure Hypertension (after development of fluid overload) Hypotension (early) Pericardial effusion Pericarditis Volume overload
Respiratory	Kussmaul's respirations Pleural effusions Pulmonary edema
Gastrointestinal	Anorexia Bleeding Constipation Diarrhea Nausea and vomiting Stomatitis
Hematological	Anemia (development within 48 hr) Defect in platelet functioning Leukocytosis ↑ Susceptibility to infection
Neurological	Asterixis Lethargy Memory impairment Seizures
Metabolic	↑ BUN ↑ Creatinine ↑ Phosphate ↑ Potassium ↓ Bicarbonate ↓ Calcium ↓ pH ↓ Sodium

BUN, blood urea nitrogen.

exposure to industrial chemicals, and preventing prolonged episodes of hypotension and hypovolemia. In the hospital, the factors that increase the risk of developing AKI are advanced age, massive trauma, major surgical procedures, extensive burns, cardiac failure, sepsis, obstetrical complications, and baseline renal insufficiency caused by hypertension or diabetes mellitus. Careful monitoring of intake and output and of fluid and electrolyte balance is essential. Extrarenal losses of fluid from vomiting, diarrhea, and hemorrhage should be assessed and recorded as well as increased insensible losses. Prompt replacement of significant fluid losses will help prevent ischemic tubular damage associated with trauma, burns, and extensive surgery. Intake and output records and the patient's weight provide valuable indicators of fluid volume status. Aggressive diuretic therapy for the patient with fluid overload resulting from any cause can lead to decreased renal blood flow.

For patients with any level of renal insufficiency—and particularly patients with diabetes or older patients with renal insufficiency—who are undergoing diagnostic studies requiring IV contrast media, special attention must be given to prevent a nephrotoxic injury secondary to the dye. Adequate hydration before and after the test is critical. The use of acetylcysteine may be helpful in providing added protection to the kidneys (Poh et al., 2018). Patients with urinary tract infections need prompt treatment and careful follow-up care. Chemotherapeutic drugs that cause hyperuricemia also can put a patient at risk for renal injury.

Individuals taking medications that are potentially nephrotoxic (see Chapter 47, Table 47.3) must have renal function monitored. Nephrotoxic medications should be used sparingly in high-risk patients. When these medications must be used, they should be given in the smallest effective doses for the shortest possible periods. The patient should be cautioned about the misuse of over-the-counter analgesics (especially nonsteroidal anti-inflammatory drugs [NSAIDs]) because some of these may worsen renal function in the patient with borderline renal insufficiency by decreasing glomerular pressure or causing interstitial nephritis. ACE inhibitors can also decrease perfusion pressure and cause hyperkalemia, and their use may be contraindicated in renal insufficiency. Industrial and agricultural chemicals and products (e.g., organic solvents, insecticides, cleaning agents) must be monitored regularly to assess their safety for employees and the general population.

ACUTE INTERVENTION. The patient with AKI is most often critically ill. Frequently, these patients have a high burden of comorbid illness (e.g., diabetes, cardiovascular disease) that also affects renal function. The nurse needs to focus on the patient holistically because they have many physical and emotional needs. Usually, the changes caused by AKI arise suddenly. Both the patient and the family need assistance in understanding that the functioning of the whole body can be disrupted by renal failure.

The nurse has an important role in managing fluid and electrolyte balance during the oliguric and diuretic phases. Observing and recording accurate intake and output are essential. It is important to measure weights daily, with the same scale and at the same time each day, to allow for the evaluation and detection of excessive gains or losses of body fluid (1 kg is equivalent to 1 000 mL of fluid). The nurse needs to be know the common signs and symptoms of hypervolemia (in the oliguric phase) or hypovolemia (in the diuretic phase) and watch for potassium and sodium disturbances as well as other electrolyte imbalances that may occur in AKI (see Chapter 19).

Because infection is the leading cause of death in AKI, meticulous aseptic technique is critical. The patient must be protected from other individuals with infectious diseases. The nurse should be alert for local manifestations of infection (e.g., swelling, redness, pain) as well as systemic manifestations (e.g., malaise, leukocytosis) but should realize that an elevated temperature may not be present. Patients with renal failure have a blunted febrile response to an infection (e.g., pneumonia). If antibiotics are used to treat an infection, the type, frequency, and dosage must be carefully considered because the kidneys are the primary route of excretion for many antibiotics. Dosages and dosing intervals need to be considered in relation to the patient's level of kidney function if the medication is primarily eliminated by the kidneys. Use of nephrotoxic medications (see Chapter 47, Table 47.3) should be avoided.

Skin care and measures to prevent pressure injuries should be performed because the patient usually develops edema as well as decreased muscle tone. Mouth care is important to prevent stomatitis, which develops when ammonia (produced by bacterial breakdown of urea) in saliva irritates the mucous membranes.

AMBULATORY AND HOME CARE. Recovery from AKI is highly variable and depends on the underlying illness, the general condition and the age of the patient, the length of the oliguric phase, and the severity of nephron damage. Good nutrition, rest, and activity are necessary. Dietary restrictions should be regulated in accordance with kidney function. Follow-up care and regular evaluation of renal function are necessary. The nurse needs to teach the patient the signs and symptoms of recurrent kidney disease. Measures to prevent the recurrence of AKI should be emphasized.

The long-term convalescence of 3 to 12 months may cause psychosocial and financial hardships for the family. The nurse should make referrals for counselling as appropriate. If the kidneys do not recover, the patient will need to transition to life on chronic dialysis or possible future transplantation.

EVALUATION

The following are expected outcomes for the patient with AKI:
- Regain and maintain normal fluid and electrolyte balance.
- Adhere to the treatment regimen.
- Experience no infectious complications.
- Have complete recovery.

AGE-RELATED CONSIDERATIONS

ACUTE KIDNEY INJURY

Older persons are more susceptible than younger adults to AKI because the number of functioning nephrons decreases with age. Impaired function of other organ systems (e.g., cardiovascular disease, impaired pancreas function) can increase the risk of developing AKI. The aging kidney is less able to compensate for changes in fluid volume, solute load, and cardiac output. Common causes of AKI in the older person include dehydration, hypotension, diuretic therapy, aminoglycoside therapy, obstructive disorders (e.g., prostatic hyperplasia), surgery, infection, and radiocontrast agents.

CHRONIC KIDNEY DISEASE

Chronic kidney disease (CKD) involves the progressive, irreversible loss of kidney function. The Kidney Disease Outcomes Quality Initiative (KDOQI) defines CKD as either kidney damage or GFR less than 60 mL/min/1.73 m² for 3 months or longer. CKD is classified as one of five stages, depending on the level of severity based on GFR (Table 49.7). CKD involves progressive, irreversible destruction of the nephrons in both kidneys. Not all people with CKD will progress to stage 5, in which RRT would be necessary; however, all those affected will require ongoing monitoring.

Identifying the stage of CKD allows for early intervention to reduce cardiovascular risk, delay progression, and prevent the need for RRT. RRTs include PD, HD, and renal transplantation.

TABLE 49.7   STAGES* AND DESCRIPTIONS OF CHRONIC KIDNEY DISEASE†

	Description	GFR (mL/min/1.73 m²)	Action‡
Stage 1	Kidney damage with normal or ↑ GFR	≥90	Diagnosis and treatment of comorbid conditions CVD risk reduction
Stage 2	Kidney damage with mild ↓ GFR	60–89	Estimation of progression
Stage 3	Moderate ↓ GFR	30–59	Evaluation and treatment of complications
Stage 4	Severe ↓ GFR	15–29	Preparation for renal replacement therapy
Stage 5	Kidney failure	<15 (or dialysis)	Renal replacement therapy (if uremia present and patient desires treatment)

CVD, cardiovascular disease; *GFR*, glomerular filtration rate.
*Stages 1 to 5 identify patients who have chronic kidney disease.
†*Chronic kidney disease* is defined as either kidney damage or GFR <60 mL/min/1.73 m² for 3 mo. *Kidney damage* is defined as pathological abnormalities or markers of damage, including abnormalities in blood or urine tests or imaging studies.
‡Includes actions from preceding stages.
Source: Reprinted from Levey, A. S., Coresh, J., Bolton, K., et al. (2002). KDOQI clinical practice guidelines for chronic kidney disease: Evaluation, classification and stratification. *American Journal of Kidney Disease 39*(2), S1–S266 (Suppl 1), with permission from Elsevier.

Stage 5 CKD, often referred to as end-stage renal disease (ESRD), is advanced kidney disease with GFR less than 15 mL/min/1.73 m², when most patients with CKD require some form of RRT. At this point, RRT (dialysis or transplantation) is usually required. In 2018, there were 6 045 new patients started on RRT in Canada. Of these, over half (54%) were older than 65 years and 62% were male (CIHI, 2019). Although there are many causes of CKD, the leading causes of CKD in Canada are diabetes mellitus (38%) and renal vascular disease (15%).

The kidneys have remarkable functional reserve. Up to 80% of the GFR (reflected in creatinine clearance measurements) may be lost with few overt changes in the functioning of the body. A person is born with about 2 million nephrons and can survive without RRT until almost 90% of the nephrons are lost. In the majority of cases, the individual passes through the early stages of CKD without recognizing the disease state because the remaining nephrons hypertrophy to compensate. The prognosis and the course of CKD are highly variable, depending on the etiology, the individual's condition and age, and the adequacy of medical follow-up. Some individuals live normal, active lives with compensated renal failure, whereas others may rapidly progress to ESRD.

Since 1973, many deaths have been prevented through the use of RRTs. Dialysis modalities remain the most common RRT for people with stage 5 CKD because of (1) a lack of donated organs, (2) medical conditions that preclude transplantation, or (3) personal reasons, in which an individual may decline transplantation as a treatment option. With the advances made in medical science, an increasing number of individuals are receiving RRTs, including older persons and those with complex medical conditions. All people with advanced CKD, regardless of age, should be offered RRT unless it is medically contraindicated.

Clinical Manifestations

As renal function progressively deteriorates, excretory, regulatory, and endocrine function are lost, and these effects are manifested in every body system, no matter what the underlying cause of CKD. These excretory, regulatory, and endocrine functional impairments are manifested in retained substances, including urea, creatinine, phenols, hormones, electrolytes, water, and many other substances. Uremia is a constellation of signs and symptoms resulting from the buildup of waste products and excess fluid associated with kidney failure. These signs and symptoms may include, but are not limited to, elevated serum creatinine and BUN, abnormal electrolytes, acidosis, anemia, fluid volume excess, nausea, loss of appetite, fatigue, decreased cognition, pruritus, and neuropathy (Figure 49.3). It is important to recognize that the manifestations of uremia vary among patients, according to the cause of the kidney disease, comorbid conditions, age, and degree of adherence to the prescribed medical regimen. Many patients are very tolerant of the changes that occur because the changes develop gradually. Uremia often occurs when the GFR is 10 mL/min/1.73 m² or lower.

Urinary System. In the early stage of CKD, polyuria results from the inability of the kidneys to concentrate urine. This happens most often at night, and the patient must arise several times to urinate (nocturia). Because of the decrease in renal concentrating ability, the specific gravity of urine gradually becomes fixed at around 1.010 (the osmolar concentration of plasma). As CKD worsens, oliguria develops, and eventually anuria (urine output 40 mL/24 hr) develops. If the patient is still producing urine, proteinuria, casts, pyuria, and hematuria could be present, depending on the cause of the kidney disease.

Metabolic Disturbances

Waste Product Accumulation. As GFR declines, the serum creatinine and BUN levels increase. Accumulation of nitrogenous waste products in advanced stages of CKD is often manifested by symptoms of nausea, vomiting, lethargy, fatigue, impaired thought processes, and headaches as a result of the multisystemic involvement of CKD.

Serum creatinine continues to be the most common biochemical parameter to estimate the GFR, but it alone is not an accurate measure of GFR (Ptáčník et al., 2019). Serum creatinine tends to be an ineffective marker of early as well as advanced kidney disease. The eGFR is a better measure of overall kidney function than creatinine or BUN. The eGFR may be calculated by the laboratory using mathematical formulas. If this method is not available, GFR calculators and tables can be used (see link to the MDRD [modification of diet in renal disease] calculator in Table 49.9, later in the chapter). The serum creatinine level in an older patient with ESRD will be lower than it is in a younger person with the same degree of renal dysfunction. Decreased muscle mass and decreased muscle activity from aging account for this finding because creatinine is an end product of muscle metabolism.

Altered Carbohydrate Metabolism. Defective carbohydrate metabolism is caused by impaired glucose use resulting from cellular insensitivity to the normal action of insulin. The exact nature of this insulin resistance is unclear, but it may be related to circulating insulin antagonists, alterations in hormone receptors, or abnormalities of transport mechanisms. Moderate hyperglycemia, hyperinsulinemia, and abnormal glucose tolerance tests may be seen. Insulin and glucose metabolism may improve (but not to normal values) after the initiation of dialysis.

Patients with diabetes who become uremic may require less insulin than before the onset of CKD. This is because insulin, which is dependent on the kidneys for excretion, remains in circulation longer. The insulin regimen must be individualized and glucose levels monitored carefully.

Elevated Triglycerides. Hyperinsulinemia stimulates hepatic production of triglycerides. Almost all patients with uremia develop dyslipidemia, with elevated very-low-density lipoproteins, normal or decreased low-density lipoproteins, and lowered high-density lipoproteins. The altered lipid metabolism is related to decreased levels of the enzyme lipoprotein lipase, which is important in the breakdown of lipoproteins.

Electrolyte and Acid–Base Imbalances

Potassium. Hyperkalemia is a serious electrolyte disorder associated with kidney disease. Fatal dysrhythmias can occur when the serum potassium level reaches 7 to 8 mmol/L. Hyperkalemia results from the decreased excretion by the kidneys, the breakdown of cellular protein, bleeding, and metabolic acidosis. The most common causes of hyperkalemia in CKD are associated with diet, dietary supplements, medications, and IV infusions.

Sodium. Sodium may be normal or low in renal failure. Because of impaired sodium excretion, sodium is retained along with water. If large quantities of body water are retained, dilutional hyponatremia occurs. Sodium retention can contribute to edema, hypertension, and heart failure. Sodium intake must be individually determined but is generally restricted to 2 g/24 hr.

Calcium and Phosphate. Calcium and phosphate alterations are in the Musculoskeletal System section, later in this chapter.

Magnesium. Magnesium is excreted primarily by the kidneys. It is sometimes used as a phosphate-binding agent in patients with CKD. Hypermagnesemia is generally not a concern unless the patient is ingesting magnesium (e.g., milk of magnesia, magnesium citrate, antacids containing magnesium). Clinical manifestations of hypermagnesemia can include absence of reflexes, decreased mental status, cardiac dysrhythmias, hypotension, and respiratory failure.

Metabolic Acidosis. Metabolic acidosis results from the impaired ability of the kidneys to excrete the acid load

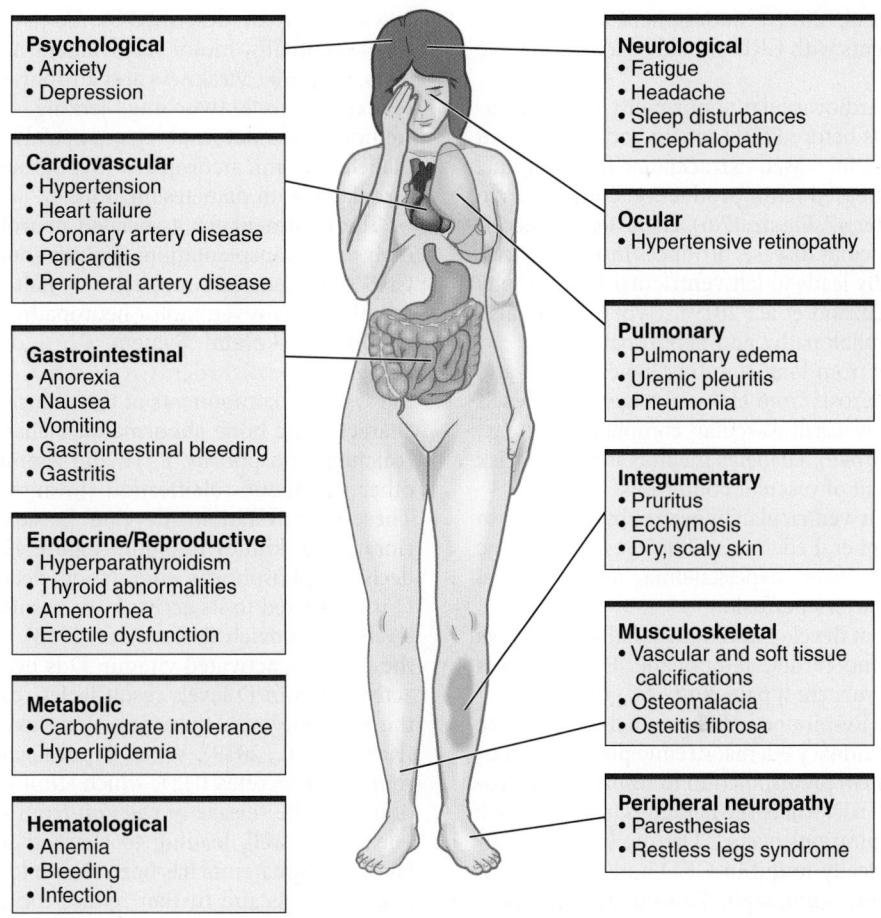

FIG. 49.3 Clinical manifestations of chronic uremia.

(primarily ammonia) and from defective reabsorption and regeneration of bicarbonate. The average adult produces 80 to 90 mmol/day of acid. In renal failure, plasma bicarbonate, which is an indirect measure of acidosis, usually falls to a new steady state at around 16 to 20 mmol/L. It generally does not progress below this level because hydrogen ion production is usually balanced by buffering from demineralization of the bone (the phosphate buffering system). Although Kussmaul's respiration is uncommon in CKD, this breathing pattern reduces the severity of acidosis by increasing carbon dioxide excretion.

Hematological System

Anemia. Anemia is very common in CKD. A normocytic, normochromic anemia is associated with CKD and is a result of decreased production of the hormone erythropoietin by the kidneys, resulting in decreased erythropoiesis by the bone marrow (Cheng et al., 2017). Erythropoietin stimulates precursor cells in the bone marrow to produce RBCs. Other factors contributing to anemia are nutritional deficiencies, decreased RBC lifespan, increased hemolysis of RBCs, frequent blood samplings, and bleeding from the GI tract. For patients receiving maintenance HD, blood loss in the dialyzer may also contribute to the anemic state. Elevated levels of PTH (produced to compensate for low serum calcium levels) can inhibit erythropoiesis, shorten survival of RBCs, and cause bone marrow fibrosis, which can result in decreased numbers of hematopoietic cells.

Sufficient iron stores are needed for erythropoiesis. Many patients with renal failure are iron deficient and require iron replacement. Folic acid, which is water soluble and essential for RBC maturation, is removed with dialysis and needs to be replaced in the diet with supplementation (1 mg/day).

Bleeding Tendencies. The most common cause of bleeding in uremia is a qualitative defect in platelet function. This dysfunction is caused by impaired platelet aggregation and impaired release of platelet factor III. In addition, alterations in the coagulation system with increased concentrations of both factor VIII and fibrinogen are found in the serum of these patients. The altered platelet function, hemorrhagic tendencies, and GI bleeding can usually be corrected with regular HD or PD.

Infection. Patients with advanced CKD have an increased susceptibility to infection. Infectious complications are caused by changes in leukocyte function and altered immune response and function. Both cellular and humoral immune responses are suppressed. Other factors contributing to the increased risk for infection include malnutrition, hyperglycemia, and external trauma (e.g., catheters, needle insertions into vascular access sites).

Cardiovascular System. Morbidity and mortality from cardiovascular disease are high in patients with CKD, and the presence of CKD worsens the outcomes of cardiovascular disease (Provenzano et al., 2019). Many patients will die from cardiovascular disease before CKD stage 5, requiring dialysis, develops (Provenzano et al., 2019). Management of cardiovascular risk factors in patients with CKD should be a focus of care (Provenzano et al., 2019).

The most common cardiovascular abnormality is hypertension, which usually exists before ESRD sets in and is worsened by sodium retention and increased extracellular fluid volume. In some individuals, increased renin production contributes to the condition (see Chapter 47, Figure 47.6). Hypertension accelerates atherosclerotic vascular disease, produces intrarenal arterial spasm, and eventually leads to left ventricular hypertrophy and heart failure (Provenzano et al., 2019). Hypertension also causes retinopathy, encephalopathy, and nephropathy.

The vascular changes from long-standing hypertension and the accelerated atherosclerosis from elevated triglyceride levels are responsible for many cardiovascular complications (e.g., myocardial infarction, stroke). Diabetes mellitus is a major risk factor for the development of vascular conditions.

Heart failure from left ventricular hypertrophy can lead to pulmonary edema. Peripheral edema is often present. Cardiac dysrhythmias may result from hyperkalemia, hypocalcemia, and decreased coronary artery perfusion.

Uremic pericarditis can develop and occasionally progresses to pericardial effusion and cardiac tamponade. Pericarditis is manifested by a friction rub, chest pain, and low-grade fever.

Respiratory System. Respiratory changes include dyspnea from fluid overload, pulmonary edema, uremic pleuritis (pleurisy), pleural effusion, and a predisposition to respiratory infections. In very advanced CKD, where the patient is in a metabolic acidosis, Kussmaul's respirations occur. "Uremic lung," or uremic pneumonitis, is typically found in CKD and shows up as interstitial edema on chest radiograph. This condition usually responds to vigorous fluid removal during dialysis treatments.

Gastrointestinal System. Every part of the GI system is affected in CKD, as a result of inflammation of the mucosa caused by excessive urea. Stomatitis with exudates and ulcerations, a metallic taste in the mouth, and *uremic fetor* (a urinous odour of the breath) are commonly found. As CKD progresses, anorexia, nausea, and vomiting caused by irritation of the GI tract by waste products may be present. Patients are also at risk for weight loss and malnutrition. Diabetic gastroparesis (delayed gastric emptying) can compound these health problems for patients with diabetes. GI bleeding is also a risk because of irritation of the mucosa by waste products, coupled with the platelet defect. Constipation may be caused by the ingestion of iron salts or calcium-containing phosphate binders, or both. Constipation can be made worse by the limited fluid intake and inactivity.

Neurological System. Neurological changes are expected as renal failure progresses. They are attributed to increased nitrogenous waste products, electrolyte imbalances, metabolic acidosis, and axonal atrophy and demyelination of nerve fibres (Renjen et al., 2018). High levels of uremic toxins have been implicated in axonal damage.

The central nervous system (CNS) becomes depressed, resulting in lethargy, apathy, decreased ability to concentrate, fatigue, irritability, and altered mental ability. Although uncommon, seizures and coma may result from a rapidly increasing BUN and hypertensive encephalopathy.

Peripheral neuropathy is initially manifested by a slowing of nerve conduction to the extremities. The patient experiences restless legs syndrome and may describe it as "bugs crawling inside the leg." Paresthesias occur most often in the feet and legs and may be described by the patient as a burning sensation. Eventually, motor involvement may lead to bilateral foot drop, muscular weakness and atrophy, and loss of deep tendon reflexes. Muscle twitching, jerking, asterixis (hand-flapping tremor), and nocturnal leg cramps also occur. In patients with diabetes, uremic neuropathy is compounded by the neuropathy associated with diabetes mellitus.

The treatment for associated neurological complications is dialysis or transplantation. Dialysis should improve the general CNS symptoms and may slow or halt the progression of neuropathies. However, motor neuropathy may not be reversible.

Musculoskeletal System. Chronic kidney disease–mineral and bone disorder (CKD–MBD) is a term used to describe the systemic components of this clinical syndrome that include characteristic bone abnormalities, changes in mineral balance (calcium, phosphorus, PTH, and vitamin D), and vascular and other soft tissue calcification (Jovanovich & Kendrick, 2018). These manifestations develop because of progressive deterioration in kidney function (Figure 49.4). As kidney function declines, phosphorus elimination decreases and less vitamin D is converted to its active form, resulting in decreased serum levels (Jovanovich & Kendrick, 2018). To absorb calcium from the GI tract, activated vitamin D is necessary. Thus, decreased active vitamin D levels result in less calcium absorption from the intestine and, therefore, decreased serum calcium levels (Kakani et al., 2019). When hypocalcemia occurs, the parathyroid gland secretes PTH, which stimulates bone demineralization with the release of calcium from the bones. Phosphate is released as well, leading to elevated serum phosphate levels. Hyperphosphatemia has been shown to directly decrease serum calcium levels and further reduce the ability of the kidneys to activate vitamin D (Jovanovich & Kendrick, 2018).

Hyperphosphatemia, decreased vitamin D level, and hypocalcemia lead to overstimulation of the parathyroid glands, resulting in excess secretion of PTH (Jovanovich & Kendrick, 2018). PTH that remains elevated for long periods of time leads to hypertrophy of the parathyroid gland and bone disease (Jovanovich & Kendrick, 2018).

CKD–MBD is a common complication of CKD and results in both skeletal (renal osteodystrophy) and extraskeletal complications (vascular and soft tissue complications). Renal osteodystrophy includes a number of skeletal disorders: (1) *osteitis fibrosa,* in which there is an increased number of osteoclasts and osteoblasts, high bone turnover, and fibrosis of the marrow; (2) *osteomalacia,* with low bone turnover and abnormal mineralized bone; (3) *adynamic bone disorder,* in which there is low bone turnover with normal mineralization; and (4) *mixed osteodystrophy,* with high bone turnover and abnormal mineralization (Kritmetapak & Pongchaiyakul, 2019).

Extraskeletal complications include vascular and soft tissue calcification (Jovanovich & Kendrick, 2018). The excess phosphate binds with calcium, leading to the formation of insoluble calcifications that are deposited in the vascular walls and soft tissue. Common sites are blood vessels, GI tract, lungs, muscles, skin, subcutaneous tissues, myocardium, and eyes (Chen et al., 2019). Cardiovascular calcification is an important contributor to cardiovascular disease in people with CKD and CKD–MBD (Chen et al., 2019), and vascular calcification is the likely cause of high cardiovascular morbidity and mortality in patients with CKD (Chen et al., 2019).

Integumentary System. Pruritus is highly prevalent in patients with CKD. It most commonly results from a combination of the

PATHOPHYSIOLOGY MAP

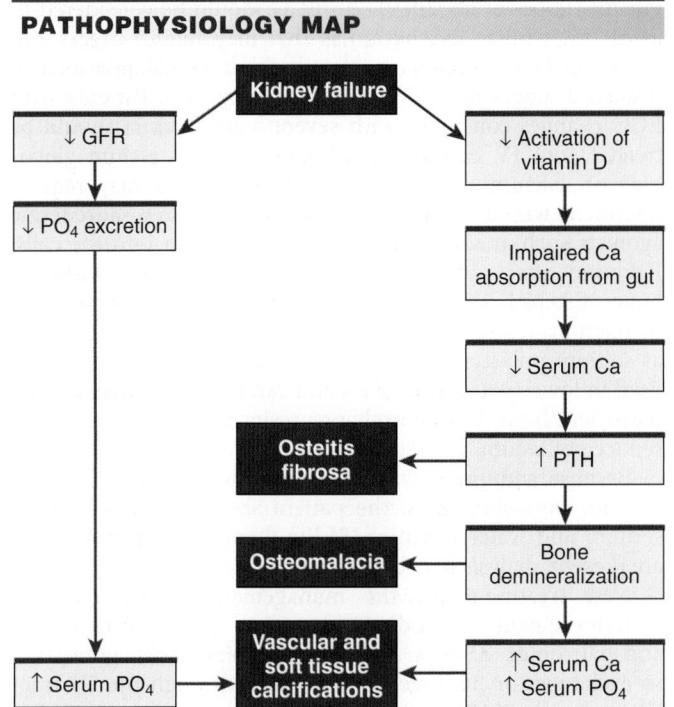

FIG. 49.4 Mechanisms of chronic kidney disease–mineral and bone disorder (CKD–MBD). *Ca*, calcium; *GFR*, glomerular filtration rate; *PO₄*, phosphate; *PTH*, parathyroid hormone.

TABLE 49.8 INTERPROFESSIONAL CARE
Management of Chronic Kidney Disease

Diagnostic
- BUN, serum creatinine, and eGFR
- CT scan
- History and physical examination
- Identification of reversible renal disease
- Protein-to-creatinine ratio in first, morning-voided specimen
- Renal biopsy
- Renal scan
- Renal ultrasound
- Serum calcium, phosphorous, albumin, and parathyroid hormone levels
- Serum electrolytes
- Serum hemoglobin level and iron indices
- Urinalysis and urine culture

Interprofessional Therapy
- Adjustment of medication dosages according to degree of renal function
- Antihypertensive therapy
- Calcium supplementation, phosphate binders, or both
- Correction of extracellular fluid volume overload or deficit
- Erythropoietin therapy
- Measures to lower potassium*
- Nutritional therapy†
- Renal replacement therapy (dialysis, kidney transplantation)

*See Table 49.5.
†See Tables 49.10 and 49.11.

dry skin, calcium–phosphate deposition in the skin, and sensory neuropathy. The itching may be so intense that it can lead to bleeding or infection secondary to scratching. Uremic frost is a rare condition in which urea crystallizes on the skin and is usually seen only when BUN levels are extremely high.

Reproductive System. Both men and women can experience infertility and a decreased libido in CKD. Women usually have decreased levels of estrogen, progesterone, and luteinizing hormone, causing anovulation and menstrual changes (usually amenorrhea). Menses and ovulation may return after dialysis is started. Men experience loss of testicular consistency, decreased testosterone levels, and low sperm counts. Sexual dysfunction in both sexes may also be caused by anemia, which leads to fatigue and decreased libido. In addition, peripheral neuropathy can cause impotence in men and anorgasmy in women. Additional factors that may result in changes in sexual function are psychological conditions (e.g., anxiety, depression), physical stress, and adverse effects of medications.

Sexual function may improve with maintenance dialysis and may become normal with successful transplantation. Pregnant patients undergoing dialysis have been able to carry a fetus to term, but there is significant risk to the mother and newborn. Pregnancy in patients undergoing transplantation is more common, but here, too, there is a risk to both mother and fetus.

Psychological Changes. Personality and behavioural changes, emotional lability, withdrawal, and depression are commonly observed. Fatigue and lethargy contribute to the feeling of illness. The changes in body image caused by edema, integumentary disturbances, and access devices (e.g., fistulas, catheters) can lead to further anxiety and depression. Decreased ability to concentrate and slowed mental activity can give the appearance of dullness and disinterest in the environment. There are

also significant changes in lifestyle, occupation, family responsibilities, and financial status that the patient must cope with. Long-term survival depends on medication therapy, dietary restrictions, dialysis, and possibly transplantation. The patient will also grieve the loss of renal function. Living with CKD can be a prolonged process for some individuals.

Diagnostic Studies

Adverse outcomes of CKD can often be prevented or delayed through early detection and treatment. Early stages of CKD can be detected through routine laboratory measurements (Table 49.8). Proteinuria is one of the most important risk factors for the progression of CKD leading to dialysis and is the earliest marker of kidney damage. Patients at high risk for kidney disease, such as those with diabetes, hypertension, vascular disease, autoimmune disease, GFR less than 60 mL/min/1.73 m², and edema, should be screened for proteinuria (Rainey, 2019). The preferred method for screening for proteinuria is measurement of the urine protein-to-creatinine ratio or the albumin-to-creatinine ratio. A dipstick evaluation for protein in the urine may be done but is not as accurate. Patients with diabetes need to have examination of their urine for microalbuminuria if none is detected on routine urinalysis. The presence of proteinuria in two or three consecutive urine samples is needed to determine persistent proteinuria. A person with persistent proteinuria (1+ protein on standard dipstick testing, two or more times, over a 3-month period) should have further assessment of risk factors and a diagnostic workup with blood and urine tests. A urine test for albumin-to-creatinine ratio provides an accurate estimate of the protein and albumin excretion rate. A ratio greater than 300 mg albumin/1 g creatinine signals CKD.

A urinalysis can detect RBCs, WBCs, protein, casts, and glucose. Imaging of the kidneys to exclude obstruction and note

TABLE 49.9	SERUM CREATININE IS A POOR INDICATOR OF KIDNEY FUNCTION	

Calculation of GFR is considered the best index to estimate kidney function, as indicated by the following example.

	Type of Patient	
Estimation of GFR	**76-Year-Old White Woman (Weight 56 kg)**	**28-Year-Old White Man (Weight 74 kg)**
SCr	155 mmol/L	155 mmol/L
GFR—estimated by the Cockcroft-Gault formula*	28.4 mL/min	65.7 mL/min
GFR—estimated by MDRD equation†	30 mL/min/1.73 m²	49 mL/min/1.73 m²

GFR, glomerular filtration rate; *MDRD*, modification of diet in renal disease; *SCr*, serum creatinine.

*Cockcroft-Gault GFR = [(140 − age) × (weight in kg) × 1.2]/SCr (mmol/L). For women, multiply the result by 0.85 (Flamant et al., 2012).

†GFR as estimated by MDRD and Cockcroft-Gault equation calculator can be accessed at http://www.mdcalc.com/mdrd-gfr-equation/.

the size of the kidneys is usually done by ultrasound. Other diagnostic studies (Table 49.8) help establish the diagnosis and cause of CKD.

Serum creatinine alone poorly reflects kidney function, and a rise in blood creatinine is observed only after significant loss of functioning nephrons (National Institute of Diabetes and Digestive and Kidney Diseases [NIDDKD], 2021). GFR is the preferred measure used to determine kidney function. Several GFR calculators are available. The two equations used most frequently to estimate GFR are the Cockcroft–Gault formula and the Modification of Diet in Renal Disease (MDRD) Study equation (Table 49.9). The National Kidney Foundation KDOQI guidelines recommend the MDRD Study equation to estimate GFR (Norton et al., 2017).

Interprofessional Management: Chronic Kidney Disease

The focus in CKD is on prevention and early identification to deter the progression of kidney disease. When a patient is diagnosed as having CKD, every effort is made to detect and treat potentially reversible causes (e.g., cardiac failure, dehydration, infections, nephrotoxins, urinary tract obstruction, renal artery stenosis). A renal biopsy may be necessary to provide a definitive diagnosis. The goals of CKD care are to preserve existing renal function, delay progression of renal disease, treat clinical manifestations, prevent complications, educate patients and families in kidney disease and options for care, and prepare patients for RRT. The care of the patient with CKD must be tailored to the stage of CKD. Early CKD care can lead to effective planning and appropriate timing of dialysis start and creation of the dialysis access. In the early stages of CKD, pharmacological and nutritional therapy and supportive care are essential components of the CKD care plan.

Medication Therapy

Hyperkalemia. There are multiple strategies for managing hyperkalemia (see Table 49.5). Every effort is made to control it with the restriction of high-potassium foods and medications. Acute hyperkalemia may require urgent intervention. The level of potassium that should be treated has not been firmly established; nonpharmacological steps be instituted for management of potassium levels above 5.5 mmol/L and pharmacological intervention at potassium levels of 6.0 mmol/L or

greater (Lopes et al., 2019). An ECG should be considered to assess for cardiac dysrhythmias that may require treatment. Common ECG changes associated with hyperkalemia include peaked T waves and widened QRS complexes. Patients with ECG changes consistent with severe hyperkalemia should be treated with IV calcium-based salts such as calcium gluconate or calcium chloride. Acute hyperkalemia may require treatment with IV glucose and insulin and/or β_2-adrenergic agonists such as salbutamol to shift potassium into the cells. Rebound after potassium-shifting therapy occurs within 2 hours if steps have not been taken to reduce potassium either through urine excretion or HD. A cation exchange resin, such as sodium polystyrene sulphonate (Kayexalate), is commonly used to lower potassium levels and can be administered on an outpatient basis. Cation exchange resins take hours to days to reduce potassium.

Because sodium polystyrene sulfonate exchanges sodium ions for potassium ions, the patient should be observed for sodium and water retention. If life-threatening dysrhythmias are present, dialysis may be required.

New treatment for the management of hyperkalemia includes the use of sodium zirconium cyclosilicate (ZS-9) and patiromer. ZS-9 is an agent that binds with potassium in exchange for hydrogen and sodium through the GI tract (Palaka et al., 2018). Patiromer binds and removes potassium, primarily through the colon. As hyperkalemia is common in ESRD and can be life-threatening, acute management is required.

Hypertension. The progression of CKD can be delayed by controlling hypertension. Treatment of hypertension consists of lifestyle modifications (e.g., exercise, weight reduction, avoidance of alcohol intake, stress management), dietary sodium and fluid restriction, and the administration of antihypertensive medications. The Canadian Hypertension Education Program (CHEP) recommends a target blood pressure (BP) for patients with nondiabetic CKD of less than 140/90 mm Hg; for those with diabetes mellitus, it should be less than 130/80 mm Hg (Nerenberg et al., 2018).

For patients with nondiabetic CKD and proteinuria, ACE inhibitors (e.g., ramipril [Altace], enalapril [Vasotec]) or ARBs (e.g., irbesartan [Avapro], losartan [Cozaar]) are recommended as initial therapy. ACE inhibitors and ARBs decrease proteinuria and delay the progression of renal failure. For additional therapy, the use of thiazide diuretics (e.g., hydrochlorothiazide) or loop diuretics (e.g., furosemide [Lasix]) for volume overload is suggested.

For patients with renovascular disease, CHEP suggests cautious use of ACE inhibitors and ARBs, as patients with bilateral disease or a solitary kidney are at increased risk for AKI (Nerenberg et al., 2018).

For patients with diabetes, CHEP suggests use of ACE inhibitors or ARBs as initial therapy (Nerenberg et al., 2018). Other antihypertensive medications commonly used include dihydropyridine calcium channel blockers (nifedipine [Adalat], amlodipine [Norvasc] and thiazide or thiazide-like diuretics).

ACE inhibitors and ARBs must be used with caution in CKD because they can further decrease the GFR and increase serum potassium levels. Most people require a number of antihypertensives to achieve target BP, and regimens must be individualized on the basis of other existing comorbidities.

BP should periodically be measured in supine, sitting, and standing positions to effectively monitor the effect of antihypertensive medications. The patient should be taught how to monitor their BP at home and taught what BP readings require immediate intervention. BP control is essential to slow atherosclerotic changes that could further impair renal function.

Chronic Kidney Disease–Mineral and Bone Disorder. Interventions for CKD–MBD include limiting dietary phosphorus, administering phosphate binders, and supplementing vitamin D. Phosphate intake is generally restricted to less than 1 000 mg/day, but usually dietary control is not adequate. Calcium-based phosphate binders such as calcium carbonate and calcium acetate are used to bind the phosphate, which is then excreted in the stool. Giving a calcium-based binder when the phosphate levels are still high (1.98 mmol/L) may cause the formation of calcium–phosphate deposits. Sevelamer (Renagel) is a phosphate binder that contains neither calcium nor aluminum.

Because dementia (aluminum toxicity) and bone disease (osteomalacia) are associated with excessive absorption of aluminum, aluminum preparations should be avoided if possible and used with caution in patients with renal failure. Magnesium-containing antacids (Maalox, Mylanta) are used in moderation because magnesium is dependent on the kidneys for excretion. Phosphate binders should be administered with each meal to be effective because most phosphate is absorbed within 1 hour after eating. Hypercalcemia may occur with calcium supplementation and is associated with increased cardiac calcifications and mortality in patients with ESRD. Calcium binders are generally limited to a maximum of 1 500 mg/day with the total daily calcium intake including diet not exceeding 2 g. Constipation is a frequent adverse effect of phosphate binders and may necessitate the use of stool softeners.

Hypocalcemia is often a concern because of the inability of the GI tract to absorb calcium in the absence of vitamin D. If hypocalcemia persists even when serum phosphate levels are controlled and supplemental calcium is given, the active form of vitamin D should be given. It is commercially available in oral preparations such as calcitriol (Rocaltrol). It is important to lower the phosphate level before administering calcium or vitamin D because these medications may contribute to soft tissue calcification if both calcium and phosphate levels are elevated. Calcimimetics such as cinacalcet (Sensipar) may be prescribed to lower PTH and may also cause hypocalcemia (Jovanovich & Kendrick, 2018).

If renal osteodystrophy remains severe despite medical management, a subtotal parathyroidectomy may be performed to decrease the synthesis and secretion of PTH. In some situations, a total parathyroidectomy is performed, and some parathyroid tissue is transplanted into the forearm. The transplanted cells produce PTH as needed. If production of PTH becomes excessive, some of the cells can be removed from the forearm under local anaesthesia.

The most common methods for evaluating the status of the bone disease are skeletal radiographs, bone scans, bone biopsy, and bone densitometry. PTH and alkaline phosphatase levels should also be measured. Alkaline phosphatase is elevated when there is demineralization of the bone but can also be increased by liver disease.

Anemia. The most important cause of anemia in CKD is a decreased production of erythropoietin. With the use of recombinant DNA technology, erythropoiesis-stimulating agents (ESAs) are available for the treatment of anemia. ESAs can be administered intravenously or subcutaneously. They have been very effective in treating anemia. A significant increase in hemoglobin is usually not seen for 2 to 3 weeks. The patient who is receiving erythropoietin has improved exercise tolerance and an enhanced quality of life.

Significant morbidity and mortality have been associated with trying to normalize hemoglobin levels. The Canadian Society of Nephrology (CSN) *Guidelines for the Management of Chronic Kidney Disease* recommend a target hemoglobin of 110 g/L, with an acceptable range between 100 and 120 g/L (Rainey, 2019). A common adverse effect of ESAs is the development or acceleration of hypertension. The underlying mechanism is related to the hemodynamic changes (e.g., increased whole blood viscosity) that occur as the anemia is corrected. Patients with significantly elevated BP should not receive ESAs.

Another adverse effect of ESA therapy is the development of functional iron deficiency resulting from the increased demand for iron to support erythropoiesis. The CSN *Guidelines for the Management of Chronic Kidney Disease* recommend a target ferritin level greater than 100 ng/mL and a transferring saturation level greater than 20%. Most patients receive iron supplements. The GI adverse effects of oral iron, including gastric irritation and constipation, may lead to nonadherence to therapy. Orally administered iron should not be taken at the same time as phosphate binders because calcium binds the iron, preventing absorption. The patient should be advised that iron may make the stool a dark colour.

Most patients on HD receive IV iron. Supplemental folic acid is usually given because it is needed for RBC formation and is removed by dialysis.

Blood transfusions should be avoided in treating anemia unless the patient experiences an acute blood loss or has symptomatic anemia (e.g., dyspnea, excess fatigue, tachycardia, palpitations, chest pain). Undesirable effects of transfusions are the suppression of erythropoiesis as a result of a decrease in the hypoxic stimulus. Although rare, the possible transmission of hepatitis B or C or human immunodeficiency virus (HIV) may occur. There is the possibility of developing antibodies that may affect transplantation, and the possibility of iron overload because each unit of blood contains about 250 mg of iron.

Dyslipidemia. There is a high prevalence of dyslipidemia among patients with CKD. Currently, good evidence-informed research is lacking to guide the management of dyslipidemia in CKD. The National Kidney Foundation KDOQI recommends the use of statins in patients with stages 1 to 3 CKD, per guidelines for the general population (Gluba-Brzozka et al., 2019).

Complications of Medication Therapy. Because the kidneys play a large role in the absorption, distribution, metabolism, and elimination of medications, people with CKD are at risk for medication-related complications that can lead to increased morbidity and mortality. Many medications are partially or totally excreted by the kidneys. Delayed and decreased elimination lead to an accumulation of medications in the body and potential for medication toxicity. Dialysis may remove or lower medication levels. Medication doses and frequency of administration must be adjusted on the basis of level of kidney function and whether or not the patient is receiving dialysis. Medications of particular concern include digoxin, oral glycemic agents (e.g., metformin, glyburide), antibiotics, and opioid medication (e.g., hydromorphone [Dilaudid], morphine).

Patients should be advised to avoid using NSAIDs. These medications block the synthesis of the renal prostaglandins that promote vasodilation. This can worsen renal hypoperfusion and cause interstitial nephritis. Many NSAIDs are available over the counter, so it is essential that the patient be cautioned. Acetaminophen can be substituted for an NSAID.

TABLE 49.10 NUTRITIONAL THERAPY

Daily Requirements for the Patient With Chronic Kidney Disease

	CKD Stages 3–4 Management	Hemodialysis	Peritoneal Dialysis
Fluid allowance	Urine output + 600 mL	Urine output + 600 mL	Often no restriction
Protein*	0.6–0.75 g/kg body weight	1.2–1.3 g/kg IBW	≥1.2–1.3 g/kg IBW
Calories	30–35 kcal/kg EDW	30–35 kcal/kg EDW†	30–35 kcal/kg IBW†
Fat	Determined by caloric requirement	Determined by caloric requirement	Determined by caloric requirement
Carbohydrate	Unlimited intake of sugars, starches; bread and cereal products limited because of protein restriction	Same as for conservative management	Dependent on individual patient needs
Iron	Variable	Variable	Variable
Potassium	2–3 g	2–3 g	3–4 g, no restrictions
Sodium	2–3 g	2–3 g	2–4 g
Phosphorus	800–1000 mg	1000 mg	1000 mg
Calcium	Variable	1000–1500 mg	1000–1500 mg
Folic acid	1-mg supplement	1-mg supplement	1-mg supplement

CKD, chronic kidney disease; *EDW*, estimated dry weight; *IBW*, ideal body weight.
*At least 50% of protein intake should be of high biological value (e.g., coming from eggs, milk, meat).
†Includes dialysate calories.

Nutritional Therapy

Protein Restriction. The diet is designed to be as normal as possible to maintain good nutrition (Table 49.10). All patients with CKD should be seen by a renal dietitian. Protein energy wasting in CKD is a strong predictor of mortality. Protein is moderately restricted because BUN is an end product of protein metabolism. For the patient who is not undergoing dialysis, one guide is to restrict protein intake to 0.6 to 0.75 g/kg of ideal body weight (IBW)/day when the creatinine clearance is less than 25 mL/min (Lee et al., 2019). This moderate restriction may slow progression of CKD for these patients. For patients with more severe renal insufficiency, low-protein diets should be used with caution because these patients are at risk of developing malnutrition.

Once the patient starts dialysis, protein intake can be increased to 1.2 to 1.3 g/kg of IBW/day. Dietary protein guidelines for PD differ from those for HD because excessive amounts of protein are lost in the dialysate. The protein intake must be high enough to compensate for the losses so that the nitrogen balance is maintained. The recommended protein intake is at least 1.2 g/kg of IBW/day and can be increased depending on the individual needs of the patient. At least 50% of protein intake should have high biological value, containing all of the essential amino acids (e.g., eggs, milk, meat, poultry).

Sufficient calories from carbohydrates and fat are needed to minimize catabolism of body protein and to maintain body weight. Therefore, 100 g of carbohydrates and an appropriate amount of fat are prescribed to maintain an intake of 30 to 35 kcal/kg body weight/day. See Table 49.10 for specific guidelines.

For patients with malnutrition or inadequate caloric intake, commercially prepared products that are high in calories and low in protein, sodium, and potassium are available.

Because the diet for CKD is deficient in vitamins, and water-soluble vitamins are lost through dialysis, multivitamins are prescribed.

Sodium and Fluid Restriction. Fluid intake for patients with CKD depends on the daily urine output and overall fluid balance. For patients not yet on dialysis, fluids are generally not restricted and diuretics and a low-sodium diet help to manage fluid retention. For patients receiving HD, fluids are generally restricted as urine output begins to decline. Generally, 600 mL (from insensible loss) plus an amount equal to the previous day's urine output is allowed for a patient receiving dialysis. Foods that are liquid at room temperature (e.g., gelatin, ice cream) should be counted as fluid intake. The fluid allotment should be spaced throughout the day so that the patient does not become thirsty. For the patient receiving long-term HD, fluid intake is adjusted so that weight gains are no more than 1 to 3 kg between dialyses.

To achieve the optimal fluid balance, sodium must also be restricted. Sodium-restricted diet allowances may vary from 2 to 4 g, depending on the degree of edema and hypertension. Sodium and salt should not be equated because the sodium content in 1 g of sodium chloride is equivalent to 400 mg of sodium. The patient should be instructed to avoid eating high-sodium foods such as cured meats, pickled foods, canned soups and stews, frankfurters, cold cuts, soy sauce, and salad dressings. Most salt substitutes should not be used because they contain potassium chloride.

Potassium Restriction. The potassium restriction depends on the ability of the kidneys to excrete this electrolyte. Dietary allowances for potassium range from about 2 to 4 g. Some patients on PD do not need potassium restrictions. Some foods with high potassium content that should be avoided are oranges, bananas, melons, tomatoes, prunes, raisins, deep green and yellow vegetables, beans, and legumes (Table 49.11).

Phosphate Restriction. CKD alters the homeostasis of calcium, phosphorus, and vitamin D (Jovanovich & Kendrick, 2018). As CKD progresses, phosphorus excretion diminishes, resulting in hyperphosphatemia. Phosphate should be limited to approximately 1000 mg/day. Foods that are high in phosphate include dairy products (e.g., milk, ice cream, cheese, yogourt) and foods containing dairy products (e.g., pudding). Most foods that are high in phosphate are also high in calcium. Restricting phosphate will restrict calcium intake.

NURSING MANAGEMENT CHRONIC KIDNEY DISEASE

NURSING ASSESSMENT

The nurse should obtain a complete history of any existing renal disease or family history of renal disease, because some renal disorders have a hereditary basis (e.g., polycystic kidney disease, Alport's syndrome). Information on long-term health conditions such as hypertension, diabetes, recurrent urinary tract infections, and systemic lupus erythematosus should be

TABLE 49.11   NUTRITIONAL THERAPY

High-Potassium Foods

Fruits and Fruit Juices	Vegetables	Cereal
• Apple juice	• Beans, white and pinto*	• All-Bran*
• Avocados*	• Broccoli	• Raisin Bran*
• Bananas*	• Carrots	**Meat and Poultry**
• Grapefruit juice	• Lima beans, cooked*	• Beef,* pork, cooked
• Honeydew melons*	• Mushrooms, fresh*	• Chicken
• Orange juice*	• Potato, baked*	• Turkey
• Oranges	• Squash, baked*	
• Prune juice*	• Spinach, cooked*	**Miscellaneous**
• Prunes*		• Chocolate
• Raisins*	**Dairy**	• Molasses
• Tomato juice*	• Milk*	• Sunflower seeds*
• Tomatoes	• Yogourt*	

*>10 mmol of potassium per serving.

obtained because these conditions can lead to CKD. Because the kidneys play a large role in the absorption, distribution, metabolism, and elimination of medications and because many medications are potentially nephrotoxic, both current and past use of prescription and over-the-counter medications must be reviewed.

The nurse should assess the patient's dietary habits and discuss any concerns. The height and weight should be measured, and any recent weight changes must be evaluated.

Clinical manifestations of CKD are apparent in multiple body systems (see Figure 49.3). Fatigue, lethargy, and pruritus are often the early symptoms of CKD. Hypertension and changes in urine characteristics are often the first signs.

CKD is a lifelong and life-limiting illness. The chronicity of renal disease and the long-term nature of treatment modalities can affect every area of a person's life, including family relationships, social and work activities, and self-image and emotional state. Support systems should be assessed. The choice of treatment modality may be related to support systems available to the patient.

It is important to respect a patient's choice not to receive treatment. Many times, patients will initiate the conversation about palliative care themselves. The discussion needs to focus on moving from the curative approach to promotion of comfort care and consideration for end-of-life care. The nurse needs to listen to the patient and caregiver, allowing them to do most of the talking, and pay special attention to their hopes and fears (Montoya, 2017). (Palliative and end of-life care is discussed in Chapter 13.)

NURSING DIAGNOSES

Nursing diagnoses for the patient with CKD in stage 4 may include but are not limited to the following:

• *Excess fluid volume* resulting from *excessive fluid intake* (impaired kidney function)
• *Potential for electrolyte imbalance* as evidenced by *excessive fluid volume* (impaired kidney function)
• *Inadequate nutrition: less than body requirements* resulting from *insufficient dietary intake* (restricted intake of nutrients, nausea, vomiting, anorexia, stomatitis)

Additional information on nursing diagnoses for the patient with CKD is presented in Nursing Care Plan (NCP) 49.1, available on the Evolve website.

PLANNING

The majority of CKD care occurs in the ambulatory care setting. The overall goals are that a patient with CKD will (1) demonstrate knowledge and ability to adhere to the therapeutic regimen, (2) participate in decision making for the plan of care and future treatment modality, (3) demonstrate effective coping strategies, and (4) continue with activities of daily living within physiological limitations.

NURSING IMPLEMENTATION

HEALTH PROMOTION. The nurse needs to identify individuals at risk for CKD, including people with a history (or a family history) of renal disease, hypertension, diabetes mellitus, and repeated urinary tract infection. These individuals should have regular checkups, including assessments of serum creatinine and BUN and urinalysis. People with diabetes should have their urine checked for microalbuminuria if routine urinalysis is negative for protein. They should be advised that any changes in urine appearance (colour, odour), frequency, or volume must be reported to the health care provider. If a patient must be prescribed a potentially nephrotoxic medication, it is important to monitor renal function with serum creatinine and BUN.

Individuals who have been identified as being at risk need to take measures to prevent or delay the progression of CKD and reduce the risk for cardiovascular disease. These measures include glycemic control for patients with diabetes (see Chapter 52), optimizing BP control, and lifestyle modifications, including smoking cessation. The nurse needs to consider that Indigenous populations may lack the support that is required for this screening and follow-up (Thomas et al., 2017).

CARE CONSIDERATIONS FOR CHRONIC KIDNEY DISEASE IN STAGES 4 TO 5. The specific nursing management of the patient with CKD in stages 4 to 5 is detailed in NCP 49.1, available on the Evolve website. It is important to teach the patient and the family because diet, medications, and follow-up medical care are the responsibilities of the patient (Table 49.12). The patient should check their weight daily, learn to take daily BPs, and be able to identify signs and symptoms of fluid overload, hyperkalemia, and other electrolyte imbalances. The patient and the family must understand the importance of strict dietary adherence. A registered dietitian should meet with the patient and the family on a regular basis for diet planning. A diet history and consideration of cultural variations will facilitate diet planning and adherence.

The patient needs a complete understanding of prescribed medications, the dosages, and the common adverse effects. It may be helpful to make a list of the medications and the times of administration that can be posted in the home. The patient must be instructed to avoid certain over-the-counter medications such as NSAIDs and natural and herbal preparations. ACE inhibitors may have to be discontinued if they are contributing to hyperkalemia or decreased GFR.

Motivation on the part of the patient to assume the primary role in the management of the disease is essential. The period of predialysis care provides an opportunity to evaluate each patient's ability to manage the disease. This knowledge will be helpful when determining the treatment modality.

AMBULATORY AND HOME CARE. The length of time that a patient with CKD can be managed without RRT is highly variable and depends on the progression of renal failure and the presence of other comorbid conditions. When RRT is required, HD, PD, and transplantation are the available treatment options.

TABLE 49.12	PATIENT & CAREGIVER TEACHING GUIDE

Chronic Kidney Disease in Stages 4 and 5

When teaching the patient and caregiver about management of chronic kidney disease, the nurse should:

1. Explain dietary (protein, sodium, potassium, phosphate) and fluid restrictions, incorporating the patient's own cultural dietary patterns.
2. Encourage discussion of difficulties in modifying diet and fluid intake.
3. Explain signs and symptoms of electrolyte imbalance, especially high potassium.
4. Teach alternative ways of reducing thirst, such as sucking on ice cubes, lemon, or hard candy.
5. Explain the rationale for prescribed medications and common adverse effects. *Examples:*
   - Phosphate binders should be taken with meals.
   - Iron supplements should be taken between meals.
6. Explain the importance of reporting any of the following:
   - Weight gain >2 kg
   - Increasing blood pressure
   - Shortness of breath
   - Edema
   - Increasing fatigue or weakness
   - Confusion or lethargy
7. Encourage the patient and caregiver(s) to share concerns about lifestyle changes, living with a chronic illness, and decisions about type of dialysis or transplantation.

Extensive and ongoing teaching and discussion about RRTs should occur early (CKD in stage 3) in order for the patient to make an informed decision about future therapies, including RRT and advanced directives.

The patient and the family need a clear explanation of what is involved in dialysis and transplantation. The patient should be informed that, if dialysis is chosen, the option of transplantation still remains, if the patient is medically suitable. It should be emphasized that, if a transplanted organ fails, the patient can return to dialysis. The patient should also be counselled that retransplantation may also be an option.

EVALUATION

The expected outcomes for the patient with CKD are presented in NCP 49.1, available on the Evolve website.

DIALYSIS

Dialysis is the movement of fluid and molecules across a semipermeable membrane from one compartment to another. Clinically, dialysis is a technique in which substances move from the blood through a semipermeable membrane (*dialyzer*) and into a dialysis solution (*dialysate*). It is used to correct fluid and electrolyte imbalances and to remove waste products in renal failure. It can also be used to treat drug overdoses. The two methods of dialysis available are PD and HD (Table 49.13). Peritoneal dialysis (PD) is a method of removing waste products and excess fluid from the blood using a natural semipermeable membrane, the peritoneum. Dialysis fluid is infused into the peritoneal cavity, and excess fluid and waste products pass across the membrane into the fluid, which is then drained and discarded. In hemodialysis (HD), waste products and excess fluid are removed from the blood using a machine to pump the blood through an artificial semipermeable membrane (usually made of cellulose-based or synthetic materials).

TABLE 49.13	COMPARISON OF PERITONEAL DIALYSIS AND HEMODIALYSIS

Peritoneal Dialysis	Hemodialysis
Advantages	**Advantages**
• Fewer dietary restrictions	• Effective potassium removal
• Home dialysis possible	• Home dialysis possible
• Less cardiovascular stress	• Less protein loss than with peritoneal dialysis
• Less complicated than hemodialysis	• Lowering of serum triglycerides
• Portable system with CAPD	• Rapid fluid removal
• Preferable for the diabetic patient	• Rapid removal of urea and creatinine
• Relatively short training time	• Temporary access can be placed at bedside
• Usable in the patient with vascular access difficulties	
Disadvantages	**Disadvantages**
• Catheter can migrate	• Added blood loss that contributes to anemia
• Contraindication in the patient with multiple abdominal surgeries, trauma, unrepaired hernia	• Dietary and fluid restrictions
	• Extensive equipment necessary
• Protein loss into dialysate	• Heparinization may be necessary
• Risk for aggravated dyslipidemia	• Hypotension during dialysis
• Risk for bacterial or chemical peritonitis	• Longer training time for home hemodialysis vs. peritoneal
• Risk for exit-site and tunnel infections	• Self-image challenges with permanent access
• Risk for hyperglycemia	• Specially trained personnel necessary (if in-centre option chosen)
• Risk for self-image challenges with catheter placement	• Surgery for permanent access placement
• Surgery for catheter placement	• Vascular access difficulties

CAPD, continuous ambulatory peritoneal dialysis.

When CKD progresses to the point that the patient's symptoms, fluid volume status, or both can no longer be managed without dialysis, dialysis therapy is initiated. Generally, dialysis is initiated when the GFR (or creatinine clearance) is less than $15 \text{ mL/min/}1.73 \text{ m}^2$. This criterion can vary widely in different clinical situations. Certain uremic complications, including encephalopathy, neuropathies, uncontrolled hyperkalemia, pericarditis, and accelerated hypertension, indicate a need for immediate dialysis.

GENERAL PRINCIPLES OF DIALYSIS

Solutes and water move across the semipermeable membrane from the blood to the dialysate or from the dialysate to the blood, in accordance with concentration gradients. The principles of diffusion, osmosis, and ultrafiltration are involved in dialysis (Figure 49.5). *Diffusion* is the movement of solutes from an area of greater concentration to an area of lesser concentration. In renal failure, urea, creatinine, uric acid, and electrolytes (potassium, phosphate) move from the blood to the dialysate with the net effect of lowering their concentration in the blood. RBCs, WBCs, and plasma proteins are too large to diffuse through the pores of the membrane. Bacteria and viruses that may be present in the dialysate are too large to migrate through the pores into the blood.

Osmosis is the movement of fluid from an area of lesser to an area of greater concentration of solutes. Glucose is added to the dialysate and creates an osmotic gradient across the membrane, pulling excess fluid from the blood.

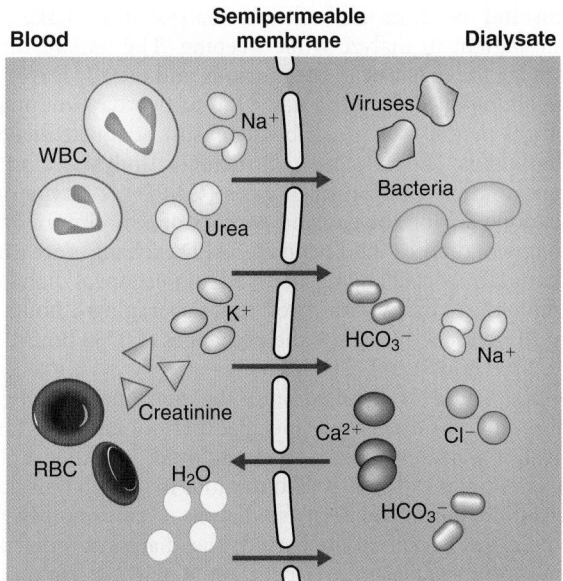

FIG. 49.5 Osmosis and diffusion across a semipermeable membrane. *Ca,* calcium; *Cl,* chlorine; *HCO₃,* bicarbonate; *H₂O,* water; *K,* potassium; *Na,* sodium; *RBC,* red blood cell; *WBC,* white blood cell.

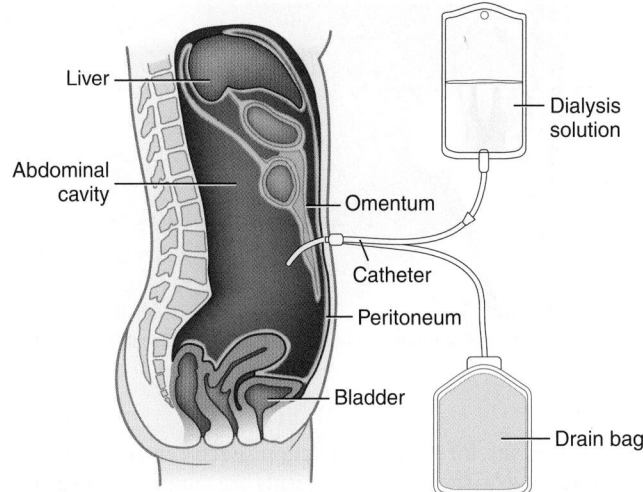

FIG. 49.6 Peritoneal dialysis showing a peritoneal catheter inserted into the peritoneal cavity.

Ultrafiltration (water and fluid removal) results when there is an osmotic gradient or pressure gradient across the membrane. In PD, excess fluid is removed by increasing the osmolality of the dialysate (osmotic gradient) with the addition of glucose. In HD, the gradient is created by increasing pressure in the blood compartment (positive pressure) or decreasing pressure in the dialysate compartment (negative pressure). Extracellular fluid moves into the dialysate because of the pressure gradient. The excess fluid is removed by creating a pressure differential between the blood and the dialysate solution, with a combination of positive pressure in the blood compartment and negative pressure in the dialysate compartment.

PERITONEAL DIALYSIS

Although PD was first used in 1923, it did not come into widespread use for chronic treatment until the 1970s with the development of soft, pliable peritoneal solution bags and the introduction of the concept of continuous PD. In Canada, in 2018, 18% of patients were receiving PD, compared with 82% who were receiving HD (CIHI, 2019).

Catheter Placement

Peritoneal access is obtained by inserting a catheter through the anterior abdominal wall (Figure 49.6). Most catheter exit sites are in the abdomen; however, some catheters are inserted using a presternal technique, where the catheter exits on the chest. The catheters vary in length and have one or two Dacron cuffs on the subcutaneous and peritoneal portions of the catheter that act as anchors and prevent the migration of microorganisms down the shaft from the skin. Within a few weeks of insertion, fibrous tissue grows into the Dacron cuff, holding the catheter in place and preventing bacterial penetration into the peritoneal cavity. The tip of the catheter rests in the peritoneal cavity and has many perforations spaced along the distal end of the tubing to allow fluid to flow in and out of the catheter. There are numerous types of PD catheters.

The technique for catheter placement varies. Although it is possible to place a permanent catheter in the peritoneal cavity at the bedside with a trocar, it is usually done via surgery so that its placement can be directly visualized, minimizing potential complications. Preparation of the patient for catheter insertion includes emptying the bladder and the bowel, weighing the patient, and obtaining a signed consent form.

In the nonsurgical (bedside) approach, an area approximately 2 cm below the umbilicus is numbed with a local anaesthetic, and a small stab wound is made. A stylet is inserted, and the abdomen is distended with dialysis solution. The catheter is then placed into the peritoneal cavity. When the patient feels pressure in the rectal area and has the urge to defecate, the catheter is in place.

In the surgical approach, a midline umbilical incision is made, and a small puncture is made to one side and below this incision. The distal end of the catheter is placed in the peritoneum, and it is tunnelled under the skin to the puncture site. The tunnel helps prevent peritonitis. After the catheter is inserted, the skin is cleaned with an antiseptic solution, and a sterile dressing is applied. Complications of catheter insertion include perforation of the bladder, the bowel, or a blood vessel and the introduction of bacteria.

The catheter is connected to a sterile tubing system and secured to the abdomen with tape. The catheter is irrigated immediately with heparinized dialysate (usually 500 mL) to clear blood and fibrin from it. Prophylactic antibiotics may also be given. Catheter placement is usually done with same-day surgery, and the patient is discharged home with a sterile dressing covering the PD catheter. The patient needs instructions on keeping the dressing dry, avoiding accidentally pulling the catheter, and receiving follow-up care.

Before starting PD, it is preferable to allow a waiting period of 7 to 14 days for proper sealing of the catheter and for tissue to grow into the cuffs. Postoperative exit-site care should be restricted to trained staff (George, 2019). About 2 to 4 weeks after catheter implantation, the exit site should be clean, dry, and free of redness and tenderness (Figure 49.7). Once the catheter incision site is healed, routine care should be performed daily or every other day. This care includes the use of antibacterial soap or mild, medical-grade disinfectants as well as examination of

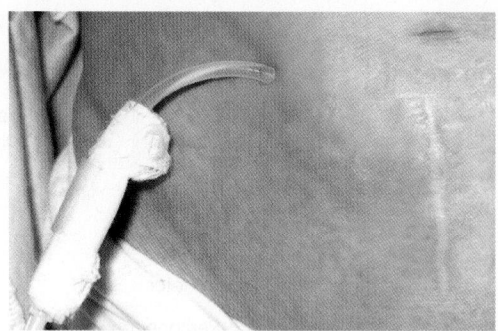

FIG. 49.7 Peritoneal catheter exit site. Source: Mediscan/Alamy Stock Photo.

the catheter site for signs of infection. Each centre will have a policy about exit-site care, and patients are taught how to examine and care for their PD catheter and exit site by the PD nursing staff.

Dialysis Solutions and Cycles

PD is accomplished by putting dialysis solution into the peritoneal space. The three phases of the PD cycle are *inflow* (fill), *dwell* (equilibration), and *drain*. The three phases are called an *exchange*. The dialysis prescription is tailored to the patient's needs. During inflow, a prescribed amount of solution, usually 2 L, is infused through an established catheter over about 10 minutes. After the solution has been infused, the inflow clamp is closed before air enters the tubing.

During the dwell phase, or equilibration phase, diffusion and osmosis occur between the patient's blood and the peritoneal cavity. The dwell time can last from 20 to 30 minutes to 8 or more hours, depending on the goals of PD.

Drain time takes 15 to 30 minutes. The cycle starts again with the infusion of another 2 L of solution. For manual PD, a period of about 30 to 50 minutes is required to complete an exchange.

Dialysis solutions vary, and the choice of exchange volume is primarily determined by the size of the peritoneal cavity. A larger person may tolerate a 3-L volume without any difficulty, whereas an average-size person usually tolerates a 2-L exchange.

Ultrafiltration (fluid removal) during PD depends on osmotic forces, with glucose being the most effective agent available. Dextrose remains the most commonly used osmotic agent available in PD solutions. It is relatively safe but has been associated with high rates of peritoneal glucose absorption leading to hypertriglyceridemia, hyperglycemia, and long-term peritoneal membrane dysfunction. The amount of dextrose in the solution varies among 0.5%, 1.5%, 2.5%, and 4.25%, depending on the fluid volume goal. Alternate osmotic agents include icodextrin and amino acid solutions.

Peritoneal Dialysis Systems

Two types of PD currently being used are automated peritoneal dialysis (APD) and continuous ambulatory peritoneal dialysis (CAPD).

Automated Peritoneal Dialysis. Automated peritoneal dialysis (APD), also called *continuous cycling peritoneal dialysis,* is a popular form of PD that is done while the patient sleeps. An automated device called a *cycler* is used to perform the dialysis exchanges (Figure 49.8). The automated cycler times and controls the fill, dwell, and drain phases. The machine cycles four or more exchanges per night, with 1 to 2 hours per exchange.

Alarms and monitors are built into the system to make it safe for the patient to dialyze while sleeping. The patient disconnects from the machine in the morning and usually leaves fluid in the abdomen during the day. One to two daytime manual exchanges may also be prescribed to ensure adequate dialysis.

Continuous Ambulatory Peritoneal Dialysis. Continuous ambulatory peritoneal dialysis (CAPD) is a type of PD that is done during the day and consists of a minimum of four exchanges of dialysis fluid per day. CAPD exchanges are carried out manually by exchanging 1.5 to 3 L of peritoneal dialysate at least four times daily, with dwell times averaging 4 hours. For example, one schedule starts the exchanges at 0700 hours, 1200 hours, 1700 hours, and 2200 hours.

Dialysis fluid is instilled into the peritoneal cavity and remains (dwells) there for a specified period, allowing for the removal of waste products and excess fluid; it is then drained and fresh fluid is instilled. It is continuous in that dialysis fluid is always in the peritoneal cavity so dialysis is continuously going on. After the equilibration period, the dialysate (effluent) is drained from the peritoneal cavity, and a new 2-L bag of dialysate solution is infused. It is critical in PD to maintain aseptic technique to avoid peritonitis. Several tubing connections and devices are commercially available to help maintain an aseptic system.

Potential contraindications for PD include the following:
1. History of multiple abdominal surgical procedures or severe abdominal pathological condition (e.g., severe pancreatitis, diverticulitis)
2. Recurrent abdominal wall or inguinal hernias
3. Excessive obesity with large abdominal wall and fat deposits
4. Pre-existing vertebral disease (e.g., chronic back pain)
5. Severe obstructive pulmonary disease

Complications of Peritoneal Dialysis

Exit-Site Infection. Infection of the peritoneal catheter exit site is most commonly caused by *Staphylococcus aureus* or *Staphylococcus epidermidis* (from skin flora). Superficial exit-site infections caused by these organisms are generally resolved with antibiotic therapy. Clinical manifestations of an exit-site infection include redness at the site, tenderness, and drainage. If not treated immediately, subcutaneous tunnel infections usually result in abscess formation and may cause peritonitis, necessitating catheter removal.

Peritonitis. Peritonitis results from contamination or from progression of an exit-site or tunnel infection. Most frequently, peritonitis occurs because of improper technique in making or breaking connections for exchanges. Less commonly, peritonitis results from bacteria in the intestine crossing over into the peritoneal cavity. Peritonitis is usually caused by *S. aureus* or *S. epidermidis.*

The primary clinical manifestation of peritonitis is a cloudy peritoneal effluent that has a WBC count of over 0.1×10^9/L (particularly neutrophils) or demonstration of bacteria in the peritoneal effluent by Gram stain or culture. GI manifestations may also be present, including diffuse abdominal pain, diarrhea, vomiting, abdominal distension, and hyperactive bowel sounds. Fever may or may not be present. Cultures, Gram stain, and a cell count with WBC differential of the peritoneal effluent are used to confirm the diagnosis of peritonitis. Antibiotics can be given by mouth or by IV or intraperitoneal route. The patient is usually treated on an outpatient basis. Repeated infections may necessitate the removal of the peritoneal catheter and

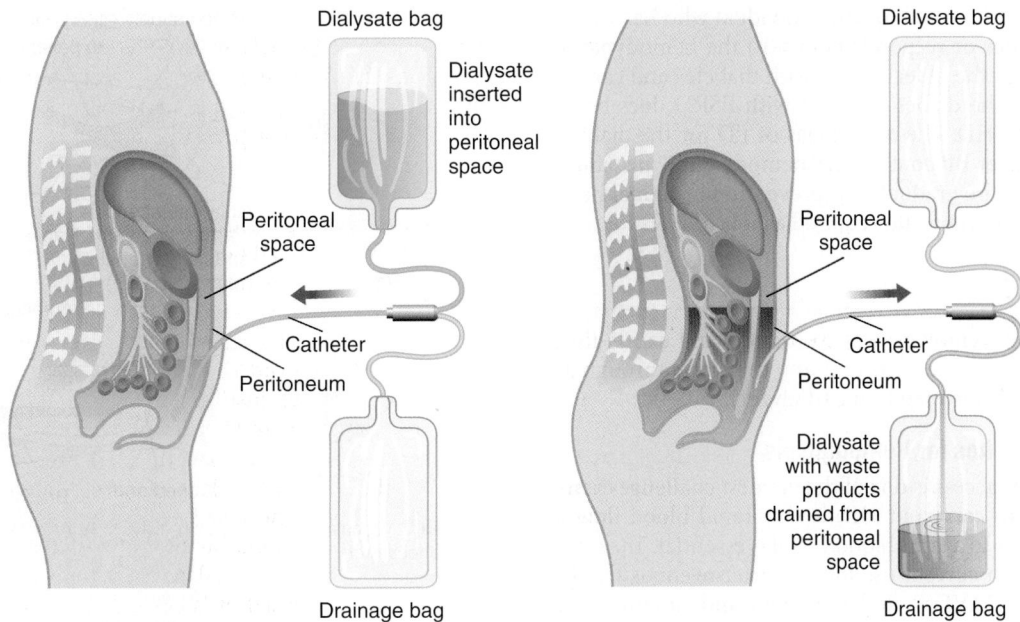

FIG. 49.8 Automated peritoneal dialysis cycler, which can be used while the patient is sleeping at night or for hospitalized patients who require frequent exchanges. Source: © Can Stock Photo/rob3000.

termination of PD. The formation of adhesions in the peritoneum can result from repeated infections and interferes with the peritoneal membrane's ability to act as a dialyzing surface.

Abdominal Pain. Although not severe, pain is a common complication, caused by the low pH of the dialysate solution, peritonitis, intraperitoneal irritation (which usually subsides in 1 to 2 weeks), and placement of the catheter. Pain can also occur when the tip of the catheter touches the bladder, the bowel, or the peritoneum. A change in the position of the catheter should correct this problem. Accidental infusion of air or infusing the dialysate too rapidly may cause referred pain in the shoulder. If the infusion rate is decreased, the pain usually subsides.

Outflow Disorders. It is expected that at least 80% of the volume instilled in the peritoneal cavity is returned when draining the cavity after an exchange. Causes of poor outflow include constipation, a kink in the catheter or transfer set, omentum wrapped around the catheter, and migration of the catheter out of the pelvic region. Laxatives and stool softeners can be used to relieve constipation and promote regular bowel movements. Outflow disorders related to omental entrapment or migration may necessitate radiological intervention, surgical manipulation of the catheter, or both.

Hernias. Because of increased intra-abdominal pressure secondary to the dialysate infusion, umbilical or inguinal hernias or diastasis recti can develop in predisposed individuals, such as multiparous women and older men. However, in most situations after hernia repair, PD can be resumed after several days, using small dialysate volumes and keeping the patient supine.

Lower Back Pain. Increased intra-abdominal pressure can cause or aggravate lower back pain. The lumbosacral curvature is increased by intraperitoneal infusion of dialysate. Orthopedic binders and a regular exercise program for strengthening the back muscles have been beneficial for some patients.

Bleeding. Effluent drained after the first few exchanges may be pink or slightly bloody because of the trauma of catheter insertion. Bloody effluent over several days or the new appearance of blood in the effluent can indicate active intraperitoneal bleeding. If this occurs, BP and hemoglobin should be checked. Blood may also be present in the effluent of women who are menstruating or ovulating; this occurrence requires no intervention.

Pulmonary Complications. Atelectasis, pneumonia, and bronchitis may occur from repeated upward displacement of the diaphragm, resulting in decreased lung expansion. The longer the dwell time, the greater the likelihood of pulmonary complications. Frequent repositioning and deep-breathing exercises can help. When the patient is lying in bed, elevation of the head of the bed may prevent these complications.

Protein Loss. The peritoneal membrane is permeable to plasma proteins, amino acids, and polypeptides. These substances are lost in the dialysate fluid. The amount of loss may be as much as 5 to 15 g/day. This loss may increase to up to 40 g/day during episodes of peritonitis as the membrane becomes more permeable. Positive nitrogen balance can be maintained with adequate protein intake.

Carbohydrate and Lipid Abnormalities. Dialysate glucose is absorbed via the peritoneum in quantities that may be as high as 100 to 150 g/day. Continuous absorption of glucose results in increased insulin secretion and increased plasma insulin levels. The hyperinsulinemia stimulates hepatic production of triglycerides.

Effectiveness of and Adaptation to Chronic Peritoneal Dialysis

Learning the self-management skills required to do PD involves a relatively short training program. PD provides independence and flexibility with treatment, and travelling is easier. A major advantage of PD is its simplicity and that it is a home-based treatment that allows the patient to be in control.

Clinically, the patient receiving PD does as well as the patient receiving HD and sometimes better. There are fewer dietary restrictions, and greater mobility is possible than with conventional HD. The major disadvantage is the possibility of developing peritonitis.

PD is especially indicated for the individual who has vascular access difficulties or responds poorly to the hemodynamic stresses of HD (e.g., the older patient with diabetes and cardiovascular disease). The diabetic patient with ESRD does better with PD than with HD. The advantages of PD for the diabetic patient include better BP control, less hemodynamic instability because fluid shifts are gradual, and prevention of retinal hemorrhage because heparin is not required as it is in HD.

HEMODIALYSIS

HD is a method of removing waste products and excess fluid from the blood using a machine to pump the blood through an artificial semipermeable membrane (dialyzer).

Vascular Access Sites for Hemodialysis

Obtaining vascular access is one of the greatest challenges associated with HD. To carry out HD, a very rapid blood flow is required, and access to a large blood vessel is essential. The types of vascular access in current use include arteriovenous fistulas (AVFs) and grafts (AVGs), and tunnelled and nontunnelled central venous catheters (CVCs). AVFs are superior to synthetic AVGs and CVCs and are associated with better long-term survival, lower infection and complication rates, and lower health care expenditure (Houck & Neumann, 2019).

Arteriovenous Fistulas and Grafts. A native arteriovenous fistula (AVF) is the preferred HD access, created by surgically connecting a vein and an artery, usually in the forearm (Houck & Neumann, 2019) (Figures 49.9, *A* and 49.10). The preferred sites for creating an AVF are the wrist (radiocephalic) and the elbow (brachiocephalic). The fistula provides for arterial blood flow through the vein. The increased pressure of the arterial blood flow through the vein causes the vein to dilate and become tough, making it amenable to repeated venipuncture. The vein is accessed using two large-gauge needles.

AVFs have the best overall patency rates and the least number of complications (e.g., thrombosis, infection) of all vascular accesses. The AVF should be created at least 3 to 4 months before starting dialysis (Debus & Grundmann, 2017). The AVF requires 4 to 6 weeks, and preferably 3 months, to mature (dilate and toughen) sufficiently for use. AVFs are more difficult to create in people with severe peripheral vascular disease, diabetes, prolonged IV drug use, or previous multiple IV procedures in the forearm. For these individuals, a synthetic graft may be required.

An arteriovenous graft (AVG) is an HD access created with a synthetic graft that is attached to an artery and a vein. It is used for people who do not have suitable vessels for an AVF. The preferred site for a synthetic graft is a forearm, using a curved loop radiocephalic graft. The graft is a surgically created anastomosis between an artery (usually radial) and a vein (usually cephalic) (see Figure 49.9, *B*). An interval of 3 to 6 weeks is usually necessary to allow the graft to heal, but some centres may use it earlier. The graft, like the fistula, is under the skin and is accessed using two large-gauge needles. The graft material is self-healing, meaning it should close over any puncture site after the needle is removed. Infections in other parts of the body can result in infection and damage to the graft and have a tendency to be thrombogenic.

Normally, a *thrill* can be felt by palpating the area of anastomosis, and a *bruit* can be heard with a stethoscope. The bruit and the thrill are created by the turbulence of arterial blood

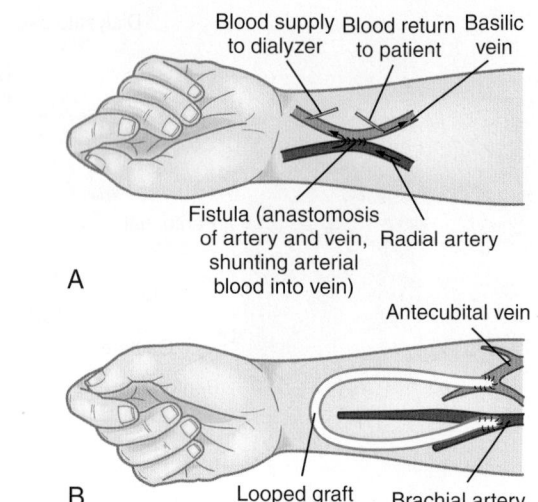

FIG. 49.9 Vascular access for hemodialysis. **A,** Arteriovenous fistula. **B,** Arteriovenous graft.

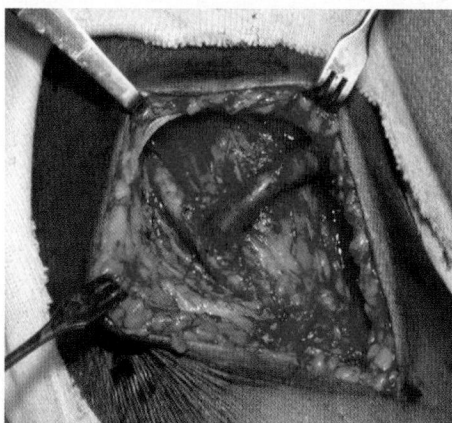

FIG. 49.10 Arteriovenous fistula created by anastomosing an artery and a vein. Source: Courtesy Dr. Stephen Van Voorst, MD.

rushing into the vein. BP measurement, IV insertion, and venipuncture should not be performed on an extremity with an AVF or AVG. This is to prevent thrombosis and infection in the vascular access. Protection of the vascular access site is of paramount importance.

An AVF is much less likely to clot and become infected than a graft. Thrombosis in AVGs is common but can often be corrected using interventional radiology techniques or a surgical procedure. AVFs and AVGs can cause the development of distal ischemia (steal syndrome) because too much of the arterial blood is being shunted or "stolen" from the distal extremity. This is usually seen soon after surgery and may require surgical correction. Aneurysms can also develop at the fistula site and can rupture if left untreated. AVG infections are not uncommon, and immediate treatment is essential to salvage the graft and prevent bacteremia. Severe AVG infections may necessitate graft removal.

Central Venous Catheters. In some situations when immediate vascular access is required, a temporary CVC is placed by percutaneous cannulation of the internal jugular or the femoral vein. Internal jugular vein cannulation is associated with a low incidence of thrombosis, which is the primary reason this method is preferred over subclavian cannulation. In

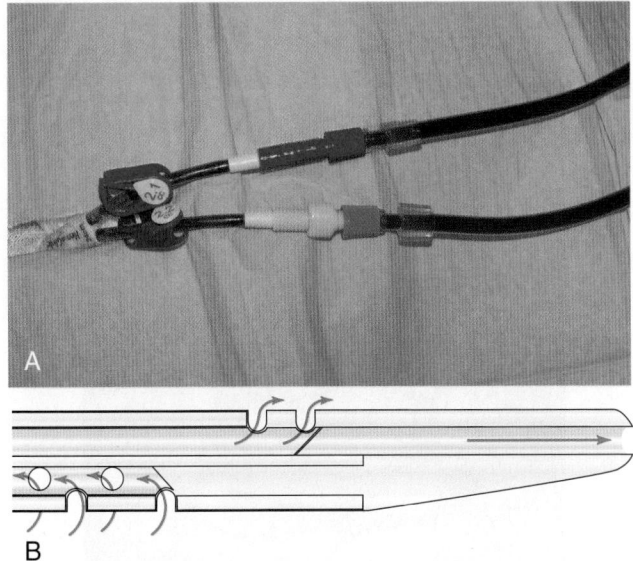

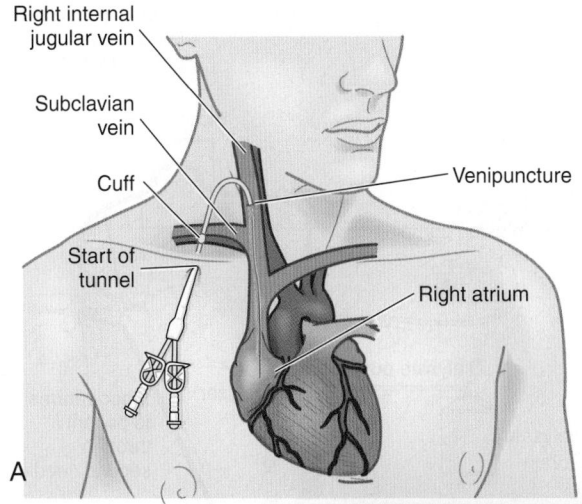

FIG. 49.11 Temporary double-lumen vascular access catheter for acute hemodialysis. **A,** Soft, flexible dual-lumen tube is attached to a Y hub. **B,** Blood is withdrawn continuously through the red lumen (upstream) and returned through the blue lumen (downstream), thus reducing recirculation. Source: *A,* © Can Stock Photo/Terrapanthera.

addition to vessel thrombosis and stenosis, subclavian vein cannulation has been associated with pneumothorax and brachial plexus; therefore, this site should be used as a last resort. A flexible Teflon, silicone rubber, or polyurethane catheter can be inserted at the bedside into the internal jugular vein and provides access to circulation without surgery (Figure 49.11, *A*). The catheters usually have a double external lumen with an internal septum separating the two internal segments (see Figure 49.11, *B*). One lumen is used for blood removal and the other for blood return. Femoral catheters should be sutured into place and can be left in place as long as there are no complications.

Disadvantages of femoral vessel cannulation include the following: (1) the location encourages catheter kinking, and (2) the groin is not a clean site. Potential complications of femoral catheterization are femoral vein thrombosis with pulmonary emboli (especially if the treatment is prolonged), infections, immobility, and inadvertent blood vessel punctures with hematoma formation. Temporary catheters are generally stiff and inflexible. They can cause trauma to the vessel, so bed rest is recommended. Temporary catheters in the internal jugular vein should be sutured in place and should be replaced as soon as possible by a tunnelled catheter that can be left in place for several weeks. Proper catheter position should be confirmed using radiography before use. Temporary catheters are generally left in place only for short periods or until a tunnelled catheter can be inserted.

Tunnelled catheters, which are soft and flexible, may be an option for patients who have exhausted all other vascular access sites. These catheters can be used as temporary access while awaiting fistula placement and development or as long-term access when other forms of access have failed. This type of catheter exits on the upper chest wall and is tunnelled subcutaneously to the internal jugular vein (Figure 49.12). The catheter tip rests in the right atrium. It has one or two subcutaneous Dacron cuffs that prevent infection from tracking along the catheter and anchor the catheter, eliminating the need for sutures.

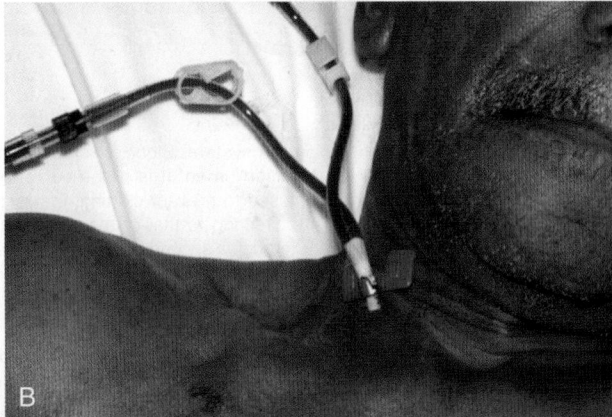

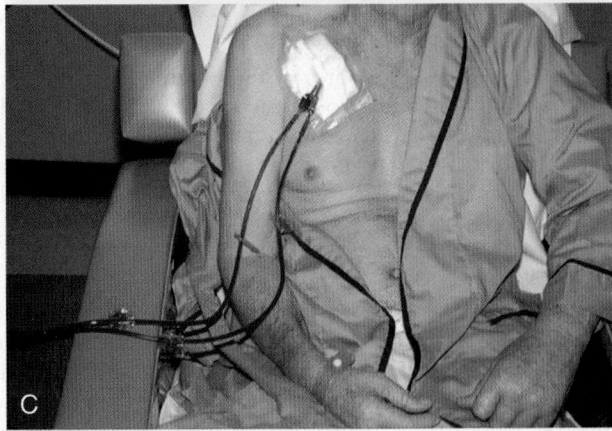

FIG. 49.12 A, Right internal jugular placement for a tunnelled, cuffed semipermanent catheter. **B,** Temporary hemodialysis catheter in place. **C,** Long-term cuffed hemodialysis catheter. Source: *B* and *C*, Courtesy Dr. Stephen Van Voorst, MD.

No medications should be administered or blood withdrawn via the catheter by staff not trained in the care and management of a CVC. This is to minimize the risk for infection, catheter loss, and accidental injection of heparin. Trained dialysis staff will instill heparin into the lumens of the catheter at the end of each treatment to ensure patency and withdraw it before the next treatment.

Dialyzers

The dialyzer is a long plastic cartridge that contains thousands of parallel hollow tubes or fibres (Figure 49.13). The fibres are

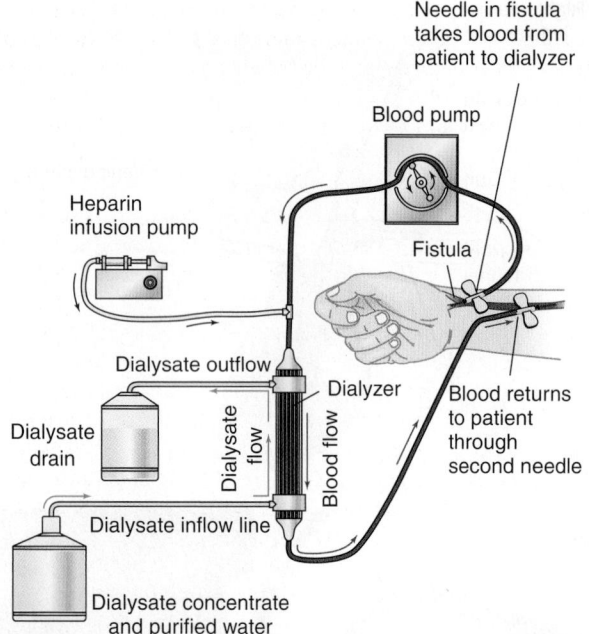

FIG. 49.13 Components of a hemodialysis system. Blood is removed via a needle inserted in a fistula or via catheter lumen. It is propelled to the dialyzer by a blood pump. Heparin is infused to prevent clotting. Dialysate is pumped in and flows in the opposite direction to that of the blood. The dialyzed blood is returned to the patient through a second needle or catheter lumen. Old dialysate and ultrafiltrate are drained and discarded.

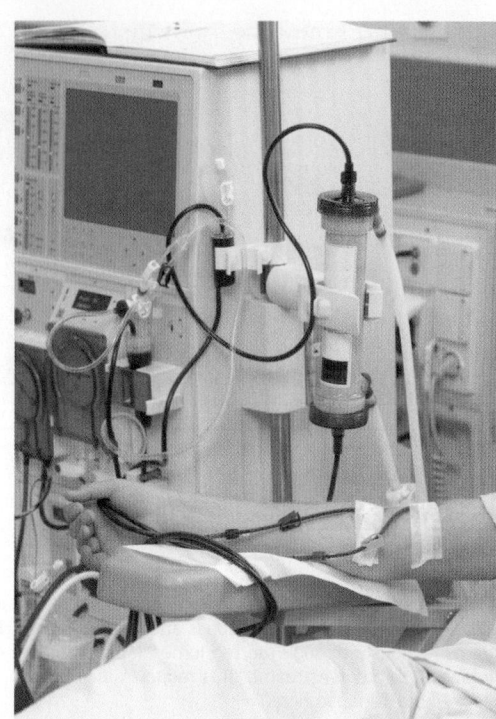

FIG. 49.14 Patient receiving in-centre hemodialysis. Source: © Can Stock Photo/PicsFive.

the semipermeable membrane, made of cellulose-based or other synthetic materials. The blood is pumped into the top of the cartridge and is dispersed into all of the fibres. Dialysis fluid (dialysate) is pumped into the bottom of the cartridge and bathes the outside of the fibres. Ultrafiltration, diffusion, and osmosis occur across the pores of this semipermeable membrane. When the dialyzed blood reaches the end of the semipermeable fibres, it converges into a single tube that returns it to the patient. Available dialyzers differ in regard to surface area, membrane composition and thickness, clearance of waste products, and removal of fluid.

Procedure

To initiate chronic dialysis in a patient with an AVG or AVF, two needles are placed in the fistula or graft. One needle is used to draw blood from the patient and circulate it through the extracorporeal circuit and dialyzer, and the other needle is used to return the blood. If the patient has a catheter, the two blood lines are attached to the two catheter lumens, and blood is circulated through the dialysis blood circuit similar to that of the AVF and is sent to the dialyzer with the assistance of a blood pump. Heparin is added to the blood as it flows into the dialyzer, because any time blood contacts a foreign substance, it has a tendency to clot. When the blood enters the extracorporeal circuit, it is propelled through the top of the dialyzer by a blood pump at a flow rate of 200 to 500 mL/min while the dialysate circulates in the opposite direction at a rate of 300 to 900 mL/min. Blood is returned from the dialyzer to the patient through the second needle or the blue (venous) catheter lumen.

In addition to the dialyzer, there is a dialysate delivery and monitoring system (Figure 49.14). This system pumps the dialysate through the dialyzer in the direction opposite that of the blood flow.

Before beginning treatment, the nurse must complete an assessment of the patient that includes fluid status (weight, BP, peripheral edema, lung and heart sounds), condition of vascular access, temperature, and general skin condition. The difference between the last postdialysis weight and the present predialysis weight represents the amount of fluid weight gained since the last treatment. This information is used to determine the ultrafiltration or the amount of fluid to be removed. Each kilogram represents approximately 1 L of fluid. Ideally, no more than 1 to 1.5 kg should be gained between treatments, to prevent the hypotension associated with the removal of larger volumes of fluid. Many patients gain 2 to 3 kg between treatments, and this volume usually can be removed if their BP is not labile. While the patient is on dialysis, vital signs should be taken at least every 30 to 60 minutes because rapid changes may occur in the BP.

Most maintenance dialysis units use reclining chairs that allow for elevation of the feet if hypotension develops. Most people sleep, read, talk, or watch television during dialysis. Treatments usually last 3 to 5 hours and are done a minimum of three times per week to achieve adequate clearance and maintain fluid balance.

Prior to sending the patient for HD, the nurse must make sure that the access site is functioning properly. The site needs to be assessed for bleeding, drainage, erythema, and pain. Any signs of infection need to be reported to the health care provider. The patient's medications need to be reviewed prior to sending the patient for HD. In collaboration with the health care provider, antihypertensive medications may be held before HD treatment. Certain medications will pass through the dialysis machine and may be held before the dialysis treatment. The health care provider should be contacted for individual orders of what medications can be administered prior to the dialysis treatment.

HD units and treatments are performed in a variety of settings. Acutely ill patients may require dialysis in the CCU setting. Most large teaching hospitals in Canada have dialysis units that accommodate patients who are in hospital, as well as a chronic outpatient population. Many satellite and outpatient clinics provide chronic HD treatments. The patient may choose to do self-care with backup support from trained personnel if needed. Self-care patients generally put in their dialysis needles, set up the machine, and monitor the course of their treatment. Patients receiving HD are able to travel if dialysis treatments can be arranged at another dialysis unit.

Dialysis done at home is an optimal option for patients requiring RRT. Treatments are more cost-effective and have many benefits for the patient (Buena et al., 2018). HD can also be done at home. In Canada, approximately 20% of those requiring dialysis receive peritoneal dialysis in their home (Blake, 2020). One of the main advantages of home HD is that it allows greater freedom in choosing dialysis times. Some modifications for a special electrical outlet, plumbing, and water treatment are necessary to accommodate the HD machine in the home setting.

Complications of Hemodialysis

Hypotension. Hypotension that occurs during HD primarily results from rapid removal of vascular volume (hypovolemia), decreased cardiac output, and decreased systemic intravascular resistance. The drop in BP during dialysis may precipitate lightheadedness, nausea, vomiting, seizures, vision changes, and chest pain from cardiac ischemia. The usual treatment for hypotension includes decreasing the volume of fluid being removed and infusion of 0.9% saline solution (100–300 mL). If a patient experiences recurrent hypotensive episodes, reassessment of dry weight and BP medications should be performed. BP medications should be held before dialysis if there are frequent episodes of hypotension during dialysis.

Muscle Cramps. Painful muscle cramps are a common symptom with HD. They result from rapid removal of sodium and water or from neuromuscular hypersensitivity. Treatment includes reducing the ultrafiltration rate and infusing hypertonic saline or a normal saline bolus. The nurse should also educate the patient about restricting salt and fluid in the diet to reduce weight gains between dialysis treatments.

Loss of Blood. Blood loss may result from blood not being completely rinsed from the dialyzer, accidental separation of blood tubing, dialysis membrane rupture, or bleeding after the removal of needles at the end of dialysis. If a patient has received too much heparin or has clotting issues, there can be significant postdialysis bleeding. It is essential to rinse back all blood, to closely monitor heparinization to prevent excess anticoagulation, and to hold firm but nonocclusive pressure on access sites until the risk of bleeding has passed.

Hepatitis. A common cause of hepatitis B and C in dialysis patients includes transmission of health care–associated infection within HD units. As blood is screened for hepatitis B and C, blood transfusions are an unlikely source for the hepatitis infection. Dialysis patients may contract the blood-borne pathogen of hepatitis B and C as the general population does, through IV drug use or unprotected sex. (See Chapter 17 for infection control precautions and Chapter 46 for a more detailed discussion on hepatitis.)

Sepsis. Sepsis is most often related to infections of vascular access sites. Bacteria can also be introduced during the dialysis treatment as a result of poor technique or interruption of blood tubing or dialyzer membranes. Bacterial endocarditis can occur because of the frequent and prolonged access to the vascular system. Aseptic technique is essential to prevent this condition. Nurses must monitor patients for signs and symptoms of sepsis, such as fever, hypotension, and an elevated WBC count. (See Chapter 69 for nursing management of septic shock.)

Disequilibrium Syndrome. *Disequilibrium syndrome* is a rare complication of HD and develops as a result of very rapid changes in the composition of the extracellular fluid (Steward, 2019). Urea, sodium, and other solutes are removed more rapidly from the blood than from the cerebrospinal fluid and the brain. This rapid removal creates a high osmotic gradient in the brain, resulting in a shift of fluid into the brain, which causes cerebral edema. Manifestations include nausea, vomiting, confusion, restlessness, headaches, twitching and jerking, and seizures. The rapid changes in osmolality may cause muscle cramps and worsen hypotension. Treatment consists of slowing or stopping dialysis and infusing hypertonic saline solution, albumin, or mannitol to draw fluid from the brain cells back into the systemic circulation. It is more commonly observed in the initial treatment of the patient when the BUN level is high. First dialysis treatment sessions are purposely short, with limited total solute removal, to prevent this rare syndrome.

Effectiveness of and Adaptation to Hemodialysis

HD is still an imperfect technique to treat stage 5 CKD. It cannot fully replace the metabolic and hormonal functions of the kidneys. It can ease many of the symptoms of CKD and, if started early, can prevent certain complications. It does not alter the accelerated atherosclerosis.

The 5-year survival rate for patients receiving maintenance HD is 44.4% (CIHI, 2019). Age and primary diagnosis are associated with survival of dialysis patients—the 5-year survival rate is 26% for those age 75 and older, whereas patients with renal vascular disease and diabetes have a 5-year survival rate of 37% and 41%, respectively.

Individual adaptation to maintenance HD varies considerably. Initially, many patients feel positive about the dialysis because it makes them feel better and keeps them alive, but there is often great ambivalence about whether it is worthwhile. Dependence on a machine is a reality, and some have dreams about being tied to the machine. In response to their illness, patients undergoing dialysis may demonstrate nonadherence to medical therapy, depression, and suicidal tendencies. The primary nursing goals are to help patients regain or maintain positive self-esteem and control of their lives and continue to be productive in society.

Continuous Renal Replacement Therapy

Continuous renal replacement therapy (CRRT) is an alternative or adjunctive method for treating AKI. It provides a means by which uremic toxins and fluids are removed from a patient who is hemodynamically unstable, while acid–base status and electrolytes are adjusted slowly and continuously. Patients selected for this treatment are usually those who do not respond to dietary interventions or pharmacological agents.

Various types of CRRT are available, such as continuous venovenous hemofiltration (CVVH), continuous venovenous hemodialysis (CVVHD), and continuous venovenous hemodiafiltration (CVVHDF) (Table 49.14). Various hybrid modalities that combine aspects of conventional HD and CRRT can be used and are determined on the basis of the patient's needs.

TABLE 49.14   TYPES OF CONTINUOUS RENAL REPLACEMENT THERAPIES

Therapies	Abbreviation	Purpose
Continuous venovenous hemofiltration*	CVVH	Solute loss via convection; hemodilution using replacement fluid
Continuous venovenous hemodialysis*	CVVHD	Solute loss via convection and diffusion
Continuous venovenous hemodiafiltration	CVVHDF	—
Slow continuous ultrafiltration	SCUF	Fluid removal via ultrafiltration
Slow low-efficiency dialysis	SLED	—

*Most commonly used therapies.

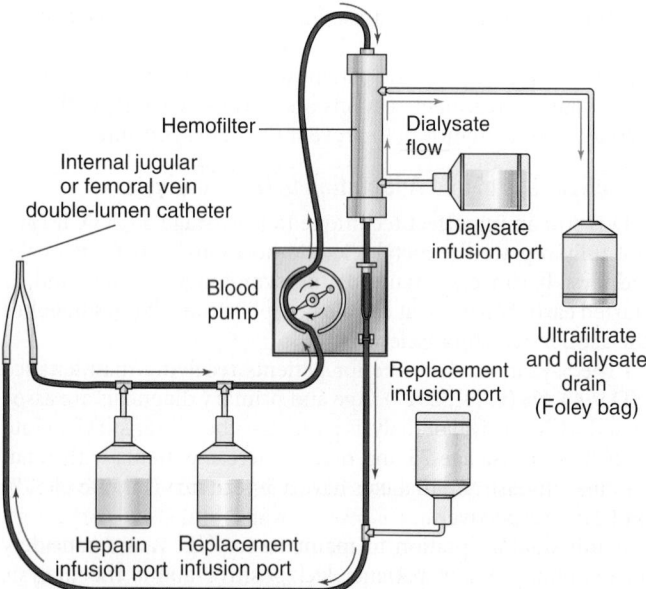

FIG. 49.15 Basic schematic of continuous venovenous therapies. Blood pump is required to pump blood through the circuit. Replacement ports are used for continuous venovenous hemofiltration (CVVH) and continuous venovenous hemodialysis (CVVHD) only; replacements can be given prefilter or postfilter. Dialysate port is used for CVVHD only. Regardless of modality, ultrafiltrate is drained via the ultrafiltration drain port.

Some common hybrid modalities include slow low-efficiency dialysis (SLED) and slow continuous ultrafiltration (SCUF) (Schell-Chaple, 2017).

Vascular access for CRRT is achieved through the use of a double-lumen catheter (as used in HD, noted in Figure 49.11, A) placed in the femoral or the jugular vein. The subclavian vein should be used only if no other access site is available, owing to the increased complication rates of pneumothorax, hemorrhage, and stenosis. Under the influence of hydrostatic pressure and osmotic pressure, water and nonprotein solutes pass out of the filter into the extracapillary space and drain through the ultrafiltrate port into a collection device (Foley bag) (Figure 49.15). The remaining fluid continues through the filter and returns to the patient via the return port of the double-lumen catheter. While the ultrafiltrate drains out of the hemofilter, fluid and electrolyte replacements can be infused into the infusion port located after the filter, as the blood returns to the patient. This fluid is

designed to replace volume and solutes such as sodium, chloride, bicarbonate, and glucose. It will also further dilute intravascular fluid, decreasing the concentration of unwanted solutes such as BUN, creatinine, and potassium. The infusion rate of replacement fluid is determined by the degree of the fluid and electrolyte imbalance. Replacement fluid may also be infused into the infusion port before the hemofilter. This method allows for greater clearance of urea and can decrease filter clotting.

Anticoagulation (e.g., heparin) is needed to prevent blood clotting during CRRT. Heparin dosage is based on the patient's activated clotting time (ACT), partial prothrombin time (PPT), or prothrombin time (PT).

Several features of CRRT differ from those of HD:
1. It is continuous rather than intermittent. Large volumes of fluid can be removed over days (24 hours to >2 weeks) instead of hours (3 to 4 hours).
2. Solute removal can occur by convection (no dialysate required) in addition to osmosis and diffusion.
3. It causes less hemodynamic instability (e.g., hypotension).
4. It does not require constant monitoring by a specialized HD nurse but does require a trained CCU nurse.
5. It does not require complicated HD equipment, but a blood pump is needed for venovenous therapies.

The type of CRRT is customized to the needs of the patient. Some types involve the use of replacement fluids. Large volumes of fluid may be removed hourly (200–800 mL), and then a portion of this fluid is replaced. The type of fluid replacement is dependent on the stability of the patient's condition and the patient's individualized needs. Ultrafiltration and convective losses occur, and solute concentrations in the blood are diluted with the replacement fluid.

CRRT can be continued as long as 30 to 40 days, but the hemofilter should be changed every 24 to 48 hours because of loss of filtration efficiency and the potential for clotting.

The nurse responsible for the care of the patient with AKI who is receiving CRRT may be a critical care nurse or a nephrology nurse specialist, working in collaboration with other health care providers. Specific nursing interventions include obtaining weights and monitoring and documenting laboratory values daily to ensure adequate fluid and electrolyte balance. Hourly intake–output measurements and monitoring of vital signs and hemodynamic status are essential. Although reductions in central venous pressure and pulmonary artery pressure are expected, there should be little change in mean arterial pressure or cardiac output. Patency of the CRRT system is assessed and maintained, and the patient's vascular access site is cared for to prevent infection. Treatment is discontinued and the vascular access is removed once the patient's AKI is resolved or there is a decision to withdraw treatment because of patient deterioration.

KIDNEY TRANSPLANTATION

Major progress has been made in organ transplantation since the first kidney transplantation was performed in 1954 in Boston between identical twins. The advances made in organ procurement and preservation, surgical techniques, tissue typing and matching, understanding of the immune system, immunosuppressant therapy, and prevention and treatment of rejection have dramatically increased the success of organ transplantation.

The disparity between the supply and the demand for organs is significant. In Canada, over 40 289 Canadians patients received dialysis in 2018, a level that has almost doubled since 2012.

Over 17 000 patients were living with a kidney transplant in 2018, almost triple the number in 1993 (CIHI, 2019). According to CIHI data, 1 706 adult patients received renal transplants in 2018. Transplantation from a deceased donor usually requires a prolonged waiting period, with median waiting times in 2018 of approximately 4 years. By province, the longest median wait time was in British Columbia (5.0 years), while the shortest median wait time was in Saskatchewan, at just 2.2 years.

Kidney transplantation is extremely successful, with 1-year graft survival rates of about 93% for deceased donor transplants and greater than 97.5% for living donor transplants (CIHI, 2019). An advantage of kidney transplantation when compared with dialysis is that when normal kidney function is restored, many of the pathophysiological changes associated with renal failure are reversed. It also eliminates the dependence on dialysis and the accompanying dietary and lifestyle restrictions. Transplantation is also less expensive than dialysis after the first year.

Kidney transplantation rates are low in the Indigenous population. The reasons for this low rate are multifactorial, including living in remote or rural areas and having to travel long distances to treatment facilities. Educational resources on organ donation and transplantation for Indigenous people can increase awareness and prevent misconceptions about transplantation.

Ethical Issues

Transplantation health care in Canada is governed by laws and statutes. It is complex and involves many people, professionals, services, functions, and levels of government. Voluntary consent must be given by the donor (Contiero & Wilson, 2019) in some provinces; one can provide advance written consent on a driver's license or in a will (although permission from the donor's legal next of kin is still required after brain death is determined). In the absence of formal written consent at death, family members or significant others can donate organs of the deceased if they had prior knowledge of the donor's intent. Kidneys may be obtained from deceased or living donors. It is illegal to buy or sell organs in Canada. (See the Ethical Dilemmas box in this chapter and in Chapter 16.)

Recipient Selection

Appropriate recipient selection is important for a successful outcome. Candidacy is determined by a variety of medical and psychosocial factors that vary among transplantation centres. A careful evaluation is completed in an attempt to identify and minimize potential complications after transplantation. Certain patients, particularly those with cardiovascular disease and diabetes mellitus, are considered high risk. With careful evaluation and monitoring, high-risk patients can achieve the same success rates as other patients. Some patients who are approaching ESRD can receive a transplant before dialysis is required if they have a living donor. This approach is most advantageous for patients with diabetes, who have a much higher mortality rate on dialysis than people who do not have diabetes.

Contraindications to transplantation include disseminated malignancies, refractory or untreated cardiac disease, chronic respiratory failure, extensive vascular disease, chronic infection, and unresolved psychosocial disorders (e.g., alcoholism, drug addiction) and nonadherence to medical regimens. The presence of hepatitis B or C is not a contraindication to transplantation.

Surgical procedures may be required before transplantation based on the results of the recipient evaluation. Coronary artery bypass graft surgery may be indicated for advanced coronary artery disease. Cholecystectomy may be necessary for patients with a history of gallstones, biliary obstruction, or cholecystitis. On rare occasions, bilateral nephrectomies may be done for patients with refractory hypertension, recurrent urinary tract infections, or grossly enlarged kidneys resulting from polycystic kidney disease.

Histocompatibility Studies

Histocompatibility testing is discussed in Chapter 16.

Donor Sources

Kidneys for transplantation may be obtained from compatible blood–type deceased donors, blood relatives, emotionally related living donors (e.g., spouses, friends), and altruistic living donors who are unknown to the recipient. Expanding the living donor pool is one of the best possibilities for decreasing the size of the deceased donor waiting list and reducing waiting times.

Living Donors. Living donors must undergo an extensive multidisciplinary evaluation to be certain they are in good health and have no history of disease that would place them at risk of developing kidney failure or operative complications. Psychosocial and financial evaluations are done as well. Crossmatches are done at the time of the evaluation and about a week before the transplantation to ensure that no antibodies to the donor are present or that the antibody titre is below the allowed level. Advantages of a living donor transplantation include better patient and graft survival rates regardless of histocompatibility match, immediate organ availability, immediate function because of minimal "cold time" (kidney out of the body and not getting blood supply), and the opportunity to have the recipient in the best possible medical condition because the surgery is elective.

The potential donor will see a nephrologist for a complete history and physical and laboratory and diagnostic studies. Laboratory studies include a 24-hour urine study for creatinine clearance and total protein, complete blood count, and chemistry and electrolyte profiles. Hepatitis B and C, HIV, and cytomegalovirus (CMV) testing is done to assess for the presence of any transmissible diseases. An ECG and chest radiography are also obtained. A renal ultrasound and a renal arteriogram or three-dimensional CT are performed to ensure that the blood vessels supplying each kidney are adequate and that there are no anomalies and to determine which kidney will be removed.

A transplantation psychologist or social worker will determine whether the individual is emotionally stable and able to cope with the issues related to organ donation. All donors must be informed about the risks and benefits of donation, the potential short- and long-term complications, and what can be expected during the hospitalization and recovery phases. Although the cost of the evaluation and surgery are covered by the recipient's insurance, there is no compensation available for lost wages during the posthospitalization recovery period. This period can last 6 weeks or longer.

Incompatibility between a potential transplant recipient and a prospective donor is a major barrier to living donor transplantations. Paired organ donation is another option that allows a living donor to donate a kidney to a different compatible recipient, with the intent that another donor will donate to the first donor's designated recipient. In 2009, the Canadian Blood Services launched a pilot project for a living donor paired exchange (LDPE) registry that is now available to every province (Canadian Blood Services, 2019). The registry is designed to facilitate transplants between recipients and living donors who have an incompatible match with other recipient donor pairs in the same situation. The recipient–donor pairs in the LDPE registry are entered in a complex computer algorithm that identifies opportunities for transplants between them.

Deceased Donors. Deceased (cadaver) kidney donors are relatively healthy individuals who have suffered an irreversible brain injury with a declaration of brain death. The most common causes of injury are cerebral trauma from motor vehicle accidents or gunshot wounds, intracerebral or subarachnoid hemorrhage, and anoxic brain damage caused by cardiac arrest. The donor must have effective cardiovascular function and be supported on a ventilator to preserve the organs. The age range of most suitable kidney donors is from 2 to 70 years. The age of the donor is less important than the quality of kidney function. The donor must be free of active IV drug use; severe hypertension; long-standing diabetes mellitus; malignancies; sepsis; and communicable diseases, including HIV, hepatitis B and C, syphilis, and tuberculosis. Permission from the donor's legal next of kin is required after brain death is determined, even if the donor carried a signed donor card.

The kidneys are removed and preserved. They can be preserved for up to 72 hours, but most transplantation surgeons prefer to transplant kidneys before the cold time reaches 24 hours. Experience has shown that prolonged cold time increases the likelihood that the kidney will not function immediately and the transplant recipient will require dialysis until the ATN from the extended cold time resolves.

In Canada, patients who receive a kidney from deceased donors are selected from provincial waiting lists that use an objective computerized point system. ABO group, human lymphocyte antigen (HLA) typing, age, antibody level, and length of time waiting are entered into the computer matching program as each candidate is listed. When a donor becomes available, the donor's HLA data, ABO type, and other key information are compared with the data of all patients awaiting transplantation locally. Donors and recipients must have the same blood type. The kidney is offered to the recipient with the most points. If there are no patients in the local area who are suitable, the organ is then offered in the region, and then to the nation. When a kidney arrives at the recipient's transplantation centre, a final crossmatch is done. The final crossmatch must be negative for the deceased donor transplantation to proceed. (Crossmatching is discussed in Chapter 16.)

Surgical Procedure

Living Donor. The donor nephrectomy is performed by a urologist or transplantation surgeon. The donor's surgery begins 1 to 2 hours before the recipient's surgery is started. The recipient is surgically prepared for the kidney transplantation in a nearby operating room.

Laparoscopic donor nephrectomy is the most common approach to removing a kidney from a living donor. (Laparoscopic nephrectomy is discussed in Chapter 48.) The laparoscopic approach significantly decreases length of hospital stay, pain, operative blood loss, debilitation, and length of time off work.

For a conventional nephrectomy, the donor is placed in the lateral decubitus position on the operating table so that the flank is presented laterally. An incision is made at the level of the eleventh rib. The rib may have to be removed to provide adequate visualization of the kidney.

Kidney Transplant Recipient. The transplanted kidney is usually placed extraperitoneally in the iliac fossa. The right iliac fossa is preferred to facilitate anastomoses and minimize the occurrence of ileus.

Before any incisions are made, a urinary catheter is placed into the bladder. An antibiotic solution is instilled to distend the bladder and decrease the risk for infection. A crescent-shaped incision is made, extending from the iliac crest to the symphysis pubis (Figure 49.16). The peritoneum is left intact. The iliac and the hypogastric vessels are dissected free.

Rapid revascularization is critical to prevent ischemic injury to the kidney. The donor artery is anastomosed to the recipient's internal iliac (hypogastric) or external iliac artery. The donor vein is anastomosed to the recipient's external iliac vein. Kidney transplants with living donors can be technically more difficult because the blood vessel lengths can be shorter than in cadaveric transplants.

When the anastomoses are complete, the clamps are released, and blood flow to the kidney is re-established. The kidney should become firm and pink. Urine may begin to flow from the ureter immediately. Mannitol or furosemide (Lasix) may be administered to promote diuresis.

The donor ureter in most cases is then tunnelled through the bladder submucosa before entering the bladder cavity and being sutured in place. This approach is called a *ureteroneocystostomy.*

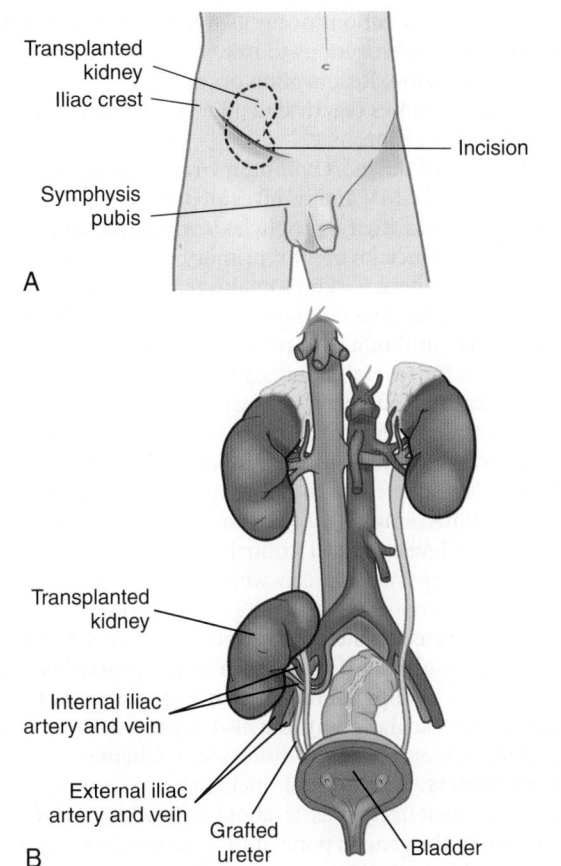

FIG. 49.16 **A,** Surgical incision for a renal transplantation. **B,** Surgical placement of a transplanted kidney.

This approach allows the bladder wall to compress the ureter as it contracts for micturition, thereby preventing reflux of urine up the ureter into the transplanted kidney. The transplantation surgery takes approximately 3 to 4 hours.

NURSING MANAGEMENT
KIDNEY TRANSPLANT RECIPIENT

The successful recovery and rehabilitation of the recipient are made possible with careful nursing assessment, diagnosis, intervention, and evaluation of all body systems. With a length of hospital stay averaging 4 to 5 days, discharge planning and teaching needs must be identified and addressed early in the hospital course.

PREOPERATIVE CARE

Nursing care of the patient in the preoperative phase includes emotional and physical preparation for surgery. Because the patient and the family may have been waiting years for the kidney transplantation, a review of the operative procedure and what can be expected in the immediate postoperative recovery period is necessary. It is important to stress that there is a chance the kidney may not function immediately and that dialysis may be required for days to weeks. The need for immunosuppressive medications and measures to prevent infection must be reviewed.

To ensure the patient is in optimal physical condition for surgery, an ECG, chest radiograph, and laboratory studies are ordered. Dialysis may be required before surgery for any

significant abnormality such as fluid overload or hyperkalemia. A patient on PD must empty the peritoneal cavity of all dialysate solution before going to surgery. Because dialysis may be required after transplantation, the patency of the vascular access must be maintained. The vascular access extremity should be labelled "dialysis access, no procedures" to prevent use of the affected extremity for BP measurement, blood drawing, or IV infusions.

POSTOPERATIVE CARE

LIVING DONOR. The usual postoperative care for the donor is similar to that following conventional or laparoscopic nephrectomy (see Chapter 48). Close monitoring of renal function, to assess for impairment, and of the hemoglobin, to assess for bleeding, is essential. The creatinine should be less than 124 mcmol/L, and the hemoglobin should be stable. The pain experienced by a donor who had a conventional nephrectomy is greater than that of the donor who had a laparoscopic procedure. Generally, donors experience more pain than the recipients. Conventional donors are ready to be discharged from the hospital in 4 to 7 days and can usually return to work in 6 to 8 weeks. Laparoscopic donors are able to be discharged from hospital in 2 to 4 days and can return to work in 4 to 6 weeks. The donor is seen by the surgeon 1 to 2 weeks after discharge.

Nurses caring for the living donor need to acknowledge the precious gift that this person has given. The donor has taken physical, emotional, and financial risks to assist the recipient. It is vital that this individual not be forgotten after surgery. The donor will need even greater support if the donated organ either does not work immediately or, for some reason, fails.

KIDNEY TRANSPLANT RECIPIENT. The first priority during this period is maintenance of fluid and electrolyte balance. In some centres, kidney transplant recipients spend the first 12 to 24 hours in the CCU because of the close monitoring required. Very large volumes of urine may be produced soon after the blood supply to the transplanted kidney is re-established. This diuresis is due to (1) the new kidney's ability to filter BUN, which acts as an osmotic diuretic; (2) the abundance of fluids administered during the operation; and (3) initial renal tubular dysfunction, which inhibits the kidney from concentrating urine normally. Urine output during this phase may be as high as 1 L/hr and gradually decreases as the BUN and creatinine levels become more normal. Urine output is replaced, millilitre for millilitre, hourly for the first 12 to 24 hours. Central venous pressure readings are essential for monitoring postoperative fluid status. Dehydration must be prevented to prevent subsequent renal hypoperfusion and renal tubular damage. Electrolyte monitoring is critical to assess for the hyponatremia and hypokalemia often associated with rapid diuresis. Treatment with potassium supplements or 0.9% normal saline solution infusion may be indicated. IV sodium bicarbonate may also be required if the patient becomes acidotic.

ATN is becoming more common because of prolonged cold times and the use of marginal deceased donors (those who are medically suboptimal)—the ischemic damage from extended cold times causes ATN. While ATN is present, dialysis may be required to maintain fluid and electrolyte balance. If high-output ATN is present, the ability to excrete fluid is intact, but not the ability to regulate metabolic wastes or electrolytes. If oliguric or anuric ATN is present, there is risk for fluid overload in the immediate postoperative period, and the patient must be assessed closely for the need for dialysis. The period of ATN can last anywhere from days to weeks, with gradually improving kidney function. Most patients experiencing ATN will be discharged from the hospital on dialysis. This can be extremely discouraging for the patient, who will need reassurance that renal function usually improves. Dialysis will be discontinued when urine output increases and kidney function begins to normalize.

A sudden decrease in urine output in the early postoperative period is a cause for concern. It may be due to dehydration, rejection, a urine leak, or obstruction. A common cause of early obstruction is a blood clot in the urinary catheter. Catheter patency must be maintained because the catheter remains in the bladder for 3 to 5 days to allow the bladder anastomosis to heal. If blood clots are suspected, gentle catheter irrigation with an order from the health care provider can re-establish patency.

Postoperative teaching should include the prevention and treatment of rejection, infection, and complications of surgery and the purpose and adverse effects of immunosuppression (Lonargáin et al., 2017). Frequent blood tests and clinic visits can help in detecting rejection early. Patient education to ensure a smooth transition from hospital to home is an integral part of nursing care.

Immunosuppressive Therapy

The goal of immunosuppression is to adequately suppress the immune response to prevent rejection of the transplanted kidney while maintaining sufficient immunity to prevent overwhelming infection. Immunosuppressive therapy is discussed in Chapter 16 and in Table 16.16).

Complications of Transplantation

Rejection. Rejection is one of the major concerns following kidney transplantation. Rejection can be hyperacute or acute or chronic. (These types of rejection are discussed in Chapter 16.) Prevention and early diagnosis of rejection is essential for long-term graft function.

Infection. Infection remains a significant cause of morbidity and mortality after transplantation. The transplant recipient is at risk for infection because of suppression of the body's normal defence mechanisms by surgery, immunosuppressive medications, and the effects of ESRD. Underlying systemic illness such as diabetes mellitus or systemic lupus erythematosus, malnutrition, and advanced age can further compound the negative effects on the immune response (Cajanding, 2018). At times, the signs and symptoms of infection can be subtle. Nurses caring for transplant recipients must be astute in their observations and assessment because prompt diagnosis and treatment of infections will improve patient outcomes.

The most common infections observed in the first month after transplantation are similar to those acquired by any postoperative patient, such as pneumonia, wound infections, IV line and drain infections, and urinary tract infections. Fungal and viral infections are not uncommon because of the patient's immunosuppressed state. Fungal infections can include *Candida, Cryptococcus, Aspergillus,* and *Pneumocystis jiroveci.* Fungal infections are difficult to treat, require prolonged treatment periods, and often involve the administration of nephrotoxic medications. Transplant recipients usually receive prophylactic antifungal medications to prevent these infections, such as nystatin, fluconazole (Diflucan), and sulphamethoxazole-trimethoprim.

Viral infections, including CMV, Epstein-Barr virus, herpes simplex virus (HSV), varicella-zoster virus, and polyomavirus (e.g., BK virus) can be primary or reactivation of existing disease. Primary infections occur as new infections after transplantation from an exogenous source, such as the donated organ or blood transfusion. Reactivation occurs when a virus exists in a patient and becomes reactivated after transplantation because of immunosuppression.

CMV is one of the most common viral infections. If a recipient has never had CMV and receives an organ from a donor with a history of CMV, antiviral prophylaxis will be administered (IV ganciclovir, valganciclovir). If a primary active CMV infection is diagnosed or there is symptomatic reactivation of CMV, IV ganciclovir will be given along with an immune globulin that contains CMV antibodies. To prevent HSV infections, oral acyclovir is given for several months after the transplantation.

Cardiovascular Disease. Transplant recipients have an increased incidence of atherosclerotic vascular disease; cardiovascular disease is the leading cause of death after renal transplantation (Kang et al., 2019). Hypertension, dyslipidemia, diabetes mellitus, smoking, rejection, infections, and increased homocysteine levels can all contribute to cardiovascular disease. Immunosuppressants can worsen hypertension and dyslipidemia. It is important that the patient be taught to control risk factors such as elevated cholesterol, triglycerides, and blood glucose and weight gain. Adherence to the prescribed antihypertensive and dyslipidemia regimen is essential not only to prevent cardiovascular events but also to prevent damage to the new kidney. (Hypertension is discussed in Chapter 35.)

Malignancies. The overall incidence of malignancies in kidney transplant recipients is about 6%, which is 100 times greater than in the general population. The primary cause of this increased incidence is the immunosuppressive therapy. Not only do immunosuppressants suppress the immune system, but they also suppress the ability to fight infection and the production of abnormal cells, such as cancer cells. The malignancies include cancers of the skin, lips, kidney, hepatobiliary system, vulva, and perineum; lymphomas; and Kaposi's sarcoma and other sarcomas. Regular screening for cancer is an important part of the transplant recipient's preventive care. The patient must also be advised to avoid sun exposure by using protective clothing and sunscreens to minimize the incidence of skin cancers and to check the skin regularly and report any suspicious lesions.

Recurrence of Original Renal Disease. Recurrence of the original disease that destroyed the native kidneys occurs in some kidney transplant recipients. It is most common with certain types of glomerulonephritis, immunoglobulin A nephropathy, diabetes mellitus, and focal segmental sclerosis. Disease recurrence can result in loss of a functioning kidney transplant. Patients must be advised before transplantation if they have a disease known to recur.

Corticosteroid-Related Complications. Aseptic necrosis of the hips, knees, and other joints can result from chronic corticosteroid therapy and renal osteodystrophy. Most transplant recipients receive calcium supplements, vitamin D, and bisphosphonates in an effort to prevent or minimize the bone disorders associated with corticosteroid use. Patient teaching should include the importance of regular bone mineral density testing, weight-bearing exercise, smoking cessation, and limiting alcohol consumption. Other significant adverse effects related to corticosteroids include peptic ulcer disease, glucose intolerance and diabetes, cataracts, dyslipidemia, and an increased incidence of infections and malignancies. In the first year after transplantation, corticosteroid doses are usually decreased to 5 to 10 mg a day. The use of tacrolimus and cyclosporin has allowed for corticosteroid doses to be much lower than they were in the past. Some patients have been successfully withdrawn from corticosteroids 1.5 to 2 years after transplantation, thus eliminating these effects. Vigilant monitoring for adverse effects of corticosteroids and early treatment are essential.

AGE-RELATED CONSIDERATIONS

CHRONIC KIDNEY DISEASE

The incidence of stage 5 CKD in Canada is increasing most rapidly in older patients. At the end of 2018, 40 289 Canadians were living with stage 5 CKD. More than half (54%) of newly diagnosed patients with CKD were 65 years of age or older (CIHI, 2019). The most common diseases leading to renal failure in older persons are diabetes and hypertension. HD is the predominant RRT for older patients starting dialysis. The average age of patients receiving a kidney transplant was 56 years, and 45.3% pf patients were age 60 and older. Expenditures can be expected to increase as the CKD-affected population ages and has a correspondingly greater number of comorbid conditions.

The care of the older person with CKD is particularly challenging, not only because of the normal physiological changes of aging that occur but also because of the number of comorbid conditions that develop. Physiological changes of clinical importance in the older patient with CKD include diminished cardiopulmonary function, bone loss, immunodeficiency, altered protein synthesis, impaired cognition, and altered medication metabolism. Malnutrition is common in the older patient with CKD for a variety of reasons, including lack of mobility, lack of understanding of basic nutritional requirements, social isolation, physical disability, impaired cognitive function, and malabsorption disorders (Balogun et al., 2017).

The older patient needs to consider the best option for treatment modality based on their health, personal preferences, and the support available. Home PD allows the patient to be more mobile and to enjoy an increased sense of control over the illness. PD causes less hemodynamic instability than HD but does require self-care or assistance from another person. The older person may not have adequate help in the home to provide assistance. Establishing vascular access for HD may be difficult in an older patient because of atherosclerotic changes. Travel to and from the HD unit may also be problematic if the patient does not drive or have access to reliable public transportation. Although transplantation is an option, older patients must be carefully screened to ensure that the benefits outweigh the risks. A living donor is preferable so that there is not a prolonged waiting time.

The most common cause of death in the older patient with CKD is cardiovascular disease (myocardial infarction, stroke), followed by withdrawal from dialysis. If a competent patient decides to withdraw from dialysis, it is essential to support the patient and the family. Ethical issues (see the Ethical Dilemmas box) to be considered in this situation include patient competency, benefit versus burden of treatment, and futility of treatment. Withdrawal from treatment is not a failure if the patient is well informed and comfortable with the decision.

The increasing number of debilitated older patients with CKD receiving dialysis has raised a number of ethical concerns about the use of scarce resources in a population with a limited life expectancy. Substantial evidence exists showing success of dialysis (especially PD) in older people. Quality of life has also been reported to be good to excellent in many older patients with CKD. There appears to be no justification for excluding older persons from dialysis programs. Rationing dialysis on the basis of age alone is not supported based on current outcome and quality-of-life data.

ETHICAL DILEMMAS
Withdrawing Treatment

Situation

A 70-year-old (pronouns he/him) with diabetes mellitus and chronic renal failure who has been receiving dialysis for 10 years tells the nurse that he wants to discontinue his dialysis. His quality of life has diminished during the past 2 years since his wife died. He is not a prospective transplantation patient.

Important Points for Consideration

- Quality of life is an important consideration for patients when evaluating whether to begin or discontinue treatment.
- Quality-of-life decisions often involve weighing the benefit of treatment against the burden of treatment. When a treatment becomes too burdensome, the patient (if competent) may request to withdraw the treatment.
- A determination must be made as to whether there is some other treatable condition, such as depression, that may be clouding the patient's judgement.
- Patient autonomy, or the patient's right to self-determination regarding treatment decisions, applies to both initiating and discontinuing treatment.
- If a decision is made to withdraw treatment, the health care team, the patient, and the family should develop an appropriate follow-up plan that includes palliative care and hospice support.

Clinical Decision-Making Questions

1. How should the nurse respond to the patient's request?
2. What is the position of the Canadian Nurses Association (CNA) on withdrawing or withholding treatment that no longer benefits the patient or causes suffering?

CASE STUDY
Chronic Kidney Disease

Patient Profile

N. B. (pronouns they/them), a 42-year-old school teacher, has been treated for type 2 diabetes mellitus since the age of 25. N. B.'s nephrologist has observed the patient for the past several years for manifestations of progressive chronic kidney disease. Eight weeks ago, N. B. had an arteriovenous fistula created in preparation for starting hemodialysis. Over the past week, they have experienced anorexia, nausea, vomiting, difficulties with concentration, and pruritus.

Subjective Data

- Complains of swelling in feet and hands
- Has gained 4.5 kg in the past 2 weeks
- Complains of dyspnea and weakness when walking

Continued

CASE STUDY

Chronic Kidney Disease—cont'd

Objective Data
Laboratory Data
- Estimated glomerular filtration rate (eGFR): 8.0 mL/min/1.73 m²
- Serum creatinine: 560 mmol/L
- Blood urea nitrogen (BUN): 32 mmol/L
- Potassium: 6 mmol/L
- Hemoglobin: 95 g/L

Chest Radiograph
- Pulmonary edema

Discussion Questions
1. Explain the basic pathophysiological changes that resulted in the development of N. B.'s diabetic nephropathy.
2. What are the indications for dialysis in this patient?

3. Identify the abnormal diagnostic study results, and explain why each would occur.
4. Explain why N. B. developed each of the clinical manifestations they experience.
5. *Priority decision:* What are the priority nursing interventions for N. B. and this patient's family?
6. *Priority decision:* Based on the assessment data provided, what are the priority nursing diagnoses? Are there any interprofessional issues?

℮volve
Answers are available at http://evolve.elsevier.com/Canada/Lewis/medsurg.

REVIEW QUESTIONS

The number of the question corresponds to the same-numbered objective at the beginning of the chapter.

1. Which of the following characterizes acute kidney injury? *(Select all that apply.)*
   a. The primary cause of death is infection.
   b. There is an abrupt decline in kidney function with a rise in serum creatinine.
   c. The disease course is potentially reversible.
   d. Cardiovascular disease is the most common cause of death.
2. The RIFLE criteria define three stages of AKI based on changes in which of the following?
   a. Blood pressure (BP) and urine osmolality
   b. Urine output and urinary creatinine
   c. Fractional excretion of urinary sodium and glomerular filtration rate (GFR)
   d. Baseline serum creatinine and urine output
3. In the oliguric phase of acute kidney injury (AKI), for which symptoms does the nurse monitor the client?
   a. Hypotension
   b. Pulmonary edema
   c. Hypernatremia
   d. Hypokalemia
4. The nurse monitors the client in the diuretic phase of AKI for which serum electrolyte imbalances?
   a. Hyperkalemia and hyponatremia
   b. Hyperkalemia and hypernatremia
   c. Hypokalemia and hyponatremia
   d. Hypokalemia and hypernatremia
5. Which systemic effect best characterizes chronic kidney disease (CKD)?
   a. Progressive irreversible damage of the kidneys
   b. Rapid decrease in urinary output with an elevated blood urea nitrogen (BUN)
   c. Progressive increase in creatinine clearance
   d. Rapid rise in serum creatinine from baseline
6. Nurses need to educate clients at risk for developing CKD. Which of the following individuals are considered to be at increased risk? *(Select all that apply.)*
   a. Older Canadians who are Black
   b. People who are older than age 60 years
   c. Clients with a history of pancreatitis
   d. Individuals with obesity

7. Clients with CKD experience an increased incidence of cardiovascular disease related to which of the following? *(Select all that apply.)*
   a. Vascular calcification
   b. Genetic predisposition
   c. Hypertension
   d. Increased high-density lipoproteins
8. Clients with CKD stages 3–4 require an interprofessional approach to care that focuses on delaying the progression of CKD by which of the following?
   a. Educating clients and caregivers about BP control
   b. Instructing clients to significantly restrict protein in their diet
   c. Instructing clients that radiocontrast agents are not harmful at this stage of CKD
   d. Educating clients to restrict their sodium intake to 3.5 g/day
9. Which of the following interventions should the nurse undertake to assess the patency of a newly placed arteriovenous graft for dialysis?
   a. Irrigate the graft daily with low-dose heparin.
   b. Monitor for any increase in blood pressure in the affected arm.
   c. Listen with a stethoscope over the graft for the presence of a bruit.
   d. Frequently monitor the pulses and the neurovascular status distal to the graft.
10. Following a kidney transplantation, which signs of rejection would the nurse include in the client education?
   a. Fever, weight loss, increased urinary output, increased blood pressure (BP)
   b. Fever, weight gain, increased urinary output, increased BP
   c. Fever, weight loss, decreased urinary output, decreased BP
   d. Fever, weight gain, decreased urinary output, increased BP

1. a, b, c; 2. d; 3. b; 4. c; 5. a; 6. a, b, d; 7. a, c; 8. a; 9. c; 10. d.

℮volve

For even more review questions, visit http://evolve.elsevier.com/Canada/Lewis/medsurg.

REFERENCES

Balogun, S. A., Balogun, R., Philbrick, J., et al. (2017). Quality of life, perceptions, and health satisfaction of older adults with end-stage renal disease: A systematic review. *Journal of the American Geriatrics Society, 65*(4), 777–785. https://doi.org/10.1111/jgs.14659

Benett, I. (2020). Key learning points: NICE acute kidney injury. *Guidelines in Practice, 23*(2), 20–24.

Blake, P. G. (2020). Global dialysis perspective: Canada. *Kidney 360, 1*(2), 115–118. https://doi.org/10.34067/KID.0000462019

Bonfield, B. (2018). Acute kidney injury: What is it and how can it be prevented? *Practice Nursing, 29*(1), 10–16. https://doi.org/10.12968/pnur.2018.29.1.10

Buena, T., Tregaskis, P., & Elliott, M. (2018). Peritoneal dialysis home visits: A review of timing, frequency and assessment criteria. *Renal Society of Australasia Journal, 14*(2), 70–77.

Cajanding, R. (2018). Immunosuppression following organ transplantation. Part 1: Mechanisms and immunosuppressive agents. *British Journal of Nursing, 27*(16), 920–927. https://doi.org/10.12968/bjon.2018.27.16.920

Canadian Blood Services. (2019). *Professional education.* https://profedu.blood.ca/en/organes-et-tissus/resources

Canadian Institute for Health Information (CIHI). (2019). *Annual statistics on organ replacement in Canada 2009 to 2018.* https://www.cihi.ca/sites/default/files/document/corr-snapshot-2019-en.pdf

Canadian Nurses Association (CNA). (2017). *Code of ethics for registered nurses.* https://hl-prod-ca-oc-download.s3-ca-central-1.amazonaws.com/CNA/2f975e7e-4a40-45ca-863c-5ebf0a138d5e/UploadedImages/documents/Code_of_Ethics_2017_Edition_Secure_Interactive.pdf

Canadian Society of Nephrology. (2018). *Enhancing vascular access education in Canada.* https://www.csnscn.ca/csnva

Chen, T. K., Knicely, D. H., & Grams, M. E. (2019). Chronic kidney disease diagnosis and management: A review. *JAMA: Journal of the American Medical Association, 322*(13), 1294–1304. https://doi.org/10.1001/jama.2019.14745

Cheng, H. W. B., Chan, K. Y., Lau, H. T., et al. (2017). Use of erythropoietin-stimulating agents (ESA) in patients with end-stage renal failure decided to forego dialysis: Palliative perspective. *American Journal of Hospice & Palliative Medicine, 34*(4), 380–384. https://doi.org/10.1177/1049909115624653

Coelho, F. U. D. A., Watanabe, M., Fonseca, C. D. D., et al. (2017). Nursing activities score and acute kidney injury. *Revista Brasileira de Enfermagem, 70*(3), 475–480. https://doi.org/10.1590/0034-7167-2016-0266

Contiero, P. P., & Wilson, D. M. (2019). Understanding ambivalence toward organ donation and transplantation: An exploratory study of nursing students. *Nurse Education Today, 76*, 191–195. https://doi.org/10.1016/j.nedt.2019.02.008

Debus, E. S., & Grundmann, R. T. (2017). *Evidence-Based Therapy in Vascular Surgery.* Springer International Publishing.

Flamant, M., Haymann, J. P., Vidal-Petiot, E., et al. (2012). GFR estimation using the Cockcroft-Gault, MDRD study, and CKD-EPI equations in the elderly. *American Journal of Kidney Diseases, 60*(5), 847–849. https://doi.org/10.1053/j.ajkd.2012.08.001

George, C. (2019). Caring for patients receiving peritoneal dialysis: Part I. *Medsurg Nursing, 28*(4), 227–233.

Gluba-Brzozka, A., Franczyk, B., & Rysz, J. (2019). Cholesterol disturbances and the role of proper nutrition in CKD patients. *Nutrients, 11*(11), 2820. https://doi.org/10.3390/nu11112820

Góes, C. R. de, Balbi, A. L., & Ponce, D. (2018). Evaluation of factors associated with hypermetabolism and hypometabolism in critical-ly ill AKI patients. *Nutrients, 10*(4), 505. https://doi.org/10.3390/nu10040505

Harrois, A., Libert, N., & Duranteau, J. (2017). Acute kidney injury in trauma patients. *Current Opinion in Critical Care, 23*(6), 447–456. https://doi.org/10.1097/MCC.0000000000000463

Houck, K., & Neumann, M. E. (2019). Revised KDOQI guidelines call for matching vascular access type with modality choice, patient goals. *Nephrology News & Issues, 33*(6), 10.

Jovanovich, A., & Kendrick, J. (2018). Personalized management of bone and mineral disorders and precision medicine in end-stage kidney disease. *Seminars in Nephrology, 38*(4), 397–409. https://doi.org/10.1016/j.semnephrol.2018.05.009

Kakani, E., Elyamny, M., Ayach, T., et al. (2019). Pathogenesis and management of vascular calcification in CKD and dialysis patients. *Seminars in Dialysis, 32*(6), 553–561. https://doi.org/10.1111/sdi.12840

Kang, A. W., Garber, C. E., Eaton, C. B., et al. (2019). Physical activity and cardiovascular risk among kidney transplant patients. *Medicine & Science in Sports & Exercise, 51*(6), 1154–1161. https://doi.org/10.1249/MSS.0000000000001886

Kidney Foundation of Canada. (2021). *Living with kidney disease.* https://kidney.ca/Kidney-Health/Living-With-Kidney-Disease

Kritmetapak, K., & Pongchaiyakul, C. (2019). Parathyroid hormone measurement in chronic kidney disease: From basics to clinical implications. *International Journal of Nephrology.* Article No. 5496710, 1–9. https://doi.org/10.1155/2019/5496710

Lee, S. W., Kim, Y.-S., Kim, Y. H., et al. (2019). Dietary protein intake, protein energy wasting, and the progression of chronic kidney disease: Analysis from the KNOW-CKD study. *Nutrients, 11*(1), 121. https://doi.org/10.3390/nu11010121

Levey, A. S., Coresh, J., Bolton, K., et al. (2002). KDOQI clinical practice guidelines for chronic kidney disease: Evaluation, classification and stratification. *American Journal of Kidney Disease, 39*(2) (Suppl 1), S1-S266. (Seminal).

Lonargáin, D. Ó., Brannigan, D., & Murray, C. (2017). The experience of receiving a kidney transplant from a deceased donor: Implications for renal services. *Psychology & Health, 32*(2), 204–220. https://doi.org/10.1080/08870446.2016.1254214

Lopes, M. B., Rocha, P. N., & Pecoits-Filho, R. (2019). Updates on medical management of hyperkalemia. *Current Opinion in Nephrology & Hypertension, 28*(5), 417–423. https://doi.org/10.1097/MNH.0000000000000530

Mercado, M. G., Smith, D. K., & Guard, E. L. (2019). Acute kidney injury: Diagnosis and management. *American Family Physician, 100*(11), 687–694.

Montoya, V. (2017). Advanced practice nurses and end-of-life care for patients with progressive chronic kidney disease and end stage renal disease. *Nephrology Nursing Journal, 44*(3), 256–259.

National Institute of Diabetes and Digestive and Kidney Diseases (NIDDKD). (2021). *Frequently asked questions: eGFR.* https://www.niddk.nih.gov/health-information/professionals/clinical-tools-patient-management/kidney-disease/laboratory-evaluation/frequently-asked-questions

Nerenberg, K. A., Zarnke, K. B., Leung, A. A., et al. (2018). Hypertension Canada's 2018 guidelines for diagnosis, risk assessment, prevention, and treatment of hypertension in adults and children. *Canadian Journal of Cardiology, 34*(5), 506–525. https://doi.org/10.1016/j.cjca.2018.02.022

Norton, J. M., Narva, A. S., Newman, E. P., et al. (2017). Improving outcomes for patients with chronic kidney disease: Part 1. *AJN American Journal of Nursing, 117*(2), 22–33. https://doi.org/10.1097/01.NAJ.0000512272.33956.8b

Palaka, E., Leonard, S., Buchanan, H. A., et al. (2018). Evidence in support of hyperkalaemia management strategies: A systematic literature review. *International Journal of Clinical Practice, 72*(2):e13052. https://doi.org/10.1111/ijcp.13052

Poh, W.-Y., Omar, M. S., & Tan, H.-P. (2018). Predictive factors for contrast-induced acute kidney injury in high-risk patients given N-acetylcysteine prophylaxis. *Annals of Saudi Medicine, 38*(4), 269–276. https://doi.org/10.5144/0256-4947.2018.269

Provenzano, M., Coppolino, G., Faga, T., et al. (2019). Epidemiology of cardiovascular risk in chronic kidney disease patients: The real silent killer. *Reviews in Cardiovascular Medicine, 20*(4), 209–220. https://doi.org/10.31083/j.rcm.2019.04.548

Ptáčník, V., Zogala, D., Skibová, D., et al. (2019). Assessment of renal function before contrast media injection: right decisions based on inaccurate estimates. *European Radiology, 29*(6), 3192–3199. https://doi.org/10.1007/s00330-018-5753-z

Rainey, H. (2019). Preventing complications and managing symptoms of CKD. *Practice Nursing, 30*(6), 276–281. https://doi.org/10.12968/pnur.2019.30.6.276

Renjen, P. N., Chaudhari, D., Sagar, G., et al. (2018). Neurology of renal disorders. *Neurology India, 66*(1), 163–167. https://doi.org/10.4103/0028-3886.222815

Schell-Chaple, H. (2017). Continuous renal replacement therapies: Raising the bar for quality care. *AACN Advanced Critical Care, 28*(1), 28–40. https://doi.org/10.4037/aacnacc2017235

Skube, S. J., Katz, S. A., Chipman, J. G., et al. (2018). Acute kidney injury and sepsis. *Surgical Infections, 19*(2), 216–224. https://doi.org/10.1089/sur.2017.261

Stevens, A., & Lowe, J. (2000). *Pathology: Illustrated review in color* (2nd ed.). Mosby. (Seminal).

Steward, C. (2019). Dialysis disequilibrium syndrome in the neurointensive care unit: A case study. *Nephrology Nursing Journal, 46*(6), 597–603.

Thomas, D. A., Huang, A., McCarron, M. C. E., et al. (2017). A retrospective study of chronic kidney disease burden in Saskatchewan's First Nations People. *Canadian Journal of Kidney Health and Disease, 5*, 1-13. https://doi.org/10.1177.2054538118799689

Ülger, F., Küçük, M. P., Küçük, A. O., et al. (2018). Evaluation of acute kidney injury (AKI) with RIFLE, AKIN, CK, and KDIGO in critically ill trauma patients. *European Journal of Trauma & Emergency Surgery, 44*(4), 597–605. https://doi.org/10.1007/s00068-017-0820-8

Williams, L. (2014). Take aim at acute kidney injury with RIFLE criteria. *Nursing, 44*(7), 50–55. (Seminal). https://doi.org/10.1097/01.NURSE.0000445730.84886.88

RESOURCES

Canadian Association of Nephrology Nurses and Technologists (CANNT)
https://cannt-acitn.ca/
Canadian Institute for Health Information
https://www.cihi.ca
Canadian Organ Replacement Register (CORR)
https://www.cihi.ca/en/canadian-organ-replacement-register-corr
Canadian Society of Nephrology (CSN)
https://www.csnscn.ca/
Hypertension Canada
https://www.hypertension.ca/
Kidney Foundation of Canada
https://www.kidney.ca/

International Society of Nephrology (ISN)
https://www.theisn.org/
International Transplant Nurses Society
https://www.itns.org
National Kidney Foundation
https://www.kidney.org
National Kidney Foundation—*Calculators for Health Care Professionals: eGFR Calculator*
https://www.kidney.org/professionals/kdoqi/gfr_calculator.cfm
RenalWEB Patient Education
http://www.renalweb.com/topics/patiented/patiented.htm
United Network for Organ Sharing (UNOS)
https://www.unos.org

evolve

For additional Internet resources, see the website for this book at http://evolve.elsevier.com/Canada/Lewis/medsurg.

Conditions Related to Regulatory and Reproductive Mechanisms

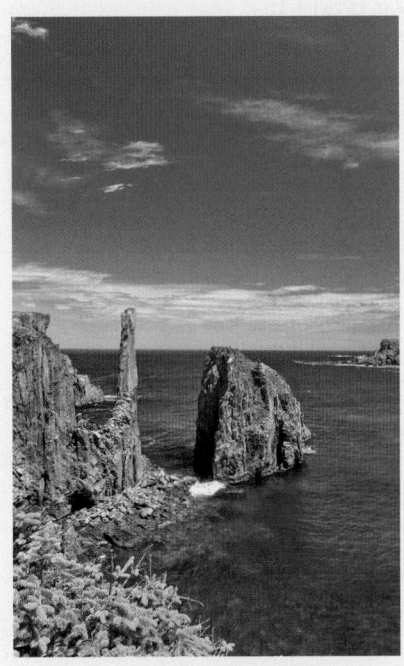

Source: © CanStock Photo / fmcginn

50

Nursing Assessment
Endocrine System

Renée Gordon
Originating US chapter by Julia A. Hitch

---

evolve WEBSITE

http://evolve.elsevier.com/Canada/Lewis/medsurg

- Review Questions (Online Only)
- Key Points
- Answer Guidelines for Case Study
- Conceptual Care Map Creator
- Audio Glossary
- Content Updates

LEARNING OBJECTIVES

1. Describe common characteristics and functions of hormones.
2. Identify endocrine gland locations.
3. Describe functions of hormones secreted by the pituitary, thyroid, parathyroid, pancreas, and adrenal glands.
4. Describe locations and roles of hormone receptors.
5. Identify significant subjective and objective assessment data related to the endocrine system.
6. Link age-related endocrine system changes to differences in assessment findings.
7. Differentiate normal from abnormal physical assessment findings of the endocrine system.
8. Describe the purpose, significance, and nursing responsibilities related to diagnostic studies of the endocrine system.

KEY TERMS

aldosterone	glucagon	thyroxine (T_4)
antidiuretic hormone (ADH)	hormones	triiodothyronine (T_3)
catecholamines	insulin	tropic hormones
corticosteroid	negative feedback	
cortisol	positive feedback	

The endocrine, nervous, and immune systems are some of the most critical communicating and coordinating systems in the body. These systems interconnect through bidirectional immune–neuroendocrine communication to regulate bodily responses to internal and external environments (Manley et al., 2018). The nervous system controls the body's activities by communicating through *nerve impulses*; the endocrine system regulates these activities by communicating through *hormones*; and when triggered, the immune system further modulates these activities by communicating through *cytokines* (Hannon & Porth, 2017). The nervous, endocrine, and immune systems are not the only organ systems which communicate. For example, the gastrointestinal (GI) microbiome communicates bidirectionally with the central nervous system (CNS) through the brain–gut–microbiome axis (Martin et al., 2018).

The endocrine system has five general functions: a role in reproductive and CNS development in the fetus, stimulating growth and development during childhood and adolescence, sexual reproduction, maintaining homeostasis, and responding to emergency demands (Brashers et al., 2018). The endocrine system includes the hypothalamus, pituitary, thyroid, parathyroids, thymus, adrenals, pancreas, ovaries, testes, and pineal gland (Figure 50.1).

Adipose tissue is considered an endocrine organ, producing and secreting adipokines and adipocytokines (adiponectin and leptin hormones) (Booth et al., 2016). In healthy states, white and brown adipose tissues maintain metabolic homeostasis (Booth et al., 2016). In obesity, hypertrophic adipocytes and adipose tissue–resident immune cells accelerate a chronic, pro-inflammatory profile with altered secretion of adipokines and lipokines, thereby exacerbating cardiometabolic disease (Booth et al., 2016) (see Chapter 52).

In addition to endocrine glands, other body organs secrete hormones. For example, the kidneys secrete erythropoietin

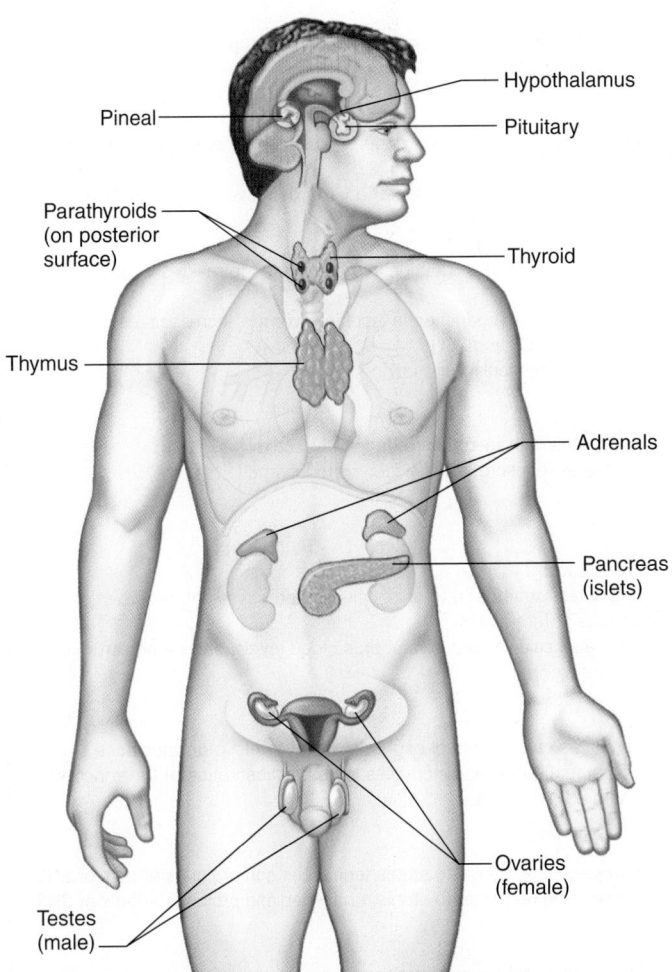

FIG. 50.1 Locations of some major endocrine glands. Source: Patton, K. (2019). *Anatomy and physiology* (10th ed., Figure 25-2). Elsevier.

Pineal
Hypothalamus
Pituitary
Parathyroids (on posterior surface)
Thyroid
Thymus
Adrenals
Pancreas (islets)
Ovaries (female)
Testes (male)

and renin, the heart secretes natriuretic peptides, bone secretes osteocalcin, and the GI tract secretes numerous peptide hormones (e.g., gastrin). These hormones are discussed in their respective assessment chapters.

STRUCTURES AND FUNCTIONS OF THE ENDOCRINE SYSTEM

Glands

Organs of the endocrine system, referred to as *glands*, produce hormones which control and regulate specific target tissues. A *target tissue* is body tissue or an organ on which the hormone has its effect (Brashers et al., 2018). For example, the thyroid (gland) synthesizes thyroxine (hormone), which affects many body tissues (target tissue). There are two types of glands. *Exocrine glands* secrete substances into ducts that empty into a body cavity or onto a surface (e.g., skin) (Betts et al., 2019). For example, salivary glands produce saliva, secreted through salivary ducts into the mouth. *Endocrine glands,* in contrast, are ductless and secrete substances directly into the blood (Betts et al., 2019). For example, the adrenal glands produce epinephrine and norepinephrine and release these chemicals into the bloodstream to regulate the body's response to stress.

Hormones

Classifications and Functions. Hormones are chemical substances synthesized and secreted by endocrine glands. Many are made in one part of the body and control and regulate distinct cells or organs in another part of the body, referred to as *endocrine action* or *signalling* (Brashers et al., 2018). Some hormones act locally on nearby cells; this is known as *paracrine* action, such as the action of sex steroids on the ovary (Hannon & Porth, 2017). A hormone may also act on the same cell that produced it; this is called *autocrine action*. For example, insulin secretion from pancreatic β cells can inhibit further insulin release from the same cells (Hannon & Porth, 2017). Most hormones have common characteristics, including secretion in small amounts at variable but predictable rates, regulation by feedback systems, and the ability to bind to specific target cell receptors (Brashers et al., 2018).

Hormones control a number of physiological activities, including reproduction, response to stress and injury, electrolyte balance, energy metabolism, growth, maturation, and aging. Hormones also play a role in regulating the nervous and immune systems (Manley et al., 2018). Catecholamines are hormones when secreted by the adrenal medulla but act as neurotransmitters when secreted by nerve cells in the brain and peripheral nervous system (Barnes et al., 2015). When the immune–neuroendocrine network is activated, numerous hormones are secreted in response, which affects many body systems and leads to corresponding changes in immune cell activity (Chapter 8 discusses this in greater detail). Hormones can also influence behaviour. For example, hypothyroidism can cause emotional lability and is responsible for depressive symptoms in 60% of cases (Talaei et al., 2017). Elevated cortisol levels contribute to depression, post-traumatic stress disorder, and anxiety (Glad et al., 2017).

Table 50.1 summarizes the major hormones and glands, tissues from which they are synthesized, target organs or tissues, and functions.

Hormones can be either endogenous or exogenous. *Endogenous* hormones are produced within the body, whereas *exogenous* hormones are introduced to the body from outside and may be of natural (e.g., plant-based *phytoestrogen*s) or synthetic origin (e.g., synthetic estrogen used in hormone replacement therapy and oral contraceptives) (Betts et al., 2019). Debate regarding the safety of long-term exposure to some exogenous hormones is ongoing, as a link to the development of chronic illness (e.g., cardiovascular disease and cancer) may exist (Hannon & Porth, 2017; McCance et al., 2018; Rosenthal & Hembree, 2018).

Hormone Transport. Hormones are classified by chemical structure as either lipid-soluble or water-soluble. *Lipid-soluble* hormones (steroids, thyroid) are bound to plasma proteins as they travel to target cells, crossing the cell membrane by diffusion (Brashers et al., 2018). *Water-soluble* protein (peptide) hormones (insulin, growth hormone, and prolactin) circulate freely in the blood and act directly on target tissues (Brashers et al., 2018).

Hormone Receptors. Hormones exert their effects by recognizing their target tissues and attaching to receptor sites in a "lock-and-key" type of mechanism. This means a hormone will act only on cells that have a receptor specific for that hormone (Figure 50.2).

Regulation of Hormonal Secretion. Specific mechanisms regulate endocrine activity by stimulating or inhibiting hormone

TABLE 50.1   MAJOR ENDOCRINE GLANDS AND HORMONES

Hormones	Target Tissue	Functions
Anterior Pituitary (Adenohypophysis)		
Growth hormone (GH) or somatotropin	All body cells	Promotes protein anabolism (growth, tissue repair) and lipid mobilization and catabolism
Thyroid-stimulating hormone (TSH) or thyrotropin	Thyroid gland	Stimulates synthesis and release of thyroid hormones, growth and function of thyroid gland
Adrenocorticotrophic hormone (ACTH)	Adrenal cortex	Fosters growth of adrenal cortex; stimulates secretion of corticosteroids
Gonadotropic hormones • Follicle-stimulating hormone (FSH) • Luteinizing hormone (LH)*	Reproductive organs	Stimulates sex hormone secretion, reproductive organ growth, reproductive processes
Melanocyte-stimulating hormone (MSH)	Melanocytes in skin	Increases melanin production in melanocytes to make skin darker in colour
Prolactin	Ovary and mammary glands in girls and women	Stimulates milk production in lactating women; increases response of follicles to LH and FSH
	Testes in men	Stimulates testicular function in men
Posterior Pituitary (Neurohypophysis)		
Oxytocin	Uterus; mammary glands	Stimulates milk secretion, uterine contractility
Antidiuretic hormone (ADH; vasopressin)	Renal tubules, vascular smooth muscle	Promotes reabsorption of water, vasoconstriction
Thyroid		
Thyroxine (T_4)	All body tissues	Precursor to T_3
Triiodothyronine (T_3)	All body tissues	Regulates metabolic rate of all cells and processes of cell growth and tissue differentiation
Calcitonin	Bone tissue	Regulates calcium and phosphorus blood levels; decreases serum Ca^{2+} levels
Parathyroids		
Parathyroid hormone (PTH), or parathormone	Bone, intestine, kidney tissues	Regulates calcium and phosphorus blood levels; promotes bone demineralization and increases intestinal absorption of Ca^{2+}; increases serum Ca^{2+} levels
Adrenal Medulla		
Epinephrine (adrenaline)	Sympathetic effectors	Increases in response to stress; enhances and prolongs effects of SNS
Norepinephrine (noradrenaline)	Sympathetic effectors	Increases in response to stress; enhances and prolongs effects of SNS
Adrenal Cortex		
Corticosteroids (e.g., cortisol, hydrocortisone)	All body tissues	Promotes metabolism, response to stress; anti-inflammatory
Androgens (e.g., dehydroepiandrosterone [DHEA], androsterone, and estradiol)	Reproductive organs	Promotes masculinization in men, growth and sexual activity in women
Mineralocorticoids (e.g., aldosterone)	Kidney	Regulates sodium and potassium balance and thus water balance
Pancreas (Islets of Langerhans)		
Insulin (from β cells)	General	Promotes movement of glucose out of blood and into cells
Amylin (from β cells)	Liver, stomach	Decreases gastric motility, glucagon secretion, and endogenous glucose release from liver; increases satiety
Glucagon (from α cells)	General	Stimulates glycogenolysis and gluconeogenesis
Somatostatin	Pancreas	Inhibits insulin and glucagon secretion
Pancreatic polypeptide	General	Influences regulation of pancreatic exocrine function and metabolism of absorbed nutrients
Gonads		
Women: Ovaries		
Estrogen	Reproductive system, breasts	Stimulates development of secondary sex characteristics, preparation of uterus for fertilization, and fetal development; stimulates bone growth
Progesterone	Reproductive system	Maintains lining of uterus necessary for successful pregnancy
Men: Testes		
Testosterone	Reproductive system	Stimulates development of secondary sex characteristics, spermatogenesis

SNS, sympathetic nervous system.

*In men, sometimes referred to as interstitial cell-stimulating hormone (ICSH).

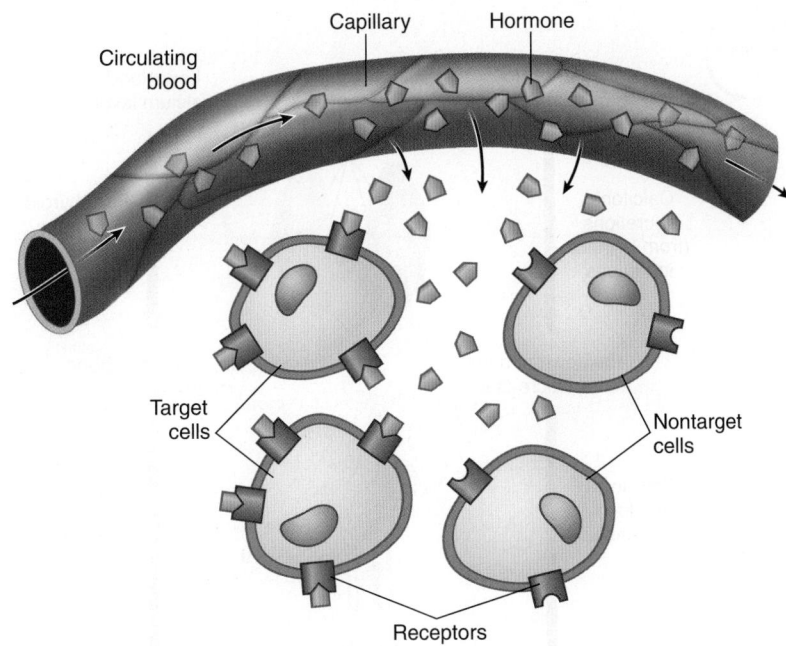

FIG. 50.2 The target cell concept. A hormone acts only on cells that have receptors specific to that hormone. The shape of the receptor determines which hormone can react with it. This is an example of the lock-and-key model of biochemical reactions. Source: Patton, K. (2019). *Anatomy and physiology* (10th ed., Figure 25-7). Elsevier.

synthesis and secretion. These include positive and negative feedback, nervous system control, and physiological rhythms (Hannon & Porth, 2017).

Feedback Regulation. The regulation of blood hormone levels depends on a highly specialized mechanism called *feedback*. Feedback is based on the blood level of a substance. The substance may be a hormone, or another chemical compound regulated by or responsive to a hormone (e.g., glucose). In nega-tive feedback, the most common feedback system, the gland responds by increasing or decreasing the secretion of a hormone (Brashers et al., 2018). Negative feedback functions like a thermostat (Hannon & Porth, 2017)—cold air activates the thermostat to release heat and warm air turns off the thermostat to prevent more hot air from entering the room. An example of negative feedback is the relationship between calcium and parathyroid hormone (PTH). Low blood levels of calcium stimulate the parathyroid gland to release PTH, which acts on bone, intestines, and kidneys to increase blood calcium levels. The increased blood calcium levels then inhibit further PTH release (Figure 50.3).

Positive feedback increases the target organ action, causing another gland to release a hormone that then stimulates further release of the first hormone (Brashers et al., 2018). Something must stop the release of the first hormone or its release will continue. The action of oxytocin during childbirth is an example. The hormone oxytocin from the posterior pituitary stimulates and increases uterine contractions. The release of oxytocin is stimulated by pressure receptors in the vagina. As the fetus enters the vagina during childbirth, the receptors sense increased pressure and signal the brain to release more oxyto-cin. Oxytocin release leads to stronger uterine contractions. When birth is finished, the stimulus to the pressure receptors in the vagina ends, and thus oxytocin secretion decreases.

Exogenous hormones may influence normal feedback mech-anisms for hormone production and release (Hannon & Porth,

2017). For example, exogenous corticosteroids may suppress the intrinsic body systems that regulate the production of these hormones.

Nervous System Control. Nervous system activity directly affects endocrine glands (Molina, 2018). Pain, emotion, sexual excitement, and stress can stimulate the nervous system to mod-ulate hormone secretion. For example, when the CNS senses or perceives stress, the sympathetic nervous system (SNS) secretes catecholamines (e.g., epinephrine), which maximize heart and lung function and vision to respond to the stress more effec-tively. Chronic exposure to some stressors can cause persistent increases in heart rate and blood pressure and changes in the endocrine system, putting individuals at risk for chronic dis-ease, such as hypertension and heart disease. Stress-related effects are discussed in Chapter 8.

Rhythms. Another regulatory mechanism affecting many hormonal secretions is the rhythm of secretions originating in the brain. A common physiological rhythm is the *circadian rhythm,* in which hormone levels fluctuate predictably over a 24-hour period based on either sleep–wake or dark–light (*diur-nal*) cycles. For example, cortisol levels typically rise early in the day, decline toward evening, and rise again toward the end of sleep to peak by morning (Figure 50.4). Growth hormone, thyroid-stimulating hormone (TSH), and prolactin levels peak during sleep. Disruption of the circadian rhythms can cause fatigue, disorientation, changes in hormone levels, and elevated mortality (Molina, 2018). Reproductive cycles are often longer than 24 hours (*ultradian*) (Rosen & Cedars, 2018). An example is the menstrual cycle. These rhythms are important to consider when interpreting laboratory results for hormone levels.

Hypothalamus

Although the pituitary has been referred to as the "master gland" of the endocrine system, most of its functions rely on an interre-lationship with the hypothalamus, which lies next to the pituitary

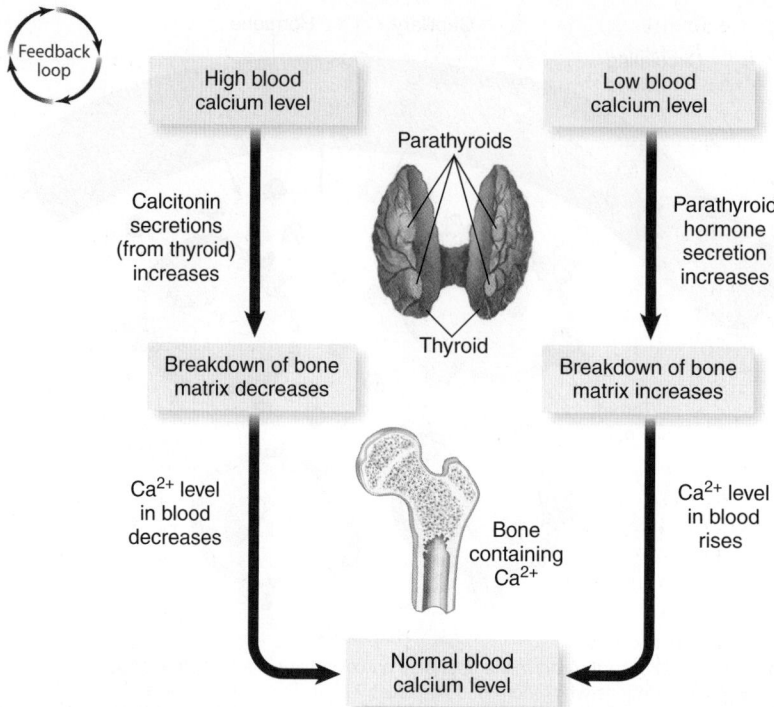

FIG. 50.3 Feedback mechanism between parathyroid hormone (PTH) and calcium. Calcitonin and parathyroid hormones have antagonistic (opposing) effects that regulate blood calcium levels. Source: Patton, K. (2019). *Anatomy and physiology* (10th ed., Figure 11-12). Elsevier.

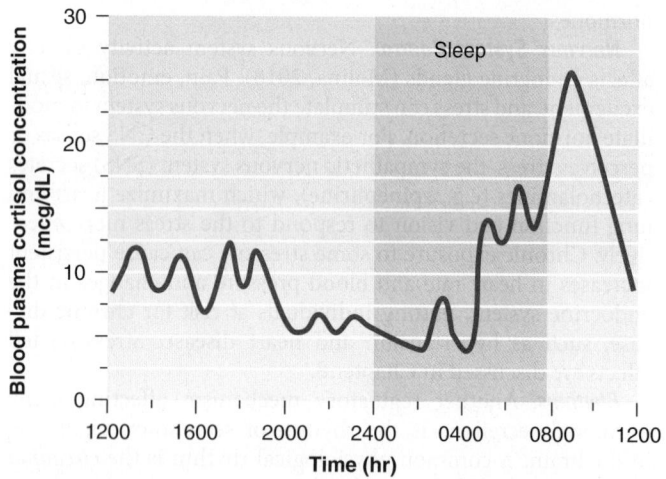

FIG. 50.4 Secretion of cortisol. As with many hormones, the amount of cortisol secreted into the blood varies chaotically throughout the day. However, pulses of increased hormone secretion occur occasionally, with the highest peaks shortly before and after waking. Pulsing secretion (in response to specific conditions in the body) with a daily, or diurnal, pattern is seen in many hormones, including all the adrenal cortical hormones. Source: Patton, K. (2019). *Anatomy and physiology* (10th ed., Figure 26-20). Elsevier.

(see Figure 50.1). The hypothalamus and pituitary integrate communication between the nervous and endocrine systems. The hypothalamus releases substances that either stimulate or inhibit production and release of hormones from the pituitary (Molina, 2018). Examples of stimulating hormones include corticotropin-releasing hormone (CRH) and thyrotropin-releasing hormone (TRH). An example of an inhibitory hormone is somatostatin, which inhibits growth hormone release (Table 50.2).

Neurons in the hypothalamus receive input from the cerebral cortex (especially the limbic area) and release hormones, translating nerve impulses into hormone secretion. Thus, the

TABLE 50.2 HORMONES OF THE HYPOTHALAMUS

The following hormones from the hypothalamus target the anterior pituitary.

Releasing Hormones
- Corticotropin-releasing hormone (CRH)
- Gonadotropin-releasing hormone (GnRH)
- Growth hormone–releasing factor (GHRH), or somatotropin-releasing hormone
- Prolactin-releasing hormone (PRF)
- Thyrotropin-releasing hormone (TRH)

Inhibiting Hormones
- Prolactin-inhibiting hormone (PIH)
- Somatostatin (inhibits growth hormone release)

hypothalamus links the nervous system to the endocrine system, creating a circuit that coordinates expression of complex behavioural responses, such as anger, fear, and pleasure (Patton, 2019).

Pituitary Gland

The pituitary (*hypophysis*) is in the sella turcica, under the hypothalamus, at the base of the brain above the sphenoid bone (see Figure 50.1). The infundibular (*hypophyseal*) stalk connects the pituitary and hypothalamus; this stalk serves as a communication mechanism between the hypothalamus and pituitary (Molina, 2018). The pituitary consists of two main parts, the *anterior* lobe (*adenohypophysis*) and the *posterior* lobe (*neurohypophysis*). A smaller intermediate lobe makes melanocyte-stimulating hormone (MSH), which stimulates the production and release of melanin (Javorsky et al., 2018).

Anterior Pituitary Gland. The anterior lobe constitutes two-thirds of the pituitary gland; the hypothalamus regulates this lobe through releasing and inhibiting hormones. The hypothalamic hormones reach the anterior pituitary through a network of capillaries known as the *hypothalamus–hypophyseal portal system* (Javorsky et al., 2018). The releasing and inhibiting hormones in turn affect the secretion of specific hormones from the anterior lobe of the pituitary (Figure 50.5).

Tropic Hormones. Tropic hormones are hormones that target other endocrine glands, in turn causing the target glands to secrete hormone. Most tropic hormones are produced and secreted by the anterior pituitary (Molina, 2018). For example, TSH stimulates the thyroid gland to secrete thyroid hormones. Adrenocorticotrophic hormone (ACTH) stimulates the adrenal cortex to secrete corticosteroids. Follicle-stimulating hormone (FSH) stimulates secretion of estrogen and the development of ova in women and sperm in men. Luteinizing hormone (LH) stimulates ovulation in women and secretion of sex hormones in both men and women.

Growth Hormone. *Growth hormone* (GH) affects the growth and development of all body tissues and has numerous biological actions. For example, GH affects multiple aspects of the immune response and plays a role in protein, fat, and carbohydrate metabolism (Molina, 2018).

Prolactin. Prolactin (*lactogenic hormone*) is a hormone that plays a role in normal development in mammary tissue and stimulates milk production and lactation after childbirth (Molina, 2018).

Posterior Pituitary Gland. The posterior pituitary gland is an extension of the hypothalamus composed of nerve. Communication between the hypothalamus and posterior lobe of the pituitary occurs through nerve tracts (*median eminence*). Hormones secreted by the posterior pituitary lobe, antidiuretic hormone (ADH) and oxytocin, are produced in the hypothalamus (Molina, 2018). These hormones travel down the nerve tracts from the hypothalamus to the posterior pituitary and are stored there until stimuli trigger their release (see Figure 50.5).

Antidiuretic Hormone. The major physiological role of ADH, also called *vasopressin*, is regulation of fluid volume by stimulating reabsorption of water in the renal tubules. ADH is also a potent vasoconstrictor, increasing vascular resistance. The most important stimulus of ADH secretion is *plasma osmolality,* a measure of solute concentration of circulating blood (Figure 50.6). Plasma osmolality increases when there is a decrease in extracellular fluid (e.g., *hypovolemia,* decreased blood volume) or an increase in solute concentration (e.g., *hypernatremia,* elevated serum sodium concentration). The increased plasma osmolality activates *osmoreceptors,* specialized neurons in the hypothalamus, which stimulate ADH release (Molina, 2018). When ADH is released, renal tubules reabsorb water, causing urine to be more concentrated. When ADH release is inhibited, renal tubules do not reabsorb water, causing urine to be more dilute.

Oxytocin. *Oxytocin* stimulates both ejection of milk into mammary ducts and contraction of uterine smooth muscle during pregnancy. Oxytocin secretion is increased by stimulation of touch receptors in the nipples of lactating women and of vaginal pressure receptors (Molina, 2018).

Pineal Gland

The pineal gland is located within the brain but has very limited neural connectedness with the brain. The gland is composed of photoreceptive cells and is primarily responsible for melatonin hormone secretion. Regulated by the SNS, melatonin secretion is increased in response to hypoglycemia and darkness. The pineal gland is believed to play a role in the regulation of circadian rhythms and reproductive systems at puberty onset (Javorsky et al., 2018).

Thyroid Gland

The thyroid gland is located in the anterior neck and is midline, straddling the trachea. It consists of two encapsulated lateral lobes connected by a narrow isthmus (Figure 50.7). The thyroid is a highly vascular organ and is regulated by TSH secreted by the anterior pituitary. The three hormones produced and secreted by the thyroid gland are thyroxine (T4), triiodothyronine (T3), and calcitonin (Jarvis et al., 2019).

Thyroxine and Triiodothyronine. Thyroid hormones exert effects on nearly every organ system, stimulating cell metabolism and activity. The thyroid gland's major function is the production, storage, and release of thyroid hormones T_4 and T_3. T_4 accounts for 90% of thyroid hormone. T_3, however, is more biologically active and has significant metabolic effects on the body. Approximately 20% of circulating T_3 is secreted directly by the thyroid gland; the remainder is obtained by peripheral conversion of T_4. Dietary iodine is necessary for thyroid hormone synthesis. T_4 and T_3 affect metabolic rate, caloric requirements, oxygen consumption, carbohydrate and lipid metabolism, growth and development, brain function, and nervous system activity. More than 99% of thyroid hormones are bound to plasma proteins, which ensures a circulating reserve, especially T_4-binding globulin synthesized by the liver. Only the unbound (i.e., free) hormones are biologically active (Molina, 2018).

Thyroid hormone production and release is regulated by a negative feedback cycle. When circulating levels of thyroid hormone are low, the hypothalamus releases TRH, which causes the anterior pituitary gland to release TSH. High levels of circulating thyroid hormone have an inhibitory effect on the secretion of both TRH from the hypothalamus and TSH from the anterior pituitary gland (Molina, 2018).

Calcitonin. Calcitonin is a hormone produced by *parafollicular* or C cells of the thyroid gland in response to high circulating calcium levels. Calcitonin inhibits calcium resorption (i.e., loss) from bone, increases calcium storage in bone, and increases renal excretion of calcium and phosphorus, thereby lowering serum calcium and phosphate levels. Although it provides a counter-mechanism to PTH, calcitonin does not play a critical role in calcium balance (Molina, 2018).

Parathyroid Glands

The parathyroid glands are small, oval structures usually arranged in two pairs, one behind each thyroid lobe, typically totaling four glands (Figure 50.8).

Parathyroid Hormone. The parathyroids secrete PTH, also called *parathormone*; its major role is to regulate the blood level of calcium. PTH acts on bone, kidneys, and, indirectly, the GI tract. In bone, PTH stimulates resorption and inhibits bone formation, which results in the release of calcium and phosphate into the blood. In the kidneys, PTH increases calcium reabsorption and phosphate excretion. In addition, PTH stimulates the renal conversion of vitamin D to its most active form (1,25-dihydroxyvitamin D_3), which is responsible for enhancing intestinal absorption of calcium (Molina, 2018). The secretion of PTH is directly regulated by a negative feedback system (see Figure 50.3). When serum calcium or magnesium levels are low, PTH secretion increases; when serum calcium or active vitamin D levels rise, PTH secretion falls.

Thymus Gland

The thymus is most active in childhood and shrinks significantly as a person ages (Nigam & Knight, 2020). Positioned just behind the sternum, the thymus can be classified as either an endocrine or lymphatic organ as it has both immune and

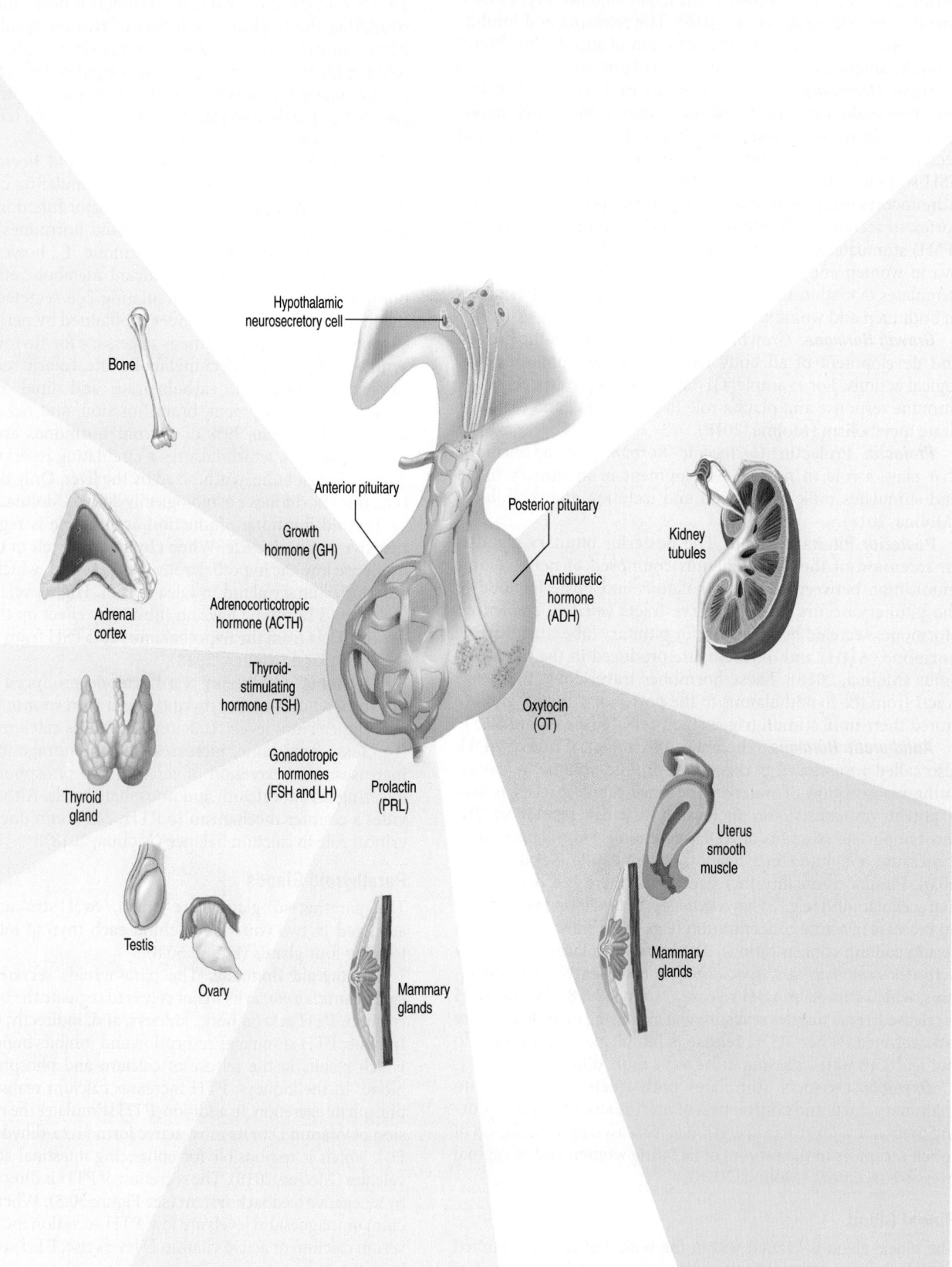

FIG. 50.5 Pituitary hormones. Some of the major hormones of the adenohypophysis and neurohypophysis and their principal target organs. Source: Patton, K. (2019). *Anatomy and physiology* (10th ed., Figure 26-3). Elsevier.

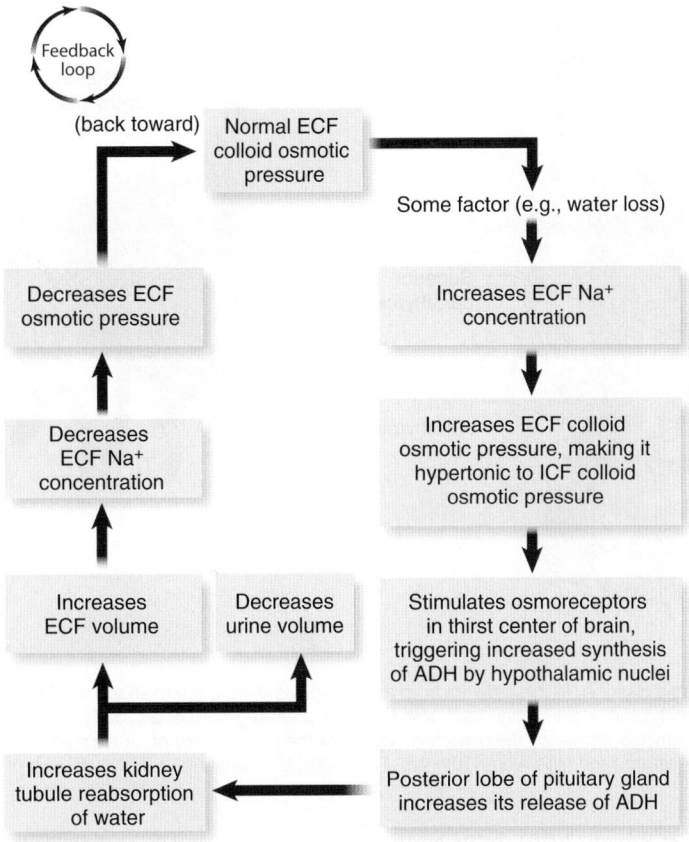

FIG. 50.6 Antidiuretic hormone (ADH) mechanism for extracellular fluid (EFC) homeostasis. The ADH mechanism helps maintain homeostasis of ECF colloid osmotic pressure by regulating its volume and, thereby, its electrolyte concentration—that is, mainly ECF sodium (Na⁺) concentration. *ICF,* intracellular fluid. Source: Patton, K. (2019). *Anatomy and physiology* (10th ed., Figure 43-15). Elsevier.

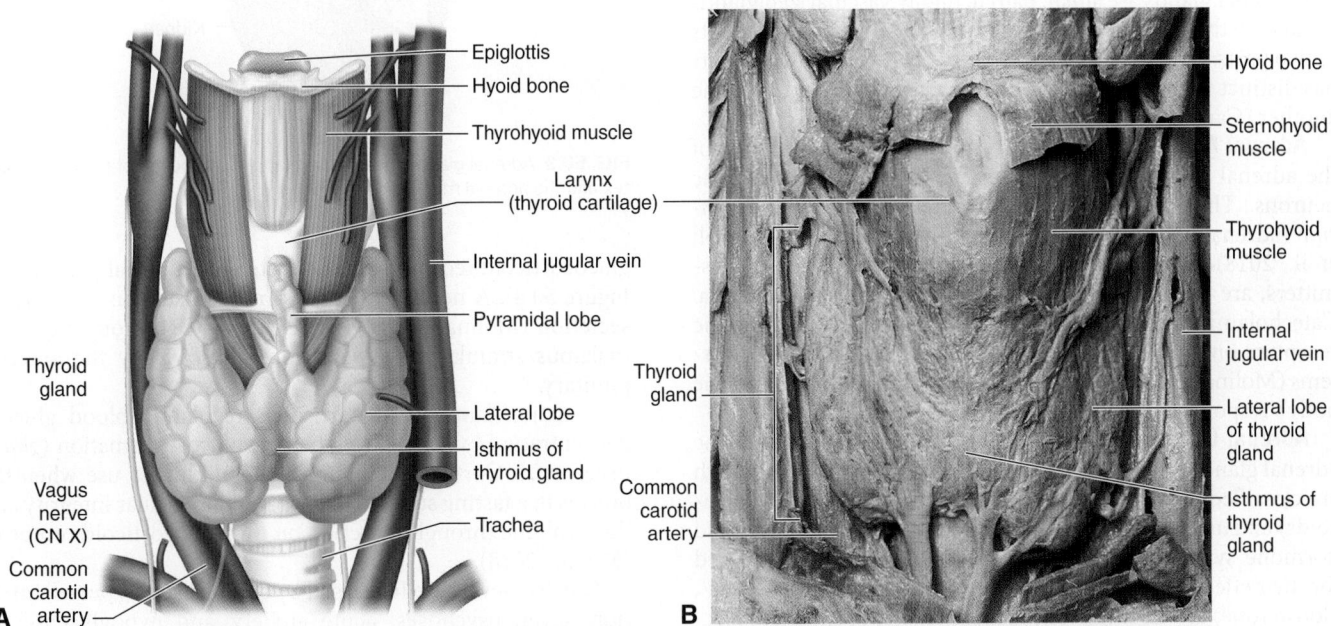

FIG. 50.7 Thyroid gland. **A,** In this drawing, the relationship of the thyroid to the larynx (voice box) and trachea is easily seen. **B,** In this photo of a dissected cadaver, the location of the thyroid relative to the carotid arteries and jugular veins is shown. Source: Patton, K. (2019). *Anatomy and physiology* (10th ed., Figure 26-9). Elsevier.

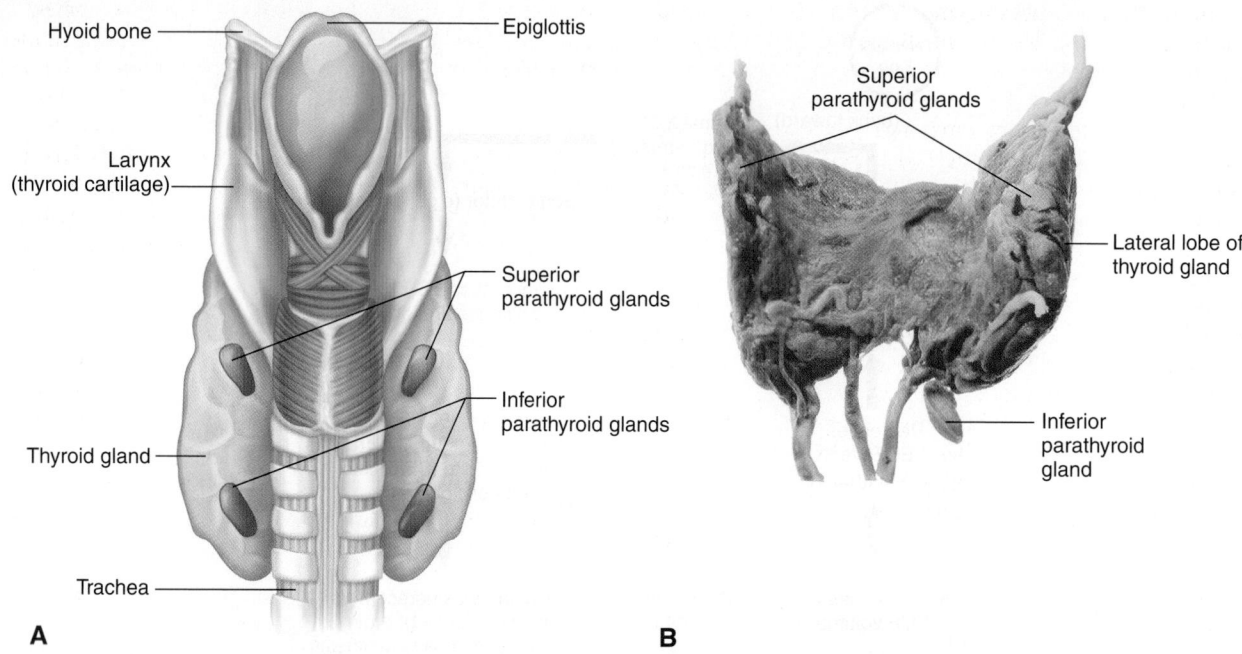

FIG. 50.8 Parathyroid gland. **A**, In this drawing from a posterior view, note the relationship of the parathyroid glands to each other, thyroid gland, larynx (voice box), and to the trachea. **B**, Photo of a cadaver dissection (also posterior view) showing parathyroid glands on the posterior surface of the lateral lobes of an isolated thyroid gland. Source: Patton, K. (2019). *Anatomy and physiology* (10th ed., Figure 26-12). Elsevier.

endocrine functions (Saghazadeh & Rezaei, 2020). In its endocrine role, the thymus produces thymosin hormones, which contribute to the immune response (Betts et al., 2019). The thymus is also thought to play a role in neuroendocrine communication (Saghazadeh & Rezaei, 2020). The immune modulating functions of the thymus are discussed further in Chapter 8.

Adrenal Glands

The adrenal glands are small, paired, highly vascularized glands located on the upper portion of each kidney; each gland consists of two parts: the medulla and the cortex (Figure 50.9). Each part has distinct functions, and the glands act independently of one another (Carroll et al., 2018).

Adrenal Medulla. The adrenal medulla is the inner part of the adrenal gland and consists of sympathetic postganglionic neurons. The medulla secretes the catecholamines *epinephrine* (adrenaline) and *norepinephrine* (noradrenaline) (Carroll et al., 2018). Catecholamines, usually considered neurotransmitters, are hormones when secreted by the adrenal medulla. Catecholamines exert their effects after binding to adrenergic receptors on cells and have widespread effects on all body systems (Molina, 2018). Catecholamines are an essential part of the body's response to stress (Chapter 8).

Adrenal Cortex. The adrenal cortex is the outer part of the adrenal gland. It secretes more than 50 steroid hormones, which are classified as *corticosteroids* (glucocorticoids, mineralocorticoids) and *androgens*. Cholesterol is the precursor for all steroid hormone synthesis. *Glucocorticoids* (e.g., cortisol) are named for their effects on glucose metabolism. *Mineralocorticoids* (e.g., aldosterone) are essential for the maintenance of fluid and electrolyte balance. Adrenal androgens are produced and secreted in small but significant amounts (Molina, 2018).

Cortisol. Cortisol, the most abundant and potent glucocorticoid, exerts multisystemic effects necessary to maintain life and protect the body from stress—virtually all cells express

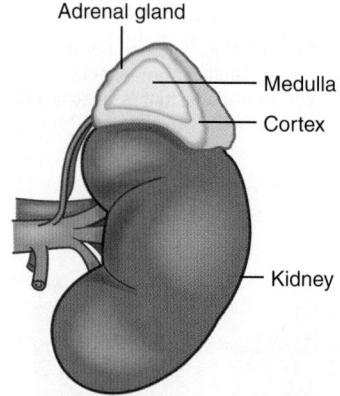

FIG. 50.9 Adrenal gland. The adrenal gland is composed of the adrenal cortex and the adrenal medulla.

glucocorticoid receptors. It is secreted in a diurnal pattern (see Figure 50.4). A negative feedback mechanism controls cortisol secretion (Molina, 2018). The release of CRH from the hypothalamus stimulates the secretion of ACTH by the anterior pituitary.

A major function of cortisol is regulating blood glucose concentration by stimulating hepatic glucose formation (*gluconeogenesis*). Cortisol inhibits peripheral glucose use when the body is in a fasting state. It helps maintain vascular integrity and fluid volume through its action on mineralocorticoid receptors (Molina, 2018).

Cortisol levels are increased by surgical stress, burns, infection, fever, psychoses, acute anxiety, and hypoglycemia. A major effect of glucocorticoids is their anti-inflammatory and supportive actions in response to stress. A marked increase in the rate of cortisol secretion by the adrenal cortex decreases the inflammatory response aiding the body in coping more effectively with stressful situations (Chapter 8). Cortisol also inhibits production of prostaglandins, thromboxanes, and leukotrienes, enhancing the cell-mediated immune response (Molina, 2018).

Aldosterone. Aldosterone is a potent mineralocorticoid that maintains extracellular fluid volume. It acts at the renal tubule to promote reabsorption of sodium and excretion of potassium and hydrogen ions (Molina, 2018). Aldosterone synthesis and secretion are stimulated by angiotensin II, hyponatremia, and hyperkalemia and inhibited by atrial natriuretic peptide (ANP) and hypokalemia (Young, 2018).

Adrenal Androgens. The adrenal cortex secretes small amounts of androgens. They are converted to sex steroids in peripheral tissues: testosterone in men and estrogen in women. The most common adrenal androgens are dehydroepiandrosterone (DHEA) and androstenedione. Because they are precursors to other sex steroids, their actions are like those of testosterone and estrogen (Carroll et al., 2018). For example, in postmenopausal women, the major source of estrogen is the peripheral conversion of adrenal androgens to estrogen. The effects of adrenal androgen in men are negligible in comparison with testosterone secreted by the testes.

Pancreas

The pancreas is a long, tapered, lobular, soft gland located behind the stomach and anterior to the first and second lumbar vertebrae. The pancreas has both exocrine and endocrine functions; the hormone-secreting portion of the pancreas is referred to as the *islets of Langerhans*. The islets account for less than 2% of the gland but receive up to 15% of the pancreatic blood flow and consist of four types of hormone-secreting cells: alpha (α), beta (β), delta (D), and gamma (F) cells (Molina, 2018). Glucagon is produced and secreted by α cells; insulin and amylin are produced and secreted by β cells; somatostatin is produced and secreted by D cells; and, pancreatic polypeptide (PP) is secreted by the F (or PP) cells (Molina, 2018).

Glucagon. Glucagon is synthesized and released from pancreatic α cells in response to low blood glucose levels, protein ingestion, and exercise. Glucagon increases blood glucose through *catabolism,* providing fuel for energy during fasting states, when ingested glucose is not readily available. Glucagon does this by stimulating *glycogenolysis* (breakdown of glycogen into glucose), *gluconeogenesis* (formation of glucose from noncarbohydrate molecules), and *ketogenesis* (breakdown of fatty acids and amino acids to produce ketone bodies) (Molina, 2018). Glucagon and insulin function in a reciprocal manner via a negative feedback loop to maintain normal blood glucose levels (Figure 50.10).

Insulin. Insulin is an essential hormone and acts as the principal regulator of metabolism and storage of ingested carbohydrates, fats, and proteins. Insulin facilitates glucose transport across cell membranes in most tissues. However, the brain, nerves, lens of the eye, hepatocytes, erythrocytes, and cells in the intestinal mucosa and kidney tubules are not dependent on insulin for glucose uptake. Insulin is responsible for how ingested nutrients are used for energy and stored (*anabolism*). An increased blood glucose level is the major stimulus for insulin synthesis and secretion (see Figure 50.10). Other stimuli to insulin secretion are increased amino acid levels and vagal stimulation (Masharani & German, 2018). Insulin secretion is usually inhibited by low blood glucose levels, glucagon, somatostatin, hypokalemia, and catecholamines (Table 50.3).

A variety of mechanisms carefully modulate insulin secretion to prevent both hypo- and hyperglycemia in the healthy individual. *Hyperinsulinemia* (chronically elevated insulin levels) is a significant predictor of cardiovascular and metabolic disease and is strongly associated with the development of type 2 diabetes mellitus (Thomas et al., 2019). Hyperinsulinemia is thought to be caused by the overconsumption of refined sugars (i.e., fructose, sucrose, and glucose). This initiates de novo lipogenesis, a process in which the liver converts excess dietary carbohydrates into fat (often in the form of triglycerides). A chronic overabundance of insulin causes the body to become resistant to its effects over time. Both insulin resistance and hyperinsulinemia can be corrected with dietary and exercise lifestyle modifications—primarily lowering simple carbohydrate and sugar consumption and decreasing visceral adipose tissue, respectively (Thomas et al., 2019).

Nurses play a critical role in health promotion and, as part of the interprofessional health care team, should provide lifestyle counselling to all patients with or at risk for these illnesses. (See Chapter 52 for more information on type 2 diabetes mellitus.)

AGE-RELATED CONSIDERATIONS

THE ENDOCRINE SYSTEM

Normal aging has many effects on the endocrine system (Table 50.4), including decreased hormone production and secretion, altered hormone metabolism and biological activity, decreased responsiveness of target tissues to hormones, and alterations in circadian rhythms. For example, GH and insulin-like growth factor both decline with aging, causing changes in reproductive and cognitive function, decreased muscle mass, decreased bone density, and increased visceral fat (Brashers et al., 2018). Assessment of the effects of aging on the endocrine system is difficult because subtle age-related changes may mimic manifestations of endocrine disorders. Endocrine disorders may manifest differently in an older person than in a younger person (Van Den Beld et al., 2018). Older people may have multiple comorbid conditions and take medications that alter the body's usual response to endocrine function. Symptoms of endocrine dysfunction such as fatigue, constipation, or mental impairment may be attributed to aging, resulting in delayed treatment (Van Den Beld et al., 2018).

ASSESSMENT OF THE ENDOCRINE SYSTEM

Hormones affect every tissue and system in the body, causing great diversity in manifestations of endocrine dysfunction. Endocrine disorders generally result from too much or too little of a specific hormone (Hannon & Porth, 2017). The onset of symptoms is often gradual. Subtle or vague symptoms are often attributed to other physiological or psychological causes. Patients may present with fluid and electrolyte imbalances, altered tissue perfusion, inadequate coping mechanisms, changes in heart rhythm, or changes in skin integrity that can be interpreted as many other conditions. Alternatively, patients may present with acute symptoms that are life-threatening and demand immediate intervention.

Subjective Data

Endocrine system assessment is predominantly captured through a thorough health history. Key questions to ask the patient with a suspected endocrine disorder are presented in Table 50.5.

Important Health Information

Past Health History. Patients with endocrine disorders often present with nonspecific symptoms. The chief complaint may relate to a group of symptoms. The most common presenting conditions include fatigue, weakness, menstrual

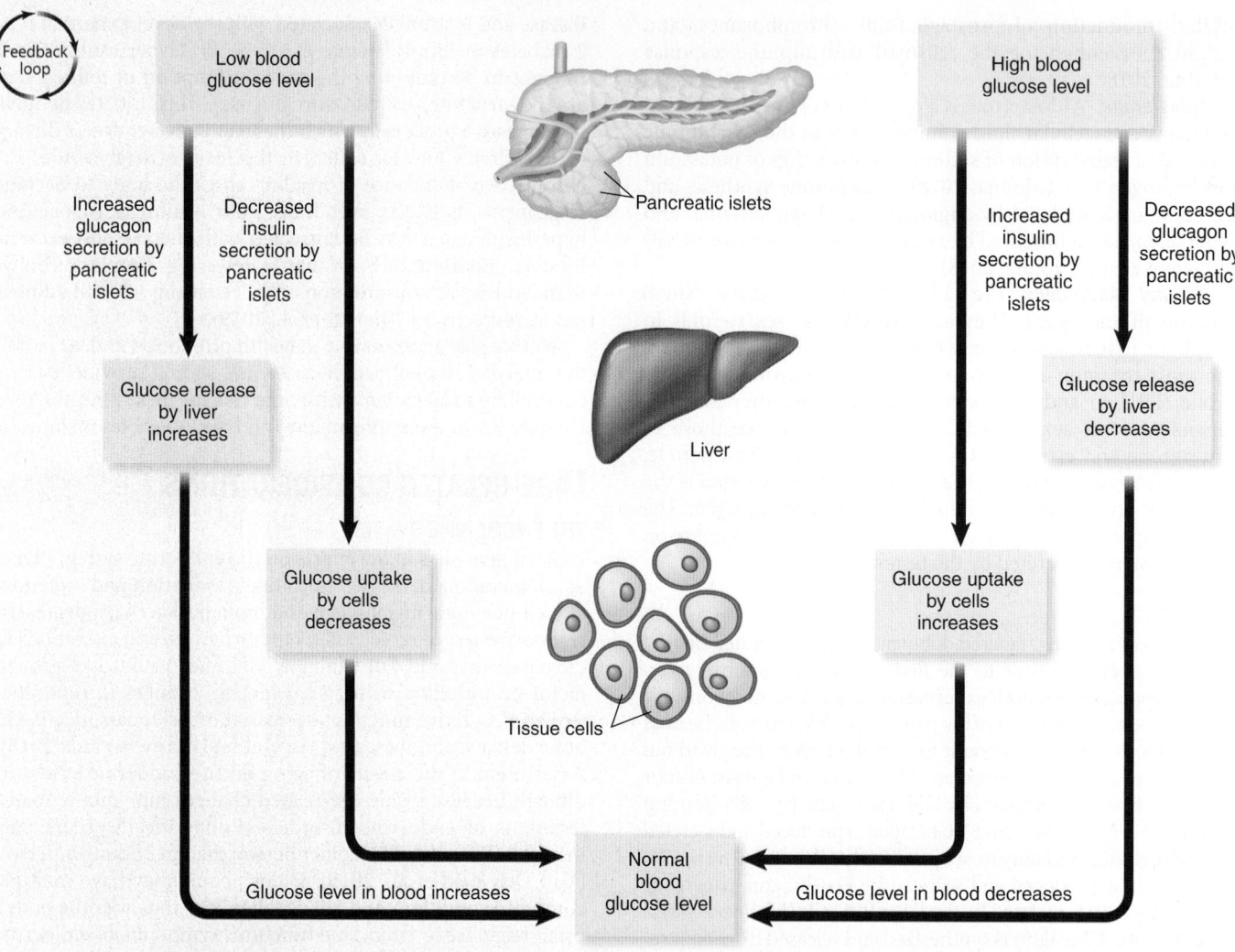

FIG. 50.10 Regulation of blood glucose levels. Insulin and glucagon, two of the major pancreatic hormones, have antagonistic (opposite) effects on glucose concentration in the blood. Many other hormones, such as growth hormone (GH) and cortisol, also influence blood glucose levels. Source: Patton, K. (2019). *Anatomy and physiology* (10th ed., Figure 26-23). Elsevier.

TABLE 50.3	FACTORS INFLUENCING SECRETION OF INSULIN
Stimulate Secretion	**Inhibit Secretion**
↑ Glucose levels	↓ Glucose levels
↑ Amino acid levels	↓ Amino acid levels
↑ Gastrointestinal hormone levels	↓ Potassium levels
↑ Vagal stimulation	↑ Corticosteroid hormone levels
↑ Fats	↑ Catecholamine levels
	↑ Somatostatin levels
	↑ Glucagon levels (usually)
	↑ Insulin levels

CASE STUDY

Patient Introduction

L. M. (pronouns she/her), 35 years old, has come to the clinic complaining of "just not feeling well." L. M. is accompanied by her partner. L. M. states she has gained a lot of weight despite monitoring her diet, and that she just seems to be getting more and more tired. Her partner voices concern about changes in L. M.'s energy level.

Critical Thinking

Throughout this assessment chapter, think about L. M.'s condition with the following questions in mind:

1. What are possible causes of L. M.'s weight gain, fatigue, and irritability?
2. What questions should the nurse ask this patient?
3. What would be the nurse's priority assessment?
4. What should be included in the physical assessment? What would the nurse be looking for?
5. What diagnostic studies might be ordered?

   L. M.'s condition will be followed throughout this assessment chapter. See Case Study: Subjective Data, Case Study: Objective Data: Physical Examination, and Case Study: Objective Data: Diagnostic Studies for more information on L. M.

evolve
Answers are available at http://evolve.elsevier.com/Canada/Lewis/medsurg.

irregularities, and weight changes (Jarvis & MacDonald-Jenkins, 2019). It is important to determine if the onset of symptoms has been gradual or sudden and what the patient has done about them.

Because some of the more general manifestations of endocrine disorders are the easiest to overlook, any reported or observed changes in weight, appetite, skin, libido, mental acuity, emotional stability, or energy levels must be evaluated.

Family History. Heredity can play a significant role in the development of endocrine conditions (Grody, 2019). The patient should be asked about first-degree relatives with

TABLE 50.4 AGE-RELATED DIFFERENCES IN ASSESSMENT

Endocrine System

Changes	Clinical Significance
Thyroid Atrophy of thyroid gland; decrease in TSH and T$_3$ secretion; increased nodules	Increased incidence of hypothyroidism with aging; however, most older persons maintain adequate thyroid function. Thyroid hormone replacement dose lower in older persons.
Parathyroid Increased secretion of PTH and increased basal level of PTH	Increased calcium resorption from bone (demineralization); hypercalcemia, hypercalciuria (may reflect defective renal mechanism)
Adrenal Cortex Adrenal cortex: more fibrotic and slightly smaller Decreased metabolism of cortisol Decreased plasma levels of adrenal androgens and aldosterone	Decreased metabolic clearance rate for glucocorticoids
Adrenal Medulla Increased secretion and basal level of norepinephrine No change in plasma epinephrine levels Decreased β-adrenergic receptor response to norepinephrine	Decreased responsiveness to β-adrenergic agonists and receptor blockers May partly explain increased incidence of hypertension with aging
Pancreas Increase in fibrosis and fatty deposits in pancreas Increased glucose intolerance and decreased sensitivity to insulin	May partly contribute to increased incidence of diabetes mellitus with advanced aging
Gonads *Women:* decline in estrogen secretion *Men:* decline in testosterone secretion	Women experience symptoms associated with menopause and have increased risk for atherosclerosis and osteoporosis. Men may or may not experience symptoms.

PTH, parathyroid hormone; *T$_3$,* triiodothyronine; *TSH,* thyroid-stimulating hormone.

diabetes mellitus or insipidus, hyperthyroidism or hypothyroidism, endocrine gland cancers, or goitre (see Table 50.5 for more examples). Such questioning frequently elicits information about a familial tendency.

Medications. The patient should be asked about the use of all medications (prescription, over-the-counter, recreational), herbs, and dietary supplements. The patient should be asked the reason for taking the medication, the dosage, and the length of time it has been taken. The patient should specifically be asked about the use of hormone replacements. Information that the patient is currently taking hormone replacements such as insulin, thyroid hormone, or corticosteroids (e.g., prednisone) can alert the nurse to potential adverse effects. For example, corticosteroids may cause bone loss with long-term use and may increase blood glucose levels in susceptible patients by increasing glycogenolysis and insulin resistance. Thyroid preparations (e.g., levothyroxine [Synthroid]) may cause tachycardia or cardiac dysrhythmias.

Medication-to- medication interactions and adverse effects of nonhormonal medications can also contribute to endocrine conditions.

Surgery and Other Treatments. The nurse should inquire about previous obstetrical history, hospitalizations, surgery, chemotherapy, and radiation therapy (especially irradiation of the neck). For example, traumatic brain injury (e.g., concussion) can cause pituitary or hypothalamic dysfunction (Lavin, 2018).

Objective Data

Most endocrine glands are inaccessible for direct examination. Except for the thyroid and male gonads, glands are deeply encased in the body, protected against injury and trauma. However, assessment can be accomplished by collecting objective data. The nurse must understand the actions of hormones in order to effectively monitor target tissue and assess the function of a gland.

CASE STUDY

Subjective Data

A focused subjective assessment of L. M. reveals the following information.

Past medical history: Denies any medical or surgical history. She has not seen a health care provider for 8 years.

Medications: None.

Overall health management: L. M. works as a paralegal for a local law firm and states that it is a great effort some days to make it through the workday.

Functional Assessment

Sleep and rest: L. M. frequently wakes up with a headache and goes to bed with the same headache, describing it as a dull, throbbing ache between the eyes. She sleeps 10+ hours at night but does not feel rested on awakening.

L. M. does not have the energy of 5 years or even 6 months ago. She used to enjoy gardening and going out with friends but now can barely manage work and coming home.

L. M. states that she has no ambition to exercise, being too tired at the end of the workday and with no energy on the weekends either. She also reports leg cramps with walking.

Nutrition, elimination, and metabolic history: L. M. reports a steady weight gain over the past 6 months, mainly in the abdominal area. She feels "bloated" and "looks pregnant" but knows it is not possible. Her appetite has decreased but she has not been able to lose any weight. L. M. also reports facial hair growth and has noticed easy bruising. Whenever she gets a bug bite, it seems to take forever to heal. She denies difficulty swallowing, hoarseness, palpitations, or tremors and denies any changes or difficulty with urination or bowel habits.

Coping and stress management: L.M. is worried about "going crazy." She is easily angered and irritable, frequently snapping at her coworkers and her partner. L. M. states that this is not usual behaviour and first thought it was because of dealing with a constant, dull headache.

Lately, she has noticed that she has blurry vision, which is making work and life even more difficult and stressful. When asked about her headache, she states it hurts between her eyes. L.M. rates the pain as a 4 on a scale of 0 to 10 and states that acetaminophen (Tylenol) or ibuprofen (Advil) does not alleviate the pain. The pain is typically worse on arising in the morning and slowly decreases during the day.

L. M. hates the way she looks—looking in the mirror, she cannot believe her image. She feels 10 years older over the past 6 months and has gained weight in her face, neck, and trunk. She is concerned about thinning scalp hair and beard growth. L.M. is beginning to wonder, "Am I turning into a man?"

She states she is finding it difficult to cope with job and relationship stresses and life in general. L. M.'s emotions are very "raw and labile," totally different from the easy-going person she has always been.

See Case Study: Patient Introduction, Case Study: Objective Data: Physical Examination, and Case Study: Objective Data: Diagnostic Studies for more information on L. M.

TABLE 50.5 HEALTH HISTORY
Endocrine System: Subjective Data

Past History
- Do you have any previous or current conditions with your endocrine system (e.g., issues with thyroid, diabetes, changes in facial or body hair)?
- Have you had any previous hospitalizations, surgical procedures, or treatments for endocrine conditions?
- Are you currently taking or have you ever taken medications for an endocrine condition such as a thyroid disorder or diabetes?

Family History
- Is there any family history of diabetes mellitus or insipidus; hyperthyroidism or hypothyroidism; goitre; hypertension or hypotension; obesity; infertility; growth challenges; pheochromocytoma (neoplastic tumour of the adrenal medulla or sympathetic ganglia); autoimmune diseases (e.g., Addison's disease); or adrenal hyperplasia?
- Have any other members of your family ever had a condition similar to your condition today?

Review of Systems
Overall Health Status
- How do you feel generally? Have you had any changes recently to your health?
- Have there been any changes in your appetite or weight?*
- Have you noticed any changes in your ability to perform your usual activities in comparison with last year? Five years ago?*
- Do you experience fatigue with or without activity?*

Eyes, Ears, Nose, Mouth, and Throat
- Have you experienced any blurring or double vision?* When was your last eye examination?
- Have you noticed any difficulty swallowing?*
- Are your shirts harder to button at the neck?

Cardiovascular System
- Do you experience heart palpitations?*

Musculoskeletal System
- Do you have difficulty holding things because of shakiness of your hands?*

Gastrointestinal System
- Describe your usual bowel pattern. Have you noted any bowel changes?*
- Do you use anything, such as laxatives, to help you move your bowels?*

Genitourinary System
- Do you have to get up at night to urinate? If so, how many times? Do you keep water by your bed at night?
- Have you ever had a kidney stone?*

Neurological System
- Do you feel more nervous than you used to? Do you notice your heart pounding or that you sweat at times when you do not think you should be sweating?
- How is your memory? Have you noticed any changes?
- How long can you concentrate on any one thing? Has this changed lately?

Endocrine System
- Do you feel that most rooms are too hot or too cold? Do you frequently have to put on a sweater, or do you feel as though you need to open windows when others in the room seem comfortable?*

Integumentary System
- Have you noticed any changes in the distribution of the hair anywhere on your body?*
- Have you noticed any changes in the colour of your skin, particularly on your face, neck, hands, or body creases?*
- Has the texture of your skin changed? For example, does it seem thicker and drier than it used to?*

Sexual and Reproductive History
Women
- When did you start to menstruate? Was this earlier or later than other women in your family? If you still menstruate, do you have scant, heavy, or irregular menstrual flows?
- How many children have you had? How much did they weigh at birth? Were you told you had diabetes during any pregnancy?*
- Were you able to nurse your children if you wanted to?
- Are you menopausal? If so, for how long?
- Are you attempting to get pregnant but cannot?* Are you in treatment to become pregnant?* Are you using birth control?*
- Are you postmenopausal? If so, do you have any vaginal bleeding?

Men
- Have you noticed any changes in your ability to have an erection?*
- Are you trying to have children but cannot?*

Functional Assessment (Including Activities of Daily Living)
Activity and Mobility
- Do you have a planned exercise program? If yes, what is it, and have you had to make any changes in this routine lately? If so, why and what kinds of changes?

Sleep and Rest
- How many hours do you sleep at night? Do you feel rested on awakening?
- Are you ever awakened by sweating during the night?*
- Do you have nightmares?*
- Does anyone in your family complain about your snoring?*

Nutrition and Elimination
- What is your weight and height?
- How much do you want to weigh?
- Have there been any changes in your appetite or weight?*

Interpersonal Relationships
- Are you in a relationship? Are you able to take care of any significant others that need your assistance? Are you able to take care of your home? If not, why not?

Coping and Stress Management
- What kind of stressors do you have?
- How do you cope with stress or problems?
- What is your support system? To whom do you turn when you have a problem?
- Do you feel sad or uninterested in life?*

Occupational Health
- Where do you work? What kind of work do you do? Are you able to do what is expected of you and what you expect of yourself?
- If you are retired, what do you do with your time? What did you do before you retired?
- If you are unemployed, are you looking for work?

Self-Care and Health Promotion Activities
- Women: Have you had a mammogram or Pap smear recently?
- Men: Have you had a prostate examination recently?
- Both: If so, what were the results and dates of these tests? How often do you have these tests?

*If yes, describe.

Source: Adapted from Jarvis, C., Browne, A. J., MacDonald-Jenkins, J., et al. (Eds.). (2019). *Physical examination and health assessment* (3rd Canadian ed., pp. 68–73). Elsevier Inc.

Physical Examination. The nurse must remember that the endocrine system affects every system in the body. Clinical manifestations of endocrine function vary significantly, depending on the gland involved. Specific clinical findings for the various endocrine conditions are discussed in Chapters 51 and 52. Regardless of the type of endocrine dysfunction, the following general examination procedure should be followed.

Vital Signs. Vital signs are measured at the beginning of the examination. Variations in temperature may be associated with thyroid dysfunction. Cardiovascular changes such as tachycardia, bradycardia, hypotension, or hypertension may occur with a variety of endocrine-related disorders (Hannon & Porth, 2017).

Height and Weight. Assessment of the endocrine system includes a history of growth and development patterns, weight distribution and changes, and comparisons of these factors with normal findings. Growth pattern abnormalities are suggestive of problems associated with growth hormone (Hannon & Porth, 2017). Changes in weight also may be associated with endocrine dysfunction; thyroid disorders and diabetes mellitus are examples of endocrine disorders that can affect body weight. Body mass index is a height-to-weight ratio used to assess nutritional status (Chapter 43, Figure 43.1).

It may also be helpful to compare the patient's current body weight to their usual body weight to assess changes. Weight change (percentage) is calculated by subtracting the current body weight from the usual weight, dividing by the usual body weight, and multiplying by 100 (Keithley, 2019).

Mental–Emotional Status. Endocrine disorders may cause changes in mental and emotional status (Hannon & Porth, 2017). Throughout the examination, the patient's orientation, alertness, memory, affect, personality, anxiety, appropriateness of dress, and speech pattern should be assessed objectively.

Integument. The nurse should note the colour and the texture of skin, hair, and nails. The overall skin colour, pigmentation, and ecchymosis (bruising) should be noted. Hyperpigmentation, or "bronzing," of the skin (particularly on knuckles, elbows, knees, genitalia, and palmar creases) is a classic finding in Addison's disease but is also present with ACTH-producing tumours and acromegaly (Jarvis et al., 2019). The nurse should palpate the skin for texture and presence of moisture. The nurse should also examine the hair distribution, not only on the head but also on the face, the trunk, and the extremities. The appearance and texture of the hair should be examined. Dull, brittle hair, excessive hair growth, or hair loss may indicate endocrine dysfunction (Hannon & Porth, 2017).

Head. The size and contour of the head are inspected. Facial features should be symmetrical. The eyes are inspected for position, symmetry, shape, movement, opacity over the lens, eyelid lag, and edema. Visual acuity should also be checked because changes may be associated with a pituitary tumour or diabetic retinopathy (Hannon & Porth, 2017). In the mouth, buccal mucosa, condition of the teeth (malocclusion and mottling), and tongue size should be inspected and fasciculations (localized, uncoordinated, uncontrollable twitching of a single muscle group) noted.

Neck. When visually inspecting the thyroid gland, the nurse should make observations first in the normal position (preferably with side lighting), then with the patient's neck in slight extension, and then as the patient swallows some water (Jarvis et al., 2019). The trachea should be midline, and the neck should appear symmetrical. Any unusual bulging over the thyroid area should be noted. Thyroid cancer is the most common endocrine malignancy and is more prevalent in women (Sousa et al., 2020). Many thyroid cancers are detected early simply by noting new neck swelling, enlargement, or nodule during inspection as part of a routine physical assessment and initiating further investigation. (See Chapter 51 for more information on thyroid cancer.)

The thyroid gland is rarely palpable. Thyroid palpation is considered an advanced practice competency, thus this assessment would typically be done by an advance practice nurse or physician. Palpation can trigger the release of thyroid hormones and should be deferred in patients with a visibly enlarged thyroid gland. If enlargement of the thyroid gland is not noticeable, palpation can be performed, noting size, consistency, symmetry, tenderness, and presence of nodules. If it is enlarged, lateral lobes should be auscultated with the stethoscope bell to determine the presence of a bruit (Jarvis et al., 2019). Nodules, enlargement, asymmetry, or hardness are abnormal and require further investigation.

Thorax. The thorax should be inspected for shape and characteristics of the skin. The presence of gynecomastia (enlarged breast tissue) in men should be noted. The nurse auscultates lung sounds and heart sounds, noting adventitious lung sounds or extra heart sounds. Signs of fluid overload or heart failure may be present in patients with syndrome of inappropriate antidiuretic hormone (SIADH) or hypothyroidism (Hannon & Porth, 2017).

Abdomen. The contour symmetry and colour of the abdomen should be noted. Cushing's syndrome (hypercortisolism) causes the skin to be fragile, resulting in purple-blue striae across the abdomen (Hannon & Porth, 2017). The nurse should also auscultate bowel sounds.

Extremities. The nurse assesses the size, shape, symmetry, and general proportion of hands and feet. The skin is inspected for changes in pigmentation and presence of lesions and edema. Muscle strength is evaluated, as are deep tendon reflexes. In the upper extremities, the nurse assesses for the presence of tremors

---

CASE STUDY

Objective Data: Physical Examination

A focused assessment of L. M. reveals the following:

L. M. is sitting on the edge of the examination table and appears anxious. Her BP is 190/80, heart rate 84, respiratory rate 20, temp 37°C. She weighs 82.6 kg and is 160 cm tall.

L. M.'s face is reddened and puffy and she appears to have a lump on the back of her neck and shoulders. She has some facial acne along with some hair growth on her upper lip and chin. Her abdomen is protruding but her arms and legs are thin. Assessment reveals +1 edema in both ankles. There are several ecchymotic areas on her upper and lower extremities, as well as purple striae (stretch marks) on her abdomen.

Throughout this chapter, consider which diagnostic studies would likely be performed for L. M.

See Case Study: Patient Introduction, Case Study: Subjective Data, and Case Study: Objective Data: Diagnostic Studies for more information on L. M.

by placing a piece of paper in the patient's outstretched fingers, palm down.

Genitalia. The nurse inspects the hair distribution pattern. A diamond pubic hair distribution pattern in women and a triangular pattern in men are abnormal findings and may indicate endocrine dysfunction. For men, the testes should be palpated; for women, any clitoral enlargement should be noted.

Common assessment abnormalities related to the endocrine system are presented in Table 50.6. A focused assessment is used to evaluate the status of previously identified endocrine conditions and to monitor for signs of new ones (Chapter 3, Table 3.6). A focused assessment of the endocrine system is described in the Focused Assessment box.

DIAGNOSTIC STUDIES OF THE ENDOCRINE SYSTEM

Accurately performed laboratory tests and radiological examinations contribute to the diagnosis of an endocrine disorder. Laboratory tests usually involve blood and urine testing. Ultrasonography and radiological tests (e.g., regular radiography, computed tomography, magnetic resonance imaging) may be used to localize endocrine growths (e.g., thyroid nodules) as required based on clinical presentation. For all diagnostic testing, the nurse is responsible for explaining the procedure to the patient and family. Diagnostic studies common to the endocrine system are described in Table 50.7.

TABLE 50.6 ASSESSMENT ABNORMALITIES

Endocrine System

Finding	Description	Possible Etiology and Significance
Integument		
Hyperpigmentation	Darkening of the skin, particularly in creases and skinfolds	Addison's disease, caused by increased secretion of melanocyte-stimulating hormone
Depigmentation (vitiligo)	Patchy areas of light skin	May be a marker of autoimmune endocrine disorders
Striae	Purplish-red marks below the skin surface, usually observed on abdomen, breasts, and buttocks (see Chapter 51, Figure 51.11)	Cushing's syndrome
Changes in skin texture	Thick, cold, dry skin	Hypothyroidism
	Thick, leathery, oily skin	Growth hormone excess (acromegaly)
	Warm, smooth, moist skin	Hyperthyroidism
Changes in hair distribution	Hair loss	Hypothyroidism, hyperthyroidism, decreased pituitary secretion
	Diminished axillary and pubic hair	Cortisol deficiency
	Hirsutism (excessive facial hair on women)	Cushing's syndrome, prolactinoma (a pituitary tumour)
Skin ulceration	Areas of ulcerated skin, most commonly observed on legs and feet	Peripheral neuropathy and peripheral vascular disease, which are contributory factors in the development of diabetic foot ulcers
Edema	Generalized edema	Mucopolysaccharide accumulation in tissue in hypothyroidism
Head and Neck		
Visual changes	Decreased visual acuity or decreased peripheral vision	Pituitary gland enlargement or tumour, which leads to pressure on optic nerve
Exophthalmos	Protrusion of eyeballs from orbits	Hyperthyroidism; results from fluid accumulation in eye and retro-orbital tissue
Moon facies	Periorbital edema and facial fullness	Increased cortisol secretion as a result of Cushing's syndrome
Myxedema	Puffiness, periorbital edema, masklike affect	Infiltration of dermis by hydrophilic mucopolysaccharides in hypothyroidism
Goitre	Generalized enlargement of thyroid gland	Hyperthyroidism, hypothyroidism, iodine deficiency
Thyroid nodule (one or more)	Localized enlargement of thyroid gland	May be benign or malignant
Cardiovascular		
Chest pain	Angina caused by increased metabolic demands	Hyperthyroidism, hypothyroidism
Dysrhythmias	Tachycardia, atrial fibrillation	Hypothyroidism or hyperthyroidism, hypoparathyroidism, or hyperparathyroidism, pheochromocytoma
Hypertension	Elevation in blood pressure caused by increased metabolic demands and catecholamines	Hyperthyroidism, pheochromocytoma, Cushing's syndrome
Musculoskeletal		
Changes in muscular strength or muscle mass	Generalized weakness, fatigue, or both	Common symptoms associated with many endocrine conditions, including pituitary, thyroid, parathyroid, and adrenal dysfunction; diabetes mellitus; diabetes insipidus
	Decreased muscle mass	Specifically observed in growth hormone deficiency and in Cushing's syndrome secondary to protein wasting
Enlargement of bones and cartilage	Coarsening of facial features; increases in size of hands and feet over a period of several years	Growth hormone excess in adults, as in acromegaly

TABLE 50.6 ASSESSMENT ABNORMALITIES

Endocrine System—cont'd

Finding	Description	Possible Etiology and Significance
Nutrition		
Changes in weight	Weight loss	Hyperthyroidism; caused by increases in metabolism, diabetic ketoacidosis
Altered glucose levels	Weight gain	Hypothyroidism, Cushing's syndrome, type 2 diabetes mellitus
	Increased serum glucose level	Diabetes mellitus, Cushing's syndrome, growth hormone excess
Neurological		
Lethargy	State of mental sluggishness or somnolence	Hypothyroidism
Tetany	Intermittent involuntary muscle spasms, usually involving the extremities	Severe calcium deficiency that can occur with hypoparathyroidism
Seizure	Sudden involuntary contraction of muscles	Consequence of a pituitary tumour; fluid and electrolyte imbalance associated with excessive antidiuretic hormone (ADH) secretion; complications of diabetes mellitus; severe hypothyroidism
Increased deep tendon reflexes	Hyper-reflexia	Hyperthyroidism, hypoparathyroidism
Gastrointestinal		
Constipation	Passage of infrequent, hard stools	Hyperthyroidism or calcium imbalances caused by hyperparathyroidism
Reproductive		
Changes in reproductive function	Menstrual irregularities, decreased libido, decreased fertility, erectile dysfunction	Various endocrine abnormalities, including pituitary hypofunction, growth hormone excess, thyroid dysfunction, and adrenocortical dysfunction
Other		
Polyuria	Excessive urinary output	Diabetes mellitus (secondary to hyperglycemia) or diabetes insipidus (associated with decreased ADH secretion)
Polydipsia	Excessive thirst	Extreme water losses in diabetes mellitus (with severe hyperglycemia) or diabetes insipidus (associated with decreased ADH)
Decreased urine output	ADH leading to reabsorption of water from kidney tubules	Syndrome of inappropriate antidiuretic hormone (SIADH)
Thermoregulation	Cold sensitivity	Hypothyroidism caused by a slowing of metabolic processes
	Heat intolerance	Hyperthyroidism caused by excessive metabolism

TABLE 50.7 DIAGNOSTIC STUDIES

Endocrine System

Study	Description and Purpose	Normal Values	Nursing Responsibility
Pituitary Studies			
Blood Studies			
Growth hormone (GH) (somatotropin)	Evaluation of GH secretion Used to identify GH deficiency or excess; GH levels are affected by time of day, food intake, and stress	Male: <5 mcg/L Female: <10 mcg/L	Make sure that patient has been fasting and has not recently been emotionally or physically stressed. Indicate patient fasting status and recent activity level on the laboratory slip. Send blood sample to laboratory immediately.
Somatomedin C (insulin-like growth factor [IGF-1])	Evaluation of GH secretion Provides an accurate reflection of mean plasma concentration of GH because it is not subject to circadian rhythm and fluctuations	5.5–14.4 nmol/L Low levels indicate GH deficiency; high levels indicate GH excess	Note if patient has fasted overnight, as overnight fasting is preferred.
Growth hormone (GH) stimulation	Needed to adequately diagnose GH deficiency Measurement of GH secretion in response to stimulation (insulin, arginine) For insulin, baseline blood levels for GH, glucose, and cortisol are obtained; insulin is then administered IV; blood samples for GH are obtained at 0, 60, and 90 min after insulin is administered; blood glucose levels are monitored at 15- to 30-min intervals; blood glucose should drop to less than 2.2 mmol/L for effective test results, and GH level should rise two-fold to three-fold over baseline levels. Response is subnormal or absent in GH deficiency.	Growth hormone levels >10 mcg/L	Ensure that patient or family understands this procedure. Patient must be on NPO status after midnight. Water is permitted on morning of the test. IV access is established for administration of medications and frequent blood sampling. Continually assess for hypoglycemia and hypotension. After test, provide a sweet snack or IV glucose infusion as physician orders.

Continued

TABLE 50.7   DIAGNOSTIC STUDIES

Endocrine System—cont'd

Study	Description and Purpose	Normal Values	Nursing Responsibility
Gonadotropins • Follicle-stimulating hormone (FSH) • Luteinizing hormone (LH)	Useful in distinguishing primary gonadal conditions from pituitary insufficiency Normal levels vary according to age and sex. Levels are low in pituitary insufficiency and high in primary gonadal failure.	*FSH* Male: <22 IU/L Female: • Follicular phase: <20 IU/L • Ovulatory peak: <40 IU/L • Luteal phase: <20 IU/L • Postmenopausal levels: 40–160 IU/L *LH* Male: 1–9 IU/L Female: • Follicular phase: 1–18 IU/L • Ovulatory peak: 20–80 IU/L • Luteal phase: 0.5–18 IU/L • Postmenopausal levels: 12–55 IU/L	There is no special preparation of the patient. Note on the laboratory slip the time of menstrual cycle or whether female patient is postmenopausal.
Water deprivation (restriction) (ADH stimulation)	Used to differentiate causes of polyuria, including neurogenic DI, nephrogenic DI, and psychogenic polydipsia ADH or vasopressin is administered subcutaneously	Neurogenic DI: >9% increase in urine osmolality Nephrogenic DI: <9% increase in urine osmolality Psychogenic polydipsia: <9% increase in osmolality	Caution: Severe dehydration may occur with neurogenic or nephrogenic DI during this test. Test lasts 6 hr, usually from 0600 to 1200 hours. Obtain baseline weight and urine and plasma osmolality. Send hourly samples for measuring urine osmolality. Discontinue test and rehydrate if patient's weight drops more than 2 kg at any time. Rehydrate with oral fluids. Check orthostatic BP and pulse after rehydration to ensure adequate fluid volume.
Prolactin level	Diagnose and monitor prolactin-secreting pituitary adenomas	Male: <20 mcg/L Female: • Nonlactating: <25 mcg/L • Pregnant: 20–400 mcg/L Levels above normal reflect potential pituitary tumour; levels below may be pituitary apoplexy	Draw blood within 3–4 hr after patient awakens. Specimen must be sent to laboratory immediately. If there is a delay, specimen is placed in water and crushed ice.
Radiology Magnetic resonance imaging (MRI)	Most common uses are visualization of the CNS, bony spine, joints, extremities, and breasts.	—	Inform patient of the need to lie as still as possible during the test; explain that tests are painless and noninvasive.
Computed tomographic (CT) scan with contrast media	Used to detect presence and size of tumour Oral or IV contrast medium (or both) may be used.	—	Inform patient of the need to lie still during the procedure. If IV contrast medium is to be used, check for iodine allergy before test.
Thyroid Studies **Blood Studies** Thyroid-stimulating hormone (TSH)	Measurement of TSH levels Considered the most sensitive method for evaluating thyroid disease Generally recommended as first diagnostic test for thyroid dysfunction	2–10 mIU/L	Explain blood collection procedure to patient. No specific preparations are necessary.
Thyroxine (T_4), total	Measurement of total serum level of T_4 Useful in evaluating thyroid function and monitoring thyroid therapy	Male: 51–154 nmol/L Female: 64–154 nmol/L	Same as for TSH measurement.
Triiodothyronine (T_3)	Measurement of serum levels of T_3 Helpful in diagnosing hyperthyroidism if T_4 levels are normal	Adult: 1.7–5.2 pmol/L	Same as for TSH measurement.
Free T_4	Measurement of active component of total T_4 Because level remains constant, this is considered a better indication of thyroid function than total T_4.	10–36 pmol/L	Same as for TSH measurement.

TABLE 50.7   DIAGNOSTIC STUDIES

Endocrine System—cont'd

Study	Description and Purpose	Normal Values	Nursing Responsibility
T_3 uptake (T_3RU)	Indirect measurement of binding capacity of thyroid-binding globulin	24–34% uptake	Same as for TSH measurement.
Thyroid antibodies (Ab) • Thyroid peroxidase (TPO) Ab • Thyroglobulin Ab • Thyroid-stimulating Ab	Measurements of levels of thyroid antibodies Assists in diagnosis of an autoimmune thyroid disease and distinguishes it from thyroiditis One or more antibody tests may be ordered, depending on symptoms.	—	Same as for TSH measurement.
Thyroglobulin	Test to identify the presence of functioning thyroid tissue or thyroid cancer cells; result is used primarily as a tumour marker for patients being treated for thyroid cancer	Male: 0.5–53 mcg/L Female: 0.5–43 mcg/L	Same as for TSH measurement.
Radiology			
Ultrasonography	Evaluation of thyroid nodule or nodules to determine whether they are fluid filled (cystic) or solid tumour	—	Explain that gel and a transducer will be used over the neck. Neither fasting nor sedation is required.
Thyroid scan and uptake	Scan: Used to evaluate nodules of the thyroid. Radioactive isotopes are given PO or IV. Scanner passes over thyroid and makes graphic record of radiation emitted. Normal thyroid scan reveals homogeneous pattern with symmetrical lobes. Benign nodules appear as warm spots because they take up the radionuclide; malignant tumours appear as cold spots because they tend not to take up the radionuclide. Radioactive iodine uptake (RAIU): Provides direct measurement of thyroid activity. Useful for evaluation of functional activity of solitary thyroid nodules. Patient is given radioactive iodine either PO or IV. Uptake by the thyroid gland is measured with a scanner at several time intervals, such as 2- to 4-hr intervals, and at 24 hr. The values of RAIU are expressed in percentage of uptake.	—	Explain procedure to the patient. Check for iodine and shellfish allergy before the test. Be sure patient understands that radioactive iodine taken orally is harmless. No special preparation is required. Patient should not have supplemental iodine for several weeks before the test. Thyroid medications interfere with test results.
Parathyroid Studies ***Blood Studies***			
Parathyroid hormone (PTH)	Measurement of PTH level in serum to evaluate hypercalcemia or hypocalcemia Results must be interpreted in terms of concomitantly measured serum calcium level.	Intact (whole): 10–65 ng/L	Fasting specimen is preferred. Inform patient that blood sample will be collected. Sample may need to be kept on ice. Apply pressure to venipuncture site.
Total serum calcium	Measurement of total serum calcium to help detect bone and parathyroid disorders Hypercalcemia can indicate primary hyperparathyroidism, and hypocalcemia can indicate hypoparathyroidism.	2.25–2.75 mmol/L	Inform patient that blood sample will be collected. Avoid prolonged tourniquet application. Apply pressure to venipuncture site.
Ionized calcium	Measurement of free form of calcium unaffected by variable serum albumin levels	1.05–1.3 mmol/L	Same as for total serum calcium.
Serum phosphate	Measurement of inorganic phosphorus Hyperphosphatemia indicates primary hypoparathyroidism or secondary causes (e.g., renal failure); hypophosphatemia indicates hyperparathyroidism Phosphorus and calcium levels are inversely related.	0.97–1.45 mmol/L	Fasting is preferred. Inform patient that blood sample will be collected. Take specimen to the laboratory immediately. Apply pressure to venipuncture site.
Adrenal Studies ***Blood Studies***			
Cortisol	Measures amount of total cortisol in serum and evaluation of status of adrenal cortex function	138–635 nmol/L at 0800 hr 83–359 nmol/L at 1600 hr	Cortisol has diurnal variation: levels are higher in the morning than in evening. Sample should be collected in the morning; evening samples may also be ordered. Mark time of blood collection on the laboratory slip. Patient's anxiety should be minimized.

Continued

TABLE 50.7 **DIAGNOSTIC STUDIES**

Endocrine System—cont'd

Study	Description and Purpose	Normal Values	Nursing Responsibility
Aldosterone	Measurement of aldosterone levels to evaluate for hyperaldosteronism	Upright posture (at least 2 hr): <0.03–1.05 nmol/L Supine position: Peak: 0.35 nmol/L Nadir: 0.14 nmol/L	Usually, a morning blood sample is preferred. On the laboratory slip, indicate patient position (supine, sitting, standing) during venipuncture.
Adrenocorticotrophic hormone (ACTH) (corticotropin)	Measurement of plasma level of ACTH Although ACTH is a pituitary hormone, it controls adrenal cortex secretion; this value helps determine whether underproduction or overproduction of cortisol is caused by dysfunction of the adrenal gland or pituitary gland.	Morning: <18 pmol/L Evening: <11 pmol/L	Patient should be on NPO status after midnight before morning blood collection. Minimize patient's stress. Diurnal levels correspond with variation of cortisol levels; that is, levels are higher in the morning, lower in the evening. ACTH is very unstable; the blood tube must be placed on ice and sent to the laboratory immediately.
ACTH stimulation with cosyntropin	Used to evaluate adrenal function Baseline plasma cortisol levels are measured; IV cosyntropin (synthetic ACTH) is administered; samples are collected 30 and 60 min after bolus.	For the rapid stimulation test, cortisol levels increase more than 267 nmol/L above baseline.	Inject cosyntropin with a plastic syringe and collect blood samples in plastic heparinized tubes. Ensure sample collection at appropriate times.
ACTH suppression (dexamethasone suppression)	Assessment of adrenal function; especially helpful if hyperactivity is suspected Useful in evaluation of Cushing's syndrome Dexamethasone is administered at 2300 hr to suppress secretion of corticotropin-releasing hormone (CRH); plasma cortisol sample is collected at 0800 hr.	Cortisol level <138 nmol/L indicates normal adrenal response (50% decrease in cortisol production)	Ensure that patient has fasted. Inform patient that blood sample will be collected. Observe venipuncture site for bleeding and hematoma formation. Do not test acutely ill patients; those under stress are not tested. ACTH may override suppression. Screen patient for medications such as estrogen and glucocorticoids, which may produce false-positive results. Ensure accurate timing of medication and sample collection.
Metanephrine	Screening for pheochromocytoma; more accurate than urinary vanillylmandelic acid (VMA) and catecholamine measurements	12–60 pg/mL Normetanephrine: 18–111 pg/mL Results may vary by laboratory	Ask about recent history of vigorous exercise, high levels of stress, or starvation (may artificially ↑ levels). Ingestion of caffeine, alcohol, levodopa, lithium, nitroglycerin, acetaminophen, and medications containing epinephrine or norepinephrine can alter test results.
Urine Studies			
17-Ketosteroids	Measurement of androgen metabolites in urine and evaluation of adrenocortical and gonadal function	Male: 20–70 mcmol/day Female: 20–60 mcmol/day	Instruct patient in 24-hr urine collection. Tell patient that specimen must be kept refrigerated or on ice during collection. Determine whether preservative is required for method used.
Aldosterone	Measurement of urinary aldosterone level to diagnose hyperaldosteronism	0.11–0.86 nmol	Ensure that patient is on an unrestricted diet with normal salt intake and no medication for 3 weeks before collection. Instruct patient in 24-hr urine collection.
Cortisol, urine (free cortisol)	Measurement of free (unbound) cortisol for patients with suspected hyper- or hypofunction of the adrenal gland Preferred test for evaluating hypercortisolism	0800 hr: 138–635 nmol/L 1600 hr: 83–359 nmol/L	Instruct patient in 24-hr urine collection and to avoid stressful situations and doing excessive physical exercise. Some medications may alter levels. Ensure that patient is on a low-sodium diet.
Vanillylmandelic acid (VMA)	Measurement of urinary excretion of catecholamine metabolite; helpful in diagnosing pheochromocytoma	<35 mcmol/24 hr Elevated values indicate pheochromocytoma	Collect specimen with a preservative. Keep it on ice. Consult with laboratory or physician about whether patient should discontinue any medications 3 days before urine collection and a VMA-restricted diet.
Radiology			
Abdominal computed tomographic (CT) scan	The radiological examination of choice for the adrenal gland Used to detect tumour and size of tumour mass or metastatic spread Oral or IV contrast medium, or both, may be used	—	Inform patient of the need to lie still during the procedure. If IV contrast medium is to be used, check for iodine and shellfish allergy before the test.

TABLE 50.7   DIAGNOSTIC STUDIES
Endocrine System—cont'd

Study	Description and Purpose	Normal Values	Nursing Responsibility
Pancreatic Studies			
Blood Studies			
Fasting blood glucose (FBG) level	Measurement of circulating glucose level	4–6 mmol/L	Ensure that patient fasts for at least 4–8 hr; water intake is permitted.
Oral glucose tolerance test (OGTT)	2-hr test: Used to diagnose diabetes mellitus if FBG result is equivocal; patient drinks 75 g of glucose. Samples for glucose are collected immediately and at 30, 60, and 120 min. 5-hr test: Used to evaluate hypoglycemia. Patient drinks 100 g of glucose; samples of glucose are collected immediately and at 30, 60, 90, 120, 180, 240, and 300 min.	<11.1 mmol/L at 30 and 60 min <7.8 mmol/L at 120 min <6.4 mmol/L at 3 and 4 hr	Instruct patient to fast (unless otherwise ordered), refrain from smoking and ingesting caffeine, and fast for 12 hr before test. Ensure that patient's diet 3 days before test included 150–300 g of carbohydrate. Simultaneously monitor glucose levels with capillary glucose monitoring if patient is symptomatic. Encourage water intake during the test. Collect urine samples hourly. Allow patient to eat after test. Administer medications as ordered, after the test.
Capillary glucose monitoring	Provides immediate glucose values with glucose oxidase or electrochemical methods	Capillary values (whole blood): 10–15% less than serum values Most capillary blood glucose meters automatically accommodate for this discrepancy.	Obtain a large drop of blood from a clean finger, touch strip to drop of blood (not finger), time accurately, and compare colours in good lighting if visual method is used. Use digital readout if it is available. Use an automatic finger-puncture device if it is available. Be sure to change section of device that touches patient's fingers between uses.
Glycosylated or hemoglobin (A1c)	Measurement of degree of glucose control during previous 3 mo (lifespan of hemoglobin molecule)	<6% for patients without diabetes <7% for patients with good diabetic control (values vary; check with laboratory)	Inform patient that fasting is not necessary and that blood sample will be collected. Observe venipuncture site for bleeding or hematoma formation.
Urine Studies			
Glucose	Estimation of amount of glucose in urine through use of an enzymatic method Dipstick is dipped into the urine and read for colour changes after 1 min.	Random: negative 24-hr: <2.78 mmol/24 hr (<0.5 g/24 hr)	Use a freshly voided urine specimen collected at appropriate time. Know that many different medications alter glucose readings and that errors are great if directions for timing are not followed exactly. Follow package directions.
Ketones	Measurement of amount of acetone excreted in urine as result of incomplete fat metabolism Tested with a dipstick as described for glucose study	Negative or trace amount of ketone is normal Positive result can indicate lack of insulin and diabetic ketoacidosis	Use a freshly voided urine specimen. The test is often performed with a glucose test. Directions must be followed exactly. Certain medications can produce false-positive and false-negative results.
Radiology			
Abdominal computed tomographic (CT) scan	The radiological examination of choice for pancreas Used to identify tumours or cysts Oral or IV contrast medium (or both) may be ordered	—	Inform patient of the need to lie still during the procedure. If IV contrast is to be used, check for iodine allergy before test.

ADH, antidiuretic hormone; *BP*, blood pressure; *CNS*, central nervous system; *DI*, diabetes insipidus; *IV*, intravenous; *NPO*, nothing by mouth; *PO*, by mouth.

Laboratory Studies

Laboratory studies used to diagnose endocrine problems may include direct measurement of the hormone level or an indirect indication of gland function by evaluation of blood or urine components affected by the hormone (e.g., electrolytes).

Hormones with constant basal levels (e.g., T_4) need be measured only once. Notation of sample time is important for hormones with circadian or sleep-related secretion (e.g., cortisol). Evaluation of other hormones may require multiple blood sampling, as in suppression tests (e.g., dexamethasone) and stimulation tests (e.g., glucose tolerance). In these situations, it is often necessary to obtain intravenous access to administer medications and fluids and to collect multiple blood samples.

FOCUSED ASSESSMENT

Endocrine System

Use this checklist to ensure the key assessment steps have been performed.

Subjective

Ask the patient about experiencing any of the following and note responses.

Excessive or increased thirst	Y	N
Excessive or decreased urination	Y	N
Excessive hunger	Y	N
Intolerance of heat or cold	Y	N
Excessive sweating	Y	N
Recent weight gain or loss	Y	N

Objective: Diagnostic

Check the following laboratory results for critical values.

Potassium level	✓
Glucose level	✓
Sodium level	✓
Glycosylated hemoglobin (A_{1C}) level	✓
Thyroid studies: TSH, (T_3, and T_4 levels [if ordered])	✓

Objective: Physical Examination

Inspect/Measure

Body temperature	✓
Height and weight	✓
Alertness and emotional state	✓
Skin, for changes in colour and texture	✓
Hair, for changes in colour, texture, and distribution	✓

Auscultate

Heart rate, blood pressure	✓

Palpate

Extremities, for edema	✓
Skin, for texture and temperature	✓
Neck, for thyroid size, shape	✓

TSH, thyroid-stimulating hormone; *T3*, triiodothyronine; *T4*, thyroxine.

CASE STUDY

Objective Data: Diagnostic Studies

The health care provider orders the following initial diagnostic studies to be drawn in the morning after 8 hours of fasting:

- Complete blood count (CBC), basic metabolic panel (electrolytes, BUN, creatinine)
- Fasting blood glucose (FBG)
- TSH, free T_4
- Plasma cortisol levels
- Plasma ACTH levels

CBC results reveal a white blood cell (WBC) count of 12.2×10^9/L and a lymphocyte count at 8×10^9/L. The rest of the CBC is within defined limits (WDL).

The fasting blood glucose (FBG) is 7.2 mmol/L. Plasma cortisol and ACTH levels are elevated. Thyroid studies are WDL. Based on these findings, the health care provider diagnoses L. M. with Cushing's syndrome. L. M. will require interprofessional care to determine the cause of and a plan of care for this new diagnosis. The primary goal is to normalize hormone secretion. (See Chapter 51 for more information on Cushing's syndrome.)

See Case Study: Patient Introduction, Case Study: Subjective Data, and Case Study: Objective Data: Physical Examination for more information on L. M.

Pituitary Studies. Disorders associated with the pituitary gland can manifest in a wide variety of ways because of the number of hormones produced. Many diagnostic studies are available to evaluate these hormones either directly or indirectly (see Table 50.7).

Thyroid Studies. A number of tests are available to evaluate thyroid function. The most sensitive and accurate laboratory test is TSH measurement; thus, it is recommended as the main diagnostic test for evaluation of thyroid function (Canadian Society of Endocrinology and Metabolism [CSEM], 2019). Common additional tests ordered in the presence of abnormal TSH levels include total serum T_4, free T_4, and total serum T_3. The Canadian Society of Endocrinology and Metabolism in conjunction with Choosing Wisely Canada has recommended that free T_4 or T_3 not be used to screen for hypothyroidism or to monitor and adjust levothyroxine (L-T_4, Synthroid) dosage in patients with known primary hypothyroidism, unless the patient has suspected or known pituitary or hypothalamic disease (CSEM, 2019).

Free T_4 is the unbound T_4, and its level is a more accurate reflection of thyroid function than total T_4. Less common tests that help differentiate various types of thyroid disease include measurement of T_3, assessment of free T_3 resin uptake, measurement of thyroid autoantibodies, thyroid scanning, ultrasonography, and biopsy. Thyroid ultrasound is not a part of routine evaluation unless palpable lumps or enlargement are noted, as overzealous use of ultrasound frequently identifies benign nodules that are unrelated to abnormal thyroid function (Choosing Wisely Canada, 2020).

Parathyroid Studies. The only hormone secreted by the parathyroid glands is PTH. Because the function of PTH is to regulate serum calcium and phosphate levels, abnormalities in PTH secretion are reflected in the calcium and phosphate levels. For this reason, diagnostic tests for the parathyroid gland typically include measurements of PTH, serum calcium, and serum phosphate.

Adrenal Studies. Diagnostic tests associated with the adrenal glands focus on the three types of hormones secreted: glucocorticoids, mineralocorticoids, and androgens. These hormone levels can be measured in both blood plasma and urine. Urine studies are usually performed as 24-hour collections. The major advantage of a 24-hour urine sample is that the short-term fluctuations in hormone levels seen in plasma samples are eliminated (Pagana & Pagana, 2019).

Pancreatic Studies. The tests found in Table 50.7 are geared toward evaluating the metabolism of glucose. They are important in the diagnosis and management of diabetes. (Diagnostic studies for diabetes are discussed in Chapter 52.)

REVIEW QUESTIONS

The number of the question corresponds to the same-numbered objective at the beginning of the chapter.

1. Which of the following is a characteristic common to all hormones?
   a. They circulate in the blood bound to plasma proteins.
   b. They influence cellular activity of specific target tissues.
   c. They accelerate the metabolic processes of all body cells.
   d. They enter cells to alter the cell's metabolism or gene expression.

2. A client is receiving radiation therapy for cancer of the kidney. The nurse monitors the client for manifestations of damage to which of the following organ(s)?
   a. Pancreas
   b. Thyroid
   c. Adrenal glands
   d. Posterior pituitary gland

3. A client has a serum sodium level of 152 mmol/L. What is the normal hormonal response to this situation?
   a. Release of ADH
   b. Release of renin
   c. Secretion of aldosterone
   d. Secretion of corticotropin-releasing hormone

4. All cells in the body are believed to have intracellular receptors for which of the following?
   a. Insulin
   b. Glucagon
   c. Growth hormone
   d. Thyroid hormone

5. When obtaining subjective data from a client during assessment of the endocrine system, the nurse asks specifically about which of the following?
   a. Energy level
   b. Intake of vitamin C
   c. Employment history
   d. Frequency of sexual intercourse

6. Why do endocrine disorders often go unrecognized in older persons?
   a. Symptoms are often attributed to aging.
   b. Older persons rarely have identifiable symptoms.
   c. Endocrine disorders are relatively rare in the older person.
   d. Older persons usually have subclinical endocrine disorders that minimize symptoms.

7. Which of the following would the nurse consider an abnormal finding during an endocrine assessment? *(Select all that apply.)*
   a. Blood pressure of 100/70
   b. Soft, formed stool every other day
   c. Excessive facial hair on a woman
   d. 1.5-kg weight gain over the last 6 months
   e. Hyperpigmented coloration in lower legs

8. A client has a total serum calcium level of 0.75 mmol/L. If this finding reflects hypoparathyroidism, what would the nurse expect further diagnostic testing to reveal?
   a. Decreased serum PTH
   b. Increased serum ACTH
   c. Increased serum glucose
   d. Decreased serum cortisol levels

1. b; 2. c; 3. a; 4. d; 5. a; 6. a; 7. c, e; 8. a.

ⓔvolve

For even more review questions, visit http://evolve.elsevier.com/Canada/Lewis/medsurg.

REFERENCES

Barnes, M. A., Carson, M. J., & Nair, M. G. (2015). Non-traditional cytokines: How catecholamines and adipokines influence macrophages in immunity, metabolism and the central nervous system. *Cytokine, 72*(2), 210–219. https://doi.org/10.1016/j.cyto.2015.01.008

Betts, J. G., Young, K. A., Wise, J. A., et al. (2019). *Anatomy and physiology*. OpenStax.

Booth, A., Magnuson, A., Fouts, J., et al. (2016). Adipose tissue: An endocrine organ playing a role in metabolic regulation. *Hormone Molecular Biology and Clinical Investigation, 26*(1), 25–42. https://doi.org/10.1515/hmbci-2015-0073

Brashers, V. L., Huether, S. E., & Power-Kean, K. (2018). Mechanisms of hormonal regulation. In M. T. El-Hussein, K. Power-Kean, S. Zettel, et al. (Eds.), *Understanding pathophysiology* (1st Canadian ed.) (pp. 443–464). Elsevier.

Canadian Society of Endocrinology and Metabolism (CSEM). (2019). *CSEM review and response: Choosing wisely Canada recommendation #3: Testing and management of primary hypothyroidism.* https://thyroid.ca/wp-content/uploads/2019/04/CSEM-Thyroid-Testing-and-Management-Response-2019.pdf

Carroll, T. B., Aron, D. C., Findling, J. W., et al. (2018). Glucocorticoids and adrenal androgens. In D. G. Gardner, & D. Shoback (Eds.), *Greenspan's basic and clinical endocrinology* (10th ed.) (pp. 299–341). Lange.

Choosing Wisely Canada. (2020). *Endocrinology and metabolism: Five things physicians and patients should question.* https://choosingwiselycanada.org/endocrinology-and-metabolism/

Glad, C. A. M., Andersson-Assarsson, J. C., Berglund, P., et al. (2017). Reduced DNA methylation and psychopathology following endogenous hypercortisolism—A genome-wide study. *Scientific Reports, 7*, 44445. https://doi.org/10.1038/srep44445

Grody, W. W. (2019). Clinical molecular endocrinology laboratory testing. In N. Lavin (Ed.), *Manual of endocrinology and metabolism* (5th ed.). Wolters Kluwer.

Hannon, R. A., & Porth, C. M. (2017). *Porth pathophysiology concepts of altered health states* (2nd Canadian ed.). Wolters Kluwer.

Jarvis, C., Browne, A. J., MacDonald-Jenkins, J., et al. (Eds.). (2019). *Physical examination & health assessment* (3rd Canadian ed.) Elsevier.

Jarvis, C., & MacDonald-Jenkins, J. (2019). Head, face, and neck, including regional lymphatic system. In C. Jarvis, A. J. Browne, J. MacDonald-Jenkins, et al. (Eds.), *Physical examination & health assessment* (3rd Canadian ed.) (pp. 271–299). Elsevier.

Javorsky, B. R., Aron, D. C., Findling, J. W., et al. (2018). Hypothalamus and pituitary gland. In D. G. Gardner, & D. Shoback (Eds.), *Greenspan's basic and clinical endocrinology* (10th ed.) (pp. 69–119). Lange.

Keithley, J. K., Vogel, E., Miller, A., et al. (2019). Nutritional assessment and nursing practice. In C. Jarvis, A. J. Browne, J. MacDonald-Jenkins, et al. (Eds.), *Physical examination & health assessment* (3rd Canadian ed.) (pp. 196–218). Elsevier.

Lavin, N. (2019). Hypopituitarism after traumatic brain injury. In N. Lavin (Ed.), *Manual of endocrinology and metabolism* (5th ed.). Wolters Kluwer.

Manley, K., Han, W., Zelin, G., et al. (2018). Crosstalk between the immune, endocrine, and nervous systems in immunotoxicology. *Current Opinion in Toxicology, 10,* 37–45. https://doi.org/10.1016/j.cotox.2017.12.003

Martin, C. R., Osadchiy, V., Kalani, A., et al. (2018). The brain–gut–microbe axis. *Cellular and Molecular Gastroenterology and Hepatology, 6,* 133–148. https://doi.org/10.1016/j.jcmgh.2018.04.003

Masharani, U., & German, M. S. (2018). Pancreatic hormones and diabetes mellitus. In D. G. Gardner, & D. Shoback (Eds.), *Greenspan's basic and clinical endocrinology* (10th ed.) (pp. 595–682). Lange.

McCance, K. L., Moktar, A., & Power-Kean, K. (2018). Alterations of the female reproductive systems. In M. T. El-Hussein, K. Power-Kean, S. Zettel, et al. (Eds.), *Understanding pathophysiology* (1st Canadian ed.) (pp. 816–867). Elsevier.

Molina, P. E. (2018). *Endocrine physiology* (5th ed.). McGraw-Hill.

Nigam, Y., & Knight, J. (2020). The lymphatic system 2: Structure and function of the lymphoid organs. *Nursing Times, 116*(11), 44–48.

Pagana, K. D., & Pagana, T. J. (2019). *Mosby's Canadian manual of diagnostic and laboratory tests* (2nd Canadian ed.). Elsevier.

Patton, K. (2019). *Anatomy and physiology* (10th ed.). Elsevier.

Rosen, M. P., & Cedars, M. I. (2018). Female reproductive endocrinology and infertility. In D. G. Gardner, & D. Shoback (Eds.), *Greenspan's basic and clinical endocrinology* (10th ed.) (pp. 443–500). Lange.

Rosenthal, S. M., & Hembree, W. C. (2018). Transgender endocrinology. In D. G. Gardner, & D. Shoback (Eds.), *Greenspan's basic and clinical endocrinology* (10th ed.) (pp. 771–782). Lange.

Saghazadeh, A., & Rezaei, N. (2020). In N. Rezaei (Ed.), *Introductory chapter: Thymus—The central self-tolerance system*. IntechOpen. Thymus (pp. 7-6).

Sousa, A., Ferreira, M., Oliveira, C., et al. (2020). Gender differential transcriptome in gastric and thyroid cancers. *Frontiers in Genetics, 11*(808), 1–11. https://doi.org/10.3389/fgene.2020.00808

Talaei, A., Rafee, N., Rafei, F., et al. (2017). TSH cut off point based on depression in hypothyroid patients. *BMC Psychiatry, 17*(1), 327. https://doi.org/10.1186/s12888-017-1478-9

Thomas, D. D., Corkey, B. E., Istfan, N. W., et al. (2019). Hyperinsulinemia: An early indicator of metabolic dysfunction. *Journal of the Endocrine Society, 3*(9), 1727–1747. https://doi.org/10.1210/js.2019-00065

Van Den Beld, A. W., Kaufman, J. M., Zillikens, M. C., et al. (2018). The physiology of endocrine systems with ageing. *The Lancet Diabetes & Endocrinology, 6*(8), 647–657. https://doi.org/10.1016/S2213-8587(18)30026-3

Young, W. F. (2018). Endocrine hypertension. In D. G. Gardner, & D. Shoback (Eds.), *Greenspan's basic and clinical endocrinology* (10th ed.) (pp. 343–357). Lange.

RESOURCES

Resources for this chapter are listed in Chapter 51 and Chapter 52.

Nursing Management
Endocrine Conditions

Heather E. Helpard
Originating US chapter by Ann Crawford

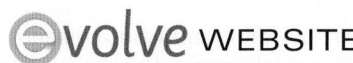 WEBSITE

http://evolve.elsevier.com/Canada/Lewis/medsurg

- Review Questions (Online Only)
- Key Points
- Answer Guidelines for Case Study
- Student Case Studies
  - Addison's Disease

- Cushing's Syndrome
- Hyperthyroidism
- Customizable Nursing Care Plans
  - Hyperthyroidism
  - Hypothyroidism

- Patient with Cushing's Syndrome
- Conceptual Care Map Creator
- Audio Glossary
- Content Updates

LEARNING OBJECTIVES

1. Describe the pathophysiology and clinical manifestations relating to an imbalance of hormones produced by the anterior pituitary gland as well as the interprofessional care and nursing management of patients with this imbalance.
2. Describe the pathophysiology and clinical manifestations relating to an imbalance of hormones produced by the posterior pituitary gland as well as the interprofessional care and nursing management of patients with this imbalance.
3. Describe the pathophysiology and clinical manifestations of thyroid dysfunction as well as the interprofessional care and nursing management of the patient with thyroid dysfunction.
4. Describe the pathophysiology and clinical manifestations of imbalance of the hormone produced by the parathyroid glands as well as the interprofessional care and nursing management of affected patients.

5. Describe the pathophysiology and clinical manifestations of an imbalance of hormones produced by the adrenal cortex as well as the interprofessional care and nursing management of affected patients.
6. Describe the pathophysiology and clinical manifestations relating to excess of hormones produced by the adrenal medulla as well as the interprofessional care and nursing management of affected patients.
7. Explain the adverse effects of corticosteroid therapy.
8. Describe common nursing assessments, interventions, rationales, and expected outcomes related to patient teaching for management of chronic endocrine conditions.

KEY TERMS

acromegaly
Addison's disease
Cushing's syndrome
diabetes insipidus (DI)
exophthalmos
goitre
Graves' disease

hyperaldosteronism
hyperparathyroidism
hyperthyroidism
hypoparathyroidism
hypopituitarism
hypothyroidism
myxedema

myxedema coma
pheochromocytoma
syndrome of inappropriate antidiuretic
  hormone (SIADH)
thyroiditis
thyrotoxicosis

DISORDERS OF THE ANTERIOR PITUITARY GLAND

ACROMEGALY

Etiology and Pathophysiology

Acromegaly is a relatively rare condition caused by excessive secretion of growth hormone (GH), which typically results from a benign GH-secreting pituitary tumour (adenoma). Hypersecretion of circulating GH leads to the secondary elevation of circulating insulin-like growth factor-1 (IGF-1) from the liver and systemic tissues, contributing to metabolic dysfunction and bone and soft tissue overgrowth, particularly in the face, hands, and feet. Acromegaly affects only adults because the condition develops after epiphyseal closure. The estimated worldwide prevalence is about 4 600 per million population, with about

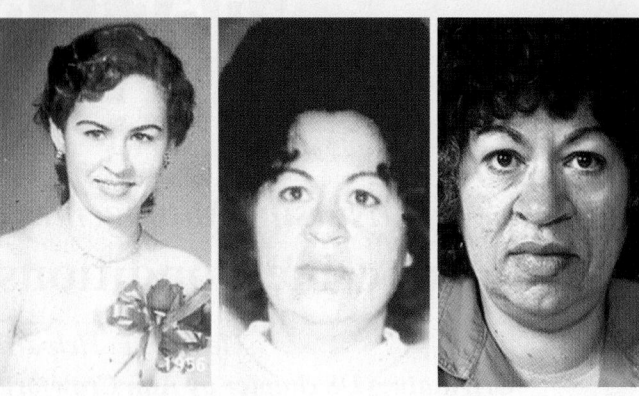

FIG. 51.1 Example of progressive changes in facial features in acromegaly. Source: Courtesy Linda Haas, Seattle, Washington.

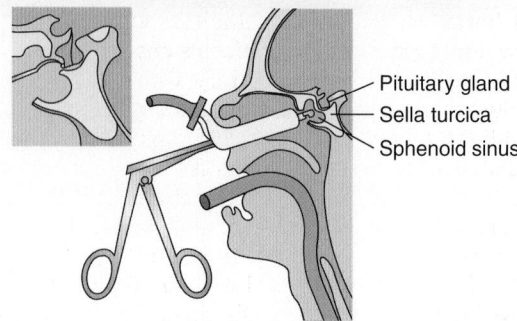

Pituitary gland
Sella turcica
Sphenoid sinus

FIG. 51.2 Surgery on the pituitary gland is most commonly performed with the trans-sphenoidal approach. An incision is made in the inner aspect of the upper lip and gingiva. The sella turcica is entered through the floor of the nose and the sphenoid sinuses.

116.9 new cases per million annually (Matyjaszek-Matuszek et al., 2018). Men and women are affected in equal numbers.

Clinical Manifestations

Manifestations of acromegaly begin insidiously, usually in the third and fourth decades of life. Delayed diagnosis often occurs 6 to 20 years after the appearance of the first symptom (Sesmilo et al., 2013). What is most noticeable is the enlargement of the hands and feet. The amplification of the bones and cartilage may cause symptoms ranging from mild joint pain to deforming, crippling arthritis. Changes in physical appearance occur, with thickening and enlargement of bony and soft tissue on the face and head (Figure 51.1). Enlargement of the mandible causes the jaw to protrude forward. The paranasal and the frontal sinuses enlarge, as does the bony tissue of the forehead. Enlargement of soft tissue around the eyes, nose, and mouth results in a coarsening of facial features. Enlargement of the tongue results in speech difficulties, and the voice deepens as a result of hypertrophy of the vocal cords.

Sleep apnea may also occur and is thought to be related to anatomical changes in bone structures and soft tissue enlargement and narrowing of the upper airway (Sesmilo et al., 2017). The skin becomes thick, leathery, and oily, with many patients experiencing peripheral neuropathy (nerve compression by hypertrophic tissue) and proximal muscle weakness. Women may develop menstrual irregularities due to higher GH levels and marked estrogen deficiency. With elevated serum GH and circulating IGF-1 levels, patients are also more likely to develop polyps in the colon and colon cancer, necessitating screening approximately every 5 years (Katznelson et al., 2014).

The enlarged pituitary gland can exert pressure on surrounding structures within the brain, leading to frequent visual disturbances and headaches. Elevated GH and IGF-1 levels predispose individuals to metabolic disturbances such as hyperinsulinemia, contributing to alterations in pancreatic β cell function, peripheral insulin resistance, decreased glucose disposal in the muscle, and hyperglycemia (Ferrau et al., 2018). Manifestations of impaired glucose intolerance or diabetes mellitus (DM) may occur, including *polydipsia* (increased thirst) and *polyuria* (increased urination). As GH mobilizes stored fat for energy, it increases free fatty acid levels in the blood, predisposing patients to atherosclerosis, coronary artery disease, left ventricular dysfunction, and cardiac arrhythmias (Ramos-Levi & Marazeula, 2019). Other systems that undergo changes include the gastrointestinal (GI), genitourinary, musculoskeletal, and nervous systems.

Diagnostic Studies

In addition to the history and physical examination, diagnosis of acromegaly requires biochemical testing. The best single test is measurement of serum IGF-1 (Katznelson et al., 2014). Unlike GH, serum IGF-1 concentrations do not vary throughout the day with food intake, exercise, or sleep and are virtually elevated in all individuals with acromegaly. If for some reason serum IGF-1 levels are ambiguous, serum GH levels should be measured in response to an oral glucose tolerance test (OGTT). Normally, GH concentration falls during an OGTT. In acromegaly, these levels do not fall (AlDallal, 2018).

Magnetic resonance imaging (MRI) with contrast administration is considered the most effective technique to identify and localize a pituitary tumour as small as 2 mm in diameter. MRI evaluation determines pituitary tumour extension into surrounding tissue and proximity to the optic chiasm. High-resolution computed tomographic (CT) scan with contrast media may also be used to localize the tumour, but it is less sensitive. A complete ophthalmological examination, including evaluation of visual fields, is performed if the tumour lies adjacent to the optic chiasm or the optic nerves (AlDallal, 2018).

Interprofessional Care

The therapeutic goal in acromegaly is to return serum GH and circulating IGF-1 levels to normal ranges appropriate for a patient's age and gender. This is accomplished by surgery, radiation therapy, medication therapy, or a combination of these therapies. The prognosis depends on age at onset, age when treatment is initiated, and tumour size. Usually, bone growth can be arrested, soft tissue hypertrophy can be reversed, and headaches and visual changes can be alleviated. However, bony abnormalities do not generally regress, and joint, sleep apnea, and diabetic and cardiac complications, while improved, may persist in spite of treatment.

Surgical Therapy. For most patients with acromegaly, *trans-sphenoidal* surgery is the treatment of choice for those with pituitary microadenomas or resectable macroadenomas (Katznelson et al., 2014; Figure 51.2). Surgery produces an immediate reduction in GH levels, followed by a drop and normalization in IGF-1 levels within 3 months (Katznelson et al., 2014). When the entire pituitary gland is removed during surgery *(hypophysectomy)*, the loss of pituitary hormones is permanent. Potential complications with macroadenoma removal may include long-term deficiency in one or more pituitary hormones, central diabetes insipidus (DI), cerebrospinal rhinorrhea, and meningitis. Rather than replacing the pituitary (tropic) hormones parenterally, the essential hormones produced by target organs (glucocorticoids, thyroid hormone, and sex hormones) can be replaced orally with lifelong hormonal medication therapy. Also, patients with macroadenomas or those with GH levels higher than 50 mcg/L may require adjuvant radiation or stereotactic radiation therapy.

Radiation Therapy. Radiation therapy is considered when (1) surgery has failed to produce complete remission and (2) patients are considered to be at high risk for surgical complications. The long delay before GH and circulating IGF-1 levels normalize limits the usefulness of radiation therapy in treating symptoms (AlDallal, 2018). Radiation therapy is usually offered in combination with medications that reduce GH and circulating IGF-1 levels or to reduce the size of a tumour before surgery. (Radiation therapy is discussed in Chapter 18.) Hypopituitarism commonly results from radiation therapy and necessitates hormone therapy.

Stereotactic radiosurgery (gamma-knife surgery, proton beam, linear accelerator) may be used for small, surgically inaccessible pituitary tumours (see Chapter 59). This procedure consists of a single dose of radiation delivered to one site from multiple angles.

Medication Therapy. Three groups of medications are used in the initial or adjuvant treatment (surgery, radiation) of acromegaly: somatostatin analogues, dopamine agonists, and GH-receptor antagonists. These medications reduce GH levels by binding to specific receptors for somatostatin and its analogues. The most common medication used for acromegaly is octreotide (Sandostatin), a somatostatin analogue given by subcutaneous injection three times a day, which reduces and normalizes GH levels in many patients. Two long-acting analogues, octreotide (Sandostatin LAR) and lanreotide (Somatuline Autogel), are available as intramuscular (IM) injections every 2 to 4 weeks. Dopamine agonists, such as oral cabergoline (Dostinex) and bromocriptine mesylate (Apo-bromocriptine), may also be used in the treatment of acromegaly to suppress GH secretion. They are not commonly used as sole therapy; rather, they are combined with somatostatin analogues. A GH receptor antagonist, pegvisomant (Somavert), delivered via daily, subcutaneous injection, directly blocks GH action, resulting in decreased circulating levels of IGF-1. With this medication, serum IGF-1 concentration should be measured every 4 to 6 weeks and the dose adjusted, in 5-mg increments to a maximum of 30 mg/day. It is recommended in patients for whom surgery, somatostatin analogues, and dopamine agonists have failed. Recently, researchers have started to favor combination pegvisomant therapy with somatostatin analogue or dopamine agonist agents, provided patients do not exhibit abnormal liver function (Strasburger et al., 2018)

NURSING MANAGEMENT
ACROMEGALY

NURSING ASSESSMENT

Signs and symptoms of acromegaly develop very slowly over time. The nurse must assess for signs and symptoms of abnormal tissue growth and evaluate changes in the physical size of each patient. Patients should be questioned about increases in hat, ring, glove, and shoe sizes, as well as changes in facial (protrusion of the brow and lower jaw) and maxillary (teeth do not line up correctly when the mouth is closed) appearance. Photographs are helpful for evaluating any changes (see Figure 51.1).

Other areas of assessment include the development of carpal tunnel syndrome, visual field defects, skin changes (thickened, oily skin, acne, excessive sweating), deepening voice, fatigue and weakness, sleep apnea, hypothyroidism, hyperglycemia, insulin resistance, dyslipidemia, hypertension, coronary artery disease, peripheral neuropathy, menstrual irregularities in women, and impotence in men.

In addition, blood tests of IGF-1 levels, growth hormone–releasing hormone (GHRH), and other pituitary hormones are needed. An OGTT may be done to see if GH drops, which will not be the case in acromegaly. Following these tests, an MRI with contrast is recommended to locate a possible pituitary tumour.

NURSING IMPLEMENTATION

PREOPERATIVE. At the time of diagnosis, the patient requires educational and emotional support. Surgical and medical treatment can reverse or improve some physical deformities, metabolic disturbances, and hormonal imbalances. Emotional support should include the exploration of coping methods, social support networks, and mental health resources to promote healthy body image and self-esteem and to reduce anxiety and depressive symptoms.

POSTOPERATIVE. After surgery, in which a *trans-sphenoidal* approach has been used, the head of the patient's bed should be elevated at a 15- to 30-degree angle at all times to prevent pressure on the sella turcica and decrease the incidence of headaches, a frequent postoperative symptom also relieved by mild analgesics. Neurological status, including pupillary response, should be monitored to detect neurological complications. Patients should be instructed to avoid vigorous coughing, sneezing, nose blowing, and straining during bowel movements (Valsalva manoeuvre), to prevent leakage of cerebrospinal fluid (CSF) from the point at which the sella turcica was entered. The nurse should perform mouth care every 4 hours to keep the surgical area clean and free of debris and to promote patient comfort. Tooth brushing should be avoided for at least 10 days to prevent disrupting the suture line and to avoid discomfort. Stool softeners are often prescribed to avoid increased intracranial pressure during defecation.

Any clear nasal drainage should be sent to the laboratory to be tested for glucose. A glucose level higher than 1.67 mmol/L indicates leakage of CSF from an open connection to the brain and puts the patient at increased risk for meningitis. Complaints of persistent and severe generalized or supraorbital headache or salty and metallic taste sensations may indicate leakage of CSF into the sinuses. A CSF leak usually resolves within 72 hours when treated with head elevation and bed rest. If the leak persists, daily spinal taps may be performed to reduce intracranial pressure. When a patient has a CSF leak, intravenous (IV) antibiotics should be administered as ordered to prevent meningitis. If the leak does not respond to treatment within 72 hours, surgical repair may be required.

If stereotactic radiosurgery is performed, the patient is usually moved from the specialized radiation centre to the neurosurgical nursing unit for overnight observation. The patient is in a stereotactic head frame with pin sites that may create discomfort. All interprofessional team members should know how to remove a stereotactic frame in case of an emergency. Vital signs, pain level, neurological status, and fluid volume status must be carefully monitored, as possible complications include increased headaches, seizures (at least 24 hours postprocedure), nausea, and vomiting. Pin site care should be performed according to institutional policy. Family members can be instructed in pin site care if the patient is discharged with pins in place.

A possible postoperative complication is transient DI. This complication may occur because of the loss of antidiuretic hormone (ADH) or because of cerebral edema related to manipulation of the pituitary gland during surgery. To assess for DI, increased, dilute urine output as well as high serum and low urine osmolality must be monitored and reported. Clinical manifestations and treatment of DI are discussed in more detail later in this chapter.

Surgery may result in permanent loss or deficiencies in follicle-stimulating hormone (FSH) and luteinizing hormone (LH), which can lead to decreased fertility for both men and women. The nurse should assist patients in working through the grieving process associated with these losses.

If a *hypophysectomy* is performed or the pituitary gland is damaged, replacement of ADH, cortisol, and thyroid hormone is necessary. These medications must be taken for life, and the need for continued medication therapy may reduce the patient's perception of independence and require considerable emotional adjustment. Somatostatin analogues, such as octreotide (Sandostatin), are usually well tolerated. If prescribed, the teaching plan should include self-administration of subcutaneous injections and discussion of potential adverse effects, such as nausea, abdominal discomfort, bloating, loose stools, and fat malabsorption during the first several weeks of therapy. For patients prescribed pegvisomant, the teaching plan should include education about monthly serum IGF-1 and liver function tests, administration of subcutaneous injections, and injection-site rotation to avoid lipohypertrophy. Issues related to the expense of ongoing medication, as well as other therapies, may be another area for nursing intervention.

For patients with acromegaly who are experiencing risks (hypertension, hyperinsulinemia, and dyslipidemia) for metabolic disorders (diabetes and cardiovascular disease), referral to cardiology and endocrinology specialists and services is recommended (Frara et al., 2016; Ramos-Levi & Marazuela, 2019). Also, for those patients at higher risk for colon polyps and colorectal cancer, screening for colon neoplasia with colonoscopy at diagnosis is suggested (Gordon et al., 2016).

The nurse must consider the emotional impact of a *hypophysectomy* when counselling patients and planning the educational program related to hormone replacement. Serial photographs to show improvement may be helpful, as well as connecting patients and their families with mental health services and social support resources.

HYPOFUNCTION OF THE PITUITARY GLAND

Hypopituitarism is a rare disorder that involves a decrease in one or more of the pituitary hormones; signs and symptoms relate to the underlying disorder and to the specific pituitary hormones that are deficient or absent. The hormone deficiencies most commonly associated with hypopituitarism involve GH and the gonadotropins (e.g., LH, FSH).

Etiology and Pathophysiology

The most common cause of pituitary hypofunction is a pituitary tumour. Autoimmune disorders, infections, pituitary infarction (Sheehan's syndrome), or destruction of the pituitary gland (as a result of trauma, irradiation, or surgical procedures) can also cause hypopituitarism. *Sheehan's syndrome* is a postpartum condition of pituitary necrosis and hypopituitarism after circulatory collapse resulting from uterine hemorrhaging.

Clinical Manifestations and Diagnostic Studies

The manifestations associated with pituitary hypofunction vary with the type and degree of dysfunction. Early manifestations associated with a space-occupying lesion include headaches, visual changes (decreased visual acuity or decreased peripheral vision), loss of smell, nausea and vomiting, and seizures.

In addition to a history and physical examination, diagnostic studies such as MRI and CT are used to identify a pituitary tumour. Laboratory tests for diagnosing hypopituitarism vary widely but generally involve the direct measurement of pituitary hormones (e.g., thyroid-stimulating hormone [TSH]) or an indirect determination of the target organ hormones (e.g., triiodothyronine [T_3], thyroxine [T_4]). (See Chapter 50 for more information regarding diagnostic studies.)

NURSING AND INTERPROFESSIONAL MANAGEMENT HYPOPITUITARISM

Treatment of hypopituitarism consists of surgery or radiation therapy for tumour removal, followed by permanent hormone replacement. Surgery and radiation therapy for pituitary tumours are discussed earlier in this chapter. Hormone therapy is carried out with the appropriate pituitary hormone (e.g., GH, corticosteroids, thyroid hormone, and sex hormones). Hormone therapies for thyroid hormone and corticosteroids are discussed later in this chapter.

A primary nursing role in anterior pituitary insufficiency is the assessment and recognition of signs and symptoms associated with hypopituitarism. Nursing management is directed at conditions that result from hormone deficiency. The nurse also plays a pivotal role in teaching patients about diagnostic procedures, the disease process, and interprofessional care options. Because the need for hormone therapy is lifelong, patient teaching must cover hormonal administration, adverse medication effects, and follow-up therapy.

DISORDERS OF THE POSTERIOR PITUITARY GLAND

The hormones secreted by the posterior pituitary—ADH and oxytocin—are actually produced in the hypothalamus and then transported to and stored in the posterior pituitary gland. ADH, also referred to as *arginine vasopressin* (AVP) or *vasopressin,* plays a major role in the regulation of water balance and serum and urine osmolality (see Chapter 50).

Overproduction or oversecretion of ADH results in the syndrome of inappropriate antidiuretic hormone (SIADH). Underproduction or undersecretion of ADH results in DI.

SYNDROME OF INAPPROPRIATE ANTIDIURETIC HORMONE

Etiology and Pathophysiology

SIADH is a disorder of impaired water excretion. Despite normal or low plasma osmolality, there is abnormal production or sustained secretion of ADH (Figure 51.3). SIADH is characterized by fluid retention, serum hypo-osmolality, dilutional

PATHOPHYSIOLOGY MAP

FIG. 51.3 Pathophysiology of syndrome of inappropriate antidiuretic hormone (SIADH). Source: Redrawn from Urden, L. D., Stacy, K. M., & Lough, M. E. (2014). *Critical care nursing: Diagnosis and management* (8th ed., p. 838, Figure 33-6). Mosby.

TABLE 51.1	CAUSES OF SYNDROME OF INAPPROPRIATE ANTIDIURETIC HORMONE
Malignant Tumours • Colorectal cancer • Lymphoid cancers (Hodgkin's disease, non-Hodgkin's lymphoma, lymphocytic leukemia) • Pancreatic cancer • Prostate cancer • Small cell carcinoma of the lung • Thymus cancer **Central Nervous System Disorders** • Brain tumours • Cerebral atrophy • Cerebrovascular injury • Guillain-Barré syndrome • Head injury (skull fracture, subdural hematoma, subarachnoid hemorrhage) • Infection (encephalitis, meningitis) • Systemic lupus erythematosus	**Medication Therapy** • Antineoplastic agents (vincristine, vinblastine, cyclophosphamide [Procytox]) • Carbamazepine (Tegretol) • Chlorpropamide • General anaesthetic agents • Opioids • Oxytocin • SSRI antidepressants • Thiazide diuretics • Tricyclic antidepressants **Miscellaneous Conditions** • Adrenal insufficiency • Chronic obstructive pulmonary disease • HIV infection • Hypothyroidism • Lung infection (pneumonia, tuberculosis, lung abscess) • Positive pressure mechanical ventilation

HIV, human immunodeficiency virus; *SSRI,* selective serotonin reuptake inhibitor.

hyponatremia, hypochloremia, concentrated urine in the presence of normal or increased intravascular volume, and normal renal function. While this syndrome occurs commonly in older persons, a higher incidence of SIADH has been reported recently in children (Jones, 2018).

The abnormal production or sustained secretion of ADH that leads to SIADH has various causes (Table 51.1). The most common cause is malignancy, especially ectopic ADH produced in small cell lung cancer. SIADH tends to be self-limiting when caused by head trauma, psychosis, or medications (e.g., carbamazepine, cyclophosphamide, selective serotonin reuptake inhibitors [SSRIs]) but is chronic in nature when associated with tumours or metabolic diseases.

Clinical Manifestations and Diagnostic Studies

Excess ADH increases both permeability of the distal tubules and collecting ducts and reabsorption of water into the circulation. Consequently, extracellular fluid volume expands, plasma osmolality declines, the glomerular filtration rate (GFR) increases, and sodium levels decline (dilutional hyponatremia) (Peri et al., 2017). SIADH is diagnosed from simultaneous measurements of urine and serum osmolality. The dilutional hyponatremia is indicated by a serum sodium level of less than 134 mmol/L, serum osmolality of less than 280 mmol/kg, and a urine specific gravity greater than 1.005. A serum osmolality much lower than the urine osmolality indicates the inappropriate excretion of concentrated urine in the presence of dilute serum.

As the serum sodium level falls (usually to less than 120 mmol/L), manifestations become more severe and include vomiting, abdominal cramps, muscle twitching, and seizures. As plasma osmolality and serum sodium levels continue to decline, cerebral edema may occur, leading to lethargy, anorexia, confusion, headache, seizures, and coma. Patients with SIADH also experience low urinary output and increased body weight (Silvera et al., 2018).

Interprofessional Care

Once SIADH is identified, treatment is directed at the underlying cause of the disorder. Medications that stimulate the release of ADH should be avoided or discontinued (see Table 51.1).

The immediate treatment goal is to restore normal fluid volume and serum osmolality. If symptoms are mild and the serum sodium level exceeds 125 mmol/L, the only treatment may be fluid restriction (between 800 and 1 000 mL/day). This restriction should result in gradual daily weight reduction, a progressive rise in serum sodium concentration and osmolality, and improvement in symptoms.

In cases of severe hyponatremia (serum sodium level <120 mmol/L) involving neurological symptoms such as seizures, IV hypertonic saline solution (3 to 5%) may be administered. Hypertonic saline must be administered very slowly on an infusion pump to avoid resultant neurological damage. A diuretic such as furosemide (Lasix) may be used to promote diuresis, but only if the serum sodium level is at least 125 mmol/L, to avoid further sodium loss. In patients with severe hyponatremia, fluid restrictions of no more than 500 mL/day are indicated, as well as supplements to offset potassium, calcium, and magnesium losses associated with diuretic therapy. In chronic SIADH, water restriction between 800 and 1 000 mL/day is recommended. Agents that block the effect of ADH on the renal tubules may be prescribed for patients who do not tolerate water restriction guidelines, thereby allowing more dilution of urine. Tolvaptan (Samsca), a vasopressin receptor antagonist, is used to treat euvolemic hyponatremia in hospitalized patients under specialist guidance and strict monitoring to prevent rapid correction of serum sodium levels.

NURSING MANAGEMENT
SYNDROME OF INAPPROPRIATE ANTIDIURETIC HORMONE

The nurse can be instrumental in the early detection and treatment of SIADH. An appropriate nursing assessment (Table 51.2) should be conducted for patients at risk for or experiencing SIADH. Specifically, the nurse should be alert for low urinary

TABLE 51.2 NURSING ASSESSMENT

Syndrome of Inappropriate Antidiuretic Hormone

Assessment
- Daily weight measurement
- Frequent measurement of intake (oral and parenteral) and output
- Frequent measurement of urine specific gravity
- Frequent measurement of vital signs
- Monitoring of heart and lung sounds
- Monitoring of level of consciousness
- Observation for signs of hyponatremia (e.g., decreased neurological function, seizures, nausea and vomiting, muscle cramping)

Management
- Frequent oral hygiene
- Frequent turning, positioning, and range of motion exercise (if patient is bedridden)
- Positioning of head of bed flat or with no more than 10 degrees of elevation to enhance venous return to heart and increase left atrial filling pressure, thereby reducing ADH release
- Protection from injury (e.g., assist with ambulation, bed alarm) because of potential alterations in mental status
- Provision of distractions to decrease the discomfort of thirst related to fluid restrictions
- Provision of support for patient and significant others regarding diagnosis and any mental status changes
- Restricting total fluid intake to no more than 1 000 mL/day (including that taken with medications)
- Seizure precautions

ADH, antidiuretic hormone.

output with a high specific gravity, a sudden weight gain, or a decline in serum sodium level. Nursing management of acute onset of SIADH is presented in Table 51.2.

When SIADH is chronic, patients must learn to self-manage prescribed treatment regimens such as fluid restriction (800 to 1 000 mL/day). Ice chips or sugarless chewing gum can help decrease thirst, and patients should be assisted with planning fluid intake to align with social occasions. Patients may be treated with a diuretic to remove excess fluid volume, and well-diluted sodium and potassium supplements are indicated at mealtimes to prevent GI irritation or damage. In addition, patients should be taught the symptoms of fluid and sodium and potassium electrolyte imbalances so that they can monitor progress during treatment (see Chapter 19).

DIABETES INSIPIDUS

Etiology and Pathophysiology

Diabetes insipidus (DI) is a group of conditions associated with a deficiency of ADH production or secretion, as well as decreased renal response to ADH caused by injury to the neurohypophyseal system. The decrease in ADH results in fluid and electrolyte imbalances caused by increased urinary output and increased plasma osmolality (Figure 51.4). Depending on the cause, DI may be transient or a chronic, lifelong condition.

Diabetes insipidus has several classifications (Table 51.3). *Central DI* is the most common form.

A comparison of the features of DI and SIADH is provided in Table 51.4.

Clinical Manifestations

DI is characterized by increased thirst (*polydipsia*), nocturia, and increased urination (*polyuria*; see Figure 51.4) (Prete et al., 2017).

PATHOPHYSIOLOGY MAP

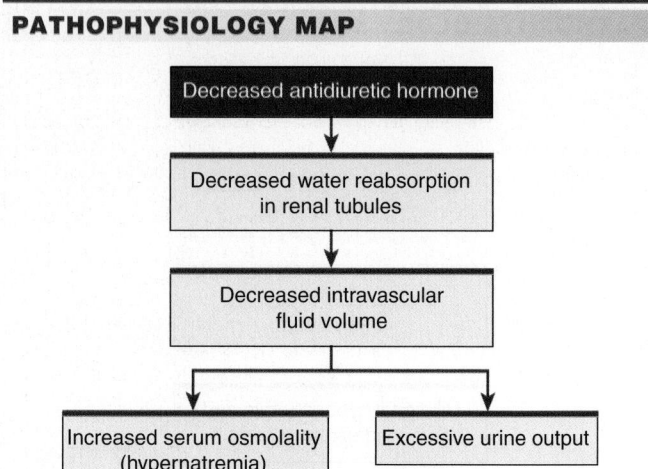

FIG. 51.4 Pathophysiology of diabetes insipidus. Source: Redrawn from Urden, L. D., Stacy, K. M., & Lough, M. E. (2014). *Critical care nursing: Diagnosis and management* (8th ed., p. 833, Figure 33-5). Mosby.

TABLE 51.3 TYPES AND CAUSES OF DIABETES INSIPIDUS

Types	Causes
Central (neurogenic) DI	Results from an interference with ADH synthesis or release. Multiple causes include brain tumour, head injury, brain surgery, and CNS infections.
Nephrogenic DI	Results from inadequate renal response to ADH despite presence in adequate levels. Causes include medication therapy (especially lithium), renal damage, or hereditary renal disease.
Primary DI	Results from excessive water intake. Causes are structural lesion in the thirst centre and psychological disorder.

ADH, antidiuretic hormone; *CNS*, central nervous system; *DI*, diabetes insipidus.

The primary characteristic of DI is the excretion of large quantities of urine (5–20 L per day) with a very low specific gravity (<1.005) and urine osmolality of less than 100 mmol/kg. Serum osmolality is elevated (usually >300 mmol/kg) as a result of hypernatremia caused by pure water loss from the kidneys. Most affected patients compensate for fluid loss by drinking great amounts of water, resulting in normal to only moderately elevated serum osmolality. Patients may be fatigued from nocturia and may experience generalized weakness.

Central DI usually occurs suddenly with excessive fluid loss. After intracranial surgery, DI usually has a triphasic pattern: the acute phase, with abrupt onset of polyuria; an interphase, in which urine volume apparently normalizes; and a third phase (10 to 14 days postoperative), in which central DI is permanent. Central DI resulting from head trauma is usually self-limiting and improves with treatment of the underlying health problem, whereas DI following cranial surgery is more likely to be permanent. Although the clinical manifestations of nephrogenic DI are similar, the onset and the amount of fluid losses are less dramatic.

If oral fluid intake cannot keep up with urinary losses, a severe fluid volume deficit results. This deficit is manifested by weight loss, constipation, poor tissue turgor, hypotension,

TABLE 51.4	COMPARISON OF DIABETES INSIPIDUS AND SIADH	
Feature	**Diabetes Insipidus**	**SIADH**
Definition	Deficiency of ADH results in inability to conserve water.	Excessive amounts of ADH are secreted from the posterior pituitary and other ectopic sources.
Pathophysiological features	With ADH deficiency, permeability of water is diminished, which results in excretion of large volumes of hypotonic fluid. Three patterns may develop: (1) transient diabetes insipidus—abrupt onset within the first few days after neurosurgery then resolves; (2) permanent diabetes insipidus—abrupt and early onset, persists for several weeks or for life; (3) triphasic diabetes insipidus—an acute phase with abrupt onset of polyuria; an interphase, in which urine volume apparently normalizes; and a third phase, in which central diabetes insipidus is permanent.	Key features of ADH excess are (a) water retention, (b) hyponatremia, and (c) hypo-osmolality. Continual release of ADH causes water retention from renal tubules and collecting ducts; extracellular fluid volume increases with dilutional hyponatremia; and hyponatremia suppresses renin and aldosterone secretions, which causes a decrease in proximal tubule reabsorption of Na⁺.
Clinical manifestations	Genitourinary: polyuria: 5 to 18 L/day; clear urine; urinary frequency; nocturia Gastrointestinal: weight loss; polydipsia (if thirst mechanism is intact) Integumentary: dry skin and mucous membranes Neurological: mentation changes as electrolyte imbalance and hypotension worsen	Related to degree of hyponatremia: confusion, lethargy, irritability, seizures, coma Gastrointestinal: decreased motility with anorexia, nausea, vomiting; abrupt weight gain *without edema* in 5–10% of affected patients

ADH, antidiuretic hormone; *SIADH,* syndrome of inappropriate antidiuretic hormone.
Source: Adapted from Black, J. M., & Hawks, J. H. (2009). *Medical-surgical nursing: Clinical management for positive outcomes* (8th ed., pp. 1058–1059). Saunders Elsevier.

tachycardia, and shock. In addition, with increasing serum osmolality and hypernatremia, affected patients show central nervous system (CNS) manifestations, ranging from irritability and mental dullness to coma. With low urine osmolality due to polyuria, patients are at significant risk for severe hydration and hypovolemic shock.

Diagnostic Studies

Because DI may be central, nephrogenic, or psychogenic in origin, an initial identification of the cause is imperative. A complete history is documented, and a thorough physical examination is performed. Primary or psychogenic DI is associated with overhydration and hypervolemia rather than dehydration and hypovolemia. A water deprivation test is usually performed to confirm the diagnosis of central DI. Prior to the water deprivation test, the patient's baseline weight, pulse, urine and plasma osmolality, specific urine gravity, and blood pressure (BP) are measured. All fluids are withheld for 8 to 16 hours. Patients may be anxious and should be observed and reassured that the test will be stopped if fluid volume deficit becomes severe. During the test, the patient's BP, weight, and urine osmolality are assessed hourly. The test continues until urine osmolality stabilizes (hourly increase of <30 mmol/kg in 3 consecutive hours), body weight declines by 3%, or orthostatic hypotension develops. At this point, ADH is then given and urine osmolality is measured 1 hour later. In central DI, it is expected that a patient's urinary osmolality will increase significantly after vasopressin administration, whereas a patient with nephrogenic DI will have no response (Bockenhauer & Bichet, 2015).

Interprofessional Care

Determining and treating the primary cause is central in the interprofessional management of DI. The therapeutic goal is maintenance of fluid and electrolyte balance.

For central DI, fluid and hormonal replacement is the cornerstone of treatment. In acute presentations of DI, hypotonic saline (0.45% normal saline [NS]) is administered intravenously and titrated to replace urinary output (Zimmerman et al., 2017). Hormone replacement is necessary because of the lack of ADH

production or secretion. Desmopressin acetate (DDAVP), an analogue of ADH, is the hormone replacement of choice for central DI. DDAVP can be administered orally, intravenously, subcutaneously, or as a nasal spray. Another medication available for ADH replacement is vasopressin. These medications can lead to water retention and hyponatremia if the urine is concentrated for most of the day. The serum sodium concentration should be checked at 24 hours after the initiation of therapy and patients educated about resultant hyponatremia symptoms.

Several medications can be used for the treatment of partial central DI to increase ADH release or enhance ADH effects on the kidney, including carbamazepine (Tegretol), nonsteroidal anti-inflammatory drugs (NSAIDs), and a low-salt diet combined with thiazide diuretics.

Hormone replacement has little effect in the treatment of nephrogenic DI because the kidney is unable to respond to ADH. Instead, the treatment for nephrogenic DI revolves around dietary measures (low-sodium diet) and thiazide diuretics. Limiting sodium intake to no more than 3 g per day is thought to help decrease urine output. Thiazide diuretics (e.g., hydrochlorothiazide) are able to slow the GFR and allow the kidneys to increase proximal sodium and water reabsorption in the loop of Henle and the distal tubules. This reabsorption diminishes water delivery to the ADH-sensitive sites in the collecting tubules and reduces urine output. When a low-sodium diet and thiazides are not effective, indomethacin (Indocin) may be prescribed. Indomethacin, an NSAID, helps increase renal responsiveness to ADH.

NURSING MANAGEMENT
CENTRAL DIABETES INSIPIDUS

Nursing management of patients with central DI revolves around (1) early detection of polyuria, nocturia, and polydipsia; (2) maintenance of adequate hydration; and (3) patient teaching regarding nutrition (i.e., low-sodium and protein diet) and pharmacological management.

Fluids are replaced orally or intravenously, depending on the patient's condition and ability to drink copious amounts of fluids. Adequate amounts of fluids should be kept at the patient's bedside. If IV glucose solutions are used, the serum glucose level should be monitored because hyperglycemia and glycosuria can lead to osmotic diuresis, increasing fluid volume deficit. Monitoring of BP, heart rate, and urine output and specific gravity is essential and, for an acutely ill patient, may be required hourly. Level of consciousness must also be monitored, as well as signs of acute dehydration, by assessing alertness, response to stimuli, mucous membranes, tachycardia, and skin turgor. Accurate records of intake and output, urine specific gravity, and daily weights are imperative to assess fluid volume status.

The initial aim of desmopressin therapy is to reduce nocturia and control diuresis during the day. Patients should be assessed for weight gain, headache, restlessness, and signs of hyponatremia and water intoxication. By monitoring fluid intake and output and the urine specific gravity, the nurse can assess the adequacy of treatment. The health care provider should be notified immediately if the patient with DI develops increased urine volume with a low specific gravity, because this may indicate the need to change the dosage of DDAVP.

The patient with chronic DI requiring long-term ADH replacement needs instruction in self-management. DDAVP can be taken orally or intranasally. Nasal irritation may result from nasal administration. Patient reports of headache, nausea, and other signs of hyponatremia may indicate overdosage, whereas failure to improve may indicate underdosage. Patients taking DDAVP should be instructed to monitor their weight daily; increases in weight may indicate fluid retention. The need for close follow-up, including laboratory studies, is an essential part of the teaching plan.

DISORDERS OF THE THYROID GLAND

Contact with perfluoroalkyl contaminants (PFAS) has been associated with alterations in thyroid hormones in children, particularly those living within Indigenous communities. This disproportionately high exposure to PFAS within Indigenous populations raises concerns about present and future endocrine disruption and poor health outcomes in these communities (Caron-Beaudoin et al., 2019).

The thyroid hormones—thyroxine (T_4) and triiodothyronine (T_3)—regulate energy metabolism, growth, and development. Disorders of the thyroid gland include enlargement, benign and malignant nodules, inflammation, and hyperfunctioning and hypofunctioning states (Figure 51.5).

GOITRE

The term **goitre** refers to an abnormal growth of the thyroid gland. Goitres can be nodular or diffuse, depending on the cause that stimulates the thyroid cells to grow. Goitres may be associated with normal (*nontoxic*), decreased (*hypothyroidism*), or increased (*hyperthyroidism*) thyroid hormone production. Goitres that are *toxic* are common in patients with conditions of hyperthyroidism such as Graves' disease (Figure 51.6). Goitre as a clinical manifestation of thyroid disorders is further discussed in the following sections.

The most common cause of goitre worldwide is a lack of iodine in the diet. In Canada, where most people use iodized salt, goitre is more often caused by (a) the overproduction or underproduction of thyroid hormones or (b) nodules that develop in the gland itself. Foods or medications that contain

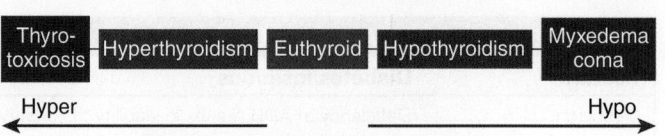

FIG. 51.5 Continuum of thyroid dysfunction.

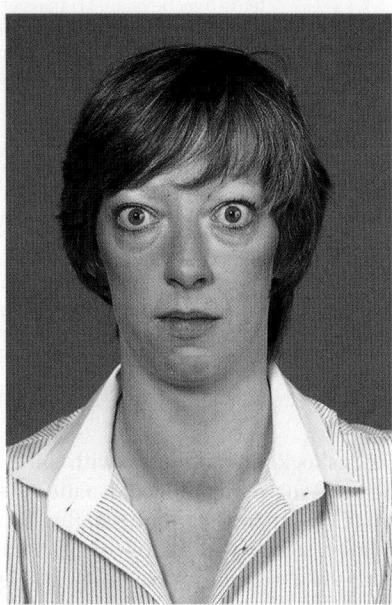

FIG. 51.6 Exophthalmos and goitre of Graves' disease. Source: Forbes, C. D., & Jackson, W. F. (2003). *Color atlas and text of clinical medicine* (3rd ed., p. 309, Figure 7.55). Mosby.

TABLE 51.5	GOITROGENS	
Thyroid Inhibitors	**Other Medications**	**Foods***
• Iodine in large doses • Methimazole (Tapazole) • Propylthiouracil	• Amiodarone • Lithium • Para-aminosalicylic acid • Salicylates • Sulphonamides	• Broccoli • Brussels sprouts • Cabbage • Cauliflower • Kale • Mustard • Peanuts • Turnips

*List is not all-inclusive.

thyroid-inhibiting substances (*goitrogens*) can cause goitre (Table 51.5).

In a person with a goitre, TSH and T_4 levels are measured to determine whether a goitre is associated with hyperthyroidism, hypothyroidism, or normal thyroid function. Thyroid antibodies are measured to assess for *thyroiditis* (inflammation of the thyroid). Treatment with thyroid hormone may prevent further thyroid enlargement in some cases. In other situations, large goitres are surgically removed.

THYROID NODULES AND CANCER

A *thyroid nodule*, a palpable deformity of the thyroid gland, may be benign or malignant. More than 95% of all thyroid nodules are benign. The incidence of thyroid nodules increases with age. Benign nodules are usually not dangerous, but they can cause tracheal compression if they become too large. Nodules should be assessed and evaluated (discussed in the section Diagnostic Studies).

Thyroid cancer is the most common endocrine-related carcinoma. In 2019, estimates projected that 8 200 Canadians (2 100 men and 6 100 women) would be diagnosed with new cases of thyroid cancer (Canadian Cancer Statistics Advisory Committee, 2019). The primary sign of thyroid cancer is the presence of a painless, palpable nodule or nodules in an enlarged thyroid gland.

Types of Thyroid Cancer

The four main types of thyroid cancer include papillary (70 to 80% of cases), follicular (10 to 15% of cases), medullary (5 to 10% of cases), and anaplastic (less than 5% of cases). *Papillary* thyroid cancer tends to grow slowly and spreads initially to lymph nodes in the neck. *Follicular* thyroid cancer tends to occur in older persons. Follicular cancer first grows into the cervical lymph nodes. Follicular cancer is more likely than papillary cancer to grow into blood vessels and, from there, spread to the lungs and bones. *Medullary* thyroid cancer is more likely to occur in families and to be associated with other endocrine disorders. It can be diagnosed through genetic testing for a proto-oncogene called *RET*. In family members of a person with medullary thyroid cancer, a positive finding of the *RET* proto-oncogene can enable early diagnosis and treatment of medullary thyroid cancer. *Anaplastic* thyroid cancer is the most advanced and aggressive thyroid cancer and the least likely to respond to treatment.

Diagnostic Studies

Radiological evaluation of a palpated mass or nodular enlargement within the thyroid gland is required. Ultrasonography is often the first radiological test used and, when indicated, CT, MRI, and ultrasonography-guided fine-needle aspiration (FNA) are other reasonable diagnostic options. FNA is indicated when a tissue sample is necessary for pathological examination, while a thyroid scan is required to identify a possible malignancy. Thyroid tumours may or may not take up radioactive iodine (RAI). Tumours that take up the RAI are called "hot" nodules and are nearly always benign. If the nodule does not take up the RAI, it appears as "cold" and has a higher risk of being malignant. Measurement of increased levels of serum calcitonin, often associated with medullary thyroid carcinoma, is also helpful in diagnosis.

NURSING AND INTERPROFESSIONAL CARE THYROID CANCER

Surgical removal of the tumour is usually indicated in the treatment of thyroid cancer. Surgical procedures may range from unilateral total lobectomy to total thyroidectomy with bilateral lobectomy. RAI may be given to some patients to destroy any remaining cancer cells after surgery but is not commonly used. In addition, many thyroid cancers are TSH dependent, and thyroid hormone in high doses is often prescribed to inhibit pituitary secretion of TSH (Haugen et al., 2015). Chemotherapy may be used in advanced disease. Nursing care for patients with thyroid tumours is similar to care for patients who have undergone thyroidectomy and should also include general nursing measures for patients with cancer. (See Chapter 18 and Nursing Care Plans 18.1 and 18.2 for the care of patients undergoing radiation and chemotherapy, available on the Evolve website.)

MULTIPLE ENDOCRINE NEOPLASIA

Multiple endocrine neoplasia is an autosomal dominant inherited condition characterized by hormone-secreting tumours (Marx, 2018). Multiple endocrine neoplasia is caused by the mutation of one of two genes, *MEN1* or *RET,* that normally control cell growth. Tumours may develop in childhood or later in life. Treatment of the tumour(s) may include conservative management (watchful waiting), medication to block the effects of excess hormone, and surgical removal of the gland or tumour (or both). It is important for patients with multiple endocrine neoplasia to have regular screening visits with their health care provider so that new tumours may be detected early and existing tumours carefully monitored.

THYROIDITIS

Thyroiditis is an inflammation of the thyroid gland that can have several causes. *Subacute granulomatous thyroiditis* is thought to be caused by a viral infection (e.g., mumps, measles, adenovirus) or post–viral inflammatory processes resulting from prior upper respiratory infections. *Acute thyroiditis* can also be caused by a bacterial or fungal infection. The thyroid gland is tender and enlarged, and the patient often experiences neck pain and fatigue (Dalugama, 2018). *Chronic autoimmune thyroiditis* (Hashimoto's thyroiditis), most common in women, can lead to hypothyroidism and goitre formation. *Hashimoto's thyroiditis* is a chronic autoimmune disease in which thyroid tissue is replaced by lymphocytes and fibrous tissue (Figure 51.7). *Silent thyroiditis,* a form of lymphocytic thyroiditis, has a variable onset and no apparent symptoms. *Postpartum thyroiditis* occurs frequently in women with a history of thyroid disease who have recently given birth. In most respects, silent and postpartum thyroiditis resemble Hashimoto's thyroiditis, except that the gland tends to recover, and thyroid hormone treatment needs to be administered for only a few weeks (Domingo et al., 2019).

T_4 and T_3 levels are initially elevated in subacute, acute, and silent thyroiditis but may become depressed over time. TSH levels are initially low and then elevated. Thyroid hormone levels are usually low in chronic Hashimoto's thyroiditis, but the TSH level is high and antithyroid antibodies are present. Radioactive iodine uptake (RAIU) is suppressed in subacute and silent thyroiditis.

Recovery from thyroiditis may be complete in weeks or months without treatment. How thyroiditis is treated depends on the type, symptoms, and phase (thyrotoxic or hypothyroid). In the thyrotoxic stage, treatment is symptomatic. If the condition is bacterial in origin, treatment may include specific antibiotics or surgical drainage. In subacute and acute forms, salicylates and NSAIDs are administered. If the patient's condition does not respond to these medications in 48 hours, corticosteroids are administered. Propranolol (Inderal) or atenolol (Tenormin) may be used for the cardiovascular symptoms of a hyperthyroid condition. Thyroid hormone replacement is indicated if a patient moves to the hypothyroid phase.

Nursing care of patients with thyroiditis involves teaching about treatment and encouraging adherence to the treatment regimen. Patients' progress should be closely monitored so that any change in symptoms can be reported immediately to the health care provider.

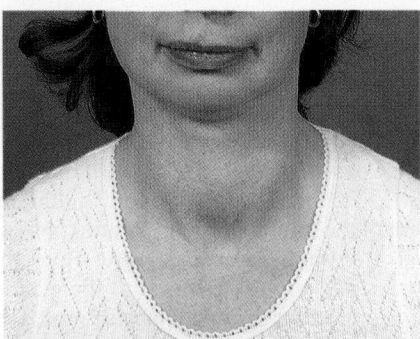

FIG. 51.7 Appearance of the neck in Hashimoto's thyroiditis. Source: Belchetz, P. E., & Hammond, P. (2003). *Mosby's color atlas and text of diabetes and endocrinology*. Mosby.

Patients with thyroiditis of autoimmune origin may be susceptible to other autoimmune disorders, such as Addison's disease, pernicious anemia, premature gonadal failure, or Graves' disease (Domingo et al., 2019). Patients should be taught the signs and symptoms of these disorders. A patient receiving thyroid hormone replacement must be taught the expected adverse effects of these medications and how to manage them. Patients treated surgically need care similar to that given to patients undergoing thyroidectomy.

HYPERTHYROIDISM

Hyperthyroidism is hyperactivity of the thyroid gland with sustained increase in synthesis and release of thyroid hormones. Thyrotoxicosis is the clinical state resulting from inappropriately high tissue thyroid levels of T_4, T_3, or both, and subsequent actions in tissues. Hyperthyroidism is a form of thyrotoxicosis and both usually occur together, as in Graves' disease (the most common form of hyperthyroidism). However, in some forms of thyroiditis, thyrotoxicosis may occur without hyperthyroidism (Taylor et al., 2018). Other causes include toxic nodular goitre, thyroiditis, exogenous iodine excess, pituitary tumours, and thyroid cancer.

Etiology and Pathophysiology

Graves' Disease. Graves' disease is an autoimmune disease of unknown etiology marked by diffuse thyroid enlargement and excessive thyroid hormone secretion. In Canada, Graves' disease accounts for 90% of the cases of hyperthyroidism and is more common in women, particularly between the ages of 20 to 40 years (Thyroid Foundation of Canada, 2016). Precipitating factors such as insufficient iodine supply, infections, and stressful life events may interact with genetic factors to cause Graves' disease. As well, cigarette smoking may correlate with increased orbital venous congestion leading to inflamed and swollen eye muscles and tissues (Sadeghi-Tari et al., 2016). Patients with this disease develop abnormal antibodies that mimic TSH, attaching to and creating false signals to the TSH receptors that stimulate the thyroid gland to release T_3, T_4, or both. The excessive release of thyroid hormones leads to the clinical manifestations associated with thyrotoxicosis (excessive sweating, heat intolerance, tachycardia, tremors). The disease is characterized by remissions and exacerbations, with or without treatment. It may progress to destruction of thyroid tissue, which causes hypothyroidism.

Toxic Nodular Goitres. Nodular goitres are characterized by thyroid hormone–secreting nodules that are independent of TSH stimulation. If associated with signs of hyperthyroidism, a nodule is termed *toxic*. A goitre may have multiple benign nodules *(multinodular goitre)* or a single benign nodule *(solitary autonomous nodule)* called *follicular adenomas.* Toxic nodular goitres occur equally in men and women. Although they can appear at any age, the frequency of toxic multinodular goitre is highest among people older than 40 years.

Clinical Manifestations

The clinical manifestations of hyperthyroidism are related to the effects of excess amounts of circulating thyroid hormones, which directly increase metabolism and tissue sensitivity to sympathetic nervous system stimulation.

The palpation or visualization of the thyroid gland may reveal a goitre. The auscultation of the thyroid gland may reveal bruits, a reflection of increased blood supply. Another common finding associated with hyperthyroidism is *ophthalmopathy*, a term used to describe abnormal eye appearance or function. A classic finding in 20 to 50% of patients with Graves' disease is exophthalmos, a bilateral, unilateral, or asymmetrical protrusion of the eyeballs from the orbits (see Figure 51.6). Exophthalmos is a type of infiltrative ophthalmopathy that results from impairment of venous drainage from the orbit, which causes increased fat deposits and fluid (edema) in the retro-orbital tissues. Because of increased pressure, the eyeballs are forced outward and protrude. In ophthalmopathy, the upper eyelids are usually retracted and elevated, with the sclera visible above the iris. When the eyelids do not close completely, the exposed corneal surfaces become dry and irritated. Serious consequences, such as corneal ulcers and eventual loss of vision, can occur. The changes in the ocular muscles result in muscle weakness, causing diplopia.

Other common manifestations of thyroid hyperfunction are summarized in Table 51.6. A patient with advanced disease may exhibit many of the manifestations, whereas a patient in the early stages of hyperthyroidism may exhibit only weight loss and increased nervousness. Manifestations of hyperthyroidism (e.g., palpitations, tremors, weight loss) in older people do not differ significantly from those in younger adults. In some instances, in which confusion and agitation are reported, dementia may be suspected and may delay the diagnosis. In Table 51.7, features of hyperthyroidism in younger and older patients are compared.

Complications

Thyrotoxic crisis (also called *thyroid storm*) is a rare, acute condition in which all hyperthyroid manifestations are intensified. Although thyrotoxic crisis is considered a life-threatening emergency, death is rare when treatment is initiated early. The cause is thought to be stressors (e.g., infection, trauma, surgery) in a patient with pre-existing hyperthyroidism, either diagnosed or undiagnosed. There is a rapid increase in serum thyroid levels, and heart and nerve tissues become more sensitive to sympathetic nervous system activation because more binding sites for epinephrine and norepinephrine are present This increased responsiveness to catecholamines enhances cellular responses to thyroid hormones.

Manifestations include severe tachycardia, heart failure, shock, hyperthermia (temperature up to 40.7°C), restlessness, agitation, seizures, abdominal pain, nausea, vomiting, diarrhea, delirium, and coma with biochemical evidence of hyperthyroidism.

TABLE 51.6 CLINICAL MANIFESTATIONS OF THYROID DYSFUNCTION

Hypofunction	Hyperfunction	Hypofunction	Hyperfunction
Cardiovascular System		**Musculoskeletal System**	
• Anemia	• Angina	• Arthralgia	• Dependent edema
• Cardiac hypertrophy	• Atrial fibrillation (more common in older persons)	• Fatigue	• Fatigue
• Decreased rate and force of cardiac contractions	• Bounding, rapid pulse	• Muscular aches and pains	• Muscle weakness
• Distant heart sounds	• Cardiac hypertrophy	• Slow movements	• Osteoporosis
• Increased capillary fragility	• Dysrhythmias	• Weakness	• Proximal muscle wasting
• Tendency to develop heart failure, angina, myocardial infarction	• Increased cardiac output		
	• Increased rate and force of cardiac contractions	**Nervous System**	
• Varied changes in blood pressure	• Palpitations	• Anxiety, depression	• Depression, fatigue, apathy (in older persons)
	• Systolic hypertension	• Apathy	• Difficulty in focusing eyes
	• Systolic murmurs	• Delayed relaxation of deep tendon reflexes	• Exhaustion
Respiratory System		• Fatigue	• Fine tremor (of fingers and tongue)
• Decreased breathing capacity	• Dyspnea on mild exertion	• Forgetfulness	• Hyper-reflexia of tendon reflexes
• Dyspnea	• Increased respiratory rate	• Hoarseness	• Inability to concentrate
		• Lethargy	• Insomnia
Gastrointestinal System		• Paresthesias	• Lability of mood, delirium
• Celiac disease	• Diarrhea, frequent defecation	• Polyneuropathy	• Nervousness
• Constipation	• Hepatomegaly	• Slow, slurred speech	• Personality changes: irritability, agitation
• Decreased appetite	• Increased appetite, thirst	• Slowed mental processes	• Restlessness
• Distended abdomen	• Increased bowel sounds	• Stupor, coma	• Stupor, coma
• Enlarged, scaly tongue	• Increased peristalsis		
• Nausea and vomiting	• Splenomegaly	**Reproductive System**	
• Weight gain	• Weight loss	• Decreased libido	• Amenorrhea
		• Infertility	• Decreased fertility
Integumentary System		• Prolonged menstrual periods or amenorrhea	• Decreased libido
• Decreased sweating	• Clubbing of fingers (thyroid acropachy)		• Erectile dysfunction in men
• Dry, sparse, coarse hair	• Diaphoresis		• Gynecomastia in men
• Dry, thick, inelastic, cold skin	• Fine, silky hair		• Menstrual irregularities
• Generalized interstitial edema	• Hair loss (may be patchy)	**Other**	
• Pallor	• Palmar erythema	• Hearing impairment	• Elevated basal temperature
• Poor turgor of mucosa	• Premature greying (in men)	• Goitre	• Exophthalmos
• Puffy face	• Pretibial myxedema (infiltrative dermopathy)	• Increased sensitivity to opioids, barbiturates, anaesthetics	• Eyelid lag, stare
• Thick, brittle nails	• Thin, brittle nails detached from nail bed (onycholysis)	• Increased susceptibility to infection	• Eyelid retraction
	• Warm, smooth, moist skin	• Intolerance of cold	• Goitre
		• Sleepiness	• Increased sensitivity to stimulant medications
			• Intolerance of heat
			• Rapid speech

TABLE 51.7 COMPARISON OF HYPERTHYROIDISM IN YOUNGER AND OLDER PERSONS

Features	Younger Adults	Older Persons
Common causes	Graves' disease in >90% of cases	Graves' disease or toxic nodular goitre
Common symptoms	Nervousness; irritability; weight loss; heat intolerance; warm, moist skin	Anorexia, weight loss, apathy, lassitude, depression, confusion
Goitre	Present in >90% of cases	Present in ~50% of cases
Ophthalmopathy	Exophthalmos present in 20–50% of cases	Occasional exophthalmos
Cardiac features	Tachycardia and palpitations common, but without heart failure	Angina, dysrhythmias (especially atrial fibrillation), or heart failure may occur

Treatment is aimed at reducing circulating thyroid hormone levels and the clinical manifestations of this disorder by appropriate medication therapy. Supportive therapy is directed at managing respiratory distress, fever reduction, fluid replacement, and elimination or management of the initiating stressor or stressors.

Diagnostic Studies

The two primary laboratory findings used to confirm the diagnosis of hyperthyroidism are decreased TSH levels and elevated free T_4 levels. Total T_3 and T_4 levels may also be assessed, but these are not as definitive. Measurements of total T_3 and T_4 include both free and bound (to protein) hormone levels. The free hormone is the only form of the hormone that is biologically active.

The RAIU test is indicated to differentiate Graves' disease from other forms of thyroiditis. The 24-hour test of radioiodine uptake in patients with Graves' disease reveals a diffuse,

TABLE 51.8   INTERPROFESSIONAL CARE

Hyperthyroidism

Diagnostic
- History and physical examination
- Electrocardiography
- Laboratory tests
- Serum free T$_4$, TSH levels
- TRH stimulation test
- Ophthalmological examination
- Radioactive iodine uptake (RAIU)

Interprofessional Therapy
Medication Therapy
- Antithyroid medications
- Methimazole (Tapazole)
- Propylthiouracil (Propyl-Thyracil)
- Iodine
- β-Adrenergic blockers (e.g., propranolol [Inderal])

Radiation Therapy
- Radioactive iodine

Surgical Therapy
- Subtotal thyroidectomy

Nutritional Therapy
- Frequent meals
- High-calorie diet
- High-protein diet

T$_4$, thyroxine; *TRH,* thyrotropin-releasing hormone; *TSH,* thyroid-stimulating hormone.

homogeneous uptake of 35 to 90%, whereas in patients with thyroiditis, the amount of uptake is less than 20%. Patients with nodular goitre demonstrate uptake in the high-normal range (see Table 51.7).

Interprofessional Care

The overall goal in the treatment of hyperthyroidism is to block the adverse effects of thyroid hormones and stop their oversecretion. The three primary treatment options for patients with hyperthyroidism are antithyroid medications, RAI therapy, and subtotal thyroidectomy (Table 51.8). However, the choice of treatment is influenced by the patient's age, the severity of the disorder, complicating features (including pregnancy), and the patient's preferences.

Medication Therapy. Medications used in the treatment of hyperthyroidism include antithyroid medications, iodine, and β-adrenergic blockers. It is important to note that although these medications are useful in the treatment of thyrotoxic states, they are not considered curative. Radiation therapy or surgery may ultimately be required.

Antithyroid Medications. The first-line antithyroid medications used in the treatment of hyperthyroidism are thionamides, such as propylthiouracil (PTU), carbimazole, and methimazole (Tapazole). These medications inhibit the synthesis of thyroid hormones. Individual response is considerably varied; however, improvement usually begins 1 to 2 weeks after the initiation of therapy, and good results are seen within 4 to 8 weeks. Therapy is usually continued for 6 months to 2 years to allow for spontaneous remission. However, only approximately 20 to 30% of patients receive a permanent remission (Ross et al., 2016). The major disadvantages of these medications are possible nonadherence to the regimen and a high rate of recurrence of hyperthyroidism when the medications are discontinued. The indications for use of antithyroid medications include Graves' disease in young patients, hyperthyroidism during pregnancy, and the need to attain a euthyroid state before surgery or radiation therapy.

Iodine. Iodine is used with other antithyroid medications in the preparation of a patient for thyroidectomy or for treatment of thyrotoxic crisis. The administration of iodine in large doses rapidly inhibits synthesis of T$_3$ and T$_4$ and blocks the release of these hormones into the circulation within hours. It also decreases the vascularity of the thyroid gland, which makes surgery safer and easier. The effect of iodine is usually maximal within 1 to 2 weeks. Because the therapeutic effect lessens, long-term iodine therapy is not effective in controlling hyperthyroidism. Iodine is available in the form of Lugol's solution, potassium iodide (KI) tablets, and saturated solution of potassium iodide (SSKI) (Ross et al., 2016).

β-Adrenergic Blockers. β-Adrenergic blockers are used for symptomatic relief of thyrotoxicosis that results from increased β-adrenergic receptor stimulation caused by excess thyroid hormones. Propranolol (Inderal) is usually administered with other antithyroid agents and rapidly provides symptomatic relief. Atenolol (Tenormin) is the preferred β-adrenergic blocker for use in hyperthyroid patients with asthma or heart disease.

Radioactive Iodine Therapy. RAI therapy is the treatment of choice for most nonpregnant adults. RAI damages or destroys thyroid tissue, thus limiting thyroid hormone secretion. Patients should be instructed that radiation-related thyroiditis and parotiditis are possible and may cause dryness and irritation of the mouth and throat. Relief may be obtained with frequent sips of water, ice chips, or the use of normal saline or a baking soda solution (e.g., 10 mL of baking soda in 250 mL of water) to gargle three or four times per day. The discomfort should subside in 3 to 4 days. If dryness and irritation persist, patients should contact the health care provider. The response to RAI is delayed, and the effect may not be maximal for 2 to 3 months. For this reason, patients are usually treated with antithyroid medications and propranolol before and during the first 3 months after the initiation of RAI therapy, until the effects of irradiation become apparent. Although this method of treatment is usually effective, there is a high incidence of posttreatment hypothyroidism, which results in the need for lifelong thyroid hormone replacement. Patients and the family or caregiver should be taught about the symptoms of hypothyroidism and instructed to seek medical help if these symptoms occur.

Surgical Therapy. Thyroidectomy is indicated when a large goitre causes tracheal compression, when patients' condition does not respond to antithyroid therapy, and in patients with thyroid cancer. In addition, surgery may be performed when an individual is not a candidate for RAI. One advantage of thyroidectomy over RAI is a more rapid reduction in T$_3$ and T$_4$ levels. A *subtotal thyroidectomy* is the preferred surgical procedure and involves the removal of a significant portion (90%) of the thyroid gland. If too much tissue is taken, the gland does not regenerate after surgery, and hypothyroidism results.

Endoscopic thyroidectomy is a minimally invasive procedure with less scarring, less pain, and a faster return to normal activity than traditional approaches. In this procedure, several small incisions are made through which an endoscope and other instruments can be passed to remove thyroid tissue or nodules. It is an appropriate procedure for patients with small nodules (<3 cm in diameter) in whom there is no evidence of malignancy. Before surgery, antithyroid medications, iodine, and β-adrenergic blockers may be administered to achieve a euthyroid state and to control symptoms. Iodine reduces vascularization of the gland, thereby reducing the risk for hemorrhage. Postoperative complications include hypothyroidism, damage to or inadvertent removal of parathyroid glands (causing hypoparathyroidism and hypocalcemia), hemorrhage, injury to the recurrent or the superior laryngeal nerve, thyrotoxic crisis, and infection.

Nutritional Therapy. The potential for nutritional deficits is high when the metabolic rate is increased. A high-calorie diet (4 000 to 5 000 kcal/day) may be ordered to satisfy hunger and prevent tissue breakdown. This is accomplished with six full meals a day and snacks high in protein, carbohydrates, minerals, and vitamins, particularly vitamin A, thiamine, vitamin B$_6$, and vitamin C. The protein allowance should be 1 to 2 g/kg of ideal body weight. Increased carbohydrates should compensate for disturbed metabolism, provide energy, and spare body protein stores. Highly seasoned and high-fibre foods should be avoided because they can further stimulate the already hyperactive GI tract. Substitutes should be provided for caffeine-containing beverages such as coffee, tea, and cola because their stimulating effects increase restlessness and sleep disturbances. The nurse should consult a dietitian for guidance in meeting the nutritional needs of a patient with hyperthyroidism.

NURSING MANAGEMENT HYPERTHYROIDISM

NURSING ASSESSMENT
Subjective and objective data that should be obtained from an individual with hyperthyroidism are presented in Table 51.9.

NURSING DIAGNOSES
Nursing diagnoses for patients with hyperthyroidism include but are not limited to the following:
- *Reduced stamina* resulting from *physical deconditioning* (fatigue, exhaustion, heat intolerance secondary to hypermetabolism)
- *Inadequate nutrition* resulting from *insufficient dietary intake* (hypermetabolism)

Additional information on nursing diagnoses for the patient with hyperthyroidism are presented in Nursing Care Plan (NCP) 51.1, available on the Evolve website.

PLANNING
The overall goals are that patients with hyperthyroidism will (a) experience relief from symptoms, (b) have no serious complications related to the disease or treatment, (c) maintain nutritional balance, and (d) adhere to the therapeutic plan.

NURSING IMPLEMENTATION
ACUTE INTERVENTION. Individuals with hyperthyroidism are usually treated in an outpatient setting. However, patients who develop acute thyrotoxicosis and those who undergo thyroidectomy require hospitalization and acute care.

Acute Thyrotoxicosis. *Acute thyrotoxicosis* refers to a state of excess circulating thyroid hormone. It is a systemic syndrome that necessitates aggressive treatment, often in a critical care unit. Medications that block thyroid hormone production and the sympathetic nervous system (see previous discussion) should be administered. Supportive therapy includes monitoring for cardiac dysrhythmias and decompensation, ensuring adequate oxygenation, and administering IV fluids to replace fluid and electrolyte losses. This is especially important in patients who develop vomiting and diarrhea.

The patient's room should be kept calm and quiet because increased metabolism causes sleep disturbances. Provision of adequate rest may be a challenge because of the patient's irritability and restlessness. Specific interventions may include (a)

TABLE 51.9 NURSING ASSESSMENT
Hyperthyroidism

Subjective Data
Important Health Information
Past health history: Pre-existing goitre; recent infection or trauma; immigration from iodine-deficient area; autoimmune disease; positive family history of thyroid or autoimmune disorders
Medications: Use of thyroid hormones or herbal therapies that may contain thyroid hormone

Symptoms
- Chest pain; dyspnea on exertion; palpitations
- Decreased libido; erectile dysfunction, gynecomastia (in men); amenorrhea (in women)
- Diarrhea; polyuria
- Emotional lability, irritability, restlessness, personality changes, delirium, nervousness
- Heat intolerance; pruritus; sweating
- Insomnia
- Insufficient iodine intake; weight loss; increased appetite or thirst; nausea
- Muscle weakness, fatigue

Objective Data
General Observation
Agitation, rapid speech and body movements; hyperthermia, enlarged or nodular thyroid gland

Eyes
Exophthalmos, eyelid retraction; infrequent blinking

Integumentary
Warm, diaphoretic, velvety skin; thin, loose nails; fine, silky hair and hair loss; palmar erythema; digital clubbing; white pigmentation of skin (vitiligo); diffuse edema of legs and feet

Respiratory
Tachypnea

Cardiovascular
Tachycardia, bounding pulse, systolic murmurs, dysrhythmias, hypertension

Gastrointestinal
Increased bowel sounds; hepatosplenomegaly

Neurological
Hyper-reflexia; diplopia; fine tremors of hands, tongue, eyelids; stupor; coma

Musculoskeletal
Muscle wasting

Reproductive
Menstrual irregularities, infertility in women; erectile dysfunction, gynecomastia in men

Possible Findings
↑ T$_3$ level, ↑ T$_4$ level; ↑ T$_3$ resin uptake; ↓ serum TSH level; chest radiograph showing enlarged heart, findings of tachycardia, atrial fibrillation on ECG

ECG, electrocardiogram; *T$_3$,* triiodothyronine; *T$_4$,* thyroxine; *TSH,* thyroid-stimulating hormone.

placing the patient in a cool room, away from very ill patients and noisy, high-traffic areas; (b) using lightweight bed coverings and changing the linen frequently if the patient is diaphoretic; (c) encouraging and assisting with exercise involving large muscle groups (tremors can interfere with small-muscle coordination) to allow the release of nervous tension and restlessness; and (d) establishing a supportive, trusting relationship to help the patient cope with aggravating events and to lessen anxiety.

Exophthalmos, when present, incurs a potential for corneal injury related to irritation and dryness, and affected patients may also have orbital pain. Nursing interventions to relieve eye discomfort and prevent corneal ulceration include applying artificial tears to soothe and moisten conjunctival membranes. Salt restriction may help reduce periorbital edema. Elevation of the patient's head promotes fluid drainage from the periorbital area—the patient should sit upright as much as possible. Dark glasses reduce glare and prevent irritation from air currents, dust, and dirt. If the eyelids cannot be closed, they should be lightly taped shut for sleep. To maintain flexibility, the patient should be taught to exercise the intraocular muscles several times a day by turning the eyes in the complete range of motion. Good grooming can be helpful in reducing the loss of self-esteem that can result from an altered body image. If the exophthalmos is severe, corticosteroids, radiation of retro-orbital tissues, orbital decompression, or corrective eyelid or muscle surgery may be helpful.

Thyroid Surgery. When subtotal thyroidectomy is the treatment of choice, patients must be adequately prepared in order to avoid postoperative complications. All patients undergoing thyroid surgery require preoperative thyroid imaging, laboratory testing (serum TSH level), and laryngeal examination (direct and indirect laryngoscopy, ultrasound, videostroboscopy). To alleviate the risk of thyrotoxicosis, β-adrenergic medication, iodine treatment, or PTU may be given before surgery. Preoperative oral Lugol's solution is given to block iodine uptake and the secretion of thyroid hormone. It may also decrease the vascularity of the thyroid gland and the risk of intraoperative bleeding (Ross et al., 2016). Iodine is mixed with water or juice and sipped through a straw after meals. The nurse assesses patients for signs of iodine toxicity, such as swelling of buccal mucosa and other mucous membranes, excessive salivation, nausea and vomiting, and skin reactions. If toxicity occurs, iodine administration should be discontinued and the health care provider notified. Another consideration is to provide vitamin D and calcium supplementation to minimize the risk of hypocalcemia in the postoperative period.

Preoperative teaching should include comfort and safety measures in which patients can participate. Coughing, deep breathing, and leg exercises should be practiced and their importance explained. Patients should be taught how to support the head manually while turning in bed because this manoeuvre minimizes stress on the suture line after surgery. Range-of-motion exercises of the neck should be completed frequently. The nurse should explain routine postoperative care such as IV infusions. Patients should be informed that talking is likely to be difficult for a short time after surgery.

SAFETY ALERT
- Airway obstruction is an emergency situation.
- Airway obstruction, although not common, may occur postoperatively.
- Oxygen, suction equipment, and a tracheostomy tray should be readily available in the patient's room.

Recurrent laryngeal nerve damage leads to vocal cord paralysis. If both cords are paralyzed, spastic airway obstruction may occur, necessitating an immediate tracheostomy.

Respiration may also become difficult because of excess swelling of the neck tissues, hemorrhage, hematoma formation, and laryngeal stridor. *Laryngeal stridor* (harsh, vibratory sound) may occur during inspiration and expiration as a result of edema of the laryngeal nerve. Laryngeal stridor may also be related to tetany, which occurs if the parathyroid glands are removed or damaged during surgery, which leads to hypocalcemia. To treat tetany, calcium salts such as calcium gluconate and calcium chloride should be readily available for IV administration. After a thyroidectomy, the patient should be cared for as follows:

1. Assessment every 2 hours for 24 hours for signs of hemorrhage or tracheal compression, such as irregular breathing, neck swelling, frequent swallowing, sensations of fullness at the incision site, choking, and blood on the dressings
2. Placement in a semi-Fowler's position, and support of the patient's head with pillows, with care to avoid flexion of the neck and any tension on the suture lines
3. Monitoring of vital signs. The nurse completes the initial assessment by checking for signs of hypocalcemia and tetany secondary to hypoparathyroidism (e.g., tingling sensation in toes, in fingers, or around the mouth; muscular twitching; apprehension) and by evaluating difficulty in speaking and hoarseness. The nurse should also check for the presence of Trousseau's and Chvostek's signs for 72 hours (see Chapter 19, Figure 19.15). Some hoarseness is to be expected for 3 to 4 days after surgery because of edema.
4. Control of postoperative pain and nausea with medication

If postoperative recovery is uneventful, patients are ambulated within hours after surgery, are permitted to take fluid as soon as tolerated, and may eat soft foods the day after surgery.

The appearance of the incision may be distressing to patients. They can be reassured that the scar will fade and eventually look like a normal neck wrinkle. A scarf, jewellery, a high collar, or other covering can effectively camouflage a fresh scar.

AMBULATORY AND HOME CARE

Postoperative Care. Patients and family members need to be aware that thyroid hormone balance should be monitored periodically to ensure that normal function has returned. Most patients experience a period of relative hypothyroidism soon after surgery because of the substantial reduction in the size of the thyroid. The remaining tissue usually hypertrophies, recovering the capacity to produce the hormone needed by the body, but this takes time. Thyroid hormone is not administered because exogenous hormone inhibits pituitary production of TSH and delays or prevents the restoration of normal gland function and thyroid tissue regeneration. As a precaution, the wound area will need to be gently supported when coughing, and patients should avoid heavy lifting of objects, overexertion (e.g., gardening), and constipation by maintaining adequate fluid intake (6 to 8 glasses of water per day). To prevent weight gain, caloric intake must be reduced substantially below the amount required before surgery. Adequate iodine is necessary to promote thyroid function, but excesses inhibit the thyroid. Intake of seafood once or twice a week or normal use of iodized salt should provide sufficient iodine intake. Regular exercise (gentle walking and light activities) stimulates the thyroid gland and should be encouraged. High environmental temperature should be avoided because it inhibits thyroid regeneration.

Regular follow-up care is necessary. If patients have difficulties swallowing or breathing, noticeable signs of infection around the wound (redness, warmth, swelling, or discharge), fever, tingling or numbness in the mouth and fingers, or progressive pain or nausea, they should return immediately to the hospital. Patients should be seen biweekly for a month and then at least semiannually to assess for the development of hypothyroidism. If a complete thyroidectomy has been performed, patients need instruction in lifelong thyroid replacement. Patients should be taught the signs and symptoms of progressive thyroid failure (fatigue, weight gain, increased sensitivity to cold, muscle weakness) and instructed to seek medical care if these develop. Hypothyroidism is relatively easy to manage with oral administration of thyroid replacement.

EVALUATION

The following are expected outcomes for patients with hyperthyroidism:

- Relief from symptoms
- No serious complications related to the disease or the treatment
- Adherence to the therapeutic plan

HYPOTHYROIDISM

Etiology and Pathophysiology

Hypothyroidism affects approximately 2 per 100 people, and its prevalence increases with age (Thyroid Foundation of Canada, 2016). Overt primary hypothyroidism is characterized biochemically by high serum levels of TSH and insufficient free circulating thyroid T_4 hormone. Subclinical hypothyroidism is characterized by a high serum TSH and a normal serum level of free circulating T_4 hormone. Hypothyroidism can be primary (related to destruction of thyroid tissue or defective hormone synthesis) or secondary (related to pituitary disease with decreased secretion of TSH or hypothalamic dysfunction with decreased secretion of thyrotropin-releasing hormone [TRH]). It may also be transient, related to thyroiditis or discontinuation of thyroid hormone therapy.

Iodine deficiency is the most common cause of hypothyroidism worldwide. In Canada, the most common cause of primary hypothyroidism in the adult is atrophy of the thyroid gland (Thyroid Foundation of Canada, 2016). This atrophy is the end result of autoimmune diseases such as Hashimoto's thyroiditis and Graves' disease, which destroy the thyroid gland. Hypothyroidism also may develop as a result of treatment for hyperthyroidism, specifically the surgical removal of the thyroid gland or RAI therapy. Medications such as amiodarone (which contains iodine) and lithium (which blocks hormone production) are known to produce hypothyroidism.

Clinical Manifestations

Regardless of the cause, hypothyroidism has common features. It has systemic effects, characterized by an insidious and nonspecific slowing of body processes. The clinical presentation can range from no symptoms to classic symptoms and physical changes easily detected on examination. Unless hypothyroidism occurs after thyroidectomy or thyroid ablation, or during treatment with antithyroid medications, the onset of symptoms may occur unnoticed over months to years. The severity of symptoms experienced depends on the degree of thyroid hormone deficiency and the long-term physiological effects of thyroid hormone deficiency. Long-term effects may involve any body system but are more pronounced in neurological, cardiovascular, GI, reproductive, and hematological systems.

Many affected patients are fatigued and lethargic and experience personality and mental changes. The mental changes observed in hypothyroidism include impaired memory, slowed speech, decreased initiative, and somnolence. Many individuals with hypothyroidism appear depressed.

Hypothyroidism is associated with decreased cardiac output and decreased cardiac contractility. The patient may experience low exercise tolerance and shortness of breath on exertion. In patients with a pre-existing cardiovascular condition, hypothyroidism may cause significant hemodynamic compromise (Rothberger et al., 2017).

Anemia is a common feature of hypothyroidism. The bone marrow is hypocellular, leading to decreased oxygen demand, low or normal erythropoietin levels, diminished platelet function, and low hematocrit levels. Other hematological conditions are related to cobalamin, iron, and folate deficiencies. These cumulative changes result in slower cellular metabolism, enhanced fatigue, and bruising tendencies. Also, increased serum cholesterol and triglyceride levels and the accumulation of mucopolysaccharides in the intima of small blood vessels can result in coronary atherosclerosis. This accumulation is seldom symptomatic (i.e., characterized by angina) because of the decreased myocardial oxygen consumption that has been observed in hypothyroidism.

GI motility is decreased in hypothyroidism, and achlorhydria (absence or decrease of hydrochloric acid) is common. Constipation, which is a common symptom, may progress to obstipation and, in rare cases, to intestinal obstruction. Other physical changes related to decreased metabolism include cold intolerance, hair loss, dry and coarse skin, brittle nails, hoarseness, muscle weakness and swelling, and weight gain.

Patients with severe, long-standing hypothyroidism may display myxedema, the accumulation of hydrophilic mucopolysaccharides in the dermis and other tissues (Figure 51.8). This mucinous edema causes the characteristic facies of hypothyroidism (i.e., puffiness, periorbital edema, and masklike affect). Individuals with hypothyroidism may describe impaired self-image in regard to their disabilities and altered appearance.

Women with hypothyroidism frequently experience menorrhagia. As circulating thyroid hormone concentrations have been found to be associated with sex steroid hormone levels in women, they may not have sufficient levels of sex steroid hormones to coordinate reproductive cycles, resulting in anovulatory cycles and potential infertility (Jacobson et al., 2018). In older persons, the typical manifestations of hypothyroidism (including fatigue, cold and dry skin, hoarseness, hair loss, constipation, and cold intolerance) may be attributed to normal aging. For this reason, these symptoms may not raise suspicion about an underlying condition. Older people who experience confusion, lethargy, and depression should be evaluated for thyroid disease.

Complications

The mental sluggishness, drowsiness, and lethargy of hypothyroidism may progress gradually or suddenly to hypothermia and a notable impairment of consciousness or coma. This situation, myxedema coma, constitutes a medical emergency. Myxedema coma in a poorly responsive patient can be recognized by the presence of a thyroidectomy scar or a history

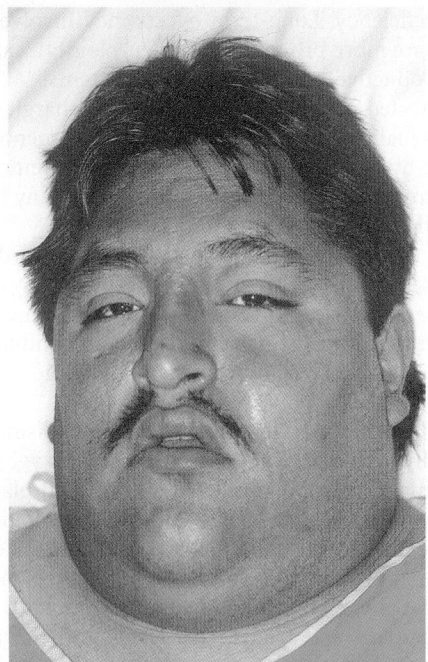

FIG. 51.8 Patient with myxedema, displaying the characteristic facies of hypothyroidism (i.e., puffiness, periorbital edema, and masklike affect). Source: Seidel, H. M., Ball, J., Dains, J., et al. (2015). *Mosby's guide to physical examination* (8th ed., p. 190, Figure 10-10). Mosby. (Originally from Lemmi, F. O., & Lemmi, C. A. E. [2000]. *Physical assessment findings.* [CD-ROM]. Saunders.)

of radioiodine therapy or hypothyroidism (Ono et al., 2017). Myxedema coma can be precipitated by infection, medications (especially opioids, tranquilizers, and barbiturates), exposure to cold, and trauma. It is characterized by subnormal temperature, hypotension, and hypoventilation. For patients experiencing myxedema to survive, vital functions must be supported, and initial serum levels of T_4, TSH, and cortisol must be drawn and analyzed. These patients must be treated aggressively with IV thyroid hormone replacement and high-dose glucocorticoid therapy until coexisting adrenal insufficiency can be excluded (Yafit et al., 2019).

Diagnostic Studies

The most common and reliable laboratory tests used to evaluate thyroid function are measurements of TSH and free T_4. These values, when correlated with symptoms evident in the history and physical examination, confirm the diagnosis. Serum TSH levels help determine the cause of hypothyroidism—they are high when the defect is in the thyroid and low when it is in the pituitary gland or hypothalamus. An increase in TSH level after injection of TRH suggests hypothalamic dysfunction, whereas no change suggests anterior pituitary dysfunction (Table 51.10). The presence of thyroid peroxidase antibodies suggests an autoimmune origin of the disorder. Other abnormal laboratory findings are elevated cholesterol and triglyceride levels, anemia, and increased creatine kinase level.

Interprofessional Care

The overall goal for treatment in a patient with hypothyroidism is restoration of a euthyroid state as safely and rapidly as possible with hormone replacement therapy. Levothyroxine (Synthroid, Eltroxin) is the medication of choice to treat

TABLE 51.10   INTERPROFESSIONAL CARE
Hypothyroidism

Diagnostic Studies	Interprofessional Therapy
• History and physical examination • Serum T_3 and serum T_4 levels (if ordered) • Serum TSH and free T_4 levels • Thyroid peroxidase antibodies • TRH stimulation test	• Monitoring thyroid hormone levels and adjusting dosage (if needed) • Nutritional therapy to promote weight loss • Patient and caregiver teaching (see Table 51.11) • Thyroid hormone replacement (e.g., levothyroxine)

T_3, triiodothyronine; *T_4,* thyroxine; *TRH,* thyrotropin-releasing hormone; *TSH,* thyroid-stimulating hormone.

hypothyroidism. In young and otherwise healthy patients, the maintenance replacement dose is adjusted according to the patients' response and laboratory findings. In older patients and in patients with compromised cardiac status, a lower initial dosage is recommended because the usual dosage may increase myocardial oxygen demand. The increased oxygen demand may cause angina and cardiac dysrhythmias. Any chest pain experienced by a patient starting thyroid replacement should be reported immediately. In patients without adverse effects, the dose is increased at 4- to 6-week intervals. It is important that patients take replacement medication regularly. Lifelong thyroid replacement therapy is usually required.

MEDICATION ALERT—Levothyroxine (Synthroid)
- Patients with cardiovascular disease who take this medication must be carefully monitored.
- Heart rate must be monitored and pulse greater than 100 beats/min or an irregular heartbeat must be reported.
- Chest pain, weight loss, nervousness, tremors, or insomnia must be promptly reported.
- Multiple levothyroxine preparations are currently available. Patients taking levothyroxine must have serum TSH levels checked 4 to 6 weeks after changing levothyroxine preparation.

NURSING MANAGEMENT HYPOTHYROIDISM

NURSING ASSESSMENT

Careful assessment of patients suspected of having hypothyroidism may reveal the early and subtle changes that indicate dysfunction. Assessment should include questions about weight gain, mental changes, fatigue, slowed and slurred speech, cold intolerance, skin changes such as increased dryness or thickening, constipation, and dyspnea. Patients should be questioned about recent introduction of iodine-containing medications. They should be assessed for bradycardia; distended abdomen; dry, thick, cold skin; thick, brittle nails; paresthesias; and muscular aches and pains.

NURSING DIAGNOSES

Nursing diagnoses for patients with hypothyroidism may include but are not limited to the following:
- *Reduced stamina* resulting from *physical deconditioning* (weakness and fatigue)
- *Constipation* resulting from *decrease in GI motility*

Additional information on nursing diagnoses for the patient with hypothyroidism is presented in NCP 51.2, available on the Evolve website.

PLANNING

The overall goals are that patients with hypothyroidism will (a) experience relief from symptoms, (b) maintain a euthyroid state, (c) maintain a positive self-image, and (d) adhere to a life-long regimen of thyroid replacement therapy.

NURSING IMPLEMENTATION

HEALTH PROMOTION. There is currently no consensus regarding thyroid function screening, particularly for those with subclinical presentations of asymptomatic hypothyroidism. Although hypothyroidism is relatively common, particularly among women older than 50, recommendations related to the screening of the general population are mixed. Research suggests that populations at high risk for thyroid dysfunction should be screened for subclinical (asymptomatic) thyroid disease since it is associated with increased cardiovascular risk, especially with regard to elevated total and low-density lipoprotein (LDL) cholesterol levels and diminished overall left-sided cardiac function. Individuals at risk include those with a family history of thyroid disease, those with a history of neck irradiation, women older than 50, and women who have just given birth (Abreu et al., 2017). In contrast, no benefits of subclinical thyroid disease screening have been found for older persons (Stott et al., 2017).

ACUTE INTERVENTION. Most individuals with hypothyroidism do not require acute nursing care. However, a patient who develops myxedema coma does require acute nursing care, often in a critical care setting. Myxedema coma is associated with a high mortality rate (30–50%), particularly in circumstances of older age, cardiac complications, reduced level of consciousness, persistent hypothermia, and sepsis (Ono et al., 2017). Mechanical respiratory support and cardiac monitoring are frequently necessary. Thyroid hormone replacement therapy and all other medications should be administered intravenously because paralytic ileus may be present with myxedema coma. If the patient is hyponatremic, hypertonic saline may be administered slowly until the serum sodium level reaches at least 130 mmol/L. Core temperature should be monitored because many patients with myxedema coma are hypothermic.

The nurse monitors a patient's progress by assessing vital signs, body weight, fluid intake and output, and visible edema. Cardiac assessment is especially important because the cardiovascular response to the hormone determines the medication regimen. Energy level and mental alertness should be noted. These should increase within 2 to 14 days and continue to rise steadily to normal levels.

AMBULATORY AND HOME CARE. Patient and caregiver teaching is essential for patients with hypothyroidism (Table 51.11). Initially, patients with hypothyroidism need more time than usual to comprehend all the necessary information. It is important to provide written instructions, repeat the information often, and assess the patient's comprehension level regularly.

The need for lifelong medication therapy must be stressed. Patients should be taught expected and unexpected adverse medication effects. Specifically, the signs and symptoms of hypothyroidism or hyperthyroidism that indicate hormone imbalance should be included in the teaching plan. Toxic symptoms

TABLE 51.11	**PATIENT & CAREGIVER TEACHING GUIDE**

Hypothyroidism

The following instructions should be included when teaching the patient and caregiver about management of hypothyroidism. The nurse should:

1. Explain the nature of thyroid hormone deficiency and self-care practices necessary to prevent complications. The patient and caregivers must understand thyroid replacement therapy. It is especially important to emphasize the need for lifelong replacement, the need to take the medication continually, and the need for regular follow-up care.
2. Emphasize the need for a comfortable, warm environment because of intolerance of cold.
3. Teach measures to prevent skin breakdown. Soap should be used sparingly and lotion applied to skin.
4. Caution patients, especially older people, to avoid use of sedatives. If sedatives must be used, suggest that the lowest dose be used. Caregivers should closely monitor the patient's mental status, level of consciousness, and respiration.
5. Discuss with the patient measures to minimize constipation. Suggestions should include a gradual increase in activity and exercise, increased fibre in diet, use of stool softeners, and maintenance of a regular bowel elimination time. Enemas should not be used because they produce vagal stimulation, which can be hazardous if cardiac disease is present.

should be clearly defined. Table 51.6 lists signs of hyperthyroidism that are the same as toxic symptoms of thyroid hormone replacement.

Patients must be taught to contact a health care provider immediately if signs of overdose—such as orthopnea, dyspnea, rapid pulse, palpitations, nervousness, or insomnia—appear. A patient with diabetes mellitus should test their capillary blood glucose level at least daily because return to the euthyroid state frequently increases insulin requirements. In addition, thyroid preparations potentiate the effects of anticoagulants and decrease the effect of digitalis compounds. Thus, the patient should be taught the toxic signs and symptoms of these medications and should remain under close medical observation until their condition is stable.

It is sometimes difficult for patients to recognize signs of overdosage or underdosage of medication therapy; therefore, a family member or friend should also receive instructions. Handouts for patients should be written in understandable language and should accompany verbal instruction. The handouts should be reviewed with the patient and the family to assess understanding, and information should be clarified when necessary.

With treatment, striking transformations occur in both appearance and mental function. In most adults, both return to normal. Cardiovascular conditions and (occasionally) psychosis may persist despite corrections of the hormonal imbalance. Relapses occur if treatment is interrupted.

EVALUATION

The following are expected outcomes for patients with hypothyroidism:

- Relief from symptoms
- Maintenance of a euthyroid state as evidenced by normal thyroid hormone and TSH levels
- Avoidance of complications of therapy
- Adherence to lifelong therapy

DISORDERS OF THE PARATHYROID GLANDS

HYPERPARATHYROIDISM

Etiology and Pathophysiology

Hyperparathyroidism is a common endocrine disorder characterized by inappropriately normal or increased secretion of parathyroid hormone (PTH). PTH helps regulate calcium and phosphate levels by stimulating bone resorption of calcium, renal tubular reabsorption of calcium, and activation of vitamin D. Thus, oversecretion of PTH is characterized by hypercalcemia (polydipsia, polyuria, diminished deep tendon reflexes, hypertension). Incidence of hyperparathyroidism is approximately 0.4 to 82 cases per 100 000 of the general population. It occurs more frequently among women, and the incidence increases with age (Walker & Silverberg, 2018).

Hyperparathyroidism is classified as primary, secondary, or tertiary. *Primary hyperparathyroidism* results from an increased secretion of PTH, which leads to disorders of calcium, phosphate, and bone metabolism. The most common cause is a benign neoplasm or a single adenoma in the parathyroid gland. Primary hyperparathyroidism usually occurs between the ages of 30 and 70 years. The incidence peaks in the fifth and sixth decades of life. Patients who have previously undergone head and neck irradiation may have an increased risk of developing a parathyroid adenoma.

Secondary hyperparathyroidism appears to be a compensatory response to states that induce or cause hypocalcemia, the main stimulus of PTH secretion. Disease conditions associated with secondary hyperparathyroidism include vitamin D deficiencies, malabsorption, chronic renal failure, and hyperphosphatemia.

Tertiary hyperparathyroidism occurs when the parathyroid glands become hyperplastic and negative feedback is lost from circulating calcium levels; thus, PTH is secreted autonomously, even with normal calcium levels. This condition is observed in patients who have undergone kidney transplantation after a long period of dialysis treatment for chronic renal failure. (Chapter 49 discusses parathyroid hormone and kidney function.)

Excessive levels of circulating PTH usually lead to hypercalcemia and hypophosphatemia, creating a multisystem effect (Table 51.12). In the skeleton, decreased bone density, cyst formation, and general weakness can occur as a result of the effect of PTH on *osteoclastic* activity (bone resorption) and *osteoblastic* activity (bone formation). In the kidneys, the excess calcium cannot be reabsorbed; as a result, levels of calcium in the urine increase *(hypercalciuria)*. This urinary calcium level, along with a large amount of urinary phosphate, can lead to calculi formation (Walker & Silverberg, 2018). In addition, PTH stimulates the synthesis of a biologically active form of vitamin D, a potent stimulator of calcium transport in the intestine. In this way, PTH indirectly increases GI absorption of calcium, contributing further to the high serum calcium levels.

Clinical Manifestations and Complications

Clinical manifestations of hyperparathyroidism range from no symptoms (the condition is diagnosed through testing for unrelated conditions) to overt symptoms. Clinical manifestations are associated with hypercalcemia and are summarized in Table 51.12. The major manifestations include muscle weakness, loss of appetite, constipation, fatigue, emotional disorders, and shortened attention span. Major signs include loss of calcium from bones *(osteoporosis)*, fractures, and kidney stones *(nephrolithiasis)*. Neuromuscular abnormalities are characterized by muscle weakness, particularly in the proximal muscles of the lower extremities. Asymptomatic cases are often identified through routine calcium screening. Serious complications of hyperparathyroidism are renal failure, pancreatitis, cardiac changes, and fractures of long bones, ribs, and vertebrae.

Diagnostic Studies

PTH levels are elevated in hyperparathyroidism. Serum calcium levels usually exceed 2.75 mmol/L. Because of its inverse relation with the calcium level, the serum phosphorus level is usually below 0.1 mmol/L. Elevations occur in other laboratory values: urine calcium, serum chloride, uric acid, creatinine, amylase (if pancreatitis is present), and alkaline phosphatase (if bone disease is present). Bone density measurements may also be used to detect bone loss. Imaging studies, such as MRI, CT, and ultrasonography, may help localize the adenoma.

Interprofessional Care

The treatment objectives for hyperparathyroidism are to relieve the manifestations and prevent complications caused by excess PTH. The choice of therapy depends on the urgency of the clinical situation, the degree of hypercalcemia, and the underlying cause of the disorder.

Surgical Therapy. The most effective treatment of primary and secondary hyperparathyroidism is surgical intervention. Parathyroidectomy leads to rapid reduction of chronically high calcium levels. Criteria for surgery include serum calcium levels higher than 0.25 mmol/L above normal level; creatinine clearance rate of less than 60 mL/min; *T*-score lower than −2.5 at any site on bone mineral density testing, previous fracture fragility, or both; and age younger than 50 years. The surgical procedure involves partial or complete removal of the parathyroid glands. The most common procedure involves use of an endoscope and is performed on an outpatient basis. Successful removal of the

TABLE 51.12	**CLINICAL MANIFESTATIONS OF PARATHYROID DYSFUNCTION**			
Hypofunction	**Hyperfunction**	**Hypofunction**	**Hyperfunction**
Cardiovascular		**Neurological**	
• Decreased cardiac output • Decreased contractility of heart muscle • Dysrhythmias • Prolongation of Q–T and ST intervals on ECG	• Dysrhythmias • Hypertension • Shortened Q–T interval on ECG	• Disorientation, confusion (in older persons) • Headache • Hyperactive deep tendon reflexes • Irritability • Memory impairment • Paresthesias of perioral area, hands, and feet • Personality changes • Positive Chvostek's or Trousseau's sign • Psychiatric manifestations of depression, anxiety, psychosis • Seizures • Tremor	• Abnormalities of gait • Delirium, confusion, coma • Emotional irritability • Headache • Hyperactive deep tendon reflexes • Memory impairment • Paresthesias • Personality disturbances • Poor coordination • Psychomotor retardation • Psychosis, depression
Gastrointestinal			
• Abdominal cramps • Fecal incontinence (in older persons) • Malabsorption	• Anorexia • Cholelithiasis • Constipation • Nausea and vomiting • Pancreatitis • Peptic ulcer disease • Vague abdominal pain • Weight loss		
Integumentary		**Renal**	
• Brittle nails, transverse ridging • Changes in developing teeth, lack of tooth enamel • Dry, scaly skin • Hair loss on scalp and body	• Moist skin • Skin necrosis	• Urinary frequency • Urinary incontinence	• Hypercalciuria • Kidney stones (nephrolithiasis) • Polyuria • Urinary tract infections
Musculoskeletal		**Other**	
• Difficulty in walking • Fatigue • Painful muscle cramps • Skeletal radiograph changes, osteosclerosis • Soft tissue calcification • Weakness	• Backache • Compression fractures of spine • Decreased muscle tone, muscle atrophy • Osteoporosis • Pain on weight bearing • Pathological fractures of long bones • Skeletal pain • Weakness, fatigue	• Eye changes, including lenticular opacities, cataracts, papilledema	• Corneal calcification on slit-lamp examination

ECG, electrocardiogram.

parathyroid glands is facilitated by preoperative nuclear scanning with technetium-99m (99mTc) (Wilhelm et al., 2016).

Autotransplantation of normal parathyroid tissue in the forearm or near the sternocleidomastoid muscle may be performed, which allows PTH secretion to continue with normalization of calcium levels. If autotransplantation is not possible, or if it fails, patients need to take calcium supplements for the rest of their lives.

Nonsurgical Therapy. A conservative approach is often used in patients who are asymptomatic or have mild symptoms of hyperparathyroidism. This approach includes an annual examination with tests for serum calcium and creatinine clearance and evaluation of bone density every 1 to 2 years. Continued ambulation and the avoidance of immobility are critical aspects of management. Dietary measures also include maintenance of a high fluid intake and a moderate calcium intake.

Phosphorus intake is usually supplemented unless this is contraindicated by an increased risk for urinary calculi formation. Several medications currently used in the treatment of hyperparathyroidism are helpful in lowering calcium levels but do not treat the underlying condition. Bisphosphonates (e.g., alendronate [Fosamax]) inhibit osteoclastic bone resorption and rapidly normalize serum calcium levels. Estrogen or progestin therapy can reduce serum and urinary calcium

levels in postmenopausal women and may slow the demineralization of the skeleton. Oral phosphate may be used to inhibit the calcium-absorbing effects of vitamin D in the intestine. Phosphates should be used only if a patient has normal renal function and low serum phosphate levels. Calcimimetic agents (e.g., cinacalcet [Sensipar]) are a class of medications that increase the sensitivity of the calcium receptor on the parathyroid gland, resulting in decreased PTH secretion and calcium blood levels and thus sparing calcium stores in the bone. Medications in this class are currently indicated for secondary hyperparathyroidism in individuals with chronic kidney disease who are undergoing dialysis, for patients with parathyroid cancer, and for patients with symptomatic hypercalcemia in primary hyperparathyroidism.

NURSING MANAGEMENT
HYPERPARATHYROIDISM

Nursing care for patients after a parathyroidectomy is similar to that for patients after a thyroidectomy. The major postoperative complications are associated with hemorrhage and fluid and electrolyte disturbances. *Tetany,* a condition of neuromuscular hyperexcitability associated with a sudden decrease in calcium levels, is another concern. It is usually apparent early in the postoperative period but may develop over several days. Mild tetany, characterized by an unpleasant tingling sensation of the hands and around the mouth, may be present but should abate without problems. If tetany becomes more severe (e.g., muscular spasms or laryngospasms develop), IV calcium may be given. IV calcium gluconate should be readily available for patients after parathyroidectomy in case acute tetany occurs.

The nurse monitors intake and output to evaluate fluid status. Calcium, potassium, phosphate, and magnesium levels are assessed frequently, as are Chvostek's and Trousseau's signs (see Chapter 19, Figure 19.15). The nurse also encourages mobility to promote bone calcification.

If surgery is not performed, treatment to relieve symptoms and prevent complications is initiated. The nurse can assist patients with hyperparathyroidism to adapt the meal plan to their lifestyle. A referral to a dietitian may be useful. Because immobility can aggravate the bone loss, the nurse must stress to patients the importance of an exercise program. Patients should be encouraged to keep regular appointments, and the tests being performed should be explained. Patients should also be instructed in the symptoms of hypocalcemia or hypercalcemia and to report them should they occur. Hypocalcemia and hypercalcemia are discussed in Chapter 19.

HYPOPARATHYROIDISM

Etiology and Pathophysiology

Hypoparathyroidism is an uncommon condition that most often occurs as a result of iatrogenic causes such as accidental removal or destruction to the vascular supply of the parathyroid glands (e.g., surgical, autoimmune). It can also be the result of abnormal parathyroid development and inadequate levels of circulating PTH. It is characterized by hypocalcemia that results from a lack of PTH to maintain serum calcium levels. PTH resistance at the cellular level may also occur (pseudohypoparathyroidism). This condition is caused by a genetic defect that results in hypocalcemia in spite of normal or high PTH levels and is often associated with hypothyroidism and hypogonadism (Lopes et al., 2016).

Idiopathic hypoparathyroidism resulting from the absence, fatty replacement, or atrophy of the glands is a rare disease that usually occurs early in life and may be associated with other endocrine disorders. Affected patients may have antiparathyroid antibodies. Severe hypomagnesemia also leads to a suppression of PTH secretion (Mutnuri et al., 2016).

Clinical Manifestations

The clinical features of acute hypoparathyroidism result from a low serum calcium level (see Table 51.12). Sudden decreases in calcium concentration cause tetany characterized by tingling sensations in the lips, the fingertips, and occasionally the feet, and by increased muscle tension, which escalates to paresthesias and stiffness. Painful tonic spasms of smooth and skeletal muscles can cause dysphagia, a constricted feeling in the throat, and laryngospasms that can compromise breathing. Patients are usually anxious and apprehensive. Abnormal laboratory findings include decreased serum calcium and PTH levels and increased serum phosphate levels. Other causes of chronic hypocalcemia include chronic renal failure, vitamin D deficiency, and hypomagnesemia.

NURSING AND INTERPROFESSIONAL MANAGEMENT HYPOPARATHYROIDISM

The primary treatment goals for a patient with hypoparathyroidism are to treat acute complications such as tetany, maintain normal serum calcium levels, correct low magnesium levels, and prevent long-term complications. Emergency treatment of tetany requires the administration of IV calcium. IV calcium chloride or calcium gluconate should be infused slowly because high blood levels of calcium can cause hypotension, serious cardiac dysrhythmias, or cardiac arrest; thus ECG monitoring is indicated when calcium is administered. IV calcium can cause venous irritation and inflammation. Extravasation may cause cellulitis, necrosis, and tissue sloughing. IV patency should be assessed before administration.

Rebreathing may partially alleviate acute neuromuscular symptoms associated with hypocalcemia, such as generalized muscle cramps or mild tetany. Patients who can cooperate should be instructed to breathe in and out of a paper bag or breathing mask. This practice reduces carbon dioxide excretion from the lungs, increases carbonic acid levels in the blood, and lowers the pH.

A lower pH (acidic environment) enhances the degree of ionization of calcium, causing an increase in the proportion of total body calcium available in the active form.

Patients with hypoparathyroidism need instruction in the management of long-term medication therapy and nutrition. Oral calcium supplements of at least 1.5 to 3 g/day in divided doses are usually prescribed. PTH replacement is not a recommended medication therapy because of the expense and the need for parenteral administration. Vitamin D is administered to patients with chronic and resistant hypocalcemia to enhance intestinal calcium absorption and bone resorption. The primary preparation is Calcitrol, which raises calcium levels rapidly and is quickly metabolized. Rapid metabolism is desired because vitamin D is a fat-soluble vitamin, and toxicity can cause irreversible renal impairment.

A high-calcium meal plan includes foods such as dark green vegetables, soybeans, and tofu. Patients should be told to avoid foods containing oxalic acid (e.g., spinach, rhubarb), phytic acid (e.g., bran, whole grains), and phosphorus (e.g., protein-rich foods such as meats, poultry, fish, nuts, beans, and dairy products) because they reduce calcium absorption.

Patients should be informed of the need for lifelong treatment and follow-up care, including the monitoring of calcium levels three to four times a year.

DISORDERS OF THE ADRENAL CORTEX

There are three main classifications of adrenal steroid hormones. *Glucocorticoids* regulate metabolism, increase blood glucose levels, and are critical in the physiological stress response. In humans, the primary glucocorticoid is cortisol. *Mineralocorticoids* regulate sodium and potassium balance. The primary mineralocorticoid is aldosterone. *Androgens* contribute to growth and development in both genders and to sexual desire and satisfaction in women. The term *corticosteroid* refers to any one of these three types of hormones produced by the adrenal cortex.

CUSHING'S SYNDROME

Etiology and Pathophysiology

Cushing's syndrome is a spectrum of clinical abnormalities characterized by endogenous hypercortisolism, which may be

TABLE 51.13	CAUSES OF CUSHING'S SYNDROME

- ACTH-secreting pituitary tumour (Cushing's disease)
- Cortisol-secreting neoplasm within the adrenal cortex that can be either carcinoma or adenoma
- Excess secretion of ACTH from carcinoma of the lung or other malignant growth outside the pituitary or the adrenal glands
- Prolonged administration of high doses of corticosteroids

ACTH, adrenocorticotrophic hormone.

difficult to recognize (Niemen, 2018). Approximately 85% of cases of endogenous Cushing's syndrome result from an adrenocorticotrophic hormone (ACTH)-secreting pituitary tumour (Cushing's disease), most commonly seen in women aged 20 to 40 years. Several conditions can cause this metabolic disorder (Table 51.13). Very common causes of Cushing's syndrome are iatrogenic administration of exogenous corticosteroids (e.g., prednisone) in large doses for several weeks or longer and the chronic and excessive production of cortisol by the adrenal cortex. Other causes include adrenal tumours and ectopic ACTH production by tumours (more common in men) outside the hypothalamic–pituitary–adrenal axis (usually of the lung or the pancreas).

Clinical Manifestations

The clinical manifestations of Cushing's syndrome can occur in most body systems and are related to excess levels of corticosteroids (Table 51.14). Corticosteroid excess causes pronounced changes in physical appearance (Figure 51.9). Weight gain, the most common feature, results from the accumulation of adipose tissue in the trunk, the face, and the cervical area (see Figure 51.9). Transient weight gain from sodium and water retention may be present because of the mineralocorticoid effects of cortisol. Hyperglycemia occurs because of glucose intolerance (associated with cortisol-induced insulin resistance) and increased gluconeogenesis by the liver.

The catabolic effects of cortisol on peripheral tissue cause protein wasting. Muscle wasting leads to muscle weakness, especially in the extremities. Loss of protein matrix in bone leads to osteoporosis with subsequent pathological fractures (e.g., vertebral compression fractures) and bone and back pain. Loss of collagen makes the skin weaker and thinner; therefore, the skin bruises more easily. Catabolic processes predominate, and wound healing is delayed. Mood disturbances (e.g., irritability, anxiety, euphoria), insomnia, irrationality, and occasionally psychosis may occur.

Mineralocorticoid excess may cause hypertension (secondary to fluid retention), whereas adrenal androgen excess may cause pronounced acne, masculinization in women, and feminization in men. Menstrual disorders and hirsutism in women and gynecomastia and erectile dysfunction in men occur more commonly with adrenal carcinomas.

The clinical presentation is the first indication of Cushing's syndrome (Figure 51.10). Of particular importance are (a) centripetal (truncal) obesity or generalized obesity; (b) so-called moon facies (fullness of the face) with facial plethora; (c) purplish red striae, which are usually depressed below the skin surface, on the abdomen, the breasts, or the buttocks (Figure 51.11); (d) hirsutism in women; (e) menstrual disorders in women; (f) hypertension; and (g) unexplained hypokalemia.

Diagnostic Studies

When Cushing's syndrome is suspected, at least two of three different screening tests are used: (1) a 24-hour urine free cortisol (UFC) excretion (see Chapter 50), (2) late-night/bedtime salivary cortisol levels, and (3) the 1-mg overnight dexamethasone suppression test (Nieman, 2018). The result of each cortisol screening test (saliva, serum, urine) is considered abnormal if it falls outside of normal reference ranges, particularly elevation in the midnight serum cortisol level, which confirms the diagnosis of Cushing's syndrome (Nieman, 2018). False-positive results can occur in patients who are (a) exercising to capacity, (b) experiencing depression, (c) experiencing acute stress and significant weight loss, and (d) misusing alcohol. CT and MRI of the pituitary and adrenal glands may be used.

Plasma ACTH levels may be low, normal, or elevated, depending on the underlying condition. High or normal levels indicate ACTH-dependent Cushing's disease, whereas low or undetectable levels indicate an adrenal or exogenous etiology. Other findings on diagnostic tests associated with but not diagnostic of Cushing's syndrome include granulocytosis, lymphopenia, eosinopenia, hyperglycemia, glycosuria, hypercalciuria, and osteoporosis. Hypokalemia and alkalosis occur in ectopic ACTH syndrome and adrenal carcinoma.

Interprofessional Care

The primary goal of treatment for Cushing's disease and Cushing's syndrome is to normalize hormone secretion. The specific treatment is dependent on the underlying cause (Table 51.15). If the underlying cause is a pituitary adenoma, the standard treatment is surgical removal of the tumour through the trans-sphenoidal approach (Lonser et al., 2017). (The trans-sphenoidal approach is discussed earlier in this chapter). Irradiation of the pituitary adenoma may be necessary if surgical outcomes are not optimal or if a patient is at high risk for surgical complications. Unilateral or, on occasion, bilateral adrenalectomy is indicated for Cushing's syndrome caused by adrenal tumours or hyperplasia. Laparoscopic adrenalectomy is considered an appropriate surgical approach except for patients with known or suspected malignant adrenal tumours. An open surgical adrenalectomy is the treatment of choice for adrenal cancer. Patients with ectopic ACTH-secreting tumours are managed by treating the primary neoplasm.

Medication therapy is used when surgery is contraindicated or as an adjunct to surgery. The goal of medication therapy is the inhibition of adrenal function (*medical adrenalectomy*). Mitotane (Lysodren) suppresses cortisol production, alters peripheral metabolism of cortisol, and decreases plasma and urine corticosteroid levels. Ketoconazole can be used to inhibit cortisol synthesis. These medications should be used with caution because they are often toxic at doses needed to reduce corticosteroid synthesis.

If Cushing's syndrome has developed during the course of prolonged administration of corticosteroids (e.g., prednisone), one or more of the following alternatives may be tried: (1) gradual discontinuance of corticosteroid therapy, (2) reduction of the corticosteroid dose, and (3) conversion to an alternate-day regimen. Gradual tapering of the corticosteroids is necessary to avoid potentially life-threatening adrenal insufficiency. An alternate-day regimen is one in which twice the daily dosage of a shorter-acting corticosteroid is given every other morning to minimize hypothalamic–pituitary–adrenal suppression, growth suppression, and altered appearance.

TABLE 51.14   CLINICAL MANIFESTATIONS: ADRENOCORTICAL HORMONE DYSFUNCTION

Category	Hypofunction (Addison's Disease)	Hyperfunction (Cushing's Syndrome)
Glucocorticoids		
Cardiovascular	Hypotension, tendency to develop refractory shock, vasodilation	Hypervolemia, hypertension, edema of lower extremities
Fluids and electrolytes	Hyponatremia, hypovolemia, dehydration, hyperkalemia	Sodium and water retention, edema, hypokalemia
Gastrointestinal	Anorexia, nausea and vomiting, cramping abdominal pain, diarrhea	Increase in secretion of pepsin and hydrochloric acid; anorexia
General appearance	Weight loss	Centripetal (truncal) obesity, thin extremities, rounding of face (moon facies), fat deposits on back of neck and on shoulders (buffalo hump)
Hematological system	Anemia, lymphocytosis	Leukocytosis, lymphopenia, polycythemia, increased coagulability
Immune system	Tendency for coexisting autoimmune diseases	Inhibition of immune response, suppression of allergic response, inhibition of inflammation
Integumentary system	Bronzed or smoky hyperpigmentation of face, neck, hands (especially creases), buccal membranes, nipples, genitalia, and scars (if pituitary function is normal); vitiligo, alopecia	Thin, fragile skin; purplish red striae (see Figure 51.11); petechial hemorrhages; bruises; florid cheeks (facial plethora); acne; poor wound healing
Mental and emotional state	Neurasthenia, depression, exhaustion or irritability, confusion, delusions	Euphoria, irritability, hypomania to depression, emotional lability
Metabolism	Hypoglycemia, insulin sensitivity, fever	Hyperglycemia, negative nitrogen balance, dyslipidemia
Musculoskeletal	Fatigability	Muscle wasting in extremities, proximal muscle weakness, fatigue, osteoporosis, awkward gait, back and joint pain, weakness
Renal/urinary	—	Glycosuria, hypercalciuria, kidney stones
Mineralocorticoids		
Cardiovascular	Hypovolemia, tendency toward shock, decreased cardiac output, decrease in heart size	Hypertension, hypervolemia
Fluids and electrolytes	Sodium loss, decreased volume of extracellular fluid, hyperkalemia, salt craving	Marked sodium and water retention, tendency toward edema, marked hypokalemia, alkalosis
Androgens		
Integumentary	Decreased axillary and pubic hair (in women)	Hirsutism, acne, hyperpigmentation
Musculoskeletal	Decrease in muscle size and tone	Muscle wasting and weakness
Reproductive	No effect in men; decreased libido in women	Menstrual irregularities and enlargement of clitoris in women; gynecomastia and testicular atrophy in men

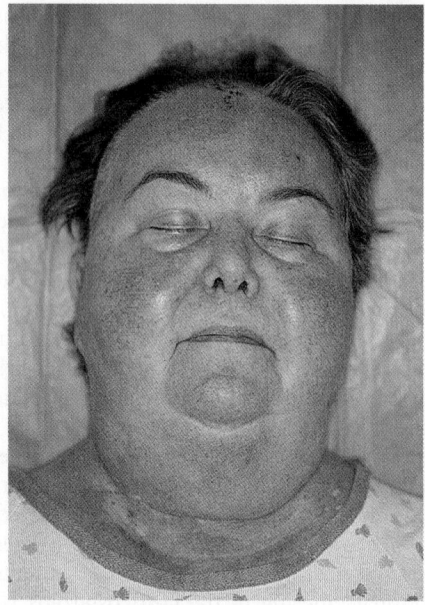

FIG. 51.9 Cushing's syndrome. Facies include a rounded face (moon facies) with thin, reddened skin. Hirsutism may also be present. Source: Seidel, H. M., Ball, J., Dains, J., et al. (2006). *Mosby's guide to physical examination* (6th ed., p. 272, Figure 10-17). Mosby.

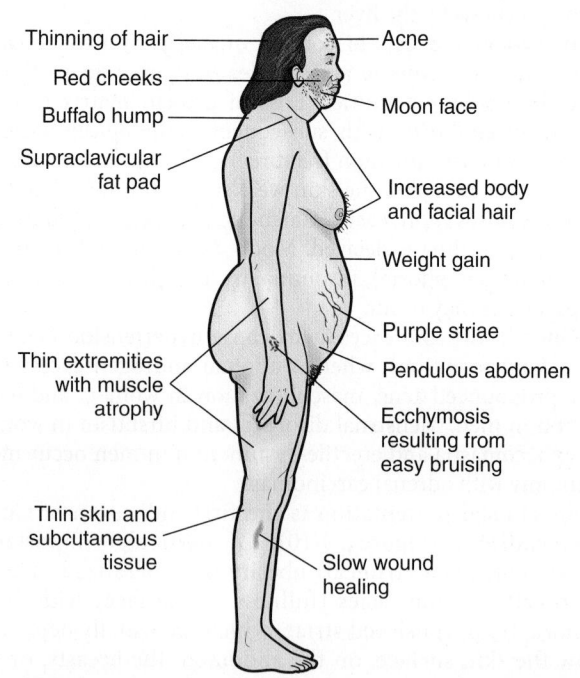

Thinning of hair — Acne
Red cheeks
Buffalo hump — Moon face
Supraclavicular fat pad
Increased body and facial hair
Weight gain
Purple striae
Thin extremities with muscle atrophy — Pendulous abdomen
Ecchymosis resulting from easy bruising
Thin skin and subcutaneous tissue
Slow wound healing

FIG. 51.10 Common characteristics of Cushing's syndrome.

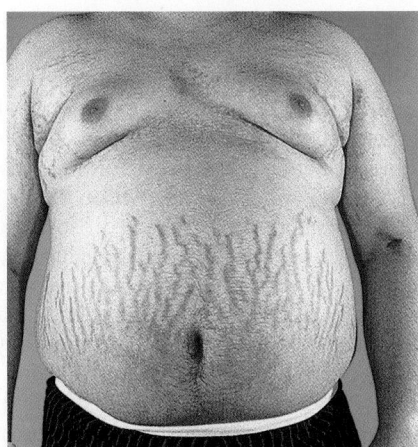

FIG. 51.11 Cushing's syndrome. Truncal obesity; broad, purple striae; and easy bruising (left antecubital fossa). Source: Chew, S. L., & Leslie, D. (2006). *Clinical endocrinology and diabetes: An illustrated colour text.* (1st ed., p. 28, Figure 2). Churchill Livingstone.

TABLE 51.15 INTERPROFESSIONAL CARE

Cushing's Syndrome

Diagnostic	Interprofessional Therapy*
• History and physical examination • 24-hour urine collection for free cortisol measurement • Blood chemistry evaluation for sodium, potassium, and glucose • Complete blood cell count • CT, MRI • Dexamethasone suppression test • Examination of visual field • Measurement of plasma ACTH level • Measurement of plasma cortisol levels for diurnal variations • Mental status examination	**Adrenocortical Adenoma, Carcinoma, or Hyperplasia** • Adrenalectomy (open or laparoscopic) • Medication therapy • Ketoconazole (Nizoral) • Mitotane (Lysodren) **Pituitary Adenoma** • Radiation therapy • Trans-sphenoidal resection **Ectopic ACTH-Secreting Tumour** • Treatment of the tumour responsible (surgical removal or radiation therapy) **Exogenous Corticosteroid Therapy** • Discontinuance of or alteration in administration of exogenous corticosteroids

ACTH, adrenocorticotrophic hormone; *CT,* computed tomographic (scan); *MRI,* magnetic resonance imaging.
*Treatment is based on underlying cause.

NURSING MANAGEMENT CUSHING'S SYNDROME

NURSING ASSESSMENT

Subjective and objective data that should be obtained from a patient with Cushing's syndrome are presented in Table 51.16.

NURSING DIAGNOSES

Nursing diagnoses for patients with Cushing's syndrome may include but are not limited to the following:
• *Potential for infection* resulting from *insufficient knowledge to avoid exposure to pathogens* (suppression of immune system)

TABLE 51.16 NURSING ASSESSMENT

Cushing's Syndrome

Subjective Data
Important Health Information
Past health history: Pituitary tumour (Cushing's disease); adrenal, pancreatic, or pulmonary neoplasms; GI bleeding; frequent infections
Medications: Use of corticosteroids

Symptoms
• Amenorrhea, erectile dysfunction, decreased libido
• Anxiety, mood disturbances, emotional lability, psychosis
• Headache; back, joint, bone, and rib pain; poor concentration and memory
• Insomnia, poor sleep quality
• Malaise, weakness, fatigue
• Negative feelings regarding changes in personal appearance
• Polyuria
• Prolonged wound healing, easy bruising
• Weight gain, anorexia

Objective Data
General
Centripetal (truncal) obesity, supraclavicular fat pads, buffalo hump, moon facies

Integumentary
Facial plethora; hirsutism of body and face, thinning of head hair; thin, friable skin; acne; petechiae; purpura; hyperpigmentation; purplish red striae on breasts, buttocks, and abdomen; edema of lower extremities

Cardiovascular
Hypertension

Musculoskeletal
Muscle wasting, thin extremities, awkward gait

Reproductive
Gynecomastia, testicular atrophy (in men); enlarged clitoris (in women)

Possible Findings
Hypokalemia, hyperglycemia, dyslipidemia; polycythemia, granulocytosis, lymphocytopenia, eosinopenia; ↑ plasma cortisol level; high, low, or normal ACTH levels; abnormal result of dexamethasone suppression test; ↑ levels of urine free cortisol and 17-ketosteroids; glycosuria, hypercalciuria; osteoporosis on radiograph

ACTH, adrenocorticotrophic hormone; *GI,* gastrointestinal.

• *Potential for overweight* as demonstrated by *energy expenditure below energy intake based on standard assessment* (increased appetite, high caloric content of foods, inactivity)
• *Disrupted body image* resulting from *alteration in self-perception* (change in appearance)
• *Disrupted skin integrity* resulting from *chemical injury agent* (excess corticosteroids)

Additional information on nursing diagnoses for the patient with Cushing's syndrome is presented in NCP 51.3, available on the Evolve website.

PLANNING

The overall goals are that the patient with Cushing's syndrome will (1) experience relief of symptoms, (2) avoid serious complications, (3) maintain a positive self-image, and (4) actively participate in the therapeutic plan.

NURSING IMPLEMENTATION

HEALTH PROMOTION. Health promotion is focused on identifying patients at risk for Cushing's syndrome. Patients receiving long-term, exogenous cortisol for a variety of diseases are at risk. Teaching patients about medication use and monitoring of adverse effects are important preventive measures.

ACUTE INTERVENTION. Patients with Cushing's syndrome are seriously ill. Because the therapeutic interventions produce many adverse medication effects, the focus of daily assessment is on signs and symptoms of hormone and drug toxicity and complicating conditions such as cardiovascular disease, diabetes mellitus, and infection. Nursing assessment should include monitoring of vital signs, daily weighing, and measuring glucose levels. Because signs and symptoms of inflammation such as fever and redness may be minimal or absent, the nurse must assess for pain, loss of function, and purulent drainage as signs of possible infection. The nurse also monitors for signs and symptoms of thromboembolic events (pulmonary emboli) such as sudden chest pain, dyspnea, or tachypnea.

Another important focus of nursing care is emotional support. Changes in appearance such as centripetal obesity, multiple bruises, hirsutism in women, and gynecomastia in men can be distressing. Patients may feel unattractive or unwanted. The nurse can help by remaining sensitive to patients' feelings and offering respect and unconditional acceptance. Patients can be reassured that the physical changes and much of the emotional lability will resolve when hormone levels return to normal.

If treatment involves surgical removal of a pituitary adenoma (in the case of Cushing disease), an adrenal tumour, or one or both adrenal glands, nursing care has an additional focus on preoperative and postoperative care.

Preoperative Care. Before surgery, the patient should be brought to optimal physical condition. Hypertension and hyperglycemia must be controlled, and hypokalemia is corrected with diet and potassium supplements. A high-protein meal plan helps correct the protein depletion. Preoperative teaching depends on the type of surgical approach planned (hypophysectomy or adrenalectomy) but should include information regarding the postoperative care that patients should anticipate. Patients should be told that in the postoperative period (for both open and laparoscopic adrenalectomy) they will probably have a nasogastric tube, urinary catheter, IV therapy, central venous pressure monitoring, and leg sequential compression devices to prevent emboli. Preoperative management for patients undergoing a hypophysectomy is discussed earlier in this chapter.

Postoperative Care. Surgery on the adrenal glands poses risks beyond those of other types of operations. Because the glands are highly vascular, the risk for hemorrhage is increased. Manipulation of glandular tissue during surgery may cause the release of large amounts of hormone into the circulation that produce marked fluctuations in the metabolic processes affected by these hormones. If large amounts of endogenous hormone have been released into the systemic circulation during surgery, hypertension is likely to develop, increasing the risk for hemorrhage. After surgery, BP, fluid balance, and electrolyte levels tend to be unstable because of these hormone fluctuations. Any significant changes in BP, respirations, or heart rate should be reported to the health care provider. Fluid intake and output should be monitored carefully and assessed for potential imbalances. The critical period for circulatory instability ranges from 24 to 48 hours after surgery.

High doses of corticosteroids (e.g., hydrocortisone [Solu-Cortef]), which increase susceptibility to infection and delay wound healing, are administered intravenously during surgery and for several days afterward to ensure adequate responses to the stress of the procedure. The dosage and the rate of flow are adjusted to the patient's clinical manifestations and fluid and electrolyte balances. Oral doses are given as tolerated. The IV may be kept in place after IV corticosteroids are discontinued, to maintain access for quick administration of corticosteroids or vasopressors. Morning urine levels of cortisol (assessed at the same time each morning) are measured to evaluate the effectiveness of the surgery. If the corticosteroid dosage is tapered too rapidly after surgery, acute adrenal insufficiency may develop. Vomiting, increased weakness, dehydration, and hypotension may indicate hypocortisolism. In addition, patients may experience painful joints, pruritus, or peeling skin and may have severe emotional disturbances. These signs and symptoms of corticosteroid imbalance should be reported so that medication doses can be adjusted. After surgery, the patient is usually maintained on bed rest until the BP stabilizes. Because the usual inflammatory responses are suppressed, the nurse must be alert for subtle signs of postoperative infections. The nurse must use meticulous care when changing the dressing and during any other procedures that necessitate access to body cavities, circulation, or areas under the skin, so that infection is prevented. A nursing care plan for patients with Cushing's syndrome (NCP 51.3) is available on the Evolve website for this chapter.

AMBULATORY AND HOME CARE. Discharge instructions are based on the patient's lack of endogenous corticosteroids and resulting inability to react to stressors physiologically. The nurse should consider a referral for a visiting nurse, especially for older persons, because of the need for ongoing evaluation and education. Patients should wear medical alert bracelets at all times and carry medical identification and instructions with them. Exposure to extremes of temperature, infections, and emotional disturbances should be avoided as much as possible. Stress may produce or precipitate acute adrenal insufficiency because the remaining adrenal tissue cannot meet an increased hormonal demand. Many patients can be taught to adjust their corticosteroid replacement therapy in accordance with their stress levels. The nurse should consult with each patient's health care provider to determine the parameters for dosage changes if this plan is feasible. If a patient cannot adjust their own medication or if weakness, fainting, fever, or nausea and vomiting occur, the patient should contact the health care provider for a possible adjustment in corticosteroid dosage. Many patients require lifetime replacement therapy; however, it may take several months to adjust the hormone dose satisfactorily, and patients should be prepared for this.

EVALUATION

The expected outcomes for patients with Cushing's syndrome are as follows:

- No signs or symptoms of infection
- Appropriate weight for height
- Increased acceptance of appearance
- Healing and maintenance of intact skin

ADRENOCORTICAL INSUFFICIENCY

Etiology and Pathophysiology

Adrenal insufficiency most often occurs in adults younger than 60 years and affects both men and women equally. However, the symptoms and signs of adrenocortical insufficiency depend on the rate and extent of adrenal function loss, the degree of stress, and whether mineralocorticoid production is preserved. This hypofunction of the adrenal cortex may have a primary cause (known as *Addison's disease*) or a secondary cause (lack of pituitary ACTH secretion). In Addison's disease, the supply of all three classes of adrenal corticosteroids (glucocorticoids, mineralocorticoids, and androgens) is reduced. In secondary adrenocortical insufficiency, levels of mineralocorticoids are most often normal and levels of corticosteroids and androgens are deficient. ACTH deficiency may be caused by pituitary disease or suppression of the hypothalamic–pituitary–adrenal axis as a result of the administration of exogenous corticosteroids. The onset of adrenocortical insufficiency is gradual and often undetectable unless precipitated by an illness or an adrenal crisis.

The most common cause of Addison's disease in industrialized nations, such as Canada, is autoimmune adrenalitis, commonly associated with increased levels of 21-hydroxylase antibodies that destroy adrenal tissue. Often, other endocrine conditions are present, and Addison's disease is considered a component of polyglandular autoimmune syndrome (Choudhury & Meeran, 2018; Yamamoto, 2018). Addison's disease, if caused by an autoimmune response, is most common in White women (Bornstein et al., 2016). Globally, tuberculosis causes Addison's disease. Other causes include infarction, fungal infections (e.g., histoplasmosis), acquired immune deficiency syndrome (AIDS), and metastatic cancer. Iatrogenic Addison's disease may be caused by adrenal hemorrhage, often related to anticoagulant therapy, antineoplastic chemotherapy, ketoconazole therapy for AIDS, or bilateral adrenalectomy.

Clinical Manifestations

Since manifestations of adrenocortical insufficiency do not usually become evident until 90% of the adrenal cortex is destroyed, the disease is often advanced before it is diagnosed. The manifestations have a very slow (insidious) onset and include progressive weakness, fatigue, weight loss, and anorexia as primary features. Skin hyperpigmentation, a striking feature, is observed primarily in sun-exposed areas of the body, at pressure points, over joints, and in skin creases (Figure 51.12); it is most likely caused by increased secretion of β-lipotropin (which contains melanocyte-stimulating hormone [MSH]). Secretion of this tropic hormone is increased because of decreased negative feedback loops and subsequent low corticosteroid levels. Other frequent manifestations of primary adrenal hypofunction are hypotension, hyponatremia, hyperkalemia, nausea and vomiting, diarrhea, irritability, and depression.

Secondary adrenocortical hypofunction shares many signs and symptoms in common with Addison's disease except hyperpigmentation, given that ACTH and related peptide levels are often low.

Complications

Adrenal crisis (addisonian crisis) refers to acute adrenal insufficiency, a life-threatening emergency caused by insufficient adrenocortical hormones or a sudden sharp decrease in these hormones. Addisonian crisis is triggered by stress (e.g., from infection, surgery, trauma, hemorrhage, or psychological distress); by sudden withdrawal of corticosteroid hormone therapy (which often occurs when a patient who lacks knowledge of the importance of replacement therapy stops following the

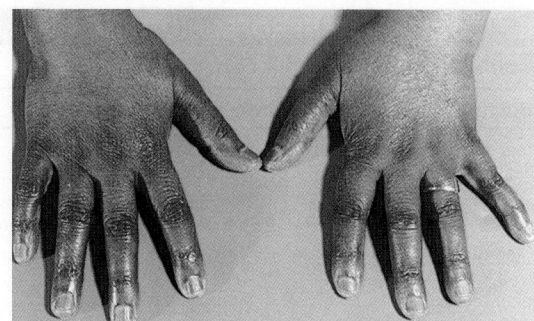

FIG. 51.12 Hyperpigmentation typically observed in Addison's disease. Source: Chew, S. L., & Leslie, D. (2006). *Clinical endocrinology and diabetes: An illustrated colour text.* Churchill Livingstone.

treatment regimen); by adrenal surgery; or by sudden pituitary gland destruction.

During acute adrenal insufficiency, manifestations of glucocorticoid and mineralocorticoid deficiencies are severe and include hypotension (particularly postural), tachycardia, dehydration, hyponatremia, hyperkalemia, hypoglycemia, fever, weakness, and confusion. Hypotension may lead to shock and circulatory collage, often unresponsive to vasopressors and fluid replacement. GI manifestations include nausea, vomiting, diarrhea, and pain in the abdomen, lower back, or the legs.

Diagnostic Studies

In addition to clinical features, cortisol levels that are subnormal or fail to rise over basal levels with an ACTH stimulation test can be diagnostic for Addison's disease. A failure of cortisol levels to rise in response to ACTH stimulation indicates primary adrenal disease. A positive response to ACTH stimulation indicates that the adrenal gland is functioning and that the probable cause is pituitary disease (see Chapter 50).

Other abnormal laboratory findings include hyperkalemia, hypochloremia, hyponatremia, hypoglycemia, anemia, and increased blood urea nitrogen levels. Urine levels of free cortisol are low, as is the urine level of aldosterone (Bornstein et al., 2016). An electrocardiogram (ECG) may show low voltage and a vertical QRS axis. In addition, peaked T-waves caused by hyperkalemia may be evident. CT and MRI are used to localize tumours or identify adrenal calcifications or enlargement (Table 51.17).

Interprofessional Care

Treatment of adrenocortical insufficiency is focused on management of the underlying cause, when possible. The mainstay of treatment for adrenocortical insufficiency is replacement therapy (see Table 51.17). Hydrocortisone, the most commonly used form of replacement therapy, has both glucocorticoid and mineralocorticoid properties. During situations associated with physiological stress, glucocorticoid dosage must be increased to prevent addisonian crisis. Mineralocorticoid replacement with fludrocortisone acetate is administered daily, along with increased salt in the diet.

Addisonian crisis is a life-threatening emergency requiring aggressive management. Treatment must be directed toward shock management and high-dose hydrocortisone replacement. Large volumes of 0.9% saline solution and 5% dextrose are administered to reverse hypotension and electrolyte imbalances until the BP returns to normal.

TABLE 51.17	**INTERPROFESSIONAL CARE**

Addison's Disease

Diagnostic	Interprofessional Therapy
• History and physical examination • ACTH stimulation test • CT, MRI • Measurement of plasma cortisol levels • Measurement of serum electrolytes • Measurement of urine cortisol and aldosterone levels	• Daily glucocorticoid (e.g., hydrocortisone) replacement (two thirds on awakening in morning, one third in late afternoon)* • Daily mineralocorticoid (fludrocortisone acetate) replacement in morning* • Increased dose of cortisol for stress situations (e.g., surgery, hospitalization) • Salt additives for excess heat or humidity

ACTH, adrenocorticotrophic hormone; *CT,* computed tomographic (scan); *MRI,* magnetic resonance imaging.
*For conditions of normal daily stress, in individuals with usual daytime activity.

NURSING MANAGEMENT
ADDISON'S DISEASE

NURSING IMPLEMENTATION

ACUTE INTERVENTION. When the patient with Addison's disease is hospitalized—whether for diagnosis, an acute crisis, or some other health problem—treatment should not be delayed while diagnostic tests such as serum cortisol, corticotropin (ACTH), aldosterone, renin, and serum chemistry are performed. Patients in an adrenal crisis should have an immediate administration of IV hydrocortisone. For IV therapy, 1 to 3 litres of 0.9% normal saline (NS) or 5% dextrose in 0.9% NS should be started to correct possible hypoglycemia, fluid volume deficit, and trends in sodium and potassium electrolyte imbalance within the first 12 to 24 hours, based on volume status, lab value analysis, and urinary output. Use of hypotonic IV 0.45% NS should be avoided because it can worsen the hyponatremia. In chronic adrenal insufficiency, nursing management focuses on adherence to prescribed glucocorticoid regimens and on maintaining fluid and electrolyte balance through regular assessments of mental status, vital signs, weight, and signs and symptoms of fluid volume deficit and electrolyte imbalance in serum glucose, sodium, and potassium. A complete medication history is obtained to determine medications that can potentially interact with corticosteroids. These medications include oral hypoglycemics, cardiac glycosides, oral contraceptives, anticoagulants, and NSAIDs.

Changes are noted in BP, weight gain, weakness, or other manifestations of Cushing's syndrome. In addition, the patient must be protected against exposure to infection and assisted with daily hygiene. The patient must also be protected from noise, light, and environmental temperature extremes—the patient cannot cope with these stresses because of the inability to produce corticosteroids.

The patient who is hospitalized because of adrenal crisis usually responds by the second day and can start oral corticosteroid replacement. The patient must be instructed about the importance of keeping scheduled follow-up appointments.

AMBULATORY AND HOME CARE. The nurse has an important role in the long-term management of Addison's disease. The serious nature of the disease and the need for lifelong replacement therapy necessitate a well-organized and carefully

TABLE 51.18	**PATIENT & CAREGIVER TEACHING GUIDE**

Addison's Disease

The following information should be included when teaching the patient and caregiver about management of Addison's disease:
1. Names, dosages, and actions of medications
2. Symptoms of overdosage and underdosage
3. Conditions necessitating increased medication (e.g., trauma, infection, surgery, emotional crisis)
4. Course of action to take in regard to changes in medication
   • Increase in dose of corticosteroid
   • Administration of large dose of corticosteroid intramuscularly, including demonstration and return demonstration
   • Consultation with health care provider
5. Prevention of infection and need for prompt and vigorous treatment of existing infections
6. Need for lifelong replacement therapy
7. Need for lifelong medical supervision
8. Need for medical identification device
9. Prevention of falls
10. Adverse effects of corticosteroid therapy and prevention techniques
11. Special instruction for patients who are diabetic, and management of blood glucose when taking corticosteroids

presented teaching plan. Table 51.18 outlines the major areas that must be included in the teaching plan.

Glucocorticoids are usually given in divided doses—two thirds in the morning and one third in the afternoon. Mineralocorticoids are given once daily, preferably in the morning. This dosage schedule reflects normal circadian rhythm in endogenous hormone secretion and decreases the intensity of adverse effects associated with corticosteroid replacement therapy. Because the aim of replacement therapy is to return hormone levels to normal, nursing care is designed to help patients maintain hormone balance and manage the medication regimen.

Because the patient with Addison's disease is unable to tolerate physical or emotional stress without additional exogenous corticosteroids, long-term care revolves around recognizing the need for extra medication and techniques for stress management. The need for corticosteroid hormone is proportional to stress levels. A patient who cannot produce endogenous hormone must adjust the dose of exogenous hormone to the stress level. Examples of situations requiring corticosteroid adjustment are fever, influenza, extraction of teeth, and rigorous physical activity, such as playing tennis on a hot day or running a marathon. Doses are usually doubled in situations of minor stress (e.g., a respiratory infection, dental work) and tripled in situations of major stress (e.g., divorce, loss of parent). When the stress level is in doubt, it is better to err on the side of over-replacement. If vomiting or diarrhea occurs, as may happen with influenza, the health care provider must be notified immediately because electrolyte replacement may be necessary. In addition, these manifestations may be early indicators of crisis. Overall, patients who take their medications consistently can anticipate a normal life expectancy.

The patient must be taught the signs and symptoms of corticosteroid deficiency and excess and to report these signs to the health care provider so that the dosage can be adjusted to the patient's needs. It is critical that patients wear a medical alert bracelet and carry a wallet card stating that they have Addison's disease so that appropriate therapy can be initiated in case of an unexpected stressful event. The patient should be instructed in

TABLE 51.19 **MEDICATION THERAPY**

Diseases and Disorders Treated With Corticosteroids

Hormone Replacement	Endocrine Diseases
• Adrenal insufficiency • Congenital adrenal hyperplasia	• Hashimoto's thyroiditis • Hypercalcemia • Thyrotoxic crisis (thyroid storm)
Therapeutic Effect **Allergic Reactions** • Anaphylaxis • Bee stings • Contact dermatitis • Medication reactions • Serum sickness • Urticaria	**Liver Diseases** • Alcohol-related hepatitis • Autoimmune hepatitis **Neurological Diseases** • Head trauma • Prevention of cerebral edema and increase in intracranial pressure
Collagen Diseases • Giant cell arteritis • Mixed connective tissue disorders • Polymyositis • Polyarteritis nodosa • Rheumatoid arthritis • Systemic lupus erythematosus	**Pulmonary Diseases** • Aspiration pneumonia • Asthma • Chronic obstructive pulmonary disease **Other Diseases and Disorders** • Immunosuppression • Inflammation • Malignancies, leukemia, lymphoma
Gastrointestinal Diseases • Celiac disease • Inflammatory bowel disease	• Nephrotic syndrome • Skin diseases

TABLE 51.20 **MEDICATION THERAPY**

Effects and Adverse Effects of Corticosteroids

- BP increases because of excess blood volume and potentiation of vasoconstrictor effects. Hypertension predisposes to heart failure.
- Fat from extremities is redistributed to trunk and face.
- Glucose intolerance predisposes to diabetes mellitus.
- Healing is delayed, and patient is at increased risk for wound dehiscence.
- Hypocalcemia related to anti–vitamin D effect may occur.
- Hypokalemia may develop.
- Manifestations of inflammation, including redness, tenderness, heat, swelling, and local edema, are suppressed.
- Mood and behaviour changes may be observed.
- Patient is predisposed to peptic ulcer disease.
- Protein depletion decreases bone formation, density, and strength; patient is thus predisposed to pathological fractures, especially compression fractures of the vertebrae (osteoporosis).
- Skeletal muscle atrophy and weakness occur.
- Suppression of pituitary ACTH synthesis occurs. Corticosteroid deficiency is likely if hormone treatment is withdrawn abruptly. Corticosteroid doses should be tapered.
- Susceptibility to infection is increased. Infection develops more rapidly and spreads more widely.

ACTH, adrenocorticotrophic hormone; *BP,* blood pressure.

and given handouts related to other medications that cause a need to increase glucocorticoid dosage (e.g., phenytoin [Dilantin], barbiturates, rifampin [Rifadin], and antacids). Estrogen inhibits steroid metabolism. The nurse should instruct patients receiving mineralocorticoid therapy (fludrocortisone acetate) (a) on how to measure their BP, (b) to increase salt intake, and (c) to report significant changes to their health care provider. Changes may indicate a need for dosage adjustment.

Patients should carry an emergency kit at all times. The kit should consist of 100 mg of IM hydrocortisone, syringes, and instructions for use. The patient and family should be instructed in how to administer an IM injection in case the replacement therapy cannot be taken orally. Patients should confirm understanding of instructions, practise administering IM injections with saline, and receive written instructions about when to alter the dose (Bornstein et al., 2016).

CORTICOSTEROID THERAPY

Corticosteroids are used to relieve the signs and symptoms associated with many diseases (Table 51.19). The long-term administration of corticosteroids in therapeutic dosages often leads to serious complications and adverse effects (Table 51.20). For this reason, corticosteroid therapy is not recommended for minor chronic conditions. Therapy should be reserved for diseases in which there is a risk for death or permanent loss of function and conditions in which short-term therapy is likely to produce remission or recovery. The potential benefits of treatment must always be weighed against the risks.

Effects of Corticosteroid Therapy

Corticosteroid therapy has multiple effects. Although these actions can prove to be beneficial and therapeutic in some situations, they can contribute to adverse effects as well.

The expected effects of corticosteroid therapy include the following:

1. *Anti-inflammatory action.* Corticosteroids decrease the number of circulating lymphocytes, monocytes, and eosinophils. They enhance the release of polymorphonuclear leukocytes from bone marrow, inhibit the accumulation of leukocytes at the site of inflammation, and inhibit the release of substances involved in the inflammatory response (e.g., kinins, prostaglandins, histamine) from the leukocytes. As a result, manifestations of inflammation, including redness, tenderness, heat, swelling, and local edema, are suppressed.
2. *Immunosuppression.* Corticosteroids cause atrophy of lymphoid tissue, suppress the cell-mediated immune responses, and decrease the production of antibodies.
3. *Maintenance of normal BP.* Corticosteroids potentiate the vasoconstrictor effect of norepinephrine and act on the renal tubules to increase sodium reabsorption and enhance potassium and hydrogen excretion. Retention of sodium (and subsequently water) increases blood volume and helps maintain BP. Mineralocorticoids have a direct effect on sodium reabsorption in the distal tubules of the kidneys; as a result, sodium retention and water retention are increased.
4. *Carbohydrate and protein metabolism.* Corticosteroids antagonize the effects of insulin and can induce glucose intolerance by increasing hepatic glycogenolysis and insulin resistance. They also stimulate the breakdown of protein for gluconeogenesis, which can lead to skeletal muscle wasting. Although corticosteroids mobilize free fatty acids and cause redistribution of fat in Cushingoid patterns, the mechanism underlying this process is unknown.

Complications Associated With Corticosteroid Therapy

A beneficial effect in one situation may be a harmful one in another. For example, the vasopressive effect of a hormone is critical in enabling the organism to function in stressful situations, but it can produce hypertension when used for medication therapy. Suppression of inflammation and the immune response may help save the life of someone experiencing anaphylaxis or receiving a transplant, but it causes reactivation of latent tuberculosis and greatly reduces resistance to other infections and cancers. In addition, corticosteroids inhibit the antibody response to vaccines.

MEDICATION ALERT—Corticosteroids
The nurse should do the following:
• Instruct patients not to discontinue therapy abruptly.
• Monitor patients for signs of infection.
• Instruct patients with diabetes to closely monitor blood glucose levels.

NURSING AND INTERPROFESSIONAL MANAGEMENT
CORTICOSTEROID THERAPY

Many patients receive corticosteroid therapy, particularly glucocorticoid therapy, for nonendocrine reasons (see Table 51.19). Thorough instruction is necessary to ensure patient adherence to the regimen. When corticosteroids are used as nonreplacement therapy, they are taken once daily or once every other day. They should be taken early in the morning with food to decrease gastric irritation. Because exogenous corticosteroid administration may suppress endogenous ACTH and therefore endogenous cortisol (suppression is time and dose dependent), the danger of abrupt cessation of corticosteroid therapy must be emphasized to patients and their families. When taken for longer than 1 week, corticosteroids suppress adrenal production, and oral steroids should be tapered. In acute care or home care situations, nurses must ensure that increased doses of steroid are prescribed with increased physical or emotional stress.

Because patients often receive corticosteroid treatment for prolonged periods (>3 months), corticosteroid-induced osteoporosis is an important concern (Bornstein et al., 2016). Therapies to reduce the resorption of bone may include increased calcium intake, vitamin D supplementation, administration of bisphosphonates (e.g., alendronate [Fosamax]), and institution of a low-impact exercise program. Further instruction and interventions to minimize the adverse effects and complications of corticosteroid therapy are listed in Table 51.21.

HYPERALDOSTERONISM

Etiology and Pathophysiology

Hyperaldosteronism is characterized by excessive aldosterone secretion. The main effects of aldosterone are retention of sodium and excretion of potassium and hydrogen ion. Thus the hallmark of this disease is hypertension with hypokalemic alkalosis. *Primary hyperaldosteronism* (PA) is most commonly caused by a small, solitary adrenocortical adenoma. On occasion, multiple lesions are involved and are associated with bilateral adrenal hyperplasia. PA affects both sexes equally and occurs most frequently between the ages of 30 and 50 years. It is estimated that approximately 1% of cases of hypertension are caused by PA. *Secondary hyperaldosteronism* occurs in response to a nonadrenal cause of elevated aldosterone levels, such as renal artery stenosis, renin-secreting tumours, or chronic renal disease.

Clinical Manifestations

Elevations in aldosterone levels are associated with retention of sodium and elimination of potassium. Sodium retention

TABLE 51.21	PATIENT & CAREGIVER TEACHING GUIDE

Corticosteroid Therapy

The following instructions should be included when teaching the patient and caregiver about management of corticosteroid therapy.
1. Plan a diet high in protein, calcium, and potassium but low in fat and concentrated simple carbohydrates such as sugar, honey, syrups, and candy.
2. Identify measures to ensure adequate rest and sleep, such as daily naps and avoidance of caffeine late in the day.
3. Develop and maintain an exercise program to help maintain bone integrity.
4. Recognize edema and ways to restrict sodium intake to less than 2 000 mg/day if edema occurs.
5. Monitor glucose levels and recognize symptoms and signs of hyperglycemia (e.g., polydipsia, polyuria, blurred vision) and glycosuria (glucose in the urine). Patients should be instructed to report hyperglycemic symptoms or capillary glucose levels higher than 10 mmol/L or urine findings that are positive for glucose.
6. Notify the health care provider if the patient is experiencing post-prandial heartburn or epigastric pain that is not relieved by antacids.
7. See an eye specialist yearly to assess possible development of cataracts.
8. Use safety measures such as getting up slowly from a bed or a chair, and use good lighting to prevent accidental injury.
9. Maintain good hygiene practices and avoid contact with people with colds or other contagious illnesses to prevent infection.
10. Inform all health care providers about long-term corticosteroid use.
11. Realize that doses of corticosteroids may need to be increased in times of physical and emotional stress.
12. Never abruptly stop taking the corticosteroids because this could lead to addisonian crisis and possibly death.

leads to hypernatremia, hypertension, and headache. Edema does not usually occur because the rate of sodium excretion increases, which prevents more severe sodium retention. The potassium wasting leads to hypokalemia, which causes generalized muscle weakness, fatigue, cardiac dysrhythmias, glucose intolerance, and metabolic alkalosis that may lead to tetany.

Diagnostic Studies

The diagnosis of hyperaldosteronism should be suspected in all hypertensive patients with hypokalemia who are not being treated with diuretics. PA is associated with elevations in plasma aldosterone levels and decreased plasma renin activity, elevated sodium levels, and decreased serum potassium levels. Adenomas are localized by means of CT or MRI. If a tumour is not found, plasma 18-hydroxycorticosterone is measured after overnight bed rest. A level higher than 1.38 nmol/L indicates the presence of an adenoma.

NURSING AND INTERPROFESSIONAL MANAGEMENT
PRIMARY HYPERALDOSTERONISM

The preferred treatment for PA is surgical removal of the adrenal gland that has the adenoma (*adrenalectomy*). A laparoscopic approach is most often used. Before surgery, patients should be treated with a low-sodium diet, potassium-sparing diuretics (spironolactone [Aldactone] or eplerenone [Inspra]), and antihypertensive agents to normalize serum potassium levels and BP. Spironolactone and eplerenone block the binding of aldosterone to the mineralocorticoid receptor in the terminal distal tubules and collecting ducts of the kidneys, thus increasing the excretion of sodium and water and the retention of potassium. Oral potassium supplements and sodium restrictions may also be necessary. Potassium supplementation and a potassium-sparing diuretic should not be started simultaneously because of the danger of hyperkalemia. Patients taking eplerenone should be instructed to avoid drinking grapefruit juice.

Patients with bilateral adrenal hyperplasia are treated with a potassium-sparing diuretic. Calcium channel blockers may also be used to control BP. Dexamethasone may be used to decrease the hyperplasia.

Nursing care includes careful assessment for signs of fluid and electrolyte imbalance (especially potassium imbalance) and monitoring of cardiovascular status. BP should be monitored frequently before and after surgery because unilateral adrenalectomy is successful in controlling hypertension in only 80% of patients with adenoma. Patients receiving maintenance therapy with spironolactone need instruction about the possible adverse effects (gynecomastia, erectile dysfunction, and menstrual disorders), as well as knowledge about the signs and symptoms of hypokalemia and hyperkalemia. Patients should be taught how to monitor their own BP and the need for frequent monitoring. The need for continued health care supervision should be stressed.

DISORDERS OF THE ADRENAL MEDULLA

PHEOCHROMOCYTOMA

Etiology and Pathophysiology

Pheochromocytoma is a rare condition characterized by a tumour of the adrenal medulla that arises from the chromaffin cells and produces excessive amounts of catecholamines (epinephrine, norepinephrine). The secretion of excessive catecholamines results in severe hypertension (Gruber et al., 2019). If left untreated, it may lead to hypertensive encephalopathy, diabetes mellitus, cardiomyopathy, and death. It is most commonly seen in young to middle-aged adults.

Clinical Manifestations

The most striking clinical features of pheochromocytoma include severe, episodic hypertension accompanied by the classic manifestations of severe, pounding headache; tachycardia with palpitations; profuse sweating; and unexplained abdominal or chest pain, lasting a few minutes to several hours. Such "attacks" may be provoked by many medications, including antihypertensives, opioids, radiological contrast media, and tricyclic antidepressants.

Diagnostic Studies

Pheochromocytoma is an uncommon cause of hypertension, accounting for only 0.1% of all cases. This condition should be considered in patients who do not respond to traditional hypertensive treatments.

The simplest and most reliable diagnostic test for pheochromocytoma is measurement of urinary fractionated metanephrines (catecholamine metabolites) and fractionated catecholamines and creatinine, usually done as a 24-hour urine collection. Serum catecholamines may be elevated during an "attack." CT scans and MRI are used for diagnosing tumours. Health care providers should avoid palpating the abdomen of a patient with suspected pheochromocytoma, since it may cause the sudden release of catecholamines and severe hypertension.

NURSING AND INTERPROFESSIONAL MANAGEMENT PHEOCHROMOCYTOMA

The primary treatment for pheochromocytoma consists of surgical removal of the tumour. Treatment with α- and β-adrenergic receptor blockers is required preoperatively to control BP and prevent an intraoperative hypertensive crisis. The α-adrenergic receptor blocker prazosin (Minipress) is given up to 2 weeks preoperatively to reduce BP and alleviate other symptoms of catecholamine excess, and calcium channel blockers may be administered (Kumar et al., 2020). After adequate α-adrenergic blockade, β-adrenergic receptor blockers (e.g., propranolol) are used to decrease tachycardia and other dysrhythmias. If β blockers are started too early, unopposed α-adrenergic stimulation could precipitate a hypertensive crisis. Sympathetic blocking agents may result in orthostatic hypotension. Patients must be advised to make postural changes with caution.

Surgery is more commonly performed via laparoscopic adrenalectomy than via open abdominal incision. Complete removal of the adrenal tumour cures the hypertension in the majority of affected individuals, but hypertension persists in approximately 10 to 30% of patients. For these individuals, BP management involves standard antihypertensive medication therapy. If surgery is not an option, medication is used to diminish catecholamine production by the tumour and simplify chronic management.

Identification of patients with pheochromocytoma is an important nursing function. Any patient with hypertension accompanied by symptoms of sympathoadrenal discharge should be referred to a health care provider for definitive diagnosis. An important part of the nursing assessment is observation of patients for the classic triad of symptoms of pheochromocytoma—severe, pounding headache; tachycardia; and profuse sweating. BP should be monitored immediately if a patient is experiencing an attack. The nurse should be prepared to check BP when any of the medications that might precipitate an attack are administered.

All diagnostic samples should be collected appropriately. Capillary blood glucose levels should be monitored to assess for diabetes mellitus. Patients need rest, nourishing food, and emotional support during this period.

Preoperative and postoperative care is similar to that for any patient undergoing adrenalectomy, except that BP fluctuations from catecholamine excesses tend to be severe and must be carefully monitored. Because hypertension may persist even when the tumour is removed, the nurse should stress the importance of follow-up care and routine BP monitoring. Patients taking catecholamine synthesis inhibitors should be instructed to rise slowly while holding on to a secure object because this medication can cause orthostatic hypotension.

CASE STUDY

Graves' Disease

Patient Profile

R. D. (pronouns she/her), 47 years old, was admitted to the hospital with a high fever. After an endocrine workup, she received a diagnosis of Graves' disease.

Subjective Data

- Reports recent job loss because of inability to cope with job stress
- Reports symptoms including fatigue, unintentional weight loss, insomnia, palpitations, and heat intolerance

Objective Data
Physical Examination

- Fever of 40°C
- BP of 150/78, pulse of 118, and respiratory rate of 24
- Hot, moist skin
- Fine tremors of the hands
- Grade 4+ deep tendon reflexes and muscle strength of grades 1 to 2

Interprofessional Care

- Subtotal thyroidectomy planned for 2 months later
- Started on propylthiouracil and propranolol (Inderal)

Discussion Questions

1. What is the cause of R. D.'s symptoms? What pathophysiological mechanisms explain the symptoms?
2. What diagnostic studies were probably ordered? What lab and diagnostic test results would the nurse expect to see in order to establish the diagnosis of Graves' disease?
3. Why was surgery delayed?
4. What was the purpose of medication therapy for R. D.?
5. *Priority decision:* What are R. D.'s priority learning needs? What teaching strategies would the nurse use if the patient was not able to read?
6. What are the nursing interventions for successful long-term management of R. D. after the subtotal thyroidectomy?
7. *Priority decision:* On the basis of the assessment data presented, what are the priority nursing diagnoses pertinent to R. D. while being hospitalized? Are there any interprofessional issues?
8. *Evidence-informed practice:* Why is R. D. counselled to give up the habit of long-standing cigarette smoking?

ⓔvolve

Answers are available at http://evolve.elsevier.com/Canada/Lewis/medsurg.

REVIEW QUESTIONS

The number of the question corresponds to the same-numbered objective at the beginning of the chapter.

1. After a hypophysectomy for acromegaly, which of the following should be the focus of postoperative nursing care?
   a. Frequent monitoring of serum and urine osmolality
   b. Parenteral administration of a GH-receptor antagonist
   c. Keeping the client in a recumbent position at all times
   d. Client teaching regarding the need for lifelong hormone therapy

2. A client with a head injury develops SIADH. Which of the following manifestations of SIADH would the nurse expect to find?
   a. Hypernatremia and edema
   b. Muscle spasticity and hypertension
   c. Low urine output and hyponatremia
   d. Weight gain and decreased glomerular filtration rate (GFR)

3. The health care provider prescribes levothyroxine (Synthroid) for a client with myxedema. After teaching regarding this medication, the nurse determines that further instruction is needed when the client says which of the following?
   a. "I can expect the medication dose may need to be adjusted."
   b. "I only need to take this medication until my symptoms are improved."
   c. "I can expect to return to normal function with the use of this medication."
   d. "I will report any chest pain or difficulty breathing to the doctor right away."

4. Which of the following symptoms would lead the nurse to suspect damage or removal of the parathyroid glands after thyroid surgery?
   a. Muscle weakness and weight loss
   b. Hyperthermia and severe tachycardia
   c. Hypertension and difficulty swallowing
   d. Laryngospasms and tingling in the hands and feet

5. Which of the following are important nursing intervention(s) when caring for a client with Cushing's syndrome? *(Select all that apply.)*
   a. Restricting protein intake
   b. Monitoring blood glucose levels
   c. Observing for signs of hypotension
   d. Administering medication in equal doses
   e. Protecting the client from exposure to infection

6. Which of the following is an important preoperative nursing intervention before an adrenalectomy for hyperaldosteronism?
   a. Monitor blood glucose levels.
   b. Restrict fluid and sodium intake.
   c. Administer potassium-sparing diuretics.
   d. Advise the client to make postural changes slowly.

7. How does the nurse instruct the client who is taking corticosteroids to control the adverse effects of medication therapy?
   a. Increase calcium intake to 1 500 mg/day.
   b. Perform glucose monitoring for hypoglycemia.
   c. Obtain immunizations due to high risk for infections.
   d. Avoid abrupt position changes because of the risk for orthostatic hypotension.

8. What does the nurse teach the client regarding the best time to take corticosteroids for replacement purposes?
   a. Once a day at bedtime
   b. Every other day on awakening
   c. On arising and in the late afternoon
   d. At consistent intervals every 6 to 8 hours

1. a; 2. c; 3. b; 4. d; 5. b, e; 6. c; 7. a; 8. c.

ⓔvolve

For even more review questions, visit http://evolve.elsevier.com/Canada/Lewis/medsurg.

REFERENCES

Abreu, I., Lau, E., de Sousa Pinto, B., et al. (2017). Subclinical hypothyroidism: To treat or not to treat, that is the question! A systemic review with meta-analysis on lipid profile. *Endocrine Connections*, 6(3), 188–199. https://doi.org/10.1530/EC-17-0028

AlDallal, S. (2018). Acromegaly: A challenging condition to diagnose. *International Journal of General Medicine*, 11, 337–343. https://doi.org/10.2147/IJGM.S169611

Bockenhauer, D., & Bichet, D. (2015). Pathophysiology, diagnosis and management of nephrogenic diabetes insipidus. *Nature Reviews Nephrology*, 11(10), 576–588. https://doi.org/10.1038/nrneph.2015.89

Bornstein, S., Allolio, B., Arlt, W., et al. (2016). Diagnosis and treatment of primary adrenal insufficiency: An endocrine society clinical practice guideline. *The Journal of Clinical Endocrinology & Metabolism*, 101(2), 364–389. https://doi.org/10.1210/jc.2015-1710

Canadian Cancer Statistics Advisory Committee. (2019). *Canadian cancer statistics 2019*. Canadian Cancer Society. https://cdn.cancer.ca/-/media/files/research/cancer-statistics/2019-statistics/canadian-cancer-statistics-2019-en.pdf

Caron-Beaudoin, E., Avotte, P., Sidi, E., et al. (2019). Exposure to perfluoroalkyl substances (PFAS) and associations with thyroid parameters in First Nation children and youth from Quebec. *Environment International*, 128, 13–23. https://doi.org/10.1016/j.envint.2019.04.029

Choudhury, S., & Meeran, K. (2018). Glucocorticoid replacement in Addison disease. *Nature Reviews Endocrinology*, 14(9), 562. https://doi.org/10.1038/s41574-018-0049-6

Dalugama, C. (2018). Asymptomatic thyroiditis presenting as pyrexia of unknown origin: A case report. *Journal of Medicine Case Reports*, 12(1), 15. https://doi.org/10.1186/s13256-018-1590-6

Ferrau, F., Albani, A., Ciresi, A., et al. (2018). Diabetes secondary to acromegaly: Physiopathology, clinical features and effects of treatment. *Frontiers in Endocrinology*, 9, 358. https://doi.org/10.3389/fendo.2018.00358

Frara, S., Maffezzoni, F., Mazziotti, G., et al. (2016). Current and emerging aspects of diabetes mellitus in acromegaly. *Trends in Endocrinology and Metabolism*, 27(7), 470–483. https://doi.org/10.1016/j.tem.2016.04.014

Gordon, M., Nakhle, S., & Ludlam, W. (2016). Patients with acromegaly presenting with colon cancer: A case series. *Case Reports in Endocrinology*, 2016(1), 1–4. https://doi.org/10.1155/2016/5156295

Gruber, L., Hartman, R., Thompson, G., et al. (2019). Pheochromocytoma characteristics and behavior differ depending on method of discovery. *The Journal of Clinical Endocrinology & Metabolism*, 104(5), 1386–1393. https://doi.org/10.1210/jc.2018-01707

Haugen, B., Alexander, E., Bible, K., et al. (2016). 2015 American Thyroid Association management guidelines for adult patients with thyroid nodules and differentiated thyroid cancer: The American Thyroid Association Guidelines Task Force on Thyroid Nodules and Differentiated Thyroid Cancer. *Thyroid*, 26(1), 1–133. https://doi.org/10.1089/thy.2015.0020

Jacobson, M., Howards, P., Darrow, L., et al. (2018). Thyroid hormones and menstrual cycle function in a longitudinal cohort of premenopausal women. *Pediatric and Perinatal Epidemiology*, 32(3), 225–234. https://doi.org/10.1111/ppe.12462

Jones, D. (2018). Syndrome of inappropriate secretion of antidiuretic hormone and hyponatremia. *Pediatrics in Review*, 39(1), 27–35. https://doi.org/10.1542/pir.2016-0165

Katznelson, L., Laws, E. R., Jr., Melmed, S., et al. (2014). Acromegaly: An Endocrine Society clinical practice guideline. *Journal of Clinical Endocrinology & Metabolism*, 99(11), 3933–3951. https://doi.org/10.1210/jc.2014-2700

Kumar, A., Gupta, N., & Gupta, A. (2020). Urapidil in the preoperative treatment of pheochromocytoma: How safe is it? *Journal of Anaesthesiology, Clinical Pharmacology*, 36(1), 55–56. https://doi.org/10.4103/joacp.JOACP_328_18

Loner, R., Nieman, L., & Oldfield, E. (2017). Cushing's disease: Pathobiology, diagnosis and management. *Journal of Neurosurgery*, 126(2), 404–417. https://doi.org/10.3171/2016.1.JNS152119

Lopes, M., Kliemann, B., Bini, I., et al. (2016). Hypoparathyroidism and pseudohypoparathyroidism: Etiology, laboratory features, and complications. *Archives of Endocrinology*, 60(6), 532–536. https://doi.org/10.1590/2359-3997000000221

Marx, S. (2018). Recent topics around multiple endocrine neoplasia type 1. *The Journal of Clinical Endocrinology & Metabolism*, 103(4), 1296–1301. https://doi.org/10.1210/jc.2017-02340

Matyjaszek-Matuszek, B., Obel, E., Lewicki, M., et al. (2018). Prevalence of neoplasms in patients with acromegaly-the need for a national registry. *Annals of Agricultural and Environmental Medicine*, 25(3), 559–561. https://doi.org/10.26444/aaem/85652

Mutnuri, S., Fernandez, I., & Kochar, T. (2016). Suppression of parathyroid hormone in a patient with severe magnesium depletion. *Case Reports Nephrology*. Article 2608538. https://doi.org/10.1155/2016/2608538

Nieman, L. (2018). Recent updates on the diagnosis and management of Cushing's syndrome. *Endocrinology & Metabolism*, 33(2), 139–146. https://doi.org/10.3803/EnM.2018.33.2.139

Ono, Y., Ono, S., Yasunaga, H., et al. (2017). Clinical characteristics and outcomes of myxedema: Analysis of a national inpatient database in Japan. *Journal of Epidemiology*, 27(3), 117–122. https://doi.org/10.1016/j.je.2016.04.002

Peri, A., Grohe, C., Berardi, R., et al. (2017). SIADH: Differential diagnosis and clinical management. *Endocrine*, 55(1), 311–319. https://doi.org/10.1007/s12020-016-0936-3

Prete, A., Corsello, S., & Salvatori, R. (2017). Current best practice in the management of patients after pituitary surgery. *Therapeutic Advances in Endocrinology and Metabolism*, 8(3), 33–48. https://doi.org/10.1177/2042018816687240

Ramos-Levi, A. M., & Marazuela, M. (2019). Bringing cardiovascular comorbidities in acromegaly to an update. How should we diagnose and manage them? *Frontiers in Endocrinology*, 10, 120. https://doi.org/10.3389/fendo.2019.00120

Ross, D., Burch, H., Cooper, D., et al. (2016). 2016 American Thyroid Association guidelines for the diagnosis and management of hyperthyroidism and other causes of thyrotoxicosis. *Thyroid*, 26(10), 1343–1421. https://doi.org/10.1089/thy.2016.0229

Rothberger, G., Gadhvi, S., Michelakis, N., et al. (2017). Non thyroidal illness syndrome. In M. McDermott (Ed.), *Management of patients with pseudo-endocrine disorders: A case-based pocket guide* (pp. 331–340). Springer.

Sadeghi-Tari, A., Jamshidian-Tehrani, M., Nabavi, A., et al. (2016). Effect of smoking on retrobulbar blood flow in thyroid eye disease. *Eye*, 30, 1573–1578. https://doi.org/10.1038/eye.2016.184

Sesmilo, G., Gaztambide, S., Venegas, E., et al. (2013). Changes in acromegaly treatment over four decades in Spain: Analysis of the Spanish Acromegaly Registry (REA). *Pituitary*, 16(1), 115–121. https://doi.org/10.1007/s11102-012-0384-x

Sesmilo, G., Resmini, E., Sambo, M., et al. (2017). Prevalence of acromegaly in patients with symptoms of sleep apnea. *PLOS One*, 12(9), e0183539. https://doi.org/10.1371/journal.pone.018539

Silveira, M., Seguro, A., da Silva, J., et al. (2018). Chronic hyponatremia due to the syndrome of inappropriate antidiuresis (SIAD)

in adult women with corpus callosum agenesis. *American Journal of Case Reports, 19*, 1345–1349. https://doi.org/10.12659/AJCR.911810

Stott, D., Rodondi, N., Kearney, P., et al. (2017). Thyroid hormone therapy for older adults with subclinical hypothyroidism. *New England Journal of Medicine, 376*(26), 2534–2544. https://doi.org/10.1056/NEJMoa1603825

Strasburger, C. J., Mattsson, A., Wilton, P., et al. (2018). Increasing frequency of combination medical therapy in the treatment of acromegaly with the GH receptor antagonist pegvisomant. *European Journal of Endocrinology, 178*(4), 321–329. doi:10.1530/EJE-17-0996.

Taylor, P. N., Albrecht, D., Scholz, A., et al. (2018). Global epidemiology of hyperthyroidism and hypothyroidism. *Nature Reviews Endocrinology, 14*(5), 301–316. doi:130.1038/nrendo.2018.18.

Thyroid Foundation of Canada. (2016). *Resource material: Information on thyroid disease.* https://thyroid.ca/resource-material/information-on-thyroid-disease/

Walker, M., & Silverberg, S. (2018). Primary hyperparathyroidism. *Nature Reviews Endocrinology, 14*(2), 115–125. https://doi.org/10.1038/nrendo.2017.104

Wilhelm, S., Wang, T., Ruan, D., et al. (2016). The American Association of Endocrine Surgeons guidelines for definitive management of primary hyperparathyroidism. *JAMA Surgical, 151*(10), 959–968. https://doi.org/10.1001/jamasurg.2016.2310

Yafit, D., Carmel-Neiderman, N. N., Levy, N., et al. (2019). Postoperative myxedema coma in patients undergoing major surgery: Case series. *Auris, Nasis, Larynx, 46*(4), 605–608. https://doi.org/10.1016/j.anl.2018.10.019

Yamamoto, T. (2018). Latent adrenal insufficiency: Concept, clues to detection, and diagnosis. *Endocrine Practice, 24*(8), 746–755. https://doi.org/10.4158/EP-2018-0114

Zimmerman, C., Leib, D., & Knight, Z. (2017). Neural circuits underlying thirst and fluid homeostasis. *Nature Reviews Neuroscience, 18*(8), 459–469. https://doi.org/10.1038/nrn.2017.71

RESOURCES

Canadian Addison Society
https://www.addisonsociety.ca
Canadian Society of Endocrinology and Metabolism
https://www.endo-metab.ca/
Thyroid Foundation of Canada
https://www.thyroid.ca

American Association of Clinical Endocrinologists (AACE)
https://www.aace.com
American Society for Bone and Mineral Research
https://www.asbmr.org
Endocrine Nurses Society (ENS)
https://www.endo-nurses.org
Endocrine Society
https://www.endocrine.org
EndocrineWeb.com
https://www.endocrineweb.com/
National Institute of Diabetes and Digestive and Kidney Disease—
Endocrine Diseases & Metabolic Diseases
https://www.niddk.nih.gov/about-niddk/research-areas/endocrine-metabolic-diseases
Pituitary Network Association
https://www.pituitary.org
Society for Endocrinology
https://www.endocrinology.org/

evolve

For additional Internet resources, see the website for this book at http://evolve.elsevier.com/Canada/Lewis/medsurg.

Nursing Management
Diabetes Mellitus

Tess Montada-Atin
Originating US chapter by Jane K. Dickinson

⊖volve WEBSITE

http://evolve.elsevier.com/Canada/Lewis/medsurg

- Review Questions (Online Only)
- Key Points
- Answer Guidelines for Case Study
- Student Case Studies
  - Patient with Type 1 Diabetes Mellitus and Diabetic Ketoacidosis
- Customizable Nursing Care Plan
  - Patient with Diabetes Mellitus
- Conceptual Care Map Creator
  - Conceptual Care Map for Textbook Case Study
- Audio Glossary
- Content Updates

LEARNING OBJECTIVES

1. Describe the pathophysiology and clinical manifestations of diabetes mellitus.
2. Describe the differences between type 1 and type 2 diabetes mellitus.
3. Describe the interprofessional care of the patient with diabetes mellitus.
4. Describe the role of nutrition and exercise in the management of diabetes mellitus.
5. Describe the nursing management of a patient with newly diagnosed diabetes mellitus.
6. Describe the nursing management of the patient with diabetes mellitus in the ambulatory and home care settings.
7. Identify the pathophysiology and clinical manifestations of acute and chronic complications of diabetes mellitus.
8. Explain the interprofessional care and nursing management of the patient with acute and chronic complications of diabetes mellitus.

KEY TERMS

diabetes mellitus (DM)
diabetic ketoacidosis (DKA)
diabetic nephropathy
diabetic neuropathy

gestational diabetes mellitus (GDM)
glycated hemoglobin (A_{1c})
glycemic index (GI)
hyperosmolar hyperglycemic state (HHS)

insulin resistance
lipodystrophy
prediabetes
Somogyi effect

▍DIABETES MELLITUS

Diabetes mellitus (DM) is a multisystem disease related to abnormal insulin production, impaired insulin utilization, or both. DM is a serious health problem throughout the world. According to the International Diabetes Federation (IDF), 537 million people have DM (IDF, 2021). By 2030, this figure is expected to top 634 million. Canadian data indicate that the estimated prevalence of diagnosed DM in adults is 9.0% (~3.6 million people) (Diabetes Canada, 2019a).

Approximately 65 to 80% of people with DM will die as a result of heart disease or stroke (Poirier et al., 2018). DM is a contributing factor in the deaths of approximately 41 500 Canadians each year. Canadian adults with DM are twice as likely as people without DM to die prematurely. For example, a 35-year-old Canadian with DM is four times more likely to die

at that age than a 35-year-old without DM. Life expectancy for people with diabetes may be shortened by 5 to 15 years (Diabetes Canada, 2019a). The financial burden of DM and its complications on people with the disease and on the Canadian health care system is enormous. In 2019, the cost of treating diabetes in Canada was nearly $30 billion dollars (Diabetes Canada, 2019b). A person with DM incurs medical costs that are three to four times higher than those of a person without DM. A person with DM can face direct costs for medication and supplies equivalent to 3% of their income.

Approximately 10% of people with DM have type 1 DM. However, the number of people with type 2 DM is increasing dramatically owing to a number of factors—in the Western world, people are living longer, obesity rates are rising, and lifestyles are becoming increasingly sedentary. There is increased immigration from high-risk populations, with one in seven

Canadians coming from populations that are at higher risk for type 2 DM. These populations include people of Hispanic, Asian, South Asian, and African descent (Diabetes Canada, 2019a) (see the Determinants of Health box). Risk levels for these groups are between two and six times higher than for White Canadians.

There are three recognized groups of Indigenous people in Canada: First Nations, Inuit, and Métis. These populations are three to five times more likely than the general population to develop type 2 DM (Diabetes Canada Clinical Practice Guidelines Expert Committee, 2018). An estimated 25% of individuals in First Nations communities on reserves who are over age 45 years have DM. According to the Diabetes Canada Clinical Practice Guidelines Expert Committee (2018), the prevalence of type 2 DM in Canadian Indigenous children 5 to 18 years of age is as high as 1%, with the highest rate being in the Plains Cree people of Central Canada. Screening every 2 years should also be considered in nonpubertal children with at least three risk factors beginning at age 8, or at least two risk factors in pubertal children (Diabetes Canada Clinical Practice Guidelines Expert Committee, 2018).

Etiology and Pathophysiology

Current theories link the causes of DM, singly or in combination, to genetic, autoimmune, viral, and environmental factors (e.g., obesity, sedentary lifestyle, stress). Regardless of its cause, DM is primarily a disorder of glucose metabolism related to absent or insufficient insulin supply or poor utilization of the insulin that is available.

Although the *Diabetes Canada 2018 Clinical Practice Guidelines* recognizes 11 different classifications of the disease, most of these types are rarely encountered in routine nursing practice (Diabetes Canada Clinical Practice Guidelines Expert Committee, 2018). The two most common types of DM are classified as type 1 and type 2 DM (Table 52.1). Gestational diabetes mellitus (GDM), prediabetes, and secondary DM (discussed later in this chapter) are other classifications of DM commonly seen in clinical practice.

Normal Insulin Metabolism. *Insulin* is a hormone produced by the β cells in the islets of Langerhans of the pancreas. Under normal conditions, insulin is continuously released into the bloodstream in small, pulsatile increments (a basal rate), with increased release (bolus) when food is ingested (Figure 52.1). The activity of released insulin lowers blood glucose and facilitates a stable, normal glucose range of approximately 4 to 6 mmol/L. The average amount of insulin secreted daily by an adult is approximately 40 to 50 units, or 0.6 units/kg of body weight.

Other hormones (glucagon, epinephrine, growth hormone, and cortisol) work to oppose the effects of insulin and are often referred to as *counter-regulatory hormones*. These hormones work to increase blood glucose levels by stimulating glucose production and output by the liver and by decreasing the movement of glucose into the cells. Insulin and these counter-regulatory hormones provide a sustained but regulated release of glucose for energy during food intake and periods of fasting and usually maintain blood glucose levels within the normal range. An abnormal production of any or all of these hormones may be present in DM.

Insulin is released from the pancreatic β cells as its precursor, *proinsulin,* and is then routed through the liver. Proinsulin is composed of two polypeptide chains, chain A and chain B, which are linked by the C-peptide chain. Insulin is formed when enzymes cleave C off, leaving the A and B chains. The presence of C peptide in serum is a useful indicator of β-cell function.

Insulin facilitates glucose transport from the bloodstream across the cell membrane to the cytoplasm of the cell. The rise in plasma insulin after a meal stimulates storage of glucose as glycogen in liver and muscle, inhibits gluconeogenesis, enhances fat deposition in adipose tissue, and increases protein synthesis. The fall in insulin level during normal overnight fasting facilitates the release of stored glucose from the liver, protein from muscle, and fat from adipose tissue. For this reason, insulin is known as the *anabolic* or *storage hormone.*

Skeletal muscle and adipose tissue have specific receptors for insulin and are considered insulin-dependent tissues. Other tissues (e.g., brain, liver, blood cells) do not directly depend on insulin for glucose transport but require an adequate glucose supply for normal function. Although liver cells are not considered insulin-dependent tissue, insulin receptor sites on the liver facilitate the hepatic uptake of glucose and its conversion to glycogen.

Type 1 Diabetes Mellitus. Formerly known as "juvenile-onset" or "insulin-dependent" DM, *type 1 DM* most often occurs in people who are younger than 30 years, with a peak onset between ages 11 and 13. The rate of type 1 DM in children is highest in Europe (Finland, Sweden, and Norway) (IDF, 2021). Most cases of type 1 DM are sporadic; only 10 to 15%

TABLE 52.1   CHARACTERISTICS OF TYPE 1 AND TYPE 2 DIABETES MELLITUS

Factor	Type 1 Diabetes Mellitus	Type 2 Diabetes Mellitus	Factor	Type 1 Diabetes Mellitus	Type 2 Diabetes Mellitus
Age at onset	More common in young people but can occur at any age	Usually ≥35 yr but can occur at any age. Incidence is increasing in children	Endogenous insulin	Minimal or absent	Possibly excessive; adequate but delayed secretion or reduced utilization; secretions diminish over time
Type of onset	Signs and symptoms abrupt, but disease process may be present for several years	Insidious; may go undiagnosed for years	Nutritional status	Thin, normal, or obese	Obese or normal
Prevalence	Accounts for 5–10% of all types of diabetes	Accounts for 90% of all types of diabetes	Symptoms	Thirst, polyuria, polyphagia, fatigue, weight loss	Frequently none, fatigue, recurrent infections
Environmental factors	Viruses, toxins	Obesity, lack of exercise	Ketosis	Prone at onset or during insulin deficiency	Resistant except during infection or stress
Primary defect	Absent or minimal insulin production due to an autoimmune process	Insulin resistance, decreased insulin production over time, and alterations in production of adipokines	Nutritional therapy	Essential	Essential
			Insulin	Required for all	Required for some
			Oral antihyperglycemic agents	Not indicated	Usually beneficial
Islet-cell antibodies	Often present at onset	Absent	Vascular and neurological complications	Frequent	Frequent

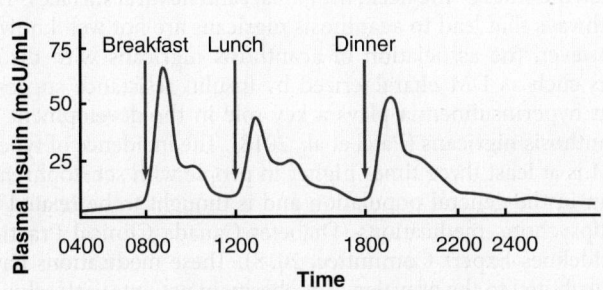

FIG. 52.1 Normal endogenous insulin secretion. In the first hour or two after meals, insulin concentrations rise rapidly in blood and peak at about 1 hour. After meals, insulin concentrations promptly decline toward preprandial values as carbohydrate absorption from the gastrointestinal tract declines. After carbohydrate absorption from the gastrointestinal tract is complete and during the night, insulin concentrations are low and fairly constant, with a slight increase at dawn.

of affected individuals have a first-degree relative with type 1 DM at the time of diagnosis. Typically, it is seen in people with a lean body type, although it can occur in people who are overweight. This form includes *latent autoimmune diabetes mellitus in adults* (LADA); the term is used to describe the small number of people with apparent type 2 DM who appear to have immune-mediated loss of pancreatic β cells (Diabetes Canada Clinical Practice Guidelines Expert Committee, 2018).

Etiology and Pathophysiology. Type 1 DM results from progressive destruction of pancreatic β cells due to an autoimmune process in susceptible individuals. Autoantibodies to the islet cells cause a reduction of 80 to 90% of normal β-cell function before hyperglycemia and other manifestations occur (Figure 52.2). A genetic predisposition and exposure to a virus are factors that may contribute to the pathogenesis of type 1 DM. Occasionally, type 1 DM may be caused by nonimmune factors of unknown (*idiopathic*) etiologies. This type of DM is known as

Type 1 Diabetes Mellitus

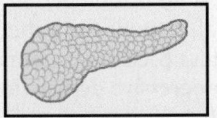

Pancreas
- Autoimmune destruction of β cells
- Autoantibodies present for months to years before clinical symptoms
- Insufficient production of insulin

Type 2 Diabetes Mellitus

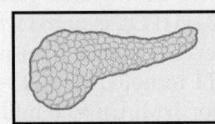

Pancreas
- Defective β cell secretion of insulin
- Insulin resistance stimulates ↑ insulin secretion
- Eventual exhaustion of β cells in many people
- ↑ Glucagon secretion

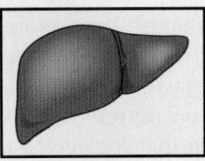

Liver
- Excess glucose production
- Inappropriate regulation of glucose production

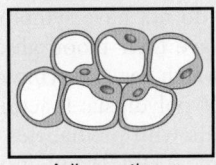

Adipose tissue
- ↓ Adiponectin and ↑ leptin
- Results in altered glucose and fat metabolism

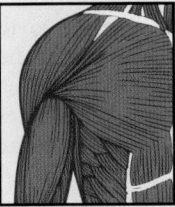

Muscle
- Defective insulin receptors
- Insulin resistance
- Decreased uptake of glucose by cells resulting in hyperglycemia

FIG. 52.2 Altered mechanisms in type 1 and type 2 diabetes mellitus.

type 1B DM. When type 1 DM is caused by an immune mechanism, the disease is known as *type 1A DM.*

Predisposition to type 1 DM is believed to be related to human leukocyte antigens (HLAs) (see Chapter 16 for a discussion of HLAs and disease associations). Theoretically, when an individual with certain HLA types is exposed to viral infections, the β cells of the pancreas are destroyed, either directly or through an autoimmune process. The HLA types associated with an increased risk for type 1 DM include HLA-DR3 and HLA-DR4 (see the Genetics in Clinical Practice box, Types 1 and 2 Diabetes Mellitus).

Onset of Disease. Type 1 DM is associated with a long preclinical period. The islet-cell autoantibodies responsible for β-cell destruction are present for months to years before the onset of symptoms. Manifestations of type 1 DM develop when the person's pancreas can no longer produce insulin. Once this occurs, the onset of symptoms is usually rapid, and the patient comes to the emergency department with impending or actual ketoacidosis. The patient usually has a history of recent and sudden weight loss as well as the classic symptoms of *polydipsia* (excessive thirst), *polyuria* (frequent urination), and *polyphagia* (excessive hunger).

The individual with type 1 DM requires a supply of insulin from an outside source *(exogenous insulin),* such as an injection, in order to sustain life. Without insulin, the patient will develop diabetic ketoacidosis (DKA), a life-threatening condition resulting in metabolic acidosis that, if untreated, could be fatal. Newly diagnosed patients with type 1 DM may experience a remission, or "honeymoon period," soon after treatment is initiated. During this time, the patient requires very little injected insulin because β-cell mass remains sufficient for glucose control as the progressive destruction continues to occur. Eventually, as more β cells are destroyed, blood glucose levels increase, more insulin is needed, and the honeymoon period ends. It is critical for the patient to monitor blood glucose very closely during this period, and frequent follow-up visits are recommended. The honeymoon period usually lasts 3 to 12 months, after which the person will require insulin on a permanent basis.

Prediabetes. Prediabetes, also known as *impaired glucose tolerance* (IGT) or *impaired fasting glucose* (IFG), is noted when a fasting or a 2-hour plasma glucose level is higher than normal (6.1–6.9 mmol/L for IFG and 7.1–11 mmol/L for IGT) but lower than that considered diagnostic for DM. Up to 6 million Canadians have prediabetes, putting them at risk of developing DM and its complications, particularly cardiovascular disease. About 50% of Canadians with prediabetes develop type 2 DM in their lifetime (Diabetes Canada Clinical Practice Guidelines Expert Committee, 2018).

Long-term damage to the body, especially the heart and blood vessels, may already be occurring in patients with prediabetes. People with prediabetes usually do not have symptoms. Individuals with prediabetes should have their blood glucose and A$_{1c}$ tested regularly and should watch for the symptoms of DM, such as polyuria, polyphagia, or polydipsia. If action is taken to manage blood glucose, patients with prediabetes can delay or prevent the development of type 2 DM. Maintaining a healthy weight, exercising regularly, eating a healthy diet, and using medication when required are measures found to reduce the risk of developing DM in people with prediabetes by almost 60% (Diabetes Canada Clinical Practice Guidelines Expert Committee, 2018).

Type 2 Diabetes Mellitus. Type 2 DM is, by far, the most prevalent type of DM, accounting for over 90% of patients with DM. Type 2 DM usually occurs in people older than 35 years, and 80 to 90% of patients are overweight at the time of diagnosis. The most powerful risk factor is believed to be obesity, specifically abdominal and visceral adiposity. Visceral adipocytes release an excess amount of free fatty acids, which are associated with insulin resistance at the level of the liver, as well as several adipocytokines, which cause insulin resistance in the muscle (Czech, 2020). Obesity has a tendency to run in families and probably has a genetic basis (see the Genetics in Clinical Practice box, Types 1 and 2 Diabetes Mellitus).

Other risk factors for type 2 DM are being in a high-risk population (e.g., people of Indigenous, Latin American, South Asian, Asian, or African descent), history of IGT or IFG, presence of complications associated with DM, vascular disease, history of GDM, and history of delivery of an infant with macrosomia. Hypertension, dyslipidemia, being overweight, abdominal obesity, polycystic ovary syndrome (PCOS), and acanthosis nigricans are associated with insulin resistance and are also risk factors for type 2 DM. Insulin resistance with compensatory hyperinsulinemia is a common feature of PCOS, in both lean and obese women. The exact mechanisms for abnormalities of insulin action in PCOS are not fully understood (Tosi et al., 2017). Acanthosis nigricans is a cutaneous sign of an underlying condition and is characterized by a velvety, light brown to black hyperpigmented thickening of the skin, usually on the back, the sides of the neck, the axillae, and flexural surfaces. The pathways that lead to acanthosis nigricans are not well known. However, the association of acanthosis nigricans with disorders such as DM characterized by insulin resistance suggests that hyperinsulinemia plays a key role in the development of acanthosis nigricans (Patel et al., 2018). The incidence of type 2 DM is at least three times higher in people with schizophrenia than in the general population and is thought to be related to antipsychotic medications (Diabetes Canada Clinical Practice Guidelines Expert Committee, 2018). These medications have contributed to the prevalence of obesity in patients with schizophrenia, which is a known risk factor for insulin resistance and type 2 DM. A systematic review and meta-analysis (Pillinger et al., 2017) found that abnormal glucose homeostasis exists at the onset of illness in schizophrenia, suggesting that patients are at increased risk of DM as a result.

Prevalence of type 2 DM increases with age, with about half of the people diagnosed being older than 55. In the past, type 2 DM was known as "adult-onset" DM. This term is no longer considered appropriate because the disease is now being seen in a rapidly growing number of children and adolescents, particularly in Indigenous populations. In a large study, people at risk for type 2 DM were able to cut that risk by 58% by exercising moderately for 30 minutes a day and by losing 5 to 7% of their body weight (Diabetes Canada Clinical Practice Guidelines Expert Committee, 2018). Other large studies have shown similar results in reducing risk.

Etiology and Pathophysiology. In type 2 DM, the pancreas usually continues to produce some *endogenous* (self-made) insulin. However, the insulin that is produced is either insufficient for the needs of the body, poorly utilized by the tissues, or both. In contrast, there is a virtual absence of endogenous insulin in type 1 DM. The presence of endogenous insulin is the major pathophysiological distinction between type 1 and type 2 DM.

Genetic mutations that lead to insulin resistance and a higher risk for obesity have been found in many people with type 2 DM. It is likely that multiple genes are involved in this complex, multifactorial disorder (see the Genetics in Clinical Practice box).

GENETICS IN CLINICAL PRACTICE

Types 1 and 2 Diabetes Mellitus

	Type 1 Diabetes Mellitus	Type 2 Diabetes Mellitus	Maturity-Onset Diabetes of the Young (MODY)
Genetic basis	Associations between specific human leukocyte antigens (HLA-DR3, HLA-DR4)	Majority of cases are polygenic	Autosomal dominant, monogenic (single gene)
	As many as 40 genes (and maybe more) influence susceptibility	As many as 25 genes influence susceptibility	Caused by mutations in any of the MODY genes (types 1–11)
Incidence	Accounts for about 5–10% of cases in Canada	Accounts for about 90% of cases in Canada	Accounts for 1–5% of people with diabetes
Risk to offspring and twins	Risk to offspring of mothers with diabetes is only 1–4% Risk to offspring of fathers with diabetes is 5–6%	Risk to offspring is 8–14%	If one parent has MODY, the offspring has a 50% chance of developing the disease. If one parent has MODY, the offspring has a 50% chance of being a carrier.
	Identical twin concordance is 30–40%	Identical twin concordance often exceeds 60–75%	
Clinical implications	Disease is a result of complex interaction of genetic, autoimmune, and environmental factors	Disease is a result of complex genetic interactions, which are modified by environmental factors such as body weight and exercise	Characterized by young age of onset (often before 25), not associated with obesity or hypertension

Four major metabolic abnormalities have a role in the development of type 2 DM. The first factor is insulin resistance in glucose and lipid metabolism, which is a condition in which body tissues do not respond to the action of insulin. This lack of response is due to insulin receptors that are unresponsive to the action of insulin, insufficient in number, or both. Most insulin receptors are located on skeletal muscle, fat, and liver cells. Insulin mediates glucose uptake into fat tissue and skeletal muscle through GLUT4 glucose transporters. Insulin resistance in fat cells is associated with a decrease in the number of GLUT4 transporters and altered activity in individuals with type 2 DM (Alam et al., 2016). When insulin is not properly used, the entry of glucose into the cell is impeded, resulting in hyperglycemia. In the early stages of insulin resistance, the pancreas responds to high blood glucose by producing greater amounts of insulin (if β-cell function is normal). This creates a temporary state of hyperinsulinemia that coexists with the hyperglycemia.

A second factor in the development of type 2 DM is a marked decrease in the ability of the pancreas to produce insulin, as the β cells become fatigued from the compensatory overproduction of insulin or when β-cell mass is lost. The resulting IFG and IGT place the individual at risk of developing DM and its complications. This does not necessarily mean that all people with prediabetes will progress to DM. A significant proportion will revert to normal blood glucose levels (Diabetes Canada Clinical Practice Guidelines Expert Committee, 2018). The underlying basis for the failure of β cells to adapt is unknown. However, it may be linked to the adverse effects of chronic hyperglycemia or high circulating free fatty acids.

A third factor is inappropriate glucose production by the liver. Instead of properly regulating the release of glucose in response to blood levels, the liver does so in a haphazard way that does not correspond to the body's needs at the time. Furthermore, there is increased secretion of glucagon from the α cells of the pancreas that stimulates glucose production by the liver, adding to the increase in blood sugar. However, this is not considered a primary factor in the development of type 2 DM.

A fourth factor is alteration in the production of hormones and cytokines by adipose tissue (adipocytokines). Adipocytokines appear to play a role in glucose and fat metabolism and are likely to contribute to the pathophysiology of type 2 DM. The two main adipocytokines believed to affect insulin sensitivity are adiponectin and leptin. Others include tumour necrosis factor α (TNF-α), interleukin-6 (IL-6), and resistin. The role of resistin in the pathogenesis of obesity-mediated insulin resistance and type 2 DM, however, remains controversial (Gurumurthy, 2018). Figure 52.2 depicts the altered mechanisms in type 1 and type 2 DM.

Metabolic syndrome (also known as *insulin resistance syndrome*) is a cluster of abnormalities that act synergistically to greatly increase the risk for cardiovascular disease. Metabolic syndrome is characterized by abdominal obesity, hypertension, dyslipidemia, insulin resistance, and dysglycemia. Patients with metabolic syndrome are at significant risk of developing DM and cardiovascular disease (Diabetes Canada Clinical Practice Guidelines Expert Committee, 2018). Healthy behaviour interventions have been shown to be highly effective in delaying or preventing the onset of DM in people with IGT. Risk factors for metabolic syndrome include but are not limited to abdominal obesity, sedentary lifestyle, urbanization and Westernization, and being of Indigenous or of Latin American or African descent. Overweight individuals with metabolic syndrome can prevent or delay the onset of DM through a program of weight loss and regular physical activity. (Metabolic syndrome is discussed in further detail in Chapter 43.)

Onset of Disease. Disease onset in type 2 DM is usually gradual. The person may go for many years with undetected hyperglycemia that might produce few, if any, symptoms. Many people are diagnosed on routine laboratory testing. If the patient with type 2 DM has marked hyperglycemia (e.g., 28–55 mmol/L), a sufficient endogenous insulin supply may prevent DKA from occurring, as DKA happens when there is an absence of insulin. However, osmotic fluid and electrolyte loss related to hyperglycemia may become severe and lead to hyperosmolar hyperglycemic state. (Complications of DM are discussed later in this chapter.)

Gestational Diabetes. Gestational diabetes mellitus (GDM) develops during pregnancy. In Canada, it occurs in about 3% of pregnancies in the non-Indigenous population, and the rates are two to three times higher in Indigenous populations (Diabetes Canada Clinical Practice Guidelines Expert Committee, 2018). It is detected between 24 and 28 weeks of gestation, using a sequential screening method with a 50-g oral glucose challenge test, followed by a 75-g oral glucose tolerance test (OGTT). A fasting blood sugar is obtained prior to each test and then 50 g or 75 g of glucose drink is given. Blood is drawn exactly 1 hour after for both and at 2 hours after for the 75 g test. Women with multiple risk factors should be offered screening at any time during pregnancy.

Treatment of GDM reduces perinatal death and neonatal complications such as birth trauma, hypoglycemia, hyperbilirubinemia, and respiratory distress syndrome (Diabetes Canada Clinical Practice Guidelines Expert Committee, 2018). Nutritional counselling is considered to be the first-line therapy. Physical activity should be encouraged as tolerated. If nutritional counselling alone does not achieve target fasting, or postprandial blood glucose levels, or both, insulin therapy is usually indicated.

Approximately 10% of patients progress to DM soon after pregnancy. Although most women with GDM will have normal glucose levels within 6 weeks postpartum, their risk of developing type 2 DM in 5 to 10 years is increased. Women should be screened postpartum to determine their glucose status. Guidelines recommend a 75-g OGTT be done between 6 weeks and 6 months postpartum (Diabetes Canada Clinical Practice Guidelines Expert Committee, 2018). Education on healthy behaviour interventions to prevent DM should continue postpartum. GDM and management of the pregnant patient with DM is a specialized area not covered in detail in this chapter. The reader is advised to consult a DM and obstetrics text for information about this subject.

Secondary Diabetes. In some people, DM occurs because of another medical condition or as a result of the treatment of a medical condition that causes abnormal blood glucose levels. Conditions that may cause secondary DM include schizophrenia, cystic fibrosis, Cushing's syndrome, hyperthyroidism, immunosuppressive therapy, and the use of parenteral nutrition. Commonly used medications that can induce DM in some people include corticosteroids (prednisone), phenytoin (Dilantin), and atypical antipsychotics (e.g., clozapine [Clozaril]). Secondary DM may resolve when the underlying condition is treated or the medication is discontinued.

Clinical Manifestations

Type 1 Diabetes Mellitus. Because the onset of type 1 DM is rapid, the initial manifestations are usually acute. The classic symptoms are *polyuria* (frequent urination), *polydipsia* (excessive thirst), and *polyphagia* (excessive hunger). The osmotic effect of glucose produces the manifestations of polydipsia and polyuria. Polyphagia is a consequence of cellular malnourishment when insulin deficiency prevents utilization of glucose for energy. Weight loss may occur because the body cannot get glucose and turns to other energy sources, such as fat and protein. Weakness and fatigue may also be experienced, because body cells lack needed energy from glucose. There may be pronounced changes in visual acuity due to

changes in the lens with hyperglycemia and fluid retention. Women may have vaginal yeast infections. Ketoacidosis, a complication associated with untreated type 1 DM, is associated with additional clinical manifestations that are discussed later in this chapter.

Type 2 Diabetes Mellitus. The clinical manifestations of type 2 DM are often nonspecific, although it is possible that an individual with type 2 DM will experience some of the classic symptoms associated with type 1. Some of the more common manifestations associated with type 2 DM include fatigue, recurrent infections, prolonged wound healing, visual acuity changes, and painful peripheral neuropathy in the feet. Unfortunately, the clinical manifestations appear so gradually that, before the person knows it, they may have complications.

Complications

Complications of DM are discussed in detail later in this chapter.

Diagnostic Studies

The guidelines (Diabetes Canada Clinical Practice Guidelines Expert Committee, 2018) recommend any one of the following four methods and their criteria for the diagnosis of DM and a repeat confirmatory test on another day in the absence of symptomatic hyperglycemia:

1. Glycated hemoglobin (A_{1c}) ≥6.5% (in adults), using a standardized, validated assay, in the absence of conditions that affect the accuracy of the A_{1c} and not for suspected type 1 DM, *or*
2. Fasting blood glucose (FBG) level ≥7.0 mmol/L (*fasting* is defined as no caloric intake for at least 8 hours), *or*
3. Random plasma glucose (RPG) measurement ≥11.1 mmol/L (*random* is defined as any time of day without regard to the interval since the last meal), *or*
4. Two-hour plasma glucose (PG) level in a 75 g OGTT ≥11.1 mmol/L

It is preferable that the same test be repeated for confirmation, but an RPG level in an asymptomatic individual should be confirmed with any of the other tests (A_{1c}, FBG, or 2-hr PG in 75-g OGTT). When overt symptoms of hyperglycemia (polyuria, polydipsia, and polyphagia) are present, the diagnosis has been made and a confirmatory test is not required before treatment is initiated.

IFG, IGT, or A_{1c} of 6.0 to 6.4% each represents an intermediate stage between normal glucose homeostasis and DM. The stage is called *prediabetes* (see discussion on prediabetes earlier in this chapter). When the FBG level is 6.1 to 6.9 mmol/L, the individual is considered to have IFG. IGT is classified when a 2-hour PG in a 75-g OGTT level is 7.8 to 11.0 mmol/L (Diabetes Canada Clinical Practice Guidelines Expert Committee, 2018). The combination of IFG and an A_{1c} of 6.0 to 6.4% is predictive of 100% progression to type 2 DM over a 5-year period.

Measurement of glycated hemoglobin (A1c), also known as the A_{1c} *test,* is not only used for diagnosing diabetes but is also useful in determining glycemic control over time. The test works by showing the amount of glucose that has been attached to hemoglobin molecules, which are attached to the red blood cell (RBC) for the life of the cell (~120 days). Therefore, an A_{1c} test indicates the overall glucose control for the previous 90 to 120 days. All patients with DM should have regular assessments of A_{1c} every 3 to 6 months. Major studies have demonstrated that people with DM who can maintain near-normal A_{1c} levels over time have a greatly reduced risk for the development of retinopathy, nephropathy, and neuropathy. For most people with

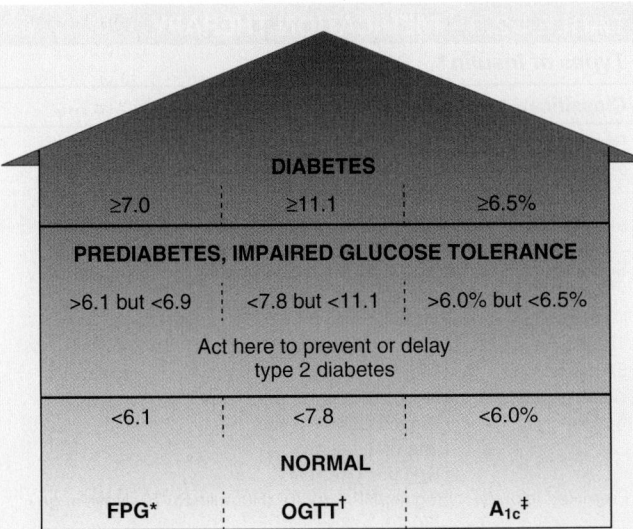

FIG. 52.3 The glucose continuum. Numbers represent blood glucose levels in millimoles per litre (mmol/L).

*The fasting plasma glucose (FPG) test: After an overnight fast, blood glucose is measured in the morning.

†The 2-hour oral glucose tolerance test (OGTT): Includes a fasting blood glucose test and glucose measurements 2 hours after drinking a glucose-containing solution.

‡The glycated hemoglobin (A_{1c}) is a 2- to 3-month average blood glucose test that can be done at any time of the day.

Note: Diabetes Canada believes that either test is appropriate to measure prediabetes (impaired glucose tolerance) and diabetes.

DM, the ideal A_{1c} goal is 7% or less; normal range is less than 6%. A target A_{1c} of less than 6.5% can be considered in some patients with type 2 DM to further lower the risk for nephropathy but must be balanced against the risk for hypoglycemia and increased mortality in those at an elevated risk for cardiovascular disease (Diabetes Canada Clinical Practice Guidelines Expert Committee, 2018). Diseases affecting RBCs (e.g., sickle cell anemia, thalassemia trait) or recent blood transfusions can affect the A_{1c} results and should be taken into consideration in the interpretation of this test result. It is important to know where an individual is on the glucose continuum (Figure 52.3).

Interprofessional Care

The goals of DM management are to promote well-being, reduce symptoms, prevent acute complications of hyperglycemia and hypoglycemia, and delay the onset and progression of long-term complications. These goals are most likely to be met when patients are able to maintain blood glucose levels as near to normal as possible. Patient and family teaching enables them to become the most active participants in their own care and is essential for a successful treatment plan. Nutritional therapy, exercise, self-monitoring of blood glucose, and medication therapy are the tools used in the management of DM (Table 52.2). All individuals with type 1 DM require insulin from the time of diagnosis. For some people with type 2 DM, healthy behaviour interventions, including healthy eating, regular physical activity, and maintenance of desirable body weight, will be sufficient to attain an optimal level of blood glucose control. For the majority, however, medication therapy with oral antihyperglycemic agents (OHAs), noninsulin injectable agents, or insulin will be necessary.

TABLE 52.2 INTERPROFESSIONAL CARE

Diabetes Mellitus

Diagnostic
- History and physical examination
- Blood pressure
- Blood tests: including FBG, postprandial blood glucose, glycated hemoglobin (A_{1c}), fasting lipid profile, serum creatinine, electrolytes, calculation of creatinine clearance, TSH
- Dental examination
- Doppler scan—ankle-brachial index (if indicated)
- ECG (if indicated)
- Foot (podiatric) examination
- Fundoscopic examination—dilated eye examination
- Monitoring of weight
- Neurological examination, including monofilament test for sensation to lower extremities
- Random urine for microalbuminuria (MAU), complete urinalysis, and acetone if indicated

Interprofessional Therapy
- Oral antihyperglycemic agents and noninsulin injectable agents (see Table 52.7)
- Angiotensin-converting enzyme (ACE) inhibitors or angiotensin II receptor blockers (ARBs) (high risk for a cardiovascular event) (see Chapter 35, Table 35.8)
- Blood pressure control
  - Target <130/80 mm Hg
- Medication therapy
  - Enteric-coated acetylsalicylic acid (ASA; Aspirin) (80 mg or 325 mg)
  - Insulin (see Figure 52.4 and Tables 52.3 and 52.4)
  - Lipid-lowering therapy (high risk for a cardiovascular event) (see Chapter 36, Table 36.5)
- Exercise therapy (see Table 52.9)
- Nutritional therapy (see Table 52.8)
- Patient and caregiver teaching and follow-up programs
- Self-monitoring of blood glucose (SMBG)
- Vascular protection

ECG, electrocardiogram; *FBG,* fasting blood glucose; *TSH,* thyroid-stimulating hormone.
Source: Diabetes Canada Clinical Practice Guidelines Expert Committee. (2018). Clinical practice guidelines for the prevention and management of diabetes in Canada. *Canadian Journal of Diabetes, 42*(Suppl. 1), S1–S325.

Medication Therapy: Insulin

Exogenous (injected) insulin is needed when a patient has inadequate insulin to meet specific metabolic needs and a satisfactory blood glucose level cannot be maintained through the combination of nutritional therapy, exercise, and OHAs and noninsulin injectable agents. Exogenous insulin is always required for the management of type 1 DM. Individuals with type 2 DM may be treated with insulin alone or with insulin in combination with OHAs or noninsulin injectable agents (Diabetes Canada Clinical Practice Guidelines Expert Committee, 2018). Insulin requirement may increase significantly during periods of severe stress, such as illness or surgery.

Types of Insulin. In Canada, beef insulin was withdrawn in 1999 but can still be bought from international sources. Human biosynthetic insulin is now the most widely used insulin. Human insulin is derived from common bacteria (e.g., *Escherichia coli*) or yeast cells using recombinant DNA technology. Insulin analogues are made by modifying the amino acid sequence of the insulin molecule (Melo et al., 2019). Insulins differ in regard to onset, peak action, and duration (Figure 52.4). The specific properties and different combinations of these insulins can be used to tailor treatment to the patient's specific patterns of blood glucose levels, lifestyle, eating, and activity. Different types of

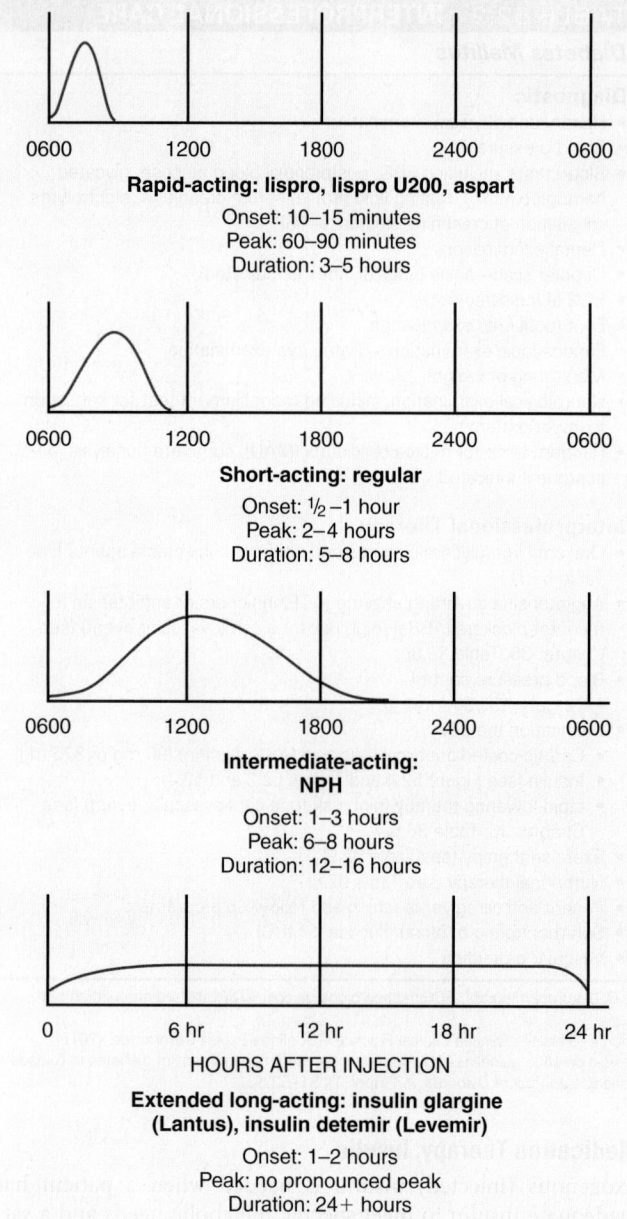

FIG. 52.4 Commercially available insulin preparations showing onset, peak, and duration of action of relative plasma insulin level. *NPH,* neutral protamine Hagedorn.

TABLE 52.3   MEDICATION THERAPY

Types of Insulin*

Classification	Examples
Rapid-acting analogue (clear)	Lispro (Humalog) Lispro U200 (Humalog) Aspart (NovoRapid) Faster-acting aspart (Fisasp) Glulisine (Apidra)
Short-acting (clear)	Regular (Novolin ge Toronto, Humulin R, Entuzity [U500])
Intermediate-acting (cloudy)	NPH (Humulin N, Novolin ge NPH)
Extended long-acting analogue (clear)	Glargine (Lantus) Glargine biosimilar (Basaglar) Glargine U300 (Toujeo) Detemir (Levemir) Degludec (Tresiba)
Premixed (cloudy)	Regular/NPH 30/70[†] (Humulin 30/70, Novolin ge 30/70) Regular/NPH 50/50 and 40/60 Lispro/lispro protamine 25/75 (Humalog Mix 25); 50/50 (Humalog Mix 50) Aspart/aspart protamine 30/70 (NovoMix 30)

*Insulin preparations are clear solutions except for NPH and protamine-containing insulin, which are cloudy.
[†]These numbers refer to percentages of each type of insulin.
NPH, neutral protamine Hagedorn.

insulin are listed in Table 52.3. Most insulin preparations start with regular insulin as a base. By adding zinc, acetate buffers, and protamine to insulin in various ways, the onset of activity, peak, and duration times can be manipulated. Zinc and protamine are added to make NPH (neutral protamine Hagedorn). In rare instances, these additives may cause an allergic reaction at the injection site. Switching the brand or the type of insulin may alleviate this localized reaction.

Health care providers should refer to the most current edition of *Compendium of Pharmaceuticals and Specialties* (Canadian Pharmacists Association, Ottawa, Ontario, Canada) and product monographs for detailed information.

Insulin Regimens. Examples of insulin regimens ranging from one to four injections per day are presented in Table 52.4. The exogenous insulin regimen that most closely mimics endogenous insulin production is the basal–bolus regimen, which uses rapid- or short-acting (bolus) insulin before meals and intermediate- or long-acting (basal) background insulin once or twice a day. The basal–bolus regimen is *intensive insulin therapy,* which consists of multiple daily injections. The goal is to achieve a near-normal glucose level of 4 to 7 mmol/L before meals, or 4 to 6 mmol/L if this can be reached safely without severe hypoglycemia. A landmark study by the Diabetes Control and Complications Trial (DCCT) Research Group demonstrated that people with type 1 DM who have tight glucose control through intensive management develop fewer and less severe complications (DCCT, 1993). Ideally, regimens should be collaboratively selected by the patient and the interprofessional health care team (Diabetes Canada Clinical Practice Guidelines Expert Committee, 2018). The criteria for selection are based on the type of DM and the required, desired, and feasible levels of glycemic control, in addition to economic factors and flexibility. Starting a multiple daily injection regimen with three to four injections per day may be overwhelming for patients. Depending on the patient's glycemic control, introducing a once or twice a day insulin regimen may be more manageable.

Mealtime Insulin (Bolus). Synthetic, rapid-acting insulins include lispro U100 (Humalog), lispro U200, aspart insulin (NovoRapid), faster-acting aspart (Fiasp), and glulisine (Apidra). They have an onset of action of approximately 10 to 15 minutes (as compared with 30 to 60 minutes for regular insulin) except for faster-acting aspart, which has an onset of action of 4 minutes. Rapid-acting insulin is considered to be the type that best mimics natural insulin secretion in response to a meal. It should be administered 10 to 15 minutes before meals and can be given up to 15 minutes after meals. However, preprandial administration achieves better postprandial glycemic control. When rapid-acting insulin is used as mealtime coverage in people with type 1 DM, an additional and longer-acting insulin must also be used as basal background insulin because the duration of rapid-acting insulin is so short. Other benefits of rapid-acting insulin include decreased postmeal hyperglycemia, decreased hypoglycemic episodes, and increased flexibility compared with regular insulin (Diabetes Canada Clinical Practice Guidelines Expert Committee, 2018).

TABLE 52.4 MEDICATION THERAPY

Common Insulin Regimens

Regimen	Type of Insulin/Frequency	Action Profile*	Comments
Once a day Single dose	Intermediate (NPH) *at bedtime* *Or*		One injection should cover night-time coverage.
	Long-acting (glargine [Lantus], glargine U300 [Toujeo], detemir [Levemir] or degludec [Tresiba]) *In morning or at bedtime*		One injection will last 24 hr with no peaks and less chance for hypoglycemia. Does not cover postprandial blood sugars.
Twice a day Split-mixed dose	NPH and regular *Or* NPH and rapid *Before breakfast and at dinner*		Two injections provide coverage for 24 hr. Patient must adhere to a set meal plan.
Three times a day Combination of mixed and single dose	NPH and regular *Or* NPH and rapid *Before breakfast* + Regular or rapid *Before dinner* + NPH *At bedtime*		Three injections provide coverage for 24 hr, particularly during early A.M. hours. Potential is reduced for hypoglycemia between 0200 and 0300 hours.
Basal-bolus Multiple dose	Regular or rapid *Before breakfast, lunch, and dinner* + NPH *Twice daily or at bedtime* *Or*		More flexibility is allowed at mealtimes and for amount of food intake. Good postprandial control. Premeal blood glucose checks and establishing and following individualized algorithms are necessary. Patients with type 1 DM will require basal insulin to cover 24 hr.
Basal-bolus Multiple dose	Regular or rapid *Before breakfast, lunch, and dinner* + Long-acting (glargine [Toujeo], detemir or degludec) *Once a day, usually at bedtime*		Four injections required per day. Most physiological approach, except for pump.

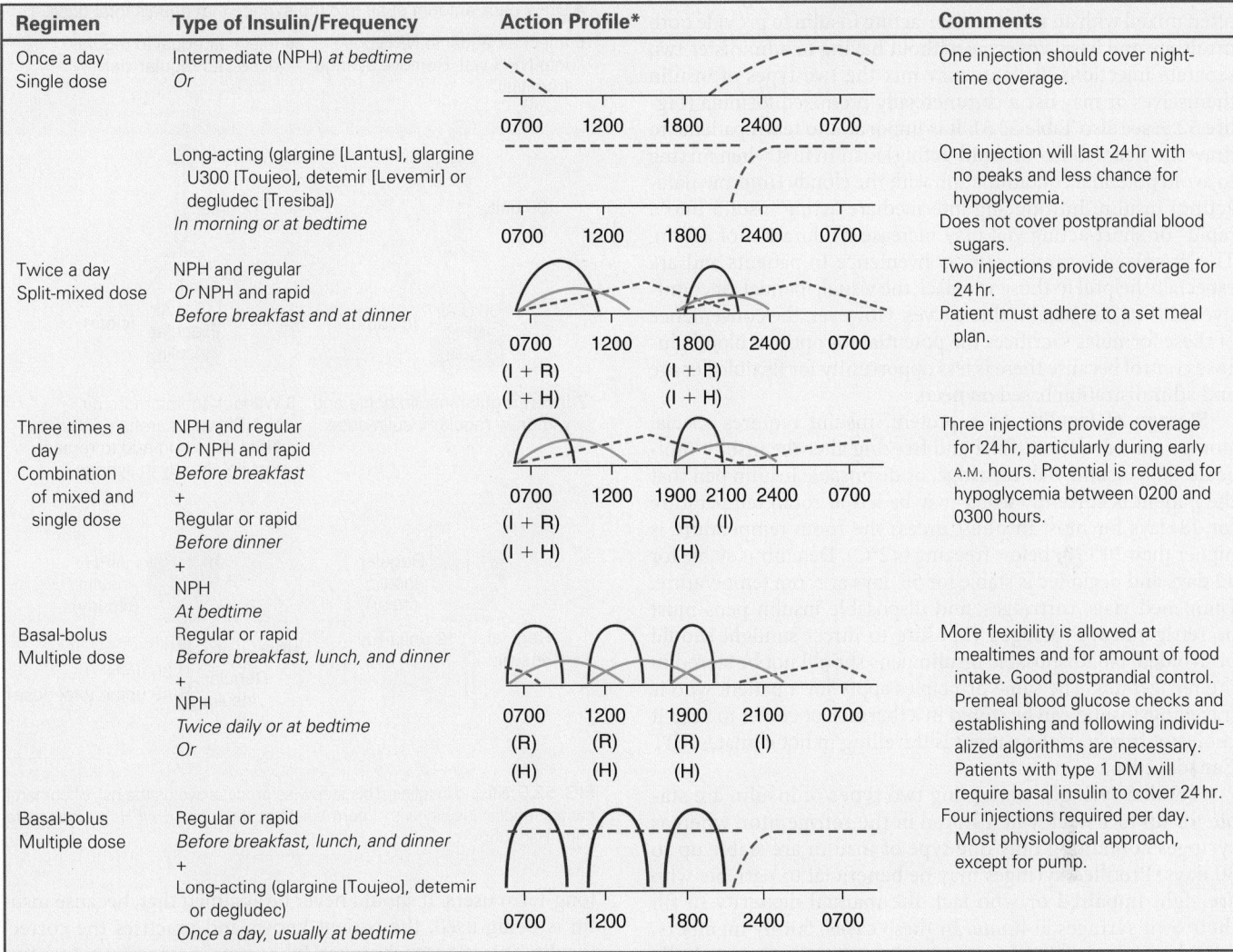

NPH, neutral protamine Hagedorn.

*Key:

————— Rapid-acting (lispro, aspart, faster-acting aspart, glulisine) insulin
————— Short-acting (regular) insulin
- - - - - - - - - Intermediate-acting (NPH) or long-acting (glargine, glargine U300, detemir, degludec) insulin

Regular insulin is also a mealtime insulin and has an onset of action of 30 to 60 minutes; it should be injected 30 to 45 minutes before a meal to ensure that the onset of action coincides with meal absorption. Because timing an injection 30 to 45 minutes before a meal can be difficult for people to incorporate into their lifestyles, the rapid-acting insulins are often preferred by people who take insulin with meals (Diabetes Canada Clinical Practice Guidelines Expert Committee, 2018).

Long- or Intermediate-Acting (Basal) Background Insulin. Insulin glargine U100 (Lantus), insulin glargine biosimilar (Basaglar), and detemir (Levemir) are extended long-acting basal insulins that are released steadily and continuously over 24 hours. The duration of insulin glargine U300 (Toujeo) is up to 30 hours, and that of degludec U100 and U200 (Tresiba) is up to 42 hours; these are ultra-long acting basal insulins. These long-acting insulins do not have a peak of action (see Figure 52.4). They may be used for once-daily subcutaneous administration at bedtime in patients with type 1 and type 2 DM who require basal (long-acting) insulin for the control of hyperglycemia. Because they lack a peak action time, the risk for hypoglycemia is greatly

reduced. They are clear, colourless insulins. The nurse should be aware of the potential danger of confusing glargine U100, glargine U300, detemir, and degludec U100 and U200 with other clear insulins (rapid- or short-acting). Glargine U100, glargine U300, glargine biosimilar, detemir, and degludec U100 and U200 must not be diluted or mixed with any other insulin or solution as this action can change the time or action profile of these long-acting analogues and cause precipitation (Eli Lilly Canada, 2021a; NovoNordisk, 2017, 2019; Sanofi-Aventis Canada, 2020, 2021). Insulin is one of the top five medications implicated in medication incidents associated with death in Canada (Kasprzak et al., 2016). Thus, when insulin is given in the hospital the standard is a two-nurse check before administration.

Intermediate-acting insulin NPH is also used as a basal insulin that has a duration of 10 to 16 hours. The disadvantage of this insulin is that it has a peak at 4 to 10 hours, which can result in hypoglycemia. It is the only basal insulin that can be mixed with the short- and rapid-acting insulins. NPH is a cloudy insulin that must be gently agitated before administration (Forum for Injection Technique [FIT] Canada, 2016).

Combination Therapy. Two different insulin types are commonly used in combination to mimic normal endogenous insulin secretion (see Table 52.4). Short- or rapid-acting insulin is often mixed with an intermediate-acting insulin to provide both mealtime and basal coverage without having to administer two separate injections. Patients may mix the two types of insulin themselves or may use a commercially premixed formula (Figure 52.5; see also Table 52.3). It is important to teach patients to draw the clear (short- or rapid-acting) insulin first when mixing to avoid potential contamination with the cloudy (intermediate-acting) insulin. Introducing intermediate-acting insulin into a rapid- or short-acting vial may increase its duration of action. The premixed formulas offer convenience to patients and are especially helpful to those who lack the visual, manual, or cognitive skills to mix insulin themselves. However, the convenience of these formulas sacrifices the potential for optimal blood glucose control because there is less opportunity for flexible dosage and administration based on need.

Storage of Insulin. As a protein, insulin requires special storage considerations. Heat and freezing alter the insulin molecule. The insulin vial, cartridge, or disposable insulin pen that the patient is currently using may be left at room temperature for 28 days for most insulins, unless the room temperature is higher than 30°C or below freezing (<2°C). Detemir is stable for 42 days and degludec is stable for 56 days at room temperature. Unopened vials, cartridges, and disposable insulin pens must be refrigerated. Prolonged exposure to direct sunlight should be avoided. Nondisposable insulin pens should not be stored in the refrigerator. The same principles apply for a patient who is travelling; insulin can be stored in a thermos or cooler to keep it cool (not frozen) if the patient is travelling in hot climates (FIT Canada, 2016).

Prefilled syringes containing two types of insulin are stable for up to 1 week when stored in the refrigerator, whereas syringes containing only one type of insulin are stable up to 30 days. Prefilled syringes may be beneficial to patients who are sight impaired or who lack the manual dexterity to fill their own syringes at home. In these cases, family members, friends, and caregivers may prefill syringes on a periodic basis. These should be stored in a vertical position with the needle pointed up to avoid clumping of suspended insulin binders in the needle. Some insulin combinations, such as insulin lispro and NPH, are not appropriate for prefilling and storage because the onset, action, and peak times of the mixture of the two can differ from those of either of the types. Pharmacy references should be consulted as needed when mixing and prefilling different types of insulin. Prefilled syringes should be gently rolled between the palms to warm the refrigerated insulin and to resuspend the particles before injecting. Lantus insulin cannot be stored in a prefilled syringe (Sanofi-Aventis, 2021).

Administration of Insulin. Because insulin is inactivated by gastric juices, it cannot be taken orally. The only route of administration currently approved for self-administration is subcutaneous injection by syringe or insulin pen or by continuous subcutaneous infusion (pump). Only regular insulin can be given intravenously and done with medical supervision when immediate onset of action is desired in the hospital setting.

Injection. The steps in administering a subcutaneous insulin injection are outlined in Table 52.5. The technique should be taught to new insulin users and reviewed periodically with

1 Wash hands.
2 Gently rotate NPH insulin bottle.
3 Wipe off tops of insulin vials with alcohol sponge.
4 Draw back amount of air into the syringe that equals total dose.

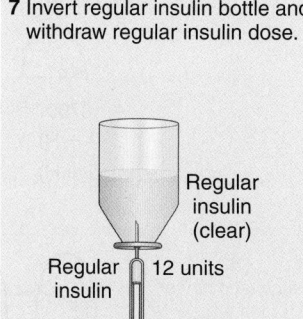

5 Inject air equal to NPH dose into NPH vial. Remove syringe from vial.

36 units

36 U Air NPH insulin (cloudy)

6 Inject air equal to regular dose into regular vial.

12 units

12 U Air Regular insulin (clear)

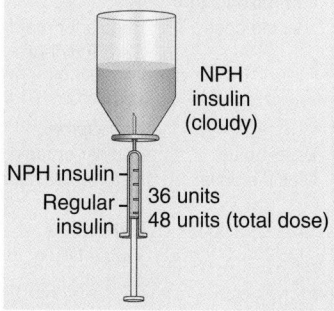

7 Invert regular insulin bottle and withdraw regular insulin dose.

Regular insulin (clear)

Regular insulin   12 units

8 Without adding more air to NPH vial, carefully withdraw NPH dose and add to regular insulin already in syringe.

NPH insulin (cloudy)

NPH insulin
Regular insulin   36 units
48 units (total dose)

FIG. 52.5 Mixing insulins. This stepwise process avoids the risk of contaminating regular insulin with intermediate-acting insulin. *NPH,* neutral protamine Hagedorn.

long-term users. It should never be assumed that, because insulin is being used, the patient knows and practises the correct insulin injection technique. Inaccurate preparation is often caused by poor eyesight. Air bubbles in the syringe may not be seen, or the scale on the syringe may be read improperly.

The patient receiving mixed insulins (e.g., regular and an intermediate-acting insulin) needs to learn the proper technique for combining both in the same syringe if commercially prepared premixed insulins are not being used (see Figure 52.5).

The speed with which peak serum concentrations are reached varies with the anatomical site used for injection. The fastest absorption is from the abdomen, followed by the arm, the thigh, and the buttock. Appropriate sites for insulin injection are noted in Figure 52.6, although the abdomen is the preferred site. The patient should be cautioned about injecting into a site that is to be exercised. For example, the patient should not inject insulin into the thigh and then go jogging. Exercise of the area containing the injection site together with the increased body heat generated by the exercise may increase the rate of absorption and speed the onset of insulin action.

Before purified human insulins were widely used, patients were advised to rotate anatomical injection sites to prevent *lipodystrophy,* a condition that produces lumps and dents in the skin from repeated injection in the same spot. The use of human insulin reduces the risk for lipodystrophy. Because of this, and because rotating sites causes variability in insulin

TABLE 52.5 PATIENT & CAREGIVER TEACHING GUIDE

Insulin Therapy

The following instructions should be included when teaching the patient and caregiver about insulin therapy.

1. Wash hands thoroughly.
2. Check insulin type and expiration date.
3. If a cloudy insulin is used, gently roll container to resuspend insulin. It should look uniformly milky.
4. Remove the cover from the needle.
5. Pull plunger down until the tip of the plunger is at the line for the number of units required. Put needle into the vial and push the air into the vial.
6. Turn vial upside down and slowly push plunger up and down to get rid of air bubbles and then pull plunger down until it is at the line for the correct dose of insulin.
7. Check that amount of insulin is correct and that there are no large air bubbles in the syringe. Remove the syringe.
8. Select proper injection site (see Figure 52.6). The use of a 6-mm needle is recommended with or without a skin lift (pinched skin) at 90 degrees (check facility policy). To prevent possible intramuscular injections, slim individuals may need to inject into the skin lift at 45 degrees when using an 8-mm needle.
9. After injecting insulin, leave the needle in place for 5 sec to ensure that all insulin has been injected and then remove needle and release skin lift.
10. Dispose of single-use syringe safely. *Note:* When instructing patient to self-inject insulin, use the following guidelines (if appropriate):
    - Inspect insulin for any changes before each use (i.e., clumping, precipitation, change in clarity or colour).
    - Aspiration does not need to be done before injection. The injection site does not need to be cleansed with alcohol.

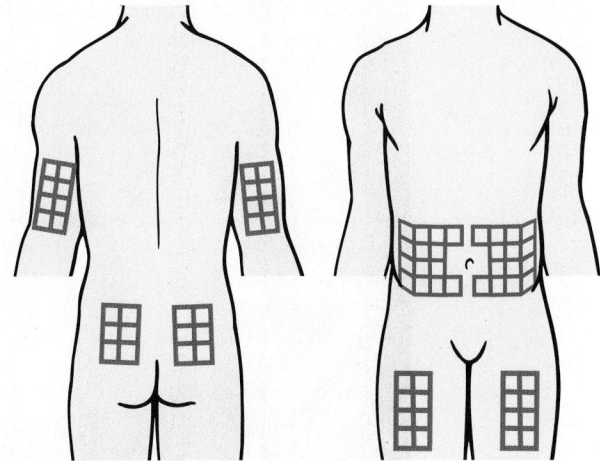

FIG. 52.6 Injection sites for insulin. The abdomen is the preferred site.

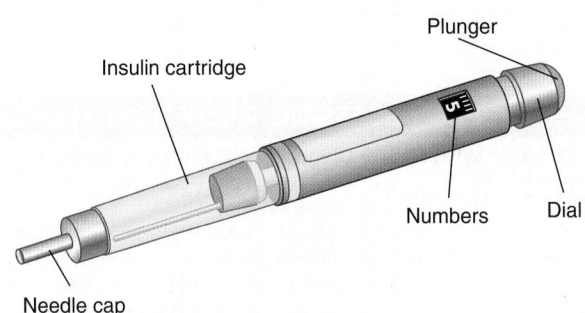

FIG. 52.7 Parts of an insulin pen.

absorption, rotation of injection sites to different anatomical sites is no longer the recommended practice. Instead, patients are advised to rotate the injection within one particular site, such as the abdomen. Sometimes, it is helpful to think of the entire abdomen as a checkerboard, with each square representing an injection site as the patient rotates sites systematically across the board.

Most commercial insulin is available as U100, indicating that 1 mL contains 100 units of insulin. U100 insulin must be used with a U100-marked syringe. Disposable, plastic insulin syringes are available in a variety of sizes, including 1, 0.5, and 0.3 mL. The 0.5-mL size may be used for doses of 50 units or less, and the 0.3-mL syringe can be used for doses of 30 units or less. Smaller syringes offer a number of advantages. The major benefit is increased accuracy and reliability when delivering smaller doses because wider line markings are easier to see. Patients should be cautioned to check dosage lines carefully when changing syringe types because some use a scale of one-unit increments and others use two-unit increments.

Recapping should be done only by the person using the syringe. The nurse must never recap a needle that has been used by a patient. The use of an alcohol swab on the site before self-injection is no longer recommended. Routine hygiene such as washing with soap and rinsing with water is adequate. This recommendation applies primarily to patient self-injection technique. When injection occurs in a health care facility, policy may dictate site preparation with alcohol to prevent hospital-acquired infection. Injection should be performed at a 45- to 90-degree angle, depending on the thickness of the patient's fat pad.

An insulin pen is a compact portable device that serves the same function as a needle and syringe but is handier to use (Figure 52.7). The insulin pen uses 300-unit cartridges, which are packaged in a box of five, for a total of 1 500 units. One of the advantages of insulin pens is that they are less "medical" looking. The insulin pen has a numerical dial-up device that clicks for each unit being dialed. The pen can dial up to a maximum of 60 to 70 units, depending on the device. This is a safer and more convenient option for most patients, especially those with visual impairment, dexterity challenges, and peripheral neuropathy. Pen-needle tips are finer than syringe tips and must be changed with every injection. They are manufactured in a variety of sizes—4, 5, 6, 8, and 12 to 12.7 mm—for a variety of body-fat types (FIT Canada, 2016).

Alternate Delivery Methods. Continuous subcutaneous insulin infusion can be administered using an insulin pump, a small battery-operated device that holds and delivers insulin (Figure 52.8). Usually worn on the belt, under clothing, or directly affixed to the body, the pump is connected to a catheter inserted into the subcutaneous tissue in the abdominal wall. Every 2 to 3 days, the insertion site is changed and the pump is refilled with insulin and reprogrammed. The device is programmed to deliver a continuous infusion of rapid-acting insulin 24 hours a day, known as the *basal rate*. Basal insulin can be temporarily increased or decreased on the basis of activity level changes or illness. At mealtime, the user programs the pump to deliver a bolus infusion of insulin appropriate to the amount of carbohydrate ingested and to bring down high premeal blood glucose, if necessary. A major advantage of the insulin pump is the

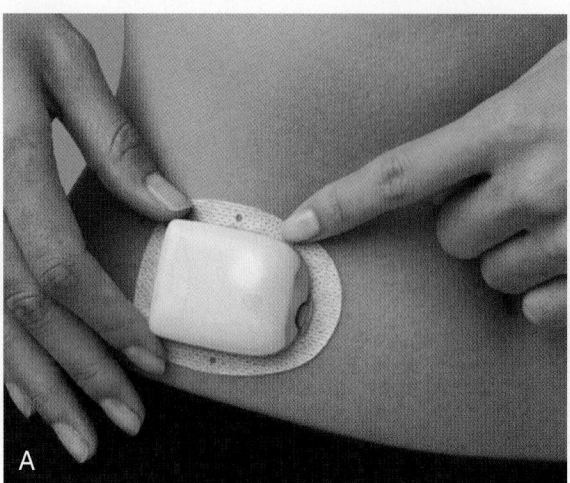
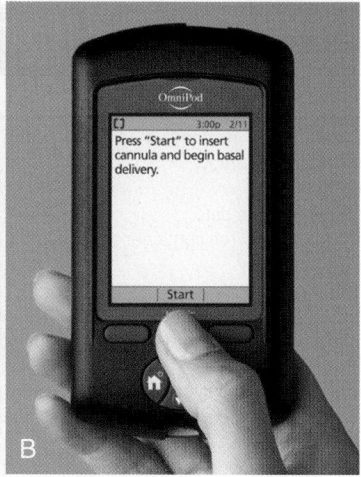

FIG. 52.8 A, The Omnipod® Insulin Management System is a tubeless, wireless, and waterproof pump that is affixed directly to the body and holds and delivers insulin. **B,** The Personal Diabetes Manager (PDM) wirelessly programs insulin delivery via the Pod. The PDM has a built-in glucose meter. Source: Courtesy Insulet Canada Corporation.

TABLE 52.6	ASSESSING THE PATIENT TREATED WITH ANTIHYPERGLYCEMIC AGENTS
For Patient With Newly Diagnosed Diabetes or Re-Evaluation of Medication Regimen	
Cognitive	Is the patient or a responsible other person able to understand that antihyperglycemic agents are being used as part of diabetes management?
	Is patient or responsible other person able to understand concepts of asepsis, combining insulins, insulin–OHA actions, and adverse effects?
	Is patient able to remember to take more than one dose per day?
	Does patient take medications at the right times in relation to meals?
Psychomotor	Is the patient or responsible other person physically able to prepare and administer accurate doses of the medication?
Affective	What emotions and attitudes are the patient and responsible others displaying in regard to the diagnosis of diabetes and antihyperglycemic treatment? Is the patient displaying acceptance of diagnosis of DM and readiness to learn?
For Follow-Up of Patient Treated With Antihyperglycemic Agents	
Effectiveness of therapy	Is the patient having symptoms of hyperglycemia or hypoglycemia?
	Does the blood glucose record show good or poor control?
	Is glycated hemoglobin (A_{1c}) consistent with glucose records?
Adverse effects of therapy	Has the patient had hypoglycemic episodes? If so, how often? What time of day? What was the precipitating event? Inconsistent meal timing, meal carbohydrate content, use of alcohol, or exercise?
	Are there reports of nightmares, night sweats, or early-morning headaches?
	Has the patient had skin rash, gastrointestinal upset, ankle edema, or weight gain since taking the antihyperglycemic agent?
	Is atrophy or hypertrophy present at injection sites?
Self-management behaviours	If the patient is having hypoglycemic episodes, how are those episodes managed? Has the patient analyzed episodes to determine the cause?
	How much insulin, OHA, or noninsulin injectable is the patient taking and at what time of day? Is the patient adjusting the medication dose? Under what circumstances and by how much?
	Has exercise pattern changed?
	Is the patient adhering to healthy eating recommendations? Are meals taken at times corresponding to peak insulin action? Is the patient performing SMBG?

DM, diabetes mellitus; *OHA,* oral antihyperglycemic agent; *SMBG,* self-monitoring of blood glucose.

reduction of hypoglycemia episodes. Pumps also offer the benefit of a more normal lifestyle, allowing users more flexibility with meal and activity patterns as insulin delivery becomes very similar to the normal physiological pattern. The insertion site should be checked daily for redness and swelling (Institute for Safe Medication Practices [ISMP] Canada, 2016).

Complications With Insulin Therapy. Hypoglycemia, allergic reactions, lipodystrophy, and Somogyi effect are the complications associated with insulin therapy. Hypoglycemia is discussed in detail later in this chapter. (Guidelines for assessing patients treated with insulin are presented in Table 52.6.)

Allergic Reactions. Local inflammatory reactions to insulin, such as itching, erythema, and burning around the injection site, may occur. Local reactions may be self-limiting within 1 to 3 months or may improve with a low dose of antihistamine. A true insulin allergy is a systemic response with urticaria and possibly anaphylactic shock, generally resulting from the use of animal insulins. Fortunately, this type of allergy is rare, particularly since human insulin has become available. Zinc and protamine—used as preservatives in the insulin and the latex rubber stoppers on the vials—have been implicated in insulin reactions.

Lipodystrophy. Lipodystrophy (hypertrophy or atrophy of subcutaneous tissue) may occur if the same injection sites are used frequently. *Hypertrophy,* a thickening of the subcutaneous tissue, eventually regresses if the patient does not use the site for at least 6 months. The use of hypertrophied sites may result in erratic insulin absorption. Lipodystrophies have been most commonly associated with beef, or beef and pork, insulin and rarely with human insulin.

Somogyi Effect and Dawn Phenomenon. Wide differences in early-morning (low) and fasting (high) glucose levels characterize the Somogyi effect. Usually occurring during the hours of sleep, the Somogyi effect is associated with a decline in blood glucose level in response to too much insulin. Counter-regulatory hormones are released, stimulating lipolysis, gluconeogenesis, and glycogenolysis, which in turn produce rebound hyperglycemia and ketosis. The danger of this effect is that, when blood glucose levels are measured in the morning, hyperglycemia is apparent, and the patient (or the health care provider) may therefore increase the insulin dose. The Somogyi effect is associated with the occurrence of undetected hypoglycemia during sleep, although it can happen at any time.

The patient may report headaches on awakening and may recall night sweats or nightmares. If the Somogyi effect is suspected as a cause for early-morning high blood glucose, the patient may be advised to check blood glucose levels between 0200 and 0400 hours to determine whether hypoglycemia is present at that time. If it is, the insulin dosage of administration affecting the early-morning blood glucose is reduced.

The *dawn phenomenon* is characterized by hyperglycemia that is present on awakening in the morning, owing to the release of counter-regulatory hormones in the predawn hours. It has been suggested that growth hormone and cortisol are possible factors in this occurrence. The dawn phenomenon affects the majority of people with DM and tends to be most severe when growth hormone is at its peak in adolescence and young adulthood.

Careful assessment is required to document each phenomenon because the treatment for each differs. The treatment for Somogyi effect is reduction of insulin dosage. The treatment for dawn phenomenon is an adjustment in the timing of insulin administration or an increase in insulin. The assessment must include insulin dose, injection sites, and variability in the time of meals or insulin administration. In addition, the patient is asked to measure and document bedtime, nighttime (between 0200 and 0400 hours), and morning FBG levels on several occasions. If the predawn levels are below 3.3 mmol/L and signs and symptoms of hypoglycemia are present, the insulin dosage should be reduced. If the 0200 to 0400–hour blood glucose level is high, the insulin dosage should be increased. In addition, the patient should be counselled on appropriate bedtime snacks (Brijesh, 2015).

Medication Therapy: Antihyperglycemic Agents

Oral antihyperglycemic agents and noninsulin injectables work to improve the mechanisms by which insulin and glucose are produced and used by the body. These medications work on three defects of type 2 diabetes: (1) insulin resistance, (2) decreased insulin production, and (3) increased hepatic glucose production. Oral antihyperglycemic agents and noninsulin injectables may be used in combination with agents from several classes or with insulin to achieve blood glucose targets. Guidelines for assessing patients receiving these medications are shown in Table 52.6.

Currently, many classes of antihyperglycemics are available to improve DM control for patients with type 2 DM (Diabetes Canada Clinical Practice Guidelines Expert Committee, 2018). These agents are listed in Table 52.7.

Insulin Secretagogues. *Sulphonylureas* have been widely used to treat type 2 DM since the 1950s. The primary action of the sulphonylureas is to increase β-cell insulin production from the pancreas. Caution must be exercised in dosage determination in older persons and patients with renal impairment because of the increased risk for hypoglycemia. Therapy with sulphonylureas is generally more effective early in the course of type 2 DM and is used as second-line therapy after metformin.

Meglitinides. Like the sulphonylureas, meglitinides (repaglinide [GlucoNorm]) increase insulin production from the pancreas. But because they are more rapidly absorbed and eliminated, they offer a reduced potential for hypoglycemia. When meglitinides are taken just before meals, pancreatic insulin production increases during and after the meal, mimicking the normal blood glucose response to eating. Patients should be instructed to take meglitinides anytime from 30 minutes before each meal right up to the time of the meal, and not to take a dose if they are not eating. They are safer to use in patients with irregular mealtimes.

Biguanides. Metformin (Glucophage) is the only biguanide glucose-lowering agent available worldwide. It can be used alone or with other OHAs, noninsulin injectables, or insulin to treat type 2 DM. The primary action of metformin is to reduce glucose production by the liver. It also enhances insulin sensitivity at the tissue level and improves glucose transport into the cells. Metformin is recommended as the first-line medication for most people with type 2 DM (Diabetes Canada Clinical Practice Guidelines Expert Committee, 2018). Besides being an effective blood glucose–lowering agent, metformin has other advantages. Unlike insulin secretagogues and insulin, metformin does not promote weight gain. It also has beneficial effects on plasma lipids. Metformin is also used to treat prediabetes, especially in individuals with obesity and who have impaired fasting glucose.

Patients who are undergoing surgery or any radiological procedures that involve the use of a contrast medium are instructed to temporarily discontinue metformin before surgery or the procedure. They should not resume the metformin until 48 hours afterward, once their serum creatinine has been checked and is found to be normal.

> **MEDICATION ALERT—Metformin**
> - Do not use in patients with stage 4 or 5 kidney disease or with an estimated glomerular filtration rate (eGFR) <30 mL/min, liver disease, or unstable heart failure. Lactic acidosis is a rare complication of metformin accumulation.
> - IV contrast media that contain iodine pose a risk for acute kidney injury, which could exacerbate metformin-induced lactic acidosis.
> - Avoid use in people who drink excessive amounts of alcohol.

α-Glucosidase Inhibitors. Also known as *starch blockers,* glucosidase inhibitors work by slowing down the absorption of carbohydrate in the small intestine. Acarbose (Glucobay) is the available medication in this class. Taken with the first bite of each main meal, they are most effective in lowering postprandial blood glucose. Effectiveness of these medications is measured by checking 2-hour postprandial glucose levels. Medications from this class are not effective against fasting hyperglycemia (Diabetes Canada Clinical Practice Guidelines Expert Committee, 2018).

TABLE 52.7 MEDICATION THERAPY

Antihyperglycemic Agents for Diabetes Mellitus

Type	Mechanism of Action	Adverse Effects
Insulin Secretagogues: Sulphonylureas		
Gliclazide (Diamicron, Diamicron MR) Glimepiride (Amaryl) Glyburide (Diabeta) (chlorpropamide and tolbutamide are available in Canada but rarely used)	Stimulate release of insulin from β cells; decrease glycogenolysis and gluconeogenesis; glimepiride may improve insensitivity in tissues	Weight gain, hypoglycemia
Meglitinide Repaglinide (GlucoNorm)	Stimulates a rapid and short-lived release of insulin from the pancreas	Less weight gain, decreased incidence of hypoglycemia compared with glyburide
Biguanide Metformin (Glucophage) Metformin ER (Glumetza)	Inhibits hepatic glucose production; increases peripheral and liver sensitivity to insulin	Nausea, upset stomach, diarrhea; less weight gain than sulphonylureas and does not cause hypoglycemia; potential lactic acidosis in renal or hepatic impairment; has to be held at the time of or before procedures and held for 48 hr after administration of IV contrast media
α-Glucosidase Inhibitors Acarbose (Glucobay)	Delays absorption of glucose and digestion of CHO in small intestine, lowering after-meal blood glucose levels	Flatulence, abdominal pain, diarrhea
Thiazolidinediones Pioglitazone (Actos) Rosiglitazone (Avandia)	↑ Glucose uptake in muscle and fat; inhibit hepatic glucose production	Edema, weight gain, heart failure; causes ovulation in premenopausal women with PCOS; not recommended for patients with heart failure
Dipeptidyl Peptidase-4 Inhibitors Sitagliptin (Januvia) Saxagliptin (Onglyza) Linagliptin (Trajenta) Alogliptin (Nesina)	Enhance the incretin system, stimulate release of insulin from pancreatic β cells, and inhibit hepatic glucose production	Upper respiratory tract infection, sore throat, headache, diarrhea
Noninsulin Injectable Agents: GLP-1 Receptor Agonists Liraglutide (Victoza) Exenatide (Byetta) Dulaglutide (Trulicity) Exenatide QW (Bydureon) Lixesenatide (Adlyxine) Semaglutide (Ozempic)	Stimulate release of insulin; decrease glucagon secretion, increase satiety, decrease gastric emptying	Nausea, vomiting, hypoglycemia, diarrhea, headache
Sodium-Glucose Cotransporter Type 2 (SGLT2) Inhibitors Canagliflozin (Invokana) Dapagliflozin (Forxiga) Empagliflozin (Jardiance) Ertugliflozin (Steglatro)	Enhance urinary glucose excretion	Genital infections, urinary tract infections, hypotension, increased lipids
Combination Therapy Avandamet (rosiglitazone [Avandia] and metformin [Glucophage]) Janumet/Janumet XR (sitagliptin [Januvia] and metformin/metformin XR [Glucophage/Glucophage XR]) Jentadueto (linagliptin [Trajenta] and metformin [Glucophage]) Kazano (alogliptin [Nesina] and metformin [Glucophage]) Komboglyze (metformin [Glucophage] and saxagliptin [Onglyza]) Oseni (alogliptin [Nesina] and pioglitazone [Actos]) Soliqua (glargine [Lantus] U100 and Lixisenatide [Adlyxine]) Xultophy (degludec [Tresiba] and liraglutide [Victoza]) Invokamet (canagliflozin [Invokana] and metformin [Glucophage]) Xigduo (Dapagliflozin [Forxiga] and metformin [Glucophage]) Glyxambi (empagliflozin [Jardiance] and linagliptin [Trajenta]) Synjardy (empagliflozin [Jardiance] and metformin [Glucophage]) Segluromet (ertugliflozin [Steglatro] and metformin [Glucophage]) Steglujan (ertugliflozin [Steglatro] and sitagliptin [Januvia])	See mechanism of action for individual medications, above	See adverse effects for individual medications, above

CHO, carbohydrates; *IV*, intravenous; *PCOS*, polycystic ovarian syndrome.

Thiazolidinediones. Sometimes referred to as *insulin sensitizers,* thiazolidinediones include pioglitazone (Actos) and rosiglitazone (Avandia). They are most effective for people who have insulin resistance. They improve insulin sensitivity, transport, and utilization at target tissues.

Because they do not increase insulin production, thiazolidinediones will not cause hypoglycemia when used alone, but the risk is still present when a thiazolidinedione is used in combination with insulin or an insulin secretagogue. Patients taking these medications may experience a secondary benefit of improved triglyceride, high-density lipoprotein (HDL), and blood pressure levels (Diabetes Canada Clinical Practice Guidelines Expert Committee, 2018).

Dipeptidyl Peptidase-4 Inhibitors. The dipeptidyl peptidase-4 (DPP-4) inhibitors includes sitagliptin (Januvia), saxagliptin (Onglyza), linagliptin (Trajenta), and alogliptin (Nesina). The incretin hormones, which are part of the physiological process that regulates glucose homeostasis, are normally inactivated by DPP-4. By inhibiting DDP-4, these medications slow the inactivation of incretin hormones. Incretin hormones are released by the intestines throughout the day, but levels increase in response to a meal. When glucose levels are normal or elevated, incretins increase insulin synthesis and release from the pancreas as well as decrease hepatic glucose production. DPP-4 inhibitors manage type 2 DM by increasing and prolonging increased incretin levels. These medications are glucose dependent (i.e., they respond to the presence of elevated glucose and result in insulin release only when needed); therefore, they lower the potential for hypoglycemia. The main benefit of these medications over other medications for DM with similar effects is the absence of weight gain as an adverse effect. These medications may be taken alone or in combination with other OHAs (Diabetes Canada Clinical Practice Guidelines Expert Committee, 2018; Merck Canada, 2021).

Sodium-Glucose Cotransporter 2 (SGLT2) Inhibitors. Canagliflozin (Invokana), dapagliflozin (Forxiga), empagliflozin (Jardiance), and ertugliflozin (Steglatro) are known as sodium-glucose cotransporter 2 (SGLT2) inhibitors. These medications work by blocking the reabsorption of glucose by the kidney, increasing glucose excretion, and lowering blood glucose levels (Lo et al., 2020). If metformin is contraindicated as first-line treatment, an SGLT2 inhibitor can be considered. These medications have shown benefit in reducing adverse cardiovascular and renal events and are recommended as second-line therapy in patients with established cardiovascular disease, heart failure, or renal disease or those over 60 years of age with two cardiovascular risk factors and whose A_{1c} is not at target (Liscombe et al, 2020).

Combination Therapy. Many combination medications are currently available. These medications combine two different classes of medications to treat DM. These agents are listed in Table 52.7. One advantage of combined therapy is improved patient adherence.

Glucagon-Like Peptide (GLP)-1 Receptor Agonists (Incretin Mimetics). Liraglutide (Victoza), exenatide (Byetta), exenatide QW (Bydureon), dulaglutide (Trulicity), lixisenatide (Adlyxine), and semaglutide (Ozempic) are the GLP-1 receptor agonists available in Canada. These medications stimulate GLP-1 (one of the incretin hormones), which is found to be decreased in people with type 2 DM. The mechanisms of action of these medications are similar to those performed by the incretin hormone it mimics. They stimulate the release of insulin from the pancreas β cells. Other mechanisms of actions are (1)

suppression of glucagon secretion from the pancreatic β cells, which reduces glucose output from the liver; (2) reduction of food intake by increasing satiety, thereby reducing caloric intake; and (3) slowing gastric emptying. GLP-1 receptor agonists are administered using a subcutaneous injection in a pre-filled pen (Eli Lilly Canada, 2021b; NovoNordisk, 2020). GLP-1 receptor agonists have demonstrated cardiovascular benefit and should be considered as second-line therapy in patients with established cardiovascular or renal disease or those over age 60 years with two cardiovascular risk factors and whose glycemic control is not yet achieved (Liscombe et al., 2020).

Other Medications Affecting Blood Glucose Levels. Both the patient and the health care provider must be aware of medication interactions that can potentiate hypoglycemic and hyperglycemic effects. For example, β-adrenergic blockers can mask symptoms of hypoglycemia and prolong the hypoglycemic effects of insulin. Thiazide and loop diuretics can potentiate hyperglycemia by inducing potassium loss, although low-dose therapy with a thiazide is usually considered safe.

Nutritional Therapy

Although nutritional therapy is the cornerstone of care for the person with DM, it is also its most challenging aspect. Nutritional therapy can reduce A_{1c} by an absolute 1 to 2% with the greatest impact at the initial stages of DM (Diabetes Canada Clinical Practice Guidelines Expert Committee, 2018). Achieving nutritional goals requires a coordinated team effort that takes into account the behavioural, cognitive, socioeconomic, cultural, and spiritual aspects of the person. Because of these complexities, it is recommended that a DM nurse educator and a registered dietitian with expertise in DM management be members of the team.

Nutritional therapy for the management of DM is based on a plan of healthy eating that is appropriate and beneficial for all members of the general population, whether they have DM or not. In an institutional setting, the prescribed diet is often labelled "diabetic diet" or "no added sugar," indicating that the meal plan follows the Canadian Diabetes Association's current nutritional recommendations.

Canada's Food Guide (see Chapter 42, Figure 42.1) summarizes and illustrates nutritional guidelines and nutrient needs. These are appropriate in guiding the food choices of people with DM. Nutritional therapy and meal planning should be individualized to accommodate the person's preferences, age, needs, culture, lifestyle, and readiness to change. Tools used to measure the effectiveness of nutritional therapy include blood glucose, A_{1c}, and lipid values; tests of renal status; and clinical measurements such as body weight, body mass index, waist circumference, and blood pressure (Diabetes Canada Clinical Practice Guidelines Expert Committee, 2018). Table 52.8 describes nutritional therapy for type 1 and type 2 DM.

Diabetes Canada provides a variety of nutrition teaching tools to assist health care providers. These are accessible online at the Diabetes Canada website or through the Diabetes Canada office. The resource entitled *Just the Basics: Healthy Eating for Diabetes Management and Prevention* is an example of such a tool (Diabetes Canada, 2018). It provides tips for healthy eating, DM prevention, and management for support until the person can see a dietitian. This tool highlights the need for the following:

1. Eating three meals per day at regular times and eating at intervals no more than 6 hours apart
2. Limiting sugars and sweets such as sugar, regular pop, desserts, candies, jam, and honey

TABLE 52.8   NUTRITIONAL THERAPY

Diabetes Mellitus

Factor	Type 1 Diabetes Mellitus	Type 2 Diabetes Mellitus
Total calories	Increase in caloric intake possibly necessary to achieve desirable body weight and restore body tissues	Reduction in caloric intake desirable for overweight or obese patient
Effect of diet	Diet and insulin necessary for glucose control	Diet alone possibly sufficient for glucose control
Distribution of calories	Equal distribution of carbohydrates through meals or adjustment of carbohydrates for insulin activity	Equal distribution recommended; low-fat diet desirable; consistency of carbohydrate at meals desirable
Consistency in daily intake	Necessary for glucose control	Desirable for weight reduction and moderation of blood glucose levels
Uniform timing of meals	Crucial for NPH insulin programs; flexibility with multidose rapid-acting insulin	Desirable but not essential, unless using insulin or sulphonylureas
Intermeal and bedtime snacks	Frequently necessary	Is based on patient's eating habits and preferences; may be necessary if using insulin or sulphonylureas
Nutritional supplement for exercise programs	Carbohydrates 20 g/hr for moderate physical activities	May be necessary if patient's blood glucose levels are controlled on sulphonylureas or insulin

NPH, neutral protamine Hagedorn.

3. Limiting the amount of high-fat food such as fried foods, chips, and pastries
4. Eating more high-fibre foods (whole-grain breads and cereals, lentils, dried beans and peas, brown rice, fruits, and vegetables)
5. Drinking water if thirsty as drink of choice
6. Adding physical activity to the lifestyle (Diabetes Canada Clinical Practice Guidelines Expert Committee, 2018)

Type 1 Diabetes Mellitus. Meal planning should be based on the individual's usual food intake and balanced with insulin and exercise patterns. The insulin regimen should be developed with the patient's eating habits and activity pattern in mind. Patients using rapid-acting insulin can make adjustments in dosage before the meal, based on the current blood glucose level and the carbohydrate content of the meal or snack. Intensified insulin therapy, such as multiple daily injections or the use of an insulin pump, allows considerable flexibility in food selection and can be adjusted for deviations from usual eating and exercise habits. All people with type 1 DM should be seen by a registered dietitian to learn about carbohydrate-counting strategies.

Type 2 Diabetes Mellitus. The emphasis for nutritional therapy in type 2 DM should be placed on achieving glucose, lipid, and blood pressure goals. Because 80 to 90% of people with type 2 DM are overweight, calorie and fat reduction is a goal. Weight loss has been shown to improve glycemic control by increasing insulin sensitivity and glucose uptake and decreasing hepatic glucose output (Diabetes Canada Clinical Practice Guidelines Expert Committee, 2018).

There is no one proven strategy or method that can be uniformly recommended. A nutritionally adequate meal plan with a reduction of total fat (especially saturated fats), an increase of fibre, and a decrease in simple sugars can bring about decreased calorie and carbohydrate consumption. Eating many small meals is another strategy that can be adopted to spread nutrient intake throughout the day. A weight loss of 5 to 7% of body weight often improves glycemic control, even if desirable body weight is not achieved. Weight loss is best attempted by a moderate decrease in calories and an increase in caloric expenditure. Regular exercise and learning new behaviours and attitudes can help facilitate long-term lifestyle changes. Monitoring of blood glucose levels, A_{1c}, lipids, and blood pressure provides feedback on how well the goals of nutritional therapy are being met.

Food Composition. DM has been called a disease of carbohydrate metabolism, but it is actually a general metabolic disorder involving three categories of energy-providing nutrients: carbohydrates, fats, and proteins. Therefore, the nutrient balance of a diabetic diet is essential to maintenance of blood glucose levels. The nutritional energy intake should be constantly balanced with the energy output of the individual, taking into account exercise and metabolic work of the body. The following are general recommendations for nutrient balance; each patient's individual meal plan should be developed with a dietitian and with their lifestyle and health goals in mind and be based on *Canada's Food Guide* (Diabetes Canada Clinical Practice Guidelines Expert Committee, 2018; Evert et al., 2019; Health Canada, 2021):

- *Protein:* 15 to 20% of energy. There is no evidence that usual protein intake (15–20% of energy) should be modified. Those with diabetic nephropathy should limit protein intake to 15% of energy and be monitored closely by a registered dietitian.
- *Fat:* less than 35% of energy. Combined saturated fats and trans-fatty acids should be reduced to less than 9% of energy intake. Polyunsaturated fat should be limited to less than 10% of energy intake. Foods rich in polyunsaturated omega-3 fatty acids and plant oils should be included.
- *Fibre:* approximately 30 to 50 g/day from a variety of food sources, including soluble and cereal fibres
- *Carbohydrate:* 45 to 60% of energy. Carbohydrates should include whole grains, fruits, vegetables, and low-fat milk. Patients should try to consume higher-fibre sources of carbohydrate. Less than 10% of daily energy should come from sucrose (sugar). Low-carbohydrate diets are not recommended for DM management.

Glycemic index (GI) is the term used to describe the rise in blood glucose levels after a person has consumed carbohydrate-containing food. The GI of foods was developed to compare the postprandial responses of the body with carbohydrate-containing foods. A GI of 100 refers to the response to 50 g of glucose or white bread in a normal person without DM. All other food with an equivalent carbohydrate value is measured against this standard. For example, the GI of an apple is 52, regular milk 27, baked potato 93, cornflake cereal 119, and baked beans 69 (American Diabetes Association [ADA], 2008) (see the Resources at the end of this chapter for an online calculator for GI).

The GI of carbohydrates should be considered when choosing them in a meal plan. Foods with a high GI (e.g., potatoes, white bread) will cause a sharp rise in blood glucose, whereas those with a low GI (e.g., brown rice) steadily increase blood glucose over a longer period. Although the GI affects blood glucose, the total amount of carbohydrates is more important than the source (Diabetes Canada Clinical Practice Guidelines Expert Committee, 2018).

Nutritive and non-nutritive sweeteners may be included in a healthy meal plan, in moderation. Non-nutritive sweeteners approved by Health Canada include the sugar substitutes, saccharin, aspartame, sucralose, acesulphame-K, steviol glycosides, tagatose, thaumatin, and cyclamate (Diabetes Canada Clinical Practice Guidelines Expert Committee, 2018).

Alcohol. Alcohol is high in calories, has no nutritive value, and can be a partner in contributing to hypertriglyceridemia. In addition, it has detrimental effects on the liver (see Chapter 46). The inhibitory effect of alcohol on glucose production by the liver can cause severe hypoglycemia in patients taking insulin or OHAs that increase insulin secretion. Hypoglycemia may occur up to 24 hours after alcohol consumption in those with type 1 DM. Because alcohol consumption can make blood glucose more difficult to control, patients should be encouraged to discuss their use of alcohol honestly with their health care providers (Diabetes Canada Clinical Practice Guidelines Expert Committee, 2018).

Alcohol can also cause other serious adverse effects when used in conjunction with certain OHAs used to treat DM. For example, there is a risk for lactic acidosis in patients with alcohol dependency and who use metformin. Alcohol consumption should be limited to less than 2 standard drinks per day (e.g., 142 mL 12% alcohol wine) and fewer than 10 per week for women and less than 3 standard drinks per day and fewer than 15 per week for men (Diabetes Canada Clinical Practice Guidelines Expert Committee, 2018). Alcohol can sometimes be incorporated into healthy eating if blood glucose is well controlled and if the patient is not on medications that will cause adverse effects. A patient can reduce the risk for alcohol-induced hyperglycemia or hypoglycemia by consuming alcohol with food, using sugar-free mixes, and drinking dry, light wines (Diabetes Canada Clinical Practice Guidelines Expert Committee, 2018).

Healthy Eating Education. Dietitians are the primary source of nutrition education. However, all members of the interprofessional team should be prepared to answer basic questions about healthy eating and DM. Access to a dietitian may not be possible for patients who live in remote areas, and nurses often assume responsibility for teaching basic dietary management. *Canada's Food Guide* (see Chapter 42, Figure 42.1) is a simple, accessible, and appropriate tool for health care team members to use to educate people with DM about nutrition.

An effective method of presenting the basics of meal planning is the *plate method*. This simple method helps the patient visualize the amount of vegetables, starch, and protein that should fill a dinner plate (Diabetes Canada Clinical Practice Guidelines Expert Committee, 2018). For lunch and dinner, one-half of the plate is filled with vegetables, one-fourth is filled with a starch, and one-fourth is filled with 60 to 90 g (2–3 oz) of lean meat or other protein source. A glass of low-fat milk and a small piece of fresh fruit complete the meal. The breakfast plate is filled halfway with starch, and one-fourth of the plate contains an optional protein. Low-fat milk and fresh fruit complete the breakfast. Assuming low-fat and nonfat foods are selected, following the plate method will provide a well-balanced diet.

Nutrition education should include the patient's family and significant others, and it is most effective to teach the person who will be cooking. However, it is important that the responsibility for making healthy food choices falls to the patient with DM. A support network of family and friends is the key to making successful and sustainable nutritional and lifestyle changes.

In an acute health care facility, the nutritional needs of the patient with DM vary slightly from the normal meal plans. Previously, standardized calorie-level meal patterns were used, but new alternatives are now being used, such as the consistent-carbohydrate DM meal plan. Under this system, meal plans are not created according to calorie levels, but instead are created with consistent carbohydrate content. For example, every day, each breakfast contains the same amount of carbohydrates as the previous day; the same method is used for lunch and dinner (Diabetes Canada Clinical Practice Guidelines Expert Committee, 2018).

Exercise

Regular, consistent exercise is considered an essential part of DM and prediabetes management. Exercise increases insulin sensitivity and can have a direct effect on lowering blood glucose levels. It also contributes to weight loss, which also decreases insulin resistance. The therapeutic benefits of regular physical activity may result in a decreased need for DM medicines in order to reach target blood glucose goals. Regular exercise may help reduce triglyceride and low-density lipoprotein (LDL) cholesterol levels, reduce blood pressure, and improve circulation (ADA, 2019; Diabetes Canada Clinical Practice Guidelines Expert Committee, 2018). Any new exercise program for the person with DM should be started only after medical clearance and should be started slowly, with gradual progression toward the desired goal. People with type 2 DM should accumulate at least 150 minutes of moderate-intensity aerobic activity—such as brisk walking, cycling, or dancing—each week, spread over at least 3 separate days. Performance of resistance exercises three times per week should also be encouraged in addition to aerobic exercise (Diabetes Canada Clinical Practice Guidelines Expert Committee, 2018).

Before starting an exercise program, all patients with DM should undergo a pre-exercise assessment by a health care provider and should be started slowly with gradual progression toward the desired goal (Diabetes Canada Clinical Practice Guidelines Expert Committee, 2018). Patients who use insulin and insulin secretagogues, such as sulphonylureas or meglitinides, are at increased risk for hypoglycemia when there is an increase in physical activity, especially if the patient exercises at the time of peak drug action or if food intake has not been sufficient to maintain adequate blood glucose levels. Hypoglycemia can also occur if a normally sedentary patient with DM has an unusually active day. The glucose-lowering effects of exercise can last up to 48 hours after the activity, so it is possible for hypoglycemia to occur during that time. It is recommended that patients who use medications that can cause hypoglycemia schedule exercise about 1 hour after a meal or have a 10- to 15-g carbohydrate snack before exercising. Several small carbohydrate snacks can be taken every 30 minutes during exercise to prevent hypoglycemia. Patients using medications that place them at risk for hypoglycemia should always carry a fast-acting source of carbohydrate, such as juice, glucose tablets, or hard candies, when exercising. Table 52.9 gives guidelines on the number of calories burned per hour for different activities. Monitoring the blood sugar level may be necessary before, during, and after exercise, especially for high-performance activities, to prevent hypoglycemia.

TABLE 52.9	ACTIVITIES THAT AFFECT CALORIC EXPENDITURE	
Light Activity (100–200 Kcal/Hr)	**Moderate Activity (200–350 Kcal/Hr)**	**Vigorous Activity (400–900 Kcal/Hr)**
• Driving a car • Fishing • Light housework • Secretarial work • Teaching • Walking casually	• Active housework • Bicycling (light) • Bowling • Dancing • Gardening • Golfing • Roller skating • Walking briskly	• Aerobic exercise • Bicycling (vigorous) • Hard labour • Ice skating • Outdoor sports • Running • Soccer • Tennis • Wood chopping

Although exercise is generally beneficial to blood glucose levels, strenuous activity can be perceived by the body as a stress, causing a release of counter-regulatory hormones, which results in a temporary elevation of blood glucose. As a result, hyperglycemia may occur in cases of poorly controlled type 2 DM or in patients with type 1 DM who exercise at a time of day when insulin action is waning. Some patients may have to inject a small bolus of rapid-acting or regular insulin if the blood glucose level is elevated before exercising to prevent progressive hyperglycemia. Furthermore, patients should exercise with caution if the blood glucose is elevated and there are no ketones. However, exercise should be postponed, and the patient should take additional insulin when the blood sugar is elevated and urine ketones are present (Diabetes Canada Clinical Practice Guidelines Expert Committee, 2018).

Monitoring Blood Glucose

Self-monitoring of blood glucose (SMBG) is a cornerstone of DM management. By providing a "real-time" blood glucose reading, SMBG enables the patient to make self-management decisions regarding diet, exercise, and medication. SMBG is also important for detecting episodic hyperglycemia and hypoglycemia.

Portable blood glucose monitors are used at the hospital bedside and by patients who perform SMBG independently. A wide variety of blood glucose monitors are available (Figure 52.9). Usually, disposable lancets are used to obtain a small drop of capillary blood (usually from a finger stick) that is placed onto a glucose testing strip. After a specified time, the monitor displays a digital reading of the blood glucose. The technology of SMBG is a rapidly changing field, with more convenient systems being introduced every year. Newer systems allow the user to collect blood from alternative sites such as the forearm or the palm but will not register rapidly changing blood glucose readings. Therefore, finger sticks are still recommended if symptoms of low blood glucose are present. The most advanced systems require 4 seconds to provide results with only 0.3 McL of capillary blood.

Continuous glucose monitoring (CGM) systems provide another route for monitoring glucose. They are used to measure glucose concentrations in the interstitial fluid. There are two devices available: the real-time CGM (personal) and the retrospective CGM (professional). There are two real-time CGM devices and one flash glucose monitor (FGM) available in Canada. The CGM system uses a sensor inserted under the skin. It displays glucose values continuously, with

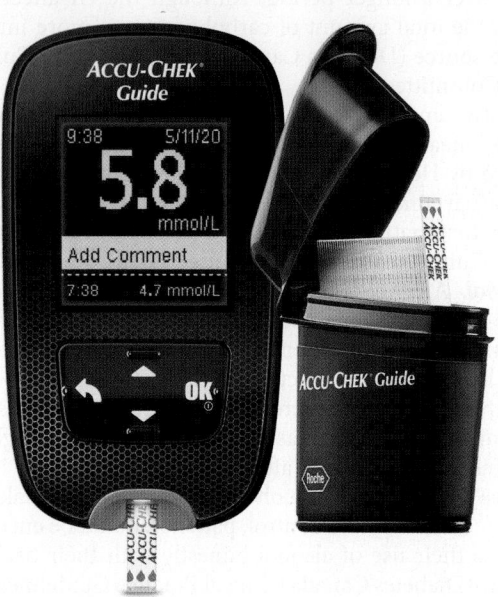

FIG. 52.9 A blood glucose monitor (Accu-Chek® Guide) is used to measure blood glucose levels. Source: Accu-Chek.

the values updating every 5 minutes. The sensor is inserted by the patient, using an automatic insertion device. Data are sent from the sensor to a transmitter, which displays the glucose value. CGMs can be used as a stand-alone device or with an insulin pump. The real-time CGMs currently available in Canada are the Medtronic Guardian Connect (stand-alone) and DexCom G6 (stand-alone or with insulin pump). The Medtronic Guardian Sensor 3 is also integrated with an insulin pump (Figure 52.10). The patient is alerted during episodes of hypoglycemia and hyperglycemia, prompting corrective action to be taken quickly. The retrospective CGM captures data but does not display them. CGM systems assist patients and health care providers in identifying trends and tracking patterns. These data are particularly useful for the management of insulin therapy. Some systems still require finger-stick measurements using a blood glucose monitor to calibrate the sensor and to make treatment decisions. The Freestyle Libre is the only FGM available in Canada. Users can wave a reader or smartphone over a subcutaneous sensor and obtain glucose readings at any time. It does not require calibrations with an SBGM as it is factory calibrated.

The blood glucose level reported by a laboratory is sometimes higher than that reported on the patient's home glucose monitor or the hospital's portable monitor. This is because some monitors give capillary blood glucose values from whole blood (via finger stick), whereas venous samples taken in the laboratory provide plasma readings. Plasma samples, or venous samples, are approximately 10 to 12% higher. Most monitors are automatically calibrated to give a "plasma" test result (even though whole blood was used for the sample) so that the home readings can be more readily compared with laboratory values. The literature accompanying a monitor will identify whether that particular monitor is calibrated to give plasma or whole blood readings.

Instructions for using a blood glucose monitor accompany each product. Because errors in monitoring technique can cause

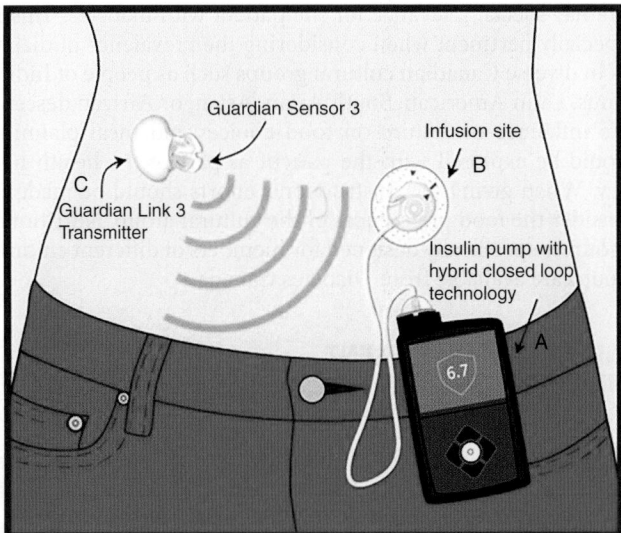

FIG. 52.10 The Medtronic MiniMed 670G Insulin Pump (A) delivers insulin through a thin plastic tubing to an infusion set, which has a cannula (B) that sits under the skin. Continuous glucose monitoring occurs through a tiny sensor (C) inserted under the skin. Sensor data are sent continuously to the insulin pump through wireless technology, giving a more complete picture of glucose levels, which can lead to better treatment decisions and better glucose control. Source: Medgadget, Inc.

TABLE 52.10	PATIENT & CAREGIVER TEACHING GUIDE

Obtaining a Capillary Sample for Blood Glucose Testing

The following instructions should be included when teaching the patient and caregiver about SMBG.

1. Wash hands with soap and warm water. It is not necessary to clean the site with alcohol, and it may interfere with test results by artificially lowering them.
2. If it is difficult to obtain an adequate drop of blood for testing, do any or all of the following: warm the hands in warm water, let the arm hang down for a few minutes before the finger puncture is made, use a new lancet with every puncture, or use a higher setting on the lancing device.
3. If the puncture is made on the finger, use the side of the finger pad rather than near the centre. There are fewer nerve endings along the side of the finger pad. If an alternative site is used (e.g., forearm), special equipment may be needed. Alternative-site testing is not recommended after a meal or for people with erratic blood glucose control experiencing hypoglycemia. Refer to manufacturer's instructions for alternative-site use.
4. The puncture should be only deep enough to obtain a sufficiently large drop of blood. Unnecessarily deep punctures may cause pain and bruising.
5. Lancets should be disposed of in designated "sharps" containers obtained from drug stores. Lancets and needles should not be placed in garbage cans, recycling bins, toilets, or glass jars.

SMBG, self-monitoring of blood glucose.

errors in management strategies, thorough patient education is crucial. Initial education should be followed up at regular intervals with reassessment. In addition, patients must be taught to use and interpret control solutions. Control solution should be used when first using a glucometer, when a new bottle of strips is used, or when there is a reason to believe that the readings are not correct. Lab-to-meter correlation should be done between SMBG and simultaneous venous FBG at least annually or when the A$_{1c}$ does not match SMBG readings, to ensure accuracy of SMBG. At blood glucose levels greater than 4.2 mmol/L, a difference of less than 20% is considered acceptable (Diabetes Canada Clinical Practice Guidelines Expert Committee, 2018). Table 52.10 lists the steps that should be taught to the patient learning to perform SMBG.

The primary advantage of SMBG is that it supplies immediate information about blood glucose levels that can be used to make adjustments in food intake, activity patterns, and medication dosages. It also produces accurate records of daily glucose fluctuations and trends and alerts the patient to acute episodes of hyperglycemia and hypoglycemia. Furthermore, SMBG provides patients with a tool for achieving and maintaining specific glycemic goals. SMBG is recommended as an essential part of daily DM management for all people using insulin or OHAs. The frequency of monitoring depends on several factors, including the patient's glycemic goals, the type of DM the patient has, the patient's ability and willingness to perform the test independently, and the treatment regimen. It is recommended that patients with type 1 DM test at least three times per day and include both preprandial and postprandial testing. Those using an insulin pump may test more frequently. People with type 2 DM treated with OHAs or lifestyle alone will have more variable and individualized testing regimens. For patients with type 2 DM treated with once-daily insulin and OHAs, monitoring at least once daily is recommended (Diabetes Canada Clinical Practice Guidelines Expert Committee, 2018).

Blood glucose testing should also be performed whenever hypoglycemia is suspected so that immediate action can be taken, if necessary. When the person with DM is ill, the blood glucose should be tested at 4-hour intervals to determine the effects of this stressor on the blood glucose level.

SMBG is an empowering tool that enables the patient to be an active partner in the treatment of DM. Achieving the desired level of patient participation can require time and effort from the health care provider. The nurse involved in this aspect of management should anticipate a close working relationship with patients as they refine their techniques and learn appropriate decision making about managing their DM. A patient who is visually impaired, cognitively impaired, or limited in manual dexterity needs careful evaluation of the degree to which SMBG can be performed independently. Nurses working in home health and outpatient settings may need to identify caregivers who can assume this responsibility. Adaptive devices are available to help patients with certain limitations. These include "talking meters" and other equipment for people who are visually impaired, as well as devices to stabilize insulin vials and syringes for those with limitations affecting dexterity.

Bariatric Surgery

Bariatric surgery may be considered for patients with type 2 diabetes who have a body mass index (BMI) greater than 40.0 kg/m^2 (class III obesity) or BMI greater than 35.0 to 39.9 kg/m^2 (class II obesity) and comorbidities, when lifestyle interventions are inadequate in achieving and maintaining healthy weight goals (Diabetes Canada Clinical Practice Guidelines Expert Committee, 2018) (see the Evidence-Informed Practice box). Patients with type 2 diabetes who have undergone bariatric surgery need lifelong monitoring and support. (Bariatric surgery is discussed in Chapter 43.)

EVIDENCE-INFORMED PRACTICE

Research Highlight

Bariatric Surgery for Adults With Type 2 Diabetes Who Are Living With Obesity

Clinical Question
In adults who are severely obese (P), what is the effectiveness and safety of bariatric surgery (I) compared with medical therapy (C) for remission from type 2 diabetes mellitus (O)?

Best Available Evidence
- Systematic review of randomized controlled trials (RCTs) and retrospective controlled cohort studies

Critical Appraisal and Synthesis of Evidence
- Systematic reviews of nine RCTs and eight retrospective controlled cohort studies (N = 32 250 participants)
- Diabetes remission (concentrations of plasma glucose, plasma insulin, and glycosylated hemoglobin return to normal without medication) within 2 years following the surgery
- One systematic review found that the diabetes remission rate was approximately six times higher in the surgical group as compared to the medical therapy group.
- Surgery significantly reduced risks for microvascular events (e.g., diabetic nephropathy, neuropathy, or retinopathy) by 48% and macrovascular events (e.g., angina, nonfatal myocardial infarction, and stroke) by 79% among patients with diabetes as compared to patients receiving only nonsurgical treatment.

Conclusion
- Bariatric surgery is a treatment option in severely obese patients with type 2 diabetes to improve diabetes control.

Implications for Nursing Practice
1. In addition to behavioural and medical approaches, bariatric surgery often normalizes blood glucose levels, reduces or avoids the need for medications, and provides a potentially cost-effective approach to treating the disease.
2. Bariatric surgery is an appropriate treatment for people with type 2 diabetes living with severe obesity who are not achieving recommended treatment targets with medical therapies, especially when there are other major comorbidities.

Reference for Evidence
Gyi, A. A. (2019). Type 2 diabetes mellitus: Bariatric metabolic surgery. *JBI Evidence Summary*, JBI21472.
P, patient population of interest; *I*, intervention or area of interest; *C*, comparison of interest or comparison group; *O*, outcomes of interest.

CULTURALLY COMPETENT CARE

DIABETES MELLITUS
The causes of diabetes are complex. Learning about the medical, social, and cultural factors is key to diabetes prevention. For example, it is important to understand the relationships between the history of colonization and the current high rates of diabetes among Indigenous peoples (Diabetes Canada Clinical Practice Guidelines Expert Committee, 2018). It is also important to involve Indigenous communities in developing diabetes prevention strategies to ensure that such strategies are culturally appropriate, promote empowerment, and are sustainable (Halseth, 2019). A key message from the 2018 Clinical Practice Guidelines regarding type 2 diabetes in Indigenous people is that a focus on building a therapeutic relationship with an Indigenous person with diabetes is essential, rather than just emphasizing obtaining management targets.

Because culture can have a strong influence on dietary preferences and meal preparation practices, culturally competent care has special relevance for the patient with diabetes. This is especially pertinent when considering the prevalence of diabetes in diverse Canadian cultural groups such as people of Indigenous, Latin American, South Asian, Asian, or African descent. The influence of culture on food choices and meal planning should be explored with the patient as part of the health history. When giving diet instructions, efforts should be made to consider the food preferences of the cultural group. Nutritional resources specifically designed for members of different cultural groups are available from Diabetes Canada.

NURSING MANAGEMENT DIABETES MELLITUS

NURSING ASSESSMENT
Table 52.11 provides initial subjective and objective data that might be obtained from a person with DM. After the initial assessment, periodic patient assessments should be done on a regular basis.

NURSING DIAGNOSES
Nursing diagnoses related to DM may include but are not limited to the following:
- *Inadequate health management* resulting from *insufficient resources* (deficient knowledge of diabetes management)
- *Potential for unstable blood glucose levels* as demonstrated by *insufficient diabetes management*
- *Potential for injury* as demonstrated by *insufficient knowledge of modifiable factors* (resulting in episodes of hypoglycemia)
- *Potential for peripheral neurovascular dysfunction* (resulting from vascular effects of diabetes)

Additional information on nursing diagnoses for the patient with diabetes is presented in Nursing Care Plan (NCP) 52.1, available on the Evolve website.

PLANNING
The overall goals for the patient with DM include the following: (a) to be an active participant in management of the DM regimen; (b) to experience few or no episodes of hypoglycemia or acute hyperglycemic emergencies; (c) to maintain blood glucose levels at normal or near-normal levels; (d) to prevent, minimize, or delay the occurrence of chronic complications of DM; and (e) to adjust their lifestyle to accommodate a DM regimen with a minimum of stress.

NURSING IMPLEMENTATION
HEALTH PROMOTION. The role of the nurse in health promotion and maintenance relates to the identification, monitoring, and education of the patient at risk for the development of DM. Obesity is the number one predictor of type 2 DM. Maintaining a healthy weight and exercising 30 to 60 minutes per day for most days of the week improve patient outcomes (Wexler, 2021).

Diabetes Canada recommends screening every 3 years in individuals 40 years of age or older or in individuals at high risk, identified by means of a risk calculator. It is important to screen earlier and more frequently in people with additional risk factors for diabetes or for those at very high risk using a risk calculator. The Canadian Diabetes Risk Assessment Questionnaire (CANRISK) is a statistically valid tool that may be suitable for diabetes risk assessment in the Canadian population and is

TABLE 52.11 NURSING ASSESSMENT

Diabetes Mellitus

Subjective Data

Important Health Information

Past health history: Mumps, rubella, coxsackievirus, or other viral infections; recent trauma, infection, or stress; pregnancy, gave birth to an infant >4 kg; chronic pancreatitis; Cushing's syndrome, acromegaly; family history of type 1 or type 2 diabetes mellitus; obesity

Date of last eye and dental examinations, adherence to diet for patients with previously diagnosed diabetes

Medications: Use of and adherence to insulin or OHA treatment; use of corticosteroids, diuretics, phenytoin (Dilantin)

Surgery or other treatments: Any recent surgery

Symptoms

- Constipation or diarrhea; frequent urination, nocturia, urinary incontinence
- Depression, irritability, apathy
- Erectile dysfunction; frequent vaginal infections; decreased libido
- Malaise
- Muscle weakness, fatigue
- Poor healing, especially involving the feet
- Thirst, hunger, nausea and vomiting
- Weight loss (type 1), weight gain (type 2)

Objective Data

Eyes

Vitreal hemorrhages; cataracts; soft, sunken eyeballs*

Integumentary

Dry, warm, inelastic skin; pigmented lesions (on legs); ulcers (especially on feet), loss of hair on toes; acanthosis nigricans

Respiratory

Rapid, deep respirations (Kussmaul's respiration)*

Cardiovascular

Hypotension*; weak, rapid pulse*, peripheral pulses diminished, feet pale and cool to touch

Gastrointestinal

Dry mouth, vomiting*, fruity breath*

Neurological

Altered reflexes, restlessness, confusion, stupor, coma, reduced sensation or vibration sense in feet

Musculoskeletal

Muscle wasting

Possible Findings

- Glucose level ≥7.0 mmol/L; glucose tolerance test ≥11.1 mmol/L; glycosylated hemoglobin ≥6.5%
- Urinalysis: glycosuria, ketonuria, microalbuminuria, or proteinuria
- Other: serum electrolyte abnormalities; acidosis; ↑ creatinine, ↑ total cholesterol, LDL, VLDL, and triglycerides; ↓ HDL; leukocytosis

*Indicates manifestations of ketoacidosis.
HDL, high-density lipoprotein; *LDL,* low-density lipoprotein; *OHA,* oral antihyperglycemic agent; *VLDL,* very-low-density lipoprotein.

TABLE 52.12 CRITERIA FOR SCREENING IN ASYMPTOMATIC, UNDIAGNOSED INDIVIDUALS

Type 1 Diabetes Mellitus

Screening presumably healthy individuals for the presence of any immune markers (e.g., HLA), outside of a clinical trial setting, is not recommended.

Type 2 Diabetes Mellitus

In asymptomatic, undiagnosed individuals, or those at high risk according to a risk calculator, screening* for diabetes should be considered in all individuals at ≥40 yr and, if normal, should be repeated at 3-yr intervals.

Screening should be considered at a younger age, or be carried out more frequently, in individuals who are at very high risk according to a risk calculator, or who have the following additional risk factors:

- Are members of a high-risk population (Indigenous or of Latin American, South Asian, Asian, or African descent)
- Are overweight, particularly with abdominal obesity
- Have a first-degree relative with type 2 diabetes
- Have a history of gestational diabetes mellitus
- Have a history of impaired fasting glucose or impaired glucose tolerance
- Have acanthosis nigricans
- Have complications associated with diabetes
- Have delivered a macrosomic infant (>4.4 kg)
- Have dyslipidemia
- Have hypertension
- Have polycystic ovary syndrome
- Have schizophrenia
- Have vascular disease

*Screening may include fasting blood glucose (FBG), glycated hemoglobin (A$_{1c}$), or both. A 75-g oral glucose tolerance test (OGTT) is indicated when the FBG is 6.1 mmol/L to 6.9 mmol/L or A$_{1c}$ is 6.0 to 6.4%, or both.
HLA, human lymphocyte antigen.
Source: Adapted from Diabetes Canada Clinical Practice Guidelines Expert Committee. (2018). Clinical practice guidelines for the prevention and management of diabetes in Canada. *Canadian Journal of Diabetes Care, 42*(Suppl 1), S17.

individuals who meet the criteria listed in Table 52.12 (Diabetes Canada Clinical Practice Guidelines Expert Committee, 2018).

ACUTE INTERVENTION. Acute situations involving the patient with DM include hypoglycemia, DKA, and hyperosmolar hyperglycemic state (HHS). Nursing management for these situations is discussed in more detail later in this chapter. Other areas of acute intervention relate to management during stress, such as during acute illness (e.g., SARS-CoV-2 infection) and surgery.

Stress of Acute Illness and Surgery. Both emotional and physical stress can increase the blood glucose level and result in hyperglycemia. Because it is impossible to totally avoid stress in life, certain situations may require more intense management, such as extra insulin, to maintain glycemic goals and prevent hyperglycemia.

Acute illness, injury, and surgery are situations that may evoke a counter-regulatory hormone response resulting in hyperglycemia. Even minor illnesses such as a viral upper respiratory infection or the flu can cause this. Studies have shown that people with diabetes and SARS-CoV-2 infection are at higher risk of developing severe symptoms and complications, including adult respiratory distress syndrome (ARDS) and pneumonia, and of dying (Diabetes Canada, 2020). When patients with DM are ill, they should continue with the regular meal plan while increasing the intake of noncarbohydrate-containing fluids, such as broth, water, and other decaffeinated beverages. They should also continue taking OHAs and insulin as prescribed and check blood

available at http://healthycanadians.gc.ca/diseases-conditions-maladies-affections/disease-maladie/diabetes-diabete/canrisk/index-eng.php.

The FBG, A$_{1c}$, or both are the preferred methods for screening in clinical settings; however, the 75-g OGTT is indicated in those with IFG or when A$_{1c}$ is 6.0 to 6.4%. Screening should be considered at a younger age or be carried out more frequently in glucose at least every 4 hours around the clock. With type 1 DM, if the glucose is greater than 14 mmol/L, urine should be tested for ketones every 3 to 4 hours. Patients should report moderate to large ketone levels to the health care provider.

When the illness causes the patient to eat less than normal, the patient should continue to take OHAs, noninsulin injectables, and insulin as prescribed, while supplementing food intake with carbohydrate-containing fluids. Examples include soups, juices, and regular decaffeinated soft drinks. The health care provider should be notified promptly if the patient vomits more than twice in 12 hours or has diarrhea causing dehydration, as the patient may need to go to the emergency department. The patient should understand that certain medication for DM, including insulin, should not be withheld during times of illness because counter-regulatory mechanisms often increase the blood glucose level dramatically. However, patients who are on metformin, sulphonylureas, or SGLT2i should not take these medications when ill and dehydrated (e.g., experiencing vomiting and diarrhea) or unable to drink enough fluid to maintain hydration, as doing so increases the risk for a decline in kidney function and adverse effects. Food intake is also important during this time because the body requires extra energy to cope with the stress of the illness. Extra insulin may be necessary to meet this demand and to prevent the onset of DKA in the patient with type 1 DM (Diabetes Canada Clinical Practice Guidelines Expert Committee, 2018).

During the perioperative period, adjustments in the DM regimen can be planned to ensure glycemic control. For patients undergoing major surgery who require insulin (type 1 or type 2 DM), intravenous (IV) fluids with dextrose and insulin are administered immediately before, during, and after surgery. For patients undergoing minor or moderate surgery who require insulin (type 1 or type 2 DM), recommendations are provided by the health care provider to reduce the insulin dosage the night before and the day of surgery. For patients taking OHAs who are undergoing major, moderate, or minor surgery, DM medications may be put on hold for as long as 24 hours before the day of surgery, and IV fluids with dextrose and insulin may be administered. The patient should understand that this is a temporary measure and is not to be interpreted as a worsening of DM. Patients who are undergoing surgery or any radiological procedures that involve the use of a contrast medium are instructed to hold their metformin (Glucophage) at the time of or before surgery or the procedure. They will also be instructed not to resume the metformin (Glucophage) until 48 hours after the surgery or procedure and after their serum creatinine has been checked and is normal (Sanofi-Aventis, 2018).

The nurse caring for an unconscious surgical patient receiving insulin must be alert for signs of hypoglycemia, such as sweating, tachycardia, and tremors. Frequent monitoring of blood glucose will prevent episodes of severe hypoglycemia in such a patient (Diabetes Canada Clinical Practice Guidelines Expert Committee, 2018).

AMBULATORY AND HOME CARE. Successful management of DM requires ongoing interaction among the patient, the family, and the health care team. It is important that a DM nurse educator be involved in the care of the patient and the family. This person provides expertise in many areas of specialized care needs.

Because DM is a complex, chronic condition, a great deal of patient contact takes place in outpatient and home settings. The major goal of patient care in these settings is to enable the patient or caregiver to reach an optimal level of independence in self-care activities. Unfortunately, many patients with DM face challenges in reaching these goals. DM increases the risk for other chronic conditions that can affect self-care activities. These include visual impairment, lower extremity conditions that affect mobility, and other functional limitations related to cardiovascular disease. Therefore, important nursing functions are to assess the ability of patients and caregivers in such activities as meal preparation, SMBG, safe administration of OHAs, and insulin injection techniques. Assistive devices for self-administration of insulin include syringe magnifiers, vial stabilizers, and dose-preparation aids for people who are visually impaired, as well as pill organizers for those taking OHAs. In some cases, the nurse will make referrals to others who can help the patient achieve the self-care goals. These may include a community health nurse, pharmacist, dietitian, occupational therapist, or social worker.

A diagnosis of DM affects the patient in many profound ways. Patients with DM must continually contend with lifestyle choices that affect the food they eat, the activities they engage in, and the demands on their time and energy. In addition, they face the prospect of the devastating complications of this disease. Careful assessment of what it means to the patient to have DM should be the starting point of patient teaching. The nurse can help patients make adjustments, by displaying an attitude that is supportive and nonjudgemental. The goals of teaching should be collaboratively determined by the patient and the nurse, based on individual needs as well as therapeutic requirements.

The patient's support system must be identified. The family or other members of the support system need to be involved in teaching so they can care for the patient when self-care is no longer possible. The family and significant others need to be encouraged to provide emotional support and encouragement as the patient comes to terms with the reality of living with a chronic disease.

Insulin Therapy. Nursing responsibilities for the patient receiving insulin include proper administration, assessment of the patient's response to insulin therapy, and education of the patient in administration of, adjustment to, and adverse effects of insulin (Table 52.13). Table 52.6 lists guidelines for the nurse assessing a patient using OHAs and insulin.

Assessment of the patient who is new to insulin administration must include an evaluation of the patient's ability to manage this therapy safely. This includes the ability to understand the interaction of insulin, diet, and activity and to be able to recognize and treat the symptoms of hypoglycemia appropriately. If the patient does not have the cognitive skills to do these things, another responsible person must be identified and educated. The patient or caregiver must also have the cognitive and the manual skills needed to prepare and inject the insulin. If the patient or family lacks these, additional resources will be needed to assist the patient.

Many patients are fearful when they first begin using insulin. Some patients find it difficult to self-inject because they are afraid of needles or the pain associated with an injection. Some are afraid they will hurt themselves by giving too much or too little insulin. And in some cases, the patient believes that using insulin is a "last ditch" effort and that they are now in the final stages of the disease process. Therefore, it is important to explore the patient's underlying fears before beginning the teaching (Allen et al., 2017; RNAO, 2009).

TABLE 52.13   PATIENT & CAREGIVER TEACHING GUIDE

General Guidelines for the Management of Diabetes Mellitus

When teaching patients and caregivers about the management of diabetes mellitus, the nurse should:

Disease Process
- Determine the patient's readiness to learn.
- Include an introduction about the pancreas and the islets of Langerhans.
- Describe how insulin is made and what affects its production.
- Discuss the relationship between insulin and glucose.
- Explain the difference between type 1 and type 2 diabetes.

Physical Activity
- Determine patient's readiness to change.
- Help the patient identify realistic goals of and barriers to physical activity.
- Discuss the importance of regular exercise on the management of blood glucose, improvement of cardiovascular function, and general health.

Menu Planning
- Individualize meal plans to accommodate the patient's age, type and duration of diabetes, concurrent medical therapies, treatment goals, values, preferences, needs, culture, lifestyle, economic status, activity level, readiness to change, and abilities.
- Educate the patient on the importance of a well-balanced diet as part of a diabetes management plan.
- Explain the impact of carbohydrates on the glycemic index and blood glucose levels.

Medication Adherence
- Ensure that the patient is well educated on the proper use of insulin (see Table 52.5), noninsulin injectables, and oral agents.
- Account for any limitations or inabilities for self-medication on the patient's part. If necessary, involve the family or caregiver in proper use of medication.
- Discuss all adverse effects and safety issues regarding medication, including sick-day management.

Monitoring Blood Glucose
- Individualize the frequency of monitoring to the patient's unique circumstances.
- Teach how to correctly monitor blood glucose levels.
- Include when blood glucose levels should be checked, how to record them, and, if appropriate, how to adjust insulin levels accordingly.
- Teach how behaviour and actions affect results.

Risk Reduction
- Ensure that the patient understands and appropriately responds to the signs and symptoms of hypoglycemia and hyperglycemia (see Table 52.15).
- Stress the importance of proper foot care (see Table 52.20), regular eye examinations, and consistent glucose monitoring.
- Inform the patient about the effect that stress can have on blood glucose.

Psychosocial
- Help the patient identify what is important to them.
- Advise the patient of resources that are available to facilitate the adjustment and to answer questions about living with a chronic condition such as diabetes (see Resources at the end of this chapter).

Follow-up assessment of the patient who has been using insulin therapy includes an inspection of injection sites for signs of lipodystrophy and other reactions; review of insulin preparation, storage, timing, and injection technique; a history of hypoglycemic episodes; and review of the patient's method for handling hypoglycemic episodes. A review of the patient's recorded blood glucose tests is also important in assessing overall glycemic control.

Oral and Noninsulin Injectable Agents. Nursing responsibilities for the patient taking OHAs and noninsulin injectables are similar to those for the patient taking insulin. Proper administration, assessment of the patient's use of and response to these medications, and education of the patient and the family about OHAs and noninsulin injectables are all part of the nurse's function.

The nurse's assessment can be extremely valuable in determining the most appropriate antihyperglycemic agent for a patient. Factors such as the patient's financial situation, cognitive status, eating habits, home environment, attitude toward DM, and medication history all play a significant role in determining the most appropriate OHA for the individual patient. For example, frail older people who live alone are at high risk for severe hypoglycemia because low blood glucose is frequently undetected and untreated in this population. This is especially true if the patient has a short-term memory deficit. In these cases, an OHA that does not cause hypoglycemia, or a shorter-acting OHA, would be most appropriate.

Patient education is an essential nursing function when caring for the patient who uses OHAs for blood glucose control. Some patients may assume that their DM is not a serious condition if they are taking "only a pill" for glycemic control. Therefore, the patient should be instructed that these agents will help keep blood glucose controlled and will help prevent serious long- and short-term complications of DM. Patients should be instructed that OHAs and noninsulin injectables are used in addition to healthy eating and activity as therapy for DM and that they should continue with their meal and activity plans. Patients should not take extra pills if overeating has occurred unless specifically instructed to do so by their health care provider. If the patient uses insulin secretagogues, instructions should be given regarding prevention, symptom recognition, and management of hypoglycemia.

The patient should also be instructed to contact a health care provider if periods of illness or extreme stress occur. During such a period, insulin therapy may be required to prevent or treat hyperglycemic symptoms and avoid an acute hyperglycemic emergency.

Personal Hygiene. The potential for microvascular complications and infections necessitates that the patient practise diligent skin and dental hygiene. Because of the susceptibility to periodontal disease, daily tooth brushing and flossing should be encouraged, in addition to regular visits to the dentist. When dental work must be done, the dentist should be informed that the patient has DM.

Routine care should include an emphasis on foot care, including daily assessment of feet (Botros et al., 2019; Diabetes Canada Clinical Practice Guidelines Expert Committee, 2018). Conditions associated with the feet and the lower extremities are presented later in this chapter. If cuts, scrapes, or burns occur, they should be treated promptly and monitored carefully. The area should be washed, and a nonabrasive or nonirritating antiseptic ointment may be applied. The area should be covered

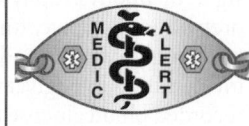

I have DIABETES

If unconscious or behaving abnormally, I may be having a reaction associated with diabetes or its treatment.

If I can swallow, give me a sweet drink, orange juice, LifeSavers, or low-fat milk.

If I do not recover promptly, call a physician or send me to the hospital.

If I am unconscious or cannot swallow, do not attempt to give me anything by mouth, but call 911 or send me to the hospital immediately.

FIG. 52.11 Medical alerts. A patient with diabetes should carry a card and wear a bracelet or necklace that indicates diabetes. If the patient with diabetes is unconscious, these measures will ensure prompt and appropriate attention.

with a dry, sterile pad. If the injury does not begin to heal within 24 hours, or if signs of infection develop, the health care provider should be notified immediately.

Medical Identification and Travel. Patients should be instructed to carry medical identification at all times indicating that they have DM (Figure 52.11). Police, paramedics, and many private citizens are aware of the need to look for this identification when working with someone who is sick or unconscious. Every person with DM should wear a medical alert bracelet or necklace. An identification card or phone app not requiring a password can supply valuable information, such as the name of the health care provider and the type and dose of insulin, non-insulin injectables, or OHA.

Travel for a patient with DM requires advance planning. The patient should have a full set of DM care supplies in the carry-on luggage when travelling by plane, train, or bus. This includes blood glucose monitoring equipment, insulin, and pen needles or syringes. When pen needles, syringes, and lancing devices are carried onto a commercial airliner, a letter from the prescribing health care provider indicating medical necessity may prevent delays at security checkpoints. Screeners should be notified if an insulin pump is used so they can inspect it while it is on the body, rather than remove it.

For patients who use insulin or an OHA that can cause hypoglycemia, snack items and a fast-acting carbohydrate source for treating hypoglycemia should be included in the carry-on luggage and on the person at all times. Extra insulin should be available in case a vial or cartridge breaks or gets lost. In addition, the patient should carry a full day's supply of food to be prepared for possibly cancelled flights, delayed meals, and closed restaurants. If the patient is planning a trip out of the country, it is wise to have a letter from the health care provider explaining that the patient has DM and requires all the materials being transported, particularly pen needles and syringes, for ongoing health care.

Some travel involves significant time changes, such as travelling coast to coast or across the International Date Line. The patient should contact the DM health care provider to plan an appropriate meal and insulin schedule. During travel, most patients find it helpful to keep watches set to the time of the city of origin until they reach their destination, and then switch to travel destination time as soon as possible. The key to travel when taking insulin is to know the type of insulin being taken, its onset of action, the anticipated peak time, and mealtimes.

Patient and Caregiver Teaching. The goals of DM self-management education are to enable the patient to become the most active participant in their own care, while matching level of self-management to the ability of the individual patient. Patients who actively manage their DM care have better outcomes than those who do not. For this reason, an educational approach that facilitates informed decision making on the part of the patient is widely advocated. Sometimes, this is referred to as the *empowerment approach* to education.

Unfortunately, patients can encounter a variety of physical, psychological, emotional, and socioeconomic barriers when it comes to effectively managing their DM. These barriers may include feelings of inadequacy about their abilities, unwillingness to make the necessary behavioural changes, ineffective coping strategies, lack of resources, and cognitive deficits. If the patient is not able to manage the disease, a family member may be able to assume part of this role. If the patient or the family cannot make decisions related to DM management, the nurse may refer the patient to a social worker or other resources within the community. These resources can assist the patient and the family in outlining a feasible treatment program that meets their capabilities. Patient and health care provider resources are listed at the end of this chapter in the Resources section.

An assessment of the patient's knowledge of DM and lifestyle preferences is useful in planning a teaching program. Tables 52.13 and 52.14 present guidelines to use for patient and caregiver teaching (See the Informatics in Practice box on using gaming for patient teaching). The nurse should assess the patient's knowledge base frequently so that gaps in knowledge or incorrect or inaccurate ideas can be quickly corrected.

Diabetes Canada offers pamphlets, booklets, and a bimonthly magazine called *Diabetes Dialogue*. Chapters of Diabetes Canada are located in all major Canadian cities, and most can be reached by accessing Diabetes Canada online. Diabetes Canada also publishes research and education materials and sponsors conferences for health care providers involved in DM education, research, and management of patients. The *Clinical Practice Guidelines for the Prevention and Management of Diabetes in Canada* (Diabetes Canada Clinical Practice Guidelines Expert Committee, 2018) are revised every 5 years (see the Resources at the end of this chapter). Prepared under the leadership of the Clinical and Scientific Section of the Canadian Diabetes Association/Diabetes Canada, the guidelines represent the contributions of more than 99 experts from a broad range of health care disciplines. These experts have evaluated and graded the international literature on the best evidence to guide screening, prevention, diagnosis, care, management, and education for Canadians living with type 1 and type 2 DM and GDM. Diabetes Canada also gives recognition to education programs that meet the international standards of DM education and can provide a list of these programs. Pharmaceutical and diagnostic companies specializing in DM-related products also have promotions and free educational materials for patients and health care providers.

EVALUATION

The expected outcomes for the patient with DM are addressed in NCP 52.1, available on the Evolve website.

TABLE 52.14 PATIENT & CAREGIVER TEACHING GUIDE

Instructions for Patients With Diabetes Mellitus

Do	Do Not	Do	Do Not
Blood Glucose • Monitor your blood glucose at home and record results in a log. • Take your insulin, OHA, or noninsulin injectable (or any combination) as prescribed. • Rotate injection site areas weekly. • Obtain an A_{1c} blood test every 3–6 mo as an indicator of your long-term blood glucose control. • Know signs and symptoms of hypoglycemia and hyperglycemia. • Carry some form of rapid-acting glucose at all times so you can treat hypoglycemia quickly. • Instruct family members in the use of glucagon administration in the case of emergencies due to severe hypoglycemia.	• Skip doses of your insulin, especially when you are sick. • Run out of insulin. • Ignore the symptoms of hypoglycemia and hyperglycemia.	**Nutrition** • Follow a healthy eating plan, and eat regular meals at regular times. • Choose foods low in saturated and trans-fats and high in fibre. • Limit the amount of alcohol you drink. • Know your cholesterol level.	• Drink excessive amounts of alcohol, because this may lead to unpredictable low blood glucose reactions and high triglycerides. • Follow a fad diet. • Drink regular pop or lots of fruit juices.
Exercise • Learn how exercise and food affect your blood glucose levels. • Begin an exercise program after approval from a health care provider.	• Forget that exercise will lower your blood glucose level. • Exercise if your blood glucose levels are very elevated. This may lead to a temporary worsening of your blood glucose levels.	**Other Guidelines** • Obtain an annual eye examination by an ophthalmologist. • Obtain annual urine testing for protein. • Examine your feet at home, daily. • Change socks daily. • Trim nails straight across. • Wear well-fitting shoes to help prevent foot injury. Break in new shoes gradually. • Always carry identification that says you have diabetes. • Have other medical conditions treated, especially high blood pressure and high cholesterol. • Quit smoking. • Have an annual influenza vaccination.	• Smoke cigarettes. • Go barefoot. • Put baby oil or lotion between your toes. • Ignore the signs of infection. • Apply hot or cold directly to your feet. • Wear tight socks, garters, or elastics or knee-highs.

OHA, oral antihyperglycemic agent.

 COMPLEMENTARY & ALTERNATIVE THERAPIES

Herbs and Supplements That May Affect Glucose Levels

Possible Hypoglycemic Herbs and Supplements*
• Aloe, α-lipoic acid, fish oils, goldenseal, bilberry eleuthero, ginseng, milk thistle, Chinese cinnamon *(Cinnamomum cassia)*, chromium, garlic, and sage

Possible Hyperglycemic Herbs and Supplements*
• St. John's wort, celery seed, rosemary, and melatonin

Nursing Implications
• It is very important that patients with diabetes consult with their health care providers before using natural health products such as herbs, probiotics, or nutritional supplements. Patients who use herbs should monitor their blood glucose levels carefully and regularly. The Diabetes Canada Clinical Practice Guidelines Expert Committee (2018) does not recommend the use of natural health products for the management of diabetes as there is insufficient evidence regarding its safety and efficacy.

*https://naturalmedicines.therapeuticresearch.com/

ACUTE COMPLICATIONS OF DIABETES MELLITUS

Acute complications of DM arise from events associated with *hyperglycemia* or *hypoglycemia*. Hypoglycemia is also referred to as an *insulin reaction* or *low blood glucose*. It is important for the health care provider to be able to distinguish between hyperglycemia and hypoglycemia because hypoglycemia worsens

---

INFORMATICS IN PRACTICE

Patient Teaching Using Gaming

• Teaching is a critical part of nursing care for patients with diabetes. It is possible to put some fun into patient teaching by using gaming applications.
• Patients can try an application with a quiz-show format. The patient answers questions about diabetes and then compares their answers in real time to those of other players. The questions (e.g., How does exercise affect insulin?) are written to help the patient learn to manage diabetes on a daily basis.
• Players in online simulations become either a caregiver to or a patient with type 1 DM. Players earn rewards by properly managing blood glucose levels.

rapidly and constitutes a serious threat if action is not immediately taken. Table 52.15 compares manifestations, causes, treatment, and prevention of hyperglycemia and hypoglycemia.

DIABETIC KETOACIDOSIS

Etiology and Pathophysiology

Diabetic ketoacidosis (DKA) is an acute metabolic complication of DM occurring when fats are metabolized in the absence of insulin. It is caused by a profound deficiency of insulin and is characterized by hyperglycemia, ketosis, metabolic acidosis, and dehydration (volume depletion). It is most likely to occur in people with type 1 DM but may be seen in type 2 DM in conditions of severe illness or stress, when the pancreas cannot

TABLE 52.15	COMPARISON OF HYPERGLYCEMIA AND HYPOGLYCEMIA		
Hyperglycemia	**Hypoglycemia**	**Hyperglycemia**	**Hypoglycemia**
Manifestations*		**Treatment**	
• Abdominal cramps • Blurred vision • Elevated blood glucose[†] • Glycosuria • Headache • Increase in appetite followed by lack of appetite • Increase in urination • Nausea and vomiting • Progression to DKA or HHS • Weakness, fatigue	• Blood glucose <4.0 mmol/L • Changes in vision • Cold, clammy skin • Emotional changes • Faintness, dizziness • Headache • Hunger • Nervousness, tremors • Numbness of fingers, toes, mouth • Rapid heartbeat • Seizures, coma • Unsteady gait, slurred speech	• Check blood glucose frequently; check urine for ketones; record results • Continuation of OHA or insulin as ordered; may need an increase in dose • Get medical care • Hourly drinking of fluids • IV fluids may be necessary	• Discussion with health care provider about insulin or OHA dosage • Follow up with a snack if regular meal is more than 1 hr away, and contact health care provider if there is no effect • Immediate ingestion of 15–20 g of simple carbohydrates • Ingestion of another 15–20 g of simple carbohydrates in 15 min if no relief obtained
Causes		**Preventive Measures**	
• Corticosteroids • Emotional, physical stress • Illness, infection • Inactivity • Poor absorption or lack of insulin • Too little or no diabetes medication • Too much food	• Alcohol intake without food • Diabetes medication or food taken at wrong time • Loss of weight without change in medication • Too little food—delayed, omitted, inadequate intake • Too much diabetic medication • Too much exercise without compensation • Use of β-adrenergic blockers interfering with recognition of symptoms	• Accurate administration of insulin, noninsulin injectables, and OHA • Adherence to sick-day rules when ill • Checking of blood for glucose as ordered • Contacting of health care provider regarding ketonuria • Maintenance of diet • Maintenance of good personal hygiene • Taking prescribed dose of medication at proper time • Wearing medical alert bracelet (diabetes)	• Ability to recognize and know symptoms and treat them immediately • Accurate administration of insulin, noninsulin injectables, and OHA • Carrying a snack of simple carbohydrates • Checking blood glucose as ordered • Education of friends, family, fellow employees about symptoms and treatment • Ingestion of all recommended foods at proper time • Provision of compensation for exercise • Taking prescribed dose of medication at proper time • Wearing medical alert bracelet (diabetes)

DKA, diabetic ketoacidosis; *HHS*, hyperosmolar hyperglycemic state; *IV*, intravenous; *OHA*, oral antihyperglycemic agent.
*There is usually a gradual onset of symptoms in hyperglycemia and a rapid onset in hypoglycemia.
[†]Specific clinical manifestations related to elevated levels of blood glucose vary according to the patient.

meet the extra demand for insulin. Precipitating factors include illness, infection, inadequate insulin dosage, insulin omission, undiagnosed type 1 DM, and poor self-management.

When the circulating supply of insulin is insufficient, glucose cannot be properly used for energy, so the body breaks down fat stores as a secondary source of fuel (Figure 52.12). Ketones are acidic by-products of fat metabolism that can cause serious health problems when they become excessive in the blood. Ketosis alters the pH balance, causing metabolic acidosis to develop. Ketonuria is a process that begins when ketone bodies are excreted in the urine. During this process, electrolytes become depleted as cations (sodium, potassium, and ammonium salts) are eliminated along with the anionic ketones in an attempt to maintain electrical neutrality.

Insulin deficiency impairs protein synthesis and causes excessive protein degradation. This condition results in nitrogen losses from the tissues. Insulin deficiency also stimulates the production of glucose from amino acids (from proteins) in the liver and leads to further hyperglycemia. But because there is a deficiency of insulin, the additional glucose cannot be used and the blood glucose level rises further, adding to the osmotic diuresis. In osmotic diuresis, this additional amount of glucose enters the renal tubules and draws a large amount of water that leads to an increase in urine output. Untreated, this condition leads to severe depletion of sodium, potassium, chloride, magnesium, and phosphate. Potassium is most affected in DKA. Acidosis causes hydrogen ions to move from the extracellular fluid to the intracellular space. Hydrogen movement into the cell promotes potassium movement out of the cell into the extracellular compartment, resulting in severe potassium depletion in the intracellular space. Most of the shifted extracellular potassium is lost in the urine because of osmotic diuresis. The serum potassium can be normal or even high, but this finding is misleading because there is an intracellular and total body loss of potassium (Diabetes Canada Clinical Practice Guidelines Expert Committee, 2018).

Vomiting caused by buildup of ketoacids in the blood or acidosis results in more fluid and electrolyte losses. Eventually, hypovolemia, followed by shock, ensues.

Renal failure may eventually occur from hypovolemic shock. This result causes the retention of ketones and glucose, and the metabolic acidosis progresses. Untreated, the patient becomes comatose as a result of dehydration, electrolyte imbalance, and acidosis. If the condition is not treated, death is inevitable.

Clinical Manifestations

Signs and symptoms of DKA include polyuria and polydipsia, leading to dehydration. Dehydration is manifested by poor skin turgor, dry mucous membranes, tachycardia, and orthostatic hypotension. Early symptoms may include lethargy and weakness. As the patient becomes severely dehydrated, the skin becomes dry and loose, and the eye sockets become sunken. Nausea and vomiting are common symptoms. Abdominal pain is occasionally seen. This may be due to dehydration of muscle tissue, delayed gastric emptying, and ileus induced by

PATHOPHYSIOLOGY MAP

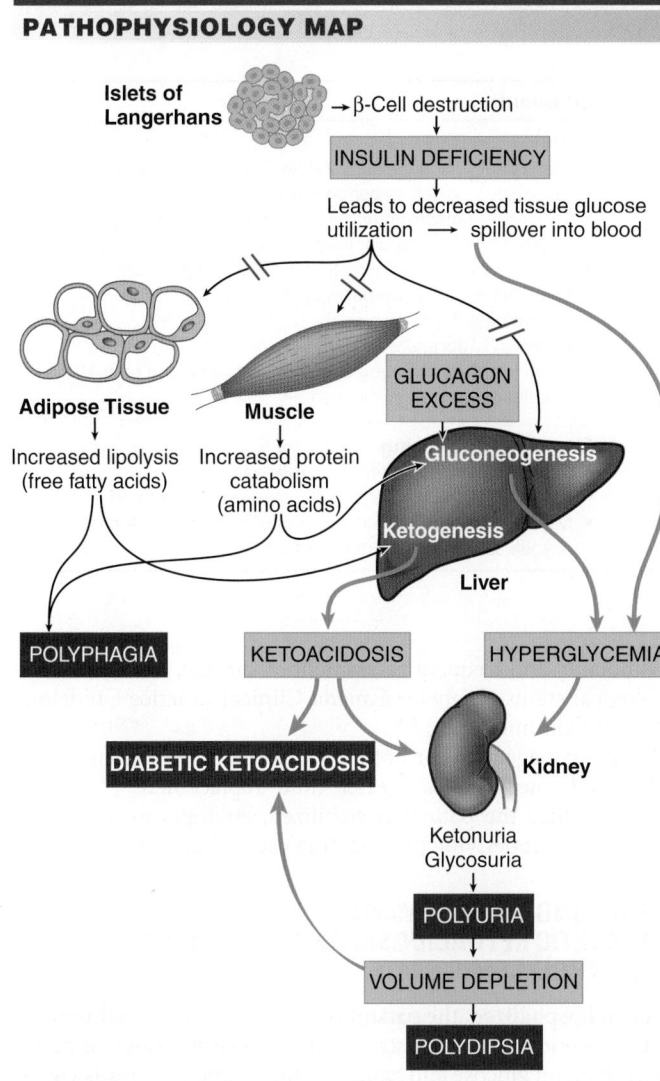

FIG. 52.12 Metabolic events leading to diabetic ketoacidosis. Source: Kumar, V., Abbas, A. K., Fausto, N., et al. (2010). *Robbins and Cotran pathologic basis of disease* (8th ed., p. 1144, Figure 24-39). Saunders.

electrolyte disturbance and metabolic acidosis (Kreider, 2018). Finally, Kussmaul's respiration (rapid, deep breathing associated with dyspnea) is the body's attempt to reverse metabolic acidosis through the exhalation of excess carbon dioxide. Acetone is noted on the breath as a sweet, fruity odour, due to high levels of ketones in the blood. (See Chapter 19 for a discussion of respiratory compensation of metabolic acidosis.) Laboratory findings include a blood glucose level above 14 mmol/L, arterial blood pH below 7.35, serum bicarbonate level less than 15 mmol/L, anion gap greater than 12 mmol/L, and ketones in the blood and urine (Diabetes Canada Clinical Practice Guidelines Expert Committee, 2018).

Interprofessional Care

Before the advent of SMBG and β-hydroxybutyrate (capillary blood ketones), all patients with DKA required hospitalization for treatment. Today, hospitalization may not be required. In instances where fluid and electrolyte imbalances are not severe and blood glucose levels can be safely monitored at home, early stages of DKA may be managed on an outpatient basis (Table 52.16). However, the decision about where the patient

TABLE 52.16 INTERPROFESSIONAL CARE

Diabetic Ketoacidosis (DKA) and Hyperosmolar Hyperglycemic State (HHS)

Diagnostic
- History and physical examination
- Blood studies, including immediate blood glucose, complete blood count, ketones, pH, electrolytes, blood urea nitrogen, arterial blood gases
- Urinalysis, including specific gravity, pH, glucose, ketones

Interprofessional Therapy
- Administration of IV fluids
- Assessment of blood and urine for ketones
- Assessment of blood glucose levels
- Assessment of cardiovascular and respiratory status
- Assessment of mental status
- Central venous pressure monitoring (if indicated)
- ECG monitoring
- Electrolyte replacement
- IV administration of short-acting insulin
- Recording of intake and output

ECG, electrocardiogram; *IV,* intravenous.

is managed must also take other factors into consideration. These factors include the presence of fever, nausea, vomiting, and diarrhea; altered mental status; nature of the cause of the ketoacidosis; and availability of frequent communication (every few hours) with the health care provider.

Regardless of the setting in which it occurs, DKA is a serious condition that proceeds rapidly and must be treated promptly. (Table 52.17 describes the emergency management of a patient with DKA.) Because fluid imbalance is potentially life-threatening, the initial goal of therapy is to establish IV access and begin fluid and electrolyte replacement. Typically, the initial fluid therapy regimen comprises an infusion of 0.45% or 0.9% NaCl IV solution at a rate to restore urine output to 30 to 60 mL/hr and to raise blood pressure. When blood glucose levels approach 14 mmol/L, 5% dextrose is added to the fluid regimen to prevent hypoglycemia (Diabetes Canada Clinical Practice Guidelines Expert Committee, 2018; Kreider 2018).

The aim of fluid and electrolyte therapy is to replace extracellular and intracellular water and to correct deficits of sodium, chloride, bicarbonate, potassium, phosphate, magnesium, and nitrogen. Early potassium replacement is essential because hypokalemia is a significant cause of preventable death during treatment of DKA. Although initial serum potassium may be normal or high, levels can rapidly decrease once therapy starts because insulin drives potassium into the cells, leading to life-threatening hypokalemia.

IV insulin administration is therapy directed toward correcting hyperglycemia and hyperketonemia. Insulin therapy is withheld until fluid resuscitation is under way and serum potassium is greater than 3.3 mmol/L, because insulin allows water and potassium to enter the cell along with glucose and can lead to a depletion of vascular volume and hypokalemia. Initially, a bolus of insulin is delivered, followed by a continuous infusion (Diabetes Canada Clinical Practice Guidelines Expert Committee, 2018).

SAFETY ALERT
- Too-rapid administration of IV fluid and a rapid lowering of serum glucose can lead to cerebral edema.

TABLE 52.17   EMERGENCY MANAGEMENT

Diabetic Ketoacidosis

Etiology	Assessment Findings	Interventions
• Change in diet, insulin, or exercise regimen • Dehydration owing to illness with vomiting or diarrhea • Inadequate treatment of existing diabetes mellitus • Infection • Insulin not taken as prescribed, or omitted • Undiagnosed diabetes mellitus	• Abdominal pain • Breath odour of acetone • Dry mouth • Eyes that appear sunken • Fever • Flushed, dry skin • Glucosuria and ketonuria • Gradually increasing restlessness, confusion, lethargy • Laboured breathing (Kussmaul's respiration) • Nausea and vomiting • Oral or vaginal *Candida albicans* (yeast infection) • Rapid, weak pulse; orthostatic hypotension • Serum glucose >14 mmol/L • Thirst • Urinary frequency	**Initial** • Administer IV sodium bicarbonate if severe acidosis (pH <7.0). • Administer oxygen as per physician's order. • Administer potassium IV to correct hypokalemia. • Begin continuous regular insulin drip 0.1 units/kg/hr, as needed. • Begin fluid resuscitation with 0.9% NaCl solution until BP is stabilized and urine output is 30–60 mL/hr. • Ensure patent airway. • Establish IV access with large-bore catheter. • Identify history of diabetes, time of last food, and time and amount of last insulin injection. **Ongoing Monitoring** • Assess breath sounds for fluid overload. • Monitor serum glucose, pH, and serum potassium. • Monitor vital signs, level of consciousness, cardiac rhythm, oxygen saturation, and urine output.

BP, blood pressure; *IV,* intravenous.

HYPEROSMOLAR HYPERGLYCEMIC STATE

Hyperosmolar hyperglycemic state (HHS) is a life-threatening syndrome that can occur in the patient with DM who is able to produce enough insulin to prevent DKA but not enough to prevent severe hyperglycemia, osmotic diuresis, and extracellular fluid depletion (Figure 52.13). HHS is less common than DKA. The main difference between HHS and DKA is that the patient with HHS usually has enough circulating insulin so that ketoacidosis does not occur. Because HHS produces fewer symptoms in the earlier stages, blood glucose levels can climb quite high before the condition is recognized. The higher blood glucose levels increase serum osmolality and produce more-severe neurological manifestations, such as somnolence, coma, seizures, hemiparesis, and aphasia. HHS often occurs in the older patient with type 2 DM and is often related to impaired thirst sensation, a functional inability to replace fluids, or both. There is usually a history of inadequate fluid intake, increasing mental depression, and polyuria. Laboratory values in HHS include blood glucose greater than 34 mmol/L and a marked increase in serum osmolality. Ketone bodies are absent or minimal in both blood and urine.

Interprofessional Care

HHS constitutes a medical emergency and has a high mortality rate. Therapy is similar to that for the treatment of DKA and includes immediate IV administration of either 0.9% or 0.45% NaCl at a rate that is dependent on cardiac status and the degree of fluid volume deficit. Regular insulin is given by IV bolus, followed by an infusion after fluid replacement therapy is instituted to aid in reducing the hyperglycemia. When blood glucose levels fall to approximately 14 mmol/L, IV fluids containing glucose are administered to prevent hypoglycemia. Electrolytes are monitored and replaced as needed. Hypokalemia is not as significant in HHS as it is in DKA, although fluid losses may result in milder potassium deficits that necessitate replacement. Vital signs, intake and output, tissue turgor, laboratory values, and cardiac monitoring are assessed to monitor the efficacy of fluid and electrolyte replacement. Patients with renal or cardiac compromise require special monitoring to avoid fluid overload during fluid replacement. This includes monitoring of serum osmolality and frequent assessment of cardiac, renal, and neurological status (Diabetes Canada Clinical Practice Guidelines Expert Committee, 2018).

The management for both DKA and HHS is similar, except that HHS necessitates greater fluid replacement (see Table 52.16). Once the patient is stabilized, attempts to detect and correct the underlying precipitating cause should be initiated.

NURSING MANAGEMENT
DIABETIC KETOACIDOSIS AND HYPEROSMOLAR HYPERGLYCEMIC STATE

When hospitalized, the patient is closely monitored with appropriate blood and urine tests. The nurse is responsible for monitoring blood glucose and urine for output and ketones as well as for using laboratory data to support care.

Nursing responsibilities include monitoring the administration of IV fluids to correct dehydration, insulin therapy to reduce blood glucose and serum ketones, and electrolytes to correct electrolyte imbalance; assessment of renal status; assessment of the cardiopulmonary status related to hydration and electrolyte levels; and monitoring of the level of consciousness.

The nurse must also monitor the signs of potassium imbalance resulting from hypoinsulinemia and osmotic diuresis (see Chapter 19). When treatment for hyperglycemia is begun with insulin, serum potassium levels may decrease rapidly because potassium moves into the cells once insulin becomes available. This movement of potassium into and out of extracellular fluid influences cardiac functioning. Cardiac monitoring is a useful aid in detecting hyperkalemia and hypokalemia because characteristic changes indicating potassium excess or deficit are observable on electrocardiogram (ECG) tracings (see Chapter 19, Figure 19.14). Vital signs should be assessed often to determine the presence of fever, hypovolemic shock, tachycardia, and Kussmaul's respiration (Kreider, 2018).

HYPOGLYCEMIA

Hypoglycemia, or low blood glucose, occurs when there is too much insulin in proportion to available glucose in the blood.

PATHOPHYSIOLOGY MAP

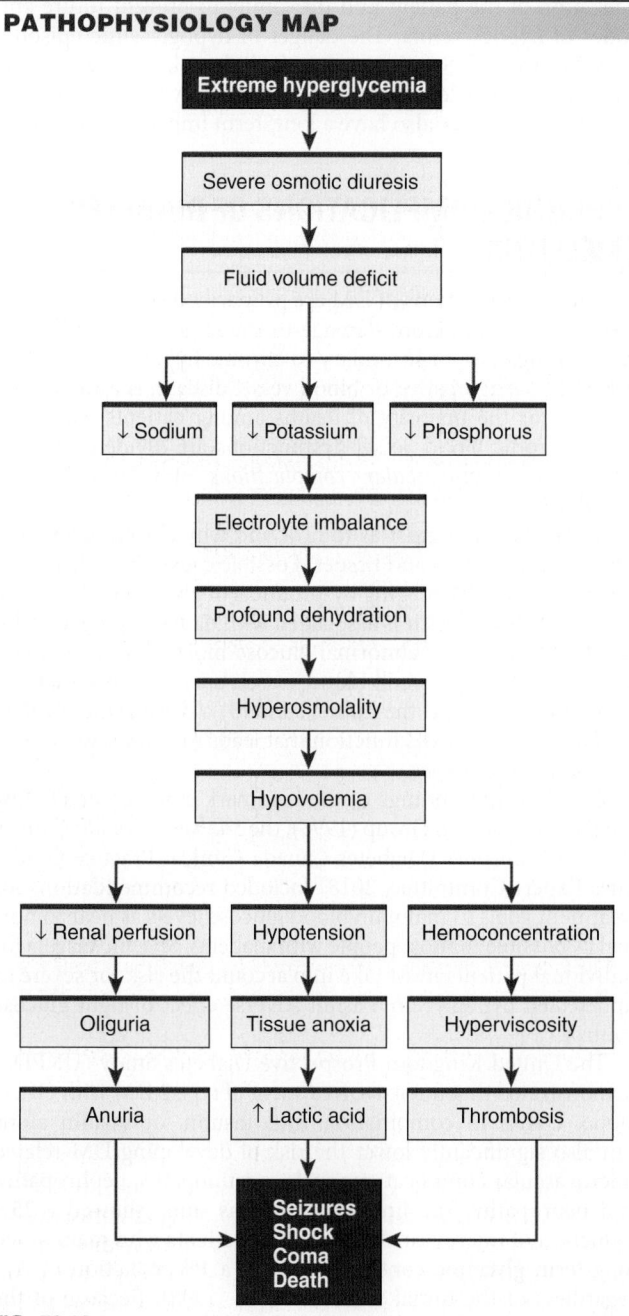

FIG. 52.13 Pathophysiology of hyperosmolar hyperglycemic state (HHS). Source: Redrawn from Urden, L. D., Stacy, K. M., & Lough, M. E. (2014). *Critical care nursing: Diagnosis and management* (7th ed., p. 828, Figure 33-4). Mosby.

This causes the blood glucose level to drop to less than 4 mmol/L. Once plasma glucose drops to this level, neuroendocrine hormones are released and the autonomic nervous system is activated. Suppression of insulin secretion and production of glucagon and epinephrine provide defence against hypoglycemia. Epinephrine release causes manifestations that include diaphoresis, tremors, hunger, nervousness, anxiety, pallor, and palpitations. As a primary energy source, the brain requires a constant supply of glucose in sufficient quantities to function properly; therefore, hypoglycemia can eventually affect cognitive functioning. These manifestations are referred to as *neuroglycopenic signs* and may include irritability, visual disturbances, difficulty speaking, stupor, confusion, and coma. Manifestations of hypoglycemia can mimic alcohol intoxication. Untreated hypoglycemia can progress to loss of consciousness, seizures, coma, and death.

Hypoglycemic unawareness (or *asymptomatic hypoglycemia*) is a condition in which patients do not experience the usual autonomic nervous system warning signs and symptoms of hypoglycemia, increasing their risk for dangerously low blood glucose levels. This condition is often related to autonomic neuropathy of DM that interferes with the secretion of counter-regulatory hormones that produce these symptoms. Older patients and patients who use β-adrenergic blockers are also at risk for hypoglycemic unawareness. For patients with risk factors for hypoglycemic unawareness, it is usually not safe to aim for tight blood glucose control because of the increased potential of hypoglycemia. They are usually managed with blood glucose goals that are somewhat higher than for patients who are able to detect and manage the onset of hypoglycemia.

Hypoglycemic symptoms may occur when a very high blood glucose level falls too rapidly—for example, a blood glucose level of 16 mmol/L falling quickly to 8 mmol/L. Although the blood glucose level is above normal by definition and measurement, the sudden metabolic shift can evoke hypoglycemic symptoms. Too-vigorous management of hyperglycemia with insulin can induce this type of situation.

Causes of hypoglycemia are often related to a mismatch in the timing of food intake and the peak action of insulin or OHAs that increase endogenous insulin secretion. The balance between blood glucose and insulin can be disrupted by the administration of too much insulin or medication, the ingestion of insufficient carbohydrates, delaying the time of eating, and performing unusual amounts of exercise. Insulin reactions can occur at any time, but most occur when the OHA or insulin is at its peak of action. Although hypoglycemia is more common with insulin therapy, it can occur with OHAs and may be severe and persist for an extended time because of the longer duration of action.

NURSING AND INTERPROFESSIONAL MANAGEMENT HYPOGLYCEMIA

Hypoglycemia can usually be quickly reversed with effective and rapid treatment. At the first sign of hypoglycemia, the blood glucose should be checked, if possible (Table 52.18). If it is below 4 mmol/L, the patient should begin treatment immediately. If the blood glucose is above 4 mmol/L, other causes of the signs and symptoms should be investigated. If the patient has manifestations of hypoglycemia and monitoring equipment is not available, hypoglycemia should be assumed and treatment should be initiated.

Hypoglycemia is treated by ingesting 15 to 20 g of a simple (fast-acting) carbohydrate, such as three or four glucose tablets, 175 mL of fruit juice or regular soft drink, or six Life Savers candies. Commercial products such as gels or tablets containing specific amounts of glucose are convenient for carrying in a purse or pocket to be used in such situations.

Treatment with sweet foods containing fat, such as chocolate bars, cookies, and ice cream, should be avoided because fat will slow down the absorption of the sugar and delay the response to treatment. Overtreatment with large quantities of simple carbohydrates should be avoided to prevent a rapid fluctuation to hyperglycemia. A prompt but moderate approach is best. Blood

TABLE 52.18   INTERPROFESSIONAL CARE

Hypoglycemia

Diagnostic
- Capillary blood glucose (evaluated and reported on an emergency basis)
- History (if possible) and physical examination

Interprofessional Therapy
- Determination of cause of hypoglycemia (after correction of condition)

Conscious Patient With Mild to Moderate Hypoglycemia
- Administration of 15–20 g of fast-acting (simple) carbohydrate (e.g., commercial dextrose products [per label instructions]; 175 mL of fruit juice or regular soft drink; 6–8 Life Savers; for patient taking acarbose: 15 mL (1 tbsp) syrup or honey, or 125–150 mL low-fat milk, or dextrose tabs (because the absorption of glucose itself is not affected)*
- Recheck of blood glucose in 15 min; if no improvement, repetition of treatment of 15–20 g of carbohydrate
- Administration of additional food or longer-acting combination such as carbohydrate plus protein or fat (e.g., crackers with peanut butter or cheese) after symptoms subside, if meal is longer than 1 hr away
- Immediate notification of health care provider or emergency service (if patient is outside hospital) if symptoms do not subside after two or three administrations of fast-acting carbohydrate

Severe Hypoglycemia or Unconscious Patient
- Intravenous administration of 20–50 mL of dextrose 50% in water (D50W) given over 1–3 min
- Subcutaneous or intramuscular injection of 1 mg or 3 mg intranasal glucagon

*Diabetes Canada Clinical Practice Guidelines Expert Committee. (2018). 2018 Clinical practice guidelines for the prevention and management of diabetes in Canada. *Canadian Journal of Diabetes Care, 42*(Suppl 1), S104–S108.

glucose should be checked 15 minutes after the initial treatment and repeated if blood glucose remains lower than 4 mmol/L. Once the blood glucose is greater than 4 mmol/L, the patient should eat a snack if the next regularly scheduled meal is more than an hour away in order to prevent hypoglycemia from recurring. Good snacks include one protein and one starch choice, such as a peanut butter sandwich, cheese and crackers, or cereal and milk. Blood glucose should also be checked again about 45 minutes after eating the snack to ensure that hypoglycemia is not recurring (Diabetes Canada Clinical Practice Guidelines Expert Committee, 2018).

If there is no significant improvement in the patient's condition after two to three doses of 15 to 20 g of simple carbohydrate or if the patient is not alert enough to swallow, 1 mg of glucagon may be administered by intramuscular or subcutaneous injection. An intranasal form of glucagon (Baqsimi) 3 mg is now available without prescription. Glucagon stimulates a strong hepatic response to convert glycogen to glucose, making glucose rapidly available. Rebound hypoglycemia is a potential adverse effect of glucagon. Having the patient ingest a starch snack after recovery may prevent this from happening. Patients with minimal glycogen stores will not respond to glucagon. These include patients with alcohol-related hepatic disease, starvation, and adrenal insufficiency. In an acute care setting, patients with hypoglycemia are treated with 20 to 50 mL of 50% dextrose by IV push.

Once the hypoglycemic episode has resolved, the nurse should explore with the patient the reasons why the situation developed. This assessment may indicate the need for additional education of the patient and the family to prevent future episodes of hypoglycemia. The danger of hypoglycemic episodes must be stressed. Safety concerns include risks such as driving a motorized vehicle or bicycle, operating heavy machinery, and falls; these episodes also have a long-term impact on memory.

CHRONIC COMPLICATIONS OF DIABETES MELLITUS

Chronic complications of DM are primarily those of end-organ disease that result from damage to the large and small blood vessels (angiopathy) secondary to chronic hyperglycemia (Figure 52.14). Angiopathy, or blood vessel disease, is estimated to account for the majority of deaths among patients with DM. These chronic blood vessel dysfunctions are divided into two categories: *macrovascular complications* and *microvascular complications.*

Several theories exist as to how and why chronic hyperglycemia damages cells and tissues. Possible causes include (1) the accumulation of damaging by-products of glucose metabolism, such as sorbitol, which is associated with damage to nerve cells; (2) the formation of abnormal glucose molecules in the basement membrane of small blood vessels such as those that circulate to the eye and the kidney; and (3) a derangement called *oxidative stress* in RBC function that leads to a decrease in oxygenation to the tissues.

Based on the findings of the landmark study completed by the DCCT Research Group (1993), the *Diabetes Canada Clinical Practice Guidelines* (Diabetes Canada Clinical Practice Guidelines Expert Committee, 2018) included recommendations for treatment goals to maintain blood glucose levels as near to normal as possible in most people with diabetes. Specific targets for individual patients must take into account the risk for severe or undetected hypoglycemia as an adverse effect of tight glucose control.

The United Kingdom Prospective Diabetes Study (UKPDS) demonstrated that intensive treatment of type 2 DM with OHAs alone, OHAs in combination with insulin, or insulin alone can also significantly lower the risk of developing DM-related microvascular complications such as retinopathy, nephropathy, and neuropathy. The findings from this study showed a 25% reduction of microvascular disease in patients who maintained long-term glycemic control, including a 1% reduction in A_{1c}, regardless of the initial value (UKPDS, 1998). Because of the devastating effects of long-term complications, patients with DM require scheduled and ongoing monitoring for the detection and prevention of chronic complications. The recommendations for ongoing evaluation are listed in Table 52.19. It is imperative that patients understand the importance of regular follow-up examinations (Diabetes Canada Clinical Practice Guidelines Expert Committee, 2018).

MACROVASCULAR COMPLICATIONS

Macrovascular complications are diseases of the large and medium-sized blood vessels; these complications occur with greater frequency and with an earlier onset in people with DM. Although atherosclerotic plaque formation is believed to have a genetic origin, its development seems to be promoted by the altered lipid metabolism common to DM. Tight glucose control may help delay the atherosclerotic process (Diabetes

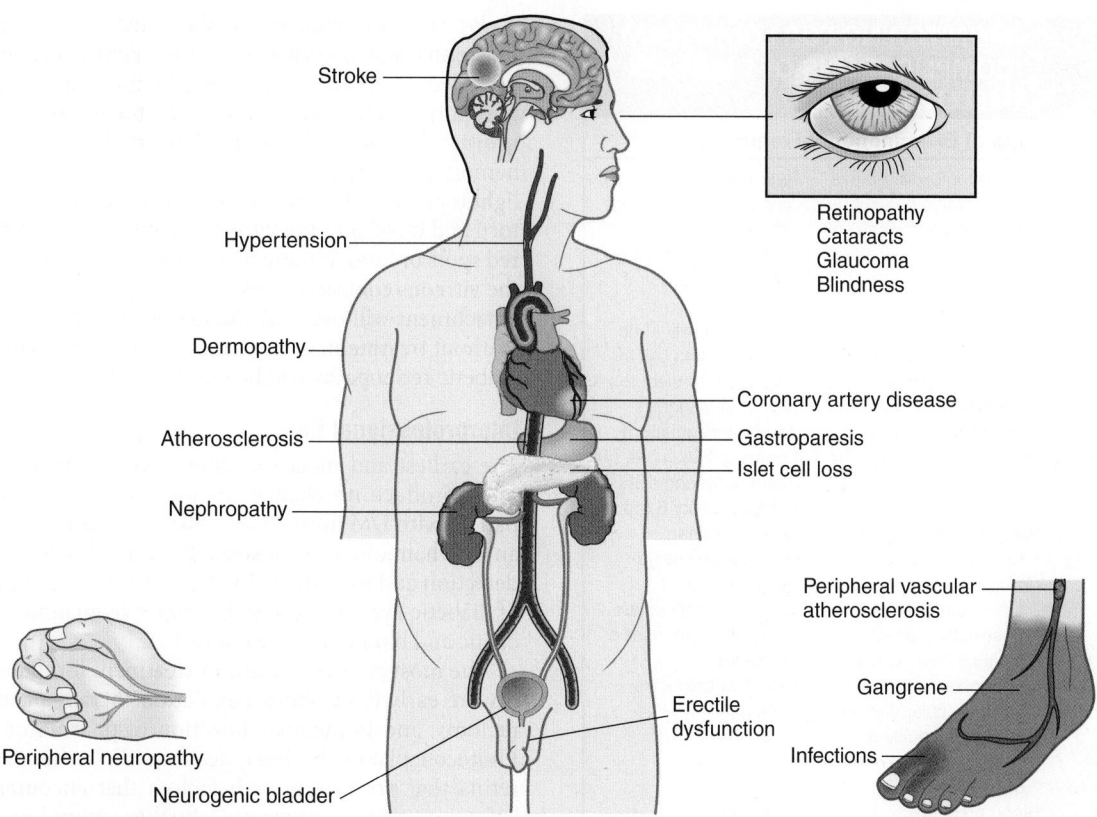

FIG. 52.14 Long-term complications of diabetes mellitus. Source: Kumar, V., Abbas, A. K., & Aster, J. (2015). *Robbins and Cotran pathologic basis of disease* (9th ed., p. 1116, Figure 24-34). Saunders.

Canada Clinical Practice Guidelines Expert Committee, 2018). Macrovascular diseases include cerebrovascular, cardiovascular, and peripheral vascular disease. Adults with DM have two to three times the risk for heart and cerebrovascular disease of those without DM (Diabetes Canada Clinical Practice Guidelines Expert Committee, 2018). Although genetic makeup cannot be altered, strategies for vascular protection are recommended and include healthy behaviour interventions such as healthy eating, weight modification, smoking cessation, and increased physical activity. Smoking is associated with significantly increased risks for total mortality, cardiovascular events, and lower extremity amputation in those with DM. The cessation of smoking reduces cardiovascular risk and the risk for renal disease and improves glycemic control (Diabetes Canada Clinical Practice Guidelines Expert Committee, 2018; Keto, et al., 2016). (Smoking is discussed in Chapter 11.) The addition of an angiotensin-converting enzyme (ACE) inhibitor, antiplatelet therapy such as acetylsalicylic acid (ASA; Aspirin), and lipid, blood pressure, and glycemic control are pharmacological interventions that protect the heart and are known to reduce mortality risk in patients with type 2 DM. Optimizing blood pressure control in patients with DM is significant for the prevention of cardiovascular and renal disease. The target blood pressure for people with DM is 130/80 mm Hg.

Insulin resistance seems to play an important role in the development of cardiovascular disease and is implicated in the pathogenesis of essential hypertension and dyslipidemia. The term *metabolic syndrome* is applied to the clinical association of insulin resistance, hypertension, and increased very-low-density lipoprotein (VLDL) and decreased HDL cholesterol concentrations. The role of insulin resistance in the pathogenesis of cardiovascular disease is not well understood, but it seems to combine with dyslipidemia in contributing to greater risk for cardiovascular disease in patients with DM. All patients with DM should be screened for dyslipidemia at the time DM is diagnosed. Most people with DM are considered at high risk for a vascular event (Diabetes Canada Clinical Practice Guidelines Expert Committee, 2018).

Lifestyle changes such as healthy eating and exercise are first-line interventions to achieve an optimal lipid profile. If unsuccessful, lipid-lowering therapy such as statins, fibrates, or both may be added to optimize lipid levels, thereby reducing risk for a vascular event.

MICROVASCULAR COMPLICATIONS

Microvascular complications result from thickening of the vessel membranes in the capillaries and arterioles in response to conditions of chronic hyperglycemia. They differ from macrovascular complications in that they are specific to DM. Although microangiopathy can be found throughout the body, the areas most noticeably affected are the eyes (retinopathy), the kidneys (nephropathy), the nerves (neuropathy), and the skin (dermopathy). Thickening of the basement membrane has been found in some people with type 2 DM before or at the time of diagnosis or before the onset of symptoms of DM. However, clinical manifestations may not appear until 10 to 20 years after the onset of DM, depending on the glycemic control over that period of time as measured by A_{1c}.

TABLE 52.19	MONITORING FOR LONG-TERM COMPLICATIONS OF DIABETES MELLITUS*	
Complication	**Type of Examination**	**Frequency**
Retinopathy	Funduscopic–dilated-eye examination by experienced professional	*Type 1:* annually, starting 5 yr after onset of diabetes *Type 2:* at diagnosis; then every 1–2 yr if normal
Nephropathy	Random urinalysis for albumin-to-creatinine ratio (ACR), serum creatinine converted to eGFR	*Type 1:* annually; if no CKD, starting 5 yr after onset of diabetes *Type 2:* at diagnosis and then annually if normal; if CKD present, ACR and eGFR at least every 6 mo
Neuropathy (foot and lower extremities)	Visual examination of foot	Daily by patient
	Comprehensive foot examination: assessment of structural abnormalities, neuropathy (monofilament, tuning fork), vascular disease (peripheral pulses), ulcerations, and evidence of infection	Every visit by health care provider *Type 1:* annually, starting 5 yr after onset of diabetes *Type 2:* at diagnosis and annually
Cardiovascular disease	Blood pressure	Every visit
	Lipid panel	At the time of diagnosis, and then every 1–3 yr
	ECG	Baseline and every 2 yr if >40 yr; >30 yr and duration >15 yr; end organ damage; cardiac risk factors

*Based on the recommendations of the Diabetes Canada Clinical Practice Guidelines Expert Committee. (2018). 2018 Clinical practice guidelines for the prevention and management of diabetes in Canada. *Canadian Journal of Diabetes Care, 42*(Suppl 1), S1–S325.
CKD, chronic kidney disease; *ECG,* electrocardiogram; *eGFR,* estimated glomerular filtration rate.

DIABETIC RETINOPATHY

Etiology and Pathophysiology

Diabetic retinopathy refers to the process of microvascular damage to the blood vessels in the retina as a result of chronic hyperglycemia, presence of nephropathy, and hypertension in patients with DM. After 15 years with DM, nearly all patients with type 1 DM and 80% with type 2 DM will have some degree of retinal disease. Diabetic retinopathy is estimated to be the most common cause of new cases of blindness in people of working age (ADA, 2019; Diabetes Canada Clinical Practice Guidelines Expert Committee, 2018).

Retinopathy can be classified as nonproliferative or proliferative. In *nonproliferative retinopathy,* the most common form, partial occlusion of the small blood vessels in the retina causes the development of microaneurysms in the capillary walls. The walls of these microaneurysms are so weak that capillary fluid leaks out, causing retinal edema and eventually hard exudates or intraretinal hemorrhages. Vision may be affected if the macula is involved.

Proliferative retinopathy, the most severe form, involves the retina and the vitreous. When retinal capillaries become occluded, the body compensates by forming new blood vessels to supply the retina with blood, a pathological process known as *neovascularization.* These new vessels are extremely fragile and hemorrhage easily, producing vitreous contraction. Eventually, light is prevented from reaching the retina as the vessels become torn and bleed into the vitreous cavity. The patient sees black or red spots or lines. If these new blood vessels pull the retina while the vitreous contracts, causing a tear, partial or complete retinal detachment will occur. If the macula is involved, vision is lost. Without treatment, more than half of patients with proliferative diabetic retinopathy will be blind.

Interprofessional Care

The earliest and most treatable stages of diabetic retinopathy often produce no changes in the vision. Because of this, the patient with DM must have regular dilated-eye examinations by an ophthalmologist or a specially trained optometrist for early detection and treatment. The best approach to the management of diabetic eye disease is to prevent it by maintaining good glycemic and blood pressure control.

The most common forms of treatment for diabetic retinopathy are early laser photocoagulation therapy of the retina, vitrectomy, and intraocular injection of pharmacological agents. Photocoagulation by laser destroys the ischemic areas of the retina that produce growth factors that encourage neovascularization, thereby preventing further vision loss, and reduces legal blindness up to 90% in people with severe nonproliferative retinopathy and proliferative retinopathy (Diabetes Canada Clinical Practice Guidelines Expert Committee, 2018). (Photocoagulation is discussed in Chapter 24.)

Vitrectomy is the aspiration of blood, membrane, and fibres from the inside of the eye through a small incision just behind the cornea. Vitrectomy is indicated in patients with advanced proliferative retinopathy with vitreous hemorrhage or retinal detachment of the macula. (Vitrectomy is discussed in Chapter 24.)

Recent research has identified the importance of vascular endothelial growth factor (VEFG) in the development of diabetic retinopathy. Three anti-VEFG medications are now widely used in Canada to treat diabetic retinopathy: aflibercept (Eylea), bevacizumab (Avastin), and ranibizumab (Lucentis) (Freige & Butcher, 2020). Bevacizumab (Avastin) is used in an expanded or off-label manner but has not been approved by Health Canada for this purpose (Diabetes Canada Clinical Practice Guidelines Expert Committee, 2018).

People with DM are also prone to other visual conditions. Glaucoma occurs as a result of the occlusion of the outflow channels, secondary to neovascularization. This type of glaucoma is difficult to treat and often results in blindness. Cataracts develop at an earlier age and progress more rapidly in people with DM.

NEPHROPATHY

Diabetic nephropathy is a microvascular complication associated with damage to the small blood vessels that supply the glomeruli of the kidney. It is the leading cause of end-stage renal disease (ESRD) in Canada. The risk for nephropathy is similar in patients with either type 1 or type 2 DM. Risk factors for the development of diabetic nephropathy include hypertension, genetic predisposition, smoking, and chronic hyperglycemia. Kidney disease can be significantly reduced when near-normal blood glucose control is achieved and maintained (Diabetes Canada Clinical Practice Guidelines Expert Committee, 2018).

Hypertension significantly accelerates the progression of diabetic nephropathy and retinopathy and the risk for stroke. Therefore, aggressive blood pressure management is indicated for all patients with DM. ACE inhibitor medications (e.g., ramipril [Altace]) and angiotensin II receptor blockers (e.g., losartan [Cozaar]) are commonly prescribed to patients with DM because they are effective blood pressure–lowering agents with few adverse effects. In addition, both of these medications are often prescribed to patients with DM even when they are not hypertensive because medications in either class have a protective effect on the kidney that prevents the progression of diabetic nephropathy independent of hypertension control (Diabetes Canada Clinical Practice Guidelines Expert Committee, 2018). (See Chapter 35 for a discussion of hypertension and Chapter 49 for a discussion of renal failure.)

Standards for the prevention and detection of nephropathy in patients with DM include yearly screening for the presence of microalbuminuria (MAU). This test is used to detect kidney damage at an earlier stage than the standard dipstick test for macroprotein in the urine. Screening for MAU should be performed using a random urine collection for albumin-to-creatinine ratio and serum creatinine for estimated glomerular filtration rate (eGFR). A 24-hour urine collection for determination of creatinine clearance and serum creatinine may be performed when there is doubt about the accuracy of an eGFR (Diabetes Canada Clinical Practice Guidelines Expert Committee, 2018).

NEUROPATHY

Diabetic neuropathy is nerve damage that occurs because of the metabolic derangements associated with DM. About 40 to 50% of patients with DM have some degree of neuropathy, with neurological complications occurring equally in type 1 and type 2 DM (Diabetes Canada Clinical Practice Guidelines Expert Committee, 2018). The most common type of neuropathy affecting people with DM is peripheral sensory neuropathy. This condition can lead to the loss of protective sensation in the lower extremities, and, coupled with other factors, peripheral sensory neuropathy significantly increases the risk for complications that can result in a lower limb amputation. Although, amputation rates for people with diabetes have decreased in the past decade, they remain very high compared with rates for people without diabetes (Diabetes Canada Clinical Practice Guidelines Expert Committee, 2018).

Etiology and Pathophysiology

The pathophysiological processes of diabetic neuropathy are not well understood. Several theories exist, including metabolic, vascular, and autoimmune elements. The prevailing theory suggests that persistent hyperglycemia leads to an accumulation of sorbitol and fructose in the nerves that causes damage by an unknown mechanism. The result is reduced nerve conduction and demyelinization. Ischemia in blood vessels damaged by chronic hyperglycemia that supply the peripheral nerves is also implicated in the development of diabetic neuropathy. Neuropathy can precede, accompany, or follow the diagnosis of DM.

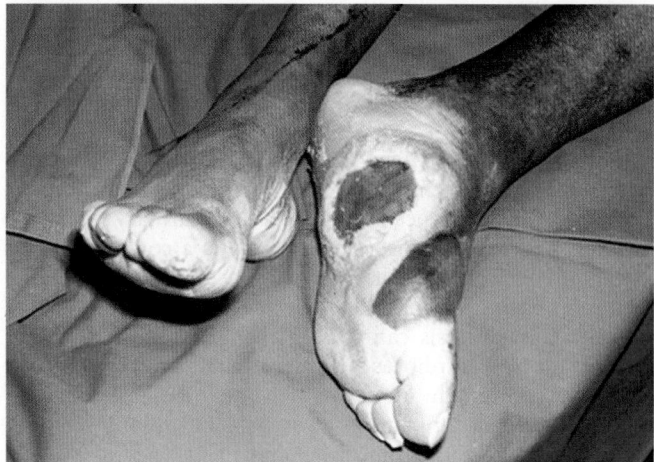

FIG. 52.15 Neuropathy: neurotrophic ulceration. Source: Urden, L. D., Stacy, K. M., & Lough, M. E. (2009). *Thelan's critical care nursing: Diagnosis and management* (6th ed.). Mosby.

Classification

The two major categories of diabetic neuropathy affect the peripheral nervous system: sensory neuropathy (which affects the somatic division) and autonomic neuropathy (which affects the autonomic division). Each of these types can take on several forms.

Sensory Neuropathy. The most common form of sensory polyneuropathy is distal symmetrical neuropathy, which affects the hands, the feet, or both, bilaterally. This condition is sometimes referred to as *stocking-glove neuropathy*. Characteristics of distal symmetrical neuropathy include paresthesias, abnormal sensations, pain, and loss of sensation. The paresthesias may be associated with tingling, burning, and itching sensations. The patient may report a feeling of walking on pillows or numb feet. At times, the skin becomes so sensitive (hyperesthesia) that even light pressure from bed sheets cannot be tolerated. Complete or partial loss of sensitivity to touch and temperature is common. The pain, which is often described as burning, cramping, crushing, or tearing, is usually worse at night and may occur only at that time. Foot injury and ulcerations can occur without the patient ever having pain (Figure 52.15). Neuropathy can also cause atrophy of the small muscles of the hands and feet, causing deformity and limiting fine movement.

Control of blood glucose is the only treatment for diabetic neuropathy. It is effective in many but not all cases. Medication therapy may be used to treat neuropathic symptoms, particularly pain. Medications commonly used include topical creams (e.g., capsaicin), tricyclic antidepressants (e.g., amitriptyline [Elavil]), selective serotonin and norepinephrine reuptake inhibitors (e.g., duloxetine [Cymbalta]), and antiseizure medications (e.g., gabapentin [Neurontin], pregabalin [Lyrica]). Capsaicin is a moderately effective topical cream made from chili peppers. It depletes the accumulation of pain-mediating chemicals in the peripheral sensory neurons. The cream is applied with gloves three to four times a day. There is usually an increase in symptoms at the start of therapy, which is followed by relief of pain in 2 to 3 weeks. Tricyclic antidepressants are also moderately effective in treating the symptoms of diabetic neuropathy. They work by inhibiting the reuptake of norepinephrine and serotonin, which are neurotransmitters believed to play a role in the transmission of pain through the spinal cord (Javed et al., 2015). Duloxetine is thought to relieve pain by increasing the levels of serotonin and norepinephrine, which improves the body's ability to regulate pain. Although gabapentin has been found to be effective in treating the pain of diabetic neuropathy, its mechanism of action is not well understood.

Autonomic Neuropathy. Autonomic neuropathy can affect nearly all body systems and lead to hypoglycemia unawareness, bowel incontinence and diarrhea, and urinary retention. Delayed gastric emptying *(gastroparesis)* is a complication of autonomic neuropathy that can produce anorexia, nausea, vomiting, gastroesophageal reflux, and persistent feelings of fullness. Gastroparesis can trigger hypoglycemia by delaying food absorption. Cardiovascular abnormalities associated with autonomic neuropathy are postural hypotension, resting tachycardia, and "silent" or painless myocardial infarction. A patient with postural hypotension should be instructed to change slowly from a lying or sitting position to a standing position.

DM can affect sexual function in men and women. Erectile dysfunction in men with diabetes is well recognized and common, often being the first manifestation of autonomic failure. Erectile dysfunction associated with DM is believed to result from damage to the sacral parasympathetic nerves. Determining whether this condition is of organic or psychological origin is an important part of the assessment. Decreased libido is a concern for some women with DM. Monilial and nonspecific vaginitis are also common. Organic erectile dysfunction or sexual dysfunction in either the male or the female patient requires sensitive therapeutic counselling for both the patient and the patient's partner (Diabetes Canada Clinical Practice Guidelines Expert Committee, 2018). (See Chapter 57 for a further discussion of erectile dysfunction.)

A neurogenic bladder may develop as sensation in the inner bladder wall decreases, causing urinary retention. A patient with retention has infrequent voiding, difficulty in voiding, and a weak stream of urine. Emptying the bladder every 3 hours in a sitting position helps prevent stasis and subsequent infection. Tightening the abdominal muscles during voiding and using Credé manoeuvre (mild massage downward over the lower abdomen and bladder) may also help with complete bladder emptying. Cholinergic agonist medications such as bethanechol (Duvoid) may be used. The patient may also have to learn self-catheterization (see Chapter 48).

COMPLICATIONS OF THE FOOT AND THE LOWER EXTREMITY

In Canada, people with diabetes are approximately 20 times more likely to be hospitalized for nontraumatic lower limb amputations than people without diabetes (Diabetes Canada Clinical Practice Guidelines Expert Committee, 2018). The development of diabetic foot complications is a multifactorial process (Botros et al., 2019). Complications result from a combination of microvascular and macrovascular diseases that place the patient at risk for injury and serious infection that may lead to amputation (Figure 52.16). Sensory neuropathy and peripheral vascular disease (PVD) are risk factors, and clotting abnormalities, impaired immune function, and autonomic neuropathy also play important roles. Smoking is deleterious to the health of lower extremity blood vessels and increases the risk for amputation.

Sensory neuropathy is a major risk factor for lower extremity amputation in the person with DM. Loss of protective sensation (LOPS) often prevents the patient from becoming aware that a foot injury has occurred. Improper footwear and injury from

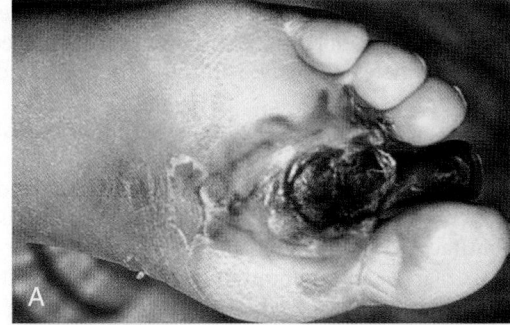
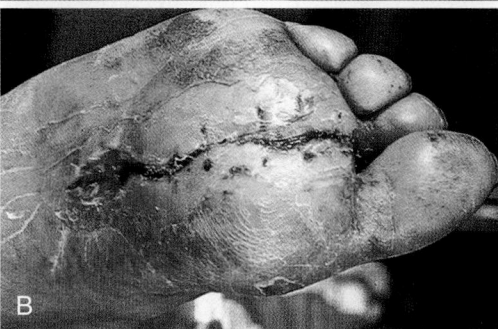

FIG. 52.16 The necrotic toe developed as a complication of diabetes. **A,** Before amputation. **B,** After amputation. Source: Chew, S. L., & Leslie, D. (2006). *Clinical endocrinology and diabetes: An illustrated colour text.* Churchill Livingstone.

stepping on foreign objects while barefoot are common causes of undetected foot injury in the person with LOPS (Armstrong et al., 2017; Botros et al., 2019). Because the primary risk factor for lower extremity amputation is LOPS, annual screening using a *monofilament* is an extremely important preventive measure. This is done by applying a thin, flexible filament to several spots on the plantar surface of the foot and toes and asking the patient to report if it is felt. Insensitivity to a 10-g Semmes-Weinstein monofilament has been shown to greatly increase the risk for diabetic foot ulcers that can lead to amputation. If the patient has LOPS, aggressive measures must be taken to teach the patient how to prevent foot ulceration. These measures include the selection of proper footwear, including prescription shoes. Other measures are to carefully avoid injury to the foot, practise diligent skin and nail care, inspect the foot thoroughly each day, and treat small health problems promptly (Botros et al., 2019; Diabetes Canada Clinical Practice Guidelines Expert Committee, 2018).

PVD increases the risk for amputation by causing a reduction in blood flow to the lower extremities. When blood flow is decreased, oxygen, white blood cells, and vital nutrients are not available to the tissues. Therefore, wounds take longer to heal and the risk for infection increases. Signs of PVD include intermittent claudication, pain at rest, cold feet, loss of hair, delayed capillary filling, and dependent rubor (redness of the skin that occurs when the extremity is in a dependent position). The disease is diagnosed by history, ankle–brachial index (ABI), and angiography. Management includes control or reduction of risk factors, particularly smoking, high saturated fat intake, and hypertension. Femoral bypass or graft surgery is indicated in some patients. Proper care of the feet is essential for patients with PVD. Guidelines for patient teaching are listed in Table 52.20.

The Doppler instrument is used to perform the ABI to diagnose the presence or degree of PVD. Similar to an electronic stethoscope, this device amplifies sound. The procedure is noninvasive and can measure blood pressure and blood flow velocity in

TABLE 52.20 PATIENT & CAREGIVER TEACHING GUIDE

Foot Care

The following instructions should be included when teaching the patient and caregiver about foot care.

1. Wash feet daily with a mild soap and warm water. Test water temperature with a thermometer or hands first.
2. Pat feet dry gently, especially between toes.
3. Examine feet daily for cuts, blisters, swelling, and red, tender areas. Do not depend on feeling sores. If eyesight is poor, have others inspect feet.
4. Use lanolin on feet to prevent skin from drying and cracking. Do not apply between toes.
5. Do not use commercial remedies or sharp blades to remove calluses or corns.
6. Cleanse cuts with warm water and mild soap, covering with a clean dressing. Do not use iodine, rubbing alcohol, or strong adhesives.
7. Report skin infections or nonhealing sores to the health care provider immediately.
8. Cut and file toenails even, with the rounded contour of the toes. Do not cut down corners. The best time to trim nails is after a shower or bath. See a foot care specialist if advice or treatment is needed.
9. Separate overlapping toes with cotton or lamb's wool.
10. Avoid open-toe, open-heel, and high-heel shoes. Leather shoes are preferred to synthetic ones. Wear slippers at home and shoes on the beach. Do not go barefoot. Shake out shoes before putting them on.
11. Wear clean, absorbent (cotton or wool) socks or stockings that have not been mended. Coloured socks must be colourfast.
12. Do not wear socks or stockings that leave impressions, hindering circulation.
13. Do not use hot water bottles or heating pads to warm feet. Wear socks for warmth.
14. Guard against frostbite.
15. Exercise feet daily either by walking or by flexing and extending feet in suspended position. Avoid prolonged sitting, standing, and crossing of legs.

Source: Diabetes Canada Clinical Practice Guidelines Expert Committee. (2018). 2018 Clinical practice guidelines for the prevention and management of diabetes in Canada. *Canadian Journal of Diabetes, 42*(Suppl.1), S222–S227.

the lower extremities. It can indicate areas of stenosis or occlusion and is useful as an indicator of the need for additional vascular tests. To determine location and extent of PVD, an angiography can be completed. Angiography is an invasive procedure and it provides information on the actual blood vessel condition.

Proper care of a diabetic foot ulcer is critical to prevention of infections. Management requires an interprofessional approach that addresses glycemic control, infection, lower extremity vascular status, and local wound care (Diabetes Canada Clinical Practice Guidelines Expert Committee, 2018). The fundamentals of good wound care involve an optimal wound environment, off-loading of the ulcer site, and in nonischemic wounds, regular debridement of nonviable tissue.

Neuropathic arthropathy, or *Charcot foot,* results in ligament softening and bony deformities that ultimately lead to joint dysfunction and foot drop. The pathogenesis of Charcot foot is not clear, but it is likely due to a combination of mechanical and vascular factors resulting from peripheral neuropathy and is mediated through an uncontrolled inflammation in the foot (Diabetes Canada Clinical Practice Guidelines Expert Committee, 2018; Schmidt & Holmes, 2018). Changes that occur with Charcot foot happen gradually and create an abnormal distribution of weight over the foot, further increasing the chances of developing an ulcer on the plantar aspect of the foot as new pressure points

emerge. Neuropathic ulcers resemble a "BB-shot" or "punched-out" wound and are usually painless. This high-risk foot complication requires immediate attention such as foot radiographic studies and referral to a high-risk foot team of chiropody, orthopedic surgery, and plastic surgery specialists. Infection and subsequent amputation is a danger and necessitates the long-term use of antibiotics and weeks of avoidance of weight bearing on the affected limb (Diabetes Canada Clinical Practice Guidelines Expert Committee, 2018). Foot deformity should be recognized early and proper footwear fitted before ulceration occurs.

INTEGUMENTARY COMPLICATIONS

The skin is often affected in patients with DM. *Acanthosis nigricans* is a dark, coarse, thickened skin predominantly seen in flexures and on the neck. Acanthosis nigricans is a risk factor for type 2 DM and is associated with hyperinsulinemia and insulin resistance (Diabetes Canada Clinical Practice Guidelines Expert Committee, 2018; Patel et al., 2018). Skin disorders such as diabetic dermopathy and necrobiosis lipoidica diabeticorum are attributed to microangiopathy. Shin spots are brown spots located on the anterior surfaces of the lower extremities. They are harmless and painless and initially measure less than 1 cm in diameter. *Necrobiosis lipoidica diabeticorum* (Figure 52.17) is believed to be the result of the breakdown of collagen in the skin. It usually appears as red-yellow lesions, with atrophic skin that becomes shiny and transparent, revealing tiny blood vessels under the surface. Because the thin skin is prone to injury, special care must be taken to protect affected areas from injury and ulceration. This condition is not common, but it may appear before other clinical signs or symptoms of DM. It is more frequently seen in young women. *Granuloma annulare,* associated mainly with type 1 DM, is probably autoimmune in nature and forms partial rings of papules, often on the dorsal surface of hands and feet.

INFECTION

A patient with DM is more susceptible to infections than other patients are. The mechanisms for this phenomenon include a defect in the mobilization of inflammatory cells and an impairment of phagocytosis by neutrophils and monocytes. Organisms such as yeast thrive in a high–blood glucose environment. Thus, recurring or persistent infections such as *Candida albicans,* as well as boils and furuncles, in the undiagnosed patient often lead the health care provider to suspect DM. Loss of sensation (peripheral neuropathy) may delay the detection of an infection in the feet.

Persistent glycosuria may predispose to bladder infections, especially in patients with a neurogenic bladder. Decreased circulation resulting from angiopathy can prevent or delay the immune response. Antibiotic therapy has prevented infection from being a major cause of death in patients with DM. The treatment of infections must be prompt and vigorous.

AGE-RELATED CONSIDERATIONS

DIABETES MELLITUS

The prevalence of DM increases with age. A major reason for this is that the process of aging is associated with a reduction in β-cell function, decreased insulin sensitivity, altered carbohydrate metabolism, and a progressive increase in A_{1c} (Diabetes Canada Clinical Practice Guidelines Expert Committee, 2018). Aging is also associated with a number of conditions

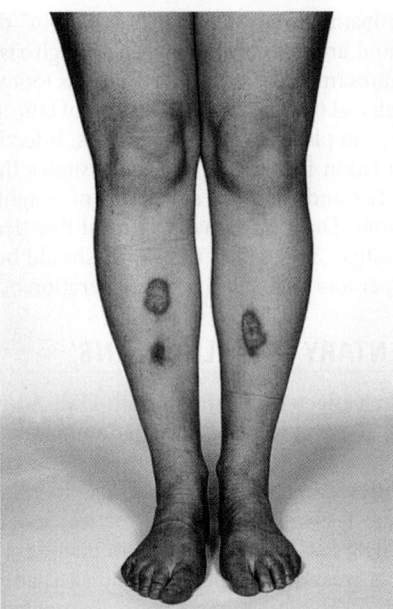

FIG. 52.17 Necrobiosis lipoidica diabeticorum. Source: Chew, S. L., & Leslie, D. (2006). *Clinical endocrinology and diabetes: An illustrated colour text.* Churchill Livingstone.

that are more likely to be treated with medications that impair insulin action (e.g., corticosteroids, antihypertensives, phenothiazines). Undiagnosed and untreated DM is more common in the older person, partly because many of the normal physiological changes of aging, such as visual changes and decreased glomerular filtration, resemble those of DM.

Although good glycemic control is important to people of all ages with DM, several factors are taken into account when determining glycemic goals for an older person. Hypoglycemia unawareness is more common in this age group, making these patients more likely to suffer adverse consequences from blood glucose–lowering therapy. They may also have delayed psychomotor function that could interfere with the ability to treat hypoglycemia. Other factors to consider in establishing

glycemic goals for the older patient include the patient's own desire for treatment and other coexisting medical conditions such as cognitive impairment. Compounding the challenge is that DM has been found to contribute to a greater rate of decline of cognitive function. Although it is generally agreed that treatment aiming for the same glycemic targets is indicated for otherwise healthy older persons as well as younger persons with DM to prevent acute complications and avoid unpleasant symptoms, strict glycemic control should be based on the degree of frailty. Patients with moderate or advanced frailty have a reduced life expectancy and thus should have a less stringent glycemic target A_{1c} of less than 8.5% (Diabetes Canada Clinical Practice Guidelines Expert Committee, 2018).

As for any group, healthy eating and exercise are recommended as therapy for older patients with DM. This plan should take into account functional limitations that may interfere with physical activity and the ability to prepare meals. Because of the physiological changes that occur with aging, the therapeutic outcome for the older person with DM who receives OHAs may be altered and priority should be prevention of hypoglycemia. Thus, sulphonylureas should be used with caution in the older person as risk of hypoglycemia increases with age. DDP4-inhibitors should be used over sulphonylureas (Diabetes Canada Clinical Practice Guidelines Expert Committee, 2018). Other OHAs described earlier in this chapter may also be used in older patients with DM. Insulin therapy may be instituted if OHAs are not effective. However, it is important to recognize that older patients are more likely to have limitations in manual dexterity and visual acuity, both of which are necessary for accurate insulin administration (Diabetes Canada Clinical Practice Guidelines Expert Committee, 2018).

Patient teaching should be based on the individual's needs, using a slower pace with simple, printed materials. It is important to include family or a support person in the teaching. The patient education issues for the older patient include those related to vision, mobility, cognitive status, memory, functional ability, financial and social situation, the effect of multiple medications, eating habits, the potential for undetected hypoglycemia, and quality of life.

CASE STUDY

Diabetic Ketoacidosis

Patient Profile
H. D. (pronouns he/him), 34 years old, was admitted to the emergency department after he was found unconscious at home by his partner.

Subjective Data (Provided by Partner)
- Was diagnosed with type 1 DM 12 months ago
- Has had difficulty coping with the diagnosis and missed his last two follow-up appointments with the diabetes team
- Was taking 50 units of insulin daily: 5 units of insulin lispro (Humalog) with breakfast, 5 units with lunch, and 10 units with dinner, plus 30 units of insulin glargine (Lantus) at bedtime
- Has history of gastroenteritis for 1 week, with vomiting and anorexia
- Stopped taking insulin 2 days ago when he was unable to eat

Objective Data
Physical Examination
- Breathing is deep and rapid
- Acetone smell on breath
- Skin flushed and dry

Diagnostic Studies
- Blood glucose level of 40.5 mmol/L
- Blood pH of 7.26

Discussion Questions
1. Briefly explain the pathophysiology of the development of diabetic ketoacidosis (DKA) in this patient.
2. What clinical manifestations of DKA does H. D. exhibit?
3. What factors precipitated the DKA?
4. ***Priority decision:*** What is the priority nursing intervention for H. D.?
5. What distinguishes this case history from one of hyperosmolar hyperglycemic state (HHS) or hypoglycemia?
6. ***Priority decision:*** What is the priority teaching that should be done with H. D. and the family?
7. What role should H. D.'s partner have in the management of H. D.'s diabetes?
8. ***Priority decision:*** Based on the assessment data presented, what are the priority nursing diagnoses? Are there any interprofessional issues?
9. ***Evidence-informed practice:*** H. D.'s partner asks if they should have administered insulin when H. D. got sick. How should the nurse respond?

ⓔvolve
Answers are available on http://evolve.elsevier.com/Canada/Lewis/medsurg.

REVIEW QUESTIONS

The number of the question corresponds to the same-numbered objective at the beginning of the chapter.

1. Polydipsia and polyuria related to diabetes mellitus are primarily caused by which of the following?
   a. The release of ketones from cells during fat metabolism
   b. Fluid shifts resulting from the osmotic effect of hyperglycemia
   c. Damage to the kidneys from exposure to high levels of glucose
   d. Changes in red blood cells resulting from attachment of excessive glucose to hemoglobin

2. Which statement would be correct for a client with type 2 diabetes mellitus who is admitted to the hospital with pneumonia?
   a. The client must receive insulin therapy to prevent the development of ketoacidosis.
   b. The client has islet-cell antibodies that have destroyed the ability of the pancreas to produce insulin.
   c. The client has minimal or absent endogenous insulin secretion and requires daily insulin injections.
   d. The client may have sufficient endogenous insulin to prevent ketosis but is at risk for development of hyperosmolar hyperglycemic state.

3. Analyze the following diagnostic findings for a client with type 2 diabetes. Which of the following results will need further assessment?
   a. A_{1c} 9.0%
   b. FBG 7.2 mmol/L
   c. BP 126/80
   d. LDL cholesterol of 2.1 mmol/L

4. Which statement by the client with type 2 diabetes is accurate?
   a. "I am supposed to have a meal or snack if I drink alcohol."
   b. "I am not allowed to eat any sweets because of my diabetes."
   c. "I do not need to watch what I eat because my diabetes is not the bad kind."
   d. "The amount of fat in my diet is not important. Only carbohydrates raise my blood sugar."

5. The nurse is caring for a client with newly diagnosed type 1 diabetes. What information is essential to include in the client teaching before discharge from the hospital? *(Select all that apply.)*
   a. Insulin administration
   b. Elimination of sugar from diet
   c. Need to reduce physical activity
   d. Use of a portable blood glucose monitor
   e. Hypoglycemia prevention, symptoms, and treatment

6. What is the priority action for the nurse to take if the client with type 2 diabetes reports blurred vision and irritability?
   a. Call the health care provider.
   b. Administer insulin as ordered.
   c. Check the client's blood glucose level.
   d. Assess for other neurological symptoms.

7. A client with diabetes has a serum glucose level of 36 mmol/L and is unresponsive. Following assessment of the client, the nurse suspects diabetic ketoacidosis (DKA) rather than hyperosmolar hyperglycemic state (HHS), based on which finding?
   a. Polyuria
   b. Severe dehydration
   c. Rapid, deep respirations
   d. Decreased serum potassium

8. Which of the following are appropriate therapies for clients with diabetes mellitus? *(Select all that apply.)*
   a. Use of diuretics to treat nephropathy
   b. Use of angiotensin-converting enzyme inhibitors to treat nephropathy
   c. Use of serotonin agonists to decrease appetite
   d. Use of laser photocoagulation to treat retinopathy
   e. Use of statins to treat dyslipidemia

1. b, 2. d, 3. a, 4. a, 5. a, d, e, 6. c, 7. c, 8. b, d, e.

evolve

For even more review questions, visit http://evolve.elsevier.com/Canada/Lewis/medsurg.

REFERENCES

Alam, F., Islam, A., Khalil, I., et al. (2016). Metabolic control of type 2 diabetes by targeting the GLUT4 glucose transporter: Intervention approaches. *Current Pharmaceutical Design, 22,* 3034. https://doi.org/10.2174/1381612822666160307145801

Allen, N. A., Zagarins, S. E., Feinberg, R. G., et al. (2017). Treating psychological insulin resistance in type 2 diabetes. *Journal of Clinical and Translational Endocrinology, 7,* 1–6.

American Diabetes Association (ADA). (2008). Nutrition recommendations and interventions for diabetes. *Diabetes Care, 31*(Suppl. 1), S61–S78. (Seminal). https://doi.org/10.2337/dc08-S061

American Diabetes Association (ADA). (2019). Standards of medical care in diabetes. *Diabetes Care, 42*(Suppl. 1), S1–S187. https://care.diabetesjournals.org/content/diacare/suppl/2018/12/17/42.Supplement_1.DC1/DC_42_S1_2019_UPDATED.pdf

Armstrong, D. G., Boulton, A., & Bus, S. (2017). Diabetic foot ulcers and their recurrence. *New England Journal of Medicine, 376,* 2367–2375. https://doi.org/10.1056/NEJMra1615439

Botros, M., Kuhnke, J., Embil, J., et al. (2019). *Best practice recommendations for the prevention and management of diabetic foot ulcers—update 2017.* Wounds Canada. https://www.woundscanada.ca/docman/public/health-care-professional/bpr-workshop/895-

wc-bpr-prevention-and-management-of-diabetic-foot-ulcers-1573r1e-final/file

Brijesh, M. (2015). Somogyi effect in a patient of type 2 diabetes mellitus. *Journal of Diabetes and Metabolism, 6,* 2. https://doi.org/10.4172/2155-6156.1000493

Czech, M. P. (2020). Mechanisms of insulin resistance related to white, beige and brown adipocytes. *Molecular Metabolism, 34,* 27–42. https://doi.org/10.1016/j.molmet.2019.12.014

Diabetes Canada. (2018). *Just the basics.* https://www.diabetes.ca/DiabetesCanadaWebsite/media/Managing-My-Diabetes/Tools%20and%20Resources/just-the-basics.pdf?ext=.pdf

Diabetes Canada. (2019a). *Diabetes charter for Canada. Diabetes in Canada.* https://www.diabetes.ca/DiabetesCanadaWebsite/media/About-Diabetes/Diabetes%20Charter/2019-Backgrounder-Canada.pdf

Diabetes Canada. (2019b). *New data shows diabetes rates and economic burden on families continue to rise in Ontario.* https://www.diabetes.ca/media-room/press-releases/new-data-shows-diabetes-rates-and-economic-burden-on-families-continue-to-rise-in-ontario--

Diabetes Canada. (2020). *Relationship between diabetes and COVID-19.* https://www.diabetes.ca/DiabetesCanadaWebsite/media/Campaigns/COVID-19%20and%20Diabetes/Relationship-between-Diabetes-and-COVID-Sept-2020.pdf

Diabetes Canada Clinical Practice Guidelines Expert Committee. (2018). Diabetes Canada 2018 clinical practice guidelines for the prevention and management of diabetes in Canada. *Canadian Journal of Diabetes, 42*(Suppl. 1), S1–S325.

Diabetes Control Complications Trial (DCCT) Research Group. (1993). The effect of intensive treatment of diabetes on the development and progression of long-term complications in insulin-dependent diabetes mellitus. *New England Journal of Medicine, 329*(14), 977–986. (Seminal).

Eli Lilly Canada. (2021a). *Product monograph: Basaglar.* Eli Lilly Canada Inc. http://pi.lilly.com/ca/basaglar-ca-pm.pdf

Eli Lilly Canada. (2021b). *Product monograph: Trulicity.* Eli Lilly Canada Inc. http://pi.lilly.com/ca/trulicity-ca-pm.pdf

Evert, A. B., Dennison, M., Gardner, C. D., et al. (2019). Nutrition therapy for adults with diabetes or prediabetes: A consensus report. *Diabetes Care, 42*(5), 731–754. https://doi.org/10.2337/dci19-0014

Forum for Injection Technique (FIT) Canada. (2016). *Recommendations for best practice in injection technique* (3rd ed.). http://www.fit4diabetes.com/files/2314/8777/6632/FIT_Recommendations_3rd_Edition_2017.pdf

Freige, C., & Butcher, R. (2020). *Anti-vascular endothelial growth factor drugs for retinal conditions: Comparative clinical effectiveness and guidelines (CADTH rapid response report: summary of abstracts).* CADTH. https://cadth.ca/sites/default/files/pdf/htis/2020/RB1415-%20Anti-VEGF%20Drugs%20V.5.4%20ABS%20corrected.pdf

Gurumurthy, R. P. (2018). Resistin: Is there any role in the mediation of obesity, insulin resistance and type-II diabetes mellitus? *Juniper Online Journal of Case Studies, 6*(3), 555686. https://doi.org/10.19080/JOJCS.2018.06.555686

Health Canada. (2021). *Canada's dietary guidelines.* https://food-guide.canada.ca/en/guidelines/what-are-canadas-dietary-guidelines/

Institute for Safe Medication Practices (ISMP) Canada. (2016). *Safe management of patients with an external subcutaneous insulin pump during hospitalization.* https://www.ismp.org/resources/safe-management-patients-external-subcutaneous-insulin-pump-during-hospitalization

International Diabetes Federation (IDF). (2021). *Diabetes atlas* (10th ed.). https://diabetesatlas.org/en/

Javed, S., Petropoulos, I. N., Alam, U., et al. (2015). Treatment of painful diabetic neuropathy. *Therapeutic Advances in Chronic Disease, 6*(1), 15–28. https://doi.org/10.1177/2040622314552071

Kasprzak, C., Ho, C., & Dan, L. (2016). *A multi-incident analysis by ISMP Canada. Insulin medication incidents in the community. Pharmacy Connection, Summer 2016.* https://www.ismp-canada.org/download/PharmacyConnection/PC2016-InsulinMedicationIncidentsintheCommunity.pdf

Keto, J., Ventola, H., Jokelainen, J., et al. (2016). Cardiovascular disease risk factors in relation to smoking behaviour and history: A population-based cohort study. *Open Heart, 3,* e000358. https://doi.org/10.1136/openhrt-2015-000358

Kreider, K. E. (2018). Updates in the management of diabetic ketoacidosis. *The Journal for Nurse Practitioners, 14*(8), 591–597. https://doi.org/10.1016/j.nurpra.2018.06.013

Liscombe, L., Butalia, S., Dasgupta, K., et al. (2020). Pharmacologic glycemic management of type 2 diabetes in adults: 2020 update. *Canadian Journal of Diabetes, 44,* 575–591. https://doi.org/10.1016/j.jcjd.2020.08.001

Lo, K. B., Gul, F., Ram, P., et al. (2020). The effects of SGLT2 inhibitors on cardiovascular and renal outcomes in diabetic patients: A systematic review and meta-analysis. *Cardiorenal Medicine, 10,* 1–10. https://doi.org/10.1159/000503919

Melo, K. F. S., Bahia, L. R., Pasinato, B., et al. (2019). Short-acting insulin analogues versus regular human insulin on postprandial glucose and hypoglycemia in type 1 diabetes mellitus: A systematic review and meta-analysis. *Diabetology & Metabolic Syndrome, 11*(2). https://doi.org/10.1186/s13098-018-0397-3

Merck Canada. (2021). *Product monograph including patient information: Januvia.* Merck Canada Inc. https://www.merck.ca/static/pdf/JANUVIA-PM_E.pdf

NovoNordisk. (2017). *Product monograph: Levemir.* NovoNordisk Canada Inc. https://www.novonordisk.ca/content/dam/Canada/AFFILIATE/www-novonordisk-ca/OurProducts/PDF/levemir-product-monograph.pdf

NovoNordisk. (2019). *Product monograph including patient information: Tresiba.* NovoNordisk Canada Inc. https://www.novonordisk.ca/content/dam/Canada/AFFILIATE/www-novonordisk-ca/OurProducts/PDF/tresiba-product-monograph.pdf

NovoNordisk. (2020). *Product monograph including patient information: Victoza.* Novo-Nordisk Canada Inc. https://www.novonordisk.ca/content/dam/Canada/AFFILIATE/www-novonordisk-ca/OurProducts/PDF/victoza-product-monograph.pdf

Patel, N. U., Roach, C., Alinia, H., et al. (2018). Current treatment options for acanthosis nigricans. *Clinical, Cosmetic and Investigational Dermatology, 11,* 407–413. https://doi.org/10.2147/CCID.S137527

Pillinger, T., Beck, K., Gobjila, C., et al. (2017). Impaired glucose homeostasis in first-episode schizophrenia: A systematic review and meta-analysis. *JAMA Psychiatry, 74*(3), 261–269. https://doi.org/10.1001/jamapsychiatry.2016.3803

Poirier, P., Bertrand, O. R., Leipsic, J., et al. (2018). Diabetes Canada 2018 clinical practice guidelines for the prevention and management of diabetes in Canada: Screening for the presence of cardiovascular disease. *Canadian Journal of Diabetes, 42* (Suppl. 1), S170–S177.

Registered Nurses' Association of Ontario (RNAO). (2009). *Nursing Best Practice Guidelines. Subcutaneous administration of insulin in adults with type 2 diabetes—Revision.* (Seminal). https://rnao.ca/sites/rnao-ca/files/BPG_for_the_Subcutaneous_Administration_of_Insulin_in_Adults_with_Type_2_Diabetes.pdf

Sanofi-Aventis Canada Inc. (2018). *Product monograph: Glucophage.* Sanofi-Aventis Inc. http://products.sanofi.ca/en/glucophage.pdf

Sanofi-Aventis Canada Inc. (2020). *Product monograph including patient information: Toujeo.* Sanofi-Aventis Canada Inc. http://products.sanofi.ca/en/toujeo-solostar.pdf

Sanofi-Aventis Canada Inc. (2021). *Product monograph including patient information: Lantus.* Sanofi-Aventis Canada Inc. http://products.sanofi.ca/en/lantus.pdf

Schmidt, B. M., & Holmes, C. M. (2018). Updates on diabetic foot and charcot osteopathic arthropathy. *Current Diabetes Reports, 18,* 74. https://doi.org/10.1007/s11892-018-1047-8

Tosi, F., Bonora, E., & Moghetti, P. (2017). Insulin resistance in a large cohort of women with polycystic ovary syndrome: A comparison between euglycaemic-hyperinsulinaemic clamp and surrogate indexes. *Human Reproduction, 32*(12), 2515–2521. https://doi.org/10.1093/humrep/dex308

United Kingdom Prospective Diabetes Study (UKPDS). (1998). Intensive blood glucose control with sulphonylureas or insulin compared with conventional treatment and risk of complications in patients with type 2 diabetes. *Lancet, 352*(9131), 837–853. (Seminal).

Wexler, D. (2021). *Initial management of blood glucose in adults with type 2 diabetes mellitus.* UpToDate. https://www.uptodate.com/contents/initial-management-of-blood-glucose-in-adults-with-type-2-diabetes-mellitus#H4090323182

RESOURCES

Diabetes Canada
https://www.diabetes.ca

Diabetes Canada—*2018 Clinical Practice Guidelines for the Prevention and Management of Diabetes in Canada*
http://guidelines.diabetes.ca/cpg

Diabetes Canada—*Financial Assistance for People With Diabetes*
https://diabetes.ca/learn-about-diabetes/your-rights/financial-assistance

Dietitians of Canada
https://www.dietitians.ca

Heart and Stroke Foundation
https://www.heartandstroke.on.ca/

Ontario Ministry of Health—*MedsCheck Diabetes Program*
https://www.health.gov.on.ca/en/pro/programs/drugs/medscheck/medscheck_diabetes.aspx

Public Health Agency of Canada—*Can I Get Help to Pay for My Diabetes Medications and Supplies?*
https://www.phac-aspc.gc.ca/cd-mc/diabetes-diabete/pay-payer-eng.php

Public Health Agency of Canada—*Diabetes in Canada*
http://www.phac-aspc.gc.ca/cd-mc/publications/diabetes-diabete/facts-figures-faits-chiffres-2011/highlights-saillants-eng.php#chp5

Registered Nurses' Association of Ontario (RNAO)—*Nursing Best Practice Guidelines*
https://rnao.ca/bpg

American Diabetes Association (ADA)
https://www.diabetes.org

Glycemic Index Calculator (University of Sydney)
https://www.glycemicindex.com

International Diabetes Federation (IDF)
https://www.idf.org

Joslin Diabetes Center
https://www.joslin.org/

National Institute of Diabetes and Digestive and Kidney Disease—*Diabetes*
https://www.niddk.nih.gov/health-information/diabetes

⊖volve

For additional Internet resources, see the website for this book at http://evolve.elsevier.com/Canada/Lewis/medsurg.

WEBSITE

http://evolve.elsevier.com/Canada/Lewis/medsurg

- Review Questions (Online Only)
- Key Points
- Answer Guidelines for Case Study

- Conceptual Care Map Creator
- Audio Glossary

- Supporting Media—Animations
  - Lymphatic Drainage of Breast
  - The Menstrual Cycle
- Content Updates

LEARNING OBJECTIVES

1. Describe the structures and functions of the reproductive systems.
2. Outline the functions of the major hormones essential for functioning of the reproductive systems.
3. Explain the physiological changes during the stages of sexual response.
4. Link the age-related changes of the reproductive systems to the differences in assessment findings.
5. Identify significant subjective and objective data related to the reproductive systems and information about sexual function that should be obtained from a patient.
6. Select the appropriate techniques to use in the physical assessment of the reproductive systems.
7. Differentiate normal from common abnormal findings of a physical assessment of the reproductive systems.
8. Describe the purpose, significance of results, and nursing responsibilities related to diagnostic studies of the reproductive systems.

KEY TERMS

amenorrhea	epididymis	menstrual cycle
clitoris	gonads	mons pubis
ductus deferens (or vas deferens)	menarche	nulliparous
dyspareunia	menopause	spermatogenesis

STRUCTURES AND FUNCTIONS OF THE MALE AND FEMALE REPRODUCTIVE SYSTEMS

The reproductive system consists of primary (or essential) organs and secondary (or accessory) organs. The primary reproductive organs are referred to as gonads. The female gonads are the ovaries; the male gonads are the testes. The primary responsibility of the gonads is secretion of hormones and production of gametes (ova and sperm). Secondary or accessory organs are responsible for (a) transporting and nourishing the ova and sperm and (b) preserving and protecting the fertilized eggs.

Male Reproductive System

The three primary roles of the male reproductive system are (1) production and transportation of sperm, (2) deposit of sperm in the female reproductive tract, and (3) secretion of hormones.

The primary reproductive organs are the testes. Secondary reproductive organs include ducts (epididymis, ductus deferens, ejaculatory duct, and urethra), sex glands (prostate gland, Cowper's glands, and seminal vesicles), and the external genitalia (scrotum and penis) (Figure 53.1).

Testes. The paired testes are ovoid, smooth, firm organs measuring 3.5 to 5.5 cm long and 2 to 3 cm wide. They are within the scrotum, which is a loose protective sac composed of a thin, loose outer layer of skin over a tough connective tissue layer. Within the testes, coiled structures known as *seminiferous tubules* form *spermatozoa* (immature sperm). The process of sperm production is called spermatogenesis. Interstitial cells of the testes lie between the seminiferous tubules and produce the male sex hormone testosterone.

Ducts. Sperm formed in the seminiferous tubules move through a series of ducts. These ducts transport the sperm from

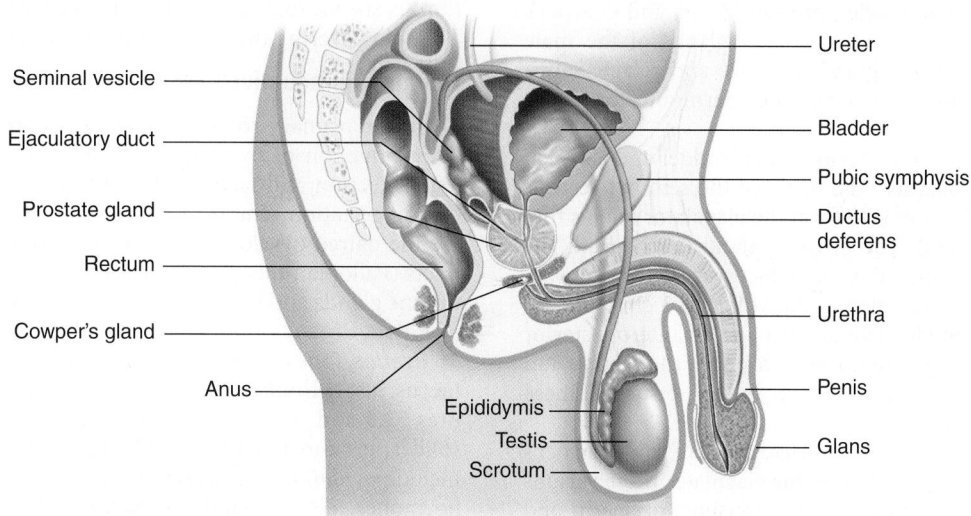

FIG. 53.1 External and internal male sex organs. Source: Patton, K. T., & Thibodeau, G. A. (2013). *Anatomy and physiology* (8th ed., p. 1045, Figure 34.1). Mosby.

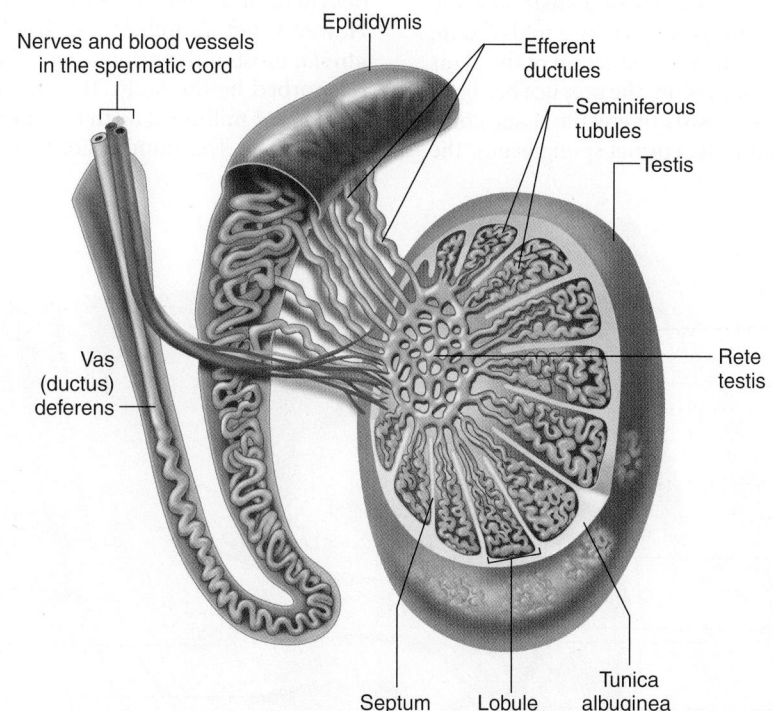

FIG. 53.2 Seminiferous tubules, testis, epididymis, and ductus (vas) deferens in the male reproductive system. Source: Patton, K. T., & Thibodeau, G. A. (2013). *Anatomy and physiology* (8th ed., p. 1046, Figure 34.3B). Mosby.

the testes to the outside of the body. As sperm exit the testes, they enter and pass through the epididymis, the ductus deferens, the ejaculatory duct, and the urethra.

The **epididymis** is a comma-shaped structure located on the posterior-superior aspect of each testis within the scrotum; it transports the sperm as they mature (Figure 53.2; see also Figure 53.1). It is a very long, tightly coiled tubular structure that measures about 6 m in length (Patton & Thibodeau, 2015). The epididymis transports the sperm as they mature. Sperm exit the epididymis through a long, thick tube known as the **ductus deferens (or vas deferens)**.

The ductus deferens is continuous with the epididymis within the scrotal sac. It travels upward through the scrotum and continues through the inguinal ring into the abdominal cavity. The spermatic cord is a connective tissue sheath that encloses the ductus deferens, arteries, veins, nerves, and lymph vessels as it ascends up through the inguinal canal (see Figure 53.2). In the abdominal cavity, the ductus deferens travels up, over, and behind the bladder. Posterior to the bladder, the ductus deferens joins the seminal vesicle to form the ejaculatory duct (see Figure 53.1).

The ejaculatory duct passes downward through the prostate gland, connecting with the urethra. The urethra extends from the bladder and through the prostate and ends in a slitlike opening (the meatus) on the ventral side of the *glans,* the tip of the penis. During the process of ejaculation, sperm travels through the urethra and out of the penis.

Glands. The seminal vesicles, prostate gland, and Cowper's (bulbourethral) glands are the accessory glands of the male reproductive system. These glands produce and secrete seminal fluid (semen), which surrounds the sperm and forms the *ejaculate.*

The seminal vesicles lie posterior to the bladder and between the rectum and the bladder. The ducts of the seminal vesicles fuse with the ductus deferens to form the ejaculatory ducts that enter the prostate gland. The prostate gland lies beneath the bladder. Its posterior surface is in contact with the rectal wall. The prostate normally measures 2 cm wide and 3 cm long and is divided into right and left lateral lobes and an anteroposterior median lobe. Cowper's glands lie on each side of the urethra and slightly posterior to it, just below the prostate. The ducts of these glands enter directly into the urethra.

Secretions from the seminal vesicles, prostate, and Cowper's glands make up most of the fluid in the ejaculate. These various secretions serve as a medium for the transport of sperm and create an alkaline, nutritious environment that promotes sperm motility and survival.

External Genitalia. The external genitalia consist of the penis and the scrotum. The penis consists of a shaft, and the tip is known as the *glans.* The glans is covered by a fold of skin, the prepuce (or foreskin), that forms at the junction of the glans and the shaft of the penis. In circumcision, the prepuce has been removed. The shaft of the penis consists of erectile tissue composed of the corpus cavernosum, the corpus spongiosum, the fibrous sheath that encases the erectile tissue, and the urethra. The skin covering the penis is thin, loose, and hairless.

Female Reproductive System

The three primary roles of the female reproductive system are (1) production of ova (eggs), (2) secretion of hormones, and (3) protection and facilitation of the development of the fetus during gestation. The primary reproductive organs in females are the paired ovaries. Secondary reproductive organs include ducts (Fallopian tubes), the uterus, the vagina, sex glands (Bartholin's glands and breasts), and the external genitalia (vulva).

Pelvic Organs

Ovaries. The ovaries are usually located on either side of the uterus, just behind and below the Fallopian (uterine) tubes (Figures 53.3 and 53.4). The almond-shaped ovaries are firm and solid, approximately 1.5 cm wide and 3 cm long. Their functions include *ovulation* and secretion of the two major reproductive hormones, *estrogen* and *progesterone*. The outer zone of the ovary contains follicles with germ cells, or *oocytes*. Each follicle contains a primordial (immature) oocyte surrounded by granulosa and theca cells. These two layers protect and nourish the oocyte until the follicle reaches maturity and ovulation occurs. However, not all follicles reach maturity. In a process termed *atresia*, most of the primordial follicles become smaller and are reabsorbed by the body. Thus the number of follicles declines from 2 to 4 million at birth to approximately 300 000 to 400 000 at menarche. This number continues to decrease throughout the

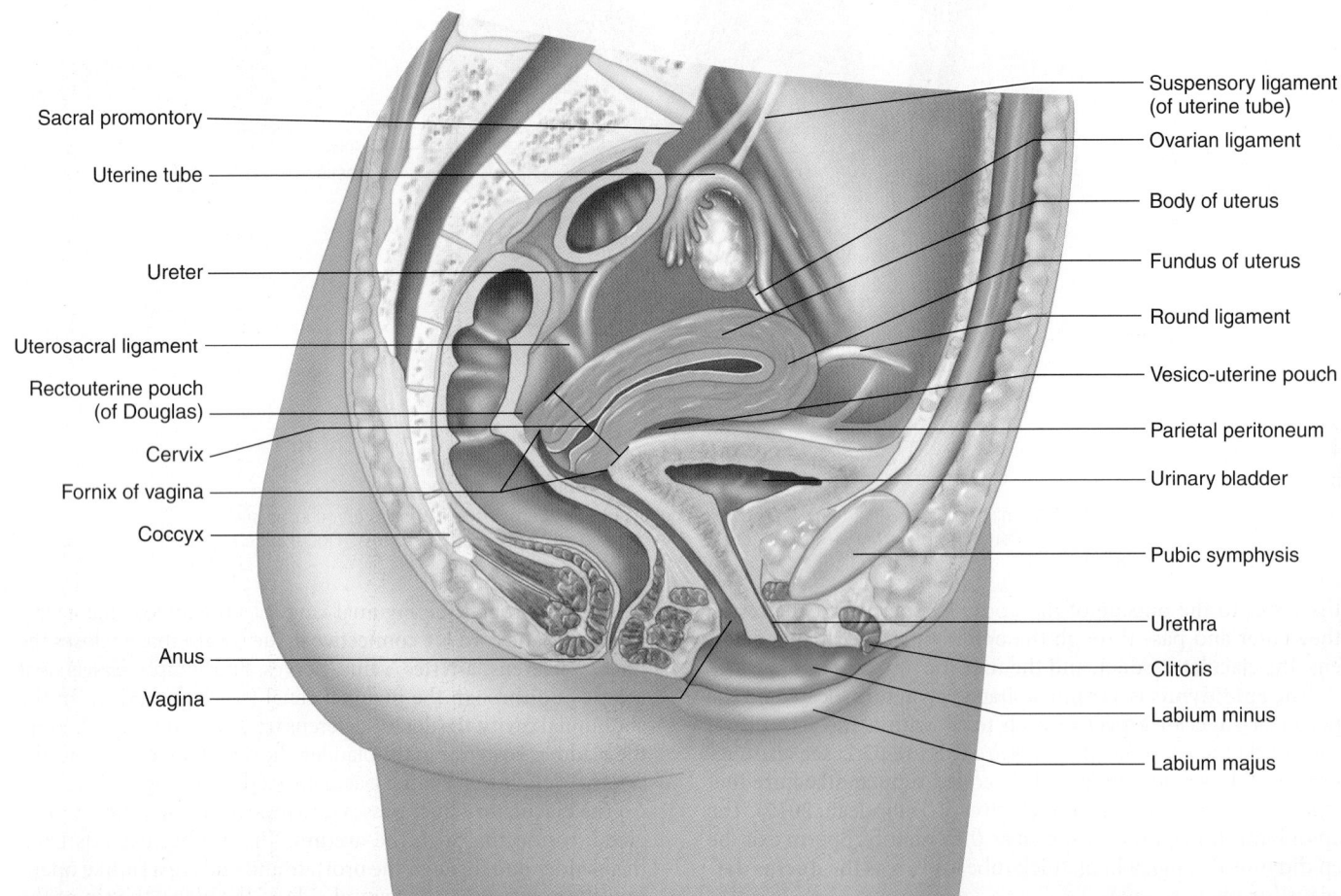

FIG. 53.3 Female reproductive tract and related organs. Source: Patton, K. T., & Thibodeau, G. A. (2013). *Anatomy and physiology* (8th ed., p. 1065, Figure 35.1A). Mosby.

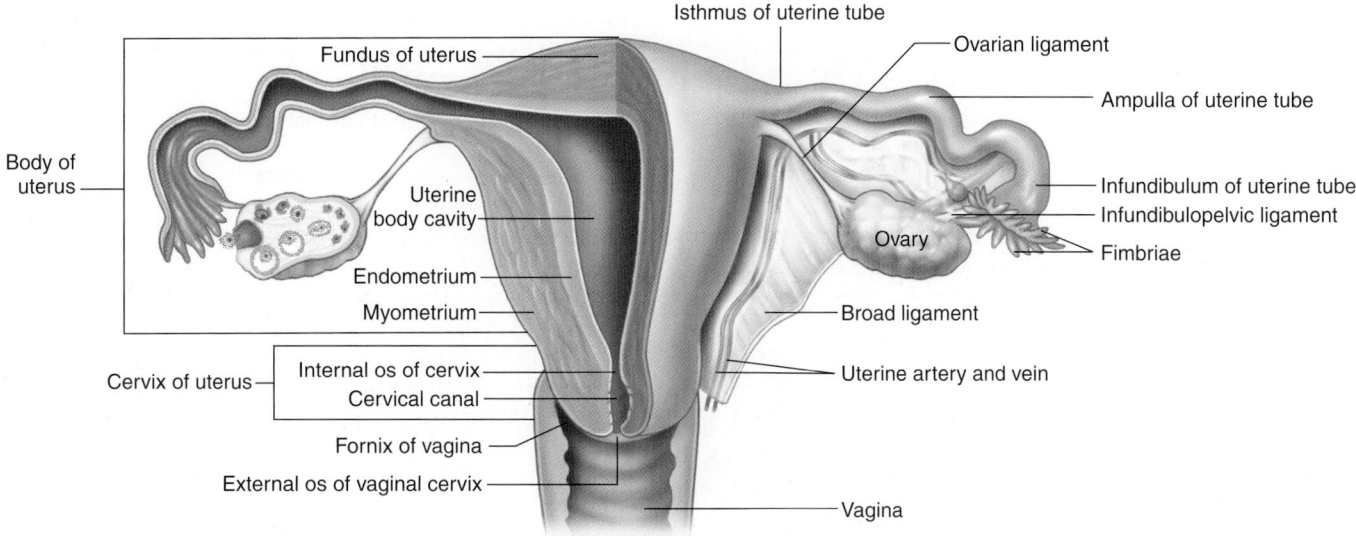

FIG. 53.4 Female reproductive tract. Source: Modified from Patton, K. T., & Thibodeau, G. A. (2013). *Anatomy and physiology* (8th ed., p. 1066, Figure 35.3A). Mosby.

reproductive years. Fewer than 500 oocytes are actually released by ovulation during the reproductive years of a normal healthy woman.

Fallopian Tubes. Normally, each month during a woman's reproductive years, one ovarian follicle reaches maturity, and the ovum is ovulated, or expelled, from the ovary through the stimulus of the gonadotropic hormones: follicle-stimulating hormone (FSH) and luteinizing hormone (LH). The ovum then travels up a Fallopian tube, where fertilization by sperm may occur. An ovum can be fertilized up to 72 hours after its release from the ovary.

The distal ends of the Fallopian tubes consist of finger-like projections called *fimbriae* that "massage" the ovaries at ovulation to help extract the mature ovum. The tubes, which average 12 cm in length, extend from the fimbriae to the superior lateral borders of the uterus. Fertilization usually takes place within the outer third of the Fallopian tubes.

Uterus. The uterus is a pear-shaped, hollow, muscular organ (see Figures 53.3 and 53.4). It is located between the bladder and the rectum. In the mature **nulliparous** (never pregnant) woman, the uterus is approximately 6 to 8 cm long and 4 cm wide. The uterine walls consist of an outer serosal layer, the *perimetrium;* a middle muscular layer, the *myometrium;* and an inner mucosal layer, the *endometrium.*

The uterus consists of the fundus, the body (or corpus), and the cervix (see Figures 53.3 and 53.4). The body makes up about 80% of the uterus and connects with the cervix at the isthmus (or neck). The cervix is the lower portion of the uterus that projects into the anterior wall of the vaginal canal. It makes up about 15 to 20% of the uterus in the nulliparous female. The cervix consists of the *ectocervix,* the outer portion that protrudes into the vagina, and the *endocervix,* the canal in the opening of the cervix. The opening of the cervix is referred to as the *cervical os* (Figure 53.5).

The ectocervix is covered with squamous epithelial cells, which give it a smooth, pinkish appearance. The endocervix contains a lining of columnar epithelial cells, which give it a rough, reddened appearance. The junction at which the two types of epithelial cells meet is termed the *squamocolumnar*

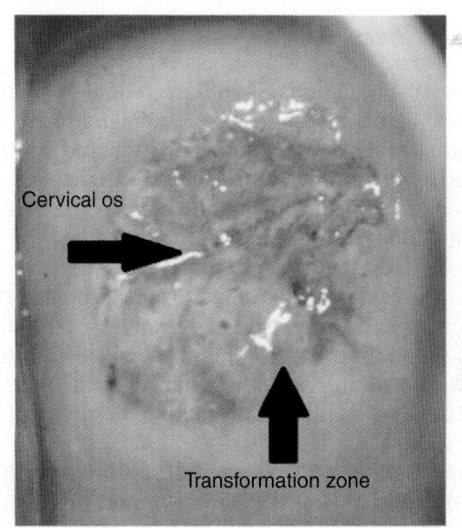

FIG. 53.5 Cervical os and squamocolumnar junction (transformation zone). Courtesy Candy Tedschi, NP, Great Neck, NY.

junction and contains the optimal types of cells needed for an accurate Papanicolaou (Pap) smear to screen for cervical cancer.

The cervical canal is 2 to 4 cm long and is relatively tightly closed. The cervix, however, allows sperm to enter the uterus and also allows menstruation to occur. The columnar epithelium, under hormonal influence, provides elasticity; thus the cervix can stretch to allow passage of a fetus during labour and the birth process. The entrance of sperm into the uterus is facilitated by mucus produced by the cervix under the influence of estrogen. Under normal conditions, the cervical mucus becomes watery, stretchy, and more abundant at ovulation. This mucus facilitates the passage of sperm into the uterus. The post-ovulatory cervical mucus, under the influence of progesterone, is thick and inhibits sperm passage.

Vagina. The vagina is a tubular structure 8 to 10 cm long that is lined with squamous epithelium. The secretions of the vagina consist of cervical mucus, desquamated epithelium, and

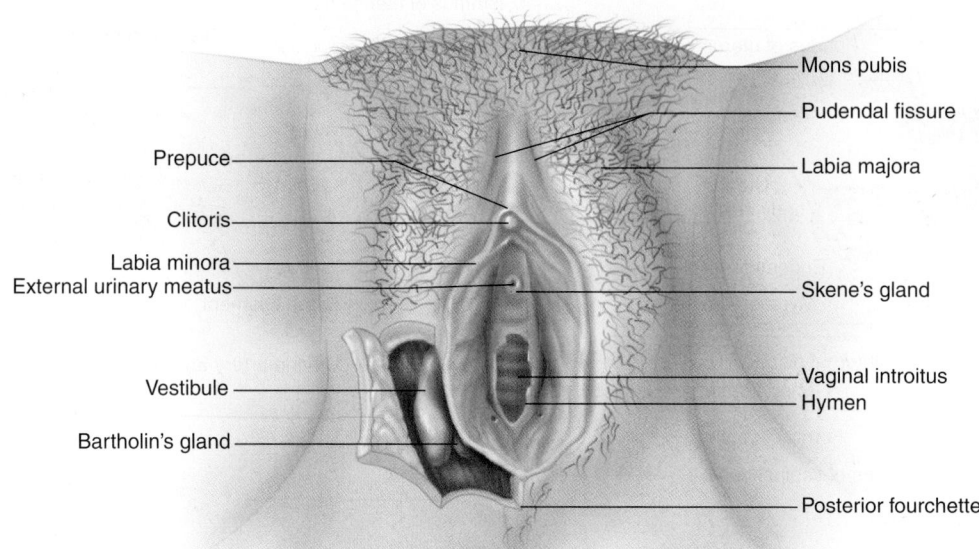

Prepuce

Clitoris

Labia minora
External urinary meatus

Vestibule

Bartholin's gland

Mons pubis

Pudendal fissure

Labia majora

Skene's gland

Vaginal introitus
Hymen

Posterior fourchette

FIG. 53.6 External female genitalia. Source: Modified from Thibodeau, G. A., & Patton, K. T. (2013). *Anatomy and physiology* (8th ed., p. 1065, Figure 35.2). Mosby.

during sexual stimulation, a watery secretion. These fluids protect against vaginal infection. The muscular and erectile tissue of the vaginal walls allows enough dilation and contraction to accommodate the passage of the fetus during labour, as well as penetration of the penis during intercourse. The anterior vaginal wall lies along the urethra and the bladder. The posterior vaginal wall is adjacent to the rectum.

Pelvis. The female pelvis consists of four bones (two pelvic bones, sacrum, and coccyx) held together by several strong ligaments. The sections of these bones that lie below the iliopectineal line play a very important role during birth: Their ability to separate is often a factor in determining the ability of a woman to deliver a child vaginally.

External Genitalia. The external portion of the female reproductive system (Figure 53.6), commonly called the *vulva,* consists of the mons pubis, labia majora, labia minora, clitoris, urethral meatus, Skene's glands, vaginal introitus (opening), and Bartholin's glands.

The **mons pubis** is a fatty layer lying over the pubic bone. In female adults, it is covered by coarse hair that lies in a triangular pattern. (The pubic hair pattern in male adults is diamond-shaped.) The labia majora are folds of adiposė tissue that form the outer borders of the vulva. The hairless labia minora form the borders of the vaginal orifice and extend anteriorly to enclose the clitoris (Gress, 2017).

The *vestibule* is a boat-shaped fossa between the labia minora, extending from the clitoris at the anterior end to the vaginal opening at the posterior end. The *perineum* is the area between the vagina and the anus. The vaginal introitus is surrounded by thin membranous tissue called the *hymen.* In female adults, the hymen usually appears as folds or hymenal tags and separates the external genitalia from the vagina. At the posterior aspect of the vagina, a tense band of mucous membrane connecting the posterior ends of the labia minora is referred to as the *posterior fourchette.*

The **clitoris** is erectile tissue that lies anterior to the urethral meatus and the vaginal orifice and becomes engorged during

sexual excitation. It lies anterior to the urethral meatus and the vaginal orifice and is usually covered by the prepuce (Gress, 2017). Clitoral stimulation is an important part of sexual activity for many women.

Ducts of the *Skene's glands* lie alongside the urinary meatus and are thought to help lubricate the urinary meatus (Gress, 2017). *Bartholin's glands,* located at the posterior and lateral aspects of the vaginal orifice, secrete a thin, mucoid material believed to contribute slightly to lubrication during sexual intercourse. These glands are not usually palpable unless sebaceous-like cysts form or an infection is present, such as sexually transmitted and blood-borne infections (STBBIs).

Breasts. The breasts are a secondary sex characteristic; they develop during puberty in response to estrogen and progesterone. Cyclical hormonal changes lead to regular changes in breast tissue to prepare it for lactation when fertilization and pregnancy occur.

The breasts extend from the second to the sixth ribs, with an area called the *tail of Spence* reaching the axilla. The fully mature breast is dome-shaped and contains a pigmented centre termed the *areola.* The areolar region contains Montgomery's tubercles, which are similar to sebaceous glands and assist in lubricating the nipple. During lactation, the alveoli secrete milk (Figure 53.7). The milk then flows into a ductal system and is transported to the lactiferous sinuses. The nipple contains 15 to 20 tiny openings through which the milk flows during breastfeeding. The fibrous and fatty tissue that supports and separates the channels of the mammary duct system primarily accounts for the varying sizes and shapes of the breasts in different individuals.

The breast has a rich lymphatic network that drains into the axillary and clavicular channels (see Chapter 54, Figure 54.7). Superficial lymph nodes are located in the axilla and are accessible to examination. This system is often responsible for the metastasis of a malignant tumour from the breast to other parts of the body.

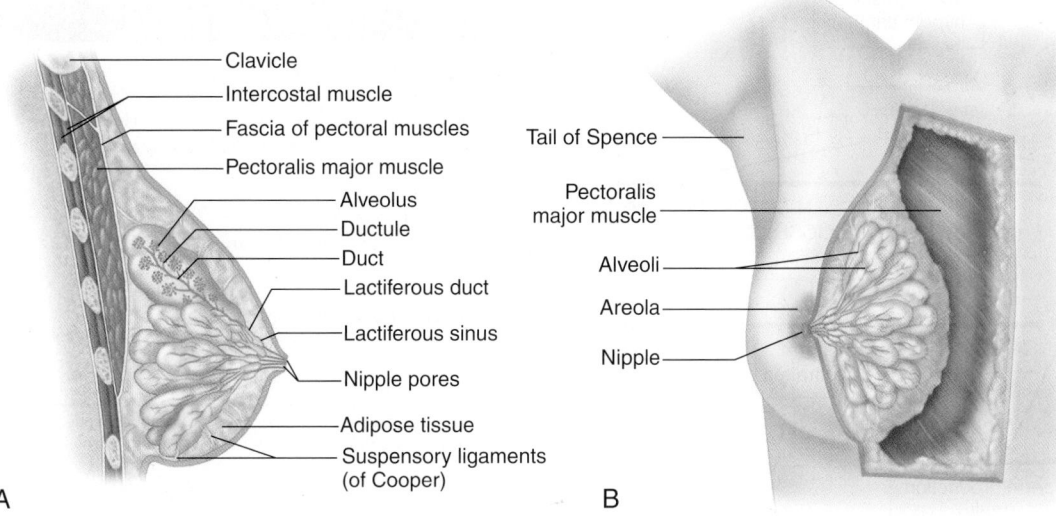

FIG. 53.7 The lactating female breast. **A,** Illustration of a sagittal section of a lactating breast. Glandular structures are anchored to the overlying skin and to the pectoral muscle by suspensory ligaments of Cooper. Each lobule of glandular tissues is drained by a lactiferous duct that eventually opens through the nipple. **B,** Illustration of the anterior view of a lactating breast. In nonlactating breasts, the glandular tissue is much less evident; adipose tissue makes up most of each breast. Source: Thibodeau, G. A., & Patton, K. T. (2013). *Anatomy and physiology* (8th ed., p. 1083, Figure 36.16). Mosby.

CASE STUDY

Patient Introduction

A. K. (pronouns she/her), 21 years old, is being evaluated for pelvic pain and irregular menstrual bleeding for the past several months. Medications include oral contraceptive pills orally once daily and naproxen as need for pain.

Discussion Questions

Throughout this chapter, think about A. K.'s concerns with the following questions in mind:
1. What are the possible causes for her irregular menstrual bleeding?
2. What would be the priority assessment questions to ask her?
3. How would the nurse individualize the assessment based on her age, ethnic or cultural background, and condition?

You will learn more about A. K. as you read through this assessment chapter. See Case Study: Subjective Data, Case Study: Objective Data: Physical Examination, and Case Study: Objective Data: Diagnostic Studies for more information on A. K.

🅔volve
Answers available at http://evolve.elsevier.com/Lewis/medsurg.

Neuroendocrine Regulation of the Reproductive System

The hypothalamus, the pituitary gland, and the gonads secrete numerous hormones (Figure 53.8). (Endocrine hormones are discussed in Chapter 50.) These hormones regulate the processes of ovulation, spermatogenesis (process of sperm production), and fertilization and the formation and function of the secondary sex characteristics. In women, the hormones secreted by the anterior pituitary gland cause cyclical changes in the ovaries. The hypothalamus secretes gonadotropin-releasing hormone (GnRH), which stimulates the pituitary gland to secrete its hormones, including FSH and LH. LH in males is sometimes called *interstitial cell–stimulating hormone* (ICSH). The gonadal hormones are estrogen, progesterone, and testosterone.

In women, FSH production by the anterior pituitary gland stimulates the growth and maturity of the ovarian follicles

necessary for ovulation (Holesh et al., 2021). The mature follicle produces estrogen, which in turn suppresses the release of FSH. Another hormone, inhibin, is also secreted by the ovarian follicles and inhibits both GnRH and FSH secretion. In men, FSH stimulates the seminiferous tubules to produce sperm.

LH contributes to the ovulatory process because it causes follicles to complete maturation and undergo ovulation. It also causes the ruptured follicle (area where the ovum exited during ovulation) to turn into a corpus luteum from which progesterone is secreted. Progesterone maintains the rich vascular state of the uterus (secretory phase) in preparation for fertilization and implantation. In men, LH (ICSH) triggers testosterone production by the interstitial cells of the testes and thus is essential for the full maturation of sperm. Prolactin has no known function in men. In women, prolactin stimulates the development and growth of the mammary glands. During lactation, it initiates and maintains milk production.

The gonadal hormones, estrogen and progesterone, are produced by the ovaries in women. Small amounts of an estrogen precursor are also produced in the adrenal cortices. Estrogen is essential to the development and maintenance of the secondary sex characteristics, the proliferative phase of the menstrual cycle immediately after menstruation, and the uterine changes essential to pregnancy. The role and importance of estrogen in men are not well understood. In men, estrogen is produced predominantly in the adrenal cortex.

Progesterone plays a major role in the menstrual cycle but most specifically in the secretory phase. Like estrogen, progesterone is involved in the bodily changes associated with pregnancy. Adequate progesterone is necessary to maintain an implanted egg.

In men, the major gonadal hormone is testosterone, which is produced by the testes. Testosterone is responsible for the development and maintenance of secondary sex characteristics, as well as for adequate spermatogenesis. In women, androgens are produced in small amounts by the adrenal glands and ovaries.

The circulating levels of gonadal hormones are controlled primarily by a *negative feedback process.* Receptors within the

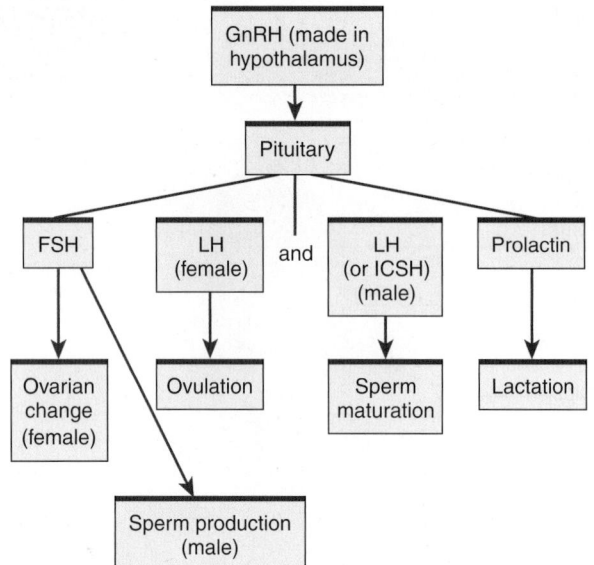

FIG. 53.8 Hypothalamic–pituitary–gonadal axis. Only the major pituitary hormone actions are depicted. *FSH,* follicle-stimulating hormone; *GnRH,* gonadotropin-releasing hormone; *ICSH,* interstitial cell–stimulating hormone; *LH,* luteinizing hormone.

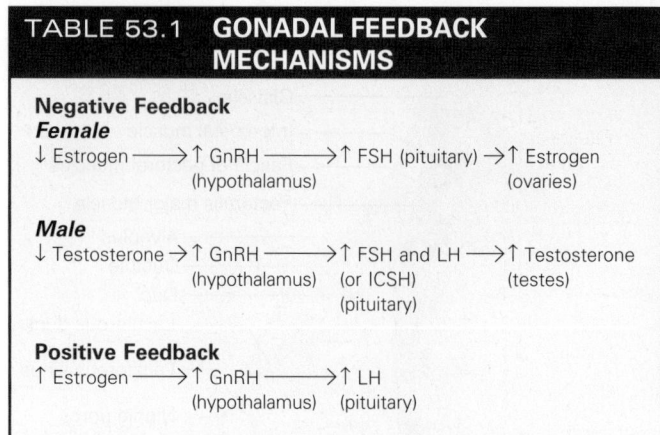

FSH, follicle-stimulating hormone; *GnRH,* gonadotropin-releasing hormone; *ICSH,* interstitial cell–stimulating hormone; *LH,* luteinizing hormone.

hypothalamus and the pituitary are sensitive to the circulating blood levels of the hormones (Table 53.1). Increased levels of hormones stimulate a hypothalamic response that decreases the high circulating levels. Likewise, low circulating levels provoke a hypothalamic response that increases the low circulating levels. For example, if the circulating level of testosterone in men is low, the hypothalamus is stimulated to secrete GnRH. This triggers the anterior pituitary gland to secrete greater amounts of FSH and LH, which in turn set off an increase in the production of testosterone. The high levels of testosterone then stimulate a decrease in the production of GnRH and thus of FSH and LH.

In women, however, this process is slightly different. The circulating levels are controlled through a combination of both a negative and a positive feedback system. The negative feedback control mechanism is similar to that described previously in men. When circulating estrogen levels are low, the hypothalamus is stimulated to increase its production of GnRH. GnRH stimulates the pituitary to secrete greater amounts of FSH and LH, which results in higher levels of estrogen production by the ovaries. Reciprocally, higher levels of circulating estrogen result in a decreasing secretion of GnRH and thus bring about a decrease in the secretion of FSH by the pituitary gland.

A positive feedback control mechanism also exists in women: With the increased levels of circulating estrogen, GnRH is produced at a higher level, which results in an increased level of LH from the pituitary, which instigates ovulation. Likewise, lowered levels of estrogen result in a lowered level of LH.

Menarche

Menarche is the first episode of menstrual bleeding and indicates that a girl has reached puberty. On average, menarche begins at 12.4 years of age (Lacroix et al., 2021). Menstrual cycles are often irregular for the first 1 to 2 years after menarche because of *anovulatory* cycles (cycles without ovulation).

Menstrual Cycle

The major functions of the ovaries are ovulation and the secretion of hormones. These functions are accomplished during the normal **menstrual cycle**, a monthly process mediated by the hormonal activity of the hypothalamus, the pituitary gland, and the ovaries. Menstruation occurs during each month in which an egg is not fertilized (Figure 53.9). The endometrial cycle is divided into three phases labelled in relation to uterine and ovarian changes: (1) the *proliferative* or *follicular phase,* (2) the *secretory* or *luteal phase,* and (3) the *menstrual* or *ischemic phase.* The length of the menstrual cycle ranges from 20 to 40 days, the average being 28 days.

The menstrual cycle begins on the first day of one menstrual period (menses), which usually lasts 4 to 6 days, and ends the day before the first day of the next. Table 53.2 provides characteristics of the menstrual cycle and related patient teaching. During this time, estrogen and progesterone levels are low, but FSH levels begin to increase. During the follicular phase, usually a single follicle matures fully under the stimulation of FSH. (The mechanism that ensures that usually only one follicle reaches maturity is not known.) The mature follicle stimulates estrogen production, causing the negative feedback that results in decreased FSH secretion.

Although the initial stage of follicular maturation is stimulated by FSH, complete maturation and ovulation occur only when LH is present. When estrogen levels peak on about the twelfth day of the cycle, there is a surge of LH, which triggers ovulation a day or two later. After ovulation (maturation and release of an ovum), LH promotes the development of the corpus luteum.

The fully developed corpus luteum continues to secrete estrogen and initiates progesterone secretion. If fertilization occurs, high levels of estrogen and progesterone continue to be secreted because of the continued activity of the corpus luteum from stimulation by human chorionic gonadotropin (hCG). If fertilization does not take place, estrogen production decreases, and progesterone secretion stops and, accordingly, menses occurs.

During the *follicular phase,* the endometrial lining of the uterus also undergoes change. As larger amounts of estrogen are produced, the endometrial lining undergoes proliferative changes, and cellular growth, including the length of blood vessels and glandular tissue, increases.

With ovulation and the resulting increased levels of progesterone, the *luteal* (or *secretory*) phase begins. If the corpus luteum regresses (i.e., fertilization does not occur) and estrogen and progesterone levels fall, the endometrial lining can no

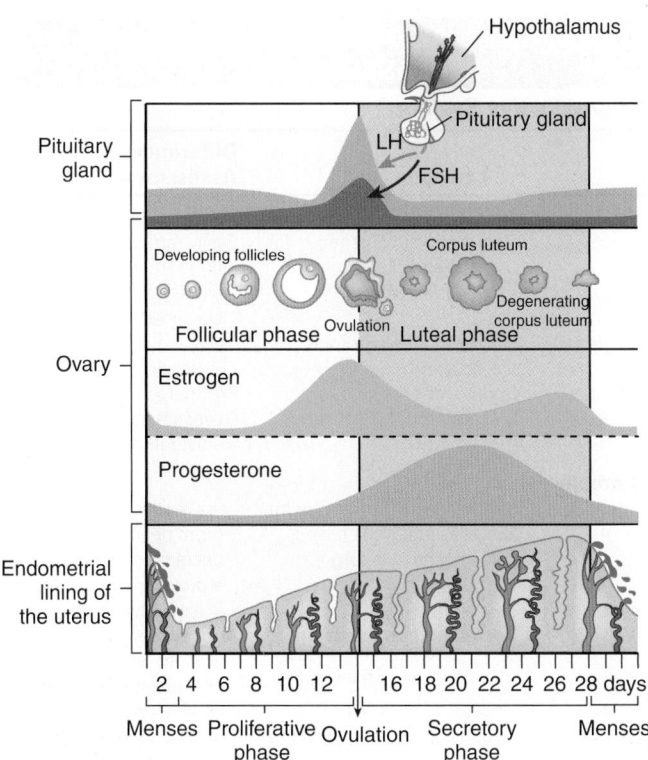

FIG. 53.9 Events of the menstrual cycle. The various *lines* depict the changes in blood hormone levels, the development of the follicles, and the changes in the endometrium during the cycle. *FSH,* follicle-stimulating hormone; *LH,* luteinizing hormone. Source: Adapted from Thibodeau, G. A., & Patton, K. T. (2013). *Anatomy and physiology* (8th ed., p. 1079, Figure 35.14). Mosby.

longer be supported. As a result, the blood vessels contract, and tissue begins to slough (fall away). This sloughing results in the menses and the start of the menstrual cycle (Rosner et al., 2021).

Menopause

Menopause is the physiological cessation of menses associated with declining ovarian function. It is usually considered complete after 1 year of amenorrhea (absence of menstruation) (Peacock & Ketvertis, 2021). (Menopause is discussed in Chapter 56.)

Phases of the Sexual Response

The sexual response is a complex interplay of psychological and physiological phenomena and is influenced by a number of variables, including daily stress, illness, and crisis. The changes that occur during sexual excitement are similar for men and women. Masters and Johnson (1966) described the sexual response in terms of excitement, plateau, orgasmic, and resolution phases.

Male Sexual Response. The penis and the urethra are essential for the transport of sperm into the vagina and the cervix during intercourse. This transport is facilitated by penile erection in response to sexual stimulation during the *excitement phase.* Erection results from the filling of the large venous sinuses within the erectile tissue of the penis. In the flaccid state, these sinuses hold only a small amount of blood, but during the erection stage, they are congested with blood. Because the penis is richly endowed with sympathetic, parasympathetic, and pudendal nerve endings, it is readily stimulated to erection. The loose skin of the penis becomes taut as a result of the intense venous congestion. This erectile tautness allows for easy insertion during intercourse.

TABLE 53.2 PATIENT & CAREGIVER TEACHING GUIDE

Characteristics of Menstruation

The following information should be included when teaching the patient and their family about menstruation.

Characteristic	Teaching
Menarche Occurs between ages 10 and 16 yr; average age at onset is 12.4 yr.	See health care provider regarding possible endocrine or developmental abnormality when menarche is delayed.
Interval Usually is 21–35 days, but regular cycles as short as 17 or as long as 45 days are considered normal if the pattern is consistent for the individual.	Keep a written record to identify own pattern of menstrual cycle. Expect some irregularity in perimenopausal period. Be aware that medications (phenothiazines, opioids, contraceptives) and stressful life events can result in missed periods.
Duration Menstrual flow generally lasts 2–8 days.	Realize that pattern is fairly constant but that wide variations do exist.
Amount Menstrual flow varies from 20 to 80 mL per menses; average is 30 mL. Amount varies among women and in the same woman at different times. It is usually heaviest first 2 days.	Count the number of pads or tampons used per day. The average tampon or pad, when completely saturated, absorbs 20–30 mL. Very heavy flow is indicated by complete soaking of two pads in 1–2 hr. IUD or medications such as anticoagulants and thiazides can produce heavy menses.
Composition Menstrual discharge is a mixture of endometrium, blood, mucus, and vaginal cells. It is dark red and less viscous than blood and usually does not clot.	Clots indicate heavy flow or vaginal pooling.

IUD, intrauterine device.

As the man reaches the *plateau phase,* the erection is maintained, and the penis increases in diameter as a result of a slight increase in vasocongestion. Testicle size also increases. Sometimes the glans penis becomes more reddish-purple.

The subsequent contraction of the penile and urethral musculature during the *orgasmic phase* propels the sperm outward through the meatus. In this process, termed *ejaculation,* sperm are released into the ductus deferens during contractions. Sperm advance through the urethra, where fluids from the prostate and the seminal vesicles are added to the sperm, forming the ejaculate. The sperm continue their path through the urethra, receiving a small amount of fluid from Cowper's glands, and are finally ejaculated through the urinary meatus. *Orgasm* is characterized by the rapid release of the vasocongestion and muscular tension (myotonia) that have developed. The rapid release of muscular tension (through rhythmic contractions) occurs primarily in the penis, prostate gland, and seminal vesicles. After ejaculation, the man enters the *resolution phase.* During this phase, the penis undergoes involution, gradually returning to its unstimulated, flaccid state.

Female Sexual Response. The changes that occur in a woman during sexual excitation are similar to those in a man. In response to stimulation, the clitoris becomes congested, and vaginal lubrication increases as a result of secretions from the cervix, Bartholin's glands, and vaginal walls. This initial response is the *excitation phase.*

As excitation is maintained in the *plateau phase,* the vagina expands and the uterus is elevated. In the *orgasmic phase,* contractions occur in the uterus from the fundus to the lower uterine segment. The cervical os relaxes slightly, which helps the sperm enter, and the vagina undergoes rhythmic contractions. Muscular tension is rapidly released through rhythmic contractions in the clitoris, the vagina, and the uterus. This phase is followed by a *resolution phase* in which these organs return to their pre-excitation state. However, women do not have to go through the resolution (refractory) recovery state before they can be orgasmic again. They can be multi-orgasmic without resolution between orgasms.

AGE-RELATED CONSIDERATIONS

THE REPRODUCTIVE SYSTEM AND SEXUAL RESPONSE

With advancing age, changes occur in the male and female reproductive systems. In women, many of these changes are related to the altered estrogen production that is associated with menopause. A reduction in circulating estrogen along with an increase in androgens in postmenopausal women is associated with breast and genital atrophy, reduction in bone mass, and increased rate of atherosclerosis. Vaginal dryness may occur, which can lead to urogenital atrophy and changes in the quantity and composition of vaginal secretions (Palacois, 2019).

A gradual decline in testosterone levels occurs in men as they age. Manifestations of this decline in men can be physical, psychological, or sexual. Some of the changes include an increase in prostate size and a decrease in testosterone level, sperm production, muscle tone of the scrotum, and size and firmness of the testicles (Touhy & Jett, 2016). Erectile dysfunction (ED) and sexual dysfunction occur in some men as a result of these changes. Age-related changes in the reproductive systems and differences in assessment findings are presented in Table 53.3.

Gradual changes resulting from advancing age occur in the sexual responses of men and women (Table 53.4). The cumulative effects of these changes, as well as the negative social attitude toward sexuality in older persons, can affect the sexual practices of older people. Nurses play a vital role in providing accurate and unbiased information about sexuality and age. Nurses should emphasize the normality of sexual activity among older persons.

ASSESSMENT OF THE MALE AND FEMALE REPRODUCTIVE SYSTEMS

Subjective Data

Important Health Information. In addition to general health information, the nurse needs to elicit information specifically relating to the reproductive system. Reproduction and sexual issues are often considered extremely personal and private. The nurse must develop trust to elicit such information. A professional demeanour is important when obtaining a sexual health history. The interview should be conducted in

TABLE 53.3 **AGE-RELATED DIFFERENCES IN ASSESSMENT**

Reproductive System

	Changes	Differences In Assessment Findings
Male		
Penis	Decreased subcutaneous fat, decreased skin turgor	Easily retractable foreskin (if uncircumcised); decrease in size; fewer sustained erections
Testes	Decreased testosterone production	Decrease in size; change in position (lower)
Prostate	Benign hyperplasia	Enlargement
Breasts	Enlargement	Gynecomastia (abnormal enlargement)
Female		
Breasts	Decreased subcutaneous fat, increased fibrous tissue, decreased skin turgor	Less resilient, looser, more pendulous tissue; decreased size; duct around nipple may feel like stringy strand
Vulva	Decreased skin turgor	Atrophy; decreased amount of pubic hair; decreased size of clitoris and labia
Vagina	Atrophy of tissue, decreased muscle tone, alkaline pH	Pale and dry mucosa; relaxation of outlet; mucosa thinning; narrowing and shortening of vagina; increased potential for infection
Urethra	Decreased muscle tone	Cystocele (protrusion of bladder through vaginal wall)
Uterus	Decreased thickness of myometrium	Decrease in size, uterine prolapse
Ovaries	Decreased ovarian function	Nonpalpable ovaries; decreased size

TABLE 53.4 **AGE-RELATED CHANGES IN SEXUAL FUNCTIONING**

Men
- Increased stimulation necessary for erection
- Decreased force of ejaculation
- Decreased ability to attain or sustain erection
- Decreased size and rigidity of the penis at full erection
- Decreased libido and interest in sex

Women
- Decreased vaginal lubrication
- Decreased sensitivity with labia shrinking and more clitoris exposed
- Difficulty in maintaining arousal
- Difficulty in achieving orgasm after stimulation
- Decreased libido and interest in sex

a safe environment that provides reassurance and confidentiality with a nonjudgemental attitude. The nurse can support patient autonomy by encouraging them to ask questions. Trauma-informed care (TIC) focuses on creating environments where patients do not experience further traumatization or re-traumatization. Trauma- and violence-informed care (TVIC) takes TIC a step beyond this to recognize and work with the broader social and structural factors that affect health, including facility policies and practices (Canadian Public Health Association [CPHA], 2017). The nurse must be sensitive, ask gender-neutral questions when asking about partners, and maintain an awareness of the patient's culture and beliefs. Indigenous people may have difficulty disclosing information about their sexual health because of shame from sexual abuse, lack of knowledge of anatomy and physiology, or embarrassment. It is helpful if the nurse begins with the least sensitive information (e.g., menstrual history) before asking questions about more sensitive issues, such as sexual practices or STBBIs. The nurse needs to pay attention to the client's body language and nonverbal cues, and refrain from making heteronormative assumptions and confirm the pronouns a client uses. The nurse should welcome and normalize disclosures of sexuality, gender identity, and gender expression.

Past Health History. The past health history should include information about major illnesses, hospitalizations, and surgeries. The nurse should inquire about any infections involving the reproductive system, including STBBIs. For women, a complete obstetrical and gynecological history should be documented.

Common pediatric illnesses that affect reproductive function are mumps and rubella. The occurrence of mumps in young men has been associated with an increase in sterility. Bilateral testicular atrophy can occur secondary to mumps-related orchitis. In the health history, the nurse should ask male patients whether they have had mumps, have been immunized with mumps vaccine, or have any indications of sterility.

Rubella is of primary concern to women of childbearing age. If rubella occurs during the first 3 months of pregnancy, the fetus is at increased risk for congenital anomalies. For this reason, nurses should encourage immunization for all women of childbearing age who have not yet been immunized for rubella or have not already had the disease. (Rubella immunity can be determined by antibody titres.) Women should not be immunized if they are already pregnant (Public Health Agency of Canada [PHAC], 2019). Women are also advised not to conceive for at least 1 month after being immunized with the combination measles–mumps–rubella vaccine (PHAC, 2019).

The nurse should also ask about the patient's current health status and the presence of any acute or chronic health problems. Conditions in other body systems are often related to disorders in the reproductive system. The nurse should ask about possible endocrine disorders, particularly diabetes mellitus, hypothyroidism, and hyperthyroidism, because these disorders directly interfere with women's menstrual cycles and with sexual performance. Men who have diabetes mellitus may experience ED and retrograde ejaculation. In women with uncontrolled diabetes mellitus, pregnancy may incur significant health risks. Many other chronic illnesses, such as cardiovascular disease, respiratory disorders, anemia, cancer, and kidney and urinary tract disorders, may affect the reproductive system and sexual functioning.

A history of stroke should be determined. In men, strokes may cause physiological or psychological ED. Men who have suffered a myocardial infarction (MI) may experience ED because of the fear that sexual activity will precipitate another heart attack. Women share this concern, both as a partners of someone who has had an MI and as patients recovering from an MI. Although most patients who have had an MI have concerns about sexual activity after an MI, many are not comfortable expressing these concerns to the nurse. Therefore, the nurse must be sensitive to this concern. Women with a history of cardiovascular disease (e.g., hypertension, thrombophlebitis, angina) have a higher incidence of morbidity and mortality with pregnancy or the use of oral contraceptives.

Family History. The nurse should inquire about history of cancer, particularly cancer of the reproductive organs. Having a first-degree relative who has had cancer of the breast, the ovaries, the uterus, or the prostate significantly increases the risk of cancer for the patient. It is also important to determine if the patient has a familial tendency for diabetes mellitus, hypothyroidism, hyperthyroidism, hypertension, stroke, angina, MI, endocrine disorders, or anemia.

Medications. The nurse should document all prescription and over-the-counter medications that the patient is taking, as well as the reasons for using the medications, the dosages, and the lengths of time that the medications have been taken. All medications taken by female patients of childbearing age should be evaluated for possible teratogenic effects. The patient should also be asked about the use of herbal products and dietary or nutritional supplements.

Particularly relevant in the assessment of the reproductive system is the use of diuretics (sometimes prescribed for premenstrual edema) and psychotropic agents (which may interfere with sexual performance). Antihypertensives, such as amlodipine, lisinopril, and propranolol, may cause ED. The nurse must also note the use of drugs such as alcohol, marijuana, barbiturates, amphetamines, and cocaine as they can affect the reproductive system.

The use of oral contraceptives or other hormone therapy should be noted. The long-term use of both estrogen and progesterone in hormone therapy appears to increase the risk of blood clots, cardiovascular disease, stroke, gallbladder disease, and breast and uterine cancer in postmenopausal women (Marcinkow et al., 2019). The short-term use of hormone therapy appears to be appropriate for certain women, depending on their risk factors. (Hormone therapy is discussed in Chapter 56.) Women who use tobacco have a much higher risk of clotting disorders than do women who do not use tobacco.

A history of cholecystitis and hepatitis is important information because these conditions may be contraindications to oral contraceptive use. Cholecystitis is often aggravated by oral contraceptives, and chronic active inflammation of the liver generally precludes the use of estrogen products because they are metabolized by the liver. Chronic obstructive pulmonary disease may be a contraindication to oral contraceptive use because progesterone thickens respiratory secretions.

Surgery or Other Treatments. Any surgical procedures should be noted in the health history. Surgical procedures involving the reproductive system are listed in Table 53.5. Therapeutic or spontaneous abortions should also be documented.

Documenting a Health History Related to a Reproductive Condition. When collecting information related to reproductive health, as stated earlier, the nurse should start with questions of lesser sensitivity, proceeding to more sensitive issues after rapport has been established. The nurse is also in a unique position to discuss general health issues and to emphasize health promotion and self-care activities. The key questions to ask a patient with a reproductive condition are presented in Table 53.6 and discussed in more detail in the paragraphs below.

Menstrual History. The menstrual history includes the date of the beginning of the most recent menstrual period, description of menstrual flow, age at menarche, and, if applicable, age at menopause. Menstrual history data are used in the detection of

CASE STUDY

Subjective Data

An assessment of A. K. reveals the following information.

Past medical history: Pap smear 2 months ago was normal. No surgical history

Family history: No significant data

Medications: Oral contraceptive pill, one tablet daily for the past 4 years

Overall health management: Indicates a perception of good health

Sexual and reproductive history: Had onset of menarche at age 14. Last menstrual period 2 weeks ago. Menses is usually every 28 days, lasting 2 days, but has noted irregular bleeding with increased pelvic pain over past few months. She denies dyspareunia.

Functional Assessment

Activity and mobility: Exercises at the gym 3 times a week

Nutrition and metabolic history: She is 163 cm tall and weighs 63.55 kg.

Elimination: Denies any changes or difficulty with urination or bowel movements

Interpersonal relationships: Single, lives with three women in off-campus housing. Sexually active with men—three lifetime partners. In a mutually monogamous relationship of 2 years duration. Practices vaginal and oral sex.

Discussion Questions

1. Which subjective assessment findings are of most concern to the nurse?
2. What should be included in the physical assessment?
   You will learn more about physical examination of the reproductive system in the next section. See Case Study: Patient Information, Case Study: Objective Data: Physical Examination, and Case Study: Objective Data: Diagnostic Studies for more information on A. K.

TABLE 53.5   SURGICAL PROCEDURES INVOLVING THE REPRODUCTIVE SYSTEM

Surgery	Description
Male	
Herniorrhaphy	Repair of hernia
Orchiectomy	Removal of one or both testes
Prostatectomy	Removal of prostate gland
Repair of testicular torsion	Correction of axial rotation of spermatic cord, which cuts off blood supply to the testicle, epididymis, and other structures
Transurethral resection of prostate (TURP)	Removal of prostate tissue via the urethra (e.g., obstructive benign prostatic hyperplasia)
Varicocelectomy	Repair of varicose vein of scrotum
Vasectomy	Removal of part of ductus (vas) deferens; can be an elective procedure for sterilization or contraception
Female	
Cryosurgery	Use of subfreezing temperature to destroy tissue, especially for treatment of abnormal cells in the cervix
Dilation and curettage (D&C)	Dilation of cervix and scraping of endometrium, performed to diagnose disease of uterus, to correct heavy or prolonged vaginal bleeding, or to empty uterus of products of conception; also used in treatment of infertility to correlate state of endometrium and time of cycle
Hysterectomy	Removal of uterus
Mastectomy	Removal of one or both breasts
Oophorectomy	Removal of one or both ovaries
Repair of cystocele	Correction of protrusion of urinary bladder into vagina
Repair of rectocele	Correction of protrusion of rectum into vagina
Salpingectomy	Removal of one or both Fallopian tubes
Tubal ligation or sterilization	Ligation of Fallopian tubes

pregnancy, infertility, and numerous other gynecological concerns. Changes in the usual menstrual pattern must be explicitly described to determine whether the change is transient and unimportant or connected with a more serious gynecological condition. *Metrorrhagia* (spotting or bleeding between menstruations), *menorrhagia* (excessive menstrual bleeding), *amenorrhea* (absence of menstruation), and *postcoital bleeding* are examples of such changes. Changes in menstrual patterns associated with the use of oral contraceptives, intrauterine devices (IUDs), birth control patches, vaginal rings, progestin-only implants, or medroxyprogesterone (Depo-Provera) injections must be identified. Oral contraceptives usually decrease the amount and duration of flow, whereas some IUDs may cause an increase in flow. Some IUDs are used for both contraception and as a nonsurgical treatment for heavy menstrual flow.

There are varying cultural views of menstruation, so it is important that the nurse clarify the patient's personal view. Some Indigenous people refer to menstruation as "moontime," a monthly cleansing that has specific behaviours and expectations (Northern College, 2020). Seclusion may be practised when women are on their moontime, which is viewed as a ceremony of life for women and a time for renewal. Daily household chores, child care, and meal preparation are completed by other family members, as this is a time for the woman to think about herself, reflect, and have a period of self-renewal, often done in self-isolation (Pember, 2019).

Obstetrical History. The obstetrical history includes the number of pregnancies, full-term births, preterm births, stillbirths, living children, and abortions (including both spontaneous [miscarriage], ectopic, or induced). Other obstetrical information should include any problems that occurred with pregnancy.

Menopause. Obtaining a menopause history includes asking the date of the beginning of the most recent menstrual period and asking about any other symptoms of menopause, such as hot flashes, heavy sweats, vaginal dryness, headaches, sleeping difficulties, mood changes, decreased libido, and urinary conditions. Women should be asked whether they are using or have ever used hormone therapy. It is also important to explore how the woman feels about menopause because the drop in estrogen levels during perimenopause and menopause can lead to depression. Women are also more prone to osteoporosis and heart disease after menopause because of the lower levels of estrogen. The nurse must discuss ways to prevent and reduce the risk of these diseases.

Nutritional History. Anemia is a common condition in women in their reproductive years, particularly during pregnancy and the postpartum period. The adequacy of the diet should be evaluated with this condition in mind. Iron-deficiency anemia is the most common cause of anemia in menstruating females.

A thorough nutritional and psychological history should be taken to assess for the presence of an eating disorder. Anorexia can cause amenorrhea and subsequent conditions, such as osteoporosis, that are related to estrogen deficiency. From early adolescence, women can be counselled regarding adequate calcium and vitamin D intake and the prevention of osteoporosis. The patient's daily calcium intake should be estimated to

TABLE 53.6 HEALTH HISTORY

Reproductive System: Questions for Obtaining Subjective Data

Past History
- Are you having any health problems in the area of your genitals?*
- Have you had treatment for such problems in the past, and how were those treated?
- Have you had any surgery on your uterus, ovaries, vagina, or prostate?*
- Any history of kidney disease, kidney stones, prostate conditions?*
- Have you had bladder infections? If so, when? How often?

Family History
- Describe the health of your family members. Any history of breast, uterine, ovarian, or prostate cancer?

Review of Systems
Overall Health Status
- How do you feel in general? Have you had any changes recently in your health?
- What is your weight and height? Have there been any changes in your appetite or weight?*

Gastrointestinal System
- Describe your usual bowel pattern. Have you noted any bowel changes?*

Genitourinary System
- Do you experience difficulties with urination (e.g., pain; burning; dribbling; inability to control urine; frequency; small amounts; urinating at night; blood in the urine; urine that is dark, cloudy, or foul smelling)? Do you urinate when you sneeze or laugh or cough?
- Do you have any discharge from your vagina or penis?*
- Have you had bladder infections? If so, when? How often?

Sexual and Reproductive History†
Women
- *Menstrual history:* When did you start to menstruate? Was this earlier or later than other women in your family? Do you have scant, heavy, or irregular menstrual flows? On what date did your most recent menstrual period begin?
- *Obstetrical history:* How many children have you had? How many times were you pregnant? How many living children, miscarriages, or abortions? Could you be pregnant now? Are you trying to become pregnant?

- *Menopausal history:* Have your periods changed or stopped? Are you experiencing any of the symptoms of menopause—hot flashes, headaches, heavy sweats, vaginal dryness? Are you taking or have you taken HT? How are you feeling about menopause?
- Are you postmenopausal? If so, do you have any bleeding from your uterus?

Men
- Have you noticed any changes in your ability to have an erection?*
- Are you trying to have children but cannot?*

Functional Assessment (Including Activities of Daily Living)
Activity and Mobility
- Do you have a planned exercise program? If yes, what is it, and have you had to make any changes in this routine lately? If so, why and what kinds of changes?

Sleep and Rest
- How many hours do you sleep at night? Do you feel rested on awakening?
- Are you ever awakened by sweating during the night?*

Nutrition
- *Women:* Have you had any problems with anemia?* Have you had problems with eating disorders?*

Interpersonal Relationships
- Are you in a relationship? Are you able to take care of your significant others and your home? If not, why not?

Self-Care and Health Promotion Activities
- *Women:* Have you noticed anything different about your breasts? Have you had a Pap test or mammography recently? If so, what were the results and dates of these tests? How often do you have these checks?
- *Men:* Have you noticed anything different about your testes? Have you had a prostate examination recently? If so, what were the results and dates of these tests?

*If yes, describe.
†See Table 53.7 for sexual health history questions.
HT, hormone therapy; Pap, Papanicolaou.
Adapted from Jarvis, C., Browne, A. J., MacDonald-Jenkins, J., & Luctkar-Flude, M. (Eds.). (2019). *Physical examination and health assessment.* (3rd Canadian ed.). Elsevier Inc.

determine whether the patient needs supplementation. Folic acid intake for women in their reproductive years should be evaluated because a deficiency can result in spina bifida and other neural tube defects in the fetus (Cordero et al., 2015).

Self-Care History. It is important to establish the patient's perception of their own health and measures that the patient takes to maintain health. Specifically, it is important to ask about self-examination practices and screenings. While regular breast self-examination is no longer recommended, women are encouraged to become familiar with their own breasts because they are often the ones who notice changes possibly indicative of breast cancer (Canadian Cancer Society, 2021a). Screening mammography according to age-specific guidelines (see Chapter 54) and Pap tests are integral to a woman's health. Sexually active women older than 21 are also advised to have regular Pap tests every 1 to 3 years, depending on provincial/territorial screening guidelines and previous test results (Canadian Cancer Society, 2021b).

While there is not enough evidence to support regular testicular self-examinations for men, it is important that men know what is normal for them because most testicular cancers are discovered first by men themselves (Canadian Cancer Society, 2021c). Men older than 50 years are advised to talk to their health care provider about their personal risk for prostate cancer and the advisability of them undergoing screening tests for early detection of prostate cancer, such as a digital rectal examination and a prostate-specific antigen (PSA) test (Canadian Cancer Society, 2020). Men at high risk for prostate cancer (i.e., Black men, men with first-degree relatives who have prostate cancer) should begin these discussions before age 50 with their health care provider (Canadian Cancer Society, 2020).

Assessment of the reproductive system is incomplete without information about the patient's lifestyle choices. The nurse should know whether a patient uses cigarettes, alcohol, caffeine, or other drugs, because these substances can be detrimental to both the mother and fetus. Cigarette smoking may initiate early menopause, delay conception, and can increase the risk of morbidity in oral contraceptive users. These substances may also adversely affect the sperm count in men and cause ED or decreased libido. Tobacco use is a known cofactor for persistence of human papillomavirus (HPV) infection for oral and anogenital cancers among men and women (deSanjose et al., 2018). HPV vaccine status should be ascertained.

The nurse should also document whether the patient is allergic to sulphonamides, penicillin, rubber, or latex. Sulphonamides and penicillin are used frequently in the treatment of reproductive and genitourinary conditions such as vaginitis and gonorrhea. Rubber and latex are commonly used in diaphragms and condoms. An allergy to these substances precludes their use as contraceptive methods.

Elimination. Many gynecological conditions can result in genitourinary conditions. Stress incontinence and urge incontinence are common in older women because the pelvic musculature relaxes as a result of multiple births or advancing age. Vaginal infections predispose patients to chronic or recurrent urinary tract infections. Metastasis of malignant tumours of the reproductive system to the genitourinary system is possible because of their proximity. Benign prostatic hyperplasia is a common condition in older men and can cause urinary retention or difficulty in initiating the urinary stream.

Sexual Health History. The extent and the depth of the interview about a patient's sexuality depend primarily on the expertise of the interviewer and on the needs and the willingness of the patient. Before obtaining a sexual history, interviewers should assess their comfort with their own sexuality, because any discomfort in questioning becomes obvious to the patient. The nurse needs to explain that a sexual health history is a routine part of history taking for all patients and ask permission to ask questions related to sexual health.

There is evidence that older people avoid seeking help for sexual concerns because of sexual stigma, including their lack of knowledge about sexual conditions, discomfort talking about sex, and beliefs that sexual activity in older persons is inappropriate (Syme & Cohn, 2016). Sexual history taking should be a routine part of periodic health examinations.

Table 53.7 outlines an approach for obtaining a sexual health history. The nurse should never make an assumption about a patient's sexual orientation, their gender identity, or the physiology of their sexual partners. Sexual orientation should not be conflated with sexual activity. The nurse should seek to normalize disclosures of all sexual activity, including sex with men, women, trans or gender-diverse persons, Two-Spirited persons, or any combination thereof (CPHA, 2017). The nurse should collect information from the patient regarding their general satisfaction with their sexuality. The patient should be asked about sexual beliefs and practices and whether they achieve orgasm. The patient's knowledge of safe sexual practices should be determined. A history of multiple sex partners and unprotected sex increases the risk of contracting an STBBI or pelvic inflammatory disease, which can compromise the ability to conceive.

People who are transgender or have had reassignment surgery may find that disclosing their sexual history is a very sensitive issue related to prior experiences of gender discrimination in health care. It is important to establish their preferred pronouns, exhibit a nonjudgemental attitude, and avoid making assumptions. Transgender people may be of any sexual orientation, and their partners may be cisgender men or women or other transgender people (Centers for Disease Control and

TABLE 53.7	SEXUAL HEALTH HISTORY FORMAT
The 5 Ps	**Questions**
1. **P**ractices	Are you currently sexually active? If not, have you ever been sexually active? • What kind of sex do you have (or have you had in the past) (e.g., vaginal sex, anal sex, oral sex, manual stimulation of the penis, vagina, anus)? • If yes to anal sex, are you the insertive or receptive partner? • Do you feel comfortable talking about consent with your partner(s) before having sex? • Have you ever shared sex toys? If yes, did you use a barrier?
2. **P**artners	• How many different people have you had sex with in the past 2 months? In the past year? (0, 1–2, 3–10, 10+)? • Do you ask about your partner's sexual health history or history of STBBIs before having sex?
3. **P**rotection from STBBIs	Can you share with me what you know about protecting yourself and your partner(s) from STBBIs? • Do you use any barriers (i.e., condoms, dental dams, split condoms/gloves) during sex? When do you use them (i.e., all the time, sometimes, never) and for what kind of sex (i.e., vaginal, oral, anal)? • Do you have any problems related to the use of barriers (e.g., cost, do not know how to use them, partner refuses to use them)?
4. **P**ast history of STBBIs	Have you ever been tested for HIV or other STBBIs? • Have you ever had an STBBI? If yes, when? How were you treated? • Have you ever had a Pap test and/or pelvic exam? If yes, when was your last Pap test? Were you screened for HPV? • Do you have any signs or symptoms that worry you—any lumps, bumps, discharge, or pain?
5. **P**regnancy	Are you pregnant now? • If not, what are you doing to prevent pregnancy? • Are you or your partner(s) trying to get pregnant? If not, are you interested in becoming pregnant in the future?

HIV, human immunodeficiency virus; *HPV,* human papillomavirus; *Pap,* Papanicolaou (test); *STBBIs,* sexually transmitted and blood-borne infections.
Source: Adapted from Canadian Public Health Association. (2017). *Discussing sexual health, substance use and STBBIs: A guide for service providers.* Author.

Prevention [CDC], 2020). Transgender people may be at any stage of the transition process when seeking health care. If medically necessary, data collection should include information about current anatomy and hormonal or surgical interventions (CDC, 2020). Any unexplained change in sexual practices or performance for reproductive issues needs to be explored. Conditions of the reproductive system can cause physiological or psychological difficulties that can lead to **dyspareunia** (painful intercourse), ED, sexual dysfunction, or infertility.

Inclusive and Appropriate Health Care. It is difficult to locate a percentage of the Canadian population that identifies as LGBTQ2+, as data are collected on one or more sexual or gender minorities rather than on all of the identified communities. Approximately 1.7% of Canadians aged 18 to 59 years identified themselves as gay or lesbian and 1.3% as bisexual (Statistics Canada, 2017). Health inequities among the LGBTQ2+ community include poorer mental health, higher rates of suicidal behaviours and self-injury, higher rates of violence and victimization, and higher rates of substance misuse (Jackman et al., 2019).

It is important for the nurse to clarify terms that the patient uses so that there is a shared understanding. The term *trans* refers to transsexual, transgender, gender-nonconforming, and gender-questioning people (Bourns, 2015). Trans people are more likely to report poor mental and physical health than their nontransgender counterparts (Meyer et al., 2017; Streed et al., 2017). Trans people also experience higher rates of multiple chronic health conditions (Dragon et al., 2017).

Nurses must understand the unique needs of LGBTQ2+ community members and provide inclusive and appropriate health care. Members of sexual- and gender-minority communities need to know that they are welcome, have rights, and are safe. The physical environment must be welcoming to LGBTQ2+ people (e.g., through signage, posters, brochures, facility literature). As stated earlier, it is important to avoid making assumptions about a person's physiology or gender identity based on appearance.

In language and facility forms and assessment tools, heterosexuality should not be assumed as the norm but individuals should be allowed to disclose their sexual identity, same-sex partnerships, and sexual behaviour without fear of discrimination. Inclusive and nonstigmatizing language should be used (e.g., *partner* instead of *husband/wife*; *significant relationships* instead of *next of kin)*, as well as a broad definition of family that goes beyond traditional concepts, to recognize as family whomever the patient considers their family to be.

Members of the LGBTQ2+ community and their families also need affirmation that their identity is acknowledged and respected. The behaviour of interprofessional health care team members must demonstrate understanding of each person's unique needs. The nurse should adopt a sex-positive approach and strive toward the provision of safe, respectful, and inclusive care for all patients (CPHA, 2017).

Objective Data

Physical Examination: Male. The examination of the male external genitalia includes inspection and palpation. An examination may be performed with the patient lying or standing. The standing position is generally preferred. The examiner should be seated in front of the standing patient and should wear gloves during examination of the male genitalia.

Pubis. The nurse observes the distribution and general characteristics of the pubic hair and the skin. Normally, the hair is in a diamond-shaped pattern and is coarser than scalp hair. The absence of hair is not a normal finding unless the man is shaving or waxing the pubic hair.

Penis. The nurse notes the size and the skin texture of the penis and any lesions, scars, or swelling. In addition, the location of the urethral meatus, as well as the presence or absence of a foreskin, should be documented. The foreskin, if present, should be retracted to note any redness, discharge, irritation, or swelling and then replaced over the glans after observation. The glans is compressed to note any discharge and, if present, its amount, colour, and odour. The examiner palpates the penile shaft for tenderness or masses and observes the ventral and dorsal aspects.

Scrotum and Testes. This part of the examination begins by performing a complete skin examination by lifting each testis to inspect all sides of the scrotal sac. The scrotum is palpated in order to note changes in consistency or the presence of masses. It is important to note whether the testes are descended. The left testis usually hangs lower than the right. An undescended testis

is a major risk factor for testicular cancer, as well as a potential cause of male infertility (Gurney et al., 2017).

Inguinal Region and Spermatic Cord. The nurse first inspects the skin overlying the inguinal regions for rashes or lesions. The patient should be asked to bear down or cough. While he is straining, the inguinal area should be inspected for the presence of a bulge. No bulging should be seen.

Examination of the inguinal area continues with palpation. Using the index or the middle finger, the nurse palpates the right and left inguinal rings. The finger should be inserted into the lower aspect of the scrotum and should follow the spermatic cord upward through the triangular, slitlike opening of the inguinal ring. At this point, the patient should be asked to bear down and cough. The nurse determines whether the strain produces a bulging of the intestines through the ring, indicating the presence of a hernia, a condition that necessitates follow-up. The inguinal lymph nodes should also be palpated. Enlargement of the lymph nodes (termed *lymphadenopathy*) could suggest a pelvic organ infection or malignancy.

Anus and Prostate. The nurse inspects the anal sphincter and the perineal region for lesions, masses, and hemorrhoids. A digital rectal examination is required for all men who have symptoms of prostate trouble, such as difficulty in initiating the flow and the urge to void frequently. This examination should be performed annually for all men 50 years of age or older by their health care provider.

Physical Examination: Female. Physical examination of female genitalia often begins with inspection and palpation of the breasts and then proceeds to the abdomen and the genitalia. Examination of the abdomen provides an opportunity to detect pain or any masses that may involve the genitourinary system. (Abdominal examination is discussed in more detail in Chapter 41.) The nurse needs to assess the patient's comfort level and obtain consent before beginning an assessment of the reproductive system. It is also important to be sensitive to the patient's questions and needs during the assessment.

Breasts. A clinical breast examination is a thorough breast assessment performed by a health care provider as a diagnostic assessment rather than as a screening examination. Clinical breast examinations and breast self-examination are not recommended as effective screening procedures for breast cancer (Klarenbach et al., 2018).

If the patient has a breast lump or breast changes, a clinical breast examination should be performed. The nurse first examines the breasts by visual inspection. With the patient seated, the breasts are observed for symmetry, size, shape, skin colour and texture, vascular patterns, dimpling, and unusual lesions. The patient is asked to put her arms at her sides and then overhead, to lean forward, and to press her hands on her hips. The nurse observes for any abnormalities during these manoeuvres. The axillae and the clavicular areas are palpated for enlarged lymph nodes.

After the patient assumes a supine position, a pillow is placed under her back on the side to be examined. The nurse should ask the patient to put her arm above and behind her head. These manoeuvres flatten breast tissue and make palpation easier. Then the nurse palpates the breast in a systematic manner, using the distal finger pads for palpation. The area palpated includes the tail of Spence (the upper outer tail of breast tissue that extends into the axilla) because this region and the upper outer quadrant are the areas where most breast malignancies develop. Finally, the nurse palpates the area around the areolae for masses. The nipple is compressed to determine the presence of discharge or any masses. The colour, consistency, and odour of any discharge are documented.

CASE STUDY

Objective Data: Physical Examination

Physical assessment of A. K. reveals the following:

BP is 118.76 mm Hg; pulse is 70 beats/min, regular. Skin is warm and dry without lesions. There is no cyanosis of lips, mucous membranes, or nail beds. Thyroid is not enlarged. Heart examination is normal. Abdomen is soft and nontender. External genitalia examination is normal. Bimanual examination by the health care provider is negative for cervical motion tenderness or uterine anomalies. Patient has pain on left side with palpation of a soft mass consistent with an ovarian cyst.

Discussion Question

1. Based on the assessment findings, what diagnostic tests would the nurse anticipate being ordered for her?
   See Case Study: Patient Information, Case Study: Subjective Data, and Case Study: Objective Data: Diagnostic Studies for more information on A. K.

External Genitalia. Gloves are used for examination of the female external genitalia. The nurse inspects the mons pubis, labia majora, labia minora, posterior fourchette, perineum, and anal region for characteristics of skin, hair distribution, and contour. Any lesions, inflammation, swelling, and discharge are documented. The nurse separates the labia to fully inspect the clitoris, the urethral meatus, and the vaginal orifice.

Internal Pelvic Examination. This part of the examination is performed by a nurse with advanced skills. During the speculum examination, the nurse observes the walls of the vagina and the cervix for inflammation, discharge, polyps, and suspicious growths. During this examination, it is possible to obtain a Pap test and collect secretions for culture and microscopic examination. After the speculum examination, the nurse performs a bimanual examination to assess the size, shape, and consistency of the uterus, the ovaries, and the tubes. The tubes are not normally palpable.

Parts of the pelvic and bimanual examinations are not included in this text because they are considered advanced skills and are not usually within the scope of the nurse generalist.

Table 53.8 provides an example of a recording format for the physical assessment findings for the male and female reproductive systems. Tables 53.9, 53.10, and 53.11 summarize common assessment abnormalities of the breasts, the female reproductive system, and the male reproductive system, respectively.

A *focused assessment* is used to evaluate the status of previously identified reproductive conditions and to monitor for signs of new ones (see Table 3.5). This evaluation is described in the Focused Assessment box.

DIAGNOSTIC STUDIES OF REPRODUCTIVE SYSTEMS

The most commonly used diagnostic studies in the assessment of the reproductive systems are summarized in Table 53.12, and select studies (Figure 53.10) are described in more detail below.

Urine Studies

Pregnancy Testing. Pregnancy is generally validated by measuring hCG in the urine (Cole & Butler, 2020). A solution containing monoclonal antibodies specific for hCG is mixed with a small amount of urine. The presence of hCG causes a change in colour of the tested urine.

TABLE 53.8   PHYSICAL ASSESSMENT OF THE REPRODUCTIVE SYSTEM: NORMAL FINDINGS

Male	Female
Breasts	
Symmetrical; no masses or tenderness behind nipple; no drainage, retraction, or lesions noted; no lymphadenopathy	Symmetrical without dimpling; no masses or tenderness behind nipple; nipples soft; no drainage, retraction, or lesions noted; no lymphadenopathy
External Genitalia	
Diamond-shaped hair distribution; no lesions or discharge noted. Scrotum symmetrical, testes descended; no masses; no inguinal hernia	Triangular hair distribution. Genitalia dark pink; no lesions, redness, swelling, or inflammation in perineal region. No vaginal discharge noted; no tenderness with palpation of Skene's ducts and Bartholin's glands
Anus	
No hemorrhoids, fissures, or lesions noted	No hemorrhoids, fissures, or lesions noted

FOCUSED ASSESSMENT

Reproductive System

Use this checklist to ensure the key assessment steps have been done.

Subjective
Ask the patient about any of the following and note responses:

Vaginal discharge/itching, unusual bleeding	Y	N
Penile pain, lesions, discharge	Y	N
Medications: oral contraceptives, antihypertensives, psychotropics, hormones	Y	N
Clinical examinations of reproductive systems (breast, pelvis, testicles, prostate) and results	Y	N
Pain in the abdomen, pelvis, or genitalia	Y	N

Objective: Diagnostic
Check the following for results and critical values:

Serum hCG	✓
Serum PSA	✓
Culture and sensitivity test results	✓
Hormone levels (testosterone, progesterone, estrogen) if done	✓
Screen for STBBIs (e.g., *Chlamydia*, gonorrhea)	✓
Laboratory reports: wet mounts, dark-field microscopy	✓
Radiograph of pelvis or breasts	✓
Ultrasound study of prostate	✓

Objective: Physical Examination
Inspect or observe for the following:

External genitalia for redness, swelling, drainage	✓
Breasts for swelling, dimpling, retraction, drainage	✓
Palpate for the following:	
Breast tissue for masses or inflammation	✓
Testicles for lumps	✓

hCG, human chorionic gonadotropin; *PSA*, prostate-specific antigen; *STBBIs*, sexually transmitted or blood-borne infections.

TABLE 53.9 ASSESSMENT ABNORMALITIES

Breast

Finding	Description	Possible Etiology and Significance
Nipple inversion or retraction	Recent onset, erythematous, pain, unilateral	Abscess, inflammation, cancer
	Recent onset (usually within past year), unilateral, lack of tenderness	Neoplasm
Nipple secretions		
• Galactorrhea (female)	Milky, no relationship to lactation, unilateral or bilateral or intermittent or consistent presentation	Medication therapy, particularly phenothiazines, tricyclic antidepressants, methyldopa
		Hypofunction or hyperfunction of thyroid or adrenal glands
		Tumours of hypothalamus or pituitary gland
		Excessive estrogen
		Prolonged suckling or breast foreplay
• Galactorrhea (male)	Milky, bilateral presentation	Chorioepithelioma of testes, manifestation of pituitary tumour
• Purulent	Grey-green or yellow	Puerperal (after birth) mastitis (inflammatory condition of breast) or abscess
	Frequent unilateral presentation	
	Association with pain, erythema, induration, nipple inversion	
	Same description as mastitis or abscess but usually without nipple inversion	Infected sebaceous cyst
• Serous discharge	Clear appearance, unilateral or bilateral or intermittent or consistent presentation	Intraductal papilloma
• Dark green or multicoloured discharge	Thick, sticky, and frequently bilateral	Ductal ectasia (dilation of mammary ducts)
• Serosanguineous or bloody drainage	Unilateral presentation	Papillomatosis (widespread development of nipple-like growths), intraductal papilloma, carcinoma (male and female)
Scaling or irritation of nipple	Unilateral or bilateral presentation, crusting, possible ulceration	Paget's disease, eczema, infection
Nodules, lumps, or masses (male and female)	Multiple, bilateral, well-delineated, soft or firm, mobile cysts; pain. Premenstrual occurrence	Fibrocystic changes
	Rubbery consistency, fluid-filled interior; pain	Ductal ectasia
	Soft, mobile, well-delineated cyst; absence of pain	Lipoma, fibroadenoma
	Erythema, tenderness, induration	Infected sebaceous cysts, abscesses
	Usually singular, hard, irregularly shaped, poorly delineated, nonmobile	Neoplasm
Dimpling of breast	Unilateral, recent onset, no pain	Neoplasm

TABLE 53.10 ASSESSMENT ABNORMALITIES

Female Reproductive System

Finding/Description	Possible Etiology and Significance	Finding/Description	Possible Etiology and Significance
Vulvar Discharge		Flat and warty appearance, non-tender	Condyloma latum
White, thick, curdy, frequent itching and inflammation, yeast-like smell or lack of odour	Candidiasis (candidal or yeast infection), vaginitis	Same as either of preceding descriptions, possible pain	Neoplasm
Thin grey or white, copious flow; malodorous or "fishy" smell; vulvar irritation	Bacterial vaginosis infection	Reddened base, vesicles, and small erosions; pain	Lymphogranuloma venereum, genital herpes, chancroid
Frothy green or yellow; malodorous	*Trichomonas vaginalis* infection	Indurated, firm ulcers; lack of pain	Chancre (syphilis), granuloma inguinale
Bloody discharge	*Chlamydia trachomatis* or *Neisseria gonorrhoeae* infection, menstruation, trauma, cancer	**Abdominal Pain or Tenderness**	
		Intermittent or consistent tenderness in right or left lower quadrant	Salpingitis (infection of Fallopian tube), ectopic pregnancy, ruptured ovarian cyst, PID, tubal or ovarian abscess
Vulvar Erythema			
Bright or beefy red colour, itching	*Candida albicans,* allergy, chemical vaginitis	Periumbilical location, consistent occurrence	Cystitis, endometritis (inflammation of endometrium), ectopic pregnancy
Reddened base, painful vesicles or ulcerations	Genital herpes	**Abnormal Vaginal Bleeding**	
Macules or papules, itching	Chancroid (STI), contact dermatitis, scabies, pediculosis	Unusual and inappropriate uterine bleeding	Dysfunctional uterine bleeding, usually anovulatory bleeding, menorrhagia (heavy menstrual bleeding), metrorrhagia (irregular, frequent bleeding), postmenopausal bleeding
Vulvar Growths			
Soft, fleshy growth; nontender	Condyloma acuminatum		

PID, pelvic inflammatory disease; *STI,* sexually transmitted infection.

TABLE 53.11   ASSESSMENT ABNORMALITIES

Male Reproductive System

Finding	Description	Possible Etiology and Significance	Finding	Description	Possible Etiology and Significance
Penile growths or masses	Indurated, smooth, dislike appearance; absence of pain; singular presentation	Chancre	Scrotal masses	Localized swelling with tenderness, unilateral or bilateral presentation	Epididymitis (inflammation of epididymis), testicular torsion, orchitis (mumps)
	Papular to irregularly shaped ulceration with pus, lack of induration	Chancroid		Swelling, tenderness	Incarcerated hernia
	Ulceration with induration and nodularity	Cancer		Unilateral or bilateral presentation; swelling without pain; translucent, cordlike or wormlike appearance	Hydrocele (accumulation of fluid in outer covering of testes), spermatocele (firm, sperm-containing cyst of epididymis), varicocele (dilation of veins that drain testes), hematocele (accumulation of blood within scrotum)
	Flat, wartlike nodule	Condyloma latum			
	Elevated, fleshy, moist, elongated projections with single or multiple projections	Condyloma acuminatum			
	Localized swelling with retracted, tight foreskin	Paraphimosis (inability to replace foreskin to its normal position after retraction), trauma		Firm, nodular testes or epididymis; frequent unilateral presentation	Tuberculosis, cancer
			Penile discharge	Clear to purulent colour, minimal to copious flow	Urethritis or gonorrhea, *Chlamydia trachomatis* infection, trauma
Vesicles, erosions, or ulcers	Painful, erythematous base; vesicular or small erosions	Genital herpes, balanitis (inflammation of glans penis), chancroid	Penile or scrotal erythema	Macules and papules	Scabies, pediculosis
	Painless, singular, small erosion with eventual lymphadenopathy	Lymphogranuloma venereum, cancer	Inguinal masses	Bulging, unilateral presentation during straining	Inguinal hernia
				1- to 3-cm nodules	Lymphadenopathy

TABLE 53.12   DIAGNOSTIC STUDIES

Male and Female Reproductive Systems

Study	Description and Purpose	Nursing Responsibility
Urine Studies		
Human chorionic gonadotropin (hCG)	Reveals pregnancy Also reveals hydatidiform mole and chorioepithelioma (in men and women) *Males and nonpregnant females*: negative	Obtain menstrual history from patient, including birth control methods. Determine presence or absence of presumptive signs of pregnancy (e.g., breast changes, increased whitish vaginal discharge).
Testosterone	Reveals tumours and developmental anomalies of the testes *Female*: 6.9–41.6 nmol/24 hr *Male*: 139–469 nmol/24 hr	Instruct patient to collect 24-hr urine specimen and to keep it refrigerated.
Follicle-stimulating hormone (FSH)	Indicates gonadal failure because of pituitary dysfunction *Female:* Follicular phase: 2–5 U/24 hr Midcycle: 8–60 U/24 hr Luteal phase: 2–10 U/24 hr Postmenopause: 35–100 U/24 hr *Male*: 3–11 U/24 hr	Instruct patient to collect 24-hr urine specimen, to indicate phase of menstrual cycle or if menopausal, and to indicate whether taking oral contraceptives or hormones.
Blood Studies		
Prolactin	Reveals pituitary dysfunction that can cause amenorrhea *Female*: <25 mcg/L *Male*: <20 mcg/L	Observe venipuncture site for bleeding or hematoma.
Prostate-specific antigen (PSA)	Reveals presence of prostate cancer Also a sensitive test for monitoring response to therapy Reference interval: <2.5 mcg/L	Inform patient that there are no food or fluid restrictions. Collect 5 mL of blood. Observe venipuncture site for bleeding.
hCG	Reveals pregnancy Can be used as a tumour marker for testicular malignancy Also used to detect hydatidiform mole *Males and nonpregnant females*: <5 IU/mL	Ask patient at which phase of menstrual cycle they are in, whether any menses were missed, and, if so, how late menses are.

TABLE 53.12   DIAGNOSTIC STUDIES

Male and Female Reproductive Systems—cont'd

Study	Description and Purpose	Nursing Responsibility
Testosterone	Indicates whether androgen levels are elevated because of testicular, adrenal, or ovarian dysfunction or pituitary tumours Serum levels also measured to assess male infertility and tumours of testicle or ovary *Male:* 9.75–38 nmol/L *Female:* <0.52–2.43 nmol/L	Collect a health history to rule out potential sources of interference with accuracy of results (e.g., use of corticosteroids or barbiturates, presence of hypothyroidism or hyperthyroidism).
Progesterone	Indicates cause of infertility Used to monitor success of medications for infertility or the effect of treatment with progesterone Indicates whether ovulation is occurring Helps diagnose conditions related to the adrenal glands and some types of cancer *Female:* Follicular phase: 1.6 nmol/L Luteal phase: 9.54–79.5 nmol/L After menopause: <1.27 nmol/L *Male:* 0.32–1.6 nmol/L	Include measurements during most recent menstrual period and trimester of pregnancy because progesterone levels vary with gestation.
Estradiol	Indicates ovarian function Useful in assessing estrogen-secreting tumours and states of precocious female puberty May be used to confirm perimenopausal status Increased serum estradiol levels in men may be indicative of testicular tumours *Female:* Follicular phase: 73.4–1284.9 pmol/L Luteal phase: 110–1652 pmol/L After menopause: ≤73.4 pmol/L *Male:* 37–183.5 pmol/L	Observe venipuncture site for bleeding or hematoma.
FSH	Indicates gonadal failure due to pituitary dysfunction Used to validate menopausal status *Female:* Follicular phase: 1.37–9.9 IU/L Ovulatory peak: 6.7–17.2 IU/L Luteal phase: 1.09–9.2 IU/L Postmenopause: 19.3–100.6 IU/L *Male:* 1.42–15.4 IU/L	Inform patient that no food or fluid restrictions are required. Ask patient at which phase of menstrual cycle they are in, whether they are experiencing menopause, or taking oral contraceptive or hormone therapy.
Venereal Disease Research Laboratory (VDRL) test (flocculation)	Nonspecific antibody tests used to screen for syphilis Readings can be positive within 1–2 wk after appearance of primary lesion (chancre) or 4–15 wk after initial infection *Reference interval:* negative or nonreactive	
Rapid plasma reagin (RPR) assay (agglutination)	Nonspecific antibody tests used to screen for syphilis *Reference interval:* negative or nonreactive	Obtain data to identify conditions such as hepatitis, pregnancy, and autoimmune diseases that may interfere with accuracy of results.
Fluorescent treponemal antibody absorption (FTA-Abs) test	Reveals syphilis antibodies Also reveals early syphilis with great accuracy Usually performed if results of aforementioned nonspecific tests are equivocal *Reference interval:* negative or nonreactive	

Cultures and Smears

Study	Description and Purpose	Nursing Responsibility
Dark-field microscopy	Direct examination of specimen obtained from potential syphilitic lesion (chancre) to detect *Treponema pallidum*	Avoid direct skin contact with open lesion.
Wet mounts	Direct microscopic examination of specimen of vaginal discharge, performed immediately after collection Indicates presence or absence and number of *Trichomonas* organisms, bacteria, white and red blood cells, and candidal buds or hyphae May reveal other clues to or causes of inflammation or infection	Explain procedure and purpose to patient. Instruct patient not to use douche before the examination. Prepare for collection of specimens (glass slide, 10–20% potassium hydroxide [KOH] solution, sodium chloride [NaCl] solution, and cotton-tipped applicators).
Cultures	Specimens of vaginal, urethral, or cervical discharge that are cultured to assess presence of gonorrhea or *Chlamydia* Rectal and throat cultures may also be obtained, depending on data in sexual history	Obtain specific contact and sexual history inclusive of oral and rectal intercourse. Instruct patient against using douche before examination. Obtain urethral specimen from men before they void. Instruct women who are sexually active with multiple partners to have at least a yearly culture for gonorrhea and *Chlamydia*. Instruct sexually active men to have any discharge evaluated immediately to rule out gonorrhea strains that do not cause classic symptoms of dysuria.

Continued

TABLE 53.12 **DIAGNOSTIC STUDIES**

Male and Female Reproductive Systems—cont'd

Study	Description and Purpose	Nursing Responsibility
Gram stain	Used for rapid detection of gonorrhea Presence of Gram-negative intracellular diplococci generally warrants initiation of treatment Not highly accurate for women Also a valid alternative for *Chlamydia* testing	Same as for cultures.
Cytological Studies		
Papanicolaou (Pap) smear	Microscopic study of exfoliated cells via special staining and fixation technique to detect abnormal cells Most commonly studies of cells obtained directly from the endocervix and ectocervix	Instruct women who are sexually active and who are between the ages of 21 and 69 to have Pap smears according to Canadian Cancer Society guidelines (every 1–3 yr, depending on provincial and territorial screening guidelines).* Instruct patients not to use douche for at least 24 hr before examination. Carefully document menstrual and gynecological history.
Nipple discharge test	Cytological study of nipple discharge	Ask whether patient is taking hormonal preparations or other medications, is breastfeeding, or has a history of amenorrhea.
Radiological Studies		
Mammography • Screening • Diagnostic	X-ray image of breast tissue on radiographic film, used to assess breast tissue Reveals benign and malignant masses Performed when patient has suspect clinical symptoms or when an abnormality is found on screening mammogram Additional views of affected breast are taken	Instruct patient about advantages of the examination. Explain that the Canadian Cancer Society recommends screening with mammography every 2 yr for women who are 50–69 yr of age (see Chapter 54 for more information).†
Ultrasonography (abdominal and transvaginal)	Used to measure and record high-frequency sound waves as they pass through tissues of variable density In women, useful in detecting masses >3 cm, such as ectopic pregnancy, IUD, ovarian cyst, and hydatidiform mole In men, used to detect testicular torsion or masses	Instruct patient that a full bladder may be required, depending on the reason for the study.
Ultrasound-guided biopsy	Use of ultrasound guidance during a biopsy, usually done as an outpatient procedure Used to direct the biopsy needle into the region of interest and obtain a sample of tissue Small tissue sample is removed to diagnose infection, inflammation, or mass	Inform patient of purpose of this procedure. It is usually done as an outpatient procedure.
Computed tomography (CT) of pelvis	Reveals tumours within the pelvis	Explain procedure to the patient. Instruct patient to lie still during the procedure. If IV contrast medium is used, check for iodine allergy.
Magnetic resonance imaging (MRI)	Use of radio waves and magnetic field to view soft tissue Useful if mammogram is abnormal or in presence of breast dysplasia Also used to diagnose abnormalities in the female and male reproductive systems	Screen patient for metal parts and pacemaker. Inform patient that the procedure is painless. Instruct patient to lie still during the procedure.
Invasive Procedures		
Breast biopsy	Histological examination of breast tissue excised either by needle aspiration or excisional biopsy	*Before biopsy:* Instruct patient about operative procedures and sedation. *After biopsy:* Perform wound care and instruct patient about breast self-examination.
Hysteroscopy	Visualization of uterine lining through hysteroscope inserted through cervix Used mainly to diagnose and treat abnormal bleeding such as that caused by fibroids or polyps Biopsy sample may be taken during the procedure	Explain purpose and method of the procedure and that it might be done in the health care provider's office. Inform patient that mild cramping and slight bloody discharge after the procedure is normal.
Hysterosalpingography	Fluoroscopy with a contrast material injected into the uterine cavity via the cervix Used to check for blocked Fallopian tubes, adhesions near ovary, or abnormalities of the uterus	Inform patient about the procedure and that it may be fairly uncomfortable. Check patient for iodine allergy.
Colposcopy	Direct visualization of cervix with binocular microscope that allows magnification and study of cellular dysplasia and cervix abnormalities Used as follow-up study for abnormal Pap test results and for examination of women exposed to DES in utero Biopsy sample from cervix may be taken during examination Valuable in decreasing number of false-negative results of cervical biopsies	Describe this outpatient procedure to the patient. Inform patient that this examination is similar to speculum examination.

TABLE 53.12 **DIAGNOSTIC STUDIES**

Male and Female Reproductive Systems—cont'd

Study	Description and Purpose	Nursing Responsibility
Conization	Removal of cone-shaped sample of squamocolumnar tissue of cervix for direct study	Explain purpose and method of the procedure and that it requires use of surgical facilities and anaesthesia. Instruct patient to avoid sexual intercourse and using tampons for about 3–4 wk. Also discuss necessity for 3-wk follow-up.
Loop electrosurgical excision procedure (LEEP)	Excision of cervical tissue via an electrosurgical instrument Helps diagnose and treat cervical dysplasia Minimizes amount of tissue removed and preserves childbearing ability	Explain purpose and method of procedure and that it may be done in the physician's office. Inform patient that slight tingling or abdominal cramping during the procedure may be felt. Inform patient that discharge, bleeding, and cramping may occur for 1–3 days after the procedure.
Culdotomy, culdoscopy, and culdocentesis	*Culdotomy:* incision made through posterior fornix of cul-de-sac that allows visualization of peritoneal cavity (i.e., uterus, tubes, and ovaries) *Culdoscopy:* used after culdotomy to closely study these structures; valuable in fertility evaluations *Culdocentesis:* withdrawal of fluid for examination	Explain purpose and method of the procedure. Prepare patient for vaginal operation with preoperative instruction and sedation. Perform assessment of bleeding and discomfort after surgery.
Laparoscopy (peritoneoscopy)	Visualization of pelvic structures via fibre-optic endoscopes inserted through small abdominal incisions Instillation of CO_2 into cavity to improve visualization Used in diagnostic assessment of uterus, tubes, and ovaries (see Figure 53.10) Can be performed in conjunction with tubal sterilization	Before surgery, instruct patient about the procedure, prepare patient's abdomen, and reassure patient about sedation. Inform patient of probability of shoulder pain due to air in the abdomen.
Dilatation and curettage (D&C)	Operative procedure dilates cervix and allows curetting of endometrial lining Used in assessment of abnormal bleeding and cytological evaluation of lining.	Before surgery, instruct patient about the procedure and sedation. Perform postoperative assessment of degree of bleeding (frequent perineal pad check during first 24 hr).
Fertility Studies		
Semen analysis	Assessment of semen for volume (2–5 mL), viscosity, sperm count (>20 million/mL), sperm motility (60% motile), and percentage of abnormal sperm (60% with normal structure)	Instruct patient to bring in a fresh specimen within 2 hr of ejaculation.
Basal body temperature assessment	Indirect indication of whether ovulation has occurred (temperature rises at ovulation and remains elevated during secretory phase of normal menstrual cycle)	Instruct woman to take her temperature with a special basal temperature thermometer (calibrated in tenths of degrees) every morning before getting out of bed. Instruct woman to record temperature on a graph.
Huhner, postcoital test	Examination of mucus sample of cervix within 2–8 hr after intercourse Assessment of total number of sperm in relation to number of live sperm Used to determine whether cervical mucus is "hostile" to passage of sperm from vagina into uterus	Instruct couples to have intercourse at estimated time of ovulation and be present for test within 2–8 hr after intercourse.
Endometrial biopsy	Use of small curette to obtain piece of endometrial lining to assess endometrial changes common to progesterone secretion after ovulation Also used to assess abnormal menstrual or postmenopausal uterine bleeding	Tell patient that the test must be performed after ovulation. Explain that the procedure should cause only a short period of uterine cramping and light, bloody vaginal discharge for about 24 hr.
Serum progesterone measurement	Same as those of blood studies.	Same as those of blood studies.
Genetic Studies		
DNA testing for *BRCA1* and *BRCA2* gene mutations (blood or saliva sample)	Testing for inherited mutations in breast cancer (*BRCA*) genes, which increase a female's susceptibility for the development of breast or ovarian cancer Recommended in cases of family history associated with an increased risk of a harmful mutation in either gene	Inform patient that results may take up to 1 month to be available. Advise genetic counselling before and after testing.

*Canadian Cancer Society. (2020). *Cervical cancer: Screening for cervical cancer.* http://www.cancer.ca/en/cancer-information/cancer-type/cervical/screening/?region=on
†Canadian Cancer Society. (2020). *Breast cancer: Screening for breast cancer.* http://www.cancer.ca/en/cancer-information/cancer-type/breast/screening/?region=on
DES, diethylstilbestrol; *IUDs,* intrauterine devices; *IV,* intravenous.

In home pregnancy test kits, the same assay principle is used. Positive results are based on the presence of hCG in urine. Some tests can detect pregnancy as early as the first day after a missed menstrual period. These tests are 99% accurate if the test is performed exactly per instructions (Cole & Butler, 2020). A second test is recommended within a week if the first test result is negative (assuming menses have not yet occurred).

Hormone Studies. Although estrogen studies are performed on urine, the results are frequently inaccurate because estrogen levels vary during the normal cycle and it is difficult to estimate the day of the cycle in women with irregular menses. Adrenal androgens are precursors of estrogens and can be measured in the urine of both men and women. For more information regarding hormone studies, see Chapter 50.

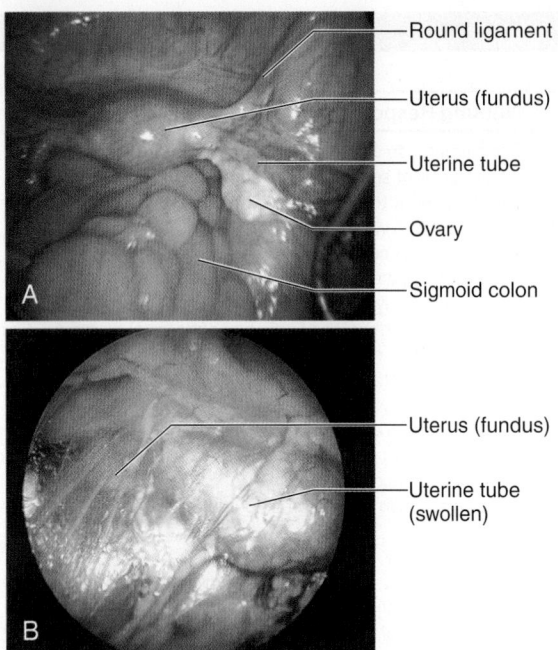

Round ligament
Uterus (fundus)
Uterine tube
Ovary
Sigmoid colon

Uterus (fundus)
Uterine tube (swollen)

FIG. 53.10 Laparoscopic views of the female pelvis. **A,** Normal appearance. **B,** Pelvic inflammatory disease. Note the reddish inflammatory membrane covering and fixing the ovary and uterus to the surrounding structures. Source: Thibodeau, G. A., & Patton, K. T. (2013). *Anatomy and physiology* (8th ed., p. 1088, Figure 35.21). Mosby.

Blood Studies

Hormone Studies. Serum assays for hCG can detect pregnancy before a woman misses her menstrual period, as early as 10 days after conception (Pagana et al., 2019). The prolactin assay is used primarily in the workup of a patient with amenorrhea. High levels of prolactin are normally associated with low levels of estrogen, such as those that occur during lactation. However, the same finding can occur with pituitary adenomas, especially with otherwise unexplained *galactorrhea* (excessive secretion of breast milk). Serum progesterone and estradiol are sometimes measured in ovarian function assessment, particularly for amenorrhea. In addition, hormonal blood studies are essential components of a thorough fertility workup.

Tumour Markers. Biological tumour markers are used to assess for malignant disease and to monitor therapy (marker levels rise as disease progresses and fall with disease regression). α-Fetoprotein, hCG, and cancer antigen 125 (CA-125) are sometimes used as tumour markers for reproductive system malignancies. A specific tumour antigen such as PSA is another type of tumour marker, frequently measured to determine the presence of prostate cancer.

Serological Tests for Syphilis. The Venereal Disease Research Laboratory (VDRL) test and the rapid plasma reagin (RPR) test are used to detect the presence of antibodies in the serum of patients thought to be infected with syphilis. These tests are inexpensive and reliable but yield high levels of false-positive results in patients with inflammatory disorders. The fluorescent treponemal antibody absorption test is a more specific treponemal assay and should be used after a positive finding on the VDRL or RPR test.

Cultures and Smears

Cultures and smears are most frequently employed in the diagnosis of STBBIs. Specimens for cultures and smears are most commonly taken from the vagina, endocervix, and rectum for females and the urethra and rectum for males. For a culture, the specimen is placed on a special culture medium. A smear involves rubbing the specimen on a slide for direct examination. Gram stain smears have been shown to be effective in the diagnosis of *Chlamydia* infection. A nucleic acid amplification test is used to screen for both gonorrhea and *Chlamydia* from a wide variety of samples, including vaginal, endocervical, urine, and urethral specimens. Dark-field microscopy involves the direct examination of a specimen obtained from a syphilitic chancre for the diagnosis of syphilis.

Cytological Studies

Cytology is the study of cells under microscopic examination. The Pap smear is a screening test to detect abnormal cells obtained from the cervix or vagina. It involves obtaining cells from the cervical canal, preferably the endocervix, as well as from the vagina. The cells are placed in a fixative for examination by a cytologist for cellular abnormalities. Screening guidelines for the Pap test (also called a *smear*) are discussed in Chapter 56.

Cytological study is also indicated for nipple discharge. Cytological examination can be used to detect the presence of malignant cells and distinguish the discharge with such cells from one associated with infection.

Radiological Studies

Mammography. Mammography, one of the most frequently used diagnostic tools to assess the reproductive system, is used to detect breast masses. Mammography and screening guidelines for mammography are discussed in Chapter 54.

CASE STUDY

Objective Data: Diagnostic Studies

The following laboratory and diagnostic test results for A. K. were obtained:
- Urine pregnancy test: negative
- Urinalysis: normal findings
- CBC: hemoglobin 132 g/L, hematocrit 36%
- TSH: 2.3 mIU/L
- Gonorrhea and chlamydia tests: negative
  The pelvic and transvaginal ultrasound revealed a 4-cm ovarian cyst.

Discussion Questions
1. Which diagnostic and laboratory test results should be of concern to the nurse?
2. What patient teaching can the nurse provide her, based on the diagnostic tests results?
   See Case Study: Patient Information, Case Study: Subjective Data, and Case Study: Objective Data: Physical Examination for more information on A. K.

Ultrasonography. Ultrasonography has many applications for diagnostic study. Pelvic ultrasonography is used to obtain images of the pelvic organs. Transvaginal ultrasonography can be used to aid in diagnosing abnormalities of the ovaries or the uterus. These types of ultrasound studies are also used to detect pregnancy in the uterus, ectopic pregnancy, ovarian cysts, and other pelvic masses. Breast ultrasonography is useful in the detection of fluid-filled masses. In men, ultrasonography is used to detect testicular masses and testicular torsion. Transrectal ultrasonography is useful in locating prostate tumours.

REVIEW QUESTIONS

The number of the question corresponds to the same-numbered objective at the beginning of the chapter.

1. Which of the following is a normal reproductive function that may be altered in a client who undergoes a prostatectomy?
   a. Sperm production
   b. Production of testosterone
   c. Production of seminal fluid
   d. Release of sperm from the epididymis

2. What does estrogen production by the mature ovarian follicle cause?
   a. Decreased secretion of follicle-stimulating hormone (FSH) and luteinizing hormone (LH)
   b. Increased production of gonadotropin-releasing hormone (GnRH) and FSH
   c. Release of GnRH and increased secretion of LH
   d. Decreased release of FSH and decreased progesterone production

3. Female orgasm is the result of which of the following? *(Select all that apply.)*
   a. Constriction of the cervical os
   b. Uterine and vaginal contractions
   c. Vaginal enlargement and uterine elevation
   d. Clitoral swelling and increased vaginal lubrication
   e. Rapid release of muscular tension in the reproductive structures

4. Which of the following is an age-related finding noted by the nurse during assessment of an older woman's reproductive system?
   a. Dyspareunia
   b. Vaginal dryness
   c. Nipple retraction
   d. Increased sensitivity of labia

5. Which of the following should be included as significant information about a client's past medical history in relation to the reproductive system?
   a. Extent of sexual activity
   b. General satisfaction with sexuality
   c. Previous sexually transmitted infections
   d. Self-image and relationships with others

6. Which of the following examination techniques is used to evaluate a client's breasts? *(Select all that apply.)*
   a. Palpation
   b. Percussion
   c. Inspection
   d. Auscultation

7. Which of the following would be considered an abnormal finding during physical assessment of the male reproductive system?
   a. Slight clear urethral discharge
   b. The glans covered with prepuce
   c. Symmetrical scrotum
   d. Descended testes

8. The nurse is caring for a client scheduled for an endometrial biopsy who is having difficulty becoming pregnant. What will the nurse explain to the woman?
   a. That the outpatient procedure is usually performed before ovulation
   b. That bleeding and discharge are common 2 to 4 days after the procedure
   c. That a small sample of tissue is obtained to diagnose and treat cervical dysplasia
   d. That common changes in endometrial cells in relation to progesterone levels will be assessed

1. c; 2. c; 3. b, c, d, e; 4. b; 5. c; 6. a, c; 7. a; 8. d.

Ⓔvolve

For even more review questions, visit http://evolve.elsevier.com/Canada/Lewis/medsurg.

REFERENCES

Bourne, A. (2019). *Sherburne's guidelines for gender-affirming primary care for trans and non-binary clients* (4th ed.). Sherbourne Health Centre. http://sherbourne.on.ca/wp-content/uploads/2014/02/Guidelines-and-Protocols-for-Comprehensive-Primary-Care-for-Trans-Clients-2015.pdf

Canadian Cancer Society. (2020). *Finding prostate cancer early*. http://www.cancer.ca/en/cancer-information/cancer-type/prostate/finding-cancer-early/?region=on

Canadian Cancer Society. (2021a). *Know your breasts*. https://www.cancer.ca/en/prevention-and-screening/reduce-cancer-risk/find-cancer-early/know-your-body/know-your-breasts/?region=qc

Canadian Cancer Society. (2021b). *Screening for cervical cancer*. https://www.cancer.ca/en/cancer-information/cancer-type/cervical/screening/?region=qc

Canadian Cancer Society. (2021c). *Testicular cancer: Finding testicular cancer early*. http://www.cancer.ca/en/cancer-information/cancer-type/testicular/finding-cancer-early/?region=on

Canadian Public Health Association (CPHA). (2017). *Discussing sexual health, substance use and STBBIs: A guide for service providers*. Author. https://www.cpha.ca/sites/default/files/assets/progs/stbbi/discussionguide_e.pdf.

Centers for Disease Control and Prevention (CDC). (2020). *Taking a sexual history*. https://www.cdc.gov/hiv/clinicians/transforming-health/health-care-providers/sexual-history.html

Cole, L., & Butler, S. (2020). *100 years of human chorionic gonadotropin: Reviews and new perspectives*. Elsevier Inc. https://doi.org/10.1016/C2019-0-00014-3

Cordero, A. M., Crider, K. S., Rogers, L. M., et al. (2015). Optimal serum and red blood cell folate concentrations in women of reproductive age for prevention of neural tube defects: World Health Organization guidelines. *Morbidity and Mortality Weekly Report (MMWR), 64*(15), 421–423. http://www.cdc.gov/mmwr/preview/mmwrhtml/mm6415a5.htm?s_cid=mm6415a5_e

deSanjose, S., Brotons, M., & Pavon, M. A. (2018). The natural history of human papillomavirus infection. *Best Practice & Research: Clinical Obstetrics & Gynaecology, 47*, 2. https://doi.org/10.1016/j.bpobgyn.2017.08.015

Dragon, C. N., Guerino, P., Ewald, E., et al. (2017). Transgender medicare beneficiaries and chronic conditions: Exploring fee-for-service claims data. *LGBT Health, 4*(6), 404–411. https://doi.org/10.1089/lgbt.2016.020

Gress, S. (2017). *Aesthetic and functional labiaplasty*. Springer. https://doi.org/10.1007/978-3-319-60222-6

Gurney, J. K., McGlynn, K. A., Stanley, J., et al. (2017). Risk factors for cryptorchidism. *Nature reviews. Urology, 14*(9), 534–548. https://doi.org/10.1038/nrurol.2017.90

Holesh, J. E., Bass, A. N., & Lord, M. (2021). *Physiology, ovulation.* StatPearls [Internet]. https://www.ncbi.nlm.nih.gov/books/NBK441996/

Jackman, K., Bosse, J., Eliason, M., et al. (2019). Sexual and gender minority health research in nursing. *Nursing Outlook, 67*(1), 21–38. https://doi.org/10.1016/j.outlook.2018.10.006

Klarenbach, S., Sims-Jones, N., Lewin, G., et al. (2018). The Canadian Task Force on Preventative Health Care. Recommendations on screening for breast cancer in women aged 40–74 years who are not at increased risk for breast cancer. *Canadian Medical Association Journal, 190*(49), E1441–E1451. https://doi.org/10.1503/cmaj.180463

Lacroix, A. E., Gondal, H., & Langaker, M. D. (2021). *Physiology, menarche.* StatPearls [Internet]. https://www.ncbi.nlm.nih.gov/books/NBK470216/

Marcinkow, A., Parkhomchik, P., Schmode, A., et al. (2019). The quality of information on combined oral contraceptives available on the Internet. *Journal of Obstetrics and Gynaecology Canada, 41*(11), 1599–1607. https://doi.org/10.1016/j.jogc.2019.01.024

Masters, W. H., & Johnson, E. (1966). *Human sexual response.* Little Brown. (Seminal).

Meyer, I. H., Brown, T. N., Herman, J. L., et al. (2017). Demographic characteristics and health status of transgender adults in select US regions: Behavioral risk factor surveillance system, 2014. *American Journal of Public Health, 107*, 582–589. https://doi.org/10.2105/AJPH.2016.303648

Northern College. (2020). *Moontime.* http://www.northernc.on.ca/indigenous/moontime/

Pagana, K. D., Pagana, T. J., & Pike-MacDonald, S. A. (2019). *Mosby's Canadian manual of diagnostic and laboratory tests* (2nd Canadian ed.). Mosby.

Palacios, S. (2019). Assessing symptomatic vulvar, vaginal, and lower urinary tract atrophy. *Climacteric, 2*(4), 348–351. https://doi.org/10.1080/13697137.2019.1600499

Patton, K. T., & Thibodeau, G. A. (2015). *Structure and function of the body* (15th ed.). Mosby.

Peacock, K., & Ketvertis, K. M. (2021). *Menopause.* StatPearls [Internet]. https://www.ncbi.nlm.nih.gov/books/NBK507826/

Pember, M. A. (2019). *"Honouring our monthly moons": Some menstruation rituals give Indigenous women hope.* Rewire News Group. https://rewire.news/article/2019/02/20/monthly-moons-menstruation-rituals-indigenous-women/

Public Health Agency of Canada (PHAC). (2019). *For health professionals: Rubella.* https://www.canada.ca/en/public-health/services/diseases/rubella/information-health-professionals-rubella.html

Rosner, J., Samardzic, T., & Sarao, M. S. (2021). *Physiology, female reproduction.* StatPearls [Internet]. https://www.ncbi.nlm.nih.gov/books/NBK537132/

Statistics Canada. (2017). *Census in brief: Same-sex couples in Canada in 2016.* https://www12.statcan.gc.ca/census-recensement/2016/as-sa/98-200-x/2016007/98-200-x2016007-eng.cfm

Streed, C. G., McCarty, E. P., & Haas, J. S. (2017). Association between gender minority status and self-reported physical and mental health in the United States. *JAMA Internal Medicine, 177*(8), 1210–1212. https://doi.org/10.1001/jamainternmed.2017.1460

Syme, M. L., & Cohn, T. J. (2016). Examining aging sexual stigma attitudes among adults by gender, age, and generational status. *Aging & Mental Health, 20*(1), 36–45. https://doi.org/10.1080/13607863.2015.1012044

Touhy, T., & Jett, K. (2016). *Ebersole & Hess' toward healthy aging: Human needs and nursing response* (9th ed.). Elsevier.

RESOURCES

Resources for this chapter are listed in Chapters 56 and 57.

Nursing Management
Breast Disorders

Jackie Hartigan-Rogers
Originating US chapter by Deena Dell

evolve WEBSITE

http://evolve.elsevier.com/Canada/Lewis/medsurg

- Review Questions (Online Only)
- Key Points
- Answer Guidelines for Case Study
- Customizable Nursing Care Plan
  - After Mastectomy or Lumpectomy
- Conceptual Care Map Creator
  - Conceptual Care Map for Textbook Case Study
- Audio Glossary
- Content Updates

LEARNING OBJECTIVES

1. Summarize screening guidelines for the early detection of breast cancer.
2. Describe the technique of breast self-awareness, including rationale and reasons for referral.
3. Explain the types, causes, clinical manifestations, interprofessional care, and nursing management of common benign breast disorders.
4. Assess the risk factors for breast cancer.
5. Describe the pathophysiology and clinical manifestations of breast cancer.
6. Describe the interprofessional care and the nursing management of patients with breast cancer.
7. Specify the physical and psychological preoperative and postoperative aspects of nursing management for patients undergoing a mastectomy.
8. Explain the indications, types, potential risks, and complications of reconstructive breast surgery and the nursing management of patients after undergoing reconstructive breast surgery.

KEY TERMS

cyst	gynecomastia	mastalgia
fibroadenoma	lumpectomy	mastectomy
fibrocystic changes	lymphedema	mastitis
galactorrhea	mammoplasty	Paget's disease

Breast disorders are a significant health concern for women. Most breast pain is of a benign nature, with the most frequently encountered breast disorders in women being nipple discharge, intraductal papilloma, duct ectasia, breast pain, and fibrocystic changes such as cysts and fibroadenomas (Sasaki et al., 2018). In men, gynecomastia is the most common breast disorder.

In Canada, there is a one in eight chance that a woman will receive a diagnosis of breast cancer in their lifetime (Canadian Cancer Society, 2021a). Whether the actual diagnosis is one of a benign condition or a malignancy, the initial discovery of a lump or change in the breast often triggers intense feelings of anxiety, fear, and denial. These feelings can be associated with both the fear of death and the possible loss of a breast. The potential loss of a breast, or part of a breast, may be devastating because of the significant psychological, social, sexual, and body image implications associated with it.

ASSESSMENT OF BREAST DISORDERS

It is critical that breast disorders be detected early, diagnosed accurately, and treated promptly. The frequency of breast examinations is determined by a woman's age, the presence of significant risk factors, and medical history. Guidelines established in Canada regarding breast surveillance practices include the following:

- Women of all ages should be familiar with their breasts and report any changes to their health care providers (Canadian Cancer Society, 2021b).
- Women aged 40 to 49 should discuss with a health care provider their individual risks for breast cancer, along with the risks and benefits of mammography.
- Women aged 50 to 74 should undergo mammography every 2 years.

- Women aged 75 or older should talk to a health care provider about an individualized screening program.
- A health care provider may also perform a physical examination of the breasts (clinical breast examination).
- Women who are at high risk for developing breast cancer should talk to their health care providers about a personal plan of testing (Canadian Cancer Society, 2021c).

It is recommended that all women discuss the risks and benefits of mammography with their health care providers (Canadian Cancer Society, 2021c). The benefits of early detection of breast cancer are well established. The use of screening mammography has significantly improved early and accurate detection of breast malignancies. Mammography can be used to identify breast abnormalities that may be cancer before physical symptoms appear. Canada's national guidelines have been established on the basis of research that women aged 50 to 74 benefit most from regular breast screening (Canadian Cancer Society, 2021c).

Current recommendations for younger women are informed by evidence review of the benefits and harms of breast cancer screening and its role in reducing rates of mortality from breast cancer (Canadian Task Force on Preventive Health Care, 2018). The emphasis now is to assist women to become aware of how their breasts normally look and feel and to understand that there is no right or wrong way for them to check their breasts (Figure 54.1). Nurses should teach women that it is important to get to know the whole area of breast tissue, including up to the collarbone and under armpits and nipples (Canadian Cancer Society, 2021b). Women should be encouraged to report any new breast changes (e.g., nipple discharge, presence of a lump) to their health care providers (Canadian Cancer Society, 2021b).

If a woman decides to practise breast self-examination (BSE) and undergo mammography screening, health care providers must ensure that the benefits and risks, as well as the woman's values and preferences, are discussed fully (Canadian Task Force on Preventive Health Care, 2018).

It is also important that nurses ensure patients' awareness of Canada's clinical practice guidelines for the care and treatment of breast cancer. All patients who have completed primary treatment for breast cancer should have regular follow-up surveillance that comprises a medical history, physical examination, and annual mammography. The frequency of visits must be adjusted according to the individual patient's needs. Special topics of concern that must be addressed with patients who have breast cancer include cognitive functioning, fatigue, physical activity, sexual functioning, and fertility (Canadian Cancer Society, 2021d).

DIAGNOSTIC STUDIES

Radiological Studies

Several techniques can be used to screen for breast disorders or provide a diagnosis of a suspect physical finding. *Mammography* is a method used to visualize the internal structure of the breast with the use of radiography (Figure 54.2). This generally well-tolerated procedure can detect suspect findings that cannot be felt by palpation. Mammography has significantly improved the early and accurate detection of breast malignancies. Improved imaging technology has also reduced the amount of radiation used in mammography. Digital mammography, in which radiographic images are digitally coded into a computer, is an addition to screening programs (Canadian Cancer Society, 2021e; see Figure 54.2). Three-dimensional (3-D) mammography provides a clearer view of overlapping breast tissue structures, which helps to accurately detect and diagnose breast cancer (Barbeau & Pillay, 2017).

Calcifications are the abnormality most easily recognized on mammograms (see Figure 54.2). These deposits of calcium crystals form in the breast for many reasons, such as inflammation, trauma, and aging. Although most calcifications are benign, they also may be associated with preinvasive cancer.

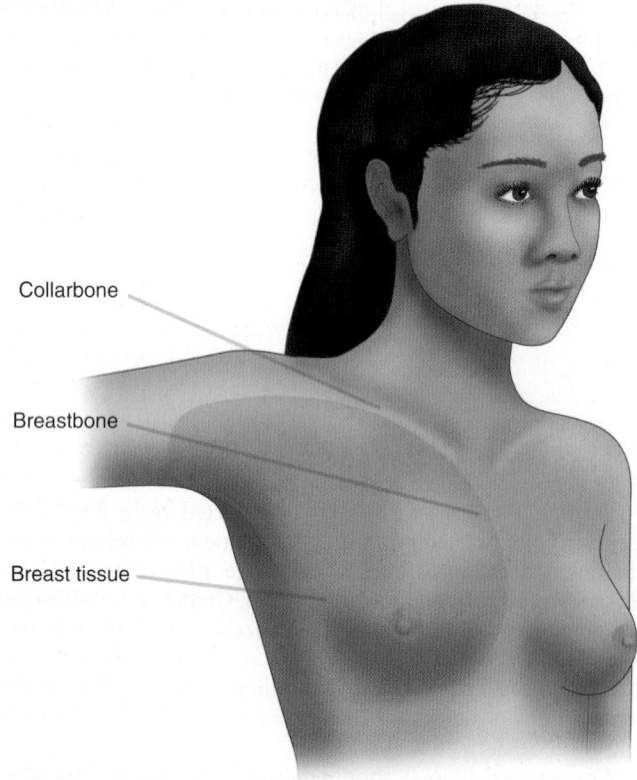

Collarbone

Breastbone

Breast tissue

FIG. 54.1 Every woman should know their breasts and be aware of what is normal by looking at and feeling their breasts any way that works best, including the whole area of breast tissue: up to the collarbone, under the armpits, and including the nipples. Source: Monica Schroeder/Science Source.

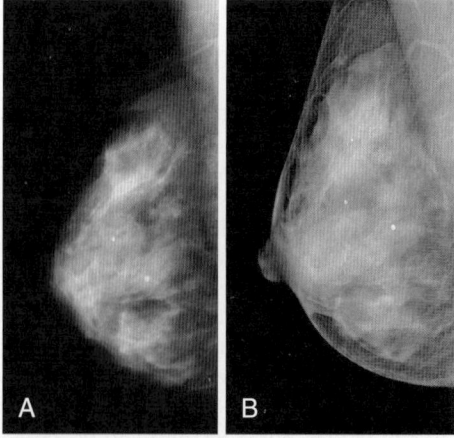

FIG. 54.2 Screening mammograms showing dense breast tissue and benign, scattered microcalcifications of a 57-year-old. **A,** Image obtained with conventional radiography. **B,** Image obtained with digital radiography. Source: Adam, A. (2008). *Grainger and Allison's diagnostic radiology* (5th ed.). Churchill Livingstone.

A comparison of current and prior mammograms may reveal early cancerous tissue changes. Because some tumours metastasize late, early detection by mammography allows for earlier treatment and the prevention of metastasis of lesions that are smaller or less aggressive. In younger women, mammography is less sensitive because of the greater density of breast tissue and because developing breast tissue is radiosensitive, resulting in more false-negative results (Barbeau & Pillay, 2017). About 10 to 15% of all breast cancers cannot be seen on mammograms and are detected only by palpation. If the clinical findings are suspect, ultrasound or magnetic resonance imaging (MRI) may be used, and biopsy may be recommended on the basis of the findings.

Ultrasonography is used in conjunction with mammography to differentiate a solid mass from a cystic mass, to evaluate a mass in a pregnant or lactating woman, or to locate and guide biopsy for a suspect lesion on breast MRI. Palpable masses should be investigated with both mammography and ultrasonography (Barbeau & Pillay, 2017).

MRI is recommended as a sensitive screening tool for patients at high risk for breast cancer, whose findings on mammography or ultrasonography are suspect for malignancy, and in whom breast cancer was previously detected by mammography. Limitations of MRI include its high cost, which may result in less frequent use of this method of screening (Barbeau & Pillay, 2017).

Biopsies

A definitive diagnosis of a suspect area is made by means of histological examination of a biopsy sample of tissue. Biopsy techniques include fine-needle aspiration (FNA), core needle, stereotactic core needle, wire localization, and surgical biopsy (also called *open biopsy*).

In *FNA biopsy,* a thin, fine needle is inserted into the lesion and cellular fluid aspirated into a syringe. Three or four passes are usually made. FNA and cytological evaluation may be helpful in making a diagnosis and planning treatment. If the results are negative but the lesion is suspect, an additional biopsy may be necessary. Biopsy results are usually available within 24 to 48 hours.

A *core needle biopsy* is commonly used as a preferred method for obtaining and diagnosing a breast tissue specimen (Canadian Cancer Society, 2021f). It involves removing samples of breast tissue using a hollow needle, which takes small cylinder-shaped (core) samples.

Stereotactic core needle biopsy is a reliable diagnostic technique for obtaining a biopsy sample of an abnormality seen on a mammogram. The use of 3-D images assists in pinpointing the exact location of a lump or suspect lesion in order to guide the needle to obtain a sample of breast tissue. Patients should be informed that the procedure is uncomfortable. The patient is positioned lying face down on a table that has an opening for the breast. The skin is anaesthetized, and a small incision is made to allow the entrance of a biopsy needle that has a special cutting device. This process is repeated several times, and the core samples are sent for pathological analysis. Larger samples of tissue can be removed using a special *vacuum-assisted device* (VAD), which uses suction to collect the tissue sample. An advantage of VAD is that the needle is inserted only once into the breast and then can be rotated, which allows for multiple samples being taken through a single needle insertion.

Minimally invasive breast biopsies have become the standard of care for diagnosing abnormalities found through either imaging or BSE. These outpatient techniques have advantages over a surgical biopsy, including minimal scarring, local anaesthesia, reduced cost, and shorter recovery time. In some cases, a *surgical biopsy* is recommended, which involves removal of part or all of a suspect lesion through an incision into the breast. If the lesion is small, deep, and difficult to locate, a *wire localization biopsy* may be used during surgery. A special fine wire is placed into the lesion under radiographic guidance, allowing the surgeon to locate the lesion.

BENIGN BREAST DISORDERS

Mastalgia

Mastalgia (breast pain) is the most common breast-related condition in women. The most common form is *cyclic mastalgia,* which coincides with the menstrual cycle (Sasaki et al., 2018). It is described as diffuse breast tenderness or heaviness. Breast pain may last 2 to 3 days or most of the month. The pain is related to hormonal sensitivity. The symptoms often decrease with menopause. *Noncyclic mastalgia* usually affects only one breast, has no relationship to the menstrual cycle, and can continue into menopause. It may be constant or intermittent throughout the month and last for several years. Symptoms include a burning sensation, aching, or soreness in the breast. The woman should be encouraged to see their health care provider for assistance in finding the cause and best treatment for new or changes in the pain experienced (Canadian Cancer Society, 2021g).

Mammography and targeted ultrasound are often performed to exclude cancer and provide etiology of mastalgia. Cyclic pain may be relieved somewhat by reductions in caffeine and dietary fat intake; by vitamin E and gamma-linolenic acid (evening primrose oil); and by continual wearing of a support bra. Massage with ice or heat, analgesics, and anti-inflammatory medications may also help. Medications that might be recommended include oral contraceptives, tamoxifen (Nolvadex), and danazol (Cyclomen). Because of the androgenic adverse effects of danazol (acne, edema, hirsutism), this therapy is unacceptable for many women.

Breast Infections

Mastitis. Mastitis is an inflammatory condition of the breast that occurs most frequently in lactating women (Table 54.1). *Lactational mastitis* manifests as a localized area that is erythematous, painful, and tender on palpation. Fever is often present. The infection develops when organisms, usually staphylococci, gain access to the breast through a cracked nipple. In its early stages, mastitis can be cured with antibiotics. Breastfeeding should continue unless an abscess is forming or a purulent drainage is noted. The person may wish to use a nipple shield or to hand-express milk from the involved breast until the pain subsides and should consult a health care provider promptly to begin a course of antibiotic therapy. Any breast that remains red, tender, and not responsive to antibiotics necessitates follow-up care and evaluation for inflammatory breast cancer (Sasaki et al., 2018).

Lactational Breast Abscess. If lactational mastitis persists after several days of antibiotic therapy, a lactational breast abscess may have developed. In this condition, the skin may become red and edematous over the involved breast, often with a corresponding palpable mass, and the patient may have a

TABLE 54.1	SELECT BENIGN BREAST DISORDERS	
Disorder	**Incidence**	**Clinical Manifestations**
Lactational mastitis	Occurs in up to 10% of postpartum lactating mothers (both primipara and multipara), usually within first 3 mo after parturition	Warm to touch, indurated, painful, often unilateral; most commonly caused by *Staphylococcus aureus*
Fibrocystic changes	Most common between ages 30 and 50	Not usually discrete masses but nodularity instead (movable, soft); usually accompanied by cyclic pain and tenderness; mass(es) often cyclic in occurrence
Cyst	Most common after age 35, incidence decreases after menopause	Palpable fluid-filled mass (movable, soft); multiple cysts can occur and recur; rarely associated with breast cancer
Fibroadenoma	Most common between ages 20 and 30	Palpable mass (movable, firm), usually 1–2 cm in size; rarely associated with breast cancer
Fat necrosis	Many women report previous history of trauma to breast	Usually a hard, very tender, mobile, indurated mass with irregular borders
Duct ectasia	Perimenopausal woman: most common in women between ages 40 and 50; may be due to duct obstruction or mastitis	Fixation of nipple, usually accompanied by nipple discharge of thick, green or black material; often associated with breast pain

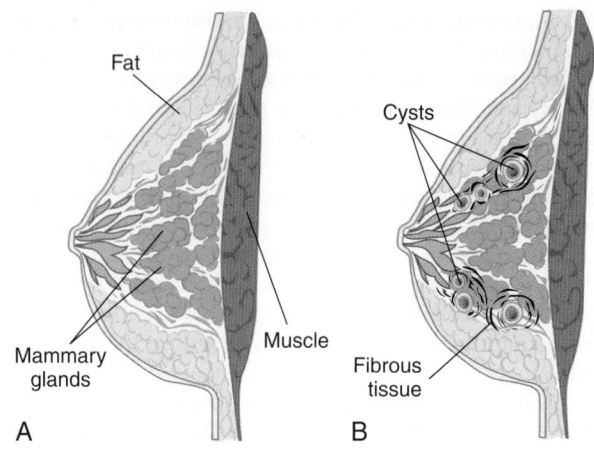

FIG. 54.3 **A,** Normal breast tissue. **B,** Fibrocystic breast tissue.

fever. Antibiotics alone constitute insufficient treatment for a breast abscess. Ultrasonography-guided drainage of the abscess or surgical incision and drainage are necessary (Sasaki et al., 2018). The drainage is cultured, sensitivities are measured, and therapy with an appropriate antibiotic is begun. Breastfeeding can continue in most cases with ongoing treatment of the abscess (MyHealth.Alberta.ca, 2019).

Fibrocystic Changes

Fibrocystic changes in the breast constitute a benign condition characterized by changes in breast tissue (Figure 54.3). The changes include the development of excess fibrous tissue, hyperplasia of the epithelial lining of the mammary ducts, proliferation of mammary ducts, and cyst formation. Pain is caused by nerve irritation from edema in the connective tissue and by fibrosis from pinching of the nerve. Fibrocystic changes are not associated with increased risk for breast cancer. Masses or nodularities can appear in both breasts. They are often found in the upper, outer quadrants and usually occur bilaterally.

Fibrocystic changes are the most frequently occurring breast disorder. They occur most often in women between 30 and 50 years of age but can begin as early as 20 years of age. Pain and nodularity often increase over time but tend to subside after menopause unless high doses of estrogen replacement are used. Fibrocystic changes are thought to result from a heightened responsiveness of breast tissue to circulating estrogen and progesterone (Canadian Cancer Society, 2021h; Sasaki et al., 2018).

Fibrocystic changes most commonly occur in women with premenstrual abnormalities, nulliparous women, women with a history of spontaneous abortion, nonusers of oral contraceptives, and women with early menarche and late menopause. Symptoms related to fibrocystic changes often worsen in the premenstrual phase and subside after menstruation.

Manifestations of fibrocystic breast changes include one or more palpable lumps that are often round, well delineated, and freely movable within the breast (see Table 54.1). Discomfort ranging from tenderness to pain may also occur. The lump is usually observed to increase in size and perhaps in tenderness before menstruation. Cysts may enlarge or shrink rapidly, becoming larger before menstruation and shrinking afterward. Nipple discharge associated with fibrocystic breasts is often milky, watery-milky, yellow, or green.

Mammography may be helpful in distinguishing fibrocystic changes from breast cancer. However, in some women, the breast tissue is so dense that it is difficult to obtain a mammographic study. In these situations, ultrasonography may be more useful in differentiating a cystic mass from a solid mass.

NURSING AND INTERPROFESSIONAL MANAGEMENT FIBROCYSTIC CHANGES

With the initial discovery of a discrete mass in the breast by the person or their health care provider, aspiration or surgical biopsy may be indicated. If the nodularity is recurrent, a wait of 7 to 10 days may be planned in order to note any changes that may be related to the menstrual cycle. For large or frequent cysts, surgical removal may be favoured over repeated aspiration. An excisional biopsy would be recommended if (a) no fluid is found on aspiration, (b) the fluid that is found is hemorrhagic, or (c) a residual mass remains after fluid aspiration. Excisional biopsy is performed in an outpatient surgery unit.

Biopsy may be indicated for persons with fibrocystic disorders who are at increased risk for breast cancer. A person with cystic changes should be encouraged to return regularly for follow-up examinations throughout life. They may also be taught BSE to self-monitor changes. Severe fibrocystic changes may make palpation of the breast more difficult. Any changes in symptoms or changes found during the BSE should be reported and evaluated.

Treatment for a fibrocystic condition is similar to that described earlier for mastalgia. The nurse's role in the care of patients with fibrocystic breast changes is primarily one of teaching. Patients should be taught that the cysts may recur in one or both breasts until menopause and that the cysts may enlarge or become painful just before menstruation. In addition, patients should be reassured that the cysts do not "turn into" cancer. Patients should be advised that any new lump that does not respond in a cyclic manner over 1 to 2 weeks should be examined by a health care provider promptly.

Fibroadenoma

Fibroadenoma is a common cause of discrete benign breast lumps in young women, generally between 20 and 30 years of age. The possible cause of fibroadenoma may be increased estrogen sensitivity in a localized area of the breast. Fibroadenomas are usually small (1 to 2 cm) but can be larger and are typically painless, round, well delineated, and very mobile. They may be soft but are usually solid, firm, and rubbery in consistency. There is no accompanying retraction or nipple discharge, and they are often painless. Fibroadenomas may appear as a single, unilateral mass, although multiple, bilateral fibroadenomas have been reported. Size is not affected by menstruation. However, pregnancy can stimulate dramatic growth.

NURSING AND INTERPROFESSIONAL MANAGEMENT FIBROADENOMA

Fibroadenomas are easily detected on physical examination and may be visible on mammography and ultrasonography. Definitive diagnosis, however, requires an image-guided core needle biopsy or excisional biopsy and tissue examination by a pathologist. Treatment of fibroadenomas can include observation with regular monitoring, after a malignancy has been ruled out, or surgical excision.

In some clinical settings, as an alternative to surgery, cryoablation can be used to remove tumours after an established diagnosis of a fibroadenoma. In *cryoablation,* a cryoprobe is inserted into the tumour under ultrasound guidance. Extremely cold gas is piped into the tumour. The frozen tumour dies and is either reduced in size or completely eliminated. Benefits include minimal scarring and quick recovery time.

The nurse needs to emphasize to patients with a fibroadenoma the benign nature of the lesion and encourage them to have follow-up examinations.

Nipple Discharge

Nipple discharge may occur spontaneously or as a result of nipple manipulation. A milky secretion constitutes inappropriate lactation (galactorrhea) and may be a result of medication therapy, endocrine conditions, or a neurological disorder, or it may be idiopathic.

Secretions can also be serous, grossly bloody, or brown to green (Li et al., 2018). These secretions may be caused by either benign or malignant disease. Cytological study of the secretion may help determine the specific disease. Diseases associated with nipple discharge include intraductal papilloma, duct ectasia, cystic disease, and malignancies. Treatment depends on identification of the cause (Li et al., 2018). In most cases, nipple discharge is not related to malignancy.

Atypical Hyperplasia. *Atypical hyperplasia* can be in either the ducts (atypical ductal hyperplasia) or in the lobules (atypical lobular hyperplasia) and usually is found during screening mammography. Both are associated with an increased risk for developing breast cancer.

Intraductal Papilloma. An *intraductal papilloma* is a benign, soft, wartlike growth found in the mammary ducts. It is usually unilateral. It is typically accompanied by a bloody discharge

from the nipple that can be intermittent or spontaneous. Most intraductal papillomas are beneath the areola and cannot be palpated. They are usually found in women aged 35 to 55 years. A single duct or several ducts may be involved. Treatment includes excision of the papilloma and the involved duct or duct system. Papillomas may be associated with an increased risk for cancer.

Duct Ectasia. *Duct ectasia* (duct dilation) is a benign breast disorder of perimenopausal and postmenopausal women that involves the ducts in the subareolar area. Several bilateral ducts are usually involved. Multicoloured, sticky discharge is the primary symptom. Duct ectasia is initially painless but may progress to causing a burning sensation, itching, and pain around the nipple, as well as swelling in the areolar area. Inflammatory signs are often present, the nipple may retract, and the discharge may become bloody in more advanced disease. Duct ectasia is not associated with malignancy. If an abscess develops, warm compresses and antibiotics are usually effective treatments. Therapy consists of close follow-up examinations or surgical excision of the involved ducts.

Gynecomastia

Gynecomastia, a transient, noninflammatory enlargement of one or both breasts, is a common noncancerous breast condition in men (Canadian Cancer Society, 2021i). Gynecomastia by itself is not an established risk factor for breast cancer. Mammography may be completed to screen for malignancy. The most common cause of gynecomastia is a disturbance of the normal ratio of active androgen to estrogen in plasma or within the breast itself.

Gynecomastia may also be a manifestation of other health conditions. It may accompany developmental abnormalities of the male reproductive organs. Gynecomastia may occur as an adverse effect of medication therapy, particularly with administration of estrogens and androgens, digitalis, ranitidine (Zantac), and spironolactone (Aldactone). Use of heroin and marihuana can also cause gynecomastia.

Senescent Gynecomastia. *Senescent gynecomastia* is frequently seen in men over 60 years of age (Swerdloff & Ng, 2019). A probable cause is the elevation in plasma estrogen in older men as the result of increased conversion of androgens to estrogens in peripheral circulation. Although initially unilateral, the tender, firm, centrally located enlargement may become bilateral. When gynecomastia is characterized by a discrete, circumscribed mass, it must be biopsied to differentiate it from the rarer breast cancer in men. Senescent gynecomastia requires no treatment and generally regresses within 6 to 12 months.

AGE-RELATED CONSIDERATIONS

BREAST CHANGES

The loss of subcutaneous fat and structural support and the atrophy of mammary glands often cause breasts to become pendulous in postmenopausal women. The nurse should encourage older women to wear a well-fitting bra. Adequate support can improve physical appearance and reduce pain in the back, shoulders, and neck. It can also prevent *intertrigo* (dermatitis caused by friction between opposing surfaces of skin). Surgical lifting of sagging breasts is possible and may be desirable when reconstruction is performed after a mastectomy (surgical removal of all or a portion of a breast).

The decrease in glandular tissue in older women makes a breast mass easier to palpate. This decreased density is probably age related and occurs to a lesser degree with women receiving hormone therapy. Rib margins may be palpable in older women and can be confused with a mass. Anxiety should decrease as a woman becomes more familiar with their breasts and is reassured about their findings. The nurse should encourage older women to continue examining their breasts and to talk to their health care providers about an individualized screening program, because of the increased incidence of breast cancer.

BREAST CANCER

Breast cancer is the most common cancer in Canadian women, excluding nonmelanoma skin cancer. It is second only to lung cancer as the leading cause of death from cancer in women. It can occur in men, although less commonly (Canadian Cancer Society, 2021a). It was estimated that, in 2019, 26 900 new cases of breast cancer were diagnosed in women in Canada and approximately 230 new cases in men. Each year in Canada, approximately 5 055 deaths (5 000 women and 55 men) occur in relation to breast cancer (Canadian Cancer Society, 2021a). The number of deaths of women from breast cancer in every age group has declined, partly as a result of increased mammography screening and decreased use of hormone therapy (Canadian Cancer Society, 2021a). It is important to acknowledge that Indigenous people in Canada experience significant inequities in cancer outcomes in terms of increased incidence and mortality rates, which have been associated with factors such as later stage of diagnosis and decreased screening (Gall et al., 2018).

The 5-year survival rate for women with breast cancer is 88% and is 80% for men (Canadian Cancer Society, 2021a).

Etiology and Risk Factors

Although the etiology is not completely understood, a number of factors are thought to contribute to breast cancer (Canadian Cancer Society, 2021j) (Table 54.2). Risk factors appear to be cumulative and interacting. Therefore, the presence of other risk factors may greatly increase the overall risk, especially for people with a positive family history. Identification of risk factors increases the need for careful clinical surveillance of a patient and for participation in cancer screening measures.

Risk Factors for Women. The identifiable risk factors most associated with breast cancer include female gender and advancing age. Women are at far greater risk than men; 99% of breast cancers occur in women. The incidence of breast cancer in women is very low before 25 years of age and increases gradually until age 60. After age 60, the incidence increases dramatically.

Hormonal regulation of the breast is related to the development of breast cancer, but the mechanisms are poorly understood. The hormones estrogen and progesterone may act as tumour promoters to stimulate breast cancer growth if malignant changes in the cells have already occurred. The Canadian Cancer Society recommends that women avoid taking hormone replacement therapy other than to relieve severe symptoms of menopause that have not responded to other treatments (Canadian Cancer Society, 2021k). Oral contraceptives that contain both estrogen and progesterone cause a slight increase in the risk of breast cancer, particularly for women who have used them for 10 years or longer (Canadian Cancer Society, 2021j). Modifiable risk factors include weight gain during adulthood,

TABLE 54.2	RISK FACTORS FOR BREAST CANCER
Increased Risk	**Comments**
Female	Women account for 99% of breast cancer cases.
Age 50 or older	The majority of breast cancers are found in postmenopausal women. After age 60, the incidence is greatly elevated.
Family history	Breast cancer in a first-degree relative—particularly when the person is premenopausal or the tumour is bilateral—increases risk. Gene mutations (*BRCA1* or *BRCA2*) play a role in 5–10% of breast cancer cases.
Hormone use	The use of estrogen, progesterone, or both as hormone therapy, especially in postmenopausal women, increases risk.
Personal history of breast cancer, colon cancer, endometrial cancer, ovarian cancer	Personal history significantly increases risk for breast cancer, risk for cancer in the other breast, and recurrence.
Early menarche (<age 12); late menopause (>age 55)	A long menstrual history increases the risk for breast cancer.
First full-term pregnancy after age 30; nulliparity	Prolonged exposure to unopposed estrogen increases risk for breast cancer.
Benign breast disorder with atypical epithelial hyperplasia, LCIS	Atypical changes in breast biopsy increase risk for breast cancer.
Dense breast tissue	Mammograms are harder to read and interpret. Dense tissue may be associated with more aggressive tumours.
Weight gain and obesity after menopause	Fat cells store estrogen, which increases the likelihood of developing breast cancer.
Exposure to ionizing radiation	Radiation (e.g., prior treatment for Hodgkin's lymphoma) damages DNA.
Alcohol consumption	Women who drink ≥1 alcoholic beverage per day have an increased risk for breast cancer.
Physical inactivity	Breast cancer risk is increased in sedentary women in comparison with physically active women.

DNA, deoxyribonucleic acid; *LCIS*, lobular carcinoma in situ.

sedentary lifestyle, obesity, smoking, and alcohol intake (Canadian Cancer Society, 2021l). Environmental factors such as radiation exposure may also play a role.

Genetic Factors. Family history is an important risk factor, especially if the involved family member also had ovarian cancer, was premenopausal, had bilateral breast cancer, and is a first-degree relative (i.e., mother, sister, daughter). Having any first-degree relative with breast cancer increases a woman's risk for breast cancer 1.5 to 3 times, depending on age. (The Determinants of Health box discusses other factors contributing to breast cancer.)

As many as 5 to 10% of all patients with breast cancer may have inherited a specific genetic abnormality contributing to the development of breast cancer (Canadian Cancer Society, 2021j). The *BRCA1* gene, located on chromosome 17, and the *BRCA2* gene, located on chromosome 11, are tumour suppressor genes that, when functioning normally, inhibit tumour development. Women with inherited *BRCA1* or *BRCA2* mutations have up to an 85% lifetime chance of developing breast cancer (Canadian Cancer Society, 2021j). These women are also at high risk for

DETERMINANTS OF HEALTH
Breast Cancer

Access to Health Services
- Geographic location and disparities to cancer services such as screening and radiography are significant barriers particularly for Indigenous populations in Canada and may explain poorer health outcomes.*
- Individuals from Indigenous populations may be concerned they will experience racism and negative healthcare experiences due to the history in Canada of colonialism, and the impact of economic, social and cultural marginalization.†
- Individuals from lesbian, gay, bisexual, transgender, queer, Two-Spirited (LGBTQ2+) communities may be concerned they will experience homophobia or biphobia during breast cancer screening.‡

Personal Health Practices and Coping Skills
- Women with a higher body mass index (BMI) (>31.1) are at an increased risk for developing breast cancer.**
- Physical inactivity increases the risk for breast cancer.**

Gender
- Breast cancer is more common in women; it can occur in men, although it is rare.††

Income
- Women with higher incomes have a slightly higher incidence of breast cancer, which may be related to having children later in life or having fewer children.**

Lifestyle
- Working at night may increase the risk of developing breast cancer.**
- Active smoking and exposure to second-hand smoke increases risk.**

References
* Chan, J., Friborg, J., Zubizarreta, E., et al. (2020). Examining geographic accessibility to radiotherapy in Canada and Greenland for indigenous populations: Measuring inequities to inform solutions. *Radiotherapy and Oncology, 146*, 1–8. https://doi.org/10.1016/j.radonc.2020.01.023
† Lavoie, J. G., Kaufert, J., Browne, A., et al. (2016). Managing Matajoosh: Determinants of First Nations' cancer care decisions. *BMC Health Services Research, 16*(402), 1–12. https://doi.org/10.1186/s12913-016-1665-2
‡ Canadian Cancer Society. (2021). *Screening in LGBTQ communities.* http://www.cancer.ca/en/prevention-and-screening/reduce-cancer-risk/find-cancer-early/screening-in-lgbtq-communities/?region=bc
** Canadian Cancer Society. (2021). *Risk factors for breast cancer.* http://www.cancer.ca/en/cancer-information/cancer-type/breast/risks/?region=on
†† Canadian Cancer Society. (2021). *Breast cancer statistics.* http://www.cancer.ca/en/cancer-information/cancer-type/breast/statistics/?region=bc

GENETICS IN CLINICAL PRACTICE
Breast Cancer

Genetic Basis
- Mutations in genes *BRCA1* and *BRCA2*
- Autosomal dominant transmission

Incidence
- Approximately 5 to 10% of breast cancers are related to *BRCA1* and *BRCA2* gene mutations.
- Women with *BRCA1* and *BRCA2* gene mutations have a 40 to 80% lifetime risk of developing breast cancer.
- *BRCA1* and *BRCA2* gene mutations are associated with early-onset breast cancer.
- Men with *BRCA1* and *BRCA2* gene mutations have an increased risk for breast and prostate cancer.
- Family history of both breast and ovarian cancer increases the risk of having a *BRCA1* mutation.

Genetic Testing
- DNA testing is available for *BRCA1* and *BRCA2* gene mutations.

Clinical Implications
- Most breast cancers (about 90–95%) are not inherited. They are associated with genetic changes that occur after a person is born *(somatic mutations)*.
- Bilateral oophorectomy, bilateral mastectomy, or both reduce the risk for breast cancer in women with *BRCA1* and *BRCA2* mutations.
- Mutations in the *BRCA1* and *BRCA2* genes increase the risk for ovarian cancer.
- Genetic counselling and testing for *BRCA* mutations should be considered for women whose personal or family history puts them at high risk for a genetic predisposition to breast cancer.

developing ovarian cancer (Canadian Cancer Society, 2021j). Routine screening for genetic abnormalities in women without evidence of a strong family history of breast cancer is not warranted (see the Genetics in Clinical Practice: Breast Cancer box). Research investigating the role of genes in the development of breast cancer continues.

Risk Factors for Men. Predisposing risk factors for breast cancer in men include hyperestrogenism, a family history of breast cancer, and radiation exposure. A thorough examination of the male breast should be a routine part of a physical examination for all men. Men in *BRCA*-positive families may consider genetic testing. Men with an abnormal *BRCA* gene also have an increased risk of developing prostate cancer.

Prophylactic Oophorectomy and Mastectomy. In women with *BRCA1* or *BRCA2* mutations, prophylactic bilateral oophorectomy can decrease the risk for breast cancer and ovarian cancer (Canadian Cancer Society, 2021l). In deciding whether and when to undergo this surgical procedure, women should receive counselling about the risks and benefits of prophylactic oophorectomy, including those related to fertility.

Women who have a high risk of developing breast cancer (i.e., related to factors such as family history and prior tissue biopsy findings) may, in consultation with their health care provider, choose to undergo prophylactic bilateral mastectomy. Research has shown that contralateral prophylactic mastectomy (mastectomy of the unaffected breast) can decrease the risk for contralateral breast cancer, but survival rates have not been determined (Canadian Cancer Society, 2021l).

Women with hereditary (non-*BRCA*) breast cancer have a higher risk of developing a secondary primary breast cancer in the unaffected (contralateral) breast. These women may also choose to have the unaffected breast removed prophylactically at the time of initial surgery for breast cancer or at a later time. The rate of contralateral prophylactic mastectomies in women has been steadily increasing despite the lack of supportive evidence (Squires et al., 2019).

Pathophysiology

Various types of breast cancer have been identified on the basis of their histological characteristics and growth patterns (Table 54.3). The main components of the breast are lobules (milk-producing glands) and ducts (milk passages that connect the lobules and the nipple). In general, breast cancer arises from the epithelial lining of the ducts *(ductal carcinoma)* or from the

TABLE 54.3	TYPES OF BREAST CANCER
Type	**Frequency of Occurrence**
Invasive/Infiltrating ductal carcinoma	80%
• Colloid (mucinous)	
• Inflammatory	
• Paget's disease	
• Medullary	
• Tubular	
Invasive/Infiltrating lobular carcinoma	10–15%
Noninvasive carcinoma	20%
• Ductal carcinoma in situ	

epithelium of the lobules *(lobular carcinoma).* Breast cancers may be *in situ* (within the duct or lobule) or *invasive* (arising from the duct or lobule and invading through the wall of the duct or lobule).

Metastatic breast cancer is breast cancer that has spread to bone, the liver, the lungs, or the brain. Cancer growth rate can range from slow to rapid. Factors that affect cancer prognosis are tumour size, axillary node involvement (the more nodes involved, the worse the prognosis), tumour differentiation, estrogen and progesterone receptor status, and human epidermal growth factor receptor 2 (HER2) status. HER2 is a transmembrane receptor that helps regulate cell growth. In many patients with breast cancer, it is overexpressed (Canadian Cancer Society, 2021m).

Breast cancer can be classified as noninvasive or invasive, and as ductal or lobular (see Table 54.3).

Noninvasive Breast Cancer. An estimated 20% of all breast cancers are noninvasive. These intraductal cancers include *ductal carcinoma in situ* (DCIS) and *lobular carcinoma in situ* (LCIS). DCIS tends to be unilateral and may progress to invasive breast cancer if left untreated.

Although the management of DCIS can be controversial, patients should discuss all treatment options with their health care provider, including local excision, mastectomy with breast reconstruction, breast-conserving surgery (lumpectomy), radiation therapy, and tamoxifen (Nolvadex-D) therapy.

The term *lobular carcinoma in situ* is somewhat misleading. Although LCIS is a risk factor for developing breast cancer, it is not known to be a premalignant lesion. Although no treatment is necessary, patients with LCIS should increase their surveillance for breast cancer. Tamoxifen may be given to some patients as a chemopreventive medication.

Invasive (Infiltrating) Ductal Carcinoma. *Invasive (infiltrating) ductal carcinoma* is the most common type of breast cancer. It starts in the milk duct and then breaks through the wall of the duct, invading the surrounding tissue. From there it may metastasize to other parts of the body.

Types of invasive (infiltrating) ductal carcinoma include *medullary carcinoma,* which most frequently occurs in women in their late 40s and 50s. *Tubular carcinoma* is usually found in women over 50 years of age and has an excellent prognosis. *Colloid (mucinous) carcinoma* usually has a favourable prognosis. These types of invasive ductal carcinoma are less common and account for fewer than 5% of all breast cancers.

Invasive (Infiltrating) Lobular Carcinoma. *Invasive (infiltrating) lobular carcinoma* begins in the lobules (milk-producing glands) of the breast. It accounts for 10 to 15% of invasive breast cancers. It usually appears as a subtle thickening in the upper

outer quadrant of the breast. Often positive for estrogen and progesterone receptors, these tumours respond well to hormone therapy.

Inflammatory Breast Cancer. *Inflammatory breast cancer,* the most malignant form of all breast cancers, is rare. It is an aggressive and fast-growing cancer with a high risk for metastasis. The skin of the breast looks red, feels warm, and has a thickened appearance that is often described as resembling an orange peel *(peau d'orange).* The inflammatory changes, often mistaken for an infection, are caused by blockage of lymph channels by cancer cells. Chemotherapy given before surgery is usually the first course of treatment, often followed by radiation. Hormonal therapy may also be indicated.

Paget's Disease. Paget's disease is a rare breast malignancy characterized by a persistent lesion of the nipple and areola with or without a palpable mass. (This is different from Paget's disease of the bone, which is discussed in Chapter 66.) Most women with Paget's disease have underlying ductal carcinoma. Only in rare cases is the cancer confined to the nipple itself. Itching, a burning sensation, bloody nipple discharge with superficial erosion, and ulceration may be present. Diagnosis of Paget's disease is confirmed by pathological examination of the erosion. Nipple changes are often diagnosed as an infection or dermatitis, which can lead to delays in proper treatment. The treatment of Paget's disease may include lumpectomy and radiation therapy or a simple or modified radical mastectomy. The prognosis is good when the cancer is confined to the nipple. The nursing care for patients with Paget's disease is the same as the care for patients with breast cancer.

Triple-Negative Breast Cancer. Breast cancer that tests negative for all three receptors (estrogen, progesterone, HER2) is *triple-negative breast cancer.* The incidence is increased in women under the age of 40 and of African or Asian ancestry. These tumours are aggressive, and chemotherapy appears to be the most successful treatment.

Clinical Manifestations

Breast cancer is detected as a lump or mammographic abnormality in the breast. It occurs most often in the upper outer quadrant of the breast because this is the location of most of the glandular tissue (Figure 54.4). Breast cancers vary in growth rate. If palpable, breast cancer is characteristically hard and may be irregularly shaped, poorly delineated, nonmobile, and nontender.

A small percentage of breast cancers cause nipple discharge. The discharge is usually unilateral and may be clear or bloody. Nipple retraction may occur. *Peau d'orange* may result from the plugging of the dermal lymphatic vessels. With large cancers, infiltration, induration, and dimpling (pulling in) of the overlying skin may also be noted.

Complications

The main complication of breast cancer is recurrence (Table 54.4). Recurrence may be local or regional (skin or soft tissue near the mastectomy site, axillary or internal mammary lymph nodes) or distant (most commonly involving bone, the lung, the brain, or the liver). However, metastatic disease can be found in any distant site.

Metastatic disease involves the growth of colonies of cancerous breast cells in parts of the body distant from the breast. Metastases primarily occur through the lymphatic vessels, principally those of the axilla (see Figure 54.7, later in the chapter).

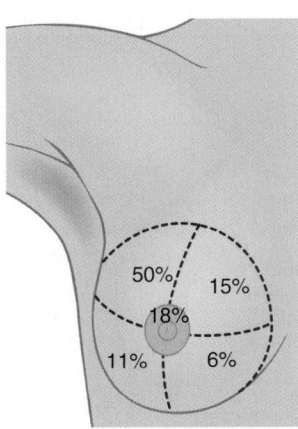

FIG. 54.4 Distribution of where breast cancer occurs.

TABLE 54.4	COMMON SITES OF BREAST CANCER RECURRENCE AND METASTASIS
Site	**Clinical Manifestations**
Local Recurrence	
Skin, chest wall	Firm, discrete nodules; occasionally pruritic, usually painless; commonly in or near a scar
Regional Recurrence	
Lymph nodes	Enlarged nodes in axilla or supraclavicular area, usually nontender
Distant Metastases	
Skeletal	Localized pain of gradually increasing intensity; percussion tenderness at involved sites; pathological fracture caused by involvement of bone cortex
Spinal cord	Progressive back pain, localized and radiating; change in bladder or bowel function; loss of sensation in lower extremities
Brain	Headache described as "different"; unilateral sensory loss; focal muscular weakness, hemiparesis, incoordination (ataxia); nausea or vomiting unrelated to medication; cognitive changes
Pulmonary (including lung nodules and pleural effusions)	Shortness of breath, tachypnea, nonproductive cough (not present in all patients)
Liver	Abdominal distension; right lower quadrant abdominal pain, sometimes with radiation to scapular area; nausea and vomiting, anorexia, weight loss; weakness and fatigue; hepatomegaly, ascites, jaundice; peripheral edema; elevated liver enzyme levels
Bone marrow	Anemia; infection; increased bleeding, bruising, petechiae; weakness and fatigue; mild confusion, light-headedness; dyspnea

However, the cancer can spread to other parts of the body without invading the axillary nodes even when the primary breast tumour is small. Even with node-negative breast cancer, there is a possibility of distant metastasis.

Diagnostic Studies

In addition to studies used to diagnose breast cancer (see discussion earlier in this chapter), other tests are useful in predicting the risk for local or systemic recurrence. These tests include axillary lymph node status, tumour size, estrogen and progesterone receptor status, and cell-proliferative indices. Results of many of these diagnostic studies are useful prognostic indicators of the disease.

Axillary lymph node involvement is one of the most important prognostic factors in breast cancer. An *axillary lymph node dissection (ALND)* is often performed to determine whether cancer has spread to the axilla on the side of the breast cancer (Canadian Cancer Society, 2021n). The more nodes involved, the higher the risk for recurrence. Patients with four or more positive nodes have the highest risk for recurrence.

Lymphatic mapping and *sentinel lymph node biopsy (SLNB)* help the surgeon identify the lymph node or nodes that drain first from the tumour site *(sentinel node)*. SLNB is less invasive than ALND (Canadian Cancer Society, 2021o). A radioisotope or blue dye is injected into the tumour site, and intraoperatively, it is determined in which sentinel lymph nodes the radioisotope or blue dye is located (Figure 54.5). A local incision is made in the axilla, and the surgeon dissects the blue-stained sentinel node or the radioactive lymph node. In general, in SLNB, one to four axillary lymph nodes are removed. The nodes are then sent for a frozen-section pathological analysis. If the results are negative, no further axillary surgery is required. If the results are positive, the surgeon may choose to remove additional lymph nodes during the same procedure or during a follow-up surgical procedure in consultation with the patient. SLNB has been associated with lower rates of lymphedema and other arm symptoms (Canadian Cancer Society, 2021o).

Tumour size is a valuable prognostic variable: The larger the tumour, the poorer the prognosis. The wide variety of histological types of breast cancer explains the heterogeneity of the disease. In general, the more well-differentiated the tumour is, the less aggressive it is. Poorly differentiated tumours appear morphologically disorganized and are more aggressive.

Another diagnostic test useful for both treatment decisions and prediction of prognosis is measurement of estrogen and progesterone receptor status. Receptor-positive tumours (a) commonly show histological evidence of being well differentiated, (b) frequently have a diploid (more normal) deoxyribonucleic acid (DNA) content and low proliferative indices, (c) have a lower chance for recurrence, and (d) are frequently hormone dependent and responsive to hormone therapy. Receptor-negative tumours (a) are often poorly differentiated histologically, (b) have a high incidence of aneuploidy (abnormally high or low DNA content) and higher proliferative indices, (c) frequently recur, and (d) are usually unresponsive to hormonal therapy.

Ploidy status correlates with tumour aggressiveness. Diploid tumours have been shown to have a significantly lower risk for recurrence than aneuploid tumours.

Cell-proliferative indices indirectly measure the rate of tumour cell proliferation. The percentage of tumour cells in the synthesis (S) phase of the cell cycle (see Chapter 18, Figure 18.1) is another important prognostic indicator.

Another prognostic indicator is the marker HER2, which is a protein that can be measured in breast tissue. Overexpression of this receptor has been associated with a greater risk for recurrence and a poorer prognosis in breast cancer. High numbers of HER2 receptors are associated with unusually aggressive tumour growth. The presence of this marker assists in the selection and sequence of chemotherapy and the prediction of a patient's response to treatment (Canadian Cancer Society, 2021p).

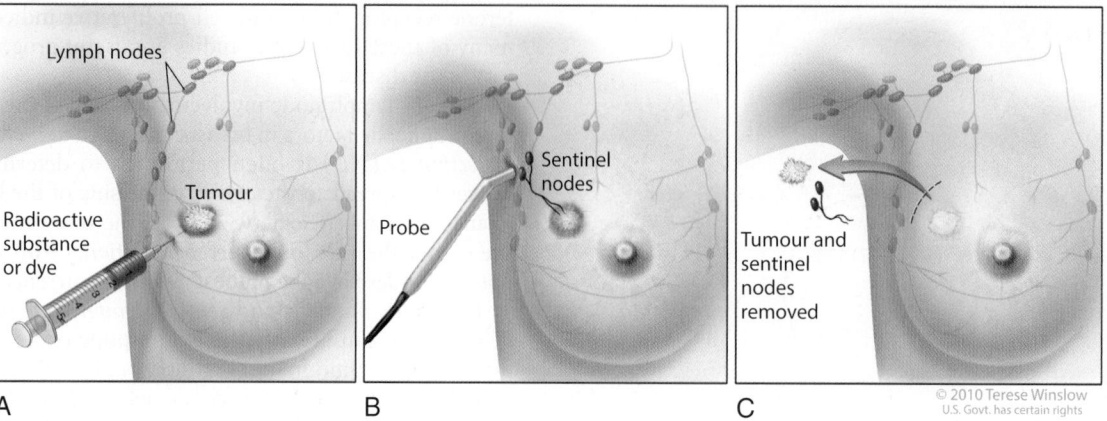

A   B   C

© 2010 Terese Winslow
U.S. Govt. has certain rights

FIG. 54.5 Sentinel lymph node biopsy of the breast. **A,** A radioactive dye or blue dye is injected near the tumour. **B,** The injected material is detected visually or with a probe that detects radioactivity. **C,** The sentinel nodes (the first lymph nodes to take up the material) are removed and checked for cancer cells. Source: Ignatavicius, D., & Workman, M. L. (2016). *Medical-surgical nursing: Patient-centered collaborative care.* (8th ed., p. 1472, Figure 70-5). Saunders.

Interprofessional Care

Currently, a wide range of treatment options are available to patients and health care providers making critical decisions about how to treat breast cancer (Tables 54.5 and 54.6). Prognostic factors are considered when treatment decisions are made about a specific breast cancer. Some of these factors also enter into the staging of breast cancer. The most widely accepted staging method for breast cancer is the American Joint Committee on Cancer's TNM system (Canadian Cancer Society, 2021q). In this system, tumour size (T), nodal involvement (N), and presence of metastasis (M) are used to determine the stage of disease. The stage of a breast cancer describes its size and the extent to which it has spread (Table 54.7).

The stages range from I to IV, with stage I being very small tumours (<2 cm) with no lymph node involvement and no metastasis. Further classification within these stages depends on the size of the tumour and the number of lymph nodes involved. Stage IV indicates the presence of metastatic spread, regardless of tumour size or lymph node involvement.

The therapeutic regimen is often dictated by the clinical stage and biology of the cancer. (Adverse medication effects and appropriate nursing management of general treatment modalities for cancer are discussed in Chapter 18 and in Nursing Care Plan [NCP] 18.1, available on the Evolve website.)

In spite of the advent of new prognostic indicators such as determination of DNA content and analysis of cell-cycle phases, the presence or absence of malignant cells in lymph nodes remains a powerful prognostic factor related to local recurrence or metastasis after primary therapy.

Surgical Therapy. Surgery is considered the primary treatment for breast cancer. Table 54.8 describes the most common surgical procedures used to treat breast cancer. Breast-conserving surgery with radiation therapy and mastectomy with or without reconstruction are currently the most common options for resectable breast cancer (Figure 54.6). Most women with a diagnosis of early-stage breast cancer (≤4 to 5 cm in size) are candidates for either treatment choice. Recent evidence has indicated better survival rates after breast-conserving surgery combined with radiation therapy compared with mastectomy (Corradini et al., 2019).

Breast-Conserving Surgery. Breast-conserving surgery (also called **lumpectomy**) involves the removal of the entire tumour

TABLE 54.5 INTERPROFESSIONAL CARE
Breast Cancer

Diagnostic
Prediagnosis
- Health history, including risk factors
- Biopsy
- Breast MRI (if indicated)
- Mammography
- Physical examination, including breast and lymph nodes
- Ultrasonography

Postdiagnosis
- Cell-proliferative indices
- Estrogen and progesterone receptor status
- Genetic assays
- HER2 marker
- Lymphatic mapping and SNLD

Staging Workup
- Bone scan (if indicated)
- Calcium and phosphate levels
- Chest radiograph
- Complete blood cell count, platelet count
- CT scan of chest, abdomen, pelvis (if indicated)
- Liver function tests
- MRI (if indicated)
- PET (if indicated)

Interprofessional Therapy
- Surgery
- Breast-conserving (lumpectomy) with SNLD, ALND, or both
- Simple (total) mastectomy (removal of entire breast) or modified radical mastectomy (may include reconstruction)
- Radiation therapy
- Primary radiotherapy
- Adjuvant radiotherapy
- High-dose brachytherapy
- Palliative radiotherapy
- Medication therapy (see Table 54.6)
- Biological and targeted therapy
- Chemotherapy
- Chemotherapy for recurrent or metastatic disease
- Hormonal therapy
- Neoadjuvant or adjuvant chemotherapy

ALND, axillary lymph node dissection; *CT,* computed tomography; *HER2,* human epidermal growth factor receptor 2; *MRI,* magnetic resonance imaging; *PET,* positron emission tomography; *SNLD,* sentinel lymph node dissection.

TABLE 54.6 MEDICATION THERAPY

Breast Cancer

Medication Class	Mechanism of Action	Indications
Hormone Therapy		
Estrogen Receptor Blockers		
Tamoxifen (Nolvadex-D)	Blocks estrogen receptors (ERs)	ER-positive breast cancer in premenopausal and postmenopausal women Used as a preventive measure in high-risk premenopausal and postmenopausal women
Fulvestrant (Faslodex)	Blocks ERs	ER-positive breast cancer in postmenopausal women only
Aromatase Inhibitors		
Anastrozole (Arimidex) Letrozole (Femara) Exemestane (Aromasin)	Prevent production of estrogen by inhibiting aromatase	ER-positive breast cancer in postmenopausal women only
Estrogen Receptor Modulator		
Raloxifene (Evista)	In breast, blocks the effect of estrogen In bone, promotes the effect of estrogen and prevents bone loss	Postmenopausal women
Biological and Targeted Therapy		
Trastuzumab emtasine (Kadcyla) Everolimus (Afinitor) Trastuzumab (Herceptin) Pertuzumab (Perjeta)	Trastuzumab combined with chemotherapy medication (DM1) Binds to mechanistic target of Rapamycin (mTOR) suppressing T-cell activation and proliferation Blocks HER2 receptor	HER2- positive breast cancer ER-positive, HER2-negative breast cancer in postmenopausal women ER-positive breast cancer in postmenopausal women only
Lapatinib (Tykerb) Palbociclib (Ibrance) Ribociclib succinate (Kisqali) Neratinib (Nerlynx)	Inhibits HER2 tyrosine kinase and EGFR tyrosine kinase Kinase inhibitors Blocks HER2 receptor	ER-positive breast cancer in postmenopausal women only ER-positive, HER2-negative breast cancer in postmenopausal women HER2 breast cancer

EGFR, epidermal growth factor receptor; *HER2*, human epidermal growth factor receptor 2.

TABLE 54.7 STAGING OF BREAST CANCER

Stage	Tumour Size	Lymph Node Involvement	Metastasis
0	TIS*	No	No
I	<2 cm	No	No
A	<2 cm	<2 mm	No
B			
II			
A	No evidence of tumour ranging to 5 cm	No, or 1–3 axillary nodes or internal mammary nodes or both	No
B	Ranging from <2 to >5 cm	No, or 1–3 axillary nodes or internal mammary nodes or both	No
III			
A	Ranging from <2 to >5 cm	Yes, 1–9 axillary nodes or internal mammary nodes or both	No
B	Any size with extension to chest wall or skin	No, 1–9 axillary nodes or internal mammary nodes or both	No
C	Any size	Yes, ≥10 axillary nodes, internal mammary nodes, infraclavicular nodes, or a combination of these	No
IV	Any size	Any type of nodal involvement	Yes

*TIS, tumour in situ.
Source: Adapted from Canadian Cancer Society. (2020). *Stages of breast cancer.* http://www.cancer.ca/en/cancer-information/cancer-type/breast/staging/?region=on; and Giuliano, A. E., Connolly, J. L., Edge, S. B., Mittenhorf, E. A., Rugo, H. S., Lawrence, J. S., Weaver, D. L., Winchester, D. J., & Hortobagyi, G. N. (2017). Breast cancer: Major changes in the American Joint Committee on Cancer eighth edition cancer staging manual. *Cancer Journal for Clinicians, 67,* 290–303. https://doi.org/10.3322/caac.21393

quadrant), diffuse calcifications in more than one quadrant, or central location of tumour near the nipple. Contraindications to radiation therapy (e.g., active lupus or prior radiation therapy in the radiation field) may make mastectomy a better surgical option.

One of the main advantages of breast-conserving surgery and radiation therapy is that the breast, including the nipple, is preserved. The goal of the combined surgery and radiation is to both maximize the benefits of the cancer treatment and the cosmetic outcome and minimize the risks. Disadvantages of this approach include the increased cost of the surgery plus radiation therapy over surgery alone and the possible adverse effects of irradiation.

Axillary Node Dissection. ALND on the same side as the breast cancer may be performed and had been the standard of care for invasive breast cancer. ALND typically involves the removal of 15 to 20 nodes. SLNB has replaced ALND for patients in whom malignant cells are not identified in the sentinel nodes (Canadian Cancer Society, 2021r) (see Figure 54.5). Examination of the lymph nodes provides prognostic information and helps determine further treatment (chemotherapy, hormone therapy, or both).

Lymphedema (accumulation of lymph in soft tissue) can occur as a result of the excision or irradiation of lymph nodes (Canadian Cancer Society, 2021s) (Figure 54.7). When the axillary nodes cannot return lymph fluid to the central circulation, the fluid accumulates in the arm, causing obstructive pressure on the veins and impeding venous return (Figure 54.8). Patients

along with a margin of normal surrounding tissue (see Figure 54.6, *B*). After surgery, radiation therapy is delivered to the entire breast, ending with a boost to the tumour bed. Depending on the staging of the disease, chemotherapy may be administered before radiation therapy. Contraindications to breast-conserving surgery include the following: breast size too small in relation to the tumour size to yield an acceptable cosmetic result, masses and calcifications that are multifocal (within the same breast quadrant), masses that are multicentric (in more than one

TABLE 54.8	SURGICAL PROCEDURES FOR BREAST CANCER			
Procedure	**Description**	**Adverse Effects**	**Complications**	**Patient Issues**
Breast-conserving surgery (lumpectomy) with radiation therapy	Wide excision of tumour, SLNB or ALND, radiation therapy	Breast soreness Breast edema Skin reactions Arm swelling Sensory changes in breast and arm	Short-term: moist desquamation,* hematoma, seroma, infection Long-term: fibrosis, lymphedema,† myositis, pneumonitis,* rib fractures*	Prolonged treatment* Impaired arm mobility† Change in texture and sensitivity of breast
Simple or modified radical mastectomy	Removal of breast, preservation of pectoralis muscle, SLNB or ALND	Tightening of chest wall, scarring Phantom breast sensations Lymphedema Sensory changes Impaired range of motion	Short-term: skin flap necrosis, seroma, hematoma, infection Long-term: sensory loss, muscle weakness, lymphedema	Loss of breast Incision Body image Need for prosthesis Impaired arm mobility
Tissue expansion and breast implants	Expander used to slowly stretch tissue; saline gradually injected into reservoir over weeks to months Insertion of implant under musculofascial layer of chest wall	Discomfort Sensation of chest wall tightness	Short-term: skin flap necrosis, wound separation, seroma, hematoma, infection Long-term: capsular contractions, displacement of implant	Body image Prolonged physician visits to expand implants Potential additional surgical procedures for nipple construction, symmetry
Breast reconstruction tissue flap procedures	TRAM flap procedure‡: a musculocutaneous flap (muscle, skin, fat, blood supply) is transposed from abdomen to the mastectomy site	Pain related to two surgical sites and extensive surgery	Short-term: delayed wound healing, infection, skin flap necrosis, abdominal hernia, hematoma	Prolonged postoperative recovery
	DIEP flap procedure: a free flap that transfers skin and fat from the abdomen to the chest; differs from TRAM flap in that no muscle is moved	Requires more time in surgery than TRAM flap Pain related to two surgical sites	If procedure fails, tissue flap may die and have to be completely removed If tissue dies, new reconstruction may not be done for 6–12 months	Patients may experience less pain and restriction of movement than with a TRAM flap

*Specific to radiation therapy.
†If ALND is performed (less likely with SLNB).
‡May be performed concurrently with mastectomy.
ALND, axillary lymph node dissection; *DIEP,* deep inferior epigastric artery perforator; *SLNB,* sentinel lymph node biopsy; *TRAM,* transverse rectus abdominis musculocutaneous.

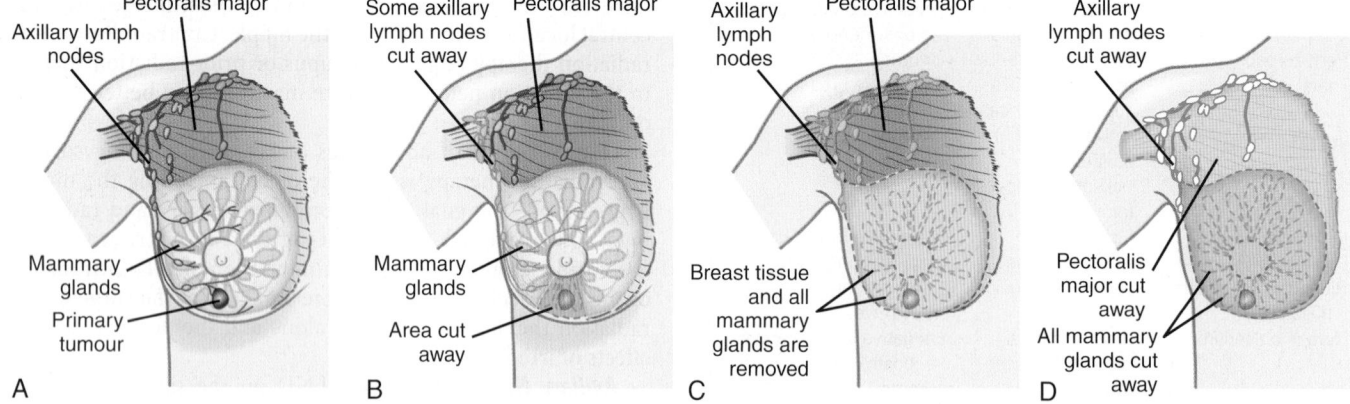

FIG. 54.6 Breast cancer surgery. **A,** Preoperative. **B,** Lumpectomy. **C,** Simple mastectomy. **D,** Modified radical mastectomy.

may experience heaviness, pain, impaired motor function in the arm, and numbness and paraesthesia in the fingers as a result of lymphedema. Cellulitis and progressive fibrosis can result from lymphedema. Although lymphedema is not always preventable, it can be controlled somewhat after surgery or radiation therapy (see discussion later in this chapter).

Modified Radical Mastectomy. A modified radical mastectomy includes removal of the breast and the axillary lymph nodes, but it spares the pectoralis major muscle. This surgery is preferred over breast-conserving surgery if the tumour is too

large to excise with adequate margins, or if it is so large that excision would produce a poor cosmetic result. Some patients may select this surgical procedure over lumpectomy when presented with a choice.

When a modified radical mastectomy is performed, patients have the option of breast reconstruction. If a patient chooses to have reconstructive surgery, it can be performed immediately after the mastectomy, or it can be delayed until postoperative recovery is complete (Canadian Cancer Society, 2021t).

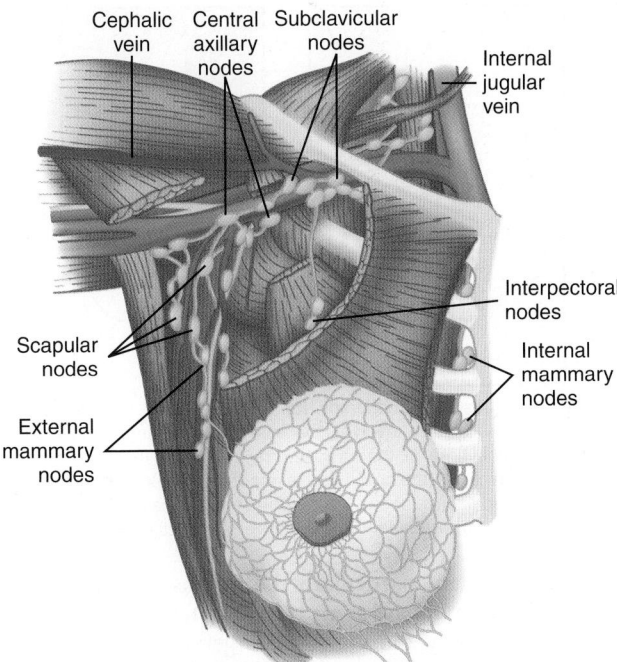

FIG. 54.7 Illustration of lymph nodes and drainage in the axilla. The sentinel lymph node is usually found in the external mammary nodes. In a complete axillary dissection, all nodes would be removed. Source: Townsend, C. M., Beauchamp, R. D., Evers, B. M., et al. (2009). *Sabiston textbook of surgery* (18th ed.). Mosby.

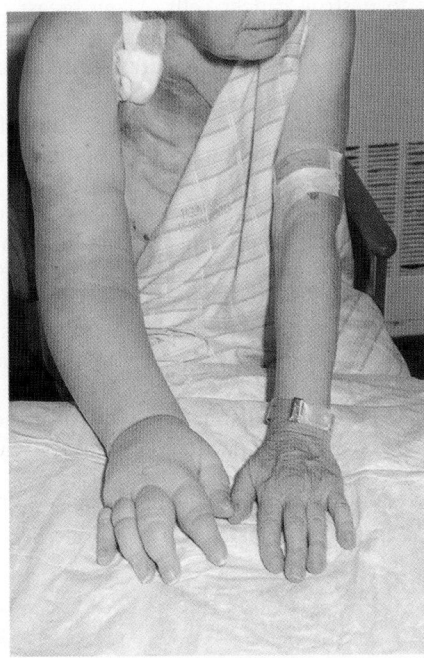

FIG. 54.8 Lymphedema. Accumulation of fluid in the tissue after excision of lymph nodes. Source: Swartz, M. H. (2010). *Textbook of physical diagnosis: History and examination* (6th ed., p. 443, Figure 15-3). W. B. Saunders.

Postmastectomy Pain Syndrome. *Postmastectomy pain syndrome (PMPS)* can occur after a mastectomy or an axillary node dissection. Common symptoms include chest and upper arm pain, tingling sensations down the arm, numbness, shooting or pricking pain, and unbearable itching that persist beyond the normal 3-month healing time. The cause most commonly theorized about the onset of this syndrome is injury

to intercostobrachial nerves, which are sensory nerves that exit chest wall muscles and provide sensation to the shoulder and the upper arm.

Treatments include nonsteroidal anti-inflammatory medications, antidepressants, topical lidocaine patches, an eutectic mixture of local anaesthetics (lidocaine and prilocaine), and anticonvulsant medications (e.g., gabapentin [Neurontin]). Other possible treatment modalities include imagery, biofeedback, physical therapy to prevent "frozen shoulder" syndrome as a result of inadequate movement, and psychological counselling with a person trained in the management of chronic pain syndromes.

Adjuvant Therapy. The decision to recommend adjuvant (additional) therapy after surgery depends on the stage of the disease (number of involved nodes and tumour size); the menstrual status, health, and age of the patient; cancer cell characteristics; and presence or absence of estrogen, progesterone, and HER2. Adjuvant therapies include local radiation therapy and systemic therapies such as chemotherapy and hormone therapy (Canadian Cancer Society, 2021u).

Radiation Therapy. Radiation therapy may be used as (a) primary treatment to prevent local breast recurrences after breast-conserving surgery (see the Evidence-Informed Practice: Translating Research Into Practice box), (b) adjuvant treatment after mastectomy to prevent local and nodal recurrences, and (c) palliative treatment for pain caused by local, regional, or distant recurrence.

⟳ EVIDENCE-INFORMED PRACTICE

Translating Research Into Practice

M. S. (pronouns she, her), 53 years old, was diagnosed with breast cancer 2 weeks ago. M. S. is recovering from a lumpectomy with negative lymph nodes. Her health care provider has recommended adjuvant therapy with radiation.

Best Available Evidence	Clinician Expertise	Patient Preferences and Values
The addition of radiation therapy to lumpectomy reduces the risk for local cancer recurrence.	Radiation is recommended even with negative lymph nodes after a lumpectomy. Many patients have minimal or no adverse effects from radiation therapy. The most common ones are fatigue, malaise, skin reactions, and ulcers or irritation of the skin.	M. S. is not sure about wanting to have radiation treatment because of fear of the adverse effects.

Decision and Action

The nurse should review the possible adverse effects and how they can be managed and then explain to M. S. the risks of not taking the radiation treatment, which can include recurrence. M. S. tells the nurse that she will discuss it with her partner and possibly reconsider. The nurse understands the patient's concerns and informs the health care provider of M. S.'s indecisiveness.

Reference for Evidence

Williams, P. A., Yang, D., Cao, S., et al. (2018). Breast cancer patients perceive psychosocial side effects of cancer radiation therapy as worse than non-breast cancer patients. *International Journal of Radiation, 102*(3), e743. https://doi.org/10.1016/j.ijrobp.2018.07.1986

Primary Radiation Therapy. When radiation therapy is the primary treatment, it is usually performed after local excision of the breast mass. The breast (and, in some cases, the regional lymph nodes) is irradiated 5 days per week over the course of approximately 3 to 4 weeks. An external beam of radiation is used to deliver an approximate total dose of 4500 to 5000 cGy (4500 to 5000 rd). During the final week or so, the patient receives a supplemental dose of radiation targeted directly to the area where the tumour was located. This dose is called a "boost" and is usually delivered in a method similar to the patient's regular radiation but to a smaller area. Fatigue, skin changes, and breast edema may be temporary adverse effects of external beam radiation therapy. To decrease the risk for axillary recurrence, irradiation of the axilla or supraclavicular nodes or both may be indicated when lymph nodes are involved. Chemotherapy may be used systemically before radiation therapy to enhance the local effects of radiation. (Nursing management of patients receiving radiation therapy is discussed in Chapter 18, and in NCP 18.1.)

The decision to use radiation therapy after mastectomy is based on the probability that local residual cancer cells are present (related to tumour size and biology and number of involved lymph nodes). Irradiating the area does not prevent the appearance of distant metastasis at a later date. The site of the radiation therapy field (lymph nodes, chest wall, or both) depends on the risk for recurrence.

High-Dose Brachytherapy. *Brachytherapy* (internal radiation) is an alternative to traditional radiation treatment for early-stage breast cancer. Internal radiation therapy had been delivered primarily through a multicatheter implant method that delivered a radioactive seed into many catheters placed in the breast to treat the target area. Currently, the most widely practised method is balloon brachytherapy, which may require only 5 days.

The MammoSite Radiation Therapy System (MammoSite RTS) is a minimally invasive method of delivering internal radiation therapy. In this technique, a balloon catheter is used to insert radioactive seeds into the breast after the tumour is removed (Figure 54.9). Radiation is emitted by a tiny radioactive seed attached by a wire on the way to an afterloader, a computer-controlled machine. The seed travels through the MammoSite RTS applicator into the inflated balloon. The radiation dose is focused on the area of the breast at highest risk for tumour recurrence. Radiation therapy with the MammoSite RTS is performed over a 1- to 5-day period on an outpatient basis. Patients typically receive treatments twice a day for 5 days. The MammoSite RTS may also be used as boost therapy in conjunction with external irradiation.

The source of radiation does not remain in the body between treatments or after the final treatment is over. The tiny radioactive seed is inserted only during treatment and then removed. Once the final session is completed, the balloon is deflated and the system is removed.

Palliative Radiation Therapy. In addition to reducing the primary tumour mass with a resultant decrease in pain, radiation therapy is used to stabilize symptomatic metastatic lesions in such sites as bone, soft tissue organs, the brain, and the chest and is successful in controlling recurrent or metastatic disease.

Systemic Therapy. The goal of systemic therapy is to destroy tumour cells that may have spread to distant sites. Systemic therapy as an adjuvant to primary local treatment (in the absence of demonstrable metastases) can decrease the rate of recurrence and increase the length of survival. Because of the high risk for recurrent disease, nearly all women with evidence

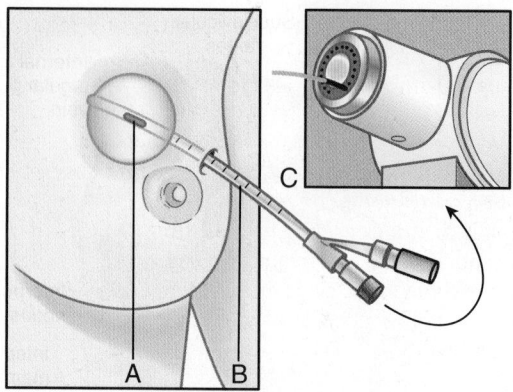

FIG. 54.9 High-dose brachytherapy for breast cancer. The MammoSite Radiation Therapy System involves the insertion of a single small balloon catheter *(B)* at the time of the lumpectomy or shortly thereafter into the tumour resection cavity (the space that is left after the surgeon removes the tumour). A tiny radioactive seed *(A)* is inserted into the balloon, connected to a machine called an *afterloader (C)*, and delivers the radiation therapy.

of node involvement, particularly those whose hormone receptor status is negative, have some type of systemic therapy. Some women, particularly those with a larger tumour or a more aggressive type of tumour, are at higher risk for recurrent or metastatic disease. Systemic therapy is often recommended for such women even when no evidence of node involvement is found. Weighing the risks and benefits of adjuvant therapy is a complex process.

Chemotherapy. *Chemotherapy* is the use of cytotoxic medications to destroy cancer cells. Many breast cancers are responsive to chemotherapy. In some patients, chemotherapy is administered preoperatively. Preoperative (neoadjuvant) chemotherapy can decrease the size of the primary tumour, possibly enabling surgery to be less extensive. Initiation of treatment in a timely manner and monitoring for response are the main goals of treatment (Simmons, 2018).

Combinations of medications yield results superior to those of a single medication. The benefits of combination treatment result from the use of medications that have different mechanisms of action and work at different parts of the cell cycle. The more common combination-therapy protocols are as follows:
- Cyclophosphamide (Procytox), methotrexate, and 5-fluorouracil (5-FU), referred to as *CMF*
- Doxorubicin and cyclophosphamide, with or without the addition of a taxane such as paclitaxel (Abraxane) or docetaxel (Taxotere)
- Cyclophosphamide, doxorubicin or epirubicin (Pharmorubicin PFS), and 5-FU, referred to as *CAF* or *CEF*

MEDICATION ALERT—Doxorubicin
- Patient should be monitored for signs of cardiotoxicity and heart failure (e.g., new onset of shortness of breath, pedal edema, decreased activity tolerance, dysrhythmias, ECG changes).
- Patient should not have immunizations without the health care provider's approval.
- Patient must avoid contact with those who recently received live virus vaccine.

Certain medications may be used alone to treat metastatic breast cancer. A medication used alone results in fewer adverse effects than do combinations. Docetaxel (Taxotere), capecitabine (Xeloda), and an albumin-bound form of paclitaxel (Abraxane) are used when metastatic breast cancer has not responded to standard chemotherapy (Canadian Cancer Society, 2021v). Vinorelbine (Navelbine), used to treat metastatic breast cancer, is better tolerated because it produces fewer and milder adverse effects than do other chemotherapeutic medications.

Because healthy cells are also affected by chemotherapy, various adverse effects accompany this treatment modality. The incidence and severity of predictable and commonly observed adverse effects are influenced by the specific medication combination, medication schedule, and medication doses. Usually, body organs with rapidly dividing cells are the most strongly affected. The most common adverse effects involve the gastrointestinal tract, bone marrow, and hair follicles, resulting in nausea, anorexia, weight gain, bone marrow suppression and subsequent fatigue, and alopecia (hair loss) (Canadian Cancer Society, 2021w).

Cognitive changes during and after treatment, especially with chemotherapy ("chemo brain"), can occur. These changes include difficulties in concentration, memory, and maintaining focus and attention (Canadian Cancer Society, 2021w).

Hormonal Therapy. Estrogen can promote the growth of breast cancer cells if the cells are estrogen receptor–positive. Hormonal therapy blocks the source of estrogen, thus promoting tumour regression (Canadian Cancer Society, 2021x). Hormonal therapy may be used as an adjuvant to primary treatment or in patients with recurrent or metastatic cancer. Two advances have increased the use of hormone therapy in breast cancer. First, hormone receptor assays, which are reliable diagnostic tests, are used to identify women who are likely to respond to hormone therapy. Both the estrogen and progesterone receptor status of the tumour can be determined. The importance of these assays is their ability to predict whether hormonal therapy is a treatment option for women with breast cancer, either at the time of initial therapy or if the cancer recurs. Second, medications have been developed that can inactivate the hormone-secreting glands as effectively as surgery or radiation. Chances of tumour regression are significantly greater in women whose tumours contain estrogen and progesterone receptors (Canadian Cancer Society, 2021x).

Estrogen deprivation can occur when ovarian function is damaged by surgery, radiation therapy, or medication therapy (see Table 54.6). Hormonal therapy can (a) block or destroy the estrogen receptors or (b) suppress estrogen synthesis through inhibiting aromatase, an enzyme needed for endogenous estrogen synthesis.

Estrogen Receptor Blockers. Tamoxifen (Nolvadex) has for many years been the hormonal agent of choice in estrogen receptor–positive women with breast cancer of all stages (Canadian Cancer Society, 2021x). Tamoxifen, an antiestrogen medication, blocks the estrogen receptor sites of malignant cells and thus inhibits the growth-stimulating effects of estrogen. It is commonly used in early-stage and advanced breast cancer and to treat recurrent disease. Tamoxifen may also be used to prevent breast cancer in individuals at high risk for its development. Adverse effects of tamoxifen may include hot flashes, mood swings, vaginal discharge and dryness, and other effects commonly associated with decreased estrogen levels. It also increases the risk for blood clots, cataracts, stroke, and endometrial cancer in postmenopausal women. Treatment with tamoxifen generally lasts 5 years (Canadian Cancer Society, 2021x).

MEDICATION ALERT—Tamoxifen (Nolvadex-D)
- Irregular vaginal bleeding or spotting may occur.
- Decreased visual acuity, corneal opacity, and retinopathy can occur in women receiving high doses (240–320 mg/day for >17 months). These conditions may be irreversible.
- Patient should be instructed to report decreased visual acuity immediately.
- Patient should be monitored for signs of deep-vein thrombosis, pulmonary embolism, and stroke, including shortness of breath, leg cramps, and weakness.

Fulvestrant (Faslodex) may be administered when advanced breast cancer no longer responds to tamoxifen. This medication slows cancer progression by destroying estrogen receptors in the breast cancer cells. Fulvestrant is given intramuscularly on a monthly basis. Common adverse effects include fatigue, hot flashes, and nausea.

Aromatase Inhibitors. Aromatase inhibitor medications interfere with the enzyme that synthesizes endogenous estrogen and are used in the treatment of breast cancer in postmenopausal women. These medications include anastrozole (Arimidex), letrozole (Femara), and exemestane (Aromasin). Aromatase inhibitors do not block the production of estrogen by the ovaries; thus they are of little benefit and may be harmful in premenopausal women.

Clinical trials have demonstrated improved disease-free survival when these medications are given after tamoxifen treatment has ended (Canadian Cancer Society, 2021r). They also appear to be more effective than tamoxifen in preventing breast cancer recurrence and possibly more effective in preventing contralateral disease. The adverse effects of aromatase inhibitors are different from those of tamoxifen. Aromatase inhibitors only rarely cause blood clots, and they do not cause endometrial cancer. Because they block the production of estrogen in postmenopausal women, osteoporosis and bone fractures may occur. These medications have also been associated with night sweats, nausea, arthralgias, and myalgias.

Raloxifene (Evista), a medication used to prevent bone loss, is used to reduce the risk for breast cancer in postmenopausal women without stimulating endometrial growth. Raloxifene may act by blocking estrogen receptors in the breast, similar to its action in the bone. (Raloxifene is discussed in the section on osteoporosis in Chapter 66.)

Less common hormone-deprivation strategies include bilateral oophorectomy, adrenalectomy, and hypophysectomy.

Biological and Targeted Therapy. Some breast cancers make excessive amounts of the HER2 protein. For patients who are HER2 positive, trastuzumab (Herceptin) is a monoclonal antibody to HER2. After the antibody attaches to the antigen, it is taken into the cancer cells and eventually kills them. It can be used alone or in combination with other chemotherapy such as docetaxel (Taxotere) or paclitaxel (Abraxane) to treat patients whose tumours overexpress the *HER2* gene. Additional genetic testing may offer information on which patients are good candidates for treatment with trastuzumab.

MEDICATION ALERT—Trastuzumab (Herceptin)
- Medication should be used with caution in women with pre-existing heart disease.
- Patient should be monitored for signs of ventricular dysfunction and heart failure.

Other medications that target HE2 protein include trastuzumab emtansine (Kadcyla), made up of the medications trastuzumab and emtansine, which is an antibody–medication combination. Pertuzumab (Perjeta) is another anti-HER2 therapy that is used for patients who have not received prior treatment for metastatic breast cancer with an anti-HER2 agent or chemotherapy.

Lapatinib (Tykerb) may be used in combination with capecitabine (Xeloda) for patients with advanced, metastatic disease whose tumours produce excessive HER2. The combination treatment is indicated for women in whom disease has become resistant to other cancer medications (Canadian Cancer Society, 2021m). Lapatinib works inside the cell by blocking the function of the HER2 protein. Adverse effects can include diarrhea, nausea, vomiting, rash, and a syndrome of numbness, tingling, swelling, and pain in the hands and feet. Cardiotoxicity has also been reported.

Advanced breast cancer in postmenopausal women who are estrogen and progesterone receptor–positive and HER2-positive may be treated with lapatinib in combination with capecitabine (Xeloda) and letrozole (Femara). Denosumab (Prolia, Xgeva), a monoclonal antibody, may be used to increase bone mass in patients with metastasis to the bone and at high risk for fracture from aromatase inhibitor therapy. (The use of biological and targeted therapies is discussed further in Chapter 18.)

Follow-Up and Survivorship Care. After surgery, patients must be monitored for the rest of their life at regular intervals. Most have professional examinations every 3 to 6 months for the first 5 years and then annually thereafter. In addition, it is recommended that these patients perform monthly examinations on both breasts or on the remaining breast and the surgical site. The most common site of local recurrence of breast cancer is at the surgical site. These patients should also undergo appropriate breast imaging at regular intervals (usually 6 months after treatment is finished to annually), as determined by their risk for recurrence and breast cancer history.

EVIDENCE-INFORMED PRACTICE

Research Highlight

What Is the Effect of Exercise for Women Receiving Adjuvant Therapy for Breast Cancer?

Clinical Question
For women with breast cancer (P) does exercise (I) improve physical and psychological outcomes (O) after receiving adjuvant therapy (T)?

Best Available Evidence
Systematic review of randomized controlled trials (RCTs)

Critical Appraisal and Synthesis of Evidence
- Sixty-three RCTs of women with breast cancer who had completed active cancer treatment. Intervention was mostly aerobic exercise. There was wide variation in types of physical activity, frequency and duration of sessions, and levels of effort.
- Breast cancer survivors who did physical activity experienced greater positive changes in social function, body fat, and muscle strength.
- Overall, physical activity interventions may have small to moderate effects on health-related quality of life and psychosocial and physical function after adjuvant therapy for women with breast cancer.

Conclusion
- Physical activity has positive effects on physical and psychological outcomes and quality of life.

Implications for Nursing
- To help patients get interested in physical activity, nurses should discuss with them their favourite forms of exercise, hobbies, and activities.
- Nurses should help patients identify physical activity resources (e.g., walking paths, swimming pool, gym).
- The patient's barriers to active participation in exercise should be assessed.
- When possible, patients should be assisted in adhering to recommended activities.

Reference for Evidence
Furmaniak, A. C., Menig, M., & Markes, M. H. (2016). Exercise for women receiving adjuvant therapy for breast cancer. *Cochrane Database of Systematic Reviews, 9*, CD005001. doi:10.1002/14651858.CD005001.pub3. *P*, patient population of interest; *I*, intervention or area of interest; *O*, outcome(s) of interest; *T*, timing (see Chapter 1).

CULTURALLY COMPETENT CARE

BREAST CANCER
Among diverse ethnic groups, differences exist in the incidence, mortality rates, and relevant care issues related to breast cancer. In addition, cultural differences may involve gender roles, health beliefs, religion, and family structure. Other differences may relate to dietary factors and disparities in the access to and use of clinical breast examinations and screening mammography. Despite universal health care, inequities in cancer care and outcomes exist among Canada's various ethnic and social groups (Sayani, 2017). Cultural values strongly influence how women respond to and cope with breast cancer and treatment. Nurses need to consider how health behaviours are influenced by cultural norms and, in particular, the cultural value of breasts and the cultural factors related to the disease of breast cancer.

Immigrants to Canada often underutilize screening and prevention services. Women may delay screening or treatment for varying reasons, including an acceptance of disease as inevitable fate or "God's will," a mistrust of Western medicine, language barriers, lack of health care access, or the stigma of a cancer diagnosis. Among Indigenous populations, survival rates after a breast cancer diagnosis are poorer than in the general population (Garvey et al., 2020). In order to understand Indigenous peoples' experience of cancer, nurses must consider the cultural contexts and social realities of their lives (Garvey et al., 2020). Holistic approaches that eliminate cultural barriers to quality cancer care are essential, including integration of person-centred care and cultural safety and responsiveness as core values, to meet the needs of racially visible and ethnically diverse patients with breast cancer (Sayani, 2017). Understanding the role and use of spirituality and traditional medicines that are individualized to the patient's survivorship needs can enhance overall well-being and quality of life in Indigenous populations in Canada (Gall et al., 2018; Gifford et al., 2019).

NURSING MANAGEMENT BREAST CANCER

NURSING ASSESSMENT
Many factors need to be considered when a nurse is assessing a patient with a breast disorder. The history of the breast disorder assists in establishing the diagnosis. The presence of nipple discharge, pain, rate of growth of the lump, breast asymmetry, and correlation with the menstrual cycle should all be investigated.

The size and location of the lump or lumps should be carefully documented. The physical characteristics of the lesion, such as consistency, mobility, and shape, should be assessed. If nipple discharge is present, the colour and consistency should be noted, as well as whether it occurs from one or both breasts.

Subjective and objective data that should be obtained from an individual with suspected or diagnosed breast cancer are presented in Table 54.9.

NURSING DIAGNOSES
Nursing diagnoses related to the care of a patient with diagnosed breast cancer vary. After diagnosis and before a treatment plan has been selected, the following diagnoses apply:
- *Personal uncertainty* resulting from *insufficient information* (treatment options and their effects)
- *Anxiety* resulting from *threat to current status, threat of death* (diagnosis of cancer)

TABLE 54.9   NURSING ASSESSMENT
Breast Cancer

Subjective Data

Important Health Information

Past health history:
- Family history of breast cancer (especially mother or sister, young age at diagnosis)
- History of abnormal mammogram findings or atypical findings in prior biopsy
- Benign breast disorders with atypical changes
- Previous unilateral breast cancer
- Menstrual history (early menarche with late menopause)
- Pregnancy history (nulliparity or first full-term pregnancy after age 30)
- Previous endometrial, ovarian, or colon cancer
- Hyperestrogenism and testicular atrophy (in men)
- Dietary habits and history of alcohol use
- Level of usual physical activity, weight, and BMI

Medications: Use of hormones, especially as postmenopausal hormone therapy and in oral contraceptives; infertility treatments

Surgeries or other treatments: Exposure to therapeutic radiation (e.g., for Hodgkin's lymphoma or thyroid cancer)

Symptoms
- Palpable change found on self-examination
- Obesity; unexplained severe weight loss (possible indicator of metastasis)
- Changes in cognition; headache; bone pain (possible indicators of metastasis)
- Unilateral nipple discharge (clear, milky, or bloody)
- Change in breast contour, size, or symmetry
- Psychological stress
- Anxiety regarding threat to self-esteem

Objective Data

General

Axillary and supraclavicular lymphadenopathy

Integumentary

Firm, discrete nodules at mastectomy site (possible indicator of local recurrence); peripheral edema (possible indicator of metastasis)

Respiratory

Pleural effusions (possible indicator of metastasis)

Gastrointestinal

Hepatomegaly, jaundice; ascites (possible indicators of liver metastasis)

Reproductive

Hard, irregular, nonmobile breast lump, most often in upper outer sector, possibly fixated to fascia or chest wall; nipple inversion or retraction, erosion; edema (*peau d'orange* appearance), erythema, induration, infiltration, or dimpling (in later stages)

Possible Diagnostic Findings

Finding of mass or change in tissue on breast examination; abnormal findings on mammography, ultrasonography, or breast MRI; positive results of FNA or surgical biopsy or similar results with needle biopsy

BMI, body mass index; *FNA,* fine-needle aspiration; *MRI,* magnetic resonance imaging.

- *Reduced self-concept* resulting from *alteration in self-perception*

If a mastectomy or lumpectomy is planned, the nursing diagnoses may include but are not limited to those presented in NCP 54.1, available on the Evolve website.

PLANNING

The overall goals are that patients with breast cancer will (a) actively participate in the decision-making process related to treatment options, (b) adhere to the therapeutic plan, (c) manage the adverse effects of adjuvant therapy, and (d) access and benefit from the support provided by significant others and health care providers.

NURSING IMPLEMENTATION

ACUTE INTERVENTION. The time between the diagnosis of breast cancer and the selection of a treatment plan can be a difficult period for a patient and their family. Although the primary health care provider has discussed treatment options, patients often rely on a nurse to clarify and expand on these options. During this often stressful time, patients may not be coping effectively. Appropriate nursing interventions are to explore the patient's usual decision-making patterns, to help accurately evaluate the advantages and disadvantages of the options, to provide information relevant to the decision, and to support the patient and family once the decision is made.

During this period, patients may exhibit signs of distress or tension—such as tachycardia, increased muscle tension, sleep disturbances, and restlessness—whenever they focus on the decision to be made. Nurses should assess the body language, motor activity, and affect of their patients during periods of high stress and indecision so that appropriate interventions can be used.

Regardless of the surgery planned, patients must be provided with sufficient information to ensure informed consent. Some patients seek extensive, detailed information, whereas others avoid information. Sensitivity to the individual's need for and type of information is essential. The information includes (a) preoperative instructions on pain control, turning, coughing, and deep breathing; (b) a review of postoperative exercises; and (c) explanation of the recovery period from the time of surgery until discharge.

Many women who undergo breast-conserving surgery have an uncomplicated postoperative course with variable pain intensity. Pain is most affected by the extent of the lymph node dissection performed. If an ALND or a mastectomy has been performed, drains are generally left in place, and patients are discharged home with them. Patients and their families need to be taught, with a return demonstration, how to manage the drains at home.

Restoring arm function on the affected side after mastectomy and ALND is a key nursing goal. The patient should be placed in a semi-Fowler's position with the arm on the affected side elevated on a pillow. Flexing and extending the fingers should begin in the recovery room, with progressive increases in activity encouraged.

Postoperative arm and shoulder exercises are instituted gradually with a surgeon's direction (Figure 54.10). These exercises are designed to prevent contractures and muscle shortening, maintain muscle tone, and improve lymph and blood circulation. The difficulty and pain encountered by the patient in performing the previously simple tasks included in the exercise program may cause frustration and depression. The goal of all exercise is a gradual return to full range of motion within 4 to 6 weeks.

The nurse can minimize postoperative discomfort by administering analgesics about 30 minutes before the patient initiates exercises. When the patient is able to shower, the warm water on the involved shoulder often has a muscle-relaxing effect and reduces joint stiffness.

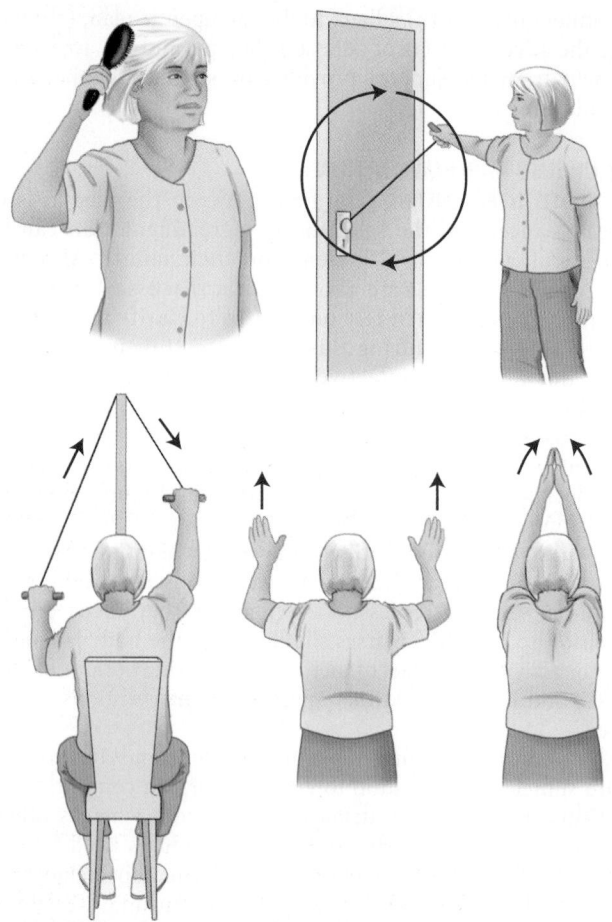

FIG. 54.10 Postoperative exercises for patient with a mastectomy or lumpectomy with axillary lymph node dissection.

The nurse must use measures to prevent or reduce lymphedema after ALND and teach these to the patient. The affected arm should not be dependent, even during sleep. Elastic bandages should not be used in the early postoperative period because they inhibit collateral lymph drainage. Patients must be instructed to protect the arm on the operative side from even minor trauma such as a pinprick or sunburn. If trauma to the arm occurs, the area should be washed thoroughly with soap and water, and a topical antibiotic ointment and a bandage or other sterile dressing should be applied. Patients must be taught to advise their surgeon of the trauma, and the site of injury must be observed closely for evidence of inflammation. Patients must understand that for the rest of their life, they are at risk of developing lymphedema.

SAFETY ALERT
- Blood pressure readings, venipunctures, and injections should not be performed on the affected arm so as to prevent lymphedema.

When lymphedema is acute (see Figure 54.8), complete decongestive therapy may be recommended (Canadian Cancer Society, 2021s). This therapy consists of a massage-like technique to mobilize the subcutaneous accumulation of fluid. This is then followed by compression bandaging and the wearing of a pneumatic compression sleeve. This sleeve intermittently applies mechanical massage to the arm and facilitates lymph drainage up toward the heart. Diuretics, isometric exercises, and elevation of the arm so that it is level with the heart may

be recommended to reduce the fluid volume in the arm. The patient may need to wear a fitted elastic pressure-gradient sleeve (a) during waking hours to maintain maximum volume reduction and (b) preventively during air travel.

PSYCHOLOGICAL CARE. Effective care includes sensitivity to the patient's efforts to cope with a life-threatening disease. A relationship in which the patient can express their authentic feelings is therapeutic. The nurse can help to meet the patient's psychological needs in the following ways:
- Providing a culturally safe environment for the expression of the full range of feelings
- Conducting a culturally appropriate needs assessment to support specific cancer needs across cultures
- Helping identify sources of support and strength, such as their partner, family, and spiritual or religious practices
- Encouraging the patient to identify and learn individual coping strengths
- Promoting communication between the patient and their family, friends, or both
- Providing accurate and complete answers to questions about the disease, treatment options, and reproductive, fertility, or lactation issues (if appropriate)
- Offering information about community resources, such as CancerConnection through the Canadian Cancer Society, CanSurmount, Look Good Feel Better, and local support organizations and groups
- Offering information about available resources for mental health counselling if needed

Nurses can promote a patient's recovery by referral to peer support resources. The Reach to Recovery program of the Canadian Cancer Society is a rehabilitation program for people who have undergone breast surgery. It is designed to help them meet their psychological, physical, and cosmetic needs. The volunteers, who have had breast cancer, can answer questions about expectations, surgery, and recovery. The Canadian Cancer Society and the Canadian Cancer Society Research Institute can provide excellent materials to assist nurses in meeting the special needs of individuals living with breast cancer.

It is important for health care providers to remain sensitive to the complex psychological effect that a diagnosis of cancer and subsequent breast surgery can have on a patient and their family (Ray & Veluscek, 2021). Diverse emotional responses are common. The nurse's accepting attitude and the offering of resources can greatly alleviate the common feelings of fear, anger, anxiety, and depression experienced by many patients.

AMBULATORY AND HOME CARE. The nurse should explain the specific follow-up routine to patients and emphasize the importance of ongoing monitoring and breast self-awareness. To address needs for individual and family support in addition to coping needs, referral to a mental health care provider may be indicated. Immediately after surgery, symptoms that should be reported to the clinician include fever, inflammation at the surgical site, erythema, postoperative constipation, and unusual swelling. Changes to report beyond the immediate postsurgical period are new back pain, weakness, shortness of breath, and confusion.

For women who have undergone mastectomy without breast reconstruction, a variety of products are available to meet specific individual needs. These include garments ranging from camisoles with soft breast prosthetic inserts to a fitted prosthesis with bra. For women who choose a breast prosthesis, a certified fitter can help them select a comfortable, more permanent

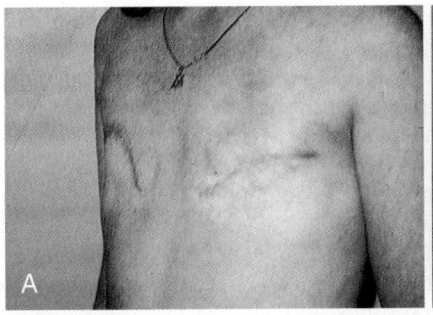 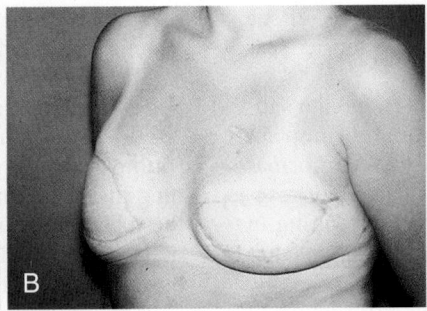 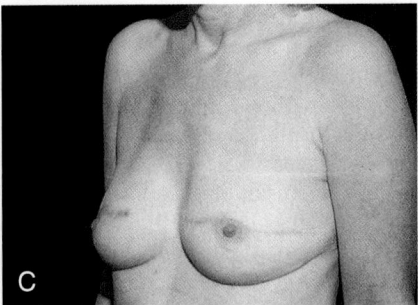

FIG. 54.11 Appearances after breast surgery. **A,** Appearance of chest after bilateral mastectomy. **B,** Postoperative breast reconstruction before nipple–areolar reconstruction. **C,** Postoperative breast reconstruction after nipple–areolar reconstruction. Source: Fortunato, N., & McCullough, S. M. (1998). *Plastic and reconstructive surgery.* Mosby. Courtesy Brian Davies, MD.

weighted prosthesis and bra, generally at 4 to 8 weeks postoperatively. The role of the nurse is to present the choices and resources without judgement.

The loss of a breast can have varying implications for a patient's sexual identity and relationships. The nurse can initiate a discussion of sexuality by inviting questions about relationships or intimacy concerns within the recovery framework (Canadian Cancer Society, 2018). To be effective sources of support for the patient, the spouse, sexual partner, or family members often need help in coping with their emotional reactions to the diagnosis and surgery. There are no physical reasons for a mastectomy to prevent sexual satisfaction. Women taking hormonal therapy, however, may have a decreased sexual drive or vaginal dryness. They may need to use lubrication to prevent discomfort during intercourse. Concerns about sexuality are often not well addressed by health care providers (Canadian Cancer Society, 2018). If difficulty in adjustment or other issues develop, counselling may be necessary to cope with the emotional component of a mastectomy and the diagnosis of cancer.

Depression and anxiety may occur with the continued stress and uncertainty of a cancer diagnosis. Patients' self-esteem and identity may also be threatened. The support of family and friends and participation in a cancer support group are important aspects of care that are often helpful in improving patient's quality of life.

EVALUATION

The expected outcomes for patients after a mastectomy or lumpectomy are presented in NCP 54.1, available on the Evolve website.

MAMMOPLASTY

Mammoplasty is the surgical change in the size or shape of the breast. It may be performed electively for cosmetic purposes to either enlarge or reduce the size of the breasts. It may also be performed to reconstruct the breast after a mastectomy.

A professional, nonjudgemental attitude and clear information about surgical breast options are most useful for patients engaged in decision making about mammoplasty. It is important that patients set realistic expectations about what mammoplasty can accomplish and about possible complications, such as hematoma formation, hemorrhage, and infection. If an implant is involved, the patient must understand that capsular contracture (complication of internal scar tissue forming a constricting capsule around a breast implant) and the resultant loss of the implant are possible (Canadian Cancer Society, 2021y).

Breast Reconstruction

Breast reconstructive surgery may be performed simultaneously with a mastectomy or some time afterward to achieve symmetry and to restore or preserve body image. The timing of reconstruction surgery should be based on the psychological needs of individual patients. Immediate breast reconstruction after mastectomy is commonly performed. The advantages of immediate reconstruction are the need for only one surgical procedure, only one anaesthesia induction, and only one recovery period; also, reconstructive surgery takes place before the development of scar tissue or adhesions. Early reconstruction does not delay or influence further treatment or adversely affect predicted survival.

Indications. The main indication for breast reconstruction is to improve a patient's self-image and help regain a sense of normality and assist in coping with the loss of the breast. Current techniques cannot restore lactation, nipple sensation, or nipple erectility. Therefore, the erotic functions of the breast are not present. Although the breast will not fully resemble its premastectomy appearance, the reconstructed appearance usually represents an improvement over the mastectomy scar (Figure 54.11). The contour of the breast is restored without the use of an external prosthesis.

Types of Reconstruction

Breast Implants and Tissue Expansion. Breast implants are placed in a pocket under the pectoralis muscle, which protects the implant and provides soft tissue coverage over it. Implants can be placed either at the time of mastectomy or later. A small magnet is embedded in most expanders to help locate the port where the fluid is injected. Therefore, a patient with a magnet in place should not undergo MRI. Because many patients who have undergone mastectomy have insufficient tissue, simple placement of an implant may lead to small breast reconstruction that is tight or firm. Autologous (one's own) tissue reconstruction may then be recommended.

A tissue expander can be used to stretch the skin and muscle at the mastectomy site before implants are inserted (Figure 54.12). The use of tissue expanders and breast implants is the most common breast reconstruction technique currently used. Placement of the expander can be performed at the time of mastectomy or at a later date. The tissue expander, which is minimally inflated at the time of surgery, is gradually filled by weekly injections of sterile water or saline solution, which stretch the skin and muscle. Once the tissue is adequately stretched and the anticipated breast size is reached, the expander is surgically removed and a permanent implant is inserted. Some expanders are designed to remain in place and become the implant, eliminating the need for a second surgical procedure. Tissue expansion does not work well in individuals with extensive scar tissue from surgery or radiation therapy.

The body's natural response to the presence of a foreign substance is the formation of a fibrous capsule around the implant (Canadian Cancer Society, 2021y). If excessive capsular formation occurs as a result of infection, hematoma, trauma, or reaction to a foreign body, a contracture can develop, resulting in deformation of the breast. Surgeons differ in their approaches to the prevention of contracture formation, although gentle manual massage around the implant is routine. Prevention of the problems that cause excessive capsule formation is critical. Other postoperative complications include skin ulceration, hypertrophic scar formation, intercostal neuralgia, and wound infection.

Tissue Flap Procedures. An additional choice for breast reconstruction is the use of autologous tissue to recreate a breast mound. If insufficient muscle is left after mastectomy or if the chest wall has been irradiated, the person's own tissue may be used to repair the soft tissue defects. Musculocutaneous flaps are most often taken from the back (latissimus dorsi muscle) or the abdomen (transverse rectus abdominis muscle). In the latissimus dorsi musculocutaneous flap, a block of skin and muscle from the patient's back is used to replace tissue removed during mastectomy. A small implant may be needed beneath the flap to

obtain reasonable breast shape and size. A disadvantage of this technique is an additional scar on the back.

The *transverse rectus abdominis musculocutaneous (TRAM) flap* is a common surgical procedure (Canadian Cancer Society, 2021y). The rectus abdominis muscles are paired flat muscles running from the rib cage down to the pubic bone. Arteries running inside the muscles provide branches at many levels, and these branches supply the fat and skin across a large expanse of the abdomen. In this technique, the surgeon elevates a large block of tissue from the lower abdominal area but leaves it attached to the rectus muscle (Figure 54.13). This tissue is then tunnelled or placed as "free flaps" under the skin up to the area where the breast will be reconstructed. Then it is moulded and fashioned to form a breast. The abdominal incision is closed, which results in an appearance similar to that of an abdominoplasty. This surgical procedure can last 2 to 8 hours, and recovery can take at least 6 to 12 weeks (Bussey et al., 2019). Complications include bleeding, seroma, hernia, infection, and low back pain. An implant may be used in addition to the flap if the flap does not provide the desired cosmetic result alone. Patients who smoke, who are too thin, or who are overweight are not good candidates for this type of procedure.

A *deep inferior epigastric artery perforator (DIEP) flap* is a version of the free flap that does not use muscle tissue. With the DIEP flap, only the skin and fat are taken from the same lower abdominal area as the TRAM flap. Patients may experience less pain and restriction of movement with this procedure.

Total skin-sparing mastectomy is the preservation of the skin of the nipple and areola with the removal of underlying breast tissue. It can be done at the same time as immediate breast reconstructive surgery.

Nipple–Areolar Reconstruction. The majority of patients who undergo breast reconstruction also receive nipple–areolar reconstruction. Nipple reconstruction gives the reconstructed breast a much more natural appearance. Nipple–areolar reconstruction is usually done a few months after breast reconstruction. Tissue to construct a nipple may be taken from the opposite

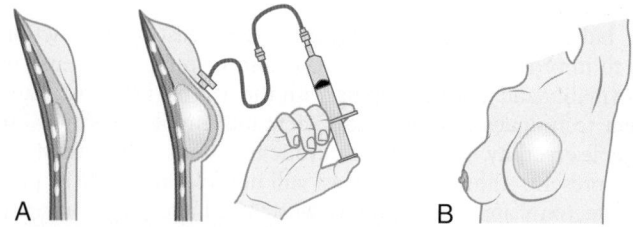

FIG. 54.12 Tissue expansion. **A,** Tissue expander with gradual expansion. **B,** Tissue expander in place after mastectomy.

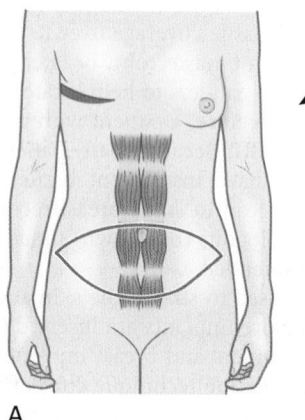
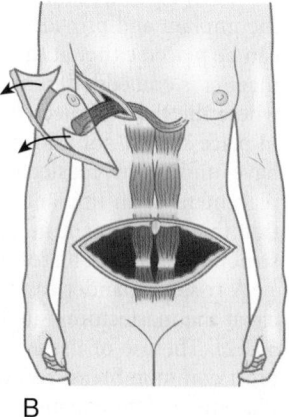
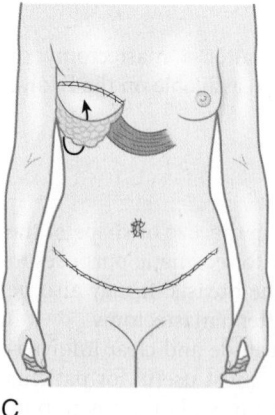
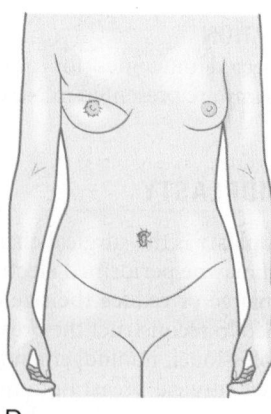

A   B   C   D

FIG. 54.13 Diagrams of the transverse rectus abdominis musculocutaneous (TRAM) flap procedure. **A,** TRAM flap is planned. **B,** The abdominal tissue, while attached to the rectus muscle, nerve, and blood supply, is tunnelled through the abdomen to the chest. **C,** The flap is trimmed to shape the breast. The lower abdominal incision is closed. **D,** Nipple and areola are reconstructed after the breast is healed.

breast or from a small flap of tissue on the reconstructed breast mound. The areola may be grafted from the labia, skin in the area of the groin, or lower abdominal skin, or it may be tattooed with a permanent pigmented dye. In some patients, a small implant may be placed under the completed nipple–areolar reconstruction to add additional projection.

Breast Augmentation

In augmentation mammoplasty (the procedure to enlarge the breasts), an implant is placed in a surgically created pocket between the capsule of the breast and the pectoral fascia or, ideally, under the pectoral muscle. Most implants are silicone envelopes filled with a fluid such as saline or silicone. Currently in Canada, two types of breast implants (saline-filled and silicone gel–filled) have the required licensing from Health Canada. All implants contain an insert that identifies all potential risks related to breast implant surgery (Health Canada, 2020).

Breast Reduction

For some patients, large breasts can be a source of physical and psychological discomfort. They can interfere with normal daily activities such as walking, typing, and driving a car. The weight of large breasts can lead to back, shoulder, and neck conditions, including degenerative nerve changes. Overly large breasts can compromise self-esteem and self-image, and the comfort in wearing some clothing may be affected. Reduction in the size of the breasts can have positive effects on both the psychological and physical health of the patient. Reduction mammoplasty is performed by resecting wedges of tissue from the upper and lower quadrants of the breast. The excess skin is removed, and the areola and nipple are relocated on the breast. Lactation can usually be accomplished if massive amounts of tissue are not removed and the nipples are left connected during surgery.

NURSING MANAGEMENT
BREAST AUGMENTATION AND REDUCTION

Breast augmentation and breast reduction may be performed in the outpatient surgical area, or they may involve overnight hospitalization. General anaesthesia is used. Drains are generally placed in the surgical site to prevent hematoma formation and then removed 2 to 3 days after surgery or when drainage is less than 20 to 30 mL per day. The drainage must be examined for colour and odour to detect postoperative infection or hemorrhage. The woman's temperature should also be monitored. Dressings should be changed as necessary, with sterile technique. After surgery, the patient should be assured that the appearance of the breast will improve once healing is complete. Depending on health care provider instructions, patients may be instructed to wear a bra that provides good support continuously for 2 to 3 days after breast reduction or augmentation. Depending on the extent of the operation, most patients can resume normal activities within 2 to 3 weeks. Strenuous exercise may not be appropriate until several weeks later.

CASE STUDY

Breast Cancer

Patient Profile

A. K. (pronouns she/her), 68 years old, has been diagnosed with breast cancer. A. K. is scheduled for surgery in the morning for a lumpectomy and sentinel lymph node biopsy (SLNB) with possible axillary dissection.

Interprofessional Care
Preoperative

- When seen in the preoperative clinic 1 week before surgery, A. K. is crying uncontrollably and says, "My partner does not want to look at me anymore. He is afraid of what I am going to look like with a flat chest."
- She states, "I cannot sleep, so I just pace the floor at night."
- She expresses concern that their two daughters (34 and 32) are going to get "this horrible disease."

Operative Procedure

- A lumpectomy and SLNB are performed.
- A. K. has cancer cells in the sentinel lymph node.
- Axillary node dissection is then done involving the removal of 15 to 20 nodes.

Postoperative

- Does not want to leave hospital; wants to stay in bed
- Fever with swelling and restricted range of motion in right arm
- Pain is not controlled well with pain medication.

Follow-Up Findings and Treatment

- Two positive lymph nodes are found.
- She is scheduled for outpatient chemotherapy followed by external beam radiation.

Discussion Questions

1. What in A. K's breast cancer–related experience with her family members might influence her coping response?
2. What information would the nurse provide to her about surgery?
3. What complication did A. K. develop after surgery?
4. Which common postoperative exercises will A. K. need to practise after surgery?
5. What community resources are available to help the patient and family adjust to this body change and to cope with the diagnosis of cancer? How can the nurse access these resources?
6. What information about breast cancer risks is important to provide to A. K. about radiation treatment and chemotherapy?
7. **Priority decision:** On the basis of the assessment data, what are the priority nursing diagnoses? Are there any interprofessional issues?
8. What information is important for the nurse to provide to A. K. and her daughters? What early-detection measures are important for them to know?
9. **Evidence-informed practice:** A. K. wants to know what the psychological benefit may be for her daughters if they decide to have a breast cancer genetic risk assessment.

evolve
Answers are available at http://evolve.elsevier.com/Canada/Lewis/medsurg.

REVIEW QUESTIONS

The number of the question corresponds to the same-numbered objective at the beginning of the chapter.

1. An occupational health nurse is planning a program on breast screening practices for employees in the company. Which method should the nurse use to promote learning and adherence among participants? (*Select all that apply.*)
   a. A recording that describes the procedure of breast self-awareness
   b. Distribution of a packet of articles from the medical literature
   c. A discussion of the value of early detection of breast cancer
   d. Written guidelines for mammography and breast self-awareness
   e. Community resources where they can obtain an ultrasound and MRI

2. Which of the following techniques is the most appropriate way to teach a client how to know their breasts?
   a. Teach palpation of cervical lymph nodes.
   b. Teach client to practise hard squeezing of the breast tissue.
   c. Teach the importance of a mammogram to evaluate breast tissue.
   d. Teach inspection of the whole area of breast tissue for any changes.

3. What explanation should the nurse provide when teaching a client with painful fibrocystic breast changes about the condition?
   a. All discrete breast lumps must be subjected to biopsy to rule out malignant changes.
   b. The symptoms will probably subside after menopause unless hormone replacement is used.
   c. The lumps will become progressively larger and more painful, eventually necessitating surgical removal.
   d. Restriction of coffee and chocolate and supplements of vitamin E can relieve the discomfort for many patients.

4. When discussing risk factors for breast cancer, which of the following should the nurse stress as the greatest known risk factor for breast cancer?
   a. Being a woman older than 60 years
   b. Experiencing menstruation for 40 years or more
   c. Using estrogen replacement therapy during menopause
   d. Having a paternal grandmother with postmenopausal breast cancer

5. A client has a lumpectomy with sentinel lymph node biopsy that yields results positive for cancer. Which of the following results supports the most favourable prognosis? (*Select all that apply.*)
   a. Well-differentiated tumour
   b. Estrogen receptor–positive tumour
   c. Involvement of two to four axillary nodes
   d. Overexpression of *HER2* cell marker
   e. Aneuploidy status from cell proliferation studies

6. A client with breast cancer has been scheduled for a modified radical mastectomy with an axillary node dissection. Which of the following should the nurse perform postoperatively to restore arm function on the affected side?
   a. Apply heating pads or blankets to increase circulation.
   b. Place daily ice packs to minimize the risk for lymphedema.
   c. Teach passive exercises with the affected arm in a dependent position.
   d. Emphasize regular exercises for the affected shoulder to increase range of motion.

7. Which of the following should the nurse implement preoperatively to meet the psychological needs of a client scheduled for a modified radical mastectomy?
   a. Discuss the limitations of breast reconstruction.
   b. Include their significant other in all conversations.
   c. Promote an environment for expression of feelings.
   d. Explain the importance of regular follow-up screening.

8. Which of the following statements is suitable to make when teaching clients how to prevent capsular formation after breast reconstruction with implants?
   a. Gently massage the area around the implant.
   b. Bind the breasts tightly with elastic bandages.
   c. Exercise the arm on the affected side to promote drainage.
   d. Avoid strenuous exercise until implant healing has occurred.

1. c, d; 2. d; 3. d, 4. a; 5. a, b; 6. d; 7. c; 8. a.

⊜volve

For even more review questions, visit http://evolve.elsevier.com/Canada/Lewis/medsurg.

REFERENCES

Barbeau, P., & Pillay, J. (2017). *Breast cancer screening: Protocol for an evidence report to reform an update of the Canadian Task Force on Preventive Health Care 2011 guidelines.* https://canadiantaskforce.ca/wp-content/uploads/2017/03/BCU-protocol-14Mar2017-FINAL.pdf

Bussey, M. D., Aldabe, D., & Jones, L. M. (2019). Reorganization of postural stability after tram flap breast reconstruction surgery: A longitudinal case report. *Journal of Women's Health Physical Therapy, 43*(3), 136–143. https://doi.org/10.1097/JWH.0000000000000134

Canadian Cancer Society. (2018). *Sex, intimacy and cancer.* https://www.cancer.ca/~/media/cancer.ca/CW/publications/Sex%20intimacy%20and%20cancer/32061-1-NO.pdf

Canadian Cancer Society. (2021a). *Breast cancer statistics.* https://cancer.ca/en/cancer-information/cancer-types/breast/statistics

Canadian Cancer Society. (2021b). *Know your breasts.* https://cancer.ca/en/cancer-information/find-cancer-early/know-your-body/know-your-breasts

Canadian Cancer Society. (2021c). *Screening for breast cancer.* https://cancer.ca/en/cancer-information/cancer-types/breast/screening

Canadian Cancer Society. (2021d). *Supportive care for breast cancer.* https://cancer.ca/en/cancer-information/cancer-types/breast/supportive-care

Canadian Cancer Society. (2021e). *Mammography.* https://cancer.ca/en/treatments/tests-and-procedures/mammography

Canadian Cancer Society. (2021f). *Core biopsy.* https://cancer.ca/en/treatments/tests-and-procedures/core-biopsy

Canadian Cancer Society. (2021g). *Breast pain.* https://cancer.ca/en/cancer-information/cancer-types/breast/what-is-breast-cancer/non-cancerous-conditions/breast-pain-mastalgia

Canadian Cancer Society. (2021h). *Fibrocystic breasts.* https://cancer.ca/en/cancer-information/cancer-types/breast/what-is-breast-cancer/non-cancerous-conditions/fibrocystic-changes

Canadian Cancer Society. (2021i). *Other non-cancerous breast conditions.* https://cancer.ca/en/cancer-information/cancer-types/breast/what-is-breast-cancer/non-cancerous-conditions/other-pon-cancerous-conditions

Canadian Cancer Society. (2021j). *Risks for breast cancer.* https://cancer.ca/en/cancer-information/cancer-types/breast/risks

Canadian Cancer Society. (2021k). *All about hormone replacement therapy (HRT).* https://cancer.ca/en/cancer-information/reduce-your-risk/understand-hormones/all-about-hormone-replacement--therapy-hrt

Canadian Cancer Society. (2021l). *Reducing your risk for breast cancer.* https://cancer.ca/en/cancer-information/cancer-types/breast/risks/reducing-your-risk

Canadian Cancer Society. (2021m). *Targeted therapy for breast cancer.* https://cancer.ca/en/cancer-information/cancer-types/breast/treatment/targeted-therapy

Canadian Cancer Society. (2021n). *Axillary lymph node dissection (ALND).* https://cancer.ca/en/treatments/tests-and-procedures/axillary-lymph-node-dissection-alnd

Canadian Cancer Society. (2021o). *Sentinel lymph node dissection (SNND).* https://cancer.ca/en/treatments/tests-and-procedures/sentinel-lymph-node-biopsy-slnb

Canadian Cancer Society. (2021p). *HER2 status test.* https://cancer.ca/en/treatments/tests-and-procedures/her2-status-test

Canadian Cancer Society. (2021q). *Stages of breast cancer.* https://cancer.ca/en/cancer-information/cancer-types/breast/staging

Canadian Cancer Society. (2021r). *Research in breast cancer.* https://cancer.ca/en/cancer-information/cancer-types/breast/research

Canadian Cancer Society. (2021s). *Lymphedema.* https://cancer.ca/en/treatments/side-effects/lymphedema

Canadian Cancer Society. (2021t). *Surgery for breast cancer.* https://cancer.ca/en/cancer-information/cancer-types/breast/treatment/surgery

Canadian Cancer Society. (2021u). *Risk of recurrence after surgery and additional treatments.* https://cancer.ca/en/cancer-information/cancer-types/breast/treatment/risk-of-breast-cancer-recurrence-and-adjuvant-therapy

Canadian Cancer Society. (2021v). *Chemotherapy for breast cancer.* https://cancer.ca/en/cancer-information/cancer-types/breast/treatment/chemotherapy

Canadian Cancer Society. (2021w). *Side effects of chemotherapy.* https://cancer.ca/en/treatments/treatment-types/chemotherapy/side-effects-of-chemotherapy

Canadian Cancer Society. (2021x). *Hormonal therapy for breast cancer.* https://cancer.ca/en/cancer-information/cancer-types/breast/treatment/hormonal-therapy

Canadian Cancer Society. (2021y). *Types of breast reconstruction.* https://cancer.ca/en/cancer-information/cancer-types/breast/reconstruction-and-prostheses/types-of-breast-reconstruction

Canadian Task Force on Preventive Health Care. (2018). *Breast cancer update.* https://canadiantaskforce.ca/guidelines/published-guidelines/breast-cancer-update/

Corradini, S., Reitz, D., Pazos, M., et al. (2019). Mastectomy or breast-conserving therapy for early breast cancer in real-life clinical practice: Outcome comparison of 7565 Cases. *Cancers, 11*(2), 160. https://doi.org/10.3390/cancers11020160

Gall, A., Leske, S., Adams, J., et al. (2018). Traditional and complementary medicine use among Indigenous cancer patients in Australia, Canada, New Zealand, and the United States: A systematic review. *Integrative Cancer Therapies, 17*(3), 568–581. https://doi:10.1177/1534735418775821

Garvey, G., Cunningham, J., Mayer, C., et al. (2020). Psychosocial aspects of delivering cancer care to Indigenous people: An overview. *JCO Global Oncology, 6,* 148–154. https://doi:10.1200/JCO.19.00130

Gifford, W., Thomas, O., Thomas, R., et al. (2019). Spirituality in cancer survivorship with First nations people in Canada. *Supportive Care in Cancer, 27,* 2969–2976. https://doi.org/10.1007/s00520-018-4609-z

Health Canada. (2020). *Breast implants.* https://www.canada.ca/en/health-canada/services/drugs-medical-devices/breast-implants.html

Li, G. Z., Wong, S. M., Lester, S., et al. (2018). Evaluating the risk of underlying malignancy in patients with pathologic nipple discharge. *The Breast Journal, 24,* 624–627. https://onlinelibrary.wiley.com/doi/abs/10.1111/tbj.13018

MyHealth.Alberta.ca. (2019). *Breast abscess: Care instructions.* https://myhealth.alberta.ca/Health/aftercareinformation/pages/conditions.aspx?hwid=uh2663

Ray, C. D., & Veluscek, A. M. (2021). Nonsupport versus varying levels of person-centered emotional support: A study of women with breast cancer. *Journal of Cancer Education, 33,* 649–652. https://doi.org/10.1007/s13187-016-1125-z

Sasaki, J., Geletzke, A., Kass, R. B., et al. (2018). Etiology and management of benign breast disease. In K. I. Bland, V. S. Klimberg, E. M. Copeland, et al. (Eds.), *The breast: Comprehensive management of benign and malignant diseases* (5th ed., pp. 79–92). Elsevier. https://doi.org/10.1016/B978-0-323-35955-9.00005-2

Sayani, A. (2017). Socially-based inequities in breast cancer care: Intersections of the social determinants of health and the cancer care continuum. *Women's Health & Urban Life, 13*(1), 24–36. http://orcid.org/0000-0001-5391-7769

Simmons, C. E. (2018). The changing role of neoadjuvant therapy in breast cancer: Considering systemic treatment for patients with operable as well as inoperable disease. *BC Medical Journal, 60*(2), 103–108. https://www.bcmj.org/articles/changing-role-neoadjuvant-therapy-breast-cancer-considering-systemic-treatment-patients

Squires, J., Simard, S., Asad, S., et al. (2019). Exploring reasons for overuse of contralateral prophylactic mastectomy in Canada. *Current Oncology, 26*(4), e439–e457. https://doi.org/10.3747/co.26.4951

Swerdloff, R. S., & Ng, C. M. (2019). Gynecomastia: Etiology, diagnosis, and treatment. In K. R. Feingold, B. Anawalt, A. Boyce, et al. (Eds.), *Endotext.* MDText.com. https://www.ncbi.nlm.nih.gov/books/NBK279105/

RESOURCES

Breast Cancer Society of Canada
    https://www.bcsc.ca
Canadian Association of Nurses in Oncology
    https://www.cano-acio.ca/
Canadian Association of Provincial Cancer Agencies (CAPCA)
    https://www.capca.ca
Canadian Breast Cancer Foundation (CBCF)
    https://www.cbcf.org
Canadian Breast Cancer Network (CBCN)
    https://www.cbcn.ca

Canadian Cancer Society
https://www.cancer.ca

Canadian Cancer Society Research Institute
https://www.cancer.ca/research

Canadian Oncology Societies (COS)
https://www.omicsonline.org/societies/canadian-oncology-society-cos/

Canadian Partnership Against Cancer
https://www.partnershipagainstcancer.ca

American Cancer Society—*Breast Cancer*
https://www.cancer.org/cancer/breastcancer/index

Living Beyond Breast Cancer
https://www.lbbc.org

National Breast Cancer Coalition
https://www.stopbreastcancer.org/

National Cancer Institute
https://www.cancer.gov

National Cancer Institute—*Breast Cancer Risk Assessment Tool*
https://bcrisktool.cancer.gov/

National Coalition for Cancer Survivorship (NCS)
https://canceradvocacy.org

National Lymphedema Network (NLN)
https://www.lymphnet.org

OncoLink (cancer information site of the Abramson Cancer Center, University of Pennsylvania)
https://www.oncolink.org

Oncology Nursing Society (ONS)
https://www.ons.org

Susan G. Komen
https://www.komen.org

ⓔvolve

For additional Internet resources, see the website for this book at http://evolve.elsevier.com/Canada/Lewis/medsurg.

Nursing Management
Sexually Transmitted Infections

Laura Fairley
Originating US chapter by Daniel P. Worrall

℮volve WEBSITE

http://evolve.elsevier.com/Canada/Lewis/medsurg

- Review Questions (Online Only)
- Key Points
- Answer Guidelines for Case Study
- Conceptual Care Map Creator
- Audio Glossary
- Content Updates

LEARNING OBJECTIVES

1. Assess the factors contributing to the high incidence of sexually transmitted infections (STIs).
2. Explain the etiology, clinical manifestations, complications, and diagnostic abnormalities of gonorrhea, syphilis, chlamydial infections, genital herpes, and genital warts.
3. Compare and contrast primary genital herpes with recurrent genital herpes.
4. Explain the interprofessional care and the medication therapy for gonorrhea, syphilis, chlamydial infections, genital herpes, and genital warts.
5. Identify the nursing assessment and the nursing diagnoses for patients who have an STI.
6. Describe the nursing role in the prevention and control of STIs.
7. Describe the nursing management of patients with STIs.

KEY TERMS

chancre	gonorrhea	syphilis
chlamydial infections	gummas	
genital herpes	sexually transmitted infections (STIs)	

SEXUALLY TRANSMITTED INFECTIONS

Sexually transmitted infections (STIs) are infectious diseases that are most commonly acquired through sexual contact with the mouth, penis, vagina, anus, sexual fluids, or sex toys of an infected person but may also be contracted by other routes, such as through blood, blood products, perinatal transmission, and autoinoculation. STIs can be caused by different agents, including bacteria, viruses, or parasites. A list of common STIs is shown in Table 55.1.

The mucosal membranes of the rectum, genitals, mouth, and throat are particularly vulnerable to the agents that cause STIs and are usually the initial site of infection. Once the agent enters the body, the disease has an incubation period, during which the affected individual is infected but asymptomatic. This allows for the continued transmission of the disease from the infected (but asymptomatic) individual to another person. The individual may go on to develop clinical signs and symptoms of the infection or may remain asymptomatic, but they will continue to be infectious whether they develop symptoms or not.

STIs remain a significant public health concern in Canada. While they are largely preventable and treatable, STIs can have long-term negative effects on both pregnancy and fertility, increase the risk of certain kinds of cancer, and make people more vulnerable to acquiring another STI. It is possible for a person to have more than one STI at the same time.

In Canada, three nationally reportable STIs—gonorrhea, syphilis, and chlamydial infection—must be reported to the Communicable Disease Division in each province and territory (Public Health Agency of Canada [PHAC], 2019). For the past 25 years, there has been a steady increase in the rates of all three of these infections, despite innovations in prevention, treatment, and surveillance methods (PHAC, 2019). While young Canadians continue to have the highest reported rates of STIs, the highest relative increases in reported rates are being experienced by middle-aged and older persons (PHAC, 2019).

TABLE 55.1 CAUSES OF SEXUALLY TRANSMITTED INFECTIONS

Cause	Infection or Condition
Bacterial	
Chlamydia trachomatis	Nongonococcal urethritis; cervicitis; lymphogranuloma venereum
Neisseria gonorrhoeae	Gonorrhea
Treponema pallidum	Syphilis
Viral	
Cytomegalovirus	Encephalitis, esophagitis, retinitis, pneumonitis in immunocompromised patients
Hepatitis B & C viruses	Hepatitis B and C (see Chapter 46)
Herpes simplex virus (HSV)	Genital herpes
Human immunodeficiency virus (HIV) (see Chapter 17)	HIV infection, acquired immune deficiency syndrome (AIDS)
Human papilloma virus (HPV)	Genital warts; cervical, vulvar, vaginal, penile, anal, and oropharyngeal cancers
Poxvirus*	Molluscum contagiosum
Other	
Trichomonas vaginalis	Trichomoniasis
Phthirus pubis (crab louse)*	Ectoparasitic infestation (pubic lice) (see Chapter 26)
Sarcoptes scabiei*	Ectoparasitic infestation (scabies) (see Chapter 26)

*Transmission through both intimate sexual and nonsexual contact.

TABLE 55.2 STI RISK FACTORS

STI Risk Factors
- Inconsistent use of barrier methods or lack of use of barrier methods
- New sexual partner or more than two sexual partners in 1 yr
- Anonymous sexual partnering
- Sex under the influence of alcohol, drugs, or both
- Sex work
- Survival sex (exchanging sex for money, shelter, food, drugs)
- Intravenous drug use
- History of previous STI
- History of sexual abuse or sexual assault

STI, sexually transmitted disease.
Source: Adapted from Public Health Agency of Canada. (2016). *Canadian guidelines on sexually transmitted infections.* http://www.phac-aspc.gc.ca/std-mts/sti-its/cgsti-ldcits/section-5-6-eng.php

FACTORS AFFECTING INCIDENCE OF SEXUALLY TRANSMITTED INFECTION

Many factors contribute to the current STI rates. Earlier reproductive maturity and increased life expectancy have resulted in a longer sexual lifespan. Other factors include (1) greater sexual freedom, (2) inconsistent or incorrect use of barrier methods (e.g., condom/dental dam) during sexual activity, (3) the media's increased emphasis on sexuality without promoting safer sex practices, (4) the judgement-impairing effects of substance use on high-risk sexual behaviors, (5) growth of the online dating industry, (6) increased international travel, and (7) lack of knowledge and awareness about STIs and safer sex practices (PHAC, 2015b). There are also particular populations that are disproportionately affected by STIs as a result of various social and economic factors. Such populations include sex workers, members of the trans community, individuals experiencing homelessness, individuals who are incarcerated, and Indigenous people (Green et al., 2015; Hackett et al., 2020). Risk factors for STIs are outlined in Table 52.2.

Condoms are considered to be the best form of protection (other than abstinence) against contracting STIs because they provide a physical barrier between the mucosal membranes of sexual partners. Despite the efficacy of condoms, they are often not used by sexually active Canadians, particularly among the younger and older age cohorts. Adolescents and young adults perceive their risk of acquiring an STI as low. For this reason, hormonal contraceptives and long-acting reversible contraceptives are more commonly used by young sexually active people than are condoms, even though such contraceptives do not protect against STIs (Shannon et al., 2018). For Indigenous youth, lower rates of condom use can also be attributed to the legacy of colonialism, in disrupting the family bonds required

for effective intergenerational sexual health education (Hackett et al., 2020). Condom use is highest among young adults, those with higher levels of education, people belonging to an equity-seeking group, and individuals who self-report as being single (Fetner et al., 2020).

Adults over the age of 50 years have been found to have low levels of condom use (McKay et al., 2017). Current STI education and prevention messaging tends to target a younger audience, reinforcing the perception among older persons that their STI risk is low. Sexual health concerns, including education and prevention, are not routinely discussed with older persons and the interprofessional health team member, despite common changes in relationship status in this life stage (separation, divorce, widowhood) that may lead to the formation of new sexual relationships and concomitant risks. Assumptions by health care providers that these patients are not engaging in high-risk sexual behaviours also lowers the likelihood that they will be screened for STIs (PHAC, 2015b), which leads to further spread of these diseases amongst sexually active older persons.

The more commonly diagnosed STIs are discussed in this chapter. Human immunodeficiency virus (HIV) infection and related conditions are discussed in Chapter 17. Hepatitis B and C infection and related conditions are discussed in Chapter 46.

BACTERIAL INFECTIONS

GONORRHEA

Gonorrhea is the second-most frequently occurring STI. Between 2007 and 2016, the rate of reported cases of gonorrhea in Canada increased by 81%, from 36.1 to 65.4 per 100 000 (PHAC, 2019). Although rates of gonorrhea increased in both sexes and across all age groups (23 708 cases reported in 2016), a greater relative rate increase was observed among females (PHAC, 2019). Continued monitoring for antimicrobial resistance is important to prevent the spread of medication-resistant gonorrhea and to ensure successful cure rates for this treatable infection. Most provinces and territories have enacted laws that permit examination and treatment of minors without parental consent.

Etiology and Pathophysiology

Gonorrhea is caused by *Neisseria gonorrhoeae*, a Gram-negative diplococcus bacterium. The infection is spread by direct physical contact with an infected host, usually during sexual activity (vaginal, oral, or anal). Mucosal tissues in the genitalia including the urethra, cervix, rectum, and oropharynx are especially sensitive to gonococcal infection. Newborns can develop gonorrhea during delivery from an infected birth parent. The delicate gonococcus is easily killed by drying, heating, or washing with an antiseptic solution. As a consequence, indirect transmission by instruments or linens is rare.

The incubation period is 3 to 8 days. The disease confers no immunity to subsequent reinfection. Gonorrhea elicits an inflammatory response that, if left untreated, leads to the formation of fibrous tissue and adhesions, which increase a patient's risk of experiencing an ectopic pregnancy (PHAC, 2020).

Clinical Manifestations

The initial site of infection in cis-gender men and nonoperative trans women is usually the urethra. Symptoms of urethritis consist of dysuria and profuse, purulent urethral discharge that develops 2 to 5 days after infection (Figure 55.1). The testicles may also become painful or swollen. Patients generally seek medical evaluation early in the infection because their symptoms are usually obvious and distressing. It is unusual for these patients with gonorrhea to be asymptomatic (PHAC, 2021).

Most cis-gender women and nonoperative trans men who contract gonorrhea are asymptomatic or have minor symptoms that are often overlooked. Some patients may experience vaginal discharge, dysuria, menstruation changes, or frequency of urination. After the incubation period, redness and swelling occur at the site of contact, which is usually the cervix or the urethra (Figure 55.2). A greenish-yellow purulent exudate often develops, with a potential for abscess formation. The infection may remain local or can spread by direct tissue extension to the uterus, fallopian tubes, and ovaries. Although the vulva and the vagina are uncommon sites for a gonorrheal infection, they may become involved when little or no estrogen is present, as is the case in prepubertal children, people taking testosterone, and postmenopausal individuals.

Anorectal gonorrhea is usually caused by anal intercourse. Symptoms may include rectal pain, pruritus, and mucopurulent anal discharge. Ulceration and erythema of the anus may be seen on inspection. In a small percentage of individuals, gonococcal pharyngitis results from orogenital sexual contact. Symptoms may include a painful, burning sensation in the throat or difficulty swallowing. Most patients with rectal infections and infections in the throat have few symptoms.

Complications

Complications for cis-gender men and nonoperative trans women that can occur include prostatitis, urethral strictures, and sterility from orchitis or epididymitis. Because cis-gender women and trans men without symptoms seldom seek treatment, complications are more common and usually constitute the reason for seeking medical attention. Pelvic inflammatory disease (PID), Bartholin abscess, ectopic pregnancy, chronic pelvic pain, and infertility are the main complications of gonorrhea that this population experiences. A small percentage of infected people may develop disseminated gonococcal infection (DGI). In DGI, the appearance of skin lesions, fever, arthralgia, arthritis, or endocarditis usually causes the patient to seek medical help.

Eye Infections in Newborns. Infants with untreated gonorrheal infection develop permanent blindness. Most provinces and territories require the instillation of a prophylactic medication such as erythromycin or tetracycline into the eyes of all newborns as a precaution (Perry et al., 2017). Gonococcal eye

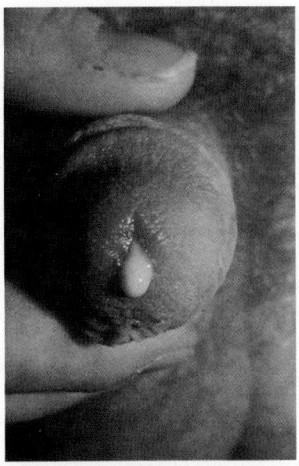

FIG. 55.1 Profuse, purulent drainage in a patient with gonorrhea. Source: Marx, K., Walls, R., & Hockberger, R. (2010). *Rosen's emergency medicine: Concepts and clinical practice* (7th ed.). Mosby.

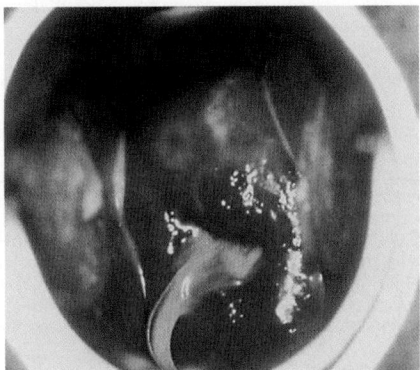

FIG. 55.2 Endocervical gonorrhea. Cervical redness and edema with discharge. Source: Morse, S., Moreland, A., & Holmes, K. (Eds.). (1996). *Atlas of sexually transmitted diseases and AIDS*. Mosby-Wolfe.

infections in newborns (ophthalmia neonatorum) are therefore relatively rare today.

Diagnostic Studies

For cis-gender men and nonoperative trans women, a presumptive diagnosis of gonorrhea is made if the client has a history of sexual contact with a new or infected partner followed within a few days by a urethral discharge. Typical clinical manifestations, combined with a positive finding in a Gram-stained smear of the purulent discharge from the penis, give an almost certain diagnosis. A culture of the discharge is indicated for clients whose smears are negative in the presence of strong clinical evidence. The nucleic acid amplification test (NAAT) (using ligase or polymerase chain reaction) is a nonculture test with sensitivity similar to that of culture tests for *N. gonorrhoeae* and can be done on a wide variety of samples, including vaginal, endocervical, urethral, and urine specimens (PHAC, 2017a).

Diagnosing gonorrhea in cis-gender women and trans men on the basis of symptoms is difficult because most infected clients are symptom-free or have symptoms that may be confused with other conditions. Smears and purulent discharge do not establish a diagnosis of gonorrhea because their genitourinary tract normally harbours a large number of organisms that resemble *N. gonorrhoeae*. A culture must be performed to confirm the diagnosis. Although the cervix is the most common

TABLE 55.3 INTERPROFESSIONAL CARE

Gonorrhea

Diagnostic
- History and physical examination
- Gram-stained smears of urethral or endocervical exudate
- Cultures for *Neisseria gonorrhoeae*
- NAAT to detect *N. gonorrhoeae*
- Testing for other STIs (syphilis, HIV, chlamydial infection)

Interprofessional Therapy
Medication Therapy
- Uncomplicated gonorrheal infections:
  - Ceftriaxone 250 mg IM in a single dose (preferred) plus azithromycin (Zithromax) 1 g PO in a single dose
  - Cefixime (Suprax) 800 mg PO in a single dose plus azithromycin (Zithromax) 1 g PO in a single dose OR
  - Alternate treatment with azithromycin (Zithromax) 2 g PO in a single dose

Other
- Also treated for chlamydial infection, unless a *Chlamydia* test result is available and negative
- Gonococcal infections reportable to the public health department in all provinces and territories
- Treatment of sexual contacts
- Instruction on abstinence from sexual intercourse and alcohol during treatment
- Re-examination if symptoms persist or recur after completion of treatment

HIV, human immunodeficiency virus; *IM,* intramuscularly; *PO,* by mouth (per os); *NAAT,* nucleic acid amplification test; *STI,* sexually transmitted infection.
Source: Modified from Centers for Disease Control and Prevention. (2015). Sexually transmitted diseases treatment guidelines, 2015. *Morbidity and Mortality Weekly Report, 64*(3), 1–138. http://www.cdc.gov/std/tg2015/tg-2015-print.pdf and from Public Health Agency of Canada. (2013, updated 2016). *Canadian guidelines on sexually transmitted infections.* http://www.phac-aspc.gc.ca/std-mts/sti-its/cgsti-ldcits/section-5-6-eng.php

site of sampling, specimens for culture may also be taken from the urethra, anus, or oropharynx. A urine specimen can reveal gonorrhea if it is present in the cervix or urethra.

Interprofessional Care

Interprofessional care for the patient with a gonorrheal infection is presented in Table 55.3.

Medication Therapy. Because of a short incubation period and high infectivity, treatment is generally instituted before culture results are available, even in the absence of any signs or symptoms. *N. gonorrhoeae* now shows resistance to six previously recommended treatment options: sulphonamides, penicillins, earlier-generation cephalosporins, tetracyclines, macrolides, and fluoroquinolones (Bodie et al., 2019). Unfortunately, strains with decreased susceptibility to cephalosporins and resistance to azithromycin are also on the rise in Canada, posing a threat to current treatment options (Choudhri et al., 2018b). Patients with coexisting syphilis are likely to be treated with the same medications used for gonorrhea.

All sexual contacts of patients with gonorrhea must be examined and treated to prevent reinfection after resumption of sexual relations. The "ping-pong" effect of re-exposure, treatment, and reinfection can cease only when infected partners are treated simultaneously. In addition, the patient should be counselled to abstain from sexual intercourse and alcohol during treatment. Sexual intercourse allows the infection to spread and can delay complete healing, and alcohol has an irritant effect on the healing urethral walls. Caution patients against squeezing

the penis to look for further discharge as this can also delay healing. Reinfection, rather than treatment failure, is the main cause for infections identified after treatment has ended.

SYPHILIS

The incidence of syphilis steadily increased in Canada by 178% between 2007 and 2016, from 3.8 to 10.6 per 100 000 (PHAC, 2019). During this same time frame, rates increased among males by 192% and increased among females by 75%, and the rate of reported cases of infectious syphilis in males was markedly higher than that in females (19.5 as compared to 1.7 per 100 000) (PHAC, 2019). In males, rates of infectious syphilis were highest among those 25 to 29 years of age; in females, rates were highest among those age 20 to 24 years. In 2016, infectious syphilis rates varied geographically, with the highest rates occurring in Nunavut (PHAC, 2019).

Etiology and Pathophysiology

Syphilis is caused by *Treponema pallidum,* a spirochete. This bacterium is thought to enter the body through very small breaks in the skin or mucous membranes. Its entry is facilitated by the minor abrasions that often occur during vaginal, oral, or anal sexual intercourse. Syphilis is a complex disease in which many organs and tissues of the body can become infected with *T. pallidum.* The infection causes the production of antibodies that also react with normal tissues. Not all people who are exposed to syphilis acquire the disease. In about one third of cases, infection is acquired after intercourse with an infected person; in addition to sexual contact, syphilis may be spread through contact with infectious lesions and sharing of needles among people who use intravenous (IV) drugs.

T. pallidum is extremely fragile and easily destroyed by drying, heating, or washing. The incubation period for syphilis ranges from 10 to 90 days (average 21 days) (HealthLinkBC, 2020). In congenital syphilis, the infection is usually transmitted to the fetus in utero from the infected pregnant parent but the newborn can also be infected by contact with an active genital lesion during delivery. When a pregnant person has infectious syphilis, they are at high risk for miscarriage, still birth, or the death of a newborn. Universal screening of pregnant people has remained the standard of care in Canada in most jurisdictions (PHAC, 2020a).

People at high risk for acquiring syphilis are also at an increased risk for acquiring HIV infection. The presence of syphilitic lesions on the genitalia enhances HIV transmission. HIV-infected patients with syphilis appear to be at greatest risk for clinically significant central nervous system (CNS) involvement and may require more intensive treatment with penicillin than other patients with syphilis do, as well as closer and longer-term follow-up. The treatment failure rate is higher in HIV-positive patients with syphilis than in HIV-negative patients who acquire syphilis (Choudhri et al., 2018c). Therefore, the assessment of all patients with syphilis should also include testing for HIV (with consent). Conversely, patients with HIV should be tested at least annually for syphilis.

Clinical Manifestations

Syphilis has a variety of signs and symptoms that can mimic those of several other diseases, which makes it harder to recognize. If it is not diagnosed and treated, specific clinical stages occur with the progression of syphilis, which are summarized in Table 55.4 and shown in Figures 55.3, 55.4, and 55.5.

TABLE 55.4 STAGES OF SYPHILIS

Manifestations	Communicability	Manifestations	Communicability
Primary Chancre (painless indurated lesion of penis, vulva, lips, mouth, vagina, and rectum) (see Figure 55.3) occurs 3 to 90 days after inoculation Regional lymphadenopathy (draining of the microorganisms into the lymph nodes) Genital ulcers *Duration of stage:* 3–8 wk	Exudate from chancre highly infectious; blood is infectious Most infectious stage, but transmission can occur at any stage if there are moist lesions	**Latent** Absence of signs or symptoms Diagnosis based on positive specific treponemal antibody test together with normal CSF and absence of clinical manifestations *Duration of stage:* Throughout life or progression to late stage	Noninfectious after 4 yr; possible placental transmission Almost 25% of persons with latent syphilis develop late syphilis, in some cases many years later.
Secondary Occurs a few weeks after chancre appears Systemic manifestations: flulike symptoms (e.g., malaise, fever, sore throat, headaches, fatigue, arthralgia, headache, generalized adenopathy) Cutaneous lesions bilateral; symmetrical rash that begins on the trunk and involves the palms and soles (see Figure 55.4); mucous patches in the mouth, tongue, or cervix; *Condylomata lata* (moist, weeping papules) in the anal and genital area Weight loss, alopecia *Duration of stage:* 1–2 yr	Exudate from skin and mucous membrane lesions highly infectious	**Late (Tertiary)*** Appearance 3–20 yr after initial infection Gummas (chronic, destructive lesions affecting any organ of the body, especially skin, bone, liver, mucous membranes) (see Figure 55.5) *Cardiovascular:* Aneurysms, aortic valve insufficiency, aortitis *Neurosyphilis:* General paresis (personality changes from minor to extreme [psychosis], tremors, physical and mental deterioration), tabes dorsalis (ataxia, areflexia, paresthesias, lightning pains, damaged joints [Charcot's joints]), speech disturbances *Duration of stage:* Chronic (without treatment), possibly fatal	Noninfectious Spinal fluid possibly containing organism

*Several forms such as cardiovascular syphilis and neurosyphilis occur together in approximately 25% of untreated cases.
CSF, cerebrospinal fluid.

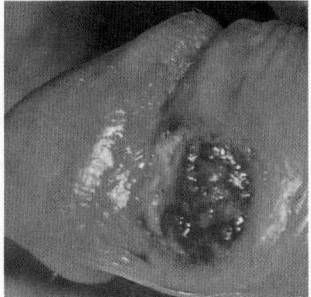

FIG. 55.3 Primary syphilis chancre. Source: Forbes, C. D., & Jackson, W. F. (2003). *Color atlas and text of clinical medicine.* (3rd ed.). Mosby.

Complications

Complications of syphilis occur mostly in the late stage of the disease. The gummas of benign late syphilis may produce irreparable damage to bone, liver, or skin but seldom result in death. In cardiovascular syphilis, the resulting aneurysm may press on structures such as the intercostal nerves, causing pain. The possibility of a rupture rises as the aneurysm increases in size. Scarring of the aortic valve results in aortic valve insufficiency and, eventually, heart failure.

Neurosyphilis causes degeneration of the brain with mental deterioration (Choudhri et al., 2018c). Conditions related to sensory nerve involvement are a result of tabes dorsalis (progressive locomotor ataxia). There may be sudden attacks of pain anywhere in the body, which can confuse the diagnosis with other conditions. Loss of vision and sense of position in the feet

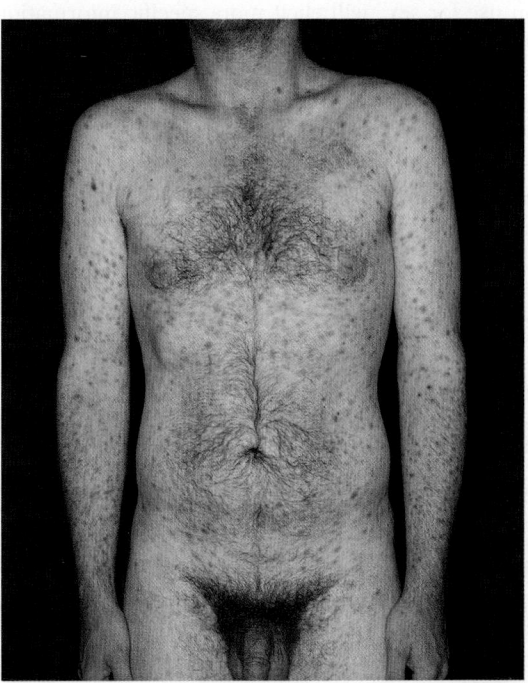

FIG. 55.4 Secondary syphilis. Bilateral, symmetrical cutaneous lesions. Source: Habif, T. (2004). *Clinical dermatology: A color guide to diagnosis and therapy* (4th ed., p. 319, Figure 10-9). Mosby.

and legs can also occur. Walking may become even more difficult as joint stability is lost. (Neurosyphilis is also discussed in Chapter 63.)

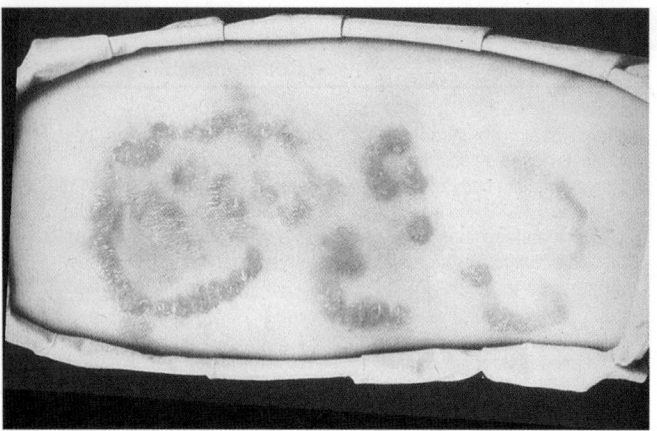

FIG. 55.5 Destructive skin gummas associated with tertiary syphilis. Source: Cohen, J., & Powderly, W. G. (2004). *Infectious diseases* (2nd ed.). Mosby.

TABLE 55.5 **INTERPROFESSIONAL CARE**	
Syphilis	
Diagnostic	**Interprofessional Therapy**

• History and physical examination
• Dark-field microscopy
• Nontreponemal or treponemal (or both) serological testing
• Testing for other STIs (HIV infection, gonorrhea, chlamydial infection)
	• Appropriate medication therapy (see Table 55.6)
	• Confidential counselling and testing for HIV infection
	• Case finding
	• Surveillance
	  • Repeat of quantitative nontreponemal tests at 6 and 12 months
	  • Examination of cerebrospinal fluid at 1 year if treatment involves alternative antibiotics or treatment failure has occurred

HIV, human immunodeficiency virus; *STIs*, sexually transmitted infections.

Diagnostic Studies

The first step in the diagnosis of syphilis is to obtain a detailed and accurate sexual history. Chapter 53 provides some guidelines for taking a sexual health history, as well as examples of sexual health history questions in Table 53.7.

When taking a sexual history, it is important that the nurse not make any assumptions about a person's gender identity, sexual orientation, or sexual practices. Care should be taken to use the individual's preferred terminology when referring to different parts of their body. Questions related to STI risk should use inclusive language that will capture the broad spectrum of sexual practices (Poteat, 2016). Asking "What parts of your body do you use for sex" will elicit more specific information than "Do you have sex with men or women or both?" Similarly, asking "What parts of your body, if any, do you insert into another person's body?" and "What parts of another person's body, if any, are inserted into your body?" minimizes the chance of miscommunication. A physical examination should be done to identify any suspicious lesions or other significant signs and symptoms.

Moreover, when completing a sexual health history and related physical examination, it is critical that the nurse take a trauma-informed approach. This involves recognizing that many individuals have experienced emotional, psychological, physical, or sexual violence, memories of which may be triggered during a sexual health examination. This is particularly true for Indigenous patients, who remain deeply affected by the legacy of colonialism, including the Indian hospitals, the residential school system, the sixties scoop, the forced sterilization program, and the millennium scoop. It is critical that the nurse is understanding and responsive to the impact of trauma on patients, emphasizing physical and psychological safety by explaining why they are asking what they are asking, informing patients about what they are going to do before they do it, collaborating on ways to do parts of the examination so that the patient feels safer, and building on the patient's strengths and skills (PHAC, 2020c).

A clinical diagnosis of syphilis can be confirmed by the presence of spirochetes on dark-field microscopic examination and direct fluorescent antibody (DFA) tests of lesion exudate or tissue. However, syphilis is more commonly diagnosed through a serological test. Tests for syphilis may be classified as those performed for screening and those performed for confirmation of a positive screening result. Nonspecific antitreponemal antibodies can be detected by tests such as the Venereal Disease Research Laboratory (VDRL) test and the rapid plasma reagin (RPR) test. These nontreponemal tests are suitable for screening purposes and usually yield positive results 10 to 14 days after the appearance of a chancre. The fluorescent treponemal antibody absorption (FTA-ABS) test and the *T. pallidum* particle agglutination (TP-PA) test detect specific antitreponemal antibodies and are suitable for confirming the diagnosis.

False-negative and false-positive results do occur with the nontreponemal tests (VDRL, RPR). A false-negative result may be obtained during primary syphilis if the test is performed before the individual has had time to produce antibodies. A false-positive finding may occur after smallpox vaccination or with other diseases or conditions such as hepatitis, infectious mononucleosis, collagen diseases (e.g., systemic lupus erythematosus), pregnancy, or aging. Positive nontreponemal test results should be confirmed by more specific treponemal tests to rule out other causes. In the cerebrospinal fluid (CSF), changes such as increased white blood cell count, increased total protein levels, and a positive result of the treponemal antibody test are diagnostic of asymptomatic neurosyphilis.

If a patient is treated with antibiotics early in the course of the disease on the basis of the history and the symptoms, the serological test may not indicate the presence of syphilis. Once a patient has positive serological findings for syphilis, indicating the presence of antibodies, these findings may remain positive for an indefinite period despite successful treatment.

Interprofessional Care

Medication Therapy. Management of syphilis is aimed at eradication of all syphilitic organisms (Table 55.5). However, treatment cannot reverse damage that is already present in the late stage of the disease. Benzathine penicillin G remains the treatment of choice for all stages of syphilis (Government of Canada, 2019). Therapy for the various stages of syphilis that is in accordance with national STI guidelines provided by the PHAC (2016) is described in Table 55.6. All stages of syphilis should be treated. When symptoms are chronic or recur after medication therapy has ended, the patient should undergo repeated treatment. All patients with neurosyphilis must be carefully monitored, with periodic serological testing, clinical evaluation at 6-month intervals, and repeat CSF examinations for at least 3 years. It is also very important that all sexual contacts in the previous 90 days be treated.

TABLE 55.6   MEDICATION THERAPY

Syphilis

Stage	Preferred Treatment	Alternative Treatment*
All nonpregnant adults: • Primary syphilis • Secondary syphilis • Early latent syphilis (<1 yr duration)	Benzathine penicillin G (Bicillin L-A) 2.4 million units IM in a single dose	• Doxycycline (Vibramycin) 100 mg PO BID for 14 days • Alternate agent (to be used in exceptional circumstances)—ceftriaxone 1 g IV or IM daily for 10 days
All nonpregnant adults • Late latent syphilis • Latent syphilis of unknown duration • Cardiovascular syphilis and other tertiary syphilis not involving central nervous system	Benzathine penicillin G (Bicillin L-A) three doses of 2.4 million units each, IM, at 1-wk intervals (total dose, 7.2 million units)	• Consider penicillin desensitization • Doxycycline (Vibramycin) 100 mg PO BID for 28 days • Alternate agent (to be used in exceptional circumstances)—ceftriaxone 1 g IV or IM daily for 10 days
All adults • Neurosyphilis	Penicillin G 3-4 million units every 4 hr IV for 10–14 days (total dose, 16–24 million units)	• Strongly consider penicillin desensitization followed by treatment with penicillin • Ceftriaxone 2 g IV or IM daily for 10–14 days

*Given when penicillin is contraindicated.
BID, twice a day; *IM,* intramuscularly; *IV,* intravenously; *PO,* by mouth (per os).
Source: © All rights reserved. *Canadian Guidelines on Sexually Transmitted Infections.* Public Health Agency of Canada, 2013. Adapted and reproduced with permission from the Minister of Health, 2017.

MEDICATION ALERT—Benzathine penicillin G (Bicillin L-A)
• Reports from some jurisdictions have indicated inappropriate use of short-acting benzylpenicillin (penicillin G) intramuscularly for the treatment of infectious syphilis rather than long-acting benzathine penicillin G (Bicillin L-A) (PHAC, 2016).
• Nurses need to be aware of the similar names of these two products to prevent and avoid inappropriate and inadequate treatment.

To treat syphilis during pregnancy, benzathine penicillin G, 2.4 million units intramuscularly weekly for one to three doses, is administered, depending on the stage of syphilis. Treatment administered in the second half of pregnancy may pose a risk for premature labour and fetal distress. Pregnant individuals receiving treatment should be advised to seek medical care if fetal movements decrease.

CHLAMYDIAL INFECTIONS

Chlamydial infections are the most prevalent bacterial STI in Canada today, with 121 244 cases reported in 2016, 60% of which occurred in women. However, between 2007 and 2016, chlamydia rates for men rose faster than for women, with a 69% increase compared to a 40% increase, respectively. In 2016, 76% of the total reported cases were among those in the age groups between 15 and 29 years (PHAC, 2019). Underreporting is substantial because most infected people have no symptoms and therefore do not seek testing. Untreated chlamydial infections are a major contributor to epididymoorchitis, PID, ectopic pregnancy, and infertility (Choudhri et al., 2018a).

Etiology and Pathophysiology

Chlamydial infections are caused by *Chlamydia trachomatis,* a Gram-negative bacterium, and can be transmitted during penetrative vaginal, anal, or oral sex. Numerous different serotypes, or strains, of *C. trachomatis* cause urogenital infections (e.g., nongonococcal urethritis [NGU] and cervicitis), ocular trachoma, and lymphogranuloma venereum. Because of the high prevalence of asymptomatic infections, screening of populations at high risk is needed to identify persons who are infected (see the Evidence-Informed Practice box).

EVIDENCE-INFORMED PRACTICE

Research Highlight

Would Home-Based Strategies Improve Screening Rates for Chlamydial and Gonorrheal Infections?
Clinical Question
In sexually active people (P), what is the effect of home-based specimen collection (I) versus clinic-based specimen collection (C) on screening rates for *Chlamydia trachomatis* or *Neisseria gonorrhoeae* (O)?

Best Available Evidence
Cochrane systematic review of randomized controlled trials (RCTs)

Critical Appraisal and Synthesis of Evidence
• Ten trials (N = 1 566) in which people were invited either to collect specimens at home or to attend a clinic for collection of specimens
• There was no evidence of a difference between home-based and clinic-based specimen collection in the proportion of people who completed testing, diagnosis, and treatment.
• A lower number of participants diagnosed in the home-based compared with the clinic-based group was found.

Conclusion
• Home-based specimen collection could result in similar levels of index case management for *Chlamydia trachomatis* or *Neisseria gonorrhoeae* infection when compared with clinic-based specimen collection.

Implications for Nursing Practice
• Chlamydial and gonorrheal infections are common and often asymptomatic.
• To increase screening rates, interventions should be tailored to meet patient needs and preferences, which may include home-based specimen collection.

Reference for Evidence
Fajardo-Bernal, L., Aponte-Gonzalez, J., Vigil, P., et al. (2015). Home-based versus clinic-based specimen collection in the management of *Chlamydia trachomatis* and *Neisseria gonorrhoeae* infections. *Cochrane Database of Systematic Reviews,* Issue 9, Art. No.: CD011317. doi:10.1002/14651858.CD011317.pub2.

P, patient population of interest; *I,* intervention or area of interest; *C,* comparison of interest or comparison group; *O,* outcomes of interest (see Chapter 1).

Clinical Manifestations and Complications

Chlamydial infection is known as a silent disease because symptoms may be absent or minor in most infected people (Choudhri et al., 2018a). Signs and symptoms in cis-gender men and nonoperative trans women include urethritis (dysuria, urethral discharge), epididymitis (unilateral scrotal pain, swelling, tenderness, fever), and proctitis (rectal discharge and pain during defecation). In cis-gender women and nonoperative trans men, signs and symptoms include cervicitis (mucopurulent discharge, hypertrophic ectopy [area that is edematous and bleeds easily]), urethritis (dysuria, frequent urination, pyuria), bartholinitis (purulent exudate), dyspareunia (pain with intercourse), and menstrual abnormalities.

Complications often develop when chlamydial infections are poorly managed, inaccurately diagnosed, or undiagnosed. Because chlamydial infections are closely associated with gonococcal infections, clinical differentiation may be difficult. Therefore, both infections are usually treated concurrently, even without diagnostic confirmation. The incubation period of 1 to 3 weeks for chlamydial infection is longer than that for gonorrhea, and the symptoms are often milder. If a pregnant individual has chlamydia, their baby may be born prematurely, have eye infections, or develop pneumonia (Choudhri et al., 2018a).

In cis-gender men and nonoperative trans women, epididymitis can lead to rare complications, including abscess, sepsis, and infertility. In cis-gender women and nonoperative trans men, chlamydial infections may result in PID and scarring of the fallopian tubes, which can result in infertility and a higher risk for ectopic or tubal pregnancies (Choudhri et al., 2018a).

Diagnostic Studies and Interprofessional Care

Chlamydial infections can be diagnosed by ruling out gonorrhea. The cervical and urethral discharge in chlamydial infections appears to be less purulent, less watery, and less painful than in gonorrhea. Culture is the preferred method of diagnosis for medicolegal purposes, and culture is recommended for throat specimens (PHAC, 2017b). NAATs are more sensitive and more specific than culture, enzyme immunoassay, and DFA assay. For nonmedicolegal purposes, NAATs should be used whenever possible for urine and for urethral or cervical specimens.

Medication Therapy. When diagnosed, chlamydial infection can be easily treated and cured. Chlamydial infections respond to treatment with doxycycline or azithromycin, with erythromycin or ofloxacin used as an alternative treatment regimen (PHAC, 2017b). Follow-up care should include advising the patient to return if the symptoms persist or recur, treatment of sex partners, and encouraging the use of condoms during all sexual contacts. The high incidence of recurrence may be due to failure to treat the sexual partners of infected people.

> **MEDICATION ALERT—Doxycycline**
> - Patients on this medication should avoid unnecessary exposure to sunlight.
> - Patients should not take this medication with antacids, iron products, or dairy products.

VIRAL INFECTIONS

GENITAL HERPES

Genital herpes is not a reportable infection in most provinces and territories, except the Atlantic provinces. The annual incidence of genital herpes in Canada is, therefore, not known.

Worldwide, 500 million people are estimated to have the herpes simplex virus (HSV) infection (PHAC, 2020b).

Etiology and Pathophysiology

Genital herpes is a sexually transmitted infection caused by the HSV, usually type 2 (HSV-2). The virus enters through the mucous membranes or breaks in the skin during contact with an infected person (Figure 55.6). HSV then reproduces inside the cell and spreads to the surrounding cells. The virus next enters the peripheral or autonomic nerve endings and ascends to the sensory or autonomic nerve ganglion, where it often becomes dormant. Viral reactivation (recurrence) may occur when the virus descends to the initial site of infection, either the mucous membranes or the skin. When a person is infected with HSV, the infection is usually chronic within the individual for life. Transmission occurs through direct contact with skin or mucous membrane or through asymptomatic viral shedding (PHAC, 2020b).

Two different strains of HSV cause infection. In general, HSV type 1 (HSV-1) causes infection above the waist, involving the gingivae, the dermis, the upper respiratory tract, and the CNS. HSV-2 most frequently causes infection of the genital tract and the perineum. However, either strain can cause disease on the mouth or the genitals. The incidence and prevalence of HSV-1 genital infection are increasing globally, particularly among college students. The majority of genital herpes cases, however, are caused by HSV-2 infection (PHAC, 2020b).

Clinical Manifestations

In the primary (initial) episode of genital herpes, the individual may experience burning, itching, or tingling at the site of inoculation. Multiple small, vesicular, and sometimes painless lesions may appear on the inner thigh, penis, scrotum, vulva, perineum, perianal region, vagina, or cervix (Groves, 2016) and contain large quantities of infectious viral particles (Figure 55.7). The lesions rupture and form shallow, moist ulcerations. Finally, crusting and epithelialization of the erosions occur. Primary infections tend to be associated with local inflammation and pain, accompanied by systemic manifestations such as fever, headache, malaise, myalgia, and regional lymphadenopathy.

Urination may be painful from the urine touching active lesions. Urinary retention may occur as a result of HSV urethritis or cystitis. A purulent vaginal discharge may develop with HSV cervicitis. The duration of symptoms is longer and the frequency of complications is greater in women. Primary lesions are generally present for 17 to 20 days, but new lesions sometimes continue to develop for 6 weeks. The lesions heal spontaneously unless secondary infection occurs.

Recurrent genital herpes occurs in about 50 to 80% of individuals during the year after the primary episode. Stress, fatigue, sunburn, general illness, immunosuppression, and menses are commonly noted triggers. Many patients can predict a recurrence by noticing the early prodrome symptoms of tingling, burning, and itching at the site where the lesions will eventually appear (CATIE, 2016). The symptoms of recurrent episodes are less severe, and the lesions usually heal within 8 to 12 days. With time, the lesions generally recur less frequently.

Complications

Although most infections are of a relatively benign nature, complications of genital herpes may involve the CNS, causing aseptic meningitis and lower motor neuron damage. Neuron damage may result in atonic bladder, erectile dysfunction, and

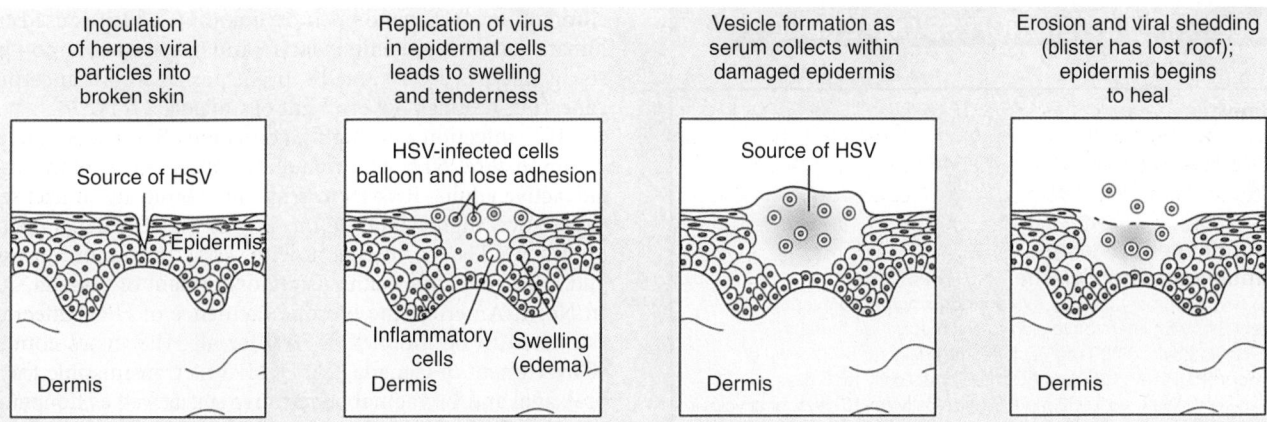

| Inoculation of herpes viral particles into broken skin | Replication of virus in epidermal cells leads to swelling and tenderness | Vesicle formation as serum collects within damaged epidermis | Erosion and viral shedding (blister has lost roof); epidermis begins to heal |

FIG. 55.6 Stages of infection with herpes simplex virus (HSV). Source: Morse, S., Moreland, A., & Holmes, K. (Eds.). (1996). *Atlas of sexually transmitted diseases and AIDS*. Mosby-Wolfe.

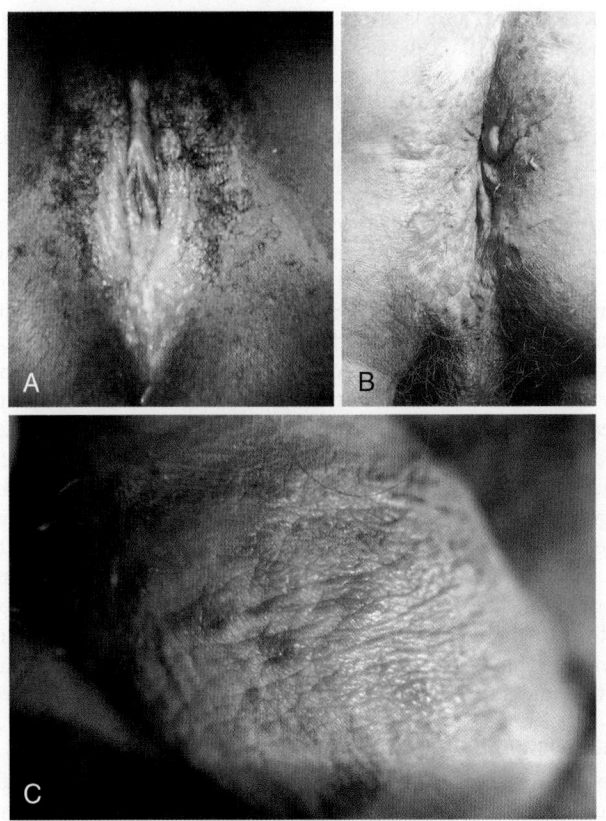

FIG. 55.7 Unruptured vesicles of herpes simplex virus type 2 (HSV-2). **A,** Vulvar area. **B,** Perianal area. **C,** Penile herpes simplex, ulcerative stage. Sources: *A* and *C*, From the Centers for Disease Control and Prevention; courtesy Susan Lindsley. *B,* From Morse, S., Moreland, A., & Holmes, K. (Eds.). (1996). *Atlas of sexually transmitted diseases and AIDS*. Mosby-Wolfe.

constipation. Another complication is *autoinoculation* of the virus to extragenital sites such as the lips, the breasts, and, most commonly, the fingers (herpetic whitlow).

Herpes Simplex Virus Infection During Pregnancy. Pregnant individuals with a primary episode of HSV near the time of delivery have the highest risk of transmitting genital herpes to the newborn (Groves, 2016). The risk for transmission is lowest for individuals who acquire HSV early in the pregnancy or have a history of recurrent HSV. An active genital lesion at the time of delivery is usually an indication for Caesarean delivery because most infections in newborns occur during birth (Groves, 2016).

Diagnostic Studies and Interprofessional Care

A diagnosis of genital herpes is usually based on the patient's symptoms and history. The diagnosis can be confirmed through isolation of the virus from active lesions by means of tissue culture, or through polymerase chain reaction assay, which is four times more sensitive than HSV culture and is 100% specific (PHAC, 2017a). Other techniques to detect HSV include direct immunofluorescence, enzyme immunoassay, and DNA amplification. These tests enable more rapid identification of HSV than a culture does. Highly accurate serological methods for detecting the HSV type are available (PHAC, 2017a).

It is important to encourage symptomatic treatment, such as using good genital hygiene and wearing loose-fitting cotton undergarments. The lesions should be kept clean and dry. To ensure complete drying of the perineal area, women may use a hair dryer set on a cool setting. Frequent sitz baths may soothe the area and reduce inflammation. Drying agents such as colloidal oatmeal (Aveeno) and aluminum salts (Burow solution) may provide some relief from the burning and itching. Techniques to reduce pain on urination include pouring a pitcher of water onto the perineal area while voiding to dilute the urine, and voiding in a warm tub of water or shower. Pain may require a local anaesthetic such as lidocaine (Xylocaine) or systemic analgesics such as codeine, ibuprofen (Advil), acetaminophen (Tylenol), or a combination of these agents.

Sexual transmission of HSV can occur during asymptomatic periods, so the use of barrier methods, especially condoms and dental dams, should be encouraged. When lesions are present, the patient should avoid sexual activity altogether because even barrier protection is not satisfactory in eliminating infection transmission.

Medication Therapy. Three antiviral agents are available for the treatment of HSV: acyclovir (Zovirax), valacyclovir (Valtrex), and famciclovir (Famvir). These medications inhibit herpetic viral replication and are prescribed for primary and recurrent infections (Table 55.7). Acyclovir, valacyclovir, and famciclovir are also used to suppress frequent recurrences (more than six episodes per year). Although not a cure, these medications shorten the duration of viral shedding and the healing time of genital lesions and reduce outbreaks by over 60% (Groves, 2016). Continued use of oral acyclovir as suppressive therapy for up to 6 years is safe and effective. Adverse

TABLE 55.7 INTERPROFESSIONAL CARE
Genital Herpes

Diagnostic
- History and physical examination
- Antibody assay for specific HSV viral type
- Viral isolation by tissue culture

Interprofessional Therapy
Treatment for First Episode
- For severe primary disease, IV acyclovir 5 mg/per kg over 60 min every 8 hr with later conversion to oral medication therapy
- Acyclovir (Zovirax) 200 mg PO five times daily for 5–10 days; or famciclovir (Famvir) 250 mg PO three times daily for 5 days; or valacyclovir (Valtrex) 1 000 mg PO twice daily for 10 days; or acyclovir 400 mg PO three times daily for 7–10 days (recommended by Centers for Disease Control and Prevention)

Treatment for Recurrent Episodes
- Acyclovir (Zovirax) 200 mg PO five times daily for 5 days or 800 mg PO three times daily for 2 days
- Valacyclovir (Valtrex) 500 mg PO twice daily or 1 g daily for 3 days; or famciclovir (Famvir) 125 mg PO twice daily for 5 days

Suppressive Therapy for Frequent Recurrence in Nonpregnant Patients
- Any of the treatments listed below:
  - Acyclovir (Zovirax) 200 mg PO three to five times daily or 400 mg PO twice daily
  - Famciclovir (Famvir) 250 mg PO twice daily
  - Valacyclovir (Valtrex) 500 mg PO daily (patients with ≤9 recurrences per year) or 1 000 mg PO daily (patients with >9 recurrences per year)

Other Considerations
- Abstinence from sexual contact while lesions are present; however, virus may be shed without lesions
- Annual Pap smear
- Confidential counselling and testing for HIV
- Identify trigger mechanisms
- Symptomatic care

HIV, human immunodeficiency virus; *HSV,* herpes simplex virus; *IV,* intravenously; *Pap,* Papanicolaou; *PO,* by mouth (per os).
Source: Modified from Public Health Agency of Canada. (2013). *Canadian guidelines on sexually transmitted infections. Section 5: Genital herpes simplex virus (HSV) infections.* http://www.phac-aspc.gc.ca/std-mts/sti-its/cgsti-ldcits/section-5-4-eng.php

reactions are mild and include headache, occasional nausea and vomiting, and diarrhea. The safety of these medications for treatment of pregnant women has not been established. Acyclovir ointment appears to have no clinical benefit in the treatment of recurrent lesions, either in speed of healing or in resolution of pain, and is not commonly recommended. IV acyclovir is reserved for severe or life-threatening infections in which hospitalization is required for the treatment of disseminated infections, CNS infections (meningitis), or pneumonitis. Nephrotoxicity has been observed with high-dose IV administration. Clinical trials are examining the effectiveness of a vaccine for HSV-2 (Chandra et al., 2019).

GENITAL HUMAN PAPILLOMA VIRUS INFECTIONS

Human papilloma virus (HPV) causes skin and mucosal infections and has a strong affinity for the moist mucosa of the anal, genital, and aerodigestive tracts. There are more than 130 types of the virus, many of which are sexually transmitted. Most types do not cause any symptoms and go away on their own. The most common low-risk genotypes are 6 and 11, which cause condylomata acuminata (genital warts), and the most common high-risk genotypes are 16 and 18, predisposing to precancerous or cancerous lesions (Government of Canada, 2021).

HPV infection is a highly contagious STI and is the most common viral STI; it is frequently observed in young, sexually active adults. Risk factors include young age at first sexual experience, higher lifetime number of sexual partners, history of other STIs, co-infection with HIV, immunosuppression, and tobacco or marijuana use (Government of Canada, 2021). In North America, the lifetime incidence of HPV infection is estimated to be more than 70% for all HPV types combined (Government of Canada, 2021). HPV is transmissible through oral, anal and/or vaginal penetrative sex as well as nonpenetrative sexual activity (such as digital vaginal/anal penetration and tribadism). The incubation period of the virus is generally 3 to 4 months but may be longer.

Prevention is hampered by a high proportion of asymptomatic infections and lack of curative treatment. In Canada, the reporting of HPV infection is not required.

Clinical Manifestations and Complications

The discussion here of clinical manifestations, complications, and care focuses on the low-risk HPV genotypes resulting in genital warts; cervical cancer is discussed in Chapter 56. Most people with HPV do not know that they are infected because they remain asymptomatic. Genital or anal warts are discrete single or multiple papillary growths that are white to grey and flesh-pink. They may grow and coalesce to form large, cauliflower-like masses. Most affected patients have from 1 to 10 genital warts. In cis-gender women and nonoperative trans men, the warts may be located on the vulva, in the vagina or the cervix, and in the perianal area. In cis-gender men and nonoperative trans women, the warts may occur on the penis and the scrotum, around the anus, or in the urethra (Figure 55.8). There are usually no other signs or symptoms. Itching may occur with anogenital warts. Bleeding on defecation may occur with anal warts.

During pregnancy, genital warts tend to grow rapidly and increase in size. An infected birth parent may transmit the condition to their newborn, but the risk of this is extremely low (Xiong et al., 2018). Caesarean delivery is not routinely indicated unless the birth canal becomes blocked by massive warts.

Diagnostic Studies and Interprofessional Care

Up to two thirds of the early lesions caused by HPV are undetectable by visual examination. Genital warts can be diagnosed on the basis of the gross appearance of the lesions. However, the warts may be confused with condylomata lata of secondary syphilis, carcinoma, or benign neoplasms. Several DNA and RNA tests are approved for use in Canada to determine HPV genotypes when required (PHAC, 2017a).

The primary goal in treating visible genital warts is the removal of symptomatic warts. The removal may or may not decrease infectivity. Genital warts are difficult to treat and often necessitate multiple office visits with a variety of treatment modalities. The therapy should be modified if a patient has not experienced improvement after three treatments or if after six treatments the warts have not completely disappeared. Treatment consists of chemical or ablative (removal with laser or electrocautery) methods. One common treatment is the use of 50 to 80% trichloroacetic acid (TCA) or bichloroacetic acid (BCA) solutions in 70% alcohol, applied directly to the wart

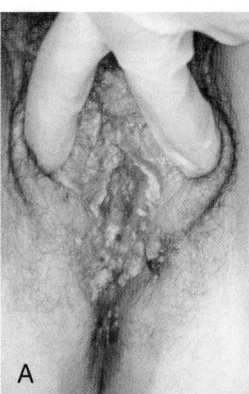 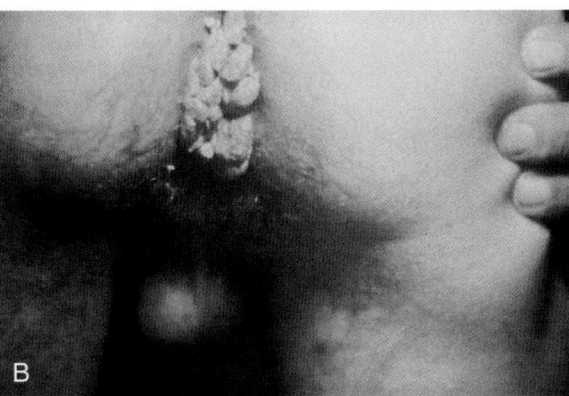 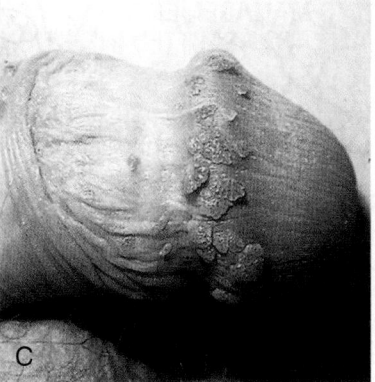

FIG. 55.8 Genital warts. **A,** Severe vulvar warts. **B,** Perineal wart. **C,** Multiple genital warts of the glans penis. Source: *A,* From the Centers for Disease Control and Prevention, courtesy Joe Millar. *B,* From the Centers for Disease Control and Prevention, courtesy Dr. Wiesner. *C,* From the Centers for Disease Control and Prevention, courtesy Susan Lindsley.

surface. Petroleum jelly is applied to the surrounding normal skin to minimize irritation before a small amount of TCA is applied to the wart with a cotton swab. A sharp, stinging pain is often felt with initial acid contact, but this quickly subsides. TCA is not washed off after treatment and is safe for use during pregnancy.

Topical treatments include imiquimod, podofilox/podophyllotoxin, podophyllin, sinecatechins, and TCA (PHAC, 2015a). With topical treatments it is important to avoid contact with mucosal tissue, eyes, tongue, lips, broken skin, and surrounding healthy skin, and patients should be instructed to refrain from sexual activity while undergoing treatment (PHAC, 2015a). Treatment may cause skin reactions such as itching, tenderness, erythema, and ulceration. TCA is the only treatment that is to be used with pregnant and lactating women (PHAC, 2015a). If topical treatments are not effective, over-the-counter, self-applied cryotherapy kits are available (PHAC, 2015a). Because treatment does not destroy the virus, merely the infected tissue, recurrences and reinfection are possible, and careful long-term follow-up is advised.

Human Papilloma Virus Immunization

HPV infection has been linked to cancers of the cervix, penis, anus, vagina, vulva, mouth, and oropharynx (PHAC, 2017a). There are currently three vaccines available to protect against HPV. A quadrivalent vaccine called Gardasil (HPV4) protects against HPV types 6, 11, 16, and 18. The bivalent vaccine called Cevarix (HPV2) offers protection against HPV types 16 and 18. A 9-valent vaccine called Gardasil 9 (HPV9) protects against HPV types 6, 11, 16, 18, 31, 33, 45, 52, and 58. Choice of vaccine depends on the goal of immunization. Canada's National Advisory Committee on Immunization currently recommends HPV2, HPV4, or HPV9 vaccine for all women aged 9 to 45 years of age, and HPV4 or HPV9 vaccine for all men aged 9 to 26 years (NACI, 2017). These vaccines are given in two or three intramuscular (IM) injections over a 6-month period and have few adverse effects. The most commonly reported adverse events following HPV vaccination are injection site pain, swelling or redness, and syncope (PHAC, 2017a). These vaccines do not treat active HPV infections. Ideally, they should be administered before the start of sexual activity to maximize their benefit, but people who are sexually active, as well as those who are infected, will still obtain protection from the HPV types they have not already acquired.

EVIDENCE-INFORMED PRACTICE
Translating Research Into Practice

F. C. (pronouns he/him) is a 19-year-old who is being seen in the health care centre for signs and symptoms of a urinary tract infection. When asked, F. C. shares with the nurse that he is sexually active. After reviewing the health history, the nurse learns that the patient has not received the human papilloma virus (HPV) vaccine. F. C. tells the nurse that the vaccine is not needed because his current partner has already gotten it.

Best Available Evidence	Clinician Expertise	Patient Preferences and Values
Males ages 9–26 years, including males who have sex with males, are advised to be vaccinated with one of the HPV vaccines available to reduce the incidence of penile, anal, and oropharyngeal cancers as well as genital warts. The majority of all HPV-associated cancers are caused by HPV types 16 or 18. Approximately 64% of invasive HPV-associated cancers are attributable to HPV 16 or 18.	Approximately 90% of anal cancers have been linked to HPV infection. Males may be unaware of the expanded recommendations for HPV vaccines, which were originally approved to prevent cervical, vulvar, and vaginal cancer caused by HPV types 6, 11, 16, and 18 in females ages 9 through 26 years.	F. C. states that he never has unprotected sex and does not like injections.

Implications for Nursing Practice
1. Why is it important to discuss the risk and benefits of the vaccine with F. C.?
2. If F. C. suggests the vaccine will not be effective because he's already sexually active, how should the nurse respond?
3. How can the nurse address F. C.'s dislike of injections?

Reference for Evidence

National Advisory Committee on Immunization (NACI). (2017). *Updated recommendations on human papillomavirus (HPV)vaccines: 9-valent HPV vaccine 2-dose immunization schedule and the use of HPV vaccines in immunocompromised populations.* https://www.canada.ca/content/dam/phac-aspc/documents/services/publications/healthy-living/updated-recommendations-human-papillomavirus-immunization-schedule-immunocompromised-populations/updated-recommendations-human-papillomavirus-immunization-schedule-immunocompromised-populationsv3-eng.pdf

NURSING MANAGEMENT
SEXUALLY TRANSMITTED INFECTIONS

NURSING ASSESSMENT

Subjective and objective data that should be obtained from a person with an STI are presented in Table 55.8.

NURSING DIAGNOSES

Nursing diagnoses for the patient with an STI include but are not limited to the following:

- *Potential for infection* resulting from insufficient knowledge to avoid exposure to pathogens (STI transmission, engaging in high-risk behaviours)
- *Anxiety* resulting from stressors, threat to current status (impact of condition on relationships, long-term effects of infection)
- *Reduced health maintenance* resulting from insufficient resources (lack of knowledge about disease process and transmission)

PLANNING

The overall goals are that the patient with an STI will (a) demonstrate understanding of the mode of transmission of STIs and the risk posed by STIs, (b) complete treatment and return for appropriate follow-up, (c) notify or assist in notification of sexual contacts about their need for testing and treatment, (d) abstain from intercourse until the infection is resolved, and (e) demonstrate knowledge of safer sex practices.

NURSING IMPLEMENTATION

HEALTH PROMOTION. Many approaches to curtailing the spread of STIs have been advocated and have met with varying degrees of success. Nurses should be prepared to discuss "safer" sex practices with all patients, not only those who are perceived to be at risk. These practices include abstinence, monogamy with an uninfected partner, engagement in low-risk sexual practices such as mutual masturbation, and use of barriers (e.g., dental dams, condoms) to limit contact with potentially infectious body fluids or lesions. Health promotion programs aimed at teaching condom use skills and improving communication and negotiation skills have been found to reduce the incidence of STIs by 30% (Petrova et al., 2015). A patient and caregiver teaching guide regarding the patient with an STI is presented in Table 55.9.

All sexually active cis-gender women and nonoperative trans men should be screened for cervical cancer using a Pap test. Individuals with a history of STIs are at greater risk for cervical cancer than those without this history. Anal Pap tests should also be done for all individuals who are recipients of anal sex. (Pap smears are discussed in Chapter 56.)

Measures to Prevent Infection. An inspection of the sexual partner's genitalia before intercourse is recommended. Discharge, sores, blisters, or rash should be viewed with concern. A person who is aware of specific signs and symptoms of infection can make the decision to continue the sexual interaction with modifications or elect not to have sexual relations. The person should remember that, when engaging in sex, there is exposure to the infections of everyone with whom the partner has ever had sex. Cis-gender men and nonoperative trans women should be told that some protection is provided if they void immediately after intercourse and wash their genitalia and the adjacent areas with soap and water. Cis-gender women

TABLE 55.8	NURSING ASSESSMENT

Sexually Transmitted Infections

Subjective Data
Important Health Information
Past health history: Contact with individuals with STIs, multiple sexual partners, pregnancy, shared needles during IV drug use, previous vaccination against HPV
Medications: Oral contraceptives; allergy to any antibiotics, especially penicillin

Symptoms
- Alopecia
- Arthralgia, headache
- Dyspareunia; vaginal discharge, menstrual abnormalities; presence of painful, burning genital or perianal lesions
- Dysuria, urinary frequency, retention; urethral discharge; tenesmus, proctitis
- Itching at infected site; lesions that cause pain or burning sensation
- Malaise; chills
- Nausea, vomiting, anorexia, pharyngitis, oral lesions

Objective Data
General
Fever, lymphadenopathy (generalized or inguinal)

Integumentary
Syphilis:
- *Primary:* painless, indurated genital, oral, or perianal lesions
- *Secondary:* bilateral, symmetrical rash on palms, soles, or entire body; mucous patches on mouth or tongue; alopecia
Genital herpes: Painful genital or anal vesicular lesions
Genital warts: Single or multiple grey or white genital or anal warts (possibly becoming massive)

Gastrointestinal
Purulent rectal discharge (indicator of gonorrhea), rectal lesions, proctitis

Urinary
Urethral discharge, erythema

Reproductive
Cervical discharge, lesions, inflamed Bartholin glands

Possible Diagnostic Findings
- *Chlamydial infection:* Positive culture or DNA amplification for *Chlamydia*
- *Genital herpes:* Positive tissue culture for HSV-1 or HSV-2; positive HSV-1 or HSV-2 antibody titre
- *Gonorrhea:* Positive Gram stain, smears, cultures, and DNA amplification for *Neisseria gonorrhoeae*
- *Syphilis:* Positive findings on VDRL and RPR tests, spirochetes on dark-field microscopy

HPV, human papilloma virus; *HSV-1,* herpes simplex virus type 1; *HSV-2,* herpes simplex virus type 2; *IV,* intravenous; *RPR,* rapid plasma reagin; *STI,* sexually transmitted infection; *VDRL,* Venereal Disease Research Laboratory.

and nonoperative trans men may also benefit from voiding and washing after intercourse. It is important to emphasize that this does not provide adequate protection against STIs after exposure to infection.

Vaginal microbicides, topical gels, or creams that contain tenofovir have been found to reduce HIV and HSV-2 acquisition in cis-gender women by 39% and 51%, respectively, but there is no evidence that other kinds of vaginal microbicides have an effect on reducing acquisition of HIV, HSV-2, or any other STI (Mpondo, 2016). These gels or creams can serve as

TABLE 55.9	PATIENT & CAREGIVER TEACHING GUIDE

Sexually Transmitted Infections

When teaching the patient with sexually transmitted infections, the nurse should carry out the following steps:

1. Instruct patient in hygienic measures, such as washing and urinating after intercourse to flush out some of the causative organisms.
2. Explain the importance of taking all antibiotics or antiviral agents (or both) as prescribed. Symptoms improve after 1 to 2 days of therapy but organisms may still be present.
3. Teach patient about the need for treatment of sexual partners to prevent transmission of disease.
4. Instruct patient to abstain from sexual intercourse during treatment and to use condoms when sexual activity is resumed to prevent spread of infection and prevent reinfection.
5. Explain the importance of follow-up examination and repeated culture at least once after treatment if appropriate, to confirm complete cure and prevent relapse.
6. Allow patient and partner to verbalize concerns to clarify areas that need explanation.
7. Instruct patient about symptoms of complications and need to report problems to ensure proper follow-up and early treatment of reinfection.
8. Explain precautions to take, such as being monogamous; asking potential partners about sexual history; avoiding sex with partners who use intravenous drugs or who have visible oral, inguinal, genital, perineal, or anal lesions; using male or female condoms or dental dams; and voiding and washing genitalia after intercourse to reduce the occurrence of reinfection.
9. Inform patient regarding state of infectivity to prevent a false sense of security, which might result in careless sexual practices and poor personal hygiene.
10. Provide information related to HPV vaccination.

HPV, human papilloma virus.

supplementary lubrication, thereby decreasing irritation and friction and chances for development of a minor laceration that could serve as an entry point for the organism. Proper use of a condom is a highly effective mechanical barrier to infection—the condom should be undamaged and correctly in place throughout all phases of sexual activity. A deterrent to condom usage is alcohol and drug use (PHAC, 2020b). Use of barrier contraceptives requires planning and motivation, both of which are impaired with alcohol or drug ingestion. The patient should be given specific verbal and written instructions on the proper use of condoms (see Chapter 17, Table 17.18). The objections to condom usage, such as interference with spontaneity and the presence of a barrier, should be discussed by the partners. Information about the mechanics of sexual arousal and incorporating the use of a condom into sexual activity can help in overcoming resistance to its use. Internal ("female") condoms are lubricated polyurethane sheaths with a ring at each end designed for vaginal use but are considerably more expensive than external ("male") condoms (see Chapter 17, Table 17.19).

Among couples with one infected partner, consistent and scrupulous barrier use can reduce transmission to the uninfected partner. Unprotected anal intercourse and other high-risk behaviours should be eliminated, and condoms should be used if sexual contact continues.

The nurse should initiate a discussion to assess the patient's risk of contracting an STI (see Table 53.7). Interpersonal skills necessary for this interview include respect, compassion, and a nonjudgemental attitude. Counselling should be tailored to the individual patient. The nurse should not assume that older people are not at risk; an increasing number of older people are acquiring STIs.

Screening Programs. Screening programs can help prevent certain STIs. For many years, there have been various screening programs to identify cases of syphilis. With the increase of infection rates across Canada, more stringent screening and follow-up treatment are required. Many institutions offer voluntary prenatal HIV and syphilis testing and counselling for pregnant women.

Screening programs have also been developed and implemented for detection of gonorrhea and chlamydial infection. These programs are targeted to cis-gender women because they are more likely to have asymptomatic gonorrhea and thereby serve as sources of infection; however, nonoperative trans men should be targeted as well. Gonorrheal and chlamydial testing during pelvic examinations and prenatal visits is becoming a major routine part of these programs. Mass application of screening programs for genital chlamydial infections, genital herpes, and HPV infections may also be possible with the advent of rapid, cost-effective tests.

Case Finding. Interviewing and case finding are other processes used to control spread of STIs. These activities are directed toward locating and examining all contacts of each known patient with an STI as soon after sexual exposure as possible so that effective treatment can be initiated. Trained interviewers may often find cases even if they are supplied with only limited information. The caseworkers, who are often nurses, are aware of the social implications of these diseases and the need for discretion. Often, sexual contacts are not informed about the origin of the information naming them as a contact, so that greater cooperation and privacy is ensured. (See the Ethical Dilemmas box on confidentiality.) *Expedited partner therapy (EPT)* is an evidence-informed approach that allows a health care provider to provide prescriptions to a patient to take to their partner, without examining the partner. This method has been found to be beneficial in high-risk and hard-to-reach populations (Schillinger et al., 2016).

Educational and Research Programs. Nurses should actively encourage people in their community to provide better education about STIs for its citizens. Teenagers, who are known to have a high incidence of infection, should be a prime target for such educational programs, as should older persons. Hotline services, reliable Internet sites, school nurses, primary care nurses, nurse practitioners, nurse midwives, and outreach programs sponsored by Canada's Health Protection Branch are effective means of providing educational programs.

Knowledge and understanding can decrease the STI epidemic. The HPV vaccine that protects against genital warts and cervical cancer should be encouraged before the start of sexual activity. Accurate and current information may help reduce parental fears related to the vaccine. Nurses should consider stressing the prevention of cancer as a reason for the vaccine, which may be more productive and less controversial, thus making the parent and adolescent more receptive. Efforts are being made to develop vaccines for syphilis, gonorrhea, genital herpes, and HIV. The development of effective vaccines is viewed by many clinicians as a prerequisite for eradication of STIs.

Harm Reduction. Behavioural interventions to promote condom use and to modify sexual risk behaviours include individual

ETHICAL DILEMMAS
Confidentiality

Situation
A nurse in a clinic gives the positive results of a test for *Chlamydia* infection to a patient and advises her to tell her sexual partners that she has this infection. The patient refuses to tell her boyfriend because he will then know that she has had sex with another partner. Should the nurse contact the boyfriend?

Important Points for Consideration
- Nurses and other health care providers have both a legal and an ethical obligation to maintain confidentiality of patient information. If confidentiality is violated, trust is eroded and patients may not share privileged information that is essential to plan effective care.
- Nurses have a legal responsibility to report three STIs in Canada: chlamydia, syphilis, and gonorrhea (and HSV in the Atlantic provinces).
- The nurse must assess if giving the patient the option to tell their partner is responsible, accountable, ethical nursing practice, as this may put the patient at risk for intimate partner violence.
- Health care providers have an obligation to maintain confidentiality unless there is a risk to the health or life of innocent third parties.
- The nurse's primary obligation is to the patient seeking care. However, there are long-term health consequences for this patient, as well as for the public in general.
- Patient teaching is one way to establish a partnership. Information should be shared about the effects of the infection being untreated, the risks for and consequences of reinfection, and the results that the infection may have on others who may not know they are infected. The patient can then be encouraged to inform all intimate partners of the diagnosis in the event that follow-up treatment is required.

Clinical Decision-Making Questions
1. What are the provincial or territorial requirements for reportable conditions?
2. What information should the nurse share with this patient regarding the transmission of chlamydial infection to increase her willingness to discuss the results with her partner?
3. What is the best way to balance the needs of an individual patient with those of the general public?

counselling, skills training, coping strategies, peer education, and social and educational support and should be integrated in harm-reduction programs and in health care settings to prevent STIs (Carvalho et al., 2017). For individuals identified as being at ongoing risk for STIs, screening is recommended at 3-month intervals for HIV, gonorrhea, syphilis, and chlamydial infection. Ongoing contact with a health care provider is an opportunity for reinforcement of safer sex practices. (Harm reduction is discussed in Chapter 11.)

ACUTE INTERVENTION
Psychological Support. The diagnosis of an STI may be met with a variety of emotions, such as shame, guilt, anger, and a desire for vengeance. Nurses should provide counselling and encourage the patient to verbalize their feelings. Couples in monogamous relationships are confronted with an added problem when an STI is diagnosed because they must face the implication of sexual activity outside the relationship. Support and counselling for the couple are needed.

A patient who has genital herpes is faced with the fact that infections can recur and that no cure is available. This can be frustrating and disruptive to the patient's physical, emotional,

social, and sexual life. The nurse should help the patient identify and avoid any factors that may precipitate the condition and inform the patient that the frequency and severity of recurrences may decrease over time.

HPV infections involve a prolonged course of treatment. The patient can become frustrated and distressed because of frequent office visits, associated costs, potential for unpleasant adverse effects as a result of treatment, and effects of the infection on future health and sexual relationships. Tremendous support and a willingness to listen to the patient's concerns are needed. Support groups are also available.

Follow-Up. A nurse working in public health facilities, clinics, or other outpatient settings may care for patients with STIs more often than a nurse in a hospital. This nurse is in a position to explain and interpret treatment measures such as the purpose and possible adverse effects of prescribed medications and the need for follow-up care.

Single-dose treatment for gonococcal infection, chlamydial infection, and syphilis helps prevent the problems associated with nonadherence to medication therapy. Patients who require multiple-dose therapy should be given special instructions in completing the prescribed regimen and should be informed about problems resulting from nonadherence. All patients should return to the treatment centre for a repeat culture from the infected sites or for serological testing at designated times to determine the effectiveness of the treatment. Explaining to the patient that cures are not always obtained on the first treatment can reinforce the need for a follow-up visit. The patient should also be advised to inform sexual partners of the need for testing and treatment, regardless of whether they are free of symptoms or are experiencing symptoms.

Hygiene Measures. The nurse must emphasize certain hygiene measures to patients with an STI. An important measure is frequent handwashing and bathing. Bathing and cleaning of the involved areas can provide local comfort and prevent secondary infection. Douching is contraindicated as it may spread the infection or undermine local immune responses. The synthetic materials used in most undergarments frequently increase or exacerbate local irritations by trapping moisture. Cotton undergarments provide better absorption and are cooler and more comfortable for the patient with an STI.

Sexual Activity. Sexual abstinence is indicated during the communicable phase of the infection. If sexual activity occurs before treatment of the patient has been completed, the use of external or internal condoms may prevent the spread of infection and reinfection. Condom usage after treatment should be encouraged to prevent future exposure to infection. The patient can also choose to relate to a partner in an intimate way that avoids both intercourse and oral–genital contact. It is important to note that even single-dose treatments can take up to 1 week to be effective, and the patient is infectious during this period.

AMBULATORY AND HOME CARE.
Because many STIs are cured with a single dose or short course of antibiotic therapy, many people are casual about the outcome of these diseases. The consequences of this attitude can include delays in treatment, nonadherence to instructions, and subsequent development of complications. The complications are serious and costly; they can result in disfigurement and destruction of important tissues and organs.

Surgery and prolonged therapy are indicated for many patients with infection-related complications. Major surgical procedures such as resection of an aneurysm or aortic valve replacement may be necessary to treat cardiovascular conditions caused by syphilis. Pelvic surgery and procedures to correct fertility conditions secondary to an STI may include lysis of adhesions, dilation of strictures, reconstructive tuboplasty, and in vitro fertilization.

EVALUATION

Expected outcomes for a patient with an STI are that the patient will do the following:

- Describe modes of transmission
- Use appropriate hygienic measures
- Experience no reinfection
- Demonstrate adherence to a follow-up protocol

CASE STUDY

Chlamydial Infection and Gonorrhea

Patient Profile

C. R. (pronouns she/her) is a 23-year-old cis-gender woman who is seen at the outpatient clinic with symptoms of a purulent yellow-white discharge and frequent urination over the past 2 weeks. C. R. is sexually active with a new partner after breaking up with her long-term boyfriend. C. R. was treated in the past for chlamydia at age 20.

Subjective Data

- Did not use condom or spermicide
- Sexual partner was recently treated for epididymitis
- Last menstrual period was 3 weeks ago
- Appears very nervous

Objective Data

- Cervical ectopy noted during Pap test
- Mucopurulent cervical discharge
- Nucleic acid amplification test is positive for *Neisseria gonorrhoeae* and *Chlamydia trachomatis*
- Urine pregnancy test is negative
- Patient is crying and very upset when informed of positive test results

Interprofessional Care

- Doxycycline, 100 mg PO twice a day for 7 days
- Ceftriaxone, 250 mg intramuscularly once

Discussion Questions

1. What were C. R.'s risk factors for acquiring chlamydial and gonococcal infections?
2. What complications could occur if these infections are not treated?
3. **Priority decision:** What is the priority of care for C. R.?
4. What instructions should C. R. receive to ensure successful treatment? To prevent reinfection? To prevent further transmission of the infection?
5. What impact is this diagnosis likely to have on C. R.'s self-image? On the sexual partner relationship?
6. **Priority decision:** Based on the assessment data presented, what are the priority nursing diagnoses? Are there any interprofessional issues?
7. **Evidence-informed practice:** C. R. asks if the spermicide nonoxynol-9 (N-9) should be used to protect against STIs. How should the nurse respond?

⊖volve
Answers are available at http://evolve.elsevier.com/Canada/Lewis/medsurg.

REVIEW QUESTIONS

The number of the question corresponds to the same-numbered objective at the beginning of the chapter.

1. Which of the following are high-risk factors for acquiring sexually transmitted infections (STIs)? *(Select all that apply.)*
   a. Survival sex
   b. Consistent use of barrier methods of contraception
   c. Anonymous sexual partnering
   d. Sex under the influence of drugs
   e. Sexual assault

2. The nurse is obtaining subjective assessment data from a nonoperative transgender man reported as a sexual contact of a cis-gender man with chlamydial infection. The nurse understands which of the following about symptoms of chlamydial infection in a transgender man?
   a. They are frequently absent.
   b. They are similar to those of genital herpes.
   c. They include a macular palmar rash in later stages.
   d. They may involve chancres hidden inside the vagina.

3. In which way(s) does a primary HSV infection differ from recurrent HSV episodes? *(Select all that apply.)*
   a. Symptoms are less severe during recurrent episodes.
   b. Only primary infections are sexually transmissible.
   c. Systemic manifestations such as fever and myalgia are more common in primary infection.
   d. Transmission of the virus to a fetus is less likely during primary infection.
   e. Lesions from recurrent HSV are more likely to transmit the virus than lesions from primary HSV.

4. Why should the nurse explain to a client with gonorrhea that treatment will include both ceftriaxone and doxycycline?
   a. Most clients need both medications to eradicate the organism.
   b. Coverage with more than one antibiotic will prevent reinfection.
   c. No single agent successfully eradicates both primary and recurrent infections.
   d. The high rate of coexisting chlamydial infection and gonorrhea indicates coverage with both medications.

5. In assessing clients for STIs, the nurse needs to know that many STIs can be asymptomatic. Which of the following STIs can be asymptomatic? *(Select all that apply.)*
   a. Syphilis
   b. Gonorrhea
   c. Genital warts
   d. Genital herpes
   e. Chlamydial infection

6. To prevent infection and the transmission of STIs, the nurse's teaching plan would include an explanation of which of the following?
   a. The appropriate use of oral contraceptives
   b. Sexual positions that can be used to avoid infection
   c. The necessity of annual Pap smears for clients with HPV
   d. Sexual practices that are considered high-risk behaviours

7. Which of the following is an appropriate nursing intervention to provide emotional support to a client with an STI?
   a. Offering information on how safer sexual practices can prevent STIs
   b. Showing concern when listening to the client who expresses negative feelings
   c. Reassuring the client that the disease is highly curable with appropriate treatment
   d. Helping the client who received an STI from their sexual partner in forgiving the partner

1. a, c, d, e; 2. a; 3. a, c; 4. d; 5. a, b, c, d, e; 6. d; 7. b.

ⓔvolve

For even more review questions, visit http://evolve.elsevier.com/Canada/Lewis/medsurg.

REFERENCES

Bodie, M., Gale-Rowe, M., Alexandre, S., et al. (2019). Addressing the rising rates of gonorrhea and drug-resistant gonorrhea: There's no time like the present. *Canada Communicable Disease Report*, 45(2/3), 54–62. https://doi.org/10.14745/ccdr.v45i23a02

Carvalho, F., Goncalves, T., Faria, E., et al. (2017). Behavioural interventions to promote condom use among women living with HIV: A systematic review update. *Cadernos de Saude Publica*, 33(1). https://doi.org/10.1590/0102-311x00202515

Chandra, J., Woo, W., Dutton, J., et al. (2019). Immune responses to a HSV-2 polynucleotide immunotherapy COR-1 in HSV-2 positive subjects: A randomized double blinded phase I/IIa trial. *PLoS One*, 14(12), e0226320. https://doi.org/10.1371/journal.pone.0226320

Choudri, Y., Miller, J., Sandhu, J., et al. (2018a). Chlamydia in Canada, 2010–2015. *Canada Communicable Disease Report (CCDR)*, 44(2), 49–54. https://doi.org/10.14745/ccdr.v44i02a03

Choudri, Y., Miller, J., Sandhu, J., et al. (2018b). Gonorrhea in Canada, 2010–2015. *Canada Communicable Disease Report (CCDR)*, 44(2), 37–42. https://doi.org/10.14745/ccdr.v44i02a01

Choudri, Y., Miller, J., Sandhu, J., et al. (2018c). Infectious and congenital syphilis in Canada, 2010–2015. *Canada Communicable Disease Report (CCDR)*, 44(2), 43–48. https://doi.org/10.14745/ccdr.v44i02a02

Community AIDS Treatment Information Exchange (CATIE). (2016). *Genital herpes: CATIE fact sheet*. https://www.catie.ca/en/fact-sheets/sti/genital-herpes

Fetner, T., Dion, M., Heath, M., et al. (2020). Condom use in penile-vaginal intercourse among Canadian adults: Results from the sex in Canada survey. *PLoS ONE*, 15(2). https://doi.org/10.1371/journal.pone.0228981. e0228981.

Government of Canada. (2019). *Canadian guidelines on sexually transmitted infections: Summary of recommendations for Chlamydia trachomatis (CT), Neisseria gonorrhoeae (NG) and syphilis.* https://www.canada.ca/en/services/health/publications/diseases-conditions/guidelines-sti-recommendations-chlamydia-trachomatis-neisseria-gonorrhoeae-syphilis-2019.html

Government of Canada. (2021). *Human papillomavirus vaccine: Canadian immunization guide.* https://www.canada.ca/en/public-health/services/publications/healthy-living/canadian-immunization-guide-part-4-active-vaccines/page-9-human-papillomavirus-vaccine.html

Green, N., Hoenigl, M., Morris, S., et al. (2015). Risk behavior and sexually transmitted infections among transgender women and men undergoing community-based screening for acute and early HIV infection in San Diego. *Medicine (Baltimore)*, 94(41):e1830. https://doi.org/10.1097/MD.0000000000001830

Groves, M. (2016). Genital herpes: A review. *American Family Physician*, 93(11), 928–934.

Hackett, L., Bidermann, M., Doria, N., et al. (2020). A rapid review of Indigenous boys' and men's sexual health in Canada. *Culture, Health & Sexuality*, 22, 1–18. https://doi.org/10.1080/13691058.2020.1722856

HealthLinkBC. (2020). *Ectopic pregnancy.* https://www.healthlinkbc.ca/health-topics/hw144921

Mckay, A., Quinn-Nilas, C., & Milhausen, R. (2017). Prevalence and correlates of condom use among single midlife Canadian women and men aged 40 to 59. *Canadian Journal of Human Sexuality*, 26(1), 38–47. https://doi.org/10.3138/cjhs.261-A6

Mpondo, B. (2016). New biomedical technologies and strategies for prevention of HIV and other sexually transmitted infection. *Journal of Sexually Transmitted Diseases*, 1–10. https://doi.org/10.1155/2016/7684768

National Advisory Committee on Immunization (NACI). (2017). *Updated recommendations on human papillomavirus (HPV) vaccines: 9-Valent HPV vaccine 2-dose immunization schedule and the use of HPV vaccines in immunocompromised populations.* PHAC. https://www.canada.ca/content/dam/phac-aspc/documents/services/publications/healthy-living/updated-recommendations-human-papillomavirus-immunization-schedule-immunocompromised-populations/updated-recommendations-human-papillomavirus-immunization-schedule-immunocompromised-populationsv3-eng.pdf

Perry, S. E., Hockenberry, M. J., Lowdermilk, D. L., et al. (Eds.). (2017). *Maternal child nursing care in Canada.* Elsevier Canada.

Petrova, D., & Garcia-Retamero, R. (2015). Effective evidence-based programs for preventing sexually-transmitted infections: A meta-analysis. *Current HIV Research*, 13(5), 432–438. https://doi.org/10.2174/1570162x13666150511143943

Poteat, T. (2016). Transgender people and sexually transmitted infections (STIs). In M. Deutsch (Ed.), *Guidelines for the primary and gender-affirming care of transgender and non-binary people* (2nd ed., pp. 90–93). University of California San Francisco. https://transcare.ucsf.edu/sites/transcare.ucsf.edu/files/Transgender-PGACG-6-17-16.pdf

Public Health Agency of Canada (PHAC). (2015a). *Canadian guidelines on sexually transmitted infections—Management and treatment of specific infections—Human papillomavirus HPV infections.* http://www.phac-aspc.gc.ca/std-mts/sti-its/cgsti-ldcits/section-5-5-eng.php

Public Health Agency of Canada (PHAC). (2015b). *Question and answers: Prevention of sexually transmitted infections and blood borne infections among older adults.* https://www.canada.ca/en/public-health/services/infectious-diseases/sexual-health-sexually-transmitted-infections/reports-publications/questions-answers-adults.html#a1

Public Health Agency of Canada (PHAC). (2016). *Canadian guidelines on sexually transmitted infections* (updated 2016 edition). http://www.phac-aspc.gc.ca/std-mts/sti-its/index-eng.php

Public Health Agency of Canada (PHAC). (2017a). *Section 3: Canadian guidelines on sexually transmitted infections—Laboratory diagnosis of sexually transmitted infections (revised January 2018).* https://www.canada.ca/en/public-health/services/infectious-diseases/sexual-health-sexually-transmitted-infections/canadian-guidelines/sexually-transmitted-infections/canadian-guidelines-sexually-transmitted-infections-18.html

Public Health Agency of Canada (PHAC). (2017b). *Section 5-2: Canadian guidelines on sexually transmitted infections—Management and treatment of specific infections—Chlamydial infections.* https://www.canada.ca/en/public-health/services/infectious-diseases/sexual-health-sexually-transmitted-infections/canadian-guidelines/sexually-transmitted-infections/canadian-guidelines-sexually-transmitted-infections-30.html

Public Health Agency of Canada (PHAC). (2019). *Update on sexually transmitted infections in Canada: 2016.* https://www.canada.ca/en/health-canada/services/publications/diseases-conditions/update-sexually-transmitted-infections-canada-2016.html

Public Health Agency of Canada (PHAC). (2020a). *Responding to syphilis in Canada (fact sheet).* https://www.canada.ca/en/public-health/services/publications/diseases-conditions/responding-syphilis-canada-fact-sheet.html

Public Health Agency of Canada (PHAC). (2020b). *Sexually transmitted infections.* https://www.canada.ca/content/dam/phac-aspc/documents/services/publications/diseases-conditions/booklet-sexually-transmitted-infections/booklet-sexually-transmitted-infections-eng.pdf

Public Health Agency of Canada (PHAC). (2020c). *Trauma and violence-informed care toolkit for reducing stigma related to sexually transmitted and blood-borne infections.* Centre for Sexuality. https://www.cpha.ca/sites/default/files/uploads/resources/stbbi/STBBI-TVIC-toolkit_e.pdf

Public Health Agency of Canada (PHAC). (2021). *Gonorrhea.* https://www.canada.ca/en/public-health/services/diseases/gonorrhea.html

Schillinger, J., Gorwitz, R., Rietmeiier, C., et al. (2016). The expedited partner therapy continuum: A conceptual framework to guide programmatic efforts to increase partner treatment. *Sexually Transmitted Diseases, 43*(2 Suppl 1), S63–S75. https://doi.org/10.1097/OLQ.0000000000000399

Shannon, C. L., & Klausner, J. D. (2018). The growing epidemic of sexually transmitted infections in adolescents: A neglected population. *Current Opinion in Pediatrics, 30*(1), 137–143. https://doi.org/10.1097/MOP.0000000000000578

Xiong, Y.-Q., Mo, Y., Luo, Q.-M., et al. (2018). The risk of human papillomavirus infection for spontaneous abortion, spontaneous preterm birth, and pregnancy rate of assisted reproductive technologies: A systematic review and meta-analysis. *Gynecologic and Obstetric Investigation, 83*, 417–427. https://doi.org/10.1159/000482008

RESOURCES

Action Canada for Sexual Health & Rights
https://www.actioncanadashr.org/

CATIE: Canada's Source for HIV and Hepatitis C Information
https://www.catie.ca/en/home

Health Canada—*Sexually Transmitted Infections (STIs)*
https://www.hc-sc.gc.ca/hc-ps/dc-ma/sti-its-eng.php

Phoenix Association—*Toronto Help*
https://www.torontoherpes.com/

Public Health Agency of Canada—*Canadian Guidelines for Sexual Health Education*
https://www.phac-aspc.gc.ca/publicat/cgshe-ldnemss/index-eng.php

Public Health Agency of Canada—*Sexual Health and Sexually Transmitted Infections*
https://www.phac-aspc.gc.ca/std-mts

Sex Information and Education Council of Canada
http://www.sieccan.org

SexualityandU.ca
https://www.sexualityandu.ca/

SexualityandU.ca—*Emergency Contraception*
https://www.sexandu.ca/contraception/emergency-contraception/

Teaching Sexual Health
https://www.teachingsexualhealth.ca/

International Herpes Resource Center
https://www.herpesresourcecenter.com/

evolve

For additional Internet resources, see the website for this book at http://evolve.elsevier.com/Canada/Lewis/medsurg.

Nursing Management
Female Reproductive Conditions

Catherine Sheffer
Originating US chapter by Kim K. Choma

⊖volve WEBSITE

http://evolve.elsevier.com/Canada/Lewis/Canada/medsurg

- Review Questions (Online Only)
- Key Points
- Answer Guidelines for Case Study

- Student Case Study
  - Patient with Endometrial Cancer and Blood Transfusion

- Customizable Nursing Care Plan
  - Abdominal Hysterectomy
- Conceptual Care Map Creator
- Audio Glossary
- Content Updates

LEARNING OBJECTIVES

1. Summarize the etiologies of infertility and the strategies for diagnosis and treatment of women who are infertile.
2. Describe the etiology, clinical manifestations, and nursing and interprofessional management of menstrual difficulties and abnormal vaginal bleeding.
3. Identify the risk factors and clinical manifestations of ectopic pregnancy and the interprofessional care of patients with ectopic pregnancy.
4. Discuss the changes related to menopause and the nursing and interprofessional management of patients with menopausal symptoms.
5. Differentiate among the common conditions that affect the vulva, vagina, and cervix and related nursing and interprofessional management.

6. Describe the assessment, interprofessional care, and nursing management of patients with pelvic inflammatory disease and endometriosis.
7. Explain the clinical manifestations of and diagnostic studies, interprofessional care, and surgical therapy for cervical, endometrial, ovarian, and vulvar cancers.
8. Summarize the preoperative and the postoperative nursing management for the patient requiring surgery of the female reproductive system.
9. Differentiate among the common conditions that occur with cystoceles, rectoceles, and fistulas and the related nursing and interprofessional management.

KEY TERMS

abortion
amenorrhea
cystocele
dysmenorrhea
ectopic pregnancy
endometriosis

hysterectomy
infertility
leiomyomas
menopause
pelvic inflammatory disease (PID)
perimenopause

postmenopause
premenstrual syndrome (PMS)
rectocele
uterine prolapse

INFERTILITY

Infertility is the inability to achieve a pregnancy after at least 1 year of regular unprotected intercourse (World Health Organization [WHO], 2021). Current evidence indicates that approximately 16% of couples (one in six) in Canada experience infertility (Public Health Agency of Canada [PHAC], 2019). Assessment and therapy measures can be invasive, expensive, and lengthy. Understandably, infertility can be both a physical and emotional crisis.

Etiology and Pathophysiology

Infertility may be caused by female, male, or combined factors. (Conditions that cause male infertility are discussed in Chapter 57.) In some cases, the cause of infertility may not be identified.

The factors usually causing female infertility include problems with ovulation (anovulation or inadequate corpus luteum), tubal obstruction or dysfunction (endometriosis or damage from pelvic infection), and uterine or cervical factors (fibroid tumours or structural anomalies). Risk factors for infertility include tobacco

TABLE 56.1 INTERPROFESSIONAL CARE

Infertility

Diagnostic
- History and physical examination of both partners, including psychosocial functioning
- Assessment of possible sexually transmitted infections
- Genetic screening
- Hormone levels
- Serum hormone levels (e.g., FSH, LH, prolactin)
- Urinary LH
- Ovulatory study
- Pap test
- Pelvic ultrasonography
- Postcoital test
- Cervical mucus
- Semen analysis
- Sperm penetration assay
- Review of menstrual and gynecological history
- Tubal patency study
- Hysterosalpingogram

Interprofessional Therapy
- Assisted reproductive technologies (ARTs)
- Medication therapy (see Table 56.2)
- Hormone supplement therapy
- Intrauterine insemination

FSH, follicle-stimulating hormone; *LH,* luteinizing hormone.

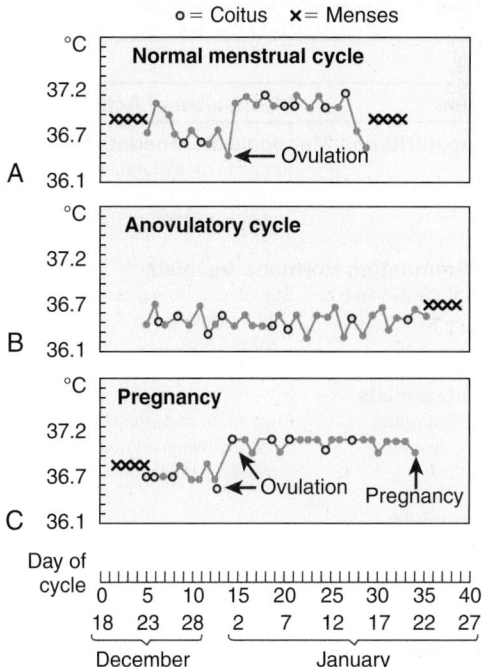

FIG. 56.1 Basal body temperature chart. **A,** Typical biphasic temperature curve indicative of ovulation and normal progesterone effect. **B,** Irregular monophasic curve characteristic of anovulatory cycles. **C,** Ovulatory curve with sustained temperature elevation following conception and the first missed period.

and illicit drug use and being obese or thin (Rossi et al., 2016). In women, the risk for infertility starts at about age 30 and increases exponentially after age 40 (Schumacher et al., 2018).

Diagnostic Studies

A detailed history and general physical examination of the patient and their partner provide the basis for selecting diagnostic studies (Table 56.1). The possibility of medical, genetic, or gynecological diseases is explored before tests are performed to determine issues affecting general health as well as fertility. These tests include hormonal levels, ovulatory studies, tubal patency studies, and postcoital studies. Other screening tests for infertility include semen analysis and pelvic ultrasound.

Ovulatory Studies. A basal body temperature record is kept to determine if there is regular ovulation (Figure 56.1). The woman is instructed to take and graph her temperature, referred to as *basal body temperature,* on awakening, before any activity. As ovulation approaches, the production of estrogen increases, which may cause a drop in temperature. When ovulation occurs, progesterone is produced, causing a rise in temperature. Thus a temperature graph helps in detecting ovulation and suggests the timing of intercourse if pregnancy is desired. Ovulation prediction kits are now available for use by women at home. Other tests for ovulation include cervical and vaginal smears, endometrial biopsy, and plasma progesterone levels.

Tubal Patency Studies. Tubal factors (occlusion or deformity) are assessed most commonly by means of hysterosalpingogram. This procedure consists of the radiographic visualization of the uterus and tubes by injecting a radiopaque dye through the cervix. Also, ultrasound is being used with increased comfort for the patient and more accurate results to evaluate tubal patency (Mardanian et al., 2018). Tubal patency, shape, and position and any distortions of the endometrial cavity can be determined. Laparoscopy may be used when a hysterosalpingogram is contraindicated or other pathological pelvic conditions appear likely.

Postcoital Studies. A postcoital test can determine whether the cervical environment is favourable for the sperm. The

couple is asked to have intercourse about the time ovulation is expected and 2 to 12 hours before the office visit. Douching or bathing should be avoided before the test. The cervical and vaginal secretions are aspirated and examined for the number and the motility of sperm present.

NURSING AND INTERPROFESSIONAL MANAGEMENT INFERTILITY

The management of infertility depends on the cause. If infertility is secondary to an alteration in ovarian function, supplemental hormone therapy (HT) to restore and maintain ovulation may be attempted. Medication therapy used to treat infertility is presented in Table 56.2. Chronic cervicitis and inadequate estrogenic stimulation are cervical factors causing infertility. Antibiotic therapy is indicated for cervicitis. Inadequate estrogenic stimulation is treated using estrogen.

When a couple has not succeeded in conceiving during infertility management, an option is intrauterine insemination (IUI) with sperm from the partner or a donor. If this technique does not succeed, assisted reproductive technologies (ARTs) may be used. ARTs include in vitro fertilization (IVF), gamete intrafallopian transfer (GIFT), zygote intrafallopian transfer (ZIFT), donor gametes, and embryo cryopreservation. IVF is the removal of mature oocytes from the patient's ovarian follicle via laparoscopy, followed by IVF of the ova with the partner's or donor's sperm. When fertilization and cleavage have occurred, the resulting embryos are transferred into the patient's uterus. The procedure requires 2 to 3 days to complete and is used in cases of Fallopian tube obstruction, diminished sperm count, and unexplained infertility. Frequently, multiple attempts are needed for successful implantation. IVF is costly and emotionally stressful (Maxwell et al., 2018).

Nurses can assist women experiencing infertility by providing information about the physiology of reproduction and infertility evaluation and by addressing the psychological and social

TABLE 56.2   MEDICATION THERAPY

Infertility

Medication	Mechanism of Action
Menotropin (Human Menopausal Gonadotropin)	
Repronex	Product made of equal amounts of FSH and LH that promotes the development and maturation of follicles in the ovaries
Follicle-Stimulating Hormone Agonists	
Follitropin alpha (Gonal-F & Gonal-F pen)	Stimulate follicle growth and maturation by mimicking the actions of the body's natural FSH
GnRH Antagonists	
Cetrorelix (Cetrotide) Ganirelix (Orgalutran)	Prevent premature LH surges and premature ovulation in women undergoing ovarian stimulation
GnRH Agonists	
Leuprolide (Lupron, Eligard) Nafarelin (Synarel)	Suppress release of LH and FSH with continuous use. May also be used in the treatment of endometriosis
Human chorionic gonadotropin (Pregnyl)	Induce ovulation by stimulating the release of eggs from follicles

FSH, follicle-stimulating hormone; *GnRH*, gonadotropin-releasing hormone; *LH*, luteinizing hormone.

distress that can accompany infertility. There is some evidence that psychological stress can have a negative effect on fertility, especially during the time of ovulation (Akhter et al., 2016).

The nurse has a major responsibility for teaching and providing emotional support throughout infertility testing and treatment. Feelings of anger, frustration, grief, and helplessness may heighten as additional diagnostic tests are performed. Infertility can generate great tension in a relationship as the couple exhausts financial and emotional resources. Few insurance carriers cover the high cost of infertility testing and treatment. Couples should be encouraged to participate in a support group for infertile couples as well as individual therapy.

ABORTION

An abortion is the loss or termination of a pregnancy before the fetus has developed to a state of viability. Abortions are classified as *spontaneous* (those occurring naturally) or *induced* (those occurring as a result of mechanical or medical intervention). *Miscarriage* is the common term for the unintended loss of a pregnancy or spontaneous abortion.

Spontaneous Abortion

Spontaneous abortion is the natural loss of pregnancy before 20 weeks of gestation. Fetal chromosomal anomalies may account for many miscarriages before 8 weeks of gestation. Other causes of spontaneous abortions include endocrine abnormalities, maternal infection, acquired anatomical abnormalities (e.g., uterine fibroids, endometriosis), immunological factors, and environmental factors. About 10 to 15% of all clinically recognized pregnancies end as a result of spontaneous abortion (Keenan-Lindsay & Mancuso, 2017).

Uterine cramping coupled with vaginal bleeding often indicates a spontaneous abortion. Cramping is usually absent if the vaginal bleeding is caused by other conditions, such as polyps. Serial measurements of serum β-human chorionic gonadotropin (β-hCG) hormone and vaginal ultrasonography

examination of the pelvis are the most reliable indicators of viability of the pregnancy.

Treatment to prevent a possible spontaneous abortion is limited. Although bed rest and avoiding vaginal intercourse are often recommended, there is no evidence that these measures improve the outcome. The patient is advised to report any bleeding to their health care provider. Most women proceed to abortion regardless of treatment. If the products of conception do not pass completely or bleeding becomes excessive, a *dilation and curettage* (D&C) procedure is generally performed (Zara, 2020). The D&C involves dilating the uterine cervix and scraping the endometrium of the uterus to empty the contents of the uterus.

Patients who are experiencing bleeding and cramping during pregnancy may be admitted to the hospital. Vital signs and estimated blood loss are monitored. Arranging for someone to stay with the patient provides important emotional support. The nurse should be aware of the grieving process that results from pregnancy loss (Özgür Köneş & Yıldız, 2020) and provide emotional support.

Induced Abortion

Induced abortion is an intentional or elective termination of a pregnancy. Induced abortion is done for personal reasons (at the request of the woman) or for medical reasons. The number of induced abortions performed in Canada in 2018 was approximately 85 195 (Canadian Institute for Health Information [CIHI], 2018).

Several techniques are used to induce abortion, including menstrual evacuation, suction curettage, dilation and evacuation (D&E), and medication therapy. Deciding which technique to use to terminate a pregnancy depends on the gestational age (length of the pregnancy) and the woman's condition and preference. Suction curettage may be performed up to 14 weeks of gestation and accounts for more than 90% of abortion procedures. D&E is conducted in the second semester. Table 56.3 lists current methods for induced abortion available in Canada.

Medication therapy using mifepristone and misoprostol is another method to induce abortion (medical abortion) early in pregnancy. These agents must be given within the first 49 days (7 weeks) of pregnancy (day 1 being the first day of the last menstrual period) (Keenan-Lindsay & Mancuso, 2017).

Once the decision is made to have an abortion, the patient and significant others need support and acceptance. The patient should be prepared for what to expect both emotionally and physically. For some women, grief and sadness can be normal emotions after an abortion. The patient needs to understand the procedure, including instructions prior to the procedure as well as afterward. The nurse's caring, nonjudgemental attitude can be a positive factor in the patient's experience.

Follow-up care includes instructions on signs and symptoms of possible complications, including abnormal vaginal bleeding, severe abdominal cramping, fever, and foul drainage. The need to avoid intercourse, use of tampons, and douching until re-examination in 2 weeks should be stressed. Contraception can be started the day of the procedure or during the patient's return visit, in accordance with her needs and desires.

CONDITIONS RELATED TO MENSTRUATION

The normal menstrual cycle is discussed in Chapter 53. The hormonal influences related to the menstrual cycle are shown in Figure 53.9. Menstruation may be irregular during

TABLE 56.3 METHODS FOR INDUCING ABORTION

Method	Length of Pregnancy	Description
Early Abortion		
Methotrexate with misoprostol	≤7 wk	Methotrexate is administered intramuscularly. Misoprostol is given intravaginally, 5–7 days later.
Menstrual extraction	Usually up to second week after first missed period	Catheter is inserted through cervix into uterus, and suction is applied. Endometrium and contents of uterus are aspirated.
Suction aspiration (curettage)	≤14 wk	Cervix is usually dilated, uterine aspirator is introduced, and suction is applied, removing endometrial tissue and implanted pregnancy.
Dilation and evacuation (D&E)	10–16 wk (approximate)	Cervix is dilated, and products of conception are removed by vacuum cannula and use of other instruments as needed.
Late Abortion		
After 20 weeks, late abortion is available in Canada only under special circumstances, such as risk to the health of the mother or serious fetal abnormalities.		

ETHICAL DILEMMAS

Abortion

Situation

A recently married, 39-year-old woman is informed that the results of her amniocentesis indicate that her fetus has major chromosomal abnormalities and is expected to have severe physical and intellectual disabilities. The patient has no children, but her husband has three children from a previous marriage. She asks the nurse what she should do. How would the nurse respond?

Important Points for Consideration

- Decisions about whether to continue a pregnancy with a child who has severe disabilities are extremely personal and emotional. The woman and her husband will need support and information to explore their options and their values.
- Pregnancy counselling is warranted about the woman's choices, her feelings about the pregnancy, her desire to have a child with her husband, her concerns about raising a child with severe disabilities, her feelings about abortion, and concerns about possible future pregnancies.
- Patient autonomy ensures that a woman decide for herself whether or not to continue a pregnancy.
- Abortion is legal in Canada. Canada is one of a small number of countries without a law restricting abortion. Abortion is governed by provincial or territorial and medical regulations and treated like any other medical procedure. In the first trimester, abortion is a private matter between a woman and her health care provider. An abortion can be obtained in a clinic or hospital in many, but not all, provinces and territories.
- The role of the health care provider in these difficult situations is to provide education and support in order to facilitate a decision consistent with the patient's values.
- Nurses are bound by core nursing values and ethical responsibilities such as providing safe, compassionate, competent, and ethical care; promoting health and well-being; promoting and respecting informed decision making; honouring dignity; maintaining privacy and confidentiality; promoting justice; and being accountable (Canadian Nurses Association, 2017).

Clinical Decision-Making Questions

1. How would the nurse's feelings about abortion affect their ability to care for this patient?
2. What type of counselling and genetic testing are available to the patient regarding genetic abnormalities?

the first few years after menarche and the years preceding menopause. Once established, a woman's menstrual cycles usually have a predictable pattern. However, considerable normal variation exists among women in cycle length as well as in the duration, amount, and character of the menstrual flow (see Table 53.2).

PREMENSTRUAL SYNDROME

Premenstrual syndrome (PMS) is a symptom complex related to the luteal phase of the menstrual cycle that resolves with menstruation (Keenan-Lindsay, 2017). The symptoms can be severe enough to impair interpersonal relationships or interfere with usual activities. Because many symptoms are associated with PMS, it is difficult to concisely define PMS. However, PMS symptoms always occur cyclically, during the luteal phase before the onset of menstruation, and are not present at other times of the month. Up to 50% of women of fertile age experience mild to moderate PMS (Ekenros et al., 2019).

Etiology and Pathophysiology

The etiology and pathophysiology of PMS are not well understood. It may have a biological trigger with compounding psychosocial factors. Neurotransmitters, such as serotonin, could also be involved. Some women may have a genetic predisposition to PMS. Other proposed causes include hormone imbalance and nutritional deficiencies. PMS occurs in 20 to 30% of women who are premenopausal. *Premenstrual dysphoric disorder* (PMDD) is the term applied to a type of PMS that affects 2 to 8% of women who are premenopausal (Ekenros et al., 2019). Risk factors for PMDD include severe mood disorders, family history of mood disorders, depression, history of sexual abuse, and history of domestic violence experiences, in addition to PMS (Keenan-Lindsay, 2017).

Clinical Manifestations

PMS is extremely variable in its clinical manifestations between women and, for an individual woman, from one cycle to another. Common physical symptoms include breast discomfort, peripheral edema, abdominal bloating, sensation of weight gain, episodes of binge eating, and migraine headache. Abdominal bloating and breast swelling are caused by fluid shifts because total body weight does not generally change. Anxiety, depression, irritability, and mood swings are some of the emotional symptoms that women may experience (Gnanasambanthan & Datta, 2019).

Diagnostic Studies and Interprofessional Care

PMS can be diagnosed only when other possible causes for the symptoms have been ruled out. A focused health history and physical examination are done to identify any underlying conditions, such as thyroid dysfunction, uterine fibroids, or depression, that may account for the symptoms. No definitive diagnostic test is available for PMS. When PMS or PMDD is a

TABLE 56.4 INTERPROFESSIONAL CARE

Premenstrual Syndrome (PMS)

Diagnostic
- History and physical examination
- Symptom diary

Interprofessional Therapy
- Aerobic exercise
- Medication therapy
- Combined oral contraceptives
- Diuretics
- Prostaglandin inhibitors (e.g., ibuprofen [Advil])
- Selective serotonin reuptake inhibitors (e.g., sertraline [Zoloft])
- Nutritional therapy
- Stress management and relaxation therapy

possible diagnosis, a patient is given a symptom diary to record symptoms prospectively for two or three menstrual cycles. Diagnosis is based on an evaluation of the patient's symptoms.

Nonpharmacological and pharmacological treatments can relieve some PMS symptoms (Table 56.4). However, no single treatment is available. The goal of treatment is to reduce the severity of symptoms and enhance the patient's sense of control and quality of life.

Several conservative approaches to managing the symptoms are considered helpful, including stress management, diet changes, exercise, education, and counselling. Techniques for stress reduction include yoga, meditation, imagery, and biofeedback (see Chapter 8). To decrease autonomic nervous system arousal, women should avoid caffeine, reduce dietary intake of refined carbohydrates, exercise on a regular basis, and practise relaxation techniques. Eating complex carbohydrates with high fibre, foods rich in vitamin B_6, and sources of tryptophan (dairy and poultry) is thought to promote serotonin production, which improves the symptoms. Vitamin B_6 may be found in such foods as pork, milk, egg yolk, and legumes.

Exercise results in a release of endorphins, leading to mood elevation. Aerobic exercise can also have a relaxing effect. Because fatigue tends to exaggerate the symptoms of PMS, adequate rest in the premenstrual period is a priority.

Explanations about PMS can help the patient understand the complexity of the disorder and ways that they can regain a better sense of control. The patient needs to be assured that the symptoms are real, that PMS exists, and that they are not imagining the problem. Acknowledgement of having PMS can itself be therapeutic. Teaching the patient's partner about the nature of PMS can help the partner to better understand the disorder and its effects.

Medication Therapy. Medication therapy is considered when symptoms persist or interfere with daily functioning. At present, no single medication can treat all the symptoms associated with PMS. One therapy may be tried for a time, and if no improvement is observed, another approach is tried. Many treatments are symptom specific. For fluid retention, diuretics such as spironolactone (Aldactone) are used. For reducing cramps, backache, and headache, prostaglandin inhibitors such as ibuprofen (Advil) are used. To improve negative mood, vitamin B_6 supplementation (50 mg daily) may be used. Calcium and magnesium supplementation may also be effective in alleviating psychological and physiological symptoms. For anxiety, buspirone taken during the luteal phase has helped some patients. Patients with PMDD may benefit from antidepressants,

including fluoxetine HCl (Prozac) and tricyclic antidepressants (e.g., amitriptyline).

Other pharmacological treatments are directed at PMS in general. Selective serotonin reuptake inhibitors (SSRIs) (e.g., sertraline [Zoloft]) have provided significant relief to women with severe PMS. Other general treatments include oral contraceptives containing estrogen and progesterone. Evening primrose oil may help some patients.

MEDICATION ALERT—Oral Contraceptives (Both Estrogen and Progesterone)
- May increase the risk for cervical, liver, and perhaps breast cancer
- May elevate blood pressure and cholesterol (related to estrogen)
- Increase risk for cardiac disease if patient is also smoking
- May have impaired effectiveness if used concurrently with certain antibiotics
- Are contraindicated in patients with migraine headaches and depression

DYSMENORRHEA

Dysmenorrhea is abdominal cramping pain or discomfort associated with menstrual flow. The degree of pain and discomfort varies with the individual. The two types of dysmenorrhea are primary (no pathology exists) and secondary (pelvic disease is the underlying cause). Dysmenorrhea is one of the most common gynecological conditions, affecting approximately 50% of all women.

Etiology and Pathophysiology

Primary dysmenorrhea is not a disease; it is caused by an excess of prostaglandin $F_{2\alpha}$ ($PGF_{2\alpha}$), an increased sensitivity to it, or both. Stimulation of the endometrium by estrogen followed by progesterone results in a dramatic increase in prostaglandin production by the endometrium. With the onset of menses, degeneration of the endometrium releases prostaglandin. Locally, prostaglandins increase myometrial contractions and constriction of small endometrial blood vessels. This combination causes tissue ischemia and increased sensitization of the pain receptors, resulting in menstrual pain. Primary dysmenorrhea begins in the first few years after menarche, typically with the onset of regular ovulatory cycles.

Secondary dysmenorrhea is acquired usually after adolescence, occurring most commonly at 30 to 40 years of age. Common pelvic conditions that cause secondary dysmenorrhea include endometriosis, chronic pelvic inflammatory disease (PID), and uterine fibroids. Because secondary dysmenorrhea is caused by multiple conditions, symptoms vary. However, painful menses are present in all situations.

Clinical Manifestations

Primary dysmenorrhea starts 12 to 24 hours before the onset of menses. The pain is most severe on the first day of menses and rarely lasts more than 2 days. Characteristic manifestations include lower abdominal pain that is colicky in nature, frequently radiating to the lower back and upper thighs. The abdominal pain is often accompanied by nausea, diarrhea, loose stools, fatigue, and headache.

Secondary dysmenorrhea occurs usually after the woman has experienced problem-free periods for some time. The pain may be unilateral and it is generally more constant and continues longer than in primary dysmenorrhea. Depending on the cause, symptoms such as *dyspareunia* (painful intercourse), painful defecation, or irregular bleeding may occur at times other than menstruation.

NURSING AND INTERPROFESSIONAL MANAGEMENT DYSMENORRHEA

Evaluation begins with distinguishing primary from secondary dysmenorrhea. A complete health history with special attention to menstrual and gynecological history should be obtained. A pelvic examination is also performed. The probable diagnosis is primary dysmenorrhea if the history reveals an onset shortly after menarche, symptoms are associated only with menses, and the pelvic examination is normal. If any specific cause of dysmenorrhea is evident, the diagnosis is secondary dysmenorrhea.

Treatment for primary dysmenorrhea includes heat, exercise, and medication therapy. Heat is applied to the lower abdomen or back. Regular exercise is thought to be beneficial because it may reduce endometrial hyperplasia and subsequently reduce prostaglandin production. The primary medication therapy is nonsteroidal anti-inflammatory drugs (NSAIDs) such as naproxen (Naprosyn, Aleve), which has antiprostaglandin activity. NSAIDs should be started at the first sign of menses and continued every 4 to 8 hours to maintain a sufficient level of the medication to inhibit prostaglandin synthesis for the usual duration of discomfort.

Oral contraceptives may also be used. They decrease dysmenorrhea by reducing endometrial hyperplasia. Acupuncture and transcutaneous nerve stimulation may be used for patients who have inadequate relief from medications or who prefer not to take medications. Patients whose condition is unresponsive to these treatments should be evaluated for chronic pelvic pain (discussed later in this chapter).

Treatment of secondary dysmenorrhea depends on the cause. Some individuals with secondary dysmenorrhea will be helped by the approaches used for primary dysmenorrhea.

Patients should be taught why dysmenorrhea occurs, as well as how to treat it. Teaching and supportive therapy can provide patients with a foundation for coping with this common occurrence and increase feelings of control and self-reliance.

Patients often ask what can be done for minor discomforts associated with menstrual cycles. They should be advised that, during acute pain, relief may be obtained by applying heat to the abdomen or the back and taking NSAIDs for analgesia. The nurse can also suggest noninvasive pain-relieving practices, such as relaxed breathing and guided imagery.

Other health care measures to reduce the discomfort of dysmenorrhea include regular exercise and proper nutritional habits. Avoiding constipation, maintaining good body mechanics, and eliminating stress and fatigue, particularly during the time preceding menstrual periods, can also decrease discomfort. Staying active and interested in activities may also help.

ABNORMAL VAGINAL BLEEDING

Abnormal vaginal or uterine bleeding is a common gynecological concern. Irregularities include *oligomenorrhea* (long intervals between menses, generally longer than 35 days), amenorrhea (absence of menstruation), *menorrhagia* (excessive or prolonged menstrual bleeding), and *metrorrhagia* (irregular uterine bleeding or bleeding between menses). The cause of abnormal bleeding may vary from anovulatory menstrual cycles to more serious causes such as ectopic pregnancy or endometrial cancer.

TABLE 56.5 CAUSES OF AMENORRHEA	
Natural Amenorrhea • Breastfeeding • Menopause • Pregnancy	**Hormonal Imbalance** • Pituitary tumours • Polycystic ovary syndrome • Premature menopause
Medications • Antidepressants • Antipsychotics • Chemotherapy	**Structural Conditions** • Damage to ovaries or uterus from radiation • Structural abnormalities of vagina • Uterine scarring
Lifestyle • Acute and chronic illness • Excessive exercise • Low body weight • Stress	

The patient's age provides direction for identifying the cause of bleeding. For example, a patient who is postmenopausal with abnormal bleeding must always be evaluated for endometrial cancer but does not need to be evaluated for possible pregnancy. For a 20-year-old patient with abnormal bleeding, the possibility of pregnancy must always be considered, and the possibility of endometrial cancer would be unlikely.

Abnormal bleeding may be caused by dysfunction of the hypothalamic–pituitary–ovarian axis, such as a pituitary adenoma. Another cause may be infection. Changes in lifestyle such as marriage, recent moves, a death in the family, financial stress, and other emotional crises can also cause irregular bleeding. Because psychological factors can influence endocrine function, they should be considered when the patient is evaluated.

Types of Irregular Bleeding

Oligomenorrhea and Amenorrhea. Once pregnancy has been ruled out, anovulation is the most common cause for missing menses. Additional causes of amenorrhea are listed in Table 56.5. *Primary amenorrhea* refers to the failure of menstrual cycles to begin by age 16 years or by age 14 years if secondary sex characteristics are present. *Secondary amenorrhea* refers to cessation of menstrual cycles once established. Women who are pregnant, breastfeeding, or in menopause are not considered to have secondary amenorrhea.

Ovulation is often erratic for several years following menarche and before menopause. Thus, oligomenorrhea due to anovulation is common for women at the beginning and end of menstruation. In anovulatory cycles, the corpus luteum that produces progesterone does not form. This may result in a situation referred to as *unopposed estrogen*. When unopposed by progesterone, estrogen can cause excessive buildup of the endometrium. Persistent overgrowth of the endometrium increases a woman's risk for endometrial cancer. To reduce this risk, progesterone or oral contraceptives are prescribed to ensure that the patient's endometrial lining will be shed at least four to six times per year.

Menorrhagia. The excessive bleeding associated with menorrhagia can be characterized as an increased duration (>7 days), increased amount (>80 mL), or both. Menorrhagia is a common condition that affects 36 to 38% of all women in the reproductive age (Kamaludin et al., 2019). Anovulatory uterine bleeding is the most common cause of menorrhagia. An unopposed estrogen state continues to build up the endometrium until it becomes unstable, resulting in menorrhagia. For young women with excessive bleeding, clotting disorders must be considered. Uterine fibroids (also called *leiomyomas*) and endometrial polyps are a common cause of menorrhagia for women in their 30s and 40s.

Metrorrhagia. Metrorrhagia, also referred to as *spotting* or *breakthrough bleeding*, is bleeding between menstrual periods. For all women of reproductive age, pregnancy complications such as spontaneous abortion or ectopic pregnancy must be considered as a possible cause. Other causes include cervical or endometrial polyps, infection, and carcinoma. Spotting is common during the first three cycles of oral contraceptives. If spotting continues beyond that, a different pill formulation can be prescribed once other causes of metrorrhagia have been ruled out. Spotting with long-acting progestin therapy (e.g., Mirena intrauterine device [IUD]) or progestin-only pills (Depo-Provera) is also common. For patients who are postmenopausal, endometrial cancer must be considered whenever spotting is experienced. In women who are postmenopausal, exogenous estrogen administration during HT is a common cause of metrorrhagia.

Diagnostic Studies and Interprofessional Care

Because abnormal vaginal bleeding has multiple causes, the diagnostic and interprofessional care varies. A health history and physical examination directed at the most likely causes of vaginal bleeding for the patient's age group is the first step. These findings will provide the basis for selecting the necessary laboratory tests and diagnostic procedures. Treatment depends on the etiology of the condition (e.g., menorrhagia, amenorrhea), the degree of threat to the patient's health, and whether the patient wishes to preserve their fertility.

Combined oral contraceptives may be prescribed for a patient with amenorrhea to ensure regular shedding of endometrium if they also want contraception. An antifibrinolytic agent, tranexamic acid (Cyklokapron), may be used to treat heavy menstrual bleeding by helping blood to clot. Adverse effects may include headache, back pain, abdominal pain, muscle and joint pain, anemia, and fatigue. Patients using hormonal contraception should take tranexamic acid only if there is a strong medical need, since there is an associated increased risk for blood clots and stroke. Estradiol valerate/dienogest (Natazia) may be given to patients with heavy menstrual bleeding who desire an oral contraceptive to prevent pregnancy.

The treatment goal for patients with menorrhagia is to minimize further blood loss. If menorrhagia is the result of anovulatory cycles, the endometrium must be stabilized by a combination of oral estrogen and progesterone.

Ablation of the endometrium is a viable, inexpensive treatment for menorrhagia, often performed on an outpatient basis. Using heat (devices filled with heated fluid, microwave energy, radiofrequency ionized argon gas) or extreme cold (cryotherapy), the endometrium is destroyed safely and effectively. When the ablative treatment is completed, the heat/cold source is removed from the uterus, and the uterine lining sloughs off in the following 7 to 10 days. Ablative therapy is contraindicated for patients desiring to maintain their fertility and for patients with suspected endometrial cancer, prior non–lower segment Caesarean birth, or myomectomy (Famuyide, 2018). With severe bleeding, hospitalization is indicated. All patients with menorrhagia should be evaluated for anemia and treated as indicated.

Surgical Therapy. Surgery may be indicated, depending on the underlying cause of the abnormal vaginal bleeding. D&C is used only in cases of acute excess bleeding or for older patients when endometrial biopsy and ultrasonography have not provided the necessary diagnostic information. Endometrial ablation for menorrhagia may be done by laser, thermal balloon, cryotherapy, or microwave energy for patients who do not want to maintain their fertility.

If menorrhagia is caused by uterine fibroids, a hysterectomy (surgical removal of the uterus) may be performed. A *myomectomy* (removal of fibroids without removal of the uterus) may be performed if uterine preservation is desired. The myomectomy is done via laparotomy, laparoscopy, or hysteroscopy. Hormonal regimens and embolization of blood vessels supplying the fibroids are other treatment options.

NURSING MANAGEMENT
ABNORMAL VAGINAL BLEEDING

Teaching patients about the characteristics of the menstrual cycle will assist them in identifying normal variations. Table 53.2 in Chapter 53 includes characteristics of the menstrual cycle and related patient teaching. This knowledge can diminish apprehension and dispel misconceptions about the menstrual cycle. If the patient's menstrual cycle pattern does not fall within the normal range, the nurse should urge her to visit her health care provider.

The selection of internal or external sanitary protection is a matter of personal preference. Tampons and menstrual cups are convenient and may make menstrual hygiene easier, whereas pads may provide better protection. Using a combination of tampons/menstrual cups and pads and avoiding prolonged use of superabsorbent tampons may decrease the risk for *toxic shock syndrome* (TSS). TSS is an acute condition caused by a toxin from *Staphylococcus aureus*. Symptoms of TSS may initially include flulike symptoms such as high fever, nausea, vomiting, diarrhea, dizziness, fainting, and disorientation. Other symptoms may include low blood pressure, shock, dehydration, sore throat, muscle pain, peeling skin, and a sunburn-like rash (Nonfoux et al., 2018).

Whenever excessive, the amount of the patient's vaginal bleeding should be assessed as accurately as possible. The patient should record and report the number and size of pads or tampons used and the degree of saturation. The patient's fatigue level, along with variations in blood pressure and pulse, should be monitored because anemia and hypovolemia may be present. If a surgical procedure is indicated, the nurse should provide appropriate preoperative and postoperative care.

ECTOPIC PREGNANCY

An ectopic pregnancy is the implantation of the fertilized ovum anywhere outside the uterine cavity (Figure 56.2). Approximately

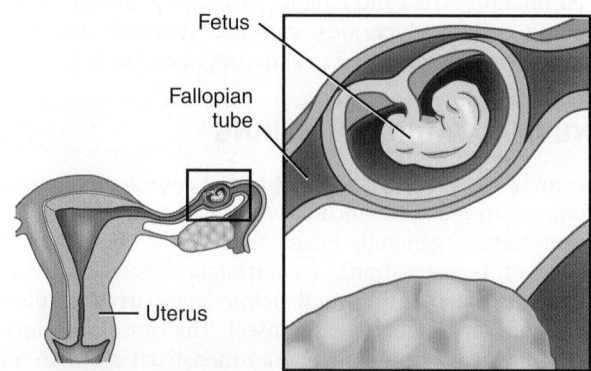

FIG. 56.2 Ectopic pregnancy occurring in the Fallopian tube.

3% of all pregnancies are ectopic, and approximately 98% of these occur in the Fallopian tube. The remaining 2 to 3% may be ovarian, abdominal, or cervical. Ectopic pregnancy is a life-threatening condition. Earlier identification has contributed to decreased mortality rates (Madhra et al., 2017).

Etiology and Pathophysiology

Any blockage of the Fallopian tube or reduction of tubal peristalsis that impedes or delays the zygote passing to the uterine cavity can result in tubal implantation. After implantation, the growth of the gestational sac expands the tubal wall. Eventually, the tube ruptures, causing acute peritoneal symptoms. Less acute symptoms usually begin within 6 to 8 weeks after the last normal menstrual period and weeks before rupture would occur.

Risk factors for ectopic pregnancy include a history of PID, prior ectopic pregnancy, current progestin-releasing IUD, progestin-only birth control failure, and prior pelvic or tubal surgery. Additional risk factors for ectopic pregnancy include procedures used in infertility treatment, including in IVF, embryo transfer, and ovulation induction.

Clinical Manifestations

The classic manifestations of ectopic pregnancy are abdominal or pelvic pain, missed menses, and irregular vaginal bleeding. Other manifestations include morning sickness, breast tenderness, gastrointestinal disturbance, malaise, and syncope. Pain is almost always present and is caused by distension of the Fallopian tube. It may start unilaterally and then spread to become bilateral. The character of the pain varies among patients and can be colicky or vague. If tubal rupture occurs, the pain is intense and may be referred to the shoulder as a result of irritation of the diaphragm by blood released into the abdominal cavity. Symptom severity does not necessarily correlate with the extent of external (vaginal) bleeding present. With rupture, the risk for hemorrhage and hypovolemic shock is present. Suspected rupture is treated as an emergency. Vaginal bleeding that accompanies ectopic pregnancy is usually described as spotting. However, it is also possible that bleeding may be heavier and can be confused with menses.

Diagnostic Studies

Ectopic pregnancy can be a diagnostic challenge because of its similarity to other pelvic and abdominal disorders, such as salpingitis, spontaneous abortion, ruptured ovarian cyst, appendicitis, and peritonitis. A serum (radioimmunoassay) pregnancy test should be performed. If the test is negative, an ectopic pregnancy is not likely. If ectopic pregnancy cannot be excluded by the pregnancy test, further evaluation is warranted. If the patient is in stable condition, a combination of serial β-hCG and transvaginal ultrasound is used (Madhra et al., 2017).

Absence of a normal intrauterine pregnancy means that the diagnosis is probably spontaneous abortion or ectopic pregnancy. With a spontaneous abortion, serial β-hCG levels will decrease over time. A complete blood cell count is obtained when there is any concern regarding the amount of blood loss or if surgery is being contemplated.

NURSING AND INTERPROFESSIONAL MANAGEMENT ECTOPIC PREGNANCY

Surgery remains the primary approach for treating ectopic pregnancies and should be performed immediately. However, medical management with intramuscular injection of methotrexate is being used with increasing success and safety in patients who are hemodynamically stable and where the size of gestation is smaller than 3 cm (Madhra et al., 2017). A conservative surgical approach limits damage to the reproductive system as much as possible. Removal of the fetus from the tube is preferred to removing the tube. Laparoscopy is preferable to laparotomy because it decreases blood loss and the length of the hospital stay. If the tube ruptures, conservative surgical approaches may not be possible. The patient may need a blood transfusion and supplemental intravenous (IV) fluid therapy to relieve shock and restore a satisfactory blood volume for safe anaesthesia and surgery. The use of laparoscopy has resulted in fewer repeated ectopic pregnancies and a higher rate of future successful pregnancies.

Nursing care depends on the patient's condition. Before the diagnosis has been confirmed, the nurse should be alert to signs of increasing pain and vaginal bleeding, which may indicate that rupture of the tube has occurred. Vital signs are monitored closely, along with observation for signs of shock. Explanations and preparation for diagnostic procedures are given when appropriate. Preparation of the patient for abdominal surgery may follow rapidly. The patient's emotional status should be assessed. Reassurance and support for the surgery should be given to the patient and family. Postoperatively, the patient may express a fear of future ectopic pregnancies and have many questions about the impact of this experience on future fertility.

PERIMENOPAUSE AND POSTMENOPAUSE

Perimenopause is a normal life transition that begins with the first signs of change in menstrual cycles and ends after cessation of menses. Menopause is a normal physiological cessation of menses associated with declining ovarian function that ends in cessation of the menstrual cycle and ovulation. Natural menopause is diagnosed retrospectively after 12 months of no periods. The average age for a woman is 52 years. The age can vary from 40 to 58 years. Induced menopause occurs after surgical intervention to remove the ovaries or from adverse effects of chemotherapy, radiation therapy, or other medications. The age at which menopause occurs is not affected by age at menarche, physical characteristics, number of pregnancies, date of last pregnancy, or oral contraceptive use. However, genetic factors, autoimmune conditions, cigarette smoking, and racial or ethnic factors have been linked to earlier age at menopause. Postmenopause refers to the time in a woman's life after menopause.

Changes within the ovary start the cascade of events that finally result in menopause. The regression of the follicles within each ovary begins at puberty and accelerates after age 35. With age, fewer follicles remain that are responsive to follicle-stimulating hormone (FSH). FSH normally stimulates the dominant follicle to secrete estrogen. When the follicles can no longer respond to FSH, ovarian production of estrogen and progesterone declines. However, women who are perimenopausal can get pregnant until menopause has occurred, since many women have long anovulatory cycles interspersed with shorter, ovulatory cycles.

With decreased ovarian function, decreased levels of estrogen cause a gradual increase in FSH and luteinizing hormone (LH) as a result of the negative feedback process. By the time menopause occurs, there is a 10- to 20-fold increase in FSH. The elevated FSH level may take several years to return to the premenopausal level. The reduced estrogen level also causes a decrease in the frequency of ovulation and results in changes in the reproductive organs and tissues (e.g., atrophy of vaginal tissue).

Clinical Manifestations

Clinical manifestations of perimenopause and postmenopause are presented in Table 56.6. Perimenopause is a time of erratic hormonal fluctuation. Irregular vaginal bleeding is common. With decreasing estrogen, hot flashes and other symptoms can begin. The signs and symptoms of diminished estrogen are listed in Table 56.7. The loss of estrogen plays a significant role in the cause of age-related alterations. Changes most critical to a woman's well-being are the increased risks for coronary artery disease (CAD) and osteoporosis (secondary to bone density loss). Other changes include a redistribution of fat, a tendency to gain weight more easily, muscle and joint pain, loss of skin elasticity, changes in hair amount and distribution, and atrophy of external genitalia and breast tissue.

Hallmarks of perimenopause include *vasomotor instability* (hot flashes) and irregular menses. A hot flash (occurs in up to 80% of all women) is described as a sudden sensation of intense heat along with perspiration and flushing (McGarry et al., 2018). These sensations last from several seconds to 5 minutes and occur most often at night, thereby disturbing sleep. The cause of hot flashes, or vasomotor instability, is not clearly understood. It has been theorized that temperature regulators in the brain are in proximity to the area where gonadotropin-releasing hormone (GnRH) is released. The lowered estrogen levels are correlated with dilation of cutaneous blood vessels, resulting in hot flashes and increased sweating. The more sudden the withdrawal of estrogen (e.g., surgical removal of the ovaries), the more likely the symptoms will be severe if no hormone replacement is provided. Symptoms usually subside over time and typically last from 5 to 10 years with or without treatment. Hot flashes can be triggered by situations that affect body temperature, such as eating a hot meal, hot weather, drinking an alcoholic beverage, stress, or warm clothing. Women who smoke are at higher risk for hot flashes because smoking affects estrogen metabolism. In the United States, Black women report the highest incidence of hot flashes, whereas Asian women report the lowest number (McNamara et al., 2015).

Atrophic vaginal changes secondary to decreased estrogen include thinning of the vaginal mucosa and disappearance of rugae. Vaginal secretions also decrease and become more alkaline. As a result of these changes, the vagina is easily traumatized and more susceptible to infection, including a higher risk for human immunodeficiency virus (HIV) infection if exposed.

Dyspareunia (painful intercourse) may also occur. This can lead to unnecessary and premature cessation of sexual activity. Dryness is a concern that can be easily corrected with water-soluble lubricants or, if needed, with hormonal creams or systemic HT.

Atrophic changes in the lower urinary tract also occur with a decrease in estrogen. Bladder capacity decreases, and the bladder and urethral tissue lose tone. These changes can cause symptoms that mimic a bladder infection (e.g., dysuria, urgency, frequency) when no infection is present.

Whether decreasing estrogen is responsible for the psychological changes associated with perimenopause is unclear. Depression, irritability, and cognitive difficulties, which are often attributed to menopause, could result from life stressors or sleep deprivation from hot flashes. Depressive symptoms appear to improve when hormone levels stabilize.

Interprofessional Care

The diagnosis of perimenopause should be made only after careful consideration of other possible causes for the patient's symptoms. Depression, thyroid dysfunction, anemia, or anxiety could be responsible for the same symptoms. An accurate history of menstrual patterns should be reviewed as part of establishing the diagnosis. Because of the hormonal fluctuations that occur before menopause, routine testing of the serum FSH level is not indicated.

Medication Therapy. Hormone therapy (HT) was once standard therapy in Canada for treating menopausal symptoms. HT includes estrogen for patients without ovaries or estrogen and progesterone for patients with a uterus. Findings from the Women's Health Initiative (WHI) clinical trials led to changes in this practice (National Institutes of Health [NIH], 2016). The data showed that women who had taken estrogen plus progestin had an increased risk for breast cancer, stroke, heart disease, and emboli. However, these women had fewer hip fractures and a lower risk of developing colorectal cancer. Women who took

TABLE 56.6	CLINICAL MANIFESTATIONS OF PERIMENOPAUSE AND POSTMENOPAUSE	
Perimenopause	**Postmenopause**
• Atrophy of genitourinary tissue with decreased support	• Atrophy of genitourinary tissue (e.g., vaginal epithelium)
• Irregular menses	• Breast tenderness
• Mood changes	• Cessation of menses
• Occasional vasomotor symptoms	• Stress and urge incontinence
• Osteoporosis	• Vasomotor instability (hot flashes and night sweats)
• Stress and urge incontinence	

TABLE 56.7	SIGNS AND SYMPTOMS OF ESTROGEN DEFICIENCY
Vasomotor	
• Hot flashes	
• Night sweats	
Genitourinary	
• Atrophic vaginitis	
• Dyspareunia secondary to poor lubrication	
• Incontinence	
Psychological	
• Change in sleep pattern	
• Decreased REM sleep	
• Emotional lability	
Skeletal	
• Increased fracture rate, especially of vertebral bodies but also of humerus, distal radius, and upper femur	
Cardiovascular	
• Decreased high-density lipoproteins (HDLs)	
• Increased low-density lipoproteins (LDLs)	
Dermatological	
• Breast tissue changes	
• Diminished collagen content of skin	

REM, rapid eye movement.

only estrogen (Premarin) had an increased risk for stroke and emboli. However, these women had decreased risk for fractures, with no increased risk for heart disease or breast or colorectal cancer.

If patients wish to consider taking HT for the short-term treatment (less than 5 years) of menopausal symptoms, the risks and benefits of therapy (e.g., minimizes bone loss, hot flashes, vaginal atrophic changes) should be considered carefully. The patient and their health care provider should thoroughly discuss the decision to take HT. If a patient chooses to use HT, the lowest effective dose should be used for the shortest amount of time to manage menopausal symptoms. Estrogen-alone HT may decrease the risk for coronary heart disease and decrease mortality in women younger than 60 years and within 10 years of menopause (Akter & Shirin, 2018).

The adverse effects of estrogen include nausea, fluid retention, headache, and breast enlargement. Adverse effects of progesterone include increased appetite, weight gain, irritability, depression, spotting, and breast tenderness. A commonly used estrogen preparation is 0.625 mg of conjugated estrogen (Premarin) daily. For symptom relief, a higher dose may be needed. To receive the protective benefit of progesterone, 5 to 10 mg of medroxyprogesterone (Provera) is indicated for 12 days of each month on a cyclical regimen or 2.5 mg if on a continuous regimen. If the estrogen is to be increased for symptom relief, the progesterone should also be increased. Other forms of progesterone include norethindrone-ethinyl estradiol (Brevicon, Synphasic) and micronized progesterone creams, dermal patches, gels, and lotions; rings placed around the cervix; and subcutaneous pellets. Vaginal creams are especially useful for urogenital symptoms (e.g., dryness). Transdermal estrogen (skin patch or spray) has the advantage of bypassing the liver but has the disadvantage of causing skin irritation (Akter & Shirin, 2018).

MEDICATION ALERT—Medroxyprogesterone (Depo-Provera, Provera)
- Report immediately the development of sudden loss of vision, severe headache, chest pain, hemoptysis, pain in calves (especially with swelling, redness), numbness in the arm or leg, and abdominal pain or tenderness.

Selective estrogen receptor modulators (SERMs), such as raloxifene (Evista), are also used in treating menopausal conditions. These medications have some of the positive benefits of estrogen, such as preventing bone loss, without the negative effects, such as endometrial hyperplasia. Raloxifene competes with estrogen for estrogen receptor sites (Vardanyan, 2017). It decreases bone loss and serum cholesterol but has minimal effects on breast and uterine tissue.

Bisphosphonates, including alendronate (Fosamax) and risedronate (Actonel/Actonel DR), are also used to decrease the risk for osteoporosis in patients who are postmenopausal. These medications enhance bone mineral density by suppressing resorption. SERMs and bisphosphonates are discussed further in Chapter 66 with respect to their role in the management of osteoporosis.

Nonhormonal Therapy. Because of the risks associated with HT, many patients try other therapies to relieve menopausal symptoms. SSRI antidepressants, including paroxetine (Paxil), fluoxetine (Prozac), and venlafaxine (Effexor XR), are an effective alternative to HT in reducing hot flashes. This effect is noted even if the user is not depressed. The mechanism of action is unknown. Gabapentin (Neurontin), an anticonvulsant,

analgesic adjunct, and mood stabilizer, has also been shown to relieve hot flashes (Kaunitz & Manson, 2015; McGarry et al., 2018).

Hot-flash frequency and severity can be reduced through measures that lead to a decrease in heat production and an increase in heat loss. Keeping a cool environment and limiting caffeine and alcohol intake lower heat production. Relaxation techniques (e.g., relaxation breathing, imagery) may also help. To promote heat loss at night when hot flashes can disrupt sleep, air circulation can be increased in the room and bedding avoided that traps the heat (e.g., heavy quilts). Loose-fitting clothes do not retain body heat, whereas clothes with tight necks and wrists do. Cool cloths applied to flushed areas also aid in heat loss.

Daily intake of vitamin E in doses up to 800 IU may also help reduce hot flashes in some women. Changing sleep patterns may be helped by avoiding alcohol use and controlling hot flashes. Relaxation techniques can promote a better night's sleep by decreasing anxiety. A regular, moderate program (three to four times per week) of aerobic and weight-bearing exercises can slow the process of bone loss and a tendency toward weight gain (McGarry et al., 2018).

Nutritional Therapy. Good nutrition can decrease the risk for cardiovascular disease and osteoporosis, in addition to assisting with vasomotor symptoms. A daily intake of about 30 kcal/kg of body weight is recommended. A decrease in metabolic rate and careless eating habits can cause the weight gain and fatigue often attributed to menopause. An adequate intake of calcium and vitamin D helps maintain healthy bones and counteracts loss of bone density. Women who are postmenopausal and are not receiving supplemental estrogen should have a daily calcium intake of at least 1500 mg, whereas those taking estrogen replacement need at least 1000 mg/day. Calcium supplements are best absorbed when taken with meals. Either dietary calcium or calcium supplements may be used (see Chapter 66, Tables 66.5 and 66.6).

The diet should be high in complex carbohydrates and vitamin B complex, especially B_6. Phytoestrogens (soy, tofu, chickpeas, sunflower seeds) may reduce menopausal symptoms. Herbal remedies, such as black cohosh, have become popular in treating menopausal symptoms (see the Complementary & Alternative Therapies box). Consultation with an experienced herbal practitioner is recommended before initiating therapy.

CULTURALLY COMPETENT CARE

Nurses caring for patients of cultures other than their own or for patients who self-identify along the lesbian, gay, bisexual, transgender, queer, or Two-Spirited (LGBTQ2+) spectrum must develop competencies in caring for these populations. Assumptions about experiences of women's health issues must be validated or clarified when caring for individuals who see these experiences differently through a cultural or gendered lens. Nurses must approach the provision of sexual and reproductive health care for these populations with respect for persons in an environment that is safe and free from judgement (Walker et al., 2016).

MENOPAUSE

Although all women experience menopause, the perception of menopause varies by culture. Different ethnic groups have different traditions and beliefs regarding menopause, including the use of complementary and alternative therapies to manage symptoms (Stanzel et al., 2018). In many cultures, menopause is considered a normal part of aging, and little emphasis is placed

🌿 COMPLEMENTARY & ALTERNATIVE THERAPIES

Herbs and Supplements for Menopause*

Herb	Scientific Evidence	Nursing Implications
Black cohosh	Mixed evidence for use in the treatment of menopausal symptoms†	Generally well tolerated in recommended doses for ≤6 months to relieve symptoms such as hot flashes. Should not be used in people with a liver disorder. Should not be combined with birth control pills, hormone therapy, or tamoxifen or used by women who are allergic to acetylsalicylic acid (ASA; Aspirin).
Soy	Mixed evidence for treatment of menopausal symptoms‡	Soy isoflavone (rather than soy protein) has shown the most promise for treatment of hot flashes. The long-term effects of a high soy diet have not been well-researched. High soy intake cannot be considered safe until more studies are done. In some women, soy causes digestive upset.

*In general, the evidence for use of these herbs as treatments for menopause symptoms is limited by a lack of well-designed, controlled trials.

†HealthLinksBC. (2015). *Black cohosh for menopause symptoms.* http://www.healthlinkbc.ca/healthtopics/content.asp?hwid=tn9522

‡HealthLinksBC. (2015). *Soy for menopause symptoms.* http://www.healthlinkbc.ca/healthtopics/content.asp?hwid=tn9521

on the physical and emotional symptoms that accompany the loss of fertility. In cultures in which older persons are revered, menopause is often seen as a liberating transition to a state of being a "wise woman." Immigrant women seeking help during the menopause may fail to access health care in Canada because of barriers including lack of eligibility for health care coverage, language incompatibility between provider and client, and diminished opportunity for or access to care provision (Silverberg et al., 2018). Persons self-identifying as LGBTQ2 experience similar barriers when seeking health care providers with knowledge of LGBTQ2 health issues (Walker et al., 2016).

North American culture is generally negative toward aging and places a high value on youth. Menopause is often considered a disorder that requires treatment. Menopausal symptoms may be viewed as troublesome, with hot flashes and mood swings needing to be treated. Numerous substances, from HT to herbal preparations, are often used to treat menopausal symptoms. Menopause is experienced by all women; however, its meaning and symptoms vary. Menopause is a milestone in a person's life that is embedded in their own personality and culture. Approaching patients who are menopausal with this understanding is important to providing culturally competent care.

NURSING MANAGEMENT
PERIMENOPAUSE AND POSTMENOPAUSE

Nurses can play a key role in helping patients understand perimenopausal changes (see Table 56.6) and options to minimize unwanted symptoms that are bothersome. Nurses can foster a positive image of perimenopause as a time of vitality and attractiveness. Perimenopause can provide women with a renewed incentive to enhance self-care and well-being. It is important to provide teaching and reassurance to patients who are perimenopausal who experience difficulty in managing their symptoms. The fact that symptoms are normal and only temporary should be discussed. Nonpharmacological approaches to managing symptoms should also be reviewed with patients who are perimenopausal.

Patients with dry skin can use moisturizing soaps and body lotions to alleviate discomfort. Kegel exercises may help decrease stress incontinence (see Table 48.19). Sexual function can continue with little change in the vast majority of women who are postmenopausal. Cessation of menstruation and ability to bear children should not be equated with cessation of sexual capability. Femininity and libido do not disappear with menopause. A water-soluble lubricant (e.g., Replens, Astroglide, K-Y Jelly) is often effective in managing atrophic changes in vaginal epithelium. An active sex life helps increase lubrication and maintains the pliability of vaginal tissues. The nurse should provide the patient with an opportunity to candidly discuss concerns related to sexual functioning.

CONDITIONS OF THE VULVA, VAGINA, AND CERVIX
Etiology and Pathophysiology

Infection and inflammation of the vagina, the cervix, and the vulva tend to occur when the natural defences of the acid vaginal secretions (maintained by sufficient estrogen levels) and the presence of *Lactobacillus* are disrupted. Women's resistance may also be decreased as a result of aging, poor nutrition, and the use of medications that alter the bacterial flora or mucosa. Organisms gain entrance to the areas through contaminated hands, clothing, douching, and intercourse. Table 56.8 presents the causes, manifestations and diagnostic methods, and interprofessional care of common inflammations and infections.

Most lower genital tract infections are related to sexual intercourse. Through intercourse, organisms can be transmitted, tissues injured, and the acid–base balance of the vagina altered. Vulvar infections caused by viruses such as herpes and genital warts can be sexually transmitted when no lesions are apparent. Oral contraceptives, antibiotics, and corticosteroids may produce changes in the vaginal pH and trigger an overgrowth of the organisms present. For example, *Candida albicans* may be present in small numbers in the vagina. An overgrowth of this organism causes vulvovaginitis.

Clinical Manifestations

Abnormal vaginal discharge and reddened vulvar lesions are common clinical manifestations. In addition to a thick, white, curdlike discharge, patients with vulvovaginal candidiasis (VVC) often experience intense itching and dysuria, which is the result of urine coming into contact with fissures and irritated areas on the vulva. The hallmark of bacterial vaginosis is the fishy odour of the discharge. Patients with cervicitis may notice spotting after intercourse.

Common vulvar lesions include herpes infection and genital warts. Initial or primary herpes infections may be extremely painful. Herpes begins as a small vesicle followed by a superficial red ulcer. Most herpes lesions are painful. Genital warts, caused by the human papilloma virus (HPV), vary in appearance. Irregularly shaped "cauliflower" lesions are common. Genital warts are painless unless traumatized. (Herpes infection and genital warts are discussed in Chapter 55.)

TABLE 56.8   INFECTIONS OF THE LOWER GENITAL TRACT

Infection/Etiology	Manifestations and Diagnostic Methods	Medication Therapy
Vulvovaginal Candidiasis (VVC) (Monilial Vaginitis)		
Candida albicans (fungus)	Commonly found in mouth, gastrointestinal tract, and vagina; pruritus, thick white, curdlike discharge; KOH microscopic examination—pseudohyphae; pH 4–4.7	Antifungal agents, over-the-counter vaginal suppository and creams (e.g., clotrimazole [Canesten], miconazole [Micozole]) Fluconazole (Diflucan)
Trichomoniasis Vaginitis		
Trichomonas vaginalis (protozoa)	Sexually transmitted; pruritus; frothy greenish or grey discharge; hemorrhagic spots on cervix or vaginal walls; saline microscopic examination—swimming trichomonads; pH >4.5	Metronidazole (Flagyl) for patient and partner
Bacterial Vaginosis		
Gardnerella vaginalis *Corynebacterium vaginale*	Mode of transmission unclear; watery discharge with fishy odour; may or may not have symptoms; saline microscopic examination—epithelial cells; pH >4.5	Oral or vaginal metronidazole (Flagyl) or clindamycin (Dalacin C) cream 2% Lactobacillus acidophilus taken orally by diet (e.g., yogourt, fermented soy products) or supplements can decrease unwanted vaginal bacteria Examine and treat partner
Cervicitis		
Chlamydia trachomatis *Neisseria gonorrhoeae*	Sexually transmitted; mucopurulent discharge with postcoital spotting from cervical inflammation; culture for *Chlamydia trachomatis* and *Neisseria gonorrhoeae*	Combination gonorrhea infection therapy (e.g., azithromycin [Zithromax] and cephalosporins [e.g., cefixime and ceftriaxone]) should be used because of increasing antimicrobial resistance. Treat partners with same medications
Severe Recurrent Vaginitis		
C. albicans (most often)	May be indicative of HIV infection; all patients whose condition is unresponsive to first-line treatment should be offered HIV testing	Medication appropriate to opportunistic organism

HIV, human immunodeficiency virus; *KOH*, potassium hydroxide.
Source: Adapted from Public Health Agency of Canada (PHAC). (2015). *Canadian guidelines on sexually transmitted infections.* http://www.phac-aspc.gc.ca/std-mts/sti-its/cgsti-ldcits/index-eng.php

Women who are postmenopausal may develop gynecological conditions such as *lichen sclerosis* (Lewis et al., 2018). This chronic inflammatory condition is associated with intense itching in the genital skin area (e.g., labia minora, clitoris). The lesions are white with a "tissue paper" appearance initially, although scratching produces changes in the appearance. The cause is unknown. Treatment of vulvar dystrophies is symptomatic because no cures are available. Treatment involves controlling the "itch–scratch cycle," preventing further secondary damage to the skin. High-potency topical corticosteroid ointment such as clobetasol propionate (Clobex) may help relieve itching.

Interprofessional Care

Genital conditions are evaluated by taking a history, performing a physical examination, and obtaining the appropriate laboratory and diagnostic studies. Because many of these conditions relate to sexual activity, a sexual history is essential. The nature of the condition determines the extent of the evaluation. Ulcerative lesions should be cultured for herpes. A blood test for syphilis may be done when ulcerative lesions are present. Genital warts are usually identified by their clinical appearance. Vulvar dystrophies may be examined via colposcopy with a biopsy taken for diagnosis.

Conditions involving vaginal discharge are evaluated by microscopy and cultures. The most common vaginal conditions (i.e., bacterial vaginosis, VVC, and trichomoniasis) are diagnosed by a procedure called a *wet mount*. The findings that are characteristic of each condition are shown in Table 56.8. To assess for cervicitis, endocervical cultures are obtained for

Chlamydia and gonorrhea. If purulent discharge is observed coming from the cervix, a sample of endocervical cells may be taken to be evaluated by Gram staining. The Gram-stained slide is examined with a microscope to identify white blood cells and Gram-negative diplococci (indicative of gonorrhea). (Sexually transmitted infections [STIs] are discussed in Chapter 55.)

Medication therapy is based on the diagnosis and is shown in Table 56.8. Antibiotics taken as directed will cure bacterial infections. Treatment duration and medications vary with specific STIs. Patients need to be taught how to properly take their medications and to follow up to verify a cure. Partners should be treated so that reinfection does not occur.

Patients with vaginal conditions or cervical infection should abstain from intercourse for at least 1 week. Douching should be avoided because it has been adversely linked to PID, STIs, and ectopic pregnancy. Sexual partners must be evaluated and treated if the patient is diagnosed with trichomoniasis, chlamydial infection, gonorrhea, syphilis, or HIV.

NURSING MANAGEMENT
CONDITIONS OF THE VULVA, VAGINA, AND CERVIX

Nurses have the opportunity to teach patients about common genital conditions and how to reduce their risks of contracting these conditions. The ability to recognize symptoms that indicate a disorder helps patients seek care in a timely manner. Discussing concerns regarding one's genitals or sexual intercourse is frequently difficult. The nurse's nonjudgemental attitude can make patients feel more comfortable and empower them to ask questions and seek accurate information.

When a patient is diagnosed with a genital condition, the nurse should ensure that they fully understand the directions for treatment. Taking the full course of medication is especially important to decrease the chance of relapse. Because genitalia are such a private area, use of graphs and models is especially helpful for patient teaching. When a patient will be using a vaginal medication for the first time, showing them the applicator and how to fill it is important. The patient should be taught where and how the applicator should be inserted, using visual aids or models. Vaginal creams should be inserted before going to bed so that the medication will remain in the vagina for a long time. Patients using vaginal creams or suppositories may wish to use panty liners during the day, when the residual medication may drain out.

PELVIC INFLAMMATORY DISEASE

Pelvic inflammatory disease (PID) is an infectious condition of the pelvic cavity that may involve the Fallopian tubes (salpingitis), ovaries (oophoritis), and pelvic peritoneum (peritonitis) (Brunham et al., 2015). A tubo-ovarian abscess may also form (Figure 56.3). The most recent statistics indicate that there are about 100 000 cases of symptomatic PID annually in Canada, but precise numbers are not known, as PID is not reportable nationally (PHAC, 2013). PID is referred to as "silent" when individuals do not perceive any symptoms; other patients with PID will be in acute distress.

Etiology and Pathophysiology

PID is often the result of untreated cervicitis. The organism infecting the cervix ascends higher into the uterus, Fallopian tubes, ovaries, and peritoneal cavity. *C. trachomatis* and *N. gonorrhoeae* are the most common causative organisms of PID. These organisms, as well as anaerobes, mycoplasma, streptococci, and enteric Gram-negative rods, gain entrance during sexual intercourse or after pregnancy termination, pelvic surgery, or childbirth. It is important to remember that not all cases of PID are the result of an STI.

Women at increased risk for chlamydial infections (younger than 24 years of age, with multiple sex partners, or with a new sex partner) should be routinely tested for *C. trachomatis*. Chlamydial infections can be asymptomatic and unknowingly

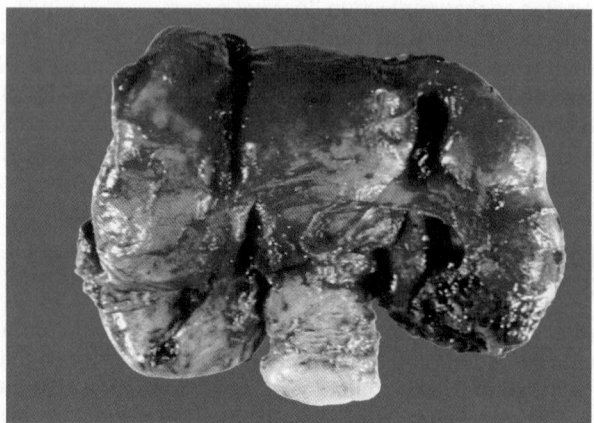

FIG. 56.3 Pelvic inflammatory disease. Acute infection of the Fallopian tubes and ovaries. The tubes and ovaries have become an inflamed mass attached to the uterus. A tubo-ovarian abscess is also present. Source: Kumar, V., Abbas, A. K., Fausto, N., et al. (2010). *Robbins and Cotran pathologic basis of disease* (8th ed., p. 1010, Figure 22-4A). Saunders.

transmitted during intercourse. Silent PID is a major cause of female infertility.

Clinical Manifestations

Women with PID usually go to a health care provider because they are experiencing lower abdominal pain. The pain typically starts gradually and then becomes constant. The intensity may vary from mild to severe. Movement such as walking can increase the pain; pain is also frequently associated with intercourse. Spotting after intercourse and purulent cervical or vaginal discharge may also be noted. Fever and chills may be present. Women with less acute symptoms notice increased cramping pain with menses, irregular bleeding, and some pain with intercourse. Women with mild symptoms may go untreated either because they did not seek care or the health care provider misdiagnosed their symptoms.

A pelvic examination assists in the diagnosis of PID. Patients with PID have pelvic organ tenderness, as indicated by adnexal tenderness (tenderness of uterine appendages such as Fallopian tubes, ovaries, and ligaments that hold the uterus in place), positive cervical motion tenderness, or uterine compression tenderness during bimanual examination (Society of Obstetricians and Gynaecologists of Canada, 2019). Additional criteria useful for diagnosis include fever and abnormal discharge (vaginal or cervical), as well as lower genital tract inflammation. Cultures for *N. gonorrhoeae* and *C. trachomatis* are also obtained, and a pregnancy test should be done to rule out ectopic pregnancy. Medication therapy begins when minimal diagnostic criteria are met. Thus, treatment is not delayed for culture results. When the patient's pain or obesity compromises the pelvic examination and a tubo-ovarian abscess may be present, vaginal ultrasonography is indicated.

Complications

Immediate complications of PID include septic shock and *Fitz–Hugh–Curtis syndrome*, which occurs when PID spreads to the liver and causes acute perihepatitis. The patient has symptoms of right upper quadrant pain, but liver function tests are normal. Tubo-ovarian abscesses may "leak" or rupture, resulting in pelvic or generalized peritonitis. As the general circulation is flooded with bacterial endotoxins from the infected areas, septic shock may result. Embolisms may occur as the result of thrombophlebitis of the pelvic veins.

PID can cause adhesions and strictures to develop in the Fallopian tubes. Ectopic pregnancy may result when a tube is partially obstructed because the sperm can pass through the stricture but the fertilized ovum cannot reach the uterus. After one episode of PID, the risk of having an ectopic pregnancy increases 10-fold. Further damage can obstruct the Fallopian tubes and cause infertility.

Interprofessional Care

PID is usually treated on an outpatient basis. The patient is given a combination of antibiotics such as cefoxitin and doxycycline to provide broad coverage against the causative organisms. With effective antibiotic therapy, the pain should subside. The patient must have no intercourse for 3 weeks. Her partner(s) must be examined and treated. An important part of care is physical rest and oral fluids. Re-evaluation in 48 to 72 hours, even if symptoms are improving, is an essential part of outpatient care.

If outpatient treatment is unsuccessful or if the patient is acutely ill or in severe pain, admission to hospital is indicated.

If a tubo-ovarian abscess is present, hospitalization is necessary. Maximum doses of parenteral antibiotics are given in the hospital. Corticosteroids may be added to the antibiotic regimen to reduce inflammation, allowing for faster recovery and improvement in subsequent fertility. Application of heat to the lower abdomen or sitz baths may be used to improve circulation and decrease pain. Bed rest in the semi-Fowler's position promotes drainage of the pelvic cavity by gravity and may prevent the development of abscesses high in the abdomen. Analgesics to relieve pain and IV fluids to prevent dehydration are also used.

Surgery is indicated for abscesses that fail to resolve with IV antibiotics. The abscess may be drained by laparoscopy or laparotomy. In extreme cases of infection or severe chronic pelvic pain, a hysterectomy may be performed. When surgery is necessary, every attempt is made to preserve fertility in patients of childbearing age.

NURSING MANAGEMENT
PELVIC INFLAMMATORY DISEASE

Subjective and objective data that should be obtained from patients with PID are presented in Table 56.9. Prevention, early recognition, and prompt treatment of vaginal and cervical infections can help prevent PID and its serious complications. Nurses should urge patients to seek medical attention for any unusual vaginal discharge or possible infection of their reproductive organs. Patients should be helped to understand that not all discharge is indicative of infection, but that early diagnosis and treatment of an infection, if present, can prevent serious complications. Patients should be informed of the methods to decrease the risk of getting STIs and to recognize the signs of infection in their partner(s).

The patient may have guilt feelings about having PID, especially if it was associated with an STI. They may also be concerned about the complications associated with PID, such as adhesions and strictures of the Fallopian tubes, infertility, and the increased incidence of ectopic pregnancy. Discussion with the patient regarding their feelings and concerns can help them cope more effectively.

For patients requiring hospitalization, nurses have an important role in implementing medication therapy, monitoring the patient's health status, and providing symptom relief and patient teaching. Vital signs and character, amount, colour, and odour of the vaginal discharge should be recorded. Explanations about the need for limited activity, maintaining a semi-Fowler's position, and increased fluid intake should increase patient cooperation. Assessing the degree of abdominal pain will provide information about the effectiveness of medication therapy.

CHRONIC PELVIC PAIN

Chronic pelvic pain refers to pain in the pelvic region (below the umbilicus and between the hips) that lasts 6 months or longer (Chen et al., 2017). It accounts for 10% of all visits to gynecologists and is the reason for 20 to 30% of all laparoscopies. Up to one third of women with PID have chronic pelvic pain (Safrai et al., 2020).

The cause of chronic pelvic pain is often hard to find. Many different conditions can cause pelvic pain. Gynecological etiologies include dysmenorrhea, endometriosis, PID, ovarian cysts, uterine fibroids, pelvic adhesions, and ectopic pregnancies. Abdominal etiologies include irritable bowel syndrome, interstitial cystitis, appendicitis, and colitis. Psychological factors

TABLE 56.9 NURSING ASSESSMENT
Pelvic Inflammatory Disease

Subjective Data
Important Health Information
Past health history: Use of IUD; previous PID, gonorrhea, or chlamydial infection; multiple sexual partners; exposure to partner with urethritis; infertility
Medications: Use of and allergy to any antibiotics
Surgery or other treatments: Recent abortion or pelvic surgery

Symptoms
- Abnormal vaginal bleeding and menstrual irregularity; vaginal discharge
- Lower abdominal and pelvic pain; low back pain; pain on fundal palpation and cervical motion; onset of pain just after a menstrual cycle; dysmenorrhea, dyspareunia, dysuria, vulvar pruritus
- Malaise
- Nausea, vomiting; chills; fever
- Urinary frequency, urgency

Objective Data
General
Fever

Reproductive
Mucopurulent cervicitis, vulvar maceration, vaginal discharge (from heavy and purulent to thin and mucoid), tenderness on motion of cervix and uterus; presence of inflammatory masses on palpation

Possible Findings
Leukocytosis; ↑ erythrocyte sedimentation rate; positive culture of secretions or endocervical fluid; pelvic inflammation and positive endometrial biopsy on laparoscopic examination; abscess or inflammation on ultrasonography

IUD, intrauterine device; *PID,* pelvic inflammatory disease.

(e.g., depression, chronic stress, history of sexual or physical abuse) may increase the risk of developing chronic pelvic pain. Emotional distress makes pain worse; living with chronic pain contributes to emotional distress.

Chronic pelvic pain has many different clinical manifestations, including severe and steady pain, intermittent pain, dull and achy pain, pelvic pressure or heaviness, and sharp pain or cramping. In addition, pain may occur during intercourse or while having a bowel movement.

Determining the cause of chronic pelvic pain often involves a process of elimination. In addition to a detailed history and physical examination (including a pelvic examination), the patient may be asked to keep a journal of the onset of symptoms and any precipitating factors.

Diagnostic tests may include cultures from the cervix or vagina (used to detect STIs), ultrasound, computed tomographic (CT) scan, or magnetic resonance imaging (MRI) to detect abnormal structures or growths. Laparoscopy may be used to visualize the pelvic organs. This procedure is especially useful in detecting endometriosis and chronic PID.

If the cause of chronic pelvic pain is found, treatment focuses on that cause. If no cause can be found, treatment involves managing the pain. Over-the-counter pain medications (e.g., acetylsalicylic acid [ASA: Aspirin], ibuprofen, acetaminophen) may provide some relief. Sometimes, stronger pain medications may be needed. Birth control pills or other hormonal medications may help relieve cyclic pelvic pain related to menstrual cycles. If an infection is the source of the pain, antibiotics are used.

Tricyclic antidepressants (e.g., amitriptyline, nortriptyline) have pain-relieving and antidepressant effects. These medications may help improve chronic pelvic pain even in patients who do not have depression. The patient may be encouraged to get counselling for any emotional issues.

ENDOMETRIOSIS

Endometriosis is the presence of endometrial epithelial cells in sites outside the uterine cavity (Peiris et al., 2018). The most frequent sites are in or near the ovaries, uterosacral ligaments, and uterovesical peritoneum (Figure 56.4). However, endometrial tissues can be in many other locations, such as the stomach, the lungs, the intestines, and the spleen. The tissue responds to the hormones of the ovarian cycle and undergoes a "minimenstrual cycle" similar to the uterine endometrium.

The typical patient with endometriosis is in her late 20s or early 30s and has never had a full-term pregnancy. Although it is not a life-threatening condition, endometriosis can cause considerable pain. It is also a common cause of infertility and increases the risk for ovarian cancer. While endometriosis is one of the most common gynecological conditions, it is difficult to know the number of women with the condition as many do not have symptoms. Current estimates suggest that 11% of women in the reproductive years have endometriosis (Peiris et al., 2018).

Etiology and Pathophysiology

Although the etiology of endometriosis is poorly understood, many theories have been proposed. A widely held view is that retrograde menstrual flow passes through the Fallopian tubes carrying viable endometrial tissues into the pelvis (Vallvé-Juanico et al., 2019). The tissue attaches to various sites, as shown in Figure 56.4. Another theory suggests that undifferentiated embryonic peritoneal cavity cells remain dormant in the pelvic tissue until the ovaries produce sufficient hormones to stimulate their growth. Other proposed causes are a genetic predisposition and altered immune function.

Clinical Manifestations

Patients with endometriosis have a wide range of clinical manifestations and severity. The magnitude of a patient's symptoms does not necessarily correlate with the clinical extent of the endometriosis. Dysmenorrhea after years of relatively pain-free menses and infertility may serve as a clue to the presence of endometriosis. The most common manifestations are secondary dysmenorrhea, infertility, pelvic pain, dyspareunia, and irregular bleeding. Less common manifestations include backache, painful bowel movements, and dysuria. With menopause, estrogen is no longer produced in the ovaries, and the symptoms may disappear.

When the ectopic endometrial tissues "menstruate," the blood collects in cystlike nodules that have a characteristic bluish-black colour. Nodules in the ovaries are sometimes called *chocolate cysts* because of the thick, chocolate-coloured material they contain. When a cyst ruptures, the pain may be acute, and the resulting irritation promotes the formation of adhesions, which fix the affected area to another pelvic structure. Endometrial adhesions may become severe enough to cause a bowel obstruction or painful micturition.

Interprofessional Care

Endometriosis may be suspected from a patient's history of the characteristic symptoms and the health care provider's palpation of firm nodular lumps in the adnexa on bimanual examination. However, laparoscopy is necessary for a definitive diagnosis. The treatment of endometriosis is influenced by the patient's age, desire for pregnancy, symptom severity, and the extent and location of the disease. When symptoms are not disruptive, a "watch-and-wait" approach is used (Table 56.10). When endometriosis is identified as a probable cause of infertility, therapy proceeds more rapidly.

Medication Therapy. Medication therapy is used to reduce symptoms. Pain may be relieved with NSAIDs such as ibuprofen (Advil) and diclofenac (Voltaren). Medications to inhibit estrogen production by the ovaries are often given to shrink the endometrial tissue. Ovulation is suppressed by progestin agents such as medroxyprogesterone. Another approach to hormonal treatment is danazol (Cyclomen), a synthetic androgen that inhibits the anterior pituitary. This medication causes atrophy of ectopic endometrial tissue. Subjective relief of symptoms is noted within 6 weeks of danazol use. The adverse effects of weight gain, acne, hot flashes, and hirsutism and the expense of this medication restrict its use.

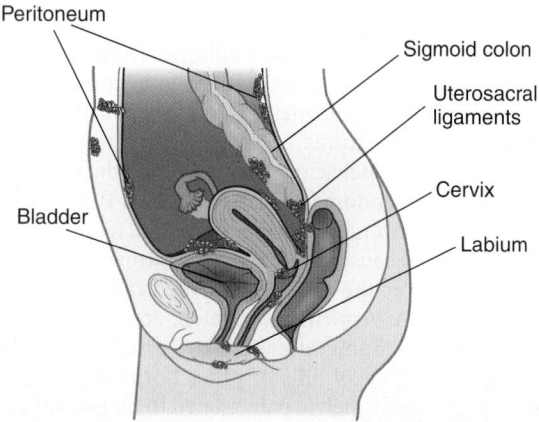

FIG. 56.4 Common sites of endometriosis.

Peritoneum

Sigmoid colon

Uterosacral ligaments

Cervix

Bladder

Labium

TABLE 56.10   INTERPROFESSIONAL CARE
Endometriosis

Diagnostic
- History and physical examination
- Laparoscopy
- MRI
- Pelvic examination
- Pelvic ultrasonography

Interprofessional Therapy
- Conservative therapy (watch and wait)

Medication Therapy
- Danazol (Cyclomen)
- GnRH agonists (e.g., leuprolide [Lupron])
- Nonsteroidal anti-inflammatory medications
- Oral contraceptives

Surgical Therapy
- Laparotomy to remove implants and adhesions
- Total abdominal hysterectomy and bilateral salpingo-oophorectomy (TAH-BSO)

GnRH, gonadotropin-releasing hormone; *MRI*, magnetic resonance imaging.

Another class of medications used is GnRH agonists (e.g., leuprolide [Lupron], nafarelin [Synarel]). These medications result in amenorrhea. Adverse effects are usually the same as those of menopause (hot flashes, vaginal dryness, emotional lability). Loss of bone density has also been reported in women who remain on the therapy longer than 6 months. Endometriosis is controlled but not cured by HT. Persistent lesions give rise to subsequent recurrences once the menstrual cycle is re-established.

> **MEDICATION ALERT—Leuprolide (Lupron)**
> - Assess patient for pregnancy before initiating therapy.
> - Monitor patient for dysrhythmias, palpitations.
> - Instruct patient to use nonhormonal contraceptive measures during therapy.

Surgical Therapy. The only cure for endometriosis is surgical removal of all the endometrial implants. Surgical therapy may be conservative or definitive. Conservative surgery is done to confirm the diagnosis or to remove implants. It involves removal or destruction of endometrial implants and lysing or excision of adhesions by means of laparoscopic laser surgery or laparotomy. GnRH agonist therapy (e.g., leuprolide) can be administered for 4 to 6 months to reduce the size of the lesions before surgery. By reducing the extent of the surgery, this preoperative medication treatment helps reduce the development of adhesions that may further threaten fertility. Laparoscopic surgery may be used to remove pelvic adhesions or endometrial tissue. As a last resort, a hysterectomy may be done. Definitive surgery involves removal of the uterus, Fallopian tubes, ovaries, and as many endometrial implants as possible.

For patients wishing to get pregnant, conservative surgical therapy is used to remove implants blocking the Fallopian tube. Adhesions are removed from the tubes, the ovaries, and the pelvic structures. Efforts are made to conserve all tissues necessary to maintain fertility.

The patient should be actively involved in making the decision about preserving part or all of the ovaries if surgically possible. The patient's feelings about maintaining their cyclical ovarian function must be explored. The health care provider should assess the patient's risk for ovarian cancer and provide this information for consideration.

NURSING MANAGEMENT
ENDOMETRIOSIS

Education of the patient and reassurance that a life-threatening situation does not exist may enable her to accept a conservative and progressive treatment. When the symptoms are less severe, teaching about nonpharmacological comfort measures may be helpful. Nurses must assist patients to understand the medications that have been ordered to treat their condition. The action of the prescribed medication should be explained as well as the possible adverse effects. Psychological support may be needed for patients experiencing severe disabling pain, sexual difficulties secondary to dyspareunia, and infertility.

If conservative surgery is the treatment selected, the nursing care is similar to the general preoperative and postoperative care of a patient undergoing laparotomy (see Nursing Care Plan [NCP] 45.2 for the patient following laparotomy, available on the Evolve website). If definitive surgery is planned, the nursing care is similar to care for the patient undergoing an abdominal hysterectomy (NCP 56.1). The nurse must know the extent of the procedure so that appropriate preoperative teaching can be done.

BENIGN TUMOURS OF THE FEMALE REPRODUCTIVE SYSTEM

LEIOMYOMAS

Etiology and Pathophysiology

Leiomyomas (uterine fibroids) are benign smooth muscle tumours that occur most commonly within the uterus (Figure 56.5). Estimates of the prevalence of fibroids in women range from 20 to 77%, but the literature provides weak evidence of the overall burden of disease posed by uterine fibroids (Stewart, 2015). The cause of leiomyomas is unknown. They appear to depend on ovarian hormones because they grow slowly during the reproductive years and undergo atrophy after menopause.

Clinical Manifestations

The majority of women with leiomyomas do not have any symptoms. When present, the most common symptoms include abnormal uterine bleeding, pain, and symptoms associated with pelvic pressure. Increased bleeding is thought to be associated with the increased endometrial surface area that is associated with leiomyomas. Pain is associated with infection or twisting of the pedicle from which the tumour is growing. Devascularization and blood vessel compression may also contribute to pain. Pressure on surrounding organs may result in rectal, bladder, and lower abdominal discomfort. Large tumours may cause a general enlargement of the lower abdomen. These tumours are sometimes associated with miscarriage and infertility.

Interprofessional Care

Clinical diagnosis is based on the characteristic pelvic findings of an enlarged uterus distorted by nodular masses. Treatment depends on the symptoms, the patient's age, her desire to preserve her fertility, and the location and size of the tumour or tumours. If the symptoms are minimal, the health care provider may elect to follow the patient closely for a time.

Persistent, heavy menstrual bleeding causing anemia and large or rapidly growing tumours are indications for surgery. The leiomyomas are removed by hysterectomy or myomectomy for patients who wish to maintain their fertility. In this case, only the fibroids are removed to preserve the uterus. Small tumours may be removed using a hysteroscope and laser resection instruments.

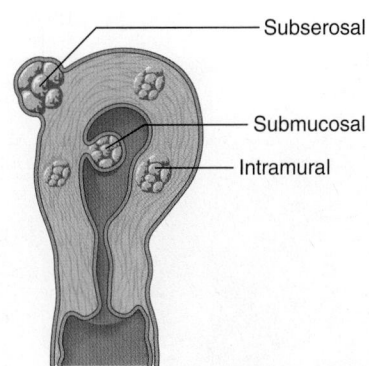

FIG. 56.5 Leiomyomas. Uterine section shows the whorl-like appearance and locations of leiomyomas, which are also called *uterine fibroids*. Source: McCance, K. L., Huether, S. E., Brashers, V. L., et al. (2014). *Pathophysiology: The biologic basis for disease in adults and children* (7th ed., p. 823, Figure 24-15A). Mosby.

Uterine artery embolization (UAE) is increasingly being used as an alternative treatment to treat fibroids. UAE is the process by which embolic material (small plastic or gelatin beads) is injected into the uterine artery. This process blocks blood flow to the uterus and shrinks the fibroid (El Shamy et al., 2020). Because the effects of UAE on future fertility are unknown, the procedure is offered to patients who no longer desire pregnancy.

Cryosurgery is another option. In cases of large leiomyomas, a GnRH agonist (e.g., leuprolide [Lupron]) may be used preoperatively to shrink the size of the tumour. However, the risks and benefits of this medication should be fully discussed, including the potential for irreversible loss of bone mass. The treatment should not be used on patients who wish to preserve their fertility. Another treatment option uses MRI-guided focused ultrasonography to target and destroy uterine fibroids. Treatment requires repeated targeting and heating of the fibroid tissue while the patient lies inside the MRI machine. The procedure can last as long as 3 hours.

CERVICAL POLYPS

Cervical polyps are benign pedunculated lesions that generally arise from the endocervical mucosa and are seen protruding through the cervical os during a speculum examination. Polyps are a characteristic bright cherry red and are soft and fragile in consistency. They are generally small, measuring less than 3 cm in length, and may be single or multiple. Their cause is unknown. Symptoms are usually not present, but metrorrhagia and bleeding after straining for a bowel movement and coitus can occur. Polyps are prone to infection. When the polyp is small, it can be excised in an outpatient procedure. If the point of attachment of the polyp cannot be identified and is not accessible to cautery, a polypectomy is performed in an operating room. All tissue removed is sent for pathological review because polyps occasionally undergo malignant changes.

BENIGN OVARIAN TUMOURS

There are many different types of benign tumours. The cause of most of them is unknown. They can be divided into cysts and neoplasms. *Cysts* are usually soft, are surrounded by a thin capsule, and may be detected during the reproductive years. Follicle and corpus luteum cysts are common ovarian cysts (Figure 56.6).

Multiple small ovarian follicles may occur in a condition called *polycystic ovary syndrome* (PCOS) (discussed in the next section). Epithelial ovarian neoplasms may be cystic or solid, small or extremely large. Cystic teratomas, or dermoid cysts, originate from germ cells and can contain bits of any type of body tissue, such as hair or teeth.

Ovarian masses are often asymptomatic until they are large enough to cause pressure in the pelvis. Constipation, menstrual irregularities, urinary frequency, a full feeling in the abdomen, anorexia, and peripheral edema may occur, depending on the size and the location of the tumour. There may be an increase in abdominal girth. Pelvic pain may be present if the tumour is growing rapidly. Severe pain results when the cyst twists on its pedicle (ovarian torsion).

In some cases, an ovarian cyst can rupture. A ruptured ovarian cyst is not only extremely painful, but it can lead to serious complications, such as hemorrhage and infection.

Pelvic examination reveals a mass or an enlarged ovary that demands further investigation. If the mass is cystic and smaller than 8 cm, the patient is asked to return for re-examination in 4 to 6 weeks. If the mass is cystic and greater than 8 cm or is solid, laparoscopic surgery or laparotomy is performed. Immediate surgery is necessary if ovarian torsion occurs, causing the ovary to rotate and cut off circulation. Surgical techniques are used to save as much of the ovary as possible.

Polycystic Ovarian Syndrome

PCOS is a chronic disorder in which many benign cysts form on the ovaries. It most commonly occurs in women younger than 30 years of age and is a cause of infertility. It affects about 5 to 10% of women of reproductive age (Trikudanathan, 2015). PCOS is caused by hormonal abnormalities in which the ovaries produce estrogen and excess testosterone but not progesterone. Fluid-filled cysts develop from mature ovarian follicles that fail to rupture (thereby releasing an egg) each month (Figure 56.7). This disorder affects both ovaries.

Clinical manifestations include irregular menstrual periods, amenorrhea, hirsutism, and obesity. Of these manifestations, obesity in particular has been associated with severe symptoms such as excess androgens, oligomenorrhea, amenorrhea, and infertility. Many women start with normal menstrual periods that, after 1 to 2 years, become irregular and then infrequent. If PCOS is left untreated, cardiovascular disease and abnormal insulin resistance with type 2 diabetes mellitus may develop (Trikudanathan, 2015).

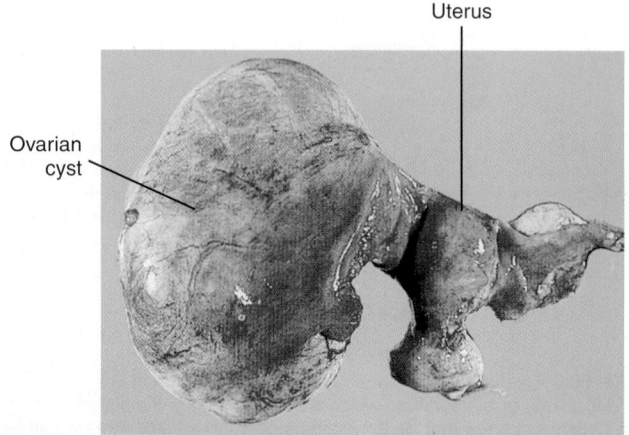

FIG. 56.6 Large ovarian cyst. Source: Symonds, E. M., & MacPherson, M. B. A. (1994). *Colour atlas of obstetrics and gynecology.* Mosby.

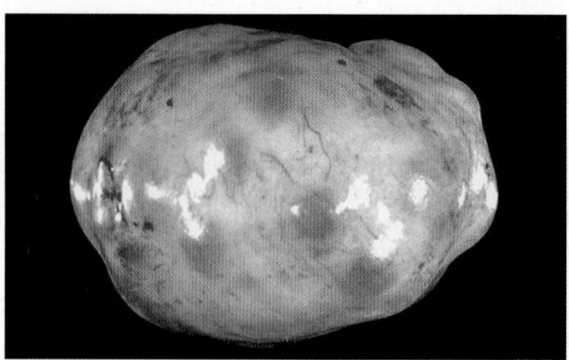

FIG. 56.7 Polycystic ovary syndrome. Multiple fluid-filled cysts in the ovary. Source: Patton, K. T. & Thibodeau, G. (2013). *Anatomy and physiology* (8th ed., p. 1089, Figure 35-23). Mosby.

Pelvic ultrasonography will reveal enlarged ovaries with multiple small cysts. Successful management includes early diagnosis and treatment to improve quality of life and decrease the risk for complications. Oral contraceptives are useful in regulating menstrual cycles. Hirsutism may be treated with spironolactone (Aldactone). Hyperandrogenism can be treated with flutamide and a GnRH agonist such as leuprolide (Lupron). Metformin (Glucophage) reduces hyperinsulinemia and has been shown to improve hyperandrogenism and restore ovulation. For women desiring to become pregnant, fertility medications may be used to induce ovulation. If all other treatments are unsuccessful, a hysterectomy with bilateral salpingo-oophorectomy may be performed.

Patient teaching for the patient with PCOS includes the importance of weight management and exercise to decrease insulin resistance. Obesity exacerbates the complications related to PCOS. Lipid profile and fasting glucose levels should be monitored. Hirsutism is cosmetically distressing for many women. It is important to support the patient as she explores measures to remove unwanted hair (e.g., depilating agents, electrolysis). Regular follow-up care is important in monitoring the effectiveness of therapy and detecting any complications.

CANCER OF THE FEMALE REPRODUCTIVE SYSTEM

CERVICAL CANCER

Cervical cancer is the second most common cancer affecting women in the world, with 80 to 85% of these cases occurring in under-resourced countries. Noninvasive cervical cancer is about four times more common than invasive cervical cancer. Based on 2012 estimates, the lifetime probability of a woman developing cervical cancer in Canada is 1 in 152, and the lifetime probability of dying from cervical cancer is 1 in 426 (Canadian Cancer Society, 2017). An increased risk for cervical cancer is associated with low socioeconomic status, early sexual activity (before 17 years of age), multiple sexual partners, infection with HPV, immunosuppression, and smoking.

The number of deaths from cervical cancer in women who undergo regular screening and follow-up has fallen steadily since the 1950s. This is attributable to better and earlier diagnosis with the widespread use of the Papanicolaou (Pap) test. In addition to being used to detect cancer, the Pap test is also used to detect precancerous changes. By treating precancerous lesions, progression to cervical cancer can be prevented.

Etiology and Pathophysiology

Risk factors for cervical cancer include (1) previous infection (e.g., high risk strains of HPV 16 and 18, HIV, STI), (2) being sexually active, (3) using oral contraceptives for a long period of time, (4) being exposed to the medication diethylstilbestrol (DES), (5) giving birth to many children, and (6) tobacco use. Use of immunosuppressant medications is a possible risk factor, but more definitive evidence is required (Canadian Cancer Society, 2021b).

The cervix is the lower third of the uterus that projects into the vagina. It is made up of glandular cells that line the uterine

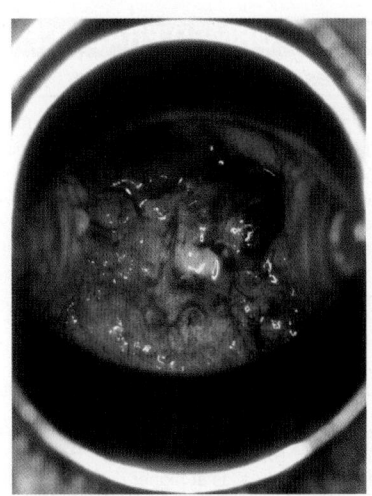

FIG. 56.8 Cervical cancer. View through a speculum inserted into the vagina. Source: Drake, R. L., Vogl, W., & Mitchell, A. W. M. (2010). *Gray's anatomy for students* (2nd ed., p. 457, Figure 5.55). Churchill Livingstone.

cavity and endocervical canal. Squamous epithelium lines the vagina and outer part of the cervix. These two cell types meet and undergo a normal physiological process known as *squamous metaplasia*. This is the transformation of columnar epithelium into squamous epithelium, which results in an area called the *transformation zone*. This process begins at puberty and continues throughout a women's reproductive life cycle. The transformation zone moves in and out the endocervical canal, depending on hormonal status and other factors. While the entire anogenital tract can be infected by HPV, the transformation zone is an area that is particularly susceptible to HPV-associated carcinogenesis.

Clinical Manifestations

Precancerous changes are asymptomatic, highlighting the importance of routine screening. An unusual discharge, abnormal uterine bleeding, or postcoital bleeding eventually occurs. The discharge is usually thin and watery but becomes dark and foul smelling as the disease advances. Vaginal bleeding first presents as spotting. As the tumour enlarges, bleeding becomes heavier and more frequent (Figure 56.8). Pain is a late symptom, followed by weight loss, anemia, and cachexia. The peak incidence of noninvasive cervical cancer is in women in their early 30s. The average age for women with invasive cervical cancer is 50.

Diagnostic Studies

Cervical cancer screening is recommended in Canada for sexually active women between the ages of 21 and 69. Some provinces or territories may offer screening at earlier or later ages. The Canadian Cancer Society (2021c) recommends that women have a Pap test every 1 to 3 years, depending on the screening guidelines in their province or territory and depending on their previous test results. After age 69, women should talk to their health care provider about the possibility of stopping the Pap test following two or three previously normal (negative) Pap results. Women who have sex with women, women who are no longer sexually active, women who have had a partial hysterectomy, and transgender men who are sexually active should follow the same cervical screening guidelines. Women

Translating Research Into Practice

H. K. (pronouns she/her) is a 38-year-old who had a tubal ligation in the outpatient surgery unit. Previous history includes a kidney transplant less than a year ago and current immunosuppressant medications to prevent rejection. In preparing for discharge, the nurse reminds H. K. about the need to have regular Pap tests to screen for cervical cancer. H.K. expresses concern over the distance required to travel to see her family doctor. H. K. does not drive and is a single parent with three young children at home. She does not remember when a Pap test was last done.

Best Available Evidence	Clinician Expertise	Patient Preferences and Values
For women after age 21 who have had three normal Pap tests, the Canadian Cancer Society recommends screening every 1 to 3 years.	The nurse knows that H. K. is at higher risk for cervical cancer because of the immunosuppression medications taken for her recent kidney transplant.	H. K. is concerned about difficulty in getting to see her family doctor. She adds that no family member has ever had cervical cancer.

Decision and Action

The nurse explains the Canadian Cancer Society recommendations and the increased risk for cervical cancer. H. K. tells the nurse that she understands and that a follow-up appointment will be scheduled, but unless some help with child care and travel costs can be found, she will probably not be able to get yearly Pap tests.

Reference for Evidence

Canadian Cancer Society. (2021). *Screening for cervical cancer.* https://cancer.ca/en/cancer-information/cancer-types/cervical/screening

with previous abnormal Pap tests may be screened more often (Canadian Cancer Society, 2021c). Patients who have had a total hysterectomy do not need to be screened for cervical cancer, unless the surgery was done for cervical precancer or cancer.

Patients with a history of cervical cancer should continue with screening for at least 20 years, as recommended by their health care provider. Patients who have been vaccinated against HPV need to continue following the screening guidelines for their age group.

The two types of HPV that have been associated with most cases of cervical cancer (types 16 and 18) can be identified through deoxyribonucleic acid (DNA) testing. HPV DNA tests help to determine if patients with abnormal Pap test results need further follow-up. Patients aged 30 to 65 who have the HPV DNA test and the Pap test (co-testing) can be screened every 5 years rather than every 3 years.

Pap tests are less than 100% accurate; there are problems with both false-positive and false-negative reports. Use of Thin-Prep, a newer, liquid-based technique for Pap tests, has reduced the number of inaccurate Pap test results.

The finding of an abnormal Pap smear indicates the need for follow-up. Patients with minor changes may be followed with a repeated Pap test in 4 to 6 months for 2 years. Up to 80% of abnormal Pap tests may revert to normal results spontaneously. Patients with more prominent changes will receive additional procedures, such as colposcopy and biopsy, before

TABLE 56.11	**STAGING AND TREATMENT OF CERVICAL CANCER**

Stage	Extent	Treatment
0	In situ	Cervical conization, hysterectomy, cryosurgery, laser surgery
I	Confinement to cervix	Radiation, radical hysterectomy
II	Spread beyond cervix to upper two thirds of vagina but not to tissues around uterus	Radiation, cisplatin-based chemotherapy, radical hysterectomy
III	Spread to pelvic wall, involvement of lower third of vagina, or has caused kidney conditions (or both of the latter two)	Radiation, cisplatin-based chemotherapy
IV	Spread to other parts of the body, such as bladder, rectum, liver, lungs, and bones	Radiation, surgery (e.g., pelvic exenteration), cisplatin-based chemotherapy

Source: Modified from National Cancer Institute (NCI). (2016). *Cancer cervical treatment: Stages of cervical cancer.* https://www.cancer.gov/cancertopics/pdq/treatment/cervical/Patient/page2

a definitive diagnosis can be made. Colposcopy is used to help identify possible epithelial abnormalities and areas for biopsy. Biopsies are sent for pathology evaluation. Colposcopy and biopsy have improved diagnosis and enable more focused treatments.

The type and the extent of the biopsy vary with the abnormality seen. A punch biopsy may be done on an outpatient basis with special punch biopsy forceps. The excision of a cone-shaped section of the cervix may be used for both diagnosis and treatment. Conization is accomplished using one of several techniques, depending on the health care provider's experience and the availability of equipment. *Cryotherapy* (freezing) and laser cone vaporization destroy the tissue. With laser cone excision and the *loop electrosurgery excision procedure* (LEEP), the identified tissue is removed for histological examination to ensure that all microinvasive tissue has been removed. These procedures can be performed as outpatient procedures with mild analgesics or sedation. Complications of these procedures include excessive bleeding and possible cervical stenosis after healing.

Interprofessional Care

Vaccines against HPV (e.g., Gardasil, Cervarix) reduce the incidence of both cervical-related neoplasia and cervical cancer caused by infection from HPV types 16 and 18. HPV types 16 and 18 together cause 70% of cervical cancers (Canadian Cancer Society, 2021a). (HPV transmission and vaccines are discussed further in Chapter 55.)

The treatment of cancer of the cervix is guided by the stage of the tumour and the patient's age and general state of health (Table 56.11). There are four procedures in which fertility can be preserved. Conization may be the only type of therapy needed for noninvasive cervical cancer if analysis of removed tissue demonstrates that a wide area of normal tissue surrounds the excised tissue. Laser treatments can be used in which a directed infrared beam is employed to destroy abnormal tissue. Cautery and cryosurgery may also be used.

Invasive cancer of the cervix is treated with surgery, irradiation, and chemotherapy as single treatments or in combination. Surgical procedures include hysterectomy, radical hysterectomy (involving adjacent structures), and rarely, pelvic exenteration. (Surgical therapy is discussed earlier in this chapter; pelvic exenteration is discussed later in the chapter.) Radiation may be external (e.g., cobalt), or internal implants (e.g., cesium, radium) may be used. Standard radiation treatment is 4 to 6 weeks of external radiation followed by one or two treatments with internal implants (brachytherapy). (Radiation therapy is discussed in Chapter 18 and in NCP 18.1, available on the Evolve website.) Cisplatin-based chemotherapy regimens benefit patients with cancer that has spread beyond the cervix.

ENDOMETRIAL OR UTERINE CANCER

Cancer of the endometrium is the most common gynecological malignancy, accounting for nearly 50% of female genital tract neoplasms. The probability of a Canadian woman developing uterine cancer in her lifetime is 1 in 40. In 2015, it was estimated that there were 6 300 new cases of endometrial cancer in Canada and that 1 050 women would die from the condition (Canadian Cancer Society Advisory Committee on Cancer Statistics, 2015). Endometrial cancer has a relatively low mortality rate since most cases are diagnosed early. The survival rate is 95% if the cancer has not spread at the time of diagnosis.

Etiology and Pathophysiology

The major risk factor for endometrial cancer is estrogen, especially unopposed estrogen (Rodriguez et al., 2019). Additional risk factors include increasing age, nulliparity (women who have never been pregnant), late menopause, obesity, smoking, diabetes mellitus, and having a personal or family history of hereditary nonpolyposis colorectal cancer (HNPCC) (see the Genetics in Clinical Practice box on HNPCC in Chapter 45). Obesity is a risk factor because adipose cells store estrogen, thus increasing endogenous estrogen. Pregnancy and oral contraceptives are protective factors.

Endometrial cancer arises from the lining of the endometrium. Most tumours are adenocarcinomas. The precursor may be a hyperplasic state that progresses to invasive carcinoma. Hyperplasia occurs when estrogen is not counteracted by progesterone. The cancer extends directly into the cervix and through the uterine serosa. As invasion of the myometrium occurs, regional lymph nodes, including the paravaginal and para-aortic, become involved. Hematogenous metastases develop concurrently. The usual sites of metastases are the lung, bones, the liver, and, eventually, the brain. Malignant cells can be found in the peritoneal cavity, probably having arrived by transport through the Fallopian tubes.

Prognostic factors include histological differentiation, myometrial invasion, peritoneal cytology, lymph node and adnexal metastases, and tumour size. Endometrial cancer grows slowly, metastasizes late, and is amenable to therapy if diagnosed early.

Clinical Manifestations

The first sign of endometrial cancer is abnormal uterine bleeding, usually in women who are postmenopausal. Because women who are perimenopausal have sporadic periods for a time, it is important that this sign not be ignored or attributed to menopause.

Pain occurs late in the disease process. Other manifestations that may arise are related to metastasis to other organs.

Metastatic spread occurs in a characteristic pattern. Spread to the pelvic and para-aortic nodes is common. When distant metastasis occurs, it most commonly involves the lungs, liver, bones, brain, and vagina.

Interprofessional Care

Endometrial biopsy is the primary diagnostic procedure for endometrial cancer and is done on an outpatient basis. Any abnormal or unexpected bleeding in a postmenopausal woman requires obtaining a tissue sample to exclude endometrial cancer. It is recommended that an endometrial biopsy be performed at menopause and then periodically in women who are at risk. The Pap test is not a reliable diagnostic tool for endometrial cancer, but it can rule out cervical cancer.

Most cases of endometrial cancer are diagnosed at an early stage, when surgery alone may result in cure. Treatment of endometrial cancer is a total abdominal hysterectomy and bilateral salpingo-oophorectomy (TAH-BSO) with lymph node biopsies. The lack of estrogen and progesterone receptors is a poor prognostic indicator. Surgery may be followed by radiation, either to the pelvis or the abdomen, externally or intravaginally, to decrease local recurrence.

No tumour markers with high sensitivity and high specificity for endometrial cancer are known at present, although carbohydrate antigen-125 (CA-125) is often used in clinical practice. CA-125 has been used in surveillance of advanced endometrial cancer. In patients who have increased CA-125 values pretreatment, this test might prove useful in post-treatment surveillance.

Treatment of advanced or recurrent disease is difficult. Progesterone HT (e.g., megestrol [Megace OS]) is the treatment of choice when the progesterone receptor status is positive and the tumour is well differentiated. Tamoxifen (Nolvadex-D), either alone or in combination with progesterone therapy, is also effective in patients with advanced or recurrent endometrial cancer. Chemotherapy is considered when progesterone therapy is unsuccessful. The most common agents used are doxorubicin, cisplatin (Cisplatin), carboplatin, and paclitaxel (Haydu et al., 2016).

OVARIAN CANCER

Ovarian cancer is a malignant neoplasm of the ovaries. In 2015, it was estimated that there were 2 800 new cases of ovarian cancer in Canada and that 1 750 women would die from the condition (Canadian Cancer Society Advisory Committee on Cancer Statistics, 2015). Ovarian cancer has the highest mortality rate of all gynecological cancers because most women have advanced disease at diagnosis (Stewart et al., 2019). In Canada, the lifetime probability of a woman dying from ovarian cancer is 1 in 91 (Canadian Cancer Society Advisory Committee on Cancer Statistics, 2015). It occurs most frequently in women between 55 and 65 years of age.

Etiology and Pathophysiology

The cause of ovarian cancer is not known. Women who have mutations of the *BRCA* genes have increased susceptibility for ovarian and breast cancer (Mainor & Isaacs, 2020). The *BRCA* genes are tumour suppressor genes that inhibit tumour growth when functioning normally. When they mutate, they lose their tumour suppressor ability. This loss results in an increased risk for women to develop ovarian or breast cancer (see the Genetics in Clinical Practice box).

GENETICS IN CLINICAL PRACTICE
Ovarian Cancer

Genetic Basis
- Mutations in genes *BRCA1* and *BRCA2*
- Autosomal dominant transmission
- Mutations can be passed down from either mother or father

Incidence
- About 10% of cases of ovarian cancer are related to hereditary factors.
- Women with *BRCA1* mutations have a 25 to 40% lifetime risk of developing ovarian cancer.
- Women with *BRCA2* mutations have a 10 to 20% lifetime risk of developing ovarian cancer.
- Family history of both breast and ovarian cancer increases the risk of having a *BRCA* mutation.
- *BRCA* mutations occur in 10 to 20% of patients with ovarian cancer who have no family history of breast or ovarian cancer.

Genetic Testing
- DNA testing is available for *BRCA1* and *BRCA2* genetic mutations.

Clinical Implications
- Bilateral oophorectomy reduces the risk for ovarian cancer in women with *BRCA1* and *BRCA2* mutations.
- Genetic counselling and testing for *BRCA* mutations should be considered for women whose personal or family history puts them at high risk for a genetic predisposition to ovarian cancer.

TABLE 56.12   INTERPROFESSIONAL CARE
Ovarian Cancer

Diagnostic
- History and physical examination
- Abdominal and transvaginal ultrasonography
- CA-125 levels
- Laparotomy for diagnostic staging
- Pelvic examination

Interprofessional Therapy
- Surgery
- Abdominal hysterectomy and bilateral salpingo-oophorectomy with pelvic lymph node biopsies
- Debulking for advanced disease
- Chemotherapy
- Adjuvant and palliative
- Radiation therapy
- Adjuvant and palliative

CA, carbohydrate antigen.

new, persistent (occur at least 12 days per month), or worsening, need to see their health care provider. Vaginal bleeding rarely occurs, and pain is not an early symptom. Later signs are increased abdominal girth, unexplained weight loss or gain, and menstrual changes.

Diagnostic Studies

No screening test exists for ovarian cancer. Because early ovarian cancer has vague symptoms, yearly bimanual pelvic examinations should be performed to identify the presence of an ovarian mass (Table 56.12). Women who are postmenopausal should not have palpable ovaries, so a mass of any size should be suspected as possible ovarian cancer. An abdominal or transvaginal ultrasonography can be used to detect ovarian masses. An exploratory laparotomy may be used to establish the diagnosis and stage the disease.

A test called *OVA1* can help detect whether a pelvic mass is benign or malignant before it is surgically removed. With OVA1 a blood sample is used to test for levels of five proteins that change because of ovarian cancer. It is not intended for ovarian cancer screening or for a definitive diagnosis of ovarian cancer.

For patients with a high risk for ovarian cancer, screening using a combination of the tumour marker CA-125 and ultrasonography is recommended in addition to a yearly pelvic examination. CA-125 is positive in 80% of patients with epithelial ovarian cancer and is used to monitor the course of the disease. However, levels of CA-125 may be elevated with other malignancies (e.g., pancreatic cancer) or with benign conditions such as fibroids or endometriosis. Currently, only 20% of ovarian cancers are diagnosed at an early stage.

Interprofessional Care

Patients identified as being at high risk for ovarian cancer on the basis of family and health history may require counselling regarding options such as prophylactic oophorectomy and oral contraceptives. It is important to note that although oophorectomy will significantly reduce the risk for ovarian cancer, it will not completely eliminate the possibility of the disease.

Ovarian cancer staging is critical for guiding treatment decisions. *Stage I* describes disease limited to the ovaries; *stage II,* disease limited to the true pelvis; *stage III,* disease limited to the abdominal cavity; and *stage IV,* distant metastatic disease. The overall survival rate is 90% with early disease, 36% with local spread, and 20% with distant metastases.

The major risk factor for ovarian cancer is family history (one or more first-degree relatives with ovarian cancer). A family history of breast or colon cancer is also a risk factor. Other risk factors include a personal history of breast or colon cancer and HNPCC (see the Genetics in Clinical Practice box on HNPCC in Chapter 45).

Nulliparity also places women at higher risk. Other risk factors include increasing age, high-fat diet, increased number of ovulatory cycles (usually associated with early menarche and late menopause), HT, and possibly the use of infertility medications. Breastfeeding, multiple pregnancies, oral contraceptive use (>5 years), and early age at first birth seem to reduce the risk for ovarian cancer. These factors may have a protective effect because they reduce the number of ovulatory cycles and, thus, reduce the exposure to estrogen.

About 90% of ovarian cancers are epithelial carcinomas that arise from malignant transformation of the surface epithelial cells. Epithelial ovarian cancer is primarily a disease of women who are postmenopausal and in the sixth or seventh decade of life (Stewart et al., 2019). Germ cell tumours account for the other 10%. Histological grading is an important prognostic determinant. Tumours are graded according to the level of differentiation, ranging from *well differentiated* (grade I), *moderately well differentiated* (grade II), and *poorly differentiated* (grade III) to *undifferentiated* (grade IV). Grade IV lesions carry a poorer prognosis than the other grades.

Intraperitoneal dissemination is a common characteristic of ovarian cancer. It metastasizes to the uterus, bladder, bowel, and omentum. In advanced disease, it can spread to the stomach, colon, liver, and other parts of the body.

Clinical Manifestations

Nonspecific symptoms that warrant further evaluation include pelvic or abdominal pain, abdominal distention, difficulty eating or feeling full quickly, and dyspnea (Goff, 2021). Women who have one or more of these symptoms, especially if they are

Most patients with ovarian cancer have widespread disease at presentation. The initial treatment for all stages of ovarian cancer is surgery, which is usually TAH-BSO with omentectomy and removal of as much of the tumour as possible (i.e., tumour debulking). Surgery facilitates chemotherapy by reducing the number of cells that the chemotherapy has to kill.

Depending on the differentiation of the cells and the stage of cancer, other treatment options include intraperitoneal and systemic chemotherapy, intraperitoneal instillation of radioisotopes, and external abdominal and pelvic radiation therapy. If a patient is clinically free of symptoms after completing treatment, a "second-look" surgical procedure is often performed to determine whether there is any evidence of disease. If no disease is found, the patient is monitored for recurrent disease.

Chemotherapy usually consists of a combination of a platinum compound, such as cisplatin or carboplatin, and a taxane, such as paclitaxel or docetaxel (Taxotere). The typical course of chemotherapy involves three to six cycles. A cycle is a schedule that allows regular doses of a medication, followed by a rest period.

Other chemotherapy agents used include topotecan (Hycamtin), etoposide (Vepesid), gemcitabine, and oxaliplatin (Eloxatin). These medications may be used to treat recurrent disease or as a palliative measure to shrink the tumour to relieve pressure and pain.

VAGINAL CANCER

Primary vaginal cancers are rare. The peak incidence is between 50 and 70 years of age. Vaginal tumours are usually secondary sites or metastases of other cancers such as cervical or endometrial carcinomas. The most common type of vaginal cancer is squamous cell carcinoma. Intrauterine exposure to DES (a synthetic form of estrogen no longer in use) places a woman at risk for clear cell adenocarcinoma of the vagina.

Treatment of vaginal cancer depends on the type of cells involved and the stage of the disease, the size of the tumour, and the location of the tumour. Squamous cell carcinomas can be treated with both surgery and radiation.

VULVAR CANCER

Cancer of the vulva is relatively rare. Similar to cervical cancer, preinvasive lesions, referred to as *vulvar intraepithelial neoplasia* (VIN), precede invasive vulvar cancer. The invasive form occurs mainly in women older than 60 years, with the highest incidence being in women in their 70s.

Patients with vulvar neoplasia may have symptoms of vulvar itching or burning, pain, bleeding, or discharge. Women who are immunosuppressed or have diabetes mellitus, hypertension, or chronic vulvar dystrophies are at a higher risk of developing vulvar cancers. Several subtypes of HPV have been identified in some but not all vulvar cancers.

Diagnosis of vulvar cancer is determined by the pathology report on the biopsy of the suspicious lesion. VIN can be treated topically with imiquimod cream (Aldara) or surgery.

Laser therapy may be used to kill cancer cells. Surgery is the most common treatment for cancer of the vulva. The goal of surgery is to remove all the cancer without any loss of the patient's sexual function. A local excision with removal of the lesion and surrounding tissue may be done. For more extensive lesions, vulvectomy may be done (various types of vulvectomies are presented in Table 56.13). If the cancer is extensive, a pelvic exenteration may be done. The patient may have chemotherapy or radiation therapy after surgery, as adjuvant measures.

TABLE 56.13	SURGICAL PROCDURES INVOLVING THE FEMALE REPRODUCTIVE SYSTEM
Type of Surgery	**Description**
Abdominal Hysterectomy	
Total hysterectomy	Uterus and cervix removed using large abdominal incision (bikini cut)
Total abdominal hysterectomy and bilateral salpingo-oophorectomy (TAH-BSO)	Uterus, cervix, Fallopian tubes, and ovaries removed using large abdominal incision
Radical hysterectomy	Panhysterectomy, partial vaginectomy, and dissection of lymph nodes in pelvis
Vaginal Hysterectomy	Uterus and cervix removed through a cut in the top of vagina
Laparoscopic Hysterectomy	Laparoscope (video camera and small surgical instruments)
Laparoscopic-assisted vaginal hysterectomy (LAVH)	Incision made at top of vagina; uterus and cervix removed through the vagina; laparoscope inserted into abdomen to assist in the procedure
Laparoscopic supra-cervical hysterectomy	Uterus removed using only laparoscopic instruments; cervix is left intact
Robot-Assisted Surgery	Robot (special machine) used to do surgery through small abdominal incisions; most often used when a patient has cancer or is very overweight and vaginal surgery is not safe
Vulvectomy	Surgical procedure to remove part or all of the vulva
Skinning vulvectomy	Removal of top layer of vulvar skin where the cancer is found; skin grafts from other parts of the body may be needed to cover the area
Simple vulvectomy	Entire vulva is removed
Radical vulvectomy	Entire vulva, including clitoris, labia majora and minora, and nearby tissue, is removed; nearby lymph nodes may also be removed
Vaginectomy	Removal of vagina
Pelvic Exenteration	Radical hysterectomy, total vaginectomy, removal of bladder with diversion of urinary system and resection of colon and rectum with colostomy

SURGICAL PROCEDURES: FEMALE REPRODUCTIVE SYSTEM

A variety of surgical procedures are performed when benign or malignant tumours of the genital tract are found (Table 56.13). A *hysterectomy* (removal of the uterus) is the type of surgery performed for excision of cancerous tumours of the female reproductive system. A hysterectomy may be done abdominally, vaginally, or laparoscopically. The abdominal route is used when large tumours are present and the pelvic cavity is to be explored or when the tubes and ovaries are to be removed at the same time (Figure 56.9). The abdominal route can present more postoperative complications because it involves an incision and the opening of the abdominal cavity.

A vaginal route is often used when vaginal repair is done in addition to removal of the uterus. In both vaginal and abdominal hysterectomies, the ligaments that support the uterus are attached to the vaginal cuff to maintain the normal depth of the vagina. Laparoscopic procedures may have the advantage of quicker recovery time and fewer complications, but vaginal hysterectomy is more cost effective (Mohammed et al., 2017).

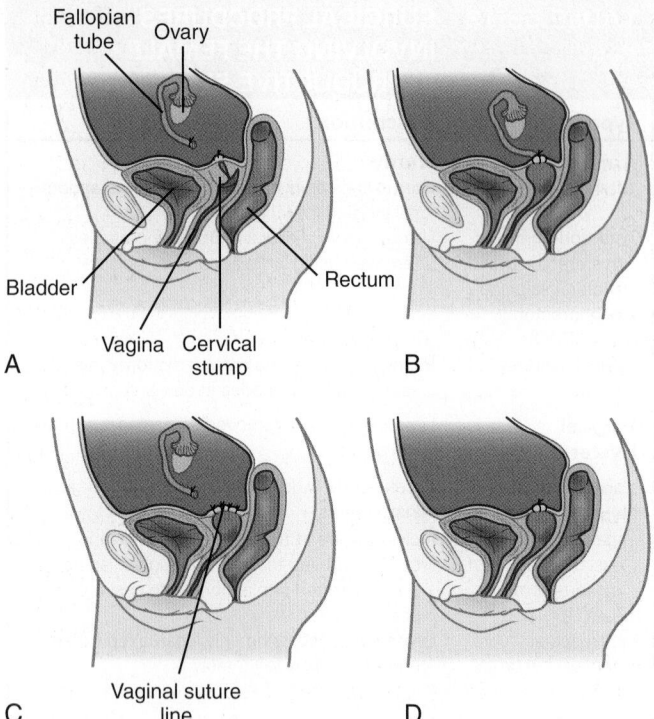

FIG. 56.9 A, Cross-section of subtotal hysterectomy. Note that the cervical stump, Fallopian tubes, and ovaries remain. **B,** Cross-section of total hysterectomy. Note that the Fallopian tubes and ovaries remain. **C,** Cross-section of vaginal hysterectomy. Note that the Fallopian tubes and ovaries remain. **D,** Total hysterectomy, salpingectomy, and oophorectomy. Note that the uterus, Fallopian tubes, and ovaries are completely removed.

RADIATION THERAPY: CANCERS OF THE FEMALE REPRODUCTIVE SYSTEM

Radiation is used to cure or control or as a palliative measure for cancers of the female reproductive system, either alone or in combination with other treatments. The goal of radiation therapy is to deliver a specific amount of high-energy (or ionizing) radiation to the cancer with minimal damage to the normal surrounding tissue. Radiation therapy may be external or internal (brachytherapy).

External Radiation Therapy

With external radiation therapy, a source outside of the body delivers electromagnetic radiation in the form of waves. (External radiation therapy and related nursing care are discussed in Chapter 18 and in NCP 18.1, available on the Evolve website.)

Internal Radiation Therapy (Vaginal Brachytherapy)

Vaginal brachytherapy allows the radiation to be placed near or into the tumour. This method can deliver a high dose of radiation directly to the tumour. The dose decreases sharply as distance from the source increases, causing less damage to the surrounding normal tissue. A variety of forms are used to deliver the therapy, including wires, capsules, needles, tubes, and seeds. Brachytherapy is used in the management of cervical and endometrial cancer because of the accessibility of these body parts and the favourable results obtained. Radium and cesium are two commonly used isotopes (Hass et al., 2018).

To prepare the patient for the treatment, the nurse gives a cleansing enema to prevent straining at stool, which could cause displacement of the isotope. An in-dwelling catheter is inserted to prevent a distended bladder from coming into contact with the radioactive source.

A variety of applicators have been developed for intrauterine treatment. Applicators are inserted into the endometrial cavity and the vagina in the operating room. When the applicator contains the radioactive material, this is known as *preloading*. In *afterloading*, the applicator is implanted in the operating room but is not loaded with the radioactive material until its correct placement is verified and the patient has been returned to her room.

Radiation exposure to the patient is precisely controlled. The radiation exposure to the health care provider and other personnel involved in the implantation is reduced when the afterload technique is used. The applicator is secured with vaginal packing and is left in place for 24 to 72 hours.

During the treatment, the patient is placed in a lead-lined private room, on absolute bed rest. The patient may be turned from side to side. The presence of an intrauterine applicator produces uterine contractions that may require analgesics. The destruction of cells results in a foul-smelling vaginal discharge; thus use of a deodorizer is helpful. Nausea, vomiting, diarrhea, and malaise may develop as a systemic reaction to the radiation.

At the end of the prescribed period of radiation, the radioactive material and the catheter are removed. The patient is allowed off bed rest and is discharged from the hospital when stable. Late complications that may arise include fistulas (vesicovaginal, ureterovaginal), cystitis, phlebitis, hemorrhage, and fibrosis. If fibrosis occurs, the vaginal wall becomes smaller in diameter and shorter. Dilation of the vagina through intercourse or the use of sequentially sized dilators may be indicated. The patient is urged to report any unusual symptoms to the health care provider. (Brachytherapy and related nursing care are discussed in Chapter 18.)

NURSING MANAGEMENT
CANCERS OF THE FEMALE REPRODUCTIVE SYSTEM

NURSING ASSESSMENT

Malignant tumours of the female reproductive system can be found in the cervix, endometrium, ovaries, vagina, and vulva. The patient with any of these malignant tumours may experience a variety of clinical manifestations, including leukorrhea, other types of vaginal discharge, irregular vaginal bleeding, increase in abdominal pain and pressure, bowel and bladder dysfunction, and vulvar itching and burning. Assessment for these signs and symptoms is an important nursing responsibility.

NURSING DIAGNOSES

Nursing diagnoses for the female patient with cancer of the reproductive system include but are not limited to the following:
- *Anxiety* resulting from *threat to current status, threat of death* (cancer diagnosis)
- *Acute pain* resulting from *biological injury agent* (enlarging tumour)
- *Disrupted body image* resulting from *alteration in self-perception* (loss of body part, loss of good health)
- *Inadequate sexuality pattern* resulting from *insufficient knowledge about alternatives related to sexuality* (physiological limitations, fatigue)
- *Potential grieving* as a result of a *poor prognosis of advanced disease*

PLANNING

The overall goals are that the patient with cancer of the female reproductive system will (1) actively participate in treatment decisions, (2) achieve satisfactory pain and symptom management, (3) recognize and report health problems promptly, (4) maintain their preferred lifestyle as long as possible, and (5) continue to practise cancer detection strategies.

NURSING IMPLEMENTATION

HEALTH PROMOTION. Through their contact with patients in a variety of settings, nurses can teach patients the importance of routine screening for cancers of the reproductive system. Cancer may be prevented when screening reveals precancerous conditions of the vulva, cervix, endometrium, and, rarely, the ovaries. Also, routine screening increases the chance that a cancer will be identified in its early stage. When cancer is identified earlier, treatment can be more conservative and the patient's prognosis improves. Regular pelvic examinations and Pap tests (as indicated) will enable the health care provider to detect lesions on the vulva or any uterine or ovarian irregularities and screen for cervical cancer. Nurses can assist patients to view routine cancer screening and vaccination against cervical cancer as important self-care activities.

Educating patients about risk factors for cancers of the reproductive system is also important. Limiting sexual activity during adolescence, using condoms, having fewer sexual partners, and not smoking reduce the risk for cervical cancer. When high-risk behaviours are identified, nurses should assist patients to identify lifestyle changes to decrease risk.

ACUTE INTERVENTION RELATED TO SURGERY. All patients experience a degree of anxiety when surgery is contemplated, but the prospect of major gynecological surgery increases these concerns. Some patients may experience guilt, anger, or embarrassment. Still others may focus on the effect the surgery will have on their reproductive and sexual functions. Some patients view the whole process as annoying, whereas others are relieved by the thought of no longer having menstrual periods or becoming pregnant. The nurse should try to understand the patient's fears and concerns. Each patient needs to be assessed as an individual. Being willing to listen can provide considerable psychological support for patients.

Physically, the patient is prepared preoperatively for surgery with the standard perineal or abdominal preparation. A vaginal douche and enemas may be given (based on the surgeon's preference). The bladder should be emptied before the patient is sent to the operating room. An in-dwelling catheter is sometimes inserted preoperatively (see Chapter 20 for discussion of general preoperative patient care).

Hysterectomy. Postoperatively, the patient who has had a hysterectomy will have an abdominal dressing (abdominal hysterectomy) or a sterile perineal pad (vaginal hysterectomy). (See NCP 56.1, on the Evolve site, for care of the patient after a total abdominal hysterectomy. See Chapter 22 for potential surgical complications, wound care, and other postoperative care.) The dressing should be observed frequently for any sign of bleeding during the first 8 hours after surgery.

The patient may experience urinary retention postoperatively because of temporary bladder atony resulting from edema or nerve trauma. At times, an in-dwelling catheter is used for 1 to 2 days postoperatively to maintain constant drainage of the bladder and prevent strain on the suture line. If an in-dwelling catheter is not used, catheterization may be necessary if the patient has not urinated for 8 hours postoperatively. If residual urine is suspected after the removal of an in-dwelling catheter, intermittent catheterization is done to prevent bladder infection caused by pooling of urine. Accidental ligation of a ureter is a serious surgical complication. Any signs of backache or decreased urine output should be reported to the surgeon.

Abdominal distension may develop from the sudden release of pressure on the intestines when a large tumour is removed or from paralytic ileus secondary to anaesthesia and manipulation of the bowel. Food and fluids may be restricted if the patient is nauseated. Early ambulation is encouraged to relieve abdominal pain related to flatus and to prevent abdominal distension.

Special care must be taken to prevent the development of deep venous thrombosis (DVT). Frequent changes of position, avoidance of the high Fowler's position, and avoidance of pressure under the knees minimize stasis and pooling of blood. Leg exercises should be encouraged to promote circulation.

The loss of the uterus may bring about a grief response in some patients, similar to any significant personal loss. The ability to bear children may be associated with the perception of womanhood. Grief from this loss is normal. Eliciting the patient's feelings and concerns about the surgery will provide the needed information to give understanding care.

When the ovaries are removed as well through surgery, patients experience surgical menopause. Estrogen is no longer available from the ovaries, so symptoms of estrogen deficiency will arise. To counter this, HT may be initiated in the early postoperative period.

Discharge teaching should prepare the patient for what to expect following surgery (e.g., they will not menstruate). Teaching should include specific activity restrictions. Intercourse should be avoided until the wound is healed (~4 to 6 weeks). If a vaginal hysterectomy is performed, the patient needs to know that there may be a temporary loss of vaginal sensation. They should be reassured that sensation will return in several months.

Physical restrictions are limited for a short time. Heavy lifting should be avoided for 6 to 8 weeks. The patient should be assured that once healing is complete, all previous activity can be resumed.

Salpingectomy and Oophorectomy. Postoperative care of the patient who has undergone removal of a Fallopian tube (salpingectomy) or an ovary (oophorectomy) is similar to that for any patient having abdominal surgery. However, if a large ovarian cyst is removed, there may be abdominal distension caused by the sudden release of pressure in the intestines. An abdominal binder may provide relief until the distension subsides.

When both ovaries are removed (bilateral oophorectomy), surgical menopause results. The symptoms are similar to those of regular menopause but may be more severe because of the sudden withdrawal of hormones. Attempts may be made to leave at least a portion of an ovary.

Vulvectomy. Although cancer of the vulva is relatively uncommon, it is important that the nurse recognize the extent of the vulvectomy and the significant effect it is likely to have on the patient's life. An honest, open attitude with the patient and their partner preoperatively can be most helpful in the postoperative period.

After a vulvectomy (see Table 56.13), the patient returns to the unit with a wound in the perineal area extending to the groin. The wound may be covered or left exposed and frequently has drains attached to portable suction (e.g., Hemovac, Jackson-Pratt). Often, a heavy pressure dressing is in place for the first 24 to 48 hours. The wound is cleaned with normal saline solution, twice daily. The normal saline can be applied with an aseptic bulb syringe or a Water Pik machine. A heat lamp or a hair dryer may be used to dry the area. Wound care must be meticulous to prevent infection, which results in delayed healing.

Special attention to bowel and bladder care is needed. A low-residue diet and stool softeners prevent straining and wound contamination. An in-dwelling catheter is used to provide urinary drainage. Great care is taken not to dislodge the catheter because extensive edema makes its reinsertion difficult. Heavy, taut sutures are often used to close the wounds, resulting in severe discomfort for the patient. In other instances, the wound may be allowed to heal by granulation. Analgesics may be required frequently to control pain. Careful positioning of the patient through the use of strategically placed pillows provides comfort. Anticoagulant therapy to prevent DVT is common.

Because the surgery causes mutilation of the perineal area and the healing process is slow, the patient is likely to become discouraged. Opportunities for the patient to express their feelings and concerns about the operation should be provided. The patient needs specific instructions in self-care before being discharged. The patient should be told to report any unusual odour, fresh bleeding, breakdown of incision, or perineal pain. Home care nursing can benefit the patient during the adjustment period.

Sexual function is often retained. Whether clitoral sensation is retained may be critical to some patients, particularly if it was a primary source of orgasmic satisfaction. A discussion of alternative methods of achieving sexual satisfaction may also be indicated.

Pelvic Exenteration. When other forms of therapy fail to control the spread of cancer and no metastases have been found outside of the pelvis, pelvic exenteration may be performed. This radical surgery usually involves removal of the uterus, ovaries, Fallopian tubes, vagina, bladder, urethra, and pelvic lymph nodes. In some situations, the descending colon, rectum, and anal canal may also be removed. Candidates for this procedure are selected on the basis of their likelihood of surviving the surgery and their ability to adjust to and accept the resulting limitations.

Postoperative care is similar to that of a patient who has had a radical hysterectomy, an abdominal perineal resection, and an ileostomy or colostomy. The physical, emotional, and social adjustments to life on the part of the patient and their family are great. There are urinary or fecal diversions in the abdominal wall, a reconstructed vagina, and the onset of menopausal symptoms.

The patient's rehabilitative process should keep pace with their acceptance of the situation. Much understanding and support is needed from the nursing staff during a long recovery period. The patient should be gently encouraged to regain their independence. The patient needs to verbalize their feelings about altered body structure. Inclusion of the family in the plan of care is important.

The patient will need to return to their health care provider at specified intervals. Early recurrence of the cancer may be identified and treated. At this time, the patient's physical and emotional adjustment to the changes in body image produced by the surgery and their ability to carry out any treatment measures can also be assessed. Additional teaching and counselling can then be provided.

ACUTE INTERVENTION WITH RADIATION THERAPY. When the patient is to receive external radiation, they should be told to urinate immediately before the treatment to minimize radiation exposure to the bladder. The patient should be advised about radiation adverse effects, including enteritis and cystitis. These are natural reactions to radiotherapy and do not indicate an overdose. The patient should be fully informed of the possible adverse effects and measures to use to reduce their impact.

Nursing management of the patient receiving brachytherapy requires special considerations. Efficient organization of nursing care is essential so that the nurse does not stay in the immediate area of the patient any longer than is necessary to give proper care and attention. No individual nurse should attend the patient for more than 30 minutes per day. The nurse should stay at the foot of the bed or at the entrance to the room to minimize radiation exposure. Visitors need to be told to stay about 2 m away from the bed and limit visits to less than 3 hours a day. The reasons for these precautions must be explained fully to the patient and visitors. (A more detailed discussion of nursing care of the patient receiving brachytherapy is given in Chapter 18.)

EVALUATION

The expected outcomes are that the patient with cancer of the female reproductive system will do the following:

- Actively participate in treatment decisions
- Achieve satisfactory pain and symptom management
- Recognize and report health problems promptly
- Maintain preferred lifestyle as long as possible
- Continue to practise cancer-detection strategies

CONDITIONS WITH PELVIC SUPPORT

The most commonly occurring conditions with pelvic support are uterine prolapse, cystocele, and rectocele. Pelvic organ prolapse (POP) is a common condition involving the loss of fibromuscular support of the pelvic viscera, causing the descent or herniation of the pelvic organs into the vagina. The general prevalence of POP is thought to be 41% of parous women, with the prevalence of cystocele varying from 25 to 34%, rectocele varying from 13 to 19%, and uterine prolapse varying from 4 to 14% (American Urogynecologic Society, 2019).

Although vaginal birth increases the risk for these conditions, they can occur in women who have never experienced childbirth. Obesity, chronic coughing, and straining during bowel movements can increase the likelihood of these conditions. The decreased estrogen that normally accompanies perimenopause also reduces some connective tissue support.

UTERINE PROLAPSE

Uterine prolapse is the downward displacement of the uterus into the vaginal canal as a result of impaired pelvic support (Gray & Radley, 2020) (Figure 56.10). Prolapse is rated by degrees. In *first-degree* prolapse, the cervix rests in the lower part of the vagina. *Second-degree* prolapse means the cervix is at the vaginal opening. *Third-degree* prolapse means the uterus protrudes through the introitus (entrance to the vaginal canal).

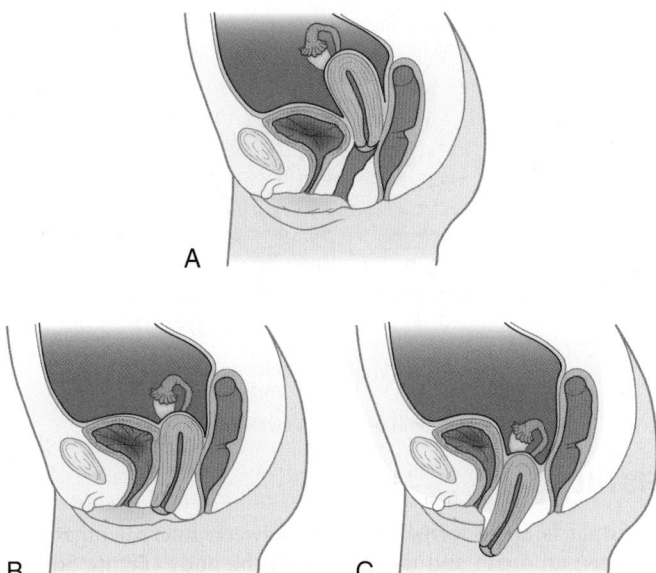

FIG. 56.10 Uterine prolapse. **A,** First-degree prolapse. **B,** Second-degree prolapse. **C,** Third-degree prolapse.

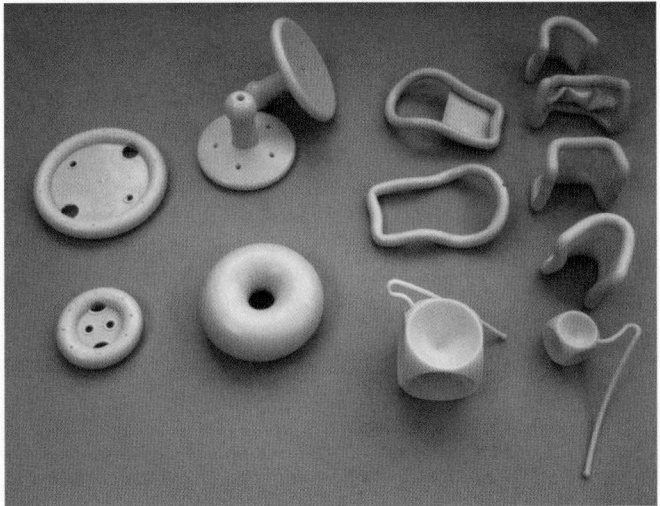

FIG. 56.11 Various types of pessaries. Source: Huckfinne/Wikimedia Commons.

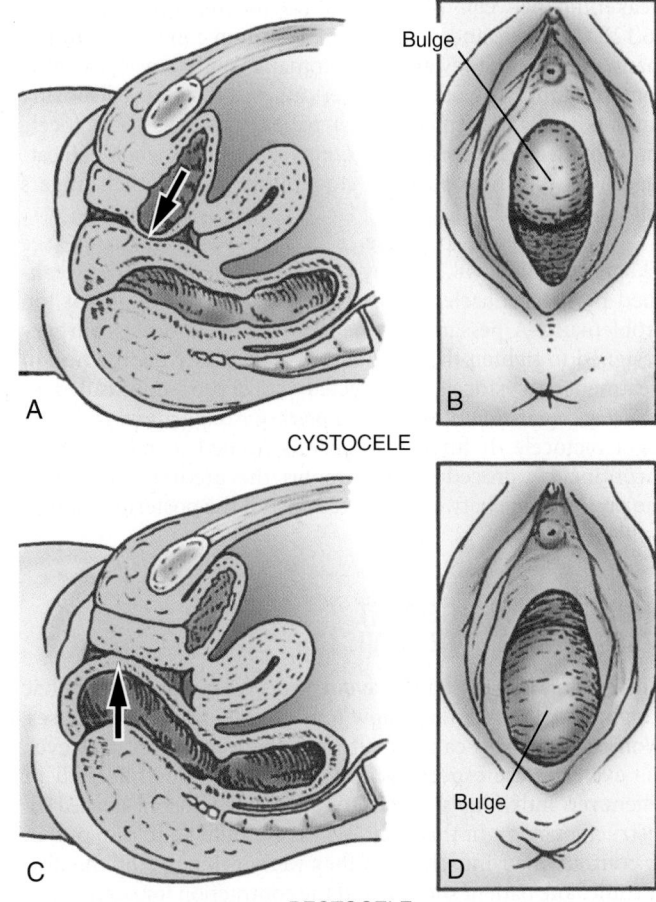

CYSTOCELE

RECTOCELE

FIG. 56.12 **A,** Cystocele. Note the bulging of the anterior vaginal wall. The urinary bladder is displaced downward. **B,** The cystocele pushes the anterior vaginal wall downward into the vagina. **C,** Rectocele. Note the bulging of the posterior vaginal wall. **D,** The rectocele pushes the posterior vaginal wall into the vagina. Source: Black, J. M., & Hawks, J. H. (2009). *Medical-surgical nursing: Clinical management for positive outcomes* (8th ed., p. 930, Figure 39-7). Saunders.

Symptoms vary with the degree of prolapse. The patient may describe a feeling of "something coming down." They may have dyspareunia, a dragging or heavy feeling in the pelvis, backache, and bowel or bladder disorders if cystocele or rectocele is also present. Stress incontinence is a common and troubling problem. When third-degree uterine prolapse occurs, the protruding cervix and vaginal walls are subjected to constant irritation, and tissue changes may occur.

Therapy depends on the degree of prolapse and how much the patient's daily activities have been affected. Pelvic floor muscle training (PFMT) or Kegel exercises may be effective for some patients (see Chapter 48, Table 48.19). There is some evidence that proper training and consistent interpersonal support from health care providers increases the effectiveness of PFMT (Hagen & Thakar, 2015). If PFMT does not provide improvement, a pessary may be used. A *pessary* is a device that is placed in the vagina to help support the uterus (Figure 56.11). The pessary can help prevent worsening of the POP, decrease the frequency or severity of symptoms, and delay need for surgical intervention. A wide variety of pessary shapes exist, including rings, arches, and balls. They can be made from materials such as rubber, clear plastic, soft plastic with metal reinforcements, or silicone. When a patient first receives a pessary, they need instructions for its cleaning and for follow-up. Pessaries that are left in place for long periods are associated with erosion, fistulas, and an increased incidence of vaginal carcinoma.

If more conservative measures are not successful, surgery is indicated. Surgery generally involves a vaginal hysterectomy with anterior and posterior repair of the vagina and the underlying fascia.

CYSTOCELE AND RECTOCELE

Cystocele, or anterior wall prolapse, occurs when support between the vagina and the bladder is weakened (Figure 56.12). Similarly, a rectocele or posterior wall prolapse results from weakening between the vagina and the rectum (see Figure 56.12). Cystocele and rectocele are common conditions, and in many individuals they are asymptomatic. With large cystoceles, complete emptying of the bladder can be difficult, predisposing patients to bladder infections. A patient with a large rectocele may not be able to completely empty the rectum when defecating unless they help push the stool out by putting their fingers in the vagina.

As with uterine prolapse, PFMT or Kegel exercises (see Chapter 48, Table 48.19) may be used to strengthen the weakened perineal muscles if the cystocele or rectocele is not too problematic. A pessary may be helpful for cystoceles. Surgery designed to tighten the vaginal wall is generally the method of treatment. A cystocele is corrected with a procedure called an *anterior colporrhaphy*, whereas a *posterior colporrhaphy* is done for a rectocele. If further surgery is needed to relieve stress incontinence, procedures to support the urethra and restore the proper angle between the urethra and the posterior bladder wall are used.

NURSING MANAGEMENT
DIFFICULTIES WITH PELVIC SUPPORT

Nurses can assist patients to avoid or decrease issues with pelvic support by teaching them how to do PFMT or Kegel exercises. Women of all ages can benefit from these exercises. However, the exercises are especially important following childbirth or whenever individuals begin to experience incontinence. To instruct a patient in this exercise, they should be told to pull in or contract their muscles as if they were trying to stop the flow of urine. The patient should hold the contraction for several seconds and then relax. Sets of 5 to 10 contractions each should be done, several times daily.

If vaginal surgery is necessary, the preoperative preparation may include a cleansing douche the morning of surgery. A cathartic and a cleansing enema are usually given when a rectocele repair is scheduled.

In the postoperative period, the goals of care are to prevent wound infection and pressure on the vaginal suture line. This necessitates perineal care at least two to three times per day and after each urination or defecation. An ice pack applied locally may relieve the initial perineal discomfort and swelling. Later, sitz baths may be used.

After an anterior colporrhaphy, often an in-dwelling catheter is left in the bladder for 2 to 3 days to allow the local edema to subside. Alternatively, a suprapubic catheter can be inserted at the time of surgery. The catheter keeps the bladder empty, preventing strain on the sutures. The amount of urine left in the bladder after voiding is checked for the first few voidings to make sure it is less than 150 mL. This is checked by intermittent catheterization after the patient has voided (postresidual) or by using a bladder scanner or by opening the valve on the suprapubic catheter. After posterior colporrhaphy, straining at stool is avoided by means of a low-residue diet and daily stool softeners to prevent constipation.

Discharge instructions should be reviewed before the patient leaves the hospital. They include the use of a mild laxative as needed; restriction of heavy lifting and prolonged standing, walking, or sitting; and avoidance of intercourse until the health care provider gives permission. There may be a temporary loss of vaginal sensation, which can last for several months.

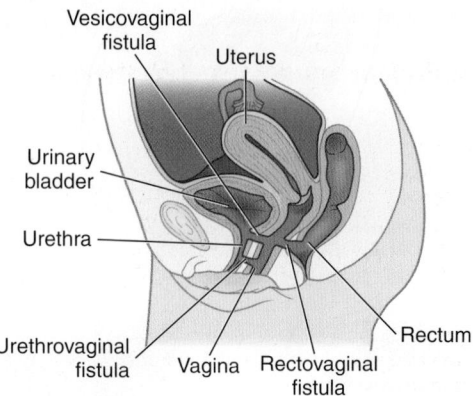

FIG. 56.13 Common fistulas involving the vagina.

FISTULA

A *fistula* is an abnormal opening between internal organs or between an organ and the exterior of the body (Figure 56.13). Gynecological procedures cause most urinary tract fistulas. Other causes include injury during childbirth and disease processes, such as cancer. Fistulas may develop between the vagina and the bladder, the urethra, the ureter, or the rectum. When *vesicovaginal* fistulas (between the bladder and the vagina) develop, some urine leaks into the vagina, whereas with rectovaginal fistulas (between the rectum and the vagina), flatus and feces escape into the vagina. In both instances, excoriation and irritation of the vaginal and vulvar tissues occur and may lead to severe infections. In addition to wetness, offensive odours may develop, causing embarrassment and severely limiting socialization.

Because small fistulas may heal spontaneously within a matter of months, treatment may not be needed. If the fistula does not heal, surgical excision is required. Inflammation and tissue edema must be eliminated before surgery is attempted. This may involve a wait of up to 6 months for the surgery. The fistulectomy may result in the patient's having an ileal conduit or temporary colostomy.

NURSING MANAGEMENT
FISTULAS

Perineal hygiene is of great importance, both preoperatively and postoperatively. The perineum should be cleansed every 4 hours. Warm sitz baths should be taken three times daily if possible. Perineal pads should be changed frequently. The patient should be encouraged to maintain an adequate fluid intake. Encouragement and reassurance are needed to help the patient cope with symptoms.

Postoperatively, nursing care emphasis is on avoidance of stress on the repaired areas and prevention of infection. Care should be taken so that the in-dwelling catheter, usually in place for 7 to 10 days, is draining at all times. Oral fluids should be urged to provide for internal catheter irrigation. Minimal pressure and strict asepsis are used if catheter irrigation becomes necessary. The first stool after bowel surgery may be purposely delayed to prevent contamination of the wound. Later, stool softeners or mild laxatives may be given. (See Chapter 48 and NCP 48.3, available on the Evolve website, for care of a patient with an ileal conduit, and Chapter 45 and NCP 45.4 for care of a patient with a colostomy.) Surgical repair of fistulas is not always effective, even in the best conditions. Therefore, supportive nursing care for the patient and their significant others is especially important.

CASE STUDY

Uterine Prolapse and Vaginal Hysterectomy

Patient Profile

T. P. (pronouns she/her), 62 years old, has developed lower pelvic discomfort and stress incontinence. She has a history of type 2 diabetes mellitus and hypertension. She has four children. A second-degree uterine prolapse is diagnosed. Conservative treatment was instituted with a pessary, but her symptoms did not improve. T. P. comes to the hospital for a vaginal hysterectomy and anteroposterior vaginal repair.

Subjective Data

- Was initially reluctant about surgery
- Concerned about dyspareunia and partner's reaction to the surgery
- Concerned she may have uterine cancer
- States she has stress incontinence and pelvic discomfort

Objective Data

Physical Examination

- Second-degree uterine prolapse on vaginal examination
- Blood pressure (BP) 150/100 mm Hg, pulse 110 beats/min, respirations 20 breaths/min

Laboratory Studies

- Hemoglobin 100 g/L
- Hemoglobin A$_{1c}$ 9%

Postoperative Status

- Returned to room with suprapubic urinary catheter in place
- Vaginal packing in place
- Sequential compression devices on lower extremities
- Patient-controlled analgesia (PCA) pump for pain management

Discussion questions

1. What are the common causes of uterine prolapse?
2. T. P. asks about the effect of the surgery on sexuality. How would the nurse respond?
3. *Priority decision:* What are the priorities of care for T. P.?
4. What possible complications (including reasons for their development) can arise after vaginal hysterectomy?
5. What does T. P. need to be taught before discharge related to diabetes mellitus and hypertension?
6. *Priority decision:* Based on the assessment data presented, what are the priority nursing diagnoses? Are there any interprofessional issues?

Ⓔvolve
Answers are available at http://evolve.elsevier.com/Canada/Lewis/medsurg.

▌ REVIEW QUESTIONS

The number of the question corresponds to the same-numbered objective at the beginning of the chapter.

1. A couple will be undergoing infertility assessment. Which of the following facts should the nurse mention when discussing what the couple should expect during the assessment?
   a. Ovulatory studies can help determine tube patency.
   b. A hysterosalpingogram is a common diagnostic study.
   c. The cause will remain unexplained for 40% of couples.
   d. If postcoital studies are normal, tests for infection will be done.

2. Which of the following is the most appropriate question to ask the client with painful menstruation, to differentiate primary from secondary dysmenorrhea?
   a. "Does your pain become worse with activity or overexertion?"
   b. "Have you had a recent personal crisis or change in your lifestyle?"
   c. "Is your pain relieved by nonsteroidal anti-inflammatory medications?"
   d. "When in your menstrual history did the pain with your period begin?"

3. The nurse is caring for a client after an ectopic pregnancy was surgically removed. What should the nurse advise the recovering client?
   a. She has an increased risk for salpingitis.
   b. Bed rest must be maintained for 12 hours to assist healing.
   c. Having one ectopic pregnancy increases her risk for another.
   d. Intrauterine devices and infertility treatments should be avoided.

4. The nurse is teaching a client who chooses not to take hormone therapy how to prevent or decrease age-related changes that occur after menopause. Which of the following is the most important self-care measure that the nurse should teach?
   a. Maintaining usual sexual activity
   b. Increasing the intake of dairy products
   c. Performing regular aerobic, weight-bearing exercise
   d. Taking vitamin E and B-complex vitamin supplements

5. The client has a history indicating thick, white, and curdlike vaginal discharge and vulvar pruritus. What are these symptoms most consistent with?
   a. Trichomoniasis
   b. Monilial vaginitis
   c. Bacterial vaginosis
   d. Chlamydial cervicitis

6. Why does the nurse caring for a client with pelvic inflammatory disease place her in a semi-Fowler's position?
   a. To relieve severe pain
   b. To promote drainage to prevent abscesses
   c. To improve circulation and promote healing
   d. To prevent complication of bowel obstruction

7. Which of the following is a nursing responsibility related to the care of the client receiving brachytherapy for endometrial cancer?
   a. Maintaining absolute bed rest
   b. Keeping the client in high Fowler's position
   c. Allowing visitors to stay if they remain 1 m from the bed
   d. Limiting direct nurse-to-client contact to 30 minutes per shift

8. Postoperative goals in caring for the client who has undergone an abdominal hysterectomy include which of the following? *(Select all that apply.)*
   a. Monitoring urine output
   b. Changing position frequently
   c. Restricting all food for 24 hours
   d. Observing perineal pad for bleeding
   e. Encouraging leg exercises to promote circulation

9. Which of the following are included in the postoperative nursing care for the patient with a gynecological fistula? *(Select all that apply.)*
   a. Ambulation
   b. Bladder training
   c. Warm sitz baths
   d. Perineal hygiene
   e. Use of stool softeners

1. b; 2. d; 3. c; 4. c; 5. b; 6. b; 7. a; 8. a, b, e; 9. c, d.

Ⓔvolve
For even more review questions, visit http://evolve.elsevier.com/Canada/Lewis/medsurg.

REFERENCES

Akhter, S., Marcus, M., Kerber, R. A., et al. (2016). The impact of periconceptional maternal stress on fecundability. *Annals of Epidemiology*, 26(10), 710–716. https://doi.org/10.1016/j.annepidem.2016.07.015

Akter, M., & Shirin, E. (2018). Latest evidence on using hormone replacement therapy in the menopause. *Journal of Bangladesh College of Physicians and Surgeons*, 36(1), 26–32. https://doi.org/10.3329/jbcps.v36i1.35508

American Urogynecologic Society. (2019). Pelvic organ prolapse. *Female Pelvic Medicine & Reconstructive Surgery*, 25(6), 397–408. https://doi.org/10.1097/SPV.0000000000000794

Brunham, R. C., Gottlieb, S. L., & Paavonen, J. (2015). Pelvic inflammatory disease. *New England Journal of Medicine*, 372(21), 2039–2048. https://doi.org/10.1056/NEJMra1411426

Canadian Cancer Society. (2017). *Canadian cancer statistics 2017*. https://cancer.ca/en/research/cancer-statistics/canadian-cancer-statistics

Canadian Cancer Society. (2021a). *Human papillomavirus: All about vaccines*. https://cancer.ca/en/cancer-information/reduce-your-risk/get-vaccinated/human-papillomavirus-hpv

Canadian Cancer Society. (2021b). *Risk factors for cervical cancer*. https://cancer.ca/en/cancer-information/cancer-types/cervical/risks#Sexual_activity

Canadian Cancer Society. (2021c). *Screening for cervical cancer*. https://cancer.ca/en/cancer-information/cancer-types/cervical/screening

Canadian Cancer Society Advisory Committee on Cancer Statistics. (2015). *Canadian cancer statistics 2015*. https://www.cancer.ca/en/cancer-information/cancer-type/cervical/statistics/?region=on

Canadian Institute for Health Information (CIHI). (2018). *Induced abortions reported in Canada in 2018*. https://www.cihi.ca/sites/default/files/document/induced-abortion-2018-en-web.xlsx

Canadian Nurses Association (CNA). (2017). *Code of ethics for registered nurses*. https://www.cna-aiic.ca/html/en/Code-of-Ethics-2017-Edition/files/assets/basic-html/page-1.html#

Chen, I., Thavorn, K., Shen, M., et al. (2017). Hospital associated costs of chronic pelvic pain in Canada: A population based descriptive study. *Journal of Obstetrics and Gynaecology Canada*, 39(3), 174–180.

Ekenros, L., Bäckström, T., Hirschberg, A., et al. (2019). Changes in premenstrual symptoms in women starting or discontinuing use of oral contraceptives. *Gynecological Endocrinology*, 35(5), 422–426. https://doi.org/10.1080/09513590.2018.1534097

El Shamy, T., Amer, S., Mohamed, A., et al. (2020). The impact of uterine artery embolization on ovarian reserve: A systematic review and meta-analysis. *AOGS: Acta Obstetrica Gynecologica Scandinavica*, 99, 16–23. https://doi.org/10.1111/aogs.13698

Famuyide, A. (2018). Endometrial ablation. *Journal of Minimally Invasive Gynecology*, 25(2), 299–307. https://doi.org/10.1016/j.jmig.2017.08.656

Gnanasambanthan, S., & Datta, S. (2019). Premenstrual syndrome. *Obstetrics, Gynaecology and Reproductive Medicine*, 29(10), 281–285. https://doi.org/10.1016/j.ogrm.2019.06.003

Goff, B. (2021). *Early detection of epithelial ovarian cancer: Role of symptom recognition*. UpToDate. https://www.uptodate.com/contents/early-detection-of-epithelial-ovarian-cancer-role-of-symptom-recognition/print

Gray, T., & Radley, S. (2020). Pelvic organ prolapse. In C. Chapple, W. Steers, & C. Evans (Eds.), *Urologic principles and practice*. Springer. https://doi.org/10.1007/978-3-030-28599-9_29

Hagen, S., & Thakar, R. (2015). Conservative management of pelvic organ prolapse. *Obstetrics, Gynaecology and Reproductive Medicine*, 25(4), 91–95. https://doi.org/10.1016/j.ogrm.2015.01.006

Hass, P., Seinsch, S., Eggemann, H., et al. (2018). Vaginal brachytherapy for endometrial cancer. *Journal of Cancer Research and Clinical Oncology*, 144, 1523–1530. https://doi-org.ezproxy.library.dal.ca/10.1007/s00432-018-2659-8

Haydu, C., Black, J., Schwab, C., et al. (2016). An update on the current pharmacotherapy for endometrial cancer. *Expert Opinion on Pharmacotherapy*, 17(4), 489–499. https://doi.org/10.1517/14656566.2016.1127351

Kamaludin, S., Zhang, X., & Shorey, S. (2019). Perspectives of women experiencing menorrhagia: A descriptive qualitative study. *Journal of Clinical Nursing*, 28, 2659–2668. https://doi.org/10.1111/jocn.14856

Kaunitz, A. M., & Manson, F. E. (2015). Management of menopausal symptoms. *Obstetrics and Gynecology*, 126(4), 859–876. https://doi.org/10.1097/AOG.0000000000001058

Keenan-Lindsay, L. (2017). Reproductive health. In S. Perry, M. Hockenberry, D. Lowdermilk, et al. (Eds.), *Maternal child nursing care in Canada* (2nd ed., pp. 104–143). Elsevier.

Keenan-Lindsay, L., & Mancuso, P. (2017). Infertility, contraception, and abortion. In S. Perry, M. Hockenberry, D. Lowdermilk, et al. (Eds.), *Maternal child nursing care in Canada* (2nd ed., pp. 144–175). Elsevier.

Lewis, F., Tatnall, F., Velangi, S., et al. (2018). British Association of Dermatologists guidelines for the management of lichen sclerosus, 2018. *British Journal of Dermatology*, 178, 839–853. https://doi.org/10.1111/bjd.16241

Madhra, M., Otify, M., & Horne, A. (2017). Ectopic pregnancy. *Obstetrics, Gynaecology and Reproductive Medicine*, 27(8), 245–250. https://doi.org/10.1016/j.ogrm.2017.06.004

Mainor, C., & Isaacs, C. (2020). Risk management for *BRCA1/BRCA2* mutation carriers without and with breast cancer. *Current Breast Cancer Reports*. https://doi.org/10.1007/s12609-019-00350-2

Mardanian, F., Rouholamin, S., & Nazemi, M. (2018). Evaluation of efficacy of transvaginal sonography with hysteroscopy for assessment of tubal patency in infertile women regarding diagnostic laparoscopy. *Advanced Biomedical Research*, 7, 101. https://doi.org/10.4103/abr.abr_71_17

Maxwell, E., Mathews, M., & Mulay, S. (2018). The impact of access barriers on fertility treatment decision making: A qualitative study from the perspectives of patients and service providers. *Journal of Obstetrics and Gynaecology Canada*, 40(2), 334–341. https://doi.org/10.1016/j.jogc.2017.08.025

McGarry, K., Geary, M., & Gopinath, V. (2018). Beyond estrogen: Treatment options for hot flashes. *Clinical Therapeutics*, 40(10), 1778–1786. https://doi.org/10.1016/j.clinthera.2018.08.010

McNamara, M., Batur, P., & DeSapri, K. T. (2015). Perimenopause. *Annals of Internal Medicine*, 162(3), ITC1–ITC15. https://doi.org/10.7326/AITC201502030

Mohammed, W., Salama, F., Tharwat, A., et al. (2017). Vaginal hysterectomy versus laparoscopically assisted vaginal hysterectomy for large uteri between 280 and 700 g: A randomized controlled trial. *Archives of Gynecology and Obstetrics*, 296, 77–83. https://doi.org/10.1007/s00404-017-4397-6

National Institutes of Health (NIH). (2016). *Menopausal hormone therapy information*. https://www.nih.gov/health-information/menopausal-hormone-therapy-information

Nonfoux, L., Chiaruzzi, M., Badiou, C., et al. (2018). Impact of currently marketed tampons and menstrual cups on *Staphylococcus aureus* growth and toxic shock syndrome toxin 1 production in vitro. *Applied and Environmental Microbiology, 84*(12), e00351–e00358. https://doi.org/10.1128/AEM.00351-18

Özgür Köneş, M., & Yıldız, H. (2020). The level of grief in women with pregnancy loss: A prospective evaluation of the first three months of perinatal loss. *Journal of Psychosomatic Obstetrics & Gynecology, 6,* 1–10. https://doi.org/10.1080/016748 2X.2020.1759543

Peiris, A., Chaljub, E., & Medlock, D. (2018). Endometriosis. *Journal of the American Medical Association, 320*(24), 2608. https://doi.org/10.1001/jama.2018.17953

Public Health Agency of Canada (PHAC). (2013). *Pelvic inflammatory disease (PID). Canadian guidelines on sexually transmitted infections. Section 4—Management and treatment of specific syndromes.* https://www.phac-aspc.gc.ca/std-mts/sti-its/cgsti-ldcits/section-4-4-eng.php

Public Health Agency of Canada (PHAC). (2019). *Fertility.* https://www.canada.ca/en/public-health/services/fertility/fertility.html

Rodriguez, A., Blanchard, Z., Maurer, K., et al. (2019). Estrogen signaling in endometrial cancer: A key oncogenic pathway with several open questions. *Hormones and Cancer, 10,* 51–63. https://doi.org/10.1007/s12672-019-0358-9

Rossi, B., Abusief, M., & Missmer, S. (2016). Modifiable risk factors and infertility: What are the connections? *American Journal of Lifestyle Medicine, 10*(4), 220–231. https://doi.org/10.1177/1559827614558020

Safrai, M., Rottenstreich, A., Shushan, A., et al. (2020). Risk factors for recurrent pelvic inflammatory disease. *European Journal of Obstetrics & Gynecology and Reproductive Biology, 244,* 40–44. https://doi.org/10.1016/j.ejogrb.2019.11.004

Schumacher, B., Jukic, A., & Steiner, A. (2018). Antimullerian hormone as a risk factor for miscarriage in naturally conceived pregnancies. *Fertility and Sterility, 109*(6), 1065–1071. https://doi.org/10.1016/j.fertnstert.2018.01.039

Silverberg, S., Harding, L., Spitzer, R., et al. (2018). The who, what, why and when of gynaecological referrals for refugee women. *Journal of Immigrant and Minority Health, 20*(6), 1347–1354. https://doi.org/10.1007/s10903-018-0733-6

Society of Obstetricians and Gynaecologists of Canada. (2019). Indications for pelvic examination. *Journal of Obstetrics and Gynaecology Canada, 41*(8), 1221–1234. https://doi.org/10.1016/j.jogc.2018.12.007

Stanzel, K., Hammarberg, K., & Fisher, J. (2018). Experiences of menopause, self-management strategies for menopausal symptoms and perceptions of health care among immigrant women: A systematic review. *Climacteric, 21*(2), 101–110. https://doi.org/10.1080/13697137.2017.1421922

Stewart, C., Ralyea, C., & Lockwood, S. (2019). Ovarian cancer: An integrated review. *Seminars in Oncology Nursing, 35*(2), 151–156. https://doi.org/10.1016/j.soncn.2019.02.001

Stewart, E. (2015). Uterine fibroids. *New England Journal of Medicine, 372*(17), 1646–1655. https://doi.org/10.1056/NEJMcp1411029

Trikudanathan, S. (2015). Polycystic ovarian syndrome. *Medical Clinics of North America, 99*(1), 221–235. https://doi.org/10.1016/j.mcna.2014.09.003

Vallvé-Juanico, J., López-Gil, C., Ballesteros, A., et al. (2019). Endometrial stromal cells circulate in the bloodstream of women with endometriosis: A pilot study. *International Journal of Molecular Science, 20*(15), 3740. https://doi.org/10.3390/ijms20153740

Vardanyan, R. (2017). *Piperidine-based drug discovery* (1st ed.). Elsevier.

Walker, K., Arbour, M., & Waryold, J. (2016). Educational strategies to help students provide respectful sexual and reproductive health care for lesbian, gay, bisexual, and transgender persons. *Journal of Midwifery and Women's Health, 61*(6), 737–743. https://doi.org/10.1111/jmwh.12506

World Health Organization (WHO). (2021). *Health topics: Infertility.* https://www.who.int/health-topics/infertility#tab=tab_1

Zara, I. (2020). Overview on abortion. *Journal of Biochemistry, Biotechnology and Allied Fields, 5*(1), 45–51. https://www.idosr.org/wp-content/uploads/2020/05/IDOSR-JBBAF-5145-512020.pdf

RESOURCES

Canadian Cancer Society
https://www.cancer.ca

Canadian Fertility and Andrology Society
https://www.cfas.ca/

Ovarian Cancer Canada
https://www.ovariancanada.org

SexandU.ca
https://www.sexandu.ca/

Society of Obstetricians and Gynaecologists of Canada
https://sogc.org/index.html

Society of Obstetricians and Gynaecologists of Canada—*Endometriosis*
https://www.yourperiod.ca/endometriosis/

Women's Health Matters
https://www.womenshealthmatters.ca/

American Cancer Society
https://www.cancer.org

American College of Obstetricians and Gynecologists
https://www.acog.org

American Urological Association
https://www.auanet.org

Hysterectomy Educational Resources and Services (HERS) Foundation
https://www.hersfoundation.org/

National Ovarian Cancer Coalition (NOCC)
https://ovarian.org/

North American Menopause Society
https://www.menopause.org

SIECUS: Sex Ed for Social Change
https://www.siecus.org

⊘volve

For additional Internet resources, see the website for this book at http://evolve.elsevier.com/Canada/Lewis/medsurg.

Nursing Management
Male Reproductive Conditions

Catharine R. Simpson and Shelley L. Cobbett
Originating US chapter by Anthony Lutz

evolve WEBSITE

http://evolve.elsevier.com/Canada/Lewis/medsurg

- Review Questions (Online Only)
- Key Points
- Answer Guidelines for Case Study

- Student Case Study
  - Benign Prostatic Hyperplasia
- Customizable Nursing Care Plan
  - Prostate Surgery

- Conceptual Care Map Creator
- Audio Glossary
- Content Updates

LEARNING OBJECTIVES

1. Describe the pathophysiology, clinical manifestations, and interprofessional management of benign prostatic hyperplasia.
2. Discuss the nursing care of patients with benign prostatic hyperplasia.
3. Describe the pathophysiology, clinical manifestations, and interprofessional management of prostate cancer.
4. Explain the nursing care of patients with prostate cancer.
5. Specify the pathophysiology, clinical manifestations, and nursing and interprofessional management of prostatitis and conditions of the penis and scrotum.

6. Explain the clinical manifestations and interprofessional management of testicular cancer.
7. Describe the pathophysiology, clinical manifestations, and nursing and interprofessional management of conditions related to male sexual function.
8. Summarize the psychological and emotional implications related to male reproductive conditions.

KEY TERMS

benign prostatic hyperplasia (BPH)
epididymitis
epispadias
erectile dysfunction (ED)
hydrocele
hypospadias

orchitis
paraphimosis
phimosis
prostate-specific antigen (PSA)
prostatitis
radical prostatectomy

spermatocele
testicular torsion
transurethral resection of the prostate
    (TURP)
varicocele
vasectomy

Conditions of the male reproductive system can involve a variety of structures, including the prostate, the penis, the urethra, the ejaculatory duct, the scrotum, the testes, the epididymis, the vas deferens, and the rectum (Figure 57.1).

CONDITIONS OF THE PROSTATE GLAND

BENIGN PROSTATIC HYPERPLASIA

Benign prostatic hyperplasia (BPH) is a condition involving the increase in size of the prostate gland leading to a disruption of urine outflow from the bladder through the urethra. BPH is present in 10% of men by 40 years of age and increases with age. Half of men have some signs of BPH by the age of 50. BPH

with lower urinary tract symptoms (LUTS) does not lead to an increased risk of prostate cancer (Jarvis, 2019).

Etiology and Pathophysiology

There are several potential factors that play a role in the development and progression of BPH. Hormonal changes associated with aging are a contributing factor. Dihydroxytestosterone (DHT), one of several sex hormones, stimulates prostate cell growth (Hannon & Porth, 2017). Excess amounts of DHT can cause overgrowth of prostate tissue. As men age, a decrease in testosterone occurs; however, DHT accumulates, resulting in prostate enlargement. Another possible cause is an increased proportion of estrogen as compared to testosterone. A higher amount of estrogen within the prostate gland increases the

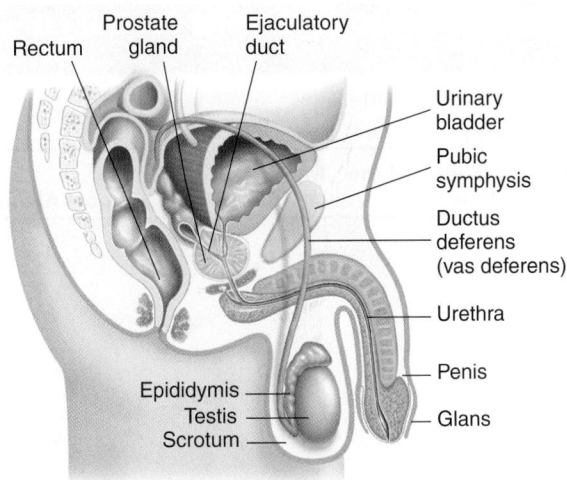

FIG. 57.1 Areas of the male reproductive system in which health problems are likely to develop.

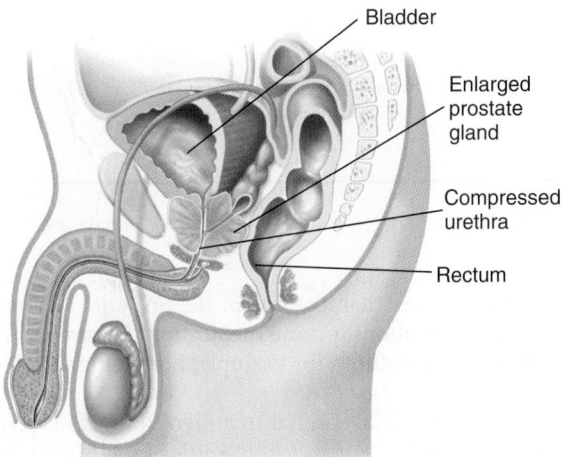

FIG. 57.2 Benign prostatic hyperplasia. The enlarged prostate compresses the urethra.

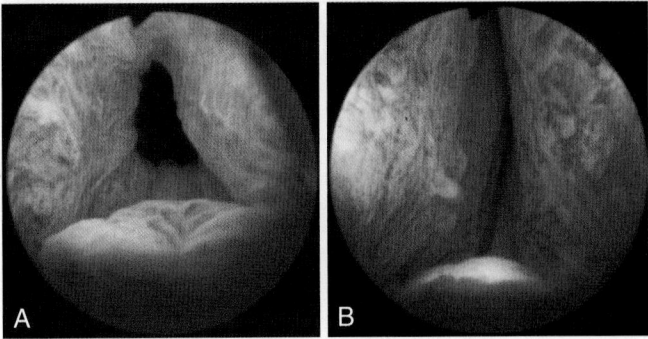

FIG. 57.3 Views of the prostate by cystoscopy. **A,** Normal appearance. **B,** Moderate benign prostatic hyperplasia with urethral obstruction. Source: Townsend, C. M., Beauchamp, R. D., Evers, B. M., et al. (2012). *Sabiston textbook of surgery* (19th ed.). Saunders.

activity of substances (including DHT) that promote prostate cell growth.

BPH usually develops in the inner part of the prostate, called the *transition zone*. Prostate cancer is more likely to develop in the *peripheral zone*, the outer portion. As the transition zone enlarges, it gradually compresses the urethra, leading to partial or complete obstruction (Figure 57.2). This compression leads to the development of clinical manifestations. There is no direct relationship between overall prostate size and the severity of manifestations or degree of obstruction (Figure 57.3).

Risk factors for BPH include aging, obesity (especially increased waist circumference), lack of physical activity, smoking, and diabetes (Trumble et al., 2015). A family history of BPH in a first-degree relative also may be a risk factor.

Clinical Manifestations

Manifestations of BPH result from urinary obstruction. Symptoms are usually gradual and not noticed until prostatic enlargement has been present for some time. Early symptoms are usually minimal because the bladder can compensate for a small amount of resistance to urine flow. As the severity of urethral obstruction increases, symptoms gradually worsen.

Symptoms can be divided into two groups: obstructive and irritative. *Obstructive symptoms* include a decrease in the calibre and force of the urinary stream, difficulty in initiating voiding, intermittency of urine while voiding, and dribbling at the end of urination. *Irritative symptoms,* which include urinary frequency, urgency, dysuria, bladder pain, nocturia, and incontinence, are associated with inflammation and infection. Nocturia is often the first symptom the patient notices. The American Urological Association (AUA) Symptom Index for BPH (Table 57.1) is a widely used tool to assess voiding symptoms associated with obstruction (Barry et al., 1992). Although this tool is not diagnostic, it is useful in determining the degree of symptoms. Higher scores on this tool indicate greater symptom severity.

Complications

Complications of urinary obstruction are relatively uncommon in BPH. Acute urinary retention is a complication manifested by the sudden and painful inability to urinate. Treatment involves the insertion of a catheter to drain the bladder. Surgery may also be indicated.

Another common complication is urinary tract infection (UTI) and, potentially, sepsis secondary to UTI. Incomplete bladder emptying (associated with partial obstruction) results in residual urine, providing a favourable environment for bacterial growth. Calculi (stones) may develop in the bladder because of the alkalinization of the residual urine. Although bladder stones are more common in men with BPH, the risk for renal calculi is not significantly increased. Additional complications include renal failure caused by hydronephrosis (distension of the pelvis and the calyces of the kidney by urine that cannot flow through the ureter to the bladder), pyelonephritis, and bladder damage if treatment for acute urinary retention is delayed.

Diagnostic Studies

The primary methods used to diagnose BPH include a history and physical examination. The prostate can be palpated by digital rectal examination (DRE) to estimate its size, symmetry, and consistency. In BPH, the prostate is symmetrically enlarged, firm, and smooth.

A blood test for **prostate-specific antigen (PSA)**, a glycoprotein found only in the epithelial cells of the prostate, may be offered to patients who have at least a 10-year life expectancy and when knowledge of prostate cancer would change health management (Nickel et al., 2018). Elevated PSA levels indicate a pathological condition of the prostate, although not necessarily prostate cancer. PSA levels may be slightly elevated in patients

TABLE 57.1   AMERICAN UROLOGICAL ASSOCIATION SYMPTOM INDEX TO DETERMINE SEVERITY OF PROSTATIC CONDITIONS

			American Urological Association (AUA) Symptom Score*			
			(Circle one number on each line.)			
Questions to Be Answered	Not at All	Less Than 1 Time in 5	Less Than Half the Time	About Half the Time	More Than Half the Time	Almost Always
Over the past month: 1. How often have you had a sensation of not emptying your bladder completely after you finished urinating?	0	1	2	3	4	5
2. How often have you had to urinate again <2 hr after you finished urinating?	0	1	2	3	4	5
3. How often have you found you stopped and started again several times when you urinated?	0	1	2	3	4	5
4. How often have you found it difficult to postpone urination?	0	1	2	3	4	5
5. How often have you had a weak urinary stream?	0	1	2	3	4	5
6. How often have you had to push or strain to begin urination?	0	1	2	3	4	5
7. How many times did you most typically get up to urinate from the time you went to bed at night until the time you got up in the morning?	0 (None)	1 (1 time)	2 (2 times)	3 (3 times)	4 (4 times)	5 (≥5 times)
Sum of circled numbers (AUA Symptom Score):* _____						

*Score is interpreted as 0–7, mild; 8–19, moderate; 20–35, severe.

Source: Reprinted from *Journal of Urology, 148*(5), Barry, M. J., Fowler, F. J., Jr., O'Leary, M. P., et al., The American Urological Association symptom index for benign prostatic hyperplasia, pp. 1549–1557, Copyright 1992, with permission from Elsevier.

with BPH. The following diagnostics are not mandatory; however, they may be completed with diagnostic uncertainty or when rationale warrants further investigation. Optional diagnostics include serum creatinine, urine cytology, uroflowmetry, postvoid residual urine volumes, voiding diary, and sexual function questionnaire (Nickel et al., 2018). Uroflowmetry, a study that measures the volume of urine expelled from the bladder per second, is helpful in determining the extent of urethral blockage and thus the type of treatment needed. Postvoid residual urine volume is often measured to determine the degree of urine flow obstruction.

The following diagnostics are only required in patients with DRE abnormalities, uncertain diagnosis, or poor response to medical therapy; for preoperative planning; and in patients with a definite indication (such as hematuria): cytology, cystoscopy, urodynamics, radiological evaluation of the upper urinary tract, prostate ultrasound, and prostate biopsy. These diagnostics are unnecessary in the routine initial evaluation of patients with BPH and LUTS (Nickel et al., 2018).

Transrectal ultrasonography (TRUS) allows for accurate assessment of prostate size and is helpful in differentiating BPH from prostate cancer. Biopsies can be taken during the ultrasonography procedure. Cystoscopy, a procedure enabling internal visualization of the urethra and the bladder, is performed if the diagnosis is uncertain and in patients scheduled for prostatectomy.

Interprofessional Care

The goals of interprofessional care are to restore bladder drainage, relieve the patient's symptoms, and prevent or treat the complications of BPH. Treatment is generally based on the degree to which the symptoms bother the patient or the presence of

complications rather than the size of the prostate. Alternatives to surgical interventions include medication therapy and minimally invasive procedures, for example, holmium laser enucleation (Das et al., 2019).

The most conservative initial treatment for BPH is referred to as *active surveillance* or *watchful waiting* (Table 57.2). When there are no symptoms or only mild ones (AUA symptom scores <7), a wait-and-see approach is taken. Because symptoms may come and go, a conservative approach has value. Dietary changes (decreasing intake of caffeine, artificial sweeteners, and spicy or acidic foods), avoiding medications such as decongestants and anticholinergics, and restricting evening fluid intake may improve symptoms. A timed voiding schedule may reduce or eliminate symptoms, thus negating the need for further intervention. If the patient begins to have signs or symptoms that indicate an increase in obstruction, further treatment is indicated.

Medication Therapy. The primary medical management of BPH and LUTS involves the use of α blockers (α-adrenergic receptor blockers) and 5-α-reductase inhibitors (5α-reductase inhibitors) (Nickel et al., 2018).

5α-Reductase Inhibitors. These medications work by reducing the size of the prostate gland. Finasteride (Proscar) blocks the enzyme 5α-reductase, which is necessary for the conversion of testosterone to DHT, the principal intraprostatic androgen. This medication causes regression of hyperplastic tissue through suppression of androgens. Finasteride is an appropriate treatment option for individuals who score between 12 and 26 on the AUA Symptom Index (see Table 57.1). Although more than 50% of patients who are treated with the medication show symptom improvement, it takes about 6 months to be effective, and the medication must be taken on a continuous

TABLE 57.2   INTERPROFESSIONAL CARE
Benign Prostatic Hyperplasia

Diagnostic
- History and physical examination
- Digital rectal examination (DRE)
- Urinalysis with culture
- Serum creatinine
- Prostate-specific antigen (PSA)
- Postvoid residual
- Uroflowmetry
- Transrectal ultrasonography (TRUS)
- Cystourethroscopy

Interprofessional Therapy
- Conservative therapy (active surveillance or "watchful waiting")

Medication Therapy
- 5α-Reductase inhibitors
- α-Adrenergic receptor blockers
- Erectogenic medications

Invasive Therapy*
- Open prostatectomy
- Transurethral incision of the prostate (TUIP)
- Transurethral resection of the prostate (TURP)

Minimally Invasive Therapy*
- Intraprostatic urethral stents
- Laser prostatectomy
- Transurethral electrovaporization of the prostate (TUVP)
- Transurethral microwave thermotherapy (TUMT)
- Transurethral needle ablation (TUNA)

*See Table 57.3.

basis to maintain therapeutic results. Serum PSA levels decrease by almost 50% when taking finasteride. Therefore, PSA levels should be doubled when comparing the patient's current levels to premedication levels.

Dutasteride (Avodart) is a dual inhibitor of 5α-reductase types 1 and 2 isoenzymes. (Finasteride inhibits only the type 2 isoenzyme.) The combination of a 5α-reductase inhibitor (dutasteride) and an α-adrenergic receptor blocker (tamsulosin) is available in a single oral medication (Jalyn). Adverse effects of 5α-reductase inhibitors include decreased libido, decreased volume of ejaculate, and erectile dysfunction (ED).

MEDICATION ALERT—Finasteride (Proscar)
- Patient should be aware of the increased risk for orthostatic hypotension with concomitant use of ED medications.
- Women who may be or are pregnant should not handle finasteride tablets because of the potential risk to the male fetus (anomaly).

α-Adrenergic Receptor Blockers. α-Adrenergic receptor blockers are another medication treatment option for BPH. These agents selectively block α1-adrenergic receptors, which are abundant in the prostate and are increased in hyperplastic prostate tissue. Although α-adrenergic blockers are more commonly used for treatment of hypertension, these medications promote smooth muscle relaxation in the prostate, facilitating urinary flow through the urethra. These agents demonstrate a 50 to 60% efficacy in improvement of symptoms, which occurs within 2 to 3 weeks.

Several α-adrenergic blockers, including silodosin (Rapaflo), alfuzosin (Xatral), prazosin, doxazosin (Cardura), terazosin, and tamsulosin, are currently being used. Adverse effects include postural hypotension, dizziness, fatigue, retrograde

ejaculation, and nasal congestion. It must be pointed out that, although these medications offer symptomatic relief of BPH, they do not treat hyperplasia.

Erectogenic Medications. Tadalafil (Cialis) has been used in men who have symptoms of BPH alone or in combination with ED. The medication has shown effectiveness in reducing symptoms for both of these conditions (Roehrborn et al., 2015) (see Erectile Dysfunction section later in this chapter).

Herbal Therapy. Plant-based herbal preparations appeal to some patients for the management of LUTS associated with BPH. Some examples of herbal formations include saw palmetto (*Serenoa repens*), *Pygeum africanum* (African plum bark), and *Urtica dioica* (stinging nettle). Numerous studies report no significant difference in results between herbal therapies and placebos. Herbal therapies are not recommended for the treatment of LUTS and BPH (Nickel et al., 2018).

Minimally Invasive Therapy. Minimally invasive therapies are becoming more common as an alternative to watchful waiting and invasive treatment (Table 57.3). They generally do not require hospitalization or catheterization and are associated with few adverse events.

Transurethral Microwave Thermotherapy. Transurethral microwave thermotherapy (TUMT) is an outpatient procedure that involves the delivery of microwaves directly to the prostate through a transurethral probe to raise the temperature of the prostate tissue to about 45°C. The heat causes death of tissue, thus relieving the obstruction. A rectal temperature probe is used during the procedure to ensure that the temperature is kept below 43.5°C to prevent rectal tissue damage. The procedure takes about 90 minutes.

Postoperative urinary retention is a common complication. Thus, the patient is generally sent home with an in-dwelling catheter for 2 to 7 days to maintain urinary flow and to facilitate the passing of small clots or necrotic tissue. Antibiotics, pain medication, and bladder antispasmodic medications are used to treat and prevent postprocedural complications. The procedure is not appropriate for patients with rectal conditions. Anticoagulant therapy should be stopped 10 days before treatment. Mild adverse effects include occasional problems of bladder spasm, hematuria, dysuria, and retention.

Transurethral Needle Ablation. Transurethral needle ablation (TUNA) is another procedure that increases the temperature of prostate tissue, causing localized necrosis. TUNA differs from TUMT in that low-wave radiofrequency is used to heat the prostate. Only prostate tissue in direct contact with the needle is affected, thus allowing greater precision in removal of the target tissue. The extent of tissue removed by this process is determined by the amount of tissue contact (needle length), amount of energy delivered, and duration of treatment. The majority of patients undergoing TUNA have an improvement in symptoms.

This procedure is performed in an outpatient unit or health care provider's office using local anaesthesia and IV or oral sedation. The TUNA procedure lasts approximately 30 minutes. The patient typically experiences little pain with an early return to regular activities. Complications include urinary retention, UTI, and irritative voiding symptoms (e.g., frequency, urgency, dysuria). Some patients require a urinary catheter for a short time. Patients often have hematuria for up to a week.

Laser Prostatectomy. The use of laser therapy through visual or ultrasound guidance is an effective alternative to transurethral resection of the prostate (TURP) in treating BPH. The laser beam is delivered transurethrally through a fibre instrument

TABLE 57.3   TREATMENT FOR BENIGN PROSTATIC HYPERPLASIA

Description	Advantages	Disadvantages
Minimally Invasive		
Transurethral Microwave Thermotherapy (TUMT)		
Use of microwave radiating heat to produce coagulative necrosis of the prostate	Outpatient procedure Erectile dysfunction, urinary incontinence, and retrograde ejaculation are rare.	Potential for damage to surrounding tissue Urinary catheter needed after procedure
Transurethral Needle Ablation (TUNA)		
Low-wave radiofrequency used to heat the prostate, causing necrosis	Outpatient procedure Erectile dysfunction, urinary incontinence, and retrograde ejaculation are rare. Precise delivery of heat to desired area Very little pain experienced	Urinary retention common Irritative voiding symptoms Hematuria
Laser Prostatectomy		
Use of a laser beam to cut or destroy part of the prostate Techniques available: • Visual laser ablation of prostate (VLAP) • Contact laser • Photovaporization of prostate (PVP) • Interstitial laser coagulation (ILC)	Short procedure Comparable results to TURP Minimal bleeding Fast recovery time Rapid symptom improvement Very effective	Catheter (up to 7 days) needed after procedure because of edema and urinary retention Delayed sloughing of tissue Takes several weeks to reach optimal effect Retrograde ejaculation
Transurethral Electrovaporization of Prostate (TUVP)		
Electrosurgical vaporization and desiccation used together to destroy prostatic tissue	Minimal risks Minimal bleeding and sloughing	Retrograde ejaculation Intermittent hematuria
Intraprostatic Urethral Stents		
Insertion of self-expandable metallic stent into the urethra, where enlarged area of prostate occurs	Safe and effective Low risk	Stent may move Long-term effect unknown
Invasive (Surgery)		
Transurethral Resection of Prostate (TURP)		
Use of excision and cauterization to remove prostate tissue cystoscopically Remains the standard for treatment of BPH	Erectile dysfunction unlikely	Bleeding Retrograde ejaculation
Transurethral Incision of Prostate (TUIP)		
Involves transurethral incisions into prostatic tissue to relieve obstruction Effective for men with small to moderate prostates	Outpatient procedure Minimal complications Low occurrence of erectile dysfunction or retrograde ejaculation	Urinary catheter needed after procedure
Open Prostatectomy		
Surgery of choice for men with large prostates, bladder damage, or other complicating factors Involves external incision with two possible approaches (see Figure 57.6)	Complete visualization of prostate and surrounding tissue	Erectile dysfunction Bleeding Postoperative pain Risk for infection

and is used for cutting, coagulation, and vaporization of prostatic tissue. There are a variety of laser procedures using different sources, wavelengths, and delivery systems. Retreatment rates are comparable to those of TURP (Chughtai et al., 2015). Laser techniques available include visual laser ablation of the prostate (VLAP), contact laser techniques, photovaporization of the prostate (PVP), and interstitial laser coagulation (ILC).

Intraprostatic Urethral Stents. Symptoms from obstruction in patients who are poor surgical candidates can be relieved with intraprostatic urethral stents. The stents are placed directly into the prostatic tissue. Complications include chronic pain, infection, and encrustation. The long-term effects are not known.

Invasive Therapy (Surgery). Invasive treatment of symptomatic BPH involves surgery. The choice of the treatment approach depends on the size and location of the prostatic enlargement and patient factors such as age and surgical risk. Invasive treatments are summarized in Table 57.3.

Invasive therapy is indicated when the decrease in urine flow is enough to cause discomfort, persistent residual urine, acute urinary retention because of obstruction with no reversible precipitating cause, or hydronephrosis. Intermittent catheterization or insertion of an in-dwelling catheter can temporarily reduce symptoms and bypass the obstruction. However, long-term catheter use should be avoided because of the increased risk for infection.

Transurethral Resection of the Prostate. Transurethral resection of the prostate (TURP) is a surgical procedure involving the removal of prostate tissue using a resectoscope inserted through the urethra. TURP has long been considered the primary standard surgical treatment for moderate to severe BPH (Nickel et al., 2018). TURP is performed under a spinal or general anaesthetic. No external surgical incision is made. Instead, a resectoscope is inserted through the urethra to excise and cauterize obstructing prostatic tissue (Figure 57.4). A large

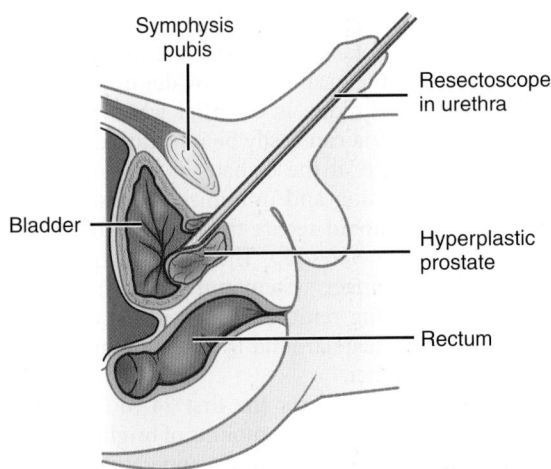

Symphysis
pubis

Resectoscope
in urethra

Bladder

Hyperplastic
prostate

Rectum

FIG. 57.4 Transurethral resection of the prostate.

three-way in-dwelling catheter with a 30-mL balloon is inserted into the bladder after the procedure to provide hemostasis and to facilitate urinary drainage. Usually for the first 24 hours, the bladder is irrigated, either continuously or intermittently, to prevent obstruction from mucus and blood clots.

The outcome for 80 to 90% of patients is excellent, with marked improvements in symptoms and urinary flow rates. TURP is a surgical procedure with relatively low risk. Postoperative complications include bleeding, clot retention, bladder spasms, and dilutional hyponatremia associated with irrigation. Because bleeding is a common complication, patients taking acetylsalicylic acid (ASA; Aspirin) or warfarin (Coumadin) or other anticoagulants must discontinue these medications several days before surgery.

Transurethral Incision of the Prostate. *Transurethral incision of the prostate* (TUIP) is a surgical procedure that is indicated for patients with moderate to severe symptoms and small prostates who are poor surgical candidates. It is done under local anaesthesia and is as effective as TURP in symptom relief.

Prostatectomy. Prostatectomy is the surgery of choice for large prostates and is discussed later in this chapter.

NURSING MANAGEMENT
BENIGN PROSTATIC HYPERPLASIA

Because the nurse is most directly involved in the care of patients with BPH who are having invasive procedures, the focus of nursing management in this section is on preoperative and postoperative care.

NURSING ASSESSMENT
Subjective and objective data that should be obtained from a patient with BPH are presented in Table 57.4.

NURSING DIAGNOSES
Nursing diagnoses for a patient with BPH preoperatively may include but are not limited to the following:

- *Acute pain* resulting from *biological injury agent* (bladder distention secondary to enlarged prostate)
- *Potential for infection* resulting from *insufficient knowledge to avoid pathogens, stasis of body fluid* (in-dwelling catheter, urinary stasis)

TABLE 57.4 NURSING ASSESSMENT
Benign Prostatic Hyperplasia

Subjective Data
Important Health Information
Past health history: Family history of BPH; obesity; diet high in fat or zinc
Medications: Estrogen or testosterone supplementation
Surgeries or other treatments: Previous treatment for BPH

Symptoms
- Voluntary fluid restriction; urinary urgency; urinary dysuria; diminution in calibre and force of urinary stream; hesitancy in initiating voiding; postvoid dribbling; urinary retention; incontinence; nocturia; bladder discomfort; anxiety about sexual functioning

Objective Data
General
Older male

Urinary
Distended bladder on palpation
Smooth, firm, elastic enlargement of prostate on rectal examination (Advanced Nursing Competency)

Possible Findings
Enlarged prostate on ultrasonography; vesicle neck obstruction on cystoscopy; residual urine with postvoiding catheterization; presence of WBCs, bacteria, or microscopic hematuria with infection; ↑ serum creatinine levels with renal involvement

BPH, benign prostatic hyperplasia; *WBCs,* white blood cells.

Nursing diagnoses for a patient with BPH who has invasive therapy (surgery) are presented in Nursing Care Plan (NCP) 57.1, available on the Evolve website.

PLANNING
The overall preoperative goals for patients having invasive procedures are (a) restoration of urinary drainage, (b) treatment of any UTI, and (c) an understanding of the upcoming procedure, the implications for sexual functioning, and urinary control. The overall postoperative goals are (a) no complications, (b) restoration of urinary control, (c) complete bladder emptying, and (d) the ability for satisfying sexual expression.

NURSING IMPLEMENTATION
HEALTH PROMOTION. The cause of BPH is largely attributed to the aging process. Health promotion focuses on early detection and treatment. Prostate cancer screening is a controversial issue, with varying recommendations on PSA screening, with no consensus (Rendon et al., 2017). Some patients may be interested in PSA screening despite the advice of their health care provider about personal risk of developing prostate cancer and the benefits and risks of having a PSA test. A PSA is only completed if life expectancy is greater than 10 years. Men with average risk can be screened at 50 years of age and men at increased risk can be screened at 45 years of age. The results of the PSA indicate the timeline of subsequent PSAs (Rendon et al., 2017).

Some patients find the ingestion of alcohol and caffeine increases prostatic symptoms because diuretic effects of these substances increase bladder distension. Compounds found in common cough and cold remedies such as pseudoephedrine (e.g., Sudafed) and phenylephrine (e.g., Dimetapp) often worsen the symptoms of BPH. These medications are α-adrenergic agonists that cause smooth muscle contraction.

Patients with obstructive symptoms should be advised to urinate every 2 to 3 hours and when first feeling the urge. Doing so will minimize urinary stasis and acute urinary retention. Fluid intake should be maintained at a normal level to prevent dehydration or fluid overload. The patient may believe if fluid intake is restricted, symptoms will be less severe, but this increases the chances of infection. However, if the patient increases their intake too rapidly, bladder distension can develop because of the prostatic obstruction.

ACUTE INTERVENTION. The following discussion focuses on preoperative and postoperative care for the patient undergoing a TURP.

Preoperative Care. Urinary drainage must be restored before surgery. Prostatic obstruction may result in acute retention or inability to void. A urethral catheter such as a coudé (curved-tip) catheter may be needed to restore drainage. In many health care settings, 10 mL of sterile 2% lidocaine gel is injected into the urethra before insertion of the catheter. The lidocaine gel not only acts as a lubricant but also provides local anaesthesia and helps open the urethral lumen. If a sizable obstruction of the urethra exists, the urologist may insert a filiform catheter with sufficient rigidity to pass the obstruction. Aseptic technique is important at all times to avoid introducing bacteria into the bladder. (Urinary catheters are discussed in Chapter 48.)

Antibiotics are usually administered before any invasive procedure. Any infection of the urinary tract must be treated before surgery. Restoring urine drainage and encouraging a high fluid intake (2 to 3 L/day unless contraindicated) are also helpful in managing the infection.

Patients are often concerned about the impact of the impending surgery on sexual functioning. Patients and their partners should be provided an opportunity to express their concerns. They should be informed that surgery may affect sexual function and that most types of prostatic surgery result in some degree of retrograde ejaculation. The patient should know that the amount of ejaculate may decrease or be totally absent. As a result, orgasmic sensations felt during ejaculation may decrease. Retrograde ejaculation is not harmful because the semen is eliminated during the next urination.

Postoperative Care. The main complications following surgery are hemorrhage, bladder spasms, urinary incontinence, and infection. The plan of care should be adjusted to the type of surgery, the reasons for surgery, and the patient's response to surgery.

After surgery, the patient will have a standard catheter or a triple-lumen catheter. Bladder irrigation is typically done to remove clotted blood from the bladder and to ensure drainage of urine. The bladder is irrigated either manually on an intermittent basis or, more commonly, as continuous bladder irrigation (CBI) with sterile normal saline solution or another prescribed solution. If manual irrigation of the bladder is ordered, 50 mL of irrigating solution (commonly normal saline) is instilled, and then withdrawn with a syringe to remove clots that may be in the bladder and catheter. Painful bladder spasms often occur as a result of manual irrigation. With CBI, irrigating solution is continuously infused and drained from the bladder. The rate of infusion is based on the colour of drainage. Ideally, the urine drainage should be light pink without clots. The inflow and outflow of irrigant must be continuously monitored. If outflow is less than inflow, the bladder should be assessed immediately,

and the catheter patency checked. If the outflow is blocked and patency cannot be re-established by manual irrigation, the CBI must be stopped and the health care provider notified.

Careful aseptic technique is essential when irrigating the bladder because bacteria can easily be introduced into the urinary tract. Proper care of the catheter is also important. To prevent urethral irritation and minimize the risk for bladder infection, the nurse should secure the catheter to the patient's leg with tape or a catheter strap. The catheter should be connected to a closed drainage system and should not be disconnected unless it is being removed, changed, or irrigated. The secretions that accumulate around the meatus can be cleansed daily with soap and water.

Blood clots are expected for the first 24 to 36 hours after prostate surgery. However, large amounts of bright-red blood in the urine can indicate hemorrhage. Postoperative hemorrhage may occur from displacement of the catheter, dislodgement of a large clot, or increases in abdominal pressure. Release or displacement of the catheter dislodges the balloon that provides counter-pressure on the operative site. Traction on the catheter may be applied to provide counter-pressure (tamponade) on the bleeding site in the prostate, thereby decreasing bleeding. Such traction can result in local necrosis if pressure is applied for too long. Therefore, pressure should be relieved on a scheduled basis by qualified personnel. Activities that increase abdominal pressure, such as sitting or walking for prolonged periods and straining to have a bowel movement (Valsalva manoeuvre), should be avoided in the postoperative recovery period.

Bladder spasms are a distressing complication for patients after transurethral procedures. They occur as a result of irritation of the bladder mucosa from the insertion of the resectoscope, presence of a catheter, or clots leading to obstruction of the catheter. Patients should be instructed not to urinate around the catheter because it increases the likelihood of spasm. If bladder spasms develop, the catheter should be checked for clots. Any clots discovered should be removed by irrigation so that urine can flow freely. Antispasmodics (e.g., belladonna and opium suppositories, oxybutynin [Oxytrol]), along with relaxation techniques, are used to relieve the pain and decrease spasm. The catheter is often removed 2 to 4 days after surgery. The patient should urinate within 6 hours after catheter removal. If they cannot, a catheter is reinserted for a day or two. If the problem continues, the nurse may need to instruct the patient in clean intermittent self-catheterization (see Chapter 48).

Sphincter tone may be poor immediately after catheter removal, resulting in urinary incontinence or dribbling. This is a common but distressing situation for patients. Sphincter tone can be strengthened with Kegel exercises (pelvic floor muscle technique) practised 10 to 20 times per hour while awake (see Table 48.19 in Chapter 48). Patients should be encouraged to practise starting and stopping the stream several times during urination. This facilitates learning of the pelvic floor exercises. It usually takes several weeks to achieve urinary continence. In some instances, control of urine may not be fully regained. Continence can improve for up to 12 months. If continence has not been achieved by that time, patients may be referred to a continence clinic. A variety of methods, including biofeedback, have been used to achieve positive results. Patients can also be instructed to use a penile clamp, condom catheter, or incontinence pads or briefs to avoid embarrassment from dribbling. In severe cases, an occlusive cuff that serves as an artificial sphincter can be surgically implanted to restore continence. The nurse should assist the patient in finding ways to manage incontinence so the patient can engage in social interactions without embarrassment.

Patients should be observed for signs of postoperative infection. If an external wound is present (from an open prostatectomy), the nurse should assess the area for erythema (redness), heat, swelling, and purulent drainage. Special care must be taken if a perineal incision is present because of the proximity of the anus. Rectal procedures, such as taking rectal temperatures and administering enemas, should be avoided. The insertion of well-lubricated belladonna and opium suppositories is acceptable.

Dietary intervention and stool softeners are important measures in the postoperative period to prevent patients from straining while having bowel movements. Straining increases the intra-abdominal pressure, which can lead to bleeding at the operative site. Adequate fluid intake and a diet high in fibre facilitate the passage of stool.

AMBULATORY AND HOME CARE. Discharge planning and home care issues are important aspects of care after prostate surgery. Instructions patients will need include those for (a) caring for an in-dwelling catheter (if one is left in place); (b) managing urinary incontinence; (c) maintaining oral fluids between 2 000 and 3 000 mL/day; (d) observing for signs and symptoms of UTI and wound infection; (e) preventing constipation; (f) avoiding heavy lifting (>4.5 kg); and (g) refraining from driving or having intercourse after surgery as directed by the health care provider.

Patients may experience a change in sexual functioning following surgery, for example, retrograde ejaculation or physiological ED (if the nerves are cut or damaged during surgery). Patients may experience anxiety over the change because of a perceived loss of sex role, lower self-esteem, or perceived decrease in the quality of sexual interaction with a partner. The nurse should discuss these changes with the patient and their partner and allow them to ask questions and express their concerns. Sexual counselling and treatment options may be necessary if ED becomes a chronic or permanent condition (ED is discussed later in this chapter.) Although some patients experience concerns regarding change in sexual functioning, this is not a universal concern. It may take up to 1 year for complete sexual functioning to return.

The bladder may take up to 2 months to return to its normal capacity. Patients should be instructed to drink at least 2 to 3 L of fluid per day and to urinate every 2 to 3 hours to flush the urinary tract. The nurse should also teach the patient to avoid or limit the intake of bladder irritants such as caffeine products, citrus juices, and alcohol. Because the patient may be experiencing incontinence or dribbling, they may incorrectly believe that decreasing fluid intake will relieve this problem. Urethral strictures may result from instrumentation or catheterization. Treatment may include intermittent clean self-catheterization (which will need to be taught to the patient) or a urethral dilation.

Patients who have had any procedure other than complete removal of the prostate will need to continue having yearly DREs because hyperplasia or cancer can occur in the remaining prostatic tissue.

EVALUATION

Expected outcomes for a patient with BPH are presented in NCP 57.1, available on the Evolve website.

PROSTATE CANCER

Prostate cancer is a malignant tumour of the prostate gland. In 2017, it was estimated that 21 300 new cases of prostate cancer were diagnosed in Canada that year and that 4 100 men would die of it (Canadian Cancer Society's Advisory Committee on Cancer Statistics, 2017), meaning that, on average, 59 Canadians are diagnosed with prostate cancer each day and 11 men die from it. The lifetime probability of a man developing prostate cancer in Canada is 1 in 7 (Canadian Cancer Society's Advisory Committee on Cancer Statistics, 2017). Prostate cancer is the most common cancer among men, excluding skin cancer. Among the Canadian Indigenous population, lower mortality and poorer survival rates are concurrently observed in men with prostate cancer (Wong & Kapoor, 2017). The majority (>75%) of cases occur in men older than age 65. However, many cases occur in younger men, who sometimes have a more aggressive type of cancer.

There were peaks in the incidence of newly diagnosed cases of prostate cancer in 1993 and 2001. These peaks were followed by a decline. These increases were attributed to the widespread use of PSA as a screening procedure and were in fact linked to two waves of intense screening. The age-standardized incidence rate has been in decline since 2001 (1.6% per year) (Canadian Cancer Society's Advisory Committee on Cancer Statistics, 2017).

Etiology and Pathophysiology

Prostate cancer is an androgen-dependent adenocarcinoma that is usually slow growing. It can spread by three routes: (1) through direct extension, (2) through the lymph system, or (3) through the bloodstream. Spread by direct extension involves the seminal vesicles, the urethral mucosa, the bladder wall, and the external sphincter. The cancer later spreads through the lymphatic system to the regional lymph nodes. The veins from the prostate seem to be the mode of spread to the pelvic bones, the head of the femur, the lower lumbar spine, the liver, and the lungs.

Age, ethnicity, and family history are three nonmodifiable risk factors for prostate cancer. Men over the age of 65 are at a greater risk for developing prostate cancer (Jarvis, 2019). Men of Asian ancestry have lower rates of prostate cancer, while men of African ancestry have a higher risk of developing prostate cancer (Canadian Cancer Society, 2020). See the Determinants of Health box for other risk factors.

Clinical Manifestations and Complications

Prostate cancer is usually asymptomatic in the early stages. Eventually, the patient may have symptoms similar to those of BPH, including dysuria, hesitancy, dribbling, frequency, urgency, hematuria, nocturia, retention, interruption of urinary stream, and inability to urinate. Pain in the lumbosacral area that radiates down to the hips or the legs, when coupled with urinary symptoms, may indicate metastasis.

Early recognition and treatment are required to control growth, prevent metastasis, and preserve quality of life. The tumour can spread to pelvic lymph nodes, bones, bladder, lungs, and liver. Once the tumour has spread to distant sites, the major concern becomes the management of pain. As the cancer spreads to the bones (a common site of metastasis), pain can become severe, especially in the back and the legs because of compression of the spinal cord and destruction of bone (Figure 57.5).

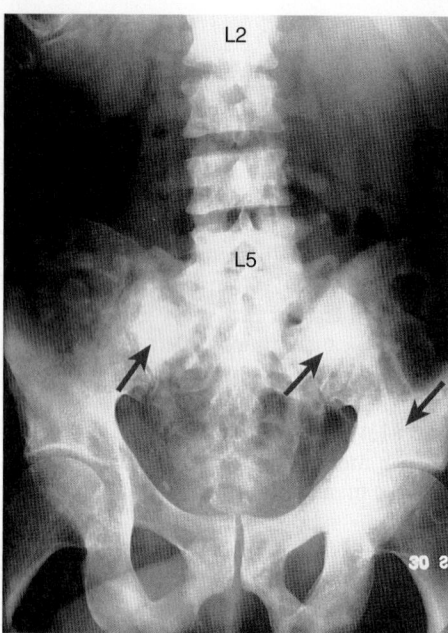

FIG. 57.5 Metastasis *(arrows)* of prostate cancer to the pelvis and lumbar spine. Source: Mettler, F. (2004). *Essentials of radiology* (2nd ed.). Saunders.

DETERMINANTS OF HEALTH

Prostate Cancer

Biology, Genetic Endowment, and Culture

- One of the strongest risk factors for prostate cancer is age, as the majority of diagnoses occur in men over 55 years of age.
- Canadian men of African descent have the highest rates of prostate cancer, while Canadians of Asian descent have the lowest rates.
- Men of African descent are diagnosed at a younger age, have more aggressive tumours, and are diagnosed at a more advanced stage than White men.
- Indigenous men (including First Nations, Métis, and Inuit) in Canada have a higher risk of developing prostate cancer than non-Indigenous men.*
- There is a genetic link to the development of prostate cancer, especially if a first-degree relative has a history of the disease.
- The *BRCA2* gene, linked with breast cancer, is also linked with prostate cancer.
- Long-term exposure to high levels of testosterone dihydroxytestosterone (DHT) may increase the risk for prostate cancer.

Personal Health Practices and Coping Skills

- Eating a diet high in fat increases the risk for prostate cancer.
- Consuming large amounts of dairy products increases the risk, as calcium is linked to prostate cancer.
- Consuming red meat (e.g., beef, pork) cooked at high temperatures and processed meat (e.g., bacon, hot dogs) increases the risk for prostate cancer.
- Being overweight or obese is linked to being diagnosed with advanced or aggressive prostate cancer.

Physical Environment; Employment/Working Conditions

- Occupational exposure to chemical carcinogens such as insecticides, cadmium, or rubber manufacturing is linked to prostate cancer.

References

Canadian Cancer Society. (2021). *Risk factors for prostate cancer.* http://www.cancer.ca/en/cancer-information/cancer-type/prostate/risks/?region=on

*Wong, E., & Kapoor, A. (2017). Epidemiology of prostate and kidney cancer in the Aboriginal population of Canada: A systematic review. *Canadian Urological Association Journal, 11*(5), E222–E232. doi:10.5489/cuaj.4185.

Diagnostic Studies

The primary screening tool for prostate cancer is a DRE. On DRE, an abnormal prostate may feel hard, nodular, and asymmetrical. The DRE is not a definitive diagnostic test for prostate cancer. If the DRE is abnormal, biopsy of the prostate tissue is indicated and necessary to confirm diagnosis of prostate cancer. The biopsy is typically done using TRUS because it allows the health care provider to visualize the prostate and pinpoint abnormalities. When a suspicious area is located, a biopsy needle is inserted into the prostate to obtain a tissue sample. A pathological examination of the specimen is done to assess for malignant changes.

The PSA test is no longer recommended for routine screening as the risks may outweigh the benefits (Nickel et al., 2018). Although specific recommendations regarding PSA screening vary, there is general agreement that patients should talk to their health care provider about their personal risk of developing prostate cancer and the potential risks (e.g., subsequent evaluation and treatment that may be unnecessary) and benefits (early detection of prostate cancer) of PSA screening before being tested.

PSA is used to monitor the success of treatment. When treatment for prostate cancer has been successful, PSA levels should fall to undetectable levels. Regular measurement of PSA levels following treatment is important to evaluate the continuing effectiveness of treatment and the possible recurrence of prostate cancer.

An elevated level of prostatic isoenzyme of serum acid phosphatase (prostatic acid phosphatase [PAP]) is an indicator of prostate cancer, especially if there is extracapsular spread. In advanced prostate cancer, serum alkaline phosphatase is increased as a result of bone metastasis.

A recent development in the diagnosis of prostate cancer is the discovery of the gene *prostate cancer associated 3* (non–protein coding) (*PCA3*) that is specific to prostate cancer cells and, if present in the urine, indicates prostate cancer. The *PCA3* test is more accurate than the PSA test because benign enlargement of the prostate will not cause an increase in *PCA3*, whereas it can cause an increase in the PSA test. The *PCA3* test offers a potential solution to the clinical diagnostic challenge posed by the PSA test.

Once a diagnosis of prostate cancer is confirmed, other tests used to determine the location and the extent of the spread of the cancer may include bone scan, computed tomography (CT), and magnetic resonance imaging (MRI) using an endorectal probe.

Interprofessional Care

Early-stage prostate cancer is curable in most patients. The prostate cancer is staged and graded on the basis of findings from diagnostic studies. Two common classification systems for staging prostate cancer, the Whitmore–Jewett and tumour–nodes–metastasis (TNM) systems, are both based on the size (volume) of the tumour and spread (Table 57.5). Both classification systems are used in Canada, with description and treatment based on the Whitmore–Jewett classification (e.g., stage A, B, C, or D) and description of the extent of the cancer based on the TNM system (see Chapter 18). Approximately 80% of patients with prostate cancer are diagnosed when cancer is in either a local or a regional stage.

Grading of the tumour is done on the basis of tumour histology using the *Gleason scale*. With this scale, tumours are graded

TABLE 57.5 WHITMORE–JEWETT STAGING CLASSIFICATION OF PROSTATE CANCER

Stage A: Clinically Unrecognized

A_1 <5% of prostatic tissue neoplastic

A_2 >5% of prostatic tissue neoplastic, all high-grade tumours

Stage B: Clinically Intracapsular

B_1 Nodule <2 cm and surrounded by palpably normal tissue

B_2 Nodule >2 cm or multiple nodules

Stage C: Clinically Extracapsular

C_1 Minimal extracapsular extension

C_2 Large tumours involving seminal vesicles, adjacent structures, or both

Stage D: Metastatic Disease

D_1 Pelvic lymph node metastases or ureteral obstruction causing hydronephrosis

D_2 Distant metastases to bone, viscera, or other soft tissue structures

TABLE 57.6 INTERPROFESSIONAL CARE

Prostate Cancer

Diagnostic
- History and physical examination
- Digital rectal examination (DRE)
- Prostatic acid phosphatase
- Transrectal ultrasonography
- Biopsy of prostate and lymph nodes
- CT scan, MRI, bone scan (to evaluate for metastatic disease)

Interprofessional Therapy

Active Surveillance
- Watchful waiting with annual physical exam including DRE

Surgery
- Radical prostatectomy
- Cryotherapy
- Orchiectomy (for metastatic disease)

Radiation Therapy
- External beam for primary, adjuvant, and recurrent disease
- Brachytherapy

Medication Therapy
- Androgen deprivation therapy
- Chemotherapy for metastatic disease

CT, computed tomography; *MRI*, magnetic resonance imaging.

from 1 to 5 based on the degree of glandular differentiation. Grade 1 represents the most well differentiated (most like the original cells), and grade 5 represents the most poorly differentiated (undifferentiated). Gleason grades are given to the two most commonly occurring patterns of cells and added together. The *Gleason score* is a number from 2 to 10. This scale is used to predict how quickly the cancer will progress.

The interprofessional care of the patient with prostate cancer depends on the stage of the cancer and the overall health of the patient. At all stages, there is more than one possible treatment option. The decision of which treatment course to pursue is made jointly by the patient and the health care team on the basis of a careful analysis of the facts and the patient's preference (Canadian Cancer Society, 2021b). Table 57.6 summarizes the various treatment options available.

Conservative Therapy. Prostate cancer is relatively slow growing, and an active surveillance approach to the management of prostate cancer is indicated. This strategy is appropriate when the patient has (a) a life expectancy of less than 10 years (low risk of dying of the disease), (b) serious coexisting medical conditions, and (c) a low-grade, low-stage tumour. These patients are typically followed with frequent PSA measurements, along with DRE, to monitor progress of the disease. A significant change in either PSA or DRE or the development of symptoms warrants a re-evaluation of treatment options.

Surgical Therapy

Radical Prostatectomy. With **radical prostatectomy**, the entire prostate gland, the seminal vesicles, and part of the bladder neck (ampulla) are surgically removed. The entire prostate is removed because the cancer tends to be in many different locations within the gland. In addition, a retroperitoneal lymph node dissection is usually done as a separate procedure. Surgery is usually not considered an option for advanced-stage disease (except to relieve symptoms associated with obstruction) because metastasis has already occurred. The two most common approaches for radical prostatectomy are retropubic and perineal resection (Figure 57.6). With the *retropubic* approach, a low midline abdominal incision is made to access the prostate gland, and the pelvic lymph nodes then can be dissected. With the *perineal* resection, an incision is made between the scrotum and the anus.

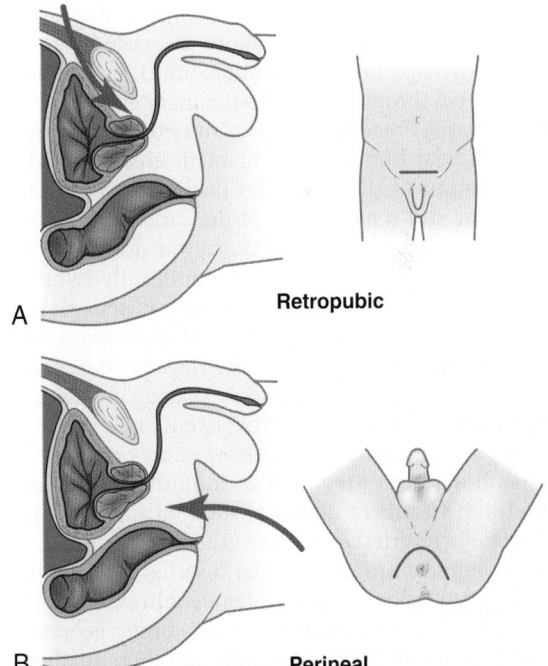

FIG. 57.6 Common approaches used to perform a prostatectomy. **A,** Retropubic approach involves a midline abdominal incision. **B,** Perineal approach involves an incision between the scrotum and the anus.

A *laparoscopic* approach to prostatectomy is being used in some settings. In this method, four small incisions are made into the abdomen. It results in less bleeding, less pain, and a faster recovery compared with other approaches.

A *robotic-assisted* (e.g., da Vinci system) prostatectomy is a type of laparoscopy in which the surgeon sits at a computer console while controlling high-resolution cameras and microsurgical instruments. Robotic-assisted prostatectomy has lower estimated blood loss and shorter hospital stays; however, there is conflicting evidence regarding its impact on functional outcomes (Chandrasekar & Tilki, 2018).

After surgery, the patient has a large in-dwelling catheter with a 30-mL balloon placed in the bladder via the urethra. This catheter is typically left in place for 1 to 2 weeks. A drain is left in the surgical site to aid in the removal of drainage from the area. This drain is typically removed after a couple of days. Because the perineal approach has a higher risk for postoperative infection (because of the location of the incision related to the anus), careful dressing changes and perineal care after each bowel movement are important to promote comfort and prevent infection. Depending on the type of surgery, the length of hospital stay postoperatively ranges from 1 to 3 days.

Two adverse outcomes following a radical prostatectomy are ED and urinary incontinence. ED may be permanent or temporary, with recovery being up to a couple of years. Incontinence is temporary, but approximately 10% of patients will continue to have stress incontinence, and 2 to 3% of patients suffer from long-term incontinence (Canadian Cancer Society, 2021b). The incidence of ED depends on the patient's age, preoperative sexual functioning, whether nerve-sparing surgery was performed, and the surgeon's expertise. Difficulties with urinary control occur in nearly all patients for the first few months following surgery because the bladder must be reattached to the urethra after the prostate is removed. Over time, the bladder adjusts, and most patients regain control (Mandel et al., 2017). Kegel exercises strengthen the urinary sphincter and may help improve incontinence. Other common complications associated with surgery include hemorrhage, urinary retention, infection, wound dehiscence, deep vein thrombosis, and pulmonary emboli.

Nerve-Sparing Procedure. In proximity to the prostate gland are neurovascular bundles that maintain erectile functioning. The preservation of these bundles during a prostatectomy is possible while still removing all of the cancer. This procedure is not indicated for patients with cancer outside of the prostate gland. Although the risk for ED is significantly reduced with this procedure, there is no guarantee that potency will be maintained. However, most patients younger than 50 years with good preoperative erectile function and low-stage prostate cancer can expect a return of potency after nerve-sparing prostatectomy.

Cryosurgery. Cryotherapy (cryoablation) is a surgical technique for prostate cancer that destroys cancer cells by freezing the tissue. It has been used both as an initial treatment and as a second-line treatment after radiation treatment failures. A TRUS probe is inserted to visualize the prostate gland. Probes containing liquid nitrogen are then inserted into the prostate. Liquid nitrogen delivers freezing temperatures, destroying the tissue. The treatment takes about 2 hours under general or spinal anaesthesia and does not involve an abdominal incision. Possible complications of prostatic cryosurgery include damage to the urethra and, in rare cases, a urethrorectal fistula (an opening between the urethra and the rectum) or a urethrocutaneous fistula (an opening between the urethra and the skin). Tissue sloughing, ED, urinary incontinence, prostatitis, and hemorrhage have also been reported.

Radiation Therapy. Radiation therapy is a common treatment option for prostate cancer, especially for patients older than 70, patients who are poor surgical risks, or those who wish to avoid surgery. Radiation therapy may be offered as the only treatment, or it may be offered in combination with surgery or with hormonal therapy. Salvage radiation therapy given for cancer recurrence after a radical prostatectomy may improve survival in some patients.

External Beam Irradiation. External beam irradiation is the most widely used method of delivering radiation treatments in patients with prostate cancer. This therapy can be used to treat patients with prostate cancer confined to the prostate or surrounding tissue. Patients are treated on an outpatient basis 5 days a week for 4 to 8 weeks. Each treatment lasts only a few minutes. Adverse effects from radiation can be acute (occurring during treatment or within 90 days following) or delayed (occurring months or years after treatment). Common adverse effects may involve gastrointestinal conditions, urinary symptoms, sexual dysfunction, fatigue, fractures, and secondary malignancies (DiBiase & Roach, 2021).

These effects usually resolve 2 to 3 weeks after the completion of radiation therapy. In patients with localized prostate cancer, cure rates using external beam radiation are comparable to those using radical prostatectomy.

Brachytherapy. Brachytherapy involves the placement of radioactive seeds directly into the prostate gland, allowing higher radiation doses directly in the impacted tissue. Brachytherapy minimizes the exposure of radiation to normal tissues. Brachytherapy is indicated for patients with localized prostate cancer without metastasis (Roach & DiBiase, 2020). The radioactive seeds are placed in the prostate gland with a needle through a grid template guided by TRUS (Figure 57.7). The grid template and ultrasonography ensure accurate placement of the seeds. Because brachytherapy is a one-time outpatient procedure, it is more convenient than external beam radiation treatment. The most common adverse effect is the development of urinary irritative or obstructive conditions. The AUA Symptom Index (see Table 57.1) can be used to measure urinary function

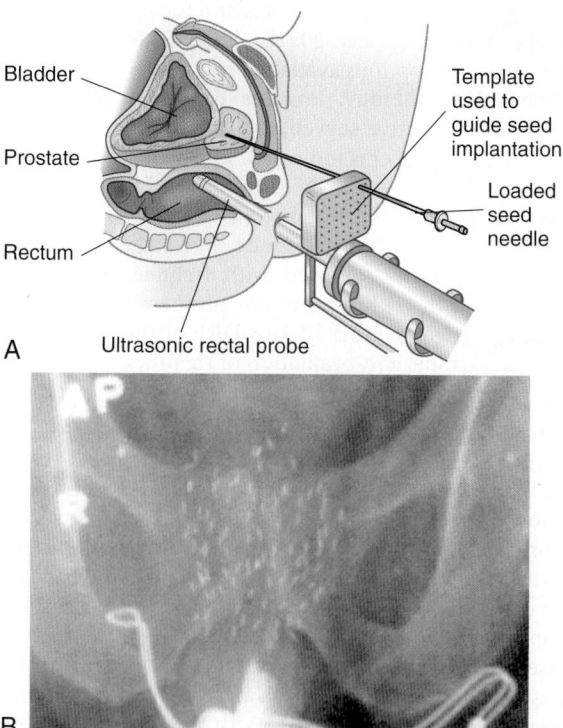

FIG. 57.7 A, Prostate brachytherapy. Implantation of seeds with a needle guided by ultrasonography and a template grid. **B,** Radioactive seeds. Source: *B,* Abeloff, M., Armitage, J. O., Niederhuber, J. D., et al. (Eds.). (2008). *Abeloff's clinical oncology* (4th ed., Figure 88-12A). Churchill Livingstone.

for patients undergoing brachytherapy and can be incorporated into postoperative nursing management. For patients with more advanced tumours, brachytherapy is combined with external beam radiation (Roach & DiBiase, 2020). (Brachytherapy is discussed further in Chapter 18.)

Medication Therapy. The forms of medication therapy available for the treatment of prostate cancer are androgen deprivation (hormone) therapy, chemotherapy, or a combination of both.

Androgen Deprivation Therapy. Prostate cancer growth is largely dependent on the presence of androgens. Androgen deprivation therapy (ADT) reduces the levels of circulating androgens to diminish the tumour's growth. Androgen deprivation can be produced by inhibiting androgen production or blocking androgen receptors (Table 57.7). One of the biggest challenges with ADT is that almost all tumours treated become resistant to this therapy *(hormone refractory)* within a few years. An elevated PSA level is often the first sign that this therapy is no longer effective. Adverse effects of ADT include sexual dysfunction, osteoporosis, cardiovascular disease, diabetes, decreased muscle, increased fat, hot flashes, fatigue, decreased cognitive performance, and changes in body image (Smith, 2021). ADT should not be the standard treatment for localized prostate cancer. There are multiple studies indicating increased mortality and shorter survival rates when ADT is provided as the primary treatment (Wright & Lange, 2021).

TABLE 57.7 MEDICATION THERAPY

Androgen Deprivation Therapy for Prostate Cancer

Therapy	Mechanism of Action	Adverse Effects
Androgen Synthesis Inhibitors		
LH-RH Agonists		
Goserelin (Zoladex)	Reduce secretion of LH and FSH	Hot flashes, gynecomastia, decreased libido, ED
Leuprolide (Lupron, Eligard)	Decrease testosterone production	Depression and mood changes
Buserelin (Suprefact)		
Triptorelin (Trelstar)		
LH-RH Antagonist		
Degarelix (Firmagon)	Block LH receptors Immediately suppress testosterone	Pain, redness, and swelling at injection site Elevated liver enzymes
CYP17 Enzyme Inhibitor		
Abiraterone (Zytiga)	Inhibits CYP17, an enzyme needed for production of testosterone Inhibits testosterone synthesis from the testes, adrenal glands, and prostate cancer cells	Joint swelling, fluid retention, muscle discomfort, hot flashes, diarrhea
Androgen Receptor Blockers		
Bicalutamide (Casodex)	Block the action of testosterone by competing with receptor sites	Loss of libido, ED, and hot flashes Breast pain and gynecomastia may also occur
Flutamide		
Nilutamide (Anandron)		
Enzalutamide (Xtandi)		

CYP17, cytochrome P450 17α–hydroxy/17,20-lyase; *ED,* erectile dysfunction; *FSH,* follicle-stimulating hormone; *LH,* luteinizing hormone; *LH-RH,* luteinizing hormone–releasing hormone.

Androgen Synthesis Inhibitors. Luteinizing hormone–releasing hormone (LH-RH) is released from the hypothalamus to stimulate the anterior pituitary to produce luteinizing hormone (LH) and follicle-stimulating hormone (FSH). LH stimulates the testicular Leydig cells to produce testosterone. LH-RH agonists stimulate the pituitary, ultimately resulting in down-regulation of the LH-RH receptors, leading to a refractory condition in which the anterior pituitary is unresponsive to LH-RH. These medications cause an initial transient increase in LH and testosterone called a "flare," and a worsening of symptoms may occur during this time. However, with continued administration, LH and testosterone levels decrease. LH-RH agonists include leuprolide (Lupron, Eligard), goserelin (Zoladex), buserelin (Suprefact), and triptorelin (Trelstar). These medications essentially produce a chemical castration similar to the effects of an orchiectomy. They are administered by subcutaneous or intramuscular injections on a regular basis, and they must be taken indefinitely.

Degarelix (Firmagon) is an LH-RH antagonist that lowers testosterone levels. Unlike the LH-RH agonists, degarelix does not cause a testosterone flare because it acts directly to block LH and FSH receptors. It is given as a subcutaneous injection.

Abiraterone (Zytiga) works by inhibiting an enzyme, CYP17, which is needed for the production of testosterone. This medication is given orally.

Androgen Receptor Blockers. Another classification of anti-androgens is medications that compete with circulating androgens at the receptor sites. Flutamide, nilutamide (Anandron), enzalutamide (Xtandi), and bicalutamide (Casodex) are androgen receptor blockers. They are often used in combination with an LH-RH agonist (e.g., goserelin, leuprolide), resulting in a combined androgen blockade.

Orchiectomy. Testosterone, produced by the testes, stimulates growth of the prostate cancer. A bilateral orchiectomy is the surgical removal of the testes that may be done alone or in combination with prostatectomy. An orchiectomy is one treatment option for cancer control in patients in an advanced stage of prostate cancer. Another possible benefit of this procedure is the rapid relief of bone pain associated with advanced tumours. Orchiectomy may also induce sufficient shrinkage of the prostate to relieve urinary obstruction in later stages of disease when surgery is not an option.

Adverse effects of orchiectomy include hot flashes, ED, loss of sex drive, osteoporosis, and irritability. Weight gain and loss of muscle mass, which are also common, can alter a patient's physical appearance, possibly affecting self-esteem and leading to grief and depression. Because this procedure is permanent, many patients prefer medication therapy to orchiectomy.

Chemotherapy. The use of chemotherapy has primarily been limited to treatment for patients with hormone-resistant prostate cancer (HRPC) in late-stage disease. In HRPC the cancer progresses despite treatment. This progression occurs in patients who have taken an antiandrogen for a certain period of time. The goal of chemotherapy is mainly palliation. Some of the more commonly used chemotherapeutic agents include docetaxel (Taxotere), mitoxantrone, cyclophosphamide (Procytox), idarubicin, cabazitaxel (Jevtana), and paclitaxel (Abraxane).

Radiotherapy. Radium-223 dichloride (Xofigo) can be used in the treatment of patients with castration-resistant prostate cancer, symptomatic bone metastases, and no known visceral metastatic disease. It is an α particle–emitting radiotherapy medication that mimics calcium and forms complexes with hydroxyapatite at areas of increased bone turnover, such as bone metastases.

CULTURALLY COMPETENT CARE

PROSTATE CANCER

Nurses need to be aware of ethnic and cultural considerations when providing information about the risk for prostate cancer and screening recommendations. They must consider not only the ethnic differences in the incidence of prostate cancer but also differences in health-promotion practices.

Although exposure to electronic and print media is successful in informing some patients about prostate cancer, significant differences of effectiveness exist based on demographic variables such as ethnicity, age, education level, and socioeconomic level. Nurses should consider patients individually and determine the best method to communicate this information in order to achieve the greatest degree of understanding and participation in prostate cancer screening.

NURSING MANAGEMENT
PROSTATE CANCER

NURSING ASSESSMENT

Subjective and objective data that should be obtained from a patient with prostate cancer are presented in Table 57.8.

NURSING DIAGNOSES

Nursing diagnoses for the patient with prostate cancer depend on the stage of the cancer. General nursing diagnoses may include the following:

- *Decisional conflict* resulting from *conflicting information sources, inexperience with decision-making* (numerous alternative treatment options)

- *Acute pain* resulting from *biological injury agent, physical injury agent* (prostatic enlargement, surgery)
- *Inadequate urinary elimination* resulting from *multiple causality* (obstruction of the urethra by the prostate, loss of bladder tone)
- *Sexual dysfunction* resulting from *vulnerability* (effects of treatment)
- *Anxiety* resulting from *threat to current status, threat of death* (effect of treatment on sexual function, uncertain outcome of disease process)

PLANNING

The overall goals are that the patient with prostate cancer will (a) be an active participant in the treatment plan, (b) have satisfactory pain control, (c) follow the therapeutic plan, (d) understand the effect of the therapeutic plan on sexual function, and (e) find a satisfactory way to manage the impact on bladder or bowel function.

NURSING IMPLEMENTATION

HEALTH PROMOTION. One of the nurse's most important roles in relation to prostate cancer is to encourage patients, in consultation with their health care providers, to have annual health checkups, including a DRE, starting at age 50 (or younger if risk factors are present).

TABLE 57.8 NURSING ASSESSMENT

Prostate Cancer

Subjective Data

Important Health Information

Past health history: Family history of prostate cancer; diet high in fat
Medications: Use of testosterone supplements or any other medications affecting urinary tract, such as morphine, anticholinergics, monoamine oxidase inhibitors, and tricyclic antidepressants
Surgeries or other treatments: History of urinary tract infections or prostate conditions

Symptoms

- *Urinary:* Hesitancy or straining to start stream; weak stream; urinary urgency or frequency; dysuria; retention with dribbling; hematuria; nocturia
- *Other:* Low back pain radiating to legs or pelvis; bone pain (possible indicators of metastasis); anorexia, weight loss (possible indicators of metastasis); increasing fatigue and malaise; anxiety related to self-concept or sexuality

Objective Data
General
Older male; pelvic lymphadenopathy (late sign)

Urinary
Distended bladder on palpation; unilaterally hard, enlarged, fixed prostate on rectal examination

Musculoskeletal
Pathological fractures (metastasis)

Possible Findings
↑ Serum PSA; ↑ serum PAP (metastasis); nodular and irregular prostate on ultrasonography, positive biopsy results; anemia

PAP, prostatic acid phosphatase; *PSA,* prostate-specific antigen.

🗘 EVIDENCE-INFORMED PRACTICE

Translating Research Into Practice

G. N. (pronouns he/him) is a 56-year-old who has gone to the occupational health nurse for a regular blood pressure check. G. N.'s father and uncle have a history of prostate cancer and relocated to Canada from Africa 70 years ago. The patient tells the nurse that screening for prostate cancer has been "all over the news." G. N. has been getting a blood test for prostate-specific antigen (PSA) yearly and asks if this needs to continue.

Best Available Evidence	Clinician Expertise	Patient Preferences and Values
PSA screening saves lives when performed appropriately in men at *high risk* of developing prostate cancer.	The nurse knows G. N. is in a high-risk category for prostate cancer. G. N. has African ancestry, is over 50 years old, and has first-degree relatives with prostate cancer. Based on these risk factors, the nurse encourages G. N. to have an annual health examination, including DRE and a *PCA3* urine test.	G. N. wants the best preventive measures to screen for prostate cancer. G. N. was involved in the care of both his father and uncle when they were sick, and he does not want what happened to them to happen to him.

Decision and Action
The nurse encourages G. N. to discuss any concerns about annual PSA testing with the health care provider and to have a thorough discussion about the use of *PCA3* testing to screen for prostate cancer. The nurse also discusses the potential influence of risk factors and diet on developing prostate cancer and teaches G. N. about foods to avoid or limit (e.g., red meat, high-fat dietary products) and those to increase (e.g., vegetables, fruits).

Reference for Evidence

Canadian Cancer Society. (2020). *Finding prostate cancer early.* http://www.cancer.ca/en/cancer-information/cancer-type/prostate/finding-cancer-early/?region=on

ACUTE INTERVENTION. Preoperative and postoperative phases of radical prostatectomy are similar to surgical procedures for BPH (see Nursing Management: Benign Prostatic Hyperplasia). Nursing interventions for a patient who undergoes radiation therapy and chemotherapy are discussed in Chapter 18. An additional consideration is the psychological response of the patient to a diagnosis of cancer. The nurse should provide sensitive, caring support for the patient and family to help them cope with the diagnosis of cancer. Prostate support groups are available for patients and their families to encourage them to be active, informed participants in their own care.

AMBULATORY AND HOME CARE. The nurse should teach appropriate catheter care if the patient is discharged with an in-dwelling catheter. The patient should be instructed to clean the urethral meatus with soap and water once a day; maintain a high fluid intake; keep the collecting bag lower than the bladder at all times; keep the catheter securely anchored to the inner thigh or the abdomen; and report any signs of bladder infection, such as bladder spasms, fever, or hematuria. If urinary incontinence is a concern, patients should be encouraged to practise pelvic floor muscle exercises (Kegel exercises) at every urination and throughout the day. Continuous practice during the 4- to 6-week healing process improves the success rate. Products for incontinence specifically designed for men are available through home care product catalogues and many retail stores.

Palliative and end-of-life care are often appropriate and beneficial to the patient and family (see Chapter 13). Common conditions experienced by patients with advanced prostate cancer include fatigue, bladder outlet obstruction and ureteral obstruction (caused by compression of the urethra or ureters, or both, from tumour mass or lymph node metastasis), severe bone pain and fractures (caused by bone metastasis), spinal cord compression (from spinal metastasis), and leg edema (caused by lymphedema, deep vein thrombosis, or another medical condition). Nursing interventions must focus on all of these conditions. However, management of pain is one of the most important aspects of nursing care for these patients. Pain control involves ongoing pain assessment, administration of prescribed medications (both opioid and nonopioid agents), and nonpharmacological methods of pain relief (e.g., relaxation breathing). (Pain management is discussed further in Chapter 10.)

EVALUATION

The expected outcomes for the patient with prostate cancer are that they will:
- Be an active participant in the treatment plan
- Have satisfactory pain control
- Follow the therapeutic plan
- Understand the effect of the treatment on sexual function
- Find a satisfactory way to manage the impact on bladder or bowel function

PROSTATITIS

Etiology and Pathophysiology

Prostatitis is a broad term that describes a group of acute or chronic inflammatory conditions affecting the prostate gland, usually as a result of infection. It is the most common urological condition in men younger than 50 years, and nearly 50% of men will have some form of prostatitis in their lifetime (Canadian Cancer Society, 2021c). Classifications for prostatitis include four categories: (1) acute bacterial prostatitis, (2) chronic bacterial prostatitis, (3) chronic prostatitis–chronic pelvic pain syndrome, and (4) asymptomatic inflammatory prostatitis (Canadian Cancer Society, 2021c).

Both acute and chronic bacterial prostatitis generally result from organisms reaching the prostate gland by one of the following routes: ascending from the urethra, descending from the bladder, or invading via the bloodstream or the lymphatic channels. Common causative organisms are *Escherichia coli, Klebsiella, Pseudomonas, Enterobacter, Proteus, Chlamydia trachomatis, Neisseria gonorrhoeae,* and group D streptococci. Chronic bacterial prostatitis differs from acute prostatitis in that it involves recurrent episodes of infection.

Chronic prostatitis–chronic pelvic pain syndrome describes a syndrome with prostate and urinary pain in the absence of an obvious infectious process. The etiology of this syndrome is not known. It may occur after a viral illness, or it may be associated with sexually transmitted infections, particularly in younger adults. A culture reveals no causative organisms. However, leukocytes may be found in prostatic secretions.

Asymptomatic inflammatory prostatitis is usually diagnosed in individuals who have no symptoms but are found to have an inflammatory process in the prostate. These patients are usually diagnosed during the evaluation of other genitourinary tract conditions. Leukocytes are present in the seminal fluid from the prostate, but the cause of this process is unclear.

Clinical Manifestations and Complications

Clinical manifestations of acute bacterial prostatitis include fever, chills, malaise, myalgia, and urinary symptoms such as dysuria, urinary frequency, urgency, urge incontinence, and cloudy urine. Swelling of the prostate may lead to acute urinary retention. With DRE, the prostate is extremely swollen, very tender, and firm. The complications of prostatitis are epididymitis, chronic bacterial prostatitis, bacteremia, prostatic abscess, and metastatic infection urine (Meyrier & Fekete, 2021).

Chronic bacterial prostatitis and chronic prostatitis–pelvic pain syndrome manifest with similar symptoms that are generally milder than those in acute bacterial prostatitis. These include irritative voiding symptoms (frequency, urgency, dysuria), backache, perineal or pelvic pain, and ejaculatory pain. Obstructive symptoms are uncommon unless the patient has coexisting BPH. With DRE, the prostate feels enlarged and firm (often described as "boggy") and is slightly tender with palpation. Chronic prostatitis can predispose the patient to recurrent UTIs.

The clinical features of prostatitis can mimic those of a UTI. However, acute cystitis (inflammation of the bladder associated with bacterial infection) is not common in men.

Diagnostic Studies

Because patients with prostatitis have urinary symptoms, a urinalysis and urine culture are indicated; often white blood cells and bacteria are present. Elevated white blood cell count and PSA support the diagnosis of bacterial prostatitis (Meyrier & Fekete, 2021).

Microscopic evaluation and culture of expressed prostate secretion are considered useful in the diagnosis of prostatitis. Expressed prostate secretion is obtained using a premassage and postmassage test (HealthLinkBC, 2020). The patient is asked to void into a specimen cup just before and just after a vigorous prostate massage. Prostatic massage (for expressed prostate secretion) should be avoided if acute bacterial prostatitis is suspected because compression is extremely painful and can increase the risk for bacteria spread. TRUS has not been particularly useful in the diagnosis of prostatitis. However, transabdominal ultrasonography or MRI may be done to rule out an abscess on the prostate.

NURSING AND INTERPROFESSIONAL MANAGEMENT PROSTATITIS

Antibiotics commonly used for acute and chronic bacterial prostatitis include trimethoprim–sulphamethoxazole (Septra) and ciprofloxacin (Cipro). Doxycycline or tetracycline may be prescribed for patients who have multiple sex partners. Antibiotics are usually given orally for up to 4 weeks for acute bacterial prostatitis. However, if the patient has high fever or other signs of impending sepsis, hospitalization and intravenous antibiotics are prescribed. Patients with chronic bacterial prostatitis are given oral antibiotic therapy for 4 to 12 weeks. A short course of oral antibiotics is usually prescribed for those with chronic prostatitis–chronic pelvic pain syndrome. However, antibiotic therapy often is ineffective for patients whose prostatitis is not caused by bacteria.

Although patients with acute and chronic bacterial prostatitis tend to experience a great amount of discomfort, the pain resolves as the infection is treated. Pain management for patients with chronic prostatitis–chronic pelvic pain syndrome is more difficult because the pain persists for weeks to months. Anti-inflammatory agents are the most common medications used for pain control in prostatitis, but these provide only moderate pain relief. Opioid pain medications can be used, but if the pain is chronic in nature, multimodal therapies should be considered. Relaxation of muscle tissue in the prostate using α-adrenergic blockers has been shown to be effective in reducing discomfort for some patients (Azoulay et al., 2015).

Acute urinary retention can develop in acute prostatitis, necessitating bladder drainage with suprapubic catheterization. Passage of a catheter through the inflamed urethra in acute prostatitis is contraindicated. Repetitive prostatic massage may be recommended as adjunct therapy for prostatitis for men. This measure relieves congestion within the prostate by squeezing out excess prostatic secretions, thus providing pain relief. Prostatic massage is performed by using the index finger of a gloved hand and pressing down on the prostate, covering the entire gland's surface in longitudinal strokes. Measures to stimulate ejaculation (masturbation and intercourse) help drain the prostate and provide some relief.

Because the prostate can serve as a source of bacteria, patients experiencing prostatitis should maintain a high fluid intake. The nurse should encourage the patient to drink plenty of fluids. This is especially important for those with acute bacterial prostatitis because of the increased fluid needs associated with fever and infection. Management of fever is also an important nursing intervention.

CONDITIONS OF THE PENIS

Health problems of the penis are rare if sexually transmitted infections are excluded (see Chapter 55). Conditions of the penis may be classified as congenital, conditions of the prepuce, problems with the erectile mechanism, and cancer.

CONGENITAL CONDITIONS

Hypospadias is a urological abnormality in which the urethral meatus is located on the ventral surface of the penis anywhere from the corona to the perineum. Hormonal influences in utero, environmental factors, and genetic factors are possible causes. Surgical repair of hypospadias may be necessary if it is associated with *chordee* (a painful downward curvature of the penis during erection) or if it prevents intercourse or normal urination. Surgery may be done for cosmetic reasons or emotional well-being.

Epispadias, an opening of the urethra on the dorsal surface of the penis, is a complex birth defect that is usually associated with other genitourinary tract defects. Corrective surgery to place the urethra in a normal position in the penis is usually done in early childhood.

CONDITIONS OF THE PREPUCE

Conditions of the prepuce are rare in Canada because, up until the 1990s, circumcision was a routine procedure for most male infants. Circumcision, the surgical removal of the foreskin of the penis, is a procedure done to male infants for religious or cultural reasons.

Phimosis is a constriction of the uncircumcised foreskin around the head of the penis, making retraction over the glans penis difficult. It is caused by edema or inflammation of the foreskin, usually associated with poor hygiene techniques that allow bacterial and yeast organisms to become trapped under the foreskin (Figure 57.8, *A*). The goal of treatment is to return the foreskin to its natural position over the glans penis through manual reduction. One strategy involves pushing the glans back through the prepuce by applying constant thumb pressure while the index fingers pull the prepuce over the glans. Ice, hand compression, or both on the foreskin, glans, and penis may be used before this technique to reduce edema. Topical corticosteroid cream applied two or three times daily to the exterior and interior of the tip of the foreskin may also be effective.

Paraphimosis is narrowing or edema of the retracted uncircumcised foreskin, preventing normal return over the glans and causing strangulation. This can occur when the foreskin is pulled back for cleansing, for the use of a urinary catheter, or during intercourse and is not returned to the forward position. Antibiotics, warm soaks, and sometimes circumcision or dorsal slitting of the prepuce may be required. Careful cleaning followed by replacement of the foreskin generally prevents these problems (see Figure 57.8, *B*).

CONDITIONS OF ERECTILE MECHANISM

Priapism is a persistent erection of the penis that is not linked to sexual desire or stimulation (Deveci, 2021). Causes of priapism

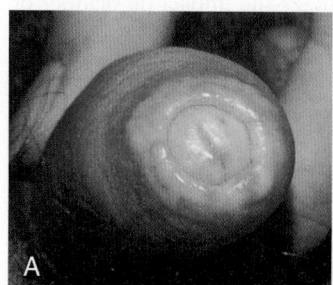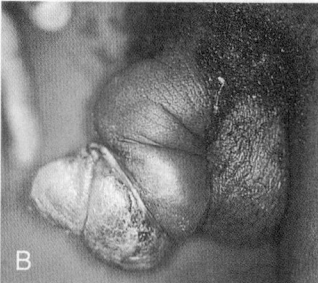

FIG. 57.8 A, Phimosis: inability to retract the foreskin due to secondary lesions on the prepuce. **B,** Paraphimosis: ulcer with edema from foreskin remaining contracted over the prepuce.

include thrombosis of the corpus cavernosal veins, leukemia, sickle cell anemia, diabetes mellitus, degenerative lesions of the spine, neoplasms of the brain or spinal cord, prolonged foreplay, injection of vasoactive medications into the corpus cavernosa, and use of certain medications and cocaine. Treatment may include sedatives, injection of smooth muscle relaxants directly into the penis, aspiration and irrigation of the corpora cavernosa with a large-bore needle, and the surgical creation of a shunt to drain the corpora. Complications may include penile tissue necrosis caused by lack of blood flow or hydronephrosis from bladder distension. With immediate medical treatment, the risk for permanent ED is low.

Peyronie's disease, sometimes referred to as *curved* or *crooked penis,* is caused by plaque formation in one of the corpora cavernosa of the penis. The palpable, nontender, hard plaque formation is usually found on the posterior surface. It may result from trauma to the penile shaft or may occur spontaneously. The plaque prevents adequate blood flow into the spongy tissue, which results in a curvature during erection. The condition is not dangerous but can result in painful erections, ED, or embarrassment. Patients may improve over time, stabilize, or need surgery.

CANCER OF THE PENIS

Cancer of the penis is rare. Major risk factors include human papilloma virus, phimosis, not being circumcised, poor genital hygiene, weakened immune system, and treatment of ultraviolet light therapy in psoriasis (Canadian Cancer Society, 2021a). The tumour may appear as a superficial ulceration or a pimple-like nodule. The nontender warty lesion may be mistaken for a venereal wart. Most malignancies (95%) are well-differentiated squamous cell carcinomas. Treatment in the early stages is laser removal of the growth. A radical resection of the penis may be done if the cancer has spread. Surgery, radiation, or chemotherapy may be tried, depending on the extent of the disease, lymph node involvement, or metastasis.

CONDITIONS OF THE SCROTUM AND TESTES

INFLAMMATORY AND INFECTIOUS CONDITIONS

Skin Conditions

The skin of the scrotum is susceptible to a number of common skin diseases. The most common conditions of the scrotal skin are fungal infections, dermatitis (neurodermatitis, contact dermatitis, seborrheic dermatitis), and parasitic infections (scabies, lice). These conditions involve discomfort for the patient but are associated with few, if any, severe complications (see Chapter 26).

Epididymitis

Epididymitis is an inflammation of the epididymis (Figure 57.9), usually secondary to an infectious process (sexually or nonsexually transmitted) and rarely as a result of trauma or urinary reflux down the vas deferens from the urethra. Swelling may progress to the point that the epididymis and the testis are indistinguishable. In men younger than 40 years of age, the most common cause is gonorrhea or chlamydial infection. UTI and prostatitis are common causes in older men. The use of antibiotics is important for both partners if the transmission is through sexual contact. Patients should be encouraged to refrain from

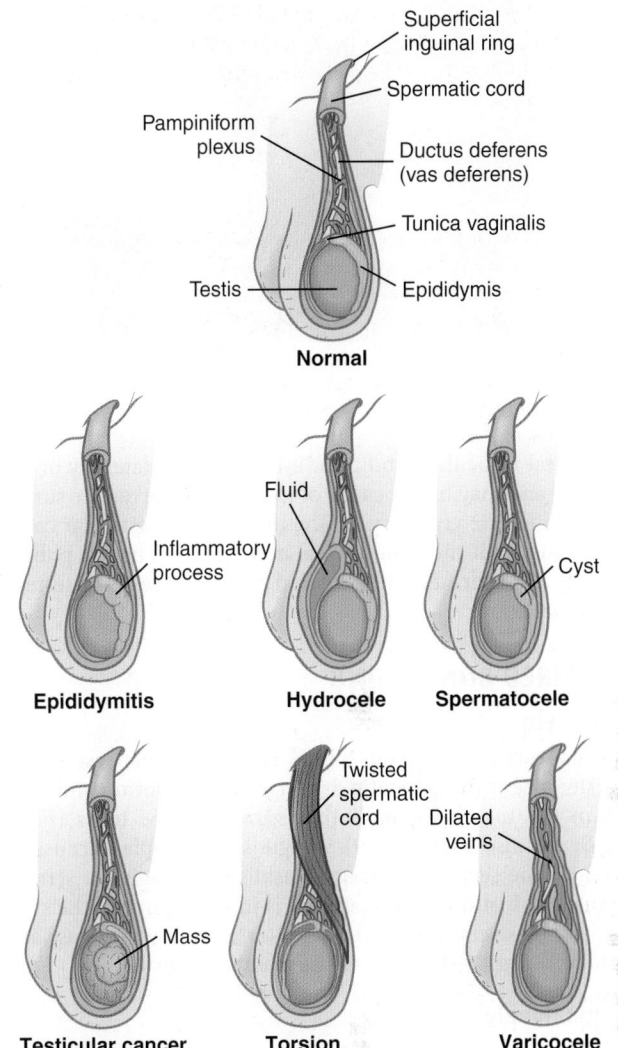

FIG. 57.9 Scrotal masses.

sexual intercourse during the acute phase. If they do engage in intercourse, a condom should be used. Conservative treatment consists of bed rest with elevation of the scrotum, use of ice packs, and analgesics. Ambulation places the scrotum in a dependent position and increases pain. Most tenderness subsides within 1 week, although swelling may last for weeks or months.

Orchitis

Orchitis refers to an acute inflammation of the testis. In orchitis, the testis is painful, tender, and swollen. It generally occurs after an episode of bacterial or viral infections such as mumps, pneumonia, tuberculosis, or syphilis. It can also be caused by epididymitis, prostatectomy, trauma, infectious mononucleosis, influenza, catheterization, or complicated UTI. Mumps orchitis is a condition contributing to infertility, and its incidence could easily be decreased by childhood vaccination against mumps. Treatment involves the use of antibiotics (if the organism is known), pain medications, or bed rest with the scrotum elevated on an ice pack.

CONGENITAL CONDITIONS

Cryptorchidism (undescended testes) is failure of the testes to descend into the scrotal sac before birth. It is the most common

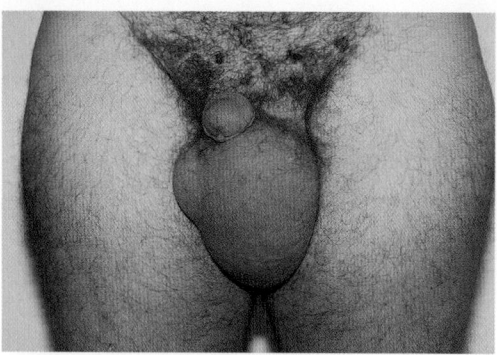

FIG. 57.10 Hydrocele. Source: Swartz, M. H. (2010). *Textbook of physical diagnosis: History and examination* (6th ed., p. 537, Figure 18-28). Saunders.

congenital testicular condition. It may occur bilaterally or unilaterally and may be the cause of infertility if corrective surgery is not done by 2 years of age. The incidence of testicular cancer is also higher if the condition is not corrected before puberty. Surgery is performed to locate and suture the testis or testes to the scrotum.

ACQUIRED CONDITIONS

Hydrocele

A hydrocele is a nontender, fluid-filled mass that results from interference with lymphatic drainage of the scrotum and swelling of the tunica vaginalis that surrounds the testis (Figure 57.10; see also Figure 57.9). Diagnosis is simple because the mass can be seen by shining a flashlight through the scrotum (transillumination). No treatment is indicated unless the swelling becomes very large and uncomfortable, in which case aspiration or surgical drainage of the mass is performed.

Spermatocele

A spermatocele is a firm, sperm-containing, painless cyst of the epididymis that may be visible with transillumination (see Figure 57.9). The cause is unknown, and surgical removal is the treatment. It is important for patients to see their doctor if they feel any scrotal lumps.

Varicocele

A varicocele is a dilation of the veins that drain the testes (see Figure 57.9). The scrotum feels wormlike when palpated. The cause of the condition is unknown. The varicocele is usually located on the left side of the scrotum because of retrograde blood flow from the left renal vein. Most varicoceles do not require intervention; however, surgery is indicated for patients who desire fertility. Repair of the varicocele may be through injection of a sclerosing agent or by surgical ligation of the spermatic vein.

Testicular Torsion

Testicular torsion is a surgical emergency involving the twisting of the spermatic cord that supplies blood to the testes and epididymis, causing an interruption to the blood supply (see Figure 57.9). It is most common in males younger than 20 years of age. Clinical manifestations include severe scrotal pain, swelling, nausea, and vomiting. Urinary symptoms, fever, and white blood cells or bacteria in the urine are absent. The pain does not subside with rest or elevation of the scrotum. Nuclear technetium scan of the testes or Doppler ultrasonography is typically

performed to assess blood flow within the testicle. The cremasteric reflex is absent on the side of the swelling, and a decrease in or absence of blood flow confirms the diagnosis. Unless the torsion resolves spontaneously, surgery to untwist the cord and restore the blood supply must be performed immediately. If blood supply to the affected testicle is not restored within 4 to 6 hours, ischemia to the testis will occur, leading to necrosis and the possible need for removal.

TESTICULAR CANCER

Etiology and Pathophysiology

Testicular cancer is relatively rare, accounting for less than 1% of all cancers found in males. It has a 5-year survival rate of 96% (Canadian Cancer Society, 2021e). Testicular cancer is the most common type of cancer in young men between 15 and 29 years of age (Canadian Cancer Society, 2021d). Testicular tumours are also more common in males who have had undescended testes (cryptorchidism), a family history of testicular cancer or anomalies, or Klinefelter's syndrome (Canadian Cancer Society, 2021d). Other predisposing factors include orchitis, human immunodeficiency virus (HIV) infection, maternal exposure to diethylstilbestrol (DES), and testicular cancer in the contralateral testis.

Most testicular cancers develop from embryonic germ cells. The two types of germ cell cancers are seminomas and nonseminomas. Although seminoma germ cell cancers are the most common, they are the least aggressive. Nonseminoma testicular germ cell tumours are rare but aggressive. Non–germ cell tumours arise from other testicular tissue and include Leydig cell and Sertoli cell tumours. These account for less than 10% of testicular cancers.

Clinical Manifestations and Complications

Testicular cancer may have a slow or rapid onset depending on the type of tumour. The patient may notice a painless lump in the scrotum as well as scrotal swelling and a feeling of heaviness. The scrotal mass usually is nontender and very firm. Some patients experience a dull ache or heavy sensation in the lower abdomen, the perianal area, or the scrotum. Acute pain is the presenting symptom in about 10% of patients. Manifestations associated with advanced disease are varied and include lower back or chest pain, cough, and dyspnea.

Diagnostic Studies

Palpation of the scrotal contents is the first step in diagnosing testicular cancer. A cancerous mass is firm and does not transilluminate. Ultrasonography of the testes is indicated whenever testicular cancer is suspected (e.g., palpable mass) or when persistent or painful testicular swelling is present. If a testicular neoplasm is suspected, blood is obtained to determine the serum levels of α-fetoprotein, lactate dehydrogenase, and human chorionic gonadotropin. (α-Fetoprotein is discussed in Chapter 18.) A chest radiograph and CT scan of the abdomen and pelvis are done to detect metastasis. Anemia may be present, and liver function may be elevated in metastatic disease.

NURSING AND INTERPROFESSIONAL MANAGEMENT TESTICULAR CANCER

TESTICULAR SELF-EXAMINATION

The scrotum is easily examined and beginning tumours are usually palpable. Every male from the age of 15 years of age should

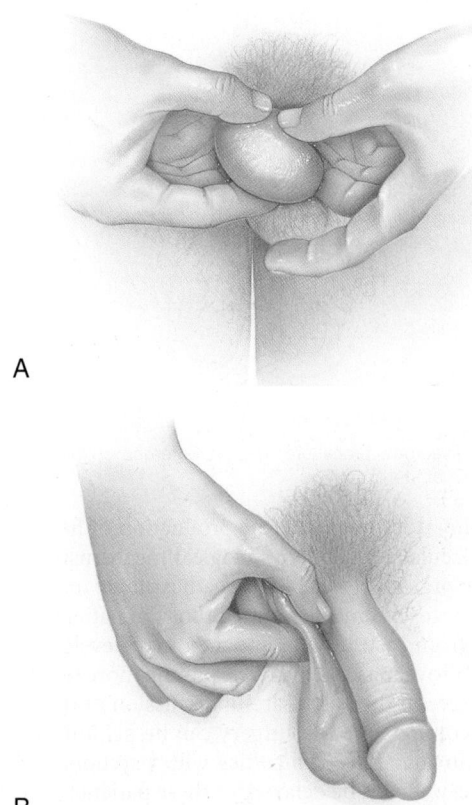

A

B

FIG. 57.11 Testicular self-examination. **A,** The testicle is checked for smoothness by rolling it between the thumb and the fingers. **B,** The spermatic cord or vas deferens can be felt toward the back of the testicle and should feel soft and tender. Source: *The wellness way: Testicular examination.* Copyright 1987, 1994, 2000, 2001, 2002. The StayWell Company.

be taught and encouraged to perform a monthly testicular self-examination (TSE) so that he knows what is normal for his testicles and can notice changes. Male patients, especially those with a history of undescended testis or a previous testicular tumour, should be taught how to perform TSE.

Guidelines for TSE of the scrotum are presented in Table 57.9 and Figure 57.11. The procedure is not difficult. Some patients may indicate reluctance to examine their own genitals, but with encouragement, they can learn this simple procedure. They should be encouraged to perform TSEs frequently until they are comfortable with the procedure and then examine the scrotum once a month.

Videotapes and illustrations on shower hangers are available as teaching aids and ideally should be introduced during high school or college health classes. Free information is available through the Canadian Cancer Society.

INTERPROFESSIONAL CARE

Interprofessional care of testicular cancer generally involves an orchiectomy or a radical orchiectomy (surgical removal of the affected testis, the spermatic cord, and regional lymph nodes). Postorchiectomy treatment involves surveillance, radiation therapy, or chemotherapy, depending on the stage of the cancer. Chemotherapy protocols use combination therapy: bleomycin, etoposide (Vepesid), and cisplatin; or etoposide (Vepesid), ifosfamide (Ifex), and cisplatin. (Testicular germ cell tumours are more sensitive to systemic chemotherapy than any other adult solid tumour.)

If testicular cancer is detected early, the cure rate is approximately 100% (Jarvis, 2019b). As a result of treatment successes, most patients with testicular cancer become long-term survivors. Treatment-related toxicity, however, is a significant issue. All patients with testicular cancer, regardless of pathological condition or stage, require follow-up, regular physical examinations, chest radiographic examinations, CT scans, and assessment of human chorionic gonadotropin and α-fetoprotein. The goal is to detect relapse when the tumour burden is minimal. Secondary malignancies that occur as a result of chemotherapy and radiation are described in Chapter 18 and in the NCPs 18.1 and 18.2, available on the Evolve website.

Patients with testicular cancer should have the opportunity to discuss fertility and sperm banking before any treatment. The nurse should be sensitive to any psychosocial challenges this type of cancer can have on a patient's feelings of self-worth or sexual performance. Treatment has the potential to interfere with erections and fertility.

SEXUAL FUNCTIONING

VASECTOMY

Vasectomy is the bilateral surgical ligation or resection of the vas deferens performed for the purpose of sterilization (Figure 57.12). The procedure requires 15 to 30 minutes and is performed on an outpatient basis with the patient under local anaesthesia. Vasectomy is considered a permanent form of sterilization, although some successful reversals (*vasovasotomy*) have been reported.

After vasectomy, the patient should not notice any difference in the look or feel of the ejaculate because its major component is seminal and prostatic fluid. The patient will need to use an alternative form of contraception until semen examination reveals no sperm. This usually requires at least 10 ejaculations or 6 weeks, until sperm distal to the surgical site are evacuated. Sperm cells continue to be produced by the testes but are absorbed by the body rather than being passed through the vas deferens. Occasionally, postoperative hematoma and swelling of the scrotum occur.

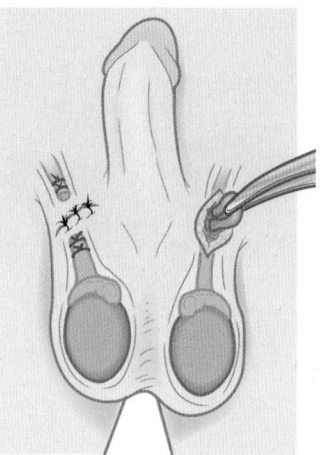

FIG. 57.12 Vasectomy procedure. The vas deferens is ligated or resected for the purpose of sterilization.

Vasectomy does not affect the production of hormones, the ability to ejaculate, or the physiological mechanisms related to erection or orgasm. Psychological adjustment may be a concern after surgery. It may be difficult for the patient to separate vasectomy from castration. Some men may develop ED or feel the need to prove masculinity by becoming more sexually active than they were in the past. Careful discussion of the procedure and its outcome before the surgery can be helpful in detecting patients who may have difficulties with psychological adjustment. Surgery should be delayed for these patients. (The Ethical Dilemmas box discusses sterilization.)

ETHICAL DILEMMAS

Sterilization

Situation

A 43-year-old patient is requesting a vasectomy and informs the nurse that this has not been discussed with his partner. The health care provider's policy is to have the partner sign a form acknowledging the patient's desire to be sterilized. This patient explains that, although his partner wants to have more children, the one they already have is all he wants.

Important Points for Consideration

- Patient autonomy suggests matters of reproduction are left to the privacy and discretion of the individual. Competent adults may legally choose to be sterilized for medical reasons or for convenience.
- To prevent possible future harm, this patient should include his partner in the decision to permanently eliminate the ability to procreate.
- In most provinces and territories, women can terminate a pregnancy without proof that their partners are aware of their intentions. Sterilization, conversely, can be considered a more permanent decision that has consequences for individuals in the relationship.
- This health care provider's standard is to have evidence of the partner's knowledge of the intent for sterilization. The nurse should inform the man of the standard in this physician's practice and encourage a discussion between the partners.
- If the patient remains unwilling to discuss the matter with his partner, either the nurse or the health care provider should reinforce the health care provider's practice of obtaining evidence from both partners about their intent for sterilization and direct the patient to another health care provider.

Clinical Decision-Making Questions

1. How should the nurse approach this situation?
2. Should the nurse tell the patient's partner of their intention for sterilization?
3. Are there ever circumstances in which deception of a patient or family would be justified?

TABLE 57.10	RISK FACTORS FOR ERECTILE DYSFUNCTION

Vascular • Atherosclerosis • Hypertension • Peripheral vascular disease	**Genitourinary** • Radical prostatectomy • Prostatitis • Renal failure
Drug-Induced • Alcohol • Antiandrogens • Antilipidemic agents • Antihypertensives • Diuretics (chlorothiazide, spironolactone [Aldactone]) • Major tranquilizers (diazepam [Valium], alprazolam [Xanax]) • Marijuana, cocaine • Nicotine • Tricyclic antidepressants (e.g., amitriptyline [Elavil])	**Neurological** • Parkinson's disease • Cerebrovascular disease • Trauma to the spinal cord • Tumours or transection of spinal cord **Psychological** • Anxiety • Depression • Fear of failure to perform • Stress **Other** • Aging • Gout
Endocrine • Diabetes mellitus • Obesity • Testosterone deficiency	

ERECTILE DYSFUNCTION

Erectile dysfunction (ED) is the inability to attain or maintain an erect penis that allows satisfactory sexual performance. Although sexual function is a topic many individuals are uncomfortable discussing, health care providers must be able and willing to address ED. Treatment may include phosphodiesterase type 5 (PDE5) inhibitors, a class of medications used to treat ED, including tadalafil (Cialis), vardenafil (Levitra), and sildenafil (Viagra).

The effects of ED can lead to anxiety and depression as well as potentially interfere with a person's self-esteem, confidence, relationships, and overall sense of well-being. ED is a condition that is significant because of its prevalence; it is estimated that its prevalence among men in Canada aged 40 to 88 is 49.4%, with estimates that approximately 3 million Canadians over the age of 40 years are affected by ED (Bella et al., 2015). The condition is increasing in all segments of the sexually active male population and affects both the man and his partner. In younger men, the increase is attributed to substance use, such as recreational drugs and alcohol. Middle-aged men are affected by medical conditions such as diabetes, hypertension, renal disease, organ transplants, coronary artery bypass graft surgeries, and cancer or the therapy for these conditions. Men are living longer and expect to remain sexually active, regardless of any existing medical conditions.

Etiology and Pathophysiology

ED can result from several factors in two general categories: physiological (organic) and psychological (Table 57.10). Causes of ED are related to vascular, endocrine, and neurological disease as well as situational, end organ (e.g., penile deformity, trauma), and mixed causes (underlying physiological causes can lead to anxiety, stress, and depression as a result of ED). Risk factors of ED are like cardiovascular disease risk factors and should be identified during evaluation (Bella et al., 2015). Patients with ED without obvious cause should be screened for cardiovascular disease. Treating cardiovascular risk factors with lifestyle modifications sometimes prevents ED or reduces need for treatment (Rosen & Khera, 2021).

EVIDENCE-INFORMED PRACTICE
Research Highlight

Do Lifestyle Interventions Aid in the Management of Sexual Dysfunction?
Clinical Question
For patients with sexual dysfunction (P), what is the effect of lifestyle interventions (I) on severity of erectile dysfunction (O)?

Best Available Evidence
- Joanna Briggs Institute Evidence Summary including expert opinion, cross-sectional analysis, randomized controlled trial, and meta-analysis

Critical Appraisal and Synthesis of Evidence
- A meta-analysis (n = 89 studies) examined the magnitude of association of six lifestyle interventions (e.g., tobacco use, alcohol use, caffeine intake, cannabis use, physical activity, and diet) and sexual dysfunction (lack of desire, ED, reduced pleasure).
- Tobacco and cannabis use were found to be a risk factor for sexual dysfunction.
- A diet high in fruit and vegetables and physical activity was associated with a decreased risk of ED.
- Moderate alcohol intake (1–3 drinks/day) was associated with a lower risk of ED as compared to a higher alcohol intake (>3 drinks/day).
- There was no association found between caffeine use and risk for ED.
- Lifestyle interventions such as physical activity, smoking cessation, and diet modification should be considered as the first option to prevent or treat ED.

Implications for Nursing Practice
- Emphasize the importance of a healthy diet high in fruits and vegetables for the prevention and treatment of ED.
- Encourage physical activity by collaborating with the patient to create an individualized activity plan.

Reference for Evidence
Pamaiahgari, P. (2018). *Evidence summary. Sexual dysfunction (men): Lifestyle interventions* [evidence summary]. The Joanna Briggs Institute EBP Database JBI12004.

P, patient population of interest; *I,* intervention or area of interest; *O,* outcomes of interest (see Chapter 1).

Normal physiological age-related changes are associated with changes in erectile function and may be an underlying cause of ED. Table 53.4 in Chapter 53 lists age-related changes in sexual function. The nurse should be able to explain these age-related changes to reassure an anxious older patient regarding changes in sexual abilities. (The male sexual response is discussed in Chapter 53.)

Clinical Manifestations and Complications
The typical symptom of ED is a patient's self-report of difficulties associated with sexual performance. The patient usually describes an inability to attain or maintain an erection. The symptoms may occur occasionally, may be continual with a gradual onset, or may occur with a sudden onset. A gradual onset of symptoms is usually associated with physiological factors, whereas a sudden or rapid onset of symptoms may be associated with psychological issues.

A man's inability to perform sexually may cause distress in interpersonal relationships and interfere with self-concept. Difficulties with ED can lead to several personal issues, including anger, anxiety, and depression.

Diagnostic Studies
The first step in diagnosis and management of ED begins with a thorough sexual, health, and psychosocial history.

TABLE 57.11 INTERPROFESSIONAL CARE
Erectile Dysfunction

Diagnostic
- History and physical examination
- Nocturnal penile tumescence and rigidity testing
- Serum glucose and lipid profile
- Sexual history
- Testosterone, prolactin, and thyroid hormone levels
- Vascular studies

Interprofessional Therapy
- Medication therapy (sildenafil [Viagra], vardenafil [Levitra], tadalafil [Cialis])
- Intracavernosal self-injection
- Intraurethral medication pellet
- Modify reversible causes
- Penile implants
- Sexual counselling
- Topical gels
- Vacuum constriction device (VCD)

Self-administered assessment and treatment-related questionnaires have been developed and may prove useful as primary screening tools, for example, the Erection Quality Scale (Rosen et al., 2007). Second, a physical examination should be performed that focuses on secondary sexual characteristics, including pubic hair distribution, size and appearance of the penis and scrotum, and rectal examination. A DRE should be done to assess prostate size, consistency, and presence of nodules. Assessment of blood pressure, palpation of peripheral pulses, and sensation of the genitalia should also be included.

Further examination or diagnostic testing is typically based on findings from the history and physical examination. Serum glucose and lipid profile bloodwork is recommended to rule out diabetes mellitus. Hormonal levels for testosterone, prolactin, LH, and thyroid may help identify endocrine-related conditions, and a complete blood count may be helpful in identifying unrecognized systemic diseases.

Other diagnostic tests may be conducted to diagnose ED. Nocturnal penile tumescence and rigidity testing is a noninvasive method that involves the continuous measurement of penile circumference and axial rigidity during sleep. Such measurements are used to differentiate between physiological and psychological causes of ED as well as to evaluate the effectiveness of medication therapy. Vascular studies, including penile arteriography, penile blood flow study, and duplex Doppler ultrasonography studies, are used to assess penile blood inflow and outflow. Such studies help assess vascular conditions interfering with erection.

Interprofessional Care
The goal of ED therapy is for the patient and their partner to achieve a satisfactory sexual relationship. The treatment for ED is based on the underlying cause. A variety of treatment options are available (Bella et al., 2015) (Table 57.11). The results of these interventions are usually most satisfactory when both partners are involved in the decision-making process and have realistic expectations of the treatment.

It is important to determine whether ED is reversible before treatment is started. For example, if ED appears to be an adverse effect of prescribed medications, alternative agents or treatments should be explored. When there is an established diagnosis of testicular failure (hypogonadism), androgen replacement therapy may sometimes be effective in improving erectile function. For individuals who have ED that is psychological in nature, counselling should be provided by a qualified therapist for the patient (and possibly their partner).

Erectogenic Medications. Sildenafil (Viagra), tadalafil (Cialis), and vardenafil (Levitra) are erectogenic medications (Khera, 2021). These medications are PDE5 inhibitors that cause smooth muscle relaxation and increased blood flow into the corpus cavernosum, thus promoting penile erection. They are taken orally about 30 to 60 minutes before sexual activity, but not more than once a day. These medications have been found to be generally safe and effective for the treatment of most types of ED.

Adverse effects include headaches, dyspepsia, flushing, and nasal congestion. Additional rare adverse effects are blurred or blue-green visual disturbances, sudden hearing loss, and priapism. The patient should be instructed to seek immediate medical attention if any of these rare reactions occur. Because these medications may potentiate the hypotensive effect of nitrates (e.g., nitroglycerin), they are contraindicated for individuals taking nitrates.

> **MEDICATION ALERT—Sildenafil (Viagra)**
> • Should not be used with nitrates (nitroglycerin) in any form
> • Can potentiate hypotensive effects of nitrates

Vacuum Constriction Devices. Vacuum constriction devices (VCDs) are suction devices that can be applied to the flaccid penis to produce an erection by pulling blood up into the corporeal bodies. A penile ring or constrictive band is placed around the base of the penis to retain venous blood, thereby preventing the erection from subsiding. Special care must be taken in using these devices to prevent tissue bruising.

Vasoactive Medications. Vasoactive medications can be administered as a topical gel, by injection into the penis (intracavernosal self-injection), or by insertion of a medicated pellet (alprostadil) into the urethra using an intraurethral device. These vasoactive medications enhance blood flow into the penile arteries. Current vasoactive medications include papaverine, alprostadil (Caverject), and phentolamine.

Penile Implants. Surgical implantation of semirigid or inflatable penile prostheses is shown in Figure 57.13. These surgical procedures are highly invasive and associated with potential complications. Thus, they are usually indicated only for patients with severe ED for which other interventions are ineffective.

The devices are implanted into the corporeal bodies to provide an erection firm enough for penetration. The semirigid malleable implant is displayed in Figure 57.13, *A*. The inflatable implant consists of cylinders in the penis, a small pump in the scrotum, and a reservoir in the lower abdomen (Figure 57.13, *B*). The main issues associated with penile prostheses are mechanical failure, infection, and erosions.

Sexual Counselling. Sexual counselling is often recommended before and after treatment. It should address psychological or interpersonal factors that may enhance sexual expression as well as other factors of concern. Counselling can be effective for the individual patient, but it is typically preferred to include their partner, particularly if the patient is involved in a long-term relationship. The ability for both partners to be pleased enhances a patient's satisfaction levels. Counselling should begin after the start of medical treatment for ED.

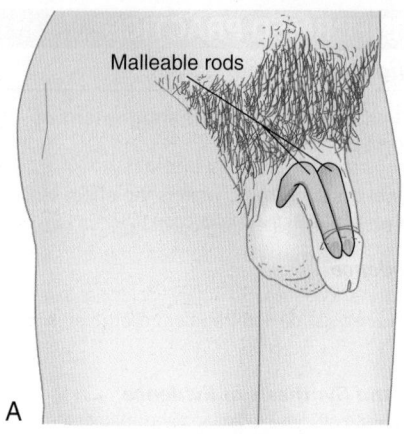

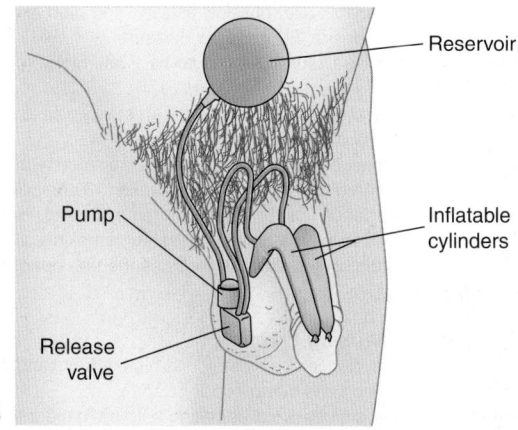

FIG. 57.13 Penile implants. **A,** A malleable implant is always erect but can be bent close to the body for concealment. **B,** An inflatable implant consists of cylinders in the penis, a small pump in the scrotum, and a reservoir in the lower abdomen. When activated, the pump fills the cylinders with fluid from the reservoir. A small release valve permits the fluid to drain back into the reservoir after intercourse.

NURSING MANAGEMENT
ERECTILE DYSFUNCTION

Patients experiencing ED require a great deal of emotional support for both themselves and their partners. Men often do not feel comfortable discussing these types of difficulties with others because of society's expectations of a man's sexual abilities. They need reassurance that confidentiality will be maintained. Men may experience and demonstrate isolation from support systems and lose self-esteem. In conjunction with medical treatment, counselling and therapy may be necessary for couples to establish realistic expectations and develop meaningful communication patterns.

Most men delay seeking medical assistance. Once they do, they are often highly motivated and expect immediate solutions. The health care team should provide a support system and accurate information as soon as possible. Nurses are in a unique position of conducting routine health assessments on men seeking any form of medical treatment. These assessments provide an opportunity to ask questions pertaining to general health as well as sexual health and function. Sexual health programs that promote traditional Indigenous knowledge and intergenerational relationships may be effective for promoting sexual health among Indigenous boys and men (Hackett et al., 2020). Given the opportunity and recognition that someone cares and can provide them with answers, men are less hesitant to answer these questions.

ANDROPAUSE

Andropause is a gradual decline in androgen secretion occurring in most men as they age and can begin as early as age 40. The primary male androgen that is reduced is testosterone. Factors determining the rate of decline are not clearly known. Clinical manifestations are associated with a decline in testosterone, including loss of libido, fatigue, decreased muscle mass and strength, depression, decreased bone mineral density, and anemia. Symptoms are often attributed to normal aging and may not be reported by the patient (Figure 57.14) (Snyder, 2020).

INFERTILITY

Infertility in a couple is defined as the inability to conceive after 1 year of frequent, unprotected intercourse. Infertility is a disorder of a couple, not of one individual. For this reason, both partners must be involved in determining the cause of infertility. In about 33% of the cases, the cause involves the man. Male infertility can be caused by disorders of the hypothalamic–pituitary system, disorders of the testes, and abnormalities of the ejaculatory system.

The physical causes are generally divided into three categories: pretesticular, testicular, and post-testicular. The *pretesticular* or endocrine causes occur 2 to 5% of the time and the *testicular* causes occur in 65 to 80% of the cases (Anawalt & Page, 2020). Other factors that influence the testes include infection (e.g., mumps virus, sexually transmitted infections, bacterial infections), congenital anomalies, medications, radiation, substance use (alcohol, nicotine, drugs), and environmental hazards. *Post-testicular* causes account for approximately 5 to 7% of the cases, with obstruction, infection, or the result of a surgical procedure being the primary causes. The remaining 40% are classified as *idiopathic,* or of unknown cause.

A careful health history and examination may reveal the cause of a patient's infertility. Thus, the history is a starting point for determining cause and treatment. The history should include age; occupation; past injury, surgery, or infections to the genital tract; lifestyle issues such as use of hot tubs, weight training, or wearing of tight undergarments; sexual practices; frequency of intercourse; and emotional factors such as stress

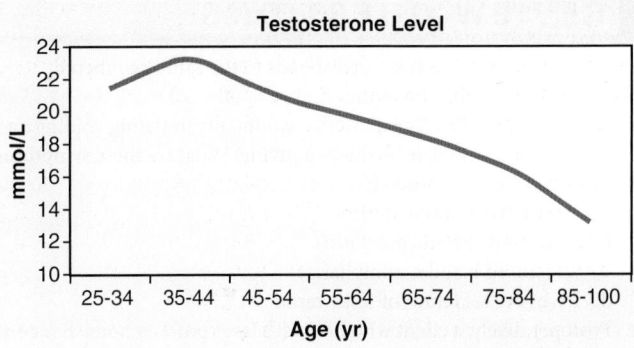

FIG. 57.14 Changes in testosterone plasma level in men as they age.

levels and the desire for children. The use of medications and drugs, such as chemotherapeutic agents, anabolic steroids (testosterone), sulphasalazine, cimetidine, and recreational drugs, should be documented because these can reduce sperm count. A physical examination can disclose a varicocele, Peyronie's disease, or other physical abnormalities.

The first test in an infertility study is a semen analysis. The test determines the sperm concentration (count >20 million/mL), forward progressive motility (at least 60% with a grade >2), and morphology (at least 60% have a normal oval head and long tail). Additional tests that may be helpful in determining the etiology include plasma testosterone and serum LH and FSH measurements. A test for sperm penetration abilities may also be done. The specific cause of infertility is often not determined.

Nurses should be concerned and tactful in dealing with male patients undergoing infertility studies. Many men equate fertility with masculinity. The nurse must be sensitive to the issue of gender identity in the infertile man.

Treatment options for men include medications, conservative lifestyle changes (e.g., avoidance of scrotal heat, substance abuse, high stress), in vitro fertilization techniques, and corrective surgery. Infertility can seriously strain a relationship, and the couple may require counselling and discussion of alternatives if conception is not achieved. (Female infertility is discussed in Chapter 56.)

CASE STUDY

Benign Prostatic Hyperplasia

Patient Profile
L. W. (pronouns he/him), 60 years old, comes to the primary health outpatient clinic because of an inability to void for the past 13 hours and pain in his lower abdomen.

Subjective Data
- Reports urge to void
- Is very restless, anxious, and agitated

Objective Data
- Prostate enlargement on digital rectal examination
- Hematuria, bacteria, and white blood cells in urine
- Tender and palpable bladder above umbilicus

Interprofessional Care
- In-dwelling catheter inserted by a urology resident
- Admitted to hospital

Discussion Questions
1. What risk factors for prostate conditions are present in L. W.?

2. Explain the etiology of the objective symptoms he exhibited.
3. Discuss the medication options available to L. W.
4. Discuss the invasive options available to L. W.
5. L. W. asks about the effect of the various treatment options on his ability to have sex. How should the nurse respond?
6. ***Priority decision:*** What are the priority nursing diagnoses based on the assessment data presented? Are there any interprofessional issues?
7. ***Priority decision:*** What is the priority nursing intervention for L. W.?
8. On further assessment, the nurse notes he has a nursing diagnosis of *decisional conflict.* How should the nurse help resolve this conflict related to treatment options?
9. ***Evidence-informed practice:*** What information should the nurse offer in response to L. W. asking if taking saw palmetto is helpful to prevent future UTIs?

evolve
Answers are available at http://evolve.elsevier.com/Canada/Lewis/medsurg.

REVIEW QUESTIONS

The number of the question corresponds to the same-numbered objective at the beginning of the chapter.

1. An older male client is experiencing difficulty initiating voiding and a feeling of incomplete bladder emptying. What are these symptoms of BPH primarily caused by?
   a. Obstruction of the urethra
   b. Untreated chronic prostatitis
   c. Decreased bladder compliance
   d. Excessive secretion of testosterone

2. Postoperatively, a client who has had a laser prostatectomy has continuous bladder irrigation with a three-way urinary catheter with a 30-mL balloon. When he complains of bladder spasms with the catheter in place, what should the nurse do?
   a. Deflate the catheter balloon to 10 mL to decrease bulk in the bladder.
   b. Deflate the catheter balloon and then reinflate to ensure that it is patent.
   c. Encourage the client to try to have a bowel movement to relieve colon pressure.
   d. Explain that this feeling is normal and that he should not try to urinate around the catheter.

3. Which factors would place a client at higher risk for prostate cancer? *(Select all that apply.)*
   a. Older than 65 years
   b. Asian or Indigenous Canadian
   c. Long-term use of an in-dwelling urethral catheter
   d. Father diagnosed and treated for early-stage prostate cancer
   e. Previous history of undescended testicle and testicular cancer

4. A client scheduled for a prostatectomy for prostate cancer expresses the fear that he will have erectile dysfunction (ED). In responding to this client, what should the nurse keep in mind?
   a. ED can occur even with a nerve-sparing procedure.
   b. Retrograde ejaculation affects sexual function more frequently than erectile dysfunction.
   c. The most common complication of this surgery is postoperative bowel incontinence.
   d. Preoperative sexual function is the most important factor in determining postoperative erectile dysfunction.

5. What should the nurse explain to the client with chronic bacterial prostatitis who is undergoing antibiotic therapy? *(Select all that apply.)*
   a. All clients require hospitalization.
   b. Pain will lessen once the infection is resolved.
   c. The course of treatment is generally 4 to 12 weeks.
   d. Long-term therapy may be indicated in immunocompromised clients.
   e. If the condition is unresolved and untreated, the client is at risk for prostate cancer.

6. Which manifestations of testicular cancer would the nurse observe for when assessing a client for this disease?
   a. Acute back spasms and testicular pain
   b. Rapid onset of scrotal swelling and fever
   c. Fertility challenges and bilateral scrotal tenderness
   d. Painless mass and sensation of heaviness in the scrotal area

7. What should the nurse explain to the client who has had a vasectomy?
   a. The procedure blocks the production of sperm.
   b. ED is temporary and will return with continued sexual activity.
   c. The ejaculate will be about half the volume it was before the procedure.
   d. An alternative form of contraception will be necessary for 6 to 8 weeks.

8. What measure should the nurse use to decrease the client's discomfort over care related to his reproductive organs?
   a. Relate his sexual concerns to his sexual partner.
   b. Arrange to have only male nurses care for the client.
   c. Maintain a nonjudgemental attitude toward his sexual practices.
   d. Use only technical terminology when discussing reproductive function.

1. b; 2. d; 3. a, d; 4. a; 5. b, c, d; 6. d; 7. d; 8. c.

evolve

For even more review questions, visit http://evolve.elsevier.com/Canada/Lewis/medsurg.

REFERENCES

Anawalt, B., & Page, S. (2020). *Causes of male infertility.* https://www.uptodate.com/contents/causes-of-male-infertility

Azoulay, L., Eberg, M., Benayoun, S., et al. (2015). 5α-reductase inhibitors and the risk of cancer-related mortality in men with prostate cancer. *Journal of the American Medical Association Oncology, 1*(3), 314–320. https://doi.org/10.1001/jamaoncol.2015.0387

Barry, M., Fowler, F., O'Leary, M., et al. (1992). The American Urologic Association Symptom Index for benign prostatic hyperplasia. *Journal of Urology, 148*(5), 1549–1557.

Bella, A., Lee, J., Carrier, S., et al. (2015). CUA Practice guidelines for erectile dysfunction. *Canadian Urological Association, 9*(1-2), 23–29. https://doi.org/10.5489/cuaj.2699

Canadian Cancer Society. (2020). *Risk factors for prostate cancer.* https://cancer.ca/en/cancer-information/cancer-types/prostate/risks

Canadian Cancer Society. (2021a). *Penile cancer.* https://cancer.ca/en/cancer-information/cancer-types/penile

Canadian Cancer Society. (2021b). *Prostate cancer.* https://cancer.ca/en/about-us/prostate-cancer

Canadian Cancer Society. (2021c). *Prostatitis.* https://cancer.ca/en/cancer-information/cancer-types/prostate/what-is-prostate-cancer/prostatitis

Canadian Cancer Society. (2021d). *Risk factors for testicular cancer.* https://cancer.ca/en/cancer-information/cancer-types/testicular/risks

Canadian Cancer Society. (2021e). *Survival statistics for testicular cancer.* https://cancer.ca/en/cancer-information/cancer-types/testicular/prognosis-and-survival/survival-statistics

Canadian Cancer Society Advisory Committee on Cancer Statistics. (2017). *Canadian cancer statistics 2017.* https://cancer.ca/en/research/cancer-statistics/canadian-cancer-statistics

Chandrasekar, T., & Tilki, D. (2018). Robotic assisted vs. open radical prostatectomy: An update to the never-ending debate. *Translational Andrology and Urology, 7*(1), 120–123. https://doi.org/10.21037/tau.2017.12.20

Chughtai, B., Simma-Chiang, V., Lee, R., et al. (2015). Trends and utilization of laser prostatectomy in ambulatory surgical procedures for the treatment of benign prostatic hyperplasia in New York State (2000–2011). *Journal of Endourology, 29*(6), 700–706.

Das, A. K., Teplitsky, S., & Humphreys, M. R. (2019). Holmium laser enucleation of the prostate (HoLEP): A review and update. *Canadian Journal of Urology, 26*(4), 13–19.

Deveci, S. (2021). *Priapism.* https://www.uptodate.com/contents/priapism

DiBiase, S., & Roach, M. (2021). *External beam radiation therapy for localized prostate cancer.* https://www.uptodate.com/contents/external-beam-radiation-therapy-for-localized-prostate-cancer

Hackett, L., Biderman, M., Doria, N., et al. (2020). A rapid review of Indigenous boys' and men's sexual health in Canada. *Journal Culture, Health & Sexuality.* https://doi.org/10.1080/13691058.2020.1722856. 2020.

Hannon, R. A., & Porth, C. M. (2017). *Porth pathophysiology: Concepts of altered health states* (2nd Canadian ed.). Wolters Kluwer.

HealthLinkBC. (2020). *Prostatitis: Examinations and tests.* https://www.healthlinkbc.ca/health-topics/hw73293#hw73394

Jarvis, C. (2019a). Anus, rectum, and prostate. In A. J. Browne, J. Macdonald-Jenkins, & M. Luctkar-Flude (Eds.), *Physical examination & health assessment* (pp. 607–624). Elsevier.

Jarvis, C. (2019b). Male genitourinary system. In A. J. Browne, J. Macdonald-Jenkins, & M. Luctkar-Flude (Eds.), *Physical examination & health assessment* (pp. 607–624). Elsevier.

Khera, M. (2021). Treatment of male sexual dysfunction. https://www.uptodate.com/contents/treatment-of-male-sexual-dysfunction

Mandel, P., Preisser, F., Graefen, M., et al. (2017). High chance of late recovery of urinary and erectile dysfunction beyond 12 months after radical prostatectomy. *European Urology, 71*(6), 484–450. https://doi.org/10.1016/j.eururo.2016.09.030

Meyrier, A., & Fekete, T. (2021). *Acute bacterial prostatitis.* https://www.uptodate.com/contents/acute-bacterial-prostatitis

Nickel, J. C., Aaron, L., Barkin, J., et al. (2018). Canadian Urological Association guidelines on male lower urinary tract symptoms/benign prostatic hyperplasia (MLUTS/BPH): 2018 update. *Canadian Urological Association Journal, 12*(10), 303–312. https://doi.org/10.5489/cuaj.5616

Rendon, R., Mason, R., Marzouk, K., et al. (2017). Canadian Urological Association recommendations on prostate cancer screening and early diagnosis. *Canadian Urological Association Journal, 11*(10), 298–309. https://doi.org/10.5489/cuaj.48

Roach, M., & DiBiase, S. (2020). *Brachytherapy for low-risk or favorable intermediate-risk, clinically located prostate cancer.* https://www.uptodate.com/contents/brachytherapy-for-low-risk-or-favorable-intermediate-risk-clinically-localized-prostate-cancer

Roehrborn, C., Casabé, A., Glina, S., et al. (2015). Treatment satisfaction and clinically meaningful symptom improvement in men with lower urinary tract symptoms and prostatic enlargement secondary to benign prostatic hyperplasia: Secondary results from a 6-month, randomized, double-blind study comparing finasteride plus tadalafil with finasteride plus placebo. *International Journal of Urology, 22*(6), 582–587. https://doi.org/10.1111/iju.12741

Rosen, R., & Khera, M. (2021). *Epidemiology and etiologies of male sexual dysfunction.* www.uptodate.com/contents/epidemiology-and-etiologies-of-male-sexual-dysfunction

Rosen, R., Wincze, J., Mollen, M., et al. (2007). Responsiveness and minimum important differences for the erection quality scale. *Journal of Urology, 178*(5), 2076–2081. https://doi.org/10.1016/j.juro.2007.07.019

Rosenberg, M., Witt, E., Miner, M., et al. (2014). A practical primary care approach to lower urinary tract symptoms caused by benign prostatic hyperplasia (BPH-LUTS). *Canadian Journal of Urology, 21*(2), 12–24.

Smith, M. R. (2021). *Side effects of androgen deprivation therapy.* https://www.uptodate.com/contents/side-effects-of-androgen-deprivation-therapy

Snyder, P. (2020). *Approach to older men with low testosterone.* https://www.uptodate.com/contents/approach-to-older-men-with-low-testosterone

Trumble, B., Stieglitz, J., Eid Rodriguez, D., et al. (2015). Challenging the inevitability of prostate enlargement: Low levels of benign prostatic hyperplasia among Tsimane forager-horticulturalists. *Journals of Gerontology. Series A: Biological Sciences & Medical Sciences, 70*(10), 1262–1268. https://doi.org/10.1093/gerona/glv051

Wong, E., & Kapoor, A. (2017). Epidemiology of prostate and kidney cancer in the Aboriginal population of Canada: A systematic review. *Canadian Urological Association Journal, 11*(5), E222–E232. https://doi.org/10.5489/cuaj.4185

Wright, J. L., & Lange, P. (2021). *Prostate cancer in older men.* https://www.uptodate.com/contents/prostate-cancer-in-older-men

RESOURCES

Canadian Cancer Society
https://www.cancer.ca

Canadian Urological Association
https://www.cua.org

CancerCare Manitoba—*Cancer and Blood Disorders*
https://www.cancercare.mb.ca/Treatments/cancer-and-blood-disorders

Ontario Men's Health—*Erectile Dysfunction*
https://www.ontariomenshealth.ca/erectile-dysfunction

Prostate Cancer Centre
https://www.prostatecancercentre.ca

Vancouver Prostate Centre
https://www.prostatecentre.com

National Cancer Institute—*Prostate Cancer*
https://www.cancer.gov/types/prostate

Prostate Calculator: Forecasting the Course of Disease (Artificial Neural Networks in Prostate Cancer Project)
http://prostatecalculator.org

evolve

For additional Internet resources, see the website for this book at http://evolve.elsevier.com/Canada/Lewis/medsurg.

Conditions Related to Movement and Coordination

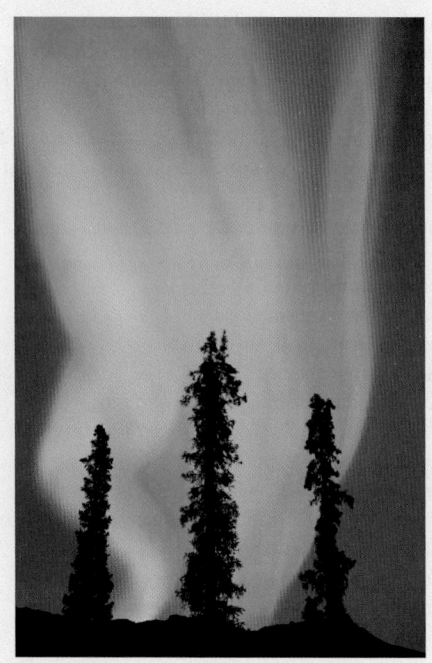

Source: CanStock Photo / PiLens

Nursing Assessment
Nervous System

Jana Lok
Originating US chapter by Tara Shaw

evolve WEBSITE

http://evolve.elsevier.com/Canada/Lewis/medsurg

- Review Questions (Online Only)
- Key Points
- Answer Guidelines for Case Study
- Conceptual Care Map Creator
- Audio Glossary

- Supporting Media—Animations
  - Motor Pathways and Clinical Evaluation of the Central Nervous System
  - Reflex Arc
  - Sensory Pathways and Clinical Evaluation of the Central Nervous System

- Content Updates

LEARNING OBJECTIVES

1. Describe the functions of neurons and glial cells.
2. Explain the electrochemical aspects of nerve impulse transmission.
3. Explain the anatomical location and functions of the cerebrum, brainstem, cerebellum, spinal cord, peripheral nerves, and cerebrospinal fluid.
4. Identify the major arteries supplying the brain.
5. Describe the functions of the 12 cranial nerves.
6. Compare the functions of the two divisions of the autonomic nervous system.
7. Describe age-related changes in the neurological system and differences in assessment findings.
8. Identify the significant subjective and objective data related to the nervous system that should be obtained from a patient.
9. Select appropriate techniques in the physical assessment of the nervous system.
10. Differentiate normal from common abnormal findings of a physical assessment of the nervous system.
11. Describe the purpose, the significance of results, and the nursing responsibilities related to diagnostic studies of the nervous system.

KEY TERMS

autonomic nervous system (ANS)
blood–brain barrier
central nervous system (CNS)
cerebrospinal fluid (CSF)
cranial nerves (CNs)

dermatome
glial cells
lower motor neurons (LMNs)
meninges
neurons

neurotransmitter
peripheral nervous system (PNS)
reflex
synapse
upper motor neurons (UMNs)

STRUCTURES AND FUNCTIONS OF THE NERVOUS SYSTEM

The human nervous system is a highly specialized system responsible for the control and integration of the body's many activities. The nervous system has two main divisions: the **central nervous system (CNS)** and the **peripheral nervous system (PNS)**. The CNS consists of the brain and spinal cord. The PNS consists of cranial nerves, spinal nerves, and the peripheral components of the autonomic nervous system (ANS).

Cells of the Nervous System

The nervous system is made up of two types of cells: neurons and glial cells. **Neurons** are the primary functional unit of the nervous system. Glial cells provide structural support and are more numerous than neurons.

Neurons. Neurons come in many different shapes and sizes, but they share three characteristics: (1) *excitability,* or the ability to generate a nerve impulse; (2) *conductivity,* or the ability to transmit an impulse; and (3) the ability to *influence* other neurons, muscle cells, and glandular cells by transmitting nerve impulses to them.

A typical neuron consists of a cell body, an axon, and several dendrites (Figure 58.1). The *cell body,* which contains the nucleus and the cytoplasm, is the metabolic centre of the neuron. *Dendrites* are short processes extending from the cell body. They receive nerve impulses from the axons of other neurons and conduct impulses toward the cell body. The nerve *axon* projects varying distances from the cell body, ranging from several micrometres to more than a metre. Its function is to carry nerve impulses to other neurons or to end organs. The end organs are smooth and striated muscles and glands. Axons may be myelinated or unmyelinated.

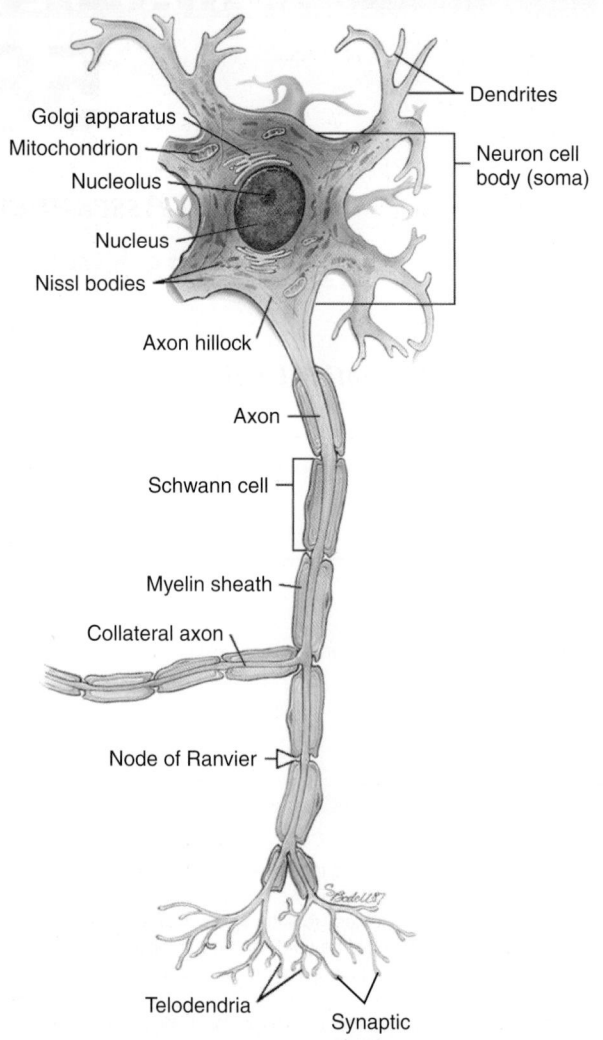

FIG. 58.1 Structural features of neurons: dendrites, cell body, and axons. Source: Adapted from Patton, K. T., & Thibodeau, G. A. (2010). *Anatomy and physiology* (7th ed., p. 379, Figure 12-5). Mosby.

Many axons present in the CNS and the PNS are covered by a segmentally interrupted myelin sheath composed of a white lipid substance that acts as an insulator for the conduction of impulses. In general, the smaller fibres are unmyelinated.

Glial Cells. Glial cells provide support, nourishment, and protection to neurons. They constitute almost half the brain and spinal cord mass and are 5 to 10 times more numerous than neurons. Different types of glial cells include astrocytes (most abundant), oligodendrocytes, ependymal cells, and microglia. *Astrocytes* provide structural and physiological support to neurons, form the blood–brain barrier with the endothelium of the blood vessels, and play a role in synaptic transmission (conduction of impulses between neurons). They are found primarily in grey matter. When the brain is injured (e.g., through trauma), causing damage to nerve cells, astrocytes act as phagocytes for neuronal debris. They help restore the neurochemical milieu and provide support for repair. Proliferation of astrocytes contributes to the formation of scar tissue (*gliosis*) in the CNS.

Oligodendrocytes are specialized cells that produce the myelin sheath of nerve fibres in the CNS and are found primarily in the white matter of the CNS. (*Schwann cells* myelinate the nerve fibres in the periphery.)

Ependymal cells line the brain ventricles and aid in the secretion of cerebrospinal fluid (CSF). *Microglia*, a type of macrophage, are relatively rare in normal CNS tissue. They are phagocytes and are important in host defence.

Neurogenesis

Neurons have long been thought to be nonmitotic—that is, after being damaged, neurons could not be replaced. The discovery of neural stem cells now demonstrates that neurogenesis can occur in adult brains after cerebral injury (Tang et al., 2020). Neuroglia are mitotic and can replicate. In general, when neurons are destroyed, the tissue is replaced by the proliferation of neuroglial cells. Most primary CNS tumours involve glial cells. Primary malignancies involving neurons are rare.

If the axon of a nerve cell is damaged, the cell attempts to repair itself. Damaged nerve cells attempt to grow back to their original destinations by sprouting many branches from the damaged ends of their axons. Unfortunately, axons in the CNS are less successful than peripheral axons in regenerating. Endogenous inhibitors (e.g., neurite outgrowth inhibitor, myelin-associated glycoprotein) decrease axon regeneration.

In the PNS (outside the brain and the spinal cord), injured nerve fibres can successfully regenerate by growing within the protective myelin sheath of the supporting Schwann cells if the cell body is intact. Nerve regeneration is a very slow process, and the final result depends on the number of axon sprouts that join with the appropriate Schwann cell columns and reinnervate appropriate end organs.

🔍 EVIDENCE-INFORMED PRACTICE

Research Highlight

Can Cell Transplantation Promote Recovery Following Spinal Cord Injury?

Clinical Question

Following spinal cord injuries (P), can transplanted cells (I) promote repair and function of the spinal cord (O)?

Best Available Evidence

- Dr. Peggy Assinck, a Canadian researcher and former national athlete, is working with a team at the University of British Columbia to explore cell transplantation as a possible therapy for spinal cord injury.
- Transplanting various types of cells (i.e., Schwann, neural stem, olfactory ensheathing, oligodendrocyte precursor, and mesenchymal stem cells) is being explored for managing spinal cord injuries.

Critical Appraisal and Synthesis of Evidence

- This research is still in its experimental stage. Research using animal models has provided insight into possible mechanisms of how cell transplantation may promote healing following spinal cord injury.

Conclusion

- Current studies are still exploring the mechanisms through which various cells promote repair and function of the spinal cord, with the goal of developing targeted therapies in the future.

Implications for Nursing Practice

1. Damage to the spinal cord is one of the more traumatic events that can affect an individual's life. Unfortunately, there are few viable treatment options.
2. This research provides new insight into future treatment options for spinal cord injuries.

Reference for Evidence

Assinck, P., Duncan, G. J., Hilton, B. J., et al. (2017). Cell transplantation therapy for spinal cord injury. *Nature Neuroscience, 20*(5), 637.

P, patient population of interest; *I,* intervention or area of interest; *O,* outcomes of interest (see Chapter 1).

Nerve Impulse

The function of a neuron is to initiate, receive, and process messages about events both within and outside the body. The initiation of a neuronal message (*nerve impulse*) involves the generation of an action potential. An *action potential* is a rapid, self-propagating and transient change in the voltage across a cell membrane (caused by the influx of Na^+ followed by an efflux of K^+). An action potential is generated when a stimulus causes the resting membrane potential (-70 mV) to depolarize (to about $+30$ mV) within a short time period (1–2 ms). Once an action potential is initiated, a series of action potentials travel along the axon. When the impulse reaches the end of the nerve fibre, it is transmitted across the junction between nerve cells (*synapse*) by a chemical interaction involving neurotransmitters. This chemical interaction generates another set of action potentials in the next neuron. These events are repeated until the nerve impulse reaches its destination.

Because of its insulating capacity, myelination of nerve axons facilitates the conduction of an action potential. Many peripheral nerve axons have gaps, termed *nodes of Ranvier,* at regular intervals in the myelin sheath surrounding them. An action potential travelling down one of these axons hops from node to node without traversing the insulated membrane segment between nodes, which makes the action potential travel much faster than it would otherwise. This process is called *saltatory* (hopping) conduction. In an unmyelinated fibre, the wave of depolarization traverses the entire length of the axon, and each portion of the membrane becomes depolarized in turn. Figure 58.2 depicts a comparison of nerve impulse transmission of myelinated and unmyelinated fibres.

Synapse. A synapse is the structural and functional junction between two neurons. It is the point at which the nerve impulse is transmitted from one neuron to another or from a neuron to glands or muscles. The essential structures of synaptic transmission are a presynaptic terminal, a synaptic cleft, and a receptor site on the postsynaptic cell (Figure 58.3). There are two types of synapses: electrical and chemical. In an *electrical* synapse, an action potential moves from neuron to neuron directly, by allowing electrical current to flow between neurons. In a *chemical* synapse, an action potential reaches the end of the axon (presynaptic terminal); then, it causes release of a chemical substance (neurotransmitter) from tiny vesicles within the axon terminal. The neurotransmitter then crosses the microscopic space (synaptic cleft) between the two neurons and attaches to receptor sites of the receiving (postsynaptic) neuron. Parts of the synapse include the neurotransmitters, the inactivators, and the receptors (see Figure 58.3).

Neurotransmitters. A neurotransmitter is a chemical agent that affects the transmission of an impulse across the synaptic cleft. Examples of neurotransmitters are presented in Table 58.1. *Excitatory* neurotransmitters activate postsynaptic receptors, causing an influx of Na^+, increasing the likelihood that an action potential will be generated. *Inhibitory* neurotransmitters activate postsynaptic receptors, causing an efflux of K^+, inhibiting the likelihood that an action potential will be generated.

Each of the hundreds to thousands of synaptic connections of a single neuron has an influence on that neuron. The net effect of the input is sometimes excitatory and sometimes inhibitory. In general, the net effect depends on the number of presynaptic neurons that are releasing neurotransmitters on the postsynaptic cell. A presynaptic cell that releases an excitatory neurotransmitter does not always cause the postsynaptic cell to

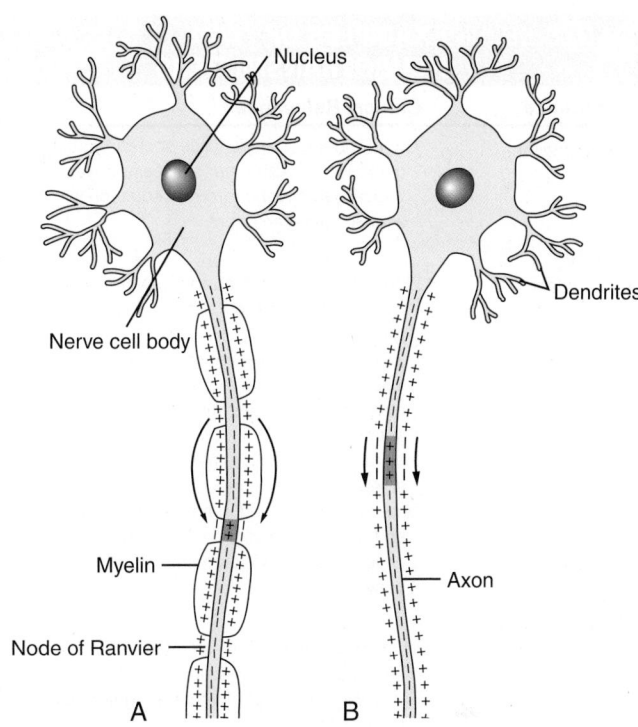

FIG. 58.2 Nerve impulse transmission. **A,** Saltatory conduction in a myelinated nerve. **B,** Depolarization in an unmyelinated fibre.

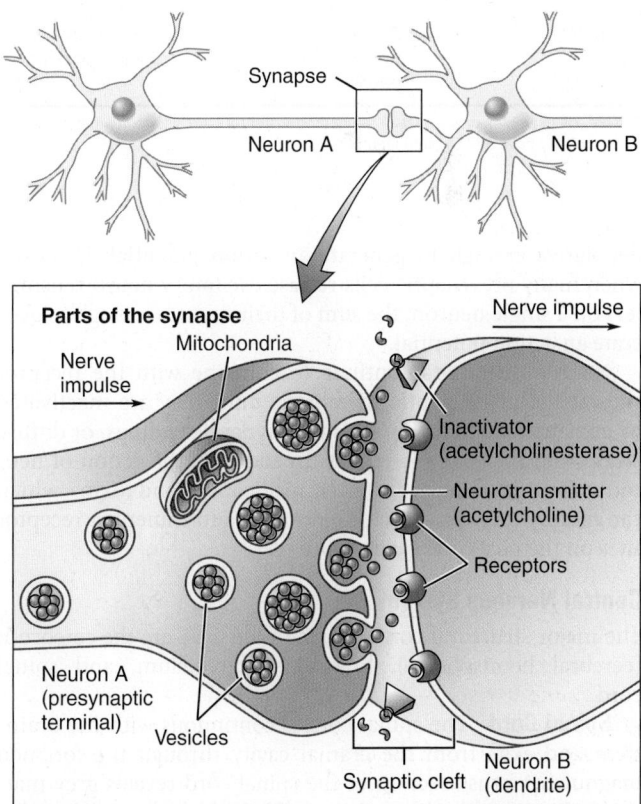

FIG. 58.3 The synapse is located in the space between neuron A and neuron B. Parts of the synapse include the neurotransmitters, the inactivators, and the receptors. The neurotransmitters are located in the vesicles of neuron A. The inactivators are located on the membrane of neuron B. The receptors are located on the membrane of neuron B. Source: Adapted from Herlihy, B. (2007). *The human body in health and illness* (3rd ed., p. 170, Figure 10-9). W. B. Saunders.

TABLE 58.1	EXAMPLES OF NEUROTRANSMITTERS
Substance	**Clinical Relevance***
Acetylcholine	The number of acetylcholine-secreting neurons decreases in Alzheimer's disease; myasthenia gravis results from a reduction in acetylcholine receptors.
Amines	
Epinephrine	Epinephrine acts as a hormone when secreted by the neurosecretory cells of the adrenal medulla.
Norepinephrine	Cocaine and amphetamines increase the release and block the reuptake of norepinephrine, resulting in overstimulation of postsynaptic neurons.
Serotonin	Serotonin is involved in moods, emotions, and sleep.
Dopamine	Dopamine is involved in emotions and moods and regulating motor control. Parkinson's disease results from destruction of dopamine-secreting neurons.
Amino Acids	
γ-Aminobutyric acid (GABA)	Medications that increase GABA function have been used to treat seizure disorders.
Glutamate and aspartate	Sustained release of glutamate triggers neuronal apoptosis.
Neuropeptides	
Endorphins and enkephalins	The opioids morphine and heroin bind to endorphin and enkephalin receptors on presynaptic neurons and reduce pain by blocking the release of neurotransmitter (see Chapter 10).
Substance P	Substance P is a neurotransmitter in pain transmission pathways; morphine blocks its release.

*These are examples only; most of the neurotransmitters are also found in other locations and may have additional functions.

depolarize enough to generate an action potential. However, when many presynaptic cells release excitatory neurotransmitters on a single neuron, the sum of their input is enough to generate an action potential.

Neurotransmitters continue to combine with the receptor sites at the postsynaptic membrane until they are inactivated by enzymes, are taken up by the presynaptic endings, or diffuse away from the synaptic region. In addition, the action of neurotransmitters can be affected by medications and toxins, which can modify their function or block their attachment to receptor sites on the postsynaptic membrane.

Central Nervous System

The major structural components of the CNS are the cerebrum (cerebral hemispheres), brainstem, cerebellum, and spinal cord.

Spinal Cord. The spinal cord is continuous with the brainstem and exits from the cranial cavity through the foramen magnum. A cross-section of the spinal cord reveals grey matter that is centrally located in an H-shape and is surrounded by white matter (Figure 58.4). The *grey matter* contains the cell bodies of voluntary motor neurons and preganglionic autonomic motor neurons, as well as cell bodies of association neurons (interneurons). The *white matter* contains the axons of the ascending sensory and the descending (suprasegmental) motor

fibres. The myelin surrounding these fibres gives them their white appearance. Specific ascending and descending pathways in the white matter can be identified. The spinal pathways or tracts are named for the point of origin and the point of destination (e.g., spinocerebellar tract [ascending], corticospinal tract [descending]).

Ascending Tracts. In general, the ascending tracts carry specific sensory information to higher levels of the CNS. This information comes from special sensory endings (receptors) in the skin, the muscles and joints, the viscera, and the blood vessels and enters the spinal cord by way of the dorsal roots of the spinal nerves. The fasciculus gracilis and the fasciculus cuneatus (together, commonly called the *dorsal* or *posterior column*) carry information and transmit impulses concerned with touch, deep pressure, vibration, position sense, and kinesthesia (appreciation of movement, weight, and body parts). The *spinocerebellar tracts* carry information about muscle tension and body position to the cerebellum for coordination of movement. The *spinothalamic tracts* carry pain and temperature sensations. Thus, the ascending tracts are organized by sensory modality as well as by anatomy. Other ascending tracts may also participate in transmission of sensory information.

Descending Tracts. Descending tracts carry impulses that are responsible for muscle movement. Among the most important descending tracts are the corticobulbar and corticospinal tracts, collectively termed the *pyramidal tract*. These tracts carry volitional (voluntary) impulses from the cortex to the cranial and the peripheral nerves. Another group of descending motor tracts carries impulses from the *extrapyramidal system,* which includes all motor systems (except the pyramidal system) concerned with voluntary movement. It includes descending pathways originating in the brainstem, basal ganglia, and cerebellum. The motor output exits the spinal cord by way of the ventral roots of the spinal nerves.

Lower Motor Neurons. Lower motor neurons (LMNs) are the final common pathway through which descending motor tracts influence skeletal muscle, the effector organ for movement. The cell bodies of LMNs, which send axons to innervate the skeletal muscles of arms, trunk, and legs, are located in the anterior horn of the corresponding segments of the spinal cord (e.g., cervical segments contain LMNs for the arms). LMNs for skeletal muscles of eyes, face, mouth, and throat are located in the corresponding segments of the brainstem. These cell bodies and their axons make up the somatic motor components of the cranial nerves. LMN lesions generally cause weakness or paralysis, denervation atrophy, hyperreflexia or areflexia, and decreased muscle tone (*flaccidity*).

Upper Motor Neurons. Upper motor neurons (UMNs) originate in the cerebral cortex and project downward. The corticobulbar tract ends in the brainstem, and the corticospinal tract descends into the spinal cord. These neurons influence skeletal muscle movement. UMN lesions generally cause weakness or paralysis, disuse atrophy, hyperreflexia, and increased muscle tone (*spasticity*).

Reflex Arc. A reflex is defined as an involuntary response to a stimulus. The components of a monosynaptic reflex arc (the simplest kind of reflex arc) are a receptor organ, an afferent neuron, an effector neuron, and an effector organ (e.g., skeletal muscle). The afferent neuron synapses with the efferent neuron in the grey matter of the spinal cord. A reflex arc is shown in Figure 58.5. In more complex (polysynaptic) reflex arcs, the effector neuron is influenced by other neurons (interneurons)

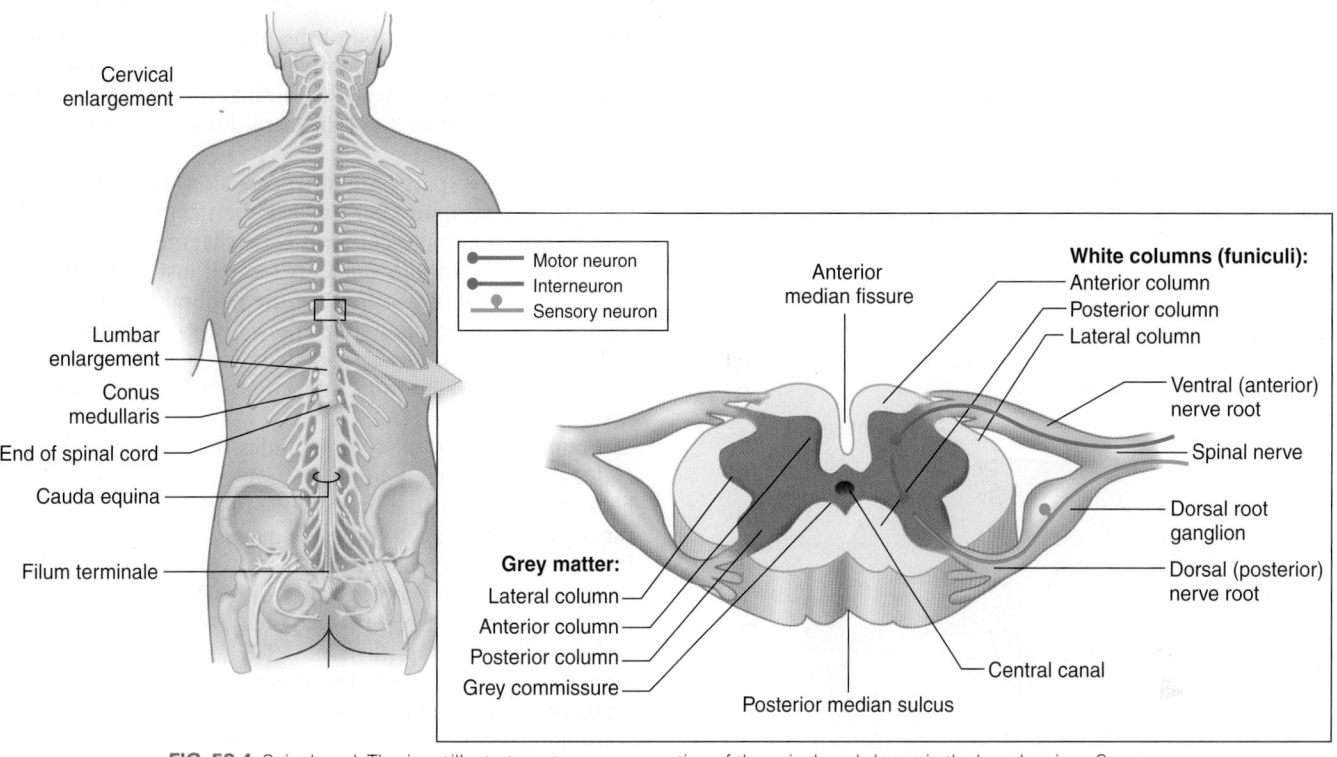

FIG. 58.4 Spinal cord. The *inset* illustrates a transverse section of the spinal cord shown in the broader view. Source: Adapted from Patton, K. T., & Thibodeau, G. A. (2013). *Anatomy and physiology* (8th ed., p. 426, Figure 14-6). Mosby.

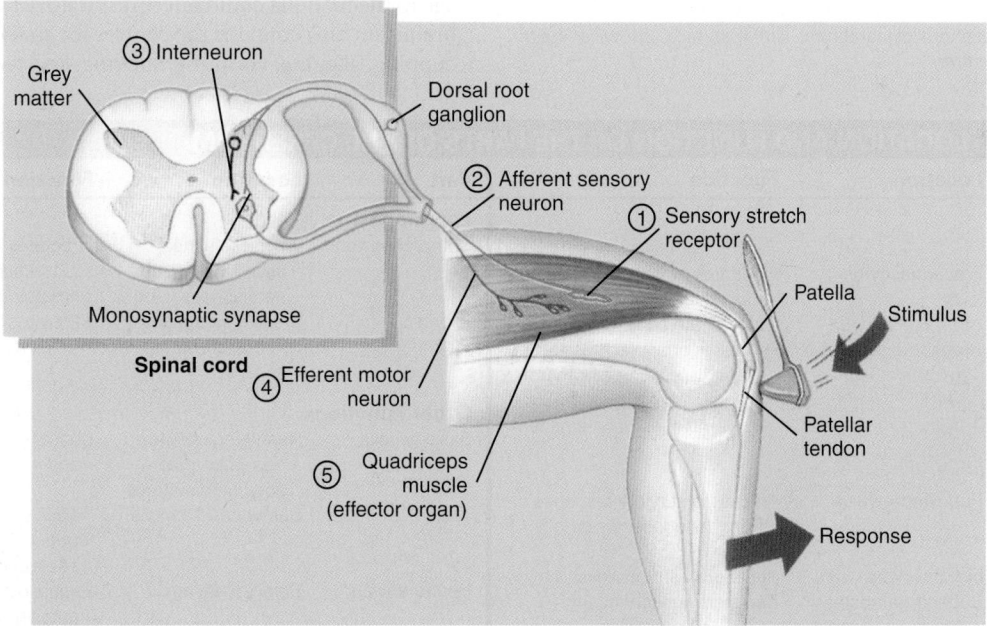

FIG. 58.5 Basic diagram of the patellar "knee-jerk" reflex arc. The impulse travels through the *(1)* sensory stretch receptor and *(2)* afferent sensory neuron, through the *(3)* interneuron, and back through the *(4)* efferent motor neuron and to the *(5)* quadriceps muscle (effector organ). Source: Adapted from Thibodeau, G. A., & Patton, K. T. (2008). *Structure and function of the body* (13th ed., p. 192, Figure 8-5). Mosby.

in addition to the afferent neuron. In the spinal cord, reflex arcs play an important role in maintaining muscle tone, which is essential for body posture.

Brain. The brain can be divided into three major components: cerebrum, brainstem, and cerebellum.

Cerebrum. The *cerebrum* is composed of the right and left cerebral hemispheres and divided into four major lobes: frontal, temporal, parietal, and occipital (Figure 58.6).

The functions of the cerebrum are multiple and complex. Specific areas of the cerebral cortex are associated with specific functions. Table 58.2 summarizes the location and function of the parts of the cerebrum. The *frontal lobe* controls higher cognitive function, memory, voluntary eye movements, voluntary movements, and, usually in the left hemisphere, expressive speech and language in Broca's area. The *temporal lobe* contains integration of somatic, visual, and auditory data and, usually in the left hemisphere, Wernicke's area, which is responsible for receptive language. The *parietal lobe* is composed of the sensory cortex and controlling and interpreting spatial information. Processing of visual data takes place in the *occipital lobe*.

The basal ganglia, the thalamus, the hypothalamus, and the limbic system are also located in the cerebrum. The *basal ganglia* are a group of paired structures located centrally in the cerebrum and the midbrain; most of them are on both sides of the thalamus. The function of the basal ganglia is to modulate initiation, execution, and completion of voluntary movements and automatic movements associated with skeletal muscle activity, such as swinging of the arms during walking, swallowing saliva, and blinking.

The *thalamus* (part of the diencephalon) lies directly above the brainstem (Figure 58.7) and is the major relay centre for sensory and other afferent (e.g., cerebellar) inputs to the cerebral cortex. The *hypothalamus* is located just inferiorly to the thalamus and slightly in front of the midbrain. It regulates the ANS and the endocrine system. The *limbic system* is located near the inner surfaces of the cerebral hemispheres (Figure 58.8) and is concerned with emotion, aggression, feeding behaviour, and sexual response.

Brainstem. The *brainstem* includes the midbrain, the pons, and the medulla (see Figure 58.7). Ascending and descending fibres pass through the brainstem between the cerebrum and the cerebellum. The cell bodies, or nuclei, of cranial nerves (CN) III through XII are in the brainstem. Also located in the brainstem is the *reticular formation,* a diffusely arranged group of neurons and their axons that extends from the medulla to the thalamus and the hypothalamus. The functions of the reticular formation include relaying sensory information, influencing excitatory and inhibitory control of spinal motor neurons, and controlling vasomotor and respiratory activity. The reticular activating system is part of the reticular formation and is the regulatory system for arousal, a component of consciousness.

The vital centres concerned with respiratory, vasomotor, and cardiac function are located in the medulla. For example, damage to the medulla could affect respiratory rate and rhythm. The brainstem also contains the centres for sneezing, coughing, hiccupping, gagging, vomiting, sucking, and swallowing.

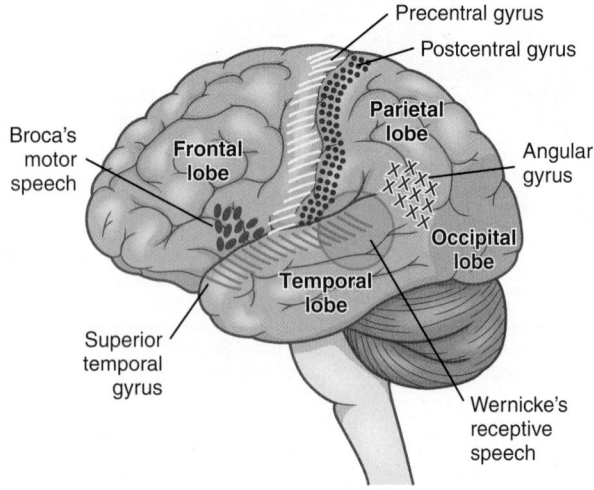

FIG. 58.6 Left hemisphere of cerebrum, lateral surface, showing major lobes and areas of the brain.

TABLE 58.2	LOCATION AND FUNCTION OF THE PARTS OF THE CEREBRUM					
Part	**Location**	**Function**		**Part**	**Location**	**Function**
Cortical Areas				**Language**		
Motor				Comprehension	Wernicke's area, usually in the left hemisphere	Integrates auditory language (understanding of spoken words)
Primary	Precentral gyrus	Facilitates motor control and movement on the opposite side of the body		Expression	Broca's area, usually in the left hemisphere	Regulates verbal expression
Supplemental	Anterior to precentral gyrus	Facilitates proximal muscle activity, including activity for stance and gait, spontaneous movement, and coordination		**Other Functions**		
				Basal ganglia	Near lateral ventricles of both cerebral hemispheres	Control and facilitate learned and automatic movements
Sensory				Thalamus	Below basal ganglia	Relays sensory and motor inputs to cortex and other parts of cerebrum
Somatic	Postcentral gyrus	Processes sensory response from the opposite side of body		Hypothalamus	Below thalamus	Regulates endocrine and autonomic functions (e.g., feeding, sleeping, emotional and sexual responses)
Visual	Occipital lobe	Registers visual images				
Auditory	Superior temporal gyrus	Registers auditory inputs				
Association areas	Parietal lobe	Integrates somatic and sensory inputs		Limbic system	Lateral to hypothalamus	Influences affective (emotional) behaviour and basic drives such as feeding and sexual behaviour
	Posterior temporal lobe	Integrates visual and auditory inputs for language comprehension				
	Anterior temporal lobe	Integrates past experiences				
	Anterior frontal lobe	Controls higher-order processes (e.g., judgement, insight, reasoning, problem solving, planning)				

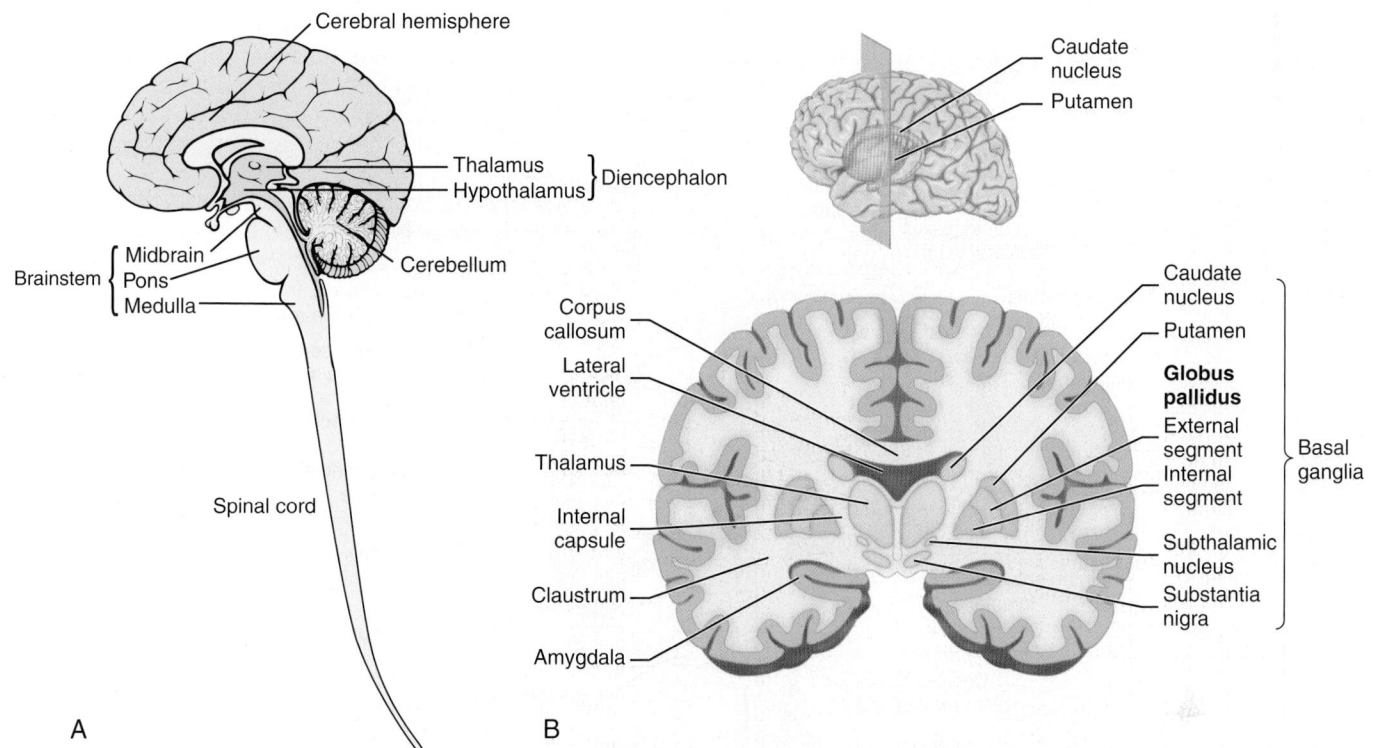

FIG. 58.7 The central nervous system. **A,** Side view of major divisions. **B,** Coronal overview of the components of the basal ganglia. Source: *B,* Based on Nieuwenhuys, Voogd, and van Huijzen, 1981.

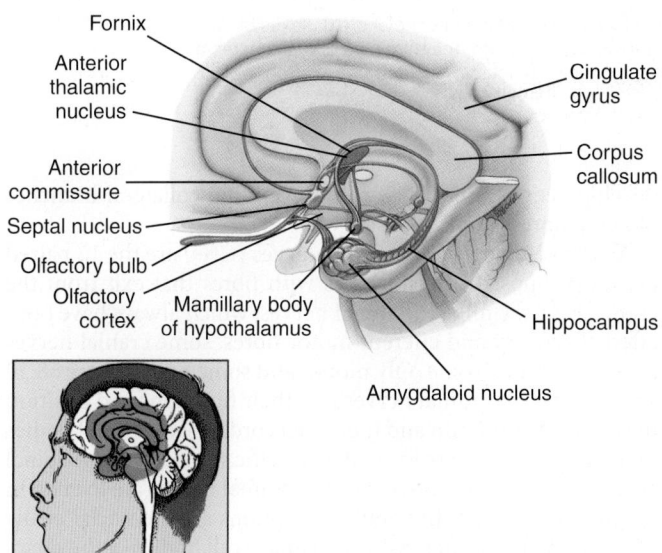

FIG. 58.8 Structures of the limbic system. Source: Adapted from Patton, K. T., & Thibodeau, G. A. (2010). *Anatomy and physiology* (7th ed., p. 436, Figure 13-22). Mosby.

Cerebellum. The *cerebellum* is located in the posterior part of the cranial fossa, inferior to the occipital lobe. The cerebellum coordinates voluntary movement and maintains trunk stability and equilibrium. To perform these functions, the cerebellum receives information from the cerebral cortex, the muscles, the joints, and the inner ear. It influences motor activity through its axonal connections to the motor cortex, the brainstem nuclei, and their descending pathways.

Ventricles and Cerebrospinal Fluid. The ventricles are four cavities within the brain, filled with CSF, that connect with one another and with the spinal canal. The lower portion of the fourth ventricle becomes the central canal in the lower part of the brainstem. The spinal canal is located in the centre of the spinal cord and extends the full length of the spinal cord. Figure 58.9 depicts the ventricles and the flow of CSF in the CNS.

Cerebrospinal Fluid. Cerebrospinal fluid (CSF) is a clear, colourless fluid similar to blood plasma and interstitial fluid (McCance et al., 2018). CSF circulates within the subarachnoid space that surrounds the brain, the brainstem, and the spinal cord. It provides cushioning for the brain and the spinal cord, allows fluid shifts from the cranial cavity to the spinal cavity, and carries nutrients. CSF is produced primarily by the choroid plexus in the lateral, third, and fourth ventricles. It flows from the lateral ventricles to the third ventricle via the interventricular foramen and then moves from the third to the fourth ventricle through the cerebral aqueduct. Finally, CSF flows into the subarachnoid space through the lateral and median foramen (see Figure 58.9). It is absorbed primarily through the *arachnoid villi* (tiny projections into the subarachnoid space), into the intradural venous sinuses, and eventually into the venous system. Although CSF is continually being formed, many physiological factors influence its rate of absorption and formation. The ventricles and the central canal are normally filled with an average of 135 mL of CSF. A disturbance in the formation, flow, or absorption of CSF can lead to hydrocephalus.

The analysis of CSF composition provides useful diagnostic information relating to certain nervous system diseases. CSF pressure is often measured in patients with actual or suspected intracranial diseases. Increases in intracranial pressure, indicated by increased CSF pressure, can lead to herniation of the brain and compression of vital brainstem structures. The signs marking this event are part of the herniation (see Chapter 59).

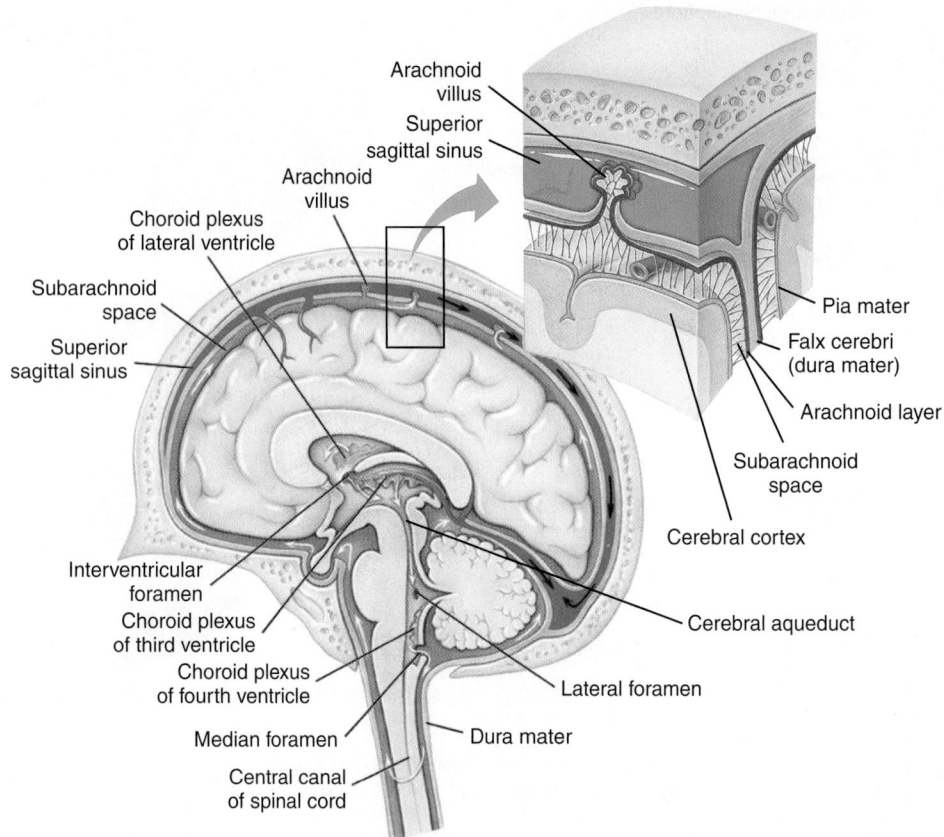

FIG. 58.9 Flow of cerebrospinal fluid (CSF). The fluid produced by filtration of blood by the choroid plexus of each ventricle flows inferiorly through the lateral ventricles, the interventricular foramen, the third ventricle, the cerebral aqueduct, the fourth ventricle, and the subarachnoid space and to the blood. Source: Adapted from Patton, K. T., & Thibodeau, G. A. (2010). *Anatomy and physiology* (7th ed., p. 417, Figure 13-5). Mosby.

Peripheral Nervous System

The PNS includes all of the neuronal structures that lie outside the CNS. It consists of the spinal and cranial nerves, their associated ganglia (groupings of cell bodies), and portions of the ANS.

Spinal Nerves. The spinal cord is a series of spinal segments, one on top of another. In addition to the cell bodies, each segment contains a pair of dorsal *(afferent)* sensory nerve fibres or roots and ventral *(efferent)* motor fibres or roots, which innervate a specific region of neck, trunk, or limbs. This combined motor–sensory nerve is called a *spinal nerve* (Figure 58.10). The cell bodies of the voluntary motor system are located in the anterior horn of the spinal cord grey matter. The cell bodies of the autonomic (involuntary) motor system are located in the anterolateral portion of spinal cord grey matter. The cell bodies of sensory fibres are located in the dorsal root ganglia just outside the spinal cord. On exiting the spinal column, each spinal nerve divides into ventral and dorsal rami, a collection of motor and sensory fibres that eventually extend to peripheral structures (e.g., skin, muscles, viscera).

A **dermatome** is the area of skin innervated by the sensory fibres of a single dorsal root of a spinal nerve. The locations of dermatomes indicate the general pattern of somatic sensory innervation by spinal segments. A *myotome* is a muscle group innervated by the primary motor neurons of a single ventral root. The dermatomes and myotomes of a given spinal segment overlap with those of adjacent segments because of the

development of ascending and descending collateral branches of nerve fibres (Figure 58.11).

Cranial Nerves. The cranial nerves (CNs) are the 12 paired nerves composed of cell bodies with fibres that exit from the cranial cavity. Unlike the spinal nerves, which always have both afferent sensory and efferent motor fibres, some cranial nerves are only sensory, some only motor, and some both. Figure 58.12 summarizes the cranial nerves and their functions and position in relation to the brain and the spinal cord. Just as the cell bodies of the spinal nerves are located in specific segments of the spinal cord, the cell bodies (nuclei) of the cranial nerves are located in specific segments of the brain. Exceptions are the nuclei of the olfactory and optic nerves. The primary cell bodies of the olfactory nerve are located in the nasal epithelium, and those of the optic nerve are in the retina.

Autonomic Nervous System. The autonomic nervous system (ANS) governs involuntary functions of cardiac muscle, smooth (involuntary) muscle, and glands.

The ANS is divided into two components, sympathetic and parasympathetic, which are anatomically and functionally different. These two systems function together to maintain a relatively balanced internal environment. The ANS is both an efferent and an afferent system. It consists of preganglionic nerves and postganglionic nerves.

The preganglionic cell bodies of the *sympathetic nervous system* (SNS) are located in spinal segments T1 through L2. The major neurotransmitter released by the postganglionic fibres of

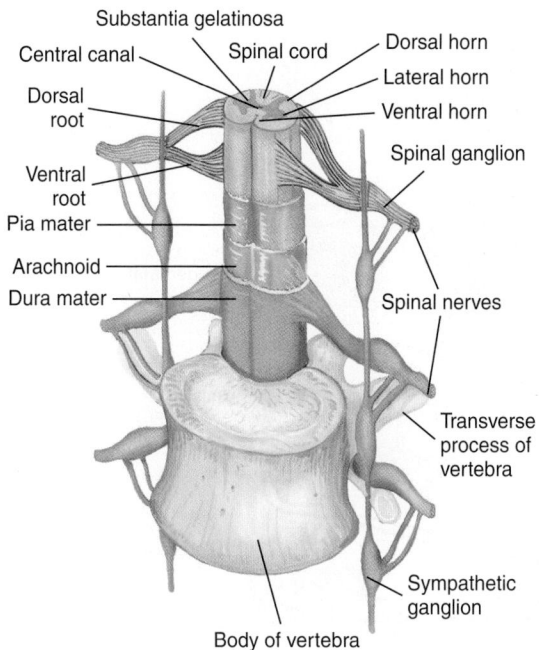

FIG. 58.10 Illustration of a cross-section of spinal cord, showing attachments of spinal nerves and coverings of the spinal cord. Source: Adapted from Thibodeau, G. A., & Patton, K. T. (2008). *Structure and function of the body* (13th ed., p. 205, Figure 8-13). Mosby.

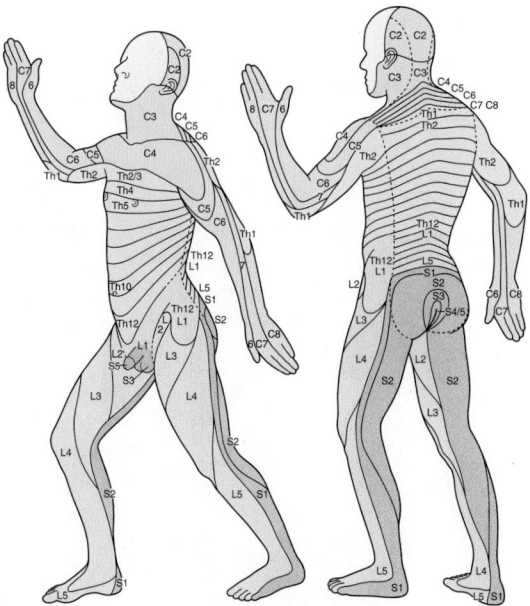

FIG. 58.11 Dermatome map, anterolateral view (*left*) and posterolateral view (*right*). Source: Salvo, S. G. (2014). *Mosby's pathology for massage therapists* (3rd ed.). Mosby. In El-Hussein, M. T., Power-Kean, K., Zettel, S., et al. (2018). *Understanding pathophysiology* (1st Canadian ed., p. 327, Figure 13-25, C). Elsevier.

the SNS is norepinephrine, and the neurotransmitter released by the preganglionic fibres is acetylcholine.

In contrast, the preganglionic cell bodies of the *parasympathetic nervous system* (PSNS) are located in the brainstem and in the sacral spinal segments (S2 through S4). Acetylcholine is the neurotransmitter released at both preganglionic and postganglionic nerve endings.

The ANS provides dual and often reciprocal innervation to many structures. For example, the SNS increases the rate and force of the heart contraction, and the PSNS decreases the rate and force. Table 58.3 lists the effects of the SNS and PSNS.

The result of SNS stimulation is activation of mechanisms required for the "fight or flight" response that occurs throughout the body. In contrast, the PSNS is geared to act in localized and discrete regions. It serves to conserve and restore the energy stores of the body.

Cerebral Circulation

Knowledge of the distribution of the major arteries of the brain and the area supplied is essential for understanding and evaluating the signs and symptoms of cerebrovascular disease and trauma. The blood supply of the brain arises from the internal carotid arteries (anterior circulation) and the vertebral arteries (posterior circulation) (Figure 58.13).

The internal carotid arteries provide blood flow to the anterior and middle portions of the cerebrum. The vertebral arteries join to form the basilar artery and provide blood flow to the brainstem, cerebellum, and posterior cerebrum. The *circle of Willis* arises from the basilar artery and the two internal carotid arteries (Figure 58.14). This vascular circle may act as a safety valve when differential pressures are present in these arteries. It also may function as an anastomotic pathway when a major artery on one side of the brain becomes occluded. Superior to the circle of Willis, three pairs of arteries supply blood to the left and right hemispheres. The anterior cerebral artery feeds the

medial and anterior portions of the frontal lobes. The middle cerebral artery feeds the outer portions of the frontal, parietal, and superior temporal lobes. The posterior cerebral artery feeds the medial portions of the occipital and inferior temporal lobes. Venous blood drains from the brain through the dural sinuses, which form channels that drain into the two jugular veins.

Blood–Brain Barrier. The blood–brain barrier is a physiological barrier between blood capillaries and brain tissue (McCance et al., 2018). This barrier protects the brain from certain potentially harmful agents while allowing nutrients and gases to enter. Because the blood–brain barrier affects the penetration of drugs, only certain ones can enter the CNS from the bloodstream. Lipid-soluble compounds (e.g., barbiturates) enter the brain quickly, whereas water-soluble and ionized medications (e.g., penicillin) enter the brain and spinal cord slowly. Damage to the blood–brain barrier (e.g., trauma) results in the penetration of medications and other substances into brain tissue.

Protective Structures

Meninges. The meninges are three layers of protective membranes that surround the brain and the spinal cord: dura mater, arachnoid, and pia mater (see Figure 58.9). The thick *dura mater* forms the outermost layer. The *falx cerebri* is a fold of the dura that separates the two cerebral hemispheres and prevents expansion of brain tissue in situations such as the presence of a rapidly growing tumour or acute hemorrhage. The *tentorium cerebelli* is a fold of dura that separates the cerebral hemispheres from the posterior fossa, which contains the brainstem and the cerebellum. Expansion of mass lesions in the cerebrum forces the brain to herniate through the opening created by the brainstem. This condition is termed *tentorial herniation* (see Chapter 59).

The *arachnoid layer* is a delicate, impermeable membrane that lies between the thick dura mater and the pia mater (the delicate, innermost layer of the meninges). The area between

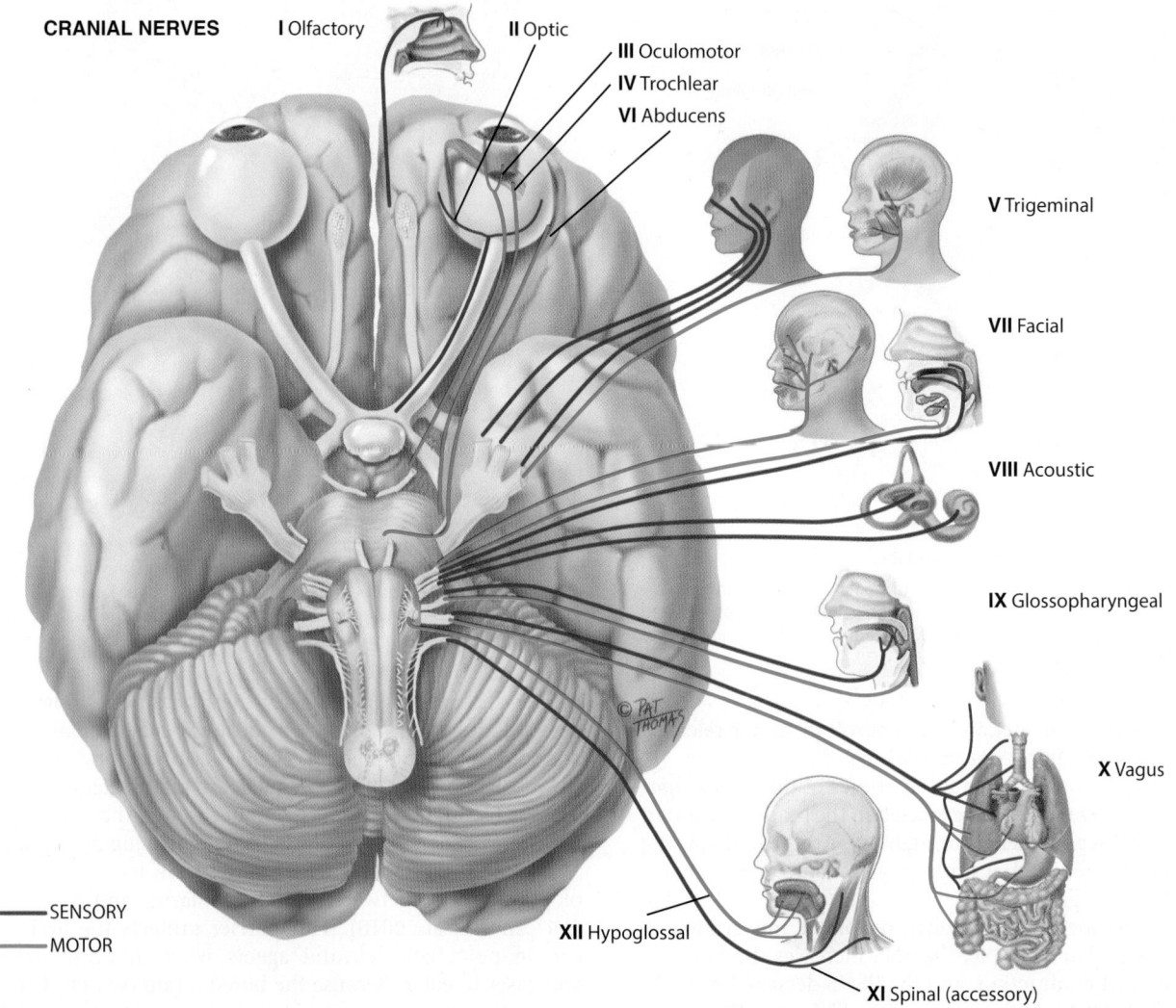

Cranial Nerve	Type	Function
I: Olfactory	Sensory	Smell
II: Optic	Sensory	Vision
III: Oculomotor	Mixed*	Motor—most EOM movement, opening of eyelids Parasympathetic—pupil constriction, lens shape
IV: Trochlear	Motor	Down and inward movement of eye
V: Trigeminal	Mixed	Motor—muscles of mastication Sensory—sensation of face and scalp, cornea, mucous membranes of mouth and nose
VI: Abducens	Motor	Lateral movement of eye
VII: Facial	Mixed	Motor—facial muscles, close eye, labial speech, close mouth Sensory—taste (sweet, salty, sour, bitter) on anterior two-thirds of tongue Parasympathetic—saliva and tear secretion
VIII: Acoustic	Sensory	Hearing and equilibrium
IX: Glossopharyngeal	Mixed	Motor—pharynx (phonation and swallowing) Sensory—taste on posterior one third of tongue, pharynx (gag reflex) Parasympathetic—parotid gland, carotid reflex
X: Vagus	Mixed	Motor—pharynx and larynx (vocalizing and swallowing) Sensory—general sensation from carotid body, carotid sinus, pharynx, viscera Parasympathetic—carotid reflex
XI: Spinal (accessory)	Motor	Movement of trapezius and sternocleidomastoid muscles
XII: Hypoglossal	Motor	Movement of tongue

*Mixed refers to a nerve carrying a combination of fibres: motor + sensory; motor + parasympathetic; or motor + sensory + parasympathetic.

FIG. 58.12 The cranial nerves and their functions. *EOM,* extraocular movement. Source: Jarvis, C., Brown, A. J., MacDonald-Jenkins, J., et al. (2019). *Physical examination & health assessment* (3rd Canadian ed., p. 692, Figure 25-7). Elsevier Inc.

TABLE 58.3	EFFECTS OF SYMPATHETIC AND PARASYMPATHETIC NERVOUS SYSTEMS	
Visceral Effector	**Effect of Sympathetic Nervous System***	**Effect of Parasympathetic Nervous System†**
Heart	Increase in rate and strength of heartbeat (β-receptors)	Decrease in rate and strength of heartbeat
Smooth muscle of blood vessels		
• Skin blood vessels	Constriction (α-receptors)	No effect
• Skeletal muscle blood vessels	Dilation (β-receptors)	No effect
• Coronary blood vessels	Dilation (β-receptors), constriction (α-receptors)	Dilation (β-receptors)
• Abdominal blood vessels	Constriction (α-receptors)	No effect
• Blood vessels of external genitals	Ejaculation (contraction of smooth muscle in male ducts [e.g., epididymis, ductus deferens])	Dilation of blood vessels, causing penile erection
Smooth muscle of hollow organs and sphincters		
• Bronchi	Dilation (β-receptors)	Constriction (α-receptors)
• Digestive tract, except sphincters	Decrease in rate of peristalsis (β-receptors)	Increase in rate of peristalsis
• Sphincters of digestive tract	Contraction (α-receptors)	Relaxation
• Urinary bladder	Relaxation (β-receptors)	Contraction
• Urinary sphincters	Contraction (α-receptors)	Relaxation
Iris	Contraction of radial muscle, dilation of pupil	Contraction of circular muscle, constriction of pupil
• Ciliary	Relaxation, accommodation for far vision	Contraction, accommodation for near vision
Hairs (pilomotor muscles)	Contraction producing goose pimples or piloerection (α-receptors)	No effect
Glands		
• Sweat	Increase in sweat (neurotransmitter, acetylcholine)	No effect
• Digestive (e.g., salivary, gastric)	Decrease in secretion of saliva; not known for others	Increase in secretion of saliva and gastric hydrochloric acid (HCl)
• Pancreas, including islets	Decrease in secretion	Increase in secretion of pancreatic juice and insulin
• Liver	Increase in glycogenolysis (β-receptors), increase in blood glucose level	No effect
• Adrenal medulla‡	Increase in epinephrine secretion	No effect

*Neurotransmitter is norepinephrine unless otherwise stated.
†Neurotransmitter is acetylcholine unless otherwise stated.
‡Sympathetic preganglionic axons terminate in contact with secreting cells of the adrenal medulla. Thus, the adrenal medulla functions as what is sometimes called a *giant sympathetic postganglionic neuron.*
Source: Adapted from Patton, K. T., & Thibodeau, G. A. (2010). *Anatomy and physiology* (7th ed., p. 483, Table 14-6). Mosby.

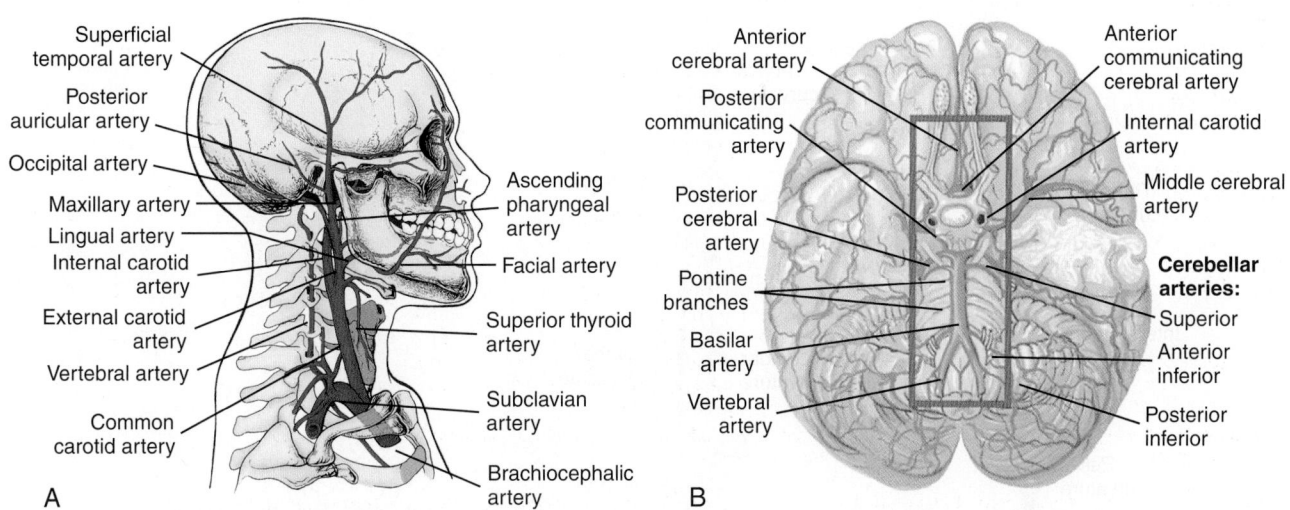

FIG. 58.13 Arteries of the head and neck. **A,** Right lateral view: brachiocephalic artery, right common carotid artery, right subclavian artery, and their branches. The major arteries to the head are the common carotid and vertebral arteries. **B,** Inferior view of the brain, showing the vertebral, basilar, and internal carotid arteries and their branches. Source: Adapted from Patton, K. T., & Thibodeau, G. A. (2010). *Anatomy and physiology* (7th ed., p. 633, Figure 18-19). Mosby.

the arachnoid layer and the pia mater is the *subarachnoid space* and is filled with CSF. Structures such as arteries, veins, and cranial nerves passing to and from the brain and the skull must pass through the subarachnoid space. A larger subarachnoid space in the region of the third and fourth lumbar vertebrae is the area used to obtain CSF during a lumbar puncture. (The spinal cord itself ends between the first and second lumbar vertebrae.)

Skull. The bony skull protects the brain from external trauma. It is composed of 8 cranial bones and 14 facial bones. Although the top and the sides of the inside of the skull are relatively smooth, the bottom surface is uneven; it has many ridges, prominences, and foramina (holes through which blood vessels and nerves enter the intracranial vault). The largest hole is the foramen magnum, through which the brainstem extends to the spinal cord. This foramen is the only major space for the expansion of brain contents when increased intracranial pressure occurs.

Vertebral Column. The vertebral column protects the spinal cord, supports the head, and provides flexibility. The vertebral column is made up of 33 individual vertebrae: 7 cervical (C), 12 thoracic (T), 5 lumbar (L), 5 sacral (S) (fused into one, the sacrum), and 4 coccygeal (fused into one, the coccyx). Each vertebra has a central opening through which the spinal cord passes. The vertebrae are held together by a series of ligaments. Intervertebral discs occupy the spaces between vertebrae. Figure 58.15 depicts the vertebral column in relation to the trunk.

AGE-RELATED CONSIDERATIONS

EFFECTS OF AGING ON THE NERVOUS SYSTEM

Several parts of the nervous system are affected by aging. In the CNS, neurons are lost in certain areas of the brainstem, the cerebellum, and the cerebral cortex. This loss is a gradual process that begins in early adulthood. With loss of neurons, the ventricles widen. Brain weight also decreases by 10 to 15% between the second and ninth decades of life (Porter, 2018). Cerebral blood flow decreases, and CSF production declines. Changes in neurotransmitters of the dopaminergic and cholinergic systems result in decreasing amounts of acetylcholine, serotonin, and catecholamines.

In general, the intellectual performance of older people who do not have brain dysfunction remains fairly consistent. A slowdown in central processing may result in needing longer to perform certain tasks. Sensory changes, including decreases in taste and smell perception, may result in decreased dietary intake in older persons. Changes in pain perception may occur. Decline in visual and auditory acuity can result in perceptual challenges. Difficulties with balance and coordination can increase older people's risk for falls and subsequent fractures. In the PNS, degenerative changes in myelin cause a decrease in nerve conduction. Coordinated neuromuscular activity, such as the maintenance of blood pressure in response to changing from a lying to a standing position, is altered with aging. As a result, older people are more likely to experience orthostatic

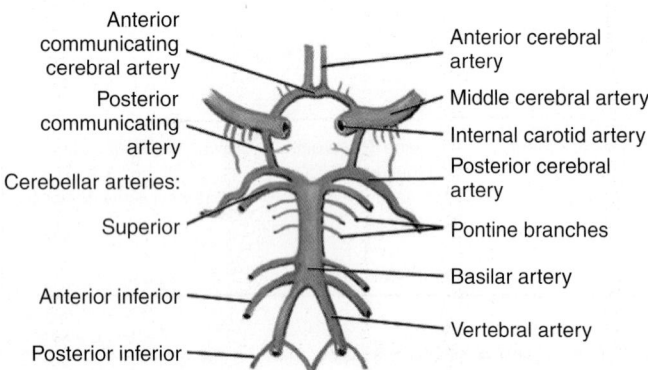

FIG. 58.14 Arteries at the base of the brain. The arteries that compose the circle of Willis are the two anterior cerebral arteries, joined to each other by the anterior communicating cerebral artery and to the posterior cerebral arteries by the posterior communicating arteries. Source: Adapted from Patton, K. T., & Thibodeau, G. A. (2010). *Anatomy and physiology* (7th ed., p. 634, Figure 18-20). Mosby.

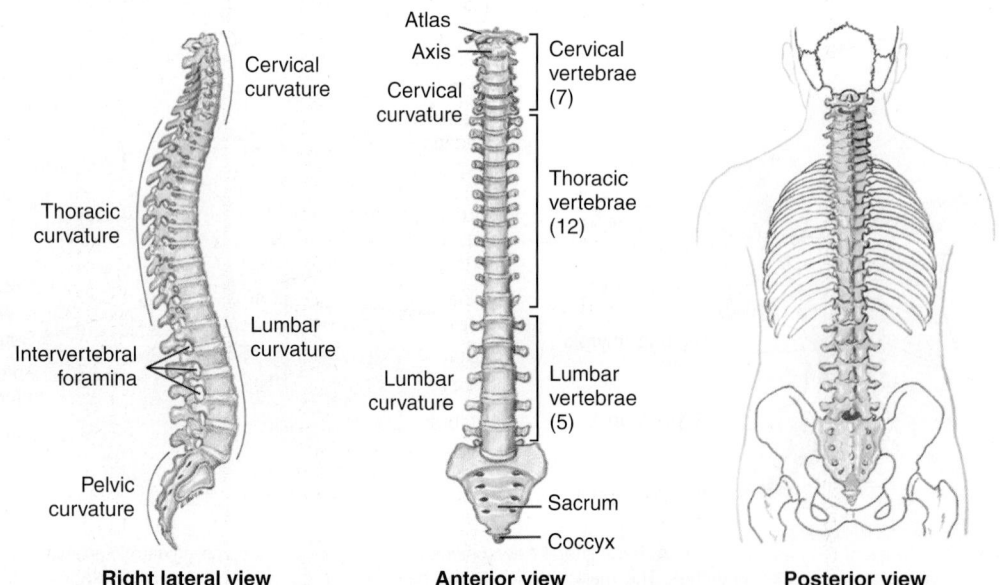

Right lateral view   **Anterior view**   **Posterior view**

FIG. 58.15 Vertebral column (three views). Source: Adapted from Patton, K. T., & Thibodeau, G. A. (2010). *Anatomy and physiology* (7th ed., p. 237, Figure 8-13). Mosby.

hypotension. Similarly, coordination of neuromuscular activity to maintain body temperature is also less efficient with aging, making older persons less able to adapt to extremes in environmental temperature and more vulnerable to both hypothermia and hyperthermia.

Changes in assessment findings result from age-related alterations in the various components of the nervous system. Age-related changes in the nervous system and differences in assessment findings are presented in Table 58.4.

ASSESSMENT OF THE NERVOUS SYSTEM

Because of the complexity of the nervous system, neurological assessment is challenging and lengthy. Involving family members in the assessment is critical because patients with neurological disorders often experience cognitive, emotional, and motivational deficits. Careful observation is an especially important nursing skill because many neurological changes are subtle.

Subjective Data

The history should begin with an open-ended and indirect inquiry that allows the patient to describe the chief complaint and current health (Jarvis et al., 2019). Three points should be considered in documenting the history of a patient with neurological conditions. First, questions about symptoms should be open-ended. It is better to ask, "What is your headache like?" rather than "Do you experience headaches?" It is also better to allow the patient to provide the details, for example, "Is there anything about your right side that bothers you?" than to ask leading questions like, "Is your headache throbbing?" or "Are you weak on the right side?" Second, the mode of onset and the course of the illness are especially important aspects of the history. The nature of a neurological disease process can often be described by these facts alone, and the nurse should obtain all pertinent data in the history of the present illness, especially data related to the characteristics and progression of the symptoms. Third, because many neurological diseases affect a patient's mental functioning, mental status must be assessed

TABLE 58.4 AGE-RELATED DIFFERENCES IN ASSESSMENT

Nervous System

Component	Changes	Differences in Assessment Findings
Central Nervous System		
Brain	Reduction in cerebral blood flow and metabolism	Alterations in certain mental functions
	Decrease in efficiency of temperature-regulating mechanism	Decrease in body temperature, impairment of ability to adapt to environmental temperature
	Decrease in neurotransmitter volume, disruption in integration as result of loss of neurons	Conduction of nerve impulses slowed, response time slowed
	Decrease in oxygen supply, changes in basal ganglia caused by vascular changes	Changes in gait and ambulation; diminished kinesthetic sense
	Cerebral tissue atrophy and increased size of ventricles	Altered balance, vertigo, syncope; increased postural hypotension; decreased proprioception; decreased sensation
Peripheral Nervous System		
Cranial and spinal nerves	Loss of myelin and decrease in conduction time in some nerves	Decrease in reaction time in specific nerves
	Cellular degeneration, death of neurons	Decrease in speed and intensity of neuronal reflexes
Functional Divisions		
Motor	Decrease in muscle bulk	Diminished strength and agility
	Decrease in electrical activity	Increased reaction and movement time
Sensory*	Decrease in sensory receptors, caused by degenerative changes and involution of fine corpuscles of nerve endings	Diminished sense of touch; inability to localize stimuli; decrease in appreciation of touch, temperature, and peripheral vibrations
	Decrease in electrical activity	Slowing of or alteration in sensory reception
	Atrophy of taste buds	Signs of malnutrition, weight loss
	Degeneration and loss of fibres in olfactory bulb	Diminished sense of smell
	Degenerative changes in nerve cells in vestibular system of inner ear, cerebellum, and proprioceptive pathways in nervous system	Poor ability to maintain balance, widened gait
Reflexes	Possible decrease in deep tendon reflexes	Below-average reflex score
	Decrease in sensory conduction velocity as result of myelin sheath degeneration	Sluggish reflexes, lengthened reaction time
Reticular Formation		
Reticular activating system	Modification of hypothalamic function, reduction in stage IV sleep	Increase in frequency of spontaneous awakening, together with tiredness, interrupted sleep, insomnia
Autonomic Nervous System		
SNS and PSNS	Morphological changes in features of ganglia, slowing of ANS responses	Orthostatic hypotension, systolic hypertension

ANS, autonomic nervous system; *PSNS*, parasympathetic nervous system; *SNS*, sympathetic nervous system.
*Specific changes related to the eye and the ear are described in Chapter 24.

accurately before the nurse assumes that the history is factual. If the patient is not considered a reliable historian, the history should be obtained from a person who has first-hand knowledge of the patient's health problems. In many cases, a complete health history cannot be obtained, and the nurse must proceed with only objective data.

Important Health Information

Past Health History. The health history helps guide the approach for the neurological examination; that is, it can direct the nurse toward the parts of the nervous system that must be closely assessed. If the patient's primary complaint is dizziness, the examination may be focused on visual, vestibular, and cerebellar functions rather than on somatic motor and sensory functions.

CASE STUDY

Patient Introduction

E. J. (pronouns she/her), 66 years old, arrives in the emergency department after falling in the middle of the night when getting up to go to the bathroom. She states that her fall happened because of her inability to control her left leg. E. J.'s partner brought her to the hospital but states that there was difficulty getting her to the car.

Critical Thinking

Throughout this assessment chapter, think about E. J.'s concerns, with the following questions in mind:

1. What are the possible causes for E. J.'s acute leg weakness?
2. What type of assessment would be most appropriate for E. J.: comprehensive, focused, or emergency? What would the priority assessment be?
3. What questions should the nurse ask E. J.?
4. What should be included in the physical assessment? What should the nurse be looking for?
5. What diagnostic studies might be ordered?

See Case Study: Subjective Data, Case Study: Objective Data: Physical Examination, and Case Study: Objective Data: Diagnostic Studies for more information on E. J.

ⓔvolve

Answers are available at http://evolve.elsevier.com/Canada/Lewis/med surg.

Medications. Special attention should be given to obtaining a careful medication history, especially the use of sedatives, opioids, tranquilizers, mood-elevating drugs, over-the-counter medications, and herbal remedies. Many medications can cause adverse neurological effects.

Surgery or Other Treatments. The nurse should inquire about any surgery involving any part of the nervous system, such as the head or brain, the spine or spinal cord, or the sensory organs. If a patient has had surgery, the date, the cause, the procedure, the recovery, and the current status should be investigated.

The perinatal history may reveal exposure to toxic agents such as viruses, alcohol, tobacco, drugs, and radiation, which are known to adversely influence the development of the nervous system. The history may reveal a difficult labour and delivery, which can cause brain damage as a result of hypoxia, forceps delivery, or Rh incompatibility.

Growth and developmental history can be important in ascertaining whether nervous system dysfunction was present at an early age. The nurse should specifically inquire about major developmental tasks such as walking and talking. Successes at school or identified problems in an educational setting are other

important developmental data to gather. Often, this information is not available when an older patient is interviewed.

Health Status. Key questions to ask a patient with a neurological condition are presented in Table 58.5.

General Health Practices. The nurse should ask about the patient's general health practices that may affect the nervous system, such as substance use and smoking, nutrition, participation in physical and recreational activities, use of seat belts and helmets, and control of hypertension. The nurse should ask about previous hospitalizations for neurological disorders. A careful family history may determine whether the neurological condition has a hereditary or congenital background.

GENETICS IN CLINICAL PRACTICE

Huntington's Disease

- Huntington's disease is a genetically transmitted, autosomal dominant disorder.
- Major neurological disorders that may have a genetic basis are multiple sclerosis, headaches, Parkinson's disease, and Alzheimer's disease. The presence of these disorders in a family history increases the likelihood of similar disorders occurring in the patient.
- A careful family history may determine whether a neurological disorder has a genetic basis.

If the patient has an existing neurological disorder, the nurse should ask about how it affects daily living and the ability to carry out self-care. After a careful review of information, and with the patient's permission, the nurse may find it helpful to ask someone who knows the patient well whether any mental or physical changes have been noticed in the patient. The patient with a neurological disorder may not be aware of it or may be unable to provide enough specific data to aid in the diagnosis.

Nutritional Challenges. Neurological disorders can result in inadequate nutrition. Challenges related to chewing, swallowing, facial nerve paralysis, or muscle coordination could make it difficult for affected patients to ingest adequate nutrients. Also, certain vitamins, such as thiamine (B_1), niacin (B_3), and pyridoxine (B_6), are essential for the maintenance and health of the CNS. Deficiencies in one or more of these vitamins could result in such nonspecific conditions as depression, apathy, neuritis, weakness, mental confusion, and irritability. Risk for cobalamin (vitamin B_{12}) deficiency is higher in older persons because they may have difficulties with vitamin absorption. Untreated, this deficiency may cause a decline in mental function (Wolffenbuttel et al., 2019).

Bowel and Bladder Disorders. Bowel and bladder disorders are often associated with neurological disorders, such as stroke, head injury, spinal cord injury, multiple sclerosis, and dementia. To plan appropriate interventions, it is important to determine whether the bowel or bladder condition was present before or after the neurological event. Incontinence of urine and feces and urinary retention are the most common elimination challenges associated with a neurological disorder or its treatment (Panicker & Sakakibara, 2020). For example, nerve root compression leads to a sudden onset of incontinence. The details of the disorder—such as number of episodes, accompanying sensations or lack of sensations, and measures taken to control the disorder—must be documented carefully.

Motor Disorders. Many neurological disorders can cause difficulties in the patient's mobility, strength, and coordination. Neurological disorders can result in changes in the patient's usual activity and exercise patterns. These problems can also

TABLE 58.5 HEALTH HISTORY

Nervous System

Headaches
- Have you had any unusually frequent or severe headaches?
- When did this start? How often does this happen?
- Show me where you feel the pain in your head.
- What do you think the headaches are caused by?

Head Injury
- Please describe any head injuries you have had.
- Which part of your head was injured?
- Did you lose consciousness? For how long?

Dizziness or Vertigo
- Have you ever felt light-headed or faint?
- When does this feeling occur? Does activity or change in position bring this on?
- Do you ever feel something called *vertigo* (a spinning sensation)? Does the room spin (objective vertigo)? Do you feel you are spinning (subjective vertigo)?

Seizures
- Have you ever had seizures or convulsions? When did they start? How often did they or do they occur?
- When a seizure starts, do you have any warning? What do you experience?
- Where in your body do the seizures begin? On one side or both? Do they travel through your body? Are your muscles tense or limp?
- Are there other signs that go along with the seizures (loss of consciousness, colour change in face or lips, eyelid fluttering, eye-rolling, lip smacking, or incontinence)?
- After the seizure, are you told that you fall asleep or experience confusion, weakness, headache, or muscle ache?
- What seems to bring on the seizures (activity, discontinuing medications, fatigue, stress)?
- Are you taking medication for the seizures?
- How have the seizures affected your daily life?

Tremors
- Have you experienced any shaking or tremors in the hands or the face? When did these start?
- Are the tremors worse with anxiety? With deliberate movement? With rest?
- Are the tremors better with rest? With activity? With alcohol?
- Do the tremors affect your daily activity?

Weakness
- Do you have any weakness or difficulty moving any body part? Is the weakness just in one body part or everywhere?
- Does this occur with any particular movement? (Example: difficulty getting out of a chair may signal proximal or large muscle weakness, whereas distal or small muscle weakness makes it difficult to open a jar or to write.)

Coordination
- Do you have any problems with coordination or balance when walking?
- Do you lean to one side?
- Do you have any problems with falling? Which way?
- Do your legs give out from under you?
- Do you have any clumsy movement?

Numbness or Tingling
- Have you experienced any numbness or tingling? Does it feel like pins and needles? When did this start? Is it worse with activity?
- Show me where you feel this.

Difficulty Swallowing
- Do you have any difficulty swallowing? Does this occur with solids or liquids?
- Have you experienced excessive salivation or drooling?

Difficulty Speaking
- Have you had any difficulties with forming words or with saying what you meant to say?
- When did this start? How long did it last?

Significant Past History
- Have you ever had a stroke, a spinal cord or head injury, meningitis, or encephalitis?
- Do you have any congenital defects?
- Have you had past problems with alcohol or drug use?

Environmental and Occupational Hazards
- Are you exposed to any environmental or occupational hazards such as insecticides, lead, or organic solvents?
- Do you use head protection for work, sporting, or leisure activities (e.g., hard hats, bicycle helmets, motorcycle helmets)?
- Are you taking any medications now, including pain medications?
- How much alcohol do you drink? Each day? Each week?
- Do you use any mood-altering drugs—marijuana, barbiturates, tranquilizers?

Additional History for Older Persons
- Have you had any increase in falls? Is this related to dizziness? Does this occur with movement (e.g., change of position) or after taking medications?
- Have you had any changes in memory or mental function? Have you felt any confusion? Has it come on suddenly or gradually?
- Have you noticed any tremors? Are they in your hands or face? Do they change with activity, rest, or use of alcohol? Do they interfere with your daily life?
- Have you had any sudden vision changes? Did this occur with weakness or loss of consciousness?

Source: Adapted from Jarvis, C., Browne, A. J., Macdonald-Jenkins, J., et al. (2019). *Physical examination & health assessment* (3rd Canadian ed., pp. 697–747). Elsevier Inc.

result in falls (Baker, 2018). Many activities of daily living, such as getting out of a bed or chair, ambulating, preparing meals, and performing personal hygiene, can be affected and should be assessed. The ability to perform fine motor tasks may be affected, which increases the possibility of personal injury.

Sleep Disorders. Sleep pattern disruptions can be both a cause of and a response to many neurologically related concerns. Discomfort from pain and inability to move and change to a position of comfort because of muscle weakness and paralysis could interfere with sound sleep. Hallucinations resulting from dementia or medications can also interrupt sleep. The nurse should carefully document the sleep disorder and the patient's methods of coping with it.

Cognition and Sensory Disorders. Because the nervous system controls cognition and sensory integration, many neurological disorders affect these functions. The nurse should assess orientation, memory, language, calculation ability, problem-solving ability, insight, and judgement. A structured mental status questionnaire is often used to evaluate these functions and provide baseline data.

Information about sensory changes related to hearing, sight, and touch should be sought. The patient should be questioned about problems with vertigo and sensitivity to heat and cold.

Ability to both use and understand language is a cognitive function that the nurse should assess. Appropriateness of responses is a useful indicator of cognitive and perceptual ability, but it is culturally determined.

Pain is a common event associated with many health conditions. Pain is often the reason why patients seek health care. A patient's pain should be assessed carefully (see Chapter 10).

Emotional Challenges. Neurological disease can drastically alter control over one's life and create dependency on others for daily needs. A patient's physical appearance and emotional control can be affected. The nurse should ask in a sensitive manner about the patient's evaluation of self-worth, perception of abilities, body image, and general emotional pattern. The physical sequelae of a neurological disorder can seriously strain the patient's coping abilities. The nurse should determine whether coping abilities are sufficient to meet the challenges faced by the patient.

Relationship Issues. The patient should be asked whether a neurological condition has resulted in changes to roles such as spouse, parent, or breadwinner. Physical impairments such as weakness and paralysis can alter or limit participation in usual roles and activities. Cognitive changes, however, can permanently change a person's ability to maintain previous roles. These changes can dramatically affect both the patient and significant others. Dependent relationships can develop.

Sexual Issues. Because many nervous system disorders can affect sexual functioning, sexual health may be an important part of the assessment for some patients. Cerebral lesions may inhibit the desire phase or the reflex responses of the excitement phase. Brainstem and spinal cord lesions may partially or completely interrupt the connections between the brain and the effector systems necessary for intercourse.

Neuropathies and spinal cord lesions that affect sensation, especially in the erotic zones, may decrease desire. Autonomic neuropathies and lesions of the sacral cord and the cauda equina may prevent reflex activities of the sexual response. The nurse should determine whether the patient and the partner are satisfied with their sexual activity. The use or need for alternative methods of achieving sexual satisfaction should be explored. Despite neurologically related changes in sexual functioning, many people can achieve satisfying expression of intimacy and affection.

CASE STUDY

Subjective Data

A subjective assessment of E. J. revealed the following information:
- **History of current illness:** States that her fall was due to sudden weakness in her left leg. States she had a brief episode of left-sided weakness and tingling of her face, arm, and hand 3 months ago. The symptoms totally resolved and no treatment was sought. Denies dizziness, change in hearing, or memory deficits. Has never been hospitalized for a neurological disorder. Is depressed and fearful. Concerned about a stroke.
- **Past health history:** Hyperlipidemia, hypertension
- **Medications:** Pravastatin 40 mg/day PO; lisinopril 10 mg/day PO
- **Functional assessment:** Has smoked one pack of cigarettes per day since age 28 years. Drinks alcohol occasionally. Hypertension controlled when on medication but has not taken lisinopril for a few weeks because did not have enough money for the refill and was waiting for next Social Assistance cheque. E. J. is 160 cm tall and weighs 73 kg. States that up until tonight she was able to walk slowly, but with pain in the knees and hips.

See Case Study: Patient Introduction, Case Study: Objective Data: Physical Examination, and Case Study: Objective Data: Diagnostic Studies for more information on E. J.

Objective Data

Physical Examination. The standard neurological examination helps determine the presence, the location, and the nature of disease of the nervous system. In this examination, six categories of functions are assessed: mental status, function of cranial nerves, motor function, cerebellar function, sensory function, and reflex function. The choice of particular parts of the examination depends on what information is needed. The nurse should develop a systematic and consistent approach to assessment.

Mental Status. Assessment of mental status (cerebral functioning) gives an indication of how the patient is functioning. It involves determination of complex and high-level cerebral functions that are governed by many areas of the cerebral cortex. Much of the mental status examination can be conducted during the routine history and may not need to be evaluated further. For example, language and memory can be assessed when the patient is asked for details of the illness and significant past events. The patient's cultural and educational background should be taken into account when mental status is evaluated.

The components of the mental status examination are as follows:

- *General appearance and behaviour:* This component includes motor activity, body posture, dress and hygiene, facial expression, and speech.
- *Level of consciousness (LOC):* This is the most sensitive indicator of changes in neurological status (McCance et al., 2018). LOC concerns arousal and wakefulness and the ability to respond to the environment. The Glasgow Coma Scale is often used to assess a patient's response to stimuli (see Chapter 59 and Table 59.4).
- *Cognition:* The nurse should note the patient's orientation to time, place, person, and situation. Further assessment of memory, intellectual ability, insight, judgement, problem solving, and calculation may be warranted (see Chapter 62). The nurse should consider whether the patient's plans and goals match the patient's physical and mental capabilities. Difficulties with memory may have implications for retention of new information, and impaired judgement and insight may jeopardize the patient's safety.
- *Mood and affect:* The nurse should note restlessness, agitation, anger, depression, or euphoria and the appropriateness of these states. The nurse should also note whether the patient's affect is appropriate for the situation.
- *Thought content:* The nurse should note the presence or report of illusions, hallucinations, delusions, or paranoia.

Function of Cranial Nerves. Testing of each cranial nerve is an essential component of the neurological examination (see Figure 58.12).

Olfactory Nerve. After determining that both nostrils are patent, the olfactory nerve (CN I) is tested by asking the patient to close one nostril, close both eyes, and sniff from a bottle containing coffee, spice, soap, or some other readily recognized odour. The same procedure is done for the other nostril. In general, olfaction is not tested unless the patient has some disturbance with smell. Chronic rhinitis, sinusitis, and heavy smoking can often decrease the sense of smell. Disturbance in ability to smell may be associated with a tumour involving the olfactory bulb, or it may be the result of a basilar skull fracture that has damaged the olfactory fibres as they pass through the delicate cribriform plate of the skull.

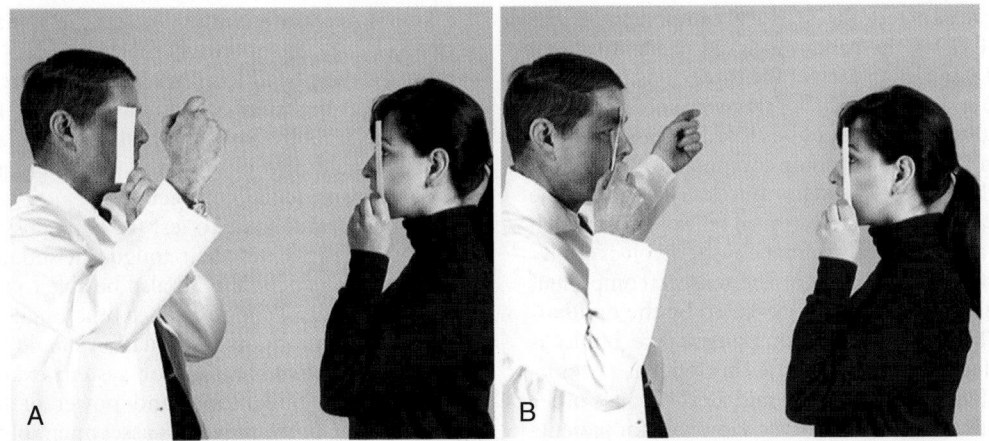

FIG. 58.16 Assessment of visual fields by gross confrontation. In gross confrontation, the target is moved in a flat plane between the nurse and the patient. The nurse's own monocular field is compared with that of that patient. **A,** Assessing left visual fields of right eye. **B,** Assessing right visual fields of right eye.

Optic Nerve. Visual fields and visual acuity are assessed to test the function of the optic nerve (CN II). Visual fields are assessed by gross confrontation. The nurse, positioned directly opposite the patient, asks the patient to close one eye, look directly at the bridge of the nurse's nose, and indicate when an object (finger, pencil tip, head of pin) presented from the periphery of each of the four visual field quadrants becomes visible (Figure 58.16). The same test is repeated for the other eye. The nurse is used as a control because both nurse and patient are sharing the same visual field. It is important to remember that the nasal side of the visual field is narrower because of the nasal bridge. Visual field defects may arise from lesions of the optic nerve, the optic chiasm, or the tracts that extend through the temporal, parietal, and occipital lobes. Visual field changes resulting from brain lesions are usually a *hemianopia* (one-half of the visual field is affected), a *quadrantanopsia* (one-fourth of the visual field is affected), or monocular (one eye is affected).

To test visual acuity, the patient reads a Snellen chart from 6 metres away. The nurse records the number of the lowest line that the patient can read accurately. The patient who wears glasses should wear them during testing, unless they are used only for reading. The eyes should be tested individually and together. If a Snellen chart is not available, the patient should be asked to read newsprint for a gross assessment of acuity. The distance from the patient to the newsprint required for accurate reading should be recorded. Acuity may not be testable by these means if the patient does not read English or has aphasia (a language disorder).

Funduscopy is used to assess the physical condition of the optic disc (head of the optic nerve), as well as that of the retina and the blood vessels. This procedure is routinely performed when the optic nerve is tested. Optic nerve atrophy and papilledema can be detected by this method.

Oculomotor, Trochlear, and Abducens Nerves. Because the oculomotor (CN III), trochlear (CN IV), and abducens (CN VI) nerves all help move the eye, they are tested together for what are termed *extraocular movements*. The patient is asked to keep the head steady and to follow the nurse's finger only with the eyes. The nurse should keep the finger back about 30 cm so that the patient can focus on it comfortably. The nurse moves the finger to each of the six positions (right and up, right, right and down, left and up, left, left and down), holds it momentarily, and then moves back to the centre (Figure 58.17). A normal response is parallel tracking of the object with both eyes.

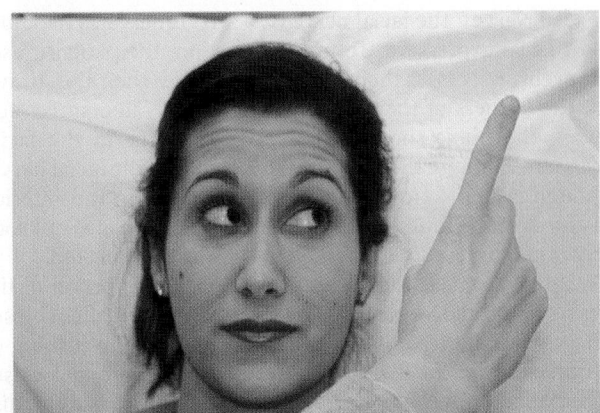

FIG. 58.17 Nurse checking extraocular movement. Normally, both eyes move together. Eye movements should be smooth and coordinated.

If weakness or paralysis is present in one of the eye muscles, the eyes do not move together, and the patient has a *disconjugate gaze*. The presence and direction of *nystagmus* (fine, rapid jerking movements of the eyes) are observed at this time, even though this condition most often indicates vestibulocerebellar disorders.

Other functions of the oculomotor nerve are tested by checking for pupillary constriction and for *convergence* (eyes turning inward) and *accommodation* (pupils constricting with near vision). To test pupillary constriction, the nurse shines a light into the pupil of one eye and looks for *ipsilateral* (same side) constriction of the same pupil and *contralateral* (consensual) constriction of the opposite eye. The size and shape of the pupils are also noted. For this reflex to occur, the optic nerve must be intact. Testing for papillary constriction is an important component of the neurological assessment of patients at risk for herniation (see Chapter 59). Because the oculomotor nerve exits at the top of the brainstem at the tentorial notch, it can be easily compressed by expanding mass lesions in the cerebral hemispheres. The result is that the pupil does not constrict in response to light; it may become dilated because the sympathetic input to the pupil acts unopposed. To test convergence and accommodation, the patient focuses on the nurse's finger as it moves toward the patient's nose. Another function of the oculomotor nerve is to keep the eyelid open. Damage to the nerve can cause *ptosis* (drooping eyelid), pupillary abnormalities, and eye muscle weakness.

Trigeminal Nerve. To test the sensory component of the trigeminal nerve (CN V), the patient is asked to identify light touch (cotton) and pinprick in each of the three divisions (ophthalmic, maxillary, and mandibular) of the nerve on both sides of the face. The patient's eyes should be closed during this part of the examination. To test the motor component, the patient clenches their teeth, and the masseter muscles, just above the mandibular angle, are palpated. The corneal reflex test, in which CN V and CN VII are evaluated simultaneously, involves applying a cotton wisp strand to the cornea. The sensory component of this reflex (corneal sensation) is innervated by the ophthalmic division of CN V. The motor component (eye blink) is innervated by the facial nerve (CN VII). This reflex is not normally tested in patients who are awake and alert because other tests are used to evaluate these two nerves. However, for patients with a decreased LOC, the corneal reflex test provides an opportunity to evaluate the integrity of the brainstem at the level of the pons because the fibres of CN V and CN VII have connections in this area.

Facial Nerve. The facial nerve (CN VII) innervates the muscles of facial expression. To test its function, the patient raises their eyebrows, closes their eyes tightly, purses their lips, draws back the corners of their mouth in an exaggerated smile, and frowns. The nurse should note any asymmetry in the facial movements because this can indicate damage to the facial nerve. Although taste discrimination of salt and sugar in the anterior two-thirds of the tongue is a function of this nerve, it is not routinely tested unless a peripheral nerve lesion is suspected.

Vestibulocochlear Nerve. To test the cochlear portion of the acoustic (vestibulocochlear) nerve (CN VIII), the patient closes their eyes and indicates when a ticking watch or the rustling of the nurse's fingertips is heard as the stimulus is brought closer to the patient's ear. Each ear is tested individually, and the distance from the patient's ear to the sound source when first heard is recorded. This test identifies only gross deficits in hearing. For more precise assessment of hearing, an audiometer (or tuning forks) can be used (see Chapter 23). The vestibular portion of this nerve is not routinely tested unless the patient reports dizziness, vertigo, or unsteadiness or has auditory dysfunction. In a patient who is unconscious, the oculocephalic reflex (movement of the eyes when the head is briskly turned to the side) may be assessed.

Glossopharyngeal and Vagus Nerves. The glossopharyngeal and vagus nerves are tested together because both innervate the pharynx. The glossopharyngeal nerve (CN IX) is primarily sensory. In the gag reflex (bilateral contraction of the palatal muscles initiated by stroking or touching either side of the posterior pharynx or soft palate with a tongue blade), the sensory component is mediated by CN IX and the major motor component by the vagus nerve (CN X). It is important to assess the gag reflex in patients who have a decreased LOC, a brainstem lesion, or a disease involving the throat musculature. If the reflex is weak or absent, the patient may be at risk of aspirating food or secretions. The strength and efficiency of swallowing are important to test in these patients for the same reason. In another test for an awake, cooperative patient, the patient phonates by saying "ah" and the nurse notes the bilateral symmetry of elevation of the soft palate. Any asymmetry can indicate weakness or paralysis. To assess swallowing, the nurse's hands are held lightly on either side of the patient's throat while the patient swallows. Any asymmetry is noted. If the patient is endotracheally intubated, the cough reflex (elicited when the suction catheter contacts the carina of the respiratory tree) is a method of assessing CN X.

Spinal Accessory Nerve. To test the spinal accessory nerve (CN XI), the patient shrugs their shoulders against resistance and turns their head to either side against resistance. The contraction of the sternocleidomastoid and trapezius muscles should be smooth. Symmetry, atrophy, or fasciculation of the muscle should also be noted. A *fasciculation* is a small, local involuntary muscular contraction.

Hypoglossal Nerve. To test the hypoglossal nerve (CN XII), the patient sticks out their tongue. It should protrude in the midline. The patient should also be able to push the tongue to either side against the resistance of a tongue blade. Again, any asymmetry, atrophy, or fasciculation should be noted.

Motor Function. The motor system examination includes assessment of bulk, tone, and power of the major muscle groups of the body, as well as assessment of balance and coordination. To test strength, the patient pushes and pulls against the resistance of the nurse's arm as it opposes flexion and extension of the patient's muscle. The patient should be asked to offer resistance at the shoulders, elbows, wrists, hips, knees, and ankles. The patient's grip strength can also be tested. To test for mild weakness of the upper extremities, the patient extends both arms forward at shoulder height with palms up while the eyes are closed. Mild weakness of the arm is demonstrated by downward drifting of the arm or pronation of the palm (*pronator drift*). Any weakness or asymmetry of strength between the same muscle groups of the right and left side should be noted.

To test tone, the limbs are passively moved through their range of motion; there should be a slight resistance to these movements. Abnormal tone is described as *hypotonia* (flaccidity) or *hypertonia* (spasticity). Involuntary movements—such as tics, tremor, *myoclonus* (spasm of muscles), *athetosis* (slow, writhing, involuntary movements of extremities), *chorea* (involuntary, purposeless, rapid motions), and *dystonia* (impairment of muscle tone)—should be noted.

To test cerebellar function, balance and coordination are assessed. A good screening test for both balance and muscle strength is to observe the patient's stance (posture while standing) and gait. The nurse should note the pace and rhythm of the gait and observe the arm swing. (The arms should move symmetrically and in the opposite direction of the leg on the same side.) The patient's ability to ambulate is a key factor in determining the amount of nursing care that is needed and the risk for injury from falling. A patient with cerebellar disease may have an *ataxic* or *staggering gait*, in which the feet are placed wide apart and the steps are unsteady.

Coordination can be easily tested in several ways. In the finger-to-nose test, the patient alternately touches their nose with their index finger and then touches the nurse's finger. The nurse repositions the finger while the patient is touching the nose so that the patient must adjust to a new distance each time the nurse's finger is touched. These movements should be performed smoothly and accurately. Other tests include asking the patient to pronate and supinate both hands rapidly and to perform a shallow knee bend, first on one leg and then on the other. Dysarthria or slurred speech should be noted because it is a sign of incoordination of the speech muscles.

In the heel-to-shin test, the patient places one heel on the opposite shin below the knee and moves the heel down the shin to the ankle. This procedure is repeated for the other leg. These movements should flow smoothly without jerking or hesitation.

Sensory Function. Several modalities are tested in the somatic sensory examination. Each modality is carried by a specific ascending pathway in the spinal cord before it reaches the sensory cortex.

There are some general guidelines for performing the sensory examination. The patient should always have their eyes closed to avoid visual clues. The nurse should avoid giving verbal cues such as, "Is this sharp?" The sensory stimulus should be applied in such a way that the patient does not expect it; that is, the nurse should avoid rhythmic application of the stimulus. In the routine neurological examination, sensory testing of the four extremities is sufficient. However, if a disturbance in sensory function of the skin is identified, the boundaries of that dysfunction should be carefully delineated along the dermatome.

Light Touch. The sensation of light touch is usually tested first. The nurse gently strokes each of the four extremities with a cotton wisp and asks the patient to indicate when the stimulus is felt by saying "touch." (The sensory examination of the trigeminal nerve may be delayed until this time because the same material for testing sensation is used.)

Pain and Temperature. Pain is tested by touching the skin with the sharp end of a safety pin. This stimulus is irregularly alternated with a simple touch stimulus with the dull end of the pin to determine whether the patient can distinguish the two stimuli.

The sensation of temperature is tested by applying tubes of warm and cold water to the skin and asking the patient to identify the stimuli with their eyes closed. If pain sensation is intact, assessment of temperature sensation may be omitted because both sensations are carried by the same ascending pathways.

Vibration Sense. To assess vibration sense, a vibrating C128 tuning fork is applied to the patient's fingernails and the bony prominences of the hands, the legs, and the feet while the patient's eyes are closed. The nurse asks the patient whether the vibration or "buzz" is felt. The nurse then asks the patient to indicate when the vibration ceases. The nurse stops the vibration with the hand as desired.

Position Sense. To assess position sense, the nurse places their thumb and forefinger on either side of the patient's forefinger or great toe and gently moves the patient's digit up or down. The patient is asked to indicate the direction in which the digit is moved.

Another test of position sense of the lower extremities is the *Romberg test.* The patient is asked to stand with their feet together and then to close their eyes. If the patient is able to maintain balance with the eyes open but sways or falls with the eyes closed (i.e., a positive result of the Romberg test), disease may be present in the posterior columns of the spinal cord or the cerebellum. It is important for the nurse to ensure the patient's safety during this test.

Cortical Sensory Functions. Several tests are used to evaluate cortical integration of sensory perceptions (which occurs in the parietal lobes). The patient's eyes should remain closed during these assessments. To assess two-point discrimination, the two points of a calibrated compass are placed on the tips of the patient's fingers and toes. The minimum recognizable separation is 4 to 5 mm in the fingertips and a greater degree of separation elsewhere. This test is important in diagnosing diseases of the sensory cortex and the PNS.

To test *graphesthesia* (ability to feel writing on skin), the patient is asked to identify numbers traced on the palm of the hands. To test *stereognosis* (ability to perceive the form and

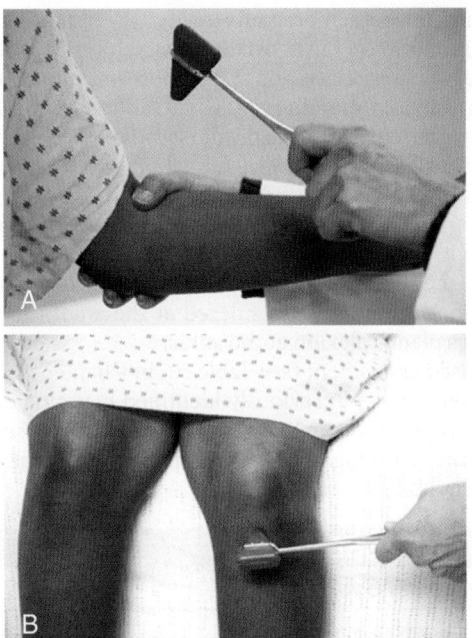

FIG. 58.18 The nurse strikes a swift blow over a stretched tendon to elicit a stretch reflex. **A,** Biceps reflex. **B,** Patellar reflex.

nature of objects), the patient is asked to identify the size and shape of easily recognized objects (e.g., coins, keys, a safety pin) placed in the hands. To evaluate sensory extinction or inattention, the nurse touches both sides of the patient's body simultaneously. An abnormal response occurs when the patient perceives the stimulus only on one side. The other stimulus is "extinguished."

Reflex Function. Tendons attached to skeletal muscles have receptors that are sensitive to stretch. A reflex contraction of the skeletal muscle occurs when the tendon is stretched. A simple muscle stretch reflex is initiated by briskly tapping the tendon of a stretched muscle, usually with a reflex hammer (Figure 58.18). The response (muscle contraction of the corresponding muscle) is measured as follows:

0	Absence of response—always abnormal
1+	Slight but definitely present response—may or may not be normal
2+	Brisk response—normal
3+	Very brisk response—may or may not be normal
4+	Repeating reflex (clonus)—always abnormal

Clonus is a continued rhythmic contraction of the muscle with continuous application of the stimulus.

In general, the biceps, triceps, brachioradialis, and patellar and Achilles tendon reflexes are tested. The nurse elicits the biceps reflex by placing their thumb over the patient's biceps tendon in the antecubital space and striking the thumb with a hammer. The nurse should support the patient's forearm so that it is partially flexed at the elbow, with the palm up and relaxed. The normal response is flexion of the arm at the elbow or contraction of the biceps muscle that can be felt by the nurse's thumb.

To elicit the triceps reflex, the nurse should support the patient's upper arm (to let the arm hang limply) and then strike the patient's triceps tendon above the elbow. The normal response is extension of the arm or visible contraction of the triceps.

To elicit the brachioradialis reflex, the nurse strikes the patient's radius 3 to 5 cm above the wrist while the patient's arm is relaxed. The normal response is flexion and supination at the elbow or visible contraction of the brachioradialis muscle.

To elicit the patellar reflex, the nurse strikes the patient's patellar tendon just below the patella. The patient can be sitting or lying as long as the leg being tested hangs freely. The normal response is extension of the leg with contraction of the quadriceps.

To elicit the Achilles tendon reflex, the nurse strikes the patient's Achilles tendon while the patient's leg is flexed at the knee and the foot is dorsiflexed at the ankle. The normal response is plantar flexion at the ankle.

A focused assessment (see Table 3.6 in Chapter 3) is used to evaluate the status of previously identified neurological conditions and to monitor for signs of new ones. A focused assessment of the neurological system is presented in the Focused Assessment box.

FOCUSED ASSESSMENT

Neurological System

Use this checklist to make sure the key assessment steps have been performed.

Subjective
Ask the patient about any of the following, and note responses:

Blackouts or loss of memory	Y	N
Weakness, numbness, tingling sensation in arms or legs	Y	N
Headaches, especially of new onset	Y	N
Loss of balance or coordination	Y	N
Orientation to person, place, and time	Y	N

Objective: Diagnostic
Check the following laboratory results for critical values:

Lumbar puncture	✓
CT or MRI of brain	✓
EEG	✓

Objective: Physical Examination
Inspect or observe the following:

General level of consciousness and orientation	✓
Oropharynx for gag reflex and soft palate movement	✓
Peripheral sensation of light touch and pinprick (face, hands, feet)	✓
Sense of smell with an alcohol wipe	✓
Eyes for extraocular movements, PERRLA, peripheral vision, nystagmus	✓
Gait for smoothness and coordination	✓

Palpate for the following:

Strength of neck, shoulders, arms, and legs; full and symmetrical	✓

Percuss for the following:

Reflexes	✓

CT, computed tomographic (scan); *EEG,* electroencephalogram; *MRI,* magnetic resonance imaging; *PERRLA,* pupils equal, round, and reactive to light and accommodation.

Table 58.6 is a listing of normal findings in a neurological assessment. Abnormal assessment findings of the neurological system are presented in Table 58.7.

Diagnostic Studies of the Nervous System

Numerous diagnostic studies are available to assess the nervous system. Table 58.8 presents the most commonly encountered studies.

TABLE 58.6 NORMAL PHYSICAL ASSESSMENT OF THE NERVOUS SYSTEM*

Mental Status
Alert and oriented, orderly thought processes, appropriate mood and affect

Cranial Nerves[†]
Sense of smell intact for soap and coffee; visual fields full to confrontation; visual acuity 20/20 in both eyes; intact extraocular movements; no nystagmus; pupils equal, round, reactive to light and accommodation; intact facial sensation for touch and pinprick; facial movements full; intact gag and swallow reflexes; symmetrical elevation of soft palate; full strength with head turning and shrugging of shoulders against resistance; midline protrusion of tongue

Motor System
Normal gait and station; normal tandem walk; negative result of Romberg test; normal and symmetrical muscle bulk, tone, strength; smooth performance of finger–nose, heel–shin movements

Sensory System
Intact sensation to light touch, position sense, vibration, pinprick, heat and cold, two-point discrimination; intact stereognosis and graphesthesia

Reflexes[‡]
Biceps, triceps, brachioradialis, patellar, and Achilles tendon reflexes 2+ bilaterally; downward-pointing toes with plantar stimulation

*If some portion of the neurological examination was not performed, this should be indicated (e.g., "Smell not tested").
[†]May also be recorded as "CNs [cranial nerves] I to XII intact."
[‡]May also be recorded as drawing of stick figure indicating reflex strength at appropriate sites.

CASE STUDY

Objective Data: Physical Examination

A physical examination of E. J. reveals the following:
- Alert, oriented, and able to answer questions appropriately but mild slowness in responding
- BP 180/110, HR 94, RR 22, T 37°C
- CNS (Canadian Neurological Scale) (see Chapter 60, Figure 60.11) score is 10
- Left-sided arm weakness (3/5) and leg weakness (4/5)

Throughout this chapter, consider diagnostic studies that may be ordered for E. J.

See Case Study: Patient Introduction, Case Study: Subjective Data, and Case Study: Objective Data: Diagnostic Studies for more information on E. J.

Cerebrospinal Fluid Analysis. CSF analysis provides information about a variety of CNS diseases. Normal CSF fluid is clear, colourless, and free of red blood cells and contains little protein. In conditions such as bacterial meningitis, the CSF may show decreased glucose, increased white blood cells, and increased protein. Normal CSF values are listed in Table 58.9.

Lumbar Puncture. Lumbar puncture is the most common method of obtaining CSF for analysis. It is contraindicated in the presence of increased intracranial pressure or infection at the site of puncture.

Nurses often assist in this procedure because it is usually performed in the patient's room. Before the procedure, the patient should empty the bladder. The patient should lie in the lateral recumbent position, with the back as near as possible to the edge of

TABLE 58.7 ASSESSMENT ABNORMALITIES

Nervous System

Finding	Description	Possible Etiology and Significance
Agnosia	Inability to determine meaning or significance of sensory stimulus	Cerebral cortex lesion
Altered consciousness	Inability to speak, obey commands, open eyes appropriately with verbal or painful stimulus	Intracranial lesions, metabolic disorder, psychiatric disorders
Anaesthesia	Absence of sensation	Lesions in spinal cord, thalamus, sensory cortex, or peripheral sensory nerve
Analgesia	Loss of pain sensation	Lesion in spinothalamic tract or thalamus, lack of or damage to sensory nerve endings
Anisocoria	Unequal pupil size	Lesion, injury, or intracranial pressure in area of midbrain; can also be normal
Anosognosia	Inability to recognize bodily defect or disease	Lesions in right parietal cortex, common in right-sided brain stroke
Aphasia	Loss of language faculty (language comprehension, language expression, or both)	Cerebral cortex lesion
Apraxia	Inability to perform learned movements; defect in motor planning	Cerebral cortex lesion
Astereognosis	Inability to recognize form of object by touch	Lesions in parietal cortex
Ataxia	Lack of coordination of movement	Lesions of sensory or motor pathways, cerebellum; anticonvulsant medication, sedative, or hypnotic drug toxicity (including alcohol)
Bladder dysfunction		
• Atonic (autonomous)	Absence of muscle tone and contractility, enlarged capacity, no discomfort, overflow with large residual, inability to voluntarily empty or empty by reflex	Early stage of spinal cord injury
• Hypotonic	More ability to empty by reflex than with atonic bladder but less than normal	Interruption of afferent pathways from bladder
• Hypertonic	Increase in muscle tone, diminished capacity, reflex emptying, dribbling, incontinence	Lesions in pyramidal tracts (efferent pathways)
Diplopia	Double vision	Lesions affecting nerves of extraocular muscles, cerebellar damage
Dysarthria	Lack of coordination in articulating speech	Lesions in cerebellum or pathway of cranial nerves (including brainstem); anticonvulsant medication, sedative, or hypnotic drug toxicity (including alcohol)
Dyskinesia	Impaired power of voluntary movement, resulting in fragmentary or incomplete movements	Disorders of basal ganglia, idiosyncratic reaction to psychotropic drugs
Dysphagia	Difficulty in swallowing	Lesions involving motor pathways of cranial nerves IX and X (including lower brainstem)
Extensor plantar response (Babinski sign)	Upward-pointing toes with plantar stimulation	Suprasegmental or upper motor neuron lesion
Hemiplegia	Paralysis on one side	Stroke and other lesions involving motor cortex
Homonymous hemianopia	Loss of vision in one side of visual field	Injury or lesions in area of optic tract or its radiations to occipital cortex
Hyperesthesia	Increase in sensation	Shingles, nerve compression, stress, or chronic pain
Hypoesthesia	Decrease in sensation	Impingement or damage of a nerve (e.g., peripheral neuropathy in diabetes)
Muscle atrophy (disuse or denervation atrophy)	Wasting away or diminution in size of muscle	Suprasegmental (upper motor neuron) lesions, segmental (lower motor neuron) lesions
Nystagmus	Jerking or bobbing of eyes as they track moving object	Lesions in cerebellum, brainstem, vestibular system; toxic effects of anticonvulsants, sedatives, hypnotics (including alcohol)
Ophthalmoplegia	Paralysis of eye muscles	Lesions in brainstem or cranial nerves III, IV, and VI
Opisthotonus	Extreme arching of back with retraction of head	Meningitis, tonic phase of grand mal seizure
Papilledema	Swelling of optic disk	Increase in intracranial pressure
Paraplegia	Paralysis of lower extremities	Spinal cord transection or mass lesion (thoracolumbar region)
Tetraplegia (quadriplegia)	Paralysis of all extremities	Spinal cord transection or mass lesion (cervical region or brainstem)

the bed. The nurse should assist the patient in drawing up the knees to the abdomen and flexing the head to the chest. This helps separate the vertebrae so that the needle can be inserted more easily.

Using sterile technique, the physician inserts a long needle below the third lumbar vertebra. This may cause some local discomfort. There is no danger of injuring the spinal cord because the cord terminates between the first and second lumbar vertebrae. However, the patient may experience some pain radiating down the leg or muscle twitching if the needle irritates the spinal root. The nurse can assure the patient that this is temporary and that they are not in danger of being paralyzed.

A manometer is attached to the needle, and CSF pressure is determined after the patient is asked to relax and extend their legs. If the patient does not relax and extend their legs,

TABLE 58.8 DIAGNOSTIC STUDIES

Nervous System

Study	Description and Purpose	Nursing Responsibility
Cerebrospinal Fluid Analysis		
Lumbar puncture	CSF is aspirated by needle insertion in L3–4 or L4–5 interspace to assess many CNS diseases (see Table 58.9).	Help patient assume and maintain lateral recumbent position with knees flexed. Ensure maintenance of strict aseptic technique. Ensure labelling of CSF specimens in proper sequence. Encourage patient to drink fluids. Monitor neurological and vital signs. Administer analgesia as needed.
Radiological		
Cerebral angiography	Serial radiographic visualization of intracranial and extracranial blood vessels can help in detecting vascular lesions and tumours of brain. Contrast medium is used (see Figure 58.19).	Assess for risk for stroke because thrombi may be dislodged during the procedure. Withhold preceding meal. Explain that patient will experience a hot flush of head and neck when contrast medium is injected. Explain need to be absolutely still during the procedure. Monitor neurological and vital signs every 15–30 min for first 2 hr, every hour for next 6 hr, then every 2 hr for 24 hr. Maintain pressure dressing and ice on injection site. Keep patient on bed rest until patient is alert and vital signs are stable. Report any signs of change in neurological status.
Computed tomography (CT)	Computer-assisted radiographic views of several levels or thin cross-sections of body parts can help in detecting conditions such as hemorrhage, space-occupying lesions, cerebral edema, brain atrophy, and other abnormalities (see Figure 58.20, *A*).	Explain that the procedure is noninvasive (if no contrast medium is used). Observe for allergic reaction, and note puncture site (if contrast medium is used). Explain appearance of scanner. Instruct patient to remain absolutely still during the procedure.
Magnetic resonance angiography (MRA)	Differential signal characteristics of flowing blood are studied to evaluate extracranial and intracranial blood vessels. The test provides both anatomical and hemodynamic information. MRA can be used in conjunction with contrast medium (contrast-enhanced MRA [cMRA]). MRA is rapidly replacing cerebral angiography for use in diagnosing cerebrovascular diseases.	Nursing responsibilities are similar to those for MRI.
Magnetic resonance imaging (MRI)	Imaging of brain, spinal cord, and spinal canal by means of magnetic energy helps in detecting infarctions, multiple sclerosis, tumours, trauma, herniation, and seizures. No invasive procedures are required (see Figure 58.20, *B*).	Screen patient for joint replacements and pacemaker in the body. Instruct patient to lie very still for up to 1 hr. Sedation may be necessary if patient is claustrophobic.
Positron emission tomography (PET)	Metabolic activity of brain regions is measured to assess cell death or damage. The test involves the use of radioactive material that shows up as a bright spot on the image.	Explain procedure to the patient. Explain that two IV lines will be inserted. Instruct patient not to take sedatives or tranquilizers and to empty their bladder before the procedure. The patient may be asked to perform different activities during the test.
Single-photon emission computed tomography (SPECT)	This method of scanning is similar to PET, but more stable substances and different detectors are used. Radiolabelled compounds are injected, and their photon emissions can be detected. Images made are an accumulation of labelled compound. SPECT is used to visualize blood flow or oxygen or glucose metabolism in the brain. It is useful in diagnosing strokes, brain tumours, and seizure disorders.	Nursing responsibilities are similar to those for PET.
Skull and spine radiographs	Simple radiographs of the skull and spinal column can help in detecting fractures, spinal misalignment, bone erosion, calcifications, or abnormal vascularity.	Explain to patient that the procedure is noninvasive. Explain positions to be assumed.
Electrographic		
Electroencephalography (EEG)	Electrical activity of the brain is recorded by scalp electrodes to evaluate cerebral disease, CNS effects of systemic diseases, and brain death.	Inform patient that the procedure is painless and without danger of electric shock. The patient may be asked to perform various activities such as hyperventilation during the test. Determine whether any medications (e.g., tranquilizers, anticonvulsant medications) should be withheld. Resume medications after test. Assist patient in washing electrode paste out of their hair.
Electromyography (EMG) and nerve conduction	Electrical activity associated with nerve and skeletal muscle is recorded by insertion of needle electrodes to detect muscle and peripheral nerve disease.	Inform patient of slight discomfort associated with insertion of needles.
Evoked potentials	Electrical activity associated with nerve conduction along sensory pathways is recorded by electrodes placed on the skin and scalp. Stimulus generates the impulse. The procedure is used to diagnose disease, locate nerve damage, and monitor function intraoperatively.	Explain procedure to patient. Instruct patient to avoid using hair spray, gel, or other hair care products and sedative medications such as benzodiazepines and barbiturates.

TABLE 58.8 DIAGNOSTIC STUDIES

Nervous System—cont'd

Study	Description and Purpose	Nursing Responsibility
Magnetoencephalography (MEG)	A sensitivity machine called a *biomagnetometer* is used to detect very small magnetic fields generated by neural activity. It can accurately pinpoint the part of the brain involved in a stroke, seizure, or other disorder or injury. Extracranial magnetic fields, as well as scalp electrical field (EEG), are measured.	MEG, a passive sensor, does not make physical contact with the patient. Explain procedure to patient.
Ultrasonography Carotid duplex studies	Sound waves are used to determine blood flow velocity, which may indicate presence of occlusive vascular disease.	Explain procedure to patient.
Transcranial Doppler ultrasonography	Technology is the same as that used for carotid duplex studies, but intracranial vessels are evaluated.	Explain procedure to patient.

CNS, central nervous system; *CSF,* cerebrospinal fluid; *IV,* intravenous; *VS,* vital signs.

TABLE 58.9 NORMAL CEREBROSPINAL FLUID VALUES

Parameter	Normal Value
Appearance	Clear, colourless
Glucose	2.8–4.2 mmol/L
Microorganisms	None
pH	7.33
Pressure	9–14 mm Hg
Protein	
• Cisternal	0.15–0.25 g/L
• Lumbar	0.15–0.45 g/L
• Ventricular	0.05–0.15 g/L
RBCs	None
Specific gravity	1.007
WBCs	Adult: 0–5 × 10⁹ WBCs/L

RBCs, red blood cells; *WBCs,* white blood cells.

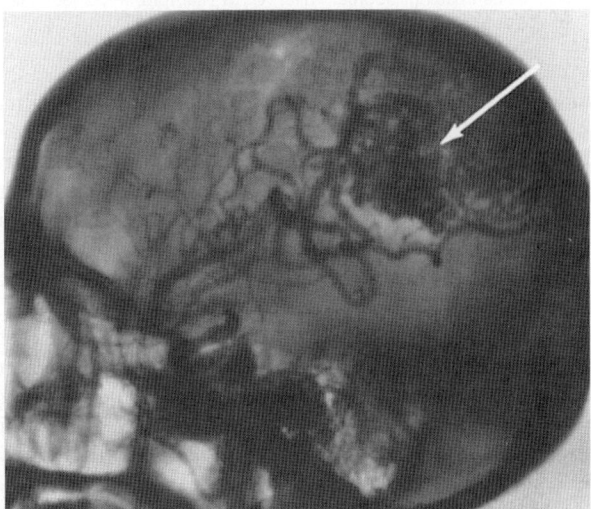

FIG. 58.19 Cerebral angiogram illustrating an arteriovenous malformation *(arrow).* Source: Chipps, E., Clanin, N., & Campbell, V. (1992). *Neurologic disorders.* Mosby.

the pressure reading is abnormally high. Normal CSF pressure is approximately 9 to 14 mm Hg (McCance et al., 2018). CSF is withdrawn in a series of tubes and sent for analysis. Some examiners believe that the patient should be kept lying flat for at least a few hours after the procedure to avoid a spinal headache, which is presumably caused by loss of the cushioning effect of CSF as a result of leakage at the puncture site. The prone position may be effective in preventing CSF leakage. Other examiners do not believe that the lying position is necessary because headache seems to develop in some patients despite precautions. Meningeal irritation (nuchal rigidity) or signs and symptoms of local trauma (e.g., hematoma, pain) may develop in some patients.

Radiological Studies

Cerebral Angiography. Cerebral angiography is indicated when vascular lesions or tumours are suspected. A catheter is inserted into the femoral (sometimes brachial) artery. It is then passed up the artery to the aortic arch and into the base of a carotid or a vertebral artery for injection of radiopaque contrast medium. Radiographs are taken in a timed sequence so that pictures of the arteries, smaller vessels, and veins can be obtained (Figure 58.19). This study can help localize and determine the presence of abscesses, aneurysms, hematomas, arteriovenous malformations, arterial spasm, and certain tumours.

Because this is an invasive procedure, adverse reactions may occur. The patient may have an allergic (anaphylactic) reaction to the contrast medium. When this reaction occurs, it is usually immediately after injection of the contrast medium and may necessitate emergency resuscitation measures in the procedure room. The most common precaution for nurses to take in caring for the patient after the return to the room is observation for bleeding at the catheter puncture site (usually the groin). A pressure dressing and ice are usually placed on the site to promote hemostasis and prevent swelling.

CASE STUDY

Objective Data: Diagnostic Studies

The emergency department health care provider immediately orders a stat CT scan of the head. The CT scan rules out a hemorrhagic stroke. Stat laboratory test results include a blood glucose of 7.5 mmol/L and a PT/INR of 12.0/1.1.

This case study is continued in Chapter 60.

See Case Study: Patient Introduction, Case Study: Subjective Data, and Case Study: Objective Data: Physical Examination for more information on E. J.

Computed Tomography. Computed tomography (CT) is a noninvasive procedure, although intravenous injection of contrast medium may be used to enhance visualization of the blood vessels and identify disruptions in the blood–brain barrier. A

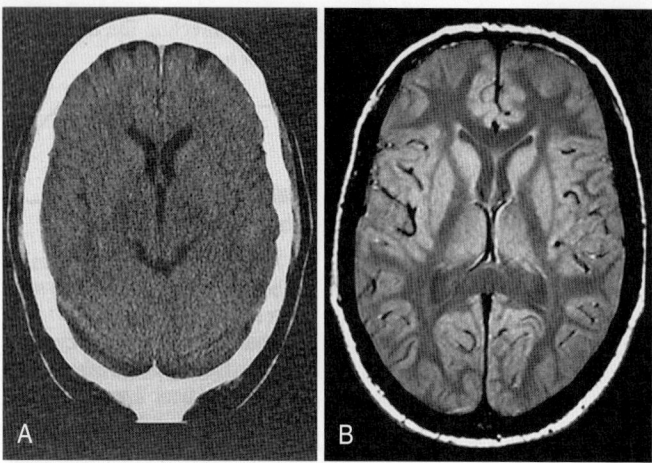

FIG. 58.20 Normal images of the brain. **A,** Computed tomography. **B,** Magnetic resonance imaging. Source: Fuller, G., & Manford, M. (2006). *Neurology: An illustrated colour text.* Churchill Livingstone.

number of radiographic scans of different levels of the brain are compiled with computer assistance and presented in a series of black-and-white pictures. These pictures, which illustrate "slices" of the brain (Figure 58.20, *A*), can show hemorrhages, tumours, cysts, edema, infarction, brain atrophy, and hydrocephalus. CT does not illustrate structures in the posterior fossa and the base of the brain as clearly as magnetic resonance imaging (MRI) does.

Magnetic Resonance Imaging. MRI provides greater detail than CT and improved resolution (detail) of the intracranial structures (see Figure 58.20, *B*). However, MRI requires a longer time to complete and may not be appropriate in life-threatening emergencies. Techniques of functional MRI (fMRI) provide time-related (temporal) images that can be used to evaluate how the brain responds to various stimuli.

MRI is useful in evaluating brain and spinal cord edema, hemorrhage, infarction, blood vessels, tumours, herniation, and bone lesions. It is used in the detection of early strokes and multiple sclerosis. Intravenous injection of gadolinium-containing contrast agents can enhance the images obtained with MRI. Because the images of soft tissue structures have greater contrast with MRI than with CT, MRI is the diagnostic test of choice for many neurological conditions and diseases.

Positron Emission Tomography. Positron emission tomography (PET) is used to determine regional metabolism in the brain. PET provides a noninvasive means of determining biochemical processes that occur in the brain. PET is increasingly used to monitor patients with stroke, Alzheimer's disease, seizure disorders, epilepsy, tumours, and Parkinson's disease.

Electrographic Studies

Electroencephalography. *Electroencephalography* (EEG) is the recording of the electrical activity of the surface cortical neurons of the brain, using 8 to 16 electrodes placed on specific areas of the scalp. This test is done to evaluate not only cerebral disease but also the CNS effects of many metabolic and systemic diseases and to determine brain death. Among the cerebral diseases and other conditions assessed with EEG are epilepsy, mass lesions (e.g., tumour, abscess, hematoma), cerebrovascular lesions, and brain injury. The procedure is noninvasive. Patients sometimes have the misconception that the recording electrodes will give them an electric shock. They should be assured that this idea is not true and that the procedure is similar to electrocardiography.

Electromyography and Nerve Conduction Studies. *Electromyography* (EMG) is the recording of electrical activity associated with innervation of skeletal muscle. The recording is displayed on a computer screen and may be played on a loudspeaker for simultaneous analysis. Needle electrodes are inserted into the muscle to record specific motor units because recording from the skin is not sufficient. Normal muscle at rest shows no electrical activity. Typical electrical activity occurs when the muscle contracts. This activity may be altered in diseases of muscle itself (e.g., myopathic conditions) or in disorders of muscle innervation (e.g., segmental or LMN lesions, peripheral neuropathic conditions). *Fibrillations* are spontaneous, independent contractions of individual muscle fibres that can be detected only by EMG. They appear on EMG 1 to 3 weeks after a muscle has lost its nerve supply.

In *nerve conduction studies,* a brief electrical stimulus is applied to a distal portion of a sensory or mixed nerve, and the resulting wave of depolarization is recorded at some point proximal to the stimulation. For example, a stimulus can be applied to the forefinger and a recording electrode placed over the median nerve at the wrist. The time between the onset of the stimulus and the initial wave of depolarization at the recording electrode is measured. The speed of this response is termed *nerve conduction velocity.* Damaged nerves have slower conduction velocities.

Evoked Potentials. *Evoked potentials* are recordings of electrical activity associated with nerve conduction along sensory pathways. The activity is generated by a specific sensory stimulus related to the type of study (e.g., checkerboard patterns for visual-evoked potentials, clicking sounds for auditory-evoked potentials, mild electrical pulses for somatosensory-evoked potentials). Electrodes placed on specific areas of the skin and scalp record the electrical activity, and these data are stored and averaged by a computerized instrument. A wave pattern appears on a screen and is printed on paper. Peaks in the wave pattern correspond to conduction of the stimulus through certain points along the sensory pathway (e.g., peripheral nerve, brainstem, cortical areas). Increases in the time from stimulus onset to a given peak (latency) indicate slowed nerve conduction or nerve damage. This technique is useful in diagnosing abnormalities of the visual or auditory systems because it reveals whether a sensory impulse is reaching the appropriate part of the brain. Purposes for these tests include evaluation of the optic nerve in conditions such as multiple sclerosis (optic neuritis) and the vestibulocochlear nerve in acoustic neuroma.

Combined Doppler and Ultrasound (Duplex) Studies

Carotid Duplex. In a *duplex study,* ultrasonography and pulsed Doppler technology are combined. A technician places a probe on the patient's skin over the carotid artery and slowly moves the probe along the course of the common carotid artery to the bifurcation of the external and internal carotid arteries. The ultrasound signal emitted from the probe reflects off the moving blood cells within the vessel. The frequency of the reflected signal corresponds to the blood flow velocity. This response is amplified and is registered on a graphic record and also as sound. The graphic record registers blood flow velocity. Increases in blood flow velocity can indicate stenosis of a vessel. Duplex scanning is a noninvasive study in which the degree of stenosis of the carotid and vertebral arteries is evaluated.

Transcranial Doppler Sonography. The same technology used in duplex studies is used in transcranial Doppler sonography, except that blood flow velocities of the intracranial blood vessels are recorded. The probe is placed on the patient's skin at various "windows" in the skull (areas in the skull that have only a thin bony covering) to register velocities of the middle cerebral artery, anterior cerebral artery, posterior cerebral artery, terminal carotid artery, and, occasionally, the anterior and posterior communicating arteries.

The temporal, orbital, and suboccipital sites are used. The ultrasound signal received is recorded graphically as a waveform. Peak blood flow velocities and systolic–diastolic ratios can be calculated from this information. Transcranial Doppler sonography is a noninvasive technique that is useful in assessing vasospasm associated with subarachnoid hemorrhage, altered intracranial blood flow dynamics associated with occlusive vascular disease, presence of emboli, and cerebral autoregulation.

REVIEW QUESTIONS

The number of the question corresponds to the same-numbered objective at the beginning of the chapter.

1. In a client with a disease that affects the myelin sheath of nerves, such as multiple sclerosis, which glial cells are affected?
   a. Microglia
   b. Astrocytes
   c. Oligodendrocytes
   d. Ependymal cells
2. A state of hypoxia alters the repeated action potentials necessary for transmission of nerve impulses. Which of the following requires energy?
   a. Repolarization of the cell membrane
   b. Creation of cell membrane permeability
   c. Movement of sodium into the nerve cell
   d. Maintenance of the resting membrane potential
3. Medications or diseases that impair the function of the extrapyramidal system may cause the loss of which of the following?
   a. Sensations of pain and temperature
   b. Regulation of the ANS
   c. Integration of somatic and special sensory inputs
   d. Automatic movements associated with skeletal muscle activity
4. Which of the following will be affected by an obstruction of the anterior cerebral arteries?
   a. Visual imaging
   b. Balance and coordination
   c. Judgement, insight, and reasoning
   d. Visual and auditory integration for language comprehension
5. Data regarding mobility, strength, coordination, and activity tolerance are important for the nurse to obtain for which of the following reasons?
   a. Many neurological diseases affect one or more of these abilities.
   b. Clients are less able to identify other neurological impairments.
   c. These are the first functions to be lost in neurological disease.
   d. Aspects of movement are the most important function of the nervous system.
6. Which of the following is a result of stimulation of the parasympathetic nervous system? *(Select all that apply.)*
   a. Constriction of the bronchi
   b. Increase in rate of peristalsis
   c. Increased secretion of insulin
   d. Increased blood glucose levels
   e. Relaxation of the urinary sphincters

7. Why should the muscle strength of older persons not be compared with that of younger adults?
   a. Stroke is more common in older persons.
   b. Nutritional status is better in young persons.
   c. Most young people exercise more than older people.
   d. Aging leads to a decrease in muscle bulk and strength.
8. A lesion of which cranial nerve would cause paralysis of the lateral gaze?
   a. Cranial nerve II
   b. Cranial nerve III
   c. Cranial nerve IV
   d. Cranial nerve VI
9. During neurological testing, the client is able to perceive pain elicited by pinprick. On the basis of this finding, which of the following tests may the nurse omit?
   a. Position sense
   b. Patellar reflexes
   c. Temperature perception
   d. Heel-to-shin movements
10. A client's eyes jerk as they follow the nurse's moving finger. How would the nurse record this finding?
    a. Nystagmus
    b. Normal tracking
    c. Ophthalmoplegia
    d. Ophthalmic dyskinesia
11. Which of the following are nursing responsibilities for lumbar puncture?
    a. Ensuring the client has a full bladder
    b. Placing the client in the lateral recumbent position
    c. Straightening the client's legs just before the puncture
    d. Having the client cough when the needle has been inserted

1. c; 2. d; 3. d; 4. c; 5. a; 6. a, b, c; 7. d; 8. d; 9. c; 10. a; 11. b.

⊖volve

For even more review questions, visit http://evolve.elsevier.com/Canada/Lewis/medsurg.

REFERENCES

Baker, J. M. (2018). Gait disorders. *American Journal of Medicine, 131*(6), 602–607. https://doi.org/10.1016/j.amjmed.2017.11.051

Jarvis, C., Browne, A. J., Macdonald-Jenkins, J., et al. (2019). *Physical examination & health assessment* (3rd Canadian ed.). Elsevier Inc.

McCance, K. L., Huether, S. E., Brashers, V. L., et al. (2018). *Understanding pathophysiology* (1st Canadian ed.). Elsevier.

Panicker, J. N., & Sakakibara, R. (2020). Lower urinary tract and bowel dysfunction in neurologic disease. *CONTINUUM: Lifelong Learning in Neurology, 26*(1), 178–199. https://doi.org/10.1212/CON.0000000000000824

Porter, R. S. (Ed.). (2018). *Merck manual of diagnosis and therapy* (20th ed.). Merck & Co.

Tang, H., Jiang, Y., & Zhang, J. H. (2020). Stem cell therapy for brain injury. *Stem Cells and Development, 29*(4), 177. https://doi.org/10.1089/scd.2020.29005.tan

Wolffenbuttel, B. H., Wouters, H. J., Heiner-Fokkema, M. R., et al. (2019). The many faces of cobalamin (vitamin B12) deficiency. *Mayo Clinic Proceedings: Innovations, Quality & Outcomes, 3*(2), 200–214. https://doi.org/10.1016/j.mayocpiqo.2019.03.002

RESOURCES

Resources for this chapter are listed in Chapters 59 to 63.

Nursing Management

Acute Intracranial Conditions

Sarah L. Johnston

Originating US chapter by Kristen Keller

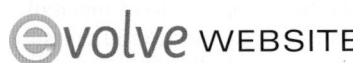
WEBSITE

---

http://evolve.elsevier.com/Canada/Lewis/medsurg

- Review Questions (Online Only)
- Key Points
- Answer Guidelines for Case Study
- Student Case Studies
  - Patient with Meningitis

- Customizable Nursing Care Plans
  - Bacterial Meningitis
  - Increased Intracranial Pressure
  - Cranial Surgery
- Conceptual Care Map Creator

- Audio Glossary
- Supporting Media Animations
  - Parts of the Brain
- Content Updates

LEARNING OBJECTIVES

1. Explain the physiological mechanisms that maintain normal intracranial pressure.
2. Describe the common etiologies and clinical manifestations of increased intracranial pressure.
3. Describe the interprofessional care and nursing management of the patient with increased intracranial pressure.
4. Differentiate between the types of head injury by mechanism of injury and clinical manifestations.

5. Describe the interprofessional care and nursing management of the patient with a head injury.
6. Explain the types, clinical manifestations, and interprofessional care of brain tumours.
7. Discuss the nursing management of the patient with a brain tumour.
8. Discuss the nursing management of the patient undergoing cranial surgery.
9. Compare the primary causes, interprofessional care, and nursing management of meningitis, encephalitis, and brain abscess.

KEY TERMS

brain abscess
cerebral edema
coma
concussion
contusion
diffuse axonal injury (DAI)

encephalitis
epidural hematoma
Glasgow Coma Scale (GCS)
head injury
intracranial pressure (ICP)
intraparenchymal or intracerebral hematoma

meningitis
nuchal rigidity
subdural hematoma
unconsciousness

Acute intracranial conditions include diseases and disorders that can increase intracranial pressure (ICP). This chapter discusses ICP, head injuries, brain tumours, and cerebral inflammatory disorders.

INTRACRANIAL PRESSURE

Understanding the mechanisms associated with ICP is important in caring for patients with many different neurological conditions. The skull is like a closed box, with three essential components constituting its volume: brain tissue, blood, and cerebrospinal fluid (CSF) (Figure 59.1). The brain compartment, made up of neurons, neuroglial cells, and intracellular

and extracellular fluids of brain tissue, makes up approximately 78% of this volume. Blood in the arterial, the venous, and the capillary networks makes up 12% of the volume, and the remaining 10% is the volume of the CSF. Under normal conditions, the volume of these three compartments is relatively stable, maintaining ICP within normal limits. Factors that influence ICP under normal circumstances are changes in (1) blood pressure (BP), (2) cardiac function, (3) intra-abdominal and intrathoracic pressure, (4) body position, (5) temperature, and (6) blood gases, particularly carbon dioxide (CO_2) levels. The degree to which these factors increase or decrease the ICP depends on the ability of the brain to accommodate to the changes.

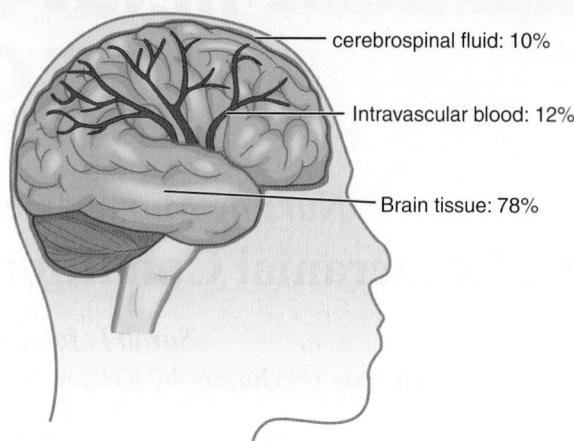

cerebrospinal fluid: 10%

Intravascular blood: 12%

Brain tissue: 78%

FIG. 59.1 Components of the brain.

Primary versus secondary injury is another important concept in understanding ICP. *Primary injury* occurs at the initial time of an injury (e.g., impact of motor vehicle accident, blunt-force trauma) that results in displacement, bruising, or damage of the three components. *Secondary injury* is the resulting hypoxia, ischemia, hypotension, edema, or increased ICP that follows the primary injury. Secondary injury, which could occur several hours to days after the initial injury, is a primary concern when managing a brain injury. Nursing management of the patient with an acute intracranial condition must include management of secondary injury and, thus, increased ICP.

Regulation and Maintenance of Intracranial Pressure

Normal Intracranial Pressure. Intracranial pressure (ICP) is the pressure exerted due to the combined total volume of the three components within the skull: brain tissue, blood, and CSF. The modified Monro–Kellie doctrine describes how a state of dynamic equilibrium is maintained by the volume relationship of these three components within the rigid skull structure. If the volume in any one of the three components increases within the cranial vault and the volume from another component is displaced, the total intracranial volume will not change (Cushing, 1925). If the volume of any one of these three components increases without a corresponding decrease in another component, the result is an elevated ICP. This hypothesis is not applicable in situations in which the skull is not rigid (e.g., in newborns, in adults with unfused skull fractures).

ICP can be measured in the ventricles, subarachnoid space, subdural space, epidural space, or brain tissue, using a pressure transducer (Harary et al., 2018). Normal ICP ranges from 5 to 15 mm Hg. A sustained pressure greater than 20 mm Hg is considered increased and must be treated.

Normal Compensatory Adaptations. Intrinsic compensatory mechanisms exist to resist increases in ICP. A major compensatory mechanism involves changes in the CSF volume. These changes are achieved primarily by the displacement of CSF into the spinal subarachnoid space or the basal subarachnoid cisterns and, to a lesser degree, by altering CSF production and absorption rates. Alterations in intracranial blood volume occur through the compression of cerebral veins and dural sinuses, regional cerebral vasoconstriction or dilation, and changes in venous outflow. Brain tissue volume compensates through distension of the dura or compression of brain tissue. Initially, an

increase in volume produces no increase in ICP as a result of these compensatory mechanisms. However, compensatory adaptations are finite, and progressive increases in volume eventually exhaust compensatory mechanisms (Cushing, 1925). The result is increased ICP, neuronal compression, and ischemia.

Cerebral Blood Flow

Cerebral blood flow (CBF) is the amount of blood in millilitres (mL) passing through 100 grams (g) of brain tissue per minute (min). In adults, this equates to approximately 50 mL of blood/min/100 g of brain tissue or approximately 750 mL/min. Unlike other organs, the brain lacks the ability to store oxygen or glucose; therefore, the maintenance of adequate blood flow to the brain is critical for neuronal functioning and survival. Although the brain accounts for only about 2% of body weight, it uses 20% of the body's oxygen and 25% of its glucose.

Autoregulation of Cerebral Blood Flow. The brain's intrinsic ability to regulate its own blood flow in response to its metabolic needs in spite of wide fluctuations in systemic arterial pressure is termed *autoregulation*. Autoregulation is the automatic alteration in the diameter of the cerebral blood vessels to maintain a constant blood flow to the brain during changes in BP. The purpose of autoregulation is to ensure adequate CBF to meet the metabolic needs of brain tissue and to maintain cerebral perfusion pressure within normal limits.

In healthy individuals, autoregulation operates within limited parameters. In cases of extreme hypotension or hypertension, autoregulation fails. If mean arterial pressure (MAP) is less than 50 mm Hg, CBF is decreased and symptoms of cerebral ischemia may occur. If MAP is greater than 150 mm Hg, the cerebral vessels are maximally constricted and further vasoconstrictor response is lost; CBF increases and intracranial hypertension may occur. MAP is discussed in Chapter 32.

Other Factors Affecting Cerebral Blood Flow. Carbon dioxide, oxygen, and hydrogen ion concentration affect cerebral vessel tone. The partial pressure of arterial carbon dioxide ($PaCO_2$) is a potent factor in vasoactive reactivity. An increase in $PaCO_2$ relaxes smooth muscle, dilates cerebral vessels, decreases cerebrovascular resistance, and increases CBF. Alternately, a decrease in $PaCO_2$ reverses this process and decreases CBF. Cerebral oxygen tension (PaO_2) below 50 mm Hg results in cerebral vascular dilation. This dilation decreases cerebral vascular resistance and increases CBF. If PaO_2 is not raised, anaerobic metabolism begins, resulting in an accumulation of lactic acid. As lactic acid increases and hydrogen ions accumulate, the cerebral environment becomes more acidic. Within this acidic environment, further vasodilation occurs in a continued attempt to increase blood flow. The combination of a severely low arterial oxygen pressure (PaO_2) and an elevated hydrogen ion concentration (acidosis), which are both potent cerebral vasodilators, may produce a state in which autoregulation is lost and compensatory mechanisms fail to meet tissue metabolic demands (Cushing, 1925).

CBF can be globally affected by cardiac or respiratory arrest, systemic hemorrhage, and other pathophysiological states (e.g., diabetic coma, encephalopathies, infections, toxicities). Regional CBF can also be affected by trauma, tumours, cerebral hemorrhage, or stroke. When regional or global autoregulation is lost, CBF is no longer maintained at a constant level but is directly influenced by changes in systemic BP, $PaCO_2$ levels, or catecholamine levels. CBF can be indirectly reflected by calculating *cerebral perfusion pressure* (CPP). CPP is the pressure

TABLE 59.1	CALCULATION OF CEREBRAL PERFUSION PRESSURE

$$CPP = MAP - ICP$$

$$MAP = DBP + \tfrac{1}{3}(SBP - DBP) \quad or \quad \frac{SBP + 2(DBP)}{3}$$

Example: Systemic blood pressure = 122/84 mm Hg

MAP = 97 mm Hg

ICP = 12 mm Hg

CPP = 85 mm Hg

CPP, cerebral perfusion pressure; *DBP,* diastolic blood pressure; *ICP,* intracranial pressure; *MAP,* mean arterial pressure; *SBP,* systolic blood pressure.

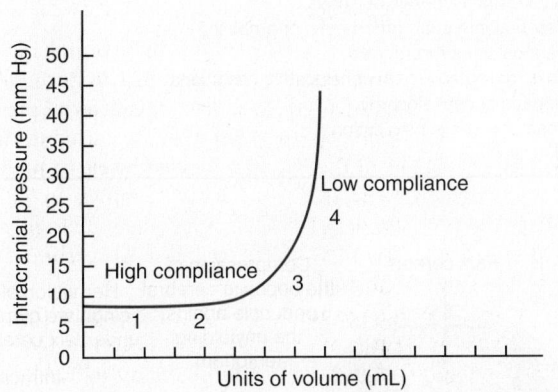

FIG. 59.2 Intracranial pressure–volume curve. (See text for descriptions of *1, 2, 3,* and *4.*)

needed to ensure adequate brain tissue perfusion. CPP is equal to the MAP minus the ICP (CPP = MAP – ICP) (see example in Table 59.1). If CPP is inadequate, brain perfusion can be improved by either decreasing ICP or increasing MAP.

As the CPP decreases, autoregulation fails and CBF decreases. Normal CPP is 70 to 100 mm Hg, and a minimum of 50 to 60 mm Hg is necessary for adequate cerebral perfusion. CPP less than 50 mm Hg is associated with cerebral ischemia. A CPP below 30 mm Hg results in cellular ischemia and is incompatible with life. Under normal circumstances, autoregulation maintains an adequate CBF and perfusion pressure primarily by cerebral vasoreactivity and metabolic adjustments that affect ICP. It is of paramount importance to maintain MAP when ICP is elevated. It should be remembered that CPP does not reflect perfusion pressure in all parts of the brain. There may be local areas of swelling and compression limiting regional perfusion pressure. Thus, for patients with these symptoms, a higher CPP may be needed to prevent localized tissue damage.

Pressure Changes. The relationship of pressure to volume is depicted in the pressure–volume curve (Figure 59.2). The curve is affected by the brain's compliance. *Compliance* is the expandability of the brain. It is represented as the volume increase for each unit increase in pressure. With low compliance, small increases in volume result in greater increases in pressure.

The pressure–volume curve can be used to represent the stages of increased ICP (see Figure 59.2). At stage 1 on the curve, there is high compliance. The brain is in total compensation, with accommodation and autoregulation intact. An increase in volume (in brain tissue, blood, or CSF) does not increase the

ICP. At stage 2, the compliance is lessening, and an increase in volume places the patient at risk for increased ICP. At stage 3, there is low compliance as compensatory mechanisms are becoming exhausted. Any small addition of volume causes a great increase in ICP. As compensatory mechanisms fail, there is a loss of autoregulation, and the patient may exhibit symptoms indicating increased ICP, such as headache, changes in level of consciousness, or pupil responsiveness.

As the patient enters stage 4, the ICP rises to lethal levels with even slight increases in volume. Here the patient is at significant risk for hypoperfusion and brain herniation and death. *Herniation* occurs as the brain tissue is forcibly shifted from the compartment of greater pressure to a compartment of lesser pressure. In this situation, intense pressure is placed on the brainstem, and if herniation continues, brainstem death is imminent.

INCREASED INTRACRANIAL PRESSURE

Increased ICP is a life-threatening situation resulting from an increase in any or all of the three components (brain tissue, blood, CSF) of the skull. Elevated ICP is clinically significant because it diminishes CPP, increasing risk for brain ischemia and infarction as well as herniation of brain tissue.

Mechanisms of Increased Intracranial Pressure

The brain tissue component of ICP can be increased by cerebral neoplasm, contusion, abscess, or cerebral edema. Conditions that increase the cerebral blood volume include intracranial hematomas or hemorrhages, metabolic and physiological factors (e.g., CO_2, O_2, fever, pain), and vascular anomalies. Increases in the CSF volume can result from CSF-secreting tumours or hydrocephalus. These cerebral insults may result in hypercapnia, cerebral acidosis, impaired autoregulation, and systemic hypertension, which promote the formation and spread of cerebral edema. This edema distorts brain tissue, further increasing the ICP, which leads to even more tissue hypoxia and acidosis. Figure 59.3 illustrates the progression of increased ICP.

Crucial to preservation of tissue is maintenance of CBF. Elevations in pressure that are more evenly distributed throughout the brain or slow increases in ICP (e.g., an enlarging brain lesion) preserve blood flow better than a rapid increase, as in primary brain injury. Sustained increases in ICP result in brainstem compression and herniation of the brain from one compartment to another.

Displacement and herniation of brain tissue cause a potentially reversible pathophysiological process to become irreversible. Ischemia and edema are further increased, compounding the pre-existing condition. Herniations force the cerebellum and the brainstem downward through the foramen magnum. If compression of the brainstem is unrelieved, respiratory arrest may occur. Compression of brain tissue, brainstem structures, cranial nerves, and vessels may be fatal. Figure 59.4 illustrates herniation. (Herniation is further described in the later section of this chapter on complications of ICP.)

Cerebral Edema

As shown in Table 59.2, there are a variety of causes of cerebral edema (increased accumulation of fluid in the extravascular spaces of brain tissue). Regardless of the cause, cerebral edema results in an increase in tissue volume that carries the potential for increased ICP. Factors that contribute to the degree of

PATHOPHYSIOLOGY MAP

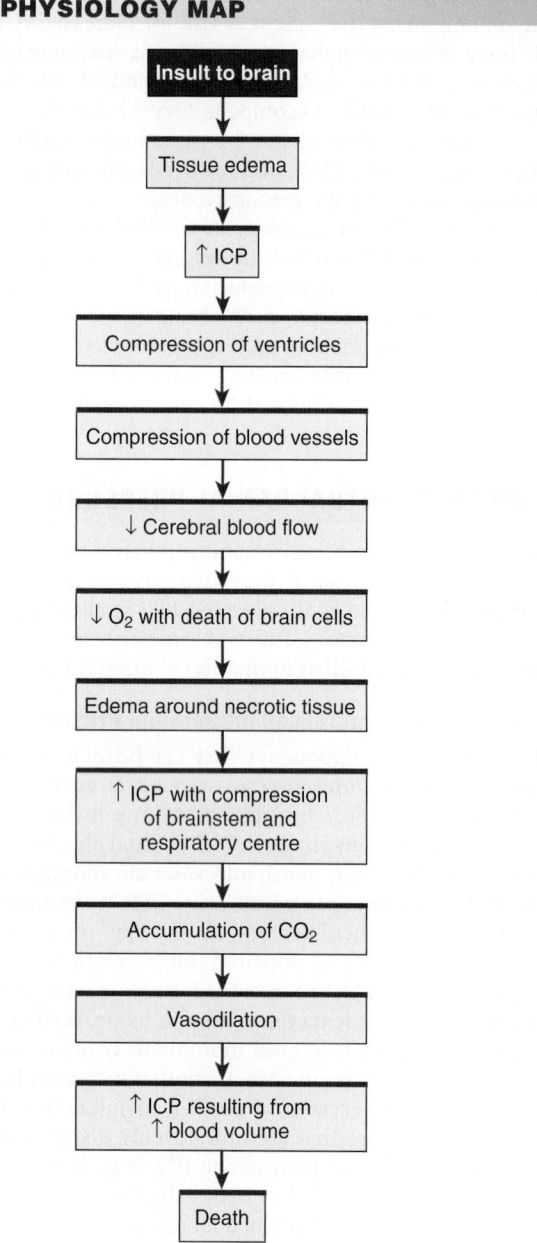

FIG. 59.3 Progression of increased intracranial pressure (ICP).

Insult to brain → Tissue edema → ↑ ICP → Compression of ventricles → Compression of blood vessels → ↓ Cerebral blood flow → ↓ O₂ with death of brain cells → Edema around necrotic tissue → ↑ ICP with compression of brainstem and respiratory centre → Accumulation of CO₂ → Vasodilation → ↑ ICP resulting from ↑ blood volume → Death

TABLE 59.2	CAUSES OF CEREBRAL EDEMA

- Mass lesions
- Brain abscess
- Brain tumour (primary or metastatic)
- Hematoma (intracerebral, subdural, epidural)
- Hemorrhage (intracerebral, cerebellar, brainstem)
- Head injuries
- Contusion
- Diffuse axonal injury
- Hemorrhage
- Post-traumatic brain swelling
- Brain surgery
- Cerebral infections
- Meningitis
- Encephalitis
- Vascular insult
- Anoxic and ischemic episodes
- Cerebral infarction (thrombotic or embolic)
- Venous sinus thrombosis
- Toxic or metabolic encephalopathic conditions
- Hepatic encephalopathy
- Lead or arsenic intoxication
- Uremia

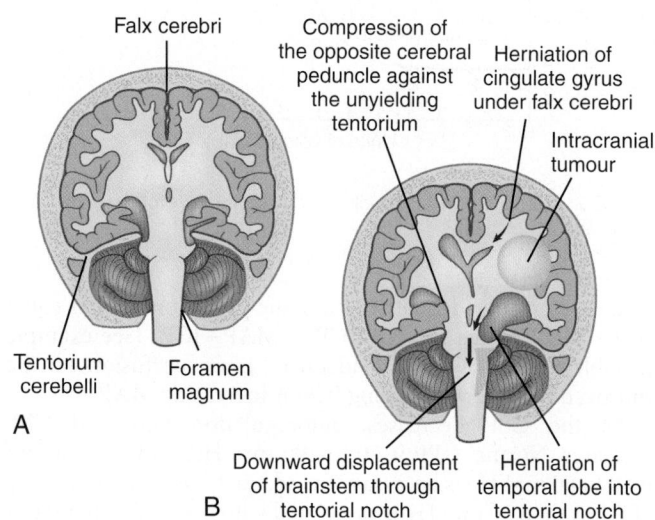

FIG. 59.4 Herniation. **A,** Normal relationship of intracranial structures. **B,** Shift of intracranial structures. Source: Adapted from McCance, K. L., & Huether, S. E. (2010). *Pathophysiology: The biologic basis for disease in adults and children* (6th ed., p. 558, Figure 16-16). Mosby.

cerebral edema are the extent and the severity of the original insult as well as the cascade of secondary cellular events that occur in the hours and days following insult or injury.

Three types of cerebral edema have been distinguished: vasogenic, cytotoxic, and interstitial. More than one type may result from a single insult in the same patient. Regardless of the cause of cerebral edema, manifestations of increased ICP result, unless compensation is adequate.

Vasogenic Cerebral Edema. *Vasogenic cerebral edema,* the most common type of edema, occurs mainly in the white matter and is attributed to changes in the endothelial lining of cerebral capillaries. These changes allow leakage of macromolecules from the capillaries into the surrounding extracellular space, resulting in an osmotic gradient that favours the flow of water from the intravascular to the extravascular space. A variety of insults, such as brain tumours, head trauma, abscesses, and

ingested toxins, may cause an increase in the permeability of the blood–brain barrier and produce an increase in the extracellular fluid volume. The speed and extent of the spread of the edema fluid are influenced by the systemic BP, the site of the brain injury, and the extent of the blood–brain barrier defect. This edema may produce a continuum of symptoms, ranging from headache and focal neurological deficits to disturbances in consciousness, including coma (profound state of unconsciousness). It is important to recognize that although a headache may seem to be a benign symptom, in cases of cerebral edema it can quickly progress to coma and death; therefore, vigilant assessment is key.

Cytotoxic Cerebral Edema. *Cytotoxic cerebral edema* results from local disruption of the functional or morphological integrity of cell membranes and occurs most often in the grey matter. It develops from destructive lesions or trauma to brain tissue that lead to cerebral hypoxia or anoxia, sodium depletion, and syndrome of inappropriate antidiuretic hormone (SIADH). Cerebral edema results as fluid and protein shift from the extracellular space directly into the cells, with subsequent swelling and loss of cellular function.

Interstitial Cerebral Edema. *Interstitial cerebral edema* is the result of periventricular diffusion of ventricular CSF in a patient with uncontrolled hydrocephalus. It can also be caused by enlargement of the extracellular space as a result of systemic water excess (hyponatremia). Fluid moves into the cells to equilibrate with the hypo-osmotic interstitial fluid.

Clinical Manifestations

The clinical manifestations of increased ICP can take many forms, depending on the cause, the location, and the rate at which the pressure increase occurs (Figure 59.5). The earlier the condition is recognized and treated, the better the prognosis.

Change in Level of Consciousness. *Level of consciousness* (LOC) is a sensitive and early indicator of the patient's neurological status. Changes in LOC are a result of impaired CBF, which deprives the cells of the cerebral cortex and the reticular activating system (RAS) of oxygen. The RAS is located in the brainstem, with neural connections to many parts of the nervous system. An intact RAS can maintain a state of wakefulness even in the absence of a functioning cerebral cortex. Interruptions of impulses from the RAS or alteration of the functioning of the cerebral hemispheres can cause unconsciousness (an abnormal state of complete or partial unawareness of self or environment).

The patient's state of consciousness is defined by both the behaviour and the pattern of brain activity recorded by an electroencephalogram (EEG). The change in consciousness may be subtle, such as a flattening of affect, confusion, or decrease in level of attention. A decrease in consciousness may be dramatic, as in coma—the deepest state of unconsciousness, when the patient does not respond to sensory stimuli. The EEG pattern demonstrates decreased neuronal activity.

Changes in Vital Signs. Changes in vital signs are caused by increasing pressure on the thalamus, the hypothalamus, the pons, and the medulla. Manifestations such as *Cushing's triad,* consisting of increasing systolic pressure (widening pulse pressure), bradycardia with a full and bounding pulse, and irregular respiratory pattern, may be present but often do not appear until ICP has been increased for some time or suddenly and markedly increases (e.g., head trauma). (Pulse pressure is discussed in Chapter 34.) Cushing's triad must always be recognized as a medical emergency, since this is a sign of brainstem compression and impending death. A change in body temperature may also be noted and is caused by associated pressure on the hypothalamus.

Ocular Signs. Compression of the oculomotor nerve (cranial nerve [CN] III) results in dilation of the pupil *ipsilateral* to (same side as) the mass or lesion, sluggish or no response to light, inability to move the eye upward, and ptosis of the eyelid. These signs can be the result of a shifting of the brain from the midline, a process that compresses the trunk of CN III, paralyzing the pupil sphincter. A fixed (unresponsive), unilaterally dilated pupil is a neurological emergency that indicates herniation of the brain.

Other cranial nerves may also be affected, such as the optic (CN II), trochlear (CN IV), and abducens (CN VI) nerves. Signs of dysfunction of these cranial nerves include blurred vision, diplopia, and changes in extraocular eye movements. Central herniation may initially manifest as sluggish but equal pupil responses. Lateral herniation of the uncus, the innermost part

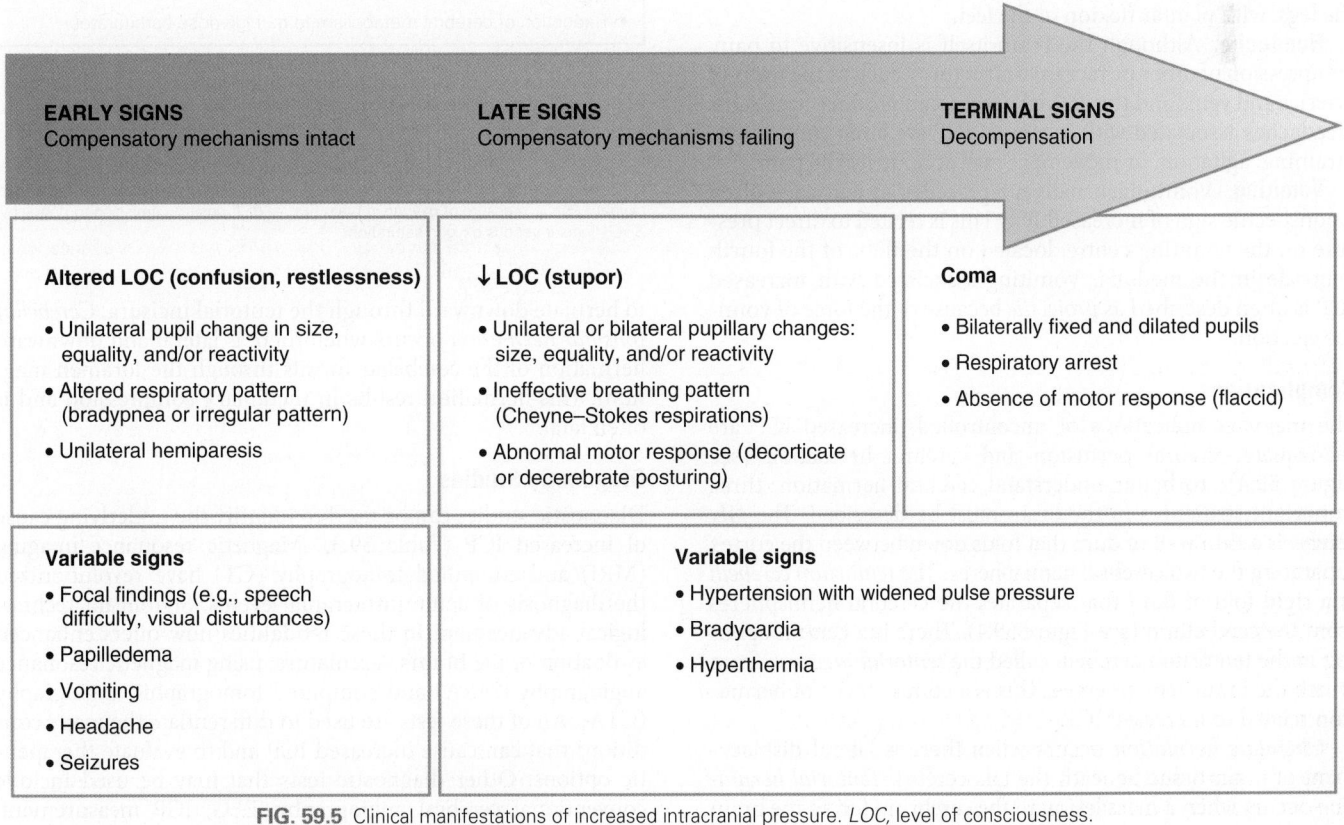

EARLY SIGNS Compensatory mechanisms intact	**LATE SIGNS** Compensatory mechanisms failing	**TERMINAL SIGNS** Decompensation
Altered LOC (confusion, restlessness) • Unilateral pupil change in size, equality, and/or reactivity • Altered respiratory pattern (bradypnea or irregular pattern) • Unilateral hemiparesis	**↓ LOC (stupor)** • Unilateral or bilateral pupillary changes: size, equality, and/or reactivity • Ineffective breathing pattern (Cheyne–Stokes respirations) • Abnormal motor response (decorticate or decerebrate posturing)	**Coma** • Bilaterally fixed and dilated pupils • Respiratory arrest • Absence of motor response (flaccid)
Variable signs • Focal findings (e.g., speech difficulty, visual disturbances) • Papilledema • Vomiting • Headache • Seizures	**Variable signs** • Hypertension with widened pulse pressure • Bradycardia • Hyperthermia	

FIG. 59.5 Clinical manifestations of increased intracranial pressure. *LOC,* level of consciousness.

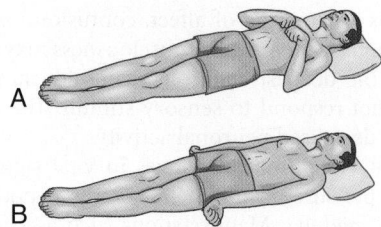

FIG. 59.6 Abnormal posturing. **A,** Abnormal flexion (decorticate posturing). Flexion of arms, wrists, and fingers with adduction in upper extremities. Extension, internal rotation, and plantar flexion in lower extremities. **B,** Abnormal extension (decerebrate posturing). All four extremities in rigid extension, with hyperpronation of forearms and plantar flexion of feet.

of the temporal lobe, may cause a dilated unilateral pupil. *Papilledema*, an edematous optic disc seen on retinal examination, is also noted and is a nonspecific sign associated with swelling of the optic nerve related to increased ICP.

Decrease in Motor Function. As the ICP continues to rise, the patient manifests changes in motor ability. A *contralateral* (opposite side of the mass lesion) hemiparesis or hemiplegia may be seen, depending on the location of the source of the increased ICP. If painful stimuli are used to elicit a motor response, the patient may exhibit localization to the stimuli or a withdrawal from the stimuli. Abnormal flexion *(decorticate posturing)* and abnormal extension *(decerebrate posturing)* may also be elicited by noxious stimuli (Figure 59.6). *Abnormal flexion* consists of internal rotation and adduction of the arms, with flexion of elbows, wrists, and fingers as a result of interruption of voluntary motor tracts. Extension of the legs may also be seen. *Abnormal extension* may indicate more serious damage and results from disruption of motor fibres in the midbrain and brainstem. In this position, the arms are stiffly extended, adducted, and hyperpronated. There is also hyperextension of the legs, with plantar flexion of the feet.

Headache. Although the brain itself is insensitive to pain, compression of other intracranial structures, such as the walls of arteries and veins and the cranial nerves, can produce headache. Headaches associated with increased ICP are often continuous. Straining, agitation, or movement may accentuate the pain.

Vomiting. Vomiting, usually not preceded by nausea, is often a nonspecific sign of increased ICP. This is related to direct pressure on the vomiting centre, located on the floor of the fourth ventricle in the medulla. Vomiting associated with increased ICP is often described as *projectile* because of the force of vomitus ejection.

Complications

The major complications of uncontrolled, increased ICP are inadequate cerebral perfusion and cerebral herniation (see Figure 59.4). To better understand cerebral herniation, three important structures in the brain must be described. The *falx cerebri* is a thin wall of dura that folds down between the cortex separating the two cerebral hemispheres. The *tentorium cerebelli* is a rigid fold of dura that separates the cerebral hemispheres from the cerebellum (see Figure 59.4). There is a central opening in the tentorium cerebelli called the *tentorial incisura*, from which the brainstem emerges. This is a common site of herniation related to increased ICP.

Cingulate herniation occurs when there is lateral displacement of brain tissue beneath the falx cerebri. *Tentorial herniation* occurs when a mass lesion in the cerebrum forces the brain

---

TABLE 59.3 INTERPROFESSIONAL CARE

Increased Intracranial Pressure

Diagnostic Tests and Neuromonitoring
- History and physical examination
- Cerebral oxygenation monitoring (Licox catheter, SjvO$_2$)
- ECG
- Infrascanner
- Laboratory studies, including CBC; coagulation profile; electrolytes; creatinine; BUN; ABGs; ammonia level; general medication and toxicology screen; CSF analysis for protein, cells, glucose*
- MRI, CT scan, MRA, CTA, EEG, angiography, EP studies, PET
- Skull and facial radiographic studies
- Transcranial Doppler studies
- Vital signs, neurological assessments, ICP measurements

Interprofessional Therapy
- Cerebral oxygenation monitoring (PbtO$_2$, SjvO$_2$)
- Medication therapy
- Anticonvulsant medications (e.g., phenytoin [Dilantin])
- Antipyretics
- Corticosteroids (dexamethasone) (for brain tumours, bacterial meningitis)
- Histamine H$_2$-receptor antagonist (e.g., ranitidine [Zantac]) or proton pump inhibitor (e.g., pantoprazole [Pantoloc]) to prevent gastrointestinal ulcers and bleeding
- Hypertonic saline
- Nutritional support
- Osmotic diuretics (mannitol)
- Stool softeners
- Elevation of head of bed to 30 degrees with head in a neutral position
- ICP monitoring
- Intubation and mechanical ventilation
- Maintenance of CPP >60 mm Hg
- Maintenance of fluid balance and assessment of osmolality
- Maintenance of PaO$_2$ at ≥100 mm Hg
- Maintenance of systolic arterial pressure between 100 and 160 mm Hg
- Reduction of cerebral metabolism (e.g., high-dose barbiturates)

*CSF sampling via lumbar puncture is contraindicated if there is suspected raised ICP because there is a possibility of cerebral herniation and death.

ABGs, arterial blood gases; *BUN,* blood urea nitrogen; *CBC,* complete blood count; *CPP,* cerebral perfusion pressure; *CSF,* cerebrospinal fluid; *CT,* computed tomography; *CTA,* computed tomography angiography; *ECG,* electrocardiogram; *EEG,* electroencephalogram; *EP,* evoked potential; *ICP,* intracranial pressure; *MRA,* magnetic resonance angiography; *MRI,* magnetic resonance imaging; *PaO$_2$,* partial pressure of arterial oxygen; *PbtO$_2$,* pressure of oxygen in brain tissue; *PET,* positron emission tomography; *SjvO$_2$,* jugular venous oxygen saturation.

---

to herniate downward through the tentorial incisura. *Cerebellar tonsillar herniation* occurs when there is lateral and downward herniation of the cerebellar tonsils through the foramen magnum. This herniation results in medullary compression and is often fatal.

Diagnostic Studies

Diagnostic studies can be used to identify the underlying cause of increased ICP (Table 59.3). Magnetic resonance imaging (MRI) and computed tomography (CT) have revolutionized the diagnosis of acute intracranial events. Significant technological advancement in these modalities now offers enhanced evaluation of the brain's vasculature, using magnetic resonance angiography (MRA) and computed tomographic angiography (CTA). All of these tests are used to differentiate the many conditions that can cause increased ICP and to evaluate therapeutic options. Other diagnostic tests that may be used include conventional cerebral angiography, EEG, ICP measurement,

TABLE 59.4 GLASGOW COMA SCALE

Appropriate Stimulus	Response	Score
Eyes Open		
Approach to bedside	Spontaneous response	4
Verbal command	Opening of eyes to name or command	3
Pain	Lack of opening of eyes to previous stimuli but opening to pain	2
	Lack of opening of eyes to any stimulus	1
	Untestable* (e.g., swollen)	U
Best Verbal Response		
Verbal questioning with maximum arousal	Appropriate orientation, conversant; correct identification of self, place, year, and month	5
	Confusion; conversant, but disorientation in one or more spheres	4
	Inappropriate or disorganized use of words (e.g., cursing), lack of sustained conversation	3
	Incomprehensible words, sounds (e.g., moaning)	2
	Lack of sound, even with painful stimuli	1
	Untestable* (e.g., endotracheal tube)	U
Best Motor Response		
Verbal command (e.g., "raise your arm, hold up two fingers")	Obedience of command	6
Pain applied centrally (e.g., sternal rub, pinching of upper third of trapezius, or supraorbital pressure)	Localization of pain, lack of obedience but presence of attempts to remove offending stimulus—purposeful movement	5
	Flexion withdrawal, flexion of arm in response to pain without abnormal flexion posture—nonpurposeful movement	4
	Abnormal flexion, flexing of arm at elbow and pronation, making a fist	3
	Abnormal extension, extension of arm at elbow usually with adduction and internal rotation of arm at shoulder	2
	Lack of response	1
	Untestable*	U

*Added to the original scale by many centres.

brain tissue oxygenation measurement via the Licox catheter (described later in this chapter), transcranial Doppler studies, and evoked potential studies. Positron emission tomography (PET) can also be used to diagnose the cause of increased ICP. In general, a lumbar puncture is not performed when increased ICP is suspected because of the possibility of cerebral herniation from the sudden release of the pressure in the skull from the area above the lumbar puncture.

A hand-held device called an Infrascanner can be used to detect life-threatening intracranial bleeding. The scanner directs a wavelength of light that can penetrate tissue and bone. Blood from intracranial hematomas absorbs the light differently from other areas of the brain.

Neuromonitoring

Measurement of Intracranial Pressure. ICP may become elevated because of head trauma, stroke, subarachnoid hemorrhage, brain tumour, inflammation or infection, hydrocephalus, or brain tissue damage from other causes. Patients with or at risk for elevated ICP usually receive invasive ICP monitoring in a critical care unit (CCU), except patients with irreversible conditions or advanced neurological disease. Goals for nursing management of elevated ICP include preservation of cerebral oxygenation and perfusion, early identification of neurological changes, and prevention of complications secondary to intracranial hypertension.

ICP monitoring is used to guide clinical care when the patient is at risk for or has elevations in ICP. ICP should be monitored in patients admitted with a Glasgow Coma Scale (GCS) score of 8 or less and an abnormal CT scan or MRI (hematomas, contusion, edema). (The GCS is presented in Table 59.4.) Multiple methods and devices are available to monitor ICP (Figure 59.7).

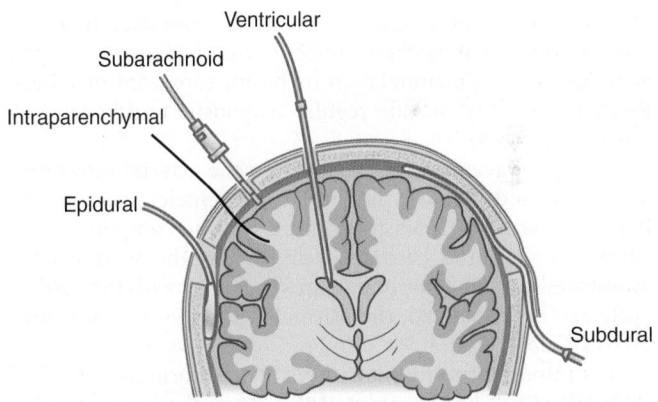

FIG. 59.7 Coronal section of the brain shows potential sites for placement of intracranial pressure monitoring devices.

The gold standard for monitoring ICP is the *ventriculostomy*, whereby a catheter is inserted into the lateral ventricle and coupled to an external transducer (Zhang et al., 2017). This technique directly measures the pressure within the ventricles and facilitates removal or sampling (or both) of CSF. Significant consideration in caring for a patient with a ventriculostomy is the constant positioning of the external transducer relative to the position of the patient's head to maintain consistent measurements. The transducer should be level with the foramen of Monro (intraventricular foramen); the reference point for this on the patient is the tragus of the ear (Figure 59.8, *A*). Another device used for monitoring ICP is the *fibre-optic catheter*, the tip of which is placed directly into the ventricle or the brain tissue. A sensor transducer located in the catheter tip provides measurement of the pressure in the brain. Lastly, the *subarachnoid bolt*

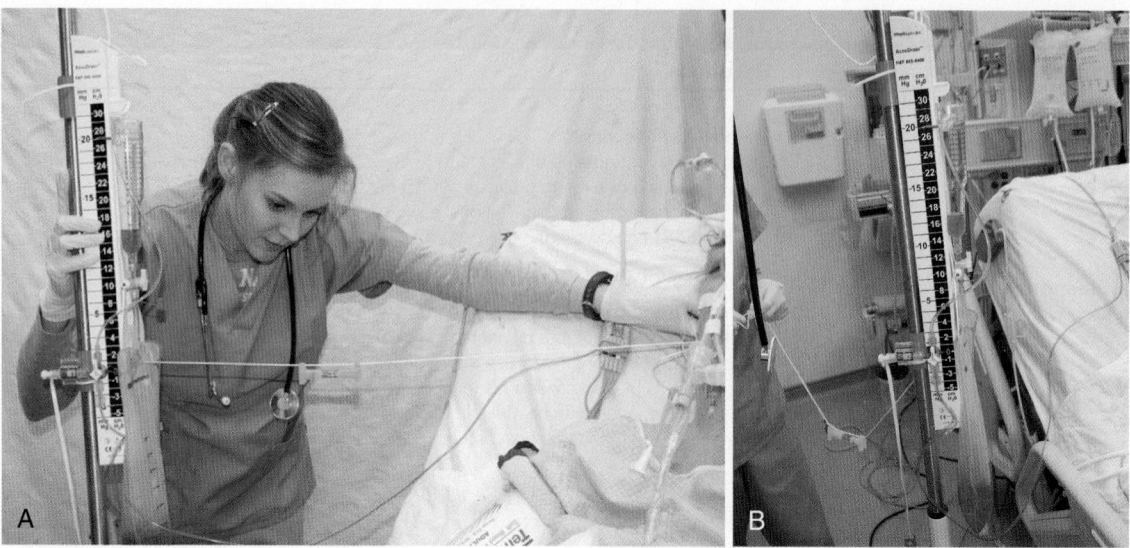

FIG. 59.8 A, Levelling a ventriculostomy. **B,** Cerebrospinal fluid is drained into a drainage system. Source: Courtesy Meg Zomorodi.

or *screw* may be placed through the skull between the arachnoid membrane and the cerebral cortex to measure ICP; this method does not allow for drainage of CSF but can be converted into a ventriculostomy if the patient's clinical condition changes to require that intervention.

Infection is a serious consideration with ICP monitoring. Prophylactic systemic antibiotics may be administered to reduce the chances of infection. Factors that contribute to the development of infection include ICP monitoring for longer than 5 days, use of a ventriculostomy, the presence of a CSF leak, a concurrent systemic infection, and improper aseptic technique during manipulation by health care team members. Routine care may include regular diagnostic testing for CSF organism growth.

The ICP waveform is derived from the arterial pulsations of the choroid plexuses in the lateral ventricles. A normal ICP waveform has a diastolic and a systolic component and correlates with the cardiac cycle. When the waveform is monitored so that components in synchrony with the cardiac cycle can be visualized, the normal ICP waveform has three phases (Table 59.5).

It is important to monitor the ICP waveform and the CPP (Figure 59.9). It has been noted that when the height of P2 is higher than P1, this represents low *compliance* and the patient is at risk for development of elevated ICP. It is important to consider both the rate at which changes occur and the patient's clinical condition. Neurological deterioration might not occur until ICP elevation is pronounced and sustained. Any indication of ICP elevation, either as a mean increase in pressure or as an abnormal waveform configuration, should be reported to the physician immediately.

Cerebrospinal Fluid Drainage. With the ventricular catheter and certain fibre-optic systems, it is possible to control elevations in ICP by removing CSF. Using a closed system (Figure 59.10), CSF is removed by gravity drainage and by adjusting the height of the drip chamber and drainage bag relative to the patient's ventricular reference point. Typically, a point 15 cm above the ear is selected (see Figure 59.8, *B*). Raising the system diminishes drainage, whereas lowering the system increases drainage volume. The physician orders the level of the ICP indicating that drainage should be initiated, the amount of fluid to be drained, the height of the system, and the frequency of

TABLE 59.5	NORMAL INTRACRANIAL PRESSURE WAVEFORMS*	
Waveform	**Meaning**
P1 Percussion wave	Represents arterial pulsations; normally the highest of the three waveforms
P2 Rebound wave	Reflects intracranial compliance or relative brain volume. When P2 is higher than P1, intracranial compliance is compromised
P3 Dicrotic wave	Follows dicrotic notch; represents venous pulsations; normally, the lowest waveform

*See Figure 59.9.

drainage (intermittent or continuous).

The two options for CSF drainage are intermittent and continuous. If *intermittent* drainage is ordered, the ventriculostomy system is opened at the indicated ICP and CSF is allowed to drain for 2 to 3 minutes. Then the stopcock is closed to return the ventriculostomy to a closed system. If *continuous* ICP drainage is ordered, careful monitoring of the volume of CSF drained is essential, keeping in mind that normal CSF production is about 20 to 30 mL/hr, with a total CSF volume of 90 to 150 mL within the ventricles and subarachnoid space.

Prevention of infection is imperative by use of strict aseptic technique during dressing changes or sampling of CSF. The system must remain intact to ensure that the ICP readings are accurate, because treatment is initiated and evaluated on the basis of the readings. It is also recommended that a sign be posted above the patient's bed to notify anyone before turning, moving, or suctioning the patient to prevent the removal of too much CSF, which can result in complications such as ventricular collapse, herniation, or subdural hematoma from rapid decompression. Although it is generally recognized that CSF removal decreases ICP and improves CPP, guidelines for CSF removal are not universally accepted but are typically based on institution or physician preference.

Cerebral Oxygenation Monitoring. Failure to adequately deliver oxygenated blood to an injured brain is a major contributor to poor outcomes. Technology is available to measure cerebral oxygenation and cerebral perfusion. Two such devices are currently being used in critical care settings: the *Licox brain tissue oxygenation catheter* and the *jugular venous bulb catheter.*

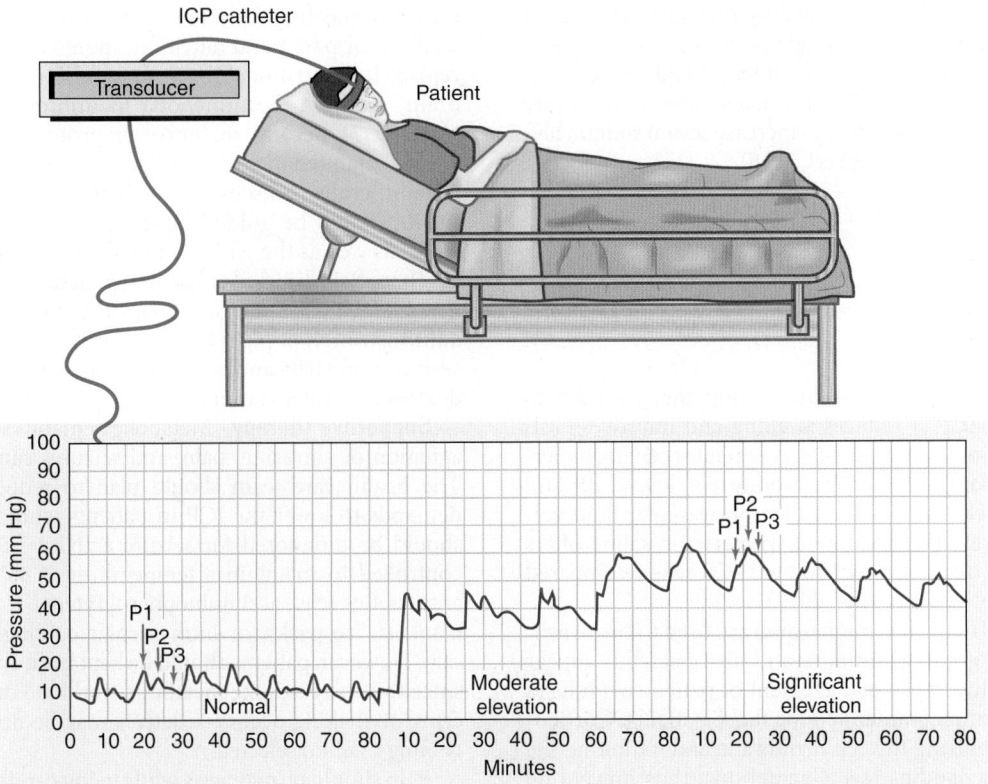

FIG. 59.9 Intracranial pressure (ICP) monitoring can be used to continuously measure ICP. The ICP tracing shows normal, elevated, and plateau waves. At high ICP, the P2 peak is higher than the P1 peak, and the peaks become less distinct and plateau. Source: Copstead-Kirkhorn, L. C., & Banasik, J. L. (2010). *Pathophysiology* (4th ed., p. 1043, Figure 44-7). Mosby.

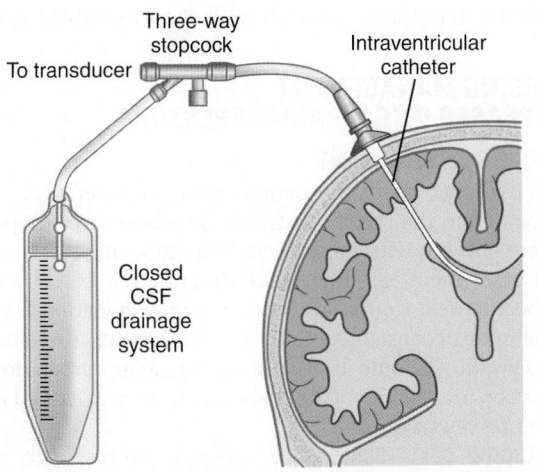

FIG. 59.10 Intermittent drainage system. Cerebrospinal fluid (CSF) is drained via a ventriculostomy when intracranial pressure (ICP) exceeds the upper pressure parameter set by the physician. Intermittent drainage involves opening the three-way stopcock to allow CSF to flow into the draining bag for brief periods (≤5 min) until the pressure is below the upper pressure parameters.

The Licox catheter is placed in the healthy white matter of the brain and provides continuous monitoring of the pressure of oxygen in brain tissue ($PbtO_2$).

The jugular venous bulb catheter is placed in the internal jugular vein and positioned so that the catheter tip is located in the jugular bulb. This catheter provides a measurement of jugular venous oxygen saturation ($SjvO_2$), which indicates total venous brain tissue extraction of oxygen as a measure of cerebral oxygen supply and demand. Neither device has the capability of monitoring ICP; therefore, an ICP monitoring device may be placed for this purpose.

Interprofessional Care

The goals of interprofessional care (see Table 59.3) are to identify and treat the underlying cause of increased ICP and to support brain function. A careful history is an important diagnostic aid that can direct the search for the underlying cause of increased ICP (usually an increase in blood [hemorrhage], brain tissue [tumour or edema], or CSF [hydrocephalus] in the brain).

Ensuring adequate oxygenation to support brain function is the first step in the management of increased ICP. An endotracheal tube or tracheostomy may be necessary to maintain adequate ventilation. Arterial blood gas (ABG) analysis guides the oxygen therapy. The goal is to maintain the PaO_2 at 100 mm Hg or greater. It may be necessary to maintain the patient on a mechanical ventilator to ensure adequate oxygenation.

If the condition is caused by a mass lesion, such as a tumour or hematoma, surgical removal of the mass is the best management (see the Brain Tumours and Cranial Surgery sections later in this chapter). Nonsurgical intervention for the reduction of tissue volume related to cerebral tissue swelling and cerebral edema includes the use of osmotic diuretics, hypertonic saline, and corticosteroids.

Medication Therapy. Medication therapy plays an important role in the management of increased ICP. Mannitol (Osmitrol), an osmotic diuretic given intravenously, can be used to decrease the ICP in acute situations. Mannitol acts to decrease ICP in two ways: plasma expansion and osmotic effect. There is an immediate plasma-expanding effect that reduces the hematocrit and blood viscosity, thereby increasing CBF and cerebral oxygen delivery.

A vascular osmotic gradient is created by mannitol. Thus, fluid moves from the tissues into the blood vessels. ICP is reduced by the decrease in the total brain fluid content. Fluid and electrolyte status must be closely monitored when osmotic diuretics are used, as multiple administrations can increase serum sodium levels and osmolality (Sacco & Delibert, 2018).

> **MEDICATION ALERT—Mannitol (Osmitrol)**
> - Careful monitoring of patients is required because of the adverse effect of fluid shift and the potential for fluid overload and pulmonary congestion.
> - Mannitol may crystallize at lower temperatures; administer intravenously using a filter.

Hypertonic saline is another medication therapy used to manage increased ICP. It reduces swelling and improves CBF, drawing water out of the brain tissue. A patient receiving hypertonic saline infusion must also be monitored closely; BP and serum sodium levels can be affected by intravascular fluid volume excess as a result of treatment. Hypertonic saline offers effective first-line treatment for elevated ICP when compared with mannitol (DeNett & Feltner, 2019).

Corticosteroids (e.g., dexamethasone) are used to treat vasogenic edema surrounding tumours and abscesses but appear to have limited value in the management of patients with head injuries and are not recommended for those patients. Corticosteroids act by stabilizing the cell membrane and inhibiting the synthesis of prostaglandins (see Chapter 14), thus preventing the formation of proinflammatory mediators. Corticosteroids are also thought to improve neuronal function by improving CBF and restoring autoregulation.

Complications associated with the use of corticosteroids include hyperglycemia, increased incidence of infections, gastrointestinal (GI) bleeding, and hyponatremia. Fluid intake and sodium and glucose levels should be monitored regularly. Patients receiving corticosteroids should concurrently be given antacids or histamine (H₂)-receptor blockers (e.g., ranitidine [Zantac]) or proton pump inhibitors (e.g., omeprazole [Losec], pantoprazole [Pantoloc]) to prevent GI ulcers and bleeding.

Medication therapy for reducing cerebral metabolism may be an effective strategy to control ICP. Sedation with propofol (Diprivan) and analgesia, along with the treatments described above, can be used to manage elevated ICP (Sacco & Delibert, 2018). The decision may be made to use high-dose barbiturates (e.g., pentobarbital sodium [Somnotol]) in patients with increased ICP that is refractory to all other treatments (Sacco & Delibert, 2018). Barbiturates dampen the effects of environmental stimuli on patients, thereby decreasing cerebral metabolism and, subsequently, ICP. Capabilities to monitor the patient's ICP, blood flow, EEG, and metabolism should be available when this treatment is used; hypotension as a result of treatment is a concern. There is not sufficient evidence to suggest that outcomes for patients with acute traumatic brain injuries are improved with this treatment (Abraham et al., 2017). Anticonvulsant medications such as phenytoin (Dilantin) may be used because seizures can further increase ICP (seizures are discussed in greater detail in Chapter 61).

Nutritional Therapy. All patients must have their nutritional needs met, regardless of their state of consciousness or health. The patient with increased ICP is in a hypermetabolic and hypercatabolic state that increases the need for glucose to provide the necessary fuel for metabolism of the injured brain. If the patient cannot maintain an adequate oral intake, other means of meeting the nutritional requirements, such as enteral feedings or parenteral nutrition, should be initiated. Feeding to replace full nutritional requirements between days 5 and 7 after brain injury is recommended to improve outcomes (Carney et al., 2017). Because malnutrition promotes continued cerebral edema, maintenance of optimal nutrition is imperative. (Nutritional therapy is discussed in Chapter 42.) Feedings or supplements should be guided by the patient's fluid and electrolyte status as well as the patient's metabolic needs.

Therapy is directed at keeping patients normovolemic. Intravenous (IV) 0.9% sodium chloride is the preferred solution for administration of piggyback medications because a lowering of serum osmolarity and an increase in cerebral edema occur if 5% dextrose in water is used.

Supportive Therapy. Metabolic demands such as fever (38°C), agitation or shivering, pain, and seizures can also increase ICP. The health care team should plan to reduce these metabolic demands to lower the ICP in patients who are at risk. Patients should be monitored for seizure activity. Fever should be well controlled to maintain a temperature of 36° to 37°C by using antipyretics (e.g., acetaminophen [Tylenol]), cool baths, cooling blankets, ice packs, or intravascular cooling devices, as necessary. However, patients should be kept from shivering or shaking, since this increases the metabolic workload on the brain. If shivering or shaking occurs, sedatives may be needed or a different cooling method selected.

Pain should be managed while being careful not to oversedate or overmedicate. Finally, the patient should remain in a quiet, calm environment with minimal noise and interruptions. The patient should be observed for signs of agitation, irritation, or frustration. Also, the caregiver and the family should be taught about decreasing stimulation, and the health care team should coordinate to minimize procedures that may produce agitation.

NURSING MANAGEMENT
INCREASED INTRACRANIAL PRESSURE

NURSING ASSESSMENT

Subjective data about the patient with increased ICP can be obtained from the patient or family members or other persons who are familiar with the patient. The nurse must learn appropriate assessment techniques and describe the LOC by noting the specific behaviours observed. When a deviation from the normal state of consciousness occurs, a more structured method of observation should be initiated. Adequate circulation and respiration are the most vital body functions and should always be the first ones assessed.

GLASGOW COMA SCALE. The Glasgow Coma Scale (GCS), developed in 1974, is a quick, practical, and standardized system for assessing the degree to which consciousness is impaired. It provides a universal language for describing altered states of consciousness. The three areas assessed in the GCS correspond to the definition of coma as the inability of a patient to speak, obey commands, or open their eyes when a verbal or painful stimulus is applied (Jennett & Teasdale, 1977). Specific assessments evaluate the patient's response to varying degrees of stimuli. Three indicators of response are evaluated: (1) eye opening, (2) best verbal response, and (3) best motor response (see Table 59.4). Specific behaviours that are seen as responses to the testing stimulus in each of these three areas are given a numeric value and can be plotted on a graph. The nurse's responsibility is to elicit the best response on each of the scales; the higher the scores, the higher the level of brain functioning. A graph can be used to determine whether the patient's condition is stable, improving, or deteriorating. The subscale scores are particularly important if a patient is untestable in one area. For example, severe periorbital edema may make eye opening impossible. The total GCS score is a sum of the numeric values assigned to each of the three areas evaluated. The highest GCS score is 15 for a fully alert person, and the lowest possible score is 3. A GCS score of 8 or less is generally indicative of coma (Teasdale & Jennett, 1974).

The GCS offers several advantages in the assessment of the unconscious patient. It is specific and structured, allowing different health care providers to arrive at the same conclusion regarding the patient's status. It saves time for the assessor because the ratings are done with numbers rather than with lengthy descriptions.

The GCS is also specific enough to discriminate between different or changing states. It is used to assess the arousal aspect of consciousness. Other components of the neurological assessment include pupillary checks, extremity strength testing, vital signs, and, if appropriate, testing of the function of specific cranial nerves.

NEUROLOGICAL ASSESSMENT. The pupils are compared with one another for size, movement, and response (Figure 59.11). If the oculomotor nerve is compressed, the pupil on the affected side (ipsilateral) becomes larger until it fully dilates. If ICP continues to increase, both pupils dilate. Pupil size is measured in millimetres before assessing the pupil response to light.

Pupillary reaction is tested with a penlight. The normal reaction is brisk constriction when the light is shone directly into the eye. A consensual response (a slight constriction in the opposite pupil) should also be noted at the same time. A sluggish reaction can indicate early pressure on CN III. A fixed pupil shows no response to light stimulus, which usually indicates increased ICP. However, there are other causes of a fixed pupil, including direct injury to CN III, previous eye surgery, administration of atropine, and use of mydriatic eye drops.

Evaluation of other cranial nerves can be included in the neurological assessment. Eye movements controlled by CNs III, IV, and VI can be examined in the patient who is awake and can be used to assess the function of the brainstem. In patients who are unconscious, eye movements can be elicited by reflex with the use of head movements (oculocephalic) and caloric

stimulation (oculovestibular). (Chapters 23 and 24 discuss assessment and conditions of the eye and ear.) Testing the corneal reflex provides clinical information regarding the function of CNs V and VII. If corneal reflexes are absent, routine eye care should be initiated to prevent corneal abrasion.

For the patient who is awake, motor strength is tested by asking the patient to squeeze the nurse's hands to compare strength in the hands. The palmar (or pronator) drift test is an excellent measure of strength in the upper extremities. With eyes closed, the patient raises their arms in front of the body with the palmar surface facing upward. If there is any weakness in the upper extremity, the palmar surface rotates inward and the arm may drift downward. The patient keeps their eyes closed to prevent being able to see the palmar drift and trying to correct the rotating hand position. Detection of a palmar drift is an early indicator of corticospinal tract compression and possible increased ICP. Asking the patient to raise their foot from the bed or to bend their knees up in bed is a good assessment of lower extremity strength. All four extremities should be tested for strength and evaluated for any asymmetry in strength or movement.

For patients who are unconscious or uncooperative, motor strength can be assessed by observation of their spontaneous movement. If no spontaneous movement is possible, a pain stimulus should be applied to the patient, and the response should be noted. Resistance to movement during passive range-of-motion exercises is another measure of strength.

Vital signs, including BP, pulse, respiratory rate, and temperature, should also be systematically recorded. Cushing's triad is a triad of changes to vital signs (increased BP with a widening pulse pressure, bradycardia, and irregular respiratory pattern). This triad indicates severe increased ICP and impending cerebral herniation. Specific respiratory patterns are associated with severely increased ICP (Figure 59.12).

Pattern	Location of Lesion	Description
1. Cheyne–Stokes	Bilateral hemispheric disease or metabolic brain dysfunction	Cycles of hyperventilation and apnea
2. Central neurogenic hyperventilation	Brainstem between lower midbrain and upper pons	Sustained, regular rapid and deep breathing
3. Apneustic breathing	Mid or lower pons	Prolonged inspiratory phase or pauses alternating with expiratory pauses
4. Cluster breathing	Medulla or lower pons	Clusters of breaths follow each other with irregular pauses between
5. Ataxic breathing	Reticular formation of the medulla	Completely irregular with some breaths deep and some shallow. Random, irregular pauses, slow rate

FIG. 59.12 Common abnormal respiratory patterns associated with coma.

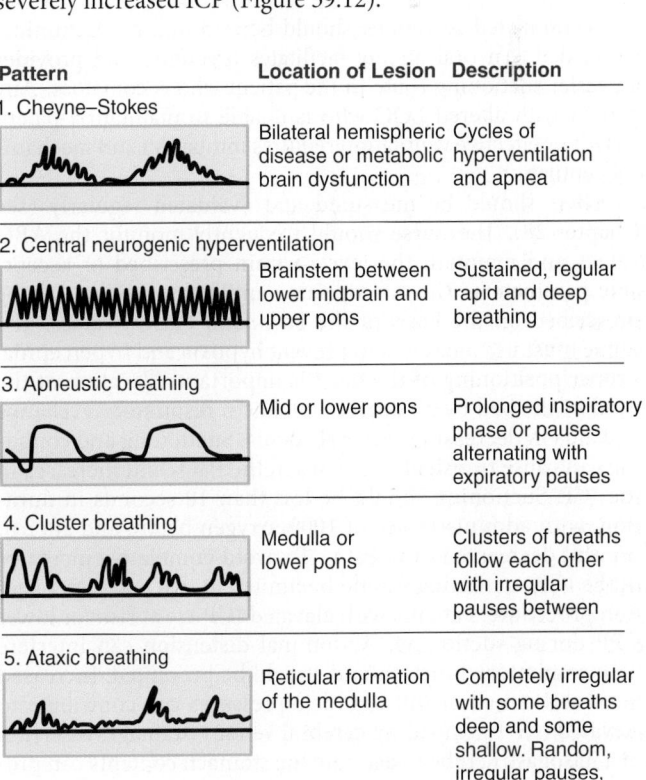

○ ○ Pupils equal and react normally

○ ○ Pupil reacts to light (slowly or briskly)

○ ○ Dilated pupil (compressed cranial nerve III)

○ ○ Bilateral dilated, fixed pupils (ominous sign)

○ ○ Pinpoint pupils (pons damage or drugs)

FIG. 59.11 Pupillary check for size and response.

NURSING DIAGNOSES

Nursing diagnoses for the patient with increased ICP include but are not limited to the following:

- *Decreased intracranial adaptive capacity* resulting from *decreased cerebral perfusion or increased ICP*
- *Potential for inadequate cerebral tissue perfusion* as demonstrated by *brain injury, brain neoplasm, cerebral aneurysm*
- *Potential for disuse syndrome* as demonstrated by *alteration in LOC, mechanical immobility, paralysis*

Additional information on nursing diagnoses for patients with increased ICP is presented in Nursing Care Plan (NCP) 59.1, available on the Evolve website.

PLANNING

The overall goals are that the patient with increased ICP will (1) maintain a patent airway, (2) have ICP within normal limits, (3) have normal fluid and electrolyte balance, and (4) have no complications secondary to immobility and decreased LOC.

NURSING IMPLEMENTATION

ACUTE INTERVENTION

Respiratory Function. Maintenance of a patent airway is critical in the patient with increased ICP and is a primary nursing responsibility. As the LOC decreases, the patient is at increased risk for airway obstruction from the tongue dropping back and occluding the airway or from accumulation of secretions. Altered breathing patterns may become evident. Airway patency can be aided by keeping the patient lying on one side, with frequent position changes.

SAFETY ALERT
- Be alert to altered breathing patterns in a patient with increased ICP.
- Snoring sounds indicate obstruction and require immediate intervention.

Accumulated secretions should be removed by suctioning, as needed. An oral airway facilitates breathing and provides an easier suctioning route in the patient who is comatose. Any patient with altered LOC who is unable to maintain a patent airway or effective ventilation requires intubation and mechanical ventilation.

ABGs should be measured and evaluated regularly (see Chapter 28). The nurse should frequently monitor the ABG values and maintain the levels within prescribed or acceptable parameters. The appropriate ventilatory support can be prescribed on the basis of the PaO_2 and $PaCO_2$ values. The nurse must use measures to prevent hypoxia and hypercapnia. Proper positioning of the head is important. Elevation of the head of the bed by 30 degrees enhances respiratory exchange and aids in decreasing cerebral edema. Suctioning and coughing can cause transient decreases in the PaO_2 and increases in the ICP. Suctioning should be less than 10 seconds in duration, with administration of 100% oxygen before and after to prevent decreases in the PaO_2. To avoid cumulative increases in the ICP, suctioning should be limited to two passes per suction procedure. Patients with elevated ICP are at risk for lower CPP during suctioning. Abdominal distension can interfere with respiratory function and should be prevented. Increased intra-abdominal or intrathoracic pressures can contribute to elevated ICP by impeding cerebral venous drainage. Insertion of a nasogastric tube to aspirate the stomach contents can prevent distension, vomiting, and possible aspiration. However, in patients with facial and skull fractures, a nasogastric tube is contraindicated, and oral insertion of a gastric tube is preferred.

Pain, anxiety, and fear from the initial injury, therapeutic procedures, or noxious stimuli can increase ICP and BP, complicating the management and the recovery of the patient with a brain injury. The appropriate choice or combination of sedatives, paralytics, and analgesics for symptom management presents a challenge to the CCU team. Administration of these agents may alter the neurological state, masking true neurological changes. It may be necessary to temporarily suspend pharmacological therapy to appropriately assess neurological status. The choice, the dosage, and the combination of agents may vary depending on the patient's history, neurological state, and overall clinical presentation.

The IV anaesthetic sedative propofol (Diprivan) has gained popularity in the management of pain and anxiety in the CCU because of its rapid onset, short half-life, and oxygen-saving properties. It has been shown to depress cerebral metabolism and oxygen consumption, offering neuroprotective benefits, and is a medication of choice for sedation and elevated ICP in the ICU setting (Oddo et al., 2016).

Dexmedetomidine (Precedex), an α_2-adrenergic agonist, is used for continuous IV sedation of patients who are intubated and mechanically ventilated in the CCU setting for up to 24 hours. It is another ideal agent for patients with neurological conditions because of the ease in obtaining a neurological assessment without altering the dose because of its anxiolytic properties. The benzodiazepine midazolam can be used for sedation and management of ICP as well (Sacco & Delibert, 2018). When using continuous IV sedatives, the nurse needs to be aware of the adverse effects of these medications, especially hypotension, since this can result in a lower CPP value.

Nondepolarizing neuromuscular blocking agents (e.g., cisatracurium) are useful for ventilatory management and treatment of refractory intracranial hypertension. Because these agents paralyze muscles without blocking pain or noxious stimuli, they are used in combination with sedatives, analgesics, or benzodiazepines. Opioids, such as morphine sulphate and fentanyl, are rapid-onset analgesics with minimal effect on CBF or oxygen metabolism.

Fluid and Electrolyte Balance. Fluid and electrolyte disturbances can have an adverse effect on ICP. IV fluids should be closely monitored with the use of a limited-volume device or a volume-control apparatus for accuracy. Intake and output, with insensible losses and daily weights taken into account, are important parameters in the assessment of fluid balance.

Electrolyte determinations should be made daily, and any abnormal values should be discussed with the physician. It is especially important to monitor serum glucose, sodium, potassium, and osmolality. Urinary output is monitored to detect conditions related to diabetes insipidus (DI) (e.g., increased urinary output related to a decrease in antidiuretic hormone secretion); SIADH, which results in decreased urinary output; and cerebral salt wasting, a form of hyponatremia caused by excessive renal sodium excretion associated with cerebral insult. Besides urinary output, the serum and urine sodium and osmolality are also used to diagnose DI, SIADH, and cerebral salt wasting. DI may result in severe dehydration unless treated. The usual treatment is fluid replacement, vasopressin, or desmopressin acetate (DDAVP). SIADH results in a dilutional hyponatremia that may produce cerebral edema, changes in LOC, seizures, and coma.

(Treatment of SIADH is described in Chapter 51.) Treatment of cerebral salt wasting consists of aggressive sodium (Na^+) and volume replacement.

Monitoring Intracranial Pressure. ICP monitoring is used in combination with other physiological parameters to guide the care of the patient and assess the patient's response to routine care. The Valsalva manoeuvre, coughing, sneezing, hypoxemia, pain, fever, and environmental stimuli are factors that can increase ICP. Nurses should be alert to these factors and attempt to keep them to a minimum.

Body Position. The patient with increased ICP should be maintained in the head-up position. The nurse must take care to prevent extreme neck flexion, which can cause venous obstruction and contribute to elevated ICP. The body position should be adjusted to decrease the ICP as much as possible and to improve the CPP. Traditional practice has been to elevate the head of the bed to 30 degrees, unless a concurrent cervical neck injury has been identified, in which case a reverse Trendelenburg position may be indicated to elevate the head while keeping the spine aligned. Elevation of the head of the bed reduces sagittal sinus pressure, promotes venous drainage from the head via the valveless jugular system, and decreases the vascular congestion that can produce cerebral edema. However, raising the head of the bed above 30 degrees may decrease the CPP. Careful evaluation of the effects of elevation of the head of the bed on both the ICP and the CPP is required—the bed should be positioned so that it lowers the ICP while maintaining the CPP and other indices of cerebral oxygenation.

Care should be taken to turn the patient with slow, gentle movements because rapid changes in position may increase the ICP. Caution should be used to prevent discomfort in turning and positioning the patient because pain or agitation also increases ICP. Increased intra-abdominal and intrathoracic pressure contribute to increased ICP by impeding the venous return. Thus, coughing, straining, and the Valsalva manoeuvre should be avoided. Extreme hip flexion should be prevented to decrease the risk of raising the intra-abdominal pressure. The patient should be turned at least every 2 hours.

Abnormal posturing (abnormal flexion and extension) is a reflex response in some patients with increased ICP (see Figure 59.6). Turning, skin care, and even passive range of motion can elicit the posturing reflexes. Attempts should be made to provide needed physical-care activities to minimize complications of immobility, such as atelectasis and contractures. In cases of severe posturing reflexes, these activities may have to be done less frequently because posturing can cause increases in ICP.

Protection From Injury. The patient with increased ICP and a decreased LOC needs protection from self-injury. Confusion, agitation, and the possibility of seizures can put the patient at risk for injury. In these cases, environmental, chemical, or physical restraints may be considered to protect the patient from harm (e.g., removing tubes, wandering). A least-restraint approach should be used and considered only after all possible alternative interventions are exhausted. Specific employer policies and procedures should help guide restraint practice. The need for restraints should be reassessed daily. If restraints are necessary, they should be secure enough to be effective, and the area under the restraints should be observed regularly for skin irritation and adequate blood circulation. Restrained extremities should be assessed at least every 2 hours for colour, warmth, sensation, and movement. Agitation may increase with the use of restraints, which indicates the need for other measures to protect the patient from injury. Light sedation with agents such as haloperidol (Haldol) or lorazepam (Ativan) may be needed. Patient history and clinical presentation may be used to guide medication choice. Having a family member stay with the patient may have a calming effect.

For the patient with seizures or the patient at risk for seizure activity, seizure precautions should be instituted. These include padded side rails, an airway at the bedside, accurate and timely administration of anticonvulsant medications, and close observation (see Chapter 61).

The patient can benefit from a quiet, nonstimulating environment. The nurse should always use a calm, reassuring approach. Touching and talking to the patient, even one who is in a coma, is always appropriate care. The nurse must create a balance between sensory deprivation and overload for the patient with increased ICP.

Psychological Considerations. In addition to providing carefully planned physical care to patients with increased ICP, the nurse must also be aware of the psychological well-being of patients and their families. Anxiety over the diagnosis and the prognosis for patients with neurological disorders can be distressing to patients and their families. The nurse's competent and assured manner in performing the care that patients need is reassuring to everyone involved. Short, simple explanations are appropriate and enable patients and their families to acquire the amount of information they desire. There is a need for support, information, and education of patients, families, and caregivers. The nurse should assess the family members' desire to assist in providing care for the patient and allow for their participation as appropriate. The nurse should encourage interdisciplinary management (social work, chaplain, etc.) of the patient and family in decision making as much as possible.

EVALUATION

The expected outcomes for the patient with ICP are addressed in NCP 59.1, available on the Evolve website.

HEAD INJURY

Head injury includes any trauma to the scalp, the skull, or the brain. The term *head trauma* is used primarily to signify craniocerebral trauma, which includes an alteration in consciousness, no matter how brief.

Statistics for head injuries are incomplete because many victims die at the scene of the accident or because the condition is considered minor and health care services are not sought. Approximately 160 000 Canadians sustain a head injury annually, and over 1.5 million live with the effects of an acquired brain injury (Brain Injury Canada [BIC], 2021). Brain injuries among Indigenous populations is estimated to be four to five times the rate of the general population, and the rate increases in more remote locations (Northern Brain Injury Association, 2021). Traumatic brain injury (TBI) continues to be one of the leading causes of death and the leading cause of disability after trauma. In Canada, the most common causes of TBI requiring hospitalizations are motor vehicle accidents and falls. Other causes include assaults, sports-related injuries, and gunshot wounds (BIC, 2021).

Head trauma has a high potential for poor outcome. Death from head trauma occurs at three time periods following an injury: immediately after the injury, within 2 hours after the injury, and approximately 3 weeks after injury. The majority of deaths after a head injury occur immediately after the injury, either from the direct head trauma or from massive hemorrhage and shock. Deaths occurring within a few hours of the trauma are caused by progressive worsening of the head injury or from internal bleeding. An immediate note of changes in neurological status and surgical intervention are critical in the prevention of deaths at this point. Deaths occurring 3 weeks or longer after injury result from multisystem failure. Expert nursing care in the weeks following the injury is crucial in decreasing mortality and optimizing patient outcomes.

Types of Head Injuries

Scalp Lacerations. *Scalp lacerations* are the most minor type of head trauma. Because the scalp contains many blood vessels with poor constrictive abilities, most scalp lacerations are associated with profuse bleeding. The major complications associated with scalp laceration are blood loss and infection.

Skull Fractures. *Skull fractures* frequently occur with head trauma. There are several ways to describe skull fractures: (1) linear or depressed; (2) simple, comminuted, or compound; and (3) closed or open (Table 59.6). Fractures may be closed or open, depending on the presence of a scalp laceration or extension of the fracture into the air sinuses or the dura. The type and severity of a skull fracture depend on the velocity, the momentum, the direction of the injuring agent, and the site of impact.

The location of the fracture alters the presentation of the manifestations (Table 59.7). For example, a specialized type of linear fracture is seen when the fracture occurs at the base of the skull—a basilar skull fracture. Manifestations include *Battle sign* (postauricular ecchymosis) (Figure 59.13) and *bilateral periorbital ecchymosis* (raccoon eyes). This fracture generally crosses a sinus and tears the dura (e.g., the frontal or temporal dura) and is associated with cranial nerve damage and leakage of CSF. *CSF rhinorrhea* (CSF leakage from the nose) or *CSF otorrhea* (CSF leakage from the ear) generally confirms that the fracture has traversed the dura (Figure 59.14). The CSF leak places these patients at high risk for meningitis.

Two methods of testing can be used to determine whether the fluid leaking from the nose or ear is CSF. The first method is to test the leaking fluid with a Dextrostix or Tes-Tape strip to determine whether glucose is present. CSF gives a positive reading for glucose. If blood is present in the fluid, testing for the presence of glucose is unreliable because blood contains glucose. In this event, the nurse should look for the *halo* or *ring sign* (see Figure 59.14, *C*). To perform this test, the nurse allows the leaking fluid to drip onto a white pad (4-cm × 4-cm) or towel and observes the drainage. Within a few minutes, the blood coalesces into the centre, and a yellowish ring encircles the blood if CSF is present. The colour, the appearance, and the amount of leaking fluid must be noted because both tests can give false-positive results.

The major potential complications of skull fractures are intracranial infections and hematoma, as well as meningeal and brain tissue damage.

Head Trauma. Brain injuries are categorized as diffuse (generalized) or focal (localized). In a *diffuse* injury (e.g., concussion, diffuse axonal injury), damage to the brain cannot be localized to one particular area. In a *focal injury* (e.g., contusion, hematoma), damage can be localized to a specific area of the brain. Brain injury can be classified as *mild* (GCS score of 13 to 15), *moderate* (GCS score of 9 to 12), and *severe* (GCS score of 3 to 8).

TABLE 59.6   TYPES OF SKULL FRACTURES

Description	Cause
Linear Break in continuity of bone without alteration of relationship of parts	Low-velocity injuries
Depressed Inward indentation of skull	Powerful blow
Simple Linear or depressed skull fracture without fragmentation or communicating lacerations	Low-to-moderate impact
Comminuted Multiple linear fractures with fragmentation of bone into many pieces	Direct, high-momentum impact
Compound Depressed skull fracture and scalp laceration with communicating pathway to intracranial cavity	Severe head injury

TABLE 59.7   CLINICAL MANIFESTATIONS OF DIFFERENT TYPES OF SKULL FRACTURES

Location	Clinical Manifestations
Frontal fracture	Exposure of brain to contaminants through frontal air sinus, possible association with air in forehead tissue, CSF rhinorrhea, or pneumocranium (air between the cranium and dura mater)
Orbital fracture	Periorbital ecchymosis (raccoon eyes), optic nerve injury
Temporal fracture	Boggy temporalis muscle because of extravasation of blood, oval bruise behind ear in mastoid region (Battle sign), CSF otorrhea, middle meningeal artery disruption, epidural hematoma
Parietal fracture	Deafness, CSF or brain otorrhea, bulging of tympanic membrane caused by blood or CSF, facial paralysis, Battle sign
Posterior fossa fracture	Occipital bruising resulting in cortical blindness, visual field defects; rare appearance of ataxia or other cerebellar signs
Basilar skull fracture	Otorrhea, bulging of tympanic membrane caused by blood or CSF, Battle sign, tinnitus or hearing difficulty, rhinorrhea, facial paralysis, conjugate deviation of gaze, vertigo, bilateral raccoon eyes

CSF, cerebrospinal fluid.

Diffuse Injury. Concussion (a sudden, transient, mechanical head injury with disruption of neural activity and a change in the LOC) is considered a mild traumatic brain injury. The patient may or may not lose total consciousness with this injury. Mild TBI is significantly underdiagnosed, and the societal impact is great.

Signs of concussion may include the following: any period of loss of or a decreased LOC less than 30 minutes; any lack of memory for events immediately before or after the injury (posttraumatic amnesia) less than 24 hours; any alteration in mental state at the time of the injury (e.g., confusion, disorientation, slowed thinking, alteration of consciousness or mental state);

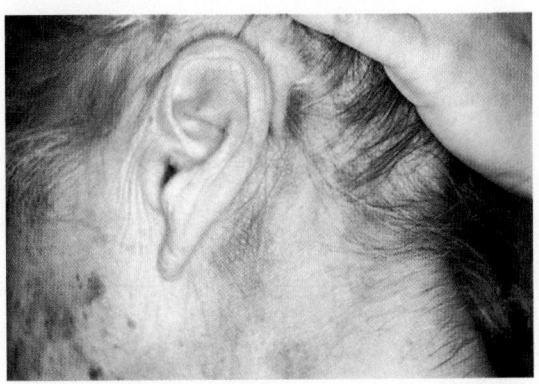

FIG. 59.13 Battle sign. Source: Bingham, B. J. G., Hawke, M., & Kwok, P. (1992). *Clinical atlas of otolaryngology.* Mosby.

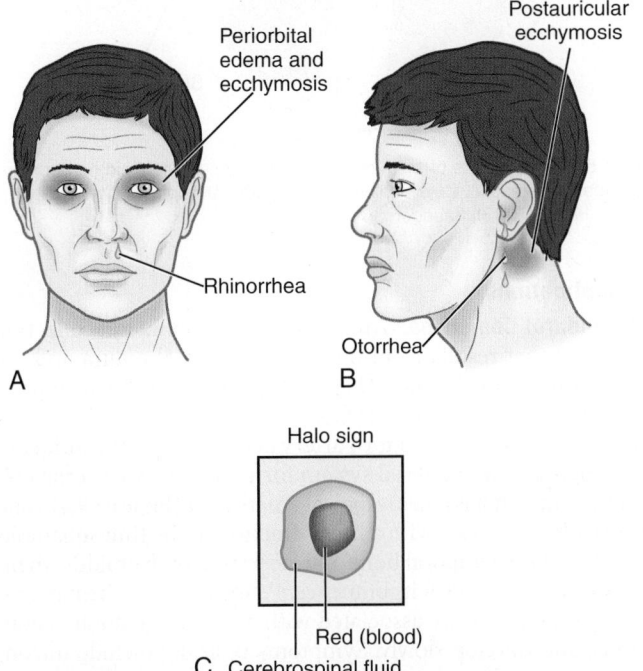

FIG. 59.14 **A,** Raccoon eyes and rhinorrhea. **B,** Battle sign (postauricular ecchymosis) with otorrhea. **C,** Halo or ring sign (see text).

and physical symptoms that include headache, weakness, loss of balance, change in vision or hearing changes, or dizziness (Marshall et al., 2018). The manifestations of concussion are generally of short duration. Patients can usually be discharged for home observation if they have a normal mental status with resolving symptoms and no additional risk factors (e.g., vomiting, severe headache, multiple injuries, intoxication) after 4 hours of observation (Marshall et al., 2018). The patient and caregiver require appropriate discharge instructions, including signs and symptoms of acute deterioration and when to notify the health care provider (Marshall et al., 2018).

Postconcussion syndrome is seen anywhere from 2 weeks to 2 months after the concussion. Symptoms include persistent headache, lethargy, personality and behavioural changes, shortened attention span, decreased short-term memory, and changes in intellectual ability. This syndrome can significantly affect the patient's abilities to perform activities of daily living.

Although concussion is generally considered benign and usually resolves spontaneously, the symptoms may be the beginning of a more serious, progressive condition that can continue for years following the injury.

Individuals with mild or moderate, sports-related concussions are more likely to have future concussive injuries. Recurrent concussions are also associated with slower recovery and may have long-term effects. Patients should be instructed to avoid contact sports until all symptoms have subsided. In addition, return to play should be gradual (Parachute, 2021).

Chronic traumatic encephalopathy (CTE) is the term used to describe degeneration in the brain from repeated concussions, including those sustained during sports. Research is ongoing to examine the link between repeated concussions and brain degeneration (Canadian Concussion Centre, 2020).

Diffuse Axonal Injury. Diffuse axonal injury (DAI) is widespread axonal damage occurring after a mild, moderate, or severe TBI. The damage occurs primarily around axons in subcortical white matter of the cerebral hemispheres, the basal ganglia, the thalamus, and the brainstem. Initially, DAI was believed to occur from the tensile forces of trauma that sheared axons, resulting in axonal disconnection. There is increasing evidence that axonal damage is not preceded by an immediate tearing of the axon from the traumatic impact, but rather that the trauma changes the function of the axon, resulting in axon swelling (axonal ballooning) and disconnection. This process takes approximately 12 to 24 hours to develop and may persist longer. The clinical signs and symptoms include a decreased LOC, increased ICP, decerebration or decortication, and global cerebral edema. Severity of DAI has been linked with unfavourable outcomes (van Eijk et al., 2018).

Focal Injury. Focal injury can be mild to severe and is localized to an area of injury. Focal injury consists of lacerations, contusions, hematomas, and cranial nerve injuries.

Lacerations involve actual tearing of the brain tissue and often occur in association with depressed and compound fractures and penetrating injuries. Tissue damage is severe, and surgical repair of the laceration is impossible because of the texture of the brain tissue.

When major head trauma occurs, many delayed responses are seen, including hemorrhage, hematoma formation, seizures, and cerebral edema. Intracerebral hemorrhage is generally associated with cerebral laceration. This hemorrhage manifests as a space-occupying lesion accompanied by unconsciousness, hemiplegia on the contralateral side, and a dilated pupil on the ipsilateral side. As the hematoma expands, symptoms of increased ICP become more severe. Prognosis is generally poor for the patient with a large intracerebral hemorrhage. Subarachnoid hemorrhage and intraventricular hemorrhage can also occur secondary to head trauma. The Ethical Dilemmas box considers a case of brain death due to severe brain injury.

A **contusion**, frequently occurring near the site of a skull fracture, is the bruising of the brain tissue within a focal area. A contusion often develops in areas of hemorrhage, infarction, necrosis, and edema. With contusion, the phenomenon of *coup–contrecoup injury* is often noted (Figure 59.15). Damage from coup–contrecoup injury occurs because of mass movement of the brain inside the skull. Contusions or lacerations occur both at the site of the direct impact of the brain on the skull *(coup)* and at a secondary area of damage on the opposite side away from the injury *(contrecoup)*, leading to multiple contused areas. Patient prognosis is dependent on the amount of bleeding around the contusion sites, which can range from minimal to

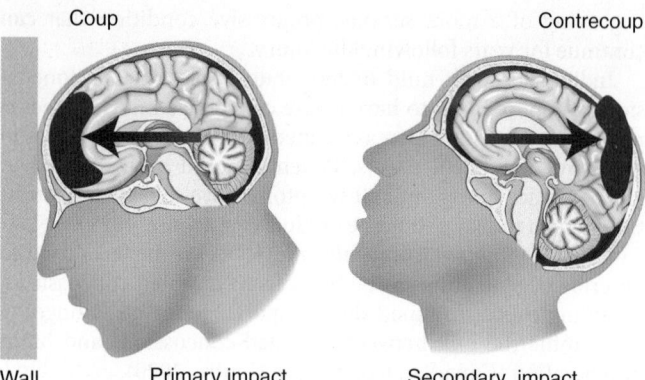

FIG. 59.15 Coup–contrecoup injury. After the head strikes the wall, a coup injury occurs as the brain strikes the skull (primary impact). The contrecoup injury (the secondary impact) occurs when the brain strikes the skull surface opposite to the site of the original impact.

ETHICAL DILEMMAS
Brain Death

Situation
The emergency nurse receives a call from emergency medical services (EMS) personnel about a young man who has been involved in a motorcycle crash. The patient was not wearing a helmet and has a large, open-skull fracture with obvious grey matter oozing from the area. Transport from the accident scene was delayed by 45 minutes as a result of a severe thunderstorm and traffic congestion. On the way to the hospital, the patient has fixed, dilated pupils and a cardiac arrest. Estimated time of arrival at the hospital is still an additional 45 minutes as a result of the severe weather. The decision is made to stop resuscitation efforts.

Important Points for Consideration
- Death, by neurological criteria, occurs when the cerebral cortex stops functioning or is irreversibly destroyed.
- Because technology has been developed that assists in supporting life, controversies have arisen related to an exact definition of *death*.
- Criteria for *brain death* include coma or unresponsiveness, absence of brainstem reflexes, and apnea. Specific assessments by a physician are required to validate each of the criteria.
- The patient's clinical manifestations indicate that brain death has occurred.
- Although there is a slight chance that the patient's heart function could be resuscitated and supported with mechanical ventilation, there is no obligation to provide medically futile care for a patient with brain death.
- Brain death criteria do not address patients in a permanent vegetative state because the brainstem activity in these patients is adequate to maintain heart and lung function.

Critical Thinking Questions
1. What might the nurse's feelings be about cessation of brain function versus cessation of heart and lung function as the criteria for death of a patient?
2. What legislation or practices are there in the nurse's province or territory about EMS personnel stopping cardiopulmonary resuscitation (CPR) efforts in the field?

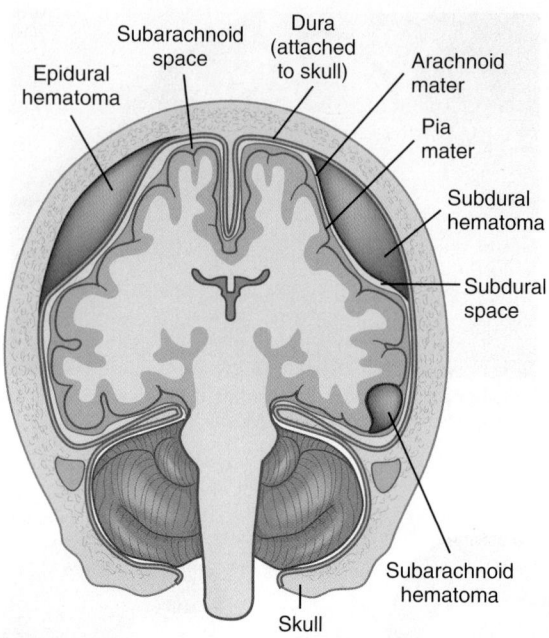

FIG. 59.16 Locations of epidural, subdural, and subarachnoid hematomas. Source: Copstead, L. C., & Banaski, J. L. (2010). *Pathophysiology* (4th ed., p. 1051, Figure 44-13). Saunders.

Complications

Epidural Hematoma. An **epidural hematoma** is a collection of blood that results from bleeding between the dura and the inner surface of the skull (Figure 59.16); it produces compression of the dura mater and thus of the brain. Epidural hematomas that are a result of a torn artery and are under the influence of a high-pressure arterial system form rapidly. An arterial epidural hematoma is a neurological emergency (Figure 59.17) and is usually associated with a linear fracture to the thin squamous portion of the temporal bone and laceration of the middle meningeal artery or one of its branches. Venous epidural hematomas are less common, are associated with a tear of the dural venous sinus, and develop slowly. Symptoms typically include unconsciousness at the scene, with a brief lucid interval followed by a decrease in LOC. Other symptoms may be a headache, nausea and vomiting, or focal findings. Rapid surgical intervention to prevent cerebral herniation dramatically improves outcomes.

Subdural Hematoma. A **subdural hematoma** is a collection of blood that results from bleeding between the dura mater and the arachnoid layer of the meningeal covering of the brain. A subdural hematoma usually results from injury to the brain substance and its parenchymal vessels (see Figure 59.16). The bridging veins that drain from the surface of the brain into the sagittal sinus are the source of most subdural hematomas. Because a subdural hematoma is usually venous in origin, the hematoma is much slower to develop into a mass large enough to produce symptoms. However, a subdural hematoma may also be caused by tearing of small cortical arteries, in which case it develops more rapidly. Subdural hematomas may be acute, subacute, or chronic (Table 59.8).

An *acute subdural hematoma* manifests signs within 48 hours of the injury. The size of the hematoma determines the patient's clinical presentation as well as prognosis. The signs and symptoms are similar to those associated with brain tissue compression in increased ICP and include decreasing LOC and headache. The patient can range from being drowsy and confused to being unconscious. The ipsilateral pupil may dilate

severe. Contusions may continue to bleed or rebleed and appear to evolve on subsequent CT scans of the brain. Contusions that continue to evolve have a poorer prognosis. Neurological assessment demonstrates focal findings and a generalized disturbance in the LOC. Seizures are a common complication of brain contusion.

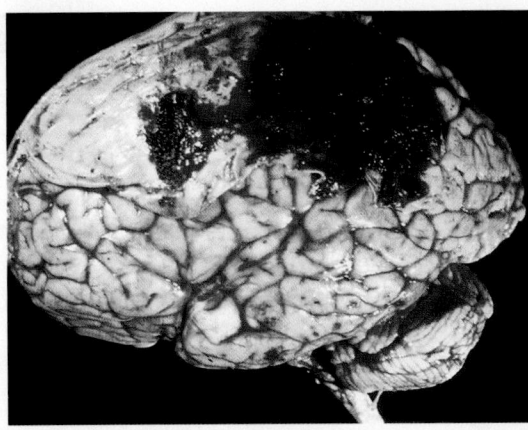

FIG. 59.17 Epidural hematoma covering a portion of the dura. Multiple small contusions are seen in the temporal lobe. Source: Kumar, V., Abbas, A. K., Fausto, N., et al. (2010). *Robbins and Cotran: Pathologic basis of disease* (8th ed., p. 1289, Figure 28-11). Saunders. Courtesy the late Dr. Raymond D. Adams, Massachusetts General Hospital, Boston.

TABLE 59.8	TYPES OF SUBDURAL HEMATOMAS	
Occurrence After Injury	**Progression of Symptoms**	**Treatment**
Acute Up to 48 hr after severe trauma	Immediate deterioration	Craniotomy, evacuation, and decompression
Subacute 48 hr to 2 wk after severe trauma	Alteration in mental status as hematoma develops; progression dependent on size and location of hematoma	Evacuation and decompression
Chronic Weeks, months, usually >20 days after injury; often, injury seemed trivial or is forgotten by patient	Nonspecific, nonlocalizing progression; progressive alteration in LOC	Evacuation and decompression, membranectomy

LOC, level of consciousness.

and become fixed if ICP is sufficiently increased. Acute subdural hematoma is most often associated with traumatic injury, and underlying brain injury may result in cerebral edema, worsening the neurological assessment. The subsequent cerebral edema contributes to increased morbidity and mortality despite surgical intervention to evacuate the hematoma.

A *subacute subdural hematoma* usually occurs within 2 to 14 days of the injury. Failure to regain consciousness may point to this possibility. After the initial bleeding, a subdural hematoma may appear to enlarge over time as the breakdown products of the blood draw fluid into the subdural space to reach isotonicity.

A *chronic subdural hematoma* develops over weeks or months after a seemingly minor head injury. The peak incidence of chronic subdural hematoma occurs to individuals in their 50s and 60s, when a potentially larger subdural space is available as a result of brain atrophy. With atrophy, the brain remains attached to the supportive structures, but tension to the bridging veins is increased and the bridging veins are subject to tearing. The larger

size of the subdural space also accounts for the presenting complaint being the focal symptoms, rather than the signs of increased ICP. People with chronic alcoholism are also prone to cerebral atrophy and subsequent development of subdural hematoma.

Delay in diagnosis of a subdural hematoma in older persons can be attributed to symptoms that mimic other health problems in people of this age group, such as vascular disease and dementia. Somnolence, confusion, lethargy, and memory loss are also associated with health conditions other than subdural hematoma.

Intraparenchymal Hematoma. Intraparenchymal or intracerebral hematoma is a collection of blood within the parenchyma that results from bleeding within the brain tissue itself and occurs in approximately 16% of head injuries. Usually, it occurs within the frontal and temporal lobes, possibly from the rupture of intracerebral vessels at the time of injury. The size and location of the hematoma are key determinants of patient outcome.

Traumatic Subarachnoid Hemorrhage. *Traumatic subarachnoid hemorrhage* is a result of traumatic forces damaging the superficial vascular structures in the subarachnoid space. The presence of a traumatic subarachnoid hemorrhage may predispose the patient to cerebral vasospasm and diminished CBF, increasing the risk for ischemic damage following brain injury.

Diagnostic Studies and Interprofessional Care

A CT scan is considered the best diagnostic test to determine craniocerebral trauma because it allows for rapid diagnosis and intervention. An MRI scan is more sensitive in detecting small DAI lesions than a CT scan because of the lack of gross pathological changes in brain tissue. Transcranial Doppler studies allow for the measurement of CBF velocity. A cervical spine radiographic study is indicated because cervical spine trauma often occurs concomitantly with head injury. In general, the diagnostic studies are similar to those used for a patient with increased ICP (see Table 59.3).

Emergency management of the patient with a head injury is presented in Table 59.9. In addition to measures to prevent secondary injury by treating cerebral edema and managing increased ICP, the principal treatment of head injuries is timely diagnosis and surgery if necessary. For the patient with concussion and contusion, observation and management of increased ICP are the primary management strategies.

The treatment of skull fractures is usually conservative. For depressed fractures and fractures with loose fragments, a craniotomy is necessary to elevate the depressed bone and remove the free fragments. If large amounts of bone are destroyed, the bone may be removed (*craniectomy*) and a cranioplasty will be needed at a later time (see the Cranial Surgery section later in this chapter).

In cases of clinically large subdural and epidural hematomas, or those associated with significant neurological impairment, the blood must be removed surgically through either a craniotomy or a burr-hole approach.

NURSING MANAGEMENT
HEAD INJURY

NURSING ASSESSMENT

The patient with a head injury is always considered to have the potential for developing increased ICP. The most important aspects of the objective data are noting the GCS score (see Table 59.4), assessing and monitoring the neurological status

+ TABLE 59.9   EMERGENCY MANAGEMENT
Head Injury

Etiology	Assessment Findings	Interventions
Blunt • Assault • Fall • Motor vehicle accident • Pedestrian event • Sports injury **Penetrating** • High-velocity projectile (e.g., gunshot wound) • Low-velocity projectile (e.g., knife, bone fragments from skull fracture)	**Surface Findings** • Bruises or contusions on face, Battle sign (bruising behind ears) • Fracture or depressions in skull • Raccoon eyes (dependent bruising around eyes) • Scalp lacerations **Respiratory** • Abnormal respiratory patterns (e.g., Cheyne–Stokes respirations) • Central neurogenic hyperventilation • Decreased O_2 saturation • Pulmonary edema **Central Nervous System** • Asymmetrical facial movements • Bowel and bladder incontinence • Combativeness • Confusion • CSF leaking from ears or nose • Decerebrate or decorticate posturing • Decreased level of consciousness • Depressed or hyperactive reflexes • Flaccidity • Glasgow Coma Scale score <12 • Incomprehensible speech, abusive speech • Involuntary movements • Seizures • Unequal or dilated pupils	**Initial** • Ensure patent airway. • Stabilize cervical spine. • Administer O_2 via nasal cannula or nonrebreather mask. • Establish IV access with two large-bore catheters to infuse normal saline or lactated Ringer's solution. • Control external bleeding with sterile pressure dressing. • Assess for rhinorrhea, otorrhea, scalp wounds. • Remove patient's clothing. **Ongoing Monitoring** • Administer fluids with caution to prevent fluid overload and increasing ICP. • Anticipate need for intubation for ineffective breathing patterns or absent gag reflex. • Assume cervical spine injury until proven otherwise. • Maintain patient warmth using blankets; warm IV fluids; overhead warming lights; warm, humidified O_2. • Monitor frequently for signs and symptoms of increased ICP or decreased cerebral perfusion. • Monitor vital signs, level of consciousness, O_2 saturation, cardiac rhythm, Glasgow Coma Scale score, pupil size and reactivity.

CSF, cerebrospinal fluid; *ICP*, intracranial pressure; *IV*, intravenous.

(see Figure 59.11), and determining whether a CSF leak has occurred. (See the Nursing Assessment section for Increased Intracranial Pressure earlier in this chapter.)

NURSING DIAGNOSES
Nursing diagnoses and potential complications for the patient who has sustained a head injury may include but are not limited to the following:
• *Potential for inadequate cerebral tissue perfusion* as demonstrated by *brain injury, brain neoplasm, cerebral aneurysm*
• *Hyperthermia* resulting from *increased metabolic rate*
• *Reduced physical mobility* resulting from *physical deconditioning* (decreased LOC)
• *Anxiety* resulting from *threat to current status, threat of death* (abrupt change in health status)
• *Potential complication: increased ICP* as a result of *cerebral edema and hemorrhage*

PLANNING
The overall goals are that the patient with an acute head injury will (1) maintain adequate cerebral perfusion; (2) remain normothermic; (3) be free from pain, discomfort, and infection; and (4) attain maximal cognitive, motor, and sensory function.

NURSING IMPLEMENTATION
HEALTH PROMOTION. One of the best ways to prevent head injuries is to prevent motor vehicle accidents. The nurse can be active in campaigns that promote driving safety and can speak to driver education classes regarding the dangers of unsafe driving and of driving after drinking alcohol or using drugs. The use of seat belts in cars and use of helmets for riding on motorcycles are the most effective measures for increasing survival after accidents. It is also recommended that lumberjacks, construction workers, miners, horseback riders, bicycle riders, snowboarders, and skydivers wear protective helmets. The use of helmets when cycling can significantly reduce serious head injury, but not all provinces and territories in Canada have legislation for helmet use (Parachute, 2019). Nurses can become involved with organizations such as Parachute that attempt to reduce the incidence of injuries among Canadian youth through education, community awareness, and public policy health initiatives.

ACUTE INTERVENTION. Management at the scene of the accident can have a significant impact on the outcome of a head injury. Emergency management of head injury is discussed in Table 59.9. The general goal of nursing management of the patient with a head injury is to maintain cerebral oxygenation and perfusion and prevent secondary cerebral ischemia. Surveillance or monitoring for changes in neurological status is critically important because the patient's condition may deteriorate rapidly, necessitating emergency surgery. Appropriate preoperative and postoperative nursing interventions are initiated if surgery is anticipated. Because of the close association between hemodynamic status and cerebral perfusion, the nurse must be aware of any coexisting injuries or conditions. In the acute injury period, treating other life-threatening conditions (e.g., hemorrhage, hypoxia) may take initial priority in nursing care.

The nurse should explain the need for frequent neurological assessments to both the patient and the caregivers. Behavioural manifestations associated with head injury can result in patients who may be frightened and disoriented, may be combative, and may resist help. The nurse's approach should be calm and gentle. A family member may be available to stay with the patient and thus prevent increasing anxiety and fear.

The nurse should perform neurological assessments at intervals based on the patient's condition. The GCS is useful in assessing the level of arousal (see Table 59.4). Indications of a deteriorating neurological state, such as a decreasing LOC, increasingly impaired motor strength, or pupillary changes, should be reported to a physician, and the patient's condition should be closely monitored.

The major focus of nursing care for patients with brain injuries relates to increased ICP (see NCP 59.1 on the Evolve website). However, there may be specific conditions that require nursing intervention.

Eye conditions may include loss of the corneal reflex, periorbital ecchymosis and edema, and diplopia. Loss of the corneal reflex may necessitate administering lubricating eye drops, taping the eyes shut, or suturing the eyelids closed to prevent abrasion. While periorbital ecchymosis and edema disappear spontaneously, cold and, later, warm compresses provide comfort and hasten the process. Diplopia can be relieved by use of an eye patch.

Hyperthermia may occur in relation to an infectious process or from injury to or inflammation of the hypothalamus. Elevations in body temperature can result in increased cerebral metabolic rate, CBF, cerebral blood volume, and ICP. Pyrexia increases cerebral metabolic rate, which increases CBF, which in turn can further increase ICP. The nurse should attempt to control hyperthermia and maintain normothermia (goal temperature of 36° to 38°C) in patients with head injuries using strategies previously discussed (see Supportive Therapy section).

If CSF rhinorrhea or otorrhea occurs, the nurse should inform the physician immediately. The head of the bed may be raised to decrease the CSF pressure so that a dural tear can seal. A loose collection pad may be placed under the nose or over the ear. No dressing should be placed into the nasal cavity or ear canal. The patient should be cautioned not to sneeze or blow their nose. Nasogastric tubes should not be used, and nasotracheal suctioning should not be performed on these patients because of the high risk for meningitis.

Nursing measures specific to the care of patients who are immobilized—such as those related to bladder and bowel function, skin care, and infection—are also indicated. Nausea and vomiting may be a concern and can be alleviated by antiemetic medications. Headache can usually be controlled with acetaminophen or small doses of codeine.

If the patient's condition deteriorates, urgent intracranial surgery may be necessary (see the Cranial Surgery section later in this chapter). A burr-hole opening or craniotomy may be indicated, depending on the underlying injury causing the symptoms.

The patient is often unconscious before surgery, making it necessary for a family member to sign the consent form for surgery. This is a difficult and frightening time for the patient's family, and the situation requires sensitive nursing management. The suddenness of the situation can make it especially difficult for the family to cope.

AMBULATORY AND HOME CARE. Once the condition has stabilized, the patient is usually transferred for acute rehabilitation management to prepare the patient for re-entry into the community. As with any craniocerebral condition, there may be chronic issues related to motor and sensory deficits, communication, memory, and cognitive functioning. Many of the principles of nursing management of patients with a stroke are appropriate (see Chapter 60). Conditions that may require nursing and interprofessional management include poor nutritional status, bowel and bladder management, spasticity, dysphagia, deep venous thrombosis, and hydrocephalus. The patient's outward appearance is not a good indicator of how well the patient will ultimately function in the home or work environment given recovery time and rehabilitation.

Post-traumatic seizure (PTS) disorders are seen in approximately 5% of patients with a nonpenetrating head injury. The time when the patient is most vulnerable to the development of PTS is during the first week after the head injury, although some patients may not develop a PTS disorder until years after the initial injury. Anticonvulsant medications may be used to decrease the risk for early PTS within 7 days of injury (Carney et al., 2017). Phenytoin (Dilantin) is the anticonvulsant medication of choice to use with PTS activity.

The cognitive and emotional sequelae of brain trauma are often the most incapacitating ones. Many patients with head injuries who have been comatose for more than 6 hours undergo some personality change. They may suffer loss of concentration and memory and defective memory processing. Personal drive may decrease; apathy and apparent laziness may increase. Euphoria and mood swings, along with a seeming lack of awareness of the seriousness of the injury, may occur. The patient's behaviour may indicate a loss of social restraint, judgement, tact, and emotional control.

Progressive recovery may continue for 6 months or more before a plateau is reached and a prognosis for recovery can be made. Specific nursing management in the post-traumatic phase depends on specific residual deficits.

In all cases, the family must be given special consideration. They need to be helped to understand what is happening and be taught appropriate interaction patterns. The nurse must give guidance and referrals for financial aid, child care, and other personal needs and must assist the family in involving the patient in family activities whenever possible. Community referrals for support should be offered. Nursing research validates the requirement of family members to have access to information and support from the health care team. Involving them early in the patient's care is also recommended (de Goumoens et al., 2019).

The family often has unrealistic expectations of the patient as the coma begins to recede. The family expects full return to pretrauma status. In reality, the patient experiences a reduced awareness and ability to interpret environmental stimuli. The nurse must prepare the family for the emergence of the patient from coma and must explain that the process of awakening often takes several weeks.

When the time for discharge planning arrives, the family and the patient may benefit from very specific posthospital instructions to avoid family–patient friction. Special "no" policies that may be appropriately suggested by the neurosurgeon, neuropsychologist, and nurse include no drinking of alcoholic beverages, no driving, no work with hazardous implements and machinery, and no unsupervised smoking. Family members, particularly spouses, go through a role transition as the role changes from spouse to caregiver.

EVALUATION

The following are expected outcomes for the patient with a head injury:

- The patient will maintain normal CPP.
- The patient will achieve maximal cognitive, motor, and sensory function.
- The patient will experience no infection or hyperthermia.
- The patient will achieve pain control.

BRAIN TUMOURS

It is estimated that 55 000 Canadians are surviving with a brain tumour, and that every day, 27 Canadians are diagnosed with one (Brain Tumour Foundation of Canada [BTFC], 2019). The brain is a frequent site for metastasis from other sites as well. The 5-year relative survival rate for brain tumours in Canada is approximately 21% (Canadian Cancer Society, 2021b).

Types

Brain tumours can occur in any part of the brain or spinal cord. Tumours of the brain may be *primary,* arising from tissues within the brain, or *secondary,* resulting from a metastasis from a malignant neoplasm elsewhere in the body. Secondary brain tumours are the most common type. Brain tumours are generally classified according to the tissue from which they arise. Meningiomas represent 34% of all primary brain tumours, making them the most common primary brain tumour (BTFC, 2021b). Most meningiomas are benign. Gliomas (a group of tumour types including astrocytoma and glioblastoma multiforme) account for 60% of all primary intracranial brain tumours and are frequently malignant. Glioblastoma multiforme is the most common primary malignant brain tumour and the most aggressive (BTFC, 2021a).

More than half of all brain tumours are malignant; they infiltrate the brain parenchyma and are not amenable to complete surgical removal. Other tumours may be histologically benign, but their location is such that complete removal is not possible. Brain tumours are more commonly seen in middle-aged persons, but they may occur at any age.

Unless treated, all brain tumours eventually cause death from increasing tumour volume leading to increased ICP. Brain tumours rarely metastasize outside the CNS because they are contained by structural (meninges) and physiological (blood–brain) barriers. Table 59.10 compares the major brain tumours. A glioblastoma and a meningioma are depicted in Figure 59.18.

Clinical Manifestations

The clinical manifestations of brain tumours depend mainly on the location, the rate of growth, and the size of the tumour. Figure 59.19 illustrates the functional areas of the cerebral cortex and can be used as a guide to correlate manifestations with the location of the tumour. Some tumours have aggressive mitotic rates and are associated with a rapid onset of symptoms. Tumours such as meningiomas are slow growing and can become quite large before clinical symptoms are noted. The rate of growth depends on the location and size of the tumour and the mitotic rate of the cells of the tissue of origin.

Wide ranges of possible clinical manifestations are associated with brain tumours. Headache is a common symptom.

TABLE 59.10	**TYPES OF BRAIN TUMOURS**	
Type	**Tissue of Origin**	**Characteristics**
Gliomas		
• Astrocytoma	Supportive tissue, glial cells and astrocytes	Can range from low-grade to moderate-grade malignancy
• Ependymoma	Ependymal epithelium	Range from benign to highly malignant; most are benign and encapsulated
• Glioblastoma multiforme	Primitive stem cell (glioblast)	Highly malignant and invasive; among the most devastating of primary brain tumours
• Medulloblastoma	Primitive neuroecto-dermal cell	Highly malignant and invasive; metastatic to spinal cord and remote areas of brain
• Oligodendroglioma	Oligodendrocytes	Benign (encapsulation and calcification)
Meningioma	Meninges	Can be benign or malignant; most are benign
Acoustic neuroma (Schwannoma)	Cells that form my-elin sheath around nerves; commonly affects cranial nerve VIII	Many grow on both sides of the brain; usually benign or low-grade malig-nancy
Pituitary adenoma	Pituitary gland	Usually benign
Hemangioblastoma	Blood vessels of brain	Rare and benign; surgery is curative
Primary central nervous system lymphoma	Lymphocytes	Increased incidence in transplant recipi-ents and patients with acquired immune deficiency syndrome (AIDS)
Metastatic tumours	Lungs, breast, kidney, thyroid, prostate	Malignant

Tumour-related headaches tend to be worse at night and may awaken the patient. The headaches are usually dull and constant but occasionally throbbing. Seizures are common in gliomas and brain metastases. Brain tumours can cause nausea and vomiting from increased ICP. Cognitive dysfunction, including memory difficulties and mood or personality changes, is another common manifestation, especially in patients with brain metastases. Muscle weakness, sensory losses, aphasia, and visuospatial dysfunction are further manifestations of brain tumours. As the brain tumour expands, it may also produce global signs of increased ICP, cerebral edema, or obstruction of the CSF pathways. Manifestations may clearly indicate the location of the tumour by an alteration in the function controlled by the affected area (Table 59.11).

Complications

If the tumour mass obstructs the ventricles or occludes the outlet, ventricular enlargement (hydrocephalus) can occur. As a tumour expands, patients may develop manifestations of increased ICP, cerebral edema, or obstruction of the CSF pathways. Unless treated, all brain tumours eventually cause death from increasing tumour volume leading to increased ICP.

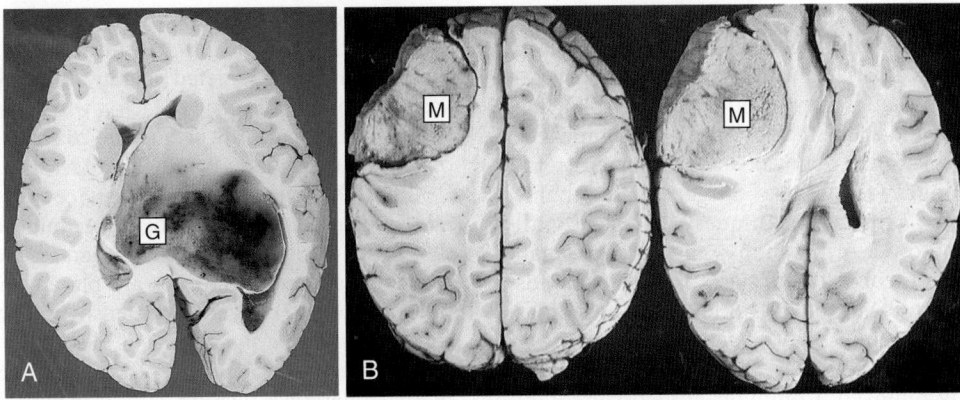

FIG. 59.18 A, Glioblastoma. A large glioblastoma *(G)* arises from one cerebral hemisphere and has grown to fill the ventricular system. **B,** Meningioma. These two different sections from different levels in the same brain show a meningioma *(M)* compressing the frontal lobe and distorting the underlying brain. Source: Stevens, A., & Lowe, J. (2000). *Pathology: Illustrated review in colour* (2nd ed.). Mosby.

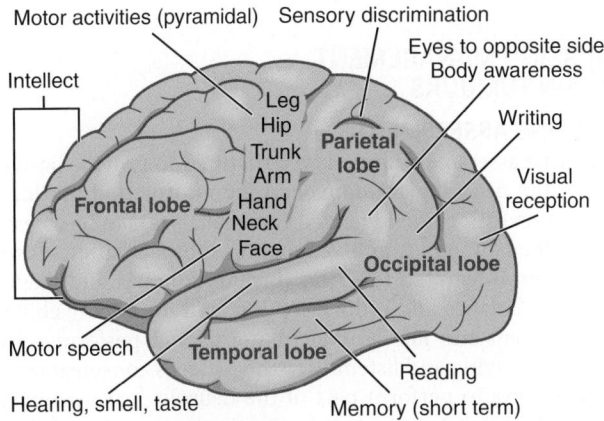

FIG. 59.19 Each area of the brain controls a particular activity.

Diagnostic Studies

An extensive history and a comprehensive neurological examination must be done in the workup of a patient with a suspected brain tumour. A careful history and physical examination may provide data concerning location. Diagnostic studies are similar to those used for a patient with increased ICP (see Table 59.3). The sensitivity of techniques such as MRI and PET scans allows for detection of very small tumours and may provide more reliable diagnostic information. CT and brain scanning are used to diagnose the location of the lesion. Other tests include magnetic resonance spectroscopy, functional MRI, and single-photon emission computed tomography (SPECT). The EEG is useful but of less importance. A lumbar puncture is seldom diagnostic and carries with it the risk for cerebral herniation. Angiography can be used to determine blood flow to the tumour and further localize the tumour. Other studies are done to rule out a primary lesion elsewhere in the body. Endocrine studies are helpful when a pituitary adenoma is suspected (see Chapter 51).

The correct diagnosis of a brain tumour can be made by obtaining tissue for histological study. In most patients, tissue is obtained at the time of surgery. Computer-guided stereotactic biopsy is also an option if surgical intervention does not appear to be the most advantageous treatment option. A smear or frozen section can be performed in the operating room for a preliminary interpretation of the histological type. With this

information, the neurosurgeon can make a better decision about the extent of surgery. In some cases, immunohistochemical stains or electron microscopy may be necessary to ascertain the correct diagnosis.

Interprofessional Care

Treatment goals are aimed at (1) identifying the tumour type and location, (2) removing or decreasing tumour mass, and (3) preventing or managing increased ICP.

TABLE 59.11	BRAIN TUMOUR LOCATIONS AND PRESENTING MANIFESTATIONS
Tumour Location	**Clinical Manifestations**
Cerebral hemisphere	
• Frontal lobe (unilateral)	Unilateral hemiplegia, seizures, memory deficit, personality and judgement changes, visual disturbances
• Frontal lobe (bilateral)	Symptoms associated with unilateral frontal lobe tumours; ataxic gait
• Occipital lobe	Vision deficits and seizures
• Parietal lobe	Speech disturbance (if tumour is in the dominant hemisphere: inability to write, spatial disorders, and unilateral neglect)
• Temporal lobe	Few symptoms; seizures, impaired speech, and memory difficulty
Subcortical	Hemiplegia; other symptoms may depend on area of infiltration
Meningeal tumours	Symptoms are associated with compression of the brain and depend on tumour location
Metastatic tumours	Headache, nausea, or vomiting because of ↑ ICP; other symptoms depend on tumour location
Thalamus and sellar tumours	Headache, nausea, vision disturbances, papilledema, and nystagmus occur from ↑ ICP; diabetes insipidus may occur
Fourth ventricle and cerebellar tumours	Headache, nausea, and papilledema from ↑ ICP; ataxic gait and changes in coordination
Cerebellopontine tumours	Tinnitus and vertigo, deafness
Brainstem tumours	Headache on awakening, drowsiness, vomiting, ataxic gait, facial muscle weakness, hearing loss, dysphagia, dysarthria, "crossed eyes" or other visual changes, hemiparesis

ICP, intracranial pressure.

Medication Therapy. Corticosteroids (dexamethasone, prednisone, or methylprednisolone [Solu-Medrol]) are useful in reducing cerebral edema associated with neoplasms. Corticosteroids are often prescribed at diagnosis and continued following surgery, until radiation and chemotherapy have been completed.

Surgical Therapy. Surgical removal is the preferred treatment for brain tumours (see Cranial Surgery, later in this chapter). Stereotactic surgical techniques are used with increasing frequency to perform a biopsy and remove small brain tumours. The outcome of surgical therapy depends on the type, size, and location of the tumour. Meningiomas and oligodendrogliomas can usually be completely removed, whereas the more invasive gliomas and medulloblastomas can be only partially removed. Computer-guided stereotactic biopsy, ultrasound, functional MRI, and cortical mapping can be used to localize brain tumours intraoperatively. Complete surgical removal is not always possible because the tumour is not always accessible and sometimes involves vital parts of the brain. Surgery can reduce tumour mass, which decreases ICP and provides relief of symptoms with an extension of survival time.

Ventricular Shunts. Hydrocephalus can be treated with the placement of a ventricular shunt. A catheter with one-way valves is placed in the lateral ventricle and then tunnelled through the skin to drain CSF into the right atrium or the peritoneum. Rapid decompression of ICP can cause total body collapse and weakness, including a headache that may be prevented by gradually introducing the patient to the upright position.

Manifestations of shunt malfunction, which are related to increased ICP, include decreasing LOC, restlessness, headache, blurred vision, or vomiting. This may necessitate shunt revision or replacement. Infection may also occur, as exhibited by high fever, persistent headache, and stiff neck. Antibiotics are used to treat the infection. In some situations the shunt must be replaced.

Radiation Therapy and Radiosurgery. Radiation therapy may be used as a follow-up measure after surgery. Radiation seeds can also be implanted into the brain. Cerebral edema and rapidly increasing ICP may be a complication of radiation therapy, but these conditions can be managed with high doses of corticosteroids (dexamethasone, prednisone, or methylprednisolone). (Radiation therapy is discussed in Chapter 18 and in NCP 18.1, available on the Evolve website.)

Stereotactic radiosurgery is a method of delivering a high, concentrated dose of radiation precisely directed at a location within the brain and may be used when conventional surgery has failed or is not an option because of the tumour location. (Radiosurgery is discussed later in this chapter.)

Chemotherapy and Targeted Therapy. The effectiveness of chemotherapy has been limited by difficulty getting medications across the blood–brain barrier, tumour cell heterogeneity, and tumour cell medication resistance. Normally, the blood–brain barrier prohibits the entry of most medications into the brain. A group of chemotherapeutic agents called the *nitrosoureas* (e.g., carmustine [BiCNU], lomustine [CeeNU]) are particularly effective in treating brain tumours. Chemotherapy-laden biodegradable wafers implanted at the time of surgery can deliver chemotherapy directly to the tumour site, and some chemotherapeutic agents can be administered intrathecally via an Ommaya reservoir (see Chapter 18) (Canadian Cancer Society, 2021a).

Bevacizumab (Avastin) is used to treat patients with glioblastoma multiforme and other central nervous system tumours. Bevacizumab is a targeted therapy that inhibits the action of vascular endothelial growth factor, which helps form new blood vessels (Canadian Cancer Society, 2021c). (Targeted therapy is discussed in Chapter 18 and Table 18.16.)

Other Therapies. A medical device system, NovoTTF-100A System, is used to treat glioblastoma multiforme that recurs or progresses after receiving chemotherapy and radiation therapy. With this system, electrodes are placed on the surface of the patient's scalp to deliver low-intensity, changing electrical fields called *tumour treatment fields* (TTFs) to the tumour site.

Many techniques to control and treat brain tumours are currently under investigation. These include local hyperthermia and biological therapy. Although progress in treatment has increased the length and quality of survival of patients with gliomas, outcomes still remain poor (Alexander & Cloughesy, 2017).

NURSING MANAGEMENT BRAIN TUMOURS

NURSING ASSESSMENT

The initial assessment should be structured to provide baseline data of the neurological status and the information needed to design a realistic, individualized care plan. Areas to be assessed include the LOC and cognitive function, motor abilities, sensory perception, integrated function (including bowel and bladder function), balance and proprioception, and the coping abilities of the patient and family. Watching a patient perform activities of daily living and listening to the patient's conversation are possible ways to perform part of the neurological assessment. Having the patient or the family explain the patient's condition and challenges can be helpful in determining the patient's limitations and can also provide the nurse with information about the patient's insight into any concerns. All initial data should be accurately recorded to provide a baseline for comparison to determine whether the patient's condition is improving or deteriorating.

Interview data are as important as the actual physical assessment. Questions should be asked concerning medical history, intellectual abilities and educational level, and history of nervous system infections and trauma. Determination of the presence of seizures, syncope, nausea and vomiting, pain, headaches, and physical limitations is important in planning care for the patient.

NURSING DIAGNOSES

Nursing diagnoses and potential complications for the patient with a brain tumour may include but are not limited to the following:

- *Potential for inadequate cerebral tissue perfusion* as demonstrated by *brain injury* (cerebral edema)
- *Acute pain* resulting from *biological injury agent, physical injury agent* (cerebral edema, increased intracranial pressure)
- *Anxiety* resulting from *threat to current status, threat of death* (diagnosis and treatment)
- *Potential complications: seizures* resulting from *abnormal electrical activity of the brain and increased ICP* as a result of the *tumour and failure of normal compensatory mechanisms*

PLANNING

The overall goals are that the patient with a brain tumour will (1) maintain normal ICP, (2) maximize neurological functioning, (3) be free from pain and discomfort, and (4) be aware of the long-term implications with respect to prognosis and cognitive and physical functioning.

NURSING IMPLEMENTATION

A primary or metastatic tumour of the frontal lobe can cause behavioural and personality changes. Loss of emotional control, confusion, disorientation, memory loss, and depression may be signs of a frontal lobe lesion. These behavioural changes are often not perceived by the patient but can be disturbing and even frightening to the family. These changes can also cause a distancing to occur between the family and the patient. The nurse has an important role in assisting the family in understanding what is happening to the patient and in emotionally supporting the family.

The patient who is confused and has behavioural instability can be a challenge. Protecting the patient from self-harm is an important part of nursing care. At times when the patient manifests rage and aggression, the nurse must also be concerned about self-protection. Close supervision of activity; use of side rails; use of restraints; padding of the rails and the area around the bed; and a calm, reassuring approach to care are all essential techniques for the care of these patients.

Perceptual disorders associated with frontal lobe and parietal lobe tumours contribute to a patient's disorientation and confusion. Minimization of environmental stimuli, creation of a routine, and use of reality orientation can be incorporated into the care plan for the patient experiencing confusion.

Seizures often occur with brain tumours. These are managed with anticonvulsant medications. Seizure precautions should be instituted for the protection of the patient. Some behavioural changes seen in the patient with a brain tumour are a result of seizure disorders and can improve with control of the seizures through medication therapy (see Chapter 61 for more information regarding seizures and anticonvulsant medication therapy).

Motor and sensory dysfunctions are conditions that interfere with the activities of daily living. Alterations in mobility must be managed, and the patient should be encouraged to provide as much self-care as physically possible. Self-image often depends on the patient's ability to participate in care within the limitations of the physical deficits.

Language deficits can also occur in patients with brain tumours. Motor (expressive) or sensory (receptive) aphasia may occur (see Chapter 60). The disturbance in communication can be frustrating for the patient and may interfere with the nurse's ability to meet the patient's needs. Attempts should be made to establish a communication system that can be used by both the patient and the staff.

Nutritional intake may be decreased because of the patient's inability to eat, loss of appetite, or loss of desire to eat. Assessing the patient's nutritional status and ensuring adequate nutritional intake are important aspects of care. The patient may need encouragement to eat or, in some cases, may have to be fed nonorally, by gastrostomy or nasogastric tube, or by parenteral nutrition. The patient with a brain tumour who undergoes cranial surgery requires complex nursing care. This care is discussed in the next section.

EVALUATION

The following are expected outcomes for the patient with a brain tumour:

- The patient will achieve control of pain, vomiting, and other discomforts.
- The patient will maintain ICP within normal limits.
- The patient will demonstrate maximal neurological function (cognitive, motor, sensory) in regard to the location and extent of the tumour.
- The patient will maintain optimal nutritional status.
- The patient will accept the long-term consequences of the tumour and its treatment.

CRANIAL SURGERY

The cause or indication for cranial surgery may be related to a brain tumour, CNS infection (e.g., abscess), vascular abnormalities, craniocerebral trauma, seizure, or intractable pain (Table 59.12).

Types

Various types of cranial surgical procedures are presented in Table 59.13.

Stereotactic Surgery. *Stereotactic surgery* involves use of a precision apparatus (often computer-guided) that assists the surgeon to target a very precise area of the brain (Figure 59.20).

Stereotactic biopsy can be performed to obtain tissue samples for histological examination. CT scanning and MRI are used to image the targeted tissue. With the patient under general or local anaesthesia, the surgeon drills a burr hole or creates a bone flap for an entry site and then introduces a probe and biopsy needle. Stereotactic procedures are used for removal of small brain tumours and abscesses, drainage of hematomas, ablative procedures for extrapyramidal diseases (e.g., Parkinson's disease), and repair of arteriovenous malformations. A major advantage of the stereotactic approach is a reduction in damage to surrounding tissue.

Stereotactic radiosurgery is a procedure that involves closed-skull destruction of an intracranial target using ionizing radiation, focused with the assistance of an intracranial guiding device. A sophisticated computer program is used while the patient's head is held still in a stereotactic frame. Radiosurgical techniques can involve use of a linear accelerator or a gamma knife. In the gamma-knife procedure, a high dose of cobalt radiation is delivered to precisely targeted tumour tissue. The dose of radiation can be delivered in a few minutes or may take up to an hour or more, depending on the size and shape of the tumour. In some situations, tumours are treated over several weeks.

In combination with stereotactic procedures to identify and localize tumour sites, surgical lasers can be used to destroy tumours. Stereotactic procedures are used to identify the tumour site. Three surgical lasers currently used include the carbon dioxide, argon, and neodymium:yttrium–aluminum–garnet (Nd:YAG) lasers. All three work by creating thermal energy, which destroys the tissue on which it is focused. Laser therapy also provides the benefit of reducing damage to surrounding tissue.

Craniotomy. Depending on the location of the pathological condition, a craniotomy may be frontal, parietal, occipital, temporal, or a combination of any of these. A set of burr holes is drilled, and a saw is used to connect the holes to remove the

TABLE 59.12	INDICATIONS FOR CRANIAL SURGERY	
Cause	Manifestations	Procedure
Brain Abscess Bacteria that caused intracranial infection	*Early findings:* stiff neck, headache, fever, weakness, seizures *Later findings:* seizures, hemiplegia, speech disturbances, ocular disturbances, change in LOC	Excision or drainage of abscess
Hydrocephalus Overproduction of CSF, obstruction to flow, defective reabsorption	*Early findings:* mental changes, disturbances in gait *Later findings:* memory impairment, urinary incontinence, increased tendon reflexes	Placement of ventriculoatrial or ventriculoperitoneal shunt
Brain Tumours Benign or malignant cell growth	Change in LOC, pupillary changes, sensory or motor deficit, papilledema, seizures, personality changes	Excision or partial resection of tumour
Intracranial Bleeding Rupture of cerebral vessels because of trauma or stroke	*Epidural:* momentary unconsciousness; lucid period, then rapid deterioration *Subdural:* headache, seizures, pupillary changes	Surgical evacuation through burr holes or craniotomy
Skull Fractures Trauma to skull	Headache, CSF leakage, cranial nerve deficit	Debridement of fragments and necrotic tissue, elevation and realignment of bone fragments
Arteriovenous Malformation (AVM) Congenital tangle of arteries and veins (frequently in middle cerebral artery)	Headache, intracranial hemorrhage, seizures, mental deterioration	Excision of malformation
Aneurysm Repair Dilation of weak area in arterial wall (usually near anterior portion of circle of Willis)	*Before rupture:* headache, lethargy, visual disturbance *After rupture:* violent headache, decreased LOC, visual disturbances, motor deficit	Dissection and clipping or coiling of aneurysm

CSF, cerebrospinal fluid; *LOC*, level of consciousness.

TABLE 59.13	TYPES OF CRANIAL SURGERY
Type	Description
Burr hole	Opening into the cranium made with a drill; used to remove localized fluid and blood beneath the dura
Craniotomy	Opening into the cranium with removal of a bone flap and opening the dura to remove a lesion, repair a damaged area, drain blood, or relieve increased ICP
Craniectomy	Excision into the cranium to cut away a bone flap
Cranioplasty	Repair of a cranial defect resulting from trauma, malformation, or previous surgical procedure; artificial material used to replace damaged or lost bone
Stereotaxis	Precision localization of a specific area of the brain using a frame or a frameless system based on three-dimensional coordinates; procedure is used for biopsy, radiosurgery, or dissection
Shunt procedures	Alternate pathway created to redirect cerebrospinal fluid from one area to another using a tube or implanted device; examples include ventriculoperitoneal shunt and Ommaya reservoir

ICP, intracranial pressure.

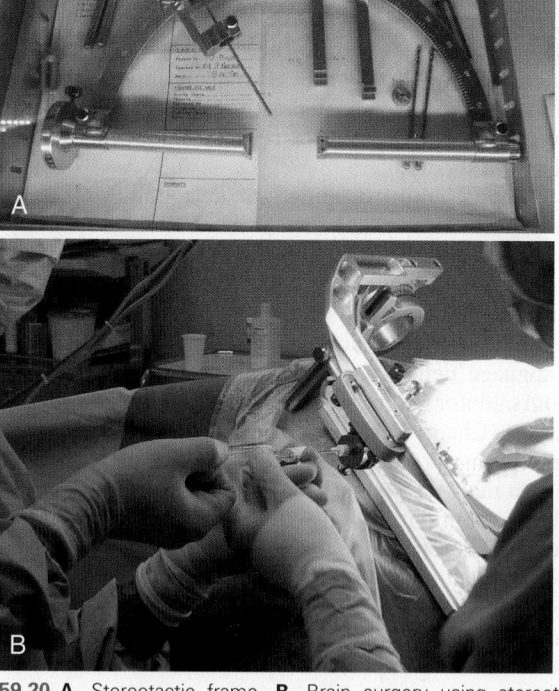

FIG. 59.20 **A,** Stereotactic frame. **B,** Brain surgery using stereotactic frame. Sources: *A,* Rodw. This file is licensed under the Creative Commons Attribution-Share Alike 4.0 International license, https://creativecommons.org/licenses/by-sa/4.0/deed.en. *B,* Dake. This file is licensed under the Creative Commons Attribution-Share Alike 2.5 Generic license, https://creativecommons.org/licenses/by-sa/2.5/deed.en.

bone flap. Sometimes operating microscopes are used to magnify the site. After surgery, the bone flap is wired or sutured. Sometimes drains are placed to remove fluid and blood. Patients are usually cared for in a CCU until stable.

In certain cases, a tumour may be infiltrating brain tissue that is involved in essential functions such as language. In these cases, an *awake craniotomy* may be performed. The patient is fully anaesthetized during the opening of the cranial vault and then brought to consciousness once the brain is exposed. Relevant areas of the brain are stimulated to assess function and determine what tissue can and cannot be safely resected. Although keeping the patient awake adds to the complexity and length of the surgery, it enhances the safety of the procedure.

NURSING MANAGEMENT
CRANIAL SURGERY

NURSING ASSESSMENT

The nursing assessment of the patient undergoing cranial surgery is similar to that for the patient with increased ICP.

NURSING DIAGNOSES

Nursing diagnoses for the patient undergoing cranial surgery are similar to those for the patient with increased ICP and may include but are not limited to the following:

- *Acute pain* resulting from *physical injury agent, biological injury agent* (tissue injury, inflammation)
- *Potential for surgical site infection* as a result of an *invasive procedure*
- *Potential for infection* resulting from an *invasive procedure* (venous or urinary catheters)

Additional information on nursing diagnoses for the patient undergoing cranial surgery are presented in NCP 59.3, available on the Evolve website.

PLANNING

The overall goals are that the patient with cranial surgery will (1) return to normal consciousness, (2) be free from pain and discomfort, (3) have maximal neuromuscular functioning, and (4) be rehabilitated to their maximal ability.

NURSING IMPLEMENTATION

ACUTE INTERVENTION. Nursing management is presented in NCP 59.1. The patient facing cranial surgery (if conscious and coherent), the caregiver, and the family will be gravely concerned about the potential physical and emotional challenges that can result from surgery. The uncertainty regarding prognosis and outcome necessitates compassionate nursing care in the preoperative period.

Preoperative teaching is important in allaying the fears of the patient and the family and also in preparing them for the postoperative period. The patient and the family should be given information regarding the operative procedure and what can be expected immediately after the surgery. Explaining that some hair may be shaved may help alleviate the patient's concern. The family should also be informed that the patient will be taken to a CCU or to a special care unit after the operation.

The primary goal of care after cranial surgery is prevention of increased ICP. (Nursing management of the patient with increased ICP is presented in the Nursing Management: Increased Intracranial Pressure section.) Frequent assessment of the patient's neurological status is essential during the first

48 hours. In addition to the neurological functions, fluids, electrolyte levels, and osmolality are monitored closely to detect changes in sodium regulation, the onset of DI, or severe hypovolemia. The turning and positioning of the patient sometimes depend on the site of the operation. To lessen postoperative cerebral edema, the patient is cared for with the head of the bed elevated 30 to 45 degrees. Maximum swelling in the operative area usually occurs within 24 to 48 hours after the surgery. If a bone flap has been removed (craniectomy), care should be taken not to have the patient positioned on the operative side.

The surgical dressing should be observed for colour, odour, and amount of drainage. The health care provider should be notified immediately of any excessive bleeding or clear drainage. Checking drains for placement and assessing the area around the dressing are also important. Scalp care should include meticulous care of the incision to prevent wound infection. The area should be cleansed and treated in accordance with hospital protocol. Once the dressing is removed, use of an antiseptic soap for washing the scalp may also be beneficial. Sutures or staples may be removed after 7 days. Incisions to the posterior fossa require sutures or staples to remain in situ for a minimum of 10 days.

The nurse needs to monitor the patient for pain and nausea (see the Evidence-Informed Practice: Research Highlight box). Although the brain itself does not possess pain receptors, patients often report headache caused by edema or pain at the incision site. Pain is controlled with short-acting opioids, and neurological status must be monitored. Nausea and vomiting are common after surgery and are usually treated with antiemetics.

The psychological impact of hair removal can be alleviated by the use of a wig, a turban, scarves, or a cap after the incision has completely healed. For the patient who is receiving radiation, use of a sunblock and head covering should be advocated if any exposure to the sun is anticipated.

AMBULATORY AND HOME CARE. The rehabilitative potential for a patient after cranial surgery depends on the reason for the surgery, the postoperative course, and the patient's general state of health. Nursing interventions must be based on a realistic appraisal of these factors. An overall goal for the nurse is to foster independence for as long as possible and to the highest degree possible.

Specific rehabilitation potential cannot be determined until cerebral edema and increased ICP subside postoperatively. Care must be taken to maintain as much function as possible through measures such as careful positioning, meticulous skin and mouth care, regular range-of-motion exercises, bowel and bladder care, and adequate nutrition.

Referrals may be made to other specialists on the health care team. For example, the speech pathologist may be helpful to the patient who has speech and language or swallowing deficits or the physiotherapist may provide an exercise plan to regain functional deficits. The needs and challenges of each patient should be addressed individually because many variables affect the plan. Mental and physical deterioration of the patient, including seizures, personality disorganization, apathy, and wasting, is difficult for both the family and health care providers to endure. Cognitive and emotional residual deficits are often more difficult for the patient and the family to accept than are motor and sensory losses. Although progress is continually being made to help the patient with a brain tumour by means of chemotherapy, conventional and interstitial radiation, and biological therapies, prognosis has not changed. The nurse can provide much help and support during the adjustment phase and in long-range planning.

Research Highlight

What Is the Optimal Pharmacological Intervention for the Prevention of Acute Postoperative Pain in Adults Following Craniotomy?

Clinical Question

In patients who have undergone craniotomy (P), do nonsteroidal anti-inflammatory drugs (NSAIDs) (I) versus a control or placebo medication (C) decrease postoperative pain (O)?

Best Available Evidence

Cochrane systematic review of blinded and nonblinded, randomized controlled trials

Critical Appraisal and Synthesis of Evidence

- 42 (n = 3 458 participants) eligible studies were reviewed
  Studies included local anaesthetic into the scalp (n = 10), local anaesthetic around scalp nerves (n = 12), NSAIDs (n = 8), dexmedetomidine (n = 4), acetaminophen (n = 4), opioid (n = 2), gabapentin (n = 3), and one study each of local anaesthetic injected into the veins, injected into the jaw, and the medication flupirtine.
  Assessment of the overall quality of the evidence was judged to be "high" for pain-reducing effects of NSAIDs; "moderate" to "low" for pain-reducing effects of dexmedetomidine, acetaminophen, pregabalin and gabapentin, and local anaesthetics injected around specific scalp nerves; and "low" to "very low" for pain-reducing effects of local anaesthetic injections around the surgical wound.

Conclusions

- NSAIDs reduce pain up to 24 hours postoperatively.
- While NSAIDs produced a reduction in pain intensity, there was no corresponding significant reduction in additional analgesia requirements.
- Dexmedetomidine was effective in the first 12 hours, and gabapentin was effective in the first 6 hours after surgery.
- Scalp blocks were effective at 12 hours and scalp infiltration at 48 hours but not at earlier time points.
- Acetaminophen did not show any benefit for pain reduction.

Implications for Nursing Practice

- This review provides an evidence base for the use of NSAIDs within the initial 24 hours for patients who are postcraniotomy.
- Nurses can use this information to advocate for best practice for reducing postoperative pain when caring for patients postcraniotomy.

Reference for Evidence

Galvin, I. M., Levy, R., Day, A. G., et al. (2019). Pharmacological interventions for the prevention of acute postoperative pain in adults following brain surgery. *Cochrane Database of Systematic Reviews, 2019*(Issue 11), Art. No.: CD011931. doi:10.1002/14651858.CD011931.pub2.

P, patient population of interest; *I*, intervention or area of interest; *C*, comparison of interest or comparison group; *O*, outcome(s) of interest (see Chapter 1).

Withholding Treatment

Situation

A 26-year-old patient in a persistent vegetative state is diagnosed with her fifteenth bladder infection. Her home care nurse must determine whether or not to seek antibiotics for this infection. The family members have expressed a concern that no heroic measures be used to extend the biological life of their daughter and sister, but they have been unwilling to withdraw the existing treatment, which is enteral nutrition through a gastrostomy tube. Should antibiotics be withheld?

Important Points for Consideration

- Patients in a persistent vegetative state do not recover.
- Providing nutrition and hydration, even if by artificial means, can have significant cultural, religious, and psychological meaning to patients and families.
- It is imperative to clarify with the family about the goals of treatment and the patient's wishes, when she was competent and if they are known. It is important to know whether treatment for an infection would be considered heroic based on the family's perspective of what the patient would want.
- The family's concerns about pain, suffering, and quality of life for the patient must be explored within the context of the overall plan of care.
- Withholding treatment is morally acceptable when a competent patient consents to it, if there is no medical benefit to the patient, if the treatment merely prolongs life, or if the burden of treatment outweighs the benefit to the patient.

Clinical Decision-Making Questions

1. How would the nurse approach the patient's family?
2. What might the nurse be feeling about providing nutrition, hydration, and treatments that will prolong life in a patient for whom there is no hope of recovery?
3. What options are available to the family for the care of their daughter once a decision is made about withholding antibiotics?

Inflammation can be caused by bacteria, viruses, fungi, and chemicals (e.g., contrast media used in diagnostic tests or blood in the subarachnoid space) (Table 59.14). CNS infections may occur via the bloodstream (e.g., insect bites), by extension from a primary site (e.g., ear infection, sinusitis, open skull fracture), or along cranial, spinal, and peripheral nerves (e.g., rabies).

BACTERIAL MENINGITIS

Etiology and Pathophysiology

Meningitis is an acute inflammation of meningeal tissues (the pia mater, arachnoid mater, and dura mater) surrounding the brain and the spinal cord. Bacterial meningitis is considered a medical emergency, and untreated meningitis has a mortality rate approaching 100%. The organisms usually gain entry to the CNS through the upper respiratory tract or the bloodstream, but they may enter by direct extension from penetrating wounds of the skull or through fractured sinuses in basal skull fractures. Cases most often occur in infants, older persons, and members of certain high-risk groups.

Meningitis usually occurs in winter or early spring and is often secondary to viral respiratory disease. *Streptococcus pneumoniae* (pneumococcus meningitis) and *Neisseria meningitidis* (meningococcal meningitis) are the leading causes of bacterial meningitis in adults. *Haemophilus influenzae* was once the most common cause. However, the use of *H. influenzae* vaccine has resulted in a significant decrease in meningitis related to this organism.

Other causes of meningitis are *Listeria monocytogenes* (commonly called *Listeria*), a bacteria found in food that can cause

---

EVALUATION

The following are expected outcomes for the patient who has had cranial surgery:

- The patient will regain cognitive, motor, and sensory function to the fullest possible extent.
- The patient will be free of infection.
- The patient's pain and discomfort will be alleviated.
- The patient will be free of seizures.
- The patient will have optimal nutritional intake.

INFLAMMATORY CONDITIONS OF THE BRAIN

Meningitis, encephalitis, and brain abscesses are the most common inflammatory conditions of the brain and spinal cord.

TABLE 59.14   COMPARISON OF CEREBRAL INFLAMMATORY CONDITIONS

	Meningitis	Encephalitis	Brain Abscess
Causative organisms	Bacteria (*Streptococcus pneumoniae*, *Neisseria meningitidis*, group B streptococcus, viruses, fungi)	Bacteria, fungi, parasites, herpes simplex virus (HSV), other viruses (e.g., West Nile virus)	Streptococci, staphylococci through bloodstream
CSF			
• Pressure (normal, <20 cm H_2O, same as SI units)	Increased	Normal to slightly increased	Increased
• WBC count (normal, $0–5 \times 10^6$/L or 0–5 cells/mcL	*Bacterial:* >1 000/mcL (mainly PMN) *Viral:* 25–500/mcL (mainly lymphocytes)	500/mcL, PMN (early), lymphocytes (later)	25–300/mcL (PMN)
• Protein (normal, 0.15–0.45 g/L)	*Bacterial:* >5 g/L *Viral:* 0.5–5 g/L	Slightly increased	Normal
• Glucose (normal, 2.8–4.2 mmol/L)	*Bacterial:* decreased *Viral:* normal or low	Normal	Low or absent
• Appearance	*Bacterial:* turbid, cloudy *Viral:* clear or cloudy	Clear	Clear
Diagnostic studies	CT scan, Gram stain, smear, culture, PCR*	CT scan, EEG, MRI, PET, PCR, IgM antibodies to virus in serum or CSF	CT scan, skull radiograph, MRI
Treatment	Antibiotics, dexamethasone, supportive care, prevention of ↑ ICP	Supportive care, prevention of ↑ ICP, acyclovir (Zovirax) for HSV	Antibiotics, incision and drainage, supportive care

CSF, cerebrospinal fluid; *CT*, computed tomography; *EEG*, electroencephalogram; *ICP*, intracranial pressure; *IgM*, immunoglobulin M; *MRI*, magnetic resonance imaging; *PCR*, polymerase chain reaction; *PET*, positron emission tomography; *PMN*, polymorphonuclear cell; *WBC*, white blood cell.
*PCR is used to detect viral RNA or DNA.

a rare and potentially fatal disease called *listeriosis*. In Canada, listeriosis is a relatively rare disease, with only a few cases each year (Meningitis Research Foundation of Canada, n.d.).

The inflammatory response to the infection of the meninges and CSF (whatever the cause) may increase CSF production, while exudate accumulation leads to blockage of the arachnoid villi, causing obstruction of CSF absorption. The resulting hydrocephalus may cause an increase in ICP. The purulent secretions that are produced spread quickly to other areas of the brain through the CSF. If this process extends into the brain parenchyma or if concurrent encephalitis is present, cerebral edema and increased ICP become more of a problem. All patients with meningitis must be observed closely for manifestations of increased ICP, which is thought to be a result of swelling around the dura, and increased CSF volume.

Clinical Manifestations

Fever, severe headache, nausea, vomiting, and nuchal rigidity (resistance to flexion of the neck) are key signs of meningitis. A positive Kernig sign (flexion of the patient's hip 90 degrees and extension of the knee cause pain), a positive Brudzinski sign (flexion of the patient's neck causes flexion of the patient's hips and knees), photophobia, a decreased LOC, and signs of increased ICP may also be present. Coma is associated with a poor prognosis and occurs in 5 to 10% of patients with bacterial meningitis. Seizures occur in one third of all cases. With meningitis, the headache becomes progressively worse and may be accompanied by vomiting and irritability. If the infecting organism is a meningococcus, early symptoms may include chills, fever, headache, malaise, rash, and petechial hemorrhage on skin and mucous membranes.

Complications

The most common acute complication of bacterial meningitis is increased ICP. Most patients with the infection will have increased ICP, and it is the major cause of altered mental status. Another complication of bacterial meningitis is residual

neurological dysfunction. Cranial nerve dysfunction in bacterial meningitis often occurs with cranial nerves III, IV, VI, VII, or VIII. The dysfunction usually disappears within a few weeks. However, hearing loss may be permanent after bacterial meningitis.

Cranial nerve irritation can have serious sequelae. The optic nerve (CN II) is compressed by increased ICP. Papilledema is often present, and blindness may occur. When the oculomotor (CN III), trochlear (CN IV), and abducens (CN VI) nerves are irritated, ocular movements are affected. Ptosis, unequal pupils, and diplopia are common. Irritation of the trigeminal nerve (CN V) is evidenced by sensory losses and loss of the corneal reflex, and irritation of the facial nerve (CN VII) results in facial paresis. Irritation of the vestibulocochlear nerve (CN VIII) causes tinnitus, vertigo, and deafness.

Hemiparesis, aphasia, and hemianopia may also occur. These signs usually resolve over time. If resolution does not occur, the presence of a cerebral abscess, subdural empyema, subdural effusion, or persistent meningitis is suggested. Acute cerebral edema may occur with bacterial meningitis, causing seizures, CN III palsy, bradycardia, hypertensive coma, and death.

A noncommunicating hydrocephalus may occur if the exudate causes adhesions that prevent the normal flow of CSF from the ventricles. CSF reabsorption by the arachnoid villi may also be obstructed by the exudate. In these cases, surgical implantation of a shunt may be necessary.

Headaches may occur for months after the diagnosis of meningitis until the irritation and inflammation have completely resolved. It is important to implement pain management for chronic headaches.

Waterhouse–Friderichsen syndrome is a complication of meningococcal meningitis. The syndrome is manifested by petechiae, disseminated intravascular coagulation (DIC), adrenal hemorrhage, and circulatory collapse. DIC and shock, which are some of the most serious complications of meningitis, are associated with meningococcemia. (DIC is discussed in detail in Chapter 33.)

Diagnostic Studies

When a patient is seen with manifestations suggestive of bacterial meningitis, a blood culture and CT scan should be done. Diagnosis is usually verified by doing a lumbar puncture and analysis of the CSF. Variations in the CSF depend on the causative organism. Protein levels in the CSF are usually elevated and are higher in bacterial than in viral meningitis. Decreased CSF glucose concentration is common in bacterial meningitis; the glucose level may be normal in viral meningitis. The CSF is purulent and turbid in bacterial meningitis; it may be the same or clear in viral meningitis. The predominant white blood cell type in the CSF during bacterial meningitis is polymorphonuclear cells (see Table 59.14). Specimens of CSF, sputum, and nasopharyngeal secretions are taken for culture before the start of antibiotic therapy to identify the causative organism. A Gram stain is done to detect bacteria. Variations in the CSF depend on the causative organism (bacterial or viral; see Table 59.14).

Radiographic studies of the skull may demonstrate infected sinuses. CT scans and MRI may be normal in uncomplicated meningitis. In other cases, CT scans may reveal evidence of increased ICP or hydrocephalus.

Interprofessional Care

Rapid diagnosis based on history and physical examination is crucial because the patient is usually in a critical state when health care is sought. When meningitis is suspected, antibiotic therapy is instituted after the collection of specimens for cultures, even before the diagnosis is confirmed (Table 59.15).

Ampicillin, vancomycin, cefotaxime (Claforan), and ceftriaxone are common medications given for treatment of meningitis. The corticosteroid dexamethasone may also be prescribed before or with the first dose of antibiotics. Although data are limited, administration of dexamethasone appears to be associated with a reduced incidence of hearing impairment in patients with bacterial meningitis (Brouwer et al., 2015).

NURSING MANAGEMENT BACTERIAL MENINGITIS

NURSING ASSESSMENT

Initial assessment should include vital signs, neurological evaluation, assessment of fluid intake and output, and evaluation of the lungs and skin (see Figure 59.12).

NURSING DIAGNOSES

Nursing diagnoses for the patient with bacterial meningitis may include but are not limited to the following:

- *Inadequate intracranial adaptive capacity* resulting from *decreased cerebral perfusion or increased ICP*
- *Potential for ineffective cerebral tissue perfusion* as demonstrated by *brain injury* (reduction of blood flow, cerebral edema)
- *Hyperthermia* resulting from *increase in metabolic rate* (infection)
- *Acute pain* resulting from *biological injury agent* (headache, muscle aches)

Additional information on nursing diagnoses for the patient with bacterial meningitis is presented in NCP 59.2, available on the Evolve website.

PLANNING

The overall goals are that the patient with bacterial meningitis

---

TABLE 59.15   INTERPROFESSIONAL CARE

Bacterial Meningitis

Diagnostic
- History and physical examination
- Analysis of CSF for protein, glucose, WBC; Gram stain; culture
- Blood culture
- CBC, coagulation profile, electrolyte levels, glucose, platelet count
- CT scan, MRI
- Skull radiograph studies

Interprofessional Therapy
- Acetaminophen (Tylenol) for temperature >38.5°C
- Clear liquids as desired or tolerated
- Codeine for headache
- Dexamethasone
- Hypothermia
- IV antibiotics
- Ampicillin, penicillin
- Cephalosporin (e.g., ceftriaxone)
- IV fluids
- IV furosemide (Lasix) or mannitol (Osmitrol) for diuresis
- IV phenytoin (Dilantin)
- Rest

CBC, complete blood cell count; *CSF,* cerebrospinal fluid; *CT,* computed tomography; *IV,* intravenous; *MRI,* magnetic resonance imaging; *WBC,* white blood cell.

---

will have (1) return to maximal neurological functioning, (2) resolution of infection, and (3) control of pain and discomfort.

NURSING IMPLEMENTATION

HEALTH PROMOTION. Prevention of respiratory infections through vaccination programs for pneumococcal pneumonia and influenza should be supported by nurses. Several meningococcal vaccine preparations are available in Canada and are recommended to protect against developing bacterial meningitis. The schedule varies by province and territory. In addition, early and vigorous treatment of respiratory and ear infections is important. People who have close contact with anyone who has bacterial meningitis should be given prophylactic antibiotics. In Canada, cases of pneumococcal meningitis must be reported to the Public Health Agency of Canada.

ACUTE INTERVENTION. The patient with bacterial meningitis is usually acutely ill. The fever is high, and headache is severe. Irritation of the cerebral cortex may result in seizures. The changes in mental status and LOC depend on the degree of increased ICP. Assessment of vital signs, neurological evaluation, monitoring of fluid intake and output, and evaluation of lung fields and skin should be performed at regular intervals, based on the patient's condition, and recorded carefully.

Head pain and neck pain secondary to movement require attention. Codeine provides some pain relief without undue sedation for most patients. The patient should be assisted to a position of comfort, often curled up with the head slightly extended. The head of the bed should be slightly elevated, when permitted after lumbar puncture. A darkened room and a cool cloth over the eyes may relieve the discomfort of photophobia.

For the patient who is delirious, additional low lighting may be necessary to decrease hallucinations. All patients with bacterial meningitis suffer some degree of mental distortion and hypersensitivity and may be frightened and misinterpret the environment. Every attempt should be made to minimize environmental stimuli and prevent injury. The presence of a familiar person at the bedside often has a calming effect. The nurse must be efficient with care but also should project an attitude of caring and of unhurried gentleness. The use of touch and a soothing voice to give simple explanations of activities is helpful. If seizures occur, appropriate observations should be made and protective measures should be taken. Anticonvulsant medications such as phenytoin (Dilantin) are administered as ordered. Conditions associated with increased ICP are also managed (see the Increased Intracranial Pressure section, earlier in this chapter).

Fever must be vigorously managed because it increases cerebral edema and the frequency of seizures. In addition, neurological damage may result from an extremely high temperature over a prolonged period of time. If the fever is resistant to antipyretics, more vigorous means may be necessary, such as an automatic cooling blanket. Care should be taken not to reduce the temperature too rapidly because shivering may result, causing a rebound effect and increasing the temperature. The extremities should be wrapped in soft towels or covered with a thin blanket to protect them from "frostbite." Skin assessment and care should be meticulous. If a cooling blanket is not available or desirable, tepid sponge baths with water may be effective in lowering the temperature. The skin must be protected from excessive drying and injury.

Because high fever greatly increases the metabolic rate and thus insensible fluid loss, the patient should be assessed for dehydration and adequacy of fluid intake. Diaphoresis further increases fluid losses. Supplemental feeding to maintain adequate nutritional intake via tube or oral feedings may be necessary. The designated antibiotic schedule must be followed to maintain therapeutic blood levels. Observations should be made for adverse effects of the medications used.

In most cases, patients with meningitis are placed in respiratory isolation for up to 48 hours of appropriate antibiotic therapy. Meningococcal meningitis is highly contagious, whereas other causes of meningitis may pose minimal to no infection risk with patient contact. Routine practices (also called *Standard Precautions*) are essential to protect the patient and the nurse.

AMBULATORY AND HOME CARE. After the acute period has passed, the patient requires several weeks of convalescence before normal activities can be resumed. In this period, good nutrition should be stressed, with an emphasis on a high-protein, high-calorie diet in small, frequent feedings.

Muscle rigidity may persist in the neck and the backs of the legs. Progressive range-of-motion exercises and warm baths are useful. Activity should be gradually increased as tolerated, but adequate bed rest and sleep should be encouraged.

Residual effects are uncommon in meningococcal meningitis, but pneumococcal meningitis can result in sequelae such as dementia, seizures, deafness, hemiplegia, and hydrocephalus. Vision, hearing, cognitive skills, and motor and sensory abilities should be assessed after recovery, with appropriate referrals made as indicated. Throughout the acute and convalescent periods, the nurse should be aware of the anxiety and stress experienced by individuals close to the patient.

▌EVALUATION

The expected outcomes for the patient with bacterial meningitis are addressed in NCP 59.2, available on the Evolve website.

VIRAL MENINGITIS

The most common causes of viral meningitis are enteroviruses, arboviruses, human immunodeficiency virus (HIV), and herpes simplex virus (HSV). Viral meningitis usually presents as a headache, fever, photophobia, and nuchal rigidity. The fever may be moderate or high. There are usually no symptoms of brain involvement.

The most important diagnostic test is examination of the CSF obtained via a lumbar puncture. The CSF can be clear or cloudy, and the typical finding is lymphocytosis (see Table 59.14). Organisms are not seen on Gram stain or acid-fast smears. Polymerase chain reaction used to detect viral-specific deoxyribonucleic acid (DNA) or ribonucleic acid (RNA) is a highly sensitive method for diagnosing CNS viral infections. Viral meningitis is managed symptomatically because the disease is self-limiting. Antiviral therapy is not used. Full recovery from viral meningitis is expected. Rare sequelae include persistent headaches, mild mental impairment, and incoordination.

ENCEPHALITIS

Etiology and Pathophysiology

Encephalitis, an acute inflammation of the brain, is a serious and sometimes fatal disease. Encephalitis is usually caused by a virus. Many different viruses have been implicated in encephalitis, some associated with seasons of the year or endemic to certain geographic areas. Ticks and mosquitoes transmit epidemic encephalitis. Examples include La Crosse encephalitis, St. Louis encephalitis, West Nile virus, and Western equine encephalitis. Nonepidemic encephalitis may occur as a complication of measles, chicken pox, or mumps. HSV encephalitis is the most common form of acute, nonepidemic, viral encephalitis. Cytomegalovirus encephalitis is one of the common complications in patients with acquired immune deficiency syndrome (AIDS).

West Nile virus was first identified in Uganda in 1937. The first human case of West Nile virus in Canada occurred in summer–fall 2001. Since that time, the number of cases annually has fluctuated. In 2017, 193 cases were reported in Canada (Public Health Agency of Canada, 2017). Advanced age is the primary risk factor for encephalitis and mortality associated with this virus. The incubation period is from 3 to 14 days. Most cases involve mild, flulike symptoms, but about 1 in 150 will result in severe neurological disease, with encephalitis more commonly seen than meningitis.

Clinical Manifestations and Diagnostic Studies

The onset of infection is typically nonspecific, with fever, headache, nausea, and vomiting. It can be acute or subacute. Signs of encephalitis appear on day 2 or 3 and may vary from minimal alterations in mental status to coma. Virtually any CNS abnormality can occur, including hemiparesis, tremors, seizures, cranial nerve palsies, personality changes, memory impairment, amnesia, and aphasia.

Early diagnosis and treatment of viral encephalitis are essential for favourable outcomes. Diagnostic findings related to viral encephalitis are shown in Table 59.14. Brain imaging techniques include CT, MRI, and PET. Polymerase chain reaction tests for HSV DNA and RNA levels in CSF allow for early detection of HSV viral encephalitis. West Nile virus should be strongly considered in adults older than 50 years who develop encephalitis or meningitis in summer or early fall. The best diagnostic test for West Nile virus is a blood test that detects viral RNA. This test is also used in screening blood, organs, cells, and tissues that have been donated.

NURSING AND INTERPROFESSIONAL MANAGEMENT VIRAL ENCEPHALITIS

To prevent encephalitis, mosquito control should be practised, including cleaning rain gutters, removing old tires, draining bird baths, and removing water where mosquitoes can breed. In addition, insect repellent should be used during mosquito season.

Interprofessional and nursing management of encephalitis, including West Nile virus infection, is symptomatic and supportive. Treatment for mild cases consists mainly of rest, adequate nutrition and fluids, acetaminophen for fever and headaches, and anticonvulsant medications for seizures, if necessary. Generally, encephalitis does not respond to antiviral medications; however, the HSV and varicella-zoster virus respond to antiviral medications such as acyclovir (Zovirax) or ganciclovir (Cytovene), and these have been shown to reduce mortality rates. For maximal benefit, antiviral agents should be started before the onset of coma. Current research is investigating the use of interferon therapy as a treatment for encephalitis caused by West Nile and St. Louis viruses; however, more studies are needed. In the initial stages, many patients require critical care.

Seizure disorders should be treated with anticonvulsant medications (see Chapter 61, Table 61.10). Prophylactic treatment with anticonvulsant medications may be used in severe cases of encephalitis. Treatment of cytomegalovirus encephalitis in patients with AIDS is discussed in Chapter 17.

BRAIN ABSCESS

Brain abscess is an accumulation of pus within the brain tissue that can result from a local or systemic infection. Direct extension from ear, tooth, mastoid, or sinus infection is the primary cause. Other causes for brain abscess formation include spread from a distant site (e.g., pulmonary infection, bacterial endocarditis), skull fracture, and a prior brain trauma or surgery. *Streptococci* and *Staphylococcus aureus* are the primary infective organisms.

Manifestations are similar to those of meningitis and encephalitis and include headache, fever, and nausea and vomiting. Signs of increased ICP may include drowsiness, confusion, and seizures. Focal symptoms may be present and reflect the local area of the abscess. For example, visual field defects or psychomotor seizures are common with a temporal lobe abscess, whereas an occipital abscess may be accompanied by visual impairment and hallucinations. CT and MRI are used to diagnose a brain abscess.

Antimicrobial therapy is the primary treatment for brain abscess, generally for a minimum of 4 to 8 weeks (Chow, 2018). Depending on the size and response of the abscess to antimicrobial treatment, the patient may require surgery to drain or remove the abscess if it is encapsulated. Other manifestations are treated symptomatically. Nursing measures are similar to those for management of meningitis or increased ICP. If surgical drainage or removal is the treatment of choice, nursing care is similar to that described for recovery from cranial surgery. Some patients may be clinically well enough after the acute surgical phase to be discharged home. The nurse must be aware of the additional discharge planning requirements of a patient going home with IV antibiotic therapy, if indicated.

CASE STUDY

Head Injury

Patient Profile
G. F. (pronouns he/him), 33 years old, was the driver of a motorcycle that ran into an automobile broadside at a high rate of speed. G. F. was sedated, paralyzed, and intubated by emergency medical personnel (EMS) at the scene before transport by helicopter. He was brought to the emergency department with a prehospital report of multiple trauma and an open skull fracture. Paramedics also reported that he was not wearing a helmet.

Subjective Data
G. F. was reportedly unresponsive at the scene, with a Glasgow Coma Scale (GCS) score of 3, hypotension, tachycardia, and shallow, irregular respirations.

Objective Data
At the Scene
- Was unresponsive, with obvious deformity to the left side of the skull
- Respirations were shallow and irregular
- O_2 saturations ranged from 88 to 90%
- Systolic BP ranged from 50 to 80 mm Hg
- Heart rate ranged from 100 to 130 beats/min

In the Emergency Department
- Right pupil, 4 mm nonreactive; left pupil, 3 mm nonreactive
- GCS score = 3
- Hypotension and tachycardia continued in spite of fluid resuscitation

Diagnostic Studies
- Computed tomography (CT) of the head showed left skull fracture, left subdural hematoma, bilateral intraventricular and subarachnoid hemorrhage, and cerebral edema.
- CT of the abdomen and pelvis showed a lacerated liver, multiple infarcts to the right kidney, fluid around the duodenum and pancreas, and multiple left pelvic fractures.
- C-spine radiograph series was negative.
- Chest radiograph showed a right lung contusion and pneumomediastinum and subcutaneous emphysema.

Discussion Questions
1. What could be the cause of G. F.'s hypoxia, hypotension, and tachycardia?
2. How could the injuries affect this neurological condition?
3. What area of the brain do his clinical manifestations suggest may be injured?
4. **Priority decision:** What are the priority nursing interventions that should be implemented?
5. **Priority decision:** Based on the assessment data presented, what are the priority nursing diagnoses? Are there any interprofessional issues?

*e*volve
Answers are available at http://evolve.elsevier.com/Canada/Lewis/medsurg.

REVIEW QUESTIONS

The number of the question corresponds to the same-numbered objective at the beginning of the chapter.

1. The nurse understands that an intracranial pressure of 12 mm Hg reflects which of the following?
   a. A severe decrease in cerebral perfusion pressure
   b. An alteration in the production of cerebrospinal fluid (CSF)
   c. The loss of autoregulatory control of intracranial pressure
   d. A normal balance between brain tissue, blood, and cerebrospinal fluid

2. Vasogenic cerebral edema increases intracranial pressure by which of the following effects?
   a. Shifting fluid in the grey matter
   b. Altering the endothelial lining of cerebral capillaries
   c. Leaking molecules from the intracellular fluid to the capillaries
   d. Altering the osmotic gradient flow into the intravascular component

3. A nurse caring for a client with increased intracranial pressure knows that the best way to position the client is which of the following?
   a. Keep the head of the bed flat.
   b. Elevate the head of the bed to 30 degrees.
   c. Maintain the client on the left side with head supported on a pillow.
   d. Use a continuous-rotation bed to continuously change the client's position.

4. The nurse is alerted to a possible acute subdural hematoma in the client who has which of the following symptoms?
   a. A linear skull fracture crossing a major artery
   b. Focal symptoms of brain damage with no recollection of a head injury
   c. Decreased level of consciousness and a headache within 48 hours of a head injury
   d. An immediate loss of consciousness with a brief lucid interval followed by decreasing level of consciousness

5. During admission of a client with a severe head injury to the emergency department, the nurse places the highest priority on assessment for which of the following?
   a. Patency of the airway
   b. Presence of a neck injury
   c. Neurological status according to the Glasgow Coma Scale
   d. Cerebrospinal fluid leakage from the ears or nose

6. A client is suspected of having an intracranial tumour. The signs and symptoms include memory deficits, visual disturbances, weakness of right upper and lower extremities, and personality changes. The nurse recognizes that the tumour is most likely located in which of the following areas?
   a. The frontal lobe
   b. The parietal lobe
   c. The occipital lobe
   d. The temporal lobe

7. Nursing management of a client with a brain tumour includes which of the following? *(Select all that apply.)*
   a. Discussing with the client methods to control inappropriate behaviour
   b. Using diversion techniques to keep the client stimulated and motivated
   c. Assisting and supporting the family in understanding any changes in behaviour
   d. Limiting self-care activities until the client has regained maximum physical functioning
   e. Planning for seizure precautions and teaching the patient and the caregiver about anticonvulsant medications

8. The nurse on the clinical unit is assigned to four clients. Which client should the nurse assess first?
   a. The client with a skull fracture whose nose is bleeding
   b. The older client with a stroke who is confused and whose daughter is present
   c. The client with meningitis who is suddenly agitated and reporting a headache of 10 on a 0–10 scale
   d. The client who had a craniotomy for a brain tumour who is now 3 days postoperative and has had continued emesis

9. Which of the following nursing measures is indicated to reduce the potential for seizures and increased intracranial pressure in the client with bacterial meningitis?
   a. Administering codeine for relief of head and neck pain
   b. Controlling fever with prescribed medications and cooling techniques
   c. Keeping the room darkened and quiet to minimize environmental stimulation
   d. Maintaining the client on strict bed rest with the head of the bed slightly elevated

1. b; 2. d; 3. b; 4. c; 5. a; 6. a; 7. c, e; 8. c; 9. b.

⟲evolve

For even more review questions, visit http://evolve.elsevier.com/Canada/Lewis/medsurg.

REFERENCES

Abraham, P., Rennert, R. C., Gabel, B. C., et al. (2017). ICP management in patients suffering from traumatic brain injury: A systematic review of randomized controlled trials. *Acta Neurochirurgica, 159,* 2279–2287. https://doi.org/10.1007/s00701-017-3363-1

Alexander, B. M., & Cloughesy, T. F. (2017). Adult glioblastoma. *Journal of Clinical Oncology, 35*(21), 2402–2409. https://doi.org/10.1200/JCO.2017.73.0119

Brain Injury Canada (BIC). (2021). *About brain injury.* https://braininjurycanada.ca/en/caregiver/about-brain-injury

Brain Tumour Foundation of Canada (BTFC). (2019). *10 Facts about brain tumours.* http://www.braintumour.ca/wp-content/uploads/2019/09/2019-Brain-Tumour-Facts.pdf

Brain Tumour Foundation of Canada (BTFC). (2021a). *Brain tumour types: Glioblastoma (GB).* https://www.braintumour.ca/brain_tumour_types/glioblastoma-gb/

Brain Tumour Foundation of Canada (BTFC). (2021b). *Brain tumour types: Meningioma.* https://www.braintumour.ca/brain_tumour_types/meningioma/

Brouwer, M. C., McIntyre, P., Prasad, K., et al. (2015). Corticosteroids for acute bacterial meningitis. *Cochrane Database of Systematic Reviews, No. 9,* Article CD004405. https://doi.org/10.1002/14651858.CD004405.pub.5.

Canadian Cancer Society. (2021a). *Chemotherapy for brain and spinal cord tumours.* https://cancer.ca/en/cancer-information/cancer-types/brain-and-spinal-cord/treatment/chemotherapy

Canadian Cancer Society. (2021b). *Survival statistics for brain and spinal cord tumours.* https://cancer.ca/en/cancer-information/cancer-types/brain-and-spinal-cord/prognosis-and-survival/survival-statistics

Canadian Cancer Society. (2021c). *Targeted therapy for brain and spinal cord tumours.* https://cancer.ca/en/cancer-information/cancer-types/brain-and-spinal-cord/treatment/targeted-therapy

Canadian Concussion Centre. (2020). *Research details of the Chronic Traumatic Encephalopathy (CTE) study at the Canadian Concussion Centre.* https://www.uhn.ca/KNC/Research/Projects/Canadian_Concussion_Centre/Pages/research.aspx

Carney, N., Totten, M. D., O'Reilly, C., et al. (2017). Guidelines for the management of severe traumatic brain injury, fourth edition. *Neurosurgery, 80*(1), 6–15. https://doi-org.myaccess.library.utoronto.ca/10.1227/NEU.0000000000001432

Chow, F. (2018). Brain and spinal epidural abscess. Neuroinfectious disease. *CONTINUUM: Lifelong Learning in Neurology, 24*(5), 1327–1348. https://doi.org/10.1212/CON.0000000000000649

Cushing, H. (1925). *Studies in intracranial physiology and surgery.* Oxford University Press. (Seminal).

de Goumoens, V., Didier, A., Mabire, C., et al. (2019). Families' needs of patients with acquired brain injury: Acute phase and rehabilitation. *Rehabilitation Nursing Journal, 44*(6), 319–327. https://doi.org/10.1097/rnj.0000000000000122

DeNett, T., & Feltner, C. (2019). Hypertonic saline versus mannitol for the treatment of increased intracranial pressure in traumatic brain injury. *Journal of the American Association of Nurse Practitioners, 33*(4), 283–293. https://doi.org/10.1097/JXX.0000000000000340

Harary, M., Dolmans, R. G. F., & Gormley, W. B. (2018). Intracranial pressure monitoring—Review and avenues for development. *Sensors, 18*(2), 465. https://doi.org/10.3390/s18020465

Jennett, B., & Teasdale, G. (1977). Aspects of coma after severe head injury. *Lancet, 1*(8017), 878–881. (Seminal). https://doi.org/10.1016/S0140-6736(77)91201-6

Marshall, S., Bayley, M., McCullagh, S., et al. (2018). *Guideline for concussion/mild traumatic brain injury and prolonged symptoms: Adults (18+ years of age)* (3rd ed.). Ontario Neurotrauma Foundation. https://braininjuryguidelines.org/concussion/fileadmin/media/Concussion_guideline_3rd_edition_final.pdf

Meningitis Research Foundation of Canada. (n.d.). *Bacterial.* https://www.meningitis.ca/en/Bacterial

Northern Brain Injury Association. (2021). *First Nations.* https://www.nbia.ca/first-nations-brain-injury/

Oddo, M., Crippa, I. A., Mehta, S., et al. (2016). Optimizing sedation in patients with acute brain injury. *Critical Care: The Official Journal of the Critical Care Forum, 20*(128). https://doi.org/10.1186/s130-54-016-1294-5

Parachute. (2019). *Cycling helmet legislation.* https://parachute.ca/en/professional-resource/policy/helmets/

Parachute. (2021). *Canadian guideline on concussion in sport.* https://parachute.ca/en/professional-resource/concussion-collection/canadian-guideline-on-concussion-in-sport/

Public Health Agency of Canada. (2017). *West Nile virus and other mosquito-borne diseases annual national surveillance report—2017.* https://www.canada.ca/content/dam/phac-aspc/documents/services/publications/diseases-conditions/west-nile-virus-surveillance/2017/annual-national-surveillance-report/annual-national-surveillance-report-en.pdf

Sacco, T. L., & Delibert, S. A. (2018). Management of intracranial pressure: Part 1. Pharmacologic interventions. *Dimensions of Critical Care Nursing, 37*(3), 12–129. https://doi.org/10.1097/DCC.0000000000000293

Teasdale, G., & Jennett, B. (1974). Assessment of coma and impaired consciousness: A practical scale. *Lancet, 2*(7872), 81–84. (Seminal). https://doi.org/10.1016/S0140-6736(74)91639-0

Thompson, K., Pohlmann-Eden, B., Campbell, L. A., et al. (2015). Pharmacological treatments for preventing epilepsy following traumatic head injury. *Cochrane Database of Systematic Reviews, No. 8,* Article CD009900. https://doi.org/10.1002/14651858.CD009900.pub2.

van Eijk, M. M., Schoonman, G. G., van der Naalt, J., et al. (2018). Diffuse axonal injury after traumatic brain injury is a prognostic factor for functional outcome: A systematic review and meta-analysis. *Brain Injury, 32*(4), 395–402. https://doi.org/10.1080/02699052.2018.1429018

Zhang, X., Medow, J. E., Iskander, B. J., et al. (2017). Invasive and noninvasive means of measuring intracranial pressure: A review. *Physiological Measurement, 38*(8), R143–R182. https://doi.org/10.1088/1361-6579/aa7256

RESOURCES

Brain Injury Canada
https://www.braininjurycanada.ca/
Brain Tumour Foundation of Canada
https://www.braintumour.ca
Canadian Cancer Society
https://www.cancer.ca
Parachute—*Preventing Injuries, Saving Lives*
https://www.parachutecanada.org
Toronto Acquired Brain Injury Network
https://www.abinetwork.ca

Inspire—*Encephalitis Global Support Group and Discussion Community*
http://www.inspire.com/groups/encephalitis-global/
National Brain Tumor Foundation
https://www.braintumor.org

evolve

For additional Internet resources, see the website for this book at http://evolve.elsevier.com/Canada/Lewis/medsurg.

Nursing Management
Stroke

Marie-Noëlle Paulin
Originating US chapter by Michelle Bussard

⊘volve WEBSITE

http://evolve.elsevier.com/Canada/Lewis/medsurg

- Review Questions (Online Only)
- Key Points
- Answer Guidelines for Case Study

- Student Case Study
  - Patient with Stroke
- Customizable Nursing Care Plan
  - Stroke

- Conceptual Care Map Creator
- Conceptual Care Map for Textbook Case Study
- Audio Glossary
- Content Updates

LEARNING OBJECTIVES

1. Describe the incidence of and risk factors for stroke.
2. Explain mechanisms that affect cerebral blood flow.
3. Differentiate the etiology and pathophysiology of ischemic and hemorrhagic strokes.
4. Correlate the clinical manifestations of stroke with the underlying pathophysiology.
5. Identify diagnostic studies performed for a patient with a stroke.

6. Describe the interprofessional care, medication therapy, and nutritional therapy for a patient with a stroke.
7. Describe the acute nursing management of a patient with a stroke.
8. Discuss the rehabilitative nursing management of a patient with a stroke.
9. Explain the psychosocial impact of a stroke on the patient, caregiver, and family.

KEY TERMS

aneurysm	embolic stroke	subarachnoid hemorrhage (SAH)
aphasia	hemorrhagic strokes	thrombotic stroke
cerebrovascular accident (CVA)	intracerebral hemorrhage	transient ischemic attack (TIA)
dysarthria	ischemic strokes	
dysphasia	stroke	

Stroke, or **cerebrovascular accident (CVA)** (the medical term for *stroke*), occurs when there is *ischemia* (inadequate blood flow) to a part of the brain or hemorrhage into the brain. Cerebral arteries carry blood to the brain. The brain needs a constant supply of oxygen to function. With a stroke, the blood flow is disrupted, and some brain cells do not get the oxygen they need. When brain cells die, it affects that area of the brain and it will not function as it did before (Heart and Stroke Foundation of Canada [HSFC], 2021d). Functions such as movement, sensation, or emotions that were controlled by the affected area of the brain are lost or impaired. The severity of the loss of function varies according to the location and extent of the brain involved. Early recognition of the clinical manifestations associated with the onset of a stroke is vital to ensure that immediate medical attention is sought, which is crucial in reducing disability and preventing death.

Stroke is a major public health concern. Each year, 62 000 persons in Canada experience a stroke (HSFC, 2016). Over 13 000 Canadians die from stroke annually, making it the third most common cause of death in Canada, behind cancer and heart disease (Statistics Canada, 2017). More than 400 000 Canadians are currently living with the effects of stroke, and it is the leading cause of adult disability (HSFC, 2017). Common long-term disabilities include *hemiparesis* (paralysis of one side of the body), inability to walk, complete or partial dependence in activities of daily living (ADLs), aphasia (total loss of comprehension and use of language or total inability to communicate), and depression. In addition to the physical, cognitive, and emotional impact of a stroke on stroke survivors and their families, stroke also has an enormous financial impact. The direct and indirect costs of strokes are estimated to be greater than $3.6 billion per year in Canada (HSFC, 2021b).

PATHOPHYSIOLOGY OF A STROKE

Anatomy of Cerebral Circulation

Blood is supplied to the brain by two major pairs of arteries: the internal carotid arteries (anterior circulation) and the vertebral arteries (posterior circulation). The carotid arteries branch to supply most of the frontal, parietal, and temporal lobes; the basal ganglia; and part of the diencephalon (thalamus and hypothalamus). The major branches of the carotid arteries are the middle cerebral and anterior cerebral arteries. The vertebral arteries join to form the basilar artery, which branches to supply the middle and lower part of the temporal lobes, the occipital lobes, the cerebellum, the brainstem, and part of the diencephalon. The main branch of the basilar artery is the posterior cerebral artery. The anterior and posterior cerebral circulation is connected at the circle of Willis by the anterior and posterior communicating arteries (Figure 60.1). (See Chapter 58, Figure 58.14, for an illustration of the arteries at the base of the brain.) Genetic variations in this area are common, and some connecting vessels may not be present.

Regulation of Cerebral Blood Flow

The brain requires a continuous supply of blood to provide the oxygen and glucose that neurons need to function. Blood flow must be maintained at 750 to 1000 mL/min (55 mL/100 g of brain tissue), or 20% of the cardiac output, for optimal brain functioning. If blood flow to the brain is totally interrupted (e.g., cardiac arrest), neurological metabolism is altered in 30 seconds, metabolism stops in 2 minutes, and cellular death occurs in 5 minutes.

The brain is normally well protected from changes in blood pressure (BP) by a mechanism known as *cerebral autoregulation* (see Chapter 59). Factors that affect blood flow to the brain include systemic BP, cardiac output, and blood viscosity. During normal activity, oxygen requirements vary considerably, but changes in cardiac output, vasomotor tone, and distribution of blood flow normally maintain adequate blood flow to the head. Cardiac output has to be reduced by one-third before cerebral blood flow is reduced. Changes in blood viscosity affect cerebral blood flow, with decreased viscosity increasing flow.

Collateral circulation may develop to compensate for a decrease in cerebral blood flow. Because of the connections between arteries at the circle of Willis, an area of the brain can potentially receive blood supply from another blood vessel if its original blood supply is cut off (e.g., because of thrombosis). Individual differences in collateral circulation partly determine the degree of brain damage and functional loss when a stroke occurs.

Intracranial pressure (ICP) also influences cerebral blood flow (see Chapter 58). Increased ICP within the fixed space of the skull may cause reduced cerebral blood flow as a compensatory mechanism.

Atherosclerosis

Atherosclerosis (hardening and thickening of arteries) is a major cause of stroke. It can lead to thrombus formation and contribute to development of emboli. (The role of atherosclerosis in thrombosis and emboli development is discussed in Chapter 36.) Initially, there is abnormal infiltration of lipids in the intimal layer of the artery. This fatty streak further develops into a plaque. Plaques often develop in areas of increased turbulence of the blood, such as at the bifurcation of an artery

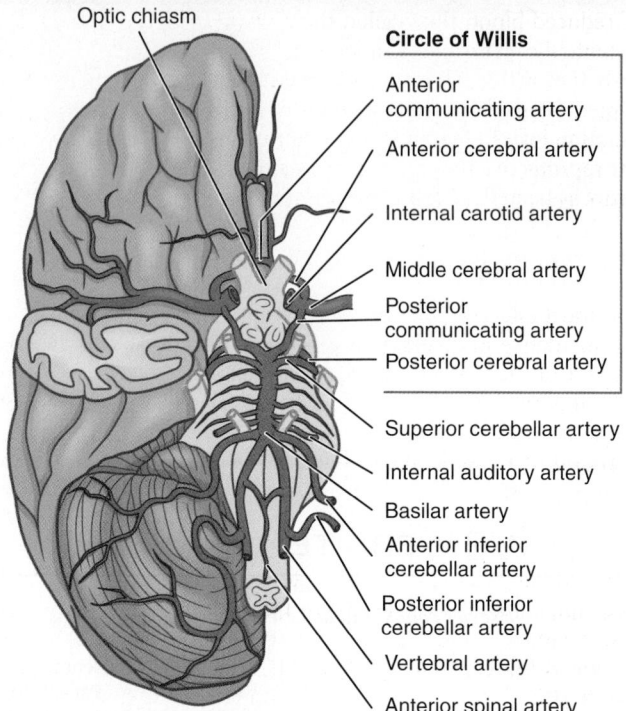

FIG. 60.1 Cerebral arteries and the circle of Willis. The tip of the temporal lobe has been removed to show the course of the middle cerebral artery.

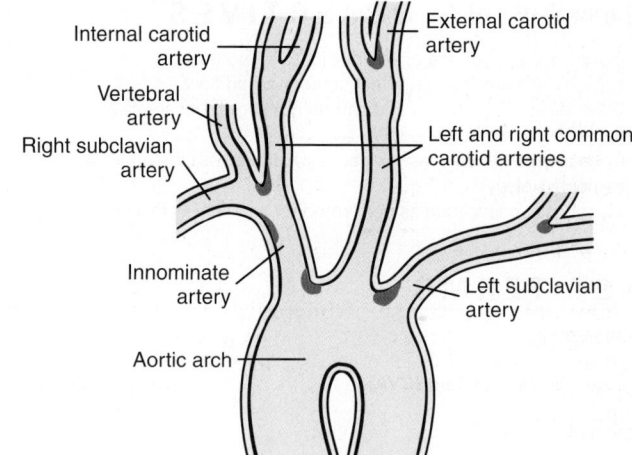

FIG. 60.2 Common sites for the development of atherosclerosis in extracranial and intracranial arteries. The main locations are just above the common carotid bifurcation (most common site) and the start of the branches from the aorta and the innominate and subclavian arteries.

or a tortuous area (Figure 60.2). Calcified, brittle plaques may rupture or fissure, leading to an inflammatory response. Platelet and fibrin are released and stick to the roughened plaque surface. Plaque may narrow or occlude the artery. Also, parts of the plaque or thrombus can break off and travel to a narrower distal artery. Cerebral infarction occurs when a cerebral artery becomes blocked and blood supply to the brain beyond the blockage is occluded.

In response to ischemia, a series of metabolic events, termed the *ischemic cascade,* occur, including inadequate adenosine triphosphate production, loss of ion homeostasis, release of excitatory amino acids (e.g., glutamate), free radical formation, and cell death. Around the core area of ischemia is a border zone of reduced blood flow called the *penumbra,* where ischemia is potentially reversible. If adequate blood flow can be restored early (i.e., within 3 hours) and the ischemic cascade can be interrupted, brain damage may be minimized and less neurological function lost. Research is ongoing to identify thrombolytic and neuroprotective therapies to re-establish blood flow and protect neurons from further ischemic damage.

RISK FACTORS FOR STROKE

The most effective way to decrease the burden of and reduce the incidence of stroke is prevention through awareness and control of modifiable risk factors. Stroke risk increases considerably in the presence of multiple risk factors. The Determinants of Health box offers more specific information on nonmodifiable and modifiable risk factors within the Canadian population.

Nonmodifiable Risk Factors

Nonmodifiable risk factors include age; sex; Indigenous, African, and South Asian heritage; family and medical history; and personal circumstances (e.g., eating healthy food, access to safe drinking water and health services) (HSFC, 2021c). Stroke risk increases with age, doubling each decade after age 55. Two-thirds of all strokes occur in individuals older than 65 years, but a stroke can occur at any age. The risk for stroke or transient ischemic attack (TIA) among younger adults is on the rise. Patients between 20 and 59 years of age comprise 19% of hospital admissions for stroke and TIA, according to recent data. More than 62 000 people suffer from a stroke in Canada each year. More than 32 000 of these strokes happen in women. Of all stroke-related deaths, 59% occur in women and 41% in men (HSFC, 2018c). Because women tend to live longer than men, they have a longer period during which to suffer a stroke. A family history of stroke, a prior TIA, or a prior stroke also increases the risk for stroke.

An *arteriovenous malformation* (AVM) is an abnormal group of tangled arteries and veins. AVMs can occur anywhere in the body; however, they pose the greatest risk in the brain, as these vessels are more likely than others to bleed. Based on the location and size of the AVM, treatment options can include embolization, radiation, or surgery (Toronto Brain Vascular Malformation Study Group, n.d.).

Modifiable Risk Factors

Modifiable risk factors are those that can potentially be altered through lifestyle changes and medical treatment, thus reducing the risk for stroke (Table 60.1).

Hypertension is the single most important, well-documented modifiable risk factor for stroke. One in four Canadians have diagnosed hypertension (DeGuire et al., 2019). Increases in systolic and diastolic BP independently increase the risk for stroke. Stroke risk can be significantly reduced through the adequate treatment and early diagnosis of hypertension (HSFC, 2021c).

Heart disease, including atrial fibrillation (AF), myocardial infarction (MI), cardiomyopathy, cardiac valve abnormalities, and congenital defects, is also a risk factor for stroke. Of these, AF is the most important modifiable cardiac-related risk factor, controlled through the use of anticoagulants. The incidence of AF increases with age. Approximately 15% of all strokes are caused by AF, and this risk is greater after the age of 60, when 33% of strokes are caused by AF (HSFC, 2021a).

DETERMINANTS OF HEALTH

Stroke

Sex

Although both sexes are at risk for strokes, the occurrence and rate of a first stroke are consistently higher among men than women. However, since women have a longer life expectancy, more women will suffer a stroke each year. The risk of stroke increases after menopause.

Biology and Genetic Endowment

Individuals of African or South Asian heritage are more likely to have high blood pressure, diabetes mellitus, or other risk factors for stroke at a younger age. Indigenous people are more likely to have high blood pressure and diabetes, which puts them at greater risk of stroke than the general population. Individuals with a family history of stroke or TIA at an early age are also at increased risk for stroke.

Personal Health Practices and Coping Skills
- Alcohol misuse and illicit drug use can lead to stroke.
- Obesity is linked to a higher risk for stroke.
- Physical inability is associated with higher risk for stroke.
- Smoking increases risk for stroke.
- An unhealthy diet increases stroke risk.
- Heart-healthy diets can reduce stroke risk by up to 80%.
- Stress is associated with increased risk for stroke.

References

Public Health Agency of Canada. (2019). Stroke in Canada: Highlights from the Canadian Chronic Disease Surveillance System. https://www.canada.ca/en/public-health/services/publications/diseases-conditions/stroke-canada-fact-sheet.html

Heart and Stroke Foundation of Canada (HSFC). (2021). Risk and prevention. https://www.heartandstroke.ca/stroke/risk-and-prevention

TABLE 60.1	MODIFIABLE RISK FACTORS FOR STROKE

- Asymptomatic carotid stenosis
- Arteriovenous malformation (in brain)
- Diabetes mellitus
- Heart disease; atrial fibrillation
- Alcohol use
- Hypercoagulability
- Illicit drugs
- Dyslipidemia
- Hypertension
- Obesity and body fat distribution
- Oral contraceptive use
- Physical inactivity
- Sleep apnea
- Smoking

Diabetes mellitus is a significant risk factor for ischemic stroke. The risk for stroke in people with diabetes mellitus is four to five times higher than in the general population. Good control of hypertension in individuals living with diabetes mellitus significantly decreases stroke risk.

Increased serum cholesterol and carotid stenosis are both risk factors for ischemic stroke. Smoking increases the risk for ischemic stroke two to four times. Fortunately, the risk associated with smoking decreases over time after smoking cessation and, in 10 to 15 years, is reduced to that of nonsmokers (World Health Organization [WHO], 2020).

The effect of alcohol on stroke risk appears to depend on the amount consumed. Light to moderate use of alcohol, in particular wine, has been linked to reduced risk for ischemic stroke. Heavier use of alcohol does increase risk for stroke. Heavy drinking is defined as five or more drinks for males, four or more for females, per occasion, at least once a month during the past year (Statistics Canada, 2019a).

About 63% of adults ages 18 and older, or 17.2 million Canadians, self-reported being overweight or obese in 2018 (Statistics Canada, 2019b). An association between physical inactivity and increased ischemic stroke risk is present in both men and women, regardless of ethnicity. Benefits of physical activity can occur with even light to moderate regular activity and may be in part related to the beneficial effect of exercise on other risk factors. Nutrition teaching is important for individuals at risk for stroke, since a diet high in fat and low in fruits and vegetables may increase stroke risk (HSFC, 2021c).

Use of illicit drugs (e.g., amphetamines, cannabis, cocaine, ecstasy, heroin, opioids) has also been associated with increased stroke risk (HSFC, 2021c).

The early forms of birth control pills that contained high levels of progestin and estrogen increased a woman's chance of experiencing a stroke, especially if the woman also smoked heavily. Newer, low-dose oral contraceptives have lower risks for stroke except in individuals who are hypertensive and smoke. Women also face a higher risk for stroke during pregnancy and when taking hormone therapy, so their other risk factors should be assessed by a health care provider (HSFC, 2021c).

Other conditions that may increase stroke risk include migraines, metabolic syndrome, sleep-disordered breathing, inflammation and infection, hypercoagulability, and hyperhomocysteinemia.

TYPES OF STROKE

Strokes are classified as ischemic or hemorrhagic on the basis of underlying pathophysiological findings (Figure 60.3 and Table 60.2).

Ischemic Stroke

Ischemic strokes result from inadequate blood flow to the brain from partial or complete occlusion of an artery and account for the majority of strokes (HSFC, 2021e). Ischemic strokes are further divided by their causality into *thrombotic* and *embolic*. A TIA is usually a precursor to ischemic stroke.

Transient Ischemic Attack. A transient ischemic attack (TIA) is a temporary episode of neurological dysfunction caused by focal brain, spinal cord, or retinal ischemia but without acute infarction of the brain. Clinical symptoms typically last less than 1 hour. In the past, TIAs were operationally defined as any focal cerebral ischemic event with symptoms lasting less than 24 hours. However, it has been demonstrated that this arbitrary time threshold was too broad because over 30% of classically defined TIAs show brain infarction on magnetic resonance imaging (MRI) (Souillard-Scemama, et al., 2015).

Most TIAs resolve. However, once a TIA starts, it is not possible to know whether it will persist and become a true stroke or resolve. Stroke risk following TIA is greatest immediately after the event; therefore, it is urgent that individuals seek medical attention immediately upon symptom onset (Khare, 2016).

TIAs may be caused by microemboli or plaque that temporarily block the blood flow. TIAs are a warning sign of progressive cerebrovascular disease (HSFC, 2021e). The signs and symptoms of a TIA depend on the blood vessel that is involved and the area of the brain that is ischemic. If the carotid system is involved, patients may have a temporary loss of vision in one eye *(amaurosis fugax),* a transient hemiparesis, numbness or loss of sensation, or a sudden inability to speak. Signs of a TIA involving the vertebrobasilar system may include tinnitus, vertigo, darkened or blurred vision, *diplopia* (double vision), *ptosis* (drooping eyelid), dysarthria (a disturbance in the muscular control of speech), *dysphagia* (difficulty swallowing), *ataxia* (loss of muscle control), and unilateral or bilateral numbness or weakness.

Thrombotic Stroke. A thrombotic stroke occurs when a blood clot forms in a diseased and narrowed blood vessel in the brain (see Figure 60.3, *A*). If the narrowed lumen of the blood vessel becomes occluded, infarction occurs. Thrombosis develops readily where atherosclerotic plaques have already narrowed blood vessels. Thrombotic stroke is the most common type of ischemic stroke. Two-thirds of thrombotic strokes are associated with hypertension or diabetes mellitus, both of which accelerate atherosclerosis. Patients experiencing a TIA have symptoms that resolve without interventions, whereas patients suffering a thrombotic stroke have symptoms that will continue to evolve if treatment is not received quickly. In 30 to 50% of individuals, TIAs have preceded thrombotic strokes.

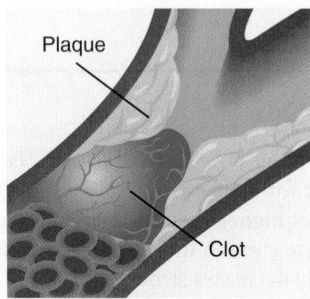

Thrombotic stroke. Cerebral thrombosis is a narrowing of the artery by fatty deposits called *plaque.* Plaque can cause a clot to form, which blocks the passage of blood through the artery.

A

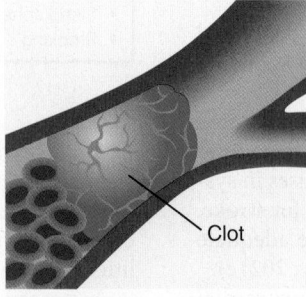

Embolic stroke. An embolus is a blood clot or other debris circulating in the blood. When it reaches an artery in the brain that is too narrow to pass through, it lodges there and blocks the flow of blood.

B

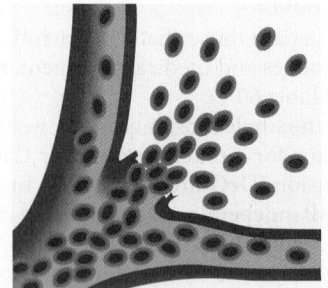

Hemorrhagic stroke. A burst blood vessel may allow blood to seep into and damage brain tissues until clotting shuts off the leak.

C

FIG. 60.3 A to **C,** Major types of stroke.

TABLE 60.2 TYPES OF STROKE

Gender/Age	Warning/Onset	Course
Ischemic		
Thrombotic Men more than women Oldest median age	*Warning:* TIA (30–50% of cases) *Onset:* Often during or after sleep	Stepwise progression, signs and symptoms develop slowly, usually some improvement, recurrence in 20–25% of survivors
Embolic Men more than women	*Warning:* TIA uncommon *Onset:* Lack of relationship to activity, sudden onset	Single event, signs and symptoms develop quickly, usually some improvement, recurrence common without aggressive treatment of underlying disease
Hemorrhagic		
Intracerebral Slightly higher in women	*Warning:* Headache (25% of cases) *Onset:* Activity (often)	Progression over 24 hr; fatality more likely with presence of coma
Subarachnoid Higher in women Youngest median age	*Warning:* Headache (common) *Onset:* Activity (often), sudden onset	Acute onset, usually single sudden event described as the "worst headache of one's life," fatality more likely with presence of coma

TIA, transient ischemic attack.

The extent of the stroke depends on the rapidity of onset, the size of the lesion, and the presence of collateral circulation. Most patients with ischemic stroke do not have a decreased level of consciousness (LOC) in the first 24 hours, unless it is due to a brainstem stroke or other conditions such as seizures, increased ICP, or hemorrhage. Ischemic stroke symptoms may progress in the first 72 hours as infarction and cerebral edema increase.

A *lacunar stroke* refers to a stroke from occlusion of a small penetrating artery that supplies blood to tissues deep within the brain. This most commonly occurs in the basal ganglia, thalamus, internal capsule, or pons. Although many lacunar strokes are asymptomatic, when present, symptoms can cause considerable deficits. These include pure motor *hemiplegia* (paralysis of one side of the body), pure sensory stroke (contralateral loss of all sensory modalities), contralateral leg and face weakness with arm and leg ataxia, and isolated motor or sensory stroke. Multiple small vessel infarcts may also result in a decrease in vascular function (e.g., vascular dementia) (see Chapter 62).

Embolic Stroke. Embolic stroke occurs when an embolus lodges in and occludes a cerebral artery, resulting in infarction and edema of the area supplied by the involved vessel (see Figure 60.3, *B*). Embolism is the second most common cause of stroke, accounting for about 24% of strokes. The majority of emboli originate in the endocardial (inside) layer of the heart, with plaque breaking off from the endocardium and entering the circulation. The embolus travels upward to the cerebral circulation and lodges where a vessel narrows or bifurcates. Heart conditions associated with emboli include valvular heart disease and valvular prosthesis MI, infective endocarditis, rheumatic heart disease, and intracardiac congenital defects such as atrial septal defects and patent foramen ovale. One-fourth of all strokes after age 40 years are caused by AF (HSFC, 2021a). Less common triggers of emboli include air and fat from long bone (femur) fractures.

The patient with an embolic stroke commonly has a rapid occurrence of severe clinical symptoms, but warning signs are less common than with thrombotic stroke. The onset of an embolic stroke is usually sudden and may or may not be related to activity. The patient usually remains conscious and may or may not experience a headache. Prognosis is related to the amount and location of brain tissue deprived of its blood supply. The effects of the emboli are initially characterized by severe neurological deficits, which can be temporary if the clot breaks up and allows blood to flow. Smaller emboli then continue to obstruct smaller vessels, which in turn involve smaller portions of the brain with fewer deficits noted. The embolic stroke often occurs rapidly, and the body does not have time to accommodate by developing collateral circulation. Recurrence of embolic stroke is common unless the underlying cause is aggressively treated.

Hemorrhagic Stroke

Hemorrhagic strokes account for approximately 15% of all strokes; they result from bleeding into the brain tissue itself (intracerebral or intraparenchymal hemorrhage) or into the subarachnoid space or the ventricles (subarachnoid hemorrhage [SAH] or intraventricular hemorrhage).

Intracerebral Hemorrhage. Intracerebral hemorrhage is bleeding within the brain caused by a rupture of a vessel; it accounts for about 10% of all strokes (see Figure 60.3, *C*). Hypertension is the most important risk factor for intracerebral hemorrhage (Figure 60.4). Other causes include cerebral amyloid angiopathy, vascular malformations, coagulation disorders, anticoagulant and thrombolytic medications, trauma, brain tumours, and ruptured aneurysms. Hemorrhage commonly occurs during periods of activity. There is most often a sudden onset of symptoms, with progression over minutes to hours because of ongoing bleeding. Symptoms include neurological deficits, headache, nausea, vomiting, decreased LOC (in about 50% of patients), and hypertension. The extent of the symptoms varies depending on the amount, location, and duration of the bleeding. A blood clot within the closed skull can result in a mass that causes pressure on brain tissue, displaces brain tissue, and decreases cerebral blood flow, leading to ischemia and infarction.

Approximately 50% of intracerebral hemorrhages occur in the putamen and the internal capsule, central white matter, thalamus, cerebellar hemispheres, and pons. Initially, patients experience a severe headache with nausea and vomiting. Clinical manifestations of bleeding within the putamen and internal capsule include weakness of one side (including face, arm, and leg), slurred speech, and deviation of the eyes. Progression of symptoms related to a severe hemorrhage includes hemiplegia, fixed and dilated pupils, abnormal body posturing, and coma. Thalamic hemorrhage results in hemiplegia with more sensory than motor loss. Bleeding into the subthalamic areas of the brain leads to difficulties with vision and eye movement. Cerebellar hemorrhages are characterized by severe headache, vomiting, loss of ability to walk, dysphagia, dysarthria, and eye movement disturbances. Hemorrhage in the pons is the most serious because basic life functions (e.g., respiration) are rapidly affected. Hemorrhage in the pons can be characterized by hemiplegia leading to complete paralysis, coma, abnormal body posturing, fixed pupils (small in size), hyperthermia, and death. It is difficult to predict the prognosis of patients with intracerebral hemorrhage. Early recognition and aggressive medical

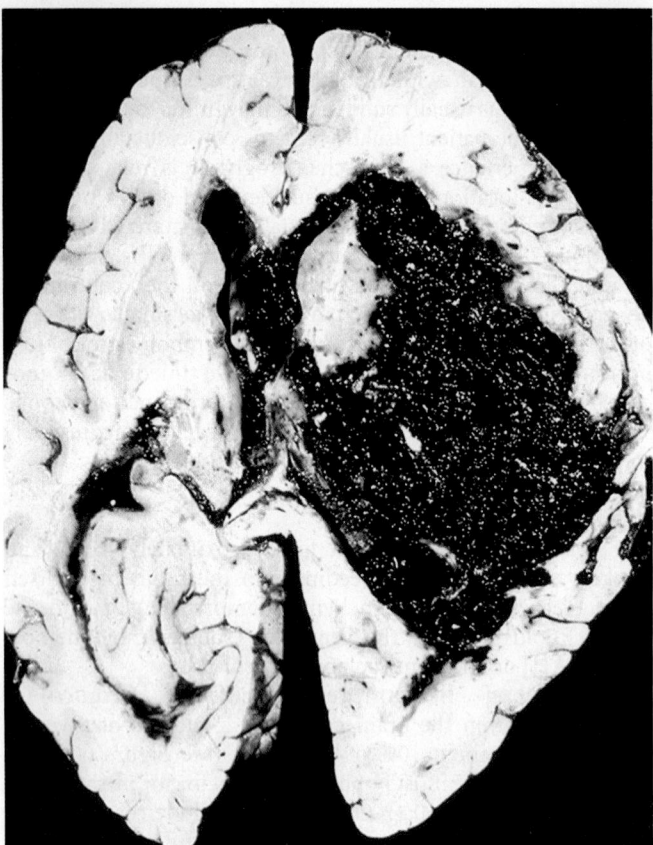

FIG. 60.4 Massive hypertensive hemorrhage rupturing into a lateral ventricle of the brain. Source: Kumar, V., Abbas, A. K., Fausto, N., et al. (2010). *Robbins and Cotran pathologic basis of disease* (8th ed., p. 1296, Figure 28-18). Saunders.

TABLE 60.3	STROKE MANIFESTATIONS RELATED TO ARTERY INVOLVEMENT
Artery	**Deficit or Syndrome**
Anterior cerebral	Motor or sensory deficit (contralateral) or both, sucking or rooting reflex, rigidity, gait problems, loss of proprioception, fine touch
Middle cerebral	*Dominant side:* Aphasia, motor and sensory deficit, *hemianopia* (blindness over half the field of vision) *Nondominant side:* Neglect, motor and sensory deficit, hemianopia
Posterior cerebral	Hemianopia, visual hallucination, spontaneous pain, motor deficit
Vertebral	Cranial nerve deficits, diplopia, dizziness, nausea, vomiting, dysarthria, dysphagia, coma

management are associated with improved outcomes. Factors such as the patient's age, initial Glasgow Coma Scale (GCS) score, and location and volume of hemorrhage play a role in decision making and prognostication (Hemphill et al., 2015).

Subarachnoid Hemorrhage. Subarachnoid hemorrhage (SAH) occurs when there is intracranial bleeding into the cerebrospinal fluid (CSF)–filled space between the arachnoid and the pia mater membranes on the surface of the brain. SAH is commonly caused by rupture of a cerebral aneurysm (congenital or acquired permanent, localized outpouching or dilation of the blood vessel wall). Aneurysms may vary in shape and can be described as saccular or berry aneurysms, ranging from a few millimetres to 20 to 30 mm in size, or fusiform atherosclerotic aneurysms. The majority of aneurysms are in the circle of Willis. Other causes of SAH include AVMs, trauma, and illicit drug (cocaine) use. About 35% of people who have a hemorrhagic stroke due to a ruptured aneurysm die, and neurological deficits are common in survivors. Contributing factors for SAH caused by a ruptured aneurysm include connective tissue disorders, family history, hypertension, and tobacco use (Chong, 2020).

The patient may have warning symptoms if the ballooning artery applies pressure to brain tissue or if an aneurysm leaks before major rupture. Overall, cerebral aneurysms are viewed as a "silent killer" because individuals usually do not have warning signs of an aneurysm until rupture has occurred.

Loss of consciousness may or may not occur. The patient's LOC may range from alert to comatose, depending on the severity of the bleed. Other symptoms include focal neurological deficits (including cranial nerve deficits), nausea, vomiting, seizures, and stiff neck. Improvements in surgical techniques and aggressive medical management of complications have led to better outcomes; however, many patients are left with significant morbidity, including cognitive difficulties.

Complications of aneurysmal SAH include rebleeding before surgery or other therapy is initiated and cerebral vasospasm (narrowing of the large blood vessels at the base of the brain), which can result in cerebral infarction. Cerebral vasospasm is most likely due to an interaction between the metabolites of blood and the vascular smooth muscle. During the lysis of subarachnoid blood clots, metabolites are released. These metabolites can cause endothelial damage and vasoconstriction. In addition, release of endothelin (a potent vasoconstrictor) may play a major role in the induction of cerebral vasospasm after SAH. Peak time for vasospasm to occur is 7 to 10 days after the initial bleed.

SAFETY ALERT
Sudden onset of a severe headache that is different from a previous headache and typically the "worst headache of one's life" is characteristic of a ruptured aneurysm, and individuals experiencing it should seek medical attention immediately.

Clinical Manifestations of Stroke

The neurological manifestations do not significantly differ between ischemic and hemorrhagic stroke. The reason for this is that destruction of neural tissue is the basis for neurological dysfunction caused by both types of stroke. The clinical manifestations are related to location of the stroke. Specific manifestations related to the type of stroke are discussed in the previous section on types of stroke.

The general clinical manifestations of ischemic and hemorrhagic stroke are discussed together in this section. A stroke can have an effect on many body functions, including motor activity, bladder and bowel elimination, intellectual function, spatial–perceptual alterations, personality, affect, sensation, and communication. The functions affected are directly related to the artery involved and the area of the brain it supplies (Table 60.3). Manifestations related to right- and left-brain damage differ somewhat and are shown in Figure 60.5.

Motor Function. Motor deficits are the most obvious effect of stroke. Motor deficits include impairment of (a) mobility, (b) respiratory function, (c) swallowing and speech, (d) gag reflex, and (e) self-care abilities. Symptoms are caused by the

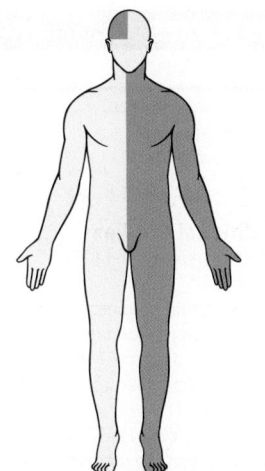 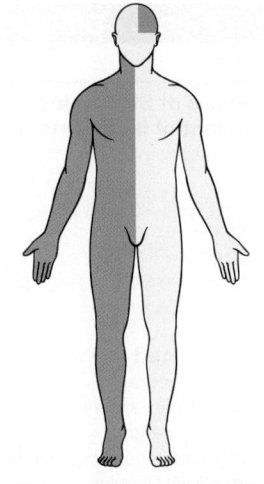

Right-brain damage
(stroke on right side of the brain)

- Paralyzed left side: hemiplegia
- Left-sided neglect
- Spatial–perceptual deficits
- Tends to deny or minimize problems
- Rapid performance, short attention span
- Impulsive; safety problems
- Impaired judgement
- Impaired time concepts

Left-brain damage
(stroke on left side of the brain)

- Paralyzed right side: hemiplegia
- Impaired speech–language (aphasias)
- Impaired right–left discrimination
- Slow performance, cautious
- Aware of deficits: depression, anxiety
- Impaired comprehension related to language, math

FIG. 60.5 Manifestations of right-brain and left-brain stroke.

destruction of motor neurons in the pyramidal pathway (nerve fibres from the brain and passing through the spinal cord to the motor cells). The characteristic motor deficits include loss of skilled voluntary movement (*akinesia*), impairment of integration of movements, alterations in muscle tone, and alterations in reflexes. The initial *hyporeflexia* (depressed reflexes) progresses to *hyper-reflexia* (hyperactive reflexes) for most patients.

Motor deficits after a stroke follow certain specific patterns. A lesion of the cortex will lead to weakness in the *contralateral* lower face only. If the injury affects the facial nerve, weakness will present in the *ipsilateral* upper and lower face (Mullen & Loomis, 2014). The arms and legs of the affected side may be weakened or paralyzed to different degrees depending on which part of and to what extent the cerebral circulation was compromised. A stroke affecting the middle cerebral artery (most common) leads to a greater weakness in the upper extremity than the lower extremity and contralateral hemiparesis affects the lower half of the face which presents as facial droop. The affected shoulder tends to rotate internally and the hip rotates externally. The affected foot is plantar flexed and inverted. An initial period of flaccidity may last from days to several weeks and is related to nerve damage. Spasticity of the muscles follows the flaccid stage and is related to interruption of upper motor neuron influence.

Communication. The left hemisphere is dominant for language skills in right-handed persons and in most left-handed persons. Language disorders involve expression and comprehension of written and spoken words. The patient may experience aphasia affecting the comprehension of language, the ability to speak, or both. It occurs when a stroke damages the dominant

hemisphere of the brain. Dysphasia refers to the impaired ability to communicate. However, in most settings, the terms *aphasia* and *dysphasia* are used interchangeably to mean the same thing, with *aphasia* often being the more common term used.

According to the National Institute of Neurological Disorders and Stroke (NINDS, 2017), there are four categories of aphasia. The first is *expressive aphasia* (also called *Broca's aphasia*), or difficulty in expressing thoughts through speech or writing. The patient cannot find the words needed but does know what they want to say. The stroke survivor's speech is reduced often to fewer than four words. The second category is *receptive aphasia* (also called *Wernicke's aphasia*), which involves difficulty understanding spoken or written language. These patients are difficult to understand. They speak without hesitation, but words may be used incorrectly and sentences may be ungrammatical. The third category is *anomic* or *amnesic aphasia*, which is the least severe form of aphasia and involves difficulty finding the correct names for specific objects, people, places, or events. *Global aphasia*, the fourth category, results in loss of all expressive and receptive function. It is usually caused by a massive stroke. Some aphasia is mixed, with impairment in both expression and understanding.

Many stroke patients also experience *dysarthria*, a disturbance in the muscular control of speech. Impairments may involve pronunciation, articulation, and phonation (use of the voice). Dysarthria does not affect the meaning of communication or the comprehension of language, but it does affect the mechanics of speech. Some patients experience a combination of aphasia and dysarthria.

Affect. Patients who have had a stroke may have difficulty controlling their emotions, and so emotional responses may be exaggerated or unpredictable. Depression, common in the first year following a stroke (HSFC, 2017), and feelings associated with changes in body image and loss of function can make this worse. Patients may also be frustrated by mobility and communication difficulties.

Intellectual Function. Both memory and judgement may be impaired as a result of stroke. These impairments can occur with strokes affecting either side of the brain. A left-brain stroke is more likely to result in memory problems related to language. Patients with a left-brain stroke often are very cautious in making judgements. The patient with a right-brain stroke tends to be impulsive and to move quickly. An example of behaviour with right-brain stroke is the patient who tries to rise quickly from the wheelchair without locking the wheels or raising the foot rests. The patient with a left-brain stroke would move slowly and cautiously from the wheelchair. Patients with either type of stroke may have difficulty making generalizations, which interferes with their ability to learn.

Spatial–Perceptual Alterations. A stroke on the right side of the brain is more likely to cause difficulties in spatial–perceptual orientation, although these issues can also occur with left-brain stroke. Spatial–perceptual disorders may be divided into four categories:

1. The patient's incorrect perception of self and illness. This deficit follows damage to the parietal lobe. Patients may deny their illnesses or their own body parts (*anosognosia*).
2. The patient's erroneous perception of self in space. The patient may neglect all input from the affected side. This may be worsened by *homonymous hemianopia*, in which blindness occurs in the same half of the visual fields of both eyes. The patient also has difficulty with spatial orientation, such as judging distances.

3. *Agnosia,* the inability to recognize an object by sight, touch, or hearing.
4. *Apraxia,* the inability to carry out learned sequential movements on command.

Patients may or may not be aware of their spatial–perceptual alterations.

Elimination. Fortunately, most difficulties with urinary and bowel elimination that occur initially are temporary. When a stroke affects one hemisphere of the brain, the prognosis for normal bladder function is excellent. At least partial sensation for bladder filling remains, and voluntary urination is present. Initially, the patient may experience frequency, urgency, and incontinence. Although motor control of the bowel is usually not a problem, patients frequently become constipated. Constipation is associated with immobility, weak abdominal muscles, dehydration, and diminished response to the defecation reflex. Urinary and bowel elimination challenges may also be related to the inability to express needs and to manage clothing.

Diagnostic Studies

When manifestations of a stroke occur, diagnostic studies are done to (a) confirm that it is a stroke and not another brain lesion, such as a subdural hematoma, and (b) identify the likely cause of the stroke (Table 60.4). Tests also guide decisions about therapy to prevent a secondary stroke. The single most important timely primary assessment tool for a stroke patient is brain imaging—either MRI or noncontrast computed tomographic (CT) scan (HSFC, 2018a). The CT scan is quick and easy to access in most facilities. It should optimally be obtained within 25 minutes and read within 45 minutes of arrival at the emergency department. The CT scan indicates the size and location of the lesion and helps to differentiate between ischemic and hemorrhagic stroke. Serial CT scans may be used to assess the effectiveness of treatment and to evaluate recovery.

Computed tomographic angiography (CTA) provides visualization of cerebral vasculature and can be performed after or at the same time as the noncontrast CT scan. CTA can provide an estimate of perfusion and be used to detect defects in the cerebral arteries.

MRI is used to determine the extent of brain injury and has greater specificity than CT in determining the location of vascular lesions and blockages. Patient preparation and access to an MRI scanner can be delayed for many reasons but should not delay the patient having alternative diagnostic studies performed. Magnetic resonance angiography (MRA) can be used to detect vascular lesions and blockages, similar to CTA.

Angiography can identify cervical and cerebrovascular occlusion, atherosclerotic plaques, and malformation of vessels. Cerebral angiography is a definitive study to identify the source of SAH. Risks of angiography include dislodging an embolus, vasospasm, inducing further hemorrhage, and allergic reaction to contrast media.

Intra-arterial digital subtraction angiography requires a smaller dose of contrast material, uses smaller catheters, and is a shorter procedure compared with conventional angiography. Digital subtraction angiography involves the injection of a contrast agent to visualize blood vessels in the neck and the large vessels of the circle of Willis. It is considered safer than cerebral angiography because less vascular manipulation is required.

Transcranial Doppler ultrasonography is a noninvasive study that measures the velocity of blood flow in the major cerebral

TABLE 60.4   DIAGNOSTIC STUDIES

Stroke

Diagnosis of Stroke (Including Extent of Involvement) • Computed tomographic (CT) scan • CT angiography (CTA) • Magnetic resonance angiography (MRA) • Magnetic resonance imaging (MRI) **Cerebral Blood Flow** • Carotid angiography • Carotid duplex scanning • Cerebral angiography • Digital subtraction angiography • Transcranial Doppler ultrasonography **Cardiac Assessment** • Cardiac markers (troponin, creatine kinase–MB) • Chest radiograph	• Echocardiography (transthoracic, transesophageal) • Electrocardiogram **Additional Studies** • Cerebrospinal fluid (CSF) analysis* • Coagulation studies: prothrombin time/international normalized ratio (PT/INR), activated partial thromboplastin time (aPTT) • Complete blood cell count (CBC) including platelets • Electrolytes, blood glucose; hemoglobin A$_{1c}$ (Hb A$_{1c}$) • Lipid profile • Renal and hepatic studies

*A lumbar puncture to obtain CSF is avoided if increased intracranial pressure is suspected, because this procedure can cause a low-pressure shunt, drawing the CSF fluid down the spinal column. As the CSF pressure decreases, CSF and brain mass may shift toward the lower pressure area, causing herniation of the brain (see Chapter 58).

arteries. Transcranial Doppler has been shown to be effective in detecting microemboli and vasospasm and is ideal for patients confirmed to have SAH. Carotid duplex scanning is used not only to detect the cause of the stroke but also to stratify patients for either medical management or carotid intervention if they have carotid stenosis.

If the suspected cause of the stroke includes emboli from the heart, diagnostic cardiac tests should be done (see Table 60.4). Blood tests are also done to help identify conditions contributing to stroke and to guide treatment (see Table 60.4).

Interprofessional Care

Prevention Therapy. Primary prevention is a priority for decreasing morbidity and mortality from stroke (Table 60.5). The goals of stroke prevention include health management for the well individual and education and management of modifiable risk factors to prevent a primary or secondary stroke. Health management focuses on (a) BP control, (b) blood glucose control, (c) diet and exercise, (d) smoking cessation, (e) limiting alcohol consumption, and (f) routine health assessments. Patients with known risk factors such as diabetes mellitus, hypertension, smoking, high serum lipids, or cardiovascular dysfunction require close management.

Medication Therapy. Measures to prevent the development of a thrombus or embolus are used in patients with TIAs because they are at risk for stroke. Antiplatelet medications are usually the chosen treatment to prevent stroke in patients who have had a TIA. ASA (Aspirin) is the most frequently used antiplatelet agent, commonly at a dose of 81 to 325 mg/day. Medication therapy may also include clopidogrel (Plavix). Oral anticoagulation using apixaban (Eliquis), dabigatran (Pradaxa), or rivaroxaban (Xarelto) is the treatment of choice for individuals with AF who have had a TIA. Patients using these anticoagulation medications need to have their renal function regularly monitored and doses adjusted accordingly. Statins (simvastatin

TABLE 60.5 INTERPROFESSIONAL CARE

Stroke

Diagnostic	Surgical Therapy

Diagnostic
- History and physical examination
- See Table 60.4

Interprofessional Therapy

Prevention
- Control of hypertension
- Control of diabetes mellitus
- Treatment of underlying cardiac problem

Lifestyle Modifications
- Limiting of alcohol intake
- Increase in exercise
- Weight loss to normalize BMI
- Reduction of sodium intake
- Smoking cessation

Medication Therapy
- Anticoagulation therapy for patients with atrial fibrillation (if indicated by use of the CHADS2 classification)
- Platelet inhibitors (e.g., acetylsalicylic acid [ASA; Aspirin])

Surgical Therapy
- Carotid endarterectomy (see Figure 60.6)
- Extracranial–intracranial bypass
- Stenting of carotid artery
- Surgical interventions for aneurysms at risk of bleeding
- Transluminal angioplasty

Acute Care
- DVT prevention with LMWH
- Fluid therapy
- Maintenance of airway
- Prevention of secondary injury
- Treatment of cerebral edema

Ischemic Stroke
- Endovascular treatment
- Tissue plasminogen activator (tPA)

Hemorrhagic Stroke
- Clipping or coiling of aneurysm
- Surgical decompression if indicated

Embolic Stroke
- Treatment of underlying cause (usually cardiac related)

BMI, body mass index; *CHADS2,* clinical prediction tool used to estimate the risk for stroke in patients with atrial fibrillation and to determine the degree of anticoagulation required; *DVT,* deep vein thrombosis; *LMWH,* low-molecular-weight heparin.

[Zocor], lovastatin) have been shown to be effective in the prevention of ischemic strokes and cardiovascular events (Tramacere et al., 2019).

MEDICATION ALERT—Clopidogrel (Plavix)
- All health care providers and dentists must be informed that this medication is being taken, especially before scheduling surgery or major dental procedures.
- Medication may need to be discontinued 10 to 14 days before surgery if antiplatelet effect is not desired.

Surgical Therapy. Surgical interventions for the patient with TIAs from carotid disease are outlined in Table 60.5. Figure 60.6 demonstrates one intervention, carotid endarterectomy.

Transluminal angioplasty is the insertion of a balloon to open a stenosed artery and improve blood flow. The balloon is threaded up to the carotid artery via a catheter inserted in the femoral artery. Stenting involves intravascular placement of a stent in an attempt to maintain patency of the artery (Figure 60.7). The stent can be inserted during an angioplasty. Once in place, the system can be used with a tiny filter that opens like an umbrella. The filter catches and removes the debris that is stirred up during the stenting procedure so that it does not float to the brain, where it can trigger a stroke. Patients' comorbidities should be carefully considered as carotid stenting is associated with cerebral infarction or hemorrhage, hyperperfusion syndrome, stent insertion site complications, and systemic complications (Park & Lee, 2018).

Extracranial-to-intracranial artery bypass involves anastomosing (surgically connecting) a branch of an extracranial

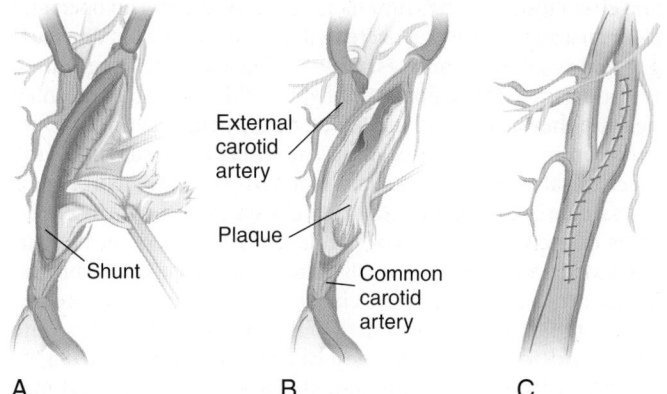

FIG. 60.6 Carotid endarterectomy is performed to prevent impending cerebral infarct. **A,** A tube is inserted above and below the blockage to reroute the blood flow. **B,** Atherosclerotic plaque in the common carotid artery is removed. **C,** Once the artery is stitched closed, the tube can be removed. A surgeon may also perform the technique without rerouting the blood flow.

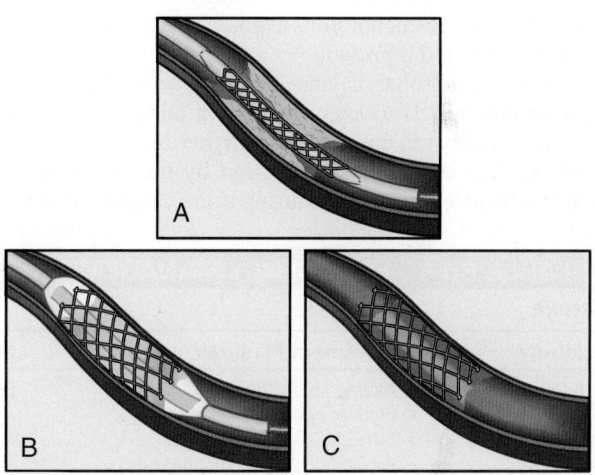

FIG. 60.7 Brain stent used to treat blockages in cerebral blood flow. **A,** A balloon catheter is used to implant the stent into an artery of the brain. **B,** The balloon catheter is moved to the blocked area of the artery and then inflated. The stent expands due to inflation of the balloon. **C,** The balloon is deflated and withdrawn, leaving the stent permanently in place holding the artery open and improving the flow of blood.

artery to an intracranial artery (most commonly, superficial temporal to middle cerebral artery) beyond an area of obstruction with the goal of increasing cerebral perfusion. This procedure is generally reserved for those patients who do not benefit from other forms of therapy.

Interprofessional Acute Care for Ischemic Stroke. The goals for interprofessional care during the acute phase are preserving life, preventing further brain damage, and reducing disability. During initial evaluation, the single most important point in the patient's history is the time of onset. Fifty-four percent of patients who seek acute care for stroke present at the emergency department, and the rest seek out their primary health care provider. The current standard for acute care treatment of stroke is that all patients with possible stroke will be assessed, have their acute health needs addressed, undergo diagnostic studies, and receive thrombolytic therapy within 4.5 hours from the onset of their symptoms. Best practice includes admission to a stroke unit or hospital ward within 4 hours of arrival (HSFC, 2018a).

Table 60.6 outlines the emergency management of patients with a stroke. Acute care begins with managing airway, breathing, and circulation. Patients may have difficulty keeping an open and clear airway because of a decreased LOC or decreased or absent gag and swallowing reflexes. Maintaining adequate oxygenation is important. Both hypoxia and hypercarbia are to be prevented because they can contribute to secondary neuronal injury. Oxygen administration, artificial airway insertion, intubation, and mechanical ventilation may be required. Baseline neurological assessment is carried out, and patients are monitored closely for signs of increasing neurological deficit. About 25% of patients will worsen in the first 24 to 48 hours. A designated interprofessional stroke team (e.g., physician, neurologist, nurse, neurosurgeons, radiologists, rehabilitation therapists, pharmacists, and social workers) provides the best care possible (HSFC, 2018a).

Elevated BP is common immediately after a stroke and may be a protective response to maintain cerebral perfusion. Immediately following ischemic stroke, use of medications to lower BP is recommended only if BP is markedly increased (mean arterial pressure >130 mm Hg or systolic BP >220 mm Hg). Intravenous (IV) antihypertensive medications such as labetalol are used in the acute phase. Although low BP immediately following stroke is uncommon, hypotension and hypovolemia should be corrected if present.

Fluid and electrolyte balance must be controlled carefully. The goal generally is to keep the patient adequately hydrated to promote perfusion and decrease further brain injury. Overhydration may compromise perfusion by increasing cerebral edema. Adequate fluid intake during acute care via oral, IV, or tube feedings should be 1500 to 2000 mL/day. Urine output should be closely monitored. If secretion of antidiuretic hormone increases in response to the stroke, urine output decreases and fluid is retained. Low serum sodium (hyponatremia) may occur. IV solutions with glucose and water should be avoided because they are hypotonic and may further increase cerebral edema and ICP. In addition, hyperglycemia may be associated with further brain damage and should be treated. In general, decisions regarding individualized fluid and electrolyte replacement therapy are based on the extent of intracranial edema, symptoms of increased ICP, central venous pressure levels, laboratory values for electrolytes, and intake and output.

Increased ICP is more likely to occur with hemorrhagic strokes but can occur with ischemic strokes. Increased ICP from cerebral edema usually peaks in 72 hours and may cause brain herniation. Management of increased ICP includes practices that improve venous drainage, such as elevating the head of the bed, maintaining the head and neck in alignment, and avoiding hip flexion. Hyperthermia, which is seen commonly following stroke, is associated with poorer outcome; patient temperature should be assessed every 4 hours for at least the initial 48 hours (HSFC, 2018a). Increased temperature contributes to increased cerebral metabolism. Medication therapies to treat hyperthermia include acetaminophen (Tylenol) or indomethacin. A temperature elevation of even 1°C can increase brain metabolism by 10% and contribute to further brain damage. Cooling blankets or IV cooling methods may be used to

---

✚ TABLE 60.6   EMERGENCY MANAGEMENT

Stroke

Etiology	Assessment Findings	Interventions
• Aneurysm • Arteriovenous malformation • Embolism • Hemorrhage • Sudden vascular compromise causing disruption of blood flow to the brain • Thrombosis • Trauma	• Altered level of consciousness • Bladder or bowel incontinence • Difficulty swallowing • Facial drooping on affected side • Hypertension • Increased or decreased heart rate • Nausea and vomiting • Respiratory distress • Seizures • Severe headache • Speech or visual disturbances • Unequal pupils • Vertigo • Weakness, numbness, or paralysis of portion of body	**Initial Care** • Evaluate airway, breathing, and circulation. • Conduct neurological examination. • Assess heart rhythm and vital signs. • Assess for presence of seizure activity. • Conduct blood work for electrolytes, random glucose, complete blood count (CBC), coagulation status (INR, aPTT), and creatinine. • Obtain CT or MRI (HSFC, 2018b). • Ensure patent airway. • Call a stroke code or the stroke team. • Remove dentures. • Perform pulse oximetry. • Maintain adequate oxygenation (SaO$_2$ >95%) with supplemental O$_2$, if necessary. • Establish IV access with normal saline. • Maintain BP according to guidelines (e.g., advanced cardiac life support). • Remove clothing. • Insert Foley catheter. • Obtain CT scan immediately. • Perform baseline laboratory tests (including blood glucose) immediately, and treat if hypoglycemic. • Position head midline. • Elevate head of bed 30 degrees if there are no symptoms of shock or suspicion of spinal cord injury. • Institute seizure precautions. • Anticipate thrombolytic therapy for ischemic stroke. • Keep patient NPO until swallow reflex is evaluated. **Ongoing Monitoring** • Monitor vital signs and neurological status, including level of consciousness (e.g., Glasgow Coma Scale or Canadian Neurological Scale or NIH Stroke Scale), motor and sensory function, pupil size and reactivity, SaO$_2$, and cardiac rhythm. • Educate and update patient and family or caregiver.

aPTT, activated partial thromboplastin time; *BP*, blood pressure; *CT*, computed tomography; *INR*, international normalized ratio; *IV*, intravenous; *MRI*, magnetic resonance imaging; *NIH*, National Institutes of Health; *NPO*, nothing by mouth; *O$_2$*, oxygen; *SaO$_2$*, arterial oxygen saturation.

lower temperature. The nurse must closely monitor the patient's temperature. Aggressive management of temperature during the first 24 hours after a stroke is most effective in preventing detrimental outcomes.

Seizures occur in 5 to 7% of stroke patients in the first 24 hours. New-onset seizures in patients with acute stroke should be treated using short-acting medications (e.g., lorazepam IV) if they are not self-limiting. Furthermore, a single, self-limiting seizure occurring at the onset, or within 24 hours after an ischemic stroke (considered an "immediate" post-stroke seizure) should not be treated with long-term anticonvulsant medications (HSFC, 2018a).

Other measures include pain management, avoidance of hypervolemia, and management of constipation. CSF drainage may be used in some patients to reduce ICP or manage hydrocephalus. Patients with elevated ICP may be treated with hyperosmolar therapy and elevation of the head of their bed (HSFC, 2018a). Additional strategies for managing ICP are found in Chapter 59.

Medication Therapy for Ischemic Stroke. Recombinant tissue plasminogen activator (tPA) is administered intravenously to re-establish blood flow through a blocked artery to prevent cell death in patients with the acute onset of ischemic stroke symptoms. Patients are screened carefully before tPA can be given. Screening includes a noncontrast CT or MRI to rule out hemorrhagic stroke; blood tests for coagulation disorders; and screening for recent history (past 3 months) of gastrointestinal bleeding, stroke, or head trauma or major surgery within the previous 14 days. Intra-arterial infusion of tPA remains an option for a subgroup of patients with large vessel occlusions primarily in the middle cerebral artery. Thrombolytic medications, such as tPA, produce localized fibrinolysis by binding to the fibrin in the thrombi. The fibrinolytic action of tPA occurs as the plasminogen is converted to plasmin, whose enzymatic action digests fibrin and fibrinogen and thus lyses the clot. Because it is clot specific in its activation of the fibrinolytic system, tPA is the only treatment indicated for acute ischemic stroke. tPA must be administered within 4.5 hours of the onset of clinical signs of ischemic stroke. The door-to-needle time for tPA remains less than 60 minutes whether the patient arrives at the hospital at 3 hours or 1 hour after the onset of clinical signs. The probability of disability-free survival decreases over time within the treatment window, and all phases of patient care should aim for the shortest process and treatment times possible (HSFC, 2018a). (Thrombolytic therapy is further discussed in Chapter 36.)

During infusion of the medication, the patient's vital signs and neurological status are monitored closely to assess for improvement or for potential deterioration related to intracerebral hemorrhage. Control of BP is critical during treatment and for 24 hours afterward. No anticoagulant or antiplatelet medications are given for 24 hours after tPA treatment because of the risk for intracranial hemorrhage.

Surgical Therapy for Ischemic Stroke. Endovascular treatment (Figure 60.8) during cerebral ischemia enables physicians to go inside the blocked artery of patients who are experiencing ischemic strokes. The retriever goes to the artery that is blocked, directly to the site of the injury, and pulls the clot out. The retriever is a tiny corkscrew device that uses a microcatheter inserted through a femoral artery balloon catheter. Once the corkscrew device reaches the clot in the brain, the device penetrates the clot, allowing it to be removed. Under radiographic guidance, the balloon catheter is manoeuvred up

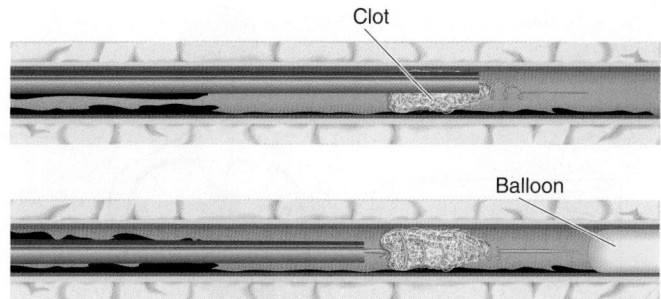

FIG. 60.8 Endovascular treatment removes blood clots in patients who are experiencing ischemic strokes. The retriever is a long, thin wire that is threaded through a catheter into the femoral artery. The wire is pushed through the end of the catheter up to the carotid artery. The wire reshapes itself into tiny loops that latch onto the clot, and the clot can then be pulled out. To prevent the clot from breaking off, a balloon at the end of the catheter inflates to stop blood flow through the artery.

to the carotid artery in the neck; a guide wire and the microcatheter are deployed through the balloon catheter and then placed just beyond the clot. The physician then deploys the retriever device to engage and ensnare the clot. Once the clot is captured, the balloon catheter is inflated to temporarily arrest forward flow while the clot is being withdrawn. The clot is pulled into the balloon catheter and completely out of the body. The balloon is then deflated, and blood flow is restored. More research is required to support endovascular treatment at reducing mortality and increasing functional outcomes (HSFC, 2018a).

Interprofessional Acute Care for Hemorrhagic Stroke

Medication Therapy. Anticoagulants and platelet inhibitors are contraindicated in patients with acute hemorrhagic strokes. The main medication therapy for patients with hemorrhagic stroke is the management of hypertension. Oral and IV agents may be used to maintain BP within a normal to high-normal range (systolic BP <160 mm Hg). Once BP is stabilized, pharmacological venous thromboembolism prophylaxis should be initiated unless contraindicated (Boulanger et al., 2018). There is no evidence to support the practice of routine reversal of anticoagulation (Boulanger et al., 2018). Seizure prophylaxis in the acute period after intracerebral hemorrhages and SAHs may be used. Prophylactic use of anticonvulsant medications in patients with acute stroke is not recommended (HSFC, 2018a).

Surgical Therapy. Surgical interventions for hemorrhagic stroke include immediate evacuation of aneurysm-induced hematomas or cerebellar hematomas larger than 3 cm. Individuals who have an AVM may experience a hemorrhagic stroke if the AVM ruptures. The treatment of AVM is surgical resection, radiosurgery (e.g., Gamma Knife), or both. Either may be preceded by interventional neuroradiology to embolize the blood vessels that supply the AVM.

SAH is usually caused by a ruptured aneurysm. Approximately 20% of patients will have multiple aneurysms. Treatment of an aneurysm involves coiling or clipping the aneurysm to prevent rebleeding (Figures 60.9 and 60.10). In the endovascular procedure known as *coiling*, a metal coil is inserted into the lumen of the aneurysm via interventional neuroradiology (see Figure 60.9). Guglielmi detachable coils provide immediate protection against hemorrhage by reducing the blood pulsations within the aneurysm. Eventually, a thrombus forms within the aneurysm and the aneurysm becomes sealed off from the parent vessel by the formation of an endothelialized layer of

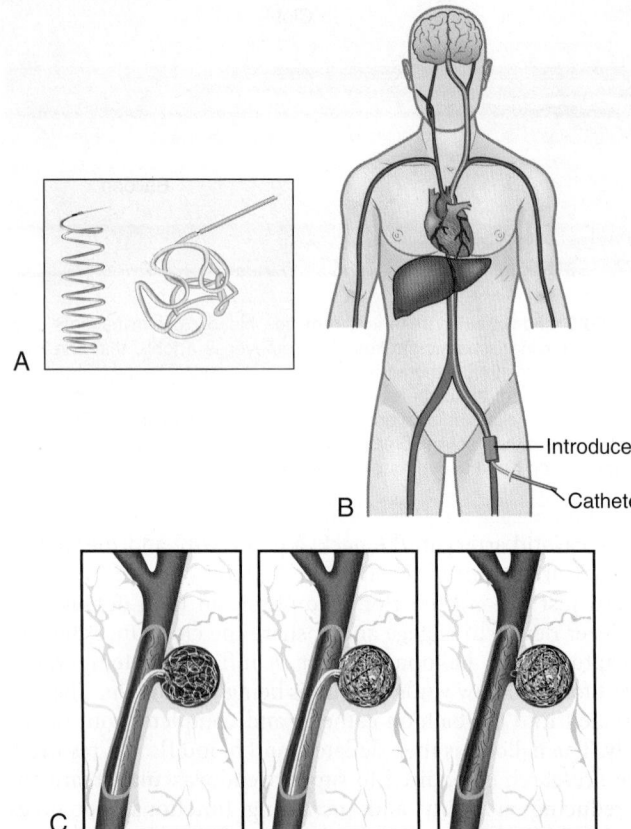

FIG. 60.9 Guglielmi detachable coil. **A,** A coil is used to occlude an aneurysm. Coils are made of soft, springlike platinum. The softness of the platinum allows the coil to assume the shape of irregularly shaped aneurysms while posing little threat of rupture of the aneurysm. **B,** A catheter is inserted through an introducer (small tube) in an artery in the leg. The catheter is threaded up to the cerebral blood vessels. **C,** Platinum coils attached to a thin wire are inserted into the catheter and then placed in the aneurysm until the aneurysm is filled with coils. Packing the aneurysm with coils prevents the blood from circulating through the aneurysm, reducing the risk for rupture.

connective tissue. Guglielmi detachable coils provide a less invasive therapy than the traditional surgical clipping of aneurysms (see Figure 60.10).

A calcium channel blocker (CCB) (e.g., amlodipine [Norvasc], nifedipine XL [Adalat XL]) is given every 2 or 4 hours from the time of aneurysmal rupture (SAH) for 21 days to decrease the effects of vasospasm and minimize cerebral damage. CCBs restrict the influx of calcium ions into cells by reducing the number of open calcium channels.

Slight neurological decline or pronator drift is an indicator of vasospasm. Assessment for these complications is important. Once vasospasm is confirmed by CTA, the goals of therapy are to use IV milrinone to promote cerebral vasodilation and to maintain homeostasis by replacing fluid losses, targeting normal parameters for glucose, electrolytes, and temperature while carefully assessing for its main adverse effect, hypotension (Liu et al., 2016).

SAH and intracerebral hemorrhage can involve bleeding into the ventricles of the brain. This situation produces hydrocephalus (enlarged ventricles), which further damages brain tissue from increased ICP. Insertion of an external ventricular drain (EVD) for CSF drainage in patients with hydrocephalus can drain excess CSF that is not draining because of lack of absorption or obstruction. CSF drainage can reduce

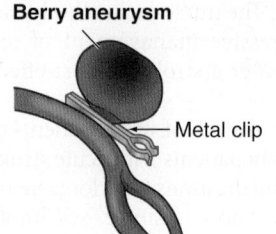

FIG. 60.10 Clipping of aneurysms.

ICP, and the patient may have an improved neurological examination.

Rehabilitation Care. After the acute stroke patient has stabilized for 12 to 72 hours, interprofessional care shifts from preserving life to lessening disability and attaining optimal function. The patient may be evaluated by a physiatrist (a physician who specializes in physical medicine and rehabilitation). It is important to remember that some aspects of rehabilitation actually begin in the acute care phase as soon as the patient is stabilized. Depending on the patient's status, other medical conditions, rehabilitation potential, and available resources, the patient may be transferred to a rehabilitation unit, discharged home for outpatient therapy, or referred to home care–based rehabilitation.

As part of the long-term interprofessional care after a stroke, various members of the health care team may be involved in the effort to promote optimal function of the patient and family. The composition of the interprofessional team depends on patient and family or caregiver needs and rehabilitation facility resources. The Evidence-Informed Practice box discusses how health care providers can assist patients and family members. It highlights the importance of utilizing evidence-informed information to maximize patient safety.

NURSING MANAGEMENT
STROKE

NURSING ASSESSMENT

Subjective and objective data that should be obtained from a person who has had a stroke are presented in Table 60.7. Primary assessment focuses on cardiac status and respiratory and neurological assessment. If the patient's condition is stable, the nursing history is obtained as follows: (a) description of the current illness with attention to initial symptoms, including onset and duration, nature (intermittent or continuous), and changes; (b) history of similar symptoms previously experienced; (c) current medications; (d) history of risk factors and other illnesses such as hypertension; and (e) family history of stroke or cardiovascular diseases. This information is gained through an interview of the patient, family members, significant others, or caregiver.

Secondary assessment should include a comprehensive neurological examination of the patient. This includes (a) LOC, using the Canadian Neurological Scale (Figure 60.11) (or a similar tool, e.g., the National Institutes of Health Stroke Scale [NIHSS]), (b) cognition, (c) motor abilities, (d) cranial nerve function, (e) sensation, (f) proprioception, (g) cerebellar function, and (h) deep tendon reflexes. Clear documentation of initial and ongoing neurological examinations is essential to note changes in patient status. The HSFC has developed best-practice guidelines and recommendations for stroke care across the continuum.

EVIDENCE-INFORMED PRACTICE

Research Highlight

How Does New Evidence Change Best Practices for the Use of Acetylsalicylic Acid (ASA) in Prevention of Vascular Events?

Background

The use of ASA for primary and secondary prevention of vascular events has been recommended practice for many years, in Canada and internationally. Based on an appraisal of available evidence of large clinical trials, the Heart and Stroke Foundation of Canada released new best practices guidelines in March 2020 related to ASA use for the prevention of vascular events. ASA increases the chance of dangerous bleeding in people who take it on a daily basis. The guidelines are about balancing risk. The new guideline confirms some past treatment directives but contradicts the use of ASA in healthy individuals; therefore, widespread education is important to maximize patient safety with ASA use.

Best Canadian Practice Guidelines

Three recommendations were developed regarding the use of ASA for the prevention of vascular events:

1. *Primary prevention:* The use of ASA is not recommended for primary prevention of a first vascular event; this pertains to individuals with and without vascular risk factors who have not had a first vascular event.
2. *Secondary prevention:* ASA is strongly recommended for secondary prevention in individuals with symptomatic cardiovascular, cerebrovascular, or peripheral arterial disease.
3. *Shared decision-making:* The interprofessional health care team should engage patients and families in discussions regarding use of ASA for primary prevention of vascular disease to ensure that the risk, benefit, value, and preference are considered in order to make an informed decision to start, continue, or stop ASA for primary prevention of vascular disease.

Conclusion

- All individuals should be advised that daily ASA is not recommended for primary prevention of vascular events because the bleeding risks potentially outweigh the benefits.
- It is important to be aware of new best practice guidelines and advocate for policy change.

Implications for Nursing Practice

- Nurses need to educate patients, families, and other health care providers of the change in use of ASA as a primary preventative measure.
- Nurses can advocate for treatment options that maximize patient safety in reducing cardiovascular risk factors. Working with individuals, groups, and communities, nurses can promote lifestyle and behavioural changes that are effective in preventing cardiovascular events.

References for Evidence

Heart and Stroke Foundation of Canada. (2020). *ASA for prevention: What you need to know.* https://www.heartandstroke.ca/articles/asa-for-prevention-what-you-need-to-know

Wein, T., Lindsay, P., Gladstone, D., et al. (2020). Canadian stroke best practice recommendations, seventh edition: Acetylsalicylic acid for prevention of vascular events. *Canadian Medical Association Journal, 192,* E302–E311. https://doi.org/10.1503/cmaj.191599

NURSING DIAGNOSES

Nursing diagnoses for a person with a stroke may include but are not limited to the following:

- *Reduced intracranial adaptive capacity* resulting from *decreased cerebral perfusion pressure of ≤50 to 60 mm Hg, baseline ICP ≥15 mm Hg, elevated systolic BP, bradycardia, widened pulse pressure, and decreasing Canadian Neurological Scale score*
- *Potential for aspiration* resulting from *barrier to elevating upper body, decrease in level of consciousness, depressed gag reflex*

TABLE 60.7 NURSING ASSESSMENT

Stroke

Subjective Data

Important Health Information

Past health history: Hypertension; previous stroke, TIA, aneurysm, trauma, cardiac disease (including recent MI), dysrhythmias, heart failure, valvular disease, infective endocarditis, polycythemia, dyslipidemia, smoking, kidney disease, diabetes, gout, family history of hypertension, diabetes, deep vein thrombosis, stroke, or coronary artery disease

Medications: Use of hormone therapy or oral contraceptives; use of and adherence to antihypertensive and diabetes regimen, antiplatelet therapy, and anticoagulant medications; use of illegal substances (e.g., cocaine)

Symptoms

- Anorexia, nausea, vomiting; dysphagia, altered sensation of taste and smell
- Change in bowel and bladder patterns
- Loss of movement and sensation; syncope; weakness on one side; mouth droop, half smile; generalized weakness, easy fatigability
- Numbness, tingling of one side of the body; loss of memory; alteration in speech, language, problem-solving ability
- Pain; headache, possibly sudden and severe (hemorrhage); visual disturbances; denial of illness

Objective Data

General

Emotional lability, lethargy, apathy or combativeness, fever

Respiratory

Loss of cough reflex, laboured or irregular respirations, tachypnea, wheezing (aspiration), airway occlusion (tongue), apnea, coughing when eating or delayed coughing

Cardiovascular

Hypertension, tachycardia, carotid bruit

Gastrointestinal

Loss of gag reflex, bowel incontinence, decreased or absent bowel sounds, constipation
Urinary
Frequency, urgency, incontinence

Neurological

Contralateral motor and sensory deficits, including weakness, paresis, paralysis, anaesthesia; unequal pupils, hand grasps; akinesia, aphasia (expressive, receptive, global), dysarthria (slurred speech), agnosias, apraxia, visual deficits, perceptual or spatial disturbances, altered level of consciousness (drowsiness to deep coma) and Babinski reflex, ↓ followed by ↑deep tendon reflexes, flaccidity followed by spasticity, amnesia, ataxia, personality change, nuchal rigidity, seizures

Possible Findings

Positive CT, CTA, MRI, MRA, or other neuroimaging scans showing size, location, and type of lesion; positive Doppler ultrasonography and angiography indicating stenosis

CT, computed tomography; *CTA,* computed tomographic angiography; *MI,* myocardial infarction; *MRA,* magnetic resonance angiography; *MRI,* magnetic resonance imaging; *TIA,* transient ischemic attack.

- *Reduced physical mobility* resulting from *decrease in muscle control, decrease in muscle strength, physical deconditioning*
- *Unilateral neglect* resulting from *visual field cut and sensory loss on one side of body and brain injury from cerebrovascular conditions*
- *Inadequate urinary elimination* resulting from *multiple causality* (impaired impulse to void, inability to reach toilet, manage tasks of voiding)

CANADIAN NEUROLOGICAL SCALE

Assess: Vital Signs and Pupils   **Vital Signs:** BP, Temp, Pulse, Respirations, Oximetry   **Pupils:** Size and reaction to light

Section A: MENTATION: LOC, Orientation, Speech

LEVEL OF CONSCIOUSNESS
CNS (Alert, Drowsy) GCS (Stuporous, Comatose)

ORIENTATION:
Place (city or hospital), Time (month and year)
*Patient can speak, write, or gesture their responses.
SCORE: Patient is Oriented, score 1.0, if they correctly state both place and correct month and year. If dysarthric, speech must be intelligible. If patient cannot state both, Disoriented, score 0.0.

SPEECH:
RECEPTIVE: Ask patient the following separately (do not prompt by gesturing):

1. Close your eyes
2. "Does a stone sink in water?"
3. Point to the ceiling

SCORE: If patient is unable to do all three, Receptive Deficit, score 0.0, go to A2.

EXPRESSIVE:

1. Show patient 3 items separately (pencil, watch, key) and ask patient to name each object.
2. Ask patient what each object is used for while holding each up again, i.e., "What do you do with a pencil?"

SCORE: If patient is able to state the name and use of all 3 objects, Normal Speech, score 1.0.

If patient is unable to state the name and use of all 3 objects, Expressive Deficit, score 0.5.

*If patient answers all questions correctly but speech is slurred and intelligible, score Normal Speech and record "SL" along with the score.

Section A1: MOTOR FUNCTION

NO RECEPTIVE DEFICIT

FACE: Ask patient to smile/grin, note weakness in mouth or nasal/labial folds.

SCORE: None/no weakness = 0.5 or Present/weakness = 0.0. Test both limbs and always record the side with the WORST deficit and indicate side by entering a R/L.

None 1.5	no weakness present
Mild 1.0	mild weakness present, full ROM, cannot withstand resistance
Significant 0.5	moderate weakness, some movement, not full ROM
Total 0.0	complete loss of movement, total weakness

SCORE:
Arm: Proximal Ask patient to lift arm 45-90 degrees. Apply resistance between shoulder and elbow.
Arm: Distal Ask patient to make fist and flex wrist backwards, apply resistance between wrist and knuckles.
Leg: Proximal In supine position, ask patient to flex hip to 90 degrees, apply pressure to mid thigh.
Leg: Distal Ask patient to dorsiflex foot, apply resistance to top of foot.

Section A2: MOTOR RESPONSE

RECEPTIVE DEFICIT PRESENT
FACE: Have patient mimic your smile. If unable, note facial expression while applying sternal pressure.
ARMS: Demonstrate or lift patient's arms to 90 degrees, score ability to maintain equal levels (>5 secs).
If unable to maintain raised arms, apply nail bed pressure to assess reflex response.
LEGS: Lift patient's hip to 90 degrees, score ability to maintain equal levels (>5 secs), If unable to maintain raised position, apply nail bed pressure to assess reflex response.

FIG. 60.11 Canadian Neurological Scale. *CNS,* central nervous system; *GCS,* Glasgow Coma Scale; *LOC,* level of consciousness; *R/L,* right/left; *ROM,* range of motion. Source: Heart and Stroke Foundation of Canada. (2015). *Stroke nurse pocket guide.* Author. Used by permission of Dr. Robert Côté, MD.

- *Inadequate swallowing* resulting from *behavioural feeding problem* (weakness, paralysis of affected muscles)
- *Reduced self-esteem* resulting from *alteration in body image, decreased control over environment*

Additional information on nursing diagnoses for the patient with stroke is presented in Nursing Care Plan (NCP) 60.1.

PLANNING

The patient, the family, and the nurse establish the goals of nursing care in a cooperative manner. Typical goals are that the patient will (a) maintain a stable or improved LOC, (b) attain maximum physical functioning, (c) attain maximum self-care abilities and skills, (d) maintain stable body functions (e.g., bladder control), (e) maximize communication abilities, (f) maintain adequate nutrition, (g) avoid complications of stroke, and (h) maintain effective personal and family coping.

NURSING IMPLEMENTATION

HEALTH PROMOTION. In any health care setting and for the population as a whole, nurses can play a major role in the promotion of a healthy lifestyle. To reduce the incidence of stroke, the nurse should focus teaching efforts on stroke prevention, particularly for persons with known risk factors (see Table 60.1). Measures to reduce risk factors for stroke are similar to those for coronary artery disease (see Table 36.2 and surrounding discussion of health promotion in Chapter 36).

One of the nurse's major roles is education about hypertension control and maintaining adherence to antihypertensive medications. Uncontrolled hypertension is the primary cause of stroke. The nurse needs to be an advocate for the monitoring and management of hypertension, including assessing financial need and prescription coverage. For patients with diabetes, it is very important that the blood glucose level be well controlled. For patients with AF, an anticoagulant such as

⊙ NURSING CARE PLAN 60.1

Stroke

| NURSING DIAGNOSIS | *Reduced intracranial adaptive capacity* (resulting from decreased cerebral perfusion pressure of ≤50–60 mm Hg, baseline ICP ≥15 mm Hg, elevated systolic BP, bradycardia, widened pulse pressure, and decreasing Canadian Neurological Scale score) |

Expected Patient Outcome	Nursing Interventions and *Rationales*
• Demonstrates signs of stable or improved cerebral perfusion	*Cerebral Perfusion Promotion*

- Consult with health care provider *to determine hemodynamic parameters and maintain hemodynamic parameters within this range.*
- Monitor neurological status *to detect changes indicative of worsening or improving condition.*
- Calculate and monitor CPP *to detect change in condition.*
- Monitor respiratory status (e.g., rate, rhythm, and depth of respirations; PaO_2, $PaCO_2$, pH, and bicarbonate levels) *because high $PaCO_2$ and a high hydrogen ion concentration (acidosis) are potent vasodilators that increase cerebral blood flow.*
- Monitor patient's ICP and neurological responses to care activities *because changes in positioning and movement can increase ICP.*
- Monitor determinants of tissue oxygen delivery (e.g., $PaCO_2$, SaO_2, hemoglobin levels, and cardiac output) *to ensure adequate cerebral oxygenation.*
- Administer and titrate vasoactive medications, as ordered, *to maintain hemodynamic parameters.*
- Avoid neck flexion or extreme hip or knee flexion *to avoid obstruction of arterial and venous blood flow.*

| NURSING DIAGNOSIS | *Potential for aspiration* as evidenced by *decreased level of consciousness, depressed gag reflex, impaired ability to swallow* |

Expected Patient Outcomes	Nursing Interventions and *Rationales*
• Demonstrates ability to swallow oral foods without aspiration • Maintains a clear airway	*Aspiration Precautions*

- A speech–language pathologist or other trained health care provider should screen for swallowing impairment using a valid screening tool before any oral intake (liquids, food, medication) is administered (HSFC, 2019a).
- Monitor level of consciousness, cough reflex, gag reflex, and swallowing ability *to determine patient's ability to swallow food without aspiration.*
- Avoid liquids or use thickening agent *to facilitate swallowing.*
- Feed in small amounts *to reduce risk for aspiration.*
- Offer foods or liquids that can be formed into a bolus before swallowing.

Airway Management

- Auscultate breath sounds, noting areas of decreased or absent ventilation and presence of adventitious sounds *to identify airway obstruction and accumulation of secretions.*
- Remove secretions by encouraging coughing or by suctioning *to clear airway.*
- Encourage slow, deep breathing; turning; and coughing *to increase airway clearance without increasing ICP.*
- Assist with incentive spirometer *to open collapsed alveoli, promote deep breathing, and prevent atelectasis.*

| NURSING DIAGNOSIS | *Reduced physical mobility* resulting from *decrease in muscle control, decrease in muscle strength, physical deconditioning* as demonstrated by *neuromuscular impairment, sensory-perceptual impairment* |

Expected Patient Outcomes	Nursing Interventions and *Rationales*
• Demonstrates increased muscle strength and ability to move • Uses adaptive equipment to increase mobility	*Exercise Therapy: Muscle Control*

- Collaborate with the interprofessional team (e.g., physiotherapist, occupational and recreational therapists) in developing and executing exercise program *to determine extent of disability and plan appropriate interventions.*
- Determine patient's readiness to engage in activity or exercise protocol *to assess expected level of participation.*
- Apply splints to achieve stability of proximal joints involved with fine motor skill activities *to prevent contractures.*
- Encourage patient to practise exercises independently *to promote patient's sense of control.*
- Reinforce instructions provided to patient about the proper way to perform exercises *to minimize injury and maximize effectiveness.*
- Provide restful environment for patient after periods of exercise *to facilitate recuperation.*

| NURSING DIAGNOSIS | *Reduced verbal communication* resulting from *central nervous system impairment* as evidenced by *difficulty speaking* |

Expected Patient Outcomes	Nursing Interventions and *Rationales*
• Uses effective oral and written communication techniques • Demonstrates congruency of verbal and nonverbal communication	*Communication Enhancement: Speech Deficit*

- Provide alternative methods of speech communication (e.g., writing tablet, flash cards, eye blinking, communication board with pictures and letters, hand signals or other gestures, and computer) *to aid and promote patient communication.*
- Provide positive reinforcement *to build self-esteem and confidence.*
- Adjust communication style (e.g., stand in front of patient when speaking, listen attentively, present one idea or thought at a time, speak slowly while avoiding shouting, use written communication, or solicit caregiver's or family's assistance in understanding patient's speech) *to meet patient's needs.*
- Maintain structured environment and routines (e.g., ensure consistent daily schedules, provide frequent reminders, and provide calendars and other environmental cues) *to promote patient's independence and self-care.*
- Collaborate with caregiver, family, or both and interprofessional team *to develop a plan for effective communication.*

Continued

◎ NURSING CARE PLAN 60.1

Stroke—cont'd

NURSING DIAGNOSIS	***Unilateral neglect*** resulting from *visual field cut and sensory loss on one side of body and brain injury from cerebrovascular conditions* as evidenced by *consistent inattention to stimuli on affected side*

Expected Patient Outcomes	**Nursing Interventions and *Rationales***
• Cares for both sides of the body appropriately • Uses strategies to minimize unilateral neglect	*Unilateral Neglect Management* • Monitor for abnormal responses to three types of stimuli—sensory, visual, and auditory—*to determine the presence of and degree to which unilateral neglect exists* (e.g., inability to see objects on affected side, leaving food on a plate that corresponds to affected side, lack of sensation on affected side). • Instruct patient to scan from left to right *to visualize the entire environment.* • Position bed in room so that individuals approach and care for patient on unaffected side. • Rearrange the environment to use the right or left visual field; position personal items, television, or reading materials within view on unaffected side *to compensate for visual field deficits.* • Touch unaffected shoulder when initiating conversation *to attract patient's attention.* • Gradually move personal items and activity to affected side as patient demonstrates an ability to compensate for neglect. • Include caregiver(s), family member(s), or both in rehabilitation process to support the patient's efforts and assist with care *to promote reintegration with the whole body.*

NURSING DIAGNOSIS	***Reduced urinary elimination*** resulting from *multiple causality* (impaired impulse to void, inability to reach toilet or manage tasks of voiding) as demonstrated by *sensory motor impairment*

Expected Patient Outcomes	**Nursing Interventions and *Rationales***
• Perceives impulse to void, removes clothing for toileting, and uses toilet • Demonstrates ability to urinate when the urge arises or with a timed schedule	*Urinary Habit Training* • Keep a continence specification record for 3 days *to establish voiding pattern and plan appropriate interventions.* • Establish interval of initial toileting schedule (based on voiding pattern and usual routine) *to initiate process of improving bladder functioning and increased muscle tone.* • Assist patient to toilet and prompt to void at prescribed intervals *to assist patient in adapting to new toileting schedule.* • Discuss daily record of continence with staff *to provide reinforcement and encourage adherence to toileting schedule.* • Give positive feedback or positive reinforcement to patient when they void at scheduled toileting times, and make no comment when patient is incontinent, *to reinforce desired behaviour.*

NURSING DIAGNOSIS	***Inadequate swallowing*** resulting from *behavioural feeding problem* (weakness, paralysis of affected muscles) as demonstrated by *brain injury* (difficulty swallowing, choking)

Expected Patient Outcome	**Nursing Interventions and *Rationales***
• Demonstrates effective swallowing without choking, coughing, or aspiration	*Swallowing Therapy* • Collaborate with interprofessional health care team (e.g., occupational therapist, speech–language pathologist, dietitian) *to provide continuity in patient's rehabilitative plan.* • Assist patient to sit in an erect position (as close to 90 degrees as possible) for feeding and exercise *to provide optimal position for chewing and swallowing without aspirating.* • Assist patient to position head in forward flexion in preparation for swallowing ("chin tuck"). • Assist patient to maintain sitting position for 30 minutes after completing meal *to prevent regurgitation of food.* • Instruct patient or caregiver on emergency measures for choking *to prevent complications in the home setting.* • Check mouth for pocketing of food after eating *to prevent collection and putrefaction of food or aspiration.* • Provide mouth care as needed *to promote comfort and oral health.* • Monitor body weight to determine adequacy of nutritional intake.

NURSING DIAGNOSIS	***Reduced self-esteem*** resulting from *decreased control over environment, alteration in body image* as demonstrated by *helplessness, purposelessness, indecisive behaviour, self-negating verbalizations*

Expected Patient Outcomes	**Nursing Interventions and *Rationales***
• Expresses positive feelings of self-worth • Participates in self-care of affected body parts	*Self-Esteem Enhancement* • Monitor patient's statements of self-worth *to determine effect of stroke on self-esteem.* • Encourage patient to identify strengths *to facilitate patient's recognition of their intrinsic value.* • Assist in setting realistic goals *to achieve higher self-esteem.* • Reward or praise patient's progress toward reaching goals. • Encourage increased responsibility for self *to promote sense of satisfaction, independence, and control and to reduce frustrations.* • Monitor levels of self-esteem over time *to determine stressors or situations that trigger low self-esteem and to teach coping mechanisms.*

BP, blood pressure; *CPP,* cerebral perfusion pressure; *ICP,* intracranial pressure; *PaCO₂,* partial pressure of carbon dioxide in arterial blood; *PaO₂,* partial pressure of oxygen in arterial blood; *SaO₂,* saturation of oxygen in arterial blood.

apixaban (Eliquis), dabigatran etexilate (Pradaxa), or rivaroxaban (Xarelto) may be used to treat the condition to prevent the risk for stroke. Because smoking is a major risk factor for stroke, the nurse needs to be actively involved in helping patients to stop smoking (see Chapter 11).

Another very important aspect of health promotion is teaching patients and families about early symptoms associated with stroke or TIA. Table 60.8 presents information on when to seek health care for these symptoms.

ACUTE INTERVENTION FOR ALL STROKE PATIENTS. Acute intervention for the stroke patient includes care of the respiratory, neurological, cardiovascular, musculoskeletal, integumentary, gastrointestinal, and urinary systems, as well as attention to the patient's nutrition.

Respiratory System. During the acute phase following a stroke, management of the respiratory system is a nursing priority. Stroke patients are particularly vulnerable to respiratory problems as it has been shown that respiratory muscle strength decreases following stroke. Pneumonia is a common diagnosis post-stroke (HFSC, 2018a).

Risk for aspiration pneumonia may be high because of impaired consciousness or dysphagia. Dysphagia after stroke is common. Airway obstruction can occur because of difficulties with chewing and swallowing, food pocketing (food remaining in the buccal cavity of the mouth), and the tongue falling back. Some patients with stroke, especially those with brainstem or hemorrhagic stroke, may require endotracheal intubation and mechanical ventilation initially or with increasing cerebral edema or ICP. Enteral tube feedings also place the patient at risk for aspiration pneumonia. All patients should be screened for their ability to swallow and for dysphagia within 48 hours of admission (HSFC, 2018a).

Nursing interventions to support adequate respiratory function are individualized to meet the needs of the patient. An oropharyngeal airway may be used in comatose patients to prevent the tongue from falling back and obstructing the airway and to provide access for suctioning. Alternatively, a nasopharyngeal airway may be used to provide airway protection and access. When an artificial airway will be required for a prolonged time, a tracheostomy may be performed. Nursing interventions include frequent assessment of airway patency and function, oxygenation, suctioning, patient mobility, positioning of the patient to prevent aspiration, and encouraging deep breathing. Patients who have an unclipped or uncoiled aneurysm may experience rebleeding, and the possibility of further ICP increases with coughing exercises.

Interventions related to maintenance of airway function are described in NCP 60.1.

Neurological System. The patient's neurological status must be monitored closely to detect slight changes suggesting extension of the stroke, increased ICP, vasospasm, or recovery from stroke symptoms. There are many neurological assessment tools, such as the Glasgow Coma Scale (GCS), National Institutes of Health Stroke Scale, and the Canadian Neurological Scale, that can be used to assist in the monitoring of a patient's neurological status. The GCS is used to measure LOC, mental status, pupillary responses, and extremity movement and strength. (The GCS is shown in Chapter 59, Table 59.4.) The GCS might not be sensitive enough for use with stroke patients who have cognitive and communication deficits (rather than impaired LOC), which would not be detected using this scale. The Canadian Neurological Scale was designed specifically for evaluating and monitoring the neurological status of patients with acute stroke

| TABLE 60.8 | **PATIENT & CAREGIVER TEACHING GUIDE** |

Warning Signs of Stroke

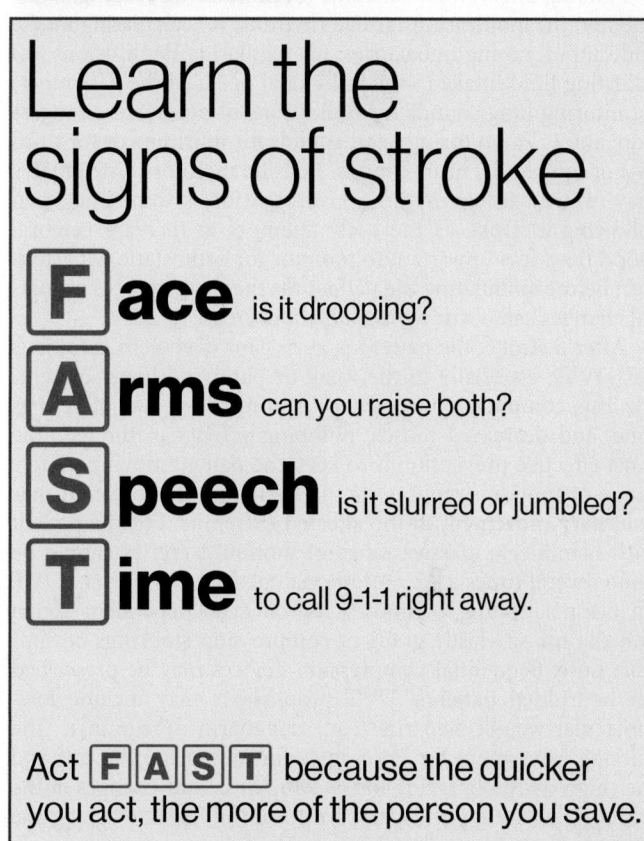

Source: © 2017, Heart and Stroke Foundation of Canada. Reproduced with the permission of the Heart and Stroke Foundation of Canada. https://www.heartandstroke.ca.

(see Figure 60.11). It is an assessment tool that measures LOC, orientation, speech, and motor responses of the face, arms, and legs and takes into account if the patient has a receptive deficit.

Additional neurological assessment includes mental status, pupillary responses, checking for pronator drift, and extremity movement and strength. Also, vital signs need to be monitored closely. A decreasing LOC may indicate increasing ICP. ICP and cerebral perfusion pressure may be monitored as well if the patient is in a critical care environment. Data from the nursing assessment are recorded on flow sheets to compare the trends over time and to communicate the evaluation of neurological status to the interprofessional team.

Cardiovascular System. Nursing goals for the cardiovascular system are aimed at maintaining homeostasis. Many patients with stroke have decreased cardiac reserves from the secondary diagnoses of cardiac diseases. Cardiac efficiency may be further compromised by fluid retention, overhydration, dehydration, BP variations, or a combination of these. Fluids are retained if there is increased production of antidiuretic hormone and aldosterone secondary to stress. Fluid retention plus overhydration can result in fluid overload. It can also increase cerebral edema and ICP. At the same time, dehydration can add to the morbidity and mortality associated with stroke, especially in patients with vasospasm. IV therapy should be carefully regulated. The nurse should closely monitor intake and output. Central venous pressure, pulmonary artery pressure, or hemodynamic monitoring may be used as indicators of fluid balance or cardiac function in the critical care unit.

Nursing interventions include (a) monitoring vital signs frequently; (b) monitoring cardiac rhythms; (c) calculating intake and output, noting imbalances; (d) regulating IV infusions; (e) adjusting fluid intake to the individual needs of the patient; (f) monitoring lung sounds for indications of pulmonary congestion; and (g) monitoring heart sounds for murmurs or for third (S_3) or fourth (S_4) heart sounds. Bedside monitors or telemetry may record cardiac rhythms. Hypertension is sometimes seen following a stroke as the body attempts to increase cerebral blood flow. It is important to monitor for orthostatic hypertension before ambulating the patient for the first time. Neurological changes can occur with a sudden decrease in BP.

After a stroke, the patient is at risk for deep vein thrombosis (DVT), especially in the weak or paralyzed lower extremity. This complication is related to immobility, loss of venous tone, and decreased muscle pumping activity in the leg. The most effective prevention is to keep the patient moving. Active range-of-motion exercises should be taught if the patient has voluntary movement in the affected extremity. For the patient with hemiplegia, passive range-of-motion exercises should be done several times a day. Additional measures to prevent DVT include positioning to minimize the effects of dependent edema and the use of elastic gradient compression stockings or support hose. Sequential compression devices may be prescribed for bedridden patients. DVT prophylaxis may include low-molecular-weight heparin (e.g., dalteparin [Fragmin]). The nursing assessment for DVT includes measuring the calf and the thigh daily, observing for swelling or colour changes of the extremities, noting unusual warmth of the leg, and asking the patient about pain in the limbs.

Musculoskeletal System. The nursing goal for the musculoskeletal system is to maintain optimal function. This is accomplished by preventing joint contractures and muscular atrophy. In the acute phase, range-of-motion exercises and positioning are important nursing interventions. Passive range-of-motion exercise is begun on the first day of hospitalization. If the stroke is caused by SAH, the movement is limited to the extremities. The patient is taught to actively exercise as soon as possible. Muscle atrophy secondary to lack of innervation and activity can develop within 1 month following stroke.

The paralyzed or weak side needs special attention when the patient is positioned. Each joint should be positioned higher than the joint proximal to it to prevent dependent edema. Specific deformities on the weak or paralyzed side that may be present in patients with stroke include internal rotation of the shoulder; flexion contractures of the hand, wrist, and elbow; external rotation of the hip; and plantar flexion of the foot. Subluxation of the shoulder on the affected side is common. Careful positioning and moving of the affected arm may prevent the development of a painful shoulder condition; immobilization of the affected upper extremity may precipitate a painful shoulder–hand syndrome.

Nursing interventions to optimize musculoskeletal function include (a) placing a trochanter roll at the hip to prevent external rotation; (b) using hand splints (not rolled washcloths) to prevent hand contractures; (c) providing arm supports with slings and lap boards to prevent shoulder displacement; (d) avoiding pulling the patient by the arm to prevent shoulder displacement;

(e) using posterior leg splints, footboards, or high-topped tennis shoes to prevent foot drop; and (f) using hand splints to reduce spasticity. The early use of splints in hemiplegic patients has been associated with improved mobility and enhanced functional recovery (Bianca et al., 2018).

Integumentary System. The skin of the patient with stroke is particularly susceptible to breakdown related to loss of sensation, decreased circulation, and immobility. This complication is compounded by patient age, poor nutrition, dehydration, edema, and incontinence. The nursing plan for prevention of skin breakdown includes (a) relieving pressure through position changes, special mattresses, or wheelchair cushions; (b) providing good skin hygiene; (c) applying emollients to dry skin; and (d) promoting early mobility. The ideal position-change schedule is side–back–side with a maximum duration of 2 hours for any position. Nurses should position the patient on the weak or paralyzed side for only 30 minutes. If an area of redness develops and does not return to normal colour within 15 minutes of pressure relief, the epidermis and dermis are damaged. The damaged area should not be massaged because massage may cause additional damage. Pressure relief is the single most important factor in both the prevention and treatment of skin breakdown. Pillows can be used under lower extremities to reduce pressure on the heels. Vigilance and good nursing care are required to prevent pressure injuries.

Gastrointestinal System. The most common bowel symptom for patients who have experienced a stroke is constipation. Patients may be prophylactically placed on stool softeners or fibre (psyllium [Metamucil]), or both. The patient who has liquid stools should also be checked for stool impaction. Depending on the patient's fluid balance status and swallowing ability, fluid intake should be 1 800 to 2 000 mL/day, and fibre intake up to 25 g/day. Physical activity also promotes bowel function. Laxatives, suppositories, or additional stool softeners may be ordered if the patient does not respond to increased fluid and fibre. Similarly, enemas are used only if suppositories and digital stimulation are ineffective, because they cause vagal stimulation and increase ICP.

Urinary System. In the acute stage of stroke, the primary urinary challenge is poor bladder control, resulting in incontinence. Efforts should be made to promote normal bladder function and avoid the use of in-dwelling catheters. If an in-dwelling catheter must be used initially, it should be removed as soon as the patient is medically and neurologically stable. Long-term use of an in-dwelling catheter is associated with urinary tract infections and delayed bladder retraining. An alternative to intermittent catheterizations is offering the opportunity for frequent toileting to patients with urinary incontinence. Male patients with urinary incontinence also have the alternative of using an external catheter.

A bladder retraining program consists of (a) adequate fluid intake with the majority given between 0800 and 1900 hours; (b) scheduled toileting every 2 hours using bedpan, urinal, commode, or bathroom; and (c) noting signs of restlessness, which may indicate the need for urination.

Nutrition. The nutritional needs of patients require quick assessment and treatment. Patients may initially receive IV infusions to maintain fluid and electrolyte balance as well as for administration of medications. Patients with severe impairment may require enteral or parenteral nutrition support. Individual assessment and planning for nutrition are necessary, and patients' needs will depend on the severity of the stroke.

Speech–language pathologists (SLPs) (if available) can perform a swallowing evaluation before patients are started on oral intake. The first oral feeding should be approached with caution because dysphagia may be present; the majority of patients will experience dysphagia after a stroke (Cohen et al., 2016). Before initiation of feeding, the gag reflex may be assessed by gently stimulating the back of the throat with a tongue blade. If a gag reflex is present, the patient will gag spontaneously. If it is absent, feeding should be deferred, and exercises to stimulate swallowing should be started. The SLP or occupational therapist is usually responsible for designing this program. However, in some clinical settings, the nurse may be called on to develop the program.

To screen for swallowing ability, the nurse should elevate the head of the bed to an upright position (unless contraindicated) and do a bedside trial of fluid (e.g., Toronto Bedside Swallowing Screening Test [TOR-BSST] or Burke test), giving the patient at least 3 tsp of water before proceeding to 50 mL of water by cup. Because of the dangers of silent aspiration, the nurse should not use any other liquid but water for this screening. If problems are experienced, the patient is not allowed anything orally and is referred to an SLP. If no problems are experienced, the patient should be placed on a modified diet and monitored during meals (HSFC, 2018a).

After careful assessment of swallowing, chewing, gag reflex, and pocketing, oral feedings can be initiated. Mouth care before feeding helps stimulate sensory awareness and salivation and can facilitate swallowing. The patient should remain in a high Fowler's position, preferably in a chair with the head flexed forward for the feeding and for 30 minutes afterward. Various dietary items may be recommended by the SLP. Foods should be easy to swallow and provide enough texture, temperature (warm or cold), and flavour to stimulate a swallow reflex. Crushed ice can be used as a stimulant. The patient should be instructed to swallow and then swallow again. Puréed foods are not usually the best choice because they are often bland and too smooth. Thin liquids are often difficult to swallow and may promote coughing. Thin fluids can be thickened with a commercially available thickening agent (e.g., Thick-It). Milk products should be avoided because they tend to increase the viscosity of mucus and increase salivation.

Food should be placed on the unaffected side of the mouth. The nurse should ensure an unrushed, nonstressful atmosphere. Feedings must be followed by scrupulous oral hygiene because food may collect on the affected side of the mouth.

Communication. During the acute stage of stroke, the nurse's role in meeting the psychological needs of the patient is primarily supportive. An alert patient is usually anxious because of lack of understanding about what has happened and because communication is difficult. The patient is assessed for the ability to both speak and understand. The patient's response to simple questions can give the nurse a guideline for structuring explanations and instructions. If the patient cannot understand words, gestures may be used to support verbal cues. It is helpful to speak slowly and calmly, using simple words or sentences to enhance communication. The nurse must give the patient extra time to comprehend and respond to communication. The

TABLE 60.9	COMMUNICATION WITH A PATIENT EXPERIENCING APHASIA
1.	Environmental stimuli that may distract and disrupt communication efforts should be avoided.
2.	When speaking, the nurse should look in the patient's direction because observance of facial expression may help the patient with aphasia to understand what the nurse is saying.
3.	The nurse should speak with normal volume and in a tone of voice suitable for communicating with an adult rather than a child.
4.	The nurse should present one thought or idea at a time.
5.	Writing out key words or drawing instructions using a thick black marker and large printed letters can help the patient to follow along.
6.	Questions should be kept simple and preferably be able to be answered with "yes" or "no."
7.	The nurse should let the patient speak and not interrupt, allowing the patient time to complete thoughts.
8.	Mimicking or making use of gestures or demonstration is an acceptable alternative form of communication. The nurse can encourage this by saying, "Show me …" or "Point to what you want."
9.	If the nurse does not understand the patient, the nurse should calmly express the lack of understanding and encourage the use of nonverbal communication or ask the person to write out what they want.
10.	The patient should be given time to process information and generate a response before a question or statement is repeated.
11.	The nurse should allow body contact (e.g., the clasp of a hand, touching) as much as possible. Touching may be the only way the patient can express feelings.
12.	The more familiar a routine, the easier it will be, so the nurse should organize the patient's day by preparing and following a schedule.
13.	The nurse should not push communication if the patient is tired or upset. Aphasia worsens with fatigue.

stroke patient with aphasia may be easily overwhelmed by verbal stimuli. (Guidelines for communicating with a patient who has aphasia are presented in Table 60.9.) Evaluation and treatment of language and communication deficits are often done by the SLP once the patient has stabilized.

Sensory–Perceptual Alterations. Homonymous hemianopia (blindness in the same half of each visual field) is a common condition after a stroke (Figure 60.12, *B*). Persistent disregard of objects in part of the visual field should alert the nurse to this possibility. Initially, the nurse can help the patient to compensate by arranging the environment within the patient's perceptual field, such as arranging the food tray so that all foods are on the right side or the left side to accommodate for field of vision (see Figure 60.12, *B*). Later, the patient learns to compensate for the visual defect by consciously attending to or scanning the neglected side (see Figure 60.12, *A*). The weak or paralyzed extremities are carefully checked for adequacy of dressing, for hygiene, and for trauma.

In the clinical situation, it is often difficult to distinguish between a visual field cut and a neglect syndrome. Both conditions may occur with strokes affecting either the right or the left side of the brain. A person may be unfortunate enough to have both homonymous hemianopia and a neglect syndrome, a combination that increases the inattention to the weak or paralyzed side. A neglect syndrome results in decreased safety awareness and thereby places the patient at high risk for injury. Immediately after the stroke, the nurse must anticipate potential safety hazards and provide protection from injury. Safety measures can include close observation of the patient, use of a sitter or

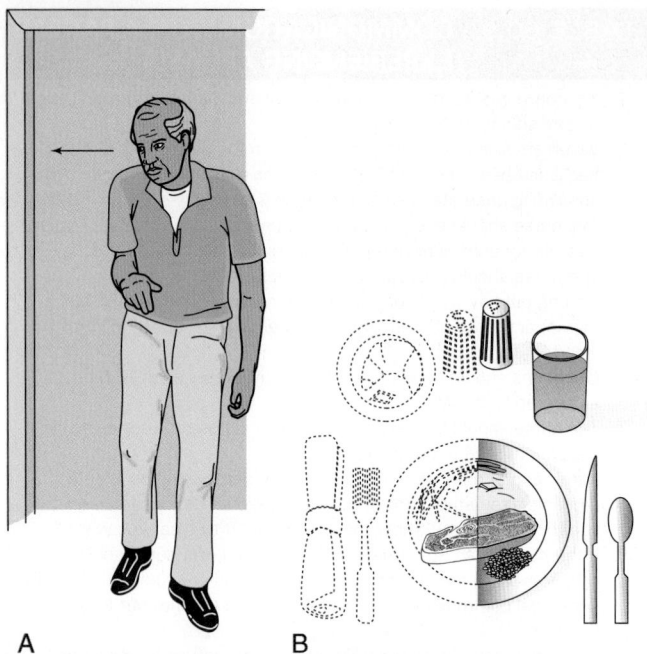

FIG. 60.12 Spatial and perceptual deficits in stroke. **A,** The patient is instructed to look toward the affected side when walking to avoid bumping into things. **B,** With homonymous hemianopia, the patient is unable to see the left side of the tray and may ignore items on that side. Source: Monahan, F. D., Neighbors, M., Sands, J. K., et al. (2007). *Phipps' medical-surgical nursing: Health and illness perspectives* (8th ed., p. 1437, Figure 49-10). Mosby.

family member, a lower bed height, and video monitors. The use of restraints and soft vests is to be avoided as they may agitate the patient.

Other visual disorders may include diplopia, loss of the corneal reflex, and ptosis, especially if the area of stroke is in the vertebrobasilar distribution. Diplopia is often treated with an eye patch. If the corneal reflex is absent, the patient is at risk for corneal abrasion and should be observed closely and protected against eye injuries. Corneal abrasion can be prevented with artificial tears or gel to keep the eyes moist and with an eye shield (especially at night). Ptosis is generally not treated because it usually does not inhibit vision.

Coping. A stroke is usually a sudden, extremely stressful event for the patient, family members, and significant others. A stroke is often a family disease, affecting the family emotionally, socially, and financially, as well as changing roles and responsibilities within the family. An older couple may perceive the stroke as a very real threat to life and to their accustomed lifestyle. Reactions to this threat vary considerably but may involve fear, apprehension, denial of the severity of stroke, depression, anger, and sorrow. During the acute phase of caring for the stroke patient and the family, nursing interventions designed to facilitate coping include providing information and emotional support.

Explanations to the patient and family about what has happened and about diagnostic and therapeutic procedures should be clear, detailed, and understandable. However, if the family is extremely anxious and upset during the acute phase, explanations may need to be repeated at a later time. Because family members usually have not had time to prepare for the illness, they may need assistance in arranging care for family members or pets and for transportation and finances. A social services referral is often helpful.

The patient's decision making and health care providers' commitment to uphold the patient's wishes during this challenging time are of utmost importance. Advance directives should be honoured and family meetings or updates should be held regularly in regard to feeding tube placement or tracheotomy.

It is particularly challenging to keep the aphasic patient adequately informed. Tone, demeanour, and touch may help to convey support. When communicating with a patient who has a communication deficit, the nurse should speak with normal volume and tone, keep questions simple, and present one thought or idea at a time. To decrease the patient's frustration, the nurse should always let the patient speak without interruption and use gestures. It is important, too, to make use of writing and communication boards (Burns et al., 2015).

AMBULATORY AND HOME CARE: STROKE RECOVERY. The patient is usually discharged from the acute care setting to home, an intermediate- or long-term care facility, or a rehabilitation facility. Ideally, discharge planning with the patient and family or caregiver starts early in the hospitalization and promotes a smooth transition from one care setting to another. The interprofessional team provides guidance for the appropriate care required after discharge. If the patient requires a short- or long-term health care facility, the team can make appropriate referrals that allow time for the family to select and arrange care. A critical factor in discharge planning is the patient's level of independence in performing ADLs. If the patient is returning home, the team can make referrals for needed equipment and services in preparation for discharge.

Nurses have an excellent opportunity to prepare the patient and family or caregiver for discharge through education, demonstration and return demonstration, practice, and evaluation of self-care skills before discharge. Total care is considered in discharge planning: medications, nutrition, mobility, exercises, hygiene, and toileting. Follow-up care is carefully planned to ensure continuing nursing care, physiotherapy, occupational therapy, and speech therapy, as well as medical care. Community resources should be identified to provide recreational activities, group support, spiritual assistance, respite care, adult day care, and home assistance based on the individual patient's needs.

Rehabilitation is the process of maximizing the patient's capabilities and resources to promote optimal functioning related to physical, mental, and social well-being. The goals of rehabilitation are to prevent deformity and to maintain and improve function. Regardless of the care setting, ongoing rehabilitation is essential to maximize the patient's abilities. During the first 3 months post-stroke, the major part of neurological recovery occurs and may continue for up to 1 year or longer (Teasell & Norhayati, 2016).

Rehabilitation requires an interprofessional team approach so the patient and family can benefit from a range of combined and expert care. The team must communicate and coordinate care to achieve the patient's and family's goals. There is strong evidence that organized post-acute inpatient stroke care delivered within the first 4 weeks by an interprofessional team of health care providers can result in a reduction in the number of deaths related to stroke. The stroke rehabilitation team generally consists of a rehabilitation nurse, neuropsychologist, occupational therapist, certified rehabilitation counsellor, physiotherapist, physician, recreational therapist, social worker, and SLP. The nurse is in a good position to facilitate rehabilitation and is often key to successful rehabilitation efforts. Physiotherapy focuses on mobility, progressive ambulation, transfer techniques, and equipment needed for mobility. Occupational therapy emphasizes retraining for ADLs such as eating, dressing, hygiene, and cooking. Occupational therapists are also skilled in cognitive and perceptual evaluation and training. Speech–language pathology focuses on speech, communication, cognition, and swallowing abilities. Combined therapy time from a physiotherapist, occupational therapist, and SLP is associated with improved functional outcomes (HSFC, 2019b).

Many of the nursing interventions outlined in NCP 60.1 for the patient who has had a stroke are initiated in the acute phase of care and continue throughout rehabilitation. Some of the interventions are independent nursing actions, whereas others involve the entire rehabilitation team.

The rehabilitation nurse assesses the patient, caregiver, and family with attention to the (a) rehabilitation potential of the patient, (b) physical status of all body systems, (c) presence of complications caused by the stroke or other chronic conditions, (d) cognitive status of the patient, (e) family resources and support, and (f) expectations of the patient and family related to the rehabilitation program.

Musculoskeletal Function. The nurse initially emphasizes the musculoskeletal functions of eating, toileting, and walking for the rehabilitation of the patient. Initial assessment consists of determining the stage of recovery of muscle function. If the muscles are still flaccid several weeks after the stroke, the prognosis for regaining function is poor, and the focus of care is on preventing additional loss. Most patients begin to show signs of spasticity with exaggerated reflexes within 48 hours following the stroke. Spasticity at this phase of the stroke denotes progress toward recovery. As improvement continues, small voluntary movements of the hip or the shoulder may be accompanied by involuntary movements in the rest of the extremity *(synergy)*. The final stage of recovery occurs when the patient has voluntary control of isolated muscle groups.

Interventions for the musculoskeletal system advance in a manner of progressive activity. Balance training is the initial step and begins with the patient sitting up in bed or dangling their legs from the edge of the bed. The nurse evaluates tolerance by noting dizziness or syncope caused by vasomotor instability. Loss of postural stability is common after a stroke. When the nondominant hemisphere is involved, walking apraxia and loss of postural control are usually apparent. The nurse needs to assess whether the patient autocorrects their posture when sitting on the edge of the bed. If the patient can straighten their posture instead of leaning to the weaker side, the patient may be ready for the next step of transferring from the bed to a chair. The chair is placed beside the bed so that the patient can lead with the stronger arm and leg. The patient sits on the side of the bed, stands, places their strong hand on the far wheelchair arm, and sits down. The nurse may either supervise the transfer or provide minimal assistance by guiding the patient's strong hand to the wheelchair arm, standing in front of the patient and blocking the patient's knees with the nurse's own knees to prevent knee buckling, and guiding the patient into a sitting position.

Constraint-induced movement therapy (CIMT) encourages the patient to use the weakened extremity by restricting movement of the unaffected extremity. This approach has demonstrated limited improvements in motor impairment and function and little effect on reducing disability (Corbetta et al., 2016). The Canadian Stroke Best Practices guidelines suggest that CIMT be considered for a select group of patients who demonstrate at least 20 degrees of active wrist extension and 10 degrees of active finger extension, with minimal sensory deficits and normal cognition (HSFC, 2019b). Patients should engage in training that is meaningful, repetitive, progressively adapted, and task- and goal-oriented to enhance and restore sensorimotor function (HSFC, 2019b). Supportive or assistive equipment, such as canes, walkers, and leg braces, may be needed on a short- or long-term basis for mobility. The physiotherapist usually selects the most appropriate supportive device(s) to meet individual needs and instructs the patient regarding use. The nurse should incorporate physiotherapy activities into the patient's daily routine for additional practice and repetition of rehabilitation efforts.

INFORMATICS IN PRACTICE

Video Games for Stroke Recovery

Patients coping with the effects of a stroke often have difficulty performing ADLs. Playing active video games (e.g., Nintendo Wii™ or Xbox Kinect™) can bring some fun into stroke recovery and may get patients to spend more time in therapy.

Gaming helps patients regain lost strength, improve motor skills, and improve problem solving and short- and long-term memory.

Patients can play with their families, including children, making gaming a way to involve others in rehabilitation.

Nutritional Therapy. After the acute phase, a dietitian can assist in determining the appropriate daily caloric intake based on the patient's size, weight, and activity level. If the patient is unable to take in an adequate oral diet, a percutaneous endoscopic gastrostomy (see Chapter 42, Figure 42.8) may be used for nutritional support if dysphagia persists. Most commercially prepared formulas provide about 1 cal/mL. (Enteral feedings are described in Chapter 42.)

The nurse and the SLP must assess the ability of the patient to swallow solids and fluids and adjust the diet appropriately. The dietitian plans the diet type, texture, calorie count, and fluids to meet the patient's nutritional needs. The occupational therapist and the nurse must evaluate the patient's ability to feed themselves and recommend assistive devices to allow for independent eating.

The inability to feed oneself can be frustrating and may result in malnutrition and dehydration. Interventions to promote self-feeding include using the unaffected upper extremity to eat; employing assistive devices such as rocker knives, plate guards, and nonslip pads for dishes (Figure 60.13); removing unnecessary items from the tray or table, which can reduce spills; and providing a nondistracting environment to decrease sensory overload and distraction. The effectiveness of the dietary program is evaluated in terms of maintenance of weight, adequate hydration, and patient satisfaction.

Bowel Function. A bowel management program is implemented for problems with bowel control, constipation, or incontinence. A high-fibre diet (see Chapter 45, Table 45.8) and adequate fluid intake (2 500–3 000 mL) are usually recommended. Patients with stroke frequently have constipation, which responds to the following dietary management:

- Fluid intake of 2 500 to 3 000 mL daily unless contraindicated
- Prune juice (120 mL) or stewed prunes daily
- Cooked vegetables or fruit three times daily
- Whole-grain cereal or bread three to five times daily

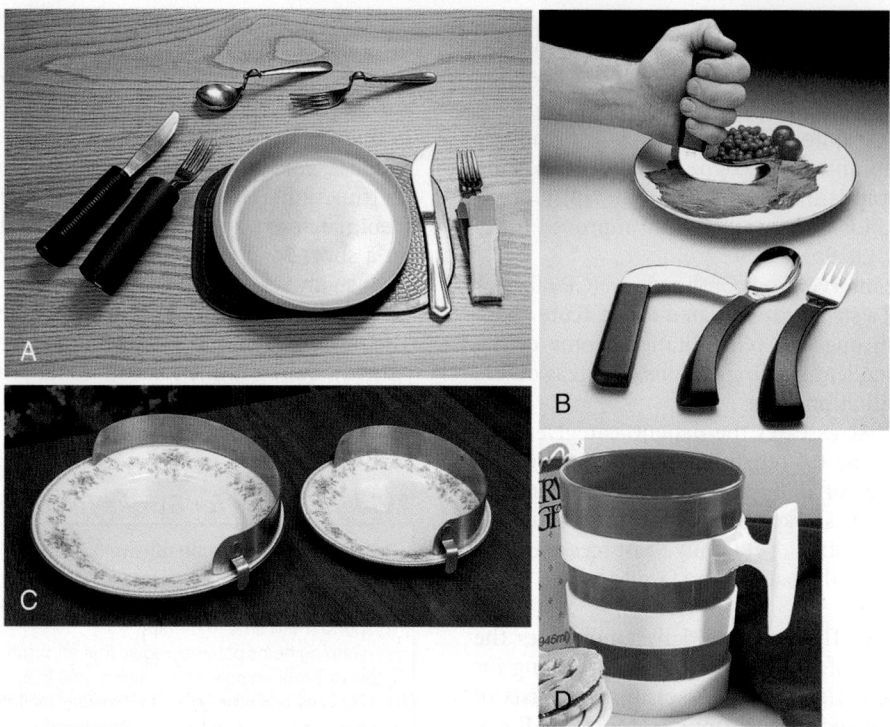

FIG. 60.13 Assistive devices for eating. **A,** The curved fork fits over the hand. The rounded plate helps keep food on the plate. Special grips and swivel handles are helpful for some persons. **B,** Knives with rounded blades are rocked back and forth to cut food. The person does not need a fork in one hand and a knife in the other. **C,** Plate guards help keep food on the plate. **D,** Cup with special handle. Source: Courtesy Sammons Preston, Bolingbrook, Illinois.

The bowel management program for incontinence consists of placing the patient on the bedpan or bedside commode or taking the patient to the bathroom at a regular time daily to re-establish bowel regularity. A good time for the bowel program is 30 minutes after breakfast because eating stimulates the gastrocolic reflex and peristalsis. The time can be adjusted for individual bowel habits and preferred timing. Sitting on the commode or toilet promotes bowel elimination through both gravity and increased abdominal pressure. Stool softeners or suppositories may be ordered if the bowel program is ineffective in re-establishing bowel regularity. A glycerin suppository can be inserted 15 to 30 minutes before evacuation time to stimulate the anorectal reflex. A bisacodyl (Dulcolax) suppository is a chemical stimulant to the bowel and is used when other measures are ineffective. Ideally, suppository use is for short-term management.

Bladder Function. The nurse assists the patient with urinary issues or incontinence that may follow a stroke. Often the patient with stroke has functional incontinence, which is associated with communication difficulties, mobility challenges, and dressing or undressing difficulties. Nursing interventions focused on urinary continence include (a) assessing for bladder distension by palpation; (b) offering the bedpan, urinal, commode, or toilet every 2 hours during waking hours and every 3 to 4 hours at night; (c) focusing the patient on the need to urinate with direct command; (d) assisting with clothing and mobility; (e) scheduling the majority of fluid intake between 0700 and 1900 hours; and (f) encouraging the usual position for urinating (standing for men and sitting for women).

Short-term interventions for urinary incontinence may include in-dwelling catheters, intermittent catheterization, frequent toileting, or incontinence briefs. These are not long-term solutions for urinary incontinence because complications such as urinary infections or skin irritation may occur.

Nurses often assess postvoid residual volume using bladder ultrasonography. The ultrasonogram measures how much urine is in the bladder after voiding. If urine remains in the bladder, incomplete emptying is a problem and may cause urinary tract infections. A coordinated program by the entire nursing staff is needed to achieve urinary continence.

Sensory–Perceptual Function. Patients who have had a stroke frequently have perceptual deficits. Patients with a stroke on the right side of the brain usually have difficulty in judging position, distance, and rate of movement. These patients are often impulsive and impatient and tend to deny problems related to strokes. They may fail to correlate spatial–perceptual disorders with the inability to perform activities, such as guiding a wheelchair through the doorway. The patient with a right-brain stroke (left hemiplegia) is at higher risk for injury because of mobility difficulties. Directions for activities are best given verbally for comprehension. The task should be broken down into simple steps for ease of understanding. Environmental control, such as removing clutter and obstacles and providing good lighting, aids in concentration and helps provide safer mobility. The patient should wear nonslip socks at all times. One-sided neglect is common for people with right-brain stroke, so the nurse may assist or remind the patient to dress the weak or paralyzed side or shave the forgotten side of the face.

Patients with a left-brain stroke (right hemiplegia) commonly are slower in organization and performance of tasks. They tend to have impaired spatial discrimination. These patients usually admit to deficits and have a fearful, anxious response to a stroke. Their behaviours are slow and cautious. Nonverbal cues and instructions are helpful for comprehension with patients who have had a left-brain stroke.

Affect. Patients who have had strokes often exhibit emotional responses that are not appropriate or typical for the situation. Patients may appear apathetic, depressed, fearful, anxious, weepy, frustrated, or angry. Some patients, especially those with a stroke on the left side of the brain, exhibit exaggerated mood swings. The patient may be unable to control emotions and may suddenly burst into tears or laughter. This behaviour is out of context and often is unrelated to the underlying emotional state of the patient. Nursing interventions for atypical emotional response are to (a) distract the patient who suddenly becomes emotional, (b) explain to the patient and family that emotional outbursts may occur after a stroke, (c) maintain a calm environment, and (d) avoid shaming or scolding the patient during emotional outbursts.

Coping. The patient with a stroke may experience many losses, including those that are sensory, intellectual, communicative, functional, role behaviour, emotional, social, and vocational. The patient, caregiver, and family often go through the process of grief and mourning associated with the losses. Some patients experience long-term depression, exhibiting symptoms such as anxiety, weight loss, loss of energy, poor appetite, and sleep disturbances. In addition, the time and energy required to perform previously simple tasks can arouse anger and frustration.

The patient, caregiver, and family need help with coping with the losses associated with stroke. The nurse may assist the coping by (a) supporting communication between the patient and the family; (b) discussing lifestyle changes resulting from stroke deficits; (c) discussing changing roles and responsibilities within the family; (d) being an active listener to enable the expression of fear, frustration, and anxiety; (e) including the family and patient in short- and long-term goal planning and patient care; and (f) supporting family conferences. Maladjusted dependence with inadequate coping occurs when the patient does not maintain optimal functioning for self-care, family responsibilities, decision making, or socialization. This situation can cause resentment from both the patient and the family with a negative cycle of interpersonal dependency and control. *Maladjusted independence* occurs when the patient overestimates personal cognitive or physical capabilities and energy levels. These patients are at risk for injury.

Family members must cope with three aspects of the patient's behaviour: (a) recognition of behavioural changes resulting from neurological deficits that are not changeable, (b) responses to multiple losses by both the patient and the family, and (c) behaviours that may have been reinforced during the early stages of stroke as continued dependency. The patient, caregiver, and family may express feelings of guilt over not living healthy lifestyles or not seeking professional help sooner. Family therapy is a helpful adjunct to rehabilitation. Open communication, information regarding the total effects of stroke, education regarding stroke treatment, and therapy are helpful. Stroke support groups within rehabilitation facilities and in the community can be useful in terms of mutual sharing, education, coping, and understanding.

Sexual Function. A patient who has had a stroke may be concerned about the loss of sexual function. Many patients are comfortable talking about their anxieties and fears regarding sexual function if the nurse is comfortable and open to the topic. The nurse may initiate the topic with the patient and partner or significant other. Common concerns about sexual activity among patients with stroke are impotence and the occurrence of another stroke during sex. Nursing interventions for sexual activity include education on (a) optimal positioning of partners, (b) timing for peak energy times, and (c) patient and partner counselling.

Community Reintegration. Traditionally, successful community integration following stroke has been difficult for the patient because of persistent problems with cognition, coping, physical deficits, and emotional lability that interfere with functioning. Older patients who have had a stroke often have more severe deficits and frequently experience multiple health problems. Failure to continue the rehabilitation regimen at home may result in deterioration and further complications.

Improved outcomes have been noted in patients suffering from severe stroke who have received inpatient rehabilitation. Results showed that these patients had lower mortality rates, stayed in hospital for shorter periods, and were more likely to return home than those receiving rehabilitation in other facilities. Best results were seen in patients treated in units that were designated as specialized stroke units (HSFC, 2019b).

Community resources can be an asset to patients and their families. The Heart and Stroke Foundation of Canada is a great resource for anyone who has been affected by or had a family member affected by a stroke. The Canadian Stroke Network provides newsletters on stroke, and After Stroke offers support to stroke survivors. Other local groups can offer more daily assistance, such as provision of meals and transportation. These resources can be identified by nurse case managers, advanced-practice nurses, community health nurses, discharge planners, and social workers. (Resources are listed at the end of the chapter.)

AGE-RELATED CONSIDERATIONS
STROKE
Stroke is a significant cause of death and disability. The highest incidence of stroke occurs among older persons. Stroke can result in a profound disruption in the life of an older person. The magnitude of disability and changes in total function can leave patients wondering if they can ever return to their prestroke life, and loss of independence may be a major concern. Performing ADLs may require many adaptive changes because of physical, emotional, perceptual, and cognitive deficits. Home management may be a particular challenge if the patient has an older spouse caretaker who also has health problems. There may be limited family members (including adult children) living nearby to provide help.

Assisting the older patient through the rehabilitative phase and to deal with the residual deficits of stroke, as well as aging, can provide a challenging nursing experience. Patients may become fearful and depressed because of the possibility of another attack, or death. The fear can become immobilizing and interfere with effective rehabilitation.

Changes may occur in the patient–partner relationship. The dependency resulting from a stroke can be threatening to the relationship. Some partners may also have chronic medical problems that affect their ability to take care of the stroke survivor. The patient may not want anyone other than the spouse or partner to provide care, placing a significant burden on the spouse or partner.

The nurse has the opportunity to assist the patient and family in the transition through acute hospitalization, rehabilitation, long-term care, and home care. The needs of the patient and the family require ongoing nursing assessment, and interventions must be adapted in response to changing needs to optimize quality of life for both the patient and the family.

CASE STUDY

Stroke

Patient Profile

E. J. (pronouns she/her), 66 years old, awoke in the middle of the night and fell, unable to control her left leg, when trying to get up to go to the bathroom (see the Chapter 58 case study). E. J.'s partner took her to the hospital, where the diagnosis was an acute right-sided ischemic stroke (right middle cerebral artery stroke). Because symptoms had awakened E. J., the actual time of onset was unknown, and she therefore is not a candidate for tissue plasminogen activator (tPA).

Subjective Data

- Left arm, leg, and face are weak and feel numb
- Feeling depressed and fearful
- Requires help with activities of daily living
- Is concerned about having another stroke
- Says has not taken medications for high cholesterol for many weeks
- Has history of a brief episode of left-sided weakness and tingling of face, arm, and hand 3 months earlier, which totally resolved and for which treatment was not sought

Objective Data

- BP: 180/110 mm Hg
- ECG is shown in the graph below
- Left-sided arm weakness (3/5) and leg weakness (4/5)
- Decreased sensation on the left side, particularly the hand
- Left homonymous hemianopsia
- 160 cm tall and weighs 73 kg; body mass index = 28.5
- Alert, oriented, and able to answer questions appropriately but has mild slowness in responding

Past Medical History

- Migraines
- Hyperlipidemia
- Hypertension
- Smoking

Discussion Questions

1. How do E. J.'s health history and current findings increase her risk for a stroke?
2. How can the nurse address E. J.'s concerns regarding having another stroke?
3. Why would her ability to drive be affected after the stroke?
4. What strategies might the nurse use to help E. J. and her family cope with her feelings of depression?
5. *Priority decision:* What priority lifestyle changes should E. J. make to reduce the likelihood of another stroke?
6. How will homonymous hemianopia affect E. J.'s hygiene, eating, driving, and community activities?
7. What factors should the nurse assess for related to outpatient rehabilitation for E. J.?
8. *Priority decision:* What are the priority nursing interventions for E. J.?
9. *Priority decision:* Based on the assessment data provided, what are the priority nursing diagnoses? Are there any interprofessional issues?
10. *Evidence-informed practice:* E. J.'s family wants to know if atrial flutter caused the stroke and, if so, what can be done to prevent additional problems resulting from her atrial flutter.

evolve

Answers are available at http://evolve.elsevier.com/Canada/Lewis/medsurg.

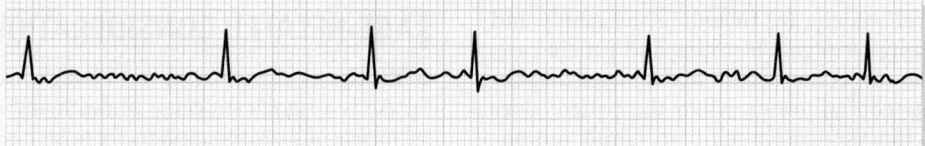

REVIEW QUESTIONS

The number of the question corresponds to the same-numbered objective at the beginning of the chapter.

1. Which health condition(s) can increase an individual's risk for stroke? *(Select all that apply.)*
   a. Pneumonia
   b. Atrial fibrillation
   c. Previous transient ischemic attack (TIA)
   d. Hypertension
   e. Migraines

2. Which of the following factors related to cerebral blood flow most often determines the extent of cerebral damage from a stroke?
   a. Amount of cardiac output
   b. Oxygen content of the blood
   c. Degree of collateral circulation
   d. Level of carbon dioxide in the blood

3. Which of the following pieces of information provided by the client would help differentiate a hemorrhagic stroke from an ischemic stroke?
   a. Sensory disturbance
   b. A history of hypertension
   c. Presence of motor weakness
   d. Sudden onset of severe headache

4. A client with right-sided hemiplegia and aphasia resulting from a stroke most likely has involvement of which of the following?
   a. Brainstem
   b. Vertebral artery
   c. Left middle cerebral artery
   d. Right middle cerebral artery

5. A client with a stroke is scheduled for angiography. Which of the following can this test detect?
   a. Presence of increased intracranial pressure
   b. Site and size of the infarction
   c. Patency of the cerebral blood vessels
   d. Presence of blood in the cerebrospinal fluid

6. A client experiencing transient ischemic attacks is scheduled for a carotid endarterectomy. What does the nurse explain to the client about the purpose of this procedure?
   a. To decrease cerebral edema
   b. To reduce the brain damage that occurs during a stroke in evolution
   c. To prevent a stroke by removing atherosclerotic plaques blocking cerebral blood flow
   d. To provide a circulatory bypass around thrombotic plaques obstructing cranial circulation

7. For a client who is suspected to have had a stroke, what is one of the most important pieces of information that the nurse can obtain?
   a. Time of the client's last meal
   b. Time at which stroke symptoms first appeared
   c. Client's hypertension history and management
   d. Family history of stroke and other cardiovascular diseases
8. What does bladder training in a male client who has urinary incontinence after a stroke include?
   a. Limiting fluid intake
   b. Keeping a urinal in place at all times
   c. Assisting the client to stand to void
   d. Catheterizing the client every 4 hours

9. What is the most common response of a client who sustained a stroke regarding the change in body image?
   a. Denial
   b. Depression
   c. Dissociation
   d. Intellectualization

1. b, c, d; 2. c; 3. d; 4. c; 5. c; 6. c; 7. b; 8. c; 9. b.

evolve

For even more review questions, visit http://evolve.elsevier.com/Canada/Lewis/medsurg.

REFERENCES

Bianca, C., Machuki, J. O., Chen, W., et al. (2018). A dynamic splint for the treatment of spasticity of the hand after stroke—recognition of its design, functionality and limitations: A narrative review article. *Journal of Neurology and Neurorehabilitation Research, 3*(2), 1–7. doi:10.35841/neurology-neurorehabilitation.3.2.1-5

Boulanger, J. M., Butcher, K., Gubitz, G., et al. (2018). *Canadian stroke best practice recommendations. Acute stroke management: Pre-hospital, emergency department, and acute inpatient stroke care* (6th ed.). https://www.heartandstroke.ca/-/media/1-stroke-best-practices/acute-stroke-management/csbpr2018-acute-stroke-module-final-17jul2018-en.ashx?rev=f57ce75409804a98a1fdd7523c73bbd7

Burns, M., Baylor, C., Dudgeon, B. J., et al. (2015). Asking the stakeholders: Perspectives of individuals with aphasia, their family members, and physicians regarding communication in medical interactions. *American Journal of Speech-Language Pathology, 24*(3), 341–357. https://doi.org/10.1044/2015_AJSLP-14-0051

Chong, J. (2020). Brain aneurysms. *Merck manual.* Professional version. https://www.merckmanuals.com/en-ca/professional/neurologic-disorders/stroke/brain-aneurysms

Cohen, D., Roffe, C., Beavan, J., et al. (2016). Post-stroke dysphagia: A review and design considerations for future trials. *International Journal of Stroke, 11*(4), 399–411. https://doi.org/10.1177/1747493016639057

Corbetta, D., Sirtori, V., Castellini, G., et al. (2016). Constraint-induced movement therapy for upper extremities in people with stroke. *Stroke, 47*, e205–206. https://doi.org/10.1161/STROKEAHA.116.013281

DeGuire, J., Clarke, J., Rouleau, K., et al. (2019). *Health reports. Blood pressure and hypertension.* Statistics Canada. https://www.doi.org/10.25318/82-003-x201900200002

Heart and Stroke Foundation of Canada (HSFC). (2016). *Mind the connection: Preventing stroke and dementia.* https://www.heartandstroke.ca/-/media/pdf-files/canada/stroke-report/hsf-stroke-report-2016.ashx?la=en&hash=B84FFD-2C434B4E3F5CF4585D9CB35713E6C406E5

Heart and Stroke Foundation of Canada (HSFC). (2017). *Different strokes: Recovery triumphs and challenges at any age.* https://www.heartandstroke.ca/-/media/pdf-files/canada/stroke-report/strokereport2017en.ashx?la=en&hash=67F86E4C3338-D5A7FE7862EA5D0DD57CA8539847

Heart and Stroke Foundation of Canada (HSFC). (2018a). *Acute stroke management* (6th ed.). https://www.strokebestpractices.ca/recommendations/acute-stroke-management

Heart and Stroke Foundation of Canada (HSFC). (2018b). *Emergency department evaluation and management of patients with acute stroke and TIA.* https://www.strokebestpractices.ca/recommendations/acute-stroke-management/emergency-department-evaluation-and-management

Heart and Stroke Foundation of Canada (HSFC). (2018c). *Lives disrupted: The impact of stroke on women.* https://www.heartandstroke.ca/-/media/pdf-files/canada/stroke-report/strokereport2018.ashx?la=en

Heart and Stroke Foundation of Canada (HSFC). (2019a). *Assessment and management of dysphagia and malnutrition following stroke* (6th ed.). https://www.strokebestpractices.ca/recommendations/stroke-rehabilitation/assessment-and-management-of-dysphagia-and-malnutrition-following-stroke

Heart and Stroke Foundation of Canada (HSFC). (2019b). Management of the upper extremity following stroke. https://www.strokebestpractices.ca/recommendations/stroke-rehabilitation/management-of-the-upper-extremity-following-stroke

Heart and Stroke Foundation of Canada (HSFC). (2021a). *Atrial fibrillation.* https://www.heartandstroke.ca/heart/conditions/atrial-fibrillation

Heart and Stroke Foundation of Canada (HSFC). (2021b). *Connected by the numbers.* https://www.heartandstroke.ca/articles/connected-by-the-numbers

Heart and Stroke Foundation of Canada (HSFC). (2021c). *Risk and prevention.* https://www.heartandstroke.ca/stroke/risk-and-prevention

Heart and Stroke Foundation of Canada (HSFC). (2021d). *Stroke and the brain.* https://www.heartandstroke.ca/stroke/what-is-stroke/stroke-and-the-brain

Heart and Stroke Foundation of Canada (HSFC). (2021e). *Types of stroke.* https://www.heartandstroke.ca/stroke/what-is-stroke/types-of-stroke

Hemphill, J. C., Greenberg, S. M., Anderson, C. S., et al. (2015). Guidelines for the management of spontaneous intracerebral hemorrhage. *Stroke, 46*(7), 1–30. https://doi.org/10.1161/STR.0000000000000069

Khare, S. (2016). Risk factors of transient ischemic attack: An overview. *Journal of Mid-life Health, 7*(1), 2–7. https://doi.org/10.4103/0976-7800.179166

Liu, Y., Qiu, H., Su, J., et al. (2016). Drug treatment of cerebral vasospasm after subarachnoid hemorrhage following aneurysms. *Chinese Neurosurgical Journal, 2*(4). https://doi.org/10.1186/s41016-016-0023-x

Mullen, M. T., & Loomis, C. (2014). Differentiating Facial Weakness Caused by Bell's Palsy vs. Acute Stroke. *Journal of Emergency Medical Services.*

Park, J. H., & Lee, J. H. (2018). Carotid artery stenting. *Korean Circulation Journal, 48*(2), 97–113. https://doi.org/10.4070/kcj.2017.0208

Public Health Agency of Canada (PHAC). (2019). *Stroke in Canada: Highlights from the Canadian Chronic Disease Surveillance System.* https://www.canada.ca/en/public-health/services/publications/diseases-conditions/stroke-canada-fact-sheet.html

Souillard-Scemama, R., Tisserand, M., Calvet, D., et al. (2015). An update on brain imaging in transient ischemic attack. *Journal of Neuroradiology, 42*(1), 3–11. https://doi.org/10.1016/j.neurad.2014.11.001

Statistics Canada. (2017). *The 10 leading causes of death, 2013.* http://www.statcan.gc.ca/pub/82-625-x/2017001/article/14776-eng.htm

Statistics Canada. (2019a). *Heavy drinking.* https://www150.statcan.gc.ca/n1/pub/82-625-x/2019001/article/00007-eng.htm

Statistics Canada. (2019b). *Overweight and obese adults, 2018.* https://www150.statcan.gc.ca/n1/en/pub/82-625-x/2019001/article/00005-eng.pdf%3Fst%3DOBRuwojR

Teasell, R., & Hussein, N. (2016). Brain reorganization, recovery and organized care. In R. Teasell, N. Hussein, R. Viana, et al. (Eds.), *Stroke rehabilitation clinician handbook* (pp. 1–34). Canadian Stroke Network. http://www.ebrsr.com/clinician-handbook

Toronto Brain VascularMalformation Study Group. (n.d.). *Embolization treatment for arteriovenous malformations (AVMs) of the brain and spinal cord.* http://brainavm.oci.utoronto.ca/malformations/embo_treat_avm_index.htm

Tramacere, I., Boncoraglio, G. B., Banzi, R., et al. (2019). Comparison of statins for secondary prevention in patients with ischemic stroke or transient ischemic attack: A systematic review and network meta-analysis. *BMC Medicine, 17,* 67. https://doi.org/10.1186/s12916-019-1298-5

World Health Organization (WHO). (2020). *Tobacco free initiative (TFI).* https://www.who.int/tobacco/quitting/benefits/en/

RESOURCES

Aphasia Institute
https://www.aphasia.ca
Canadian Association of Neuroscience Nurses (CANN)
https://www.cann.ca
Canadian Lung Association—*How to Quit Smoking*
https://www.lung.ca/quit
Canadian Stroke Network—*Life After Strokes*
https://www.canadianstrokenetwork.ca

CorHealth Ontario (formerly Cardiac Care Network of Ontario/Ontario Stroke Network)
https://www.corhealthontario.ca/
Diabetes Canada
https://www.diabetes.ca
Heart and Stroke Foundation of Canada
https://www.heartandstroke.com
Heart and Stroke Foundation of Canada—*Canadian Stroke Best Practice Recommendations*
https://www.strokebestpractices.ca
Hypertension Canada
https://www.hypertension.ca
March of Dimes Canada—*After Stroke*
https://www.afterstroke.ca/
Montreal Cognitive Assessment (MoCA)
https://www.mocatest.org
Registered Nurses' Association of Ontario—*Integrating Tobacco Interventions Into Daily Practice*
https://rnao.ca/bpg/guidelines/integrating-smoking-cessation-daily-nursing-practice
Registered Nurses' Association of Ontario—*Stroke Assessment Across the Continuum of Care*
https://rnao.ca/bpg/guidelines/stroke-assessment-across-continuum-care
Thrombosis Canada
https://thrombosiscanada.ca

American Association of Neuroscience Nurses (AANN)
https://www.aann.org
American Heart Association—*Stroke (Journal)*
https://stroke.ahajournals.org
American Stroke Association
https://www.stroke.org
Association of Rehabilitation Nurses (ARN)
https://www.rehabnurse.org
DASH Diet—*DASH Eating Plan (pp. 8–11)*
https://www.nhlbi.nih.gov/health/public/heart/hbp/dash/new_dash.pdf
National Institute of Neurological Disorders and Stroke
https://www.ninds.nih.gov
Society for Neuroscience
https://www.sfn.org
World Health Organization—*Cardiovascular Disease*
https://www.who.int/health-topics/cardiovascular-diseases/#tab=tab_1

Ⓔvolve

For additional Internet resources, see the website for this book at http://evolve.elsevier.com/Canada/Lewis/medsurg.

Nursing Management

Chronic Neurological Conditions

Denise Ouellette

Originating US chapter by Madona D. Plueger and Dottie Roberts

℮volve WEBSITE

http://evolve.elsevier.com/Canada/Lewis/medsurg

- Review Questions (Online Only)
- Key Points
- Answer Guidelines for Case Study
- Student Case Studies
  - Patient with Seizures
  - Patient with Parkinson's Disease and Hip Fracture

- Customizable Nursing Care Plans
  - Patient with Headache
  - Seizure Disorder or Epilepsy
  - Multiple Sclerosis
  - Parkinson's Disease

- Conceptual Care Map Creator
- Conceptual Care Map for Textbook Case Study
- Audio Glossary
- Content Updates

LEARNING OBJECTIVES

1. Compare and contrast the etiology, clinical manifestations, and nursing and interprofessional management of tension-type, migraine, and cluster headaches.
2. Differentiate the etiology and clinical manifestations of and the diagnostic studies, interprofessional care, and nursing management for seizure disorders, multiple sclerosis, Parkinson's disease, myasthenia gravis, and normal pressure hydrocephalus.

3. Describe the clinical manifestations and the nursing and interprofessional management of restless legs syndrome, amyotrophic lateral sclerosis, and Huntington's disease.
4. Explain the potential impact of chronic neurological disease on a patient's physical, emotional, and psychological well-being.
5. Outline the major goals of treatment for the patient with a chronic, progressive neurological disease.

KEY TERMS

absence seizure
amyotrophic lateral sclerosis (ALS)
aura
cluster headaches
epilepsy
focal onset seizures
generalized seizures

headache
Huntington's disease (HD)
migraine headache
multiple sclerosis (MS)
myasthenia gravis (MG)
myasthenic crisis
normal pressure hydrocephalus (NPH)

Parkinson's disease (PD)
prodrome
restless legs syndrome (RLS)
seizure disorder
status epilepticus
tension-type headache
tonic–clonic seizure

▌HEADACHE

Headache is probably the most common type of pain that humans experience. The majority of people have functional headaches, such as migraine or tension-type headaches. Others have organic headaches caused by intracranial or extracranial disease.

Not all tissues of the head are sensitive to pain. Pain-sensitive cranial structures include the venous sinuses, the dura, cranial blood vessels, the three divisions of the trigeminal nerve, the facial nerve, the glossopharyngeal nerve, the vagus nerve, and the first three cervical spinal nerves.

Headaches are classified as either primary or secondary. *Primary* headaches have no organic cause and include tension-type, migraine, and cluster headaches. The type of primary headache is determined using the International Headache Society (IHS) guidelines, based on characteristics of the headache (Table 61.1). *Secondary* headaches are caused by another condition or disorder, such as a sinus infection or stroke. A patient may have more than one type of headache. The history and neurological examination are keys to determining the type of headache.

MIGRAINE HEADACHE

Migraine headache (MH) is characterized by unilateral throbbing pain, a triggering event or factor, and manifestations associated with neurological and autonomic nervous system dysfunction. The effects of MH pain are dramatic, often causing

TABLE 61.1	COMPARISON OF MIGRAINE, TENSION-TYPE, AND CLUSTER HEADACHES		
	Migraine Headache	**Tension-Type Headache**	**Cluster Headache**
Site (see Figure 61.1)	Unilateral (in 60%), may switch sides, commonly anterior	Bilateral, bandlike pressure at base of skull	Unilateral, radiating up or down from one eye
Quality	Throbbing, synchronous with pulse	Constant, squeezing tightness	Severe, "bone-crushing"
Frequency	Periodic, cycles of several months to years	Cycles for many years	May have months or years between attacks
			Attacks occur in clusters: once every second day to eight times daily for weeks to months at a time
Duration	4–72 hr	30 min –7 days	15 min to 3 hr
Time and mode of onset	May be preceded by prodrome Onset after awakening Gets better with sleep	Not related to time	Nocturnal, commonly awakens patient from sleep
Associated symptoms	Nausea; vomiting; edema; irritability; sweating; photophobia; phonophobia; prodrome of sensory, motor, or psychic phenomena	Palpable neck and shoulder muscle tension, stiff neck, tenderness	Facial flushing or pallor, unilateral lacrimation, ptosis, and rhinitis

both physical and emotional disability. It has been reported that migraines are more common in women than in men and are more prevalent in adults between 35 and 45 years of age (World Health Organization [WHO], 2016).

Etiology and Pathophysiology

The exact etiology of MH remains unknown (Andreou & Edvinsson, 2019; Gupta, 2019). Recent literature points to migraines as being a functional disorder of the nervous system rather than a vascular headache (Charles, 2018). Acute migraine medication overuse, ineffective treatment of acute migraine, obesity, depression, low education level, and life stressors are all risk factors for chronic migraine (May & Schulte, 2016). Migraine has been associated with epilepsy, stroke, depression, anxiety, and irritable bowel syndrome (Gargya & Abdallah, 2019). In many cases, MHs have no known precipitating events; however, for some patients, specific factors may trigger a headache. These may include dietary factors, menses, head trauma, physical exertion, fatigue, stress, weather, and medications. Food triggers include chocolate, cheese, oranges, tomatoes, onions, monosodium glutamate, aspartame, and alcohol (particularly red wine).

Clinical Manifestations

MHs are subdivided by the IHS into categories, including those with and without **aura** (Headache Classification Committee of the IHS, 2018). *Auras* are the neurological symptoms such as visual field defects, tingling or burning sensations, paresthesia, motor dysfunction (e.g., weakness, paralysis), dizziness, confusion, and even loss of consciousness that usually precede the onset of migraine pain (Headache Classification Committee of the IHS, 2018). Clinical manifestations that might occur in MH are generalized edema, irritability, pallor, nausea, vomiting, and sweating. **Prodrome** signs, or symptoms that precede a MH, may include psychic disturbances, low mood, food cravings, frequent yawning, and stiff or painful neck (Headache Classification Committee of the IHS, 2018).

During the headache phase, some patients with MH may seek shelter from noise, light, odours, people, and stressors. The headache is described as a steady, throbbing pain that is synchronous with the pulse. However, the presentation of MH is varied in its severity. Although the headache is usually unilateral, it may switch to the opposite side in another episode. Not all MHs are disabling, and many patients do not seek health care

treatment for them. In some patients, the symptoms of MHs may become worse over time.

Diagnostic Studies

Usually, the diagnosis of MH is made on the basis of patient history. Neurological and other diagnostic examinations are often normal. There are no specific laboratory or radiological tests used to diagnose MHs. Neuroimaging techniques (e.g. computed tomographic [CT] scan or magnetic resonance imaging [MRI]) of the head are not recommended for routine evaluation of headache unless there are abnormal findings on the neurological examination. If atypical features are present, secondary headaches must be ruled out.

TENSION-TYPE HEADACHE

Tension-type headache (TTH), also called *stress headache,* is the most common type of primary headache. These headaches are characterized by their bilateral location and pressing or tightening quality. TTHs are usually of mild or moderate intensity and can last from minutes to days. TTHs are divided by frequency into episodic and chronic types (Headache Classification Committee of the IHS, 2018).

Etiology and Pathophysiology

It has long been thought that TTHs were the result of painfully sustained contraction of the muscles of the scalp and the neck; however, modern research points to the likelihood that neurobiological and genetic factors play a role in the development of TTH. Historically, TTH has been somewhat understudied compared to other headache types such as migraine. As a result, the pathophysiology of TTH is not fully understood (Mier & Dhadwal, 2018).

Clinical Manifestations

Patients usually present with a bilateral frontal–occipital headache described as a constant, dull pressure, or bandlike headache associated with neck pain and increased muscle tension. The headache may involve sensitivity to light or sound but does not involve nausea or vomiting. Increased resistance to passive movement of the head, and tenderness of the head and neck may be present. There is no prodrome, and physical activity does not aggravate symptoms. The headaches may occur

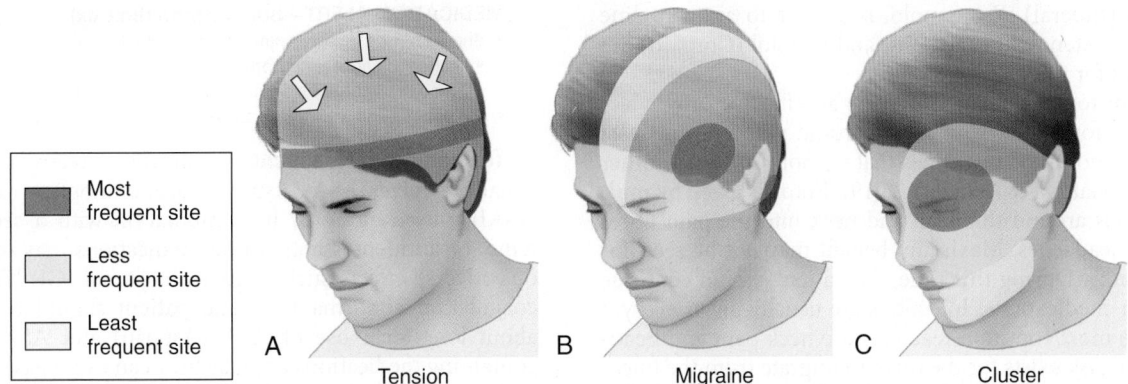

FIG. 61.1 Location of pain for common headache syndromes. **A,** Tension headache is often described as the feeling of a weight in or on the head or a band squeezing the head (or both). **B,** Migraine headache is described as an intense, throbbing, or pounding pain that involves one temple. The pain is usually unilateral, although it can be bilateral. **C,** Cluster headache pain is focused in and around one eye and is often described as sharp, penetrating, or burning.

Legend:
- Most frequent site
- Less frequent site
- Least frequent site

A — Tension
B — Migraine
C — Cluster

intermittently for weeks, months, or even years. Many patients can have a combination of migraine and TTHs, with features of both occurring simultaneously. Patients with MHs may experience TTHs between migraine attacks. Figure 61.1 shows the location of pain for common headache syndromes.

Diagnostic Studies

Generally speaking, TTH diagnosis is based on assessment of a patient's clinical symptoms and presentation. If a patient's presentation does not clearly fit the TTH picture or their usual headache pattern has changed, further diagnostic tests (e.g., CT scan and MRI) may be done to rule out secondary headache causes such as brain aneurysm, meningitis, concussion, and brain tumour.

CLUSTER HEADACHE

Cluster headaches (CHs) are a rare form of headache, affecting less than 1 in 1 000 adults (WHO, 2016). CHs are headaches that occur as frequently as one to eight times daily (in clusters) for weeks to months at a time, followed by periods of remission.

Etiology and Pathophysiology

Neither the cause nor the pathophysiological mechanism of CH is fully known. The trigeminal nerve is implicated in the production of pain, but CHs also involve dysfunction of intracranial blood vessels, the sympathetic nervous system, and pain modulation systems. Imaging studies show hypothalamic activation at the onset of CH (Hoffmann & May, 2018). Common triggers include but are not limited to alcohol, stress, hot and cold weather, sleep deprivation, bright lights, TV watching, and chocolate (Steinberg et al., 2018).

Clinical Manifestations

The CH is one of the most severe forms of headache and is characterized by intense, stabbing pain that is ipsilateral in nature and usually occurs at night or at the same time each day (Gargya & Abdallah, 2019). Other manifestations may include swelling around the eye, lacrimation (tearing), facial flushing or pallor, rhinitis, and constriction of the pupil (Buture et al., 2016). During the headache, the patient is often agitated and restless, unable to sit still or relax.

Diagnostic Studies

The diagnosis of CH is based primarily on the patient history and clinical presentation. Asking patients to keep a headache diary can be useful. CT scan, MRI, or magnetic resonance angiography (MRA) may be done to rule out an aneurysm, a tumour, or an infection. A lumbar puncture may be used to rule out other disorders that may cause similar symptoms.

OTHER TYPES OF HEADACHES

The inability to diagnose a headache as MH, TTH, or CH may indicate that the pain is a symptom of a more serious illness. Headache can accompany subarachnoid hemorrhage; brain tumours; other intracranial masses; arteritis; vascular abnormalities; trigeminal neuralgia (tic douloureux); diseases of the eyes, nose, and teeth; and systemic illness (e.g., bacteremia, carbon monoxide poisoning, mountain sickness, polycythemia vera). Given the many causes of headache, clinical evaluation should include an evaluation of personality, life adjustment, environment, and family situation as well as a comprehensive evaluation of neurological and physical status.

INTERPROFESSIONAL CARE FOR HEADACHES

If no systemic underlying disease is the cause, the type of headache guides therapy. Table 61.2 outlines the general workup for a patient with headache to rule out any intracranial or extracranial disease. Table 61.3 summarizes the current therapies for prophylaxis and symptom relief of common headaches. These therapies include medications, meditation, yoga, biofeedback, cognitive behavioural therapy, and relaxation training.

Medication Therapy

Migraine Headache. Medication treatment of the acute MH attack is aimed at terminating or decreasing the symptoms of the attack. Many people with mild or moderate MH can obtain relief with nonsteroidal anti-inflammatory drugs (NSAIDs), acetylsalicylic acid (ASA: Aspirin), or caffeine-containing combination analgesics. For moderate to severe headaches, triptans are the first line of therapy.

Triptans (e.g., sumatriptan [Imitrex]) affect selected serotonin receptors. They reduce neurogenic inflammation of the cerebral blood vessels and produce vasoconstriction. Because these medications cause constriction of coronary arteries, they must be avoided in patients with heart disease. Triptans should be taken at the first symptom of MH.

β Blockers have been effective in preventing migraine. Commonly prescribed agents include metoprolol (Lopressor) and propranolol (Inderal). Propranolol is similar to amitriptyline in its efficacy. Atenolol (Tenormin) and nadolol (Corgard) are other options for migraine prevention.

Botulinum toxin A (Botox) may be an effective prophylactic treatment for adults who have chronic migraines at least 15 days each month or migraines that do not respond to other medications (Gargya & Abdallah, 2019). Botox is given by multiple injections around the head and neck into the pain fibres involved in headaches. Maximum benefit may not be seen for up to 6 months. During this time, the patient should continue their regular medications. Injections are usually given every 3 months. The most common reactions are neck pain and headache. A slight risk exists for the toxin to migrate from the injection site to other areas of the face and neck, causing swallowing and breathing difficulties. The patient should be taught to seek immediate medical attention if this occurs.

TABLE 61.2 DIAGNOSTIC STUDIES

Headaches

- History and physical examination
- Neurological examination (often negative)
- Inspection for local infections
- Palpation for tenderness, bony swellings
- Auscultation for bruits over major arteries
- Routine laboratory studies
- CBC
- Electrolytes
- Urinalysis
- CT scan of sinuses
- Special studies (e.g., CT scan of brain, angiography, EEG, EMG, MRA, MRI, lumbar puncture)

CBC, complete blood cell count; *CT*, computed tomographic (scan); *EEG*, electroencephalography; *EMG*, electromyography; *MRA*, magnetic resonance angiography; *MRI*, magnetic resonance imaging.

MEDICATION ALERT—Sumatriptan (Imitrex)
- Should not be given to patients with a history of:
  - Ischemic cardiac, cerebrovascular, or peripheral vascular conditions
  - Uncontrolled hypertension (may increase BP)
- Excess dosage may cause tremor and decrease respirations.

Tension-Type Headache. Medication treatment for TTH usually involves ASA (Aspirin), acetaminophen (Tylenol), or NSAIDs used alone or in combination with a sedative, caffeine, or antidepressants; these medications may lead to serious adverse effects such as gastrointestinal (GI) bleeding and coagulation abnormalities. The patient should be cautioned about long-term use of ASA (Aspirin) and ASA (Aspirin)-containing medications because they can cause gastric bleeding and coagulation abnormalities in susceptible patients. Medications containing acetaminophen (Tylenol) can cause kidney damage with chronic use and liver damage when taking large doses or combined with alcohol. Antidepressants (e.g., amitriptyline [Elavil], nortriptyline [Aventyl], venlafaxine [Effexor], mirtazapine [Remeron]) and antiseizure medications (e.g., topiramate [Topamax], divalproate [Depakote]) may be prescribed.

MEDICATION ALERT—Topiramate (Topamax)
Teach patient to:
- Not abruptly stop therapy because this may cause seizures.
- Avoid tasks that require alertness (e.g., driving, operating heavy machinery) until response to the medication is known.
- Take adequate fluids to decrease risk for developing renal stones.
- Tell the health care provider if they are pregnant or want to become pregnant.

Cluster Headache. Triptans are the standard of treatment for occasional CH. Nasal administration or subcutaneous injection is appropriate. However, as discussed earlier, they are contraindicated for patients with vascular risk factors because of their vasoconstrictive effects.

TABLE 61.3 INTERPROFESSIONAL CARE

Headaches

	Migraine Headache	Tension-Type Headache	Cluster Headache
Diagnostic	• History*	• History*	• History*
Interprofessional Therapy			
Symptomatic	• Antiemetic: metoclopramide • Prokinetics: domperidone • Nonopioid analgesics: acetylsalicylic acid (ASA; Aspirin), acetaminophen (Tylenol), ibuprofen (Advil), naproxen (Naprosyn) • Sympatholytic (adrenergic blocking) agent: dihydroergotamine (DHE) via inhalation or intravenous • Triptans: sumatriptan (Imitrex), zolmitriptan (Zomig)	• Analgesic combinations: acetaminophen with caffeine, ibuprofen with caffeine • Nonopioid analgesics: acetylsalicylic acid (ASA; Aspirin), ibuprofen (Advil), acetaminophen (Tylenol) • Nonsteroidal anti-inflammatory medication: naproxen (Naprosyn)	• Oxygen • Sympatholytic (adrenergic blocking) agent: dihydroergotamine (DHE) via inhalation or intravenous • Triptans: sumatriptan (Imitrex), zolmitriptan (Zomig)
Prophylactic	• β-Adrenergic blockers: propranolol (Inderal), metoprolol (Lopresor), nadolol • Acupuncture • Anticonvulsant: valproic acid (Depakene), divalproex sodium (Epival), gabapentin (Neurontin), topiramate (Topamax) • Antidepressants: amitriptyline (Elavil), nortriptyline (Aventyl), venlafaxine (Effexor) • Biofeedback • Cognitive behavioural therapy • Relaxation therapy	• Acupuncture • Antidepressants: amitriptyline (Elavil), mirtazapine (Remeron), venlafaxine (Effexor) • Biofeedback • Cognitive behavioural therapy • Muscle relaxation training • Physiotherapy • Psychotherapy • Relaxation therapy	• Anticonvulsant: topiramate (Topamax) • Antimanic agent: lithium (Carbolith/Lithane) • Biofeedback • Calcium channel blocker: verapamil (Isoptin) • Corticosteroid: prednisone (Apo-prednisone) • Melatonin • Physiotherapy

*Magnetic resonance imaging (MRI) should be considered in patients with nonacute headache who have an unexplained abnormal neurological examination, an atypical headache or headache features, or an additional risk factor, such as immunodeficiency.

High-flow 100% oxygen by non-rebreather mask is well tolerated, safe, and effective as an alternative treatment. Oxygen delivered at a rate of 7 to 12 L/min for 15 minutes via mask (Brandt et al., 2020) may relieve headache by causing vasoconstriction and increasing synthesis of serotonin in the central nervous system (CNS). Treatment can be repeated after a 5-minute rest. A drawback to this treatment is that the patient must have continuous access to oxygen supply.

Persons with chronic CH often need preventive treatment. High-dose verapamil is the first-choice medication. It is typically given at double or more the dose used for other disorders. Because of its effects on cardiac conduction, verapamil should be started only after careful consideration of the risks. Careful monitoring is needed during treatment. For patient safety, an electrocardiogram (ECG) should be done with every dose increase and every 6 months during treatment. Other medication options may include lithium (Carbolith/Lithane), ergotamine, antiseizure medications (e.g., topiramate), and melatonin. Options for patients with refractory CHs include invasive nerve blocks, deep brain stimulation, and ablative neurosurgical procedures (e.g., percutaneous radiofrequency).

Other Headaches. Patients with frequent headaches may overuse analgesic medications. Such overuse can lead to chronic daily headache, also called *analgesic rebound headache* or *drug-induced headache*. Medications known to cause this condition are acetaminophen (Tylenol), ASA (Aspirin), NSAIDs (e.g., ibuprofen [Advil]), triptans, and opioids. Treatment can be difficult and involves gradual withdrawal, possible hospitalization, and initiation of prophylactic medications such as amitriptyline (Elavil).

NURSING MANAGEMENT HEADACHES

NURSING ASSESSMENT
Nursing assessment of a patient with headache (Table 61.4) should include data specific to the headache itself, such as the location and type of pain, onset, frequency, duration, relation to events (emotional, psychological, physical), and time of day of the occurrence. Information should also be obtained about previous illnesses, surgery, trauma, allergies, family history, and response to medication. The nurse should suggest that the patient keep a diary of headache episodes with specific details. This type of record can be of great help in determining the type of headache and the precipitating events. If the patient has a history of MH, TTH, or CH, it is important to determine if the quality of the headache has changed. This may be an important clue about the cause of the headache (Table 61.5).

NURSING DIAGNOSES
Nursing diagnoses for the patient with headache may include but are not limited to the following:
- *Acute pain* resulting from *biological injury agent*
- *Inadequate health management* resulting from *difficulty managing complex treatment regimen*

Additional information on nursing diagnoses for the patient with headache is presented in Nursing Care Plan (NCP) 61.1, Patient with Headache, available on the Evolve website.

PLANNING
The overall goals are that the patient with a headache will (1) have reduced or no pain, (2) understand triggering events and treatments, (3) use positive coping strategies to manage pain, and (4) have increased quality of life and decreased disability.

TABLE 61.4 NURSING ASSESSMENT
Headaches

Subjective Data
Important Health Information
Current health history: Pain assessment including location, characteristics, onset and duration, frequency, quality, intensity or severity of pain, and precipitating factors (nurse should use a pain scale and observation of actions for cognitively impaired individual); positive family history of headaches; history of recent ingestion of alcohol, caffeine, cheese, chocolate, monosodium glutamate, aspartame, lunch meats (nitrites in cured meats), sausage, hot dog, onion, avocado; level of hydration
Past health history: Seizures, cancer, recent fall or trauma, cranial infection, stroke; asthma or allergies; mental health disorder; relationship of headache to overwork, stress, menstruation, sexual activity, travel, bright lights, disruptions in sleep, or noxious environmental stimuli
Medications: Use of hydralazine, bromides, nitroglycerin, ergotamine (withdrawal), nonsteroidal anti-inflammatory medications, estrogen preparations, oral contraceptives, over-the-counter or prescription remedies
Surgery or other treatments: Craniotomy, sinus surgery, facial surgery, dental surgery

Symptoms
- Anorexia, nausea, vomiting (migraine prodrome)
- Vertigo, fatigue, weakness, paralysis, fainting, malaise
- *Migraine:* Aura; unilateral, severe, throbbing (possible switching of side) headache; visual disturbances; photophobia; phonophobia; dizziness; tingling or burning sensations
- *Tension-type:* Bilateral, bandlike, dull and persistent, base-of-skull headache, neck tenderness
- *Cluster:* Unilateral and severe, nocturnal headaches; nasal stuffiness, unilateral lacrimation

Objective Data
General
Anxiety, apprehension

Integumentary
Cluster: Forehead diaphoresis, pallor, unilateral facial flushing with cheek edema, conjunctivitis
Migraine: Generalized edema (prodrome), pallor, diaphoresis

Neurological
Horner syndrome (results from damage to sympathetic nerves and is signified by the following ipsilateral signs: pupillary contraction, ptosis, and a lack of facial sweating), restlessness *(cluster)*, hemiparesis *(migraine)*

Musculoskeletal
Neck stiffness (or nuchal rigidity) resulting from impaired neck flexion secondary to muscle spasms of the neck *(meningeal, tension-type)*, palpable neck and shoulder muscles *(tension-type)*

Possible Findings
Possible evidence of disease, deformity, or infection on brain imaging, cerebral angiogram, lumbar puncture, EEG, EMG; nonspecific brain imaging or laboratory tests

EEG, electroencephalography; *EMG,* electromyography.

NURSING IMPLEMENTATION
Caring for patients with headache can be challenging. Effective treatment may involve helping the patient examine the daily routine, recognize stressful situations, and develop effective coping strategies. The nurse needs to help the patient identify precipitating factors and develop ways to avoid or minimize them. Daily exercise, relaxation periods, and socialization should be encouraged as ways to decrease headaches. The nurse can suggest nonpharmacological pain control measures such as relaxation, medication, and yoga.

TABLE 61.5 COMMON SCREENING ASSESSMENT QUESTIONS TO DETERMINE TYPE OF HEADACHE

- When do the headaches occur?
- How frequent are the headaches?
- What is the duration of the headache(s)?
- Are there any known triggers for the headaches, such as environmental, food, or alcohol?
- Where do you feel the headache pain? Does the pain radiate?
- Do you experience any visual changes such as blurring or double vision?
- Do you experience any other symptoms, such as nausea, vomiting, dizziness, weakness, changes in speech, swallowing difficulty?
- What relieves the headache pain?

TABLE 61.6 PATIENT & CAREGIVER TEACHING GUIDE

Headaches

The following information should be included when teaching the caregiver about headaches.

1. Keep a diary or calendar of headaches and possible precipitating events.
2. Avoid factors that can trigger a headache:
   - Foods containing amines (cheese, chocolate), nitrites (meats such as hot dogs), vinegar, onions, or monosodium glutamate
   - Fermented or marinated foods
   - Caffeine
   - Nicotine
   - Ice cream
   - Alcohol (particularly red wine)
   - Emotional stress
   - Fatigue
   - Medications such as those containing ergot and monoamine oxidase inhibitors
3. Describe the purpose, action, dosage, and adverse effects of medications taken.
4. Be able to self-administer sumatriptan (Imitrex) subcutaneously if prescribed.
5. Use stress-reduction techniques such as relaxation.
6. Participate in regular exercise.
7. Contact the health care provider if any of the following occur:
   - Symptoms become more severe, last longer than usual, or are resistant to medication.
   - Nausea and vomiting (if severe or not typical), change in vision, or fever occurs with the headache.

The nurse must teach the patient about medications prescribed for preventive and symptomatic treatment of headache. The patient should be able to describe the purpose, action, dosage, and adverse effects of the medications. To prevent accidental overdose, the patient should be urged to make a written note of each dose of medication or headache remedy. In addition to using analgesics and analgesic combinations to relieve headache, the patient with migraines can seek a quiet, dimly lit environment. Massage and moist hot packs to the neck and head can help a patient with TTH.

For patients whose headaches are triggered by certain foods, dietary counselling by a registered dietitian should be provided. Patients are encouraged to eliminate foods that may provoke headaches. Active challenge and provocative testing with suspect foods may be necessary to determine specific causative agents. However, food triggers may change over time.

Patients should be taught to avoid smoking and exposure to triggers. CH attacks may occur at high altitudes with low oxygen levels, such as during air travel. Inhaled ergotamine may decrease the likelihood of these attacks. See Table 61.6 for a teaching guide for the patient with a headache.

The Evidence-Informed Practice box looks at evidence related to the efficacy of acupuncture in the treatment of MHs.

EVIDENCE-INFORMED PRACTICE

Research Highlight

What Is the Effectiveness of Using Acupuncture to Treat Migraine Headaches?

Clinical Question
For adults with migraine headaches (P), does acupuncture (I) versus pharmacological treatment (C) decrease migraine headache frequency or severity (O)?

Best Available Evidence
Summary evidence of randomized controlled trials (RCTs), systematic reviews, and expert opinion

Critical Appraisal and Synthesis of Evidence
- Four RCTs ($n = 965$) compared acupuncture with other treatments (e.g., botulinum toxin-A).
- Acupuncture is a traditional Chinese medicine practiced worldwide for its analgesic benefits.
- Migraine headache assessed was defined as lasting 15 or more days per month, with at least 8 days per month for at least 3 months in the absence of ongoing medication misuse.
- Acupuncture was demonstrated to reduce symptoms of migraine headache, decrease medication requirements, decrease mean number of headaches per month, and have fewer complications from treatment as compared to pharmacological intervention.
- Acupuncture may be as effective as prophylactic pharmacological treatment to prevent occurrence of migraine headache.

Conclusion
Acupuncture is beneficial for migraine headaches and should be considered as a treatment option.

Implications for Nursing Practice
- Inform patients that acupuncture can help reduce frequency of migraine headache occurrences.
- Advise patients of the mechanism of action and the minimal side effects associated with acupuncture.

Reference for Evidence
Sivapuram, M. S. (2020). The Joanna Briggs Institute (JBI) evidence summary. Migraine: Acupuncture. AN: JBI5365.

P, Patient population of interest; *I,* intervention or area of interest; *C,* comparison of interest or comparison group; *O,* outcomes of interest (see Chapter 1).

EVALUATION

Expected outcomes for the patient with headache are addressed in NCP 61.1, available on the Evolve website.

CHRONIC NEUROLOGICAL DISORDERS

SEIZURE DISORDER

Seizure disorder consists of a group of neurological diseases marked by recurring seizures. It is the fourth most common neurological disorder behind migraine, stroke, and Alzheimer's disease. A *seizure* is a transient, uncontrolled electrical discharge of neurons in the brain that interrupts normal function.

Epilepsy is a type of seizure disorder in which at least two spontaneous seizures occur more than 24 hours apart. Epilepsy affects approximately 0.6% of Canadians, with 75 to 85% of people with epilepsy receiving a diagnosis before age 18 (Epilepsy Canada, 2021).

Etiology and Pathophysiology

Approximately 50% of epilepsy cases are idiopathic (WHO, 2019). Seizures resulting from systemic and metabolic disturbances are not considered epilepsy if the seizures cease when the underlying health problem is corrected.

Often, seizures are symptoms of an underlying condition. The most common causes of seizures during the first 6 months of life are severe birth injury, CNS congenital defects, infections, and inborn metabolic disorders. In patients between 2 and 20 years of age, the primary causative factors are birth injury, infection, trauma, and genetic factors. In individuals between 20 and 30 years of age, seizure disorder usually occurs as the result of structural lesions, such as trauma, brain tumours, or vascular disease. After 50 years of age, primary causes of seizure disorders are cerebrovascular lesions and metastatic brain tumours. In adults, metabolic disturbances that provoke seizures include acidosis, electrolyte imbalances, hypoglycemia, hypoxia, alcohol and barbiturate withdrawal, dehydration, and water intoxication. Extracranial disorders that can cause seizures are heart, lung, liver, or kidney diseases; systemic lupus erythematosus; diabetes mellitus; hypertension; and septicemia.

The role of heredity in seizure disorders has been difficult to determine given the challenge of separating hereditary from environmental or acquired influences. Some families carry a predisposition to seizure disorders in the form of an inherently low threshold to seizure-producing stimuli, such as trauma, disease, and high fever.

Seizure disorder is characterized by a group of abnormal neurons that seem to fire without a clear cause. Any stimulus that causes the neuron's cell membrane to depolarize can cause this firing. It spreads by physiological pathways to involve near or distant areas of the brain. Localization of the seizure focus (the place where the seizure originates) is critical to the success of any possible surgical treatment.

Besides neuron alterations, changes in the function of astrocytes may play several key roles in recurring seizures. Activation of astrocytes by hyperactive neurons is one of the crucial factors that causes nearby neurons to generate an epileptic discharge. Researchers are also continuing to learn about abnormal neural antibodies that can cause seizures. N-methyl-d-aspartate (NMDA) receptor antibodies are present in the cerebrospinal fluid (CSF) in 80% of patients. The emerging concept of autoimmune seizure disorder may lead to better outcomes for patients whose condition is resistant to medication therapy (Gaspard, 2016).

Clinical Manifestations

The specific clinical manifestations of a seizure are determined by the site of the electrical disturbance. The International League Against Epilepsy (ILAE) Classification System is an essential tool for the interprofessional health care team (Table 61.7). Revised in 2017, this system is based on the clinical and electroencephalographic manifestations of seizures. In this system, seizures are divided into three major classes: generalized onset, focal onset, and unknown onset, with each of these classes further subdivided according to motor or nonmotor presentation. Depending on the type, a seizure may progress through several phases: (1) the *prodrome phase,* with signs or activities that precede a seizure; (2) the *aural phase,* with a sensory warning;

TABLE 61.7 INTERNATIONAL CLASSIFICATION OF SEIZURE TYPES

Focal Onset	Generalized Onset	Unknown Onset
Aware or impaired awareness Motor or nonmotor onset	Motor or nonmotor onset	Motor or nonmotor onset
Motor onset–type examples: • Automatisms • Atonic • Clonic • Epileptic spasms • Hyperkinetic • Myoclonic • Tonic	Motor onset–type examples: • Atonic • Epileptic spasms • Clonic • Myoclonic • Tonic • Tonic–clonic	Motor onset–type examples: • Epileptic spasms • Tonic–clonic
Nonmotor onset–type examples: • Autonomic • Behaviour arrest • Cognitive • Emotional • Sensory	Nonmotor (absence) onset–type examples: • Atypical • Eyelid myoclonia • Myoclonic • Typical	Nonmotor onset–type examples: • Behaviour arrest

Source: Adapted from Fisher, R. S., Cross, J. H., French, J. A., et al. (2017). Operational classification of seizure types by the International League Against Epilepsy: Position paper of the ILAE Commission for Classification and Terminology. *Epilepsia, 58*(4), 522–530.

(3) the *ictal phase,* with full seizure; and (4) the *postictal phase,* which is the period of recovery after the seizure.

Generalized Onset Seizures. Generalized seizures are characterized by bilateral synchronous epileptic discharges in the brain from the onset of the seizure. Because the entire brain is affected at the onset of the seizures, there is no warning or aura. In most cases, the patient loses consciousness for a few seconds to several minutes. There are a number of generalized seizure types. Some of the more common ones are discussed below.

Tonic–Clonic Seizures. Tonic–clonic seizure (formerly called *grand mal*) is the most common generalized onset motor seizure. It is characterized by loss of consciousness and falling to the ground if the patient is upright. The body stiffens (*tonic* phase) for 10 to 20 seconds and the extremities jerk (*clonic* phase) for another 30 to 40 seconds. Cyanosis, excessive salivation, tongue or cheek biting, and incontinence may accompany the seizure.

In the postictal phase, the patient usually has muscle soreness, feels tired, and may sleep for several hours. Some patients may not feel normal for several hours or days after a seizure. The patient has no memory of the seizure.

Other Generalized Onset Motor Seizures. Other types of generalized onset motor seizures include tonic and clonic. A *tonic seizure* involves a sudden onset of increased tone in the extensor muscles, contributing to sudden stiff movements. Tonic seizures most often occur in sleep and affect both sides of the body. Patients will fall if they are standing when the seizure occurs. Tonic seizures usually last less than 20 seconds. The patient usually stays aware. Clonic seizures begin with loss of awareness and sudden loss of muscle tone, followed by rhythmic limb jerking that may or may not be symmetrical. Clonic seizures are rare.

A generalized *atonic seizure* (or *drop attack*) involves either a tonic episode or a paroxysmal loss of muscle tone. It begins suddenly with the person falling to the ground. Seizures typically last less than 15 seconds. The person usually stays conscious and can resume normal activity immediately. Patients with atonic seizure are at great risk for head injury. They often have to wear protective helmets.

Generalized Onset Nonmotor (Absence) Seizures. Absence seizure usually occurs only in children and rarely beyond adolescence. This type of seizure may cease altogether as the child matures, or it may evolve into another type of seizure. A *typical absence seizure* is marked by a brief staring spell that resembles daydreaming. It often goes unnoticed because it lasts less than 10 seconds. Usually the patient is unresponsive when spoken to during the seizure. The electroencephalogram (EEG) has a classic spike-wave pattern with 3 per second.

In *atypical absence seizure,* the staring spell is accompanied by other signs and symptoms, such as eye blinking or jerking movements of the lips. This type of seizure often lasts more than 10 seconds (as much as 30 seconds), with a gradual beginning and end. If the patient has existing cognitive impairment, it may be hard to tell seizure activity from usual behaviour. Atypical absence seizures usually continue into adulthood. An EEG shows atypical spike-and-wave patterns, with fewer than 3 per second.

Other generalized onset nonmotor seizures include myoclonic and eyelid myoclonia. The *myoclonic absence seizure* is characterized by rhythmic arm abduction (3 movements per second) leading to progressive arm elevation. It usually lasts 10 to 60 seconds. *Eyelid myoclonia* refers to jerking of the eyelids (at least 3 per second), often with upward eye deviation.

Focal Onset Seizures. Focal onset seizures (previously known as *partial* or *partial focal seizures*) are one of the other major classes of seizures in the ILAE classification system. Focal seizures begin in a specific region of the cortex, as indicated by the EEG and the clinical manifestations. For example, if the discharging focus is located in the medial aspect of the postcentral gyrus, the patient may experience numbness and tingling in the leg on the side opposite the focus. If the discharging focus is located in the part of the brain that governs a particular function, manifestations of those functions (for example, sensory, motor, cognitive, or emotional) may occur.

Focal seizures may be confined to one side of the brain and remain partial, or focal, in nature, or they may spread to involve the entire brain, culminating in a generalized tonic–clonic seizure. Any tonic–clonic seizure that is preceded by an aura is a focal seizure that generalizes secondarily. Many tonic–clonic seizures that appear to be generalized from the outset may actually be secondary generalized seizures, but the preceding partial component may be so brief that it is undetected by the patient, by an observer, or even on the EEG. Unlike the primary generalized tonic–clonic seizure, the secondary generalized seizure may result in a transient residual neurological deficit postictally. This phenomenon is called *Todd paralysis* (focal weakness), which resolves after varying lengths of time.

Per the ILAE's updated classification system, focal seizures are further divided into (1) focal aware seizures (those with simple motor or sensory phenomena) and (2) focal impaired awareness seizures (those with complex symptoms).

Focal Aware Seizures. *Focal aware seizures* (formerly known as *simple partial seizures*) with elementary symptoms do not involve loss of consciousness and rarely last longer than 1 minute. They may involve motor, sensory, or autonomic phenomena, or a combination of these. The terms *focal motor, focal sensory,* and *jacksonian* have been used to describe seizures of the focal aware type.

Focal Impaired Awareness Seizures. In a *focal impaired awareness seizure* (previously called *complex partial seizures*), patients have a loss of consciousness or a change in their awareness, producing a dreamlike state. Their eyes are open. They make movements that may seem purposeful, but they cannot interact with observers. During a seizure, some people may do things that can be dangerous or embarrassing, such as walking into traffic or removing their clothes. They may continue an activity started before the seizure, such as counting coins or choosing items from a grocery shelf. After the seizure they do not remember the activity performed during the seizure. Seizures usually last 1 to 2 minutes. Patients may be tired or confused after the seizure and may not return to normal activity for hours.

The degree of awareness can be unspecified, and a seizure is classified as *motor* or *nonmotor*. Motor activities include *atonic* (loss of tone), *tonic* (sustained stiffening), *clonic* (rhythmic jerking), *myoclonic* (irregular, brief jerking), or *epileptic* spasms (flexion or extension of arms with flexion of trunk). Some people show strange behaviour, such as lip smacking or other repetitive, purposeless actions *(automatisms)*. With a focal nonmotor seizure, the patient can have emotional manifestations, such as fear or joy, strange feelings, or symptoms such as a racing heart, goose bumps, or waves of heat or cold.

Psychogenic Nonepileptic Seizures (PNES). Because of the close resemblance, psychogenic seizures may be misdiagnosed as seizure disorder. Proper diagnosis usually requires video-EEG monitoring to identify associated events. If the diagnosis of seizure disorder is excluded, history of emotional or physical abuse or a specific traumatic event often emerges. Some patients may have both psychogenic seizures and seizure disorder. Care provided by a specialist is essential. Once the diagnosis is made, the treatment of choice is psychological intervention.

Complications

Physical. Status epilepticus (SE) is a state of continuous seizure activity in which seizures recur in rapid succession without return to consciousness between seizures. SE is a neurological emergency and can involve any type of seizure. During repeated seizures, the brain uses more energy than can be supplied. Permanent brain damage may result. Tonic–clonic SE is the most dangerous type because it can cause ventilatory insufficiency, hypoxemia, cardiac dysrhythmias, hyperthermia, and systemic acidosis, all of which can be fatal. Airway securement via medical intervention using sedation and endotracheal intubation may be necessary to avoid life-threatening complications. Patients who lose consciousness during a seizure are at greatest risk. Death can result from head injury incurred during a fall, from drowning, or from severe burns. Perinatal seizures are associated with acute and long-term adverse outcomes to pregnant women and their babies (Razaz et al., 2017).

Psychosocial. Seizure disorders place many limitations on a patient's lifestyle. Epilepsy generally carries a social stigma, and patients diagnosed with seizure disorders may experience depression, anxiety, or anger, and relationships are often affected. The patient with epilepsy may experience discrimination in employment and educational opportunities. Obtaining a driver's license may be difficult because of legal sanctions against driving (Canadian League Against Epilepsy, 2020).

Depression is common among people with epilepsy (National Institute of Neurological Disorders and Stroke [NINDS], 2020). Not only can depression impair daily functioning, but it can also lead to increased seizure frequency through sleep deprivation and its role as an emotional stressor. Treatment for depression among patients with epilepsy should focus first on seizure control, and if depression persists in spite of this treatment, antidepressant medication and psychological therapy may be necessary.

Diagnostic Studies

The most useful diagnostic tools are accurate and comprehensive description of the seizures and the patient's health history (Table 61.8). The EEG is a useful diagnostic adjuvant to the history, but only if it shows abnormalities. Abnormal findings help determine the type of seizure and help pinpoint the seizure focus. Unfortunately, only a small percentage of patients with seizure disorders have abnormal findings on the EEG the first time the test is done. EEGs may need to be repeated often, or continuous EEG monitoring may be needed to detect abnormalities. Abnormal discharges may not occur during the 30 to 40 minutes of sampling during EEG, and the test may be negative. It is not a definitive test because some patients who do not have seizure disorders have abnormal patterns on their EEGs, whereas many patients with seizure disorders have normal EEGs between seizures. Magnetoencephalography may be done in conjunction with the EEG. This test has greater sensitivity in detecting small magnetic fields generated by neuronal activity. Video-EEG can give definitive diagnosis of seizures with impairment of consciousness.

A complete blood cell count, basic metabolic panel, studies of liver and kidney function, and urinalysis should be done to rule out metabolic disorders. A CT scan or MRI should be considered with any new-onset seizure to rule out structural abnormalities. Cerebral angiography, single-photon emission computed tomography (SPECT), magnetic resonance spectroscopy (MRS), MRA, and positron emission tomography (PET) may be used in select situations.

Interprofessional Care

Most seizures do not require professional emergency medical care because they are self-limiting and rarely cause bodily injury. However, if SE occurs, significant bodily harm occurs, or the event is a first-time seizure, medical care should be sought immediately. Table 61.9 summarizes emergency care of the patient with a generalized tonic–clonic seizure, the seizure most likely to warrant emergency medical care. The diagnostic studies and interprofessional care for seizure disorders are summarized in Table 61.8.

Medication Therapy. Seizure disorders are primarily treated with anticonvulsant medications (Table 61.10). Therapy is aimed at preventing seizures because a cure is not possible. Medications generally act by stabilizing nerve cell membranes and preventing spread of the epileptic discharge. Therapy should begin with a single medication based on the patient's age and weight and type, frequency, and cause of seizure. Dosage should be increased until seizures are under control or toxic adverse effects occur. Antiseizure medications successfully control seizures for about 70% of patients.

If seizure control is not achieved with a single medication, dosage or timing of administration may be changed or a second medication may be added. About one third of patients need a combination regimen for enough seizure control. Patients should discuss new treatments with their health care provider to provide the best control with the least amount of medication.

The therapeutic range for each medication indicates the serum level above which most patients experience toxic adverse effects and below which most continue to have seizures. Therapeutic ranges are only guides for therapy. If the patient's seizures are well controlled with a subtherapeutic level, the medication dose need not be increased. Likewise, if a medication level is above the therapeutic range and the patient has good seizure control without toxic adverse effects, the medication dose need not be decreased. Serum medication levels are monitored if seizures continue to occur, frequency increases, or medication adherence is questioned. Because they have a large therapeutic range, many newer medications do not require medication-level monitoring.

> **MEDICATION ALERT—Carbamazepine (Tegretol)**
> Patients taking carbamazepine should be instructed as follows:
> - Do not take with grapefruit juice.
> - Report visual abnormalities.
> - Be aware that abrupt withdrawal after long-term use may precipitate seizures.

For many years, the primary medications for treatment of generalized tonic–clonic and focal seizures were sodium channel blockers. Barbiturates, such as phenobarbital, also have a long history of use. Both sodium channel blockers and benzodiazepines are effective in the treatment of absence, akinetic, and myoclonic seizures.

The main medications used to treat tonic–clonic and focal onset seizures are phenytoin (Dilantin), carbamazepine (Tegretol), phenobarbital, and divalproex (Epival ECT). The medications used most often to treat generalized onset nonmotor and myoclonic seizures include ethosuximide (Zarontin), divalproex (Epival ECT), and clonazepam (Rivotril). Current medications used in seizure management are shown in Table 61.10. Some medications are effective for multiple seizure types. Pregabalin (Lyrica) is used as an additional treatment for focal aware or impaired awareness seizures not successfully controlled with one medication.

> **MEDICATION ALERT—Phenytoin (Dilantin)**
> - IV phenytoin (Dilantin) should be administered slowly to prevent acute hypotension.

TABLE 61.8 INTERPROFESSIONAL CARE	
Diagnosis of Seizure Disorders and Epilepsy	
Diagnostic	• Diagnostic studies
• History and physical examination	• CBC, urinalysis, electrolytes,
• Birth and development history	creatinine, fasting blood
• Comprehensive neurological	glucose
assessment	• CT, MRI, MRA, MRS, PET scan
• Family history	• EEG
• Febrile seizures	• Lumbar puncture
• Significant illnesses and injuries	
• Seizure history	**Interprofessional Therapy**
• Antecedent events	• Anticonvulsant medications
• Precipitating factors	(see Table 61.10)
• Seizure description (including	• Psychosocial counselling
onset, duration, frequency,	• Surgery (see Table 61.11)
postictal state)	• Vagal nerve stimulation

CBC, complete blood cell count; *CT*, computed tomographic (scan); *EEG*, electroencephalography; *MRA*, magnetic resonance angiography; *MRI*, magnetic resonance imaging; *MRS*, magnetic resonance spectroscopy; *PET*, positron emission tomography.

✚ TABLE 61.9   EMERGENCY MANAGEMENT

Tonic–Clonic Seizures

Etiology	Assessment Findings	Interventions
Head Trauma • Epidural hematoma • Subdural hematoma • Intracranial hematoma • Cerebral contusion • Traumatic birth injury **Medication-Related Processes** • Overdose • Withdrawal of alcohol, opioids, anticonvulsant medications • Ingestion, inhalation **Infectious Processes** • Meningitis • Septicemia • Encephalitis **Intracranial Events** • Brain tumour • Subarachnoid hemorrhage • Stroke • Neurodegenerative diseases • Hypertensive crisis • Increased ICP secondary to clogged shunt **Metabolic Imbalances** • Fluid and electrolyte imbalance • Hypoglycemia **Medical Disorders** • Heart, liver, lung, or kidney disease • Systemic lupus erythematosus **Other** • Cardiac arrest • Idiopathic • Psychiatric disorders • High fever • Autoimmune disease • Genetic diseases	• Aura—peculiar sensations that precede seizure • Loss of consciousness • Bowel and bladder incontinence • Tachycardia • Diaphoresis • Warm skin • Pallor, flushing, or cyanosis • *Tonic phase:* continuous muscle contractions • *Hypertonic phase:* extreme muscular rigidity lasting 5–15 sec • *Clonic phase:* rigidity and relaxation alternate in rapid succession • *Postictal phase:* lethargy, altered level of consciousness • Confusion and headache • Repeated tonic–clonic seizures for several minutes	**Initial** • Ensure patent airway (sedation may be required if teeth are clenched). • Apply oxygen as needed. • Assist ventilations if patient does not breathe spontaneously after seizure. Anticipate need for intubation if gag reflex is absent. • Suction as needed. • Stay with patient until seizure has passed. • Ensure safety at all times and protect patient from injury during seizure. *Do not restrain.* Pad side rails. • Establish IV access. • Anticipate administration of phenobarbital, phenytoin (Dilantin), or benzodiazepines (diazepam [Valium], midazolam, lorazepam [Ativan]) to control seizures. • Reposition patient to side-lying position when possible to avoid aspiration if patient vomits. • Remove or loosen tight clothing. **Ongoing Monitoring** • Monitor vital signs, level of consciousness, oxygen saturation, Glasgow Coma Scale score, pupil size and reactivity. • Reassure and orient patient after seizure. • Never force an airway between a patient's clenched teeth. • Give IV dextrose for hypoglycemia as per prescription.

ICP, intracranial pressure; *IV,* intravenous.

- Serum albumin levels should be measured along with serum phenytoin levels during therapeutic monitoring.
- Phenytoin (Dilantin) should be discontinued at the first sign of rash and anticonvulsive treatment, and therefore reassessed.
- Alcohol intake (acute and chronic) may affect phenytoin serum levels.

Adverse effects of anticonvulsant medications primarily involve the CNS and include diplopia, drowsiness, ataxia, and mental slowing. Neurological assessment for dose-related toxicity involves testing the eyes for nystagmus, hand and gait coordination, cognitive functioning, and general alertness. Abrupt discontinuation of anticonvulsant medications can precipitate seizures and can be life-threatening (Hall, 2019).

Idiosyncratic adverse effects involve organs outside the CNS, including skin (rashes), gingiva (hyperplasia), bone marrow (blood dyscrasias), liver, and kidneys. Nurses should be knowledgeable about medication adverse effects and teach patients about these effects. A common adverse effect of phenytoin is gingival hyperplasia (excessive growth of gingival tissue), especially in children and young adults. This can be limited by practising good dental hygiene. If gingival hyperplasia is extensive, the hyperplastic tissue may have to be surgically removed (gingivectomy), and phenytoin may have to be replaced by another medication. Because phenytoin can also cause hirsutism in young people, other medications are often used first.

Medication nonadherence can be a challenge among people with epilepsy because of the undesirable adverse effects. Measures should be taken to increase adherence to the prescribed medication regimens. If made aware of the issue, health care providers can work with the patient to find an acceptable medication regimen.

Surgical Therapy. Patients whose epilepsy cannot be controlled with medication therapy may be candidates for surgical intervention to remove the epileptic focus or prevent spread of epileptic activity in the brain (Table 61.11). About 30% of epilepsy patients have epilepsy that does not respond to antiseizure medications. For people with a defined site of seizure origin (epileptogenic zone), research shows the benefit of surgical resection of that focal area over continued use of different

TABLE 61.10 MEDICATION THERAPY

Epilepsy

Medication	Average Adult Daily Dosage	Possible Adverse Effects
carbamazepine (Tegretol)	800–1 200 mg	Dizziness, drowsiness, blurred or double vision, nausea, skin rashes, blood abnormalities
clobazam	30–40 mg	Drowsiness, dizziness, fatigue
clonazepam (Rivotril)	8–10 mg	Drowsiness, clumsiness, behaviour changes, tremor, appetite loss
divalproex sodium (Epival)	1 750–3 000 mg	Upset stomach, altered bleeding time, liver toxicity (rare), hair loss, weight gain, tremor
ethosuximide (Zarontin)	500 mg	Appetite loss, nausea, drowsiness, headache, dizziness, fatigue
gabapentin (Neurontin)	900–2 400 mg	Somnolence, fatigue, dizziness
lamotrigine (Lamictal)	100–500 mg	Headache, fatigue, nausea, dizziness, clumsiness, serious and life-threatening rash (rare), double or blurred vision
levetiracetam (Keppra)	1 000–3 000 mg	Dizziness, somnolence, asthenia (weakness), low hematocrit and leukocyte count (rare), depression and mood swings
oxcarbazepine (Trileptal)	1 200–2 400 mg	Somnolence, diplopia, rash, hyponatremia, ataxia and staggering gait
phenobarbital	30–600 mg	Drowsiness, irritability, hyperactivity, somnolence
phenytoin (Dilantin)	300 mg	Clumsiness, drowsiness, nausea, rash, gum overgrowth, hairiness, thickening of features
primidone	250–1 000 mg	Clumsiness, dizziness, appetite loss, fatigue, drowsiness, hyperirritability
topiramate (Topamax)	200–600 mg	Drowsiness, dizziness, weight loss, tingling, decreased alertness, kidney stones (rare)
valproic acid (Depakene)	1 750–3 000 mg	Upset stomach, altered bleeding time, liver toxicity

Source: Adapted from Epilepsy Canada. (1987 [revised 2009]). *Your medication for epilepsy* (pp. 12–13). Author. http://www.epilepsy.ca/uploads/7/0/8/6/70868839/medication-new.pdf

TABLE 61.11 SURGICAL PROCEDURES FOR SEIZURE DISORDERS AND EPILEPSY

Type of Seizure	Surgical Procedure	Results
Focal impaired awareness seizures of temporal lobe origin	Resectioning of epileptogenic tissue	Absence of seizures 5 yr postoperatively in 55–70% of patients
Focal seizures of frontal lobe origin	Resectioning of epileptogenic tissue (if in resectable area)	Absence of seizures 5 yr postoperatively in 30–50% of patients
Generalized seizures (Lennox–Gastaut syndrome or drop attacks)	Sectioning of corpus callosum	Persistence of seizures; less violent, less frequent, less disabling events
Intractable, unilateral multifocal epilepsy associated with infantile hemiplegia	Hemispherectomy or callosotomy	Reduction in seizure frequency and type, improvement in behaviour

antiseizure medications. About 80% are seizure free 5 years after surgery, with 72% still seizure free at 10 years.

For patients for whom surgery is an option, an extensive preoperative evaluation is important, including continuous EEG monitoring and other tests to ensure precise localization of the focal point. Surgical candidates must meet three requirements: (1) a confirmed diagnosis of seizure disorder, (2) an adequate trial with medication therapy without satisfactory results, and (3) a defined electroclinical syndrome (type of seizure disorder).

Alternate Therapies. *Vagal nerve stimulation* (VNS), a form of neuromodulation, is used as an adjunct to medications when an accessible focal point cannot be identified for surgical removal. The exact mechanism of action is unknown. It may increase blood flow to specific brain areas. It could raise levels of neurotransmitters important to seizure control and change EEG patterns during a seizure. In VNS, a surgically implanted electrode in the neck is programmed to deliver electrical impulses to the vagus nerve, usually on the left side. The patient activates the electrode with a magnet when they sense a seizure is imminent. Newer devices respond to an increasing heart rate, which is often associated with seizures. Adverse effects include coughing, hoarseness, dyspnea, and tingling in the neck. Battery life is 5 to 10 years, and surgical replacement is needed. Benefits of VNS can be seen within 24 months after implantation. Contraindications include a history of dysrhythmias or sleep apnea.

Responsive neurostimulation (RNS) is similar to a cardiac pacemaker. It continually monitors the EEG to detect abnormalities, then responds to seizure activity by delivering electrical stimulation to a precise location. The device is placed under the skin, outside the skull, with connections to electrodes over the area of seizure focus. The health care provider uses a programmable wand to download information about seizure activity. This is used to assess treatment efficacy and guide care. This modality is an option for persons who are not surgical candidates or have multiple areas of seizure focus.

A *ketogenic diet* is a special high-fat, low-carbohydrate diet that helps control seizures in some people (Poff et al., 2019). A person on this diet produces ketones that pass into the brain, where they replace glucose as an energy source. Meals are carefully planned to restrict the amount of protein and carbohydrate in the diet. Patients on this diet who take vitamin K antagonists (e.g., warfarin) and who therefore follow a vitamin K–restricted diet may need closer monitoring of their anticoagulation levels, especially in cases where there is a significant increase in the dietary intake of vitamin K–rich foods (Westman et al., 2018). Although health care providers are more likely to recommend the diet for children than for adults, the diet can work equally well in both age groups. Most people must continue their use of antiseizure medication but may take smaller doses or fewer medications. Seizures may worsen if the diet is stopped abruptly. Long-term effects of the diet are not clear.

Biofeedback to control seizures is aimed at teaching patients to maintain a certain brain wave frequency that is refractory to seizure activity. For patients with seizures, biofeedback involves attaching sensors to a patient's skin (e.g., to the scalp or hands) to monitor for potential signs of seizure. In a systematic review that examined the effectiveness of galvanic skin response (GSR) biofeedback in adult patients with medication-resistant epilepsy, the authors found that GSR reduced seizure frequency in over 70% of participants (Nagai et al., 2019).

NURSING MANAGEMENT SEIZURE DISORDERS AND EPILEPSY

NURSING ASSESSMENT

Data that should be obtained from a patient with a seizure disorder are presented in Table 61.12. Data related to a specific seizure episode can be obtained from a witness.

NURSING DIAGNOSES

Nursing diagnoses for the patient with seizure disorders and epilepsy may include but are not limited to the following:

- *Inadequate breathing pattern* resulting from *body position that inhibits lung expansion* (neuromuscular impairment)
- *Inadequate health management* resulting from *difficulty managing complex treatment regimen* (medication therapy and lifestyle adjustment)
- *Potential for injury* as demonstrated by *alteration in cognitive functioning, alteration in psychomotor functioning* (seizure)

Additional information on nursing diagnoses for the patient with a seizure disorder is presented in NCP 61.2, available on the Evolve website.

PLANNING

The overall goals are that the patient with seizures will (1) be free from injury during a seizure, (2) have optimal mental and physical functioning while taking anticonvulsant medications, and (3) have satisfactory psychosocial functioning.

NURSING IMPLEMENTATION

HEALTH PROMOTION. Complications such as head injury related to seizure disorders can be prevented through general safety measures such as the wearing of helmets. Optimal perinatal care facilitates reduced fetal trauma and hypoxia and, therefore, reduced brain damage leading to seizure disorders.

The patient with a seizure disorder should practise good general health habits (e.g., maintaining a proper diet, getting adequate rest, exercising). Nurses should help patients identify events or situations that precipitate seizures and provide suggestions for avoiding or managing them more effectively. The patient should be taught to reduce stressors and avoid excessive alcohol intake, fatigue, and loss of sleep.

ACUTE INTERVENTION. Nursing care of a patient who is hospitalized with seizures involves several responsibilities, including observation and treatment of the seizure, education, and psychosocial intervention. When a seizure occurs, nurses should carefully observe and record details of the event, as the diagnosis and subsequent treatment often rest solely on the seizure description. All aspects of the seizure should be noted. What events preceded the seizure? When did the seizure occur? How long did each phase last? What occurred during each phase?

Both subjective and objective data are important. Objective data should include the exact time of seizure onset; the course and nature of the seizure activity (loss of consciousness, tongue biting, automatisms, stiffening, jerking, total lack of muscle tone); the body parts involved and their sequence

---

TABLE 61.12 NURSING ASSESSMENT

Seizure Disorders and Epilepsy

Subjective Data

Important Health Information

Past health history: Previous seizures, birth defects, or injuries; anoxic episodes; CNS trauma, tumours, or infections; stroke; metabolic disorders; alcoholism; exposure to metals and carbon monoxide; hepatic or renal failure; fever; pregnancy; systemic lupus erythematosus; positive family history of seizure disorders or epilepsy

Medications: Adherence to anticonvulsant medications; barbiturate or alcohol withdrawal; use of cocaine, amphetamines, lidocaine, theophylline (Uniphyl), penicillins, lithium (Carbolith/Lithane), phenothiazines, tricyclic antidepressants, benzodiazepines

Symptoms

- Headaches, aura, mood or behavioural changes before seizure; mentation changes; abdominal pain, muscle pain (postictal)
- Anxiety, depression; loss of self-esteem, social isolation
- Decreased sexual drive, erectile dysfunction; increased sexual drive (postictal)

Objective Data

General

Precipitating factors, including severe metabolic acidosis or alkalosis, hyperkalemia, hypoglycemia, dehydration, or water intoxication

Integumentary

Bitten tongue, soft tissue damage, cyanosis, diaphoresis (postictal)

Respiratory

Abnormal respiratory rate, rhythm, or depth; apnea (ictal); absent or abnormal breath sounds, possible airway occlusion

Cardiovascular

Hypertension, tachycardia, or bradycardia (ictal)

Gastrointestinal

Bowel incontinence; excessive salivation

Urinary

Incontinence

Neurological

Generalized

Tonic–clonic: Loss of consciousness, muscle tightening, then jerking; dilated pupils; hyperventilation, then apnea; postictal somnolence

Absence: Altered consciousness, minor facial motor activity

Focal Onset

Focal aware: Aura; consciousness; focal sensory, motor, cognitive, or emotional phenomena (focal motor); unilateral "marching" motor seizure (jacksonian)

Focal impaired awareness: Altered consciousness with inappropriate behaviours, automatisms, amnesia of event

Musculoskeletal

Weakness, paralysis, ataxia (postictal)

Possible Findings

Positive toxicology screen or alcohol level; altered serum electrolytes, acidosis or alkalosis, very low blood glucose level, increased blood urea nitrogen or creatinine, liver function tests, ammonia; abnormal CT scan or MRI of head, abnormal findings from lumbar puncture; abnormal discharges on EEG.

CNS, central nervous system; *CT,* computed tomographic (scan); *EEG,* electroencephalography; *MRI,* magnetic resonance imaging.

of involvement; and the presence of autonomic signs, such as dilated pupils, excessive salivation, altered breathing, cyanosis, flushing, diaphoresis, or incontinence. Assessment of the post-ictal period should include a detailed description of level of consciousness, vital signs, memory loss, muscle soreness, speech disorders (aphasia, dysarthria), weakness or paralysis, sleep period, and the duration of each sign or symptom.

SAFETY ALERT

During a seizure, the nurse should:

- Maintain a patent airway for the patient. This may be facilitated by turning the patient to the side and ensuring the tongue falls forward so as not to block the patient's airway.
- Protect the patient's head, turn the patient to the side, loosen constrictive clothing, and ease the patient to the floor (if seated).
- Not restrain the patient.
- Not place any objects in the patient's mouth.

After the seizure, the patient may require repositioning, suctioning, and oxygen; therefore, the nurse should ensure that oxygen and suction equipment are available and in working order for patients with a history of seizures. A seizure can be a frightening experience for the patient and for others who may witness it. The nurse needs to assess their level of understanding and provide information about how and why the event occurred. This is an excellent opportunity for the nurse to dispel many common misconceptions about seizures.

AMBULATORY AND HOME CARE. Prevention of recurring seizures is the major goal of treatment. The nurse can help the patient understand that for treatment to be effective, medications must be taken regularly and consistently. The nurse should review details of the medication plan and what to do if a dose is missed. Usually, the dose should be made up if the omission is remembered within 24 hours. The patient should be cautioned to not adjust medication doses without professional guidance as this can increase seizure frequency and even cause SE. The patient should be encouraged to report any medication adverse effects and to keep regular appointments with their health care provider.

Nurses play an important role in teaching patients and caregivers. Caregivers should be taught the emergency management of tonic–clonic seizures (see Table 61.9). The nurse should remind them that it is not necessary to call an ambulance or send a person to the hospital after a single seizure unless the seizure is prolonged, another seizure immediately follows, extensive injury has occurred, or it is unknown if this was a first-time seizure. Guidelines for teaching are shown in Table 61.13.

Patients with seizure disorder also experience concerns or fears related to recurrent seizures, incontinence, and loss of self-control. The nurse can support patients through education and by helping patients use effective coping mechanisms.

Perhaps the greatest challenge that a seizure disorder presents to the patient is adjusting to the limitations imposed by the condition. Discrimination at work can be a serious problem for persons with seizure disorder. For issues relating to job discrimination, patients can be referred to the Canadian Human Rights Commission through its national or regional offices.

A variety of other resources can be offered to the patient with a seizure disorder. Patients should be informed that medical alert bracelets, necklaces, and identification cards are available through a number of North American companies specializing in identification devices (e.g., MedicAlert). If the nurse believes that associating with others who have a seizure disorder would be beneficial, the patient can be referred to Epilepsy Canada, a voluntary agency with local members'

TABLE 61.13	**PATIENT & CAREGIVER TEACHING GUIDE**

Seizure Disorders and Epilepsy

The following information should be included when teaching the patient and caregiver about seizure disorders and epilepsy:

1. Medications must be taken as prescribed. Adverse effects of medications should be reported to the health care provider. When necessary, blood work may be drawn to ensure that therapeutic medication levels are maintained.
2. Use of nonpharmacological techniques, such as diet and biofeedback training, to potentially reduce the number of seizures
3. Availability of community resources
4. Need to wear a medical alert bracelet or necklace and carry an identification card
5. Avoidance of excessive alcohol intake, fatigue, and loss of sleep
6. Regular meals and snacks in between if feeling shaky, faint, or hungry

Caregivers should be taught the following:

1. For first aid treatment of tonic–clonic seizure, it is not necessary to call an ambulance or send the patient to the hospital after a single seizure unless the seizure is prolonged, another seizure immediately follows, or extensive injury has occurred.
2. During an acute seizure, it is important to protect the patient from injury. This may involve supporting and protecting the head, turning the patient to their side, loosening constrictive clothing, and easing the patient to a lying position on the floor, if seated.

associations across the country that offer a variety of services to patients with epilepsy. Patients who are eligible veterans can be referred to Veterans Affairs Canada to explore services for which they may qualify.

Social workers and welfare agencies can help with financial difficulties and living arrangements. Provincial and territorial services for individuals with developmental disabilities include assistance with vocational assessment and training, sheltered housing, funding for special needs, and placement for patients whose seizures are not well controlled. They can also offer financial assistance for transportation and medical costs related to vocational rehabilitation or job maintenance. If psychological counselling is needed, the nurse can refer the patient to a community mental health centre.

Patients should be encouraged to learn more about epilepsy through self-education materials. Epilepsy Canada provides information pamphlets and may facilitate support groups. Many agencies that offer services to people with epilepsy, as well as many locally based epilepsy associations, have these services available.

EVALUATION

Expected outcomes for patients with seizures are addressed in NCP 61.2.

MULTIPLE SCLEROSIS

Multiple sclerosis (MS) is a chronic, progressive, degenerative, autoimmune disorder of the CNS characterized by disseminated demyelination of nerve fibres of the brain, the spinal cord, and the optic nerves. Among adults aged 20 years and older, over 77 000 Canadians live with MS, 75% of whom are women (Government of Canada, 2019). Provincial data suggest that Canada has one of highest prevalence rates of MS in the world (Gilmour et al., 2018). The usual age of onset of MS is between 20 and 50 years of age, with symptoms often first appearing at 30 to 35 years of age. People diagnosed at 50 years of age or older generally have more progressive disease.

MS is more prevalent in temperate climates (between 45 and 65 degrees of latitude), such as those found in the northern United States, Canada, and Europe. People who are born in a high-risk area and move to a low-risk area before age 15 assume the risk of their new home. It is suspected that exposure to some environmental agent before puberty may cause a person to develop MS later in life. MS is less common among Hispanics, Asians, and people of African descent. It rarely occurs in some ethnic groups, including Alaskan Natives and Indigenous people. In fact, one Canadian study found that the incidence and prevalence of MS among Indigenous Canadians is two times lower than for non-Indigenous Canadians (Marrie et al., 2018).

Etiology and Pathophysiology

While the cause of MS is not known, it is unlikely due to a single cause. It is thought that MS develops in a genetically susceptible person after an environmental exposure, such as an infection. The inherited susceptibility to MS likely involves multiple genes. Having a first-degree relative with MS increases a person's risk for developing the disease. Common genetic factors in families with more than one affected member have been found (National Multiple Sclerosis Society, 2021).

Possible precipitating factors include infection, smoking, physical injury, emotional stress, excessive fatigue, pregnancy, and a poor state of health. The role of factors such as exposure to pathogens has yet to be determined. More than a dozen viruses and bacteria have been investigated but have not been proven to cause MS.

MS is marked by three processes: chronic inflammation, demyelination, and gliosis in the CNS. The primary condition is an autoimmune process driven by activated T cells. An unknown trigger in a genetically susceptible person may start this process. The activated T cells in the systemic circulation go to the CNS and disrupt the blood–brain barrier. This may be the first event in the development of MS. Subsequent antigen–antibody reaction within the CNS activates the inflammatory response and leads to axon demyelination.

Initially, the myelin sheaths of the neurons in the brain and spinal cord are attacked (Figure 61.2, *A* and *B*). Early in the disease, the myelin sheath is damaged, but the nerve fibre is not affected and nerve impulses are still transmitted (see Figure 61.2, *C*). At this point, the patient may complain of a noticeable impairment of function (e.g., weakness). However, the myelin can regenerate, and the symptoms disappear, resulting in a remission.

In addition to myelin disruption, the axon also becomes involved (see Figure 61.2, *D*). Myelin is replaced by glial scar tissue, which forms hard, sclerotic plaques in multiple regions of the CNS (Figure 61.3). Without myelin, nerve impulses slow down, and with destruction of nerve axons, impulses are totally blocked, resulting in permanent loss of function. In many chronic lesions, demyelination continues with progressive loss of nerve function.

The average life expectancy after the onset of symptoms is more than 25 years. Death usually occurs from infectious complications of immobility (e.g., pneumonia) or because of an unrelated disease.

Clinical Manifestations

The onset of MS is often slow and gradual. Vague symptoms occur periodically over months or years. Because they do not prompt the patient to seek medical attention, MS may not be diagnosed until long after the first symptom. For some patients, MS is marked by rapid, progressive deterioration. Others have remissions and exacerbations. With repeated exacerbations, the overall trend is progressive deterioration in neurological function. Figure 61.4 provides a general overview of the effects MS can have on bodily systems.

Because changes from MS have a spotty distribution in the CNS, symptoms vary with each patient based on the areas of the CNS involved. Some patients have severe, long-lasting symptoms early in the course of the disease. Others have only occasional, mild symptoms for several years after onset. A classification scheme of MS, with four primary patterns, has been developed on the basis of clinical course (Table 61.14).

Common signs and symptoms of MS include motor, sensory, cerebellar, and emotional conditions. Motor symptoms include weakness or paralysis of the limbs, the trunk, or the head; diplopia;

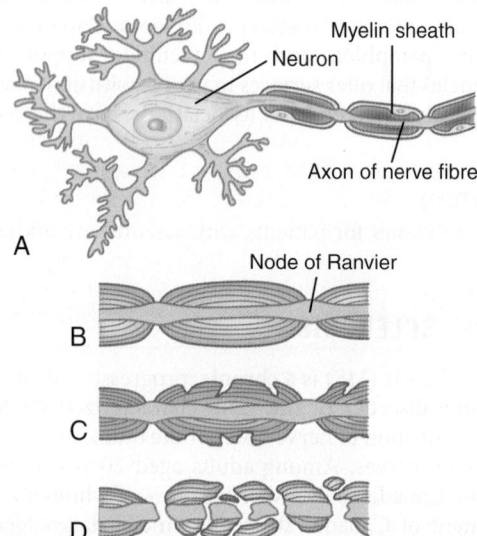

FIG. 61.2 Pathogenesis of multiple sclerosis. **A,** Normal nerve cell with myelin sheath. **B,** Normal axon. **C,** Myelin breakdown. **D,** Myelin totally disrupted; axon not functioning.

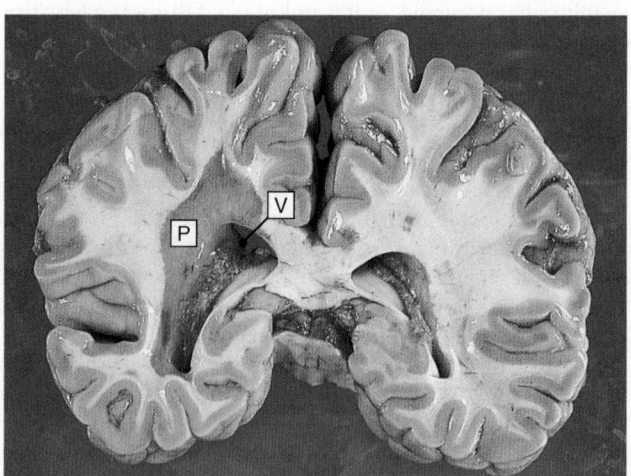

FIG. 61.3 Chronic multiple sclerosis. Demyelination plaque *(P)* at grey-white junction and adjacent partially remyelinated shadow plaque *(V)*. Source: Stevens, A., & Lowe, J. (2000). *Pathology: Illustrated review in colour* (2nd ed.). Mosby.

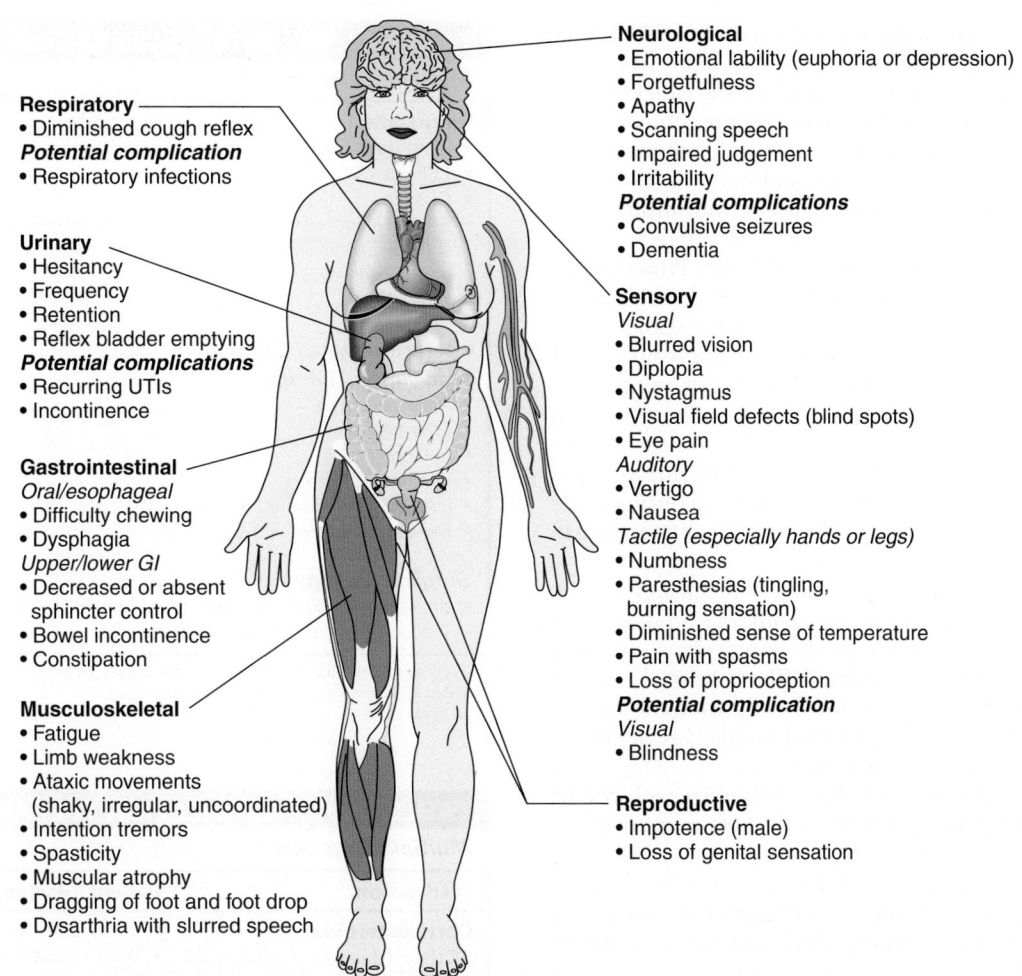

Respiratory
- Diminished cough reflex
Potential complication
- Respiratory infections

Urinary
- Hesitancy
- Frequency
- Retention
- Reflex bladder emptying
Potential complications
- Recurring UTIs
- Incontinence

Gastrointestinal
Oral/esophageal
- Difficulty chewing
- Dysphagia
Upper/lower GI
- Decreased or absent sphincter control
- Bowel incontinence
- Constipation

Musculoskeletal
- Fatigue
- Limb weakness
- Ataxic movements (shaky, irregular, uncoordinated)
- Intention tremors
- Spasticity
- Muscular atrophy
- Dragging of foot and foot drop
- Dysarthria with slurred speech

Neurological
- Emotional lability (euphoria or depression)
- Forgetfulness
- Apathy
- Scanning speech
- Impaired judgement
- Irritability
Potential complications
- Convulsive seizures
- Dementia

Sensory
Visual
- Blurred vision
- Diplopia
- Nystagmus
- Visual field defects (blind spots)
- Eye pain
Auditory
- Vertigo
- Nausea
Tactile (especially hands or legs)
- Numbness
- Paresthesias (tingling, burning sensation)
- Diminished sense of temperature
- Pain with spasms
- Loss of proprioception
Potential complication
Visual
- Blindness

Reproductive
- Impotence (male)
- Loss of genital sensation

FIG. 61.4 Common effects of multiple sclerosis on bodily systems. *GI,* gastrointestinal; *UTIs,* urinary tract infections. Source: Lemone, P. T., Burke, K. M., & Bauldoff, G. (2011). *Medical-surgical nursing: Critical thinking in patient care* (5th ed.). Reprinted by permission of Pearson Education, Inc.

TABLE 61.14	CLINICAL COURSES OF MULTIPLE SCLEROSIS (MS)
Category	**Characteristics**
Clinically isolated syndrome (CIS)	CIS is defined by a single episode of neurological symptoms reminiscent of MS.
Relapsing–remitting MS (RRMS)	Clearly defined relapses with full recovery or sequelae and residual deficit on recovery. This is the most common form of MS.
Primary-progressive MS (PPMS)	Slow and steady disease progression from onset with occasional plateaus and temporary minor improvements; no clear relapses or remissions
Secondary-progressive MS (SPMS)	A relapsing–remitting initial course, followed by progression with or without occasional relapses, minor remissions, and plateaus. Disability generally accumulates over time.
Progressive–relapsing MS (PRMS)	Progressive disease from onset, with clear acute relapses, with or without full recovery. Periods between relapses are characterized by continuing progression, occurring in approximately 5% of cases of MS.

Source: Adapted from Multiple Sclerosis Society of Canada. (2016). *Types of MS.* https://mssociety.ca/about-ms/types

scanning speech (spoken words are unintentionally slowed or injected with pauses between syllables and may be accompanied by involuntary variations in vocal tone); and spasticity of the muscles that are chronically affected. Patients with MS experience a variety of sensory abnormalities, including numbness, tingling and other paresthesias, patchy blindness (scotomas), blurred vision, vertigo, tinnitus, decreased hearing, and chronic neuropathic pain. Radicular (nerve root) pain may be present, particularly in the low thoracic and abdominal regions. *Lhermitte sign* is a transient sensory symptom described as an electric shock radiating down the spine or into the limbs with flexion of the neck. Cerebellar signs include nystagmus, ataxia, dysarthria, and dysphagia. Severe fatigue is present in many patients with MS, and it causes significant disability for some patients.

Bowel and bladder function can be affected if the sclerotic plaque is located in areas of the CNS that control elimination. Issues with defecation usually involve constipation rather than fecal incontinence. Urinary disorders are variable. A common condition in patients with MS is a *spastic* (uninhibited) bladder, indicating a lesion above the second sacral nerve, which cuts off suprasegmental inhibiting influences on bladder contractility. As a result, the bladder has a small capacity for urine, and its contractions are unchecked. This condition is accompanied by urinary urgency and frequency and results in dribbling or incontinence. A *flaccid* (hypotonic) bladder occurs with a lesion in the reflex arc controlling bladder function. The patient generally has urinary retention because there is no sensation or desire to void, no pressure, and no pain. Urgency and frequency may be present. A combination of spastic and flaccid bladder can occur. Urinary conditions can be diagnosed with urodynamic studies.

Sexual issues occur in many people with MS. Physiological erectile dysfunction may result from spinal cord involvement in men. Women may have decreased desire for sexual activity (libido), difficulty with orgasm, painful intercourse, and decreased vaginal lubrication. Decreased sensation can prevent a normal sexual response in men and women. The emotional effects of chronic illness and the loss of self-esteem can contribute to loss of sexual response. Some women with MS have remission or an improvement in their symptoms during pregnancy. Hormonal changes associated with pregnancy appear to affect the immune system.

MS has no apparent effect on the course of pregnancy, labour, delivery, or lactation. Some women with MS who become pregnant experience remission or an improvement in their symptoms during the gestation period. The hormonal changes associated with pregnancy appear to affect the immune system. However, during the postpartum period, women are at greater risk for remission relapses (Kamel, 2019).

About half of people with MS have difficulties with cognitive function. Most involve problems with short-term memory, attention, information processing, planning, visual perception, and word finding. General intellect stays unchanged and intact. This includes long-term memory, conversational skills, and reading comprehension. Symptoms can be mild and thus easily overlooked.

Diagnostic Studies

Because there is no definitive diagnostic test for MS, the history, manifestations, and results of certain diagnostic tests are important in establishing a diagnosis (Table 61.15). Imaging in MS is vital. An MRI of the brain and spinal cord may show plaques, inflammation, atrophy, and tissue breakdown and destruction. CSF analysis may show an increase in immunoglobulin G and the presence of oligoclonal banding (Thompson et al., 2018). Evoked potential responses are often delayed because of decreased nerve conduction from the eye and ear to the brain.

To be diagnosed with MS, the patient must have (1) evidence of at least two inflammatory demyelinating lesions in at least two different locations within the CNS, (2) damage or an attack occurring at different times (usually 1 month or more apart), and (3) all other possible diagnoses ruled out. If evidence exists for only one lesion, or only one clinical attack has occurred, the interprofessional team should monitor the patient for another attack or for an attack at a different site in the CNS.

Interprofessional Care

Medication Therapy. Because no cure currently exists for MS, interprofessional care is aimed at treating the disease process and providing symptomatic relief (see Table 61.15). The goal of medication therapy is to decrease the progression of the disease process and control symptoms with a variety of medications and other forms of therapy. Adrenocorticotrophic

TABLE 61.15	INTERPROFESSIONAL CARE

Multiple Sclerosis

Diagnostic
- History and physical examination
- CSF analysis
- CT scan
- Evoked response testing (also called *evoked potential testing*, e.g., somatosensory evoked potential [SSEP], auditory evoked potential [AEP], visual evoked potential [VEP])
- MRI, MRS

Interprofessional Therapy
Medication Therapy*
- Anticholinergics
- Cholinergics
- Corticosteroids
- Immunomodulators
- Immunosuppressants
- Muscle relaxants

Surgical Therapy
- Neurectomy, rhizotomy, cordotomy (unmanageable spasticity)
- Thalamotomy (unmanageable tremor)

CSF, cerebrospinal fluid; *CT*, computed tomographic (scan); *MRI*, magnetic resonance imaging; *MRS*, magnetic resonance spectroscopy.
*See Table 61.16.

TABLE 61.16	MEDICATION THERAPY

Multiple Sclerosis

Medication	Patient Teaching
Corticosteroids ACTH, prednisone, methylprednisolone (Solu-Medrol)	• Restrict salt intake. • Do not abruptly stop therapy. • Be aware of possible medication interactions.
Immunomodulators interferon beta (Betaseron, Avonex, Rebif), glatiramer acetate (Copaxone)	• Perform self-injection techniques. • Report adverse effects.
Cholinergics neostigmine	• Consult with health care provider before using other medications, including over-the-counter medications.
Anticholinergics oxybutynin (Ditropan)	• Consult health care provider before using other medications, especially sleeping aids, antihistamines (possibly lead to potentiated effect).
Muscle Relaxants diazepam (Valium), baclofen (Lioresal), tizanidine	• Avoid driving and similar activities because of sedative effects. • Do not abruptly stop therapy. • Avoid use with tranquilizers and alcohol.
Acetylcholinesterase Inhibitor donepezil (Aricept)	• Maintain adequate hydration of 2–3 L of fluid per day. • Rise slowly when getting up from a sitting or lying position. • Report persistent abdominal discomfort, increased salivation, unresolved diarrhea, increased muscle pain, visual changes, or shortness of breath.
Sphingosine-1-Phosphate Receptor Modulator fingolimod (Gilenya)	• May increase risk for infections and reduce effectiveness of influenza and tetanus boosters

ACTH, adrenocorticotrophic hormone.

hormone, methylprednisolone (Solu-Medrol), and prednisone are helpful in treating acute exacerbations of the disease, probably by reducing edema and acute inflammation at the site of demyelination (Table 61.16). These medications are used in patients with all types of MS; however, they do not affect the ultimate outcome or the degree of residual neurological impairment from the exacerbation (See Chapter 51 for effects of long-term corticosteroid therapy).

Immunosuppressive medications, such as azathioprine (Imuran), methotrexate, and cyclophosphamide (Procytox), have been shown to produce some beneficial effects in patients with progressive–relapsing, secondary-progressive, and primary-progressive MS. However, the potential benefits of these medications in patients with MS must be weighed against the potential risks.

Immunomodulator medications modify the disease process. Interferon beta-1b (Betaseron) is used for patients with relapsing–remitting MS who are ambulatory. Interferon beta-1a (Avonex) is similar to interferon beta-1b in efficacy and is used in similar patient groups with MS. These medications have antiviral effects. Glatiramer acetate (Copaxone), formerly known as copolymer-1, is unrelated to interferon.

MEDICATION ALERT—Interferon Beta Medications (Avonex, Betaseron, Rebif)
- Rotate injection sites with each dose.
- Assess for depression, suicidal ideation.
- Wear sunscreen and protective clothing while exposed to sun.
- Know that flulike symptoms are common after initiation of therapy.

Teriflunomide (Aubagio) is an emerging immunomodulatory medication that is a promising new therapy for the treatment of relapsing–remitting multiple sclerosis (RRMS). It has been shown to decrease the number of MS relapses and to reduce the progression toward disability in patients with MS (Multiple Sclerosis Society of Canada, 2021a).

Mitoxantrone is an antineoplastic agent used for the treatment of primary-progressive and progressive–relapsing MS. It is an immunosuppressant medication that reduces both B and T lymphocytes and impairs antigen presentation. Unlike the other disease-modifying medications, it has a lifetime dose limit because of cardiac toxicity. Therefore, it cannot be used for more than 2 to 3 years.

Many other medications are used to treat the various symptoms of MS. These may include medications for spasticity, fatigue, tremor, vertigo or dizziness, depression, pain, bowel and bladder conditions, sexual issues, and cognitive changes. For example, amantadine and fluoxetine (Prozac) are used to treat fatigue. Anticholinergics can treat bladder symptoms. Tricyclic antidepressants and antiseizure medications are used for chronic pain syndromes.

Alternate Therapies. A variety of alternate therapies have been used, aiming to minimize MS symptoms and decrease exacerbations. Surgical intervention may include neurectomy, rhizotomy, cordotomy, or dorsal-column electrical stimulation. Use of an intrathecal baclofen (Lioresal) pump may be required to manage spasticity. Tremors that become unmanageable with medications are sometimes treated by thalamotomy or deep brain stimulation.

Neurological dysfunction may improve with physiotherapy and speech therapy. Exercise improves the daily functioning for patients with MS not experiencing an exacerbation. Exercise decreases spasticity, increases coordination and muscle strength, and improves mobilization, gait, fatigue, and quality of life for patients with MS. The Canadian Physical Activity Guidelines for Adults with MS (Canadian Society for Exercise Physiology, 2020) is a useful resource that outlines recommendations for adults with mild to moderate disability related to MS. An especially beneficial type of physiotherapy is water exercise. Water gives buoyancy to the body and enables the patient to perform activities that would normally be too difficult because the patient has more control over their body. Other therapies may include heat therapy, massage, acupuncture, bee stings, and aromatherapy. The effectiveness of these therapies requires more research.

Stem cell therapy has shown much promise in the treatment of MS. For example, the MESCAMS (MEsenchymal Stem cell therapy for CAnadian MS patients) study is being conducted to determine whether mesenchymal stem cell (MSC) therapy can reduce brain inflammation related to MS, if it is a safe treatment option, and if it has neurorestorative properties. At the time of the release of the study's preliminary findings, it was reported that MSC was found to be a safe treatment option and that there was a trend toward a reduction in MS relapses (Multiple Sclerosis Society of Canada, 2019).

In recent years, media attention has emerged surrounding the controversial MS treatment of chronic cerebrospinal venous insufficiency (CCSVI). Zamboni and associates (2008) first proposed the theory that CCSVI may be a contributing factor in the pathology of MS. These researchers suggested that MS may be related to an immune or inflammatory reaction to iron accumulation in the CNS relating to drainage impairment of the cerebrospinal vessels. This accumulation was detected via the use of cranial ultrasound. In 2010, the American and Canadian multiple sclerosis societies contributed to the funding of several studies to investigate the link between CCSVI and MS (Multiple Sclerosis Society of Canada, 2021b). Since that time, all of these studies have shown no positive relationship between CCSVI and MS, and CCSVI surgery for patients with MS remains unavailable in Canada (Multiple Sclerosis Society of Canada, 2021b). A re-evaluation study of earlier findings concluded that although the procedure could be safely performed, it was deemed to be ineffective, and as such, the previous recommendation that the treatment be considered for patients with MS has been abandoned (Zamboni et al., 2018).

Nutritional Therapy. Various nutritional measures have been used in the management of MS, including megavitamin therapy (cobalamin [vitamin B_{12}], vitamin C), supplemental vitamin D, and diets consisting of low-fat, gluten-free food and raw vegetables. Particular dietary measures are not widely recommended, owing to insufficient evidence supporting their effectiveness.

A nutritious, well-balanced diet is essential. Although there is no standard prescribed diet, a high-protein, high-roughage diet with supplementary vitamins is often advocated. Vitamins are merely supplemental and not curative. Nutrition therapy must be adapted, depending on the patient's ability to chew and swallow.

NURSING MANAGEMENT
MULTIPLE SCLEROSIS

NURSING ASSESSMENT
Subjective and objective data that should be obtained from a patient with MS are presented in Table 61.17.

TABLE 61.17 NURSING ASSESSMENT

Multiple Sclerosis

Subjective Data

Important Health Information

Past health history: Recent or past viral infections or vaccinations, other recent infections, residence in cold or temperate climates, recent physical or emotional stress, pregnancy, exposure to extremes of heat and cold; positive family history

Medications: Use of and adherence to taking corticosteroids, immunomodulators, immunosuppressants, selective adhesion molecule inhibitor cholinergics, anticholinergics, antispasmodics, antivirals

Symptoms

- Weight loss; difficulty chewing, dysphagia
- Urinary frequency, urgency, dribbling or incontinence, retention; constipation
- Generalized muscle weakness, muscle fatigue; tingling and numbness, ataxia (clumsiness), malaise
- Eye, back, leg, joint pain; painful muscle spasms; vertigo; blurred or lost vision; diplopia; tinnitus
- Erectile and sexual dysfunction; decreased libido
- Anger, depression, euphoria, social isolation, cognitive changes, memory loss

Objective Data

General

Apathy, inattentiveness

Neurological

Scanning speech, nystagmus, ataxia, tremor, spasticity, hyper-reflexia, decreased hearing

Musculoskeletal

Muscular weakness, paresis, paralysis, spasms, foot dragging, dysarthria (may be unilateral or bilateral changes)

Possible Findings

Decreased T suppressor cells, demyelinating lesions on MRI or MRS scans, increased IgG or oligoclonal banding in cerebrospinal fluid, delayed evoked potential

IgG, immunoglobulin G; *MRI,* magnetic resonance imaging; *MRS,* magnetic resonance spectroscopy.

NURSING DIAGNOSES

Nursing diagnoses for patients with MS may include but are not limited to the following:

- *Reduced stamina* resulting from *decrease in muscle strength, decrease in muscle control, physical deconditioning*
- *Overflow urinary incontinence* resulting from *detrusor hypocontractility*
- *Inadequate health management* resulting from *difficulty managing complex treatment regimen* (knowledge deficit regarding management of MS)

Additional information on nursing diagnoses for the patient with MS is presented in NCP 61.3, available on the Evolve website.

PLANNING

The overall goals are that the patient with MS will (1) maximize neuromuscular function, (2) maintain independence in activities of daily living for as long as possible, (3) manage fatigue, (4) optimize psychosocial well-being, (5) adjust to the illness, and (6) reduce factors that precipitate exacerbations.

INFORMATICS IN PRACTICE

Phone Applications in Multiple Sclerosis

- Patients with MS, especially those who are newly diagnosed, might feel overwhelmed at the thought of living with a chronic disease and managing multiple medications.
- Smartphone applications can improve the lives of patients with MS by helping them manage their health care.
- Applications are available that send medication reminders by text message or email, track injection site rotation, and email medication reports to the health care provider. Patients can keep track of their medication inventory and be reminded to order refills.

NURSING IMPLEMENTATION

Patients with MS should be aware of triggers that may cause exacerbations or worsening of the disease. These include infection (especially upper respiratory and urinary tract infections [UTIs]), trauma, immunization, childbirth, stress, and change in climate. Each person responds differently to these triggers. The nurse should help the patient identify particular triggers and develop ways to avoid them or minimize their effects.

During the diagnostic phase, the nurse should reassure the patient that certain diagnostic studies must be done to rule out other neurological disorders, even if a tentative diagnosis of MS has been made. The nurse can help the patient manage the anxiety caused by a diagnosis of a disabling illness. The patient with recently diagnosed MS may need help with the grieving process.

During an acute exacerbation, the patient may be immobile and confined to bed. The focus of nursing interventions at this phase is to prevent complications of immobility. These include respiratory and urinary tract infections and pressure injuries.

Patient teaching is focused on measures to aid in general resistance to illness. This includes avoiding fatigue, extremes of heat and cold, and exposure to infection. Early treatment of infection is encouraged when it occurs. The nurse should teach the patient to seek a good balance of exercise and rest; minimize caffeine intake; and eat nutritious, well-balanced meals. The patient should know the treatment plan, medication adverse effects, how to identify and manage adverse effects, and medication interactions with over-the-counter (OTC) medications. The patient should consult the health care provider before taking any OTC medications.

Bladder control is a major concern for many patients with MS. Anticholinergics may help some patients to decrease spasticity. The nurse may need to teach some patients self-catheterization. Constipation is common; a diet high in fibre may help relieve constipation.

The patient with MS and their caregivers may need to make many emotional adjustments because of disease unpredictability, the need for lifestyle changes, and the challenge of avoiding or decreasing precipitating factors. The uncertainty of disease progression, along with fatigue and decreased mobility, can cause anxiety and depression.

EVALUATION

Expected outcomes for patients with MS are addressed in NCP 61.3, available on the Evolve website.

PARKINSON'S DISEASE

Parkinson's disease (PD) is named after James Parkinson, who, in 1817, wrote a classic essay on "shaking palsy," a disease whose cause is still unknown and for which no cure exists. Following Alzheimer's disease, PD is the second most common neurodegenerative disease. In 2013–2014, approximately 84 000 Canadian adults had been diagnosed with PD (Public Health Agency of Canada, 2018), 85% of whom were 65 years of age or older at the time of their diagnosis (Parkinson Canada, 2020). When a patient is 50 years of age or younger at the time of their diagnosis, they are diagnosed with early-onset PD.

PD is a progressive, neurodegenerative disease of the CNS (basal ganglia) characterized by delayed initiation and execution of movement (bradykinesia), increased muscle tone (rigidity), tremor at rest, and impaired gait changes. It is the most common form of parkinsonism, a syndrome characterized by similar symptoms.

Etiology and Pathophysiology

The exact cause of PD is unknown. In patients with PD, unusual aggregations of protein that develop inside nerve cells known as *Lewy bodies* are found within the brain. It is not known what causes Lewy bodies to form. Their presence can lead to abnormal brain functioning that can affect cognition, movements, mood, and behaviours.

Although we do not consider PD a hereditary condition, the question of whether genetics plays a role in PD has been studied. Current estimates indicate that about 10% of all cases may be genetically linked (Parkinson's Foundation, 2021). Exposure to well water, pesticides, herbicides, industrial chemicals, and wood pulp mills may also increase the risk for PD.

Many changes found in the brains of people with PD may play a part in development of the disease, including a lack of neurotransmitter dopamine. The pathological process of PD involves degeneration of the dopamine-producing neurons in the substantia nigra of the midbrain (Figure 61.5). This in turn disrupts the normal balance between dopamine and acetylcholine (ACh) in the basal ganglia. Dopamine is essential for normal functioning of the extrapyramidal motor system, including control of posture, support, and voluntary motion. Manifestations of PD do not occur until 80% of neurons in the substantia nigra are lost.

Many forms of secondary *(atypical)* parkinsonism exist other than PD. Symptoms of parkinsonism have occurred after exposure to a variety of chemicals, including carbon monoxide and manganese (among copper miners). Medication-induced parkinsonism can follow therapy with metoclopramide (Maxeran), methyldopa (Aldomet), lithium (Carbolith/Lithane), and haloperidol (Haldol). It can be seen after the use of illicit drugs, including amphetamine and methamphetamine. After stopping these drugs, symptoms of parkinsonism generally disappear. One notable exception is irreversible parkinsonism that follows exposure to the product of meperidine (Demerol) analogue synthesis (MTPT). Other causes include hydrocephalus, other neurodegenerative disorders, hypoparathyroidism, infections, stroke, tumour, and trauma.

Clinical Manifestations

The onset of PD is gradual, with an ongoing progression. Only one side of the body may be involved at first. Classic manifestations can be remembered by the mnemonic *TRAP* (**t**remor, **r**igidity, **a**kinesia, **p**ostural instability). Early in the disease, only a mild tremor, a slight limp, or a decreased arm swing may be seen. Later, the patient may have a shuffling gait and appear unable to stop. The patient's arms are flexed, and postural reflexes seem to be lost. The patient may have speech difficulties (hypokinetic *dysarthria)* that can affect communication and quality of life.

Tremor. *Tremor* is often the first sign. It may be minimal at first, so the patient is the only one who notices it. This tremor can affect handwriting, causing it to trail off, especially toward the ends of words. Parkinsonian tremor is more prominent at rest. It is worsened by emotional stress or increased concentration. The hand tremor is described as "pill rolling" because the thumb and forefinger appear to move in a rotary fashion as if rolling a pill, coin, or other small object. Tremor can involve the diaphragm, tongue, lips, and jaw. It rarely causes shaking of the head.

Unfortunately, in many people a benign *essential tremor* is mistakenly diagnosed as PD. Essential tremor occurs during voluntary movement, has a more rapid frequency than Parkinsonian tremor, and is often familial.

Rigidity. *Rigidity* is the increased resistance to passive motion when the limbs are moved through their range of motion (ROM). Parkinsonian rigidity is typified by a jerky quality *(cogwheel rigidity),* as if there were occasional catches in the passive movement of a joint. Sustained muscle contraction causes the rigidity and results in muscle soreness; feeling tired and achy; or pain in the head, upper body, spine, or legs. Slow movement is another result of rigidity because the alternating contraction and relaxation in opposing muscle groups (e.g., biceps and triceps) is inhibited.

Akinesia. *Akinesia* is the absence or loss of control of voluntary muscle movements. In PD, *bradykinesia* (slowness of movement) is especially evident in the loss of automatic movements. This occurs because of the physical and chemical change of the basal ganglia and other structures in the extrapyramidal portion of the CNS. In the unaffected patient, automatic movements are involuntary and occur subconsciously. They include blinking of the eyelids, swinging of the arms while walking, swallowing saliva, using facial and hand movements for self-expression, and making minor movements to adjust posture.

The patient with PD does not perform these movements and lacks natural activity. This accounts for the stooped posture, masked face (deadpan expression), drooling of saliva, and shuffling gait *(festination)* that are typical of a person with PD. The posture is that of a slowed, poorly postured individual, with the head and trunk bent forward and the legs constantly flexed (Figure 61.6).

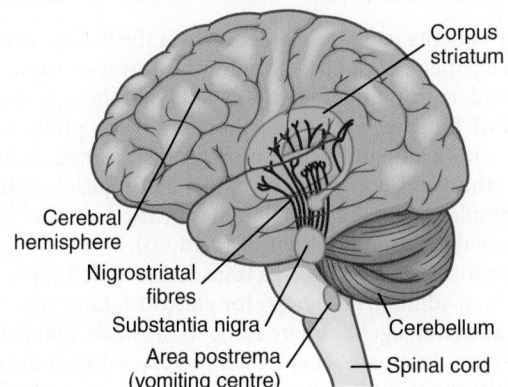

FIG. 61.5 Nigrostriatal disorders produce parkinsonism. Left-sided view of the human brain shows the substantia nigra and the corpus striatum (shaded area) lying deep within the cerebral hemisphere. Nerve fibres extend upward from the substantia nigra, divide into many branches, and carry dopamine to all regions of the corpus striatum.

Corpus striatum
Cerebral hemisphere
Nigrostriatal fibres
Substantia nigra
Area postrema (vomiting centre)
Cerebellum
Spinal cord

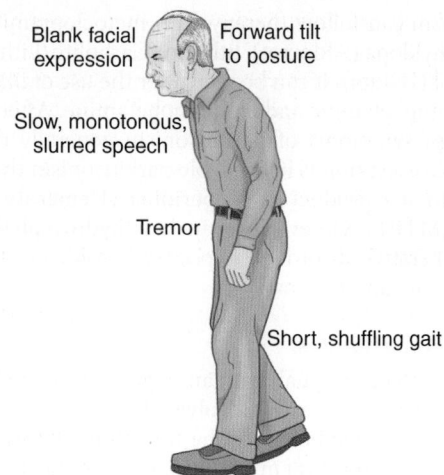

Blank facial expression
Forward tilt to posture
Slow, monotonous, slurred speech
Tremor
Short, shuffling gait

FIG. 61.6 Characteristic appearance of a patient with Parkinson's disease.

TABLE 61.18   INTERPROFESSIONAL CARE

Parkinson's Disease

Diagnostic
- History and physical examination
- Bradykinesia
- MRI
- Positive response to antiparkinsonian medications*
- Rigidity
- Rule out adverse effects of phenothiazines, benzodiazepines, haloperidol
- Tremor

Interprofessional Therapy
- Antiparkinsonian medications*
- Ablation surgery
- Deep brain stimulation

MRI, magnetic resonance imaging.
*See Table 61.19.

Postural Instability. *Postural instability* is common. Patients may describe being unable to stop themselves from going forward *(propulsion)* or backward *(retropulsion)*. Assessment of postural instability includes the "pull test." The examiner stands behind the patient and gives a tug backward on the shoulder, causing the patient to lose their balance and fall backward.

Nonmotor. Many nonmotor symptoms are common. They include depression, anxiety, apathy, fatigue, pain, urinary retention, constipation, erectile dysfunction, and memory changes. Sleep disorders are common. They include difficulty staying asleep at night, restless sleep, nightmares, and drowsiness or sudden sleep onset during the day. Rapid eye movement (REM) sleep behaviour disorder is a preparkinsonian state that occurs in about one third of patients with PD. It is characterized by violent dreams and potentially dangerous motor activity during REM sleep. It may cause harm to the patient or bed partner (Jennum et al., 2016).

Complications

As the disease progresses, complications increase. These include motor symptoms (e.g., dyskinesias [spontaneous, involuntary movements], weakness, akinesia [total immobility]), neurological conditions (e.g., dementia), and neuropsychiatric conditions (e.g., depression, hallucinations, psychosis). As PD progresses, it often results in severe dementia, which is associated with an increase in mortality.

As swallowing becomes more difficult *(dysphagia)*, malnutrition or aspiration may result. Increasing weakness may lead to pneumonia, UTIs, and skin breakdown. Orthostatic hypotension may occur in some patients and, along with loss of postural reflexes, may result in falls or other injuries. The patient's increased fall risk means caregivers must be aware of environmental conditions that may contribute to falls.

Diagnostic Studies

Because no specific diagnostic test exists for PD, diagnosis is based on the patient's history and clinical features. Clinical diagnosis requires the presence of TRAP and asymmetrical onset. Confirmation of PD is a positive response to antiparkinsonian medications (levodopa or dopamine agonist). MRI and CT have a limited role in the diagnosis of PD because they do not show a specific pathological finding; however, a diagnosis of stroke or brain tumour can be ruled out.

Interprofessional Care

Because there is no cure for PD, interprofessional care focuses on symptom management (Table 61.18).

Medication Therapy. Medication therapy for PD is aimed at correcting an imbalance of neurotransmitters within the CNS. Antiparkinsonian medications either enhance the release or supply of dopamine *(dopaminergic)* or block the effects of the overactive cholinergic neurons in the striatum *(anticholinergic)*. Levodopa with carbidopa (Sinemet) is often the first medication used. Levodopa is a precursor of dopamine and can cross the blood–brain barrier. It is converted to dopamine in the basal ganglia. Sinemet is the preferred medication because it also contains carbidopa, an agent that inhibits the enzyme dopa decarboxylase in the peripheral tissues. This enzyme breaks down levodopa before it reaches the brain. The net result of the combination of levodopa and carbidopa is that more levodopa reaches the brain, and therefore less medication is needed.

> **MEDICATION ALERT—Carbidopa–Levodopa (Sinemet)**
> - Monitor for signs of dyskinesia.
> - Monitor for short-term adverse effects of nausea, vomiting, and light-headedness.
> - Stress that effects may be delayed for several weeks to months.
> - Teach patient or caregiver to report any uncontrolled movement of face, eyelids, mouth, tongue, arms, hands, or legs; mental changes; palpitations; and difficulty urinating.
> - Do not give levodopa with food because protein reduces absorption.

Many patients receive Sinemet early in the disease course for the management of motor symptoms. However, some health care providers think that, after a few years of therapy, the effectiveness of Sinemet wears off; therefore, they prefer to start therapy with a dopamine receptor agonist, a medication that directly stimulates dopamine receptors. Pramipexole (Mirapex) is an example of a medication that may be used alone or in combination with Sinemet. Rotigotine (Neupro), another dopamine receptor agonist, is available as a transdermal patch applied once daily. It is an adjunctive therapy for patients taking Sinemet.

The antiviral agent amantadine is a weak antagonist of NMDA-type glutamate receptors. It increases dopamine release and blocks its reuptake. It may be useful as a single therapy for early PD. It can be used later with levodopa. As a single treatment, amantadine often becomes less effective after a few months (Gonzalez-Usigli, 2020). Withdrawal of amantadine even after extended therapy can worsen dyskinesia.

Anticholinergic medications, such as trihexyphenidyl, decrease the activity of ACh, providing balance between cholinergic and dopaminergic actions (Gonzalez-Usigli, 2020). Antihistamines (e.g., diphenhydramine [Benadryl]) with anticholinergic properties may be used to manage tremors.

Selegiline and rasagiline are examples of monoamine oxidase type B (MAO-B) inhibitors that are sometimes used in combination with Sinemet. By inhibiting MAO-B, the enzyme that degrades dopamine, these agents increase the levels of dopamine and prolong the half-life of levodopa. Rasagiline can be used alone as therapy in early PD. However, MAO-B inhibitors are less effective at treating motor symptoms than dopamine receptor agonists.

Entacapone (Comtan) blocks the enzyme catechol-O-methyltransferase (COMT), which breaks down levodopa in the peripheral circulation. Thus, they prolong the effect of Sinemet and are used only as adjuncts. They are often used when the patient's response to levodopa is wearing off at the end of the dosing interval.

Table 61.19 summarizes the medications commonly used in PD. The use of only one medication is preferred because fewer adverse effects occur, and the drug dosage is easier to adjust than when several medications are used. However, as PD progresses, combination therapy is often needed. Excessive amounts of dopaminergic medications can worsen rather than relieve symptoms (*paradoxical intoxication*).

Within 3 to 5 years of standard PD treatments, many patients have episodes of hypomobility (e.g., inability to rise from chair, speak, or walk; also called *off episodes*). Off episodes can occur toward the end of a dosing interval with standard medications (so-called end-of-dose wearing off) or at unpredictable times (spontaneous "on/off"). A combination of carbidopa, levodopa, and entacapone (Stalevo) is available for patients with end-of-dose wearing off. It can be prescribed to make dosing easier, with one pill substituting for three. Stalevo is typically prescribed for patients with advanced PD with intense motor fluctuations.

Genome Therapy. Genome therapy is an experimental therapy that involves the injection of genes into a patient's cells with the aim of replacing or abolishing dysfunctional genes (National Institutes of Health, 2021). While the concept of genome therapy may be theoretically promising, evidence to support its practice remains intangible. However, there is increasing evidence that this treatment may be an effective treatment for future patients living with PD (Jamebozorgi et al., 2019).

Surgical Therapy. Surgical procedures are aimed at relieving symptoms of PD and are usually used in patients who are unresponsive to medication therapy or who have developed severe motor complications. Surgical procedures fall into

TABLE 61.19   MEDICATION THERAPY

Parkinson's Disease

Medication	Symptoms Relieved	Adverse Effects and Precautions
Dopaminergic		
levodopa	Bradykinesia, tremor, rigidity	Nausea, dyskinesia, hypotension, palpitations, dysrhythmias; agitation, hallucinations, confusion (in older patient)
		Avoidance of multivitamin pills and diet high in vitamin B_6 (reversal of effect of levodopa); contraindicated in narrow-angle glaucoma
levodopa–carbidopa (Sinemet)	Same as above	Less nausea but greater chance of dyskinesia, confusion, hallucinations
		Periodic check of BUN, AST, WBCs, Hct
		Contraindicated in melanoma; narrow-angle glaucoma; combination with MAO inhibitors, methyldopa, antipsychotics
bromocriptine mesylate	Same as above	Orthostatic hypotension, nausea, vomiting, toxic psychosis, limb edema, phlebitis, dizziness, headache, insomnia
pramipexole (Mirapex)	Same as above	
ropinirole (Requip)	Same as above	
amantadine	Rigidity, akinesia	Nervousness, insomnia, confusion, hallucinations, dry mouth, nausea, edema, orthostatic hypotension
Anticholinergic		
benztropine	Tremor	Dry mouth, blurred vision, constipation, delirium, anxiety, agitation, hallucinations
procyclidine		
trihexyphenidyl		Avoidance of medications with similar actions, including over-the-counter medications containing scopolamine or antihistamines, antispasmodics, tricyclic antidepressants (e.g., amitriptyline [Elavil])
Antihistamine		
diphenhydramine (Benadryl)	Tremor, rigidity	Sedation, same precautions as for anticholinergic medications
orphenadrine		
Monoamine Oxidase Inhibitor		
selegiline	Bradykinesia, rigidity, tremor	Similar to dopaminergic medications
Catechol-O-Methyltransferase (COMT) Inhibitor		
entacapone (Comtan)	By blocking COMT, this medication slows down the breakdown of levodopa, thus prolonging the action of levodopa	Similar to dopaminergic medications; works only when used in combination with Sinemet

AST, aspartate aminotransferase; *BUN*, blood urea nitrogen; *Hct*, hematocrit; *MAO*, monoamine oxidase; *WBCs*, white blood cells.

three categories: ablation (destruction), deep brain stimulation (DBS), and transplantation.

Ablation surgery involves stereotactic ablation of areas in the thalamus (thalamotomy), globus pallidus (pallidotomy), and subthalamic nucleus (subthalamic nucleotomy). Ablative procedures have been used for PD for over 50 years, but they have been replaced recently by DBS.

DBS involves placing an electrode in the thalamus, the globus pallidus, or the subthalamic nucleus and connecting it to a generator placed in the upper chest (like a pacemaker). The device is programmed to deliver a specific current to the targeted brain location. Unlike ablation procedures, DBS can be adjusted to control symptoms better and is reversible (the device is removable). These ablative and DBS procedures work by blocking the neuronal impulses that lead to the motor symptoms seen in PD (NINDS, 2021b).

Transplantation of fetal neural tissue into the basal ganglia was designed to provide dopamine agonist–producing cells in the brains of patients with PD. Research of this therapy was largely abandoned after mixed results over several decades. In the last few years, better transplant techniques have renewed interest in this as a potential option.

Nutritional Therapy. Diet is of major importance to patients with PD because malnutrition and constipation can result from poor nutrition. Patients who have dysphagia and bradykinesia need appetizing foods that are easy to chew and swallow. The diet should contain adequate fibre and fruit to reduce constipation.

Eating six small meals a day may be less tiring than eating three large meals a day. The patient needs to plan ample time for eating to avoid frustration. Food should be cut into bite-sized pieces. Protein ingestion and vitamin B_6 can impair the absorption of levodopa. Limiting protein intake to the evening meal can decrease this problem. The interprofessional health team should be consulted about including vitamin B_6 in a multivitamin and fortified cereals.

NURSING MANAGEMENT PARKINSON'S DISEASE

NURSING ASSESSMENT

Subjective and objective data that should be obtained from a patient with PD are presented in Table 61.20.

NURSING DIAGNOSES

Nursing diagnoses for patients with PD may include but are not limited to the following:

- *Reduced stamina* resulting from *decrease in muscle control, decrease in muscle strength, physical deconditioning*
- *Inadequate nutrition* resulting from *insufficient dietary intake* (difficulty ingesting food)
- *Inadequate swallowing* resulting from *behavioural feeding problem* (neuromuscular impairment)

Additional information on nursing diagnoses for the patient with PD is presented in NCP 61.4, available on the Evolve website.

PLANNING

The overall goals are that the patient with PD will (1) experience improved symptoms, (2) maximize neurological function, (3) maintain independence in activities of daily living for as long as possible, and (4) optimize psychosocial well-being.

TABLE 61.20 NURSING ASSESSMENT

Parkinson's Disease

Subjective Data

Important Health Information

Past health history: CNS trauma, cerebrovascular disorders, exposure to metals or carbon monoxide, encephalitis; positive family history

Medications: Use of major tranquilizers, especially haloperidol and phenothiazines, methyldopa, amphetamines

Symptoms

- Excessive salivation, dysphagia; weight loss
- Constipation, incontinence; excessive sweating
- Fatigue, sleep disturbance, difficulty initiating movements; postural instability; frequent falls; loss of dexterity; micrographia (handwriting deterioration)
- Diffuse headache; pain in shoulders, neck, back, legs, and hips; muscle soreness and cramping; difficulty concentrating
- Depression, mood swings, hallucinations

Objective Data

General

Blank (masked) facies, slow and monotonous speech, infrequent blinking

Integumentary

Seborrhea, dandruff; ankle edema

Cardiovascular

Postural hypotension

Gastrointestinal

Drooling

Neurological

Tremor at rest, first in hands (pill rolling), later in legs, arms, face, and tongue; aggravation of tremor with anxiety, absence in sleep; poor coordination; subtle dementia, impaired postural reflexes

Musculoskeletal

Cogwheel rigidity, dysarthria, bradykinesia, contractures, stooped posture, shuffling gait

Possible Findings

Lack of specific tests; diagnosis on basis of history and physical findings and ruling out of other diseases

CNS, central nervous system.

NURSING IMPLEMENTATION

Because PD is a chronic, degenerative disorder with no acute exacerbations, patient teaching and nursing care are directed toward maintaining good health, encouraging independence, and avoiding complications, such as contractures and falls. Difficulties due to bradykinesia can be addressed by relatively simple measures.

Promoting physical exercise and a well-balanced diet are major concerns for nursing care. Exercise can limit the consequences of decreased mobility, such as muscle atrophy, contractures, and constipation. Parkinson Canada (www.parkinson.ca) has produced a series of booklets and videos with helpful exercises that can be used by patients, family members, and health care providers.

A physiotherapist may be consulted to design an exercise program aimed at strengthening, improving muscle tone, and stretching specific muscles. A speech–language pathologist may be consulted to strengthen the muscles involved with speaking and swallowing. Although exercise will not halt the progression of the disease, it will enhance the patient's functional ability. An occupational therapist can also assist the patient with strategies to increase self-care abilities, including eating and dressing.

Nurses should work closely with patient caregivers in exploring creative adaptations that enable maximal independence and self-care. The patient can facilitate getting out of a chair by using an upright chair with arms and placing the back legs of the chair on small (5-cm) blocks. The nurse should encourage environmental alterations, such as removing rugs and excess furniture to avoid stumbling, using an elevated toilet seat to facilitate getting on and off the toilet, and elevating the legs on an ottoman to decrease dependent ankle edema. Clothing can be simplified by the use of slip-on shoes and Velcro hook-and-loop fasteners or zippers on clothing, instead of buttons and hooks.

Effective management of sleep disorders can greatly improve the quality of life for patients with PD. Some patients find the use of satin nightwear or satin sheets beneficial. Information on teaching regarding sleep hygiene practices is presented in Chapter 9.

In the early stages of PD, many patients experience depression and anxiety. Patients need to adjust their lifestyle, including work and home responsibilities. As PD progresses, the impact on the patient's psychological well-being also increases. The nurse can assist the patient by listening, educating, gently correcting distorted thoughts, and encouraging social interactions. Psychotherapy and counselling can also be helpful. Patients with PD must receive prescribed medications on time to avoid on-off effects.

In the early stage of the disease, the patient has subtle changes in cognitive function, which may progress to dementia. This progression results in increased caregiver burden and the potential for long-term care placement. Information on care of the patient with dementia is provided in Chapter 62.

The majority of patients with PD are cared for by family caregivers. As the disease progresses, caregiver burden increases, often at the cost of the caregiver's physical and mental health. Strategies to reduce caregiver stress are described in Chapter 62, Table 62.13. Other interventions for the patient with PD are presented in NCP 61.4 (available on the Evolve website).

▌EVALUATION

The expected outcomes are that the patient with PD will:
• Maintain optimal muscle function
• Use assistive devices appropriately for ambulation and mobility
• Maintain nutritional intake adequate for metabolic needs
• Experience unimpaired swallowing of fluids and/or solids
• Use methods of communication that allow interaction with others

Additional information on expected outcomes for the patient with PD is presented in NCP 61.4 (available on the Evolve website).

MYASTHENIA GRAVIS

Myasthenia gravis (MG) is an autoimmune disease of the neuromuscular junction marked by fluctuating weakness of certain skeletal muscle groups. This weakness increases with muscle use. The prevalence of MG is approximately 3 cases per 100 000 population with an incidence most common among younger women and older men (Bourque & Breiner, 2018); however, MG is thought to be underdiagnosed and the prevalence is likely higher.

Etiology and Pathophysiology

MG is caused by an autoimmune process in which antibodies attack ACh receptors, resulting in a decreased number of ACh receptor (AChR) sites at the neuromuscular junction (Figure 61.7). This prevents ACh molecules from attaching and stimulating muscle contraction. Anti-AChR antibodies are detectable in the serum of 90% of patients with generalized MG. In patients who lack autoantibodies to AChR, muscular weakness may be related to autoantibodies to the muscle-specific receptor tyrosine kinase or to other unknown antigens (Mayo Clinic, 2019). Thymic hyperplasia and tumours are common in patients with MG, suggesting that autoantibody production occurs in the thymus (NINDS, 2021a).

Clinical Manifestations and Complications

The primary feature of MG is fluctuating weakness of skeletal muscle. Strength is usually restored after a period of rest. The muscles most often involved are those used for moving the eyes and eyelids, chewing, swallowing, speaking, and breathing. The muscles are generally the strongest in the morning and become exhausted with continued activity. Consequently, by the end of the day, muscle weakness is prominent (Myasthenia Gravis Coalition of Canada, 2021) (Table 61.21).

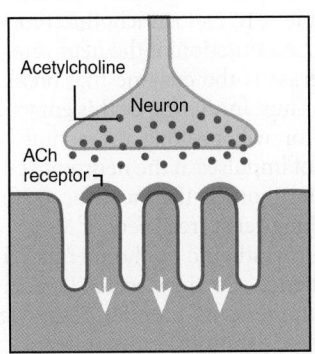
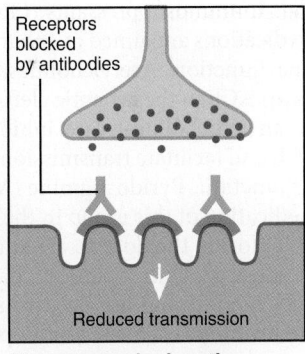

Normal neuromuscular junction

Neuromuscular junction in myasthenia gravis

FIG. 61.7 Neuromuscular junction in myasthenia gravis. *ACh,* acetylcholine. Source: Myasthenia Gravis Coalition of Canada. (2017). *What is MG?* https://www.mgcc-ccmg.org/about.asp

TABLE 61.21	CLINICAL MANIFESTATIONS OF MYASTHENIA GRAVIS

• Change in facial expression
• Chronic muscle fatigue
• Difficulty breathing
• Difficulty chewing or swallowing
• Drooping eyelid(s) (ptosis)
• Impaired or slurred speech
• Unstable or unusual gait
• Vision changes (blurred or double)
• Weakness in arms, hands, fingers, legs, and neck

Source: National Institute of Neurological Disorders and Stroke. (2020). *Myasthenia fact sheet.* https://www.ninds.nih.gov/Disorders/Patient-Caregiver-Education/Fact-Sheets/Myasthenia-Gravis-Fact-Sheet#4

The course of MG is highly variable. Some patients may have short-term remissions, and others may stabilize. Others may have severe, progressive involvement. Fatigue, pregnancy, illness, trauma, temperature extremes, stress, and hypokalemia can exacerbate MG. Certain medications, including β-adrenergic blockers, quinidine, phenytoin (Dilantin), certain anaesthetics, and aminoglycoside antibiotics, can worsen MG (Mayo Clinic, 2019).

Myasthenic crisis is an acute exacerbation of muscle weakness triggered by infection, surgery, emotional distress, pregnancy, exposure to certain medications, or beginning treatment with corticosteroids. Generally, it occurs in the first 2 years after diagnosis. The major complications of MG result from muscle weakness in areas that affect swallowing and breathing. This weakness results in aspiration, respiratory insufficiency, and respiratory infection.

Diagnostic Studies

The diagnosis of MG can be made on the basis of history, physical examination, and diagnostic testing. Diagnostic testing for MG could include testing for AChR antibodies, single-fibre electromyography (EMG) (to show the muscles' response to electrical shocks), and repetitive nerve stimulation testing. Tensilon testing is no longer performed in North America as edrophonium (Tensilon) has become obsolete. Once a diagnosis of MG is made, CT scanning of the chest may be performed to rule out thymoma (Bourque & Breiner, 2018).

Interprofessional Care

Medication Therapy. Medication therapy for MG includes anticholinesterase medications, alternate-day corticosteroids, and immunosuppressants (Table 61.22). Anticholinesterase medications are aimed at enhancing function of the neuromuscular junction. Acetylcholinesterase is the enzyme that breaks down ACh in the synaptic cleft. Thus, inhibition of this enzyme by an anticholinesterase inhibitor will prolong the action of ACh and facilitate transmission of impulses at the neuromuscular junction. Pyridostigmine (Mestinon) is the most successful medication of this group in the long-term treatment of MG.

Tailoring the dose to avoid a myasthenic or cholinergic crisis often presents a clinical challenge. Corticosteroids (specifically prednisone) are used to suppress the immune response. Medications such as azathioprine (Imuran), mycophenolate (CellCept), and cyclosporin (Sandimmune) may also be used for immunosuppression. Many patients who receive corticosteroids have complete cessation of symptoms or marked improvement. Some patients become weaker for a brief time before regaining strength. These benefits must be weighed with concerns about chronic use of these medications.

Many medications are contraindicated for use or must be used with caution in patients with MG. Classes of medication that should be cautiously evaluated before use include anaesthetics, antidysrhythmics, antibiotics, quinine, antipsychotics, barbiturates and sedative–hypnotics, cathartics, diuretics, opioids, muscle relaxants, thyroid preparations, and tranquilizers.

Surgical Therapy. Because the presence of the thymus gland in patients with MG appears to enhance the production of AChR antibodies, removal of the thymus gland results in improvement in most patients. Thymectomy is indicated for all patients with thymoma, for patients with generalized MG between puberty and about age 65 years, and for patients with purely ocular MG.

Other Therapies. Plasmapheresis and IV immunoglobulin G (IVIG) can yield a short-term improvement in symptoms and are indicated for patients in myasthenic crisis or in preparation for surgery when corticosteroids must be avoided. Plasmapheresis directly removes circulating AChR antibodies, leading to a decrease in symptoms. (Plasmapheresis is discussed in Chapter 16). Treatment decisions should be based on the patient's unique clinical presentation.

NURSING MANAGEMENT
MYASTHENIA GRAVIS

NURSING ASSESSMENT

The nurse can assess the severity of MG by asking the patient about fatigue, what body parts are affected, and how severely they are affected. Some patients become so fatigued that they are no longer able to work or even walk. The patient's coping abilities and understanding of MG must also be assessed.

Objective data should include respiratory rate and depth, oxygen saturation, arterial blood gas analyses, pulmonary function tests, and evidence of respiratory distress in patients with acute myasthenic crisis. Muscle strength of all face and limb muscles should be assessed, as should swallowing, speech (dysarthria) and voice (volume and clarity), cough and gag reflexes, and bladder function.

A thorough medication history must be obtained. As stated earlier, many medications are contraindicated or must be used with caution in patients with MG. Classes of medications that should be carefully evaluated before use include β-adrenergic blockers, quinidine, phenytoin (Dilantin), certain anaesthetics, and aminoglycoside antibiotics.

NURSING DIAGNOSES

Nursing diagnoses for patients with MG may include but are not limited to the following:

- *Inadequate airway clearance* resulting from *excessive mucus, retained secretions* (intercostal muscle weakness, impaired cough and gag reflexes)
- *Reduced stamina* resulting from *immobility, physical deconditioning* (muscle weakness, fatigue)
- *Disrupted body image* resulting from *alteration in self-perception* (inability to maintain usual lifestyle and role responsibility)

TABLE 61.22 INTERPROFESSIONAL CARE

Myasthenia Gravis

Diagnostic
- History and physical examination
- Acetylcholine receptor antibodies
- EMG
- Fatigability when upward gaze is prolonged (2–3 min)
- Muscle weakness

Interprofessional Therapy
- Medications
- Anticholinesterase agents
- Corticosteroids
- Immunosuppressive agents
- Plasmapheresis
- Surgery (thymectomy)

EMG, electromyography.

TABLE 61.23	COMPARISON OF MYASTHENIC CRISIS AND CHOLINERGIC CRISIS	
Myasthenic Crisis	**Cholinergic Crisis**
Causes	
Exacerbation of myasthenia following precipitating factors or failure to take medication as prescribed or drug dose too low	Overdose of anticholinesterase medications resulting in increased ACh at the receptor sites, remission (spontaneous or after thymectomy)
Differential Diagnosis	
Improved strength after IV administration of anticholinesterase medications	Weakness within 1 hr after ingestion of anticholinesterase
Increased weakness of skeletal muscles manifesting as ptosis, bulbar signs (e.g., difficulty in swallowing, difficulty in articulating words), or dyspnea	Increased weakness of skeletal muscles manifesting as ptosis, bulbar signs, dyspnea
	Effects on smooth muscle include papillary miosis, salivation, diarrhea, nausea or vomiting, abdominal cramps, increased bronchial secretions, sweating, or lacrimation

ACh, acetylcholine; *IV*, intravenous.

PLANNING

The overall goals are that the patient with MG will (1) have a return of normal muscle strength, (2) manage fatigue, (3) avoid complications, and (4) maintain a quality of life appropriate to the disease course.

NURSING IMPLEMENTATION

The patient with MG who is admitted to the hospital usually has a respiratory tract infection or is in an acute myasthenic crisis. Nursing care is aimed at maintaining adequate ventilation, continuing medication therapy, and watching for adverse effects of therapy. The nurse must be able to distinguish cholinergic from myasthenic crisis (Table 61.23) because the causes and treatment of the two conditions differ greatly. Features of a cholinergic crisis include involuntary muscle contraction, sweating, excessive salivation, and constricted pupils.

As with other chronic illnesses, care is focused on the neurological deficits and their impact on daily living. The nurse should teach the patient about having a balanced diet that can easily be chewed and swallowed. Semisolid foods may be easier to eat than solids or liquids. Scheduling doses of medications to reach peak action at mealtime may make eating easier. Diversional activities that need little physical effort and match the patient's interests should be arranged. The nurse can help the patient plan activities of daily living in such a way to avoid fatigue. Teaching is focused on adherence to the treatment plan, disease complications, potential adverse reactions to specific medications, complications of therapy (crisis conditions), and what to do about them. Contact with the Myasthenia Gravis Coalition of Canada or an MG support group may be helpful.

EVALUATION

The expected outcomes are that the patient with MG will:
- Maintain optimal muscle function
- Be free from adverse effects of medications
- Have no complications (myasthenic or cholinergic crises) from MG
- Maintain a quality of life appropriate to the disease course

RESTLESS LEGS SYNDROME

Etiology and Pathophysiology

Restless legs syndrome (RLS) (also known as *Willis–Ekbom disease*) is characterized by unpleasant sensory (paresthesias) and motor abnormalities of one or both legs. RLS is prevalent in 5 to 10% of the population, with a higher incidence in women over the age of 35 years (Rizek & Kumar, 2017).

There are two distinct types of RLS: primary (idiopathic) and secondary. Most people have primary RLS. Secondary RLS can occur with metabolic conditions associated with iron deficiency, renal disease and hemodialysis, and neuropathy. Sleep deprivation, sleep apnea, pregnancy (especially third trimester), and use of certain medications (e.g., antiemetics, antidepressants that increase serotonin) can cause or worsen symptoms.

The exact pathophysiology of primary RLS is unknown. It is thought to be related to a dysfunction in the brain's basal ganglia circuits that use the neurotransmitter dopamine, which controls movements. In RLS, this dysfunction causes the urge to move the legs. RLS has a genetic link. Individuals with primary RLS often report a positive family history, with symptoms that start before age 40.

Clinical Manifestations

The severity of RLS sensory symptoms ranges from infrequent minor discomfort (paresthesias, including numbness and tingling) to severe pain. Sensory symptoms often appear first. Patients describe annoying and uncomfortable (but usually not painful) sensations in the legs. Some describe the sensations like bugs crawling on the legs. The leg pain is localized within the calf muscles. Patients can also experience pain in the upper extremities and the trunk. The discomfort occurs when the patient is sedentary and is most common in the evening or at night, resulting in sleep disruption. In severe cases, patients sleep only a few hours at night, resulting in daytime fatigue and disruption of their daily routine. Physical activity, such as walking or stretching, often relieves the pain. The motor abnormalities associated with RLS consist of voluntary restlessness and stereotyped, periodic, involuntary movements (NINDS, 2021c). Fatigue further aggravates symptoms. Over time, RLS advances to more frequent and severe episodes.

Diagnostic Studies

Diagnosis of RLS can be made when the patient meets all five specific criteria: (1) overwhelming urge to move the legs, often accompanied by uncomfortable or unpleasant sensations in the legs; (2) urge to move the legs worsens during rest or inactivity; (3) urge to move the legs is partially or totally relieved by movement, as long as the activity continues; (4) urge to move the legs becomes worse in the evening or at night; and (5) these features are not due to another medical or behavioural condition (NINDS, 2021c).

The patient may have polysomnography studies done during sleep to distinguish RLS from other clinical conditions that can disturb sleep (e.g., sleep apnea). While periodic leg movements in sleep can support the diagnosis of RLS, they are not exclusive to RLS. Blood tests, such as a complete blood count, serum ferritin, and renal function tests (e.g., serum creatinine), may help exclude secondary causes of RLS. A patient with diabetes may have paresthesia caused by peripheral neuropathy related to diabetes or RLS.

NURSING AND INTERPROFESSIONAL MANAGEMENT RESTLESS LEGS SYNDROME

The goal of interprofessional management is to reduce patient discomfort and distress and to improve sleep quality. When RLS is due to renal failure or iron deficiency, treating these conditions may decrease symptoms. Lifestyle changes may help persons with mild to moderate RLS. For example, decreasing the use of alcohol or tobacco, maintaining regular sleep habits, exercising, and massaging and stretching the legs may be helpful. The patient should avoid using antihistamine-containing medications (e.g., diphenhydramine).

If nonpharmacological measures fail to provide symptom relief, medication therapy may be started. The main medications used in RLS are dopaminergic agents, opioids, and benzodiazepines. Dopaminergic agents such as carbidopa–levodopa (Sinemet) and dopamine agonists (bromocriptine, pramipexole [Mirapex]) are preferred for treating RLS. These agents are effective in managing sensory and motor symptoms.

Other agents that may be used include anticonvulsant medications such as gabapentin (Neurontin), divalproex (Epival), lamotrigine (Lamictal), and carbamazepine (Tegretol). Clonidine and propranolol (Inderal) are also effective in some patients. While quinine sulphate has been used prophylactically and as a treatment for RLS, its use is not recommended as it has been linked with serious adverse reactions such as life-threatening hematological reactions and chronic renal failure. Opioids are usually reserved for those patients with severe symptoms that fail to respond to other medications. When used, opioids given in low doses have also been found to be effective in reducing the symptoms associated with RLS.

AMYOTROPHIC LATERAL SCLEROSIS

Amyotrophic lateral sclerosis (ALS) is a rare, progressive, neurological disorder that is characterized by loss of motor neurons and by weakness and atrophy of the muscles of the hands, the forearms, and the legs, spreading to involve most of the body and the face. ALS became known as *Lou Gehrig's disease* when the famous baseball player was stricken with it in the 1940s. Approximately 3 000 Canadians are living with ALS, and 2 to 3 people die from ALS each day (Amyotrophic Lateral Sclerosis Society of Canada, 2020). ALS usually leads to death within 2 to 6 years after diagnosis.

For unknown reasons, motor neurons in the brainstem and spinal cord gradually degenerate in ALS. Dead motor neurons cannot produce or transport vital signals to muscles. Consequently, electrical and chemical messages originating in the brain do not reach the muscles to activate them.

The typical symptoms of ALS are limb weakness, dysarthria, and dysphagia. Muscle wasting and fasciculations result from the denervation of the muscles and lack of stimulation and use. Other symptoms include pain, sleep disorders, spasticity, drooling, emotional lability, depression, constipation, and esophageal reflux. Death usually results from respiratory tract infection secondary to compromised respiratory function. Unfortunately, there is no cure for ALS. Riluzole (Rilutek) slows the progression of ALS. This medication works to decrease the amount of glutamate (an excitatory neurotransmitter) in the brain.

The illness trajectory for ALS is devastating because the patient is cognitively intact while wasting away. The patient should be guided in the use of moderate-intensity, endurance-type exercises for the trunk and limbs because they may help to reduce

ALS spasticity. Nursing interventions include (1) facilitating communication, (2) reducing aspiration risk, (3) early identification of respiratory insufficiency, (4) decreasing pain from muscle weakness, (5) decreasing risk for fall-related injury, and (6) providing diversional activities, such as reading and companionship.

The patient and caregivers need to be supported emotionally, particularly with regard to grieving related to the loss of motor function and impending death. The nurse should discuss advance directives and artificial methods of ventilation with the patient and caregiver.

HUNTINGTON'S DISEASE

Huntington's disease (HD) is a progressive, degenerative brain disorder. It is a genetically transmitted, autosomal dominant disorder. The offspring of a person with HD have a 50% risk for inheriting it (see the Genetics in Clinical Practice box). The onset of HD is usually between ages 30 and 50 years. Diagnosis is often made after the affected person has had children. About 1 in 7 000 Canadians have HD (Huntington Society of Canada, 2017). It affects men and women equally.

The diagnostic process for HD begins with a review of the family history and clinical symptoms. Genetic testing confirms the disease in a person with symptoms. People who are asymptomatic but who have a positive family history of HD face the dilemma of whether to be genetically tested. If the test is positive, the person will develop HD, but when and to what extent the disease develops cannot be determined.

GENETICS IN CLINICAL PRACTICE
Huntington's Disease

Genetic Basis
- Autosomal dominant disorder
- Caused by mutation in *HTT* gene found on chromosome 4
- A single copy of altered gene (heterozygous) is enough to cause HD.
- Offspring of a person with HD have a 50% chance of inheriting the disease-causing allele.

Incidence
- 1 in 7 000 Canadians
- Higher incidence in people of European ancestry

Genetic Testing
- DNA testing is available.
- DNA testing can be done on fetal cells obtained by amniocentesis or chorionic villus sampling.
- Preimplantation genetic diagnosis can be done on embryos before implantation and pregnancy.
- No test is available to predict when symptoms will develop.

Clinical Implications
- Consider genetic counselling if there is a family history of HD.
- Because HD is an autosomal dominant disorder, those at risk have a strong motivation to seek genetic testing.
- A positive result is not considered a diagnosis because it may be obtained decades before symptoms begin.
- A negative test means that the individual does not carry the mutated gene and will not develop HD.

Social Networking in Huntington's Disease
- Many patients with HD experience social isolation and depression.
- The patient should be encouraged to participate in an online community where people with HD discuss their condition.
- Social contact and a social network with others who have HD can help patients cope better with their illness and improve their quality of life.

Like PD, the pathological process of HD involves the basal ganglia and the extrapyramidal motor system. However, instead of a deficiency of dopamine, HD involves a deficiency of the neurotransmitters ACh and γ-aminobutyric acid (GABA). The net effect is an excess of dopamine, which leads to symptoms that are the opposite of those of parkinsonism.

Manifestations include movement disorder and cognitive and psychiatric challenges. The movement disorder is marked by abnormal and excessive involuntary movements *(chorea)*. These are writhing, twisting movements of the face, limbs, and body. The movements get worse as the disease progresses. Because facial movements involving speech, chewing, and swallowing are affected, aspiration and malnutrition are likely. The gait deteriorates, and ambulation eventually becomes impossible. Eventually, all psychomotor processes, including the ability to eat and talk, are impaired.

Psychiatric symptoms are often present in the early stage of HD, even before the onset of motor symptoms. Depression is common. Other psychiatric symptoms include anxiety, agitation, impulsivity, apathy, social withdrawal, and obsessiveness. Cognitive deterioration is more variable. It involves perception, memory, attention, and learning.

The median survival rate for HD is 15 to 18 years (Genetics Education Canada–Knowledge Organization, 2019). The most common causes of death related to HD are pneumonia and suicide; however, injuries related to a fall or other complications have also been attributed to HD-related mortality.

Because there is no cure, interprofessional care is palliative. The first medication of any kind approved specifically for HD is tetrabenazine. It is used to treat the chorea and works to decrease the amount of dopamine available at synapses in the brain and thus decreases the involuntary movements of chorea.

Other medications used for the movement disorder include neuroleptics such as haloperidol (Haldol) and risperidone (Risperdal), benzodiazepines such as diazepam (Valium) and clonazepam (Rivotril), and dopamine-depleting agents. Cognitive disorders are treated as needed with nonmedication therapies (e.g., counselling, memory books). The psychiatric disorders can be treated with selective serotonin reuptake inhibitors such as sertraline (Zoloft) and paroxetine (Paxil). Antipsychotic medication, such as haloperidol or risperidone (Risperdal), may also be needed.

Given the chorea associated with HD, caloric requirements are high. Patients with HD may require as many as 5 000 calories per day to maintain body weight. As the disease progresses, meeting caloric needs becomes more challenging as the patient has difficulty swallowing and holding their head still. Depression and mental deterioration can also compromise nutritional intake. Alternative sources of nutrition may be indicated as the disease progresses.

Care of patients with HD presents a great challenge to health care providers. The goal of nursing management is to provide the most comfortable environment possible for the patient and the family by maintaining physical safety, treating physical symptoms, and providing emotional and psychological support. End-of-life issues should be discussed with the patient and caregiver. These include care in the home or long-term care facility, artificial methods of feeding, advance directives and cardiopulmonary resuscitation (CPR), use of antibiotics to treat infections, and guardianship. These topics should be readdressed throughout the course of the disease as the patient and caregiver adapt to the patient's increasing disability.

NORMAL PRESSURE HYDROCEPHALUS

Normal pressure hydrocephalus (NPH) is an abnormal increase of CSF characterized by an obstruction in the normal flow of CSF throughout the brain, spinal cord, and ventricles. NPH is a relatively uncommon disorder. Symptoms of the condition include mental impairment, dementia, urinary incontinence, and gait and balance disturbances. Meningitis, encephalitis, or head injury may cause the condition. NPH can occur at any age, although it is most common in older persons. If diagnosed early in the disease, NPH is treatable by surgery that involves a shunt insertion to divert the fluid away from the brain into the abdomen to help resolve the symptoms (NINDS, 2019).

CASE STUDY

Parkinson's Disease

Patient Profile
J. D. (pronouns he/him), a 79-year-old retiree, was diagnosed with Parkinson's disease 3 years ago after experiencing months of progressive tremor, rigidity, and bradykinesia. J. D. has been taking levodopa with carbidopa (Sinemet) since then, and symptoms had been improving until recently. When J. D.'s daughter was visiting, she noticed that he had lost a considerable amount of weight over the past month, and his speech had become slower and difficult to understand.

Subjective Data
- Reports increasing difficulty with speech and swallowing
- Dietary intake has decreased
- Reports being constipated for 2 weeks

Objective Data
Physical Examination
- Body weight has decreased by 5 kg in 1 month.
- Gait has developed a mild shuffling and propulsive quality.

- "Pill rolling" motion and tremor are observed in both hands at rest.
- "Cogwheel rigidity" is encountered during passive range-of-motion exercises.

Discussion Questions
1. What is the pathogenesis of Parkinson's disease?
2. What is the likely explanation for the progression of J. D.'s condition?
3. What teaching plan should be developed for J. D.?
4. *Priority decision:* What are the priority nursing interventions for J. D.?
5. *Priority decision:* What are the priority nursing diagnoses based on the assessment data presented for J. D.?

🅔volve
Answers are available at http://evolve.elsevier.com/Canada/Lewis/medsurg.

REVIEW QUESTIONS

The number of the question corresponds to the same-numbered objective at the beginning of the chapter.

1. What of the following is the nurse most likely to recognize as a symptom of a client with a migraine headache?
   a. Withdraws from stimuli
   b. Acts out with bizarre behaviour
   c. Seeks out the company of others
   d. Experiences painful facial spasms and tearing

2. What are the classic symptoms the nurse would expect to find during assessment of the client with Parkinson's disease?
   a. Spasticity, diplopia, tremor, ataxia
   b. Tremor, rigidity, ataxia, postural instability
   c. Ataxia, drowsiness, dysarthria, tremor
   d. Diplopia, tremor, bradykinesia, postural instability

3. What would the nurse expect to find during an assessment of the client with amyotrophic lateral sclerosis?
   a. Emotional lability
   b. Mental deterioration
   c. Muscle weakness and wasting
   d. Sensory loss in the extremities

4. Social effects of a chronic neurological disease include which of the following? (Select all that apply.)
   a. Divorce
   b. Job loss
   c. Depression
   d. Role changes
   e. Loss of self-esteem

5. What is a major goal of treatment for the client with a chronic, progressive neurological disease?
   a. Reversal of pathophysiological features
   b. Total remission of the disease
   c. Continuation of usual lifestyle
   d. Adaptation by client and family to the disease

1. a; 2. b; 3. c; 4. a, b, c, d, e; 5. d.

ⓔvolve

For even more review questions, visit http://evolve.elsevier.com/Canada/Lewis/medsurg.

REFERENCES

American Migraine Foundation. (2016). *Migraine and common co-morbidities.* https://americanmigrainefoundation.org/resource-library/migraine-and-common-co-morbidities/

American Migraine Foundation. (2019). *Understanding cluster headache.* https://americanmigrainefoundation.org/resource-library/cluster-headache-2/

Amyotrophic Lateral Sclerosis Society of Canada. (2020). *ALS, MS and MD: How do they differ?.* https://als.ca/wp-content/uploads/2021/05/Fact-Sheet-ALS-MS-and-MD_FINAL.pdf

Andreou, A. P., & Edvinsson, L. (2019). Mechanisms of migraine as a chronic evolutive condition. *The Journal of Headache and Pain,* 20(1), 1–17.

Becker, W. J., Findlay, T., Moga, C., et al. (2015). Guideline for primary care management of headache in adults. *Canadian Family Physician,* 61(8), 670–679.

Bourque, P. R., & Breiner, A. (2018). Myasthenia gravis. *CMAJ: Canadian Medical Association Journal,* 190(38), E1141.

Brandt, R. B., Doesborg, P. G., Haan, J., et al. (2020). Pharmacotherapy for cluster headache. *CNS Drugs,* 34(2), 171–184. https://doi.org/10.1007/s40263-019-00696-2

Buture, A., Gooriah, R., Nimeri, R., et al. (2016). Current understanding on pain mechanism in migraine and cluster headache. *Anesthesiology and Pain Medicine,* 6(3) e35190.

Canadian League Against Epilepsy. (2020). *Safety measures.* https://claegroup.org/Safety-Measures

Canadian Society for Exercise Physiology. (2020). *Canadian physical activity guidelines for adults with multiple sclerosis.* https://csepguidelines.ca/guidelines/multiple-sclerosis/

Charles, A. (2018). The pathophysiology of migraine: Implications for clinical management. *The Lancet Neurology,* 17(2), 174–182.

Epilepsy Canada. (2021). *What is epilepsy?.* https://www.epilepsy.ca/what-is-epilepsy

Fisher, R. S., Cross, J. H., French, J. A., et al. (2017). Operational classification of seizure types by the International League Against Epilepsy: Position paper of the ILAE Commission for Classification and Terminology. *Epilepsia,* 58(4), 522–530.

Gargya, A., & Abdallah, R. (2019). Migraine headaches. In A. Abd-Elsayed (Ed.), *Pain.* Springer. https://link.springer.com/chapter/10.1007/978-3-319-99124-5_121

Gaspard, N. (2016). Autoimmune epilepsy. *CONTINUUM: Lifelong Learning in Neurology,* 22(1), 227–245.

Genetics Education Canada–Knowledge Organization. (2019). *Huntington disease.* https://geneticseducation.ca/educational-resources/gec-ko-on-the-run/huntington-disease/

Gilmour, H., Ramage-Morin, P. L., & Wong, S. L. (2018). *Multiple sclerosis: Prevalence and impact.* Statistics Canada. https://www150.statcan.gc.ca/n1/pub/82-003-x/2018001/article/54902-eng.htm

Gonzalez-Usigli, H. A. (2020). *Parkinson disease.* https://www.merckmanuals.com/professional/neurologic-disorders/movement-and-cerebellar-disorders/parkinson-disease#section_15

Government of Canada. (2019). *Multiple sclerosis in Canada.* https://www.canada.ca/en/public-health/services/publications/diseases-conditions/multiple-sclerosis-infographic.html

Gupta, V. K. (2019). Pathophysiology of migraine: An increasingly complex narrative to 2020. *Future Neurology,* 14(2), FNL12.

Hall, W. (2019). Psychiatric medication withdrawal: Survivor perspectives and clinical practice. *Journal of Humanistic Psychology,* 59(5), 720–729. https://doi.org/10.1177/0022167818765331

Headache Classification Committee of the International Headache Society (IHS). (2018). The International Classification of Headache Disorders, 3rd edition. *Cephalgia: An International Journal of Headache,* 38(1), 1–211.

Hoffmann, J., & May, A. (2018). Diagnosis, pathophysiology, and management of cluster headache. *The Lancet Neurology,* 17(1), 75–83.

Huntington Society of Canada. (2017). *Living at-risk for Huntington disease.* https://www.huntingtonsociety.ca/wp-content/uploads/2017/03/Living-At-Risk-Mar-2017.pdf

Jamebozorgi, K., Taghizadeh, E., Rostami, D., et al. (2019). Cellular and molecular aspects of Parkinson treatment: Future therapeutic perspectives. *Molecular Neurobiology, 56,* 4799–4811. https://doi.org/10.1007/s12035-018-1419-8

Jennum, P., Christensen, J. A., Zoetm Jennum, P., et al. (2016). Neurophysiological basis of rapid eye movement sleep behavior disorder: Informing future drug development. *Nature and Science of Sleep, 8,* 107–120. https://doi.org/10.2147/NSS.S99240

Kamel, F. O. (2019). Factors involved in relapse of multiple sclerosis. *Journal of Microscopy and Ultrastructure, 7*(3), 103.

Marrie, R. A., Leung, S., Yu, N., et al. (2018). Lower prevalence of multiple sclerosis in First Nations Canadians. *Neurology: Clinical Practice, 8*(1), 33–39.

May, A., & Schulte, L. H. (2016). Chronic migraine: Risk factors, mechanisms and treatment. *Nature Reviews Neurology, 12*(8), 455.

Mayo Clinic. (2019). *Myasthenia gravis.* https://www.mayoclinic.org/diseases-conditions/myasthenia-gravis/symptoms-causes/syc-20352036

Mier, R. W., & Dhadwal, S. (2018). Primary headaches. *Dental Clinics, 62*(4), 611–628.

Multiple Sclerosis Society of Canada. (2019). *Update: Preliminary results of the mesenchymal stem cell study for the treatment of multiple sclerosis.* https://mssociety.ca/research-news/article/update-mescams

Multiple Sclerosis Society of Canada. (2021a). *Aubagio.* https://mssociety.ca/managing-ms/treatments/medications/disease-modifying-therapies-dmts/aubagio

Multiple Sclerosis Society of Canada. (2021b). *Chronic cerebrospinal venous insufficiency (CCSVI).* https://mssociety.ca/hot-topics/chronic-cerebrospinal-venous-insufficiency-ccsvi

Myasthenia Gravis Coalition of Canada. (2021). *Signs and symptoms of MG.* http://mgcc-ccmg.org/about.asp

Nagai, Y., Jones, C. I., & Sen, A. (2019). Galvanic skin response (GSR)/electrodermal/skin conductance biofeedback on epilepsy: A systematic review and meta-analysis. *Frontiers in Neurology, 10,* 377. https://doi.org/10.3389/fneur.2019.00377

National Institute of Neurological Disorders and Stroke (NINDS). (2019). *Normal pressure hydrocephalus information page.* https://www.ninds.nih.gov/Disorders/All-Disorders/Normal-Pressure-Hydrocephalus-Information-Page

National Institute of Neurological Disorders and Stroke (NINDS). (2020). *The epilepsies and seizures: Hope through research.* https://www.ninds.nih.gov/Disorders/Patient-Caregiver-Education/Hope-Through-Research/Epilepsies-and-Seizures-Hope-Through

National Institute of Neurological Disorders and Stroke (NINDS). (2021a). *Myasthenia gravis fact sheet.* https://www.ninds.nih.gov/Disorders/Patient-Caregiver-Education/Fact-Sheets/Myasthenia-Gravis-Fact-Sheet#4

National Institute of Neurological Disorders and Stroke (NINDS). (2021b). *Parkinson's disease: Hope through research.* https://www.ninds.nih.gov/Disorders/Patient-Caregiver-Education/Hope-Through-Research/Parkinsons-Disease-Hope-Through-Research

National Institute of Neurological Disorders and Stroke (NINDS). (2021c). *Restless legs syndrome fact sheet.* www.ninds.nih.gov/Disorders/Patient-Caregiver-Education/Fact-Sheets/Restless-Legs-Syndrome-Fact-Sheet

National Institutes of Health (NIH). (2021). *What is gene therapy?* https://ghr.nlm.nih.gov/primer/therapy/genetherapy

National Multiple Sclerosis Society. (2021). *What causes MS?.* https://www.nationalmssociety.org/What-is-MS/What-Causes-MS

Parkinson Canada. (2020). *Infographic.* https://www.parkinson.ca/wp-content/uploads/infographic.pdf

Parkinson's Foundation. (2021). *FAQ's: Genetics & Parkinson's.* https://www.parkinson.org/understanding-parkinsons/causes/genetics/faqs

Poff, A., Rho, J., & D'Agostino, D. (2019). Ketone administration for seizure disorders: History and rationale for ketone esters and metabolic alternatives. *Frontiers in Neuroscience, 13,* ART. 1041. https://doi.org/10.1177/0022167818765331

Public Health Agency of Canada. (2018). *Parkinsonism in Canada, including Parkinson's disease.* https://www.canada.ca/en/public-health/services/publications/diseases-conditions/parkinsonism.html

Razaz, N., Tomson, T., Wikström, A. K., et al. (2017). Association between pregnancy and perinatal outcomes among women with epilepsy. *JAMA Neurology, 74*(8), 983–991.

Rizek, P., & Kumar, N. (2017). Restless legs syndrome. *Canadian Medical Association Journal, 189*(6) E245-E245.

Steinberg, A., Fourier, C., Ran, C., et al. (2018). Cluster headache—Clinical pattern and a new severity scale in a Swedish cohort. *Cephalalgia, 38*(7), 1286–1295.

Thompson, A. J., Banwell, B. L., Barkhof, F., et al. (2018). Diagnosis of multiple sclerosis: 2017 revisions of the McDonald criteria. *The Lancet Neurology, 17*(2), 162–173.

Westman, E. C., Tondt, J., Eberstein, J., et al. (2018). Use of a low-carbohydrate, ketogenic diet to treat obesity. *Primary Care Reports, 24*(10).

World Health Organization (WHO). (2016). *Headache disorders.* https://www.who.int/news-room/fact-sheets/detail/headache-disorders

World Health Organization (WHO). (2019). *Epilepsy.* https://www.who.int/news-room/fact-sheets/detail/epilepsy

Zamboni, P., Galeotti, R., Menegatti, E., et al. (2008). Chronic cerebrospinal venous insufficiency in patients with multiple sclerosis. *Journal of Neurology, Neurosurgery, and Psychiatry, 80*(4), 392–399. (Seminal). https://doi.org/10.1136/jnnp.2008.157164

Zamboni, P., Tesio, L., Galimberti, S., et al. (2018). Efficacy and safety of extracranial vein angioplasty in multiple sclerosis: A randomized clinical trial. *JAMA Neurology, 75*(1), 35–43.

RESOURCES

Amyotrophic Lateral Sclerosis Society of Canada
https://www.als.ca

Canadian Association of Neuroscience Nurses (CANN)
https://www.cann.ca

Canadian Human Rights Commission
https://www.chrc-ccdp.ca

Canadian Institute of Health Research
https://www.cihr-irsc.gc.ca

Epilepsy Canada
https://www.epilepsy.ca

Huntington Society of Canada
https://www.huntingtonsociety.ca/

Multiple Sclerosis Society of Canada
https://www.mssociety.ca

Myasthenia Gravis Coalition of Canada
http://www.mgcc-ccmg.org

Parkinson Canada
https://www.parkinson.ca

Veterans Affairs Canada
https://www.veterans.gc.ca

American Migraine Foundation
https://americanmigrainefoundation.org/

Association of Rehabilitation Nurses (ARN)
https://www.rehabnurse.org
Myasthenia Gravis Foundation of America
https://www.myasthenia.org
National Headache Foundation
https://www.headaches.org
National Institute of Neurological Disorders and Stroke (NINDS)
https://www.ninds.nih.gov

Restless Legs Syndrome Foundation
https://www.rls.org

(e)volve

For additional Internet resources, see the website for this book at
http://evolve.elsevier.com/Canada/Lewis/medsurg.

Nursing Management

Delirium, Alzheimer's Disease, and Other Dementias

Lynn McCleary

⊜volve WEBSITE

http://evolve.elsevier.com/Canada/Lewis/medsurg

- Review Questions (Online Only)
- Key Points
- Answer Guidelines for Case Study
- Student Case Study
  - Patient with Alzheimer's Disease

- Customizable Nursing Care Plans
  - Dementia
  - Family Caregivers

- Conceptual Care Map Creator
- Audio Glossary
- Content Updates

LEARNING OBJECTIVES

1. Describe the etiology, the pathophysiology, and the clinical manifestations of delirium.
2. Describe the diagnostic studies and the interprofessional management of delirium.
3. Define dementia and describe its effect on society.
4. Compare and contrast etiologies of different types of dementia.
5. Describe the clinical manifestations, the diagnostic studies, and the interprofessional management of dementia.
6. Describe the clinical manifestations of mild cognitive impairment.
7. Describe the nursing management of patients with dementia.

KEY TERMS

Alzheimer's disease (AD)
amyloid plaques
behavioural and psychological symptoms of
   dementia (BPSDs)
Confusion Assessment Method
Creutzfeldt–Jakob disease (CJD)

delirium
dementia
dementia with Lewy bodies (DLB)
familial Alzheimer's disease
frontotemporal dementia (FTD)
mild cognitive impairment (MCI)

neurofibrillary tangles
responsive behaviours
self-protective behaviours
sundowning
vascular dementia

The three most common cognitive conditions to occur in adults are delirium, dementia, and depression. These conditions often manifest with overlapping clinical features and may coexist in an older person (Registered Nurses Association of Ontario [RNAO], 2016). It is important to identify the distinguishing characteristics because the treatment for each condition is different. This chapter focuses on delirium and dementia. Dementia is also known as *major neurocognitive disorder* (Moore, 2021), but the term *dementia* will be used in this chapter. The reader should consult a mental health nursing textbook for additional information about depression.

DELIRIUM

Delirium, an acute brain dysfunction resulting in impaired attention, awareness, and cognition, is a medical emergency. It is one of the most common life-threatening conditions in older individuals and preventable in more than 30% of cases (RNAO, 2016). Nurses are at the front line for prevention and early detection of delirium. However, like other health care providers, nurses often fail to recognize delirium. The prevalence of delirium is highest among hospitalized older persons. More than half of hospitalized older patients develop delirium, with rates of up to 50% after fractures or surgery and 82% in the critical care unit. Rates are even higher among patients with pre-existing dementia (Hshieh et al., 2018). Delirium is associated with longer hospitalizations, decline in cognition and functioning, higher rates of institutionalization, and higher rates of mortality (Hshieh et al., 2018).

Etiology and Pathophysiology

The pathophysiology of delirium is related to multiple processes. Inflammation, hypoxia, and other biological and physiological factors are thought to cause neurotransmitter imbalance, particularly acetylcholine deficiency and dopamine excess. Other neurotransmitters, including γ-aminobutyric acid (GABA), serotonin, norepinephrine, and glutamate, are also implicated and may account for the different subtypes of delirium (Mulkey et al., 2018).

Delirium is usually the result of interaction between the patient's underlying condition and a precipitating event. Delirium can occur after a relatively minor insult in a vulnerable patient. For example, patients with underlying health problems such as heart failure, cognitive impairment, or sensory limitations may develop delirium after a relatively minor change (e.g., a single dose of a sleeping medication). In less vulnerable patients, it may take a combination of factors (e.g., anaesthesia, major surgery, infection, prolonged sleep deprivation) to precipitate delirium (Hshieh et al., 2018). Delirium can also be a symptom of a serious medical illness such as bacterial meningitis. Knowing which factors increase vulnerability to delirium (*predisposing factors*) or precipitate delirium (*precipitating factors*) facilitates prevention of delirium and effective intervention. These factors are listed in Table 62.1.

Delirium occurs in children and adults, but older people are at higher risk. They are more likely to have one of more of the risk factors for delirium. Normal age-related changes (see Chapter 7) limit older persons' abilities to compensate for physiological insults such as hypoxia, hypoglycemia, and dehydration and increase their susceptibility to medication-induced delirium. Patients with dementia are at risk on two fronts: Their risk for developing delirium is higher, and the probability that the delirium will be identified is lower (Morandi et al., 2015).

Clinical Manifestations

The core features of delirium are (a) disturbance of attention and of awareness of the environment; (b) a change in cognition (such as memory deficit, disorientation, language disturbance, perceptual disturbance) that is not due to neurocognitive disorder such as dementia; and (c) development of the disturbance over a short time (usually hours to days) and a tendency for it to fluctuate during the course of the day (American Psychiatric Association, 2013).

There are three subtypes of delirium: *hyperactive delirium*, which is characterized by restlessness, psychomotor agitation, and hypervigilance; *hypoactive delirium*, which is characterized by lethargy, drowsiness, and decreased motor activity; and *mixed delirium*, which has features of both hypoactive and hyperactive delirium. Other common symptoms include hallucinations, illusions, disturbed sleep–wake cycle, and disorientation to person, place, situation, and time (Shaji et al., 2018). Hypoactive delirium is more common in older persons and is potentially more serious because this form is often not identified. It may be overlooked because the patient is quiet, or it may be mistaken for depression.

Delirium is often mistaken for dementia. A key distinction between delirium and dementia is the *sudden* development of symptoms of delirium over a short time period. (A comparison of delirium and dementia is presented in Table 62.2.) To distinguish between dementia and delirium superimposed on dementia, the nurse may need collateral information from a reliable informant about baseline mental status and changes in cognition.

When effectively treated, delirium usually resolves within 4 to 7 days. However, it can recur, and it may persist for weeks to months after hospital discharge. Patient safety must be considered in discharge planning preparations.

TABLE 62.1   RISK FACTORS FOR DELIRIUM

Predisposing Factors
- Age over 75 years
- Alcohol misuse
- Comorbid or severe illness
- Dementia
- Depression
- Functional impairment
- History of cerebrovascular incident
- History of delirium
- Pain
- Sensory impairment

Precipitating Factors
- Abnormal physiological indices (i.e., electrolytes, BUN, serum urea, serum albumin)

- Bladder catheter
- Coma
- Medications
- Multiple medications prescribed
- Psychoactive medications
- Sedatives or hypnotics
- Iatrogenic event
- Infection
- Physiological (increased serum urea or BUN; creatinine ratio; abnormal serum albumin, glucose, or potassium; metabolic acidosis)
- Overstimulating or understimulating environment
- Physical restraints
- Surgery
- Trauma
- Urgent admission

BUN, blood urea nitrogen.
Source: Adapted from Hshieh, T. T., Inouye, S. K., & Oh, E. S. (2018). Delirium in the elderly (Table 4). *Psychiatric Clinics of North America, 41*(2018), 1–17. https://doi.org/10.1016/j.psc.2017.10.001; and Tullmann, D. F., Blevins, C., & Fletcher, K. (2016). Delirium: Prevention, early recognition, and treatment. In M. Boltz, et al. (Eds.), *Evidence-based geriatric nursing protocols for best practice* (5th ed., pp. 252–261). Springer.

TABLE 62.2   COMPARISON OF CLINICAL FEATURES OF DELIRIUM, DEMENTIA, AND DEPRESSION

Feature	Delirium	Dementia	Depression
Onset	Acute	Insidious	Variable
Duration	Days to weeks	Months to years	Variable
Course	Fluctuating	Slowly progressive	Diurnal variation (worse in morning, improves during day)
Consciousness	Impaired, fluctuating	Clear until late in course of the illness	Unimpaired
Attention and memory	Inattentiveness Poor memory	Poor memory without marked inattention	Difficulty concentrating: memory intact/minimally impaired
Affect	Variable	Variable	Depressed; loss of interest and pleasure in usual activities

Source: Canadian Coalition for Seniors' Mental Health (CCSMH). (2006). *National guidelines for seniors' mental health: The assessment and treatment of delirium* (p. 23, Table 1.1). Author.

Diagnostic Studies

Delirium is diagnosed on the basis of behavioural observation and the results of mental status examination. There are several valid ways for nurses to screen for the presence of delirium. The Recognizing Acute Delirium As part of your Routine (RADAR) approach can easily be incorporated in routine nursing assessment and care (Voyer et al., 2017). It is a very brief approach (7 seconds) consisting of three questions in relation to the patient interaction: (1) Was the patient drowsy? (2) Did the patient have trouble following directions? (3) Were the patient's movements slowed down? Screening is positive if the answer is yes to any of these questions. If the RADAR screen is positive, then the Confusion Assessment Method (CAM) or 4 A's Test (4AT) should be completed. The CAM is a widely used, 5- to 10-minute screening assessment and diagnostic aid (Inouye et al., 1990). Delirium is difficult to detect in patients with moderate to severe dementia because of overlap of symptoms of inattention. The 4AT is a brief delirium assessment that is validated with patients who have dementia, available in English and French (Gagné et al., 2018).

When delirium is diagnosed, identification and treatment of the underlying causes is urgent. The patient's history and physical examination findings, medication history, laboratory test results, additional diagnostic investigation as indicated, and environmental risk factors must be evaluated. Usual investigations include complete blood cell count; biochemistry evaluations (measurements of calcium, albumin, magnesium, phosphate, creatinine, urea, electrolytes, and glucose levels; liver function tests); thyroid function tests; blood, urine, and sputum cultures; oxygen saturation measurement; urinalysis; chest radiography; and electrocardiography (ECG) (Hshieh et al., 2018). If meningitis or encephalitis is suspected, a lumbar puncture may be performed (see Chapter 59). If the patient's history includes head injury, appropriate radiographic examinations or scans may be ordered. Brain imaging studies such as computed tomography (CT) and magnetic resonance imaging (MRI) are performed if the patient has a known or suspected head injury or brain lesion.

NURSING AND INTERPROFESSIONAL MANAGEMENT DELIRIUM

The priority for nursing care is prevention of delirium. The priorities when a patient has delirium are to identify and treat underlying cause or causes, to maintain physiological stability, and to ensure the patient's safety (RNAO, 2016; Tullmann et al., 2016). Prevention involves recognition of patients at high risk for delirium (see Table 62.1) and providing care that targets each patient's risk factors. Among older persons, most of the precipitating factors for delirium during hospitalization are influenced by nursing interventions (e.g., physical restraints, polypharmacy).

The Canadian Patient Safety Institute (2016) recommends that hospitals develop delirium prevention and management protocols and enable staff to implement them. There is strong research evidence that proactive multicomponent interventions reduce incidence of new cases of delirium and improve outcomes for patients with delirium (RNAO, 2016; Tullman et al., 2016). The Hospital Elder Life Program (HELP) is a well-researched multicomponent program (Hshieh et al., 2018). Components of the program are listed in Table 62.3. Details about the program are available on the HELP website (see the Resources at the end of this chapter).

Additional strategies to eliminate or minimize risk factors are listed in Table 62.4. It is important to maintain the patient's physiological stability. Many medications can contribute to delirium. Categories of medications to use with caution are antipsychotics, anticholinergics, H_2-blocking agents, opioids, sedative hypnotics, tricyclic antidepressants, and dihydropyridine calcium channel blockers (Hshieh et al., 2018; Lau et al., 2019). The Beers Criteria for Potentially Inappropriate Medication Use in Older Adults can be used to identify medication that should be avoided in treatment of older patients (American Geriatrics Society Beers Criteria® Update Expert Panel, 2019). Resources for using it are available on the Canadian Patient Safety Institute and the American Geriatrics Society websites (see Resources at the end of this chapter).

Adequate pain management is important because under-treated pain significantly increases risk for delirium. However, analgesics can also increase risk for delirium. Thus, interventions that minimize the use of opioids are recommended (Devlin et al., 2018).

TABLE 62.3 COMPONENTS OF THE HOSPITAL ELDER LIFE PROGRAM (HELP)

1. Systematic screening to identify patients at risk for developing delirium
2. Tailored interventions developed by an interprofessional team that consists of a geriatric nurse specialist, elder life specialist, and trained volunteers. Interventions include the following:
   - Daily orientation
   - Cognitive stimulation and therapeutic activities three times per day
   - Sleep enhancement and sleep deprivation prevention
   - Ambulation three times a day and minimization of immobilizing equipment (e.g., bladder catheters)
   - Visual aids
   - Hearing support
   - Avoiding dehydration
   - Feeding assistance
   - Preventing falls
3. Interdisciplinary rounds twice a week
4. Geriatrician and interdisciplinary team consultations
5. Community liaison and postdischarge telephone follow-up

Source: Adapted from Hsieh, T. T., Yang, T., Gartaganis, S. L., et al. (2018). Hospital Elder Life Program: Systematic review and meta-analysis of effectiveness. *Geriatric Psychiatry, 26*, 1015–1033. https://doi.org/10.1016/j.jagp.2018.06.007

TABLE 62.4 STRATEGIES TO ELIMINATE OR MINIMIZE RISK FACTORS FOR DELIRIUM

- Adequate nutrition
- Assessment and treatment of pain
- Judicious use of medication, elimination of nonessential medication, use of the lowest possible dose, avoidance of medications that contribute to delirium
- Optimized oxygenation
- Prevention and prompt treatment of dehydration and electrolyte imbalance
- Prevention and prompt treatment of infections
- Regulation of bowel and bladder function
- Use of sensory aids

Source: Adapted from Tullmann, D. F., Blevins, C., & Fletcher, K. (2016). Delirium: Prevention, early recognition, and treatment. In M. Boltz, et al. (Eds.), *Evidence-based geriatric nursing protocols for best practice* (5th ed., pp. 252–261). Springer; and Registered Nurses' Association of Ontario (RNAO). (2016). *Delirium, dementia, and depression in older adults: Assessment and care* (2nd ed.). Author. https://rnao.ca/sites/rnao-ca/files/bpg/RNAO_Delirium_Dementia_Depression_Older_Adults_Assessment_and_Care.pdf

TABLE 62.5	THERAPEUTIC ENVIRONMENT FOR PATIENTS WITH DELIRIUM OR RISK FOR DELIRIUM
Strategy	**Examples**
Foster orientation	• Explain all activities • Frequent reassurance and orientation (unless this causes agitation), avoiding confrontation about delusional beliefs • Use of hearing aids and eye glasses • Visible calendars, clocks, and staff identification
Provide appropriate stimulation	• Avoid overstimulation or sensory deprivation • Cognitively stimulating activities (e.g., family visits, familiar activities, reminiscence) • Adequate light • Music as preferred by the patient • Noise reduction • One task at a time • Quiet room
Facilitate sleep	• Back massage, warm milk, or herbal tea at bedtime • Reduce nighttime noise • Plan care to avoid disturbing sleep • Provide light during the day and reduce light at night • Relaxation music
Foster familiarity	• Bring familiar objects from home • Encourage family or friends to stay with patient • Minimize relocation • Provide consistent nursing staff
Maximize mobility	• Ambulate or provide range-of-motion exercises three times a day • Avoid use of medical devices (e.g., intravenous lines, bladder catheters) • Avoid use of restraints
Communicate clearly	• Convey warmth, kindness, and calmness • One question or direction at a time • Simple explanations
Reassure and educate patient and family	• Acknowledge emotions • Manage stigma • Provide post-delirium education • Provide written and verbal information and education about delirium and family role in management

Sources: Adapted from Tullmann, D. F., Blevins, C., & Fletcher, K. (2016). Delirium: Prevention, early recognition, and treatment. In M. Boltz, et al. (Eds.), *Evidence-based geriatric nursing protocols for best practice* (5th ed., pp. 252–261). Springer; and Registered Nurses' Association of Ontario (RNAO). (2016). *Delirium, dementia, and depression in older adults: Assessment and care* (2nd ed.). Author. https://rnao.ca/sites/rnao-ca/files/bpg/RNAO_Delirium_Dementia_Depression_Older_Adults_Assessment_and_Care.pdf

Strategies to provide a therapeutic environment for patients with delirium or who are at risk for delirium are provided in Table 62.5. Frequent assessment is required. Mental status should be assessed every shift, with delirium screening being the "sixth vital sign" for patients who have delirium or are at risk for delirium (Voyer et al., 2016). Close observation is required, especially for patients with hyperactive delirium. Use of invasive procedures should be minimized (Tullmann et al., 2016).

Medication Therapy

Medication therapy is not recommended for patients with delirium, except when there is severe agitation that interferes with needed medical therapy (e.g., fluid replacement, intubation) or presents a danger. In these instances, antipsychotics are the recommended medication therapy. Haloperidol, the first-line treatment, is started at low doses (0.25–0.5 mg once or twice a day) and slowly titrated upward, if necessary. Adverse effects of haloperidol include sedation, hypotension, extrapyramidal medication effects, muscle tone changes, and anticholinergic effects. Newer antipsychotics, including risperidone (Risperdal), olanzapine (Zyprexa), aripiprazole (Abilify), and quetiapine (Seroquel), may be used. Although these medications produce fewer adverse effects than does haloperidol, the adverse effects are significant; antipsychotics may worsen the delirium. Close monitoring is required. Medication therapy should be limited to the shortest time needed to manage the symptoms. Benzodiazepines (e.g., lorazepam [Ativan]) are contraindicated, except for treatment of delirium caused by withdrawal from either alcohol or sedative-hypnotics (Boland et al., 2019).

DEMENTIA

Dementia is a collection of symptoms caused by various diseases affecting the brain. Cognitive functioning in multiple areas declines progressively. In addition to impairing memory, dementia affects the individual's judgement, reasoning, and abilities to communicate, to carry out purposeful movements, and to recognize common objects and familiar people. Mood and behaviour are commonly affected. Ultimately, these challenges lead to inability to work, carry out social and family responsibilities, and perform activities of daily living (ADLs). The multiple effects on cognition and slow gradual decline differentiate dementia from delirium, which has a sudden onset.

In Canada in 2020, approximately 663 000 people were estimated to be living with dementia, and this number is expected to increase to 987 000 by 2033 (Chambers et al., 2016). Dementia occurs most often in older persons and is more common in women than in men. Among those between the ages of 65 and 69 years, the prevalence is 1.9% of males and 2.8% of females. Prevalence rises with increasing age; up to 28.7% of males and 37.1% of females older than 85 are living with dementia (Chambers et al., 2016). Among Indigenous people, prevalence of dementia is higher than in the general population, has a younger age of onset, and affects men more than women (Walker & Jacklin, 2019). This pattern may be related to social determinants of health that are associated with dementia risk, such as lower level of education, history of head injury, poverty, and stressors, and to physiological risk factors such as diabetes mellitus and hypertension (MacDonald et al., 2018; Walker & Jacklin, 2019).

The cost of dementia in Canada is high (Chambers et al., 2016). In 2011, family members and friends provided approximately 19.2 million hours of informal unpaid caregiver time to people with dementia, and this number is expected to double by 2031. The economic burden of dementia, including health care costs and out-of-pocket expenses for persons with dementia and their families is estimated to be $11.2 billion per year in 2021. When indirect costs, such as lost wages and lost productivity are included, the cost is about three times greater. The four most common types of dementia are Alzheimer's disease (approximately 70%), vascular dementia (approximately 10%), dementia with Lewy bodies (approximately 5%), and frontotemporal dementia (approximately 5%) (Fiest et al., 2016; Hogan et al., 2016; Salthouse et al., 2019). Mixed dementia, in which more than one type of dementia is present, occurs in between 10 and 20% of cases of dementia (Custodio et al., 2017). Dementia is also part of the later stages of Parkinson's disease and Huntington's disease. In individuals with Down syndrome, the prevalence of dementia is significantly greater than in the general population and age of onset is younger. Another type of dementia is caused by Creutzfeldt–Jakob disease (CJD), a very rare, fatal, infectious brain disorder thought to be the result of accumulation in the brain of an abnormally folded prion protein.

Etiology and Pathophysiology

In a small number of patients, dementia symptoms are secondary to a treatable condition such as delirium, depression, subdural hematoma, cerebral tumours, normal-pressure hydrocephalus, heavy metal neurotoxicity, Wilson's disease, and infections such as bacterial meningitis and viral encephalitis. The diagnostic workup for dementia includes ruling out other causes of cognitive impairment (Merino & Wright, 2018).

Dementia is not a normal part of aging. Old age and family history are risk factors for the most common types of irreversible dementias. There are more women than men who have dementia because women have a longer life expectancy and dementia is more prevalent in women than in men. This may be due to effects of sex hormones on the brain in older age and in brain development (Pike, 2017). Etiology and pathophysiology of each of the most common types of dementia are described separately as follows.

Alzheimer's Disease. Alzheimer's disease (AD) is a chronic, progressive, degenerative disease of the brain. The exact etiology of AD is unknown. As in other forms of dementia, age is the most important risk factor for developing AD. Only a small percentage of people younger than 60 years develop AD. When AD develops in someone younger than 60 years old, it is referred to as familial Alzheimer's disease (also known as *early-onset AD*). AD that begins after age 60 is called *late-onset AD*. Early-onset AD has a stronger genetic basis than does late-onset AD. The pathogenesis is similar in both forms of AD.

In knowing the modifiable risk factors for AD, nurses can advise individuals on how to reduce their risk of developing AD (Table 62.6). Mild cognitive impairment, discussed later in this chapter, is a risk factor for developing AD.

Characteristic findings of AD are related to changes in the brain's structure and function: (a) amyloid plaques, (b) neurofibrillary tangles, and (c) loss of connections between cells, as well as cell death (National Institute on Aging, 2017). Figure 62.1 depicts the pathological changes in AD.

In AD, amyloid plaques are present in the brain in abnormal quantities. These plaques consist of clusters of insoluble deposits of a protein called *β-amyloid*, other proteins, remnants of neurons, non-nerve cells such as microglia (cells that surround and digest damaged cells or foreign substances), and other cells, such as astrocytes. β-Amyloid is cleaved from amyloid precursor protein, which is associated with the cell membrane (Figure 62.2). The normal function of amyloid precursor protein is unknown. In AD, plaques develop first in areas of the brain used for memory and cognitive function. Eventually, AD attacks the cerebral cortex, especially the areas responsible for language and reasoning.

Neurofibrillary tangles are abnormal collections of twisted protein threads inside nerve cells seen in the areas of the brain most affected by AD. The main component of these structures is a protein called *tau*. Tau proteins in the central nervous system are involved in intracellular structure through their support of microtubules. Tau proteins hold the microtubules together. In AD, the tau protein is altered in a way that causes the

TABLE 62.6 DEMENTIA PREVENTION	
Modifiable Risk Factors	**Reducing Risk**
Medical conditions • Type 2 diabetes • Stroke and transient ischemic attack • Hyperlipidemia • Hypertension • Obesity • Chronic inflammatory conditions (e.g., arthritis)	• Healthy lifestyle choices to reduce the risk of developing these conditions (maintaining healthy weight, regular physical activity, healthy balanced diet, not smoking, stress management, moderate or no alcohol consumption) • Appropriate treatment when such conditions are present
Head injury	• Use of recreational or sport helmets • Fall and concussion prevention • Use of seat belts
Late-life clinical depression	• Identification and appropriate treatment of depression • Healthy lifestyle choices and appropriate support for traumatic experiences and stressful life events (may reduce risk for depression)
Social isolation	• Active social life • Volunteering • Participation in intellectual activities (reading, playing cards, solving puzzles, playing chess, learning new skills, hobbies)
Educational attainment	• Policies and programs to support young adults' completion of secondary and post-secondary education • Lifelong learning programs
Midlife hearing impairment	• Reduce occupational noise exposure • Reduce smoking • Use auditory amplification, including hearing aids or cochlear implants

Sources: Adapted from Alzheimer Society of Canada. (2020). *Risk factors.* https://alzheimer.ca/en/Home/About-dementia/Alzheimer-s-disease/Risk-factors; Alzheimer Society of Canada. (2019). *Brain health.* https://alzheimer.ca/en/Home/About-dementia/Brain-health; Jafari, Z., Kolb, B. E., & Mohajerani, M. H. (2019). Age-related hearing loss and tinnitus, dementia risk, and auditory amplification. *Aging Research Reviews, 56.* https://doi.org/10.1016/j.arr.2019.100963; and Livingston, G., Sommerland, A., Orgeta, V., et al. (2017). Dementia prevention, intervention, and care. *The Lancet, 390*(10113), 2673–2743. https://doi.org/10.1016/S0140-6736(17)31363-6

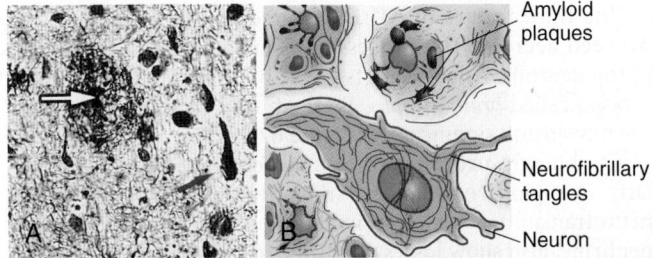

FIG. 62.1 Pathological changes in Alzheimer's disease. **A,** Senile plaque with central amyloid core *(white arrow)* next to a neurofibrillary tangle *(red arrow)* on histological specimen from a brain autopsy. **B,** Schematic representation of neuritic plaque and neurofibrillary tangles. Source: *A,* Damjanov, I., & Linder, J. (Eds.). (1996). *Anderson's pathology* (10th ed.). Mosby.

microtubules to twist together in a helical manner (see Figure 62.2). This twisting ultimately forms the neurofibrillary tangles observed in the neurons of persons with AD.

Plaques and neurofibrillary tangles are not unique to patients with AD. They are also found in the brains of individuals without evidence of cognitive impairment. However, they are more plentiful in the brains of individuals with AD.

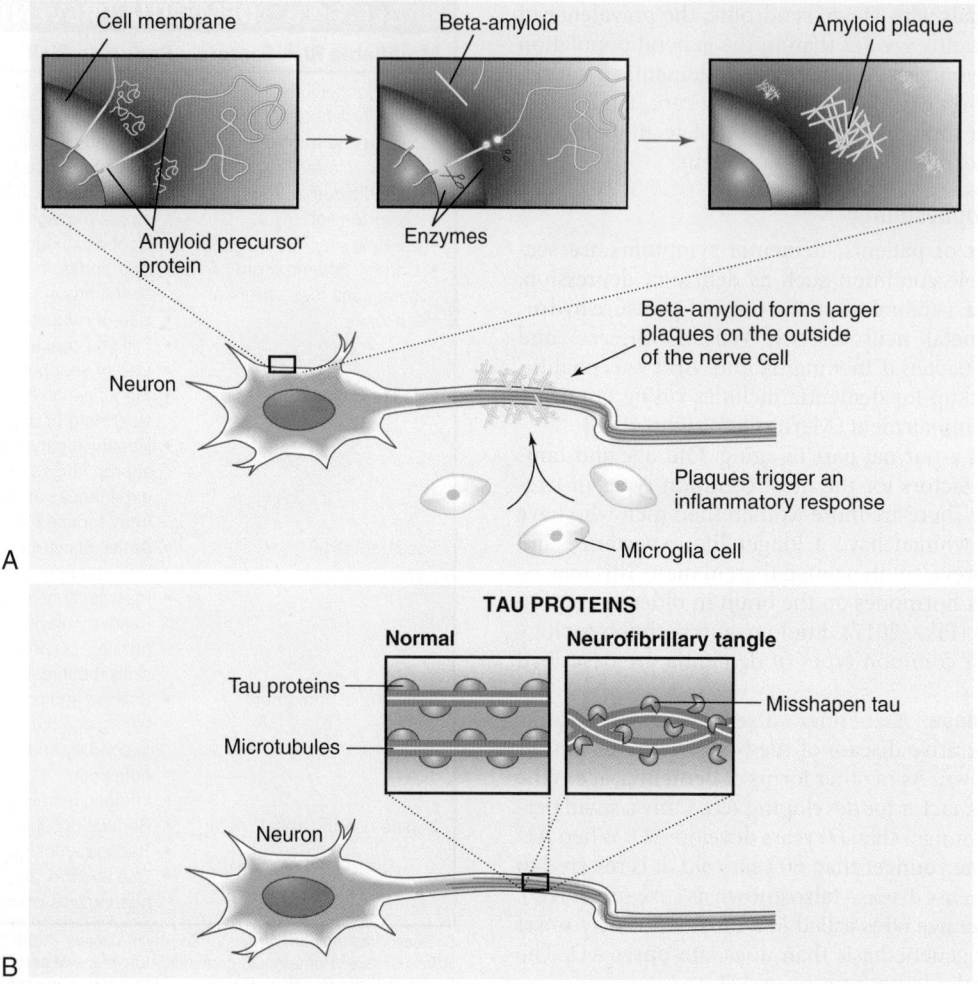

FIG. 62.2 Current etiological theories for the development of Alzheimer's disease. **A,** Abnormal amounts of β-amyloid are cleaved from the amyloid precursor protein (APP) and released into the circulation. The β-amyloid fragments clump together to form plaques that attach to the neuron. Microglia react to the plaque, and an inflammatory response results. **B,** Tau proteins provide structural support for the neuron microtubules. Chemical changes in the neuron produce structural changes in tau proteins. This results in twisting and tangling of the microtubules (neurofibrillary tangles).

The third feature of AD is the gradual loss of connections between neurons. This process leads to damage and then death of the neurons. Affected parts of the brain begin to shrink in a process called *brain atrophy*. By the final state of AD, brain tissue has shrunk significantly (Figure 62.3).

Cholinergic neurons are lost in people with AD, particularly in regions essential for memory and cognition. Other neurotransmitter systems, including serotonin and norepinephrine, also show losses over time in patients with AD. Such neurotransmitter changes are the basis of current medication therapies for AD.

Vascular Dementia. Vascular dementia, also called *multiinfarct dementia,* is a type of dementia that results from ischemic, ischemic-hypoxic, or hemorrhagic brain damage caused by cardiovascular disease. When these events occur, blood and oxygen supply to brain tissues is blocked, which results in cell death. Vascular dementia may be caused by a single stroke (infarct) or by multiple strokes. As with AD, risk for vascular dementia increases with older age. Other risk factors are smoking, hypertension, cardiac diseases, diabetes mellitus, hypercholesterolemia, coronary artery disease, and atrial fibrillation.

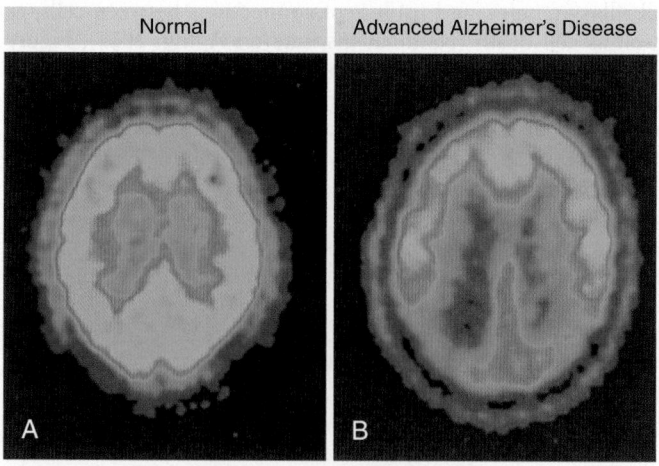

FIG. 62.3 The effects of Alzheimer's disease (AD) on the brain, shown by positron emission tomography (PET). In PET, radioactive fluorine is applied to glucose (fluorodeoxyglucose), and the yellow areas indicate metabolically active cells. **A,** A normal brain. **B,** Advanced AD, evidenced by hypometabolism that indicates cell death in many areas of the brain. Source: Stuart, G. W. (2009). *Principles and practice of psychiatric nursing* (9th ed., p. 398, Figure 22-4, A & D). Mosby.

TABLE 62.7   THE EIGHT *A*'S OF DEMENTIA

Deficit	Definition	Possible Effects on Behaviour
Amnesia	Initially, loss of recall of recent events, but eventually, loss of long-term memory	• Repeated questions • Disorientation • Misplaces items
Aphasia	Loss of ability to express and comprehend spoken and written language	• Social withdrawal • Loss of ability to communicate in a second language • Misunderstandings • Inability to communicate needs
Agnosia	Inability to recognize common objects or faces of familiar people (including one's own face)	• Using wrong objects • Suspiciousness • Mistaking self in the mirror for someone else
Apraxia	Loss of ability to initiate purposeful movement	• Difficulty understanding terms such as *back, front, up,* and *down* • Difficulty performing activities of daily living • Inability to perform previously learned tasks
Altered perception	Misinterpretation of sensory information, loss of depth perception, visual distortions	• Fear when walking down stairs or sitting down • Misinterpreting objects • Bumping into things • Falls
Apathy	Loss of drive or initiative	• Sitting in one place for long periods of time • Inability to initiate conversation or activities, but participates when invited by someone else
Anosognosia	Loss of ability to realize that there is a problem with memory and functioning	• Resistance to care • Self-protective behaviours • Irritability
Attentional deficits	Decreased ability to pay attention and focus	• Inability to complete a conversation • Easily distracted

Source: Adapted from Baycrest Center for Geriatric Care. (2018). *Dementia simulation toolkit. Version 2.0.* https://clri-ltc.ca/files/2018/07/Dementia-Simulation-Toolkit-2.0.pdf

Dementia With Lewy Bodies. Dementia with Lewy bodies (DLB) is characterized by the presence of Lewy bodies (deposits of α-synuclein protein) throughout the cortex as well as in the brainstem and autonomic structures (amygdala, medulla, pons). The α-synuclein protein is also linked to dementia in Parkinson's disease. DLB has features of both AD and Parkinson's disease (changes in thinking and reasoning, confusion, memory loss, balance problems, and muscle rigidity) (Salthouse et al., 2019).

Frontotemporal Dementia. Frontotemporal dementia (FTD) is characterized by degeneration of the frontal lobe, temporal lobe, or both. There are four subtypes of FTD and the two most common types are the behavioral variant and the language variant, associated with effects to the frontal lobe and temporal lobe, respectively. Nerve cells die because of abnormal accumulation of proteins in the neurons. The proteins most commonly found are ubiquitin and transactive response DNA binding protein 43 (TDP-43). Tau proteins are present in approximately 40% of cases. Approximately 10% of patients with FTD have an inherited form of the disorder, and 30 to 50% have a family history of FTD. The typical age at onset is between 52 and 56 years, making it the most common type of dementia among those aged 60 or younger (Caceres et al., 2016; Wilfong et al., 2016).

Clinical Manifestations

The onset of symptoms of dementia is usually gradual, with progressive deterioration. Vascular dementia, however, may have a sudden onset after a cerebrovascular event. In vascular dementia, mental decline is typically stepwise: Deterioration is followed by stabilization, then deterioration again. The rate of deterioration in AD is highly variable from individual to individual, and the course ranges in duration from 3 to 20 years.

AD may be preceded by mild neurocognitive disorder (mNCD) also known as mild cognitive impairment (MCI).

mNCD is cognitive decline that is not severe enough to interfere with ADLs. The diagnosis of mNCD is made in the presence of (a) evidence of modest change in cognition; (b) concern about the decline on the part of the affected individual, a knowledgeable informant, or a clinician; (c) preservation of the ability to independently perform ADLs and independent ADLs; and (d) absence of delirium or another condition that explains the symptoms (American Psychiatric Association, 2013). Many patients with mNCD eventually develop dementia. Between 5 and 30% of people who have mNCD develop dementia within a year of the onset of mNCD (Chen et al., 2017).

The symptoms of dementia can be classified according to the *eight A's of dementia* (Baycrest Center for Geriatric Care, 2018): **a**nosognosia, **a**gnosia, **a**phasia, **a**praxia, **a**ltered perception, **a**mnesia, **a**pathy, and **a**ttentional deficits (Table 62.7). By recognizing these symptoms, the nurse can understand why and how dementia affects the patient's ability to function. These symptoms are common, although patients with dementia do not necessarily exhibit all of them.

The initial changes of dementia may be difficult to recognize. Many people mistakenly think that they are part of normal aging. It can take up to 4 years after the onset of symptoms until patients and their family members seek health care. Reasons for this delay include lack of knowledge about dementia, lack of knowledge about services for dementia, attributing the changes to normal aging, linguistically and culturally inaccessible services, and stigma (Koehn, 2020; MacDonald et al., 2018).

As time goes on, the dementia affects more areas of the brain. Cognitive abilities and functioning are progressively lost. Clinical manifestations of dementia are classified as mild, moderate, and severe, corresponding to the early, middle, and late stages of the disorder (Table 62.8).

The early clinical manifestations of FTD differ from those of AD. Early in FTD, social conduct and personality are profoundly

TABLE 62.8   CLINICAL MANIFESTATIONS OF DEMENTIA

Early (Mild)

- Anxiety
- Confusion about location of familiar places (may become lost)
- Difficulty finding the right word
- Difficulty recognizing what numbers mean, trouble handling money and paying bills
- Loss of initiative and interests
- Mild forgetfulness and misplacing items
- Poor judgement
- Short-term memory impairment, especially for learning new information
- Taking longer than usual to accomplish daily tasks

Middle (Moderate)

- Anxiety, mood swings, suspiciousness, jealousy, irritability
- Difficulty completing tasks that involve a sequence of steps; interference with activities of daily living
- Difficulty learning new things or coping in new and unexpected situations
- Difficulty recognizing family members and friends
- Difficulty with language and understanding, and problems with reading, writing, and working with numbers
- Difficulty with logic and organizing thoughts
- Flat affect
- Hallucinations and delusions
- Impaired attention
- Increasing memory loss, including some loss of remote memory
- Loss of impulse control (e.g., undressing at inappropriate times or places, vulgar language)

- Loss of interest in hygiene
- Loss of remote memory
- Poor insight and decision making, need for supervision and cuing
- Sleep disturbances
- Wandering, getting lost

Late (Severe)

- Behaviours that may appear aggressive (verbal [e.g., swearing, screaming, shouting, making threats] or physical [e.g., hitting, pinching, scratching, hair-pulling, biting]) but are communicating a need (relief from, e.g., physical discomfort, social isolation, lack of stimulation, emotional distress, confusion, frustration)
- Difficulty eating, swallowing
- Hallucinations, delusion, agitation
- Inability to perform self-care activities
- Inability to understand words
- Incontinence
- Loss of appetite and weight loss
- Loss of most memories, inability to process new information
- Loss of social skills
- Progression to loss of facial expression, primitive reflexes, loss of voluntary movement, loss of speech, recurrent infections
- Repetitious words or sounds
- Responding to short, simple communication
- Seizures
- Sexual disinhibition

Source: Adapted from National Institute on Aging. (2017). *What are the signs of Alzheimer's disease?* https://www.nia.nih.gov/health/what-are-signs-alzheimers-disease; and Vancouver Health Authority. (2010). *Clinical stages of Alzheimer disease.* http://geropsychiatriceducation.vch.ca/docs/edu-downloads/dementia/clinical_stages_CPS-MMSE_comparison.pdf

altered, but memory loss is minimal or nonexistent. If the temporal lobe is affected first, the patient experiences difficulties with speech and language and, eventually, the inability to communicate (Wilfong et al., 2016). Eventually all areas of the brain are involved diffusely and the symptoms resemble those of AD.

The core feature of DLB is fluctuating cognition, from hour to hour or over days or weeks. Another feature of DLB is parkinsonian symptoms (extrapyramidal signs such as bradykinesia, rigidity, and rest tremor). About 80% of patients experience visual hallucinations and rapid eye movement (REM) sleep behaviour disorder. Severe sensitivity to antipsychotic medications is common, as is severe autonomic dysfunction. Swallowing difficulties in later stages can lead to impairment in nutrition and pneumonia. Affected patients are at risk for falls because of syncope and impaired mobility and balance (McKeith et al., 2017; Salthouse et al., 2019).

Behavioural and Psychological Symptoms of Dementia. Some of the clinical manifestations of dementia are called **behavioural and psychological symptoms of dementia (BPSDs).** These behaviours are often responses to something in the patient's environment or to a perceived threat and are thus referred to as **responsive behaviours** or **self-protective behaviours.** Behavioural symptoms include appetite changes, slowed or excessive movements and speech, agitation, pacing, wandering, exit seeking, constant requests for help, grabbing on to people, cursing, screaming, socially inappropriate behaviours, sexual disinhibition, and hoarding. Psychological symptoms include anhedonia (loss of pleasure from activities that are usually pleasurable), worry, depressed mood, euphoria, fear, apprehension, panic, tension, irritability, labile mood, psychosis (hallucinations, delusions, illusions), and sleep

disturbances (Walaszek, 2020). These symptoms cause distress to patients and their families and negatively affect patients' functioning. They are caused by a combination of biological factors (e.g., changes in brain functioning, medical conditions, pain, adverse effects of medication, hearing or visual impairment), environmental factors (e.g., changes in routine, changes in environment), and social factors (e.g., inadequate support for the patient or family caregiver). These behaviours may be mistakenly interpreted. For example, the grasp reflex may appear in patients in middle to late stages because of frontal lobe damage. Reflexive grasping of care providers or objects on contact may be misinterpreted as intentional. Dementia affects patients' abilities to communicate. Sometimes, these behaviours are the only way in which the affected person can communicate an unmet need.

> **SAFETY ALERT**
> A sudden change in behaviour should trigger a search for underlying causes, including possible delirium.

Diagnostic Studies

The diagnostic process includes making a clinical diagnosis based on the history, interviews with the patient and a caregiver or family member, physical examination, and brief cognitive tests. The next step is laboratory tests to identify treatable medical conditions. Routine laboratory tests include complete blood cell count and measurements of thyroid-stimulating hormone; serum electrolytes; and serum calcium, serum fasting glucose, and serum vitamin B_{12} levels. Measurements of serum folic acid or red blood cell folate levels are optional. Neuropsychological testing and neuroimaging are performed only when certain symptoms are present. None of the diagnostic procedures can identify whether the underlying pathological change in the brain is present (e.g., plaques and tangles in AD). This determination can be made only by microscopic examination of brain tissue after the person dies.

Related Assessments. Mental status testing is an important component of assessment. Patients with mild dementia may be able to compensate, which makes it difficult to evaluate cognitive function through conversation alone. Cognitive testing is focused on evaluating memory, attention, ability to perform calculations, language, visuospatial skills, and degree of alertness. The Mini-Mental State Examination (MMSE; Folstein et al., 1975) is the most commonly used tool for brief assessment of cognitive functioning. It cannot be used to diagnose dementia, but it is useful for monitoring change over time. However, the MMSE is not sensitive to very early stages of dementia and mNCD. The Montreal Cognitive Assessment (MoCA) is a brief cognitive screening tool that has good sensitivity for detecting early dementia (Nasreddine et al., 2005). Culturally and linguistically inappropriate diagnostic tools contribute to lack of recognition of dementia in Indigenous communities (MacDonald et al., 2018). The Canadian Indigenous Cognitive Assessment (CICA) is a validated cognitive screening tool (Blind & Pitawanakwat, 2019; Jacklin et al., 2020; Pitawanakwat et al., 2016). The CICA tool and training videos are available in English and Anishanaabemowin through the I-CAARE website (see Resources section at the end of this chapter). The https://hign.org/consultgeri-resources/try-this-series website includes two-page *Try This* summaries of research about three cognitive screening tools (Borson et al., 2000; Kennedy, 2012; Mezey & Maslow, 2016), copies of the tools, articles about how to use them, and videos that demonstrate and explain how to use them.

Depression is often mistaken for dementia in older persons and, conversely, dementia for depression. Late-life depression is a risk factor for dementia, may proceed it, and is comorbid with dementia in as many as 40% of dementia cases. Furthermore, there is symptom overlap. Symptoms of depression include excessive sadness, difficulty thinking and concentrating, fatigue, apathy, feelings of despair, and inactivity. When the depression is severe, concentration and attention may be poor, which manifests as memory and functional impairment. Depression, alone or in combination with dementia, is treatable. The Cornell Scale for Depression in Dementia (Alexopolous et al., 1998) and the Hamilton Depression Rating Scale (Hamilton, 1960) work well to detect depression in patients living with dementia (Goodarzi et al., 2017).

Risk Modification

Many of the risk factors for AD and vascular dementia are modifiable, and there is some evidence that incidence of dementia may be decreasing, possibly in response to healthy lifestyles and higher education levels. Some research suggests that as many as 30% of cases of dementia could be prevented by targeting modifiable risk factors such as education, obesity, hypertension, diabetes, and physical inactivity (Yaffe, 2018) Table 62.6 lists strategies that may reduce risk for dementia. The federal government's *National Dementia Strategy* (Public Health Agency of Canada, 2021) identifies dementia prevention as a priority for Canada. Preventing dementia or delaying its onset would substantially reduce the economic and caregiver burden of dementia.

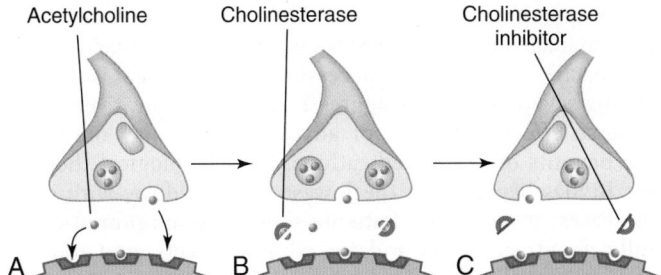

FIG. 62.4 Mechanism of action of cholinesterase inhibitors. Acetylcholine **(A)** is released from the nerve synapses and carries a message across the synapse. Cholinesterase **(B)** breaks down acetylcholine. Cholinesterase inhibitors **(C)** block cholinesterase, which gives acetylcholine more time to transmit the message.

Interprofessional Care

There is no cure for any of the forms of dementia. The goals of interprofessional management of dementia are to slow decline in cognition, maintain and maximize functioning and quality of life of the person with dementia, and support family caregivers.

Medication Therapy. Medications used for dementia do not cure or reverse the progression of the disease. They are not effective for mNCD. They may slow decline of some forms of dementia, but the effects are modest. AD is the only form of dementia for which medications that affect cognitive decline are approved by Health Canada. However, some experts recommend prescribing these medications for dementia associated with Parkinson's disease and for DLB as well (Livingston et al., 2017). There are no medications that slow cognitive decline in other types of dementia. Cholinesterase inhibitors block cholinesterase, the enzyme responsible for the breakdown of acetylcholine in the synaptic cleft (Figure 62.4). Cholinesterase inhibitors include donepezil (Aricept), rivastigmine (Exelon), and galantamine (Reminyl). These medications may stabilize or improve cognitive function in AD and enhance the patient's functional abilities. They can be used at any stage of dementia. Cholinesterase inhibitors increase risk for bradycardia and syncope—and associated falls (Haake et al., 2020). The bradycardia may be difficult to detect because it is often transient. Other adverse effects include nausea, vomiting, diarrhea, vivid dreams, and leg cramps.

MEDICATION ALERT—Galantamine
The extended-release formulation of galantamine (Reminyl) may cause severe skin reactions. Its use should be discontinued if skin rash is observed.

Memantine (Ebixa), an *N*-methyl-D-aspartate (NMDA) receptor antagonist, may be prescribed if cholinesterase inhibitors are ineffective. Memantine appears to protect the brain's nerve cells against excess amounts of glutamate, which is released in large amounts by cells damaged by AD. Memantine is recommended for moderate to severe AD. Adverse effects include diarrhea, agitation, and insomnia.

Medications for AD are prescribed until their clinical benefit can no longer be demonstrated. They should be tapered and discontinued for patients who have taken them for at least 1 year and experience either (1) significant decreases in cognition or functioning, (2) no benefit over the year of taking the medication, or (3) end-stage dementia (bedridden, noncommunicative, cannot perform ADLs) (Reeve et al., 2019).

Antipsychotic medications should only be used for the management of BPSDs when nonpharmacological approaches alone are not successful and the patient is experiencing severe psychosis, aggression, or agitation. Even then, adverse effects and risk of adverse events may outweigh the benefits of these medications. Pharmacological therapy for BPSDs begins with the lowest possible dose, with slow increases, if necessary. Patients should be monitored carefully for effectiveness and for adverse effects, and routine assessment must be conducted to taper and discontinue the medication (Livingston et al., 2017).

If antipsychotic medications are prescribed, atypical antipsychotic medications are preferred. Conventional antipsychotic medications (e.g., haloperidol) should not be administered because of extrapyramidal and anticholinergic adverse effects. Adverse medication effects for patients with dementia who are prescribed antipsychotics include cerebrovascular events, significantly increased risk of mortality, cardiac and metabolic disturbance, extrapyramidal adverse effects (akathisia, bradykinesia, tremor, rigidity), gait disturbance, sedation, increased cognitive impairment, and anticholinergic effects. Antipsychotic agents are not used in patients with DLB because they produce severe adverse effects (Livingston et al., 2017).

MEDICATION ALERT—Risperidone

Risperidone (Risperdal) is not recommended for patients with dementia other than AD.

BPSDs without psychosis can be treated selective serotonin reuptake inhibitors such as sertraline (Zoloft), fluvoxamine (Luvox), and citalopram (Celexa). However, these medications have risks that may outweigh benefits, including prolonged QT, falls, and hyponatremia. Like antipsychotics, they carry risk for extrapyramidal symptoms (Livingston et al., 2017). Benzodiazepines should not be used. They produce adverse effects such as disinhibition and increase the risk for falls and delirium. In urgent situations, very low doses of short-acting benzodiazepines such as lorazepam (Ativan) may be used with caution. Valproate should not be used (Walaszek, 2020).

MEDICATION ALERT

- Do not give antipsychotics to patients who have dementia with Lewy bodies.
- Psychiatric medications increase the risk of delirium.

For patients who have depression in addition to dementia, the depression may be treated with a combination of pharmacological and nonpharmacological approaches. Potential underlying causes, such as pain or social isolation should be addressed first. For patients with moderate depression symptoms, antidepressants may be considered if there is no response to psychosocial approaches after 4 to 6 weeks. For patients with severe depression symptoms, an antidepressant may be prescribed in addition to psychosocial approaches. Antidepressants are commonly prescribed. However, evidence of their effectiveness for patients with dementia and depression is equivocal and the risk of adverse effects may outweigh the possible benefits (Livingston et al., 2017). For patients with a history of depression that responded to antidepressants, the first choice of medications is selective serotonin reuptake inhibitors such as venlafaxine (Effexor), mirtazapine (Remeron), or bupropion (Wellbutrin). Tricyclic antidepressants are not recommended because of the negative effects on cognition associated with anticholinergic adverse effects (American Geriatrics Society 2019 Beers Criteria®

Update Expert Panel, 2019). The patient must be carefully monitored for effectiveness and adverse effects.

NURSING MANAGEMENT DEMENTIA

Person-centred care is the cornerstone of nursing care for patients with dementia and their families. The focus is on the person's experience and their uniqueness. Principles and values associated with person-centred care include holism, choice, dignity, self-determination, purpose, respect, and meaning (Fazio et al., 2018).

NURSING ASSESSMENT

Comprehensive assessment is necessary to provide patient-centred care. Assessment should focus on the patient, their family or caregivers, and the physical and social environment. Assessment includes mental status, cognition, neurological symptoms, psychiatric symptoms, and functional assessment of ADLs and instrumental ADLs. Many patients with dementia lack awareness of their condition, and communication deficits are frequent. Thus, collateral information should be obtained from people who know the patient well. Assessment of communication abilities can help the nurse adapt assessment approaches to the patient's abilities. Objective data from observation are important.

Data that should be obtained are listed in Table 62.9. Articles and the website that provide cognitive and standardized assessment tools are listed in Table 62.10. A number of assessment tools are provided as appendices to the RNAO's (2016) nursing best practice guideline, *Delirium, Dementia, and Depression in Older Adults: Assessment and Care.*

NURSING DIAGNOSES

Nursing diagnoses for dementia may include but are not limited to the following:

- *Self-neglect* resulting from *deficient executive function* (memory deficit, cognitive impairment)
- *Potential for injury* resulting from *alteration in cognitive functioning* (impaired judgement, gait instability, sensory/perceptual alteration)
- *Wandering* resulting from *altered physiological state* (cognitive impairment)

Additional information on nursing diagnoses for the patient with dementia is presented in Nursing Care Plan (NCP) 62.1, available on the Evolve website.

PLANNING

The overall goal is that patients with dementia will have a dignified quality of life. Specific goals are maintaining physical health, retaining functional abilities as long as possible, enhancing or stabilizing cognition, eliminating pain, preventing or minimizing responsive and self-protective behaviours, and supporting emotional and psychological well-being (Fletcher, 2016; RNAO, 2016). The goals for the family caregiver of a patient with dementia are to reduce caregiver stress and maintain health and well-being (Fletcher, 2016; RNAO, 2016). Partnership and collaboration with patients and families is essential.

NURSING IMPLEMENTATION

HEALTH PROMOTION. Strategies to prevent dementia are described earlier in this chapter. The Alzheimer Society of

TABLE 62.9   NURSING ASSESSMENT
Patient With Dementia

Subjective Data
Important Information
Past health history: Head trauma, falls, history of previous delirium or psychiatric illness
Medications: All medications, including cholinesterase inhibitors, psychotropic medications, and nonprescription medications

Symptoms
- Activities of daily living (e.g., dressing, feeding, using the toilet, performing personal hygiene)
- Instrumental activities of daily living (e.g., managing money, performing household chores, cooking, using transportation)
- Mental status examination (mood, perceptions and beliefs, thinking, orientation, memory and recall, concentration, insight, hallucinations, delusions, apathy)
- Pain
- Response to stressful situations
- Strength and mobility
- Symptoms according to mild, moderate, and severe stages of dementia (see Table 62.8)

Impact on Family
- Coping resources, including finances and social support
- Self-care practices
- Caregiving self-efficacy
- Understanding of dementia and prognosis
- Physical health
- Mental health

Objective Data
- Appearance and behaviour
- Neurological symptoms (tremors, gait, tone, akathisia, dystonia)
- Symptoms according to mild, moderate, and severe stages of dementia
- Retained abilities and strengths
- Behavioural changes
- Trends and patterns of behaviour change in relation to potential internal or environmental triggers

TABLE 62.10   EVIDENCE-INFORMED DEMENTIA ASSESSMENT & CARE RESOURCES: *TRY THIS ®:* TOOLS

Amella, E. J., & Lawrence, J. F. Eating and feeding issues with older adults with dementia: Part II: Interventions (Issue D11.2).
Conedera, F., & Kingston, L. Therapeutic activity kits (Issue D4).
Cotter, V. T., & Evans, L. K. Avoiding restraints in patients with dementia (Issue D1).
Debrzuski, C. Communication difficulties: Assessment and interventions (Issue D7).
Fick, D., & Mion, L. Assessing and managing delirium in persons with dementia (Issue D8).
Horgas, A. L. Assessing pain in persons with dementia (Issue D2).
Maslow, K. Working with families of hospitalized older adults with dementia (Issue D10).
Silverstein, N. M., & Flaherty, G. Wandering in the hospitalized older adult (Issue D6).
Mezey, M., & Maslow, K. Recognition of dementia in hospitalized older adults (Issue D5).

Source: These tools are available at https://consultgeri.org/tools/try-this-series. This website includes demonstrations of how to use many of the tools.

Canada's *Brain Health* Web page provides helpful information about healthy lifestyle choices for long-term brain health (see the Resources at the end of this chapter).

TABLE 62.11   NURSING HEALTH PROMOTION INTERVENTIONS

- Promote activities that are important and meaningful to the person
- Socializing
- Promote independence by modifying the living environment
- Adapt activities and the physical environment for safety
- Healthy lifestyle
- Cognitive stimulation
- Exercise
- Establish routines
- Adopt dementia-friendly designs in private and public spaces

Sources: Adapted from Bowes, A., & Dawson, A. (2019). *Designing environments for people with dementia: A systematic review of the literature.* Emerald Publishing Limited; Lam, F. M. H., Huang, M-Z., Liao, L-R., et al. (2018). Physical exercise improves strength, balance, mobility, and endurance in people with cognitive impairment and dementia: A systematic review. *Journal of Physiotherapy, 64*(1), 4–15. https://doi.org/10.1016/j.jphys.2017.12.001; Registered Nurses' Association of Ontario (RNAO). (2016). *Delirium, dementia, and depression in older adults: Assessment and care* (2nd ed.). Author. https://rnao.ca/sites/rnao-ca/files/bpg/RNAO_Delirium_Dementia_Depression_Older_Adults_Assessment_and_Care.pdf; and Travers, C., Brooks, D., Hines, S., et al. (2016). Effectiveness of meaningful occupation interventions for people living with dementia in residential aged care: A systematic review. *JBI Database of Systematic Reviews and Implementation Reports, 14*(12), 163–225.

Dementia must be recognized early so that patients with dementia and their families can have time to make treatment decisions and plan for the future. Sometimes dementia is first identified when patients are admitted to an acute care facility for another condition (Koehn, 2020). As stated earlier, lack of recognition and diagnosis of dementia is a problem in Indigenous communities. Reasons for this include lack of awareness of dementia and lack of access to specialty health care providers and services (MacDonald et al., 2018).

Health promotion can improve quality of life for patients with dementia and for family caregivers. Exercise programs for patients with dementia may improve the patient's ability to perform ADLs, delay cognitive decline, reduce symptoms, and reduce caregiver burden (de Almeida et al., 2020). Yoga may improve physical health, mental health, and behaviours for patients with dementia (Brenes et al., 2019). Other interventions that support quality of life and promote health are listed in Table 62.11.

ACUTE INTERVENTION. The diagnosis of dementia can be traumatic for both the patient and the family. It is not unusual for patients to experience depressed mood, denial, anxiety and fear, isolation, and grieving. The nurse is in an important position to assess for depression and suicidal ideation and to provide support and referral. The nurse must assess the abilities of family members to accept and cope with the diagnosis.

Ongoing assessment of the patient and caregiver is required as the dementia progresses and the patient's functioning changes. An important nursing responsibility is to work in partnership with the patient and the caregiver to effectively manage clinical manifestations as they change over time. Effective partnership is enhanced when the nurse provides support, education, and collaboration with a focus on enabling meaningful caregiving roles in all settings. The patient with dementia and the caregiver have overlapping but unique challenges. To aid in identifying challenges the caregiver may experience, see NCP 62.2, Family Caregivers of the Patient with Dementia, available on the Evolve website.

Patients with dementia may be hospitalized for other health problems. Approximately 20 to 40% of patients in hospitals have dementia. This dementia is not necessarily documented on their health record (Butcher, 2018). They are at much higher risk than other older patients for negative outcomes, including delirium, avoidable functional decline, longer admissions, and death (McGilton & Lemay, 2020). Interventions to prevent delirium, described earlier in the chapter, are important for preventing many of these negative outcomes.

SAFETY ALERT
Patients with dementia who are admitted to hospital are at risk for delirium, falls, dehydration, inadequate nutrition, untreated pain, medication-related conditions, pneumonia, urinary tract infections, sepsis, wandering, behavioural symptoms, and preventable functional decline.

Patients may be unable to accurately communicate their symptoms and health problems, making it important to engage families in assessment and care planning. Nurses cannot rely on patients to pass on information to family members. Effective communication skills are important to compensate for patients' impaired ability to communicate (Table 62.12). Patients with dementia who are hospitalized in acute care settings should be observed more closely because of concerns for safety. Consistent assignment of nursing staff, frequent reassurance, and orientation to place and time may reduce anxiety and prevent behavioural symptoms.

Access to rehabilitation after acute care is an issue for patients with dementia because of false assumptions that rehabilitation is not possible. However, an approach that incorporates interprofessional care, intensive rehabilitation, delirium and dementia management, and staff and family education results in positive

TABLE 62.12 STRATEGIES FOR COMMUNICATING WITH PATIENTS WHO HAVE DEMENTIA

Verbal	• Adapt to the patient's abilities. • Introduce yourself and repeatedly address the person by their name. • Use active listening techniques (paraphrasing, clarifying). • Use empathetic statements. • Use short sentences and closed-ended questions. • Rephrase. • Give one-step and step-by-step instructions. • Avoid arguments and correcting misstatements. • Do not use elderspeak "baby talk" (i.e., diminutives; pronoun substitution; exaggerated intonation, pitch, and volume; slowed rate). • Engage through reminiscence. • Respond to validate emotions. • Respond to underlying needs.
Nonverbal	• Approach from the front and make eye contact. • Use an open stance. • Respect personal space. • Maintain a calm demeanor. • Maintain eye contact. • Give the patient time to respond. • Minimize environmental distractions. • Use gestures to demonstrate. • Recognize patient behaviour as communication.

Sources: Alzheimer Society of Canada. (n.d.). *10 communication tips.* https://archive.alzheimer.ca/sites/default/files/files/national/for-hcp/10-communication-tips.pdf?_ga=2.97982620.2018651171.1601907243-979569958.1586808641; James, I. A., & Gibbons, L. (2019). *Communication skills for effective dementia care: A practical guide to communication and interaction training (CAIT).* Jessica Kingsley Publishers; and Registered Nurses' Association of Ontario (RNAO). (2016). *Delirium, dementia, and depression in older adults: Assessment and care* (2nd ed.). Author. https://rnao.ca/sites/rnao-ca/files/bpg/RNAO_Delirium_Dementia_Depression_Older_Adults_Assessment_and_Care

functional outcomes and shorter length of admission (McGilton & Lemay, 2020).

AMBULATORY AND HOME CARE. Most persons with dementia live in their homes, supported and cared for by family members or friends. The most typical caregiver is a spouse or an adult child. Patients with dementia progress through the stages at variable rates, and care needs change as the disease progresses. Regular assessment, monitoring, and support for the patient and family are necessary. Regardless of the setting, cognition and functioning decline, and the amount of care required intensifies over time.

In the phase of mNCD, memory aids (e.g., calendars) may be beneficial. Patients may develop depression in this phase. Depression may occur because of the neurochemical changes in the brain. Depression may be related to adjusting to a diagnosis of an incurable disorder, as well as the effect of dementia on the person's life (e.g., restricted driving, difficulties socializing with friends, impaired participation in hobbies or recreational activities).

After the initial diagnosis of dementia, patients need to be aware that the progression of the disease is variable. Anticipating and planning for changes and transitions, such as loss of ability to drive, loss of financial autonomy, requiring family support, and moving, can make these transitions more positive. An important nursing role is providing anticipatory guidance and support before and during these transitions.

The patient, family members, and the health care team should collaborate in making decisions related to care early in the disease. The patient and family should be supported to discuss decision making for health care and advance care planning while the patient still has the capacity to do so. Discussion guides are available online (see Resources section at the end of this chapter).

Adult day care programs are an option for patients in early and middle stages of dementia. These programs provide respite for the family and support the patient to live in the community for as long as possible Services include assistance with ADLs, therapeutic recreation, cognitive stimulation, and transportation to the program. Patients return home more relaxed, content, less frustrated, and ready to be with their family. The respite from the demands of care allows the caregiver to be more responsive to the patient's needs. Other respite options include home visits from community respite workers, overnight care provided by community nursing services, and short-term (1–2 weeks) admission to a long-term care facility.

As the disease progresses, the demands on the caregiver may eventually exceed the resources or there may not be a caregiver, and the person with dementia may have to move to an assisted-living residence or long-term care facility. Patients in the final stages of dementia require total care. Even in long-term care facilities, often family caregivers continue to provide personal care, preserve the dignity of the person with dementia, share their unique knowledge of the person with staff, and monitor quality of care.

Specific issues related to the care of the patient with dementia span all phases of the disease. Brief, evidence-informed guides to effective nursing intervention can help with care planning (see Table 62.10). These issues are described in the following sections.

Behavioural Changes. BPSDs occur in approximately 50 to 60% of patients with dementia. BPSDs are more common in middle and late stages, and most patients with dementia demonstrate BPSDs at some time. Often, the behaviours are not persistent.

Health care providers need to be aware that these behaviours are not intentional. Behaviours are a way of communicating. It is up to the nurse to try to understand the meaning of the behaviour and what is being communicated. Behaviours may communicate emotions. By responding to these emotions, the nurse validates the patient's feelings (Pizzacalla et al., 2015). BPSDs may worsen in acute care settings when behaviour is influenced by delirium, pain, changes in routine, and the unfamiliar environment. BPSDs often contribute to the decision to move patients to a long-term care facility. See the following Evidence-Informed Practice box, which describes how training nurses in acute care hospitals to use gentle-persuasive approaches can be helpful to patients.

EVIDENCE-INFORMED PRACTICE

Research Highlight

What Is the Effect of Training Staff in Acute Care Hospital Settings to Use Gentle-Persuasive Approaches?

Clinical Question

In nursing staff working in acute care hospitals (P), does education and training to use gentle-persuasive approaches (I), in comparison with no training (C), increase competencies in behavioural management with cognitively impaired patients (O)?

Best Available Evidence

- Quasi-experimental studies

Critical Appraisal and Synthesis of Evidence

- Staff in acute care settings report lack of understanding of BPSD and skills and confidence to use person-centred interventions for patients with dementia experiencing responsive or self-protective behaviours.
- One-day workshops on the principles of gentle-persuasive approaches (an approach that had been previously shown to be effective in long-term care settings) was provided to 468 staff.
- The training focused on the following:
  - Person-centred care and understanding the meaning of behaviour as communication
  - Effect of dementia and delirium on the brain and how that relates to behaviour
  - Communication techniques to use with patients with delirium or dementia
  - Respectful self-protective techniques to use when encountering responsive behaviours
- The staff who received this training noted that their confidence in working with patients was significantly improved after the training. They found the training useful in practice.
- Most participants recommended training for colleagues.

Conclusions

- Staff who receive training and education to understand the reasons for responsive behaviours improve their competence to provide effective, safe care to patients with delirium and dementia.

Implications for Nursing Practice

- Hospital administrators should provide education to staff members who work with patients with dementia or delirium and should support them in using their learning in practice.
- Further examination of effects for patients is needed.

Reference for Evidence

Schindel Martin, L., Gillies, L., Coker, E., et al. (2016). An education intervention to enhance staff self-efficacy to provide dementia care in an acute care hospital in Canada: A nonrandomized controlled study. *American Journal of Alzheimer's Disease & Other Dementias, 31*, 664–677. https://doi.org/10.1177/1533317516668574

P, patient population of interest; *I*, intervention or area of interest; *C*, comparison of interest or comparison group; *O*, outcome(s) of interest (see Chapter 1).

Behaviours do not occur in a vacuum; they are often in response to a precipitating factor (e.g., pain, frustration, temperature extremes, anxiety, perceived danger). The first step to identifying precipitating factors is to assess the patient's physical status. Environmental assessment to identify factors that could trigger behaviours is the next step. When the patient is agitated by the environment, either the patient or the stimulus should be moved. The patient can be assisted to call family members if this is reassuring. When a patient resists or pulls at tubes or dressings, these items can be covered with stretch tube gauze or removed from the visual field. The patient should be reassured that the nurse is present to provide safety and protection. Orientation to place and person can be used, depending on the patient's cognitive abilities. The nurse should avoid asking challenging "why" questions, especially if the patient is anxious or agitated. Communication strategies are listed in Table 62.12.

When nurses communicate effectively with patients during care, patients are less anxious and agitation is reduced. To communicate effectively, it is important that the nurse (a) stay near the patient during care, sit beside the patient, and use touch as appropriate; (b) recognize the patient's rhythm and adapt the pace of care to it; and (c) focus on care beyond the task by acknowledging the patient's personal experience and providing reassurance (McGilton & Lemay, 2020).

Other strategies to manage behaviour include redirection, distraction, and reassurance. For a patient who is restless or agitated, redirecting would involve changing the patient's focus by having them perform activities such as sweeping, raking, or dusting. Effective strategies to distract the agitated patient might include snacks, car rides, favourite music, looking at family photographs, or walking. Repetitive activities, songs, poems, massage, aromas, or a favourite object can be soothing to some patients.

When nonpharmacological therapies are ineffective and patient safety is threatened, medications may be used with caution for a short time. However, the medications do not treat the unmet needs such as pain, social isolation, or boredom that are often the underlying cause of symptoms such as agitation. Adverse effects should be monitored carefully.

Some patients have a pattern of behavioural disturbance that occurs in the late afternoon. This is often referred to as **sundowning**. According to some experts, BPSDs are more disruptive to staff when they occur in the evening and are thus more noticeable to them, resulting in the sundowning label for BPSD. Others point out that the symptoms are characteristic of delirium, related to disruption of circadian rhythm. Behaviour should be assessed for the underlying cause. Maximizing exposure to light during the day, ensuring quiet and uninterrupted nighttime sleep, implementing other sleep hygiene interventions (see Chapter 9), and engaging the patient in activities during the day may be helpful (Boronat et al, 2019).

Safety. The person with dementia is at risk for several situations related to personal safety. These include injury from falls, wandering in unsafe areas, injury to others and self with sharp objects or from fire and other heat sources, impaired judgement and decision making, and vulnerability to elder abuse (see Chapter 7). Care must be taken to minimize risk and provide appropriate supervision in the home environment. As cognitive function declines over time, patients with dementia may have difficulty navigating physical spaces and interpreting environmental cues. The Alzheimer Society of Canada website (see the Resources at the end of this chapter) has a home safety checklist that nurses can assist families to use. Examples of environmental modifications include improving lighting; removing tripping hazards; installing stairway handrails with the end of rail shaped differently to alert the patient that it is the end of the stairway; storing dangerous materials and items in a secure place; using child-proof locks; wiping wet areas on the floors; removing snow and ice; and using grip bars and nonskid surfaces in showers and bathtubs (Alzheimer Society of Canada, 2021a).

People with dementia have a higher risk of falling than other older persons do. This risk is present at home, in hospitals, and in long-term care facilities. The rate of falls-related hospital admission for people with dementia is twice that of older people who do not have dementia (Dudevich et al., 2018). Fall risk should be assessed. Effective fall prevention programs include multiple components such as staff training, environmental modification, and exercise (RNAO, 2017).

Wandering is a major safety concern. Wandering may be the expression of a physical or emotional need or may result from cognitive loss, adverse effects of medications, restlessness, curiosity, or stimuli that trigger memories of earlier routines. The nurse should observe for factors or events that may precipitate wandering. For example, patients may be sensitive to stress and tension in the environment. In such cases, wandering may reflect an attempt to leave the environment. Patients with dementia can be registered with the Alzheimer Society of Canada's MedicAlert® Safely Home Registry. The registry includes identification products (e.g., bracelets, necklaces, watches) that allow police and emergency responders to identify the person quickly and return them home (Alzheimer Society of Canada, 2021b).

Pain Management. Pain management is complex. Pain from comorbid musculoskeletal disorders associated with aging is common among patients with dementia. Often, this pain is not recognized by health care providers. Because of dementia-associated difficulties with language and communication, patients with moderate or severe dementia may have difficulty expressing physical complaints, including pain. The nurse must rely on other behavioural cues and signs of distress such as breathing changes, vocalizations, facial expression, body language, and consolability (Horgas, 2018). If nurses cannot determine the reasons for BPSDs, they should suspect and treat pain and monitor the patient's response. Acetaminophen (Tylenol) is recommended. Low doses of long-acting opioids with slow titration to higher doses is recommended when trials of acetaminophen (Tylenol) are ineffective (Walaszek, 2020). The *Try This* series on the https://hign.org/consultgeri-resources/try-this-series website includes tools for pain assessment in patients with dementia. See Chapter 10 for information about pain assessment and management.

Eating and Swallowing Difficulties. Loss of interest in food and decreased ability to feed oneself *(feeding apraxia)*, as well as comorbid conditions, can result in significant nutritional deficits and possible dehydration in patients with dementia. In long-term care and acute care settings, inadequate assistance with eating may further add to the problem.

Individualized nursing interventions should be based on assessment of the patient's needs and abilities (see Table 62.9). Puréed foods, thickened liquids, and nutritional supplements can be used when chewing and swallowing become problematic for patients. Patients may need to be reminded to chew their food and to swallow. A quiet and unhurried environment for eating is essential. Distractions at mealtimes, including television, should be avoided. Creation of a normal social environment for meals provides supportive cues for patients with dementia. If self-feeding is difficult, finger foods, verbal cuing, demonstrating eating motions, and hand-over-hand techniques can initiate self-feeding. Liquids should be offered frequently.

When oral feeding is not possible, alternative routes may be explored. Nutritional support therapies are described in Chapter 42.

Oral Care. Ability to perform oral self-care declines as dementia progresses. With decreased toothbrushing and flossing, dental problems are likely to occur. Food may become lodged in pockets in the mouth because of swallowing difficulties, which increases the potential for tooth decay. Dental caries and tooth abscesses cause discomfort and pain, potentially increasing responsive behaviours. The mouth should be inspected regularly and mouth care provided for patients unable to perform self-care.

Infection Prevention. Urinary tract infection and pneumonia are the most common infections in patients with dementia. Such infections are ultimately the cause of death in many patients with dementia. Patients with dementia are at risk for aspiration pneumonia because of feeding and swallowing difficulties. See Chapters 30 and 48 for additional information about these infections. Manifestations of infection—including changes in behaviour, delirium, fever, cough (pneumonia), and pain on urination (bladder)—need to be evaluated and appropriately treated. See Chapter 7 for information about normal changes of aging that diminish signs of infection.

Skin Care. It is important to monitor the patient's skin. Rashes, areas of redness, and skin breakdown should be noted and treated appropriately. In the late stages of dementia, incontinence along with immobility and undernutrition can increase patients' risk for skin breakdown. The nurse must keep the patient's skin dry and clean and change the patient's position regularly to prevent the creation of pressure areas over bony prominences.

Elimination Problems. During the middle and late stages of dementia, urinary and fecal incontinence become more common. Multifaceted individualized nursing care to reduce incontinence should include regular toileting (with prompting and reminders if necessary), changing incontinence products, increasing fluid and fibre intake, and ensuring that the toilet is accessible.

Constipation is also a common problem. Causes may include immobility, dietary intake, and decreased fluid intake. Management of constipation is discussed in Chapter 45.

Caregiver Support. Dementia is a disease that disrupts all aspects of personal and family life. Individuals caring for the person with dementia frequently describe such care as stressful. Caregivers of patients with dementia often experience negative effects on their work and family roles and on their mental and physical health. Caregiver strain is common. Family caregivers can support the patient's well-being through activities suggested in Table 62.11. The nurse should provide education and support about adapting communication with the patient with dementia (see Table 62.12). Strategies for reducing caregiver stress are listed in Table 62.13.

As the disease progresses, the relationship of the caregiver to the patient changes. Family roles may be altered or reversed.

Decisions that must be made include when the patient must stop driving or performing activities that might be dangerous, when to ask for assistance, and when to use respite care services or long-term care facilities. Nurses can support families by helping them know what to expect through these transitions. Family members may assume that the person with dementia cannot be involved in decisions related to these transitions. However, nurses can support families to understand the patient's preferences and maintain their autonomy as much as possible. This approach can result in better transition experiences for the person living with dementia and for their family.

Sexual relations for couples are also seriously affected by dementia. As dementia progresses, sexual interest may decline for both the patient and their partner. Several reasons account for this, including caregiver fatigue (when the partner is the caregiver), as well as memory impairment, apraxia, and episodes of incontinence in the patient with AD. It is also possible for patients to become sexually disinhibited as the disease progresses.

The nurse needs to work with the caregiver to identify stressors and determine coping strategies to reduce the burden of caregiving. Establishing what the caregiver views as most disruptive or distressful can help in identifying priorities for care. Risk to the safety of the patient and the caregiver is given high priority. It is also important to assess the caregiver's expectations regarding the patient's behaviour: Are the expectations reasonable in view of the progression of the disease? The nurse must work with the caregiver to identify risk factors for complications, including behavioural problems.

Support groups for caregivers and family members can provide emotional support and information about dementia and related topics such as safety and legal, ethical, and financial issues. These groups are often facilitated by nurses, social workers, or occupational therapists. The Alzheimer Society of Canada has many educational and support systems available to help family caregivers. Other strategies related to stress management are discussed in Chapters 8 and 12.

Legal Matters and Personal Care Planning. In the early stage of dementia, while the patient is still capable of making decisions and signing legal papers, it is important for the patient to be part of the decision making about their financial and legal affairs. Some important legal documents that must be put in place as soon as possible are a will; an enduring power of attorney (a document naming a substitute decision maker) for financial and legal matters, as well as for future health care decisions; and an advance care plan or advance directive. The names and the required content of these documents vary among the provinces and territories, and the local chapter of the Alzheimer Society of Canada can help locate this information for persons with dementia and their families. Chapters 7 and 13 provide more information about these documents. Conversation guides and written information about the expected course of dementia make it possible to engage patients with dementia in advance care planning discussions, even when the patient's communication is impaired (Sussman et al., 2017; see Resources at the end of this chapter).

EVALUATION

Expected outcomes for patients with dementia are addressed in NCP 62.1, available on the Evolve website. See NCP 62.2 for expected outcomes for the caregiver of a patient with dementia.

TABLE 62.13	**10 WAYS TO REDUCE CAREGIVER STRESS**

1. Learn about the disease.
2. Be realistic about the disease.
3. Be realistic about how much you can do.
4. Accept your feelings.
5. Share information and feelings with others.
6. Be positive.
7. Look for humour.
8. Take care of yourself.
9. Get help, both practical help and support.
10. Plan for the future.

Source: Alzheimer Society of Canada. (2015). *Reducing caregiver stress.* http://www. alzheimer.ca/en/Living-with-dementia/Caring-for-someone/Self-care-for-the-caregiver/Reducing-caregiver-stress

CASE STUDY

Alzheimer's Disease

Patient Profile
Y. B. (pronouns he/him), 80 years old, received a diagnosis of AD 3 years ago. Today, Y. B.'s 78-year-old partner brings him to the emergency department because he wandered away from home, fell, and injured his left hip.

Subjective Data
- Can state name
- Is disoriented regarding place and time
- Cannot recall wandering or falling
- Is agitated, trying to get up
- Denies pain

Objective Data
Physical Examination
- Left leg shorter than right leg
- Patient is tense and anxious
- Grimacing

Diagnostic Studies
- Radiographic study of left hip indicates a fracture.
- Mini-Mental State Examination shows cognitive impairment.

Discussion Questions
1. What is the pathogenesis of AD?
2. What precipitating factors may have resulted in Y. B.'s fall?
3. ***Priority decision:*** What are the priority nursing interventions for Y. B.?
4. What precautions must be taken regarding the inpatient care of Y. B.?
5. What teaching plan should be developed for Y. B. and his partner?
6. ***Priority decision:*** Based on the assessment data presented, what are the priority nursing diagnoses? Are there any interprofessional issues?
7. ***Evidence-informed practice:*** Y. B.'s partner asks whether Y. B. should take ginkgo to help with his memory. How should the nurse respond?

evolve
Answers are available at http://evolve.elsevier.com/Canada/Lewis/medsurg.

REVIEW QUESTIONS

The number of the question corresponds to the same-numbered objective at the beginning of the chapter.

1. Which of the following clients is most at risk for developing delirium?
   a. A 50-year-old woman with cholecystitis
   b. A 19-year-old man with a fractured femur
   c. A 42-year-old woman having an elective hysterectomy
   d. A 78-year-old man admitted to the medical unit with complications related to congestive heart failure

2. Which of the following symptoms are the hallmarks of delirium?
   a. Inattention, fluctuating course, hyperactivity, and altered level of consciousness
   b. Disorganized thinking, insidious onset, inattention, and altered level of consciousness
   c. Acute onset, fluctuating course, memory loss, and altered level of consciousness
   d. Acute onset, fluctuating course, inattention or disorganized thinking, and altered level of consciousness

3. Which of the following descriptions best characterizes dementia?
   a. Syndrome that results only in memory loss
   b. Disease associated with abrupt changes in behaviour
   c. Disease that is always due to reduced blood flow to the brain
   d. Syndrome characterized by cognitive dysfunction and loss of memory

4. Which of the following is associated with vascular dementia?
   a. Transient ischemic attacks
   b. Bacterial or viral infection of neuronal tissue
   c. Cognitive changes secondary to cerebral ischemia
   d. Abrupt changes in cognitive function that are irreversible

5. On which of the following findings is the clinical diagnosis of dementia based?
   a. Brain biopsy
   b. Electroencephalography
   c. Patient history and cognitive assessment
   d. Computed tomography or MRI

6. Which statement(s) accurately describe(s) mild cognitive impairment? *(Select all that apply.)*
   a. Always progresses to AD
   b. Caused by a variety of factors and may progress to AD
   c. Should be aggressively treated with acetylcholinesterase medications
   d. Caused by vascular infarcts that, if treated, will delay progression to AD
   e. Client is usually not aware that there is a problem with their memory

7. What is a major goal of treatment for the client with dementia?
   a. Maintain safety
   b. Maintain or increase body weight
   c. Return to a higher level of self-care
   d. Enhance functional ability over time

1. d; 2. d; 3. d; 4. c; 5. c; 6. b; 7. a.

Ⓔvolve

For even more review questions, visit http://evolve.elsevier.com/Canada/Lewis/medsurg.

REFERENCES

Alexopoulos, G. S., Abrams, R. C., Young, R. C., et al. (1998). Cornell Scale for Depression in Dementia. *Biological Psychiatry, 23,* 271–284. https://doi.org/10.1037/t20968-000

Alzheimer Society of Canada. (2021a). *Making your environment safe.* https://alzheimer.ca/en/help-support/im-caring-person-living-dementia/ensuring-safety-security/making-your-environment-safe

Alzheimer Society of Canada. (2021b). *MedicAlert® Safely Home®.* https://alzheimer.ca/en/Home/Living-with-dementia/Day-to-day-living/Safety/Safely-Home?_ga=2.89031067.1646362266.1583690766-165643703.1572200436

American Geriatrics Society 2019 Beers Criteria® Update Expert Panel. (2019). American Geriatrics Society 2019 updated AGS Beers Criteria® for potentially inappropriate medication use in older adults. *Journal of the American Geriatric Society, 67,* 674–694. https://doi.org/10.1111/jgs.15767

American Psychiatric Association. (2013). *Diagnostic and statistical manual of mental disorders* (5th ed.). Author.

Baycrest Center for Geriatric Care. (2018). *Dementia simulation toolkit.* Version 2.0. https://clri-ltc.ca/files/2018/07/Dementia-Simulation-Toolkit-2.0.pdf

Bellelli, G., Morandi, A., Davis, D. H. J., et al. (2014). Validation of the 4AT, a new instrument for rapid delirium screening: A study in 234 hospitalized older people. *Age and Ageing, 43,* 496–502. https://doi.org/10.1186/isrctn53388093

Blind, M., & Pitawanakwat, K. (2019). *Adapting and validating a culturally appropriate cognitive assessment tool: The Canadian Indigenous Cognitive Assessment (CICA). Presented at Dementia Care 2019.* Winnipeg, MB. March 4-5, 2019.

https://alzheimer.mb.ca/wp-content/uploads/2019/03/2A-Adapting-Validating-a-Culturally-Appropriate-Cognitive-Assessment-Tool.pdf

Boland, J. W., Lawlor, P. G., & Bush, S. H. (2019). Delirium: Nonpharmacological and pharmacological management. *BMJ Supportive & Palliative Care, 9,* 482–484. https://doi.org/10.1136/bmjspcare-2019-001966

Boronat, A. C., Ferreira-Maia, A. P., & Wang, Y.-P. (2019). Sundown syndrome in older persons: A scoping review. *JAMDA: Journal of the American Medical Directors Association, 20,* 664–671. https://doi.org/10.1016/j.jamda.2019.03.001

Borson, S., Scanlan, J., Brush, M., et al. (2000). The Mini-Cog: A cognitive "vital signs" measure for dementia screening in multi-lingual elderly. *International Journal of Geriatric Psychiatry, 15,* 1021–1027. (Seminal). https://doi.org/10.1002/1099-1166(200011)15:11%3C1021::AID-GPS234%3E3.0.CO;2-6

Brenes, G. A., Soh, S., Wells, R. E., et al. (2019). The effects of yoga on patients with mild cognitive impairment and dementia: A scoping review. *American Journal of Geriatric Psychiatry, 27*(2), 188–197. https://doi.org/10.1016/j.jagp.2018.10.013

Butcher, L. (2018). Caring for patients with dementia in the acute care setting. *British Journal of Nursing, 27*(7), 358–362. https://doi.org/10.12968/bjon.2018.27.7.358

Caceres, B. A., Frank, M. O., Jun, J., et al. (2016). Family caregivers of patients with frontotemporal dementia: An integrative review. *International Journal of Nursing Studies, 55,* 71–84.

Canadian Patient Safety Institute (CPSI). (2016). *Hospital harm improvement resource: Delirium.* https://www.patientsafetyinstitute.ca/en/toolsResources/Hospital-Harm-Measure/Documents/Resource-Library/HHIR%20Delirium.pdf

Chambers, L. W., Bancej, C., & McDowell, I. (Eds.). (2016). *Prevalence and monetary costs of dementia in Canada.* Alzheimer Society of Canada. https://alzheimer.ca/sites/default/files/files/national/statistics/prevalenceandcostsofdementia_en.pdf

Chen, Y., Denny, K. G., Harvey, D., et al. (2017). Progression from normal cognition to mild cognitive impairment in a diverse clinic-based and community-based elderly cohort. *Alzheimer's & Dementia, 13*(4), 399–405. https://doi.org/10.1016/j.jalz.2016.07.151

Custodio, N., Montesinos, R., Lira, D., et al. (2017). Mixed dementia: A review of the evidence. *Dementia Neuropsychologia, 11*(4), 365–370. https://doi.org/10.1590/1980-57642016dn11-040005

de Almeida, S. I. L., Da Silva, M. G., & Marques, A. S. P. D. (2020). Home-based physical activity programs for people with dementia: Systematic review and meta-analysis. *The Gerontologist, 60*(8), 600–608. https://doi.org/10.1093/geront/gnz176

Devlin, J., Skrobik, Y., Gélinas, C., et al. (2018). Clinical Practice Guidelines for the Prevention and Management of Pain, Agitation/Sedation, Delirium, Immobility, and Sleep Disruption in Adult Patients in the ICU. *Critical Care Medicine, 46*(9), 1532–1548.

Dudevich, A., Husak, L., Johnson, T., et al. (2018). Safety and quality of care for seniors living with dementia. *Healthcare Quarterly, 21*(3), 12–15. https://doi.org/10.12927/hcq.2018.25708

Fazio, S., Pace, D., Flinner, J., et al. (2018). The fundamentals of person-centered care for individuals with dementia. *The Gerontologist, 58*(S1), S10–S19. https://doi.org/10.1093/geront/gnx122

Fiest, K. M., Roberts, J. I., Maxwell, C. J., et al. (2016). The prevalence and incidence of dementia due to Alzheimer's disease: A systematic review and meta-analysis. *Canadian Journal of Neurological Sciences, 43*, S51–S82. https://doi.org/10.1017/cjn.2016.36

Fletcher, K. (2016). Dementia: A neurocognitive disorder. In M. Boltz, T. T. Fullmer, E. Capezuti, et al. (Eds.), *Evidence-based geriatric nursing protocols for best practice* (5th ed., pp. 233–250). Springer.

Folstein, M. F., Folstein, S. E., & McHugh, P. R. (1975). "Mini-mental state": A practical method for grading the cognitive state of patients for the clinician. *Journal of Psychiatric Research, 12*, 189–198. (Seminal). https://doi.org/10.1016/0022-3956(75)90026-6

Gagné, A., Voyer, P., Boucher, V., et al. (2018). Performance of the French version of the 4AT for screening the elderly for delirium in the emergency department. *Canadian Journal of Emergency Medicine, 20*, 903–910. https://doi.org/10.1017/cem.2018.367

Goodarzi, Z. S., Mele, B. S., Roberts, D. J., et al. (2017). Depression case findings in individuals with dementia: A systematic review and meta-analysis. *Journal of the American Geriatrics Society, 65*. 937–348. https://doi.org/10.1111/jgs.14713

Haake, A., Nguyen, K., Friedman, L., et al. (2020). An update on the utility and safety of cholinesterase inhibitors for the treatment of Alzheimer's disease. *Expert Opinion on Drug Safety, 19*(2), 147–157. https://doi.org/10.1080/14740338.2020.1721456

Hamilton, M. (1960). A rating scale for depression. *Journal of Neurology, Neurosurgery, and Psychiatry, 23*, 56–62. https://doi.org/10.1136/jnnp.23.1.56

Hogan, D. B., Jetté, N., Fiest, K. M., et al. (2016). The prevalence and incidence of frontotemporal dementia: A systematic review. *Canadian Journal of Neurological Sciences, 43*, S96–S109. https://doi.org/10.1017/cjn.2016.25

Horgas, A. L. (2018). Assessing pain in older adults with dementia. Try This: *Best Practices in Nursing Care to Older Adults With Dementia*, Issue Number D2. Hartford Institute for Geriatric Nursing. https://hign.org/sites/default/files/2020-06/Try_This_Dementia_2.pdf

Hshieh, T. T., Inouye, S. K., & Oh, E. S. (2018). Delirium in the elderly. *Psychiatric Clinics of North America, 41*(1), 1–17. https://doi.org/10.1016/j.psc.2017.10.001

Inouye, S. K., van Dyck, C. H., Alessi, C. A., et al. (1990). Clarifying confusion: The Confusion Assessment Method, a new method for detecting delirium. *Annals of Internal Medicine, 113*, 941–948. (Seminal). https://doi.org/10.7326/0003-4819-113-12-941

Jacklin, K., Pitawanakwat, K., Blind, M., et al. (2020). Developing the Canadian Indigenous Cognitive Assessment for use with Indigenous older Anishinaabe adults in Ontario, Canada. *Innovation in Aging, 4*(4). https://doi.org/10.1093/geroni/igaa038

Kennedy, G. J. (2012). Brief evaluation of executive dysfunction: An essential refinement in the assessment of cognitive impairment. *Try This Series: Best Practices in Nursing Care to Older Adults With Dementia,* Issue Number D3. https://consultgeri.org/try-this/dementia/issue-d3.pdf

Koehn, S. (2020). "It is not a disease, only memory loss": Exploring the complexity of access to a diagnosis of dementia in a cross-cultural sample. In L. Garcia, L. McCleary, & N. Drummond (Eds.), *Evidence informed approaches for managing dementia transitions: Riding the waves* (pp. 29–52). Academic Press, Elsevier Inc. https://doi.org/10.1016/B978-0-12-817566-8.00002-4

Lau, T., Kozyra, E., & Cheng, C. (2019). Delirium: Risk factors, contributors, identification, work-up, and treatment. In H. H. Fenn, A. Hategan, & J. A. Bourgeois (Eds.), *Inpatient geriatric psychiatry.* Springer International Publishing.

Livingston, G., Sommerland, A., Orgeta, V., et al. (2017). Dementia prevention, intervention, and care. *The Lancet, 390*(10113), 2673–2743. https://doi.org/10.1016/S0140-6736(17)31363-6

MacDonald, J. P., Ward, V., & Halseth, R. (2018). Alzheimer's disease and related dementias in Indigenous populations in Canada: Prevalence and risk factors. *National Collaborating Centre for Aboriginal Health.* https://www.nccih.ca/docs/emerging/RPT-Alzheimer-Dementia-MacDonald-Ward-Halseth-EN.pdf

McGilton, K. S., & Lemay, G. (2020). Hospitalization of persons with dementia. In L. Garcia, L. McCleary, & N. Drummond (Eds.), *Evidence informed approaches for managing dementia transitions: Riding the waves* (pp. 109–135). Academic Press, Elsevier Inc. https://doi.org/10.1016/B978-0-12-817566-8.00005-X

McKeith, I. G., Boeve, B. F., Dickson, D. W., et al. (2017). Diagnosis and management of dementia with Lewy bodies: Fourth consensus report of the DLB Consortium. *Neurology, 89*, 88–100. https://doi.org/10.1212/WNL.0000000000004058

Merino, J. G., & Wright, C. B. (2018). Diagnosis of potentially preventable dementias. In V. Hachinski (Ed.), *Treatable and potentially preventable dementias* (pp. 23–41). Cambridge University Press.

Mezey, M., & Maslow, K. (2016). Recognition of dementia in hospitalized older adults. Try This: *Best Practices in Nursing Care to Older Adults With Dementia*, Issue Number D5. https://hign.org/sites/default/files/2020-06/Try_This_Dementia_5.pdf

Moore, M. (2021). *Symptoms of major neurocognitive disorder.* PsychCentral. https://psychcentral.com/disorders/symptoms-of-major-neurocognitive-disorder/

Morandi, A., Davis, D., Bellelli, G., et al. (2017). The diagnosis of delirium superimposed on dementia: An emerging challenge. *Journal of the American Medical Directors Association, 18*(2017), 12–18. https://doi.org/10.1016/j.jamda.2016.07.014

Morandi, A., Lucchi, E., Turco, R., et al. (2015). Delirium superimposed on dementia: A quantitative and qualitative evaluation of informal caregivers and health care staff experience. *Journal of Psychosomatic Research, 79,* 272–280. https://doi.org/10.1016/j.jpsychores.2015.06.012

Mulkey, M. A., Hardin, S. R., Olson, D., et al. (2018). Pathophysiology review: Seven neurotransmitters associated with delirium. *Clinical Nurse Specialist, 32*(4), 195–211. https://doi.org/10.1097/NUR.0000000000000384

Nasreddine, Z. S., Phillips, N. A., Bédirian, V., et al. (2005). The Montreal Cognitive Assessment, MoCA: A brief screening tool for mild cognitive impairment. *Journal of the American Geriatrics Society, 53,* 695–699. (Seminal). https://doi.org/10.1111/j.1532-5415.2005.53221.x

National Institute on Aging. (2017). *What happens to the brain in Alzheimer's disease?* https://www.nia.nih.gov/health/what-happens-brain-alzheimers-disease

Pike, C. J. (2017). Sex and the development of Alzheimer's disease. *Journal of Neuroscience Research, 95,* 671–680. https://doi.org/10.1002/jnr.23827

Pitawanakwat, K., Jacklin, K., Blind, M., et al. (2016). Adapting the Kimberley Indigenous Cognitive Assessment for use with Indigenous older adults in Canada. *Alzheimer's & Dementia, 12*(7Suppl), P311. https://doi.org/10.1016/j.jalz.2016.06.564

Pizzacalla, A., Montemuro, M., Coker, E., et al. (2015). Gentle persuasive approaches: Introducing an educational program on an orthopaedic unit for staff caring for patients with dementia and delirium. *Orthopaedic Nursing, 34*(2), 101–107. https://doi.org/10.1097/NOR.0000000000000127

Public Health Agency of Canada. (2021). *A dementia strategy for Canada: Together we aspire.* https://www.canada.ca/en/public-health/services/publications/diseases-conditions/dementia-strategy.html

Reeve, E., Farrell, B., Thompson, W., et al. (2019). Deprescribing cholinesterase inhibitors and memantine in dementia: Guideline summary. *Medical Journal of Australia, 210*(4), 174–179. https://doi.org/10.5694/mja2.50015

Registered Nurses' Association of Ontario (RNAO). (2016). *Delirium, dementia, and depression in older adults: Assessment and care* (2nd ed.). Author. https://rnao.ca/sites/rnao-ca/files/bpg/RNAO_Delirium_Dementia_Depression_Older_Adults_Assessment_and_Care.pdf

Registered Nurses' Association of Ontario (RNAO). (2017). *Preventing falls and reducing injury from falls* (4th ed.). Author. https://rnao.ca/sites/rnao-ca/files/bpg/FALL_PREVENTION_WEB_1207-17.pdf

Salthouse, O., Bradshaw, J., & Saling, M. (2019). Dementia with Lewy bodies. In D. R. Hocking, J. L. Bradshaw, & J. Fielding (Eds.), *Degenerative disorders of the brain* (pp. 186–198). Routledge: Taylor & Francis Group.

Shaji, K. S., Sivakumar, P. T., Rao, G. P., et al. (2018). Clinical practice guidelines for management of dementia. *Indian Journal of Psychiatry, 60*(Suppl 3), S312–S328. https://doi.org/10.4103/0019-5545.224472

Shea, Y.-F., Chu, L.-W., Chan, A., et al. (2016). A systematic review of familial Alzheimer's disease: Differences in presentation of clinical features among three mutated genes and potential ethnic differences. *Journal of the Formosan Medical Association, 115,* 67–75. https://doi.org/10.1016/j.jfma.2015.08.004

Sussman, T., Kaasalainen, S., & Bui, M. (2017). "Now I don't have to guess": Using pamphlets to encourage residents and families/friends to engage in advance care planning in long-term care. *Gerontology & Geriatric Medicine, 3,* 1–11. https://doi.org/10.1177/2333721417747323

Tullmann, D. F., Blevins, C., & Fletcher, K. (2016). Delirium: Prevention, early recognition, and treatment. In M. Boltz, T. T. Fullmer, E. Capezuti, et al. (Eds.), *Evidence-based geriatric nursing protocols for best practice* (5th ed., pp. 252–261). Springer.

Voyer, P., Champoux, N., Desrosiers, J., et al. (2016). RADAR: A measure of the sixth vital sign? *Clinical Nursing Research, 25*(1), 9–29. https://doi.org/10.1177/1054773815603346

Voyer, P., Émond, M., Boucher, V., et al. (2017). RADAR: A rapid detection tool for signs of delirium (6th vital sign) in emergency departments. *Canadian Journal of Emergency Nursing, 40*(2), 35–43.

Walaszek, A. (2020). *Behavioral and psychological symptoms of dementia.* American Psychiatric Association Publishing.

Walker, J., & Jacklin, K. (2019). Current and projected dementia prevalence in First Nations Populations in Canada. In W. Hulko, D. Wilson, & J. E. Balestrery (Eds.), *Indigenous peoples and dementia: New understandings of memory loss and memory care.* UBC Press.

Wilfong, L., Edwards, N. E., Yehle, K. S., et al. (2016). Frontotemporal dementia: Identification and management. *The Journal for Nurse Practitioners–JNP, 12*(4), 277–282. https://doi.org/10.1016/j.nurpra.2015.08.006

Yaffe, K. (2018). Modifiable risk factors and prevention of dementia: What is the latest evidence? *JAMA Internal Medicine, 178*(2), 281–282. https://doi.org/10.1001/jamainternmed.2017.7299

RESOURCES

Acute Care Geriatric Nurse Network
http://acgnn.ca/
Alzheimer Society of Canada
https://www.alzheimer.ca
Alzheimer Society of Canada—*Brain Healthy Tips to Reduce Your Dementia*
https://alzheimer.ca/en/Home/About-dementia/Brain-health
Alzheimer Society of Canada—*Making Your Environment Safe*
https://alzheimer.ca/en/help-support/im-caring-person-living-dementia/ensuring-safety-security/making-your-environment-safe
BrainXchange
https://brainxchange.ca/
Canadian Academy of Geriatric Psychiatry (CAGP)
http://www.cagp.ca
Canadian Association of Retired Persons (C.A.R.P.)
https://www.carp.ca
Canadian Coalition for Seniors' Mental Health
https://www.ccsmh.ca
Canadian Geriatrics Society
https://www.canadiangeriatrics.ca
Canadian Gerontological Nursing Association (CGNA)
https://www.cgna.net
Carers Canada
https://www.carerscanada.ca/
Indigenous Cognition & Aging Awareness Research Exchange
https://www.i-caare.ca/cica
Island Health—*Delirium*
https://www.islandhealth.ca/learn-about-health/seniors/delirium
National Initiative for the Care of the Elderly (NICE)
https://www.nicenet.ca
Registered Nurses' Association of Ontario (RNAO)—*Nursing Best Practice Guidelines (BPG)*
https://www.rnao.org/bestpractices

Confusion Assessment Method (CAM) Training Manual and Coding Guide
http://www.hospitalelderlifeprogram.org/uploads/disclaimers/CAM_Training_Manual_(Long_CAM)_9-23-14.pdf

Hartford Institute for Geriatric Nursing—*eLearning*
https://hign.org/consultgeri-resources/elearning

Hospital Elder Life Program (HELP) for Prevention of Delirium
https://help.agscocare.org/

The Conversation Project—*Your Conversation Starter Guide*
https://theconversationproject.org/wp-content/uploads/2017/02/ConversationProject-StarterKit-Alzheimers-English.pdf

evolve

For additional Internet resources, see the website for this book at http://evolve.elsevier.com/Canada/Lewis/medsurg.

Nursing Management
Peripheral Nerve and Spinal Cord Conditions

Janet MacIntyre
Originating US chapter by Cindy Sullivan

evolve WEBSITE

http://evolve.elsevier.com/Canada/Lewis/medsurg

- Review Questions (Online Only)
- Key Points
- Answer Guidelines for Case Study

- Customizable Nursing Care Plan
  - Spinal Cord Injury
- Student Case Study
  - Patient with Spinal Cord Injury

- Audio Glossary
- Content Updates

LEARNING OBJECTIVES

1. Explain the etiology, clinical manifestations, and nursing management of trigeminal neuralgia and Bell's palsy and the related interprofessional care.
2. Explain the etiology, clinical manifestations, and nursing management of Guillain-Barré syndrome, botulism, tetanus, and neurosyphilis and the related interprofessional care.
3. Describe the classification of spinal cord injuries and associated clinical manifestations.
4. Describe the clinical manifestations and nursing management of spinal cord injury and interprofessional care of patients with spinal cord injury.

5. Explain the correlation between the severity and location of spinal cord injury and disruption of bodily function and the functional goals for rehabilitation.
6. Describe the nursing management of the major physical and psychological challenges of patients with a spinal cord injury.
7. Describe the effects of spinal cord injury on older persons.
8. Explain the types, clinical manifestations, and nursing management of spinal cord tumours and the interprofessional care of patients with spinal cord tumours.
9. Describe the pathophysiology, clinical manifestations, and nursing and interprofessional management of postpolio syndrome.

KEY TERMS

autonomic dysreflexia
Bell's palsy
botulism
Brown-Séquard syndrome
Guillain-Barré syndrome (GBS)

neurogenic bladder
neurogenic shock
neurosyphilis
paraplegia
poikilothermism

postpolio syndrome (PPS)
spinal shock
tetanus
tetraplegia
trigeminal neuralgia (TN)

▌CRANIAL NERVE DISORDERS

Cranial nerve disorders are commonly classified as peripheral neuropathies. The 12 pairs of cranial nerves are considered the peripheral nerves of the brain. The associated disorders usually involve the motor or sensory (or both) branches of a single nerve *(mononeuropathies)*. Causes of cranial nerve disorders include tumours, trauma, infections, inflammatory processes, and idiopathic (unknown) causes. Two cranial nerve disorders that will be discussed in this chapter are trigeminal neuralgia and Bell's palsy.

TRIGEMINAL NEURALGIA

Etiology and Pathophysiology

Trigeminal neuralgia (TN), also known as *tic douloureux,* is a relatively uncommon cranial nerve disorder. The annual incidence of TN is 5 in 100 000 in Canada (Trigeminal Neuralgia Association of Canada [TNAC], 2015). The average age of onset is 60 years; it is rarely diagnosed in individuals under 40 and develops slightly more often in women than in men (Keskinruzgar et al., 2019).

The trigeminal nerve is the fifth cranial nerve (cranial nerve [CN] V) and has both motor and sensory branches (TNAC, 2015). In TN, the sensory, or afferent, branches, primarily the maxillary and mandibular branches, are involved (Figure 63.1).

The pathophysiology of TN is not fully understood. One theory is that blood vessels, the superior cerebellar artery in particular, are compressed. This compression results in chronic irritation of the trigeminal nerve at the root entry zone. This irritation results in increased firing of the afferent or sensory fibre, commonly referred to as *classical TN. Symptomatic TN* is typically caused by a structural, nonvascular lesion (benign tumours, aneurysms, multiple sclerosis) (Al-Quliti, 2015). Other factors that may result in neuralgia include herpesvirus infection, infection of gums and jaw, and a brainstem infarct. The effectiveness of anticonvulsant medication therapy in reducing pain may be related to the ability of these medications to stabilize the neuronal membrane and decrease paroxysmal afferent impulses of the nerve (Al-Quliti, 2015).

Clinical Manifestations

The classic feature of TN is an abrupt onset of paroxysms of flashing, stabbing pain radiating along the course of a branch of the trigeminal facial nerve from the angle of the jaw, described as a burning, knifelike, or lightning-like shock in the lips, the upper or lower gums, the cheek, the forehead, or the side of the nose. Intense pain, twitching, grimacing, and frequent blinking and tearing of the eye occur during the acute attack (hence the term *tic douloureux*). Some patients may experience facial sensory loss. The attacks are usually brief, lasting only seconds to 2 or 3 minutes, and are generally unilateral. Recurrences are unpredictable; they may occur several times a day or weeks or months apart. After the refractory (pain-free) period, a phenomenon known as *clustering* can occur. Clustering is characterized by a cycle of pain and refractoriness that continues for hours.

The painful episodes are usually initiated by a triggering mechanism of light cutaneous stimulation at a specific point *(trigger zone)* along the distribution of the nerve branches. Precipitating stimuli include chewing, brushing teeth, a hot or cold blast of air on the face, washing the face, yawning, and even talking. Touch and tickle seem to predominate as causative triggers, rather than pain or changes in temperature. As a result, the patient may eat improperly, neglect hygienic practices, wear a cloth over their face, and withdraw from interaction with other individuals. The patient may sleep excessively as a means of coping with the pain.

Although this condition is considered benign, the severity of the pain and the disruption of lifestyle can result in almost total physical and psychological dysfunction or even suicide.

Diagnostic Studies

It is important to rule out other conditions with similar manifestations, such as other forms of facial and cephalic neuralgias and pain arising from the sinuses, the gums, and the jaws. In most patients with bilateral facial pain, magnetic resonance imaging (MRI) is performed to rule out lesions, vascular abnormalities, and multiple sclerosis (TNAC, 2015). A complete neurological assessment is performed, including audiological evaluation, although results are usually normal. Electromyography (EMG) can be performed to help distinguish between symptomatic and classical TN. Once the diagnosis is made, the goal of treatment is relief of pain by either medical or surgical intervention (Table 63.1).

Interprofessional Care

Medication Therapy. Carbamazepine (Tegretol) is considered the first-line therapy in patients with newly diagnosed TN (Keskinruzgar et al., 2019). By acting on sodium channels,

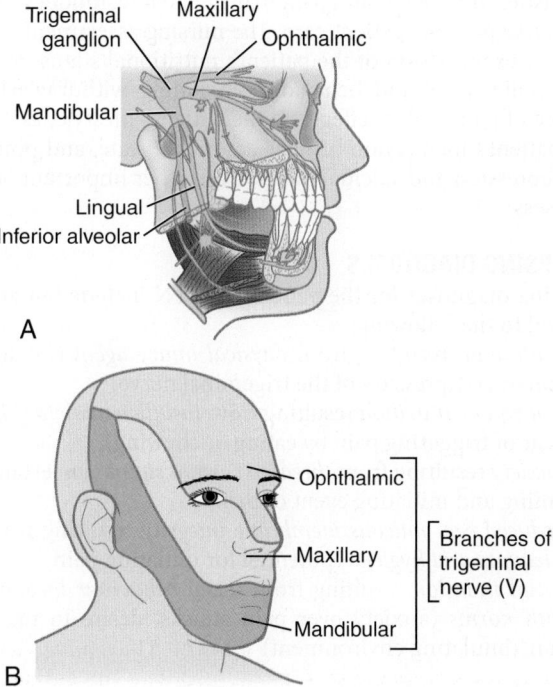

FIG. 63.1 A, Trigeminal nerve (fifth cranial nerve) and its three main divisions: the ophthalmic, maxillary, and mandibular nerves. **B,** Sensory fibres of the trigeminal nerve for three branch nerves (ophthalmic, maxillary, and mandibular nerves), each of which conducts information from a different region of the face. Source: Modified from Patton, K. T., & Thibodeau, G. A. (2016). *Anatomy and physiology* (9th ed., p. 491, Figure 21-11). Mosby.

TABLE 63.1   **INTERPROFESSIONAL CARE**
Clinical Management of Trigeminal Neuralgia

Diagnostic
- EMG studies
- Evaluation for symptomatic TN
- MRI of brain to assess for secondary causes
- Normal neurological examination
- Paroxysmal lancinating facial pain in distribution of trigeminal nerve (classic TN)

Interprofessional Therapy
Medication Therapy
- First-line: carbamazepine (Tegretol), oxcarbazepine (Trileptal)
- Second-line: baclofen (Lioresal), lamotrigine (Lamictal)
- Third-line: gabapentin (Neurontin), pregabalin (Lyrica), topiramate (Topamax)

Surgical Options
- Percutaneous
- Glycerol rhizotomy
- Radiofrequency rhizotomy
- Intracranial
- Gamma Knife radiosurgery
- Microvascular decompression

EMG, electromyography; *MRI,* magnetic resonance imaging.

carbamazepine and other anticonvulsant medications lengthen the time needed for neuron repolarization, which results in decreased neuron firing. Adverse effects of carbamazepine may include bone marrow suppression, which leads to blood abnormalities. Therefore, routine complete blood cell (CBC) counts are required. Baclofen (Lioresal), an antispasmodic agent, has demonstrated efficacy in reducing pain from TN. Baclofen works synergistically with carbamazepine and can therefore be used as a monotherapy or in conjunction with carbamazepine if pain relief is incomplete. Other anticonvulsant medications that may be used in the management of TN are listed in Table 63.1. These anticonvulsant medications may prevent an acute attack or promote a remission of symptoms. Because medication therapy may not provide permanent pain relief, some patients may seek continued help and make numerous visits to otolaryngologists for assessment or may attempt alternative therapies such as acupuncture and megavitamins.

Conservative Therapy. Local anaesthetics can be used to block nerves. Local nerve blocking results in complete anaesthesia of the area supplied by the injected branches. Relief of pain is temporary, lasting from 6 to 18 months.

Biofeedback is another strategy that may be helpful for some patients. In addition to controlling the pain, the patient may experience a strong sense of personal control by mastering the technique and altering certain body functions. (Biofeedback is discussed in Chapter 12.)

Surgical Therapy. If a conservative approach, including medication therapy, is not effective, surgical therapy is available. *Glycerol rhizotomy* is a percutaneous procedure that consists of an injection of glycerol through the foramen ovale into the trigeminal cistern (Figure 63.2). Glycerol injections produce immediate pain relief in 90% of patients, but by 5 years, approximately 50% experience recurrence of pain (Al-Quliti, 2015).

Percutaneous radiofrequency rhizotomy (electrocoagulation) and microvascular decompression provide the greatest relief of pain. In *percutaneous radiofrequency rhizotomy,* a

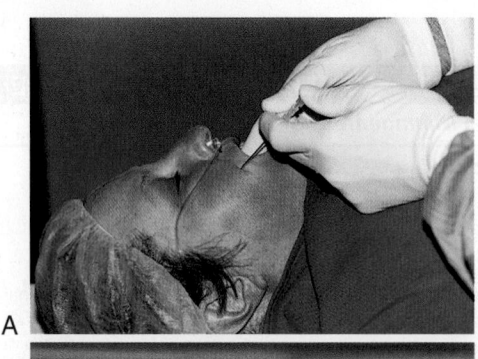
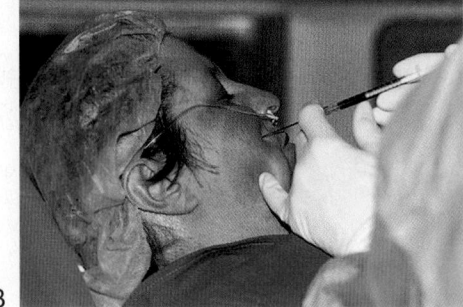

FIG. 63.2 Glycerol rhizotomy. **A,** Needle placed in face of patient with trigeminal neuralgia. **B,** Physician injecting glycerol. Source: Courtesy Joe Rothrock, Media, PA.

needle is inserted into the trigeminal rootlets that are adjacent to the pons, and the area is destroyed by means of a radiofrequency current. This can result in facial numbness (although some degree of sensation may be retained), corneal anaesthesia, and trigeminal motor weakness. This procedure is easily performed with few complications and minimal risk to the patient and essentially exchanges pain for numbness. It is usually performed on an outpatient basis. It is tolerated well by older patients and avoids a major operative procedure, which is beneficial for patients at high risk for surgical complications (Al-Quliti, 2015).

Microvascular decompression of the trigeminal nerve, another commonly used procedure, is accomplished by displacing and repositioning blood vessels that appear to be compressing the nerve at the root entry zone where it exits the pons. This procedure relieves pain without residual sensory loss. Microvascular decompression has a long-term success rate equal or superior to that of percutaneous procedures, and the rate of permanent neurological outcomes such as numbness is lower (National Institute of Neurological Disorders and Stroke [NINDS], 2021).

Gamma Knife radiosurgery is another surgical treatment that is used to alleviate TN. Radiosurgery with the Gamma Knife provides precise radiation of the proximal trigeminal nerve identified on high-resolution imaging. This approach has been useful both for patients with persistent pain after other surgical procedures and as a primary surgical option (Al-Quliti, 2015).

NURSING MANAGEMENT
TRIGEMINAL NEURALGIA

NURSING ASSESSMENT

Assessment of the attacks—including triggering factors, characteristics, frequency, and pain management techniques—helps the nurse plan for patient care. The nursing assessment should include examination of the patient's nutritional status, hygiene (especially oral), and behaviour (including withdrawal). The degree of pain and its effects on the patient's lifestyle, as well as the patient's medication history, emotional state, and potential for depression and suicidal ideation are other important factors to assess.

NURSING DIAGNOSES

Nursing diagnoses for the patient with TN include but are not limited to the following:

- *Acute pain* resulting from *physical injury agent* (inflammation or compression of the trigeminal nerve)
- *Inadequate nutrition* resulting from *insufficient dietary intake* (fear of triggering pain by eating or chewing)
- *Anxiety* resulting from *threat to current status* (uncertainty of timing and initiating event of pain)
- *Reduced oral mucous membrane integrity* resulting from *inadequate oral hygiene* (potential for initiating pain)
- *Social isolation* resulting from *social behaviour incongruent with norms* (anxiety over pain attacks, desire to maintain nonstimulating environment)

PLANNING

The overall goals are that the patient with TN will (a) be free of pain, (b) maintain adequate nutritional and oral hygiene status, (c) have minimal to no anxiety, and (d) return to their usual or previous socialization and occupational activities.

NURSING IMPLEMENTATION

HEALTH PROMOTION. Because the etiology of TN remains unknown, health promotion is directed at reducing recurrent episodes in patients with TN. Awareness and reduction of triggering events may be possible for some patients.

ACUTE INTERVENTION. Patients with TN are usually treated on an outpatient basis. Pain relief is obtained primarily by the administration of the recommended medication therapy. The nurse monitors the patient's response to therapy and notes any adverse effects. Alternative pain relief measures, such as biofeedback, should be explored for patients who are not surgical candidates and whose pain is not controlled by other therapeutic measures. A thorough assessment of pain with a valid and reliable tool, which includes the history of the pain and effectiveness of pain relief measures, can assist in selecting appropriate pain management interventions.

The nurse should review with the patient the importance of nutrition, hygiene, and oral care and teach methods to achieve all of this self-care if neglect is apparent. For cleansing the face, the nurse should provide lukewarm water and soft cloths or cotton saturated with solutions that do not require rinsing. A small, soft-bristled toothbrush or a warm mouthwash assists in promoting oral care. Hygiene activities are best performed when pain is managed and analgesic effectiveness is at its peak. Environmental management is essential during an acute period to lessen triggering stimuli.

Food should be high in protein and calories and easy to chew. It should be served lukewarm and offered frequently. When oral intake is sharply reduced and the patient's nutritional status is compromised, a nasogastric tube can be inserted on the unaffected side for enteral feedings.

The patient will probably not engage in extensive conversation during the acute period. Alternative communication methods, such as paper and pencil, should be provided.

The nurse should provide information or instructions related to diagnostic studies used to rule out other disorders—such as multiple sclerosis, dental or sinus conditions, and neoplasms—and for preoperative teaching if surgery is planned. The nurse may also have to clarify expectations related to postoperative outcomes. Appropriate teaching related to postoperative activities depends on the type of procedure planned (e.g., percutaneous, intracranial). The patient needs to know that they will be awake during local procedures so that they can cooperate when corneal and ciliary reflexes and facial sensations are checked. Patients should be informed about the potential risk of postoperative facial numbness.

After the procedure, the patient's pain is compared with the preoperative level. The corneal reflex, extraocular muscles, hearing, sensation, and facial nerve function are evaluated frequently (see Chapter 58). If the corneal reflex is impaired, special attention must be paid to eye protection. This includes the use of artificial tears or eye shields. General postoperative nursing care after a craniotomy is appropriate if intracranial surgery is performed. (Nursing care related to craniotomy is discussed in Chapter 59.) Caloric intake and ambulation should be increased according to the patient's progress or specific orders.

After a percutaneous radiofrequency electrocoagulation procedure, an ice pack is applied to the jaw on the operative side for 3 to 5 hours. To avoid injuring the mouth, the patient should not chew on the operative side until sensation has returned.

AMBULATORY AND HOME CARE. Regular follow-up care should be planned. The patient needs instruction regarding the dosage and adverse effects of medications. Although relief of pain may be complete, the patient should be encouraged to keep environmental stimuli to a moderate level and to use stress-reduction methods. The patient may have developed protective practices to prevent pain and may need counselling or psychiatric assistance in the readjustment, especially in re-establishing personal relationships. Herpes simplex infection (cold sores) can occur as a result of manipulation of the gasserian ganglion. Treatment consists of antiviral agents such as acyclovir (Zovirax) (see Chapter 26).

Long-term management after surgical intervention depends on the residual effects of the type of procedure. If hypesthesia (decreased sensitivity to stimulation, excluding the special senses) is present or the corneal reflex is altered, the patient should be taught to (a) chew on the unaffected side; (b) avoid hot foods or beverages, which can burn the mucous membranes; (c) check the oral cavity after meals to remove food particles; (d) practise meticulous oral hygiene and continue with semi-annual dental visits; (e) protect the face against extremes of temperature; (f) use an electric razor; and (g) wear a protective eye shield.

EVALUATION

The following are expected outcomes for patients with TN:
- Relief or decreased pain
- Appearing more comfortable and less anxious
- Normal facial sensation or expected paresthesias and anaesthesias
- Return to previous socialization, or improved socialization, and occupational activities

BELL'S PALSY

Etiology and Pathophysiology

Bell's palsy (peripheral facial paralysis, acute benign cranial polyneuritis) is a disorder characterized by a disruption of the motor branches of the facial nerve (cranial nerve VII) on one side of the face in the absence of any other disease such as a stroke. Bell's palsy is an acute, peripheral facial paresis of unknown cause. Average annual incidence rates of Bell's palsy are similar throughout the world, ranging between 11.5 and 40.2 per 100 000. It affects males and females equally and has a slightly higher incidence in mid- to later life (Eviston et al., 2015).

Although the exact etiology is not known, there is evidence associating immune, infective, and ischemic mechanisms as potential contributors. The reactivation of the herpes simplex virus infection is one example. The reactivation causes an inflammatory response with subsequent demyelination of the nerve, causing alterations in motor and sensory function (Eviston et al., 2015).

Bell's palsy is considered benign; the majority of patients make a complete recovery. Improvement in facial function occurs in 85% of people within 3 weeks of onset. Patients with complete facial paralysis at onset who have not experienced some recovery within the first 3 to 4 months are more likely to have incomplete recovery. Chronic facial palsy can be a disabling condition that has an impact on social function, emotional expression, and quality of life (Eviston et al., 2015).

Clinical Manifestations

The characteristic findings of Bell's palsy are acute onset of unilateral facial paralysis affecting muscles of the upper and

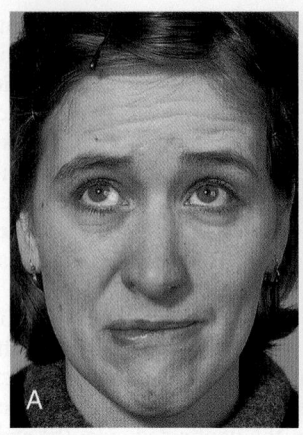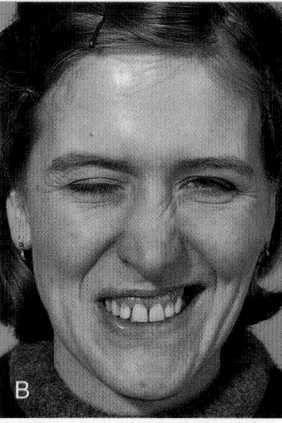

FIG. 63.3 Facial characteristics of Bell's palsy. **A,** At rest the face may look almost normal, but the patient is not able to wrinkle her forehead on the affected (right) side, and the right corner of the mouth droops. **B,** When she tries to close her eyes and show her teeth, the differences between the affected and unaffected sides become more obvious. Source: Forbes, C. D., & Jackson, W. F. (2003). *Color atlas and text of clinical medicine* (3rd ed., p. 453, Figures 11.15 and 11.16). Mosby.

lower face reaching a peak within 72 hours, resulting in facial drooping, an inability to close the eyelid, or an inability to frown or smile (Figure 63.3). Decreased muscle movement may alter chewing ability. Some patients may experience a loss of or excessive tearing. The muscle weakness causes the lower eyelid to turn out, allowing overflow of normal tear production. These symptoms are frequently accompanied by neck, mastoid, or ear pain; distortion in sense of taste; and altered facial sensation.

Diagnostic Studies

The diagnosis of Bell's palsy is based on clinical presentation. The diagnosis and prognosis are indicated by observation of the typical pattern of onset of symptoms. In situations with complete facial paralysis, neurophysiological testing (EMG studies) is helpful in predicting potential nerve recovery. A computed tomographic (CT) scan or MRI may be performed to rule out stroke or other neurological disease (Eviston et al., 2015).

Interprofessional Care

Nonpharmacological treatments for Bell's palsy include eye protection for patients with incomplete closure of their eyes. Prolonged irritation and drying can cause keratitis and ulceration and potentially impair eyesight. Eye protection includes barrier protection, lubrication, and taped closure at night. Oral care may include use of a straw for drinking. A change in diet texture toward soft foods may be necessary, and mastication techniques may need to change in order to avoid mucous membrane trauma (Eviston et al., 2015).

Medication Therapy. Treatment with corticosteroids (prednisone) should be commenced within 72 hours of onset of symptoms. Steroids are given over a 2- to 3-week period with tapering doses after approximately 10 days. Usually, the corticosteroid treatment decreases the edema and pain, but analgesics can be used if necessary to manage pain. Combining prednisone with an antiviral medication such as acyclovir (Zovirax) or valacyclovir (Valtrex) can improve the rate of recovery given that the herpes simplex virus can be a causal factor (Eviston et al., 2015). The length of treatment with antiviral medications

is usually between 5 and 10 days. It is important to review with the patient and the family the medications that have been prescribed for the treatment of Bell's palsy, including any potential adverse effects.

NURSING MANAGEMENT
BELL'S PALSY

NURSING ASSESSMENT

Early recognition of the possibility of Bell's palsy is important. Because herpes simplex virus is a possible etiological factor, any person who is prone to herpes simplex should be alerted to seek health care if pain occurs in or around the ear. A complete assessment of CN VII, which includes the facial muscles, should be completed, with careful attention to any signs of weakness; patients should be asked to close their eyes, show their teeth, puff their cheeks, and smile (Taylor, 2021).

NURSING DIAGNOSES

The nursing diagnoses for the patient with Bell's palsy may include but are not limited to the following:
- *Acute pain* resulting from *physical injury agent* (inflammation of CN VII—facial nerve)
- *Inadequate nutrition* resulting from *insufficient dietary intake* (inability to ingest food secondary to muscle weakness)
- *Potential for corneal injury* as demonstrated by *blinking less than five times per minute*
- *Disrupted body image* resulting from *alteration in self-perception* (change in facial appearance)

PLANNING

The overall goals are that the patient with Bell's palsy will (a) be pain free or be able to manage pain, (b) maintain adequate nutritional status, (c) maintain appropriate oral hygiene, (d) not experience injury to the eye, (e) return to normal or previous perception of body image, and (f) be optimistic about disease outcome.

NURSING IMPLEMENTATION

Bell's palsy is treated on an outpatient basis. The following interventions are used throughout the course of the disease. Mild analgesics can relieve pain. Hot wet packs can reduce the discomfort of herpetic lesions if present, aid circulation, and relieve pain. The face should be protected from cold and drafts because trigeminal *hyperesthesia* (increased sensitivity to stimulation such as touch) may accompany the syndrome. Maintenance of good nutrition is important. The patient should be taught to chew on the unaffected side of the mouth to avoid trapping food and to enjoy the taste of food. Thorough oral hygiene must be carried out after each meal to prevent the development of parotitis, caries, and periodontal disease from accumulated residual food.

Dark glasses may be worn for protective and cosmetic reasons. Artificial tears (methyl cellulose) should be instilled frequently during the day to prevent drying of the cornea. The eye should be inspected for the presence of eyelashes. Ointment and an impermeable eye shield can be used at night to retain moisture. In some patients, taping the lids closed at night may be necessary to provide protection. The patient is taught to report ocular pain, drainage, or discharge.

A facial sling may be helpful to support affected muscles, improve lip alignment, and facilitate eating. The facial sling is usually made and fitted by a physiotherapist or occupational therapist. Vigorous massage can break down tissues, but gentle upward massage has psychological benefits even if physical effects, other than the maintenance of circulation, are questionable. When function begins to return, active facial exercises are performed several times a day.

The change in physical appearance as a result of Bell's palsy can be devastating. Affected patients must be reassured that a stroke did not occur and that chances for a full recovery are good. A patient's need for privacy should be respected, especially during meals, but the nurse's assistance in the patient's adjustment to the physical changes should not be delayed. Enlisting support from family and friends is important. It is important to inform the patient that most patients with Bell's palsy recover within about 6 weeks of the onset of symptoms.

EVALUATION

The following are expected outcomes for the patient with Bell's palsy:

- Freedom from pain
- No complications (e.g., corneal abrasion)
- Appropriate nutritional intake
- Minimal adverse effects associated with corticosteroid treatment
- Return to previous perception of body image

POLYNEUROPATHIES

GUILLAIN-BARRÉ SYNDROME

Etiology and Pathophysiology

Guillain-Barré syndrome (GBS), also known as *Landry–Guillain-Barré–Strohl syndrome, postinfectious polyneuropathy,* and *ascending polyneuropathic paralysis,* is an acute, rapidly progressing, and potentially fatal form of polyneuritis. GBS affects the peripheral nervous system and results in loss of myelin (segmental demyelination), edema, and inflammation of the affected nerves. GBS manifests as a symmetrical ascending paralysis. The incidence is 1 to 2 cases per 100 000 per year. The disease is present worldwide and affects individuals of all age groups (Top et al., 2015).

The etiology of this disorder is unknown, but it is believed to be a cell-mediated immunological reaction directed at the peripheral nerves. About two-thirds of the diagnosis is preceded by either an upper respiratory or a gastrointestinal infection (Babazadeh et al., 2019). A possible link between vaccinations and the occurrence of GBS has been proposed, although the evidence indicates that this is a very rare event and poses minimal risk (Babazadeh et al., 2019). *Campylobacter jejuni* is the organism most recognized to be associated with GBS (Ansar & Valadi, 2015). Other potential pathogens include *Mycoplasma pneumoniae,* cytomegalovirus, Epstein-Barr virus, varicella-zoster virus, and vaccines (rabies, swine influenza). These stimuli are thought to cause an alteration in the immune system, resulting in sensitization of T lymphocytes to the patient's myelin and, ultimately, myelin damage. Demyelination occurs, and the transmission of nerve impulses is stopped or slowed down. The muscles innervated by the damaged peripheral nerves undergo denervation and atrophy. In the recovery phase, remyelination occurs slowly, and neurological function returns in a proximal-to-distal pattern.

Clinical Manifestations

GBS symptoms range from mild to severe and typically progress over the course of hours to several days. GBS is characterized by relatively symmetrical muscle weakness, mild distal sensory symptoms of paresthesias (first in the feet, then in the hands) with absent or depressed deep tendon reflexes. Weakness develops classically in an ascending pattern involving the lower limbs first, then the upper extremities, followed by the face and respiratory muscle; weakness may progress to complete paralysis (Rubin, 2020).

Four main subtypes of GBS include (1) acute inflammatory demyelinating polyneuropathy (AIDP) (80–90%); (2) acute motor axonal neuropathy and (3) acute sensorimotor axonal neuropathy (5–10%); and (4) Miller Fisher syndrome (5%), a rare disorder characterized by ataxia, areflexia, and *ophthalmoplegia* (weakness or paralysis of the muscles controlling eye movements). In GBS, autonomic nervous system dysfunction results from alterations in both the sympathetic and the parasympathetic nervous systems. Autonomic disturbances are usually observed in patients with severe muscle involvement and respiratory muscle paralysis. The most dangerous autonomic dysfunctions include life-threatening blood pressure fluctuations, cardiac arrhythmias, gastrointestinal stasis, urinary retention, and pupillary changes (Rubin, 2020). Affected patients may also have the syndrome of inappropriate antidiuretic hormone secretion (SIADH, discussed in Chapter 51). Progression of GBS to include the lower brainstem involves the facial, abducens, oculomotor, hypoglossal, trigeminal, and vagus nerves (CNs VII, VI, III, XII, V, and X, respectively). This involvement manifests through facial weakness, difficulties with extraocular eye movement, dysphagia, and paresthesia of the face.

Pain is a common symptom in patients with GBS, secondary to the neuropathy that is occurring. The pain can be categorized as neuropathic pain and is described as prickling (paresthesia), burning, shooting, or stabbing. Pain appears to be worse at night. Pain may lead to a decrease in appetite and may interfere with sleep. Management of pain can include the use of analgesics such as nonsteroidal anti-inflammatory medications, opioids, and medications used to treat neuropathic pain (gabapentin, pregabalin, and carbamazepine). Nonpharmacological measures such as positioning, range-of-motion exercises, massage, and distraction can also be used to help manage pain. Pain management measures should be adapted on the basis of assessment findings and evaluation of the pain management plan.

Complications. The most serious complication of this syndrome is respiratory failure, which occurs as the paralysis progresses to the nerves that innervate the thoracic area. Constant monitoring of the respiratory system by checking respiratory rate, depth, forced vital capacity, and negative inspiratory force provides information about the need for immediate intervention, including intubation and mechanical ventilation. Urinary tract infections (UTIs) or respiratory tract infections may occur. Fever is generally the first sign of infection, and treatment is directed at the infecting organism. Immobility from the paralysis can cause complications such as paralytic ileus, muscle atrophy, contractures, deep vein thrombosis (DVT), pulmonary emboli (PEs), skin breakdown, orthostatic hypotension, and nutritional deficiencies.

Diagnostic Studies

Diagnosis is based primarily on the patient's history and clinical signs. Cerebrospinal fluid (CSF) is normal or has a low protein content initially, but after 7 to 10 days, the protein level is elevated and the white blood cell count is normal. Results of EMG and nerve conduction studies are markedly abnormal and show evidence of demyelination in about two thirds of patients (Rubin, 2020).

Interprofessional Care

Management is aimed at supportive care, particularly ventilatory support, during the acute phase. Prevention of DVT and PE through prophylactic anticoagulation with heparin or low-molecular-weight heparin (LMWH) is routine. Practice guidelines endorse the use of plasma exchange or intravenous administration of immune globulin (IVIG) within 4 weeks of symptom onset in nonambulatory patients and within 2 weeks in ambulatory patients (Ansar & Valadi, 2015). Treatment results in distinct reductions in the length of hospital stay, length of time on a ventilator, and time required to resume walking. IVIG has also been shown to be as effective as plasma exchange (plasmapheresis) and has the advantage of immediate availability and greater safety. However, patients receiving IVIG need to be well hydrated and have adequate renal function. (Plasmapheresis is discussed in Chapter 16.) Once 3 weeks pass after disease onset, plasma exchange and IVIG therapies have little value. A review of the use of corticosteroids in the treatment of GBS has not shown them to be of any benefit (Ansar & Valadi, 2015).

NURSING MANAGEMENT
GUILLAIN-BARRÉ SYNDROME

NURSING ASSESSMENT

Assessment of patients with GBS is the most important aspect of nursing care during the acute phase. The nurse must monitor for ascending paralysis; assess respiratory function; monitor arterial blood gas (ABG) levels; and assess the gag, corneal, and swallowing reflexes during the routine assessment. Reflexes are usually decreased or absent.

Monitoring blood pressure and cardiac rate and rhythm is also important during the acute phase because transient cardiac dysrhythmias may occur as a result of autonomic dysfunction. Orthostatic hypotension secondary to muscle atony may occur in severe cases. Vasopressor agents and volume expanders may be needed to treat the low blood pressure. However, if SIADH is present, fluid restriction may be required.

NURSING DIAGNOSES

Nursing diagnoses for patients with GBS may include but are not limited to the following:

- *Reduced spontaneous ventilation* resulting from *respiratory muscle fatigue*
- *Potential for aspiration* as demonstrated by *depressed gag reflex, impaired ability to swallow*
- *Acute pain* resulting from *physical injury agent* (paresthesias, muscle aches and cramps, hyperesthesias)
- *Reduced verbal communication* resulting from environmental barrier (intubation)
- *Anxiety* resulting from threat to current status (uncertain outcome and seriousness of the disease)
- *Reduced self-care* (bathing, dressing, feeding, toileting) resulting from *fatigue, weakness, pain*
- *Potential for impaired skin integrity* resulting from *pressure over bony prominences* (decreased mobility)

PLANNING

The overall goals are that the patient with GBS will (a) maintain adequate ventilation, (b) be free from aspiration, (c) be able to manage pain, (d) maintain an acceptable method of communication, (e) maintain adequate nutritional intake, and (f) return to usual physical functioning.

NURSING IMPLEMENTATION

The objective of therapy is to support body systems until the patient recovers. In the acute phase, patients are often cared for in the critical care unit (CCU). Respiratory failure and infection are serious threats. Monitoring the vital lung capacity and ABG values is essential. Patients would benefit from interprofessional collaboration with a respiratory therapist. If the vital capacity drops to less than 800 mL (15 mL/kg, or two thirds of the patient's normal vital capacity) or the ABG levels deteriorate, endotracheal intubation or tracheostomy may be performed so that the patient can be mechanically ventilated (see Chapter 70). Meticulous suctioning technique is needed to prevent infection if the patient has an endotracheal tube or tracheostomy. Thorough bronchial hygiene and chest physiotherapy help clear secretions and prevent respiratory deterioration. If fever develops, sputum cultures should be obtained to identify the pathogen. Appropriate antibiotic therapy is then initiated.

Fear and anxiety are common feelings for both the patient and the family. These feelings often result from lack of knowledge regarding the disease progression. Answering the patient's and family's questions, clarifying misconceptions, and keeping the patient and the family informed can help reduce this fear. Collaboration with other members of the interprofessional team, including occupational therapists and speech–language pathologists, is essential. At the peak of a severe episode, the patient may be incapable of communicating, and this can add to the patient's fear. A communication system must be established according to the patient's available abilities. Communication, however, remains extremely difficult if the disease progresses to involve the cranial nerves. The nurse must explain all procedures before performing them and reassure the patient that muscle function will return.

Urinary retention is common for a few days. Intermittent catheterization is preferred to an in-dwelling catheter to decrease the incidence of UTIs. However, for acutely ill patients receiving a large volume of fluids (>2.5 L/day), in-dwelling catheterization may be safer because it reduces overdistension of a temporarily flaccid bladder and prevents vesicoureteral reflux. Physiotherapy is indicated early to help prevent problems related to immobility. Passive range-of-motion exercises and attention to body position help maintain function and prevent contractures. Patients who develop facial paralysis must receive meticulous eye care to prevent corneal irritation or damage *(exposure keratitis)*. Artificial tears should be instilled frequently during the day to prevent drying of the cornea. The eyes should be inspected for the presence of eyelashes. Ointment and an impermeable eye shield can be used at night to retain moisture.

Nutritional needs must be met despite possible problems associated with delayed gastric emptying, paralytic ileus, and potential for aspiration if the gag reflex is lost. In addition to checking for the gag reflex, nurses should note drooling and other difficulties with secretions, which may be more indicative of an inadequate gag reflex. Initially, tube feedings or parenteral nutrition may be used to ensure adequate caloric intake. Because of delayed gastric emptying, residual volumes of the feedings should be assessed at regular intervals or before feedings (see Chapter 42). Fluid and electrolyte therapy must be monitored carefully to prevent electrolyte imbalances. A bowel program should be initiated because constipation is a common problem related to diet changes, immobility, and decreased gastrointestinal motility.

Nutritional intake can be compromised in patients with GBS. During the acute phase, patients may experience difficulty swallowing because of cranial nerve involvement. Mild dysphagia can be managed by placing patients in an upright position and flexing the head forward during feeding. For more severe dysphagia, tube feedings may be required. Patients who experience paralytic ileus or intestinal obstruction may require total parenteral nutrition. Later in the course of the disease, motor paralysis or weakness continues to affect the ability to self-feed. Patients' nutritional status, including body weight, serum albumin levels, and calorie counts, must be evaluated at regular intervals.

Pain assessment should be completed at least daily with a valid and reliable tool and the patient's self-report. A method of assessing pain without the patient's self-report may have to be established if the patient is unable to communicate verbally.

Patients with GBS who are experiencing paralysis are prone to skin breakdown as a result of immobility and decreased sensation. Patients should be assisted or encouraged to turn frequently; a turning schedule can be helpful in this regard. Skin and wound assessment should be performed daily. Specialty pressure-relieving beds can be used to decrease the potential for skin breakdown in these patients.

Throughout the course of the illness, the nurse must provide support and encouragement to the family and the patient. Residual symptoms and relapses are uncommon except in the chronic form of the disease. Complete recovery can be anticipated, although many patients continue to have a degree of residual pain and fatigue, requiring them to change their work and daily activities. Recovery is a slow process that takes months (3–6 on average), with most of the recovery occurring within the first year. Further recovery can be seen even up to 3 years after disease onset (Willison et al., 2016).

EVALUATION

The following are expected outcomes for the patient with GBS:
- Return to usual level of physical functioning
- Freedom from pain and discomfort
- Maintenance of nutritional status

BOTULISM

Etiology and Pathophysiology

Botulism is an acute neurological disorder that causes potentially life-threatening neuroparalysis due to a neurotoxin produced by the spore-forming bacterium *Clostridium botulinum*, which is present naturally throughout the environment and can be found in soil, water, and household dust and on surfaces of many foods. There are three main clinical presentations: foodborne botulism, infant botulism, and wound botulism. Botulism, a reportable disease, is rare in Canada. Indigenous people are at higher risk of botulism related to the consumption of raw meat (e.g., walrus, caribou), which poses a health risk from pathogens normally destroyed by proper cooking, traditional fermentation processes, and access to safe drinking water (Jung & Skinner, 2017). All forms of botulism can cause paralysis and be fatal. It is thought that the botulism neurotoxin destroys or inhibits the neurotransmission of acetylcholine at the myoneural junction, resulting in disturbed muscle innervation. The classic syndrome of botulism is a symmetrical, descending motor paralysis in an alert patient, with no sensory deficits (Population and Public Health Division, 2017).

Clinical Manifestations

Symptoms of foodborne botulism generally begin 12 to 36 hours after ingesting contaminated food; however, onset can begin as soon as 6 hours after exposure, or as long as 10 days later. Neurological manifestations develop rapidly over 2 to 4 days. Early symptoms for all types of botulism include fatigue, weakness, dizziness, double or blurred vision, difficulty speaking and swallowing, dry mouth, and headache. Symptoms associated with foodborne botulism include nausea, vomiting, and abdominal cramps. Paralysis typically starts in the shoulders and arms and progresses down the body. The course of the disease depends on the amount of toxin absorbed. If only a small amount is absorbed, symptoms are mild and recovery is complete. When large amounts are absorbed, death may occur from circulatory failure, respiratory paralysis, or development of pulmonary complications. With proper early treatment, the fatality rate of botulism cases in Canada is less than 5% (Ministry of Health and Long-term Care, 2019).

Medication Therapy

The initial treatment of botulism is intravenous (IV) administration of botulinum antitoxin. Botulism antitoxin may be readministered in 2 to 4 hours if symptoms persist and again at 12- to 24-hour intervals if required.

The gastrointestinal tract is purged by high colonic enemas, gastric lavage, and laxatives that do not contain magnesium, to decrease the absorption of the toxin. Magnesium is contraindicated because it worsens toxin-induced neuromuscular blockade.

Most people recover if diagnosed and treated quickly. Recovery can take several weeks to months. Severe botulism can require intensive medical and nursing care. If not diagnosed and treated, botulism can lead to death from respiratory failure within 3 to 10 days.

TETANUS

Etiology and Pathophysiology

Tetanus (lockjaw) is an extremely severe polyradiculitis (inflammation of the nerve roots) and polyneuritis (inflammation of nerves) affecting spinal and cranial nerves. It results from the effects of a potent neurotoxin produced by *Clostridium tetani*. The toxin interferes with the function of the reflex arc by blocking inhibitory transmitters at the presynaptic sites in the spinal cord and the brainstem. The spores of the bacillus are present in soil, garden mould, and manure. Thus *C. tetani* enters the body through contamination of a traumatic wound that provides an appropriate low-oxygen environment for the organisms to mature and produce toxin. The incubation period for tetanus is usually 3 to 21 days, with a range of 1 day to several months.

Tetanus is very rare in Canada thanks to routine immunizations. Over the years, the death rate has fallen to almost zero. Only six deaths had been reported in Canada between 2000 and 2014, with the last death reported in 2010 (Government of Canada, 2014).

Clinical Manifestations

Initial manifestations of generalized tetanus include a feeling of stiffness in the jaw *(trismus)* or the neck, fever, and other symptoms of general infection; these symptoms then descend. Generalized tonic spasms occur because of the lack of reciprocal innervation. As the disease progresses, the neck muscles, the back, the abdomen, and the extremities become progressively rigid. In severe forms, continuous tonic convulsions may occur with *opisthotonos* (extreme arching of the back and retraction of the head). Laryngeal and respiratory spasms cause apnea and anoxia. Additional effects are manifested by overstimulation of the sympathetic nervous system, including profuse diaphoresis, labile hypertension, episodic tachycardia, hyperthermia, and dysrhythmias. The slightest noise, jarring motion, or bright light can set off a seizure. These seizures are agonizing. Mortality rates are highest in infants and older persons, and death is usually attributable to asphyxia or heart failure resulting from constantly recurring spasms. Residual injury—such as vertebral fracture, muscle contracture, and brain damage secondary to hypoxia—may be long-term consequences.

Medication Therapy

The management of tetanus includes administration of tetanus and diphtheria toxoid booster and tetanus immune globulin (TIG) before the onset of symptoms to neutralize circulating toxins (see Chapter 71, Table 71.6). A much larger dose of TIG is administered to patients with manifestations of clinical tetanus. Control of spasms is essential and is managed by deep sedation and skeletal muscle relaxation, usually with diazepam (Valium), barbiturates, and, in severe cases, neuromuscular blocking agents such as rocuronium bromide that act to paralyze skeletal muscles. Opioid analgesics such as morphine or fentanyl are also indicated for pain management. A 10- to 14-day course of penicillin, metronidazole, tetracycline, or doxycycline is recommended to inhibit further growth of *C. tetani*.

Because of laryngospasm and the potential need for neuromuscular blocking medications, a tracheostomy is usually performed early, and the patient is maintained on mechanical ventilation. Sedative agents and opioid analgesics are given concomitantly to all patients who are pharmacologically paralyzed. Any recognized wound should be debrided, and any abscess drained. Antibiotics may be given to prevent secondary infections. Nutrition is maintained through parenteral nutrition or nasogastric feeding.

As stated earlier, the mortality rate associated with tetanus is declining. For patients who recover, convalescence is long and includes extensive physiotherapy.

NURSING MANAGEMENT
TETANUS

Health teaching is aimed at ensuring tetanus prophylaxis, which is the most important factor influencing the incidence of this disease. Tetanus prevention and immunization protocols are summarized in Table 71.6 in Chapter 71. Adults should receive a tetanus and diphtheria toxoid booster every 10 years. The patient should be taught that immediate, thorough cleansing of all wounds with soap and water is important to the prevention of tetanus. If a patient sustains an open wound and has not been immunized within the previous 5 years, the health care provider should be contacted so that the patient can receive a tetanus booster.

The acute nursing management of the patient with tetanus is aimed at supportive care based on the treatment of clinical manifestations. The patient should be placed in a quiet, darkened room that is insulated against noise. Sedation should be induced judiciously. Nursing care should be administered with the utmost caution to avoid triggering spasms. Nursing care related to tracheostomy and mechanical ventilation is given as appropriate. An in-dwelling urinary catheter may be used to prevent bladder distension and urinary reflux in the presence of spasms in the muscles of the pelvic floor. Attention is also given to skin care. The patient needs emotional support during the acute phase because of the fear of death. The family also needs support and education.

NEUROSYPHILIS

Neurosyphilis is an infection of any part of the nervous system by the organism *Treponema pallidum* (see Chapter 55). The organism can invade the central nervous system within a few months of the original infection, and the disease can be fatal if not treated. Neurosyphilis is often referred to incorrectly as "tertiary syphilis," but it can occur at any time in the course of syphilis and occurs in about 30% of untreated cases (Marra, 2015). Except for causing some changes in the CSF, including increases in the white blood cell count and protein levels and positive serological reaction, *T. pallidum* lies dormant for years. Late neurosyphilis results from degenerative changes in the spinal cord *(tabes dorsalis)* and the brainstem *(general paresis)*. *Tabes dorsalis* (progressive locomotor ataxia) is characterized by vague, sharp pains in the legs; ataxia; "slapping" gait; loss of proprioception and deep tendon reflexes; and zones of hyperesthesia. *Charcot joints,* which are characterized by enlargement, bone destruction, and hypermobility, also occur as a result of joint effusion and edema. Other manifestations of neurosyphilis include seizures and difficulties with vision and hearing.

Neurological symptoms associated with neurosyphilis are numerous and, in many cases, nonspecific. Neurosyphilis is a differential diagnosis for patients with neurological and psychiatric symptoms. *Dementia paralytica* is an ongoing spirochetal meningoencephalitis that causes a general dissolution of mental and physical capabilities. It may mimic a number of major or minor psychoses. Management includes treatment with penicillin, symptomatic care, and protection from physical injury.

SPINAL CORD CONDITIONS
SPINAL CORD INJURY

Spinal cord injuries (SCIs) have a devastating effect on health and well-being. The physical effects of SCI, as well as the complications and comorbid conditions associated with SCI, significantly affect quality of life and can even be life-threatening. Associated economic burdens result not only from health care costs but also from physical morbidity and premature mortality that affect productivity at a societal level. SCI is divided into *traumatic* (result of external physical impact) and *nontraumatic* (result of disease, infection, or tumour) categories.

It is estimated that Canada has 4 529 new cases of SCI each year, with 1 786 as a result of traumatic injury (Spinal Cord Injury BC, 2021). It is anticipated that this number will increase over the next couple of decades, and Canada's aging population is anticipated to contribute to this increase. The current economic burden of traumatic SCI is approximately $3.6 billion

(Spinal Cord Injury BC, 2021). Indigenous people are more likely to experience a traumatic SCI than other Canadians (Ahmed et al., 2020).

Older persons with traumatic injuries experience more complications, are hospitalized longer, and have a higher rate of mortality. Injuries are most common in the cervical spine, and such injuries are associated with the most devastating neurological impairments.

The most common causes of premature death in the patient with **tetraplegia** (formerly called *quadriplegia* and used interchangeably; paralysis of both arms and legs and the trunk, which occurs with spinal cord damage at C8 or above) are usually related to compromised respiratory function (pneumonia), impaired renal function (UTI), and impaired skin integrity (pressure injuries). Any combination of these will certainly increase risk for mortality.

Because of the potential for disruption of individual growth and development, altered family dynamics, economic loss in terms of absence from work, and the high cost of rehabilitation and long-term health care, spinal cord trauma is a major event. Although many people with SCIs can care for themselves independently, those with the highest level of injury may require round-the-clock care at home or in a long-term care facility.

Etiology and Pathophysiology

Common causes of traumatic SCI include motor vehicle and motorcycle crashes, which account for 50% of SCI cases, and falls and work-related injuries (30–40%). Falls are more typically causes of SCI in the older person, whereas motor vehicle crashes are a more common cause among young adults. Almost half of new traumatic injuries occur in people (mainly male) 15 to 39 years of age as a result of motor vehicle accidents, sporting accidents, and other external causes (Spinal Cord Injury BC, 2021).

Initial Injury. SCI can result from cord compression by bone displacement, tumour, or abscess or from interruption of blood supply to the cord. The spinal cord is wrapped in tough layers of dura and is rarely torn or transected by direct trauma. Penetrating trauma, such as gunshot and stab wounds, can result in tearing and transection. The pathophysiology of SCI is best described as *biphasic*. The initial mechanical injury *(primary injury)* with failure of the spinal column (fracture or dislocation) imparts force to the spinal cord, disrupting axons, blood vessels, and cell membranes. This process is followed by a second phase *(secondary injury)* involving vascular dysfunction, edema, ischemia, electrolyte shifts, inflammation, free radical production, and apoptotic cell death (Witiw & Fehlings, 2015).

At the molecular level, *apoptosis* (cell death) occurs and may continue for weeks or months after the initial injury. Thus the complete cord damage in severe trauma is related to autodestruction of the cord. This autodestruction is confirmed by observations that, shortly after the injury, petechial hemorrhages occur in the central grey matter of the cord. This hemorrhaging further leads to microvascular disruption and hemorrhage in surrounding white matter. Cord ischemia develops and may extend for many segments above and below the injury (Witiw & Fehlings, 2015). By 24 hours or less after injury, the development of edema above and below the level of injury as a result of ischemic damage may cause permanent cord damage. This ongoing destructive process is dominant early on; therefore, it is crucial that the initial care and management of the patient with an SCI limit further activation of these processes.

Figure 63.4 illustrates the cascade of events causing secondary injury after traumatic SCI. The resulting hypoxia reduces

PATHOPHYSIOLOGY MAP

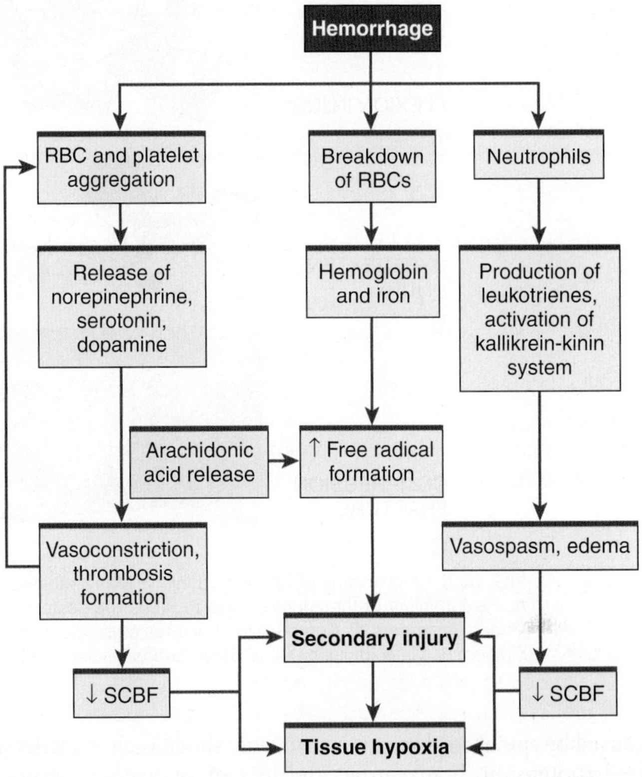

FIG. 63.4 Cascade of metabolic and cellular events that leads to spinal cord ischemia and the hypoxia of secondary injury. *RBC,* red blood cell; *SCBF,* spinal cord blood flow. Source: Redrawn from Marciano, F. F., Greene, K., Apostolides, P. J., et al. (1995). Pharmacologic management of spinal cord injury. *BNI Quarterly, 11*(2), 6; and from McCance, K. L., & Huether, S. E. (2006). *Pathophysiology: The biologic basis for disease in adults and children* (5th ed.). Mosby.

the oxygen tension below the level that meets the metabolic needs of the spinal cord. Lactate metabolites and an increase in vasoactive substances—including norepinephrine, serotonin, and dopamine—are noted. At high levels, these vasoactive substances cause vasospasms and hypoxia, leading to subsequent necrosis. Unfortunately, the spinal cord has minimal ability to adapt to vasospasm.

The extent of the neurological damage caused by an SCI results both from primary injury or damage (actual physical disruption of axons) and from secondary injury damage (ischemia, hypoxia, microhemorrhage, and edema) (Witiw & Fehlings, 2015). Because secondary injury processes occur over time, the extent of injury and the prognosis for recovery are most accurately determined at 72 hours or longer after injury.

Spinal and Neurogenic Shock. About 50% of people with acute SCI experience a temporary neurological syndrome known as **spinal shock** that is characterized by decreased reflexes, loss of sensation, and flaccid paralysis below the level of the injury (Chin, 2018). This syndrome lasts days to months and may mask postinjury neurological function. Active rehabilitation may begin in the presence of spinal shock.

Neurogenic shock, in contrast, is caused by SCI at the fifth thoracic (T5) vertebra or above. It is a hemodynamic syndrome of massive vasodilation without compensation that results from the loss of sympathetic nervous system vasoconstrictor tone

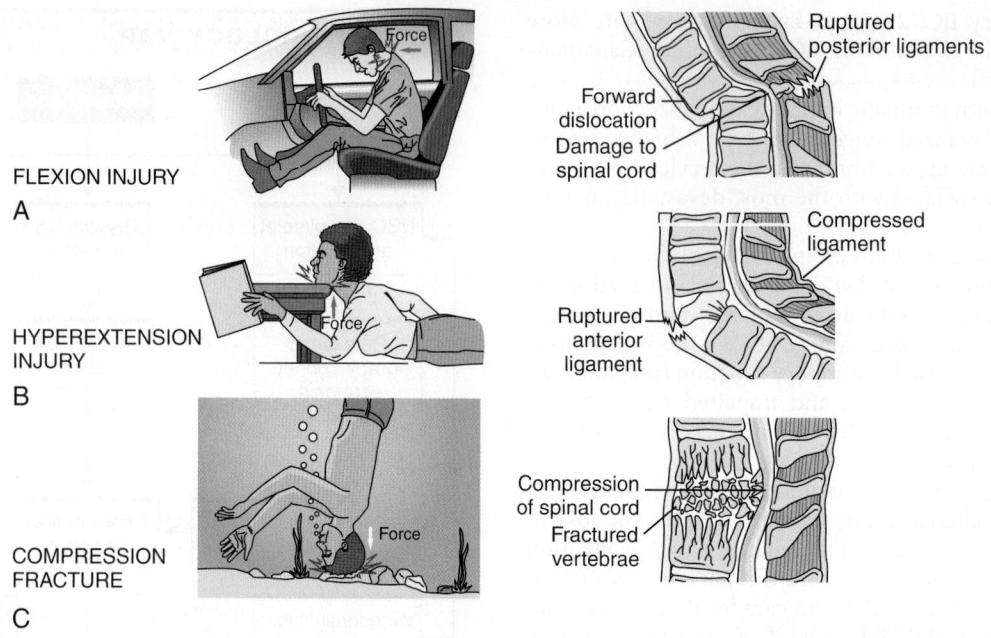

FIG. 63.5 Mechanisms of spinal cord injury. Many situations can produce these injuries. This figure shows only some examples. **A,** Flexion injury of the cervical spine ruptures the posterior ligaments. **B,** Hyperextension injury of the cervical spine ruptures the anterior ligaments. **C,** Compression fractures crush the vertebrae and force bony fragments into the spinal canal. Source: Copstead-Kirkhorn, L. C., & Banasik, J. L. (2014). *Pathophysiology* (5th ed., p. 937, Figure 45-12). W. B. Saunders.

caused by spinal cord injury. Neurogenic shock is characterized by hypotension, bradycardia, and loss of sympathetic innervation, which produces peripheral vasodilation, venous pooling, and a decreased cardiac output (Chin, 2018). Chapter 69 includes information related to the nursing management of shock.

Classification of Spinal Cord Injury. SCIs are classified according to the mechanism of injury, the skeletal and neurological level of injury, and the completeness or degree of injury.

Mechanisms of Injury. The major mechanisms of injury are flexion, hyperextension, flexion-rotation, extension-rotation, and compression (Figure 63.5). The flexion-rotation injury is the most unstable of all injuries because the ligamentous structures that stabilize the spine are torn. This injury is most often implicated in severe neurological deficits.

Level of Injury. The *skeletal level* of injury is the vertebral level where damage to vertebral bones and ligaments is most extensive. The *neurological level* of injury is the lowest segment of the spinal cord at which sensory and motor function on both sides of the body are normal. The level of injury may be cervical, thoracic, or lumbar. Cervical and lumbar injuries are most common because these levels are associated with the greatest flexibility and movement. If the cervical cord is involved, paralysis of all four extremities *(tetraplegia)* occurs. If the thoracic cord or conus in the lumbar spine is damaged, the result is paraplegia. Figure 63.6 shows affected structures and functions at different levels of cord injury.

Degree of Injury. The degree of spinal cord involvement may be either complete or incomplete (partial). *Complete cord involvement* (American Spinal Injury Association [ASIA] grade A) results in total loss of sensory and motor function below the level of the lesion (injury). *Incomplete cord involvement* (ASIA grades B–D) results in a mixed loss of motor and sensory function (Figure 63.7). The degree of sensory and motor loss

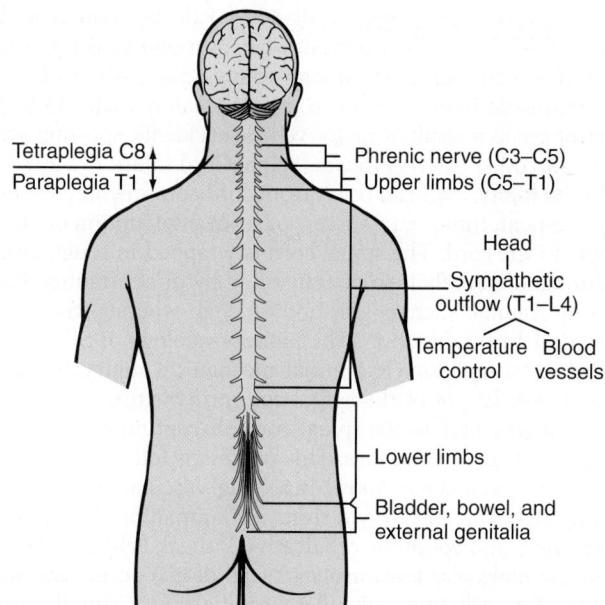

FIG. 63.6 Results of spinal cord injury, depending on location. Symptoms, degree of paralysis, and potential for rehabilitation depend on the level of the lesion.

varies depending on the level of the lesion and reflects the specific nerve tracts damaged. Six syndromes are associated with incomplete lesions: central cord syndrome, anterior cord syndrome, Brown-Séquard syndrome, posterior cord syndrome, cauda equina syndrome, and conus medullaris syndrome.

American Spinal Injury Association Impairment Scale. The ASIA Impairment Scale is the gold-standard assessment scale used for classifying the severity of impairment resulting from SCI. It combines assessments of motor and sensory function of various myotomes and dermatomes to determine neurological

ASIA Impairment Scale (AIS)

A = Complete. No sensory or motor function is preserved in the sacral segments S4-5.

B = Sensory Incomplete. Sensory but not motor function is preserved below the neurological level and includes the sacral segments S4-5 (light touch or pin prick at S4-5 or deep anal pressure) AND no motor function is preserved more than three levels below the motor level on either side of the body.

C = Motor Incomplete. Motor function is preserved at the most caudal sacral segments for voluntary anal contraction (VAC) OR the patient meets the criteria for sensory incomplete status (sensory function preserved at the most caudal sacral segments S4-S5 by LT, PP or DAP), and has some sparing of motor function more than three levels below the ipsilateral motor level on either side of the body.
(This includes key or non-key muscle functions to determine motor incomplete status.) For AIS C – less than half of key muscle functions below the single NLI have a muscle grade ≥3.

D = Motor Incomplete. Motor incomplete status as defined above, with at least half (half or more) of key muscle functions below the single NLI having a muscle grade ≥3.

E = Normal. If sensation and motor function as tested with the ISNCSCI are graded as normal in all segments, and the patient had prior deficits, then the AIS grade is E. Someone without an initial SCI does not receive an AIS grade.

Using ND: To document the sensory, motor and NLI levels, the ASIA Impairment Scale grade, and/or the zone of partial preservation (ZPP) when they are unable to be determined based on the examination results.

FIG. 63.7 International standards for neurological classification of spinal cord injury. *DAP,* deep anal pressure; *ISNCSCI,* international standards for neurological classification of spinal cord injury; *LT,* light touch; *ND,* not determined; *NLI,* neurological injury; *PP,* pin prick. Source: American Spinal Injury Association: *International standards for neurological classification of spinal cord injury,* revised 2019. Richmond, VA.

level and completeness of injury. The strength of key muscle groups is graded on a scale of 0 to 5 and is tested bilaterally. Sensation is documented as *absent, impaired,* or *normal.* An ASIA grade (A–E) is then determined on the basis of assessment findings (Figure 63.8). This grading establishes whether the findings indicate complete or incomplete SCI or are normal. Various incomplete cord syndromes are also defined with this classification system and have been discussed previously. In addition, this scale is useful for recording changes in neurological status and identifying appropriate functional goals for rehabilitation.

Central Cord Syndrome. Damage to the central spinal cord is termed *central cord syndrome.* It occurs most commonly in the cervical cord region and is common with hyperextension injuries. Motor weakness and sensory loss are present in both the upper and the lower extremities; the upper extremities are more affected than the lower ones.

Anterior Cord Syndrome. *Anterior cord syndrome* is caused by damage to the anterior spinal artery. It typically results from acute compression of the anterior portion of the spinal cord, often from a flexion injury. Manifestations include motor paralysis and loss of pain and temperature sensation below the level of injury. Because the posterior cord tracts are not injured, sensations of touch, position, vibration, and motion remain intact.

Brown-Séquard Syndrome. Brown-Séquard syndrome is a result of damage to half of the spinal cord. This syndrome is characterized by a loss of motor function (spastic paralysis), sense of position (proprioception), and sense of vibration on the same *(ipsilateral)* side as the lesion. The opposite *(contralateral)* side has loss of pain and temperature sensation below the level of the lesion.

Posterior Cord Syndrome. *Posterior cord syndrome* results from compression or damage to the posterior spinal artery. It is a very rare condition. In general, the dorsal columns are damaged, which results in loss of proprioception. However, pain, temperature sensation, and motor function below the level of the lesion remain intact.

Conus Medullaris Syndrome and Cauda Equina Syndrome. *Conus medullaris syndrome* and *cauda equina syndrome* result from damage to the very lowest portion of the spinal cord *(conus)* and the lumbar and sacral nerve roots *(cauda equina).* Injury to the conus results in motor and sensory impairment, as well as bladder and bowel dysfunction. Injury to the cauda equina results in nerve root symptoms dependent on the level of the lesion; bowel and bladder function are typically affected.

Clinical Manifestations

The manifestations of SCI are generally the direct result of trauma that causes cord compression, ischemia, edema, and, rarely, cord transection. Manifestations of SCI are related to the level and the degree of injury. A patient with an incomplete lesion may demonstrate a mixture of symptoms. The higher the injury, the more serious the sequelae because of the proximity of the cervical cord to the medulla and the brainstem. Movement and functional goals related to specific locations of the SCI are described in Table 63.2. In general, sensory function closely parallels motor function at all levels.

Immediate postinjury care includes maintaining patency of the airway, adequate ventilation, and adequate circulating blood volume and blood pressure to minimize extension of spinal cord damage (secondary injury).

Respiratory System. Respiratory complications closely correspond to the level of the injury (Mao, 2021). Cervical injury above the level of C4 presents special challenges because of the total loss of respiratory muscle function. Mechanical ventilation is required to keep the patient alive. Injury or fracture below the level of C4 spares diaphragmatic breathing if the phrenic nerve is functioning. Even if the injury is below C4, spinal cord edema and hemorrhage can affect the function of the phrenic nerve and cause respiratory insufficiency. Hypoventilation almost always occurs with diaphragmatic respirations because of the decrease in vital capacity and tidal volume, which occurs as a result of impairment of the intercostal muscles.

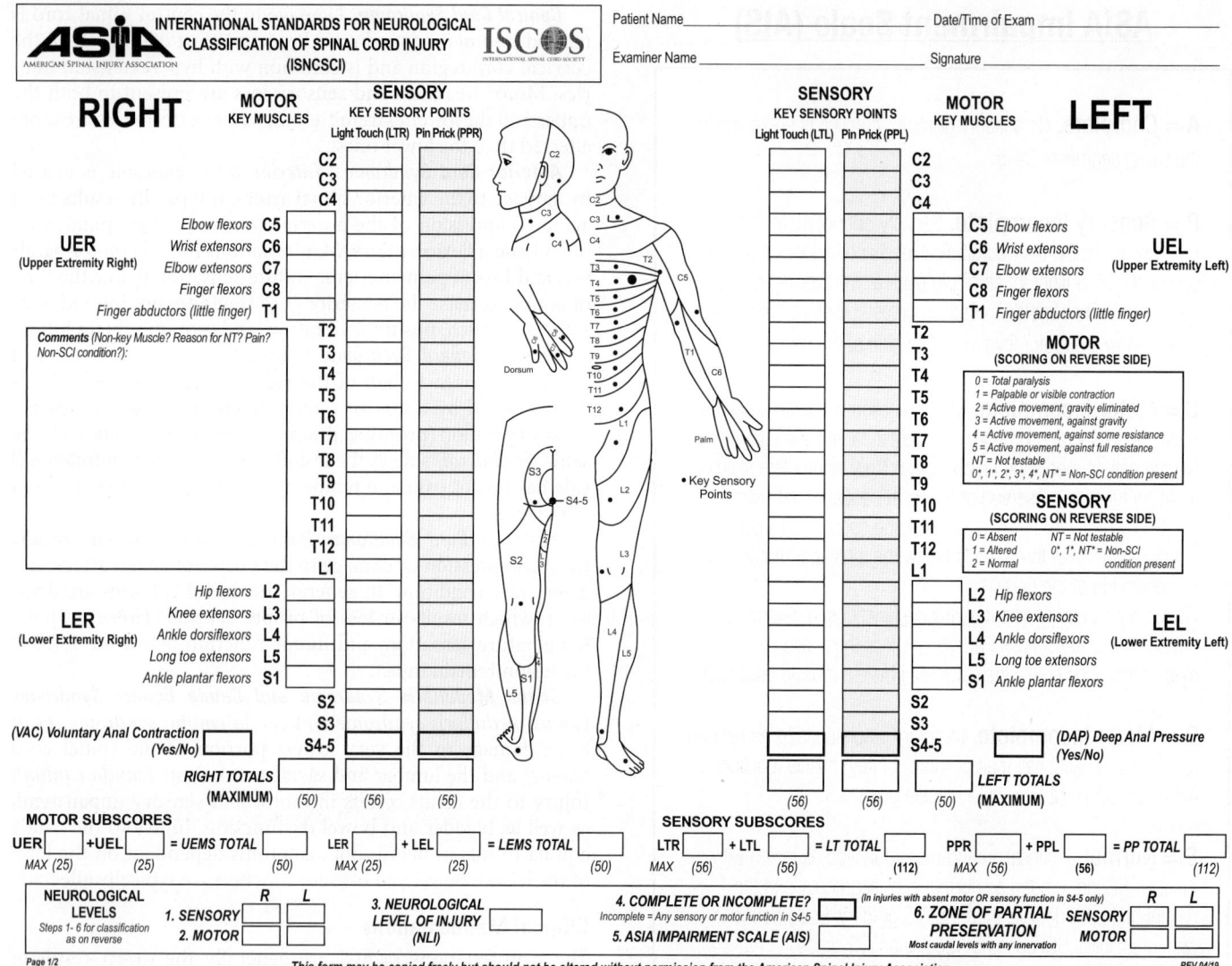

FIG. 63.8 International standards for neurological classification of spinal cord injury. Source: American Spinal Injury Association: *International standards for neurological classification of spinal cord injury,* revised 2019. Richmond, VA.

Cervical and thoracic injuries cause paralysis of abdominal muscles and, often, of intercostal muscles. Therefore, the patient cannot cough effectively enough to remove secretions, which can lead to atelectasis and pneumonia. An artificial airway such as an endotracheal or tracheostomy tube provides direct access for pathogens; thus bronchial hygiene and chest physiotherapy to reduce infection are extremely important. Neurogenic pulmonary edema, which is caused by an increase in pulmonary interstitial and alveolar fluid, may occur secondary to a dramatic increase in sympathetic nervous system activity at the time of injury. In addition, pulmonary edema may occur in response to fluid overload.

Cardiovascular System. Any SCI above the level of T6 greatly decreases the influence of the sympathetic nervous system, thereby resulting in bradycardia. Peripheral vasodilation results in hypotension. A relative hypovolemia exists because of the increase in venous capacitance. Cardiac monitoring is necessary. In marked bradycardia (heart rate <40 beats/min), appropriate medications (atropine) to increase the heart rate are necessary. Peripheral vasodilation reduces the venous return of blood to the heart and subsequently decreases cardiac output,

which results in hypotension. IV fluids or vasopressor medications may be needed to support blood pressure and maintain a mean arterial pressure of 85 mm Hg to adequately perfuse the spinal cord.

Urinary System. Urinary retention occurs in acute SCIs and spinal shock. During spinal shock, the bladder is atonic and becomes overdistended. An in-dwelling urinary catheter is inserted to drain the bladder. After the acute phase, the bladder may become hyperirritable, with a loss of inhibition from the brain, which results in reflex emptying. Once the patient is medically and hemodynamically stable and large quantities of IV fluids are no longer required, the in-dwelling catheter should be removed and intermittent catheterization should begin as early as possible. Removal of the in-dwelling catheter helps to maintain bladder tone and decrease the risk for infection. (Intermittent catheterization is discussed later in this chapter and in Chapter 48.)

Gastrointestinal System. If the cord injury has occurred above the level of T5, the primary gastrointestinal concerns are related to hypomotility. Decreased gastrointestinal motor activity contributes to the development of paralytic ileus and gastric

TABLE 63.2   FUNCTIONAL GOALS WITH SPINAL CORD INJURY

Level of Injury	Movement and Deficits	Functional Goal	Assistance Needs
C1–4	• Absence of independent respiratory function • Loss of innervation to diaphragm • Movement in neck and above	Breathing Personal care Nutritional needs Transfers Mobility Environmental control Housing	May necessitate ventilator or other devices Attendant services Assistance required Attendant services Motorized wheelchair Devices to control lights, phone, door entry, voice- activated computer Supportive living services
C5	• Decreased respiratory reserve • Full neck • Gross elbow • Inability to roll over or use hands • Partial shoulder and biceps	Breathing Personal care Nutritional needs Transfers Mobility Environmental control Housing	No assistance needed Attendant services Assistance to meet needs (devices) Attendant services Motorized or manual wheelchair Devices to control lights, phone, door entry, voice- activated computer Supportive living services
C6	• Full biceps to elbow flexion • Rotation at shoulder • Shoulder and upper back abduction • Weak grasp of thumb • Wrist extension	Personal care Transfers Mobility	Independent with most activities (eating, washing, dressing upper body) Attendant services for some dressing, toileting Devices to assist sitting up and rolling over in bed Minimal assistance Independent in manual wheelchair; may be able to drive with adaptation to vehicle
C7	• Elbow extension • Finger extensors and flexors • Good grasp with some decreased strength	Personal care Transfers Mobility	Independent with most self-care activities Independent with transfers Independent in wheelchair
C8–T1	• Same as for C7	Personal care Transfers Mobility Driving Housing	Independent with all self-care activities Independent Independent Adaptations to vehicle required Independent living
T2–6	• Decreased trunk stability • Full movement of upper extremities • Full strength and dexterity of grasp • Intrinsic muscles of hand	Personal care Mobility	Independent with all self-care activities May be able to stand in long leg braces with supports
T7–12	• Full, stable thoracic muscles and upper back • Functional intercostal muscles and therefore increased respiratory reserve	Personal care Mobility	Independent with all self-care activities May walk for limited distances with long leg braces and crutches, using swing-through gait
L1–2	• Some instability of lower back • Varying control of legs and pelvis	Personal care Mobility	Independent May require assistance with bowel and bladder functioning Good sitting balance Independent use of wheelchair May walk for limited distances with long leg braces
L3–4	• Absence of hamstring function • Flail ankles • Quadriceps and hip flexors	Personal care Mobility	Independent Independent ambulation with assistive devices

Source: Adapted from Sarro, A. (2012). Pediatric and adult spine. In *Navigating neuroscience nursing: A Canadian perspective* (Chapter 4). Pappin Communications.

distension. A nasogastric tube for intermittent suctioning may relieve the gastric distension. Metoclopramide may be used to treat delayed gastric emptying. The development of stress ulcers is common because of excessive release of hydrochloric acid in the stomach. Histamine H_2-receptor blockers (such as raniti-dine [Zantac] and famotidine [Pepcid AC]) and proton pump inhibitors (e.g., omeprazole [Losec] or lansoprazole [Prevacid]) are frequently administered to prevent the occurrence of stress ulcers during the initial phase. Intra-abdominal bleeding may occur and is difficult to diagnose because the patient exhibits no subjective signs, such as pain, tenderness, or guarding. Continued hypotension, despite vigorous treatment and decreased hemoglobin and hematocrit, may be indications of bleeding. The girth of the abdomen may also expand.

Loss of neurological control over the bowel results in a *neurogenic bowel*. In the early period after injury when spinal shock is present and for patients with an injury level of T12 or below, the bowel is areflexic and sphincter tone is decreased. As reflexes return, the bowel becomes reflexic, sphincter tone is enhanced, and reflex emptying occurs. Both types of neurogenic bowel can be managed successfully with a regular bowel program coordinated with the gastrocolic reflex to minimize untimely incontinence.

Integumentary System. A major consequence of lack of movement is the potential for skin breakdown over bony prominences in areas of decreased or no sensation. Pressure injuries can occur quickly and can lead to major infection or sepsis. See Chapter 14 for further information on pressure injuries.

Thermoregulation. Poikilothermism is the adjustment of the body temperature to the room temperature. It occurs in patients with SCIs because the interruption of the sympathetic nervous system prevents peripheral temperature sensations from reaching the hypothalamus. The ability to sweat or shiver is also decreased below the level of the lesion, which affects the ability to regulate body temperature. The degree of poikilothermism depends on the level of injury. Patients with high cervical injuries have a greater loss of the ability to regulate temperature than do those with thoracic or lumbar injuries.

Metabolic Needs. Nasogastric suctioning may lead to metabolic alkalosis, and decreases in tissue perfusion may lead to acidosis. Electrolyte levels can be altered by gastric suctioning and must be monitored until suctioning is discontinued and normal nutritional requirements are met. Loss of body weight (10% or more) is common, and nitrogen excretion mirrors weight loss (Welch-West et al., 2019). Nutritional needs are much greater than what would be expected for an immobilized person. A positive nitrogen balance, which may not occur for more than 2 months after the injury, and a high-protein diet can help prevent skin breakdown and infections and decrease the rate of muscle atrophy.

Peripheral Vascular Conditions. Thromboembolism is a common condition accompanying SCI, with the highest incidence occurring during the first 2 weeks following injury and peak occurrence between days 7 and 10 (McKinney, 2021). It is more difficult to detect in a person with an SCI because the patient does not exhibit the usual signs and symptoms, such as pain and tenderness. PE is one of the leading causes of death in patients with SCI. Techniques for assessment of thromboembolism include Doppler ultrasound examination and measurement of leg and thigh girth.

Diagnostic Studies

Complete spine radiography may be performed initially to assess for vertebral fracture. MRI for imaging neurological tissues, including the spinal cord, is usually completed first (Mao, 2021). It is recommended that MRI be used to direct clinical decision making. MRI is performed to assess spinal cord compression and soft tissue injuries (Mao, 2021). CT may be used to assess the degree of bony injury and the degree of spinal canal compromise. A comprehensive neurological examination is performed, along with assessment of the head, the chest, and the abdomen for additional injuries or trauma. In patients with cervical injuries who demonstrate altered mental status, vertebral angiography may also be needed to rule out vertebral artery damage.

Interprofessional Care

The initial goals for the patient with an SCI are to sustain life and prevent further cord damage. Table 63.3 outlines the emergency management of a patient with an SCI. Systemic and neurogenic shock must be treated to maintain blood pressure. For injury at the cervical level, all body systems must be maintained until the full extent of the damage can be evaluated.

Interprofessional care during the acute phase for a patient with a cervical injury is described in Table 63.4. The systemic support required by the patient is less intense for SCIs of the thoracic and lumbar vertebrae. Respiratory compromise is not as severe, and bradycardia is not a concern. Specific conditions are treated symptomatically. After stabilization at the injury scene, the patient is transferred to a medical facility, where further assessment, both clinical and radiological, is completed. A thorough assessment is performed to specifically evaluate the degree of deficit and to establish the level and the degree of injury. A history is obtained, with emphasis on how the accident

---

✚ TABLE 63.3 EMERGENCY MANAGEMENT
Spinal Cord Injury

Etiology

Blunt Injury
- Compression, flexion, extension, or rotational injuries to spinal column
- Diving
- Falls
- Motor vehicle accidents
- Pedestrian accidents

Penetrating Injury
- Gunshot
- Stab wounds
- Stretched, torn, crushed, or lacerated spinal cord

Assessment Findings
- Alterations in sensation: temperature, light touch, deep pressure, proprioception
- Bowel and bladder incontinence
- Cuts; bruises; open wounds over head, face, neck, or back
- Difficulty breathing
- Diminished rectal sphincter tone
- Neurogenic shock: hypotension; bradycardia; dry, flushed skin
- Numbness, paresthesias
- Pain, tenderness, deformities, or muscle spasms adjacent to vertebral column
- Priapism
- Spinal shock
- Urinary retention
- Weakness or heaviness in limbs
- Weakness, paralysis, or flaccidity of muscles

Interventions

Initial
- Administer oxygen via nasal cannula or nonrebreather mask.
- Assess for other injuries.
- Control external bleeding.
- Ensure patency of airway.
- Establish intravenous access with two large-bore catheters to infuse normal saline or lactated Ringer's solution, as appropriate.
- Insert Foley catheter.
- Stabilize cervical spine with hard collar or sandbags if indicated.

Ongoing Monitoring
- Anticipate need for intubation if gag reflex is absent or respiratory function declines.
- Keep patient warm.
- Monitor vital signs, level of consciousness, oxygen saturation, cardiac rhythm, and urine output.

---

occurred and the extent of injury as perceived by the patient immediately after the accident. Assessment involves testing muscle groups rather than individual muscles. Muscle groups should be tested with and against gravity, alone and against resistance, and on both sides of the body. Spontaneous movement should be noted. The patient should be asked to move legs and then hands, spread fingers, extend wrists, and shrug shoulders. After assessment of motor status, a sensory examination, including assessment of touch and pain, should be carried out, starting at the toes and working upward. If time and conditions permit, position sense can also be assessed.

The types of injury mechanisms that cause spinal cord trauma, especially those involving the cervical cord, may also result in brain injury. The patient should therefore be assessed for history of unconsciousness, signs of concussion, and increased intracranial

TABLE 63.4 INTERPROFESSIONAL CARE

Cervical Cord Injury

Diagnostic
- History and physical examination, including complete neurological examination
- Anteroposterior, lateral, and odontoid spinal radiographs
- Arterial blood gas measurements
- CT, MRI
- Electrolyte measurements, glucose level, coagulation studies, hemoglobin and hematocrit levels
- Serial bedside pulmonary function testing
- Urinalysis

Interprofessional Therapy

Acute Care
- Administration of intravenous fluids
- Administration of O_2 by high-humidity mask
- Bowel and bladder monitoring and initiation of training when hemodynamically stable
- High-dose methylprednisolone therapy if ordered
- Insertion of nasogastric tube and attachment to suction
- Intubation if indicated
- Maintenance of heart rate (e.g., with atropine) and blood pressure (e.g., with dopamine)
- Placement and maintenance of halo traction if necessary
- Placement of in-dwelling urinary catheter
- Prophylaxis for deep vein thrombosis
- Prophylaxis for stress ulcers
- Use of pressure-relieving surface

Rehabilitation and Home Care
- Bowel and bladder training
- Occupational therapy (activities of daily living training)
- Patient and caregiver education
- Physiotherapy
- Chest physiotherapy
- Mobility training
- Muscle strengthening
- Range-of-motion exercises
- Prevention of autonomic dysreflexia
- Prevention of pressure injuries
- Recreation therapy

CT, computed tomography; *MRI*, magnetic resonance imaging; O_2, oxygen.

🔍 EVIDENCE-INFORMED PRACTICE

Research Highlight

What Is the Effect of Robot-Assisted Gait Training for Patients With Spinal Cord Injury?

Clinical Question

In patients with spinal cord injury (SCI) *(P)*, what is the effect of robot-assisted gait training (RAGT) *(I)* versus other training modalities or no training *(C)* on patient spasticity, pain, lower extremity motor control, and walking *(O)*?

Best Available Evidence

Meta-analysis comparing the effects of RAGT with other treatments or no treatment. Primary outcomes were spasticity (Ashworth scale) and pain (visual analogue scale), and secondary outcome measures were lower extremity motor score and walking ability.

Seven randomized controlled trials (RCTs) (*n* = 222) and 11 non-RCTs (*n* = 79) were included in the analysis.

Clinical Appraisal and Synthesis of Evidence
- The 30- to 60-minute intervention of RAGT was done three to five times per week, for 4 to 12 weeks. The protocol for the non-RCT studies was 30 to 90 minutes, two to five times per week, for 1 to 12 weeks. Findings indicated that, in some of the studies, there was a significant decrease in spasticity.
- The trend favoured pain reduction but there were no significant differences between treatment groups.
- Lower extremity motor scores and walking distance were significantly increased in the RAGT group.

Conclusions
- RAGT decreased spasticity and improved walking ability in individuals with SCI. The level of pain showed no change after RAGT.

Implications for Nursing Practice
- It is important for nurses working with patients who have experienced SCI to provide education related to treatment options.
- Rehabilitation of patients with SCI have many goals of treatment, including walking ability in those patients with incomplete injury. The nurse should collaborate with the interprofessional team to develop a person-centred exercise program.

Reference for Evidence

Fang, C., Tsai, J., Li, G., et al. (2020). Effects of robot-assisted gait training in individuals with spinal cord injury: A meta-analysis. *BioMed Research International*, *2020*, Art. 2102785. https://doi.org/10.1155/2020/2102785

P, patient population of interest; *I*, intervention or areas of interest; *C*, comparison of interest; *O*, outcomes of interest (see Chapter 1).

pressure (see Chapter 59). In addition, a careful assessment for musculoskeletal injuries and trauma to internal organs should be performed. Because the patient may have no muscle, bone, or visceral sensations, the only clue to internal trauma with hemorrhage may be rapidly falling hematocrit levels or persistent hypotension. Urinary output is examined for volume and hematuria, another indication of internal injuries.

To prevent further injury, the patient must be moved in alignment as a unit, as in log-rolling, during transfers and when repositioned. Respiratory, cardiac, urinary, and gastrointestinal functions should be monitored closely. The patient may undergo surgery directly after initial immobilization and stabilization or be taken to the CCU for monitoring and management.

Nonoperative Stabilization. Nonoperative treatments focus on stabilization and realignment of the injured spinal segment through traction. Stabilization methods eliminate damaging motion at the injury site. They are intended to prevent secondary spinal cord damage caused by repeated contusion or compression.

Surgical Therapy. The decision to perform surgery on a patient with an SCI often depends on the preference of the physician and the availability of surgical services. Surgery is used to stabilize, realign, and decompress the spinal column. There is evidence that early surgical intervention is safe and feasible and that it can improve clinical and neurological outcomes and reduce health care costs. Recent research suggests the use of robot-assisted gait training as part of a rehabilitation program (see the Evidence-Informed Practice: Research Highlight box). Other criteria used in the decision for early surgery include (a) evidence of cord compression, (b) progressive neurological deficit, (c) compound fracture of the vertebrae, (d) bony fragments (may dislodge and penetrate the cord), and (e) penetrating wounds of the spinal cord or surrounding structures.

The more common surgical procedures include decompression, realignment, and stabilization with instrumentation. These procedures are performed either posteriorly or anteriorly, depending on the level of injury and the area of cord compression (i.e., anterior versus posterior). If instability is considered severe enough, both anterior and posterior stabilization may be considered.

Medication Therapy. Corticosteroid administration, starting within 8 hours after SCI, has traditionally been used to improve patient outcomes, but multiple clinical trials in adults have demonstrated that there is no clinical benefit. Furthermore, an increased risk of wound infection, PE, sepsis, and death was reported with its use (Mao, 2021). Thus, corticosteroid use is no longer recommended in patients with SCI.

Treatments under ongoing investigation include measures to promote nerve regeneration and minimize scar tissue formation—for example, implantation of a polymer scaffold at the level of the injury, injections of autologous incubated macrophages, and stem cell research. Vasopressor agents such as dopamine and norepinephrine are administered in the acute phase as adjuvants to treatment. These agents are used to maintain the mean arterial pressure at a level greater than 85 mm Hg to improve spinal cord perfusion and reduce incidence of hypotensive episodes (Mao, 2021).

Pharmacological agents are administered to treat specific autonomic dysfunctions, such as bradycardia, orthostatic hypotension, gastrointestinal hypoactivity, inadequate emptying of the bladder, and autonomic dysreflexia (discussed later in this chapter). The nurse must know the intended effects of such medications, observe responses, and provide specific interventions when adverse reactions are seen.

NURSING MANAGEMENT SPINAL CORD INJURY

NURSING ASSESSMENT

Subjective and objective data that should be obtained from a patient with a recent SCI are presented in Table 63.5.

NURSING DIAGNOSES

Nursing diagnoses for patients with an SCI depend on the severity of the injury and the level of dysfunction. The nursing diagnoses for patients with an SCI may include but are not limited to the following:

- *Inadequate breathing pattern* resulting from *respiratory muscle fatigue, body position that inhibits lung expansion, fatigue*
- *Inadequate nutrition* resulting from *insufficient dietary intake* (paralytic ileus, metabolic demands of body)
- *Inadequate peripheral tissue perfusion* resulting from *sedentary lifestyle* (lack of mobility)
- *Reduced skin integrity* resulting from *pressure over bony prominence* (immobility)
- *Reduced urinary elimination* resulting from multiple causality (spinal injury, limited fluid intake)
- *Constipation* resulting from *irregular defecation habits* (neurogenic bowel, immobility)

Additional information on nursing diagnoses for the patient with SCI is presented in Nursing Care Plan (NCP) 63.1, available on the Evolve website.

PLANNING

The overall goals are that the patient with an SCI will (a) maintain optimal level of neurological functioning; (b) have minimal or no complications of immobility; (c) learn new skills, gain new knowledge, and acquire new behaviours to be able to care for themselves or successfully direct others to do so; and (d) return home and to the community at an optimal level of functioning.

TABLE 63.5 NURSING ASSESSMENT

Spinal Cord Injury

Subjective Data
Important Health Information
Past health history: Motor vehicle accident, sports injury, industrial accident, gunshot or stabbing injury, falls
Current medical history: Use of alcohol or recreational drugs; risk-taking behaviours

Symptoms
- Dyspnea, inability to breathe adequately ("air hunger")
- Fear, denial, anger, depression
- Loss of strength, movement, and sensation below level of injury
- Presence of tenderness, pain at or above level of injury; numbness, tingling sensation, burning sensation, twitching of extremities

Objective Data
General
Poikilothermism (inability to regulate body heat)

Integumentary
Warm, dry, flushed extremities below level of injury (neurogenic shock)

Respiratory
Lesions at C1–3: apnea, inability to cough
Lesions at C4: poor cough, diaphragmatic breathing, hypoventilation
Lesions at C5–T6: decreased respiratory reserve

Cardiovascular
Lesions above T5: bradycardia, hypotension, postural hypotension, absence of vasomotor tone

Gastrointestinal
Decreased or absent bowel sounds (paralytic ileus in lesions above T5), abdominal distension, constipation, fecal incontinence, fecal impaction

Urinary
Retention (for lesions between T1 and L2); flaccid bladder (acute stages); spasticity with reflex bladder emptying (later stages)

Reproductive
Priapism, loss of sexual function

Neurological
Complete: Flaccid paralysis and anaesthesia below level of injury that results in tetraplegia (for lesions above C8) or paraplegia (for lesions below C8); hyperactive deep tendon reflexes; bilaterally positive response to Babinski test (after resolution of spinal shock)
Incomplete: Mixed loss of voluntary motor activity and sensation

Musculoskeletal
Muscle atony (in flaccid state), contractures (in spastic state)

Possible Findings
Spinal radiography: location of level and type of bony involvement
CT: bony destruction and compression
MRI: lesions and edema

CT, computed tomography; *MRI,* magnetic resonance imaging.

NURSING IMPLEMENTATION

HEALTH PROMOTION. Nursing interventions for injury prevention include identification of at-risk populations, counselling, and education. Support of local legislation related to seat belt use in cars, helmets for motorcyclists and bicyclists, child safety seats, and tougher penalties for drunk driving offences is a professional responsibility. Parachute Canada is a national charitable organization that is dedicated to preventing injuries and saving lives. It has partnered with organizations including ThinkFirst Canada, Safe Communities Canada, SMARTRISK, and Safe Kids Canada to develop injury-prevention programs.

It is important that the nurse emphasize the importance of other health promotion measures and health screening in addition to SCI care. After injury, health-promoting behaviours can have a significant effect on the health and well-being of the individual with SCI. Nursing interventions include education; counselling and referral to programs such as smoking cessation classes, recreation and exercise programs, and alcohol treatment programs; and maintenance of routine physical examinations for non-neurological conditions. Outpatient health care requires that screening and prevention programs be accessible to people with SCIs. Nurses in these settings should facilitate the availability of wheelchair-accessible examination rooms, adjustable-height examination tables, and scheduling that allows extra time if needed.

ACUTE INTERVENTION. Regardless of the mechanism of injury and resultant spinal column damage, care of patients with SCIs is similar. Interventions for care are discussed in this section and may need to be modified on an individual basis.

Immobilization. Proper immobilization of the neck involves maintenance of a neutral position with correct body alignment. A blanket or rolled towel, a hard cervical collar, and a backboard can be used to stabilize the neck to prevent lateral rotation of the cervical spine. There is debate as to whether spinal immobilization for all patients following SCI should be the standard of care (Sharwood et al., 2018). The widespread use of the Canadian C-Spine Rule for alert and stable trauma patients by paramedics, emergency department health care providers, and triage nurses can help to minimize adverse patient outcomes (Vaillancourt et al., 2020). Because of the controversy in best practice standard of care, the nurse must always follow facility policy related to spinal immobilization for patients with SCI.

For cervical injuries, cervical traction is used less frequently. Traction should not be used unless the patient can communicate any changes in clinical status during application and subsequent assessments. When cervical traction is used, realignment or reduction of the injury is the goal. Halo traction involves the placement of a halo ring or crown, secured into the skull with four pins, with subsequent additions of weight to aid in spinal realignment. Traction is provided by a rope that is extended from the centre of the halo crown over a pulley and has weights attached at the end. Traction must be maintained at all times. The initial weight is typically 4.5 to 6.8 kg and thereafter approximately 2.2 kg per level of SCI (e.g., 2.2 kg for C1, 4.4 kg for C2, 6.6 kg for C3), with continual neurological monitoring. Additional weights are added until alignment is achieved, neurological changes occur, or overdistraction within the disc space is noted. Once proper alignment has been established, a halo vest is applied to provide ongoing immobilization of the cervical spine. The halo vest stabilizes the injured area and allows ambulation if the patient is neurologically intact (Figure 63.9). Special care of the halo pin sites and halo vest is important for preventing infection and skin breakdown (Royal College of Nursing, 2021) (Table 63.6).

Infection at the sites of pin insertion is a potential concern. Preventive care includes assessing once per shift and cleansing the sites twice a day with normal saline solution. The development of redness or crusting could indicate looseness of pins, and the health care provider should be informed. The preventive care of insertion sites may vary (check facility policy) (Royal College of Nursing, 2021).

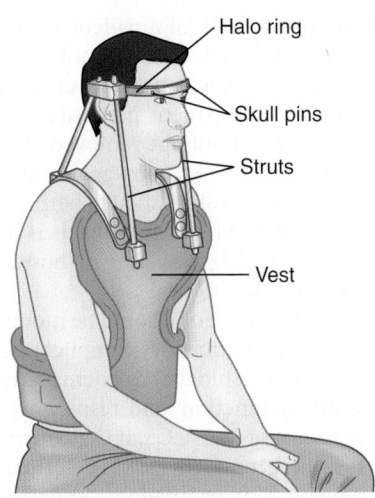

FIG. 63.9 Halo vest. The halo traction brace immobilizes the cervical spine, which allows the patient to ambulate and perform self-care. Source: Urden, L. D., Stacy, K. M., & Lough, M. E. (2012). *Priorities in critical care nursing* (6th ed., p. 525, Figure 25-6). Mosby.

TABLE 63.6	PATIENT & CAREGIVER TEACHING GUIDE

Halo Vest Care

The following are teaching guidelines for a patient with a halo vest:
1. Visually inspect the pin sites on the halo ring on a regular basis. Report to the health care provider if pins are loose or if there are signs of infection, including redness, tenderness, swelling, or drainage at the insertion sites.
2. Assess pin sites once per shift. Wet sterile gauze with normal saline (patients may use clean technique at home) and gently clean around each pin. Use a new gauze for each pin site. Work in a circular pattern.
3. If crusting is present, wrap the pin site with normal saline–soaked gauze for 15–20 minutes and then remove. Using a gentle rolling motion, the crust can then be removed with a cotton-tipped applicator that has been soaked in normal saline.
4. Do not use any ointments or antiseptics on the pin sites unless prescribed by the health care provider.
5. To provide skin care, position patient flat on their side. Loosen one side of the vest and place a towel against the sheepskin to protect it from getting wet. Mark the buckle position on the strap before removing. Inspect skin integrity. Wash the patient's chest and back with soap and water. Dry the skin thoroughly, and resecure buckle straps. Turn the patient onto the opposite side and repeat the steps.
6. In case of an emergency, the halo spanner for the bolts should be attached to the vest at all times.

Source: Royal College of Nursing. (2021). *Traction: Principles and application.* https://www.rcn.org.uk/professional-development/publications/pub-004721

Specialized beds or mattresses are often used in the management of patients with SCI to help prevent development of pressure injury. Many products are available and are often institution dependent. Mattress overlays often use gel as mediums. Specialized beds are typically dynamic and use a power source to alternate air currents and pressure against the body.

Cervical collars for postsurgical stabilization are used on the basis of the surgeon's preference. With new techniques and better surgical stabilization, a collar is not required postoperatively. Patients with thoracic or lumbar spine injuries are stabilized with a custom thoraco-lumbar-sacral orthosis (TLSO brace), which controls spinal flexion, extension, and rotation, or with a Jewett brace, which restricts forward flexion.

Immobilization of the neck of a patient with SCI may prevent further injury, but the effects of immobility are profound. Meticulous skin care is critical because decreased sensation and circulation render the patient particularly susceptible to skin breakdown. Patients should be removed from backboards as soon as possible to prevent coccygeal and occipital area skin breakdown. Cervical collars should be properly fitted or replaced with other forms of stabilization. It is important that areas under the halo vest, braces, and orthoses be inspected regularly to assess skin condition.

Respiratory Dysfunction. Patients should be monitored in a special care unit to minimize pulmonary complications. During the first 48 hours after injury, spinal cord edema may increase the level of spinal cord dysfunction, and respiratory distress may occur. If the injury is at or above C3, if the patient is exhausted from laboured breathing, or if ABG levels deteriorate (indicating inadequate oxygenation or ventilation), endotracheal intubation and mechanical ventilation should be initiated. Respiratory arrest is a possibility that necessitates careful monitoring of the respiratory system and prompt action. Pneumonia and atelectasis are potential complications because of reduced vital capacity and the loss of intercostal and abdominal muscle function, which can result in diaphragmatic breathing, pooling of secretions, and ineffectiveness of cough (Mao, 2021). In addition to the neurological injury, predictive factors of potential respiratory complications include tachypnea on admission, older age, and previous respiratory disease. Older persons have a more difficult time responding to hypoxia and hypercapnia and are extremely intolerant of hypoxia caused by lack of reserve. Therefore, aggressive chest physiotherapy, adequate oxygenation, and proper pain management are essential for maximizing respiratory function and gas exchange. Other concerns include nasal stuffiness and bronchospasm.

The nurse must regularly assess (a) breath sounds, (b) ABG levels, (c) tidal volume, (d) vital capacity, (e) skin colour, (f) breathing patterns (especially the use of accessory muscles), (g) subjective comments about the ability to breathe, and (h) the amount and colour of sputum. Partial pressure of oxygen in arterial blood (PaO_2) above 60 mm Hg and partial pressure of carbon dioxide in arterial blood ($PaCO_2$) below 45 mm Hg are acceptable values in a patient with uncomplicated tetraplegia. A patient who is unable to count to 10 out loud without taking a breath needs immediate attention.

In addition to monitoring, the nurse can intervene in maintaining ventilation. Oxygen is administered until ABG levels stabilize. Chest physiotherapy and assisted coughing facilitate the expulsion of secretions. Assisted or augmented coughing simulates the action of the ineffective abdominal muscles during the expiratory phase of a cough. The nurse places the heels of both hands just below the patient's xiphoid process and exerts firm upward pressure to the area, timed with the patient's efforts to cough (see discussion of augmented coughing in Chapter 70). Tracheal suctioning should be performed if crackles or wheezes are present. Incentive spirometry is an additional technique that can be used to improve the patient's respiratory status.

Cardiovascular Instability. Because of unopposed vagal response, the heart rate slows, often to less than 60 beats per minute. Any increase in vagal stimulation, such as turning or suctioning, can result in cardiac arrest. Loss of sympathetic tone in peripheral vessels results in chronic low blood pressure with potential postural hypotension. Lack of muscle tone to aid venous return can result in sluggish blood flow and predispose the patient to thromboembolism or PE.

Vital signs should be assessed frequently. If bradycardia is symptomatic, an anticholinergic medication such as atropine is administered. A temporary pacemaker may be inserted. Hypotension is managed with a vasopressor agent, such as dopamine or norepinephrine (Levophed), and fluid replacement.

In older persons, the presence of cardiovascular disease must be considered. The cardiovascular system becomes less able to handle the stress of traumatic injury because heart contractions weaken, and cardiac output decreases. Maximum heart rate is also reduced.

Gradient compression stockings can be used to prevent thromboemboli and to promote venous return. The stockings must be removed every 8 hours for skin care. The use of pneumatic compression devices for the calves is advocated, and they must be applied as soon as possible after injury and maintained throughout the hospitalization. Venous duplex studies may be performed before compression devices are applied. The nurse should also help the patient perform range-of-motion exercises and stretch regularly. The thighs and calves of the legs should be assessed every shift for signs of DVT.

Administration of LMWH is recommended for thromboprophylaxis in the acute care phase following an SCI once there is no evidence of active bleeding. The use of low-dose or adjusted-dose unfractionated heparin is not recommended unless LMWH is contraindicated (Consortium for Spinal Cord Medicine, 2016).

If blood loss has resulted from other injuries, hemoglobin and hematocrit levels should be monitored, and blood should be administered according to protocol. The nurse should also monitor the patient for indications of hypovolemic shock secondary to hemorrhage.

Fluid and Nutritional Maintenance. During the first 48 to 72 hours after the injury, the gastrointestinal tract may stop functioning (paralytic ileus), and a nasogastric tube must be inserted. Because the patient cannot have oral intake, fluid and electrolyte needs must be carefully monitored. Specific solutions and additives are ordered on the basis of individual requirements. Once bowel sounds are present or flatus is passed, oral food and fluids can gradually be introduced. Because of severe catabolism, a high-protein, high-calorie diet is necessary for energy and tissue repair. In patients with cervical cord injuries, swallowing must be evaluated before oral feedings are started. Enteral feeding is the optimal route after SCI. When oral feeding is not possible, nasogastric, followed by nasojejunal and then percutaneous, endoscopic gastrostomy is suggested. The acute stage of injury is characterized by a reduction in metabolic activity, as well as a negative nitrogen balance that cannot be corrected, even with aggressive nutritional support. Metabolic demands need to be accurately monitored to avoid overfeeding (Welch-West et al., 2019).

Some patients experience anorexia, which can result from psychological depression, boredom with institutional food, or discomfort with being fed. Some patients have a normally small appetite. On occasion, refusal to eat is used as a means of maintaining control over the environment because of diminished or absent control over one's body (see the Ethical Dilemmas box). If the patient is not eating adequately, the cause should be thoroughly assessed. On the basis of this assessment, a contract may be made in which the patient and the nurse set mutual goals regarding the diet. This gives the patient increased control of the situation and often results in improved nutritional intake. General measures such as providing a pleasant eating environment, allowing adequate time to eat (including any self-feeding that the patient can achieve), encouraging the family to bring

EVIDENCE-INFORMED PRACTICE

Translating Research Into Practice

A nurse working in the rehabilitation unit for patients recovering from SCI is assigned to K. T. (pronouns he/him), a 26-year-old who suffered an SCI after an all-terrain vehicle accident. K. T. has an areflexic bladder. The nurse has discussed with him the various options for bladder management. K. T. tells the nurse that the in-dwelling catheter is preferred because it would be the least disruptive to his daily activities.

Best Available Evidence	Clinician Expertise	Patient Preferences and Values
Patients using in-dwelling catheters (ICs), compared with those using clean intermittent catheters (CICs), have similar satisfaction with life and perceived health status. Use of an IC increases the risks for urological and renal complications. Fewer adverse bladder symptoms are associated with a CIC as compared to those using an IC or other voiding methods. Unless contraindicated (e.g., quadriplegia), clean intermittent catheterization is the preferred method of bladder emptying in SCI patients.	The nurse knows that a neurogenic bladder is best managed with either an in-dwelling catheter or intermittent catheterization. The nurse also knows that patients may hesitate to select clean intermittent catheterization for a variety of reasons (e.g., they believe the procedure is painful, they are afraid of performing the procedure incorrectly and possibly hurting themselves, they do not want their lives interrupted by the need to drain their bladder 5–6 times per day). In addition, in-dwelling catheters are most commonly used in the acute phase of treatment and not recommended for long-term use because of the risk of more complications unless intermittent catheterization is contraindicated.	After reviewing all the information, K. T. indicates that an in-dwelling catheter is preferred to intermittent catheterization as the method to self-manage his bladder.

Decision and Action

The nurse respects and supports K. T.'s decision, knowing that treatment should be specific and individualized to each patient. The nurse prepares a teaching plan for K. T. and his caregiver about how to obtain the necessary supplies and how to care for the catheter once K. T. is discharged.

References for Evidence

Hsieh, J., Ethans, K., Benton, B., et al. (2020). Bladder management following spinal cord injury. In J. J. Eng, R. W. Teasell, W. C. Miller, et al. (Eds.), *Spinal cord injury rehabilitation evidence* (pp. 1–274) Version 7.0. http://scireproject.com/evidence/rehabilitation-evidence/bladder-management/

Myers, J., Lenherr, S., Stoffel, A., et al. (2019). Patient reported bladder related symptoms and quality of life after spinal cord injury with different bladder management strategies. *The Journal of Urology*, 202(3), 574–584. https://doi.org/10.1097/JU.0000000000000270

ETHICAL DILEMMAS

Right to Refuse Treatment

Situation

A 25-year-old patient (pronouns he/him) suffered an SCI to C7–T1 after a motorcycle accident. Anterior cord syndrome was diagnosed, and the patient has motor paralysis, which may prevent him from riding motorcycles again. He has become extremely depressed and no longer wishes to live. Because of his emotional state, he is now refusing to eat. Can the patient be forced to receive enteral nutrition (tube feeding)?

Important Points for Consideration

- Withholding treatment in a newly injured but otherwise healthy young adult may present an ethical dilemma for health care providers. It may be viewed as assisted suicide and believed that it violates the ethical principles of beneficence and nonmaleficence.
- Approximately 20 to 30% of people with a new SCI experience a major depressive disorder as a result of the sudden loss of bodily control and feelings of helplessness.
- A thorough mental health and psychological evaluation is warranted; treatment of depression is necessary before determining the patient's capacity to make decisions.
- Most people (more than 90%) with an SCI who receive health care and have access to appropriate resources report a good quality of life. Therefore, requests to withhold treatment soon after SCI should be scrutinized.
- If, after adequate evaluation of and treatment for pain, depression, or other medical conditions, the patient persists in requests to withhold treatment, their ability to make an informed choice must be reassessed.
- A competent adult can decide to withhold treatment. If possible, action on the request should be delayed to ensure adequate informed consent is obtained and to determine whether quality of life is adequate.

Clinical Decision-Making Questions

1. How might the nurse feel about requests to withhold treatment for a young person with a newly acquired disability?
2. What resources are available to help the patient and the staff work through this emotionally charged and ethically complex situation?

---

in special foods, and planning social rewards for eating may be useful. A calorie count should be kept and the patient's daily weight recorded as a means of evaluating progress. If feasible, the patient should participate in recording calorie intake. Dietary supplements may be necessary to meet nutritional needs. Increased dietary fibre should be included to promote bowel function. The nurse should avoid allowing the patient's nutritional intake to become a basis for a power struggle.

Bladder and Bowel Management. Immediately after injury, urine is retained because of the loss of autonomic and reflex control of the bladder and the sphincter. Because the patient has no sensation of fullness, overdistension of the bladder can result in reflux into the kidneys, with eventual renal failure. Bladder distension may even result in rupture of the bladder. Consequently, an in-dwelling catheter is usually inserted as soon as possible after injury. Its patency must be ensured by frequent inspection and irrigation if necessary. Strict aseptic technique for catheter care is essential to avoid introducing infection.

After patients are stabilized, the best means of managing urinary function is assessed. Usually, an intermittent catheterization program is started. As well as having been shown to reduce UTIs in comparison with use of an in-dwelling catheter, intermittent catheterization is the safest method of bladder management for protecting the kidneys. Many patients are maintained on fluid restriction of 1 800 to 2 000 mL/day to facilitate a bladder training program, and urinary output is monitored closely.

UTIs are a common concern. The best method for preventing UTIs is regular and complete bladder drainage. Catheterization should be performed to prevent bladder volume from exceeding 500 mL. A typical regimen would be to catheterize every 4 hours for volumes of 300 to 500 mL, every 3 hours for volumes greater than 500 mL, and every 6 hours for volumes less than 300 mL. If the appearance or odour of the urine is suspect or if the patient develops symptoms of a UTI (e.g., chills, fever, malaise), a urine specimen is sent for culture.

Age-related changes in renal function should be considered. Older persons are more likely to develop renal calculi, and older men may have prostatic hyperplasia, which may interfere with urinary flow and complicate management of urinary problems.

Constipation is generally a problem during spinal shock because no voluntary or involuntary (reflex) evacuation of the bowels occurs. A bowel program should be started during acute care. This consists of a rectal stimulant (suppository or mini-enema) to be inserted daily at a regular time of day, followed by gentle digital stimulation or manual evacuation performed by the nurse until evacuation is complete. Initially, the program may be performed in bed in the side-lying position, but as soon as the patient has resumed sitting, it should be performed in the upright position on a padded bedside commode chair.

Temperature Control. Temperature control is largely external to the patient because there is no vasoconstriction, piloerection, or heat loss through perspiration below the level of injury. The nurse must monitor the environment closely to maintain an appropriate temperature. Body temperature should be monitored regularly. The patient should not be overloaded with covers or unduly exposed (such as during bathing). If an infection with high fever develops, more extensive means of temperature control, such as a cooling blanket, may be necessary.

Stress Ulcers. Stress ulcers are a concern for the patient with an SCI because of the physiological response to severe trauma, psychological stress, and high-dose corticosteroids if used. The incidence of ulcers peaks 6 to 14 days after injury. Histamine H_2-receptor blockers, such as ranitidine (Zantac) and famotidine (Pepcid AC), or proton pump inhibitors, such as omeprazole (Losec) or pantoprazole (Prevacid), may be given prophylactically to decrease the secretion of hydrochloric acid.

Sensory Deprivation. To prevent sensory deprivation, the nurse must compensate for the patient's absence of sensations by stimulating the patient above the level of injury. Conversation, music, strong aromas, and flavours interesting to the patient should be a part of the nursing care plan. Every effort should be made to prevent the patient from withdrawing from the environment.

Patients with SCIs often report altered sensorium and vivid dreams during the acute phase of their treatment. Whether this is caused by medications used to manage pain and anxiety is not known. Patients may also experience disrupted sleep patterns as a result of the hospital environment or post-traumatic stress disorder.

Reflexes. Once spinal cord shock is resolved, the return of reflexes may complicate rehabilitation. In the absence of control from the higher brain centres, reflexes are often hyperactive, and responses may be exaggerated. Penile erections can result from a variety of stimuli, causing embarrassment and discomfort. Spasms ranging from mild twitches to convulsive movements below the level of the lesion may also occur. This reflex activity may be interpreted by the patient or family as a return of function, and the nurse must tactfully explain the reason for the activity. The patient may be informed of the positive use of these reflexes in sexual, bowel, and bladder retraining. Spasms may be controlled with the use of antispasmodic medications.

Most commonly prescribed are baclofen (Lioresal), dantrolene (Dantrium), and tizanidine. Botulism toxin injections may also be given to treat severe spasticity.

Autonomic Dysreflexia. The return of reflexes after the resolution of spinal shock means that patients with an injury level at T6 or higher may develop autonomic dysreflexia. Autonomic dysreflexia (also known as *autonomic hyper-reflexia*) is a massive, uncompensated cardiovascular reaction mediated by the sympathetic nervous system. It occurs in response to visceral stimulation once spinal shock is resolved in patients with spinal cord lesions. This condition is a life-threatening situation that requires immediate resolution. If resolution does not occur, this condition can lead to status epilepticus, stroke, myocardial infarction, or even death.

The most common precipitating cause is distension of the bladder or rectum, although any sensory stimulation may cause autonomic dysreflexia. Contraction of the bladder or the rectum, stimulation of the skin, or stimulation of the pain receptors may also cause autonomic dysreflexia. Manifestations include hypertension (up to 300 mm Hg systolic), throbbing headache, marked diaphoresis or flushing of skin above the level of the lesion, bradycardia (30 to 40 beats per minute), piloerection (erection of body hair) as a result of pilomotor spasm, blurred vision or spots in the visual fields, nasal congestion, anxiety, and nausea. It is important to measure blood pressure when a patient with an SCI complains of a headache (Allen & Leslie, 2021). A normal blood pressure for a patient with tetraplegic SCI is a systolic blood pressure of 90 to 100 mm Hg. Any pressure higher than this should be considered hypertensive.

The pathology of autonomic dysreflexia involves the stimulation of sensory receptors below the level of the cord lesion. The intact autonomic nervous system below the level of the lesion responds to the stimulation with a reflex arteriolar vasoconstriction that increases blood pressure. Baroreceptors in the carotid sinus and the aorta detect the hypertension and stimulate the parasympathetic system. This stimulation results in a decrease in heart rate, but the visceral and peripheral vessels do not dilate because efferent impulses cannot pass through the cord lesion.

In this serious emergency, nursing interventions include elevating the head of the bed 45 degrees or sitting the patient upright, notifying the health care provider, and assessing the patient to determine the cause. The most common cause is bladder distension. Immediate catheterization to relieve bladder distension may be necessary. Lidocaine jelly should be instilled in the urethra before catheterization. If a catheter is already in place, it should be checked for kinks or folds. If it is plugged, small-volume irrigation should be performed slowly and gently to open the catheter, or a new catheter may be inserted. Stool impaction can also result in autonomic dysreflexia. A digital rectal examination should be performed only after application of an anaesthetic ointment to decrease rectal stimulation and to prevent an increase of symptoms. If neither bladder nor bowel distension is determined to be causative, the nurse should remove all skin stimuli, such as constrictive clothing, tight shoes, and splints. Blood pressure should be monitored frequently during the episode. If symptoms persist after the source has been relieved, an α-adrenergic blocker or an arteriolar vasodilator (e.g., nifedipine) is administered. Careful monitoring must continue until the vital signs stabilize.

TABLE 63.7 PATIENT & CAREGIVER TEACHING GUIDE

Autonomic Dysreflexia

The following information should be included in the teaching plan for a patient at risk for autonomic dysreflexia:

1. Signs and symptoms
   - Sudden onset of acute headache
   - Elevation in blood pressure, reduction in pulse rate, or both
   - Flushed face and upper chest (above the level of the lesion) and pale extremities (below the level of the lesion)
   - Sweating above the level of the lesion
   - Nasal congestion
   - Feeling of apprehension
2. Immediate interventions
   - Raise the patient to a sitting position.
   - Remove the stimulus (fecal impaction, distended bladder, tight clothing).
   - Call the health care provider if these actions do not relieve the signs and symptoms.
3. Measures to suppress the incidence of autonomic dysreflexia
   - Maintain regular bladder and bowel function.
   - If manual rectal stimulation is used to promote bowel function, local anaesthetics may prevent autonomic dysreflexia from occurring.
   - Wear a medical alert bracelet indicating a history of autonomic dysreflexia.

The patient and caregivers should be taught the causes and symptoms of autonomic dysreflexia (Table 63.7). They must understand the life-threatening nature of this dysfunction and know how to relieve the cause.

SAFETY ALERT
- The most common stimulus that causes autonomic dysreflexia in patients with an SCI is from a urological source (e.g., UTI, bladder distension) and bowel distension.
- Prompt recognition and treatment (e.g., raising head of the bed or sitting patient upright, bladder emptying, urinary catheter irrigation) of autonomic dysreflexia can be immediately lifesaving.

REHABILITATION AND HOME CARE. The physiological and psychological rehabilitation of patients with SCI is complex and involved. With physical and psychological care and intensive and specialized rehabilitation, patients with SCI learn to function at the highest level of wellness. It is recommended that all patients with a new SCI receive comprehensive inpatient rehabilitation in a rehabilitation unit or centre that specializes in SCIs.

Many of the problems identified in the acute period become chronic and continue throughout life. It is important to understand the type of pain the patient may be experiencing and its cause to determine the most appropriate treatment. Pregabalin, gabapentin, and amitriptyline are recommended as first-line treatment for neuropathic pain in patients with SCI (Guy et al., 2016). Rehabilitation focuses on refined retraining of physiological processes and on extensive patient and caregiver teaching on how to manage the physiological and life changes resulting from injury.

Rehabilitation requires an interprofessional team approach. Team members can include rehabilitation nurses, physicians, respiratory therapists, physiotherapists, occupational therapists, speech–language pathologists, vocational counsellors, psychologists, therapeutic recreation specialists, prosthetists, orthotists, and dietitians. Rehabilitation care is organized around the individual patient's goals and needs. During rehabilitation, patients are expected to be involved in therapies and to learn self-care for several hours each day. Such intensive work at a time when the patient is coping with the sudden change in health and functional status can be very stressful. Progress may be slow, and frequent encouragement may be required. The rehabilitation nurse has a pivotal role in providing encouragement, specialized nursing care, and patient and caregiver teaching, and in helping to coordinate the efforts of the rehabilitation team.

Respiratory Rehabilitation. The patient with high cervical SCI may have greatly increased mobility with phrenic nerve stimulators or electronic diaphragmatic pacemakers. These devices are not appropriate for all ventilator-dependent patients but may be helpful for those with an intact phrenic nerve. Currently, ventilators are reasonably portable, and ventilator-dependent tetraplegic patients can be mobile and somewhat independent. Patients and caregivers should be taught all aspects of home ventilator care, and referrals should be made to appropriate community agencies. Patients with injuries at the cervical level who are not ventilator dependent should be taught assisted coughing and regular use of incentive spirometry or deep-breathing exercises.

Neurogenic Bladder. A neurogenic bladder is any type of bladder dysfunction related to abnormal or absent bladder innervation. After spinal cord shock resolves, depending on the completeness of the SCI, patients usually have some degree of neurogenic bladder. Normal voiding requires nervous system coordination of urethral and pelvic floor relaxation with simultaneous contraction of the detrusor muscle. Depending on the lesion, a neurogenic bladder may have no reflex detrusor contractions (*areflexic*, flaccid), may have hyperactive reflex detrusor contractions (*hyper-reflexic*, spastic), or may lack coordination between detrusor contraction and urethral relaxation (*dyssynergia*). Common conditions with a neurogenic bladder include urgency, frequency, incontinence, inability to void, and high bladder pressures that cause reflux of urine into the kidneys.

Neurogenic bladder can be classified according to reflex detrusor activity, intravesical filling pressure, and continence function. Types of neurogenic bladder are outlined in Table 63.8. Diagnostic and interprofessional care of patients with a neurogenic bladder is described in Table 63.9. Patients with SCI and a neurogenic bladder require a comprehensive program to manage bladder function.

After the patient's overall condition is stable and there is evidence of neurological reflexes, urodynamic testing and a urine culture are performed to aid in determining the type of neurogenic bladder dysfunction experienced. The method used for urinary drainage depends on the type of neurogenic bladder dysfunction, the preference of the patient, and availability of a family member or caregiver, the physician, and the nursing staff. Numerous drainage methods are possible. Surgical options include sphincterectomy, implantation of a functional electrical stimulation device, and urinary diversion.

Many factors are considered when a bladder management strategy is selected, including upper extremity function, caregiver burden, and lifestyle choices. The type of bladder dysfunction also defines treatment goals and management options. For a reflexic bladder with detrusor and sphincter dyssynergia, interventions must enable low-pressure storage, low-pressure voiding, and adequate emptying. Anticholinergic medications (e.g., oxybutynin [Oxytrol], tolterodine [Detrol]) may be used

TABLE 63.8 TYPES OF NEUROGENIC BLADDER

Type	Characteristics	Causes	Clinical Manifestations
Reflexic (spastic, uninhibited, upper motor neuron)	No inhibitions influence time and place of voiding; bladder empties in response to stretching of bladder wall	Corticospinal tract lesion; observed in spinal cord injury, stroke, multiple sclerosis, brain tumour, brain trauma	Incontinence, frequency, urgency; voiding is unpredictable and incomplete
Areflexic (autonomous, flaccid, lower motor neuron)	Bladder acts as if all motor functions are paralyzed, fills without emptying	Lower motor neuron lesion caused by trauma involving S2–4; observed in lesions of cauda equina, pelvic nerves	If sensory function is intact, patient feels bladder distension and hesitancy; no control of micturition results in overdistension of bladder and overflow incontinence
Sensory	Lack of sensation of need to urinate	Damage to sensory limb of bladder spinal reflex arc; observed in multiple sclerosis, diabetes mellitus	Poor bladder sensation, infrequent voiding of large residual volume

TABLE 63.9 INTERPROFESSIONAL CARE

Neurogenic Bladder

Diagnostic
- History and physical examination, including neurological examination
- Urodynamic testing
- Urine culture

Interprofessional Therapy
- Medication therapy
  - Relaxation of urethral sphincter (α-adrenergic blockers)
  - Suppression of bladder contractions (anticholinergics)
  - Suppression of pelvic floor spasticity (baclofen [Lioresal])
- Fluid intake of 1 800–2 000 mL/day
- Surgery
- Electrical stimulation
- Sphincterotomy
- Urinary diversion
- Urine drainage
- In-dwelling catheter
- Intermittent catheterization
- Voluntary or reflex voiding

to suppress bladder contraction. α-Adrenergic blockers (e.g., terazosin, alfuzosin, doxazosin [Cardura]) may be used to decrease outflow resistance at the bladder neck, and antispasmodic medications (e.g., baclofen [Lioresal]) may be used to decrease spasticity of pelvic floor muscles.

Drainage options include intermittent catheterization, placement of an external catheter (condom catheter), or placement of an in-dwelling catheter. A reflexic bladder with detrusor hyper-reflexia may be treated with anticholinergic medications, intravesical capsaicin, or botulinum A toxin. An areflexic bladder is usually managed with intermittent catheterization or an in-dwelling catheter.

The long-term use of an in-dwelling catheter should be carefully evaluated because of the associated high incidence of UTI, fistula formation, and diverticula. However, for some patients, it is the best option. Adequate fluid intake and patency of the catheter should be ensured. The frequency of routine catheter changes ranges from 1 week to 1 month, depending on the type of catheter used and institutional policy.

Intermittent catheterization is the most commonly recommended method of bladder management (see Chapter 48). Nursing assessment is important in selecting the time interval between catheterizations. Catheterization should be performed to prevent bladder volume from exceeding 500 mL. A typical regimen would be to catheterize every 4 hours for volumes of 300 to 500 mL, every 3 hours for volumes greater than 500 mL, and every 6 hours for volumes less than 300 mL. An overdistended bladder can cause ischemia of the bladder wall, which may predispose tissues to bacterial invasion and infection. Patients often experience diuresis at a regular time during a 24-hour period. The number of intermittent catheterizations per day is usually five or six.

Urinary diversion surgery may be necessary if a patient has repeated UTIs with renal involvement or repeated stones, or if therapeutic intervention has been unsuccessful (see Chapter 48). Surgical treatment of neurogenic bladder includes bladder neck revision (sphincterotomy), bladder augmentation (augmentation cystoplasty), penile prosthesis, artificial sphincter, perineal ureterostomy, cystotomy, vesicotomy, and anterior urethral transplantation.

Regardless of which bladder management strategy is selected, the nurse must teach the patient and the family or caregivers how to accomplish successful self-management, including management techniques, how to obtain necessary supplies, care of supplies and equipment, and when to seek related health care. Resources and referrals for supplies and ongoing care must be arranged.

Neurogenic Bowel. Careful management of bowel evacuation is necessary in patients with SCIs because voluntary control of this function may be lost. The usual measures for preventing constipation include a high-fibre diet and adequate fluid intake (see Chapter 45, Table 45.9). Patient and caregiver teaching guidelines related to bowel management are presented in Table 63.10. However, these measures by themselves may not be adequate to stimulate evacuation. In addition, suppositories (bisacodyl [Dulcolax] or glycerin) or small-volume enemas and digital stimulation by the nurse or patient may be necessary. In patients with an upper motor neuron lesion, digital stimulation is necessary to relax the external sphincter to promote defecation. A stool softener such as docusate sodium (Colace) can be used to regulate stool consistency. Oral stimulant laxatives should be used only if absolutely necessary for a day or two and not on a regular basis.

Valsalva manoeuvre and manual stimulation are useful in patients with lower motor neuron lesions. Valsalva manoeuvre requires intact abdominal muscles, so it is used in patients with injuries below T12.

In general, a bowel movement every other day is considered adequate. However, preinjury patterns should be considered. Incontinence can result from too much stool softener or fecal impaction.

Careful recording of bowel movements, including amount, time, and consistency, is important to overall success. Timing

TABLE 63.10 PATIENT & CAREGIVER TEACHING GUIDE

Bowel Management After Spinal Cord Injury

The following information should be included when teaching the caregiver and patient with a spinal cord injury:

1. Optimal nutritional intake includes three well-balanced meals each day in accordance with the recommendations from *Canada's Dietary Guidelines*.*
2. Daily fibre intake should be approximately 20 to 30 g. The amount of fibre eaten should be increased gradually over 1 to 2 weeks.
3. Three litres of fluid per day should be consumed, unless contraindicated. Water or fruit juices should be used, and caffeinated beverages such as coffee, tea, and cola should be avoided. Fluid softens hard stools; caffeine stimulates fluid loss through urination.
4. Foods that produce gas (e.g., beans) or upper gastrointestinal upset (spicy foods) should be avoided.
5. *Timing:* A regular schedule for bowel evacuation should be established. A good time is 30 minutes after the first meal of the day.
6. *Position:* If possible, an upright position with feet flat on the floor or on a step stool enhances bowel evacuation. Staying on the toilet, commode, or bedpan for longer than 20 to 30 minutes may cause skin breakdown. Depending on the patient's stability, someone may need to stay with the patient.
7. *Activity:* Exercise is important for bowel function. In addition to improving muscle tone, it increases gastrointestinal transit time and increases appetite. Muscles should be exercised. Exercise includes stretching, range of motion, position changing, and functional movement.
8. *Medication treatment:* Suppositories may be necessary to stimulate a bowel movement. Manual stimulation of the rectum may also be helpful in initiating defecation. Stool softeners and oral laxatives may be used as needed to regulate stool consistency.

*Health Canada. (2020). *Canada's dietary guidelines*. https://food-guide.canada.ca/en/guidelines/

TABLE 63.11 PATIENT & CAREGIVER TEACHING GUIDE

Skin Care for Patients With Spinal Cord Injury

Skin breakdown is a potential condition after spinal cord injury. The following information should be included when teaching the caregiver how to decrease this possibility:

Frequent Change of Position
- Patient in a wheelchair: lift self up and shift weight every 15 to 30 minutes.
- Patient in a bed: follow a regular turning schedule (at least every 2 hours) that includes sides, back, and abdomen.
- Use special mattresses and wheelchair cushions.
- Use pillows to protect bony prominences when in bed.

Monitor Skin Condition
- Inspect skin frequently for areas of redness, swelling, and breakdown.
- Keep fingernails trimmed to avoid scratches and abrasions.
- If a wound develops, follow standard wound care management procedures.

of defecation may also be an important factor. If bowel evacuation is planned for 30 to 60 minutes after the first meal of the day, success may be enhanced by taking advantage of the gastrocolic reflex induced by eating. Again, patient and family education is required to promote successful independent bowel management.

Neurogenic Skin. Prevention of pressure injuries and other types of injury to insensitive skin is essential for every patient with SCI. The 2013 *Canadian Best Practice Guidelines for the Prevention and Management of Pressure Ulcers in People with Spinal Cord Injury* (Houghton et al., 2013) provides an updated resource for health care providers and considers the unique challenges of pressure injury management. The guidelines take a comprehensive approach to pressure management, including self-management and telehealth approaches. Nurses in rehabilitation care are responsible for teaching these skills and providing patients information about daily skin care. A comprehensive visual and tactile examination of the skin should be performed twice daily, with special attention to areas over bony prominences. The areas most vulnerable to breakdown include the ischia, the trochanters, the heels, and the sacrum. Careful positioning and repositioning should be performed every 2 hours, with gradual increases in the times between turns if no redness over bony prominences is apparent at the time of turning. Pressure-relieving cushions must be used in wheelchairs, and special mattresses may also be needed. Movement during turns and transfers should be performed carefully to avoid shear

(stretching and folding of soft tissues), friction, or abrasion (Houghton et al., 2013).

Nutritional status should be assessed regularly. Both loss and gain in body weight can contribute to skin breakdown. Adequate intake of protein is essential for skin health. Measurement of total protein and albumin can help in identifying inadequate protein intake. The importance of nutrition to skin health should be stressed to the patient and caregivers.

Protection of the skin also requires avoidance of thermal injury. Burns can be caused by hot food or liquids, bath or shower water that is too warm, radiators, heating pads, and uninsulated plumbing. Thermal injury also can result from extreme cold (frostbite). Injuries may not be noticed until severe damage is done. Anticipatory guidance about potential risks is essential. Patient and caregiver education related to skin care is provided in Table 63.11.

Sexuality. The effects of an SCI on sexual functioning, ability to engage in sexual activities, sexual intimacy and relationships, sexual self-view, and fertility and reproductive health vary with each individual. Sexual health is a significant component of a person's overall health and well-being. Most individuals who have experienced an SCI retain their desire for sexual activity.

Male fertility after SCI is often compounded by the difficulties of erectile dysfunction, ejaculatory dysfunction, and abnormal semen quality (Ibrahim et al., 2016). Erectile dysfunction often causes erections that are unreliable or inadequate for sexual intercourse because of difficulties in maintaining an erection. Medications or surgical procedures are available to help overcome this issue. Semen may be obtained through medically assisted ejaculation methods (e.g., penile vibratory stimulation, prostate massage) and then used for intravaginal or intrauterine insemination or other assisted reproductive technology.

Female fertility appears to be unaffected by SCI. Amenorrhea can occur following SCI and last from 4 to 5 months. Women with an SCI are still able to conceive, carry, and deliver a baby, although they tend to have more complications during pregnancy, labour, and delivery than women in the general population (Spinal Outreach Team, 2017). Bladder disorders, spasticity, pressure sores, autonomic dysreflexia, and difficulties with mobility can pose a threat to the pregnant woman with SCI. A pre-emptive epidural prior to delivery is used to manage autonomic dysreflexia, which otherwise can become uncontrolled.

Because sexual health has been identified as a priority among persons with SCI, it is important to have a comprehensive and holistic rehabilitation program that normalizes sexual health concerns and questions for patients with an SCI (Giurleo et al., 2020). Sexual rehabilitation for all patients should begin informally after the acute phase of the injury has passed. Questions such as "Have you had an erection since your accident?" and "Have your menstrual periods continued since the accident?" are nonthreatening ways to introduce the topic of sexual functioning.

Open discussion with the patient is essential. A nurse or other rehabilitation professional with expertise in sexual counselling can work with the patient and partner to provide support, with an emphasis on open communication. The nurse's educational role requires respect for every couple's religious beliefs and cultural norms. Alternative methods of obtaining sexual satisfaction, such as oral–genital sex (cunnilingus and fellatio), may be suggested. Explicit video material may also be used, such as a movie demonstrating the sexual activities of a patient with paraplegia with a nondisabled partner. Graphic materials should be used with caution because they may be too limiting or focus too much on the mechanics of sex rather than on the relationship.

Sexual activities may require more planning and be less spontaneous than before the injury. For example, an attendant may have to undress the patient and remove equipment. A relaxed atmosphere with music may create an attractive environment. Ample time for intimacy (e.g., caressing, fondling, kissing) is essential. The partners should be encouraged to explore each other's erogenous areas, such as lips, neck, and ears, which can arouse psychogenic erection or orgasm. Few demands should be made initially.

Care should be taken not to dislodge an in-dwelling catheter during sexual activity. If an external catheter is used, it should be removed before sexual activity, and the patient should refrain from drinking fluids. The bowel program should include evacuation the morning after sexual activity. The partner should be informed that incontinence is always possible. The woman with an SCI may need a water-soluble lubricant to supplement diminished vaginal secretions and facilitate vaginal penetration.

Grief and Depression. Patients with SCI may feel an overwhelming sense of loss. They may temporarily lose control over everyday life activities and must depend on others for activities of daily living and for life-sustaining measures. Patients may believe that they are useless and burdens to their families. At a stage when independence is often of greatest importance, they may be totally dependent on others.

The patient's and family's response and recovery differ in some important aspects from those of patients experiencing loss from amputation or terminal illness. First, regression can and does occur at different stages. Working through grief is a difficult, lifelong process for which the patient needs support and encouragement. With advances in rehabilitation, it is common for the patient to be independent physically and discharged from the rehabilitation centre before they have completed the grief process. The goal of recovery is related more to adjustment than to acceptance. Adjustment implies the ability to go on living with certain limitations. Although some patients may be cooperative and accepting and thus are easier to treat, the nurse should expect a wide fluctuation of emotions from all patients with SCIs. Depression may not be a component of a

TABLE 63.12   MOURNING PROCESS AND NURSING INTERVENTIONS IN SPINAL CORD INJURY

Patient Behaviour	Nursing Intervention
Shock and Denial Struggle for survival, complete dependence, excessive sleep, withdrawal, fantasies, unrealistic expectations	• Employ meticulous nursing care. • Provide honest information. • Use simple diagrams to explain injury. • Encourage patient to begin process of recovery. • Establish agreement to use and improve all current abilities while not denying the possibility of future improvement.
Anger Refusal to discuss paralysis, decreased self-esteem, manipulation, hostile and abusive language	• Coordinate care with patient and encourage self-care. • Support family members; prevent them from alleviating their guilt by supporting the patient's dependency. • Use humour appropriately. • Allow patient outbursts of emotion. • Do not allow fixation on injury.
Depression Sadness, pessimism, anorexia, nightmares, insomnia, agitation, psychomotor retardation, "blues," suicidal preoccupation, refusal to participate in any self-care activities	• Encourage family involvement and use of available resources. • Plan graded steps in rehabilitation to give success with minimal opportunity for frustration. • Give cheerful and willing assistance with activities of daily living. • Avoid expressing sympathy. • Use firm kindness.
Adjustment Planning for future, active participation in therapy, finding of personal meaning in experience and continuation of growth, return to preinjury personality	• Remember that patients have individual personalities. • Balance support systems to encourage independence. • Set goals in collaboration with the patient. • Emphasize potentials.

patient's recovery process. Societal norms allow depression after severe loss, and persons confronted with death or radical lifestyle changes are almost expected to become depressed. However, not every patient may experience depression.

The nurse's role in grief work is to enable mourning as a component of the rehabilitation process. Table 63.12 summarizes the mourning process and appropriate nursing interventions. Maintaining hope is an important strategy during the grieving process and should not be interpreted as denial (Dorsett et al., 2017). During the stage of shock and denial, the nurse can reassure the patient and stress the expertise of the entire health care team. During the anger stage, the nurse can assist the patient in achieving control over their environment, particularly by allowing the patient's input into the plan of care. The nurse should not respond to anger or manipulation or become involved in a power struggle with the patient. As self-care abilities increase, the patient's independence will increase.

Peer support groups can be useful in helping individuals and their families begin to cope with the injury and adjust to life with an SCI. For instance, Spinal Cord Injury Ontario connects people living with SCIs to fully trained volunteers who can share their experience and knowledge. They can also connect family members with others who have gone through this journey. Support groups complement professional services provided in acute care hospitals, rehabilitation centres, and community-based health and social service agencies.

The patient's caregiver and family also require counselling to avoid promoting dependency in the patient through guilt or misplaced sympathy. The family and caregiver are also experiencing an intense grieving process. A support group consisting of family members and friends of patients with SCIs can help increase the patient's family members' participation in the grieving process, as well as their knowledge of physical difficulties, the rehabilitation plan, and the meaning of the disability in society (Dorsett et al., 2017).

During the stage of depression, the nurse must be patient and persistent and maintain a sense of humour; sympathy is not helpful. The patient should be treated in an adult manner and be involved in decision making about their care. A primary nurse relationship is helpful. Interprofessional team sessions in which members can express their feelings are helpful in providing consistency of care.

To achieve the stage of adjustment, the patient needs continual support throughout the rehabilitation process in the forms of acceptance, affection, and caring. The nurse must be attentive when the patient needs to talk and sensitive to needs at the various stages of the grief process. Patients with greater hope demonstrate better psychosocial adjustment outcomes, higher levels of self-efficacy, greater life satisfaction, higher self-rated adjustment, and significantly lower levels of depression and perceived problems in their lives as compared to patients who are experiencing hopelessness (Dorsett et al., 2017). If the patient becomes clinically depressed, a psychiatric consultation may be warranted.

EVALUATION

Expected outcomes for patients with SCIs are presented in NCP 63.1, available on the Evolve website.

AGE-RELATED CONSIDERATIONS

SPINAL CORD INJURY

The demographics of patients living with SCI are changing. The fact that persons with SCI now have longer lifespans has contributed to the increasing number of older persons living with an SCI. Moreover, increasing numbers of older persons sustain SCIs later in life as a result of falls. Aging is also associated with an increased likelihood of other chronic illnesses that may have a serious effect on older persons with an SCI. As patients with SCI age, both individual aging changes and duration since injury affect functional ability. For example, bowel and bladder dysfunction can increase with duration and severity of SCI.

Health promotion and screening are important health care measures for older patients with SCI. Daily skin inspections, UTI prevention measures, monthly breast examinations for women, and regular prostate cancer screening for men are recommended. Cardiovascular disease is the most common cause of morbidity and mortality among persons with SCIs. The lack of sensation, including that of angina, in patients with high-level injuries may mask acute myocardial ischemia. Altered autonomic nervous system function and decreases in physical activity can increase the risk for cardiovascular conditions, including hypertension.

At the same time, because of increased work and recreational activities of older people, an increasing number of older people are experiencing SCI. Health promotion to decrease injury risk includes fall prevention strategies (e.g., using a stepstool or a grab bar to reach high shelves, handrails on stairs). Rehabilitation for older persons with SCIs may take longer because of other pre-existing illnesses and poorer health status at the time of the initial injury. Studies show that older persons with SCIs can gain the same degree of neurological recovery as those who are younger at the time of injury, but this does not necessarily translate into meaningful functional outcomes. An interprofessional team approach to tailored rehabilitation to match specific needs of older individuals is needed to maximize their potential for recovery and reintegration into the community.

SPINAL CORD INJURY RESEARCH IN CANADA

The Rick Hansen Foundation is a Canadian organization committed to accelerating the translation of discoveries and best practices into improved treatments for individuals with SCIs. Its four distinct programs focus on *cure, care, commercialization,* and *consumers* and support research from the lab to clinical application in an effort to improve the lives of individuals with SCI (see Resources at the end of this chapter).

SPINAL CORD TUMOURS

Etiology and Pathophysiology

Spinal cord tumours account for 0.5 to 1% of all neoplasms. These tumours are classified as *primary* (arising from some component of cord, dura, nerves, or vessels) or *secondary* (from primary growths in other places in the body that have metastasized to the spinal cord). Spinal cord tumours are further classified as *extradural* (outside the spinal cord), *intradural extramedullary* (within the dura but outside the actual spinal cord), and *intradural intramedullary* (within the spinal cord itself) (Figure 63.10 and Table 63.13). Intradural intramedullary tumours are usually astrocytomas or ependymomas. Approximately 90% of all spinal tumours are extradural. Extradural tumours are usually

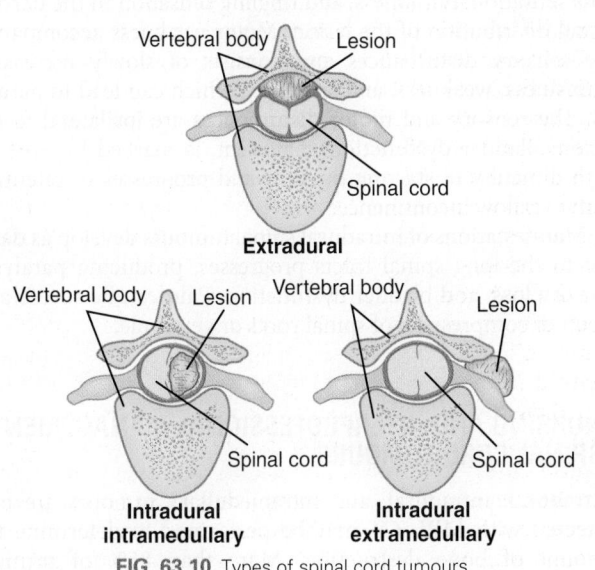

FIG. 63.10 Types of spinal cord tumours.

TABLE 63.13	**CLASSIFICATION OF SPINAL CORD TUMOURS**		
Type	**Incidence**	**Treatment**	**Prognosis**
Extradural: from bones of spine, in extradural space, or in paraspinal tissue	20–50% of all intraspinal tumours; mostly malignant metastatic lesions	Relief of cord pressure by surgical laminectomy, radiation, chemotherapy, or combination approach	Dependent on tumour type and stage; benign tumour excellent with resection; metastatic tumour poor, treatment usually palliative
Intradural extramedullary: within dura mater, outside spinal cord	Most frequent of intradural tumours (40%), mostly benign meningiomas and neurofibromas	Complete surgical removal of tumour (if possible), partial removal followed by radiation	Usually very good if no damage to cord from compression
Intradural intramedullary: within spinal cord	Least frequent of intradural tumours (5–10%); mostly benign	Complete surgical removal of tumour (if possible), partial surgical removal, radiation therapy (resulting in only temporary improvement)	Dependent on neurological function before and after decompression; usually very good if no damage to cord from compression

metastatic and most often arise in the vertebral bodies. These metastatic lesions can invade intradurally and compress the spinal cord. Tumours that commonly metastasize to the spinal epidural space are those that spread to bone, such as prostate, breast, lung, and kidney cancer. Spinal intradural extramedullary tumours account for two-thirds of all intraspinal neoplasms and consist mainly of meningiomas and schwannomas.

Because many of these tumours are slow growing, their symptoms stem from the mechanical effects of bone destruction, slow compression and irritation of nerve roots, displacement of the cord, or gradual obstruction of the vascular supply. The slow growth does not cause autodestruction (secondary injury), as occurs with traumatic lesions. Therefore, partial to complete functional restoration may be possible when the tumour is removed.

Clinical Manifestations

Both sensory and motor deficits may result; the location and extent of the tumour determine the severity and the distribution of the condition. The most common early symptom of an extradural spinal cord tumour is back pain. Radicular pain may occur as the tumour compresses nerve roots. The location of the pain depends on the level of compression. The pain worsens with activity, coughing, and straining. Some relief may occur with lying down, but there is usually a baseline of pain even in this position secondary to the inflammatory changes within the bone structure. Sensory disruption is manifested by pain, coldness sensation, numbness, and tingling sensation in the dermatomal distribution of the lesion. Motor weakness accompanies the sensory disturbances and consists of slowly increasing clumsiness, weakness, and spasticity, which can lead to paralysis. The sensory and motor disturbances are ipsilateral to the lesion. Bladder dysfunction, if present, is marked by urgency with difficulty in starting the flow and progresses to retention with overflow incontinence.

Manifestations of intradural spinal tumours develop as damage to the long spinal tracts progresses, producing paralysis, sensory loss, and bladder dysfunction. Pain can be severe as a result of compression of spinal roots or vertebrae.

NURSING AND INTERPROFESSIONAL MANAGEMENT SPINAL CORD TUMOURS

Extradural, intradural, and intramedullary tumours are best detected with MRI. CT may be performed to determine the amount of bone destruction. More than 85% of primary neoplasms are benign and can be completely resected; 90% of such patients recover without residual problems.

Compression of the spinal cord is an emergency. Relief of the ischemia related to the compression is the goal of therapy. Dexamethasone is usually used to treat edema, often in large doses (100 mg as a bolus dose). Surgical decompression can involve various approaches (anterior, posterior, or a combination of both), followed by reconstruction and stabilization. The standard treatment for spinal cord compression caused by metastatic cancer is surgery as initial treatment, followed by radiotherapy (Boussios et al., 2018).

Treatment for nearly all spinal cord tumours is surgical removal. The exception is the metastatic tumour that is sensitive to chemotherapy or radiation and that has caused only minimal neurological deficits (e.g., multiple myeloma). In general, extradural and intradural extramedullary tumours can be completely removed surgically. Intradural intramedullary tumours have a less favourable prognosis. However, exploration and removal are usually attempted.

Standard radiation therapy after surgical decompression is considered if the tumour is radiosensitive. Treatment is started approximately 3 to 4 weeks after surgery and usually consists of five doses. In a newer therapy, intensity-modulated radiotherapy, higher doses of radiation are delivered to the tumour site, which minimizes injury to surrounding normal spinal and paraspinal tissues. Chemotherapy has also been used in conjunction with radiation therapy.

Relief of pain and prevention of continued neurological decline are the ultimate goals of treatment. Nurses must be aware of the neurological status of the patient before and after treatment. Ensuring that the patient receives analgesics to manage pain is an important nursing responsibility. Depending on the amount of neurological dysfunction exhibited, the patient may need to be cared for as though they were recovering from an SCI. Rehabilitation of patients with spinal cord tumours is similar to rehabilitation of patients with SCIs.

POSTPOLIO SYNDROME

Polio, also known as *poliomyelitis*, is an infectious viral disease transmitted through the oral route by ingestion of contaminated water or food or by contact with infected sources such as unwashed hands. The virus is shed in the feces of infected individuals for as long as 6 weeks. The disease produces a range of manifestations from influenza-like symptoms (abortive poliomyelitis) that resolve in 24 to 36 hours (nonparalytic) to paralytic poliomyelitis that attacks the motor neurons in the anterior horn of the spinal cord, the brainstem, or both. Polio ravaged North American communities during the 1930s, 1940s, and 1950s. Polio was effectively eradicated in North America by the development of the Salk injectable polio vaccine in 1954 and the Sabin oral polio vaccine in 1961. It is still a threat in developing countries because of a lack of effective immunization programs. Polio survivors who recovered from the disease decades ago, notably those who had paralytic poliomyelitis, are now experiencing a recurrence of neuromuscular symptoms as they age. These late effects of polio are collectively referred to as postpolio syndrome (PPS). On the basis of criteria for diagnosis of PPS, the incidence and prevalence can range from 10 to 40% (Kedlaya, 2021).

Etiology and Pathophysiology

The etiology of PPS is not completely clear. The most commonly accepted theory is that enlarged distal motor neurons that had recovered after polio degenerate and subsequently begin to fail (Kedlaya, 2021). It appears that cellular damage caused by the effects of the polio virus may lead to exhaustion and premature failure of the motor neurons. The result is slowly progressive muscle weakness and fatigue. Factors thought to contribute to PPS include age-related motor neuron loss, musculoskeletal overuse and disuse, weight gain, pain, and other neuromuscular or systemic illnesses. There is no evidence to support the theory that PPS is caused by reactivation of the original polio virus.

Clinical Manifestations and Diagnostic Studies

PPS is manifested by a new onset of joint and muscle weakness, easy fatigability, generalized fatigue, and pain. In uncommon cases, individuals may also exhibit speech, swallowing, and respiratory difficulties. Patients should undergo thorough diagnostic testing to rule out other medical conditions that may produce similar symptoms. Criteria used to establish the diagnosis of PPS include a history of polio in the abortive, nonparalytic, or paralytic forms; recovery from polio; a lengthy period of stability of at least 10 to 20 years' duration; and clinical manifestations of PPS that are not associated with other medical disorders. Disabilities caused by PPS can have a significant effect on the patient's quality of life.

NURSING AND INTERPROFESSIONAL MANAGEMENT POSTPOLIO SYNDROME

Management approaches for PPS are targeted at controlling symptoms, particularly fatigue, weakness, and pain. An interprofessional team approach is essential for management of the patient. The cornerstone of management is lifestyle modification to conserve energy and support performance of activities of daily living.

During the polio epidemic, polio victims were subjected to rigorous therapy to regain muscle function. A particular challenge may be helping the patient understand that aggressive or strenuous therapy to strengthen muscles is now considered counterproductive and that overexertion can worsen fatigue and weakness. It is important to promote pacing of activities to prevent feelings of fatigue. Planning to include rest periods, as well as using assistive devices such as scooters, canes, and wheelchairs may be beneficial. Adaptive equipment can be helpful to patients who experience difficulty with self-care. Other strategies include arranging for a handicapped licence plate or sticker to facilitate parking close to shops and public buildings, shopping on the Internet to avoid walking, and enlisting the support of family and friends to perform necessary tasks. Physiotherapy can support mobility and fitness in view of the patient's limitations. Weight loss interventions should be considered for affected individuals who are overweight or obese.

Effective pain management through both pharmacological and nonpharmacological approaches with the health care provider or pain management team can enable an individual to remain active and achieve a greater sense of well-being. Nonpharmacological measures include massage, relaxation strategies, and guided imagery (see Chapter 12). Protection from the cold can also aid in pain relief since the individual with PPS may be especially sensitive to a cold environment. For affected individuals with speech, swallowing, or respiratory difficulties, it is important to take measures to prevent aspiration, maintain airway patency, and promote optimal nutrition. Nursing interventions for these conditions are similar to those described for patients with GBS and SCI.

Experiencing the re-emergence of symptoms related to polio can have a devastating effect on a patient's psychosocial well-being. Memories of paralysis and the challenges of recovery can cause fear when PPS is diagnosed. The patient may experience anxiety and depression, as well as difficulties with coping. The nurse can assist the individual by actively listening to concerns, providing information about PPS and available resources (e.g., respite care), and referring the patient to support groups or counselling when necessary. Gaining a sense of control through active participation in lifestyle modifications and therapy may improve the patient's ability to cope with PPS.

CASE STUDY

Spinal Cord Injury

Patient Profile: Acute Phase

S. D. (pronouns he\him), 24 years old, is admitted to the emergency department with the diagnosis of a cervical SCI. While swimming at a neighbour's backyard pool, he dove into the shallow end, striking his head on the bottom of the pool. Friends noticed that S. D. did not resurface. They rescued him and brought him to the side of the pool. They maintained neck immobilization until the rescue crews arrived.

Subjective Data

- Is awake and alert
- Has complaints of neck pain
- Is anxious and asking why he is unable to move legs and has weak arms
- Is asking to see family members

Objective Data
Physical Examination

- Weak biceps movement bilaterally
- No triceps movement bilaterally
- Gross elbow movement present bilaterally
- No movement bilaterally in lower extremities
- Decreased sensation from the shoulders down
- Loss of anal sphincter contraction
- BP: 85/50 mm Hg; pulse: 56; respirations: 32 and laboured

CASE STUDY

Spinal Cord Injury—cont'd

Diagnostic Studies
- CT of cervical spine shows subluxation and compression fracture at C5–6
- MRI of cervical spine shows a severe spinal cord compression at C5–6

Interprofessional Care
- Intubated in the emergency department
- Started on mechanical ventilation
- Placed in halo traction on arrival in the CCU
- Further went on to have surgical decompression and stabilization

Discussion Questions: Acute Phase
1. **Priority decision:** What nursing activities would be a priority upon S. D.'s arrival in the CCU?
2. What physiological conditions are causing S. D. to have hypotension and bradycardia?
3. What would the first line of treatment be for S. D.'s hypotension and bradycardia?
4. What signs and symptoms would indicate respiratory distress, and what physiological condition would cause respiratory distress in S. D.'s injury state?
5. What can the nurse do to decrease S. D.'s anxiety?
6. **Priority decision:** Based on the assessment data provided, what are the priority nursing diagnoses or problem statements? Are there any interprofessional issues?

Patient Profile: Rehabilitation Phase
One month after the injury, S. D. is at a local inpatient SCI rehabilitation facility. He has since been extubated and uses a wheelchair to mobilize. He eats three meals a day with assistance and is on a strict bowel and bladder program.

Subjective Data
- Awake and alert but anxious
- Complaining of severe headache, blurred vision, and nausea

Objective Data
Physical Examination
- Flushed and diaphoretic above the level of injury
- No bowel movement for 2 days
- BP: 180/90 mm Hg; pulse: 32 beats/min; respirations: 30 breaths/min and laboured

Discussion Questions: Rehabilitation Phase
1. **Priority decision:** What initial priority nursing interventions would be appropriate?
2. What physiological condition is causing S. D.'s hypertension and bradycardia?
3. Once the health care provider has been notified, what other interventions would be appropriate?
4. **Priority decision:** Based on the assessment data provided, what are the priority nursing diagnoses?
5. **Evidence-informed practice:** S. D. and his family are concerned about the risk for autonomic dysreflexia. What effective strategies to prevent autonomic dysreflexia could the nurse discuss with the patient and family?

(e)volve
Answers are available at http://evolve.elsevier.com/Canada/Lewis/medsurg.

REVIEW QUESTIONS

The number of the question corresponds to the same-numbered objective at the beginning of the chapter.

1. What should the nurse do during assessment of a client with trigeminal neuralgia?
   a. Inspect all aspects of the mouth and teeth.
   b. Lightly palpate the affected side of the face for edema.
   c. Test for temperature and sensation perception on the face.
   d. Ask the client to describe factors that initiate an episode.

2. During routine assessment of a client with GBS, the nurse finds the client to be short of breath. What is the cause of the client's respiratory distress?
   a. Elevated protein levels in the CSF
   b. Immobility resulting from ascending paralysis
   c. Degeneration of motor neurons in the brainstem and the spinal cord
   d. Paralysis ascending to the nerves that stimulate the thoracic area

3. A client is admitted to the CCU with a C7 SCI, and Brown-Séquard syndrome is diagnosed. What would the nurse probably find on physical examination?
   a. Upper extremity weakness only
   b. Complete motor and sensory loss below C7
   c. Loss of position sense and vibration in both lower extremities
   d. Ipsilateral motor loss and contralateral sensory loss below C7

4. A client is admitted to the hospital with SCI after an automobile accident. The nurse recognizes that the pathophysiology of secondary SCI involves which of the following?

   a. Initial infarction of the white matter of the spinal cord
   b. Mechanical transection of the cord by the trauma
   c. Necrotic destruction of the cord from hemorrhage and edema
   d. Release of epinephrine leading to massive vasodilation of spinal cord vessels

5. Goals of rehabilitation for the client with an injury at the C6 level include which of the following? *(Select all that apply.)*
   a. Stand erect with leg brace
   b. Feed self with hand devices
   c. Drive a motorized wheelchair
   d. Assist with transfer activities
   e. Control bowel and bladder function

6. A client with a C7 SCI undergoing rehabilitation tells the nurse he must have the flu because he has a bad headache and nausea. What should the nurse's initial action be?
   a. Call the health care provider.
   b. Check the client's temperature.
   c. Take the client's blood pressure.
   d. Elevate the head of the bed to 90 degrees.

7. For a 65-year-old female client who has lived with a T1 SCI for 20 years, what health teaching information would the nurse emphasize?
   a. A mammogram is needed every 2 years.
   b. Bladder function tends to improve with age.
   c. Heart disease is not common in persons with SCI.
   d. As a person ages, the need to change body position is less important.

8. What is the most common early symptom of a spinal cord tumour?
   a. Urinary incontinence
   b. Back pain that worsens with activity
   c. Paralysis below the level of involvement
   d. Impaired sensation of pain, temperature, and light touch
9. Which of the following descriptions best characterizes PPS?
   a. Autoimmune disease of motor neurons triggered by polio virus
   b. Reactivation of poliomyelitis resulting in acute musculoskeletal disease
   c. Degeneration of enlarged motor neurons many years after poliomyelitis
   d. Disorder characterized by active viral destruction of the upper motor neurons

1. d; 2. d; 3. d; 4. c; 5. b, c, d; 6. c; 7. a; 8. b; 9. c.

Ⓔvolve

For even more review questions, visit http://evolve.elsevier.com/Canada/Lewis/medsurg.

REFERENCES

Ahmed, S. U., Humphreys, S., Rivers, C., et al. (2020). Traumatic spinal cord injuries among Aboriginal and non-Aboriginal populations of Saskatchewan: A prospective outcomes study. *Canadian Journal of Surgery, 63*(3), E315–E320. https://doi.org/10.1503/cjs.012819

Allen, K. J., & Leslie, S. W. (2021). Autonomic dysreflexia. *StatPearls.* https://www.ncbi.nlm.nih.gov/books/NBK482434/

Al-Quliti, K. W. (2015). Update on neuropathic pain treatment for trigeminal neuralgia. The pharmacological and surgical options. *Neurosciences, 20*(2), 107–114. https://doi.org/10.17712/nsj.2015.2.20140501

Ansar, V., & Valadi, N. (2015). Guillain-Barré syndrome. *Primary Care: Clinics in Office Practice, 42*(2), 189–193. https://doi.org/10.1016/j.pop.2015.01.001

Babazadeh, A., Mohseni Afshar, Z., Javanian, M., et al. (2019). Influenza vaccination and Guillain-Barré syndrome: Reality or fear? *Journal of Translational Internal Medicine, 7*(4), 137–142. https://doi.org/10.2478/jtim-2019-0028

Boussios, S., Cooke, D., Hayward, C., et al. (2018). Metastatic spinal cord compression: Unraveling the diagnostic and therapeutic challenges. *International Journal of Cancer Research and Treatment, 38*(9), 4987–4997. https://doi.org/10.21873/anticanres.12817

Chin, L., Mesfin, F., & Dawodu, S. (2018). *Spinal cord injuries.* https://emedicine.medscape.com/article/793582-overview#a4

Consortium for Spinal Cord Medicine. (2016). Prevention of venous thromboembolism in individuals with spinal cord injury: Clinical practice guidelines for health care providers (3rd ed.). *Topics in Spinal Cord Injury Rehabilitation, 22*(3), 209–240. https://doi.org/10.1310/sci2203-209

Dorsett, P., Geraghty, T., Sinnott, A., et al. (2017). Hope, coping and psychosocial adjustment after spinal cord injury. *Spinal Cord Series and Cases, 3*, 17046. https://doi.org/10.1038/scsandc.2017.46

Eviston, T., Croxson, G., Kennedy, P., et al. (2015). Bell's palsy: Aetiology, clinical features and multidisciplinary care. *Journal of Neurology, Neurosurgery, and Psychiatry, 86*(12), 1356–1361. https://doi.org/10.1136/jnnp-2014-309563

Giurleo, C., McIntyre, A., Kras-Dupuis, A., et al. (2020). Addressing the elephant in the room: Integrating sexual health practice in spinal cord injury rehabilitation. *Disability and Rehabilitation.* https://doi.org/10.1080/09638288.2020.1856949

Government of Canada. (2014). *Tetanus toxoid: Canadian immunization guide.* https://www.canada.ca/en/public-health/services/publications/healthy-living/canadian-immunization-guide-part-4-active-vaccines/page-22-tetanus-toxoid.html

Guy, S. D., Mehta, S., Casalino, A., et al. (2016). The CanPain SCI clinical practice guidelines for rehabilitation management of neuropathic pain after spinal cord: Recommendations for treatment. *Spinal Cord, 54*, S14–S23. https://doi.org/10.1038/sc.2016.90

Houghton, P. E., Campbell, K. E., & Panel, C. P. G. (2013). *Canadian best practice guidelines for the prevention and management of pressure ulcers in people with spinal cord injury: A resource handbook for clinicians.* https://onf.org/wp-content/uploads/2019/04/Pressure_Ulcers_Best_Practice_Guideline_Final_web4.pdf

Ibrahim, E., Lynne, C., & Brackett, N. (2016). Male fertility following spinal cord injury: An update. *Andrology, 4*(1), 13–26. https://doi.org/10.1111/andr.12119

Jung, J. K. H., & Skinner, K. (2017). Foodborne and waterborne illness among Canadian Indigenous populations: A scoping review. *Canada Communicable Disease Report (CCDR), 43*(1), 7–13. https://doi.org/10.14745/ccdr.v43i01a02

Kedlaya, D. (2021). *Postpolio syndrome.* https://emedicine.medscape.com/article/306920-overview

Keskinruzgar, A., Yavuz, Y., Koparal, M., et al. (2019). Evaluation of biochemical variables in patients with trigeminal neuralgia. *British Journal of Oral and Maxillofacial Surgery, 57*(1), 72–75. https://doi.org/10.1016/j.bjoms.2018.11.012

Mao, G. (2021). *Spinal trauma.* Merck Manual. https://www.merckmanuals.com/en-ca/professional/injuries-poisoning/spinal-trauma/spinal-trauma?query=Injuries%20of%20the%20Spinal%20Cord%20and%20Vertebrae

Marra, C. M. (2015). Neurosyphilis. *Neuroinfectious Diseases, 21*(6), 1714–1728. https://doi.org/10.1212/CON.0000000000000250

McKinney, D. (2021). *Prevention of thromboembolism in spinal cord injury.* https://emedicine.medscape.com/article/322897-overview

Ministry of Health and Long-Term Care. (2019). *Infectious disease protocol. Appendix A: Disease-specific chapters. Botulism.* https://www.health.gov.on.ca/en/pro/programs/publichealth/oph_standards/docs/botulism_chapter.pdf

National Institute of Neurological Disorders and Stroke [NINDS]. (2021). *Trigeminal neuralgia fact sheet.* https://www.ninds.nih.gov/disorders/patient-caregiver-education/fact-sheets/trigeminal-neuralgia-fact-sheet

Population and Public Health Division. (2017). *Botulism guide for health care professionals.* https://www.health.gov.on.ca/en/pro/publications/disease/docs/botulism.pdf

Royal College of Nursing. (2021). *Traction: Principles and application.* https://www.rcn.org.uk/professional-development/publications/traction-principles-and-application-uk-pub-009-816

Rubin, M. (2020). Guillain-Barre syndrome. *Merck Manual* https://www.merckmanuals.com/en-ca/professional/neurologic-disorders/peripheral-nervous-system-and-motor-unit-disorders/guillain-barr%C3%A9-syndrome-gbs

Sharwood, L., Dhaliwal, S., Ball, J., et al. (2018). Emergency and acute care management of traumatic spinal cord injury: A survey of current practice among senior clinicians across Australia. *BMC Emergency Medicine, 18*(57), 1–8. https://doi.org/10.1186/s12873-018-0207-0

Spinal Cord Injury BC. (2021). *About spinal cord injury.* https://sci-bc.ca/info-centre/spinal-cord-injury/

Spinal Outreach Team. (2017). *The impact of a spinal cord injury on pregnancy, labour and delivery: What you need to know.* Queensland Health https://www.health.qld.gov.au/__data/assets/pdf_file/0027/425772/pregnancy-sci.pdf

Taylor, D. (2021). *Bell palsy clinical presentation.* https://emedicine.medscape.com/article/1146903-clinical#b3

Top, K., Desai, S., Moore, D., et al. (2015). Guillain–Barré syndrome after immunization in Canadian children (1996–2012). *The Pediatric Infectious Disease Journal, 34*(12), 1411–1413. https://doi.org/10.1097/INF.0000000000000903

Trigeminal Neuralgia Association of Canada (TNAC). (2015). *About trigeminal neuralgia.* http://tnac.org/tnac/about-us/

Vaillancourt, C., Charette, M., Taljaard, M., et al. (2020). Pragmatic strategy empowering paramedics to assess low-risk trauma patients with the Canadian C-Spine Rule and selectively transport them without immobilization: Protocol for a stepped-wedge cluster randomized trial. *JMIR Research Protocol, 9*(6), e16966. https://doi.org/10.2196/16966

Welch-West, P., Faltynek, P., Harnett, A., et al. (2019). Dysphagia, aspiration, and nutritional interventions for patients with acquired brain injury. In R. Teasell, N. Cullen, S. Marshall, et al. (Eds.), *Evidence-based review of moderate to severe acquired brain injury* (pp. 1–65) Version 13.0.

Willison, H., Jacobs, B. C., & van Doorn, P. A. (2016). Guillain-Barré syndrome. *The Lancet, 388*(10045), 717–727. https://doi.org/10.1016/S0140-6736(16)00339-1

Witiw, C. D., & Fehlings, M. G. (2015). Acute spinal cord injury. *Journal of Spinal Disorders & Techniques, 28*(6), 202–210. https://doi.org/10.1097/BSD.0000000000000287

RESOURCES

Canadian Association of Neuroscience Nurses (CANN)
https://www.cann.ca
Canadian Spinal Research Organization (CSRO)
https://www.csro.com
Canadian Spine Society
https://spinecanada.org/
Parachute Canada
https://parachutecanada.org
Rick Hansen Foundation
https://www.rickhansen.com/
SCI Action Canada Lab
https://sciactioncanada.ok.ubc.ca/
Spinal Cord Injury Alberta
https://www.sci-ab.ca
Spinal Cord Injury Canada
https://sci-can.ca
Spinal Cord Injury Ontario
https://www.sciontario.org
Spinal Cord Injury Prince Edward Island
https://www.sci-pei.ca
Spinal Cord Injury Research Evidence (SCIRE)
https://www.scireproject.com
Trigeminal Neuralgia Association of Canada (TNAC)
https://www.tnac.org

Academy of Spinal Cord Injury Professionals
https://test.academyscipro.org/aboutscin
Christopher and Dana Reeve Foundation
https://www.christopherreeve.org/
Guillain-Barré Syndrome–Chronic Inflammatory Demyelinating Polyneuropathy (GBS/CIDP) Foundation International
https://gbs-cidp.org
National Institute of Neurological Disorders and Stroke (NINDS)
https://www.ninds.nih.gov
National Rehabilitation Information Center (NARIC)
https://www.naric.com

⊘volve

For additional Internet resources, see the website for this book at http://evolve.elsevier.com/Canada/Lewis/medsurg.

Nursing Assessment
Musculoskeletal System

Danielle L. Byrne
Originating US chapter by Colleen Walsh

⊖volve WEBSITE

http://evolve.elsevier.com/Canada/Lewis/medsurg

- Review Questions (Online Only)
- Key Points
- Answer Guidelines for Case Study

- Supporting Media—Animations:
  - Classification of Joints: Condyloid Joint
  - Classification of Joints: Gliding Joint—Hand
  - Classification of Joints: Hinge Joint

- Conceptual Care Map Creator
- Audio Glossary
- Content Updates

LEARNING OBJECTIVES

1. Describe the gross anatomical and microscopic composition of bone.
2. Explain the classification system of joints and movements at diarthrodial joints.
3. Describe the types and structure of muscle tissue.
4. Describe the functions of cartilage, muscles, ligaments, tendons, fascia, and bursae.
5. Describe age-related changes in the musculoskeletal system and differences in assessment findings.
6. Identify the significant subjective and objective data related to the musculoskeletal system that should be obtained from a patient.
7. Describe the appropriate techniques used in the physical assessment of the musculoskeletal system.
8. Differentiate normal from abnormal findings of a physical assessment of the musculoskeletal system.
9. Describe the purpose, significance of results, and nursing responsibilities related to diagnostic studies of the musculoskeletal system.

KEY TERMS

ankylosis
arthrocentesis
arthroscopy
contracture

crepitation
isometric contractions
isotonic contractions
kyphosis

lordosis
scoliosis

The unique structures of the musculoskeletal system allow human beings to complete complex movements. The dexterity of the upper extremities enables an individual to perform complicated technical tasks, whereas stronger lower extremities enable mobility for varied activities. The musculoskeletal system is composed of voluntary muscle and five types of connective tissue: bones, cartilage, ligaments, tendons, and fascia (Patton & Thibodeau, 2020). Resilient bone and cartilage absorb energy from any impact, minimizing the risk of injury to other body structures. However, this characteristic ability makes the musculoskeletal system itself particularly vulnerable to injury from external forces. Any damage to bone and related soft tissues can cause functional disruption for an individual. Deformity, alteration in body image, alteration in mobility, pain, or permanent disability may result from musculoskeletal injury.

STRUCTURES AND FUNCTIONS OF THE MUSCULOSKELETAL SYSTEM

Bone

Function. The main functions of bone are support, movement, protection of the body's internal structures, blood cell production, and mineral storage (Huether et al., 2018). Bones provide the supporting framework that keeps the body from collapsing and allow the body to bear weight. Bones serve as a point of attachment for muscles, which are connected to bones by tendons. Bones act as a lever for muscles, and movement occurs as a result of muscle contractions applied to these levers. Bones also protect underlying vital organs and tissues. For example, the skull encloses the brain, the vertebrae surround the spinal cord, and the rib cage covers the lungs and heart. Bones contain hematopoietic tissue for the production of red and white blood cells. Bones also serve as a site for storage of inorganic minerals such as calcium and phosphorus.

Bone is a dynamic tissue that continually changes form and composition. It contains both organic material (i.e., collagen) and inorganic material (i.e., calcium, phosphate). The internal and external growth and remodelling of bone are ongoing processes.

Microscopic Structure. Bone is classified according to structure as *cortical* (compact and dense) or *cancellous* (spongy). In *cortical bone*, cylinder-shaped structural units called *osteons* (Haversian systems) fit closely together to form a dense bone structure (Figure 64.1, *A*). Within the systems, the Haversian canals run parallel to the bone's long axis and contain the blood vessels that travel to the bone's interior from the periosteum.

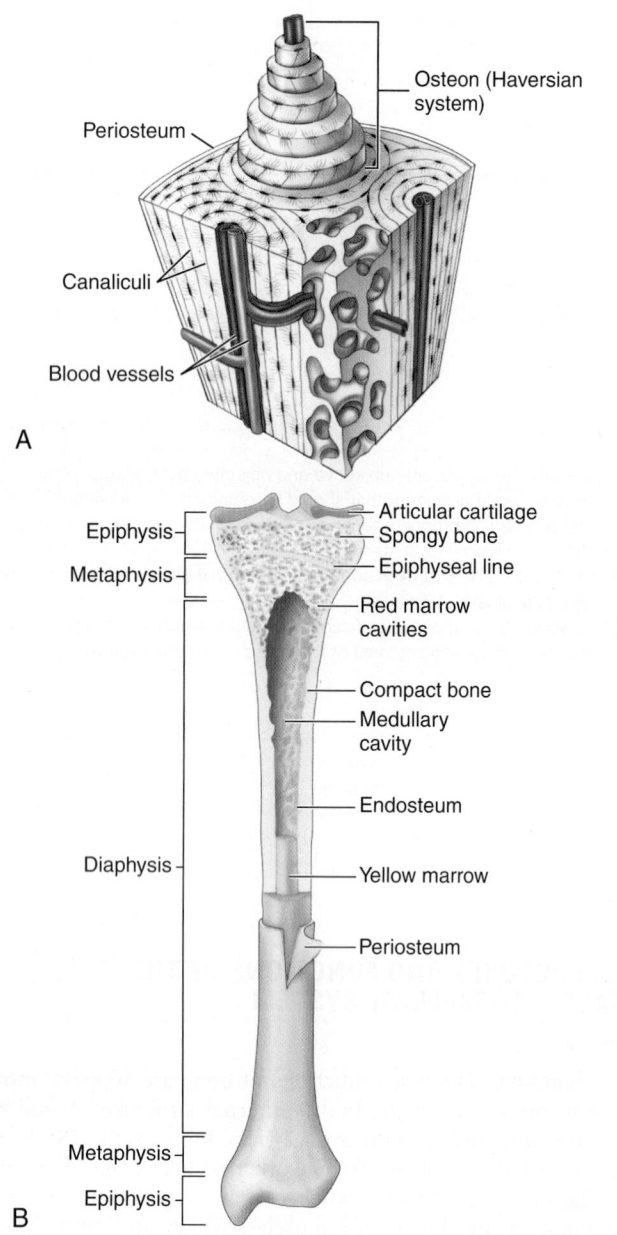

FIG. 64.1 Illustrations of bone structure. **A,** Cortical (compact) bone showing numerous structural units called *osteons.* **B,** Anatomy of a long bone (tibia), showing cancellous and compact bone. Sources: *A,* Herlihy, B. (2011). *The human body in health and illness* (4th ed.). Philadelphia: Saunders. *B,* Patton, K. T., & Thibodeau, G. A. (2020). *Structure & function of the body* (16th ed., p. 120, Figure 7-1). Elsevier.

Surrounding each *osteon* are concentric rings known as *lamellae,* which characterize mature bone. Smaller canals *(canaliculi)* extend from the Haversian canals to the *lacunae,* where mature bone cells are embedded. Cancellous (spongy) bone lacks the organized structure of cortical (compact) bone. The lamellae are arranged not in concentric rings but rather along the lines of maximum stress placed on the bone. Cancellous bone tissue is filled with red or yellow marrow, and blood reaches the bone cells by passing through spaces in the marrow.

The three types of bone cells are osteoblasts, osteocytes, and osteoclasts (Huether et al., 2018). *Osteoblasts* synthesize organic bone matrix (collagen) and are the basic bone-forming cells. *Osteocytes* are the mature bone cells. *Osteoclasts* participate in bone remodelling by assisting in the breakdown of bone tissue. *Bone remodelling* is the removal of old bone by osteoclasts *(resorption)* and the deposition of new bone by osteoblasts *(ossification).* The inner layer of bone is primarily made up of osteoblasts with a few osteoclasts.

Gross Structure. The anatomical structure of bone is best represented by a typical long bone such as the tibia (see Figure 64.1, *B*). Each long bone consists of the epiphysis, the diaphysis, and the metaphysis. The *epiphysis,* the widened area found at each end of a long bone, is composed primarily of cancellous bone. The width of the epiphysis allows for greater weight distribution and provides stability for the joint. The epiphysis is also the location of muscle attachment. Articular cartilage covers the ends of the epiphysis to provide a smooth surface for joint movement. The *diaphysis* is the main shaft of the bone. It provides structural support and is composed of compact bone. The tubular structure of the diaphysis allows it to more easily withstand bending and twisting forces. The *metaphysis* is the flared area between the epiphysis and the diaphysis. Like the epiphysis, it is composed of cancellous bone. The *epiphyseal plate,* or growth plate, is the cartilaginous area between the epiphysis and the metaphysis. It actively produces bone to allow longitudinal growth in children. Injury to the epiphyseal plate in a growing child can lead to development of a shorter extremity, which can cause significant functional problems. In the adult, the metaphysis and the epiphysis become joined as this plate hardens to become mature bone.

The *periosteum* is composed of fibrous connective tissue that covers the bone. Tiny blood vessels penetrate the periosteum to provide nutrition to underlying bone. Musculotendinous fibres anchor to the outer layer of the periosteum. The inner layer of the periosteum is attached to the bone by bundles of collagen. No periosteum exists on the articular surfaces of long bones. These bone ends are covered by articular cartilage.

The *medullary* (marrow) cavity is in the centre of the diaphysis and contains either red or yellow bone marrow (Patton & Thibodeau, 2020). In a growing child, red bone marrow is actively involved in blood cell production (hematopoiesis). In the adult, the medullary cavity of long bones contains yellow bone marrow, which is mainly adipose tissue. Yellow marrow is involved in hematopoiesis only in times of great blood cell need. In adults, red marrow is found mainly in the flat bones, such as the pelvis, skull, sternum, cranium, ribs, vertebrae, and scapulae and in the cancellous (spongy) material at the epiphyseal ends of long bones such as the femur and the humerus.

Types. The skeleton consists of 206 bones, which are classified according to shape as long, short, flat, or irregular.

Long bones are characterized by a central shaft (diaphysis) and two widened ends (epiphyses) (see Figure 64.1, *B*).

Examples include the femur, humerus, and radius. *Short bones* are composed of cancellous bone covered by a thin layer of compact bone. Examples include the carpals in the hand and the tarsals in the foot.

Flat bones have two layers of compact bone separated by a layer of cancellous bone. Examples include the ribs, skull, scapula, and sternum. The spaces in the cancellous bone contain bone marrow. *Irregular bones* appear in a variety of shapes and sizes. Examples include the vertebrae, sacrum, and ear ossicles.

Joints

A *joint* (articulation) is a place where the ends of two bones are in proximity and move in relation to each other. Joints are classified according to the degree of movement that they allow.

The most common joint is the freely movable *diarthrodial* (synovial) type. Each joint is enclosed in a capsule of fibrous connective tissue that joins the two bones together to form a cavity (Figure 64.2). The capsule is lined by a synovial membrane, which secretes thick synovial fluid to lubricate the joint and reduce friction. The end of each bone is covered with articular (hyaline) cartilage. Supporting structures (i.e., ligaments, tendons) reinforce the joint capsule and provide limits to joint movement (Patton & Thibodeau, 2020). Types of diarthrodial joints are shown in Figure 64.3.

Cartilage

Cartilage is a rigid connective tissue that serves as a support for soft tissue and provides the articular surface for joint movement. It protects underlying tissues. The cartilage in the epiphyseal plate is also involved in the growth of long bones before physical maturity is reached. Because articular cartilage is relatively avascular, it must receive nourishment by the diffusion of material from the synovial fluid. The lack of a direct blood supply contributes to the slow metabolism of cartilage cells, which is the reason why cartilage tissue heals slowly.

Hyaline cartilage, containing a moderate amount of collagen fibres, is the most common type of cartilage. It is found in the trachea, bronchi, nose, epiphyseal plate, and articular surfaces of bones. *Elastic cartilage*, which contains both collagen and elastic fibres, is more flexible than hyaline cartilage. It is found in the ear, epiglottis, and larynx. *Fibrocartilage* consists mostly of collagen fibres and is a tough tissue that often functions as a shock absorber. It is found between the vertebral discs and also forms a protective cushion between the bones of the pelvic girdle, knee, and shoulder.

Muscle

Types. The three types of muscle tissue are *cardiac* (striated, involuntary), *smooth* (nonstriated, involuntary), and *skeletal* (striated, voluntary) muscle. Cardiac muscle is found in the heart. Its spontaneous contractions propel blood through the circulatory system. Smooth muscle occurs in the walls of hollow structures such as airways, arteries, gastrointestinal tract, urinary bladder, and uterus. Smooth muscle contraction is modulated by neuronal and hormonal influences. Skeletal muscle, which requires neuronal stimulation for contraction, accounts for about half of a human being's body weight. It is the focus of the following discussion.

Structure. The skeletal muscle is enclosed by the *epimysium,* a continuous layer of deep fascia. The epimysium helps muscles slide over nearby structures. Connective tissue surrounding and extending into the muscle can be subdivided into fibre bundles, or *fasciculi.* These bundles are covered by perimysium and an innermost connective tissue layer called the *endomysium* that surrounds each fibre (Figure 64.4).

The structural unit of muscle is the muscle cell or muscle fibre, which is highly specialized for contraction. Skeletal muscle fibres are long, multinucleated cylinders that contain many mitochondria to support their high metabolic activity. Muscle fibres are composed of *myofibrils,* which in turn are made up of contractile filaments (protein).

The *sarcomere* is the contractile unit of the myofibrils (Huether et al., 2018). Each sarcomere consists of *myosin* (thick) filaments and *actin* (thin) filaments. The arrangement of the thick and thin filaments accounts for the characteristic banding of muscle when it is seen under a microscope. Muscle contraction occurs as thick and thin filaments slide past each other, causing the sarcomeres to shorten.

Contractions. Skeletal muscle contractions enable posture maintenance, movement, and facial expressions. Isometric contractions increase the tension within a muscle but do not produce movement. Repeated isometric contractions make muscles grow larger and stronger. Isotonic contractions shorten a muscle to produce movement. Most contractions are a combination of tension generation (isometric) and shortening (isotonic). Muscle atrophy (wasting of muscle and subsequent decrease in its size) occurs with the absence of contraction that results from immobility, whereas increased muscular activity leads to *hypertrophy* (increase in size).

Skeletal muscle fibres are divided into two groups according to the type of activity they demonstrate. *Slow-twitch muscle fibres* support prolonged muscle activity such as marathon running. Because they also support the body against gravity, they assist in posture maintenance. *Fast-twitch muscle fibres* are used for rapid muscle contraction required for activities such as blinking the eye, jumping, or sprinting. Fast-twitch fibres tend to tire more quickly than slow-twitch fibres.

Neuromuscular Junction. Skeletal muscle fibres require a nerve impulse to contract. A nerve fibre and the skeletal muscle fibres it stimulates are called a *motor end plate*. The junction

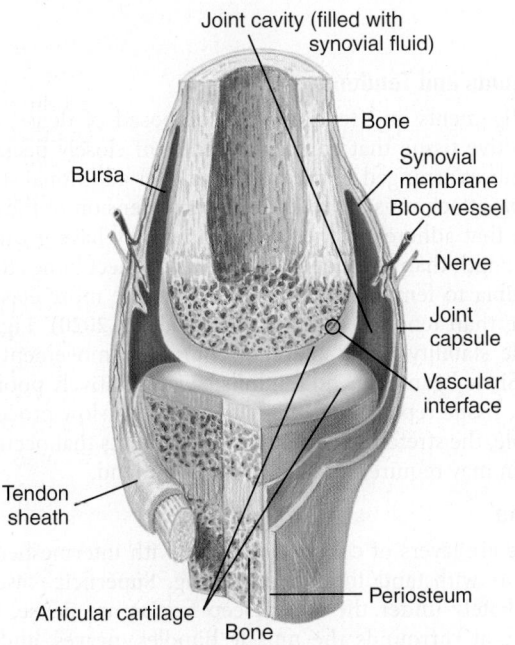

Joint cavity (filled with synovial fluid)

Bone

Bursa

Synovial membrane

Blood vessel

Nerve

Joint capsule

Vascular interface

Tendon sheath

Articular cartilage

Bone

Periosteum

FIG. 64.2 Structure of a diarthrodial (synovial) joint.

Joint	Movement	Examples	Illustration
Hinge joint	Flexion, extension	Elbow joint (shown), interphalangeal joints, knee joint	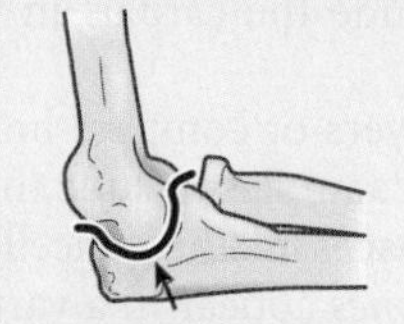
Ball and socket (spheroidal)	Flexion, extension; adduction, abduction; circumduction	Shoulder (shown), hip	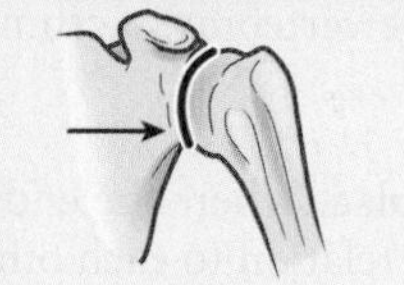
Pivot (rotary)	Rotation	Atlas-axis, proximal radioulnar joint (shown)	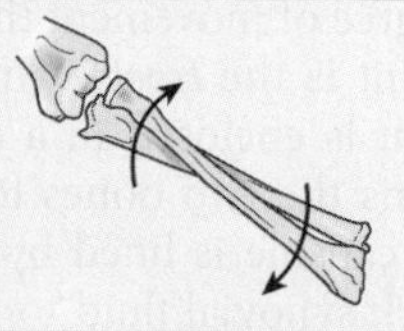
Condyloid	Flexion, extension; abduction, adduction; circumduction	Wrist joint (between radial and carpals) (shown)	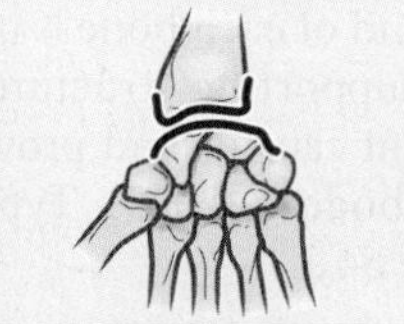
Saddle	Flexion, extension; abduction, adduction; circumduction, thumb-finger opposition	Carpometacarpal joint of thumb (shown)	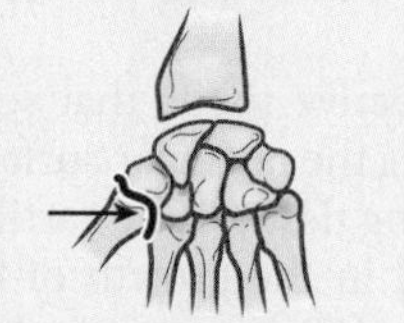
Gliding	One surface moves over another surface	Between tarsal bones, sacroiliac joint, between articular processes of vertebrae, between carpal bones (shown)	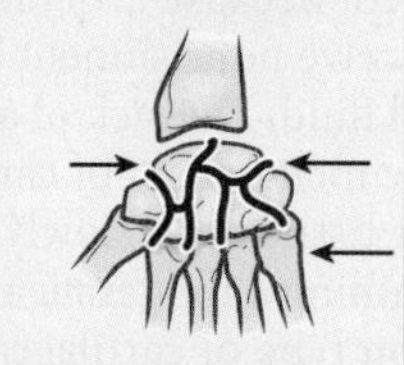

FIG. 64.3 Types of diarthrodial (synovial) joints.

between the axon of the nerve cell and the adjacent muscle cell is called the *myoneural* or *neuromuscular junction* (Figure 64.5).

Acetylcholine is released from the motor end plate of the neuron and diffuses across the neuromuscular junction to bind with receptors on the muscle fibre. In response to this stimulation, the sarcoplasmic reticulum releases calcium ions into the cytoplasm, which triggers the contraction in the myofibrils. When calcium is low, *tetany* (involuntary contractions of skeletal muscle) can occur.

Energy Source. The direct energy source for muscle fibre contractions is adenosine triphosphate (ATP). ATP is synthesized by cellular oxidative metabolism in numerous mitochondria located close to the myofibrils. It is rapidly depleted through conversion to adenosine diphosphate and must be rephosphorylated. Phosphocreatine provides a rapid source for the resynthesis of ATP, but it is in turn converted to creatine and must be recharged. Glycolysis can serve as a source of ATP when the oxygen supply is inadequate for the metabolic needs of the muscle tissue. Glucose is broken down to pyruvic acid, which can be further converted to lactic acid to make more oxygen available. An accumulation of lactic acid in tissues leads to fatigue and pain.

Ligaments and Tendons

Both ligaments and tendons are composed of dense, fibrous connective tissue that contains bundles of closely packed collagen fibres arranged in the same plane for additional strength. *Tendons* attach muscles to bones as an extension of the muscle sheath that adheres to the periosteum. They have greater tensile strength than ligaments. *Ligaments* connect bones to bones (e.g., tibia to femur at knee joint). They are more elastic and flexible than tendons (Patton & Thibodeau, 2020). Ligaments provide stability while enabling controlled movement at the joint. Since ligaments and tendons have a relatively poor blood supply, tissue repair after injury to them is a slow process. For example, the stretching or tearing of ligaments that occurs with a sprain may require weeks to months to mend.

Fasciae

Fasciae are layers of connective tissue with intermeshed fibres that can withstand limited stretching. Superficial fasciae lie immediately under the skin. Deep fasciae are dense, fibrous tissue that surrounds the muscle bundles, nerves, and blood vessels. Deep fasciae also enclose individual muscles, allowing them to act independently and to glide over each other during contraction. In addition, they provide strength to muscle tissues.

Bursae

Bursae are small sacs of connective tissue lined with synovial membrane and containing synovial fluid. They are typically located at bony prominences or joints to relieve pressure and prevent friction between moving parts (Jarvis et al., 2019). For example, bursae are found between the patella and the skin *(prepatellar bursa)* and between the greater trochanter of the proximal femur and the skin *(trochanteric bursa). Bursitis* is an inflammation of a bursa sac.

AGE-RELATED CONSIDERATIONS

THE MUSCULOSKELETAL SYSTEM

Many of the functional difficulties experienced by older people are related to changes in the musculoskeletal system. Although some changes begin in early adulthood, obvious signs of musculoskeletal impairment may not appear until later adulthood. Alterations may affect an older person's ability to complete self-care tasks and pursue other usual activities. Effects of musculoskeletal changes may range from mild discomfort and decreased ability to perform activities of daily living to severe, chronic pain and immobility. The risk for falls also increases in older persons as a result of a loss of strength, change in balance, and change in *proprioception* (awareness of self in relation to the environment).

The bone remodelling process changes as adults age. Bone resorption increases and bone formation decreases; these events cause a loss of bone density, contributing to development of osteopenia and osteoporosis (see Chapter 66). Muscle mass and strength also decrease with aging. Tendons and ligaments become less flexible, and joints and limbs become more rigid. Joints in aging adults are also more likely to be affected by osteoarthritis (see Chapter 67).

In addition to the usual musculoskeletal assessment with an emphasis on functional and activity status, the nurse should determine the effect of age-related musculoskeletal changes on an older patient's psychosocial well-being and quality of life.

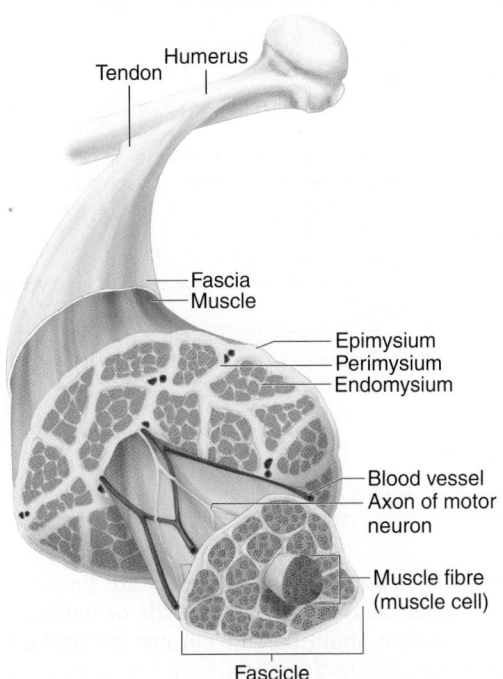

FIG. 64.4 Structure of a muscle. Source: Patton, K. T., Thibodeau, G. A., & Douglas, M. M. (2012). *Essentials of anatomy and physiology* (p. 188, Figure 10-1). Mosby.

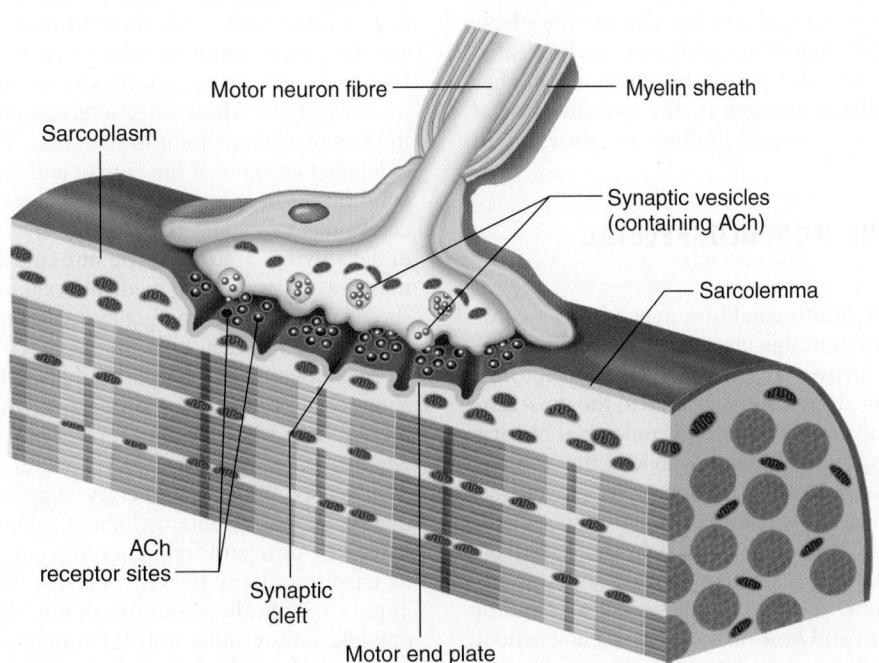

FIG. 64.5 Neuromuscular junction. Illustration of a side view of the neuromuscular junction. Note how the distal end of a motor neuron fibre forms a synapse, or "chemical junction," with an adjacent muscle fibre. Neurotransmitter molecules (specifically, acetylcholine [ACh]) are released from the neuron's synaptic vesicles and diffuse across the synaptic cleft. There they stimulate receptors in the motor end plate region of the sarcolemma. Source: Patton, K. T., & Thibodeau, G. A. (2013). *Anatomy and physiology* (8th ed., p. 353, Figure 12-7). Mosby.

TABLE 64.1   AGE-RELATED DIFFERENCES IN ASSESSMENT

Musculoskeletal System

Changes	Differences in Assessment Findings
Muscle	
Decreased number and diameter of muscle cells, replacement of muscle cells by fibrous connective tissue	Decreased muscle strength and bulk, abdominal protrusion, flabby muscle
Loss of elasticity in ligaments and cartilage	Decreased fine motor dexterity, decreased agility
Reduced ability to store glycogen; decreased ability to release glycogen as quick energy during stress	Slowed reaction times and reflexes as a result of slowing of impulse conduction along motor units; earlier fatigue with activity
Joints	
Increased risk for cartilage disruption that contributes to direct contact between bone ends and overgrowth of bone around joint margins	Joint stiffness, possible crepitation on movement; pain with motion, weight bearing, or both
Loss of water from discs between vertebrae; narrowing of intervertebral spaces	Loss of height from disc compression; posture change
Bone	
Decrease in bone density	Loss of height from vertebral compression, back pain; deformity such as kyphosis (dowager's hump) caused by vertebral compression

Older persons can use various strategies to prevent musculoskeletal conditions (see Chapter 65, Table 65.7).

Diseases such as osteoarthritis and osteoporosis are not the normal consequences of growing old; rather, they are the effects of disease in an aging adult. Symptoms of disease can be treated in many cases, helping the older person to return to a higher functional level. Age-related changes in the musculoskeletal system and differences in assessment findings are presented in Table 64.1.

ASSESSMENT OF THE MUSCULOSKELETAL SYSTEM

Correct diagnosis of any health condition depends on a complete patient history and a thorough physical examination. Musculoskeletal assessment focuses on good analyses of symptoms, functional assessment, medical history specific to the musculoskeletal system, family history, and personal and social history. The most common symptoms of musculoskeletal impairment include pain, weakness, deformity, limitation of movement, stiffness, and joint crepitation (described later in Table 64.6). Neurovascular structures are often affected by musculoskeletal conditions, and muscular disorders may be manifestations of neurological conditions. A neurological system assessment (discussed in Chapter 58) and head-to-toe physical assessment are often conducted simultaneously.

Subjective Data

Important Health Information. Appropriate questions to ask during a musculoskeletal assessment are listed in Table 64.2.

CASE STUDY

Patient Introduction

T. K. (pronouns he/him) is a 78-year-old brought to the emergency department by ambulance after a fall on a patch of ice outside his home. The patient was outside in the cold for 2 hours before neighbours heard his calls for help. T. K. is accompanied by his partner, who was asleep when the fall occurred. The patient is pale, diaphoretic, and reporting excruciating pain in his left hip. The paramedics applied O_2 at 2 L via nasal cannula.

Critical Thinking

Throughout this assessment chapter, think about T. K.'s symptoms with the following questions in mind:

1. What is the most likely cause for T. K.'s acute hip pain?
2. What type of assessment would be most appropriate to perform: comprehensive, focused, or emergency? What should the nurse's priority assessment(s) be?
3. What questions should the nurse ask T. K.?
4. What should be included in the physical assessment? What would the nurse be looking for?
5. What diagnostic studies might be ordered?

See Case Study: Subjective Data, Case Study: Objective Data: Physical Examination, and Case Study: Diagnostic Studies for more information on T. K.

evolve

Answers available at http://evolve.elsevier.com/Canada/Lewis/medsurg.

Past Health History. Certain illnesses are known to affect the musculoskeletal system either directly or indirectly. Questioning the patient about past or chronic medical conditions can uncover conditions associated with low bone density (e.g., rickets, osteomalacia, parathyroid problems, diabetes mellitus [DM], systemic lupus erythematosus [SLE]); neuromuscular disabilities (e.g., poliomyelitis); joint injury, pain, or inflammation (e.g., hemophilia, gout, psoriasis, SLE); and osteomyelitis (e.g., tuberculosis, DM, fungal infections). The nurse should ask the patient about possible sources of a secondary bacterial infection, such as the ears, tonsils, teeth, sinuses, lungs, or genitourinary tract. These infections can enter the bones, resulting in osteomyelitis or joint destruction. The nurse should obtain a detailed account of the course and treatment of any of these conditions. In addition, past or developing musculoskeletal conditions can affect the patient's overall health and activities of daily living. Trauma to the musculoskeletal system is a common reason for seeking medical evaluation; therefore, the nurse should review past emergency treatment records for any musculoskeletal injuries.

Medications. The nurse should carefully question the patient about use of prescription drugs, over-the-counter drugs, herbal products, and nutritional supplements (especially calcium and vitamin D; refer to Chapter 12, Tables 12.5 and 12.6, for commonly used herbs and dietary supplements). Detailed information should be obtained about each treatment, including its name, the dose and frequency, the length of time it was taken, its effects, and any possible adverse effects. The nurse should inquire specifically about use of any skeletal muscle relaxants, opioids, nonsteroidal anti-inflammatory drugs, and systemic and topical corticosteroids. A patient who has taken anti-inflammatory drugs should be questioned about gastrointestinal distress or signs of bleeding.

In addition to drugs taken for treatment of a musculoskeletal condition, the patient should be questioned about medications

TABLE 64.2 HEALTH HISTORY

Musculoskeletal System: Questions for Obtaining Subjective Data

Joints
- Do you have any problems with your joints?*
- Do you have any pain?* (If so, ask patient to describe location, quality, severity, onset, timing, frequency; aggravating and relieving factors; refer to Chapter 10 for pain assessment.)
- Is the joint pain associated with fever, recent infection, trauma, or repetitive activity?*
- Have you noticed any stiffness, swelling, heat, or redness in your joints?*
- Do you have any limitations in movement or function of any joint?* Which activities give you difficulties?

Muscles
- Do you have any problems with your muscles (pain, cramping)?* Is the pain widespread and associated with fatigue?
- Do you have any pain in your calf muscles?* With walking? Does it go away with rest?
- Are your muscle aches associated with fever, chills, or the "flu"?
- Do you have any muscular weakness?* Where? How long have you noticed the weakness? Do the muscles look smaller there?

Bones
- Do you have any bone pain?* Is it affected by movement? How do you manage the pain?
- Do you have any deformity of any bone or joint? What is the cause? Does it affect range of motion?*
- Have any accidents or trauma ever affected your bones or joints? When? What was the treatment? Have any ongoing limitations resulted?*

Functional Assessment (Activities of Daily Living)
- Do your joint, muscle, or bone conditions limit any of your usual daily activities?*
- Bathing: getting in and out of tub, turning faucets
- Toileting: voiding, defecating, getting on or off toilet, wiping self

- Dressing: fastening buttons, zippers, pulling clothes over head, pulling up pants or skirt, tying shoes
- Grooming: shaving, brushing teeth, fixing hair, applying makeup
- Eating: preparing meals, pouring liquids, cutting up foods, bringing food to mouth, drinking
- Mobility: walking up and down stairs, getting in and out of bed, getting out of the house
- Communicating: talking, using phone, writing

Self-Care Behaviours
- Are there any occupational hazards that could affect your muscles and joints? Does your work involve heavy lifting or repetitive motion?*
- Do you use any mechanical assistive devices or prosthetic or orthotic devices?*
- Describe your exercise pattern (frequency, warm-up, type of exercise, any pain).
- Have you had any recent weight gain or loss?* What is your usual daily diet? What dietary supplements do you take? (Ask specifically about calcium, vitamin D supplements, and herbal products.) Are you taking any medications for the musculoskeletal system (anti-inflammatory, pain reliever)?*
- How do you deal with problems (such as pain or immobility) that have resulted from your musculoskeletal condition?
- Has your illness affected your interaction with friends, family, or the way you view yourself?

Additional History for the Aging Adult
- Have you noticed any change in strength or weakness over the past weeks or months?*
- Have you been falling or stumbling more often over the past weeks or months?*
- Do you use any mobility aids to help you get around (cane, walker)?*

*If yes, ask patient to describe.
Source: Based on Jarvis, C., Browne, A. J., MacDonald-Jenkins, J., et al. (2019). *Physical examination & health assessment* (3rd Canadian ed., pp. 636–638). Elsevier Inc.

🧬 GENETICS IN CLINICAL PRACTICE

Autoimmune Diseases
- Many autoimmune diseases of the musculoskeletal system have a genetic basis involving human leukocyte antigens.
- Autoimmune diseases include ankylosing spondylitis, rheumatoid arthritis, and systemic lupus erythematosus (see in Chapter 67).

Osteoporosis
- Genetic factors contribute to osteoporosis by influencing not only bone mineral density but also bone size, bone quality, and bone turnover.

Osteoarthritis, Gout, and Scoliosis
- A genetic predisposition is a contributing risk factor in all these diseases.

Muscular Dystrophy
- The most common types of muscular dystrophy are X-linked recessive disorders.

  The nurse should obtain a family history related to rheumatoid arthritis, systemic lupus erythematosus, ankylosing spondylitis, osteoarthritis, gout, osteoporosis, and scoliosis because a patient may have a genetic predisposition to these or other musculoskeletal disorders.

that can have detrimental effects on this system. Such medications and their potential adverse effects include anticonvulsant medications (osteomalacia), phenothiazines (gait disturbances), corticosteroids (avascular necrosis, decreased bone and muscle mass), and potassium-depleting diuretics (muscle cramps and weakness). Women should be questioned about their menstrual history; episodes of amenorrhea can contribute to early development of osteoporosis. The nurse should ask postmenopausal women about their use of hormone therapy.

Surgery or Other Treatments. Information about past hospitalizations related to a musculoskeletal condition should be obtained. The nurse documents the reason for hospitalization, the date and the duration, and the treatment, including ongoing rehabilitation. The nurse should obtain specific information about any surgical procedure and the postoperative course. If the patient experienced a period of prolonged immobilization, the development of osteoporosis and muscle atrophy should be considered.

Objective Data

Physical Examination. Examination of the musculoskeletal system involves inspection, palpation, motion, and muscular assessment. The nurse should conduct a general overview, while

Subjective Data

A focused subjective assessment of T. K. by the nurse revealed the following information:

- **History of current illness:** Rates left hip pain at a 9 on a scale of 0–10. Describes pain as sharp spasms that increase in intensity with any movement. Is asking for pain medicine "as strong as you can give me." Denies any history of musculoskeletal conditions.
- **Past health:** Type 2 diabetes for 11 yr; COPD for 15 yr; 40 pack-year smoking history
- **Medications:** metformin (Glucophage), 500 mg PO bid; glyburide (DiaBeta), 5 mg/day PO; fluticasone and salmeterol combination (Advair), 250/50 mcg, 1 inhalation bid; salbutamol (Ventolin), 2 puffs q4h PRN as rescue inhaler
- **Functional assessment:** Until this current fall, has been able to perform ADLs without assistance. Currently smokes 2 to 3 packs of cigarettes per day. Is trying to quit but finding it difficult. Drinks alcohol at night. Is 188 cm tall and weighs 88 kg. Does not take any nutritional supplements and tends to shy away from milk and other dairy products because they make him "gassy." Leads a sedentary lifestyle because of dyspnea on exertion.

See Case Study: Patient Introduction, Case Study: Objective Data: Physical Examination, and Case Study: Diagnostic Studies for more information on T. K.

ADLs, activities of daily living; *COPD,* chronic obstructive pulmonary disease.

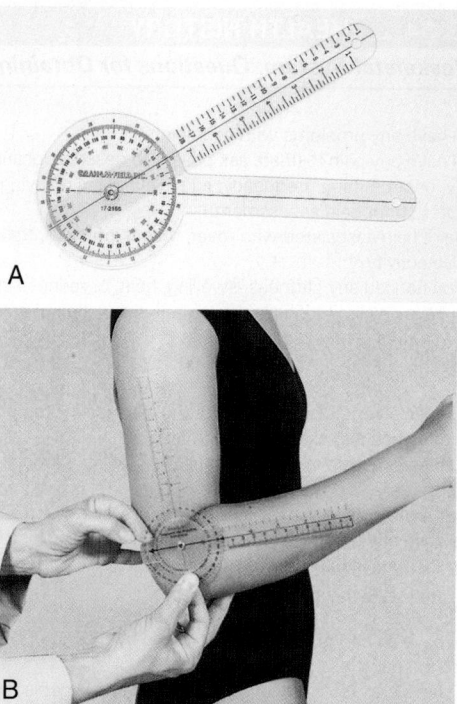

FIG. 64.6 Measurement of joint motion with a goniometer. Sources: *A,* Wilson, S. F., & Giddens, J. F. (2013). *Health assessment for nursing practice* (5th ed., p. 34, Figure 3-23). Mosby; *B,* Patton, K. T., & Thibodeau, G. A. (2013). *Anatomy and physiology* (8th ed., p. 286, Figure 10-15). Mosby.

obtaining data in a careful health history to provide guidance in choosing areas on which to concentrate during the local examination. Specific measurements should be taken as indicated by the results of the local examination.

Inspection. Inspection begins during the nurse's initial contact with the patient. The nurse notes the use of an assistive device such as a walker or cane. The nurse also observes general body build, muscle configuration, and symmetry of joint movement. If the patient is able to move independently, the nurse should assess posture and gait by watching the patient walk, stand, and sit. Musculoskeletal and neurological conditions can result in changes from a normal gait.

A systematic inspection is performed, starting at the head and neck and proceeding to the upper extremities, lower extremities, and trunk. The skin is inspected for general colour, scars, or other overt signs of previous injury or surgery. The nurse notes any swelling, deformity, nodules or masses, and discrepancies in limb length or muscle size. The patient's opposite-side body part is observed for comparison when an abnormality is suspected.

Palpation. Any area that has aroused concern because of a subjective complaint or appears abnormal on inspection should be carefully palpated. Palpation usually proceeds from head to toe to examine neck, shoulders, elbows, wrists, hands, back, hips, knees, ankles, and feet. Both superficial and deep palpation are usually performed, one after the other. The nurse's hands should be warm to prevent muscle spasm, which can interfere with identification of essential landmarks or soft tissue structures. Palpation allows for evaluation of skin temperature, local tenderness, swelling, crepitation, and presence of nodules. Muscles are palpated during active and passive motion for tone, strength, and ease of movement.

Motion. When assessing the patient's joint mobility, the nurse must carefully evaluate both passive and active ranges of joint motion. Measurements should be similar for both. *Active range of motion* means the patient takes their own joints through all movements without assistance. *Passive range of motion* occurs

when someone else moves the patient's joints without the patient's participation. The nurse should be cautious in performing passive range of motion because of the risk of injury to underlying structures. Manipulation must cease immediately if pain or resistance is encountered. If deficits in active or passive range of motion are noted, the nurse must also assess functional range of motion to determine whether performance of activities of daily living has been affected by joint changes. In this assessment, the patient is asked whether activities such as eating and bathing must be performed with assistance or cannot be done at all.

Range of motion is most accurately assessed with a *goniometer,* which measures the angle of the joint (Figure 64.6). Specific degrees of range of motion of all joints are usually not measured unless a musculoskeletal disorder has been identified. A less exact but valuable assessment method is to compare the range of motion of one extremity with the range of motion on the opposite side. The most common movements that occur at the diarthrodial joints are described in Table 64.3.

Muscle Strength Testing. The nurse grades the strength of individual muscles or groups of muscles during contraction (Table 64.4). The patient should be instructed to apply resistance to the force exerted by the nurse. For example, if the examiner tries to pull the patient's bent arm down, the patient tries to raise it. Muscle strength should also be compared with the strength of the opposite extremity. Subtle variations in muscle strength may be noted when the patient's dominant side is compared with the nondominant side.

Measurement. When length discrepancies or subjective issues are noted, the nurse obtains limb length and circumferential muscle mass measurements. For example, leg length should be measured when gait disorders are observed. The affected limb is measured between two bony prominences, and that measurement is compared with the corresponding

TABLE 64.3	MOVEMENT AT DIARTHRODIAL JOINTS
Movement	**Description**
Abduction	Movement of part away from midline of body
Adduction	Movement of part toward midline of body
Circumduction	Combination of flexion, extension, abduction, and adduction that results in circular motion of a body part
Dorsiflexion*	Flexing of toes and foot upward
Eversion	Turning of sole outward away from midline of body
Extension	Straightening of joint that increases angle between two bones
External rotation	Movement along longitudinal axis away from midline of body
Flexion	Bending of joint that results in decreased angle between two bones
Hyperextension	Extension in which angle exceeds 180° or beyond a joint's normal range of motion
Internal rotation	Movement along longitudinal axis toward midline of body
Inversion	Turning of sole inward toward midline of body
Opposition	Moving the thumb tip to meet the tip of each finger
Plantar flexion*	Flexing toes and foot downward
Pronation	Turning of palm downward
Supination	Turning of palm upward

*Active range of motion (ROM) only.

TABLE 64.4	MUSCLE STRENGTH SCALE
0	No detection of muscular contraction
1	A barely detectable flicker or trace of contraction with observation or palpation
2	Active movement of body part with elimination of gravity
3	Active movement against gravity only and not against resistance
4	Active movement against gravity and some resistance
5	Active movement against full resistance without evident fatigue (normal muscle strength)

measurement of the opposite extremity. Muscle mass is measured circumferentially at the largest area of the muscle. When recording measurements, the nurse documents the exact location at which the measurements were obtained (e.g., the quadriceps muscle is measured 15 cm above the patella). This informs the next examiner of the exact area to be measured and ensures consistency during reassessment.

Other. Assessment of reflexes is discussed in Chapter 58. Table 64.5 lists the elements of a normal physical assessment of the musculoskeletal system. Abnormal assessment findings of the musculoskeletal system are presented in Table 64.6.

DIAGNOSTIC STUDIES OF THE MUSCULOSKELETAL SYSTEM

Diagnostic studies provide important objective data that aid the nurse in monitoring the patient's condition and planning appropriate interventions. Table 64.7 lists diagnostic studies commonly used to evaluate the musculoskeletal system. In some situations, Canadians can expect to wait for diagnostic studies. For example, the average wait time in Canada for a magnetic resonance imaging (MRI) scan is 9.3 weeks, which may delay receiving medically necessary treatment (Barua & Moir, 2019). Tests must be carefully chosen to enhance or clarify information gained from the patient's history and physical examination.

TABLE 64.5	EXAMPLE OF A NORMAL PHYSICAL ASSESSMENT OF THE MUSCULOSKELETAL SYSTEM

- Full range of motion of all joints without pain or laxity (hypermobility)
- No joint swelling, deformity, or crepitation
- Normal spinal curvatures
- No tenderness on palpation of spine
- No muscle atrophy or asymmetry
- Muscle strength of 5

FOCUSED ASSESSMENT

Musculoskeletal System

Use this checklist to ensure that the key assessment steps have been done.

Subjective
Ask the patient about any of the following and note responses:

Joint pain or stiffness	Y	N
Muscle weakness	Y	N
Bone pain	Y	N

Objective: Diagnostic
Check the following laboratory results for critical values:

Radiograph results	✓
Bone scans	✓
Erythrocyte sedimentation rate	✓

Objective: Physical Examination
Inspect and palpate:

Skeleton and extremities (and compare sides) for alignment, contour, symmetry, size, and gross deformities	✓
Joints for range of motion, tenderness or pain, heat, crepitus, and swelling	✓
Muscles (and compare sides) for size, symmetry, tone, and tenderness or pain	✓
Bones for tenderness or pain	✓

CASE STUDY

Objective Data: Physical Examination

A physical examination of T. K. reveals the following:
- BP, 166/94; heart rate, 98; respiratory rate, 36; temperature, 35.8°C; O_2 saturation rate, 91% on 2 L of O_2
- Alert and oriented × 3
- Left leg shortened and externally rotated. No external bruising noted
- + 1 Pedal pulses bilaterally. Lungs with bibasilar crackles and expiratory wheezing

In continuing to read this chapter, consider diagnostic studies the nurse would anticipate being performed for T. K. See Case Study: Patient Introduction, Case Study: Subjective Data, and Case Study: Diagnostic Studies for more information on T. K.

BP, blood pressure.

Radiography

The *radiograph* is the diagnostic study most commonly used to assess musculoskeletal conditions and to monitor the effectiveness of treatment. The X-ray beam produces an image on a photographic film; the image appears dark if the X-rays penetrate the body tissues (e.g., lungs) and white if the transmission is partially blocked (e.g., by bones). Radiographs are two-dimensional, and multiple views may be necessary to facilitate

TABLE 64.6   ASSESSMENT ABNORMALITIES

Musculoskeletal System

Finding	Description	Possible Etiology
Achilles tendinitis	Pain in posterior leg initially during running or walking; can progress to pain at rest	Cumulative stress on Achilles tendon, resulting in inflammation
Ankylosis	Stiffness or fixation of a joint, usually resulting from destruction of articular cartilage and subchondral bone with subsequent tissue scarring	Chronic joint inflammation
Antalgic gait	Shortened stride with as little weight bearing as possible on the affected side	Pain or discomfort in the lower extremity on weight bearing; can be related to trauma or other disorders
Ataxic gait	Staggering, uncoordinated gait, often with sway	Neurogenic disorders (e.g., spinal cord lesion)
Atrophy	Decrease in the size of a tissue or organ caused by a reduction in the number or size of the individual cells; characterized by decreased circumference and flabby appearance and leading to decreased function and tone	Muscle denervation, contracture, and prolonged disuse as a result of immobilization
Contracture	Abnormal, usually permanent flexion and fixation of a muscle or joint; resistance to movement is a result of fibrosis of supporting soft tissues	Shortening of muscle or ligaments, tightness of soft tissue, incorrect positioning of immobilized extremity
Crepitation (crepitus)	Crackling sound or grating sensation as a result of friction between bones, broken bone, or cartilage bits in joint	Fracture, dislocation, chronic inflammation, osteoarthritis
Dislocation	Displacement of bone from its normal joint	Trauma, disorders of surrounding soft tissues
Hypertrophy	Increase in size of muscle as a result of enlargement of existing cells	Exercise or other increased stimulation, increased androgens
Kyphosis (dowager's hump)	Forward bending of thoracic spine: exaggerated thoracic curvature	Poor posture, tuberculosis, arthritis, osteoporosis, growth disturbance of vertebral epiphyses
Limited range of motion (ROM)	Failure of joint to achieve the expected degrees of motion	Injury, inflammation, contracture
Lordosis (swayback)	Lumbar spinal deformity that results in exaggerated lumbar curvature	Secondary to other spinal deformities, muscular dystrophy, obesity, flexion contracture of hip, congenital dislocation of hip
Muscle spasticity	Increased muscle tone (rigidity) with sustained muscle contractions (spasms); stiffness or tightness may interfere with gait, movement, speech	Neuromuscular disorders such as multiple sclerosis or cerebral palsy
Myalgia	General muscle tenderness and pain	Chronic rheumatic syndromes (e.g., fibromyalgia)
Paresthesia	Numbness and tingling, often described as a "pins and needles" sensation	Compromised sensory nerves, often owing to edema in a closed space such as a cast or bulky dressing
Pes planus (flatfoot)	Abnormal flatness of the sole and arch of the foot	Hereditary, muscle paralysis, mild cerebral palsy, early muscular dystrophy, injury to posterior tibial tendon
Plantar fasciitis	Burning, sharp pain on sole of foot; worse in the morning	Chronic degenerative–reparative cycle that results in inflammation
Scoliosis	Deformity resulting from lateral S-shaped curvature of the thoracic and lumbar spine	Idiopathic or congenital condition, fracture or dislocation, osteomalacia
Subluxation	Partial dislocation of joint	Instability of joint capsule and supporting ligaments (e.g., as a result of trauma, arthritis)
Swan neck deformity	Hyperextension of the PIP joint with flexion of the MCP and DIP joints of the fingers (see Chapter 67, Figure 67.4)	Deformity typical of rheumatoid and psoriatic arthritis, caused by contracture of muscles and tendons
Swelling	Enlargement, often of a joint, owing to fluid collection; generally leads to pain, stiffness	Trauma or inflammation
Torticollis (wry neck)	Twisting of neck in unusual position to one side	Prolonged contraction of neck muscles, congenital or acquired
Ulnar deviation (ulnar drift)	Displacement of fingers to ulnar side of forearm (see Chapter 67, Figure 67.4)	Typical deformity of rheumatoid arthritis due to tendon contracture
Valgum deformity (genu valgum; knock knees)	Condition in which the space between the medial malleoli >2.5 cm when knees are together	Poliomyelitis, congenital deformity, arthritis
Varum deformity (genu varum; bowleg)	Condition in which the space between the knees >2.5 cm when the medial malleoli are together	Arthritis, congenital deformity

DIP, distal interphalangeal; *MCP*, metacarpophalangeal; *PIP*, proximal interphalangeal.

diagnosis (e.g., anteroposterior [front-to-back], lateral [side], oblique [45-degree angle]). The contours and shades of the structures on these images provide useful information, such as showing the presence of deformity, joint congruity, calcification in soft tissue, and bone fractures. Radiographs are also useful in the evaluation of hereditary, developmental, infectious, inflammatory, neoplastic, metabolic, and degenerative disorders.

Magnetic Resonance Imaging

MRI can be useful for the early diagnosis of soft tissue disorders, including cartilage or ligament tears and herniated discs, as well as bone disorders such as avascular necrosis, tumours, and multiple myeloma. The body is composed primarily of hydrogen, which possesses magnetic properties that can be scanned by the powerful magnetic fields and radiofrequency waves. Contrast

TABLE 64.7   DIAGNOSTIC STUDIES

Musculoskeletal System

Study	Description and Purpose	Nursing Responsibility
Radiological Studies		
Standard radiography (X-ray study)	• Helps determine density of bone • Used to evaluate structural or functional changes of bones and joints • One-dimensional image provided by anteroposterior view because X-ray beam passes from front to back • Two-dimensional image provided by lateral position	• Instruct patient to avoid excessive exposure of themselves to radiation. • Remove any radiopaque objects that can interfere with results. • Explain procedure to patient. • Instruct patient to remain still. • Pregnancy is a contraindication to X-ray studies; however, sometimes the benefits outweigh the risks.
Computed tomography (CT)	• Three-dimensional radiography provided by use of an X-ray beam with a computer • Used to identify soft tissue abnormalities, bony abnormalities, and various musculoskeletal trauma • Iodinated dye often used for better visualization	• Same as for radiography. • Also, assess for adverse reactions to iodinated dye. • Patients with kidney disease or diabetes require adequate hydration to flush out the dye.
Magnetic resonance imaging (MRI)	• Viewing of soft tissue with use of radiofrequency waves and magnetic field • Especially useful in the diagnosis of avascular necrosis, disc disease, tumours, osteomyelitis, ligament tears, and cartilage tears • Patient placed inside scanning chamber • Gadolinium-based contrast dyes used to enhance visualization of the structures, may be injected into a vein • In open MRI, no requirement for placing patient inside a chamber	• MRI is contraindicated in patients with metallic implants. • Ensure that patient has no metal on clothing (e.g., snaps, zippers, jewellery, credit cards). • Inform patient that procedure is painless, and emphasize importance of remaining still throughout examination. • Claustrophobic patients may require antianxiety agents if indicated and ordered. • Open MRI may be indicated for patients with large chest and abdominal girth or severe claustrophobia.
Arthrography	• Radiography in which contrast medium or air is injected into joint cavity, enabling visualization of joint structures • Joint movement assessed with series of radiographic images	• Same as for radiography. • Assess patient for possible allergy to contrast medium. • Inform patient that procedure is painless.
Discography	• Radiography of cervical or lumbar intervertebral disc, performed after injection of contrast dye into nucleus pulposus • Enables visualization of intervertebral disc abnormalities	• Same as for arthrography.
Bone Mineral Density (BMD) Measurements		
Dual-energy X-ray absorptiometry (DEXA)	• Used to measure bone mass of spine, femur, forearm, and total body • Allows assessment of bone density with minimal radiation exposure • Used to diagnose metabolic bone disease and to monitor changes in bone density with treatment • Widely available; free screening test	• Same as for radiography. • Inform patient that procedure is painless.
Quantitative ultrasonography (QUS)	• Helps evaluate density, elasticity, and strength of bone through the use of ultrasound waves rather than radiation	• Inform patient that procedure is painless.
Radioisotope Studies		
Bone scan	• Radiography in which radioisotope (usually technetium-99m) is injected and taken up by bone • Isotope uptake is uniform when bones are normal • Uptake increased in osteomyelitis, osteoporosis, primary and metastatic malignant lesions of bone, and certain fractures • Uptake decreased in areas of avascular necrosis	• Pregnancy and lactation are usually contraindicated. • The technician gives a calculated dose of radioisotope 2 hr before procedure. • The patient's bladder is emptied before the procedure. • The procedure requires 1 hr while patient lies supine. • Increase patient's fluid intake after the examination. • Isotopes are excreted from the body within 6–24 hr.
Endoscopy		
Arthroscopy	• Procedure in which an arthroscope is inserted into the joint (usually knee) for visualization of structure and contents • Can be used for exploratory surgery (removal of loose bodies and biopsy) and for diagnosing abnormalities of meniscus, articular cartilage, ligaments, or joint capsule • Other structures that can be visualized through the arthroscope: shoulder, elbow, wrist, jaw, hip, and ankle	• Inform patient that procedure can be performed in an outpatient setting and that local or general anaesthesia may be used. • Patient is on NPO status after midnight on the day of the test. • After procedure, cover the wound with sterile dressing. • Explain postprocedure care.

Continued

TABLE 64.7   DIAGNOSTIC STUDIES
Musculoskeletal System—cont'd

Study	Description and Purpose	Nursing Responsibility
Mineral Metabolism		
Alkaline phosphatase (ALP)	• Enzyme produced by osteoblasts of bone; needed for mineralization of organic bone matrix • Levels elevated in healing fractures, bone cancers, osteoporosis, osteomalacia, and Paget's disease • *Normal:* 40–160 IU/L (age dependent)	• Inform patient that fasting is preferred but not required. • Note any medications that may affect test results.*
Calcium	• Stored primarily in bone • Provides bone with rigid consistency • Serum level decreased in osteomalacia, renal disease, and hypoparathyroidism • Level increased in hyperparathyroidism, some bone tumours; varies with level of albumin • *Normal:* total calcium 2.10–2.50 mmol/L (age dependent)	• Inform patient that fasting is not required. • Note any medications that may affect test results. • Excessive milk ingestion and prolonged tourniquet application may increase calcium levels.*
Phosphate (phosphorus)	• Amount that is present indirectly related to calcium metabolism • Level decreased in osteomalacia • Level increased in chronic renal disease, healing fractures, osteolytic metastatic tumour • *Normal:* 1.0–1.5 mmol/L (age dependent)	• Recent carbohydrate intake (including IV glucose) causes decrease in phosphorus levels. • Patient should be on NPO status after midnight on the day of the test. • Note any medications that may affect test results. • Avoid hemolysis of the blood sample because this can elevate phosphate levels.*
Serological Studies		
Rheumatoid factor (RF)	• Study to assess presence of autoantibody (RF) in serum • Factor not specific for rheumatoid arthritis; present in other connective tissue diseases, as well as in a small percentage of normal population • *Normal:* negative or <60 IU/mL by nephelometric method	• Inform patient that fasting is not required. • In older persons, results are often falsely positive. • False-positive results also occur with hemolysis or lipemia.*
Erythrocyte sedimentation rate (ESR)	• Nonspecific index of inflammation • Used to measure rapidity with which red blood cells settle out of unclotted blood in 1 hr • Results influenced by physiological factors as well as by diseases • Levels elevated with any inflammatory process (especially rheumatoid arthritis, rheumatic fever, osteomyelitis, and respiratory infections) • *Normal:* male, ≤15 mm/hr; female, ≤20 mm/hr (age dependent)	• Numerous interfering factors can affect test results (e.g., pregnancy, menstruation, anemias, medications). • Withhold medications that may affect results, if indicated.*
Antinuclear antibody (ANA)	• Used to assess presence of antibodies capable of destroying nucleus of body's tissue cells • Finding positive in 95% of patients with systemic lupus erythematosus and may also be positive in individuals with systemic sclerosis (scleroderma) or rheumatoid arthritis and in a small percentage of normal population • *Normal:* negative at 1:40 dilution	• Inform patient that fasting is not required. • Note any medications that may affect test results. • Assess for signs of infection at the venipuncture site in patients with autoimmune diseases.*
C-reactive protein (CRP)	• Used to diagnose inflammatory diseases, infections, and active widespread malignancy • CRP synthesized by the liver and present in large amounts in serum 18–24 hr after onset of tissue damage • *Normal:* negative or ≤10 mg/L	• Fasting may sometimes be required (laboratory specific). • Note any medications that may affect test results.*
Uric acid	• End product of purine metabolism that is normally excreted in urine • Levels not specific to gout but are usually elevated in patients with gout • *Normal:* male, 240–501 Mcmol/L; female, 160–430 Mcmol/L (age dependent)	• Fasting may sometimes be required (laboratory specific).*
Human leukocyte antigen–B27 (HLA-B27)	• Antigen present in disorders such as ankylosing spondylitis and rheumatoid arthritis • *Normal:* negative	• Inform patient that fasting or other preparation is not needed.*
Muscle Enzymes		
Creatine kinase (CK)	• Concentration highest in skeletal muscle • Values increased in progressive muscular dystrophy, polymyositis, and traumatic injuries • *Normal:* men, 20–215 IU/L; women, 20–160 IU/L (age and exercise dependent)	• Inform patient that procedure does not necessitate fasting. • Values can be increased after strenuous exercise, recent surgery, and intramuscular injections and with certain medications.*

TABLE 64.7   DIAGNOSTIC STUDIES

Musculoskeletal System—cont'd

Study	Description and Purpose	Nursing Responsibility
Serum potassium (K⁺)	• Values sometimes increased with muscle trauma because cell destruction releases this electrolyte into the serum (depends on renal function) • *Normal:* 3.5–5.1 mmol/L (age dependent)	• Monitor patients in trauma unit for cardiac dysrhythmias related to hypokalemia or hyperkalemia. • Note any medications that may affect test results. • Hemolysis of the blood sample and prolonged tourniquet application can elevate potassium levels.*
Invasive Procedures Arthrocentesis	• Procedure in which a needle is inserted into the joint cavity to aspirate synovial fluid, blood, or pus or to instill medications • Local anaesthesia and aseptic technique required • Useful in diagnosis of joint inflammation, infection, and subtle fractures	• Inform patient that procedure is usually done at bedside or in examination room. • Send samples of synovial fluid to laboratory for examination (if indicated). • After procedure, apply pressure dressing. • Observe dressing for leakage of blood or fluid.
Electromyography (EMG)	• Used to evaluate electrical potential associated with skeletal muscle contraction • Involves insertion of small-gauge needles into certain muscles • Needle probes are attached to leads that feed information to EMG machine; recordings of electrical activity of muscle are traced on audio transmitter, as well as on oscilloscope and recording paper • Study useful in providing information related to lower motor neuron dysfunction and primary muscle disease	• Inform patient that procedure is usually done in an EMG laboratory while patient lies supine on a special table. • Keep patient awake to participate in voluntary movement. • Inform patient that procedure involves some discomfort from needle insertion. • Contraindications include anticoagulant therapy and extensive skin infection. • Fasting is not required, but some laboratories may restrict intake of stimulants (e.g., coffee, cigarettes) 2–3 hr before procedure.
Miscellaneous Thermography	• Infrared detector is used to measure degree of heat radiating from skin surface • Useful in investigation of cause of joint inflammation and in following up patient's response to anti-inflammatory drug therapy	• Inform patient that procedure is painless and noninvasive.
Somatosensory evoked potential (SEP)	• Used to evaluate evoked potential of muscle contractions • Electrodes are placed on skin and provide recordings of electrical activity of muscle • Useful in identifying subtle dysfunction of lower motor neuron and primary muscle disease • Possible to measure nerve conduction along pathways not accessible by EMG	• Inform patient that procedure is similar to EMG but does not involve needles. • Electrodes are applied to the skin.

IV, intravenous; *IU*, international units; *NPO*, nothing by mouth.
*Blood samples are obtained by venipuncture. The nurse should observe venipuncture site for bleeding or hematoma formation.

material may be necessary to enhance the images. MRI is contraindicated in patients who have implanted metal objects (e.g., pacemaker, aneurysm clips, prosthesis, implanted cardioverter–defibrillator, electronic devices, hearing aids, shrapnel).

Arthroscopy

A small fibre-optic tube called an *arthroscope* is inserted into a joint and used to directly examine or operate on the interior of the joint cavity in a procedure known as arthroscopy (see Table 64.7). Arthroscopy is performed under sterile conditions. After local anaesthetic has been administered, a large-bore needle is inserted into the joint, and the joint is distended with fluid or air (Figure 64.7). The arthroscope enables extensive, accurate visualization of the joint cavity. Photographs or video recordings can be made through the arthroscope, and a biopsy of the synovium or cartilage can be obtained. Torn tissue can be repaired through arthroscopic surgery, which eliminates the need for a larger incision and greatly decreases the recovery time.

Arthrocentesis and Synovial Fluid Analysis

Arthrocentesis, or joint aspiration, is a procedure in which an incision or puncture is made in a joint capsule, usually to obtain samples of synovial fluid from within the joint cavity for a synovial fluid analysis. It may also be used to instill medications for a patient with septic arthritis or to remove excess fluid from joints to relieve pain. After the skin has been cleaned, a local anaesthetic is instilled. An 18-gauge or larger needle is inserted into the joint, and fluid is withdrawn. The appropriate sterile container should be readily available to receive the aspirated fluid, which must be transported immediately to the laboratory. The fluid is examined grossly for volume, colour, clarity, viscosity, and mucin clot formation. Normal synovial fluid is transparent, colourless (or straw-coloured), scant in amount, and of low viscosity. Fluid from an infected joint may be purulent and thick or grey and thin. In gout, the fluid may be whitish yellow. Blood may be aspirated in cases of hemarthrosis because of injury or a bleeding disorder. The *mucin clot test* indicates the character of the protein portion of the synovial fluid. Normally a white,

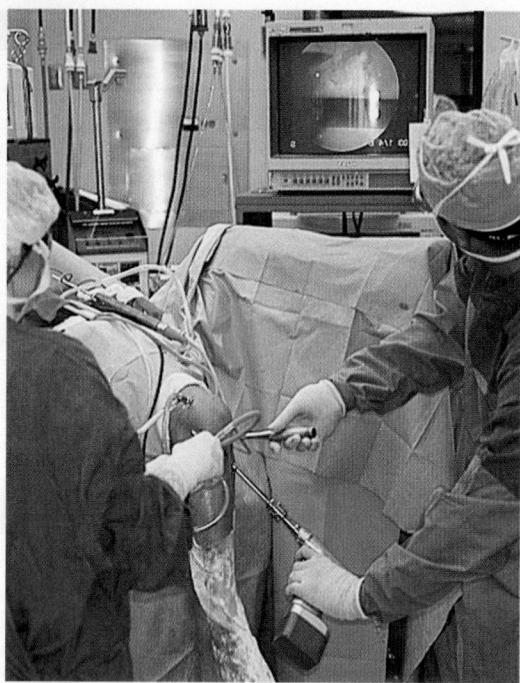

FIG. 64.7 Knee arthroscopy in progress. Notice the monitor in the background. Source: Miller, M. D., Howard, R. F., & Plancher, K. D. (2003). *Surgical atlas of sports medicine*. Saunders.

ropelike mucin clot is formed. In the presence of an inflammatory process, the clot breaks apart and easily fragments. The fluid is examined grossly for floating fat globules, which indicate bone injury.

The fluid is examined microscopically for cell count and identification. Infection would be suspected with an elevated white blood cell count and an increase in polymorphonuclear cells (i.e. neutrophils). Protein content is elevated, and the glucose level is considerably decreased in septic arthritis. The presence of uric acid crystals suggests a diagnosis of gout (Pagana et al., 2019). Specimens for a Gram stain and culture may also be obtained in arthrocentesis.

Muscle Enzymes

Muscle enzymes are released from injured or dead muscle cells. Determinations of muscle enzyme values are used to distinguish between muscle weakness caused by innervation problems and that caused by dystrophic disease of the muscle itself. The level of enzymes reflects the progress of the disorder and the effectiveness of treatment. Creatine kinase is a reliable measure of muscle damage.

Serological Studies

In approximately 80% of people with rheumatoid arthritis and related diseases, an autoantibody known as *rheumatoid factor* (RF) is present in the serum. RF is an autoantibody directed against immunoglobulin G. RF titres are higher during periods of increased disease activity. Elevated erythrocyte sedimentation rate and C-reactive protein level are nonspecific indicators of active inflammation.

CASE STUDY

Diagnostic Studies

The nurse collaborates with the emergency department health care provider immediately to discuss the assessment findings. The nurse receives the following diagnostic studies orders for T. K.:
- Radiograph of left hip
- Chest radiograph
- CBC, electrolytes, aPTT, PT/INR
- Arterial blood gases (ABGs)

The nurse arranges for T. K. to have the diagnostic studies completed. The radiograph of his left hip reveals an extracapsular fracture. The chest radiographic findings are consistent with COPD without any evidence of pneumonia at present. Hematocrit is 43%; hemoglobin, 140 mmol/L; and WBC is 15.1 × 10⁹/L. The remainder of CBC, electrolytes, aPTT, and PT/INR are WNL. The ABGs demonstrate compensated respiratory acidosis.

See Case Study: Patient Introduction, Case Study: Subjective Data, and Case Study: Objective Data: Physical Examination in this chapter for more information on T. K. This case is continued in Chapter 65.

aPTT, activated partial thromboplastin time; *CBC*, complete blood cell count; *COPD*, chronic obstructive pulmonary disease; *INR*, international normalized ratio; *PT*, prothrombin time; *WNL*, within normal limits. The Appendix contains a list of normal laboratory values.

■ REVIEW QUESTIONS

The number of the question corresponds to the same-numbered objective at the beginning of the chapter.

1. What are the bone cells that function in the breakdown of bone tissue (resorption) called?
   a. Osteoids
   b. Osteocytes
   c. Osteoclasts
   d. Osteoblasts
2. While performing passive range-of-motion exercises for a client, the nurse puts the ankle joint through the movements of which of the following? *(Select all that apply.)*
   a. Flexion and extension
   b. Inversion and eversion
   c. Pronation and supination
   d. Abduction, and adduction
   e. Dorsiflexion and plantar flexion
3. To prevent muscle atrophy, the nurse teaches the client with a leg immobilized in traction to perform which of the following manoeuvres?
   a. Flexion contractions
   b. Isotonic contractions
   c. Isometric contractions
   d. Extension contractions
4. A client with bursitis of the shoulder asks the nurse what the bursa does. What does the nurse tell the client about the function of the bursa?
   a. Bursae connect bone to bone.
   b. Bursae separate muscle from muscle.
   c. Bursae lubricate joints with synovial fluid.
   d. Bursae relieve friction between moving parts.

5. Why are many older people at increased risk for falls? *(Select all that apply.)*
   a. Changes in balance
   b. Decrease in bone mass
   c. Loss of ligament elasticity
   d. Loss of strength
   e. Erosion of articular cartilage

6. While the nurse is obtaining subjective assessment data related to the musculoskeletal system, which of the following conditions requires the nurse to ask about family history?
   a. Osteomyelitis
   b. Osteomalacia
   c. Low back pain
   d. Rheumatoid arthritis

7. When a nurse grades muscle strength with a score of 2, what does that indicate?
   a. Active movement against gravity
   b. A barely detectable flicker of contraction
   c. Active movement with elimination of gravity
   d. Active movement against full resistance without evident fatigue

8. Which of the following is a normal finding in the assessment of the musculoskeletal system?
   a. Muscle strength of 4
   b. A lateral curvature of the spine
   c. Angulation of bone toward midline
   d. Full range of motion of all joints without pain

9. Which of the following are nursing considerations for a client undergoing magnetic resonance imaging (MRI)? *(Select all that apply.)*
   a. Ensuring that the client has no metal on clothing
   b. Informing the client that the procedure is painless
   c. Checking for history of claustrophobia
   d. Ensuring that the client is on NPO status at least 8 hours before the study
   e. Administering a fluid bolus immediately before the study

1. c, 2, a, b; 3. c; 4. d; 5. a, b, c, d; 6. d; 7. c; 8. d; 9. a, b, c.

ⓔvolve

For even more review questions, visit http://evolve.elsevier.com/Canada/Lewis/medsurg.

REFERENCES

Barua, B., & Moir, M. (2019). *Waiting your turn. Wait times for health care in Canada, 2019 report.* Fraser Institute. https://www.fraserinstitute.org/studies/waiting-your-turn-wait-times-for-health-care-in-canada-2019

Huether, S. E., Power-Keen, K., El-Hussein, M., et al. (2018). *Understanding pathophysiology* (Canadian ed.). Elsevier.

Jarvis, C., Browne, A. J., MacDonald-Jenkins, J., et al. (2019). *Physical examination & health assessment* (3rd Canadian ed.). Elsevier Inc.

Pagana, K. D., Pagana, T. J., & Pike-MacDonald, S. A. (2019). *Mosby's Canadian manual of diagnostic and laboratory tests* (2nd Canadian ed.). Mosby.

Patton, K. T., & Thibodeau, G. A. (2020). *Structure & function of the body* (16th ed.). Elsevier.

RESOURCES

Resources for this chapter are listed in Chapters 65 to 67.

65

Nursing Management

Musculoskeletal Trauma and Orthopedic Surgery

Danielle L. Byrne
Originating US chapter by Matthew C. Price

evolve WEBSITE

http://evolve.elsevier.com/Canada/Lewis/medsurg

- Review Questions (Online Only)
- Key Points
- Answer Guidelines for Case Study

- Student Case Studies
  - Patient with Musculoskeletal Trauma
  - Patient with Parkinson's Disease and Hip Fracture

- Customizable Nursing Care Plans
  - Fracture
  - Orthopedic Surgery
- Conceptual Care Map Creator
- Audio Glossary
- Content Updates

LEARNING OBJECTIVES

1. Explain the etiology, pathophysiology, clinical manifestations, and interprofessional care of soft tissue injuries, including strains; sprains; dislocations; subluxations; bursitis; repetitive strain injury; carpal tunnel syndrome; and injuries to the rotator cuff, meniscus, and anterior cruciate ligament.
2. Relate the sequential events involved in fracture healing.
3. Compare closed reduction, cast immobilization, open reduction, and traction regarding purpose, complications, and nursing management.
4. Describe a neurovascular assessment for a patient with an injured extremity.

5. Explain common complications associated with a fracture and fracture healing.
6. Describe the interprofessional and nursing management of patients with specific fractures.
7. Describe the indications for and the interprofessional and nursing management of the patient with an amputation.
8. Describe the types of joint replacement surgery associated with arthritis and connective tissue diseases.
9. Describe the preoperative and postoperative management of the patient having joint replacement surgery.

KEY TERMS

arthrodesis
arthroplasty
avascular necrosis (AVN)
bursitis
carpal tunnel syndrome (CTS)
compartment syndrome

dislocation
fat embolism syndrome (FES)
fracture
osteotomy
phantom limb sensation
repetitive strain injury (RSI)

sprain
strain
subluxation
synovectomy
traction

Musculoskeletal conditions resulting from trauma, along with common orthopedic surgical procedures, are discussed in this chapter. The nurse's role in the prevention of complications and in the promotion of function in patients with fractures and orthopedic surgery is emphasized. The most common cause of musculoskeletal injuries is a traumatic event resulting in fracture, dislocation, and associated soft tissue injury. The assessment, diagnosis, and treatment of and recovery from musculoskeletal injuries require interprofessional collaboration among many team members, such as health care providers (e.g., emergentologist, anaesthesiologist, orthopedic surgeon, primary care practitioners [medical doctor or nurse practitioner]),

nurses, physiotherapists, occupational therapists, pharmacists, dietitians, and designated support people and the patient.

Although most of these injuries are not fatal, the cost in terms of pain, disability, medical expense, and lost wages is enormous. In 2019, British Columbia's First Nations Health Authority (FNHA) published a survey in which Northern Region adult participants ($n = 602$) "were asked whether they had experienced an injury serious enough to limit their normal activities the next day" (p. 65). The survey indicated that 21% of adults reported being injured in the past year, with 26% citing major sprains or strains and 20% reporting broken bones (FNHA, 2019). Injury is a serious public health issue that has a major impact on the lives of many Canadians. According to Statistics Canada (2018), unintentional injury is the leading cause of death for Canadians between the ages of 1 and 34 years and is an important cause of hospitalization (Canadian Institute for Health Information [CIHI], 2018b). Adolescent males are the age group injured most frequently, mainly while participating in sports (CIHI, 2018b). Unintentional falls requiring hospitalization occur predominantly either at home or in residential institutions (CIHI, 2018b). For all ages, unintentional injuries are exceeded only by cancer, heart disease, and stroke as a leading cause of death (Statistics Canada, 2018).

The nurse has an important role in educating the public about the basic principles of safety and of accident prevention. Such teaching should be provided to high-risk individuals (e.g., people with gait instability or visual or cognitive impairment). The morbidity associated with accidents can be significantly reduced if people are aware of and minimize environmental hazards (e.g., removal of throw rugs), use existing safety equipment, and apply safety and traffic rules. In the occupational and industrial setting, the nurse can teach employees and employers about the use of proper safety equipment and avoidance of hazardous working situations. With older patients, the nurse can suggest ways to prevent common musculoskeletal conditions in this age group (see Table 65.7 later in this chapter).

SOFT TISSUE INJURIES

Soft tissue injuries include sprains, strains, dislocations, and subluxations. These common injuries are usually caused by trauma. Sprains and strains are the most common injury (51%), with fractures and broken bones accounting for 17% of injuries (Statistics Canada, 2015a). The increasing number of people involved in a fitness program or participating in sports has contributed to the higher incidence of soft tissue injuries. Common sports-related injuries are summarized in Table 65.1. In Canada, 35% of injuries occur during participation in sports or exercise (Statistics Canada, 2015b).

Sprains and Strains

Sprains and strains are common injuries from abnormal stretching or twisting forces that may occur during vigorous activities. These injuries tend to occur around joints and in the spinal musculature.

A **sprain** is an injury related to the ligamentous structures surrounding a joint, usually caused by a wrenching or twisting motion. Most sprains occur in the ankles, knees, or wrists (Crowther-Radulewicz & McCance, 2017). A sprain is classified according to the degree of tearing in the ligament fibres. A *first-degree (mild) sprain* involves tears in only a few fibres, resulting in mild tenderness and minimal swelling. A *second-degree (moderate) sprain* is a partial tearing of the ligament, with more swelling and tenderness. A *third-degree (severe) sprain* is a complete tearing of the ligament in association with moderate to severe swelling. A gap in the muscle may be apparent or palpated through the skin if the muscle is torn. Because areas around joints are rich in nerve endings, the injury can be extremely painful.

A **strain** is an excessive stretching of a muscle, a muscle's fascial sheath, or a tendon. Most strains occur in the foot, leg (typically hamstrings), knee, wrist, or back (Crowther-Radulewicz & McCance, 2017). Strains may also be classified as *first-degree*

Injury	Definition	Treatment
Anterior cruciate ligament tear	Traumatic tearing of ligament by deceleration forces together with pivoting or odd positions of the knee or leg	• Physiotherapy with rehabilitation, knee brace • If knee instability or continued injuries, reconstructive surgery may be done.
Impingement syndrome	Entrapment of soft tissue structures under coracoacromial arch of shoulder	• NSAIDs; rest until symptoms decrease, and then gradual ROM and strengthening exercises
Ligament injury	Tearing or stretching of ligament; usually occurs as a result of inversion, eversion, shearing, or torque applied to a joint. Characterized by sudden pain, swelling, and instability	• Rest, ice, elevation of extremity if possible, NSAIDs; protection of affected extremity by use of brace • If symptoms persist, surgical repair may be necessary.
Meniscus injury	Injury to fibrocartilage of the knee, characterized by popping, clicking, tearing sensation, effusion, and swelling	• Rest, ice, elevation of extremity if possible, NSAIDs; gradual return to regular activities • If symptoms persist, MRI to diagnose meniscal injury and possible arthroscopic surgery
Rotator cuff tear	Tear within muscle or tendinoligamentous structures around shoulder	• *If minor tear:* rest, NSAIDs, and gradual mobilization with ROM and strengthening exercises • *If major tear:* surgical repair
Shin splints	Inflammation along anterior aspect of calf from periostitis caused by wearing improper shoes, overuse, or running on hard pavement	• Rest, ice, NSAIDs, proper shoes; gradual increase in activity • If pain persists, radiographic study to rule out stress fracture of tibia
Tendinitis	Inflammation of tendon as a result of overuse or incorrect use	• Rest, ice, NSAIDs; gradual return to sport activity; protective brace (orthosis) may be necessary if symptoms recur

MRI, magnetic resonance imaging; *NSAIDs*, nonsteroidal anti-inflammatory drugs; *ROM*, range of motion.

(mild or slightly pulled muscle), *second-degree* (moderate or moderately torn muscle), or *third-degree* (severely torn or ruptured muscle).

The clinical manifestations of sprains and strains are similar and include pain, edema, decrease in function, and bruising. Pain aggravated by continued use is common. Edema develops in the injured area because of the local inflammatory response.

Mild sprains and strains are usually self-limiting, with full function returning within 3 to 6 weeks. A severe sprain can result in a concomitant *avulsion fracture*, in which the ligament pulls loose a fragment of bone. Alternatively, the joint structure may become unstable and result in subluxation or dislocation. At the time of injury, *hemarthrosis* (bleeding into a joint space or cavity) or disruption of the synovial lining may occur.

Radiographs of the affected part are usually ordered to rule out a fracture or widening of the joint structure. However, some health care providers use an assessment protocol called the *Ottawa Rules* (or *Ottawa Guidelines*) for the examination of an injured ankle or knee before ordering radiographs (Murphy et al., 2020). These rules determine when radiographic studies are necessary after an injury on the basis of age, capability of flexion, location of tenderness, and inability to bear weight. Surgical repair may be necessary if the injury is significant enough to produce severe disruption of ligamentous or muscle structures, fracture, or dislocation.

NURSING AND INTERPROFESSIONAL MANAGEMENT SPRAINS AND STRAINS

NURSING IMPLEMENTATION

HEALTH PROMOTION. Doing warm-up exercises before exercising and vigorous activity, followed by stretching, significantly reduces the risk for sprains and strains. Strength, balance, and endurance exercises are also important. Strengthening exercises involve working against resistance. These exercises build up muscle strength and bone density. Balance exercises, which may overlap with some strengthening exercises, help to prevent falling. Endurance exercises should be started at a low level of effort. The person progresses gradually to a moderate level of activities. Age-dependent 24-hour movement and activity guidelines can be helpful (Canadian Society for Exercise Physiology [CSEP], 2020). For example, adults ages 18 to 64 should accumulate at least 150 minutes of moderate-to-vigorous intensity aerobic physical activity per week, in bouts of 10 minutes or more. Exercise instructions for these types of physical activity are available online at the Canadian Society for Exercise Physiology (CSEP) website (see the Resources at the end of this chapter).

ACUTE INTERVENTION. If an injury occurs, immediate care focuses on (1) stopping the activity and limiting movement, (2) application of ice compresses to the injured area, (3) compression of the involved extremity, (4) elevation of the extremity, and (5) providing analgesia as necessary (Table 65.2). The *RICE* (**R**est, **I**ce, **C**ompression, **E**levation) protocol has been found to decrease local inflammation and pain for most musculoskeletal injuries. Movement should be limited and the extremity rested as soon as pain is felt. Unless the injury is severe, prolonged rest is usually not necessary.

Cold *(cryotherapy)* in several forms can be used to produce hypothermia in the involved part. The cold induces physiological changes in soft tissue, including vasoconstriction and reduction in the transmission and perception of nerve pain impulses. In addition to pain relief, these changes reduce muscle spasms, inflammation, and edema. Cold is most useful when applied immediately after the injury has occurred. Ice applications should not exceed 20 to 30 minutes per application, and ice should not be applied directly to the skin.

An elastic compression bandage can be wrapped around the injured part. To prevent edema and encourage fluid return, the bandage should be wrapped starting distally (at the point farthest from the midline of the body) and progress proximally (toward the midline of the body). If numbness is felt below the area of compression or if there is additional pain or swelling beyond the edge of the bandage, the bandage is too tight. The bandage can be left in place for 30 minutes and then removed for 15 minutes. However, some elastic bandages are left on during training, athletic, and occupational activities.

The injured part should be elevated above the heart level to help mobilize excess fluid from the area and impede further edema. The injured part should be elevated even during sleep. Mild analgesics such as nonsteroidal anti-inflammatory drugs (NSAIDs) may be necessary to manage patient discomfort.

After the acute phase (usually lasting 24 to 48 hours), warm, moist heat can be applied to the affected part to reduce swelling and provide comfort. Heat applications should not exceed 20 to 30 minutes, and a "cool-down" time should be used between applications. NSAIDs may be recommended to decrease edema and pain. The patient is encouraged to use the limb, provided that the joint is protected by means of casting, bracing, taping, or splinting. Movement of the joint maintains nutrition to the cartilage, and muscle contraction improves circulation and resolution of the contusion and swelling.

AMBULATORY AND HOME CARE. Most sprains and strains are treated in an outpatient setting. The patient should be instructed to use ice and elevation for 24 to 48 hours after the injury to reduce edema. The use of mild analgesics to promote comfort should be encouraged. Use of an elastic bandage may provide

---

✚ TABLE 65.2 EMERGENCY MANAGEMENT

Acute Soft Tissue Injury

Etiology	Assessment Findings	Interventions
• Falls • Crush injury • Direct blows • Motor vehicle accidents • Sports injuries	• Decreased movement • Decreased pulse, coolness, and capillary refill >2 sec • Decreased sensation with severe edema • Ecchymosis, contusion • Edema • Inability to bear weight when lower extremity involved • Limited or decreased function with upper extremity involvement • Muscle spasms • Pain, tenderness • Pallor • Shortening or rotation of extremity	**Initial** • Ensure airway, breathing, and circulation. • Assess neurovascular status of involved limb. • Elevate involved limb. • Apply compression bandage unless dislocation is present. • Apply ice packs to the affected area. • Immobilize affected extremity in the position found. Do not attempt to realign or reinsert protruding bones. • Anticipate radiographs of injured extremity. • Give analgesia as necessary. • Administer tetanus prophylaxis if skin integrity is breached or there is an open fracture. • Administer antibiotic prophylaxis for open fracture, large tissue defects, or mangled extremity injury. **Ongoing Monitoring** • Monitor for changes in neurovascular status. • Eliminate weight bearing when lower extremity is involved. • Anticipate compartment pressure monitoring if neurovascular status changes and compartment syndrome is suspected.

additional support during activity. The patient should learn proper measures of strengthening and conditioning to prevent reinjury (Silva et al., 2018).

The physiotherapist may help in providing pain relief by means of modalities such as ultrasonography. The therapist may also teach the patient exercises to perform for improving flexibility and strength.

DISLOCATION AND SUBLUXATION

A dislocation is a severe injury of the ligamentous structures around a joint that results in the complete displacement of the bone from its normal position. A subluxation is a partial or incomplete displacement of the joint surface. The clinical manifestations and treatment of a subluxation are similar to those of a dislocation, but they are less severe and may require less healing time.

Dislocations characteristically result from overwhelming forces transmitted to the joint that cause a disruption of the soft tissue support structure surrounding the joint. The joints most frequently dislocated in the upper extremity include the thumb, elbow, and shoulder. In the lower extremity, the hip is vulnerable to dislocation occurring as a result of severe trauma, often associated with motor vehicle accidents (Figure 65.1). The patella may dislocate because of a sharp blow to the kneecap or after a sudden twisting inward motion while the planted foot is pointed outward (Salati et al., 2017).

The most obvious clinical manifestation of a dislocation is deformity. For example, if a hip is dislocated in a posterior (or backward) direction, the limb can be shorter and is often internally rotated on the affected side. Additional manifestations include local pain, tenderness, loss of function of the injured part, and swelling of the soft tissues in the region of the joint. The major complications of a dislocated joint are open joint injuries, intra-articular fractures, avascular necrosis (AVN) (bone cell death as a result of inadequate blood supply), and damage to adjacent neurovascular tissue.

Radiographic studies are performed to determine the extent of displacement of the involved structures. The joint may also be aspirated to determine the presence of hemarthrosis or fat cells. Fat cells in the aspirate indicate a probable intra-articular fracture.

NURSING AND INTERPROFESSIONAL MANAGEMENT DISLOCATION

ACUTE INTERVENTION

A dislocation requires prompt attention and is considered an orthopedic emergency. The longer the joint remains unreduced, the greater the possibility of AVN. Compartment syndrome (see the Compartment Syndrome section) may also occur after dislocation, and dislocation is often associated with significant vascular injury. The hip joint is particularly susceptible to AVN. Neurovascular assessment is critical (see the Neurovascular Assessment section).

The first goal of management is to realign the dislocated portion of the joint in its original anatomical position. This can be accomplished by a closed reduction, which may be performed under local or general anaesthesia or intravenous conscious sedation. Anaesthesia is often necessary to produce muscle relaxation so that the bones can be manipulated. In some situations, surgical open reduction (joint visualized through surgical

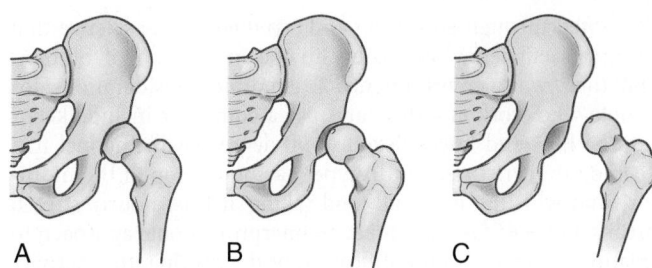

FIG. 65.1 Soft tissue injury of the hip, causing subluxation or dislocation. **A,** Healthy (before injury). **B,** Subluxation (partial dislocation). **C,** Dislocation.

incision) may be necessary. After reduction, the extremity is usually immobilized by bracing, splinting, taping, or using a sling to allow the torn ligaments and capsular tissue time to heal. Nursing management is directed toward relief of pain and support and protection of the injured joint.

After the joint has been reduced and immobilized, motion is usually restricted. In collaboration with physiotherapy, a carefully regulated rehabilitation program can prevent fracture instability and joint dysfunction. Gentle range of motion (ROM) may be started if the joint is stable and the affected joint is well supported. An exercise program slowly restores the joint to its original ROM without causing another dislocation. The patient should gradually return to their usual activities. A patient who has dislocated a joint may be at greater risk for repeated dislocations because of loose ligaments. Activity restrictions of the affected joint may be imposed to decrease the risk for repeated dislocation.

REPETITIVE STRAIN INJURY

Repetitive strain injury (RSI) and *cumulative trauma disorder* are terms used to describe injuries resulting from prolonged force or repetitive movements and awkward postures. RSI is also reported as *repetitive trauma disorder, nontraumatic musculoskeletal injury, overuse syndrome* (sports medicine), *regional musculoskeletal disorder,* and *work-related musculoskeletal disorder.* The exact cause of these disorders is unknown. There are no specific diagnostic tests, and diagnosis is often difficult.

Almost two million Canadians suffer from RSIs and more than half of these are work-related injuries (Canadian Centre for Occupational Health and Safety [CCOHS], 2016). People at risk for RSI include musicians, dancers, butchers, grocery clerks, vibratory tool workers, and those who frequently use technology such as a smartphone, computer mouse, and keyboard (Short et al., 2020). Competitive athletes and poorly trained athletes may also develop RSI. Swimming, overhead throwing (e.g., baseball), weightlifting, gymnastics, tennis, skiing, and kicking sports (e.g., soccer) require repetitive motion, and overtraining compounds the effects of RSI. Other factors related to RSI include poor posture and positioning, poor workspace ergonomics, badly designed workplace equipment (e.g., computer keyboard), and repetitive lifting of heavy workloads without sufficient muscle rest. The CCOHS (2021) reports that musculoskeletal disorders, like RSI, are the most frequent type of lost-time injury and single largest source of lost-time costs in Canada.

Symptoms of RSI include pain, weakness, numbness, or impairment of motor function in the muscles, tendons, and nerves of the neck, shoulder, forearm, and hand. RSI can be prevented through education and *ergonomics* (the science that promotes efficiency and safety in the interaction of humans and their work environment). Ergonomic considerations for people who work at a desk and use a computer include keeping the hips and knees flexed to 90 degrees with the feet flat, keeping the wrist straight to type, having the top of the monitor even with the forehead, and taking at least hourly stretch breaks. Once RSI is diagnosed, an interprofessional approach to treatment consists of identification of the precipitating activity (occupational therapist assessment); modification of equipment or activity; pain management, including heat or cold application and NSAIDs; rest; physiotherapy for strengthening and conditioning exercises; and lifestyle changes.

CARPAL TUNNEL SYNDROME

Carpal tunnel syndrome (CTS) is an RSI caused by compression of the median nerve, which enters the hand through the narrow confines of the carpal tunnel (Figure 65.2). The carpal tunnel is formed by ligaments and bones in the wrist. CTS is the most common compression neuropathy in the upper extremity. This syndrome is associated with hobbies or occupations that require continuous wrist movement (e.g., musicians, painters, carpenters, computer operators).

This condition often is caused by pressure from trauma or edema resulting from inflammation of a tendon (tenosynovitis), neoplasm, rheumatoid arthritis (RA), or soft tissue masses such as ganglia. Estrogen and progesterone may be involved, as initial manifestations often occur during the premenstrual period, pregnancy, and menopause. People with diabetes mellitus or other metabolic disorders have a higher incidence of CTS (National Institute of Neurological Disorders and Stroke [NINDS], 2020). Women are more likely than men to develop CTS, possibly because they have a smaller carpal tunnel.

The clinical manifestations of CTS are weakness (especially of the thumb), burning pain (causalgia), numbness or impaired sensation in the distribution of the median nerve, and clumsiness in performing fine hand movements. Numbness and tingling may awaken the patient at night. Shaking the hands will often relieve these symptoms.

Manifestations of CTS include a positive Tinel sign and Phalen sign. The *Tinel sign* can be elicited by tapping over the median nerve as it passes through the carpal tunnel in the wrist (see Figure 65.2). A positive response is a sensation of tingling in the distribution of the median nerve over the hand. The *Phalen sign* can be elicited by allowing the wrists to fall freely into maximum flexion and maintaining the position for longer than 60 seconds. A positive response is a sensation of tingling in the distribution of the median nerve over the hand. In late stages, there is atrophy of the thenar muscles around the base of the thumb, resulting in recurrent pain and eventual dysfunction of the hand.

NURSING AND INTERPROFESSIONAL MANAGEMENT CARPAL TUNNEL SYNDROME

HEALTH PROMOTION

Prevention of CTS involves educating patients, employees, and employers to identify risk factors. Adaptive devices such as wrist splints may be worn to hold the wrist in slight extension to relieve pressure on the median nerve. Special keyboard pads and mice that help prevent repetitive pressure on the median nerve are available for use at computers. Other ergonomic changes include workstation modifications, change in body

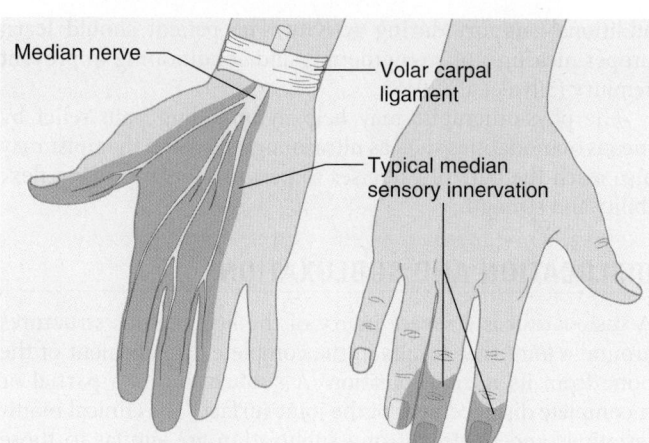

FIG. 65.2 Wrist structures involved in carpal tunnel syndrome. Median nerve distribution. *Shaded areas* depict the locations of pain in carpal tunnel syndrome. Source: Buttaravoli, P. (2012). *Minor emergencies (3rd ed.).* Saunders.

positions, and frequent breaks from work-related activities. The occupational therapist can assess and make recommendations to improve workstations both at home and at work (Canadian Association of Occupational Therapists, 2016).

ACUTE INTERVENTION

Interprofessional management of the patient with CTS is directed toward relieving the underlying cause of the nerve compression. The early symptoms associated with CTS can usually be relieved by stopping the aggravating movement and by placing the hand and wrist at rest by immobilizing them in a hand splint. Splints worn at night help keep the wrist in a neutral position and may reduce night pain and numbness. Physiotherapy with hand and wrist exercises may lessen symptom severity. Injection of a corticosteroid medication directly into the carpal tunnel may provide short-term relief. The patient may need to consider a change in occupation because of discomfort and sensory changes.

Carpal tunnel release is generally recommended if symptoms last for more than 6 months. Surgery involves severing the band of tissue around the wrist to reduce pressure on the median nerve (see Figure 65.2). Surgery is done under local anaesthesia and does not require an overnight hospital stay. The types of carpal tunnel release surgery include open-release and endoscopic surgery (Vershinin et al., 2018). In *open-release surgery,* an incision is made in the wrist and then the carpal ligament is cut to enlarge the carpal tunnel. *Endoscopic carpal tunnel release* is performed through one or more small puncture incisions in the wrist and palm. A camera is attached to a tube, and the carpal ligament is cut. The endoscopic approach may allow faster functional recovery and less postoperative discomfort than traditional open-release surgery.

Although symptoms may be relieved immediately after surgery, full recovery may take months. After surgery, the neurovascular status of the hand is assessed before discharge. The patient is instructed about wound care and the appropriate assessments to perform at home.

ROTATOR CUFF INJURY

The *rotator cuff* is a complex of four muscles in the shoulder: the supraspinatus, infraspinatus, teres minor, and subscapularis muscles. These muscles act to stabilize the humeral head in the glenoid fossa while assisting with ROM of the shoulder joint and rotation of the humerus. A tear in the rotator cuff may occur as a gradual, degenerative process resulting from aging, repetitive stress (especially overhead arm motions), or injury to the shoulder while falling. The rotator cuff can tear as a result of sudden adduction forces applied to the cuff while the arm is held in abduction. In sports, repetitive overhead motions, such as in swimming, weightlifting, and swinging a racquet (e.g., tennis, racquetball), often cause injury. Other causative factors include (a) falling onto an outstretched arm and hand, (b) a blow to the upper arm, (c) heavy lifting, or (d) repetitive work motions.

Manifestations of a rotator cuff injury include shoulder weakness and pain and decreased ROM. The patient usually experiences severe pain when the arm is abducted between 60 and 120 degrees (the painful arc). The *drop arm test,* in which the arm falls suddenly after the patient is asked to slowly lower the arm to the side after it has been abducted 90 degrees, is another sign of rotator cuff injury. A radiograph alone is usually not beneficial in the diagnosis. A tear can be confirmed by magnetic resonance imaging (MRI).

NURSING AND INTERPROFESSIONAL MANAGEMENT
ROTATOR CUFF INJURY

The patient with a partial tear or cuff inflammation may be treated conservatively with rest, ice and heat, NSAIDs, corticosteroid injections into the joint, and physiotherapy. If the patient does not respond to conservative treatment in 3 to 6 months or if a complete tear is present, a surgical repair may be necessary. Most surgical repairs are performed through arthroscopy (Figure 65.3). If an extensive tear is present, *acromioplasty* (surgical removal of part of the acromion to relieve compression of the rotator cuff during movement) may be necessary. A sling or, more commonly, a shoulder immobilizer may be used immediately after surgery. Shoulder immobilization for extended periods of time may cause a buildup of scar tissue creating arthrofibrosis or "frozen" shoulder to occur. Pendulum exercises and physiotherapy begin the first postoperative day. Restrictions for lifting weights are usually given, with full recovery taking up to 6 months.

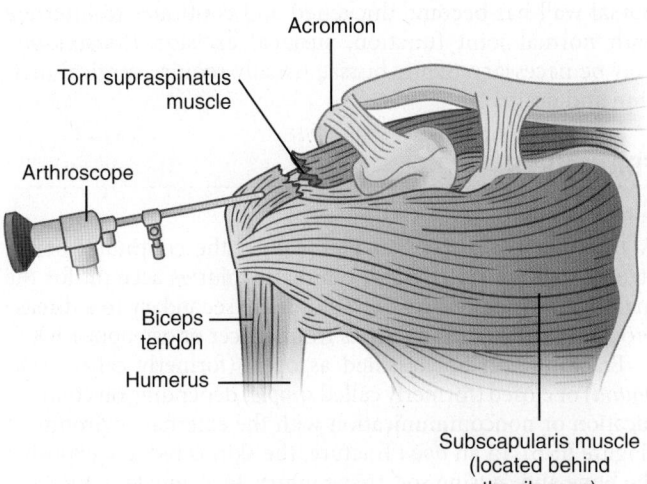

FIG. 65.3 A torn rotator cuff is repaired using arthroscopic surgery.

MENISCUS INJURY

The *menisci* are crescent-shaped pieces of fibrocartilage in the knee. Menisci are also found in other joints, including the acromioclavicular (AC), sternoclavicular, and temporomandibular joints. Meniscus injuries are closely associated with ligament sprains, commonly occurring in athletes engaged in sports such as basketball, football, soccer, and hockey (Gee et al., 2020). These activities produce rotational stress when the knee is in varying degrees of flexion and the foot is planted or fixed. A blow to the knee can cause the meniscus to be sheared between the femoral condyles and the tibial plateau, resulting in a torn meniscus. Individuals in occupations that require squatting or kneeling, as well as older persons, may be at higher risk for meniscus injuries.

Meniscus injuries alone do not usually cause significant edema because most of the cartilage is avascular. However, an acutely torn meniscus may be suspected when localized tenderness, pain, and effusion are noted (Figure 65.4). Pain is elicited by flexion, internal rotation, and then extension of the knee (called the *McMurray test*). The usual clinical picture is the patient feeling that the knee is unstable and a report that the knee may "click," "pop," "lock," or "give way." Quadriceps atrophy may be evident if the injury has been present for some time. Traumatic arthritis may occur from repeated meniscal injury and chronic inflammation.

MRI is beneficial for confirming the diagnosis before arthroscopy. The degree of knee pain and dysfunction, occupation, sport activities, and age may affect the patient's decision to have or postpone surgery.

NURSING AND INTERPROFESSIONAL MANAGEMENT
MENISCUS INJURY

Because meniscal injuries are commonly caused by sports-related activity, athletes should be taught to do warm-up activities. Examination of the acutely injured knee should occur

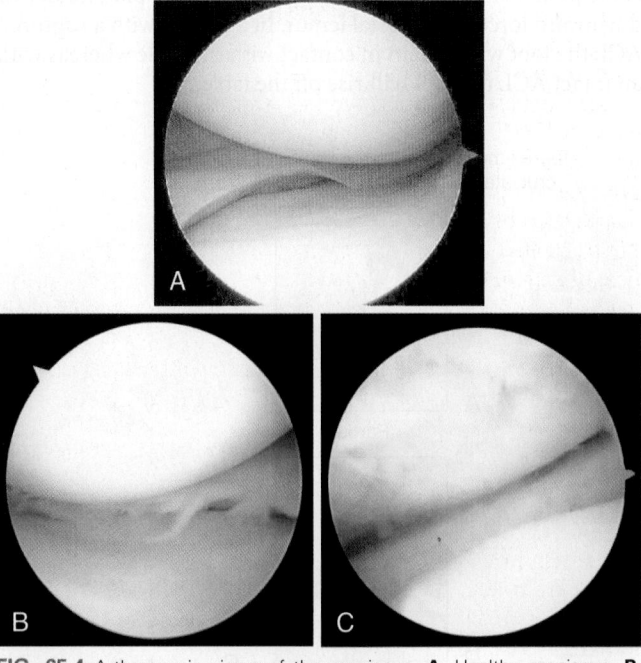

FIG. 65.4 Arthroscopic views of the meniscus. A, Healthy meniscus. B, Torn meniscus. C, Surgically repaired meniscus. Source: A, David Lintner, MD, Houston; http://www.drlintner.com. B and C, Courtesy Peter Bonner, San Antonio, TX.

within 24 hours of injury. Initial care of this type of injury involves application of ice, immobilization, and partial weight bearing with crutches. Most meniscal injuries are treated in an outpatient setting. Use of a knee brace or immobilizer during the first few days after the injury protects the knee and offers some pain relief. After acute pain has decreased, physiotherapy can help the patient regain knee flexion and muscle strength to assist in returning to full function. In patients with degenerative meniscus tears, physiotherapy and exercise treatments may improve neuromuscular function and muscle strength (Safran-Norton et al., 2019).

Surgical repair or excision of part of the meniscus *(meniscectomy)* may be necessary. Meniscal surgery is performed by arthroscopy. Pain relief may include use of NSAIDs or other analgesics. Rehabilitation starts soon after surgery, including quadriceps- and hamstring-strengthening exercises and ROM. When the patient's strength is back to its preinjury level, their usual activities may be resumed (Wiley et al., 2020).

ANTERIOR CRUCIATE LIGAMENT (ACL) INJURY

Knee injuries account for over 50% of all sport injuries. The most commonly injured knee ligament is the anterior cruciate ligament (ACL). ACL injuries usually occur from noncontact when the athlete pivots, lands from a jump, or slows down when running. Patients often report coming down on the knee, twisting, and hearing a pop, followed by acute knee pain and swelling. Athletes usually cannot continue playing, and the knee may feel unstable. An injury to the ACL can result in a partial tear, a complete tear, or an *avulsion* (tearing away) from the bone attachments that form the knee (Figure 65.5).

Examination of the knee with an ACL tear may produce a positive *Lever sign test* (McQuivey et al., 2019). This test is performed while the patient is supine with knees fully extended on the examination table. The examiner places a fist under the tibial tuberosity of the affected knee. This causes a slight flexion at the joint. With the other hand, the examiner applies moderate downward force to the distal femur. In a patient with a ruptured ACL the foot will remain in contact with the table whereas with an intact ACL the foot will rise off the table.

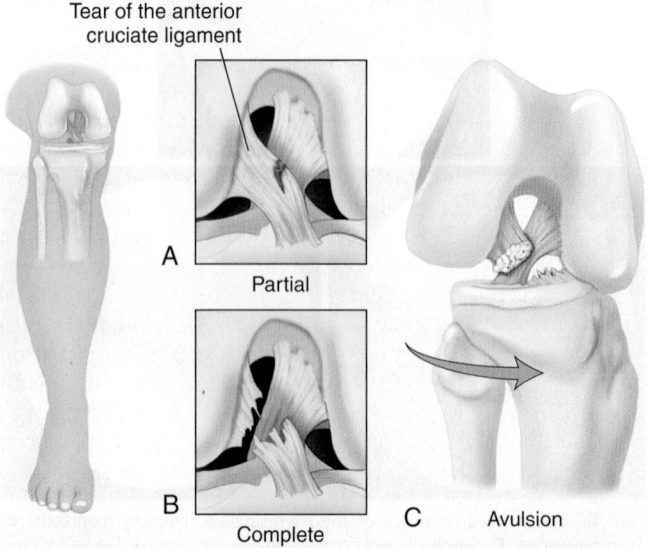

FIG. 65.5 Anterior cruciate ligament injury. **A,** Partial tear. **B,** Complete tear. **C,** Avulsion.

NURSING AND INTERPROFESSIONAL MANAGEMENT ANTERIOR CRUCIATE LIGAMENT INJURY

Prevention programs have been shown to significantly reduce ACL injuries in athletes. Conservative treatment for an intact ACL injury includes rest, ice, NSAIDs, elevation, and ambulation as tolerated with crutches. If there is a tight, painful effusion, it may be aspirated. A knee immobilizer or hinged knee brace may be helpful in supporting the knee. Often, physiotherapy assists the patient in maintaining knee joint motion and muscle tone.

Reconstructive surgery is usually recommended in physically active patients who have sustained severe injury to the ligament and meniscus. In reconstruction, the torn ACL tissue is removed and replaced with autologous or allograft tissue (Shea et al., 2015). ROM exercises are encouraged soon after surgery and the knee is placed in a brace or immobilizer. Rehabilitation with physiotherapy is critical, with progressive weight bearing determined by the degree of surgical repair. A safe return to the patient's prior level of physical functioning may take 6 to 8 months.

BURSITIS

Bursitis (inflammation of a bursa) results from repeated or excessive trauma or friction, gout, RA, or infection. The primary clinical manifestations of bursitis are warmth, pain, swelling, and limited ROM in the affected part. Sites at which bursitis commonly occurs include the hand, knee, greater trochanter of the hip, shoulder, and elbow. Improper body mechanics, repetitive kneeling (e.g., among carpet layers, coal miners, gardeners), jogging in worn-out shoes, and prolonged sitting with crossed legs are common precipitating activities.

NURSING AND INTERPROFESSIONAL MANAGEMENT BURSITIS

Attempts are made to determine and correct the cause of the bursitis. Rest is often the only treatment needed. Icing the area will decrease pain and may reduce inflammation. The affected part may be immobilized in a compression dressing or splint. NSAIDs may be used to reduce inflammation and pain (Foran, 2018a). Aspiration of the bursal fluid and intra-articular injection of a corticosteroid may be necessary. If the bursal wall has become thickened and continues to interfere with normal joint function, surgical excision *(bursectomy)* may be necessary. Septic bursae usually require surgical incision and drainage.

FRACTURES

Classification

A fracture is a disruption or break in the continuity of the structure of bone. Although traumatic injuries account for the majority of fractures, some fractures are secondary to a disease process (pathological fractures from cancer or osteoporosis).

Fractures can be classified as open (formerly called *compound*) or closed (formerly called *simple*) depending on communication or noncommunication with the external environment (Figure 65.6). In an *open* fracture, the skin is broken, exposing the bone and causing soft tissue injury. In a *closed* fracture, the skin has not been ruptured and remains intact.

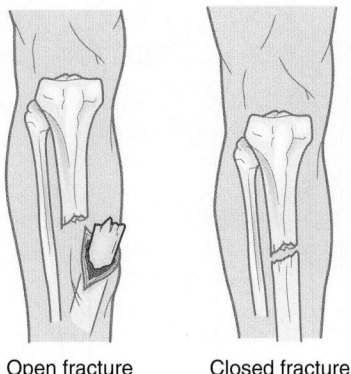

Open fracture   Closed fracture

FIG. 65.6 Fracture classification according to communication with the external environment.

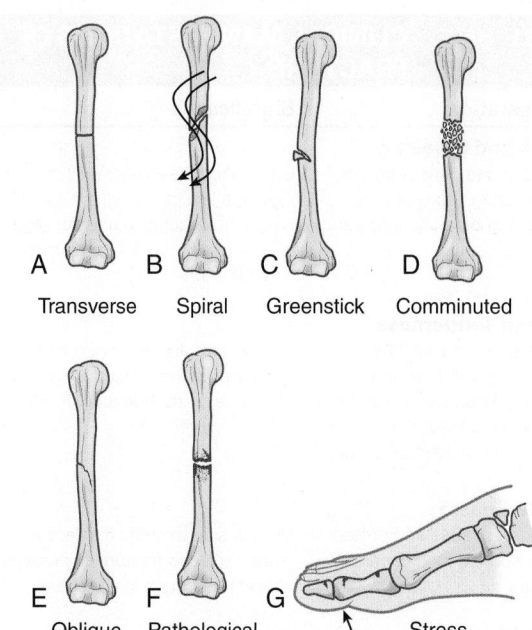

A   B   C   D
Transverse Spiral Greenstick Comminuted

E   F   G
Oblique Pathological   Stress

FIG. 65.7 Types of fractures. **A,** Transverse fracture: the line of the fracture extends across the bone shaft at a right angle to the longitudinal axis. **B,** Spiral fracture: the line of the fracture extends in a spiral direction along the shaft of the bone. **C,** Greenstick fracture: an incomplete fracture with one side splintered and the other side bent. **D,** Comminuted fracture: fracture with more than two fragments. The smaller fragments appear to be floating. **E,** Oblique fracture: the line of the fracture extends in an oblique direction. **F,** Pathological fracture: a spontaneous fracture at the site of a bone disease. **G,** Stress fracture: occurs in healthy or abnormal bone that is subject to repeated stress, such as from jogging or running.

Fractures can also be classified as complete or incomplete. Fractures are termed *complete* if the break is completely through the bone and described as *incomplete* if the fracture occurs partly across a bone shaft but the bone is still in one piece. An incomplete fracture is often the result of bending or crushing forces applied to a bone.

Fractures are also described and classified according to the direction of the fracture line. Types include linear, oblique, transverse, longitudinal, and spiral fractures (Figure 65.7). Fractures can also be classified as displaced or nondisplaced. In a *displaced* fracture, the two ends of the broken bone are separated from one another and out of their normal positions. Displaced fractures are usually *comminuted* (more than two fragments) or *oblique* (see Figure 65.7). In a *nondisplaced* fracture, the periosteum is intact across the fracture and the bone is still in alignment. Nondisplaced fractures are usually transverse, spiral, or greenstick (see Figure 65.7).

Clinical Manifestations

The clinical manifestations of a fracture include immediate localized pain, decreased function, and inability to bear weight on or use the affected part (Table 65.3). The patient guards and protects the extremity against movement. Obvious bone deformity may not be present. If a fracture is suspected, the extremity is immobilized in the position in which it is found. Unnecessary movement increases soft tissue damage and may convert a closed fracture to an open fracture or create further injury to adjacent neurovascular structures.

Fracture Healing

It is important to understand the principles of bone healing (Figure 65.8) to provide appropriate therapeutic interventions. Bone goes through a remarkable reparative process of self-healing (termed *union*) that occurs in the following stages (Hardy & Feehan, 2020):

1. *Fracture hematoma.* When a fracture occurs, bleeding creates a hematoma, which surrounds the ends of the fragments. The hematoma is extravasated blood that changes from a liquid to a semisolid clot. This hematoma formation occurs in the initial 72 hours after injury.
2. *Granulation tissue.* During this stage, active phagocytosis absorbs the products of local necrosis. The hematoma converts to granulation tissue. Granulation tissue (consisting of new blood vessels, fibroblasts, and osteoblasts) produces the basis for new bone substance called *osteoid* during days 3 to 14 after injury.

3. *Callus formation.* As minerals (calcium, phosphorus, and magnesium) and new bone matrix are deposited in the osteoid, an unorganized network of bone is formed that is woven about the fracture parts. Callus is composed primarily of cartilage, osteoblasts, calcium, and phosphorus. It usually appears by the end of the second week after injury. Evidence of callus formation can be verified by radiography.
4. *Ossification.* Ossification of the callus occurs from 3 weeks to 6 months after the fracture and continues until the fracture has healed. Callus ossification is sufficient to prevent movement at the fracture site when the bones are gently stressed. However, the fracture is still evident on a radiograph. During this stage of *clinical union,* the patient may be allowed limited mobility or the cast may be removed.
5. *Consolidation.* As callus continues to develop, the distance between bone fragments diminishes and eventually closes. During this stage, ossification continues. It can be equated with *radiological union,* which occurs when there is radiographic evidence of complete bony union. This phase can occur up to 1 year following injury.
6. *Remodelling.* Excess bone tissue is reabsorbed in the final stage of bone healing and union is completed. Gradual return of the injured bone to its preinjury structural strength and shape occurs. Bone remodels in response to physical loading stress, or *Wolff's law.* Initially, stress is provided through exercise. Weight bearing is gradually introduced. New bone is deposited in sites subjected to stress and resorbed at areas where there is little stress.

Many factors influence the time required for complete fracture healing, including displacement and site of the fracture, blood supply to the area, immobilization, and internal fixation

TABLE 65.3   CLINICAL MANIFESTATIONS OF FRACTURE

Manifestation	Significance
Edema and Swelling Disruption and penetration of bone through skin or soft tissues, or bleeding into surrounding tissues	Unchecked bleeding, swelling, and edema in a closed space can occlude circulation and damage nerves (i.e., risk for compartment syndrome).
Pain and Tenderness Muscle spasm as a result of involuntary reflex action of muscle, direct tissue trauma, increased pressure on nerves, movement of fracture parts	Pain and tenderness encourage splinting of musculature around the fracture, with reduction in motion of the injured area.
Muscle Spasm Irritation of tissues and protective response to injury and fracture	Muscle spasms may displace a nondisplaced fracture or prevent it from reducing spontaneously.
Deformity Abnormal position of extremity or part as result of original forces of injury and action of muscles pulling fragment into abnormal position; seen as a loss of normal bony contours	Deformity is a cardinal sign of fracture; if uncorrected, it may result in problems with bony union and restoration of function of the injured part.
Ecchymosis or Contusion Discoloration of skin as a result of extravasation of blood into subcutaneous tissues	Ecchymosis may appear immediately after injury and may appear distal to the injury. Patient should be reassured that the process is normal and that discoloration will eventually resolve.
Loss of Function Disruption of bone or joint, preventing functional use of limb or part	Fracture must be managed properly to ensure restoration of function to the limb or part.
Crepitation Grating or crunching together of bony fragments, producing palpable or audible crunching or popping sensation	Crepitation may increase the chance for nonunion if bone ends are allowed to move excessively. Micromovement of bone-end fragments (postfracture) assists in osteogenesis (new bone growth).

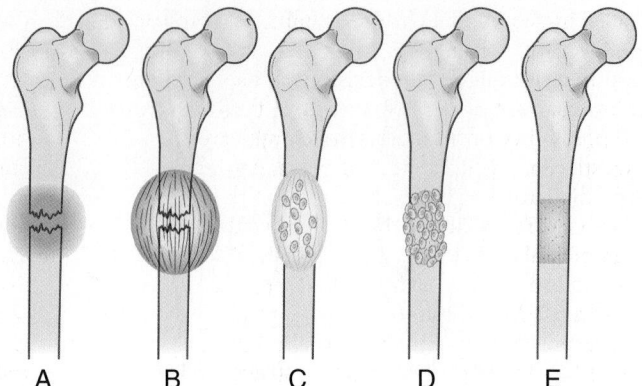

FIG. 65.8 Bone healing (schematic representation). **A,** Bleeding at broken ends of the bone with subsequent hematoma formation. **B,** Organization of hematoma into fibrous network. **C,** Invasion of osteoblasts, lengthening of collagen strands, and deposition of calcium. **D,** Callus formation: new bone is built up as osteoclasts destroy dead bone. **E,** Remodelling is accomplished as excess callus is reabsorbed and trabecular bone is laid down.

TABLE 65.4   COMPLICATIONS OF FRACTURE HEALING

Problem	Description
Delayed union	Fracture healing progresses more slowly than expected; healing eventually occurs
Nonunion	Fracture fails to heal properly despite treatment; no radiographic evidence of callus formation
Malunion	Fracture heals in expected time but in unsatisfactory position, possibly resulting in deformity or dysfunction
Angulation	Fracture heals in abnormal position in relation to midline of structure (type of malunion)
Pseudoarthrosis	Type of nonunion occurring at fracture site in which a false joint is formed with abnormal movement at site
Refracture	New fracture occurs at original fracture site
Myositis ossificans	Deposition of calcium in muscle tissue at the site of significant blunt muscle trauma or repeated muscle injury

devices (e.g., screws, pins). The ossification process may be arrested by inadequate reduction and immobilization, excessive movement of the fracture fragments, infection, poor nutrition, and systemic disease. Healing time for fractures increases with age. For example, an uncomplicated midshaft fracture of the femur heals in 3 weeks in a newborn and in 20 weeks in an adult. Smoking also increases fracture healing time. Fracture healing may not occur in the expected time (*delayed union*) or may not occur at all (*nonunion*). Table 65.4 summarizes complications of fracture healing.

Interprofessional Care

The overall goals of fracture treatment are (a) anatomical realignment of bone fragments (*reduction*), (b) immobilization to maintain realignment, and (c) restoration of normal or near-normal function of the injured part, which will require an interprofessional approach. Once the health care provider has realigned the bone fragments, nurses, physiotherapists, and occupational therapists are instrumental in maintaining alignment and restoring functioning. Pharmacists can help prevent complications by recommending appropriate pain management and antibiotic therapy, while dietitians promote bone healing through nutritional counselling.

Fracture Reduction

Closed Reduction. *Closed reduction* is a nonsurgical, manual realignment of bone fragments to their previous anatomical position. Traction and countertraction are manually applied to the bone fragments to restore position, length, and alignment. Usually, closed reduction is performed with the patient under local or general anaesthesia. After reduction, traction, casting, external fixation, splints, or orthoses (braces), the injured part is immobilized to maintain alignment until healing occurs.

Open Reduction. *Open reduction* is the correction of bone alignment through a surgical incision. It often includes internal fixation of the fracture with the use of wire, screws, pins, plates, intramedullary rods, or nails. The type and location of the fracture, patient age, and the presence of concurrent disease may influence the decision to use open reduction. The main disadvantages of this form of fracture management are the possibility of infection, the complications associated with anaesthesia, and the effect of pre-existing medical conditions (e.g., diabetes).

If open reduction with internal fixation (ORIF) is used for intra-articular fractures, early initiation of active ROM of the joint is indicated. Machines that provide continuous passive motion (CPM) to various joints (e.g., knee, shoulder) are used to prevent extra-articular and intra-articular adhesions. The use of CPM results in faster reconstruction of the subchondral (beneath cartilage) bone plate, more rapid healing of the articular cartilage, and decreased incidence of post-traumatic arthritis. ORIF facilitates early ambulation, thus decreasing the risk for complications related to prolonged immobility.

Traction. Traction is the application of a pulling force to an injured or diseased part of the body or extremity. Traction is used to (a) prevent or reduce pain and muscle spasm associated with low back pain or cervical sprain (e.g., whiplash), (b) immobilize a joint or part of the body, (c) reduce a fracture or dislocation, and (d) treat a pathological joint condition (e.g., tumour, infection). Traction is also indicated to (a) provide immobilization to prevent soft tissue damage, (b) promote active and passive exercise, (c) expand a joint space during arthroscopic procedures, and (d) expand a joint space before major joint reconstruction.

Traction devices apply a pulling force on a fractured extremity to attain realignment, while *countertraction* pulls in the opposite direction. The two most common types of traction are skin traction and skeletal traction. *Skin traction* is generally used for short-term treatment (48–72 hours) until skeletal traction or surgery is possible. Tape, boots, or splints are applied directly to the skin to maintain alignment, assist in reduction, and help diminish muscle spasms in the injured extremity. The traction weights are usually limited to 2.3 to 4.5 kg. A *Buck traction* boot is a type of skin traction used to immobilize a fracture, prevent hip flexion contractures, and reduce muscle spasms (Figure 65.9) (Matullo et al., 2016). Pelvic or cervical skin traction may require heavier weights applied intermittently. In skin traction, assessment of the skin is a priority, since pressure points and skin breakdown may develop quickly. Key pressure points are assessed every 2 to 4 hours.

Skeletal traction, generally in place for longer periods than skin traction, is used to align injured bones and joints or to treat joint contractures and congenital hip dysplasia. It provides a long-term pull that keeps the injured bones and joints aligned. To apply skeletal traction, the health care provider inserts a pin or wire into the bone, either partially or completely, to align and immobilize the injured body part (Witmer et al., 2017). Weight for skeletal traction ranges from 2 to 20 kg. The use of too much weight can result in delayed union or nonunion. The major disadvantages of skeletal traction are risk for infection in the area of the bone where the skeletal pin has been inserted and the consequences of prolonged immobility.

When traction is used to treat fractures, the forces are usually exerted on the distal fragment to obtain alignment with the proximal fragment. Several types of traction can be used for this purpose. One of the more common types of skeletal traction is balanced suspension traction (Figure 65.10). Fracture alignment depends on the correct positioning and alignment of the patient while the traction forces remain constant. For extremity traction to be effective, forces must be pulling in the opposite direction (countertraction). Countertraction is commonly supplied by the patient's body weight or by weights pulling in the opposite direction and may be augmented by elevating the end of the bed. It is imperative to maintain traction continuously and keep the weights off the floor and moving freely through the pulleys.

Fracture Immobilization. Fracture immobilization can be done using casts (including air casts), braces, splints, immobilizing devices, and external and internal fixation devices.

Casts. A *cast* is a temporary circumferential immobilization device commonly used following a closed reduction. The health care provider applies a cast to an extremity and generally incorporates the joints above and below a fracture. Immobilization above and below a joint restricts tendon and ligament movement, thus assisting with joint stabilization while the fracture heals. It allows the patient to perform many normal activities of daily living (ADLs) while providing sufficient immobilization to ensure stability. Cast materials are natural (plaster of

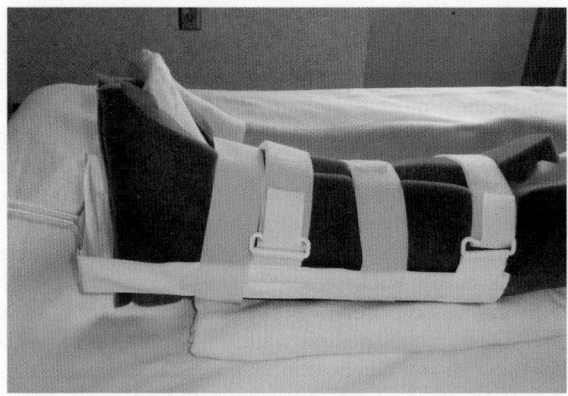

FIG. 65.9 Buck traction is most commonly used for fractures of the hip and femur. Source: Courtesy Mary Wollan, RN, BAN. Spring Park, MN.

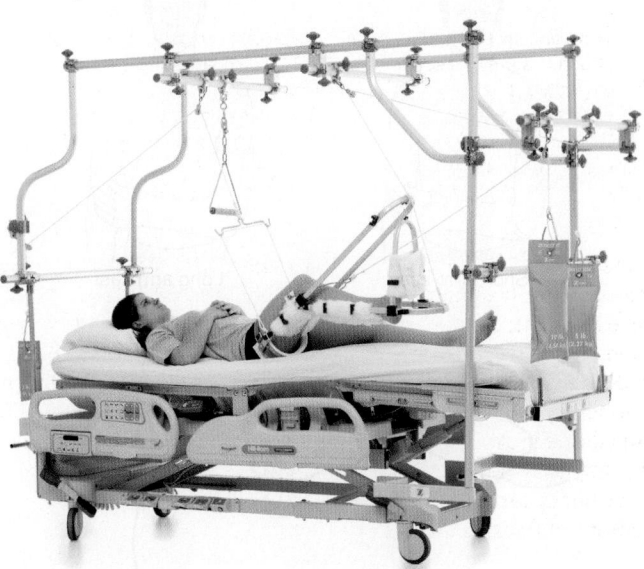

FIG. 65.10 Balanced suspension skeletal traction. This is most commonly used for fractures of the femur, hip, and lower leg. Source: Courtesy Zimmer, Inc.

Paris) or synthetic acrylic; fibreglass-free, latex-free polymer; or a hybrid of materials. Stockinette and padding are placed over the extremity with extra padding over bony prominences before casting (Szostakowski et al., 2017).

Plaster of Paris is usually immersed in warm water, then wrapped and moulded around the affected part setting in 15 minutes. Even though patients may move around without difficulty, the cast is not strong enough for weight bearing until about 24 to 72 hours after application. The decision about weight bearing is determined by the health care provider. The patient is instructed to never cover a fresh plaster cast because air cannot circulate, heat builds up in the cast that may cause a burn, and drying is delayed. During the drying period, the nurse needs to avoid direct pressure on the cast and handle it gently with an open palm to avoid denting. Once the cast is thoroughly dry, the edges may need to be smoothed with strips of tape *(petalling)*, ensuring a smooth cast edge to prevent skin irritation from rough edges and to prevent plaster of Paris debris from falling into the cast and causing irritation or pressure necrosis.

Casts made of fibreglass are being used more often than those made of plaster because they are lightweight, relatively waterproof, stronger and faster-drying than plaster, and porous (less risk for skin problems) and allow for almost immediate mobilization (Szostakowski et al., 2017). Synthetic casting materials (thermolabile plastic, thermoplastic resins, polyurethane, and fibreglass) are activated by submersion in cool or tepid water. Then they are moulded to fit the torso or the extremity.

Upper Extremity Injuries. Immobilization of an acute fracture or soft tissue injury of the upper extremity is often accomplished by use of a (a) sugar-tong splint, (b) posterior splint, (c) short arm cast, or (d) long arm cast (Figure 65.11).

The *sugar-tong splint* is typically used for acute wrist injuries or injuries that may result in significant swelling. Plaster splints are applied over a well-padded forearm, beginning at the phalangeal joints of the hand, extending up the dorsal aspect of the forearm around the distal humerus, and then extending down the volar aspect of the forearm to the distal palmar crease. The splinting material is wrapped with either elastic bandage or bias stockinette. The sugar-tong posterior splint accommodates for postinjury swelling in the fractured extremity.

The *short arm cast* is often used for the treatment of stable wrist or metacarpal fractures. An aluminum finger splint can be fabricated into the short arm cast for concurrent treatment of phalangeal injuries. The short arm cast is a circular cast extending from the distal palmar area to the proximal forearm. This cast provides wrist immobilization and permits unrestricted elbow motion.

The *long arm cast* is commonly used for stable forearm or elbow fractures and unstable wrist fractures. It is similar to the short arm cast but extends to the proximal humerus, restricting motion in the wrist and the elbow. Nursing measures should be directed toward supporting the extremity and reducing the effects of edema by maintaining extremity elevation with a sling. However, when a hanging arm cast is used for a proximal humerus fracture, elevation or a supportive sling is contraindicated because hanging provides traction and maintains fracture alignment.

When a sling is used, the nurse must ensure that the axillary area is well padded to prevent skin excoriation and maceration associated with direct skin-to-skin contact. Placement of the sling should not put undue pressure on the posterior neck. Movement of the fingers (unless contraindicated) should be encouraged to enhance the pumping action of vascular and soft tissue structures to decrease edema. The nurse should also encourage the patient to actively move nonimmobilized joints of the upper extremity to prevent stiffness and contractures.

Vertebral Injuries. The *body jacket brace* is often used for immobilization and support for stable spine injuries of the thoracic or lumbar spine. This brace goes around the chest and abdomen and extends from above the nipple line to the pubis. After application of the cast, the nurse must assess the patient for the development of superior mesenteric artery syndrome *(cast syndrome)*. This condition occurs if the body cast is applied too tightly and compresses the superior mesenteric artery against the duodenum. The patient generally experiences abdominal pain, abdominal pressure, nausea, and vomiting. The abdomen should be assessed for decreased bowel sounds (a window in the brace may be left over the umbilicus). Treatment includes gastric decompression with a nasogastric tube and suction. Nursing assessment also includes observation of respiratory status, bowel and bladder function, and areas of pressure over the bony prominences, especially the iliac crest. The brace may need to be adjusted or removed if any complications occur.

Lower Extremity Injuries. Injuries to the lower extremity are often immobilized by a long leg cast, short leg cast, cylinder cast, Jones dressing, or prefabricated splint or immobilizer. The usual indications for applying a *long leg cast* are an unstable ankle fracture, soft tissue injuries, a fractured tibia, and knee injuries. The cast usually extends from the base of the toes to the groin and the gluteal crease. The *short leg cast* can be used for a variety of conditions, but primarily for stable ankle and foot injuries. A *cylinder cast,* which is used for knee injuries or fractures, extends from the groin to the malleoli of the ankle. A *Jones dressing* is composed of bulky padding materials (absorption dressing and cotton sheet wadding), splints, and an elastic wrap or bias-cut stockinette.

After application of a lower extremity cast or dressing, the extremity should be elevated on pillows above the heart level

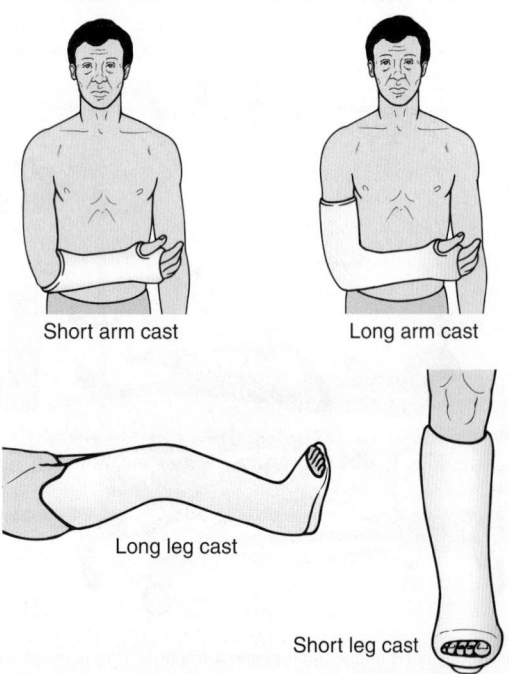

Short arm cast   Long arm cast

Long leg cast

Short leg cast

FIG. 65.11 Common types of casts.

for the first 24 hours. After the initial phase, the casted extremity should not be placed in a dependent position because of the possibility of excessive edema. After cast application, the patient should be observed for signs of compartment syndrome (see the Compartment Syndrome section) and increased pressure, especially in the heel, anterior tibia, head of the fibula, and malleoli. This increased pressure is manifested by pain or a burning feeling in these areas.

Prefabricated knee and ankle splints and immobilizers are being used in many settings. This type of immobilization is easy to apply and remove, which permits close observation of the affected joint for signs of swelling and skin breakdown. Depending on the injury, removal of the splint or immobilizer facilitates ROM of the affected joint and a faster return to function.

The *hip spica cast* is now used mainly for femur fractures in children. The purpose of the hip spica cast is to immobilize the affected extremity and the trunk. The cast extends from above the nipple line to the base of the foot (single spica) and may include the opposite extremity up to an area above the knee (spica and a half) or both extremities (double spica). The patient with a hip spica cast should be assessed for the same conditions that are associated with the body jacket brace.

External Fixation. An *external fixator* is a metallic device composed of metal pins that are inserted into the bone and attached to external rods to stabilize the fracture while it heals. It can be used to apply traction or to compress fracture fragments and to immobilize reduced fragments when the use of a cast or other traction is not appropriate. The external device holds fracture fragments in a manner similar to a surgically implanted internal device. The external fixator is attached directly to the bones by percutaneous transfixing pins or wires (Figure 65.12). External fixation is indicated in closed fractures, complex fractures with extensive soft tissue damage, correction of bony defects (congenital), nonunion or malunion, and limb lengthening.

Often, external fixation is used in an attempt to salvage extremities that otherwise might require amputation. Because the use of an external device is a long-term process, assessment for pin loosening and infection is critical. Infection—signalled by exudate, erythema, tenderness, and pain—may necessitate removal of the device. The nurse should instruct the patient and caregivers about meticulous pin care. Although each health care provider has a protocol for pin care cleaning, chlorhexidine is often used (Walker, 2018).

Internal Fixation. Internal fixation devices (pins, plates, intramedullary rods, and metal and bioabsorbable screws) are surgically inserted at the time of realignment (Figure 65.13). These metal devices are biologically inert and made from stainless steel, vitallium, or titanium. Proper alignment is evaluated by radiographs at regular intervals.

Electrical Bone Growth Stimulation. Electrical bone growth stimulation is used to facilitate the healing process for certain types of fractures, especially those with nonunion or delayed healing. The mechanism of action of electrical bone growth stimulation may include (a) increasing the calcium uptake of bone, (b) activating intracellular calcium stores, and (c) increasing the production of bone growth factors (Khalifeh et al., 2018).

Noninvasive, semi-invasive, and invasive methods of electrical bone growth stimulation are used. Noninvasive stimulators use direct current or pulsed electromagnetic fields (PEMFs) to generate a weak electrical current. Electrodes are placed over the patient's skin or cast and are used 10 to 12 hours each day, usually while the patient is sleeping. Semi-invasive or percutaneous

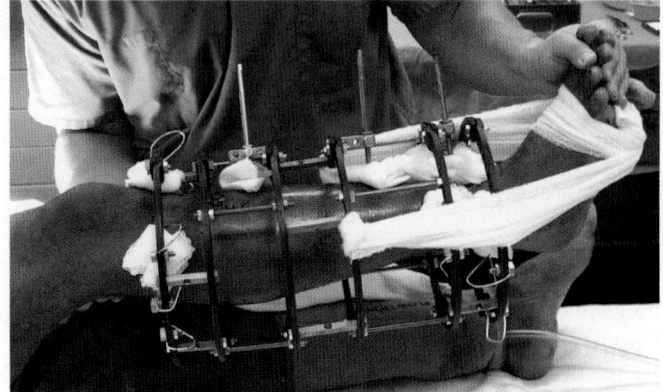

FIG. 65.12 External fixators. Stabilization of a tibial fracture. Source: Canale, S.T., &, Beatty, J. H. (2013). *Campbell's operative orthopaedics* (12th ed.). Mosby.

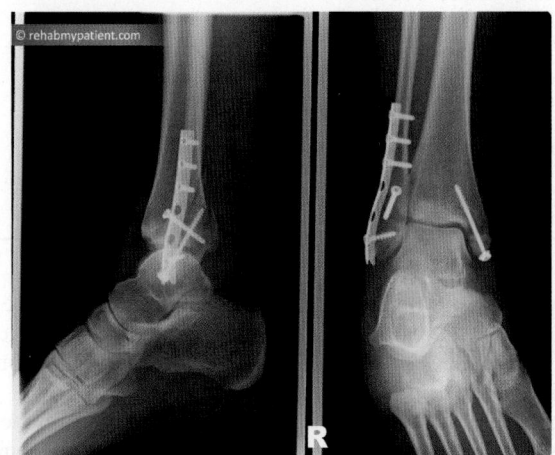

FIG. 65.13 Views of internal fixation devices to stabilize a fractured tibia and fibula. Source: Courtesy and © www.rehabmypatient.com.

bone growth stimulators use an external power supply and electrodes that are inserted through the skin and into the bone. Invasive stimulators require surgical implantation of a current generator in an intramuscular or subcutaneous space. An electrode is implanted in the bone fragments.

Medication Therapy. Pharmacists play an integral role on the interprofessional health care team in pain and infection prevention and management. Patients with fractures often experience varying degrees of pain associated with muscle spasms. Involuntary reflexes that result from edema following muscle injury cause these spasms. Central and peripheral muscle relaxants, such as cyclobenzaprine or methocarbamol (Robaxin), may be prescribed for relief of pain associated with muscle spasms.

In an open fracture, the threat of tetanus occurring can be reduced with tetanus and diphtheria toxoid or tetanus immunoglobulin for the patient who has not been previously immunized. Bone-penetrating antibiotics (such as cefazolin) are used prophylactically before surgery.

Nutritional Therapy. Proper nutrition is an essential component of the reparative process in injured tissue; thus a referral to the dietitian is needed. An adequate energy source is required to promote muscle strength and tone, build endurance, and enhance ambulation and gait-training skills. The patient's dietary intake must include ample protein (e.g., 1 g/kg of body weight); vitamins (especially B, C, and D); and calcium,

TABLE 65.5   EMERGENCY MANAGEMENT

Fractured Extremity

Etiology	Assessment Findings	Interventions
Blunt • Motor vehicle accident • Pedestrian event **Falls** • Direct blows • Forced flexion or hyperextension • Twisting forces **Penetrating** • Blast • Gunshot **Other** • Crush injury • Pathological conditions • Violent muscle contractions (seizures)	• Deformity (loss of normal bony contours) or unnatural position of affected limb • Edema and ecchymosis • Grating (crepitus) • Loss of function • Muscle spasm • Numbness, tingling, loss of distal pulses • Open wound over injured site, exposure of bone • Tenderness and pain • Warmth at site	**Initial** • Treat life-threatening injuries first. • Ensure airway, breathing, and circulation. • Control external bleeding with direct pressure or sterile pressure dressing and elevation of the limb. • Check neurovascular status distal to injury before and after splinting. • Elevate injured limb if possible. • Do *not* attempt to straighten fractured or dislocated joints. • Do *not* manipulate protruding bone ends. • Apply ice packs to affected area. • Obtain radiographs of affected limb. • Administer tetanus and diphtheria prophylaxis if there is a break in skin integrity. • Mark location of pulses to facilitate repeat assessment. • Splint fracture site, including joints above and below fracture site. **Ongoing Monitoring** • Monitor vital signs, level of consciousness, oxygen saturation, peripheral pulses, and pain. • Monitor for compartment syndrome, characterized by excessive pain, pain with passive stretch of the affected extremity muscles, pallor, paresthesia, and late signs of paralysis and pulselessness. • Monitor for signs and symptoms of a fat embolism (e.g., dyspnea, chest pain, temperature elevation).

phosphorus, and magnesium to ensure optimal soft tissue and bone healing. Low serum protein levels and vitamin C deficiencies interfere with tissue healing. Immobility and callus formation increase calcium needs.

Three well-balanced meals a day will usually provide the necessary nutrients. The well-balanced meal should be supplemented by a fluid intake of 2 000 to 3 000 mL/day to promote optimal bladder and bowel function. Adequate fluid and a high-fibre diet with fruits and vegetables will prevent constipation. If immobilized in bed with skeletal traction or in a body jacket brace, the patient should be instructed to eat six small meals to avoid overeating and thus abdominal pressure and cramping.

NURSING MANAGEMENT
FRACTURES

NURSING ASSESSMENT

A brief history of the traumatic episode, the mechanism of injury, and the position in which the patient was found can be obtained from the patient or witnesses. As soon as possible, the patient should be transported to an emergency department, where a thorough assessment and treatment can be initiated (Table 65.5). Subjective and objective data that should be obtained from an individual with a fracture are presented in Table 65.6.

Special emphasis must be placed on the region distal to the site of injury. Clinical findings must be documented before fracture treatment is initiated, to prevent doubts about whether a condition discovered later was missed during the original examination or was caused by the treatment.

NEUROVASCULAR ASSESSMENT. Musculoskeletal injuries have the potential to cause changes in the neurovascular status of an injured extremity. With musculoskeletal trauma, application of a cast or constrictive dressing, poor positioning, and the physiological response to the traumatic injury can cause nerve or vascular damage, usually distal to the injury.

The neurovascular assessment should consist of a *peripheral vascular assessment* (colour, temperature, capillary refill, peripheral pulses, and edema) and a *peripheral neurological assessment* (sensation, motor function, and pain). Throughout the neurovascular assessment, both extremities are compared to obtain an accurate assessment.

An extremity's colour (pale, cyanotic) and temperature (hot, warm, cool, cold) in the area of the affected extremity are assessed. Pallor or a cool to cold extremity below the injury could indicate arterial insufficiency. A warm, cyanotic extremity could indicate poor venous return. A capillary refill (blanching of the nail bed) of less than 3 seconds indicates good arterial perfusion.

Pulses on both the unaffected and the injured extremity are compared to identify differences in rate or quality. Pulses are described as strong, diminished, audible by hand-held Doppler transducer, or absent. A diminished or absent pulse distal to the injury can indicate vascular dysfunction and insufficiency. In adults older than 45 years of age, occasionally either the dorsalis pedis or posterior tibial pulse may be difficult to locate, but not both on the same foot (Jarvis, 2020). Peripheral edema is also assessed, and pitting edema may be present with severe injury.

Sensation and motor innervation in the upper extremity are assessed by evaluating the ulnar, median, and radial nerves. Neurovascular status can be assessed by abduction and adduction of the fingers, opposition of the fingers, and supination and pronation of the hand. In the lower extremity, dorsiflexion and plantar flexion provide information about motor function of the peroneal and tibial nerves. Sensory innervation is evaluated for the peroneal nerve on the dorsal part of the foot between the web space of the great and the second toes. Tibial nerve assessment is performed by stroking the plantar surface (sole) of the foot. Contralateral evaluation is critical. The patient may report *paresthesia* (abnormal sensation [e.g., numbness, tingling]) and

TABLE 65.6 NURSING ASSESSMENT
Fracture

Subjective Data
Important Health Information
Past health history: Traumatic injury; long-term repetitive forces (stress fracture); bone or systemic diseases, prolonged immobility (pathological fracture), osteopenia, osteoporosis
Medications: Corticosteroids (osteoporotic fractures), analgesics, hormone therapy, calcium supplementation
Surgery or other treatments: First aid treatment of fracture, previous musculoskeletal surgeries

Symptoms
- Loss of motion or weakness of affected part; muscle spasms
- Sudden and severe pain in affected area; numbness, tingling, loss of sensation distal to injury; chronic pain that increases with activity (stress fracture)

Objective Data
General
Apprehension, guarding of injured site

Integumentary
Skin lacerations, pallor and cool skin or bluish and warm skin distal to injury; ecchymosis, hematoma, edema at site of fracture

Cardiovascular
Reduced or absent pulse distal to injury, decreased skin temperature, delayed capillary refill

Neurological
Paresthesias, decreased or absent sensation, hypersensation

Musculoskeletal
Restricted or lost function of affected part; local bony deformities; abnormal angulation; shortening, rotation, or crepitation of affected part; muscle weakness

Possible Findings
Identification and extent of fractures on radiograph, bone scan, CT scan, or MRI

CT, computed tomographic (scan); *MRI,* magnetic resonance imaging.

TABLE 65.7 PATIENT & CAREGIVER TEACHING GUIDE
Prevention of Musculoskeletal Injuries and Conditions in the Older Person

The following instructions should be included when teaching older patients and their caregivers how to prevent musculoskeletal injuries and conditions.
- Use ramps in buildings and at street corners instead of steps to prevent falls.
- Remove scatter rugs in the home.
- Treat pain and discomfort from osteoarthritis.
  - Rest in a reclining position to decrease discomfort.
  - Discuss use of medication for pain with health care provider.
- Use a walker or cane to help with walking to prevent falls.
- Eat the amount and kind of foods needed to prevent excess weight gain because obesity adds stress to joints, which may predispose to osteoarthritis.
- Get regular and frequent exercise.
  - ADLs provide ROM exercises. Tai chi may also be helpful.
  - Hobbies (e.g., jigsaw puzzles, needlework, model building) exercise finger joints and prevent stiffness.
  - Performing weight-bearing exercise (e.g., walking) is essential and should be done on a daily basis.
- Wear shoes with good support to provide for safety and promote comfort.
- Gradually initiate activities to promote optimal coordination. Rise slowly to a standing position to prevent dizziness, falls, and fractures.
- Avoid walking on uneven surfaces and wet floors.

ADLs, activities of daily living; *ROM,* range of motion.

- *Potential for peripheral neurovascular complications* as demonstrated by *fracture* (vascular insufficiency and nerve compression, mechanical compression by traction, splints, or casts)
- *Pain* as a result of *physical injury agent* (edema, movement of bone fragments, muscle spasms)

Additional information on nursing diagnoses for the patient with a fracture is presented in Nursing Care Plans (NCPs) 65.1 and 65.2 (on the Evolve website).

PLANNING
The overall goals are that the patient with a fracture will (a) have healing with no associated complications, (b) obtain satisfactory pain relief, and (c) achieve maximal rehabilitation potential.

NURSING IMPLEMENTATION
HEALTH PROMOTION. The public should be taught to take appropriate safety precautions to prevent injuries while at home, at work, when driving, and when participating in sports. Nurses should be advocates for personal actions known to reduce injuries, such as regular use of seat belts, driving within posted speed limits, stretching and warming up muscles before exercise, use of protective athletic equipment (helmets and knee, wrist, and elbow pads), use of safety equipment at work, and not driving under the influence of alcohol or drugs.

Individuals (especially older people) should be encouraged to participate in moderate exercise to aid in the maintenance of muscle strength and balance. To reduce falls, they should wear adequate footwear and assess their living environment for safety (e.g., remove scatter rugs, maintain good lighting, clear paths to the bathroom for nighttime use) (Table 65.7). The nurse should also stress the importance of adequate calcium and vitamin D intake.

hyperesthesia (hypersensation). Partial or full loss of strength or movement (paresis or paralysis) may be a late sign of neurovascular damage. Reduced motion or strength in an injured extremity can alert the nurse to potential limb-threatening complications or disability.

Pain is the final element of the neurovascular assessment. The nurse must carefully assess the location, quality, and intensity of the pain (see Chapter 10). Current best practice in pain management is to ask the patient to rate their level of pain on a scale of 0 to 10, with 0 being no pain and 10 being the worst pain ever experienced. Increasing pain unrelieved by medication therapy and out of proportion to the injury can be an indication of compartment syndrome.

Patients should be instructed to report any changes in their neurovascular status. Patients need to verbalize and demonstrate a thorough understanding of all elements before they are discharged from the treatment setting.

NURSING DIAGNOSES
Nursing diagnoses for the patient with a fracture may include but are not limited to the following:
- *Reduced mobility* as a result of *joint stiffness, pain*

ACUTE INTERVENTION. Patients with fractures may be treated in an emergency department or a health care provider's office and discharged to home care, or they may require hospitalization for varying amounts of time. Specific nursing measures depend on the setting and type of treatment used.

Preoperative Management. If surgical intervention is required to treat the fracture, patients will need preoperative preparation. In addition to the usual preoperative nursing measures (see Chapter 20), the nurse should inform patients of the type of immobilization and assistive devices that will be used and the expected activity limitations after surgery. Assurance that pain medication will be available, if needed, is often beneficial (see Chapter 10).

Postoperative Management. In general, postoperative nursing care and management are directed toward monitoring vital signs and applying the general principles of postoperative nursing care (see Chapter 22). Frequent neurovascular assessments of the affected extremity are necessary to detect early and subtle neurovascular changes. Any limitations of movement or activity related to turning, positioning, and extremity support should be monitored closely. Additional nursing responsibilities depend on the type of immobilization used. Pain and discomfort can be minimized through proper alignment and positioning.

Dressings or casts should be carefully observed for any overt signs of bleeding or drainage. A significant increase in size of the drainage area should be reported. If a wound drainage system is in place, the volume of drainage should be regularly measured and the patency of the system assessed using aseptic technique to avoid contamination. A blood salvage and reinfusion system that allows for recovery and reinfusion of the patient's own blood may be used. The blood is retrieved from a joint space or cavity, and the patient receives this blood in the form of an autotransfusion. (Autotransfusion is discussed in Chapter 33.) Additional nursing measures for the patient who has undergone orthopedic surgery are discussed in NCP 65.2, available on the Evolve website.

Other Measures. Patients often have reduced mobility as a result of the fracture. The nurse must plan care to prevent the many complications associated with immobility. Constipation can be prevented by activity and maintenance of a high-fluid intake (>2500 mL/day unless contraindicated by the patient's health status) and a diet high in bulk and roughage (fresh fruit and vegetables). If these measures are not effective in maintaining the patient's usual bowel pattern, warm fluids, stool softeners, laxatives, or suppositories may be necessary. Maintaining a regular time for elimination helps to promote regularity.

Renal calculi can develop as a result of bone demineralization. The hypercalcemia from demineralization causes a rise in urine pH and stone formation resulting from the precipitation of calcium. Unless contraindicated, a fluid intake of 2500 mL/day is recommended. (Renal calculi are discussed in Chapter 48.)

Rapid deconditioning of the cardiopulmonary system can occur as a result of prolonged bed rest, resulting in orthostatic hypotension and decreased lung capacity. Unless contraindicated, these effects can be diminished by permitting the patient to sit on the side of the bed, allowing the patient's lower limbs to dangle over the bedside, and having the patient perform standing transfers. When the patient is allowed to increase activity, careful evaluation should be made to assess for orthostatic hypotension. Patients must also be assessed for venous

---

TABLE 65.8 INTERPROFESSIONAL CARE

Caring for the Patient With a Cast or in Traction

Nursing Management
- Perform neurovascular assessment on the affected extremity; report any changes to health care provider.
- Monitor pain intensity and give prescribed analgesics.
- Determine correct body alignment to enhance traction.
- Position casted extremity above heart level.
- Apply icepack to cast to help reduce edema.
- Monitor skin integrity around cast, support sling and at traction pin sites.
- Monitor cast during drying for denting or flattening.
- Assist patient with passive and active ROM exercises.
- Teach patient and caregiver about cast care or traction and measures to prevent complications (e.g., ROM exercises).
- Assess for complications associated with immobility (e.g., constipation, VTE, kidney stones, atelectasis) and develop a plan to minimize those complications.

Collaborate With Physiotherapist
- Assess patient's current mobility and need for assistance.
- Teach safe ambulation with assistive device based on patient's weight-bearing restrictions.
- Establish exercise plan and teach patient to perform exercises safely.
- Coordinate physiotherapy with nurse so that patient can receive timely analgesia.
- Discuss home environment with patient and identify modifications to promote safety (e.g., stair training).

Collaborate With Occupational Therapist
- Assess impact of patient's condition on ability to perform ADLs.
- Teach patient use of assistive devices (e.g., long-handled reacher, shoe donner) to promote self-care while maintaining activity restrictions.

ADLs, activities of daily living; *ROM,* range of motion; *VTE,* venous thromboembolism.

---

thromboembolism (VTE). (Deep vein thrombosis [DTV] and pulmonary embolism are discussed in Chapter 40 and pulmonary embolism is discussed in Chapter 30.)

Traction. When slings are used with traction, the nurse should inspect exposed skin areas regularly. Pressure over a bony prominence created by the wrinkling of sheets or bedclothes may cause pressure necrosis. Persistent skin pressure may impair blood flow, causing injury to the peripheral neurovascular structures. Skeletal traction or external fixation pin sites should be inspected for signs of infection. Pin-site care varies but usually includes regular cleansing with chlorhexidine, rinsing pin sites with sterile saline, and drying of the area with sterile gauze.

External rotation of the hip can occur when skin traction is used on the lower extremity. The nurse can help prevent the external rotation by placing a pillow or rolled-up towels (called a *trochanter roll*) along the greater trochanteric region of the femur. Generally, the patient should be in the centre of the bed, in a supine position. Incorrect alignment can result in increased pain, nonunion, or malunion. Table 65.8 summarizes interprofessional care for the patient with a cast or in traction.

To offset some of the complications associated with prolonged immobility, the nurse should discuss activity of each patient with the health care provider. If exercise is permitted, the nurse should encourage the patient's participation in a simple exercise regimen within activity restrictions. Activities that the patient should participate in include frequent position changes,

ROM exercises of unaffected joints, deep-breathing exercises, isometric exercises, and use of the trapeze bar (if permitted) to raise themselves off the bed for linen changes and use of the bedpan. These activities should be performed several times each day. The nurse should encourage and help the hospitalized patient to stay connected with friends and family through social media resources (see the Informatics in Practice box).

INFORMATICS IN PRACTICE

Staying Connected While Immobilized

A patient in traction or other immobilization devices for a long period may feel lonely or isolated. There are a number of ways to use a computer, electronic tablet, or smartphone to ease separation anxiety and help the patient reconnect with family and friends.

The patient can set up a video chat. The nurse should encourage the patient to maintain personal contact through text messaging and email and have the patient catch up on the latest news and blogs on social networking sites.

AMBULATORY AND HOME CARE

Cast Care. Because many fractures are treated in an outpatient setting, the patient often requires only a short hospitalization or none at all. Regardless of the type of cast material, a cast can interfere with circulation and nerve function from being applied too tightly or because of excessive edema after application. Thus, frequent neurovascular assessments of the immobilized extremity are critical. The patient must be taught about signs of cast complications so that they can be reported promptly. Elevation of the extremity above the level of the heart to promote venous return, and applications of ice to control or prevent edema, are frequently used measures during the initial phase. (If compartment syndrome is suspected, the extremity should not be elevated above the heart.) The nurse should instruct the patient to exercise joints above and below the cast. Pulling out cast padding and scratching or placing foreign objects inside the cast is forbidden because doing so can predispose the patient to skin breakdown and infection. For itching, the patient should be instructed that a hair dryer set on a cool setting can be directed under the cast.

Patient and caregiver teaching is an important nursing responsibility to prevent complications. In addition to providing specific instructions for cast care and recognition of complications, the nurse should encourage the patient to contact the clinic or health care provider if questions arise. Table 65.9 summarizes patient and caregiver instructions for cast care. The nurse should validate the patient's and caregivers' understanding of these instructions before discharging the patient from inpatient and ambulatory settings. Follow-up phone contact is appropriate, and home care nursing visits are warranted, especially with body or spica casts.

Cast removal is done in the outpatient setting. Patients often fear being cut by the oscillating blade of the cast saw. The nurse should reassure the patient that their skin will not be cut. More importantly, the nurse should educate the patient about possible alterations in the appearance of the extremity (e.g., dry, wrinkled skin, atrophied muscle) beneath the cast. The patient may also have anxiety related to using the injured extremity after the cast is removed.

Psychosocial Problems. Short-term rehabilitative goals are directed toward the transition from dependence to independence in performing simple ADLs and preserving or increasing strength and endurance. Long-term rehabilitative goals are

TABLE 65.9 PATIENT & CAREGIVER TEACHING GUIDE

Cast Care

After a cast is applied, include the following instructions when teaching the patient and the caregiver about cast care.

Do
- Apply ice directly over fracture site for first 24 hr (avoid getting cast wet by keeping ice in a plastic bag and protecting cast with cloth).
- Check with health care provider before getting fibreglass cast wet.
- Dry cast thoroughly after exposure to water.
  - Blot dry with towel.
  - Use hair dryer on low setting until cast is thoroughly dry.
- Elevate extremity above level of heart for first 48 hr.
- Move joints above and below cast regularly.
- Use hair dryer on cool setting for itching.
- Report signs of possible complications to health care provider:
  - Increasing pain despite elevation, ice, and analgesia
  - Swelling associated with pain and discoloration of toes or fingers
  - Pain during movement
  - Burning or tingling under cast
  - Sores or foul odour under cast
- Keep appointment to have fracture and cast checked.

Do Not
- Get plaster cast wet.
- Remove any padding.
- Insert any objects inside cast.
- Bear weight on new cast for 48 hr (not all casts are made for weight bearing; check with health care provider if unsure).
- Cover cast with plastic if it will be wet for long periods of time.

aimed at preventing conditions associated with musculoskeletal injury (Table 65.10). An important part of nursing care during the rehabilitative phase is assisting the patient to adjust to any difficulties caused by the injury (e.g., separation from family, financial impact of medical care, loss of income from inability to work, potential for lifetime disability). The nurse has an important role in offering support and encouragement while actively listening to the patient's and the caregiver's concerns.

Ambulation. The nurse must know the overall goals of physiotherapy in relation to the patient's abilities, needs, and tolerance. Mobility training and instruction in the use of assistive aids (cane, crutches, walker) constitute major areas of responsibility of the physiotherapist. The patient with lower extremity dysfunction is usually started in mobility training when able to sit in bed and dangle their feet over the side. This activity should be done two or three times a day for 10 to 15 minutes, with the nurse assisting as necessary. Collaboration of the nurse and physiotherapist to coordinate pain management and thus increase patient participation at therapy sessions is critical.

When the patient begins to ambulate, the nurse should know the patient's weight-bearing status and the correct technique if the patient is using an assistive device. Weight-bearing ambulation occurs in different degrees: (a) non–weight-bearing (NWB) ambulation (no weight on affected leg), (b) touch-down weight-bearing ambulation (TDWB) or toe-touch weight-bearing ambulation (TTWB) (contact with floor only for balance; no weight on affected leg), (c) partial weight-bearing ambulation (PWB) (directions given by the health care provider), (d) weight bearing as tolerated (WBAT) (dictated by patient's pain and tolerance), and (e) full weight-bearing (FWB) ambulation (no limitations) (Knott et al., 2019).

TABLE 65.10	CONDITIONS ASSOCIATED WITH MUSCULOSKELETAL INJURIES	
Condition	**Description**	**Nursing Considerations**
Muscle atrophy	• Decreased muscle mass normally occurs as a result of disuse following prolonged immobilization. • Loss of nerve innervation can precipitate muscle atrophy.	• Isometric muscle-strengthening exercise regimen within the confines of the immobilization device assists in reducing the amount of atrophy. • Muscle atrophy interferes with and prolongs the rehabilitation process.
Contracture	• Abnormal condition of joint characterized by flexion and fixation • Caused by atrophy and shortening of muscle fibres or by loss of normal elasticity of skin over a joint	• It can be prevented by frequent position change, correct body alignment, and doing active and passive range-of-motion exercises several times a day. • Intervention requires gradual and progressive stretching of the muscles or ligaments in the region of the joint.
Footdrop	• Plantar-flexed position of the foot (footdrop) occurs when the Achilles tendon in the ankle shortens because it has been allowed to assume an unsupported position. • Peroneal nerve palsy (a compression neuropathy) also causes footdrop.	• Management of the patient with long-term injuries must include supporting the foot in a neutral position. • Once footdrop has developed, ambulation and gait training may be significantly hindered. • The patient may require a splint to keep the foot or feet in a neutral position. • High-top athletic shoes may also help.
Pain	• Pain is frequently associated with fractures, edema, and muscle spasm. • Pain varies in intensity from mild to severe and is usually described as aching, dull, burning, throbbing, sharp, or deep.	• Causes of pain include incorrect positioning and alignment of the extremity, incorrect support of the extremity, sudden movement of the extremity, immobilization devices that are applied too tightly or in an incorrect position, constrictive dressings, and motion occurring at the fracture site. • Determine causes of pain so that corrective nursing action can be taken.
Muscle spasms	• Caused by involuntary muscle contraction after fracture, muscle strain, or nerve injury; these may last as long as several weeks. • Pain associated with muscle spasms is often intense and can last from several seconds to several minutes.	• Measures to reduce the intensity of the muscle spasms are similar to the corrective actions for pain control. • Do not massage muscle spasms. • Thermotherapy, especially heat, may reduce muscle spasm.

Assistive Devices. Devices for ambulation range from a cane, which can relieve up to 40% of the weight normally borne by a lower limb, to a walker or crutches, which may allow for complete non–weight-bearing ambulation. The decision about which device is appropriate for a patient involves weighing the need for maximum stability and safety versus manoeuvrability, which is required in small spaces such as bathrooms. It is essential to discuss with patients the requirements of their lifestyles and to determine the device with which each patient feels most secure and independent.

The technique for using assistive devices varies. The involved limb is usually advanced at the same time or immediately after the advance of the device. The uninvolved limb is advanced last. In almost all cases, canes are held in the hand opposite the involved extremity.

A transfer belt can be placed around the patient's waist to provide stability during the learning stages. The nurse should discourage the patient from reaching for furniture or relying on another person for support. When there is inadequate upper limb strength or crutches are ill fitted, the patient bears weight at the axilla rather than at the hands, endangering the neurovascular bundle that passes across the axilla. If verbal coaching does not correct the problem, the patient should be instructed in another form of ambulation until strength is adequate (e.g., platform crutches, walker).

Patients who must ambulate without weight bearing require sufficient upper limb strength to lift their own weight at each step. Because the muscles of the shoulder girdle are not accustomed to this work, they require vigorous and diligent training in preparation for this task. Push-ups, pull-ups using the overhead trapeze bar, and lifting weights develop the triceps and biceps. Straight-leg raises and quadriceps-setting exercises strengthen the quadriceps.

Counselling and Referrals. During the rehabilitative process, the patient's caregiver assumes an important role in the provision and follow-through of long-term care plans. The caregiver should be instructed in the techniques of strength and endurance exercises, assistance with mobility training, and promotion of activities that enhance the quality of daily living. The nurse should also evaluate patients for post-traumatic stress disorder. This is especially important if significant injury to others or fatalities were associated with the patient's injuries.

▌EVALUATION

The following are expected outcomes for the patient with a fracture:

- Report satisfactory relief of pain
- Demonstrate appropriate care of cast or immobilizer
- Experience no peripheral neurovascular complications
- Experience uncomplicated bone healing

COMPLICATIONS OF FRACTURES

The majority of fractures heal without complications. If death occurs after a fracture, it is usually the result of damage to underlying organs and vascular structures or from complications of the fracture or immobility. Complications of fractures can be either direct or indirect. *Direct* complications include problems with bone infection, bone union, and AVN. *Indirect* complications are associated with blood vessel and nerve damage resulting in conditions such as compartment syndrome, VTE, fat embolism, rhabdomyolysis (breakdown of skeletal muscle), and hypovolemic shock. Although most musculoskeletal injuries are not life-threatening, open fractures, fractures accompanied by severe blood loss, and fractures that damage vital organs (e.g., lung, heart) are medical emergencies requiring immediate attention.

Infection

Open fractures and soft tissue injuries resulting from high-energy trauma have a high incidence of infection (Samai & Vilella, 2018). Massive or blunt soft tissue injury often has more serious consequences than the fracture. Damage to the surrounding soft tissue and blood vessels impedes the body's natural defence mechanisms to respond to infective microorganisms (Zalavras, 2017). Necrotic and contaminated tissue provides an ideal medium for many common pathogens, including gas-forming (anaerobic) bacilli such as *Clostridium tetani*. Prophylactic antibiotic treatment for infection may be warranted to prevent the costs associated with extended length of care and osteomyelitis (Samai & Vilella, 2018). (See Chapter 66 for a discussion of osteomyelitis.)

Interprofessional Care. Open fractures require aggressive surgical debridement. The wound is initially cleansed with a sterile saline solution via low-pressure lavage, in the operating room. Gross contaminants are irrigated or mechanically removed. Contused, contaminated, and devitalized tissue such as muscle, subcutaneous fat, skin, and fragments of bone are surgically excised *(debridement)*. The extent of the soft tissue damage determines whether the wound is closed at the time of surgery and whether it requires repeat debridement, closed suction drainage, and skin grafting. Depending on the location and extent of the fracture, reduction may be maintained by external fixation or traction. During surgery, the open wound may be irrigated with antibiotic solution. Antibiotic-impregnated beads may also be placed in the surgical site. During the postoperative phase, the patient will have antibiotics administered intravenously for at least 3 days (Zalavras, 2017). Use of antibiotics, in conjunction with aggressive surgical management, has greatly reduced the occurrence of infection.

Compartment Syndrome

Compartment syndrome is a condition in which swelling and increased pressure within a limited space (a compartment) press on and compromise the function of blood vessels, nerves, and tendons that run through that compartment. Compartment syndrome causes capillary perfusion to be reduced below a level necessary for tissue viability (Limbert & Santy-Tomlinson, 2017). Compartment syndrome (acute, subacute, or chronic) usually involves the leg but can also occur in the arm, shoulder, and buttock.

Thirty-eight compartments are located in the upper and lower extremities. Two basic causes of compartment syndrome are (1) decreased compartment size resulting from restrictive dressings, splints, casts, excessive traction, or premature closure of fascia and (2) increased compartment contents related to bleeding, edema, chemical response to snakebite, or intravenous infiltration.

Edema can create sufficient pressure to obstruct circulation and cause venous occlusion, which further increases edema. Eventually, arterial flow is compromised, resulting in inadequate arterial circulation *(ischemia)* to the extremity. As ischemia continues, muscle and nerve cells are destroyed over time, and fibrotic tissue replaces the healthy tissue. Contracture,

disability, and loss of function can occur. Delay in diagnosis and treatment can result in irreversible muscle and nerve ischemia, resulting in a functionally useless or severely impaired extremity.

Compartment syndrome is usually associated with trauma, fractures (especially of the long bones), extensive soft tissue damage, and crush injury. Fractures of the distal humerus and proximal tibia are the most common fractures associated with compartment syndrome. Compartment injury can also occur following knee or leg surgery. Prolonged pressure on a muscle compartment may occur when someone is trapped under a heavy object or a person's limb is trapped beneath the body because of an obtunded state such as drug or alcohol overdose. In the upper extremity, this condition is referred to as *Volkmann ischemic contracture,* and in the lower extremity, it is known as *anterior tibial compartment syndrome,* although the underlying pathophysiological mechanism is similar.

Clinical Manifestations. Compartment syndrome may occur initially from the body's physiological response to the injury, or it may be delayed for several days after the original insult or injury. Ischemia can occur within 4 to 8 hours after the onset of compartment syndrome.

The "six P's" are a neurovascular assessment mnemonic that can be used to assess for impending compartment syndrome: (1) **p**ain distal to the injury that is not relieved by opioid analgesics and pain on passive stretch of muscle travelling through the compartment; (2) increasing **p**ressure in the compartment; (3) **p**aresthesia (numbness and tingling); (4) **p**allor, coolness, and loss of normal colour of the extremity; (5) **p**aralysis or loss of function; and (6) **p**ulselessness or diminished or absent peripheral pulses (Limbert & Santy-Tomlinson, 2017).

Interprofessional Care. Prompt, accurate diagnosis of compartment syndrome is critical. Prevention or early recognition is key. Regular neurovascular assessments should be performed and documented on all patients with fractures but especially those with injury of the distal humerus or proximal tibia or soft tissue disruption in these areas.

The nurse needs to carefully assess the location, quality, and intensity of the pain (see Chapter 10). Pain should be rated on a scale of 0 to 10. Pain unrelieved by medication therapy and out of proportion to the level of injury and pain on passive muscle stretch appear to be the most effective clinical observations (Limbert & Santy-Tomlinson, 2017) and some of the first indications of impending compartment syndrome. Pulselessness and paralysis in particular are later signs of compartment syndrome. The health care provider should be notified immediately of a patient's changing condition.

Because of the possibility of muscle damage (rhabdomyolysis), urine output should be assessed. Myoglobin released from damaged muscle cells precipitates as a gel-like substance and causes obstruction in renal tubules. This condition results in acute tubular necrosis and acute kidney injury. Common signs are dark, reddish-brown urine and clinical manifestations associated with acute kidney injury (see Chapter 49).

Elevation of the extremity may lower venous pressure and slow arterial perfusion; thus, the extremity should not be elevated above heart level. Similarly, the application of cold compresses may result in vasoconstriction and exacerbate compartment syndrome. It may also be necessary to remove or loosen the bandage and bivalve or split the cast in half. A reduction in traction weight may also decrease external circumferential pressures.

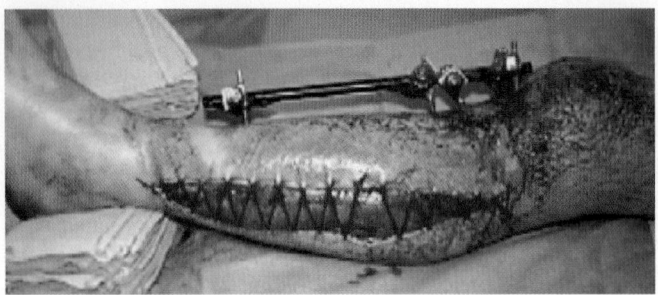

FIG. 65.14 Fasciotomy associated with compartment syndrome. Stabilization of fracture with external fixator. Source: Browner, B. D., Jupiter, J. B., Levine, A. M., et al. (2009). *Skeletal trauma: Fractures, dislocations, ligamentous injuries* (4th ed.). Saunders.

Surgical decompression (e.g., fasciotomy) of the involved compartment may be necessary (Figure 65.14). The fasciotomy site is left open for several days to ensure adequate soft tissue decompression. Infection resulting from delayed wound closure is a potential complication following a fasciotomy. In severe cases of compartment syndrome, an amputation may be required.

Venous Thromboembolism

The veins of the lower extremities and the pelvis are highly susceptible to thrombus formation after fracture, especially a hip fracture. VTE may also occur after total hip or total knee replacement surgery. In patients with limited mobility, venous stasis is aggravated by inactivity of the muscles that normally assist in the pumping action of venous blood returning to the extremities.

Because of the high risk for VTE in the orthopedic surgical patient, prophylactic anticoagulant medications should be given for at least 10 to 14 days (Lieberman & Heckmann, 2017). In addition to wearing compression gradient stockings (anti-embolism hose) and using sequential compression devices, the patient should be instructed to move (dorsiflex and plantar flex) the fingers or toes of the affected extremity against resistance and to perform ROM exercises on the unaffected lower extremities. (Assessment and management of VTE are discussed in Chapter 40.)

Fat Embolism Syndrome

Fat embolism syndrome (FES) is characterized by the presence of systemic fat globules from fractures that are distributed into tissues and organs after a traumatic skeletal injury. The fractures that most often cause FES are those of the long bones, ribs, and pelvis. FES has also been known to occur following total joint replacement, spinal fusion, liposuction, crush injuries, and bone marrow transplantation (Fukumoto & Fukumoto, 2018). Two theories about fat embolism exist. The *mechanical* theory is that fat is released from the marrow of injured bone and enters the systemic circulation, where the fat droplets become lodged in small blood vessels of organs (e.g. lungs, brain), causing local ischemia and inflammation. The *biochemical* theory is that hormonal changes caused by trauma or sepsis stimulate the systemic release of free fatty acids such as chylomicrons, which form the fat emboli.

Clinical Manifestations. Early recognition of FES is crucial in preventing a potentially lethal course. Most patients manifest symptoms within 24 to 48 hours after injury. Severe forms have occurred within hours of injury. The fat emboli in the lungs cause a hemorrhagic interstitial pneumonitis that produces signs and symptoms of acute respiratory distress syndrome (ARDS), such as chest pain, tachypnea, cyanosis, dyspnea, apprehension, tachycardia, and decreased partial pressure of arterial oxygen (PaO_2) (Fukumoto & Fukumoto, 2018). All of these symptoms are caused by poor oxygen exchange. Because they are frequently the first symptoms to manifest, changes in the patient's mental status as a result of hypoxemia are important to recognize. Memory loss, restlessness, confusion, elevated temperature, and headache must prompt further investigation so that central nervous system involvement is not mistaken for alcohol withdrawal or acute head injury. The continued change in level of consciousness and petechiae located around the neck, anterior chest wall, axilla, buccal membrane, and eye conjunctiva help distinguish fat emboli from other conditions. Intravascular thromboses caused by hypoxemia results in petechiae, which occur in 20 to 60% of cases but may fade before they are noticed (Fukumoto & Fukumoto, 2018).

The clinical course of a fat embolus may be rapid and acute. Frequently, the patient expresses a feeling of impending disaster. In a short time, skin colour changes from pallid to cyanotic, and the patient may become comatose. No specific laboratory examinations are available to aid in the diagnosis. However, certain diagnostic abnormalities may be present. These include fat cells in the blood, urine, or sputum; a decrease of the PaO_2 to less than 60 mm Hg; ST-segment changes on the electrocardiogram; a decrease in the platelet count and hematocrit levels; and high erythrocyte sedimentation rate. A chest radiograph may reveal areas of diffuse bilateral patchy infiltrates (Kosova et al., 2015).

Interprofessional Care. Treatment for fat embolism is directed at prevention. Early and careful immobilization of a long bone fracture is probably the most important element in the prevention of fat embolism. The patient should be repositioned as little as possible before fracture immobilization or stabilization because of the danger of dislodging more fat droplets into the general circulation.

Management of FES is essentially symptom related and supportive. Treatment includes fluid resuscitation to prevent hypovolemic shock, correction of acidosis, and replacement of blood loss (Fukumoto & Fukumoto, 2018). Use of corticosteroids to prevent or treat fat embolism is controversial. Oxygen is administered to treat hypoxia. Intubation or intermittent positive-pressure breathing may be considered if a satisfactory PaO_2 cannot be obtained with supplemental oxygen alone. Some patients may develop pulmonary edema, ARDS, or both, leading to an increased mortality rate. Most patients survive FES with few sequelae.

TYPES OF FRACTURES

COLLES FRACTURE

A *Colles fracture* is a fracture of the distal radius and is one of the most common fractures in adults (Figure 65.15). The styloid process of the ulna may be involved as well. Usually, the injury occurs when the patient attempts to break a fall with an outstretched hand (Sanderson et al., 2020). This type of fracture most often occurs in patients over 50 years old whose bones are osteoporotic. A younger person with a Colles fracture caused by a low-energy force should be referred for an osteoporosis evaluation.

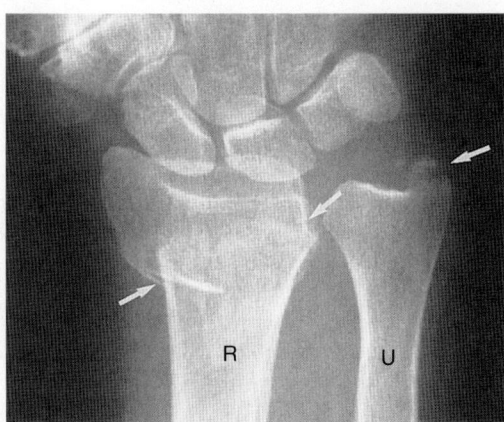

FIG. 65.15 Colles fracture. Fracture of the distal radius *(R)* and ulnar *(U)* styloid from patient falling on the outstretched hand. Source: Mettler, F. A. (2005). *Essentials of radiology* (2nd ed.). Saunders.

The clinical manifestations of a Colles fracture are pain in the immediate area of injury, pronounced swelling, and dorsal displacement of the distal fragment (silver-fork deformity). This may appear as an obvious deformity on the wrist. The major complication associated with a Colles fracture is vascular insufficiency as a result of edema. CTS can be a later complication.

A Colles fracture is usually managed by closed manipulation of the fracture and immobilization by either a splint or a cast or, if displaced, by external fixation. The wrist must be immobilized to prevent wrist supination and pronation. Nursing management should include frequent neurovascular assessments and measures to prevent or reduce edema. Support and protection of the extremity should be provided, along with encouragement of active movement of the thumb and fingers. This type of movement helps reduce edema and increases venous return. The patient should be instructed to perform active movements of the shoulder to prevent stiffness or contracture.

FRACTURE OF THE HUMERUS

Fractures involving the shaft of the humerus are a common injury among young and middle-aged adults. The most common clinical manifestations are an obvious displacement of the humerus shaft, shortened extremity, abnormal mobility, and pain. The major complications associated with fracture of the humerus are radial nerve injury and vascular injury to the brachial artery as a result of laceration, transection, or muscle spasm.

The treatment for a fracture of the humerus depends on the location and displacement of the fracture. Nonoperative treatment may include a hanging arm cast, a shoulder immobilizer, or the sling and swathe, which is a type of immobilization that prevents glenohumeral movement. The swathe encircles the trunk and the humerus as an additional binder. It is often used for surgical repairs and shoulder dislocation.

When these devices are used, the head of the bed should be elevated to assist gravity in reducing the fracture. The arm should be allowed to hang freely when the patient is sitting and standing. Nursing care should include measures to protect the axilla and prevent skin maceration by placing absorbable composite dressing pads (i.e., ABD pads) in the axilla and changing them twice daily or as needed. Skin or skeletal traction may be used for purposes of reduction and immobilization.

During the rehabilitative phase, an exercise program geared toward improving strength and motion of the injured extremity is extremely important. This program should include assisted motion of the hand and fingers. The shoulder can also be exercised if the fracture is stable. This helps prevent stiffness secondary to frozen shoulder or fibrosis of the shoulder capsule.

FRACTURE OF THE PELVIS

Pelvic fractures range from benign to life-threatening, depending on the mechanism of injury and associated vascular insult. Although only a small percentage of all fractures are pelvic fractures, this type of injury is associated with the highest mortality rate. Preoccupation with more obvious injuries at the time of a traumatic event may result in an oversight of pelvic injuries.

Pelvic fractures may cause serious intra-abdominal injury, such as paralytic ileus; hemorrhage; and laceration of the urethra, the bladder, or the colon (Brown & Yuan, 2020). Pelvic fractures can cause acute pelvic compartment syndrome. Patients may survive the initial pelvic injury, only to die from sepsis, FES, or VTE complications.

Physical examination of the abdomen demonstrates local swelling, tenderness, deformity, unusual pelvic movement, and ecchymosis. The neurovascular status of the lower extremities and manifestations of associated injuries should be assessed. Pelvic fractures are diagnosed by radiography and computed tomographic (CT) scan (Brown & Yuan, 2020).

Treatment of a pelvic fracture depends on the severity of the injury. Stable, nondisplaced fractures require limited intervention, and early mobilization is encouraged (Baumagartner et al., 2018). More complex fractures may be treated with pelvic sling traction, skeletal traction, external fixation, open reduction, or a combination of these methods. ORIF of a pelvic fracture may be necessary if the fracture is displaced. Extreme care in handling and moving the patient is important to prevent serious injury from a displaced fracture fragment. The patient should be turned only when ordered by the health care provider. Because a pelvic fracture can lead to damage to other organs, assessment of bowel and urinary tract function and distal neurovascular status are important nursing measures. Back care should be provided while the patient is raised from the bed either by independent use of the trapeze or with adequate assistance. Pelvic fractures can be extremely painful and require the appropriate assessment and management of pain to promote recovery and participation in rehabilitation.

FRACTURE OF THE HIP

Hip fractures are common in older persons and are serious injuries. Women older than 75 years are the most likely to experience a fractured hip (Beaupre, Sobolev, et al., 2019). Hip fractures require one of the longest hospital stays, averaging more than 12 days (CIHI, 2018b). Timely access to care is critical, as longer wait times have been associated with a higher risk for mortality, especially in the older population. In 2018, 87% of patients were treated within the benchmark time of 48 hours (8% higher than in 2015) (CIHI, 2019a).

A *fracture of the hip* (Figure 65.16) refers to a fracture of the proximal third of the femur, which extends up to 5 cm below the lesser trochanter. Fractures that occur within the hip joint capsule are called *intracapsular fractures*. Intracapsular (femoral neck) fractures are further identified by a name derived from

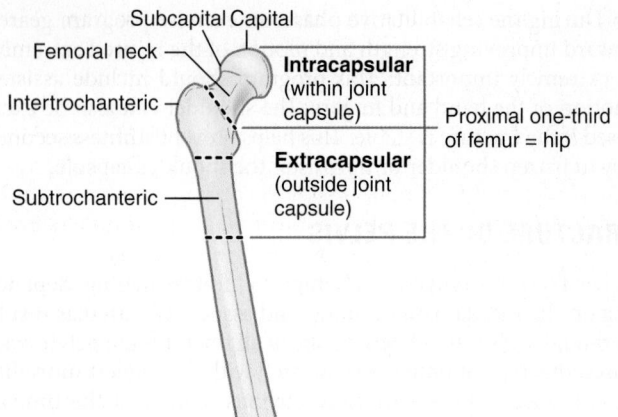

FIG. 65.16 Femur with location of various types of fracture.

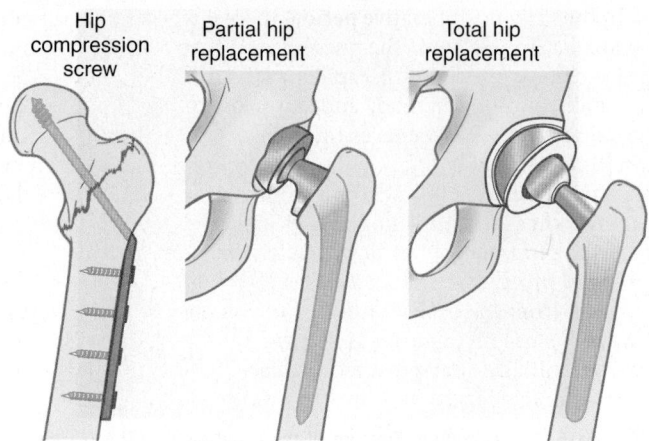

FIG. 65.17 Types of surgical repair for a hip fracture.

specific locations: (a) *capital* (fracture of the head of the femur), (b) *subcapital* (fractures just below the head of the femur), and (c) *transcervical* (fractures of the neck of the femur). These fractures are often associated with osteoporosis and minor trauma. *Extracapsular fractures* occur outside the joint capsule. They are termed *intertrochanteric* if they occur in a region between the greater and the lesser trochanter or *subtrochanteric* if they occur in the region below the lesser trochanter. Extracapsular fractures are usually caused by severe direct trauma or a fall.

Clinical Manifestations

The clinical manifestations of hip fractures are external rotation, muscle spasm, shortening of the affected extremity, and severe pain and tenderness in the region of the fracture site. Displaced femoral neck fractures cause serious disruption of the blood supply to the femoral head, which can result in AVN of the femoral head.

Interprofessional Care

Initially, the affected extremity may be temporarily immobilized by Buck traction (see Figure 65.9) until the patient's physical condition is stabilized and surgery can be performed. Buck traction relieves painful muscle spasms and is used for up to 24 to 48 hours.

Surgical treatment of hip fractures permits early mobilization and decreases the risk for major complications. The type of surgery depends on the location and severity of the fracture and the person's age. Surgical options include (a) repair with internal fixation devices (e.g., hip compression screw, intramedullary devices) (Figure 65.17), (b) replacement of part of the femur with a prosthesis (partial hip replacement) (see Figure 65.17), and (c) total hip replacement (involves both the femur and acetabulum) (see Figures 65.17 and 65.18).

NURSING MANAGEMENT
HIP FRACTURE

NURSING IMPLEMENTATION

PREOPERATIVE MANAGEMENT. The majority of people with hip fractures are older persons. When planning treatment of the hip fracture, consider the patient's chronic health problems (e.g., diabetes mellitus, cardiac disease, and pulmonary disease). The clinical benchmark for timing of surgical intervention for hip fracture is within 48 hours. In one study, increased time to surgery, especially for patients age 85 years or older, increased the mortality (Beaupre, Khong, et al., 2019).

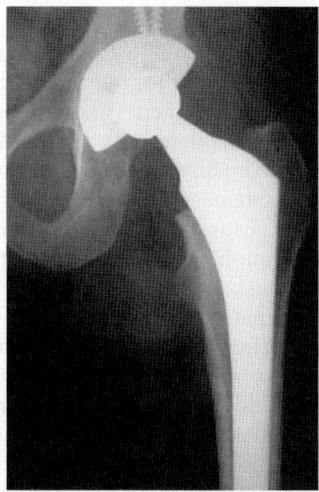

FIG. 65.18 Total hip replacement (arthroplasty) with a cementless femoral prosthesis of metal alloy with a plastic acetabular socket.

Before surgery, in addition to the usual preoperative nursing measures (see Chapter 20), severe muscle spasms may increase pain. Appropriate analgesics or muscle relaxants, comfortable positioning (unless contraindicated), and properly adjusted traction (if used) can help in managing the spasms.

Often, teaching is done in the emergency department because quick surgical intervention is the standard of care today. When possible, the patient can be taught the method and frequency for exercising the unaffected leg and both arms. The patient should also be encouraged to use the overhead trapeze bar and the opposite side rail to assist in changing positions. A physiotherapist can begin to teach out-of-bed and chair transfers. The family or caregiver must also be informed about the patient's weight-bearing status after surgery. Plans for discharge begin as the patient enters the hospital because the length of stay postoperatively will be only a few days.

POSTOPERATIVE MANAGEMENT. The initial postoperative management of a patient following ORIF of a hip fracture is similar to that for any older patient undergoing surgery. The nurse must monitor vital signs, intake, and output; supervise respiratory activities, such as deep breathing and coughing; provide pain management through pharmacological and non-pharmacological methods (see Chapter 10); and observe the dressing and incision for signs of bleeding and infection.

In the early postoperative period, there is a potential for neurovascular impairment. The nurse assesses the patient's extremity for colour, temperature, capillary refill, distal pulses, edema, sensation, motor function, and pain. Edema is alleviated by elevation of the leg whenever the patient is in a chair. The pain resulting from poor alignment of the affected extremity can be reduced by keeping pillows (or an abductor splint) between the patient's knees when turning to either side.

If the hip fracture has been treated by insertion of a femoral head prosthesis with a *posterior approach* (accessing the hip joint from the back), measures to prevent dislocation must always be used (Table 65.11). Extremes in flexion must be avoided initially after prosthetic replacement from a posterior approach. The patient and the caregiver must be fully aware of positions and activities that predispose the patient to dislocation (more than 90 degrees of flexion, adduction across the

midline [crossing of legs and ankles], internal rotation). Many daily activities may reproduce these positions, including putting on shoes and socks; crossing the legs or feet while seated; assuming the side-lying position incorrectly; standing up or sitting down while the body is flexed more than 90 degrees relative to the chair; and sitting on low seats, especially low toilet seats. The patient should be taught to avoid these activities until the soft tissue capsule surrounding the hip has healed sufficiently to stabilize the prosthesis (usually for at least 6 weeks).

Elevated toilet seats and chair alterations (e.g., raising the seat with pillows, maintaining a straight back) are necessary. Towel rolls (i.e., trochanter rolls) or pillows placed on the lateral side of the leg are also used to prevent external rotation. If a foam abduction pillow is used, it should be placed between the legs to prevent dislocation of the new joint (Figure 65.19). The nurse should ensure that the top straps are above the knee to avoid placing pressure on the peroneal nerve at the lateral tibial tubercle.

In addition to teaching the patient and caregiver how to prevent prosthesis dislocation, the nurse should also (a) place an abductor pillow or several pillows between the patient's legs when turning and (b) avoid turning the patient on the affected side until this has been approved by the health care provider. Also, some health care providers prefer that the patient keep the leg abductor pillow on except when bathing and walking.

Taking a tub bath and driving a car are not allowed for 4 to 6 weeks. An occupational therapist may teach the patient how to use assistive devices, such as reachers or grabbers, to avoid bending over to pick up something off the floor, long-handled shoehorns, or sock assists. The knees must be kept apart. The patient should be instructed to never cross their legs or twist to reach behind.

When the hip fracture is accessed during surgery with an *anterior* or *anterolateral approach* (joint reached from front of body), the hip muscles are left intact. This approach generally results in a more stable hip in the postoperative period, with a lower rate of complications (e.g., infection, dislocation). Precautions for the patient related to motion and weight bearing are few and may include instructions to avoid hyperextension.

Usually, the physiotherapist supervises exercises for the affected extremity and ambulation when the health care provider has approved this. The patient is usually out of bed on the first postoperative day. In collaboration with the physiotherapist, the nurse monitors the patient's ambulation status for proper use

TABLE 65.11   PATIENT & CAREGIVER TEACHING GUIDE

Femoral Head Prosthesis*

The following information should be included when teaching the patient and caregiver about a femoral head prosthesis.

Do
- Use an elevated toilet seat.
- Place a chair inside the shower or tub and remain seated while washing.
- Use a pillow between the legs for first 8 wk after surgery when lying on the side recommended by surgeon or when supine.
- Keep hip in a neutral, straight position when sitting, walking, or lying.
- Notify surgeon if severe pain, deformity, or loss of function occurs.
- Inform dentist of presence of prosthesis before dental work is done so that prophylactic antibiotics can be given if indicated.

Do Not
- Force hip into greater than 90 degrees of flexion (e.g., sitting in low chairs or on low toilet seats).
- Force hip into adduction.
- Force hip into internal rotation.
- Cross legs at knees.
- Put on own shoes or stockings without adaptive device (e.g., long-handled shoehorn or stocking-helper) until 8 wk after surgery.
- Sit on chairs without arms. They are needed to aid rising to a standing position.

*For patients having surgery by a posterior approach.

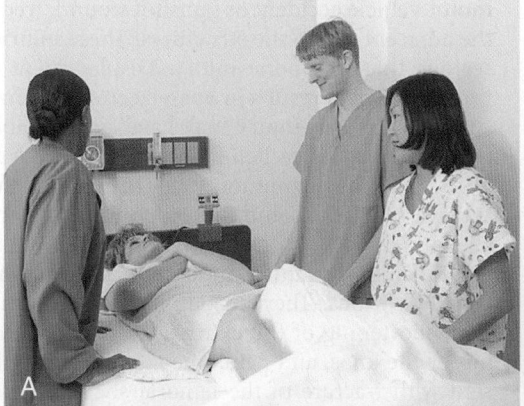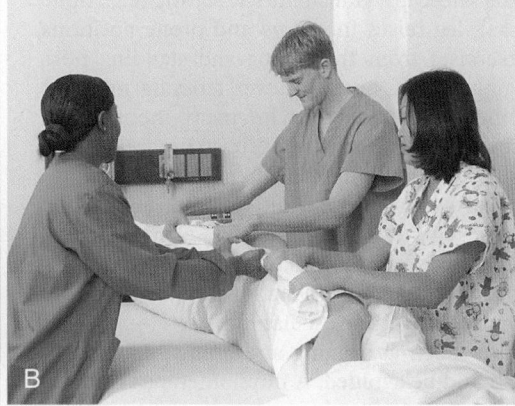

FIG. 65.19 Log rolling a patient. Source: Perry, A. G., Potter, P. A., & Ostendorf, W. R. (2016). *Nursing interventions and clinical skills* (6th ed., p. 418). Elsevier.

of crutches or a walker. For the patient to be discharged home, the nurse should have the patient demonstrate the proper use of crutches or a walker, the ability to transfer into and from a chair and bed, and the ability to ascend and descend stairs.

Weight bearing on the involved extremity varies. Weight bearing of especially fragile fractures may be restricted until radiological examination indicates adequate healing, usually 6 to 12 weeks.

Complications associated with femoral neck fracture include nonunion, AVN, dislocation, and degenerative arthritis. As a result of an intertrochanteric fracture, the affected leg may be shortened. A cane or built-up shoe may be required for safe ambulation. Sudden, severe pain; a lump in the buttock; limb shortening; and external rotation indicate prosthesis dislocation. Dislocation requires a closed reduction with conscious sedation or open reduction to realign the femoral head in the acetabulum. If it occurs (regardless of the setting), the patient should be kept on nothing-by-mouth (NPO) status in anticipation of a possible surgical intervention (Riemen & Munro, 2019).

The nurse assists both the patient and caregiver in adjusting to the restrictions and dependence imposed by the hip fracture. Anxiety and depression can easily occur, but creative nursing care and awareness of potential problems can help to prevent these states. The nurse should inform the patient and caregiver about community referral services that can assist in the postdischarge rehabilitation phase.

AMBULATORY AND HOME CARE. Hospitalization averages 3 or 4 days. Patients frequently require care in a subacute unit, at a skilled nursing facility, or in a rehabilitation facility for a few weeks before returning home. Regular follow-up care should be arranged for after discharge, including home health nursing.

Home care considerations include ongoing assessment of pain management, monitoring for infection, and prevention of VTE. The incision may be closed with metal staples, which are removed at the health care provider's office. If warfarin is used to decrease the high risk for VTE, prothrombin times are determined weekly and anticoagulation adjusted accordingly. Alternatives to warfarin include enoxaparin (Lovenox), fondaparinux (Arixtra), and rivaroxaban (Xarelto). These newer anticoagulants require less monitoring than warfarin does. The patient who is receiving an anticoagulant should be taught to immediately report signs of bleeding to the health care provider.

Exercises to restore strength and muscle tone in the quadriceps and muscles of the hip area are essential to improve function and ROM. These exercises include quadriceps setting (e.g., tightening the kneecap), gluteal muscle setting (e.g., tightening the buttocks), leg raises in supine and prone positions, and abduction exercises from the supine and standing positions (e.g., swinging the leg out but never crossing midline). The patient continues these exercises for many months after discharge. It is important to teach the exercise program to the caregiver who will be encouraging the patient at home.

A physiotherapist assesses ROM, ambulation, and adherence to the exercise regimen. The patient gradually increases the number of repetitions of exercises, adds weights to ankles, may swim, and may eventually use a stationary bicycle to tone quadriceps and improve cardiovascular fitness. High-impact exercises and sports, such as jogging and tennis, may loosen the implant and should be avoided. A physiotherapist or occupational therapist may perform a home assessment to identify hazards that may cause the patient to be at risk for falling.

EVALUATION
The following are expected outcomes for the patient with a fracture of the hip:
- Report satisfactory pain relief
- Participate in exercise therapy
- Understand prescribed treatment plan

AGE-RELATED CONSIDERATIONS
HIP FRACTURE
Factors that increase the risk for a hip fracture in older persons include a tendency to fall, inability to correct a postural imbalance, inadequacy of local tissue shock absorbers (e.g., fat, muscle bulk), and reduced skeletal strength. Factors that increase the older person's risk of falling include gait and balance problems, impaired vision and hearing, slowed reflexes, orthostatic hypotension, and medication use. Leading hazards of falls in the home include throw rugs and loose, worn or deep pile carpets; electrical cords in walkways; raised door sills; cluttered floors; poor lighting; slippery floors; poorly designed tubs, toilets, and fixtures in the bathroom; no aids or poorly installed aids such as grab bars or hand rails; and pets that get under foot (Public Health Agency of Canada [PHAC], 2016).

Many falls are associated with getting in or out of a chair or bed. Falls to the side, the most common type seen in frail older persons, are associated with a higher risk of injury, in particular hip fractures (Gratza et al., 2019). External hip protectors may help prevent hip fractures in the frail older patient (Hall et al., 2019). Older women often have osteoporosis and accompanying low bone density, which increases their risk for hip and other types of fractures.

Calcium and vitamin D supplementation, estrogen replacement, and bisphosphonate medication therapy decrease bone loss or increase bone density and thus reduce the likelihood of fracture, especially in patients with osteoporosis. (Osteoporosis is discussed in Chapter 66.) Nurses must be vigilant in planning interventions for the older person that are known to reduce the incidence of falls and hip fractures (Registered Nurses' Association of Ontario [RNAO], 2017).

FEMORAL SHAFT FRACTURE
Femoral shaft fracture occurs with a severe direct force because the femur can bend slightly before an actual fracture occurs. Young adults have a higher incidence of this type of fracture. The force exerted to cause the fracture, such as from a motor vehicle accident or gunshot wound, frequently damages the adjacent soft tissue structures. These injuries may be more serious than the bone injury. Displacement of the fracture fragments often results in open fracture and increased soft tissue damage. This injury may have considerable blood loss (1 to 1.5 L), leading to hemorrhagic anemia (Wertheimer et al., 2018). The most common types of femoral shaft fracture are transverse, spiral, comminuted, oblique, and open (see Figures 65.6 and 65.7).

The clinical manifestations of a femoral shaft fracture are usually obvious. They include marked deformity and angulation, shortening of the extremity, inability to move either the hip or the knee, and pain. The common complications associated with fracture of the femoral shaft include fat embolism, nerve and vascular injury, and problems associated with bone union, open fracture, and soft tissue damage.

Initial management of a femoral shaft fracture is directed toward stabilization of the patient and immobilization of the fracture. Traction may be used as a temporary measure before surgical treatment or in patients unable to undergo surgery. The method of treatment most often used for a femoral shaft fracture is *intramedullary nailing* (Witmer et al., 2017). A metal rod is placed into the marrow canal of the femur. The rod passes across the fracture to keep it in position. Internal fixation is preferred because it reduces the hospital stay and the complications associated with prolonged bed rest.

The initial postoperative management of a patient with femoral shaft fracture is similar to that for any patient undergoing surgery and involves monitoring for the above complications (see Chapter 22). The patient should be taught to carefully follow the health care provider's instructions for weight bearing. Promotion and maintenance of strength in the affected extremity usually include gluteal and quadriceps isometric exercises. The nurse should ensure that the patient performs ROM and strengthening exercises for all uninvolved extremities in preparation for ambulation. The patient may be allowed to begin non–weight-bearing activities with an ambulatory assistive device (e.g., walker, crutches). Full weight bearing is usually restricted until there is radiological evidence of union of the fracture fragments.

FRACTURE OF THE TIBIA

Although the tibia is vulnerable to injury because it lacks anterior muscle covering, strong force is required to produce a fractured tibia. As a result, soft tissue damage, devascularization, and open fracture are frequent. The tibia is one of the more common sites of a stress fracture. Complications associated with tibial fractures are compartment syndrome, FES, conditions associated with bony union, and possible infection associated with open fracture.

The recommended management for closed tibial fracture is closed reduction followed by immobilization in a long leg cast. ORIF with intramedullary rods, plate fixation, or external fixation is indicated for complex fractures and those with extensive soft tissue damage. Locking plates (screw and plate system) are another type of surgical device (see Figure 65.13). In both types of reduction, emphasis is placed on maintaining the strength of the quadriceps.

The neurovascular status of the affected extremity must be assessed at least every 2 hours during the first 48 hours. Patients are instructed to perform active ROM exercises with all uninvolved extremities, as well as exercises for the upper extremities, to build the strength required for crutch walking. When the health care provider has determined that the patient is ready for gait training, the patient is instructed in the principles of crutch walking. The patient may be on non–weight-bearing status for 6 to 12 weeks, depending on healing. Home nursing visits can be initiated to augment outpatient appointments and monitor the patient's progress.

STABLE VERTEBRAL FRACTURES

Stable fractures of the vertebral column are usually caused by motor vehicle accidents, falls, diving, or other athletic injuries. A *stable fracture* is one in which the fracture or the fragment is not likely to move or cause spinal cord damage. This type of injury is frequently confined to the anterior element (vertebral body) of the spinal column in the lumbar region and involves the cervical and thoracic regions less frequently. The vertebral bodies are usually protected from displacement by the intact spinal ligaments.

Most patients with spinal fractures have stable fractures and experience only brief periods of disability. However, if the ligamentous structures are significantly disrupted, dislocation of the vertebral structures may occur, resulting in instability and injury to the spinal cord (*unstable fracture*). These injuries generally require surgery. The most serious complication of vertebral fractures is fracture displacement, which can cause damage to the spinal cord (see Chapter 63). Although stable vertebral fractures are not associated with pathological spinal cord conditions, all spinal injuries should initially be considered unstable and potentially serious until diagnostic tests are done and the health care provider determines that the fracture is stable.

Usually, the patient experiences pain and tenderness in the affected region of the spine. Sudden loss of function below the level of the fracture indicates spinal cord impingement and paraplegia. Stable compression fractures are associated with a *kyphotic deformity* (flexion angulation of several vertebrae). This deformity may be noted during the physical examination. In patients with a stable vertebral fracture secondary to osteoporosis, several vertebral levels may be involved, as evidenced by a *dowager's hump* (abnormal curvature of the thoracic spine) or *lumbar lordosis* (extreme inward curve). The cervical spine may also be involved. Bowel and bladder dysfunction may be an indication of an interruption of the autonomic nervous system or injury to the spinal cord.

The overall goal in management of stable vertebral fractures is to keep the spine in good alignment until union has been accomplished. Many nursing interventions are aimed at assessing for the possibility of spinal cord trauma. Vital signs and bowel and bladder function should be evaluated regularly. The nurse should also monitor the motor and sensory status of the peripheral nerves distal to the injured region. Any deterioration in the patient's neurovascular status should be promptly reported.

Treatment includes pain medication followed by early mobilization and bracing. If hospitalized, the patient is usually placed in a standard hospital bed with firm support from the mattress. The aim is to support the spinal column, relax muscles, and prevent any potential compression on nerve roots. When turning, the patient should be taught to keep the spine straight by turning shoulders and pelvis together. Nursing assistance is necessary for the patient to learn the technique of "log rolling" (see Figure 65.19). Several days after the initial injury, the health care provider may apply a specially constructed orthotic device (e.g., Milwaukee, Jewett, or Taylor brace), a jacket cast, or a removable corset if there is no evidence of neurological deficit.

Vertebral compression fractures (which are often caused by osteoporosis) can be treated with two outpatient procedures: vertebroplasty or kyphoplasty. *Vertebroplasty* involves use of radioimaging to guide the injection of bone cement into the fractured vertebral body. The cement (when hardened) serves to stabilize and prevent further vertebral compression. *Kyphoplasty* initially involves inserting a balloon into the vertebral body and then inflating it. This procedure creates a cavity that is filled with bone cement under low pressure. Kyphoplasty results in a lower leakage of bone cement than with vertebroplasty and helps restore the height of the vertebral body. Vertebroplasty and kyphoplasty result in improved healing, better pain relief, and decreased complications compared to conservative treatment (Savage & Anderson, 2020).

If the fracture is in the cervical spine, the patient may wear a hard cervical collar. Some cervical fractures are immobilized by use of a halo vest (see Chapter 63, Figure 63.9). The halo vest consists of a plastic jacket or cast fitted around the chest and attached to a halo that is held in place by skeletal pins inserted into the cranium. These devices immobilize the spine in the fracture area but allow patient mobility.

The patient is discharged after regaining ambulation skills, learning care of the cast or orthotic device, and learning how to cope with the safety and security imposed by injury and treatment. Unstable vertebral fractures and spinal cord injuries are discussed in Chapter 63.

FACIAL FRACTURES

Any bone of the face can be fractured as a result of trauma, such as a motor vehicle accident, assault, or fall (Povolotskiy et al., 2019). The primary concern after facial injury is to establish and maintain a patent airway and to provide adequate ventilation. Suctioning may be necessary. An alternative airway (tracheostomy) may be needed if a patent airway cannot be maintained.

Concurrent facial fractures and cervical spine injuries are common. All patients with facial injuries should be treated as if they have a cervical injury until proven otherwise by examination and imaging studies (e.g., CT scan, radiographs). Table 65.12 describes the clinical manifestations of common facial fractures.

Associated soft tissue injury often makes assessment of a facial injury difficult. Oral and facial examinations are performed after the patient has been stabilized and any life-threatening conditions have been treated. Careful assessment is made of the ocular muscles and cranial nerve involvement (cranial nerves III, IV, and VI). Radiographs are used to determine the extent of the injury. CT scanning helps differentiate between bone and soft tissue (Kinsella et al., 2020).

Injury to the eye should be suspected when a facial injury occurs, particularly if the injury is near the orbit. If an eye-globe rupture is suspected, the examination should be stopped and a protective shield should be placed over the eye. Signs of globe rupture include the extrusion of vitreous humor or brown tissue (iris or ciliary body) on the surface of the globe or penetrating through a laceration with an eccentric or teardrop-shaped pupil.

Specific treatment depends on the site and extent of the facial fracture and the associated soft tissue injury. Immobilization or surgical stabilization may be necessary. A patent airway and adequate nutrition must be maintained throughout the recovery period. The nurse needs to be sensitive about the alterations in the patient's appearance that may occur after a facial fracture. The changes may be drastic. Edema and discoloration subside with time, but concurrent soft tissue injuries may result in permanent scarring.

Mandible Fracture

Mandibular fracture may result from trauma to the face or the jaws. Maxillary fractures may also occur, but they are less common than mandibular fractures. The fracture may be closed, with no bone displacement, or it may involve loss of tissue and bone. The fracture may require immediate and sometimes long-term treatment to ensure survival and restore satisfactory appearance and function.

A mandibular fracture may also be therapeutically performed to correct an underlying malocclusion problem that cannot be corrected by orthodontic procedures alone. The mandible is resected during surgery and manipulated forward or backward, depending on the occlusion condition.

Surgery consists of immobilization, usually by wiring the jaws (*intermaxillary fixation*). Internal fixation may be done with screws and plates. In a closed fracture with no loss of teeth, the lower jaw is wired to the upper jaw. Wires are placed around the teeth, and then cross-wires or rubber bands are used to hold the lower jaw tight against the upper jaw (Figure 65.20). Arch bars may be placed on the maxillary and mandibular arches of the teeth. Vertical wires are placed between the arch bars holding the jaws together. If teeth are missing or bone is displaced, other forms of fixation, such as metal arch bars in the mouth or insertion of a pin in the bone, may be needed. Bone grafting may also be required. Immobilization is usually necessary for only 4 to 6 weeks because the fractures often heal rapidly.

NURSING MANAGEMENT MANDIBULAR FRACTURE

NURSING IMPLEMENTATION

PREOPERATIVE MANAGEMENT. The patient undergoing mandibular surgery should be told preoperatively about the surgical procedure, including what it involves, how the face will look, and alterations caused by the surgery. The patient must be reassured about the ability to breathe normally, speak, and swallow liquids. Usually, hospitalization is brief unless there are other injuries or problems.

POSTOPERATIVE MANAGEMENT. Postoperative care should focus on a patent airway, oral hygiene, communication, pain

TABLE 65.12	**MANIFESTATIONS OF FACIAL FRACTURES**
Fracture	**Clinical Manifestation**
Frontal bone	Rapid edema that may mask underlying fractures
Mandible	Tooth fractures, bleeding, limited motion of mandible
Maxilla	Segmental motion of maxilla and alveolar fracture of teeth
Nasal bone	Displacement of nasal bones, epistaxis
Periorbital bone	Possible frontal sinus involvement, entrapment of ocular muscles
Zygomatic arch	Depression of zygomatic arch and entrapment of ocular muscles

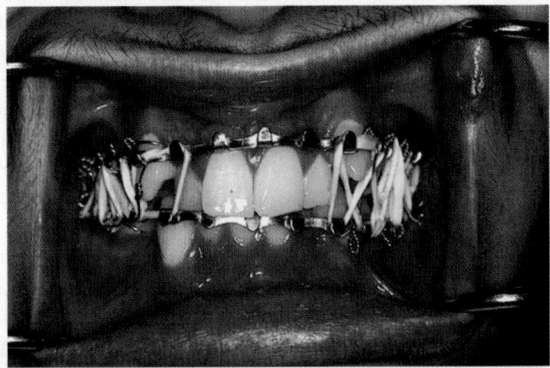

FIG. 65.20 Intermaxillary fixation. Source: Courtesy R. A. Weinstein, Denver, CO.

management, and adequate nutrition. Two major potential complications in the immediate postoperative period are airway obstruction and aspiration of vomitus. Because the patient cannot open their jaw, measures to ensure an airway are essential. The nurse must observe for signs of respiratory distress (e.g., dyspnea; alterations in rate, quality, and depth of respirations). The patient should be placed on their side with the head slightly elevated immediately after surgery.

Wire cutters or scissors (for rubber bands) must be taped to the head of the bed and sent with the patient on all appointments and examinations away from the bedside. The wire cutter or scissors may be used to cut the wires or elastic bands in case of an emergency (e.g., cardiac arrest or respiratory distress) requiring access to the pharynx or lungs. Information, including a picture showing the appropriate wires to cut, should be included in the care plan. In some cases, cutting the wires may cause the entire facial and upper jaw structure to shift or collapse and worsen the problem. A tracheostomy or endotracheal tray should always be available.

If the patient begins to vomit or choke, the nurse should try to clear the mouth and airway either by (1) having the patient bend their head over or to the side to allow the vomitus to flow out of the mouth and nose or (2) using a suction catheter to clear the mouth and nose. When suctioning is necessary, it can be performed by the nasopharyngeal or oral route, depending on the extent of injury and the type of repair. A nasogastric tube may be used for decompression to remove fluids and gas from the stomach in an effort to help prevent aspiration. This technique also helps prevent vomiting. Antiemetic medications may also be administered.

Oral hygiene is an important part of the nursing care. The mouth should be rinsed frequently, particularly after meals and snacks, to remove food debris. Warm normal saline solution or water may be used. A soft, rubber catheter or a Water-Pik is effective for a thorough oral cleansing. The nurse should inspect the mouth several times a day to see that it is clean. A flashlight is necessary, and a tongue depressor is used to retract the cheeks. The lips and corners of the mouth as well as the buccal mucosa should be kept moist. Dental wax may be used to cover any sharp edges of the wires to prevent irritation of the buccal mucosa.

Communication may be a challenge, particularly in the early postoperative period. An effective way of communicating must be established preoperatively (e.g., use of dry erase board, pad and pencil). Usually, the patient can speak well enough to be understood, especially after the first few postoperative days.

Ingestion of sufficient nutrients poses a challenge because the diet must be liquid. The patient easily tires of sucking through a straw or laboriously using a spoon. The diet must be planned to include adequate calories, protein, and fluids. Liquid protein supplements may be helpful for improving the nutritional status. The nurse needs to work with the dietitian and the patient to ensure adequate nutrition. The low-bulk, high-carbohydrate diet and the intake of air through the straw can contribute to constipation and flatus. Ambulation, prune juice, and bulk-forming laxatives may help relieve these conditions.

Usually, the patient is discharged with the wires in place. The nurse should encourage the patient to verbalize feelings about their altered appearance. Discharge teaching should include oral care, techniques of handling secretions, diet, how and when to use wire cutters, and when to notify the health care provider about concerns and complications.

AMPUTATION

An *amputation* is the removal of a body extremity by trauma or surgery. People in the middle and older age groups have the highest incidence of amputation because of the effects of peripheral vascular disease (PVD), atherosclerosis, and vascular changes related to diabetes mellitus. Based on the National Rehabilitation Reporting System, annually there are approximately 1 400 admissions related to amputation rehabilitation. The majority of patients are 55 years of age and older (CIHI, 2019b). Ontario First Nations populations with vascular changes associated with diabetes mellitus have a rate of lower-extremity amputation that is three to five times higher than that for other populations in Ontario (Shah et al., 2019). This higher incidence may be due to either underdiagnosed or undertreated PVD among First Nations people and to not seeking or having the ability to access medical treatment until irreversible tissue damage has occurred (Shah et al., 2019). Amputation in the younger population is usually secondary to trauma (e.g., motor vehicle accidents, land mines, farming-related injuries). Major advances in surgical amputation techniques, prosthetic design, and rehabilitation programs are enabling people with amputations to return to productive and satisfying social roles.

Clinical Indications

Most amputations are performed because of PVD, especially in older patients with diabetes mellitus (Botros et al., 2019). In Canada, the number of individuals living with diabetes mellitus was estimated at 4.2 million in 2020. These patients often experience peripheral neuropathy that progresses to trophic ulcers and subsequent gangrene. Careful monitoring by patients at home and nurses with validated screening tools can help with early recognition of situations that can lead to amputation (Rickards & Cornish, 2018). Other common reasons for amputation are trauma and thermal injuries, tumours, osteomyelitis, and congenital limb disorders. Although pain is often present, it is not usually the primary reason for an amputation.

Diagnostic Studies

The types of diagnostic studies performed depend on the underlying condition that makes the amputation necessary (Table 65.13). Test results that show an elevated white blood cell count with abnormal differential may indicate infection. Vascular studies such as arteriography, Doppler studies, and venography provide information about the circulatory status of the extremity.

Interprofessional Care

Whether amputation is considered "elective" or necessary, the patient's general health is carefully assessed. Chronic illnesses and the presence of infection are important considerations. The patient and family should be helped to understand the need for the amputation and be assured that rehabilitation can result in an active, useful life. If the amputation is done on an emergency basis as a result of trauma, the management is physically and emotionally more complicated.

The goal of amputation surgery is to preserve extremity length and function while removing all infected, pathological, or ischemic tissue. (Levels of amputation of upper and lower extremities are illustrated in Figure 65.21.) The type of amputation depends on the reason for the surgery. A closed amputation is performed to create a weight-bearing *residual limb*. An

TABLE 65.13   INTERPROFESSIONAL MANAGEMENT

Amputation

Diagnostic	Interprofessional Therapy
• History and physical examination	**Medical**
• Physical appearance of soft tissues	• Appropriate management of underlying disease
• Presence of peripheral pulses	• Stabilization of patient with trauma
• Sensory function	**Surgical**
• Skin temperature	• Selective type of amputation
• Arteriography	• Residual limb management
• Plethysmography	• Immediate prosthetic fitting
• Transcutaneous ultrasonic Doppler recordings	• Delayed prosthetic fitting
• Venography	**Rehabilitation**
	• Coordination of prosthesis-fitting and gait-training activities with occupational therapist and physiotherapist
	• Coordination of muscle-strengthening and physiotherapy regimens

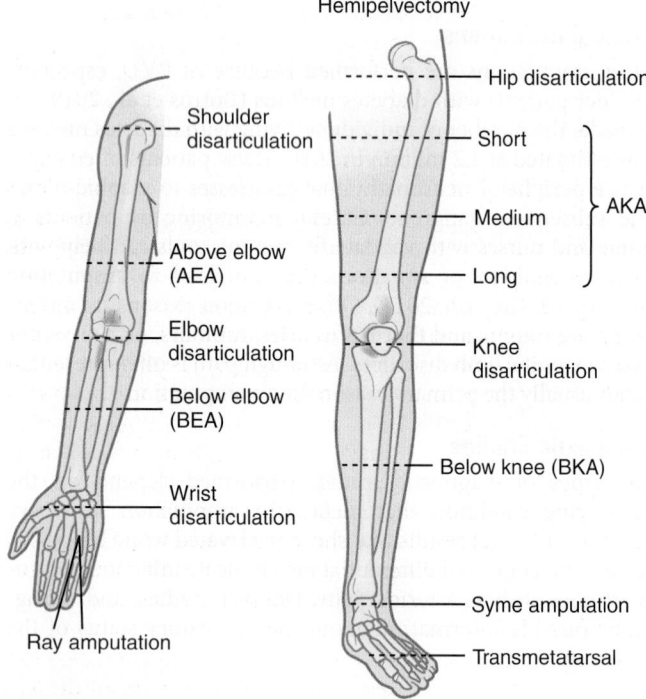

FIG. 65.21 Location and description of amputation sites of the upper and lower extremities. *AKA*, above-the-knee amputation.

anterior skin flap with dissected soft tissue padding covers the bony part of the residual limb. The skin flap is sutured posteriorly so that it will not be positioned in a weight-bearing area. Special care is necessary to prevent accumulation of drainage, which can produce pressure and harbour bacteria that may cause infection.

Disarticulation is an amputation performed through a joint. A *Syme amputation* is a form of disarticulation at the ankle. An open amputation leaves a surface on the residual limb that is not covered with skin. This type of surgery is generally indicated for control of actual or potential infection. The wound is usually closed later by a second surgical procedure or by skin traction

surrounding the residual limb. This type of amputation is often called a *guillotine amputation*.

NURSING MANAGEMENT AMPUTATION

NURSING ASSESSMENT

Pre-existing illnesses must be adequately assessed because most amputations are performed as a result of vascular disorders. Assessment of the vascular and neurological status is an important part of this assessment process (see Chapters 34 and 58).

NURSING DIAGNOSES

Nursing diagnoses for the patient with an amputation may include but are not limited to the following:

- *Altered body image* as a result of *change in self-perception* (amputation, impaired mobility)
- *Reduced tissue integrity* as a result of *pressure over bony prominence* (improperly fitted prosthesis)
- *Pain* as a result of *a surgical incision, emotional distress, nerve compression* (phantom limb sensation/pain)
- *Reduced mobility* as a result of *pain, physical deconditioning* (amputation of lower limb)

PLANNING

The overall goals are that the patient with an amputation will (a) have adequate relief from the underlying health problem, (b) have satisfactory pain control, (c) reach maximum rehabilitation potential with the use of a prosthesis (if indicated), (d) cope with the body image changes, and (e) make satisfying lifestyle adjustments.

NURSING IMPLEMENTATION

HEALTH PROMOTION. Control of causative illnesses such as PVD, diabetes mellitus, chronic osteomyelitis, and pressure injuries can eliminate or delay the need for amputation (Botros et al., 2019). Patients with these conditions should be taught to carefully examine their lower extremities daily for signs of potential problems. If the patient cannot assume this responsibility, a caregiver should be instructed in the procedure. The patient and their caregiver should be instructed to report symptoms such as a change in skin colour or temperature, decrease or absence of sensation, tingling, pain, or the presence of a lesion to the health care provider. Review of safety precautions in recreation and in the performance of hazardous work is an important nursing responsibility, especially for occupational health nurses.

ACUTE INTERVENTION. The nurse must recognize the tremendous psychological and social implications of an amputation for the patient. The alteration in body image caused by an amputation often causes a patient to go through psychological stages similar to those of the grieving process (see Chapter 13). Allowing the patient to go through a grieving process or period of depression and recognizing it as a normal consequence may do much to aid the patient's acceptance of the amputation. The patient's family must also be helped to work through the process to arrive at a realistic and positive attitude about the future. The reasons for an amputation and the rehabilitation potential depend on age, diagnosis, occupation, personality, resources, and support systems.

Preoperative Management. Before surgery, in addition to the usual preoperative nursing measures (see Chapter 20), the nurse should reinforce information that the patient and family have received about the reasons for the amputation, the proposed prosthesis, and the mobility training program. To meet the patient's educational needs, the nurse must know the level of amputation, the type of post-surgical dressing to be applied, and the type of prosthesis to be used. The patient should receive instruction in the performance of upper extremity exercises such as push-ups in bed or the wheelchair to promote arm strength. This instruction is essential for later crutch walking and gait training. General postoperative nursing care should be discussed, including positioning, support, and residual limb care. If a compression bandage is to be used after surgery, the patient should be instructed in its purpose and how it will be applied. If an immediate prosthesis is planned, the general ambulation program should be discussed.

The patient should be warned that they may feel as though the amputated limb is still present after surgery. This phenomenon is termed **phantom limb sensation** (any sensation of the missing limb except pain). Different sources have reported the incidence of phantom limb sensation as anywhere between 60 and 100% in individuals with amputations (Jerath et al., 2015). This sensation can cause patients grave concern unless they are forewarned. It can take various forms, such as the feeling that someone is touching the missing limb, pressure on the missing limb, cold, wetness, itching, tickle, or fatigue. *Phantom limb pain* (any painful sensations that are referred to the absent limb) often begins immediately after surgery. The pain can be described as shooting, burning, crushing, or severe and agonizing. It is more common for the pain to be intermittent, with short episodes (seconds to minutes) of severe pain occurring several times a day. There is some evidence that the pain present preoperatively may be mimicked in the phantom limb.

Postoperative Management. General postoperative care for the patient who has undergone an amputation depends largely on the patient's general state of health, the reason for the amputation, and the patient's age. Individuals who undergo amputation as a result of a traumatic injury need to be monitored for post-traumatic stress disorder because they had no time to prepare or perhaps even participate in the decision to have a limb amputated.

Prevention and detection of complications are important nursing responsibilities during the postoperative period. Careful monitoring of the patient's vital signs and dressing can alert the nurse to hemorrhage in the operative area. Careful attention to sterile technique during dressing changes reduces the potential for wound infection.

If an *immediate* postoperative prosthesis has been applied, the nurse must monitor vital signs carefully because the surgical site is heavily covered and may not be visible. A surgical tourniquet must always be available for emergency use. If excessive bleeding occurs, the health care provider should be notified immediately.

The *delayed* prosthetic fitting may be the best choice for patients who have had amputations above the knee or below the elbow, for older persons, for individuals who are debilitated, and for patients with infection. The appropriate time for use of a prosthesis depends on satisfactory healing of the residual limb as well as on the general condition of the patient. A temporary prosthesis may be used for partial weight bearing once the sutures are removed. Barring any complications, patients can bear full weight on permanent prostheses by approximately 3 months after their amputation.

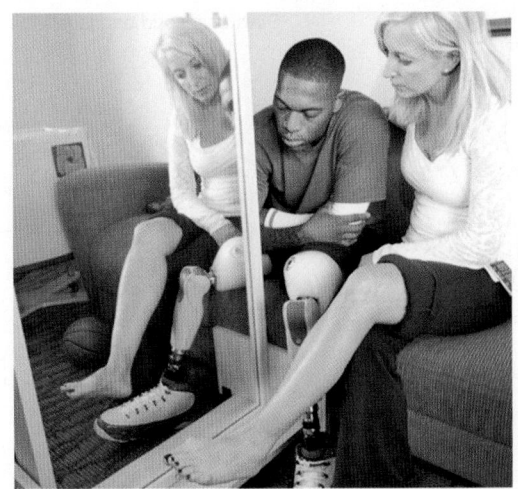

FIG. 65.22 A physiotherapist demonstrates mirror therapy, a type of treatment that may reduce phantom limb sensation and pain. Source: US Navy photo courtesy Mass Communication Specialist Seaman Joseph A. Boomhower.

Not all patients are candidates for a prosthesis. People who are seriously ill or debilitated may not have the upper body strength and energy required to use a lower extremity prosthesis. Mobility with a wheelchair may be the most realistic goal for patients who are not candidates for prostheses.

Often, patients may be anxious about phantom limb sensation because they still perceive pain in the missing portion of the limb. As recovery and ambulation progress, phantom limb sensation and pain usually subside, although the pain may become chronic. The patient may also experience shooting, burning, or crushing pain and feelings of coldness, heaviness, and cramping. Mirror therapy reduces phantom limb sensation and pain in some patients (Ambron et al., 2018) (Figure 65.22). The mirror is thought to provide visual information to the brain, replacing the sensory feedback expected from the missing limb. However, it is unknown why looking in the mirror at the unaffected limb would decrease phantom limb sensation and pain. Mirror therapy may also improve patient functioning after a stroke.

Success of the rehabilitative program depends on the physical and emotional health of the patient. Chronic illness and deconditioning complicate aggressive rehabilitation efforts. Both physiotherapy and occupational therapy must be an integral component of the patient's overall plan of care.

Flexion contractures may delay the rehabilitation process. The most common and debilitating contracture is hip flexion. Hip adduction contracture is rare. Patients should avoid sitting in a chair for more than 1 hour with hips flexed, or having pillows under the surgical extremity, to prevent flexion contractures. Unless specifically contraindicated, patients should lie on their abdomen for 30 minutes, three to four times each day, and position the hip in extension while prone.

Proper residual limb bandaging fosters shaping and moulding for eventual prosthesis fitting (Figure 65.23). The health care provider usually orders a compression bandage to be applied immediately after surgery to support the soft tissues, reduce edema, hasten healing, minimize pain, and promote residual limb shrinkage and maturation. This bandage may be an elastic roll applied to the residual limb or a residual limb shrinker, which is an elastic stocking that fits tightly over the residual limb and lower trunk area.

Start of second bandage

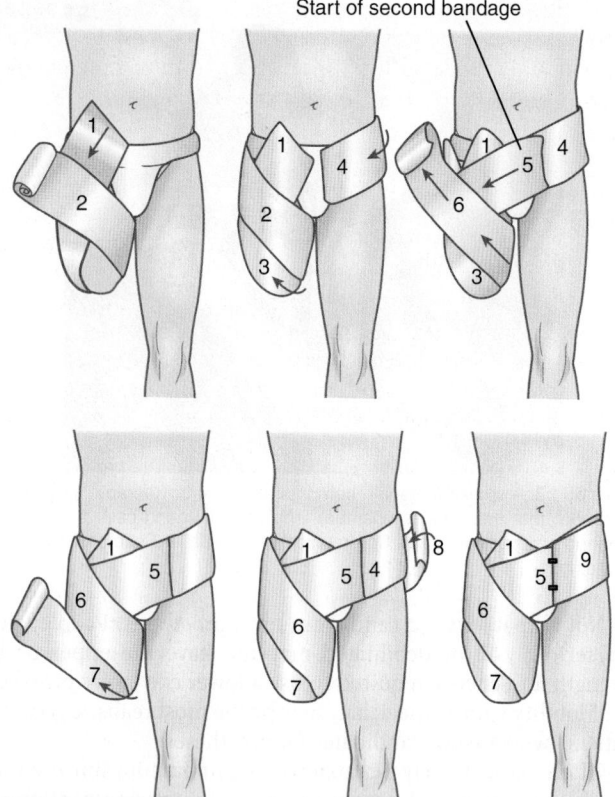

FIG. 65.23 Bandaging for the above-the-knee amputation residual limb. Figure-of-eight style covers progressive areas of the residual limb. Two elastic wraps are required.

TABLE 65.14	**PATIENT & CAREGIVER TEACHING GUIDE**

Following an Amputation

After an amputation, patient and caregiver teaching should include the following information:
- Inspect the residual limb daily for signs of skin irritation, especially erythema, excoriation, and odour. Pay particular attention to areas prone to pressure.
- Discontinue use of the prosthesis if an irritation develops. Have the area checked before resuming use of the prosthesis.
- Wash residual limb thoroughly each night with warm water and a bacteriostatic soap. Rinse thoroughly and dry gently. Expose the residual limb to air for 20 min.
- Do not use any substance such as lotions, alcohol, powders, or oil on the residual limb unless prescribed by the health care provider.
- Wear only a residual limb sock that is in good condition and supplied by the prosthetist.
- Change residual limb sock daily. Launder in a mild soap, squeeze, and lay flat to dry.
- Use prescribed pain management techniques.
- Perform ROM to all joints daily. Perform general strengthening exercises, including the upper extremities, daily.
- Do not elevate the residual limb on a pillow.
- Lie prone with hip in extension for 30 min, three to four times daily.

ROM, range of motion.

The compression bandage is initially worn at all times except during physiotherapy and bathing. The bandage is taken off and reapplied several times daily, and care is taken so that it is applied snugly but not so tightly as to interfere with circulation. Shrinker bandages should be washed and changed daily. After healing has occurred, the residual limb is bandaged only when the patient is not wearing the prosthesis. The patient should be instructed to avoid dangling the residual limb over the bedside to minimize edema formation.

As the patient's overall condition improves, an exercise regimen is normally started under the supervision of the health care provider and the physiotherapist. Active ROM exercises of all joints should be started as soon after surgery as the patient's pain level and medical status permit. In preparation for mobility, the patient should increase triceps and shoulder strength and lower limb support and learn balance of the altered body. The loss of the weight of a limb necessitates adaptation of the patient's proprioceptive and coordination mechanisms to prevent falls and injury.

Crutch walking is started as soon as patients are physically able. After an immediate postsurgical fitting, orders related to weight bearing must be carefully followed to avoid injury to the skin flap and delay of the healing process. Before discharge, the patient and caregiver need careful instruction related to residual limb care, ambulation, prevention of contractures, recognition of complications, exercise, and follow-up care. Table 65.14 outlines patient and caregiver teaching following an amputation.

AMBULATORY AND HOME CARE. When healing has occurred satisfactorily and the residual limb is well moulded, the patient is ready for fitting of a prosthesis. A prosthetist initially makes a mould of the residual limb and measures landmarks for fabrication of the prosthesis. The moulded limb socket allows the residual limb to fit snugly into the prosthesis. The limb is covered with a stocking to ensure good fit and prevent skin breakdown. The limb may continue to shrink, causing a loose fit, in which case a new socket has to be fabricated. The patient may need to have the prosthesis adjusted to prevent rubbing and friction between the residual limb and the socket. Excessive movement of a loose prosthesis can cause severe skin irritation and breakdown.

Artificial limbs become an integral part of the patient's body image. Proper care ensures their long life and useful functioning. The patient should be instructed to clean the prosthesis socket daily with a mild soap and rinse thoroughly to remove irritants. The leather and metal parts of the prosthesis should not get wet. The patient should be encouraged to have regular maintenance of the prosthesis. Consideration of the condition of the shoe is also necessary. A badly worn shoe alters the gait and may cause damage to the prosthesis.

SPECIAL CONSIDERATIONS IN UPPER LIMB AMPUTATION. The emotional implications of an upper limb amputation are often more devastating than those for lower limb amputation. The enforced dependency brought about by one-handedness may be both frustrating and difficult for the patient. Because most upper extremity amputations result from trauma, often the patient has not had the opportunity to adjust psychologically to an amputation or to participate in the decision-making process about amputation.

Both immediate and delayed prosthetic fittings are possible for the person with a below-the-elbow amputation. Prosthetic fitting is delayed for the person with an above-the-elbow amputation. The usual functional prosthesis is the arm and hook. A cosmetic hand is available but has limited functional value. As with the lower limb prosthesis, patient motivation and endurance are major factors contributing to a satisfactory outcome. Technological advances to improve the functionality of upper limb prostheses are an active area of research (Pierrie et al., 2018).

Many companies are also experimenting with 3D printing to make less expensive prosthetic limbs that also take less time to develop and produce.

EVALUATION

The following are expected outcomes for the patient with an amputation:

- Accept changed body image and integrate changes into their lifestyle
- Have no evidence of skin breakdown
- Have reduction or absence of pain
- Become mobile within limitations imposed by amputation

AGE-RELATED CONSIDERATIONS

AMPUTATION

If a lower limb amputation has been performed on an older person, the patient's previous ability to ambulate may affect the extent of recovery. Use of a prosthesis requires a significant amount of energy for ambulation. Walking with a below-the-knee prosthesis requires 40% additional energy, and an above-the-knee prosthesis requires 60% more energy than walking on two legs. Older people whose general health is weakened by disorders such as cardiac or pulmonary conditions may not be candidates for prosthesis use. These patients' ability to ambulate will be limited. If possible, this should be discussed with the patient and their family before surgery so that realistic expectations can be set.

COMMON JOINT SURGICAL PROCEDURES

Surgery plays an important role in the treatment and rehabilitation of patients with various forms of joint disease. Surgery is aimed at relieving chronic pain, improving joint motion, correcting deformity and malalignment, and removing intra-articular erosion. Joint replacement surgery is the most common orthopedic operation performed on older persons. If decreased functional ability of the joint is not corrected, contractures with permanent limitation of motion often occur. Limitation of motion at the joint can be demonstrated on physical examination and by joint-space narrowing on radiological examination.

Indications for hip or knee arthroplasty include arthritis, connective tissue disease, failed prior procedures, sepsis, tumours, Paget's disease, congenital hip dysplasia, severe varus or valgus deformity, and spondyloarthropathies.

TYPES OF JOINT SURGERIES

Synovectomy

Synovectomy (removal of synovial membrane) is used as a prophylactic measure and as a palliative treatment of rheumatoid arthritis (RA). Removal of the synovial membrane, thought to be the location of the basic pathological changes in joint destruction, helps prevent further progression of joint damage. A synovectomy is best performed early in the disease process to prevent serious destruction of joint surfaces. Removal of the thickened synovium prevents extension of the inflammatory process into the adjacent cartilage, ligaments, and tendons.

It is impossible to surgically remove all the synovium in a joint. The underlying disease process is still present and will again affect the regenerating synovium. However, the disease appears to be milder after synovectomy, and definite improvement in

pain, weight bearing, and ROM can be expected. Common sites for this surgery include the elbow, wrist, and fingers. Synovectomy in the knee is done less frequently because knee joint replacement techniques are usually performed.

Osteotomy

An osteotomy is performed by removing or adding a wedge or slice of bone to change alignment (joint and vertebral) and to shift weight bearing, thereby correcting deformity and relieving pain. Cervical osteotomy may be used to correct deformity in some patients with ankylosing spondylitis. Halo and body jackets are worn until fusion occurs (at 3–4 months). Subtrochanteric or femoral osteotomy may provide some relief of pain and improve motion in selected patients with hip osteoarthritis (OA). Osteotomy has proved ineffective in patients with inflammatory joint disease. Osteotomy of the knee (tibia) provides relief of pain in selected patients, but advanced joint destruction is usually corrected by joint replacement surgery (Saltzman et al., 2017).

The postoperative care for osteotomy is similar to the treatment of an internal fixation of a fracture at a comparable site (see Nursing Management: Fractures). Internal wires, screws and plates, bone grafts, or an external fixator usually fix the bone in place.

Debridement

Debridement is the removal of degenerative debris such as loose bodies, osteophytes, joint debris, and degenerated menisci from a joint. This procedure is usually performed on the knee or the shoulder, using a fibre-optic arthroscope. Usually, the procedure is done on an outpatient basis. A compression dressing is applied postoperatively. Weight bearing is permitted following knee arthroscopy. Patient education includes monitoring for signs of infection, managing pain, and restricting excessive activity for 24 to 48 hours.

Arthroplasty

Arthroplasty is the reconstruction or replacement of a joint to relieve pain, improve or maintain ROM, and correct deformity. There were 59 000 hip and 70 000 knee replacements in Canada for 2017–2018, representing an increase of 17.4% and 17%, respectively, over the previous 5 years (CIHI, 2019a).

Reducing wait times for hip and knee replacement surgeries is a top health care priority in Canada. All provinces are now collecting and reporting wait time data for joint replacements through the Canadian Joint Replacement Registry (CIHI, 2019a). The national trend in meeting the 182-day benchmark between 2014 and 2018 is declining for hip and knee replacements, and the number of patients included in the wait-time calculation is increasing annually (CIHI 2018a).

The most common uses of arthroplasty are for patients with OA, RA, AVN, congenital deformities or dislocations, and other systemic problems. There are several types of arthroplasty, including surgical reshaping of the bones of the joints, replacement of part of a joint (hemiarthroplasty), and total joint replacement. Replacement arthroplasty is available for elbow, shoulder, phalangeal joints of the fingers, wrist, hip, knee, ankle, and foot.

Minimally invasive surgery is available in many centres in Canada for hip and knee replacements. Minimally invasive surgery involves less dissection and smaller incisions (5 to 10 cm in the hip and 10 to 12.7 cm in the knee) and a shorter hospital stay. It is technically demanding and requires extra education for the surgeon. There is an initial quicker recovery with less rehabilitation and a quicker return to performing ADLs for the patient. Minimally invasive surgery also results in less blood loss and less need for transfusions.

Hip Arthroplasty. Total hip arthroplasty (THA) provides significant relief of pain and improvement of function for patients with OA, RA, and other conditions. Partial and total hip replacements are also used to treat hip fractures.

In THA, the prosthesis (implant) replaces the ball and socket joint and upper shaft of the femur (see Figure 65.18). The socket can be bonded to the bone (i.e., cemented) with polymethyl methacrylate. Alternatively, cementless THAs may provide longer-term prosthesis stability by facilitating biological ingrowth of new bone tissue into the porous surface coating of the prosthesis. Cementless devices are most often recommended for younger, more active patients and patients with good bone quality, where bone ingrowth into the components can be readily achieved.

The nursing care for a patient who has a THA is discussed in the section on nursing management of a patient with a hip fracture (see Nursing Management: Hip Fracture).

Hip Resurfacing. An alternative to hip replacement is hip resurfacing, which allows the femoral head to be preserved and reshaped rather than replaced. The resurfaced femoral head (ball) is then capped by a metal prosthesis (Foran, 2018b). The metal appears to have a lower rate of wear, and thus the prosthesis may have a longer lifetime. Hip resurfacing is a more favourable option for younger, active patients. After surgery, there is generally a 6-month waiting period before doing strenuous activity, until strong muscles are built around the joint. Patients receiving a smaller femoral head (including many women) have a higher failure rate with a resurfaced implant compared with patients receiving a THA.

Knee Arthroplasty. Unremitting pain and instability as a result of severe destructive deterioration of the knee joint is the main indication for total knee arthroplasty (TKA) or total knee replacement (TKR). Osteoporosis may necessitate bone grafting to augment defects and to correct bone deficiencies. Either part or all of the knee joint may be replaced with a metal and plastic prosthetic device. For a TKA, the procedure can be done cementless or cemented. Cementless prosthesis is textured to allow the bone to grow into and adhere over time, whereas the cemented prosthesis uses bone cement to affix the prosthesis to the bone (Chen & Li, 2019). A compression dressing is used to immobilize the knee in extension immediately after the operation. This is usually removed within 24 hours and may be replaced with a knee immobilizer such as a Zimmer immobilizer splint or posterior plastic shell, which stabilizes the knee and maintains extension during ambulation and at rest for about 4 weeks. Knee immobilizers are removed for various portions of physiotherapy. Dislocation is not typical with TKA.

After surgery, emphasis is placed on pain management (see Chapter 10) and physiotherapy. Managing pain decreases the patient's risk of complications and enables continuation of the exercise program (McDonald et al., 2016). Isometric quadriceps setting begins the first day after surgery. The patient progresses to straight-leg raises and gentle ROM to increase muscle strength and obtain 90-degree knee flexion. Active flexion exercises or passive flexion exercises through the use of a CPM machine postoperatively may promote joint mobility. Full weight bearing is begun before discharge. An active home exercise program involves progressive ROM with muscle strengthening and flexibility exercises. Following TKA, many older patients with advanced OA have shown significant improvement in mobility, motor function tests, and ability to complete daily tasks.

Finger Joint Arthroplasty. A silicone rubber arthroplastic device is used to help restore function in the fingers of the patient with RA. Ulnar deviation is often present, which results in severe functional limitations of the hand. The goal of hand surgery is primarily to restore function related to grasp, pinch, stability, and strength rather than to correct cosmetic deformity. Before surgery, the patient is instructed in hand exercises, including flexion, extension, abduction, and adduction of the fingers.

Postoperatively, the hand is kept elevated with a bulky dressing in place. Neurovascular assessment is conducted postoperatively, and the nurse assesses for signs of infection. The success of the surgery depends largely on the postoperative treatment plan, which is often carried out under the direction of an occupational therapist. Once the dressing is removed, a guided splinting program is initiated. The patient is discharged with splints to use while sleeping and hand exercises to perform for 10 to 12 weeks, at least three or four times a day. The patient is also instructed to avoid lifting heavy objects.

Elbow and Shoulder Arthroplasty. Although available, total replacement of elbow and shoulder joints is not as common as other forms of arthroplasty. Shoulder replacements are used in patients with severe pain because of RA, OA, AVN, or a previous trauma. Shoulder replacement is usually considered if the patient has adequate surrounding muscle strength and bone stock. If joint replacement is necessary for both the elbow and shoulder, the elbow is usually done first because a severely painful elbow interferes with the shoulder rehabilitation program.

Significant pain relief has been achieved following arthroplasty, with most patients having no pain at rest or minimal pain with activity. Functional improvements have resulted in better hygiene and increased ability to perform ADLs for most patients. Rehabilitation is longer and more difficult than with other joint surgeries.

Ankle Arthroplasty. Total ankle arthroplasty (TAA) is indicated for RA, OA, AVN, and trauma. Although the use of TAA is not widespread, it is becoming a viable alternative to fusion for the treatment of advanced ankle arthritis in selected patients. Devices available include several fixed-bearing devices and a mobile-bearing cementless prosthesis. This device more closely imitates natural ankle function.

Ankle fusion is often selected over arthroplasty, although the use of TAA has increased dramatically over the past decade (Marx & Mizel, 2015). With fusion the patient is left with a stiff foot and the inability to change heel height. TAA is advantageous because it achieves a more normal gait pattern (Marx & Mizel, 2015). Postoperatively, the patient may not bear weight for 6 weeks, must elevate the extremity to reduce and prevent edema, must be extremely careful to prevent postoperative infection, and must maintain immobilization as directed by the health care provider.

Arthrodesis

Arthrodesis is the surgical fusion of a joint. This procedure is indicated only if articular surfaces are too severely damaged or infected to allow joint replacement or if reconstructive surgery fails. Arthrodesis relieves pain and provides a stable but immobile joint. The fusion is usually accomplished by removal of the articular hyaline cartilage and the addition of bone grafts across the joint surface. The affected joint must be immobilized until bone healing has occurred. Common areas of fusion are wrist, ankle, cervical spine, lumbar spine, and metatarsophalangeal (MTP) joint of the great toe.

Complications of Joint Surgery

Infection is a serious complication of joint surgery, particularly joint replacement surgery (Bohsali et al., 2017). The most common causative organisms are Gram-positive aerobic streptococci and staphylococci. Infection almost always leads to pain and loosening of the prosthesis, generally necessitating extensive surgery. Efforts to reduce the incidence of infection include the use of specially designed self-contained operating suites, operating rooms with laminar airflow, and prophylactic antibiotic administration. Current recommendations for perioperative antibiotic prophylaxis in elective joint arthroplasty include stopping therapy after 24 hours (Siddiqi et al., 2019).

VTE is another potentially serious complication after joint surgeries, particularly those involving the lower extremities. Prophylactic measures such as warfarin, low-molecular-weight heparin (LMWH), and sequential compression devices of the legs are usually instituted. Patients may be followed postoperatively with venous Doppler ultrasonography to detect DVT, the source of most pulmonary emboli.

Interprofessional Care

Preoperative Management. The primary goal of preoperative assessment is to identify risk factors associated with postoperative complications so that nursing strategies can be implemented to promote optimal positive outcomes. A careful history will include previous medical diagnoses and complications such as diabetes and thrombophlebitis, pain tolerance and preferences for managing pain, current functional status, expectations following surgery, and level of social support and home care needs after discharge. The patient should be free from evidence of infection and acute joint inflammation.

If lower extremity surgery is planned, upper extremity muscle strength and joint function are assessed to determine the type of assistive devices needed postoperatively for ambulation and ADLs. A preoperative physiotherapist consult and teaching can inform the patient and family of the expected hospital course and postoperative management at home (e.g., stairs, bathroom, width of doors). In addition, such teaching prepares the patient to maximize the usefulness and longevity of the prosthesis. Patients also need to realize that recovery does not happen quickly. It can be helpful for patients and their families or significant others to speak with individuals who have had a total joint arthroplasty so that they better understand the reality of rehabilitation.

Postoperative Management. Postoperatively, neurovascular assessment is performed to assess nerve function and circulatory status. Anticoagulation therapy, analgesia, and parenteral antibiotics are administered. In general, the affected joint is exercised, and ambulation is encouraged as early as possible to prevent complications of immobility. Specific protocols vary according to patient, type of prosthesis, and health care provider preference. Pain management postoperatively may involve use of epidural or intrathecal analgesia, femoral nerve block (knee only), patient-controlled analgesia (PCA), intravenous injections, and oral opioids or NSAIDs.

The hospital stay after arthroplasty is 3 to 5 days, depending on the patient's course and need for physiotherapy. Physiotherapy and ambulation enhance mobility, build muscle strength, and reduce the risk for thrombus formation. If the patient is taking warfarin, therapy starts on the day of surgery and continues for 3 weeks, with an international normalized ratio (INR) assessed on a regular basis. For patients taking LMWH (e.g., enoxaparin), therapy starts after surgery and continues for 2 weeks postoperatively. Daily monitoring of the patient's coagulation status is not necessary with LMWH.

NURSING MANAGEMENT
JOINT SURGERY

The nursing management of the patient undergoing joint surgery begins with preoperative teaching and realistic goal setting. It is important that the patient understand and accept the limitations of the proposed surgery and that they realize that in some cases, surgery will not remove or treat the underlying disease. Postoperative procedures such as turning, deep breathing, use of a bedpan and high bedside commode, and use of abductor pillows should be explained and opportunities for practice provided. The patient should be reassured that pain relief will be available; PCA can be helpful. During a preoperative visit from a physiotherapist, the patient can practise postoperative exercises and be measured for crutches or other assistive devices.

Discharge planning begins immediately on admission to the hospital. The duration of the hospital stay and the expected postoperative events should be discussed because the patient and caregiver must plan ahead. The home environment must be assessed for safety (e.g., presence of scatter rugs and electrical cords) and accessibility. Are the bathroom and bedroom on the first floor? Are door frames wide enough to accommodate a walker? Social support must also be assessed. Is a friend or family member available to assist the patient in the home, or will the patient need extra assistance? Will the patient require a homemaker or meal services? The older patient may need the rehabilitation services of a subacute or long-term care facility for a few weeks postoperatively to progressively develop independent living skills. Specific nursing interventions related to the patient having orthopedic surgery are summarized in NCP 65.2, available on the Evolve website.

Patient teaching includes instructions on reporting complications, including infection (e.g., fever, increased pain, drainage) and dislocation of the prosthesis (e.g., pain, loss of function, shortening or misalignment of an extremity). The home care nurse acts as the liaison between the patient and the health care provider, monitoring for postoperative complications, assessing comfort and ROM, and facilitating improvements in functional performance.

CASE STUDY

Hip Fracture Surgery

Patient Profile

T. K. (pronouns he/him), 78 years old, is admitted to the hospital through the emergency department. Based on the team's assessment, the patient sustained a fracture to his left hip (see Chapter 64 Case Study). The patient is scheduled for a surgical hip repair in the morning.

Subjective Data

See the Case Study in Chapter 64.

Interprofessional Care
Preoperative

- Pain not relieved by morphine.
- The patient's partner is at his bedside crying and anxious, causing T. K.'s anxiety to also increase.

Operative Procedure

- Left hip repair using hip compression plate and bone screws

Postoperative

- Cefazolin 1g IV q8hr
- Intake and output for 48 hr
- Morphine via patient-controlled analgesia (PCA) pump

Discussion Questions

1. How do his pre-existing medical conditions predispose T. K. to postoperative complications?
2. What actions could be taken to help decrease T. K.'s partner's anxiety?

3. **Priority decision:** As care is planned for T. K., what are the preoperative and postoperative priority nursing interventions?
4. What are the most likely postoperative complications that T. K. could develop?
5. **Priority decision:** On assessment of the patient on the second postoperative day, an irregular pulse is noted, which is a new finding. His pulse rate is 66 and his ECG tracing is shown below. Which dysrhythmia is this? What is the priority action at this time?

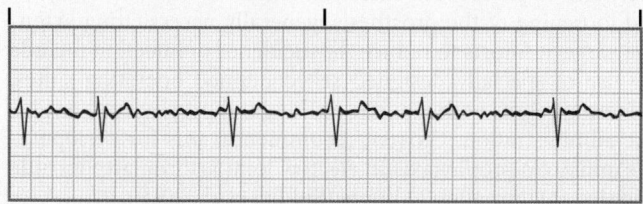

6. **Priority decision:** What are the priority teaching interventions that should be done before discharge?
7. **Evidence-informed practice:** Why is satisfactory pain relief an important nursing goal in the postoperative period for T. K.?

ⅇvolve

Answers are available at http://evolve.elsevier.com/Canada/Lewis/medsurg.

REVIEW QUESTIONS

The number of the question corresponds to the same-numbered objective at the beginning of the chapter.

1. When would the nurse suspect an ankle sprain for the client being seen at the urgent care centre?
   a. Client was hit by another soccer player on the field.
   b. Client has ankle pain after sprinting around the track.
   c. Client dropped a 4.5-kg weight on his lower leg at the health club.
   d. Client had a twisting injury while running bases during a baseball game.

2. The nurse explains to a client with a distal tibial fracture returning for a 3-week checkup that healing is indicated by which of the following?
   a. Callus formation
   b. Complete bony union
   c. Hematoma at the fracture site
   d. Presence of granulation tissue

3. A client with a comminuted fracture of the femur is to have an open reduction with internal fixation (ORIF) of the fracture. In which of the following situations is an ORIF indicated?
   a. The client is able to tolerate prolonged immobilization.
   b. The client cannot tolerate the surgery for a closed reduction.
   c. A temporary cast would be too unstable to provide normal mobility.
   d. Adequate alignment cannot be obtained by other nonsurgical methods.

4. Which of the following indicates a neurovascular condition during the nurse's assessment of a client with a fracture?
   a. Exaggeration of extremity movement
   b. Increased redness and heat below the injury
   c. Decreased sensation distal to the fracture site
   d. Purulent drainage at the site of an open fracture

5. A client with a stable, closed fracture of the humerus caused by trauma to the arm has a temporary splint with bulky padding applied with an elastic bandage. For which of the following symptoms would the nurse suspect compartment syndrome and notify the health care provider?
   a. Increasing edema of the limb
   b. Muscle spasms of the lower arm
   c. Rebounding pulse at the fracture site
   d. Pain when passively extending the fingers

6. Which of the following symptoms should the nurse be monitoring for in a client with pelvic fracture?
   a. Changes in urinary output
   b. Petechiae on the abdomen
   c. A palpable lump in the buttock
   d. Sudden increase in blood pressure

7. During the postoperative period, what should the client with an above-the-knee amputation be told about the negative effect of routinely elevating the residual limb?
   a. The flexed position can promote hip flexion contracture.
   b. This position reduces the development of phantom pain.
   c. This position promotes clot formation at the incision site and thigh.
   d. Unnecessary movement of the extremity can cause wound dehiscence.

8. A client with rheumatoid arthritis is scheduled for an arthroplasty. How should the nurse explain the purpose of this procedure? *(Select all that apply.)*
   a. To fuse the joint
   b. To replace the joint
   c. To prevent further damage
   d. To improve or maintain ROM
   e. To decrease the amount of destruction in the joint

9. What should the nurse teach a client recovering from a total hip replacement to avoid?
   a. Sleeping on the abdomen
   b. Sitting with the legs crossed
   c. Abduction exercises of the affected leg
   d. Bearing weight on the affected leg for 6 weeks

1. d; 2. a; 3. d; 4. c; 5. d; 6. a; 7. a; 8. b, d; 9. b.

Ⓔvolve

For even more review questions, visit http://evolve.elsevier.com/Canada/Lewis/medsurg.

REFERENCES

Ambron, E., Miller, A., Kuchenbecker, K. J., et al. (2018). Immersive low-cost virtual reality treatment for phantom limb pain: Evidence from two cases. *Frontiers in Neurology, 9*(67), 1–7. https://doi.org/10.3389/fneur.2018.00067

Baumgartner, R. E., Billow, D. G., & Olson, S. A. (2018). Pelvic ring injury. In M. K. Sethi, W. T. Obremskey, & A. A. Jahangir (Eds.), *Orthopedic traumatology: An evidence-based approach* (2nd ed., pp. 171–179). Springer.

Beaupre, L., Khong, H., Smith, C., et al. (2019). The impact of time to surgery after hip fracture on mortality at 30 and 90 days: Does a single benchmark apply to all? *Injury, 50*(4), 950–955. https://doi.org/10.1016/j.injury.2019.03.031

Beaupre, L., Sobolev, B., Guy, P., et al. (2019). Discharge destination following hip fracture in Canada among previously community-dwelling older adults 2004–2012: Database study. *Osteoporosis International, 30*(7), 1338–1394. https://doi.org/10.1007/s00198-019-04943-6

Bohsali, K. I., Bois, A. J., & Wirth, M. A. (2017). Complications of shoulder arthroplasty. *Journal of Bone and Joint Surgery, 99*(3), 256–269. https://doi.org/10.2106/JBJS.16.00935

Botros, M., Kuhnke, J., Embil, J., et al. (2019). *Foundations of best practice for skin and wound management: Best practice recommendations for the prevention and management of diabetic foot ulcers.* Wounds Canada. https://www.woundscanada.ca/docman/public/health-care-professional/bpr-workshop/895-wc-bpr-prevention-and-management-of-diabetic-foot-ulcers-1573r1e-final/file

Brown, J. V., & Yuan, S. (2020). Traumatic injuries of the pelvis. *Emergency Medicine Clinics of North America, 38*(1), 125–142. https://doi.org/10.1016/j.emc.2019.09.011

Canadian Association of Occupational Therapists. (2016). What is occupational therapy? https://www.caot.ca/site/aboutot/whatisot?nav=sideba

Canadian Centre for Occupational Health and Safety (CCOHS). (2016). Preventing repetitive strain injuries—A message worth repeating. *CCOHS Health and Safety Report, 14*(2). https://www.ccohs.ca/newsletters/hsreport/issues/2016/02/ezine.html

Canadian Centre for Occupational Health and Safety (CCOHS). (2021). *Repetitive strain injury awareness day: Educate and prevent.* https://www.ccohs.ca/events/rsi/

Canadian Institute of Health Information (CIHI). (2018a). *Benchmark for treatment and wait time in Canada.* http://waittimes.cihi.ca/All#trend

Canadian Institute for Health Information (CIHI). (2018b). *Injury and trauma emergency department and hospitalization statistic 2017–2018.* [data set]. https://www.cihi.ca/en/injury-and-trauma-emergency-department-and-hospitalization-statistics-2017-2018

Canadian Institute of Health Information (CIHI). (2019a). *Hip and knee replacements in Canada 2017–2018: Canadian Joint Replacement Registry annual report.* https://www.cihi.ca/sites/default/files/document/cjrr-annual-report-2019-en-web_0.pdf

Canadian Institute for Health Information (CIHI). (2019b). *Quick stats: Demographic characteristics of inpatient rehabilitation clients.* https://www.cihi.ca/en/rehabilitation#_Databases_and_Data

Canadian Society for Exercise Physiology (CSEP). (2020). *Canadian 24-hour movement guidelines.* https://csepguidelines.ca/

Chen, C., & Li, R. (2019). Cementless vs cemented total knee arthroplasty in young patients: A meta-analysis of randomized controlled trials. *Journal of Orthopaedic Surgery and Research, 14,* 262–273. https://doi.org/10.1186/s13018-019-1293-8

Crowther-Radulewicz, C., & McCance, K. (2017). Alterations of musculoskeletal function. In S. Huether, & K. McCance (Eds.), *Understanding pathophysiology* (6th ed.) (pp. 991–1035). Elsevier.

First Nations Health Authority (FNHA). (2019). *First Nations regional health survey phase 3 (2015–17): Northern Region.* British Columbia. https://www.fnha.ca/Documents/FNHA-First-Nations-Regional-Health-Survey-Phase-3-2015-2017-Northern-Region.pdf

Foran, J. R. (2018a). *Hip bursitis. OrthoInfo.* https://orthoinfo.aaos.org/en/diseases--conditions/hip-bursitis

Foran, J. R. (2018b). *Hip resurfacing. OrthoInfo.* https://orthoinfo.aaos.org/en/treatment/hip-resurfacing/

Fukumoto, L. E., & Fukumoto, K. D. (2018). Fat embolism syndrome. *Nursing Clinics of North America, 53*(3), 335–347. https://doi.org/10.1016/j.cnur.2018.04.003

Gee, S. M., Tennent, D. J., Cameron, K. L., et al. (2020). The burden of meniscus injury in young and physically active populations. *Clinics in Sports Medicine, 39*(1), 13–27. https://doi.org/10.1016/j.csm.2019.08.008

Gratza, S., Chocano-Bedoya, P., Orav, E., et al. (2019). Influence of fall environment and fall direction on risk of injury among pre-frail and frail adults. *Osteoporosis International, 30,* 2205–2215. https://doi.org/10.1007/s00198-019-05110-7

Hall, A., Boulton, E., & Stanmore, E. (2019). Older adults' perception of wearable technology hip protectors: Implications for further research and development strategies. *Disability & Rehabilitation: Assistive Technology, 14*(7), 663–668. https://doi.org/10.1080/17483107.2018.1491647

Hardy, M., & Feehan, L. M. (2020). Fracture healing: An evolving perspective. In T. M. Skirven, A. L. Osterman, J. M. Fedorczyk, et al. (Eds.), *Rehabilitation of the hand and upper extremity* (7th ed., Vol. 1, pp. 264–275). Elsevier.

Jarvis, J. (2020). *Physical examination and health assessment* (8th ed). Elsevier.

Jerath, R., Crawford, M., & Jenson, M. (2015). Etiology of phantom limb syndrome: Insights from a 3D default space consciousness model. *Medical Hypotheses, 85*(2015), 153–159. https://doi.org/10.1016/j.mehy.2015.04.025

Khalifeh, J. M., Zohny, Z., MacEwan, M., et al. (2018). Electrical stimulation and bone healing: A review of current technology and clinical applications. *IEEE Review in Biomedical Engineering, 11*(99), 217–232. https://doi.org/10.1109/RBME.2018.2799189

Kinsella, S. D., Tobert, D. G., & Harris, M. B. (2020). Initial evaluation of spine in trauma patients. In B. D. Browner, J. B. Jupiter, C. Krettek, et al. (Eds.), *Skeletal trauma: Basic science, management and reconstruction* (6th ed., pp. 356–372). Elsevier.

Knott, C., Hampton, L., Lowe, R., et al. (2019). *Weight bearing.* Physiopedia. https://www.physio-pedia.com/index.php?title=Weight_bearing&oldid=208133

Kosova, E., Bergmark, B., & Piazza, G. (2015). Fat embolism syndrome. *Circulation, 131*(3), 317–320. https://doi.org/10.1161/CIRCULATIONAHA.114.010835

Lieberman, J. R., & Heckmann, N. (2017). Venous thromboembolism prophylaxis in total hip arthroplasty and total knee arthroplasty patients: From guidelines to practice. *Journal of American Academy of Orthopedic Surgeons, 25*(12), 789–798. https://doi.org/10.5435/JAAOS-D-15-00760

Limbert, E., & Santy-Tomlinson, J. (2017). Acute limb compartment syndrome in the lower leg following trauma: Assessment in the intensive care unit. *Nursing Standard, 31*(34), 61–70. https://doi.org/10.7748/ns.2017.e10708

Marx, R. C., & Mizel, M. S. (2015). What's new in foot and ankle surgery. *Journal of Bone & Joint Surgery, 97*(10), 862–868. https://doi.org/10.2106/JBJS.O.00126

Matullo, K. S., Gangavalli, A., & Nwachuku, C. (2016). Review of lower extremity traction in current orthopedic trauma. *Journal of American Academy of Orthopaedic Surgeons, 24*(9), 600–606. https://doi.org/10.5435/JAAOS-D-14-00458

McDonald, L. T., Corbiere, N. C., DeLisle, J. A., et al. (2016). Pain management after total joint arthroplasty. *Association of perioperative Registered Nurses, 103*(6), 605–616. https://doi.org/10.1016/j.aorn.2016.04.003

McQuivey, K. S., Christopher, Z. K., Chung, A. S., et al. (2019). Implementing the Lever sign in the emergency department: Does it assist in acute anterior cruciate ligament rupture diagnosis? A pilot study. *Journal of Emergency Medicine, 57*(6), 805–811. (0736-4679). https://doi-org.ezproxy.library.dal.ca/10.1016/j.jemermed.2019.09.003

Murphy, J., Weiner, D. A., Kolter, J., et al. (2020). Utility of Ottawa ankle rules in an aging population: Evidence for addition of an age criterion. *Journal of Foot & Ankle Surgery, 59*(1), 286–290. https://doi.org/10.1053/j.jfas.2019.04.017

National Institute of Neurological Disorders and Stroke (NINDS). (2020). *Carpal tunnel syndrome fact sheet.* https://www.ninds.nih.gov/Disorders/Patient-Caregiver-Education/Fact-Sheets/Carpal-Tunnel-Syndrome-Fact-Sheet

Pierrie, S. N., Gaston, R. G., & Loeffler, B. J. (2018). Current concepts in upper-extremity amputation. *Journal of Hand Surgery, 43*(7), 657–667. https://doi.org/10.1016/j.jhsa.2018.03.053

Povolotskiy, R., Youssef, P., Kaye, R., et al. (2019). Facial fractures in young adults: A national retrospective study. *Annals of Otology, Rhinology & Laryngology, 128*(6), 516–523. https://doi.org/10.1177/0003489419830114

Public Health Agency of Canada (PHAC). (2016). *How to lower your fall risk.* https://www.canada.ca/en/public-health/services/publications/healthy-living/how-lower-your-fall-risk.html

Registered Nurses' Association of Ontario (RNAO). (2017). *Best practice guideline: Preventing fall and reducing injury form falls* (4th ed.). https://rnao.ca/bpg/guidelines/prevention-falls-and-fall-injuries

Rickards, T., & Cornish, T. (2018). Reaching out to diabetic soles: Outreach foot care pilot project. *SAGE Open Medicine, 6.* https://doi.org/10.1177/2050312118820030

Riemen, A. H., & Munro, C. (2019). Complication in hip surgery. *Orthopaedics and Trauma, 33*(6), 365–371. https://doi.org/10.1016/j.mporth.2019.10.003

Safran-Norton, C., Sullivan, J., Irrgang, J., et al. (2019). A consensus-based process for identifying physical therapy and exercise treatments for patients with degenerative meniscal tears and knee OA: The TeMPO physical therapy interventions and home exercise program. *BMC Musculoskeletal Disorders, 20*, 514. https://doi.org/10.1186/s12891-019-2872-x

Salati, U., Doody, O., Munk, P. L., et al. (2017). Evaluation of knee pain in athletes: A radiologist's perspective. *Canadian Association of Radiologists Journal, 68*(1), 27–40. https://doi.org/10.1016/j.carj.2016.04.003

Saltzman, B. M., Rao, A., Erickson, B. J., et al. (2017). A systematic review of 21 tibial tubercle osteotomy studies and more than 1000 knees: Indications, clinical outcomes, complications and reoperations. *American Journal of Orthopedics, 46*(6), E398–E407.

Samai, K., & Vilella, A. (2018). Update in therapeutics: Prophylactic antibiotics in open fractures. *Society of Trauma Nurses, 25*(2), 83–86. https://doi.org/10.1097/JTN.0000000000000348

Sanderson, M., Mohr, B., & Abraham, M. K. (2020). The emergent evaluation and treatment of hand and wrist injuries: An update. *Emergency Medicine Clinics of North America, 38*(1), 61–79. https://doi.org/10.1016/j.emc.2019.09.004

Savage, J. W., & Anderson, P. A. (2020). Osteoporotic spinal fractures. In B. D. Browner, J. B. Jupiter, C. Krettek, et al. (Eds.), *Skeletal trauma: Basic science, management and reconstruction* (6th ed., pp. 1073–1085). Elsevier.

Shah, B. R., Frymire, E., Jacklin, K., et al. (2019). Peripheral arterial disease in Ontario First Nations people with diabetes: A longitudinal population-based cohort study. *Canadian Medical Association Journal Open, 7*(4), E700–E705. https://doi.org/10.9778/cmajo.20190162

Shea, K. G., Carey, J. L., Richmond, J., et al. (2015). The American Academy of Orthopaedic Surgeons evidence-based guideline on management of anterior cruciate ligament injuries. *Journal of Bone and Joint Surgery, 97*(8), 672–674. https://doi.org/10.2106/JBJS.N.01257

Short, N., Blair, M., Crowell, C., et al. (2020). Mobile technology and cumulative trauma symptomology among millennials. *Hand Therapy, 25*(1), 11–17. https://doi.org/10.1177/1758998319871075

Siddigi, S., Forte, S., Doctor, S., et al. (2019). Perioperative antibiotic prophylaxis in total joint arthroplasty: A systematic review and meta-analysis. *The Journal of Bone and Joint Surgery, 101*(9), 828–842. https://doi.org/10.2106/JBJS.18.00990

Silva, P. V., Kamper, S. J., & da Cunha Menezes Costa, L. (2018). Exercise-based intervention for prevention of sports injuries. *British Journal of Sports Medicine, 52*(6), 408–409. https://doi.org/10.1136/bjsports-2017-098474

Statistics Canada. (2015a). *Health at a glance. Injuries in Canada: Insights from the Canadian Community Health Survey.* http://www.statcan.gc.ca/pub/82-624-x/2011001/article/11506-eng.htm

Statistics Canada. (2015b). *Canadian Community Health Survey: Combined data, 2013/2014.* http://www.statcan.gc.ca/daily-quotidien/150624/dq150624b-eng.htm

Statistics Canada. (2018). *Table 13-10-0394-01: Leading causes of death, total population, by age group (data set).* https://doi.org/10.25318/1310039401-eng.

Szostakowski, B., Smitham, P., & Khan, W. S. (2017). Plaster of Paris: Short history of casting and injured limb immobilization. *Open Orthopedic Journal, 11,* 291–296. https://doi.org/10.2174/1874325001711010291

Vershinin, A. V., Guscha, A. O., Arestov, S. O., et al. (2018). Surgical treatment of the carpal tunnel syndrome with the application of endoscopic and electrophysiology monitoring. *Human Physiology, 44*(8), 912–916. https://doi.org/10.1134/S0362119718080145

Walker, J. (2018). Assessing and managing pin sites in patients with external fixation. *Nursing Times, 114*(1), 18–21. https://www.nursingtimes.net/clinical-archive/tissue-viability/assessing-and-managing-pin-sites-in-patients-with-external-fixation-18-12-2017/

Wertheimer, A., Olaussen, A., Perera, S., et al. (2018). Fractures of the femur and blood transfusions. *Injury, 49*(4), 846–885. https://doi.org/10.1016/j.injury.2018.03.007

Wiley, T. J., Lemme, N. J., Macaccio, S., et al. (2020). Return to play following meniscal repair. *Clinics of Sports Medicine, 39*(1), 185–196. https://doi.org/10.1016/j.csm.2019.08.002

Witmer, D. K., Marshall, S. T., & Browner, B. D. (2017). Emergency care of musculoskeletal injuries. In C. Townsend, R. Beauchamp, M. Evers, et al. (Eds.), *Sabiston textbook of surgery: The biological basis of modern surgical practice* (20th ed., pp. 462–504). Elsevier.

Zalavras, C. G. (2017). Prevention of infection in open fractures. *Infectious Disease Clinics of North America, 31*(2), 339–352. https://doi.org/10.1016/j.idc.2017.01.005

RESOURCES

About Face
https://www.aboutface.ca

Amputation Coalition of Canada
http://amputeecoalitioncanada.org/

Arthritis Community & Network
https://www.arthritisnetwork.ca

Arthritis Society
https://www.arthritis.ca

Canadian Academy of Sport and Exercise Medicine
https://www.casm-acms.org

Canadian Centre for Occupational Health and Safety
https://www.ccohs.ca

Canadian Orthopaedic Association
https://www.coa-aco.org

Canadian Orthopaedic Foundation
https://whenithurtstomove.org/

Canadian Orthopaedic Nurses Association
https://www.cona-nurse.org

Canadian Society for Exercise Physiology (CSEP)
https://www.csep.ca/home

GTA Rehab Network
http://www.gtarehabnetwork.ca/

Osteoporosis Canada
https://www.osteoporosis.ca

The War Amps
https://www.waramps.ca/home/

American Academy of Orthopaedic Surgeons (AAOS)
https://www.aaos.org

American Association for Hand Surgery
https://www.handsurgery.org

American College of Sports Medicine (ACSM)
https://www.acsm.org

Amputee Coalition of America (ACA)
https://www.amputee-coalition.org

National Association of Orthopaedic Nurses (NAON)
http://www.orthonurse.org

National Center on Health, Physical Activity and Disability (NCHPAD)
https://www.nchpad.org/

National Institute on Aging—*Exercise and Physical Activity*
https://www.nia.nih.gov/health/exercise-physical-activity

National Institute of Arthritis and Musculoskeletal and Skin Diseases (NIAMS)
https://www.niams.nih.gov/

OrthoInfo
https://orthoinfo.aaos.org/

ⓔvolve

For additional Internet resources, see the website for this book at http://evolve.elsevier.com/Canada/Lewis/medsurg.

CHAPTER

66

Nursing Management

Musculoskeletal Conditions

Danielle L. Byrne
Originating US chapter by Diane Ryzner

---

evolve WEBSITE

http://evolve.elsevier.com/Canada/Lewis/medsurg

- Review Questions (Online Only)
- Key Points
- Answer Guidelines for Case Study

- Customizable Nursing Care Plans
  - Low Back Pain
  - Patient with Osteomyelitis

- Conceptual Care Map Creator
- Audio Glossary
- Content Updates

LEARNING OBJECTIVES

1. Describe the pathophysiology and clinical manifestations of osteomyelitis and the interprofessional care and nursing management of patients with osteomyelitis.
2. Describe the etiology, pathophysiology, and clinical manifestations of and interprofessional care of patients with osteoporosis and Paget's disease.
3. Differentiate between the causes and characteristics of acute and chronic low back pain.

4. Explain the conservative and surgical therapy of patients with herniated intervertebral disc.
5. Describe the postoperative nursing management of a patient who has undergone spinal surgery.
6. Explain the etiology and the nursing management of patients with common foot disorders.
7. Describe the types, pathophysiology, and clinical manifestations of bone cancer and the interprofessional care of patients with bone cancer.

KEY TERMS

degenerative disc disease (DDD)
Ewing sarcoma family of tumours (ESFT)
herniated intervertebral disc
low back pain (LBP)

osteoclastoma
osteomyelitis
osteoporosis
osteosarcoma

Paget's disease of the bone
sarcoma

Acute and chronic musculoskeletal conditions are a common source of pain and disability leading to changes in mobility that affect a person's mental, physical, and social well-being. Such changes can restrict patients from fully participating in activities of daily living. A variety of conditions unrelated to trauma that affect the musculoskeletal system are presented in this chapter, including osteomyelitis, metabolic bone diseases, low back pain, foot disorders, and bone cancer. An interprofessional team approach is essential in assessing pain and functional abilities along with initiating interventions to prevent injury and maintain mobility. The nurse plays an integral role throughout all phases to manage and maintain patient mobility.

OSTEOMYELITIS

Etiology and Pathophysiology

Osteomyelitis is a severe infection of the bone, bone marrow, and surrounding soft tissue. The most common infecting microorganism is *Staphylococcus aureus*. A variety of microorganisms can cause osteomyelitis (Kavanagh et al., 2018) (Table 66.1). Aerobic Gram-negative bacteria, alone or mixed with Gram-positive organisms, are often found. The widespread use of antibiotics in conjunction with surgical treatment has significantly reduced the mortality rate and complications associated with osteomyelitis.

The infecting microorganisms can invade by indirect or direct entry. The *indirect (hematogenous) entry* of microorganisms most frequently affects children because the metaphyseal (growing) regions of long bones are highly vascular and susceptible to even minor trauma (Thakolkaran & Shetty, 2019). Adults with vascular insufficiency disorders (e.g., caused by diabetes mellitus) or genitourinary or respiratory infections are at higher risk for a primary infection to spread via the blood to the bone. The pelvis and the vertebrae, which consist of vascular-rich bone, are the most common sites of infection (Schmitt, 2017). *Direct-entry* osteomyelitis can occur at any age, when there is an open wound (e.g., fractures, penetrating wounds) and microorganisms gain entry to the body. Osteomyelitis may also occur in the presence of a foreign body such as an implant or an orthopedic prosthetic device (e.g., plate, total joint prosthesis), with leg or foot ulcers related to vascular insufficiency, or with pressure-related injuries (Kavanagh et al., 2018). In the case of diabetic foot infections, 20 to 60% are associated with bone involvement (Senneville et al., 2020).

After gaining entrance to the bone by way of the blood, the microorganisms then lodge in an area of the bone where circulation slows, usually the metaphysis. The microorganisms grow, resulting in an increase in pressure because of the nonexpanding nature of most bone. This increasing pressure within the rigid bone structure leads to ischemia and vascular compromise of the periosteum. Eventually, the infection spreads through the bone cortex and the marrow cavity, ultimately resulting in cortical devascularization, necrosis, and bone death. The area of devitalized bone eventually separates from the surrounding living bone, forming *sequestra* (sing., *sequestrum*). The part of the periosteum that continues to have a blood supply forms new bone, called *involucrum* (Figure 66.1).

Once formed, a sequestrum continues to be an infected island of dead bone surrounded by purulent drainage. It is difficult for bloodborne antibiotics or white blood cells to reach the sequestrum. A sequestrum may serve as a reservoir for microorganisms that spread to other sites, including the lungs and brain. The sequestrum can move out of the bone and into the soft tissue. Once outside of the bone, the sequestrum may revascularize and then undergo removal by the body's normal immune processes. The sequestrum can also be surgically removed through debridement of the necrotic bone. If the necrotic sequestrum is not resolved naturally or surgically, it may develop a sinus tract, resulting in a chronic, purulent cutaneous drainage (see Figure 66.1).

Despite advances in the identification of pathogens, current use of antibiotics, and surgical debridement, acute osteomyelitis becomes chronic in 10 to 30% of cases and is difficult to treat. In recent years, understanding of bacterial virulence and host defence has improved through emerging research of bacterial biofilm models (Mifsud & McNally, 2019). A *biofilm* is a cluster of bacterial cells that form a matrix (three-dimensional structure) that requires necrotic tissue and bone. This matrix functions as a barrier, offering the bacteria protection from mechanical influences, antibiotics, and the host's defence cells. The pathogens pass from a planktonic phase to maturation. The biofilm essentially functions as a permanent source of virulent pathogens insensitive to the body's own immune system and antibiotics. Surgical excision of the sequestrum and biofilm is thus required.

Clinical Manifestations

Acute osteomyelitis refers to the initial infection or an infection of less than 1 month in duration. The clinical manifestations of acute osteomyelitis are both systemic and local. Systemic manifestations include fever, night sweats, chills, restlessness, nausea, and malaise. Local manifestations include constant bone pain that is unrelieved by rest and worsens with activity; swelling, tenderness, and warmth at the infection site; and restricted movement of the affected part. Later signs include drainage from sinus tracts to the skin or the fracture site.

Chronic osteomyelitis refers to a bone infection that persists for longer than 1 month or an infection that has failed to respond to the initial course of antibiotic therapy. Chronic osteomyelitis is either a continuous, persistent condition (a result of inadequate acute treatment) or a process of exacerbations and remissions (Figure 66.2). Systemic signs may be diminished; local signs of infection, including constant bone pain and swelling, tenderness, and warmth at the infection site, are more common. Over time, granulation tissue turns to scar tissue. This avascular scar tissue provides an ideal site for continued microorganism growth and is impenetrable by antibiotics. Long-term and rare complications of osteomyelitis include septicemia, septic arthritis, pathological fractures, and amyloidosis (a condition in which abnormal protein called *amyloid* builds up in tissues and organs and can cause organ failure).

TABLE 66.1	ORGANISMS CAUSING OSTEOMYELITIS
Organism	**Predisposing Condition**
Staphylococcus aureus	Pressure injury, penetrating wound, open fracture, orthopedic surgery, vascular insufficiency disorders (e.g., atherosclerosis; diabetes)
Staphylococcus epidermidis	In-dwelling prosthetic devices (e.g., joint replacements, fracture fixation devices)
Streptococcus viridans	Abscessed tooth, gingival disease
Escherichia coli	Urinary tract infection
Mycobacterium tuberculosis	Tuberculosis
Neisseria gonorrhoeae	Gonorrhea
Pseudomonas species	Puncture wounds, intravenous drug use
Salmonella species	Sickle cell disease
Fungi, *Mycobacteria* species	Immunocompromised host

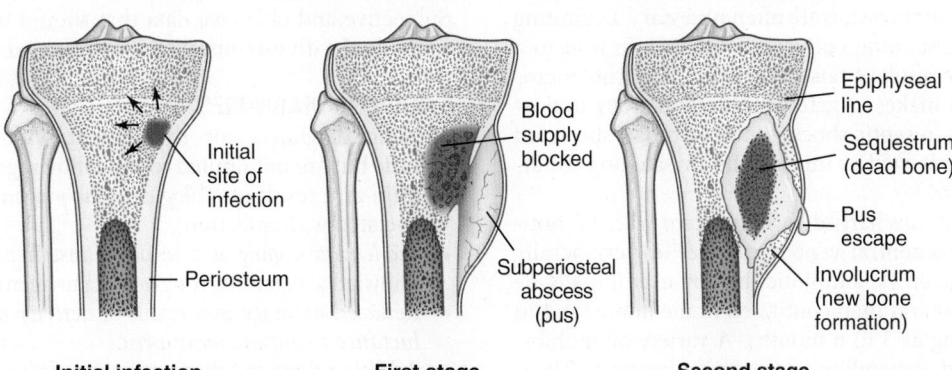

FIG. 66.1 Development of osteomyelitis infection with involucrum and sequestrum. Source: McCance, K. L., Huether, S. E., Brashers, V. L., et al. (2014). *Pathophysiology: The biologic basis for disease in adults and children* (7th ed., p. 1559, Figure 44-15). Mosby.

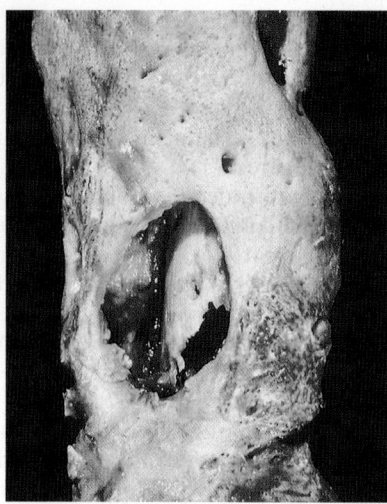

FIG. 66.2 Resection of femur due to osteomyelitis. Source: Patton, K. T., & Thibodeau, G. A. (2014). *The human body in health and disease.* (6th ed., p. 199, Figure 8-34). Mosby.

Diagnostic Studies

A bone or soft tissue biopsy is the definitive way to determine the causative microorganism. Once the causative organism is identified, antibiotic treatment can be adjusted. The patient's blood, wound cultures, or both are frequently positive for the presence of microorganisms. Elevation in the white blood cell count, erythrocyte sedimentation rate, and C-reactive protein may be found. Radiological signs suggestive of osteomyelitis usually do not appear until 10 days to weeks after the appearance of clinical symptoms, by which time the disease will have progressed. Radionuclide bone scans (gallium and indium) are helpful in diagnosis and are usually positive in the area of infection. Magnetic resonance imaging (MRI) (preferred) and computed tomographic (CT) scans may be used to help identify the extent of the infection, including soft tissue involvement (Simpfendorfer, 2017).

Interprofessional Care

Vigorous and prolonged intravenous (IV) antibiotic therapy is the treatment of choice for acute osteomyelitis, provided bone ischemia has not yet occurred. The health care provider and pharmacist will collaborate on selection, dosage, and monitoring of antibiotic effectiveness based on the cultures. Cultures or a bone biopsy should be done, if possible, before medication therapy is initiated. If antibiotic therapy is delayed, surgical debridement and decompression are often necessary. Beginning antibiotics prior to obtaining cultures or biopsy can lead to a false-negative culture result. A false-negative culture (no microorganism identified) makes targeted antibiotic therapy impossible. If the patient is in septic shock, however, broad-spectrum antibiotics should be started as this is a life-threatening condition (see Chapter 69).

Often, patients are discharged to home care with IV antibiotics delivered via a central venous catheter or peripherally inserted central catheter. IV antibiotic therapy may initially be started in the hospital and then continued in the home for 4 to 6 weeks or for as long as 3 to 6 months. A variety of antibiotics may be prescribed, depending on the microorganism. These medications include penicillin, cefazolin, gentamicin (Garamycin), and vancomycin (Vancocin).

MEDICATION ALERT—Gentamicin
- Patients should be assessed for dehydration before starting therapy.
- Renal function testing must be done before starting therapy, especially in older patients.
- Peak and trough levels must be monitored for therapeutic effect and to minimize renal and inner ear toxicity (Burchum & Rosenthal, 2019).
- Patients should be instructed to notify the health care provider if any visual, hearing, or urinary disorders develop.

In adults with chronic osteomyelitis, the choice between a curative, palliative, and alternative approach should be considered (Marais et al., 2016).

A *curative* approach involves surgical debridement (removal of the poorly vascularized tissue and dead bone or infected prosthetic device) with or without reconstructive procedures and extended use of antibiotics. Antibiotic-impregnated spacers, cement, or acrylic bead chains may be implanted at this time to aid in combating the infection (Klinder et al., 2019; Mifsud & McNally, 2019). After debridement of the devitalized and infected tissue, the wound may be closed and a suction irrigation system inserted. Intermittent surgical irrigation and debridement of the affected bone may continue. Negative pressure over the site of the infection may be used (vacuum-assisted closure). (Negative-pressure wound therapy is presented in Chapter 14.) Orthopedic prosthetic devices, if a source of chronic infection, must be removed. Muscle flaps or skin grafting provide wound coverage over the dead space (cavity) in the bone. Bone grafts may help to restore blood flow. The limb or surgical site may be protected with a cast or brace during this time, which may be fitted by an occupational therapist.

A *palliative* approach involves long-term antibiotic therapy with minimal surgical intervention. In adults, oral antibiotic therapy for 4 to 6 weeks may also be given after acute IV therapy is complete to ensure resolution of the infection (Schmitt, 2017). The patient's response to medication therapy is monitored through various imaging methods (bone scan, CT, MRI) and by monitoring erythrocyte sedimentation rate and C-reactive protein. Hyperbaric oxygen therapy with 100% oxygen may be administered as adjunct therapy in refractory cases of chronic osteomyelitis. This therapy is thought to stimulate circulation and healing in the infected tissue (see Chapter 14).

Alternatively, amputation of the affected limb may be indicated to preserve an individual's life or improve quality of life when there is extensive bone destruction due to chronic osteomyelitis (Marais et al., 2016).

NURSING MANAGEMENT OSTEOMYELITIS

NURSING ASSESSMENT

Subjective and objective data that should be obtained from an individual with osteomyelitis are presented in Table 66.2.

NURSING DIAGNOSES

Nursing diagnoses for the patient with osteomyelitis may include but are not limited to the following:

- *Pain* as a result of *biological injury agent* (inflammation associated with infection)
- *Inadequate coping* as a result of *insufficient resources* (lack of knowledge regarding long-term management of osteomyelitis)
- *Reduced mobility* as a result of *activity intolerance, pain, reluctance to initiate movement*

Additional information on nursing diagnoses for the patient with osteomyelitis is presented in Nursing Care Plan (NCP) 66.2 on the Evolve website.

TABLE 66.2 NURSING ASSESSMENT
Osteomyelitis

Subjective Data
Important Health Information
Past health history: Bone trauma, open fracture, open or puncture wounds, other infections (e.g., genitourinary and respiratory infections); vascular insufficiency disorders (e.g., arising from diabetes mellitus); adults who are immunocompromised
Medications: Analgesics or antibiotics
Surgery or other treatments: Bone surgery, especially implantation of an orthopedic prosthetic device (e.g., plate, total joint prosthesis)

Symptoms
Constant bone pain that is unrelieved by rest and worsens with activity; restricted movement of the affected part; malaise

Objective Data
General
Restlessness; fever, chills, night sweats

Integumentary
Diaphoresis; erythema, warmth, edema at infected bone
Later signs include drainage from sinus tracts to the skin or the fracture site

Musculoskeletal
Restricted movement; wound drainage; spontaneous fractures

Possible Findings
Leukocytosis, positive blood or wound cultures, ↑ erythrocyte sedimentation rate; presence of sequestrum and involucrum on radiographs, radionuclide bone scans, CT, and MRI

CT, computed tomography; *MRI,* magnetic resonance imaging.

PLANNING

The overall goals are that the patient with osteomyelitis will (a) have satisfactory pain and fever control, (b) not experience any complications associated with osteomyelitis, (c) cooperate with the treatment plan, and (d) maintain a positive outlook on the outcome of the disease.

NURSING IMPLEMENTATION

HEALTH PROMOTION. The control of infections already in the body (e.g., urinary, respiratory tract) is important in preventing osteomyelitis. Individuals susceptible to osteomyelitis are those who (alone or in combination) are immunocompromised, have orthopedic prosthetic devices, or have vascular insufficiencies. These patients should be instructed in the local and systemic manifestations of osteomyelitis. Families should also be aware of their role in monitoring the patient's health. Symptoms of bone pain, fever, swelling, and restricted limb movement should be reported immediately to the health care provider.

ACUTE INTERVENTION. Some immobilization of the affected limb (e.g., splint) is usually indicated to decrease pain. The involved limb should be handled carefully and excessive manipulation avoided as it increases pain and may cause pathological fracture. An important nursing responsibility is to assess the patient's pain. Nonsteroidal anti-inflammatory drugs (NSAIDs), opioid analgesics, and muscle relaxants may be prescribed to provide patient comfort. Nonpharmacological approaches to pain management (e.g., guided imagery, relaxation breathing) should be encouraged (Chapters 10 and 12).

Dressings are used to absorb the exudate from draining wounds and debride dead tissue from the wound bed. Sterile technique is essential when changing the dressing. Soiled dressings should be handled carefully to prevent cross-contamination of the wound or spread of the infection to other patients.

If the patient is on bed rest, proper body alignment and frequent position changes prevent complications associated with immobility and promote comfort. Flexion contracture, especially of the hip or knee, is a common sequela of osteomyelitis of the lower extremity because the patient frequently positions the affected extremity in a flexed position to promote comfort. Footdrop can develop quickly if the foot is not correctly supported in the neutral position by a splint or if there is excessive pressure on the peroneal nerve, which can occur with an improperly fitted splint. The nurse needs to collaborate with the health care provider about moving the affected limb to prevent footdrop and with the physiotherapist to select active or passive ROM or strengthening exercises.

The nurse must teach the patient about potential adverse and toxic reactions associated with prolonged and high-dose antibiotic therapy. These reactions include hearing impairment, fluid retention, and neurotoxicity—which can occur with the aminoglycosides (e.g., tobramycin [Nebcin])—and jaundice, colitis, and photosensitivity from the extended use of the cephalosporins (e.g., cefazolin). Tendon rupture (especially the Achilles tendon) can occur with use of the fluoroquinolones (e.g., ciprofloxacin [Cipro]). Peak and trough blood levels of most antibiotics must be carefully monitored throughout the course of therapy by the pharmacist to prevent these adverse effects. Lengthy antibiotic therapy can also result in an imbalance of normal flora and create an environment for overgrowth of opportunistic pathogens (e.g., *Candida albicans* and *Clostridium difficile*) in the genitourinary tract and oral cavities, especially in patients who are immunosuppressed and in older patients. The patient needs to be instructed to report any whitish, yellowish, curdlike lesions or frequent, watery diarrhea to the health care provider. The patient and family are often frightened and discouraged because of the serious nature of the disease, the uncertainty of the outcome, and the lengthy course of treatment. Thus continued psychological and emotional support is an integral part of nursing management for patients with osteomyelitis.

AMBULATORY AND HOME CARE. With the introduction of various intermittent venous access devices, IV antibiotics can be administered to the patient in the home setting via home nursing agencies. The nurse must instruct the patient and family on the proper care and management of the venous access device, the antibiotic schedule, antibiotic administration, and the need for follow-up laboratory testing. The importance of taking antibiotics even after the symptoms have subsided should be stressed.

If there is an open wound, dressing changes are often necessary. The patient and family may require supplies and instruction in the technique. If the osteomyelitis becomes chronic, patients need physical and psychological support for a prolonged period. Periodic home nursing visits for IV medication administration or dressing changes provide the family with support, which can help reduce anxiety.

EVALUATION

The expected outcomes are that the patient with osteomyelitis will:
- Have satisfactory pain relief
- Follow the recommended treatment regimen
- Verbalize confidence in the ability to implement the treatment regimen at home
- Demonstrate a consistent increase in mobility and range of motion

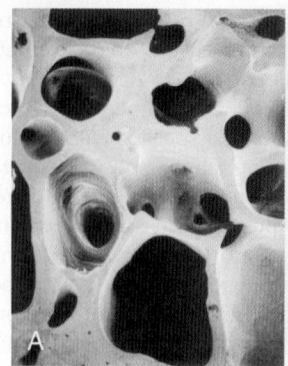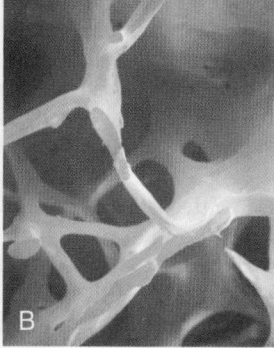

FIG. 66.3 A, Healthy bone. **B,** Osteoporotic bone. Source: Patton, K. T., & Thibodeau, G. A. (2016). *Anatomy and physiology* (7th ed., p. 277, Figure 11-25, B and C). Mosby.

METABOLIC BONE DISEASES

Normal bone metabolism is affected by hormones, nutrition, and hereditary factors. When there is dysfunction in any of these factors, a generalized reduction in bone mass and strength may result. Examples of metabolic bone diseases include osteoporosis and Paget's disease.

OSTEOPOROSIS

Osteoporosis, or porous bone (Figure 66.3), is a chronic, progressive metabolic bone disease. It is characterized by low bone mass and structural deterioration of bone tissue, leading to increased bone fragility, which predisposes the individual to bone fractures at the hip, wrist, and spine. Osteoporosis is known as the "silent thief" because it slowly and insidiously, over many years, robs the skeleton of its banked resources.

According to Statistics Canada (2021) Health Survey on Seniors, 13.8% of persons 65 years or older have a diagnosis of osteoporosis. Osteoporotic fractures result in significant morbidity and mortality. It is estimated that 28% of women and 37% of men will suffer a hip fracture due to osteoporosis and die within the following year (Osteoporosis Canada, n.d.). The estimated burden of illness from osteoporosis and subsequent fractures to Canadian society is estimated to be $4.3 billion (Hopkins et al., 2016). Many provincial, national, and international organizations are focused on initiatives to prevent fractures and develop models of post-fracture care associated with osteoporosis in efforts to minimize the economic burden of the illness. Resources are listed at the end of the chapter.

Residents of long-term care facilities need special consideration as many are frail, suffer from dementia, and are at high risk for delirium. They have a fracture rate two to four times greater than that of similar-aged adults living in the community; one third of patients with hip fractures are long-term care residents (Papaioannou et al., 2015). They also have a 30% rate of moderate to severe vertebral fractures. Papaioannou and colleagues (2015) developed Fracture Prevention for Long-Term Care Residents, which includes osteoporosis prevention, assessment, and nutritional and medication therapy recommendations.

Osteoporosis is more common in women than in men for several reasons: (1) women tend to have lower calcium intake than men (men between 15 and 50 years of age consume twice as much calcium as women); (2) women have less bone mass because of their generally smaller frame; (3) bone resorption

begins at an earlier age in women and is accelerated at menopause; (4) pregnancy and breastfeeding deplete a woman's skeletal reserve unless calcium intake is adequate; and (5) longevity increases the likelihood of osteoporosis—women live longer than men. The Determinants of Health box lists other factors that contribute to risk for osteoporosis.

Etiology and Pathophysiology

Evaluation of osteoporosis has shifted from simply treating low bone mineral density (BMD) to that of an integrated approach for patients with certain clinical factors that place them at increased risk for a fragility fracture. As such, indications for measuring BMD have shifted slightly, as shown in Table 66.3. Decreased risk is associated with regular weight-bearing exercise and calcium and vitamin D ingestion. Low testosterone levels are a risk factor in men.

Peak bone mass (maximum bone tissue) is mainly achieved before age 20 and is determined by a combination of four major factors: heredity, nutrition, exercise, and hormone function. Heredity may be responsible for up to 70% of a person's peak bone mass. Bone loss from midlife (age 35–40 years) onward is inevitable, but the rate of loss varies. At menopause, women experience rapid bone loss when the decline in estrogen production is sharpest. This rate of loss then slows and eventually matches the rate of bone lost by men at 65 to 70 years old.

Bone is continually being deposited by osteoblasts and resorbed by osteoclasts, a process called *remodelling.* Normally, the rates of bone deposition and resorption are equal to each other so that the total bone mass remains constant (Hardy & Feehan, 2020). In osteoporosis, bone resorption exceeds bone deposition. Although resorption affects the entire skeletal system, osteoporosis occurs most commonly in the bones of the spine, hips, and wrists. Over time, wedging and fractures of the vertebrae produce gradual loss of height and a humped back, known as *dowager's hump*, or *kyphosis* (Figure 66.4). The usual first signs of osteoporosis are back pain or spontaneous fractures. The loss of bone substance causes the bone to become mechanically weakened and prone to either spontaneous fractures or fractures from minimal trauma. Specific diseases and conditions associated with absorption of calcium or disturbing the remodelling process include inflammatory bowel disease, intestinal malabsorption, kidney disease, rheumatoid arthritis, hyperthyroidism, chronic alcoholism, cirrhosis of the liver, hypogonadism, and diabetes mellitus.

TABLE 66.3	INDICATIONS FOR MEASURING BONE MINERAL DENSITY
Older Persons (Age ≥50 yr)	**Younger Adults (Age <50 yr)**
• Age ≥65 yr (both women and men) • Clinical risk factors for fracture (menopausal women, men age 50–64 yr) • Fragility fracture after age 40 yr • Prolonged use of glucocorticoids* • Use of other high-risk medications† • Parental hip fracture • Vertebral fracture or osteopenia identified on radiography • Current smoking • High alcohol intake • Low body weight (<60 kg) or major weight loss (>10% of body weight at age 25 yr) • Rheumatoid arthritis • Other disorders strongly associated with osteoporosis	• Fragility fracture • Prolonged use of glucocorticoids* • Use of other high-risk medications† • Hypogonadism or premature menopause (age <45 yr) • Malabsorption syndrome • Primary hyperparathyroidism • Other disorders strongly associated with rapid bone loss, fracture, or both

*At least 3 months cumulative therapy in the previous year at a prednisone-equivalent dose ≥7.5 mg daily.
†Osteoporosis Canada. (2017). *Fast facts.* https://osteoporosis.ca/about-the-disease/fast-facts/
Source: Papaioannou, A., Morin, S., Cheung, A. M., et al. (2010). 2010 clinical practice guidelines for the diagnosis and management of osteoporosis in Canada: Summary. *Canadian Medical Association Journal 182*(17), 1864–1873, Table 1, p. 1865. https://doi.org/10.1503/cmaj.100771. Copied under licence from Access Copyright. Further reproduction, distribution or transmission is prohibited except as otherwise permitted by law.

Many medications can interfere with bone metabolism, including corticosteroids, anticonvulsant medications (e.g., phenytoin [Dilantin]), aluminum-containing antacids, heparin, certain cancer treatments, and excessive thyroid hormones. At the time a medication is prescribed, the patient should be informed of this possible adverse effect. Long-term corticosteroid use is a major contributor to osteoporosis. When a corticosteroid is taken, there is a disproportionate loss of bone, resulting from the inhibition of new bone formation.

Clinical Manifestations

Osteoporosis is often called the "silent disease" because bone loss occurs slowly, without symptoms. People may not know they have osteoporosis until their bones become so weak that a sudden strain, bump, or fall causes a hip, vertebra, or wrist fracture. Collapsed vertebrae may initially manifest as back pain, loss of height, or spinal deformities such as kyphosis or severely stooped posture.

Diagnostic Studies

Osteoporosis often goes unnoticed because it cannot be detected by conventional radiography until more than 25 to 40% of calcium in the bone is lost. Serum calcium, phosphorus, and alkaline phosphatase levels usually are normal, although alkaline phosphatase may be elevated after a fracture.

BMD measurements (e.g., dual-energy X-ray absorptiometry [DEXA] and quantitative ultrasonography [QUS]) are typically used to measure bone density, which in turn is used to assess the mass of bone per unit volume, or how tightly the bone is packed (see Chapter 64, Table 64.7). DEXA studies are also useful to evaluate changes in bone density over time and to assess the effectiveness of treatment.

DEXA results are frequently reported as T-scores. A T-score of −1 or higher indicates normal bone density. Osteoporosis is quantitatively defined as a BMD T-score at least 2.5 or more below the mean BMD of young adults. *Osteopenia* is defined as bone loss that is greater than normal (a T-score greater than a range of −1 to −2.5 standard deviations [SDs] below the mean) but not yet at the level for a diagnosis of osteoporosis. In addition to the BMD T-score, the patient's risk factors are included in determining a 10-year absolute fracture risk. This risk changes with advancing age and the development of new risk factors. Those patients with low risk are assessed in 5 to 10

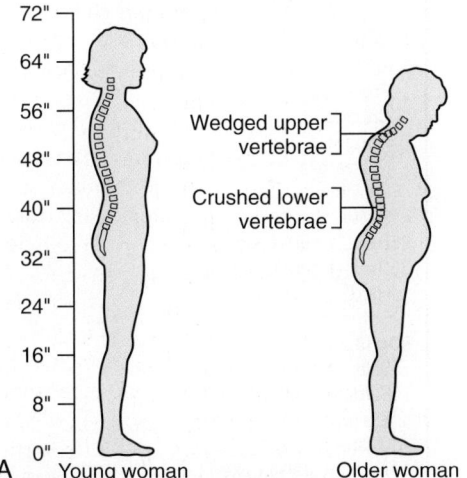
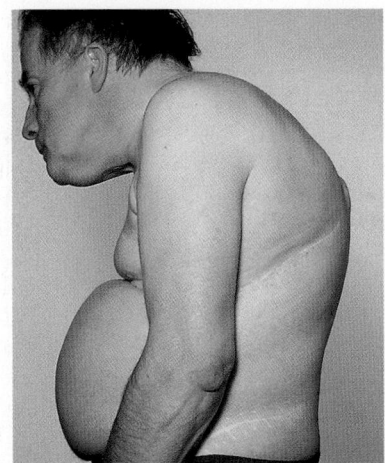

FIG. 66.4 The effects of osteoporosis. **A,** Comparison of a young woman with an older woman. **B,** Severe fixed kyphosis, producing a question-mark appearance. Source: A, Phillips, N. (2013). *Berry & Kohn's operating room technique.* (12th ed.). Mosby. B, Courtesy of Mir, M. A. In J. J. Kanski. (2006). *Clinical diagnosis in ophthalmology* (8th ed., p. 405, Figure 11.10). Mosby.

years, whereas those with moderate risk are assessed in 1 to 5 years. QUS may be considered for assessment of fracture risk when DEXA is not available, but it is not precise enough to be used for follow-up BMD testing.

There are many fracture risk prediction tools. The FRAX tool is well calibrated to predict the level of risk for major fractures (Kanis et al., 2017). FRAX tools have been individualized by each country as fracture rates are different. FRAX is used to calculate the 10-year risk for hip fracture and the 10-year risk for a major osteoporotic fracture (spine, forearm, hip, or shoulder). Osteoporosis Canada Best Practice Guidelines (Papaioannou et al., 2010) include the FRAX as a tool to assess for osteoporosis. The tool can be completed by the health care provider or the individual as it includes personal risk factors (e.g., smoking, fracture history) as well as BMD at the hip.

NURSING AND INTERPROFESSIONAL MANAGEMENT OSTEOPOROSIS

The reduced quality of life for persons with osteoporosis can be enormous. Osteoporosis can result in disfigurement, lowered self-esteem, reduction in or loss of mobility, and decreased independence. Interprofessional care of osteoporosis focuses on proper nutrition, calcium supplementation, exercise, prevention of fractures, and medication (Table 66.4). Osteoporosis Canada's *Clinical Practice Guideline for Diagnosis and Management of Osteoporosis* recommends that women who are postmenopausal and men age 50 or older be considered for treatment of osteoporosis if presenting with any of the following: (1) a hip or vertebral fracture, (2) a DEXA hip (femoral neck) or spine T-score of 1.0 to –2.5, or (3) a FRAX score of 3% or higher at the hip or 20% or higher at other sites (Papaioannou et al., 2010); Gates and colleagues (2019) suggest the need to update the 2010 guidelines to include a recommendation for screening in primary care settings adults older than 40 years of age for fragility fractures.

Prevention and treatment of osteoporosis focus on adequate calcium intake (1 000 mg/day in women between the ages 19

and 50 and men between the ages 19 and 70; and 1 200 mg in women >50 years of age and men >70 years of age). If dietary intake of calcium is inadequate, supplemental calcium should be taken (Health Canada, 2020). Foods high in calcium content include whole and skim milk, yogourt, cottage cheese, ice cream, spinach, almonds, and sardines (Table 66.5). The amount of elemental calcium varies in different calcium preparations (Table 66.6). Calcium supplementation inhibits age-related bone loss; however, it does not stimulate the formation of new bone.

Vitamin D is important in calcium absorption and function and may have a role in bone formation. Reasonable sun exposure of extremities, abdomen, and back lasting 5 to 15 minutes two to three times per week causing mild pinkish skin for fair-skinned people or 25-minute exposure for brown-skinned people equates to taking 7 000 to 10 000 IU vitamin D (Sakamoto, 2019). Most Canadians do not get enough vitamin D from their diet or naturally through synthesis in the skin from exposure to sunlight. Supplemental vitamin D for all adults year round is recommended by Osteoporosis Canada (Vatanparast, 2019). For adults who are healthy and between 19 and 50 years of age, 400–1 000 IU of vitamin D daily is required. For adults over 50 years of age and for younger adults at high risk (e.g., with osteoporosis, multiple fractures, or conditions affecting vitamin D absorption), 800–2 000 IU daily is recommended (Papaioannou et al., 2010).

Regular physical activity is important for building up and maintaining bone mass. Exercise also increases muscle strength, coordination, and balance. The best exercises are weight-bearing exercises that force an individual to work against gravity. These include walking, hiking, weight training, stair climbing, tennis, and dancing. Walking is preferred to high-impact aerobics or running, both of which may put too much stress on the bones, resulting in stress fractures. Walking for 30 minutes, three times a week, is recommended.

TABLE 66.4 INTERPROFESSIONAL CARE

Osteoporosis

Diagnostic
- History and physical examination
- Serum calcium, phosphorus, and alkaline phosphatase levels
- Bone mineral densitometry
- Dual-energy X-ray absorptiometry (DEXA)
- Quantitative ultrasonography (QUS)

Interprofessional Therapy
- Diet high in calcium (see Table 66.5)
- Calcium supplements (see Table 66.6)
- Vitamin D supplements
- Exercise program
- Estrogen replacement therapy
- Bisphosphonates
- Alendronate (Fosamax)
- Etidronate
- Risedronate (Actonel)
- Zoledronic acid (Aclasta)
- Selective estrogen receptor modulator (SERM)
- Raloxifene (Evista)
- Teriparatide (Forteo)
- Salmon calcitonin (Calcimar)

TABLE 66.5 NUTRITIONAL THERAPY

Sources of Calcium

Food	Calcium (mg)
250 mL (1 cup) milk	
Whole	291
Low-fat	300
Skim	302
30 g (1 oz) cheese	
Processed	174
Cheddar	130
Cottage	130
Mozzarella	207
Parmesan	390
Swiss	272
250 mL (1 cup) yogourt	415
250 mL (1 cup) ice cream	
Hard	176
Soft-serve	272
90 g (3 oz) seafood	
Salmon	167
Sardines with bones	372
Shrimp	98
Oysters	113
1 medium stalk cooked broccoli	158
250 g (1 cup) cooked spinach	200
250 g (1 cup) almonds	304

TABLE 66.6	ELEMENTAL CALCIUM CONTENT OF VARIOUS ORAL CALCIUM PREPARATIONS	
Calcium Preparation	**Elemental Calcium Content**
Calcium carbonate (Tums 500)	500 mg/tablet
Calcium carbonate + 5 mcg vitamin D2 (Os-Cal 250)	250 mg/tablet
Calcium gluconate	40 mg/500 mg
Calcium carbonate	400 mg/g
Calcium lactate	80 mg/600 mg
Calcium citrate	40 mg/300 mg

Cigarette smoking and excess alcohol intake are risk factors for osteoporosis. Regular consumption of 60 to 90 mL of alcohol a day may increase the degree of osteoporosis, even in young men and women. Patients should be instructed to quit smoking and cut down on alcohol intake to decrease the likelihood of losing bone mass (Papaioannou et al., 2010).

Although loss of bone cannot be significantly reversed, further loss can be prevented if the patient follows a regimen of calcium and vitamin D supplementation, exercise, estrogen replacement, and alendronate (Fosamax) or raloxifene (Evista), if indicated. Efforts should be made to keep patients with osteoporosis ambulatory to prevent further loss of bone substance as a result of immobility.

MEDICATION THERAPY

Hormone therapy should be considered as first-line treatment for preventing bone loss and fractures in early menopausal women who are symptomatic (e.g., vasomotor, urogenital, and psychological symptoms). It is believed that estrogen inhibits osteoclast activity, leading to decreased bone resorption and preventing both cortical and trabecular bone loss. Estrogen therapy (for women who have had a hysterectomy) and estrogen–progesterone therapy (for women who have not had a hysterectomy) provide significant protection against osteoporotic fractures. Despite earlier concerns raised by a number of studies, it now appears that women who are younger and recently postmenopausal do not have an increased cardiovascular risk with estrogen or estrogen–progesterone therapy. Considering the risk–benefit profile of hormone therapy, the North American Menopause Society states that the extended use of hormone therapy is suitable for women at risk for osteoporotic fractures who also have moderate to severe menopausal symptoms. As with any medication therapy, doses and regimens must be individualized according to the patient's needs. (See Chapter 56 for further discussion of hormone therapy.)

Calcitonin is secreted by the thyroid gland and inhibits osteoclastic bone resorption by directly interacting with active osteoclasts. Salmon calcitonin (Calcimar) is available in intramuscular, subcutaneous, and intranasal forms. The nasal form is easy to administer, and patients should be taught to alternate nostrils daily. Nasal dryness and irritation are the most frequent adverse effects. Administration of the intramuscular or subcutaneous form of the medication at night has been shown to decrease the adverse effects of nausea and facial flushing. Nausea does not occur with the nasal spray. When calcitonin is used, calcium supplementation is necessary to prevent secondary hyperparathyroidism.

Bisphosphonates inhibit osteoclast-mediated bone resorption, thereby increasing BMD and total bone mass. This group of medications has been shown to increase BMD by 5%. Common adverse effects are anorexia, weight loss, and gastritis. Effective osteoporosis treatment has been shown to reduce mortality in older persons and in individuals who are frail and at high risk for a fracture. The most commonly used bisphosphonate medication in treating osteoporosis is alendronate (Fosamax). Patients should be instructed in the proper administration of alendronate to aid in its absorption. It should be taken with a full glass of water after rising in the morning. The patient should not eat or drink anything for 30 minutes after taking it. The patient should also be instructed not to lie down after taking the medication. These precautions have been shown to decrease gastrointestinal adverse effects (especially esophageal irritation) and increase absorption. Alendronate is also available as a once-per-week oral tablet. Zoledronic acid (Aclasta) is approved for a once-yearly IV infusion and can prevent osteoporosis for 2 years after a single infusion. One potential adverse effect of bisphosphonates is atypical femur fractures and osteonecrosis of the jaw (Goode et al., 2020).

MEDICATION ALERT—Bisphosphonates
Patients should be instructed to do the following:
- Take with full glass of water
- Take 30 min before food or other medications
- Remain upright for at least 30 min after taking

Another type of medication used in treating osteoporosis is raloxifene (Evista), a selective estrogen receptor modulator. This medication mimics the effect of estrogen on bone by reducing bone resorption without stimulating the tissues of the breast or uterus. Raloxifene in women who are postmenopausal significantly increases BMD. The most commonly reported adverse effects are leg cramps, hot flashes, and blood clots. Raloxifine may decrease breast cancer risk. Similar to tamoxifen, it blocks the estrogen receptor sites of cancer sites.

Teriparatide (Forteo) is used for the treatment of osteoporosis in men and in women who are postmenopausal and at high risk for fractures. Teriparatide is a recombinant form of human parathyroid hormone and works by increasing the action of osteoblasts. It is the first medication approved for the treatment of osteoporosis that stimulates new bone formation. Most medications used to treat osteoporosis prevent further bone loss. Teriparatide is administered by subcutaneous injection, once a day. Adverse effects include leg cramps and dizziness. Denosumab (Prolia) may be used for women with osteoporosis who are postmenopausal and at high risk for fractures. It is a monoclonal antibody that binds to a protein (RANKL) involved in the formation and function of osteoclasts. Denosumab is given as a subcutaneous injection every 6 months.

Current guidelines clearly advocate for pharmacological treatment in patients who are at high risk for fractures and are diagnosed with osteoporosis. However, there is no clear guidance about when treatment should be stopped (Goode et al., 2020).

Medical management of patients receiving corticosteroids includes prescribing the lowest possible dose of the medication as well as calcium and vitamin D supplementation. If osteopenia is evident on bone densitometry, treatment with bisphosphonate agents, such as alendronate (Fosamax), should be considered.

EVIDENCE-INFORMED PRACTICE

Translating Research Into Practice

R. F. (pronouns she/her), 76 years old, fell in her home and sustained a hip fracture. Recent laboratory work shows a vitamin D deficiency. The nurse discusses options for improving this deficiency, including special considerations for the patient's current vegetarian diet. R. F. tells the nurse, "I'm moving to Arizona to be with family and I plan to spend many hours in the sun every day."

Best Available Evidence	Clinician Expertise	Patient Preferences and Values
Women who are post-menopausal should receive 1 200 mg of calcium and 800 IU of vitamin D daily. Dietary sources and supplements should be used to meet these requirements.	The nurse has worked with many patients recovering from fractures related to osteoporosis. The nurse reviews R. F.'s usual diet and determines that it is deficient in calcium and vitamin D.	The patient prefers sun exposure over changing her vegetarian diet or taking supplements.

Action and Decision

The nurse discusses the risks associated with daily sun exposure and points out that sun exposure will not correct a calcium deficiency. The patient tells the nurse she understands but wants to try before taking "any more pills." The nurse explains the importance of adding foods high in calcium to her diet. The nurse provides a list of some choices that meet R. F.'s vegetarian diet restrictions.

Reference for Evidence

Mangels, R. (2018). *Calcium in the vegan diet.* http://www.vrg.org/nutrition/calcium.php

Sakamoto, R. R. (2019). Sunlight in vitamin D deficiency: Clinical implications. *The Journal for Nurse Practitioners, 15*(4), 282–285. https://doi.org/10.1016/j.nurpra.2019.01.014

Statistics Canada. (2015). *Health at a glance—Vitamin D blood levels of Canadians.* http://www.statcan.gc.ca/pub/82-624-x/2013001/article/11727-eng.htm

PAGET'S DISEASE

Paget's disease of the bone (*osteitis deformans*) is a chronic skeletal bone disorder in which there is excessive bone resorption followed by replacement of normal marrow by vascular, fibrous connective tissue. The new bone is larger, disorganized, and structurally weaker. The regions of the skeleton commonly affected are the pelvis, long bones, spine, ribs, sternum, and cranium. The etiology of Paget's disease is unknown, although there is evidence that the rate of Paget's disease is influenced by genetic and environmental factors (Singer, 2015). Up to 40% of all patients with Paget's disease have at least one relative with the disorder. Men are affected at a rate of two to one compared to women, and Paget's disease is rarely seen in people younger than 40 years. Viral etiology remains controversial, as no specific virus has been isolated thus far.

In milder forms of Paget's disease, patients may remain free of symptoms, and the disease may be discovered incidentally on radiography or serum chemistry. The initial clinical manifestations are usually insidious development of bone pain (which may progress to severe, intractable pain), fatigue, and progressive development of a waddling gait. Patients may report that they are becoming shorter or that their heads are becoming larger. Headaches, dementia, visual deficits, and

hearing impairment can result, with an enlarged, thickened skull. Increased bone volume in the spine can cause spinal cord or nerve root compression. Pathological fracture is the most common complication of Paget's disease and may be the first indication of the disease. Other complications include osteosarcoma, fibrosarcoma, and osteoclastoma (giant cell) tumours.

Serum alkaline phosphatase levels are markedly elevated (indicating high bone turnover) in advanced forms of the disease. Radiographs may demonstrate that the normal contour of the affected bone is curved and the bone cortex is thickened and irregular, especially the weight-bearing bones and cranium. Bone scans using a radiolabelled biphosphate demonstrate increased uptake in the skeletal areas affected.

Interprofessional care of Paget's disease is usually limited to symptomatic and supportive care and correction of secondary deformities by either surgical intervention or braces. Bisphosphonate medications are the preferred treatment in individuals at risk for pathological fracture(s) since bisphosphonates reduce bone turnover (Appleman-Dijkstra & Papapoulos, 2018). Often, calcium and vitamin D are given to decrease hypocalcemia, a common adverse effect with these medications. Medication effectiveness may be monitored by serum alkaline phosphatase levels.

Calcitonin therapy is recommended for patients who cannot tolerate bisphosphonate medications. Human calcitonin inhibits osteoclastic activity, prevents bone resorption, relieves acute symptoms, and lowers the serum alkaline phosphatase levels. This medication is available as a subcutaneous injection. Salmon calcitonin can also be used as a subcutaneous or intramuscular injection for treating Paget's disease. Salmon calcitonin has a longer half-life and greater milligram potency than human calcitonin. Response to calcitonin therapy is not permanent and often stops when therapy is discontinued. Pain from Paget's disease is usually managed by NSAIDs or acetaminophen. Orthopedic surgery for fractures, hip and knee replacements, and knee realignment may be necessary.

A firm mattress should be used to provide back support and to relieve pain. The patient may be required to wear a corset or light brace to relieve back pain and provide support when in the upright position. The patient should be proficient in the correct application of such devices and know how to regularly examine areas of the skin for friction damage. Activities such as lifting and twisting should be discouraged. Physiotherapy may increase muscle strength. Good body mechanics are essential. A properly balanced nutritional program is important in the management of metabolic disorders of bone, especially pertaining to vitamin D, calcium, and protein, which are necessary to ensure the availability of the components for bone formation. Prevention measures such as patient education, use of an assistive device, and environmental changes should be actively pursued to prevent falls and subsequent fractures.

SAFETY ALERT

The risk for patient harm resulting from falls can be reduced as follows:
- Patients should be evaluated for fall risk.
- High-risk factors should be identified, including medications that increase risk for falls.
- Action should be taken to address any identified risks.
- Patients at risk should be encouraged to attend a fall-prevention class.

AGE-RELATED CONSIDERATIONS

METABOLIC BONE DISEASES

Osteoporosis and Paget's disease are common in older persons. Patients should be instructed in proper nutritional management to prevent further bone loss such as that occurring from osteoporosis.

Since metabolic bone disorders increase the possibility of pathological fractures, extreme caution should be used when turning or moving patients with such disorders. Hip fractures in particular can adversely affect quality of life and may lead to admission to a long-term care facility. It is important to keep patients as active as possible to slow demineralization of bone resulting from disuse or extended immobilization. A supervised exercise program is an essential part of the treatment program. If the patient's condition permits, ambulation without causing fatigue must be encouraged.

Protection from falls is paramount for prevention of osteoporotic fracture among older persons. Osteoporosis-related fractures cause considerable morbidity and an enormous financial burden through the use of health services. In Canada, one in three older people will experience a fall each year, and half of these individuals will fall more than once. Falls are the leading cause of injury among older Canadians and the cause of 95% of all hip fractures; also, 85% of falls are the cause of injury-related hospitalizations (Public Health Agency of Canada [PHAC], 2016). The frequency of falls increases dramatically with age, with women being more likely to fall than men.

Medical conditions, medications, and environmental factors have been implicated as predisposing factors to injurious falls among older persons. Best Practice Guidelines (Registered Nurses' Association of Ontario [RNAO], 2017) should be implemented to prevent falls and fall injuries in older people, who may already have bone mass below the threshold for fracture. Fall prevention could have a significant impact on the incidence of fracture in this susceptible population.

LOW BACK PAIN

Etiology and Pathophysiology

Chronic back pain is a prevalent and costly public health issue. The incidence of back pain does not differ significantly across social or demographic groups. Back pain continues to be the leading overall cause of lost productivity in the workplace (Fatoye et al., 2019) with incidence of chronic low back pain ranging from 34 to 59% (Lacasse et al., 2017).

Low back pain (LBP) is a common condition because the lumbar region (1) bears most of the weight of the body, (2) is the most flexible region of the spinal column, (3) contains nerve roots that are vulnerable to injury or disease, and (4) has an inherently poor biomechanical structure. Several risk factors are associated with LBP, including lack of muscle tone and excess body weight, poor posture, cigarette smoking, and stress. Jobs that require repetitive heavy lifting, operation of vibrating machinery, or prolonged periods of sitting are also associated with LBP.

The causes of LBP of musculoskeletal origin include (a) acute lumbosacral strain, (b) instability of the lumbosacral bony mechanism, (c) osteoarthritis of the lumbosacral vertebrae, (d) degenerative disc disease (DDD), and (e) herniation of an intervertebral disc (Traeger et al., 2017).

The nursing profession has a higher prevalence of LBP than the general population. LBP among nurses is related to the nature of nursing activities (patient handling and body movements involving bending, lifting or twisting) and length of shift (Ibrahim et al., 2019).

ACUTE LOW BACK PAIN

Acute low back pain usually lasts 6 weeks or less. Most LBP is caused by trauma or some type of activity that causes undue stress (often hyperflexion) of the lower back. Often, symptoms of LBP do not appear at the time of injury but develop later because of a gradual increase in pressure on the nerve by an intervertebral disc. Symptoms may range from muscle ache to shooting or stabbing pain, limited flexibility or range of motion, or an inability to stand straight.

Few definitive diagnostic abnormalities are present with nerve irritation and muscle strain. Diagnostic imaging, including radiography, MRI, and CT scans, are generally not done unless there are red flags, such as focal neurological deficits, trauma, or systemic disease (e.g., cancer, spinal infection) (Institute of Health Economics, 2017).

Interprofessional Care

If the acute muscle spasms and accompanying pain are not severe and debilitating, the patient is treated with analgesics such as NSAIDs or muscle relaxants. Severe pain may require a short course of opioid analgesics. A brief period (1 to 2 days) of rest at home may be necessary for some people, but most do better with a continuation of their regular activities (Institute of Health Economics, 2017). Bed rest provides no benefit to patients who have acute LBP, with or without sciatica (see Evidence-Informed Practice box). The aim of motor control

EVIDENCE-INFORMED PRACTICE

Research Highlight

Should Patients With Acute Low Back Pain Do Motor Control Exercises?

Clinical Question
In patients with acute low back pain (LBP) (P), do motor control exercises (I) as compared to other forms of exercise or doing nothing (C) improve recovery (O)?

Best Available Evidence
Systematic review of randomized controlled trials (RCTs)

Critical Appraisal and Synthesis of Evidence
- 29 randomized trials (*n* = 2431); the impact of using motor control exercises as a treatment for lower back pain was compared to other forms of exercise or doing nothing.
- Acute LBP was defined as pain lasting <6 wk.
- People who used motor control exercises for 20 days to 12 weeks, 1–5 days per week, experienced improvements, especially in pain and disability.
- Targeting the strength and coordination of muscles that support the spine through motor control exercise provided an alternative treatment for LBP. It is unclear how motor control exercise compares with other forms of exercise long term.

Conclusions
- Motor control exercises are as effective as other types of exercise, so the choice of exercise should account for factors such as patient or therapist preferences, cost, and availability.
- There is no evidence that staying active is harmful.

Implications for Nursing Practice
- Patients with acute LBP should be encouraged to continue daily activities and use motor control exercises within their limitations of pain.
- Patients should be instructed on the potential harm of extended bed rest.
- Research on the effects of staying active for chronic LBP is needed.

Reference for Evidence
Saragiotto, B. T., Maher, C. G., Yamato, T. P., et al. (2016). Motor control exercise for chronic non-specific low back pain. *Cochrane Database of Systematic Reviews (1)*, CD012004. doi:10.1002/14651858.CD012004.
P, patient population of interest; *I,* intervention or area of interest; *C,* comparison of interest or comparison group; *O,* outcome(s) of interest (see Chapter 1).

exercise is to restore strength and control of the muscles that support the spinal column (Saragiotto et al., 2016). Evidence suggests that staying active rather than resting in bed results in sooner return to work, improved functional status, and less pain (Institute of Health Economics, 2017). Patients who are unable to return to normal activities may have short-term benefits from spinal manipulation, but this may be no more effective than usual care. Multidisciplinary rehabilitation programs in occupational settings may be an option for workers with sick leave of more than 4 to 8 weeks.

The patient should be taught about the cause of the pain and ways to prevent further episodes. Collaborating with physiotherapy for muscle stretching and strengthening exercises may be part of the management plan. Patients experiencing acute nonspecific LBP should avoid bed rest for prolonged periods and activities that aggravate the pain, including lifting, bending, twisting, and prolonged sitting. Most cases spontaneously improve within 2 to 6 weeks.

CHRONIC LOW BACK PAIN

Chronic low back pain is low back pain that lasts more than 3 months or is a repeated incapacitating episode. Causes include (a) degenerative conditions such as arthritis or disc disease; (b) osteoporosis or other metabolic bone diseases; (c) prior injury (scar tissue weakens the back); (d) chronic strain on the lower back muscles from obesity, pregnancy, or job-related stooping, bending, or other stressful postures; and (e) congenital abnormalities in the spine.

Spinal Stenosis

Spinal stenosis is a narrowing of the vertebral canal or nerve root canals caused by encroachment of bone on the space. The stenosis may be inherited or acquired through degenerative or traumatic changes to the spine. Common acquired causes include osteoarthritis, rheumatoid arthritis, spinal tumours, Paget's disease, and trauma. Inherited conditions that lead to spinal stenosis include congenital spinal stenosis and scoliosis.

Arthritic changes (bone spurs, calcification of spinal ligaments, degeneration of discs) narrow the space around the spinal canal and nerve roots, eventually leading to compression. Inflammation caused by the compression results in pain, weakness, and numbness.

The pain associated with lumbar spinal stenosis often starts in the low back and then radiates to the buttock and the leg. It worsens with walking and particularly when standing without walking. Numbness, tingling, weakness, and heaviness in the legs and buttocks may also be present. In most cases, the stenosis slowly progresses and does not cause paralysis.

NURSING AND INTERPROFESSIONAL MANAGEMENT CHRONIC LOW BACK PAIN

Chronic LBP is not a clinical entity but a symptom in patients with very different stages of impairment, disability, and chronicity. Treatment for chronic LBP is much the same as for acute LBP. Cold, damp weather tends to aggravate back pain, but this can be relieved with rest and local heat application. Complementary and alternative therapies such as biofeedback, acupuncture, and yoga may help reduce pain (Institute of Health Economics, 2017). Relief of pain and stiffness by the

use of mild analgesics, such as NSAIDs, is integral to the daily comfort of people with chronic LBP. Weight reduction, sufficient rest periods, local heat or cold application, and exercise and activity throughout the day help to keep the muscles and joints mobilized. Tricyclic antidepressants (e.g., amitriptyline [Elavil]) and selective serotonin reuptake inhibitors (e.g., sertraline [Zoloft]) have been shown to improve the chronic symptoms of LBP.

Surgical intervention may be indicated in patients with severe chronic LBP whose condition does not respond to conservative care or who have continued neurological deficits. (Surgery for low LBP is discussed under Nursing Management: Vertebral Disc Surgery.)

NURSING MANAGEMENT NONSPECIFIC LOW BACK PAIN

NURSING ASSESSMENT
Subjective and objective data that should be obtained from the patient with LBP are summarized in Table 66.7.

NURSING DIAGNOSES
Nursing diagnoses for the patient with LBP may include but are not limited to the following:

TABLE 66.7 **NURSING ASSESSMENT**
Low Back Pain
Subjective Data
Important Health Information
Past health history: Acute or chronic lumbosacral strain or trauma, osteoarthritis, degenerative disc disease, obesity; metabolic, circulatory, gynecological, or urological conditions
Occupation requiring heavy lifting, vibrations, or extended driving
Medications: Opioid and nonopioid analgesics; muscle relaxants; NSAIDs; corticosteroids; antidepressants; anticonvulsant medications; over-the-counter remedies, including herbal products and nutritional supplements
Surgery or other treatments: Previous back surgery, epidural corticosteroid injections
Symptoms
• Pain in back, buttocks, or leg, associated with walking, turning, straining, coughing, leg raising
• Numbness or tingling of legs, feet, toes; muscle spasms
• Activity intolerance
• Interrupted sleep
Objective Data
General
Guarded movement
Neurological
Depressed or absent Achilles tendon reflex or patellar tendon reflex; positive straight leg–raising test, positive crossover straight leg–raising test, positive Trendelenburg test
Musculoskeletal
Tense, tight paravertebral muscles on palpation, decreased range of motion of spine; poor posture
Possible Findings
Localization of site of lesion or disorder on myelogram, CT scan, or MRI; determination of nerve root impingement on electromyography

CT, computed tomography; *MRI,* magnetic resonance imaging; *NSAIDs,* nonsteroidal anti-inflammatory drugs.

- *Episodic pain* as a result of *physical injury agent* (mechanical disorders or nonmechanical diseases and ineffective comfort measures)
- *Reduced mobility* as a result of *pain, reluctance to initiate movement*
- *Persistent pain* as a result of *injury agent* (progressive degenerative changes of the muscles and skeletal structures of the back)
- *Inadequate coping* as a result of *insufficient sense of control* (persistent pain)
- *Inadequate health management* as a result of *insufficient knowledge of therapeutic regimen*

Additional information on nursing diagnoses for the patient with LBP is presented in NCP 66.1, available on the Evolve website.

PLANNING

The overall goals are that the patient with LBP will (a) have satisfactory pain relief, (b) avoid constipation secondary to medication and immobility, (c) learn back-sparing practices, and (d) return to the previous level of activity within prescribed restrictions.

NURSING IMPLEMENTATION

HEALTH PROMOTION. Patients should be advised to maintain appropriate body weight. Excess body weight places extra stress on the lower back and weakens the abdominal muscles that support the lower back. Flat shoes or shoes with low heels (<2.5 cm) and shock-absorbing shoe inserts are recommended for women.

The position assumed while sleeping is also important in preventing LBP. Sleeping in a prone position should be avoided because it produces excessive lumbar lordosis, placing excessive stress on the lower back. A firm mattress is recommended. The patient should sleep in either a supine or a side-lying position, with the knees and hips flexed to prevent unnecessary pressure on support muscles, ligamentous structures, and lumbosacral joints. Patients should be educated about the need to avoid or cease smoking. Nicotine has been shown to decrease circulation to the vertebral discs, and a causal relationship exists between smoking and some types of LBP (Micheletti et al., 2019).

ACUTE INTERVENTION. The primary nursing responsibilities in acute LBP are to assist the patient in maintaining activity limitations, promote comfort, and educate the patient about the health condition and appropriate exercises. Other nursing interventions are summarized in NCP 66.1 on the Evolve website. The use of analgesics, NSAIDs, muscle relaxants, antidepressants, anticonvulsant medications, and thermotherapy (ice and heat), while avoiding continued bed rest, is incorporated into the plan of care.

Muscle stretching and strengthening exercises may be part of the management plan. Exercises can help to strengthen the back as a preventive measure (Suh et al., 2019). Although the actual exercises are often taught by a physiotherapist, it is the nurse's responsibility to ensure that the patient understands the type and frequency of exercise prescribed, as well as the rationale for the program.

As a role model, the nurse should use proper body mechanics at all times. The nurse should assess the patient's use of body mechanics and offer advice when activities that could produce back strain are performed (Table 66.8).

TABLE 66.8   PATIENT & CAREGIVER TEACHING GUIDE

Low Back Conditions

The following instructions should be included when teaching the patient how to manage low back conditions.

Do
- Prevent lower back from straining forward by placing a foot on a step or stool during prolonged standing.
- Sleep in a side-lying position with knees and hips bent.
- Sleep on back with a lift under knees and legs or on back with 25-cm–high pillow under knees to flex hips and knees.
- Exercise 15 minutes in the morning and 15 minutes in the evening, regularly; begin exercises with a 2- or 3-minute warm-up period by moving arms and legs; alternate relaxing and tightening muscles; exercise slowly, with smooth movements, as directed by a physiotherapist.
- Carry light items close to your body.
- Maintain appropriate body weight.
- Use local heat and cold application.
- Use a lumbar roll or pillow for sitting.
- Use proper body mechanics to avoid low back strain (e.g., when lifting objects, bend at the knees, not at the waist; stand up slowly with the object close to your body).

Do Not
- Lean forward without bending knees.
- Lift anything above level of your elbows.
- Stand in one position for a prolonged time.
- Sleep on abdomen or on back or side with legs out straight.
- Exercise without consulting your health care provider if you are having severe pain.
- Exceed prescribed amount and type of exercises without consulting your health care provider.

AMBULATORY AND HOME CARE. The goal of management is to make an episode of acute LBP an isolated incident. If the lumbosacral mechanism is unstable, repeated episodes can be anticipated. The lumbosacral spine may be unable to meet the demands placed on it without strain because of factors such as obesity, poor posture, poor muscular support, advancing age, or local trauma. Intervention is aimed at strengthening the supporting muscles through exercise. A corset limits extremes of movement and may be useful in decreasing pain and the use of pain medication.

Persistent use of poor body mechanics may also result in repeated episodes of LBP. If the strain is work related, occupational counselling may be necessary. The frustration, pain, and disability imposed on the patient with LBP require emotional support from and understanding care by the nurse.

EVALUATION

The expected outcomes for the patient with LBP are presented in NCP 66.1 (available on the Evolve website.)

INTERVERTEBRAL DISC DISEASE

Etiology and Pathophysiology

An intervertebral disc is interposed between the vertebrae from the cervical axis to the sacrum. Structural degeneration of the lumbar disc is often caused by degenerative disc disease (DDD). This progressive degeneration is a normal process of aging and results in the intervertebral discs losing their elasticity, flexibility, and shock-absorbing capabilities. Thinning of the discs occurs as the nucleus pulposus (gelatinous centre of the disc) starts to dry out and shrink. These changes limit the ability of the discs to distribute pressure loads between the vertebrae. The once-normal central loading of the intervertebral discs then changes, and the load now is transferred to the annulus fibrosis (strong outside portion of the intervertebral disc), causing structural deterioration. The annulus is now torn or stretched, which allows the nucleus pulposus to herniate or bulge outward between the vertebrae. This phenomenon is called a herniated intervertebral disc (slipped disc) (Figure 66.5).

An acute herniated intervertebral disc (slipped disc) can be the result of natural degeneration with age or repeated stress and trauma to the spine. Herniation of the nuclear material from the intervertebral disc may compress or place tension on a cervical, lumbar, or sacral spinal nerve root, causing acute back pain. The most common sites of rupture are the lumbosacral discs, specifically, L4–5 and L5–S1. Disc herniation may also occur at C5–6 and C6–7.

The spinal nerves emerge from the spinal column through an opening (intervertebral foramen) between adjacent vertebrae. Herniated discs can press against these nerves ("pinched nerve"), causing radiculopathy (radiating pain, numbness, tingling, and diminished strength or range of motion). Additionally, nerve and vascular ingrowth into the disk and exposure of these nerves to inflammatory mediators contribute to lower back pain (Kim et al., 2020).

Osteoarthritis of the spine is associated with DDD and the stresses placed on the vertebrae. The joints, which are not adequately lubricated, rub against each other, leading to damage of the protective cartilage and the formation of painful bone spurs, which are one of the changes found in osteoarthritis.

Clinical Manifestations

The most common clinical manifestation of *lumbar disc disease* is LBP. Radicular pain that radiates down the buttock and below the knee, along the distribution of the sciatic nerve, generally indicates disc herniation. (Specific manifestations for lumbar disc herniation are summarized in Table 66.9). The straight-leg raise test may be positive, indicating nerve root irritation. Back or leg pain may be reproduced by raising the leg and flexing the foot at 90 degrees. LBP from other causes may not be accompanied by leg pain. Reflexes may be depressed or absent, depending on the spinal nerve root involved. Paresthesia or muscle weakness in the legs, feet, or toes may be reported by the patient. Multiple nerve root (*cauda equina*) compression from a herniated disk, a tumour, or an epidural access may manifest as bowel and bladder incontinence or erectile dysfunction. This condition is a medical emergency.

In *cervical disc disease*, there is often pain radiating into the arms and hands, following the pattern of the nerve involved. Reflexes may or may not be present, and there is often weakness of the hand grips.

Diagnostic Studies

Radiographic studies are done to note any structural defects. A myelogram, MRI, or CT scan is helpful in localizing the damaged site. An epidural venogram or discogram may be necessary if other methods of diagnosis are unsuccessful. An electromyogram of the extremities can be performed to determine the severity of nerve irritation or to rule out other pathological conditions, such as peripheral neuropathy.

Interprofessional Care

The patient with suspected disc damage is usually managed first with conservative therapy (Table 66.10). A physiotherapist can work with patients to limit extremes of spinal movement (brace, corset, or belt), local heat or ice, ultrasonography and massage, traction, and transcutaneous electrical nerve stimulation. Medication therapy includes NSAIDs, short-term opioids, muscle relaxants, anticonvulsant medications, and antidepressants (Wu et al., 2020). Epidural corticosteroid injections may be effective in reducing inflammation and relieving acute pain. If the underlying cause remains, the pain tends to recur. Once the symptoms subside, back-strengthening exercises are done twice a day and are encouraged for a lifetime. The patient is taught the principles of good body mechanics. Extremes of flexion and torsion are strongly discouraged. Most patients heal with a conservative (nonoperative) plan after 6 months.

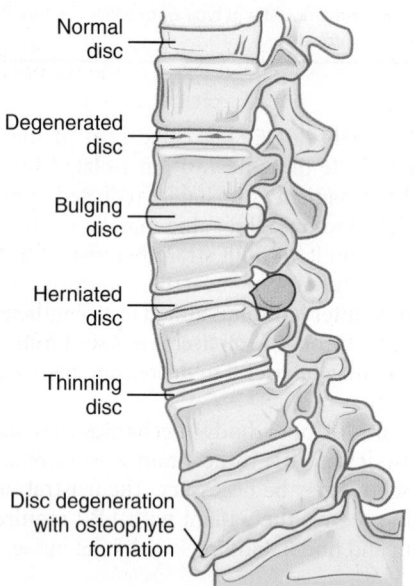

Normal disc

Degenerated disc

Bulging disc

Herniated disc

Thinning disc

Disc degeneration with osteophyte formation

FIG. 66.5 Common causes of degenerative disc damage.

TABLE 66.9	CLINICAL MANIFESTATIONS BASED ON LEVEL OF DISC HERNIATION*				
Intervertebral Level	Subjective Pain	Affected Reflex	Motor Function	Sensation	
L3–4	Back to buttocks to posterior thigh to inner calf	Patellar	Quadriceps, anterior tibialis	Inner aspect of lower leg, anterior part of thigh	
L4–5	Back to buttocks to dorsum of foot and big toe	None	Anterior tibialis, extensor hallucis longus, gluteus medius	Dorsum of foot and big toe	
L5–S1	Back to buttocks to sole of foot and heel	Achilles	Gastrocnemius, hamstring, gluteus maximus	Heel and lateral foot	

*A disc herniation can involve pressure on more than one nerve root.

TABLE 66.10 INTERPROFESSIONAL CARE

Intervertebral Disc Disease

Diagnostic
- History and physical examination
- Radiography
- CT scan
- MRI
- Myelogram
- Discogram
- EMG

Interprofessional Therapy
Conservative
- Restricted activity for several days, limit total bed rest
- Medication
- Analgesics
- Muscle relaxants
- NSAIDs
- Local ice or heat
- Physiotherapy
- Epidural corticosteroid injections

Surgical
- Intradiscal electrothermoplasty (IDET)
- Radiofrequency discal nucleoplasty
- Interspinous process decompression system (X Stop)
- Laminectomy with or without spinal fusion
- Discectomy
- Percutaneous laser discectomy
- Artificial disc replacement
- Spinal fusion with or without instrumentation (e.g., plates, screws)

CT, computed tomography; *EMG*, electromyogram; *MRI*, magnetic resonance imaging; *NSAIDs*, nonsteroidal anti-inflammatory drugs.

Surgical Therapy. If conservative treatment is unsuccessful, radiculopathy becomes progressively worse, or loss of bowel or bladder control (cauda equina) occurs, surgery may then be indicated. Surgery for a damaged disc is generally performed when diagnostic tests indicate the condition is not responding to conservative treatment and the patient is in constant pain or has a persistent neurological deficit. Surgery should be carefully considered because for some patients, for unknown reasons, their condition does not improve and symptoms may actually worsen after surgery.

Wait times for specific surgical procedures can vary across Canada. For example, Ontario reports meeting the target time of 182 days for 56% of patients waiting for low-priority lumbar disc surgery once the surgical decision was made (Health Quality Ontario, 2021), whereas in Nova Scotia, the combined wait time of surgical consult and surgery could be a little under 2 years (Nova Scotia Department of Health and Wellness, 2021). Wait times for surgical consults and actual surgery can severely affect the quality of life for the patient from a mental, physical, and social perspective.

Intradiscal electrothermoplasty (IDET) is a minimally invasive outpatient procedure that may help in treating back and sciatica pain. The procedure involves the insertion of a needle into the affected disc with radiological guidance. A wire is then threaded down through the needle and into the disc. The wire is then heated, which denervates the small nerve fibres that have grown into the cracks and invaded the degenerating disc. The heat also partially melts the annulus fibrosus, which triggers the body to generate new reinforcing proteins in the fibres of the annulus.

Another outpatient technique is *radiofrequency discal nucleoplasty* (coblation nucleoplasty). A needle is inserted into the disc in a manner similar to IDET. Instead of a heating wire, a special radiofrequency probe is used. The probe generates energy that breaks up the molecular bonds of the gel in the nucleus. The result is that up to 20% of the nucleus is removed, which decompresses the disc and reduces the pressure on both the disc and the surrounding nerve roots. Relief from pain varies among patients.

A third procedure involves use of an *interspinous process decompression system* (X Stop). This device is made of titanium and fits onto a mount that is placed on vertebrae in the lower back. The X Stop is used in patients with pain from lumbar spinal stenosis. The device works by lifting the vertebrae off the pinched nerve. The effect is similar to and less invasive than a laminectomy.

The most common surgical procedure for lumbar disc disease is a *laminectomy*. It involves the surgical excision of part of the posterior arch of the vertebra (referred to as the *lamina*) to gain access to the protruding disc to remove it. A minimal hospital stay is usually required after the procedure. Laminectomy is a safe and viable option, compared with decompression and fusion, for older patients whose condition has not improved with conservative therapy and for patients with significant comorbidities.

A *discectomy* is another common type of surgical procedure that may be performed to decompress the nerve root. Microsurgical discectomy is a version of the standard discectomy in which the surgeon uses a microscope to allow better visualization of the disc and disc space during surgery to aid in removal of the damaged portion. This procedure helps maintain the bony stability of the spine.

A *percutaneous discectomy* is an outpatient surgical procedure in which a tube is passed through the retroperitoneal soft tissues to the disc with local anaesthesia and the aid of fluoroscopy. A laser is then used on the damaged portion of the disc. Small stab wounds are made, and minimal blood loss occurs during the procedure. The procedure is effective and safe, and it decreases rehabilitation time.

Total disc replacement is used in patients with disc damage associated with DDD. This artificial disc consists of a high-density core sandwiched between two cobalt-chromium end plates (Figure 66.6). This device is surgically placed in the spine

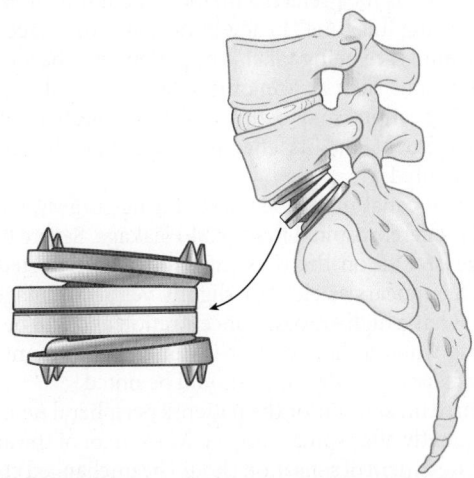

FIG. 66.6 The Charité artificial disc used in degenerative disc disease to replace a damaged intervertebral disc. The Charité artificial disc consists of two cobalt-chromium alloy end plates sandwiched around a movable high-density plastic core. The design of the disc helps align the spine and preserve its natural ability to move.

through a small incision below the umbilicus after the damaged disc is removed. The disc allows for movement at the level of the implant (Salzmann et al., 2017).

A *spinal fusion* may be performed if the spine is unstable. Spinal stabilization is created by an *ankylosis* (fusion) of contiguous vertebrae with a bone graft from the patient's fibula or iliac crest or from donated cadaver bone. Metal fixation with rods, plates, or screws may be implanted at the time of spinal surgery to provide more stability and decrease vertebral motion. A posterior lumbar interbody fusion may be performed in patients to provide extra support for bone grafting or a prosthetic device.

Bone morphogenetic protein (BMP), a genetically engineered protein, may be used to stimulate bone growth of the graft in spinal fusions (Lowery & Rosen, 2018). A dissolvable sponge soaked with BMP is implanted into the spine. The protein on the sponge stimulates the body's own cells to become active and produce bone. BMP begins the process of fusion, which continues even after the protein and sponge dissolve, leaving living bone behind.

NURSING MANAGEMENT
VERTEBRAL DISC SURGERY

Postoperative nursing interventions focus on maintaining proper alignment of the spine at all times until healing has occurred. Depending on the type and extent of surgery and the surgeon's preference, the patient may be able to dangle their legs at the side of the bed, stand, or even ambulate the first day after surgery.

After lumbar fusion, pillows can be used under the thighs of each leg when the patient is supine and between the legs when in side-lying positions, to provide comfort and ensure alignment. Often, the patient fears turning or any movement that increases pain by straining the surgical area. The patient needs to reassured that the proper technique is being used to maintain body alignment. Sufficient staff should be available to move the patient without undue pain or strain on staff members or the patient.

Postoperatively, most patients will require opioids such as morphine, intravenously, for 24 to 48 hours. Patient-controlled analgesia (PCA) or epidural analgesia allows for optimal analgesic levels and is the preferred method of continued pain management during this time (Ezhevskaya et al., 2019) (see Chapter 22). Once fluids are being taken, the patient may be switched to oral medications such as acetaminophen with codeine or oxycodone. Medications may be prescribed for muscle relaxation. Pain management and its effectiveness should be monitored and documented.

The spinal canal may be entered during surgery, so there is potential for cerebrospinal fluid (CSF) leakage. Severe headache or leakage of CSF on the dressing should be reported immediately. CSF appears as clear or slightly yellow drainage on the dressing. It has a high glucose concentration and will be positive for glucose when a dipstick test is done. The amount, colour, and characteristics of drainage should be noted.

The nurse must monitor the patient's peripheral neurological signs frequently after spinal surgery. Movement of the arms and legs and assessment of sensation should be unchanged compared with the preoperative status. Table 66.11 summarizes a lumbar laminectomy assessment appropriate for the patient who has undergone back surgery. These assessments are repeated every 2 to 4 hours during the first 48 hours after surgery, and findings

TABLE 66.11	POSTOPERATIVE ASSESSMENT FOLLOWING LUMBAR SURGERY

Sensation*
Assess sensation of extremities for paresthesia in all appropriate dermatomes.

Movement*
Assess ability to move all extremities.

Muscle Strength*
Assess for any weakness of the extremities.

Wound
Assess dressing for drainage, and note amount, colour, and characteristics.

Pain
- Document location of the pain.
- Ask patient to rate the pain on a scale of 0 to 10, with 0 being no pain and 10 being the worst pain.
- Evaluate pain after analgesia has been administered.

*Postoperative findings should be compared with preoperative assessments. It is not unusual for the patient to continue to experience these symptoms after surgery. Symptoms gradually decrease over several months.

are compared with the preoperative assessment. Paresthesias, such as numbness and tingling, may not be relieved immediately after surgery. Any new muscle weakness or paresthesias should be documented and reported to the surgeon immediately. Extremity circulation should be assessed by temperature, capillary refill, and pulses.

Paralytic ileus and interference with bowel function may occur for several days and may manifest as nausea, abdominal distension, and constipation. The nurse needs to assess if the patient is passing flatus, has bowel sounds in all quadrants, and has a flat, soft abdomen. A bowel protocol should be initiated to prevent constipation.

Adequate bladder emptying may be altered because of activity restrictions, opioids, or anaesthesia. If allowed by the surgeon, male patients should be encouraged to dangle their legs or stand to urinate. Patients should use the commode or ambulate to the bathroom when allowed, to promote adequate emptying of the bladder. The nurse needs to ensure that privacy is maintained. Intermittent catheterization or an in-dwelling catheter may be necessary for patients who have difficulty urinating.

Loss of sphincter tone or bladder tone may indicate nerve damage. Incontinence or difficulty evacuating the bowel or bladder must be monitored closely and reported to the surgeon.

In addition to the nursing care appropriate for a patient who has undergone a laminectomy, there are other nursing responsibilities if the patient has also had a spinal fusion. A bone graft is usually involved, so postoperative healing time may be longer than with a laminectomy. Reduced activity for an extended time may be necessary. A rigid orthosis (thoraco-lumbar-sacral orthosis or chairback brace) is often used during this period. Some surgeons require that the patient be taught to put the orthosis on and take it off by log-rolling in bed, whereas others allow their patients to apply the brace in a sitting or standing position. The nurse needs to verify the preferred method before initiating this activity.

In addition to the primary surgical site, the donor site for the bone graft must be regularly assessed. The posterior iliac crest is the most commonly used donor site, although the fibula may also be used. The donor site usually causes greater postoperative pain than the fused area. The donor site is bandaged with a pressure dressing to prevent excessive bleeding. If the donor site is the fibula, neurovascular assessments of the extremity are a postoperative nursing responsibility.

After a spinal fusion, the patient may experience some immobility of the spine at the fusion site. Instruction in proper body mechanics is essential and should be evaluated during the hospital stay. The patient is instructed to avoid sitting or standing for prolonged periods, while activities such as walking, lying down, and shifting weight from one foot to the other when standing are encouraged. The nurse should encourage the patient to think through an activity before starting any potentially injurious task, such as bending, lifting, or stooping. Any twisting movement of the spine is contraindicated. The patient needs to use the thighs and knees, rather than the back, to absorb the shock of activity and movement. Use of a firm mattress or bed board is essential.

NECK PAIN

Neck pain may occur almost as frequently as LBP. Neck pain may be the result of many conditions, both benign (e.g., poor posture) and serious (e.g., traumatic injury).

Cervical neck sprains and strains occur from hyperflexion and hyperextension injuries. Patients have symptoms of stiffness and neck pain and possible pain radiating into the arm and hand. Pain may also radiate into the head, anterior chest, thoracic spine region, and shoulders. Cervical nerve root compression from stenosis, DDD, or herniation may be indicated by weakness or paresthesia of the arm and hand. The cause of neck pain is determined by health history, physical examination, radiography, MRI, CT scan, and electromyography. An electromyogram of the upper extremities is performed to diagnose cervical radiculopathy.

Conservative treatment for neck pain in patients without an underlying disorder includes head support via soft cervical collars, heat and ice applications, massage, rest until symptoms subside, physiotherapy, ultrasound, and NSAIDs. Therapeutic neck exercises and acupuncture may also be used for pain relief. Most neck pain resolves without surgical intervention. Indications for cervical spine surgery are similar to those for the lower back.

Types of surgery are also similar, including discectomy, laminectomy, and spinal fusion. If surgery is done on the cervical spine, the nurse must be alert for symptoms of spinal cord edema, such as respiratory distress and a worsening neurological status of the upper extremities. An orthosis or halo may be necessary after surgery, depending on the degree of spine stabilization. After surgery, the patient's neck is immobilized in either a soft or a hard cervical collar.

Nurses can educate patients in how to prevent benign neck pain that occurs from everyday activities, such as avoiding prolonged sitting at a computer or television, not sleeping in nonaligned spinal positions, or not making jarring movements during exercise. Preventive strategies include encouraging patients to practise good posture and maintain neck flexibility (Table 66.12).

FOOT DISORDERS

The foot is the platform that provides support for the weight of the body and absorbs considerable shock in ambulation. It is a

TABLE 66.12	**PATIENT & CAREGIVER TEACHING GUIDE**

Neck Exercises

The following instructions should be included when teaching the patient about neck exercises.
- Bend your head backward until you are looking up at the ceiling. Repeat slowly five times. Stop if experiencing dizziness.
- Bring your head forward so that your chin touches your chest and your face is looking down at the floor. Repeat slowly five times.
- Keep your head facing forward, and bend your ear down toward one shoulder. Alternate this movement with your other ear. Repeat slowly five times on each side.
- Turn your head slowly around to one side as far as it will go. Repeat toward the other side. Repeat exercise five times on each side.
- Without tipping your head in any direction, pull your chin and head straight back. Relax the chin forward to its neutral position. Repeat slowly five times.

complicated structure, composed of bony structures, muscles, tendons, and ligaments. It can be affected by congenital conditions, structural weakness, traumatic injuries, and systemic conditions such as diabetes mellitus and rheumatoid arthritis. Much of the pain, deformity, and disability associated with foot disorders can be directly attributed to or accentuated by improperly fitting shoes, which cause crowding and angulation of the toes and inhibition of the normal movement of foot muscles.

The purposes of footwear are to (a) provide support, foot stability, protection, shock absorption, and a foundation for orthoses; (b) increase friction with the walking surface; and (c) treat foot abnormalities. Table 66.13 summarizes common foot disorders. One of the most common forefoot disorders is a bunion (Figure 66.7). A lateral deviation of the great toe, termed *hallux valgus*, occurs with a bunion (Buldt & Menz, 2018).

NURSING MANAGEMENT FOOT DISORDERS

NURSING IMPLEMENTATION

HEALTH PROMOTION. Well-constructed and properly fitting shoes are essential for healthy, pain-free feet. Instead of considerations of comfort and support, fashion styles, especially for women, often influence selection of footwear. Patient teaching should stress the importance of wearing shoes that conform to the foot rather than only to current fashion trends. Shoes must be long enough and wide enough to prevent crowding of the toes and forcing of the great toe into a position of hallux valgus. At the metatarsal head, the width of shoes should be sufficient to allow free movement of the foot muscles and permit bending of the toes. The shank (narrow part of sole under the instep) of the shoes should be rigid enough to give optimal support. The height of the heels should be realistic in relation to the purpose for which the shoes are worn. Ideally, the heels of the shoes should not rise more than 2.5 cm higher than the forefoot support.

Effective strategies for preventing foot injuries are also required at the workplace. Prolonged standing, especially on hard, unyielding floors, can cause the joints of bones of the feet to become misaligned and inflamed. Special antislip flooring or matting can reduce slipping accidents that can result in sprained ankles or broken foot bones.

TABLE 66.13 COMMON FOOT DISORDERS

Disorder	Description	Treatment
Forefoot		
Hallux valgus (bunion)	Painful deformity of great toe consisting of lateral angulation of great toe toward second toe, bony enlargement of medial side of first metatarsal head, swelling of bursa and formation of callus over bony enlargement (see Figure 66.7)	Conservative treatment includes wearing shoes with wide forefoot or "bunion pocket" and use of bunion pads to relieve pressure on bursal sac. Surgical treatment is removal of bursal sac and bony enlargement and correction of lateral angulation of great toe; this may include temporary or permanent internal fixation.
Hallux rigidus	Painful stiffness of first MTP joint, caused by osteoarthritis or local trauma	Conservative treatment includes intra-articular corticosteroids and passive manual stretching of first MTP joint. A shoe with a stiff sole decreases pain in the joint during walking. Surgical treatment is joint fusion or arthroplasty with silicone rubber implant.
Hammer toe	Deformity of second through fifth toes, including dorsiflexion of MTP joint, plantar flexion of PIP joint, and callus on dorsum of PIP joint and end of involved toe; symptoms related to hammer toe include burning on bottom of foot and pain and difficulty in walking when wearing shoes	Conservative treatment consists of passive manual stretching of PIP joint and use of metatarsal arch support. Surgical correction consists of resection of base of middle phalanx and head of proximal phalanx and bringing raw bone ends together. Kirschner wire maintains straight position.
Morton's neuroma (Morton's toe or plantar neuroma)	Neuroma in web space between third and fourth metatarsal heads, causing sharp, sudden attacks of pain and burning sensations	Surgical excision is the usual treatment.
Midfoot		
Pes planus (flat-foot)	Loss of metatarsal arch, causing pain in foot or leg	Symptoms are relieved by use of resilient, longitudinal arch supports. Surgical treatment consists of triple arthrodesis or fusion of subtalar joint.
Pes cavus	Elevation of longitudinal arch of foot resulting from contracture of plantar fascia or bony deformity of arch	Treatment is manipulation and casting (in patients <6 yr of age); surgical correction is necessary if it interferes with ambulation (in patients ≥6 yr of age).
Hindfoot		
Painful heels	Heel pain with weight bearing; common causes include plantar bursitis, plantar fasciitis, or bone spur in adults	Corticosteroids are injected locally into inflamed bursa, and a sponge rubber heel cushion is used; surgical excision of bursa or spur is performed. For plantar fasciitis, stretching exercises, NSAIDs, and corticosteroids are used.
Other Disorders		
Corn	Localized thickening of skin caused by continual pressure over bony prominences, especially metatarsal head, frequently causing localized pain	The corn is softened with warm water or preparations containing salicylic acid and trimmed with a razor blade or scalpel. Pressure on bony prominences caused by shoes is relieved.
Soft corn	Painful lesion caused by bony prominence of one toe pressing against adjacent toe; usual location in web space between toes; softness caused by secretions keeping web space relatively moist	Pain is relieved by placing cotton between toes to separate them. Surgical treatment is excision of projecting bone spur (if present).
Callus	Similar formation to corn but covers wider area and usual location is on weight-bearing part of foot	Same as for corn.
Plantar wart	Painful papillomatous growth caused by virus that may occur on any part of skin on sole of foot; tend to cluster on pressure points	Remedies containing salicylic acid; liquid nitrogen; excision with electrocoagulation or surgical removal; ultrasonography may also be used. Many disappear without treatment.

MTP, metatarsophalangeal; *NSAIDs,* nonsteroidal anti-inflammatory drugs; *PIP,* proximal interphalangeal.

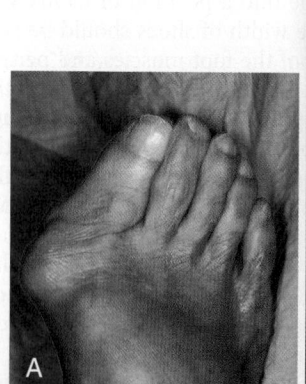
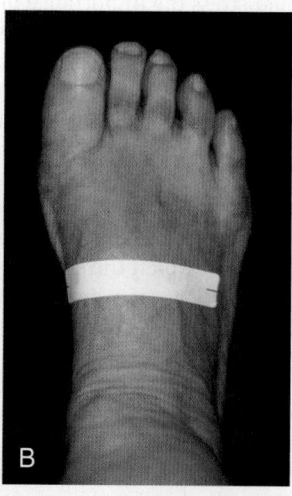

FIG. 66.7 A, Severe hallux valgus with bursa formation. **B,** Postoperative correction. Source: Canale, S., & Beaty, J. (Eds.). (2013). *Campbell's operative orthopaedics* (12th ed.). Saunders.

All jurisdictions in Canada mandate that workers wear adequate protection against workplace hazards. Workers who are exposed to high foot-hazard risk (e.g., those in the construction industry) are required to use footwear certified by the Canadian Standards Association.

ACUTE INTERVENTION. Many foot conditions require referral to a podiatrist, who specialize in diagnosing and treating conditions associated with the foot's anatomy and function. Depending on the condition, conservative therapies are usually tried first (see Table 66.13). These therapies include NSAIDs, icing, physiotherapy, alterations in footwear, stretching, warm soaks, orthotics, ultrasonography, and corticosteroid injections. If these methods do not offer relief, surgery may then be recommended.

Depending on the type of surgery, pins or wires (hardware) may extend through the toes, or a protective splint that extends over the end of the foot may be put in place. Postoperatively, the foot is usually immobilized by a bulky dressing, short leg cast, slipper (plaster) cast, or a platform "shoe" that fits over the dressing and has a rigid sole (known as a *bunion boot*). The foot should be elevated with the heel off the bed to help reduce discomfort and prevent edema. Neurovascular status should be assessed frequently during the immediate postoperative period. Care must be taken to protect hardware as impact or movement cause pain. The hardware may interfere with or preclude assessment for movement. Sensation may be difficult to evaluate because postoperative pain can interfere with the patient's ability to differentiate pain caused by the surgical procedure from pain resulting from nerve pressure or circulatory impairment.

The type and extent of surgery determine the degree of ambulation allowed. Crutches, a walker, a kneeler scooter, or a cane may be necessary. The patient may experience pain or a throbbing sensation when starting ambulation. The nurse should reinforce instructions given by the physiotherapist and ensure that the patient does not develop a faulty gait pattern, such as walking on the heels, in an attempt to avoid excessive pain or pressure. The nurse must also ensure that the patient walks with an erect posture and with proper weight distribution. Dysfunction of gait or continued pain should be reported to the health care provider. The patient should be instructed on the importance of frequent rest periods with the foot elevated.

AMBULATORY AND HOME CARE. Foot care should include carrying out daily hygienic care and wearing clean socks, which should be long enough to prevent wrinkling and the development of pressure areas. Trimming toenails straight across helps prevent ingrown toenails and reduces the possibility of infection. People with impaired circulation or diabetes mellitus require detailed instruction in how to prevent serious complications associated with blisters, pressure areas, and infections. (See Chapter 52, Table 52.20 for guidelines on foot care.)

AGE-RELATED CONSIDERATIONS

FOOT CONDITIONS

The older person is prone to developing foot conditions because of poor circulation, atherosclerosis, and decreased sensation in the lower extremities. This tendency is especially true for older patients with diabetes mellitus (Embil et al., 2018). A patient may develop an open wound but not feel it because of altered sensation, possibly as a result of peripheral vascular disease or diabetic neuropathy. Older patients should be instructed to inspect their feet daily and report any open wounds or breaks in the skin to the health care provider (Embil et al., 2018). If left untreated, wounds may become infected, lead to osteomyelitis, and require surgical debridement. If the infection becomes widespread, lower limb amputation may be necessary. The caregiver of an older person who needs assistance with hygiene practices should be taught the importance of carefully assessing the feet at regular intervals.

BONE TUMOURS

Primary benign and malignant bone tumours are rare in adults and occur most often during childhood through young adulthood. Metastatic bone cancer, in which the cancer has spread from another site, is a more common occurrence. The name given to a bone tumour is based on the area of the bone and surrounding tissue that is affected and on the type of cells forming the tumour. In 2016, 240 new cases of primary bone/joint cancer

occurred in Canada (excluding Quebec), and there were 183 related deaths in the same year (Canadian Cancer Society, 2021a).

Clinical Manifestations

Persistent nonmechanical bone pain in any bone lasting more than a few weeks is cause for concern and should undergo further evaluation and investigation. Diagnosis of a suspected bone tumour is related to age, family history, presence and location of swelling, patient's mobility, and the presence of enlarged regional or local lymph nodes (Ferguson & Turner, 2018). Recent injury does not rule out a tumour, and the patient should undergo the appropriate diagnostic procedures.

Diagnostic Studies

Conventional radiographs should always be the first investigation when a patient presents with bone pain. If the diagnosis of tumour cannot be excluded with certainty, the next step is to arrange for an MRI. A CT scan is helpful in visualizing calcification, periosteal bone formation, cortical destruction, or soft tissue involvement. In order to definitely identify and characterize the tumour, a biopsy for histology and pathology needs to be obtained by either a radiologist (radiology-guided biopsy) or surgeon (open-surgical biopsy). Once the biopsy material has been reviewed and identified, discussions about diagnosis, staging assessment, and treatment can occur with the patient and their family.

BENIGN TUMOURS

Benign bone tumours are more common than primary malignant tumours. The main types of benign bone tumours are osteochondroma, osteoclastoma, and enchondroma. These types of tumours are often removed by surgery.

Osteochondroma

Osteochondroma is the most common primary benign bone tumour. It is characterized by an overgrowth of cartilage and bone near the end of the bone, at the growth plate. It is more commonly found in the long bones of the leg, pelvis, or scapula.

Clinical manifestations include a painless, hard, immobile mass; lower-than-normal height for age; soreness of muscles in close proximity to the tumour; one leg or arm longer than the other; and pressure or irritation with exercise. Patients may also be asymptomatic. No treatment is necessary for asymptomatic osteochondroma. If the tumour is causing pain or neurological symptoms because of compression, surgical resection is usually done. Patients should have regular screening examinations for early detection of malignant transformation.

Osteoclastoma

Osteoclastoma *(giant-cell tumour)* is a destructive tumour that arises in the cancellous ends of long bones in young adults. Most (98%) of these variant, giant-cell tumours are benign, but about 10% of the time they can be locally aggressive and spread to the lungs. Giant-cell tumours most commonly occur in women between the ages of 20 and 35. Common tumour sites are in the epiphysis of the distal femur, the proximal tibia, and the distal radius. Clinical manifestations are usually swelling, local pain, and some disturbances in joint function. Radiographic evidence of giant-cell tumours usually reveals local areas of bone destruction and eventual expansion of the bone ends (Figure 66.8).

After diagnosis, surgical curettage of the tumour is usually done, followed by bone grafting or bone cement; however, this treatment has been associated with high recurrence rates.

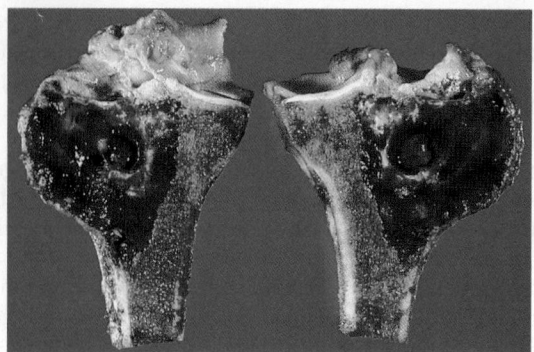

FIG. 66.8 Osteoclastoma (giant-cell tumour) in a long bone. Source: Damjanov, I., & Linder, J. (1996). *Anderson's pathology* (10th ed.). Mosby.

Additional treatments with adjuvants such as zinc chloride, bisphosphonates, phenol, liquid nitrogen, and alcohol are often used to reduce recurrence (Wallace, 2020). Recurrent giant-cell tumours may have to be treated with amputation and prosthesis.

ENCHONDROMA

Enchondroma are medullary cavity tumours usually found in a single hand or foot bone as a result of a pathological fracture or trauma (Williams et al., 2019). Clinical manifestations are usually localized pain. After diagnosis, surgical curettage of the tumour is done with bone grafting. Recurrence is rare.

MALIGNANT BONE TUMOURS

A sarcoma is a malignant tumour in the connective tissues of the body (fat, muscles, blood vessels, nerves, bones, or cartilage). The most common types of malignant bone tumours are osteosarcoma, chondrosarcoma (Figure 66.9, *B*), and Ewing sarcoma. Primary malignant tumours occur most often during childhood and young adulthood. They are characterized by their rapid metastasis and bone destruction.

Osteosarcoma

Osteosarcoma is a malignant primary bone tumour that is extremely aggressive and is characterized by rapid growth and metastasis. It usually occurs in the metaphyseal region of the long bones of the extremities, particularly in the regions of the distal femur, proximal tibia, and proximal humerus as well as the pelvis (see Figure 66.9, *A*). Osteosarcoma is the most common malignant bone tumour affecting children and young adults; the highest incidence is in boys and men 10 to 25 years of age. Secondary osteosarcoma is known to occur in adults older than age 60 and is most commonly associated with Paget's disease.

Clinical manifestations of osteosarcoma are usually associated with a gradual onset of pain and swelling, especially around the knee. The neoplasm grows rapidly and can restrict joint motion if the tumour is close to a joint structure. Metastasis is present in 10 to 20% of individuals on diagnosis, with the lung being the most frequent site.

Canadian Terry Fox was diagnosed with osteosarcoma at 18 years of age and underwent an above-knee amputation in early 1977. Influenced by his experience, Terry decided in 1980 to run across Canada to raise money and awareness about cancer. Since then, more than $700 million has been raised worldwide for cancer research in Terry's name, through the annual Terry Fox Run held across Canada and around the world (Terry Fox Foundation, 2021). Fortunately, major advances continue to be made in the treatment of osteosarcoma.

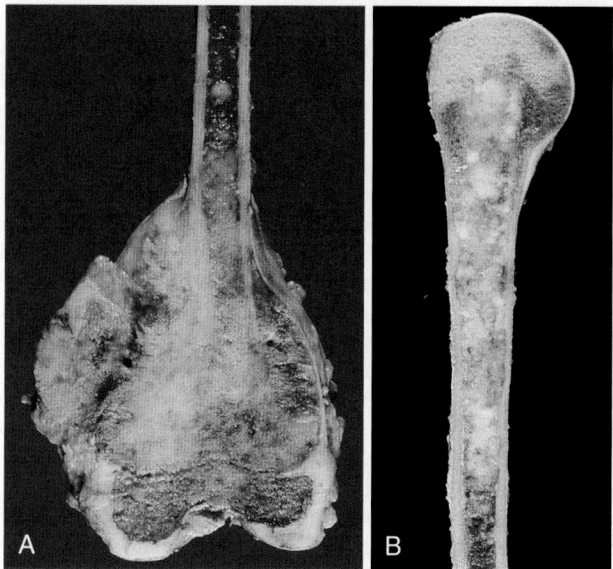

FIG. 66.9 A, Osteosarcoma. **B,** Chondrosarcoma. Source: Damjanov, I., & Linder, J. (1996). *Anderson's pathology.* (10th ed.). Mosby.

Preoperative chemotherapy is used to decrease tumour size, and limb-salvage procedures (e.g., wide surgical resection of the tumour) are being used more often if a clear (no cancer present) 6- to 7-cm margin surrounds the lesion. Limb salvage is contraindicated if there is major neurovascular involvement, pathological fracture, infection, skeletal immaturity, or extensive muscle involvement. Quality-of-life considerations also factor into the decision regarding limb salvage or amputation. The introduction of multiagent chemotherapy has improved the outcomes for these patients. Chemotherapeutic agents used include methotrexate (Rheumatrex), doxorubicin (Myocet), cisplatin (Platinol-AQ), dactinomycin (Cosmegen), and ifosfamide (Ifex) (Canadian Cancer Society, 2021b).

Ewing Sarcoma Family of Tumours

Ewing sarcoma family of tumours (ESFT) is one of the most common primary malignant neoplasms of bone and soft tissue. It occurs most often in adolescents or young adults, the majority of whom are younger than 30 years of age.

ESFT is characterized by rapid growth within the medullary cavity of long bones, especially the femur, humerus, pelvis, and tibia. Metastasis occurs early, and the most frequent site is the lungs. Common manifestations are progressive local pain, swelling, palpable soft tissue mass, noticeable increase in size of the affected part, fever, and leukocytosis. Multimodal treatment strategies combining local therapy (radiotherapy, surgery) and systemic chemotherapy have improved survival rates; however, for persons with disseminated disease or recurrent disease, prognosis is still unfavourable. Chemotherapeutic agents commonly used are vincristine, ifosfamide (Ifex), doxorubicin, and etoposide (VePesid). The 5-year disease-free survival rate for localized Ewing sarcoma treated with radiation, surgical resection, and multiagent chemotherapy is 65 to 76%. Hopefully, as new biology-driven treatment options emerge, the odds of survival can begin to improve (Ferguson & Turner, 2018).

METASTATIC BONE CANCER

The most common type of malignant bone tumour occurs as a result of metastasis from a primary tumour located at another site. Common sites for the primary tumour include breast, prostate, gastrointestinal tract, lungs, kidney, ovary, and thyroid. The bone is the third-most common site for metastatic disease. Metastatic cancer cells travel from the primary tumour via the lymph and blood supply to other sites in the body. Metastatic bone lesions are commonly found in vertebrae, pelvis, femur, humerus, or ribs. Pathological fractures at the site of metastasis are common because of weakening of the involved bone. High serum calcium levels result as calcium is released from damaged bones.

Once a primary lesion has been identified, often, radionuclide bone scans are done to detect the presence of metastatic lesions before they are visible on radiography. Metastatic bone lesions may occur at any time (even years later) following diagnosis and treatment of the primary tumour. Metastasis to the bone should be suspected in any patient who has local bone pain and a past history of cancer. Treatment may be palliative and consists of pain management and radiation (see Chapter 18). Neurosurgical or orthopedic surgical interventions may include prophylactic fixation at sites of impeding fracture, stabilization after pathological fracture, and stabilization or decompression of spinal cord and nerve roots for spinal instability (Khodabukus et al., 2018). Prognosis depends on the primary type of cancer and the extent of metastasis throughout the body.

NURSING MANAGEMENT
BONE CANCER

Patients with bone cancer should be assessed for location and severity of pain. The tumour site is also assessed for swelling, changes in circulation, and joint function, movement, and sensation. The patient is monitored for weakness caused by anemia and decreased mobility.

The overall goals are that the patient with bone cancer will (a) have satisfactory pain relief; (b) maintain preferred activities as long as possible; (c) demonstrate acceptance of body image changes resulting from chemotherapy, radiation, and surgery;

(d) remain free from injury; and (e) verbalize a realistic idea of disease progression and prognosis.

Nursing care of the patient with a malignant bone neoplasm does not differ significantly from the care given to a patient with a malignant disease of any other body system (see Chapter 18). These patients are at high risk for injury because of the nature of their disease as well as the medications they may be taking, so they require special attention and safety precautions while in the hospital. Careful handling and support of the affected extremity, and log-rolling for those on bed rest, are important measures to prevent pathological fractures. Often, patients suffer from fatigue and weakness. They are often reluctant to participate in activities because of fear of pain and of falling and fracturing a bone. Regular rest periods should be provided between activities. Plans should be discussed for home safety, including wearing nonslip footwear, ensuring a well-lit environment, and removing throw rugs and cords from the floor (Goldberg et al., 2018).

The pain associated with bone cancer can be severe. Often, the pain is caused by the tumour pressing against nerves and other organs near the bone. The patient's pain should be carefully monitored and the nurse should ensure that the patient has adequate pain medication. Sometimes, radiation therapy is used as a palliative therapy to shrink the tumour and decrease the pain.

The patient and family should be assisted in accepting the guarded prognosis associated with bone neoplasms. Inability to accomplish age-specific developmental tasks can increase the frustrations with this condition. General principles related to cancer nursing are applicable (see Chapter 18 and NCPs 18.1 and 18.2, available on the Evolve website). Special attention is necessary for the difficulties of pain and disability, chemotherapy, adverse effects of chemotherapy, and postoperative care after surgery, such as for spinal cord decompression or amputation. As with all types of cancer, the nurse should stress the importance of follow-up examinations.

CASE STUDY

Osteoporosis

Patient Profile

A. R. (pronouns she/her) is a 56-year-old retired librarian who had a total hysterectomy and salpingo-oophorectomy for removal of a benign ovarian cyst 4 years ago. She also has a history of a seizure disorder since childhood and Addison's disease.

Subjective Data

- Acute, severe lumbar pain and tenderness that radiate to the right hip and lateral thigh after falling and landing on buttocks last week
- Walking and bending increases pain
- Stress fracture in wrist 6 months ago
- Reports no noticeable loss of height
- Maternal history of osteoporosis
- Taking corticosteroids and mineralocorticoids for past 6 years for Addison's disease
- Taking phenytoin (Dilantin) every evening
- Drinks two alcoholic beverages every evening
- Dislikes dairy products

Objective Data

- 167 cm tall, 72 kg

Diagnostic Studies

- Bone mass measurement tests show decreased bone mineral density at spine and hip
- Lumbar spine radiographs reveal a slightly displaced L4 compression fracture
- Normal serum calcium, phosphorus, and alkaline phosphatase levels

Interprofessional Care

- L4 vertebroplasty
- Thoraco-lumbar-sacral orthosis (TLSO) brace postoperatively
- Alendronate (Fosamax) 70 mg once weekly PO
- Total calcium intake of 1 200 mg/day PO (supplement + dietary intake)
- High-calcium diet
- Reduction in alcohol intake
- Regular, low-impact weight-bearing exercise program

Discussion Questions

1. What factors place A. R. at risk of developing osteoporosis?
2. Why do walking and bending increase the patient's pain?
3. What is the purpose of the TLSO brace prescribed for A. R.?
4. *Priority decision:* What are the priority teaching needs for A. R.?
5. How might the nurse assist A. R. in increasing calcium intake?
6. Why would regular exercise be important for A. R.?
7. *Priority decision:* Based on the assessment data presented, what are the priority nursing diagnoses? Are there any interprofessional issues?
8. *Evidence-informed practice:* The patient asks why taking corticosteroids increases her risk of developing osteoporosis. How should the nurse respond to A. R.?

ⓔvolve

Answers are available at http://evolve.elsevier.com/Canada/Lewis/medsurg.

REVIEW QUESTIONS

The number of the question corresponds to the same-numbered objective at the beginning of the chapter.

1. A client with osteomyelitis is treated with surgical debridement with implantation of antibiotic beads. When the client asks why the beads are used, how should the nurse answer? *(Select all that apply.)*
   a. The beads are used to directly deliver antibiotics to the area of the infection.
   b. There are no effective oral or IV antibiotics to treat most cases of bone infection.
   c. This is the safest method of delivering long-term antibiotic therapy for a bone infection.
   d. The beads are used for deep infections in addition to removing the damaged tissue and oral and IV antibiotics.
   e. The lack of blood flow and the bone death that occur with osteomyelitis make IV antibiotics less effective.

2. The nurse is teaching a client with osteopenia. What is important to include in the teaching plan?
   a. Lose weight.
   b. Stop smoking.
   c. Eat a high-protein diet.
   d. Start swimming for exercise.

3. Which of the following individuals does the nurse identify as being at high risk for low back pain? *(Select all that apply.)*
   a. A 63-year-old man who is a long-distance truck driver
   b. A 36-year-old construction worker who is 190 cm tall and weighs 118 kg
   c. A 28-year-old female yoga instructor who is 170 cm tall and weighs 59 kg
   d. A 30-year-old male nurse who works on an orthopedic unit and smokes
   e. A 44-year-old female chef with prior compression fracture of the spine

4. What is the primary nursing responsibility in caring for a client with a suspected disc herniation who is experiencing acute pain and muscle spasms?
   a. Encourage total bed rest for several days.
   b. Teach the principles of back-strengthening exercises.
   c. Stress the importance of straight-leg raises to decrease pain.
   d. Promote the use of cold and hot compresses and pain medication.

5. When caring for a client after a spinal fusion, which of the following symptoms would the nurse immediately report to the physician?
   a. The client experiences a single episode of emesis.
   b. The client is unable to move the lower extremities.
   c. The client is nauseated and has not voided in 4 hours.
   d. The client reports pain at the bone graft donor site.

6. What instructions should the nurse give the client who is being discharged from same-day surgery after surgical correction of bilateral hallux valgus?
   a. Rest frequently, with the feet elevated.
   b. Soak the feet in warm water several times a day.
   c. Expect the feet to be numb for several days postoperatively.
   d. Expect continued pain in the feet, since this is not uncommon.

7. A client has been diagnosed with osteosarcoma of the humerus. Which of the following statements would indicate that he has an understanding of his treatment options?
   a. "I accept that I have to lose my arm with surgery."
   b. "The chemotherapy before surgery will shrink the tumour."
   c. "This tumour is related to the melanoma I had 3 years ago."
   d. "I'm glad they can take out the cancer with such a small scar."

1. a, d; 2. b; 3. a, b, d, e; 4. d; 5. b; 6. a; 7. b.

⊝volve

For even more review questions, visit http://evolve.elsevier.com/Canada/Lewis/medsurg.

REFERENCES

Alswat, K. A. (2017). Gender disparities in osteoporosis. *Journal of Clinical Medicine Research, 9*(5), 382–287. https://doi.org/10.14740/jocmr2970w

Appleman-Dijkstra, N. M., & Papapoulos, S. E. (2018). Paget's disease of bone. *Best practice & Research: Clinical Endocrinology & Metabolism, 32*(5), 657–668. https://doi.org/10.1016/j.beem.2018.05.005

Buldt, A. K., & Menz, H. B. (2018). Incorrectly fitted footwear, foot pain and foot disorders: A systematic search and narrative review of the literature. *Journal of Foot and Ankle Research, 11*, 43. https://doi.org/10.1186/s13047-018-0284-z

Burchum, J., & Rosenthal, L. (2019). *Lehne's pharmacology for nursing care* (10th ed.). Saunders.

Canadian Cancer Society. (2021a). *Bone cancer statistics.* https://www.cancer.ca/en/cancer-information/cancer-type/bone/statistics/?region=on

Canadian Cancer Society. (2021b). *Treatments for osteosarcoma.* https://www.cancer.ca/en/cancer-information/cancer-type/bone/treatment/osteosarcoma/?region=qc

Embil, J. M., Albalawi, Z., Bowering, K., et al. (2018). Clinical practice guideline: Foot care. *Canadian Journal of Diabetes, 42*(2018), S222–S227. https://doi.org/10.1016/j.jcjd.2017.10.020

Ezhevskaya, A. A., Ovechkin, A. M., Prusakova, Z. B., et al. (2019). Relationship among anesthesia technique, surgical stress, and cognitive dysfunction following spinal surgery: A randomized trial. *Journal of Neurosurgery: Spine, 31*(6), 894–901. https://doi.org/10.3171/2019.4.SPINE184

Fatoye, F., Gebrye, T., & Odeyemi, I. (2019). Real-world incidence and prevalence of low back pain using routinely collected data. *Rheumatology International, 39*, 619–626. https://doi.org/10.1007/s00296-019-04273-0

Ferguson, J. L., & Turner, S. P. (2018). Bone cancer: Diagnosis and treatment principles. *American Academy of Family Physicians, 98*(4), 205–213. https://www.aafp.org/afp/2018/0815/p205.html

Gates, M., Pillay, J., Thériault, G., et al. (2019). Screening to prevent fragility fractures among adults 40 years and older in primary care: Protocol for a systematic review. *Systematic Reviews, 8*, 216. https://doi.org/10.1186/s13643-019-1094-5

Goldberg, J. L., Burhenn, P. S., & Ginex, P. K. (2018). Nursing education: Review of assessment, clinical care and implications for practice regarding older adult patients with cancer. *Clinical Journal of Oncology Nursing, 22*(6), 19–25. https://doi.org/10.1188/18.CJON.S2.19-25

Goode, S. C., Wright, T. F., & Lynch, C. (2020). Osteoporosis screening and treatment: A collaborative approach. *The Journal for Nurse Practitioners, 16*(1), 60–63. https://doi.org/10.1016/j.nurpra.2019.10.017

Hardy, M., & Feehan, L. M. (2020). Fracture healing: An evolving perspective. In (7th ed.) T. M. Skirven, A. L. Osterman, J. M. Fedorczyk, et al. (Eds.), *Rehabilitation of the hand and upper extremity* (Vol. 1) (pp. 264–275). Elsevier.

Health Canada. (2020). *Vitamin D and calcium: Updated dietary reference intakes.* https://www.canada.ca/en/health-canada/services/food-nutrition/healthy-eating/vitamins-minerals/vitamin-calcium-updated-dietary-reference-intakes-nutrition.html

Health Quality Ontario. (2021). *System performance: Time from decision to having surgery or procedure—Neurosurgery: Lumbar disc surgery.* https://www.hqontario.ca/System-Performance/Wait-Times-for-Surgeries-and-Procedures/Wait-Times-for-Other-Surgeries-and-Procedures/Time-from-Decision-to-Having-Surgery-or-Procedure

Hopkins, R. B., Burke, N., Von Keyserlingk, C., et al. (2016). The current economic burden of illness of osteoporosis in Canada. *Osteoporosis International, 27*(10), 3023–3032. https://doi.org/10.1007/s00198-016-3631-6

Ibrahim, M. I., Zubair, I. U., Yaacob, N. M., et al. (2019). Low back pain and its associated factors among nurses in public hospitals of Penang Malaysia. *International Journal of Environmental Research and Public Health, 16*(21), 4254. https://doi.org/10.3390/ijerph16214254

Institute of Health Economics. (2017). *Evidence-informed primary care management of low back pain* (3rd ed.). https://www.ihe.ca/research-programs/hta/aagap/lbp

Kanis, J. A., Harvey, N. C., Johansson, H., et al. (2017). Overview of fracture prediction tools. *Journal of Clinical Densitometry, 20*(3), 444–450. https://doi.org/10.1016/j.jocd.2017.06.013

Kavanagh, N., Ryan, E. J., Widaa, A., et al. (2018). Staphylococcal osteomyelitis: Disease progression, treatment challenges, and future directions. *Clinical Microbiology Reviews, 31*(2), e00084-17. https://doi.org/10.1128/CMR.00084-17

Khodabukus, A. F., Debattista, M., Reynolds, J., et al. (2018). *Guidelines for the prevention of pathological fractures in palliative care.* Cheshire & Merseyside Palliative & End of Life Care Strategic Clinical Network. https://www.nwcscnsenate.nhs.uk/files/2514/2789/9749/Guidelines_for_the_Prevention_of_Pathological_Fracture_in_Palliative_Care_Final_March_30_2015.pdf?PDFPATHWAY=PDF

Kim, H. S., Wu, P. W., & Jang, I. (2020). Lumbar degenerative disease part 1: Anatomy and pathophysiology of intervertebral discogenic pain and radiofrequency ablation of basivertebral and sinuvertebral nerve treatment for chronic discogenic back pain: A prospective case series and review of literature. *International Journal of Molecular Sciences, 21*(4), 1483. https://doi.org/10.3390/ijms21041483

Klinder, A., Zaatreh, S., Ellenrieder, M., et al. (2019). Antibiotics release from cement spacers used for two-stage treatment of implant-associated infections after total joint arthroplasty. *Journal of Biomedical Materials Research. Part B, Applied Biomaterials, 107*(5), 1587–1597. https://doi.org/10.1002/jbm.b.34251

Lacasse, A., Roy, J. S., Parent, A. J., et al. (2017). The Canadian minimum dataset for chronic low back pain research: Cross-cultural adaptation of the National Institute of Health Task Force research standards. *Canadian Medical Association Journal Open, 5*(1), E237–E248. https://doi.org/10.9778/cmajo.20160117

Lane, G., Nisbet, C., Whiting, S. J., et al. Canadian newcomer children's bone health and vitamin D. *Applied Physiology, Nutrition and Metabolism, 44*(7), 796–803. https://doi.org/10.1139/apnm-2018-0705

Lowery, J. W., & Rosen, V. (2018). Bone morphogenetic protein-based therapeutic approaches. *Cold Spring Harbor Perspectives in Biology, 10*(4), a022327. https://doi.org/10.1101/cshperspect.a022327

Mangels, R. (2018). *Calcium in the vegan diet.* http://www.vrg.org/nutrition/calcium.php

Marais, L. C., Ferreira, N., Aldous, C., et al. (2016). The outcome of treatment of chronic osteomyelitis according to an integrated approach. *Strategies in Trauma and Limb Reconstruction, 11*(2), 135–142. https://doi.org/10.1007/s11751-016-0259-1

Micheletti, J. K., Blafoss, R., Sundstrup, E., et al. (2019). Association between lifestyle and musculoskeletal pain: Cross-sectional study among 10,000 adults from the general working population. *Biomed Central Musculoskeletal Disorders, 20*(1), 1–8. https://doi.org/10.1186/s12891-019-3002-5

Mifsud, M., & McNally, M. (2019). Local delivery of antimicrobials in the treatment of bone infections. *Orthopaedics and Trauma, 33*(3), 160–165. https://doi.org/10.1016/j.mporth.2019.03.007

Nova Scotia Department of Health and Wellness. (2021). *Healthcare wait times: Back surgery (adult).* https://waittimes.novascotia.ca/procedure/back-surgery-adult#waittimes

Osteoporosis Canada. (n.d.). About the disease. https://osteoporosis.ca/about-the-disease/

Papaioannou, A., Morin, S., Cheung, A. M., et al. (2010). 2010 clinical practice guidelines for the diagnosis and management of osteoporosis in Canada: Summary. *Canadian Medical Association Journal, 182*(17), 1864–1873. https://doi.org/10.1503/cmaj.100771

Papaioannou, A., Santesso, N., Morin, S. N., et al. (2015). Recommendations for preventing fracture in long-term care. *Canadian Medical Association Journal, 187*(15), 1135–1144. https://doi.org/10.1503/cmaj.141331

Public Health Agency of Canada (PHAC). (2016). *You CAN prevent falls!.* https://www.canada.ca/en/public-health/services/health-promotion/aging-seniors/publications/publications-general-public/you-prevent-falls.html

Registered Nurses' Association of Ontario (RNAO). (2017). *Preventing fall and reducing injury form falls: Best practice guideline* (4th ed.). https://rnao.ca/bpg/guidelines/prevention-falls-and-fall-injuries

Sakamoto, R. R. (2019). Sunlight in vitamin D deficiency: Clinical implications. *The Journal for Nurse Practitioners, 15*(4), 282–285. https://doi.org/10.1016/j.nurpra.2019.01.014

Salzmann, S. N., Plais, N., Shue, J., et al. (2017). Lumbar disc replacement surgery—Successes and obstacles to widespread adoption. *Current Reviews in Musculoskeletal Medicine, 10*(2), 153–159. https://doi.org/10.1007/s12178-017-9397-4

Saragiotto, B. T., Maher, C. G., Yamato, T. P., et al. (2016). Motor control exercise for chronic non-specific low back pain. *The Cochrane Database of Systematic Reviews, 1,* CD012004. https://doi.org/10.1002/14651858.CD012004

Schmitt, S. K. (2017). Osteomyelitis. *Infectious Disease Clinics of North America, 31*(2), 325–338. https://doi.org/10.1016/j.idc.2017.01.010

Senneville, E. M., Lipsky, B. A., van Asten, S. A. V., et al. (2020). Diagnosing diabetic foot osteomyelitis. *Diabetes/Metabolism Research and Reviews, 36*(S1), e3250. https://doi-org.ezproxy.library.dal.ca/10.1002/dmrr.3250

Simpfendorfer, C. S. (2017). Radiological approach to musculoskeletal infections. *Infectious Disease Clinics of North America, 31*(2), 299–324. https://doi.org/10.1016/j.idc.2017.01.004

Singer, F. R. (2015). Paget's disease of bone—Genetic and environmental factors. *Nature Reviews. Endocrinology, 11*(11), 662–671. https://doi.org/10.1038/nrendo.2015.138

Statistics Canada. (2015). *Health at a glance—Vitamin D blood levels of Canadians.* http://www.statcan.gc.ca/pub/82-624-x/2013001/article/11727-eng.htm

Statistics Canada. (2021). *Table 13-10-0788-01: Chronic conditions among seniors aged 65 and older, Canadian Health Survey on Seniors.* https://doi.org/10.25318/1310078801-eng

Suh, J. H., Kim, H., Jung, G. P., et al. (2019). The effect of lumbar stabilization and walking exercises on chronic low back pain: A randomized controlled trial. *Medicine, 98*(26), e16173. https://doi.org/10.1097/MD.0000000000016173

Terry Fox Foundation. (2021). *Terry Fox and the foundation.* https://terryfox.org/

Thakolkaran, N., & Shetty, A. K. (2019). Acute hematogenous osteomyelitis in children. *Ochsner Journal, 19*(2), 116–122. https://doi.org/10.31486/toj.18.0138

Traeger, A., Buchbinder, R., Harris, I., et al. (2017). Diagnosis and management of low-back pain in primary care. *Canadian Medical Association Journal, 189*(45), E1386–E1395. https://doi.org/10.1503/cmaj.170527

Vatanparast, H. (2019). Vitamin D in summer: Sun. *food, supplement.* Osteoporosis Canada https://osteoporosis.ca/vitamin-d-in-summer-sun-food-supplement/

Wallace, M. T. (2020). Active and aggressive benign bone lesions in children and young adults. In M. T. Wallace, & F. J. Frassica (Eds.), *Handbook of musculoskeletal tumors* (pp. 91–104). SLACK Incorporated.

Williams, M., Temperley, D., & Murali, R. (2019). Radiology of the hand. *Orthopaedics and Trauma, 33*(1), 45–52. https://doi.org/10.1016/j.mporth.2018.11.006

Wu, P. H., Kim, H. S., & Jang, I.-T. (2020). Intervertebral disc diseases—Part 2: A review of the current diagnostic and treatment strategies for intervertebral disc disease. *International Journal of Molecular Sciences, 21*(6), 2135. https://doi.org/10.3390/ijms21062135

RESOURCES

Canadian Academy of Exercise and Sport Medicine
https://www.casm-acms.org
Canadian Cancer Society
https://www.cancer.ca/
Canadian Centre for Occupational Health and Safety
https://www.ccohs.ca
Canadian Orthopaedic Association
https://www.coa-aco.org
Canadian Orthopaedic Foot & Ankle Society
https://coa-aco.org/foot-ankle-cofas/
Canadian Orthopaedic Nurses Association
https://www.cona-nurse.org/
Canadian Podiatric Medical Association
https://www.podiatrycanada.org
Easter Seals Canada
https://www.easterseals.ca
Osteoporosis Canada
https://www.osteoporosis.ca

International Osteoporosis Foundation—Capture the Fracture
www.capturethefracture.org
National Association of Orthopaedic Nurses (NAON)
http://www.orthonurse.org
NIH Osteoporosis and Related Bone Diseases National Resource Center
https://www.niams.nih.gov/Health_Info/Bone

evolve
For additional Internet resources, see the website for this book at http://evolve.elsevier.com/Canada/Lewis/medsurg.

Nursing Management
Arthritis and Connective Tissue Diseases

Erica Cambly
Originating US chapter by Dottie Roberts

evolve WEBSITE

LEARNING OBJECTIVES

1. Outline the sequence of events leading to joint destruction in osteoarthritis and rheumatoid arthritis.
2. Detail the clinical manifestations and nursing management of osteoarthritis and rheumatoid arthritis and the interprofessional care for patients with osteoarthritis and rheumatoid arthritis.
3. Describe the pathophysiology, clinical manifestations, and interprofessional management of gout, Lyme disease, and septic arthritis.
4. Discuss the pathophysiology, clinical manifestations, and interprofessional and nursing management of ankylosing spondylitis, psoriatic arthritis, and reactive arthritis.

5. Differentiate the pathophysiology, clinical manifestations, interprofessional care, and nursing management related to systemic lupus erythematosus, scleroderma, myositis, and Sjögren syndrome.
6. Explain the medication therapy and related nursing management associated with arthritis and connective tissue diseases.
7. Relate possible causes, clinical manifestations, interprofessional care, and nursing management of fibromyalgia and systemic exertion tolerance disease.

KEY TERMS

ankylosing spondylitis (AS)
arthritis
CREST
dermatomyositis
fibromyalgia
gout
Lyme disease

myofascial pain syndrome
myositis
osteoarthritis (OA)
polymyositis
psoriatic arthritis
Raynaud's phenomenon
rheumatoid arthritis (RA)

scleroderma
septic arthritis
Sjögren syndrome
spondyloarthropathies
systemic exertion intolerance
    disease (SEID)
systemic lupus erythematosus (SLE)

This chapter discusses *rheumatic diseases,* which primarily affect body joints, tendons, ligaments, muscles, and bones. These diseases are often characterized by inflammation, pain, and loss of function in one or more of the body's connecting or supporting structures. The patient may be challenged by limited function and fatigue, loss of self-esteem, altered body image, and fear of disability. There are more than 100 kinds of rheumatic diseases, affecting approximately 6 million Canadians (Arthritis Society, 2021a).

ARTHRITIS

Arthritis involves inflammation of a joint or joints. Most forms of arthritis affect women more frequently than men (Arthritis Society, 2021a). Arthritic conditions may be up to 1.6 times more prevalent in Indigenous populations, and Indigenous people often experience higher rates of disability (Thurston et al., 2014). Osteoarthritis is the most common chronic condition of the joints. Other forms include rheumatoid arthritis, fibromyalgia, systemic lupus erythematosus, and gout.

OSTEOARTHRITIS

Osteoarthritis (OA) is a slowly progressive noninflammatory disorder of the diarthrodial (synovial) joints. Currently, OA affects more than 5 million Canadians, and the numbers are expected to increase greatly as the population ages (Arthritis Society, 2021c).

Etiology and Pathophysiology

OA involves the gradual loss of articular cartilage with formation of bony outgrowths (spurs or osteophytes) at the joint margins (Arthritis Society, 2021c). OA is not considered a normal part of the aging process, but aging is one risk factor for disease development (Arthritis Society, 2021c). Cartilage destruction may begin between ages 20 and 30 years and the majority of adults are affected by age 40. Few patients experience symptoms until after age 50 or 60, but more than half of those older than 65 years have radiographic evidence of the disease in at least one joint.

OA may be caused by a known event or condition that directly damages cartilage or causes joint instability (Table 67.1). However, for many persons with OA, no single cause may be identified. In these situations, various genetic traits may contribute to the development of cartilage defects.

Decreased estrogen at menopause may contribute to the increased incidence of OA in aging women. Obesity is a modifiable risk factor, which contributes to hip and knee OA. Regular moderate exercise, which also helps with weight control, decreases the risk for disease development and progression. Anterior cruciate ligament injury associated with quick stops and pivoting in some sports is linked to an increased risk for knee OA (Hunter & Bierma-Zeinstra, 2019). Occupations that require frequent kneeling and stooping also increase the risk for knee OA.

The development of OA is complex. Genetic, metabolic, and local factors interact and cause cartilage deterioration from damage at the level of the chondrocytes. OA results from cartilage damage that triggers a metabolic response at the level of the chondrocytes (Figure 67.1). The normally smooth, white, translucent articular cartilage becomes dull, yellow, and granular. Affected cartilage steadily becomes softer, less elastic, and less able to resist wear with heavy use.

TABLE 67.1	CAUSES OF OSTEOARTHRITIS
Cause	**Effects on Joint Cartilage**
Medications	Medications such as indomethacin, colchicine, and corticosteroids can stimulate collagen-digesting enzymes in joint synovium.
Hematological or endocrine disorders	Chronic hemarthrosis (e.g., hemophilia) can contribute to cartilage deterioration.
Inflammation	Release of enzymes in response to local inflammation can affect cartilage integrity.
Joint instability	Damage to supporting structures causes instability, placing uneven stress on articular cartilage.
Mechanical stress	Repetitive physical activities (e.g., sports) cause cartilage deterioration.
Neurological disorders	Pain and loss of reflexes from neurological disorders, such as diabetic neuropathy, and in Charcot's joint cause abnormal movements that contribute to cartilage deterioration.
Skeletal deformities	Congenital or acquired conditions such as Legg–Calvé–Perthes disease or dislocated hip contribute to cartilage deterioration.
Trauma	Dislocations or fractures may lead to avascular necrosis or uneven stress on cartilage.

The body's attempts at cartilage repair cannot keep up with the destruction. As the collagen structure in the cartilage changes, articular surfaces become cracked and worn. While central cartilage becomes thinner, cartilage at the joint edges becomes thicker and osteophytes form. Joint surfaces become uneven, affecting the distribution of stress across the joint and causing reduced motion.

Although inflammation is not characteristic of OA, secondary synovitis may occur when phagocytes try to rid the joint of small pieces of cartilage torn from the joint surface. These changes cause the early pain and stiffness of OA. Pain in later disease occurs when articular cartilage is lost, and bony joint surfaces rub against each other.

Clinical Manifestations

Joints. Joint pain is the predominant symptom and the typical reason that affected patients seek medical attention. Manifestations of OA range from mild discomfort to significant disability, and pain generally worsens with joint use. In early stages of OA, joint pain is relieved by rest. However, in advanced disease, patients may experience pain with rest or sleep disruptions caused by increasing joint discomfort.

As OA progresses, increasing pain can contribute significantly to disability and loss of function. The pain of OA may be referred to the groin, buttock, or outside of the thigh or knee. Sitting down becomes difficult, as does rising from a chair when the hips are lower than the knees. As OA develops in the intervertebral (apophyseal) joints of the spine, localized pain and stiffness are common.

Unlike pain, which typically worsens with activity, joint stiffness occurs after periods of rest or static position. Early morning stiffness is common but generally resolves within 30 minutes. This distinguishes OA from inflammatory joint disorders such as RA. Overactivity can cause a mild joint swelling that temporarily increases stiffness. *Crepitation*, a grating sensation caused by loose particles of cartilage in the joint cavity, can cause stiffness. Crepitation is common in patients with knee OA.

OA usually affects joints on one side of the body rather than in pairs. The distal interphalangeal (DIP) and proximal interphalangeal (PIP) joints of the fingers and the metacarpophalangeal (MCP) joint of the thumb are often affected. Weight-bearing joints (hips, knees), the metatarsophalangeal (MTP) joint of the foot, and the cervical and lower lumbar vertebrae are often involved (Figure 67.2).

Deformity. Deformity or instability associated with OA is specific to the involved joint. For example, *Heberden's nodes* occur on the DIP joints due to osteophyte formation and loss of joint space (see Figure 67.1). These nodes can appear in patients as early as age 40 and tend to be seen among family members. *Bouchard's nodes* on the PIP joints indicate similar disease involvement. Heberden's and Bouchard's nodes are often red, swollen, and tender. Although these bony enlargements do not usually cause significant loss of function, patients may be distressed by the visible disfigurement.

Knee OA often leads to obvious joint deformity due to cartilage loss in the joint compartment. For example, the patient becomes bow-legged (varus deformity) in response to medial joint arthritis. Lateral joint arthritis causes a knock-kneed appearance (valgus deformity). In advanced hip OA, one leg may become shorter as the joint space narrows.

Systemic. Fatigue, fever, and organ involvement are not present in OA. This is an important distinction between OA and inflammatory joint disorders such as RA.

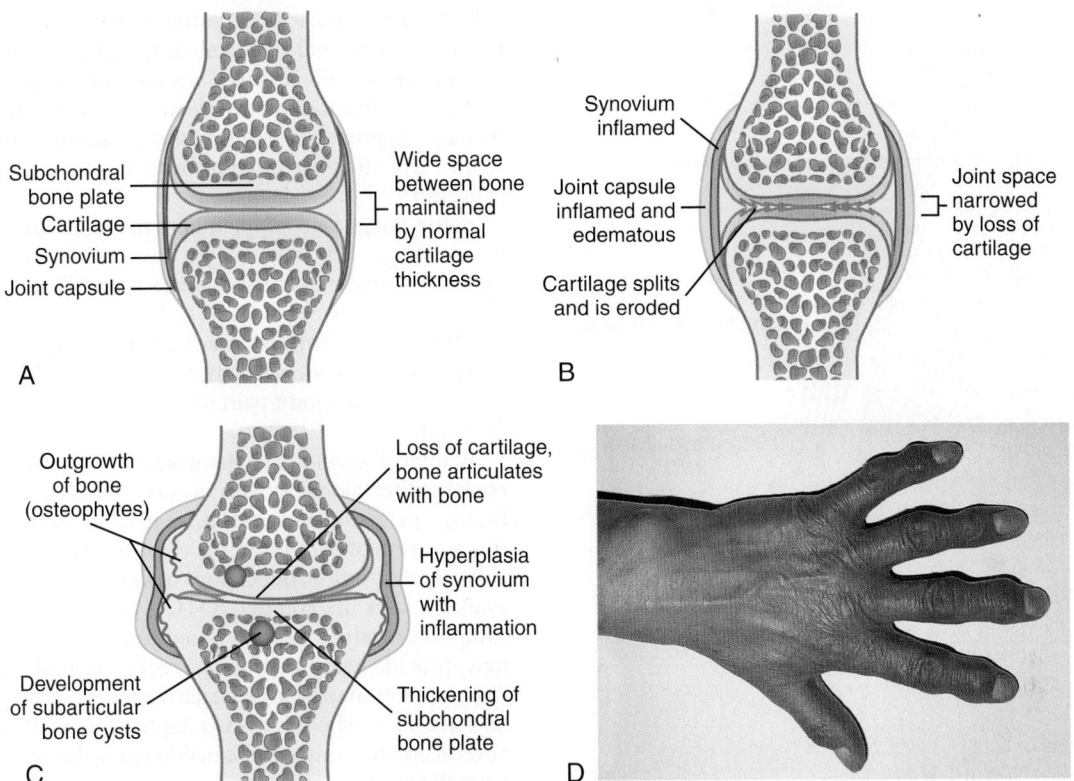

FIG. 67.1 Pathological changes in osteoarthritis. **A,** Healthy synovial joint. **B,** Early change in osteoarthritis is destruction of articular cartilage and narrowing of the joint space. Inflammation and thickening of the joint capsule and synovium occur. **C,** With time, thickening of subarticular bone is caused by constant friction of the two bone surfaces. Osteophytes form around the periphery of the joint by irregular outgrowths of bone. **D,** In osteoarthritis of the hands, osteophytes on the interphalangeal joints of the fingers, termed *Heberden nodes,* appear as small nodules. Source: D, Stevens, A., & Lowe, J. (2000). *Pathology: Illustrated review in colour* (2nd ed.). Mosby.

Diagnostic Studies

A bone scan, computed tomographic (CT) scan, or magnetic resonance imaging (MRI) may be used for diagnosing OA because of the sensitivity of these tests in detecting early joint changes. Radiological studies help confirm disease and stage of joint damage. As OA progresses, radiographs often show joint space narrowing and osteophyte formation. However, these changes do not always reflect the degree of pain that the patient experiences. Despite significant radiological indications of disease, a patient may be relatively free of symptoms. Another patient may have severe pain with only minimal radiographic changes.

No laboratory tests or biomarkers can be used to diagnose OA. The erythrocyte sedimentation rate (ESR) is normal except for slight increases during acute inflammation. Other routine blood tests (e.g., complete blood cell count [CBC], renal and liver function tests) are useful only in screening for related conditions or for establishing baseline values before the initiation of therapy. Synovial fluid analysis allows differentiation between OA and other forms of inflammatory arthritis. In OA, the fluid is clear yellow with little or no sign of inflammation.

Interprofessional Care

Because OA has no cure, interprofessional care focuses on managing pain and inflammation, preventing disability, and maintaining and improving joint function (Table 67.2). Nonpharmacological interventions are the foundation for OA management and should be maintained throughout a patient's treatment period. Medications supplement nonpharmacological treatments.

Rest and Joint Protection. Patients with OA should be taught to balance rest and activity. Rest of the affected joint is encouraged during periods of acute inflammation. Joints can be kept in a functional position with splints or braces if necessary. Immobilization should not exceed 1 week because of the risk for joint stiffness with inactivity. Patients may need to modify their usual activities to decrease stress on affected joints. The nurse should teach patients with knee OA to avoid prolonged periods of standing, kneeling, or squatting. Using an assistive device such as a cane, walker, or crutches can also help decrease stress on arthritic joints.

Heat and Cold Applications. Applications of heat and cold may help reduce pain and stiffness. Although ice is not used as often as heat in the treatment of OA, it can be appropriate if patients experience acute inflammation. Heat therapy—including hot packs, whirlpool baths, ultrasound, and paraffin wax baths—is especially helpful for stiffness.

Nutritional Therapy and Exercise. If a patient is overweight, a weight-reduction program is a critical part of the treatment plan. The nurse should help the patient evaluate the current diet to make appropriate changes. (Chapter 42 describes ways to assist patients in attaining and maintaining a healthy body weight.) Since mobilizing the joint preserves articular cartilage health, exercise is a fundamental part of OA management (Arthritis Society, 2021c). Aerobic conditioning, range-of-motion

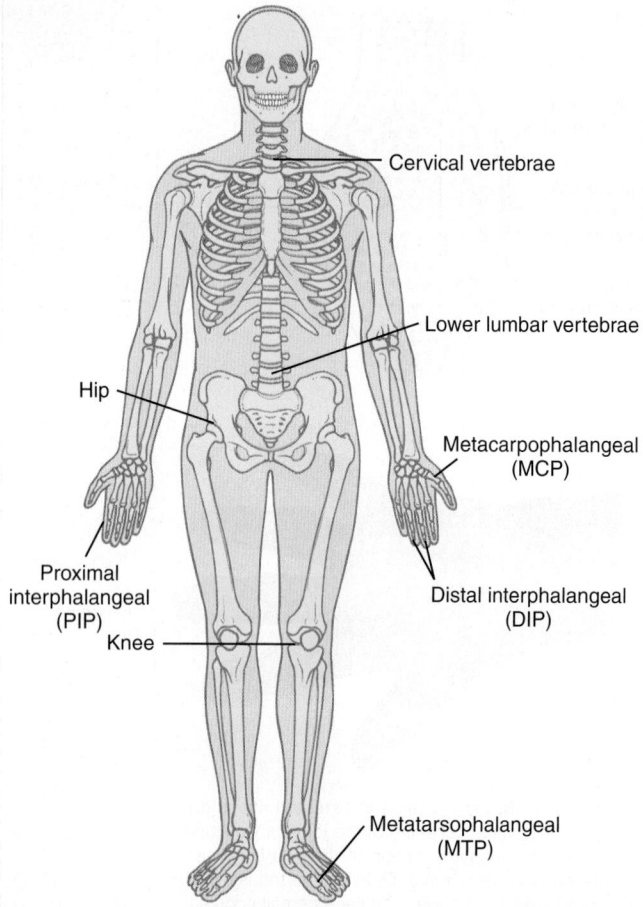

- Cervical vertebrae
- Lower lumbar vertebrae
- Hip
- Metacarpophalangeal (MCP)
- Proximal interphalangeal (PIP)
- Distal interphalangeal (DIP)
- Knee
- Metatarsophalangeal (MTP)

FIG. 67.2 Joints most frequently involved in osteoarthritis.

TABLE 67.2	INTERPROFESSIONAL CARE

Osteoarthritis

Diagnostic
- History and physical examination
- Radiological studies of involved joints (e.g. radiographs, CT scan, MRI, bone scan)
- Synovial fluid analysis

Interprofessional Therapy
- Nutritional and weight management counselling
- Rest and joint protection, use of assistive devices
- Therapeutic exercise
- Heat and cold applications
- Complementary and alternative therapies
  - Herbs and nutritional supplements (e.g., glucosamine)

- Movement therapies (e.g., yoga, tai chi)
- Transcutaneous electrical nerve stimulation (TENS)
- Acupuncture
- Medication therapy*
  - Acetaminophen
  - Nonsteroidal anti-inflammatory medications
  - Antibiotics
  - Intra-articular hyaluronic acid
  - Intra-articular corticosteroids
  - Opioid analgesics
  - Reconstructive joint surgery

CT, computed tomographic (scan); *MRI*, magnetic resonance imaging.
*See Table 67.3.

(ROM) exercises, and programs for strengthening the muscles around the affected joint have been beneficial for many patients.

Complementary and Alternative Therapies. Complementary and alternative therapies for symptom management of arthritis are popular with patients who have not found relief through traditional medical care. The nurse should teach patients to carefully research any alternative therapies and avoid replacing conventional OA treatments with unproven complementary approaches. Acupuncture, massage, and tai chi may reduce arthritic pain and improve joint mobility (Giannitrapani et al., 2019).

Some nutritional supplements may have anti-inflammatory effects (e.g., fish oil, ginger, turmeric/curcumin, SAM-e). (See the Complementary & Alternative Therapies box in this chapter.)

Medication Therapy. Medication therapy is based on the severity of the patient's symptoms (Table 67.3). Patients with mild to moderate joint pain may get relief from acetaminophen (Tylenol).

A topical agent such as capsaicin cream may also be beneficial, either alone or with acetaminophen. It blocks pain by locally interfering with substance P, which is responsible for the transmission of pain impulses. A concentrated product is available by prescription, but creams of 0.025 to 0.075% capsaicin are available over the counter (OTC). OTC products that contain camphor, eucalyptus oil, and menthol (e.g., BenGay, Arthricare) may provide temporary pain relief. Topical salicylates (e.g., Aspercreme) may be an alternative for patients who are able to take acetylsalicylic acid (ASA; Aspirin)–containing medication. Several applications may be needed daily because topical agents have short-acting effects.

If a patient does not obtain adequate pain management with acetaminophen, has moderate to severe OA pain, or has signs of joint inflammation, a non-steroidal anti-inflammatory drug (NSAID) may be more effective. NSAID therapy is typically initiated in low-dose OTC strengths (e.g., ibuprofen [Motrin, Advil]) of 200 mg, up to four times daily. The dosage may be increased if needed. If a patient is at risk for or develops gastrointestinal (GI) effects with an NSAID, adding a protective agent such as misoprostol (Cytotec) may be indicated. Arthrotec, a combination of misoprostol and the NSAID diclofenac, is also available. Diclofenac gel may be applied to the affected joint. The patient who is taking an oral NSAID should be taught to avoid the use of a topical NSAID because of increased risk of adverse effects.

🌿 **COMPLEMENTARY & ALTERNATIVE THERAPIES**

Tai Chi

Tai chi is an ancient Chinese tradition that is a form of exercise combining yoga and meditation. It involves a series of movements preformed in a slow, focused manner.

Scientific Evidence*
- Tai chi brought short-term improvements in pain and stiffness in knee OA.
- Some studies found improved balance or decreased depression.
- In a study comparing tai chi to physiotherapy, patients in both groups had improved pain for a full year.
- Temporary increase of knee pain may occur in patients with knee OA.

Nursing Implications
- Tai chi is generally considered to be a safe practice.
- Avoid overuse of affected joints.

*Source: National Center for Complementary and Integrative Health. (2016). *Osteoarthritis: in depth.* https://www.nccih.nih.gov/health/osteoarthritis-in-depth

TABLE 67.3   MEDICATION THERAPY
Arthritis and Connective Tissue Disorders

Medication	Mechanism of Action	Adverse Effects	Nursing Considerations
Salicylates ASA (Aspirin, Asaphen)	Analgesic Anti-inflammatory Antipyretic Inhibits prostaglandin synthesis	Exacerbation of asthma (ASA [Aspirin]-sensitive asthma) GI irritation (dyspepsia, nausea, ulcer, hemorrhage) Prolonged bleeding time Tinnitus, dizziness with repeated large doses	Administer medication with food, milk, antacids as prescribed, or full glass of water; enteric-coated. ASA (Aspirin) may be administered. Report signs of bleeding (e.g., tarry stools, bruising, petechiae, nosebleeds).
Nonsteroidal Anti-Inflammatory Drugs (NSAIDs) Celecoxib (Celebrex) Diclofenac (Voltaren) Ibuprofen (Motrin, Advil) Indomethacin Ketoprofen Ketorolac tromethamine (Toradol) Meloxicam (Mobicox) Nabumetone (Apo-Nabumetone) Naproxen (Naprosyn, Aleve) Piroxicam (Teva-Piroxicam) Sulindac (Teva-Sulindac)	Analgesic Anti-inflammatory Antipyretic Inhibits prostaglandin synthesis	Acute renal insufficiency and other renal medullary changes Exacerbation of asthma (cross-reactivity with ASA [Aspirin]) GI irritation (dyspepsia, nausea, ulcer, hemorrhage) Headache, tinnitus Prolonged bleeding time Rash	Administer medication with food, milk, or antacids as prescribed. Report signs of bleeding (e.g., tarry stools, bruising, petechiae, nosebleeds), edema, skin rashes, persistent headaches, visual disturbances. Monitor BP for elevations related to fluid retention. Medication must be administered regularly for maximal effect.
Antibiotics Doxycycline Minocycline	Antirheumatic effect, possibly related to immunomodulatory or anti-inflammatory properties Decreases action of enzymes on cartilage degradation	Dizziness GI effects (nausea and vomiting, diarrhea, stomach cramps) Monilial vaginitis, sensitivity to direct sunlight or ultraviolet light, nonspecific GI irritation Photosensitivity (severe)	This is a possible treatment alternative for mild disease.
Topical Analgesics Capsaicin cream	Depletes substance P from nerve endings, interrupting pain signals to the brain	Erythema Localized burning sensation Rash Urticaria	Medication must be administered regularly over time for maximal effect. Aloe vera cream may modify burning sensation. Advise patient not to use cream with external heat source (heating pad) because of risk for burns. Available in OTC and prescription strengths.
Diclofenac diethylamine (Voltaren Emulgel)	Anti-inflammatory Analgesic	Adverse GI effects similar to those of systemic NSAIDs Skin irritation	Advise patient to avoid sun and ultraviolet exposure. Medication should not be used in combination with other oral NSAIDs or ASA (Aspirin) because of potential for increased adverse effects.
Corticosteroids ***Intra-Articular Injections*** Methylprednisolone acetate (Depo-Medrol) Triamcinolone	Analgesic Anti-inflammatory Inhibit synthesis and release of mediators of inflammation	Dermal or subdermal changes leading to depression at injection site Local osteoporosis Neuropathic arthropathy from frequent injection Possibility of local infection Tendon rupture	Use strict aseptic technique for joint fluid aspiration or corticosteroid injection. Inform patient that joint may feel worse immediately after injection. Inform patient that improvement lasts weeks to months after injection. Advise patient to avoid overusing affected joint after injection.

Continued

TABLE 67.3 MEDICATION THERAPY

Arthritis and Connective Tissue Disorders—cont'd

Medication	Mechanism of Action	Adverse Effects	Nursing Considerations
Systemic Dexamethasone (Apo-dexamethasone) Hydrocortisone sodium succinate (Cortef) Methylprednisolone sodium succinate (Solu-Medrol) Prednisone Triamcinolone	Analgesic Anti-inflammatory Inhibit synthesis and release of mediators of inflammation	Acne Bruising Cushing's syndrome (including fluid retention) Diabetes mellitus GI irritation Hirsutism Hypertension Insomnia Menstrual irregularities Osteoporosis Risk for antibiotic-resistant infection Steroid psychosis	Use only in life-threatening exacerbation or when symptoms persist after treatment with less potent anti-inflammatory medications. Administer for limited time only, tapering dose slowly. Be aware that symptom exacerbation occurs with abrupt withdrawal of medication. Monitor BP, weight, CBC, and potassium level. Limit sodium intake. Have patient report signs of infection to health care provider.
Disease-Modifying Antirheumatic Drugs (DMARDs) Methotrexate	Antimetabolite Inhibits DNA, RNA, and protein synthesis	Hepatotoxicity (occurs more often with frequent small doses than with large intermittent doses); symptoms related to medication's antineoplastic activity (e.g., GI and skin toxicity, bone marrow depression, neuropathy); smaller dose and different administration schedule for RA decrease likelihood that these adverse effects will develop	Monitor CBC and hepatic and renal function. Advise patient to report signs of anemia (fatigue, weakness). Keep patient well hydrated. Because of teratogenic potential, medication should not be administered to children or women of childbearing age. Inform patient that contraception should be used during and for 3 months after treatment.
Sulphasalazine (Salazopyrin)	Anti-inflammatory Blocks prostaglandin synthesis Sulphonamide	Bleeding, bruising, jaundice GI effects (anorexia, nausea and vomiting) Headache Rash, urticaria, pruritus	Advise patient that medication may cause orange-yellow discoloration of urine or skin. Space doses evenly around the clock, administering medication with 250 mL water after meals. Treatment may be continued even after symptoms are relieved. Monitor CBC.
Leflunomide (Arava)	Anti-inflammatory Immunomodulatory agent that inhibits proliferation of lymphocytes	Alopecia Diarrhea Hepatotoxicity (especially if patient is also taking methotrexate or has history of prior alcohol abuse) Nausea Rash Respiratory tract infection	Evaluate for relief of pain, swelling, and stiffness and for increase in joint mobility. Advise women of childbearing age to avoid pregnancy.
D-penicillamine (Cuprimine)	Anti-inflammatory Exact mechanism of action in RA unknown, but may suppress cell-mediated immune response	GI irritation (nausea and vomiting, anorexia, diarrhea) Iron deficiency (especially in menstruating women) Proteinuria, hematuria Rash Reduced or altered taste	Monitor WBCs, platelets, urinalysis. Advise patient to take medication 1 hr before or 2 hr after meals or at least 1 hr before or after any other medication, food, or milk. Advise women of childbearing age to avoid pregnancy.
Gold Compounds Oral (auranofin [Ridaura]) Parenteral (gold sodium aurothiomalate [Myochrysine])	Alters immune responses, suppressing synovitis of active RA Antirheumatic	Decreased hemoglobin Leukopenia, thrombocytopenia Proteinuria, hematuria Stomatitis	Rule out pregnancy before beginning treatment. Monitor CBC, urinalysis, and hepatic and renal function. Advise patient that therapeutic response may not occur for 3 to 6 mo. Advise patient to immediately report pruritus, rash, sore mouth, indigestion, or metallic taste.

TABLE 67.3   MEDICATION THERAPY
Arthritis and Connective Tissue Disorders—cont'd

Medication	Mechanism of Action	Adverse Effects	Nursing Considerations
Antimalarials Hydroxychloroquine (Plaquenil)	Antirheumatic action unknown, but may suppress formation of antigens	Ocular toxicity (retinopathy) may progress even after medication is discontinued. Ototoxicity Peripheral neuritis, neuromyopathy, hypotension, electrocardiographic changes with prolonged therapy	Monitor CBC and hepatic function. Advise patient that therapeutic response may not occur for up to 6 mo. Advise patient to immediately report visual difficulties, muscular weakness, and decreased hearing or tinnitus.
Immunosuppressants Azathioprine (Imuran) Cyclophosphamide (Procytox)	Inhibit DNA, RNA, and protein synthesis	GI irritation (nausea and vomiting; anorexia with large doses) Rash	Evaluate for relief of pain, swelling, and stiffness and for increase in joint mobility. Advise patient to immediately report unusual bleeding or bruising. Advise patient that therapeutic response may take up to 12 wk. Advise women of childbearing age to avoid pregnancy.
JAK (Janus Kinase) Inhibitors Tofacitinib (Xeljanz)	Inhibits action of the JAK enzymes, which are signaling pathways inside the cell and have an important role in the inflammation involved in RA		Patients are at increased risk for serious infections, including opportunistic infections. Monitor patient for any sign or symptom of infection so it can be treated early.
Biological and Targeted Therapies ***Tumour Necrosis Factor (TNF) Inhibitors*** Adalimumab (Humira) Certolizumab (Cimzia) Etanercept (Enbrel) Golimumab (Simponi) Infliximab (Remicade)	Bind to TNF, blocking its interaction with TNF cell surface receptors to decrease inflammatory and immune responses	Abdominal pain, vomiting Dizziness, headache Injection site reaction including erythema, pain, itching, swelling Rhinitis, pharyngitis, cough	Evaluate for relief of pain, swelling, and stiffness and for increase in joint mobility. Advise patient of increased risk for tuberculosis (TB). Advise patient to have yearly TB skin test. Monitor for infection, bleeding, and emergence of malignancies. Advise patient that psoriasis may worsen. Advise patient that injection site reaction generally occurs in first month of treatment and decreases with continued therapy. Advise patient not to receive live-virus vaccines during treatment.
Interleukin-1 Receptor Antagonist Anakinra (Kineret)	Blocks action of interleukin-1 and thus decreases the inflammatory response	Abdominal pain Headache Injection site reaction Leukopenia Rash	Evaluate for relief of pain, swelling, and stiffness and for increase in joint mobility. Advise patient that injection site reaction generally occurs during first month of treatment and decreases with continued therapy. Evaluate renal function. Monitor for infection. Do not administer medication with other TNF inhibitors.
Interleukin-6 Receptor Antagonist Tocilizumab (Actemra)	Blocks action of interleukin-6	↑ BP ↑ liver enzyme levels Headache Inflammation of nose or nasal passage Upper respiratory tract infections	Administered to patients with RA in whom other therapies have failed. Monitor BP and for infection. Advise patient of adverse GI effects (e.g., perforation). Monitor liver enzyme and LDL levels.

Continued

TABLE 67.3 MEDICATION THERAPY

Arthritis and Connective Tissue Disorders—cont'd

Medication	Mechanism of Action	Adverse Effects	Nursing Considerations
T-Cell Activation Inhibitor			
Abatacept (Orencia)	Modulates T-cell activation; suppresses immune response	Headache Injection site reaction Nausea Sore throat Upper respiratory infection	Not recommended for concomitant use with TNF inhibitors. Evaluate for relief of pain, swelling, and stiffness and for increase in joint mobility.
B-Cell Depleting Agent			
Rituximab (Rituxan)	Monoclonal antibody that targets B cells	Difficulty breathing Dizziness Fever Itching Palpitations Sore throat	Administer in combination with methotrexate. Monitor for infection and bleeding. Advise patient to not receive live-virus vaccines during treatment. Monitor for low BP if patient is also taking antihypertensives.
Tocilizumab (Actemra)	Blocks action of interleukin-6	↑ BP ↑ Liver enzyme levels Headache Inflammation of nose or nasal passage Upper respiratory tract infections	Administered to patients with RA in whom other therapies have failed. Monitor BP and for infection. Advise patient of adverse GI effects (e.g., perforation). Monitor liver enzyme and LDL levels.

BP, blood pressure; *CBC*, complete blood cell count; *GI*, gastrointestinal; *LDL*, low-density lipoprotein; *OTC*, over-the-counter; *RA*, rheumatoid arthritis; *TNF-α*, tumour necrosis factor–alpha; *WBC*, white blood cell.

All NSAIDs inhibit the production of cyclo-oxygenase–1 (COX-1) and cyclo-oxygenase–2 (COX-2). These enzymes convert arachidonic acid into prostaglandins. Inhibiting COX-1 causes many of the untoward effects of NSAIDs, including the risk for bleeding and GI irritation (Bannuru et al., 2019). Patients taking an anticoagulant (e.g., warfarin [Coumadin]) and an NSAID are at high risk of bleeding. Long-term NSAID treatment may affect cartilage metabolism, especially in older patients, who may have poor cartilage integrity. As an alternative to traditional NSAIDs, treatment with the COX-2 inhibitor celecoxib (Celebrex) may be considered in patients with a low risk of cardiovascular complications.

When given in equivalent dosages, all NSAIDs are considered comparably effective but vary widely in cost. Individual responses to NSAIDs also vary. Some patients still prefer ASA (Aspirin), but it is no longer a common treatment. It should be used with caution when used with NSAIDs because both inhibit platelet function and prolong bleeding time. Intra-articular injections of corticosteroids may be needed for patients with local inflammation and swelling. Four or more injections without relief suggest the need for additional intervention. Systemic use of corticosteroids is not indicated and may actually accelerate the disease process.

Injection of hyaluronic acid (*viscosupplementation*) has been a common treatment of knee OA. However, its effectiveness is not clear (Arthritis Society, 2021c). Research on the long-term effects continues.

Medications thought to slow the progression of OA or support joint healing are known as *disease-modifying osteoarthritis drugs (DMOADs)*. To date, no medications have been approved to modify OA progression, despite numerous clinical trials. A variety of molecular targets are under investigation, including the use of anticatabolic agents to stimulate new cartilage growth and slow OA progression (Bannuru et al., 2019).

Surgical Therapy. Symptoms of disease are often managed conservatively for many years, but the patient's loss of joint function and unrelieved pain may lead to consideration of surgery. Patients with knee OA used to undergo arthroscopy to remove loose bodies from the joint. However, it may not have any benefit over physiotherapy and medical treatment (Arthritis Society, 2021c). Reconstructive surgical procedures (e.g., hip and knee replacements) are discussed in Chapter 65.

NURSING MANAGEMENT OSTEOARTHRITIS

NURSING ASSESSMENT

The nurse should carefully assess and document the type, location, severity, frequency, and duration of the patient's joint pain and stiffness and the extent to which these symptoms affect the ability to perform activities of daily living (ADLs). The nurse should review the patient's pain management practices and question the patient about the duration and success of each treatment. Tenderness, swelling, limitation of movement, and crepitation of affected joints should be assessed. The nurse can compare an involved joint with the contralateral joint if it is not affected.

NURSING DIAGNOSES

Nursing diagnoses for patients with OA may include but are not limited to the following:

- *Acute and chronic pain* resulting from *painful physical activity, disease process*

- *Reduced physical mobility* resulting from *activity intolerance, decrease in muscle strength, joint stiffness*
- *Difficulty coping* resulting from *inadequate confidence in ability to cope with situation*

PLANNING

The overall goals are that patients with OA will (a) maintain or improve joint function through a balance of rest and activity, (b) use joint protection measures (Table 67.4) to improve activity tolerance, (c) achieve independence in self-care and maintain optimal role function, and (d) use pharmacological and non-pharmacological strategies to manage pain satisfactorily.

NURSING IMPLEMENTATION

HEALTH PROMOTION. Prevention of OA is possible in some cases. Community education should focus on altering modifiable risk factors. The patient should be encouraged to maintain a healthy weight, eat a balanced diet, exercise regularly (including strength and endurance training), and avoid cigarette smoking. Occupational or recreational hazards should be reduced, and athletic instruction and physical fitness programs should include safety measures that protect and reduce trauma to the joints. Traumatic joint injuries should be treated promptly to decrease the risk of OA.

ACUTE INTERVENTION. Patients with OA are usually treated on an outpatient basis, often by an interprofessional team of health care providers that includes a primary health care provider, a rheumatologist, a nurse, an occupational therapist, and a physiotherapist. Often, health assessment questionnaires are used to pinpoint areas of decreased function. Questionnaires are repeated at regular intervals to document disease and treatment progression. Treatment goals can be developed on the basis of data from the questionnaires and the physical examination, with specific interventions to target identified problems. Usually, patients are hospitalized only if joint surgery is planned (see Chapter 65).

Medications are administered for the treatment of pain and inflammation. Nonpharmacological strategies to decrease pain and disability may include massage, the application of heat (thermal packs) or cold (ice packs), relaxation, tai chi, and yoga (Arthritis Society, 2021c). Splints may be prescribed to rest and stabilize painful or inflamed joints.

Once an acute flare has subsided, a physiotherapist can provide valuable assistance in planning an exercise program. The nurse should stress the importance of warming up before any exercise to decrease risk for injury.

Patient and caregiver teaching related to OA is an important nursing responsibility. The nurse needs to provide information about the nature and treatment of the disease, pain management, correct posture and body mechanics, correct use of assistive devices such as a cane or walker, principles of joint protection and energy conservation (see Table 67.4), nutritional choices and weight and stress management, and an exercise program.

The nurse should assure the patient that OA is a localized disease and that severe deforming arthritis is not the usual course. Patients can also obtain support and understanding of the disease process through community resources such as the Arthritis Society's Online Learning Modules (Arthritis Society, 2021b).

AMBULATORY AND HOME CARE. Home management goals should be individualized to meet the patient's needs. The caregiver, family members, and significant others should be included in goal setting and teaching. The nurse needs to discuss home and work environment modification for patient safety, accessibility, and self-care. Measures include removing throw rugs, providing rails at stairs and bathtub, using nightlights, and wearing well-fitting supportive shoes. Assistive devices such as canes, walkers, elevated toilet seats, and grab bars reduce the load on the affected joint(s) and promote safety. The nurse needs to assess access to health care services, medical equipment, and pharmacotherapeutics particularly when working with Indigenous patients in urban, rural, and remote locations. Patients should be urged to continue all prescribed therapies at home and be open to new approaches to symptom management.

Sexual counselling may help the patient and their partner enjoy physical closeness by introducing the idea of alternate positions and timing for sexual activity. Discussion also increases awareness of each partner's needs. The nurse should encourage the patient to take analgesics or a warm bath to decrease joint stiffness before sexual activity.

EVALUATION

The expected outcomes are that the patient with OA will:
- Experience adequate rest and activity
- Achieve acceptable pain management
- Maintain joint flexibility and muscle strength through joint protection and therapeutic exercise

RHEUMATOID ARTHRITIS

Rheumatoid arthritis (RA) is a chronic, systemic autoimmune disease characterized by inflammation of connective tissue in the diarthrodial (synovial) joints. It is the most common chronic inflammatory joint disease (Widdifield et al., 2015). RA is typically marked by periods of remission and exacerbation and is frequently accompanied by extra-articular manifestations. RA has long been considered one of the most disabling forms of arthritis. Symptoms and outcomes can vary greatly. Without adequate treatment, patients may need mobility aids or joint reconstruction. They may have loss of independence and self-care ability.

RA occurs globally, affecting all ethnic groups. It can occur at any time of life, but incidence increases with age, peaking between ages 30 and 50. An estimated 300 000 Canadians are affected by RA. The disease affects two to three times as many

TABLE 67.4	**PATIENT & CAREGIVER TEACHING GUIDE**

Joint Protection and Energy Conservation

The following should be included when teaching patients with arthritis how to protect joints and conserve energy:
- Avoid forceful repetitive movements.
- Avoid positions of joint deviation and stress.
- Develop organizing and pacing techniques for routine tasks.
- Maintain appropriate weight.
- Modify home and work environment to create less stressful ways to perform tasks.
- Seek assistance with necessary tasks that may cause pain.
- Use assistive devices, if indicated.
- Use good posture and proper body mechanics.

women as men (Arthritis Society, 2017a). Indigenous patients may have higher disease activity and a lower incidence of remission when compared to non-Indigenous patients (Barnabe et al., 2018).

Etiology and Pathophysiology

Although the exact cause of RA is unknown, it likely results from a combination of genetics and environmental triggers. An autoimmune etiology that is currently the most widely accepted theory suggests that changes associated with RA begin when a genetically susceptible person has an initial immune response to an antigen. Although a bacterium or virus has been proposed as a possible antigen, to date, no infection or organism has been identified.

The antigen, which is probably not the same in all affected patients, triggers the formation of an abnormal immunoglobulin G (IgG). RA is characterized by the presence of autoantibodies against this abnormal IgG. The autoantibodies, known as *rheumatoid factor* (RF), combine with IgG to form immune complexes that initially deposit on synovial membranes or superficial articular cartilage in the joints. Immune complex formation leads to the activation of complement and to an inflammatory response. (Complement activation is discussed in Chapter 14, and immune complex formation is discussed in Chapter 16.)

Neutrophils are attracted to the site of inflammation, where they release proteolytic enzymes that damage articular cartilage and cause the synovial lining to thicken (Figure 67.3). Other

inflammatory cells include T helper (CD4) cells, which stimulate cell-mediated immune responses. Activated CD4 cells stimulate monocytes, macrophages, and synovial fibroblasts to secrete the proinflammatory cytokines interleukin-1 (IL-1), interleukin-6 (IL-6), and tumour necrosis factor (TNF). These cytokines drive the inflammatory response in RA.

Genetic Factors. Genetic predisposition is important in the development of RA. The strongest evidence for a genetic influence is the role of human leukocyte antigens (HLA), especially the HLA-DR4 and HLA-DR1 antigens. Smoking increases the risk for RA for people who are genetically predisposed to the disease and may make successful treatment more difficult (Arthritis Society, 2021d).

Clinical Manifestations

Joints. The onset of RA is typically subtle. Nonspecific manifestations such as fatigue, anorexia, weight loss, and generalized stiffness may precede the onset of joint symptoms. Stiffness becomes more localized in the following weeks to months.

Specific joint involvement is marked by pain, stiffness, limitation of motion, and signs of inflammation such as heat, swelling, and tenderness. Joint symptoms occur symmetrically and frequently affect the small joints of the hands (PIP and MCP joints) and feet (MTP joints). Larger peripheral joints such as wrists, elbows, shoulders, knees, hips, ankles, and the jaw may also be involved. The cervical spine may be affected, but the axial skeleton (the spine and the bones connected to

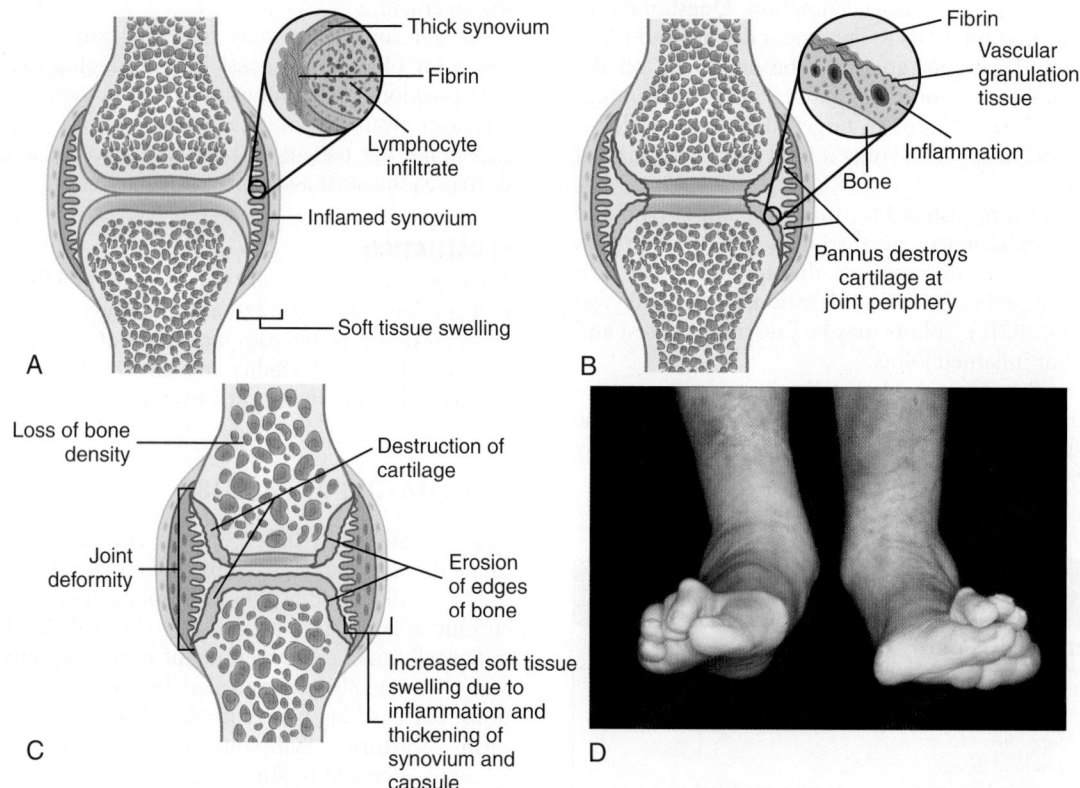

FIG. 67.3 Rheumatoid arthritis. **A,** Early pathological change in rheumatoid arthritis is rheumatoid synovitis. The synovium is inflamed. Lymphocytes and plasma cells increase greatly. **B,** With time, articular cartilage destruction occurs, vascular granulation tissue grows across the surface of the cartilage (pannus) from the edges of the joint, and the articular surface shows loss of cartilage beneath the extending pannus, most marked at the joint margins. **C,** Inflammatory pannus causes focal destruction of bone. At the edges of the joint, there is osteolytic destruction of bone, responsible for erosions seen on radiographs. This phase is associated with joint deformity. **D,** Multiple deformities of the foot associated with rheumatoid arthritis. Source: *D*, Canale, S. T., & Beaty, J. H. (2013). *Campbell's operative orthopaedics* (12th ed.). Mosby.

it) is generally spared. Table 67.5 compares features of RA and OA.

Patients characteristically experience joint stiffness after periods of inactivity. Morning stiffness may last from 60 minutes to several hours or more, depending on disease activity. MCP and PIP joints are typically swollen. In early disease, the fingers may become spindle-shaped from synovial hypertrophy and thickening of the joint capsule (see Figure 67.3). Joints become tender, painful, and warm to the touch. Joint pain increases with motion, varies in intensity, and may not be proportional to the degree of inflammation. Tenosynovitis frequently affects the extensor and flexor tendons around the wrists, producing manifestations of carpal tunnel syndrome and making it difficult for patients to grasp objects.

As the disease progresses, inflammation and fibrosis of the joint capsule and supporting structures may lead to deformity and disability. Muscle atrophy and tendon destruction cause one joint surface to slip past the other (*subluxation*). Metatarsal head dislocation and subluxation in the feet may cause pain and walking disability. Ulnar drift ("zigzag deformity"),

swan-neck, and boutonnière deformities are common in the hands (Figure 67.4).

Extra-articular Manifestations. RA can affect nearly every system in the body (Figure 67.5). Extra-articular manifestations are more likely to occur in people with high levels of biomarkers such as RF.

Rheumatoid nodules develop in 20% of all patients with RA (Arthritis Society, 2017a). Rheumatoid nodules appear subcutaneously as firm, nontender masses. They are often found on bony areas exposed to pressure, such as fingers and elbows. Nodules at the base of the spine and the back of the head are common in older persons. Treatment is usually not needed. However, these nodules can break down, like pressure injuries. Cataracts and vision loss can result from scleral nodules. Nodular myositis and muscle fiber degeneration can cause pain like that of vascular insufficiency. In later disease, nodules in the heart and lungs can cause pleurisy, pleural effusion, pericarditis, pericardial effusion, and cardiomyopathy.

Sjögren syndrome can occur by itself or with other arthritic disorders such as RA and systemic lupus erythematosus (SLE). The inflammation of RA can damage the tear-producing (lacrimal) glands, making the eyes feel dry and gritty (Arthritis Society, 2017h). Affected patients may have photosensitivity. (Sjögren syndrome is discussed later in this chapter [see Sjögren Syndrome].)

Felty's syndrome is rare but can occur in those with long-standing RA. It is characterized by an enlarged spleen and low white blood cell (WBC) count. Patients with Felty's syndrome are at increased risk for infection and lymphoma (Arthritis Society, 2020).

Flexion contractures and hand deformities cause decreased grip strength and affect the patient's ability to perform self-care tasks. The patient may experience depression. However, it is unclear if the patient becomes depressed from struggling with chronic pain and disability or if depression is part of the autoimmune disease process. Levels of C-reactive protein (CRP), a marker of inflammation, are higher in patients with depression than in those with no symptoms of depression (Chamberlain et al., 2019).

TABLE 67.5   COMPARISON OF RHEUMATOID ARTHRITIS AND OSTEOARTHRITIS

Parameter	Rheumatoid Arthritis	Osteoarthritis
Affected joints	Small joints first (PIP, MCP, and MTP joints), wrists, elbows, shoulders, knees; usually bilateral, symmetrical joint involvement	Weight-bearing joints (knees, hips); small joints (MCP, DIP, and PIP); cervical and lumbar spine; often asymmetrical
Age at onset	Young to middle age	Usually >40 yr of age
Disease	Systemic disease with exacerbations and remissions	Localized disease with variable, progressive course
Effusions	Common	Uncommon
Gender	Female-to-male ratio is 2:1 or 3:1; less marked difference after age 60	Before age 50, more men than women; after age 50, more women than men
Laboratory findings	RF positive in 80% of patients. Elevated ESR and CRP level indicative of active inflammation	RF negative. Transient elevation in ESR related to synovitis
Nodules	Present, especially on extensor surfaces	Heberden nodes (DIP joints) and Bouchard nodes (PIP joints)
Pain characteristics	Stiffness lasts from 1 hr to all day and may decrease with use; pain is variable, may disrupt sleep	Stiffness occurs on arising but usually subsides after 30 min; pain gradually worsens with joint use and disease progression, relieved with rest
Radiographs	Joint space narrowing, erosion, subluxation with advanced disease; osteoporosis related to corticosteroid use	Joint space narrowing, osteophytes, subchondral cysts, sclerosis
Synovial fluid	WBC count >2 × 10⁹/L with mostly neutrophils	WBC count <2 × 10⁹/L (mild leukocytosis)
Weight	Lost or maintained weight	Often overweight

CRP, C-reactive protein; *DIP*, distal interphalangeal; *ESR*, erythrocyte sedimentation rate; *MCP*, metacarpophalangeal; *MTP*, metatarsophalangeal; *PIP*, proximal interphalangeal; *RF*, rheumatoid factor; *WBC*, white blood cell.

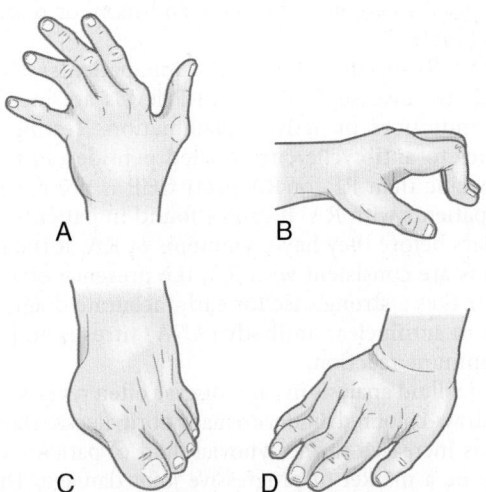

FIG. 67.4 Typical deformities of rheumatoid arthritis. **A,** Ulnar drift. **B,** Boutonnière deformity. **C,** Hallux valgus. **D,** Swan-neck deformity.

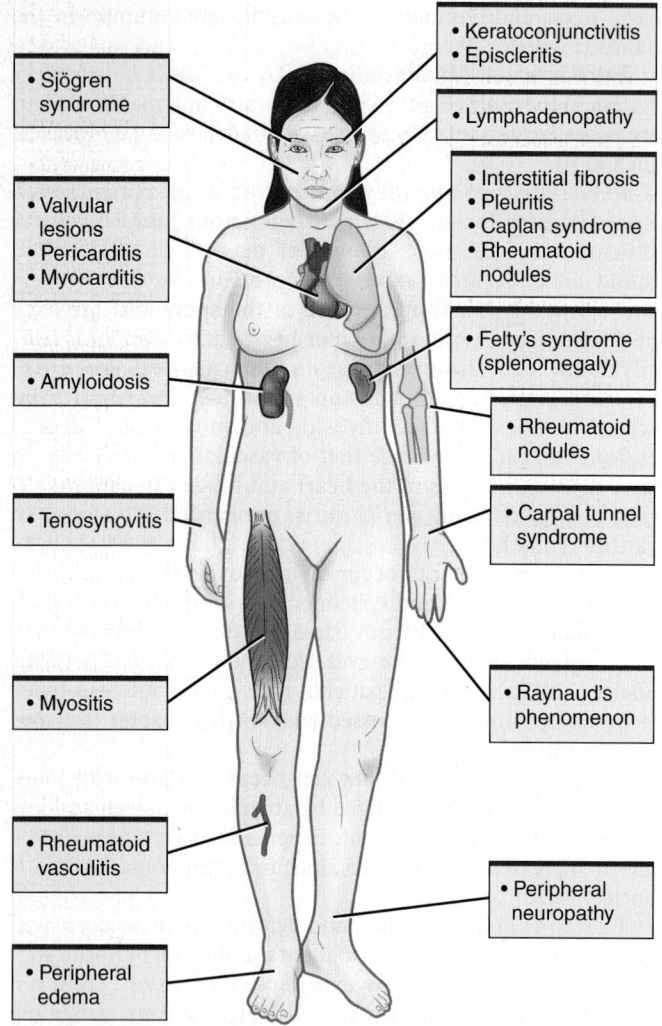

- Sjögren syndrome
- Keratoconjunctivitis
- Episcleritis
- Lymphadenopathy
- Valvular lesions
- Pericarditis
- Myocarditis
- Interstitial fibrosis
- Pleuritis
- Caplan syndrome
- Rheumatoid nodules
- Amyloidosis
- Felty's syndrome (splenomegaly)
- Rheumatoid nodules
- Tenosynovitis
- Carpal tunnel syndrome
- Myositis
- Raynaud's phenomenon
- Rheumatoid vasculitis
- Peripheral neuropathy
- Peripheral edema

FIG. 67.5 Extra-articular manifestations of rheumatoid arthritis.

TABLE 67.6 DIAGNOSTIC CRITERIA FOR RHEUMATOID ARTHRITIS

Patients should be tested for RA if they are initially seen with the following signs:
- At least one joint with definite clinical synovitis
- Synovitis not better explained by another disease

Criterion	Score*
A. Joint Involvement	
1 large joint	0
2–10 large joints	1
1–3 small joints (with or without involvement of large joints)	2
4–10 small joints (with or without involvement of large joints)	3
>10 joints (at least 1 small joint)	5
B. Serology (at Least One Test Result Needed)	
Negative RF and negative ACPA	0
Low-positive RF or low-positive ACPA	2
High-positive RF or high-positive ACPA	3
C. Acute-Phase Reactants (at Least One Test Result Needed)	
Normal CRP and normal ESR	0
Abnormal CRP or abnormal ESR	1
D. Duration of Symptoms	
<6 weeks	0
≥6 weeks	1

ACPA, anti-citrullinated peptide antibodies; *CRP,* C-reactive protein; *ESR,* erythrocyte sedimentation rate; *RF,* rheumatoid factor.
*Scoring: Add score of categories A–D. Possible scores range from 0 to 10. A score of ≥6 indicates the definitive presence of RA.
Source: Aletaha, D., Neogi, T., Silman, A., et al. (2010). 2010 rheumatoid arthritis classification criteria. *Arthritis and Rheumatism, 62*(9), 2569–2581. https://doi.org/10.1002/art.27584. Copyright © 2010 by the American College of Rheumatology.

Diagnostic Studies

Accurate diagnosis is essential to prompt initiation of treatment to decrease the risk of disability. A diagnosis is often based on history and physical findings. Criteria for diagnosis of RA in a newly presenting patient are described in Table 67.6. Laboratory tests are used to confirm diagnosis and monitor disease progression (Table 67.7).

Positive RF occurs in 80% of adult patients. Titres rise during active disease. ESR and CRP levels are increased as general indicators of active inflammation. Testing for the antibodies to anti-cyclic citrullinated peptide (anti-CCP) is more specific than RF for RA. Anti-CCP is present in 60 to 80% of patients with RA. It can be found in patients' blood 5 to 10 years before they have symptoms of RA. If the patient's symptoms are consistent with RA, the presence of anti-CCP and RF makes a strong case for early, accurate diagnosis. An increase in antinuclear antibody (ANA) titres is an indicator of autoimmune reaction.

Synovial fluid analysis in early disease often reveals a slightly cloudy, straw-coloured fluid with many fibrin flecks. The enzyme MMP-3 is increased in the synovial fluid of patients with RA and may be a marker of progressive joint damage. The WBC count of synovial fluid is increased. Inflammatory changes in the synovium can be confirmed by tissue biopsy.

TABLE 67.7 INTERPROFESSIONAL CARE

Rheumatoid Arthritis

Diagnostic
- History and physical examination
- Laboratory studies
  - Complete blood cell (CBC) count
  - Erythrocyte sedimentation rate (ESR)
  - Rheumatoid factor (RF)
  - Anti-citrullinated protein antibody (ACPA)
  - Antinuclear antibody (ANA)
  - C-reactive protein (CRP)
- Radiological studies of involved joints
- Analysis of synovial fluid

Interprofessional Therapy
- Nutritional and weight management counselling
- Therapeutic exercise
- Psychological support

- Rest, joint protection, and use of assistive devices
- Heat and cold applications
- Complementary and alternative therapies
  - Herbal products
  - Acupuncture
  - Movement therapies
- Medication therapy (see Table 67.3)
  - Disease-modifying antirheumatic drugs (DMARDs)
  - Intra-articular or systemic corticosteroids
  - Nonsteroidal anti-inflammatory drugs (NSAIDs)
  - Biological and targeted therapy
- Reconstructive surgery (e.g., arthroplasty)

Radiological studies alone are not diagnostic of RA. They may show only soft tissue swelling and possible bone demineralization in early disease. A narrowed joint space, articular cartilage destruction, erosion, subluxation, and deformity are seen in later disease. Baseline radiographs may be used to monitor disease progression and treatment effectiveness. Bone scans are more useful in detecting early joint changes and confirming a diagnosis so that RA treatment can be initiated.

Interprofessional Care

An individualized treatment plan considers disease activity, joint function, age, gender, family and social roles, and response to previous treatment (see Table 67.7). Treatment advances have improved the prognosis for patients with newly diagnosed RA. The progression of joint damage can be slowed or stopped with aggressive, early treatment (Agency for Healthcare Research and Quality, 2018). A caring, long-term relationship with an interprofessional health care team can promote the patient's self-esteem and positive coping.

Medication Therapy
Disease-Modifying Antirheumatic Drugs. Medication remains the cornerstone of RA treatment (see Table 67.3). Irreversible joint changes can occur as early as the first year of RA, so health care providers now aggressively prescribe disease-modifying antirheumatic drugs (DMARDs). These medications may slow disease progression and decrease risk for joint erosion and deformity. The choice of medication is based on disease activity, the patient's level of function, and lifestyle considerations, such as the wish to become pregnant.

Methotrexate is preferred for early treatment of patients diagnosed with RA (Agency for Healthcare Research and Quality, 2018). It has a lower risk for toxicity compared to other medications. Rare but serious adverse effects include bone marrow suppression and hepatotoxicity. Methotrexate therapy requires frequent laboratory monitoring, including CBC and blood chemistry, as adverse effects may include anemia, neutropenia, and bone marrow depression. The patient begins to see therapeutic effects within 4 to 6 weeks. However, not everyone gets adequate relief from methotrexate alone. It can be given with other DMARDs or biological response modifiers.

Sulphasalazine (Salazopyrin) and the antimalarial medication hydroxychloroquine (Plaquenil) may be effective DMARDs for mild to moderate disease. They are rapidly absorbed, relatively safe, and well tolerated. The patient taking sulphasalazine should be taught to drink adequate fluids to avoid crystal formation in the urine. The patient must also be urged to wear sunscreen with sun exposure. For patients taking hydroxychloroquine, a baseline eye examination with follow-up every 6 to 12 months is needed because of the risk of vision impairment.

The synthetic DMARD leflunomide (Arava) blocks immune cell overproduction. Its efficacy and adverse effects are similar to those of methotrexate and sulphasalazine. Because the medication is teratogenic, the possibility of pregnancy must be excluded before therapy is initiated.

Tofacitinib (Xeljanz), a JAK (Janus kinase) inhibitor, is used to treat moderate to severe active RA. The medication interferes with JAK enzymes that contribute to joint inflammation in RA (see Medication Alert).

Biological Response Modifiers. *Biological response modifiers (BRMs)* (also called *biologics* or *immunotherapy*) are used to slow disease progression in RA. BRMs are classified on the basis of their mechanism of action (see Table 67.3). They can be used to treat patients with moderate to severe disease whose condition has not responded to DMARDs. They can be used alone or in combination therapy with a DMARD such as methotrexate (Agency for Healthcare Quality and Research, 2018).

TNF inhibitors include etanercept (Enbrel), infliximab (Remicade), adalimumab (Humira), certolizumab (Cimzia), and golimumab (Simponi). Etanercept is a biologically engineered copy of the TNF cell receptor. It binds to TNF in circulation before TNF can bind to the cell surface receptor. By inhibiting binding of TNF, etanercept inhibits the inflammatory response. This medication is given as a subcutaneous injection.

Infliximab and adalimumab are monoclonal antibodies that bind to TNF, preventing it from binding to TNF receptors on cells. Infliximab is given intravenously in combination with methotrexate. Adalimumab is administered subcutaneously.

Certolizumab and golimumab are TNF inhibitors that improve symptoms in patients with moderate to severe RA. Both medications are given in combination with methotrexate.

> **MEDICATION ALERT—Tofacitinib (Xeljanz)**
> - It has an increased incidence of thrombosis and should not be used in patients who are at risk for thrombosis.
> - Live vaccinations should not be administered to patients receiving tofacitinib.

> **MEDICATION ALERT—Tumour Necrosis Factor Inhibitors**
> - Perform a tuberculin test and chest radiograph before initiation of therapy.
> - Monitor for signs of infection. Stop the medication temporarily and notify the health care provider if acute infection develops.
> - Teach patient to avoid getting live vaccination while taking the medication.
> - Bruising, bleeding, or persistent fever and other signs of infection should be reported to the health care provider.

Anakinra (Kineret) is a recombinant version of IL-1 receptor antagonist (IL-1Ra) created from new combinations of genetic material. It blocks the biological activity of IL-1 by competitively inhibiting the binding of IL-1 to the IL-1 receptor. It is given as a subcutaneous injection. Anakinra is used to reduce the pain and swelling associated with moderate to severe RA. It can be used in combination with DMARDs but not with TNF inhibitors. Concurrent use of anakinra and TNF inhibitors can cause serious infection and neutropenia.

Tocilizumab (Actemra) and sarilumab (Kevzara) block the action of IL-6, a cytokine that contributes to inflammation. They are used to treat patients with moderate to severe RA who cannot tolerate other medications or whose condition has not adequately responded to other medications for the disease.

Abatacept (Orencia) blocks T-cell activation. It is recommended for patients whose condition has had an inadequate response to DMARDS and TNF inhibitors. It is given intravenously. Like anakinra, it should not be used concomitantly with TNF inhibitors.

Rituximab (Rituxan) is a monoclonal antibody that targets B cells. It may be used in combination with methotrexate for patients with moderate to severe RA that is not responding to TNF inhibitors (e.g., etanercept, infliximab). It is given intravenously.

Other Medication Therapy. Other DMARDs include immunosuppressants (azathioprine [Imuran]), penicillamine (Cuprimine), and gold preparations. These medications are used less often because they are weak treatments compared to other DMARDs and biologics.

Corticosteroid therapy can be used for symptom control. Intra-articular injections may temporarily reduce the pain and inflammation associated with disease flare-ups. Low-dose oral corticosteroids may be used for a limited time to decrease disease activity until the effects of DMARDs or biologics are seen.

However, they are inadequate as a sole therapy because they do not affect disease progression. Their long-term use should not be a mainstay of RA treatment because of the risk for complications, including osteoporosis and avascular necrosis.

Various NSAIDs and salicylates are used to treat arthritis pain and inflammation. Enteric-coated ASA (Aspirin) may be used in doses of 3 to 4 g per day in three to four doses. Blood salicylate levels should be monitored in a patient taking more than 3 600 mg daily. NSAIDs have anti-inflammatory and analgesic effects. The patient may be able to better follow the treatment plan if using an anti-inflammatory medication that can be taken only once or twice a day (see Table 67.3). Celecoxib (Celebrex), the only available COX-2 inhibitor, is effective in RA as well as OA. All nonaspirin NSAIDs can increase the risk for blood clots, heart attack, and stroke.

Nutritional Therapy. Although there is no special diet for RA, balanced nutrition is important. Foods that lower inflammation and boost immune function (e.g., fish, berries, and leafy green vegetables) should be included in the patient's diet (Philippou et al., 2021). Fatigue, pain, and depression may cause a loss of appetite. Limited endurance or mobility may interfere with the patient's ability to shop for and prepare food. Weight loss may result. An occupational therapist can help the patient modify their home environment and use assistive devices to make food preparation easier.

Corticosteroid therapy and decreased mobility secondary to pain may result in unwanted weight gain. Corticosteroids increase the appetite, leading to a higher caloric intake. A sensible weight loss program with balanced nutrition and exercise reduces stress on affected joints. The patient taking corticosteroids may become distressed as signs and symptoms of Cushing's syndrome—including moon facies and the redistribution of fatty tissue to the trunk—change the physical appearance. The patient should be encouraged to continue to eat a balanced diet and not to alter the dose or stop therapy abruptly. Weight slowly adjusts to normal several months after cessation of therapy.

Surgical Therapy. Occasionally, surgery is needed to relieve severe pain and improve the function of severely deformed joints. Removal of the joint lining (synovectomy) is one type of surgical therapy. Total joint replacement (arthroplasty) can be done for many different joints in the body. Joint surgery is discussed in Chapter 65.

NURSING MANAGEMENT RHEUMATOID ARTHRITIS

NURSING ASSESSMENT
Subjective and objective data that should be obtained from patients with RA are presented in Table 67.8. The nurse begins with a physical assessment (e.g., joint pain, swelling, ROM, general health status). Psychosocial needs (e.g., family support, sexual satisfaction, emotional stress, financial constraints, vocational and career limitations) also are assessed. The nurse should assess for environmental concerns (e.g., transportation, home or work modification). After identifying the patient's problems, the nurse carefully plans a program for rehabilitation and education with the interprofessional care team.

NURSING DIAGNOSES
Nursing diagnoses for patients with RA may include but are not limited to the following:

TABLE 67.8 **NURSING ASSESSMENT**

Rheumatoid Arthritis

Subjective Data
Important Health Information
Past health history: Recent infections; precipitating factors such as emotional upset, infections, overwork, childbirth, surgery; pattern of remissions and exacerbations
Family history: Family history of rheumatoid arthritis or other autoimmune diseases
Medications: Use of ASA (Aspirin), NSAIDs, corticosteroids, DMARDs
Surgery or other treatments: Any joint surgery

Symptoms
- Symmetrical joint pain and aching that increases with motion or stress on joint; stiffness and joint swelling; muscle weakness, difficulty walking; paresthesias of hands and feet; numbness, tingling, loss of sensation
- Dry mucous membranes of mouth and pharynx; anorexia, weight loss; fatigue, malaise

Objective Data
General
Lymphadenopathy, fever

Integumentary
Keratoconjunctivitis; subcutaneous rheumatoid nodules on forearm, elbows; skin ulcers; shiny, taut skin over involved joints; peripheral edema

Cardiovascular
Symmetrical pallor and cyanosis of fingers (Raynaud's phenomenon); distant heart sounds, murmurs, dysrhythmias

Respiratory
Chronic bronchitis, tuberculosis, histoplasmosis, fibrosing alveolitis

Gastrointestinal
Splenomegaly (Felty's syndrome)

Musculoskeletal
Symmetrical joint involvement with swelling, erythema, heat, tenderness, and deformities; enlargement of proximal phalangeal and MCP joints; limitation of joint movement; muscle contractures, muscle atrophy

Possible Diagnostic Findings
Positive rheumatoid factor, ↑ ESR, anemia; ↑ WBC count in synovial fluid; evidence of joint space narrowing and of bone erosion and deformity on radiograph (osteoporosis with advanced disease)

DMARDs, disease-modifying antirheumatic drugs; *ESR,* erythrocyte sedimentation rate; *MCP,* metacarpophalangeal; *NSAIDs,* nonsteroidal anti-inflammatory drugs; *WBC,* white blood cell.

- *Reduced physical mobility* resulting from *pain* (joint pain, stiffness and deformity)
- *Chronic pain* resulting from *injury agent* (joint inflammation, overuse of joints, and ineffective pain or comfort measures)
- *Disrupted body image* resulting from *alteration in self-perception* (chronic disease activity, long-term treatment, deformities, stiffness, and inability to perform usual activities)

Additional information on nursing diagnoses for the patient with RA is presented in Nursing Care Plan (NCP) 67.1, available on the Evolve website.

PLANNING
The overall goals are that patients with RA will (a) have acceptable pain management, (b) have minimal loss of function of the

affected joints, (c) participate in planning and implementing the treatment plan, (d) maintain a positive self-image, and (e) perform self-care to the maximum extent possible.

NURSING IMPLEMENTATION

HEALTH PROMOTION. Prevention of RA is not possible. Early treatment can help prevent further joint damage. Community education programs should focus on symptom recognition to promote early diagnosis and treatment. The Arthritis Society offers many publications, classes, and support activities to assist people who are affected by RA (see the Resources at the end of this chapter).

ACUTE INTERVENTION. Patients who are newly diagnosed with RA are usually treated on an outpatient basis. Hospitalization may be necessary for the patient who has systemic complications or who needs surgery for decreased functional ability. The nurse works closely with the interprofessional health team to help the patient regain function and adjust to living with a chronic illness.

AMBULATORY AND HOME CARE. Care of the patient with RA includes a broad program of medication therapy, balance of rest and activity with joint protection, exercise, and patient and caregiver teaching. Nonpharmaceutical management may include the use of therapeutic heat and cold, rest, relaxation techniques, joint protection (see Table 67.4, Table 67.9), biofeedback, transcutaneous electrical nerve stimulation (see Chapter 10), and hypnosis. The patient and their caregiver should be allowed to choose therapies that promote optimal comfort and fit their lifestyle.

Rest. Alternating scheduled rest periods with activity throughout the day helps relieve fatigue and pain. The amount of rest needed varies according to the severity of the disease and the patient's limitations. Patients should rest before becoming exhausted. Total bed rest is rarely necessary and should be avoided, to prevent stiffness and other effects of immobility. However, even a patient with mild disease may require daytime rest in addition to 8 to 10 hours of sleep at night. The nurse can help the patient to identify ways to modify daily activities to avoid overexertion that can lead to fatigue and an exacerbation of disease activity. For example, a patient may tolerate meal preparation more easily while sitting on a high stool in front of the sink.

The patient should be taught to maintain good body alignment during rest through use of a firm mattress or bed board. Positions of extension should be encouraged, and positions of flexion should be avoided. To decrease the risk for joint contracture, pillows should never be placed under the knees. A small, flat pillow may be used under the head and shoulders.

Joint Protection. Protecting joints from stress is important. The nurse can help the patient identify ways to modify tasks to put less stress on joints (see Table 67.9). Energy conservation requires careful planning. The emphasis is on work simplification techniques. Work should be done in short periods with scheduled rest breaks to avoid fatigue (pacing). Activities should be organized to avoid going up and down stairs repeatedly. Carts should be used to carry supplies, and materials that are used often can be stored in a convenient, easily reached area. Time-saving joint protective devices (e.g., electric can opener) should be used whenever possible. Tasks can also be delegated to other family members.

An occupational therapist can help the patient maintain upper extremity function and should encourage use of splints or

---

TABLE 67.9   PATIENT & CAREGIVER TEACHING GUIDE

Protection of Small Joints

The following instructions should be included when teaching the patient with arthritis how to protect small joints.

1. Maintain joint in a neutral position to minimize deformity.
   - Press water from a sponge instead of wringing.
2. Use the strongest joint available for any task.
   - When rising from a chair, push with the palms rather than fingers.
   - Carry laundry basket in both arms rather than with fingers.
3. Distribute weight over many joints instead of stressing a few.
   - Slide objects instead of lifting them.
   - Hold packages close to the body for support.
4. Change positions frequently.
   - Do not hold a book or grip a steering wheel for long periods without resting.
   - Avoid grasping pencils or cutting vegetables with a knife for extended periods.
5. Avoid repetitious movements.
   - Do not knit for long periods.
   - Rest between rooms when vacuuming.
   - Modify home environment to include faucets and doorknobs that are pushed rather than turned.
6. Modify chores to avoid stress on joints.
   - Avoid heavy lifting.
   - Sit on a stool instead of standing during meal preparation.

---

other assistive devices for joint protection. Lightweight splints may be prescribed to rest an inflamed joint and prevent deformity from muscle spasms and contractures. After assessment and supportive care, splints are reapplied as prescribed.

Occupational therapy may increase patient independence through use of assistive devices that simplify tasks (e.g., built-up utensils, buttonhooks, modified drawer handles, lightweight plastic dishes, and raised toilet seats). Wearing shoes with Velcro fasteners and clothing with snaps or a zipper down the front can make dressing easier. A cane or a walker offers support and relief of pain when walking.

Heat and Cold Therapy and Exercise. Heat and cold applications can help relieve stiffness, pain, and muscle spasm. Heat and cold can be used several times a day as needed. Ice is especially beneficial during periods of disease exacerbation. Cold application should not exceed 10 to 15 minutes at a time. Plastic bags of frozen vegetables (peas or corn), which can easily mould around the shoulder, wrists, or knees, are an effective home treatment. Patients can use ice cubes or small paper cups of frozen water to massage areas proximal or distal to a painful joint. Moist heat offers better relief of chronic stiffness. Superficial heat sources such as heating pads, moist hot packs, paraffin baths, and warm baths or showers can relieve stiffness to enable participation in therapeutic exercises. However, heat application should not exceed 20 minutes at one time. The patient should be alerted to the risk for a burn and to avoid using a heat-producing cream (e.g., Capsaicin) with an external heat device. Sitting or standing in a warm shower, sitting in a tub with warm towels around the shoulders, or simply soaking the hands in a basin of warm water may relieve joint stiffness and allow the patient to perform ADLs more comfortably.

Individualized exercise is an integral part of the treatment plan. A physiotherapist may develop a therapeutic exercise program to improve the flexibility and strength of the affected joints and the patient's overall endurance. The nurse can encourage program participation and reinforce correct performance of the exercises. Progressive joint immobility and muscle weakness can occur if the patient does not move their joints. Overaggressive exercise can result in increased pain, inflammation, and joint damage. The nurse needs to emphasize that participating in a recreational exercise program (e.g., walking, swimming) or performing usual daily activities does not eliminate the patient's need for therapeutic exercise to maintain adequate joint motion.

Gentle ROM exercises are usually performed daily to keep joints functional. The patient should have the opportunity to practise the exercises with supervision. Aquatic exercises in warm water (25°C to 30°C) allow easier joint movement because of the buoyancy and warmth of the water. At the same time, although movement seems easier, water provides two-way resistance that makes muscles work harder than they would in the air. During acute inflammation, exercises should be limited to one or two repetitions.

Patient and Caregiver Teaching. Care of the patient with RA begins with a thorough program of education and medication therapy. The nurse needs to teach the patient and caregiver about the disease process and home management strategies. Inflammation may be managed through administration of NSAIDs, DMARDs, and BRMs. Careful timing of medication administration is critical to maintain a therapeutic drug level and reduce early morning stiffness. The nurse should discuss the action and adverse effects of each prescribed medication and any needed laboratory monitoring. Many patients with RA take several different medications, so the medication regimen should be made as understandable as possible. The nurse can encourage patients to develop a way to remember to take their medications (e.g., pill container).

Psychological Support. For effective self-management and adherence to an individualized home treatment program, the nurse should help the patient understand the nature and course of RA and the goals of therapy. In doing so, the nurse needs to consider the patient's value system and perception of the disease.

The nurse should discuss changes in sexuality with the patient. Chronic pain or loss of function may make the patient vulnerable to claims of false advertising about unproven or even dangerous remedies. The nurse can help the patient to recognize fears and concerns faced by people who live with chronic illness.

The nurse needs to evaluate the family support system. Financial planning may be necessary. Community resources such as a home care nurse, homemaker services, and vocational rehabilitation should be considered. Self-help groups are beneficial for some patients.

Living with chronic pain may lead to depression. To decrease depressive symptoms, the nurse can suggest activities such as listening to music, reading, exercising, and counselling. Hypnosis and biofeedback may useful.

▎AGE-RELATED CONSIDERATIONS
ARTHRITIS
The prevalence of arthritis among older persons is high, and the disease is accompanied by complications unique to this age group. Areas of concern for older people include the following:
- The high incidence of OA in older persons may keep the health care provider from considering the presence of other types of arthritis.
- Age alone causes changes that make interpretation of laboratory values such as RF and ESR more difficult. Medications taken for comorbid conditions can also affect laboratory values.

- Musculoskeletal pain syndromes and weakness may have no physical cause. Instead, they may be related to depression and physical inactivity.
- Diseases such as SLE, which commonly occur in younger adults, can develop in a milder form in older persons.

Physical and metabolic changes of aging may increase the older patient's sensitivity to both therapeutic and toxic effects of some medications. Older persons who take NSAIDs have an increased risk for adverse effects, particularly GI bleeding and renal toxicity. Using NSAIDS with a shorter half-life may require more frequent dosing and have fewer adverse effects in older patients with altered medication metabolism.

Polypharmacy in the older person is a concern. Use of medications in RA treatment may increase the chance of unexpected medication interactions. The medication regimen should be as simple as possible to increase adherence (e.g., limited number of medications with decreased frequency of administration), particularly for patients who do not receive regular assistance.

Osteopenia from corticosteroid use can worsen the occurrence of decreased bone density from aging and inactivity. The risk of pathological fractures is increased, especially compression fractures of vertebrae. Corticosteroid-related myopathy can be minimized by use of an age-appropriate exercise program. An adequate support system for older persons is critical to the ability to follow a treatment plan.

GOUT

Gout is a type of arthritis characterized by elevation of uric acid (*hyperuricemia)* and the deposit of uric acid crystals in one or more joints. Sodium urate crystals may be found in articular, periarticular, and subcutaneous tissues. Unlike other forms of arthritis, gout is marked by painful flares lasting days to weeks followed by long periods without symptoms. Gout affects approximately 5.2% of adult men and 2.4% of adult women in Canada (Arthritis Society, 2017b).

Obesity in men has been shown to increase the risk for gout. Hypertension, diuretic use, and excessive alcohol consumption are additional risk factors. A diet high in purine-rich foods (e.g., shellfish such as crab and shrimp; vegetables such as lentils, asparagus, and spinach; meats such as beef, chicken, and pork) will not cause gout but can trigger an acute attack if a person is susceptible to gout.

Etiology and Pathophysiology
Uric acid is the major end product of purine catabolism and is excreted primarily by the kidneys. Gout occurs when either the kidneys cannot excrete enough uric acid or there is too much being made for the kidneys to handle effectively.

Hyperuricemia may be classified as primary or secondary. *Primary hyperuricemia* is genetic. A hereditary error of purine metabolism leads to the overproduction or retention of uric acid. *Secondary hyperuricemia* may be caused by conditions that increase uric acid production or decrease uric acid excretion or by medications that inhibit uric acid excretion (e.g., loop diuretics, β blockers). Organ transplant recipients receiving immunosuppressive agents are at risk for hyperuricemia (Table 67.10).

Gout is likely caused by the interaction of several factors. The most important is metabolic syndrome (obesity, insulin resistance, hypertension, hyperlipidemia). High uric acid may result from prolonged fasting or excessive alcohol use because they increase the production of keto acids, which inhibit uric acid excretion.

Not everyone with high uric acid levels develops gout. Two processes are essential for a person to develop gout: crystallization and inflammation. As urate levels increase and saturate the synovial fluid or soft tissues, the excess urate coalesces into crystals through phagocytosis. This causes the release of inflammatory mediators into the surrounding areas, causing more inflammation and tissue damage (Harding, 2016).

Clinical Manifestations and Complications

In the acute phase, gout may occur in one or more joints but usually fewer than four. Inflammation of the great toe *(podagra)* is the most common initial symptom. Other affected joints may include the midtarsal area of the foot, the ankle, the knee, and the wrist. Olecranon bursae may be involved. Affected joints may appear dusky or cyanotic and are extremely tender. Acute gout arthritis is usually triggered by events such as trauma, surgery, alcohol ingestion, or systemic infection. Symptoms typically begin at night, with sudden swelling and excruciating pain; peak within several hours; and are often accompanied by low-grade fever. Individual attacks usually subside, treated or untreated, in 2 to 10 days. The affected joint returns to normal, and patients are often free of symptoms between attacks.

Chronic gout is characterized by multiple joint involvement and visible deposits of sodium urate crystals, called *tophi*. They are typically seen in subcutaneous tissue, synovial membranes, tendons, and soft tissues (Figure 67.6). Tophi generally occur many years after the onset of the disease.

The severity of gout arthritis varies. The clinical course may involve infrequent mild attacks or multiple severe episodes (up to 12 per year) marked by slowly progressive disability. In general, the higher the serum uric acid level, the earlier the appearance of tophi and the greater the tendency toward more frequent, severe episodes of acute gout. Chronic inflammation may result in joint deformity, and cartilage destruction may lead to secondary OA. Large urate crystal deposits may perforate overlying skin, producing draining sinuses that often become infected.

Excessive uric acid excretion may lead to kidney or urinary tract stone formation. Pyelonephritis associated with sodium urate deposits and obstruction may contribute to renal disease.

Diagnostic Studies

In gout, serum uric acid levels are usually elevated; however, hyperuricemia is not specifically diagnostic of gout because serum values may be normal during an acute gout attack (Harding, 2016). Increased uric acid may be related to various medications or an asymptomatic abnormality in the general population. A 24-hour urine uric acid test can be used to determine if the disease is caused by decreased renal excretion or overproduction of uric acid.

The gold standard for diagnosis of gout is synovial fluid aspiration. Affected fluid contains needle-like monosodium urate crystals. This procedure is done in only a small number of patients because diagnosis can typically be made on clinical symptoms alone. However, it is the only reliable way to distinguish gout from septic arthritis or *pseudogout* (calcium phosphate crystal formation). Aspiration may decrease pain by relieving pressure in a swollen joint capsule.

Radiographs appear normal in the early stages of gout. In chronic disease, tophi may appear as eroded areas in the bone.

Interprofessional Care and Nursing Management

Goals for care of patients with gout (Table 67.11) include ending an acute attack with an anti-inflammatory agent, such as colchicine (Colcrys). Hyperuricemia and gout are chronic

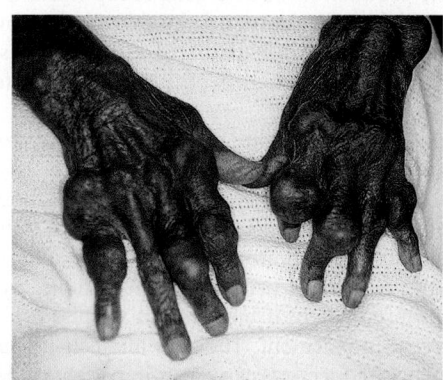

FIG. 67.6 Tophi associated with chronic gout. Nodules are painless and filled with uric acid crystals. Source: Courtesy John Cook, MD. From Goldstein, B. G., & Goldstein, A. E. (1997). *Practical dermatology.* (2nd ed.). Mosby.

TABLE 67.10 CAUSES OF HYPERURICEMIA
• Acidosis or ketosis
• Alcohol use, especially beer and red wine
• Cancer
• Chemotherapy medications
• Diabetes
• Medication-induced renal impairment
• Hyperlipidemia
• Hypertension
• Lead exposure
• Metabolic syndrome
• Myeloproliferative disorders
• Obesity
• Renal insufficiency
• Sickle cell anemia
• Starvation
• Use of certain common medications (aspirin, ACE inhibitors, β blockers, loop or thiazide diuretics, niacin)

ACE, angiotensin-converting enzyme.

TABLE 67.11 INTERPROFESSIONAL CARE
Gout

Diagnostic	**Medication therapy**
• History and physical examination	• Adrenocorticotrophic hormone (ACTH)
• Elevated serum uric acid levels	• Allopurinol (Zyloprim)
• Elevated uric acid levels in 24-hr urine collection	• Colchicine
• Family history of gout	• Corticosteroids (prednisone)
• Presence of sodium urate crystals in synovial fluid	• Febuxostat (Uloric)
• Radiographic studies	• Intra-articular corticosteroids (methylprednisolone acetate)
Interprofessional Therapy	• Nonsteroidal anti-inflammatory drugs (e.g., naproxen [Naprosyn])
• Dietary avoidance of food and fluids with high purine content (e.g., anchovies, liver, wine, beer)	• Probenecid (Benuryl)
• Joint aspiration and intra-articular corticosteroids	• Joint immobilization
	• Local application of heat or cold

conditions that can be controlled with effective patient education and adherence to a treatment program. Medication therapy is the primary therapy used in treating acute and chronic gout.

Medication Therapy. Acute gout is treated with colchicine and NSAIDs. Because colchicine has anti-inflammatory effects but no analgesic properties, an NSAID is added to the treatment regimen for pain management. Colchicine generally produces dramatic pain relief when given within 12 hours of an attack. This helps in diagnosis because good response is further evidence of gout.

Future attacks of gout are prevented in part by a maintenance dose of urate-lowering medications such as a xanthine oxidase inhibitor (allopurinol [Zyloprim]) or a uricosuric medication (probenecid [Benuryl]). Febuxostat (Uloric), a selective inhibitor of xanthine oxidase, is given for long-term management of hyperuricemia in people with chronic gout.

Corticosteroids, given either orally or by intra-articular injection, can be helpful in treating acute attacks of gout. Systemic corticosteroids may be used only if routine therapies are contraindicated or ineffective. Adrenocorticotrophic hormone (ACTH) may also be used for treating acute gout in patients for whom NSAIDs, colchicine, or steroids may be problematic.

Future attacks of gout are prevented in part by a maintenance dose of a xanthine oxidase inhibitor. These medications decrease the production of uric acid. Allopurinol is the most commonly used medication and the first choice for therapy. It is used for patients with uric acid kidney stones or renal impairment. Serious adverse effects limit the use of febuxostat (Uloric).

For many years, the standard therapy for hyperuricemia caused by urate underexcretion has been uricosuric medications such as probenecid, which inhibit renal tubular reabsorption of urates. ASA (Aspirin) inactivates the effect of uricosurics, resulting in urate retention, and should be avoided while patients are taking uricosuric medications. Acetaminophen can be used safely if analgesia is required. Uricosurics can cause renal impairment. They are ineffective when creatinine clearance is reduced, as can occur in patients older than 60 years and patients with renal impairment. Uricosurics should be taken in the morning with food and water. Patients should be instructed to stay well hydrated and to drink about 2 L of liquid a day when taking the medication.

The angiotensin II receptor antagonist losartan (Cozaar) may be especially useful in the treatment of older patients with both gout and hypertension. Losartan promotes uric acid secretion and may normalize serum urate levels. Combination therapy with losartan and allopurinol may be used.

Serum uric acid levels must be checked regularly to monitor treatment effectiveness. The nurse should explain the importance of medication therapy and the need for regular assessment of serum uric acid. Dietary restrictions that limit alcohol and foods high in purine can help minimize uric acid production (see Table 67.11). Adequate urine volume with normal renal function (2–3 L/day) must be maintained to prevent precipitation of uric acid in the renal tubules. A patient with obesity should be encouraged to participate in a carefully planned weight-reduction program. The patient should be taught about other factors that may cause attacks, including fasting, medications (e.g., diuretics), and major medical events (e.g., surgery, heart attack).

NURSING MANAGEMENT
GOUT

Nursing interventions for the patient with acute gout include supportive care of the inflamed joints. The nurse should avoid causing pain by careless handling of an inflamed joint. Bed rest may be appropriate to immobilize affected joints as needed. A cradle or footboard can be used to protect a painful lower extremity from the weight of bed linens. The nurse needs to assess motion limitations and degree of pain.

LYME DISEASE

Lyme disease is a spirochetal infection caused by the bacteria *Borrelia burgdorferi*. In 2017, over 2 000 Canadians tested positive for Lyme disease. It is transmitted by the bite of an infected blacklegged or deer tick, which appears in the southeastern or south-central regions of Canada, or the western blacklegged tick, in British Columbia (Government of Canada, 2017). Ticks typically feed on mice, dogs, cats, cows, horses, deer, and humans. Wild animals do not exhibit the illness, but clinical Lyme disease does occur in domestic animals. Person-to-person transmission does not occur.

The peak season for infection in humans is during spring and summer. The number of infected ticks continues to rise in Canada. The most prevalent areas in Canada include southern British Columbia; southeastern and south-central Manitoba; southern, eastern, and northwestern Ontario; southern Quebec; southern New Brunswick and Grand Manan Island; and all of Nova Scotia (Government of Canada, 2017). For information about removing a tick, see Chapter 71, Figure 71.5.

Symptoms of Lyme disease can mimic those of other diseases, such as multiple sclerosis, mononucleosis, and meningitis. The most characteristic clinical symptom of early localized disease is erythema migrans (EM), a skin lesion at the site of the tick bite that occurs in 70 to 80% of people who are infected, within 3 to 30 days after exposure (Figure 67.7). The lesion begins as a red macule or papule that slowly expands to form a large round lesion of up to 30 cm with a bright red border and central clearing ("bull's eye rash"). The EM lesion is often accompanied by acute flulike symptoms, such as low-grade fever, chills, headache, stiff neck, fatigue, swollen lymph nodes, and migratory joint and muscle pain. Symptoms usually occur within a week but may be delayed for up to 30 days. The flulike symptoms generally resolve over a period of weeks or months, even if untreated.

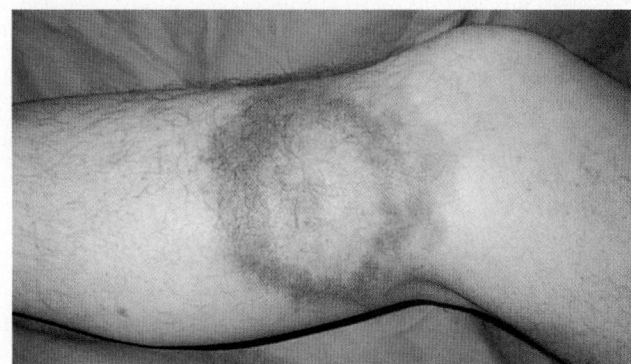

FIG. 67.7 Erythema migrans of Lyme disease. Source: Swartz, M. H. (2010). *Textbook of physical diagnosis: History and examination* (6th ed., p. 186, Figure 8-112). W. B. Saunders.

If not treated, the spirochete can disseminate within several weeks or months to the heart, joints, and central nervous system (CNS). About 60% of people with untreated infection develop chronic arthritic pain and swelling in the large joints. Cardiac symptoms may require hospitalization. Bell's palsy is the most common neurological effect. Other symptoms include short-term memory loss, cognitive impairment, shooting pains, and numbness and tingling in the feet.

A diagnosis of Lyme disease is often based on clinical manifestations, particularly the EM lesion, and a history of exposure in an endemic area. CBC count and ESR are usually normal. A two-step laboratory testing process is recommended to confirm diagnosis (Government of Canada, 2017). The first step is the enzyme immunoassay (EIA), a test that yields positive results for most people with Lyme disease. If the EIA result is positive or inconclusive, a Western blot test is done to confirm the infection. Cerebrospinal fluid should be examined in individuals with neurological involvement.

Active lesions can be treated with oral antibiotic therapy. Doxycycline, cefuroxime (Ceftin), and amoxicillin are often effective in early stages of infection and in prevention of later stages of the disease. Short-term therapy of 10 to 21 days of doxycycline is preferred. It treats both Lyme disease and human granulocytic anaplasmosis, which can be transmitted as a co-infection with a single tick bite. While other antibiotics can be used for patients who cannot tolerate any of these medications, they are all less effective. Patients with certain neurological or cardiac complications may need intravenous therapy with ceftriaxone or penicillin.

A small number of persons treated with antibiotics may have lingering fatigue or joint and muscle pain. Antibiotic treatment should be extended as needed because the risks of untreated Lyme disease outweigh those of long-term antibiotic therapy.

Reducing exposure to ticks is the best way to prevent Lyme disease (Public Health Agency of Canada, 2020). Teaching of patients and caregivers who live in endemic areas is outlined in Table 67.12. Currently, no vaccine is available for Lyme disease.

SEPTIC ARTHRITIS

Septic arthritis (infectious or bacterial arthritis) is caused by microorganisms invading the joint cavity. Bacteria can travel through the bloodstream from another site of active infection, resulting in hematogenous seeding of the joint. Organisms can also be introduced directly through trauma or surgical incision.

Any infectious agent can cause septic arthritis (bacteria, viruses, mycobacteria, fungi), especially in the immunocompromised patient. *Staphylococcus aureus* is the most common causative organism. Factors that increase the risk for infection include diseases with decreased host resistance (e.g., RA, SLE), treatment with corticosteroids or immunosuppressive medications, and debilitating chronic illness (e.g., diabetes).

Large joints, such as the knee and the hip, are most frequently involved. Inflammation of the joint cavity causes severe pain, erythema, and swelling. Septic arthritis of the hip can cause avascular necrosis. Because infection has often spread from a primary site elsewhere in the body, fever or shaking chills often accompany articular manifestations. A diagnosis may be made by aspiration of the joint (arthrocentesis) and culture of the synovial fluid. WBC counts may be low early in the infectious process, especially in persons who are immunosuppressed, so diagnosis is not possible solely on the basis of WBC counts. Blood cultures for aerobic and anaerobic organisms should be obtained.

TABLE 67.12	**PATIENT & CAREGIVER TEACHING GUIDE**

Prevention and Early Treatment of Lyme Disease

The following instructions should be included when teaching patients and caregivers how to prevent Lyme disease:
- Avoid walking through tall grasses and low brush and sitting on logs.
- Mow grass. Remove brush around paths, buildings, and campsites to create "tick-safe zones."
- Move woodpiles and bird feeders away from the house. Discourage deer (main source of food for adult ticks) from being in the area.
- Wear long pants or nylon tights of tightly woven, light-coloured fabric so that ticks can be easily seen.
- Tuck pants into boots or long socks, tuck long-sleeved shirts into pants, and wear closed shoes when hiking.
- Check often for ticks crawling from pant legs to open skin.
- Thoroughly inspect and wash clothes. Placing clothing in the dryer on high heat effectively kills ticks.
- Spray insect repellent containing DEET sparingly on skin or apply permethrin to boots and clothes (especially on lower extremities) and camping gear.
- Have pets wear tick collars, inspect them often, and do not allow pets on furniture or beds.

The following instructions should be included when teaching patients and caregivers living in endemic areas:
- Remove attached ticks with tweezers (not fingers). Grasp tick's mouth parts as close to skin as possible and gently pull straight out. Do not twist or jerk. Avoid folk solutions such as painting the tick with nail polish or petroleum jelly.
- Wash bitten area with soap and water and apply antiseptic. Wash hands.
- See a health care provider immediately if flulike symptoms or a bull's eye rash appears within 3 to 30 days after removal of tick.

DEET, diethyltoluamide.
Source: Adapted from Public Health Agency of Canada. (2020). *Enjoy the outdoors, without a tick.* https://www.canada.ca/en/public-health/services/publications/diseases-conditions/lyme-pamphlet.html

Septic arthritis requires prompt treatment to prevent joint destruction and bone loss. Broad-spectrum antibiotics against Gram-negative organisms, pneumococci, and staphylococci are often started before the causative organism is identified. Once the organism is determined, the treatment can become specific. Infections may respond to treatment within 2 weeks or may take as long as 4 to 8 weeks, depending on the causative organism. Local aspiration and surgical drainage may be required.

Nursing intervention includes assessment and monitoring of joint inflammation, pain, and fever. To manage pain, resting splints or traction can be used to immobilize affected joints. Local hot compresses can decrease pain. Gentle ROM exercises should be initiated as soon as tolerated to prevent muscle atrophy and joint contractures. The need for antibiotics and the importance of their continued use until the infection is resolved should be explained to the patient. The patient who requires arthrocentesis or operative drainage requires support. Strict aseptic technique should be used in assisting with joint aspiration.

SPONDYLOARTHROPATHIES

The spondyloarthropathies are a group of multisystem inflammatory disorders that affect the spine, the peripheral joints, and periarticular structures. These disorders include ankylosing spondylitis, psoriatic arthritis, and reactive arthritis. These disorders are all negative for RF and thus are often referred to as *seronegative arthropathies.*

Inheritance of HLA-B27 is strongly associated with these diseases. Both genetic and environmental factors play a role in their development. (HLAs and their relationship to autoimmune diseases are discussed in Chapter 16.)

The spondyloarthropathies share clinical and laboratory characteristics that make it difficult to distinguish among them in early stages of disease. These characteristics include absence of antibodies in the serum, peripheral joint involvement predominantly of the lower extremities, low back pain *(sacroiliitis)*, pain and redness of the eyes *(uveitis)*, gastrointestinal and genitourinary infection, and psoriasis (Sen et al., 2021).

ANKYLOSING SPONDYLITIS

Ankylosing spondylitis (AS) is a chronic inflammatory disease that affects primarily the axial skeleton, including the sacroiliac joints, the intervertebral disc spaces, and the costovertebral articulations. As many as 300 000 Canadians are affected by AS (Arthritis Society, 2019). The usual age at onset is 15 to 30 years, and three times more men than women develop AS.

Etiology and Pathophysiology

Genetic predisposition appears to play an important role in the disease pathogenesis, but the precise mechanisms are unknown. HLA-B27 antigen is found in about 90% of people with AS. Inflammation in the joints and adjacent tissue causes the formation of granulation tissue *(pannus)* and dense fibrous scars that can cause joint fusion. Inflammation can affect the eyes, the lungs, the heart, the kidneys, and the peripheral nervous system.

Clinical Manifestations and Complications

AS is characterized by symmetrical sacroiliitis and progressive inflammatory arthritis of the axial skeleton. Symptoms of inflammatory spine pain are the first clues to the diagnosis. Affected patients typically report low back pain, stiffness, and limitation of motion that is worse during the night and in the morning but improves with mild activity. In affected women, early symptoms of disease may be pain and stiffness in the neck rather than the lower back. Uveitis is the most common nonskeletal symptom. It can appear as an initial manifestation of the disease years before arthritic symptoms develop. Patients with AS may also experience chest pain and sternal or costal cartilage tenderness that can be distressing.

Severe postural abnormalities and deformity can lead to significant disability for patients with AS (Figure 67.8). Impaired spinal ROM and fusion, along with altered visual function, raise concerns about safe ambulation. Aortic insufficiency and pulmonary fibrosis are frequent complications. Cauda equina syndrome can also occur, contributing to lower extremity weakness and bladder dysfunction. In addition, affected patients are at risk for spinal fracture because of associated osteoporosis.

Diagnostic Studies

Radiological studies are essential for the diagnosis and follow-up of AS. However, radiographs are limited in detecting early sacroiliitis or subtle changes in posterior vertebrae. MRI can be useful in assessing early cartilage abnormalities, while a CT scan is appropriate in specific situations (e.g., cases with subtle radiographic changes). Changes on later spinal radiographs include the appearance of "bamboo spine," which is the result of calcifications *(syndesmophytes)* that bridge from one vertebra to another. An increased ESR and mild anemia may be present.

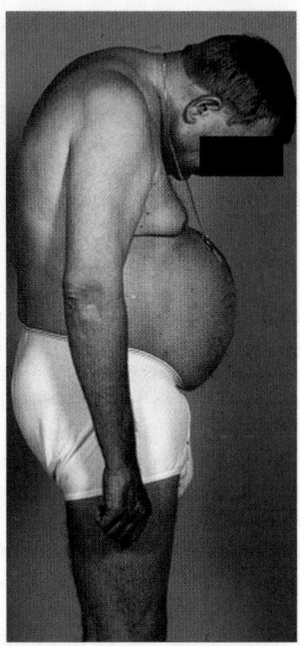

FIG. 67.8 Advanced ankylosing spondylitis. Kyphotic posture causes many patients to have a protuberant abdomen secondary to pulmonary restriction. Source: Kim, D. H., Henn, J., Vaccaro, A. R., et al. (Eds.). (2006). *Surgical anatomy and techniques to the spine.* W. B. Saunders.

When the suspicion of AS is high, the presence of HLA-B27 antigen increases the likelihood of this diagnosis.

Interprofessional Care

Prevention of AS is not possible. Families with other diagnosed HLA-B27–positive rheumatic diseases (e.g., psoriatic arthritis, juvenile spondyloarthritis) should be alert to signs of low back pain for early identification and treatment of AS.

Care of the patient with AS is aimed at maintaining maximal skeletal mobility while decreasing pain and inflammation. Heat applications can help in relief of local symptoms. NSAIDs and salicylates are commonly prescribed. DMARDs such as sulphasalazine (Salazopyrin) or methotrexate have little effect on spinal disease but may help with peripheral joint disease. Local corticosteroid injections may be beneficial in relieving symptoms.

TNF, which promotes inflammation, is found in elevated levels in the blood and certain tissues of patients with AS. Etanercept (Enbrel), a biological and targeted therapy medication, binds TNF and inhibits its action. Etanercept reduces active inflammation and improves spinal mobility. Additional anti-TNF inhibitors (infliximab, adalimumab, golimumab) may be effective.

Once pain and stiffness are managed, exercise is essential. Postural control is important for minimizing spinal deformity. The exercise regimen should include back, neck, and chest stretches. Hydrotherapy has also been shown to decrease pain and facilitate spinal extension. Surgery may be indicated for severe deformity and mobility impairment. Spinal osteotomy and total joint replacement are the most commonly performed procedures (see Chapter 65).

NURSING MANAGEMENT
ANKYLOSING SPONDYLITIS

A key nursing responsibility for patients with AS is education about the disease and principles of therapy. The home management program should include regular exercise and attention to posture, local moist heat applications, and knowledgeable use of medications.

The nurse assesses chest expansion (using breathing exercises) as part of a baseline ROM assessment. Smoking cessation should be encouraged, to decrease the risk for lung complications in patients with reduced chest expansion. Ongoing physiotherapy includes gentle, graded stretching and strengthening exercises to preserve ROM and improve thoracolumbar flexion and extension.

Excessive physical exertion during flare-ups of the disease should be discouraged. Proper positioning at rest is essential. The mattress should be firm, and patients should sleep on their back with a flat pillow, avoiding positions that encourage flexion deformity. Postural training emphasizes avoiding spinal flexion (e.g., leaning over a desk), heavy lifting, and prolonged walking, standing, or sitting. Participation in sports that facilitate natural stretching, such as swimming and racquet games, should be encouraged. Family counselling and vocational rehabilitation are important measures.

PSORIATIC ARTHRITIS

Psoriatic arthritis (PsA) is a progressive inflammatory disease that affects approximately 10 to 30% of people with psoriasis (Arthritis Society, 2017c). *Psoriasis* is a common, benign, inflammatory skin disorder characterized by red, irritated, and scaly patches. Both PsA and psoriasis appear to have a genetic link with the HLA antigens in many patients. Although the exact cause of PsA is unknown, a combination of immune, genetic, and environmental factors is suspected.

PsA can occur in different forms. *Distal arthritis* mainly involves the ends of the fingers and toes, with pitting and colour changes in the fingernails and toenails. *Asymmetric arthritis* involves different joints on each side of the body. *Symmetric psoriatic arthritis* resembles RA. It affects joints on both sides of the body at the same time and accounts for about 50% of cases. *Spinal psoriatic spondylitis* is marked by pain and stiffness in the spine and neck. *Arthritis mutilans* affects about 5% of people with PsA. It is the most severe form of the disease, causing complete destruction of small joints (Arthritis Society, 2017c).

On radiographs, the cartilage loss and erosion resemble that of RA. Many patients with advanced cases of PsA have widened joint spaces. A "pencil-in-cup" deformity is common at the DIP joints as a result of osteolysis. In this deformity, the narrowed end(s) of the metacarpals or phalanges insert into the expanded end of the other (adjacent) bone sharing the joint. Elevated ESR, mild anemia, and elevated blood uric acid levels are present in some patients; therefore, gout must be ruled out.

Treatment includes splinting, joint protection, and physiotherapy. NSAIDs given early in the course of the disease may help with inflammation. Medication therapy also includes DMARDs such as methotrexate, which are effective for both cutaneous and articular manifestations. Sulphasalazine (Salazopyrin) and cyclosporin may be used for treating PsA. In addition, biological and targeted therapy, such as etanercept, golimumab, adalimumab, and infliximab, may also be used.

REACTIVE ARTHRITIS

Reactive arthritis *(Reiter's syndrome)* occurs more commonly in young men. It is associated with a symptom complex that includes urethritis, conjunctivitis, and mucocutaneous lesions. Although the exact etiology is unknown, reactive arthritis appears to occur after exposure to specific genitourinary or GI tract infections. *Chlamydia trachomatis* is most often implicated in sexually transmitted reactive arthritis. Reactive arthritis is also associated with GI infections with *Shigella, Salmonella, Campylobacter,* or *Yersinia* species and other microorganisms (Arthritis Society, 2017d).

Individuals who are positive for HLA-B27 are at increased risk of developing reactive arthritis after sexual contact or exposure to certain enteric pathogens. This finding supports the likelihood of a genetic predisposition.

Urethritis develops within 1 to 2 weeks after sexual contact or GI infection. In women, symptoms include cervicitis. Low-grade fever, conjunctivitis, and arthritis may occur over the next several weeks. This type of arthritis tends to be asymmetrical, frequently involving the large joints of the lower extremities and the toes. Lower back pain may occur with severe disease. Mucocutaneous lesions commonly manifest as small, painless, superficial ulcerations on the tongue, the oral mucosa, and the glans penis. Soft tissue manifestations commonly include Achilles tendinitis or plantar fasciitis. Few laboratory findings are abnormal, although the ESR may be elevated.

Most patients recover within a few months of initial symptoms. Because reactive arthritis is often associated with *C. trachomatis* infection, treatment of patients and their sexual partners with doxycycline is widely recommended. Conjunctivitis and lesions require no treatment, but topical ophthalmic corticosteroids are typically prescribed for treatment of uveitis. Medication therapy may also include NSAID and DMARDs if joint symptoms do not resolve. Physiotherapy may be helpful during disease recovery.

Most patients have complete remission with restoration of full joint function. Some patients may develop chronic arthritis, but this condition is often mild. Radiographic changes in chronic disease closely resemble those of AS. Treatment is based on symptoms.

OTHER CONNECTIVE TISSUE DISORDERS

SYSTEMIC LUPUS ERYTHEMATOSUS

Systemic lupus erythematosus (SLE) is a multisystem, inflammatory, autoimmune disease. It is a complex disorder of multifactorial origin resulting from interactions among genetic, hormonal, environmental, and immunological factors. SLE typically affects the skin, joints, and serous membranes (pleura, pericardium), along with the renal, hematological, and neurological systems. SLE is characterized by a chronic, unpredictable course marked by alternating periods of exacerbation and remission.

The overall incidence of SLE in Canada is approximately 1 per 2 000 people. SLE can occur at any age, although it is much less common in the very young or the very old. Approximately 90% of people with SLE are women (Arthritis Society, 2017e).

Etiology and Pathophysiology

The etiology of the abnormal immune response in SLE is unknown. Because of the high prevalence of SLE among family members, a genetic influence is suspected. Multiple susceptibility genes from the HLA complex, including HLA-DR2 and HLA-DR3, show associations with SLE.

Hormones are known to play a role in the etiology of SLE. Onset or exacerbation of disease symptoms sometimes occurs after the onset of menses, with the use of oral contraceptives, and during and after pregnancy. The disease tends to worsen in the immediate postpartum period.

Environmental factors are believed to contribute to the occurrence of SLE; sun exposure and burns are the most common environmental triggers. Infectious agents may serve as a stimulus for immune hyperactivity. SLE may also be precipitated or aggravated by certain medications, such as procainamide, hydralazine (Apresoline), and a number of anticonvulsant agents.

SLE is characterized by the production of a large variety of autoantibodies against nucleic acids (e.g., single- and double-stranded DNA), erythrocytes, coagulation proteins, lymphocytes, platelets, and many other self-proteins. Autoimmune reactions characteristically are directed against constituents of the cell nucleus (ANAs), particularly DNA.

Circulating immune complexes containing antibodies against DNA are deposited in the basement membranes of capillaries in the kidneys, the heart, the skin, the brain, and the joints. Complement is activated and inflammation occurs. The overaggressive antibody response is also related to activation of B and T cells. The specific manifestations of SLE depend on which cell types or organs are involved. (SLE is a type III hypersensitivity response [see Chapter 16].)

Clinical Manifestations and Complications

The severity of SLE is extremely variable, ranging from relatively mild to rapidly progressive and affecting many organ systems (Figure 67.9). The progressive organ involvement of SLE has no characteristic pattern. Any organ can be affected by an accumulation of circulating immune complexes. The most commonly affected tissues are the skin and muscle, the lining of the lungs, the heart, nervous tissue, and the kidneys. Indigenous people tend to have a higher incidence of arthritis and renal disease related to SLE (Hurd & Barnabe, 2017). Generalized symptoms such as fever, weight loss, arthralgia, and excessive fatigue may precede an exacerbation of disease activity.

Dermatological Manifestations. Cutaneous vascular lesions can appear in any location but are most likely to develop in sun-exposed areas. Severe skin reactions can occur in people who are photosensitive. The classic "butterfly rash" over the cheeks and bridge of the nose occurs in 50% of patients with SLE (Figure 67.10). About 20% of patients have *discoid* (round, coin-shaped) lesions. A small number of patients have persistent lesions, photosensitivity, and mild systemic disease, in a syndrome referred to as *subacute cutaneous lupus.*

Ulcers of the oral or the nasopharyngeal membranes occur in up to one third of patients with SLE. Alopecia is also common, with or without underlying scalp lesions. The hair may grow back during remission, but hair loss may be permanent over lesions. The scalp becomes dry and scaly and atrophied.

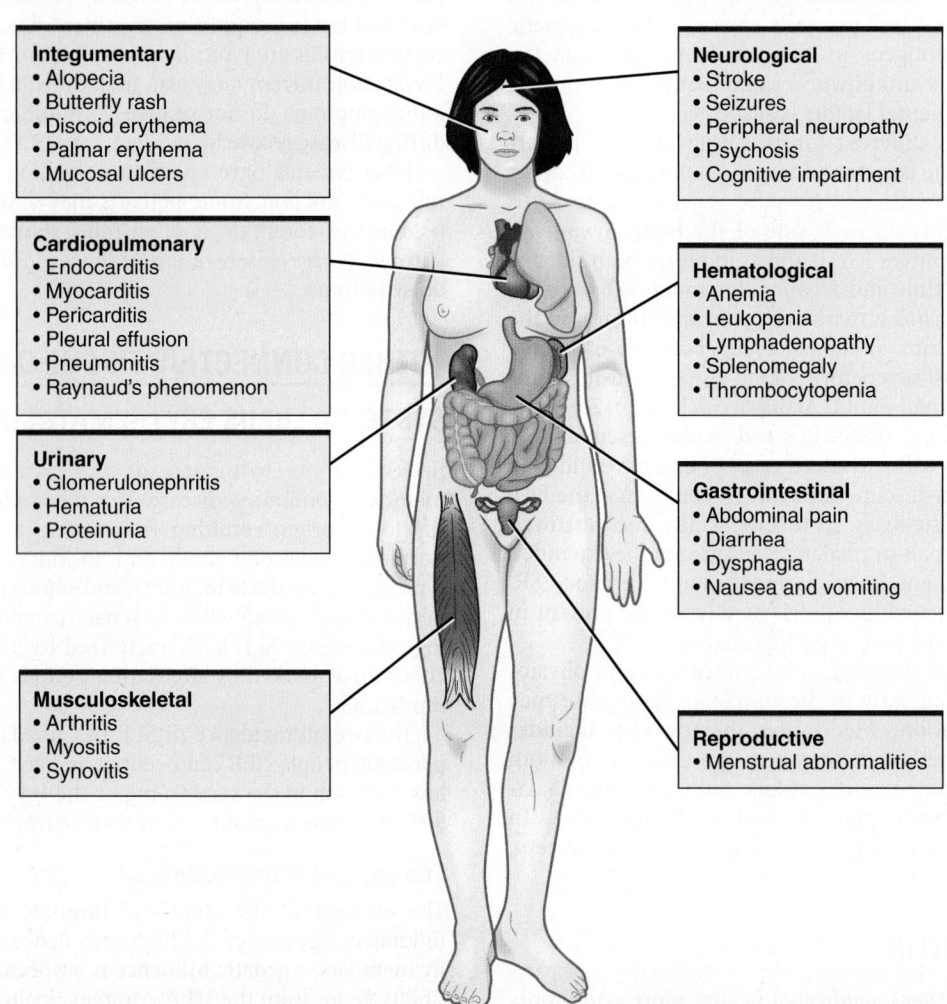

Integumentary
• Alopecia
• Butterfly rash
• Discoid erythema
• Palmar erythema
• Mucosal ulcers

Cardiopulmonary
• Endocarditis
• Myocarditis
• Pericarditis
• Pleural effusion
• Pneumonitis
• Raynaud's phenomenon

Urinary
• Glomerulonephritis
• Hematuria
• Proteinuria

Musculoskeletal
• Arthritis
• Myositis
• Synovitis

Neurological
• Stroke
• Seizures
• Peripheral neuropathy
• Psychosis
• Cognitive impairment

Hematological
• Anemia
• Leukopenia
• Lymphadenopathy
• Splenomegaly
• Thrombocytopenia

Gastrointestinal
• Abdominal pain
• Diarrhea
• Dysphagia
• Nausea and vomiting

Reproductive
• Menstrual abnormalities

FIG. 67.9 Multisystem involvement in systemic lupus erythematosus.

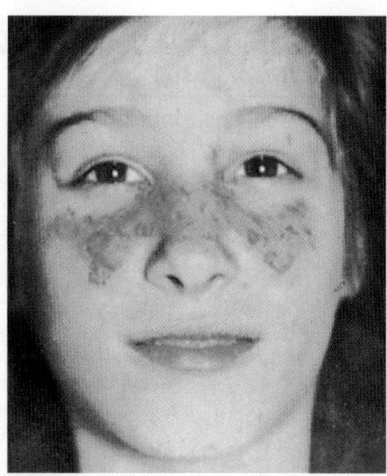

FIG. 67.10 Butterfly rash manifestation of systemic lupus erythematosus. Source: Kliegman, R. M., Stanton, B. F., St. Geme III, J. W., et al. (Eds.). (2011). *Nelson textbook of pediatrics* (19th ed., Figure 152-1, A). W. B. Saunders.

Musculoskeletal Conditions. Arthritis occurs in more than 90% of patients with SLE. Polyarthralgia with morning stiffness is often the patient's first symptom and may precede the onset of multisystem disease by many years. Diffuse swelling is accompanied by joint and muscle pain, and some stiffness may be experienced. Lupus-related arthritis is generally nonerosive, but it may cause deformities such as swan-neck appearance of the fingers (see Figure 67.4, *D*), ulnar deviation, and subluxation with hyperlaxity of the joints. Patients with SLE have an increased risk for bone loss and fracture.

Cardiopulmonary Conditions. Tachypnea and cough in patients with SLE are suggestive of lung disease. Pleurisy is also possible. Cardiac involvement may include dysrhythmias that result from fibrosis of the sinoatrial and atrioventricular nodes. This is an ominous sign of advanced disease, contributing significantly to the morbidity and mortality seen in SLE. Pericarditis can also occur. Clinical factors such as hypertension and hypercholesterolemia require aggressive therapy and careful monitoring. In addition, people with SLE are at risk for secondary antiphospholipid syndrome (APS), a disorder of coagulation that leads to clots in the arteries and veins, with associated risk for stroke, gangrene, and heart attack.

Renal Conditions. Approximately 40% of patients with SLE develop kidney conditions that need medical evaluation and treatment. Renal involvement is usually evident within 5 years after symptoms of SLE appear. Manifestations vary from mild proteinuria to rapid, progressive glomerulonephritis. Scarring and permanent damage can lead to end-stage renal disease (ESRD).

The primary goal is to slow the progression of nephropathy and preserve renal function by managing the underlying disease. The need for a renal biopsy is debated, but findings can help guide treatment. Effective treatments typically include corticosteroids, cytotoxic agents (cyclophosphamide [Procytox]), and immunosuppressive agents (azathioprine [Imuran], cyclosporin [Neoral], mycophenolate mofetil [CellCept]). Oral prednisone or pulsed IV methylprednisolone may also be used, especially in the initial treatment period, when cytotoxic agents have not yet taken effect.

Nervous System Conditions. Neuropsychiatric manifestations are prevalent in SLE. Generalized or focal seizures are the most common manifestation involving the CNS and occur in as many as 15% of patients with SLE by the time of diagnosis.

Seizures are generally controlled by corticosteroids or anticonvulsant medications. Peripheral neuropathy can also occur, leading to sensory and motor deficits.

Cognitive dysfunction may result from the deposit of immune complexes within the brain. There may be disordered thought processes, disorientation, and memory deficits. Various psychiatric conditions may occur, including depression, mood disorders, anxiety, and psychosis. SLE may cause a stroke or aseptic meningitis. Headaches are common and can become severe during exacerbation of the disease.

Hematological Conditions. Blood conditions are common because of the formation of antibodies against blood cells. Anemia, leukopenia, thrombocytopenia, and coagulation disorders are often present (Felz & Wickam, 2016). Many patients benefit from high-intensity treatment with warfarin (Coumadin).

Infection. Patients with SLE appear to have increased susceptibility to infections, possibly in relation to defects in the ability to phagocytize invading bacteria, deficiencies in production of antibodies, and the immunosuppressive effect of many anti-inflammatory medications. Pneumonia is the most common infection. Fever may indicate an underlying infectious process rather than lupus activity alone. Vaccinations are generally safe for patients with SLE. The exception is the need to avoid live virus vaccines in patients who are being treated with corticosteroids or cytotoxic agents.

Diagnostic Studies

The diagnosis of SLE is based on the presence of distinct criteria revealed through patient history, physical examination, and laboratory findings (Table 67.13). No specific test is diagnostic for SLE, but a variety of abnormalities may be present in the blood. SLE is marked by the presence of ANA in 97% of people with the disease.

Other antibodies include anti-DNA, antineuronal, anticoagulant, anti-WBC, anti–red blood cell (RBC), antiplatelet, antiphospholipid, and anti–basement membrane antibodies.

TABLE 67.13	CRITERIA FOR DIAGNOSIS OF SYSTEMIC LUPUS ERYTHEMATOSUS*

- Antinuclear antibodies
- Arthritis: nonerosive, involvement of two or more joints characterized by tenderness, swelling, and effusion
- Discoid rash
- Hematological disorder: hemolytic anemia, leukopenia, lymphopenia, or thrombocytopenia
- Immunological disorder: positive result of LE preparation; anti-DNA antibody or antibody to Sm nuclear antigen; or false-positive result of serological tests for syphilis
- Malar rash
- Neurological disorder: seizures or psychosis
- Oral ulcers
- Photosensitivity
- Renal disorder: persistent proteinuria or cellular casts in urine
- Serositis: pleuritis or pericarditis

LE, lupus erythematosus; *Sm*, Smith.

*Systemic lupus erythematosus is diagnosed if four or more of the criteria are present, serially or simultaneously, during any interval of observation. Revised criteria by a subcommittee of the American College of Rheumatology are used for the purpose of classification in population surveys, not for the diagnosis in individual patients. Sources: Tan, E. M., Cohen, A. S., Fries, J. F., et al. (1982). The 1982 revised criteria for the classification of systemic lupus erythematosus. *Arthritis and Rheumatism*, 25(11), 1271–1277. doi:10.1002/art.1780251101; and Hochberg, M. C. (1997). Updating the American College of Rheumatology revised criteria for the classification of systemic lupus erythematosus [Letter]. *Arthritis and Rheumatism*, 40(9), 1725. https://doi.org/10.1002/art.1780400928

Anti-double-stranded DNA antibodies are found in half of all people with SLE. The anti-Smith (Sm) antibodies are found in 30 to 40% of people with lupus and are almost always considered diagnostic. The lupus erythematosus (LE) cell prep test is a nonspecific test for SLE and is positive in other rheumatic diseases. ESR and CRP levels are not diagnostic of SLE but may be used to monitor disease activity and effectiveness of therapy.

Interprofessional Care

A major challenge in the treatment of SLE is to manage the active phase of the disease while preventing complications of treatments. Survival is influenced by several factors, including age, race, sex, socioeconomic status, comorbid conditions, and the severity of disease. The prognosis of SLE can be improved with early diagnosis, prompt recognition of serious organ involvement, and effective therapeutic regimens.

Medication Therapy. NSAIDs continue to be an important intervention, especially for patients with mild polyarthralgias or polyarthritis. Because prolonged therapy is likely, patients must be monitored carefully for GI and renal effects from NSAID use.

Antimalarial agents such as hydroxychloroquine (Plaquenil) and chloroquine are often used to treat fatigue and moderate skin and joint conditions. Unlike the rapid response noted with corticosteroids, effects of antimalarial therapy may not be noticed for several months. Flares may also be prevented with these medications. Funduscopic and visual field examinations must be performed by an ophthalmologist every 6 to 12 months when patients are on hydroxychloroquine. Retinopathy can develop with high-dosage use of these medications, but it generally reverses when they are discontinued. If patients cannot tolerate an antimalarial agent, an antileprosy medication such as dapsone may be used.

The use of corticosteroids should be limited to the lowest dose for the shortest possible time. For example, steroids can be used for a few weeks until a slower-acting medication becomes effective. The patient's dose of steroid should be tapered slowly rather than stopping the medication abruptly. High doses of corticosteroids may be appropriate for patients with very severe cutaneous SLE.

Immunosuppressive medications such as azathioprine (Imuran) and cyclophosphamide (Procytox) may be prescribed to reduce the need for long-term corticosteroid therapy. Close monitoring is necessary to minimize medication toxicity and other adverse effects. Because blood clots can be a life-threatening complication of SLE, anticoagulants such as warfarin may be prescribed. Belimumab (Benlysta) is a β-lymphocyte stimulator that inhibits the inflammation of SLE.

Disease management is most appropriately monitored by serial anti-DNA titres and serum complement levels (Table 67.14). Simpler and less costly tests such as ESR or CRP measurement may also help in monitoring treatment effectiveness.

NURSING MANAGEMENT
SYSTEMIC LUPUS ERYTHEMATOSUS

NURSING ASSESSMENT

Subjective and objective data that should be obtained from patients with SLE are presented in Table 67.15. In particular, the extent to which pain and fatigue influence ADLs must be evaluated.

TABLE 67.14 INTERPROFESSIONAL CARE

Systemic Lupus Erythematosus

Diagnostic	Interprofessional Therapy
• History and physical examination • Antibody titres (e.g., anti-DNA, anti-Sm, ANA) • Chest radiograph • Complete blood cell count • ECG to determine extra-articular involvement • LE cell prep • Radiographic examination of affected joints • Serum complement levels • Urinalysis	• Antimalarials (e.g., hydroxychloroquine [Plaquenil]) • Corticosteroids for exacerbations and severe disease • Immunosuppressive medications (e.g., cyclophosphamide [Procytox], mycophenolate [CellCept]) • NSAIDs for mild disease • Steroid-sparing medications (e.g., methotrexate)

ANA, antinuclear antibody; *DNA,* deoxyribonucleic acid; *ECG,* electrocardiogram; *LE,* lupus erythematosus; *NSAIDs,* nonsteroidal anti-inflammatory drugs; *Sm,* Smith.

NURSING DIAGNOSES

Nursing diagnoses for the patient with SLE may include but are not limited to the following:

- *Fatigue* resulting from *physical deconditioning* (chronic inflammation and altered immunity)
- *Reduced comfort* resulting from *insufficient situational control* (symptoms of illness, treatment adverse effects, variable and unpredictable disease progression)

Additional information on nursing diagnoses for patients with SLE is presented in NCP 67.2, available on the Evolve website.

PLANNING

The overall goals are that patients with SLE will (a) have acceptable pain management, (b) demonstrate awareness of and avoid activities that cause disease exacerbation, (c) adhere to therapeutic regimen to achieve maximum symptom management, and (d) maintain optimal role function and a positive self-image.

NURSING IMPLEMENTATION

ACUTE INTERVENTION. The unpredictable nature of SLE presents many challenges to the patient and caregiver. Physical, psychological, and sociocultural issues associated with the long-term management of SLE require the varied approaches and skills of the interprofessional team.

During an exacerbation of SLE, a patient may become abruptly and dramatically ill. The nurse assesses fever pattern, joint inflammation, limitation of motion, location and degree of discomfort, and fatigue. The nurse should also monitor the patient's weight and fluid intake and output if corticosteroids are prescribed because of the fluid-retention effect of these medications and the possibility of acute kidney injury. Collection of 24-hour urine samples for protein and creatinine clearance may be ordered. The nurse should observe for signs of bleeding that result from medication therapy, such as pallor, skin bruising, petechiae, or tarry stools.

Careful assessment of neurological status includes observation for visual disturbances, headaches, personality changes, seizures, and forgetfulness. Psychosis may indicate CNS disease or may be an adverse effect of corticosteroid therapy. Irritation of the nerves of the extremities (peripheral neuropathy) may

TABLE 67.15   NURSING ASSESSMENT

Systemic Lupus Erythematosus

Subjective Data

Important Health Information

Past health history: Exposure to ultraviolet radiation, medications, chemicals, viral infections; stress (physical or psychological); states of increased estrogen activity (including early onset of menarche; pregnancy and postpartum period); pattern of remissions and exacerbations

Medications: Oral contraceptives, procainamide, hydralazine (Apresoline), isoniazid (INH), anticonvulsant medications, antibiotics (possibly precipitating symptoms of SLE), corticosteroids, NSAIDs

Symptoms

- Weight loss; nausea and vomiting; xerostomia (salivary gland dryness); oral and nasal ulcers; dysphagia; diarrhea or constipation; decreased urine output.
- Morning stiffness; joint swelling and deformity; polyarthralgia; painful, throbbing cold fingers with numbness and tingling; photosensitivity with rash; chest pain (pericardial, pleuritic); abdominal pain; shortness of breath, dyspnea
- Visual disturbances: vertigo; headache; excessive fatigue, insomnia
- Amenorrhea; irregular menstrual periods; frequent infections
- Depression; withdrawal

Objective Data

General

Fever, lymphadenopathy, periorbital edema

Integumentary

Alopecia; dry, scaly scalp; keratoconjunctivitis, malar "butterfly" rash, palmar or discoid erythema, urticaria, periungual erythema, purpura, or petechiae; leg ulcers

Respiratory

Pleural friction rub, decreased breath sounds

Cardiovascular

Vasculitis; pericardial friction rub; hypertension, edema, dysrhythmias, murmurs; bilateral, symmetrical pallor and cyanosis of fingers (Raynaud's phenomenon)

Gastrointestinal

Oral and pharyngeal ulcers; splenomegaly

Neurological

Facial weakness, peripheral neuropathies, papilledema, dysarthria, confusion, hallucination, disorientation, psychosis, seizures, aphasia, hemiparesis

Musculoskeletal

Myopathy, myositis, arthritis

Urinary

Proteinuria

Possible Findings

Presence of anti-DNA, anti-Sm, and antinuclear antibodies; anemia, leukopenia, thrombocytopenia; ↑ ESR; positive result of LE cell prep; ↑ serum creatinine; microscopic hematuria, cellular casts in urine; pericarditis or pleural effusion evident on chest radiograph

DNA, deoxyribonucleic acid; *ESR,* erythrocyte sedimentation rate; *LE,* lupus erythematosus; *NSAIDs,* nonsteroidal anti-inflammatory drugs; *SLE,* systemic lupus erythematosus; *Sm,* Smith.

TABLE 67.16   PATIENT & CAREGIVER TEACHING GUIDE

Systemic Lupus Erythematosus

The following instructions should be included in the teaching plan for a patient with systemic lupus erythematosus and their caregiver:

- Avoidance of drying soaps, powders, household chemicals
- Avoidance of exposure to individuals with infection
- Avoidance of physical and emotional stress
- Community resources and health care agencies
- Disease process
- Energy conservation and pacing techniques
- Couples and pregnancy counselling as needed
- Names of medications, actions, adverse effects, dosage, administration
- Pain management strategies
- Regular medical and laboratory follow-up
- Therapeutic exercise, use of heat therapy (for arthralgia)
- Use of sunscreen protection (at least SPF 15), with minimal sun exposure between the hours of 1100 and 1500

SPF, sun protection factor.

use, proper administration, and adverse effects (Table 67.16). Patients need to understand that abruptly stopping a medication may worsen disease activity. Emotional support for the patient and family is essential, especially during an exacerbation.

AMBULATORY AND HOME CARE. Nursing interventions must emphasize the importance of patient cooperation for successful home management. The nurse should help patients understand that even strong adherence to the treatment plan is not a guarantee against exacerbation because the course of the disease is unpredictable. A variety of factors may increase disease activity, such as fatigue, sun exposure, emotional stress, infection, medications, and surgery. Nursing interventions should be directed toward assisting patients and their families in eliminating or minimizing exposure to precipitating factors.

SYSTEMIC LUPUS ERYTHEMATOSUS AND PREGNANCY. Because SLE is most common in women of childbearing age, treatment during pregnancy must be considered. The woman's primary health care provider (or rheumatologist) and obstetrician should thoroughly discuss with the woman her desire to become pregnant. Infertility may have already resulted from renal involvement and the use of high-dose corticosteroid and chemotherapy agents. Patients with SLE should understand that spontaneous abortion, stillbirth, and intrauterine growth restriction are common complications during pregnancy. They occur because of deposits of immune complexes in the placenta and because of inflammatory responses in the placental blood vessels.

The renal, cardiovascular, and pulmonary systems and the CNS may be especially affected during pregnancy. Women who already demonstrate serious SLE involvement in these systems should be counselled against pregnancy. For the best outcome, pregnancy should be planned at a time when the disease activity is minimal. Exacerbation is common during the postpartum period. Therapeutic abortion offers the same risk for postdelivery exacerbation as that of carrying the fetus to term.

PSYCHOSOCIAL ISSUES. Patients with SLE may have to confront many psychosocial issues. Disease onset and symptoms may be vague, and SLE may remain undiagnosed for a long period. Supportive therapies may become as important as medical treatment in helping patients cope with the disease. The nurse should inform patients and their families that SLE has a good prognosis for most people.

produce numbness, tingling sensation, and weakness of the hands and feet.

The nurse should also explain the nature of the disease, modes of therapy, and all diagnostic procedures. When teaching about medications the nurse needs to include indications for

Families often worry about hereditary aspects of the disease, and patients with SLE want to know whether their children will also have SLE. Many couples require pregnancy and sexual counselling. Individuals making decisions about relationships and careers worry about how SLE will interfere with their plans. The nurse may have to educate teachers, employers, and co-workers about the impact of SLE.

Pain and fatigue may interfere with quality of life. Pacing techniques and relaxation therapy can help the patient remain involved in day-to-day activities. The nurse should stress the importance of planning both recreational and occupational activities. Young adults may find physical limitations and restrictions of sun exposure particularly difficult to follow. Nursing interventions should assist patients in developing and accomplishing reasonable goals for improving or maintaining mobility, energy levels, and self-esteem.

EVALUATION

Following are the expected outcomes for the patient with SLE:
- Use energy-conservation techniques
- Adapt lifestyle to energy level
- Maintain skin integrity with the use of topical treatments
- Prevent exacerbations with the use of sunscreens and limited sun exposure

Additional information on expected outcomes for patients with SLE is presented in NCP 67.2, on the Evolve website.

SCLERODERMA

Scleroderma, or *systemic sclerosis,* is a rare disorder of connective tissue characterized by fibrotic, degenerative, and occasionally inflammatory changes in skin, blood vessels, synovium, skeletal muscle, and internal organs.

Although symptoms may begin at any time, the usual age at onset is between 30 and 50 years. Scleroderma affects up to five times more women than men (Arthritis Society, 2017f).

Two types of disease exist: the more common *localized scleroderma,* which affects the skin only, and *systemic scleroderma,* which affects organs throughout the body as well. Systemic disease can be further broken down into limited and diffuse scleroderma. Skin changes of localized disease are usually limited to a few places on the skin or muscle without involvement of the trunk or internal organs. The prognosis of patients with localized disease is better than for those with systemic disease (Arthritis Society, 2017f).

Etiology and Pathophysiology

The exact cause of scleroderma is unknown. Immunological dysfunction and vascular abnormalities are believed to play a role in the development of widespread systemic disease. Other risk factors associated with skin thickening include environmental occupational exposure to coal, plastics, and silica dust.

In scleroderma, *collagen*—the protein that gives normal skin its strength and elasticity—is overproduced (Figure 67.11). Excessive production of collagen leads to progressive tissue fibrosis and occlusion of blood vessels. Proliferation of collagen disrupts the normal functioning of internal organs, such as the lungs, the kidneys, the heart, and the GI tract.

The vascular alterations, which primarily involve the small arteries and arterioles, are almost always present in scleroderma. These changes are some of the earliest alterations in scleroderma.

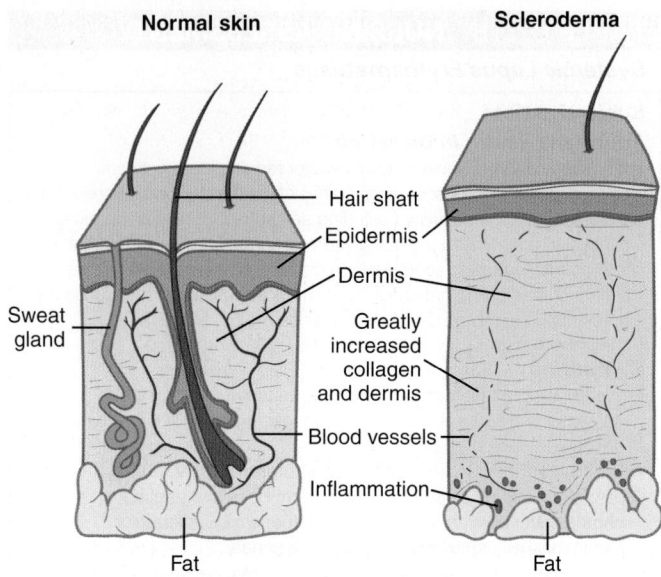

FIG. 67.11 Skin changes in scleroderma.

Clinical Manifestations

Manifestations of scleroderma range from benign limited skin disease to a diffuse skin thickening with rapidly progressive and widespread organ involvement. Limited disease is often marked by the **CREST** syndrome:

Calcinosis: painful deposits of calcium in the skin of fingers, forearms, and pressure points

Raynaud's phenomenon: intermittent vasospasm in fingertips in response to cold or stress

Esophageal dysfunction: difficulty with swallowing, caused by internal scarring

Sclerodactyly: tightening of the skin on the fingers and toes

Telangiectasia: red spots on the hands, forearms, palms, face, and lips from capillary dilation

Raynaud's Phenomenon. Raynaud's phenomenon (sudden vasospasm within the digits) is the most common initial symptom in limited scleroderma. Blood flow to these extremities is diminished on exposure to cold (blanching or white phase), followed by cyanosis as hemoglobin releases oxygen to the tissues (blue phase) and then erythema during rewarming (red phase). The colour changes are often accompanied by numbness and tingling. Raynaud's phenomenon may precede the onset of systemic disease by months, years, or even decades. (Raynaud's phenomenon is described in more detail in Chapter 40.)

Skin and Joint Changes. Symmetrical, painless swelling or thickening of the skin of the fingers and hands may progress to diffuse scleroderma of the trunk. In limited disease, skin thickening does not generally extend above the elbow or above the knee, although in some individuals the face is affected. In more diffuse disease, the skin loses elasticity and becomes taut and shiny, producing the typical expressionless face with tightly pursed lips. Skin changes in the face may also contribute to reduction in ROM in the temporomandibular joint. The hands may be affected by *sclerodactyly,* in which the fingers are in a semiflexed position, with tightened skin up to the wrist. Reduced peripheral joint function may occur as an early symptom of polyarthritis.

Internal Organ Involvement. About 20% of people with scleroderma develop secondary Sjögren syndrome, a condition associated with dry eyes and mouth. Dysphagia, gum disease, and dental caries can result. Frequent reflux of gastric acid can result from esophageal fibrosis. If swallowing becomes difficult, patients often decrease food intake and lose weight. Additional GI effects include constipation, which results from colonic hypomotility, and diarrhea, caused by malabsorption from bacterial overgrowth.

Lung involvement includes pleural thickening, pulmonary fibrosis, and pulmonary function abnormalities. Affected patients develop a cough and dyspnea. Pulmonary arterial hypertension and interstitial lung disease can occur. Pulmonary hypertension is treated with medications such as extended-release nifedipine (Adalat), bosentan, and ambrisentan. (Pulmonary hypertension is discussed in Chapter 30.) Lung disease is the main cause of death in patients with scleroderma.

Primary heart disease consists of pericarditis, pericardial effusion, and cardiac dysrhythmias. Myocardial fibrosis that results in heart failure occurs most frequently in patients with diffuse disease.

Renal disease was previously a major cause of death in diffuse scleroderma. Because malignant hypertension in association with rapidly progressive and irreversible renal insufficiency may occur, early recognition of renal involvement and initiation of therapy are critical. Improvements in dialysis, bilateral nephrectomy in patients with uncontrollable hypertension, and kidney transplantation have offered some hope to patients with renal failure. In particular, use of angiotensin-converting enzyme (ACE) inhibitors (e.g., lisinopril [Prinivil]) has markedly improved the treatment of renal disease.

Diagnostic Studies

Laboratory findings in scleroderma are relatively normal. Blood studies may show mild hemolytic anemia from RBC damage in diseased small vessels. Anticentromere antibodies related to CREST syndrome are found in about 45 to 50% of people with localized scleroderma. They are rare in people with systemic disease. Antibodies to topoisomerase-1 are present in about 30% of people with diffuse disease. Presence of either antibody is highly specific for diagnosis. If renal involvement is present, urinalysis may reveal proteinuria, microscopic hematuria, and casts. Serum levels of creatinine may be elevated. Radiographic evidence of subcutaneous calcification, distal esophageal hypomotility, or bilateral pulmonary fibrosis is diagnostic of scleroderma. Pulmonary function studies reveal decreased vital capacity and lung compliance.

Interprofessional Care

The interprofessional care of scleroderma (Table 67.17) offers no specific long-term treatment. Supportive care is directed toward attempts to prevent or treat secondary complications of involved organs. Physiotherapy helps maintain joint mobility and preserve muscle strength. Occupational therapy assists patients in maintaining functional abilities.

Medication Therapy. Vasoactive agents are often prescribed for early stages of the disease, and calcium channel blockers (nifedipine [Adalat] and diltiazem) and the angiotensin II blocker losartan are common treatments for Raynaud's phenomenon. Prazosin, an α-adrenergic blocking agent, increases blood flow to the fingers. Bosentan (Tracleer), an endothelin-receptor antagonist, and epoprostenol (Flolan), a vasodilator, may improve blood flow to the lungs. NSAIDs and topical agents may provide some relief from joint pain. Capsaicin cream may be useful, not only as a local analgesic but also as a

TABLE 67.17   INTERPROFESSIONAL CARE
Scleroderma

Diagnostic	Interprofessional Therapy
• History and physical examination • Anticentromere antibody titre • Antinuclear antibody titre • Electrocardiography • Microscopic study of nail bed capillaries • Pulmonary function test • Radiographic studies of chest and hands • Skin or visceral biopsy • Urinalysis (proteinuria, hematuria, casts)	• Physiotherapy and occupational therapy • Medication therapy • Angiotensin-converting enzyme (ACE) inhibitors (lisinopril [Prinivil]) • Calcium channel blockers (diltiazem [Cardizem], nifedipine [Adalat]) • Immunosuppressive medications (e.g., cyclophosphamide [Procytox]; mycophenolate mofetil [CellCept]) • Vasoactive agents: bosentan (Tracleer); epoprostenol (Flolan)

vasodilator. Other therapies are prescribed to address specific systemic problems, such as tetracycline for diarrhea caused by bacterial overgrowth, histamine H_2-receptor blockers (e.g., cimetidine) and proton pump inhibitors (e.g., omeprazole [Losec]) for esophageal symptoms, antihypertensive agents (e.g., captopril, propranolol [Inderal]), methyldopa for hypertension with renal involvement, and immunosuppressive medications (e.g., cyclophosphamide [Procytox], mycophenolate mofetil [CellCept]).

NURSING MANAGEMENT SCLERODERMA

Nursing intervention often begins during hospitalization for diagnostic purposes. The nurse assesses vital signs, weight, intake and output, respiratory and bowel function, and joint ROM at regular intervals, as indicated by specific symptoms, to plan appropriate care. Emotional stress and cold ambient temperatures may aggravate Raynaud's phenomenon. Patients with scleroderma should not undergo finger-stick blood testing because of compromised circulation and poor healing of the fingers.

Health teaching is an important nursing intervention as patients and their families begin to live with this disease. Obvious changes in the face and the hands often lead to compromised self-image and the loss of mobility and function. Patients must actively complete therapeutic exercises at home to prevent skin retraction and promote vascularization. Mouth excursion (opening the mouth widely, as in yawning) is a good exercise to help with temporomandibular joint function. Isometric exercises are most appropriate if the patient has *arthropathy* (disease of the joint), because no joint movement occurs. The nurse should encourage the use of moist heat applications or paraffin baths to promote skin flexibility in the hands and feet. Patients should use assistive devices as appropriate and organize activities to preserve strength and reduce disability.

Hands and feet should be protected from cold exposure and possible burns or cuts that might heal slowly. Smoking should be avoided because of its vasoconstricting effect. Signs of infection should be promptly reported. Lotions may help alleviate skin dryness and cracking, but they must be rubbed in for an unusually long time because of the thickness of the skin.

Dysphagia may be reduced by eating small, frequent meals, chewing carefully and slowly, and drinking fluids with food. Heartburn may be minimized with the use of antacids 45 to 60 minutes after each meal and by sitting upright for at least 2 hours after eating. Use of additional pillows or raising the head of the bed on blocks may help reduce nocturnal gastroesophageal reflux.

Job modifications are often necessary because stair climbing, using a computer, writing, and cold exposure may pose particular challenges. Patients may become socially withdrawn as skin tightening alters the appearance of the face and the hands. Dining out may become a socially embarrassing event because of the patient's restricted opening of their mouth, difficulty swallowing, and reflux. Some individuals with scleroderma wear gloves to protect fingertip ulcers and to provide extra warmth. Daily oral hygiene must be emphasized; neglect may lead to increased tooth and gingival complications. Patients need a dentist who is familiar with scleroderma and can work with a small mouth opening.

Psychological support, biofeedback training, and relaxation techniques can reduce stress and improve sleeping habits. Sexual dysfunction resulting from body changes, pain, muscular weakness, limited mobility, decreased self-esteem, erectile dysfunction, and decreased vaginal secretions may require sensitive counselling.

MYOSITIS

Myositis refers to diffuse, idiopathic, inflammatory myopathies of the connective tissues, especially striated muscle, that produce bilateral weakness, usually most severe in the proximal or limb-girdle muscles. Myositis was previously divided into two types (**dermatomyositis** and **polymyositis**); however, other forms have now been recognized, including immune-mediated necrotizing myopathy, overlap myositis, and inclusion-body myositis (Aggarwal & Oddis, 2019). These diseases are rare, with approximately one to five new cases per year in 100 000 people. Although they can occur at any age, they are most commonly seen in middle-aged adults. Women are affected more often than men. However, inclusion-body myositis is more common in men over the age of 50 (Arthritis Society, 2017g).

Etiology and Pathophysiology

The exact cause of myositis is unknown. Evidence suggests an autoimmune origin with T-cell–mediated destruction of unidentified muscle antigens. A combination of genetic and environmental factors is likely involved, including viral and bacterial infection, certain medications, and occupational exposure (Arthritis Society, 2017g).

Clinical Manifestations and Complications

Muscular. Patients with myositis experience weight loss and increasing fatigue, with gradually developing weakness of the muscles that leads to difficulty in performing routine activities. The muscles most commonly affected are those of the shoulders, the legs, the arms, and the pelvic girdle. Patients may have difficulty rising from a chair or bathtub, climbing stairs, combing their hair, or reaching into a high cupboard. Neck muscles may become so weak that patients are unable to raise their head from the pillow. Muscle discomfort or tenderness is uncommon. Muscle examination reveals an inability to

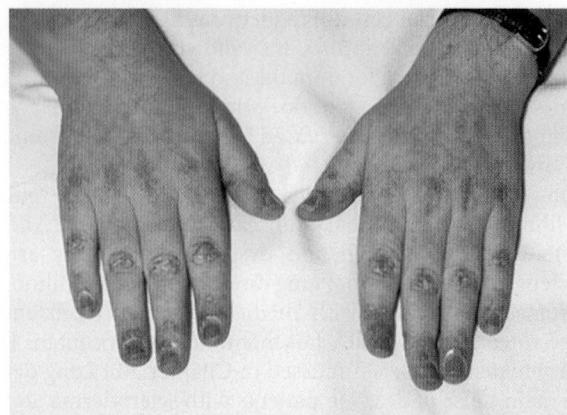

FIG. 67.12 Dermatomyositis skin changes. Gottron papules. Source: Firestein, G. S., Budd, R. C., Gabriel, S. E., et al. (2012). *Kelley's textbook of rheumatology.* (9th ed.). Saunders.

move against resistance or even gravity. Weakness of the pharyngeal muscles may result in dysphagia and dysphonia (nasal or hoarse voice).

Dermal. Rashes are typical of dermatomyositis. Skin changes include a classic violet-coloured, cyanotic, or erythematous symmetrical rash *(heliotrope rash)* with edema around the eyelids. Violet-coloured or erythematous papules *(Gottron papules)* and small plaques develop over the DIP or MCP areas and at elbow or knee joints in about 70% of patients with dermatomyositis (Figure 67.12). Because of these early skin changes, dermatomyositis is usually recognized earlier than polymyositis, in which a rash does not appear. Reddened, smooth, or scaly patches appear with the same symmetrical distribution but sparing the interphalangeal spaces (Gottron sign); they can be confused with psoriasis or seborrheic dermatitis. An erythematous scaling rash *(poikiloderma)* may develop as a late finding on the back, buttocks, and a V-shaped area of the anterior neck and chest. Hyperemia and telangiectasias are often present at the nail beds. Calcium nodules (calcinosis cutis), which can develop throughout the skin, are especially common in longstanding dermatomyositis.

Other Manifestations. Joint redness, pain, and inflammation often occur and contribute to limitations in joint ROM. Contractures and muscle atrophy may occur with advanced disease. Weakening of the pharyngeal muscles can lead to a poor cough effort, difficulty swallowing, and increased risk for aspiration pneumonia in both disorders. Interstitial lung disease occurs in up to 65% of all affected patients. People with dermatomyositis also have an increased risk for cancer, which may be present at the time of diagnosis. These diseases may be associated with other connective tissue disorders (e.g., scleroderma).

Diagnostic Studies

Biopsy is the gold standard for diagnosis of myositis after other neuromuscular disorders are excluded. Muscle biopsy shows necrosis, degeneration, regeneration, and fibrosis with pathological findings. MRI or electromyogram (EMG) can be used to identify areas of inflammation and guide the biopsy site selection (Arthritis Society, 2017g). Laboratory tests are helpful, but they are not diagnostic of disease. Increased muscle enzymes (e.g., creatine kinase, myoglobin) reflect muscle damage but will decrease to normal or near normal with treatment.

NURSING AND INTERPROFESSIONAL MANAGEMENT MYOSITIS

Myositis is initially treated with high-dose corticosteroids, with the dose tapered on the basis of patient response. Most patients respond well to treatment. Long-term corticosteroid therapy may be needed because relapses are common when the medication is withdrawn.

Immunosuppressive medications (methotrexate, azathioprine, tacrolimus, cyclophosphamine) may be used in combination with steroids or as a second-line therapy if the patient's condition does not respond well to steroids. Intravenous immunoglobulin may be given with corticosteroids or immunosuppressants, but it is not a first-line treatment.

Physiotherapy can be helpful and should be tailored to the activity of the disease. Massage and passive movement are appropriate during active disease. More aggressive exercises should be reserved for periods when disease activity is minimal, as evidenced by low serum enzyme levels.

Nursing interventions should include a thorough explanation of the disease, the prescribed therapies, all diagnostic tests, and the importance of regular medical care. It is important for patients to understand that the benefits of therapy are often delayed. For example, weakness may increase during the first few weeks of corticosteroid therapy. Special attention is paid to patient safety. Use of assistive devices should be encouraged as a fall prevention strategy. To prevent aspiration, patients should be encouraged to rest before meals, maintain an upright position when eating, and choose a diet of easily swallowed foods.

The nurse should assist patients in organizing activities and using pacing techniques to conserve energy. The nurse should encourage the patient to perform daily ROM exercises to prevent contractures. When active inflammation is not evident, muscle-strengthening (repetitive) exercises may be started. Home care and bed rest may become necessary during the acute phase of polymyositis because profound muscle weakness renders patients unable to carry out ADLs.

MIXED CONNECTIVE TISSUE DISEASE

Patients with a combination of clinical features of several rheumatic diseases are described as having *mixed connective tissue disease*. The term is used to describe a disorder with features of SLE, scleroderma, and polymyositis. This disease occurs most often in women in their 20s and 30s.

SJÖGREN SYNDROME

Sjögren syndrome is a relatively common autoimmune disease that targets moisture-producing exocrine glands, leading to the common symptoms of *xerostomia* (dry mouth) and *keratoconjunctivitis sicca* (dry eyes) (Arthritis Society, 2017h). The nose, the throat, the airways, and the skin can also become dry. The disease can affect other glands as well, including those in the stomach, the pancreas, and the intestines (extraglandular involvement). The disease is usually diagnosed in people older than 40 years but can be found in all age groups. Women are 10 times more likely than men to have Sjögren syndrome.

In primary Sjögren syndrome, symptoms can be traced to dysfunction of the lacrimal and the salivary glands. However, up to 40% of patients have extended disease affecting the lungs, liver, kidneys, and skin. This occurrence increases the risk for non-Hodgkin's lymphoma (Papageorgiou et al., 2015).

Sjögren syndrome appears to be caused by genetic and environmental factors. Several genes seem to be involved. The trigger may be a viral or bacterial infection that adversely stimulates the immune system. In Sjögren syndrome, lymphocytes attack and damage the lacrimal and salivary glands.

Dry eyes are characterized by decreased tearing, which leads to a "gritty" sensation in the eyes, burning sensation, blurred vision, and photosensitivity. Dry mouth leads to buccal membrane fissures, altered sense of taste, dysphagia, and increased frequency of mouth infections or dental caries. Dry skin and rashes, joint and muscle pain, and thyroid conditions may also be present. Other exocrine glands can be affected. For example, vaginal dryness may lead to dyspareunia (painful intercourse).

Autoimmune thyroid disorders, including Graves' disease and Hashimoto thyroiditis, are common with Sjögren syndrome. Histological study reveals lymphocyte infiltration of salivary and lacrimal glands. The disease may become more generalized and involve the lymph nodes, the bone marrow, and the visceral organs (pseudolymphoma). Ophthalmological examination (Schirmer test for tear production), measures of salivary gland function, and lower lip biopsy of minor salivary glands aid in the diagnosis.

The treatment for Sjögren syndrome is based on symptoms, including (a) instillation of preservative-free artificial tears as necessary to maintain adequate hydration and lubrication, (b) surgical punctal occlusion, and (c) increased fluids with meals. Dental hygiene is also important. Pilocarpine (Salagen) can be used to treat symptoms of dry mouth. Increased humidity in the home may reduce respiratory infections. Vaginal lubrication with a water-soluble product may increase comfort during intercourse.

SOFT TISSUE RHEUMATIC SYNDROMES

MYOFASCIAL PAIN SYNDROME

Myofascial pain syndrome is a chronic form of muscle pain. It is characterized by musculoskeletal pain and tenderness, typically in the chest, neck, shoulders, hips, and lower back. Referred pain from these muscle groups can also travel to the buttocks, hands, and head, causing severe headaches. Temporomandibular joint pain may also originate in myofascial pain. Regions of pain are often within the taut bands and fascia of skeletal muscles. When activated by pressure, trigger points are thought to activate a characteristic pattern of pain that can worsen with activity or stress.

Myofascial pain syndrome occurs most often in middle-aged adults and more often in women than in men. Affected patients describe the pain as deep and aching, accompanied by a sensation of burning, stinging, and stiffness.

Physiotherapy is one treatment used for myofascial pain syndrome. A typical exercise is the "spray and stretch" method, in which the painful area is iced or sprayed with a coolant such as ethyl chloride and then stretched. Positive results have been achieved by injection of the trigger points with a local anaesthetic (e.g., 1% lidocaine). Massage, acupuncture, biofeedback, and ultrasound therapy have also been shown to benefit some patients.

TABLE 67.18	COMMONALITIES BETWEEN FIBROMYALGIA AND SYSTEMIC EXERTION INTOLERANCE DISEASE
Commonality	**Description**
Clinical manifestations	Generalized musculoskeletal pain, malaise and fatigue, cognitive dysfunction, headaches, sleep disturbances, depression, anxiety, fever
Interprofessional therapy	Treatment is symptomatic and may include antidepressant medications such as amitriptyline (Elavil) and fluoxetine (Prozac). Other measures are heat, massage, regular stretching, biofeedback, stress management, and relaxation training. Patient and caregiver teaching is essential.
Course of disease	Variable intensity of symptoms; fluctuates over time
Diagnosis	No definitive laboratory tests or joint and muscle examinations; mainly a diagnosis of exclusion
Etiology (theories)	Infectious trigger, dysfunction in HPA axis, alteration in CNS
Occurrence	Previously healthy, young, and middle-aged women

CNS, central nervous system; *HPA,* hypothalamic–pituitary–adrenal.

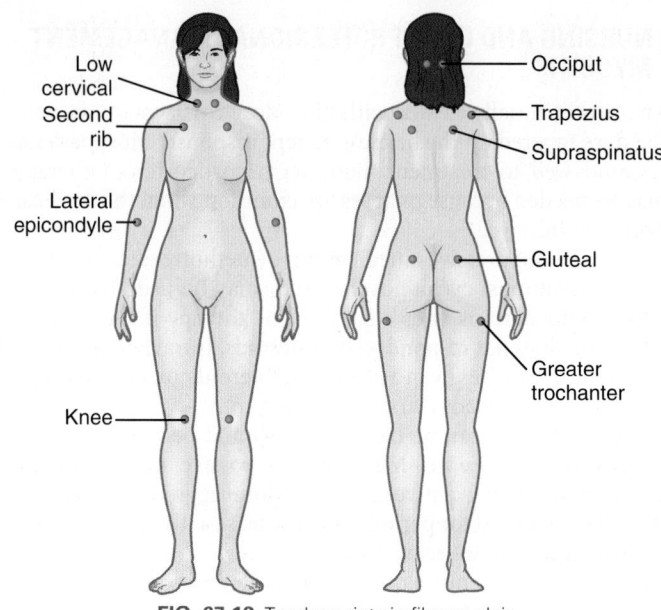

FIG. 67.13 Tender points in fibromyalgia.

FIBROMYALGIA

Fibromyalgia is a chronic disorder characterized by widespread, nonarticular musculoskeletal pain and fatigue with multiple tender points. People with fibromyalgia also typically experience nonrestorative sleep, morning stiffness, irritable bowel syndrome, and anxiety. Fibromyalgia is a commonly diagnosed musculoskeletal disorder and a major cause of disability that affects approximately 2% of Canadians, with 80 to 90% being women (Arthritis Society, 2017i). Fibromyalgia and systemic exertion intolerance disease (SEID) share many commonalities (Table 67.18).

Etiology and Pathophysiology

Fibromyalgia involves abnormal central processing of nociceptive pain input. The increased pain is due to abnormal sensory processing in the CNS. Multiple physiological abnormalities have been found, including increased levels of substance P in the spinal fluid, low levels of blood flow to the thalamus, dysfunction of the hypothalamic–pituitary–adrenal (HPA) axis, low levels of serotonin and tryptophan, and abnormalities in cytokine function. Serotonin and substance P play a role in mood regulation, sleep, and pain perception. Changes in the HPA axis can also negatively affect a person's physical and mental health, leading to an increased incidence of depression and a decreased response to stress. Genetic factors also contribute to the etiology of fibromyalgia, as a familial tendency exists. A recent illness or trauma may serve as a trigger in susceptible people.

Clinical Manifestations and Complications

Patients with fibromyalgia experience a widespread burning pain that worsens and improves throughout the course of a day. It is often difficult for patients to discriminate whether pain occurs in the muscles, the joints, or soft tissues. Head or facial pain often results from stiff or painful neck and shoulder muscles. The pain can accompany temporomandibular joint dysfunction, which affects an estimated one third of patients with fibromyalgia.

Physical examination characteristically reveals point tenderness at 11 or more of 18 identified sites (Figure 67.13). Patients with fibromyalgia are sensitive to painful stimuli throughout the body and not merely at the identified tender sites. In addition, point tenderness can vary from day to day. On some occasions, the patient may respond to fewer than 11 tender points. At other times, palpation of all sites may elicit pain.

Cognitive effects range from difficulty concentrating to memory lapses and a feeling of being overwhelmed when dealing with multiple tasks. Many individuals report migraine headaches. Depression and anxiety often occur and may require medication therapy. Stiffness, nonrefreshing sleep, fatigue, and numbness or tingling sensation in the hands or feet (paresthesia) often accompany fibromyalgia. Restless legs syndrome is also typical, with patients describing an irresistible urge to move their legs when at rest or lying down.

Irritable bowel syndrome with manifestations of constipation, diarrhea, or both; abdominal pain; and bloating is common. Patients with fibromyalgia may also experience difficulty swallowing, perhaps because of abnormalities in esophageal smooth-muscle function. Increased frequency of urination and urinary urgency, in the absence of a bladder infection, are typical symptoms. Women with fibromyalgia may experience more difficult menstruation, with a worsening of disease symptoms during this time.

Diagnostic Studies

A definitive diagnosis of fibromyalgia is often difficult to establish. Lack of knowledge among health care providers may also cause delays in diagnosis and treatment.

Laboratory results in most cases serve to rule out other disorders suspected on the basis of the patient's history and physical examination. Muscle biopsy may reveal a nonspecific moth-eaten appearance or fiber atrophy. The American College of Rheumatology classifies an individual as having fibromyalgia if the following two criteria are met: (1) pain is experienced in 11 of the 18 tender points on palpation (see Figure 67.13) and

(2) a history of widespread pain for at least 3 months is documented (Wolfe et al., 2016). In Canada, these guidelines may be used initially to validate a clinical diagnosis (Fitzcharles et al., 2012). *Widespread pain* is defined as occurring on both sides of the body and above and below the waist. In addition, fatigue, cognitive symptoms, and extensive somatic symptoms are considered in establishing a diagnosis. These symptoms vary over time.

Interprofessional Care

The treatment of fibromyalgia is symptomatic and requires a high level of patient motivation. The nurse can play a key role in teaching patients to be active participants in the therapeutic regimen. Rest can help pain, aching, and tenderness.

Medication treatment for the chronic widespread pain associated with fibromyalgia includes pregabalin (Lyrica) and duloxetine (Cymbalta). Low-dose tricyclic antidepressants, selective serotonin reuptake inhibitors (SSRIs), or benzodiazepines (e.g., diazepam [Valium]) may also be prescribed. SSRI antidepressants (e.g., sertraline [Zoloft], paroxetine [Paxil]) tend to be reserved for affected patients who also experience depression. SSRIs may need to be prescribed at higher doses than when used to treat depression. Both antidepressants and muscle relaxants have sedative effects that can help in improving nighttime rest for patients with fibromyalgia.

Long-acting opioids are generally not recommended unless fibromyalgia is refractory to other therapies. In some patients, pain may be managed with OTC analgesics such as acetaminophen (Tylenol), ibuprofen (Motrin, Advil), or naproxen (Aleve).

NURSING MANAGEMENT
FIBROMYALGIA

Because of the chronic nature of fibromyalgia, patients need consistent support from the nurse and other members of the health care team. Massage is often combined with ultrasound therapy or the application of alternating heat and cold packs to soothe tense, sore muscles and increase blood circulation. Gentle stretching can be performed by a physiotherapist or practised by the patient at home to relieve muscle tension and spasm. Yoga and tai chi are often appropriate. Low-impact aerobic exercise, such as walking, can help prevent muscle atrophy.

Often, dietitians urge patients with fibromyalgia to limit their consumption of sugar, caffeine, and alcohol because these substances have been shown to be muscle irritants. Vitamin and mineral supplements may be appropriate to combat stress, correct deficiencies, and support the immune system. However, unproven "miracle diets" or supplements should be carefully investigated by patients and discussed with the health care provider before any of them is used. Patients should understand that some foods and supplements may cause serious and even dangerous adverse effects when taken along with certain medications.

Pain and the related symptoms of fibromyalgia can cause significant stress. Patients with fibromyalgia may not cope well with stress. Effective relaxation strategies include biofeedback, mindfulness meditation, and cognitive behavioural therapy. Patients need to receive initial training for these interventions so that they can continue to practise them on their own. Psychological counselling (individual or group) may also prove

beneficial for some patients. (Stress and stress management are discussed in Chapter 8.)

SYSTEMIC EXERTION INTOLERANCE DISEASE

Systemic exertion intolerance disease (SEID), formerly known as *chronic fatigue syndrome (CFS) or myalgic encephalomyelitis,* is a serious, complex, multisystem disease in which exertion of any sort (physical, emotional, cognitive) is impaired and accompanied by profound fatigue. SEID is a poorly understood condition that can have a devastating effect on the lives of patients and their families. More women are affected than men. SEID occurs in all ethnic and socioeconomic groups. The true prevalence of SEID is unknown because many people with the disease have not been diagnosed.

Etiology and Pathophysiology

Despite efforts to determine the etiology and the pathology of SEID, the precise mechanisms remain unknown. However, there are many theories about the cause of SEID. Neuroendocrine abnormalities that have been implicated involve a hypofunction of the HPA axis and the hypothalamic–pituitary–gonadal (HPG) axis, which together regulate the stress response and reproductive hormone levels. Several microorganisms have been investigated as etiological agents, including herpes viruses (e.g., Epstein Barr virus, cytomegalovirus), retroviruses, enteroviruses, *Candida albicans,* and mycoplasma. Because many patients with the disease have cognitive deficits (e.g., decreased memory, attention, concentration), changes in the CNS have been suggested as the cause of SEID.

Clinical Manifestations

Diagnosis of SEID requires that the patient have the following three symptoms:
1. Impaired function with profound fatigue lasting at least 6 months
2. Postexertional malaise: total exhaustion after even minor physical or mental exertion that patients sometimes describe as a "crash"
3. Unrefreshing sleep
   At least one of the following two manifestations is also required:
1. Cognitive impairment ("brain fog," confusion)
2. Orthostatic intolerance (lightheadedness, dizziness, imbalance, fainting)
   SEID is often difficult to distinguish from fibromyalgia because many clinical features are similar (see Table 67.18). In about half the cases, SEID develops insidiously, or patients may have intermittent episodes that gradually become chronic. Severe fatigue is the most common symptom of SEID and causes patients to seek health care.

In other situations, SEID arises suddenly in a previously active, healthy individual. An unremarkable influenza-like illness or other acute stress is often identified as a triggering event. Associated symptoms may fluctuate in intensity over time.

Patients may become angry and frustrated with the inability of health care providers to diagnose a disease. The disorder may have a major effect on work and family responsibilities. Some patients may need help with ADLs.

Diagnostic Studies

Physical examination and diagnostic studies can be used to rule out other possible causes of a patient's symptoms. No laboratory test is available to diagnose SEID or measure its severity. SEID generally remains a diagnosis of exclusion.

NURSING AND INTERPROFESSIONAL MANAGEMENT SYSTEMIC EXERTION INTOLERANCE DISEASE

Because there is no definitive treatment for SEID, supportive management is essential. Patients should be informed about what is known about the disease, and all symptoms should be taken seriously.

NSAIDs can be used to treat headaches, muscle and joint aches, and fever. Because many patients with SEID also have allergies and sinusitis, antihistamines and decongestants can be used to treat allergic symptoms. Tricyclic antidepressants (e.g., doxepin [Sinequan], amitriptyline [Elavil]) and SSRIs (e.g., fluoxetine [Prozac], paroxetine [Paxil]) can improve mood and sleep problems. Clonazepam (Rivotril) can also be used to treat sleep disturbances and panic disorders. The use of low-dose hydrocortisone to decrease fatigue and disability is being studied.

Total rest is not advised because it can potentiate the self-image of being an invalid. On the other hand, strenuous exertion can exacerbate the exhaustion. Therefore, it is important to plan a carefully graduated exercise program. A well-balanced diet that includes fibre and fresh, dark-coloured fruits and vegetables for antioxidant action is essential in treatment. Behavioural therapy may be used to promote a positive outlook, as well as to improve overall disability, fatigue, and other symptoms.

One of the major problems facing many patients with SEID is loss of livelihood and economic security. When the illness strikes, they cannot work or must decrease the amount of time working. Obtaining disability benefits can be frustrating because of the difficulty in establishing a diagnosis of SEID. Patients with SEID may experience substantial occupational and psychosocial impairments and loss, including the social pressure and isolation from being characterized as lazy or having a mental illness.

SEID does not appear to progress. Although most patients recover or experience at least gradual improvement over time, some do not show substantial improvement. Recovery is more common in individuals with a sudden onset of SEID.

CASE STUDY

Rheumatoid Arthritis

Patient Profile

G. K. (pronouns she/her), 42 years old, is seen at the rheumatology clinic because of swelling and stiffness in the small joints of both hands.

Subjective Data

- Is a concert pianist
- Has experienced joint pain and stiffness in both hands for the past 6 weeks
- Experiencing fatigue, anorexia, and morning stiffness
- Gave birth to her first child 2 months ago

Objective Data
Physical Examination

- Swelling and tenderness of third and fourth MCP joints of both hands
- Mild pain with neck motion

Diagnostic Studies

- Elevated ESR, positive RF and ACPA
- Evidence of moderate bone demineralization on bilateral hand radiographs

Interprofessional Care

- Diagnosis: RA
- Therapy: started on methotrexate, 7.5 mg PO once per week; etanercept (Enbrel), 50 mg subcutaneously once per week; and prednisone, 10 mg daily

Discussion Questions

1. How might the nurse explain the pathophysiology of RA to G. K.?
2. How might G. K.'s recent childbirth have influenced the symptoms she is currently experiencing?
3. What are some home and work modifications that the nurse can suggest to G. K. that will reduce the symptoms?
4. What suggestions can the nurse make to G. K. about coping with fatigue?
5. ***Priority decision:*** On the basis of the assessment data presented, what are the priority nursing diagnoses? Are there any interprofessional problems?
6. ***Evidence-informed practice:*** Why is an exercise program important in the treatment plan for G.K.?

ⓔvolve

Answers are available at http://evolve.elsevier.com/Canada/Lewis/medsurg.

REVIEW QUESTIONS

The number of the question corresponds to the same-numbered objective at the beginning of the chapter.

1. Which of the following would the nurse understand as causing damage to the joints of a client with rheumatoid arthritis?
   a. The development of Heberden nodes in the joint capsule
   b. The deterioration of cartilage by the enzyme hyaluronidase
   c. Invasion of pannus into the joint capsule and subchondral bone
   d. Bony ankylosis after inflammation of the joints in HLA-B27–positive individuals

2. A client with rheumatoid arthritis is experiencing articular involvement of the joints. The nurse recognizes that these characteristic changes include which of the following? (*Select all that apply.*)
   a. Bamboo-shaped fingers
   b. Metatarsal head dislocation in feet
   c. Noninflammatory pain in large joints
   d. Asymmetrical involvement of small joints
   e. Morning stiffness lasting 60 minutes or more

3. Which of the following would the nurse teach to a client with anky-losing spondylitis?
   a. Avoid extremes in environmental temperatures.
   b. Continue with physical activity during flare-ups.
   c. Apply cool compresses for relief of local symptoms.
   d. Maintain proper posture and engage in regular exercise.
4. When the nurse administers medications to clients with gout, which of the following would the nurse recognize as a treatment for acute disease?
   a. Colchicine
   b. Sulphasalazine
   c. Allopurinol
   d. Cyclosporin
5. The nurse is teaching a client with SLE about the disorder. The nurse understands that the pathophysiology of SLE includes which of the following?
   a. Circulating immune complexes formed from IgG autoantibod-ies reacting with IgG
   b. An autoimmune T-cell reaction that results in destruction of the deep dermal skin layer
   c. Immunological dysfunction leading to chronic inflammation in the cartilage and bones
   d. The production of a variety of autoantibodies directed against constituents of the cell nucleus

6. The nurse is caring for a client with Sjögren syndrome. Which of the following autoimmune disorders may the client also develop?
   a. Uveitis
   b. Ulcerative colitis
   c. Glomerulonephritis
   d. Hashimoto thyroiditis
7. Which of the following should be considered in the management of systemic exertion intolerance disease (SEID)? *(Select all that apply.)*
   a. Dark green vegetables in diet
   b. DMARDs to reduce symptoms
   c. Total rest during acute exacerbations
   d. SSRIs or tricyclic antidepressants
   e. Behavioural therapy

1. c; 2. b, e; 3. d; 4. a; 5. d; 6. d; 7. a, d, e.

ⓔvolve

For even more review questions, visit http://evolve.elsevier.com/Canada/Lewis/medsurg.

REFERENCES

Agency for Healthcare Research and Quality. (2018). *Drug therapy for early rheumatoid arthritis: A systematic review update.* https://effectivehealthcare.ahrq.gov/products/rheumatoid-arthritis-medicine-update/final-report-update-2018

Aggarwal, R., & Oddis, C. (Eds.). (2019). *Managing myositis: A practical guide.* Springer.

Arthritis Society. (2017a). *Rheumatoid arthritis.* https://arthritis.ca/about-arthritis/arthritis-types-(a-z)/types/rheumatoid-arthritis

Arthritis Society. (2017b). *Gout.* https://arthritis.ca/about-arthritis/arthritis-types-(a-z)/types/gout

Arthritis Society. (2017c). *Psoriatic arthritis.* https://arthritis.ca/about-arthritis/arthritis-types-(a-z)/types/psoriatic-arthritis

Arthritis Society. (2017d). *Reactive arthritis.* https://arthritis.ca/about-arthritis/arthritis-types-(a-z)/types/reactive-arthritis

Arthritis Society. (2017e). *Systemic lupus erythematosus.* https://arthritis.ca/about-arthritis/arthritis-types-(a-z)/types/systemic-lupus-erythematosus

Arthritis Society. (2017f). *Scleroderma.* https://arthritis.ca/about-arthritis/arthritis-types-(a-z)/types/scleroderma

Arthritis Society. (2017g). *Myositis (dermatomyositis, polymyositis).* https://arthritis.ca/about-arthritis/arthritis-types-(a-z)/types/myositis-(dermatomyositis,-polymyositis

Arthritis Society. (2017h). *Sjögren syndrome.* https://arthritis.ca/about-arthritis/arthritis-types-(a-z)/types/sjogren-syndrome

Arthritis Society. (2017i). *Fibromyalgia.* https://arthritis.ca/about-arthritis/arthritis-types-(a-z)/types/fibromyalgia

Arthritis Society. (2019). *Ankylosing spondylitis.* https://arthritis.ca/about-arthritis/arthritis-types-(a-z)/types/ankylosing-spondylitis

Arthritis Society. (2020). *Felty's syndrome.* https://arthritis.ca/about-arthritis/arthritis-types-(a-z)/types/felty-s-syndrome

Arthritis Society. (2021a). *Arthritis facts and figures.* https://arthritis.ca/about-arthritis/what-is-arthritis/arthritis-facts-and-figures

Arthritis Society. (2021b). *Online learning modules.* https://arthritis.ca/support-education/online-learning

Arthritis Society. (2021c). *Osteoarthritis.* https://arthritis.ca/about-arthritis/arthritis-types-(a-z)/types/osteoarthritis

Arthritis Society. (2021d). *Risk factors.* https://arthritis.ca/about-arthritis/arthritis-risk-factors

Bannuru, R., Osani, M., Vaysbrot, E., et al. (2019). OARSI guidelines for the non-surgical management of knee, hip, and polyarticular osteoarthritis. *Osteoarthritis and Cartilage, 27,* 1578–1589. https://doi.org/10.1016/j.joca.2019.06.011

Barnabe, C., Zheng, Y., Ohinmaa, A., et al. (2018). Effectiveness, complications, and costs of rheumatoid arthritis treatment with biologics in Alberta: Experience of Indigenous and non-Indigenous patients. *Journal of Rheumatology, 45*(10), 1344–1352. https://doi.org/10.3899/jrheum.17077914

Chamberlain, S., Cavanagh, J., de Boer, P., et al. (2019). Treatment-resistant depression and peripheral C-reactive protein. *The British Journal of Psychiatry, 214*(1), 11–19. https://doi.org/10.1192/bjp.2018.66

Felz, M., & Wickman, M. (2016). Systemic lupus erythematosus: The devastatingly deceptive disease. *Semantic Scholar.* Corpus ID: 44073785. https://www.semanticscholar.org/paper/Systemic-Lupus-Erythematosus-The-Devastatingly-Felz-Wickham/6bacc75abd84d133f18ab18748f9e9f99f088d34#references

Fitzcharles, M.-A., Ste-Marie, P. A., Goldenberg, D. L., et al. (2012). *Canadian guidelines for the diagnosis and management of fibromyalgia syndrome.* Canadian Rheumatology Association. https://rheum.ca/wp-content/uploads/2017/11/2012CanadianFMGuidelines_17August2012.pdf

Giannitrapani, K., Holliday, J., Miake-Lue, I., et al. (2019). Synthesizing the strength of evidence of complementary and integrative health therapies for pain. *Pain Medicine, 20*(9), 1831–1840. https://doi.org/10.1093/pm/pnz068

Government of Canada. (2017). *Causes of Lyme disease.* https://www.canada.ca/en/public-health/services/diseases/lyme-disease/causes-lyme-disease.htm

Harding, M. (2016). An update on gout for primary care providers. *The Nurse Practitioner, 17*(14), 14–21. https://doi.org/10.1097/01.NPR.0000481510.32360.fa

Hitchon, C., Khan, S., Elias, B., et al. (2020). Prevalence and incidence of rheumatoid arthritis in Canadian first Nations and non-first Nations people. *Journal of Clinical Rheumatology, 26*(5), 169–175.

Hunter, D., & Bierma-Zeinstra, S. (2019). Osteoarthritis. *Lancet, 393,* 1745–1759.

Hurd, K., & Barnabe, C. (2017). Systematic review of rheumatic disease phenotypes and outcomes in the Indigenous populations of Canada, the USA, Australia and New Zealand. *Rheumatology International, 37,* 503–521. https://doi-org.myaccess.library.utoronto.ca/10.1007/s00296-016-3623-z

Papageorgiou, A., Ziogas, D., Mavragani, C., et al. (2015). Predicting the outcome of Sjögren's syndrome–associated non-Hodgkin's lymphoma patients. *PLoS One, 10*(2), e0116189. https://doi.org/10.1371/journal.pone.0116189

Philippou, E., Petersson, S. D., Rodomar, C., et al. (2021). Rheumatoid arthritis and dietary interventions: Systematic review of clinical trials. *Nutrition Reviews, 79*(4), 410–428. https://doi.org/10.1093/nutrit/nuaa033

Public Health Agency of Canada. (2020). *Enjoy the outdoors, without a tick.* https://www.canada.ca/en/public-health/services/publications/diseases-conditions/lyme-pamphlet.html

Sen, R., Goyal, A., Bansal, P., et al. (2021). *Seronegative spondyloarthropathy.* StatPearls. https://www.ncbi.nlm.nih.gov/books/NBK459356/

Thurston, W., Coupal, S., Jones, A., et al. (2014). Discordant Indigenous and provider frames explain challenges in improving access to arthritis care: A qualitative study using constructivist grounded theory. *International Journal for Equity in Health, 13*(46). https://doi.org/10.1186/1475-9276-13-46

Widdifield, J., Bernatsky, S., Bombardier, C., & Paterson, M. (2015). Rheumatoid arthritis surveillance in Ontario: Monitoring the burden, quality of care and patient outcomes through linkage of administrative health data. *Healthcare Quarterly, 18,* 7–10. https://doi.org/10.12927/hcq.2015.24439

Wolfe, F., Clauw, D., Fitzcharles, M., et al. (2016). 2016 Revisions to the 2010/2011 fibromyalgia diagnostic criteria. *Seminars in Arthritis and Rheumatism, 46,* 319–329. https://doi.org/10.1016/j.semarthit.2016.08.012

RESOURCES

Arthritis Research Canada
https://www.arthritisresearch.ca

Arthritis Society
https://www.arthritis.ca

Canadian Arthritis Community & Network
https://www.arthritisnetwork.ca

Canadian Lyme Disease Foundation (CanLyme)
https://www.canlyme.com

Canadian Organization for Rare Disorders (CORD)
https://www.raredisorders.ca

Canadian Rheumatology Association (CRA)
https://rheum.ca

Canadian Spondylitis Association (CSA)
https://www.spondylitis.ca

FM-CFS Canada
https://www.fm-cfs.ca/

Lupus Canada
https://www.lupuscanada.org

National ME/FM Action Network
https://www.mefmaction.com/

Scleroderma Society of Canada
https://www.scleroderma.ca

⊝volve

For additional Internet resources, see the website for this book at http://evolve.elsevier.com/Canada/Lewis/medsurg.

Nursing Care in Specialized Settings

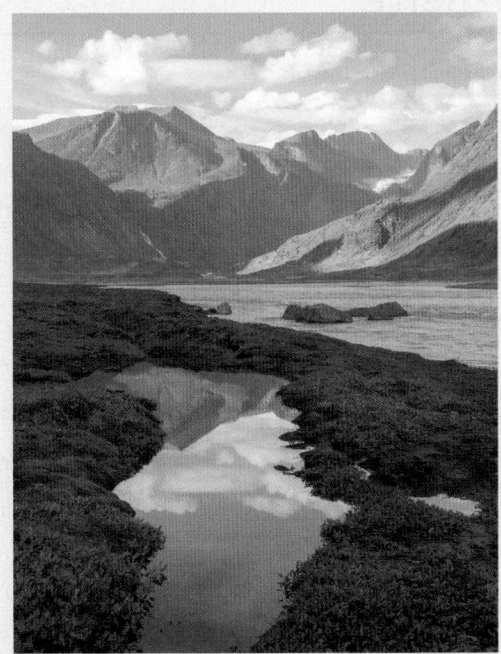

Source: © CanStock Photo / Manu_75

68

Nursing Management

Critical Care Environment

Brandi Vanderspank-Wright and Sarah Crowe
Originating US chapter by Megan Ann Brissie

evolve WEBSITE

http://evolve.elsevier.com/Canada/Lewis/medsurg

- Review Questions (Online Only)
- Key Points
- Answer Guidelines for Case Study

- Student Case Study
  - Pulmonary Embolism and Respiratory Failure
- Customizable Nursing Care Plan
  - Patient on Mechanical Ventilation

- Conceptual Care Map Creator
- Audio Glossary
- Content Updates

LEARNING OBJECTIVES

1. Describe the critical care certification process available to critical care nurses in Canada as well as advanced-practice roles such as those of the clinical nurse specialist and the acute-care nurse practitioner.
2. Select appropriate nursing interventions to manage common conditions and needs of critically ill patients.
3. Develop effective strategies to manage issues related to the families and caregivers of critically ill patients.

4. Apply the principles of hemodynamic monitoring and the interprofessional care and nursing management of the patient receiving this intervention.
5. Differentiate the indications for and contrast the modes of mechanical ventilation.
6. Select appropriate nursing interventions related to the care of an intubated patient.
7. Relate the principles of mechanical ventilation to the interprofessional care and nursing management of patients receiving this intervention.

KEY TERMS

arterial pressure–based cardiac output (APCO)
endotracheal (ET) intubation
hemodynamic monitoring

mechanical ventilation
negative-pressure ventilation
phlebostatic axis
positive end-expiratory pressure (PEEP)

positive-pressure ventilation (PPV)
pressure-support ventilation (PSV)
weaning

CRITICAL CARE NURSING

Critical Care Units

According to the Canadian Association of Critical Care Nurses (CACCN), critical care nursing is "a specialty which exists to care for patients who are experiencing life-threatening health crises within a patient-/family-centred model of care" (CACCN, 2017, p. 1). Critical care nurses care for patients with acute and unstable physiological conditions as well as for their caregivers. Their role involves assessing life-threatening conditions, initiating appropriate interventions, and evaluating the outcomes of these interventions (CACCN, 2017).

While the delivery of critical care exists in a variety of contexts, *critical care units* (CCUs) are specifically designed to meet the special needs of critically ill patients. Care in the CCU is provided by a large interprofessional team that includes but is not limited to specially trained physicians (e.g., intensivists), respiratory therapists, pharmacists, social workers, and physiotherapists, in addition to the critical care nurse who assumes a primary role. Because of the complexity of care, nurse-to-patient ratios in the CCU are kept as close as possible to 1:1. Staffing levels should be regularly assessed to ensure that they reflect the acuity of patients in the unit and the experience level of the nursing staff (CACCN, 2019).

In many acute care settings, the concept of critical care has expanded from delivering care in a standard unit to bringing critical care to patients wherever they might be. The electronic or virtual CCU is designed to augment the bedside critical care

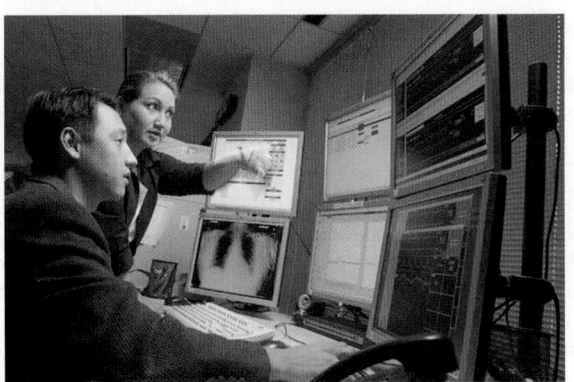

FIG. 68.1 Electronic critical care unit team members monitor patients from a remote site. Source: Amelung, P. J., & Doerfler, M. E. (2013). VISICU and the e ICU program. In P. D. Le Roux, J. Levine, & W. A. Kofke. *Monitoring in neurocritical care.* Elsevier.

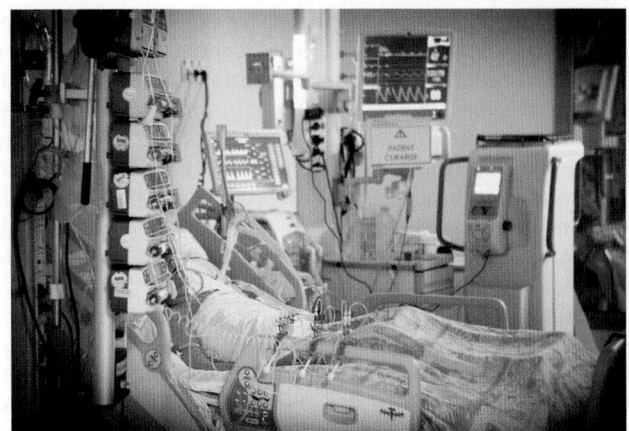

FIG. 68.2 Typical critical care unit. Source: Amélie Benoist/Science Source.

team by monitoring the patient from a remote location (Figure 68.1). Similarly, some acute care settings have established rapid response teams that provide advanced care within the hospital but outside of the CCU setting (e.g., on hospital units or floors). Rapid response teams are typically made up of specialized health care providers, usually including a critical care nurse, a respiratory therapist, and a critical care physician. These teams may either be formal or informal positions depending on the hospital. Rapid response teams ensure immediate care to unstable patients in noncritical units (Maharaj et al., 2015). Patients often exhibit subtle early signs of deterioration (e.g., changes in respiratory rate, oxygen saturation, heart rate, blood pressure, level of consciousness) 6.5 hours in advance, and these early signs may go unrecognized (Canadian Patient Safety Institute [CPSI], 2021a) without diligent observation and assessment by clinicians in both critical care and other contexts of care (in hospital and in the community).

The technology available in the CCU is extensive and always evolving. It is possible to continuously monitor the electrocardiogram (ECG), blood pressure (BP), oxygen (O_2) saturation, cardiac output (CO), intracranial pressure, and temperature. More advanced monitoring devices can provide measures of cardiac index (CI), stroke volume (SV), ejection fraction, end-tidal carbon dioxide (CO_2), and tissue O_2 consumption. Patients may receive ongoing support from mechanical ventilators, intra-aortic balloon pumps (IABPs), circulatory assist devices (CADs), and/or dialysis machines. Figure 68.2 shows a typical CCU.

Other settings such as *progressive care units* (PCUs) or *high-acuity units (HAU)*, also called *intermediate care units* or *step-down units,* provide a transition between the CCU and the general care unit or discharge (Prin & Wunsch, 2014). Generally, patients admitted to these units are at risk for serious complications, but their risk is lower than that of CCU patients. Examples of patients found in PCUs include those scheduled for interventional cardiac procedures (e.g., stent placement), patients awaiting heart transplant, those receiving stable doses of vasoactive intravenous (IV) medications, or those being weaned from prolonged mechanical ventilation. Examples of monitoring capabilities in these units typically include continuous ECG, arterial BP, and O_2 saturation. PCUs enable nursing care for at-risk populations in a more cost-effective environment.

Critical Care Nurse

In a recent position statement developed by the CACCN, a *critical care nurse* is a registered nurse with additional education in critical care (CACCN, 2019). A critical care nurse has in-depth knowledge of anatomy, physiology, pathophysiology, pharmacology, and advanced assessment skills as well as the ability to use advanced technology (CACCN, 2017). Critical care nurses perform frequent assessments to monitor trends (patterns) in the patient's physiological parameters (e.g., BP, ECG). This level of observation enables the nurse to rapidly recognize, assess, and manage complications while fostering healing and recovery. The nurse also provides psychosocial support to the patient and their caregivers. To be effective, the critical care nurse must be able to communicate and collaborate with all members of the interprofessional health care team (e.g., physician, dietitian, social worker, respiratory therapist, and occupational therapist). The CACCN has developed *Standards for Critical Care Nursing Practice* as a resource for best nursing practice in the critical care environment (CACCN, 2017).

Specialization in critical care nursing usually initially requires comprehensive theoretical preparation and a preceptored orientation or internship (Innes & Calleja, 2018). Hiring practices vary across individual unit settings, but generally speaking, new graduate nurses are hired into critical care environments. New graduates hired into critical care require support for a successful transition into their new role (Innes & Calleja, 2018). The Canadian Nurses Association (CNA) offers critical care certification (CNCC(C)) in adult critical care nursing. The designation requires that a registered nurse have practice experience in critical care nursing and have successfully completed a comprehensive written examination set to established competencies. Detailed information regarding the process for certification offered through the CNA Certification Program is available at www.cna-aiic.ca/en/certification.

Continued critical care practice and retesting or continuing education activities are required for recertification at 5-year intervals. In Canada, registered nurses may also choose to complete critical care certification through classroom or online education, typically combined with preceptored clinical experience.

Advanced Nursing Practice in Critical Care. Advanced practice nurses have a graduate degree (master's or doctorate) (Canadian Nurses Association, 2019) and assume a variety of responsibilities (e.g. education, consultation, administration, researchers, and expert-level clinical practice). In critical care, two advanced practice roles include the *clinical nurse specialist* and the *acute-care nurse practitioner* (ACNP). Clinical nurse specialists typically function in one or more of the previous listed roles but have a primary responsibility for direct clinical practice. ACNPs provide comprehensive care to select critically ill patients and their families. They conduct comprehensive assessments, order and interpret diagnostic tests, manage health problems and disease-related symptoms, prescribe treatments, and coordinate care during transitions in settings. ACNPs may practise independently (e.g., providing comprehensive care to the chronically critically ill) or interprofessionally (e.g., providing symptom management in conjunction with physicians). (See position statements published by the CACCN, all available at www.caccn.ca.)

Spotlight on Critical Care. Critical care nurses require extensive knowledge of normal and abnormal anatomy and physiology, and must acquire complex assessment and technical skills. It can take years before a critical care nurse transitions to autonomous and consistently proficient practice. Critical care patients may be medically unstable and can experience prolonged and complicated trajectories. They may have unfamiliar medical conditions and/or complex psychosocial needs. When combined with the continuously evolving body of scientific knowledge, new and experienced critical care nurses need support to succeed.

A critical care clinical nurse specialist (CC-CNS) draws on master's or doctoral education in nursing and prior critical care expertise (CNA, 2014). CC-CNSs promote high-quality care by operationalizing the four clinical nurse specialist competencies within their unique clinical environment. Clinical care may be provided through just-in-time clinical support, consultation, coordination of interdisciplinary care plans, and direct involvement with patient or family care. System leadership is displayed by role-modelling professional behaviours, embracing a culture of safety, and facilitating quality patient- and family-centred care and end-of-life care. Advancement of nursing practice is promoted through formal and informal teaching, in-the-moment clinical support, coaching and mentoring, and the development of evidence-informed practice tools or resources. Evaluation and research must be intertwined within all domains of the CC-CNS role, and a personal commitment to lifelong learning is required. The CC-CNS evaluates patient outcome data and monitors emerging research evidence, using findings to lead and support quality improvement initiatives and knowledge translation. CC-CNSs support ongoing research initiatives and engage in the conduct of critical care research as appropriate.

Nursing knowledge and a desire to learn hold the key to the development of critical thinking skills. Much of the clinical nurse specialist role is carried out subtly or behind the scenes, providing infrastructure and patient-specific support to help frontline nurses develop and excel independently. It can be a privilege to play a role in advancing nursing practice and to have a job that allows one to learn something new every day. Clinical nurse specialists have the opportunity to inspire other critical care nurses to be the best they can be and to share their passion for critical care nursing.

Critical Care Patients

Patients are admitted to the CCU for a variety of reasons, all of which require frequent and often constant monitoring. For example, a patient may be physiologically unstable, requiring advanced and sophisticated clinical judgements by a nurse, health care provider, or both. A patient may be at risk for serious complications and require frequent and often invasive interventions. Further, a patient may require intensive and complicated

nursing support related to the use of IV polypharmacy (e.g., neuromuscular blockade, thrombolytics, medications requiring titration) and advanced technology (e.g., hemodynamic monitoring, mechanical ventilation, intracranial pressure monitoring, and continuous renal replacement therapy).

CCUs can themselves be specialized. For example, patients with medical emergencies (e.g., septic shock, drug overdoses, or diabetic ketoacidosis) are often treated in a medical CCU. CCUs can also have a surgical focus (e.g. cardiac surgery, neurosurgery, major organ transplantation). In some instances, patients with trauma or burns can be cared for in trauma and burn CCUs. In most instances, CCUs are a combination of all of these areas, and CCU clinicians care for a variety of critically ill patients. Further, patients can be clustered by age group in neonatal, pediatric, and adult CCUs.

Common Problems of Critically Ill Patients. Patients admitted to the CCU are at risk for numerous complications and special conditions in both the short and long term. As a result, emphasis has been placed on preventing complications and on facilitating CCU survivorship. The PADIS Guidelines focus on the prevention and management of **p**ain, **a**gitation and sedation, **d**elirium, **i**mmobility, and **s**leep disruption within the context of adult patients admitted to CCUs (Devlin et al., 2018).

Pain. The recognition, assessment, and management of pain in a CCU patient is paramount. Critically ill patients experience pain, both at rest and during routine care and procedures, in the CCU at an incidence of up to 50% (Balas et al., 2018; Devlin et al., 2018). Self-report, which is considered the gold standard of pain assessment, is not always possible for CCU patients for a variety of reasons, including endotracheal intubation and sedation. For CCU patients who are unable to self-report, other validated and reliable tools are available. The Critical-Care Pain Observation Tool (CPOT) is frequently used. The CPOT consists of four components: facial expression, body movements, muscle tension, and compliance with the ventilator (for intubated patients) or vocalization (for nonintubated patients) (Gélinas et al., 2006) (Table 68.1). The Behavioral Pain Scale (BPS) is another validated and reliable tool that may be used (Payen et al., 2001). The BPS has three components: facial expression, upper limb movement, and compliance with ventilation (Table 68.2). A CPOT score of greater than 3 or a BPS score of greater than 5 is indicative of significant pain (Gélinas, 2018). Pain assessment itself is multifactorial, and standard approaches to assessment are applicable within the CCU context (see Chapter 10). Recently published guidelines recommend a variety of approaches to pain management in the critically ill patient and include opioid, adjuvant, and nonpharmacological measures. Common opioid analgesics are fentanyl, hydromorphone, and morphine. Nonopioid analgesics used are acetaminophen, nefopam, and ketamine. Nonopioid considerations for neuropathic pain include gabapentin, carbamazepine, and pregabalin. Nonpharmacological measures include massage, music therapy, cold therapy (e.g., an ice pack applied for 10 minutes, wrapped in gauze applied prior to chest tube removal), and relaxation techniques (Devlin et al., 2018).

Pain management is a significant issue among critically ill patients and with poor assessment can result in serious physical and psychological consequences (Georgiou et al., 2015). Inadequate pain control is often linked to agitation and anxiety and is known to contribute to the stress response.

Agitation and Sedation. The use of sedatives is a common practice in the CCU environment for a variety of indications, including

TABLE 68.1   CRITICAL CARE PAIN OBSERVATION TOOL (CPOT)

Indicator	Score		Description
Facial expression	Relaxed, neutral	0	No muscle tension observed
	Tense	1	Presence of brow lowering, orbit tightening, and levator contraction or any other change (e.g., opening eyes or tearing during nociceptive procedures)
	Grimacing	2	All previous facial movements plus eyelid tightly closed (the patient may present with mouth open biting the endotracheal tube)
Body movements	Absence of movements or normal position	0	Does not move at all (does not necessarily mean absence of pain) or normal position (movements not aimed toward the pain site or not made for the purpose of protection)
	Protection	1	Slow, cautious movements, touching or rubbing the pain site, seeking attention through movements
	Restlessness/agitation	2	Pulling tube, attempting to sit up, moving limbs/thrashing, not following commands, striking at staff, trying to climb out of bed
Compliance with the ventilator (intubated patients) *or* vocalization (nonintubated patients)	Tolerating ventilator or movement	0	Alarms not activated, easy ventilation
	Coughing but tolerating	1	Coughing, alarms may be activated but stop spontaneously
	Fighting ventilator	2	Asynchrony: blocking ventilation, alarms frequently activated
	Talking in normal tone or no sound	0	Talking in normal tone or no sound
	Sighing, moaning	1	Sighing, moaning
	Crying out, sobbing	2	Crying out, sobbing
Muscle tension	Relaxed	0	No resistance to passive movement
	Tense, rigid	1	Resistance to passive movements
	Very tense or rigid	2	Strong resistance to passive movements, incapacity to complete them
Total		/8	

1. The patient must be observed at rest for 1 min to obtain a baseline value of the CPOT.
   1.1 Observation of patient at rest (baseline)
The nurse looks at the patient's face and body to note any visible reactions for an observation period of 1 min. The nurse gives a score for all items except for muscle tension. At the end of the 1-min period, the nurse holds the patient's arm in both hands: The nurse places one hand at the elbow and uses the other one to hold the patient's hand. Then the nurse performs a passive flexion and extension of the upper limb and feels any resistance the patient may exhibit. If the movements are performed easily, the patient is found to be relaxed with no resistance (score 0). If the movements can still be performed but with more strength, it is concluded that the patient is showing resistance to movements (score 1). If the nurse cannot complete the movements, strong resistance is felt (score 2). This can be observed in patients whose movements are spastic.
2. Then the patient should be observed during painful procedures (e.g., turning, wound care) to detect any changes in the patient's behaviours.
   2.2 Observation of patient during a painful procedure
While performing a procedure known to be painful, the nurse looks at the patient's face to note any reactions, such as brow lowering or grimacing. These reactions may be brief or can last longer. The nurse also watches for body movements. For instance, the nurse looks for protective movements, such as the patient trying to reach or touching the pain site (e.g., surgical incision, injury site). In the mechanically ventilated patient, the nurse pays attention to alarms and if they stop spontaneously or require that the nurse intervene (e.g., provide reassurance, administer medication). It is important that the nurse auscultate the patient to check for position of the endotracheal tube and the presence of secretions, as these factors may influence this item without being indicative of pain. According to muscle tension, the nurse can feel if the patient is resisting against the movement or not. A score of 2 is given when the patient is resisting against the movement and attempts to get on their back.
3. The patient should be evaluated before and at the peak effect of an analgesic agent to assess whether the treatment was effective or not in relieving pain.
4. The patient should be attributed the highest score observed during the observation period.
5. The patient should be attributed a score for each behaviour included in the CPOT. Muscle tension should be evaluated last as it may lead to behavioural reactions not necessarily related to pain but more to the actual stimulation. According to compliance with the ventilator, the nurse must check that the endotracheal tube is well positioned and for the presence of secretions, which could lead to higher scores for this item.

Source: Urden, L. D., Stacy, K. M., & Lough, M. E. (Eds.). (2018). *Critical care nursing: Diagnosis and management* (8th ed., Chapter 8, Table 8.2). Elsevier.

to relieve anxiety, minimize the stress of being on a mechanical ventilator, and prevent harm or injury that can be induced by agitation (Devlin et al., 2018). Anxiety, for example, is a common issue for CCU patients. Primary sources of anxiety include the perceived or anticipated threat to physical health, actual loss of control of body functions, pain or perceived anticipation of pain, and placement in a foreign environment. Many patients feel uncomfortable in the CCU environment with its complex equipment, high noise and light levels, isolation from family, and intense pace of activity. Pain and sleeplessness enhance anxiety, as do immobilization, loss of control, and impaired communication.

To help reduce anxiety, the nurse should encourage patients and caregivers to express concerns, ask questions, and state their needs. Patients and caregivers should be included in all conversations and have the purpose of equipment and procedures explained to them. The nurse should structure the patient's environment in such a way as to decrease anxiety, if possible, and encourage caregivers to bring in photographs and personal items. Sedatives frequently used in the CCU environment include propofal, dexmedetomidine, and midazolam (Devlin et al., 2018).

Despite the relative frequency of sedative use, critical care nursing practice must include the use of valid and reliable measures to assess whether or not a sedative is indicated and to evaluate the effectiveness of the sedative after it has been administered. The PADIS guidelines include recommendations based on the use of the Richmond Agitation-Sedation Scale (RASS) (Devlin et al., 2018). Current best practice is to promote the use of light rather than deep sedation. While a consensus definition for light sedation is lacking, the studies evaluated in the PADIS guidelines used a RASS score of –2 to +1 as the range for light

sedation (Figure 68.3). Some evidence suggests that the use of light sedation contributes to a shorter time to extubation (i.e., a shorter time on the mechanical ventilator) and a decreased tracheotomy rate (Devlin et al., 2018).

Because of the frequent use of sedatives in the CCU, daily sedation interruption is a recommended practice whereby a patient's sedative is interrupted or discontinued in order to allow them to "wake up." This practice enables a patient to become alert and is reflected by their ability to follow simple commands (e.g., opening their eyes to voice) or achieving a RASS score between –1 and +1 (i.e., between drowsy and restless). The practice of daily sedation interruption allows for in-depth assessment of the patient's pain (e.g., enabling self-report), appropriate titration of sedatives to achieve a desired level of sedation, neurological examination, and assessment of readiness for weaning from the mechanical ventilator (Devlin et al., 2018). Critical care nurses assume a primary role in evaluating and initiating a daily sedation interruption when ordered and appropriate.

Delirium. *Delirium* is defined as an acute state of mental confusion and is considered a medical emergency (see Chapter 62) and is common in CCU patients. In critically ill patients, delirium is associated with worse outcomes as well as high CCU and hospital length of stay and costs (Devlin et al., 2018). (General risk factors for the development of delirium are outlined in Chapter 62, Table 62.1.) Predisposing and precipitating factors for CCU patients include both modifiable and nonmodifiable considerations. Modifiable factors include the use of benzodiazepines and blood transfusions. Nonmodifiable factors include older age, dementia, prior coma, pre-CCU emergency surgery, trauma, and increasing Acute Physiology and Chronic Health Evaluation (APACHE) scores. APACHE is a tool used for estimating CCU mortality (Etland, 2018). Current evidence supports the use of validated predictive models specific to delirium development in CCU patients. Two examples of predictive models include the PRE-DELIRIC and the Early (E)-PRE-DELIRIC. The PRE-DERILIC consists of 10 predictors: age, APACHE-II score, admission group, urgent admission, infection, coma, sedation, morphine use, urea level, and metabolic acidosis. The E-PRE-DELIRIC includes nine predictors: age, history of cognitive impairment, history of alcohol misuse, blood urea nitrogen, admission category, urgent admission, mean arterial BP, use of corticosteroids, and respiratory failure.

TABLE 68.2	**BEHAVIOURAL PAIN SCALE**	
Item	**Description**	**Score**
Facial expression	Relaxed	1
	Partially tightened (e.g., brow lowering)	2
	Fully tightened (e.g., eyelid closing)	3
	Grimacing	4
Upper limbs	No movement	1
	Partially bent	2
	Fully bent with finger flexion	3
	Permanently retracted	4
Compliance with ventilation	Tolerating movement	1
	Coughing but tolerating ventilation for most of the time	2
	Fighting ventilator	3
	Unable to control ventilation	4
Total		3–12

Source: Urden, L. D., Stacy, K. M., & Lough, M. E. (Eds.). (2018). *Critical care nursing: Diagnosis and management* (8th ed., Table 8.3). Elsevier.

RICHMOND AGITATION-SEDATION SCALE (RASS)

Step

1 Sedation Assessment

Scale	Label	Description
+4	COMBATIVE	Combative, violent, immediate danger to staff
+3	VERY AGITATED	Pulls to remove tubes or catheters; aggressive
+2	AGITATED	Frequent nonpurposeful movement, fights ventilator
+1	RESTLESS	Anxious, apprehensive, movements not aggressive
0	ALERT & CALM	Spontaneously pays attention to caregiver
−1	DROWSY	Not fully alert, but has sustained awakening to voice (eye opening & contact >10 sec)
−2	LIGHT SEDATION	Briefly awakens to voice (eyes open & contact <10 sec)
−3	MODERATE SEDATION	Movement or eye opening to voice (no eye contact)

FIG. 68.3 Richmond Agitation-Sedation Scale: sedation assessment. Source: Urden, L. D., Stacy, K. M., & Lough, M. E. (Eds.). (2018). *Critical care nursing: Diagnosis and management* (8th ed., Figure 9.2). Elsevier.

CONFUSION ASSESSMENT METHOD FOR THE ICU (CAM-ICU)

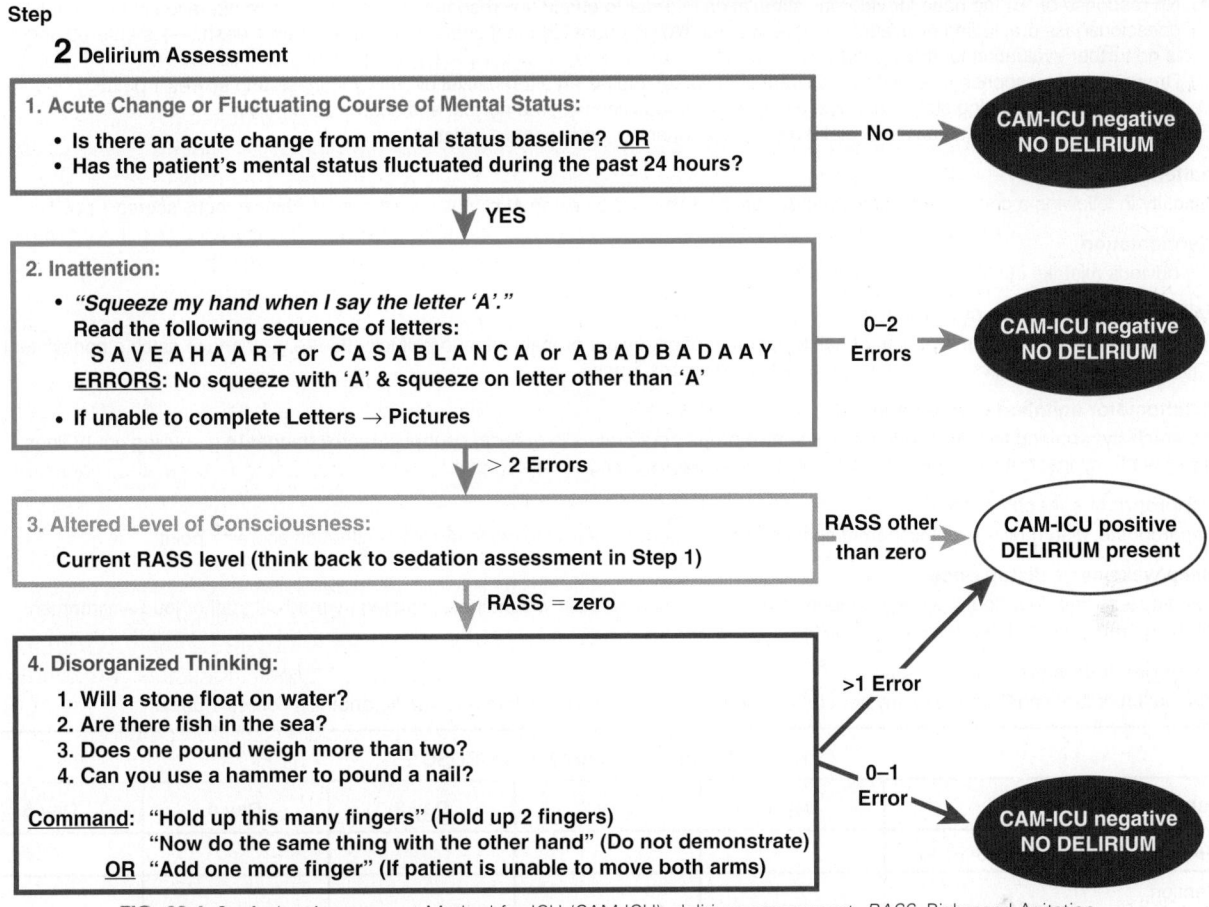

Step

2 Delirium Assessment

1. Acute Change or Fluctuating Course of Mental Status:
- **Is there an acute change from mental status baseline? OR**
- **Has the patient's mental status fluctuated during the past 24 hours?**

No → **CAM-ICU negative NO DELIRIUM**

↓ **YES**

2. Inattention:
- *"Squeeze my hand when I say the letter 'A'."*
  Read the following sequence of letters:
  S A V E A H A A R T or C A S A B L A N C A or A B A D B A D A A Y
  ERRORS: No squeeze with 'A' & squeeze on letter other than 'A'
- **If unable to complete Letters → Pictures**

0–2 Errors → **CAM-ICU negative NO DELIRIUM**

↓ **> 2 Errors**

3. Altered Level of Consciousness:
Current RASS level (think back to sedation assessment in Step 1)

RASS other than zero → **CAM-ICU positive DELIRIUM present**

↓ **RASS = zero**

4. Disorganized Thinking:
1. Will a stone float on water?
2. Are there fish in the sea?
3. Does one pound weigh more than two?
4. Can you use a hammer to pound a nail?

Command: "Hold up this many fingers" (Hold up 2 fingers)
"Now do the same thing with the other hand" (Do not demonstrate)
OR "Add one more finger" (If patient is unable to move both arms)

>1 Error → **CAM-ICU positive DELIRIUM present**

0–1 Error → **CAM-ICU negative NO DELIRIUM**

FIG. 68.4 Confusion Assessment Method for ICU (CAM-ICU): delirium assessment. *RASS,* Richmond Agitation-Sedation Scale. Source: Urden, L. D., Stacy, K. M., & Lough, M. E. (Eds.). (2018). *Critical care nursing: Diagnosis and management* (8th ed., Figure 9.2). Elsevier.

All CCU patients should be regularly screened for delirium; this is part of critical care nurses' patient assessments. The Confusion Assessment Method–ICU (CAM-ICU) is a valid and reliable tool that is frequently and easily used by critical care nurses (Figure 68.4). The CAM-ICU is organized into four features that are scored: (1) acute onset or fluctuating course, (2) inattention, (3) altered level of consciousness, and (4) disorganized thinking. Delirium is defined as positive in Feature 1 and Feature 2 and either Feature 3 or Feature 4 (Figure 68.5). A second delirium screening tool for critical care is the Intensive Care Delirium Screening Checklist (ICDSC) (Figure 68.6). The ICDSC consists of eight evaluative components that are scored: altered level of consciousness; inattention; disorientation; hallucination, delusion, or psychosis; psychomotor agitation or retardation; inappropriate speech or mood; sleep–wake cycle disturbance; and symptom fluctuation.

Current guideline recommendations are that pharmacological agents (e.g., haloperidol, dexmedetomidine) *not* be used prophylactically. The use of haloperidol for treatment of delirium in critical care patients is also *not* recommended. Instead, dexmedetomidine is recommended for mechanically ventilated patients in whom delirium-induced agitation is preventing weaning from the ventilator or extubation. Multicomponent, nonpharmacological prevention strategies aimed at reducing modifiable risk factors are also recommended (e.g., early mobilization, reorientation and

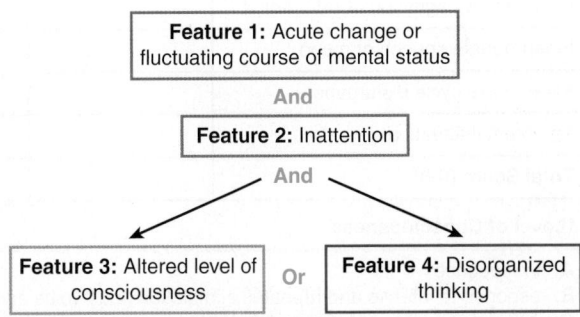

Feature 1: Acute change or fluctuating course of mental status

And

Feature 2: Inattention

And

Feature 3: Altered level of consciousness | Or | **Feature 4:** Disorganized thinking

FIG. 68.5 Confusion Assessment Method for ICU (CAM-ICU): positive features. Source: Urden, L. D., Stacy, K. M., & Lough, M. E. (Eds.). (2018). *Critical care nursing: Diagnosis and management* (8th ed., Figure 9.1). Elsevier.

cognitive stimulation treatment, ensuring patients have visual and hearing aids) (Devlin et al., 2018).

Immobility. In recent years, increased emphasis has been placed on early mobilization of CCU patients. Such measures are important in mitigating serious and long-term consequences of CCU admissions, including but not limited to CCU-acquired muscle weakness. Evidence suggests that CCU-acquired weakness is present in 25 to 50% of critically ill patients and can affect their long-term survival (post-CCU), overall physical functioning, and quality of life (Devlin et al., 2018). Efforts to mobilize

The Intensive Care Delirium Screening Checklist (ICDSC)

1. Altered level of consciousness

(A) No response or (B) the need for vigorous stimulation in order to obtain any response signified a severe alteration in the level of consciousness precluding evaluation. If there is coma (A) or stupor (B) most of the time period, then a dash (—) is entered and there is no further evaluation for that period.

(C) Drowsiness or response to a mild to moderate stimulation implies an altered level of consciousness and scores 1 point.

(D) Wakefulness or sleeping state that could easily be aroused is considered normal and scores zero points.

(E) Hypervigilance is rated as an abnormal level of consciousness and scores 1 point.

2. Inattention

Difficulty in following a conversation or instruction, easily distracted by external stimuli, or difficulty in shifting focus scores 1 point.

3. Disorientation

Any obvious mistake in time, place, or person scores 1 point.

4. Hallucination, delusion, or psychosis

The unequivocal clinical manifestation of hallucination or of behaviour probably due to hallucination (e.g., trying to catch a nonexistent object) or delusion or gross impairment in reality testing scores 1 point.

5. Psychomotor agitation or retardation

Hyperactivity requiring the use of additional sedative drugs or restraints in order to control potential danger (e.g., pulling out IV lines, hitting staff), hypoactivity, or clinically noticeable psychomotor slowing scores 1 point.

6. Inappropriate speech or mood

Inappropriate, disorganized, or incoherent speech or inappropriate mood related to events or situation scores 1 point.

7. Sleep/wake cycle disturbance

Sleeping less than four hours, waking frequently at night (do not consider wakefulness initiated by medical staff or loud environment), or sleeping during most of the day scores 1 point.

8. Symptom fluctuation

Fluctuation of the manifestation of any item or symptom over 24 hours (e.g., from one shift to another) scores 1 point.

How to Calculate a Score for the ICDSC*

Patient Evaluation	Day 1	Day 2	Day 3	Day 4	Day 5
Altered level of consciousness (A-E)*					
Inattention					
Disorientation					
Hallucination, delusion, psychosis					
Psychomotor agitation or retardation					
Inappropriate speech or mood					
Sleep-wake cycle disturbance					
Symptom fluctuation					
Total Score (0-8)					

*Level of Consciousness	Score
A: no response	–
B: response to intense and repeated stimulation (loud voice and pain)	–
C: response to mild or moderate stimulation	1
D: normal wakefulness	0
E: exaggerated response to normal stimulation	1
If **A** or **B**, do not complete patient evaluation for the period.	

Scoring System

The scale is completed based on information collected from each 8-hour shift or from the previous 24 hours. Obvious manifestation of an item = 1 point. No manifestation of an item or no assessment possible = 0 points. The score of each item is entered in the corresponding space and is 0 or 1. A total score of ≥4 on any given day has a 99% sensitivity for correlation with a psychiatric diagnosis of delirium.

*The ICDSC is also used in tandem with the RASS to assess sedation-agitation in addition to delirium.

FIG. 68.6 The Intensive Care Delirium Screening Checklist (ICDSC). *RASS,* Richmond Agitation-Sedation Scale. Source: Urden, L. D., Stacy, K. M., & Lough, M. E. (Eds.). (2018). *Critical care nursing: Diagnosis and management* (8th ed., Figure 9.3). Elsevier.

patients and engage in rehabilitative practices should consider the stability of the patient, including their cardiovascular, respiratory, and neurological status. Early mobilization practices are possible even when a patient is mechanically ventilated. Mobilizing patients (particularly those who are intubated and mechanically ventilated) requires careful assessment and planning and involves other members of the interprofessional CCU team, such as respiratory therapists, physiotherapists, and occupational therapists. Many sites use algorithms for assessing and progressing levels of mobility in critically ill patients. Additionally, because critically ill patients are usually immobile, they are at risk for venous thromboembolism and skin breakdown (see Chapter 26).

Sleep. Nearly all CCU patients experience sleep disturbances. Patients may have difficulty falling asleep or have disrupted sleep because of noise, anxiety, pain, frequent monitoring, or treatment procedures, all of which have an impact on an individual's circadian rhythm. Sleep disturbance is a significant stressor in the CCU, contributing to delirium and possibly affecting recovery (Delaney et al., 2015; Devlin et al., 2018). The nurse can structure the environment to promote the patient's sleep–wake cycle. Strategies for achieving this include clustering activities, scheduling rest periods, dimming lights at nighttime, opening curtains during the daytime, obtaining physiological measurements without disturbing the patient, limiting noise, and providing comfort measures (e.g., back rubs). If necessary, pharmacological therapy may be needed to induce and maintain sleep. (Sleep and sleep disorders are discussed in Chapter 9.)

Other Considerations

Nutrition. Patients are often admitted to CCUs with conditions that result in either hypermetabolic states (e.g., burns, trauma, sepsis) or catabolic states (e.g., acute kidney injury). Other times, patients may be admitted in severely malnourished states (e.g., chronic heart, pulmonary, or liver disease). In general, malnutrition has been linked to increased mortality and morbidity.

Whom to feed, what to feed, when to feed, and how to feed (e.g., route of administration) are crucial questions that the nurse must ask when caring for a critically ill patient. The nurse must collaborate with the physician and the dietitian to determine how best to meet the nutritional needs of CCU patients.

The primary goal of nutritional support is to prevent or correct nutritional deficiencies. This is usually accomplished by the early provision of enteral nutrition (i.e., delivery of calories via the gastrointestinal [GI] tract) or parenteral nutrition (i.e., delivery of calories intravenously). Enteral nutrition preserves the structure and function of the gut mucosa and prevents the movement of gut bacteria across the intestinal wall and into the bloodstream. In addition, early enteral nutrition is associated with fewer complications and shorter hospital stays and is less expensive than parenteral nutrition (Critical Care Nutrition, 2021; McClave et al., 2016; Patel et al., 2017). Parenteral nutrition is used when the enteral route cannot provide adequate nutrition or is contraindicated. Examples of conditions that may preclude enteral feeding include paralytic ileus, diffuse peritonitis, intestinal obstruction, pancreatitis, GI ischemia, intractable vomiting, and severe diarrhea. (Enteral and parenteral nutrition are discussed in Chapter 42.)

Impaired Communication. Inability to communicate can be distressing for patients who are unable to speak because of the use of sedative or paralyzing medications or an endotracheal tube. As part of any procedure, the nurse should explain what will happen or is happening to the patient. When the patient cannot speak, the nurse should explore alternative methods of communication, including the use of devices such as picture boards, notepads, magic slates, electronic tablets, cell phones

(with instant messaging applications), or computer keyboards. When speaking with the patient, the nurse should look directly at the patient and use hand gestures when appropriate. For patients who do not speak English, an approved interpreter must be used (see Chapter 2 and Tables 2.5 and 2.6).

Nonverbal communication is also important. A large amount of procedure-related touch and much less comfort-related touch often characterize the CCU environment. Patients have different levels of tolerance for being touched, usually related to cultural background and personal history. It may be appropriate to provide comforting touch, with ongoing evaluation of the patient's response. If appropriate, the nurse can encourage caregivers to touch and talk with the patient even if the patient is unresponsive or comatose.

HEMODYNAMIC MONITORING

Hemodynamic monitoring is the measurement of pressure, flow, and oxygenation within the cardiovascular system. Both invasive (internally placed devices) and noninvasive (external devices) hemodynamic measurements are made in the CCU. With the use of multiple invasive devices, such as central venous catheters, patients may be predisposed to health care–associated infections. Diligent observation by the critical care nurse for early signs of sepsis (e.g., tachypnea, altered mentation and hypotension) is important (see Chapter 69). There is variability in the availability of hemodynamic technologies across CCU settings and with respect to patient acuity (Lough, 2018). Values commonly measured include systemic arterial BP, oxygen saturation of the hemoglobin of arterial blood (SaO_2), central venous pressure, and mixed venous blood (SvO_2). Other hemodynamic measurements such as CO, CI, SV, stroke volume index (SVI), pulmonary artery pressure (PAP), and pulmonary artery occlusive pressure (PAOP) are indicated in certain clinical situations and are often obtained using invasive monitoring devices. From these measurements, CCU clinicians are able to calculate several values, including the resistance of the systemic and pulmonary arterial vasculature as well as oxygen content, delivery, and consumption. When these data are integrated with clinical assessment data, the critical care nurse can derive a picture of the patient's hemodynamic status and the effectiveness of therapy. All measures need to be made with attention to technical accuracy. False or inaccurate data can result in unnecessary and inappropriate treatment.

Hemodynamic Terminology

Cardiac Output and Cardiac Index. *Cardiac output* (CO) is the volume of blood pumped by the heart in 1 minute. *Cardiac index* (CI) is the measurement of the CO adjusted for body size and is a more precise measurement of the efficiency of the pumping action of the heart. Although minor beat-to-beat changes may occur, generally the left and right ventricles pump the same volume. The volume pumped with each heartbeat is the *stroke volume* (SV). Like CI, *stroke volume index* (SVI) is the measurement of SV adjusted for body size. CO and the forces opposing blood flow determine BP, the force exerted by blood on the vessel wall. The opposition to blood flow offered by the vessels is called *systemic vascular resistance* (SVR) or *pulmonary vascular resistance*. Preload, afterload, and contractility (see Chapter 34) determine SV (and thus CO and BP) (Lough, 2018). It is essential that the critical care nurse understand these concepts and their relationships. Additionally, the nurse must understand the effects of manipulation of each of these variables. The formulas and normal values for common hemodynamic parameters are given in Table 68.3.

TABLE 68.3	COMMON HEMODYNAMIC PARAMETERS	
Indicators		**Normal Range**
Preload		
Right atrial pressure (RAP) or central venous pressure (CVP)		2–8 mm Hg
Pulmonary artery wedge pressure (PAWP) or left atrial pressure (LAP)		6–12 mm Hg
Pulmonary artery diastolic pressure (PADP)		4–12 mm Hg
Right ventricular end-diastolic volume (RVEDV) = $\dfrac{\text{Stroke volume (SV)}}{\text{Right ventricular ejection fraction (RVEF)}}$		100–160 mL
Afterload		
Pulmonary vascular resistance (PVR) = $\dfrac{(\text{Pulmonary artery mean pressure [PAMP]} - \text{PAWP}) \times 80}{\text{Cardiac output (CO)}}$		<250 dynes/sec/cm^{-5}
Pulmonary vascular resistance index (PVRI) = $\dfrac{(\text{PAMP} - \text{PAWP}) \times 80}{\text{Cardiac index (CI)}}$		160–380 dynes/sec/cm^{-5}/m^2
Systemic vascular resistance (SVR) = $\dfrac{(\text{Mean arterial pressure [MAP]} - \text{CVP}) \times 80}{\text{CO}}$		800–1200 dynes/sec/cm^{-5}
Systemic vascular resistance index (SVRI) = $\dfrac{(\text{MAP} - \text{CVP}) \times 80}{\text{CI}}$		1970–2390 dynes/sec/cm^{-5}/m^2
*MAP = $\dfrac{\text{Systolic blood pressure} + 2\,(\text{Diastolic blood pressure})}{3}$		70–105 mm Hg
Other		
Stroke volume = $\dfrac{\text{CO}}{\text{Heart rate}}$		60–150 mL/beat
Stroke volume index (SVI) = $\dfrac{\text{CI}}{\text{Heart rate}}$		30–65 mL/beat/m^2
Stroke volume variation (SVV) = $\dfrac{SV_{max} - SV_{min}}{SV_{mean}}$		<13%
Heart rate (HR)		60–100 beats/min
CO = SV × HR		4–8 L/min
CI = $\dfrac{\text{CO}}{\text{Body surface area (BSA)}}$		2.2–4 L/min/m^2
RVEF = $\dfrac{\text{SV}}{\text{RVEDV} \times 100}$		40–60%
Arterial hemoglobin O$_2$ saturation		95–100%
Mixed venous hemoglobin O$_2$ saturation		60–80%
Venous hemoglobin O$_2$ saturation		70%

*These formulas are approximations because they do not take into consideration the heart rate. The monitor looks at the area under the pressure curve, as well as the heart rate, to calculate MAP.

Preload. *Preload* is the volume within a cardiac chamber at the end of diastole. Unfortunately, chamber volume measurements are difficult to obtain. Instead, various pressures are used to estimate volume. Left ventricular preload is called *left ventricular end-diastolic pressure.* PAOP reflects left ventricular end-diastolic pressure under normal conditions (i.e., when there is no mitral valve pathological condition, intracardiac defect, or dysrhythmia). Central venous pressure (CVP), measured in the right atrium or in the vena cava close to the heart, is the right ventricular preload or *right ventricular end-diastolic pressure* under normal conditions.

The effects of preload are explained by Frank-Starling's law, which states that the more a myocardial fibre is stretched during filling, the more it shortens during systole and the greater the force of the contraction to a physiological limit. As preload increases, force generated in the following contraction increases; thus, SV and CO increase. The greater the preload, the greater the myocardial (heart muscle) stretch and greater the oxygen requirement of the myocardium. Hence, increases in CO via increased preload require increased delivery of oxygen to the myocardium. It should be remembered that the change in SV with preload comes about because of stretching of the heart muscle. However, the clinical measurement made is not a direct measurement of the muscle

TABLE 68.4	MEASUREMENT OF BLOOD PRESSURE WITH INVASIVE LINES

1. The nurse explains the procedure to the patient.
2. The nurse positions the patient supine and flat or, if appropriate, with the head of the bed elevated up to 45 degrees.
3. The nurse confirms that the zero reference (port of the stopcock nearest the transducer) is placed at the level of the phlebostatic axis (see Figure 68.8). If the reference stopcock is not taped to the patient's chest, a carpenter's level should be used to position the stopcock on a bedside pole at the point level with the phlebostatic axis.
4. The nurse observes the monitor tracing, assesses the quality of the tracing, and performs a dynamic response test.
5. The nurse obtains an analogue printout, if available, and measures the systolic and diastolic pressures at end-expiration. If no printout is available, the nurse freezes the tracing on the oscilloscope screen and uses the cursor to measure the pressures at end-expiration.
6. The nurse records the pressure measurements promptly, including (if available) the printout marked to identify the points read.

length; the measurement made is pressure at the time of the peak stretch (end diastole) (Table 68.4). This pressure indirectly indicates the amount of stretch and the volume. This pressure is also important to measure because it indicates pressure in the blood vessels of the lung or in the blood returning to the heart. Preload can be increased by fluid administration and decreased by diuresis (Lough, 2018).

Afterload. *Afterload* refers to the forces opposing ventricular ejection. These forces include systemic arterial pressure, the resistance offered by the aortic valve, and the mass and density of the blood to be moved. Clinically, although the measures fail to include all the components of afterload, SVR and arterial pressure are indexes of left ventricular afterload. Similarly, pulmonary vascular resistance and PAP are indexes of right ventricular afterload. Increased afterload often results in a decreased CO. CO can be restored by decreasing afterload (i.e., decreasing forces opposing contraction). When afterload is reduced, myocardial oxygen needs are decreased. Thus, when CO is increased, myocardial oxygen requirements are decreased. Medication therapy directed at reducing afterload (e.g., nitroglycerine) is often used in the management of heart failure (see Chapter 37).

Vascular Resistance. *Systemic vascular resistance* (SVR) is the resistance of the systemic vascular bed. *Pulmonary vascular resistance* is the resistance of the pulmonary vascular bed. Both of these measures reflect afterload as described earlier and can be adjusted for body size (see Table 68.3).

Contractility. *Contractility* describes the strength of contraction. Contractility is said to increase when preload is not changed yet the heart contracts more forcefully. Epinephrine, norepinephrine, isoproterenol, dopamine, dobutamine, digitalis-like medications, calcium, and milrinone (Primacor) increase contractility. These agents are termed *positive inotropes*. Contractility is diminished by *negative inotropes*, such as acidosis and certain drugs and medications (e.g., barbiturates, alcohol, procainamide, calcium channel blockers, β-adrenergic blockers). Increased contractility results in increased SV and increased myocardial oxygen requirements. There are no direct clinical measures of cardiac contractility. To indirectly determine contractility, the nurse measures the patient's preload (PAOP or wedge pressure) and CO and graphs the results. If preload, heart rate, and afterload remain constant yet CO changes, contractility is altered.

Principles of Invasive Pressure Monitoring

Invasive lines, including central venous catheters (inserted into large upper thoracic veins, the subclavian or internal jugular) and, less frequently, pulmonary artery (PA) catheters, are used in the CCU to measure systemic and pulmonary pressures. Components of a typical invasive arterial pressure monitoring system are illustrated in Figure 68.7. To accurately measure pressure, equipment must be referenced and zero-balanced and dynamic response characteristics optimized. *Levelling* means positioning the transducer so that the zero reference point is at the level of the atria of the heart. The stopcock nearest the transducer is usually the zero reference for the transducer (see Figure 68.7). To place this level with the atria, the nurse uses an external landmark, the phlebostatic axis. To identify the phlebostatic axis, two imaginary lines are drawn with the patient supine (Figure 68.8, A). The first line, a horizontal line, is drawn through the midchest, halfway between the outermost anterior and the outermost posterior surfaces. The second line, a vertical line, is drawn through the fourth intercostal space at the sternum. The phlebostatic axis is the intersection of these two imaginary lines. Once the phlebostatic axis is identified, it should be marked on the patient's chest with a permanent marker. The port of the stopcock nearest the transducer must be positioned level with the phlebostatic axis.

Zeroing confirms that when pressure within the system is zero, the equipment reads zero. This is accomplished by opening the reference stopcock to room air and observing the monitor for a

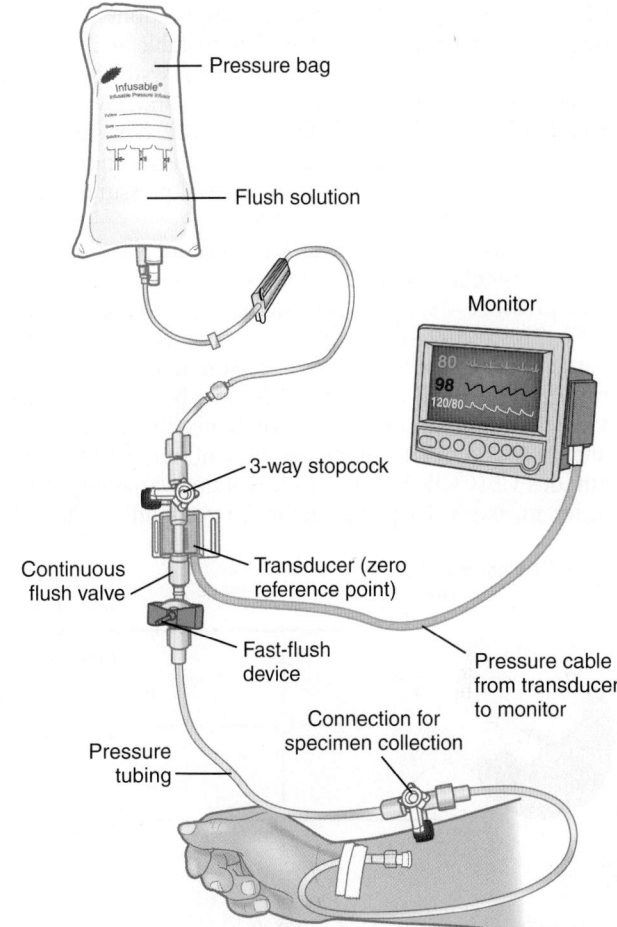

FIG. 68.7 Components of a pressure monitoring system. The cannula, shown entering the radial artery, is connected via pressure (nondistensible) tubing to the transducer. The transducer converts the pressure wave into an electronic signal. The transducer is wired to the electronic monitoring system, which amplifies, conditions, displays, and records the signal. Stopcocks are inserted into the line for specimen withdrawal and for referencing and zero-balancing procedures. A flush system, consisting of a pressurized bag of intravenous fluid, tubing, and a flush device, is connected to the system. The flush system provides continuous, slow (≈3 mL/hr) flushing and provides a mechanism for fast flushing of lines.

reading of zero. Zeroing the transducer is recommended during initial setup, immediately after insertion of the arterial line, when the transducer has been disconnected from the pressure cable or the pressure cable has been disconnected from the monitor, and when the accuracy of the measurements is questioned, and it should be done according to the manufacturer's guidelines.

Accurate readings are best obtained at the end of expiration. Initial readings are made with the patient lying flat. Unless the patient's BP is extremely sensitive to orthostatic changes, values at modest degrees of backrest elevation (≤45 degrees) are generally equivalent to measurements with the patient lying flat. It is not necessary to reposition the patient for each pressure reading. However, it is necessary to move the zero reference stopcock to keep it positioned at the phlebostatic axis (see Figure 68.8, B).

Types of Invasive Pressure Monitoring

Arterial Blood Pressure. Continuous arterial pressure monitoring is indicated for patients in many situations, including acute hypertension and hypotension, respiratory failure, shock, neurological injury, coronary interventional procedures, continuous infusion of vasoactive medications, and frequent arterial blood gas (ABG) sampling. Complications of arterial blood pressure monitoring are described in Table 68.5.

The nurse can use the arterial line to obtain systolic, diastolic, and mean arterial pressure (MAP). High- and low-pressure alarms should be set, based on the patient's current status, and activated. Measurements are obtained at end-expiration to limit the effect of the respiratory cycle on arterial pressure (Shaffer, 2011).

For patients who have an arterial line in place and who would also benefit from or require cardiac output monitoring, arterial pressure–based cardiac output (APCO) monitoring is possible. This technology involves use of a specialized sensor that attaches to a standard arterial pressure line and a monitor (Figure 68.9). APCO is a minimally invasive technique that provides real-time information to CCU health care providers to determine and trend continuous BP, continuous CO (CCO)/ continuous CI (CCI), SV, and stroke volume variability (SVV) in order to assess a patient's ability to respond to fluids by increasing SV (preload or fluid volume responsiveness) (Lough, 2018). APCO is indicated only in adult patients and cannot be used in patients who are on IABP therapy (Kern, 2011).

Pulmonary Artery Pressure Monitoring. The PA catheter is the most invasive technology for obtaining hemodynamic measurements. The PA catheter is frequently referred to as the *Swan-Ganz catheter* (named for its inventors) and may also be referred to as a *right heart catheter* (Figure 68.10). The infrequency of its use is due in part to the risks associated with the technology (e.g., infection, PA rupture, and infarction) and the development of less invasive techniques (e.g., APCO monitoring). PA catheter use is most common during and after cardiac surgery (Lough, 2018). Table 68.6 lists other possible indications for use of a PA catheter. Despite the infrequency of its use, PA diastolic pressure and PAOP are sensitive indicators of fluid volume status and cardiac function. Monitoring PAPs can enable precise therapeutic manipulation of preload, which allows CO to be maintained without placing the patient at risk for pulmonary edema. The critical care nurse plays an active role during PA catheter insertion and in monitoring a patient with a PA catheter postinsertion. It is imperative that wave forms for PA catheters be always transduced and monitored. More detailed information

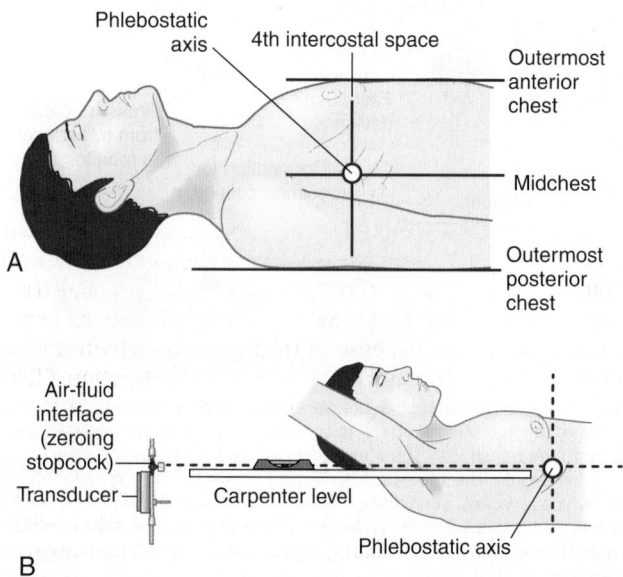

FIG. 68.8 Identification of the phlebostatic axis. **A,** Phlebostatic axis is an external landmark used to identify the level of the atria in the supine patient. It is defined as the intersection of two imaginary lines: one drawn horizontally from the midchest, midway between the anterior and posterior chest walls, and the other drawn vertically through the fourth intercostal space along the lateral chest wall. **B,** Air–fluid interface (zeroing the stopcock) is level with the phlebostatic axis using a carpenter's or laser level.

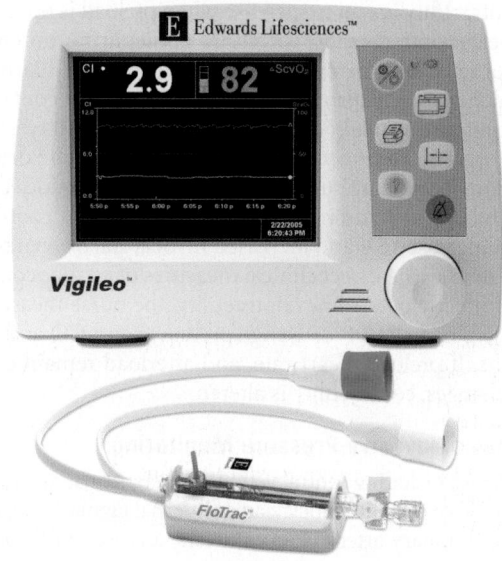

FIG. 68.9 FloTrac sensor and Vigileo monitor. Source: Courtesy Edwards Lifesciences LLC, Irvine, California. FloTrac, Vigileo, and Swan Ganz are trademarks of Edwards Lifesciences.

TABLE 68.5	ARTERIAL LINE COMPLICATIONS	
Complication	**Possible Cause**	**Prevention/Trouble Shooting**
Hemorrhage	Catheter dislodgement or disconnection	• Use Luer-LokTM system to secure connections. • Verify waveforms. • Activate monitor alarms. • Ensure continuous monitoring.
Infection	Risk associated with placement of any invasive line	• Inspect insertion site for local signs of inflammation. • Monitor patient for signs of systemic infection. • Pressure tubing and transducer should be changed every 96 hr or as per institutional policies.
Circulatory impairment	Thrombus formation around the catheter or release of an embolus, spasm, or occlusion of circulation by the catheter	• Perform Allen Test prior to catheter insertion. • To maintain line patency and limit thrombus formation, assess the continuous flush system every 1 to 4 hr to determine that (a) the pressure bag is inflated to 300 mm Hg, (b) the flush bag contains fluid, and (c) the system is delivering 3 to 6 mL/hr. • Evaluate neurovascular status distal to the arterial insertion site hourly. • Ensure circulation distal to the arterial insertion site is warm and well perfused with capillary refill time less than 3 sec. • Monitor for symptoms of neurological impairment (e.g., paresthesia, pain, paralysis).

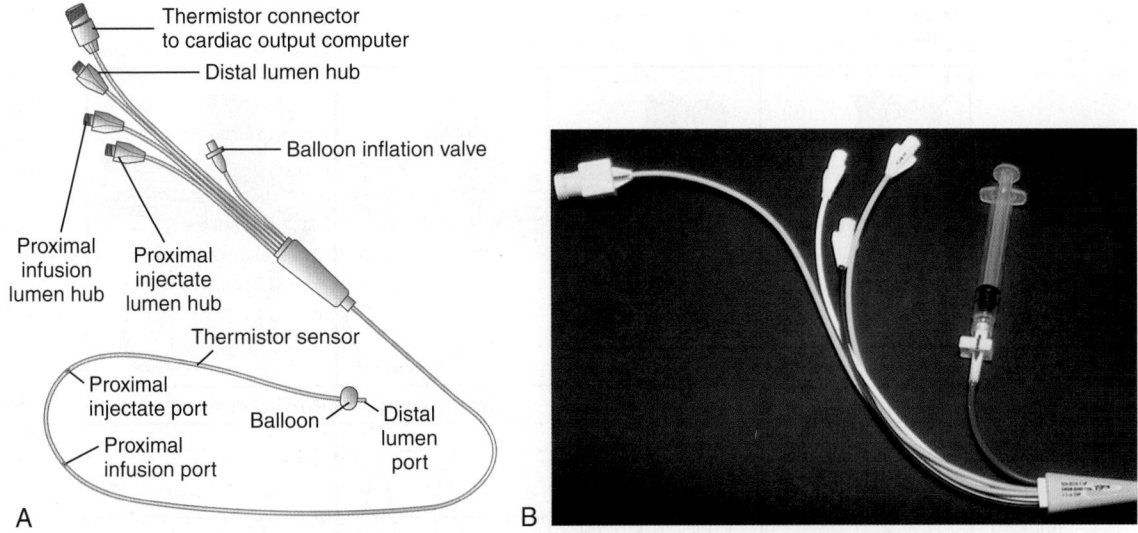

FIG. 68.10 Pulmonary artery (PA) catheter. **A,** Illustrated catheter has five lumens. When properly positioned, the distal lumen port is in the PA, and the proximal lumen ports are in the right atrium and the right ventricle. The distal port and one of the proximal ports are used to measure PA and central venous pressures, respectively. A balloon surrounds the catheter near the distal end. The balloon inflation valve is used to inflate the balloon with air to allow reading of the PA wedge pressure. A thermistor located near the distal tip senses PA temperature and is used to measure thermodilution cardiac output when solution cooler than body temperature is injected into a proximal port. **B,** Photograph of a catheter. Source: *B,* Courtesy Edwards Lifesciences LLC, Irvine, CA. Edwards Critical Care Division, Baxter Healthcare Corporation, Santa Ana, California. FloTrac, Vigileo, and Swan Ganz are trademarks of Edwards Lifesciences.

TABLE 68.6	CLINICAL INDICATIONS FOR PULMONARY ARTERY CATHETERIZATION

- Acute respiratory distress syndrome
- Acute respiratory failure in patients with chronic obstructive pulmonary disease
- Cardiac tamponade
- Complex fluid imbalance (e.g., trauma, burns, sepsis)
- Evaluation of circulatory syndromes (e.g., heart failure, mitral valve regurgitation, intraventricular shunts)
- Intra-aortic balloon pump therapy
- Myocardial infarction with complications (e.g., left ventricular failure, cardiogenic shock, ventricular septal rupture)
- Perioperative fluid imbalance in high-risk patients (e.g., cardiac history)
- Shock states (e.g., cardiogenic, septic, hypovolemic)
- Vasoactive medication therapy support

regarding PAPs, insertion procedures, and invasive hemodynamic monitoring is available in the report by Urden et al. (2018). See Figure 68.11 for positioning of the PA flow-directed catheter during progressive stages of insertion with corresponding pressure waveforms.

Central Venous or Right Atrial Pressure Measurement. CVP is a measurement of right ventricular preload and is often used to trend fluid status. It can be measured with a central venous catheter placed in the internal jugular or subclavian vein or a PA catheter. CVP is measured as a mean pressure at the end of expiration. Although the measurements of PA diastolic pressure and the wedge pressure are more sensitive indicators of fluid volume status, CVP can also be useful and a less invasive reflection of fluid volume concerns. An elevated CVP indicates right ventricular failure or volume overload. A low CVP indicates hypovolemia (Lough, 2018).

Venous Oxygen Saturation. Both CVP and PA catheters can include sensors to measure O_2 saturation of hemoglobin of venous blood. Either $ScvO_2$ (O_2 saturation of venous blood from the CVP catheter) or SvO_2 (venous O_2 saturation from the

PA catheter) are useful in determining the adequacy of tissue oxygenation. $ScvO_2/SvO_2$ reflects the dynamic balance between oxygenation of the arterial blood, tissue perfusion, and tissue oxygen consumption. $ScvO_2/SvO_2$ is useful in assessing hemodynamic status and response to treatments or activities when considered in conjunction with arterial O_2 saturation (Table 68.7). Normal $ScvO_2/SvO_2$ at rest is 60 to 80% (Lough, 2018).

Sustained decreases and increases in $ScvO_2/SvO_2$ must be analyzed carefully. Decreased SvO_2 may indicate (a) decreased arterial oxygenation, (b) low CO, (c) low hemoglobin, or (d) increased O_2 consumption. If the $ScvO_2/SvO_2$ falls, the nurse needs to determine which of these four factors has changed. The nurse observes for changes in arterial oxygenation by monitoring pulse oximetry results or ABGs. By noting any changes in level of consciousness, strength and quality of peripheral pulses, urine output, and skin colour and temperature, the nurse can generally assess CO and tissue perfusion. If arterial oxygenation, CO, and hemoglobin are unchanged, a fall in SvO_2 indicates increased O_2 consumption, which could result from an increased metabolic rate, pain, movement, or fever. If O_2 consumption increases without a comparable increase in O_2 delivery, more O_2 is extracted from the blood, and $ScvO_2/SvO_2$ will continue to fall (Lough, 2018). Increased $ScvO_2/SvO_2$ is also clinically significant and may indicate a clinical improvement (e.g., increased SaO_2, improved perfusion, decreased metabolic rate) or disorders (e.g., sepsis, ventricular septal defect). In sepsis, O_2 may not be extracted properly at the tissue level, resulting in increased mixed SvO_2 (Lough, 2018).

In many cases, as activity or metabolism increases, heart rate and CO increase, and SvO_2 remains constant or varies slightly. However, it is not uncommon for critically ill patients to have conditions that prevent substantial increases in CO. For example, such an increase could occur in the patient with heart failure, shock, dysrhythmias, or cardiac transplantation. In these cases, $ScvO_2/SvO_2$ can provide a useful indicator of the balance between O_2 delivery and consumption. Nursing interventions may be guided by changes in $ScvO_2/SvO_2$. The nurse might note

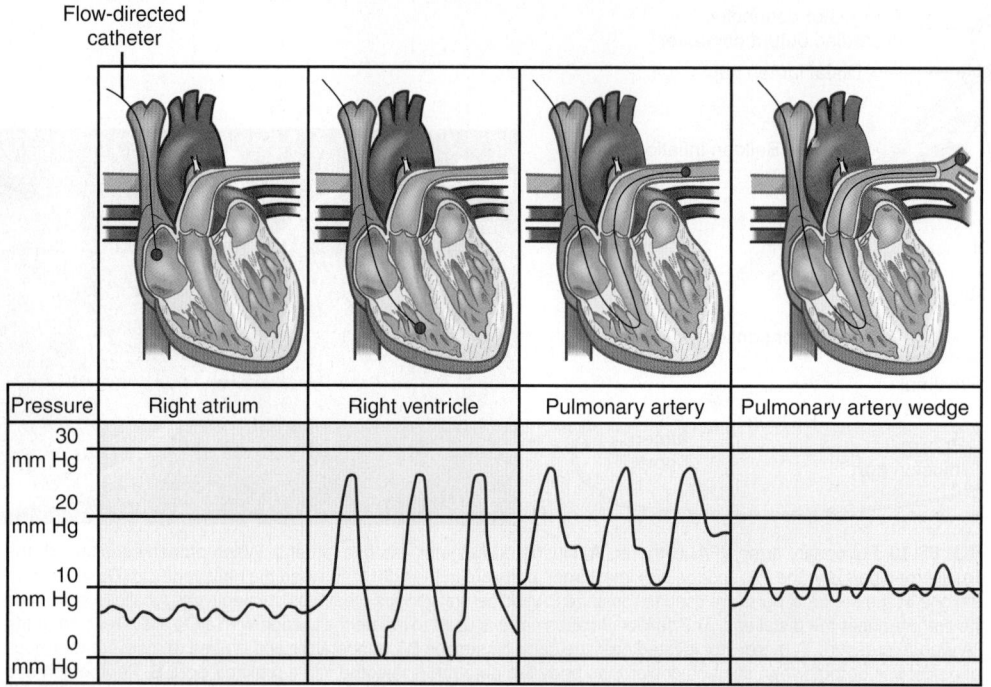

FIG. 68.11 Position of the pulmonary artery flow-directed catheter during progressive stages of insertion with corresponding pressure waveforms. Source: Adapted from Urden, L. D., Stacy, K. M., & Lough, M. E. (2010). *Critical care nursing: Diagnosis and management* (6th ed., p. 348, Figure 18-18). Mosby.

Pressure	Right atrium	Right ventricle	Pulmonary artery	Pulmonary artery wedge

TABLE 68.7 CLINICAL INTERPRETATION OF SvO₂ MEASUREMENTS

SvO₂ Measurement	Physiological Basis for Change in SvO₂	Clinical Diagnosis and Rationale
High SvO₂ (80–95%)	Increased oxygen supply Decreased oxygen demand	• Patient receiving more oxygen than required by clinical condition • Anaesthesia, which causes sedation and decreased muscle movement • Hypothermia, which lowers metabolic demand (e.g., with cardiopulmonary bypass) • Sepsis caused by decreased ability of tissues to use oxygen at the cellular level • False high-positive because pulmonary artery catheter is wedged in a pulmonary capillary
Normal SvO₂ (60–80%)	Normal oxygen supply and metabolic demand	• Balanced oxygen supply and demand
Low SvO₂ (<60%)	Decreased oxygen supply caused by: • Low hemoglobin • Low arterial saturation (SaO₂) • Low cardiac output • Increased oxygen consumption (VO₂)	• Anemia or bleeding with compromised cardiopulmonary system • Hypoxemia resulting from decreased oxygen supply or lung disease • Cardiogenic shock caused by left ventricular pump failure • Metabolic demand exceeds oxygen supply in conditions increasing metabolic rate, including physiological states such as shivering, seizures, and hyperthermia and nursing interventions that increase muscle movement, such as obtaining bed scale weight and repositioning

Source: Urden, L. D., Stacy, K. M., & Lough, M. E. (2018). *Critical care nursing: Diagnosis and management* (8th ed., p. 230, Table 13.6). Elsevier.

that the patient's heart rate increased moderately during repositioning but that the ScvO₂/SvO₂ remained stable. In this case, the nurse might conclude that the position change was tolerated. A drop in the ScvO₂/SvO₂ would be an indication to stop the activity until the SvO₂ returns to the previous level (Lough, 2018).

Noninvasive Arterial Oxygenation Monitoring. *Pulse oximetry* is a noninvasive and continuous method of determining arterial oxygenation (SpO₂), and monitoring SpO₂ may reduce how often ABG sampling is needed (see Chapter 28). In critically ill patients, SpO₂ is used to evaluate the effectiveness of O₂ therapy and to monitor how the patient tolerates decreases in fraction of inspired oxygen (FiO₂) and responds to changes in position and treatments. For example, the nurse might note that SpO₂ falls when the patient is positioned in a left lateral recumbent position. The nurse could then plan position changes that pose less risk for the patient. Additionally, accurate

SpO₂ measurements may be difficult to obtain in patients who are hypothermic, receiving IV vasopressor therapy (e.g., norepinephrine [Levophed]), or experiencing hypoperfusion (e.g., shock). The usual location for placement of the oximetry probe is a finger; alternative locations for probe placement may have to be considered (e.g., forehead, earlobe) during periods of hypoperfusion (Maiden, 2018).

NURSING MANAGEMENT HEMODYNAMIC MONITORING

Assessment of hemodynamic status requires integration of data from many sources and comparison of the data over time. Thorough, basic nursing observations provide important clues about the patient's hemodynamic status. The nurse should begin by obtaining baseline data regarding the patient's general

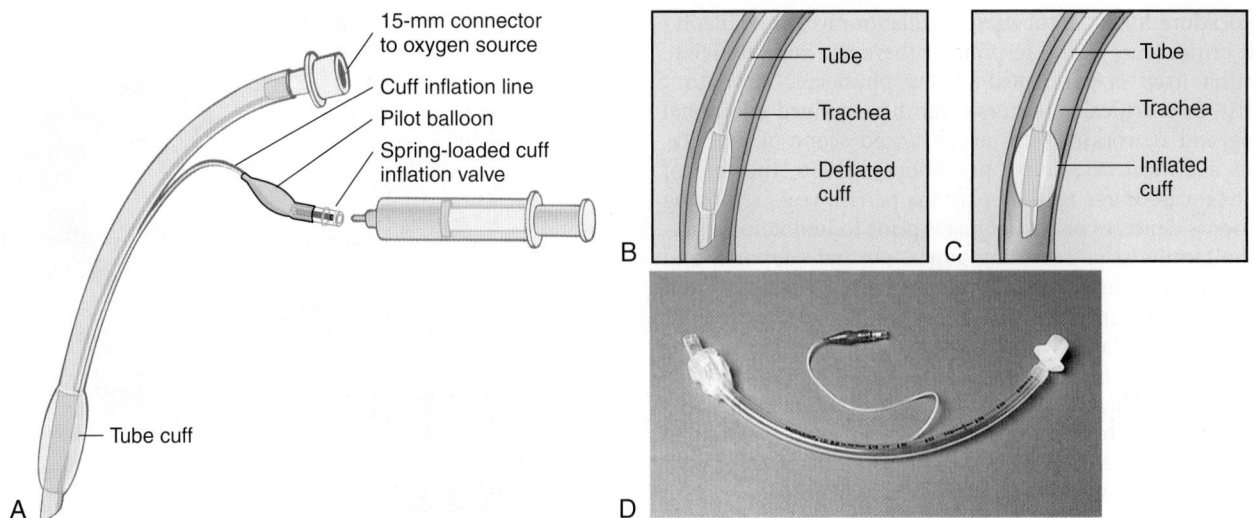

FIG. 68.12 Endotracheal tube. **A,** Parts of an endotracheal tube. **B,** Tube in place with the cuff deflated. **C,** Tube in place with the cuff inflated. **D,** Photograph of the tube before placement. Source: *A,* Beare, P. G., & Myers, J. L. (1998). *Adult health nursing* (3rd ed.). Mosby.

appearance, level of consciousness, skin colour and temperature, vital signs, peripheral pulses, and urine output. Does the patient appear tired, weak, or exhausted? There may be too little cardiac reserve to sustain even minimal activity. Pallor, cool skin, and diminished pulses may indicate decreased CO. Changes in mental clarity may reflect problems with cerebral perfusion or oxygenation. Monitoring urine output reflects the adequacy of perfusion to the kidneys. The patient with diminished perfusion to the GI tract may develop hypoactive or absent bowel sounds. If the patient is bleeding and developing shock, BP might initially be relatively stable, yet the patient may become increasingly pale and cool from peripheral vasoconstriction. Conversely, the patient experiencing septic shock may remain warm and pink yet develop tachycardia and BP instability. Although heart rates of 100 beats per minute are common among stressed, compromised, critically ill patients with sustained tachycardia, this condition greatly increases myocardial oxygen demand and may result in diminished CO (Lough, 2018).

The critical care nurse correlates observational data with data obtained from biotechnology (e.g., ECG; arterial pressure, CVP, CO, CI, SvO_2). Single hemodynamic values are rarely significant. The nurse must evaluate the whole clinical picture with the goals of recognizing early clues and intervening before critical conditions escalate.

ARTIFICIAL AIRWAYS

Patients in the CCU often need mechanical assistance to maintain airway patency. Inserting a tube into the trachea, bypassing upper airway and laryngeal structures, creates an artificial airway. The tube is placed into the trachea via the mouth or nose past the larynx (endotracheal [ET] intubation) or through a stoma in the neck *(tracheotomy)* (Stacy, 2018). ET intubation is more common than a tracheotomy in CCU patients. It is performed quickly at the bedside. Indications for ET intubation include (a) upper airway obstruction (e.g., secondary to burns, tumour, bleeding), (b) apnea, (c) respiratory distress, and (d) inability to maintain or protect the airway (e.g., ineffective clearance of secretions, altered or decreased level of consciousness). Figure 68.12 shows the parts of an ET tube (Stacy, 2018).

A *tracheotomy* is a surgical procedure that is performed when the need for an artificial airway is expected to be long term, or if there is a contraindication or inability to intubate the mouth (Stacy, 2018). There is ongoing debate regarding the timing of a tracheotomy in the patient requiring an ET tube. Research suggests that early tracheotomy (2–10 days) may have advantages over delayed tracheotomy, particularly when mechanical ventilation is predicted to be needed for longer than 10 to 14 days (Meng et al., 2016; Villwock & Jones, 2014). The situation varies with the patient, health care provider, and institution. (Chapter 29 discusses tracheostomy tubes and related nursing management.)

Endotracheal Tubes

In *oral intubation,* the ET tube is passed through the mouth and vocal cords and into the trachea with the aid of a laryngoscope or a bronchoscope. In *nasal ET intubation,* the ET is placed blindly (i.e., without seeing the larynx) through the nose, nasopharynx, and vocal cords. Oral ET intubation is preferred for most emergencies because the airway can be secured rapidly and a larger-diameter tube is used. A larger-bore ET tube reduces the work of breathing because of less airway resistance. It is easier to remove secretions and perform fiber-optic bronchoscopy if needed (Stacy, 2018). Nasal ET intubation is rarely used but may be necessary in special circumstances.

There are risks associated with oral ET intubation. It is difficult to place an oral tube if head and neck mobility is limited (e.g., suspected spinal cord injury). Teeth can be chipped or accidentally removed during the procedure. Salivation is increased and swallowing is difficult. Patients can obstruct the ET tube by biting down on it. A bite block may be used to avoid this. The ET tube and bite block (if used) should be secured (separately) to the face. Mouth care is a challenge because of limited space in the oral cavity, but it is still important and completed regularly.

Endotracheal Intubation Procedure

Unless ET intubation is emergent, consent for the procedure needs to be obtained. The patient and caregiver must be told the reason for ET intubation, the steps in the procedure, and the patient's role in the procedure (if indicated). It should also be explained that, while intubated, the patient will not be able to speak but that other means of communication will be provided.

The procedure for ET intubation is collaborative effort involving the critical care nurse, respiratory therapist, and physician. Intubation itself is performed by the physician, respiratory therapist, or a critical care nurse who has received additional training and is working with an advanced scope of practice, such as a critical care nurse practitioner. Often, the role of the critical care nurse is to prepare the patient (e.g., removing the patient's dentures or partial plates prior to intubation), prepare the family (e.g., providing education and support), and prepare and administer medications as ordered. Premedication varies depending on the patient's level of consciousness (e.g., wake or comatose) and the nature of the procedure (e.g., emergent or nonemergent). A self-inflating *bag valve mask* (BVM) should be available and attached to O_2, suctioning equipment should be ready at the bedside, and IV access should be obtained prior to starting. The BVM contains a reservoir that is filled with O_2 so that concentrations of 90 to 95% are delivered.

Rapid-sequence intubation (RSI) is the rapid, concurrent administration of both a sedative and a paralytic agent during emergency airway management to decrease the risks for aspiration and injury to the patient. RSI is not indicated in patients who are in cardiac arrest or are known to have a difficult airway (Stollings et al., 2014). A sedative–hypnotic–amnesic (e.g., midazolam, propofol) is used to induce unconsciousness, along with a rapid-onset opioid (e.g., fentanyl) to blunt the pain of the procedure. A paralytic medication (e.g., succinylcholine) is then given to produce skeletal muscle paralysis. The patient's oxygenation status must be monitored during the procedure using pulse oximetry (Stacy, 2018).

For oral intubation, the patient is placed supine with the head extended and the neck flexed, also known as the "sniffing position." This position enables visualization of the vocal cords. Before intubation is started, the patient should be preoxygenated using the BVM and 100% O_2 for 3 to 5 minutes. Each intubation attempt is limited to less than 30 seconds, and the patient should be ventilated between successive attempts using the BVM and 100% O_2.

After intubation, the cuff should be inflated and placement of the ET tube confirmed while the patient is manually ventilated using the BVM with 100% O_2. An end-tidal CO_2 detector is used to confirm proper placement by noting the presence of exhaled CO_2 from the lungs. The detector should be placed between the BVM and the ET tube, and the nurse should observe for either a colour change (indicating the presence of CO_2) or a number. If no CO_2 is detected, the tube is in the esophagus and needs to be reinserted (Stacy, 2018). The lungs must be auscultated for bilateral breath sounds, and the epigastrium for the absence of air sounds. The nurse should observe the chest for symmetrical chest wall movement. In addition, SpO_2 should be stable or improved.

If the findings support proper ET tube placement, the tube is then connected to an O_2 source and secured per employer policy (Figure 68.13). The nurse should suction the ET tube and pharynx and insert a bite block as needed. A chest radiograph is done immediately to confirm tube location (2 to 6 cm above the carina in the adult). This position allows the patient to move their neck without moving the tube or causing it to enter the right mainstem bronchus. Once proper positioning is confirmed with radiography, the nurse should record and mark the position of the tube at the lip or teeth or nose. Excess tubing is cut to reduce dead air space.

The ET tube is connected to either humidified air, O_2, or a mechanical ventilator. ABGs are obtained immediately after

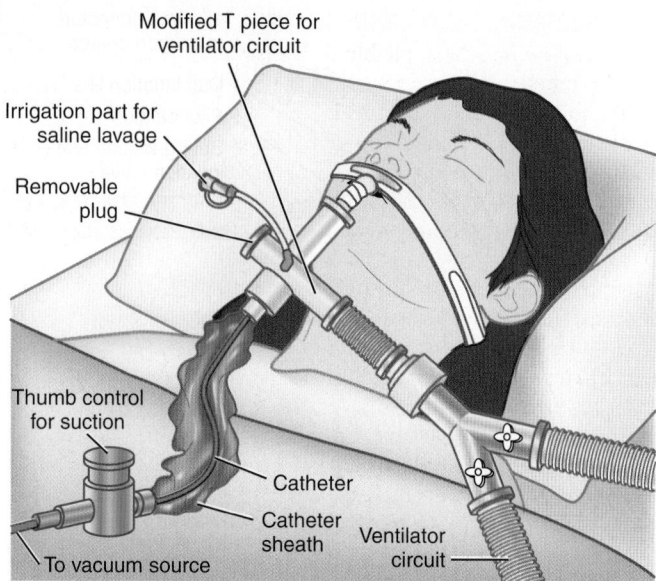

Modified T piece for ventilator circuit

Irrigation part for saline lavage

Removable plug

Thumb control for suction

To vacuum source

Catheter

Catheter sheath

Ventilator circuit

FIG. 68.13 Closed tracheal suction system.

intubation to determine baseline oxygenation and ventilation status. ABG values are reviewed and used to guide oxygenation and ventilation changes. Continuous pulse oximetry and end-tidal CO_2 monitoring provide valuable data related to arterial oxygenation and ventilation.

NURSING MANAGEMENT ARTIFICIAL AIRWAY

Management of a patient with an artificial airway is often a shared responsibility between the nurse and the respiratory therapist, with specific management tasks determined by employer policy. Nursing responsibilities for the patient with an artificial airway may include some or all of the following: (a) maintaining correct tube placement, (b) maintaining proper cuff inflation, (c) monitoring oxygenation and ventilation, (d) maintaining tube patency, (e) assessing for complications, (f) providing oral care and maintaining skin integrity, and (g) fostering comfort and communication (Stacy, 2018).

MAINTAINING CORRECT TUBE PLACEMENT

The patient with an ET tube should be continuously monitored to ensure the tube remains in place. A tube that is dislodged could end up in the pharynx or enter the esophagus or the right mainstem bronchus (thus ventilating only the right lung).

SAFETY ALERT—Endotracheal Tube Placement
- Proper ET tube position can be maintained by placing an "exit mark" on the tube.
- The mark must remain constant while the patient is at rest and during patient care, repositioning, and transport.

The chest wall must be observed for symmetrical movement and auscultated to confirm bilateral breath sounds. If the ET tube is not positioned properly, it is an emergency. The nurse should stay with the patient, maintain the airway, support ventilation, and call for the appropriate help to immediately reposition the tube. It may be necessary to remove the ET tube and ventilate the patient with a BVM and 100% O_2. If a dislodged tube is not repositioned, minimal or no O_2 is delivered to the lungs or the entire volume is delivered to one lung. This places the patient at risk for pneumothorax.

MAINTAINING PROPER CUFF INFLATION

The cuff is an inflatable, pliable sleeve encircling the outer wall of the ET tube (see Figure 68.12). The high-volume, low-pressure cuff stabilizes and "seals" the ET tube within the trachea and prevents escape of ventilating gases. However, excess volume in the cuff can damage the tracheal mucosa. To avoid this, once the cuff is inflated with air, the cuff pressure should be measured and monitored. To ensure adequate tracheal perfusion, cuff pressure should be maintained at 20 to 25 cm H_2O (Stacy, 2018). It will need to be measured and recorded after intubation and on a routine basis (e.g., every 8 hours) using the *minimal occluding volume* (MOV) *technique* or *the minimal leak technique* (MLT).

The steps in the MOV technique for cuff inflation are as follows: (a) for the mechanically ventilated patient, a stethoscope is placed over the trachea and the cuff inflated to MOV by adding air until no air leak is heard at peak inspiratory pressure (end of ventilator inspiration); (b) for the spontaneously breathing patient, the cuff is inflated until no sound is heard after a deep breath or after inhalation with a BVM; (c) a manometer is used to verify that cuff pressure is between 20 and 25 cm H_2O; and (d) cuff pressure is recorded in the chart. If adequate cuff pressure cannot be maintained or larger volumes of air are needed to keep the cuff inflated, there could be a leak in the cuff or tracheal dilation at the cuff site. In these situations, the nurse should notify the physician to reposition or change the ET tube.

The procedure for MLT is similar with one exception: A small amount of air is removed from the cuff until a slight air leak is auscultated at peak inflation. The aim of both techniques is to prevent the risk for tracheal damage from high cuff pressures.

MONITORING OXYGENATION AND VENTILATION

The patient with an ET tube must be vigilantly monitored for adequate oxygenation through assessments of clinical findings, ABGs, and SpO_2. The nurse should assess for signs of hypoxemia, such as a change in mental status (e.g., confusion), anxiety, dusky skin, and dysrhythmias. Periodic ABGs (specifically partial pressure of oxygen in arterial blood [PaO_2]) and continuous SpO_2 provide objective data regarding oxygenation (Stacy, 2018). Indicators of ventilation include clinical findings, partial pressure of carbon dioxide in arterial blood ($PaCO_2$), and continuous end-tidal CO_2 ($ETCO_2$). The nurse should assess the patient's respirations for rate, rhythm, and use of accessory muscles. $PaCO_2$ is the best indicator of alveolar hyperventilation (e.g., decreased $PaCO_2$, increased pH indicates respiratory alkalosis) or hypoventilation (e.g., increased $PaCO_2$, decreased pH indicates respiratory acidosis).

$ETCO_2$ monitoring *(capnography)* is done by analyzing exhaled gas directly at the ventilator circuit *(mainstream sampling)* or by transporting a sample of gas via small-bore tubing to a bedside monitor *(sidestream sampling)*. Continuous $ETCO_2$ monitoring can be used to assess the patency of the airway and the presence of breathing. In addition, gradual changes in $ETCO_2$ values may accompany an increase in CO_2 production (e.g., sepsis, hypoventilation, neuromuscular blockade) or a decrease in CO_2 production (e.g., hypothermia, decreased CO, metabolic acidosis). In patients with normal ventilation-to-perfusion ratios (see Chapter 70), $ETCO_2$ can be used as an estimate of $PaCO_2$, with $ETCO_2$ generally 1 to 5 mm Hg lower than $PaCO_2$.

MAINTAINING TUBE PATENCY

A patient should not be routinely suctioned; rather, the nurse should assess the patient regularly to determine if suctioning is needed. Indications for suctioning include (a) visible secretions in the ET tube, (b) sudden onset of respiratory distress, (c) suspected aspiration of secretions, (d) increase in peak airway pressures, (e) auscultation of adventitious breath sounds over the trachea or bronchi, (f) increase in respiratory rate or sustained coughing, and (g) sudden or gradual decrease in PaO_2 or SpO_2.

Table 68.8 describes two recommended suctioning methods: the closed-suction technique (CST) and the open-suction technique (OST). The CST involves use of a suction catheter that is enclosed in a plastic sleeve connected directly to the ventilator circuit (see Figure 68.13). With the CST, oxygenation and ventilation are maintained during suctioning, and exposure to the patient's secretions is reduced. The CST should be used for patients who (a) require high levels of positive end-expiratory pressure (greater than 10 cm H_2O), (b) have high levels of FiO_2, (c) have bloody or infected pulmonary secretions, (d) require frequent suctioning, or (e) experience clinical instability with the OST (Seckel, 2017).

Potential complications associated with suctioning include hypoxemia, bronchospasm, increased intracranial pressure, dysrhythmias, hypertension, hypotension, mucosal damage, pulmonary bleeding, pain, and infection. The patient must be assessed closely before, during, and after the suctioning procedure. If the patient does not tolerate suctioning (e.g., decreased SpO_2, increased or decreased BP, sustained coughing, development of dysrhythmias), the procedure should be stopped and the patient hyperoxygenated until equilibration occurs before attempting another suction pass. Hypoxemia can be prevented by hyperoxygenating the patient before and after each suctioning pass and limiting each pass to 10 seconds or less (see Table 68.8). Both the ECG and SpO_2 should be assessed before, during, and after the suctioning procedure.

Causes of dysrhythmias during suctioning include (a) hypoxemia resulting in myocardial ischemia; (b) vagal stimulation caused by tracheal irritation; and (c) sympathetic nervous system stimulation caused by anxiety, discomfort, or pain. Dysrhythmias include tachydysrhythmias and bradydysrhythmias, premature beats, and asystole. If any new dysrhythmias develop, suctioning should be stopped. Excessive suctioning must be avoided in patients with severe hypoxemia or bradycardia.

Tracheal mucosal damage may occur because of excessive suction pressures (>120 mm Hg), overly vigorous catheter insertion, or the characteristics of the suction catheter itself. Blood streaks or tissue shreds in aspirated secretions may indicate that mucosal damage has occurred. Mucosal damage increases the risk for infection and bleeding, particularly if the patient is receiving anticoagulants (Seckel, 2017). Trauma to the mucosa can be prevented by following the steps described in Table 68.8.

Secretions may be thick and difficult to suction because of inadequate hydration, inadequate humidification, infection, or inaccessibility of the left mainstem bronchus or lower airways. Adequately hydrating the patient (e.g., oral or IV fluids) and providing supplemental humidification of inspired gases may assist in thinning secretions. Instillation of normal saline into the ET tube is discouraged and may be harmful. If infection is the cause of thick secretions, the patient must receive appropriate antibiotics. Mobilization, postural drainage, percussion, and turning of the patient every 2 hours may help move secretions into larger airways.

PROVIDING ORAL CARE AND MAINTAINING SKIN INTEGRITY

When an oral ET tube is in place, the patient's mouth is always open. The nurse should moisten the lips, tongue, and gums with saline or water swabs to prevent mucosal drying. Proper oral care provides comfort and prevents injury to the gums and plaque formation (Table 68.9). Meticulous care is required to

TABLE 68.8   SUCTIONING PROCEDURES FOR A PATIENT ON A MECHANICAL VENTILATOR

General Measures

1. Gather all equipment.
2. Wash hands and don personal protective equipment.
3. Explain procedure and patient's role in assisting with secretion removal by coughing.
4. Monitor patient's cardiopulmonary status (e.g., vital signs, SpO_2, SvO_2, $ScvO_2$, ECG, level of consciousness) before, during, and after the procedure.
5. Turn on suction and set vacuum to 100 to 120 mm Hg.
6. Pause ventilator alarms.

Open-Suction Technique

1. Open sterile catheter package using the inside of the package as a sterile field. *Note:* Suction catheter should be no wider than half the diameter of the ET tube (e.g., for a 7-mm ET tube, select a 10-French suction catheter).
2. Fill the sterile solution container with sterile normal saline or water.
3. Don sterile gloves.
4. Pick up sterile suction catheter with the dominant hand. Using the nondominant hand, secure connecting tube (to suction) to the suction catheter.
5. Check equipment for proper functioning by suctioning a small volume of sterile saline solution from the container. (Go to step 7.)

Closed-Suction Technique

6. Connect suction tubing to the closed-suction port.
7. Hyperoxygenate patient for 30 sec using one of the following methods:
   - Activate the suction hyperoxygenation setting on ventilator using the nondominant hand.
   - Increase FiO_2 to 100%. *Note:* FiO_2 must be returned to baseline level at completion of the procedure if not done automatically after preset time by ventilator.
   - Disconnect ventilator tubing from the ET tube and manually ventilate patient with 100% O_2 using a BVM device.* Administer five or six breaths over 30 sec. *Note:* Use of a second person to deliver the manual breaths will significantly increase the tidal volume delivered.
8. With suction off, gently and quickly insert catheter using the dominant hand. When resistance is met, pull back 1 cm.
9. Apply continuous or intermittent suction using the nondominant thumb. Withdraw catheter within 10 sec or less.
10. Hyperoxygenate for 30 sec as described in step 7.
11. If secretions remain and the patient has tolerated the procedure, perform two to three suction passes as described in steps 8 and 9. *Note:* Rinse suction catheter with sterile saline solution between suctioning passes as needed.
12. Reconnect patient to ventilator (open-suction technique).
13. At completion of ET tube suctioning, rinse the catheter and connecting tubing with sterile saline solution.
14. Suction oral pharynx. *Note:* A separate catheter must be used for this step when using the closed-suction technique.
15. Discard suction catheter, and rinse the connecting tubing with sterile saline solution (open-suction technique).
16. Reset FiO_2 (if necessary) and ventilator alarms.
17. Reassess patient for signs of effective suctioning.

BVM, bag valve mask; *ECG,* electrocardiogram; *ET,* endotracheal; *FiO2,* fraction of inspired oxygen; *PEEP,* positive end-expiratory pressure; *ScvO2,* central venous oxygen saturation; *SpO2,* oxygen saturation; *SvO2,* venous oxygen saturation.
*Attach a PEEP valve to the BVM for patients on >5 cm H_2O PEEP.
Source: Adapted from Seckel, M. A. (2017). Suctioning: Endotracheal or tracheostomy tube. In D. L. Wiegand (Ed.), *AACN procedure manual for critical care* (7th ed.). Elsevier.

prevent skin breakdown on the face, lips, tongue, and nares due to pressure from the ET tube or bite block or the method used to secure the ET tube to the patient's face. Regular mouth care also helps to decrease the bacterial burden in the mouth, to help prevent ventilator-associated pneumonia (VAP) from aspiration of contaminated oral secretions (Chacko et al., 2017). The ET tube should be repositioned and retaped every 24 hours and as needed. This practice may be shared between the nurse and respiratory therapist or limited to the respiratory therapist.

The nurse should remove the bite block (if present) and the old tape or ties. After providing oral hygiene, the nurse repositions the ET tube to the opposite side of the mouth, replaces the bite block (if appropriate), and reconfirms proper cuff inflation and tube placement. The ET tube is then secured again per employer policy. If a manufactured tube holder is used, the straps should be loosened, the area under the straps massaged, and then the straps reapplied. Two staff members should perform the repositioning procedure to prevent accidental dislodgement. The patient must be monitored for any signs of respiratory distress throughout the procedure.

FOSTERING COMFORT AND COMMUNICATION

Intubation is a major stressor for the patient and family (Wade et al., 2013). The intubated patient may experience anxiety from not being able to talk or not knowing what to expect.

TABLE 68.9   ORAL CARE PROCEDURES FOR A PATIENT ON A MECHANICAL VENTILATOR

General Measures

1. Gather all equipment.
2. Wash hands and don personal protective equipment.
3. Explain procedure to the patient and the family, if present.
4. Perform oral care using pediatric or adult soft toothbrushes at least twice a day by gently brushing to clean and remove plaque.
5. Use oral swabs with a 1.5% hydrogen peroxide solution q2–4h. *Note:* Postoperative cardiac surgery patients are the only population in which use of 2% chlorhexidine gluconate is recommended twice a day.
6. Apply mouth moisturizer to oral mucosa and lips with each cleaning.
7. Suction oral cavity and pharynx frequently. See Figure 68.15 for an example of an endotracheal tube that can provide continuous subglottic suctioning.

Note

- All oral suction equipment and suction tubing should be changed q24h.
- The nondisposable oral suction apparatus should be rinsed with sterile normal saline after each use and placed on a dry paper towel.

Source: Adapted from Vollman, K. M., & Sole, M. L. (2011). Endotracheal tube and oral care. In D. L. Wiegand (Ed.), *AACN procedure manual for critical care* (6th ed., pp. 33–37). Elsevier.

The physical discomfort associated with ET intubation and mechanical ventilation often requires regular analgesic and, possibly, sedation until the ET tube is no longer required. The patient may need morphine, propofol, or other sedatives to blunt the anxiety and discomfort related to intubation. The nurse should evaluate the medications' effectiveness in achieving an acceptable level of patient comfort. In addition, relaxation techniques (e.g., music therapy) should be considered to accompany medication therapy.

COMPLICATIONS OF ENDOTRACHEAL INTUBATION

Two major complications of ET intubation are unplanned extubation and aspiration. Unplanned *extubation* (i.e., removal of the ET tube from the trachea) can be a catastrophic event and usually complicates the patient's recovery. Unplanned extubation can be due to patient removal of the ET tube or accidental removal during movement or a procedure. Usually the unplanned extubation is obvious (the patient is holding the ET tube). Other times, the tip of the ET tube is in the hypopharynx or esophagus and the extubation is not so obvious.

SAFETY ALERT—Unplanned Extubation
The nurse should observe for signs of unplanned extubation, which can be a life-threatening event:
• Patient talking
• Activation of the low-pressure ventilator alarm
• Diminished or absent breath sounds
• Respiratory distress
• Gastric distension

The nurse is responsible for preventing unplanned extubation by ensuring that the ET tube is secured and observing and supporting the ET tube during repositioning, procedures, and patient transfers. Should an unplanned extubation occur, the nurse should stay with the patient and call for help. Interventions are aimed at maintaining the patient's airway, supporting ventilation (e.g., manually ventilating the patient with a BVM and 100% O_2), securing the appropriate assistance to immediately reintubate the patient (if necessary), and providing psychological support to the patient.

Aspiration is another potential hazard for the patient with an ET tube. The ET tube passes through the epiglottis, splinting it in an open position. Thus, the intubated patient cannot protect the airway from aspiration. The high-volume, low-pressure ET or tracheal cuff cannot totally prevent the trickle of oral or gastric secretions into the trachea. Further, secretions collect above the cuff. When the cuff is deflated, those secretions can move into the lungs. Some ET tubes provide continuous suctioning of secretions above the cuff.

Oral intubation increases salivation, yet swallowing is difficult, so the nurse should suction the patient's mouth frequently using a suction catheter. Other factors contributing to aspiration include improper cuff inflation, patient positioning, and tracheoesophageal fistula. Patients with an ET tube are at risk for aspiration of gastric contents. Even when the cuff is properly inflated, precautions should be taken to prevent vomiting, which can lead to aspiration. Often, a nasogastric (NG) or an orogastric (OG) tube is inserted and connected to low, intermittent suction when a patient is first intubated. An OG tube is preferred over an NG tube to reduce the risk for sinusitis. All patients who are intubated or receiving enteral feedings must have the head of the bed elevated a minimum of 30 to 45 degrees unless medically contraindicated (Stacy, 2018).

MECHANICAL VENTILATION

Mechanical ventilation is the process by which ventilation and oxygenation is supported or conducted by a machine. Mechanical ventilation is not curative; it is a means of supporting patients until they recover the ability to breathe independently (Stacy, 2018). Mechanical ventilation can be invasive, via an ET tube or tracheostomy tube, or noninvasive, via a face or nasal mask. It can also serve as a bridge to long-term mechanical ventilation or to a decision being made to withdraw ventilatory support. Indications for mechanical ventilation include (a) apnea or impending inability to breathe or protect the airway, (b) acute respiratory failure (see Chapter 70), (c) severe hypoxia, and (d) respiratory muscle fatigue (Burns, 2011a).

Patients with life-limiting illnesses, such as chronic pulmonary disease, and their caregivers should be given the opportunity to discuss mechanical ventilation before end-stage respiratory disease develops. The nurse should encourage all patients, particularly those with chronic illnesses, to discuss the subject with their families and health care providers. Patients should then record and place the results of these discussions in an advance directive. The decision to use, withhold, or withdraw mechanical ventilation must be made carefully, respecting the wishes of the patient and caregiver or family.

Types of Mechanical Ventilation

The two major types of mechanical ventilation are noninvasive and invasive ventilation. Noninvasive ventilation requires use of a mask (e.g., facemask, nasal mask, nasal pillows) and a machine to help deliver breaths, whereas invasive ventilation involves use of an ET tube or tracheotomy, as described earlier. There are two main types of ventilation, negative-pressure and positive-pressure ventilation; positive-pressure ventilation is the most commonly used. Among positive-pressure ventilation modes there are many different variations (Stacy, 2018).

Negative- and Positive-Pressure Ventilation. Negative-pressure ventilation involves the use of chambers that encase the chest or body and surround it with intermittent subatmospheric (or negative) pressure. The "iron lung," developed during the polio epidemic, was the first form of negative-pressure ventilation. Intermittent negative pressure around the chest wall causes the chest to be pulled outward, reducing intrathoracic pressure. Air rushes in via the upper airway, which is outside the sealed chamber. Expiration is passive. The machine cycles off, allowing chest retraction. This type of ventilation is similar to normal ventilation in that decreased intrathoracic pressures produce inspiration, and expiration is passive. Negative-pressure ventilation is delivered by noninvasive ventilation and does not require an artificial airway.

Positive-pressure ventilation (PPV) is the primary method used with acutely ill patients (Figure 68.14). During inspiration, the ventilator pushes air into the lungs under positive pressure. Unlike spontaneous ventilation, intrathoracic pressure is raised during lung inflation rather than lowered. Expiration occurs passively as in normal expiration. Modes of PPV can be categorized into two groups: invasive and noninvasive ventilation (Stacy, 2018).

Noninvasive Ventilation. Noninvasive positive-pressure ventilation (NPPV), in addition to being commonly used for obstructive sleep apnea, can be used in a variety of situations commonly associated with critical care, such as cardiogenic pulmonary edema and acute or chronic respiratory failure. NPPV can also be used in instances where invasive ventilation is not

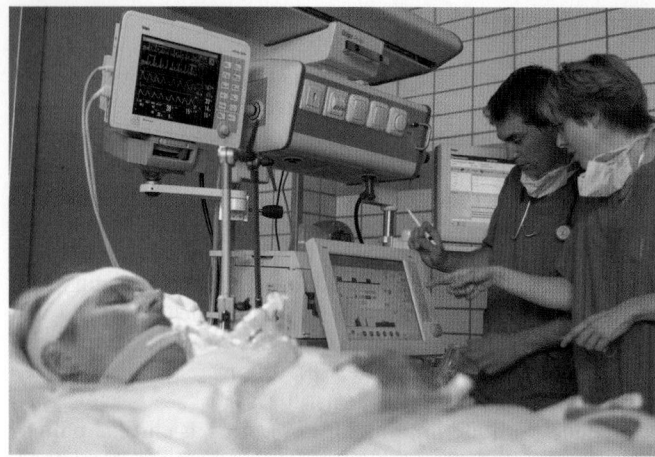

FIG. 68.14 Patient receiving mechanical ventilation. Source: Courtesy Draeger Medical.

TABLE 68.10   SETTINGS OF MECHANICAL VENTILATION

Parameter	Description
High-pressure limit	Regulates the maximal pressure the ventilator can generate to deliver the V_T; when the pressure limit is reached, the ventilator terminates the breath and spills the undelivered volume into the atmosphere; usual setting is 10–20 cm H_2O above peak inspiratory pressure
I:E ratio	Duration of inspiration (I) to duration of expiration (E); usual setting is 1:2 to 1:1.5 unless IRV is desired
Inspiratory flow rate and time	Speed with which the V_T is delivered; usual setting is 40–80 L/min and time is 0.8–1.2 sec
Oxygen concentration	Fraction of inspired oxygen (FiO_2) delivered to patient; may be set between 21% (essentially room air) and 100%; usually adjusted to maintain PaO_2 level >60 mm Hg or SpO_2 level >90%
Positive end-expiratory pressure (PEEP)	Positive pressure applied at the end of expiration of ventilator breaths; usual setting is 5 cm H_2O
Pressure support	Positive pressure used to augment patient's inspiratory pressure; usual setting is 6–18 cm H_2O
Respiratory rate (f)	Number of breaths the ventilator delivers per minute; usual setting is 6–20 breaths/min
Sensitivity	Determines the amount of effort the patient must generate to initiate a ventilator breath; it may be set for pressure triggering or flow triggering; usual setting for a pressure trigger is 0.5–1.5 cm H_2O below baseline pressure and for a flow trigger is 1–3 L/min below baseline flow
Tidal volume (V_T)	Volume of gas delivered to patient during each ventilator breath; usual volume is 6–10 mL/kg

IRV, inverse ratio ventilation; *PaO_2,* partial pressure of oxygen in arterial blood; *SpO_2,* oxygen saturation value obtained by pulse oximetry.
Source: Urden, L. D., Stacy, K. M., & Lough, M. E. (2010). *Critical care nursing: Diagnosis and management* (6th ed., p. 655, Table 25.6). Mosby.

desired and can provide temporizing care at the end of life.

There are two general ways in which noninvasive ventilation is provided: (1) continuous positive airway pressure (CPAP) and (2) bilevel positive airway pressure (BiPAP). CPAP provides one set pressure to help keep the airways and alveoli open. It is commonly used for sleep-disordered breathing (e.g., obstructive sleep apnea). The pressure keeps the airways open during inspiration and expiration and prevents collapse, thereby allowing for improved ventilation. BiPAP has two different pressure settings: inspiratory positive airway pressure (I-PAP) or pressure-support ventilation (PSV), and expiratory positive airway pressure (E-PAP) or positive end-expiratory pressure (PEEP). I-PAP helps to improve ventilation (e.g., if the patient is not strong enough and needs more help bringing air in and out of the lungs) and is evaluated using PCO_2 levels or respiratory rate. E-PAP helps improve oxygenation and is evaluated using PO_2. BiPAP is intended as a temporary measure, and if the patient does not stabilize quickly, invasive ventilation should be considered (Burns, 2011b). The use of NPPV may be precluded in patients with status asthmaticus, hemodynamic instability, inadequate airway protection, encephalopathy or coma, excessive secretions, severe agitation, or high FiO_2 requirements (Burns, 2011b).

Invasive Ventilation. There are many different modes of PPV. One way to classify the different modes is to divide them into spontaneous and control modes. In spontaneous modes of ventilation, the patient is able to determine the respiratory rate and the ventilator assists the patient, whereas in control modes, the number of breaths, the size of the breaths, and, at times, the pressure generated are all controlled and preset.

Settings of Mechanical Ventilators

Choosing the settings for mechanical ventilation is based on a number of different factors, including the patient' status (e.g., ABGs, ideal body weight, level of consciousness, muscle strength), illness acuity, and goals of care. Respiratory therapists assume a key role in determining optimal ventilator settings. The different settings that can be adjusted include rate, depth, and spontaneous versus full control (Table 68.10). The ventilator is adjusted to match the patient's needs, pattern of breathing, and comfort. Settings are evaluated and adjusted frequently until the patient achieves optimal ventilation. Some settings serve as a fail-safe mechanism, alerting staff to problems with ventilation. It is important that the nurse check that all ventilator alarms

are always on. Alarms alert the staff to potentially dangerous situations such as mechanical malfunction, apnea, unplanned extubation, or patient asynchrony with the ventilator. On many ventilators, the alarms can be temporarily suspended or silenced for up to 2 minutes for suctioning or testing while a staff member is in the room. After that time, the alarm system automatically becomes functional again. Common ventilator modes are outlined in Table 68.11.

Other Ventilatory Manoeuvres

Positive End-Expiratory Pressure. Positive end-expiratory pressure (PEEP) is a ventilatory manoeuvre in which positive pressure is applied to the airway during exhalation. Normally during exhalation, airway pressure drops to zero, and exhalation occurs passively. With PEEP, exhalation remains passive, but pressure falls to a preset level, often 3 to 20 cm H_2O. Lung volume during expiration and between breaths is greater than normal with PEEP. This increases functional residual capacity (FRC) and often improves oxygenation with restoration of lung volume that normally remains at the end of passive exhalation. The mechanisms by which PEEP increases FRC and oxygenation include increased aeration of patent alveoli, aeration of previously collapsed alveoli, and prevention of alveolar collapse throughout the respiratory cycle.

PEEP is titrated to the point that oxygenation improves without compromising hemodynamics. Often, 5 cm H_2O PEEP (referred to as *physiological PEEP*) is used prophylactically to replace the glottic mechanism, help maintain a normal FRC, and prevent alveolar

TABLE 68.11 MODES OF MECHANICAL VENTILATION

Mode	Purpose	Settings That Can Be Adjusted
Assist-control ventilation (ACV)	This is a control mode of ventilation, often used early in acute illness. The ventilator does all the work; however, the patient can breathe faster than the preset rate.	Tidal volume (V_T) Respiratory rate (RR) Positive end-expiratory pressure (PEEP) Fractioned inspired oxygen (FiO_2)
Pressure-control ventilation	This is a control mode of ventilation often used early in acute illness. For patients in whom managing pressures or comfort is challenging with ACV, this is often used as an alternative.	Pressure control (PC) PEEP RR
Pressure-support ventilation (PSV)	This is a spontaneous mode of ventilation. It is often used as the patient's status improves and is one mode of weaning from the ventilator. *Note:* The patient must be able to initiate and maintain work of breathing. A back-up rate may be programmed for safety depending on the individual ventilator.	Pressure support (PS) PEEP

There are other modes of mechanical ventilation, including synchronized intermittent mandatory ventilation (SIMV), airway pressure release ventilation (APRV), tube compensation trials, and more. For more information on additional types of the mechanical ventilation, see Stacy (2018).

Source: Modified from Burns, S. M. (2011). Ventilatory management: Volume and pressure modes. In D. L. Wiegand (Ed.), *AACN procedure manual for critical care* (6th ed., p. 266, Table 35-2). Mosby.

collapse. PEEP of 5 cm H_2O is also used for patients with a history of alveolar collapse during weaning. PEEP improves gas exchange, vital capacity, and inspiratory force when used during weaning. In contrast, *auto-PEEP* is not purposely set on the ventilator but is a result of inadequate exhalation time. Auto-PEEP is additional PEEP over what is set by the health care provider. For more information on auto-PEEP, see Stacy (2018). In general, the major purpose of PEEP is to maintain or improve oxygenation while limiting risk for O_2 toxicity. FiO_2 can often be reduced when PEEP is used. PEEP is indicated in lungs with diffuse disease, severe hypoxemia unresponsive to FiO_2 greater than 50%, and loss of compliance or stiffness. It is used in pulmonary edema to provide a counter-pressure opposing fluid extravasation. The classic indication for PEEP therapy is acute respiratory distress syndrome (ARDS) (see Chapter 70). PEEP is contraindicated or used with extreme caution in patients with highly compliant lungs (e.g., COPD), unilateral or nonuniform disease, hypovolemia, and low CO. In these cases, the adverse effects of PEEP may outweigh any benefits.

Nitric Oxide. *Nitric oxide* (NO) is a gaseous molecule that is made intravascularly and participates in the regulation of pulmonary vascular tone. Inhibition of NO production results in pulmonary vasoconstriction, and administration of continuous inhaled NO results in pulmonary vasodilation. NO may be administered via an ET tube, a tracheotomy, or a face mask. Currently, NO is used in ARDS, as a diagnostic screening tool for pulmonary hypertension during a cardiac catheterization, and during or after cardiac surgery (Haynes, 2018; Papazian et al., 2019).

Prone Positioning. *Prone positioning* is the repositioning of a patient from a supine or lateral position to a prone position (on the stomach, face down). This repositioning improves lung recruitment (re-expansion) through various mechanisms. Gravity reverses the effects of fluid in the dependent parts of the lungs as the patient is moved from supine to prone. The heart rests on the sternum, away from the lungs, contributing to an overall uniformity of pleural pressures. The prone position is a relatively safe (although nurse-intensive), supportive therapy used to improve oxygenation in critically ill patients with acute lung injury or ARDS (Barton et al., 2016; Henderson et al., 2014).

Extracorporeal Membrane Oxygenation. *Extracorporeal membrane oxygenation* (ECMO) is an alternative form of pulmonary support for the patient with severe respiratory failure. It is used more frequently in the pediatric and neonatal populations but is increasingly being used in adults. ECMO is a modification of cardiac bypass and involves partially removing blood

from a patient with large-bore catheters, infusing O_2, removing CO_2, and returning the blood to the patient. This intensive therapy requires systemic anticoagulation and is a time-limited intervention. A skilled team of specialists, including a perfusionist, is required continuously at the bedside (Combes et al., 2014).

Complications of Positive-Pressure Ventilation

Although PPV may be essential to maintain ventilation and oxygenation, it can cause adverse effects. Some of these complications include *barotrauma, volutrauma, pneumothorax* and *pneumomediastinum,* and *ventilator-associated pneumonia* (VAP).

Barotrauma. As lung inflation pressures increase, risk of *barotrauma* increases. Patients with compliant lungs (e.g., COPD) are at greater risk for barotrauma, which results when the increased airway pressure distends the lungs and possibly ruptures fragile alveoli or emphysematous blebs. Patients with stiff lungs (e.g., ARDS) who are given high inspiratory pressures and high levels of PEEP (greater than 5 cm H_2O) and patients with lung abscesses resulting from necrotizing organisms (e.g., staphylococci) are also susceptible to barotrauma (Burns, 2011a).

Volutrauma. The concept of *volutrauma* in PPV relates to the lung injury that occurs when a large tidal volume (V_T) is used to ventilate noncompliant lungs. Volutrauma results in alveolar fractures and movement of fluids and proteins into the alveolar spaces. Low-volume ventilation rather than pressure ventilation should be used in patients with ARDS to protect their lungs (Burns, 2011a).

Pneumothorax. Air can escape into the pleural space from alveoli or interstitium and become trapped. Pleural pressure increases and collapses the lung, causing *pneumothorax.* (Chapter 30 discusses the clinical manifestations of pneumothorax.) The lungs receive air during inspiration but cannot expel it during expiration. Respiratory bronchioles are larger on inspiration than expiration. They may close on expiration, and air becomes trapped. With PPV, a simple pneumothorax can become a life-threatening tension pneumothorax. The mediastinum and contralateral lung are compressed, reducing CO. Immediate treatment of the pneumothorax is required. For some patients, chest tubes are placed prophylactically (Burns, 2011a).

Pneumomediastinum usually begins with rupture of alveoli into the lung interstitium. Progressive air movement occurs into the mediastinum and subcutaneous neck tissue, and a pneumothorax often follows. New, unexplained subcutaneous emphysema is an indication for immediate chest radiography. Pneumomediastinum and subcutaneous emphysema may be too small to detect on a radiograph or to appear clinically before the development of a pneumothorax (Burns, 2011a).

Ventilator-Associated Pneumonia. The risk for health care–associated pneumonia is highest in patients requiring mechanical ventilation because the ET or tracheostomy tube bypasses normal upper airway defences. In addition, a poor nutritional state, immobility, and the underlying disease process (e.g., immunosuppression, organ failure) make the patient more prone to infection. *VAP* is pneumonia that occurs 48 hours to 72 hours after ET intubation (Stacy, 2018). It occurs in 9 to 27% of all intubated patients, with half of cases developing within the first 4 days of mechanical ventilation. In addition, patients who develop VAP have significantly longer hospital stays and higher mortality rates than those who do not.

In patients with early VAP (within 96 hours of mechanical ventilation), sputum cultures often grow Gram-negative bacteria (e.g., *Escherichia coli, Klebsiella, Streptococcus pneumoniae, Haemophilus influenzae*). Organisms associated with late VAP include antibiotic-resistant organisms such as *Pseudomonas aeruginosa* and oxacillin-resistant *Staphylococcus aureus*. These organisms are abundant in the hospital environment. They can spread in a number of ways, including through contaminated respiratory equipment, inadequate hand hygiene, adverse environmental factors such as poor room ventilation and high traffic flow, and decreased patient ability to cough and clear secretions. Colonization of the oropharynx tract by Gram-negative organisms predisposes the patient to Gram-negative pneumonia (Sachdev & Napolitano, 2012).

Clinical evidence suggesting VAP includes fever, elevated white blood cell count, purulent or odorous sputum, crackles or rhonchi on auscultation, and pulmonary infiltrates noted on chest radiograph. The patient is treated with antibiotics after appropriate cultures are taken by tracheal suctioning or bronchoscopy and when infection is evident.

In an effort to prevent and reduce the incidence of VAP, bundled recommendations have been established. The major components of the VAP bundle include (a) elevating the head of the bed a minimum of 30 to 45 degrees unless medically contraindicated, (b) assessing and evaluating a patient's readiness for extubation on a daily basis, (c) using ET tubes with subglottic secretion drainage (Figure 68.15), (d) performing meticulous oral care using chlorohexidine, and (e) initiation of safe enteral nutrition within 24 to 48 hours of admission to the CCU (CPSI, 2021b).

Recent evidence suggests some uncertainty regarding the use of chlorohexidine in different patient populations. Chlorohexidine has been found to be effective for the prevention of nosocomial pneumonia, VAP, and bloodstream infections in an adult patient population admitted to cardiothoracic CCUs (i.e., within the adult, cardiac surgery patient population). However, the evidence is unclear whether this practice has any benefit in medical or noncardiac surgery CCU patient populations (Tran & Butcher, 2019).

VAP prevention also includes strict hand hygiene before and after suctioning, after touching ventilator equipment, and after contact with any respiratory secretions (see Nursing Management: Artificial Airway, earlier in this chapter). The nurse must always wear gloves when in contact with the patient and change gloves between activities (e.g., emptying urinary catheter drainage, hanging an IV medication). Finally, the nurse must always drain the water as it collects in the ventilator tubing, keeping it away from the patient.

Psychosocial Needs in the Mechanically Ventilated Patient. The patient receiving mechanical ventilation often experiences

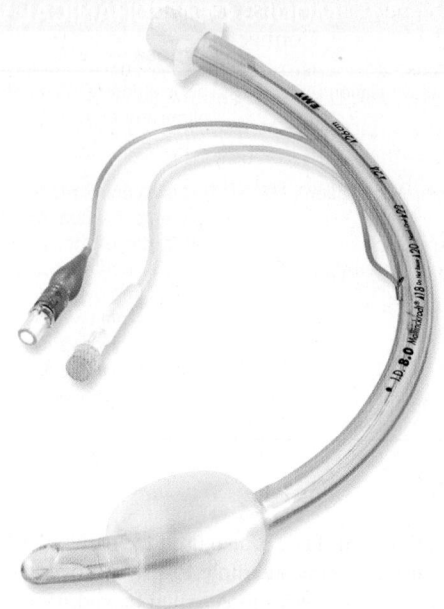

FIG. 68.15 Continuous subglottal suctioning can be provided by the Hi-Lo Evac Tube. A dorsal lumen above the cuff allows for suctioning of secretions from the subglottic area. Source: © 2017 Medtronic. All rights reserved. Used with the permission of Medtronic.

physical and emotional stress. In addition to the health challenges of critical care patients discussed at the beginning of this chapter, the patient supported by a mechanical ventilator is unable to speak, eat, move, or breathe normally. Tubes and machines can cause pain, fear, and anxiety. Usual activities of daily living such as eating, elimination, and coughing are extremely complicated. The nurse should thus involve patients and caregivers in decision making as much as possible. Many patients have few memories of their time in the CCU, whereas others remember vivid details. Although appearing to be asleep, sedated, or paralyzed, patients may be aware of their surroundings, so health care providers should always address them as if they were awake and alert.

Patients receiving PPV usually require analgesia, sedation, or both to facilitate optimal ventilation. Before initiating analgesia or sedation in the mechanically ventilated patient who is agitated or anxious, the nurse should identify the cause of distress. Common conditions or situations that can result in patient agitation or anxiety include PPV, nutritional deficits, pain, hypoxemia, hypercapnia, medications, and environmental stressors (e.g., sleep deprivation). Delirium is an acute change in mental status and is a marker of cerebral insufficiency. Delirium is associated with longer hospital stays and higher mortality rates. CCU patients are particularly vulnerable to delirium; thus the nurse must make every effort to assess and treat it (Devlin et al., 2018).

In some situations, the decision is made to paralyze the patient with a neuromuscular blocking agent to provide more effective synchrony with the ventilator and improve oxygenation. See Stacy (2018) for more information.

Trouble-Shooting Mechanical Ventilation

Machine Disconnection or Malfunction. Mechanical ventilators may become disconnected or malfunction. When turned on and operative, alarms alert the nurse to problems (Table 68.12). Most deaths from accidental ventilator disconnection occur while the alarm is off, and most accidental disconnections in critical care settings are discovered by low-pressure alarms.

The most frequent site for disconnection is between the tracheal tube and the adapter. Connections should be pushed together and then twisted to ensure they are secure. Alarms should be set at all times, and the nurse should chart that this is the case. Alarms can be paused (not inactivated) during suctioning or removal from the ventilator but must be reactivated before the nurse leaves the patient's bedside.

TABLE 68.12   INTERPRETING MECHANICAL VENTILATION ALARMS

Alarm	Possible Causes
Apnea	Change in patient condition
	Loss of airway (e.g., total or partial extubation)
	Oversedation
	Respiratory arrest
High tidal volume, minute ventilation, or respiratory rate	Change in patient condition
	Excess condensate (water) in tubing (i.e., false reading)
	Pain, anxiety
High-pressure limit	Condensate in tubing
	Decreased compliance (e.g., pulmonary edema, pneumothorax)
	Increased resistance (e.g., bronchospasm)
	Kinked or compressed tubing (e.g., patient biting on ET tube)
	Patient fighting ventilator (ventilator asynchrony)
	Secretions, coughing, or gagging
Low tidal volume or minute ventilation	Change in patient's breathing efforts (e.g., rate and volume)
	ET tube or tracheal cuff leak (e.g., patient speaking, grunting)
	Insufficient gas flow
	Patient disconnection, loose connection, or leak in circuit
Low-pressure limit	ET tube or tracheal cuff leak (e.g., patient speaking, grunting)
	Loss of airway (e.g., total or partial extubation)
	Total or partial ventilator disconnect
Ventilator inoperative or low battery	Machine malfunction
	Unplugged, power failure, or internal battery not charged

ET, endotracheal.
Source: Adapted from Pierce, L.N. (2007). *Management of the mechanically ventilated patient* (2nd ed.). Saunders.

Weaning From Positive-Pressure Ventilation and Extubation

Weaning is the process of reducing ventilator support and resuming spontaneous ventilation. Preparation for weaning begins when PPV is initiated and involves a team approach (e.g., nurse, health care provider, patient, caregiver, dietitian, respiratory therapist, physiotherapist). Patients are assessed each day to determine their readiness to wean. Table 68.13 highlights both respiratory and nonrespiratory factors that are considered indicators for weaning. Weaning assessment parameters should include criteria to assess muscle strength and endurance. In addition, the patient's lungs should be reasonably clear on auscultation and chest radiograph. Nonrespiratory factors include the patient's neurological status; hemodynamics; fluid, electrolytes, and acid–base balance; nutrition; and hemoglobin. It is important to have an alert, well-rested, and well-informed patient relatively free from pain and anxiety who can participate in the weaning plan (Stacy, 2018). A *spontaneous breathing trial* (SBT) is recommended for patients who demonstrate weaning readiness (Stacy, 2018). An SBT should be at least 30 minutes but no more than 120 minutes. It may be done with low levels of CPAP, low levels of PSV, or a T-piece. Tolerance of the trial may lead to extubation. Failure to tolerate an SBT should prompt a search for reversible or complicating factors and a return to a nonfatiguing ventilator modality for the patient. The SBT should be attempted again the next day.

The use of a weaning policy decreases the number of ventilator days. The parts of a policy are not as important as the use of a policy to prevent delays in weaning. PSV is thought to provide gentle, slow respiratory muscle conditioning. It may be especially beneficial for patients who are deconditioned or have heart conditions. Some patients may be weaned by simply providing humidified oxygen (T-piece or flow-by method) (Stacy, 2018).

Weaning may be tried at any time of day, although it is usually done during the day, with the patient ventilated at night in a rest mode. The rest mode should be a stable, nonfatiguing, and comfortable form of support for the patient. Regardless of the weaning mode selected, all health care team members should be familiar with the weaning plan. Additionally, it is important to allow the patient's respiratory muscles to rest between weaning trials. Once the respiratory muscles become fatigued, they may require 12 to 24 hours to recover. Importantly, the patient

TABLE 68.13   INDICATORS FOR WEANING

Weaning Readiness

Patients receiving mechanical ventilation for respiratory failure should undergo a formal assessment of weaning potential if the following are satisfied*:

1. Reversal of the underlying cause of respiratory failure
2. Adequate oxygenation:
   PaO_2 >80–100 (on ABG)
   FiO_2 ≤40%–50%
   PEEP ≤5–8 cm H_2O
   pH ≥7.25 (on ABG)
3. Hemodynamic stability:
   Absence of clinically significant hypotension (low-dose or no vasopressor therapy)
   Absence of myocardial ischemia
4. Patient ability to initiate an inspiratory effort

Spontaneous tidal volume (V_T)	Amount of air exchanged during normal breathing at rest; measure of muscle endurance	7–9 mL/kg	≥5 mL/kg
Vital capacity (VC)	Maximum inspiration and then measurement of air during maximal forced expiration; measure of respiratory muscle endurance or reserve or both; requires patient cooperation	65–75 mL/kg	≥10–15 mL/kg

ABG, arterial blood gas; *FiO₂*, fraction of inspired oxygen; *PaO₂*, partial pressure of oxygen in arterial blood; *PEEP*, positive end-expiratory pressure.
*The decision to use these criteria must be individualized to the patient.
Sources: Adapted from MacIntyre, N. R., Cook, D. J., Ely E. W., Jr., et al. (2001). Evidence-based guidelines for weaning and discontinuing ventilatory support. *Chest, 120*(6 Suppl), 375S–395S; and Burns, S. M. (2011). Weaning process. In D. L. Wiegand (Ed.), *AACN procedure manual for critical care* (6th ed., pp. 291–300). Elsevier.

being weaned and the caregiver need ongoing emotional support. The nurse should explain the weaning process to them and keep them informed of progress (Stacy, 2018).

Chronic Mechanical Ventilation

Some patients will experience disease processes that do not allow for weaning from the ventilator. In some circumstances, patients may continue to live on mechanical ventilators indefinitely. Some long-term ventilated patients will be cared for either in a residential care facility or at home. The decision to pursue long-term mechanical ventilation is an important decision and should not be rushed. Frequent meetings between the health care team and the patient and family are important before this decision is made. Careful consideration of the patient's quality of life and values must be ensured. Once the decision has been made to pursue long-term ventilation, careful planning and training are required for the family and caregivers if the home is the preferred destination.

NURSING MANAGEMENT
MECHANICAL VENTILATION

See Nursing Care Plan (NCP) 68.1, available on the Evolve website, for information regarding care of the patient receiving mechanical ventilation.

🔍 EVIDENCE-INFORMED PRACTICE

Research Highlight

Timing of Tracheotomy in Critically ill Patients: a Meta-Analysis

Clinical Question

In critically ill patients (P), does tracheotomy at an earlier stage (I) versus later-stage tracheotomy (C) have significant benefits for important outcomes (O)?

Best Available Evidence

Systematic review and meta-analysis of randomized controlled trials (RCTs)

Critical Appraisal and Synthesis of Evidence

- In nine RCTs ($n = 2\ 072$) of critically ill adult patients, 1 033 patients received early tracheotomy and 1 039 patients received late tracheotomy/prolonged intubation.
- Primary outcomes were mortality; all nine studies ($n = 2\ 023$ patients) reported short-term mortality.
- Of 1 002 patients in the early tracheotomy group, 322 died, compared to 359 deaths among 1 021 patients in the late-tracheotomy/prolonged-intubation group.
- Secondary outcomes were duration of mechanical ventilation, length of stay in the CCU, and ventilator-associated pneumonia (VAP).

Conclusion

- In patients who required longer-term mechanical ventilation, early tracheotomy showed no significant clinical outcomes over those for the late-tracheotomy/prolonged-intubation group.

Implications for Nursing Practice

- The optimal tracheotomy timing (early vs. late) for patients on prolonged mechanical ventilation is not really known.
- Benefits of tracheotomy (e.g., increased patient comfort, improved oral hygiene) and the risks and complications (e.g., bleeding, wound infection, tracheal stenosis) need to be considered and weighed against the risks and benefits of prolonged endotracheal intubation.

Reference for Evidence

Huang, H., Li, Y., Ariani, F., et al. (2014). Timing of tracheostomy in critically ill patients: A meta-analysis. *PlosOne, 9*(3), e92980–e92981.
P, patient population of interest; *I*, intervention or area of interest; *C*, comparison of interest or comparison group; *O*, outcomes of interest (see Chapter 1).

PATIENT- AND FAMILY-CENTRED CARE IN CRITICAL CARE

The position of the CACCN is that patients and their families are "essential members of the health care team" who are "respected as collaborative partners who contribute to the critical care experience" (CACCN, 2018, p. 1). Critical illness can have an extensive impact on both the patient and their family members; it can be disruptive to established family routines and activities of daily living and it can significantly affect roles and responsibilities (e.g., changes in household responsibilities, loss of employment). As a result: "Responses to critical illness can manifest as acute anxiety and feeling of helplessness, as well as grief, depression, emotional distress and post-traumatic stress disorder" that can persist long after the conclusion of the critical illness itself (CACCN, 2018, p.1). In recent years, concepts like post–intensive care syndrome (PICS) (Rawal et al., 2017) and postintensive care syndrome–family (PICS-F) (Davidson et al., 2012) readily acknowledge the need to think beyond the critical illness itself and explore in greater depth the needs of patients and families that stem from their experiences of critical illness and that are inextricably linked with guideline recommendations for incorporating patient- and family-centred care in critical care.

Family members contribute to the patient's well-being by:
- Providing a link to the patient's personal life and helping CCU clinicians come to know the patient more holistically (e.g., news of family, job)
- Advising the patient in health care decisions or functioning as decision makers when the patient cannot
- Helping with activities of daily living (e.g., bathing, oral suctioning)
- Providing positive, loving, and caring support

To be effective in caring for their loved one, caregivers need the nurse's guidance and support. The experience of having a friend or family member as a patient in the CCU is physically and emotionally difficult, often to the point of exhaustion. Anxiety about the patient's condition and prognosis and concerns regarding the patient's pain and other discomforts are some of the issues caregivers confront. In addition, it is common for caregivers to experience anxiety about financial issues related to the provision of care during a critical illness. Consulting with the case manager or social worker is helpful in these instances.

Caregivers typically experience disruption of their daily routines to support the patient. They may be far from their own home and supportive friends and family members. Ultimately, caregivers of the critically ill patient are considered to be in crisis; thus family-centred care is essential. To provide family-centred care effectively, the nurse must be skilled in crisis intervention. The nurse should conduct a family assessment and intervene as necessary. Such interventions can include active listening, reduction of anxiety, and support of persons who become upset or angry (Davidson et al., 2017).

The nurse should acknowledge the caregivers' feelings and accept and support their decisions. The nurse should consult other health care team members (e.g., chaplains, psychologists, patient representatives) as necessary to assist caregivers in adjusting. The extent to which family-centred care is provided can affect the patient's clinical course in the CCU. The nurse can identify a spokesperson for the family so that information between the health care team and the family is coordinated.

Caregivers need reassurance about the way in which the patient's care is managed and decisions are made. To this end, the nurse can invite the caregivers to meet the health care team members and also evaluate the appropriateness of including caregivers in interprofessional rounds and patient care conferences. The nurse should provide the caregiver with the opportunity to participate in decision making. When patients are incapable of making their own health care decisions, they may have designated a durable power of attorney for health care, and this person should also be involved in the patient's plan of care. If the patient has an advance directive or a living will, the caregiver will need to see that the patient's wishes are followed.

Caregivers are better able to accept and cope with problems if they observe that the health care team is hopeful, caring, and competent; decisions are deliberate; and their input is valued. Caregivers of critically ill patients need the convenience of access to the patient. Limiting visitation does not protect the patient from adverse physiological consequences (Davidson et al., 2017). In addition, flexible visiting hours for family members align with a family-centred approach. The first time that caregivers visit, it is important for the nurse to prepare them for the experience, by briefly describing the patient's appearance and the physical environment (e.g., equipment, noise). The nurse should accompany the caregivers as they enter the room and observe the responses of both the patient and the caregivers and invite the caregivers to participate in the patient's care, if they desire. In some CCUs, visitation includes animal-assisted therapy or pet visitation. The positive benefits of these interventions (e.g., decreases in BP and anxiety) far outweigh the risks (e.g., transmission of infection from animal to patient), and they should be a part of the visitation policy.

Indigenous Care in Critical Care

The provision of culturally safe care ought to be ubiquitous within health care and, as such, should be a central tenet of care provided in critical care contexts. Unfortunately, from a Canadian adult critical-care perspective, in research specific to the experiences of Indigenous people in CCUs there is a notable gap between the literature and the much needed area of research and scholarship.

That being said, however, culturally safe care is prefaced on reflection and acknowledgement of beliefs, attitudes, and practices of health care providers, as well as those of patients and their families (Pauly et al., 2015). Cultural safety also prompts individuals, including health care providers, to consider "the ways in which history, social relations, and politics continue to shape people's responses, needs, access and health" (Pauly et al., 2015, p. 123). Importantly, cultural safety can be "enacted in clinical contexts to mitigate marginalization, stigma and discrimination" (Pauly et al., 2015, p. 123).

In the provision of critical care, CCU nurses should be keenly aware of their own beliefs and attitudes and be particularly cognizant of discriminatory practices (both at the level of the individual and of the larger health care system). The structure of the CCU, for example, may not be conducive to large family gatherings, thus negatively affecting Indigenous patients and their families, for whom community is fundamental. Further, discriminatory practices that include black humour and stereotypes about Indigenous people are evident in critical care. Recently, the harms of culturally unsafe care have been made explicit in the Canadian media (see, for example, the case of Joyce Echaquan, in Joliette, Québec). Also, given that many critical

care patients are admitted for postoperative monitoring and care, it is important to consider the ways in which Indigenous patients admitted to the CCU have been affected by historical trauma related to lack-of-consent procedures and experimentation. There is a recognized need for continuous consent, clear instructions, and sufficient opportunity for patients and their family members to ask questions and seek information. It is also important to consider how traditional healing practices are integrated into their critical care experience. Indigenous patients and their families must feel safe, respected, and cared for, with kindness and compassion, in CCUs.

Please see previous chapters for more information specific to assessment issues, including trauma triggers, reluctance to disclose, and traditional medicines.

End-of-Life Care in the Critical Care Context

While advances in critical care have made it possible to intervene during critical illness with improved overall outcomes and decreased mortality rates, many patients inevitably succumb to critical illness and die. Overall mortality rates vary across critical care settings, but in general they range between 10 and 30% (Coombs et al., 2012; Wennberg et al., 2004). The use of life-sustaining measures in the CCU (e.g., mechanical ventilators, cardiac assist devices, vasoactive medications, renal replacement therapies) creates a clinical context in which death and dying are discussed, and decisions are made within the context of the withdrawal of life-sustaining measures (WLSM). Historically, practices specific to WLSM were physician dependent and often variable across critical care settings. Recently, however, efforts across Canada have focused on standardizing WLSM practices, while remaining necessarily flexible and consistent with patient- and family-centred care principles (Downar et al., 2016). Notably, it is ideal if patients' wishes regarding the use of life-sustaining measures can be known prior to the introduction of such measures, but this is not always the reality. Efforts to foster advance care planning in Canada, such as Speak Up (see https://www.advancecareplanning.ca), have been encouraged. It is also important to recognize that when a patient is experiencing critical illness that is unanticipated, determining goals of care can be difficult. A useful process for critical care clinicians engaging in discussions regarding goals of care and decision making within the context of critical illness is available. (See *Navigating Medical Emergencies: Goals of Care*, co-authored by Canadian critical care nurses and physicians [Vanderspank-Wright et al., 2017] and available at https://navme.royalcollege.ca.)

Critical care nurses play a primary role in caring for patients at the end of life in the CCU and their families. In a systematic review of qualitative evidence, Vanderspank-Wright et al. (2018) aimed to synthesize existing evidence specific to the experiences of critical care nurses who had cared for patients and families throughout the process of WLSM. The authors remarked that critical care nurses can experience tension and conflict stemming from situations in which communication is poor (e.g., between the health care team members themselves or between the health care team and families) or there is a lack of clear guidance and WLSM practices. While the comfort and care of patients is paramount, critical care nurses also care for families during this time. Nurses share information with families and facilitate their understanding of complex critical illness and WLSM procedures (e.g., what it might look like when mechanical ventilation is discontinued, or how nurses and family members can work together to assess the patient's level of comfort). Critical care nurses also play a pivotal role in facilitating family presence at the bedside and involving them in patient care in ways they are comfortable with (e.g., brushing a loved one's hair or washing their face). Despite the challenges that can be associated with WLSM, nurses have emphasized that working with patients and families at the end of life is a privileged aspect of their role (Vanderspank-Wright et al., 2018).

Cultural Considerations Related to Death and Dying in Critical Care. The cultural dimensions of the meaning of sickness and health, pain, dying and death, and grief need to be considered when caring for critically ill patients and their families across the critical illness trajectory—from admission to discharge from the CCU, or to death and bereavement. (Chapter 2 discusses cultural issues.)

Cultural perspectives on dying and death are complex. For example, for some patients, telling them that they are dying, as a way of letting them prepare for death, may be considered an infringement on the role of the family. Others may view a discussion about advance directives as a legal device to deny care. Customs surrounding dying and death vary widely. The nurse caring for the dying patient must make every attempt to understand and accommodate the family's cultural traditions. It is important that communication with families be open, honest, and respectful. One helpful tool for critical care clinicians can be accessed through the Royal College of Physicians and Surgeons of Canada e-book *Navigating Medical Emergencies*. The section Establishing Therapeutic Relationships was co-authored by Canadian critical care nurses and physicians (Roze des Ordon et al., 2017).

The expressions of grief that follow the loss of a loved one are highly individualized and influenced by several factors, including the relationship between the grieving person and the deceased, whether the loss is sudden or anticipated, the support systems available to the grieving person, the person's past experiences with loss, and the person's religious and cultural beliefs. It is of utmost importance that the critical care nurse proceed with sensitivity when caring for patients facing death and for their families. Asking patients "What do you want to know?" and "Who do you want with you when discussing options?" is a good starting point (CACCN, 2020). (Chapter 13 provides additional information about end-of-life care.)

Family Presence in Critical Care

In addition to traditional visiting, research has shown that caregivers of patients undergoing invasive procedures (e.g., central line insertion) and cardiopulmonary resuscitation want the option of being present at the bedside during these events. Even when the outcomes are not favourable, being present can help caregivers relieve doubts about the patient's condition, decrease their anxiety and fear, facilitate the need to be together and to support their loved one, and support the grief process when death occurs. The Canadian Critical Care Society encourages CCUs to develop policies and procedures that provide for the option of family presence during invasive procedures and cardiopulmonary resuscitation (Oczkowski et al., 2015). Importantly, when patient outcomes are poor (e.g., death has occurred or is imminent), the focus on CCU clinicians is paramount. Family members of individuals who have died in the CCU are at higher risk of severe or complicated grief (Kentish-Barnes & Prigerson, 2016). As a result, recent attention has focused on exploring bereavement support and bereavement support interventions for family members who have experienced the death of a loved one in critical care (Downar et al., 2014).

Critical Care Survivorship and Post–Critical Care Unit Syndrome

The goal of critical care is to provide care for patients and families experiencing life-threatening illness or injury. Beyond simply stabilizing patients, the purpose of critical care is to return patients to a state of optimal quality of life following their critical illness. A constellation of symptoms associated with a critical care illness include poor nutrition, muscle weakness, delirium, and depression or anxiety, among others, which can continue for months or years post–critical care. Many of the issues raised in this chapter (e.g. pain, agitation, delirium management, early mobilization) are important aspects of improving the overall health and well-being of the critical care survivor. The goal is no longer to simply survive the critical care stay but to also have quality of life beyond critical care. Increasing awareness of the complexities, challenges, and issues faced by critical care survivors is one way that nurses can continue to care and advocate for patients. Recent research has coined the term *post–intensive care unit syndrome* (PICS), which includes any new or worsening impairment in physical, cognitive, or mental health status that occurs following a critical illness (Kiernan, 2017). Learning to identify the symptoms of PICS can help health care providers improve outcomes and provide ongoing care for survivors. Continuing the care plans and preventative measures initiated in the CCU (e.g., delirium prevention, day/night routine, mobilization, and physiotherapy) is important to patients' well-being after critical care, throughout hospitalization and into the community (Kiernan, 2017).

OTHER CRITICAL CARE CONTENT

Table 68.14 lists additional critical care content presented in other chapters of this book.

TABLE 68.14	CROSS-REFERENCES TO OTHER CRITICAL CARE CONTENT
Topic	**Discussed in Chapter**
Acute coronary syndrome	36
Acute heart failure	37
Acute respiratory distress syndrome	70
Acute respiratory failure	70
Burns	27
Cardiac dysrhythmias	38
Cardiac pacemakers	38
Cardiac surgery	36
Central venous access device	19
Continuous renal replacement therapy	49
Delirium	62
Emergencies	71
End-of-life care	13
Enteral nutrition	42
Head injury, including ICP monitoring	59
Heart failure, including ventricular assist devices and intra-aortic balloon pumps	37
Multiple-organ dysfunction syndrome	69
Myocardial infarction	36
Oxygen delivery	31
Pain management	10
Pulmonary edema	37
Renal dialysis	49
Shock	69
Stroke	60
Parenteral nutrition	42
Tracheotomy	29
Trauma	71

ICP, intracranial pressure.

CASE STUDY

Critical Care and Mechanical Ventilation

Patient Profile

R. K. (pronouns he/him) is a 72-year-old who collapsed on the street. R. K. was unresponsive on admission and remains in the same state. He has an oral endotracheal (ET) tube in place and is receiving mechanical ventilation. The patient's weight is 90 kg. A subclavian central line was placed to monitor CVP and administer fluids.

Subjective Data

None; patient is unresponsive to painful stimuli

Objective Data

Physical Examination

- Noninvasive BP is 100/75 mm Hg; heart rate is 128 (atrial fibrillation with a rapid ventricular response); temperature is 38.8°C; SpO_2 is 98%
- Purulent secretions via endotracheal (ET) tube
- Breath sounds: coarse crackles bilaterally, decreased breath sounds on the right

Diagnostic Studies

- Chest radiography reveals right lower lung consolidation.
- ABGs: pH 7.48; PaO_2: 94 mm Hg; $PaCO_2$: 30 mm Hg; bicarbonate (HCO_3) 34 mmol/L
- Computed tomography (CT) scan is positive for massive cerebrovascular accident.

Interprofessional Care

- Positive-pressure ventilation, assist-control mode
- Settings: FiO_2 70%, V_T 700 mL, respiratory rate 16 breaths/min, PEEP 5 cm H_2O
- Enteral feeding at 25 mL/hr via small-bore feeding tube
- In-dwelling urinary catheter to bedside drainage
- Head of bed elevated at 40 degrees
- Position change every 2 hr
- Chest physiotherapy performed every 2 to 4 hr
- Azithromycin (Zithromax) 500 mg intravenously q24h
- Cefotaxime (Claforan) 2 g intravenously q6h
- 5% dextrose in normal saline (D_5NS) with potassium chloride (KCl) 20 mmol/L at 100 mL/hr

Discussion Questions

1. Identify two reasons for intubating and providing mechanical ventilation for R. K.
2. What do R. K.'s ABGs indicate, and which ventilator setting(s) should be changed?
3. What is R. K.'s PaO_2/FiO_2 ratio and what does it signify?
4. The patient's BP drops to 80 mm Hg, and R. K. remains in atrial fibrillation with a ventricular rate of 158. He is started on a norepinephrine infusion. What would be the purpose of hemodynamic monitoring (in addition to CVP monitoring) in this patient?
5. What interventions have been put in place for R. K. to prevent a ventilator-assisted pneumonia? Based on the data presented, what are the actual and potential conditions that the nurse can identify in this patient?
6. **Evidence-informed practice**: R. K.'s family wants to know why tube feedings are being given. What should the nurse tell the family? What is the evidence to support the use of tube feedings?
7. After 4 days, R. K. remains unresponsive and has developed renal failure. The physician believes the patient will not recover and wishes to discuss goals of care with the patient's caregiver. What would be the nurse's role in this meeting?

ⓔvolve

Answers are available at http://evolve.elsevier.com/Canada/Lewis/medsurg.

REVIEW QUESTIONS

The number of the question corresponds to the same-numbered objective at the beginning of the chapter.

1. What does a certification in critical care by the Canadian Nurses Association indicate?
   a. Has earned a master's degree in the field of providing advanced critical care nursing
   b. Is an advanced-practice nurse in the care of acutely ill clients
   c. May practise independently to provide symptom management for the critically ill
   d. Has practised in critical care and successfully completed a test of critical care knowledge

2. What are the appropriate nursing interventions for the client with delirium in the CCU? *(Select all that apply.)*
   a. Use clocks and calendars to maintain orientation.
   b. Encourage round-the-clock presence of caregivers at the bedside.
   c. Sedate the client with appropriate medications to protect the client from harmful behaviours.
   d. Silence all alarms, reduce overhead paging, and avoid conversations around the client.
   e. Identify physiological factors that may be contributing to the client's confusion and irritability.

3. What is the most ideal plan for family involvement in the CCU?
   a. Having a family member at the bedside at all times
   b. Allowing family at the bedside at brief intervals
   c. Devising an individual plan with family involved in care and comfort measures
   d. Restricting visitation in the CCU because the environment is overwhelming to visitors

4. In hemodynamic monitoring, what does *zeroing* refer to, and which one of the following does the nurse zero to?
   a. Cardiac output (CO) monitoring system to the level of the left ventricle
   b. Pressure monitoring system to the level of the catheter tip located in the client
   c. Pressure monitoring system to the level of the atrium, identified as the midaxillary line
   d. Pressure monitoring system to the level of the atrium, identified as the phlebostatic axis

5. What nursing management should be included for the client with an artificial airway?
   a. Routine suctioning of the tube at least every 2 hours
   b. Observing for cardiac dysrhythmias during suctioning
   c. Maintaining endotracheal tube cuff pressure at 30 cm H_2O
   d. Preventing tube dislodgement by limiting mouth care to lubrication of the lips

6. What is the purpose of adding positive end-expiratory pressure to positive-pressure ventilation?
   a. To increase functional residual capacity and improve oxygenation
   b. To increase fraction of inspired oxygen in an attempt to wean the client and avoid oxygen toxicity
   c. To determine whether the client is able to be weaned and avoid the risk of pneumomediastinum
   d. To determine whether the client is in synchrony with the ventilator or needs to be paralyzed

7. For what should the nurse monitor the client with positive-pressure mechanical ventilation?
   a. Paralytic ileus because pressure on the abdominal contents affects bowel motility
   b. Diuresis and sodium depletion because of increased release of atrial natriuretic peptide
   c. Signs of cardiovascular insufficiency because pressure in the chest impedes venous return
   d. Respiratory acidosis in a client with chronic obstructive pulmonary disease because of alveolar hyperventilation and increased arterial partial pressure of oxygen levels

e**volve**

For even more review questions, visit http://evolve.elsevier.com/Canada/Lewis/medsurg.

1. d; 2. a, c; 3. c; 4. d; 5. b; 6. a; 7. c.

REFERENCES

Balas, M. C., Weinhouse, G. L., Denehy, L., et al. (2018). Interpreting and implementing the 2018 pain, agitation/sedation, delirium, immobility, and sleep disruption clinical practice guideline. *Critical Care Medicine, 46*(1), 1464–1470. https://doi.org/10.1097/CCM.0000000000003307

Barton, G., Vanderspank-Wright, B., & Shea, J. (2016). Optimizing oxygenation in the mechanically ventilated patient: Nursing practice implications. *Critical Care Nursing Clinics of North America, 28,* 425–435. https://doi.org/10.1016/j.cnc.2016.07.003

Burns, S. M. (2011a). Invasive mechanical ventilation: Volume and pressure modes. In D. L. Wiegand (Ed.), *AACN procedure manual for critical care* (6th ed.) (pp. 262–284). Elsevier. (Seminal).

Burns, S. M. (2011b). Noninvasive positive pressure ventilation: Continuous positive airway pressure (CPAP) and bilevel positive airway pressure (BiPap). In D. L. Wiegand (Ed.), *AACN procedure manual for critical care* (6th ed.) (pp. 225–234). Elsevier. (Seminal).

Canadian Association of Critical Care Nurses (CACCN). (2017). *Standards for critical care nursing practice.* https://caccn.ca/publications/standards-for-critical-care-nursing-practice/

Canadian Association of Critical Care Nurses (CACCN). (2018). *Patient- and family-centred care.* https://caccn.ca/wp-content/uploads/2019/10/PS062018PSPFCCare.pdf

Canadian Association of Critical Care Nurses (CACCN). (2019). *Models of nursing care in the critical care unit.* https://caccn.ca/wp-content/uploads/2019/10/PS1903ModelsNursingCare.pdf

Canadian Association of Critical Care Nurses (CACCN). (2021). *Providing end of life care in critical care.* (Seminal). https://caccn.ca/wp-content/uploads/2020/04/PS2003EndofLifeICU.pdf

Canadian Nurses Association (CNA). (2014). *Pan Canadian competencies for the clinical nurse specialist.* (Seminal). https://hl-prod-ca-oc-download.s3-ca-central-1.amazonaws.com/CNA/2f975e7e-4a40-45ca-863c-5ebf0a138d5e/UploadedImages/documents/Clinical_Nurse_Specialists_Convention_Handout_e.pdf

Canadian Nurses Association (CNA). (2019). *Advanced practice nursing: A pan-Canadian framework.* https://hl-prod-ca-oc-download.s3-ca-central-1.amazonaws.com/CNA/2f975e7e-4a40-45ca-863c-5ebf0a138d5e/UploadedImages/documents/Advanced_Practice_Nursing_framework_EN.pdf

Canadian Patient Safety Institute (CPSI). (2021a). *Leaders: Deteriorating patient condition.* https://www.patientsafetyinstitute.ca/en/toolsResources/Deteriorating-Patient-Condition/Leaders/Pages/default.aspx

Canadian Patient Safety Institute (CPSI). (2021b). *Measures: Ventilator-associated pneumonia.* https://www.patientsafetyinstitute.ca/en/toolsResources/psm/Pages/VAP-measurement.aspx

Chacko, R., Rajan, A., Lionel, P., et al. (2017). Oral decontamination techniques and ventilator-associated pneumonia. *British Journal of Nursing, 26*(11), 594–599. https://doi.org/10.12968/bjon.2017.26.11.594

Combes, A., Brodie, D., Bartlett, R., et al. (2014). Position paper for the organization of extracorporeal membrane oxygenation programs for acute respiratory failure in adult patients. *American Journal of Respiratory and Critical Care Medicine, 190*(5), 488–496. (Seminal). https://doi.org/10.1164/rccm.201404-0630CP

Coombs, M. A., Addlington-Hall, J., & Long-Sutehall, T. (2012). Challenges in transition from intervention to end of life care in intensive care: A qualitative study. *International Journal of Nursing Studies, 49*(5), 519–527. (Seminal). https://doi.org/10.1016/j.ijnurstu.2011.10.019

Critical Care Nutrition. (2021). *2021 systematic reviews.* [See 1.0 *The use of enteral nutrition vs parenteral nutrition* and 2.0 *Early vs delayed nutrient intake.*] https://www.criticalcarenutrition.com/systematic-reviews

Davidson, J. E., Aslakson, R. A., Long, A. C., et al. (2017). Guidelines for family-centered care in the neonatal, pediatric, and adult ICU. *Critical Care Medicine, 45*(1), 103–128. https://doi.org/10.1097/CCM/.0000000000002169

Davidson, J. E., Jones, C., & Bienvenu, O. J. (2012). Family response to critical illness: Post-intensive care syndrome—family. *Critical Care Medicine, 40*(2), 618–624. (Seminal). https://doi.org/10.1097/CCM.0b013e318236ebf9

Delaney, L., Van Haren, F., & Lopez, V. (2015). Sleeping on a problem: The impact of sleep disturbance on ICU patients—A clinical review. *Annals of Intensive Care, 5,* 3. https://doi.org/10.1186/s13613-015-0043-2

Devlin, J. W., Skrobik, Y., Gélinas, C., et al. (2018). Clinical practice guidelines for the prevention and management of pain, agitation/sedation, delirium, immobility, and sleep disruption in adult patients in the ICU. *Critical Care Medicine, 46*(9), e825–e873. https://doi.org/10.1097/CCM.0000000000003299

Downar, J., Barua, R., & Sinuff, T. (2014). The desirability of an intensive care unit (ICU) clinician-led bereavement screening and support program for family members of ICU decedents (ICU Bereave). *Journal of Critical Care, 29,* 311e9–311e16. (Seminal). https://doi.org/10.1016/j.jcrc.2013.11.024

Downar, J., Delaney, J. W., Hawryluck, L., et al. (2016). Guidelines for the withdrawal of life-sustaining measures. *Intensive Care Medicine, 42*(6), 1003–1017. https://doi.org/10.1007/s00134-016-4330-7

Etland, C. (2018). End-of-life. In L. D. Urden, K. M. Stacy, & M. E. Lough (Eds.), *Critical care nursing: Diagnosis and management* (8th ed., pp. 147–160). Elsevier.

Gélinas, C. (2018). Pain and pain management. In L. D. Urden, K. M. Stacy, & M. E. Lough (Eds.), *Critical care nursing: Diagnosis and management* (8th ed., pp. 114–136). Elsevier.

Gélinas, C., Fillion, L., Puntillo, K. A., Viens, C., et al. (2006). Validation of the critical-care pain observation tool in adult patients.

American Journal of Critical Care, 15(4), 420–427. (Seminal). https://doi.org/10.4037/ajcc2006.15.4.420

Georgiou, E., Hadjibalassi, M., Lambrinou, E., et al. (2015). The impact of pain assessment on critically ill patient outcomes: A systematic review. *BioMed Research International.* https://doi.org/10.1155/2015/503830

Haynes, A. (2018). Cardiovascular disorders. In L. D. Urden, K. M. Stacy, & M. E. Lough (Eds.), *Critical care nursing: Diagnosis and management* (8th ed., pp. 290–358). Elsevier.

Henderson, W. R., Griesdale, D. E., Dominelli, P., et al. (2014). Does prone positioning improve oxygenation and reduce mortality in patients with acute respiratory distress syndrome? *Canadian Respiratory Journal, 21*(4), 213–215. (Seminal). https://doi.org/10.1155/2014/472136

Huang, H., Li, Y., Ariani, F., et al. (2014). Timing of tracheostomy in critically ill patients: A meta-analysis. *PlosOne, 9*(3), e92980–e92981. (Seminal). https://doi.org/10.1371/journal.pone.0092981

Innes, T., & Calleja, P. (2018). Transition support for new graduate and novice nurses in critical care settings: An integrative review of the literature. *Nurse Education in Practice, 30*, 62–72. https://doi.org/10.1016/j.nepr.2018.03.001

Kentish-Barnes, N., & Prigerson, H. G. (2016). Is this bereaved relative at risk of prolonged grief? *Intensive Care Medicine, 42*(8), 1279–1281. https://doi.org/10.1007/s00134-015-4182-6

Kern, M. (2011). Arterial pressure-based cardiac output monitoring. In D. L. Wiegand (Ed.), *AACN procedure manual for critical care* (6th ed., pp. 548–554). Elsevier. (Seminal).

Kiernan, F. (2017). Care of ICU survivors in the community: A guide for GPs. *British Journal of General Practice, 67*(633), 477–478. http://doi10.3399/bjgp17X693029

Lough, M. E. (2018). Cardiovascular diagnostic procedures. In L. D. Urden, K. M. Stacy, & M. E. Lough (Eds.), *Critical care nursing: Diagnosis and management* (8th ed., pp. 199–289). Elsevier.

Maharaj, R., Raffaele, I., & Wendon, J. (2015). Rapid response systems: A systematic review and meta-analysis. *Critical Care, 19*, 254. https://doi.org/10.1186/s13054-015-0973-y

Maiden, J. M. (2018). Pulmonary diagnostic procedures. In L. D. Urden, K. M. Stacy, & M. E. Lough (Eds.), *Critical care nursing: Diagnosis and management* (8th ed., pp. 445–455). Elsevier.

McClave, S. A., Taylor, B. E., Martindale, R. G., et al. (2016). Guidelines for the provision and assessment of nutrition support therapy in the adult critically ill patient: Society of Critical Care Medicine (SCCM) and American Society for Parenteral and Enteral Nutrition (A.S.P.E.N.). *Journal of Parenteral and Enteral Nutrition, 40*(2), 159–211. https://doi.org/10.1177/0148607115621863

Meng, L., Wang, C., Li, J., et al. (2016). Early vs late tracheostomy in critically ill patients: A systematic review and meta-analysis. *The Clinical Respiratory Journal, 10*(6), 684–692. https://doi.org/10.1111/crj.12286

Oczkowski, S. J., Mazzetti, I., Cupido, C., et al. (2015). Family presence during resuscitation: A Canadian Critical Care position paper. *Canadian Respiratory Journal, 22*(4), 201–205. https://doi.org/10.1155/2015/532721

Papazian, L., Aubron, C., Brochard, L., et al. (2019). Formal guidelines: Management of acute respiratory distress syndrome. *Annals of Intensive Care, 9*(69). https://doi.org/10.1186/s13613-019-0540-9

Patel, J. J., Lemieux, M., McClave, S. A., et al. (2017). Critical care nutrition support best practices: Key differences between Canadian and American guidelines. *Nutrition in Clinical Practice, 32*(5), 633–644. https://doi.org/10.1177/0884533617722165

Pauly, B., McCall, J., Browne, A. J., et al. (2015). Toward cultural safety. *Advances in Nursing Science, 38*(2), 121–135. https://doi.org/10.1097/ANS.0000000000000070

Payen, J. F., Bru, O., Bosson, J. L., et al. (2001). Assessing pain in critically ill sedated patients by using a behavioural pain scale. *Critical Care Medicine, 29*(12), 2258–2263. (Seminal). https://doi.org/10.1097/00003246-200112000-00004

Prin, M., & Wunsch, H. (2014). The role of stepdown beds in hospital care. *American Journal of Respiratory and Critical Care Medicine, 190*(11), 1210–1216. (Seminal). https://doi.org/10.1164/rccm.201406-1117PP

Rawal, G., Yadav, S., & Kumar, R. (2017). Post-intensive care syndrome: An overview. *Journal of Translational Internal Medicine, 5*(2), 90–92. https://doi.org/10.1515/jtim-2016-0016

Roze des Ordons, A., Vanderspank-Wright, B., et al. (2017). Introduction to establishing therapeutic relationships. In P. Cardinal, T. Witter, & S. Yamashita (Eds.), *Navigating medical emergencies: An interactive guide to patient management.* Royal College of Physicians and Surgeons of Canada.

Sachdev, G., & Napolitano, L. M. (2012). Postoperative pulmonary complications: Pneumonia and acute respiratory failure. *Surgical Clinics of North America, 92*(2), 321–344. (Seminal). https://doi.org/10.1016/j.suc.2012.01.013

Seckel, M. A. (2017). Suctioning: Endotracheal or tracheostomy tube. In D. L. Wiegand (Ed.), *AACN procedure manual for critical care* (7th ed., pp. 79–87). Elsevier.

Shaffer, R. B. (2011). Arterial catheter insertion (assist), care, and removal. In D. L. Wiegand (Ed.), *AACN procedure manual for critical care* (6th ed., pp. 534–547). Elsevier. (Seminal).

Stacy, K. M. (2018). Pulmonary therapeutic management. In L. D. Urden, K. M. Stacy, & M. E. Lough (Eds.), *Critical care nursing: Diagnosis and management* (8th ed., pp. 487–519). Elsevier.

Stollings, J. L., Diedrich, D. A., Oyen, L. J., et al. (2014). Rapid-sequence intubation: A review of the process and considerations when choosing medications. *Annals of Pharmacotherapy, 48*(1), 62–76. (Seminal). https://doi.org/10.1177/1060028013510488

Tran, K., & Butcher, R. (2019). *Chlorhexidine for oral care: A review of clinical effectiveness and guidelines.* Canadian Agency for Drugs and Technologies in Health. https://www.ncbi.nlm.nih.gov/books/NBK541430/

Urden, L. D., Stacy, K. M., & Lough, M. E. (2018). *Critical care nursing: Diagnosis and management* (8th ed). Elsevier.

Vanderspank-Wright, B., Efstathiou, N., & Vandyk, A. (2018). Critical care nurses' experiences of withdrawal of treatment: A systematic review of qualitative evidence. *International Journal of Nursing Studies, 77*, 15–26. https://doi.org/10.1016/j.ijnurstu.2017.09.012

Vanderspank-Wright, B., Roze des Ordons, A., & Hartwick, M. (2017). Introduction to goals of care. In P. Cardinal, T. Witter, & S. Yamashita (Eds.), *Navigating medical emergencies: An interactive guide to patient management.* Royal College of Physicians and Surgeons of Canada.

Villwock, J. A., & Jones, K. (2014). Outcomes of early versus late tracheostomy: 2008–2010. *The Laryngoscope, 124*(8), 1801–1806. (Seminal). https://doi.org/10.1002/lary.24702

Wade, D., Hardy, R., Howell, D., et al. (2013). Identifying clinical and acute psychological risk factors for PTSD after critical care: A systematic review. *Minerva Anestesiologica, 79*(8), 944–963. (Seminal).

Wennberg, J. E., Fisher, E. S., Stukel, T. A., et al. (2004). Use of hospitals, physician visits, and hospice care during last six months of life among cohorts loyal to highly respected hospitals in the United States. *British Medical Journal, 328*, 1–5. (Seminal). https://doi.org/10.1136/bmj.328.7440.607

RESOURCES

Canadian Association of Critical Care Nurses (CACCN)
https://www.caccn.ca
Canadian Critical Care Society
https://www.canadiancriticalcare.org
Canadian Patient Safety Institute—*Patient Safety Right Now*
https://www.patientsafetyinstitute.ca/en/About/Patient-Safety-Right-Now/Pages/default.aspx

American Association of Critical-Care Nurses (AACN)
https://www.aacn.org

Australian College of Critical Care Nurses (ACCCN)
https://www.acccn.com.au
Society of Critical Care Medicine (SCCM)
https://www.sccm.org
World Federation of Critical Care Nurses (WFCCN)
https://wfccn.org

evolve

For additional Internet resources, see the website for this book at
http://evolve.elsevier.com/Canada/Lewis/medsurg.

Nursing Management

Shock, Sepsis, and Multiple-Organ Dysfunction Syndrome

Evan Keys
Originating US chapter by Helen Miley

evolve WEBSITE

LEARNING OBJECTIVES

1. Relate the pathophysiology to the clinical manifestations of the different types of shock: cardiogenic, hypovolemic, distributive, and obstructive.
2. Compare the effects of shock, sepsis, and multiple-organ dysfunction syndrome on the major body systems.
3. Compare the interprofessional care, medication therapy, and nursing management of patients experiencing different types of shock.
4. Describe the nursing management of a patient experiencing multiple-organ dysfunction syndrome.

KEY TERMS

anaphylactic shock
cardiogenic shock
hypovolemic shock

multiple-organ dysfunction syndrome (MODS)
obstructive shock
neurogenic shock

sepsis
septic shock
shock

Shock, sepsis, and multiple-organ dysfunction syndrome (MODS) are serious and interrelated conditions (Figure 69.1). This chapter provides an overview of shock, sepsis, as well as MODS and explores their management.

SHOCK

Shock is a syndrome characterized by decreased tissue perfusion and impaired cellular metabolism. This results in an imbalance between the supply of and the demand for oxygen and nutrients. The exchange of oxygen and nutrients at the cellular level is essential for life. When cells experience hypoperfusion, the demand for oxygen and nutrients exceeds the supply at the microcirculatory level. Ischemia can result, leading to cell injury and death. Thus, shock of any kind can be life-threatening.

Classification of Shock

The four main categories of shock are cardiogenic, hypovolemic, distributive, and obstructive (Table 69.1). Although the cause, initial presentation, and management vary for each type, the physiological responses to cellular hypoperfusion are similar.

Shock Caused by Low Blood Flow

Cardiogenic Shock. Cardiogenic shock occurs when either systolic or diastolic dysfunction of the heart's pumping occurs, resulting in reduced stroke volume (SV), cardiac output (CO) (<4 L/min), and blood pressure (BP). These changes depress myocardial function and compromise myocardial and systemic perfusion. Cardiogenic shock has a 50% mortality rate and is a leading cause of death following a myocardial infarction (MI) (Vahadatpour et al., 2019).

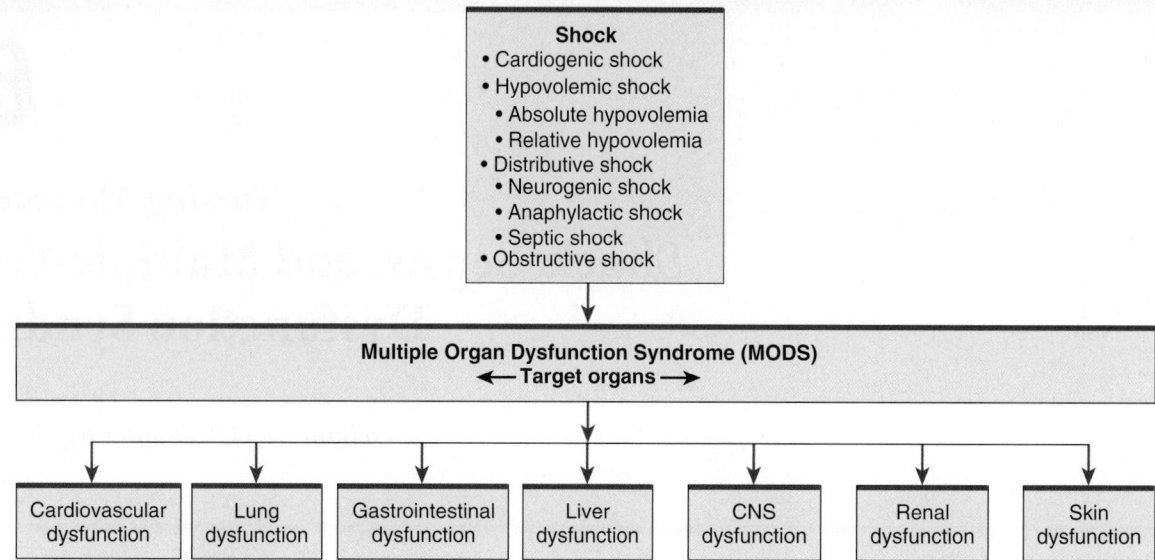

FIG. 69.1 Relationship of shock and multiple-organ dysfunction syndrome. *CNS,* central nervous system. Source: Modified from Harding, M., Kwong, J., Roberts, D., et al. (2020). *Lewis's medical-surgical nursing* (11th ed., p. 1567, Figure 66.1). Elsevier.

Systolic dysfunction is the heart's inability to pump blood forward. *Diastolic dysfunction* is the heart's inability to adequately fill during diastole. Causes of systolic and diastolic dysfunction are listed in Table 69.1. When either condition affects the right side of the heart, blood flow through the pulmonary circulation is compromised. When either condition affects the left chambers of the heart, blood flow through the systemic circulation is compromised.

Figure 69.2 describes the pathophysiology of cardiogenic shock. Whether the initiating event is myocardial ischemia, a structural issue (e.g., ventricular septal rupture, tension pneumothorax), or dysrhythmias, the physiological responses are similar: Tissue perfusion and cellular metabolism are impaired.

The early presentation of cardiogenic shock is similar to that of acute decompensated heart failure (see Chapter 37). The patient may exhibit tachycardia and hypotension. Their pulse pressure may be narrowed because of the heart's inability to pump blood forward during systole and increased volume during diastole. An increase in systemic vascular resistance (SVR) increases the workload of the heart, increasing myocardial oxygen consumption.

On examination, the patient may be tachypneic and have crackles on auscultation of breath sounds due to pulmonary congestion (Table 69.2). They may exhibit an increase in pulmonary artery wedge (or occlusive) pressure (PAWP), stroke volume variation (SVV), and pulmonary vascular resistance.

Signs of peripheral hypoperfusion include cyanosis, pallor, diaphoresis, weak peripheral pulses, cool and clammy skin, and delayed capillary refill. Decreased renal blood flow results in sodium and water retention and decreased urine output. Anxiety, confusion, and agitation may develop as cerebral perfusion is impaired. Diagnostic workup for cardiogenic shock includes laboratory studies, electrocardiography (ECG), chest radiography, and echocardiography (Table 69.3). The overall clinical presentation of a patient with cardiogenic shock is described in Table 69.4.

Hypovolemic Shock. Hypovolemic shock occurs from inadequate fluid volume in the intravascular space to support adequate perfusion. The volume loss may be either an absolute or relative volume loss. *Absolute hypovolemia* results when fluid is lost through hemorrhage, gastrointestinal (GI) loss (e.g.,

vomiting, diarrhea), fistula drainage, diabetes insipidus, hyperglycemia, or diuresis. *Relative hypovolemia* develops when fluid moves out of the vascular space into the extravascular space (e.g., interstitial or intracavitary space). This type of fluid shift is called *third spacing.* One mechanism of relative volume loss is leakage of fluid from the vascular space into the interstitial space from increased capillary permeability, occurring in sepsis or burns (see Chapter 27). Table 69.1 provides other examples of hypovolemic shock.

In hypovolemic shock, the size of the vascular compartment remains unchanged, but the volume of blood or plasma decreases. Whether the loss of intravascular volume is absolute or relative, the physiological consequences are similar. The reduced intravascular volume results in decreased venous return to the heart, decreased preload, decreased SV, and decreased CO (see Table 69.2). A cascade of events results in decreased tissue perfusion and impaired cellular metabolism—hallmarks of shock (Figure 69.3).

The patient's response to acute volume loss is dependent on a number of factors, including the extent of the patient's injury or insult, their age, and their general state of health; however, the clinical presentation of hypovolemic shock is consistent (see Table 69.4). An overall assessment of physiological reserves may indicate the patient's ability to compensate. A patient may compensate for a loss of up to 15% of the total blood volume (approximately 750 mL) (Good & Kirkwood, 2017). Further loss of volume (15 to 30%) results in a sympathetic nervous system (SNS)–mediated response (Good & Kirkwood, 2017). This response results in increases in heart rate, CO, and respiratory rate and depth. The SV and PAWP are decreased because of the decreased circulating blood volume.

The patient may appear anxious, and urine output begins to decrease. If hypovolemia is corrected by crystalloid fluid replacement at this time, tissue dysfunction is generally reversible. If volume loss is greater than 30%, compensatory mechanisms may fail, and replacement with blood products should be initiated (Good & Kirkwood, 2017). With loss of more than 40% of the total blood volume, autoregulation in the microcirculation is lost, and irreversible tissue destruction occurs

TABLE 69.1	CLASSIFICATION OF SHOCK STATES
Types and Causes	**Examples**
Cardiogenic Shock	
Diastolic dysfunction: inability of the heart to fill	Cardiac tamponade, ventricular hypertrophy, cardiomyopathy
Dysrhythmias	Bradydysrhythmias, tachydysrhythmias
Structural factors	Valvular stenosis or regurgitation, ventricular septal rupture, tension pneumothorax
Systolic dysfunction: inability of the heart to pump blood forward	Myocardial infarction, cardiomyopathy, blunt cardiac injury, severe systemic or pulmonary hypertension, myocardial depression from metabolic problems
Hypovolemic Shock	
Absolute Hypovolemia	
External loss of whole blood	Hemorrhage from trauma, surgery, gastrointestinal bleeding
Loss of other body fluids	Vomiting, diarrhea, excessive diuresis, diabetes insipidus, diabetes mellitus
Relative Hypovolemia	
Fluid shifts	Burn injuries, ascites
Internal bleeding	Fracture of long bones, ruptured spleen, hemothorax, severe pancreatitis
Massive vasodilation	Sepsis
Pooling of blood or fluids	Bowel obstruction
Distributive Shock	
Neurogenic Shock	
Hemodynamic consequence of spinal cord injury or disease at or above T5	Severe pain, medications, hypoglycemia, injury
Spinal anaesthesia	
Vasomotor centre depression	
Anaphylactic Shock	
Hypersensitivity (allergic) reaction to a sensitizing substance	Contrast media, blood or blood products, medications, insect bites, anaesthetic agents, food or food additives, vaccines, environmental agents, latex
Septic Shock	
At-risk patients	Older persons, patients with chronic diseases (e.g., diabetes mellitus, chronic kidney disease, heart failure), patients receiving immunosuppressive therapy or who are malnourished or debilitated
Infection	Pneumonia, peritonitis, urinary tract, invasive procedures, in-dwelling lines and catheters
Obstructive Shock	
Physical obstruction impeding cardiac filling or outflow, resulting in reduced cardiac output	Cardiac tamponade, tension pneumothorax, superior vena cava syndrome, abdominal compartment syndrome, pulmonary embolism

PATHOPHYSIOLOGY MAP

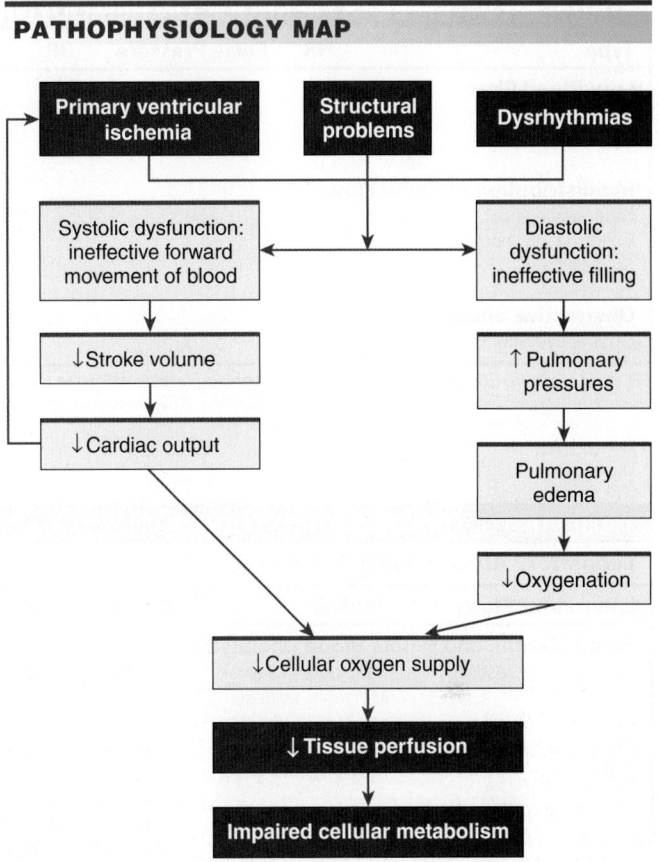

FIG. 69.2 The pathophysiology of cardiogenic shock. Source: Modified from Urden, L. D., Stacy, K. M., & Lough, M. E. (2010). *Critical care nursing: Diagnosis and management* (6th ed.). Mosby.

Shock Caused by Maldistribution of Blood Flow

Neurogenic Shock. Neurogenic shock is a hemodynamic phenomenon that can occur within 30 minutes of a spinal cord injury at the fifth thoracic (T5) vertebra or above and lasts up to 6 weeks. The injury results in a massive vasodilation without compensation that is caused by the loss of SNS vasoconstrictor tone (Taylor et al., 2017). This massive vasodilation leads to a pooling of blood in the blood vessels, tissue hypoperfusion, and impairment of cellular metabolism (Figure 69.4).

In addition to spinal cord injury, spinal anaesthesia can block transmission of impulses from the SNS. Depression of the vasomotor centre of the medulla from medications (e.g., benzodiazepines, opioids) can decrease the vasoconstrictor tone of the peripheral blood vessels, resulting in neurogenic shock (see Table 69.1).

Classic clinical manifestations are hypotension (from the massive vasodilation) and bradycardia (from unopposed parasympathetic stimulation) (Taylor et al., 2017). The patient may be unable to regulate body temperature, and in combination with massive vasodilation, severe heat loss can result. Initially, the patient's skin warms as a result of the massive dilation; however, as the heat dissipates, the risk for hypothermia escalates. Later, the patient's skin may be cool or warm, depending on the ambient temperature, due to poikilothermia (the taking on of the temperature of the environment). In either case, the skin is usually dry. Tables 69.2, 69.3, and 69.4 further describe the clinical presentation of a patient with neurogenic shock.

(Good & Kirkwood, 2017). Common laboratory studies with hypovolemic shock include serial measurements of hemoglobin and hematocrit levels, urine specific gravity, serum electrolytes, arterial and venous blood gases, and serum lactate (see Table 69.3).

TABLE 69.2 EFFECTS OF SHOCK ON HEMODYNAMIC PARAMETERS*

Type	HR	Pulse Pressure	BP	SVR	PVR	CVP	PAP	PAWP	CO	SvO₂/ScvO₂
Low Blood Flow										
Cardiogenic shock	↑	↓	↓	↑	↑	≈, ↑	↑	↑	↓	↓
Hypovolemic shock	↑	↓	↓	↑	↑	↓	↓	↓	↓	↓
Maldistribution of Blood Flow										
Neurogenic shock	↓	↓	↓	↓	≈	↓	↓	↓	↓	↓
Anaphylactic shock	↑	↓	↓	↓	≈, ↑	↓	↓	↓	↓	↓
Septic shock	↑	↓	↓	↓	≈, ↑	↓	↑, ≈, ↓	↓	↑, ≈, ↓	↑, ≈, ↓
Obstructive Shock										
Obstructive Shock	↑	↓	↓	↑	↑	↑	↑	↑	↓	↓

BP, blood pressure; *CO*, cardiac output; *CVP*, central venous pressure; *HR*, heart rate; *PAP*, pulmonary artery pressure; *PAWP*, pulmonary artery occlusive pressure; *PVR*, pulmonary vascular resistance; *ScvO₂*, central venous oxygen saturation; *SvO₂*, venous oxygen saturation; *SVR*, systemic vascular resistance.
*Hemodynamic effects in some illnesses are highly variable.
↓, decrease; ↑, increase; ≈, no change.

TABLE 69.3 DIAGNOSTIC STUDIES

Laboratory Abnormalities in Shock

Laboratory Study	Finding	Significance of Finding
Blood, Serum, and Whole Blood Chemistries		
Arterial blood gases	Respiratory alkalosis	In early shock, occurs secondary to hyperventilation
	Metabolic acidosis	In later shock, occurs when lactic acid accumulates in blood as a result of anaerobic metabolism
Base deficit	≥6	Acid production secondary to hypoxia
Blood cultures	Growth of organisms	May occur in patients who are in septic shock
BUN	Increased	Impaired kidney function as a result of hypoperfusion from severe vasoconstriction, or secondary to cell catabolism (e.g., in trauma, infection)
Creatinine	Increased	Indicates impaired kidney function caused by hypoperfusion secondary to severe vasoconstriction
		More sensitive indicator of renal function than BUN
Creatine kinase	Increased	Trauma and/or MI, increases in response to cellular damage and/or hypoxia
DIC screen		Acute DIC can develop within hours to days after an initial assault on the body (e.g., shock)
D-dimer	Increased	
Fibrin split products	Increased	
Fibrinogen level	Decreased	
Platelet count	Decreased	
PTT and INR	Prolonged	
Thrombin time	Increased	
Glucose	Increased	In early shock, increases because of release of liver glycogen stores in response to SNS stimulation and cortisol
		Insulin insensitivity develops
	Decreased	Decreases because of depleted glycogen stores, with hepatocellular dysfunction as shock progresses
Lactate	Increased	Usually increases once significant hypoperfusion and impaired oxygen use at the cellular level have occurred
		Byproduct of anaerobic metabolism
Liver enzymes (ALT, AST, GGT)	Increased	Liver cell destruction in progressive stage of shock
Potassium	Increased	Increases when cellular death liberates intracellular potassium, in AKI, and in the presence of acidosis
	Decreased	In early shock, decreases because of increased secretion of aldosterone, which causes renal excretion of potassium
RBC count, hematocrit, hemoglobin	Normal	Remains within normal limits (a) in shock because of relative hypovolemia and pump failure and (b) in hemorrhagic shock before fluid resuscitation
	Decreased	In hemorrhagic shock, decreases after fluid resuscitation when fluids other than blood are used
	Increased	In nonhemorrhagic shock, increases as a result of actual hypovolemia when fluid lost does not contain erythrocytes
Sodium	Increased	In early shock, increases because of increased secretion of aldosterone, causing renal retention of sodium
	Decreased	May occur iatrogenically when excessive hypotonic fluid is administered after fluid loss
Troponin	Increased	Myocardial ischemia
WBC count	Increased	Infection
Urine		
Specific gravity	Increased	Occurs secondary to the action of ADH
	Fixed at 1.010	Occurs in renal failure

ADH, antidiuretic hormone; *AKI*, acute kidney injury; *ALT*, alanine aminotransferase; *AST*, aspartate aminotransferase; *BUN*, blood urea nitrogen; *DIC*, disseminated intravascular coagulation; *GGT*, γ-glutamyl transferase; *INR*, international normalized ratio; *MI*, myocardial infarction; *PTT*, partial thromboplastin time; *RBC*, red blood cell; *SNS*, sympathetic nervous system; *WBC*, white blood cell.

TABLE 69.4   CLINICAL PRESENTATION IN THE MAJOR TYPES OF SHOCK

Cardiogenic Shock	Hypovolemic Shock	Neurogenic Shock	Anaphylactic Shock	Septic Shock	Obstructive Shock
Cardiovascular System					
Tachycardia	Tachycardia	Bradycardia	Tachycardia	Tachycardia	Tachycardia
↓ BP	↓ Preload	↓ BP	↑ CO	↓/↑ Temperature	↓ BP
↓ SV, CO	↓ CO, CVP, PAWP	↓ CO, CVP, SVR	↓ CVP, PAWP	Myocardial dysfunction	↓ Preload
↑ SVR, PAWP, CVP	↑ SVR	↓/↑ Temperature	Chest pain	Biventricular dilation	↓ CO
↓ Capillary refill	↓ Capillary refill		Third spacing of fluid	↓ Ejection fraction	↑ SVR, CVP
Respiratory System					
Tachypnea	Tachypnea → bradypnea	Dysfunction related to	Shortness of breath	Hyperventilation	Tachypnea → bradyp-
Crackles	(late)	level of injury	Edema of larynx and	Crackles	nea (late)
Cyanosis			epiglottis	Respiratory alkalosis →	Shortness of breath
			Wheezing	respiratory acidosis	
			Stridor	Hypoxemia	
			Rhinitis	Respiratory failure	
				ARDS	
				Pulmonary hyperten-	
				sion	
Renal System					
↑ Na⁺ and H₂O reten-	↓ Urine output	Bladder dysfunction	Incontinence	↓ Urine output	↓ Urine output
tion					
↓ Renal blood flow					
↓ Urine output					
Skin					
Pallor	Pallor	↓ Skin perfusion	Flushing	Warm and flushed →	Pallor
Cool, clammy	Cool, clammy	Cool or warm	Pruritus	cool and mottled	Cool, clammy
		Dry	Urticaria	(late)	
			Angioedema		
Neurological System					
↓ Cerebral perfusion:	↓ Cerebral perfusion:	Flaccid paralysis below	Anxiety	Change in mental sta-	↓ Cerebral perfusion:
Anxiety	Anxiety	level of the lesion	Feeling of impending	tus (e.g., confusion)	Anxiety
Confusion	Confusion	Loss of reflex activity	doom	Agitation	Confusion
Agitation	Agitation		Confusion	Coma (late)	Agitation
			↓ LOC		
			Metallic taste		
Gastrointestinal System					
↓ Bowel sounds	Absent bowel sounds	Bowel dysfunction	Cramping	GI bleeding	↓ To absent bowel
Nausea, vomiting			Abdominal pain	Paralytic ileus	sounds
			Nausea		
			Vomiting		
			Diarrhea		
Diagnostic Findings					
↑ Cardiac biomarkers	↓ Hematocrit		Sudden onset	↑/↓ WBC	Specific to cause of
↑ b-Type natriuretic	↓ Hemoglobin		History of allergies	↓ Platelets	obstruction
peptide (BNP)	↑ Lactate		Exposure to contrast	↑ Lactate	
↑ Blood glucose	↑ Urine specific gravity		media	↑ Blood glucose	
↑ BUN	Changes in electrolytes			↑ Procalcitonin	
ECG (e.g., dysrhyth-				↑ Urine specific gravity	
mias)				↓ Urine Na⁺	
Echocardiogram (e.g.,				Positive blood cultures	
left ventricular dys-					
function					
Chest X-ray (e.g., pul-					
monary infiltrates)					

ARDS, acute respiratory distress syndrome; *BP,* blood pressure; *BUN,* blood urea nitrogen; *CO,* cardiac output; *CVP,* central venous pressure; *ECG,* electrocardiogram; *GI,* gastrointestinal; *LOC,* level of consciousness; *MVO₂,* myocardial oxygen consumption; *PAWP,* pulmonary artery wedge pressure; *SV,* stroke volume; *SVR,* systemic vascular resistance; *WBC,* white blood cell.

Although spinal shock and neurogenic shock often occur in the same patient, they are not the same disorder. *Spinal shock* is a transient condition that is present after an acute spinal cord injury (see Chapter 63) (Taylor et al., 2017). A patient with spinal shock experiences an absence of all voluntary and reflex neurological activity below the level of the injury.

PATHOPHYSIOLOGY MAP

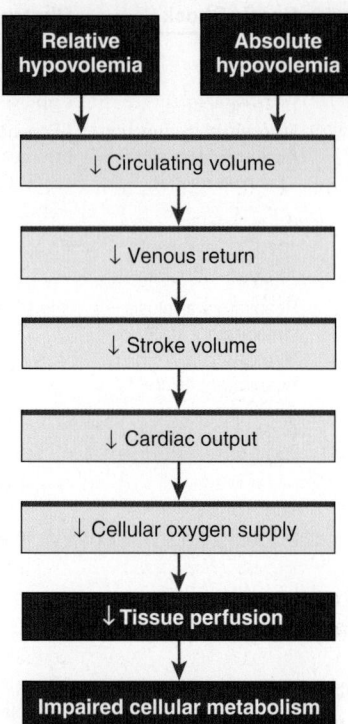

FIG. 69.3 The pathophysiology of hypovolemic shock. Source: Modified from Urden, L. D., Stacy, K. M., & Lough, M. E. (2010). *Critical care nursing: Diagnosis and management* (6th ed.). Mosby.

Anaphylactic Shock. Anaphylactic shock is an acute, life-threatening hypersensitivity (allergic) reaction to a sensitizing substance (e.g., medication, chemical, vaccine, food, insect venom) (Loverde et al., 2018). Usually an immediate reaction causes massive vasodilation, release of vasoactive mediators, and an increase in capillary permeability. As capillary permeability increases, fluid leaks from the vascular space into the interstitial space.

Anaphylactic shock can lead to airway swelling (pharyngeal and laryngeal edema, stridor, hoarse voice), breathing difficulties (shortness of breath, increased respirations, fatigue, confusion as a result of hypoxia), and circulation complications (hypotension; tachycardia; pale, clammy skin; faintness; and even loss of consciousness). A patient may become anxious and experience a sense of impending doom. Without prompt treatment, respiratory or cardiac arrest may develop.

A patient can develop a severe allergic reaction, possibly leading to anaphylactic shock, after contact with or inhalation, ingestion, or injection of an antigen (allergen) to which the person has previously been sensitized (see Table 69.1). Parenteral administration of the antigen (allergen) is the route most likely to cause anaphylaxis; however, oral, topical, and inhalation routes can also cause anaphylactic reactions. Tables 69.2, 69.3, and 69.4 describe the clinical presentation of anaphylactic shock. Quick and decisive action by the nurse is crucial for preventing the progression of an anaphylactic reaction to anaphylactic shock. (Anaphylaxis is discussed in Chapter 16.)

Septic Shock. Sepsis is a life-threatening syndrome that arises when the body's response to infection injures its own tissues and organs (Table 69.5). In as many as 30% of patients who develop sepsis, the causative organism is unknown. Globally, 48.9 million

PATHOPHYSIOLOGY MAP

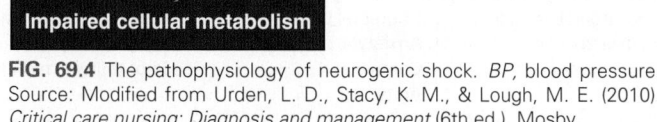

FIG. 69.4 The pathophysiology of neurogenic shock. *BP,* blood pressure. Source: Modified from Urden, L. D., Stacy, K. M., & Lough, M. E. (2010). *Critical care nursing: Diagnosis and management* (6th ed.). Mosby.

cases and 11 million deaths are reported annually (Rudd et al., 2020). This accounts for 20% of all-cause mortality worldwide (Rudd et al., 2020). In Canada, 1 in 18 deaths can be linked to sepsis, with 2 515 primary-cause deaths and 10 985 contributing-cause deaths reported in 2011 (Navaneelan et al., 2016).

Septic shock is a subset of sepsis and is characterized by persistent hypotension, despite adequate fluid resuscitation, and inadequate tissue perfusion resulting in tissue hypoxia (Singer et al., 2016). It has an increased mortality risk due to profound circulatory, cellular, and metabolic abnormalities. The primary organisms that induce sepsis are Gram-negative and Gram-positive bacteria. Parasites, fungi, and viruses can also lead to the development of sepsis and septic shock. Figure 69.5 presents the pathophysiology of septic shock.

When an antigen (microorganism) enters the body, the normal immune and inflammatory responses are initiated to destroy the antigen; however, in sepsis and septic shock, the body's response to the microorganism is exaggerated. Both proinflammatory and anti-inflammatory responses are activated, coagulation increases, and fibrinolysis decreases. Endotoxins from the microorganism cell wall stimulate the release of cytokines and other proinflammatory mediators that act through secondary mediators (see Chapter 14). The release of platelet-activating factor results in the formation of microthrombi and obstruction of the microvasculature. The combined effects of the mediators cause damage to the endothelium, vasodilation,

TABLE 69.5 DIAGNOSTIC CRITERIA FOR SEPSIS

Infection, documented or suspected, as well as one or more of the following:

General Variables
- Altered mental status
- Fever (temperature >38.3°C)
- Heart rate >90 beats/min
- Hyperglycemia (blood glucose >7.77 mmol/L) in the absence of diabetes
- Hypothermia (core temperature <36°C)
- Significant edema or positive fluid balance (>20 mL/kg over 24 hr)
- Tachypnea (respiratory rate ≥22)

Inflammatory Variables
- Elevated C-reactive protein
- Elevated procalcitonin
- Leukocytosis (WBC count >12 × 10⁹/L)
- Leukopenia (WBC count <4 × 10⁹/L)
- Normal WBC count with >10% immature forms

Hemodynamic Variables
- Arterial hypotension (SBP <90 mm Hg, MAP <70 mm Hg, or a decrease in SBP >40 mm Hg)

Organ Dysfunction Variables
- Acute oliguria (urine output <0.5 mL/kg/hr for at least 2 hr despite adequate fluid resuscitation)
- Arterial hypoxemia (PaO_2/FiO_2 <300)
- Coagulation abnormalities (INR >1.5 or PTT >60 sec)
- Hyperbilirubinemia (total bilirubin >68.4 mcmol/L)
- Ileus (absent bowel sounds)
- Serum creatinine increase >44.2 mcmol/L
- Thrombocytopenia (platelet count <100 × 10⁹/L)

Tissue Perfusion Variables
- Decreased capillary refill or mottling
- Hyperlactatemia (>1 mmol/L)

FiO₂, fraction of inspired oxygen; *INR*, international normalized ratio; *MAP*, mean arterial pressure; *PaO₂*, partial pressure of arterial oxygen; *PTT*, partial thromboplastin time; *SBP*, systolic blood pressure; *WBC*, white blood cell.
Source: Singer, M., Deutschman, C., Seymour, C., et al. (2016). The third international consensus definitions for sepsis and septic shock (Sepsis-3). *Journal of the American Medical Association, 315*(8), 801–810. https://doi.org/10.1001/jama.2016.0287

increased capillary permeability, and neutrophil and platelet aggregation and adhesion to the endothelium. With these changes, the intravascular volume leaks into the interstitial space, reducing SVR. If CO cannot increase further to compensate, septic shock develops.

The current clinical criteria for identifying septic shock are hypotension, elevated lactate level, and a sustained need for vasopressor therapy (Singer et al., 2016) (see Table 69.5). Affected patients usually experience an initial hyperdynamic state, characterized by increased CO and decreased SVR, causing tachycardia and tachypnea. Persistence of high CO and low SVR beyond 24 hours are ominous findings and are often associated with increased development of hypotension leading to MODS. Patients may be euvolemic, but because of acute vasodilation and shifting of fluids out of the intravascular space, relative hypovolemia and hypotension occur.

Respiratory failure is common. Affected patients initially hyperventilate as a compensatory mechanism, resulting in respiratory alkalosis. Once the patient can no longer compensate, respiratory acidosis develops. Acute respiratory distress syndrome (ARDS) develops in 14% of patients, and 45% of these patients will die (Bellani et al., 2016; Iriyama et al., 2020). Other clinical signs of septic shock include alteration in neurological

status, decreased urine output, and GI dysfunction, such as GI bleeding and paralytic ileus. Tables 69.2 and 69.4 further delineate the clinical presentation of septic shock.

Coronavirus Disease 2019 (COVID-19). Clinically, most patients infected by the SARS-CoV-2 virus present with mild symptomatology. But almost 5% of patients will suffer severe lung injury, MODS, or both. As a result of virus infection and, in some cases, MODS, many patients with severe COVID-19 meet sepsis criteria (Singer et al., 2016). Sepsis is the second leading cause of death among COVID-19 patients (Zhou et al., 2020), with mortality of those admitted to the critical care unit (CCU) between 8 and 38% (Beltrán-Garcia et al., 2020). The Surviving Sepsis Campaign COVID-19 has issued several statements and recommendations regarding COVID-19 and its relationship to sepsis. All recommendations, and their level of empirical support, are detailed in the report by Alhazzani et al. (2020) and relate to infection control, laboratory diagnosis and specimens, supportive care, and therapy to treat COVID-19.

Obstructive Shock. Obstructive shock develops when a physical obstruction to blood flow occurs, resulting in decreased CO (Figure 69.6). This can be caused by restricted diastolic filling of the right ventricle from compression (e.g., cardiac tamponade, tension pneumothorax). Other causes include *abdominal compartment syndrome,* in which increased abdominal pressures compress the inferior vena cava, decreasing venous return to the heart. Pulmonary embolism and right ventricular thrombi cause an outflow obstruction as blood leaves the right ventricle through the pulmonary artery. This leads to decreased blood flow to the lungs and decreased blood return to the left atrium.

Affected patients have a decreased CO, increased afterload, and variable left ventricular filling pressures depending on the obstruction. Other signs include jugular venous distention and pulsus paradoxus (see Table 69.2). Rapid assessment and treatment are crucial to prevent further hemodynamic compromise and possible cardiac arrest.

Stages of Shock

While it is important for health care providers to understand the underlying pathogenesis of the type of shock the patient is experiencing, it is equally important for them to understand which stage of the shock "continuum" the patient is in. Shock is categorized into four overlapping stages: (1) initial, (2) compensatory, (3) progressive, and (4) refractory.

Initial Stage. The continuum begins with the *initial stage* of shock at a cellular level. This stage is typically not clinically apparent. Metabolism changes at the cellular level, from aerobic to anaerobic, cause lactic acid buildup. Lactic acid is a waste product and must be removed by the liver. However, this process requires oxygen, which is unavailable because of decreased tissue perfusion.

Compensatory Stage. In the *compensatory stage,* the body activates neural, hormonal, and biochemical compensatory mechanisms in an attempt to overcome the increasing consequences of anaerobic metabolism and to maintain homeostasis. The clinical presentation begins to reflect the body's responses to the imbalance in oxygen supply and demand (Table 69.6).

A classic clinical sign of shock is hypotension, occurring from a decrease in CO and a narrowing pulse pressure. The baroreceptors in the carotid and aortic bodies immediately respond by activating the SNS. The SNS stimulates vasoconstriction and the release of potent vasoconstrictors—epinephrine and norepinephrine. Blood flow to the heart and brain is maintained,

PATHOPHYSIOLOGY MAP

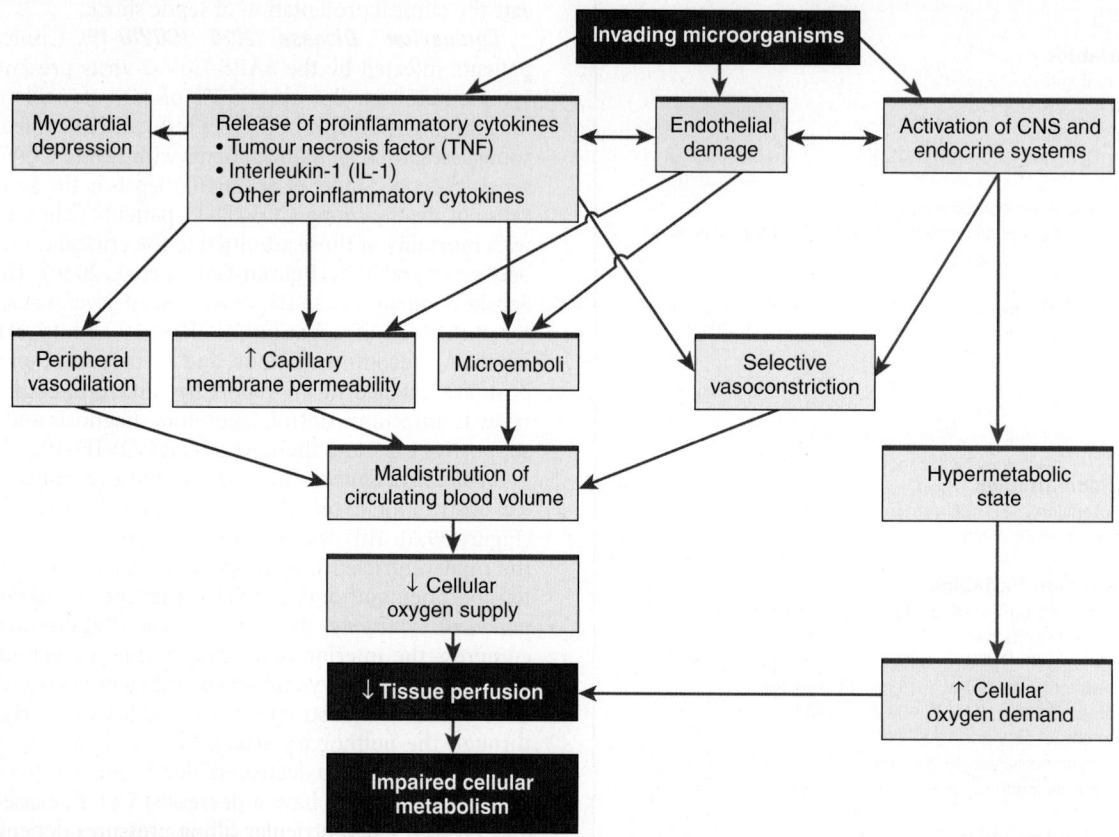

FIG. 69.5 The pathophysiology of septic shock. *CNS,* central nervous system. Source: Modified from Urden, L. D., Stacy, K. M., & Lough, M. E. (2010). *Critical care nursing: Diagnosis and management* (6th ed.). Mosby.

PATHOPHYSIOLOGY MAP

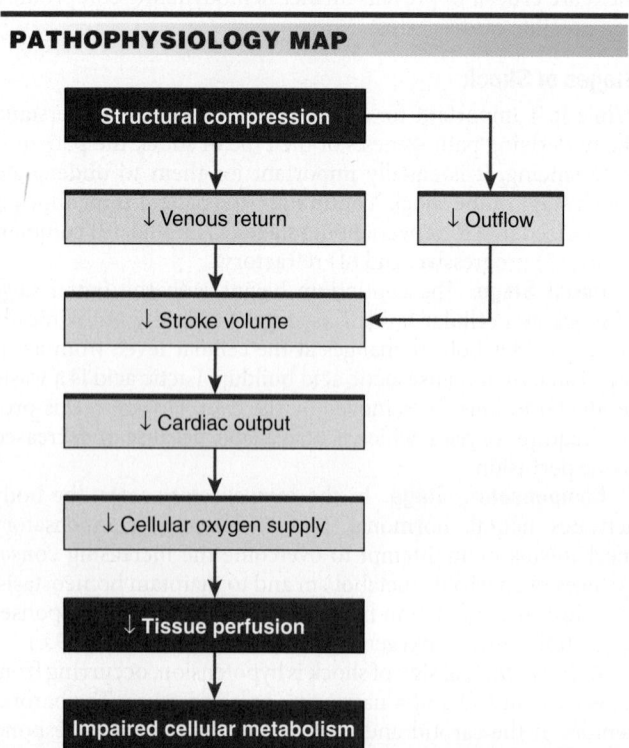

FIG. 69.6 The pathophysiology of obstructive shock. Source: Modified from Urden, L. D., Stacy, K. M., & Lough, M. E. (2010). *Critical care nursing: Diagnosis and management* (6th ed.). Mosby.

whereas blood flow to the nonvital organs (i.e., kidneys, GI tract, skin, lungs) is diverted or shunted.

The myocardium responds to the SNS stimulation and the increase in oxygen demand by increasing the heart rate and contractility. Increased contractility increases myocardial oxygen consumption (MVO_2). The coronary arteries dilate in an attempt to meet the increased oxygen demands of the myocardium.

Decreased blood flow to the kidneys activates the renin–angiotensin system. Renin is released, which activates angiotensinogen to produce angiotensin I, which is then converted to angiotensin II (see Chapter 47, Figure 47.6). Angiotensin II is a potent vasoconstrictor that causes both arterial and venous vasoconstriction. The net result is an increase in venous return to the heart and an increase in BP. Angiotensin II stimulates the adrenal cortex to release aldosterone, which results in sodium and water reabsorption and in potassium excretion by the kidneys. The increase in sodium reabsorption raises the serum osmolality and stimulates the release of antidiuretic hormone (ADH) from the posterior pituitary gland. ADH increases water reabsorption by the kidneys, further increasing blood volume. The increase in total circulating volume results in increases in CO and BP.

Shunting of blood from the GI tract leads to decreased motility and paralytic ileus. Typically, the skin is cold and clammy from low distribution of blood flow during shock; however, during septic shock the skin can initially be warm and dry.

TABLE 69.6   CLINICAL MANIFESTATIONS OF THE STAGES OF SHOCK

Compensatory Stage	Progressive Stage	Refractory Stage
Neurological System		
Oriented to person, place, time	↓ Cerebral perfusion pressure	Unresponsive
Restless, apprehensive, confused	↓ Cerebral blood flow	Areflexia (loss of reflexes)
Change in level of consciousness	↓ Responsiveness to stimuli	Pupils nonreactive and dilated
	Delirium	
Cardiovascular System		
Sympathetic nervous system response:	↑ Capillary permeability → systemic interstitial edema	Profound hypotension
• Release of epinephrine/norepinephrine (vasoconstriction)	↓ CO → ↓ BP and ↑ HR	↓ CO
• ↑ MVO$_2$	MAP <60 mm Hg (or 40 mm Hg drop in BP from baseline)	Bradycardia, irregular rhythm
• ↑ Contractility	↓ Coronary perfusion → dysrhythmias, myocardial	↓ BP inadequate to perfuse vital
• ↑ HR	ischemia, MI	organs
• Coronary artery dilation	↓ Peripheral perfusion → ischemia of distal extremities,	
• Narrowed pulse pressure	↓ pulses, ↓ capillary refill	
• ↓ BP		
Respiratory System		
↓ Blood flow to the lungs:	ARDS:	Severe refractory hypoxemia
• ↑ Physiological dead space	• ↑ Capillary permeability	Respiratory failure
• ↑ Ventilation-perfusion mismatch	• Pulmonary vasoconstriction	
• Hyperventilation	• Pulmonary interstitial edema	
• ↑ Minute ventilation (V$_E$)	• Alveolar edema	
• Tachypnea	• Diffuse infiltrates	
	• Tachypnea	
	• ↓ Compliance	
	• Moist crackles	
Gastrointestinal System		
↓ Blood supply	Vasoconstriction and ↓ perfusion → ischemic gut (e.g.,	Ischemic gut
↓ GI motility	stomach, small and large intestines, gallbladder,	
Hypoactive bowel sounds	pancreas):	
↑ Risk for paralytic ileus	• Erosive ulcers	
	• GI bleeding	
	• Translocation of GI bacteria	
	• Impaired absorption of nutrients	
Renal System		
↓ Renal blood flow	Renal tubules become ischemic → acute tubular necrosis	Anuria
↑ Renin resulting in release of angiotensin (vasoconstrictor)	↓ Urine output	
↑ Aldosterone resulting in Na$^+$ and H$_2$O reabsorption	↑ BUN-to-creatinine ratio	
↑ Antidiuretic hormone resulting in H$_2$O reabsorption	↑ Urine sodium	
	↓ Urine osmolality and specific gravity	
	↓ Urine potassium	
	Metabolic acidosis	
Hepatic System		
	Failure to metabolize medications and waste products	Metabolic changes from ac-
	Cell death (↑ liver enzymes)	cumulation of waste products
	Jaundice (↓ clearance of bilirubin)	(e.g., NH$_3$, lactate, CO$_2$)
	↑ NH$_3$ (ammonia) and lactate	
Hematological System		
	DIC:	DIC progresses
	• Thrombin clots in microcirculation	
	• Consumption of platelets and clotting factors	
Temperature		
Normal or abnormal	Hypothermia or hyperthermia	Hypothermia
Skin		
Pale and cool	Cold and clammy	Mottled, cyanotic
Warm and flushed		
Key Laboratory Findings		
↑ Blood glucose	↑ Bleeding times	↓ Blood glucose
↓ PaO$_2$	↑ Liver enzymes: ALT, AST, GGT	Metabolic acidosis
↓ PaCO$_2$	Thrombocytopenia	↑ NH$_3$, lactate, and K$^+$
↑ pH		

ALT, alanine aminotransferase; *ARDS,* acute respiratory distress syndrome; *AST,* aspartate aminotransferase; *BP,* blood pressure; *BUN,* blood urea nitrogen; *CO,* cardiac output; *DIC,* disseminated intravascular coagulation; *GGT,* γ-glutamyl transferase; *GI,* gastrointestinal; *HR,* heart rate; *K$^+$,* potassium ions; *MAP,* mean arterial pressure; *MI,* myocardial infarction; *MVO$_2$,* myocardial oxygen consumption; *Na$^+$,* sodium ions; *NH$_3$,* ammonia; *PaCO$_2$,* partial pressure of arterial carbon dioxide; *PaO$_2$,* partial pressure of arterial oxygen.

Shunting blood away from the lungs increases the patient's physiological dead space (the amount of air that does not reach gas-exchanging units) and any inspired air that cannot participate in gas exchange. The clinical result of an increase in dead space is a ventilation–perfusion (VQ) mismatch. Some areas of the lungs participating in ventilation are not perfused because of the decreased blood flow to the lungs. Arterial oxygen levels decrease, and the rate and depth of respirations increase to compensate.

During the compensatory stage, the body can compensate for the changes in tissue perfusion. If the perfusion deficit is corrected, the patient recovers with few or no residual consequences. If the perfusion deficit is not corrected and the body is unable to compensate, the patient enters the progressive stage of shock.

Progressive Stage. The *progressive stage* of shock begins as compensatory mechanisms fail. Continued decreased cellular perfusion and resulting altered capillary permeability are the distinguishing features of this stage. As a result of altered capillary permeability, fluid and protein leak out of the vascular space into the surrounding interstitial space. Fluid leakage from the vascular space also affects the solid organs (e.g., liver, spleen, GI tract, lungs) and peripheral tissues by further decreasing perfusion. Changes in the patient's mental status become apparent in this stage. Capillary permeability continues to increase, enhancing the movement of fluid from the vascular space into the interstitial space. Sustained hypoperfusion results in weakening of peripheral pulses and ischemia of the distal extremities. In this stage, aggressive interventions are necessary to prevent the development of MODS.

The pulmonary system is often the first to display signs of critical dysfunction. In response to the decreased blood flow and the SNS stimulation, the pulmonary arterioles constrict, resulting in increased pulmonary artery (PA) pressure. As the pressure within the pulmonary vasculature increases, blood flow to the pulmonary capillaries decreases, and V/Q mismatch worsens. Another key response in the lungs is the movement of fluid from the pulmonary vasculature into the interstitial space. As capillary permeability increases, the movement of fluid to the interstitial spaces results in interstitial edema, bronchoconstriction, and a decrease in functional residual capacity. With further increases in capillary permeability, the fluid moves to the alveoli, with resultant alveolar edema and a decrease in surfactant production. The combined effects of pulmonary vasoconstriction and bronchoconstriction are impaired gas exchange, decreased compliance, and worsening V/Q mismatch. Clinical manifestations are tachypnea, crackles, and overall increased work of breathing.

The cardiovascular system is profoundly affected. CO begins to fall, resulting in hypotension and decreased coronary, cerebral, and peripheral artery perfusion. Myocardial dysfunction from decreased perfusion results in dysrhythmias, myocardial ischemia, and, potentially, MI.

The effect of prolonged hypoperfusion on the kidneys is renal tubular ischemia. The resulting acute tubular necrosis may lead to the development of acute kidney injury (AKI), which can be worsened by nephrotoxic medications (e.g., certain antibiotics, anaesthetics, and diuretics) (see Chapter 49). The patient has decreased urine output and increased blood urea nitrogen (BUN) and serum creatinine. Metabolic acidosis results from an inability to excrete acids (namely lactic acid) and reabsorb bicarbonate.

The GI system is also affected by prolonged hypoperfusion. The normally protective mucosal barrier becomes ischemic. This ischemia predisposes the patient to ulcers and GI bleeding (see Chapter 44), increasing the potential risk for bacterial translocation from the GI tract to the blood. The decreased perfusion to the GI tract leads to a decrease in the ability to absorb nutrients.

The loss of the functional ability of the liver leads to the liver failing to metabolize medications and waste products (e.g., ammonia, lactate). Jaundice results from an accumulation of bilirubin. As the liver cells die, enzyme levels elevate, particularly those of alanine aminotransferase (ALT), aspartate aminotransferase (AST), and γ-glutamyl transferase (GGT). The liver also loses its ability to function as an immune organ. Bacteria may translocate from the GI system and cannot be scavenged by Kupffer cells. Instead, they are released into the bloodstream, increasing the possibility of bacteremia.

Dysfunction of the hematological system adds to the complexity of the clinical picture. The patient is at risk for disseminated intravascular coagulation (DIC). In DIC, the platelets and the clotting factors are consumed, and secondary fibrinolysis develops, resulting in clinically significant bleeding from many orifices (see Chapter 33). Numerous blood laboratory values are altered (see Chapter 33, Table 33.21; see Tables 69.3 and 69.6).

Refractory Stage. In the final stage of shock, the *refractory stage*, decreased perfusion from peripheral vasoconstriction and decreased CO exacerbate anaerobic metabolism. The accumulation of lactic acid contributes to increased capillary permeability and dilation. Increased capillary permeability allows fluid and plasma proteins to leave the vascular space and move to the interstitial space. Blood pools in the capillary beds because of the constricted venules and dilated arterioles. The loss of intravascular volume worsens hypotension and tachycardia and decreases coronary blood flow. Decreased coronary blood flow leads to worsening myocardial depression and a further decline in CO. Cerebral blood flow cannot be maintained and cerebral ischemia results.

Patients in this stage of shock demonstrate profound hypotension and hypoxemia. The failure of the liver, the lungs, and the kidneys results in an accumulation of waste products, such as lactate, urea, ammonia, and CO_2. The failure of one organ system affects several other organ systems. Recovery is unlikely at this stage. The organs are in failure and the body's compensatory mechanisms are overwhelmed (see Table 69.6).

Diagnostic Studies

Establishing a diagnosis begins with a physical examination, a thorough medical and surgical history, and findings of recent medical events (e.g., upper respiratory tract infection, surgery, chest pain, trauma). Numerous laboratory studies must be collected initially and serially.

Decreased tissue perfusion in shock initially leads to an elevation of lactate levels (>4 mmol/L) and a high base deficit (the amount needed to bring the pH back to normal). These laboratory changes reflect an undesirable increase in anaerobic metabolism. Other laboratory values found in shock are summarized in Table 69.3.

Additional diagnostic studies include 12-lead ECG, continuous cardiac monitoring, chest radiography, continuous pulse oximetry, and hemodynamic monitoring (e.g., arterial pressure monitoring, central venous or PA pressure monitoring).

Interprofessional Care: General Measures

The management of shock and MODS is an interprofessional collaborative effort. The response needs to be coordinated, timely, and effective, with each member of the team contributing in accordance to their provincial scope of practice and institutional guidelines. All members of the health care team should recognize that patients experiencing shock have a high potential for instability and must be vigilant to detect changes in patient status. Nurses are expected to seek consultation and collaboration in the event a patient's condition deteriorates and the care required exceeds their scope of practice. Astute assessment skills and urgent communication with a rapid response team may prevent the decline to the progressive or refractory stage. Successful management includes (a) identification of patients at risk for the development of shock; (b) integration of the patient's history, physical examination, and clinical findings to establish a diagnosis; (c) interventions to control or eliminate the cause of the decreased perfusion; (d) protecting target and distal organs from dysfunction; and (e) providing multisystem supportive care.

Table 69.7 provides an overview of the initial assessment findings and interventions for the emergency care of patients in shock.

Oxygen and Ventilation. The nurse must ensure that the patient's airway is patent. Once the airway is established, either naturally or with an endotracheal tube, oxygen delivery must be optimized. Supplemental oxygen and mechanical ventilation may be required to maintain an arterial oxygen saturation of 90% or higher (PaO_2 >60 mm Hg) to avoid hypoxemia. The mean arterial pressure (MAP) and the circulating blood volume are optimized with fluid replacement and medication therapy. Oxygen delivery depends on CO, available hemoglobin, and arterial oxygen saturation (SaO_2). Methods to optimize oxygen delivery are directed at increasing supply and decreasing demand. Supply can be increased by (a) optimizing CO with medication therapy, fluid replacement, or both; (b) increasing hemoglobin through transfusion of whole blood or packed red blood cells (PRBCs); and (c) increasing the SaO_2 with supplemental oxygen or mechanical ventilation.

The nurse needs to plan care in such a way as to avoid disrupting the balance of oxygen supply and demand. Activities that increase oxygen consumption (e.g., endotracheal suctioning, position changes) need to be spaced appropriately for oxygen conservation. Continuous monitoring of central venous oxygen saturation ($ScvO_2$) by a central venous catheter or of mixed venous oxygen saturation (SvO_2) by a PA catheter is helpful. Both reflect the dynamic balance between oxygen supply and demand. These values need to be considered in conjunction with the SaO_2, CO, hemoglobin, and oxygen consumption to evaluate the patient's response to treatments or activities (see Chapter 68).

TABLE 69.7 EMERGENCY MANAGEMENT

Shock

Etiology*	Assessment Findings	Interventions
Surgical • Aortic dissection • GI bleeding • Postoperative bleeding • Rupture from ectopic pregnancy or of ovarian cyst • Rupture of organ or vessel • Vaginal bleeding **Medical** • Addisonian crisis • Dehydration • Diabetes insipidus • Diabetes mellitus • MI • Pulmonary embolus • Sepsis **Trauma** • Burns • Fractures, spinal injury • Multisystem or multiorgan injury • Rupture or laceration of vessel or organ (e.g., spleen)	• Anxiety • Chills • Confusion • Cool, clammy skin (warm skin in early stages of septic and neurogenic shock) • Cyanosis • Decreased level of consciousness • Decreased O_2 saturation • Dysrhythmias • Extreme thirst • Hypotension • Narrowed pulse pressure • Nausea and vomiting • Obvious hemorrhage or injury • Pallor • Rapid, weak, thready pulses • Restlessness • Sensation of impending doom • Tachypnea, dyspnea, or shallow, irregular respirations • Temperature dysregulation • Weakness	**Initial** • Administer humidified, high-flow oxygen (100%) by nonrebreather mask or bag–valve–mask device. • Anticipate need for intubation and mechanical ventilation. • Assess for life-threatening injuries (e.g., pericardial tamponade, liver laceration, tension pneumothorax). • Collect blood for laboratory studies (e.g., blood cultures, lactate measurement, WBC count). • Consider vasopressor therapy only after hypovolemia has been corrected. • Control any external bleeding with direct pressure or pressure dressing. • Establish and maintain patency of airway. • Establish IV access with two large-bore catheters, and begin fluid resuscitation with isotonic or hypertonic crystalloids (e.g., normal saline solution). • Insert an in-dwelling bladder catheter and nasogastric tube. • Institute antibiotic therapy if sepsis is suspected. • Stabilize cervical spine as appropriate. • Treat dysrhythmias. **Ongoing Monitoring** • Cardiac rhythm • Level of consciousness • Respiratory status • Urine output • Vital signs, including pulse oximetry, peripheral pulses, capillary refill

GI, gastrointestinal; *IV*, intravenous; *MI*, myocardial infarction; *WBC*, white blood cell.
*See Table 69.1 for additional causes of shock.

TABLE 69.8 FLUID THERAPY FOR SHOCK

Fluid Type	Mechanism of Action	Type of Shock	Nursing Implications
Crystalloids			
Isotonic			
0.9% NaCl (NS) most commonly used Lactated Ringer's solution	Fluid remains primarily in the intravascular space, increasing intravascular volume.	Used with caution for initial volume replacement in most types of shock	Patient is monitored closely for circulatory overload. Lactated Ringer's solution is contraindicated in patients with liver failure.
Hypertonic			
1.8%, 3%, or 5% NaCl	Fluid remains in the intravascular space, producing rapid volume expansion.	May be used for initial volume expansion in hypovolemic shock	Patient is monitored closely for signs of hypernatremia (e.g., disorientation, convulsions). Central line is required to limit damage to veins.
Blood/Blood Products			
Whole blood or packed RBCs Fresh-frozen plasma	These replace blood loss and increase oxygen-carrying capability. They also replace coagulation factors.	All types of shock if hemoglobin is <120 g/L or if the patient does not respond to crystalloids	Same precautions as for any blood administration (see Chapter 33).
Colloids			
Human serum albumin (5%, 25%), plasma protein fraction (5% albumin in 500 mL of NS)	This can increase plasma colloid osmotic pressure and produces rapid volume expansion.	All types of shock except cardiogenic and neurogenic shock	Patient is monitored for circulatory overload. Mild adverse effects of chills, fever, and urticaria may develop. Use 5% for hypovolemia. Use 25% for patients with fluid and sodium restrictions.
Dextran; dextran 40; dextran 70	This is a hyperosmotic glucose polymer; similar degrees of volume expansion are achieved with dextran, dextran 40, and dextran 70; duration of action is longer with dextran 70.	Limited use because of adverse effects, including reducing platelet adhesion, diluting clotting factors	Increases risk of bleeding. Patient is monitored for allergic reactions and AKI.

AKI, acute kidney injury; *NS,* normal saline solution; *RBCs,* red blood cells.

Fluid Resuscitation. The cornerstone of therapy for septic, hypovolemic, and anaphylactic shock is volume expansion with prompt and aggressive fluid resuscitation to restore tissue perfusion. Fluid resuscitation should begin with one or two large-bore (e.g., 14- or 16-gauge) IV catheters, intraosseous access devices, or a central venous catheter. Both crystalloids and colloids may have a role in fluid resuscitation (Table 69.8; see Chapter 19).

Crystalloids are the initial fluid of choice for severe hypovolemia. The exact ideal fluid is still debated. Currently, normal saline (NS) is the most often used in the initial resuscitation of shock; however, large-volume resuscitation with NS can lead to hyperchloremic metabolic acidosis.

Colloids have not been shown to improve patient outcomes, with the exception of PRBCs to correct for hypovolemia due to exsanguination (Winters et al., 2017).

Fluid responsiveness is determined by clinical assessment of vital signs, cerebral and abdominal perfusion pressures, capillary refill, skin temperature, and urine output. Hemodynamic parameters, such as CO, are also used. Trends in BP are monitored with an automatic BP cuff or an arterial catheter to assess the patient's response. An in-dwelling urinary catheter is used to monitor urine output during resuscitation.

The goal of fluid resuscitation is to restore tissue perfusion. Central venous pressure (CVP) monitoring is useful in monitoring hemodynamic status during acute fluid resuscitation. However, an assessment of end-organ perfusion (e.g., urine output, neurological function, peripheral pulses) provides more relevant data.

SAFETY ALERT
- Warm crystalloid and colloid solutions during massive fluid resuscitation. Fluids are warmed to prevent hypothermia and increase colloid aggregation. Warming is done with a rapid infuser with inline warmer, typically found in the emergency department, critical care unit, or operating room.
- When administering large volumes of packed red blood cells, remember they do not contain clotting factors. Replace these factors, via IV administration, on the basis of the clinical situation and results of laboratory studies.

Medication Therapy. The goal of medication therapy for shock is the correction of decreased tissue perfusion. Many of these medications have vasoconstrictor properties and are harmful if leaked into the tissues (i.e., extravasation); therefore, medications given to improve perfusion in shock are generally given intravenously via an infusion pump and central venous line (Table 69.9).

Sympathomimetic Medications. Many of the medications used in the treatment of shock have an effect on the SNS. Medications that mimic the action of the SNS are termed *sympathomimetic*. The effects of these medications are mediated through their binding to α- or β-adrenergic receptors. The various medications have different relative α-adrenergic and β-adrenergic effects (see Chapter 35, Table 35.1).

TABLE 69.9 MEDICATION THERAPY

*Shock**

Mechanism of Action	Hemodynamic Effects	Type of Shock	Nursing Implications
Dobutamine ↑ Myocardial contractility ↓ Ventricular filling pressures	↑ CO, stroke volume, and CVP ↑/↓ HR ↓ SVR and PAWP	Used for cardiogenic shock with severe systolic dysfunction Used for septic shock with normal CO that is not meeting metabolic demands	Hypovolemia is corrected. Should not be administered in the same catheter with $NaHCO_3$. Administration via central catheter is recommended (infiltration leads to tissue sloughing). HR and BP are monitored (hypotension may worsen, necessitating addition of a vasopressor). Patient is monitored for tachydysrhythmias.
Dopamine Precursor to epinephrine and norepinephrine Hemodynamic effects from release of norepinephrine Positive inotropic effects: ↑ Myocardial contractility ↑ Automaticity ↑ Atrioventricular conduction Low doses: ↑ blood flow to renal, mesenteric, and cerebral circulation High doses: can cause progressive vasoconstriction	↑ BP ↑ CO ↑ HR	Cardiogenic shock: • ↑ HR • ↑ Mean arterial pressure • ↑ MVO_2	Hypovolemia is corrected. Administer via central catheter (infiltration leads to tissue sloughing); should not be administered in same catheter with $NaHCO_3$. Patient is monitored for tachydysrhythmias. Patient is monitored for peripheral vasoconstriction at moderate to high doses (e.g., paresthesias, coldness in extremities).
Epinephrine (Adrenalin) Low doses: β-adrenergic agonist (cardiac stimulation, bronchial dilation, peripheral vasodilation) High doses: α-adrenergic agonist (peripheral vasoconstriction)	↑ HR, contractility, and CO ↓ SVR ↑ Stroke volume ↑ SVR ↑ Systolic BP, ↓ diastolic BP, widened pulse pressure ↑ CVP, PAWP	Cardiogenic shock combined with afterload reduction Anaphylactic shock Cardiac arrest, pulseless ventricular tachycardia, ventricular fibrillation, asystole	Hypovolemia is corrected if necessary. Patient is monitored for HR >110 beats/min. Patient is monitored for dyspnea and pulmonary edema. Patient is monitored for renal failure secondary to ischemia. Patient is monitored for chest pain, dysrhythmias secondary to ↑ MVO_2.
Hydrocortisone Decreases inflammation; reverses increased capillary permeability	↑ BP, HR	Septic shock necessitating vasopressor therapy, despite fluid resuscitation, to maintain adequate BP Anaphylactic shock if hypotension persists past initial therapy	Patient is monitored for hypokalemia and hyperglycemia.
Norepinephrine (Levophed) β₁-Adrenergic agonist (cardiac stimulation) α-Adrenergic agonist (peripheral vasoconstriction) Renal and splanchnic vasoconstriction	↑ BP, MAP ↑ CVP, PAWP ↑ SVR ↑ or ↓ CO	Cardiogenic shock after MI Septic shock: works by increasing vascular tone	Used for hypotension unresponsive to adequate fluid resuscitation. Administered via a central catheter (infiltration leads to tissue sloughing). Patient is monitored for dysrhythmias secondary to ↑ MVO_2 requirements.
Phenylephrine α-Adrenergic agonist Vasoconstriction: renal, mesenteric, splanchnic, cutaneous, and pulmonary vessels	↑ HR ↑ BP ↑ SVR ↑↓ CO	Neurogenic shock	Patient is monitored for reflex bradycardia, headache, restlessness. Patient is monitored for renal failure secondary to ↓ renal blood flow. Administered via central catheter (infiltration leads to tissue sloughing).
Nitroglycerin Venous dilation Dilates coronary arteries ↓ Preload ↓ MVO_2	↓ SVR ↓ BP	Cardiogenic shock	Patient is continuously monitored for BP and for reflex tachycardia. Use glass bottles for storage of medication.

Continued

TABLE 69.9   MEDICATION THERAPY

Shock—cont'd

Mechanism of Action	Hemodynamic Effects	Type of Shock	Nursing Implications
Sodium Nitroprusside (Nipride)			
Arterial and venous vasodilation	↓ BP	Cardiogenic shock with ↑ SVR	BP is continuously monitored.
↓ Preload, afterload	↑↓ CO		Solution should be protected from light; infusion bottle should be wrapped with opaque covering.
	↓ CVP, PAWP		Administered with D_5W only.
			Patient is monitored for cyanide toxicity (e.g., tinnitus, hyper-reflexia, confusion, seizures).
Vasopressin			
ADH, nonadrenergic vasoconstrictor	↑ MAP	Shock states (most commonly septic shock) refractory to other vasopressors	Low dose usually administered.
	↓ Need for other vasopressors		Hemodynamic pressures and urine output are monitored.
	↑ Urine output		

ADH, antidiuretic hormone; *BP*, blood pressure; *CO*, cardiac output; *CVP*, central venous pressure; D_5W, 5% dextrose in water; *HR*, heart rate; *MAP*, mean arterial pressure; *MI*, myocardial infarction; MVO_2, myocardial oxygen consumption; $NaHCO_3$, sodium bicarbonate; *PAWP*, pulmonary artery wedge pressure; *SVR*, systemic vascular resistance.
*Individual facility's guidelines, pharmacist, pharmacology references, and medication manufacturer's administration materials should be consulted for additional information and dosage recommendations.

Many of these medications cause peripheral vasoconstriction and are referred to as *vasopressor medications* (e.g., dopamine, epinephrine, norepinephrine). These medications can cause severe peripheral vasoconstriction and an increase in SVR, further jeopardizing tissue perfusion. The increased SVR increases the workload of the heart and can be detrimental to a patient in cardiogenic shock by causing further myocardial damage and increasing risk for dysrhythmias. Use of vasopressor medications is generally reserved for patients whose condition has been unresponsive to fluid resuscitation. Adequate fluid resuscitation must be achieved before the use of any vasopressors because peripheral vasoconstrictor effects in patients with low blood volume cause further reduction in tissue perfusion.

The goal of vasopressor therapy is to achieve and maintain a MAP of at least 65 mm Hg (Stratton et al., 2017). The nurse must continuously monitor end-organ perfusion (e.g., urine output, level of consciousness, serum lactate levels) to ensure tissue perfusion is adequate.

Vasodilator Medications. Some patients in shock show evidence of excessive vasoconstriction and poor tissue perfusion in spite of fluid replacement and normal or even high systemic BP. This is especially true of patients in cardiogenic shock. Although generalized sympathetic vasoconstriction is a useful compensatory mechanism for maintaining systemic pressure, excessive constriction can reduce tissue blood flow and increase the workload of the heart. Patients in cardiogenic shock have decreased myocardial contractility, and vasodilators may be needed to decrease afterload. The rationale for using vasodilator therapy for a patient in shock is to break the harmful cycle of widespread vasoconstriction, which causes a decrease in CO and BP, resulting in further SNS-induced vasoconstriction.

The goal of vasodilator therapy, as in vasopressor therapy, is to maintain a MAP greater than 65 mm Hg. Other hemodynamic parameters (e.g., CVP) are also monitored so that fluids can be increased or vasodilator therapy decreased if CO or BP falls dramatically. The vasodilator agent most often used in cardiogenic shock is nitroglycerin. Vasodilation may be enhanced with nitroprusside in noncardiogenic shock.

Nutritional Therapy. Protein–calorie malnutrition common in shock is due to hypermetabolism. Good nutrition is vital to decreasing morbidity. Enteral nutrition to enhance perfusion of the GI tract and help maintain the integrity of the gut mucosa should be initiated within the first 24 hours. Slow, continuous enteral feedings are started for the first week and advanced only as tolerated. Parenteral nutrition is often required when enteral nutrition is contraindicated or not meeting the patient's nutritional needs. However, it must be used with caution because the dextrose can cause hyperglycemia, and the lipids can have an immunosuppressive effect (McClave et al., 2016) (see Chapter 42).

The patient should be weighed on the same scale at the same time of day. If significant weight loss is noted, dehydration must be ruled out before additional calories are provided. Large weight gains are common because of third spacing of fluids. Therefore, daily weight measurements serve as a better indicator of fluid status than caloric needs and balance. Serum protein, nitrogen balance, BUN, serum glucose level, and serum electrolyte values are all used to assess nutritional status.

Special consideration should be given when access to care is limited, as in rural or remote parts of Canada or on reserve, where tertiary care may be unavailable. Timely transfer of patients to specialized care facilities is best practice and a human right.

Interprofessional Care: Specific Measures

Cardiogenic Shock. For a patient in cardiogenic shock, the overall goal is to restore heart function by increasing perfusion of the myocardium through restoring the balance between oxygen supply and demand. Specific measures to restore blood flow include thrombolytic therapy, angioplasty with stent implantation, emergency revascularization, and valve replacement (see Chapter 36). Cardiac catheterization should be performed as soon as possible after the initial insult. Coronary angioplasty with or without stent implantation may be performed during cardiac catheterization. Until these interventions are performed, SV and CO must be optimized to facilitate optimal perfusion (Table 69.10; see also Table 69.9).

The aim of hemodynamic management is to reduce the workload of the heart through medication therapy, mechanical interventions, or both. Early recognition and prompt revascularization through percutaneous coronary intervention or coronary artery bypass grafting substantially improve survival rates.

| TABLE 69.10 | **INTERPROFESSIONAL CARE** |

Specific Strategies for the Treatment of Shock

Oxygenation	Circulation	Medication Therapies	Supportive Therapies
Cardiogenic Shock • Provide supplemental O_2 (e.g., nasal cannula, nonrebreather mask) • Intubation and mechanical ventilation, if needed • Monitor $ScvO_2$ or SvO_2	• Restore blood flow with angioplasty with stenting, emergent coronary revascularization • Reduce workload of heart with circulatory assist devices: IABP, VAD	• Nitrates (e.g., nitroglycerin) • Inotropes (e.g., dobutamine) • Diuretics (e.g., furosemide) • β-Adrenergic blockers (contraindicated with ↓ ejection fraction)	Treat dysrhythmias
Hypovolemic Shock • Provide supplemental O_2 • Monitor $ScvO_2$ or $ScvO_2$	• Rapid fluid replacement using two large-bore (14–16 gauge) peripheral IV lines, an intraosseous access device, or central venous catheter • Restore fluid volume (e.g., blood or blood products, crystalloids) • End points of fluid resuscitation: • CVP 15 mm Hg • PAWP 10–12 mm Hg	No specific medication therapy	• Correct the cause (e.g., stop bleeding, GI losses) • Use warmed IV fluids, including blood products (if appropriate)
Septic Shock • Provide supplemental O_2 • Intubation and mechanical ventilation, if needed • Monitor $ScvO_2$ or SvO_2	• Aggressive fluid resuscitation (e.g., 30 mL/kg of crystalloids repeated if hemodynamic improvement is noted) • End points of fluid resuscitation are based on the following: Focused physical examination including vital signs, cardiopulmonary assessment, capillary refill, peripheral pulses, and skin or any two of the following: • $ScvO_2$ >70 or SvO_2 >65 • CVP 8–12 mm Hg • Cardiovascular ultrasound • Assessment of fluid responsiveness with passive leg raise or fluid challenge	• Antibiotics as ordered • Vasopressors (e.g., norepinephrine) • Inotropes (e.g., dobutamine) • Anticoagulants (e.g., low-molecular-weight heparin)	• Obtain cultures (e.g., blood, wound) before beginning antibiotics • Monitor temperature • Control blood glucose • Stress ulcer prophylaxis
Neurogenic Shock • Maintain patent airway • Provide supplemental O_2 • Intubation and mechanical ventilation (if needed)	Cautious administration of fluids	• Vasopressors (e.g., phenylephrine) • Atropine (for bradycardia)	• Minimize spinal cord trauma with stabilization • Monitor temperature
Anaphylactic Shock • Maintain patent airway • Optimize oxygenation with supplemental O_2 • Intubation and mechanical ventilation, if needed	Aggressive fluid resuscitation with colloids	• Epinephrine (IM or IV) • Antihistamines (e.g., diphenhydramine) • Histamine (H_2)-receptor blockers (e.g., ranitidine [Zantac]) • Bronchodilators: nebulized (e.g., albuterol) • Corticosteroids (if hypotension persists)	• Identify and remove offending cause • Prevent through avoidance of known allergens • Premedicate with history of prior sensitivity (e.g., contrast media)
Obstructive Shock • Maintain patent airway • Provide supplemental O_2 • Intubation and mechanical ventilation, if needed	• Restore circulation by treating cause of obstruction • Fluid resuscitation may provide temporary improvement in CO and BP	No specific medication therapy	• Treat cause of obstruction (e.g., pericardiocentesis for cardiac tamponade, needle decompression or chest tube insertion for tension pneumothorax, embolectomy for pulmonary embolism)

CVP, central venous pressure; *GI*, gastrointestinal; *IABP*, intra-aortic balloon pump; *IM*, intramuscular; *IV*, intravenous; *PAWP*, pulmonary artery wedge pressure; *ScvO₂*, central venous oxygen saturation; *SvO₂*, venous oxygen saturation; *VAD*, ventricular assist device.
Source: Harding, M., Kwong, J., Roberts, D., et al. (2020). *Lewis's medical-surgical nursing* (11th ed., p. 1580, Table 66.9). Elsevier.

Fibrinolytic therapy is another option for reperfusion. Inotropes and vasopressors in low doses are effective pharmacological agents. Medications are used to decrease the workload of the heart by dilating coronary arteries (e.g., nitrates) and reducing preload (e.g., diuretics), afterload (e.g., vasodilators), and heart rate and cardiac contractility (e.g., β-adrenergic blockers).

Patients may also benefit from treatment with a circulatory assist device such as an intra-aortic balloon pump (IABP) or a ventricular assist device (VAD) (see Chapter 68). The goal of IABP is to increase coronary blood flow and thus decrease left ventricular workload. The VAD is used when cardiogenic shock is refractory to the IABP or fibrinolytic therapy. It is a temporary measure for patients who are in cardiogenic shock or awaiting cardiac transplantation. Cardiac transplantation is an option for a small, select group of patients with cardiogenic shock.

Hypovolemic Shock. The underlying principles of managing hypovolemic shock focus on stopping the loss of fluid and restoring the circulating volume. Fluid resuscitation in hypovolemic shock initially is calculated according to a 3:1 rule (3 mL of isotonic crystalloid for every 1 mL of estimated blood loss). Table 69.8 delineates the different types of fluid used for volume resuscitation, the mechanisms of action, and specific nursing implications for each fluid type.

Septic Shock. Patients in septic shock need to be identified early and to receive aggressive fluid resuscitation (≥30 mL/kg crystalloid fluid) in order to achieve hemodynamic improvement (Levy et al., 2018). Predetermined end points of fluid resuscitation are suggested in Table 69.10. To optimize and evaluate large-volume fluid resuscitation, hemodynamic monitoring with a central venous catheter and arterial pressure monitoring may be necessary. If fluid resuscitation is unsuccessful, vasopressor medication therapy may be added. Vasodilation and low CO, or vasodilation alone, can cause low BP in spite of adequate volume resuscitation. Norepinephrine is the first-choice vasopressor to initially increase MAP (Timmerman, 2016). Vasopressin, an ADH, may be given for patients whose condition is refractory to norepinephrine (Timmerman, 2016). Exogenous vasopressin is used to replace the stores of physiological vasopressin that are often depleted in septic shock.

MEDICATION ALERT—Vasopressin
- Infuse at low doses (e.g., 0.03 U/min).
- Do not titrate infusion.
- Use with caution in patients with coronary artery disease.

Vasopressor medications may increase BP but may also decrease SV. Often, an inotropic agent (e.g., dobutamine) is added to offset the decrease in SV (see Table 69.9). Corticosteroids are not recommended; however, IV corticosteroids (e.g., hydrocortisone 200 mg/day) may be used, only when hemodynamic status is not improving despite fluid resuscitation attempts and vasopressor therapy. In an attempt to meet the increasing tissue demands coupled with a low SVR, the patient initially demonstrates normal or high CO. If the patient is unable to achieve and maintain adequate CO and has unmet tissue oxygen demands, CO may have to be increased through medication therapy (e.g., dopamine). The adequacy of CO can be assessed with SvO_2 monitoring. The SvO_2 (normal, 65–75%) is a reflection of the balance between oxygen delivery and consumption (see Chapter 68). If the balance is maintained, the tissue demands are met.

Antimicrobial therapy is an important and early component of therapy. Broad-spectrum antibiotics should be administered within the first hour of sepsis or septic shock (Levy et al., 2018). However, before definitive treatment for the infection can begin, the cause of the infection must be identified. Therefore, cultures (e.g., blood, wound exudate, urine, stool, sputum) are obtained before antimicrobial medications are started. Broad-spectrum antimicrobials (e.g., antibiotics, antifungals, antivirals) are given initially, followed by more specific medication once the organism has been identified (Levy et al., 2018).

Glucose levels should be maintained at less than 10 mmol/L (Gunst & Van den Berghe, 2017). Stress ulcer prophylaxis with histamine H_2-receptor blockers (e.g., famotidine [Pepcid]) or proton pump inhibitors (e.g., pantoprazole) are recommended for patients with risk of bleeding. Deep venous thrombosis prophylaxis using low-molecular-weight heparin (e.g., enoxaparin) is recommended (Rhodes et al., 2017).

Neurogenic Shock. The specific treatment of neurogenic shock depends on the cause. If the cause is spinal cord injury, general measures to promote spinal stability (e.g., spinal precautions, cervical stabilization with a collar) are initially used. Once the spine is stabilized, treatment of the hypotension and bradycardia is essential to prevent further spinal cord damage. Treatment involves the use of vasopressors (e.g., phenylephrine) to maintain BP and organ perfusion (see Table 69.9). Bradycardia may be treated with atropine. Fluids are administered with caution because the cause of the hypotension is not related to fluid loss.

The patient with a spinal cord injury also needs to be monitored for hypothermia because of hypothalamic dysfunction (see Table 69.10). Although corticosteroids do not have an effect in neurogenic shock, methylprednisolone (Solu-Medrol) is used for patients with a spinal cord injury to prevent secondary spinal cord damage caused by the release of chemical mediators (see Chapter 63).

Anaphylactic Shock. The first strategy in managing patients at risk of developing anaphylactic shock is prevention. The clinical presentation of anaphylactic shock is dramatic and requires immediate intervention. The World Allergy Organization anaphylaxis guidelines (2015) recommend epinephrine as the first line of treatment (Simons et al., 2015). Ideally, an intramuscular (IM) epinephrine auto-injector dose is self-administered at the onset of an event, prior to hospitalization. IV epinephrine is used with anaphylactic shock and must not be delayed. Overdosing of epinephrine can lead to detrimental cardiovascular effects, such as hypertension, stroke, and even death; however, the benefits far outweigh the risks.

The second line of treatment includes H_1-antihistamines (e.g., diphenhydramine [Benadryl]) and H_2-antihistamines (e.g., Zantac), which block the histamine receptors. IV glucocorticoids are used to prevent further episodes or anaphylaxis. These medications should be used in combination with epinephrine.

Maintaining a patent airway is important because the patient can quickly develop airway compromise from laryngeal edema or bronchoconstriction. Nebulized bronchodilators are highly effective. Aerosolized epinephrine can also be used to treat laryngeal edema. Endotracheal intubation or cricothyroidotomy may be necessary to secure and maintain airway patency. Hypotension results from leakage of fluid out of the intravascular space into the interstitial space because of increased vascular permeability and vasodilation. Aggressive fluid resuscitation, predominantly with crystalloids, is necessary (see Tables 69.9 and 69.10).

NURSING MANAGEMENT SHOCK

NURSING ASSESSMENT

The initial assessment should be focused on the ABCs: **a**irway, **b**reathing, and **c**irculation. Further assessment includes evaluation of vital signs, level of consciousness, peripheral pulses, capillary refill, skin (e.g., temperature, colour, moisture), and urine output. As shock progresses, the patient's skin becomes cooler and mottled, urine output decreases, peripheral pulses diminish, and neurological status deteriorates.

To understand the complexity of the patient's clinical status, the nurse must integrate all of the assessment data. It is essential to obtain a brief history from the patient or a substitute decision maker. This information should include a description of the events leading to the shock condition, time at onset and duration of symptoms, and a health history (e.g., past medical history, allergies, medications, date of last tetanus vaccination, recent travel). In addition, the nurse must obtain details regarding any care the patient received prior to hospitalization.

NURSING DIAGNOSES

Nursing diagnoses for the patient in shock may include but are not limited to the following:

- *Inadequate peripheral tissue perfusion, potential for decreased cardiac tissue perfusion, inadequate cerebral tissue perfusion, and potential for reduced liver function*
- *Anxiety* resulting from *threat of death, threat to current status* (severity of condition)

Additional information on nursing diagnoses for the patient with shock is presented in Nursing Care Plan (NCP) 69.1, available on the Evolve website. Many other diagnoses are relevant, and examples appear in other chapters.

PLANNING

The overall goals for patients in shock include (a) restoration of adequate tissue perfusion; (b) normal vital signs, specifically a MAP greater than 65 mm Hg; (c) recovery of organ function; and (d) prevention of progression toward further complications related to prolonged states of hypoperfusion.

NURSING IMPLEMENTATION

HEALTH PROMOTION. Nurses have a vital role in identifying patients at risk of developing shock. In general, patients who are older, those with debilitating illnesses, and those who are immunocompromised are at increased risk. Any person who sustains surgical or accidental trauma is at high risk for shock as a result of hemorrhage, spinal cord injury, and other conditions (see Table 69.1). Any patient who is at risk for decreased oxygen delivery or tissue hypoxia is also at risk for the development of shock.

Planning is essential to help prevent shock after a susceptible individual has been identified. For example, a patient diagnosed with an acute anterior MI is at risk for cardiogenic shock. The primary goal in this scenario is to limit the size of the infarction. The infarct size can be limited by restoring coronary blood flow through thrombolytic therapy, percutaneous coronary intervention, or surgical revascularization. Rest, analgesics, and sedation can reduce the myocardial demand for oxygen. The patient's

environment should be modified to provide care intermittently so that the patient's oxygen demand is not increased. For example, if the patient becomes fatigued or anxious during bathing, this care can be done at a time that does not interfere with tests or other activities that may also increase oxygen demand.

A person with a severe allergy to such substances as medications, shellfish, and insect bites is at increased risk of developing anaphylactic shock. This risk can be decreased if the patient is carefully questioned regarding allergies before a medication is administered or before the patient undergoes diagnostic procedures involving the use of contrast media. If a patient's condition warrants receiving a medication to which they are at high risk for an allergic reaction (e.g., contrast media), institutions may have a prophylactic premedication policy involving diphenhydramine, methylprednisolone, or both. Patients with severe allergies should wear a medical alert bracelet or identifier that identifies their allergies. Patients and persons close to them should always have an epinephrine auto-injector available.

Careful monitoring of fluid balance can help prevent hypovolemic shock. This involves ongoing assessment of intake and output and daily weight measurements. In addition, monitoring the patient's clinical status is essential; identifying trends in clinical findings is more meaningful than any single piece of clinical information.

All patients need to be monitored carefully for infection. Progression from an infection to sepsis and septic shock depends on the patient's host defence mechanisms. Patients who are immunocompromised or immunosuppressed are at especially high risk for opportunistic infections. These patients may be ventilated or have numerous invasive lines. Strategies to decrease the risk for nosocomial or health care–associated infections (HAIs) include decreasing the number of in-dwelling catheters (e.g., central lines, urinary catheters), using aseptic technique during invasive procedures, and paying strict attention to hand hygiene. All equipment must be thoroughly cleaned, or discarded, according to institutional policy. Evidence-informed guidelines are available to reduce the risk of HAIs (e.g., ventilator-associated pneumonia, central-line infections, and catheter-associated urinary tract infections) (see the Resources at the end of Chapter 71). These guidelines, called *bundles*, outline key interventions aimed at reducing infections (Table 69.11).

ACUTE INTERVENTION. The nurse's role in caring for patients with shock involves (a) monitoring the patient's ongoing physical and emotional status, (b) planning and quickly implementing nursing interventions and therapy, (c) evaluating the patient's response to therapy, (d) identifying trends to detect

TABLE 69.11	SURVIVING SEPSIS CAMPAIGN CARE BUNDLE*

To Be Completed Within 1 Hour

1. Measure lactate level. Remeasure if initial lactate is >2 mmol/L.
2. Obtain blood cultures prior to administration of antibiotics.
3. Administer broad-spectrum antibiotics.
4. Administer 30 mL/kg crystalloid for hypotension or lactate level ≥4 mmol/L.
5. Apply vasopressors if patient is hypotensive during or after fluid resuscitation to maintain MAP ≥65 mm Hg.

*Targets for quantitative resuscitation included in the guidelines are central venous pressure (CVP) of ≥8 mm Hg, central venous oxygen saturation (ScvO₂) of ≥70%, and normalization of lactate.
Source: Levy, M., Evans, L., & Rhodes, A. (2018). The surviving sepsis campaign bundle: 2018 update. *Intensive Care Medicine, 44*, 925–928. 10.1007/s00134-018-5085-0.

changes in the patient's condition, (e) providing emotional support to the patient and family, and (f) collaborating with other members of the health care team to coordinate care (see NCP 69.1 on the Evolve website).

Neurological Status. Neurological status, including orientation and level of consciousness, should be assessed every 1 to 2 hours. The patient's neurological status is the best indicator of cerebral blood flow. The nurse needs to be aware of neurological clinical manifestations such as changes in behaviour, restlessness, hypervigilance, blurred vision, confusion, and paresthesia. Any subtle changes in the patient's mental status (e.g., mild agitation) must be noted.

The patient should be oriented to time, place, person, and events. If the patient is in a critical care unit, orientation to the environment is particularly important. The nurse should reduce noise and light levels to control sensory input. A day–night cycle of activity and rest should be maintained as much as possible. Sensory overload and disruption of the patient's circadian cycle may contribute to delirium.

Cardiovascular Status. Most therapy for shock is based on information about the patient's cardiovascular status. If the patient is unstable, the nurse needs to carefully assess the heart rate, BP, CVP, and the PA pressures, including continuous CO (if available). (Hemodynamic monitoring is discussed in Chapter 68.) Monitoring trends in hemodynamic parameters yields more important information than individual values. Integration of hemodynamic data with physical assessment data is essential in planning strategies to manage patients with shock.

Patients with shock classically exhibit hypotension, which should be treated with fluid resuscitation, medications, or a combination of these, after the type of shock has been identified. The Trendelenburg position should be avoided as the patient could experience compromised pulmonary function and increased intracranial pressure.

The patient's ECG should be monitored continuously to detect dysrhythmias. Heart sounds should be assessed for the presence of an S_3 or S_4 sound or new murmurs. An S_3 sound in an adult may indicate heart failure. The frequency of monitoring can be decreased as the patient's condition improves.

In addition to monitoring the patient's cardiovascular status, the nurse must administer the prescribed therapy to correct the dysfunctions of the cardiovascular system. The patient's response to fluid and medication administration is assessed and titrated as often as every 5 to 15 minutes. Changes in temperature, pallor, flushing, cyanosis, diaphoresis, and piloerection may indicate hypoperfusion. Once tissue perfusion is restored and the patient is stabilized, the frequency of monitoring can be decreased, and the patient is slowly weaned off medications that support BP and tissue perfusion.

Respiratory Status. The respiratory status of the patient in shock must be frequently assessed to ensure adequate oxygenation, detect complications early, and provide data regarding the patient's acid–base status. The rate, depth, and rhythm of respirations are initially monitored as frequently as every 15 to 30 minutes. Increased rate and depth provide information regarding the patient's attempts to correct metabolic acidosis. Breath sounds should be assessed every hour for any changes that may indicate fluid overload or accumulation of secretions.

Pulse oximetry is used to continuously monitor oxygen saturation; however, pulse oximetry using a patient's finger or toe may not be accurate in an advanced state of shock because of poor peripheral circulation. In this situation, the probe should

be attached to the nose, the ear, or the forehead (according to the manufacturer's guidelines). Arterial blood gasses (ABGs) provide information on ventilation and oxygenation status and on acid–base balance. Initial interpretation of ABGs is often the nurse's responsibility. A PaO_2 below 60 mm Hg (in the absence of chronic lung disease) indicates the presence of hypoxemia and the need for administration of higher oxygen concentrations or for a different mode of oxygen administration. Low partial pressure of arterial carbon dioxide ($PaCO_2$) with a low pH and low bicarbonate level may indicate that the patient's respiratory system is attempting to compensate for metabolic acidosis.

A rising $PaCO_2$ with a persistently low pH and PaO_2 may indicate the need for advanced pulmonary management. Many patients in shock are intubated and provided mechanical ventilation. Maintaining airway patency and monitoring for ventilator-related complications is critical. (Artificial airways and mechanical ventilation are discussed in Chapter 68.)

Renal Status. Hourly measurements of urinary output are essential to assess the adequacy of renal perfusion. An indwelling bladder catheter is inserted to facilitate measurements. Urine output of less than 0.5 mL/kg/hour may indicate inadequate perfusion of the kidneys. BUN and serum creatinine values are additional indicators used to assess renal function; however, serum creatinine is a better indicator of renal function because BUN levels can be influenced by the catabolic state of the patient.

Body Temperature. When temperature is normal, it should be monitored every 4 hours. If it is elevated or subnormal, tympanic or pulmonary arterial temperatures should be monitored hourly. If the temperature rises above 38.3°C and the patient becomes uncomfortable or experiences cardiovascular compromise, the fever may be managed with nonsteroidal anti-inflammatory drugs (NSAIDs) (e.g., ibuprofen [Advil]), with acetaminophen (Tylenol), or by removing some of the patient's bed covers. A cooling device may be considered if fever persists despite treatment.

Skin Integrity. The patient's skin should be monitored for temperature, pallor, flushing, cyanosis, diaphoresis, and piloerection. In addition, capillary refill should be assessed as an indicator of peripheral perfusion.

Gastrointestinal Status. Bowel sounds should be auscultated at least every 4 hours, and abdominal distension should be assessed. If a nasogastric tube is inserted, drainage should be measured and checked for occult blood. Stools should also be checked for occult blood.

Personal Hygiene. Hygiene is especially important for patients in shock because impaired tissue perfusion predisposes the skin to breakdown and infection. However, bathing and other nursing measures must be carried out judiciously because of difficulties with oxygen delivery to tissues. The nurse must use clinical judgement to determine priorities of care, to limit the demands for increased oxygen.

Passive range-of-motion exercises should be performed three to four times per day to maintain joint mobility. The patient should be turned at least every 1 to 2 hours and positioned in good body alignment to help prevent pressure injuries. A pressure-relieving mattress or a specialty bed may also be needed. If possible, oxygen consumption (e.g., SvO_2 or $ScvO_2$) should be monitored during all nursing interventions to monitor the patient's tolerance of activity.

Oral care is essential because mucous membranes may become dry and fragile in the state of volume depletion. In addition, patients who are intubated usually have difficulty swallowing, which results in pooled secretions in the mouth. A water-soluble lubricant applied to the lips prevents drying and cracking. Moist swabbing of the tongue and oral mucosa with saline solution or diluted mouthwash is also beneficial.

Emotional Support and Comfort. The nurse must recognize that the patient and family are faced with a critical, life-threatening situation and may experience reactions such as anxiety, fear, and pain. The nurse should address these responses, as such symptoms may aggravate respiratory distress and increase the release of catecholamines. Medications to decrease anxiety and pain are common modes of therapy. Continuous infusions of a benzodiazepine (e.g., lorazepam) and an opioid or anaesthetic (e.g., morphine, propofol) are helpful in decreasing anxiety, pain, and oxygen demand.

Goals of care and prognosis should be discussed as early as feasible, with consideration of end-of-life care planning and palliative care principles where appropriate. The nurse must not overlook the patients' spiritual needs. Patients may want a visit from a chaplain, priest, rabbi, or minister. One way to provide support is to offer to call a spiritual member of the patient's community rather than wait for the patient or caregiver to express a wish for spiritual counselling. Special consideration should be given when caring for Indigenous people. Requests for spiritual care, such as from an Indigenous Elder, Medicine Man, priest, or minister, are to be accommodated whenever possible. Requested spiritual items must not be moved, thrown out, or otherwise disrespected. It is important to recognize that Indigenous patients may have a mixture of traditional and contemporary beliefs. Consulting with patients and caregivers about meeting their cultural needs is required for practising cultural competence. If staff are asked to attend ceremonies, every effort should be made for someone to attend. Please refer to Chapter 2 for further information regarding cultural competence and how it relates to nursing care for critically ill patients.

The patient's caregivers need to be kept informed of the patient's condition. The nurse needs to give the patient and caregiver simple explanations of all procedures before carrying them out and provide information regarding the plan of care. If they ask questions about progress and prognosis, simple and honest answers should be provided.

When possible, the same nurse(s) should continually care for the patient. This practice can decrease anxiety, limit conflicting information, and increase trust. If the prognosis becomes grave, the nurse needs to support the patient and their caregiver(s) when making tough decisions, such as withdrawing life support. The interprofessional care team must promote realistic expectations and outcomes. Compassion is as essential as scientific and technical expertise in the total care of the patient and caregiver.

The nurse must ensure that the caregiver can spend time with the patient, provided the patient perceives this time as comforting. The nurse should explain in simple terms the purpose of any tubes and equipment attached to or surrounding the patient. Caregivers should be told what they may and may not touch. If possible, the patient's hands and arms should be placed outside the sheets to encourage therapeutic touch. The nurse can encourage caregivers to perform simple comfort measures if desired. Privacy should be provided as much as possible, and the nurse should assure the patient and caregiver that help is readily available should it be needed. The call light should always be positioned within reach of the patient or caregiver.

AMBULATORY AND HOME CARE. Rehabilitation of a patient who has experienced critical illness requires correction of the precipitating cause, prevention and treatment of subsequent complications, and education focused on disease management and prevention of recurrence. An interprofessional approach involving allied health services on discharge is necessary for success. The nurse should continue to monitor the patient for complications throughout the recovery period. Complications may include decreased range of motion, decreased physical endurance, renal failure after acute tubular necrosis (see Chapter 49), and the development of fibrotic lung disease as a result of ARDS (see Chapter 70). Thus, patients recovering from shock may require diverse services on discharge. These may include admission to transitional care units (e.g., for weaning from mechanical ventilation), rehabilitation centres (inpatient or outpatient), and home health care agencies. The nurse should start planning for the patient's safe transition from hospital to home as soon as the patient is admitted to the hospital.

Additional consideration should be given for patients returning to rural or remote parts of Canada, including an Indigenous reserve. There may be a lack of or insufficient access to home care services, equipment, or medications. It is important to find out if there is a nursing station on reserve or in the community. Also, food insecurity and access to clean water may pose a significant barrier to discharge, depending on where the patient lives. The patient's disposition and ability to continue to recover at home should be considered when planning discharge timelines.

EVALUATION

Expected outcomes for the patient with shock are addressed in NCP 69.1, available on the Evolve website.

SEPSIS, SEPTIC SHOCK, AND MULTIPLE-ORGAN DYSFUNCTION SYNDROME

Sepsis is life-threatening organ dysfunction caused by a dysregulated host response to infection (Singer et al., 2016). In lay terms, *sepsis* is a life-threatening condition that arises when the body's response to an infection injures its own tissues and organs. As stated earlier, *septic shock* is a subset of sepsis, in which underlying circulatory and cellular and metabolic abnormalities are profound enough to substantially increase mortality.

Multiple-organ dysfunction syndrome (MODS), often referred to as *multisystem organ failure,* is the failure of two or more organ systems in an acutely ill patient such that homeostasis cannot be maintained without intervention (Gourd & Nikitas, 2019). Mortality increases as a greater number of systems fail (Gourd & Nikitas, 2019).

Organ and Metabolic Dysfunction. When the inflammatory response is not controlled, the consequences include the release of mediators, direct damage to the endothelium, and hypermetabolism. Vasodilation becomes excessive and leads to decreased SVR and hypotension. In addition, vascular permeability increases, allowing mediators and proteins to leak out of the endothelium and into the interstitial space. White blood cells (WBCs) begin to phagocytize foreign debris, and the coagulation cascade is activated. Hypotension, decreased systemic perfusion, microemboli, and redistributed or shunted blood flow eventually compromise organ perfusion.

The respiratory system is commonly the first system to show signs of dysfunction in MODS. Inflammatory mediators have a direct effect on the pulmonary vasculature. The endothelial damage from the release of inflammatory mediators causes increased capillary permeability and facilitates movement of proteinaceous fluid from the pulmonary vasculature into the pulmonary interstitial spaces. The fluid then moves to the alveoli, causing alveolar edema. Type I pneumocytes (alveolar cells) are destroyed. Type II pneumocytes become dysfunctional, and surfactant production decreases. The alveoli collapse, leading to an increase in *shunt* (blood flow to the lungs that does not participate in gas exchange) and a worsening of the VQ mismatch. The end result is ARDS. Patients with ARDS require aggressive pulmonary management with mechanical ventilation (see Chapter 70).

Cardiovascular changes in MODS include myocardial depression and massive vasodilation in response to increasing tissue demands. Vasodilation results in decreased SVR and BP. The baroreceptor reflex causes release of *inotropic* (increase force of contraction) and *chronotropic* (increase heart rate) factors that enhance CO. To compensate for hypotension, CO rises through an increase in heart rate and SV. Increases in capillary permeability cause a shift of albumin and fluid out of the vascular space, further diminishing venous return and thus preload. The patient becomes warm and tachycardic, with a high CO and a low SVR. Other signs of MODS include decreased capillary refill, skin mottling, increases in CVP and PAWP, and dysrhythmias. SvO_2 may be abnormally high because the patient is perfusing areas not consuming much oxygen (e.g., skin, nonworking muscle). Other areas may be having blood shunted away from them. Eventually, either perfusion of vital organs becomes insufficient or the cells are unable to use oxygen and their function is further compromised.

Neurological dysfunction from MODS commonly manifests as mental status changes. Acute alteration can be an early sign of MODS. The patient may become confused and agitated, combative, disoriented, lethargic, or comatose. These changes may be caused by hypoxemia, the direct effect of the inflammatory mediators, or impaired perfusion.

AKI is frequent in MODS. Hypoperfusion and the effect of the mediators can cause AKI. When kidney perfusion is decreased, the SNS and the renin–angiotensin system are activated. Stimulation of the renin–angiotensin system causes systemic vasoconstriction and aldosterone-mediated sodium and water reabsorption. Another risk factor for the development of AKI is the use of nephrotoxic medications. Antibiotics used to treat Gram-negative bacteria (e.g., aminoglycosides) can be nephrotoxic. Careful monitoring of medication levels is essential to avoid the nephrotoxic effects.

The GI tract is highly affected during the development of MODS. GI motility is often decreased in critical illness, and this condition results in abdominal distension and paralytic ileus. In the early stages of MODS, blood is shunted away from the GI mucosa; thus the mucosa is highly vulnerable to ischemic injury. Decreased perfusion leads to a breakdown of this normally protective mucosal barrier, thus increasing the risk for ulceration and GI bleeding and the potential for bacterial translocation from the GI tract into the systemic circulation.

Metabolic changes are pronounced in MODS. MODS triggers a hypermetabolic response. Glycogen stores are rapidly converted to glucose (*glycogenolysis*). Once glycogen is depleted, amino acids are converted to glucose (*gluconeogenesis*), which reduces protein stores. Fatty acids are mobilized for fuel. Catecholamines and glucocorticoids are released, causing hyperglycemia and insulin resistance. The net result is a catabolic state, and lean body mass (muscle) is lost.

The hypermetabolism associated with MODS may last for several days and results in liver dysfunction. Liver dysfunction may exist long before it is clinically evident. Protein synthesis is impaired, leading to the liver being unable to synthesize albumin, one of the key proteins that has an essential role in maintaining plasma oncotic pressure. Consequently, plasma oncotic pressure is altered, and fluid and protein leak from the vascular spaces to the interstitial space. Administration of albumin does not normalize oncotic pressure in this situation.

As the state of hypermetabolism persists, the patient's body becomes unable to convert lactate to glucose, and lactate accumulates (lactic acidosis). Despite increases in glycogenolysis and gluconeogenesis, eventually the liver cannot maintain an adequate glucose level, and the patient becomes hypoglycemic.

DIC, or simultaneous microvascular clotting and bleeding, may occur because of the depletion of clotting factors and platelets in addition to excessive fibrinolysis (see Chapter 33).

Electrolyte imbalances are common and result from hormonal and metabolic changes and fluid shifts. These changes exacerbate mental status changes, neuromuscular dysfunction, and dysrhythmias. The release of ADH and aldosterone results in sodium and water retention. Aldosterone increases urinary potassium loss, and catecholamines cause potassium to move into the cell, which results in hypokalemia. Hypokalemia is associated with dysrhythmias and muscle weakness. Metabolic acidosis results from impairment in tissue perfusion, hypoxia, and a shift to anaerobic metabolism with a resultant increase in hydrogen ion production. This process increases lactate levels. Progressive renal dysfunction also contributes to metabolic acidosis. Hypocalcaemia, hypomagnesemia, and hypophosphatemia are common.

Clinical Manifestations

The clinical manifestations of MODS are presented in Table 69.12 and are important to consider when evaluating patients for shock and MODS.

Clinical Criteria for Identifying Patients With Sepsis and Septic Shock. Sepsis is identified through use of the Quick Sequential [Sepsis-Related] Organ Failure Assessment (qSOFA) and the Sequential [Sepsis-Related] Organ Failure Assessment (SOFA). The qSOFA comprises three variables to identify patients with sepsis and septic shock: respiratory rate, mental status, and systolic blood pressure. The SOFA has seven variables used to identify patients with sepsis and septic shock: PaO_2/FiO_2 ratio, Glasgow Coma Scale score, MAP, administration of vasopressors with type and dose rate of infusion, serum creatinine or urine output, bilirubin, and platelet count. The qSOFA is meant to be used as a rapid assessment outside of the critical care unit (e.g., prehospital paramedicine, emergency department), and the SOFA is meant to be calculated in the critical care unit.

NURSING AND INTERPROFESSIONAL MANAGEMENT MULTIPLE-ORGAN DYSFUNCTION SYNDROME

Without early, goal-directed therapy, the prognosis for patients with MODS is poor. Mortality rates range from about 40% with two systems involved to 100% with seven systems involved (Gourd & Nikitas, 2019). While sepsis is not the only precursor for MODS (e.g., cardiogenic shock), the most common cause of death is related to sepsis.

A critical component of the nursing role is vigilant assessment and ongoing monitoring to detect early signs of deterioration or organ dysfunction. Interprofessional care for patients with MODS focuses on (a) prevention and treatment of infection, (b) maintaining tissue oxygenation, (c) nutritional and

TABLE 69.12 MULTIPLE-ORGAN DYSFUNCTION SYNDROME

Clinical Manifestations and Management

Clinical Manifestations of Organ Failure	Management	Clinical Manifestations of Organ Failure	Management
Cardiovascular System Biventricular failure ↓ Ejection fraction, contractility ↑ HR, ↑ SVR, ↓ CO ↓ MAP ↓ Stroke volume Myocardial depression Systolic, diastolic dysfunction	Balancing O_2 supply and demand • Supplemental O_2 • Continuous SvO_2 monitoring Circulatory assist devices • Intra-aortic balloon pump • Ventricular assist devices Continuous ECG monitoring Hemodynamic monitoring • Arterial pressure catheter • Central venous or PA catheter • PAWP readings • Maintaining MAP >65 mm Hg Maintaining CO • Volume management • Vasopressors, inotropes, vasodilators VTE prophylaxis	**Hematological System** ↑ Bleeding times, ↑ PT, ↑ PTT, ↑ INR ↑ D-dimer test results ↑ Fibrin split products ↓ Platelet count (thrombocytopenia)	Minimizing traumatic interventions (e.g., intramuscular injections, multiple venipunctures) Observation for bleeding from obvious and occult sites Replacement of factors being lost (e.g., platelets)
		Hepatic System Bilirubin >34 mcmol/L ↑ Liver enzymes (ALT, AST, GGT) ↑ Serum NH_3 ↓ Serum albumin, prealbumin, transferrin Jaundice Hepatic encephalopathy	Maintenance of adequate tissue perfusion Nutritional support (e.g., enteral feedings) Judicious use of hepatically metabolized medications
Central Nervous System Acute change in neurological status Confusion, disorientation Failure to wean, prolonged rehabilitation Fever Hepatic encephalopathy Seizures	Evaluation for hepatic and metabolic encephalopathy Optimization of cerebral blood flow ↓ Cerebral oxygen requirements Prevention of secondary tissue ischemia • Calcium channel blockers (reduce cerebral vasospasm) Prevention of further compromise	**Renal System** Prerenal: renal hypoperfusion • BUN/creatinine ratio >20:1 • ↓ Urine Na^+ level to <40 mmol/L • ↑ Urine specific gravity to >1.020 • ↑ Urine osmolality Intrarenal: ATN BUN/creatinine ratio <10:1–15:1 • ↑ Urine Na^+ level to >40 mmol/L • ↓ Urine osmolality • Urine specific gravity (≈1.010)	Diuretics • Loop diuretics (e.g., furosemide [Lasix]) • May need to increase dose because of ↓ glomerular filtration rate Dopamine (Intropin) • Enhances renal blood flow • Improves renal perfusion • Increases urine output (if volume resuscitated) • May work synergistically with diuretics Continuous renal replacement therapy (see Chapter 49)
Endocrinological System Hyperglycemia → hypoglycemia	Continuous infusion of insulin and glucose to maintain blood glucose at <8.33 mmol/L		
Gastrointestinal System Mucosal ischemia • ↓ Intramucosal pH • Potential translocation of gut bacteria Hypoperfusion → ↓ peristalsis, paralytic ileus Mucosal ulceration on endoscopy GI bleeding	Dietary consultation Enteral feedings • Provide essential nutrients and optimal calories • Stimulate mucosal activity Stress ulcer prophylaxis • Antacids (e.g., Maalox) • Histamine H_2-receptor blockers (e.g., famotidine [Pepcid]) • Proton pump inhibitors (e.g., omeprazole) • Sucralfate	**Respiratory System** Development of ARDS (see Chapter 70): • Severe dyspnea • PaO_2/FiO_2 ratio <200 • Bilateral fluffy infiltrates on chest radiograph • PAWP <18 mm Hg • Ventilation–perfusion mismatch • Pulmonary hypertension • Increased minute ventilation • Increased respiratory rate • Decreased compliance • Refractory hypoxemia	Prevention Optimizing oxygen delivery, minimizing oxygen consumption Mechanical ventilation (see Chapter 68) • Positive end-expiratory pressure • Lung protective modes (e.g., pressure control or inverse ratio ventilation, low tidal volumes) • Permissive hypercapnia Positioning (e.g., continuous lateral rotation therapy, prone positioning)

ALT, alanine aminotransferase; *ARDS,* acute respiratory distress syndrome; *AST,* aspartate aminotransferase; *ATN,* acute tubular necrosis; *BUN,* blood urea nitrogen; *CO,* cardiac output; *ECG,* electrocardiograph; *FiO2,* fraction of inspired oxygen; *GGT,* γ-glutamyl transferase; *GI,* gastrointestinal; *HR,* heart rate; *INR,* international normalized ratio; *MAP,* mean arterial pressure; *PA,* pulmonary artery; *PaO2,* partial pressure of arterial oxygen; *PAWP,* pulmonary artery occlusive pressure; *PT,* prothrombin time; *PTT,* partial thromboplastin time; *SvO2,* venous oxygen saturation; *SVR,* systemic vascular resistance; *VTE,* venous thromboembolism.

metabolic support, and (d) appropriate support of individual failing organs. Table 69.12 summarizes the management for patients with MODS.

PREVENTION AND TREATMENT OF INFECTION

Aggressive infection control strategies are essential to decrease the risk for HAIs. Strict asepsis practice can help decrease infections related to intra-arterial lines, endotracheal tubes, urinary catheters, IV lines, and other invasive devices or procedures. Daily

assessment of the ongoing need for invasive lines is an important strategy to mitigate HAIs. Aggressive pulmonary management, including early ambulation, can reduce the risk for infection.

Despite these strategies, infection may develop. Once an infection is suspected, interventions to control the source must be instituted. Appropriate cultures should be taken, and broad-spectrum antibiotic therapy should be initiated. Early, aggressive surgery is recommended to remove necrotic tissue (e.g., early debridement of burn tissue) that may provide a culture medium for microorganisms. Once a specific organism is identified, therapy should be modified, if necessary.

MAINTENANCE OF TISSUE OXYGENATION

Hypoxemia frequently occurs because patients have greater oxygen needs and decreased oxygen supply to the tissues. Interventions that decrease oxygen demand and increase oxygen delivery are essential. Analgesia, sedation, mechanical ventilation, and rest may decrease oxygen demand and should be considered. Oxygen delivery may be optimized by maintaining normal levels of hemoglobin (e.g., transfusion of PRBCs) and PaO_2 (80–100 mm Hg), using individualized tidal volumes with positive end-expiratory pressure (PEEP), increasing preload or myocardial contractility to enhance CO, or reducing afterload to increase CO. Treating fever, chills, and pain decreases oxygen demand.

NUTRITIONAL AND METABOLIC NEEDS

Hypermetabolism can result in profound weight loss, cachexia, and further organ failure. Protein–calorie malnutrition is a primary manifestation of hypermetabolism. Total energy expenditure is often increased to 1.5 to 2.0 times the normal metabolic rate. Because of their relatively short half-life, plasma transferrin and prealbumin levels are monitored to assess hepatic protein synthesis.

The goal of nutritional support is to preserve organ function. Providing early and optimal nutrition decreases morbidity and mortality rates. Ideally, the patient consumes intake orally. If the patient is unable to do so, the enteral route is initiated slowly and increased as tolerated. If enteral nutrition is not meeting caloric needs, parenteral nutrition should be initiated or added. (Enteral and parenteral nutrition are discussed in Chapter 42.) Tight glycemic control (blood glucose level of <10 mmol/L) with the use of insulin guidelines is important in these patients (Gunst & Van den Berghe, 2017).

SUPPORT OF FAILING ORGANS

Support of any failing organs is a primary goal of therapy. For example, the patient with ARDS requires aggressive oxygen therapy and mechanical ventilation (see Chapter 70). DIC should be treated appropriately (e.g., blood products) (see Chapter 33). Renal failure may necessitate dialysis. Continuous renal replacement therapy is better tolerated than hemodialysis, especially in a patient with hemodynamic instability (see Chapter 49).

Given the poor prognosis for MODS, withdrawal of life support may need to be considered when all resuscitative attempts fail. Clear communication between the health care team and the patient's substitute decision maker(s) about realistic goals and likely outcomes is crucial. It is important to ensure that advance directives are clearly indicated and that the team follows the patient's wishes regarding end-of-life care.

CASE STUDY

Shock

Patient Profile
K. M. (pronouns he/him), 25 years old, was not wearing his seat belt when the car he was driving was involved in a motor vehicle accident. The windshield was broken, and K.M. was found 5 metres from his car. He was lying face down, conscious, and moaning. K. M.'s partner and daughter were found in the car with their seat belts on. They sustained no serious injuries but were upset. All passengers were taken to the emergency department (ED). The following information pertains to K. M.

Subjective Data
- States, "I can't breathe"
- Cries out when abdomen is palpated

Objective Data
Physical Examination
- Cardiovascular: BP 80/56 mm Hg; apical pulse 138 but no palpable radial or pedal pulses; carotid pulse present but weak
- ECG as follows:

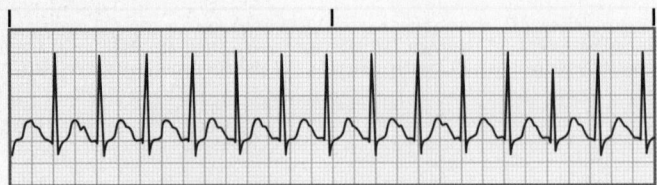

- Lungs: respiratory rate 38 breaths/min, laboured breathing with shallow respirations, asymmetrical chest wall movement, absence of breath sounds on left side
- Musculoskeletal: open compound fracture of the lower left leg
- Trachea deviated slightly to the right
- Abdomen is slightly distended and left upper quadrant painful on palpation

Diagnostic Studies
- Chest radiograph: Hemothorax and six rib fractures on left side
- Hematocrit: 0.28 volume fraction

Interprofessional Care (in the ED)
- Left chest tube placed, draining bright red blood
- IV access obtained via two peripheral lines and a right subclavian central line
- Fluid resuscitation started with crystalloids
- High-flow oxygen via nonrebreather mask

Surgical Procedure
- Repair of compound fracture
- Repair of torn intercostal artery
- Splenectomy

Discussion Questions
1. What types of shock is K. M. experiencing? What clinical manifestations did he display that support this answer?
2. What were the causes of K. M.'s shock states? What are other causes of these types of shock?
3. *Priority decision:* What are the priority nursing responsibilities for K. M.?
4. *Priority decision:* What ongoing nursing assessment parameters are essential for this patient?
5. What are K. M.'s potential complications?
6. *Priority decision:* Based on the assessment data presented, what are the priority nursing diagnoses?
7. *Evidence-informed practice:* The nurse is orienting a new graduate RN. The graduate asks why crystalloids are used instead of colloids for fluid resuscitation. What should the nurse's response be?

evolve
Answers are available at http://evolve.elsevier.com/Canada/Lewis/medsurg.

REVIEW QUESTIONS

The number of the question corresponds to the same-numbered objective at the beginning of the chapter.

1. A client has a spinal cord injury at T4. Vital signs include hypotension with bradycardia. The nurse recognizes that the client is experiencing which of the following?
   a. Relative hypervolemia
   b. Absolute hypovolemia
   c. Neurogenic shock–induced low blood flow
   d. Neurogenic shock–induced massive vasodilation

2. A 78-year-old client has confusion and a temperature of 40°C. The client has a medical history of diabetes and has a wound with purulent drainage to the right heel. After an infusion of 3 L of normal saline solution, assessment findings are BP 84/40 mm Hg; heart rate 110; respiratory rate 42 and shallow; CO 8 L/min; and PAWP 4 mm Hg. This client's symptoms are most likely indicative of which of the following?
   a. Neurogenic shock
   b. Cardiogenic shock
   c. Septic shock
   d. Multiple-organ dysfunction syndrome

3. Treatment modalities for the management of cardiogenic shock include which of the following? *(Select all that apply.)*
   a. Dobutamine to increase myocardial contractility
   b. Vasopressors to increase systemic vascular resistance
   c. Circulatory assist devices such as an intra-aortic balloon pump
   d. Trendelenburg positioning to facilitate venous return and increase preload

4. The most accurate assessment parameters for the nurse to use to determine adequate tissue perfusion in the client with MODS are which of the following?
   a. Blood pressure, pulse, and respirations
   b. Breath sounds, blood pressure, and body temperature
   c. Pulse pressure, level of consciousness, and pupillary response
   d. Level of consciousness, urine output, as well as skin colour and temperature

1. d; 2. b; 3. a, c; 4. d.

ⓔvolve

For even more review questions, visit http://evolve.elsevier.com/Canada/Lewis/medsurg.

REFERENCES

Alhazzani, W., Hylander Møller, M., Arabi, Y. M., et al. (2020). Surviving sepsis campaign: Guidelines on the management of critically ill adults with coronavirus disease 2019 (COVID-19). *Intensive Care Medicine, 46*, 854–887. https://doi.org/10.1007/s00134-020-06022-5

Bellani, G., Laffey, J., Pham, T., et al. (2016). Epidemiology, patterns of care, and mortality for patients with acute respiratory distress syndrome in intensive care units in 50 countries. *Journal of the American Medical Association, 315*(8), 788–800. https://doi.org/10.1001/jama.2016.0291

Beltrán-Garcia, J., Osca-Verdegal, R., Pallardó, F., et al. (2020). Sepsis and coronavirus disease 2019: Common features and anti-inflammatory therapeutic approaches. *Critical Care Medicine.* https://doi.org/10.1097/CCM.0000000000004625. https://doi.org/10.1097/CCM.0000000000004625

Good, V., & Kirkwood, P. (2017). *Advanced critical care nursing* (2nd ed.). Elsevier.

Gourd, N., & Nikitas, N. (2019). Multiple organ dysfunction syndrome. *Journal of Intensive Care Medicine, 35*(12), 1564–1575. https://doi.org/10.1177/0885066619871452

Gunst, J., & Van den Berghe, G. (2017). Blood glucose control in the ICU. How tight? *Annals of Translational Medicine, 5*(4), 76–78. https://doi.org/10.21037/atm.2017.01.45

Iriyama, H., Abe, T., Kushimoto, S., et al. (2020). Risk modifiers of acute respiratory distress syndrome in patients with non-pulmonary sepsis: A retrospective analysis of the FORECAST study. *Journal of Intensive Care, 8*(7), 1–9. https://doi.org/10.1186/s40560-020-0426-9

Levy, M., Evans, L., & Rhodes, A. (2018). The surviving sepsis campaign bundle: 2018 update. *Intensive Care Medicine, 44*, 925–928. https://doi.org/10.1007/s00134-018-5085-0

Loverde, D., Iweala, O., Eginli, A., et al. (2018). Anaphylaxis. *Chest, 153*(2), 528–543. https://doi.org/10.1016/j.chest.2017.07.033

McClave, S., Taylor, B., Martindale, R., et al. (2016). Guidelines for the provision and assessment of nutrition support therapy in the adult critically ill patient: Society of Critical Care Medicine (SCCM) and American Society for Parenteral and Enteral Nutrition (A.S.P.E.N.). *Journal of Parenteral and Enteral Nutrition, 40*(2), 159–211. https://doi.org/10.1177/0148607115621863

Navaneelan, T., Alam, S., Peters, P., et al. (2016). *Health at a glance: Deaths involving sepsis in Canada.* http://www.statcan.gc.ca/pub/82-624-x/2016001/article/14308-eng.htm

Rhodes, A., Evans, L., Alhazzani, W., et al. (2017). Surviving sepsis campaign. International guidelines for management of sepsis and septic shock (2016). *Intensive Care Medicine, 43*, 304–377. https://doi.org/10.1007/s00134-017-4683-6

Rudd, K., Johnson, S., Agesa, K., et al. (2020). Global, regional, and national sepsis incidence and mortality, 1990–2017: Analysis for the Global Burden of Disease Study. *The Lancet, 395*(10219), 200–211. https://doi.org/10.1016/S0140-6736(19)32989-7

Simons, F., Ebisawa, M., Sanchez-Borges, M., et al. (2015). 2015 update of the evidence base: World Allergy Organization anaphylaxis guidelines. *World Allergy Organization Journal, 8*, 1–16. https://doi.org/10.1186/s40413-015-0080-1

Singer, M., Deutschman, C., Seymour, C., et al. (2016). The third international consensus definitions for sepsis and septic shock (Sepsis-3). *Journal of the American Medical Association, 315*(8), 801–810. https://doi.org/10.1001/jama.2016.0287

Stratton, L., Verlin, D., & Arbo, J. (2017). Vasopressors and inotropes in sepsis. *Emergency Medicine Clinics of North America, 35*(1), 75–91. https://doi.org/10.1016/j.emc.2016.09.005

Taylor, M., Wrenn, P., & O'Donnell, A. (2017). Presentation of neurogenic shock within the emergency department. *Emergency Medicine Journal, 34*(3), 157–162. https://doi.org/10.1136/emermed-2016-205780

Timmerman, R. (2016). Managing vasoactive infusions to restore hemodynamic stability. *Critical Care Nursing, 11*(2), 35–43. https://doi.org/10.1097/01.CCN.0000480748.85354.b3

Vahadatpour, C., Collins, D., & Goldberg, S. (2019). Cardiogenic shock. *Journal of the American Heart Association, 8*(8), 1–12. https://doi.org/10.1161/JAHA.119.011991

Winters, M., Sherwin, R., Vilke, G., et al. (2017). What is the preferred resuscitation fluid for patients with severe sepsis and septic shock? *Journal of Emergency Medicine, 53*(6), 928–939. https://doi.org/10.1016/j.jemermed.2017.08.093

Zhou, F., Yu, T., Du, R., et al. (2020). Clinical course and risk factors for mortality of adult patients with COVID-19 in Wuhan, China: A retrospective cohort study. *The Lancet, 395*(10229), 1054–1062. https://doi.org/10.1016/S0140-6736(20)30566-3

RESOURCES

Resources for this chapter are listed in Chapter 71.

Nursing Management
Respiratory Failure and Acute Respiratory Distress Syndrome

Debbie Rickeard
Originating US chapter by Eugene Mondor

⊖volve WEBSITE

http://evolve.elsevier.com/Canada/Lewis/medsurg

- Review Questions
  (Online Only)
- Key Points
- Answer Guidelines for Case
  Study

- Student Case Studies
  - Acute Respiratory Failure and Ventilatory
    Management
  - Pulmonary Embolism and Respiratory
    Failure

- Customizable Nursing Care Plan
  - Acute Respiratory Failure
- Conceptual Care Map Creator
- Audio Glossary
- Content Updates

LEARNING OBJECTIVES

1. Compare the pathophysiological mechanisms that result in hypoxemic and hypercapnic respiratory failure.
2. Differentiate between early and late clinical manifestations of acute respiratory failure.
3. Describe the nursing and interprofessional management of a patient with hypoxemic or hypercapnic respiratory failure.
4. Explain how the pathophysiological mechanisms that result in acute respiratory distress syndrome are related to the clinical manifestations of this syndrome.

5. Describe the nursing and interprofessional management of a patient with acute respiratory distress syndrome.
6. Identify complications that may result from acute respiratory failure or acute respiratory distress syndrome and measures to prevent or reverse these complications.

KEY TERMS

acute respiratory distress syndrome (ARDS)	hypercapnia	hypoxemic respiratory failure
alveolar hypoventilation	hypercapnic respiratory failure	hypoxia
diffusion limitation	hypoxemia	refractory hypoxemia

The normal function of the respiratory system is to facilitate gas exchange. Without an adequate exchange of oxygen (O_2) and carbon dioxide (CO_2), the metabolic demands of the tissues would not be met, and body systems would begin to rapidly fail. The management of patients in acute respiratory distress or failure revolves around the improvement of oxygenation and ventilation, treatment of the underlying disease state, reduction of anxiety, and prevention and management of complications. Acute respiratory failure and acute respiratory distress syndrome (ARDS) represent important and costly public health conditions. The global effect of ARDS is difficult to estimate.

The in-hospital rate of mortality from ARDS has remained high since it was first described; current mortality rates range from 40 to 50% (Virani et al., 2019). Patients with ARDS require critical nursing assessments and interprofessional management to improve their outcomes, which is the focus of this chapter.

ACUTE RESPIRATORY FAILURE

The major function of the respiratory system is gas exchange, which involves the transfer of O_2 and CO_2 between the atmosphere and the blood (Figure 70.1; Urden et al., 2020). *Respiratory failure* is the state in which one or both gas-exchanging

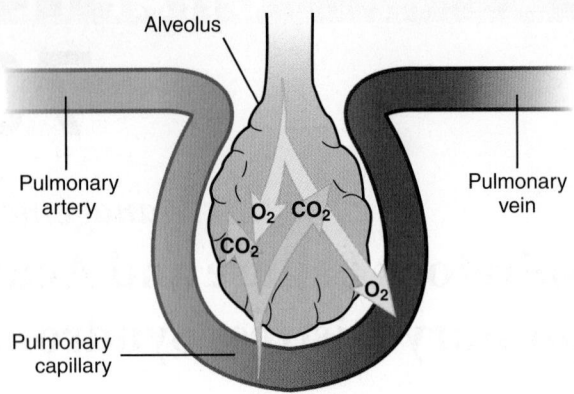

FIG. 70.1 Normal gas-exchange unit in the lung.

TABLE 70.1	ABBREVIATIONS OF COMMON PULMONARY TERMS
Arterial Blood Monitoring	
ABGs	Arterial blood gases
pH	Negative log of the free hydrogen ion [H$^+$]
PaO$_2$	Partial pressure of oxygen in arterial blood
PaCO$_2$	Partial pressure of carbon dioxide in arterial blood
SaO$_2$	Oxygen saturation in arterial blood as measured by ABGs
SpO$_2$	Oxygen saturation in arterial blood as measured by pulse oximetry
Oxygen and Lung Function Monitoring	
FiO$_2$	Fraction of inspired oxygen concentration
FRC	Functional residual capacity (volume of air in lung at end of expiration)
PEEP	Positive end-expiratory pressure (pressure in lungs at end of expiration)
PEFR	Peak expiratory flow rate (maximum airflow during a forced expiration)
VQ	Ventilation–perfusion ratio (relationship of ventilation to perfusion in the lungs)
V$_E$	Minute ventilation (tidal volume × respiratory rate)
V$_T$	Tidal volume (volume of air inspired with each breath)

functions are inadequate: Either the amount of O$_2$ transferred to the blood is insufficient or the amount of CO$_2$ removed from the lungs is inadequate. Clinical states that interfere with O$_2$ transfer result in **hypoxemia**—a state of low oxygen tension in the blood (partial pressure of oxygen in arterial blood [PaO$_2$] <60 mm Hg), characterized by a variety of nonspecific clinical signs and symptoms—and a decrease in arterial oxygen saturation (SaO$_2$) as determined by measurements of arterial blood gases (ABGs). Insufficient CO$_2$ removal results in **hypercapnia**, the presence of excessive amounts of CO$_2$ in the blood; also called *hypercarbia*, it is manifested by an increase in partial pressure (or tension) of carbon dioxide in arterial blood (PaCO$_2$; Brashers & Huether, 2018). ABGs can be measured to intermittently assess changes in pH, PaO$_2$, PaCO$_2$, bicarbonate, and SaO$_2$, and oxygen saturation can be assessed intermittently or continuously with pulse oximetry (SpO$_2$). Pulse oximetry offers advantages of noninvasiveness and real-time values; however, the accuracy of readings depends on correct application of the sensor to a well-perfused digit, usually a middle or ring finger. When the SpO$_2$ is 90%, the PaO$_2$ is approximately 60 mm Hg, if factors such as temperature, PaCO$_2$, and pH are normal (Virani et al., 2019). Data should be interpreted alongside clinical assessment findings and the patient's baseline values. For example, an individual with chronic lung disease may have a baseline PaCO$_2$ higher than what is considered the "normal" range. (To assist the reader, Table 70.1 summarizes abbreviations used in this chapter.)

Respiratory failure is not a disease; it is a condition that occurs as a result of one or more diseases involving the lungs or other body systems (Tables 70.2 and 70.3). It is classified as hypoxemic or hypercapnic (Figure 70.2). *Hypoxemic respiratory failure* is also referred to as *oxygenation failure* because the primary problem is inadequate O$_2$ transfer between the alveoli and the pulmonary capillary bed. Although no universal definition exists, **hypoxemic respiratory failure** is commonly defined as a PaO$_2$ of 60 mm Hg or less when the patient is receiving inspired oxygen at a fractional concentration (FiO$_2$) of 60% or greater. This definition incorporates two important concepts: (1) the PaO$_2$ level indicates inadequate O$_2$ saturation of hemoglobin, and (2) this PaO$_2$ level exists despite administration of supplemental O$_2$ at a percentage (60%) that is three times that in room air (21%). Disorders that interfere with O$_2$ transfer into the blood include pneumonia, pulmonary edema, pulmonary emboli, alveolar injury related to inhalation of toxic gases (e.g., smoke inhalation), and ventilator-induced lung injury. In addition, states of low cardiac output (e.g., heart failure, shock) can also cause hypoxemic respiratory failure (Urden et al., 2020).

TABLE 70.2	TYPES OF RESPIRATORY FAILURE AND COMMON CAUSES*
Hypoxemic Respiratory Failure	
Respiratory system	Acute respiratory distress syndrome (ARDS)
	Pneumonia
	Toxic inhalation (smoke inhalation)
	Hepatopulmonary syndrome (low-resistance flow state, ventilation–perfusion [VQ] mismatch)
	Massive pulmonary embolism (e.g., thrombus emboli, fat emboli)
Cardiac system	Anatomical shunt (e.g., ventricular septal defect)
	Cardiogenic pulmonary edema
	Shock (decreasing blood flow through pulmonary vasculature)
Hypercapnic Respiratory Failure	
Respiratory system	Asthma
	Chronic obstructive pulmonary disease (COPD)
	Cystic fibrosis
Central nervous system	Brainstem infarction
	Sedative and opioid (Fentanyl) overdose
	Spinal cord injury
	Severe head injury
Chest wall	Thoracic trauma (e.g., flail chest)
	Kyphoscoliosis
	Pain
	Morbid obesity
Neuromuscular system	Myasthenia gravis
	Critical illness polyneuropathy
	Acute myopathy
	Toxic ingestion (e.g., tree tobacco)
	Amyotrophic lateral sclerosis
	Phrenic nerve injury
	Guillain-Barré syndrome
	Poliomyelitis
	Muscular dystrophy
	Multiple sclerosis

*This list is not all-inclusive.

Hypercapnic respiratory failure is referred to as *ventilatory failure* because the primary problem is insufficient CO$_2$ removal. **Hypercapnic respiratory failure** is commonly defined as a PaCO$_2$ above normal (>45 mm Hg) in combination with acidemia (arterial pH <7.35). This definition incorporates three important concepts:

TABLE 70.3   PREDISPOSING FACTORS FOR ACUTE RESPIRATORY FAILURE

Predisposing Factors	Mechanisms of Respiratory Failure
Airways and Alveoli	
Acute respiratory distress syndrome (ARDS) • *Direct lung injury:* Aspiration; severe, disseminated pulmonary infection; near-drowning; toxic gas inhalation; airway contusion • *Indirect lung injury:* Sepsis or septic shock, severe nonthoracic trauma, cardiopulmonary bypass	Fluid enters the interstitial space and the alveoli, markedly impairing gas exchange. The result is an initial ↓ in PaO_2 and a later ↑ in $PaCO_2$. A low-flow state to pulmonary capillaries can result in ischemic injury to lung tissues with loss of integrity of the alveolar–capillary membrane.
Asthma	Bronchospasm escalates in severity rather than responding to therapy. Bronchospasm, edema of the bronchial mucosa, and plugging of small airways with secretions greatly reduce airflow. Work of breathing increases, causing respiratory muscle fatigue. ↓ in PaO_2 and ↑ in $PaCO_2$ (see Chapter 31).
Chronic obstructive pulmonary disease (COPD)	Alveoli are destroyed by protease–antiprotease imbalance or respiratory infection, or an exacerbation of COPD escalates in severity rather than responding to therapy. Secretions obstruct airflow. Work of breathing increases and causes respiratory muscle fatigue. ↓ in PaO_2 and ↑ in $PaCO_2$.
Cystic fibrosis	Abnormal Na^+ and Cl^- transport results in secretions that are viscous, poorly cleared, and therefore foci for infection. Over time, the airways become clogged with copious, purulent sputum. Secretions obstruct airflow. Repeated infections destroy alveoli. Work of breathing increases, causing respiratory muscle fatigue. ↓ in PaO_2 and ↑ in $PaCO_2$.
Central Nervous System	
Overdose of opioid or other CNS depressant	Respirations are slowed by medication effect. Insufficient CO_2 is excreted, resulting in ↑ $PaCO_2$.
Brainstem infarction, head injury	Medulla cannot alter respiratory rate in response to changes in $PaCO_2$.
Chest Wall	
Severe soft tissue injury, flail chest, rib fracture, pain	Structural dysfunction and pain prevent normal rib cage expansion, resulting in inadequate gas exchange.
Kyphoscoliosis	Change in spinal configuration compresses the lungs and prevents normal expansion of the chest wall, resulting in inadequate gas exchange.
Morbid obesity	Weight of the chest and abdominal contents prevents normal rib cage movement, resulting in inadequate gas exchange.
Neuromuscular Conditions	
Cervical cord injury, phrenic nerve injury	Neural control is lost, preventing use of the diaphragm, the major muscle of respiration. Consequently, the patient inspires a smaller tidal volume, which predisposes to an ↑ in $PaCO_2$.
Amyotrophic lateral sclerosis (ALS), Guillain-Barré syndrome, muscular dystrophy, multiple sclerosis (MS), poliomyelitis, myasthenia gravis, myopathy, critical illness polyneuropathy, prolonged use of neuromuscular blocking agents	Respiratory muscle weakness or paralysis occurs, preventing normal CO_2 excretion. Dysfunction may be progressive (muscular dystrophy, MS), progressive with no potential of recovery (ALS), rapid with good expectation of recovery (Guillain-Barré syndrome), or stable for extended periods (poliomyelitis, myasthenia gravis).

CNS, central nervous system; *PaCO₂,* partial pressure of carbon dioxide in arterial blood; *PaO₂,* partial pressure of oxygen in arterial blood.

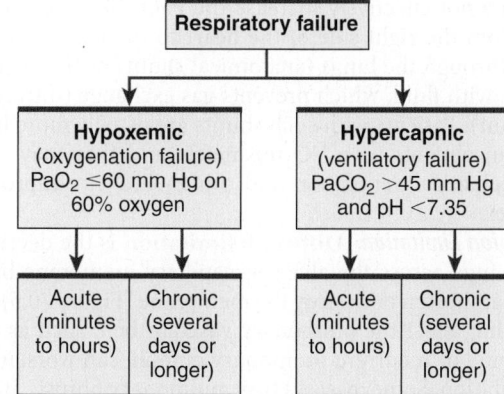

FIG. 70.2 Classification of respiratory failure. *PaCO₂,* partial pressure of carbon dioxide in arterial blood; *PaO₂,* partial pressure of oxygen in arterial blood.

(1) the $PaCO_2$ is higher than normal, (2) there is evidence of the body's inability to compensate for this increase (acidemia), and (3) the pH is at a level at which a further decrease may lead to severe acid–base imbalance. (See Chapter 19 for a discussion of acid–base balance.) Conditions that compromise lung ventilation and subsequent CO_2 removal include drug overdoses with central nervous system (CNS) depressants, neuromuscular diseases (e.g.,

myasthenia gravis), and trauma or diseases involving the spinal cord and its role in lung ventilation. Many patients experience both hypoxemic and hypercapnic respiratory failure.

Etiology and Pathophysiology

Hypoxemic Respiratory Failure. Common diseases and conditions that cause hypoxemic respiratory failure are listed in Table 70.2. Four physiological mechanisms may cause hypoxemia and subsequent hypoxemic respiratory failure: (1) mismatch between ventilation (V) and perfusion (Q), commonly referred to as *VQ mismatch*; (2) shunting; (3) diffusion limitation; and (4) hypoventilation. The most common causes are VQ mismatch and shunting.

Ventilation–Perfusion Mismatch. In normal lungs, the volume of blood perfusing the lungs each minute (4 to 5 L) approximates the amount of fresh gas that reaches the alveoli each minute (4 to 5 L). In a perfectly matched system, each portion of the lung would receive approximately 1 mL of air for each 1 mL of blood flow. This match of ventilation and perfusion would result in a VQ ratio of 1:1 (e.g., 1 mL of air per 1 mL of blood), which is expressed as VQ = 1; thus ventilation volume would be identical to perfusion volume. Although this example implies that the ideal situation is that ventilation and perfusion are matched in all areas of the lung,

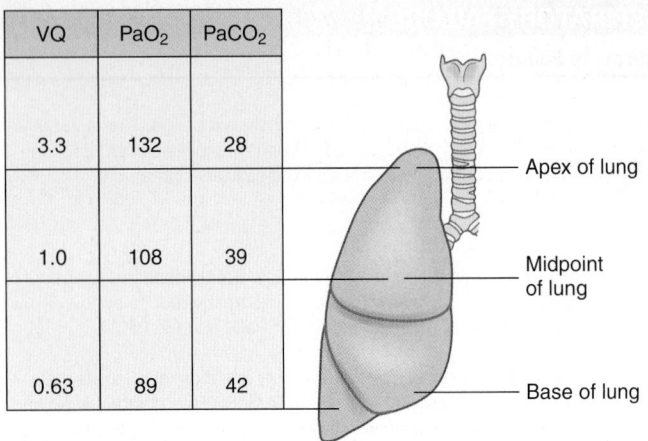

VQ	PaO$_2$	PaCO$_2$
3.3	132	28
1.0	108	39
0.63	89	42

FIG. 70.3 Regional ventilation–perfusion (VQ) differences in the normal lung. At the lung apex, the VQ ratio is 3.3; at the midpoint, it is 1.0; and at the base, it is 0.63. This difference causes the arterial partial pressure of oxygen (PaO$_2$) to be higher at the apex of the lung and lower at the base. Values for arterial partial pressure of carbon dioxide (PaCO$_2$) are the opposite (i.e., lower at the apex and higher at the base). Blood that exits the lung has a mixture of these values.

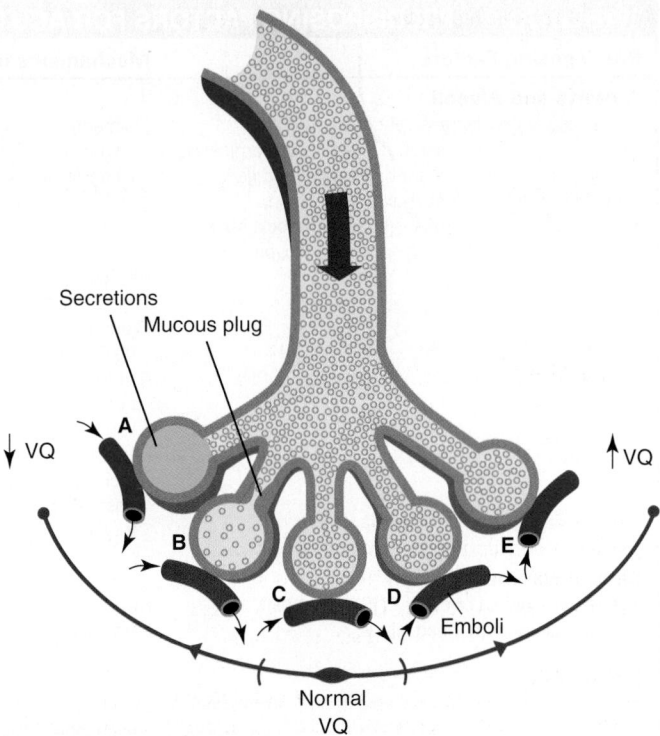

FIG. 70.4 Range of ventilation–perfusion (VQ) relationships. **A,** Absolute shunt: no ventilation as a result of fluid filling the alveoli. **B,** VQ mismatch in which ventilation is partially compromised by secretions in the airway. **C,** Normal lung unit. **D,** VQ mismatch in which perfusion is partially compromised by emboli obstructing blood flow. **E,** Dead space: no perfusion as a result of obstruction of the pulmonary capillary.

this situation does not normally exist. In reality, there is some regional mismatch even under normal conditions. At the lung apex, VQ ratios are greater than 1 (more ventilation than perfusion). At the lung base, VQ ratios are less than 1 (less ventilation than perfusion). Because changes at the lung apex balance changes at the base, the net effect is a close overall match (Figure 70.3).

Many diseases and conditions alter overall VQ matching and thus cause VQ mismatch (Figure 70.4). The most common are those in which increased secretions are present in the airways (as in chronic obstructive pulmonary disease [COPD]) or the alveoli (as in pneumonia) and when bronchospasm is present (as in asthma). VQ mismatch may also result from alveolar collapse (atelectasis) or from pain. Uncontrolled pain interferes with chest and abdominal wall movement, compromising lung ventilation. In addition, pain increases muscle and motor tension, which leads to generalized muscle rigidity, causes systemic vasoconstriction and activation of the stress response, and increases O$_2$ consumption and CO$_2$ production (Virani et al., 2019). All of these conditions may increase both metabolic demands (for O$_2$) and ventilatory demands, and, at the same time, airflow (ventilation) to alveoli is limited. Because no effect on blood flow (perfusion) to the gas-exchange units is exerted to balance the equation, the consequence is VQ mismatch. A pulmonary embolus affects the perfusion portion of the VQ relationship. The embolus limits blood flow but has no effect on airflow to the alveoli, which again causes VQ mismatch (see Figure 70.4).

Oxygen therapy is an appropriate first step to reverse hypoxemia caused by VQ mismatch because not all gas-exchange units are affected. Oxygen therapy increases the PaO$_2$ in blood leaving normal gas-exchange units, thus causing the PaO$_2$ to be higher than normal. The well-oxygenated blood mixes with poorly oxygenated blood, which raises the overall PaO$_2$ of blood leaving the lungs. Optimal treatment for hypoxemia caused by VQ mismatch is directed at the cause.

Shunt. *Shunting* is the situation in which blood exits the heart without having participated in gas exchange. A shunt can be viewed as an extreme VQ mismatch (see Figure 70.4). There

are two types of shunts. In an *anatomical shunt,* blood passes through an anatomical channel in the heart (e.g., ventricular septal defect), bypassing the lungs. In an *intrapulmonary shunt,* blood flows through the pulmonary capillaries without participating in gas exchange. Intrapulmonary shunt occurs in conditions in which alveoli fill with fluid (e.g., ARDS, pneumonia, pulmonary edema). In hypoxemia due to shunt, O$_2$ therapy alone may not effectively increase the PaO$_2$ because (a) blood passes from the right side of the heart to the left side without passing through the lungs (anatomical shunt) or (b) the alveoli are filled with fluid, which prevents gas exchange (intrapulmonary shunt). Patients with such shunts are usually more hypoxemic than patients with VQ mismatch, and they may require both mechanical ventilation and a high FiO$_2$ to improve gas exchange.

Diffusion Limitation. Diffusion limitation is the decrease in gas exchange across the alveolar–capillary membrane by processes that thicken or destroy the membrane (Figure 70.5). Conditions that affect the pulmonary vascular bed, such as severe emphysema or recurrent pulmonary emboli, can worsen diffusion limitation. Some diseases (e.g., pulmonary fibrosis, interstitial lung disease, ARDS) cause the alveolar–capillary membrane to become thicker (fibrotic), which slows gas transport. Diffusion limitation is more likely to cause hypoxemia during exercise than at rest. During exercise, blood moves more rapidly through the lungs. Because the transit rate is increased, red blood cells are in the lungs for a shorter time, limiting opportunity for diffusion of O$_2$ across the alveolar–capillary membrane. The classical sign of diffusion limitation is hypoxemia that is present during exercise but not at rest.

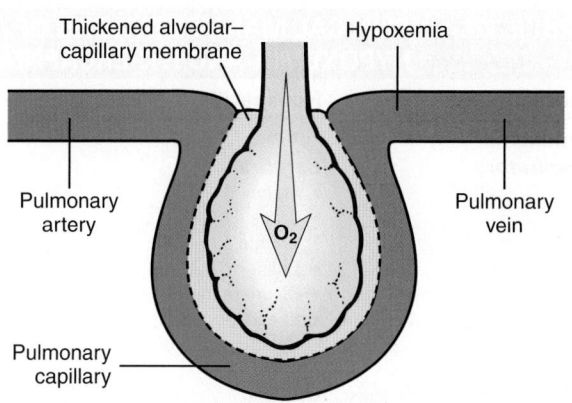

Thickened alveolar–capillary membrane

Hypoxemia

Pulmonary artery

O_2

Pulmonary vein

Pulmonary capillary

FIG. 70.5 Diffusion limitation. Exchange of CO_2 and O_2 cannot occur because of the thickened alveolar–capillary membrane.

Alveolar Hypoventilation. Alveolar hypoventilation is a decrease in ventilation that results in an increase in $PaCO_2$ and a consequent decrease in PaO_2. Alveolar hypoventilation may result from restrictive lung disease, CNS disease, chest wall dysfunction, or neuromuscular disease. Although primarily a mechanism of hypercapnic respiratory failure, alveolar hypoventilation is mentioned here because it also causes hypoxemia.

Interrelationship of Mechanisms. Frequently, hypoxemic respiratory failure is caused by a combination of two or more of the following: VQ mismatch, shunting, diffusion limitation, and hypoventilation. Patients with acute respiratory failure secondary to pneumonia may have a combination of VQ mismatch and shunting because inflammation, edema, and the hypersecretion of exudate within the bronchioles and the terminal respiratory units obstruct the airways (VQ mismatch) and fill the alveoli with exudate (shunt). In addition, shunting may be increased because of improper positioning (affected lung down). Patients with cardiogenic pulmonary edema or ARDS may have a combination of shunting and VQ mismatch because some alveoli are completely filled with fluid from edema (shunting) and others are partially filled with fluid (VQ mismatch).

Hypoxemia resulting from shunting does not respond to increases in supplemental oxygen because the capillary bed surrounding the affected alveoli is never exposed to oxygen-rich gas. As a result, hypoxemia that results from shunting is difficult to treat (Brashers & Huether, 2018).

Hypercapnic Respiratory Failure. Hypercapnic respiratory failure results from an imbalance between ventilatory supply and ventilatory demand. *Ventilatory supply* is the maximum ventilation (gas flow in and out of the lungs) that the patient can sustain without developing respiratory muscle fatigue. *Ventilatory demand* is the amount of ventilation needed to keep the $PaCO_2$ normal. Normally, ventilatory supply far exceeds ventilatory demand. As a consequence, individuals with normal lung function can engage in strenuous exercise, which increases CO_2 production without an elevation in $PaCO_2$. Patients with preexisting lung disease (e.g., severe emphysema) do not have this advantage and cannot effectively increase lung ventilation in response to exercise or metabolic demands. Typically, considerable dysfunction is present before ventilatory demand exceeds supply.

When ventilatory demand does exceed supply, a normal $PaCO_2$ cannot be sustained and hypercapnia occurs, which reflects substantial lung dysfunction. Hypercapnic respiratory failure is sometimes called *ventilatory failure* because it

represents primarily an inability of the respiratory system to clear sufficient CO_2 and maintain a normal $PaCO_2$.

The associated respiratory acidosis that accompanies hypercapnia can result in dysrhythmias, somnolence, and even coma. There are changes in intracranial pressure associated with high levels of CO_2. Hypoventilation may be overlooked because the ventilator rate and pattern may appear normal initially (Virani et al., 2019).

Diseases involving respiratory failure can be grouped into four categories: (1) abnormalities of the airways and alveoli, (2) abnormalities of the CNS, (3) abnormalities of the chest wall, and (4) neuromuscular conditions (see Table 70.3).

Airways and Alveoli. Patients with asthma, emphysema, chronic bronchitis, and cystic fibrosis are at high risk for hypercapnic respiratory failure because the underlying pathophysiology of these conditions results in airflow obstruction and air trapping.

Central Nervous System. A variety of situations may suppress the drive to breathe. Commonly, overdose of an opioid or other CNS depressant medication decreases CO_2 reactivity in the brainstem, which allows arterial CO_2 levels to rise. A brainstem infarction or severe head injury may also interfere with normal function of the respiratory centre in the medulla. Affected patients are at risk for respiratory failure because the medulla does not alter the respiratory rate in response to changes in $PaCO_2$. Independent of direct brainstem dysfunction, brain injury resulting in significant CNS depression or loss of consciousness may impair the patient's ability to protect the airway. CNS dysfunction may also include high-level spinal cord injuries that limit innervation of the respiratory muscles.

Chest Wall. Various conditions prevent normal chest wall movement, thereby limiting lung expansion. In patients with flail chest, the rib cage cannot expand normally because of painful fractures, mechanical restriction, and muscle spasm. In patients with kyphoscoliosis, changes in spinal configuration compress the lungs, preventing normal chest wall expansion. In patients with massive obesity, the weight of the chest and abdominal contents may limit lung expansion. Patients with these conditions are at risk for respiratory failure because these dysfunctions limit lung expansion or diaphragmatic movement and, consequently, gas exchange.

Neuromuscular Conditions. Various types of neuromuscular diseases may result in respiratory muscle weakness or paralysis (see Table 70.2). For example, patients with Guillain-Barré syndrome, muscular dystrophy, myasthenia gravis (acute exacerbation), or multiple sclerosis are at risk for respiratory failure because the respiratory muscles are weakened or paralyzed. Therefore, they are unable to maintain normal $PaCO_2$ levels.

Note that respiratory failure occurs in three of these categories (CNS, chest wall, neuromuscular conditions) even if the lungs are normal. Affected patients may have no damage to lung tissue but are unable to inspire sufficient tidal volume to expel CO_2 from the lungs.

Tissue Oxygen Needs. Even though respiratory failure is determined by the PaO_2 and $PaCO_2$, the major threat is the inability of the lungs to meet the oxygen demands of the tissues, whether as a result of inadequate O_2 delivery or because the tissues are unable to use the O_2 delivered to them. Respiratory failure may also occur as a result of the stress response and dramatic increases in tissue oxygen consumption (Virani et al., 2019). Tissue O_2 delivery is determined by the amount of O_2 carried in the hemoglobin, as well as by cardiac output. Therefore, respiratory failure increases risk if the patient has coexisting cardiac conditions or anemia. Failure of O_2 utilization most commonly occurs as a result of septic shock. In this situation, adequate O_2 may be delivered to the tissues, but an abnormally high amount of O_2 returns in the venous blood, which indicates that it is not being extracted and used at the tissue level. (Shock is discussed in Chapter 69.) Acid–base alterations (e.g., alkalosis, acidosis) may also interfere with oxygen delivery to peripheral tissues (see Chapter 28).

Clinical Manifestations

Respiratory failure may develop suddenly or gradually over several days or longer. A sudden decrease in PaO_2 or a rapid rise in $PaCO_2$ implies a serious condition, which can rapidly become a life-threatening emergency. An example is the development of severe bronchospasm and a marked decrease in airflow in a patient with asthma, which can result in respiratory arrest. A more gradual change in PaO_2 and $PaCO_2$ is better tolerated because compensation can occur. An example is the development of a progressive increase in $PaCO_2$ over several days after the onset of a respiratory infection in a patient with COPD. Because the change occurs gradually over several days, there is time for renal compensation (e.g., retention of bicarbonate), which minimizes the change in arterial pH. The patient has compensated respiratory acidosis (Urden et al., 2020). (See Chapter 19 for a discussion of renal compensation for acid–base disorders.)

Manifestations of respiratory failure are related to the extent of change in PaO_2 or $PaCO_2$, the rapidity of change (acute versus chronic), and the ability to compensate or overcome this change. When the patient's compensatory mechanisms fail, respiratory failure occurs. Because clinical manifestations are variable, it is important to monitor trends in ABGs and pulse oximetry to evaluate the extent of change. These measurements cannot substitute for clinical assessment and should be interpreted within the context of clinical assessment findings. Frequently, the initial indication of respiratory failure is a change in the patient's mental status. The cerebral cortex is very sensitive to variations in oxygenation and acid–base balance, and mental status changes occur early and frequently before ABG results show change. Restlessness, confusion, agitation, and combative behaviour suggest inadequate delivery of O_2 to the brain and should be investigated.

The nurse may detect manifestations of respiratory failure that are specific (arise from the respiratory system) or nonspecific (arise from other body systems; Table 70.4). An understanding of these manifestations is critical for detecting the onset of respiratory failure and effective treatment.

Tachycardia and mild hypertension can also be early signs of respiratory failure. They may indicate an attempt by the heart to compensate for decreased O_2 delivery. A severe morning headache may suggest that hypercapnia occurred during the night, increasing cerebral blood flow by vasodilation. At night, the respiratory rate is slower, and the lungs of patients at risk for respiratory failure may remove less $PaCO_2$. Rapid, shallow breaths suggest that the tidal volume may be inadequate to remove CO_2 from the lungs. Cyanosis is an unreliable indicator of hypoxemia and is a late sign of respiratory failure because it does not occur until hypoxemia is severe ($PaO_2 \leq 45$ mm Hg).

Consequences of Hypoxemia and Hypoxia. *Hypoxemia* occurs when the amount of O_2 in arterial blood is less than the normal value (see Chapter 28). Hypoxia is the condition in which the PaO_2 has fallen sufficiently to cause signs and

TABLE 70.4	**CLINICAL MANIFESTATIONS OF HYPOXEMIA AND HYPERCAPNIA***
Specific	**Nonspecific**
Hypoxemia	
Respiratory	***Cerebral***
• ↓ SpO_2 (<80%)	• Agitation
• Dyspnea	• Coma (late)
• Intercostal muscle retraction	• Confusion
	• Delirium
• Prolonged expiration (ratio of length of inspiration to that of expiration: 1:3, 1:4)	• Disorientation
	• ↓ Level of consciousness
	• Restlessness, combativeness
• Tachypnea	
• Use of accessory muscles in respiration	***Cardiac***
	• Dysrhythmias (late)
• Cyanosis (late)	• Hypertension
• Paradoxical chest or abdominal wall movement with respiratory cycle (late)	• Hypotension (late)
	• Skin cool, clammy, and diaphoretic
	• Tachycardia
	Other
	• Fatigue
	• Inability to speak without pausing to breathe
Hypercapnia	
Respiratory	***Cerebral***
• Dyspnea	• Coma (late)
• ↓ Minute ventilation	• Disorientation
• ↓ Respiratory rate or ↑ rate with shallow respirations	• Morning headache
	• Progressive somnolence
• ↓ Tidal volume	
	Cardiac
	• Bounding pulse
	• Dysrhythmias
	• Hypertension
	• Tachycardia
	Neuromuscular
	• ↓ Deep tendon reflexes
	• Muscle weakness
	• Tremor, seizures (late)
	Other
	• Pursed-lip breathing

SpO_2, oxygen saturation in arterial blood as measured by pulse oximetry.
*This list is not all-inclusive.

symptoms of inadequate oxygenation (see Table 70.4). Hypoxemia can lead to hypoxia if not corrected. If hypoxia or hypoxemia is severe, cell metabolism shifts from aerobic to anaerobic. Anaerobic metabolism entails the use of more fuel, produces less energy, and is less efficient than aerobic metabolism. The waste product of anaerobic metabolism, lactic acid, is more difficult to remove from the body than CO_2 because lactic acid must be buffered with sodium bicarbonate. When the body does not have adequate sodium bicarbonate to buffer the lactic acid produced by anaerobic metabolism, metabolic acidosis and cell death may result.

Hypoxia and metabolic acidosis have adverse effects on the vital organs and systems, especially the heart and the CNS. To compensate for decreased O_2 in the blood, the heart rate and cardiac output increase. A cardiovascular hyperdynamic state may also occur as a result of catecholamine release in association with the physiological stress response. This response can occur fairly rapidly. As the PaO_2 decreases and acidosis increases, the heart muscle may become dysfunctional, and cardiac output may decrease. In addition, angina and dysrhythmias may occur. All of these consequences result in a further decrease in oxygenation. Permanent brain damage may occur because of O_2 deprivation. Renal function may also be impaired, and sodium retention, edema formation, acute tubular necrosis, and uremia may occur. Gastrointestinal system alterations include tissue ischemia, increased permeability of the intestinal wall, and possible translocation of bacteria from the gastrointestinal tract into the circulation.

Specific Clinical Manifestations. A patient in respiratory failure may have several clinical findings indicating distress, such as rapid, shallow breathing or a respiratory rate slower than normal. Both changes predispose to insufficient CO_2 removal. The patient may increase the respiratory rate in an effort to blow off accumulated CO_2. This breathing pattern requires a substantial amount of work and predisposes to respiratory muscle fatigue. A change from a rapid rate to a slower rate in a patient in acute respiratory distress suggests extreme fatigue and possible impending respiratory arrest.

The position that the patient assumes is an indication of the effort associated with breathing. The patient may be able to lie down (mild distress), be able to lie down but prefer to sit (moderate distress), or be unable to breathe unless sitting upright (severe distress). A common position is to sit with the arms propped on the overbed table. This position, called the *tripod position,* helps decrease the work of breathing because propping the arms increases the anterior–posterior diameter of the chest and changes pressure in the thorax. The patient may use pursed-lip breathing (see Chapter 31) because it increases SaO_2 by slowing respirations, allowing more time for expiration and preventing the small bronchioles from collapsing, thus facilitating air exchange. Another assessment parameter is the number of pillows the patient requires in order to breathe comfortably when resting. The degree of dyspnea that the patient experiences when lying flat is termed *orthopnea,* documented as one-, two-, three-, or four-pillow orthopnea.

A person experiencing dyspnea is working hard to breathe and may be able to speak only a few words between breaths. The degree to which the patient is able to speak without pausing to breathe is an indication of the severity of dyspnea. The patient may speak in sentences (mild or no distress), phrases (moderate distress), or words (severe distress). The patient may have "two-word" or "three-word" dyspnea, signifying that only two or three words can be said before pausing to breathe. When walking, the patient may also experience earlier onset of fatigue. An additional assessment parameter is how far the patient is able to walk without stopping to rest.

There may be a change in the *inspiratory-to-expiratory (I:E) ratio.* Normally, the I:E ratio is 1:2, meaning expiration is twice as long as inspiration. In respiratory distress, the ratio may increase to 1:3 or 1:4, which signifies airflow obstruction, and more time is necessary to empty the lungs.

The nurse may observe *retraction* (inward movement) of the intercostal spaces or the supraclavicular area and use of the accessory muscles during inspiration or expiration, which signifies moderate distress. Paradoxical breathing indicates severe distress. Normally, the thorax and the abdomen move outward on inspiration and inward on exhalation. During *paradoxical breathing,* the abdomen and the chest move in the opposite manner: outward during exhalation and inward during inspiration. Paradoxical breathing results from maximal use of the accessory muscles of respiration. The patient may also be diaphoretic from the work associated with breathing.

Auscultation should be performed in order to assess the patient's baseline breath sounds, as well as any changes from baseline. The nurse should note the presence and the location of any adventitious breath sounds. Crackles and wheezes may indicate pulmonary edema or emphysema. Absence of or diminished breath sounds may indicate atelectasis or pleural effusion. Bronchial breath sounds over the lung periphery often result from lung consolidation, as occurs with pneumonia. A pleural friction rub may also be heard in the presence of pneumonia that has involved the pleura.

A thorough nursing assessment may result in early detection of manifestations associated with respiratory insufficiency, which allows therapy to be instituted before the patient experiences respiratory failure. Patients with end-stage (severe) chronic lung disease may have low PaO_2 values or elevated $PaCO_2$ values and crackles as their "normal" baseline. It is especially important to monitor specific and nonspecific signs of respiratory failure in patients with COPD or other pre-existing chronic diseases because a small change can cause significant decompensation (see Table 70.4). Any deterioration in mental status, such as agitation, combative behaviour, confusion, or decreased level of consciousness, should be reported immediately because this may indicate deterioration in clinical status and the need for mechanical ventilation.

Diagnostic Studies

After physical assessment, the diagnostic studies most commonly used to determine respiratory failure are ABG analysis and chest radiographic studies. ABG measurements are used to determine the levels of $PaCO_2$, PaO_2, bicarbonate, and pH. An arterial line may be inserted into a peripheral artery for monitoring systemic blood pressure and obtaining ABG measurements. Pulse oximetry is used for monitoring oxygenation but reveals little about ventilation. In respiratory failure, ABG measurements are necessary to determine both oxygenation (PaO_2) and ventilation ($PaCO_2$) status, as well as obtain information related to acid–base balance (Burns & Delgado, 2019). Chest radiographic examination helps identify possible causes of respiratory failure (e.g., atelectasis, pneumonia). In patients with respiratory failure that does not require acute intervention, pulmonary function tests may be performed.

Other diagnostic studies that may be done include a complete blood cell count (CBC), serum electrolyte measurements, urinalysis, and electrocardiography. Sputum and blood cultures are obtained if infection is likely. If pulmonary embolus is suspected, a VQ lung scan or pulmonary angiography may be done. For a patient requiring endotracheal intubation, end-tidal CO_2 is measured to assess tube placement immediately after intubation and during ventilator management to assess trends in lung ventilation.

In severe respiratory failure, a pulmonary artery catheter may be inserted to measure pressures on the right side of the heart and cardiac output, as well as mixed venous oxygen saturation. This information is helpful in determining the adequacy of tissue perfusion and the patient's response to treatment. Pulmonary artery, pulmonary artery wedge (occlusion), and left atrial pressures are monitored to determine whether the accumulation of fluid in the lungs is the result of cardiac or pulmonary problems. These parameters are also monitored to determine the response of the lungs and heart to hypoxemia and the patient's response to therapy. Pulmonary arterial pressure monitoring can also provide feedback about the physiological effects of mechanical ventilation on hemodynamic status. (See Chapter 68 for a discussion of hemodynamic monitoring.)

NURSING AND INTERPROFESSIONAL MANAGEMENT ACUTE RESPIRATORY FAILURE

Because many different conditions cause respiratory failure, care of affected patients varies. This section is a discussion of general assessment and interprofessional treatments that apply to patients with acute respiratory failure. In acute care settings, there is often an overlap of function between nursing and other members of the health care team. Aside from the interprofessional health care team, family members play a valuable role in the patient's care and recovery. Further discussion of issues related to the family and caregivers can be found in Chapter 68.

NURSING ASSESSMENT

Subjective and objective data that should be obtained from patients with acute respiratory failure are listed in Table 70.5.

NURSING DIAGNOSES

Nursing diagnoses for the patient with acute respiratory failure include but are not limited to the following:
- *Inadequate gas exchange* (as a result of alveolar hypoventilation, intrapulmonary shunting, VQ mismatch, and diffusion impairment)
- *Inadequate airway clearance* as a result of *excessive mucus, retained secretions*
- *Inadequate breathing pattern* as a result of *neuromuscular impairment of respirations, pain, anxiety, decreased level of consciousness, respiratory muscle fatigue, and bronchospasm*

Additional information on nursing diagnoses for the patient with acute respiratory failure is presented in Nursing Care Plan (NCP) 70.1, available on the Evolve website.

PLANNING

The overall goals for patients in acute respiratory failure are to restore baseline (a) ABG values, (b) breath sounds, (c) breathing patterns, and (d) ability to clear secretions.

PREVENTION

Prevention and early recognition of respiratory distress are important aspects of care for any patient at risk for respiratory failure. Prevention involves a thorough physical assessment and history (to identify patients at risk for respiratory failure) followed by appropriate nursing interventions. For example, a patient at risk for respiratory failure should receive teaching regarding coughing, deep breathing, incentive spirometry, and ambulation as appropriate. Prevention of atelectasis, pneumonia, and complications of immobility, as well as optimizing hydration and nutrition, can potentially decrease the risk of respiratory failure in acute or critically ill patients.

TABLE 70.5 NURSING ASSESSMENT
Acute Respiratory Failure

Subjective Data
Important Health Information
Past health history: Chronic lung disease; potential occupational exposures to lung toxins; smoking (pack-years); childhood illnesses, previous hospitalizations related to lung disease; thoracic or spinal cord trauma; extreme obesity; altered consciousness; age (physiological and chronological); use or misuse of alcohol, other drugs; medication allergies, recent travel, SARS
Medications: Use of oxygen, inhalers (bronchodilators), home nebulization, over-the-counter medications; immunosuppressant (corticosteroid) therapy, CNS depressants; vitamin and herbal supplements
Surgery or other treatments: Previous intubation and mechanical ventilation; recent thoracic or abdominal surgery

Symptoms
- Anorexia, bloatedness, heartburn; weight gain or loss; decreased appetite
- Anxiety, depression
- Changes in sleep pattern
- Dyspnea at rest or with activity; wheezing or cough (productive or nonproductive); sputum (volume, colour, viscosity)
- Fatigue, dizziness; diaphoresis
- Headache, chest pain or tightness
- Palpitations, swollen feet

Objective Data
General
Restlessness, agitation

Integumentary
Pale, cool, clammy skin or warm flushed skin; peripheral and central cyanosis; peripheral dependent edema

Respiratory
Shallow, increased respiratory rate progressing to decreased rate; use of accessory muscles with evidence of retractions, altered I:E ratio; increased diaphragmatic excursion or asymmetrical chest expansion; asynchronous respirations; tactile fremitus, crepitus, or deviated trachea on palpation; resonant, hyper-resonant, or dull percussion note; absence of, diminished, or adventitious breath sounds; bronchial or bronchovesicular sounds heard in other than normal location, inspiratory stridor, pleural friction rub

Cardiovascular
Tachycardia progressing to bradycardia, dysrhythmias, extra heart sounds (S_3, S_4); bounding pulse; hypertension progressing to hypotension; pulsus paradoxus; jugular vein distension; pedal edema

Gastrointestinal
Abdominal distension with tympany; ascites, epigastric tenderness, hepatojugular reflex

Neurological
Somnolence, confusion, slurred speech, restlessness, delirium, agitation, tremors, seizures, coma; asterixis, decreased deep tendon reflexes; papilledema

Possible Laboratory Findings
↑ or ↓ pH, ↑ or ↓ $PaCO_2$, ↓ PaO_2, ↑ or ↓ bicarbonate, ↓ SaO_2, ↓ PEFR, ↓ tidal volume, ↓ forced vital capacity, ↓ minute ventilation, ↓ negative inspiratory force; altered serum electrolyte values, hemoglobin, white blood cells, and hematocrit; abnormal findings on chest radiograph; abnormal pulmonary artery and pulmonary artery wedge pressures

CNS, central nervous system; *I:E*, inspiratory to expiratory; *PaCO₂*, partial pressure of carbon dioxide in arterial blood; *PaO₂*, partial pressure of oxygen in arterial blood; *PEFR*, peak expiratory flow rate; *SaO₂*, oxygen saturation in arterial blood as measured by arterial blood gases; *SARS*, severe acute respiratory syndrome.

RESPIRATORY THERAPY

The major goals of care for acute respiratory failure include maintaining adequate oxygenation and ventilation. This is accomplished by collaboration among the nursing, medical, and respiratory care teams. The respiratory therapist works in collaboration with the interprofessional teams to provide various respiratory interventions. The interventions used include O_2 therapy, mobilization of secretions, and positive-pressure ventilation (Table 70.6).

OXYGEN THERAPY. The primary goal of O_2 therapy is to correct hypoxemia. If hypoxemia is secondary to VQ mismatch, supplemental O_2 administered at 1 to 3 L/min by nasal cannula or at 24 to 32% by simple face mask or Venturi mask should improve the PaO_2 and SaO_2. Hypoxemia secondary to intrapulmonary shunt is usually not responsive to high O_2 concentrations, and affected patients usually require positive-pressure ventilation (PPV). PPV helps provide O_2 therapy and humidification, decrease the work of breathing, and reduce respiratory muscle fatigue. In addition, the positive pressure may assist in opening collapsed airways and decreasing shunting. PPV may be provided via an endotracheal tube (most frequently) or noninvasively by means of a tight-fitting mask (Ding et al., 2020). (See Chapter 68 for an overview of mechanical ventilation.)

The type of O_2 delivery system chosen for a patient in acute respiratory failure should (a) be tolerated by the patient, inasmuch as feelings of claustrophobia related to the face mask may prompt the patient to remove it, and (b) maintain PaO_2 at 55 to 60 mm Hg or more and SaO_2 at 90% or more at the lowest O_2 concentration possible. High O_2 concentration is associated with adverse effects. Intubated patients who receive more than 50% FiO_2 for more than 24 hours are at greatest risk to develop O_2 toxicity (Urden et al., 2020). Toxic O_2 free radicals are a metabolite of O_2 metabolism; in the setting of extended exposure to high concentrations, the supply of enzymes responsible for neutralizing those radicals is exhausted, which results in in acute lung injury. Absorption atelectasis can also occur when excess O_2 displaces the nitrogen normally present in alveoli, causing alveolar collapse (Virani et al., 2019). The effects of prolonged exposure to high levels of O_2 include increased pulmonary microvascular permeability, decreased surfactant production and surfactant inactivation, and fibrotic changes in the alveoli. (Oxygen delivery devices are discussed in Chapter 31.)

Additional risks of O_2 therapy are specific to patients with chronic hypercapnia, such as those with COPD. Chronic hypercapnia may blunt the response of chemoreceptors in the medulla. In this situation, respirations are stimulated by hypoxia. If the PaO_2 is suddenly increased, the patient is no longer hypoxemic, the stimulus to breathe is decreased, and respiratory arrest may occur. Patients with chronic hypercapnia should receive O_2 through a low-flow device such as a nasal cannula at 1 to 2 L/min or a Venturi mask at a volume of 24 to 28%. Close monitoring for changes in mental status and of respiratory rate and ABG results is essential until PaO_2 levels have reached their baseline value.

MOBILIZATION OF SECRETIONS. Retained pulmonary secretions may cause or exacerbate acute respiratory failure by blocking both movement of O_2 into the alveoli and the pulmonary capillary blood and removal of CO_2 during the respiratory cycle. Secretions can be mobilized through effective coughing, adequate hydration and humidification, chest physiotherapy, and tracheal suctioning.

Effective Coughing and Positioning. If secretions are obstructing the airway, the patient should be encouraged to cough. Patients with a neuromuscular weakness from a disease or exhaustion may not be able to generate sufficient airway pressures to produce an effective cough. *Augmented coughing (quad coughing)* may be of benefit to such patients. Augmented coughing is performed by placing the palm of the hand or hands on the abdomen below the xiphoid process (Figure 70.6). As the patient ends a deep inspiration and begins the expiration, the hands should

TABLE 70.6   INTERPROFESSIONAL CARE

Acute Respiratory Failure

Diagnostic	Medication Therapy
• History and physical examination • ABG measurements • Blood and sputum cultures (if indicated) • Chest radiography • Complete blood cell count • Electrocardiography • O_2 saturation • Pulmonary artery pressure, pulmonary artery occlusive (wedge) pressure, and left atrial pressure • Serum electrolyte measurements and urinalysis	• Reduction of airway inflammation (corticosteroids) • Reduction of anxiety and restlessness (e.g., lorazepam [Ativan]) • Reduction of pulmonary congestion (e.g., furosemide [Lasix]) • Relief of bronchospasm (e.g., salbutamol) • Treatment of pulmonary infections (e.g., antibiotics)
Interprofessional Therapy **Respiratory Therapy** • Airway suctioning • Chest physiotherapy • Effective coughing • Hydration and humidification • Incentive spirometry • Intubation with mechanical ventilation • Mobilization of secretions • Noninvasive positive-pressure ventilation • O_2 therapy • Positive-pressure ventilation	**Medical Supportive Therapy** • Maintenance of adequate cardiac output • Maintenance of adequate hemoglobin concentration • Management of underlying cause of respiratory failure **Nutritional Therapy** • Enteral nutrition support • Parenteral nutrition support

ABG, arterial blood gas.

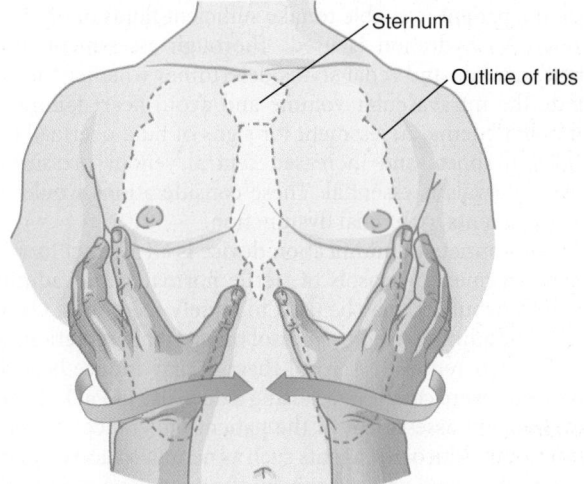

FIG. 70.6 Augmented coughing is performed by placing one or both hands over the anterolateral base of the lungs. After the patient takes a deep inspiration and at the beginning of expiration, the hand or hands are moved forcefully upward. This increases abdominal pressure and aids in producing a forceful cough.

be moved forcefully upward, increasing abdominal pressure and facilitating the cough. This measure helps increase expiratory flow and thereby facilitates secretion clearance. Health care providers need to receive appropriate training before using augmented coughing techniques.

Some patients may benefit from therapeutic cough techniques. *Huff coughing* is a series of coughs performed while saying the word "huff." This technique prevents the glottis from closing during the cough. Patients with COPD generate higher flow rates with a huff cough than they can with a normal cough. The huff cough is effective in clearing only the central airways, but it may assist in moving secretions upward. The *staged cough* also assists secretion mobilization. To perform the staged cough, the patient sits in a chair, breathes three or four times in and out through the mouth, and coughs while bending forward and pressing a pillow inward against the diaphragm.

Body positioning can be optimized for VQ matching. Positioning the patient either by elevating the head of the bed at least 45 degrees or with a reclining chair or chair bed may help maximize thoracic expansion, thereby decreasing dyspnea and improving secretion mobilization. A sitting position improves pulmonary function and assists in venous pooling in dependent body areas such as the lower extremities. When lungs are upright, ventilation and perfusion are best in the lung bases. Lateral or side-lying positioning, termed *good lung down,* may be used in patients with disease involving only one lung and allows for improved VQ matching in the affected lung (Wieslander et al., 2019). Pulmonary blood flow and ventilation are optimal in dependent lung areas. This positioning also allows for secretions to drain out of the affected lung to the point at which they may be removed by suctioning. For example, in patients with significant right-sided pneumonia, optimal positioning would be to place them on their left side to maximize ventilation and perfusion in the "good" lung and facilitate secretion removal from the affected lung (postural drainage). All patients should be lying on their side if there is any possibility that the tongue will obstruct the airway or that aspiration may occur. Equipment to create an oral or nasal airway should be kept at the bedside for use if necessary.

Hydration and Humidification. Thick and viscous secretions should be thinned to facilitate removal. Adequate fluid intake (2 to 3 L/day) is necessary to keep secretions thin and easy to expel. If a patient is unable to take sufficient fluids orally, intravenous (IV) hydration is used. Thorough assessment of the patient's cardiac and renal status determines whether they can tolerate the intravascular volume and avoid heart failure and pulmonary edema. Assessment for signs of fluid overload (e.g., crackles, dyspnea, and increased central venous pressure) at regular intervals is essential. These considerations would also apply to patients with renal dysfunction.

An appropriate humidification device is an adjunct in secretion management. Aerosols of sterile normal saline, administered by a nebulizer, may be used to liquefy secretions. Oxygen may also be administered by aerosol mask to thin secretions and facilitate their removal. Aerosol therapy may induce bronchospasm and severe coughing, causing a decrease in PaO_2. In such cases, frequent assessment of the patient's tolerance of therapy is paramount. Mucolytic agents such as nebulized acetylcysteine (Mucomyst) mixed with a bronchodilator may be used to thin secretions; however, as an adverse effect, such mixtures may also cause airway erythema and bronchospasm. Therefore, they are used only in special situations (e.g., during bronchoscopy to remove thick, copious secretions).

Chest Physiotherapy. Chest physiotherapy is indicated in patients who produce more than 30 mL of sputum per day or have evidence of severe atelectasis or pulmonary infiltrates. If tolerated, postural drainage, percussion, and vibration to the affected lung segments may assist in moving secretions to the larger airways, where they may be removed by coughing or suctioning. Because positioning may affect oxygenation, patients may not tolerate head-down or lateral positioning as a result of extreme dyspnea or hypoxemia caused by VQ mismatch. (Chest physiotherapy is discussed in Chapter 31.)

Airway Suctioning. If the patient is unable to expectorate secretions, then nasopharyngeal, oropharyngeal, or nasotracheal suctioning (blind suctioning without a tracheal tube in place) is indicated. Suctioning through an artificial airway, such as endotracheal or tracheostomy tubes, may also be performed (see Chapters 29 and 68). A mini-tracheostomy (commonly called a "mini-trach") may be used to perform suction in patients who have difficulty mobilizing secretions and when blind suctioning is difficult or ineffective. The *mini-tracheostomy* is a 4-mm in-dwelling plastic cuffless cannula inserted through the cricothyroid membrane. It is used to instill sterile normal saline solution to elicit a cough and to perform suctioning with a size 10 or smaller French catheter. Contraindications for a mini-tracheostomy include absence of the gag reflex, a history of aspiration, and the need for long-term mechanical ventilation.

POSITIVE-PRESSURE VENTILATION. If intensive measures fail to improve ventilation and oxygenation and the patient continues to exhibit acute respiratory failure, ventilatory assistance may be initiated. PPV may be provided invasively through endotracheal or nasotracheal intubation or noninvasively through a nasal or face mask. Patients who require PPV are typically cared for in a critical care unit. (See Chapter 68 for a discussion of artificial airways and mechanical ventilation.)

Noninvasive positive-pressure ventilation (NIPPV) may be used to treat patients with acute or chronic respiratory failure. During NIPPV, a mask is placed over the patient's nose or nose and mouth while the patient breathes spontaneously (Figure 70.7). With NIPPV, it is possible to decrease the work of breathing without the use of invasive endotracheal intubation. Bilevel positive airway pressure ventilation is a form of NIPPV in which different

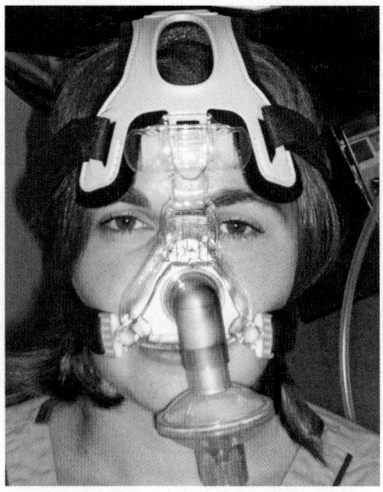

FIG. 70.7 Noninvasive bilevel positive airway pressure ventilation. A mask is placed over the nose or the nose and mouth. Positive pressure from a mechanical ventilator assists the patient's breathing efforts, decreasing the work of breathing. Source: Courtesy Richard Arbour, RN, MSN, CCRN, CNRN, CCNS, FAAN, and Anna Kirk, RN, MSN.

positive-pressure levels are set for inspiration and expiration (see Figure 70.7). In continuous positive airway pressure, another form of NIPPV, the positive pressure delivered to the airway is constant during inspiration and expiration (Urden et al., 2020).

NIPPV is most useful in managing chronic respiratory failure in patients with chest wall and neuromuscular disease (see Table 70.3). NIPPV has been used in patients with hypoxemic respiratory failure (e.g., those with ARDS, cardiogenic pulmonary edema) but with less success. NIPPV may also be used for patients who refuse endotracheal intubation but still desire some palliative ventilatory support (e.g., patients with end-stage COPD). NIPPV is not appropriate for the patient who has no spontaneous respirations, excessive secretions, decreased level of consciousness, high O_2 requirements, facial trauma, or hemodynamic instability (Urden et al., 2020).

MEDICATION THERAPY

Goals of medication therapy for patients in acute respiratory failure include relief of bronchospasm, reduction of airway inflammation and pulmonary congestion, treatment of pulmonary infection, and reduction of severe anxiety and restlessness.

RELIEF OF BRONCHOSPASM. Alveolar ventilation will be increased with relief of bronchospasm. To reverse bronchospasm, short-acting *bronchodilators,* such as fenoterol hydrobromide and salbutamol, are frequently administered through either a hand-held nebulizer or a metered-dose inhaler (MDI) with a spacer (Chao et al., 2019). For acute bronchospasm, these medications may be given at 15- to 30-minute intervals until a response can be determined. If severe bronchospasm continues, IV aminophylline may be administered. The bronchodilator effects of all of these medications can sometimes cause a worsening of arterial hypoxemia by redistributing the inspired gas to areas of decreased perfusion. Administering the bronchodilator with an O_2-enriched gas mixture usually alleviates this effect. (See Chapter 31 for nursing management related to bronchodilators.) In addition to bronchodilators, IV magnesium sulphate may be beneficial in cases of severe asthma and asthma refractory to conventional treatment (Conway & Friedman, 2020).

REDUCTION OF AIRWAY INFLAMMATION. Corticosteroids (e.g., methylprednisolone [Solu-Medrol]) may be used in conjunction with bronchodilating medications when bronchospasm and inflammation are present. They may be administered intravenously, orally, or as aerosols. In acute exacerbations, high-dose IV steroids such as methylprednisolone are used. The dosage is then tapered as tolerated by the patient. Because long-term regimens of oral steroids are associated with systemic adverse effects, their use should be avoided if possible. Instead, inhaled steroids such as fluticasone (Flovent) or budesonide (Pulmicort) are used to reduce the risk of those systemic adverse effects (Calzetta et al., 2019).

REDUCTION OF PULMONARY CONGESTION. Pulmonary interstitial fluid can accumulate as a consequence of direct or indirect injury to the alveolar capillary membrane (as in ARDS) or from right- or left-sided heart failure and can therefore be either cardiac or noncardiac in origin. The result is decreased alveolar ventilation and hypoxemia. IV diuretics (e.g., furosemide [Lasix]) and nitroglycerine are used to decrease the pulmonary congestion caused by heart failure. If atrial fibrillation is also present, calcium channel blockers (e.g., diltiazem) and β-adrenergic blockers (e.g., metoprolol) may be used to decrease heart rate and improve cardiac output. (See Chapter 37 for discussion of heart failure.)

TREATMENT OF PULMONARY INFECTIONS. Pulmonary infections (pneumonia, acute bronchitis) result in excessive mucus production, fever, and increased oxygen consumption, and alveoli become inflamed or fluid filled or collapse. Alveoli that are fluid filled or collapsed cannot participate in gas exchange. Pulmonary infections can either cause or exacerbate acute respiratory failure. IV antibiotics, such as vancomycin (Vancocin) or ceftriaxone, are frequently administered to inhibit bacterial growth. Chest radiographic examinations are performed to determine the location and the extent of a suspected infectious process. Sputum cultures are used to determine the type of organisms causing the infection and their sensitivity to antimicrobial medications (Blakeborough & Watson, 2019).

REDUCTION OF SEVERE ANXIETY, PAIN, AND AGITATION. Anxiety, restlessness, and agitation result from cerebral hypoxia. In addition, fear caused by the inability to breathe and a sense of loss of control may exacerbate anxiety. Anxiety, pain, and agitation increase O_2 consumption, which may worsen the degree of hypoxemia. Increase in anxiety and agitation can affect ventilator management. Administration of sedatives, opioids, or muscle relaxants may be necessary to provide adequate oxygenation and ventilation. Several nursing strategies can assist the patient in reducing the level of anxiety and pain (see NCP 70.1, available on the Evolve website).

Sedation and analgesia with medication therapy such as benzodiazepines (e.g., lorazepam [Ativan], midazolam) and opioids (e.g., morphine, fentanyl) may decrease anxiety, agitation, and pain. Continued agitation increases the patient's work of breathing, O_2 consumption, CO_2 production, and risk of injury (e.g., accidental extubation). In the critical care setting, sedatives and analgesics are commonly administered, and patients must be monitored closely for cardiovascular and respiratory depression. Of importance is that agitation is best characterized as a *symptom* and may be caused by pain, hypoxemia, electrolyte imbalance, evolution of structural or metabolic brain injury, and adverse medication reactions; therefore, potentially reversible causes should always be assessed and treated. Sedative and analgesic medications may have prolonged duration of action in critically ill patients. This may contribute to increased length of stay and prolonged time on a ventilator (Greene et al., 2020). Patients receiving these medications are best managed with a research-based, protocol-driven plan of care.

Sedation protocols can be used to guide the level of sedation. Most patients in whom oxygenation is difficult require heavy sedation (4 to 5 on the Richmond Agitation Sedation Scale). Patients who breathe asynchronously with mechanical ventilation may also benefit from titration of ventilator settings, as well as having underlying causes of agitation addressed.

Once complete sedation is achieved, if the patient is still hypoxic, the use of neuromuscular blockade may be indicated with agents such as vecuronium, cisatracurium, or rocuronium. Neuromuscular blockade produces skeletal muscle relaxation and synchrony with mechanical ventilation. These medications may also decrease the patient's risk of lung injury related to excessive intrathoracic pressures and promote optimal ventilatory support. Patients receiving neuromuscular blockade should receive sedation and analgesia to the point of unconsciousness, for comfort, pain relief, and elimination of the awareness of being paralyzed, which is a terrifying experience (Stawicki & Gessner, 2018). The level of pharmacological paralysis is monitored with a peripheral nerve stimulator and clinical correlation to achieve absence of respiratory effort.

Daily interruption of sedative medication infusions decreases the duration of mechanical ventilation and length of stay in the critical care unit.

MEDICAL SUPPORTIVE THERAPY

Interventions to maximize O_2 delivery and treat the underlying cause of respiratory failure are essential for improving the patient's oxygenation and ventilation status. The primary goal is to treat the underlying cause of the respiratory failure. Other goals include maintaining an adequate cardiac output and hemoglobin concentration.

TREATING THE UNDERLYING CAUSE. Interventions are directed toward reversing the disease process that resulted in the development of acute respiratory failure. Patients with hypoventilation can be diagnosed and treated rapidly. Patients with VQ mismatch, shunting, or diffusion limitation are managed differently depending on the underlying cause. In all patient situations, monitoring treatment effects, including trends in ABGs and changes in respiratory status, is a continuous process.

MAINTAINING ADEQUATE CARDIAC OUTPUT. Cardiac output reflects the blood flow reaching the tissues. Blood pressure and mean arterial pressure are important indicators of the adequacy of cardiac output and should be interpreted within the context of the overall assessment to determine adequacy of cardiac output and tissue perfusion. Usually, a systolic blood pressure of 90 mm Hg or higher and a mean arterial pressure of 60 mm Hg or higher is adequate to maintain perfusion to the vital organs; therefore, changes in mental status can usually be attributed to the level of O_2 and CO_2, rather than to decreased cerebral perfusion, when these pressures are maintained. Patients with chronic, uncontrolled hypertension may require higher systemic arterial pressures and mean arterial pressures to prevent episodes of brain ischemia.

Decreased cardiac output is treated by administration of IV fluids, medications, or both. (See Chapter 69 for a discussion of medications used to treat decreased cardiac output and shock.) Cardiac output may also be decreased by changes in intrathoracic or intrapulmonary pressures from PPV. Patients experiencing exacerbation of COPD or asthma and those receiving controlled ventilation are at risk of alveolar hyperinflation, increased right ventricular afterload, and excessive intrathoracic pressures. These alterations in thoracic pressure dynamics may cause an increase in right ventricular afterload, which limits blood flow from the right side of the heart through the pulmonary vasculature to the left side of the heart; dramatic hemodynamic compromise may result. In addition, blood return from the systemic circulation to the right side of the heart may be impaired, decreasing preload (Urden et al., 2020). Each of these physiological consequences can potentially compromise hemodynamics. Consequently, clinical indicators of adequate cardiac output and tissue perfusion should be monitored alongside initiation or titration of mechanical ventilation by mask or endotracheal intubation.

MAINTAINING ADEQUATE HEMOGLOBIN CONCENTRATION. Hemoglobin is the primary carrier when blood delivers O_2 to the tissues. In patients who are anemic, tissue O_2 delivery is compromised. A hemoglobin concentration of 6 mmol/L or greater typically ensures adequate O_2 saturation of the hemoglobin. Patients should be monitored for sites of blood loss and receive transfusions of packed red blood cells if an adequate hemoglobin concentration cannot be maintained.

NUTRITIONAL THERAPY

Maintenance of protein and energy stores is especially important in patients with acute respiratory failure because nutritional depletion causes loss of muscle mass, including the respiratory muscles, and may prolong recovery. During the acute manifestations of respiratory failure, the risk of aspiration typically prevents oral intake; therefore, enteral or parenteral nutrition may be administered until symptoms subside and the patient tolerates oral intake. A multitude of nutritional supplements are available (Korwin & Honiden, 2019). The prescription of a high-carbohydrate diet should be based on individual patient needs (Frankenfield, 2019). It may be avoided in patients who retain CO_2, because carbohydrates metabolize into CO_2, further increasing CO_2 load. However, the hypermetabolic state present in critical illness can dramatically increase caloric requirements.

EVALUATION

The expected outcomes for the patient with acute respiratory failure are presented in NCP 70.1, on the Evolve website.

AGE-RELATED CONSIDERATIONS

RESPIRATORY FAILURE

The older population is the fastest growing age group in North America, and this trend is reflected within acute and critical care settings. Of importance is that older persons are more vulnerable to delirium, hospital-acquired infections, and medication effects. Multiple factors contribute to an increased risk of respiratory failure in older persons, including the reduction in ventilatory capacity that accompanies aging, especially if risk factors are present. Physiological aging of the lung may produce alveolar dilation, diminish elastic recoil within the airways, decrease chest wall compliance, and decrease respiratory muscle strength. In older persons, the PaO_2 falls further and the $PaCO_2$ rises to a higher level before the respiratory system is stimulated to alter the rate and the depth of breathing. This delayed response can contribute to the development of respiratory failure. In addition, smoking is a risk factor that accelerates age-related respiratory changes. Poor nutritional status predisposes to decreased muscle mass, and less physiological reserve in cardiovascular, respiratory, and autonomic nervous systems increases the risk of additional diseases such as pneumonia and cardiac disease that may compromise respiratory function and precipitate respiratory failure (Killien et al., 2019).

Assessment parameters should be adjusted for age. For example, heart rate and blood pressure generally increase with age and with changes in the cardiovascular system. Therefore, determination of baseline vital signs and using them as a basis for comparison of physical assessment findings is most appropriate in evaluating changes in cardiopulmonary function in older persons.

ACUTE RESPIRATORY DISTRESS SYNDROME

Acute respiratory distress syndrome (ARDS) is a sudden and progressive form of acute respiratory failure in which the alveolar–capillary membrane becomes damaged and more permeable by intravascular fluid (Figure 70.8). The alveoli fill with fluid, which results in severe dyspnea, hypoxemia refractory to supplemental O_2, reduced lung compliance, and diffuse pulmonary infiltrates (Urden et al., 2020). Despite the fact that ARDS

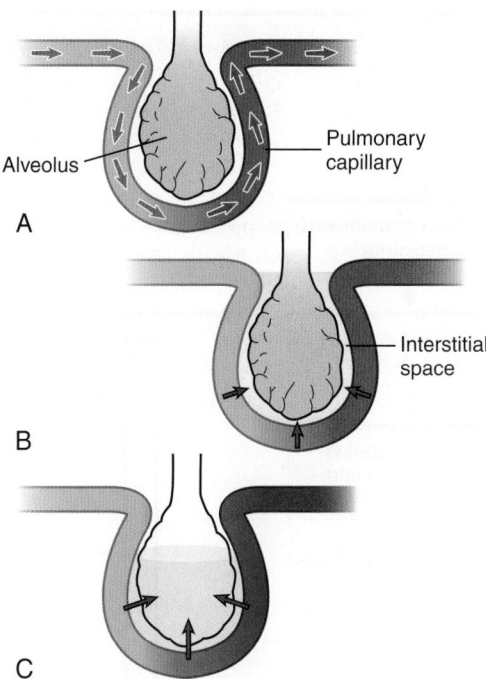

FIG. 70.8 Stages of edema formation in acute respiratory distress syndrome. **A,** Normal alveolus and pulmonary capillary. **B,** Interstitial edema occurs with increased flow of fluid into the interstitial space. **C,** Alveolar edema occurs when the fluid crosses the blood–gas barrier.

TABLE 70.7	CONDITIONS PREDISPOSING TO ACUTE RESPIRATORY DISTRESS SYNDROME	
Direct Lung Injury		**Indirect Lung Injury**
Common Causes		
• Aspiration		• Sepsis (especially Gram-negative infection)
• Viral or bacterial pneumonia		• Severe massive trauma
Less Common Causes		
• Chest trauma		• Acute pancreatitis
• Embolism: fat, air, amniotic fluid		• Anaphylaxis
• Inhalation of toxins		• Blood transfusions
• Near-drowning		• Cardiopulmonary bypass
• O_2 toxicity		• Disseminated intravascular coagulation
• Radiation pneumonitis		• Opioid overdose (e.g., heroin)
		• Nonpulmonary systemic diseases
		• Severe head injury
		• Shock

has been the focus of extensive clinical research, survival rates have not significantly improved. Despite supportive therapy, the rate of mortality from ARDS is approximately 50% (Virani et al., 2019). Patients who have both Gram-negative septic shock and ARDS have a significantly higher rate of mortality.

Etiology and Pathophysiology

Table 70.7 lists conditions that predispose patients to the development of ARDS. The most common cause of ARDS is sepsis. Patients with multiple risk factors are three to four times more likely to develop ARDS than are those without risk factors. Community-acquired pneumonia is another common cause of ARDS that develops outside of the hospital community. Common pathogens include *Streptococcus pneumoniae,* *Legionella pneumophila,* and a variety of respiratory viruses. Nosocomial (health care–related) pneumonias, including ventilator-associated pneumonia, can also progress to ARDS (see Chapter 68).

Patients may develop ARDS in the setting of influenza infection; ARDS is a fatal complication of influenza infection. Direct lung injury may cause ARDS (Figure 70.9), or ARDS may develop as a consequence of the systemic inflammatory response syndrome (see Chapter 69, Figure 69.1). This syndrome may have an infectious or a noninfectious etiology and is characterized by widespread inflammation or clinical responses to inflammation after a variety of physiological insults, including severe trauma, gut ischemia, lung injury, and sepsis (Urden et al., 2020). ARDS may also develop as a consequence of multiple-organ dysfunction syndrome, which results from organ system dysfunction that progressively increases in severity and ultimately results in multisystem organ failure. (Multiple-organ dysfunction syndrome is discussed in Chapter 69.)

In the initial injury to the lungs, the alveolar–capillary membrane is damaged. This activates complement and stimulates platelet aggregation and intravascular thrombus formation. Platelets release substances that attract and activate neutrophils (Brashers & Huether, 2018). The neutrophils cause a release of biochemical, humoral, and cellular mediators (Table 70.8) that produce changes in the lung, including increased pulmonary capillary membrane permeability, destruction of elastin and collagen, formation of pulmonary microemboli, and pulmonary artery vasoconstriction (see Figure 70.9). (Mediators are discussed in Chapters 14 and 16.) The pathophysiological changes in ARDS are divided into three phases: (1) injury or exudative phase, (2) reparative or proliferative phase, and (3) fibrotic phase.

Injury or Exudative Phase. The *injury or exudative phase* occurs approximately 1 to 7 days (usually 24 to 48 hours) after the initial direct lung injury or host insult. Neutrophils adhere to the pulmonary microcirculation, causing damage to the vascular endothelium and increased capillary permeability. In the earliest phase of injury, the peribronchial and perivascular interstitial spaces become engorged with fluid, which produces interstitial edema (Huppert et al., 2019). Next, fluid from the interstitial space crosses the alveolar epithelium and enters the alveolar space. Intrapulmonary shunting develops because the alveoli fill with fluid, and blood passing through them cannot be oxygenated (see Figures 70.4 and 70.8).

Type I and type II alveolar cells (which produce surfactant) are damaged by the changes caused by ARDS. This damage, in addition to further fluid and protein accumulation, results in surfactant dysfunction. The function of *surfactant* is to maintain alveolar stability by decreasing alveolar surface tension and preventing alveolar collapse. Decreased synthesis of surfactant and inactivation of existing surfactant cause the alveoli to become unstable and collapse (atelectasis). Widespread atelectasis further decreases lung compliance, compromises gas exchange, and contributes to hypoxemia.

During this stage, hyaline membranes begin to line the alveoli. These membranes are composed of necrotic cells, protein, and fibrin, and they lie adjacent to the alveoli wall. They are thought to result from the exudation of high-molecular-weight

PATHOPHYSIOLOGY MAP

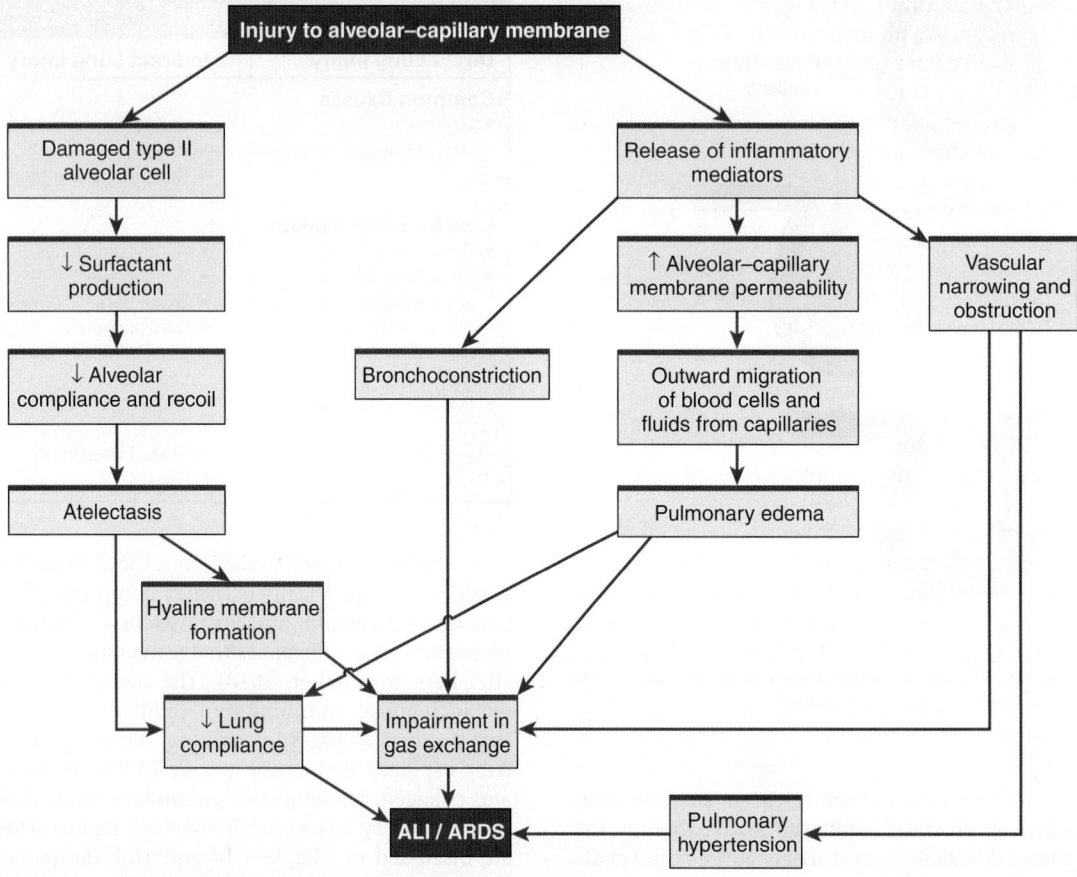

FIG. 70.9 Pathophysiology of acute respiratory distress syndrome (ARDS). *ALI,* acute lung injury.

TABLE 70.8	MEDIATORS OF ACUTE LUNG INJURY

- Arachidonic acid metabolites, including prostaglandins and leukotrienes
- Coagulation products, including kallikreins, kinins, fibrin degradation products, and plasminogen-activating factor
- Collagenase
- Complement component C5a
- Elastase
- Histamine
- Monocyte and macrophage products, including tumour necrosis factor, interleukin-1, and colony-stimulating factor
- Neutrophil products, including proteases and O_2 radicals
- Serotonin endotoxin

substances (particularly fibrinogen) in the edematous fluid. Hyaline membranes contribute to the development of fibrosis and atelectasis, which lead to a decrease in gas-exchange capability and lung compliance.

The primary pathophysiological changes that characterize the injury or exudative phase of ARDS are interstitial and alveolar edema (noncardiogenic pulmonary edema) and atelectasis (Huppert et al., 2019). Severe VQ mismatch and shunting of pulmonary capillary blood result in hypoxemia unresponsive to increasing concentrations of O_2 (termed refractory hypoxemia). Diffusion limitation, caused by hyaline membrane formation, further contributes to the severity of the hypoxemia. As

the lungs become less compliant ("stiffer") because of decreased surfactant, pulmonary edema, and atelectasis, the patient must generate higher airway pressures to inflate them. Reduced lung compliance greatly increases the patient's work of breathing. During ventilator management at this stage, a progressive increase in plateau and inspiratory pressures may be noted as lung compliance worsens.

Hypoxemia and the stimulation of juxtacapillary receptors in the stiff lung parenchyma (the juxtacapillary [J] reflex) initially cause an increase in respiratory rate and a decrease in tidal volume. This breathing pattern increases CO_2 removal, which leads to respiratory alkalosis. Cardiac output increases in response to hypoxemia, a compensatory effort to increase pulmonary blood flow. However, as atelectasis, pulmonary edema, and pulmonary shunting increase, compensation fails, and hypoventilation, a decrease in cardiac output, and a decrease in tissue O_2 perfusion eventually occur.

Reparative or Proliferative Phase. The *reparative or proliferative phase* of ARDS begins 1 to 2 weeks after the initial lung injury. During this phase, the inflammatory response includes an influx of neutrophils, monocytes, and lymphocytes, together with fibroblast proliferation. The injured lung has an immense regenerative capacity after acute lung injury. The proliferative phase is complete when the diseased lung becomes characterized by dense, fibrous tissue. Increased pulmonary vascular resistance and pulmonary hypertension may occur in this stage because fibroblasts and inflammatory cells destroy the pulmonary vasculature. Lung compliance continues to decrease as a result of interstitial fibrosis. Hypoxemia worsens because of the thickened alveolar membrane, causing diffusion limitation and shunting. If the reparative phase persists, widespread fibrosis results. If the reparative phase is arrested, the lesions resolve (Huppert et al., 2019).

Fibrotic Phase. The *fibrotic phase* of ARDS, also called the *chronic* or *late phase*, occurs approximately 2 to 3 weeks after the initial lung injury. During this time, the lung is completely remodelled by sparsely collagenous and fibrous tissues. Diffuse scarring and fibrosis further decrease lung compliance. In addition, the surface area for gas exchange is significantly reduced because the interstitium is fibrotic and, therefore, hypoxemia continues. Pulmonary hypertension results from pulmonary vascular destruction and fibrosis.

Clinical Progression

Progression of ARDS varies among patients. Some people survive the acute phase of lung injury; pulmonary edema resolves, and complete recovery occurs in a few days. The chance for survival is poor in patients who enter the fibrotic (chronic or late) phase, which necessitates long-term mechanical ventilation. It is not known why injured lungs repair and recover in some patients whereas ARDS progresses in others. Several factors seem to be important in determining the course of ARDS, including the nature of the initial injury, the extent and the severity of coexisting diseases, and pulmonary complications (Huppert et al., 2019).

Clinical Manifestations

The initial presentation of ARDS is often insidious. At the time of the initial injury, and up to 48 hours afterward, the patient may exhibit only dyspnea, tachypnea, cough, and restlessness. Chest auscultation may be normal or reveal fine, scattered crackles. ABG measurements usually indicate mild hypoxemia and respiratory alkalosis caused by hyperventilation. Respiratory alkalosis results from tachypnea, hypoxemia, and the stimulation of juxtacapillary receptors. The chest radiograph may be normal or exhibit evidence of minimal scattered interstitial infiltrates. Bilateral infiltrates become visible on the radiographs as ARDS progresses. As ARDS progresses, symptoms worsen because of increased fluid accumulation and decreased lung compliance. Respiratory distress becomes evident as the work of breathing increases. Tachypnea and intercostal and suprasternal retractions may be present. Pulmonary function tests in ARDS reveal decreased compliance and decreased lung volumes, particularly a decreased functional residual capacity. Tachycardia, diaphoresis, changes in sensorium with decreased mentation, cyanosis, and pallor may be present. Chest auscultation usually reveals scattered to diffuse crackles and wheezes. Chest radiographs demonstrate diffuse and extensive bilateral interstitial and alveolar infiltrates. A pulmonary artery catheter may need to be inserted. Pulmonary artery wedge pressure does not increase in ARDS because the cause is noncardiogenic (not related to cardiac function).

Hallmarks of ARDS include hypoxemia and a PaO_2/FiO_2 ratio below 200 despite increased FiO_2 by mask, cannula, or endotracheal tube. ABG measurements may initially demonstrate a normal or decreased $PaCO_2$ despite severe dyspnea and hypoxemia. Hypercapnia signifies that hypoventilation is occurring, and the patient is no longer able to maintain the level of ventilation needed to provide optimum gas exchange.

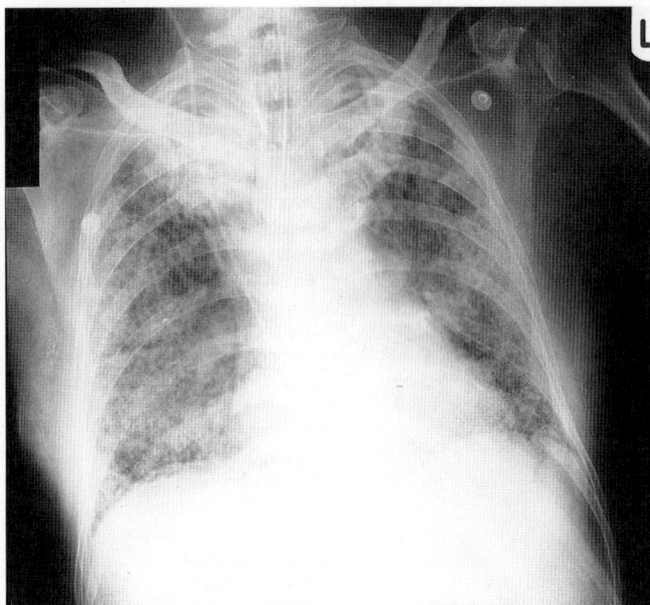

FIG. 70.10 Chest radiograph of a patient with acute respiratory distress syndrome. The image shows new, bilateral diffuse, homogeneous pulmonary infiltrates without cardiac failure, fluid overload, chest infection, or chronic lung disease. Source: Cohen, J., & Powderly, W. G. (2004). *Infectious diseases* (2nd ed.). Mosby.

TABLE 70.9	DIAGNOSTIC FINDINGS IN ACUTE RESPIRATORY DISTRESS SYNDROME
Chest radiograph	New bilateral interstitial and alveolar infiltrates
Predisposing condition	Identification of a predisposing condition for ARDS within 48 hr of clinical manifestations
Pulmonary artery wedge pressure	≤18 mm Hg and no evidence of heart failure
Refractory hypoxemia	PaO_2 <50 mm Hg, with an FiO_2 >40% and with PEEP >5 cm H_2O PaO_2/FiO_2 ratio <200

ARDS, acute respiratory distress syndrome; *FiO_2,* fraction of inspired oxygen; *PaO_2,* partial pressure of oxygen in arterial blood; *PEEP,* positive end-expiratory pressure.

As ARDS progresses, it is associated with profound respiratory distress that necessitates endotracheal intubation and PPV. The chest radiograph (Figure 70.10) shows what is often termed *whiteout* or *white lung* because consolidation and coalescing infiltrates are widespread throughout the lungs, leaving few recognizable air spaces. Pleural effusions may also be present. Severe hypoxemia, hypercapnia, and metabolic acidosis, with symptoms of target organ or tissue hypoxia, may ensue if therapy is not instituted promptly.

No precise criteria define ARDS. ARDS is considered to be present if (a) the patient has refractory hypoxemia, (b) a chest radiograph shows new bilateral interstitial or alveolar infiltrates, (c) the pulmonary artery wedge pressure is 18 mm Hg or less with no evidence of heart failure, and (d) a predisposing condition for ARDS develops within 48 hours of clinical manifestations (Table 70.9).

Complications

Complications may develop as a result of ARDS or its treatment. (Table 70.10 lists the common complications of ARDS.) The

TABLE 70.10	COMPLICATIONS ASSOCIATED WITH ACUTE RESPIRATORY DISTRESS SYNDROME
Cardiac complications	Decreased cardiac output
	Dysrhythmias
Endotracheal intubation complications	Laryngeal ulceration
	Tracheal malacia
	Tracheal stenosis
	Tracheal ulceration
Gastrointestinal complications	Hypermetabolic state, dramatically increased nutritional requirements
	Paralytic ileus
	Pneumoperitoneum
	Stress ulceration and hemorrhage
Hematological complications	Anemia
	Disseminated intravascular coagulation
	Thrombocytopenia
Infection	Catheter-related infection
	Hospital-acquired pneumonia
	Sepsis (bacteremia)
Renal complications	Acute kidney injury
Respiratory complications	O_2 toxicity
	Pulmonary barotraumas (e.g., pneumothorax, pneumomediastinum, subcutaneous emphysema)
	Pulmonary emboli
	Pulmonary fibrosis
	Ventilator-associated pneumonia

TABLE 70.11   INTERPROFESSIONAL CARE

Acute Respiratory Distress Syndrome

Diagnostic
See Table 70.9.

Interprofessional Therapy
Respiratory Therapy
- High-frequency oscillation
- Lateral rotation therapy
- Mechanical ventilation with PEEP
- O_2 administration
- Prone positioning

Supportive Therapy
- Diuretics
- Dobutamine
- Dopamine
- Hemodynamic monitoring
- Identification and treatment of underlying cause
- Inotropic or vasopressor medications
- IV fluid administration (fluid resuscitation early and less fluid later)

IV, intravenous; *PEEP*, positive end-expiratory pressure.

major cause of death in ARDS is multiple-organ dysfunction syndrome, often accompanied by sepsis. The vital organs most commonly involved are the kidneys, liver, and heart. The organ systems most often involved are the CNS and the hematological and gastrointestinal systems.

Hospital-Acquired Pneumonia. A frequent complication of ARDS is hospital-acquired pneumonia, occurring in as many as 68% of patients with ARDS. Risk factors include impaired host defences, contaminated medical equipment, invasive monitoring devices, aspiration of gastrointestinal contents, and prolonged mechanical ventilation, as well as colonization of the respiratory tract. Strategies to prevent hospital-acquired pneumonia include infection control measures (e.g., strict hand hygiene and sterile technique during endotracheal suctioning) and elevating the head of the bed 45 degrees or more to prevent aspiration (Urden et al., 2020). (See Chapter 30 for discussion of pneumonia.)

Barotrauma. *Barotrauma* may result from rupture of over-distended alveoli during mechanical ventilation. The high airway pressures necessary to ventilate patients with ARDS predispose to this complication. Barotrauma results in the presence of alveolar air in locations where it is not usually found. This can lead to pulmonary interstitial emphysema, pneumothorax, subcutaneous emphysema, pneumoperitoneum, pneumomediastinum, and tension pneumothorax. (See Chapter 30 for discussion of pneumothorax.)

To avoid barotrauma, patients with ARDS are ventilated with smaller tidal volumes. Different approaches to lung-protective ventilation are in current clinical use. Ventilation protocol include the use of small tidal volumes (e.g., 6 mL/kg) and varying amounts of positive end-expiratory pressure (PEEP) while the $PaCO_2$ gradually rises above normal (*permissive hypercapnia*), with the pH supported at 7.2 to 7.25 or above (Young et al., 2019). Permissive hypercapnia is commonly accepted as a consequence of lung-protective ventilation in ARDS. High-frequency

oscillation uses a constant mean airway pressure to maintain the alveoli in a recruited state while low tidal volumes are oscillated at a fast rate. Ventilation is achieved by the generation of extremely rapid pressure oscillations, usually in the range of 300 to 900 cycles/minute (Sklar et al., 2019).

Volutrauma. Volutrauma, or volupressure trauma, can occur in patients with ARDS when large tidal volumes (10 to 15 mL/kg) are used to ventilate noncompliant lungs. Volutrauma results in alveolar fractures and movement of fluids and proteins into the alveolar spaces. To limit this complication, it is recommended that smaller (lower) tidal volumes or pressure ventilation be used in patients with ARDS (see Chapter 68). Ventilation with low tidal volume reduces the damaging, excessive stretch of lung tissue that results in volutrauma.

Stress Ulcers. Critically ill patients with acute respiratory failure are at high risk for stress ulcers. Bleeding from stress ulcers occurs in 30% of patients with ARDS who require PPV, a higher incidence than for patients with other causes of acute respiratory failure. Management strategies include correction of predisposing conditions such as hypotension, shock, and acidosis. Prophylactic management includes antiulcer agents (e.g., famotidine [Pepcid], omeprazole [Losec], sucralphate [Sulcrate]) and early initiation of enteral nutrition (see Chapters 42 and 68).

Renal Failure. The kidneys have a close functional relationship with the lungs. The combination of ARDS and renal failure results in a greater mortality rate for these patients (Malek et al., 2018). Renal failure results from decreased renal tissue oxygenation due to hypotension, hypoxemia, or hypercapnia and from administration of nephrotoxic medications (e.g., aminoglycosides).

NURSING AND INTERPROFESSIONAL MANAGEMENT ACUTE RESPIRATORY DISTRESS SYNDROME

The interprofessional care for patients with acute respiratory failure (see Table 70.6) and the nursing care plan for acute respiratory failure (see NCP 70.1, available on the Evolve website) are applicable to ARDS. The following section is a discussion of additional interprofessional care measures for patients with ARDS (Table 70.11). Patients with ARDS are commonly cared for in critical care units.

NURSING ASSESSMENT

Because ARDS causes acute respiratory failure, the subjective and objective data that should be obtained from a patient with ARDS are the same as those for acute respiratory failure (see Table 70.5). Abnormal findings on physical examination are indications that ARDS has progressed beyond the initial stages.

NURSING DIAGNOSES

Nursing diagnoses for patients with ARDS may include but are not limited to those described for acute respiratory failure (see also NCP 70.1, available on the Evolve website).

PLANNING

With appropriate therapy, the overall goals for the patient with ARDS are a PaO_2 of at least 60 mm Hg and adequate lung ventilation to maintain normal pH. After recovery from ARDS, (a) the patient's PaO_2 should be within normal limits for age or baseline values on room air (FiO_2 of 21%), (b) the SaO_2 should be greater than 90%, (c) the patient's airway should be patent, and (d) on auscultation, the lungs should sound clear.

RESPIRATORY THERAPY

OXYGEN ADMINISTRATION. The primary goal of O_2 therapy is to correct hypoxemia. Use of a simple face mask or nasal cannula is usually inadequate to treat refractory hypoxemia associated with ARDS. Masks with high-flow systems that deliver higher O_2 concentrations are initially used to maximize O_2 delivery, and O_2 saturation is monitored continuously to assess their effectiveness. The standard for O_2 administration is to administer the lowest concentration that results in a PaO_2 of 60 mm Hg or higher so as to minimize the risk of O_2 toxicity.

Early noninvasive ventilation application may be extremely helpful in immunocompromised patients with pulmonary infiltrates, in whom intubation dramatically increases the risk of infection, pneumonia, and death. Overall, because of the high rate of failure with noninvasive ventilation, noninvasive ventilation should be used with caution in patients with acute lung injury or ARDS. Prompt intubation is required if signs of noninvasive ventilation failure emerge. Patients with ARDS commonly need intubation with mechanical ventilation because the PaO_2 cannot otherwise be maintained at acceptable levels.

MECHANICAL VENTILATION. Endotracheal intubation and mechanical ventilation provide additional respiratory support. However, FiO_2 of 50% or greater may still be necessary to maintain the PaO_2 at 60 mm Hg or higher. During mechanical ventilation, it is common to apply PEEP at 5 cm H_2O to compensate for loss of glottic function caused by the presence of the endotracheal tube. In patients with ARDS, higher levels of PEEP (e.g., 10–20 cm H_2O) may be used to increase functional residual capacity and recruit (open up) collapsed alveoli. PEEP is typically applied in increments of 3 to 5 cm H_2O until oxygenation is adequate with FiO_2 of 60% or lower. PEEP may improve VQ in respiratory units that collapse at low airway pressures, thus allowing the FiO_2 to be lowered.

PEEP, however, is not a benign therapy. The additional intrathoracic and intrapulmonic pressures can compromise venous return to the right side of the heart, thereby decreasing preload, cardiac output, and blood pressure. PEEP can also cause hyperinflation of the alveoli, compression of the pulmonary capillary bed, a reduction in blood return to the left side of the heart, and a dramatic reduction in blood pressure. In addition, PEEP and excessive inspiratory pressures can contribute to barotrauma and volutrauma (van der Zee & Gommers, 2019).

If hypoxemia persists despite high PEEP, alternative modes and therapies may be used. These include pressure-support ventilation, pressure-release ventilation, pressure-control ventilation, inverse-ratio ventilation, high-frequency oscillation, and permissive hypercapnia. (Additional information on mechanical ventilation and PEEP is provided in Chapter 68.)

In extracorporeal membrane oxygenation (ECMO) and extracorporeal carbon dioxide ($ECCO_2$) removal, blood passes across an external gas-exchanging membrane, is oxygenated, and returns to the body (Figure 70.11). These interventions are referred to as *extracorporeal life support*. Despite the use of various strategies, severe forms of ARDS do not respond and are associated with a high mortality rate (Aretha et al., 2019). Although ECMO has not been clearly demonstrated to

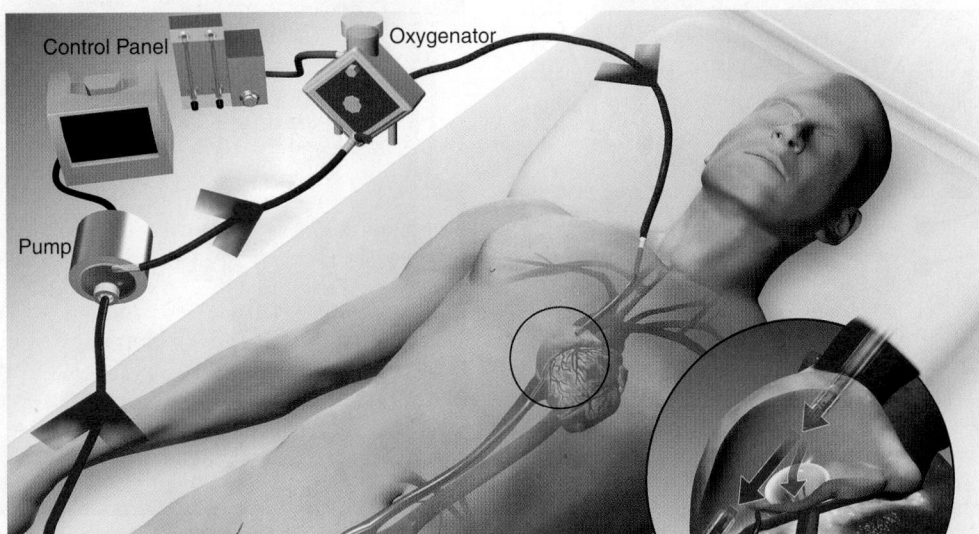

FIG. 70.11 Extracorporeal membrane oxygenation (ECMO). Blood is oxygenated outside the body (or extracorporeally) by a circuit that takes over the function of lungs or, in some cases, heart and lungs. Source: Reprinted with permission from Columbia University Irving Medical Center, Department of Surgery.

be better than the standard of care for ARDS, referral to a specialized centre with ECMO experience should be considered a therapy option for patients with severe hypoxemic ARDS (Aretha et al., 2019).

POSITIONING STRATEGIES. Some patients with ARDS demonstrate an improvement in PaO_2 when turned from the supine to prone position with no change in FiO_2. The response may be sufficient to allow a reduction in FiO_2 or PEEP.

In early ARDS, fluid moves freely throughout the lung. Because of gravity, this fluid pools in dependent lung regions in such a way that some alveoli are fluid filled (dependent areas), whereas others are air filled (nondependent areas). In addition, when the patient is supine, the mediastinal contents place more pressure on the lungs than in the prone position, which changes pleural pressure and predisposes to atelectasis. If the patient is turned to the prone position, air-filled, nonatelectic alveoli in the ventral (anterior) lung become dependent. Perfusion may be better matched to ventilation, causing less VQ mismatch. Prone positioning is typically reserved for patients with refractory hypoxemia, but not all patients respond with an increase in PaO_2. When prone positioning is used, there must be a plan for immediate repositioning for cardiopulmonary resuscitation in the event of a cardiac arrest (Sklar et al., 2019). The Roto-Prone Therapy System (Figure 70.12) is a bed that is designed for a patient placed in the prone position and provides kinetic therapy in which the patient is turned side to side to any angle between 40 and 62 degrees.

Other positioning strategies used in ARDS are lateral rotation therapy and kinetic therapy. The purpose of this therapy is to provide continuous, slow, side-to-side turning of the patient by rotation of the bed frame. Lateral movement of the bed is maintained for 18 hours daily to simulate postural drainage and help mobilize secretions. In addition, the bed may also contain a vibrator pack that can provide chest physiotherapy to further assist with secretion removal (Figure 70.13). The patient's pulmonary status (e.g., respiratory rate and rhythm, breath sounds, ABGs, SpO_2) should be assessed before initiation of the therapy and continuously throughout therapy.

MEDICAL SUPPORTIVE THERAPY

MAINTENANCE OF CARDIAC OUTPUT AND TISSUE PERFUSION. Patients receiving PPV and PEEP frequently experience decreased cardiac output in relation to impaired contractility, decreased preload, decreased venous return, or some combination of these conditions, as a result of PEEP-induced increases in intrathoracic pressure. Continuous hemodynamic monitoring is essential for detecting changes and titrating therapy. An arterial catheter is inserted for continuous blood pressure monitoring and ABG sampling. A pulmonary artery catheter enables monitoring of pulmonary artery pressures, pulmonary artery wedge pressures (which reflect the fluid status of the left side of the heart), mixed venous oxygen saturation, and cardiac output. If the cardiac output falls, it may be necessary to administer fluids or to lower the PEEP. Use of inotropic medications, such as dobutamine or dopamine, may also be necessary. (See Chapter 68 for discussion of hemodynamic monitoring.)

The hemoglobin is usually kept above 6 mmol/L with an O_2 saturation of 90 or higher (when $PaO_2 \geq 60$ mm Hg). Packed red blood cells may be administered to increase hemoglobin and thus the O_2-carrying capacity of the blood.

MAINTENANCE OF NUTRITION AND FLUID BALANCE. Maintenance of nutrition and fluid balance is challenging in patients with ARDS. Nutrition consultations can determine optimal caloric needs. Attaining access and initiating enteral nutrition should be considered as soon as fluid resuscitation is completed and the patient is hemodynamically stable. A "window of opportunity" exists in the first 24 to 72 hours after the patient's admission or the onset of a hypermetabolic insult. Omega-3 fatty acids might improve the clinical outcomes of patients undergoing ARDS (Dushianthan et al., 2020). However, current research has shown that the use of enteral omega-3 fatty acids did not significantly reduce all-cause 28-day mortality rates. Further investigations based on concentrations of omega-3 are needed to support further findings. Increased pulmonary capillary permeability

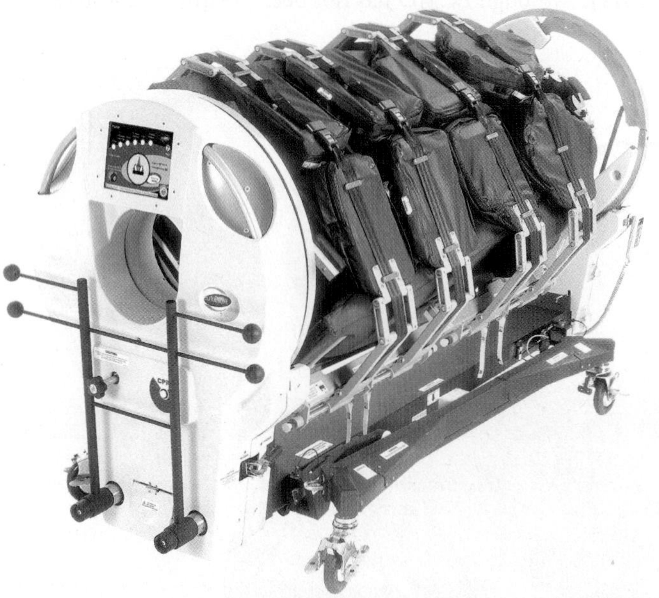

FIG. 70.12 RotoProne bed. The RotoProne Delta Therapy System allows clinicians to place patients in the prone position, safely and effectively. This product is not specifically indicated for the treatment of acute respiratory distress syndrome or ventilator-associated pneumonia. Source: Photo courtesy Arjo Inc.

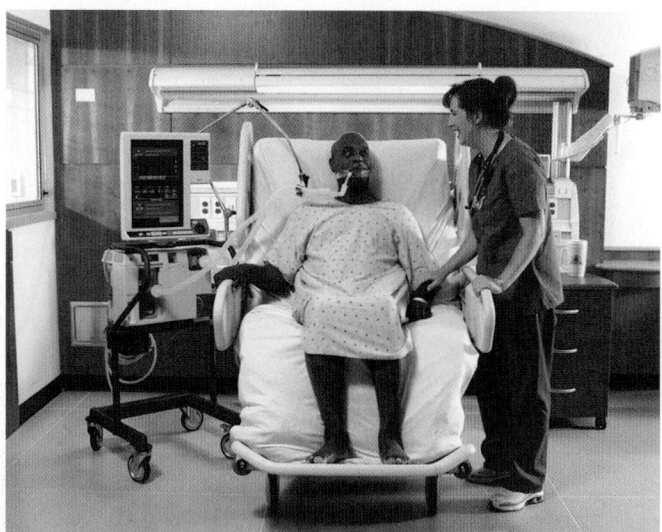

FIG. 70.13 TotalCare SpO₂RT Bed System offers continuous lateral rotation therapy and percussion and vibration therapies. Patients can be repositioned easily and quickly. Source: © 2006 Hill-Rom Services, Inc. Reprinted with permission. All rights reserved.

results in pulmonary edema. However, the patient may be volume depleted, hypotensive, and prone to decreased cardiac output from mechanical ventilation and PEEP. Pulmonary artery wedge pressures, daily weights, and intake and output are monitored to assess fluid status. Fluid replacement with crystalloids or colloids is still being debated. Critics of colloid use believe that proteins in colloid solutions leak into the pulmonary interstitium, exacerbating the movement of proteinaceous fluid into the alveoli. Advocates of colloids as replacement believe that colloids help keep fluid from leaking into the alveoli (Casey et al., 2019). The pulmonary artery wedge pressure is kept as low as possible without impairing cardiac output in order to limit pulmonary edema. Fluids are usually restricted mildly, with diuretics administered as needed (Urden et al., 2020).

EVALUATION

The expected outcomes for patients with ARDS are similar to those for patients with acute respiratory failure and are presented in NCP 70.1, available on the Evolve website.

SEVERE ACUTE RESPIRATORY SYNDROME

Severe acute respiratory syndrome (SARS) is a serious, acute respiratory infection caused by a coronavirus. Coronaviruses, a large family of viruses named for their spiked surfaces that resemble crowns, can cause a range of symptoms from the common cold to severe acute respiratory illness. The new coronavirus disease, abbreviated COVID-19, is highly contagious. The virus is spread through small droplets from the nose or mouth when a person with the disease coughs or exhales. There were two other outbreaks of coronaviruses that originated in animals and subsequently infected people: severe acute respiratory syndrome (SARS-CoV), in 2002, and Middle East respiratory syndrome (MERS-CoV), in 2012.

The 2019 novel coronavirus is termed SARS-CoV-2 because of its similar genetic makeup to SARS-CoV (World Health Organization [WHO], 2021). The virus can cause COVID-19, with symptoms such as fever, dry cough, shortness of breath, breathing difficulties, body aches, nasal congestion, sore throat, and diarrhea (WHO, 2021). Symptoms may be mild and appear in as few as 2 days or as long as 14 days after exposure (Centers for Disease Control and Prevention [CDC], 2021). Most people (80%) will fully recover without needing special treatment, whereas one out of six people will become seriously ill (WHO, 2021). Older individuals and persons with comorbidities such as cardiac disease, lung disorders, or diabetes are at a higher risk of developing serious illness.

Measures to prevent spread of the COVID-19 include staying 2 metres (6 feet) away from any person who is sick, frequent hand hygiene with soap and water or an alcohol-based hand rub, and avoiding touching one's eyes, nose, mouth, and face with unwashed hands (WHO, 2021). Multiple vaccines for the prevention of COVID-19 have been developed and became available to the public in early 2021. Vaccination and vigilant infection-control practices coupled with early identification and treatment can assist in preventing the spread of this virus and potentially decrease associated morbidity and mortality.

COVID-19 may result in pneumonia leading to ARDS (Grieco et al., 2020). Whether ARDS is from COVID-19 or other etiologies, the differences in the resulting ARDS appear to be negligible. However, further research is emerging. Until other data emerge, patients with ARDS related to COVID-19 should be treated following current ARDS treatment guidelines.

CASE STUDY

Acute Respiratory Distress Syndrome

Patient Profile

F. H. (pronouns he/him) is a 55-year-old admitted to a surgical critical care unit (CCU) 72 hr ago after undergoing bowel resection. The surgery was extensive to repair a perforated colon, irrigate the abdominal cavity, and provide hemostasis. During surgery, F. H.'s systolic blood pressure (BP) dropped to 70 mm Hg. Seven units of packed red blood cells and 4 L of normal saline were administered to restore blood loss and circulating volume. F. H. is currently receiving 60% FiO$_2$ through an aerosol face mask and has continuous cardiac monitoring and O$_2$ saturation in place. He is receiving 0.9% normal saline at 125 mL/hr through a central line. A urinary catheter is in place.

Subjective Data
- Reports shortness of breath, inability to lie flat, and diffuse abdominal pain.
- F. H.'s partner and two adult children are at the bedside voicing concerns and asking questions about his condition.

Objective Data
Physical Assessment
- *General:* Alert, well nourished, appears restless and anxious; head of bed elevated 30 degrees; skin cool, moderate diaphoresis
- *Respiratory:* No accessory muscle use, retractions, or paradoxical breathing; respiration rate, 28 breaths/min; SpO$_2$, 85%; fine crackles at lung bases
- *Cardiovascular:* BP, 90/60 mm Hg; sinus tachycardia at 130 beats/min; equal apical–radial pulse; temperature, 38°C orally

- *Gastrointestinal:* No bowel sounds heard; surgical dressing dry and intact
- *Urological:* Catheter draining concentrated urine at <30 mL/hr

Diagnostic Findings
- ABG results: pH, 7.35; PaO$_2$, 55 mm Hg; PaCO$_2$, 27 mm Hg; bicarbonate level, 16 mmol/L; SaO$_2$, 86%
- Chest radiograph: new scattered interstitial infiltrates compatible with ARDS

Discussion Questions
1. How does the pathophysiology of ARDS predispose to the development of refractory hypoxemia?
2. What clinical manifestations does F. H. exhibit that support a diagnosis of ARDS?
3. What are the possible causes of ARDS in F. H.?
4. What are the possible complications that F. H. is at risk for developing secondary to ARDS?
5. **Evidence-informed practice:** A new nurse who is being oriented asks why F. H.'s family was offered the opportunity to stay at his bedside while the chest tube was placed. How should the nurse respond?
6. **Priority decision**: What priority interventions should be implemented to improve F. H.'s respiratory status and hypoxemia?
7. **Priority decision:** On the basis of the assessment data presented, what are the priority nursing diagnoses?
8. What information should the nurse provide to the caregivers, in view of F. H.'s decline in cardiopulmonary function?

Evolve
Answers are available at http://evolve.elsevier.com/Canada/Lewis/medsurg.

REVIEW QUESTIONS

The number of the question corresponds to the same-numbered objective at the beginning of the chapter.

1. Which signs and symptoms differentiate hypoxemic respiratory failure from hypercapnic respiratory failure? *(Select all that apply.)*
   a. Cyanosis
   b. Tachypnea
   c. Morning headache
   d. Paradoxical breathing
   e. Use of pursed-lip breathing

2. What is an early sign of acute respiratory failure?
   a. Coma
   b. Cyanosis
   c. Restlessness
   d. Paradoxical breathing

3. Which type of oxygen delivery system should be chosen for clients in acute respiratory failure?
   a. A low-flow device, such as a nasal cannula
   b. One that should correct the partial pressure of oxygen in arterial blood (PaO_2) to a normal level as quickly as possible
   c. Positive-pressure ventilation to prevent CO_2 narcosis
   d. One that should maintain the PaO_2 at 60 mm Hg or higher at the lowest fraction of inspired oxygen (FiO_2) possible

4. What are the early clinical manifestations of ARDS?
   a. Dyspnea and tachypnea
   b. Cyanosis and apprehension
   c. Hypotension and tachycardia
   d. Respiratory distress and frothy sputum

5. How is fluid balance maintained in clients with ARDS?
   a. Hydration with colloids
   b. Administration of surfactant
   c. Mild fluid restriction and diuretics as necessary
   d. Keeping the hemoglobin at levels of 9.5 mmol/L (15 g/dL)

6. Which of the following is designed to prevent barotrauma in clients with ARDS?
   a. Increasing positive end-expiratory pressure (PEEP)
   b. Increasing the tidal volume
   c. Permissive hypercapnia
   d. Pressure support ventilation

1. a, b, d; 2. c; 3. d; 4. a; 5. c; 6. c.

ⓔvolve

For even more review questions, visit http://evolve.elsevier.com/Canada/Lewis/medsurg.

REFERENCES

Aretha, D., Fligou, F., Kiekkas, P., et al. (2019). Extracorporeal life support: The next step in moderate to severe ARDS—a review and meta-analysis of the literature. *BioMed Research International*, 1–11. https://doi.org/10.1155/2019/1035730

Blakeborough, L., & Watson, J. S. (2019). The importance of obtaining a sputum sample and how it can aid diagnosis and treatment. *British Journal of Nursing*, 28(5), 295–298. https://doi.org/10.12968/bjon.2019.28.5.295

Brashers, V., & Huether, S. E. (2018). Alterations of pulmonary function. In K. L. McCance, & S. E. Huether (Eds.), *Pathophysiology: The biologic basis for disease in adults and children* (8th ed., pp. 1248–1289). Elsevier Mosby.

Burns, S. M., & Delgado, S. A. (2019). *AACN essentials of critical care nursing* (4th ed.). McGraw-Hill.

Calzetta, L., Matera, M. G., Cazzola, M., et al. (2019). Optimizing the development strategy of combination therapy in respiratory medicine: From isolated airways to patients. *Advances in Therapy*, 36(12), 3291–3298. https://doi.org/10.1007/s12325-019-01119-w

Casey, J. D., Semler, M. W., & Rice, T. W. (2019). Fluid management in acute respiratory distress syndrome. *Seminars in Respiratory and Critical Care Medicine*, 40(1), 57–65. https://doi.org/10.1055/s-0039-1685206

Centers for Disease Control and Prevention (CDC). (2021). *Symptoms of COVID-2019*. https://www.cdc.gov/coronavirus/2019-ncov/symptoms-testing/symptoms.html

Chao, K.-Y., Lin, Y.-W., Chiang, C.-E., et al. (2019). Respiratory management in smoke inhalation injury. *Journal of Burn Care and Research*, 40(4), 507–512. https://doi.org/10.1093/jbcr/irz043

Conway, J., & Friedman, B. (2020). Intravenous magnesium sulfate for acute asthma exacerbation in adults. *Academic Emergency Medicine*, 27(10), 1061–1063. https://doi.org/10.1111/acem.14066

Ding, L., Wang, L., Ma, W., et al. (2020). Efficacy and safety of early prone positioning combined with HFNC or NIV in moderate to severe ARDS: A multi-center prospective cohort study. *Critical Care*, 24(1), 1–8. https://doi.org/10.1186/s13054-020-2738-5

Dushianthan, A., Cusack, R., Burgess, V. A., et al. (2020). Immunonutrition for adults with ARDS: Results from a Cochrane systematic review and meta-analysis. *Respiratory Care*, 65(1), 99–110. https://doi.org/10.4187/respcare.06965

Frankenfield, D. C. (2019). Impact of feeding on resting metabolic rate and gas exchange in critically ill patients. *JPEN - Journal of Parenteral and Enteral Nutrition*, 43(2), 226–233. https://doi.org/10.1002/jpen.1420

Greene, M. T., Gilmartin, H. M., & Saint, S. (2020). Psychological safety and infection prevention practices: Results from a national survey. *American Journal of Infection Control*, 48(1), 2–6. https://doi.org/10.1016/j.ajic.2019.09.027

Grieco, D. L., Bongiovanni, F., Chen, L., et al. (2020). Respiratory physiology of COVID-19-induced respiratory failure compared to ARDS of other etiologies. *Critical Care*, 24, 1–11. https://doi.org/10.1186/s13054-020-03253-2

Huppert, L. A., Matthay, M. A., & Ware, L. B. (2019). Pathogenesis of acute respiratory distress syndrome. *Seminars in Respiratory and Critical Care Medicine*, 40(1), 31–39. https://doi.org/10.1055/s-0039-1683996

Killien, E. Y., Mills, B., Vavilala, M. S., et al. (2019). Association between age and acute respiratory distress syndrome development and mortality following trauma. *Journal of Trauma & Acute Care Surgery*, 86(5), 844–852. https://doi.org/10.1097/TA.0000000000002202

Korwin, A., & Honiden, S. (2019). Reconsidering nutritional support in critically ill patients. *Seminars in Respiratory and Critical Care Medicine*, 40(5), 580–593. https://doi.org/10.1055/s-0039-1697967

Malek, M., Hassanshahi, J., Fartootzadeh, R., et al. (2018). Nephrogenic acute respiratory distress syndrome: A narrative review on pathophysiology and treatment. *Chinese Journal of Traumatology*, 21(1), 4–10. https://doi.org/10.1016/j.cjtee.2017.07.004

Sklar, M. C., Patel, B. K., Beitler, J. R., et al. (2019). Optimal ventilator strategies in acute respiratory distress syndrome. *Seminars in Respiratory and Critical Care Medicine, 40*(1), 81–93. https://doi.org/10.1055/s-0039-1683896

Stawicki, N., & Gessner, P. (2018). Residual neuromuscular blockade in the critical care setting. *AACN Advanced Critical Care, 29*(1), 15–24. https://doi.org/10.4037/aacnacc2018384

Urden, L. D., Stacy, K. M., & Lough, M. E. (2020). *Priorities in critical care nursing* (8th ed.). Mosby.

Virani, A., Ma, K., Leap, J., et al. (2019). Acute respiratory distress syndrome definition, causes, and pathophysiology. *Critical Care Nursing Quarterly, 42*(4), 344–348. https://doi.org/10.1097/CNQ.0000000000000274

Wieslander, B., Ramos, J. G., Ax, M., et al. (2019). Supine, prone, right and left gravitational effects on human pulmonary circulation. *Journal of Cardiovascular Magnetic Resonance, 21*(1). https://doi.org/10.1186/s12968-019-0577-9. Article no. 69.

World Health Organization (WHO). (2021). *Coronavirus disease (COVID-19).* https://www.who.int/health-topics/coronavirus

Young, M., DiSilvio, B., Rao, S., et al. (2019). Mechanical ventilation in ARDS. *Critical Care Nursing Quarterly, 42*(4), 392–399. https://doi.org/10.1097/CNQ.0000000000000279

van der Zee, P., & Gommers, D. (2019). Recruitment maneuvers and higher PEEP, the so-called open lung concept, in patients with ARDS. *Critical Care, 23*(1), 73. https://doi.org/10.1186/s13054-019-2365-1

RESOURCES

Resources for this chapter are listed in Chapter 71.

Nursing Management

Emergency Care Situations

Jane Tyerman

Originating US chapter by Cathy Edson and Amy Meredith

⊖volve WEBSITE

http://evolve.elsevier.com/Canada/Lewis/medsurg

- Review Questions (Online Only)
- Key Points
- Answer Guidelines for Case Study
- Student Case Study
  - Musculoskeletal Trauma
- Conceptual Care Map Creator
- Audio Glossary
- Content Updates

LEARNING OBJECTIVES

1. Apply the steps in triage, the primary survey, and the secondary survey to assess a patient in a medical, surgical, or traumatic emergency.
2. Relate the pathophysiology of clinical manifestations to the assessment and interprofessional care of patients experiencing select environmental emergencies.
3. Relate the pathophysiology of clinical manifestations to the assessment and interprofessional care of patients experiencing select toxicological emergencies.
4. Select appropriate nursing interventions for victims of violence.
5. Summarize the clinical manifestations of sexual assault and the appropriate nursing and interprofessional management of the patient who has been sexually assaulted.

KEY TERMS

drowning
family and intimate partner violence (IPV)
family presence
frostbite
heat cramps

heat exhaustion
heatstroke
hypothermia
primary survey
rapid-sequence intubation

secondary survey
sexual assault
submersion injury
triage

Emergency care nursing is a unique specialty that requires a solid understanding of basic nursing concepts and specific approaches to patient health problems. Nurses unaccustomed to the emergency department (ED) often describe the flow as chaotic and uncertain. Certainly, it may have this appearance. The challenge of the ED is that the nurse does not know what emergency situation or health problem the patient will present with when they come through the doors. The trained ED nurse must be prepared to meet this challenge.

Many patients report to the ED for less urgent conditions, often because they do not have access to a health care provider. Emergency nurses care for patients of all ages with a variety of health conditions, especially in the areas of health promotion and prevention and chronic disease management. Some EDs specialize in certain patient populations, such as pediatric patients, or certain conditions, such as trauma.

Nursing roles within the ED include patient care, research, and management. The National Emergency Nurses Association (NENA) is the Canadian specialty nursing organization aimed at advancing emergency nursing practice. NENA publishes standards of care for nurses working in the ED and endorses the Canadian Nurses Association (CNA) certification process to become a certified emergency nurse, ENC(C). This certification validates the knowledge and skills that a nurse needs in order to provide competent care in emergency settings (CNA, 2021; NENA, 2020).

Specific emergency management of patients with various medical, surgical, and traumatic emergencies is described throughout this book (Table 71.1). This chapter focuses on initial assessment and management of patients with trauma and emergency conditions not addressed elsewhere in this book. These include heat- and cold-related emergencies, submersion injuries, bites, stings, poisonings, abuse, and violence.

CARE OF THE EMERGENCY PATIENT

Recognizing life-threatening illness or injury is one of the most important goals of emergency nursing. Initiating interventions to reverse or prevent a crisis is often a priority before making a medical diagnosis. This process begins with the nurse's first contact with a patient. Prompt identification of patients who need immediate treatment and determining appropriate interventions are essential nurse competencies.

For instance, with the advent of the COVID-19 pandemic, care provided during emergency situations needed to be adjusted to minimize exposure risk to patients and health care workers. Comprehensive infection, prevention, and control (IPC) practices were developed to prevent or minimize the transmission of COVID-19 during care. National organizations, such as the Heart and Stroke Foundation of Canada, adjusted

current algorithms that prioritized oxygenation and ventilation strategies, reduced provider exposure, and emphasized goals of care focusing on the appropriateness of resuscitation (Heart and Stroke Foundation of Canada, 2021).

TRIAGE

Triage, a French word meaning "to sort," refers to the process of rapidly determining patient acuity. It is one of the most important assessment skills needed by ED nurses. Most often, the nurse will confront multiple patients who have a variety of health conditions. The process is based on the premise that patients who have a threat to life, limb, or vision should be treated before other patients. Unique to the ED, the triage nurse performs a brief patient assessment to categorize and prioritize the needs of each patient seeking care. This categorization is facilitated by use of the Canadian Triage and Acuity Scale (CTAS). The CTAS is used in the ED as well as by community paramedics to define the urgency of a patient's presenting condition (Bullard et al., 2017; Ding et al., 2019).

The CTAS is a five-level scale consisting of the following categories: resuscitation, emergency, urgent, less urgent, and nonurgent (Table 71.2). Patients who are assigned a high triage level (level I: resuscitation) are allocated the most health care resources and are assessed immediately. Patient assigned to a low triage level (e.g., level V: nonurgent) wait longer for nurse and physician assessment, unless they experience a deterioration in clinical status while they wait (Bullard et al., 2017). The CTAS has four major components: (1) five *triage levels* (ranging from nonurgent to resuscitation); (2) a *time to nurse and physician assessment*, which is based on the assigned triage level; (3) *usual presentation of the patient* (e.g., head injury, alert, with no vomiting; sore throat with no respiratory symptoms), which is based on the patient's reports and presentation; and (4) a *sentinel diagnosis* (e.g., head injury; upper respiratory infection).

The emergency nurse must complete an initial assessment to determine the presence of actual or potential threats to life and then rapidly initiate interventions appropriate for the patient's condition. Simultaneously, the nurse collects a history. A systematic approach to the initial assessment of the patient decreases the time required to identify potential threats and keeps to a minimum the risk of missing a life-threatening condition. Two systematic approaches initially developed for use with patients with trauma, a primary and a secondary survey, can be applied to emergency assessment.

✚ TABLE 71.1 EMERGENCY MANAGEMENT

Emergency Management Tables

Subject	Chapter
Abdominal trauma	45
Acute abdominal pain	45
Acute soft-tissue injury	65
Anaphylactic shock	16
Chemical burns	27
Chest pain	36
Chest trauma	30
Cocaine and amphetamine toxicity	11
Depressant drugs, overdose of	11
Diabetic ketoacidosis	52
Electrical burns	27
Eye injury	24
Fractured extremity	65
Head injury	59
Hyperthermia	71
Hypothermia	71
Inhalation injury	27
Sexual assault	71
Shock	69
Spinal cord injury	63
Stroke	60
Submersion injuries	71
Thermal burns	27
Thoracic injuries	30
Tonic–clonic seizures	61

TABLE 71.2 THE CANADIAN EMERGENCY DEPARTMENT TRIAGE AND ACUITY SCALE

Consideration	Resuscitation (Level I)	Emergency (Level II)	Urgent (Level III)	Less Urgent (Level IV)	Nonurgent (Level V)
Condition	Threat to life or limb; immediate assessment required Example: cardiac or respiratory arrest, major trauma, shock state, severe dehydration	Potential threat to life, limb, or function Example: altered mental state, head injury, cardiac chest pain, stroke, core temperature 39°C–41°C	Potential to progress to serious condition Example: asthma, GI bleed, acute pain	May progress to urgent status Example: headache, corneal foreign body, chronic back pain	Acute or chronic but nonurgent Example: sore throat, mild abdominal pain that is chronic or recurring
Time to nurse and health care provider assessment	Immediate	15 min	30 min	60 min	120 min
Recommended re-evaluation	Continuous	Every 15 min	Every 30 min	Every 60 min	Every 120 min

GI, gastrointestinal.

Source: Adapted from Bullard, M. J., Unger, B., Spence, J., et al. (2008). Revisions to the Canadian Triage and Acuity Scale (CTAS) adult guidelines. *Canadian Journal of Emergency Medicine, 10*(2), 137.

TABLE 71.3   PRIMARY SURVEY OF A PATIENT IN AN EMERGENCY

Assessment	Interventions
Airway With Cervical Spine Stabilization and/or Immobilization	
• Assess for catastrophic external bleeding. • Assess for respiratory distress. • Assess airway for patency. • Check for loose teeth and foreign objects. • Assess for bleeding, vomitus, or edema.	• Control bleeding with direct pressure and pressure dressings. • Open airway using jaw-thrust manoeuvre. • Remove or suction any foreign objects. • Insert oropharyngeal or nasopharyngeal airway, tracheostomy. • Initiate rapid sequence intubation (see Chapter 68). • Immobilize cervical spine using rigid cervical collar and cervical immobilization device.
Breathing	
• Assess ventilation. • Chest scan for signs of breathing • Observe for paradoxical movement of the chest wall during inspiration and expiration. • Observe for use of accessory muscles or abdominal muscles. • Observe and count respiratory rate. • Note colour of nail beds, mucous membranes, and skin. • Auscultate lungs. • Assess for jugular venous distension and position of trachea.	• Administer supplemental O_2 via appropriate delivery system (e.g., nonrebreather mask). • Ventilate with bag valve mask device with 100% O_2 if respirations are inadequate or absent. • Prepare to intubate patient if respiratory distress is severe (e.g., agonal breaths, respiratory arrest). • Have suction available. • If breath sounds are absent, prepare for needle thoracostomy and chest tube insertion.
Circulation	
• Check of carotid or femoral pulse • Palpate pulse for quality and rate. • Assess skin colour, temperature, and moisture. • Check of capillary refill	• If pulse is absent, initiate cardiopulmonary resuscitation and advanced life-support measures. • If shock symptoms are present, insert two large-bore (14- to 16-gauge) IV catheters and initiate infusions of normal saline or lactated Ringer's solution. • Consider intraosseous or central venous access if IV access cannot be rapidly obtained. • Administer blood products, if ordered.
Disability: Brief Neurological Assessment	
• Assess level of consciousness by determining response to verbal stimuli, painful stimuli, and motor response (e.g., Glasgow Coma Scale). • Assess pupils for size, shape, equality, and reactivity.	• Periodically reassess level of consciousness, mental status, and pupil size and reactivity.
Exposure and Environmental Control	
• Assess full body for determination of additional or related injuries. • Assess environment.	• Remove clothing for adequate examination. • Stabilize any impaled objects. • Keep patient warm with blankets, warmed IV fluids, overhead lights to prevent heat loss, if appropriate. • Maintain privacy.
Full Set of Vital Signs and Family Presence	
• Assess vital signs and pulse oximetry. • Determine caregiver's desire to be present during invasive procedures and/or cardiopulmonary resuscitation.	• Obtain bilateral BPs if patient has sustained or is suspected of having sustained chest trauma, or if the BP is abnormal. • Assign health team member to support caregiver(s). • Provide emotional support to patient and caregiver.
Get Resuscitation Adjuncts	
• Determine need for adjunct measures for monitoring the patient's condition.	• Obtain laboratory tests, such as type and crossmatch, CBC and metabolic panel, blood alcohol, toxicology screening, ABGs, coagulation profile, cardiac biomarkers, pregnancy. • Continuously monitor ECG. • Insert NG tube; insert orogastric tube in a patient with significant head or facial trauma. • Monitor oxygenation and ventilation (e.g., continuous pulse oximetry, capnography). • Manage pain with pharmacological (e.g., NSAIDs, IV opioids) and nonpharmacological (e.g., distraction, positioning, music) pain management strategies. • Provide comfort measures as appropriate (e.g., ice, position of comfort, warm blanket).

IV, intravenous; *O_2*, oxygen.

PRIMARY SURVEY

The **primary survey** (Table 71.3) focuses on **a**irway, **b**reathing, **c**irculation (ABC), **d**isability, **e**xposure, **f**acilitation of adjuncts and family, and **g**etting other resuscitation aids (DEFG). If uncontrolled bleeding is noted, the usual ABC assessment may be reprioritized to <C>ABC (Sweet, 2018). The <C> stands for uncontrolled bleeding or catastrophic hemorrhage. If present,

control of blood loss must be prioritized through the application of direct pressure and/or a pressure dressing.

The primary survey serves to help identify life-threatening conditions, potential causes (Table 71.4), and the appropriate interventions to be initiated (see Table 71.3). The nurse may identify life-threatening conditions related to ABCs at any point during the primary survey. When this occurs, interventions need to be started immediately, before moving to the next step of the survey.

TABLE 71.4	CAUSES OF LIFE-THREATENING CONDITIONS IDENTIFIED DURING THE PRIMARY SURVEY*
Airway • Inhalation injury • Obstruction, partial or complete, by foreign bodies, debris (e.g., vomitus), or tongue • Penetrating wounds, blunt trauma, or both to the upper airway structures **Breathing** • Anaphylaxis • Flail chest with pulmonary contusion • Hemothorax • Pneumothorax (e.g., open, tension)	**Circulation** • Direct cardiac injury (e.g., myocardial infarction, trauma) • Pericardial tamponade • Shock (e.g., massive burns, hypovolemia) • Uncontrolled external hemorrhage • Hypothermia **Disability** • Head injury • Stroke

*This list is not all-inclusive.

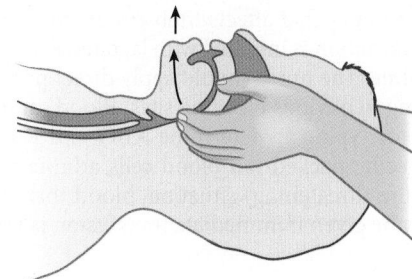

FIG. 71.1 The jaw-thrust manoeuvre is the only widely recommended procedure for use on an unconscious patient with possible neck or spinal injuries. The patient should be lying supine, and the rescuer should kneel at the top of the patient's head. The rescuer carefully reaches forward and gently places one hand on each side of the patient's chin at the lateral angles of the lower jaw. The patient's head should be stabilized by the rescuer's forearms; then the rescuer applies pressure with the index fingers to push the patient's jaw forward.

A = Alertness and Airway

Nearly all immediate deaths from trauma occur because of airway obstruction. Saliva, bloody secretions, vomitus, laryngeal trauma, facial trauma, fractures, and the tongue can obstruct the airway. Patients at risk for airway compromise include those who have experienced seizures, near-drowning, anaphylaxis, foreign body obstruction, or cardiopulmonary arrest. If an airway is not maintained, airflow is obstructed, and hypoxia, acidosis, and death result.

Primary signs and symptoms in a patient with a compromised airway include dyspnea, inability to vocalize, gasping (agonal) breaths, foreign body in the airway, and trauma to the face or neck. The patient's alertness level is a crucial factor in choosing the right airway interventions. The nurse determines level of consciousness by assessing the patient's response to verbal or painful stimuli. A simple mnemonic to remember is AVPU: **A** = alert, **V** = responsive to voice, **P** = responsive to pain, and **U** = unresponsive (Sweet, 2018).

Airway maintenance should progress rapidly from the least to the most invasive method. One treatment method is to open the airway by means of the jaw-thrust manoeuvre, in which the rescuer uses forearms to stabilize the patient's head (while avoiding neck hyperextension) and then applies pressure with the index fingers to push the patient's jaw forward (Figure 71.1). Other treatment methods include suctioning and removal of foreign objects, insertion of a nasopharyngeal or oropharyngeal airway (which causes a conscious patient to gag), and endotracheal intubation. If the patient cannot be intubated because of airway obstruction, an emergency cricothyroidotomy or tracheotomy should be performed (see Chapter 29). Patients should be ventilated with 100% oxygen (O_2) through a bag valve mask (BVM) device before intubation or cricothyroidotomy (Goto et al., 2019).

Rapid-sequence intubation is the preferred procedure for securing an unprotected airway in the ED. The patient is given a rapid-acting sedative (e.g., midazolam) and a paralyzing neuromuscular blocking agent (e.g., succinylcholine) to facilitate intubation and minimize the risk for aspiration and airway trauma (Zdravkovic et al., 2019).

If the patient has a suspected spinal cord injury and is not already immobilized, the cervical spine must be stabilized at the same time as the assessment of the airway. This can be done with manual stabilization or the use of a rigid cervical collar (C collar). The bed must be kept flat, and the nurse continues to monitor airway patency and breathing effectiveness.

B = Breathing

Adequate airflow through the upper airway does not ensure adequate ventilation. Breathing alterations are caused by many conditions, including fractured ribs, pneumothorax, penetrating injuries, allergic reactions, pulmonary emboli, and asthma attacks. Patients may exhibit a variety of signs and symptoms, including dyspnea (e.g., pulmonary emboli), stridor, accessory muscle use, paradoxical or asymmetrical chest wall movement (e.g., flail chest), decreased or absent breath sounds on the affected side (e.g., pneumothorax), visible wound to the chest wall (e.g., penetrating injury), cyanosis (e.g., asthma), tachycardia, and hypotension.

Every critically injured or ill patient has increased metabolic and oxygen demands and should receive supplemental O_2. The nurse should administer high-flow O_2 (100%) via a nonrebreather mask and monitor the patient's response. Life-threatening conditions (e.g., tension pneumothorax, flail chest) can severely compromise ventilation. Interventions in these situations include BVM ventilation with 100% O_2, intubation, needle decompression, and treatment of the underlying cause. In patients with established chronic obstructive pulmonary disease, carbon dioxide retention and level of consciousness must be monitored.

C = Circulation

An effective circulatory system includes the heart, intact blood vessels, and adequate blood volume. Uncontrolled internal or external bleeding increases the risk for hemorrhagic shock (see Chapter 69). Because peripheral pulses may be absent as a result of direct injury or vasoconstriction, the central (e.g., carotid) pulse should be checked. Palpating the pulse allows for assessment of the quality, rate, and regularity. The nurse should also assess skin for colour, temperature, and moisture. A capillary refill delay longer than 3 seconds and altered mental status are the most significant signs of shock. Care must be taken when capillary refill is evaluated in cold environments because the cold can cause vasoconstriction, which delays refill.

Two large-bore (14- to 16-gauge) intravenous (IV) catheters should be inserted into veins in the upper extremities unless this location is contraindicated—for example, because of a massive fracture or an injury that affects limb circulation—and aggressive fluid resuscitation is initiated with lactated Ringer's solution or normal saline. The nurse should apply direct pressure with a sterile dressing to obvious bleeding sites. Blood samples should be obtained for typing to determine ABO and Rh group and then type-specific packed red blood cells administered. In an emergency (life-threatening) situation, blood that is not crossmatched may be given if immediate transfusion is warranted.

D = Disability

A brief neurological examination completes the primary survey. The degree of disability is measured by level of consciousness. The Glasgow Coma Scale (GCS) and the Canadian Neurological Scale are used to assess the patient's consciousness. (The GCS is further discussed in Chapter 59, and the Canadian Neurological Scale is discussed in Chapter 60.) This allows for consistent communication among the interprofessional care team. It is important to remember that the GCS is not accurate for intubated or aphasic patients. Pupils should be also assessed for size, shape, equality, and response or reactivity to light.

E = Exposure and Environmental Control

Any patient who has suffered trauma should have their clothes removed so that a thorough physical assessment can be performed. Impaled objects (e.g., knife) should not be removed, as removing them could result in serious bleeding and further injury. Once the patient is exposed, it is important to limit heat loss and prevent hypothermia by using warming blankets, overhead warmers, and warmed IV fluids.

F = Full Set of Vital Signs and Family Presence

A complete set of vital signs, including blood pressure (BP), heart rate, respiratory rate, and temperature, should be taken after the patient's clothes have been removed. BP should be obtained in both arms if the patient has sustained or is suspected of having chest trauma.

Research supports the benefits for patients, caregivers, and staff of allowing family presence, or the attendance of one or more family members or significant others in a place where they can have visual or physical contact with the patient during resuscitation or invasive procedures (Barreto et al., 2019; Tomlinson et al., 2010; Walker & Gavin, 2019). Patients report that caregivers provide comfort, serve as advocates for them, and help remind the care team of their "personhood." Caregivers who wish to be present during invasive procedures and resuscitation view themselves as active participants in the care process. They believe that they comfort the patient and that it is their right to be with the patient. For health care providers, family presence has been shown to enhance communication, humanize the patient, and support the grieving process (Toronto & LaRocco, 2019). It is essential to assign an interprofessional team member to explain the care being delivered and answer questions if a caregiver is present during resuscitation or invasive procedures.

G = Get Resuscitation Adjuncts

Adjunct measures should be started for monitoring the patient's condition, if not already done. The mnemonic LMNOP can be used to remember these resuscitation aids:

L: Laboratory tests, such as type and crossmatch, complete blood count (CBC) and metabolic panel, blood alcohol, toxicology screening, ABGs, coagulation profile, cardiac biomarkers, pregnancy test, and urinalysis

M: Monitor ECG for heart rate and rhythm.

N: Nasogastric tube to decompress and empty the stomach, reduce the risk for aspiration, and test the contents for blood. Place an orogastric tube in a patient with significant head or facial trauma since a nasogastric tube could enter the brain.

O: Oxygenation and ventilation assessment. Continuously monitor O_2 saturation and end-tidal CO_2 ($EtCO_2$) if the patient is intubated (see Chapter 68).

P: Pain assessment and management

Most patients who come to the ED report pain (Wissman et al., 2020). Providing comfort measures is critical when caring for patients in the ED. Many EDs have pain management policies for nurses to use to treat pain early, beginning at triage. Pain management strategies should include a combination of pharmacological and nonpharmacological measures. The nurse is the advocate for ensuring that comfort measures for the patient are carried out.

SECONDARY SURVEY

After each step of the primary survey is addressed and any necessary life-saving interventions are initiated, the secondary survey begins. The secondary survey is a brief, systematic process that is aimed at identifying *all* injuries and continues the ABCDEFG mnemonic through HI: **h**istory and **h**ead-to-toe assessment; and **i**nspection of the posterior surfaces (Table 71.5).

H = History and Head-to-Toe Assessment

The history of the incident, injury, or illness provides clues to the cause of the crisis and suggests specific assessment and intervention needs. The patient may be unable to provide a history; however, family, friends, witnesses, and personnel involved before arrival at the hospital can frequently provide important information. Prehospital information should focus on the mechanism and the pattern of injury, injuries suspected, vital signs, treatment initiated, and the patient's responses.

Details of the incident are extremely important because the mechanism of injury and injury patterns can help predict specific injuries. For example, a front-seat passenger with a seat belt may have a head injury from hitting the steering wheel; knee, femur, or hip fractures or dislocation from striking the dashboard; and an abdominal injury from the seat belt. If other victims were dead at the scene, the patient has a high chance of significant injury.

Patients who jump from buildings or bridges may have bilateral calcaneal (heel) fractures, wrist fractures, or lumbar spine compression fractures, and they may be at risk for aortic tears. In older patients who have climbed ladders and fallen, a stroke or myocardial infarction (MI) may have led to the fall.

Prehospital personnel often provide a detailed description of the patient's general condition, level of consciousness, and apparent injuries. An experienced ED team can complete a history within 5 minutes of the patient's arrival. If the patient's condition is classified by triage as resuscitative, a thorough history is obtained from family or friends after the patient is taken to the treatment area. The history should include the following questions:

1. What is the chief complaint? What caused the patient to seek attention?
2. What are the patient's subjective reports?
3. What is the patient's description of pain (e.g., location, duration, quality, character)?

TABLE 71.5	SECONDARY SURVEY OF A PATIENT IN AN EMERGENCY
Assessment	**Interventions**
History and Head-to-Toe Assessment	
• History	• Obtain details of the incident or illness, mechanism and pattern of injury, length of time since incident occurred, injuries suspected, treatment provided and patient's response, and level of consciousness. • Use the mnemonic **SAMPLE** to determine **s**ymptoms associated with injury or illness; **a**llergies, including tetanus status; **m**edication history; **p**ast health history (e.g., pre-existing medical or psychiatric conditions, last menstrual period); **l**ast meal or oral intake; and **e**vents/**e**nvironment preceding illness or injury.
• Head, neck, face	• Note general appearance, including skin colour. • Assess face and scalp for lacerations, bone or soft-tissue deformity, tenderness, bleeding, foreign bodies. • Inspect eyes, ears, nose, and mouth for bleeding, foreign bodies, drainage, pain, deformity, bruising, lacerations. • Palpate head for depressions of cranial or facial bones, contusions, hematomas, areas of softness, bony crepitus. • Assess neck for stiffness, pain in cervical vertebrae, tracheal deviation, distended neck veins, bleeding, edema, difficulty swallowing, bruising, subcutaneous emphysema, bony crepitus.
• Chest	• Observe rate, depth, and effort of breathing, including chest wall movement and use of accessory muscles. • Palpate for bony crepitus and subcutaneous emphysema. • Auscultate breath sounds. • Obtain 12-lead ECG and chest X-ray. • Inspect for external signs of injury: petechiae, bleeding, cyanosis, bruises, abrasions, lacerations, old scars.
• Abdomen and flanks	• Look for symmetry of abdominal wall and bony structures. • Inspect for external signs of injury: bruises, abrasions, lacerations, punctures, old scars. • Auscultate for bowel sounds. • Palpate for masses, guarding, femoral pulses. • Note type and location of pain, rigidity, or distension of abdomen.
• Pelvis and perineum	• Gently palpate pelvis. • Assess genitalia for blood at the meatus, priapism, bruising, rectal bleeding, anal sphincter tone. • Determine ability to void.
• Extremities	• Inspect for signs of external injury: deformity, bruising, abrasions, lacerations, swelling. • Observe skin colour and palpate skin for pain, tenderness, temperature, and crepitus. • Evaluate movement, strength, and sensation in arms and legs. • Assess quality and symmetry of peripheral pulses.
Inspection of Posterior Surfaces	• Log-roll patient and inspect and palpate back for deformity, bleeding, lacerations, bruises. Maintain cervical spine immobilization, if appropriate.

ABGs, arterial blood gases; *BP,* blood pressure; *CBC,* complete blood count; *ECG,* electrocardiogram; *IV,* intravenous; *NG,* nasogastric; *NSAIDs,* nonsteroidal anti-inflammatory drugs; O_2, oxygen.

4. What are witnesses' (if any) descriptions of the patient's behaviour since the onset of illness or symptoms?
5. What is the patient's health care history? The mnemonic AMPLE helps:

A Allergies
M Medication history
P Past health history (e.g., pre-existing medical conditions, previous hospitalizations and surgeries, smoking history, recent use of drugs or alcohol, tetanus immunization, most recent menstrual period)
L Last meal
E Events or environment preceding illness or injury

Head, Neck, and Face. The patient should be assessed for general appearance, skin colour, and temperature, and the eyes should be checked for extraocular movements. A disconjugate gaze is an indication of neurological damage. Periorbital ecchymosis ("raccoon eyes") is usually caused by a basilar skull fracture. The tympanic membranes and the external canals are checked for blood and cerebrospinal fluid. Cerebrospinal fluid is allowed to flow freely because the leak usually resolves in 2 to 10 days (see Chapter 59).

The nurse should assess the airway for foreign bodies, bleeding, edema, and loose or missing teeth; check for the ability to open the mouth and swallow; examine the neck for bruising, edema, bleeding, pain, or distended neck veins; and palpate the trachea to determine whether it is in the midline. A deviated trachea may signal a life-threatening tension pneumothorax. Subcutaneous emphysema may indicate laryngotracheal disruption. A stiff or painful cervical spine area may signify a fracture of a cervical vertebra. The cervical spine should be protected with a rigid collar and supine positioning, and patients with cervical spine injuries must be log-rolled when movement is necessary.

Chest. The chest should be inspected for paradoxical chest movements and large, sucking chest wounds and assessed for pain on palpation, respiratory distress, decreased breath sounds, distant or muffled heart sounds (e.g., pericardial tamponade), and distended neck veins. Palpation of the sternum, the clavicles, and the ribs can reveal any deformity or point tenderness. In addition to tension and open pneumothorax, the patient should be evaluated for rib fractures, pulmonary contusion, blunt cardiac injury, and simple pneumothorax. A 12-lead ECG should be obtained to detect dysrhythmias and evidence of ischemia or infarction, particularly for an older patient or a patient with suspected heart disease.

Abdomen and Flanks. Assessment of the abdomen and the flanks is more difficult. Frequent evaluation for subtle changes in the abdominal examination is essential. Motor vehicle collisions and assaults can cause blunt trauma. Penetrating trauma (stabbing, gunshot wounds) tends to injure specific organs. Decreased bowel sounds may indicate a temporary paralytic ileus. Bowel sounds in the chest may indicate a diaphragmatic rupture. The abdomen is percussed for distension (e.g., tympany [excessive air] and dullness [excessive fluid]) and palpated for peritoneal irritation.

If the patient has blunt abdominal trauma or if intra-abdominal hemorrhage is suspected, a *focused abdominal sonography for trauma (FAST)* should be performed (Johnson & Raychaudhuri, 2020). This procedure can be used to identify blood in the peritoneal space and assess cardiac function. It is noninvasive and can be performed quickly at the bedside. However, a FAST cannot rule out a retroperitoneal bleed. If one is suspected, a computed tomography (CT) scan is usually done.

Pelvis and Perineum. The nurse inspects and gently palpates the pelvis. The nurse should not rock the pelvis. Pain may indicate a pelvic fracture and the need for imaging. Bladder distention, hematuria, dysuria, or inability to void need to be assessed. The health care provider may perform a rectal examination to check for blood, prostate gland conditions, and loss of sphincter tone (e.g., spinal cord injury).

Extremities. The upper and the lower extremities are assessed for point tenderness, crepitus, and deformities. Injured extremities are splinted above and below the injury to decrease the occurrence of further soft tissue injury and pain. Grossly deformed, pulseless extremities should be realigned and splinted. Pulses are checked before and after movement or splinting. A pulseless extremity represents a time-critical vascular or orthopedic emergency. The nurse needs to assess extremities for *compartment syndrome*. This occurs over several hours as pressure and swelling increase inside a muscle compartment of an extremity, compromising the viability of the muscles, nerves, and arteries. Potential causes include crush injuries, fractures, edema, and hemorrhage.

Injured extremities should be elevated and have ice applied. Fractures necessitate splinting, and patients may need pain control with analgesics. Prophylactic antibiotics are administered for open fractures.

I = Inspect the Posterior Surfaces

All patients who have suffered trauma should be turned using spinal precautions to inspect the posterior surfaces. The back is inspected for ecchymosis, abrasions, puncture wounds, cuts,

and obvious deformities. The entire spine is palpated for misalignment, deformity, and pain.

ACUTE CARE AND EVALUATION

Once the secondary survey is complete, all findings are recorded. Patients should be evaluated to determine their need for tetanus prophylaxis. It is not uncommon for older patients to have an outdated tetanus status. Information is needed about previous vaccinations and the condition of any wounds to make an appropriate decision (Table 71.6).

Regardless of the patient's chief complaint, ongoing monitoring and evaluation are critical in an emergency situation. The nurse is responsible for providing appropriate interventions and assessing the patient's response. The evaluation of airway patency and the effectiveness of breathing always assume highest priority. The nurse monitors O_2 saturation and ABGs to help determine the patient's progress. Level of consciousness, vital signs, quality of peripheral pulses, urine output, and skin temperature, colour, and moisture provide key information about circulation and perfusion.

Depending on the patient's injuries or illness, the patient may be (a) transported for diagnostic tests (e.g. CT scan, radiography, angiography) to the operating room for immediate surgery, (b) admitted to a general or critical care unit, or (c) transferred to another facility. The emergency nurse is responsible for monitoring the patient during transport and notifying the team if the patient's condition changes from baseline. Nurses accompanying critically ill patients must be competent in advanced life-support measures.

Cardiac Arrest and Targeted Temperature Management

Many patients arrive at the ED in cardiac arrest. Patients with nontraumatic, out-of-hospital cardiac arrest benefit from a

TABLE 71.6	PROPHYLAXIS AGAINST TETANUS IN WOUND MANAGEMENT	
	Type of Wound	
Vaccination History	**Clean, Minor Wounds**	**All Other Wounds**
Age 11–64 Yr*		
Unknown or <3 doses of tetanus toxoid–containing vaccine	Tdap and recommend catch-up vaccination	Tdap and recommend catch-up vaccination TIG
≥3 doses of tetanus toxoid–containing vaccine *and* <5 yr since last dose	No indication	No indication
≥3 doses of tetanus toxoid–containing vaccine *and* 5–10 yr since last dose	No indication	Tdap preferred (if not yet received) or Td
≥3 doses of tetanus toxoid–containing vaccine *and* >10 yr since last dose	Tdap preferred (if not yet received) or Td	Tdap preferred (if not yet received) or Td
Age ≥65 Yr		
Unknown or <3 doses of tetanus toxoid–containing vaccine	Td or Tdap and recommend catch-up vaccination. Tdap preferred if patient has close contact with children <12 mo of age	Td or Tdap and recommend catch-up vaccination. Tdap preferred if patient has close contact with children <12 mo of age TIG
≥3 doses of tetanus toxoid–containing vaccine *and* <5 yr since last dose	No indication	No indication
≥3 doses of tetanus toxoid–containing vaccine *and* 5–10 yr since last dose	No indication	Td or Tdap. Tdap preferred if patient has close contact with children <12 mo of age
≥3 doses of tetanus toxoid–containing vaccine *and* >10 yr since last dose	Tdap preferred (if not yet received) or Td	Td or Tdap. Tdap preferred if patient has close contact with children <12 mo of age

Td, tetanus–diphtheria toxoid absorbed (adult use); *Tdap*, tetanus toxoid, reduced diphtheria toxoid, and acellular pertussis vaccine; *TIG*, tetanus immune globulin (human).
*Pregnant women: As part of standard wound management care to prevent tetanus, a tetanus toxoid–containing vaccine might be recommended for wound management in a pregnant woman if ≥5 yr has elapsed since last receiving Td. If a tetanus booster is indicated for a pregnant woman who previously has not received Tdap, Tdap should be administered (at any gestational age).
Source: Centers for Disease Control and Prevention (CDC). (2019). *Tetanus: Prevention.* https://www.cdc.gov/tetanus/about/prevention.html

combination of good chest compressions and rapid defibrillation, targeted temperature management (TTM), and supportive care. TTM for at least 24 hours after the return of spontaneous circulation (ROSC) decreases mortality rates and improves neurological outcomes in many patients (Mody et al., 2019). TTM is recommended for all patients who are comatose or who do not follow commands after ROSC.

TTM, also called *therapeutic hypothermia,* involves three phases: induction, maintenance, and rewarming. The induction phase begins in the ED. The goal core temperature is 32°C to 36°C (89.6°F to 96.8°F). A variety of methods can be used to cool patients, including cold saline infusions and surface cooling devices (Mody et al., 2019). Patients need intubation, mechanical ventilation, and invasive monitoring and require continuous assessment. Policies often direct the care of these patients.

Mandatory Reporting of Gunshot and Stab Wounds

Most provinces have legislation that requires mandatory reporting of gunshot and stab wounds by health care agencies. Emergency staff must be familiar with their specific provincial law.

Reporting of Abuse of Children

Mandatory reporting of suspected or confirmed child abuse and maltreatment is a strategy to address violence against children. Therefore, health care providers and nurses must be aware of the legislation that governs their jurisdiction. In Canada, the Canadian Child Welfare Research Portal website (see the Resources at the end of the chapter) provides provincial and territorial policies and legislation. Professional organizations collaborate to align reporting policies for health care providers. For example, the Ontario Association of Children's Aid Societies and the College of Nurses of Ontario mandate that nurses be vigilant and accountable in reporting abuse concerns:

1. If the nurse suspects that a child is being abused or neglected, it is the nurse's legal duty to report the situation to the local Children's Aid Society.
2. Maltreatment may be in the form of physical or sexual abuse. It can also be in the form of neglect: failure to meet a child's basic needs for food, clothing, shelter, sleep, medical attention, education, and protection from harm.
3. Unexplained injuries, fear of a specific adult, difficulty trusting others or making friends, sudden changes in eating or sleeping patterns, poor hygiene, secrecy, and inappropriate sexual behaviour may be signs of abuse.

DEATH IN THE EMERGENCY DEPARTMENT

Unfortunately, a number of patients in the ED do not survive, despite the skill, expertise, and technology available in the ED. It is important for the emergency nurse to be able to cope with their own feelings about sudden death so that the nurse can help families and loved ones begin the grieving process. The nurse may require debriefing when dealing with traumatic deaths.

The emergency nurse should recognize the importance of rituals in preparing the bereaved to grieve, such as multicultural differences, the collection of belongings, coroner considerations, arranging for autopsy, viewing of the body, and the making of mortuary arrangements. The emergency nurse plays a significant role in providing comfort to and advocacy for the surviving loved ones after a death. Collaborations with clergy

and social workers are valued enhancements to the team's crisis management and grief work.

Organ and Tissue Donation

Transplantation is a critical component of the health care system. Many patients who die in the ED are potential candidates for tissue and organ donation. In 2018, over 4 300 Canadians were waiting for organ transplants, 2 782 organs were transplanted, and 223 Canadians died waiting for a transplant (Government of Canada, 2020). Solid organs that can be procured include the heart, lungs, liver, pancreas, and kidney. Certain tissues and organs, including corneas, heart valves, skin, bone, and kidneys, can be harvested from patients after death. Everyone is a potential donor, regardless of age, if the organs and the tissue are healthy at the time of death. Organ and tissue recovery is carried out with confidentiality, respect, and dignity and does not interfere with funeral practices.

Approaching families about donation after an unexpected death is distressing to both the staff and the family. For many families, however, the act of donation may be the first positive step in the grieving process. Studies show that donating the organs and tissue of a loved one who has died can provide immediate comfort and lasting consolation to family members in their grieving (Trillium Gift of Life Network, 2021). Before families are made aware of the option for donation, they must be told that the patient has died, and they must accept the fact that death has occurred. Once the family has accepted the patient's death, then the nurse can provide the family with the choice to donate, offer information, and support the family's decision.

Careful assessment of patients with standardized criteria is necessary to make an accurate determination of death. Neurological determination of death is defined as "a permanent loss of all brain function" (BC Transplant, 2021). Once this determination is complete, the donor is screened to ensure that only viable organs are recovered for transplantation. *Organ donor coordinators* are available in most institutions to assist in the process of screening potential donors, counselling donor families, obtaining informed consent, and retrieving organs from patients who have died in the ED.

The organ donor who is on a mechanical ventilator is often hemodynamically unstable, with many fluid and electrolyte imbalances. The nurse carries out interventions in an attempt to stabilize the patient's condition until the organs can be retrieved. Nursing care may consist of administration of fluids (crystalloids and colloids) and medications (vasopressors and hormones); promotion of normothermia; maintenance of ventilation and oxygenation through ventilator manipulation; and review of laboratory values such as electrolytes, blood urea nitrogen, creatinine, hematological studies, ABGs, liver function studies, and cardiac enzymes. (Transplantation is discussed in Chapter 16.)

EMERGENCY DEPARTMENT WAIT TIMES

Prolonged wait times and overcrowding, often experienced in the ED, are associated with poorer patient outcomes and increased mortality (Shen & Lee, 2018). In the period 2017 to 2018, Canadians made more than 15 million visits to EDs (Canadian Institute for Health Information [CIHI], 2019). The most common reasons for seeking emergency care included abdominal and pelvic pain, chest and throat pain, acute upper respiratory infections, and back pain. The amount of time that people spent in the ED varied according to the severity of their illness, the patient's age, how many other patients were being cared for, and the time of day the visit took place. Admitted patients spent more than five times longer in the ED (35.5 hours per visit) than patients not admitted (6.4 hours per visit). The remaining time involved waiting for an inpatient bed to become available (CIHI, 2019). Individuals aged 65 years and older spent more time in the ED and were more likely to be admitted (CIHI, 2019).

Although reducing wait times in the ED remains challenging, innovative strategies have been shown to increase patient flow. Effective strategies include creating fast-tract care pathways for patients with low acuity conditions, designating mental health specialty areas, improving interprofessional team communication (e.g., daily team huddle), ensuring adequate staffing based on patient volume, and including executive leadership involvement (Chang et al., 2018; Mercer et al., 2019).

AGE-RELATED CONSIDERATIONS

EMERGENCY CARE

The proportion of the population older than 65 is growing; most older people lead active lives. Regardless of a patient's age, aggressive interventions are warranted for all injuries or illnesses, unless the patient is known to have a pre-existing terminal illness, an extremely low probability of survival, or an advance directive indicating a different course of action.

The older population is at high risk for injury because of many anatomical and physiological changes that occur with aging (e.g., reduced visual acuity, limited neck rotation, slower gait, reduced reaction time).

Of the injury-related admissions of people aged 65 or older, many are for fractures resulting from falls; falls are the leading cause of injury (National Council on Aging, 2021). The most common causes of falls among older persons are generalized weakness, environmental hazards, syncope, and orthostatic hypotension. When assessing a patient who has experienced a fall, the nurse must determine whether the physical findings may have caused the fall or may have been caused by the fall. For example, a patient may exhibit acute confusion (delirium). The confusion may be the result of an acute MI that caused the patient to lose consciousness and fall, or the patient may have suffered a head injury as a result of a fall from tripping.

Knowledge of the concepts of aging improves the care delivered to older persons in the ED (see Chapter 7). Older patients and their conditions must be fully investigated because of atypical presentations and comorbid conditions. The expertise of advanced-practice nurses, such as nurse practitioners or clinical nurse specialists, should be put to use in caring for this complex population to improve access to care. In Ontario, geriatric emergency medicine (GEM) nurse clinicians focus on the older population in the ED and have been found to improve care and clinical outcomes (Wilding et al., 2015).

ENVIRONMENTAL EMERGENCIES

Increased interest in outdoor activities such as running, hiking, cycling, skiing, sailing, and swimming has resulted in more environmental emergencies seen in the ED. Illness or injury may be caused by the activity, exposure to weather, or attack from various animals or humans. Specific environmental emergencies discussed in this section include heat-related emergencies, cold-related emergencies, submersion injuries, bites, and stings.

TABLE 71.7 RISK FACTORS FOR HEAT-RELATED EMERGENCIES

Age	Prescription Drugs
• Extremely young age	• Anticholinergics
• Older age	• Antihistamines
	• Antiparkinsonian drugs
Environmental Conditions	• Antispasmodics
• High environmental temperature	• β-Adrenergic blockers
• High relative humidity	• Butyrophenones
• Low wind	• Diuretics
	• Phenothiazines
Pre-Existing Illness	• Tricyclic antidepressants
• Cardiovascular disease	
• Cystic fibrosis	**Street Drugs**
• Dehydration	• Amphetamines
• Diabetes	• Jimson weed
• Obesity	• Lysergic acid diethylamide (LSD)
• Previous stroke or other central nervous system lesion	• 3,4-Methylenedioxy-methamphetamine (MDMA, Ecstasy)
• Skin disorders (e.g., large burn scars)	• Phencyclidine (PCP)
	Alcohol

Source: Emergency Nurses Association. (2010). *Sheehy's emergency nursing: Principles and practice* (6th ed., p. 537, Box 40-1) (L. Newberry, Ed.). Mosby.

HEAT-RELATED EMERGENCIES

Brief exposure to intense heat or prolonged exposure to less intense heat leads to *heat stress*. Thermoregulatory mechanisms such as sweating, vasodilation, and increased respirations cannot compensate for such exposure to increased ambient temperatures. Ambient temperature is a product of environmental temperature and humidity. Strenuous activities in hot or humid environments, clothing that interferes with perspiration, high fevers, and pre-existing illnesses predispose individuals to heat stress (Table 71.7). Effects can be mild (heat rash and heat edema) or severe (heat exhaustion and heatstroke). The management of heat-related emergencies is summarized in Table 71.8.

Heat rash (miliaria or prickly heat) is a fine, red, papular rash that occurs on the torso and the neck and in skin folds. The rash occurs when sweat ducts are obstructed and become inflamed so that sweat excretion does not occur. The rash usually occurs in warm weather, but it has also been reported in cold weather as a result of clothing.

Heat syncope is associated with prolonged standing and heat exposure. Manifestations include dizziness, orthostatic hypotension, and syncope. Inadequate vasomotor tone associated with aging increases older people's risk for heat syncope.

Heat Cramps

Heat cramps are severe cramps in large muscle groups fatigued by heavy work. Cramps are brief and intense and tend to occur during rest after exercise or heavy labour. Nausea, tachycardia, pallor, weakness, and profuse diaphoresis are often present. The condition occurs most often in healthy, acclimated athletes with inadequate fluid intake. Cramps resolve rapidly with rest and oral or parenteral replacement of sodium and water. Elevation, gentle massage, and analgesia keep pain to a minimum. The patient should avoid strenuous activity for at least 12 hours after the development of heat cramps. Education should emphasize salt replacement during strenuous exercise in hot, humid

✚ TABLE 71.8 EMERGENCY MANAGEMENT

Hyperthermia

Etiology	Assessment Findings	Interventions
Environmental • Lack of acclimatization • Physical exertion, especially during hot weather • Prolonged exposure to extreme temperatures **Trauma** • Head injury • Spinal cord injury **Metabolic** • Dehydration • Diabetes • Thyrotoxicosis **Drugs** • Antihistamines • Cocaine • Diuretics • Ethanol • Phenothiazines • Tricyclic antidepressants	**Heat Cramps** • Excessive thirst • Severe muscle contractions in muscles subjected to exertion **Heat Exhaustion** • Altered mental status (e.g., irritability) • Fatigue, weakness • Hypotension • Pale, ashen complexion • Profuse sweating • Tachycardia • Temperature >37.5°C to <41°C • Weak, thready pulse **Heatstroke** • Altered mental status (e.g., ranging from confusion to coma) • Hot, dry skin • Hypotension • Tachycardia • Temperature >41°C • Weakness	**Initial** • Manage and maintain ABCs. • Provide high-flow O_2 via nonrebreather mask or BVM device. • Establish IV access, and begin fluid replacement for significant heat injury. • Place patient in a cool environment. • For patient with heatstroke, initiate rapid cooling measures: remove patient's clothing, place wet sheets over patient, and place patient in front of fan; immerse in ice-water bath; administer cool IV fluids or perform lavage with cool fluids. • Obtain ECG. • Obtain blood specimens for electrolytes and CBC. • Insert urinary catheter. **Ongoing Monitoring** • Monitor ABCs, vital signs, level of consciousness. • Monitor cardiac rhythm, O_2 saturation, electrolyte levels, and urinary output. • Replace electrolytes as needed. • Monitor clotting studies for development of disseminated intravascular coagulation. • Monitor urine for development of myoglobinuria.

ABCs, airway, breathing, and circulation; *BVM*, bag valve mask; *CBC*, complete blood cell count; *ECG*, electrocardiogram; *IV*, intravenous; *O2*, oxygen.

environments. Commercially prepared electrolyte solutions and sports drinks are recommended.

Heat Exhaustion

Prolonged exposure to heat over hours or days leads to heat exhaustion, a clinical syndrome characterized by fatigue, light-headedness, nausea, vomiting, diarrhea, and a sensation of impending doom (see Table 71.8). Tachypnea, hypotension, tachycardia, elevated body temperature, dilated pupils, mild confusion, ashen colour, and profuse diaphoresis are also present. Hypotension and mild to severe temperature elevation (37.5°C to 40°C) are caused by dehydration (Armstrong, 2020). Heat exhaustion usually occurs in individuals engaged in strenuous activity in hot, humid weather, but it also occurs in sedentary individuals.

Treatment begins with placing the patient in a cool area and removing constrictive clothing. The patient is monitored for ABCs, including cardiac dysrhythmias. Oral and parenteral fluid replacement should correspond to clinical and laboratory parameters. Salt tablets are not recommended because of potential gastric irritation and hypernatremia. A 0.9% normal saline solution is initiated intravenously when oral solutions are not tolerated. An initial fluid bolus may be used to correct hypotension. Admission is considered for affected older persons, chronically ill patients, and those whose condition does not improve within 4 hours.

Heatstroke

Heatstroke, the most serious form of heat stress, results from failure of the central thermoregulatory mechanisms and is considered a medical emergency. Table 71.7 lists risk factors for heat-related emergencies. Increased sweating, vasodilation, and increased respiratory rate, which occur in an attempt to lower temperature, deplete fluids and electrolytes. Eventually, sweat glands stop functioning, and core temperature increases

rapidly. The patient exhibits a core temperature higher than 41°C, altered mentation, absence of perspiration, and circulatory collapse. The skin is hot, dry, and ashen. Because the brain is extremely sensitive to thermal injuries, a range of neurological symptoms occur, such as hallucinations, combativeness, and loss of muscle coordination. Cerebral edema and hemorrhage may occur as a result of direct thermal injury to the brain and decreased cerebral blood flow.

The development of heatstroke is a potentially fatal disorder that directly relates to the amount of time that the patient's core body temperature remains elevated from either activity or the external environment (Sweet, 2018). Prognosis is affected by age, baseline health status, and length of exposure. Older persons and individuals with diabetes mellitus, chronic renal disease, cardiovascular disease, pulmonary disease, or other physiological compromise are vulnerable.

Interprofessional Care. Treatment of heatstroke focuses on stabilizing the patient's ABCs and rapidly reducing the core temperature. Administration of 100% O_2 to compensate for the patient's hypermetabolic state should be considered. Ventilation with a BVM device or intubation and mechanical ventilation may be required. Fluid and electrolyte imbalances are corrected, and continuous cardiac monitoring for dysrhythmias is initiated.

The patient is placed in a cool environment. Various cooling methods are available, such as removing clothing, covering with wet sheets, and placing the patient in front of a large fan (evaporative cooling); immersing the patient in cold water (conductive cooling); and administering cool fluids or performing lavage with cool fluids (Sweet, 2018). Whatever method is selected, the nurse is responsible for closely monitoring the patient's temperature and controlling shivering. Shivering increases core temperature and is associated with heat generated by muscle activity, which complicates cooling efforts. Aggressive temperature reduction should continue until core temperature reaches

38.9°C. Antipyretics are not recommended because they have no effect on the nonfunctioning thermoregulatory mechanisms.

The patient is also monitored for signs of *rhabdomyolysis,* a fatal disease characterized by the breakdown of skeletal muscle. Muscle breakdown leads to myoglobinuria, which increases the risk for acute kidney injury or failure. Therefore, urine should be carefully monitored for colour, amount, pH, and myoglobin. Finally, clotting studies are performed to monitor the patient for signs of disseminated intravascular coagulation (DIC). (Clotting studies are discussed in Chapter 32, and DIC is discussed in Chapter 33.)

Patient and caregiver teaching focuses on how to avoid future episodes of heatstroke. Providing essential information regarding proper hydration during hot weather and physical exercise is imperative. Patients should also be instructed in the early signs of and interventions for heat-related stress.

COLD-RELATED EMERGENCIES

Cold-related injuries may be localized (frostbite) or systemic (hypothermia). Contributing factors include age, duration of exposure, environmental temperature, homelessness, preexisting conditions (e.g., diabetes), medications that suppress shivering (opioids, heroin, psychotropic agents, and antiemetics), and alcohol intoxication, which causes peripheral vasodilation, increases sensations of warmth, and depresses shivering. People who smoke have an increased risk for cold-related injury as a result of the vasoconstrictive effects of nicotine.

Frostbite

Frostbite can be described as "true tissue freezing," which results in the formation of ice crystals in the tissues and cells. Peripheral vasoconstriction is the initial response to cold stress and results in a decrease in blood flow and vascular stasis. As cellular temperature decreases and ice crystals form in intracellular spaces, intracellular sodium and chloride levels increase, the cell membrane is destroyed, and organelles are damaged. These alterations result in edema. The depth of frostbite is the result of ambient temperature, length of exposure, type and condition of clothing (wet or dry), and contact with metal surfaces. Other factors that affect severity include skin colour (dark-skinned people are more prone to frostbite), lack of acclimatization, previous episodes, exhaustion, and poor peripheral vascular status.

Superficial frostbite involves skin and subcutaneous tissue, usually the ears, the nose, the fingers, and the toes. The skin appearance ranges from pale and blue to mottled, and the skin feels crunchy and frozen. The patient may experience tingling, numbness, or a burning sensation. Injured tissue is easily damaged, and so the area should be handled carefully and never squeezed, massaged, or scrubbed. Clothing and jewellery should be removed because they may constrict the extremity and decrease circulation. The affected area should be immersed in a water bath of 37°C to 40°C (Zafren & Mechem, 2021). Warm soaks may be used for the face. The patient often experiences a warm, stinging sensation as tissue thaws. Blisters form within a few hours (Figure 71.2). Nonhemorrhagic blisters should be drained, debrided, and covered with a sterile dressing. Use of heavy blankets and clothing should be avoided because friction and weight can lead to sloughing of damaged tissue. Rewarming is extremely painful. Residual pain may last for weeks or even years. Analgesics should be administered, and tetanus prophylaxis

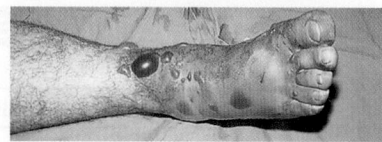

FIG. 71.2 Edema and blister formation 24 hours after frostbite injury occurring in an area covered by a tightly fitted boot. Source: Courtesy Cameron Bangs, MD. From Auerbach, P. S., Donner, H. J., & Weiss, E. A. (2007). *Wilderness medicine* (5th ed., p. 201, Figure 8-2, *A*). Mosby.

should be provided as appropriate (see Table 71.6). The patient should be evaluated for systemic hypothermia.

Deep frostbite involves muscle, bone, and tendon. The skin is white, hard, and insensitive to touch and involves complete tissue necrosis. The area has the appearance of deep thermal injury with mottling gradually progressing to gangrene (see Figure 14.1 in Chapter 14). After rewarming, significant edema may begin within 3 hours, with blistering in 6 hours to days. IV analgesia is always required in severe frostbite because of the pain associated with tissue thawing. Tetanus prophylaxis should be given (see Table 71.6), and the patient should be evaluated for systemic hypothermia. Amputation may be required if the injured area is untreated or if treatment is unsuccessful. It may take as long as 90 days to determine the final necrotic area. The patient may be admitted to the hospital for observation with bed rest, elevation of the injured part, and prophylactic antibiotics if the wound is at risk for infection.

Hypothermia

Hypothermia, defined as a core temperature lower than 35°C, occurs when heat loss exceeds production. Up to 60% of all body heat is lost as radiant energy; the loss is greatest from the head, the thorax, and the lungs (with each breath). Wet clothing increases evaporative heat loss five times greater than normal; immersion in cold water (e.g., near-drowning) increases evaporative heat loss 25 times greater than normal. Environmental exposure to freezing temperatures, cold winds, and wet, damp terrain in the presence of physical exhaustion, inadequate clothing, or inexperience predisposes individuals to hypothermia. Near-drowning and water immersion are also associated with hypothermia.

Older people are more prone to hypothermia because of decreased body fat, diminished energy reserves, decreased basal metabolic rate, decreased shivering response, decreased sensory perception, chronic medical conditions, and medications that alter body defences. In addition, certain drugs, alcohol, and diabetes are considered risk factors for hypothermia.

Hypothermia mimics cerebral or metabolic disturbances, causing ataxia, confusion, and withdrawal, and so the condition may be misdiagnosed. Peripheral vasoconstriction is the body's first attempt to conserve heat. As cold temperatures persist, shivering and movement are the body's only mechanisms for producing heat. Death usually occurs when core temperature falls below 25.6°C.

Core temperature below 30.6°C is severe and potentially life-threatening. Assessment findings in hypothermia are variable and dependent on core temperature (Table 71.9). Patients with *mild hypothermia* (33.9°C to 35°C) exhibit shivering, lethargy, confusion, minor heart rate changes, slurred speech, and incoordination. *Moderate hypothermia* (30°C to 33.9°C) causes rigidity, bradycardia, slowed respiratory rate, BP obtainable only by Doppler, metabolic and respiratory acidosis, and hypovolemia. *Severe hypothermia* (≤30°C) causes coma, hypotension, arrhythmias, and muscle rigidity (Sweet, 2018).

✚ TABLE 71.9 EMERGENCY MANAGEMENT

Hypothermia

Etiology	Assessment Findings	Interventions

Environmental
• Inadequate clothing for environmental temperature
• Prolonged exposure to cold
• Prolonged immersion or near-drown
 	
Metabolic
• Hypoglycemia
• Hypothyroidism
• Health care associated
• Administration of neuromuscular blocking agents
• Blood administration
• Cold IV fluids
• Inadequate warming or rewarming in the ED or operating room
 	
Other
• Alcohol
• Barbiturates
• Phenothiazines
• Shock
• Trauma
	• Core body temperature:
	  • Mild hypothermia: 33.9°–35°C
	  • Moderate hypothermia: 30°–33.9°C
	  • Severe hypothermia: ≤30°C
	• Altered mental status (ranging from confusion to coma)
	• Areflexia (absence of reflexes)
	• Dysrhythmias: bradycardia, atrial fibrillation, ventricular fibrillation, asystole
	• Fixed, dilated pupils
	• Hypotension
	• Hypoventilation
	• Blue, white, or frozen extremities
	• Pale, cyanotic skin
	• Shivering (diminished or absent at core body temperature ≤30°C)
		Initial
		• Remove patient from cold environment.
		• Manage and maintain ABCs.
		• Provide high-flow O_2 via nonrebreather mask or BVM device.
		• Anticipate intubation if gag reflex is diminished or absent.
		• Establish IV access with two large-bore catheters for fluid resuscitation.
		• Rewarm patient:
		  • *Passive external warming:* Remove wet clothing, apply dry clothing and warm blankets, and radiant lights.
		  • *Active external warming:* Apply heating devices (e.g., air-filled warming blankets) or warm-water immersion.
		  • *Active core warming:* Administer warmed IV fluids; heated, humidified O_2. Extracorporeal circulation (e.g., cardiopulmonary bypass, rapid fluid infuser, hemodialysis).
		• Obtain 12-lead ECG.
		• Anticipate need for defibrillation.
		• Warm central trunk first in patients with moderate or severe hypothermia to limit rewarming shock.
		• Assess for other injuries.
		• Treat patient gently to avoid increased cardiac irritability.
		
		Ongoing Monitoring
		• Monitor ABCs, level of consciousness, temperature, and vital signs.
		• Monitor O_2 saturation and cardiac rate and rhythm.
		• Monitor electrolyte and glucose levels.

ABCs, airway, breathing, and circulation; *BVM,* bag valve mask; *ED,* emergency department; *ECG,* electrocardiogram; *IV,* intravenous; *O₂,* oxygen.
NOTE: Medications and defibrillation may not be effective with core temperatures <30°C.

As core temperature drops, basal metabolic rate decreases two to three times. The cold myocardium is extremely irritable, making it vulnerable to dysrhythmias (e.g., ventricular fibrillation). Decreased renal blood flow decreases glomerular filtration rate, which impairs water reabsorption and leads to dehydration. Hematocrit increases as intravascular volume decreases. Cold blood becomes viscous and acts as a thrombus, increasing the patient's risk for stroke, MI, pulmonary emboli, acute tubular necrosis, and renal failure. Decreased blood flow leads to lactic acid accumulation from anaerobic metabolism and subsequent metabolic acidosis.

In *severe hypothermia* (≤30°C), the person may appear dead and is in a potentially life-threatening situation. Metabolic rate, heart rate, and respirations are so slow that they may be difficult to detect. Reflexes are absent, and the pupils are fixed and dilated. Profound bradycardia, asystole, or ventricular fibrillation may be present. Every effort is made to warm the patient to at least 30°C before the person is pronounced dead. The cause of death is usually refractory ventricular fibrillation.

Interprofessional Care. Treatment of hypothermia focuses on managing and maintaining ABCs, rewarming the patient, correcting dehydration and acidosis, and treating dysrhythmias. Passive or active external rewarming is used for mild hypothermia. Mildly hypothermic patients may be rewarmed with passive and active external measures since their risk for dysrhythmia is low. Those with more severe hypothermia need active internal rewarming measures.

Core temperature should be carefully monitored during rewarming procedures. Warming places the patient at risk for *afterdrop,* a further drop in core temperature, which occurs when cold peripheral blood returns to the central circulation. Rewarming

shock can produce hypotension and dysrhythmias. Thus, in patients with moderate to profound hypothermia, the core should be warmed before the extremities. Active rewarming should be discontinued once the core temperature reaches 32.2°C to 35°C.

Patient teaching should focus on how to avoid future cold-related conditions. Essential education includes dressing in layers for cold weather, covering the head, carrying high-carbohydrate foods for extra calories, and developing a plan for survival should an injury occur.

SUBMERSION INJURIES

Submersion injury results when a person becomes hypoxic as a result of submersion in a liquid, usually water (Sweet, 2018). The primary risk factors for submersion injury include inability to swim, inadequate adult supervision, use of alcohol or drugs, trauma, seizures, and hypothermia. Aggressive resuscitation efforts (e.g., airway and ventilation management), especially in the prehospital phase, improve survival of drowning victims.

Drowning is death from suffocation after submersion in water or another fluid medium. *Near-drowning* is defined as survival from potential drowning. *Immersion syndrome* occurs with immersion in cold water, which leads to stimulation of the vagus nerve and potentially fatal dysrhythmias (e.g., bradycardia).

Most drowning victims do not aspirate any liquid because of laryngospasm. If liquid is aspirated, it is in small amounts. Drowning victims who do aspirate water develop pulmonary edema, which can cause acute respiratory distress syndrome (see Chapter 70).

The osmotic gradient that results from aspirated fluid causes fluid imbalances. Figure 71.3 shows the pulmonary effects of salt water and fresh water aspiration. Hypotonic fresh water is rapidly absorbed into the circulatory system through the alveoli. Fresh water is often contaminated with chlorine, mud, and algae, which cause the breakdown of lung surfactant, fluid seepage, and pulmonary edema.

Hypertonic salt water draws protein-rich fluid from the vascular space into the alveoli, impairing alveolar ventilation and resulting in hypoxia. The body attempts to compensate for hypoxia by shunting blood to the lungs. As a result, pulmonary pressures increase and respiratory status deteriorates. More and more blood is shunted through the alveoli; however, it is not adequately oxygenated, and so the hypoxemia worsens. This can result in cerebral injury, edema, and brain death.

Interprofessional Care

Treatment focuses on correcting hypoxia and fluid imbalances, supporting basic physiological functions, and rewarming when hypothermia is present. Initial evaluation and interventions involve assessment of airway, cervical spine, breathing, and circulation (Table 71.10). Mechanical ventilation with positive end-expiratory pressure or continuous positive airway pressure may be used to improve gas exchange across the alveolar–capillary membrane when significant pulmonary edema is present. Ventilation and oxygenation are the primary techniques for treating respiratory failure (see Chapter 70).

Deterioration of neurological status is suggestive of cerebral edema, increased hypoxia, or profound acidosis. Drowning victims may also have head and neck injuries that cause alterations in level of consciousness. Complications can develop in patients who are free of symptoms immediately after the drowning episode. Consequently, all victims of drowning need to be

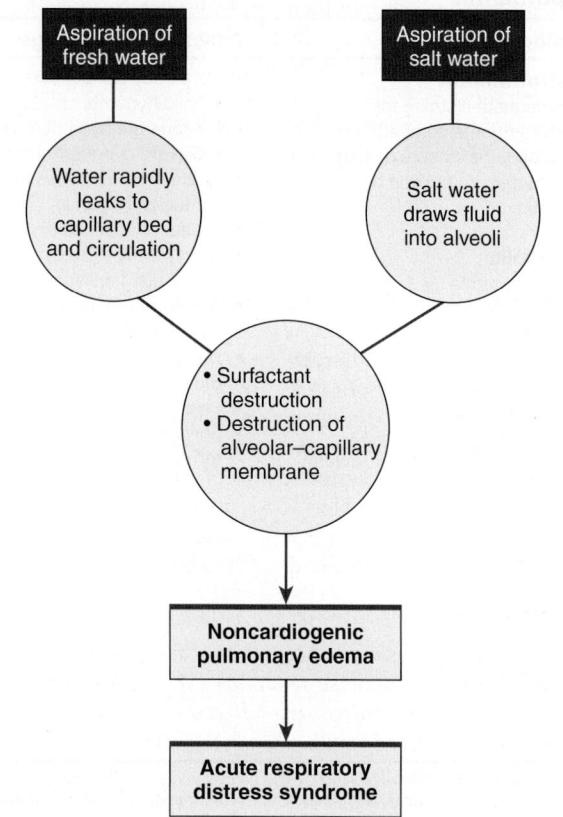

PATHOPHYSIOLOGY MAP

FIG. 71.3 Pathophysiology of submersion injury.

✚ TABLE 71.10 **EMERGENCY MANAGEMENT**

Submersion Injuries

Etiology	Assessment Findings	Interventions
• Inability to swim or exhaustion while swimming • Entrapment in or entanglement with objects in water • Loss of ability to move secondary to trauma, stroke, hypothermia, acute MI • Poor judgement as a result of alcohol or drugs • Seizure while in water	**Pulmonary** • Cough with pink, frothy sputum • Crackles, wheezes • Cyanosis • Dyspnea • Ineffective breathing • Respiratory distress/arrest **Cardiac** • Bradycardia • Cardiac arrest • Dysrhythmia • Hypotension • Tachycardia **Other** • Coexisting illness (e.g., MI) or injury (e.g., cervical spine injury) • Coma • Core temperature slightly elevated or below normal depending on water temperature and length of submersion • Exhaustion • Panic	**Initial** • Manage and maintain ABCs. • Assume cervical spine injury in all drowning victims, and stabilize or immobilize cervical spine. • Provide 100% O$_2$ via nonrebreather mask or BVM device. • Anticipate need for intubation if gag reflex is absent. • Establish IV access with two large-bore catheters for fluid resuscitation and infuse warmed fluids if appropriate. • Assess for other injuries. • Remove wet clothing and cover with warm blankets. • Measure temperature, and begin rewarming if needed. • Obtain cervical spine and chest radiographs. • Insert gastric tube. **Ongoing Monitoring** • Monitor ABCs, vital signs, and level of consciousness. • Monitor O$_2$ saturation and cardiac rhythm. • Monitor temperature, and maintain normothermia. • Monitor for signs of acute respiratory failure. • Monitor for signs of secondary drowning.

ABCs, airway, breathing, and circulation; *BVM,* bag valve mask; *IV,* intravenous; *MI,* myocardial infarction; *O$_2$,* oxygen.

observed in a hospital for a minimum of 23 hours. Additional observation is needed for patients with comorbidities.

Patient teaching should focus on water safety and minimizing the risks for drowning. Swimming pool gates should be locked, life jackets should be used on all watercraft and tubes, and water survival skills (i.e., swimming lessons and the buddy system) should be learned. The dangers of combining alcohol and drugs with swimming and other water sports should be emphasized.

BITES AND STINGS

Animals, spiders, and insects cause injury and even death by biting or stinging. Morbidity is a result of either direct tissue damage or lethal toxins. Direct tissue damage is a result of animal size, characteristics of the animal's teeth, and strength of the jaw. Tissue may be lacerated, crushed, or chewed, and toxins that are released through teeth, fangs, stingers, spines, or tentacles provoke local or systemic effects. Death associated with animal bites is caused by blood loss, allergic reactions, or lethal toxins. Injuries caused by insects, spiders, ticks, snakes, dogs, cats, rodents, and humans are described below.

Hymenopteran Stings

The *Hymenoptera* family includes bees, yellow jackets, hornets, and wasps. Stings can cause reactions ranging from mild discomfort to life-threatening anaphylaxis (see Chapter 16 and 69). Venom may be cytotoxic, hemolytic, allergenic, or vasoactive. Symptoms may begin immediately or may be delayed up to 48 hours. Most hymenopterans sting repeatedly and reactions are more severe with multiple stings. However, the honeybee stings only once, usually leaving the stinger in the skin so that the release of venom continues. A scraping motion with a fingernail, knife, or credit card is recommended for removing the stinger. Tweezers should not be used because they may squeeze the stinger and release more venom. Rings, watches, or any restrictive clothing around the sting site should be removed.

Manifestations vary and range from stinging, burning sensation, swelling, and itching to edema, headache, fever, syncope, malaise, nausea, vomiting, wheezing, bronchospasm, laryngeal edema, and hypotension. Treatment depends on the severity of the reaction. Mild reactions are treated with elevation, cool compresses, antipruritic lotions, and oral antihistamines. More severe reactions necessitate intramuscular or IV antihistamines (diphenhydramine [Benadryl]), subcutaneous epinephrine, and corticosteroids. Allergic reactions and anaphylaxis are discussed in Chapter 16.

Spider Bites (Arachnid)

Although there are 20 000 species of venomous spiders in the world, only 50 species cause illness. The venomous black widow spider is found in southern parts of Canada and also has been found in imported grapes. The venom can provoke responses ranging from a localized reaction to systemic anaphylaxis. Tarantulas look more dangerous than they actually are; their bite causes only localized stinging and pain. Other types of spiders release venom when they bite and may cause allergic reactions in some individuals, but they are not considered poisonous.

Black Widow Spiders. Black widow spiders are found in parts of British Columbia, Manitoba, and Ontario near the southern Canada–US border. They usually are found among fallen branches and firewood and under objects such as

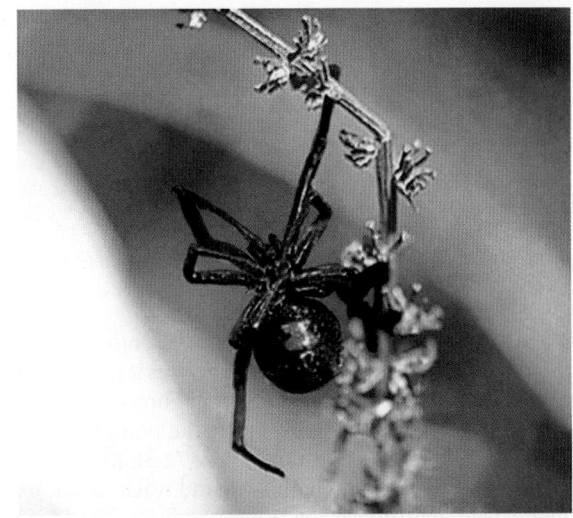

FIG. 71.4 Female black widow spider. Source: Auerbach, P. S., Donner, H. J., & Weiss, E. A. (2003). *Field guide to wilderness medicine* (2nd ed.). Mosby.

furniture, outhouse seats, and garbage. The fully grown female is about 1.2 cm long and is jet black, with an hourglass-shaped red mark on the underside of the abdomen (Figure 71.4). Males have four pairs of red dots along the sides of the abdomen.

The female's venom is poisonous and neurotoxic. When bitten, the patient feels a pinprick-like sensation, and a tiny, red bite mark appears. Approximately 15 to 60 minutes later, the patient experiences severe pain that increases over the next 12 to 48 hours. Systemic symptoms develop 30 minutes after *envenomation* (introduction of poisonous venom into the body by a bite or sting). These symptoms can include nausea, vomiting, abdominal cramping, hypertension, dyspnea, paresthesias, and tachycardia. Symptoms usually peak 2 to 3 hours after onset; however, muscle spasms and hypertension can recur for 12 to 24 hours. Chest and abdominal pain, seizures, and shock can also occur. Bites on the lower body cause abdominal rigidity, whereas bites on the upper body lead to chest, back, and shoulder rigidity. A black widow spider bite is not prominent and can be easily missed. In patients not aware of the bite, the envenomation can be misdiagnosed because symptoms mimic those of a perforated ulcer, appendicitis, pancreatitis, or other abdominal emergency.

Treatment includes IV access and O_2 administration as needed. The wound should be cleaned and tetanus prophylaxis given as appropriate. Muscle spasms are treated with benzodiazepines such as lorazepam. Pain medication may be required either orally or parentally. Intravenously administered antivenin may be used to reduce the duration of symptoms (Warrell, 2019).

Tick Bites

Ticks are found in various parts of Canada. Emergencies associated with tick bites include Rocky Mountain spotted fever, Lyme disease, and tick paralysis. Disease is caused by an infected tick or by the release of neurotoxin. Ticks transmit pathogens that cause disease through their feeding process. The infected tick attaches to its host and can slowly feed for up to several days. During this time, saliva from the tick can be transferred to the host. Tick saliva may harbour pathogens acquired by the tick from a prior host. Ticks release a neurotoxic venom for the duration that the tick head is attached to the body (White,

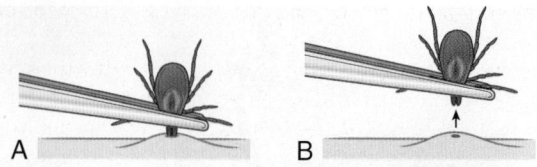

FIG. 71.5 Tick removal. **A,** Use tweezers to grasp the tick close to the skin. **B,** With a steady motion, pull the tick's body up and away from the skin. Do not be alarmed if the tick's mouthparts remain in the skin. Once the mouthparts are removed from the rest of the tick, it can no longer transmit disease.

2017). Early removal of the attached tick is essential for effective treatment, ideally within less than 24 hours, as it greatly reduces the risk for tickborne illness transmission. Forceps may be used to safely remove the tick by grasping at the point of entry and pulling upward in a steady motion (Figure 71.5). After the tick is removed, the skin is cleaned with soap and water. A hot match, petroleum jelly, nail polish, or other products should not be used to remove the tick. These measures may cause a tick to salivate, thus increasing the risk for infection. Additional information and instructional videos can be found on the Canadian Lyme Disease Foundation website (see the Resources at the end of this chapter).

Lyme disease, an arthropod-borne disease, is becoming more prevalent in Canada. Most of the reported Canadian cases have occurred in Ontario and Quebec (Government of Canada, 2019; Infection Prevention and Control Canada, 2020). It develops from a bite from the *Ixodes* tick and results from exposure to the spirochete *Borrelia burgdorferi,* which is found on the tick. Symptoms range from mild to severe and can occur in overlapping stages: early localized Lyme disease, early disseminated Lyme disease, and late Lyme disease. The initial stage of this disease is characterized by nonspecific influenza-like symptoms (e.g., headache, stiff neck, fatigue) and a characteristic bull's-eye rash—an expanding circular area of redness that is 5 cm in diameter or more. Monoarticular arthritis, meningitis, and neuropathies occur days or weeks after the initial symptoms. Chronic arthritis and myocarditis characterize the later stage of the disease, which can develop several months to 2 years after the initial skin lesion. When symptoms include a bull's-eye rash, oral antibiotic treatment is recommended. (Lyme disease is discussed in Chapter 67.)

Rocky Mountain spotted fever, caused by *Rickettsia rickettsii,* has an incubation period of 2 to 14 days. The bacterium is found among fallen branches and firewood and under objects such as furniture, outhouse seats, and garbage. A pink, macular rash appears on palms, wrists, soles, feet, and ankles within 10 days of exposure. Other symptoms include fever, chills, malaise, myalgias, and headache. It is hard to diagnose in the early stages. Antibiotic therapy with doxycycline is the treatment of choice.

Animal and Human Bites

Children are at greatest risk for animal bites. The most significant associated health problems are infection and mechanical destruction of skin, muscle, tendons, blood vessels, and bone. The bite may cause a simple laceration or be associated with a crush injury, puncture wound, or tearing or avulsion of tissue. The severity of injury depends on animal size, victim size, and anatomical location of the bite. Animal bites from cats and dogs are common; dog bites account for the majority of the bite injuries that are treated in the ED. All animal bites should be reported to the local public health unit.

Dog bites usually occur on the extremities; however, facial bites are common in small children. Cat bites cause deep puncture wounds that can involve tendons and joint capsules and result in a greater incidence of infection than with dog bites. Septic arthritis, osteomyelitis, and tenosynovitis can occur. The most common causative organisms of infections from cat and dog bites are from species of the genus *Pasteurella* (e.g., *P. canis*). Most healthy cats and dogs carry this organism in their mouths.

Human bites may result in puncture wounds, lacerations, crush injury, and soft tissue tearing. The hands, fingers, ears, nose, vagina, and penis are the most common sites of human bites and are frequently a result of violence or sexual activity. There is a high risk for infection from oral bacterial flora, most often *Staphylococcus aureus, Streptococcus* organisms, and hepatitis virus. Infection rates are as high as 50% when victims do not seek medical care within 24 hours of injury.

Interprofessional Care. Initial treatment for animal and human bites includes cleaning with copious irrigation, debridement, tetanus prophylaxis, and analgesics as needed. Prophylactic antibiotics are used for animal and human bites at risk for infection, such as wounds over joints, wounds more than 6 to 12 hours old, puncture wounds, and bites of the hand or foot. Individuals at greatest risk for infection are infants, older persons, immunosuppressed patients, people with alcohol use disorder, people with diabetes, and people taking corticosteroids.

Puncture wounds are left open, whereas lacerations are loosely sutured. Wounds over joints are splinted. Initial closure is reserved only for facial wounds. The patient often receives prophylactic antibiotics and may require IV antibiotic therapy if cellulitis, osteomyelitis, or septic arthritis develops.

Consideration of rabies prophylaxis is an essential component in management of animal bites. A neurotoxic virus found in the saliva of some mammals causes rabies. If untreated, the condition is fatal in humans. Rabies exposure should be considered if an animal attack was not provoked, involved a wild animal, or involved a domestic animal not immunized against rabies.

Rabies prophylaxis is always given when the animal cannot be found or when a carnivorous wild animal causes the bite. The prophylaxis regimen begins with an injection of rabies immune globulin (RabIg) to provide passive immunity. If possible, the calculated dose of RabIg is given via infiltration around the wound edges and the remaining volume of RabIg administered intramuscularly at a site distant from the vaccine site (e.g., gluteal site for bite wounds on the arm). This is followed by a series of five injections of human diploid cell vaccine (HDCV) on days 0, 3, 7, 14, and 28 to provide active immunity (Government of Canada, 2021). Dosage is based on the patient's weight and should be administered intramuscularly in the deltoid.

Since rabies is nearly always fatal, management efforts are directed at preventing the transmission and onset of the disease. Although death from rabies is significant worldwide, it is rare in Canada. Public health agencies should be notified for any suspected cases.

POISONINGS

A *poison* is any chemical that harms the body. In 2017, these were an estimated 4 392 deaths from accidental poisoning in Canada (Statistics Canada, 2019). Poisonings can be accidental, occupational, recreational, or intentional. Natural or manufactured toxins can be ingested, inhaled, injected, splashed in the eye, or absorbed through the skin. Common poisons are reviewed in Table 71.11. Other poisonings related to the use of illegal drugs such as amphetamines, opioids, and hallucinogens are discussed in Chapter 11. Poisoning may also be caused by toxic plants or contaminated foods. (Food poisoning is discussed in Chapter 44.)

The severity of the poisoning depends on the type, concentration, and route of exposure (see Table 71.11). Toxins can affect every tissue of the body, and so symptoms can be manifested by any body system. Specific management of toxins involves decreasing absorption, enhancing elimination, and implementing toxin-specific interventions. Provincial and territorial poison control centres are available 24 hours a day and should be consulted for the most current treatment-specific protocols.

Skin and ocular decontamination involves copious amounts of water or saline. Most toxins can be safely removed with water or saline. As a general rule, dry substances are brushed from the skin and clothing before water is used. Powdered lime should not be removed with water; it should just be brushed off. Health care providers and nurses should wear personal protective

equipment (gloves, gowns, goggles, and respirators) for decontamination to prevent secondary exposure.

Decontamination procedures are usually performed by professionals specially trained in hazardous material decontamination and are done before the patient arrives at the hospital. Personal protective equipment (PPE) for decontamination is worn to prevent secondary exposure. Decontamination takes priority over all interventions except basic life-support techniques. In some cases, decontamination is done again at the hospital, if needed. Resources such as the Workplace Hazardous Materials Information System are part of mandatory unit/hospital orientation.

Education for toxic emergencies focuses on how the poisoning occurred. Patients who experience poisoning because of a suicide attempt or related to substance abuse should be evaluated by a mental health care provider and referred for alcohol or drug detoxification, if required. Patients who have been exposed to poison in their jobs should be made aware of Canadian Centre for Occupational Health and Safety measures for a safe work environment.

TABLE 71.11 COMMON POISONS

Substance	Manifestations	Treatment
Acetaminophen (Tylenol)	*Phase 1* (within 24 hr of ingestion): malaise, diaphoresis, nausea, and vomiting *Phase 2* (24–28 hr after ingestion): right upper quadrant pain, ↓ urine output, ↓ nausea; increase in LFTs *Phase 3* (72–96 hr after ingestion): nausea and vomiting; malaise; jaundice; hypoglycemia; enlarged liver; possible coagulopathies, including DIC *Phase 4* (7–8 days after ingestion): recovery, resolution of symptoms or permanent liver damage; LFTs remain high	Activated charcoal N-acetylcysteine (oral form may cause vomiting; IV form can be used)
Acetylsalicylic acid (ASA; Aspirin) and ASA-containing medications	Tachypnea, tachycardia, hyperthermia, seizures, pulmonary edema, occult bleeding or hemorrhage, metabolic acidosis	Activated charcoal, gastric lavage, urine alkalinization, hemodialysis for severe acute ingestion, intubation and mechanical ventilation, supportive care
Acids and alkalis • *Acids:* toilet bowl cleaners, antirust compounds • *Alkalis:* drain cleaners, dishwashing detergents, ammonia	Excess salivation, dysphagia, epigastric pain, pneumonitis; burns of mouth, esophagus, and stomach	Immediate dilution (water, milk); corticosteroids (for alkali burns), induced vomiting is contraindicated
Alcohol, barbiturates, benzodiazepines, cocaine, hallucinogens, stimulants	See Chapter 11	See Chapter 11
Bleaches	Irritation of lips, mouth, and eyes; superficial injury to esophagus; chemical pneumonia and pulmonary edema	Washing of exposed skin and eyes, dilution with water and milk, gastric lavage, prevention of vomiting and aspiration
Carbon monoxide	Dyspnea, headache, tachypnea, confusion, impaired judgement, cyanosis, respiratory depression	Removal from source; administration of 100% O₂ via nonrebreather mask, BVM device, or intubation and mechanical ventilation; hyperbaric oxygen therapy a consideration
Cyanide	Almond odour to breath, headache, dizziness, nausea, confusion, hypertension, bradycardia followed by hypotension and tachycardia, tachypnea followed by bradypnea and respiratory arrest	Amyl nitrate (nasally), IV sodium nitrate, IV sodium thiosulfate, supportive care
Ethylene glycol	Sweet aromatic odour to breath, nausea and vomiting, slurred speech, ataxia, lethargy, respiratory depression	Gastric lavage, activated charcoal, supportive care
Iron	Vomiting (often bloody), diarrhea (often bloody), fever, hyperglycemia, lethargy, hypotension, seizures, coma	Gastric lavage, chelation therapy (deferoxamine [Desferal])
Nonsteroidal anti-inflammatory drugs	Gastroenteritis, abdominal pain, drowsiness, nystagmus, hepatic and renal damage	Gastric lavage, activated charcoal, supportive care
Tricyclic antidepressants (e.g., amitriptyline [Elavil])	*In low doses:* anticholinergic effects, agitation, hypertension, tachycardia *In high doses:* CNS depression, dysrhythmias, hypotension, respiratory depression	Multidose activated charcoal, gastric lavage, serum alkalinization with sodium bicarbonate, intubation and mechanical ventilation, supportive care Never induce vomiting

BVM, bag valve mask; *DIC,* disseminated intravascular coagulation; *IV,* intravenous; *LFTs,* liver function tests; *O₂,* oxygen.

VIOLENCE

Violence is the acting out of the emotions of fear or anger to cause harm to someone or something. It may be the result of organic disease (e.g., temporal lobe epilepsy), psychosis (e.g., schizophrenia), or antisocial behaviour (e.g., assault, murder). Violence can take place in a variety of settings, including the home, community, and workplace.

EDs have been identified as high-risk areas for *workplace violence* (Sachdeva et al., 2019). Violence within the ED that puts staff, patients, and visitors at risk for harm includes physical attacks, verbal abuse, and intimidating behaviour. Violent incidents are often under-reported by nurses; however, without reports being made, the implementation of safe policies and practices are hindered. Measures to protect staff include the use of on-site security personnel and police officers, metal detectors, surveillance cameras, self-defence training, and locked access doors. EDs should have in place comprehensive workplace violence prevention plans (Canadian Association of Emergency Physicians [CAEP], 2020).

Family and Intimate Partner Violence

Monitoring for family and intimate partner violence (IPV), along with the possibility of a patient being a victim or perpetrator of human trafficking, is a critical part of the ED nurse's role. Violence can take place in a variety of settings, including the home, community, and workplace. The patient cared for in the ED may be the victim or the perpetrator of violence.

Elder abuse (physical, psychological, and financial) is any action by someone in a relationship of trust that causes harm or distrust in an older person (Government of Canada, 2016). Because the older person rarely self-reports abuse, it is often identified and reported by health care providers. (See Chapter 7 for a discussion of elder abuse.)

IPV and human trafficking are patterns of coercive behaviour in a relationship that involves fear, humiliation, intimidation, neglect, or intentional physical, emotional, financial, or sexual injury or assault; or it is a combination of these (sexual assault is discussed here separately). Trafficking can involve being kidnapped or even being sold by family members. It may also involve coercion of runaways into a "safe" situation that results in anything but safety.

IPV occurs in all professions, cultures, socioeconomic groups, age groups, and genders. Although men can be victims of family violence and IPV, most victims are women, children, and older persons. IPV is often hidden and undiagnosed (Barrett et al., 2020).

It is recommended that all patients arriving at the ED be screened to determine whether they are victims of IPV. Barriers to conducting effective screening include limited privacy for screening, lack of time, and lack of knowledge about how to inquire about IPV. The development and implementation of policies, procedures, and education programs can improve the practices of ED staff in screening for IPV. Screening should begin by creating a safe and supportive environment in which to talk with the patient. Privacy must be provided, and the patient should not be questioned in the presence of the possible abuser. While several instruments have been developed for screening, research has shown that a few short questions are the most realistic for health care providers (Nelson et al., 2012). The Partner Violence Screen includes the following three questions:

1. Have you been hit, kicked, punched, or otherwise hurt by someone within the past year? If so, by whom?
2. Do you feel safe in your current relationship?
3. Is there a partner from a previous relationship who is making you feel unsafe?

In addition to questioning the patient, the nurse must assess for risk factors such as injuries consistent with abuse; fearfulness of caregivers, including health care providers; withdrawn behaviour; regular ED use; and mental health and sleep disorders (Hammond & Zimmermann, 2013). If the assessment reveals physical and behavioural findings suggestive of abuse, a more detailed assessment should be completed. A caring, nonjudgemental, and respectful approach should be used to facilitate patient disclosure. Detailed documentation and preservation of forensic evidence may be necessary, and appropriate interventions should be initiated, such as making referrals, providing emotional support, and informing victims about their options (e.g., safe plan, safe house, legal rights). Some EDs have an affiliated sexual assault care centre or domestic violence centre to facilitate ED and community referrals and linkages and to support discharged patients into the community.

Sexual assault is the forcible perpetration of a sexual act on a person without their consent. It can include any of the following actions: sodomy (anal or oral copulation with a person of the same or opposite sex), forced vaginal intercourse, assault with a foreign object, and serial battery. Sexual assault may be committed by a stranger or by an intimate partner.

Clinical Manifestations

Physical. Many women and men who seek help immediately will not have any evidence of physical trauma. Evidence of trauma may be limited because survivors do not resist for fear of physical danger and injury. When present, physical injuries may include bruising and lacerations to the perineum, hymen, vulva, vagina, cervix, and anus. Fractures, subdural hematomas, cerebral concussions, and intra-abdominal injuries may have resulted in the need for hospitalization. Sexual assault also places survivors at risk for sexually transmitted infections (STIs), and women survivors at risk for pregnancy.

Psychological. Immediately after the assault, survivors may show shock, numbness, denial, or withdrawal. Some may seem unnaturally calm; others may cry or express anger. Feelings of humiliation, degradation, embarrassment, anger, self-blame, and fear of another assault are commonly expressed. These symptoms usually decrease after 2 weeks, and survivors may appear to have adjusted. Yet, any time from 2 to 3 weeks to months to years after the assault, symptoms may return and become more severe.

Rape trauma syndrome is a classification of post-traumatic stress disorder. Flashbacks, intrusive recall, sleep disturbances, gastrointestinal symptoms, and numbing of feelings are common initial symptoms. Survivors of assault will often feel embarrassment, self-blame, and powerlessness. Later symptoms include mood swings, irritability, and anger. Feelings of despair, shame, and hopelessness are often the cause of the anger. These feelings may be internalized and expressed as depression. Suicidal ideation may also occur.

Interprofessional Care

In the acute care of an assault survivor, ensuring the patient's emotional and physical safety has the highest priority. Table 71.12 outlines the emergency management of the patient who

✚ TABLE 71.12   EMERGENCY MANAGEMENT

Sexual Assault

Etiology	Assessment Findings	Interventions
• Assault involving genitalia (male or female) without consent • Sexual molestation • Sodomy	• Agitation • Anger • Crying • Anger • Decreased level of consciousness • Emotional or physical manifestations of shock • Extragenital injuries • Hyperventilation • Hysteria • Oral, vaginal, and rectal injuries • Pain in genital area or extragenital area • Silence	**Initial** • Treat shock and other urgent medical conditions (e.g., head injury, hemorrhage, wounds, fractures). • Assess emotional state. • Contact support person (e.g., social worker, rape advocate, sexual assault nurse examiner). • Do *not* clean the patient until all evidence is collected. Make sure the patient does not wash, douche, urinate, brush teeth, or gargle. • Place sheet on floor. Then have patient stand on sheet to remove clothing. Place sheet with clothing in a paper bag. • SANE will collect forensic evidence per local protocol (i.e., body hair, nail scrapings, tissue, dried semen, vaginal washing, blood samples). • Maintain chain of evidence for all legal specimens. Clearly label evidence and keep in a locked cabinet until given to law enforcement agency. • Obtain baseline HIV, syphilis, and other STI screening. • Obtain toxicology sample to evaluate drug-facilitated sexual assault. • Determine method of contraception, date of last menstrual period, and date of last tetanus immunization. • Consider tetanus prophylaxis if lacerations contain soil or dirt. • Vaccinate for hepatitis B if not already done. **Ongoing Monitoring** • Monitor vital signs and emotional status. • Provide clothing as needed. • Counsel patient regarding confidential HIV and STI testing.

HIV, human immunodeficiency virus; *SANE,* sexual assault nurse examiner; *STI,* sexually transmitted infection.

TABLE 71.13   EVALUATION OF ALLEGED SEXUAL ASSAULT

1. Medicolegal
- Valid written consent for examination, photographs, laboratory tests, release of information, and laboratory samples
- Appropriate "chain of evidence" documentation

2. History
- History of assault (who, what, when, where)
- Penetration, ejaculation, extragenital acts
- Activities since assault (e.g., changed clothes, bathed, douched)
- Current symptoms
- Emotional status
- Inquiries about safety
- Medical history
- Menstrual and contraceptive history

3. General Physical Examination
- Vital signs and general appearance
- Cuts, bruises, scratches (photographs taken)
- Extragenital trauma—mouth, breasts, neck

4. Pelvic Examination (Females)
- Adnexa, especially hematomas
- Matted hairs or free hairs
- Uterine size
- Vaginal examination with unlubricated speculum for discharge, blood, lacerations
- Vulvar trauma, erythema; hymen, anal, and rectal status

5. Laboratory Samples
- Blood samples—VDRL serology, pregnancy test; serological testing for HIV and hepatitis B infection
- Clipping of matted pubic hairs
- Cultures—cervix and other areas (if indicated) for gonorrhea and chlamydial infection
- Fingernail scrapings
- Serum sample frozen for later testing
- Oral or rectal swabs and smears, if indicated
- Pubic hair scrapings
- Vaginal smears—microscope evaluation for trichomonads and semen
- Vaginal vault content sampling

6. Treatment
- Care of injuries and emotional trauma
- Prophylaxis for STIs, tetanus, and hepatitis B (see Chapters 55, 63, and 46, respectively)
- If appropriate, consider levonorgestrel (Plan B) emergency contraceptive pill up to 72 hr after assault; follow-up for pregnancy test in 2–3 wk
- Follow-up for pregnancy test in 2–3 wk (if appropriate)
- Testing for HIV, syphilis, and hepatitis B may be done at 6–8 wk
- Protection of legal rights
- Recommendation of continued follow-up and services of rape crisis centre

HIV, human immunodeficiency virus; *STIs,* sexually transmitted infections; *VDRL,* Venereal Disease Research Laboratory.

has been sexually assaulted. Most EDs have identified personnel who have received special training to work with people who have been assaulted.

Each province and territory has created the position of sexual assault nurse examiner (SANE). The SANE is a registered nurse who is certified to provide care to survivors of sexual assault while ensuring evidence is safeguarded. Special procedures are followed in taking the history and conducting the examination in order to preserve all evidence in case of future prosecution.

When the survivor of an assault is admitted to the ED or clinic, a specific chain of events occurs (Table 71.13). A signed informed consent is obtained before any data are collected. All materials gathered are well documented, labelled, and given to the appropriate person, such as a pathologist or a police officer. The materials are handled by as few people as possible, and signatures of all responsible for keeping and handling the data are obtained. Many items can be used as evidence if the survivor chooses to file a complaint. Consequently, the integrity of the material must be maintained. The nurse's involvement in the medicolegal process depends on the policies of the individual institution and provincial or territorial law.

A gynecological and sexual history and an account of the assault (who, what, when, and where), as well as a general physical and pelvic examination, add further information about the incident. In the case of female survivors, laboratory tests are done primarily to look for sperm in the vagina and to identify any existing STIs or pregnancy.

Follow-up physical and psychological care is essential. Survivors of assault should return weekly for the first month following the assault. This time period is when psychological reactions may be most severe. Health care providers should have the telephone numbers and names of contact people for local resources for sexual assault survivors, including rape crisis centres, legal and law enforcement authorities, and human services.

NURSING MANAGEMENT
SEXUAL ASSAULT

Nurses can assist people to become aware of sexual assault prevention tactics (Table 71.14). They should also be encouraged to learn some basic self-defence techniques. Various organizations and martial arts organizations offer self-defence classes. Practicing the various techniques with a friend builds a person's confidence in their ability to fight back. Learning self-defence can make a person feel less vulnerable and more self-reliant.

TABLE 71.14   PATIENT & CAREGIVER TEACHING GUIDE

Sexual Assault Prevention

The following suggestions should be included when discussing ways to prevent sexual assault:
- Avoid walking alone in deserted areas. Walk to the parking lot with a friend; be sure you see each other leave.
- Be aware of date-rape drugs (e.g., gamma-hydroxybutyrate [GHB], flunitrazepam [Rohypnol], ketamine). Do not leave your beverage unattended or accept a drink from an open container.
- Be proactive and take a self-defence class.
- Carry a loud whistle and use it when you think you are in danger.
- Consume alcohol in moderation if you drink. Many sexual assaults involve the use of alcohol by the offender, the survivor, or both.
- Do not advertise that you live alone. List only your initials with your last name in the telephone directory or on the mailbox. Never reveal to a caller that you are home alone.
- Have your keys ready as you approach your car or home.
- Keep all doors locked and windows up when driving.
- Keep your residence doors locked, and do not open them to a stranger; ask for identification if a service person comes to the door.
- Never get on an elevator with a person behaving suspiciously or furtive. Pretend you have forgotten something and get off.
- Place and maintain lights at all entrances to your home.
- Proceed with caution in online correspondence.
- Say what you mean in social situations. Be sure your voice and body language reflect your response.
- Yell "fire" if you are attacked, and run toward a lighted area.

When a sexual assault survivor is brought to the clinic or ED, a quiet, private area should be used for the initial assessment and the examinations that follow. The patient should not be left alone. Whenever possible, the same nurse should remain with the person throughout the hospital stay and provide needed emotional support. The patient's actions and words while describing the incident may be inconsistent, confused, and inappropriate. The nurse should maintain a nonjudgemental attitude.

The patient usually has many feelings and thoughts about the assault and generally wants to talk about them. Talking may help the patient feel better and gain an understanding of their reactions to the incident. When the nurse listens carefully, the patient may feel less alone and better able to gain control over the situation.

The nurse should assess the patient's stress before preparing them for the various procedures that will follow. The patient's coping mechanisms are supported when they know what to expect and what is expected as well as why a particular procedure must be done. Because the pelvic examination may trigger a flashback of the attack for survivors, the nurse should answer all related questions before the examination and be a supportive presence during the examination.

After the examinations, the patient's physical comfort needs should be considered. The patient will need a change of clothing because original garments may have been torn or soiled or may need to be kept as evidence. Most people who have been sexually assaulted feel dirty and would appreciate a place to wash as well as to use a mouthwash, especially if oral sex was involved. Food and drink may also provide comfort to the survivor.

For female survivors of sexual assault, the possibility of pregnancy should be discussed, and the patient can be offered emergency contraception (sold as levonorgestrel [Plan B or Option 2] in Canada) to prevent an unintended pregnancy. It is similar to birth control pills but taken in different doses and can be used up to 3 to 5 days after unprotected sex, reducing the risk of getting pregnant by approximately 75 to 89%. The effectiveness of emergency contraception is highest when taken within 24 hours after unprotected sexual intercourse and declines over time. A high body weight (body mass index [BMI] >25) may decrease the effectiveness of emergency contraception (Society of Obstetricians and Gynecologists of Canada, 2021).

When the patient is discharged, the nurse should make certain the patient has transportation home. If friends or family members are not available, the hospital or clinic should make arrangements with an appropriate community resource. The patient should not be sent home alone. The survivor's partner and family have a tremendous potential for both negative and positive influence. If the partner is the perpetrator of the assault, consultation with the risk management department and law enforcement is necessary to protect the patient.

Many communities have crisis centres. These public service organizations have trained professional and nonprofessional volunteers who provide an emotional support system for survivors on request. Their programs provide advocacy to ensure dignified treatment throughout the medical and police procedures, short-term counselling for survivors and their families, and court assistance and public education on rape-related issues.

CASE STUDY

Trauma

Patient Profile

L. W. (pronouns she/her), 30 years old, is brought to the ED in an ambulance. She was the driver in a motor vehicle collision and was not wearing a seat belt. Two unrestrained children in the car were pronounced dead at the scene. The paramedics stated that there was significant damage to the car on the driver's side.

Subjective Data

- L.W. asks, "What happened? Where am I? Where are the children?"
- Complains of shortness of breath and abdominal pain

Objective Data
Physical Examination

- Vital signs: blood pressure, 85/40 mm Hg; heart rate 140 beats/min; respiratory rate, 36 breaths/min; O_2 saturation 85% with 100% nonrebreather mask
- Asymmetrical chest movement
- Decreased breath sounds on left side of chest
- Glasgow Coma Score of 14; pupils slightly unequal
- Badly deformed right lower leg with significant swelling; a pedal pulse detectable only by Doppler
- One 4-cm head laceration; bleeding controlled

Discussion Questions

1. What life-threatening injury does L. W. probably have?
2. *Priority decision:* What is the priority of care for L. W.?
3. *Priority decision:* What interventions are needed immediately?
4. What other interventions should the nurse consider?
5. *Interprofessional care:* What activities could the nurse delegate to unlicensed assistive personnel (UAP)?
6. *Patient-centered care:* Several family members have arrived in the ED, including the mother of one of the children who died. The second child who died was L. W.'s child. How should the nurse approach the family of the first child?
7. *Priority decision:* Based on the assessment data presented, what are the priority nursing diagnoses? Are there any interprofessional issues?

Ⓔvolve
Answers are available at http://evolve.elsevier.com/Canada/Lewis/medsurg.

REVIEW QUESTIONS

The number of the question corresponds to the same-numbered objective at the beginning of the chapter.

1. An older man arrives at triage disoriented and dyspneic. He has hot, dry skin. His partner states that he was fine earlier today. What is the nurse's next *priority* action?
   a. Assess his vital signs.
   b. Obtain a brief medical history from his partner.
   c. Administer supplemental O_2 and have the health care provider assess him.
   d. Ask about advance directives.

2. A client has a core temperature of 32°C. Which of the following is the most appropriate rewarming technique?
   a. Passive rewarming with warm blankets
   b. Active internal rewarming using warmed IV fluids
   c. Passive rewarming using air-filled warming blankets
   d. Active external rewarming by submersion in a warm bath

3. Effective interventions to decrease absorption or increase elimination of an ingested poison include which of the following? *(Select all that apply.)*
   a. Hemodialysis
   b. Eye irrigation
   c. Hyperbaric O_2
   d. Gastric lavage
   e. Activated charcoal

4. An older woman ambulates to the ED alone reporting severe pain in her right shoulder. The nurse notes her clothes are oversized, she is poorly groomed, and appears tearful and anxious. She tells the nurse that she lives with her son and that she "fell." She asks if she can be admitted. What possibility should the nurse consider?
   a. Dementia
   b. Possible cancer
   c. Family violence
   d. Orthostatic hypotension

5. Which of the following would be the first nursing intervention for the client who has been sexually assaulted?
   a. Treat urgent medical conditions.
   b. Contact a support person for the client.
   c. Provide supplies for the client to cleanse themselves.
   d. Document bruises and lacerations of the perineum and the cervix.

1. a; 2. b; 3. a, d, e; 4. c; 5. a.

Ⓔvolve
For even more review questions, visit http://evolve.elsevier.com/Canada/Lewis/medsurg.

REFERENCES

Armstrong, L. E. (2020). Heat exhaustion. In *Exertional heat illness.* Springer, Cham.

Barreto, M. D. S., Garcia-Vivar, C., Matsuda, L. M., et al. (2019). Presence of the family during emergency care: Patient and family living. *Texto & Contexto-Enfermagem, 28.* https://doi.org/10.1590/1980-265x-tce-2018-0150

Barrett, B. J., Peirone, A., & Cheung, C. H. (2020). Help seeking experiences of survivors of intimate partner violence in Canada: The role of gender, violence severity, and social belonging. *Journal of Family Violence, 35*(1), 15–28. https://doi.org/10.1007/s10896-019-00086-8

BC Transplant. (2021). *Neurological determination of death.* http://www.transplant.bc.ca/health-professionals/organ-donation-resources/neurological-determination-of-death

Bullard, M. J., Musgrave, E., Warren, D., et al. (2017). Revisions to the Canadian emergency department triage and acuity scale (CTAS) guidelines 2016. *Canadian Journal of Emergency Medicine, 19*(S2), S18–S27. https://doi.org/10.1017/cem.2017.365

Canadian Association of Emergency Physicians (CAEP). (2020). *CAEP position statement on violence in the emergency department.* https://caep.ca/wp-content/uploads/2020/01/CAEP-ED-VF2-ACRLJan-16-VIOLENCE-DRAFT-Ver-2-3.pdf

Canadian Institute for Health Information (CIHI.). (2019). *NACRS emergency department visits and length of stay, 2018-2019.* https://www.cihi.ca/en/access-data-reports/results/date?f[0]=field_primary_theme:2053&f[1]=field_primary_theme:2065&f[2]=field_primary_theme:2050&f[3]=field_primary_theme:2057&

Canadian Nurses Association (CNA). (2021). *Certification nursing practice specialties.* https://www.cna-aiic.ca/en/certification/get-certified/certification-nursing-practice-specialties

Chang, A. M., Cohen, D. J., Lin, A., et al. (2018). Hospital strategies for reducing emergency department crowding: A mixed-methods study. *Annals of Emergency Medicine, 71*(4), 497–505. https://doi.org/10.1016/j.annemergmed.2017.07.022

Ding, Y., Park, E., Nagarajan, M., et al. (2019). Patient prioritization in emergency department triage systems: An empirical study of the Canadian triage and acuity scale (CTAS). *Manufacturing & Service Operations Management, 21*(4), 723–741. https://doi.org/10.1287/msom.2018.0719

Goto, T., Goto, Y., Hagiwara, Y., et al. (2019). Advancing emergency airway management practice and research. *Acute Medicine & Surgery, 6*(4), 336–351. https://doi.org/10.1002/ams2.428

Government of Canada. (2016). *Elder abuse: It's time to face the reality.* https://www.canada.ca/en/employment-social-development/campaigns/elder-abuse/reality.html

Government of Canada. (2019). *Lyme disease.* https://www.canada.ca/en/public-health/services/diseases/lyme-disease.html

Government of Canada. (2020). *Blood, organ and tissue donation.* https://www.canada.ca/en/public-health/services/healthy-living/blood-organ-tissue-donation.html

Government of Canada. (2021). *Rabies vaccine: Canada immunization guide.* https://www.canada.ca/en/public-health/services/publications/healthy-living/canadian-immunization-guide-part-4-active-vaccines/page-18-rabies-vaccine.html

Hammond, B. B., & Zimmermann, P. G. (Eds.). (2013). *Sheehy's manual of emergency care* (7th ed.). Mosby. (Seminal).

Heart and Stroke Foundation of Canada. (2021). *Updated CPR algorithms in COVID-19 patients.* https://cpr.heartandstroke.ca/s/article/COVID-19-Interim-CPR-Algorithms?language=en_US

Infection Prevention and Control Canada. (2020). *Lyme disease.* https://ipac-canada.org/lyme-disease.php

Johnson, E. S., & Raychaudhuri, C. (2020). Role of focused assessment sonography trauma (FAST) and CT scan in abdominal trauma. *International Journal of Scientific Research, 8*(12). https://doi.org/10.36106/ijsr.

Mercer, M. P., Singh, M. K., & Kanzaria, H. K. (2019). Reducing emergency department length of stay. *Journal of the American Medical Association, 321*(14), 1402–1403. https://doi.org/10.1001/jama.2018.21812

Mody, P., Kulkarni, N., Khera, R., et al. (2019). Targeted temperature management for cardiac arrest. *Progress in Cardiovascular Diseases, 62*(3), 272–278. https://doi.org/10.1016/j.pcad.2019.05.007

National Council on Aging. (2021). *Get the facts on falls prevention.* https://www.ncoa.org/article/get-the-facts-on-falls-prevention

National Emergency Nurses Association (NENA). (2020). *Certification.* https://nena.ca/courses/

Nelson, H. D., Bougatsos, C., & Blazina, I. (2012). Screening women for intimate partner violence: A systematic review to update the U.S. Preventive Services Task Force recommendation. *Annals of Internal Medicine, 156*(11), 796–808. (Seminal). https://doi.org/10.7326/0003-4819-156-11-201206050-00447

Sachdeva, S., Jamshed, N., Aggarwal, P., et al. (2019). Perception of workplace violence in the emergency department. *Journal of Emergencies, Trauma, and Shock, 12*(3), 179. https://doi.org/10.4103/JETS.JETS_81_18

Shen, Y., & Lee, L. H. (2018). Improving the wait time to consultation at the emergency department. *BMJ Open Quality, 7*(1), e000131. https://doi.org/10.1136/bmjoq-2017-000131

Society of Obstetricians and Gynecologists of Canada. (2021). *Emergency contraception.* https://www.sexandu.ca/contraception/emergency-contraception/#:~:text=A%20second%20morning%20after%20pill,who%20have%20a%20higher%20BMI

Statistics Canada. (2019). *Trends in deaths due to accidental poisonings, falls and transport accidents, Canada, 2000 to 2017.* https://www150.statcan.gc.ca/n1/daily-quotidien/190530/cg-c001-png-eng.htm

Sweet, V. (2018). *Emergency nursing core curriculum* (7th ed.). Elsevier.

Tomlinson, K. R., Golden, I. J., Mallory, J. L., et al. (2010). Family presence during adult resuscitation: A survey of emergency department registered nurses and staff attitudes. *Advanced Emergency Nursing Journal, 32*(1), 46–58.

Toronto, C. E., & LaRocco, S. A. (2019). Family perception of and experience with family presence during cardiopulmonary resuscitation: An integrative review. *Journal of Clinical Nursing, 28*(1–2), 32–46. https://doi.org/10.1111/jocn.14649

Trillium Gift of Life Network. (2021). *Resources for health care professionals.* https://www.giftoflife.on.ca/en/professionals.htm

Walker, W., & Gavin, C. (2019). Family presence during resuscitation: A narrative review of the practices and views of critical care nurses. *Intensive and Critical Care Nursing, 52*, 15–22. https://doi.org/10.1016/j.iccn.2019.04.007

Warrell, D. A. (2019). Venomous bites, stings, and poisoning: An update. *Infectious Disease Clinics, 33*(1), 17–38. https://doi.org/10.1016/j.idc.2018.10.001

White, J. (2017). Clinical toxicology of tick bites. In *Handbook of clinical toxicology of animal venoms and poisons.* CRC Press, 191–203.

Wilding, L., Gilsenan, R., Dalziel, B., et al. (2015). Promising best practice: The Champlain geriatric emergency management Plus (GEM Plus) program. *Canadian Geriatric Journal of CME, 5*(1), 6–9. (Seminal).

Wissman, K. M., Cassidy, E., D'Amico, F., et al. (2020). Improving pain reassessment and documentation rates: A quality improvement project in a teaching hospital's emergency department. *Journal of Emergency Nursing, 46*(4), P505–P510. https://doi.org/10.1016/j.jen.2019.12.008

Zafren, K., & Mechem, C. C. (2021). *Frostbite.* http://www.uptodate.com/contents/frostbite

Zdravkovic, M., Berger-Estilita, J., Sorbello, M., et al. (2019). An international survey about rapid sequence intubation of 10,003 anaesthetists and 16 airway experts. *Anaesthesia, 75*, 313–322. https://doi.org/10.1111/anae.14867

RESOURCES

Canadian Association of Emergency Physicians (CAEP)
https://www.caep.ca

Canadian Association of Poison Control Centres
http://www.capcc.ca/en

Canadian Centre for Occupational Health and Safety
https://www.ccohs.ca

Canadian Child Welfare Research Portal
https://cwrp.ca/policy-legislation
Canadian Forensic Nurses Association (CFNA)
https://forensicnurse.ca
Canadian Institute for Health Information
https://www.cihi.ca
Canadian Lyme Disease Foundation—*Tick Removal*
https://canlyme.com/lyme-basics/tick-removal
Canadian Nurses Association
https://www.cna-aiic.ca
Canadian Red Cross
https://www.redcross.ca
Centre for Research & Education on Violence Against Women & Children
https://www.learningtoendabuse.ca/
Child Safe Canada
https://childsafecanada.com/
Health Canada
https://www.canada.ca/en/health-canada.html
Heart and Stroke Foundation of Canada—*ACLS*
https://cpr.heartandstroke.ca/s/acls?language=en_US

National Emergency Nurses Association (NENA)
https://www.nena.ca
National Trauma Registry Metadata
https://www.cihi.ca/en/national-trauma-registry-metadata
Parachute: Preventing Injuries, Saving Lives
https://parachutecanada.org
Public Health Agency of Canada
https://www.canada.ca/en/public-health.html
Public Health Agency of Canada—*Stop Family Violence*
https://www.canada.ca/en/public-health/services/health-promotion/stop-family-violence.html
Trauma Association of Canada
https://www.traumacanada.org

Institute for Healthcare Improvement—*Evidence-Based Care Bundles*
http://www.ihi.org/Topics/Bundles/Pages/default.aspx

evolve
For additional Internet resources, see the website for this book at
http://evolve.elsevier.com/Canada/Lewis/medsurg.

Emergency Management and Disaster Planning

Shelley L. Cobbett and Dawn Pittman

⊝volve WEBSITE

http://evolve.elsevier.com/Canada/Lewis/medsurg

- Review Questions (Online Only)
- Key Points
- Answer Guidelines for Case Study
- Conceptual Care Map Creator
- Audio Glossary
- Content Updates

LEARNING OBJECTIVES

1. Differentiate between an emergency and a disaster situation.
2. Identify the roles and responsibilities of individuals, communities, and select provincial or territorial and federal agencies in emergency planning and disaster management.
3. Define and describe the characteristics of disaster nursing.
4. Outline the components of a comprehensive emergency management program.
5. Describe the four phases of disaster management and the nursing role in each phase.
6. Describe the application of the Incident Command System (ICS) and the roles of command centre team members.
7. Describe the differences between daily emergency department triage and triage in disaster situations.
8. Outline the components of START triage and its application in disaster situations.
9. Classify the major types of disasters based on their characteristics and describe their consequences.
10. Identify those agents most likely to be used in a terrorist attack and their health impact.
11. Describe key differences between chemical-biological-radiological-nuclear-explosive (CBRNE) events and the relevance of casualty decontamination in health care settings.
12. Describe the difference between epidemics, endemics, and pandemics and discuss the importance of pandemic planning.

KEY TERMS

bioterrorism
CBRNE event
critical incident stress management (CISM)
   or debriefing
decontamination
disaster
disaster nursing
emergency

emergency/disaster management
emergency management and disaster
   planning
endemic
epidemic
hazards
outbreak management
pandemic

pandemic influenza
quarantine
strategic emergency management plan
   (SEMP)
terrorism
triage

Daily media coverage has enabled the world to witness first-hand the depth and overwhelming impact that natural and human-made or human-induced (anthropogenic) disasters can have on the population of affected areas. The increasing frequency of disasters globally emphasizes the need for advanced planning, collaboration, and effective use of health care resources to mitigate impact and manage negative outcomes. Disasters have extensive history within the human experience and have resulted in premature death, diminished quality of life, and altered health status (Veenema, 2019b). Natural disasters include the recent forest fires in Fort McMurray, Alberta (2016) and Australia (2020); Hurricanes Katrina (2005) and Dorian (2019); and the coronavirus (SARS-CoV-2) pandemic (2020)

that has swept the planet, while anthropogenic disasters include wars, terrorist attacks, and mass shootings. The far-reaching impact of disasters and the critical need for broad-scale planning, prevention, response, and recovery mechanisms requires the development of emergency preparedness competencies in nurses (International Council of Nurses [ICN], 2019a).

Nurses, as the largest sector of the health care workforce in Canada, can expect to be on the front lines of an emergency or disaster, and regardless of work environment, nurses everywhere are affected by large-scale disasters such as the COVID-19 pandemic. In recent years, nurses have played a pivotal role in responding to emergency situations nationally and internationally and have contributed to large-scale health surveillance and education. They have also had a role in the assessment of health needs and service and resource allocation (Canadian Nurses Association [CNA], 2018). Nurses are a vital part of disaster prevention, preparedness, response, and recovery strategies. The unique knowledge, skills, and abilities possessed by nurses allow them to exercise a strategic role in promoting collaboration among health and social sectors, as well as governmental and nongovernmental agencies (ICN, 2019b). It is an expectation that all nurses demonstrate an awareness of emergency planning and disaster prevention, mitigation, preparedness, response, and recovery interventions. Nurses must work collaboratively to implement strategies to prevent illness and injuries that are a result of community disasters and global health issues (CNA, 2018; ICN, 2019a).

EMERGENCY MANAGEMENT AND DISASTER PLANNING

Emergency management and disaster planning involve advanced preparation for a variety of potential situations, including mass casualty incidents, natural or biological events, technological failures, human conflicts, and acts of terrorism. Advanced planning, when done in a comprehensive and diligent manner, decreases the impact that an emergency or disaster situation has on individuals, organizations, and communities. When discussing emergency management and disaster planning, it is important to differentiate between the terms. According to the United Nations, a *disaster* is an event that seriously disrupts the functioning of a community or society and causes widespread human, material, or environmental losses and impacts that exceed the affected community's ability to cope with those negative impacts (ICN, 2019a). Disasters are often defined by governments, humanitarian groups, and other agencies, reflecting the mission and needs of that agency. While events may be labelled as "disasters" by the communities affected and by the media, many events are more accurately classified as *emergencies*.

An emergency may be described as a present or imminent event that requires a rapid and skilled response to protect the health, safety, and wellness of individuals and to limit damage to property or the environment (Public Safety Canada [PSC], 2017a). Typically, emergency situations can be quickly managed without requiring the support and resources of other communities but require urgent intervention to prevent worsening of the situation. A disaster is the outcome of a natural hazard or event (e.g., hurricane, flood, earthquake) or a result of human action or error, whether malicious (e.g., terrorist attacks, use of biological warfare) or unintentional (e.g., an accidental chemical spill), that seriously disrupts the functioning of a community or society (PSC, 2017). Disasters typically occur suddenly and can result in mass casualties (i.e., large numbers of people injured); loss of human life and materials; and significant destruction of property, the environment, and critical infrastructure (e.g., government, water, power, food supply) (Veenema, 2019b). A disaster, because of its scale and impact, exceeds the capacity of a community to cope and respond with existing resources, and the community may require "outside" assistance from trained responders, government, nongovernmental organizations; humanitarian relief agencies; or some combination of all of these (ICN, 2019b; PSC, 2021).

Two approaches used in disaster planning initiatives are an *agent-specific approach,* in which planning efforts are directed at

those threats most likely to take place within a single geographic location (e.g., earthquakes in California), and, more commonly, an *all-hazards approach,* a comprehensive strategy in which vulnerabilities to both natural and human-induced hazards are considered to be possibilities even if they have never happened or are unlikely to ever occur (PSC, 2021; Veenema, 2019b). An all-hazards approach to emergency management is used across all jurisdictions in Canada and helps to ensure that managing one type of risk does not increase vulnerability to other risks. Hazards are defined as anything that has the potential to cause harm or loss. Hazards can be substances, human activities, or physical events that may cause injury or loss of life, threaten the delivery of critical services, cause social and economic disruption, or cause property or environmental damage (PSC, 2017). Disasters occur when a hazard interacts with a vulnerable area to produce serious adverse consequences that may exceed a community's or society's ability to cope for an unknown period of time.

Individual and Government Responsibilities

To be successful, emergency and disaster planning initiatives must be done at a variety of levels, specifically the individual and family; local, community, or municipal; provincial or territorial; and federal levels. Emergency management and disaster planning involve having plans of action, supplies, and resources in place to respond in a timely and efficient manner to inevitable events.

Preparedness starts at an individual level and requires that individuals and families assume responsibility for taking appropriate steps to ensure that they have the basics of what might be required for short-term survival. This level of preparation requires stockpiling items that would be needed to be self-sufficient for a period of at least 72 hours, as well as a detailed plan that takes into account risks to the region, knowledge of safe exits and evacuation routes, advanced identification of emergency contacts and meeting places for reunification, and awareness of where to find household fire extinguishers, water and gas valves, floor drains, and electrical control panels (Canadian Red Cross, 2021; Government of Canada, 2021b). Emergency workers focus on community members with the most urgent needs, and search and rescue efforts for casualties take precedence in the first 72 hours of an emergency event. Critical infrastructure (e.g., water and power) could be interrupted for an extended period of time, reflecting the need for advanced planning and availability of basic survival resources. Table 72.1 details items that should be included in an individual or family emergency preparedness kit.

Most emergencies in Canada are local in nature and are managed by municipalities and, when required, with provincial or territorial support. Accountability for emergency planning and response in Canada is held by individual municipalities, the underlying principle being that communities possess the greatest knowledge of their individual needs and thus are in a strategic position to most effectively plan for and manage local events (PSC, 2018; 2021). Local first responders (fire, police, and paramedics) are typically the first to respond to an emergency and are a vital component of the municipal emergency plan. While most situations can be effectively handled by a community, different levels of organizations are introduced progressively if the situation escalates and as additional help and resources are needed. When a community is unable to provide required response efforts because of the scope of the situation or because

TABLE 72.1   INDIVIDUAL OR FAMILY EMERGENCY PREPAREDNESS KIT

Meeting Places
Safe meeting place near home: _____
Safe meeting place outside immediate neighbourhood: _____
Evacuation routes from neighbourhood: _____

Basic Emergency Kit Items to Include
Food and drinking water: Have at least a 3-day (72-hr) supply of food and water on hand
Food: Ready-to-eat foods that will not spoil, such as canned food, energy bars, and dried foods (replace food and water once per year)
Drinking water: At least 2 L of water per person per day (include small water bottles that can be carried easily)

Equipment for Emergency Survival
☐ A copy of emergency plan and contact information and numbers
☐ Cash (include smaller bills, such as $10 bills and change for pay phones)
☐ Extra keys for car and house
☐ First-aid kit
☐ Wind-up or battery-powered flashlight (with extra batteries)
☐ Wind-up or battery-powered radio (with extra batteries)

Additional Supplies That Should Be Considered
☐ Additional bottles of water (2 L per person) for cooking and cleaning
☐ Backpack or duffel bag (in case of evacuation)
☐ Blankets or sleeping bags for each household member
☐ Candles in a deep can; matches or lighter
☐ Change of clothing and footwear (one change of clothes per person)
☐ Duct tape and basic tools (hammer, pliers, wrench, screwdriver, pocket knife)
☐ Garbage bags
☐ Important papers (identification, personal documents)
☐ Manual can opener, bottle opener
☐ Playing cards and games
☐ Small, fuel-operated stove and fuel
☐ Toiletries, hand sanitizer
☐ Utensils, disposable cups and plates
☐ Warning light or road flares
☐ Whistle (to attract attention)

Any Special Needs Family Members Might Have
☐ Equipment for people with disabilities
☐ Infant formula, diapers
☐ Personal prescription medications, including allergy medications
☐ A record of details about medical conditions, allergies, medication, family medical history, recent vaccinations, health screenings, and surgeries
☐ Pet food

Source: Adapted from Government of Canada. (2021). *Get prepared: Your emergency preparedness guide.* http://www.getprepared.gc.ca/cnt/rsrcs/pblctns/yprprdnssgd/index-en.aspx

of inadequate personnel or equipment, a "community emergency" is declared and the province or territory is contacted for support (PSC, 2017).

The *Emergency Management Act* (EMA) was developed with the goal of strengthening emergency management efforts in this country. The Act sets out clear roles and responsibilities for all stakeholders within Canada's emergency management system and is directed at ensuring that the country and its jurisdictions are engaged in disaster mitigation and response activities (PSC, 2021). All provinces and territories have an *Emergency Management Organization* (EMO) that is responsible for the development, coordination, training, and response operations in their jurisdiction. EMOs typically manage large-scale emergencies, providing assistance to municipal or community response teams (PSC, 2017; 2021). Recognizing the potential for emergencies to escalate rapidly in scope and severity, cross jurisdictional lines, and have an international impact, the provincial–territorial EMO will notify the federal government for assistance when required. Federal assistance is most commonly dispatched in disaster situations—for example, in those involving mass casualties or wide-scale damage, or in areas under federal authority, such as nuclear safety, national defence, and border security (PSC, 2017; 2018; 2021).

Public Safety Canada (PSC) is the department of the federal government accountable for Canadian safety and protection. PSC was created after the terrorist events of September 11, 2001, when two of four hijacked planes crashed into the World Trade Center towers in New York City, the others crashing into the Pentagon in Washington, DC, and in a field near Shanksville, Pennsylvania. PSC plays a role in the development of national policy, response systems, and standards and is responsible for providing guidance to federal government institutions on the development of emergency management plans. This approach strengthens the Canadian government's capacity to prevent, protect against, respond to, and recover from major disasters and other emergencies (PSC, 2018; 2019a; 2021).

PSC also plays a critical role by establishing partnerships across sectors with key organizations in Canada (e.g., provincial–territorial EMOs, Canadian Border Services Agency, Canadian Security Intelligence Services, Integrated Threat Assessment Centre, Royal Canadian Mounted Police) and international partners (e.g., US Department of Homeland Security, UK Resilience) as a means of managing national risks, reducing vulnerabilities to hazards, and strengthening the resilience of critical infrastructure (PSC, 2020). *Critical infrastructure* consists of physical and information technology facilities, networks, services, and assets that are considered to be essential to the health, safety, security, and economic well-being of Canadians and to the continued functioning of the country as a whole. Examples of critical infrastructure include power, water, government, and sewage services. As the COVID-19 pandemic demonstrated in 2020, Internet access was a critical infrastructure resource for children and adults to continue with their education, for health and social services to continue to provide care and support, and for employees to work from their homes. Several federal departments work alongside PSC to provide emergency response resources. For example, Health Canada plays a role in implementing strategies aimed at reducing risks to individual health and the overall environment. The Department of National Defence coordinates the Canadian Forces Disaster Assistance Response Team (DART), a multidisciplinary military organization designed to deploy on short notice anywhere in the world in response to situations ranging from natural disasters to complex humanitarian emergencies (Government of Canada, 2020).

Around the world, many government and *nongovernmental organizations* (NGOs) deliver expert humanitarian aid programs and services in response to areas of human need caused by disasters. NGOs are an important component of the emergency response system. These nonprofit agencies offer assistance with disaster prevention and preparedness, response, and recovery. The Canadian Red Cross, St. John Ambulance, and the Salvation Army are examples of NGOs that provide resources that support emergency response (equipment, supplies, and human resources) and that address basic human needs (food, clothing, shelter, emotional support, and family reunification).

Disaster Response in Indigenous Communities

Indigenous communities need to be actively involved in the development and implementation of emergency plans that address the specific local needs of people living in those communities. Indigenous communities are disproportionally affected by disasters and may experience further issues related to disaster response due to lack of trust, logistical and technical difficulties, reliance on the ecosystem for food and resources, and pre-existing social and health inequities (National Collaborating Centre for Environmental Health, n.d.). When an emergency occurs in an Indigenous community, it is the responsibility of the chief and council to use all available resources to respond to the situation. As is true of other communities, if the situation extends beyond the capacity and resources of the community and their ability to respond, additional support is requested. The critical need for municipal, provincial–territorial, and federal governments to include Indigenous communities in their emergency response plan was highlighted in the Fort McMurray forest fire disaster (2016) that negatively affected local Indigenous communities through poor planning, lack of clear communication, and no established protocols to follow (Weber, 2018; Workeye et al., 2018).

Disaster response in First Nations communities involves a collaborative agreement between Indigenous and Northern Affairs Canada (INAC) and provincial–territorial governments, ensuring community access to comparable emergency assistance services available to other residents in their respective provinces or territories. Through these agreements, INAC provides funding to cover eligible costs related to emergency assistance, while the provincial or territorial government provides the service (INAC, 2017). INAC also collaborates with provinces and territories to manage situations on reserves that have the potential to affect communities, lands, assets, and the environment (INAC, 2017).

EMERGENCY/DISASTER MANAGEMENT

Emergency/disaster management is a process that includes a series of steps, from the anticipation of a hazardous event, to minimizing the risks from such an event, to responding to and recovering from an emergency or disaster. The emergency management continuum in Canada includes four integrated functions: prevention and mitigation, preparedness, response, and recovery (PSC, 2019a) (Figure 72.1). This system ensures that prevention and preparedness efforts are in place to respond to and recover from an incident. In the centre are the main elements that influence the development of a strategic emergency management plan (SEMP), including environmental scan, leadership engagement, all-hazards risk assessment, training, exercise, capability improvement process, and performance assessment.

Prevention and Mitigation

Prevention and mitigation, a critical first step to emergency management, eliminates or reduces the impacts and risks of hazards through proactive measures taken before an emergency or disaster occurs (PSC, 2019a). Prevention and mitigation may be considered independently, or one may include the other. Prevention strategies are aimed at actively avoiding or preventing a disaster from occurring, while mitigation involves reducing the impact of disasters on communities (PSC, 2021). Prevention and mitigation strategies begin with an assessment of potential risks. A *risk* is defined as the combination of the likelihood that a hazard or event will occur and the consequences that may result

if it does (PSC, 2017). As stated earlier, emergency management takes an all-hazards approach that involves looking at all potential risks and impacts, natural and human-made, to ensure decisions made to mitigate against one risk do not increase vulnerability to other risks (PSC, 2019a). *Vulnerabilities* are conditions determined by physical, social, economic, and environmental factors that increase the susceptibility of communities to suffer the negative impact of a hazard and are a measure of how prepared and equipped a community is to cope with or minimize the impact of hazard (PSC, 2017). Examples of vulnerabilities include poor construction and design of buildings, lack of public information systems, and inadequate preparation.

The goal of mitigation is to identify and implement in advance long-term strategies to reduce, deflect, or altogether avoid the consequences a hazard might have on human health, organizational or community function, and critical infrastructure (PSC, 2017; 2018). Undertaking prevention and mitigation actions reduces vulnerability and increases resiliency (PSC, 2017). Examples of mitigation strategies within a community include structural mitigative measures (e.g., construction of floodways or dykes) and nonstructural mitigative measures (e.g., building codes, land-use planning) (PSC, 2017). In the hospital setting, mitigation might include ensuring the availability of essential equipment (e.g., personal protective equipment, portable medical gases), as well as the availability of backup emergency generators to maintain the functioning of critical equipment, thereby decreasing the impact on patients should critical infrastructure fail (Markenson & Losinski, 2019; Veenema, Corley, et al., 2019). Nurses play a pivotal role in mitigation activities across acute care and community settings. Nurses' knowledge of community needs, available resources, populations at risk, and workforce issues is essential in preparing an organization or a community for emergency situations (ICN, 2019b).

Preparedness

Preparedness is a proactive activity that involves preplanning for emergency situations that could occur within an organization, a community, or a jurisdiction. Preparedness is closely tied to emergency response and involves delineation of "what should happen, when" and "who does what, where," at the time of an emergency, and "with what resources." Preparedness includes the knowledge and capacity developed by individuals, organizations, communities, governments, and response organizations to anticipate, respond to, and recover from the impact of a hazard (PSC, 2017). Nurses play an important role in preparedness by educating individuals and communities on disaster readiness; working to reduce hazards in the home, in work settings, and within communities; participating in drills and training exercises; and developing emergency operations plans and protocols (ICN, 2019b). Within the hospital setting, the nursing role is one of leadership and advocacy, through participation on unit- and corporate-based committees and task forces and in the development of disaster protocols and exercises.

Strategic Emergency Management Plan

A **strategic emergency management plan (SEMP)** is an overarching plan that provides a comprehensive and coordinated approach to emergency management planning and preparation (see Figure 72.1). The SEMP components include an environmental scan, leadership engagement, all-hazards risk assessment, training, practice exercises, capability improvement process, and performance assessment (PSC, 2017).

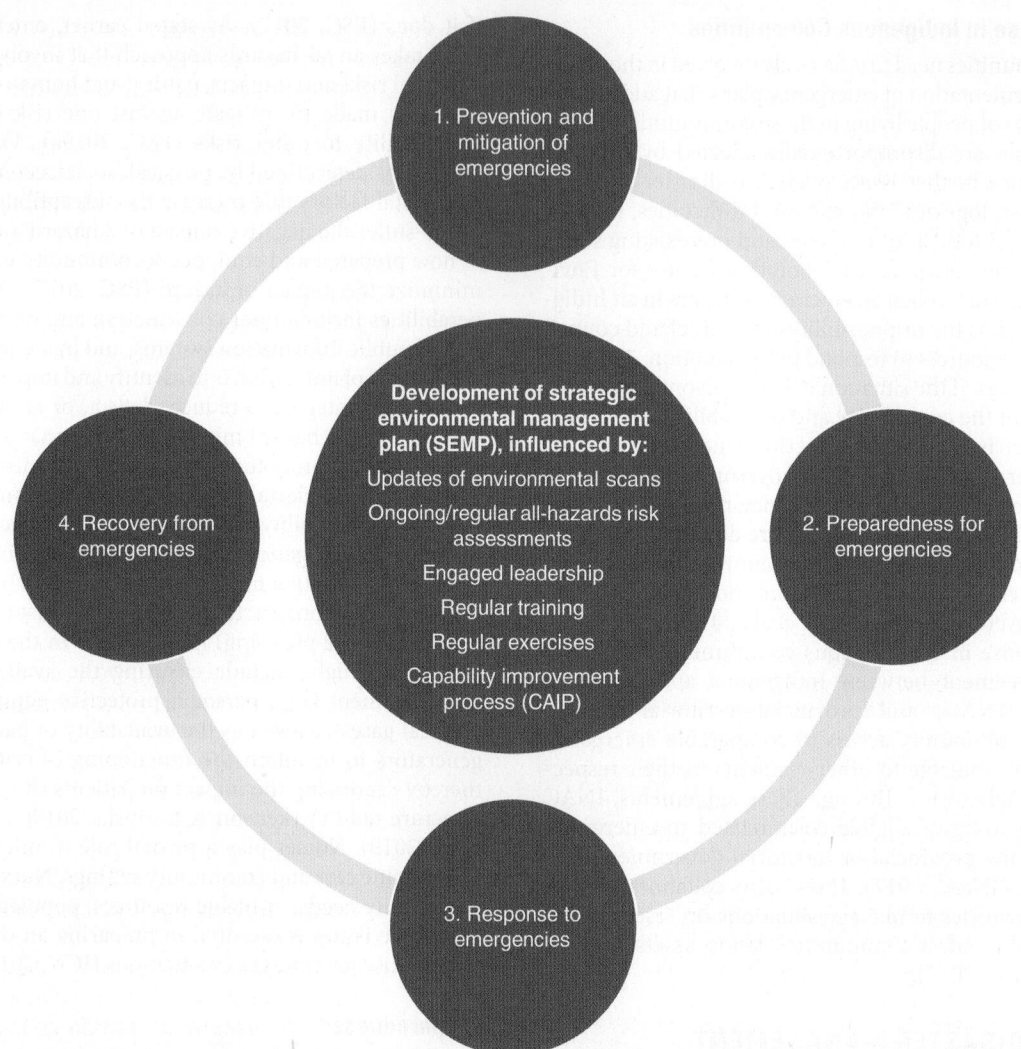

FIG. 72.1 Emergency management continuum. Source: Public Safety Canada. (2018). *Emergency management planning guide 2010–2011* (Figure 1, p. 5). https://www.publicsafety.gc.ca/cnt/rsrcs/pblctns/mrgnc-mngmnt-pnnng/mrgnc-mngmnt-pnnng-eng.pdf

Emergency Response Plan. An *emergency response plan (ERP)* is a concise description of the overall emergency organization and a designation of assigned responsibilities, actions, and procedures required in the event of an emergency. There are several names used to describe these provincial, territorial, and local plans in Canada—for example, *emergency operation plan, emergency and disaster response, emergency management plan*. Regardless of the title, the plan is to reflect the principles of emergency management in Canada (Table 72.2). These principles support the development, implementation, evaluation, and ongoing plan revisions (PSC, 2017).

Internal and External Disasters. *Internal disasters* refer to any situation that threatens or disrupts the daily, routine services of a company, organization, or building, such as a health care facility. Internal disaster situations in hospitals present a potential danger to patients and staff and may or may not occur at the same time as an external event (Veenema, 2019b). Some of the causes of internal disasters include bomb threats, chemical or radiological accidents, fire, spills, power and water loss, unavailability of staff, outbreaks of communicable disease, and violence. Internal disasters have the potential to result in a series of outcomes, including patient and staff evacuation, decreased

levels of service, diversion of transportation (e.g., ambulance and air transport), and reallocation of patient care (Gebbie & Qureshi, 2019; Veenema, 2019b).

External disasters are a result of events that originate outside of a facility. This type of disaster has the potential to threaten a facility when the consequences of the event create a demand for service that exceeds what is routinely available (Gebbie & Qureshi, 2019). External disasters may be the result of *mass casualty incidents*, which involve an influx of patients from a single incident and that exceed the capacity of a system to manage within its current resources. A health care organization can be affected by an external disaster during an influx of patients who have been injured or wounded, or exposed to a hazardous material, such as during a chemical-biological-radiological-nuclear-explosive (CBRNE) event.

Combined external–internal disasters occur as a result of external situations or events that trigger a subsequent response within the internal environment of a facility (Gebbie & Qureshi, 2019). In Canada, for example, severe weather conditions (e.g., snowstorms) can result in a combined external–internal disaster. The inability of staff to travel to work, coupled with an increased volume of trauma patients that can occur with disasters related

TABLE 72.2 PRINICPLES OF EMERGENCY MANAGEMENT

Principle	Description
Responsibility	Shared by all levels of government, communities, and individual citizens
Comprehensive	A proactive approach that integrates risk-based measures, all-hazards, partners for all parts of society to coordinate efforts across the four functions of EM
Partnerships	All Canadians are involved; whole-of-society partnerships based on effective collaboration, coordination, and communication
Coherency of action	Concerted efforts at all levels to facilitate timely and effective measures; relies on clear and appropriate roles and is based on understanding and support
Risk-based	A risk management approach is flexible and effective, allowing EM activities, programs, and systems to be individualized to particular environments, depending on identified risks.
All-hazards	This approach addresses vulnerabilities exposed by both natural and human-induced hazards and disasters.
Resilience	The capacity of a system to adapt, built through a process of empowering members of society to adapt to alterations from hazards to maintain or regain an acceptable level of living
Clear communications	Clear communications by appropriate authorities are a critical and continuous process before, during, and after an emergency.
Continuous improvement	A systematic approach is used to learn lessons from the experience, increase effectiveness, and improve EM practices and processes.
Ethical	EM decisions made by FPT governments are guided by ethics and values that accept the primacy of human life and human dignity.

EM, emergency management; *FPT,* federal/provincial/territorial.
Adapted from Public Safety Canada. (2017). *An emergency management framework for Canada* (3rd ed.). https://www.publicsafety.gc.ca/cnt/rsrcs/pblctns/2017-mrgnc-mngmnt-frmwrk/2017-mrgnc-mngmnt-frmwrk-en.pdf

to a winter storm, can precipitate a staffing crisis in the internal hospital setting. Consequently, remaining staff resources may be unable to address demands because of increased volumes and acuity in patients needing care.

Health Care Emergency Response Plans. Accreditation Canada requires health care organizations to have policies and processes in place to respond to internal emergencies as well as those arising external to the organization that, because of their size and impact, have the potential to affect day-to-day operations and patient care. Most disaster response activities occur in the hospital setting. An effective ERP uses an all-hazards approach to ensure preparedness for any event and that can be implemented almost automatically in an emergency or disaster situation (Markenson & Losinski, 2019). A hospital ERP must be flexible and scalable to the situation and take into consideration actions required for emergencies that are a result of internal, external, or a combination of external–internal circumstances. Some plans further delineate disaster responses according to the level to which the organization is able to respond. Furin (2018) describes a three-phase classification system that reflects the magnitude of a disaster relative to an organization's ability to respond:

Level 1 Disaster: The organization or community is able to effectively respond to the event using its own resources.

Level II Disaster: The emergency or disaster situation requires support and assistance from sources external to the organization that can be attained through nearby agencies or communities.

Level III Disaster: The emergency or disaster situation exceeds the ability and resources available in the community, requiring support from provincial–territorial or federal-level organizations.

The ERP starts with a risk assessment that evaluates the likelihood of disasters for the organization or community. Potential hazards to consider include weather patterns; geographic location, age, and condition of the facility; industries in close proximity (nuclear plants or factories); and large-scale public events (Gebbie & Qureshi, 2019). The assessment also includes an evaluation of staffing resources needed under various situations and supplies considered to be essential. Stockpiles of medications (analgesics, sedatives, vaccines, and antidotes), required personal protective equipment (PPE) (masks, splash suits, chemical-resistant gloves), and medical supplies (stretchers, ventilators, bandages, dressings) to support patient care should be identified, along with processes for acquisition developed. Information technology requirements may include computers (for documentation and patient registration), televisions and radios (for external coverage of emergency events), telephones, two-way radios, and fax machines. Space and needed resources for emergency response (emergency operations centre, media centre, staffing and patient–family information centres, and patient surge locations) should also be included in the plan. Basic human-needs requirements (nonperishable food, water, accommodations, and rest areas) for staff and family members who stay and work for prolonged periods should be identified as essential resources.

Numerous challenges have been identified in the management of disaster situations. These include communication difficulties; lack of leadership, planning, and clear lines of accountability; inadequate surge capacity, casualty triage, transportation, and evacuation processes; poor safety, security, and control of entry points; patient identification and data-tracking processes; management of resources; and resistance to planning initiatives (Andress, 2010). Addressing these challenges in advance in the ERP will facilitate effective management. Components of a health care ERP (WHO, 2011) are as follows:

1. *Command and control.* Activate the hospital incident command system (ICS). This includes designating individuals for each of the key components of an ERP and communicating clear roles and levels of command.
2. *Communication.* Clear, timely, and accurate communications is vital to the making of informed decisions, effective interprofessional and intersectoral collaboration and cooperation, and public awareness and trust. Appoint a public information spokesperson for public, media, and health authority communication. The availability of reliable and sustainable primary and backup communication systems and current contact information is important.
3. *Safety and security.* Well-developed procedures are required to maintain hospital functioning and for incident response operations during a disaster. Appoint a security team and prioritize security needs (e.g., identify areas where increased vulnerability is anticipated, for example, entry/exit points). Ensure that any public health directives are followed by everyone who enters the facility. Procedures for instating *lockdown status,* a process that involves restricting access to

entry points to a health care facility, should be developed. This process is of particular importance to control flow through the organization, accounting for patients and staff should evacuation be required; to prevent acts of violence or terrorism; and to avert entry of potentially contaminated patients into the hospital (Markenson & Losinski, 2019). For example, in cases where there is chemical, biological, radiological, or nuclear exposure, lockdown will assist in redirecting contaminated patients to a single designated point of entry, where decontamination can occur before entry to common areas.

4. *Triage.* Maintaining patient triage operations is essential for organization of patient care. Designate a triage officer to oversee all triage operations. Identify triage area and enter/exit routes. A contingency plan should be in place for receipt and triage of mass casualties and an alternate area for the walking wounded. Important patient information that requires documentation in a disaster includes demographic data, brief medical history, medications and allergies, type of illness or injury, treatment provided, and patient disposition (Veenema, Arbon, et al., 2019). Depending on the disaster, triage tags for patients may be used, as well as a system of classifying patients based on acuity.

5. *Surge capacity.* Surge capacity reflects an organization's ability to manage an unanticipated increase in patient numbers, with higher demands on the skills of the staff involved (Veenema, Arbon, et al., 2019). Surge planning involves a calculation of the number of available beds and potential care locations (including potential transfers and discharges) and the availability of multidisciplinary staff and supplies (backboards, ventilators, medications) (Puett., 2019). Hospitals should prepare for the transfer of care of noncritical patients to appropriate alternative treatment sites as well as create a plan for postmortem care and morgue facilities. Identify potential gaps in care and provide a contingency plan in the event of a surge in capacity. The prioritization and cancellation of nonessential services, when necessary, can allow for the reallocation of services.

6. *Continuity of essential services.* The availability of essential health care services needs to continue in parallel with the activation of the hospital ERP. Have an inventory of all hospital services, ranking them in order of priority, and the resources required to maintain them. A systematic and deployable evacuation plan that seeks to safeguard continuity of critical care is required.

7. *Human resources.* It is essential to have adequate staff capacity and the continuity of essential operations during any incident that increases the demand. Ensure contact information is up-to-date and monitor staff absenteeism and wellness. Prioritize staffing requirements and recruit and train staff as required. Address liability, insurance, and temporary licensing issues as required. Identify domestic support measures (e.g., child care) for staff and education related to deployment to areas requiring assistance. Ensure the availability of psychosocial support for patients, families, and staff. If working in an epidemic or pandemic with a respiratory-prone illness, immunizations related to national, provincial, territorial, or agency-based guidelines should be provided as required.

8. *Logistics and supply management.* Continuity of the supply-and-demand delivery chain is often an underestimated challenge during a disaster, thus requiring attentive contingency planning and response preparedness. Identify essential supplies and stockpile them in accordance with national guidelines. The amount of equipment required in an emergency situation must be assessed on a regular basis, and a process for monitoring expiration dates and ensuring circulation of supplies before their expiration should be a component of planning activities (Markenson & Losinski, 2019).

9. *Post-disaster recovery.* Planning for this phase should begin at the onset of response activities. Prompt implementation of recovery measures can help to mitigate long-term impact on the hospital's operations and services. Determine criteria for incident demobilization and system recovery. If physical damage occurred, arrange for integrity and safety assessment prior to using the building or area, or equipment. Prepare a post-action report that includes an incident summary, response assessment, and an expense report. Organize debriefing sessions for staff within 24 to 72 hours after the incident and establish a post-disaster employee recovery assistance program. Drills and mock-disaster exercises should be held on a regular basis. Organizations and staff respond to and recover from disaster situations based on their level of preparation, the culture of the organization, past experiences in dealing with emergencies, and the nature or scale of the situation (Markenson & Losinski, 2019; Veenema, Arbon, et al., 2019). Testing exercises are a key component of emergency management and are done to promote preparation, evaluate an organization's level of readiness, identify process gaps and alternate strategies, and assist in training staff in understanding and enacting response roles. Responders require an understanding of the core competencies of emergency preparedness, incident command, risk communication, and roles relative to other responders (ICN, 2019a).

Response

Response is next on the disaster management continuum, either upon impact of an event (e.g., explosion, fire) or upon an imminent event (e.g., hurricane, tornado). The ERP is critical in this stage because it provides details and information as to how response initiatives should occur. Response involves execution of the plan, where trained and exercised staff are in place, and possessing the knowledge of where they need to be and the skill to do what they need to do when confronted with an emergency situation. The goal of response is to save lives, reduce health impacts, ensure public safety, and meet the needs of individuals affected by the event (Gebbie & Qureshi, 2019). It is in the response phase that the ICS is initiated and triage of patients occurs.

The nursing role is most visible in the response phase of a disaster. Nurses provide care in a variety of areas, including patient triage, emergency and trauma care, critical care, infection control and occupational health and safety, supportive and palliative care, and public health. Nurses are also pivotal in acute care inpatient settings in disaster response because they receive the casualties who may require care on a longer-term basis as they recover from their injuries. It is critical that nurses provide support for the social challenges posed by disasters that place people at risk of experiencing mental health and psychosocial challenges (ICN, 2019b). Nurses and their families are often disproportionately affected during disaster management and response because of the need for nurses to be part of the first response and recovery teams. The daily physical and psychological demands on nurses may be greater because of frequent and

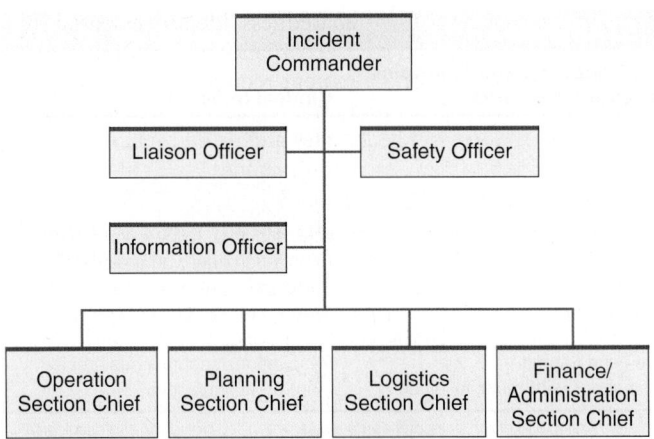

FIG. 72.2 Incident organization chart. Source: Adapted from Incident Command System Canada (2017). *Incident organization chart.* http://www.icscanada.ca/images/upload/forms/2017%20Forms%20207.pdf

first-hand exposure to human tragedy. At times they are providing care with scarce resources and working in unsafe environments (ICN, 2019b).

The Incident Command System

The ICS used in Canada consists of procedures for controlling personnel, facilities, equipment, and communications. It is a system designed to be applied from the time an incident occurs until the requirement for management and operations no longer exists, throughout the entire response period. ICS has been used by response organizations in Canada since the mid-1990s (ICS Canada, 2019). ICS, an integrated and flexible framework that identifies disaster response roles, ensures that effective communication, incident command, and control are maintained during disaster response.

While the ICS organizational chart differs for every hospital, there are main areas that are required (ICS Canada, 2019) (Figure 72.2). Some charts may have one or two roles under each main section chief, while others may have several, depending on the size of the agency and the magnitude of the disaster. ICS command roles are filled by individuals with knowledge of the tasks required to successfully address the emergency situation in each of the nine areas of an ERP (WHO, 2011).

Triage

Triage involves the sorting or ranking of casualties to prioritize health care needs and to provide direction in the allocation of scarce resources. It is a process that ensures "the right patient is in the right place, at the right time, so they may receive the right level of care" (Gilboy, 2019, p. 58). The Canadian Triage and Acuity Scale (CTAS) is used in emergency departments (EDs) in nonemergency or nondisaster situations (see Chapter 71, Table 71.2). Using this five-level scale, care providers assign a CTAS score to individuals depending on the seriousness of their condition, reported signs and symptoms, and how long they can safely wait for further assessment and intervention (Canadian Association of Emergency Physicians, 2017). The highest priority, CTAS 1, is assigned to those who are most critically ill. Daily ED triage is described with greater detail in Chapter 71.

Triage in Disaster Situations. Effective and timely prehospital triage during a disaster situation is pivotal to human survival and helps to ensure equitable distribution of patients to appropriate services and facilities throughout the health care system. Although

several mass casualty triage systems exist, there is no general or universal consensus on how triage should be performed (Bazyar et al., 2019). One of the more common types used in Canada, *simple triage and rapid treatment* (START), offers a systematic approach to triage that may be used to rank the seriousness of casualty injuries in a mass casualty incident (MCI) (Table 72.3). An MCI exists when the number of injured patients exceed the resources available to properly care for them (VandenBerg & Davidson, 2015). MCIs can be as simple as an overturned bus with five passengers or as severe as a collapsed building, a terrorist explosion, a pandemic, or a chemical or biological event. START is used at the disaster scene by first responders and involves rapid assessment and sorting of casualties by a *triage officer*. The system is used to assess all injured adults in 60 seconds or less (preferably 30 seconds) for their ability to walk, respiratory rate, capillary refill, radial pulse, and ability to obey commands (Bazyar et al., 2019). These parameters are referred to as *RPM* (respirations, perfusion, and mental status) (Romig & Lerner, 2019).

Triage is followed by tagging and transportation to a medical facility or the provision of life-saving interventions (e.g., intubation, defibrillation) by members of the first-response team. *Patient tagging* involves a system of coloured tags (Figure 72.3) that are used to designate both the seriousness of the injury and the likelihood of survival (Romig & Lerner, 2019; USDHHS-REMM, 2021b). A green tag using the START approach indicates a *minor* injury (i.e., walking wounded: sprains, lacerations) and is used for patients who may be able to assist with their own care. A yellow tag indicates a non–life-threatening injury for which transport can be delayed (e.g., open fractures, soft tissue wounds). A red tag is used to indicate a life-threatening injury requiring immediate intervention (e.g., shock, airway obstruction, unstable wounds). These patients require immediate intervention and transport for survival. A black tag is used to identify those casualties who are deceased or who are unlikely to survive as a result of their injuries (e.g., profound shock with multiple injuries, severe traumatic brain injury) (Markenson & Losinski, 2019; Romig & Lerner, 2019; USDHHS-REMM, 2021b). Triage of children, or people who look like children, is done using the *JumpSTART* framework, which addresses the physiological differences between children and adults (USDHHS-REMM, 2021a).

Disaster Triage in the Hospital Setting. Triage of casualties in the hospital setting during a disaster situation differs from routine emergency triage processes. Disaster response is dependent on the size of the organization, the number of staff and amount of resources available, and past experience in dealing with large-scale events. All health care organizations must be able to implement disaster triage with minimal notice (Romig & Lerner, 2019).

When an emergency occurs in the community, hospitals are typically notified by emergency medical services in the field, and the facility prepares for a potential influx of patients. This preparation includes gathering necessary equipment, including first-aid supplies, PPE, and medications (e.g., analgesics, antidotes). As patients are triaged, they are given a preassigned medical record number, allowing care to be provided immediately, without formal registration. Disaster charts should include a prestamped triage slip, a patient identification band with medical identification number, interprofessional health care team documentation forms, and laboratory and radiographic examination requisitions and labels. Chart numbers should be entered onto a log so patient allocation and destination can be tracked (Romig & Lerner, 2019).

TABLE 72.3 SIMPLE TRIAGE AND RAPID TREATMENT (START)

START Category/ Triage Tag Colour	Type of Injury	Patient Condition and Examples of Presenting Features	Clinical Indicators
Green "MINOR"	MINOR injuries Walking wounded; minor injuries	Sprains Lacerations	Able to ambulate
Yellow "DELAYED"	DELAYED Transport can be delayed; non–life-threatening	Open fractures Soft tissue wounds	Respiration rate: <30 breaths/min Perfusion: <2 sec Mental status: follows commands
Red "IMMEDIATE"	Unstable; immediate transport needed; life-threatening, requiring immediate intervention	Shock Airway obstruction Unstable wounds	Respiration rate: >30 breaths/min Perfusion: capillary refill >2 sec Mental status: does not follow commands
Black "EXPECTANT"	Deceased or expected to die from injuries	Massive head trauma Profound shock with multiple injuries	Respirations/spontaneous breathing: not breathing/apnea

Source: Adapted from Romig, L., & Lerner, B. (2019). Disaster triage. In T. G. Veenema (Ed.), *Disaster nursing and emergency preparedness for chemical, biological, and radiological terrorism and other hazards* (4th ed.). Springer; U.S. Department of Health and Human Services (USDHHS). (2019). *START adult triage algorithm.* http://www.remm.nlm.gov/startadult.htm; and Critical Illness and Trauma Foundation (CITF). (2001). *START: Simple triage and rapid treatment.* http://citmt.org/Start/default.htm.

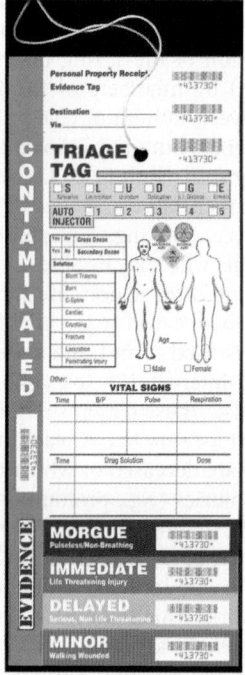

FIG. 72.3 Triage tag. Source: Copyright © 2004, Steve Mann. This picture is released under the Shared Experience License, http://eyetap.org/sel.txt.

As patients enter the ED, they are greeted by a triage team. In MCIs, several triage teams may be used, usually consisting of one to two experienced triage nurses, a physician or nurse practitioner (the triage officer), a porter (who assists with patient transportation), and a registration clerk (who assists with patient banding and data entry on the tracking form) (Romig & Lerner, 2019). Disaster triage in the hospital setting must be rapid and should be conducted in less than 15 seconds per patient. Following this rapid assessment, patients assigned with higher levels of acuity are directed to a treatment location in the ED. In situations in which patient volume is high and ED space is limited, another predesignated area of the facility to accommodate surge may be used for the care of less acute casualties.

Recovery

Recovery takes place after a response to a disaster and includes repairing or restoring conditions to an acceptable level (PSC, 2017). There is a strong connection between long-term

sustainable recovery and prevention and mitigation of future disasters. Recovery programs are designed to develop and implement strategies to strengthen resilience when responding to future disasters (PSC, 2017, p. 8). Forward-seeking recovery measures enable communities to recover from recent disasters and to build back better to overcome past vulnerabilities. Services have typically been disrupted during the disaster response; the goal is to return to a state of "normal." This includes the restoration of vital services normally provided by an organization, within a community, or by local government, rebuilding infrastructure and meeting the needs of the population served (Markenson & Losinski, 2019). Nurses are critical members of the interprofessional team in the recovery and rehabilitation phase and in re-establishing health care infrastructure. Nurses must consider the psychosocial impact of a disaster on its survivors. Nursing functions related to the care and coordination of health care services, case management, identification, and implementation of casualty referrals (e.g., social services) are essential for return to normal activities. Nurses play a key role in the documentation, review, and evaluation of the disaster response, as well as in championing changes to ERPs and to corporate, municipal, and provincial or territorial policy (ICN, 2019b).

Critical Incident Stress Management. The massive effort put forth by health care workers in response to a catastrophic event is critical to a community's recovery. Health care workers, who are already at risk of experiencing high levels of stress and burnout, are at increased risk following participation in a disaster event (Mattei et al., 2017). A critical incident is a situation faced by individuals involved in a disaster that causes them to experience strong emotional reactions that have the potential to interfere with their ability to return to a normal state of functioning at work and at home during or after the event (McMahon, 2010; Public Health Agency of Canada [PHAC], 2011). Multiple deaths; inadvertent exposure to hazardous materials; exposure to shocking sights, sounds, or smells; and incidents with high media coverage are examples of critical incidents. Challenging triage decisions, the volume of seriously injured people, limited resources, ethical issues that accompany disasters, concern for personal safety and liability, lack of sleep, heavy workload, time pressures and unmet basic needs, and political and organizational pressures also significantly contribute to the stress and an individual's resilience in the aftermath of a disaster event (Carlson, Coyne-Plum, et al., 2019; McMahon, 2010; PHAC, 2011).

All disasters have the potential to cause psychological stress to the individuals involved. This stress can persist for an extended period and is influenced in part by the nature of the event and the individual's age, pre-existing coping mechanisms, role in the event, and prior medical and psychological history (Carlson, Coyne-Plum, et al., 2019). Although the psychological trauma that results from involvement in a critical incident varies, common symptoms range from insomnia to excessive sleeping, from loss of appetite to overeating, and a loss of interest in activities normally considered pleasurable (PHAC, 2011). Post-traumatic stress disorder (PTSD) is a response to a specific, identifiable stressor that severely affects an individual's ability to function at a normal level. The diagnosis is given to individuals who have experienced or witnessed situations involving death or serious injury or a threat to self or others. PTSD can result in the development of symptoms in the first few weeks or months, or up to years following an event. Symptoms include avoidance, numbing, or the individual re-experiencing the event, causing significant impairment in function (Carlson, Meeker, et al., 2019; McMahon, 2010). PTSD requires ongoing psychological counselling, psychiatric support, or both.

Critical incident stress management (CISM) or debriefing is a comprehensive approach to preventing and managing the emotional trauma that can result from involvement in a disaster response. Strategies may include pre-incident education; individual crisis intervention and on-the-scene support; defusing and debriefing sessions; support services for families and children; and follow-up professional intervention (Carlson, Meeker, et al., 2019; McMahon, 2010). Debriefing occurs as a part of the incident review within the first 24 to 72 hours, particularly among police officers, firefighters, and medical first responders. *Defusing sessions* should occur within a few hours of the incident and may be offered as a group discussion prior to staff going off duty. This process involves brief discussion of the incident and assistance with stress management (Carlson, Meeker, et al., 2019).

THE ROLE OF NURSING LEADERSHIP IN DISASTER PREPAREDNESS AND RESPONSE

Leadership at all levels is essential for a positive outcome after a disaster event. Leadership in times of disaster involves recognition of the uncertainty created during the response and requires open, consistent communication, flexibility, and creative problem solving. Nurses who hold formal leadership roles have extended responsibilities to ensure the delivery of safe care at all stages of the disaster management continuum. However, there remains a paucity of evidence-informed leadership literature available to guide nursing leaders throughout disaster management (Veenema et al., 2017). Nurses exercise vital roles in disaster management—for example, providing patient care, health surveillance, education, assessing needs and allocating resources, evaluating response measures, coordination of the nursing response, communication, legal and ethical awareness and consideration, and patient advocacy. Nursing leadership also involves advocating for individual and community needs and services during disaster recovery, including policies at the local, national, and international levels (ICN, 2019b).

DISASTERS

A *disaster* can be defined in numerous ways, but the term is generally interpreted to mean a destructive event that disrupts the normal functioning of a community. There are two general classifications of disasters: *natural disaster* and *human-made* or *human-induced disasters*. Disease outbreaks and epidemics are usually considered to be "natural" events, but they can also be classified as "human-made" disasters when disease-causing organisms are used as an agent of terrorism with the goal of inducing large-scale epidemics. Because of these variations, disease outbreaks, epidemics, endemics, and pandemics are described in a separate section of this chapter. Table 72.4 presents a timeline of notable disasters in Canadian history.

Natural Disasters

Given its size and geographic location, Canada is vulnerable to a range of threats. Its landforms and variation in weather patterns makes severe weather and the threat of natural hazards a significant reality for Canadians. *Natural disasters* are caused by nature or the environment, are often unpredictable, and can happen at a rapid or a slow rate. Natural disasters include extreme natural events such as forest fires, avalanches, landslides, storm surges, cold or heat waves, hurricanes, tsunamis, floods, drought, earthquakes, and volcanic eruptions (PSC, 2017). Human-caused damage to the environment and the resultant climate change have also altered the intensity, pattern, and distribution of natural forces, contributing to an increase in the number of natural disasters (Veenema, Corley, et al., 2019).

Human-Made or Human-Induced Disasters

Human-made, also referred to as *human-induced disasters,* can be accidental or deliberate and can cause injuries, deaths, and long-term consequences for individuals and communities. *Accidental human-made disasters* include industrial accidents, chemical spills, inadvertent release of nuclear energy, explosions (e.g., from hazardous materials such as chemicals, nuclear materials, fuel), contamination, fires, structural collapse, large transportation accidents, and power outages. *Deliberate human-made disasters* include warfare, civil unrest, and acts of terrorism. Computer viruses or cyber-attacks are classified as human-made disasters because of their cost and potential impact on critical infrastructure.

Natural and human-made disasters can trigger one another, with both having the ability to elicit secondary disasters. These events, referred to as *synergistic disasters*, often occur simultaneously. As an example, an earthquake causes an explosion at a nuclear plant, requiring large-scale evacuation and causing illness and population displacement. The synergistic effects are exacerbated by death and devastation created by each event (Veenema, 2019b).

Terrorism

Terrorism involves intentional and overt actions that are committed to cause fear, panic, destruction, injury, and death in service of political, religious, or ideological goals. The intent of a terrorist event is to intimidate the public or to compel a specific person, government, or international organization to take specific action. Terrorist events include threats, assassinations, kidnappings, hijackings, bomb scares and bombings, and computer cyber-attacks. The use of chemical or biological agents as the element of a terrorist attack is referred to as *chemical terrorism* or bioterrorism, respectively (Croddy & Ackerman, 2019). In both cases, the terms refer to a type of terrorist event involving the deliberate spreading of microbes or chemical toxins with the intent of causing disease or death in animals, plants,

TABLE 72.4   BEST-KNOWN CANADIAN DISASTERS

Year	Disaster and Place	Approximate # of Fatalities	Injured/Infected	Evacuated
1862	Smallpox epidemic (nationwide)	20 000		0
1885	Smallpox epidemic, Montreal, Quebec	6000	9600	0
1917	Harbour explosion, Halifax, Nova Scotia	2000	9000	6000
1918	Spanish influenza pandemic (Spanish flu) across Canada	50 000	2 000 000	0
1974	Airplane crash, Rea Point, Northwest Territories	32	0	0
1985	Airplane crash, Gander, Newfoundland	256	0	0
1986	Train derailment, Hinton, Alberta	23	71	0
1987	Tornado, Edmonton, Alberta	27	600	1700
1992	Westray mining accident, Plymouth, Nova Scotia	26	0	0
1996	Floods, Saguenay, Quebec	10	0	15 825
1998	Plane crash, Peggy's Cove, Nova Scotia	230	0	0
2000	Contaminated water, Walkerton, Ontario	7	2300	0
2000	Tornado, Pine Lake, Alberta	12	140	1000
2003	Severe acute respiratory syndrome (SARS), Toronto, Ontario	44	375	0
2005	Legionnaire's disease outbreak, Toronto, Ontario	23	112	0
2008	Listeriosis outbreak across Canada	22	57	0
2009–2010	New strain of pandemic influenza	425	8582	0
2011	Slave Lake wildfire, Slave Lake, Alberta	1	0	12 055
2011	First Air Flight 6560 crash near Resolute Bay, Nunavut	12	0	3
2012	Legionnaire's disease epidemic, Quebec, Quebec	13	180	0
2012	Train derailment, Burlington, Ontario	3	45	0
2013	Alberta floods, Calgary, Alberta	4	0	100 000
2013	Rail disaster, Lac-Mégantic, Quebec	47	0	2000
2014	Nursing home fire, near L'Isle-Verte, Quebec	32	15	0
2014	Terrorist shooting, Ottawa, Ontario	2	0	0
2014	Wildfire due to heatwave, British Columbia	0	0	4500
2016	School shooting, La Loche, Saskatchewan	4	0	0
2016	Forest fire, Fort McMurray, Alberta	0	0	90 000
2017	Quebec City, Mosque shooting	6	19	0
2020	COVID-19 global pandemic*	30 957	2 624 787	—
2020	Portapique, Nova Scotia, Mass shooting	23		

*Statistics are current as of January 12 2022. (Government of Canada. (2022). *COVID-19 daily epidemiology update.* https://health-infobase.canada.ca/covid-19/epidemiological-sum-mary-covid-19-cases.html)

Sources: Adapted from Stanhope, M., Lancaster, J., Jessup-Falcioni, H., et al. (2011). *Community health nursing in Canada* (Table 16-2, p. 506). Mosby; and PSC. (2015e). *The Canadian disaster database.* http://www.publicsafety.gc.ca/cnt/rsrcs/cndn-dsstr-dtbs/index-eng.aspx

and humans (Croddy & Ackerman, 2019). Plans for dealing with each type of event, coupled with advanced training exercises and availability of necessary PPE, are essential to a safe, expedient response. Terrorist attacks across several public sites in Paris, France (2015) and in a nightclub in Orlando, Florida, (2016) illustrate the far-reaching impact of terrorism and the critical need for emergency planning. Acts of terrorism are criminal acts as defined by the *Criminal Code of Canada* and the *Security Offences Act* (Government of Canada, 2013).

Chemical-Biological-Radiological-Nuclear-Explosive Events. A CBRNE event refers to any situation in which weapons of a *chemical, biological, radiological, nuclear,* or *explosive* nature are used with the goal of causing harm. *Weapons of mass destruction* refers to a broad range of weapons that have the potential to affect the health and well-being of a large population.

In the absence of clear evidence that suggests an intentional threat, the response to a CBRNE event begins as a hazardous materials (HazMat) response (Government of Canada, 2013). Under ideal circumstances, decontamination following a CBRNE event will occur in the field, prior to the casualties' arrival to hospital. A response in the field may not occur when exposure is a result of a terrorist event, as casualties are likely to flee the site, not knowing they have been contaminated and pose a risk to others. People may arrive at health care facilities in large or small numbers and without advanced notice or may delay seeking treatment until they become symptomatic or once public information has been shared about potential exposure

(Ponampalam, 2019). Consequently, CBRNE events have significant implications for the health and safety of people who come into contact with casualties and, to ensure public safety, health care staff should assume, until it has been proven otherwise, that all individuals presenting to the hospital have *not* undergone adequate decontamination (Koenig et al., 2008; Veenema, 2019a). Hospitals must have plans in place to address CBRNE exposure, which requires advanced planning and input from the interprofessional health care team, HazMat teams, and health and safety team members (Moore et al., 2015). The use of evidence-informed protocols and systems for triage and decontamination, combined with the application of appropriate PPE, is essential for safe response, not only for first responders in the field but also for health care workers in hospital settings (Ponampalam, 2019). Despite significant focus over the last decade on emergency planning and preparation, there is still broad discomfort across the health care sector regarding inadequate addressing of and responding to these types of events (Moore et al., 2015).

Early identification, diagnosis, and treatment of people exposed to CBRNE substances is essential to preventing secondary injury and avoiding contamination of the public, staff, and the health care facility (Croddy & Ackerman, 2019; Rihl-Pryor, 2019); people need to be decontaminated *before* medical care or surgical intervention is provided. Decontamination is the process of removing or neutralizing a hazardous agent from the environment, property, equipment, or a life form through the use of water, cleansers, or neutralizers (Moore et al., 2015;

Veenema, 2019a). Decontamination decreases the absorption and toxicity of the agent and reduces contamination of other people and equipment.

For a safe response in the hospital setting, it is necessary to have decontamination teams and advanced preparation for activation of a decontamination area, complete with showers, scrubbing instruments, and ventilation (Holland & Cawthon, 2015; Moore et al., 2015). Decontamination is a multidisciplinary strategy that includes participation from the interprofessional health care team, security and housekeeping, engineering and occupational health and safety members, and porters. Participation in casualty decontamination requires significant education and training before a potential event in the application and use of PPE, activation of decontamination equipment (showers, tents, etc.), set-up of operation zones, and decontamination and scrubbing processes, through regular, full-scale hospital drills (Moore et al., 2015). Hospitals need to ensure that they have adequate amounts of antidotes, adequate numbers of showers and decontamination tents, appropriate availability of PPE, and staff trained to participate in response (Veenema, 2019a).

Casualties should be segregated from other patient populations until appropriate decontamination takes place, and security must be in place to prevent inadvertent contamination (Holland & Cawthon, 2015). Similar to decontamination in the field, decontamination in hospital settings requires activation of *operation or decontamination zones*. Typically, these zones are created through the use of barricades to determine points of entry from one area to the next. Crowd control, safety, and security are of primary concern—first responders, health care workers, and other patients who have physical contact with contaminated casualties, their belongings, or both without appropriate protection may also require decontamination (Holland & Cawthon, 2015; Koenig et al., 2008). Lockdown of entry points to a health care facility, with the exception of a designated access point for persons who require decontamination, is one strategy to prevent inadvertent exposure of patients and staff to the contaminant (Markenson & Losinski, 2019).

Three operation zones—hot, warm, and cold—support triage and decontamination activities. The *hot zone* is the area farthest from hospital entry and requires all responders to don full PPE. Minimal triage is provided in this area and is limited to life-saving measures and administration of antidotes. The *warm zone* is typically adjacent to the ED and is the location where staff in full PPE provide decontamination of casualties. Non-ambulatory patients will be scrubbed by staff through the use of hoses, trailers, or tents, using conveyor belts and trolley systems, whereas ambulatory patients will be directed to remove contaminated clothing and then assist with personal scrubbing and decontamination, using hoses and warm showers. Patients with the most severe symptoms receive priority for decontamination. The *cold zone* is the treatment location adjacent to the warm zone and is the location where patients, once decontaminated, enter. All staff who have worked in hot or warm zones also require decontamination prior to entering the cold zone. A more thorough triage occurs in the cold zone, following which people are directed to treatment areas (Veenema, 2019a).

The health and safety of health care providers is essential in a CBRNE event. A combination of respirators and protective gear (goggles, boots, full-facepiece respirators, protective suits, chemically resistant gloves) must be used (Holland & Cawthon, 2015; Veenema, 2019a). Because of the equipment that is required to be worn, workers must undergo medical screening or surveillance (including a full set of vital signs) when donning and taking off protective gear. Staff who have higher-than-normal blood pressure; rashes, open sores, or wounds; a previous history of nausea, vomiting, or diarrhea; an upper respiratory infection or history of respiratory illness (e.g., asthma); allergies; or sensitivities or phobias (e.g., claustrophobia) or who are potentially or known to be pregnant may not participate in the decontamination process. Time in decontamination gear is usually limited to 30 minutes or less because extreme heat, poor ventilation, and the heavy weight of the suit cause fatigue and other common adverse effects (Veenema, 2019a). These risks also make it necessary to monitor hydration status before and after protective gear is donned.

Biological Agents of Terrorism. Biological terrorism involves the deliberate use of microbial pathogens or toxins, the effects of which may not be known until many hours or days after exposure. Terrorist attacks using biological agents represent challenges for health care providers because these agents can be difficult to detect and can have a prolonged impact on health care facilities. Contaminants can range from accidental releases of biohazardous waste to intentional exposure from bioweapons (Rihl-Pryor, 2019). People exposed in a bioterrorist attack typically do not require decontamination (the exception being exposure to anthrax spores), and most agents are noncontagious (Croddy & Ackerman, 2019). Hospitals should have access to a variety of antidotes for biological agents and should have plans that include means for urgent acquisition of antidotes from other sources (Moore et al., 2015). Table 72.5 summarizes general information regarding biological agents of terrorism.

Chemical Agents of Terrorism. Typically, a chemical event is overt, with a sudden onset in a localized area, and has potential for vast spread with large numbers of individuals affected, making rapid containment and decontamination essential (Rihl-Pryor, 2019). These events are most likely to cause significant limitations of health care personnel, time, equipment, and space and have potential to cause major disruptions in clinical services because of their rarity and the physical and psychological impact on both casualties and responders (Croddy & Ackerman, 2019; Moore et al., 2015).

Radiological and Nuclear Agents of Terrorism. Radiological and nuclear substances can also be categorized as agents of terrorism. Radiological dispersal devices (RDDs), or "dirty bombs," consists of chemical explosives mixed with radioactivity (Karam, 2019). When an RDD is detonated, the blast is likely to lead to widespread radioactive contamination through dispersed dust, smoke, and other material into the surrounding environment (Centers for Disease Control and Prevention [CDC], 2018). Health care personnel will confront large volumes of patients, some with high levels of radioactivity contamination and many others with high levels of anxiety without presenting illness from exposure (Karam, 2019). The main danger of an RDD results from the explosion itself, with those patients suffering traumatic injury combined with significant exposure to radiation having a substantially worse prognosis (Karam, 2019). Because radiation cannot be seen, has no scent, and is unable to be felt or tasted, measures to limit contamination, like covering the patient's nose and mouth and prompt decontamination (e.g., through the use of a decontamination shower), are best initiated in a timely manner (CDC, 2018).

TABLE 72.5   BIOLOGICAL AGENTS OF TERRORISM

Pathogen and Description	Clinical Manifestations	Transmissibility	Treatment
Anthrax (Bacillus anthracis) **Inhalation** • Bacterial spores multiply in the alveoli • High mortality rate • Toxins cause hemorrhage and destruction of lung tissue	• Incubation period: 1–7 days; can be delayed up to 60 days (2 months) • Abrupt onset • Dyspnea • Diaphoresis • Fever • Cough • Chest pain • Septicemia • Shock • Meningitis • Respiratory failure • Widened mediastinum (seen on chest radiograph)	• No person-to-person spread • Found in nature; most commonly infects wild and domestic hoofed animals • Spread through direct contact with bacterium and its spores • Spores are dormant, encapsulated bacteria that become active when they enter a living host	• Antibiotics prevent systemic manifestations • Effective only if treated early • Ciprofloxacin (Cipro) is the treatment of choice • Penicillin • Doxycycline • Post-exposure prophylaxis for 30 days (if vaccine available) or 60 days (if vaccine not available) • Vaccine has limited availability
Cutaneous • 95% of anthrax infections • Least lethal form • Spores enter skin through cuts or abrasions • Handling of contaminated animal skin products • Toxins destroy surrounding tissue	• Incubation period: 2–6 days • Small papule resembles an insect bite • Advances to a depressed, black ulcer • Swollen lymph nodes in adjacent areas • Edema	—	—
Gastrointestinal • Ingestion of contaminated, undercooked meat • Intestinal lesions in ileum or cecum • Acute inflammation of intestines	• Abdominal pain • Anorexia • Ascites • Diarrhea • Hematemesis • Incubation period: 3–7 days • Nausea • Sepsis • Vomiting	—	—
Smallpox (Variola Major and Minor Viruses) • Canada ended routine vaccination in 1972 • Global eradication declared in 1980	• Incubation period: 7–17 days • Sudden onset of symptoms • Fever • Headache • Myalgia • Lesions that progress from macules to papules to pustular vesicles • Malaise • Back pain	• Direct person-to-person spread • Highly contagious • Transmitted by handling contaminated materials • Transmitted in air droplets	• Cidofovir (Vistide) under testing • Isolation for containment • No known cure • Vaccine available for those exposed • Vaccinia immune globulin (VIG) available
Botulism (Clostridium botulinum) • Spore-forming anaerobe • Found in soil • Seven different toxins • Lethal bacterial neurotoxin • Can die within 24 hr	• Incubation period: 12–36 hr • Abdominal cramps • Diarrhea • Nausea • Vomiting • Cranial nerve palsies (diplopia, dysarthria, dysphonia, dysphagia) • Skeletal muscle paralysis • Respiratory failure	• Spread through air or food • No person-to-person spread • Improperly canned foods • Contaminated wound	• Induce vomiting • Enemas • Antitoxin • Mechanical ventilation • Penicillin • No vaccine available • Toxin can be inactivated by heating food or drink to 100°C for at least 10 min

Continued

TABLE 72.5	BIOLOGICAL AGENTS OF TERRORISM—cont'd		
Pathogen and Description	**Clinical Manifestations**	**Transmissibility**	**Treatment**
Plague (Yersinia pestis) • Bacteria found in rodents and fleas **Forms** • Bubonic (most common) • Pneumonic • Septicemic (most deadly)	• Incubation period: 2–4 days • Hemoptysis • Cough • High fever • Chills • Myalgia • Headache • Respiratory failure • Lymph node swelling	• Direct person-to-person spread • Transmitted through flea bites • Ingestion of contaminated meat	• Antibiotics only effective if administered immediately • Drug of choice: streptomycin or gentamicin • Vaccine under development • Hospitalization • Isolation for containment
Tularemia (Francisella tularensis) • Bacterial infectious disease of animals • Mortality rate about 35% without treatment	• Incubation period: 3–10 days • Sudden onset • Fever • Swollen lymph nodes • Fatigue • Sore throat • Weight loss • Pneumonia • Pleural effusion • Ulcerated sore from tick bite	• No person-to-person spread • Aerosol or intradermal route • Spread by rabbits and ticks • Contaminated food, air, water	• Gentamicin treatment of choice • Streptomycin, doxycycline, and ciprofloxacin are alternatives • Vaccine in developmental stage
Hemorrhagic Fever • Caused by several viruses, including Marburg, Ebola, Lassa fever, yellow fever, and Rift Valley fever	• Fever • Conjunctivitis • Headache • Malaise • Prostration • Hemorrhage of tissues and organs • Nausea • Vomiting • Hypotension • Organ failure	• Carried by rodents and mosquitoes • Direct person-to-person spread by body fluids • Virus can be aerosolized	• No intramuscular injections • No anticoagulants • Isolation for containment • Ribavirin (Virazole) effective in some cases • Supportive treatment only, for most • Vaccine available for yellow fever only

Source: Adapted from Lewis, S. L., Heitkemper, M. M., Dirksen, S. R., et al. (2011). *Medical-surgical nursing: Assessment and management of clinical problems* (8th ed., Table 69-12). Mosby.

Explosive Agents of Terrorism. Injuries that are a result of terrorist attacks with explosives typically involve younger civilian casualties, with critical severity, requiring longer hospitalization and surgical interventions, and result in higher mortality rates (Sacco, 2019). Whether the result of an accident or terrorist event, the use of explosion devices (TNT, dynamite) in acts of terrorism results in blunt, crush, penetrating, and burn injuries as well as injuries from the blast itself (Sacco, 2019). *Blast injuries* occur from the supersonic overpressurization shock wave that results from the explosion, having the potential to cause mass injury to multiple body systems. This shock wave primarily causes damage to the lungs, gastrointestinal tract, and middle ear; the injuries are the result of casualties being blown by the blast wind against objects and structures. *Crush injuries* (i.e., blunt trauma) often ensue from explosions that occur in confined spaces and result from structural collapse (e.g., falling debris). Some explosive devices contain materials that are projected during the explosion (e.g., shrapnel), leading to *penetrating injuries*.

Outbreaks, Epidemics, Pandemics, and Endemics

Nurses are required to have an understanding of the etiology and impact of communicable disease, whether a consequence of a natural disaster (e.g., contaminated water during flooding) or a result of a deliberate act (e.g., bioterrorism) (CNA, 2018). Morbidity, mortality, and disruption from an infectious disease epidemic can overwhelm a community and its infrastructure. Lessons learned as a result of severe acute respiratory syndrome (SARS) (2003), H1N1 virus (2009), and, most recently, COVID-19 (2020) infectious disease outbreaks highlight the enormous toll taken on individuals, communities, populations, and health care workers and the need for advanced planning.

Communicable diseases may occur in an individual or a group of individuals. The term *outbreak* refers to an illness occurring among a cluster of individuals. When the number of cases of a communicable disease affects a large number of people within a defined region and exceeds the normal expected occurrence during a given period, it is referred to as an **epidemic**. The Zika virus outbreak of 2015–2016 (WHO, 2019) and HIV/AIDS are considered epidemics, with almost 38 million people living with HIV/AIDS (WHO, 2020b). If transmission of the disease is widespread and affects large numbers of people across several countries or continents or globally, it is considered to be a **pandemic**. A way to remember this difference is to think of the *p* in pandemic—meaning it has a passport and crosses country borders (Intermountain Healthcare, 2020). For example, when the SARS-CoV-2 virus was limited to Wuhan, China, it was an epidemic; once the virus crossed borders and was evident in other countries and then globally, the same virus became a pandemic. An **endemic** is something that applies to a group of people or a region or country and has a constant presence (e.g., malaria in some areas of Africa, Dengue fever in Asia). An endemic can lead to an outbreak—for example, the outbreak of malaria in Hawaii (2016), as malaria is not endemic in Hawaii. The investigation and management of an outbreak require recognition; investigation of the source, mode of transmission, and risk factors for infection; and implementation of appropriate infection-control measures (Veenema, 2019b). Nurses are actively involved in outbreak, epidemic, endemic, and pandemic responses through telephone and onsite assessment centres, health promotion and education, testing facilities, contact tracing measures, and caring for ill patients.

Coronaviruses. Coronaviruses are a very large family of viruses, with some causing illness in people and others causing illness in animals (Government of Canada, 2021a). Seven strains have been identified that cause illness in humans (PHAC, 2020). Three commonly known coronaviruses that have spread from animals to humans, causing severe illness, are severe acute respiratory syndrome coronavirus (SARS CoV), Middle East respiratory syndrome coronavirus (MERS CoV), and severe acute respiratory syndrome coronavirus 2 (SARS-CoV-2).

Severe Acute Respiratory Syndrome (SARS). *Severe acute respiratory syndrome* refers to an outbreak that occurred primarily in Canada and Asia in 2003 and is caused by the SARS coronavirus. SARS is a highly contagious, severe, febrile respiratory illness characterized by a fever of 38°C or higher, chills, headache, muscular stiffness, loss of appetite, malaise, dry cough, and shortness of breath or breathing difficulties (Canadian Centre for Occupational Health and Safety [CCOHS], 2020).

The SARS outbreak was a critical juncture in Canadian emergency management because it demonstrated the tremendous impact a communicable disease outbreak could have on individuals, communities, and the economy (PSC, 2019b). SARS cost millions of dollars across Canada as a result of its impact on health care, critical infrastructure, trade, and tourism and served as a wake-up call for health care institutions, governments, and health care providers, highlighting Canada's inadequacies in responding to public health threats.

Severe Acute Respiratory Syndrome Coronavirus 2 (SARS-CoV-2). SARS-CoV-2 infection, commonly referred to as *COVID-19*, is a new infectious disease discovered in 2019 that had not previously been identified in humans and was the cause of a global pandemic beginning in 2020. The most current epidemiological information indicates that human-to-human transmission of COVID-19 can occur when a person is in close contact with another person who has the virus (PHAC, 2020). It is most commonly spread from an infected person through respiratory or airborne droplets; close, prolonged personal contact; and touching an infected area and then touching the mouth, nose, or eyes before performing hand hygiene (PHAC, 2020). Possible symptoms include a temperature of 38°C or higher, cough, difficulty breathing, and pneumonia in both lungs (CCOHS, 2020). In severe cases, infection can lead to

death. Symptoms may take up to 14 days to appear after exposure to the virus. Evidence suggests that transmission is possible in presymptomatic patients (not yet developed symptoms) and asymptomatic patients (never develop symptoms).

Outbreak Management. Studies of pandemics across numerous countries have provided insight into the need for diligent infection-control practices and disease monitoring. The effects of globalization and the ease of air travel have led not only to the "shrinking" of the world but also to the global mobility of people, food, viruses, and bacteria. The strategies used to prevent and contain communicable diseases are fundamental, and nurses play an essential role in understanding common outbreak management strategies. This knowledge helps nurses working in acute and chronic care and within community settings to implement containment interventions and to understand how best to protect themselves and their patients.

Outbreak Management Strategies. Outbreak management refers to the strategies used to prevent the spread of communicable disease among clusters of people. Management of outbreaks within health care facilities begins with recognition of potentially exposed patients by trained staff or through public health notification. Case-finding, early detection, contact tracing, and treatment strategies not only improve the health of the infected individuals but also prevent transmission to others.

Contact tracing is an important intervention in stopping the spread of communicable diseases in communities. When an individual tests positive for the infectious agent, a public health nurse interviews them to identify individuals they may have been in contact with. For example, in the case of COVID-19, only contacts who may have been exposed to respiratory droplets from coughing, sneezing, or speaking are identified. A person who tests positive for COVID-19 can tell others about their result, but they cannot do their own contract tracing. Public health nurses will ask the identified contacts about applicable symptoms. Contacts with symptoms are sent for testing, whereas those individuals without symptoms are asked to self-isolate for up to 14 days and monitor at least daily for symptoms. When any contact of an infected person tests positive, contact tracing is started on that individual as well. Contact tracing enables earlier diagnosis and reduction in the transmission of the virus by self-isolation (British Columba Centre for Disease Control, 2021).

Surveillance is the ongoing and systematic process of gathering, analyzing, and disseminating data on communicable diseases or events to detect changes in trends or distribution of diseases. In the case of disease outbreaks, surveillance involves gathering the data that epidemiologists analyze to determine the *who, what, when, where,* and *why* behind the outbreak (Stanhope et al., 2017). There have been major efforts across Canada to develop and strengthen early-warning mechanisms at the local and global levels. The Public Health Agency of Canada (PHAC) operates a number of national surveillance systems on public health concerns that range from chronic diseases and congenital anomalies to the Respiratory Virus Detection Surveillance System, the Coronavirus (COVID-19) app and website, and FluWatch. These systems are in place to observe and scrutinize changes in the number of febrile and respiratory illnesses across the country. Many communicable diseases are considered to be reportable or notifiable diseases and must be reported to local public health units (PHAC, 2016). Nurses are often involved, both formally and informally, in different levels

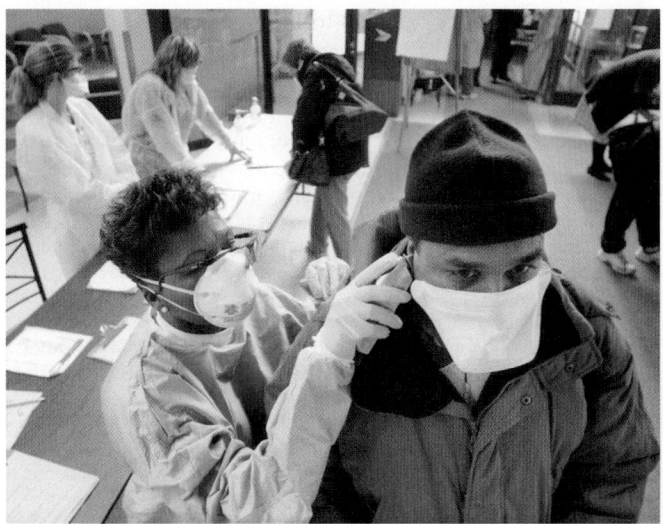

FIG. 72.4 A critical strategy in managing respiratory pandemics is screening patients for possible signs of the disease. Source: The Canadian Press/J. P. Moczulski.

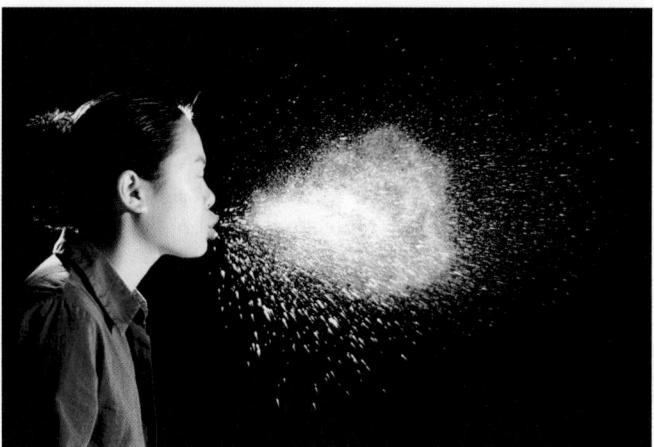

FIG. 72.5 Particle mist created upon sneezing. Source: Photo by Andrew Davidhazy/RIT.

of the surveillance system, being the first to detect an outbreak through abnormal clusters of illness among populations, for example, in a school setting.

Isolation is an outbreak management strategy that separates infected people from those assumed to be unaffected during a period of the disease's communicability (Figure 72.4). In Canada, the COVID-19 pandemic demonstrated how rapidly infectious diseases can spread, especially among vulnerable groups, such as older persons (CCOHS, 2020). Infected individuals may be confined to a hospital room or unit or to their home and may have varying types of isolation depending on the severity of their disease, its route of transmission, and the period of communicability.

Quarantine involves the isolation of people who have been exposed or potentially exposed to an infection or contagious disease but who are not yet sick or showing signs of illness. These individuals are assumed to have been exposed to the disease and may be infectious to other people before they display symptoms. During the COVID-19 outbreak, hundreds of thousands of people were advised to self-isolate at home for 14-day periods, the incubation period for SARS-CoV-2, if returning home from outside of Canada or if travelling from one province or territory to another in Canada, if they had had close contact with someone who had COVID-19 or were directed by the public health authority that exposure may have occurred (CCOHS, 2020). Each jurisdiction had their own provincial or territorial entry regulations, and these directives changed over the course of the pandemic in direct response to the incidence of SARS-CoV-2-positive individuals in any given geographic area. For example, during the pandemic, from July until November 2020, travel within the "Atlantic bubble" was not restricted (New Brunswick, Nova Scotia, Prince Edward Island, and Newfoundland); however, travel into this bubble required a 14-day self-isolation period. At the height of the pandemic, many provinces and territories had declared states of emergency and limited cross-border travel within Canada to essential services and supplies only.

Pandemic Planning. Pandemic planning is a focus of the PHAC, with the majority of past planning focusing on pandemic influenza preparedness. Pandemic influenza is a highly infectious outbreak of influenza that spreads rapidly around the world with much more serious consequences than the usual effects of seasonal influenza. There are two primary routes by which the influenza virus exits the respiratory tract of an infected person: (1) expulsion of the virus into the air through sneezing (Figure 72.5), coughing, speaking, or breathing or through aerosol-generating medical procedures, and (2) by direct transfer of respiratory secretions to another person or surface. More recently, the COVID-19 pandemic has demonstrated a need for pandemic planning that extends beyond that for seasonal influenza. The fact that these viruses can be transmitted before an infected person is symptomatic make it essential that nurses use appropriate infection-control techniques to prevent the spread of influenza and COVID-19 (see the Evidence-Informed Practice box).

🔍 EVIDENCE-INFORMED PRACTICE

Research Highlight

Early Lessons Learned from COVID-19: Behavioural Considerations and Impact on Personal Protective Equipment
A high prevalence of cutaneous irritation is associated with the use of N95 masks as part of personal protection equipment (PPE). There is evidence that face touching and surface contact transmission occur in addition to direct inhalation of droplets as a means of spreading viral disease (e.g., COVID-19). With hand-to-face contact playing a role in disease transmission, it is important to adhere to strict PPE protocols when donning and taking off masks. The presence of mild abrasions on the face may increase hand-to-face contact when not using PPE and may require careful consideration when using masks in an effort to reduce or eliminate facial irritation.

Preventative Measures to Reduce Risk of Facial Skin Irritation When Using Protective Masks
1. Educate all members of the interprofessional team to ensure proper donning and doffing of PPE, along with the expectation of mild facial skin irritation with prolonged use.
2. If topical agents are used to reduce irritation, great care in application is required; use a sterile cotton-tipped applicator to apply ointment.
3. Those individuals with a sensitivity may need to explore using a full-face shield rather than masks and goggles, provided these items are readily available.
4. There is no evidence to support the use of prophylactic dressings to mitigate skin irritation with the use of PPE; the potential impact of their use on PPE efficacy is unknown.

Reference for Evidence
Kantor, J. (2020). Behavioral considerations and impact on personal protective equipment use: Early lessons from the coronavirus (COVID-19) pandemic. *Journal of the American Academy of Dermatology, 82*(5), 1087–1088. https://doi.org/10.1016/j.jaad.2020.03.013

In June 2009, the beginning of a global influenza pandemic was confirmed as the illness was identified across 74 countries, raising the World Health Organization (WHO) alert from a 5 (widespread human transmission) to a 6 (pandemic phase) (Slepski, 2010). The impact of pandemic influenza is vast and far-reaching and continues to be an annual public health concern. On March 11, 2020, the WHO declared a global pandemic related to the SARS-CoV-2 infection. Given public health concerns and the need for vigilant monitoring of communicable illness in humans, the WHO monitors the risk as determined by its experts and an analysis of the situation in countries around the world. For further information about the current phase of pandemic alert and a detailed explanation of the phases of pandemic alert, follow the WHO link in the Resources at the end of this chapter.

Ethical Issues During a Disaster or Pandemic. Whether in connection to natural or human-made disasters or to pandemics, nurses have raised tough ethical questions regarding patient care and disease prevention. Such questions address who gets access to critical care unit services, ventilators, and respiratory support in the hospital, and which sectors of the population should be given priority to receive vaccines and antivirals during a pandemic. During a disaster situation, the primary health focus shifts from obtaining the best possible health outcomes for the individual patient (ethical principles of beneficence, autonomy, nonmaleficence, and justice) to protecting the health and safety of the population as a whole, the greatest good for the greatest number (ethical principle of utilitarianism) (Wagner et al., 2015). Many of these ethical dilemmas are about balancing the best interests of the entire population, which is referred to as the "public good," with the rights of the individual. The duty to provide care, when care poses a risk to self and loved ones, highlights the ethical implications for all health care providers (see the Ethical Dilemmas box). Nurses and other health care workers have expressed the conflict they feel between their professional and legal obligations to their patients and their responsibilities to themselves and their families (CNA, 2017). A number of ethical frameworks, articles, and resources are available that provide guidance for nurses, other health care workers, and decision makers in health care and government settings. Many of these resources can be found in the Resources section at the end of this chapter.

Vulnerable Individuals and Populations. Special attention, in all the phases of a disaster or emergency, must be given to vulnerable individuals and marginalized groups. Failure to address the physical and psychological impact of a disaster in a timely and comprehensive manner can lead to long-term challenges and mental health issues. Individuals with pre-existing health conditions, children, pregnant individuals, malnourished people, those individuals who are immunocompromised, and older persons are among the more vulnerable people of the population and are at higher risk for suffering the negative impacts of a disaster (WHO, 2020a). Poverty often leads to malnutrition, homelessness, poor housing, and destitution, which are major contributing factors to vulnerability during disasters (WHO, 2020a). Where possible, these populations should be pre-identified as a part of emergency preparation, with the creation of specific plans to address their unique needs. Vulnerable populations often have limited resources, and their ability to recover is affected by their culture, support systems, and previous experiences. In the aftermath of a disaster, nurses are key to offering reassurance, education, and referral to needed resources to

ETHICAL DILEMMAS
Duty to Provide Care During a Pandemic

Situation

A senior undergraduate nursing student is in the last semester of their nursing program. The Centre for Emergency Preparedness and Response, part of the Public Health Agency of Canada (PHAC), has declared a provincial state of emergency in the midst of the initial wave of a pandemic. Universities across the country have implemented remote teaching to maintain educational program progression wherever possible. Senior nursing students are being provided the option of completing their final clinical practicum during the pandemic. The students' parents are worried about ongoing safety and are urging their children to defer their final clinical practice placement. The student is unsure of what to do because they want to complete the program and to graduate.

Important Points for Consideration

There will be a massive need for health care workers during a pandemic given the number of people who are ill and in need of care; health care workers will also be ill. Many provincial and territorial pandemic influenza plans discuss the utilization of health science students in response to the overwhelming need for health care human resources. During this pandemic, universities are implementing emergency preparedness and pandemic plans and have developed contingency plans for students who are unable to move out of the student residence or cannot travel to their home communities during a pandemic because of travel restrictions. Nursing programs have begun developing specific guidelines and decision-making protocols for use during a pandemic because nursing students are participating in the health care system.

Clinical Decision-Making Questions

1. What guidance is provided by the Canadian Nurses Association (CNA) *Code of Ethics* to help nurses address their ethical dilemmas about providing care during a pandemic?
2. What guidance is provided by the provincial/territorial regulatory standards of nursing practice related to providing care during a pandemic?
3. The student is not yet a registered nurse. What are the legal obligations, as a student, during a pandemic?
4. What is the registered nurse's duty to provide care during a pandemic? What are the ethical considerations?

these higher-risk populations. An understanding of stress and the impact of stress, while offering strategies to cope, is a key component of the nursing role.

Disaster Nursing

With an increasing number of global disasters has come recognition of the need for increased health care preparedness. Disaster nursing involves the provision of nursing care, advocacy, and health promotion within the context of a disaster situation. Nurses, because of their position and numbers, are essential in disaster prevention and mitigation, preparedness, response, and recovery (CNA, 2018; ICN, 2019b). Nurses fill a variety of roles throughout the disaster management continuum. The ICN (2019b) has called on individual nurses in their roles as clinicians, educators, researchers, policy influencers, or executives to actively engage in disaster management committees and policy making for disaster risk reduction, response, and recovery. Nurses must be competent to provide disaster relief and meet the health needs of the population according to the specific disaster and the given situation.

When disaster strikes, the demand for nurses is much greater than for other health care providers. Opportunities for nursing abroad in countries affected by disaster also exist through humanitarian networks and volunteer agencies. Disaster nursing, irrespective of the location of the disaster, requires application of basic nursing knowledge and skills in difficult environments with scarce resources, rapidly changing conditions, and large volumes of patients. Disaster nursing involves collaboration with the interprofessional health care team, first responders, and individuals not commonly worked with, requiring an ability to shift focus in care while working within the parameters of the laws in place in the area of work. The ICN has a mission to advance nurses and to bring nursing together

worldwide (ICN, 2019a). Recognizing the valuable role that nurses play in disaster responses and the exponentially expanding literature available on effective disaster and emergency response, the ICN revised the initial *Framework of Disaster Nursing Competencies* (ICN, 2019a). The framework includes three levels of nurses needing competency in disaster nursing at increasing levels of complexity, among eight domains. The revised framework has been included in the Resources section at the end of this chapter.

CASE STUDY

Pepper Spray

Profile

It is 1636 hours on a Thursday in the month of May, in the emergency department of a downtown hospital in a major Canadian city. It has been an extremely busy day, and the triage nurse is working with the corridors fully occupied by patients, many of whom have been waiting a day or longer for inpatient beds. Several ambulances are waiting to off-load their patients from stretchers. The nurse receives a call from emergency medical services informing of the need to be prepared for the potential arrival of patients from a nearby protest rally. The nurse is told that the protesters breached the security fences and the police intervened by using significant amounts of pepper spray. On-site first responders (emergency medical services) have conducted some decontamination on site; however, many of the protesters fled on foot before decontamination.

Subjective Data

- Patients arrive within 6 minutes, with the following complaints:
  - Eye burning; some patients have temporary blindness
  - "Skin is burning"

Objective Data

- High levels of panic and anxiety
- Runny nose and watery eyes
- Severe coughing; some patients with shortness of breath

Interprofessional Care

- Decontamination shower and scrubbing are ordered before any medical intervention.

Discussion Questions

1. What risk factors do patients who require decontamination pose to an emergency department?
2. **Priority decision:** Identify priority actions the nurse will need to take in order to prepare for potential patient arrival.
3. Who should the nurse inform regarding the potential arrival of these patients?
4. What actions must be taken to manage patients who have been contaminated?
5. What equipment might be needed to care for contaminated patients?
6. **Priority decision:** What are the primary concerns of a triage nurse in this situation?
7. What information will the nurse need to obtain from contaminated patients?
8. What actions should the nurse take to ensure the safety of staff and patients currently in the emergency department?

evolve

Answers are available at http://evolve.elsevier.com/Canada/Lewis/medsurg.

REVIEW QUESTIONS

The number of the question corresponds to the same-numbered objective at the beginning of the chapter.

1. A chemical spill has occurred at a nearby industrial site. The first responders report that approximately 20 people have been affected and that they need to be transported to the emergency department after decontamination at the site. What is this scenario an example of?
   a. An emergency
   b. A natural disaster or hazard
   c. A human-made disaster
   d. An emergency response plan

2. Individuals and families must assume responsibility for taking appropriate steps to ensure they have the basics of what might be required following an emergency or disaster. Which list of items should be included in an individual emergency preparedness kit?
   a. Batteries, fresh fruits and vegetables, cups and plates
   b. Canned soups and stews, can opener, 2 L of water per day per person
   c. Fresh bread, frozen vegetables, lighter or matches
   d. 1 L of water per day per person, utensils, blankets, and sleeping bags

3. Which of the following statements *best* describes disaster nursing?
   a. Provision of nursing care, advocacy, and health promotion
   b. Provision of medical care and teaching
   c. Development and review of emergency operations plan and policy
   d. Provision of nursing care and coordination of health care interventions

4. Which of the following is a component of a comprehensive emergency response plan?
   a. Closure guidelines
   b. Safety and security strategies
   c. Pandemic plan
   d. Ethical directives

5. Which activity is correlated with the recovery phase?
   a. Development of an emergency plan
   b. Conducting emergency exercises and drills
   c. Conducting critical incident debriefing with responders
   d. Completing construction to build a flood-resistant emergency department

6. Which of the following statements best describes the incident command system (ICS)?
   a. ICS is an administrative structure that can be used in large-scale emergency situations.
   b. ICS involves a circular organizational structure where all participants are interlinked.
   c. ICS involves a modular organizational structure that can be used in small- and large-scale situations.
   d. ICS may be activated only by municipal or federal agencies.

7. Which of the following statements related to disaster triage in hospitals is correct?
   a. Hospital and emergency department disaster triage is conducted by first responders.
   b. The Canadian Triage and Acuity Scale was specifically designed for disaster triage.
   c. Disaster triage should be done in 2 minutes or less according to the START or JumpSTART algorithm.
   d. Disaster triage involves a triage team composed of one to two nurses, a physician or nurse practitioner, a porter, and a registration clerk.

8. A nurse is assisting first responders during a mass casualty incident involving a bus rollover in an isolated rural community. Using the colour triage codes outlined in the START algorithm, place the following casualties in order of highest to lowest priority:
   a. A 38-year-old female who is obese and dyspneic and has an upper thigh deformity
   b. A 40-year-old male, minimally responsive, with shallow respirations, bleeding from the mouth
   c. An older adult female, unresponsive, with a large scalp wound and a large amount of blood noted
   d. A 14-year-old female, screaming, with lower back pain
   e. A 10-year-old male, crying, with bloody gauze to the forehead

9. Which of the following is an example of a human-made disaster?
   a. A terrorist attack
   b. A pandemic
   c. A hurricane
   d. A severe ice storm

10. Which of the following biological agents of bioterrorism has no effective treatment?
    a. Anthrax
    b. Botulism
    c. Smallpox
    d. Hemorrhagic fever

11. Which of the following situations is an example of a chemical-biological-radiological-nuclear-explosive (CBRNE) event?
    a. Dissemination of anthrax spores to a department in an office building
    b. A train derailment
    c. An outbreak of seasonal influenza
    d. Forest fires

12. Which of the following examples meets the criteria for a pandemic?
    a. A cluster of clients on an inpatient unit with diarrhea
    b. Acquired immune deficiency syndrome (AIDS)
    c. A school that has been closed as a result of flulike symptoms in children in three classrooms
    d. COVID-19 illnesses globally

1. c; 2. b; 3. a; 4. b; 5. c; 6. c; 7. d; 8. b, c, a, e, d; 9. a; 10. d; 11. a; 12. d.

⊜volve

For even more review questions, visit http://evolve.elsevier.com/Canada/Lewis/medsurg.

REFERENCES

Andress, K. (2010). Healthcare facility preparedness. In R. Powers, & E. Daly (Eds.), *International disaster nursing*. Cambridge University Press. (Seminal).

Bazyar, J., Farrokhi, M., & Khankeh, H. (2019). Triage systems in mass casualty incidents and disasters: a review study with a worldwide approach. *Macedonian Journal of Medical Sciences, 7*(3), 482–494. https://doi.org/10.3889/oamjms.2019.119

British Columbia Centre for Disease Control. (2021). *Contact tracing.* http://www.bccdc.ca/health-info/diseases-conditions/covid-19/self-isolation/contact-tracing

Canadian Association of Emergency Physicians. (2017). *CTAS: Implementation guidelines.* http://ctas-phctas.ca/?page_id=294

Canadian Centre for Occupational Health and Safety (CCOHS). (2020). *Severe acute respiratory syndrome (SARS).* https://www.ccohs.ca/oshanswers/diseases/sars.html

Canadian Nurses Association (CNA). (2017). *Code of ethics for registered nurses.* https://www.cna-aiic.ca/html/en/Code-of-Ethics-2017-Edition/files/assets/basic-html/page-1.html#

Canadian Nurses Association (CNA). (2018). *Position statement: Emergency preparedness and response.* https://hl-prod-ca-oc-download.s3-ca-central-1.amazonaws.com/CNA/2f975e7e-4a40-45ca-863c-5ebf0a138d5e/UploadedImages/documents/Emergency_Preparedness_and_Response_position_statement_Dec_2018.pdf

Canadian Red Cross. (2021). *Get an emergency kit.* https://www.redcross.ca/how-we-help/emergencies-and-disasters-in-canada/be-ready-emergency-preparedness-and-recovery/get-an-emergency-kit

Carlson, S., Coyne-Plum, K. C., & Meeker, E. C. (2019). Understanding the psychosocial impact of disasters. In T. G. Veenema (Ed.), *Disaster nursing and emergency preparedness for chemical, biological, and radiological terrorism and other hazards* (4th ed.). Springer.

Carlson, S., Meeker, E. C., Coyne-Plum, K., et al. (2019). Management of the psychosocial effects of disasters. In T. G. Veenema (Ed.), *Disaster nursing and emergency preparedness for chemical, biological, and radiological terrorism and other hazards* (4th ed.). Springer.

Centers for Disease Control and Prevention (CDC). (2018). *Frequently asked questions (FAQs) about dirty bombs.* https://emergency.cdc.gov/radiation/dirtybombs.asp

Croddy, E., & Ackerman, G. (2019). Biological and chemical terrorism: A unique threat. In T. G. Veenema (Ed.), *Disaster nursing and emergency preparedness for chemical, biological, and radiological terrorism and other hazards* (4th ed.). Springer.

Furin, M. A. (2018). *Disaster planning: Categorizing disasters.* https://emedicine.medscape.com/article/765495-overview#a2

Gebbie, K. M., & Qureshi, K. (2019). Disaster management. In T. G. Veenema (Ed.), *Disaster nursing and emergency preparedness for chemical, biological, and radiological terrorism and other hazards* (4th ed.). Springer.

Gilboy, N. (2019). Triage. In V. Sweet, & A. Foley (Eds.), *Sheehy's emergency nursing: Principals and practice* (7th ed.). Mosby. (Seminal).

Government of Canada. (2013). *Building resilience against terrorism. Canada's counter-terrorism strategy.* https://www.publicsafety.gc.ca/cnt/rsrcs/pblctns/rslnc-gnst-trrrsm/rslnc-gnst-trrrsm-eng.pdf

Government of Canada. (2020). *The Disaster Assistance Response Team (DART).* https://www.canada.ca/en/department-national-defence/services/operations/military-operations/types/dart.html

Government of Canada. (2021a). *Animals and COVID-19.* https://www.canada.ca/en/public-health/services/diseases/2019-novel-coronavirus-infection/prevention-risks/animals-covid-19.html

Government of Canada. (2021b). *Get prepared: Your emergency preparedness guide.* http://www.getprepared.gc.ca/cnt/rsrcs/pblctns/yprprdnssgd/index-en.aspx

Holland, M. G., & Cawthon, D. (2015). Personal protective equipment and decontamination of adults and children. *Emergency Medicine Clinics of North America, 33*(1), 51–68. https://doi.org/10.1016/j.emc.2014.09.006

Incident Command System (ICS) Canada. (2019). *ICS Canada curriculum and training standards.* http://www.icscanada.ca/images/upload/docs/ICS%20Canada%202019v1.2.pdf

Indigenous and Northern Affairs Canada. (2017). *Indigenous and Northern Affairs Canada (INAC) national on-reserve emergency management plan.* https://www.sac-isc.gc.ca/DAM/DAM-ISC-SAC/DAM-EMPL/STAGING/texte-text/emergency_plan_1496943857348_eng.pdf

Intermountain Healthcare. (2020). *What's the difference between a pandemic, an epidemic, an endemic and an outbreak?.* https://intermountainhealthcare.org/blogs/topics/live-well/2020/04/whats-the-difference-between-a-pandemic-an-epidemic-endemic-and-an-outbreak/

International Council of Nurses (ICN). (2019a). *Core competencies in disaster nursing version 2.0.* https://www.icn.ch/sites/default/files/inline-files/ICN_Disaster-Comp-Report_WEB.pdf

International Council of Nurses (ICN). (2019b). *Position statement: Nurses and disaster risk reduction, response and recovery.* https://www.icn.ch/sites/default/files/inline-files/PS_E_Nurses_and_disaster_risk_reduction_response_and_recovery.pdf

Karam, A. (2019). Radiological incidents and emergencies. In T. G. Veenema (Ed.), *Disaster nursing and emergency preparedness for chemical, biological, and radiological terrorism and other hazards* (4th ed.). Springer.

Koenig, K. L., Boatright, C. J., Hancock, J. A., et al. (2008). Health care facility–based decontamination of victims exposed to chemical, biological and radiological materials. *American Journal of Emergency Medicine, 26*(1), 71–80. (Seminal). https://doi.org/10.1016/j.ajem.2007.07.004

Markenson, D., & Losinski, S. (2019). Hospital and emergency department preparedness. In T. G. Veenema (Ed.), *Disaster nursing and emergency preparedness for chemical, biological, and radiological terrorism and other hazards* (4th ed.). Springer.

Mattei, A., Fiasca, F., Mazzei, M., et al. (2017). Stress and burnout in health-care workers after the 2009 L'Aquila earthquake: A cross-sectional observational study. *Frontiers in Psychiatry, 8*, 98. https://doi.org/10.3389/fpsyt.2017.00098

McMahon, M. M. (2010). Hospital impact: Emergency department. In R. Powers, & E. Daly (Eds.), *International disaster nursing.* Cambridge University Press. (Seminal).

Moore, B. L., Geller, R. J., & Clark, C. (2015). Hospital preparedness for chemical and radiological disasters. *Emergency Medicine Clinics of North America, 33*(1), 37–49. https://doi.org/10.1016/j.emc.2014.09.005

National Collaborating Centre for Environmental Health. (n.d.). *Indigenous disaster response.* https://ncceh.ca/environmental-health-in-canada/health-agency-projects/indigenous-disaster-response

Ponampalam, R. (2019). A novel hospital-based mass casualty decontamination facility for hazardous material disasters. *Toxicology and Forensic Medicine, 4*(1), 18–23. https://doi.org/10.17140/TFMOJ-4-129

Public Health Agency of Canada (PHAC). (2011). *Self-care for caregivers.* https://www.canada.ca/en/public-health/services/reports-publications/responding-stressful-events/self-care-caregivers.html

Public Health Agency of Canada (PHAC). (2016). *Infectious diseases.* https://www.canada.ca/en/public-health/services/infectious-diseases.html

Public Health Agency of Canada (PHAC). (2020). Update. Coronavirus disease (COVID-19). *Canadian Communicable Disease Report, 46*(4), 98. https://www.canada.ca/content/dam/phac-aspc/documents/services/reports-publications/canada-communicable-disease-report-ccdr/monthly-issue/2020-46/issue-4-april-2-2020/ccdrv46i04-eng.pdf

Public Safety Canada (PSC). (2017). *An emergency management framework for Canada: Ministers responsible for emergency management* (3rd ed.). https://www.publicsafety.gc.ca/cnt/rsrcs/pblctns/2017-mrgnc-mngmnt-frmwrk/index-en.aspx

Public Safety Canada (PSC). (2018). Canada's national disaster mitigation strategy. http://www.publicsafety.gc.ca/cnt/rsrcs/pblctns/mtgtn-strtgy/index-eng.aspx

Public Safety Canada (PSC). (2019a). *Emergency management planning.* https://www.publicsafety.gc.ca/cnt/mrgnc-mngmnt/mrgnc-prprdnss/mrgnc-mngmnt-plnnng-en.aspx

Public Safety Canada (PSC). (2019b). *The Canadian disaster database.* https://www.publicsafety.gc.ca/cnt/rsrcs/cndn-dsstr-dtbs/index-en.aspx

Public Safety Canada (PSC). (2020). Critical infrastructure partners. https://www.publicsafety.gc.ca/cnt/ntnl-scrt/crtcl-nfrstrctr/crtcl-nfrstrtr-prtnrs-en.aspx

Public Safety Canada (PSC). (2021). *Emergency management.* https://www.publicsafety.gc.ca/cnt/mrgnc-mngmnt/index-en.aspx

Puett, L. (2019). Management of burn mass casualty incidents. In T. G. Veenema (Ed.), *Disaster nursing and emergency preparedness for chemical, biological, and radiological terrorism and other hazards* (4th ed.). Springer.

Rihl-Pryor, E. (2019). Surveillance systems for detection of biological events. In T. G. Veenema (Ed.), *Disaster nursing and emergency preparedness for chemical, biological, and radiological terrorism and other hazards* (4th ed.). Springer.

Romig, L., & Lerner, B. (2019). Disaster triage. In T. G. Veenema (Ed.), *Disaster nursing and emergency preparedness for chemical, biological, and radiological terrorism and other hazards* (4th ed.). Springer.

Sacco, T. L. (2019). Traumatic injury due to explosives and blast effects. In T. G. Veenema (Ed.), *Disaster nursing and emergency preparedness for chemical, biological, and radiological terrorism and other hazards* (4th ed.). Springer.

Slepski, L. A. (2010). Pandemic planning. In R. Powers, & E. Daly (Eds.), *International disaster nursing.* Cambridge University Press. (Seminal).

Stanhope, M., Lancaster, J., Jakubec, S. L., et al. (2017). *Community health nursing in Canada* (3rd ed.). Elsevier.

U.S. Department of Health and Human Services: Radiation Emergency Medical Management (USDHHS-REMM). (2021a). *JumpSTART pediatric triage algorithm.* https://remm.hhs.gov/startpediatric.htm

U.S. Department of Health and Human Services: Radiation Emergency Medical Management (USDHHS-REMM). (2021b). *START adult triage algorithm.* https://remm.hhs.gov/startadult.htm

VandenBerg, S., & Davidson, S. (2015). Preparation for mass casualty incidents. *Critical Care Nursing Clinics of North America, 27*(2), 157–166. https://doi.org/10.1016/j.cnc.2015.02.008

Veenema, T. G. (2019a). Decontamination and personal protective equipment. In T. G. Veenema (Ed.), *Disaster nursing and emergency preparedness for chemical, biological, and radiological terrorism and other hazards* (4th ed.). Springer.

Veenema, T. G. (2019b). Essentials of disaster planning. In T. G. Veenema (Ed.), *Disaster nursing and emergency preparedness for chemical, biological, and radiological terrorism and other hazards* (4th ed.). Springer.

Veenema, T. G., Arbon, P., & Hutton, A. (2019). Emergency medical consequence planning for special events, mass gatherings, and mass casualty incidents. In T. G. Veenema (Ed.), *Disaster nursing and emergency preparedness for chemical, biological, and radiological terrorism and other hazards* (4th ed.). Springer.

Veenema, T. G., Corley, A., & Thornton, C. P. (2019). Natural disasters. In T. G. Veenema (Ed.), *Disaster nursing and emergency preparedness for chemical, biological, and radiological terrorism and other hazards* (4th ed.). Springer.

Veenema, T. G., Losinski, S., Newton, S., et al. (2017). Exploration and development of standardized nursing leadership competencies during disasters. *Health Emergency and Disaster Nursing, 4*, 26–38. https://doi.org/10.24298/hedn.2015-0016

Wagner, J. M., Dahnke, M. D., & Pomona, N. J. (2015). Nursing ethics and disaster triage: Applying utilitarian ethical theory. *Journal of Emergency Nursing, 41*(4), 300–306. https://doi.org/10.1016/j.jen.2014.11.001

Weber, B. (2018, October 30). First Nations left out of Fort McMurray fire response, Indigenous-led report says. *Globe and Mail.* https://www.theglobeandmail.com/canada/article-first-nations-left-out-of-mcmurray-fire-response-indigenous-led/

Workeye, H., Sandy Lake First Nation, McGee, T. K., et al. (2018). Evacuation preparedness and the challenges of emergency evacuation in Indigenous communities in Canada: The case of Sandy Lake First Nation, Northern Ontario. *International Journal of Disaster Risk Reduction, 34*, 55–56. https://doi.org/10.1016/j.ijdrr.2018.11.005

World Health Organization (WHO). (2011). *Hospital emergency response checklist. An all-hazards tool for hospital administrators and emergency managers.* https://www.who.int/docs/default-source/documents/publications/hospital-emergency-response-checklist.pdf

World Health Organization (WHO). (2019). *Zika epidemiology update.* https://www.who.int/news/item/02-07-2019-zika-epidemiology-update

World Health Organization (WHO). (2020a). *Environmental health in emergencies. Vulnerable groups.* https://www.who.int/environmental_health_emergencies/vulnerable_groups/en/

World Health Organization (WHO). (2020b). *HIV/AIDS data and statistics.* https://www.who.int/hiv/data/en/

RESOURCES

Canadian Pandemic Influenza Preparedness: Planning Guidance for the Health Sector
https://www.phac-aspc.gc.ca/cpip-pclcpi/

Canadian Red Cross
https://www.redcross.ca/

Canadian Virtual Hospice—*COVID-19 Resources*
https://www.virtualhospice.ca/covid19/

COVID-19 Resources Canada
https://covid19resources.ca/

Government of Canada—*Coronavirus Disease (COVID-19)*
https://www.canada.ca/en/public-health/services/diseases/coronavirus-disease-covid-19.html

Government of Canada—*Emergency Management Organizations*
https://www.getprepared.gc.ca/cnt/rsrcs/mrgnc-mgmt-rgnztns-eng.aspx

Government of Canada—*Get Prepared*
https://www.getprepared.gc.ca/index-en.aspx

Infection and Prevention Control Canada—*Coronavirus (COVID-19) SARS-CoV-2*
https://ipac-canada.org/coronavirus-resources.php

International Council of Nurses—*Core Competencies in Disaster Nursing Version 2.0*
https://www.icn.ch/sites/default/files/inline-files/ICN_Disaster-Comp-Report_WEB.pdf

International Council of Nurses—*Position Statement: Nurses and Disaster Risk Reduction, Response and Recovery*
https://www.icn.ch/sites/default/files/inline-files/PS_E_Nurses_and_disaster_risk_reduction_response_and_recovery.pdf

Mental Health Commission of Canada—*Mental Health and Wellness During the COVID-19 Pandemic*
https://www.mentalhealthcommission.ca/English/mhcc-covid-19-resources

Ontario Ministry of Health and Long-Term Care— *Ontario Health Plan for an Influenza Pandemic 2013*
https://www.health.gov.on.ca/en/pro/programs/emb/pan_flu/pan_flu_plan.aspx

Public Health Agency of Canada
https://www.phac-aspc.gc.ca/index-eng.php

Public Health Agency of Canada—*Chemical, Biological, Radiological and Nuclear Resource Links*
https://www.phac-aspc.gc.ca/cepr-cmiu/ophs-bssp/links_index-eng.php

Public Safety Canada
https://www.publicsafety.gc.ca

Salvation Army of Canada
https://www.salvationarmy.ca

St. John Ambulance Canada
https://www.sja.ca/

Centers for Disease Control and Prevention (CDC)
https://www.cdc.gov/

Federal Emergency Management Agency (FEMA)
https://www.fema.gov/

World Health Organization
https://www.who.int/en/

evolve

For additional Internet resources, see the website for this book at http://evolve.elsevier.com/Canada/Lewis/medsurg.

Laboratory Values

Sarah Ibrahim, RN, MN, PhD, CHSE

The tables in this appendix list some of the most common tests, their normal values, and possible etiologies of abnormal values. Laboratory values are expressed in the Système International d'Unités (SI) units, which are used in Canada. Conventional units, used in the United States, are presented after the SI units in parentheses. Laboratory values may vary with different techniques and in different laboratories. Possible etiologies are presented in alphabetical order. SI abbreviations and other symbols appearing in the tables are defined as follows:

<	=	less than
>	=	greater than
≥	=	greater than or equal to
≤	=	less than or equal to
AU	=	arbitrary unit
cm H₂O	=	centimetres of water
dL	=	decilitre
EU	=	Ehrlich unit
fL	=	femtolitre
g	=	gram
IU	=	international unit
kPa	=	kilopascal
k	=	kilo
L	=	litre
mcg	=	microgram (one millionth [10^{-6}] of a gram)
mcIU	=	micro–international unit (one millionth [10^{-6}] of an international unit)

mcL	=	microlitre
mcmol	=	micromole
mEq	=	milliequivalent
mg	=	milligram (one thousandth [10^{-3}] of a gram)
McU	=	microunit
mL	=	millilitre
mm	=	millimetre
mm Hg	=	millimetre of mercury
mmol	=	millimole
mOsm	=	milliosmole
mU	=	milliunit (one hundredth [10^{-2}] of a unit)
nmol	=	nanomole (one billionth [10^{-9}] of a mole)
ng	=	nanogram (one billionth [10^{-9}] of a gram)
pg	=	picogram (one trillionth [10^{-12}] of a gram)
pmol	=	picomole (one trillionth [10^{-12}] of a mole)
U	=	unit

TABLE A.1 SERUM, PLASMA, AND WHOLE BLOOD CHEMISTRIES

Test	Normal Values (SI Units [Conventional Units])	Possible Etiology Higher Values	Possible Etiology Lower Values
Acetone • Quantitative • Qualitative	 <200 mcmol/L (<1.16 mg/dL) Negative (negative)	Diabetic ketoacidosis, high-fat diet, low-carbohydrate diet, starvation	—
Alanine aminotransferase (ALT; formerly known as serum glutamate pyruvate transferase [SGPT])	5–35 U/L (same as in SI units)	Liver disease, shock	—
Albumin	35–55 g/L (3.5–5.5 g/dL)	Dehydration	Malnutrition, pregnancy, liver disease, protein-losing enteropathies, protein-losing nephropathies, third-space losses, inflammatory disease, familial idiopathic dysproteinemia
Aldolase	<8.0 mU/L (3–8.2 Sibley-Lehninger U/dL)	Muscular disease, muscular dystrophy, dermatomyositis, polymyositis, muscle injury, muscular trauma, gangrenous/ischemic processes, hepatocellular disease, hepatitis, cirrhosis, MI, infection	Hereditary fructose intolerance, late muscular dystrophy, muscle wasting diseases, renal disease
α₁-Antitrypsin	0.85–2.13 g/L (85–213 mg/dL)	Acute and chronic inflammatory disorders, infections (i.e., thyroid infections), malignancy, stress	Chronic lung disease (early onset of emphysema), neonatal respiratory distress syndrome, cirrhosis (in children), end-stage cancer, malnutrition, nephrotic syndrome, protein-losing enteropathy, hepatic failure

Continued

TABLE A.1	**SERUM, PLASMA, AND WHOLE BLOOD CHEMISTRIES—cont'd**		
	Normal Values (SI Units [Conventional Units])	**Possible Etiology**	
Test		**Higher Values**	**Lower Values**
α-Fetoprotein	0–40 mcg/L (<40 ng/mL)	Cancers of testes, lymphoma, stomach, colon, breasts and ovaries; liver cell necrosis (i.e., cirrhosis, hepatitis); carcinoma of liver; fetal death; fetal distress or congenital abnormalities; neural tube defects (i.e., anencephaly, spina bifida) or multiple pregnancies in pregnant women	In pregnant women, fetal trisomy 21 (Down syndrome) or fetal wastage
Ammonia	6–47 mcmol/L (10–80 mcg/dL)	GI bleeding and obstruction with mild liver disease, genetic metabolic disorder of urea cycle, hemolytic disease of newborn, hepatic encephalopathy and hepatic coma, portal hypertension, Reye syndrome, primary hepatocellular disease, asparagine intoxication, severe heart failure or congestive hepatomegaly	Essential or malignant hypertension, hyperornithinemia
Amylase	25–125 U/L	Acute and chronic pancreatitis, GI disease, acute cholecystitis, mumps (salivary gland disease), perforated ulcers, ruptured ectopic pregnancy, renal failure, diabetic ketoacidosis, pulmonary infarction	Acute alcoholism, cirrhosis of liver, extensive destruction of pancreas
Aspartate aminotransferase (AST) (formerly known as serum glutamic oxaloacetic transferase [SGOT])	0–35 U/L (same as SI units)	Acute hepatitis, liver disease, MI, skeletal muscle disease, acute hemolytic anemia, acute pancreatitis	Acute renal disease, chronic renal dialysis, diabetic ketoacidosis, beriberi, pregnancy
B-type (brain-type) natriuretic peptide	<100 mcg/L (<100 ng/mL)	Cor pulmonale, heart failure, heart transplant rejection, hypertension, MI	—
Bicarbonate	23–29 mmol/L (23–29 mEq/L)	Use of mercurial diuretics, aldosteronism, compensated respiratory acidosis, metabolic alkalosis	Acute kidney injury, compensated respiratory alkalosis, diarrhea, metabolic acidosis, starvation, chronic use of loop diuretics
Bilirubin • Total • Indirect • Direct	3–22 mcmol/L (0.2–1.3 mg/dL) 3.4–12 mcmol/L (0.2–0.8 mg/dL) 1.7–5.1 mcmol/L (0.1–0.3 mg/dL)	**Direct Bilirubin:** Gallstones, extrahepatic duct obstruction (tumour, inflammation, gallstone, scarring, surgical trauma), extensive liver metastasis, cholestasis from medications, Dubin-Johnson syndrome, Rotor syndrome **Indirect Bilirubin:** Erythroblastosis fetalis, transfusion reaction, sickle cell anemia, hemolytic jaundice, hemolytic anemia, pernicious anemia, large-volume blood transfusion, resolution of large hematoma, hepatitis, cirrhosis, sepsis, neonatal hyperbilirubinemia, Crigler-Najjar syndrome, Gilbert syndrome **Increased Urine Levels of Bilirubin:** Gallstones, extrahepatic duct obstruction (tumour, inflammation, gallstone, scarring, surgical trauma), extensive liver metastasis, cholestasis from medications, Dubin-Johnson syndrome, Rotor syndrome	—
Blood gases* • Arterial pH • Venous pH • Partial pressure of carbon dioxide in arterial blood ($PaCO_2$) • Partial pressure of oxygen in arterial blood (PaO_2) • Partial pressure of oxygen in venous blood (PvO_2)	7.35–7.45 (same as SI units) 7.35–7.45 (same as SI units) 35–45 mm Hg (same as SI units) 80–100 mm Hg (same as SI units) 40–50 mm Hg (same as SI units)	Alkalosis Alkalosis Compensated metabolic alkalosis, respiratory acidosis Administration of high concentration of oxygen	Acidosis Acidosis Compensated metabolic acidosis, respiratory alkalosis Chronic lung disease, decreased cardiac output
Calcium	Adult: 2.10–2.750 mmol/L (8.4–10.6 mg/dL) Total calcium: <1.65 mmol/L or >3.25 mmol/L (13 mg/dL)	Hyperparathyroidism, nonparathyroid PTH-producing tumour (e.g., lung or renal carcinoma), Metastatic tumour to bone, Paget's disease of bone, prolonged immobilization, milk-alkali syndrome, vitamin D intoxication, lymphoma, granulomatous infections such as sarcoidosis and tuberculosis, Addison's disease, acromegaly, hyperthyroidism	Hypoparathyroidism, renal failure, hyperphosphatemia secondary to renal failure, rickets, vitamin D deficiency, osteomalacia, hypoalbuminemia, malabsorption, pancreatitis, fat embolism, alkalosis

TABLE A.1 SERUM, PLASMA, AND WHOLE BLOOD CHEMISTRIES—cont'd

Test	Normal Values (SI Units [Conventional Units])	Possible Etiology	
		Higher Values	**Lower Values**
Calcium, ionized	Adult: 1.15–1.35 mmol/L (4.6–5.1 mg/dL) Ionized calcium: <0.80 mmol/L or >1.58 mmol/L (7 mg/dL)	—	—
Carbon dioxide (CO_2 content)	21–28 mmol/L (21–28 mEq/L)	COPD, metabolic alkalosis, severe vomiting, high-volume gastric suction, use of mercurial diuretics	Chronic use of loop diuretics, DKA, metabolic acidosis, renal failure, shock, starvation
Chloride	98–106 mmol/L (98–106 mEq/L)	Dehydration, excessive infusion of normal saline solution, metabolic acidosis, renal tubular acidosis, Cushing's syndrome, kidney dysfunction, hyperparathyroidism, eclampsia, respiratory alkalosis	Overhydration, SIADH, heart failure, vomiting or prolonged gastric suction, chronic diarrhea or high-output GI fistula, chronic respiratory acidosis, metabolic alkalosis, salt-losing nephritis, Addison's disease, diuretic therapy, hypokalemia, aldosteronism, burns
Cholesterol	<5.2 mmol/L (<200 mg/dL) age dependent	Familial hypercholesterolemia, familial hyperlipidemia, hypothyroidism, uncontrolled diabetes mellitus, nephrotic syndrome, pregnancy, high-cholesterol diet, xanthomatosis, hypertension, MI, atherosclerosis, biliary cirrhosis, extrahepatic biliary, stress, nephrotic syndrome renal disease	Malabsorption, malnutrition, advanced cancer, hyperthyroidism, cholesterol-lowering medication, pernicious anemia, hemolytic anemia, sepsis/stress, liver disease, acute MI
• High-density lipoproteins (HDL)	>0.91 mmol/L (>35 mg/dL)		
• Low-density lipoproteins (LDL)	<3.4 mmol/L (<130 mg/dL)		
Cholinesterase (RBC)	5–10 U/L (same as SI units)	Reticulocytosis, hyperlipidemia, nephrosis, diabetes	Poisoning from organic phosphate insecticides, hepatocellular disease, individuals with congenital enzyme deficiency, malnutrition and other forms of hypoalbuminemia
Copper	11–22 mcmol/L (70–140 mcg/dL)	Cirrhosis, contraceptive use by female patient	Wilson's disease
Cortisol		Adrenal adenoma, Cushing's syndrome, hyperthyroidism, pancreatitis, stress, ectopic ACTH-producing tumours, obesity	Addison's disease, adrenal insufficiency, hypopituitary states, hypothyroidism, liver disease
• 0800 hours	170–635 nmol/L (6–23 mcg/dL)		
• 1600 hours	82-413 nmol/L (3–53 mcg/dL)		
Creatine		Active rheumatoid arthritis, biliary obstruction, hyperthyroidism, renal disease, severe muscle disease	Diabetes mellitus
Creatine kinase (CK)		Diseases or injury affecting the heart muscle, skeletal muscle, and brain	—
• Male	20–215 U/L (same as SI units)		
• Female	20–160 U/L (same as SI units)		
Creatine kinase isozyme of heart (CK-MB [CK-2])		Acute MI, cardiac aneurysm surgery, cardiac defibrillation, myocarditis, ventricular arrhythmias, cardiac ischemia: Any disease or injury to the myocardium causes CK-MB to spill out of the damaged cells and into the bloodstream, producing elevations in CK-MB levels.	—
• Male	20–215 U/L (same as SI units)		
• Female	20–160 U/L (same as SI units)		
Creatine kinase mass fraction	0–6%	—	—
Creatinine		Severe renal disease, rhabdomyolysis, acromegaly, gigantism	Diseases with decreased muscle mass (e.g. muscular dystrophy, myasthenia gravis)
• Male	53–106 mcmol/L (0.6–1.2 mg/dL)		
• Female	44–97 mcmol/L (0.5–1.1 mg/dL)		
Ferritin (serum)		Hemochromatosis, hemosiderosis, megaloblastic anemia, hemolytic anemia, alcoholic/inflammatory hepatocellular disease, inflammatory disease, advanced cancers, chronic illnesses such as leukemias, cirrhosis, chronic hepatitis, or collagen-vascular diseases	Iron-deficiency anemia, severe protein deficiency, hemodialysis
• Male	20–200 mcg/L (20–200 ng/mL)		
• Female	20–150 mcg/L (20–150 ng/mL)		
Folic acid (folate)	11–57 mmol/L (5–25 ng/mL)	Pernicious anemia, vegetarianism, recent massive blood transfusion	Malnutrition, malabsorption syndrome, pregnancy, folic acid deficiency (megaloblastic) anemia, hemolytic anemia, malignancy, liver disease, chronic renal disease
Gamma-glutamyltranspeptidase (GGT)		Liver diseases (e.g., hepatitis, cirrhosis, hepatic necrosis, hepatic tumour or metastasis, hepatotoxic medications, cholestasis, jaundice), MI, alcohol ingestion, pancreatic disease, Epstein–Barr virus	—
• Male	8–38 U/L (same as SI units)		
• Female	5–27 U/L (same as SI units)		
Glucose, fasting	3.9–6.1 mmol/L (70–110 mg/dL)	Diabetes mellitus, acute stress response, Cushing's syndrome, pheochromocytoma, chronic renal failure, glucagonoma, acute pancreatitis, diuretic therapy, corticosteroid therapy, acromegaly	Insulinoma, hypothyroidism, hypopituitarism, Addison's disease, extensive liver disease, insulin overdose, starvation

Continued

TABLE A.1 SERUM, PLASMA, AND WHOLE BLOOD CHEMISTRIES—cont'd

Test	Normal Values (SI Units [Conventional Units])	Possible Etiology Higher Values	Lower Values
Glucose, 2-hr oral glucose tolerance testing (OGTT)		Diabetes mellitus	Hyperinsulinism
• Fasting	4–6 mmol/L (70–110 mg/dL)		
• 1 hr	<11.1 mmol/L (<200 mg/dL)		
• 2 hr	<7.8 mmol/L (<140 mg/dL)		
Haptoglobin	0.5–2.2 g/L (50–220 mg/dL)	Collagen-rheumatic diseases, infection (e.g., pyelonephritis, urinary tract infection, pneumonia), tissue destruction (e.g., MI), nephritis, ulcerative colitis, neoplasia, biliary obstruction	Hemolytic anemia, transfusion reactions, prosthetic heart valves, primary liver disease, hematoma, tissue hemorrhage
Homocysteine		Cardiovascular disease, cerebrovascular disease, cystinuria, folate deficiency, malnutrition, peripheral vascular disease, vitamin B$_6$ or B$_{12}$ deficiency, malnutrition	—
• 0–30 years	4.6–8.1 mcmol/L (same as SI units)		
• 30–59 years			
• Male	6.13–11.2 mcmol/L (same as SI units)		
• Female	4.5–7.9 mcmol/L (same as SI units)		
• >59 years	5.8–11.9 mcmol/L (same as SI units)		
Insulin	43–186 pmol/L (6–26 microU/mL)	Insulinoma, Cushing's syndrome, acromegaly, obesity, fructose or galactose intolerance	Diabetes mellitus, hypopituitarism
Iron		Hemosiderosis or hemochromatosis, iron poisoning, hemolytic anemia, massive blood transfusions, hepatitis or hepatic necrosis, lead toxicity	Insufficient dietary iron, chronic blood loss (irregular menses, uterine cancer, GI cancer, inflammatory bowel disease, diverticulosis, urological tract [hematuria] cancer, hemangioma, arteriovenous malformation), inadequate intestinal absorption of iron, pregnancy (late), iron-deficiency anemia, neoplasia
• Male	13–31 mcmol/L (75–175 mcg/dL)		
• Female	5–29 mcmol/L (28–162 mcg/dL)		
Total iron-binding capacity (TIBC)	45–73 mcmol/L (250–410 mcg/dL)	Estrogen therapy, pregnancy (late), polycythemia vera, iron-deficiency anemia	Malnutrition, hypoproteinemia, inflammatory diseases, cirrhosis, hemolytic anemia, pernicious anemia, sickle cell anemia
Lactic acid (venous blood)	0.6–2.2 mmol/L (5–20 mg/dL)	Shock, tissue ischemia, carbon monoxide poisoning, severe liver disease, genetic errors of metabolism, diabetes mellitus (nonketotic)	
Lactic dehydrogenase (LDH)	45–90 U/L (same as SI units)	MI, pulmonary disease (e.g., embolism, infarction, pneumonia, heart failure), hepatic disease (e.g., hepatitis, active cirrhosis, neoplasm), RBC disease, skeletal muscle disease and injury, renal parenchymal disease, intestinal ischemia and infarction, neoplastic states, testicular tumours (seminoma, dysgerminomas), lymphoma and other reticuloendothelial system (RES) tumours, advanced solid tumour malignancies, pancreatitis, diffuse disease or injury (e.g., heat stroke, collagen disease, shock, hypotension)	—
Lactic dehydrogenase isoenzymes			
• LDH$_1$	0.17–0.27 (17–27%)	MI, pernicious anemia, strenuous exercise	—
• LDH$_2$	0.27–0.37 (27–37%)	Exercise, pulmonary embolus, sickle cell crisis	—
• LDH$_3$	0.18–0.25 (18–25%)	Malignant lymphoma, pulmonary embolus	—
• LDH$_4$	0.03–0.08 (3–8%)	Systemic lupus erythematosus, pancreatitis, pulmonary infarction, renal disease	—
• LDH$_5$	0.0–0.05 (0–5%)	Heart failure, hepatitis, pulmonary embolus and infarction, skeletal muscle damage, strenuous exercise	—
Lipase	0–160 U/L (same as SI units)	Pancreatic diseases, biliary diseases, renal failure, intestinal diseases, salivary gland inflammation or tumour, peptic ulcer disease	—
Magnesium	0.65–1.05 mmol/L (1.2–2.1 mEq/L)	Renal insufficiency, ingestion of magnesium-containing antacids or salts, Addison's disease, hypothyroidism	Chronic alcoholism, hyperparathyroidism, hyperthyroidism, hypoparathyroidism, malnutrition, severe malabsorption, chronic renal tubular disease

TABLE A.1   SERUM, PLASMA, AND WHOLE BLOOD CHEMISTRIES—cont'd

Test	Normal Values (SI Units [Conventional Units])	Possible Etiology — Higher Values	Possible Etiology — Lower Values
Myoglobin	1.0–5.3 nmol/L (<90 ng/mL)	MI, myositis, malignant hyperthermia, muscular dystrophy, skeletal muscle ischemia or trauma, rhabdomyolysis, seizures	Polymyositis
Osmolality	285–295 mmol/kg (280–295 mOsm/kg)	Hypernatremia; hyperglycemia; hyperosmolar nonketotic hyperglycemia; ketosis; azotemia; dehydration; mannitol therapy; ingestion of ethanol, methanol, or ethylene glycol; uremia; diabetes insipidus; renal tubular necrosis; severe pyelonephritis	Overhydration, SIADH secretion, paraneoplastic syndromes associated with carcinoma (lung, breast, colon)
Oxygen saturation • Arterial • Venous	95–100% (same as SI units) 60–80% (same as SI units)	Increased inspired oxygen, polycythemia, hyperventilation	Anemia, mucous plug, bronchospasm, atelectasis, pneumothorax, pulmonary edema, acute respiratory distress syndrome (ARDS), restrictive lung disease, atrial or ventricular cardiac septal defects, emboli, inadequate O_2 in inspired air (suffocation), severe hypoventilation states, such as oversedation or neurological somnolence
pH	*See* Blood gases		
Phenylalanine		Phenylketonuria	—
Phosphatase, acid	<30 ng/mL (<3.0 mcg/L)	Prostatic carcinoma, benign prostatic hypertrophy, prostatitis, multiple myeloma, Paget's disease, hyperparathyroidism, metastasis to the bone, multiple myeloma, sickle cell crisis, thrombocytosis, lysosomal disorders (e.g., Gaucher's disease), renal diseases, liver diseases (such as cirrhosis), rape or sexual intercourse	—
Phosphatase, alkaline (ALP)	40–160 U/L (same as SI units)	Primary cirrhosis, intrahepatic or extrahepatic biliary obstruction, primary or metastatic liver tumour, metastatic tumour to the bone, healing fracture, hyperparathyroidism, osteomalacia, Paget's disease, rheumatoid arthritis, rickets, intestinal ischemia or infarction, MI, sarcoidosis	Hypophosphatemia, hypophosphatasia, malnutrition, milk-alkali syndrome, pernicious anemia, scurvy (vitamin C deficiency)
Phosphorus, phosphate	1.0–1.5 mmol/L (3.0–4.5 mg/dL)†	Hypoparathyroidism, renal failure, increased dietary or IV intake of phosphorus, acromegaly, bone metastasis, sarcoidosis, hypocalcemia, acidosis, rhabdomyolysis, advanced lymphoma or myeloma, hemolytic anemia	Inadequate dietary ingestion of phosphorus, chronic antacid ingestion, hyperparathyroidism, hypercalcemia, chronic alcoholism, vitamin D deficiency (rickets), treatment of hyperglycemia, plasminogen, hyperinsulinism (childhood), malnutrition, alkalosis, Gram-negative sepsis
Potassium	3.5–5.1 mmol/L (3.5–5.1 mEq/L)	Excessive dietary intake, excessive IV intake, acute or chronic renal failure, Addison's disease, hypoaldosteronism, aldosterone-inhibiting diuretics (e.g., spironolactone, triamterene), crush injury to tissues, hemolysis, transfusion of hemolyzed blood, infection, acidosis, dehydration	Deficient dietary intake, deficient IV intake, burns, GI disorders (e.g., diarrhea, vomiting, villous adenomas), diuretics, hyperaldosteronism, Cushing's syndrome, renal tubular acidosis, licorice ingestion, alkalosis, insulin administration, glucose administration, ascites, renal artery stenosis, cystic fibrosis, trauma/surgery/burns
Prostate-specific antigen (PSA)	0–4 mcg/L (0–4 ng/mL)	Benign prostatic hypertrophy, prostate cancer, prostatitis	—
Proteins • Total • Albumin • Globulin	64–83 g/L (6.4–8.3 g/dL) 35–50 g/L (3.5–5 g/dL) 23–34 g/L (2.3–3.4 g/dL)	Burns, cirrhosis (globulin fraction), dehydration	Congenital agammaglobulinemia, increased capillary permeability, inflammatory disease, liver disease, malabsorption, malnutrition
• Albumin/globulin ratio	1.5:1–2.5:1 (same as SI units)	Multiple myeloma (globulin fraction), shock, vomiting	Malnutrition, nephrotic syndrome, proteinuria, renal disease, severe burns
Pseudocholinesterase (serum)	8–18 U/mL (same as SI units)	Reticulocytosis, hyperlipidemia, nephrosis, diabetes	Poisoning from organic phosphate insecticides, hepatocellular disease, individuals with congenital enzyme deficiency, malnutrition and other forms of hypoalbuminemia

Continued

TABLE A.1 SERUM, PLASMA, AND WHOLE BLOOD CHEMISTRIES—cont'd

Test	Normal Values (SI Units [Conventional Units])	Possible Etiology	
		Higher Values	**Lower Values**
Renin		Essential hypertension, malignant hypertension, renovascular hypertension, chronic renal failure, sodium-losing GI disease (vomiting or diarrhea), Addison's disease, renin-producing renal tumour, Bartter syndrome, cirrhosis, hyperkalemia, hemorrhage	Primary hyperaldosteronism, steroid therapy, congenital adrenal hyperplasia
• Upright position, sodium depleted (sodium-restricted diet)	20–39 years: 2.9–24 mcg/L/hr (2.9–24 ng/mL/hr) >40 years: 2.9–10.8 mcg/L/hr (2.9–10.8 ng/mL/hr)		
• Upright position, sodium replaced (normal-sodium diet)	20–39 years: 0.1–4.3 mcg/L/hr (0.1–4.3 ng/mL/hr) >40 years: 0.1–3 mcg/L/hr (0.1–3 ng/mL/hr)		
Sodium	136–145 mmol/L (136–145 mEq/L)	Corticosteroid therapy, dehydration, impaired renal function, increased dietary or IV intake, primary aldosteronism	Addison's disease, decreased dietary or IV intake, diabetic ketoacidosis, diuretic therapy, excessive loss from GI tract, excessive perspiration, water intoxication
Testosterone		Idiopathic sexual precocity, pinealoma, encephalitis, congenital adrenal hyperplasia, adrenocortical tumour, testicular or extragonadal tumour, hyperthyroidism, testosterone resistance syndromes	Klinefelter's syndrome, cryptorchidism, primary and secondary hypogonadism, trisomy 21, orchiectomy, hepatic cirrhosis
• Male	9.5–30 nmol/L (275–875 ng/dL)		
• Female	0.8–2.6 nmol/L (23–875 ng/dL)	Ovarian tumour, adrenal tumour, congenital adrenocortical hyperplasia, trophoblastic tumour, polycystic ovaries, idiopathic hirsutism	—
Thyroid-stimulating hormone (TSH)	0.4–4.8 mIU/L (0.4–4.8 mIU/L)	Primary hypothyroidism (thyroid dysfunction), thyroiditis, thyroid agenesis, congenital cretinism, large doses of iodine, radioactive iodine injection, surgical ablation of thyroid, severe and chronic illnesses, pituitary TSH-secreting tumour	Secondary hypothyroidism, hyperthyroidism, suppressive doses of thyroid medication, factitious hyperthyroidism
Thyroxine (T_4), total		Primary hyperthyroid states (e.g., Graves' disease, Plummer disease, toxic thyroid adenoma), acute thyroiditis, familial dysalbuminemic hyperthyroxinemia, factitious hyperthyroidism, struma ovarii TBG increase (e.g., as occurs in pregnancy, hepatitis, congenital hyperproteinemia)	Hypothyroid states (e.g., cretinism, surgical ablation, myxedema), pituitary insufficiency, hypothalamic failure, protein malnutrition and other protein-depleted states (e.g., nephrotic syndrome), iodine insufficiency, nonthyroid illnesses (e.g., renal failure, Cushing's disease, cirrhosis, surgery, advanced cancer)
• Adult male	51–154 nmol/L (4–12 mcg/dL)		
• Adult female	64–154 nmol/L (5–12 mcg/dL)		
• Adult >60 years	64–142 nmol/L (5–11 mcg/dL)		
Thyroxine (T_4), free	13–27 pmol/L (1.0–2.1 ng/dL)	Primary hyperthyroid states (e.g., Graves' disease, Plummer disease, toxic thyroid adenoma), acute thyroiditis, factitious hyperthyroidism, struma ovarii	Hypothyroid states (e.g., cretinism, surgical ablation, myxedema), pituitary insufficiency, hypothalamic failure, iodine insufficiency, nonthyroid illnesses (e.g., renal failure, Cushing's disease, cirrhosis, surgery, advanced cancer)
Triglycerides		Glycogen storage disease (von Gierke disease), familial hypertriglyceridemia, apoprotein C-II deficiency, hyperlipidemias, hypothyroidism, high-carbohydrate diet, poorly controlled diabetes, nephrotic syndrome, chronic renal failure	Hyperthyroidism, malabsorption syndrome, malnutrition, abetalipoproteinemia
• Male	0.45–1.71 mmol/L (40–150 mg/dL)		
• Female	0.40–1.52 mmol/L (35–135 mg/dL)		
Triiodothyronine (T_3)	1.1–2.9 mmol/L (70–190 ng/dL)	Primary hyperthyroid states (e.g., Graves' disease, Plummer disease, toxic thyroid adenoma), acute thyroiditis, factitious hyperthyroidism, struma ovarii, pregnancy, hepatitis, congenital hyperproteinemia	Hypothyroid states (e.g., cretinism, surgical ablation, myxedema), pituitary insufficiency, hypothalamic failure, protein malnutrition and other protein-depleted states (e.g., nephrotic syndrome), iodine insufficiency, nonthyroid illnesses (e.g., renal failure, Cushing's disease, cirrhosis, surgery, advanced cancer), hepatic diseases
Triiodothyronine (T_3) uptake	24–34 AU (24–34%)	Hyperthyroidism, hypoproteinemia (e.g., protein malnutrition, protein-losing enteropathy, nephropathy), familial dysalbuminemic hyperthyroxinemia, nonthyroid conditions (e.g., renal failure, Cushing's disease, cirrhosis, surgery, advanced cancer), factitious hyperthyroidism, struma ovarii	Hypothyroid states (e.g., cretinism, surgical ablation, pituitary insufficiency, hypothalamic failure, myxedema), hepatitis and cirrhosis, pregnancy, congenital hyperproteinemia
Troponin T (cTnT)	<0.1 mcg/L (<0.1 ng/mL)	Cardiac muscle damage (resulting from MI, myocarditis, or pericarditis), chronic renal failure, multiorgan failure, severe heart failure	—
Troponin I (cTnI)	<0.35 mcg/L (<0.35 ng/mL)		—

TABLE A.1 SERUM, PLASMA, AND WHOLE BLOOD CHEMISTRIES—cont'd

Test	Normal Values (SI Units [Conventional Units])	Possible Etiology	
		Higher Values	**Lower Values**
Urea nitrogen, blood (blood urea nitrogen [BUN], serum urea nitrogen)	2.9–8.2 mmol/L (8–23 mg/dL)	Prerenal causes, hypovolemia, shock, burns, dehydration, heart failure, MI, GI bleeding, excessive protein ingestion (alimentary tube feeding), excessive protein catabolism, starvation, sepsis, renal disease (e.g., glomerulonephritis, pyelonephritis, acute tubular necrosis), renal failure, nephrotoxic medications, ureteral obstruction from stones, tumour, or congenital anomalies, bladder outlet obstruction from prostatic hypertrophy or cancer or bladder/urethral congenital anomalies, postrenal azotemia	Liver failure, overhydration because of fluid overload in the SIADH secretion, negative nitrogen balance (e.g., malnutrition, malabsorption), pregnancy, nephrotic syndrome
Uric acid • Male • Female	 240–501 mcmol/L (4.0–8.5 mg/dL) 160–430 mcmol/L (2.7–7.3 mg/dL)	Increased ingestion of purines, genetic inborn error in purine metabolism, metastatic cancer, multiple myeloma, leukemias, cancer chemotherapy, hemolysis, rhabdomyolysis (e.g., heavy exercise, burns, crush injury, epileptic seizure, MI)	Wilson disease, Fanconi's syndrome, lead poisoning, yellow atrophy of liver
Vitamin B$_{12}$	118–701 pmol/L (160–950 pg/mL)	Leukemia, polycythemia vera, severe liver dysfunction, myeloproliferative disease	Pernicious anemia, malabsorption syndromes (e.g., inflammatory bowel disease, sprue, Crohn's disease), intestinal worm infestation, atrophic gastritis, Zollinger-Ellison syndrome, large proximal gastrectomy, resection of terminal ileum, achlorhydria, pregnancy, vitamin C deficiency, folic acid deficiency
Zinc protoporphyrin (ZPP)	0–69 mcmol ZPP/mol heme	Lead poisoning, vanadium exposure, iron deficiency, anemia of chronic illness, sickle cell anemia, sideroblastic anemia	—

COPD, chronic obstructive pulmonary disease; *DKA*, diabetic ketoacidosis; *GI*, gastrointestinal; *IV*, intravenous; *MI*, myocardial infarction; *PTH*, parathyroid hormone; *RBC*, red blood cell; *SIADH*, syndrome of inappropriate antidiuretic hormone; *TBG*, thyroxine-binding globulin.
*Because arterial blood gases are influenced by altitude, the values for PaCO$_2$, PaO$_2$, and PvO$_2$ decrease as altitude increases. The lower values are normal for an altitude of 1.6 km (1 mile).
†Values for older persons are significantly lower than those for younger adults.

TABLE A.2 HEMATOLOGY

Test	Normal Values (SI Units [Conventional Units])	Possible Etiology	
		Higher Values	**Lower Values**
Activated coagulation time or automated clotting time (ACT)	70–120 sec (same as SI units)	Heparin administration, clotting factor deficiencies, cirrhosis of the liver, Coumadin administration, lupus inhibitor	Thrombosis
Activated partial thromboplastin time (aPTT)	25–40 sec* (same as SI units)	Congenital clotting factor deficiencies (e.g., von Willebrand's disease, hemophilia, hypofibrinogenemia), cirrhosis of liver, vitamin K deficiency, DIC, heparin administration, Coumarin administration	Early stages of DIC, extensive cancer (e.g., ovarian, pancreatic, colon)
D-dimer	<3.0 nmol/L (<0.4 mcg/mL)	DIC, primary fibrinolysis, during thrombolytic or defibrination therapy, deep vein thrombosis, pulmonary embolism, arterial thromboembolism, sickle cell anemia with or without vaso-occlusive crisis, pregnancy, malignancy, surgery	—
Erythrocyte count† (RBC count [altitude dependent]) • Male • Female	 4.7–6.2 × 10^{12}/L 4.2–5.4 × 10^{12}/L	Erythrocytosis, congenital heart disease, severe COPD, polycythemia vera, severe dehydration (e.g., severe diarrhea or burns), hemoglobinopathies, thalassemia trait	Anemia, hemoglobinopathy, cirrhosis, hemolytic anemia (as in erythroblastosis fetalis, hemoglobinopathies, medication-induced reactions, transfusion reactions, paroxysmal nocturnal hemoglobinuria), hemorrhage, dietary deficiency, bone marrow failure, prosthetic valves, renal disease, normal pregnancy, rheumatoid/collagen-vascular diseases (e.g., rheumatoid arthritis, lupus, sarcoidosis), lymphoma, multiple myeloma, leukemia, Hodgkin's disease

Continued

TABLE A.2   HEMATOLOGY—cont'd

Test	Normal Values (SI Units [Conventional Units])	Possible Etiology	
		Higher Values	**Lower Values**
Erythrocyte sedimentation rate (ESR), Westergren method • Male • Female	 ≤15 mm/hr (same as SI units) ≤20 mm/hr (same as SI units)	*Moderate increase:* Acute hepatitis, MI, rheumatoid arthritis, chronic renal failure (e.g., nephritis, nephrosis), malignant diseases (e.g., multiple myeloma, Hodgkin's disease, advanced carcinomas), bacterial infection, inflammatory diseases, necrotic diseases, diseases associated with increased protein levels, severe anemias (e.g., iron deficiency or vitamin B_{12} deficiency)	Sickle cell disease, spherocytosis, hypofibrinogenemia, polycythemia vera
Fibrin split (degradation) products	<10 mg/L (<10 mcg/mL)	DIC, heart or vascular surgery, thromboembolism, thrombosis, advanced malignancy, severe inflammation, postoperative states, massive trauma, deficiency in protein S and protein C, antithrombin III deficiency	Anticoagulation therapy
Fibrinogen	5.8–11.8 mcmol/L (200–400 mg/dL)	Acute inflammatory reactions (e.g., rheumatoid arthritis, glomerulonephritis), trauma, acute infection such as pneumonia, coronary heart disease, stroke, peripheral vascular disease, cigarette smoking, pregnancy	Liver disease (hepatitis, cirrhosis), DIC, fibrinolysins, congenital afibrinogenemia, advanced carcinoma, malnutrition, large-volume blood transfusion
Hematocrit (altitude dependent)[†] • Male • Female	 0.42–0.52 volume fraction (42–52%) 0.37–0.47 volume fraction (37–47%)	Erythrocytosis, congenital heart disease, polycythemia vera, severe dehydration (e.g., severe diarrhea, burns), severe COPD	Anemia, hemoglobinopathy, cirrhosis, hemolytic anemia, hemorrhage, dietary deficiency, bone marrow failure, prosthetic valves, renal disease, normal pregnancy, rheumatoid/collagen-vascular diseases, lymphoma, multiple myeloma, leukemia, Hodgkin's disease
Hemoglobin (altitude dependent)[†] • Male • Female	 140–180 g/L (14–18 g/dL) 120–160 g/L (12–16 g/dL)	Erythrocytosis, congenital heart disease, polycythemia vera, severe dehydration (e.g., severe diarrhea, burns), severe COPD	Anemia, hemoglobinopathy, cirrhosis, hemolytic anemia, hemorrhage dietary deficiency, bone marrow failure, prosthetic valves, renal disease, normal pregnancy, rheumatoid/collagen-vascular diseases (e.g., rheumatoid arthritis, lupus), lymphoma, multiple myeloma, leukemia, Hodgkin's disease
Hemoglobin, glycosylated or glycated (hemoglobin A_{1c} [HbA_{1c}])	4–5.9% (adult/child without diabetes)	Newly diagnosed diabetes, poorly controlled diabetes, nondiabetic hyperglycemia, patients with splenectomy, pregnancy	Hemolytic anemia, chronic blood loss, chronic renal failure
International normalized ratio (INR)	0.9–1.1	Same as for PT	—
Mean corpuscular hemoglobin (MCH) [Hb/RBC]	27–31 pg (same as SI units)	Macrocytic anemia	Microcytic anemia, hypochromic anemia
Mean corpuscular hemoglobin concentration (MCHC) [Hb/Hct]	27–31 pg (same as SI units)	Spherocytosis, intravascular hemolysis, cold agglutinins	Iron-deficiency anemia, thalassemia
Mean corpuscular volume (MCV) [Hct/RBC]	76–100 fL (76–100 mm³)	Pernicious anemia (vitamin B_{12} deficiency), folic acid deficiency, antimetabolite therapy, alcoholism, chronic liver disease	Iron-deficiency anemia, thalassemia, anemia of chronic illness
Partial thromboplastin time (PTT)	60–70 sec (same as SI units)	Congenital clotting factor deficiencies, cirrhosis of liver, vitamin K deficiency, DIC, heparin administration, Coumarin administration	Early stages of DIC, extensive cancer (e.g., ovarian, pancreatic, colon)
Platelet count (thrombocytes)	150–400 × 10⁹/L (150 000–400 000/mm³)	Malignant disorders (leukemia, lymphoma, solid tumours such as of the colon), polycythemia vera, rheumatoid arthritis, iron-deficiency anemia or following hemorrhagic anemia	Hypersplenism, hemorrhage, immune thrombocytopenia (e.g., idiopathic thrombocytopenia, neonatal, post-transfusion, or medication-induced thrombocytopenia), leukemia and other myelofibrosis disorders, thrombotic thrombocytopenia, Graves' disease, inherited disorders (e.g., Wiskott-Aldrich, Bernard-Soulier, Zieve syndromes), DIC, systemic lupus erythematosus, pernicious anemia, hemolytic anemia, cancer chemotherapy, infection
Prothrombin time (PT; Protime)	11–12.5 sec	Liver disease (e.g., cirrhosis, hepatitis), hereditary factor deficiency, vitamin K deficiency, bile duct obstruction, Coumarin ingestion, DIC, massive blood transfusion, salicylate intoxication	—

TABLE A.2 HEMATOLOGY—cont'd

Test	Normal Values (SI Units [Conventional Units])	Possible Etiology	
		Higher Values	Lower Values
Red cell distribution width (RDW)	11–14.5% (same as SI units)	Iron-deficiency anemia, B_{12} vitamin or folate-deficiency anemia, hemoglobinopathies (e.g., sickle cell disease or protein C disease), hemolytic anemias: fragmentation increases RDW variation, posthemorrhagic anemias	—
Reticulocyte count (manual)	0.5–2% total number of RBCs	Hemolytic anemia (e.g., immune hemolytic anemia, hemoglobinopathies, hypersplenism, trauma from a prosthetic heart valve), hemorrhage (3 to 4 days later), hemolytic disease of the newborn, treatment for deficiency in iron, vitamin B_{12}, or folate	Pernicious anemia and folic acid deficiency, iron-deficiency anemia, aplastic anemia, radiation therapy, malignancy, marrow failure, adrenocortical hypofunction, anterior pituitary hypofunction, chronic diseases
Sickle cell solubility	0%	Sickle cell anemia	
WBC count†	$3.5–12.0 \times 10^9$/L ($3\,500–12\,000$/mm^3)	Infection, leukemic neoplasia or other myeloproliferative disorders, other malignancy, trauma, stress, or hemorrhage, tissue necrosis, inflammation, dehydration, thyroid storm, steroid use	Medication toxicity, bone marrow failure, overwhelming infections, dietary deficiency (e.g., vitamin B_{12} deficiency, iron deficiency), congenital bone marrow aplasia, bone marrow infiltration (e.g., myelofibrosis), autoimmune disease, hypersplenism
WBC differential			
• Band neutrophils	$0–1 \times 10^9$/L (0–9%)	Acute infections	—
• Basophils	$0.01–0.05 \times 10^9$/L (15–50/mm^3; 0.5–1%)	Basophilia, myeloproliferative disease (e.g., myelofibrosis, polycythemia rubra vera), leukemia	Basopenia, acute allergic reactions, hyperthyroidism, stress reactions
• Eosinophils	$0.00–0.25 \times 10^9$/L (50–250/mm^3; 1–4%)	Eosinophilia, parasitic infections, allergic reactions, eczema, leukemia, autoimmune diseases	Eosinopenia, increased adrenosteroid production
• Lymphocytes	$1.5–3.0 \times 10^9$/L ($1\,500–3\,000$/mm^3; 20–40%)	Lymphocytosis, chronic bacterial infection, viral infection (e.g., mumps, rubella), lymphocytic leukemia, multiple myeloma, infectious mononucleosis, radiation, infectious hepatitis	Lymphocytopenia, leukemia, sepsis, immunodeficiency diseases, lupus erythematosus, later stages of human immunodeficiency virus infection, medication therapy: adrenocorticosteroids, antineoplastics; radiation therapy
• Monocytes	$0.3–0.5 \times 10^9$/L (300–500/mm^3; 2–8%)	Monocytosis, chronic inflammatory disorders, viral infections (e.g., infectious mononucleosis), tuberculosis, chronic ulcerative colitis, parasites (e.g., malaria)	Monocytopenia, aplastic anemia, hairy cell leukemia, medication therapy: prednisone
• Neutrophils	$3.0–5.8 \times 10^9$/L (300–5 800/mm^3; 55–70%)	Neutrophilia, physical or emotional stress, acute suppurative infection, myelocytic leukemia, trauma, Cushing's syndrome, inflammatory disorders (e.g., rheumatic fever, thyroiditis, rheumatoid arthritis), metabolic disorders (e.g., ketoacidosis, gout, eclampsia)	Neutropenia, aplastic anemia, dietary deficiency, overwhelming bacterial infection (especially in older persons), viral infections (e.g., hepatitis, influenza, measles), radiation therapy, Addison's disease, medication therapy: myelotoxic agents (as in chemotherapy)

COPD, chronic obstructive pulmonary disease; *DIC*, disseminated intravascular coagulation; *MI*, myocardial infarction; *RBC*, red blood cell; *WBC*, white blood cell.
*For patients receiving anticoagulant therapy, aPTT is 1.5–2.5 times control value in seconds; PT is 1.5–2.0 times control value in seconds.
†Components of complete blood count (CBC).

TABLE A.3 SEROLOGY–IMMUNOLOGY

Test	Normal Values (SI Units [Conventional Units])	Possible Etiology	
		Higher Values	Lower Values
Antinuclear antibody (ANA)	Negative at 1:40 dilution (same as SI units)	SLE, rheumatoid arthritis, periarteritis (polyarteritis) nodosa, dermatomyositis, polymyositis, scleroderma, Sjögren syndrome, Raynaud's phenomenon, other immune diseases, leukemia, infectious mononucleosis, myasthenia gravis, cirrhosis, chronic hepatitis,	—
Anti-DNA antibody	Negative <70 U/mL (same as SI units)	Collagen-vascular diseases, other autoimmune diseases, such as rheumatic fever; chronic hepatitis, infectious mononucleosis, biliary cirrhosis	—
Anti-RNP (ribonucleoprotein)	Negative (negative)	Mixed connective tissue disease (MCTD), SLE, discoid lupus scleroderma	—
Anti-Sm (Smith)	Negative (negative)	SLE	—

Continued

TABLE A.3 SEROLOGY–IMMUNOLOGY—cont'd

| Test | Normal Values (SI Units [Conventional Units]) | Possible Etiology | |
		Higher Values	Lower Values
Anti-streptolysin-O titre (ASO titre)	≤160 Todd units/mL (same as SI units)	Streptococcal infection, acute rheumatic fever, bacterial endocarditis, acute glomerulonephritis, scarlet fever, streptococcal pyoderma	—
C-reactive protein (CRP)	<10 mg/L (<1.0 mg/dL)	Acute, noninfectious inflammatory reaction, collagen-vascular diseases, tissue infarction or damage, bacterial infections such as postoperative wound infection, urinary tract infection, or tuberculosis, malignant disease, bacterial infection, increased risk for cardiovascular ischemic events	—
Carcinoembryonic antigen (CEA)	<5 mcg/L (5 ng/mL)	Cancer (gastrointestinal, breast, lung, pancreatic, hepatobiliary), inflammation (colitis, cholecystitis, pancreatitis, diverticulitis), cirrhosis, Crohn's disease, peptic ulcer	—
Complement assay components • Total • C3 • C4	30–75 kU/L (30–75 U/mL) 0.75–1.75 g/L (75–175 mg/dL) 0.22–0.45 g/L (22–45 mg/dL)	Rheumatic fever (acute), MI (acute), ulcerative colitis, inflammatory illnesses, stress, and trauma, cancer	Hereditary angioedema, severe liver diseases such as hepatitis or cirrhosis, autoimmune disease (SLE, glomerulonephritis, lupus nephritis, rheumatoid arthritis [severe and active], Sjögren syndrome), serum sickness, renal transplant rejection (acute), protein malnutrition, anemia, malnutrition, infection such as Gram-negative sepsis or bacterial endocarditis, glomerulonephritis
Direct antihuman globulin test (DAT) or direct Coombs' test	Negative (negative) (no agglutination)	Hemolytic disease of the newborn, incompatible blood transfusion reaction, lymphoma, autoimmune hemolytic anemia, mycoplasmal infection, infectious mononucleosis, hemolytic anemia after heart bypass, adult hemolytic anemia (idiopathic)	—
Fluorescent treponemal antibody absorption (FTAAbs)	Negative (nonreactive)	Syphilis	—
Hepatitis A antibody	Negative (negative)	Hepatitis A	—
Hepatitis B surface antigen (HBsAg)	Negative (negative)	Hepatitis B	—
Hepatitis C antibody	Negative (negative)	Hepatitis C	—
Immunoglobulins (Igs) • IgA	0.85–3.85 g/L (85–385 mg/dL)	Chronic liver diseases (e.g., primary biliary cirrhosis), chronic infections, inflammatory bowel disease	Ataxia, telangiectasia, congenital isolated deficiency, hypoproteinemia (e.g., nephrotic syndrome, protein-losing enteropathies), medication immunosuppression (steroids, dextran), AIDS
• IgD	Minimal	Chronic infection, connective tissue disease	—
• IgE	Minimal	Anaphylactic shock, atopic disease (allergies), parasite infections	—
• IgG	5.65–17.65 g/L (565–1765 mg/dL)	Chronic granulomatous infections (e.g., tuberculosis, Wegener granulomatosis, sarcoidosis), hyperimmunization reactions, chronic liver disease, multiple myeloma, autoimmune diseases, intrauterine devices	Wiskott-Aldrich syndrome, agammaglobulinemia, AIDS, hypoproteinemia (e.g., nephrotic syndrome, protein-losing enteropathies), medication immunosuppression (steroids, dextran), non-IgG multiple myeloma, leukemia
• IgM	0.55–3.75 g/L (55–375 mg/dL)	Waldenström macroglobulinemia, chronic infections (e.g., hepatitis, mononucleosis, sarcoidosis), autoimmune diseases (e.g., SLE, rheumatoid arthritis), acute infections, chronic liver disorders (e.g., biliary cirrhosis)	Agammaglobulinemia, AIDS, hypoproteinemia (e.g., nephrotic syndrome, protein-losing enteropathies), medication immunosuppression (steroids, dextran), IgG or IgA multiple myeloma, leukemia
Monospot or Mono-Test	Negative (<1:28 titre)	Infectious mononucleosis, chronic EBV infection, chronic fatigue syndrome, Burkitt lymphoma, some forms of chronic hepatitis	—
Rheumatoid factor (RA factor)	Negative or <60 IU/mL by nephelometric testing	Rheumatoid arthritis, other autoimmune disease (e.g., SLE, Sjögren syndrome, scleroderma), chronic viral infection, subacute bacterial endocarditis, tuberculosis, chronic active hepatitis, dermatomyositis, infectious mononucleosis, leukemia, biliary cirrhosis, syphilis, renal disease	—

TABLE A.3 SEROLOGY–IMMUNOLOGY—cont'd

Test	Normal Values (SI Units [Conventional Units])	Possible Etiology	
		Higher Values	**Lower Values**
RPR (rapid plasma reagin) test	Negative or nonreactive (same as SI units)	—	—
Thyroid antibodies	Titre <9 IU/mL	Chronic thyroiditis (Hashimoto thyroiditis): Antimicrosomal antibodies attack the microsome in the thyroid cells. The immune complex creates an inflammatory and destructive process in the gland, which is mediated through the complement system. Rheumatoid arthritis, rheumatoid-collagen disease: The association with other autoimmune diseases is well known. The mechanism of this association, however, is not well known. Pernicious anemia: APCAs have been associated with the presence of antimicrosomal antibodies. Thyrotoxicosis, hypothyroidism, thyroid carcinoma: Microsomes leak out of the thyroid as a result of the presence of these destructive diseases; they stimulate the immune system to produce antimicrosomal antibodies. Myxedema: Antithyroid microsomal antibodies destroy the thyroid cell, which results in hypofunction of the gland.	—
VDRL (Venereal Disease Research Laboratory) test	Negative or nonreactive (same as SI units)	Syphilis	—

AIDS, acquired immune deficiency syndrome; *APCAs,* antiparietal cell antibodies; *EBV,* Epstein–Barr virus; *IV,* intravenous; *MI,* myocardial infarction; *SLE,* systemic lupus erythematosus.

TABLE A.4 URINE CHEMISTRY

Test	Specimen	Normal Values (SI Units [Conventional Units])	Possible Etiology	
			Higher Values	**Lower Values**
Acetone (ketones)	Random	Negative (negative)	Diabetes mellitus, high-fat and low-carbohydrate diets, starvation states	—
Aldosterone	24 hr	17–70 nmol/24 hr (2–26 mcg/24 hr)	*Primary aldosteronism:* Aldosterone-producing adrenal adenoma (Conn disease), adrenal cortical nodular hyperplasia, Bartter syndrome *Secondary aldosteronism:* Hyponatremia, hyperkalemia, diuretic ingestion resulting in hypovolemia and hyponatremia, laxative abuse, stress, malignant hypertension, poor perfusion states (e.g., heart failure), decreased intravascular volume (e.g., cirrhosis, nephrotic syndrome), renal arterial stenosis, pregnancy and oral contraceptives, hypovolemia or hemorrhage, Cushing's disease	Renin deficiency, steroid therapy, Addison's disease, patients on a high-sodium diet, hypernatremia, Addison's disease, antihypertensive therapy, aldosterone deficiency
Amylase	24 hr	25–125 U/L (same as SI units)	Acute pancreatitis, chronic relapsing pancreatitis, peptic ulcer penetrating into the pancreas, GI disease, acute cholecystitis, parotiditis (mumps), ruptured ectopic pregnancy, renal failure, diabetic ketoacidosis, pulmonary infarction, after endoscopic retrograde pancreatography	—
Bence-Jones protein	Random	Kappa total light chain: <0.68 mg/dL Lambda total light chain <0.40 mg/dL Kappa/lambda ratio: 0.7–6.2	Multiple myeloma (plasmacytoma), chronic lymphocytic leukemia, lymphoma, metastatic colon, breast, lung, or prostate cancer, amyloidosis, Waldenström macroglobulinemia	—
Bilirubin	Random	3–22 mcmol/L (0.2–1.3 mg/dL)	Gallstones, extrahepatic duct obstruction (tumour, inflammation, gallstone, scarring, surgical trauma), extensive liver metastasis, cholestasis from medications, Dubin-Johnson syndrome, Rotor syndrome	—

Continued

TABLE A.4   URINE CHEMISTRY—cont'd

Test	Specimen	Normal Values (SI Units [Conventional Units])	Possible Etiology Higher Values	Lower Values
Calcium	24 hr	2.10–2.7 mmol/day (8.4–10.6 mg/dL)	Hyperparathyroidism, nonparathyroid PTH-producing tumour (e.g., lung or renal carcinoma): PTH or a similar hormone mobilizes calcium stores from the bone to the blood. Metastatic tumour to bone, Paget's disease of bone, prolonged immobilization: Bone destruction or thinning causes calcium to leak from the bone and into the blood. Milk-alkali syndrome: With increased ingestion of milk products or antacids (which contain calcium), the serum calcium level can be elevated. Vitamin D intoxication: Vitamin D works synergistically with PTH to increase serum calcium level. Lymphoma, granulomatous infections such as sarcoidosis and tuberculosis: These diseases are associated with enhanced levels of vitamin D, which works synergistically with PTH to increase serum calcium level. Addison's disease: Glucocorticosteroids inhibit vitamin D activity. When steroid activity is decreased, vitamin D action is enhanced. Vitamin D works synergistically with PTH to increase serum calcium levels. Acromegaly, hyperthyroidism	Hypoparathyroidism: PTH acts to increase serum calcium levels. If PTH levels are reduced, serum calcium levels decline. Renal failure, hyperphosphatemia secondary to renal failure: Excess anions, present in patients with renal failure, bind serum calcium. Rickets, vitamin D deficiency: Vitamin D acts synergistically with PTH. PTH acts to increase serum calcium levels. Without that synergism, calcium levels decline. Osteomalacia, hypoalbuminemia, malabsorption: Less calcium is available to the blood. Pancreatitis, fat embolism: Pancreatitis is associated with saponification (binding of calcium to fats) of the peripancreatic tissue. This reduces calcium levels in the blood. Alkalosis: High pH in the blood drives the calcium to intracellular spaces. Blood levels decline.
Catecholamines	24 hr	<590 mmol/day (<100 mcg/24 hr)	Pheochromocytomas, neuroblastomas, ganglioneuromas, ganglioblastomas, severe stress, strenuous exercise, acute anxiety	—
• Epinephrine		<109 nmol/day (<20 mcg/24 hr)		
• Norepinephrine		<590 nmol/day (<100 mcg/24 hr)		
Chloride	24 hr	98–106 mmol/L (98–106 mEq/L)	Dehydration, excessive infusion of normal saline solution, metabolic acidosis, renal tubular acidosis, Cushing's syndrome, kidney dysfunction, hyperparathyroidism, eclampsia, respiratory alkalosis	Overhydration, syndrome of inappropriate secretion of antidiuretic hormone, heart failure, vomiting or prolonged gastric suction, chronic diarrhea or high-output GI fistula, chronic respiratory acidosis, metabolic alkalosis, salt-losing nephritis, Addison's disease, diuretic therapy, hypokalemia, aldosteronism
Coproporphyrin	24 hr		Lead poisoning, oral contraceptive use, poliomyelitis	—
• Male		15–167 nmol/24 hr (10–109 mcg/24 hr)		
• Female		5–86 nmol/24 hr (3–56 mcg/24 hr)		
Creatine	24 hr		Diseases or injury affecting the heart muscle, skeletal muscle, and brain	—
• Male		20–215 U/L (same as SI units)		
• Female		20–160 U/L (same as SI units)		
Creatinine	24 hr		Diseases affecting renal function, such as glomerulonephritis, pyelonephritis, acute tubular necrosis, urinary tract obstruction, reduced renal blood flow (e.g., shock, dehydration, congestive heart failure, atherosclerosis), diabetic nephropathy, nephritis, rhabdomyolysis, acromegaly, gigantism	Debilitation, decreased muscle mass (e.g., muscular dystrophy, myasthenia gravis)
• Male		53–106 mcmol/L (0.6–1.2 mg/dL)		
• Female		44–97 mcmol/L (0.5–1.1 mg/dL)		

TABLE A.4 URINE CHEMISTRY—cont'd

Test	Specimen	Normal Values (SI Units [Conventional Units])	Possible Etiology Higher Values	Lower Values
Creatinine clearance			Exercise, pregnancy, high cardiac output syndromes	Impaired kidney function (e.g., renal artery atherosclerosis, glomerulonephritis, acute tubular necrosis), conditions causing decreases in GFR (e.g., heart failure, cirrhosis with ascites, shock, dehydration)
• Male		1.78–2.32 mL/sec (107–139 mL/min)		
• Female		1.45–1.78 mL/sec (87–107 mL/min)		
Estriol	24 hr		Feminization syndromes, precocious puberty, ovarian tumour, testicular tumour, adrenal tumour, normal pregnancy, hepatic cirrhosis, liver necrosis, hyperthyroidism	A failing pregnancy, Turner's syndrome, hypopituitarism, primary and secondary hypogonadism, Stein-Leventhal syndrome, menopause, anorexia nervosa
• Female				
• Ovulatory phase		13–54 mcg/24 hr (104–370 nmol/L)		
• Luteal phase		4–100 mcg/24 hr (15–37 nmol/L)		
• Pregnancy		First trimester: 0–800 mcg/24 hr (0–2 900 nmol/L) Second trimester: 800–1 200 mcg/24 hr (2 900–4 4000 nmol/L) Third trimester: 5 000–12 000 mcg/24 hr (18 000–180 000 nmol/L)		
• Menopause		1.4–19.6 mcg/24 hr (5.2–72.5 nmol/L)		
• Male		1–11 mcg/24 hr (18–67 nmol/L)	—	—
Glucose	Random	Random: negative Fasting: <6.1 mmol/L (70–11 mg/dL)	Diabetes mellitus, acute stress response, Cushing's syndrome, pheochromocytoma, chronic renal failure, glucagonoma, acute pancreatitis, diuretic therapy, corticosteroid therapy, acromegaly	Insulinoma, hypothyroidism, hypopituitarism, Addison's disease, extensive liver disease, insulin overdose, starvation
Hemoglobin	Random		Erythrocytosis, congenital heart disease, severe chronic obstructive pulmonary disease, polycythemia vera, severe dehydration (e.g., severe diarrhea, burns)	—
• Male		140–180 mmol/L (14–18 g/dL)		
• Female		120–160 (12–16 g/dL)		
5-Hydroxyindole-acetic acid (5-HIAA)	24 hr	10–40 mcmol/day (2–8 mg/24 hr)	Carcinoid tumour of the appendix, bowel, lung, breast, or ovary; noncarcinoid illness, cystic fibrosis, intestinal malabsorption	Depression, migraine
Ketone bodies	Random	Negative (negative)	Poorly controlled diabetes mellitus, starvation, alcoholism, weight-reduction diets, prolonged vomiting, anorexia, fasting, high-protein diets, glycogen storage diseases, febrile illnesses in infants and children, hyperthyroidism, severe stress or illness, excessive aspirin ingestion	—
Lead	24 hr	<0.48 mcmol/day (<10 mcg/day)	Lead exposure	—
Metanephrine	24 hr	12–60 pg/mL	Pheochromocytoma	—
Myoglobin	Random	1.0–5.3 nmol/L (<90 ng/mL)	Myocardial infarction, skeletal muscle inflammation (myositis), malignant hyperthermia, muscular dystrophy, skeletal muscle ischemia, skeletal muscle trauma, rhabdomyolysis seizures	Polymyositis

Continued

TABLE A.4   URINE CHEMISTRY—cont'd

Test	Specimen	Normal Values (SI Units [Conventional Units])	Possible Etiology Higher Values	Lower Values
pH	Random	4.6–8.0 (average, 6.0)	Alkalemia, urinary tract infections, gastric suction, vomiting, renal tubular acidosis	Acidemia, diabetes mellitus, starvation, respiratory acidosis
Porphobilinogen	Random 24 hr	Negative (negative) 0–6.6 mg/24 hr (0–2 mg/24 hr)	Acute intermittent porphyria, congenital erythropoietic porphyria, hereditary coproporphyria, variegate porphyria, lead poisoning	—
Potassium	24 hr	25–100 mmol/day (25–100 mEq/L/day)	Chronic renal failure, renal tubular acidosis, starvation, Cushing's syndrome, hyperaldosteronism, excessive intake of licorice, alkalosis, diuretic therapy	Dehydration, Addison's disease, malnutrition, vomiting, diarrhea, malabsorption, acute renal failure
Protein (dipstick)	Random	Negative (negative)	Heart failure, nephritis, nephrosis, physiological stress	—
Protein (qualitative) • At rest • During exercise	24 hr	0–8 mg/dL <50–80 mg/24 hr (0.05–0.08 g/day) <250 mg/24 hr (<0.25 g/day)	Nephrotic syndrome, glomerulonephritis, malignant hypertension, diabetic glomerulosclerosis, polycystic kidney disease, systemic lupus erythematosus, Goodpasture's syndrome, heavy-metal poisoning, bacterial pyelonephritis, nephrotoxic medication therapy, trauma, macroglobulinemia, multiple myelomas, pre-eclampsia, heart failure, orthostatic proteinuria, severe muscle exertion, renal vein thrombosis: Congestion of the kidneys is associated with proteinuria. Bladder tumour, urethritis or prostatitis, amyloidosis	—
Sodium, blood	24 hr	136–145 mmol/L (136–145 mEq/L)	Increased dietary intake, excessive sodium in intravenous fluids	Cushing's syndrome, hyperaldosteronism
Specific gravity	Random	1.005–1.030 (usually, 1.010–1.025)*	Dehydration, pituitary tumour or trauma, decreased renal blood flow (as in heart failure, renal artery stenosis, or hypotension), glycosuria and proteinuria, water restriction, fever, excessive sweating, vomiting, diarrhea	Overhydration, diabetes insipidus, renal failure, diuresis
Uric acid • Male • Female		240–501 mcmol/L (4.0–8.5 mg/dL) 160–430 mcmol/L (2.7–7.3 mg/dL) (250–750 mg/24 hr)	Increased ingestion of purines, genetic inborn error in purine metabolism, metastatic cancer, multiple myeloma, leukemias, cancer chemotherapy, hemolysis, rhabdomyolysis	Idiopathic, chronic renal disease, acidosis (ketotic [diabetic or starvation] or lactic), hypothyroidism, toxemia of pregnancy, hyperlipoproteinemia, alcoholism, shock or chronic blood volume depletion states, Wilson disease, Fanconi's syndrome, lead poisoning, yellow atrophy of liver
Urobilinogen	24 hr	0.5–4.0 mg/24 hr (0.5–4.0 Ehrlich units/24 hr)	Hemolytic anemia, pernicious anemia, hemolysis because of medications, hematoma, excessive ecchymosis	Biliary obstruction, cholestasis
Uroporphyrin • Male • Female	24 hr	10–53 nmol/24 hr (8–44 mcg/24 hr) 10–26 nmol/24 hr (4–22 mcg/24 hr)	Acute intermittent porphyria, congenital erythropoietic porphyria, hereditary coproporphyria, variegate porphyria, lead poisoning	—
Vanillylmandelic acid	24 hr	<35 mcmol/day (<6.8 mg/24 hr)	Pheochromocytomas, neuroblastomas, ganglioneuromas, ganglioblastomas, severe stress, strenuous exercise, acute anxiety	—

GFR, glomerular filtration rate; *GI*, gastrointestinal; *PTH*, parathyroid hormone.
*Values decrease with age.

TABLE A.5   GASTRIC ANALYSIS

Test	Normal Values (SI Units [Conventional Units])	Possible Etiology Higher Values	Lower Values
Basal Total acidity	15–45 mmol/L (15–45 mEq/L)	Gastric and duodenal ulcers, Zollinger-Ellison syndrome	Gastric carcinoma, severe gastritis
Post-stimulation Free hydrochloric acid Total acidity	10–130 mmol/L (10–130 mEq/L) 20–150 mmol/L (20–150 mEq/L)	— —	— —

TABLE A.6 FECAL ANALYSIS

Test	Normal Values (SI Units [Conventional Units])	Possible Etiology	
		Higher Values	Lower Values
Blood*	Negative (negative)	Anal fissures, hemorrhoids, inflammatory bowel disease, malignant tumour, peptic ulcer	—
Colour			
• Brown		Various shades, depending on diet	—
• Clay		Biliary obstruction or presence of barium sulphate	—
• Tarry		More than 100 mL of blood in GI tract	—
• Red		Blood in large intestine	—
• Black		Blood in upper GI tract or iron medication	—
Fecal fat	7–21 mmol/day (2–6 g/24 hr)	Cystic fibrosis, malabsorption secondary to sprue, celiac disease, Whipple's disease, Crohn's disease (regional enteritis), or radiation enteritis, maldigestion secondary to obstruction of the pancreatobiliary tree (e.g., cancer, stricture, gallstones), short-gut syndrome secondary to surgical resection, surgical bypass, or congenital anomaly	—
Mucus	Negative (negative)	Mucous colitis, spastic constipation	—
Pus	Negative (negative)	Chronic bacillary dysentery, chronic ulcerative colitis, localized abscesses	—
Urobilinogen	51–372 mcmol/100 g of stool (30–220 mg/100 g of stool)	Hemolytic anemias	Complete biliary obstruction

GI, gastrointestinal.

*Ingestion of meat may produce false-positive results. Patient may be placed on a meat-free diet for 3 days before the test.

TABLE A.7 CEREBROSPINAL FLUID ANALYSIS

Test	Normal Values (SI Units [Conventional Units])	Possible Etiology	
		Higher Values	Lower Values
Blood	Negative (negative)	Intracranial hemorrhage	—
Cell count (age dependent)			
• White blood cells (WBCs)	0–5 × 10^6 WBCs/L (0–10 cells/mcL)	Inflammation or infections of CNS	—
• Red blood cells (RBCs)	0		—
Chloride	116–122 mmol/L of CSF (116–122 mEq/L of CSF)	Uremia	Bacterial infections of CNS (meningitis, encephalitis)
Glucose	2.8–4.2 mmol/L of CSF (50–75 mg/dL of CSF) or 60–70% of blood glucose level	Diabetes mellitus, viral infections of CNS	Bacterial infections and tuberculosis of CNS
Protein	0.15–0.45 g/L of CSF (15–45 mg/dL of CSF)		
• Lumbar	0.15–0.45 g/L (15–45 mg/dL)	Guillain-Barré syndrome, poliomyelitis, traumatic tap	—
• Cisternal	—	Cerebral neoplasm, brain abscess, cerebral hemorrhage, cancer metastasis to the brain: These pathological conditions are associated with disruption in the blood–brain barrier, which results in increased uptake of radionuclide in the cerebral cortex. Acute cerebral infarction: In the first few days to weeks after a stroke, the scan may appear normal. After a few weeks, however, the blood–brain barrier has been disrupted and cortical uptake occurs. This appearance is pathognomonic of stroke. Subdural hematoma: The cortex/subcortical tissue and meninges may become distorted and lateralized. Cerebral thrombosis, cerebrovascular occlusive disease, hematoma, arteriovenous malformation, aneurysm, CSF leakage, hydrocephalus	—
• Ventricular	0.05–0.15 g/L (5–15 mg/dL)	Acute meningitis, brain tumour, chronic CNS infections, multiple sclerosis	—
Pressure	100–200 mm Hg H2O	Hemorrhage, intracranial tumour, meningitis	Head injury, spinal tumour, subdural hematoma

CNS, central nervous system; *CSF*, cerebrospinal fluid.

Note: The content of this appendix is based on the values presented in Pagana, K. D., Pagana, T. J., & Pike-MacDonald, S. A. (2019). *Mosby's Canadian manual of diagnostic and laboratory tests* (2nd Cdn. ed.). Elsevier.

GLOSSARY

A

abortion The loss or termination of a pregnancy before the fetus has developed to a state of viability. Ch. 56

absence seizure Type of seizure typically characterized by a brief staring spell that resembles daydreaming and lasts less than 10 seconds; occurs most commonly in children and may cease altogether or evolve into another type of seizure as the child matures. Ch. 61

absorption Transfer of the end products of digestion across the intestinal wall to the circulation. Ch. 41

absorption atelectasis Absorption of oxygen into the bloodstream and collapse of the alveoli as a result of airway obstruction. Ch. 31

accommodation The convergence of the eyes and the constriction of the pupils when the eyes focus from a far to near object. Ch. 23

acculturation A multidimensional process in which individuals undergo stages of adjustment, as well as changes in domains such as language, socioeconomic status, values, and attitudes, that result in increased similarity between two cultures. Ch. 2

achalasia Absence of peristalsis of the lower two-thirds smooth muscle of the esophagus. Ch. 44

acidosis A condition in which the blood pH drops below 7.35. Ch. 19

acne vulgaris An inflammatory disorder of the sebaceous glands most common in adolscents. Noninflammatory lesions include open comedones (blackheads) and closed comedones (whiteheads); inflammatory lesions include papules, pustules, and cysts. Ch. 26

acoustic neuroma A unilateral benign tumour that occurs where the vestibulocochlear nerve (cranial nerve [CN] VIII) enters the internal auditory canal. Ch. 24

acquired immune deficiency syndrome (AIDS) End stage of chronic HIV infection; a syndrome involving a defect in cell-mediated immunity that has a long incubation period and is manifested by various opportunistic infections and cancers. Ch. 17

acromegaly A condition caused by excessive secretion of growth hormone and characterized by an overgrowth of the bones and soft tissues in the hands, feet, and face; occurs most often as a result of a benign pituitary tumour (adenoma). Ch. 51

actinic keratosis (AK) The most common premalignant skin lesion; manifests as flat or elevated, dry hyperkeratotic papules and plaques occurring on sun-exposed areas; also known as *solar keratosis*. Ch. 26

action potential The electrical impulse created and transported by the conduction system (specialized nerve tissue); it initiates depolarization and, subsequently, cardiac contraction. Ch. 34

active transport A process requiring energy in which molecules move against the concentration gradient. Ch. 19

acupuncture The insertion of fine needles into the circulation of qi underneath the skin's surface to correct disruptions in the flow of qi. Ch. 12

acute arterial ischemia A sudden interruption in the arterial blood supply to a tissue, organ, or extremity that, if left untreated, can result in tissue death. Ch. 40

acute bronchitis An inflammation of the bronchi in the lower respiratory tract that is usually caused by infection. Ch. 30

acute coronary syndrome (ACS) Syndrome encompassing the spectrum of unstable angina, non–ST-segment elevation myocardial infarction, and ST-segment elevation myocardial infarction; develops when myocardial ischemia is prolonged and not immediately reversible. Ch. 36

acute illness Illness typically characterized by a sudden onset, with signs and symptoms related to the disease process itself. Ch. 5

acute kidney injury (AKI) An abrupt decline in kidney function, leading to a rise in serum creatinine or a reduction in urine output or both; the severity of dysfunction can range from a small increase in serum creatinine or reduction in urine output to the development of azotemia. (Previously known as *acute renal failure [ARF]*.) Ch. 49

acute liver failure (ALF) A clinical condition characterized by rapid deterioration of liver function resulting in encephalopathy and coagulopathy in persons with no known history of liver disease. Ch. 46

acute pancreatitis An acute inflammation of the pancreas, ranging from mild edema to severe hemorrhagic necrosis. Ch. 46

acute renal failure (ARF) Former term for *acute kidney injury (AKI)*. Ch. 49

acute respiratory distress syndrome (ARDS) A sudden and progressive form of acute respiratory failure in which the alveolar–capillary membrane becomes damaged and more permeable by intravascular fluid. Ch. 70

acute retroviral syndrome (seroconversion illness) A flulike syndrome of fever, swollen lymph glands, sore throat, headache, malaise, nausea, muscle and joint pain, diarrhea, or a diffuse rash, or some combination of these. Ch. 17

acute rheumatic fever (ARF) A complication that occurs as a delayed sequela (usually after 2–3 weeks) of group A streptococcal pharyngitis. Ch. 39

acute tubular necrosis (ATN) Necrosis of renal tubular epithelial cells caused by ischemia, nephrotoxins, or sepsis; the most common intra-renal cause of acute kidney injury. Ch. 49

Addison's disease A disease that causes adrenocortical insufficiency (hypofunction of the adrenal cortex) and in which the supply of all three classes of adrenal corticosteroids (glucocorticoids, mineralocorticoids, and androgens) is reduced. Ch. 51

adhesions Bands of scar tissue that form between or around organs. Ch. 14

advance care planning A process of thinking about and sharing one's wishes for future health and personal care; a means by which an individual can tell others what would be important if they were ill and unable to communicate. Ch. 13

advance directives Legal documents specifying an individual's decisions regarding end-of-life care and specifying alternative decision makers as required. Ch. 13

advanced practice nursing (APN) Clinical nursing practice at a level that requires graduate education and attainment and advancement of in-depth nursing knowledge and expertise in complex decision-making to meet the health needs of individuals, families, groups, communities, and populations. Ch. 1

adventitious sounds Additional breath sounds that are abnormal. Ch. 28

afterload The peripheral resistance against which the left ventricle must pump. Ch. 34

ageism Negative attitude based on age, leading to discrimination and disparities in the care of older people. Ch. 7

age-related macular degeneration (AMD) An eye disease that begins after age 60 that progressively destroys the macula (the central portion of the retina), causing irreversible central vision loss. Ch. 24

alarm reaction First stage of the stress response; it stimulates the central nervous system and mobilizes bodily defences in a fight-or-flight response to the acute stress. Ch. 8

alcohol-associated liver disease (ALD) Liver injury, resulting from alcohol use, that ranges from liver fat (steatosis) to alcohol-associated steato-hepatitis, alcoholic hepatitis, and alcohol-associated cirrhosis; disease progression is dependent on continued heavy alcohol use and other cofactors, such as genetic susceptibility, diet, and comorbid liver disease. Ch. 46

aldosterone A potent mineralocorticoid that maintains extracellular fluid volume. Ch. 50

alkalosis A condition in which the blood pH is greater than 7.45. Ch. 19

allele One of two or more alternative forms of a gene that can occupy a particular chromosomal locus. Ch. 15

allergic rhinitis Inflammation of the nasal mucosa due to a specific allergen. Ch. 29

allostasis The process of achieving homeostasis in the presence of a challenge. Ch. 8

alopecia Partial or complete lack of hair resulting from normal aging, endocrine disorder, medication reaction, anticancer medication, or skin disease. Ch. 25

α_1-antitrypsin (AAT) deficiency The only known genetic abnormality that leads to chronic obstructive pulmonary disease; AAT, the major antiprotease in plasma, inhibits neutrophil elastase and the action of proteolytic enzymes from neutrophils and macrophages. Ch. 31

alveolar hypoventilation A decrease in ventilation that results in an increase in partial pressure of arterial carbon dioxide ($PaCO_2$) and a consequent decrease in partial pressure of arterial oxygen (PaO_2). Ch. 70

Alzheimer's disease (AD) A chronic, progressive, degenerative disease of the brain. Ch. 62

amblyopia Reduced or no vision in an affected eye; also termed "lazy eye." Ch. 24

ambulatory surgery Also called *same-day surgery*; refers to surgery conducted in emergency departments, endoscopy clinics, health care providers' offices, and outpatient surgery units in hospitals, after which the patient can be discharged on the same day. Ch. 20

amenorrhea Absence of menstruation. Chs. 53, 56

amyloid plaques Clusters of insoluble deposits of a protein called *β-amyloid*, other proteins, remnants of neurons, non-nerve cells such as microglia (cells that surround and digest damaged cells or foreign substances), and other cells, such as astrocytes; present in abnormal quantities in the brains of persons with Alzheimer's disease. Ch. 62

amyotrophic lateral sclerosis (ALS) A rare, progressive neurological disorder characterized by loss of motor neurons and by weakness and atrophy of the muscles of the hands, the forearms, and the legs, spreading to involve most of the body and the face. Ch. 61

anaesthesia care team An anaesthesiologist-led care model in which anaesthesiologists practise among a team of other professionals such as nurse practitioners–anaesthesia, anaesthesia assistants, registered nurses, and respiratory therapists. Ch. 21

anaesthesiologist Physician who is responsible for the administration of anaesthetic agents; an expert in administering potent medications used to deliver general and regional anaesthesia and in ensuring absence of pain during surgery. Ch. 21

anal fissure A skin ulcer or a crack in the lining of the anal wall that is caused by trauma, local infection, or inflammation. Ch. 45

anal fistula An abnormal tunnel leading out from the anus or the rectum, which may extend to the outside of the skin, the vagina, or the buttocks. Ch. 45

analgesic ceiling A dosage at which no additional analgesia is produced regardless of further dosage increases. Ch. 10

anaphylactic shock An acute, life-threatening hypersensitivity (allergic) reaction to a sensitizing substance, such as a medication, chemical, vaccine, food, or insect venom. Ch. 69

anaplasia Cell differentiation to a more immature or embryonic form. Ch. 14

andragogy The theoretical basis of adult learning. Ch. 4

anemia A deficiency in the number of erythrocytes (red blood cells [RBCs]), the quantity or quality of hemoglobin, the volume of packed RBCs (hematocrit), or a combination of these. Ch. 33

anergy Immunodeficient condition characterized by lack of or diminished reaction to an antigen or a group of antigens. Ch. 16

aneurysm A permanent, localized outpouching or dilation of the blood vessel wall (either congenital or acquired). Chs. 40, 60

angina Chest pain that is the clinical manifestation of reversible myocardial ischemia. Ch. 36

anions Negatively charged ions. Ch. 19

ankylosing spondylitis (AS) A chronic inflammatory disease that affects primarily the axial skeleton, including the sacroiliac joints, intervertebral disc spaces, and costovertebral articulations. Ch. 67

ankylosis Stiffness or fixation of a joint, usually resulting from destruction of articular cartilage and subchondral bone with subsequent tissue scarring. Ch. 64

anorexia nervosa A serious, often chronic, and life-threatening eating disorder characterized by self-imposed weight loss, endocrine dysfunction, and a distorted psychopathological attitude toward weight and eating. Ch. 42

antidiuretic hormone (ADH) A potent vasoconstrictor whose major physiological role is the regulation of fluid volume by stimulating reabsorption of water in the renal tubules; also called *vasopressin*. Ch. 50

antigen A substance that elicits an immune response. Ch. 16

aortic dissection Not a type of aneurysm; rather, a dissection that results from the creation of a false lumen (between the intima and the media) through which blood flows. Ch. 40

aortic stenosis A narrowing or stricture of the aortic valve resulting in obstruction of the blood flow from the left ventricle to the aorta during systole; causes left ventricular hypertrophy and increased myocardial oxygen consumption. Ch. 39

aortic valve regurgitation (AR) Retrograde blood flow from the ascending aorta into the left ventricle when the valve should be closed, resulting in volume overload. Ch. 39

aphasia Total loss of comprehension and use of language or total inability to communicate. Ch. 60

apheresis A procedure in which components of the blood are separated and then one or more of those components is removed. Ch. 16

aplastic anemia A disease in which the patient has peripheral blood pancytopenia (decrease of all blood cell types—red blood cells, white blood cells, and platelets) and hypocellular bone marrow. Ch. 33

apoptosis Programmed cell death. Ch. 14

appendicitis An inflammation of the appendix. Ch. 45

aqueous humor A clear, watery fluid that fills the anterior and posterior chambers of the anterior cavity of the eye. Ch. 23

arterial blood pressure (BP) A measure of the pressure exerted by blood against the walls of the arterial system. Ch. 34

arterial pressure–based cardiac output (APCO) A technique for determining continuous cardiac output/continuous cardiac index, used to assess a patient's ability to respond to fluids by increasing stroke volume (preload or fluid volume responsiveness). Ch. 68

arteriovenous fistula (AVF) The preferred hemodialysis access, created by the surgical connection of a vein and an artery, usually in the forearm. Ch. 49

arteriovenous graft (AVG) A hemodialysis access created with a synthetic graft that is attached to an artery and vein; used for people who do not have suitable vessels for an arteriovenous fistula. Ch. 49

arthritis A condition involving inflammation of a joint or joints; it takes the form of osteoarthritis, rheumatoid arthritis, fibromyalgia, systemic lupus erythematosus, and gout. Ch. 67

arthrocentesis A procedure in which an incision or puncture is made in a joint capsule, usually to obtain samples of synovial fluid from within the joint cavity for a synovial fluid analysis. Ch. 64

arthrodesis The surgical fusion of a joint. Ch. 65

arthroplasty The reconstruction or replacement of a joint to relieve pain, improve or maintain range of motion, and correct deformity. Ch. 65

arthroscopy A procedure in which a small fibre-optic tube called an *arthroscope* is inserted into a joint and used to directly examine or to operate on the interior of the joint cavity. Ch. 64

Aschoff bodies Tiny, rounded or spindle-shaped nodules formed by a reaction to myocardial inflammation with accompanying swelling and fragmentation of collagen fibres. Ch. 39

ascites The accumulation of serous fluid in the peritoneal or the abdominal cavity. Ch. 46

assessment The collection of subjective and objective information about the patient. Ch. 1

assisted-living facilities (ALFs) Residential care facilities that provide housing and personal care. Ch. 7

asterixis Flapping tremors (liver flap) commonly affecting the arms and hands; a manifestation of hepatic encephalopathy. Ch. 46

asthma A chronic inflammatory disorder of the airways; inflammation causes varying degrees of obstruction in the airways, which leads to recurrent episodes of wheezing, breathlessness, chest tightness, and cough, particularly at night and in the early morning. Ch. 31

astigmatism An imperfection in the curvature of the cornea or in the shape of the eye's lens that causes blurred or distorted vision for both near and far objects. Chs. 23, 24

asystole The total absence of ventricular electrical activity. Ch. 38

atelectasis A complete or partial collapse of a lung or segment of a lung that occurs when the alveoli become deflated. Chs. 22, 30

atherosclerosis A disease characterized by deposits of lipids within the intima of the artery; major cause of coronary artery disease. Ch. 36

atrial fibrillation A cardiac dysrhythmia characterized by a total disorganization of atrial electrical activity resulting in loss of effective atrial contraction. Ch. 38

atrial flutter An atrial tachydysrhythmia identified by recurring, regular, sawtooth-shaped flutter waves. Ch. 38

atrial kick During the final phase of atrial systole, a contraction of the atria that ejects a bolus of blood into the ventricles and contributes more blood to cardiac output. Ch. 34

atrophy Decrease in the size of a tissue or organ as a result of a reduction in the number or size of the individual cells. Ch. 14

aura Neurological symptoms such as visual field defects, tingling or burning sensations, paresthesias, motor dysfunction (e.g., weakness, paralysis), dizziness, confusion, and even loss of consciousness that usually precede the onset of migraine pain. Ch. 61

auscultation The act of listening for sounds produced by the body to assess normal conditions and deviations from normal; particularly useful in evaluating the heart, lungs, abdomen, and vascular system. Ch. 3

autoimmunity An immune reaction to self-proteins: the immune system no longer differentiates self from nonself. Ch. 16

automated peritoneal dialysis (APD) A popular form of peritoneal dialysis that is done while the patient sleeps, using a device called a *cycler*. (Also called *continuous cycling peritoneal dialysis*.) Ch. 49

automatic external defibrillators (AEDs) Defibrillators that have rhythm detection capability and the ability to advise the operator to deliver a shock with hands-free defibrillator pads. Ch. 38

automaticity A property of specialized cells of the heart found in the sinoatrial (SA) node, parts of the atria, the atrioventricular (AV) node, and the His–Purkinje system that are able to discharge spontaneously. Ch. 38

autonomic dysreflexia A massive, life-threatening, uncompensated cardiovascular reaction mediated by the sympathetic nervous system that occurs in patients with spinal cord lesions in response to visceral stimulation; also known as *autonomic hyper-reflexia*. Ch. 63

autonomic nervous system (ANS) The division of the nervous system that governs involuntary functions of cardiac muscle, smooth (involuntary) muscle, and glands. Ch. 58

autosome Any chromosome that is not a sex chromosome. Ch. 15

avascular necrosis (AVN) Bone cell death as a result of inadequate blood supply. Ch. 65

azotemia An accumulation of nitrogen waste products (urea nitrogen, creatinine) in the blood. Ch. 49

B

bacteria One-celled microorganisms that are found virtually everywhere on earth and are involved in fermentation, putrefaction, infectious diseases, and nitrogen fixation. Ch. 17

bariatric surgery An invasive procedure used to treat morbid obesity. Ch. 43

baroreceptors Specialized nerve cells located in the carotid sinus at the bifurcation of the external and internal carotid arteries and the arch of the aorta; they are sensitive to stretching and, when stimulated by an increase in blood pressure, send inhibitory impulses to the sympathetic vasomotor centre in the brainstem. Ch. 35

Barrett's esophagus A condition in which the normal squamous epithelium of the esophagus is replaced with columnar epithelium; it is a precancerous lesion and increases the risk for esophageal cancer. Ch. 44

basal cell carcinoma (BCC) A locally invasive malignancy arising from epidermal basal cells; the most common type of skin cancer but the least deadly. Ch. 26

behavioural and psychological symptoms of dementia (BPSDs) The behavioural manifestations (e.g., appetite changes, slowed or excessive movements and speech, agitation, pacing, wandering) and psychological manifestations (e.g.,

anhedonia, worry, depressed mood, euphoria, fear) of dementia. Ch. 62

Bell's palsy A disorder characterized by the disruption of the motor branches of the facial nerve (cranial nerve VII) on one side of the face in the absence of any other disease. Ch. 63

benign neoplasms Well-differentiated tumours that are usually encapsulated, do not metastasize, have slight vascularity, and rarely recur. Ch. 18

benign paroxysmal positional vertigo (BPPV) A common cause of vertigo in which free-floating debris ("ear rocks") in the semicircular canal produces symptoms of dizziness, vertigo, light-headedness, loss of balance, and nausea with specific head movements. Ch. 24

benign prostatic hyperplasia (BPH) A condition involving increase in size of the prostate gland leading to a disruption of urine outflow from the bladder through the urethra; thought to be caused by an excessive accumulation of dihydroxytestosterone or an increased proportion of estrogen as compared to testosterone. Ch. 57

bereavement The period after the death of a loved one during which grief is experienced and mourning occurs. Ch. 13

best buys Actions that should be undertaken immediately to produce accelerated results in terms of lives saved, diseases prevented, and heavy costs avoided. Ch. 5

bilirubin A pigment derived from the breakdown of aged red blood cells. Ch. 41

biological therapy Treatment involving the use of biological agents such as interferons, interleukins, monoclonal antibodies, and growth factors to modify the relationship between the host and the tumour. Ch. 18

bioterrorism The use of biological agents as the element of a terrorist attack; involves the deliberate spreading of microbes or toxins with the intent of causing disease or death in animals, plants, and humans. Ch. 72

blebs Air-filled alveolar dilations less than 1 cm in diameter on the edge of the lung at the apex of the upper lobe or superior segment of the lower lobe. Ch. 30

blood–brain barrier A physiological barrier between blood capillaries and brain tissue that protects the brain from certain potentially harmful agents while allowing nutrients and gases to enter. Ch. 58

blood pressure (BP) The force exerted by the blood against the walls of blood vessels; must be adequate for tissue perfusion to be maintained during activity and rest. Ch. 35

body mass index (BMI) A ratio of weight to height calculated by dividing weight (in kilograms) by height (in metres squared); higher ranges are associated with increased health risk. Ch. 43

bone marrow transplantation Life-saving procedure for patients with a number of malignant and nonmalignant diseases; cells are allogeneic (from nonmonozygotic twin donor), autologous (from self), or syngeneic (from healthy monozygotic twin). Ch. 18

botulism An acute neurological disorder that causes potentially life-threatening neuroparalysis

due to a neurotoxin produced by *Clostridium botulinum*. Ch. 63

brachytherapy "Close" radiation delivery system in which radioactive materials are implanted or inserted directly into the tumour or close to the tumour. Ch. 18

brain abscess An accumulation of pus within the brain tissue that can result from a local or systemic infection. Ch. 59

brain reward system A mechanism involving the mesolimbic system of the brain; responsible for creating the sensation of pleasure or meaning in reaction to certain behaviours that are required for survival of the human species, such as eating and sex. Ch. 11

breakthrough pain Moderate to severe pain that occurs despite treatment. Ch. 10

bronchiectasis A condition of the lungs characterized by permanent, abnormal dilation of one or more large bronchi. Ch. 30

Brown-Séquard syndrome A syndrome resulting from damage to half of the spinal cord; characterized by a loss of motor function, sense of position, and sense of vibration on the same side as the lesion. Ch. 63

buffers Fast-acting regulatory mechanisms that act chemically to change strong acids into weaker acids or to bind acids to neutralize their effect. Ch. 19

bulimia nervosa An eating disorder characterized by periods of food restriction, followed by binge eating, with recurrent compensatory behaviours such as purging or restriction, accompanied by feelings of loss of control over eating and a persistent concern with body image. Ch. 42

burn An injury to the tissues of the body caused by heat, chemicals, electric current, or radiation. Ch. 27

bursitis Inflammation of a bursa. Ch. 65

C

calculus An abnormal stone formed in body tissues by an accumulation of mineral salts. Ch. 48

cancer A group of more than 200 diseases characterized by uncontrolled and unregulated growth of cells. Ch. 18

carcinogens Cancer-causing agents capable of producing cellular alterations. Ch. 18

carcinoma in situ A lesion with all the histological features of cancer except invasion; becomes invasive if left untreated. Ch. 18

carcinomas Malignant tumours that originate from embryonal ectoderm (skin and glands) and endoderm (mucous membrane linings of the respiratory, gastrointestinal, and genitourinary tracts). Ch. 18

cardiac index A measure of the cardiac output divided by the body mass index. Ch. 34

cardiac output (CO) The amount of blood pumped by the ventricle in 1 minute, reflecting the heart's mechanical ability; can be described as the stroke volume (SV, or amount of blood pumped out of the left ventricle per beat [~70 mL]) multiplied by the heart rate (HR) over 1 minute. Chs. 34, 35

cardiac pacemaker An electronic device used to pace the heart when the normal conduction pathway is damaged or diseased. Ch. 38

cardiac reserve The ability of the heart to respond to increased demands on the cardiovascular system by increasing cardiac output as much as three-fold or four-fold. Ch. 34

cardiac tamponade A condition that develops as fluid accumulates in the pericardial sac (pericardial effusion), causing an increase in intrapericardial pressure and producing compression of the heart. Ch. 39

cardiac transplantation Transfer of a heart from one person to another. Ch. 37

cardiogenic shock Shock occurring when either systolic or diastolic dysfunction of the pumping action of the heart results in reduced stroke volume, cardiac output, and blood pressure. Ch. 69

cardiomyopathy A group of diseases that directly affect the structural or functional ability of the myocardium. Ch. 39

caregiver burden The level of multifaceted strain perceived by the caregiver from providing care to a family member or loved one over time. Ch. 5

carpal tunnel syndrome (CTS) A repetitive strain injury caused by compression of the median nerve, which enters the hand through the narrow confines of the carpal tunnel, located in the wrist. Ch. 65

carrier An individual who carries a copy of a mutated gene for a recessive disorder. Ch. 15

cataplexy A brief and sudden loss of skeletal muscle tone or muscle weakness. Manifestations range from a brief episode of muscle weakness to complete postural collapse and falling to the ground. Ch. 9

cataract An area of opacity within the lens. Ch. 24

catecholamines Substances that are usually considered neurotransmitters but are hormones when secreted by the adrenal medulla; they include epinephrine, norepinephrine, and dopamine. Catecholamines are an essential part of the body's response to stress. Ch. 50

cations Positively charged ions. Ch. 19

CBRNE event Any situation in which weapons of a **c**hemical, **b**iological, **r**adiological, **n**uclear, or **e**xplosive nature are used with the goal of causing harm. Ch. 72

ceiling effect A phenomenon in which increasing the dose of a given medication beyond an upper limit provides no greater analgesia. Ch. 10

celiac disease An autoimmune disease characterized by damage to the small intestinal mucosa from the ingestion of wheat, barley, and rye in genetically susceptible individuals. Ch. 45

cell-mediated immunity Immune responses that are initiated through specific antigen recognition by T cells. Ch. 16

cellulitis A deep inflammation of subcutaneous tissues. Ch. 26

central nervous system (CNS) The division of the nervous system that consists of the brain and the spinal cord. Ch. 58

cerebral edema Increased accumulation of fluid in the extravascular spaces of brain tissue. Ch. 59

cerebrospinal fluid (CSF) A clear, colourless fluid that provides cushioning for the brain and the spinal cord, allows fluid shifts from the cranial cavity to the spinal cavity, and carries nutrients. Ch. 58

cerebrovascular accident (CVA) The medical term for *stroke*. Ch. 60

certification of death A legal medical document stating that the patient is dead, which is usually required within 24 hours of a death. Ch. 13

chancre A painless, indurated lesion found on the penis, vulva, lips, mouth, vagina, or rectum; a primary manifestation of syphilis. Ch. 55

chemical burns Burns that result from contact with acids, alkalis, and organic compounds. Ch. 27

chemoreceptor A receptor in the medulla that responds to a change in the chemical composition (partial pressure of arterial carbon dioxide [$PaCO_2$] and pH) of the fluid around it. Ch. 28

chest physiotherapy Airway clearance technique for reducing mucus; consists of percussion, vibration, and postural drainage. Ch. 31

Cheyne–Stokes respiration An irregular pattern of breathing characterized by alternating periods of apnea and deep breathing. Ch. 13

chlamydial infections A superficial mucosal infection, caused by *Chlamydia trachomatis*, that can be transmitted during vaginal, anal, or oral sex; the most prevalent bacterial sexually transmitted infection in Canada today. Ch. 55

cholecystitis Inflammation of the gallbladder. Ch. 46

cholelithiasis Stones in the gallbladder. Ch. 46

chronic bronchitis The presence of chronic productive cough for 3 months in 2 successive years. Ch. 31

chronic disease management The use of elements and tools within the health care system (e.g., information systems, decision support tools, self-management promotion, and realignment of health services) and within the community (e.g., a supportive environment, health policy, and strengthened community action) to help patients living with chronic diseases; includes strategies to reduce risk factors. Ch. 6

chronic illness Health conditions that persist over extended periods and that are often (but not always) associated with participation and activity limitations (disability). Ch. 5

chronic kidney disease (CKD) The progressive, irreversible destruction of the nephrons in both kidneys, leading to loss of kidney function; classified at one of five stages, depending on level of severity based on glomerular filtration rate. Ch. 49

chronic kidney disease–mineral and bone disorder (CKD–MBD) A clinical syndrome with systemic components that include characteristic bone abnormalities, changes in mineral balance, and vascular and other soft tissue calcification. Ch. 49

chronic obstructive pulmonary disease (COPD) A preventable disease characterized by persistent airflow limitation that is usually progressive; associated with enhanced chronic inflammatory response in the airways and lungs, caused primarily by cigarette smoking and other noxious particles and gases. Ch. 31

chronic pancreatitis Progressive destruction of the pancreas as it is replaced with fibrotic tissues. Ch. 46

chronic stable angina Chest pain that occurs intermittently over a long period with the same pattern of onset, duration, and intensity of symptoms. Ch. 36

chronic venous insufficiency (CVI) A condition in which leg veins and valves fail to keep blood moving forward. Ch. 40

chylothorax Presence of lymphatic fluid in the pleural space caused by a leak in the thoracic duct. Ch. 30

circadian rhythms The biological rhythms of behaviour and physiology that fluctuate within a 24-hour period. Ch. 9

circadian rhythm sleep–wake disorders (CRSWDs) A group of sleep disorders that result in a person having good-quality sleep at the wrong time of day. Ch. 9

circulating nurse A perioperative nurse who is not scrubbed, gowned, or gloved and remains in an unsterile field. Ch. 21

cirrhosis The final stage of chronic liver disease; a condition (not disease) that results from chronic liver inflammation; characterized by extensive fibrosis and regenerative nodules that occur from the liver's attempt to repair itself, leading to permanent distortion in the liver architecture. Ch. 46

clinical (critical) pathway A plan outlining daily care goals for select health care problems; includes a nursing care plan, specific interventions for each day of hospitalization, and a documentation tool. Ch. 1

clitoris Erectile tissue in women that lies anterior to the urethral meatus and the vaginal orifice and becomes engorged during sexual excitation. Ch. 53

clubbing A distortion of the nail angle at the cuticle, caused by chronic hypoxemia, resulting in bulbous-appearing nails and fingertips. Ch. 25

cluster headaches A rare form of headache that involves repeated headaches that can occur for weeks to months at a time, followed by periods of remission; characterized by intense, stabbing pain that is ipsilateral in nature and usually occurs at night or at the same time each day. Ch. 61

collaborative problems Potential or actual complications of disease or of treatment that nurses manage together with other health care providers. Ch. 1

collateral circulation Arterial connections within the coronary circulation; development depends on (1) the inherited predisposition to develop new blood vessels and (2) the presence of chronic ischemia. Ch. 36

colorectal cancer A malignant disease of the colon, the rectum, or both; the second-most common cause of cancer death in Canada. Ch. 45

coma A profound state of unconsciousness. Ch. 59

community-acquired pneumonia (CAP) A lower respiratory tract infection of the lung parenchyma with onset in the community or during the first 2 days of hospitalization. Ch. 30

comorbidity The presence of two or more chronic illnesses that are not directly related to each other in a person at the same time. Ch. 5

compartment syndrome A condition in which swelling and increased pressure within a limited space (a compartment) press on and compromise the function of blood vessels, nerves, and tendons that run through that compartment. Ch. 65

complementary and alternative therapies An umbrella term used to describe a broad range of healing philosophies, therapies, and health care approaches that either accompany or are used instead of conventional biomedical practices dominant in Canada and other Western cultures. Ch. 12

complete heart block A type of heart block in which no impulses from the atria are conducted to the ventricles; also called *third-degree AV heart block*. Ch. 38

compliance A measure of the elasticity of the lungs and thorax. Ch. 28

concussion A sudden, transient, mechanical head injury, with disruption of neural activity and a change in the level of consciousness; considered a mild traumatic brain injury. Ch. 59

Confusion Assessment Method A widely used, validated screening assessment and diagnostic aid that is effective in identifying the presence of delirium. Ch. 62

conjunctiva A transparent mucous membrane that covers the inner surfaces of the eyelids (the palpebral conjunctiva) and extends over the sclera (the bulbar conjunctiva), forming a "pocket" under each eyelid. Ch. 23

conjunctivitis An infection or inflammation of the conjunctiva caused by bacteria or viruses or exposure to allergens or chemical irritants. Ch. 24

constipation A decrease in frequency of bowel movements from what is usual for the individual; hard, difficult-to-pass stools; a decrease in stool volume; and retention of feces in the rectum; or some combination of these symptoms. Ch. 45

continuing competence The ongoing ability to perform one's duties skillfully, safely, and ethically. Ch. 1

continuous ambulatory peritoneal dialysis (CAPD) A type of peritoneal dialysis that is done during the day and consists of a minimum of four exchanges of dialysis fluid over a 24-hour period. Ch. 49

continuous positive airway pressure (CPAP) A treatment for severe apnea or hypopnea in which a nasal mask attached to a high-flow blower is applied to maintain sufficient positive pressure in the airway during inspiration and expiration to prevent airway collapse. Ch. 9

continuous renal replacement therapy (CRRT) An alternative or adjunctive method for treating acute kidney injury that provides a means by which uremic toxins and fluids are removed from patients who are hemodynamically unstable, while acid–base status and electrolytes are adjusted slowly and continuously. Ch. 49

contracture An abnormal, usually permanent condition of a muscle or joint, characterized by flexion and fixation. Chs. 27, 64

contusion Bruising of the brain tissue within a focal area. Ch. 59

coping A person's cognitive and behavioural efforts to manage specific external or internal stressors that seem to exceed available resources. Ch. 8

coping resources Internal or external assets, characteristics, or actions that a person draws on to manage stress. Ch. 8

cor pulmonale A hypertrophy of the right side of the heart, with or without heart failure, resulting from pulmonary hypertension. Diseases of the lung or thorax or changes in pulmonary circulation can lead to pulmonary hypertension. Chs. 30, 31

coronary angiography Imaging with left-sided heart catheterization in which the catheter is positioned at the origin of the coronary arteries and contrast medium is injected into the arteries; images identify the location and severity of any coronary blockages. Ch. 34

coronary artery disease (CAD) A blood vessel disorder that may affect the heart's arteries and produce various pathological effects, especially the reduced flow of oxygen and nutrients to the myocardium. Ch. 36

coronary revascularization An intervention that restores blood flow to the affected myocardium. Ch. 36

corticosteroid Any of the steroid hormones synthesized by the adrenal cortex (excluding androgens). Ch. 50

cortisol The most abundant and potent glucocorticoid; one of its major functions is the regulation of blood glucose concentration. Ch. 50

costovertebral angle A physical examination landmark used to locate the kidneys, formed by the rib cage and the vertebral column. Ch. 47

cough variant asthma A type of asthma in which cough is the only symptom. Ch. 31

crackles Short, low-pitched sounds caused by the passage of air through an airway intermittently occluded by mucus, unstable bronchial wall, or fold of mucosa. Ch. 28

cranial nerves (CNs) The 12 paired nerves composed of cell bodies with fibres that exit from the cranial cavity. Ch. 58

creatinine A waste product produced by protein breakdown (primarily body muscle mass); clearance of creatinine by the kidney approximates the glomerular filtration rate. Ch. 47

crepitation Crackling sound or grating sensation as a result of friction between bones, broken bone, or cartilage bits in joint. Ch. 64

CREST An acronym used to describe the clinical manifestations of systemic sclerosis (scleroderma): **c**alcinosis, **R**aynaud's phenomenon, **e**sophageal dysfunction, **s**clerodactyly, and **t**elangiectasia. Ch. 67

Creutzfeldt–Jakob disease (CJD) A very rare, fatal, infectious brain disorder thought to be caused by accumulation in the brain of an abnormally folded prion protein. Ch. 62

critical incident stress management (CISM) or debriefing A comprehensive approach to preventing and managing the emotional trauma that can be a result of involvement in a disaster response. Ch. 72

critical limb ischemia A condition characterized by chronic ischemic rest pain lasting more than 2 weeks, arterial leg ulcers, or gangrene of the leg as a result of peripheral artery disease. Ch. 40

critical thinking The art of analyzing and evaluating thinking with a view to improving it. Ch. 1

Crohn's disease A chronic, inflammatory bowel disease of unknown origin that can affect any part of the gastrointestinal tract, from the mouth to the anus. Ch. 45

cross-tolerance The development of resistance to one or more effects of a medication as a result of tolerance developed to a similar medication; an increased dose is required for effect. Ch. 11

cryosurgery The use of subfreezing temperatures to destroy epidermal lesions. Ch. 26

cultural competence A process whereby practitioners recognize the need for the knowledge and skills to modify assessment and intervention strategies in order to achieve equity in health quality and outcomes. Ch. 2

cultural imposition The situation in which a person's own cultural beliefs and practices are, intentionally or unintentionally, imposed on another person or group of people. Ch. 2

cultural safety A concept that focuses on the impact of colonialism and power imbalances that lead to a disregard for health and illness beliefs of Indigenous people and nondominant cultures and to a privileging of the dominant cultural values. Ch. 2

culture Shared patterns that individuals share with others in a group and can be described as commonly **u**nderstood **l**earned **t**raditions and **u**nconscious **r**ules of **e**ngagement. Ch. 2

cultured epithelial autograft (CEA) Skin grafts grown from biopsy specimens obtained from the patient's own unburned skin. Ch. 27

curettage The removal and scooping away of tissue using an instrument (curette) with a circular cutting edge attached to a handle. Ch. 26

Cushing's syndrome A spectrum of clinical abnormalities characterized by endogenous hypercortisolism; most common causes are iatrogenic administration of exogenous corticosteroids (e.g., prednisone) in large doses for several weeks or longer and excessive production of cortisol by the adrenal cortex. Ch. 51

cyanosis Bluish colouration of the skin or mucous membranes, resulting from hypoxia. Ch. 25

cyst Palpable, fluid-filled mass. Ch. 54

cystic fibrosis An autosomal recessive, multi-system disease characterized by altered function of the exocrine glands, involving primarily the lungs, the pancreas, and the sweat glands. Ch. 31

cystitis An inflammatory condition of the urinary bladder, characterized by pain, urgency and frequency of urination, and hematuria. Ch. 48

cystocele Herniation or protrusion of the urinary bladder through the wall of the vagina; occurs when support between the vagina and the bladder is weakened; also known as *anterior wall prolapse*. Ch. 56

cystometrography A urodynamic study used to evaluate the compliance (elastic property) and stability of the detrusor muscle of the bladder and to evaluate bladder tone, sensations of filling, and bladder (detrusor) stability. Ch. 47

cystoscopy A radiological bladder procedure in which contrast material is instilled into the bladder to enable inspection of the interior of the bladder and evaluation of the vesicoureteral reflux using a tubular lighted instrument called a *cystoscope*. Ch. 47

cytokines Soluble factors secreted by white blood cells and a variety of other cells in the body. Ch. 16

D

database All the health information about a patient, including the data from the nursing history and physical examination, the data from the medical history and physical examination, results of laboratory and diagnostic tests, and information contributed by other health care providers. Ch. 3

death The state of when all vital organs and body systems cease to function; irreversible cessation of cardiovascular, respiratory, and brain function. Ch. 13

debridement Removal of necrotic tissue from a wound to prevent infection and promote healing. Ch. 27

decontamination The process of removing or neutralizing a hazardous agent from the environment, property, equipment, or a life form, through the use of water, cleansers, or neutralizers. Ch. 72

deep vein thrombosis (DVT) A disorder involving a thrombus in a deep vein, most commonly the iliac and femoral veins. Ch. 40

defecation The discharge of feces from the rectum. Ch. 41

degenerative disc disease (DDD) Progressive degeneration that results in intervertebral discs losing their elasticity, flexibility, and shock-absorbing capabilities; thinning of the discs also occurs. A normal process of aging. Ch. 66

deglutition The process of swallowing. Ch. 41

dehiscence Separation and disruption of previously joined wound edges. Ch. 14

delayed awakening Longer-than-expected duration of postoperative unconsciousness, usually caused by prolonged medication action or, rarely, by neurological injury. Ch. 22

delayed sleep phase disorder (DSPD) Difficulty falling asleep (staying awake until 0100–0300 hours) and typically sleeping later into the morning. Ch. 9

delirium An acute brain dysfunction resulting in impaired attention, awareness, and cognition; it is a medical emergency. Ch. 62

dementia A collection of symptoms caused by various diseases affecting the brain. Ch. 62

dementia with Lewy bodies (DLB) A type of dementia characterized by the presence of Lewy bodies (deposits of α-synuclein protein) throughout the cortex as well as in the brainstem and autonomic structures (amygdala, medulla, pons). Ch. 62

demonstration–return demonstration Strategy commonly used by nurses in which the patient is shown how to perform a motor skill–based task and the patient returns the demonstration with the nurse as observer. Ch. 4

deoxyribonucleic acid (DNA) A nucleic acid that contains the instructions in cells that drive most cellular processes by synthesizing specific proteins; genes are made up of DNA. Ch. 15

dermatomes Areas on the skin that are innervated primarily by a single spinal cord segment. Chs. 10, 58

dermatomyositis An inflammatory myopathy that presents with characteristic skin changes along with the symptoms of polymyositis (diffuse, idiopathic, inflammatory myopathies of the connective tissues, especially striated muscle, that produce bilateral weakness, usually most severe in the proximal or the limb-girdle muscles). Ch. 67

dermis Connective tissue below the epidermis. Ch. 25

determinants of health Factors that influence the health of individuals and groups. Ch. 1

deviated septum A misalignment of the normally straight nasal septum. Ch. 29

diabetes insipidus (DI) A group of conditions associated with a deficiency of production or secretion of antidiuretic hormone (ADH) or with a decreased renal response to ADH; caused by injury to the neurohypophyseal system. Ch. 51

diabetes mellitus (DM) A multisystem disease related to abnormal insulin production, impaired insulin utilization, or both. Ch. 52

diabetic ketoacidosis (DKA) An acute metabolic complication of diabetes mellitus occurring when fats are metabolized in the absence of insulin; caused by a profound deficiency of insulin and characterized by hyperglycemia, ketosis, metabolic acidosis, and dehydration (volume depletion). Ch. 52

diabetic nephropathy A microvascular complication of diabetes mellitus associated with damage to the small blood vessels that supply the glomeruli of the kidney; the leading cause of end-stage renal disease in Canada. Ch. 52

diabetic neuropathy Nerve damage that occurs because of the metabolic derangements associated with diabetes mellitus. Ch. 52

dialysis The movement of fluid and molecules across a semipermeable membrane from one compartment to another; a clinical technique in which substances move from the blood through a semipermeable membrane (dialyzer) and into a dialysis solution (dialysate), used to correct fluid and electrolyte imbalances and to remove waste products in renal failure. Ch. 49

diarrhea The frequent passage of loose, watery stools; a symptom, not a disease. Ch. 45

diastole Relaxation of the myocardium. Ch. 34

diastolic blood pressure (DBP) The residual pressure of the arterial system during ventricular relaxation. Ch. 34

diffuse axonal injury (DAI) Widespread axonal damage occurring after a mild, moderate, or severe traumatic brain injury. Ch. 59

diffusion The movement of molecules from an area of high concentration to one of low concentration. Ch. 19

diffusion limitation Decrease in gas exchange across the alveolar–capillary membrane caused by processes that thicken or destroy the membrane. Ch. 70

digestion The physical and chemical breakdown of food into absorbable substances; involves both mechanical digestion (mastication) and chemical digestion. Ch. 41

dilated cardiomyopathy (DCM) A disease characterized by a diffuse inflammation and rapid degeneration of myocardial fibres that result in ventricular dilation, impairment of systolic function, atrial enlargement, and stasis of blood in the left ventricle. Ch. 39

disability Any of a range of mental or physical impairments that limit a person's functioning in society and may result in their interacting with socially constructed barriers. Ch. 5

disaster The outcome of a natural hazard or event (e.g., hurricane, flood, earthquake) or a result of human action or error, whether malicious (e.g., terrorist attacks, use of biological warfare) or unintentional (e.g., an accidental chemical spill), that seriously disrupts the functioning of a community or society. Ch. 72

disaster nursing The provision of nursing care, advocacy, and health promotion within the context of a disaster situation. Ch. 72

disease A condition that a practitioner views from a pathophysiological model. Ch. 5

dislocation A severe injury of the ligamentous structures that surround a joint that results in the complete displacement of the bone from its normal position. Ch. 65

disseminated intravascular coagulation (DIC) A serious bleeding and thrombotic disorder resulting from the abnormally initiated and accelerated clotting and anticlotting processes that occur in response to disease or injury. Ch. 33

distress A negative response to stress that occurs when demands made exceed a person's normal coping ability. Ch. 8

diversity Presence of persons with differences from the majority or dominant group that is assumed to be the norm. Ch. 2

diverticulum An outpouching of the mucosa through the circular smooth muscle of the intestinal wall; may occur at any point within the gastrointestinal tract but is most commonly found in the sigmoid colon. Ch. 45

drowning Death from suffocation after submersion in water or another fluid medium. Ch. 71

dry gangrene Necrosis of an appendage as a result of degenerative changes that occur with chronic diseases such as atherosclerosis or diabetes, when the blood supply to the lower extremities is gradually reduced. Ch. 14

ductus deferens (or vas deferens) A long, thick tube through which sperm exit the epididymis. Ch. 53

dysarthria A disturbance in the muscular control of speech. Ch. 60

dysmenorrhea Abdominal cramping pain or discomfort associated with menstrual flow. Ch. 56

dyspareunia Pain during sexual intercourse. Ch. 53

dysphagia Difficulty swallowing. Ch. 44

dysphasia Impaired ability to communicate; often used interchangeably with *aphasia*. Ch. 60

dysplasia Abnormal differentiation of dividing cells that results in changes in their size, shape, and appearance. Ch. 14

dysplastic nevi (DN) Atypical moles that are larger than usual and have irregular borders and various shades of colour. Ch. 26

dyspnea Shortness of breath. Ch. 28

dysrhythmias Abnormal cardiac rhythms. Ch. 38

E

ecchymosis Bruising. Ch. 32

ectopic pregnancy The implantation of the fertilized ovum anywhere outside the uterine cavity. Ch. 56

ejection fraction (EF) The percentage of end-diastolic blood volume that is ejected during systole. Ch. 34

elastic recoil The tendency for the lungs to recoil after being stretched or expanded. Ch. 28

elder abuse Any action, or lack of appropriate action, by someone in a relationship of trust, that causes harm or distress to an older person. Ch. 7

elder mistreatment An act of commission (elder abuse) or omission (elder neglect) that harms or threatens to harm an older person's health or welfare. Ch. 7

elective surgery Surgery that is planned. Ch. 20

electrical burns Burns that result from intense heat generated from an electric current. Ch. 27

electrocardiogram (ECG) A graphic tracing of the electrical impulses produced in the heart. Ch. 38

electrolytes Substances whose molecules dissociate or split into ions when placed in solution. Ch. 19

electronic health records (EHRs) Computerized records of patient information that are shared among all health care team members involved in a patient's care and that move with the patient to other providers and across care settings. Ch. 1

embolic stroke A stroke that occurs when an embolus lodges in and occludes a cerebral artery, resulting in infarction and edema of the area supplied by the involved vessel. Ch. 60

embolus A piece of material that causes a blockage within the arterial blood supply, such as a clot (thrombus). Ch. 40

emergence delirium A reversible neurological alteration that occurs in some patients awakening from anaesthesia after surgery, manifesting as restlessness, agitation, disorientation, thrashing, and shouting. Ch. 22

emergency A present or imminent event that requires a rapid and skilled response to protect the health, safety, and wellness of individuals and to limit damage to property or the environment. Ch. 72

emergency management and disaster planning Advanced preparation for a variety of potential situations, including mass casualty incidents, natural or biological events, technological failures, human conflicts, and acts of terrorism. Ch. 72

emergency surgery Surgery that is unexpected and urgent. Ch. 20

emerging infectious disease An infectious disease whose incidence has recently increased or threatens to increase in the immediate future. Ch. 17

emotion-focused coping Coping strategies that involve managing the emotions an individual feels when a stressful event occurs (e.g., meditation, yoga, prayer); useful when a person

needs respite from overthinking about a stressful situation. Ch. 8

empathy The quality that allows one person to enter into the world of another so as not to judge, sympathize, or correct but to establish mutual understanding. Ch. 4

emphysema Destruction of the alveoli. Ch. 31

empirical therapy Therapy based on observation and experience, implemented when the condition's exact cause is not known. Ch. 30

empyema A pleural effusion that contains pus. Ch. 30

encephalitis Acute inflammation of the brain. Ch. 59

endemic A communicable disease that applies to a group of people or a region or country and that has a constant presence (e.g., malaria in some areas of Africa, Dengue fever in Asia). Ch. 72

end-of-life care Care provided during the last months, weeks, and days for a person with a life-limiting illness. Ch. 13

endometriosis The presence of endometrial epithelial cells in sites outside the uterine cavity. Ch. 56

endomyocardial biopsy (EMB) A technique that involves removing several small pieces of myocardial tissue percutaneously from the right ventricle and microscopically examining the samples. Ch. 39

endoscopy The direct visualization of a body structure through a lighted fibre-optic instrument (endoscope). Ch. 41

endotracheal (ET) intubation Insertion of a tube into the trachea, bypassing the upper airway and laryngeal structures, to create an artificial airway. Ch. 68

end-stage renal disease (ESRD) Advanced kidney disease with glomerular filtration rate less than 15 mL/min/1.73 m², when most patients with chronic kidney disease require some form of renal replacement therapy; also referred to as *stage 5 CKD.* Ch. 49

enteral nutrition (EN) Nutrition (e.g., a nutritionally balanced liquefied food or formula) delivered through the gastrointestinal tract distal to the oral cavity via a tube, catheter, or stoma. Ch. 42

enucleation Removal of the eye. Ch. 24

epidemic An occurrence of the number of cases of a communicable disease exceeding the normal expected occurrence during a given period. Ch. 72

epidermis The thin, avascular outer layer of the skin; made up of an outer, dead portion that serves as a protective barrier and a deeper, living portion that folds into the dermis. Ch. 25

epididymis A comma-shaped structure located on the posterior-superior aspect of each testis within the scrotum; transports the sperm as they mature. Ch. 53

epididymitis An inflammation of the epididymis, usually secondary to an infectious process and rarely as a result of trauma or urinary reflux down the vas deferens from the urethra. Ch. 57

epidural analgesia The infusion of pain-relieving medications through a catheter placed into the epidural space surrounding the spinal cord. Ch. 22

epidural block Injection of a local anaesthetic into the epidural (extradural) space via either a thoracic or a lumbar approach. Ch. 21

epidural hematoma A collection of blood that results from bleeding between the dura mater and the inner surface of the skull; produces compression of the dura mater and thus of the brain. Ch. 59

epilepsy A type of seizure disorder in which at least two spontaneous seizures occur more than 24 hours apart; often caused by an underlying pathology. Ch. 61

epispadias A congenital opening of the urethra on the dorsal surface of the penis; usually associated with other genitourinary tract defects. Ch. 57

epistaxis Nosebleed. Ch. 29

equianalgesic dose A dose of one analgesic that produces pain-relieving effects equivalent to those of another analgesic. Ch. 10

erectile dysfunction (ED) The inability to attain or maintain an erect penis that allows satisfactory sexual performance. Ch. 57

erythema Skin redness occurring in patches of variable size and shape, caused by heat, certain medications, alcohol, ultraviolet rays, and conditions that cause dilation of blood vessels to the skin. Ch. 25

erythropoiesis The process of red blood cell production. Ch. 32

escharotomy Scalpel or electrocautery incision into necrotic tissue from a severe burn; performed when circulation to extremities is compromised. Ch. 27

esophageal cancer A rare malignant neoplasm of the esophagus; the two main types are squamous cell carcinoma and adenocarcinoma. Ch. 44

esophageal diverticula Saclike outpouchings of one or more layers of the esophagus. Ch. 44

esophageal speech A method of swallowing air, trapping it in the esophagus, and releasing it to create sound. Ch. 29

esophageal varices Complexes of tortuous veins at the lower end of the esophagus; they are enlarged and swollen as a result of portal hypertension; ruptured esophageal varices are a medical emergency. Ch. 46

esophagitis Inflammation of the esophagus. Ch. 44

ethnicity Characteristics of a group whose members share a common social, cultural, linguistic, or religious heritage and often implies a geographic or national affiliation. Ch. 2

ethnocentrism A tendency of people to believe that their way of viewing and responding to the world is the most correct, natural, and superior one. Ch. 2

ethnogeriatrics A specialty area of providing culturally competent care for older people who are identified with a particular ethnic group. Ch. 7

eustress Stress that is a positive protective and adaptative reaction that motivates people to overcome challenges. Ch. 8

evaluation Process of determining whether identified outcomes have been met. Ch. 1

evidence-informed nursing Nursing that employs best practices as determined by the most current reliable research. Ch. 1

evisceration   Protrusion of intestines through a wound when wound edges separate to a certain extent. Ch. 14

Ewing sarcoma family of tumours (ESFT)   One of the most common primary malignant neoplasms of bone and soft tissue; characterized by rapid growth within the medullary cavity of long bones, especially the femur, humerus, pelvis, and tibia. Ch. 66

excision and grafting   Procedure during which eschar is removed down to the subcutaneous tissue or fascia, depending on the degree of injury, and a graft is then placed on clean, viable tissue to achieve good adherence. Ch. 27

exophthalmos   A bilateral, unilateral, or asymmetrical protrusion of the eyeballs from the orbits; a type of infiltrative ophthalmopathy that results from impairment of venous drainage from the orbit, which causes increased fat deposits and fluid (edema) in the retro-orbital tissues. Ch. 51

expected patient outcomes   Goals that articulate what is desired or expected as a result of care. Ch. 1

explanatory model   Set of beliefs regarding what causes the disease or illness and the methods that would potentially best treat the condition. Ch. 2

external otitis   Inflammation or infection of the epithelium of the auricle and ear canal. Ch. 24

extravasation   The infiltration of medications into tissues surrounding the infusion site. Ch. 18

F

facilitated diffusion   Diffusion that involves the use of a protein carrier in the cell membrane (e.g., glucose transport into cell). Ch. 19

facilitator   Someone who helps a group of people share insights about a common problem and keeps information moving among group members. Ch. 4

familial Alzheimer's disease   Alzheimer's disease that develops in someone younger than 60 years old; also known as *early-onset AD*. Ch. 62

family and intimate partner violence (IPV)   A pattern of coercive behaviour in a relationship that involves fear, humiliation, intimidation, neglect, or intentional physical, emotional, financial, or sexual injury or assault; or it is a combination of these. Ch. 71

family care conferences   Conferences that provide opportunities for the patient, their caregivers, and members of the interprofessional health care team to identify care needs, evaluate care goals, and assist with health care matters. Ch. 4

family-centred care   An approach to nursing care that involves patients and families in the planning, delivery, and evaluation of health care and emphasizes dignity and respect, information sharing, participation, and collaboration. Ch. 6

family presence   The attendance of one or more family members or significant others in a place where they can have physical or visual contact with the patient during resuscitation or invasive procedures. Ch. 71

fat embolism syndrome (FES)   A syndrome characterized by the presence of systemic fat globules that are distributed into tissues and organs after a traumatic skeletal injury involving fractures. Ch. 65

fatigue   A subjective and complex condition that prevents functioning at normal capacity because of a feeling of exhaustion. Ch. 5

fecal impaction   An accumulation of hardened feces in the rectum or the sigmoid colon that the individual is unable to move. Ch. 45

fecal incontinence   The involuntary passage of stool. Ch. 45

fetor hepaticus   A musty, sweet odour of the patient's breath resulting from the accumulation of digestive byproducts that the liver is unable to degrade. Ch. 46

fibrinolysis   A means of maintaining blood in its fluid form; a continual process that results in the dissolution of fibrin and thus clots. Ch. 32

fibroadenoma   A common cause of discrete benign breast lumps in young women; painless, round, well delineated, and very mobile. Ch. 54

fibroblasts   Immature connective tissue cells that migrate into the healing site and secrete collagen. Ch. 14

fibrocystic changes   A benign condition of the breasts characterized by development of excess fibrous tissue, hyperplasia of the epithelial lining of the mammary ducts, proliferation of mammary ducts, and cyst formation. Ch. 54

fibromyalgia   A chronic disorder characterized by widespread, nonarticular musculoskeletal pain and fatigue with multiple tender points. Ch. 67

fistula   An abnormal passage that forms between organs or between a hollow organ and the skin. Ch. 14

flail chest   A condition resulting from multiple rib fractures, causing instability of the chest wall. Ch. 30

fluid spacing   Distribution of body water in different body compartments. Ch. 19

focal seizures   One of the major classes of seizures; caused by electrical activity that begins in a specific region of the cortex, as indicated by the electroencephalogram and the clinical manifestations. (Previously known as *partial seizures*.) Ch. 61

food security   The ready availability of enough nutritious food to meet the daily requirements and food preferences for health and well-being. Ch. 42

fracture   A disruption or break in the continuity of the structure of bone. Ch. 65

frailty   A medical condition with the presence of three or more of the following: unplanned weight loss, weakness, poor endurance and energy, slowness, and low activity. Ch. 7

frontotemporal dementia (FTD)   A type of dementia characterized by degeneration of the frontal lobe, temporal lobe, or both. Ch. 62

frostbite   True tissue freezing, which results in the formation of ice crystals in the tissues and cells. Ch. 71

full-thickness burn   Destruction of all skin elements and subcutaneous tissues, with possible involvement of muscles, tendons, and bones. Ch. 27

fulminant hepatitis   An acute clinical syndrome that results in severe impairment or necrosis of liver cells and potential liver failure. Ch. 46

fungi   Organisms similar to plants but lacking in chlorophyll. Ch. 17

G

galactorrhea   A milky secretion from the nipple caused by inappropriate lactation. Ch. 54

gastric cancer   Adenocarcinoma of the stomach wall; also called *stomach cancer*; the third-most frequent cause of cancer death worldwide. Ch. 44

gastritis   Inflammation of the gastric mucosa. Ch. 44

gastroenteritis   An inflammation of the mucosa of the stomach and the small intestine. Ch. 45

gastroesophageal reflux disease (GERD)   A syndrome presenting as any clinically significant symptomatic condition or histopathological alteration presumed to be secondary to reflux of gastric contents into the lower esophagus. Ch. 44

general anaesthesia   An altered physiological state characterized by reversible loss of consciousness, skeletal muscle relaxation, amnesia, and analgesia. Ch. 21

general survey statement   Statement of the health care provider's general impression of a patient, including behavioural observations. Ch. 3

generalized seizures   Seizures characterized by bilateral synchronous epileptic discharges in the brain from the onset, with no warning or aura; in most cases, the patient loses consciousness for a few seconds to several minutes. Ch. 61

gene therapy   A technique used to treat the underlying cause of a disease; to supply a missing gene, avoid the missing gene's role, or enhance treatment of a disease. Ch. 15

genetic counsellor   A health care provider with specialized training and experience in the areas of medical genetics and counselling who provides information and support to individuals and families. Ch. 15

genetics   The study of genes and their role in inheritance. Ch. 15

genital herpes   A sexually transmitted infection caused by the herpes simplex virus (HSV), usually HSV-2; results in painful genital or anal vesicular lesions. Ch. 55

genotype   The genetic makeup of a person. Ch. 15

geragogy   The method and practice of educating older people. Ch. 4

gerontological nursing   A nursing specialty that revolves around the care of older people. Ch. 7

gestational diabetes mellitus (GDM)   Diabetes mellitus that develops during pregnancy; glucose intolerance first recognized in pregnancy. Ch. 52

Glasgow Coma Scale (GCS)   A quick, practical, and standardized system for assessing the degree to which consciousness is impaired. Ch. 59

glaucoma   A group of disorders characterized by elevated intraocular pressure and its consequences, including optic nerve atrophy and peripheral visual field loss. Ch. 24

glial cells   The cells in the nervous system that provide support, nourishment, and protection to neurons. Ch. 58

glomerular filtration rate (GFR)   The amount of blood filtered by the glomeruli in a given time. Ch. 47

glomerulonephritis An immune-related inflammation of the glomeruli characterized by proteinuria, hematuria, decreased urine production, and edema. Ch. 48

glomerulus A capillary network within the kidneys that comprises up to 50 capillaries. Ch. 47

glucagon A hormone synthesized and released from pancreatic α cells in response to low blood glucose levels, protein ingestion, and exercise; increases blood glucose by stimulating glycogenolysis, gluconeogenesis, and ketogenesis. Ch. 50

glycated hemoglobin (A$_{1c}$) The amount of glucose that has been attached to hemoglobin molecules, which are attached to the red blood cell for the life of the cell (approximately 120 days). Ch. 52

glycemic index (GI) The rise in blood glucose levels after a person has consumed carbohydrate-containing food. Ch. 52

goitre An abnormal growth of the thyroid gland; the thyroid cells are stimulated to grow, which may result in an overactive thyroid (hyperthyroidism) or an underactive one (hypothyroidism). Ch. 51

gonads The primary reproductive organs (i.e., ovaries in the female and testes in the male). Ch. 53

gonorrhea The second-most frequently occurring sexually transmitted infection, caused by *Neisseria gonorrhoeae*, which spreads by direct physical contact with an infected host, usually during sexual activity (vaginal, oral, or anal). Ch. 55

Goodpasture's syndrome An autoimmune disease characterized by the presence of circulating antibodies against the glomerular and alveolar basement membranes. Ch. 48

gout A type of arthritis characterized by elevation of uric acid and the deposit of uric acid crystals in one or more joints; characteristic deposits of sodium urate crystals occur in articular, periarticular, and subcutaneous tissues. Ch. 67

Graves' disease An autoimmune disease of unknown etiology marked by diffuse thyroid enlargement and excessive thyroid hormone secretion. Ch. 51

grief A normal reaction to loss that may manifest in both psychological and physiological ways. Ch. 13

guided imagery The use of directed thoughts or suggestions to generate mental images to positively influence an individual's health and well-being. Ch. 8

Guillain-Barré syndrome (GBS) An acute, rapidly progressing, and potentially fatal form of polyneuritis believed to be caused by a cell-mediated immunological reaction directed at the peripheral nerves. Ch. 63

gummas Chronic, destructive lesions associated with late syphilis and affecting any organ of the body, especially the skin, bones, liver, and mucous membranes. Ch. 55

gynecomastia A transient, noninflammatory enlargement of one or both breasts in men. 54

H

hazards Anything that has the potential to cause harm or loss; can be substances, human activities, or physical events that may cause injury or loss of life, threaten the delivery of critical services, cause social and economic disruption, or cause property or environmental damage. Ch. 72

headache Probably the most common type of pain that humans experience. The majority of people have functional headaches, such as migraine or tension-type headaches; others have organic headaches caused by intracranial or extracranial disease. Ch. 61

head injury Any trauma to the scalp, the skull, or the brain. Ch. 59

health A state encompassing the physical, mental, and social aspects of well-being rather than one solely defined by the absence of disease. Ch. 5

health equity A situation of creating equal opportunities for good health for everyone by decreasing the negative effect of the social determinants of health and improving services to enhance access and reduce exclusion. Ch. 2

health-related hardiness (HRH) A personality resource characterized by a sense of control, commitment, and challenge and an ability to withstand a high degree of stress without falling ill. Ch. 5

health-related quality of life (HRQL) At an individual level, perceptions of physical and mental health status; at a community level, resources, conditions, policies, and practices that influence a population's health perceptions and functional status. Ch. 5

heart failure (HF) An abnormal clinical syndrome involving impaired cardiac pumping or filling, or both. Ch. 37

heart failure with mid-range ejection fraction (HFmEF) Heart failure with a left ventricular ejection fraction of 41 to 49%; a term that applies to patients transitioning to and from heart failure with preserved ejection fraction (HFpEF). Ch. 37

heart failure with preserved ejection fraction (HFpEF) The inability of the ventricles to relax and fill during diastole. Ch. 37

heart failure with reduced ejection fraction (HFrEF) Heart failure that results from an inability of the heart to pump blood effectively; the most common form of HF. Ch. 37

heat cramps Severe cramps in large muscle groups fatigued by heavy work. Ch. 71

heat exhaustion A clinical syndrome characterized by fatigue, light-headedness, nausea, vomiting, diarrhea, and a sensation of impending doom, caused by prolonged exposure to heat over hours or days. Ch. 71

heatstroke The most serious form of heat stress, resulting from failure of the central thermoregulatory mechanisms. Ch. 71

heaves Sustained lifts of the chest wall in the precordial area that can be seen or palpated. Ch. 34

hematemesis Vomiting of blood, which indicates bleeding in the upper gastrointestinal tract. Ch. 41

hematopoiesis Blood cell production. Ch. 32

hemochromatosis An iron overload disorder caused primarily by a genetic defect or occurring secondary to diseases such as sideroblastic anemia or liver disease. Ch. 33

hemodialysis (HD) A type of dialysis that uses a machine to remove waste products and excess fluid from the blood by pumping the blood through an artificial semipermeable membrane. Ch. 49

hemodynamic monitoring The measurement of pressure, flow, and oxygenation within the cardiovascular system. Ch. 68

hemoglobin A complex compound composed of heme (an iron compound) and globin (a simple protein) that binds with oxygen and carbon dioxide. Ch. 32

hemolysis Destruction of red blood cells. Ch. 32

hemolytic anemia A condition caused by the destruction or hemolysis of red blood cells at a rate that exceeds production. Ch. 33

hemophilia An X-linked recessive genetic disorder caused by defective or deficient coagulation factor. Ch. 33

hemorrhagic stroke A stroke that results from bleeding into the brain tissue itself or into the subarachnoid space or the ventricles. Ch. 60

hemorrhoids Varicosities in the lower rectum or the anus caused by congestion in the veins of the hemorrhoidal plexus. Ch. 45

hemothorax An accumulation of blood in the intrapleural space. Ch. 30

hepatic encephalopathy A neuropsychiatric manifestation of advanced liver disease, resulting from ammonia crossing the blood–brain barrier; manifested as changes in neurological and mental responsiveness; impaired consciousness; inappropriate behaviour; and fluctuating levels of consciousness, ranging from sleep disturbances to deep coma. Ch. 46

hepatitis Inflammation of the liver. Ch. 46

hepatocytes Specialized hepatic cells. Ch. 41

hepatorenal syndrome (HRS) A serious complication of decompensated cirrhosis; it occurs in two forms: HRS-AKI, characterized by rapidly progressive renal failure in the setting of multiorgan failure, and HRS-AKD, characterized by gradual kidney dysfunction. Ch. 46

herbal therapy The use of individual herbs or combinations of herbs for therapeutic benefit; also known as *botanical medicine* or *phytotherapy*. Ch. 12

hernia A protrusion of a viscus through an abnormal opening or a weakened area in the wall of the cavity in which it is normally contained. Ch. 45

herniated intervertebral disc Herniation of nuclear material from the intervertebral disc that may compress or place tension on a cervical, lumbar, or sacral spinal nerve root, causing acute back pain; also called a *slipped disc*. Ch. 66

herpes zoster (shingles) Varicella-zoster virus infection, characterized by an eruption of grouped vesicles on erythematous base; usually unilateral on trunk, face, and lumbosacral areas. Ch. 26

heterozygous Having two different alleles for one given gene. Ch. 15

hiatal hernia Herniation of a portion of the stomach into the esophagus through an opening, or hiatus, in the diaphragm. Ch. 44

hirsutism Male-pattern distribution of hair in women, caused by an abnormality of ovaries or adrenal glands, decrease in estrogen level, or heredity. Ch. 25

histological grading A categorization of tumours in which the appearance of cells and the degree of differentiation are evaluated pathologically; four grades are used. Ch. 18

Hodgkin's lymphoma A malignant condition characterized by proliferation of abnormal, giant, multinucleated cells, called *Reed–Sternberg cells*, which are located in lymph nodes; also called *Hodgkin's disease*. Ch. 33

holding area Also called the *preoperative holding area*; an admission and waiting area inside or adjacent to the surgical suite. Ch. 21

holistic nursing Nursing practice based on the philosophies of holism and humanism that integrates mind–body–spirit principles into the development of caring and therapeutic relationships with patients that support healing and well-being. Ch. 12

home health nursing A specialized area of nursing practice rooted in community health nursing in which nursing care is delivered in the residence of the patient. Ch. 6

homeostasis The state of equilibrium in the internal environment of the body, naturally maintained by adaptive responses that promote healthy survival. Ch. 19

homozygous Having two identical alleles for one given gene. Ch. 15

hordeolum An infection of the sebaceous glands in the eyelid margin; commonly called a *stye*. Ch. 24

hormones Chemical substances synthesized and secreted by endocrine glands; most hormones have common characteristics, including secretion in small amounts at variable but predictable rates, regulation by feedback systems, and the ability to bind to specific target cell receptors. Ch. 50

hospice palliative care Term describing the convergence of hospice and palliative care; care is aimed at improving the quality of life of patients with life-threatening illness and of their families through the relief of pain and suffering. Ch. 13

hospital-acquired pneumonia (HAP) Pneumonia occurring 48 hours or longer after hospital admission and not incubating at the time of hospitalization. Ch. 30

human immunodeficiency virus (HIV) Retrovirus that causes AIDS. Ch. 17

human leukocyte antigen (HLA) system A series of linked genes that occur together on the sixth chromosome in humans that plays an important part in the body's immune response to foreign substances. Ch. 16

humoral immunity Antibody-mediated immunity. Ch. 16

Huntington's disease (HD) A genetically transmitted, autosomal dominant, progressive, degenerative brain disorder that affects both men and women; characterized by chronic loss of all neurological function, resulting in movement disorder, cognitive and psychiatric challenges, and eventually impairment of all psychomotor processes. Ch. 61

hydrocele A nontender, fluid-filled mass that results from interference with lymphatic drainage of the scrotum and swelling of the tunica vaginalis that surrounds the testis. Ch. 57

hydronephrosis Dilation or enlargement of the renal pelvis and the calyces resulting from increased bladder pressure and backflow of urine to the kidney caused by obstruction in the lower urinary tract. Ch. 48

hydrostatic pressure The force within a fluid compartment. Ch. 19

hydroureter Dilation of the renal pelvis caused by backflow of urine. Ch. 48

hyperaldosteronism A condition characterized by excessive aldosterone secretion. Ch. 51

hypercapnia The presence of excessive amounts of carbon dioxide in the blood; also called *hypercarbia*. Ch. 70

hypercapnic respiratory failure A partial pressure of arterial carbon dioxide ($PaCO_2$) above normal (>45 mm Hg) in combination with acidemia (arterial pH <7.35). Ch. 70

hyperopia A condition in which an affected person can see distant objects clearly (farsightedness) but near objects appear blurred. Chs. 23, 24

hyperosmolar hyperglycemic state (HHS) A life-threatening syndrome that can occur in the patient with diabetes mellitus who is able to produce enough insulin to prevent diabetic ketoacidosis but not enough to prevent severe hyperglycemia, osmotic diuresis, and extracellular fluid depletion. Ch. 52

hyperparathyroidism A condition involving increased secretion of parathyroid hormone (PTH). Ch. 51

hyperplasia Multiplication of cells as a result of increased cellular division. Ch. 14

hypersensitivity reaction An overreactive immune response against foreign antigens or a reaction against one's own tissue that may result in tissue damage. Ch. 16

hypertension Sustained elevation of systemic arterial blood pressure; in adults, exists when systolic blood pressure (SBP) is equal to or greater than 140 mm Hg or diastolic blood pressure (DBP) is equal to or greater than 90 mm Hg. Ch. 35

hypertensive crisis A severe and abrupt elevation in blood pressure, arbitrarily defined as a diastolic blood pressure above 120 to 130 mm Hg. Ch. 35

hyperthyroidism Hyperactivity of the thyroid gland with sustained increase in synthesis and release of thyroid hormones. Ch. 51

hypertonic Solutions in which solutes are more concentrated than they are in cells. Ch. 19

hypertrophic cardiomyopathy (HCM) Asymmetrical left ventricular hypertrophy without ventricular dilation. Ch. 39

hypertrophic scar An inappropriately large, red, raised, and hard scar. Ch. 14

hypertrophy Expansion in the size of cells, which results in increased tissue mass without cell division. Ch. 14

hypoparathyroidism An uncommon condition associated with abnormal parathyroid development and inadequate levels of circulating parathyroid hormone (PTH); characterized by

hypocalcemia that results from a lack of PTH to maintain serum calcium levels. Ch. 51

hypopituitarism A rare disorder that involves a decrease in one or more of the pituitary hormones. Ch. 51

hypospadias A urological abnormality in which the urethral meatus is located on the ventral surface of the penis anywhere from the corona to the perineum. Ch. 57

hypothermia A core temperature of less than 35°C; occurs when heat loss exceeds heat production. Chs. 22, 71

hypothyroidism Insufficient circulation of thyroid hormone as a result of various abnormalities; can be primary or secondary. Ch. 51

hypotonic Solutions in which solutes are less concentrated than they are in cells. Ch. 19

hypovolemic shock Shock that occurs from inadequate fluid volume in the intravascular space to support adequate perfusion. Ch. 69

hypoxemia Low oxygen tension in the blood (partial pressure of oxygen in arterial blood [PaO_2] <60 mm Hg), characterized by a variety of nonspecific clinical signs and symptoms. Ch. 70

hypoxemic respiratory failure A condition in which the partial pressure of oxygen in arterial blood (PaO_2) is 60 mm Hg or less when the patient is receiving inspired oxygen at a fractional concentration (FiO_2) of 60% or greater. Ch. 70

hypoxia The condition in which the partial pressure of oxygen in arterial blood (PaO_2) has fallen sufficiently to cause signs and symptoms of inadequate oxygenation. Ch. 70

hysterectomy Surgical removal of the uterus. Ch. 56

I

ileal conduit Urinary diversion procedure; ureters are anastomosed into a segment of ileum that is converted into a conduit for urinary drainage; the other end of the bowel is brought out through the abdominal wall to form a stoma. Ch. 48

illness The human experience of symptoms and suffering; specifically, how the disease is perceived, lived with, and responded to by individuals and their families. Ch. 5

illness behaviour The varying ways individuals respond to physical symptoms: how they monitor internal states, define and interpret symptoms, make attributions, take remedial actions, and use various sources of informal and formal care. Ch. 5

illness trajectory An experiential pathway along which the person with an illness progresses; it includes three phases: crisis phase, chronic phase, and terminal phase. Ch. 5

immunity The body's ability to resist disease. Ch. 16

immunocompetence The ability of the body's immune system to identify and inactivate or destroy foreign substances. Ch. 16

immunodeficiency The inability of the immune system to protect the body adequately. Ch. 16

immunological surveillance The response of the immune system to antigens of the malignant cells. Ch. 18

immunosuppressive therapy Therapy with the goal of adequately suppressing the immune response to prevent rejection of a transplanted organ and yet maintain sufficient immunity to prevent overwhelming infection; also used to treat autoimmune disorders. Ch. 16

impetigo A condition caused by group A β-hemolytic streptococci, staphylococci, or a combination of both and characterized by pruritus and an eruption of vesiculopustular lesions with a honey-coloured crust surrounded by erythema. Ch. 26

implementation The use of nursing interventions to carry out the nursing care plan. Ch. 1

Indigenous health An approach to health care involving a balance of spiritual, emotional, physical, mental, and social aspects of life in order to achieve harmony with all things; illness or disease occurs when this life equilibrium is upset. Ch. 12

infective endocarditis (IE) An infection of the heart valves or the endocardial surface of the heart; previously called *bacterial endocarditis*. Ch. 39

infertility The inability to achieve a pregnancy after at least 1 year of regular unprotected intercourse. Ch. 56

inflammatory bowel disease (IBD) An autoimmune disease characterized by idiopathic inflammation and ulceration; includes two disorders of the gastrointestinal tract—Crohn's disease and ulcerative colitis. Ch. 45

inflammatory response A biological response to cell injury caused by pathogens, irritants, or chronic health conditions that neutralizes and dilutes the inflammatory agent, removes necrotic materials, and establishes an environment suitable for healing and repair. Ch. 14

informal caregiver A person who provides care without pay to support an individual with diminishing physical ability, a debilitating cognitive condition, or a chronic life-limiting illness. Ch. 5

informed consent An active decision-making process between the surgeon and the patient that allows the patient to assess information and make an informed decision; a written, signed, and witnessed surgical consent protects the patient, surgeon, hospital, and the health care team. Ch. 20

ingestion The intake of food. Ch. 41

insomnia Difficulty falling asleep, difficulty staying asleep, waking up too early, or poor quality of sleep. Ch. 9

inspection The visual examination of a part or region of the body to assess normal conditions or deviations. Ch. 3

insulin The principal regulator of the metabolism and storage of ingested carbohydrates, fats, and proteins; facilitates glucose transport across cell membranes in most tissues. Ch. 50

insulin resistance A condition in which body tissues do not respond to the action of insulin; caused by insulin receptors that are unresponsive to the action of insulin, insufficient in number, or both. Ch. 52

integrated palliative approach An approach to care that focuses on meeting a person's and family's full range of needs—physical, psychosocial, and spiritual—at all stages of illness, not just at the end of life. Ch. 13

integrins Cell receptors that mediate attachment between endothelial cells and surrounding tissues; involved in leukocyte extravasation during the immune response. Ch. 14

intermittent claudication An ischemic muscle ache or pain that is precipitated by exercise, resolves with rest, and is reproducible. Ch. 40

intersectionality A framework for understanding how multiple social identities such as ethnicity, gender, sexual orientation, and economic status interact with each other to reflect interlocking systems of privilege and oppression. Ch. 2

interstitial cystitis (IC) A chronic, painful inflammatory disease of the bladder characterized by symptoms of urgency, frequency, and pain in the bladder, pelvis, or both. Ch. 48

intertriginous Describing an area where opposing skin surfaces overlap and rub on each other, such as skin folds of groin, axilla, abdomen, or breast. Ch. 25

intestinal obstruction Partial or complete obstruction of the intestine, preventing intestinal contents from passing through the gastrointestinal tract; may be classified as mechanical or nonmechanical. Ch. 45

intracerebral hemorrhage A type of hemorrhagic stroke in which bleeding occurs within the brain, caused by a rupture of a blood vessel. Ch. 60

intracranial pressure (ICP) Pressure exerted because of the combined total volume of the three components within the skull: brain tissue, blood, and cerebrospinal fluid. Ch. 59

intraparenchymal or intracerebral hematoma A collection of blood within the parenchyma that results from bleeding within the brain tissue itself and occurs in approximately 16% of head injuries. Ch. 59

intravenous pyelography (IVP) A diagnostic study that enables visualization of the urinary tract; an intravenous contrast medium is injected, which circulates in the blood and is excreted by the kidneys into the urine; used to evaluate the presence, position, size, and shape of the kidneys, the ureters, and the bladder. Ch. 47

ions Electrically charged molecules. Ch. 19

iron-deficiency anemia A microcytic hypochromic anemia caused by inadequate supplies of the iron needed to synthesize hemoglobin; it is the most common nutritional disorder in the world. Ch. 33

irritable bowel syndrome (IBS) A chronic functional disorder characterized by intermittent and recurrent abdominal pain associated with an alteration in bowel function (diarrhea, constipation, or both). Ch. 45

ischemic strokes Strokes that result from inadequate blood flow to the brain from partial or complete occlusion of an artery. Ch. 60

isolated systolic hypertension (ISH) A sustained elevation in systolic blood pressure equal to or greater than 140 mm Hg with a diastolic blood pressure less than 90 mm Hg. Ch. 35

isometric contractions Muscular contractions that increase tension within a muscle but do not produce movement. Ch. 64

isotonic State in which the fluid that surrounds a cell has the same osmolality as the cell interior. Ch. 19

isotonic contractions Muscular contraction that shortens a muscle to produce movement. Ch. 64

J

Janeway's lesions Flat, painless, small, red spots that may be found on the palms and the soles of patients with infective endocarditis. Ch. 39

jaundice A yellowish discoloration of the skin and/or sclera resulting from an abnormal increase in the concentration of bilirubin in the blood. Chs. 25, 46

K

keloid A protrusion of scar tissue that extends beyond the wound edges and may form tumour-like masses. Ch. 14

keratinocytes Cells synthesized from epidermal cells in the basal layer; they produce a fibrous protein, called *keratin*, which is vital to the skin's protective barrier function. Ch. 25

keratitis An inflammation or infection of the cornea that can be caused by a variety of microorganisms or by other factors. Ch. 24

Korotkoff sounds Sounds of turbulent blood flow through a compressed artery. Ch. 34

Korsakoff syndrome An irreversible form of amnesia caused by thiamine deficiency and characterized by loss of short-term memory and an inability to learn. Ch. 11

Kupffer cells A type of macrophage found in the liver that removes bacteria and toxins from the blood. Ch. 41

kyphosis Forward bending of thoracic spine: exaggerated thoracic curvature. Ch. 64

L

lacrimal puncta A small opening on the summits of the lacrimal papillae, seen on the margins of the eyelids at the lateral extremity of the lateral lake; there are two lateral puncta (singular: *punctum*) in the medial (inside) portion of each eyelid.

lactase deficiency A condition in which the lactase enzyme is deficient or absent. Ch. 45

lapses Very short periods of substance use followed by quick return to maintaining nonuse. Ch. 11

laryngeal mask airway (LMA) A supraglottic airway device that is easily placed and used as a method of elective ventilation. Ch. 21

learning The act of a person acquiring knowledge, skills, or attitudes that may result in a permanent change. Ch. 4

learning needs The new knowledge and skills that an individual must acquire to be able to meet an objective or a goal. Ch. 4

learning outcomes The achieved results of what was learned; competencies and the knowledge that the patient has achieved and can demonstrate successfully. Ch. 4

learning style The way in which each individual understands and responds to a learning situation;

may be visual, auditory, or physical or kinetic. Ch. 4

leiomyomas Benign smooth muscle tumours that occur most commonly within the uterus; also known as *uterine fibroids*. Ch. 56

lens A biconvex structure located behind the iris and supported in place by small fibres, collectively called the *suspensory ligament* (also called the *zonule*), that connect the lens to the ciliary body; the primary function of the lens is to bend light rays, which enables them to fall onto the retina. Ch. 23

lethal injury Irreversible cell injury that causes cell death. Ch. 14

leukemia A broad term given to a group of malignant diseases that affect the blood and blood-forming tissues of the bone marrow, lymph system, and spleen. Ch. 33

leukocytosis Elevations in white blood cell count. Ch. 32

leukopenia An abnormal decrease in the total white blood cell count to less than 4×10^9/L. Ch. 32

leukoplakia A whitish precancerous lesion on the mucosa of the mouth or tongue that results from chronic irritation, especially from smoking. Ch. 44

lichenification A thickening of epidermis with exaggerated markings resembling a washboard, caused by chronic scratching or rubbing of the skin. Ch. 26

lifestyle The health choices made by individuals and the influence of social, economic, and environmental factors on the decisions people make about their health. Ch. 5

lipectomy Procedure performed to remove unsightly loose folds of adipose tissue for cosmetic reasons; also called *adipectomy*. Ch. 43

lipodystrophy A condition that produces lumps and dents in the skin—hypertrophy or atrophy of subcutaneous tissue; caused by repeated injection in the same spot. Ch. 52

lithotripsy The use of sound waves to break renal stones into small particles that can be eliminated from the urinary tract. Ch. 48

local anaesthesia The loss of sensation without loss of consciousness; induced topically or via intracutaneous or subcutaneous infiltration. Ch. 21

long-term care (LTC) facilities Placement alternatives for people who can no longer live alone, who need continuous supervision, who have three or more disabilities involving activities of daily living, or who are frail. Ch. 7

lordosis Lumbar spinal deformity resulting in exaggerated lumbar curvature; also called *swayback*. Ch. 64

low back pain (LBP) A condition most often due to a musculoskeletal condition caused by (a) acute lumbosacral strain, (b) instability of the lumbosacral bony mechanism, (c) osteoarthritis of the lumbosacral vertebrae, (d) degenerative disc disease, or (e) herniation of an intervertebral disc. Ch. 66

lower motor neurons (LMNs) The final common pathway through which descending motor tracts influence skeletal muscle, the effector organ for movement. Ch. 58

lumpectomy Breast-conserving surgery that involves the removal of the entire tumour along with a margin of normal surrounding tissue. Ch. 54

lung abscess A pus-containing lesion of the lung parenchyma that gives rise to a cavity. Ch. 30

Lyme disease A spirochetal infection caused by *Borrelia burgdorferi* and transmitted by the bite of an infected blacklegged or deer tick; the most characteristic clinical symptom of early localized disease is migrans, a skin lesion at the site of the tick bite that occurs within 3 to 30 days in 70 to 80% of people who are infected. Ch. 67

lymphedema Accumulation of lymph in soft tissue that results from the excision or irradiation of lymph nodes. Ch. 54

lymphomas Cancers originating in the bone marrow and lymphatic structures resulting in the proliferation of lymphocytes. Ch. 33

M

malabsorption syndrome The impaired absorption of nutrients from the gastrointestinal tract. Ch. 42

malignant hyperthermia (MH) A rare, potentially fatal metabolic disease characterized by hyperthermia with rigidity of skeletal muscles. Ch. 21

malignant melanoma A tumour arising in melanocytes, the cells producing melanin. Ch. 26

malignant neoplasms Tumours that have the ability to invade and metastasize; can be undifferentiated. Ch. 18

Mallory–Weiss tear A tear in the esophageal mucosa at the junction of the esophagus and the stomach and results in severe bleeding; usually caused by severe retching and vomiting. Ch. 44

malnutrition A deficit, excess, or imbalance of the essential components of a balanced diet. Ch. 42

mammoplasty Surgical change in the size or shape of the breast. Ch. 54

massage therapy Therapy involving the manipulation of soft tissues and joints of the body to improve health and promote healing. Ch. 12

mastalgia Breast pain; most common breast-related condition in women. Ch. 54

mastectomy Surgical removal of all or a portion of a breast. Ch. 54

mastitis An infl ammatory condition of the breast that occurs most frequently in lactating women; usually caused by staphylococcal infection. Ch. 54

mean arterial pressure (MAP) A measurement related to blood pressure; calculated by adding the systolic blood pressure to twice the diastolic pressure and dividing this amount by three. Ch. 34

mechanical receptors Receptors located in the lungs, upper airways, chest wall, and diaphragm that are stimulated by a variety of physiological factors, such as irritants, muscle stretching, and alveolar wall distortion. Ch. 28

mechanical ventilation The process by which ventilation and oxygenation is supported or conducted by a machine. Ch. 68

Medical Assistance in Dying (MAiD) The legal, safe, and intentional ending of the life of an adult, at their request, through the prescription or administration of medications. Ch. 13

medical-surgical nursing A type of nursing that involves caring for acutely ill adults experiencing complex variations in health. Ch. 1

megaloblastic anemias A group of disorders caused by impaired DNA synthesis and characterized by the presence of large red blood cells. Ch. 33

melanocytes Cells contained in the deep, basal layer (*stratum germinativum*) of the epidermis that contain melanin, a pigment that gives colour to the skin and hair and protects the body from damaging ultraviolet sunlight. Ch. 25

melena Abnormal, black, tarry stool containing digested blood. Ch. 41

menarche The first episode of menstrual bleeding; indicates that a girl has reached puberty. Ch. 53

Ménière's disease A condition characterized by symptoms caused by inner ear disease, including episodic vertigo, tinnitus, fluctuating sensorineural hearing loss, and a sense of aural fullness; results in an excessive accumulation of endolymph in the membranous labyrinth; also called *endolymphatic hydrops*. Ch. 24

meninges Three layers of protective membranes that surround the brain and the spinal cord: dura mater, arachnoid, and pia mater. Ch. 58

meningitis An acute inflammation of meningeal tissues (the pia mater, arachnoid mater, and dura mater) surrounding the brain and the spinal cord. Ch. 59

menopause The physiological cessation of menses associated with declining ovarian function. Chs. 53, 56

menstrual cycle A monthly process mediated by the hormonal activity of the hypothalamus, the pituitary gland, and the ovaries (during which the major functions of the ovaries are ovulation and the secretion of hormones). Ch. 53

metabolic syndrome A collection of risk factors that increase an individual's chance of developing cardiovascular disease and diabetes mellitus. Ch. 43

metaplasia Transformation of one cell type into another in response to a change in physiological condition or to an external irritant. Ch. 14

metastasis Spread of cancer to a distant site. Ch. 18

migraine headache A type of headache characterized by unilateral throbbing pain, a triggering event or factor, and manifestations associated with neurological and autonomic nervous system dysfunction; the effects of migraine headache pain are dramatic, often causing both physical and emotional disability. Ch. 61

mild cognitive impairment (MCI) A state of cognitive decline that is not severe enough to interfere with activities of daily living; also known as *mild neurocognitive disorder* (mNCD). Ch. 62

mitral valve prolapse (MVP) A structural abnormality of the mitral valve leaflets and the papillary muscles or chordae that allows the leaflets to prolapse, or buckle, back into the left atrium during ventricular systole. Ch. 39

moderate sedation Also known as *procedural sedation,* a mild depression of consciousness that results from administration of intravenous sedatives, analgesics, or both so patients can tolerate minor procedures yet still maintain airway control and minimize cardiopulmonary complications. Ch. 21

modifiable risk factors Factors such as behaviour that can be changed to reduce the risk of developing an illness. Ch. 5

modulation The activation of descending pathways that exert inhibitory or facilitatory effects on the transmission of pain. Ch. 10

mole (nevus) Benign overgrowth of melanocytes, occurring as a defect of development; excessive numbers of large, irregular moles are often hereditary. Ch. 25

monoclonal antibodies Homogeneous populations of identical antibody molecules produced by specialized tissue cell culture lines. Ch. 16

mons pubis A fatty layer lying over the pubic bone that is covered in coarse hair after puberty (in a triangular pattern in women and a diamond pattern in men). Ch. 53

morbidity Rates of disease in a population. Ch. 5

morbidly obese Classification describing individuals with a body mass index greater than 40 kg/m^2. Ch. 43

mortality Rates of death in a population. Ch. 5

motivational interviewing A collaborative, person-centred counselling approach using non-confrontational techniques to motivate patients to resolve their ambivalence and, ultimately, change behaviour. Ch. 11

multimorbidity The simultaneous occurrence of two to five or more chronic medical conditions in the same person. Ch. 5

multiple myeloma A condition in which cancerous plasma cells infiltrate the bone marrow and destroy bone. Ch. 33

multiple-organ dysfunction syndrome (MODS) In a patient who is acutely ill, the failure of two or more organ systems to such a degree that homeostasis cannot be maintained without intervention. Ch. 69

multiple sclerosis (MS) A chronic, progressive, degenerative autoimmune disorder of the central nervous system characterized by disseminated demyelination of nerve fibres of the brain, the spinal cord, and the optic nerves. Ch. 61

murmurs Sounds produced by turbulent blood flow through the heart or the walls of large arteries. Ch. 34

mutation A change in the DNA sequence of a gene, affecting the original expression of the gene. Ch. 15

myasthenia gravis (MG) An autoimmune disease of the neuromuscular junction characterized by fluctuating weakness of certain skeletal muscle groups. Ch. 61

myasthenic crisis An acute exacerbation of muscle weakness triggered by infection, surgery, emotional distress, pregnancy, exposure to certain medications, or beginning treatment with corticosteroids. Ch. 61

myelodysplastic syndrome (MDS) A group of related hematological disorders characterized by a change in the quantity and the quality of bone marrow elements. Ch. 33

myocardial infarction (MI) Irreversible myocardial cell death (necrosis) caused by sustained ischemia. Ch. 36

myocarditis A focal or diffuse inflammation of the myocardium. Ch. 39

myofascial pain syndrome A chronic form of muscle pain; characterized by musculoskeletal pain and tenderness, typically in the chest, neck, shoulders, hips, and lower back. Ch. 67

myopia A condition in which an affected person can see near objects clearly (nearsightedness) but objects in the distance appear blurred. Chs. 23, 24

myositis Diffuse, idiopathic, inflammatory myopathies of the connective tissues, especially striated muscle, that produce bilateral weakness, usually most severe in the proximal or limb-girdle muscles. Ch. 67

myxedema The accumulation of hydrophilic mucopolysaccharides in the dermis and other tissues; causes the characteristic facies of hypothyroidism (i.e., puffiness, periorbital edema, and masklike affect). Ch. 51

myxedema coma A medical emergency in which the mental sluggishness, drowsiness, and lethargy of hypothyroidism progresses gradually or suddenly to a notable impairment of consciousness or coma. Ch. 51

N

nadir The lowest level of the peripheral blood cell counts that occurs secondary to bone marrow depression. Ch. 18

naloxone An opioid antagonist medication that binds to opioid receptors and is used to reverse an opioid overdose. Ch. 11

narcolepsy A chronic degenerative neurological disorder caused by the brain's inability to regulate sleep–wake cycles normally. Ch. 9

nasal fracture Fracture of nasal bones, most often caused by trauma of substantial force to the middle of the face; classified as unilateral, bilateral, or complex. Ch. 29

nasal polyps Benign mucous membrane masses that form slowly in response to repeated inflammation of the sinus or the nasal mucosa. Ch. 29

nausea A feeling of discomfort in the epigastrium with a conscious desire to vomit. Ch. 44

necrosis Tissue death that occurs as a result of a traumatic injury, infection, or exposure to a toxic chemical that causes a local inflammatory response. Ch. 14

negative feedback A highly specialized mechanism in the regulation of hormone levels; the most common type of feedback system, in which the gland responds by increasing or decreasing the secretion of a hormone. Ch. 50

negative-pressure ventilation Noninvasive ventilation (i.e., not requiring an artificial airway) delivered through the use of chambers that encase the chest or body and surround it with intermittent subatmospheric (or negative) pressure. Ch. 68

nephrolithiasis The formation of stones in the urinary tract. Ch. 48

nephron The functional unit of the kidney; each kidney has about 1 million nephrons. Ch. 47

nephrosclerosis A vascular disease of the kidney characterized by sclerosis of the small arteries and arterioles of the kidney, resulting in renal tissue destruction. Ch. 48

nephrotic syndrome A clinical course associated with a number of disease conditions of the kidney; characterized by peripheral edema, massive proteinuria, dyslipidemia, and hypoalbuminemia. Ch. 48

neuraxial blocks Regional anaesthesia (epidural or spinal) that blocks pain transmission during surgery. Ch. 21

neurofibrillary tangles Abnormal collections of twisted protein threads inside nerve cells seen in the areas of the brain most affected by Alzheimer's disease. Ch. 62

neurogenic bladder A bladder dysfunction related to abnormal or absent bladder innervation. Ch. 63

neurogenic shock A hemodynamic syndrome of massive vasodilation without compensation that results from the loss of sympathetic nervous system vasoconstrictor tone caused by spinal cord injury at the fifth thoracic (T5) vertebra or above; characterized by hypotension, bradycardia, and loss of sympathetic innervation. Chs. 63, 69

neurons The primary functional units of the nervous system; they share three characteristics: excitability, conductivity, and the ability to influence other neurons, muscle cells, and glandular cells. Ch. 58

neuropathic pain Pain caused by damage to nerve cells or changes in the central nervous system, typically described as burning, shooting, stabbing, or electrical in nature. Ch. 10

neurosyphilis An infection of any part of the nervous system by the organism *Treponema pallidum.* Ch. 63

neurotransmitter A chemical agent that affects the transmission of an impulse across the synaptic cleft. Ch. 58

neutropenia An abnormal reduction of the neutrophil count to less than $1 \times 10^9/L$ to $1.5 \times 10^9/L$. Chs. 32, 33

nociception The activation of the primary afferent nociceptors with peripheral terminals (free nerve endings) that respond differently to noxious (tissue-damaging) stimuli. Ch. 10

nociceptive pain Pain caused by damage to somatic or visceral tissue. Ch. 10

nonalcoholic fatty liver disease (NAFLD) A spectrum of disease that ranges from simple fatty liver that causes no hepatic inflammation to severe liver scarring; characterized by accumulation of fat in liver cells, not associated with alcohol use. Ch. 46

nonalcoholic steatohepatitis (NASH) A condition characterized by the accumulation of fat in the liver cells, causing inflammation and liver cell injury resulting in fibrosis; occurs in people who drink little or no alcohol. Ch. 46

non-Hodgkin's lymphomas (NHLs) A heterogeneous group of cancers of primarily B-, T-, natural killer, histiocytic, and dendritic cell origin that can affect people of all ages. Ch. 33

nonmodifiable risk factors Factors such as age, sex, and genetic makeup that contribute to the development of an illness and cannot be changed. Ch. 5

normal pressure hydrocephalus (NPH) An abnormal increase of cerebrospinal fluid, characterized by an obstruction in the normal flow of cerebrospinal fluid throughout the brain, spinal cord, and ventricles; a relatively uncommon disorder. Ch. 61

NSTEMI Abbreviation for non–ST-segment elevation myocardial infarction; acute coronary syndrome resulting from the partial occlusion of an unstable atherosclerotic plaque by a thrombus. Ch. 36

nuchal rigidity Resistance to flexion of the neck. Ch. 59

nulliparous Never pregnant. Ch. 53

nursing diagnosis The process of the nurse's identifying and labelling human responses to actual or potential health problems; also, the product of this process as articulated in standard terminology. Ch. 1

nursing history Information used to determine the patient's strengths and responses to a health condition that is diagnosed and treated by nurses. Ch. 3

nursing informatics The integration of nursing science, computer science, and information technology to manage and communicate data, information, and knowledge in nursing practice. Ch. 1

nursing intervention A single nursing action, treatment, procedure, activity, or service designed to achieve an outcome of a nursing or medical diagnosis for which the nurse is accountable. Ch. 1

nursing leadership An attitude and approach in which lifelong learning and a commitment to excellence in practice are valued. Ch. 1

nursing process An assertive, problem-solving approach to the identification and treatment of patient health conditions; a framework to organize the knowledge, judgements, and actions that nurses supply in patient care. Ch. 1

nutrition The process by which the body uses food for energy, growth, maintenance, and repair of body tissues. Ch. 42

nystagmus Abnormal eye movements that may be observed by other people as twitching of the eyeball or may be described by the patient as a blurring of vision with head or eye movement. Ch. 23

O

obese Classification used to describe individuals with body mass index value of 30 to 40 kg/m². Ch. 43

obesity A complex, chronic, multifactorial disease that develops from the interaction between genetics and the environment; manifests as an abnormal increase in the proportion of fat cells in the body. Ch. 43

objective data Data relating to the patient's condition that can be observed and measured; also called *signs*. Ch. 3

obstructive shock Shock that develops when a physical obstruction to blood flow occurs, resulting in decreased cardiac output. Ch. 69

obstructive sleep apnea (OSA) Partial or complete obstruction of the upper airway during sleep. Ch. 9

oliguria A urine output of less than 400 mL in 24 hours. Ch. 49

oncogenes Tumour-inducing genes that interfere with normal cell expression under some conditions, causing the cell to become malignant. Ch. 18

oncotic pressure Osmotic pressure exerted by colloids in solution. Ch. 19

operating room (OR) A unique acute care setting specially designed for surgery that, in a hospital, is usually adjacent to the postanaesthesia care unit and the surgical critical care unit. Ch. 21

opiates Substances that are directly derived from the opium poppy, such as morphine and codeine. Ch. 11

opioid agonists Chemicals that activate opioid receptors in the brain and exert effects; they include both prescribed medications such as morphine or methadone and nonprescribed substances such as heroin. Ch. 11

opioids Umbrella term that includes both the opiates and the many semisynthetic and synthetic narcotic agents used as analgesics. Ch. 11

opportunistic diseases Infections and cancers that occur in immunosuppressed patients that can lead to disability, disease, and death. Ch. 17

optimal nutritional status State achieved when nutrients consumed meet daily requirements and metabolic demands. Ch. 42

oral hairy leukoplakia An Epstein-Barr virus infection that causes painless, white, raised lesions on the lateral aspect of the tongue. Ch. 17

orchitis An acute inflammation of the testis. Ch. 57

organ transplantation The transfer of a whole or partial organ from one individual to another for the purpose of replacing the recipient's damaged or failing organ with a functioning one. Ch. 16

orthostatic hypotension A decrease of 20 mm Hg (or more) in systolic blood pressure or a decrease of 10 mm Hg (or more) in diastolic blood pressure that occurs when an individual assumes a standing position. Ch. 35

Osler's nodes Painful, tender, red or purple, pea-sized lesions that may be found on the fingertips or toes of patients with infective endocarditis; last only 1 or 2 days. Ch. 39

osmolality A measure of the osmotic force of solute per unit of weight of solvent. Ch. 19

osmolarity A measure of the total milliosmoles of solute per unit of total volume of solution. Ch. 19

osmosis The movement of water between two compartments separated by a semipermeable membrane, one that allows the movement of water but not solute. Ch. 19

osmotic pressure The amount of pressure necessary to stop the osmotic flow of water. Ch. 19

osteoarthritis (OA) A slowly progressive, non-inflammatory disorder of the diarthrodial (synovial) joints; the most common chronic condition of the joints. Ch. 67

osteoclastoma A destructive tumour that arises in the cancellous ends of long bones in young adults; also called a *giant-cell tumour*. Ch. 66

osteomyelitis A severe infection of the bone, bone marrow, and surrounding soft tissue, most commonly caused by *Staphylococcus aureus*. Ch. 66

osteoporosis A chronic, progressive metabolic bone disease characterized by low bone mass and structural deterioration of bone tissue, leading to increased bone fragility, which predisposes the individual to bone fractures at the hip, wrist, and spine. Ch. 66

osteosarcoma A malignant primary bone tumour that is extremely aggressive and is characterized by rapid growth and metastasis. Ch. 66

osteotomy Surgery to remove or add a wedge or slice of bone to change alignment (joint and vertebral) and to shift weight bearing, thereby correcting a deformity and relieving pain. Ch. 65

ostomy A surgical procedure in which an opening is made to allow passage of urine from the bladder, or intestinal contents from the bowel, to an incision or stoma surgically created in the wall of the abdomen. Ch. 45

otosclerosis A hereditary autosomal dominant disease in which spongy bone develops from the bony labyrinth, causing immobilization of the footplate of the stapes in the oval window; most common cause of hearing loss in young adults. Ch. 24

outbreak management Strategies used to prevent the spread of communicable disease among a cluster of people. Ch. 72

overnutrition A state that results from the consumption of nutrients—most frequently, calories, sodium, and fat—in excess of requirements. Ch. 42

overweight Classification used to describe individuals with a body mass index value of 25 to 29.9 kg/m². Ch. 43

oxygen toxicity A condition of oxygen overdosage. Ch. 31

P

Paget's disease A rare breast malignancy characterized by a persistent lesion of the nipple and areola with or without a palpable mass. Ch. 54

Paget's disease of the bone A chronic skeletal bone disorder in which there is excessive bone resorption followed by replacement of normal marrow by vascular, fibrous connective tissue and new bone that is larger, disorganized, and structurally weaker; also called *osteitis deformans*. Ch. 66

pain A subjective and unpleasant sensation caused by actual or potential tissue damage. Ch. 10

pain perception Recognition of, definition of, and response to pain by the individual experiencing it. Ch. 10

paired organ donation An option for organ donation that allows a living donor to donate an organ (e.g., kidney) to a different compatible recipient, with the intent that another donor will donate to the first donor's designated recipient. Ch. 49

pallor Unusually light or ashen skin colour when compared to a patient's baseline complexion, typically caused by narrowing of blood vessels (vasoconstriction), hypoxia, or anemia. Ch. 25

palpation Examination of the body through the use of touch. Ch. 3

pancytopenia Marked decrease in the number of red blood cells, white blood cells, and platelets. Ch. 32

pandemic The occurrence of a communicable disease being widespread and affecting large numbers of people across several countries or continents or globally. Ch. 72

pandemic influenza A highly infectious outbreak of influenza that spreads rapidly around the world, with much more serious consequences than the usual effects of seasonal influenza. Ch. 72

paracentesis A sterile procedure in which a catheter is used to withdraw fluid from the abdominal cavity; also used to diagnose a medical condition, rule out infection in the fluid, or relive pressure. Ch. 46

paralytic ileus Impairment of intestinal motility (ileus that persists for more than 2 to 3 days) postoperatively. Ch. 22

paraphimosis Narrowing or edema of the retracted uncircumcised foreskin, preventing normal return over the glans and causing strangulation. Ch. 57

paraplegia Paralysis and loss of sensation in the lower limbs and the trunk; occurs when the thoracic cord or conus in the lumbar spine is damaged. Ch. 63

parasomnias Unusual and often undesirable behaviours that occur during sleep or during arousal from sleep (e.g., abnormal movements; dream-related behaviours, emotions, and perceptions). Ch. 9

parenteral nutrition (PN) The administration of nutrients by a route other than the gastrointestinal tract (e.g., the bloodstream). Ch. 42

Parkinson's disease (PD) A progressive neurodegenerative disease of the central nervous system (basal ganglia) characterized by delayed initiation and execution of movement (bradykinesia), increased muscle tone (rigidity), tremor at rest, and impaired gait changes. Ch. 61

paroxysmal nocturnal dyspnea A disorder that occurs when the patient is asleep; characterized by awakening in a panic with feelings of suffocation and a strong desire to sit or stand up; caused by the reabsorption of fluid from dependent body areas when the patient is flat. Ch. 37

partial-thickness burn Varying degrees of epidermal and dermal skin injury, with some skin elements remaining viable for regeneration. Ch. 27

patient-centred approach An approach that focuses on respectful and responsive care to patient preferences, needs, and values, ensuring they are involved in care decisions. Ch. 1

patient-controlled analgesia (PCA) An infusion system that allows the patient to self-administer a dose of opioid through a pump when needed. Ch. 10

patient safety The absence of preventable harm to a patient while receiving health care and the unnecessary harm associated with health care. Ch. 1

peer teaching Teaching that is conducted within the setting of a peer group, such as a self-help or support group. Ch. 4

pelvic inflammatory disease (PID) An infectious condition of the pelvic cavity that may involve the fallopian tubes (salpingitis), ovaries (oophoritis), and pelvic peritoneum (peritonitis). Ch. 56

peptic ulcer disease (PUD) A condition characterized by erosion of the gastrointestinal mucosa that results from the digestive action of hydrochloric acid and pepsin. Ch. 44

percussion Technique in physical examination of tapping the body directly or indirectly with the fingertips or fist to produce a sound and vibration to obtain information about the underlying area. Ch. 3

percutaneous coronary intervention (PCI) An intervention to treat coronary artery disease in which a catheter equipped with an inflatable balloon tip is inserted into a narrowed coronary artery and the balloon is inflated; a common elective procedure and also used in emergent situations. Ch. 36

pericardial effusion An accumulation of excess fluid in the pericardium. Ch. 39

pericardial friction rub A scratching, grating, high-pitched sound believed to arise from friction between the roughened pericardial and the epicardial surfaces; hallmark finding in acute pericarditis. Ch. 39

pericardiocentesis Procedure in which a 16- to 18-gauge needle is inserted into the pericardial space to remove fluid for analysis and to relieve cardiac pressure. Ch. 39

pericarditis A condition caused by inflammation of the pericardial sac. Ch. 39

perimenopause A normal life transition that begins with the first signs of change in menstrual cycles and ends after cessation of menses. Ch. 56

perioperative The period of time that encompasses the total surgical episode. Ch. 20

peripheral artery disease (PAD) A condition that involves thickening of artery walls, which results in a progressive narrowing of the arteries of the upper and lower extremities. Ch. 40

peripheral nervous system (PNS) The division of the nervous system that consists of cranial nerves, the spinal nerves, and the peripheral components of the autonomic nervous system. Ch. 58

peritoneal dialysis (PD) A type of dialysis that uses a natural semipermeable membrane, the peritoneum; dialysis fluid is infused into the peritoneal cavity, and excess fluid and waste products pass across the membrane into the fluid, which is then drained and discarded. Ch. 49

peritonitis A localized or generalized inflammatory process of the peritoneum. Ch. 45

pernicious anemia A disease caused by the absence of intrinsic factor (IF); the gastric mucosa does not secrete IF because of either gastric mucosal atrophy or autoimmune destruction of parietal cells and possibly also because of IF itself. Ch. 33

PERRLA Acronym that stands for **p**upils are **e**qual, **r**ound, and **r**eactive to **l**ight and **a**ccommodation (a description of normal pupil function). Ch. 23

petechiae Small, purplish-red lesions. Ch. 32

pH H$^+$ concentration, usually expressed as a negative logarithm. Ch. 19

phagocytosis A process by which white blood cells ingest or engulf an unwanted organism and then digest and kill it. Ch. 32

phantom limb sensation Phenomenon whereby the patient feels as though the amputated limb is still present after surgery; describes any sensation of the missing limb except pain. Ch. 65

pharmacogenetics The study of how human genes affect medication metabolism. Ch. 15

pharmacogenomics The field of genetics that studies how medications affect and interact with the genome and output expression. Ch. 15

pheochromocytoma A rare condition characterized by a tumour of the adrenal medulla that produces excessive amounts of catecholamines (epinephrine, norepinephrine), resulting in severe hypertension. Ch. 51

phimosis A constriction of the uncircumcised foreskin around the head of the penis, making retraction over the glans penis difficult. Ch. 57

phlebostatic axis A landmark used to establish the zero reference point at the level of the atria of the heart for positioning the stopcock nearest the transducer; located at the intersection of two imaginary lines, one through the fourth intercostal space at the sternum and one through midchest, halfway between the outermost anterior and the outermost posterior surfaces. Ch. 68

physical dependence An expected physiological response to ongoing exposure to pharmacological agents such that an abrupt decrease in its use results in a withdrawal syndrome. Ch. 10

physical examination The systematic assessment of a patient's physical status. Ch. 3

physiological stress ulcer A form of erosive gastritis; multiple superficial erosions result, which may bleed. Ch. 44

pilonidal sinus A small tract under the skin between the buttocks, in the sacrococcygeal area; may have several openings and is lined with epithelium and hair. Ch. 45

planning Setting goals and expected outcomes with the patient and, when feasible, the patient's family and determining strategies for accomplishing the goals. Ch. 1

pleural effusion A collection of fluid in the pleural space. Ch. 30

pleural friction rub A creaking or grating sound that occurs when roughened, inflamed surfaces of the pleura rub together; evident during inspiration, expiration, or both; does not change with coughing. Ch. 28

pleurisy (pleuritis) Inflammation of the pleura. Ch. 30

pneumoconiosis A general term for lung diseases caused by the inhalation and retention of dust particles, literally meaning "dust in the lungs." Ch. 30

pneumonia Acute inflammation of the lung parenchyma caused by a microbial agent. Ch. 30

pneumothorax Presence of air in the pleural space. Ch. 30

poikilothermism The adjustment of the body temperature to the room temperature. Ch. 63

point of maximal impulse (PMI) The site of strongest pulsation; lies within the midclavicular line in the fifth intercostal space. Ch. 34

polycystic kidney disease (PKD) A genetic kidney disorder in which the cortex and the medulla are filled with thin-walled cysts that enlarge and destroy surrounding tissue by compression. Ch. 48

polycythemia An abnormal condition characterized by increased red blood cells. Chs. 32, 33

polymyositis Diffuse, idiopathic, inflammatory myopathies of the connective tissues, especially striated muscle, that produce bilateral weakness, usually most severe in the proximal or the limb-girdle muscles. Ch. 67

polypharmacy Use of multiple medications by a person who has more than one health condition. Ch. 7

portal hypertension Hypertension characterized by increased venous pressure in the portal circulation, as well as by splenomegaly, large collateral veins, ascites, systemic hypertension, and esophageal varices. Ch. 46

positive end-expiratory pressure (PEEP) A ventilatory manoeuvre in which positive pressure is applied to the airway during exhalation. Ch. 68

positive feedback A second method of regulation of hormone secretion; increases the target organ action, causing another gland to release a hormone that then stimulates further release of the first hormone. Ch. 50

positive-pressure ventilation (PPV) A ventilatory mode in which the ventilator pushes air into the lungs under positive pressure; the primary method used with acutely ill patients. Ch. 68

posterior cavity Also called the *vitreous cavity,* the space that lies between the posterior lens and the retina of the eye and that contains the vitreous humour. Ch. 23

postmenopause The time in a woman's life after menopause. Ch. 56

postpolio syndrome (PPS) Recurrence of neuromuscular symptoms of polio in disease survivors as they age. Ch. 63

post-thrombotic syndrome A condition that results in chronic venous hypertension caused by vein wall and vein valve damage (from acute inflammation and thrombus reorganization), venous valve reflux, and persistent venous obstruction; occurs in 20 to 50% of patients with venous thromboembolism. Ch. 40

postural drainage An airway clearance technique in which gravity is used to assist in bronchial drainage. Ch. 31

potentiation A medication interaction causing a response greater than the sum of the individual responses to each medication. Ch. 11

prayer A form of intentional communication with a higher God, or deity. Ch. 12

prediabetes A condition in which a fasting or a 2-hour plasma glucose level is higher than normal but lower than that considered diagnostic for diabetes mellitus; places the individual at risk of developing diabetes mellitus and its complications. (Also known as *impaired glucose tolerance [IGT]* or *impaired fasting glucose [IFG].*) Ch. 52

preload The volume of blood in the ventricles at the end of diastole, before the next contraction. Ch. 34

premature atrial contraction (PAC) Contraction originating from an ectopic focus in the atrium in an area other than the sinus node before the next expected beat. Ch. 38

premature ventricular contraction (PVC) A contraction originating in an ectopic focus in the ventricles. Ch. 38

premenstrual syndrome (PMS) A symptom complex related to the luteal phase of the menstrual cycle that resolves with menstruation. Ch. 56

presbycusis Hearing impairment associated with aging; includes the loss of peripheral auditory sensitivity, a decline in word recognition ability, and associated psychological and communication issues. Chs. 23, 24

presbyopia A normal aging change in which the lens of the eye loses its elasticity and flexibility, resulting in an inability to focus on near objects, usually beginning at approximately age 40. Chs. 23, 24

pressure-support ventilation (PSV) A spontaneous mode of ventilation often used as the patient's status improves and is one mode of weaning from the ventilator. Ch. 68

pressure injury A localized injury to the skin or underlying soft tissue, usually over a bony prominence, as a result of excessive or prolonged pressure, shear, and tissue deformation; can be caused by a medical or other device such as catheters. Ch. 14

primary care Historically, a term used to describe clinicians responsible for providing the majority of an individuals' health needs over a continued period of time; a facet of primary health care that focuses on health promotion, disease prevention, diagnosis, and treatment. Ch. 6

primary (essential) hypertension Elevated blood pressure without an exact identified cause but considered to be due to a complex interaction between genes and the environment; accounts for the majority of cases of hypertension. Ch. 35

primary health care A philosophy and strategy to deliver health care that focuses on a system-wide partnership between health, social services, housing, and the environment. Ch. 6

primary survey A systematic approach to emergency assessment that focuses on **a**irway, **b**reathing, **c**irculation (ABC), disability, exposure, facilitation of adjuncts and family, and other resuscitation aids and serves to identify life-threatening conditions. Ch. 71

Prinzmetal's angina Angina that occurs at rest, usually in response to spasm of a major coronary artery; also called *variant angina.* Ch. 36

problem-focused coping Purposeful, active, task-oriented approaches that are used to reduce stress (e.g., setting priorities, collecting information, seeking advice). Ch. 8

prodrome Signs or symptoms that may precede a migraine headache, including psychic disturbances, low mood, food cravings, frequent yawning, and stiff or painful neck. Ch. 61

pronouncement of death Verification of the absence of an apical pulse and respirations and that the pupils are fixed and dilated. Ch. 13

prostate-specific antigen (PSA) A glycoprotein found only in the epithelial cells of the prostate that, when elevated, indicates a pathological condition of the prostate, although not necessarily prostate cancer. Ch. 57

prostatitis A group of acute or chronic inflammatory conditions affecting the prostate gland, usually as a result of infection. Ch. 57

protein–calorie malnutrition (PCM) The most common form of undernutrition. Ch. 42

proto-oncogenes Normal genes that are regulators of normal cellular processes; promote growth. Ch. 18

protozoa Single-cell, animal-like microorganisms that normally live in soil and bodies of water but, when introduced into the human body, can cause infection; include amoebas, ciliates, flagellates, and sporozoa. Ch. 17

pruritus Itching. Ch. 25

pseudocyst An accumulation of fluid, pancreatic enzymes, tissue debris, and inflammatory exudates surrounded by a wall next to the pancreas. Ch. 46

pseudo-obstruction An apparent mechanical obstruction of the intestine without demonstration of obstruction by radiological methods. Ch. 45

psoriasis A common inherited benign disorder that is characterized by the eruption of reddish, silver-scaled maculopapules, predominantly on the elbows, knees, scalp, and trunk. Ch. 26

psoriatic arthritis A progressive inflammatory disease that affects approximately 10 to 30% of people with psoriasis (a skin disorder); has a genetic link with the HLA antigens in many patients. Ch. 67

psychoneuroimmunology Interdisciplinary science in which investigators study the interactions among psychological, neurological, and immune responses that affect human health and behaviour. Ch. 8

public health nursing A specialized area of nursing practice in which the nurse combines knowledge from public health science, primary health care, nursing science, and the social sciences and focuses on promoting, protecting, and preserving the health of populations. Ch. 6

pulmonary edema An abnormal, life-threatening accumulation of fluid in the alveoli and the interstitial spaces of the lungs. Chs. 30, 37

pulmonary embolism (PE) The blockage of pulmonary arteries by a thrombus, fat or air embolus, or tumour tissue. Ch. 30

pulmonary hypertension Elevated pulmonary pressure resulting from an increase in pulmonary vascular resistance to blood flow through small arteries and arterioles. Ch. 30

pulse pressure The difference between the systolic blood pressure and the diastolic blood pressure. Ch. 34

purpura Purplish-red rash. Ch. 32

pursed-lip breathing A breathing exercise (breathing in through the nose and then breathing out through pursed lips); used to prolong exhalation, prevent bronchiolar collapse and air trapping, and assist with dyspnea. Ch. 31

pyelonephritis Inflammation (usually caused by infection) of the renal parenchyma and the collecting system. Ch. 48

pyrosis Heartburn; burning in epigastric or substernal area. Ch. 41

Q

quality of life A subjective evaluation of both the positive and negative aspects of life. Ch. 5

quarantine The isolation of people who have been exposed, or potentially exposed, to an infection or contagious disease but who are not yet sick or showing any signs of illness. Ch. 72

R

race A biological and social construct that is sometimes used to highlight biological differences and physical characteristics such as skin colour, bone structure, or blood group. Ch. 2

racialization Social processes of categorization of groups according to race to denote superiority and inferiority, which leads to discrimination. Ch. 2

radiation The emission and distribution of energy through space or a material medium. Ch. 18

radical prostatectomy Surgical removal of the entire prostate gland, the seminal vesicles, and part of the bladder neck (ampulla). Ch. 57

rapid-sequence intubation The preferred procedure for securing an unprotected airway; the patient is given a rapid-acting sedative and a neuromuscular blocking agent to facilitate intubation and minimize the risk for aspiration and airway trauma. Ch. 71

Raynaud's phenomenon An overarching term that encompasses Raynaud disease and Raynaud syndrome; episodic vasospastic disorder of small cutaneous arteries, most frequently involving the fingers and toes; most common initial symptom in limited scleroderma. Chs. 40, 67

recessive allele An allele that has no noticeable effect on the phenotype in a heterozygous individual. Ch. 15

rectocele Herniation or protrusion of the rectum through the wall of the vagina; results from weakening between the vagina and the rectum; also known as *posterior wall prolapse*. Ch. 56

reflex An involuntary response to a stimulus. Ch. 58

refractive error A defect in which light rays focus either in front of or behind the retina, causing images to be out of focus. Ch. 24

refractory hypoxemia Hypoxemia unresponsive to increasing concentrations of oxygen. Ch. 70

regeneration Replacement of lost cells and tissues with cells of the same type. Ch. 14

regional anaesthesia Reversible loss of sensation to a region of the body without loss of consciousness, achieved by blocking nerve fibres with the administration of a local anaesthetic. Ch. 21

regulated health care professions Health care professions that are governed by a legislative framework and required to obtain an annual license to practise in their respective province or territory. Ch. 1

regurgitation Incomplete closure of the valve leaflets, resulting in the backward flow of blood; also called *valvular incompetence* or *insufficiency*. Ch. 39

relapse A return to substance use after a period of abstinence. Ch. 11

relief craving The intense desire for a substance, usually experienced after decreased use, resulting from the memory aspect related to the brain reward pathway. Ch. 11

renal arteriography A radiological study performed by injecting contrast material into the renal artery via a catheter inserted into the femoral artery; the purpose is to visualize renal blood vessels. Ch. 47

renal artery stenosis A partial occlusion of one or both renal arteries and their major branches; a major cause of abrupt-onset hypertension. Ch. 48

renal biopsy Procedure to obtain renal tissue for examination to establish a diagnosis or to monitor progress of renal disease; may be an open biopsy or, more commonly, a skin (percutaneous) biopsy conducted through needle insertion into the lower lobe of the kidney. Ch. 47

renal osteodystrophy A disorder of the bones associated with chronic kidney disease that includes a number of skeletal disorders: osteitis fibrosa, osteomalacia, adynamic bone disorder, and mixed osteodystrophy. Ch. 49

renal replacement therapy (RRT) All forms of life-supporting therapies for renal failure, including hemodialysis, peritoneal dialysis, hemofiltration, and renal transplantation. Ch. 49

renal vein thrombosis An embolus occurring in the renal vein. Ch. 48

repair Healing as a result of lost cells being replaced by connective tissue. Ch. 14

repetitive strain injury (RSI) Injury resulting from prolonged force or repetitive movements and awkward postures; also called *cumulative trauma disorder, repetitive trauma disorder, nontraumatic musculoskeletal injury, overuse syndrome* (sports medicine), *regional musculoskeletal disorder,* and *work-related musculoskeletal disorder.* Ch. 65

resilience The ability to be resourceful, be flexible, and recover from exposure to stressful situations and return to prior levels of functioning. Ch. 8

responsive behaviours In patients with dementia, behaviours that are responses to something in the patient's environment. Ch. 62

restless legs syndrome (RLS) Syndrome characterized by unpleasant sensory (paresthesias) and motor abnormalities of one or both legs; also known as *Willis–Ekbom disease.* Ch. 61

retina The innermost layer of the eye that extends and gives rise to the optic nerve; responsible for converting images into a form that the brain can understand and process as vision. Ch. 23

retinal detachment A separation of the sensory retina and the underlying pigment epithelium, with fluid accumulation between the two layers. Ch. 24

retinopathy The process of microvascular damage to the retina. Ch. 24

retrograde pyelography Radiographic visualization of the kidneys, the ureter, and the bladder after direct injection of a contrast material into the kidney. Ch. 47

retroviruses Viruses that carry a single-stranded RNA as its genetic material and replicate in a "backward" manner (transcribing their RNA and DNA after entering a cell). Ch. 17

reverse transcriptase An enzyme made by HIV and other retroviruses that helps transcribe viral RNA into a double strand of viral DNA. Ch. 17

reward craving A craving that occurs when in the presence of people, places, or things that have been previously associated with taking the substance. Ch. 11

rheumatic fever A disease that causes inflammation in connective tissues; commonly affects the heart, the brain, the joints, or the skin. Ch. 39

rheumatic heart disease A chronic condition resulting from rheumatic fever that is characterized by scarring and deformity of the heart valves. Ch. 39

rheumatoid arthritis (RA) A chronic, systemic autoimmune disease characterized by inflammation of connective tissue in the diarthrodial (synovial) joints, typically with periods of remission and exacerbation. Ch. 67

rhinoplasty Surgery performed on the nose to remodel or reconstruct the external nose. Ch. 29

ribonucleic acid (RNA) A single-stranded nucleic acid that transfers the genetic information obtained from DNA to the proper location for protein synthesis. Ch. 15

S

same-day admission Admission to hospital on the day that surgery will take place. Ch. 20

sarcoma A malignant tumour originating in the connective tissue of the body (fat, muscles, blood vessels, nerves, bones, or cartilage). Chs. 18, 66

SBAR (situation, background, assessment, and recommendation) A means for members of the health care team to talk about a patient's condition in a predictable, structured manner. Ch. 1

sclera The bulbar conjunctiva, composed of collagen fibres meshed together to form an opaque structure commonly referred to as the "white" of the eye; helps protect the intraocular structures. Ch. 23

scleroderma A disorder of connective tissue characterized by fibrotic, degenerative, and occasionally inflammatory changes in skin, blood vessels, synovium, skeletal muscle, and internal organs; also called *systemic sclerosis.* Ch. 67

scoliosis A deformity resulting from lateral S-shaped curvature of the thoracic and lumbar spine. Ch. 64

scrub nurse A practical nurse who performs surgical hand asepsis, is gowned and gloved in sterile attire, and remains in the sterile field assisting the surgical team. Ch. 21

sebaceous glands Oil-producing glands that secrete sebum, which waterproofs and lubricates the skin and hair. Ch. 25

secondary hypertension Elevated blood pressure with a specific cause that often can be identified and corrected; accounts for about 5 to 10% of hypertension in adults and more than 80% of hypertension in children. Ch. 35

secondary survey A brief, systematic process that is aimed at identifying all injuries (follows primary survey and life-saving interventions). Ch. 71

seizure disorder A group of neurological diseases marked by recurring seizures; a *seizure* is a transient uncontrolled electrical discharge of neurons in the brain that interrupts normal function. Often, seizures are symptoms of an underlying illness. Ch. 61

selectins Cell surface carbohydrate-binding proteins that mediate cell adhesion; involved in leukocyte extravasation during the immune response. Ch. 14

self-efficacy A person's sense of confidence in their ability to perform a set of actions. Ch. 4

self-management A person's ability to live with the medical, role, and emotional consequences of a chronic condition in partnership with their social network and health care providers. Ch. 5

self-protective behaviours In patients with dementia, behaviours that are responses to a perceived threat. Ch. 62

sense of coherence An individual's ability or capacity to cope with everyday life stressors; indicators include comprehensibility, manageability, and meaningfulness. Ch. 8

sepsis A life-threatening syndrome that arises when the body's response to infection injures its own tissues and organs. Ch. 69

septic arthritis An infection caused by microorganisms that invade the joint cavity; also called *infectious* or *bacterial arthritis*. Ch. 67

septic shock A subset of sepsis, characterized by persistent hypotension, despite adequate fluid resuscitation, and inadequate tissue perfusion resulting in tissue hypoxia. Ch. 69

septoplasty Rhinoplasty in addition to reconstruction and remodelling of the nasal septum. Ch. 29

sex-linked gene A gene located on a sex chromosome. Ch. 15

sexual assault The forcible perpetration of a sexual act on a person without their consent. Ch. 71

sexually transmitted infections (STIs) Infectious diseases that are commonly acquired through sexual contact but may also be contracted by other routes, such as through blood, blood products, perinatal transmission, and autoinoculation; can be caused by bacteria, viruses, or parasites. Ch. 55

shared decision making A decision-making process engaged in jointly by patients and their health care providers. Ch. 5

shearing force Pressure exerted on the skin when it adheres to the bed and the underlying skin layers slide in the direction of body movement. Ch. 14

shift work sleep disorder Insomnia, sleepiness, and fatigue often experienced by people who work a permanent night shift or rapidly rotating shifts. Ch. 9

shock A syndrome characterized by decreased tissue perfusion and impaired cellular metabolism that results in an imbalance between the supply of and the demand for oxygen and nutrients. Ch. 69

short bowel syndrome (SBS) Syndrome resulting from extensive resection of the small intestine and characterized by rapid intestinal transit, impaired digestive and absorption processes, and fluid and electrolyte losses. Ch. 45

sickle cell disease (SCD) A group of inherited, autosomal recessive disorders characterized by

the presence of an abnormal form of hemoglobin in the red blood cell. Ch. 33

signs Objective manifestations of a condition. Ch. 5

silent ischemia Ischemia that occurs in the absence of clinical symptoms such as chest pain. Ch. 36

Sjögren syndrome A relatively uncommon autoimmune disease that targets moisture-producing exocrine glands, leading to the common symptoms of xerostomia (dry mouth) and keratoconjunctivitis sicca (dry eyes). Ch. 67

sleep A state during which an individual lacks conscious awareness of environmental surroundings and from which the individual can be easily aroused. Ch. 9

sleep disorders Conditions that specifically affect the quality of sleep and wake behaviour. Ch. 9

sleep-disordered breathing Abnormal respiratory patterns associated with sleep, such as snoring, apnea, and hypopnea, characterized by increased respiratory effort that leads to frequent arousals. Ch. 9

sleep disturbances Situations of poor quality sleep. Ch. 9

sleep hygiene A variety of different practices that are important for normal, quality nighttime sleep and daytime alertness. Ch. 9

sleep terrors A sudden awakening from sleep along with a loud cry and signs of panic; includes an intense autonomic response, including increased heart rate, increased respiration, and diaphoresis. Ch. 9

smoke and inhalation injuries Damage to the tissues of the respiratory tract as a result of the inhalation of hot air or noxious chemicals. Ch. 27

Somogyi effect An effect characterized by wide differences in early-morning (low) and fasting (high) glucose levels. Usually occurs during the hours of sleep and produces a decline in blood glucose level in response to too much insulin; counter-regulatory hormones are released, stimulating lipolysis, gluconeogenesis, and glycogenolysis, which in turn produce rebound hyperglycemia and ketosis. Ch. 52

spermatocele A firm, sperm-containing, painless cyst of the epididymis. Ch. 57

spermatogenesis The process of sperm production. Ch. 53

spider angiomas Small, dilated blood vessels of the skin that have a bright-red centre and spider-like branches; occur on nose, cheeks, upper trunk, neck, and shoulders. Ch. 46

spinal anaesthesia The injection of a local anaesthetic into the cerebrospinal fluid found in the subarachnoid space, usually below the level of L2. Ch. 21

spinal shock A temporary neurological syndrome experienced after spinal cord injury and characterized by decreased reflexes, loss of sensation, and flaccid paralysis below the level of the injury. Ch. 63

spirituality Beliefs, values, and practices that relate to the search for existential meaning and purpose; may or may not include belief in a higher power. Ch. 13

spondyloarthropathies A group of interrelated, multisystem inflammatory disorders that affect the spine, the peripheral joints, and the periarticular structures. Ch. 67

sprain An injury related to the ligamentous structures surrounding a joint, usually caused by a wrenching or twisting motion. Ch. 65

squamous cell carcinoma (SCC) A malignant neoplasm of keratinizing epidermal cells that frequently occurs on sun-exposed skin. Ch. 26

stage of exhaustion Final stage of general adaptation syndrome, which occurs when all of the energy for adaptation has been expended; usually results in illness and can result in death without external sources of adaptive energy, such as medication or psychotherapy. Ch. 8

stage of resistance Second stage of general adaptation syndrome, in which physiological reserves are mobilized to increase the resistance to stress and so that adaptation can occur. Ch. 8

stages of behavioural change The six stages of change identified by Prochaska and Velicer (1997) in their transtheoretical model of behaviour change: precontemplation, contemplation, preparation, action, maintenance, and termination. Ch. 4

staging Classifying the extent and spread of disease. Ch. 18

standard of practice An authoritative statement describing nurses' accountabilities to support the safe and ethical provision of care; intended to promote, guide, direct, and regulate professional nursing practice. Ch. 1

status asthmaticus The most extreme form of an acute asthma attack, characterized by hypoxia, hypercapnia, and acute respiratory failure. Ch. 31

status epilepticus A state of continuous seizure activity in which seizures recur in rapid succession without the person returning to consciousness between seizures. It is a neurological emergency and can involve any type of seizure. Ch. 61

steatorrhea Passage of large amounts of fat as bulky, fatty, frothy, foul-smelling, yellow-grey, greasy stools with putty-like consistency; results from failure to digest and absorb fat. Ch. 41

stem cell An immature blood cell that is able to self-renew and to differentiate into hematopoietic progenitor cells. Ch. 32

STEMI Abbreviation for ST-segment elevation myocardial infarction; acute coronary syndrome resulting from the total occlusion of an unstable atherosclerotic plaque by a thrombus. Ch. 36

stereotyping The assumption that members of a specific culture, race, or ethnic group are automatically assumed to have associated characteristics that are imposed on individuals without further exploration of what the individuals are actually like. Ch. 2

stigmatization Being regarded by others as unworthy or disgraceful. Ch. 5

strabismus A condition in which the patient cannot consistently focus both eyes simultaneously on the same object. Ch. 24

strain An excessive stretching of a muscle, a muscle's fascial sheath, or a tendon; most occur in the foot, leg (typically hamstring), knee, wrist, or back. Ch. 65

strategic emergency management plan (SEMP) An overarching plan that provides a comprehensive and coordinated approach to emergency management planning and preparation; components include an environmental scan, leadership engagement, an all-hazards risk assessment, training, practice exercises, a capability improvement process, and a performance assessment. Ch. 72

stress An individualized reaction or response to a stimulus, when real or perceived demands exceed the available coping resources. Ch. 8

stressors Any demand, situation, internal stimulus, or circumstance that endangers a person's personal well-being or integrity. Ch. 8

stricture An abnormal temporary or permanent narrowing of the lumen of a hollow organ such as the ureter or the urethra. Ch. 48

stroke Death of brain cells as a result of ischemia to a part of the brain or hemorrhage into the brain. Ch. 60

subarachnoid hemorrhage (SAH) A stroke resulting from intracranial bleeding into the cerebrospinal fluid–filled space between the arachnoid and the pia mater membranes on the surface of the brain. Ch. 60

subdural hematoma A collection of blood that results from bleeding between the dura mater and arachnoid layer of the meningeal covering of the brain; usually results from injury to the brain substance and its parenchymal vessels. Ch. 59

subjective data What the person tells the nurse either spontaneously or in response to a direct question; also called *symptoms*. Ch. 3

sublethal injury Cell injury that alters function without causing cell destruction. Ch. 14

subluxation A partial or incomplete displacement of the joint surface. Ch. 65

submersion injury Injury resulting when a person becomes hypoxic as a result of submersion in a liquid, usually water. Ch. 71

substance use disorder Disorder resulting from the prolonged effects of psychoactive substances on the brain; severity categorized as mild, moderate, or severe. Ch. 11

sudden cardiac death (SCD) Unexpected death resulting from various causes, including cardiac arrest. Ch. 36

suffering Distress that occurs in association with events that threaten the biopsychosocial integrity of an individual. Ch. 10

sundowning A pattern of behavioural disturbance that occurs in the late afternoon. Ch. 62

sun protection factor (SPF) A method of measuring the effectiveness of a sunscreen in filtering and absorbing ultraviolet B light (UVB) radiation. Ch. 26

superficial vein thrombosis (SVT) The formation of a thrombus in a superficial vein, usually the greater or lesser saphenous vein. Ch. 40

surfactant A lipoprotein that lowers the surface tension in the alveoli, reduces the amount of pressure needed to inflate the alveoli, and decreases the tendency of the alveoli to collapse. Ch. 28

surgeon A physician who performs surgical procedures. Ch. 21

surgical suite A controlled environment designed to maximize infection control and provide a seamless flow of patients, personnel, and operative instruments, equipment, and supplies; it is divided into unrestricted, semi-restricted, and restricted areas. Ch. 21

symptoms The subjective reports of the patient. Ch. 5

synapse The structural and functional junction between two neurons; the point at which the nerve impulse is transmitted from one neuron to another or from a neuron to glands or muscles. Ch. 58

syncope Fainting that may occur with decreased cardiac output, fluid deficits, defects in cerebral perfusion, or orthostatic hypotension. Ch. 22

syndrome of inappropriate antidiuretic hormone (SIADH) A condition in which there is abnormal production or sustained secretion of antidiuretic hormone; characterized by fluid retention, serum hypo-osmolality, dilutional hyponatremia, hypochloremia, concentrated urine in the presence of normal or increased intravascular volume, and normal renal function. Ch. 51

synovectomy Removal of the synovial membrane; used as a prophylactic measure or as a palliative treatment for rheumatoid arthritis. Ch. 65

syphilis A sexually transmitted infection caused by *Treponema pallidum*; may also be spread through contact with infectious lesions and sharing of needles among people who use intravenous drugs. Ch. 55

systemic exertion intolerance disease (SEID) A serious, complex, multisystem disease in which exertion of any sort (physical, emotional, cognitive) is impaired and accompanied by profound fatigue; also known as *chronic fatigue syndrome (CFS)*. Ch. 67

systemic lupus erythematosus (SLE) A multisystem, inflammatory, autoimmune disease that typically affects the skin, the joints, and the serous membranes (pleura, pericardium), along with the renal, hematological, and neurological systems. Ch. 67

systemic vascular resistance (SVR) The force opposing the movement of blood within the blood vessels; the radius of the small arteries and arterioles is the principal factor determining vascular resistance. Ch. 35

systole Contraction of the myocardium. Ch. 34

systolic blood pressure (SBP) The peak pressure exerted against the arteries when the heart contracts. Ch. 34

T

tactile fremitus A palpable vibration, generated when sounds from the larynx are transmitted through the bronchi and through the lung parenchyma to the chest wall. Ch. 28

teach-back strategy A method of patient teaching in which the patient repeats back, in their own words, the health information being taught, demonstrating their level of understanding of the information. Ch. 4

teaching A process of deliberately planning experiences and sharing knowledge to meet learner outcomes in the cognitive, affective, and psychomotor domains. Ch. 4

teaching plan A learner-centred approach for action to achieve the goals and learning outcomes agreed on by the patient and nurse. Ch. 4

teaching process The development and implementation of a plan that includes assessment, diagnosis, the setting of patient outcomes or objectives, intervention, and evaluation. Ch. 4

telehomecare The delivery of health care and information through digital technologies, including high-speed Internet, wireless, satellite, and video communications. Ch. 1

tenesmus Spasmodic contraction of the anal sphincter with pain and persistent desire to empty the bowel; painful and ineffective straining at stool. Ch. 41

tension pneumothorax A pneumothorax with rapid accumulation of air in the pleural space, causing severely high intrapleural pressures with resultant tension on the heart and great vessels. Ch. 30

tension-type headache The most common type of primary headache, characterized by bilateral location and pressing or tightening quality; usually of mild or moderate intensity and lasting from minutes to days. (Also called *stress headache*.) Ch. 61

terrorism Intentional and overt actions that are committed to cause fear, panic, destruction, injury, and death in service of political, religious, or ideological goals. Ch. 72

testicular torsion A condition involving a twisting of the spermatic cord that supplies blood to the testes and epididymis, causing an interruption to the blood supply. Ch. 57

tetanus An extremely severe polyradiculitis and polyneuritis affecting spinal and cranial nerves that results from the effects of a potent neurotoxin released by *Clostridium tetani*; also called *lockjaw*. Ch. 63

tetany Condition of sustained muscle contraction. Ch. 19

tetraplegia Paralysis of the arms, the legs, and the trunk occurring with spinal cord damage at the eighth cervical (C8) vertebra or above; formerly called *quadriplegia*. Ch. 63

thalassemia A group of diseases involving inadequate production of normal hemoglobin; caused by an absent or reduced globulin protein. Ch. 33

therapeutic touch A method of detecting, balancing, and repatterning the human energy field. Ch. 12

thermal burns Burns caused by flame, flash fire, scald, or contact with hot objects. Ch. 27

thoracentesis A procedure to remove fluid from the pleural space. Ch. 30

thoracotomy Surgical opening into the thoracic cavity. Ch. 30

thromboangiitis obliterans (TAO) A non-atherosclerotic, segmental, recurrent inflammatory disorder of the small and medium-sized arteries and veins of the upper and lower extremities; also known as *Buerger's disease*. Ch. 40

thrombocytopenia A reduction of platelets to an amount below 150×10^9/L. Chs. 32, 33

thrombocytosis A condition characterized by excessive levels of platelets; a disorder that occurs with inflammation and some cancers. Ch. 32

thrombotic stroke A stroke resulting from the formation of a blood clot in a diseased and narrowed blood vessel in the brain. Ch. 60

thrombus A blood clot that develops in and partially occludes a vein, which can further develop into an embolus that largely blocks blood flow. Ch. 40

thyroiditis An inflammation of the thyroid gland; can have several causes. Ch. 51

thyrotoxicosis The clinical syndrome of hypermetabolism resulting from inappropriately high tissue thyroid levels of thyroxine, triiodothyronine, or both. Ch. 51

thyroxine (T$_4$) The most abundant hormone produced by the thyroid gland and the precursor to triiodothyronine. Ch. 50

tidal volume Volume of air exchanged with each breath. Ch. 28

tinnitus The perception of ringing in the ears. Ch. 23

titration Dosage adjustment based on assessment of the adequacy of analgesic effect versus the adverse effects produced. Ch. 10

tolerance The need for a larger dose of a substance to obtain the original effects. Ch. 11

tonic–clonic seizure The most common type of generalized seizure, characterized by loss of consciousness and falling to the ground if the patient is upright, followed by stiffening of the body (tonic phase) for 10 to 20 seconds and subsequent jerking of the extremities (clonic phase) for another 30 to 40 seconds. Ch. 61

tracheostomy A stoma (opening) that results from a tracheotomy. Ch. 29

tracheotomy A surgical incision into the trachea for the purpose of establishing an airway. Ch. 29

traction The application of a pulling force to an injured or diseased part of the body or extremity, while counter-traction pulls in the opposite direction. Ch. 65

traditional Chinese medicine (TCM) A group of treatment modalities used to replenish and smooth the flow of qi, or the fundamental life force; interventions include acupressure, acupuncture, Chinese herbal medicine, Chinese massage, cupping, moxibustion, and meditative physical exercise. Ch. 12

transcription The creation of a messenger RNA (mRNA) from a single-stranded DNA. Ch. 15

transduction The conversion of a mechanical, thermal, or chemical stimulus to a neuronal action potential. Ch. 10

transient ischemic attack (TIA) A temporary episode of neurological dysfunction caused by focal brain, spinal cord, or retinal ischemia but without acute infarction of the brain. Ch. 60

translation The process through which the codon sequence is converted into amino acids. Ch. 15

transmission The movement of pain impulses from the site of transduction to the brain. Ch. 10

transtheoretical model of change A framework of behaviour change that provides a contextual approach for clinicians; the stages of change include precontemplation, contemplation, preparation, action, maintenance, and termination. Ch. 11

transurethral resection of the prostate (TURP) A surgical procedure involving the removal of prostate tissue using a resectoscope inserted through the urethra. Ch. 57

triage The process of rapidly determining patient acuity; the sorting or ranking of casualties to prioritize health care needs and to provide direction in the allocation of scarce resources. Chs. 71, 72

trigeminal neuralgia (TN) Uncommon cranial nerve disorder affecting cranial nerve V; characterized by paroxysms of flashing, stabbing pain radiating along the course of a branch of the trigeminal facial nerve from the angle of the jaw; also called *tic douloureux*. Ch. 63

trigger point A circumscribed hypersensitive area within a tight band of muscle that is caused by acute or persistent muscle strain. Ch. 10

triiodothyronine (T$_3$) A potent hormone produced by the thyroid gland that regulates the metabolic rate of all cells and processes of cell growth and tissue differentiation. Ch. 50

tropic hormones Several hormones secreted by the anterior pituitary gland that target other endocrine glands, in turn causing the target glands to secrete hormone. Ch. 50

tuberculosis (TB) An infectious disease caused by *Mycobacterium tuberculosis*; usually involves the lungs but also occurs in the larynx, the kidneys, the bones, the adrenal glands, the lymph nodes, and the meninges and can be disseminated throughout the body. Ch. 30

tumour angiogenesis The process of the formation of blood vessels within the tumour itself. Ch. 18

tumour-associated antigens Cell surface antigens on some cancer cells that have changes as a result of malignant transformation. Ch. 18

tumour suppressor genes Normal genes that are regulators of normal cellular processes; suppress growth. Ch. 18

U

ulcerative colitis (UC) A chronic inflammatory bowel disease characterized by inflammation and ulceration of the rectum and colon. Ch. 45

unconsciousness An abnormal state of complete or partial unawareness of self or environment. Ch. 59

undernutrition A state that occurs when nutritional reserves become depleted or when nutrient intake is inadequate to meet daily requirements or metabolic demands. Ch. 42

unregulated care providers Paid employees who are not licensed or registered by a regulatory body, who have no legally defined scope of practice, who may or may not have mandatory education or practice standards, who provide care under the direct or indirect supervision of a nurse, and who are accountable for their own actions and decisions. Ch. 1

unstable angina (UA) Chest pain that is new in onset, occurs at rest, or has a worsening pattern. Ch. 36

upper motor neurons (UMNs) The classification of motor pathways that originate in the cerebral cortex and project downward; the corticobulbar tract ends in the brainstem, and the corticospinal tract descends into the spinal cord. Ch. 58

uremia A constellation of signs and symptoms resulting from the buildup of waste products and excess fluid associated with kidney failure; these signs and symptoms may include but are not limited to elevated serum creatinine and blood urea nitrogen, abnormal electrolytes, acidosis, anemia, fluid volume excess, nausea, loss of appetite, fatigue, decreased cognition, pruritus, and neuropathy. Ch. 49

urethritis Inflammation of the urethra. Ch. 48

urinalysis A general examination of urine for routine and microscopic findings; may establish baseline information, provide information about possible abnormalities, indicate what further studies need to be done, and supply information on the progression of a diagnosed disorder. Ch. 47

urinary incontinence (UI) An uncontrolled leakage of urine that is of sufficient magnitude to be a problem. Ch. 48

urinary retention The inability to empty the bladder despite micturition, or the accumulation of urine in the bladder because of an inability to urinate. Ch. 48

urodynamics testing A set of studies designed to measure urinary tract function—the storage of urine within the bladder and the flow of urine through the urinary tract to the outside of the body. Ch. 47

urticaria An eruption of spontaneously occurring, raised or irregularly shaped wheals; usually an allergic phenomenon. Ch. 26

uterine prolapse The downward displacement of the uterus into the vaginal canal as a result of impaired pelvic support. Ch. 56

V

valence The electrical charge of an ion. Ch. 19

Valsalva manoeuvre A manoeuvre that involves contraction of the chest muscles on a closed glottis with simultaneous contraction of the abdominal muscles; used during straining. Ch. 41

varicocele A dilation of the veins that drain the testes. Ch. 57

varicose veins Dilated, tortuous subcutaneous veins most commonly found in the saphenous vein system. Ch. 40

vascular dementia A form of dementia that results from ischemic, ischemic–hypoxic, or hemorrhagic brain damage caused by cardiovascular disease; also called *multi-infarct dementia*. Ch. 62

vasectomy The bilateral surgical ligation or resection of the vas deferens performed for the purpose of sterilization. Ch. 57

venous thromboembolism (VTE) Condition in which a thrombus forms in association with inflammation of the vein; also known as *venous thrombosis*. Ch. 40

ventilation Inspiration (movement of air into the lungs) and expiration (movement of air out of the lungs). Ch. 28

ventricular fibrillation A severe derangement of the heart rhythm characterized by irregular undulations of varying shapes and amplitude on the electrocardiogram (ECG). Ch. 38

ventricular tachycardia (VT) The occurrence of three or more premature ventricular contractions in succession; occurs when an ectopic focus or foci fire repetitively and the ventricle takes control as the pacemaker. Ch. 38

vertigo A sense that the person or objects around the person are moving or spinning; usually stimulated by movement of the head. Ch. 23

vesicants Agents that cause severe local tissue breakdown and necrosis when accidentally infiltrated into the skin. Ch. 18

villi Functional units present throughout the entire small intestine, they are minute, finger-like projections in the mucous membrane of the small intestine, containing goblet cells that secrete mucus and epithelial cells that produce the intestinal digestive enzymes. Ch. 41

viral load The number of HIV (or other virus) particles in the blood. Ch. 17

Virchow's triad Three important factors in the etiology of venous thrombosis: (1) venous stasis, (2) damage of the endothelium (inner lining of the vein), and (3) hypercoagulability of the blood. Ch. 40

viremia Large amounts of virus in the blood. Ch. 17

virtual care Any interaction between a patient and their care team that occurs remotely. Ch. 6

viruses Infectious agents consisting of either RNA or DNA and a protein envelope; can reproduce only in the cells of a living organism. Ch. 17

vitiligo Total loss of melanin (pigment), resulting in a chalky white patch of skin. Ch. 25

vitreous humor A transparent, gel-like substance located in the posterior (vitreous) cavity of the eye. Ch. 23

vomiting The forceful ejection of partially digested food and secretions (*emesis*) from the upper gastrointestinal tract. Ch. 44

W

waist-to-hip ratio (WHR) A method of describing the distribution of both subcutaneous and visceral adipose tissue; calculated by dividing the waist measurement by the hip measurement. Ch. 43

wake behaviour Behaviour associated with an activated cortical brain wave (electroencephalogram [EEG]) pattern. Ch. 9

weaning The process of reducing ventilator support and resuming spontaneous ventilation. Ch. 68

Wernicke's encephalopathy An inflammatory, hemorrhagic, degenerative condition of the brain caused by a thiamine deficiency; associated with long-term heavy alcohol use. Ch. 11

wet gangrene Ischemic necrosis of an appendage as a result of a sudden, rapid elimination of blood flow, such as that seen in a severe burn or traumatic crash injury. Ch. 14

wheezes Continuous high-pitched squeaking sound caused by rapid vibration of bronchial walls. Ch. 28

window period The time between exposure to HIV infection and when the test yields an accurate result. Ch. 17

windup A pain process that results in an increase in the firing of specialized dorsal horn neurons and that is dependent on the activation of *N*-methyl-D-aspartate receptors. Ch. 10

withdrawal Constellation of physiological and psychological responses that occur upon abrupt cessation or reduced intake of a substance on which an individual is physiologically dependent. Ch. 11

withdrawal management Interventions and processes aimed at addressing the physiological and psychological symptoms that occur in response to stopping a substance on which physiological and psychological dependence has developed. Ch. 11

worldview A paradigm or a set of assumptions, values, concepts, and practices that influences how people perceive, interpret, and relate to the world around them. Ch. 2

A

Abatacept (Orencia), for rheumatoid arthritis, 1677
Abdomen
  emergency assessment of, 1779–1780
  inflammatory disorders of, 1048–1051
  physical examination of, 44t, 46t, 939–941, 941f
  quadrants of, 939f, 940t
  structures of, 940t
Abdominal aortic aneurysms (AAAs), 907, 909f, 910. *See also* Aortic aneurysms
Abdominal compartment syndrome, 1735
Abdominal distention, 1062, 1173
Abdominal pain. *See* Acute abdominal pain; Chronic abdominal pain
Abdominal paradox, 558t–559t
Abdominal trauma, 1047–1048, 1047t
Abdominal ultrasonography, 944t–947t, 947, 947f
Abducens nerve, 1443
ABO blood groups, 695t
Aboriginal Canadians. *See* Indigenous Canadians
Abortion, 1374, 1375b
  induced, 1374, 1375t
  spontaneous, 1374
Absence seizure, 1518
Absolute hypovolemia, 1730
Absorption, 930, 932–933
Absorption atelectasis, 662
Acalculous cholecystitis, 1112
Acanthosis nigricans, 1303
Accommodation, 431, 450
Acculturation, 22
Acetylcholinesterase inhibitors, for multiple sclerosis, 1526t
Achalasia, 1010, 1010f
Achilles tendinitis, 1600t
Acid, 360t
Acid-base imbalances
  assessment of, 364–365
  causes of, 359–363, 361t
  chronic kidney disease and, 1188–1189
  kinds of, 362f
  respiratory acidosis, 362
  ROME mnemonic for, 364t
Acid-base regulation, 360–361
Acidemia, 360t
Acid-fast smear and culture, 561t–562t
Acidosis, 360, 360t, 550. *See also* Metabolic acidosis; Respiratory acidosis
Acne (comedone), 490t

Acne vulgaris, 505f, 506t
Acoustic neuroma, 473
Acquired hemolytic anemia, 714–715. *See also* Anemia
Acquired immunity, 253, 253t
Acquired immunodeficiency syndrome (AIDS), 285–286, 289–290, 289f, 290t, 467
Acquired thrombocytopenia, 720–721
Acrochordons (skin tags), 496–497, 506t
Acromegaly, 1237–1239, 1238f
  clinical manifestations of, 1238
  diagnostic studies of, 1238
  etiology and pathophysiology of, 1237–1238
  interprofessional care of, 1238–1239
  medication therapy for, 1239
  nursing management of, 1239–1240
  postoperative surgery for, 1239–1240
  preoperative surgery for, 1239
  radiation therapy for, 1239
  surgical therapy for, 1238–1239
Acromioplasty, 1611
ACTH. *See* Adrenocorticotrophic hormone
Actigraphy, 124, 124f
Actinic keratosis (solar keratosis), 484, 494, 497, 499t
Actinomycosis, 600t
Action potential, 137, 138f, 752, 850, 1429
Active acquired immunity, 253, 253t
Active listening, 58, 210
Active range of motion, 1598
Active transport, 344
Activities of daily living (ADLs), 78, 92
Activity-exercise pattern, 41
Acupressure, 197
Acupuncture, 126, 197, 1516b
Acute abdominal pain, 1044–1045, 1045t
Acute alcohol intoxication, 174
Acute angle-closure glaucoma, 465, 465t. *See also* Glaucoma
Acute arterial ischemia, 904
Acute asthma exacerbation, 640–641
Acute blood loss, 710–711
Acute bronchitis, 589
Acute chest syndrome, 713
Acute coronary syndrome (ACS)
  acute intervention for, 818–822
  ambulatory and home care of, 819, 823
  assessment of, 819t
  electrocardiographic changes with, 867–868, 867f, 867t
  emotional and behavioural responses to, 822t
  health promotion of, 818
  interprofessional care of, 814–818
  manifestations of, 811
  medication therapy of, 810t

Acute coronary syndrome (ACS) *(Continued)*
  nursing care plan for, 820b–821b
  overview of, 811–826
  patient teaching for, 823–824, 823t
  rehabilitation after, 821t
Acute decompensated heart failure (ADHF), 832, 833f, 841b. *See also* Heart failure
Acute exacerbation of chronic bronchitis (AECB), 589
Acute exacerbations of COPD (AECOPD), 654–655
Acute gastritis, 1012. *See also* Gastritis
Acute hemolytic reaction, 744, 745t–746t
Acute illness, characteristics of, 64, 64t
Acute infectious diarrhea, 1037t, 1039–1040
Acute intracranial conditions, 1453–1484
  brain tumours, 1472–1474
  cranial surgery, 1475–1477
  head injury, 1465–1469
  intracranial pressure, 1453–1455, 1454f
Acute kidney injury (AKI), 1180–1212, 1181f, 1181t
  age-related considerations, 1187
  clinical manifestations, 1182–1184
  diagnostic studies for, 1184
  etiology and pathophysiology, 1181–1182, 1182t
  evaluation, 1187
  initiation phase of, 1182
  interprofessional care, 1184–1185, 1184t–1185t
  maintenance phase of, 1182–1183
  nursing assessment, 1185, 1186t
  nursing diagnoses, 1185
  nursing implementation, 1185–1187
  nursing management, 1185–1187
  nutritional therapy for, 1185
  planning, 1185
  recovery phase of, 1184
Acute liver failure, 1102–1103
Acute low back pain, 1651–1652, 1651b
Acute lung injury, 1766t
Acute lymphocytic leukemia (ALL), 731t, 732, 733t. *See also* Leukemia
Acute myelogenous leukemia (AML), 730–731, 731t, 733t. *See also* Leukemia
Acute osteomyelitis, 1643
Acute otitis media (AOM), 470
Acute pain, 141t, 142, 183
Acute pain services (APS), 158–159
Acute pancreatitis, 1105–1107, 1106f, 1107t–1108t
Acute pericarditis, 877–879, 878f, 879t. *See also* Pericarditis
Acute pharyngitis, 575
Acute poststreptococcal glomerulonephritis (APSGN), 1152, 1152t

Page numbers followed by "f" indicate figures, "b" indicate boxes, and "t" indicate tables.

1853

SPECIAL FEATURES

CASE STUDIES

Assessment

INTERPROFESSIONAL CARE TABLES

MEDICATION THERAPY TABLES

EVIDENCE-INFORMED PRACTICE BOXES

Translating Research Into Practice

Topic	Chapter	Page
Adverse Effects of Hypertension Medication	35	791
Annual PSA Screening	57	1414
Extreme Exercise and Chemotherapy	33	739
Heart Failure: Hawthorn Versus Biventricular Pacing	37	841
HIV and Unprotected Sex	17	295
Human Papilloma Vaccine	55	1365
Importance of Yearly Pap Tests	56	1390
Location for Enoxaparin Injections	40	919
NPO Order for Preoperative Patient	20	384
Patient Reluctant to Take Warfarin	38	859
Physical Activity and COPD	31	657
Post-Bariatric Surgery Support Groups	43	989
Radiation Therapy for Breast Cancer	54	1343
Skin Cancer and Indoor Tanning	26	495
Spinal Cord Injury and Bladder Management	63	1579
Stage 1 Pressure Injury	14	237
Vitamin D Deficiency	66	1650

HEALTH HISTORY TABLES

Table Title	Table Number	Page
Auditory System	Table 23.8	442
Cardiovascular System	Table 34.2	757
Endocrine System	Table 50.5	1226
Gastrointestinal System	Table 41.8	939
Hematological System	Table 32.5	688
Musculoskeletal System	Table 64.2	1597
Nervous System	Table 58.5	1441
Patient About to Undergo Surgery	Table 20.3	380
Reproductive System	Table 53.6	1319
Integumentary System	Table 25.3	486
Urinary System	Table 47.4	1130
Visual System	Table 23.2	433

FOCUSED ASSESSMENT BOXES

Box Title	Chapter	Page
Auditory System	23	444
Cardiovascular System	34	762
Endocrine System	50	1234
Gastrointestinal (GI) System	41	943
Hematological System	32	691
Integumentary System	25	489
Musculoskeletal System	64	1599
Neurological System	58	1446
Reproductive System	53	1322
Respiratory System	28	558
Urinary System	47	1134
Visual System	23	438

INFORMATICS IN PRACTICE

Box Title	Chapter	Page
Chest Drainage System	30	615
Communication Devices for Patients With Laryngectomy	29	580
Computer Monitoring of Antibiotic Safety	49	1187
Digital Images	14	237
Discharge Teaching	22	423
Heart Surgery Video or CD	39	888
Managing Symptoms of Cancer	18	318
Monitoring Blood Pressure	35	791
Patient Teaching Using Gaming	52	1293
Phone Applications in Multiple Sclerosis	61	1528
Responsible Use of Social Media	1	9
Sleep Apnea Diagnosis and Monitoring	9	129
Staying Connected While Immobilized	65	1621
Texting for Patients With Chronic Obstructive Pulmonary Disease (COPD)	31	664
Use of Internet and Mobile Devices to Manage Human Immunodeficiency Virus Infection	17	298
Video Games for Stroke Recovery	60	1505
Wireless ECG Monitoring	38	852

GENETICS IN CLINICAL PRACTICE BOXES

Box Title	Chapter	Page
α1-Antitrypsin (AAT) Deficiency	31	651
Autoimmune Diseases	64	1597
Boxes Throughout This Text	15	245
Breast Cancer	54	1337
Familial Adenomatous Polyposis (FAP)	45	1064
Familial Hypercholesterolemia	36	798
Hemochromatosis	33	715
Hemophilia A and B	33	722
Hereditary Nonpolyposis Colorectal Cancer	45	1064
Huntington's Disease	58, 61	1440, 1536
Ovarian Cancer	56	1392
Polycystic Kidney Disease	48	1162
Sickle Cell Disease	33	714
Skin Malignancies	25	487
Types 1 and 2 Diabetes Mellitus	52	1273

All plans are available in customizable format from the Evolve website at *http://evolve.elsevier.com/Canada/Lewis/medsurg*. Seven plans are also provided in this text at the page numbers listed in this table.